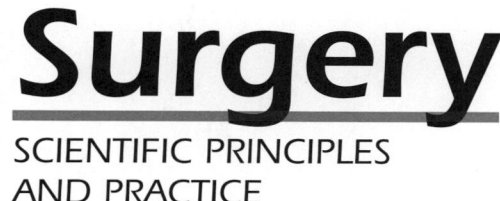

Surgery

SCIENTIFIC PRINCIPLES
AND PRACTICE

Surgery
THIRD EDITION
SCIENTIFIC PRINCIPLES AND PRACTICE

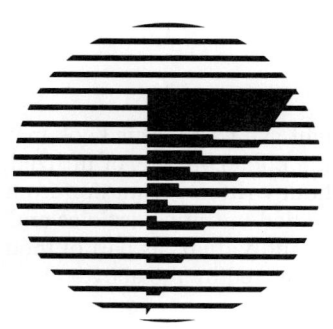

EDITOR-IN-CHIEF

Lazar J. Greenfield, MD
Frederick A. Coller Distinguished Professor of Surgery
Chairman, Department of Surgery
University of Michigan Medical School
Surgeon-in-Chief
University of Michigan Hospitals
Ann Arbor, Michigan

ASSOCIATE EDITORS

Michael W. Mulholland, MD, PhD
Section Head, General Surgery
Department of Surgery
University of Michigan Medical School
University of Michigan Hospitals
Ann Arbor, Michigan

Keith T. Oldham, MD
Surgeon-in-Chief and Marie Z. Uihlein Chair
Department of Pediatric Surgery
Medical College of Wisconsin
Milwaukee, Wisconsin

Gerald B. Zelenock, MD
Chairman, Department of Surgery
Chief, Surgical Services
William Beaumont Hospital
Royal Oak, Michigan

Keith D. Lillemoe, MD
Professor and Vice-Chairman
Department of Surgery
Johns Hopkins University School of Medicine
Johns Hopkins Hospital
Baltimore, Maryland

With 203 contributors

Illustrations by Holly R. Fischer, MFA

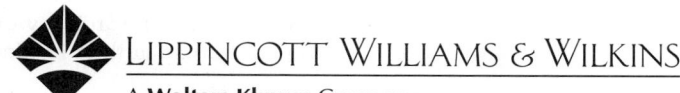

LIPPINCOTT WILLIAMS & WILKINS
A **Wolters Kluwer** Company

Philadelphia • Baltimore • New York • London
Buenos Aires • Hong Kong • Sydney • Tokyo

Acquisitions Editor: Lisa McAllister
Developmental Editor: Delois Patterson
Production Editor: Thomas Boyce
Manufacturing Manager: Benjamin Rivera
Cover Designer: Christine Jenny
Compositor: Lippincott Williams & Wilkins Desktop Division
Printer: Quebecor/World Color

Illustrations new to this edition were rendered by Holly R. Fischer, MFA.
Some radiographs in this book were electronically modified to enhance clarity.

© 2001 by LIPPINCOTT WILLIAMS & WILKINS
530 Walnut Street
Philadelphia, PA 19106 USA
LWW.com

Printed in the USA

Library of Congress Cataloging-in-Publication Data

Surgery : scientific principles and practice / editor-in-chief, Lazar J. Greenfield ;
associate editors, Michael W. Mulholland ... [et al.].— 3rd ed.
    p. ; cm.
  Includes bibliographical references and index.
  ISBN 0-7817-2254-3
  1. Surgery. 2. Medicine. I. Greenfield, Lazar J., 1934- II. Mulholland, Michael W.
  [DNLM: 1. Surgery. 2. Surgical Procedures, Operative. WO 100 S9617 2001]
RD31 .S922 2001
617—dc21

00-047793

10 9 8 7 6 5 4 3 2 1

Contributing Authors

Keith D. Aaronson, MD, MS
Assistant Professor
Department of Internal Medicine
Division of Cardiology
University of Michigan Medical Center
Ann Arbor, Michigan

C. W. Acher, MD
Assistant Professor
Department of Surgery
University of Wisconsin Medical School
Madison, Wisconsin

N. Scott Adzick, MD
Surgeon-in-Chief
Department of Surgery
Children's Hospital of Philadelphia
Philadelphia, Pennsylvania

John Aiken, MD
Department of Pediatric Surgery
Medical College of Wisconsin
Milwaukee, Wisconsin

Subodh Arora, MD
Chief, Vascular Surgery
Department of Surgery
Veterans' Administration Medical Center
Washington, D.C.

William G. Austen, Jr., MD
Edward D. Churchill Professor of Surgery
Harvard Medical School
Boston, Massachusetts

Robert H. Bartlett, MD
Professor of Surgery
University of Michigan Medical Center
Ann Arbor, Michigan

Stephen T. Bartlett, MD
Professor of Surgery and Medicine
Joseph and Corrine Schwartz Division of
    Transplantation
University of Maryland School of Medicine
Baltimore, Maryland

Barbara Lee Bass, MD
Professor and Vice Chair
Department of Surgery
University of Maryland School of Medicine
Baltimore, Maryland

B. Timothy Baxter, MD
Professor of Surgery
Department of Surgery
University of Nebraska Medical Center
Omaha, Nebraska

R. Daniel Beauchamp, MD
Section of Surgical Sciences
Vanderbilt University Medical Center
Nashville, Tennessee

James M. Becker, MD
Surgeon-in-Chief
Department of Surgery
Boston University Medical Center
Boston, Massachusetts

Hugh G. Beebe, MD
Director
Jobst Vascular Center
The Toledo Hospital
Toledo, Ohio

Bryce D. Beseth, MD
Resident, Department of Surgery
UCLA School of Medicine
Westwood, California

Timothy R. Billiar, MD
George Vance Foster Professor and Chair
Department of Surgery
University of Pittsburgh School of Medicine
Pittsburgh, Pennsylvania

Christopher J. Blewett, MD
Department of Pediatric Surgery
Penn State Children's Hospital
Milton S. Hershey Medical Center
Hershey, Pennsylvania

C. Richard Boland, MD
Professor of Medicine
University of California, San Diego
School of Medicine
San Diego, California

Steven F. Bolling, MD
Professor of Cardiac Surgery
University of Michigan Medical Center
Ann Arbor, Michigan

Edward L. Bove, MD
Head, Section of Cardiac Surgery
Director, Pediatric Cardiovascular Surgery
University of Michigan Medical Center
Ann Arbor, Michigan

Scott M. Bradley, MD
Associate Professor
Department of Surgery
Medical University of South Carolina
Charleston, South Carolina

Robert S. Bresalier, MD
Director, Gastrointestinal Oncology
Department of Medicine
Henry Ford Health Sciences Center
Detroit, Michigan

Robert E. Bristow, MD
Assistant Professor
Department of Gynecology and Obstetrics
Johns Hopkins University
Baltimore, Maryland

Jonathan S. Bromberg, MD, PhD
Professor
Surgery, Gene Therapy, and Molecular Medicine
Mt. Sinai School of Medicine
New York, New York

Jamie Brown, MD
Associate Professor
Department of Surgery
University of Maryland Hospital
Baltimore, Maryland

F. Charles Brunicardi, MD
Professor and Chairman
Michael E. DeBakey Department of Surgery
Baylor College of Medicine
Houston, Texas

Steven R. Buchman, MD
Assistant Professor
Section of Plastic and Reconstructive Surgery
University of Michigan Medical Center
Ann Arbor, Michigan

Timothy G. Buchman, MD, PhD
Edison Professor of Surgery
Professor of Anesthesiology and of Medicine
Washington University School of Medicine
St. Louis, Missouri

Arthur L. Burnett, MD
Associate Professor
Department of Urology
Johns Hopkins Hospital
Baltimore, Maryland

David R. Byrd, MD
Associate Professor
Department of Surgery
University of Washington
Seattle, Washington

John L. Cameron, MD
Department of Surgery
Johns Hopkins Hospital
Baltimore, Maryland

Robert B. Cameron, MD
Chief, Thoracic Oncology
Department of Surgery
Division of Cardiothoracic Surgery
UCLA School of Medicine
Los Angeles, California

Darrell A. Campbell, Jr., MD
Professor of Surgery
University of Michigan Medical Center
Ann Arbor, Michigan

Paul S. Cederna, MD
Assistant Professor
Section of Plastic and Reconstructive Surgery
University of Michigan Medical Center
Ann Arbor, Michigan

William F. Chandler, MD
Professor
Department of Surgery
University of Michigan Medical Center
Ann Arbor, Michigan

Alfred E. Chang, MD
Professor of Surgery
Chief, Division of Surgical Oncology
University of Michigan Medical Center
Ann Arbor, Michigan

Randall M. Chesnut, MD
Department of Neurological Surgery-L472
Oregon Health Sciences University
Portland, Oregon

Kyung J. Cho, MD
Professor of Radiology
University of Michigan Medical Center
Ann Arbor, Michigan

Kevin C. Chung, MD, MS
Assistant Professor
Section of Plastic and Reconstructive Surgery
University of Michigan Medical Center
Ann Arbor, Michigan

Robert E. Cilley, MD
Department of Pediatric Surgery
Penn State Children's Hospital
Milton S. Hershey Medical Center
Hershey, Pennsylvania

G. Patrick Clagett, MD
Chairman, Division of Vascular Surgery
University of Texas Southwestern Medical Center
Dallas, Texas

Alexander W. Clowes, MD
Professor of Surgery
Department of Surgery
University of Washington
Seattle, Washington

Raul Coimbra, MD, PhD
Associate Professor of Surgery
Department of Surgery
University of California, San Diego
San Diego, California

Lisa M. Colletti, MD
Associate Professor
Department of Surgery
University of Michigan Medical Center
Ann Arbor, Michigan

Jack L. Cronenwett, MD
Professor of Surgery
Dartmouth-Hitchcock Medical Center
Lebanon, New Hampshire

Henry Magill Cryer III, MD, PhD
Department of Surgery
University of California Medical Center
Los Angeles, California

Geoff Cundiff, MD
Department of Gynecology and Obstetrics
Johns Hopkins Medical Institutes
Baltimore, Maryland

Michael C. Dalsing, MD, FACS
Director of Vascular Surgery
Department of Surgery
Indiana University Medical School
Indianapolis, Indiana

Ben D. Davis, MD
Fellow, Division of Thoracic Surgery
Brigham and Women's Hospital
Department of Surgery
Harvard Medical School
Boston, Massachusetts

James W. Davis, MD, FACS
Chief of Trauma
Department of Surgery
University Medical Center
Fresno, California

David C. Dawson, PhD
Professor and Chair
Department of Physiology and Pharmacology
Oregon Health Sciences University
Portland, Oregon

Tom R. DeMeester, MD
Professor and Chairman
Department of Surgery
University of Southern California School of Medicine
Chief of Surgery
University of Southern California Hospital
Los Angeles, California

Peter W. Dillon, MD
Department of Pediatric Surgery
Penn State Children's Hospital
Milton S. Hershey Medical Center
Hershey, Pennsylvania

Verdi J. DiSesa, MD
Department of Cardiovascular-Thoracic Surgery
Rush Presbyterian-St. Luke's Medical Center
Chicago, Illinois

Gerard M. Doherty, MD
Associate Professor
Department of Surgery
Washington University School of Medicine
Barnes-Jewish Hospital
St. Louis, Missouri

Jeffrey Drebin, MD, PhD
Assistant Professor of Surgery
Johns Hopkins Hospital
Baltimore, Maryland

David L. Dunn, MD
Professor of Surgery
University of Minnesota
Minneapolis, Minnesota

Jean C. Emond, MD
Thomas S. Zimmer Professor of Surgery
Columbia College of Physicians and Surgeons
New York, New York

Sandra L. Engelhardt, MD
Department of Surgery
University of California, San Diego
San Diego, California

Alex Esquivel, MD
Assistant Professor of Surgery
Department of Surgery
University of Nebraska Medical Center
Omaha, Nebraska

Mark F. Fillinger, MD
Associate Professor of Surgery
Dartmouth-Hitchcock Medical Center
Lebanon, New Hampshire

Neil A. Fine, MD, FACS
Assistant Professor of Surgery
Division of Plastic and Reconstructive Surgery
Northwestern University Medical School
Chicago, Illinois

William E. Fisher, MD
Assistant Professor
Michael E. DeBakey Department of Surgery
Baylor College of Medicine
Houston, Texas

Robert J. Fitzgibbons, Jr.
Dr. Harry E. Stuckenhoff Professor of Surgery
Creighton University School of Medicine
Omaha, Nebraska

Yuman Fong, MD
Attending Surgeon
Department of Surgery
Memorial Sloan-Kettering Cancer Center
New York, New York

Douglas L. Fraker, MD
Associate Professor
Department of Surgery
University of Pennsylvania Medical Center
Philadelphia, Pennsylvania

Julie Ann Freischlag, MD
Chief, Division of Vascular Surgery
UCLA Medical Center
Los Angeles, California

Joseph Giglia, MD
Department of Surgery
University of Cincinnati Medical Center
Cincinnati, Ohio

Toby Gordon, ScD
Associate Professor (Joint Appointment)
Department of Surgery and Health Policy Management
Johns Hopkins University
Baltimore, Maryland

Robert C. Gorman, MD
Assistant Professor of Surgery
Department of Cardiothoracic Surgery
University of Pennsylvania Medical Center
Philadelphia, Pennsylvania

Linda M. Graham, MD
Department of Vascular Surgery
The Cleveland Clinic Foundation
Cleveland, Ohio

Lazar J. Greenfield, MD
Frederick A. Coller Distinguished Professor of Surgery
Chairman, Department of Surgery
University of Michigan Medical School
Surgeon-in-Chief
University of Michigan Hospitals
Ann Arbor, Michigan

John W. Hallett, Jr., MD
Professor of Surgery
Division of Vascular Surgery
Mayo Medical School
Mayo Clinic
Rochester, Minnesota

Mark R. Harrigan, MD
Lecturer
Department of Surgery
University of Michigan Medical Center
Ann Arbor, Michigan

Mary T. Hawn, MD, MPH
Fellow
Department of Surgery
Oregon Health Sciences University
Portland, Oregon

Peter K. Henke, MD
Assistant Professor
Department of Surgery
Section of Vascular Surgery
University of Michigan Medical Center
Ann Arbor, Michigan

Jennifer C. Hirsch, MD
Resident in Surgery
Department of Surgery
University of Michigan Medical Center
Ann Arbor, Michigan

Kim J. Hodgson, MD
Professor and Chairman
Division of Vascular Surgery
Southern Illinois University School of Medicine
Springfield, Illinois

Richard A. Hodin, MD
Vice-Chairman
Department of Surgery
Beth Israel Deaconess Medical Center
Boston, Massachusetts

Julian T. Hoff, MD
Professor
Department of Surgery
Section of Neurology
University of Michigan Medical Center
Ann Arbor, Michigan

David B. Hoyt, MD
Professor of Surgery
Department of Surgery
University of California, San Diego
San Diego, California

Thomas S. Huber, MD, PhD
Associate Professor
Department of Surgery
University of Florida College of Medicine
Gainesville, Florida

Roger D. Hurst, MD
Assistant Professor of Clinical Surgery
Department of Surgery
University of Chicago
Pritzker School of Medicine
Chicago, Illinois

Lloyd A. Jacobs, MD
University of Michigan Medical Center
Ann Arbor, Michigan

Eric Jacobsohn, MBChB, FRCPC
Associate Professor
Department of Anesthesiology and of Surgery
Washington University School of Medicine
St. Louis, Missouri

Thomas W. Jarrett, MD
Associate Professor
Department of Urology
Johns Hopkins Hospital
Baltimore, Maryland

Raymond J. Joehl, MD, FACS
James R. Hines Professor of Surgery
Northwestern University Medical School
Chicago, Illinois

Timothy M. Johnson, MD
Associate Professor
Department of Dermatology
University of Michigan Medical Center
Ann Arbor, Michigan

Gregory J. Jurkovich, MD, FACS
Chief of Trauma
Department of Surgery
Harborview Medical Center
Seattle, Washington

Kim U. Kahng, MD
Associate Professor of Surgery
Vice Chairman, Administrative Affairs
Medical College of Pennsylvania and
Hahnemann University School of Medicine
Philadelphia, Pennsylvania

Larry R. Kaiser, MD
The Eldridge L. Eliason Professor of Surgery
University of Pennsylvania Medical Center
Philadelphia, Pennsylvania

Karthikeshwar Kasirajan, MD
Department of Vascular Surgery
University of New Mexico School of Medicine
Albuquerque, New Mexico

Lawrence T. Kim, MD
Assistant Professor
Department of Surgery
University of Texas Southwestern Medical Center
Dallas, Texas

M. Margaret Knudson, MD
Associate Professor
Department of Surgery
University of California, San Francisco
San Francisco, California

Alexander S. Krupnick, MD
Resident in Surgery
Department of Surgery
Hospital of the University of Pennsylvania
Philadelphia, Pennsylvania

William M. Kuzon, MD, PhD
Associate Professor
Section of Plastic and Reconstructive Surgery
University of Michigan Medical Center
Ann Arbor, Michigan

Gregory J. Landry, MD
Assistant Professor
Department of Surgery
Division of Vascular Surgery
Oregon Health Sciences University
Portland, Oregon

Michael P. LaQuaglia, MD, FACS, FAAP
Professor of Surgery
Chief, Pediatric Surgery
Memorial Sloan-Kettering Cancer Center
New York, New York

Steven D. Leach, MD
The Paul K. Neumann Professor in Pancreatic Cancer
Departments of Surgery and Oncology
Johns Hopkins University
Baltimore, Maryland

Keith D. Lillemoe, MD
Professor and Vice-Chairman
Department of Surgery
Johns Hopkins University School of Medicine
Johns Hopkins Hospital
Baltimore, Maryland

Ricardo V. Lloyd, MD, PhD
Professor of Pathology
Mayo Clinic
Rochester, Minnesota

Michael R. Lucey, MD, FRCPI
Professor of Medicine
University of Pennsylvania Medical Center
Philadelphia, Pennsylvania

Robert C. Mackersie, MD, FACS
Department of Surgery
San Francisco General Hospital
San Francisco, California

John C. Magee, MD
Assistant Professor of Surgery
University of Michigan Medical Center
Ann Arbor, Michigan

David K. Magnuson, MD
Department of Pediatric Surgery
Cleveland Clinic Foundation
Cleveland, Ohio

Jocelyne Martin, MD
Fellow, Thoracic Surgery
Department of Surgery
Memorial Sloan-Kettering Cancer Center
New York, New York

Michael R. Marvin, MD
Transplant Surgery Fellow
Department of Surgery
Columbia University
New York Presbyterian Hospital
New York, New York

Jeffrey B. Matthews, MD
Chief
Division of General and Gastrointestinal Surgery
Beth Israel Deaconess Medical Center
Boston, Massachusetts

Robert M. Merion, MD
Associate Professor of Surgery
University of Michigan Medical Center
Ann Arbor, Michigan

Louis M. Messina, MD
Professor of Surgery
Department of Surgery
University of California, San Francisco
San Francisco, California

Fabrizio Michelassi, MD
Professor of Surgery
University of Chicago
Pritzker School of Medicine
Chicago, Illinois

Eugene Minevich, MD
Department of Surgery
University of Cincinnati Medical Center
Division of Pediatric Urology
Children's Hospital Medical Center
Cincinnati, Ohio

R. Scott Mitchell, MD
Professor of Cardiovascular Surgery
Stanford University School of Medicine
Stanford, California

H. David Moehring, MD
Professor of Clinical Orthopaedics
Department of Orthopaedic Surgery
University of California
Davis Medical Center
Sacramento, California

F. J. Montz, MD
Professor
Department of Gynecology and Obstetrics
Johns Hopkins University
Baltimore, Maryland

Monica Morrow, MD
Department of Surgery
Lynn Sage Breast Center
Northwestern Memorial Hospital
Chicago, Illinois

Ralph S. Mosca, MD
Assistant Professor of Surgery
C. S. Mott Children's Hospital
University of Michigan Medical Center
Ann Arbor, Michigan

James J. Mulé, PhD
Maude T. Lane Professor
Department of Surgery
University of Michigan Medical Center
Ann Arbor, Michigan

Michael W. Mulholland, MD, PhD
Section Head, General Surgery
Department of Surgery
University of Michigan Medical School
University of Michigan Hospitals
Ann Arbor, Michigan

Kenric M. Murayama, MD, FACS
Associate Professor
Department of Surgery
Northwestern University Medical School
Chicago, Illinois

Michel M. Murr, MD
Assistant Professor of Surgery
University of South Florida
Tampa General Hospital
Tampa, Florida

Isha A. Mustafa, MD
Department of Surgery
Rhode Island Hospital
Providence, Rhode Island

Thomas A. Mustoe, MD, FACS
Professor of Surgery
Chief, Division of Plastic Surgery
Northwestern University Medical School
Chicago, Illinois

Attila Nakeeb, MD
Assistant Professor
Department of Surgery
Johns Hopkins Hospital
Baltimore, Maryland

H. H. Newsome, Jr., MD
Dean, School of Medicine
Professor of Surgery
Virginia Commonwealth University
Richmond, Virginia

Santhat Nivatvongs, MD
Consultant in Colon and Rectal Surgery
Department of Surgery
Mayo Clinic
Rochester, Minnesota

James Norman, MD
Professor of Surgery
University of South Florida
Tampa General Hospital
Tampa, Florida

Keith T. Oldham, MD
Surgeon-in-Chief and Marie Z. Uihlein Chair
Department of Pediatric Surgery
Medical College of Wisconsin
Milwaukee, Wisconsin

Lisa A. Orloff, MD
Associate Professor
Department of Surgery
University of California, San Diego
Medical Center
San Diego, California

Mark B. Orringer, MD
Head, Section of Thoracic Surgery
Department of Surgery
University of Michigan Medical Center
Ann Arbor, Michigan

Mary F. Otterson, MD, MS
Associate Professor
Department of Surgery and Physiology
Medical College of Wisconsin
Milwaukee, Wisconsin

Kenneth Ouriel, MD
Department of Vascular Surgery
Cleveland Clinic Foundation
Cleveland, Ohio

C. Keith Ozaki, MD
Chief of Vascular Surgery
Department of Surgery
Malcolm Randall Veterans' Administration
    Medical Center
Gainesville, Florida

Francis D. Pagani, MD, PhD
Assistant Professor of Cardiac Surgery
Department of Surgery
University of Michigan Hospitals
Ann Arbor, Michigan

A. Scott Pearson, MD
Assistant Professor
Department of Surgery
Vanderbilt University
Nashville, Tennessee

Jeffrey H. Peters, MD
Chief, Division of General Surgery
Department of Surgery
University of Southern California
University Hospital
Los Angeles, California

Richard N. Pierson III, MD
Associate Professor of Surgery
Vanderbilt University
Nashville, Tennessee

Iraklis I. Pipinos, MD
Fellow, Vascular Surgery
Department of Surgery
Henry Ford Hospital
Detroit, Michigan

John M. Porter, MD
Professor
Department of Surgery
Division of Vascular Surgery
Oregon Health Sciences University
Portland, Oregon

Carol Pross, MD
Department of Surgery
UCLA Medical Center
Los Angeles, California

Jeffrey D. Punch, MD
Assistant Professor of Surgery
University of Michigan Medical Center
Ann Arbor, Michigan

Thomas H. Quinn, PhD
Professor of Anatomy and Surgery
Department of Biomedical Sciences
Creighton University School of Medicine
Omaha, Nebraska

Steven E. Raper, MD
Associate Professor
Department of Surgery
University of Pennsylvania
Philadelphia, Pennsylvania

Todd E. Rasmussen, MD
Division of Vascular Surgery
Mayo Medical School
Mayo Clinic
Rochester, Minnesota

Daniel J. Reddy, MD
Head, Vascular Surgery
Department of Surgery
Henry Ford Hospital
Detroit, Michigan

Riley S. Rees, MD
Professor of Surgery
University of Michigan Medical Center
Ann Arbor, Michigan

Alan T. Richards, MD, BCH, FACS, FRCS, FCS(SA)
Staff Surgeon
Department of Surgery
Saint Joseph Hospital
Omaha, Nebraska

Ronald Rodriguez, MD, PhD
Assistant Professor
Department of Urology, Medical Oncology, Cellular and
    Molecular Medicine
Johns Hopkins Medical School
Baltimore, Maryland

Michael J. Rohrer, MD
Department of Surgery
University of Massachusetts Memorial Medical Center
Worcester, Massachusetts

Ori D. Rotstein, MD
Professor of Surgery
Department of Surgery
University of Toronto
Toronto, Ontario
Canada

Grace S. Rozycki, MD, FACS
Associate Professor
Department of Surgery
Emory University School of Medicine
Atlanta, Georgia

Steven M. Rudich, MD, PhD
Assistant Professor of Surgery
University of Michigan Medical Center
Ann Arbor, Michigan

Valerie W. Rusch, MD
Chief, Thoracic Division
William G. Cahan Chair of Surgery
Department of Surgery
Memorial Sloan-Kettering Cancer Center
New York, New York

Timothy W. Rutter, MBBS, FFARCS
Clinical Associate Professor
Department of Anesthesiology
University of Michigan Medical Center
Ann Arbor, Michigan

Sergio X. Salles-Cunha, PhD
Clinical Research Director
Jobst Vascular Center
The Toledo Hospital
Toledo, Ohio

Rajabrata Sarkarf, MD, PhD
Assistant Professor of Surgery
Department of Surgery
University of California, San Francisco
San Francisco, California

Thomas T. Sato, MD
Assistant Professor of Surgery
Medical College of Wisconsin
Attending Staff
Division of Pediatric Surgery
Children's Hospital of Wisconsin
Milwaukee, Wisconsin

Luke O. Schoeniger, MD, PhD
Assistant Professor
Department of Surgery
University of Rochester School of Medicine and
    Dentistry
Rochester, New York

Margaret L. Schrieber, MD
Visiting Assistant Professor
Department of Surgery
University of Maryland School of Medicine
Baltimore, Maryland

Vaishali Dixit Schuchert, MD
Chief Resident
Department of Surgery
University of Pittsburgh
Pittsburgh, Pennsylvania

James M. Seeger, MD
Professor of Surgery
Department of Surgery
University of Florida College of Medicine
Gainesville, Florida

Steven R. Shackford, MD, FACS
Department of Surgery
The Given Building
University of Vermont
Burlington, Vermont

Curtis A. Sheldon, MD
Professor of Surgery
Director, Pediatric Urology
University of Cincinnati Medical Center
Children's Hospital Medical Center
Cincinnati, Ohio

Alexander D. Shepard, MD
Senior Staff Vascular Surgeon
Department of Surgery
Henry Ford Hospital
Detroit, Michigan

Robert L. Sheridan, MD
Associate Professor of Surgery
Harvard Medical School
Cambridge, Massachusetts

Anton N. Sidawy, MD
Chief, Surgical Services
Department of Surgery
Veterans' Affairs Medical Center
Washington, D.C.

Diane M. Simeone, MD
Assistant Professor of Surgery
University of Michigan Medical Center
Ann Arbor, Michigan

Richard K. Simons, MB, BChir, FACS
Trauma Director
Vancouver Hospital and Health Sciences Centre
Vancouver, British Columbia
Canada

Michael J. Sise, MD
Department of Surgery
Division of Trauma
Scripps-Mercy Hospital
San Diego, California

James V. Sitzmann, MD
Seymour I. Schwartz Professor and Chair
Department of Surgery
University of Rochester School of Medicine and
    Dentistry
Rochester, New York

J. Stanley Smith, Jr., MD, FACS, FCCM
Professor of Surgery
Penn State College of Medicine
Hershey Medical Center
Hershey, Pennsylvania

Iva A. Smolens, MD
Lecturer, Section of Cardiac Surgery
University of Michigan Medical Center
Ann Arbor, Michigan

Vernon K. Sondak, MD
Associate Professor of Surgery
Department of General Surgery
University of Michigan Medical Center
Ann Arbor, Michigan

Wiley W. Souba, MD, DSc, MBA
Chair
Department of Surgery
Penn State College of Medicine
Hershey Medical Center
Hershey, Pennsylvania

David I. Soybel, MD
Staff Surgeon
Department of Surgery
Boston Veterans' Administration Healthcare System
West Roxbury, Massachusetts

James C. Stanley, MD
Department of Surgery
Section of Vascular Surgery
University of Michigan Medical Center
Ann Arbor, Michigan

Steven Strasberg, MD
Pruett Professor of Surgery
Head, HPB Surgery
Washington University School of Medicine
St. Louis, Missouri

Arthur F. Stucchi, PhD
Associate Research Professor
Department of Surgery
Boston University School of Medicine
Boston, Massachusetts

David J. Sugarbaker, MD
Vice-Chair, Department of Surgery
Chief, Division of Thoracic Surgery
Brigham and Women's Hospital
Professor of Surgery
Harvard Medical School
Boston, Massachusetts

Harvey J. Sugerman, MD
David M. Hume Professor
Chief, General/Trauma Surgery Division
Medical College of Virginia of
Virginia Commonwealth University
Richmond, Virginia

John F. Sweeney, MD
Assistant Professor of Surgery
University of Michigan Medical Center
Ann Arbor, Michigan

Lloyd M. Taylor, Jr., MD
Professor
Department of Surgery
Division of Vascular Surgery
Oregon Health Sciences University
Portland, Oregon

Theodoros N. Teknos, MD
Assistant Professor
Department of Otolaryngology-Head and Neck Surgery
University of Michigan Medical Center
Ann Arbor, Michigan

Gordon L. Telford, MD
Attending Surgeon
Department of Surgery
Froedtert Memorial Lutheran Hospital
Milwaukee, Wisconsin

Ronald G. Tompkins, MD, ScD
Associate Professor of Surgery
Harvard Medical School
Visiting Surgeon
Massachusetts General Hospital
Boston, Massachusetts

Kevin K. Tremper, MD, PhD
Professor and Chairman
Department of Anesthesiology
University of Michigan Medical Center
Ann Arbor, Michigan

Richard H. Turnage, MD
Associate Professor and Vice-Chairman
Department of Surgery
University of Texas Southwestern Medical School
Dallas, Texas

Robert Udelsman, MD, MSB, MBA
Richard Bennett Darnall Professor of Surgery
Department of Surgery
Johns Hopkins Hospital
Baltimore, Maryland

Gilbert R. Upchurch, Jr., MD
Assistant Professor
Department of Surgery
Section of Vascular Surgery
University of Michigan Medical Center
Ann Arbor, Michigan

Richard B. Wait, MD, PhD
Department of Surgery
Baystate Medical Center
Springfield, Massachusetts

Thomas W. Wakefield, MD
Professor of Surgery
Department of Surgery
Section of Vascular Surgery
University of Michigan Medical Center
Ann Arbor, Michigan

Sharon Weber, MD
Surgical Fellow
Department of Surgery
Memorial Sloan-Kettering Cancer Center
New York, New York

Glenn J. R. Whitman, MD
Medical College of Pennsylvania
Philadelphia, Pennsylvania

Edwin G. Wilkins, MD, MS
Associate Professor
Section of Plastic and Reconstructive Surgery
University of Michigan Medical Center
Ann Arbor, Michigan

David M. Williams, MD
Professor of Radiology
University of Michigan Medical Center
Ann Arbor, Michigan

John A. Williams, MD, PhD
Professor and Chair
Department of Physiology
University of Michigan Medical Center
Ann Arbor, Michigan

Robert J. Winchell, MD
Department of Surgery
Division of Trauma
University of California, San Diego
Medical Center
San Diego, California

David H. Wisner, MD
Department of Surgery
University of California, Davis
Medical Center
Sacramento, California

M. M. Wynn, MD
Associate Professor
Department of Anesthesiology
University of Wisconsin Medical School
Madison, Wisconsin

Alan M. Yahanda, MD
Assistant Professor of Surgery
Department of Surgery
University of Michigan Medical Center
Ann Arbor, Michigan

James S. T. Yao, MD, PhD
Magerstadt Professor of Surgery
Chief, Division of Vascular Surgery
Northwestern University Medical School
Vice Chair, Department of Surgery
Northwestern Memorial Hospital
Chicago, Illinois

Charles J. Yeo, MD
Professor of Surgery and Oncology
Johns Hopkins University School of Medicine
Johns Hopkins Hospital
Baltimore, Maryland

Gerald B. Zelenock, MD
Chairman, Department of Surgery
Chief, Surgical Services
William Beaumont Hospital
Royal Oak, Michigan

Lambros Zellos, MD
Fellow, Division of Thoracic Surgery
Brigham and Women's Hospital
Department of Surgery
Harvard Medical School
Boston, Massachusetts

Preface

Now that we have entered a new millennium and an information age that provides vast educational resources at the click of a mouse, what is the role of a textbook? For those students of surgery whose education was not automated, a reference text is a familiar and comfortable resource that explains and illustrates important concepts. A textbook may not, however, contain the latest information, which represents both a weakness and a potential strength. The very best surgical textbooks contain current information filtered for quality and importance through a knowledgeable author. The editors of *Surgery: Scientific Principles and Practice* have accepted the incremental challenge of the third edition to provide the reader with the optimal balance of new science and technology with surgical practice. To fulfill our original commitment to use active investigators in the field, we have introduced over 100 new authors of over 200 total contributors. A new chapter on evidence-based surgery has been introduced. The consistency of the illustrations and highlighting that characterized the first two editions has been maintained and enhanced by selected color plates.

On behalf of the editors, we express our appreciation for the excellent efforts of the authors, whose scholarship makes our job easier. We are fortunate to have maintained our synergistic working relationship with Lippincott Williams & Wilkins medical editor, Lisa McAllister, and to have the support of Delois Patterson as managing editor and Thomas Boyce as production editor. We dedicate this book to our mentors, residents, and students, who form the ongoing chain of the legacy of *Surgery* in which we are privileged to provide a link.

LAZAR J. GREENFIELD, MD
Editor-in-Chief

Preface to the First Edition

Our predecessors in surgery would be amazed at the scope and sophistication of the current practice of surgery. Yet those who have witnessed this impressive expansion of clinical science are also acutely aware of the exponential growth of knowledge in the basic sciences. Surgical research has undergone a transformation from physiologic to cellular investigation, and we have now entered the era of molecular biology. These developments are changing the fundamental ways in which we think about injury and disease. The accelerated rate of scientific progress demands not only an expanded vocabulary but also a willingness to adopt new ideas and strategies and to readjust basic biologic concepts. Without this approach, future surgeons would be in danger of becoming surgical technicians and would fail their heritage as major contributors to medical progress.

These challenges prompted us to develop a new textbook of surgery that would balance scientific principles and clinical practice. The classic textbooks of past decades served their purpose well, emphasizing the rich heritage of clinical surgery. But new knowledge dictates new approaches to the integration of the basic sciences and clinical surgery. Therefore, *Surgery: Scientific Principles and Practice* begins with a major section devoted to basic topics such as cell biology, metabolism, inflammation, immunology, and wound healing. On this foundation we have added organ system chapters designed to include normal physiology and anatomy. Our commitment to clinical practice is demonstrated by the comprehensive list of topics, the emphasis on modern approaches to diagnosis and management, and descriptions of surgical techniques. We expect this book to be as useful to experienced practitioners as to students and residents in surgery.

In a departure from the customary approach, we have selected many younger authors who are scientifically sophisticated and currently active contributors to the field. Many are the authors of seminal papers in their disciplines and are joining a textbook of surgery for the first time. Their fresh and pragmatic approaches enhance both the substance and the readability of the book.

Because surgery is a very visual craft, we have aspired to set a new standard for illustration by having one group of artists provide all the line drawings. This commitment, along with the color highlighting, ensures a uniformity of presentation for maximal teaching effectiveness and clinical usefulness.

The final and perhaps most important concept of *Surgery: Scientific Principles and Practice* is that we have tried to anticipate future developments. In choosing authors who are active investigators, we have endeavored to synthesize current concepts and to look ahead to the most promising areas for future progress. Armed with these concepts and the comprehensive state-of-the-art knowledge that this book provides, students and practitioners of surgery will be well prepared for the new challenges of the 21st century.

LAZAR J. GREENFIELD, MD
Editor-in-Chief

Contents

SECTION N   VENOUS AND LYMPHATIC SYSTEMS

SECTION O   PEDIATRICS

ONE

SCIENTIFIC PRINCIPLES

SURGERY: SCIENTIFIC PRINCIPLES AND PRACTICE, Third Edition, edited by
Lazar J. Greenfield, Michael W. Mulholland, Keith T. Oldham, Gerald B. Zelenock,
and Keith D. Lillemoe. Lippincott Williams & Wilkins Publishers, Philadelphia, © 2001.

CHAPTER 1

CELL STRUCTURE AND FUNCTION

JOHN A. WILLIAMS AND DAVID C. DAWSON

Clinical medicine is in the midst of a revolution. The explosive growth in basic biologic science during the past two decades has provided unprecedented insights into normal physiology and disease processes. The bases of human illness are understood increasingly in cellular and molecular terms, and novel approaches to treatment have resulted. The pace of scientific advancement is likely to accelerate. This new knowledge requires that future surgeons learn a new scientific vocabulary. All clinicians must understand the tenets of cellular and molecular biology to appreciate both the power and the limitations of these approaches.

CELL STRUCTURE

The human body, like all living organisms, is composed of cells. Individual cells express widely differing shapes and functions, but all possess common structural and functional elements that allow the cell to use energy, maintain homeostasis, grow, and divide (1,2). Cells become differentiated for specific functions by expressing particular, specialized elements. For example, all cells possess membrane proteins that act as ion channels and participate in the maintenance of the intracellular ionic milieu, but in nerve cells, these ion channels have diversified and are highly voltage dependent, providing the basis for information transmission in the form of electrical impulses.

In many cases, proteins do not function as individual molecules but within larger structures specialized for specific functions. These structures, when visible by light and electron microscopy, are termed *organelles* (Fig. 1.1). In most cases, organelles compartmentalize the cell; they are surrounded by a biologic membrane based on a lipid bilayer that is structurally similar to the plasma membrane. This section reviews the structure of the major cell organelles as well as that of the cytoskeleton, a collection of structural proteins that form large, supramolecular aggregates.

Membranes and Organelles

Plasma Membrane

The plasma membrane defines the boundary of the cell and serves to contain and concentrate enzymes and the other macromolecular constituents (3). The plasma membrane is composed of amphipathic molecules, mainly phospholipids, sphingolipids, and proteins, that contain distinct regions that are either insoluble in water (hydrophobic) or soluble in water (hydrophilic). By orienting themselves so that their hydrophobic portions are in contact with each other, phospholipids can spontaneously form closed vesicles and planar lipid bilayers, within which proteins and hydrophobic components such as cholesterol are embedded (Fig. 1.2). Individual lipid molecules are able to diffuse in the bilayer. Embedded proteins can also move, although their movement is slower and

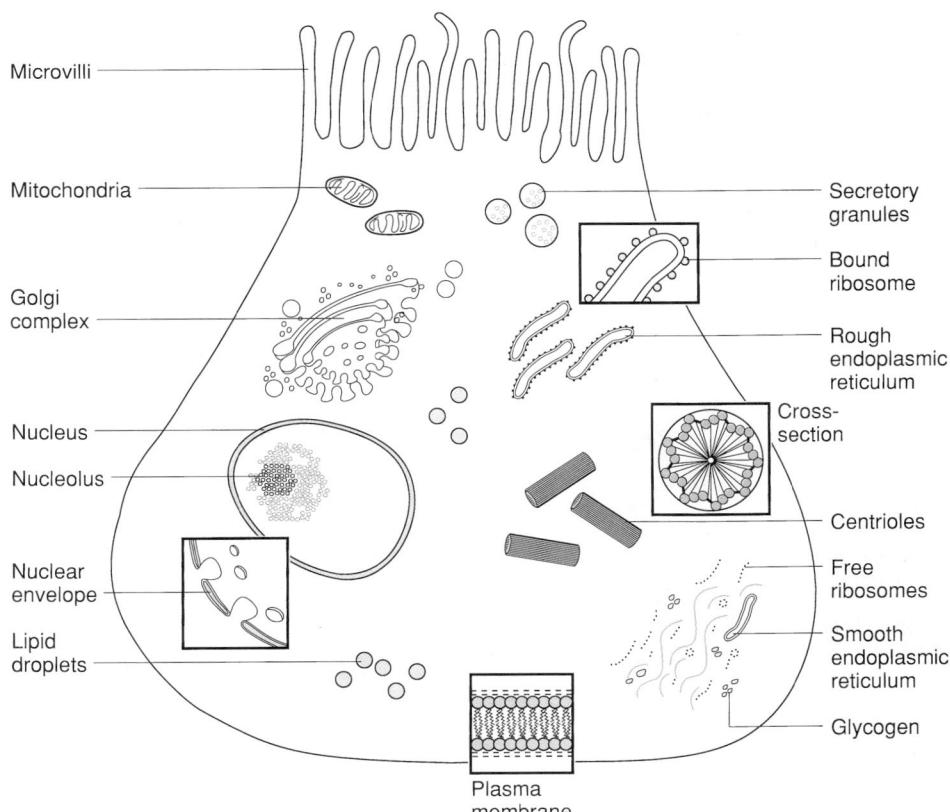

Figure 1.1. Schematic diagram of a typical epithelial cell, showing the common internal organelles.

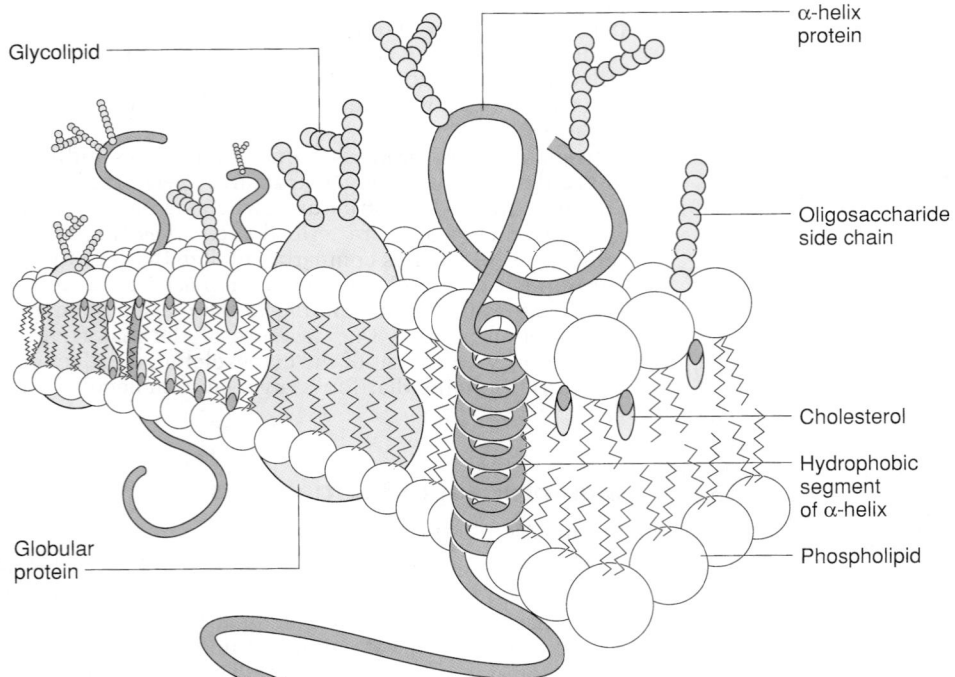

Figure 1.2. Structure of the cell membrane as a fluid mosaic consisting of a phospholipid bilayer that contains cholesterol and embedded proteins.

often restricted by cytoskeletal attachment. The lateral mobility of lipids and proteins can be quantitated by fluorescence recovery after photobleaching. The plasma membrane forms a continuous barrier between the aqueous extracellular and intracellular fluids. In addition to physically restraining macromolecules within the cell, the hydrophobic core of the lipid bilayer presents a barrier to small, charged molecules such as ions, amino acids, and adenosine triphosphate (ATP). This arrangement allows specialized transport proteins in the membrane, which act as regulated channels or transporters, to maintain an intracellular ionic milieu that is clearly different from extracellular fluid. Transport proteins and receptors are usually transmembrane proteins whose hydrophobic regions in the lipid bilayer are most often present in an α-helical configuration. Other membrane proteins on the inside of the plasma membrane, such as Ras, are attached by fatty acid

chains or isoprenyl derivatives, whereas some proteins on the external face are linked to phosphatidylinositol (PI) situated in the outer leaflet of the bilayer. Most plasma membrane proteins extending externally bear carbohydrate moieties primarily as oligosaccharide chains, which contribute to the cell coat or glycocalyx. Finally, cells can restrict lipid and protein components to specific membrane domains. This is especially prominent in ion-transporting epithelial cells of gut and kidney, which have distinct apical and basolateral domains, and in cells with specialized secretory regions such as neurons.

Nucleus

The largest of the cellular organelles is the nucleus, usually 3 to 8 μm in diameter. The nucleus is defined by an envelope consisting of two membranes, the inner and outer nuclear membranes (Fig. 1.3). Just inside the inner

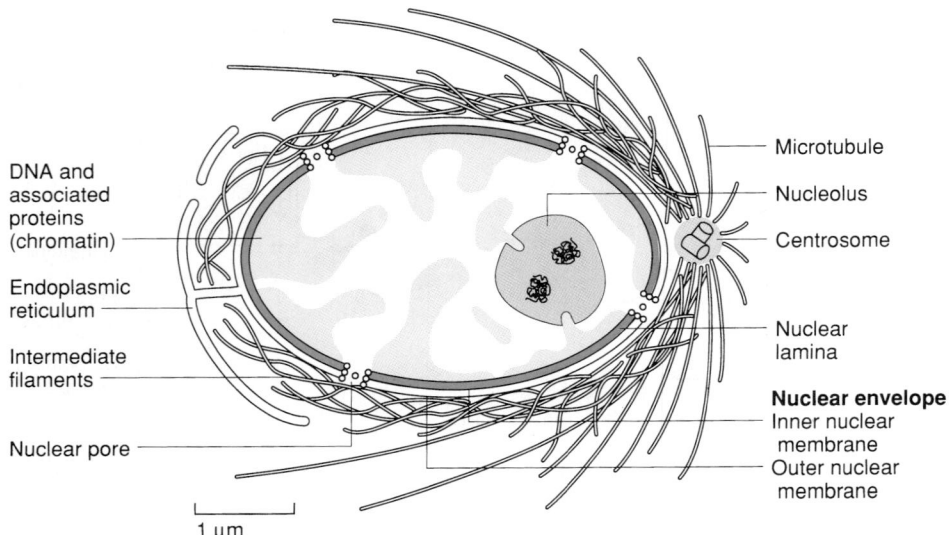

Figure 1.3. Detailed structure of the cell nucleus.

nuclear membrane is a supporting meshwork of intermediate filaments, the nuclear lamina. The outer membrane is continuous with the rough endoplasmic reticulum (ER) and is studded with ribosomes. All of the chromosomal DNA is contained in the nucleus in association with a specialized class of acidic proteins, termed *histones*. Histones and DNA exist together as chromatin fibers. The contents of the nucleus communicate with the cytoplasm by means of openings in the nuclear envelope, called *nuclear pores*. These ringlike pores are composed of specialized proteins that function as energy-dependent channels to regulate the movement of material between nucleus and cytoplasm. The nucleus also contains a specialized region, the nucleolus, where ribosomes are assembled.

The remainder of the cell, external to the nucleus and contained by the plasma membrane, is termed *cytoplasm*. Cytoplasm is composed of a nonparticulate "soup," or cytosol, as well as a number of membranous organelles and the filamentous cytoskeleton.

Mitochondria

Mitochondria are sausage-shaped organelles, 0.2 to 0.5 μm in diameter and up to several micrometers in length. They are defined by a smooth outer membrane and an inner membrane characterized by infoldings, called cristae, which protrude into the central matrix (Fig. 1.4). Mitochondria are the major source of energy production in eukaryotic cells. The enzymes involved with electron transport and oxidative phosphorylation exist in an ordered array of small, stalked particles protruding inward from the inner membrane. Enzymes involved in the final oxidation of sugars and lipids are present in the matrix space, which also contains granules of mitochondrial DNA and a few ribosomes. Mitochondria contain the genetic codes for and synthesize some of their own proteins. They also divide by fission, consistent with the notion that mitochondria originated from captive or symbiotic bacteria. Both mitochondrial membranes have unique characteristics. The outer membrane contains porins, proteins forming large channels that render the membrane permeable to molecules of up to 10 kd. The inner mitochondrial membrane is almost entirely protein, with the lowest lipid content of common biologic membranes. Oxidative phosphorylation at the inner membrane generates an electrochemical proton gradient, and the downhill movement of H⁺ through adenosine triphosphatase (ATPase) molecules provides energy to synthesize ATP.

Endoplasmic Reticulum

The ER is a network of interconnected membranes forming closed vesicles, tubules, and saccules. The ER has a number of functions and is primarily involved in the synthesis of protein and lipids. The ER is divided into rough ER, which is studded with ribosomes and involved in the synthesis of exportable proteins (Fig. 1.5), and smooth ER, which lacks ribosomes and is involved in the synthesis of fatty acids and lipids (Fig. 1.6). Rough ER is especially prominent in cells such as pancreatic acinar cells and plasma cells that secrete large amounts of protein; its functional role in protein synthesis is discussed later. Smooth ER is especially prominent in cells producing lipid derivatives such as the adrenal cortex and in the hepatocyte. Smooth ER also contains enzymes that modify or detoxify endogenous metabolites and foreign molecules such as drugs and pesticides.

Golgi Complex

Adjacent to the rough ER and functionally involved in the sorting and packaging of secreted protein is the Golgi complex (Figs. 1.1, 1.5). Each complex consists of a series of flattened membrane sacs, or cisternae, surrounded by a number of vesicles. These vesicles are transport containers that shuttle proteins destined for secretion from the rough ER to the Golgi complex. During this process, secretory proteins are modified or processed, for example, by addition of sugar residues. The Golgi complex is also the compartment involved in directing secretory proteins into either lysosomes, small vesicles that rapidly move to the periphery of the cell and release their contents, or larger secretory granules, where the contents condense and are stored to await a regulatory signal that initiates fusion with the plasma membrane and secretion (see section on Intracellular Synthesis, Transport, and Organization of Macromolecules).

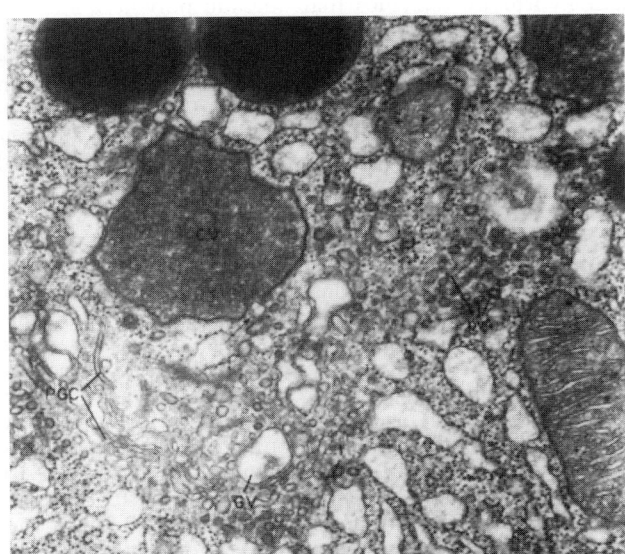

Figure 1.5. Electron photomicrograph of a portion of a pancreatic acinar cell showing endoplasmic reticulum, Golgi apparatus, and forming secretory granules. There is an abundance of small transport vesicles, which shuttle secretory proteins between the various membrane-limited organelles. CV, condensing vacuole; PGC, post-Golgi cisternae; PV, peripheral vesicles; GV, Golgi vacuole; t, transition element of the RER. (Courtesy of J. Jamieson, Yale University, New Haven, CT.)

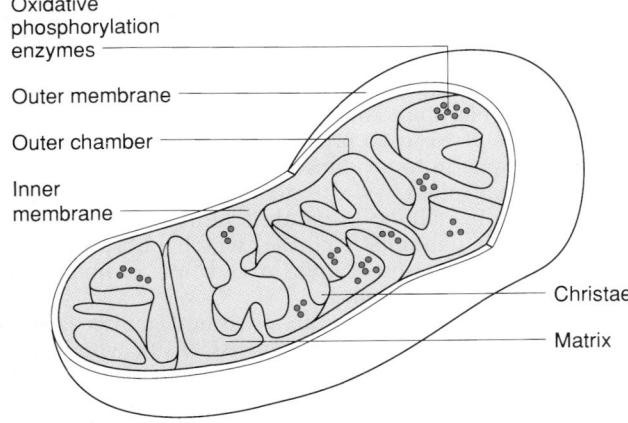

Oxidative phosphorylation enzymes

Outer membrane

Outer chamber

Inner membrane

Christae

Matrix

Figure 1.4. Schematic structure of a typical mitochondrion.

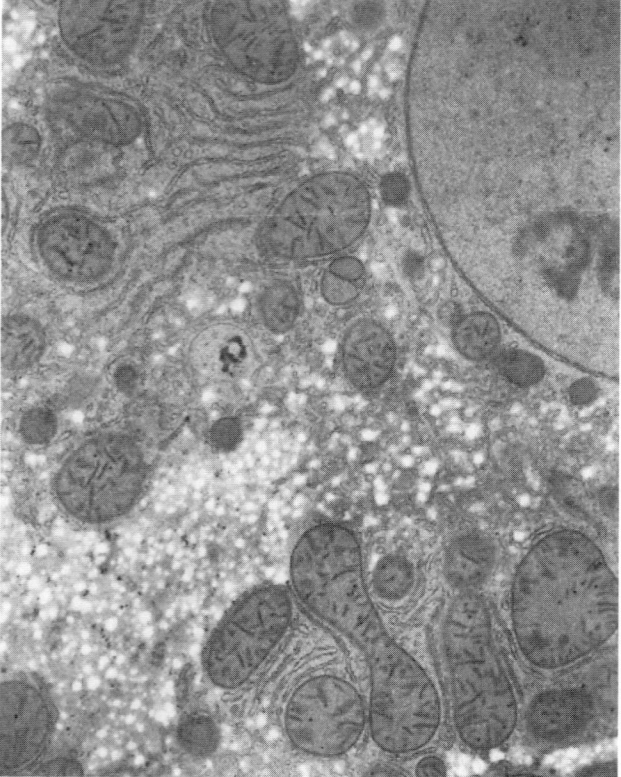

Figure 1.6. Electron photomicrograph of a portion of a hepatocyte, showing a nucleus, mitochondria, and smooth and rough endoplasmic reticulum. (Courtesy of A.K. Christensen, University of Michigan, Ann Arbor, MI.)

Lysosomes and Peroxisomes

Lysosomes are membrane-limited organelles containing acid hydrolytic enzymes that degrade polymers such as proteins, carbohydrates, and nucleic acids (4). Lysosomal enzymes all work best at an acid pH. The interior of the lysosome is maintained at a pH of approximately 5.0 by an H^+-transporting ATPase located in the lysosomal membrane in conjunction with a Cl^- channel protein. This enzyme uses ATP hydrolysis to pump H^+ into the lysosomal lumen. Lysosomes are frequently classified as primary lysosomes, small, spherical structures containing only hydrolytic enzymes, or secondary lysosomes, larger and irregularly shaped, containing membranes or particles that are being digested. Secondary lysosomes result from the fusion of primary lysosomes with engulfed or abnormal organelles or with endocytotic vesicles that are bringing extracellular material into the cell for degradation. The cell is normally protected from lysosomal enzymes by their sequestration in a membrane-limited compartment. In addition, if the lysosome ruptures into the cytoplasmic compartment, the digestive enzymes have little activity because cytoplasmic pH is maintained near 7.0. The lysosomal membrane is permeable to amino acids, monosaccharides, and other similarly sized molecules that are released after hydrolysis. These molecules can be reused by the cell.

Peroxisomes are small (≈ 0.2 to 1 µm), membrane-bounded organelles that contain enzymes involved in the oxidation of fatty acids (5). They are involved in degrading various toxic molecules. Their name is derived from the fact that they generate and degrade large amounts of hydrogen peroxide.

Cytoskeleton

The cytoskeleton is a collection of filamentous protein structures that allows cells (a) to assume and maintain a variety of shapes, (b) to produce directed movement of organelles within the cell, and (c) to effect movement of the entire cell relative to other cells (6,7). Thus, the cytoskeleton is involved with the movement of organelles in cells, the movement of cells such as leukocytes on a substrate, muscle contraction, and the changes in cell shape that occur during development. These multiple activities depend on three main types of filaments—actin filaments, intermediate filaments, and microtubules. Each type of filament is formed from protein monomers and a variety of accessory proteins that serve to cross-link individual filaments or to attach them to membranes. Additional accessory proteins regulate polymerization, that is, assembly and disassembly of filaments or movement, as in muscle and cilia.

Actin-based Filaments

Actin filaments are threadlike structures, about 8 nm in diameter, composed of a tight helix of actin monomers (Fig. 1.7). Actin filaments are polar structures with two different ends that are in equilibrium with free monomers. In muscle cells, most actin exists in stable filaments (F-actin) made from the globular subunits (G-actin). In nonmuscle cells, about half of the actin is in the free monomer pool, and filaments can form by addition of subunits to the positive end. Disassembly occurs by deletion from the negative end. This equilibrium is also regulated by a number of cytosolic actin-binding proteins, including thymosin and profilin which bind G-actin. Polymerization is also regulated by cell surface receptors acting through heterotrimeric and small guanosine triphosphate (GTP)-binding proteins of the Rho family (8).

In skeletal muscle, actin forms a regular array of thin filaments, each with the positive end attached to a Z disk. The other major protein of skeletal muscle, myosin II, contains two heavy chains, each of molecular weight 230 kd, which together form two globular heads, a hinge region, and a coiled, rodlike tail (Fig. 1.7). Also attached to each head are two distinct light chains of approximately 20 kd molecular weight. In skeletal and cardiac muscle, 300 to 400 of these myosin dimers pack together by interaction between their rodlike tails to form a bipolar aggregate, called the *thick filament*. The protruding heads of the thick filament myosin bundles interact with actin in an ATP-dependent manner to create movement by ratcheting the myosin head down the actin filament toward the positive end. This movement causes the thick and thin filaments to overlap and the muscle to shorten. Other proteins, including troponins and tropomyosin, are involved in the regulation of this interaction. One of the troponins (troponin C) binds Ca^{2+}, leading to activation of the myosin ATPase. In smooth muscle and nonmuscle cells, myosin is not as abundant or as well organized, but bipolar filaments of 15 to 20 myosin molecules exist and can interact with actin to produce movement. In this case, activation is controlled by Ca^{2+} interaction with the calcium-binding protein, calmodulin. Calmodulin activates the enzyme, myosin light-chain kinase, which phosphorylates one of the light chains of myosin and thus promotes the actin–myosin interaction.

Nonmuscle cells also contain a distinct, smaller form of myosin, termed *minimyosin* or *myosin I* (9), which does not form filaments. Rather, its smaller tail is attached to membranes or organelles, whereas its single head, which is similar to that of regular myosin, can interact with and move along an actin filament. When the actin is fixed, this

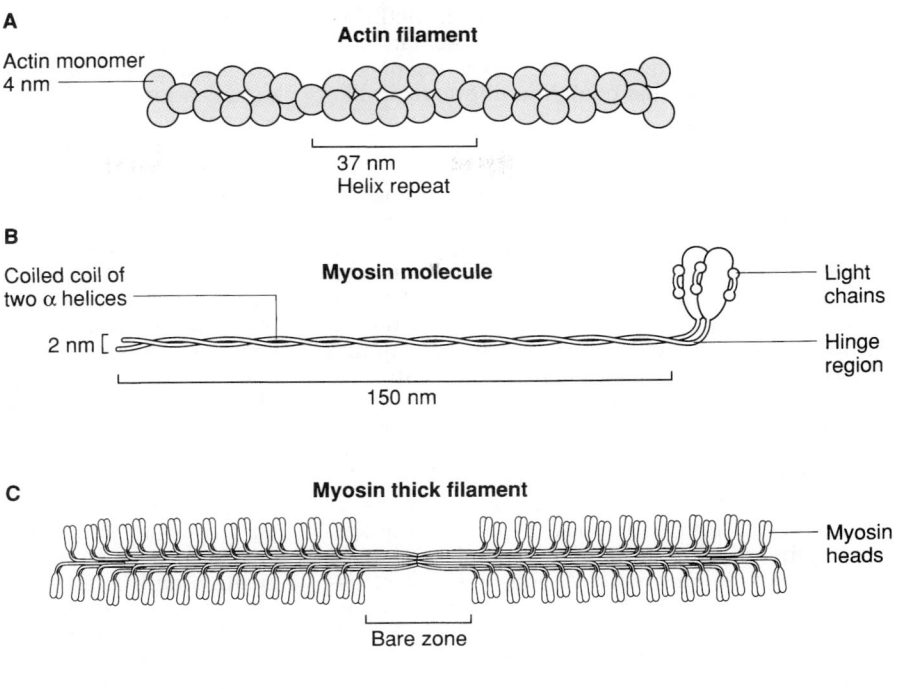

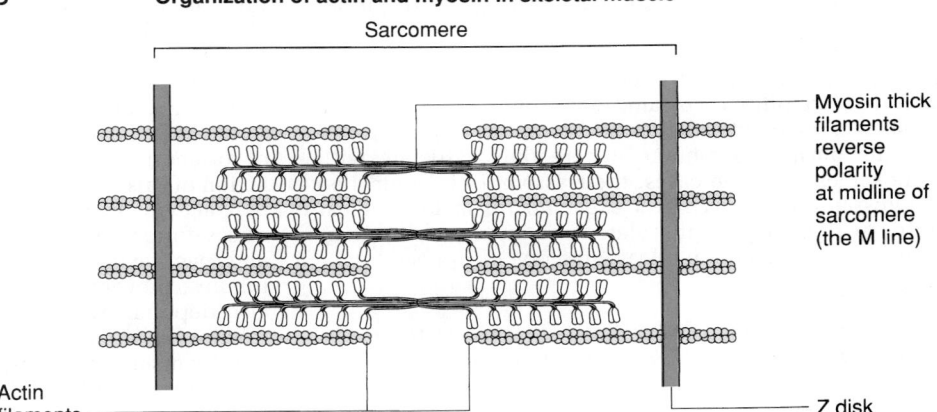

Figure 1.7. Structures of actin and myosin, their organization into filaments, and the organization of actin thin filaments and myosin thick filaments in striated muscle.

can lead to organelle movement, as in cytoplasmic streaming. Other isoforms of myosin exist but are less well characterized.

Muscle-like bundles of actin and myosin can form transiently in nonmuscle cells and can be involved in specialized functions. An example of such a temporary cellular structure is the contractile ring that leads to the separation of the two daughter cells during cell division. The contractile ring contains actin and myosin, and its formation constricts the middle of a cell. When cell division is complete, the ring disappears. Other, less transitory assemblies of actins and myosin are involved in the folding of epithelial cell sheets and in the maintenance of epithelial polarity. The latter is maintained by a belt of filaments running circumferentially around the apical end of the cell. The filaments attach to junctional complexes that connect adjacent cells.

Actin filaments are also involved in the maintenance of cell shape. An especially dense network of actin, sometimes termed the *cell web,* is present just beneath the plasma membrane. The cell web consists of a three-dimensional network of actin filaments stabilized by crosslinking proteins, one of the most abundant of which is fil-

amen (10). Filamen exists as a dimer joined head-to-head with each tail possessing an actin-binding site. The loose actin network is also connected to the plasma membranes by other proteins, including spectrin and fodrin. Because the network must disassemble to allow secretion or endocytosis, it is not surprising that actin-severing proteins also exist. When activated by Ca^{2+}, one of these, gelsolin, severs and forms a cap on the new positive end of the actin filament, thereby leading to a local and usually transient disappearance of the network. Another, cofilin, is regulated by reversible phosphorylation. Actin filaments are also stabilized by capping proteins such as CapZ and tropomodulin.

Another example of a specialized structure based on an actin-containing cytoskeleton are the microvilli found on many cells but especially on intestinal enterocytes. In the intestine, microvilli serve to increase absorptive surface area. The core of each microvillus contains a bundle of 20 to 30 parallel actin filaments attached at the tip by the positive end and extending down to anchor in a specialized cortex at the apical pole of the cell. The actin filaments are held together by several small actin-binding proteins, such as fimbrin and villin. Fimbrin contains two actin-binding sites on a single polypeptide chain such that the actin filaments are tied into a compact bundle with regular spacing. The bundle is also connected to the overlying plasma membrane by lateral arms that contain a minimyosin-like molecule.

Intermediate Filaments

Intermediate filaments are a heterogeneous class of tough protein fibers named for their thickness (≈10 nm), which is intermediate between the thin and thick filaments of muscle cells (11). These structural elements usually form a basket around the nucleus and extend out to the cell periphery. Intermediate filaments are formed from fibrous proteins that associate side to side in overlapping arrays to form long, tough, stable filaments. In contrast to actin filaments and microtubules, which are made up of unique subunits, intermediate filaments are made up of a variety of subunit proteins with homology to one another in the fiber-forming domain of each molecule.

Intermediate filaments are classified on the basis of amino acid structure into four types. Type I are the keratins, found primarily in epithelial cells and sometimes subdivided into acidic and basic. A large number of tissue-specific classes of keratin exist and can be used to distinguish the cell type of origin for certain tumors. Type II intermediate filaments include vimentin, desmin, and glial fibrillary protein. Type III are neurofilaments and are restricted to neurons. Type IV proteins are nuclear lamins that form a two-dimensional sheet just inside the inner nuclear membrane (Fig. 1.3).

Intermediate filaments are believed to be structural elements designed to resist stress and provide support. As such, they are often associated with other, more dynamic cytoskeletal elements such as microtubules (Fig. 1.8), and with the plasma membrane, where they associate with desmosomes. In some cases, their assembly is controlled by phosphorylation. This is especially true for nuclear lamins, which are phosphorylated and disassemble during mitotic division as the nuclear envelope disappears.

Microtubules

Microtubules are found in all cells except erythrocytes. Structurally, they are hollow fibers 24 nm in diameter that vary in length from less than one up to hundreds of micrometers. Their basic structure consists of 13 parallel rows, or protofilaments, each composed of globular subunits (Fig. 1.9). Chemically, microtubules contain two re-

lated major proteins, α- and β-tubulin, each with a molecular weight of approximately 50 kd. In the cell, these subunits exist as an ab heterodimer called tubulin. Tubulin dimers arranged αβ–αβ–αβ make up the protofilament. As a result of this organization, microtubules are oriented with a positive and a negative end, and all structures that contain microtubules are polarized. Specialized cellular structures based on microtubules include cilia, neuronal axons, and the mitotic spindle.

Microtubules are frequently associated with a specialized organelle, the centriole (Fig. 1.1). A centriole is a short, cylindric structure composed of nine groups of triplet microtubules. Centrioles usually exist in pairs oriented at right angles to each other. All cells contain at least one pair of centrioles near the nucleus, surrounded by a cloud of amorphous material, called the *microtubule-organizing center*. The centriole divides during DNA replication. After forming the organizing center for each pole of the mitotic spindle, one centriole remains with each daughter cell. Because microtubules always have their negative pole associated with a centriole or microtubule-organizing center, and because growth occurs faster on the positive end, microtubules can be observed to grow out from the organizing center. Cilia are made up of an ordered array of microtubules, and each is attached to a modified centriole, termed the *basal body*.

Within the cell, microtubules exist in a dynamic state in which they are continually forming and dissociating as tubulin subunits are added to or removed from the ends (12). This dynamic equilibrium involves the conversion of GTP bound to tubulin to guanosine diphosphate (GDP). Each tubulin molecule possesses a binding site for colchicine, and binding of this drug prevents microtubule formation. Colchicine binding leads to the disappearance of formed microtubules and is the basis of the antimitotic action of this class of compounds. Other antimitotic agents that act on microtubules include vinblastine, which induces formation of paracrystalline aggregates of tubulin, and paclitaxel (Taxol), which stabilizes formed microtubules, preventing their depolymerization. Microtubules also depolymerize at low temperatures. Although microtubules in dividing or motile cells such as leukocytes rapidly disappear in response to colchicine or low temperature, microtubules in organized parenchymal or epithelial cells disappear more slowly, and some microtubules, such as those in cilia, appear resistant. This difference, which is related to the function of the organelle (i.e., whether it

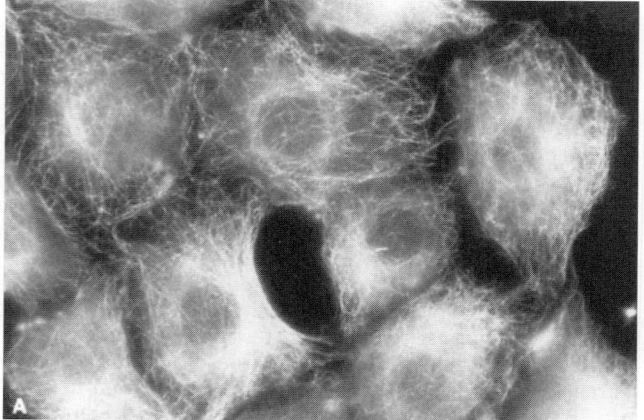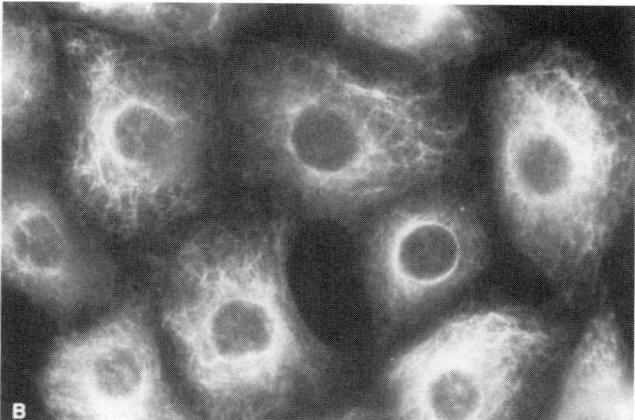

Figure 1.8. The distribution of cytoskeletal elements in pulmonary endothelial cells as detected by fluorescence-specific antibodies. Although surrounded by a cytoskeletal network, the nuclei are unstained. *(A)* Antitubulin stain. *(B)* Antivimentin stain. (Courtesy of M.J. Welsh, University of Michigan, Ann Arbor, MI.)

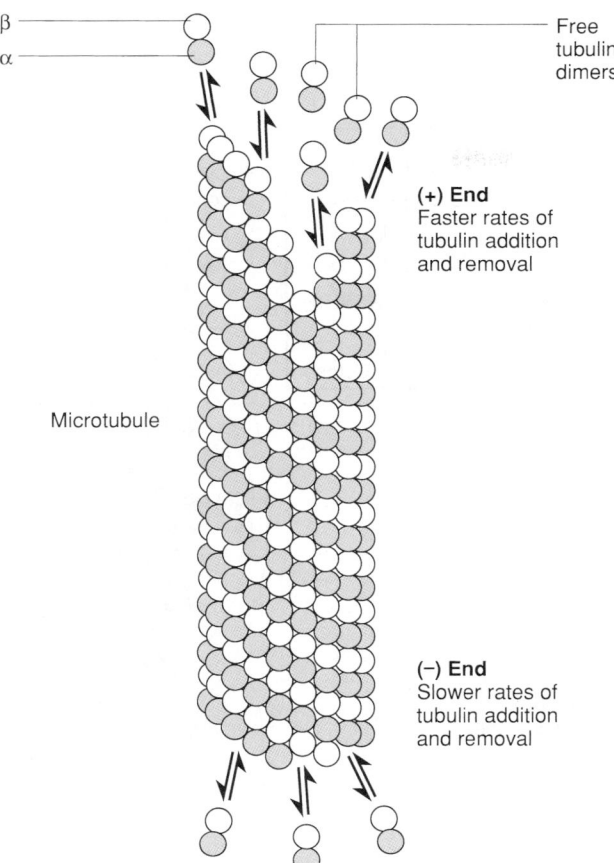

Figure 1.9. Diagram of a microtuble composed of longitudinal rows of tubulin dimers. The α- and β-tubulin dimers add to or dissociate from the two ends.

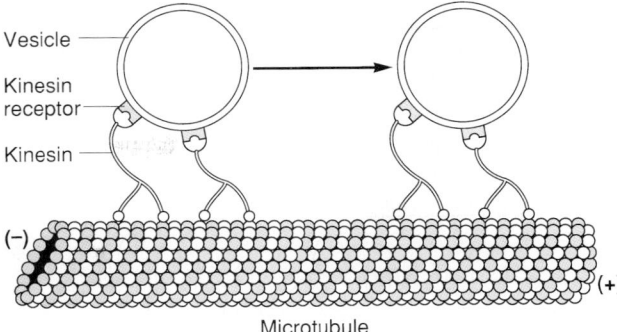

Figure 1.10. Model of kinesin-mediated transport of vesicles along a microtubule. The kinesin molecules move along the microtubule by interacting with tubulin in an adenosine triphosphate-requiring manner.

needs to be stable or dynamic), is due in large part to other associated proteins, termed *microtubule-associated proteins* (MAPs). The MAPs are responsible for holding microtubules together in permanent arrays, attaching them to other organelles, including membrane vesicles, and generating the force that is involved in microtubule-based movement. Many MAPs are high-molecular-weight proteins or complexes of proteins. One prominent lower-molecular-weight class is termed *tau protein*; it acts to facilitate microtubule polymerization.

The transport of organelles in cytoplasm is usually associated with microtubules. The most specialized case is axonal flow, whereby vesicles move at rates of 3 μm/s (250 mm/d) along the axon. When viewed in the electron microscope, a cross-bridge structure exists, connecting the moving particle to the microtubule. A motor protein, kinesin, has been isolated that mediates movement along microtubules in the negative-to-positive direction and is responsible for antegrade rapid axonal transport (13). Kinesin is composed of heavy-chain subunits, which bind tubulin and possess ATPase activity, and light chains, which attach to cellular organelles. When ATP is hydrolyzed, the kinesin moves along the microtubule, transporting the bound vesicle (Fig. 1.10). Kinesin is now known to belong to a family of motor proteins that include cytosolic kinesins responsible for vesicle and organelle transport, spindle kinesins that participate in spindle assembly and chromosomal movement during mitosis, and cytosolic dyneins, which are the primary negative end-directed motor proteins.

A specialized form of microtubule-based motility is the beating cilium. Each cilia has a basic structure of nine microtubule doublets surrounding a central microtubule pair. The entire structure, called an *axoneme,* also contains other linker proteins that hold the unit together and a specialized MAP protein, dynein, which makes contact with the adjacent microtubule doublet. Dynein is a large protein (400 kd) with ATPase activity and, like kinesin, generates force on the adjacent microtubule in one direction. Because the microtubules are attached to one another, what would otherwise be a sliding motion is converted into a bending or whiplike motion. Cilia are especially prominent in the respiratory tract, where they generate movement of mucus out of the bronchial system.

CELL–CELL INTERACTION

All cells must interact with their neighbors, and most are arranged in assemblies called *tissues.* The cells in a tissue are in contact with the extracellular matrix, which in cases such as connective tissue may surround the cells. In other cases, epithelial cells are directly attached to each other and the extracellular matrix is reduced to a thin layer, the basal lamina, which underlies the cellular sheet. Although cells such as neurons and endocrine cells influence other cells by specialized secretions, this section considers direct physical interactions mediated by molecules in the cell membrane and by the cytoskeleton.

Cell Junctions

Cell junctions were originally identified and classified by their structure as observed using the electron microscope. Functionally, cell junctions can be classified as occluding, anchoring, or communicating (2). The major occluding junction is the tight junction or zonula occludens, which connects cells in epithelia and thereby allows epithelia to serve as selective permeability barriers. As discussed later, epithelia are almost always engaged in transcellular transport. Tight junctions make this possible both by preventing backflux between cells of transported molecules and by maintaining distinct apical and basal membrane proteins. Tight junctions are normally located near the apical pole of the cell and form a belt that completely encircles the cell (Fig. 1.11). In transmission electron microscopy, the junction appears as a series of focal contacts between the outer leaflets of adjacent plasma membrane. In freeze-fracture electron microscopy, the junction appears as an anastomosing network of sealing strands. Although all tight junctions are impermeable to

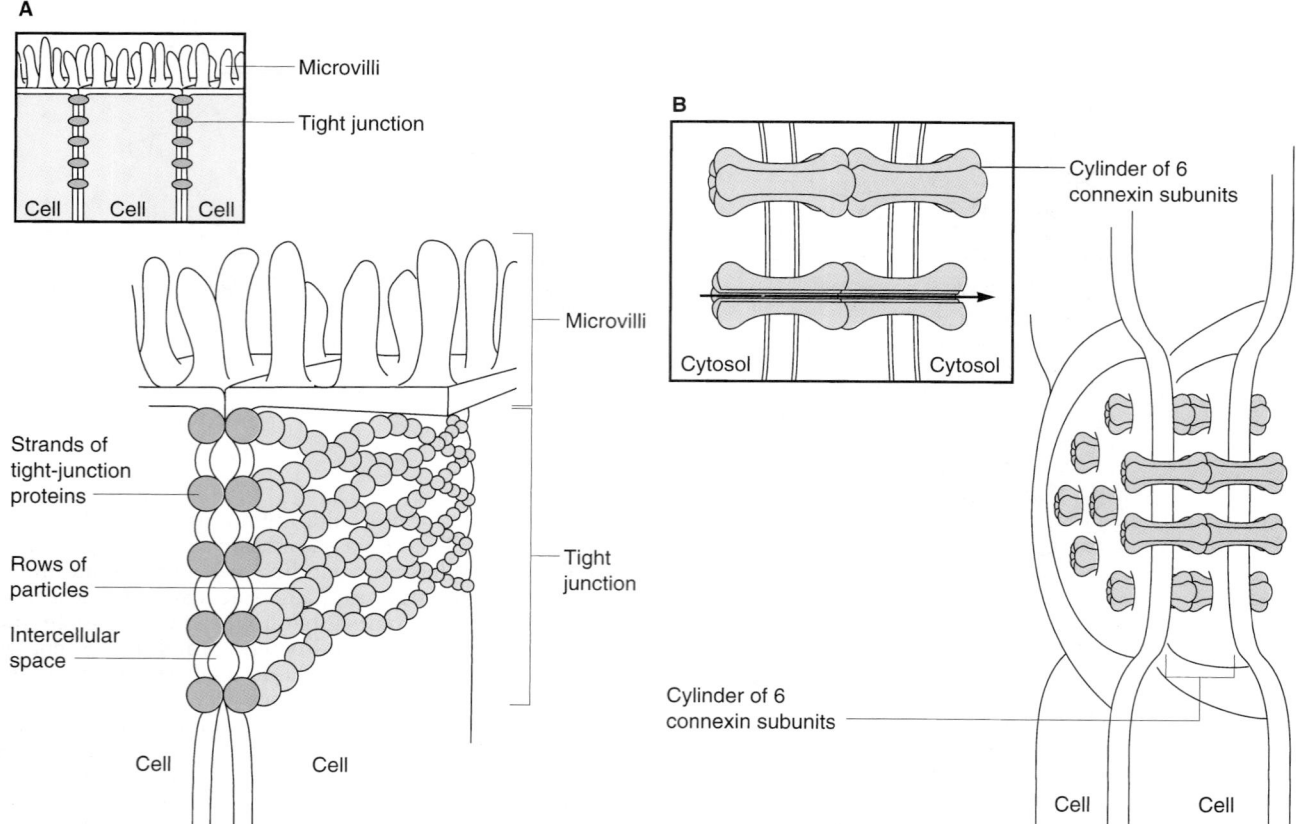

Figure 1.11. Schematic view of two intracellular junctions.

macromolecules, the barrier to ions and water is related to the number of sealing strands. The strands are composed of long rows of transmembrane proteins, occludin and claudin (14). Attached to their cytosolic domains are the proteins ZO-1, ZO-2, and ZO-3, which are also bound to actin.

Anchoring junctions connect the cytoskeleton of the cell to extracellular matrix or neighboring cells (15). Morphologically, these are adherens junctions or desmosomes. Adherens junctions occur in epithelia as a continuous adhesion belt, the zonula adherens, located just below the tight junction. Morphologically, this consists of a long stretch of continuous contact between cell membranes. The membranes are held together by a linker protein, E-cadherin, also called *uvomorulin*. E-cadherin is a single-pass transmembrane glycoprotein with four extracellular Ca^{2+}-binding domains and a terminal domain that binds to the same domain on another cadherin molecule. The properties of this molecule account for the Ca^{2+} dependence of cell adhesion. Within the cell, the adhesion belt is attached by the cytoplasmic end of cadherin molecules to contractile bundles of actin filaments by a set of intracellular linker proteins, including catenins, vinculin, and α-actinin. In nonepithelial cells, adherens junctions are localized as focal contacts or adhesion plaques where bundles of actin filaments terminate and serve primarily as attachment sites to the extracellular matrix. In addition to participating in anchoring junctions in adult cells, the cadherin family of cell-adhesion molecules, along with the structurally distinct nerve-cell adhesion molecule (N-CAM), intercellular adhesion molecule (ICAM) and selectins, play important roles in morphogenesis and in the adhesion of leukocytes to endothelial cells during inflammation.

The other type of anchoring junction is the desmosome. Desmosomes are button-like points of attachment with a prominent intracellular plaque that weld together adjacent cells by serving as anchoring sites for intermediate filaments in the cell. The particular type of intermediate filament depends on the cell type, and is keratin in most epithelial cells and desmin in cardiac muscle cells. The transmembrane-linker proteins in desmosomes are cadherins that, as discussed earlier, bind each other by a Ca^{2+}-dependent mechanism. Hemidesmosomes, or half-desmosomes, are morphologically similar to desmosomes but are chemically and functionally distinct and are considered in the next section (Cell–Matrix Adhesion).

The third functional type of cell junction is the gap junction (16,17), which is specialized for cell communication (Fig. 1.11B). In conventional electron micrographs, it appears as a patch where adjacent membranes are separated by a uniform narrow gap of approximately 20 nm. This gap, however, is spanned by protein molecules that form an array of channels through which ions and small molecules up to approximately 1,000 daltons can pass. Thus, the junction mediates both electrical and chemical coupling. This is most dramatic in cardiac and smooth muscle, but also plays an important role in embryogenesis. Gap junctions are formed from transmembrane proteins called *connexins*. Multiple connexins have been identified, each of which contains four transmembrane domains and a variable cytoplasmic domain; many of these are identified by their apparent mass (i.e., connexin-32, connexin-26), and are expressed in a tissue-specific manner. A ring of six identical connexins forms a *connexon*, with a central aqueous pore. The connexons protrude from the membrane and, when aligned with a connexon on an adjacent cell, both hold the two membranes at the characteristic distance and form a channel. These channels are not continuously open but regulated by Ca^{2+}, intracellular pH, and protein phosphorylation.

Cell–Matrix Adhesion

Extracellular matrix is a meshwork of negatively charged polysaccharide glycosaminoglycan chains and protein fibers. The protein fibers are mainly structural, such as collagen and elastin, or adhesive, such as fibronectin and laminin. The principal protein molecules in the plasma membrane that serve as receptors for matrix molecules are the integrins (18). Integrins are so named to indicate that they integrate the extracellular matrix and the cytoskeleton. Evidence is now emerging that integrins are functional as well as structural integrators and that they are involved in bidirectional signaling across the plasma membrane.

Integrins are noncovalently attached heterodimeric glycoproteins composed of α and β subunits. So far, 17 α and 8 β subunits have been identified. Different cell types express and synthesize different $\alpha\beta$ complexes, with the combination of α and β determining the ligand specificity. For example, $\alpha_5\beta_1$ is a fibronectin receptor, whereas $\alpha_6\beta_1$ is a laminin receptor; both are expressed on most cells. By contrast, β_2 chains are primarily expressed on white blood cells and mediate cell–cell interactions (e.g., between white blood cells and vascular endothelium). A significant amount of redundancy occurs; most integrins bind several adhesive glycoproteins, and most adhesive glycoproteins bind to more than one protein.

Each integrin subunit spans the membrane once with a large extracellular domain and a small cytoplasmic domain. Divalent cation-binding motifs are present in both subunits near the presumed ligand-binding site. Most integrins are clustered into focal adhesion plaques and attach to actin through linker proteins, particularly talin and α-actinin (19). In fibroblasts, these focal adhesions colocalize with the termination of stress fibers. Other proteins in the adhesion plaque include a 125-kd tyrosine kinase termed p125[FAK] (focal adhesion kinase). By virtue of this connection to the cytoskeleton, cells can orient the matrix macromolecules they secrete, and in turn, matrix macromolecules can organize the cytoskeleton. A special case is the integrin found in hemidesmosomes $\alpha_6\beta_4$, which connects intracellularly to intermediate filaments by distinct linker proteins. Whereas keratin filaments associated with desmosomes have lateral attachments to the desmosome, many filaments associated with hemidesmosomes end in the plaque.

Integrins are components of inside-out signal transduction. Various β_2-integrins on monocytes and neutrophils are stimulated (i.e., show an increased binding affinity) in response to inflammatory mediators. Platelet activation induces its integrins to bind fibrinogen. In other cases, phosphorylation of a β_1-integrin during mitosis inhibits binding of fibronectin, allowing the cell to round up or detach. Integrins also mediate outside-in signaling. The binding of antibodies or glycoproteins to integrins can affect intracellular pH and Ca^{2+} as well as tyrosine phosphorylation and lead to cellular differentiation, activation, or proliferation. An integrin-associated protein appears to function as a Ca^{2+} channel. The protein p125[FAK] can be activated by both integrins and peptide growth factors, although its role in cell function remains to be determined.

MEMBRANE TRANSPORT

The plasma membrane physically defines the boundaries of the cell and acts as a dynamic interface that medi-

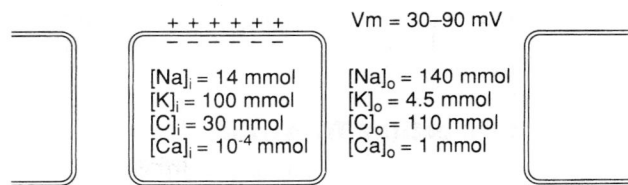

Figure 1.12. Intracellular ionic composition differs markedly from that of the surrounding extracellular fluid. Representative values for intracellular and extracellular ion concentrations are shown.

ates all interactions of the cell with the extracellular environment. The survival of the cell requires that cytosolic composition be maintained within narrow limits, despite the constant influx of nutrients and the simultaneous outflow of waste. This section focuses on the membrane transport mechanisms that enable the cell to maintain its unique composition despite the continual turnover of its contents.

A striking feature of living cells is the marked difference between the composition of the cytosol, the fluid within the cell, and the fluid of the extracellular milieu, as illustrated in Fig. 1.12. The most familiar example is the distribution of sodium (Na^+) and potassium (K^+). Cells are typically rich in K^+ and contain relatively little Na^+, despite the fact that they are constantly bathed by a fluid with precisely the opposite composition. Even more impressive is the distribution of ionized (as opposed to bound) Ca^{2+}. The extracellular concentration of this ion is typically of the order of 10^{-3} mol/L (1 mmol/L), whereas that of the cytosol is typically 10^{-7} mol/L (10^{-4} mmol/L), a 10,000-fold gradient. These and many other examples establish the fact that the cell and its environment are not in equilibrium. Such nonequilibrium ion distributions are all the more remarkable in light of the fact that the plasma membrane is, to varying degrees, leaky to ions such as Na^+, K^+, and Ca^{2+}. The key to understanding the ability of the cell to maintain nonequilibrium cellular composition is found in two fundamental properties of the plasma membrane—selectivity and energy conversion.

Selectivity and Its Modulation

The plasma membrane is leaky to a variety of substances, but it exhibits an astounding ability to discriminate, or select, one substance over another. For example, the plasma membrane of many cells is 10 to 100 times more leaky to K^+ than Na^+. Even more spectacular is the selectivity for some organic compounds: D-glucose is often favored over the L-isomer by 1,000-fold. The molecular basis for this selectivity lies in the properties of membrane-spanning proteins, which exhibit an enzyme-like specificity for particular molecules and can thus catalyze their selective transport across the plasma membrane. Much of the research in the field of membrane transport is devoted to identifying and characterizing the specific membrane proteins that constitute highly selective transport pathways.

The selectivity of biologic membranes can be altered drastically as a result of regulatory or signaling processes that occur in the cell. In nerve and muscle cells, for example, the resting membrane is 10- to 100-fold selective for K^+ over Na^+, but in a matter of milliseconds, at the peak of an action potential, this selectivity can be completely reversed so that the membrane becomes 100-fold selective for Na^+ over K^+. In the appropriate cell types, insulin can cause a 30-fold increase in the leakiness to glucose. This modulated selectivity is the basis for cellular signaling as well as regulatory processes that protect the integrity of individual cells and act as crucial elements in epithelial transport processes.

Energy-converting Transport

The selectivity of the plasma membrane, although impressive, cannot account for the nonequilibrium composition of living cells. A cell can be maintained in a nonequilibrium state only by the continual expenditure of energy. The maintenance of steady-state, nonequilibrium cellular composition is possible because the plasma membrane is the site of energy converters, membrane proteins that function as biologic transport machines using the energy derived from metabolic processes to perform transport work. The archetype for the biologic transport machine is the Na^+-K^+-ATPase, a membrane protein that hydrolyzes cytosolic ATP and couples the resulting free energy to the transport of Na^+ and K^+. The catalytic cycle involves the binding of internal Na and external K in such a way that the hydrolysis of one molecule of ATP is associated with the movement of exactly three Na^+ out of and two K^+ into the cell.

The energy conversion that occurs in the Na^+-K^+-ATPase is often referred to as an example of primary active transport, whereby energy is derived directly from ATP hydrolysis. A second and equally important type of energy-converting transporter is one in which the energy inherent in a transmembrane ion gradient, usually that of Na^+, can be used to drive the transport of a second species (e.g., protons, calcium, amino acids, or glucose). Such secondary active transport processes are extremely important to the cell because they allow energy that has been invested in the transmembrane Na gradient by the Na^+-K^+-ATPase to be used to perform various kinds of transport work (Fig. 1.13).

Cell composition is determined by the interaction of energy converters and selective leak pathways. This can be seen in Fig. 1.14. Two cells are diagrammed, one a symmetric cell and the other a polarized cell, such as is found in an epithelial cell layer. Mechanisms for Na transport are diagrammed for both cells. In either case, a steady-state, intracellular Na concentration is achieved by a balance between the net inflow of Na and the net efflux of Na. In the case of the symmetric cell, Na is shown entering by a variety of mechanisms, Na channels, Na-dependent cotransport, and countertransport. Na leaves the cell through the Na^+-K^+-ATPase. The balance between these opposing processes determines the level of intracellular Na. Simi-

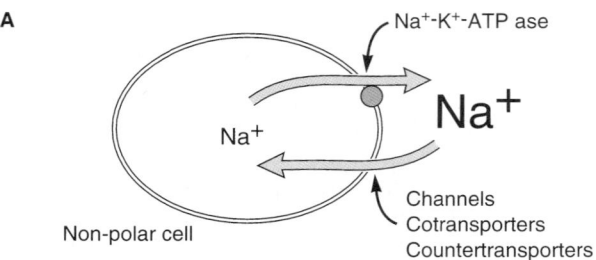

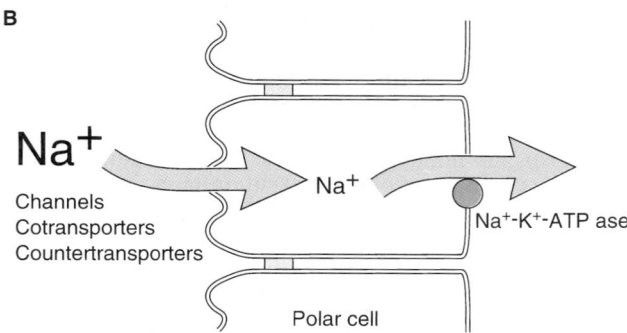

Figure 1.14. Cytosolic composition is maintained in a steady state by balancing pumps and leaks. Shown here are mechanisms that maintain low intracellular Na^+ concentration in two cells, one a symmetric cell *(A)* and the other a polar, epithelial cell *(B).* In the symmetric cell, Na^+ efflux by the pump is balanced by the sum of all the Na^+ leaks into the cell. In the polar cell, Na^+ influx at the apical (lumen-facing) side is balanced by active Na^+ efflux at the basolateral (blood-facing) side. The rates of Na^+ transport are typically much greater for the polar cell, which is designed to effect the net transcellular movement of Na^+ that is important for the function of the kidney and gastrointestinal tract.

larly, in the polarized cell, net transcellular Na transport is achieved by the serial arrangement of apical Na entry and basolateral Na exit, so that the level of intracellular Na is determined by the balance between these two processes. Despite similarities, these two cellular processes may differ significantly with regard to one important variable, the turnover rate. The symmetric cell is typically designed to maintain static gradients at a minimum rate of turnover; that is, leak rates are low, so pump rates are low. In contrast, the polarized cell is specialized for throughput. Entry and exit rates are elevated to produce significant transcellular Na transport that is important, for example, in the function of the airways, kidney, and gastrointestinal tract.

Membrane Composition: Implications for Selectivity and Energy Conversion

Plasma membranes are mosaic structures, consisting of a matrix of lipid in which are embedded the membrane proteins responsible for the specialized transport properties of the cell interface (Fig. 1.2). It is instructive to consider some of the general features of the lipid and protein regions of the plasma membrane, as an introduction to the molecular basis for membrane selectivity.

Lipid is a major component of the plasma membrane. Membrane phospholipids, being amphipathic molecules with polar and nonpolar ends, exhibit a strong tendency to organize into a stable, bimolecular layer (Fig. 1.15). The hydrocarbon layer formed by the fatty acid tails of phospholipids exhibits the transport properties that are expected for a layer of oil. Substances can penetrate this

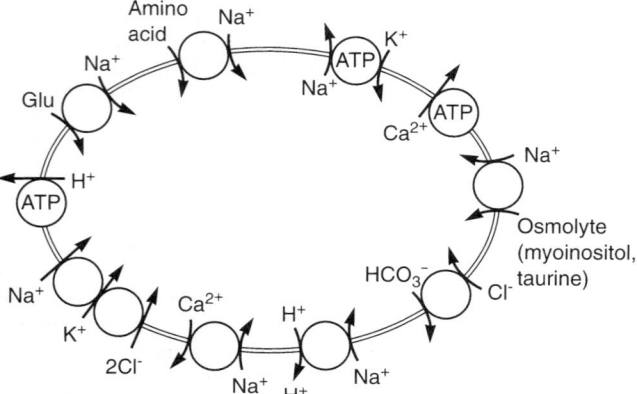

Figure 1.13. The plasma membrane contains a variety of energy-converting transporters, which function to maintain intracellular composition away from equilibrium.

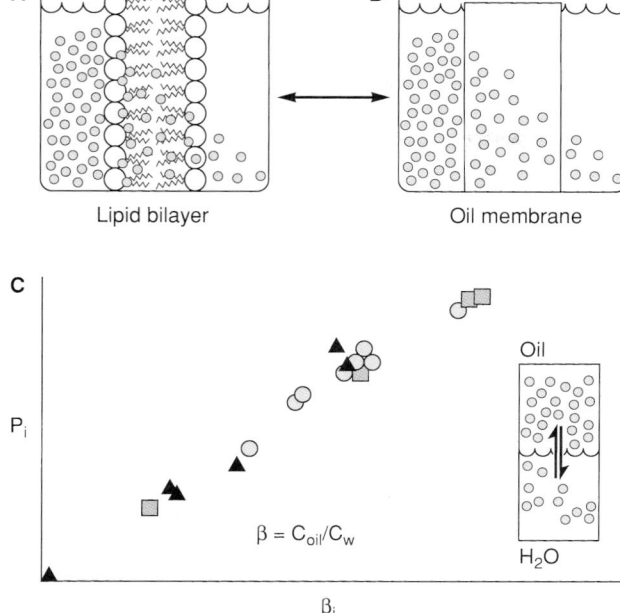

Figure 1.15. Lipophilic substances can cross a lipid bilayer by solubility diffusion. The lipid bilayer *(A)* can be approximated by a layer of oil *(B)*, and the permeability of the oil membrane to various substances is expected to be proportional to β_i, the oil–water partition coefficient or solubility of the substance in oil *(C)*. The *inset* illustrates the determination of β_i as an oil–water partition coefficient.

layer by a process of solubility–diffusion, that is, dissolving into the hydrocarbon and diffusing across. A model based on the simple notion of dissolving (partitioning) and diffusion predicts the transport properties of a lipid bilayer with amazing accuracy, and the tenet that plasma membranes are in general permeable to lipophilic molecules remains one of the most useful generalizations in cell biology.

The planar nature of the bimolecular lipid layer, combined with the physical properties of the fatty acid hydrocarbon tails of the phospholipids, has led to the concept of the plasma membrane as a "two-dimensional fluid." Experiments with labeled molecules indicate that individual phospholipids can move about relatively freely within the plane of each monolayer, but the polar head groups anchor the molecules so effectively in the aqueous phase that movement from one monolayer to another is relatively rare. Another reflection of the fluidity of the lipid bilayer is that some membrane proteins exhibit lateral mobility; that is, they can move about within the plane of the bilayer. The degree of fluidity exhibited by a lipid bilayer is affected by the type of phospholipid (particularly the degree of unsaturation of the fatty acid side chains) and the cholesterol content. Cholesterol intercalates between phospholipids and decreases membrane fluidity.

Membrane Proteins: Specific Transport Pathways

The movement of substances like glucose and ions across the plasma membrane requires specialized permeation pathways, which are formed by membrane-spanning proteins. In the earlier literature, a variety of transmembrane transport processes were attributed to components referred to as "carriers." The word *carrier* naturally evokes a picture of a mobile membrane component that could bind the transported substance and shuttle it back and forth across the lipid bilayer. Some antibiotic molecules, such as valinomycin, facilitate transmembrane ion movement in precisely this way. There is little doubt, however, that the endogenous mediators of specific transmembrane transport processes are proteins that span the bilayer to provide a path from one side to the other, which is a hospitable environment for non-lipid-soluble (hydrophilic) moieties such as ions, sugars, and amino acids. These transport proteins can be divided into two broad categories: channels and carriers. In the former, the protein forms a pore that can open and close and provides a mechanism for passive flow of solutes or water across membranes. In the latter, the protein is likely to form a porelike structure, but translocation is coupled to specific conformational changes in the protein (see later).

The transport function of membrane-spanning proteins requires that they have a dual nature chemically—they must interact both with the hydrocarbon of the bilayer and the transported substrate. Accordingly, such proteins are amphiphilic, with a hydrophobic portion that permits the protein to pass through the lipid layer and hydrophilic portions that are stable in the aqueous environments of the cytoplasm and the extracellular fluid. The functional, three-dimensional structure of such a protein may require that it cross the membrane as many as 10 or 12 times. Such proteins may consist of alternating hydrophilic and hydrophobic regions (Fig. 1.16). If the amino acid sequence is known, as a result of cloning the cDNA, it is possible to estimate the relative ability of various portions of the protein to interact with the bilayer. Stretches of amino acids that are highly hydrophobic (or hydropathic) are more likely to reside in the bilayer. A plot of the hydropathy index versus the position of the amino acids in the primary sequence (Fig. 1.16) is used to identify regions of the protein that are likely to be associated with the membrane. This hydropathy plot provides a valuable first guess as to the number of membrane-spanning regions of the protein and points to possible large intracellular or extracellular domains. In the case of transport proteins, one expectation is that the membrane-spanning region is associated with the transport process *per se,* whereas large cytoplasmic or extracellular regions may be involved in regulatory functions, such as the binding of second messengers or hormones.

A membrane-spanning polypeptide chain usually adopts an α-helical conformation. This conformation is dictated by the fact that, in the absence of water, the polar peptide bonds tend to form hydrogen bonds with each other. The α-helical conformation maximizes the number of such bonds and usually forms in such a way as also to enable nonpolar amino acid side chains to interact with the lipid bilayer matrix. An important tertiary structure thought to be common to ion channel proteins is the juxtaposition of a number of membrane-spanning α helices, arranged like barrel staves, to form a central pore that is highly polar and thus a hospitable environment for ion conduction (Fig. 1.16B).

Transport: Energetics and Mechanism

All transport mechanisms, regardless of their complexity, can be viewed as consisting of three steps: (a) the entry of the transported substance into the membrane on one side, (b) a translocation event that conveys the substance to the other side, and (c) the exit of the substance from the membrane and into the aqueous compartment. Understanding the mechanism for this process means comprehending the physical processes that govern each of these three steps. A complementary approach to understanding

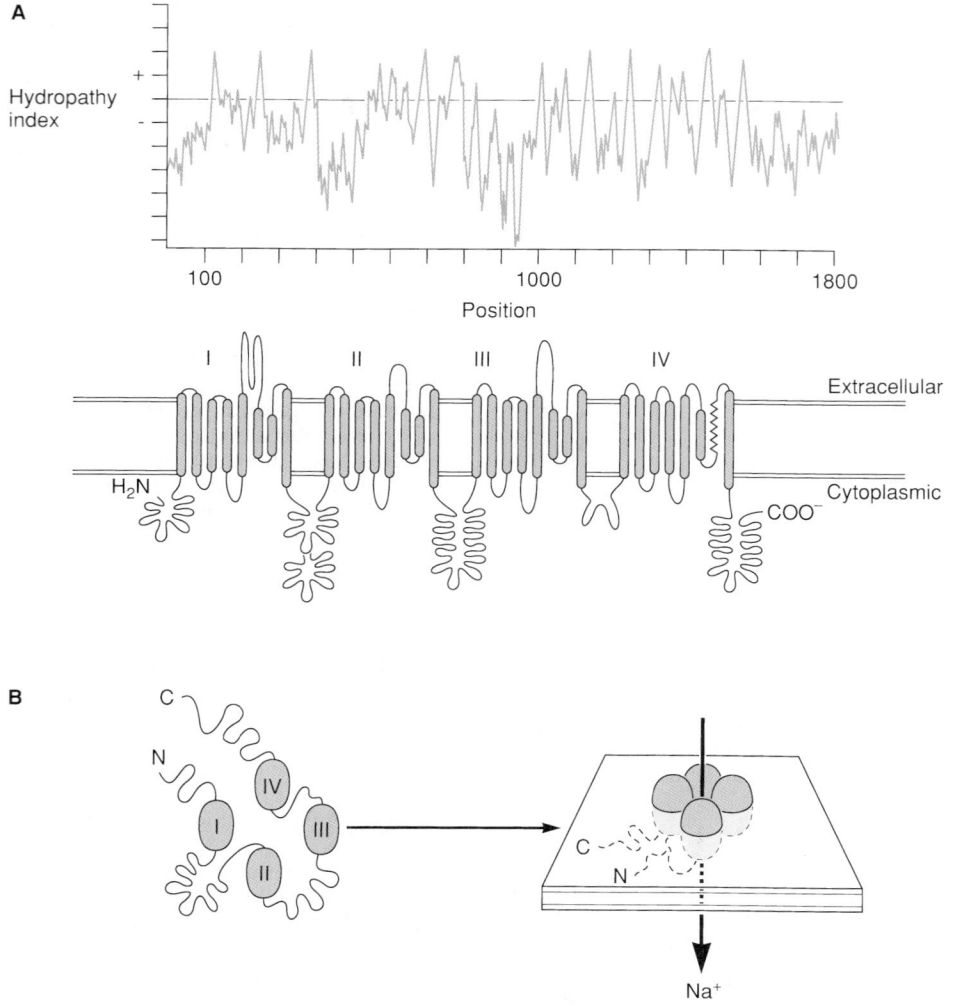

Figure 1.16. *(A)* The amino acid sequence of a sodium channel protein derived from the cDNA can be analyzed by plotting the hydropathy index versus the position of the amino acid. *(B)* Regions predicted to be hydrophobic (+) are represented in the diagram as putative membrane-spanning domains. The four repeated motifs are shown as folding around a central pore to form an ion channel. (After Trimmer JS, Agnew WS. Molecular diversity of voltage-sensitive Na channels. *Annu Rev Physiol* 1989;51:401.)

transport mechanisms is to inquire about the energetics of the transport process. Is the transporter a passive leak pathway, or does the transport event involve energy conversion?

The basis for energetic analysis of transport processes is the concept of equilibrium (20,21). If the distribution of any substance, say glucose, Na, or K, is not at equilibrium, then flow of that substance is expected to be in a direction so as to restore equilibrium. If the distribution is maintained away from equilibrium, this means that some process is moving the substance "uphill," and such a process must involve energy conversion. For uncharged substances, the analysis is particularly simple. Consider, for example, the distribution of glucose across a cell membrane (Fig. 1.17). The equilibrium condition is [glucose]$_{in}$ = [glucose]$_{out}$. In this condition, there is no net flow of glucose through a simple glucose leak pathway. If [glucose]$_{in}$ is less than [glucose]$_{out}$, net passive glucose flow through a leak pathway is into the cell. If [glucose]$_{in}$ is greater than [glucose]$_{out}$, glucose leaves the cell through such a transporter. Because this is a leak pathway (non-energy con-

verting), glucose flow can only be "downhill," from a high glucose concentration to a low glucose concentration.

It is useful to analyze equilibrium for such a solute in terms of free energy, rather than concentration. To do this, we define the difference in chemical potential for glucose across the membrane, $\Delta\mu_{glu}$, as follows:

$$\Delta\mu_{glu} \text{ (in J/mol)} = RT \ln \frac{(glucose)_i}{(glucose)_o}$$

where R = the universal gas constant, and T = the absolute temperature.

In terms of free energy, the equilibrium condition is specified by $\Delta\mu_{glu} = 0$. If $\Delta\mu_{glu} \neq 0$, there is a driving force for net flow, and the flow occurs in a direction so as to restore equilibrium.

Ion flow through a channel can be driven by either an ion concentration gradient or an electrical potential difference (Fig. 1.18). To express both of these driving forces in the same units, the electrochemical potential difference, $\Delta\bar{\mu}_i$ can be defined. For K ions, $\Delta\bar{\mu}_K$ is given by the following equation:

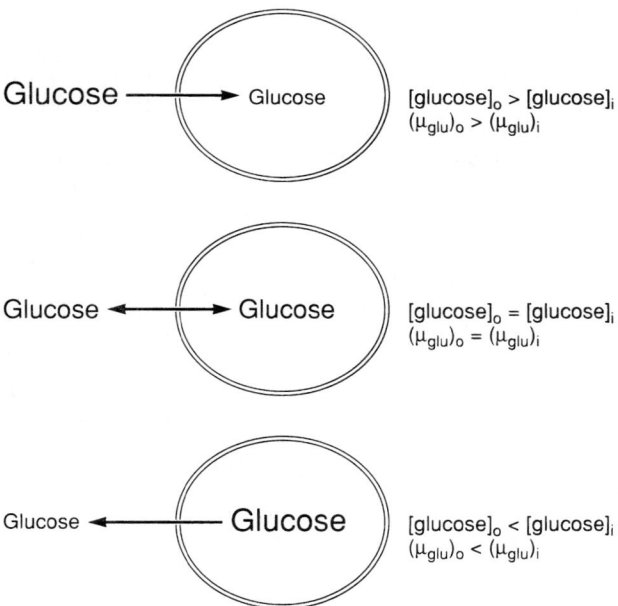

Figure 1.17. For a substance that moves by a non-energy-dependent transport mechanism, the direction of the net flow is determined by the passive driving force. In this example, the movement of glucose is determined by the orientation of the concentration gradient (the chemical potential gradient).

$$\Delta\overline{\mu}_K = RT \ln ([K]_i/[K]_o) + zFV_m$$

where $[K]_i$ and $[K]_o$ = K concentrations; z = the valence; F = the Faraday constant; and V_m = the membrane potential.

If $\Delta\overline{\mu}_K = 0$, the driving force for ion flow is zero and the ion is distributed at equilibrium. If $\Delta\overline{\mu}_K \neq 0$, there is a driving force for ion flow. The total driving force, $\Delta\overline{\mu}_K$, is the sum of two parts—one due to the K concentration gradient $[RT \ln ([K]_i/[K]_o)]$, and the other due to the electrical potential (zFV_m). The electrochemical potential difference can be regarded as a generalized potential function that encompasses driving forces due to both concentration gradients and electrical potential. $\Delta\overline{\mu}_K$ enables one to express the driving forces due to a concentration gradient and an electrical potential in the same units. This is perhaps most obvious as illustrated in Fig. 1.18, in which all terms are expressed using electrical units (i.e., millivolts), so that the driving force for K^+ flow can be written as follows:

$$\frac{\Delta\overline{\mu}_K}{zF} = V_m - E_K$$

where $E_K = RT/zF \ln ([K]_o/[K]_i)$, a measure of the driving force due to the potassium concentration gradient in electrical units.

Driving Force for Water Flow

The energetics of water movement across cell membranes is simplified by the fact that water moves only passively owing to gradients of hydrostatic pressure or water concentration. Hydrostatic pressure is an important driving force only for certain specialized cells—the capillary endothelium and the glomerulus of the kidney. For most of the cells in the body, the transmembrane hydrostatic pressure is zero (owing to membrane elasticity),

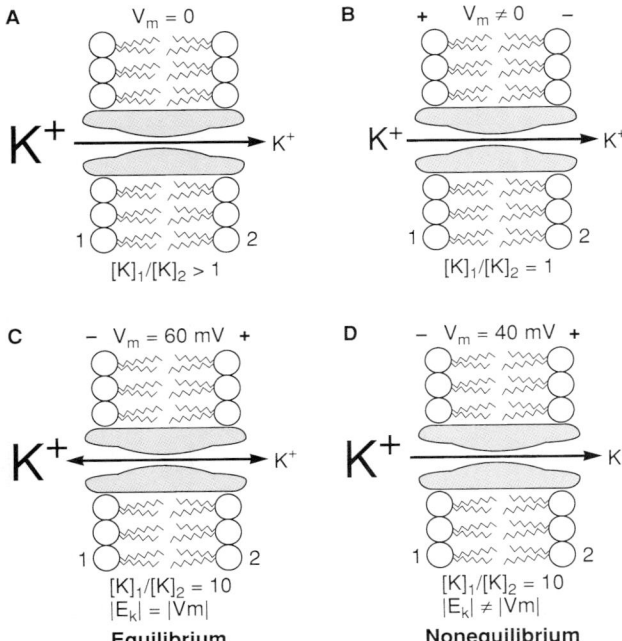

Figure 1.18. The direction of passive ion flow is determined by the *electrochemical potential gradient*. The total driving force is the sum of that due to the K concentration gradient *(A)* and that due to the electrical potential difference *(B)*. If the driving force due to the concentration gradient is equal in magnitude and opposite in direction to the electrical potential *(C)*, the total passive force is zero (i.e., the ion is distributed at equilibrium). *(D)* A net driving force exists because there is an imbalance between E_k and V_m.

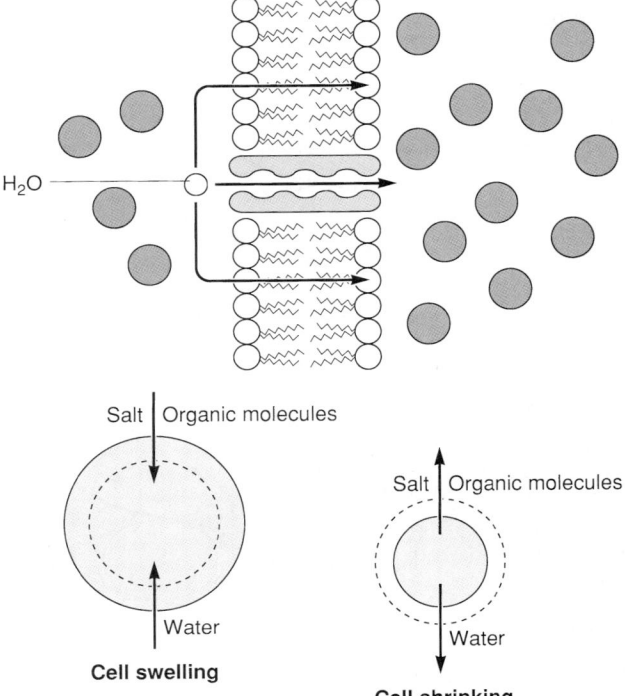

Figure 1.19. Water permeates the plasma membrane by means of *solubility–diffusion* through the lipid bilayer and, in some cells, through specialized water channels. Cell volume is normally determined by *solute* distribution because plasma membrane water permeability is high and cells tend to approach osmotic equilibrium.

and water moves only in response to water concentration gradients.

Because the concentration of water is determined by the amount of dissolved solute, the difference in water concentration is typically expressed as a function of the difference in solute concentration or, as it is more commonly known, osmotic pressure difference (Fig. 1.19). Because there are no specialized, energy-converting transport mechanisms for water, water is distributed at equilibrium. Water distribution is determined entirely by solute distribution. If a cell gains solute, it swells by gaining water. If a cell loses solute, it shrinks because of the obligatory efflux of water.

Active Transport: Conservation of Energy

Transport processes can be conceptualized in terms of the relation between work available and work done, as suggested by Fig. 1.20, which illustrates an example of a coupled transport process: Na^+–H^+ antiport or Na^+–H^+ exchange. From this perspective, the function of an Na^+–H^+ antiporter is to use the energy available in the transmembrane Na^+ gradient to drive protons out of the cell. This available energy has been invested in the Na^+ gradient by the action of the Na^+-K^+-ATPase. The work done moving protons is given by the electrochemical potential difference for protons multiplied by the number of protons (or moles of protons) moved per cycle. Similarly, the work *available* is given by the electrochemical potential difference for Na^+ times the mole number.

What would happen if we were artificially to *increase* ΔpH by acidifying the solution bathing the cell in Fig. 1.20 so that ΔH^+ exceeds ΔNa^+? Like any chemical reaction, the antiporter would run backward. Protons would enter the cell and drive Na^+ out. The energetics of any coupled transporter is an important experimental test for the coupling process.

Transport Mechanisms

The composition of the lipid bilayer suggests that its transport properties should be those of a layer of oil or, more accurately, a layer of hydrocarbon, formed by the fatty acid side chains of the phospholipids. To penetrate the lipid bilayer, a substance must enter the bilayer by dissolving, or partitioning, into it. Movement across the bilayer occurs by diffusion. The overall process is referred to as *solubility–diffusion* and is the mechanism of membrane transport for moderately lipophilic solutes and water. Cells may also have specialized transport proteins called aquaporins (22) that function as water channels, but for most cells, water movement across the plasma membrane can be accounted for by simple solubility–diffusion of H_2O across the lipid bilayer. The coexistence in some cells of two pathways for water movement is a bit puzzling, but the implied redundancy is highlighted by the observation that congenital absence of aquaporin 1 is not associated with any clinical phenotype.

At equilibrium, the partitioning of a solute between the aqueous and hydrocarbon phases can be described by an oil–water partition coefficient, β_{oil}, expressed as C_{oil}/C_{water}, the ratio of the concentration of the substance in oil to that

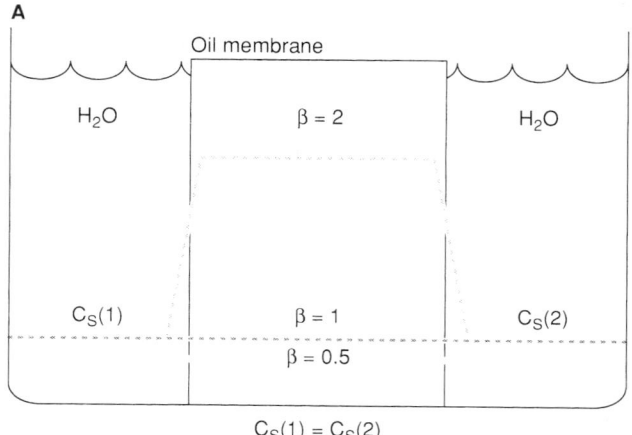

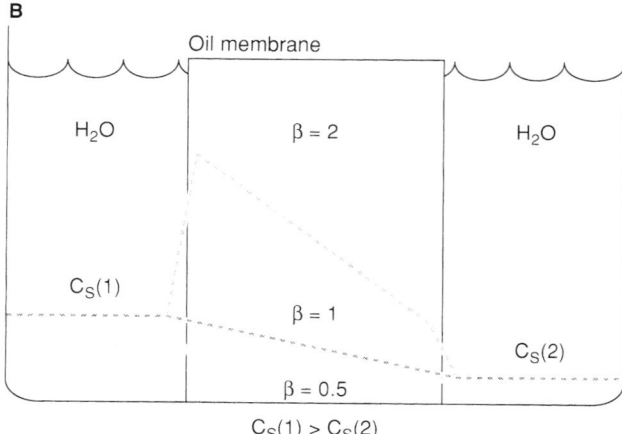

Figure 1.21. Moderately lipophilic solutes can cross the plasma membrane by solubility diffusion through the lipid bilayer, modeled here as an oil membrane. Three hypothetical solutes are depicted as having oil–water partition coefficients (β_i) of 0.5, 1, and 2. The concentration profiles in the absence *(A)* and in the presence *(B)* of a concentration gradient are shown. The dominant factor in the determination of permeability is the partition coefficient β_i.

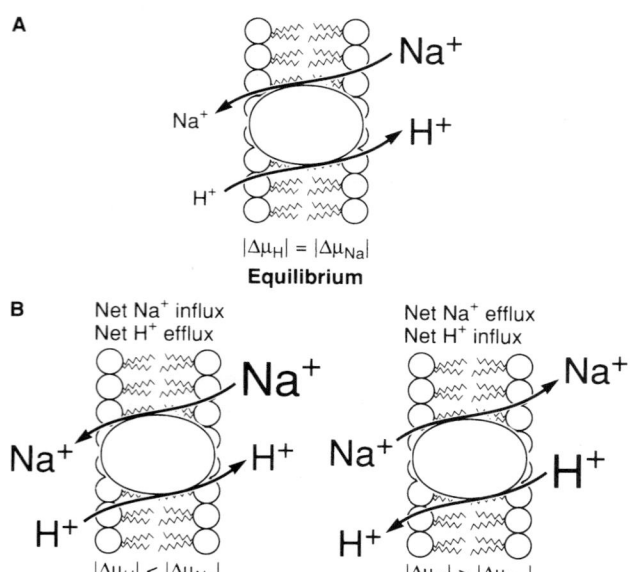

Figure 1.20. The Na^+–H^+ exchanger is an example of a *countertransporter,* a mechanism by which energy invested in the Na gradient can be used to drive protons out of the cell. The direction of turnover of the exchange process is determined by the balance of the chemical potential gradients for Na^+ and H^+.

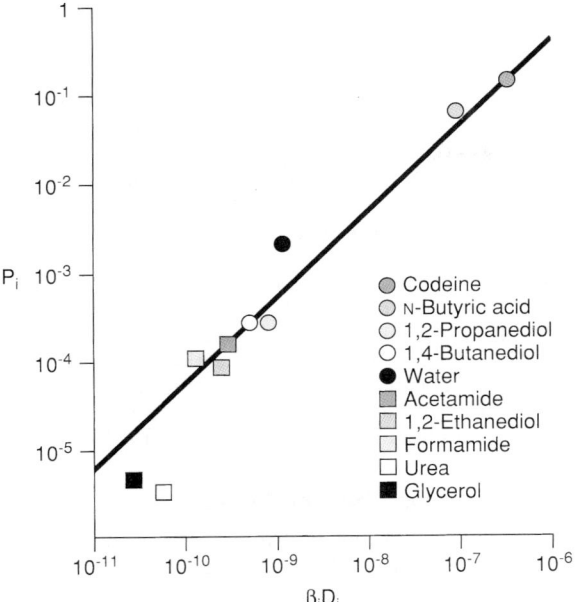

Figure 1.22. The permeability of a planar lipid bilayer to a series of lipophilic solutes is highly correlated with the product of the oil–water partition coefficient and the diffusion coefficient (i.e., $\beta_i D_i$).

in water. This equilibrium partitioning is illustrated in Fig. 1.21A for a solute that is present at the same concentration on both sides of an oil membrane. The concentration profile is shown as the concentration of the solute in the aqueous and oil phases plotted versus distance along the y-axis. Concentration profiles are illustrated for three hypothetical solutes exhibiting three different partition coefficients, $\beta = 0.5$, 1, and 2. In this case, because the concentration is identical on both sides of the membrane ($C_1 = C_2$), there is no flow across the membrane. The diffusion of lipophilic nonelectrolytes is a purely passive leak process; if there is no concentration gradient, there is no driving force for net flow. Figure 1.21B shows the concentration profiles in the presence of a concentration gradient ($C_1 > C_2$), illustrating the influence of the partition coefficient on the amount of solute in the membrane. The permeability of lipid membranes to moderately lipophilic solutes is highly correlated with the value of the oil–water partition coefficient. Figure 1.22 illustrates the correlation using data from a planar lipid bilayer. Note the position of water in this plot.

Ion Channels

Ion channels are transmembrane proteins that form pores that can conduct ions across the plasma membrane. The lipid portion of the plasma membrane is virtually impermeable to small ions such as Na^+, K^+, Cl^-, and Ca^{2+}. The inability of ions to cross a hydrophobic layer results from the enormous energy required to move an ion from a highly polar aqueous environment into the relatively nonpolar region formed by the hydrocarbon tails of the phospholipids. Ion channels are formed by membrane-spanning peptides that are arranged so that polar moieties line a central pore, as suggested in Fig. 1.16B. These polar groups take the place of the water of hydration, which stabilizes an ion in an aqueous solution. The polar groups create, in essence, a water-like environment into which the ion can partition and move in the presence of an ap-

propriate driving force. The recent crystal structure obtained for the bacterial K channel showed that when a K^+ ion enters the channel, four of its inner sphere waters of hydration are "replaced" by interactions with a halo of four carbonyl oxygen ligands (23).

The movement of an ion through a channel implies the movement of charge or current flow and hence is referred to as a *conductive process.* The physical interactions that underlie the conduction process determine both the rate at which ions can traverse the channel and the selectivity of the channel, the degree to which the channel discriminates between ions. The size of the single-channel conductance and the selectivity of the channel provide important criteria for distinguishing one channel from another on the basis of function. For example, most cells contain a variety of channels that are selective for specific ions (e.g., Na^+, K^+, Cl^- Ca^{2+}, HCO_3^-). Selectivity provides a broad classification of channels. Most cells contain several subtypes of selective channels, which are often distinguished on the basis of the size of the single-channel conductance. It is likely that channels differentiated on the basis of function reflect the properties of distinctly different membrane proteins. The existence of channel diversity suggests that different channel proteins may play different roles in the life of the cell.

Gating of Ion Channels

Ion channels are permissive transport elements: ions flow through a channel only in the presence of an appropriate driving force. Records of the current flowing through single channels (Fig. 1.23) show clearly that even in the presence of a driving force, an ion channel does not conduct all of the time. Rather, the form of the single-channel current record suggests that the channel protein undergoes conformational changes between conducting (open) states and nonconducting (closed) states. These conformational changes are collectively referred to as *gating.* Gating of ion channels is crucial to the survival of cells and organisms because gating is the basis for the regulation of ion flow through membrane channels.

The simplest model for the gating process recognizes two states of the ion channel protein—closed (nonconducting) and open (conducting), which can be represented as a reversible chemical reaction:

$$\text{closed} \underset{\alpha}{\overset{\beta}{\rightleftharpoons}} \text{open}$$

The gating process can be envisioned as being the result of the incessant thermal vibration, or "twitching," of the protein. Occasionally, one such thermal twitch has enough energy to precipitate a change in the conformation of the protein, a change from closed to open, for example. The rate coefficients, α and β, are a measure of the likelihood of these conformational changes. The relative values of α and β determine the fraction of time that the channel spends in one state or another, or, more accurately, the probability of finding the channel in a particular state. For example, if $\alpha = \beta$, then, regardless of the individual values of α and β, the channel conducts half the time. In general, the probability of finding the channel in the open state would be given by the following equation:

$$P_o = \beta/(\alpha + \beta)$$

Channel gating provides the molecular basis for exquisite regulation of the rate of ion flow across a membrane. For example, consider the rate of K flow through a population, or ensemble, of a particular type of K channel. The total conductance due to the population is given by g_K using the formula:

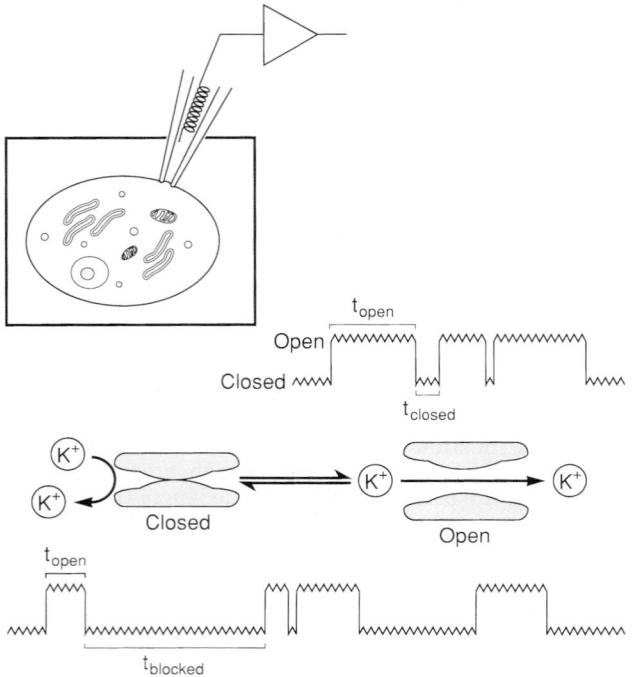

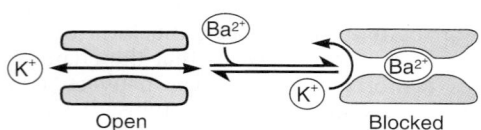

Figure 1.23. The patch-clamp method permits the recording of the currents that flow through a single open ion channel. The gating (opening and closing) of the channel is reflected in the changes in the single-channel current between two values—zero and the open-channel value. A channel blocker such as barium can induce long, nonconducting intervals because it binds in the channel and blocks ion flow.

$$g_K = \gamma_K(N_K)_o$$

where γ_K = conductance of a single K channel, and $(N_K)_o$ = average number of open channels. $(N_K)_o$, however, is given by the formula

$$(N_K)_o = N_K P_o$$

where N_K = *total* number of channels in the cell membrane (counting open *and* closed), and P_o = probability of finding any one channel in the open state.

Combining, this relation is obtained:

$$g_K = \gamma_K N_K P_o$$

This important equation relates the macroscopic conductance, g_K, to the properties of individual channel proteins. Contained within the three parameters γ_K, N_K, and P_o is the basis for the regulation of ion transport. The conductance, or leakiness, of a membrane to a particular ion can be modulated by altering P_o, N_K, or γ_K.

Ion Channel Conduction Can Be Blocked

The conduction process can be blocked by ions or organic compounds that enter the channel, bind there, and occlude the pore. Typically, channel blockade is a re-versible binding reaction, so that the efficacy of the blocker is determined by the affinity of the blocker for the binding site; this affinity determines how long the blocking molecule remains in the pore. Figure 1.23 shows the blockage of a K channel by the divalent ion, barium. The recording of the single-channel current allows us to resolve a single blocking event—that is, the interaction of one blocker molecule with a single-channel protein. The blocking events are clearly discernible as long, nonconducting intervals in the record of single-channel current.

Channel blockade is an important mechanism of action for toxins and some therapeutic agents. For example, the deadly toxin of the puffer fish, tetrodotoxin, acts by blocking the Na^+ channels that are responsible for the conduction of the nerve impulse. The diuretic, amiloride, acts by blocking the Na channels that inhibit the apical membrane of the epithelial cells of the distal nephron. Local anesthetics such as lidocaine (Xylocaine) act by blocking ion channels.

Modulation of Ion Channel Gating

Two of the most important mechanisms that operate to gate ion channels are voltage and ligand binding. Voltage-gated ion channels are the molecular basis for excitability in nerve and muscle and the conduction of the nerve impulse (action potential) from the cell body along the axon to the synaptic terminus. Voltage-dependent gating of Na and K channels is the basis of the action potential. Because Na-selective channels open more rapidly than K-selective channels, the initial effect of a depolarizing stimulus is to increase an inward Na current and further depolarize V_m. Subsequently, K channels are opened by the depolarization, and the increased K conductance tends to repolarize V_m. During an action potential, the Na conductance of the axon membrane can increase by 100-fold in less than 1 second. During this change, the number of channels in the membrane does not increase; the increase in Na conductance is due solely to a dramatic increase in the probability that an Na channel is open.

The mechanism of voltage-dependent gating is not completely understood, but data suggest that in voltage-gated channels the conformational change from closed to open is associated with the movement of a charged group on the protein. Depolarization of the membrane reduces the free energy (work) required to open the channel by reducing the work required to move this so-called gating charge. Several voltage-gated channels have been cloned, and a region has been identified that has properties appropriate for a voltage sensor. Interestingly, this region appears to be highly conserved in Na, K, and Ca channels (Fig. 1.24).

The term *ligand-gated channels* refers to a broad class of channels that can be opened (or closed) in response to the binding of some ligand to the channel protein. The ligand can be a neurotransmitter, such as acetylcholine, or an intracellular messenger, such as calcium. The binding of a ligand can increase membrane conductance by favoring the open configuration of the channel (Fig. 1.25).

Water Channels

The plasma membrane of most cells is highly permeable to water because water can cross the lipid bilayer at significant rates by means of solubility–diffusion. A few cells in the body are specialized so that they can exhibit a highly regulated water permeability. These cells include epithelial cells found in the distal tubule of the mammalian kidney. In such cells, the water permeability can be exquisitely regulated by antidiuretic hormone (ADH). ADH is a peptide hormone that binds to receptors located in the basolateral membranes of epithelial cells and, by

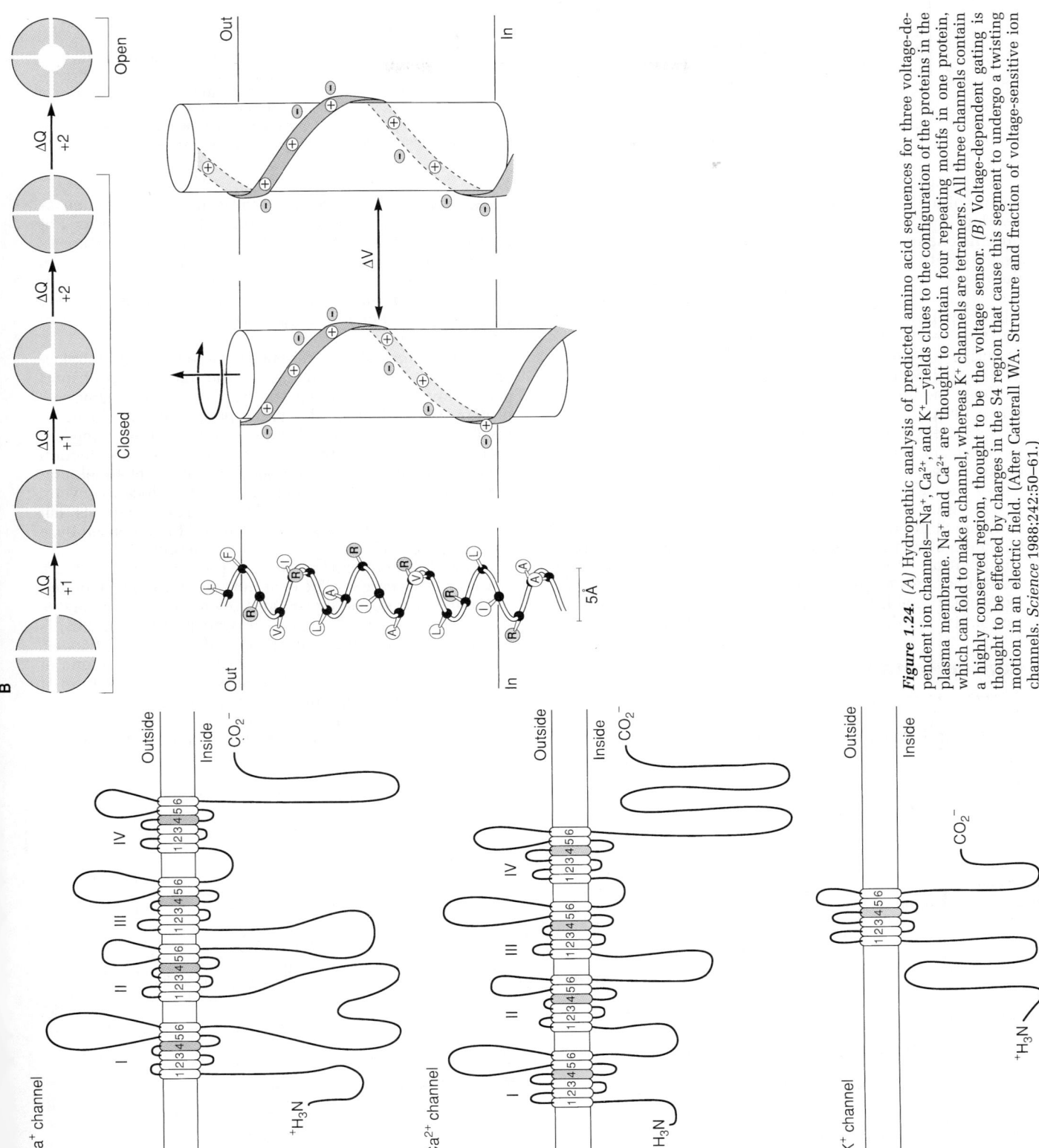

Figure 1.24. (*A*) Hydropathic analysis of predicted amino acid sequences for three voltage-dependent ion channels—Na$^+$, Ca^{2+}, and K$^+$—yields clues to the configuration of the proteins in the plasma membrane. Na$^+$ and Ca^{2+} are thought to contain four repeating motifs in one protein, which can fold to make a channel, whereas K$^+$ channels are tetramers. All three channels contain a highly conserved region, thought to be the voltage sensor. (*B*) Voltage-dependent gating is thought to be effected by charges in the S4 region that cause this segment to undergo a twisting motion in an electric field. (After Catterall WA. Structure and fraction of voltage-sensitive ion channels. *Science* 1988;242:50–61.)

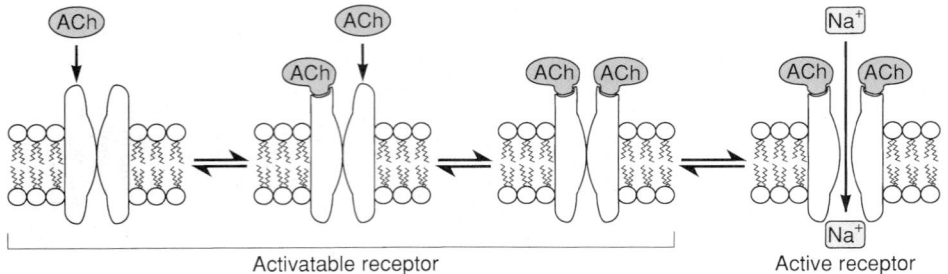

Figure 1.25. The acetylcholine receptor is an example of a ligand-gated channel. Two molecules of acetylcholine must bind before the channel can reach the open (conducting) conformation.

means of a cyclic adenosine monophosphate (cAMP)-dependent mechanism, leads to the insertion of water-conducting channels in the apical membrane. Regulated water permeability requires that two basic conditions be met: (a) there must be a regulatable pathway for water transport (i.e., water channels); and (b) the background, or non-ADH-dependent water permeability of the membrane, must be relatively low. The apical membranes of ADH-sensitive epithelia are specialized in both of these ways. The resting water permeability (or hydraulic conductivity) of these membranes is relatively low, so that in the absence of ADH, even a substantial osmotic gradient produces little water flow. ADH can effect a dramatic increase in water permeability by inducing the insertion of water-conducting channels into the apical membrane of such cells. The ADH-sensitive water channel has been identified as aquaporin 2, and congenital absence of this protein can contribute to nephrogenic diabetes insipidus (22). To be an effective instrument for the regulation of body fluid composition, these channels must be selective for water. If water channels exhibited significant ion permeability, for example, the ability of the kidney to regulate body fluid osmolality would be compromised by salt flows.

Carrier Proteins

Most transport proteins appear to function as carriers rather than as channels. Membrane carriers are a broad class of transmembrane proteins that include simple leaks as well as energy-converting mechanisms such as the ATPases, countertransporters, and cotransporters. For membrane carriers, the mechanism of translocation is probably more complicated than for an open channel. Although the details of the mechanisms are not well understood, important distinctions can be made between carrier-type and channel-type mechanisms on the basis of transport kinetics.

The most important difference between a channel mechanism and a carrier mechanism is the role in the transport event played by conformational changes in the membrane protein. For a channel, the gating process is envisioned as involving a conformational change between conducting and nonconducting states that operates like a gate. Conduction is associated only with the open state of the channel, and the gating process is not coupled to the translocation event. In a carrier mechanism, available information suggests that the translocation event is directly linked to, or caused by, a conformational change in the membrane protein.

Figure 1.26 compares the transport mechanism for a channel and a carrier. The channel (Fig. 1.26A) is depicted as having two states, closed and open, so that it operates like a switch. In contrast, carrier transport (Fig. 1.26B) is envisioned as requiring a cycle of conformational changes. In the absence of substrate, the carrier can assume one of two conformations, which are distinguished by location of the substrate binding site, an inward-facing and an outward-facing conformation. Binding of substrate permits or initiates a conformational change that translocates the site,

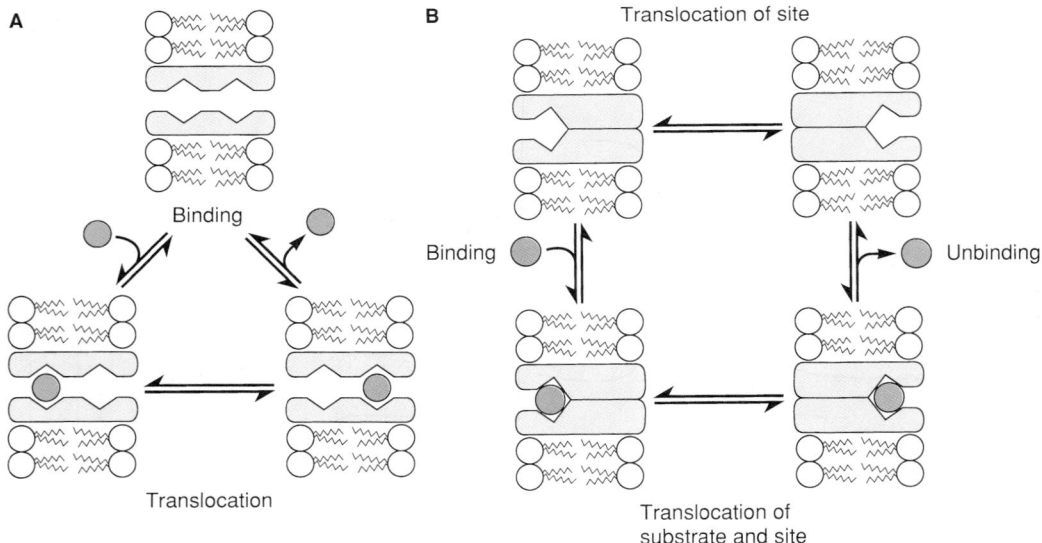

Figure 1.26. *(A)* Ion translocation through an open channel can be envisioned as involving a binding step, followed by translocation and unbinding of the ion. *(B)* In contrast, carrier-mediated flow involves binding followed by a conformational change that is coupled to the translocation of the substrate. In this model, the unbound site can translocate.

and the bound substrate, from one side to the other. The unoccupied site can then revert to the inward-facing form, and the cycle can be repeated. The transport of one molecule of substrate requires one complete cycle of the carrier. This sort of analysis suggests that carriers can be distinguished from channels based on the accessibility of the binding site. In a channel mechanism, binding sites within the open pore are equally accessible from either side of the membrane, whereas in a carrier mechanism, the binding site is available only on one side of the membrane at any instant.

The cyclic nature of the carrier transport mechanism has several important consequences. First, the linkage of transport to conformational changes renders the process slower than that of a channel by approximately one order of magnitude. A distinguishing feature of channel-mediated ion transport is the high rate of transport, of the order of 10^6 ions/s. A second consequence of the conformational cycling in carriers is that the conformation of the carrier can be strongly influenced by the transmembrane distribution of the transported substrate. This creates a mechanism for the coupling of the flows of two substrates. The intimate link between conformational change and translocation makes it possible to envision a variety of mecha-

nisms for the coupling of the flow of one substrate to that of a second substrate flow or to a chemical reaction (an ATPase). These mechanisms are diagrammed in Fig. 1.27. A cotransporter (e.g., Na$^+$–glucose) is envisioned as one in which the translocation event requires the binding of both Na and glucose (Fig. 1.26A). In one scheme, the binding of Na to one site would increase the affinity of a second site for glucose. Thus, an Na$^+$ gradient creates a net flow of glucose by favoring inward glucose flow. The fact that the Na$^+$ binds with its charge means that the inside negative membrane potential represents another force, which drives the cycle so as to favor inward glucose flow.

If the conformational changes of the unbound site are disallowed, the resulting mechanism is an exchanger or antiporter because the only possible transport event is the obligatory exchange, or swapping, of one substrate molecule for another. This process is presumed to be the basis for the energy-converting countertransport that occurs, for example, in Na$^+$–H$^+$ exchange (Fig. 1.26A). Here, the imposition of an Na$^+$ gradient can drive protons out of the cell. Because of the Na$^+$ gradient, Na$^+$ dominates the out-to-in portion of the cycle, whereas H$^+$ dominates the in-to-out portion of the cycle. There is evidence for an activation site on the cytoplasmic face of the Na$^+$–H$^+$ antiporter,

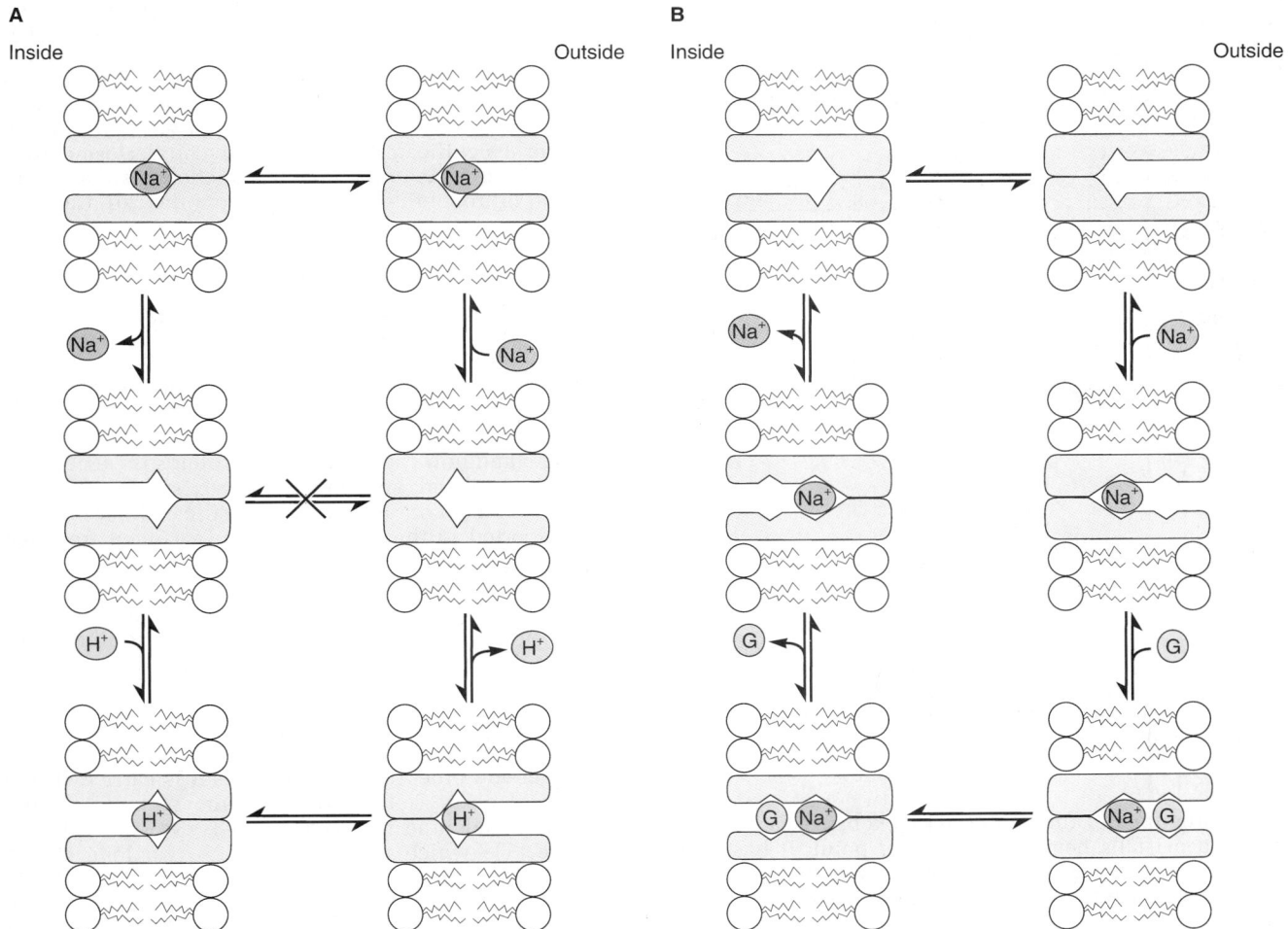

Figure 1.27. *(A)* An exchanger, or antiporter, is created by disallowing the translocation of the unbound site. For example, the catalytic cycle diagrammed here leads to the exchange of Na$^+$ for H$^+$ (i.e., Na$^+$–H$^+$ antiport). *(B)* An obligatory cotransporter is created by permitting only two forms of the protein to undergo translatory conformational changes—the doubly bound and the unbound. Here, the binding of Na$^+$ facilitates the subsequent binding of glucose, leading to the Na$^+$-dependent cotransport of Na$^+$ and glucose.

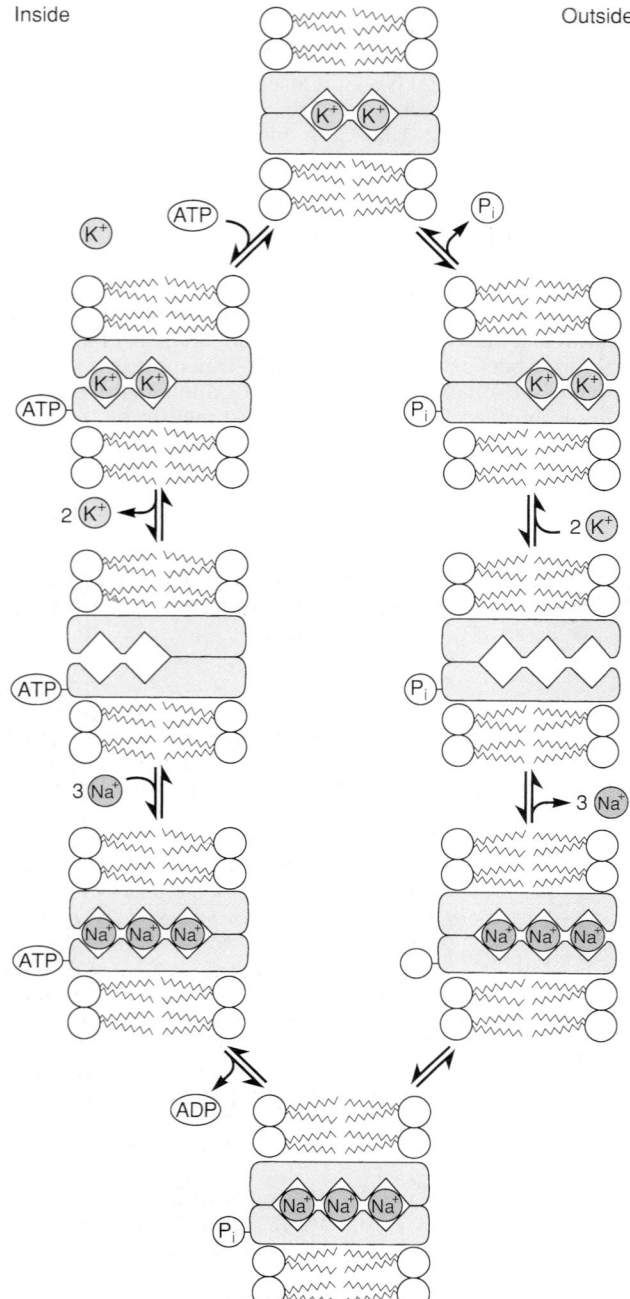

Inside   Outside

Figure 1.28. The Na$^+$-K$^+$-adenosine triphosphatase (ATPase) has a complicated catalytic cycle that involves not only the binding and unbinding of Na$^+$ and K$^+$ but the binding of ATP, phosphorylation of the protein, and subsequent dephosphorylation, so that one ATP is hydrolyzed per transport cycle.

which functions to turn on Na$^+$–H$^+$ exchange only when cytosolic pH falls below a certain set point. It has been suggested that hormones and growth factors that influence Na$^+$–H$^+$ exchange do so in part by modulating the activating site.

The archetype for biologic pumps is the Na$^+$-K$^+$-ATPase. For this transporter, the biochemical events in the catalytic cycle have been examined in great detail, although the exact nature of the translocation events still is not well understood. Figure 1.28 illustrates how the inclusion of a phosphorylation event in the catalytic cycle

could result in the coupling of the free energy of hydrolysis of ATP to the translocation of ions, in this case, the exchange of Na$^+$ for K$^+$ in the ratio of three Na$^+$ to two K$^+$. This unequal stoichiometry results in the transfer of net charge during the catalytic cycle, so that the normal pumping mode is associated with an outwardly directed membrane current.

Volume Regulation

One important function of the solute transport mechanisms that inhabit the plasma membrane is the maintenance and regulation of cell volume. Water distribution, as noted earlier, is determined in most cells entirely by solute distribution. Thus, the volume of a cell is determined by the same mechanisms that maintain the steady-state solute composition of the cell. Many, if not all, cells have the capacity to respond actively to a perturbation in cell volume—that is, they are capable of volume regulation. Volume regulatory responses are based on membrane transporters that enable the cell to undergo a net loss or a net gain of solute and hence lose or gain water. For example, if a cell is swollen by exposure to a hypotonic medium, the permeability of the cell membrane to K$^+$ and Cl$^-$ is markedly increased, such that a net efflux of salt and water occurs, bringing about a regulatory volume decrease (Fig. 1.29). Similarly, shrinking a cell by exposing it to an impermeant solute activates mechanisms for solute entry, usually NaCl. Another type of volume regulatory mechanism involves the movements of organic solutes such as taurine or myoinositol. These solutes are accumulated by cells through Na-dependent cotransporters and can account for a significant fraction of intracellular osmolality. Cell swelling leads to the opening of channels that mediate rapid efflux of these osmolytes from the cell, thus initiating a regulatory volume decrease.

INTRACELLULAR SYNTHESIS, TRANSPORT, AND ORGANIZATION OF MACROMOLECULES

Cell structure and function are ultimately determined by the proteins present in a particular cell type and their spatial arrangement in distinct organelles. It is important to understand how the synthesis of proteins is carried out, how it is regulated, and how the newly synthesized proteins are directed or targeted to a specific cellular location or transported to the cell surface and secreted from the cell. Because protein structure is coded for by DNA, this section initially reviews how genetic information is stored in DNA, transcribed into RNA, and then translated into unique proteins (1,2,24). After this, the intracellular targeting and transport of proteins are discussed.

DNA, RNA, and Protein Synthesis

The genetic blueprint of an organism is carried in the nucleus of every cell, encoded by the sequence of the four bases—adenine (A), guanine (G), cytosine (C), and thymine (T)—which together make up two long chains bound together by hydrogen bonds to form a DNA double helix. Bases in opposite strands of the double helix are specifically paired by hydrogen bonding. A is paired with T by two hydrogen bonds, and C is paired with G by three hydrogen bonds. This base-pair complementarity is the central principle on which DNA replication, RNA transcription, and protein synthesis are based.

A gene is a segment of DNA that is transcribed into a corresponding RNA molecule that either codes for a pro-

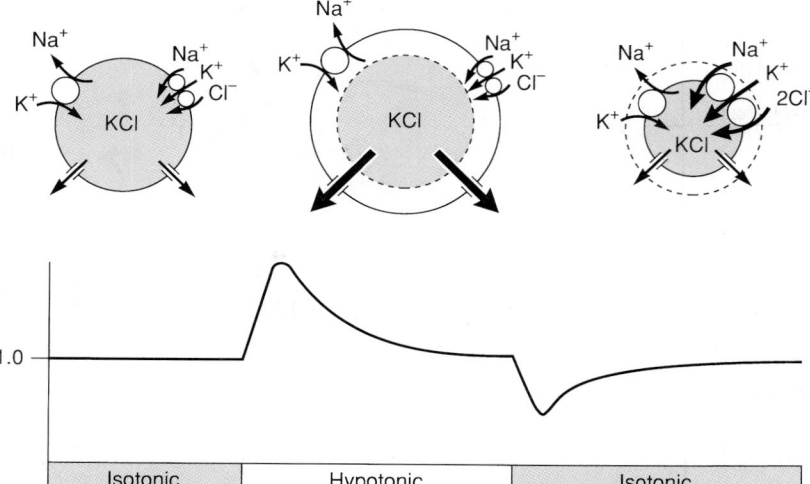

Figure 1.29. Many cells actively regulate their volume by turning on and off specific transport pathways. A hypotonic solution is shown here as causing cell swelling and activating channels for K^+ and Cl^- so that salt leaves the cell, promoting shrinkage. A return to isotonic conditions leads to water efflux and cell shrinkage, which activates a coupled, Na^+-K^+-$2Cl^-$ entry process that results in a gain of salt and water and a return to normal volume.

tein or forms a structural RNA molecule (Fig. 1.30). Genes are commonly between 10,000 and 100,000 base pairs in length and include, in addition to the coding sequence, flanking regions and intervening sequences, called *introns.* Introns are removed from the primary RNA transcript by a process called *splicing.* Each strand of DNA has polarity, and information is read from the 5′ to the 3′ direction, with the numbers referring to the free hydroxyl group on the deoxyribose moiety. The basic unit of information is the codon, a sequence of three bases or a triplet. The four nucleotide bases arranged as triplets lead to 64 possible codons. Sixty-one of these code for the 20 known amino acids, and 3 are termination signals called *stop codons.* The code is degenerate in that some amino acids are specified by up to six codons.

When cells divide, the two DNA chains that constitute the double helix separate, and each serves as a template for synthesis of a complementary strand directed by the enzyme DNA polymerase (1). One of the new double helices goes to each daughter cell, so that the amount and sequence of DNA in each new cell is the same as that of the parent cell. To direct the synthesis of protein, the DNA sequence has to be transcribed into three types of RNA—messenger RNA (mRNA), transfer RNA (tRNA), and ribosomal RNA (rRNA). RNA contains the nucleoside uridine (U) instead of thymidine and usually exists as a single-stranded, linear polymer. RNA synthesis is directed by an

RNA polymerase enzyme that makes an RNA copy of DNA. Eukaryotic cells contain three types of RNA polymerase—termed I, II, and III—each of which catalyzes the formation of a different type of RNA. RNA polymerase II directs the formation of mRNA.

Transcription of a gene begins at an initiation site associated with a specific DNA sequence, called a *promotor region.* Recognition of this region by the polymerase is aided by specific proteins, called *transcription factors,* which bind to the DNA, and by *initiation factors,* which bind to the polymerase. Some transcription factors determine tissue specificity, whereas others, such as steroid hormone receptors, are regulatory and act in various cells to increase or decrease transcription rates of specific genes. After binding to DNA, the RNA polymerase opens up a short region of the double helix to expose the nucleotides. Once the two strands of DNA are separated, the strand containing the promoter acts as a template to which ribonucleoside triphosphates base pair by hydrogen bonds. Nucleotides are then joined together with elongation, proceeding in a 5′ to 3′ direction as the RNA polymerase moves stepwise along the DNA (Fig. 1.31). Behind the polymerase, the DNA double helix reforms, displacing the nascent RNA polymer. When a termination signal is reached, the polymerase releases both the template and the newly made RNA strand and is free to rebind to another promoter region. The average length of the RNA

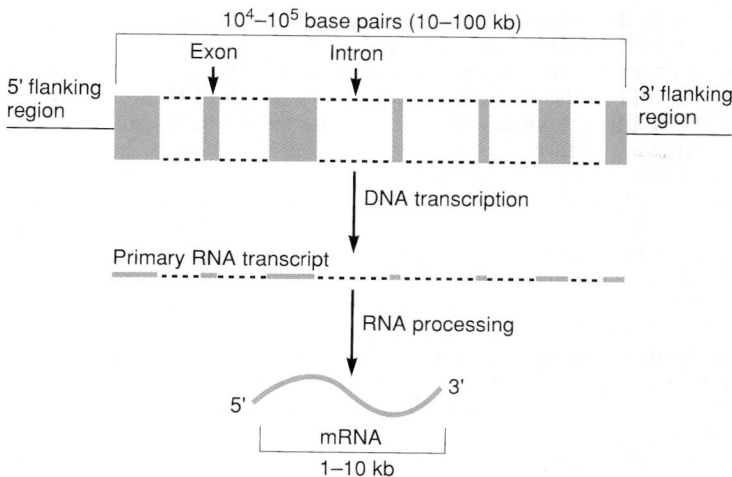

Figure 1.30. Structure of a typical gene, its primary RNA transcript, and the resulting mature mRNA. The entire coding region of the gene is initially transcribed, and the regions coded for introns are then spliced out during processing. The mature mRNA is then an RNA copy of the exon regions of the gene.

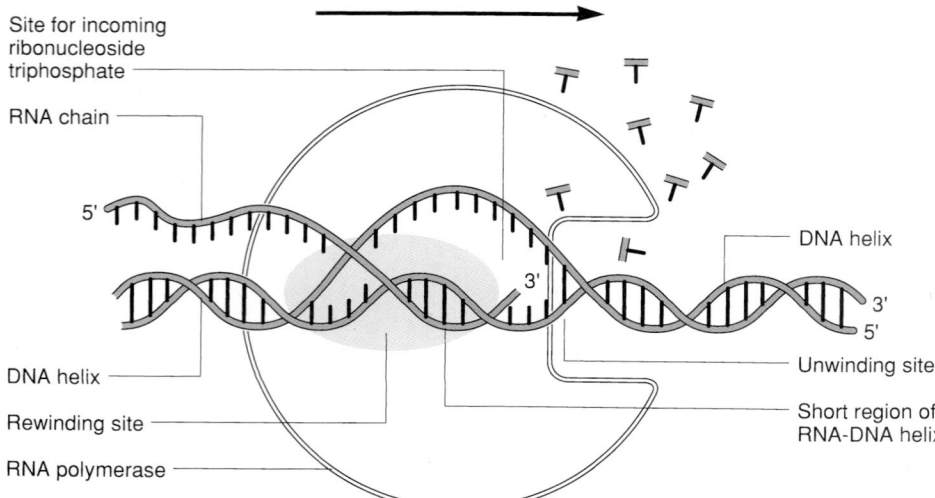

Figure 1.31. Transcription of DNA. RNA polymerase acts to unwind the DNA helix, catalyzes the formation of a transient RNA–DNA helix, and then releases the RNA as a single-strand copy while the DNA rewinds. In the process, the polymerase moves along the DNA from a start sequence to a stop sequence.

transcript is approximately 8,000 nucleotides, although much longer molecules are common.

The initial products of RNA polymerase II are known as heterogeneous nuclear RNA because of their large size variation. These primary transcripts are then processed to form mRNA. Processing includes addition of a methylguanosine to the 5′ end as a cap, addition of a long sequence of adenosine bases to the 3′ end as a tail, and removal of a number of long nucleotide sequences. As mentioned earlier, these sequences, or introns, are present in the gene but not in mature RNA (Fig. 1.30). The gene regions represented in mRNA are termed *exons,* for expressed regions. The joining of coding regions on either side of an intron sequence, or splicing, accounts for mature mRNA being much shorter than nuclear RNA. Moreover, alternative splicing can lead to the production of different mRNA molecules and, in some cases, different proteins from the same gene. mRNA is exported from the nucleus only after processing is complete. A typical mammalian cell can contain as few as 1 or 2 or up to 10,000 copies of each mRNA molecule at any one time. Although the number of copies is primarily a function of the rate of transcription (synthesis), mature mRNA is degraded in the cytoplasm, and the rate of degradation of each species also contributes to its relative abundance. mRNA species that need to be rapidly regulated probably carry a sequence that tags them for more rapid destruction.

The synthesis of protein involves conversion from a 4-letter nucleotide language to one of 20 chemically distinct amino acids. Accordingly, this process is referred to as *translation.* There is no mechanism for direct chemical recognition between specific nucleic acid bases and specific amino acids. Instead, an adapter molecule, tRNA, is used. tRNAs are small RNA molecules of 70 to 90 nucleotides, traditionally represented as a cloverleaf (Fig. 1.32). The loop on one end contains an anticodon nucleotide triplet that lines up with the complementary sequence of the mRNA, whereas the other end binds the amino acid specified by the mRNA codon. Each tRNA carries only one amino acid and must be recognized by a distinct enzyme, termed an *aminoacyl tRNA synthetase,* which catalyzes the covalent attachment of the carboxyl terminus of the amino acid to the 3′ of the tRNA in a process using ATP. Covalent attachment to the tRNA allows amino acids to be added to a growing protein in the sequence specified by the nucleic acid code. The attachment to tRNA also activates the amino acid by generating

a high-energy intermediate. This energy is used to drive the reaction by which the amino acid is added to the nascent protein.

Protein synthesis occurs by the formation of a peptide bond between the carboxyl terminus of the growing polypeptide chain and the free amino group of the activated amino acid tRNA. This event does not occur in free solution, but within ribosomes. Ribosomes are protein-synthesizing machines that bring all the necessary components together in the correct sequence and spatial orientation (25). Each ribosome is a complex of more than 80 proteins and RNA molecules arranged into 2 subunits, a small and a large, with an aggregate molecular mass of approximately 4 million. Each ribosome contains three RNA-binding sites, one for mRNA and two for tRNA (Fig. 1.33). One of the latter, termed the *P-site,* holds the tRNA attached to the last amino acid added to the growing polypeptide chain, whereas the other, the A-site, holds the aminoacyl tRNA carrying the next amino acid to be added to the chain. After formation of each new peptide bond, the resulting peptidyl tRNA is transferred from the A-site to the P-site. The free tRNA produced in the P-site is released, and a new aminoacyl tRNA can enter the A-site to begin a new cycle. In the process, the ribosome moves exactly three nucleotides along the mRNA molecule. Protein synthesis consumes a great deal of energy because four high-energy phosphate bonds must be split to make each peptide bond.

Protein synthesis requires identification of the appropriate starting and ending points on the mRNA (26). The synthesis of all eukaryotic proteins begins with a methionine coded for by an AUG triplet. Only one specific methionine tRNA can initiate synthesis. This initiator tRNA, charged with methionine, forms a complex with the small ribosomal subunit and a protein, eukaryotic initiation factor 2. This complex then binds to an mRNA, which is in most cases identified as such by its 5′ 7-methylguanosine cap, and is then joined by other proteins (initiation factors). The small ribosomal subunit moves along the RNA until its initiating tRNA reaches the start site defined by the AUG sequence. At this time, some of the initiating factors dissociate, and a large ribosomal subunit joins the complex. Chain elongation can then occur by the binding of a free aminoacyl tRNA. Chain termination occurs when the ribosome reaches one of three different stop codons. Termination involves additional proteins, called *release factors,* which catalyze the addition of a water molecule rather than an amino acid to the carboxyl terminus of the

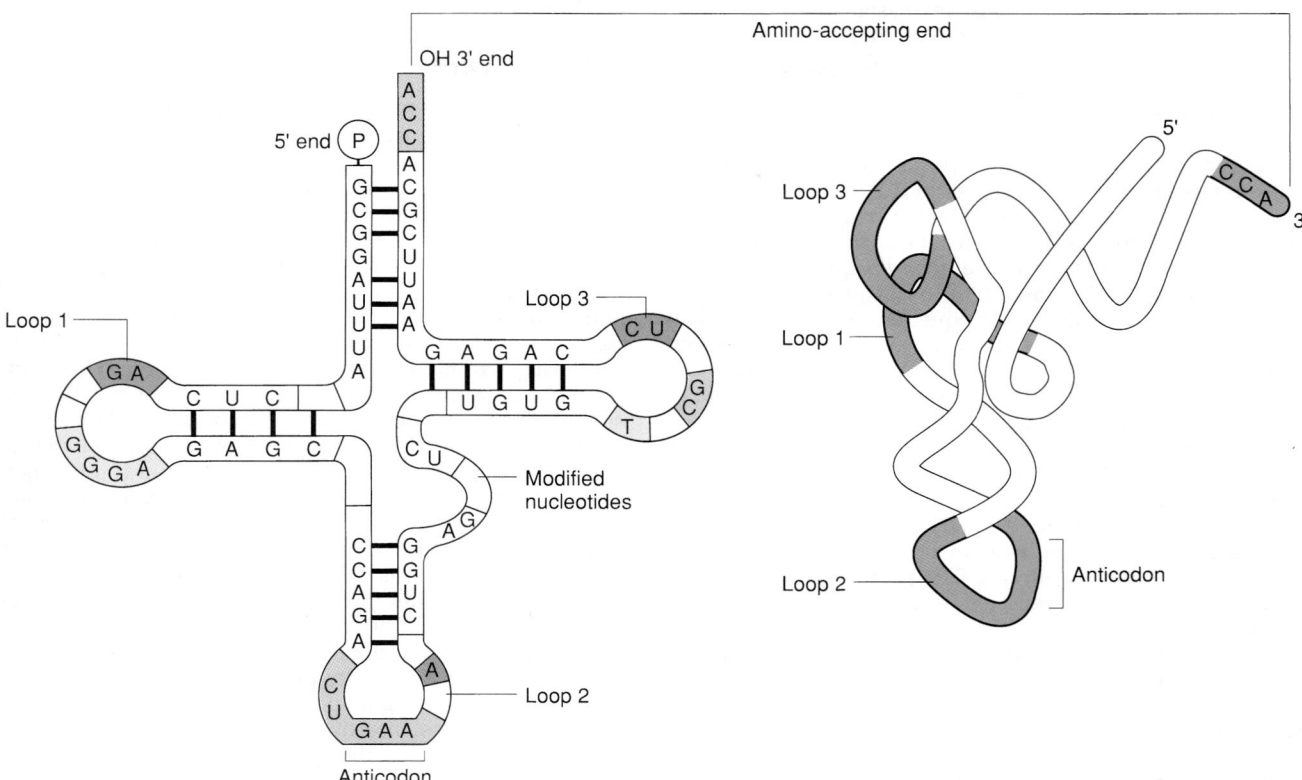

Figure 1.32. Structure of a transfer or tRNA molecule. The structure is shown as a stylized clover-leaf *(left)* and as it is believed to exist in three dimensions *(right).* Note the opposite regions for binding an amino acid and the anticodon that forms a base pair with mRNA.

polypeptide chain. At this point, there is no longer attachment to a tRNA, and the completed polypeptide is released into the cytoplasm. The ribosome then dissociates into its two subunits and releases the mRNA.

The complete synthesis of a single protein takes 30 seconds to a few minutes, but multiple ribosomes can initiate

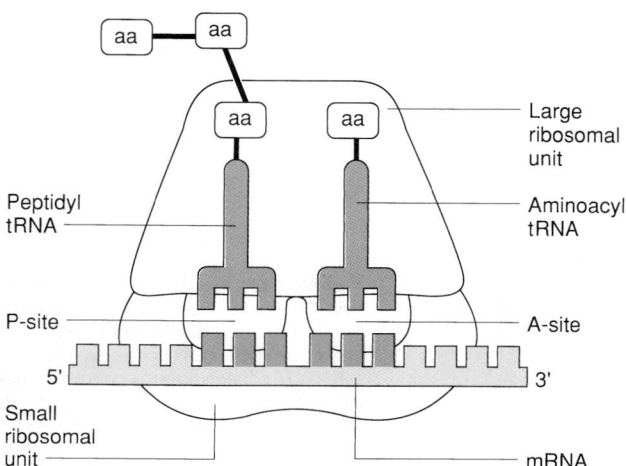

Figure 1.33. Schematic view of the elongation phase of protein synthesis on a ribosome. As the ribosome moves along the mRNA, incoming aminoacyl–tRNA complexes bind to the A-site on the ribosome, after which a new peptide bond is formed with the nascent polypeptide chain previously attached to the peptide tRNA. The ribosome then moves, ejecting the now-empty tRNA and opening the A-site for the next aminoacyl–tRNA complex.

translation and be moving down the mRNA molecule simultaneously, thus increasing the rate of protein synthesis. This complex of multiple ribosomes on an mRNA molecule is called a *polyribosome.* Protein synthesis can be blocked by a number of antibiotic molecules. Some, such as tetracyclines and streptomycin, selectively block prokaryotic protein synthesis and are therefore therapeutic agents for bacterial infections. Others, such as puromycin and cycloheximide, which act on eukaryotic protein synthesis, are useful as experimental tools. All of these inhibitors block specific steps in the complex sequence of initiation and elongation.

Targeting of Newly Synthesized Protein

After synthesis, a new protein molecule must be directed or targeted to its appropriate location in the cell. Many proteins also undergo posttranslational processing, such as the removal of some amino acids, blockage of the amino or carboxyl terminus, or the addition of carbohydrate, lipid, or phosphate residues. In the process of targeting, all proteins, except those destined to remain cytosolic, must be inserted into or cross a membrane. Posttranslational processing may occur simultaneously with this transmembrane transport or after the new protein resides in a specialized subcellular compartment possessing the necessary enzymes.

Cytosolic proteins fold rapidly and spontaneously into a structure containing most secondary structure such as α helices and β sheets. Further attainment of the final three-dimensional configuration involves helper proteins called *chaperones* (27). Most chaperones are heat-shock proteins because their synthesis is greatly increased after brief exposure to elevated temperature; they are identified by size in kilodaltons, for example, hsp60 and hsp70. These proteins bind and hydrolyze ATP and, by binding to exposed hydrophobic regions, "massage" the protein into a mature state.

Information specifying intracellular protein targeting resides in the sequence or structure of the protein and interaction with a receptor capable of recognizing that sequence. The targeting information usually resides in a sequence of 15 to 40 amino acids, termed a *signal sequence* or *signal peptide* (28). The sole function of this sequence is to direct targeting, and the sequence is frequently removed after that function is complete. In other cases, targeting information resides in a signal patch of amino acid residues, which are adjacent after protein folding but are located at different regions in the primary sequence. The definition of signal areas on proteins is evolving, and only some of the better-understood examples are presented.

After protein synthesis, the first "decision" in the targeting process is whether a newly synthesized protein is to enter the secretory pathway or remain in the cell in the cytoplasm or other organelles. The secretory pathway includes proteins to be secreted from the cell as well as those destined to reside in the plasma membrane or lysosomes or destined to remain permanently within the lumen or membranes of the ER or Golgi. Secretory pathway proteins are known to be synthesized on ribosomes bound to the ER, whereas other proteins are synthesized on cytoplasmic free ribosomes. All protein synthesis originates on ribosomes in the cytosol, but proteins destined for the secretory pathway rapidly bind to the ER. The elucidation of the process by which secretory proteins are directed into the ER lumen provided the first understanding of targeting mechanisms.

Secretory Pathway Targeting

Proteins targeted for the secretory pathway most commonly contain an amino-terminal signal sequence (Fig. 1.34). Characteristically, this sequence has a positively charged amino acid near the amino terminus, followed by a stretch of hydrophobic amino acids. When protein synthesis is studied in vitro in the presence of microsomes (fragmented ER), the protein ends up within the lumen, and the signal sequence has been removed. The enzyme responsible for this cleavage is called *signal peptidase* and is located in the ER lumen. If in vitro synthesis is completed without microsomes, the full length, or a "preprotein," results, which usually is incapable of entering subsequently added microsomes.

Insertion into the ER lumen involves a ribonucleoprotein complex, termed the *signal recognition particle* (SRP), and a receptor on the ER, called the *SRP receptor* or *docking protein* (28). The SRP is a complex of six polypeptide chains and a 300-nucleotide RNA molecule that binds to the nascent signal peptide emerging from the ribosome after the synthesis of approximately 70 amino acids (Fig. 1.34). After this interaction, translational arrest occurs until the ribosome SRP complex binds to an SRP receptor. The SRP receptor is an integral membrane protein of two polypeptide subunits exposed on the cytosolic surface of the ER membrane. At this point, translation resumes, the ribosome is passed on to bind to a ribosomal receptor protein, and SRP dissociates. Next, the signal peptide binds to another multiprotein complex termed the *translocon,* which makes up a protein-lined channel through which the nascent secretory protein is extruded (29). In the absence of a ribosome, the translocon is closed at the cytoplasmic end. In the most common case, the secretory protein is completely extruded into the lumen, the signal peptide is cleaved off, and the ribosome dissociates. Insertion of the nascent peptide through the membrane requires the hydrolysis of bound GTP. Energy released by the spontaneous folding of the secretory protein in the ER lumen may also help to pull it across. Translocation and folding are also assisted by the intraluminal binding protein, BiP, which is related to hsp70 proteins.

Lysosomal proteins are similarly inserted into the ER and later sorted into their appropriate organelles. As is the case for many other secretory proteins, lysosomal enzymes are glycosylated on certain asparagine residues as protein synthesis is occurring (30). This process involves the transfer of a preformed oligosaccharide-containing glucose, mannose, and N-acetylglucosamine from a lipid-linked dolichol phosphate (Fig. 1.35). While still in

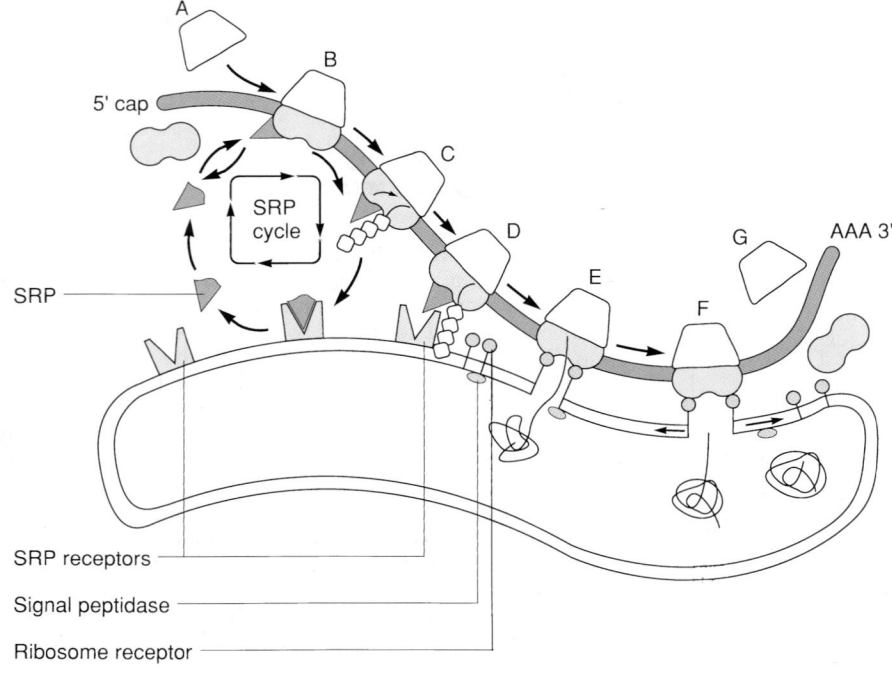

Figure 1.34. Synthesis and sequestration of secretory protein. Synthesis begins on the left as ribosomal subunits aggregate *(A)* and begin to translate mRNA *(B).* The signal-recognition particle (SRP) binds to the complex *(C)* and arrests peptide-chain elongation until SRP binds to a receptor in the endoplasmic reticulum membrane *(D).* The nascent polypeptide is then extruded into the lumen *(E and F)* with the aid of ribosome receptors, and SRP is released to recycle. The amino-terminal sequence may be cleaved by a signal peptidase. On chain termination, the ribosome dissociates *(G),* and its subunits can recycle.

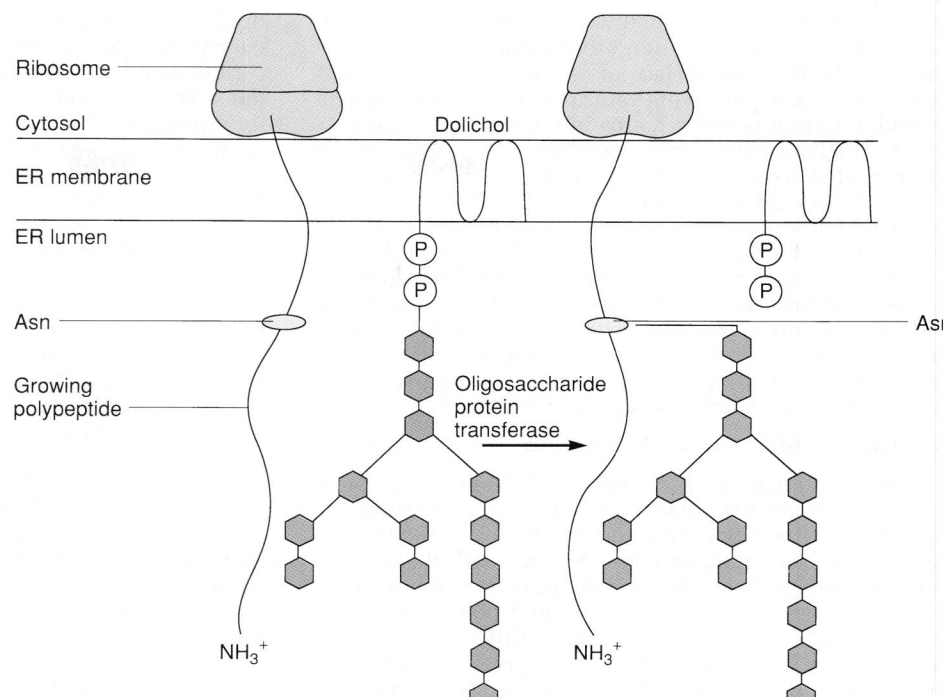

Figure 1.35. Biosynthesis of an asparagine-linked glycoprotein in the endoplasmic reticulum (ER) lumen. The sugar core is transferred as a preformed unit from a carrier lipid, dolichol phosphate, to the protein as it is being synthesized.

the ER, the glucose is removed, exposing mannose. The oligosaccharide moiety is then further processed in the Golgi.

Proteins destined to reside in the plasma membrane or in the ER membrane (such as ribosome receptor) have to stop part way through their transmembrane passage (31) (Fig. 1.36). This placement is directed by another amino acid sequence in the nascent protein, termed a *stop transfer* or *membrane anchor sequence*. In the simplest case,

the amino terminus of the molecule is extruded through the membrane, the process stops at the anchor sequence, and synthesis of the carboxyl terminus continues in the cytosol. An example of such a protein is the low-density lipoprotein (LDL) receptor. Because the lumen of the ER corresponds topologically to the outside of the cell, after vesicular transport through the Golgi to the surface, the amino terminus of the LDL receptor ends up on the external surface of the plasma membrane. This portion of the

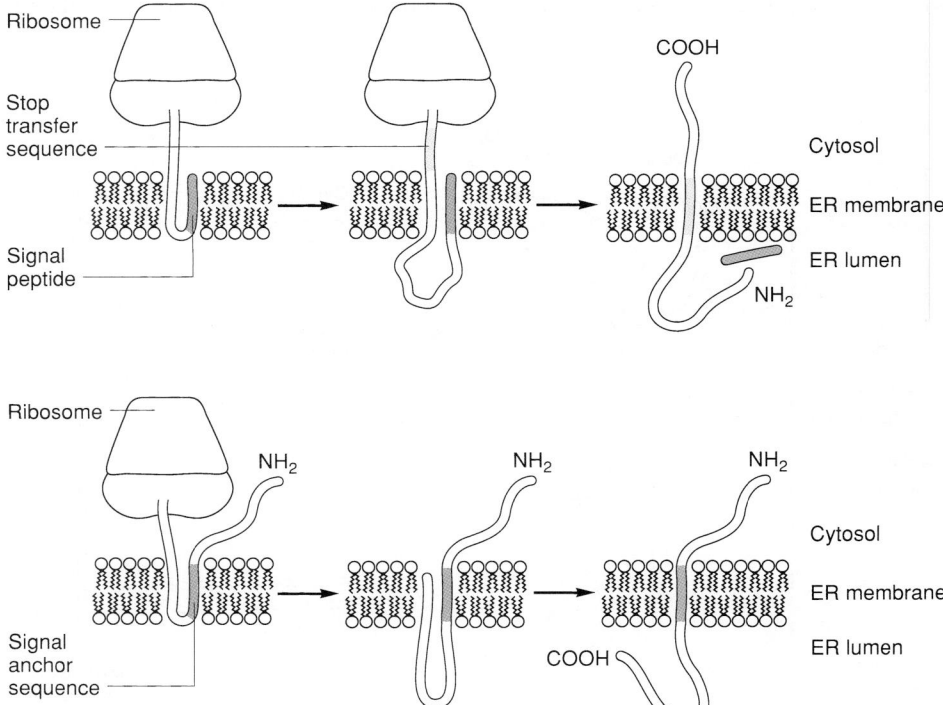

Figure 1.36. The topology of membrane proteins is the result of signals in the primary sequence. In this case, the two proteins end up with their opposite ends external. The occurrence of multiple signal anchor sequences can result in multiple transmembrane domains.

molecule may be glycosylated within the ER and Golgi lumina, with the result that the carbohydrate residues are located on the external surface of the plasma membrane. A more complex sequence of events occurs for proteins with an amino terminus that remains in the cytoplasm, such as the asialoglycoprotein and transferrin receptors, or for proteins that have multiple membrane-spanning regions. Both are thought to involve internal signal–anchor sequences. These internal sequences usually form α helices and are thought to insert into the bilayer as a hairpin loop (Fig. 1.36). In the case of membrane proteins that span the bilayer multiple times, this process must be repeated with a separate insertion for each extracellular loop. Examples of such proteins are heterotrimeric G-protein-coupled receptors that contain seven membrane-spanning segments and many ion channels and transporters.

Nuclear and Mitochondrial Targeting

Nuclear proteins, such as histones, DNA and RNA polymerases, and gene regulatory proteins, are synthesized on cytoplasmic free ribosomes and must then enter the nucleus through the nuclear pores. Studies with fluorescent-labeled proteins have shown free passage through these pores by polypeptides with a size cutoff point of approximately 60 kd, consistent with a water-filled pore approximately 9 nm in diameter. This pore serves to keep cytoplasmic organelles and large proteins out of the nucleus, except those specifically targeted. Entry of large proteins into the nucleus is energy dependent and involves use of ATP and interaction with proteins of the nuclear pore complex. Nuclear targeting is specified by a short amino acid sequence rich in positively charged lysine and arginine residues and usually containing proline. The sequence can occur anywhere in the molecule and is not cleaved after entry. The nuclear localization sequence binds to cytoplasmic proteins termed *importins*, and then interacts with the nuclear pore complex. Both nuclear import and export also involve the small GTPase Ran (32). In contrast to secretory proteins, which are targeted only once, long-lived nuclear proteins may have to be targeted multiple times because the nuclear envelope breaks down and reforms during each mitosis, after which nuclear proteins must reaccumulate. The

nuclear pore complex is also involved in regulation of nucleocytoplasmic transport of pre-mRNA.

Mitochondria contain DNA and synthesize some proteins, but most mitochondrial proteins are imported from the cytoplasm (Fig. 1.37). Translocation of matrix proteins must occur across two membranes, the outer and inner mitochondrial membranes, and with the protein in an unfolded state (33). Cytosolic chaperone proteins of the hsp70 family bind the precursor protein as it is released from the ribosome and prevent it from folding spontaneously before it binds to a receptor protein on the mitochondria. Protein import is believed to occur at points of contact where the two membranes appear to be joined. Mitochondrial proteins have a signal sequence at their amino terminus. Molecular genetic studies have shown that the signal sequence can be as short as 12 amino acids, and, if engineered onto the amino terminus of a cytosolic protein, the sequence causes its insertion into the mitochondria. The signal sequence contains positively charged amino acids every third or fourth residue and forms an amphipathic α helix that is recognized by a specific import receptor. This receptor is part of a multisubunit complex termed Tom (*transport across outer membrane*) proteins. Some of these proteins appear to form a channel. Once the protein has moved through this channel across the outer membrane, it crosses the inner membrane driven by the mitochondrial membrane potential and ATP hydrolysis through a complex of Tim proteins. Once within the mitochondrial matrix, the signal peptide is cleaved, and the protein folds to assume its mature configuration. This also involves mitochondrial matrix chaperones such as Hsc70 and Hsc60.

Secretory Pathway

Once secretory proteins have been translocated across a lipid bilayer into the lumen of the ER, they must fold properly and form disulfide bonds, with the latter process being aided by the enzyme protein disulfide isomerase (34) and several ER resident chaperones. Then they pass through a number of compartments, including the Golgi, where they are further processed and sorted and end up in a secretory vesicle or lysosome (35,36) (Fig. 1.38). This

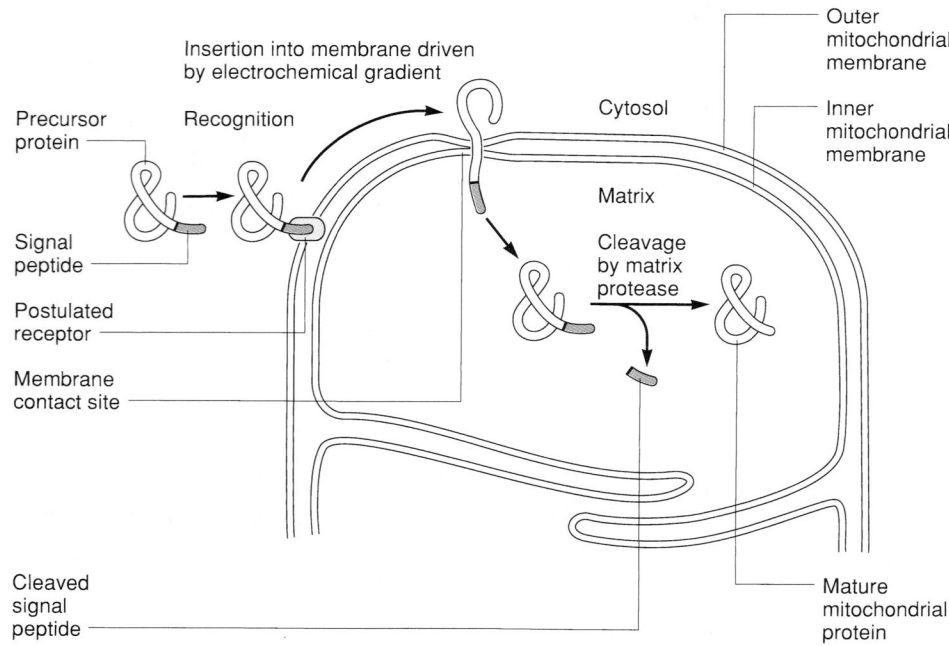

Figure 1.37. Insertion of newly synthesized protein into the mitochondrion is specified by a terminal signal peptide that interacts with a postulated receptor. These proteins are originally synthesized on free ribosomes and released into the cytoplasm, from which they insert into the mitochondrion.

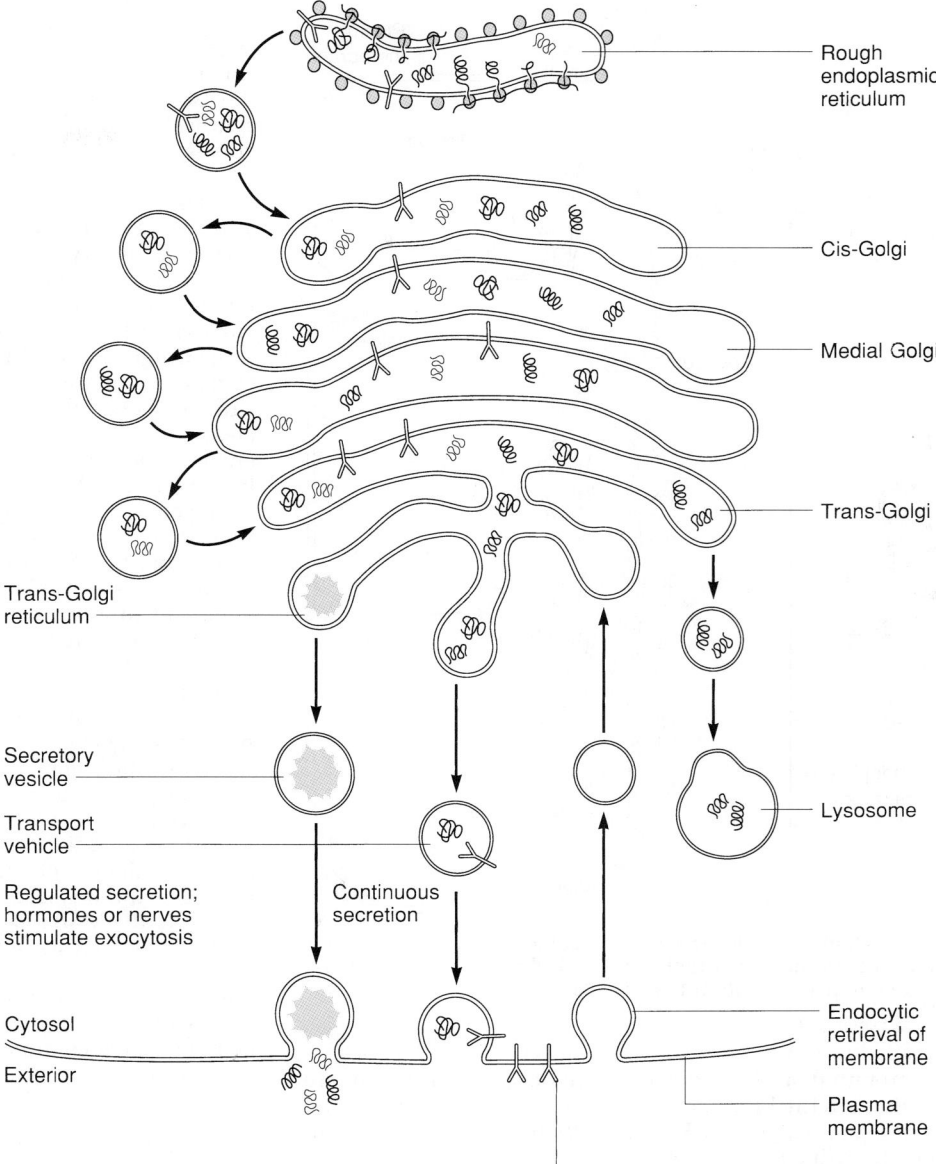

Figure 1.38. Intracellular transport and sorting of proteins destined for secretion, insertion into the plasma membrane, or targeting to the lysosome. After insertion into the endoplasmic reticulum lumen, movement from one compartment to another is by vesicular transport, which buds off one compartment and fuses with the next. Sorting signals intrinsic to the newly synthesized proteins specify the pathway to be taken.

passage involves movement by a distinct process, that of vesicular transport. In this mechanism, the proteins do not cross membranes but are transferred between the lumina of compartments. A small vesicle buds off from one compartment such as ER and then fuses with another—in this case, the Golgi. In some cases, vesicular transport is a bulk movement of all luminal contents; in other cases, it is selective, with vesicular receptors binding only certain proteins in the luminal fluid.

The first vesicular transport event in the secretory pathway is movement of newly synthesized protein from ER to Golgi (37). The Golgi apparatus, which is made up of flattened saccules, can be subdivided into *cis,* medial, and *trans* elements, *cis* being adjacent to the ER. Vesicles approximately 50 nm in diameter bud off from smooth areas of ER, called *transitional elements,* by an ATP-requiring process and fuse with the *cis*-Golgi cisternae. These vesicles are coated, that is, they have a protein visible in electron micrographs that surrounds the vesicle. The coat is composed of

coat proteins called *COPs;* these are distinct from the first identified coat protein, clathrin. Low-molecular-weight GTP-binding (LMWG) proteins, which are related to the protooncogene *ras,* serve as molecular switches in that they are active when binding GTP and inactive when binding GDP. Coat assembly is initiated by the LMWG protein ARF binding to a receptor that initiates COP binding, coat assembly, and budding. Transport vesicles also contain membrane-targeting proteins called *v-SNARES.* After GTP hydrolysis and uncoating, the v-SNARE binds to a docking protein in the target membrane termed the *t-SNARE* (Fig. 1.39), a process that also requires additional cytosolic proteins. Another large family of LMWG proteins, the Rab proteins, also appear to be involved in imposing specificity because different Rab species are associated with different membrane compartments in the cell; for example, Rab1 is associated with ER-to-Golgi transport (38).

The transport event moves both content and membrane proteins. Proteins destined to reside in the ER lumen, such

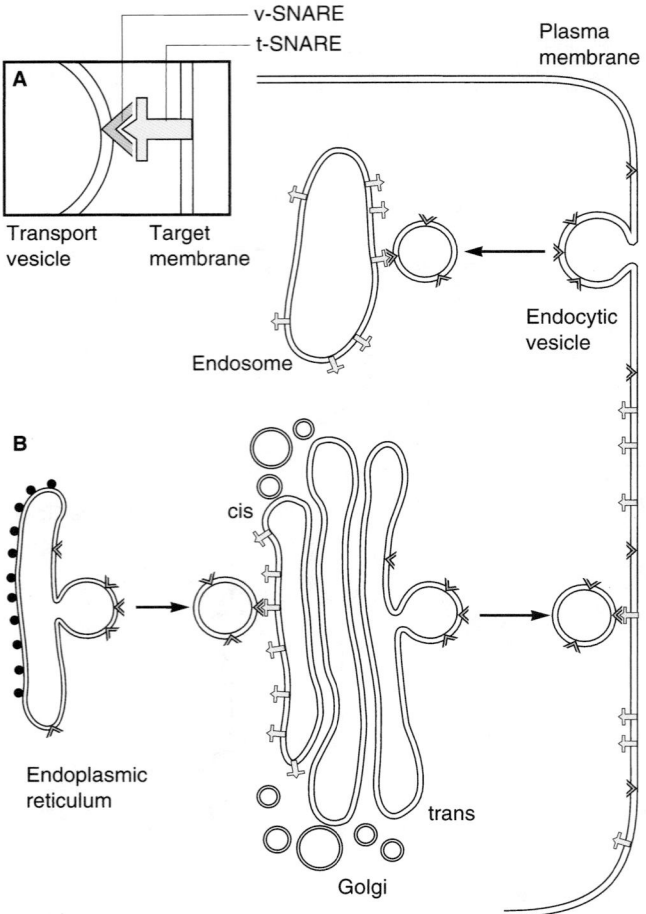

Figure 1.39. Vesicular transport is guided by distinct proteins termed *SNARES*. (After Rothman JE. Mechanisms of intracellular protein transport. *Nature* 1994;372:55.)

as protein disulfide isomerase, are not transported but are retained in the ER lumen by virtue of a specific four-amino acid signal sequence, KDEL, in their C-terminus that interacts with a receptor in the ER.

The Golgi apparatus is structurally and functionally divided. Each cisterna constitutes a functional compartment. This compartmentation is demonstrated by the localization of specific enzymes to separate compartments. The functional corollary of Golgi compartmentation is that different processing steps occur in distinct regions. For example, phosphate is added to mannose residues of future lysosomal enzymes in the *cis*-Golgi cisternae. In the processing of secreted glycoproteins, the removal of mannose residues occurs in the medial cisternae, whereas the addition of sialic acid occurs in the *trans*-Golgi cisternae. Such events have been used to develop in vitro models demonstrating vesicular transport from one Golgi compartment to another, which occurs similarly to transport from ER to Golgi. Coated vesicles bud from cisternal rims, uncoat, and then fuse selectively with the next compartment. Although all secretory proteins flow unidirectionally from *cis*- to medial to *trans*-Golgi compartments, other vesicles with a distinct coat protein move retrograde and serve to retrieve ER resident proteins that have migrated to the Golgi. From the *trans* cisternae, secretory proteins move directly into a tubular network, called the *trans-Golgi network*. It is here that sorting takes place between secretory proteins and lysosomal enzymes.

The Golgi complex is especially prominent in exocrine cells, such as pancreatic and parotid acinar cells, and in endocrine cells, such as the islets of Langerhans or anterior pituitary. In goblet and other mucus-secreting cells, the Golgi is also prominent and is where proteoglycan synthesis takes place on the nascent protein core. This involves the addition of large glycosaminoglycan polymers to serine residues on the protein core. In a later step in the *trans*-Golgi cisternae, sulfate is added. The same process, albeit to a lesser extent, takes place in many cell types that secrete proteoglycan basement membrane components.

In endocrine cells and neurons, many polypeptide hormones and neuropeptides are synthesized as larger precursors and then cleaved or processed beginning in the *trans*-Golgi and continuing in the secretory granule. In some cases, more than one biologically active peptide results. Although the rationale for this process is not always clear, it allows production of small peptides, such as enkephalins (five amino acids), that otherwise would be too small to be handled by the secretory pathway.

The biosynthesis of lysosomes (36) involves the production of both lysosomal enzymes and specific lysosomal membrane proteins such as the H[+]-transporting vacuolar ATPase; these proteins separate from other secretory proteins and proteins destined for the plasma membrane in the *trans*-Golgi network (Fig. 1.40). The sorting signal for lysosomal hydrolases is known to be mannose-6-phosphate (M6P) groups. Phosphate is added in the *cis*-Golgi, where the responsible enzymes must distinguish nascent lysosomal hydrolases from other secretory glycoproteins. Once phosphorylated, the M6P can interact with an M6P receptor protein to concentrate these enzymes in a region of the *trans*-Golgi network. These regions then bud off into vesicles coated with the protein clathrin. The coat is then shed, and the vesicle fuses with a lysosome. Once exposed to acid pH, the lysosomal acid hydrolase rapidly dissociates from the M6P receptor, which then cycles back to the *trans*-Golgi network, again by means of coated vesicles. In some cells, M6P receptors are also present on the plasma membrane, where they concentrate any lysosomal enzymes released into the extracellular medium. These receptors are concentrated in coated pits that bud off and return to the *trans*-Golgi network as a scavenger pathway.

Transport to the Cell Surface: Exocytosis

Transport vesicles that bud off from the *trans*-Golgi network carry both material to be secreted from the cell and proteins destined to become components of the plasma membrane (Fig. 1.38). These vesicles can fuse with the plasma membrane. This process, termed *exocytosis*, results in the release of vesicle content and the incorporation of the vesicle membrane into the plasma membrane with the former internal surface of the vesicle now facing the outside of the cell.

Vesicular transport to the cell surface can be divided into two components—constitutive and regulated secretion (39). Constitutive secretion involves small, coated vesicles that rapidly move to the plasma membrane and fuse. This mechanism, which occurs in all cells, is probably analogous to vesicular transport from ER to Golgi and that between Golgi cisternae. In the absence of a specific sorting mechanism, secretory and plasma membrane proteins take this route, which can be thought of as a default pathway. This pathway appears to transport basement membrane components that are secreted by all cells and also delivers membrane proteins such as Na[+]-K[+]-ATPase to the plasma membrane. Liver cells exhibit an active constitutive secretion of serum proteins, such as albumin and clotting factors.

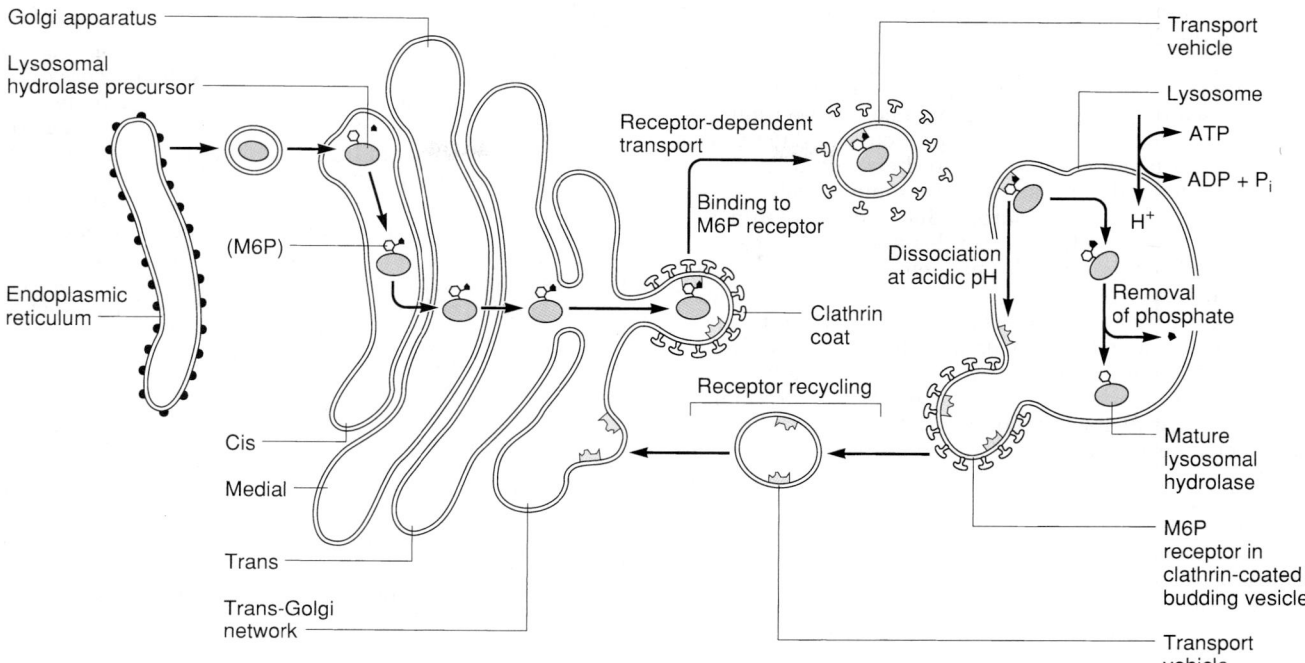

Figure 1.40. Biosynthesis of lysosomal proteins. Targeting is specified by phosphorylation of mannose and interaction with a mannose-6-phosphate receptor. The role of clathrin in the budding-off of transport vesicles is also illustrated.

Regulated secretion occurs in cells secreting digestive enzymes, hormones, and other regulatory molecules and neurotransmitters. In regulated secretion, the material to be secreted is sorted into a storage vesicle or granule; fusion with the plasma membrane and exocytosis then takes place in response to external stimulation.

In the case of digestive enzymes and protein and polypeptide hormones, there must be a signal sequence or patch on the molecules that directs it into the regulated pathway. When, for example, a pituitary cell is genetically engineered to synthesize trypsinogen or insulin, the foreign protein is packaged into secretory granules along with endogenous pituitary hormones. The production of secretory granules involves budding of clathrin-coated vesicles from the *trans*-Golgi network, which then fuse to form a large vesicle of dilute content. This vesicle, sometimes termed a *condensing vacuole,* concentrates secretory proteins and, in some cases, completes the processing of the secretory protein. In the case of insulin, its precursor, proinsulin, is cleaved to yield insulin and C peptide in the condensing vacuoles. In the process of condensation, secretory proteins may form complexes with ions such as Ca^{2+} or Zn^{2+} and may even assume a crystalline array. This process is facilitated by other packaging or organizing proteins attached to the inner face of the granule membrane and by an H^+-ATPase in the granule membrane that acidifies the granule content. Most secretory granule membranes contain a relatively limited set of specialized proteins.

In the case of some neurons and mast cells, newly formed secretory granules do not contain secretory material but rather contain transporters and enzymes necessary for the uptake or synthesis of small molecules such as histamine and norepinephrine. These molecules are then condensed with counter-ions and proteins and are stored until regulated secretion is triggered.

Regulated secretion is triggered in most cases by a hormone or neurotransmitter (Fig. 1.41). The ensuing process

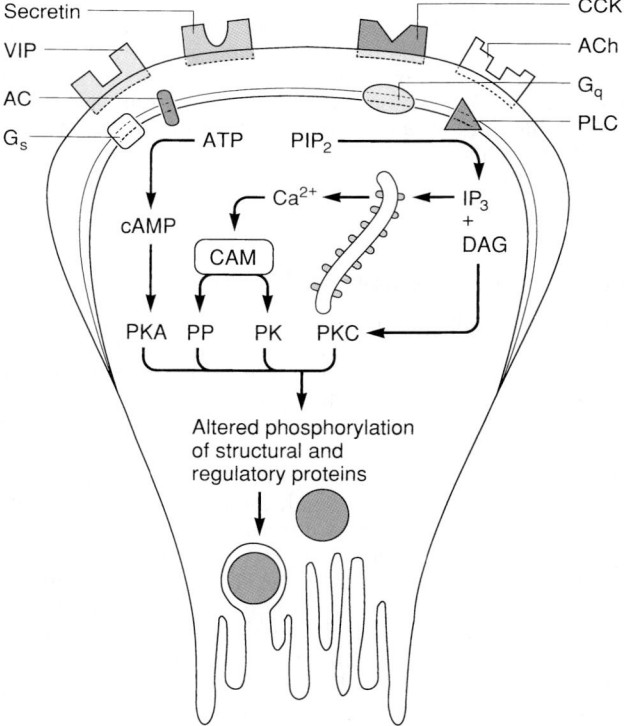

Figure 1.41. Scheme for control of regulated secretion for pancreatic acinar cells that secrete digestive enzymes. Vasoactive intestinal peptide (VIP) and secretin activate adenylate cyclase (AC) to promote adenosine monophosphate (AMP) formation, whereas cholecystokinin (CCK) and acetylcholine (ACh) activate phospholipase C (PLC), leading to production of inositol trisphosphate (IP$_3$) and diacylglycerol (DAG). IP$_3$ releases intracellular Ca^{2+}, which interacts with calmodulin (CAM). These second messengers (cAMP, Ca^{2+}, DAG) activate a battery of protein kinases (PK) and protein phosphatases (PP), which then induce secretion.

is called *stimulus–secretion coupling.* In most cases, the coupling involves an increase in the cytoplasmic concentration of Ca^{2+}, but it may also involve generation of 1,2-diacylglycerol (DAG) or production of cAMP, which activate kinases or phosphatases. Evidence has accumulated invoking a role for Rab proteins, particularly Rab3 in this process, in a manner analogous to their role in vesicular fusion in intracellular transport. In some secretory cells, such as mast cells and neurons that secrete within seconds, secretory vesicles or granules are prepositioned or "docked" adjacent to the plasma membrane and may need only an increase in Ca^{2+} to fuse. In other cases, granules are dispersed in the cytoplasm and must be continually moved to the membrane over minutes or hours. Such a process, as occurs in pancreatic acinar cells after a meal, involves the cytoskeleton and particularly microtubules. The fusion event itself involves protein–protein interactions between the outside of the granule membrane and the cytosolic face of the plasma membrane. This interaction generates a small fusion pore, which then widens by flow of membrane lipids. At this point, decondensation of secretory granule contents occurs, facilitated by a flow of ions and water across the granule membrane.

The protein machinery involved in mediating docking and fusion (40) is best known for synaptic vesicles and involves proteins functioning as v-SNARES and t-SNARES, which are believed to be synaptobrevin and syntaxin, respectively. Other proteins such as n-Sec1 block the SNARE interaction until triggering. Synaptic vesicle fusion is triggered directly by Ca^{2+} entering the cell through gated channels in the plasma membrane and binding to a Ca^{2+} sensor protein, probably synaptotagmin.

Because fusion of secretory granules with the plasma membrane greatly increases membrane surface area, there may be a transient increase in plasma membrane surface area. This increase is compensated for by an increase in endocytosis, by which coated vesicles bud from the plasma membrane and return to the *trans*-Golgi network. Endocytosis also serves a recycling function because components of the secretory granule membrane can be reused without requiring resynthesis.

Polarized Secretion in Epithelial Cells

Many cells are polarized with two distinct membrane domains. Polarization is especially prominent in epithelial cells, such as those that compose the renal tubule or the intestinal epithelium. Tight junctional complexes form a connecting belt around and between epithelial cells near their apical borders and allow apical and basolateral membranes to maintain distinct protein and even lipid composition. For example, in the small intestinal absorptive cell, the Na^+-coupled glucose transporter and digestive enzymes such as sucrase are localized exclusively in the apical membrane, whereas Na^+-K^+-ATPase is present exclusively in the basolateral membrane. Generation of cell polarity is a complex morphogenetic event, and its maintenance requires the continual resupply of specific membrane components. In polarized secretory cells, such as goblet cells and pancreatic acinar cells, the regulated secretory pathway is usually structurally polarized. The fact that acinar cell granules fuse only with the apical membrane and not with the lateral membrane implies specificity in the proteins controlling fusion. Epithelial cells may need to secrete one set of components apically and another basally. That such sorting can occur is shown by the fact that, after viral infection, some viral proteins move to one membrane, whereas in the same cell, a distinct viral protein may bud from the other side of the cell.

Endocytosis

Opposite in direction to secretion of macromolecules but occurring by similar mechanisms is the process of endocytosis. A portion of the membrane invaginates and pinches off to form an intracellular vesicle containing both membrane proteins and ingested material. As in the secretory pathway, the ingested macromolecules do not mix with the cytoplasm and are transferred within the cell by budding and fusion of vesicles. The process of endocytosis or pinocytosis, which involves the formation of small vesicles, is mechanistically distinct from phagocytosis, by which specialized cells take up larger particles, such as bacteria or erythrocytes (Fig. 1.42).

All cells continually take up portions of their cell membranes in the form of small endocytic or pinocytic vesicles. Pinocytosis, or "cell drinking," refers to the capture of surrounding fluid in the vesicle. The recovery of membrane molecules and any attached ligands is more important functionally. Endocytosis begins at a specialized region, the coated pit, which appears in electron micrographs as a depression of the membrane. The coated pit is further identified by a bristle-like coating on the cytoplasmic surface. This coating is composed of the protein clathrin, whose individual unit is a three-armed structure called a *triskelion.* Triskelions assemble into a basket-like lattice, and this assembly is believed to provide the force resulting in the invagination. The lifetime of a coated pit is short; the pit pinches off within minutes to form a coated vesicle (41). Dynamin, a large cytosolic GTPase protein, is essential for the pinching off process, which requires the hydrolysis of bound GTP. After formation, coated vesicles rapidly shed their coats, which can be reused at the membrane. The vesicle moves into the cell, guided by microtubules, to a perinuclear area near the *trans*-Golgi network. At this point, the vesicles fuse to form a larger structure, the endosome. Specific LMWG Rab proteins, particularly Rab4 and Rab5, are involved in this process. Unless specifically sorted and removed, the contents of the endosome are passed on to lysosomes, where they are digested.

Many membrane receptor molecules have a cytoplasmic portion that allows them to localize in coated pits (Fig. 1.43). This may occur spontaneously, as with the LDL receptor, or after binding of ligand, as is the case for the epidermal growth factor (EGF) receptor. Concentration of receptors in coated pits allows their selective uptake, a process called *receptor-mediated endocytosis.* In the case of the LDL receptor, this is the major mechanism whereby cells take up cholesterol. A more specialized case is the asialoglycoprotein receptor, expressed only on hepatocytes, which take up plasma glycoproteins lacking terminal sialic acid residues. Other examples of receptor-mediated endocytosis are the uptake of transferrin with its bound iron and the uptake by absorptive cells of the ileum of vitamin B_{12}.

Ligand–receptor complexes are sorted in the endosome. The contents of the endosome are maintained at an acidic pH of approximately 5.0 as a result of a specific vacuolar H^+-ATPase that transports H^+ into the endosomal lumen. Many ligand–receptor interactions are pH sensitive. The ligands dissociate in the endosome, after which the dissociated ligand is transported to lysosomes and digested. The freed receptor is sorted and buds off as part of a transport vesicle that returns to the cell membrane, where the receptor can undergo another round of endocytosis. This sequence occurs for the LDL and asialoglycoprotein receptors. Some receptors, such as the EGF receptor, do not recycle but are degraded in the lysosome, resulting in a reduced number of cell surface receptors. This process is re-

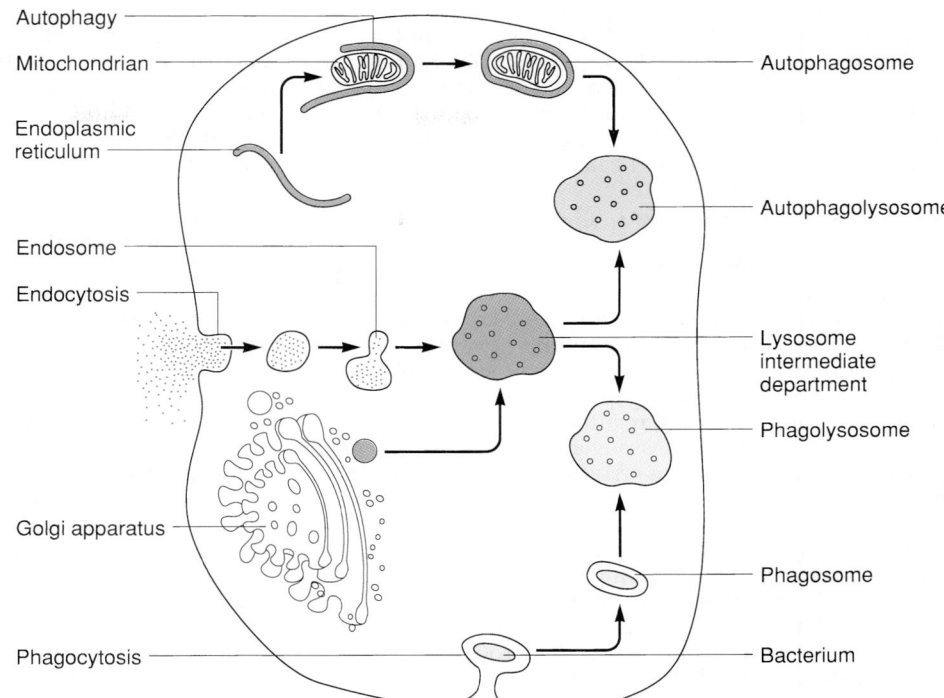

Figure 1.42. Formation of lysosomes by combination of transport vesicles from the Golgi-containing lysosomal enzymes with material that has been phagocytosed, endocytosed, or internalized by autophagy.

ferred to as *receptor down-regulation.* In the case of transferrin, the low pH of the endosome separates Fe from transferrin, and the binding protein recycles to the cell surface and is released.

Phagocytosis is a specialized form of endocytosis by which large particles are internalized by specialized cells, primarily macrophages and neutrophils (Fig. 1.42). To be phagocytosed, particles must bind to the surface of the phagocytic cell, usually as a result of specific antibody coating the particle. The phagocytic cell then extends pseudopods to engulf the particle. This event is followed by membrane fusion and a pinching off. This process does not involve clathrin but rather actin. Cytochalasin, a drug that inhibits actin polymerization, inhibits phagocytosis. After internalization, the engulfed particle, called a phagosome, fuses with lysosomes to form a phagolysosome, a type of secondary lysosome. In this terminology, the primary lysosomes are the structures budded off from the

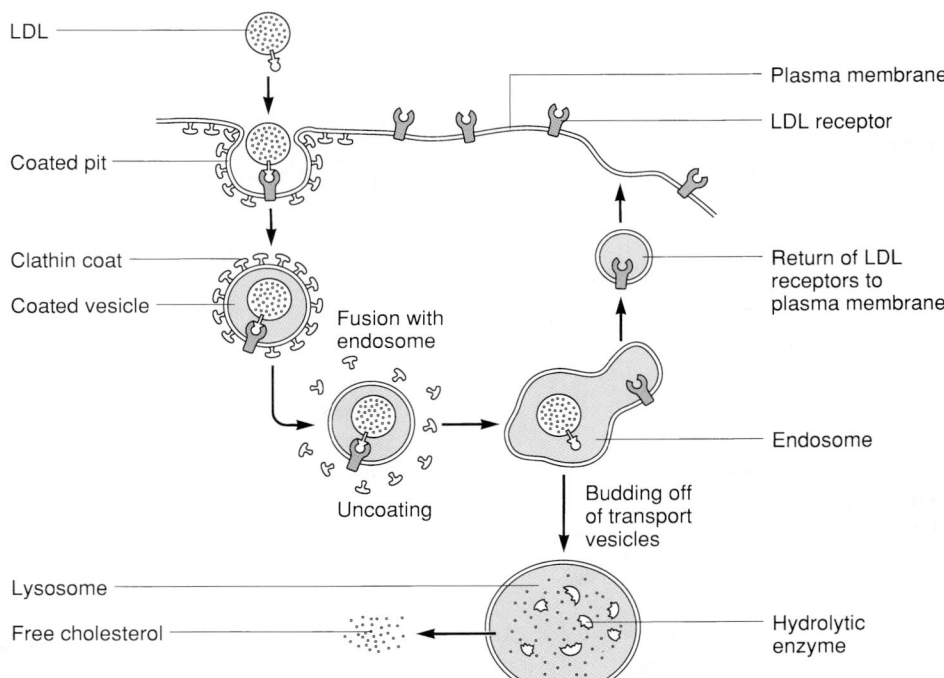

Figure 1.43. Receptor-mediated endocytosis of low-density lipoprotein (LDL), with resultant degradation of the endocytosed LDL and recycling of the receptor.

trans-Golgi network containing lysosomal enzymes or, in the case of neutrophils, specialized storage granules containing lysosomal enzymes. A physiologically relevant site of phagocytosis is the thyroid gland, where thyroid follicular cells phagocytose and digest thyroglobulin from the lumen of the thyroid follicle, thereby releasing the thyroid hormones thyroxine and triiodothyronine.

REGULATION OF CELL FUNCTION

The growth, differentiation, and function of all cells are highly regulated events. Cell regulation can be thought of as the effector side of cell communication. Communication can occur in a number of ways, including direct physical contact or passage of small molecules from cell to cell through gap junction channels (Fig. 1.11). Most commonly, cell regulation occurs by means of extracellular chemical messengers. Depending on how the extracellular messenger arrives, cell regulation can be classified as paracrine, endocrine, or neurocrine (Fig. 1.44). In paracrine regulation, a chemical messenger or mediator is produced and acts locally. This restricted domain of action is due to the limitations of diffusion and to the fact that the mediators are taken up or inactivated by target cells. Examples of paracrine regulators include histamine released from gastric enterochromaffin-like cells, prostaglandins that are made by cells in all mammalian tissues, nitric oxide (NO), and certain brain–gut peptide regulators such as somatostatin. In endocrine regulation, the extracellular messengers (hormones) are released into the blood and act on target cells anywhere in the body that possess appropriate receptors. In neurocrine regulation, neurons secrete transmitters into a highly localized region, the synaptic cleft, so that regulation depends on a physical connection between the neuron and the target cell and on the presence of a specific receptor.

In almost all cases of cell regulation, the extracellular signal or stimulus is restricted to being an informational molecule. This information is received by a receptor on or in the target cell, which usually has an affinity for the signal molecule such that changes in its concentration result in changes in the fraction of receptors that are occupied.

Hormone receptors in general have an affinity (K_d) for the ligand (a generic term for the molecule that binds to the receptor) of the order of 10^{-11} to 10^{-9} mol/L, whereas receptors for neurotransmitters usually display lower affinities, ranging from 10^{-7} to 10^{-4} mol/L. Besides exhibiting high affinity for appropriate ligands, receptors must be selective and discriminate a specific extracellular mediator from all other extracellular molecules. Most receptors are protein molecules, existing either in the plasma membrane or intracellularly. Clearly, one important determinant of cell regulation is the nature of the specific complement of receptors and receptor subtypes expressed by a particular cell. Another major determinant of the cell response is its genetic programming. Thus, the same regulator may have different actions on different tissues. For example, adrenal corticosteroids such as cortisol cause cytolysis of lymphocytes but induce the synthesis of enzymes necessary for the production of glucose in the liver.

Most hormones, local mediators, and neurotransmitters are water soluble and cannot readily cross plasma membranes. They vary in size from small amines, such as histamine and norepinephrine, to medium-sized glycoproteins, such as follicle-stimulating hormone and thyroid-stimulating hormone. Receptors for these mediators are localized on the cell membrane and transduce hormone binding into altered levels of intracellular messengers. The ligand itself, particularly polypeptide hormones, may enter the cell by receptor-mediated endocytosis, but intracellular actions of internalized peptides have not been convincingly documented. Another group of regulators, including steroid and thyroid hormones, are lipophilic. These molecules are usually carried in the plasma, bound to specific binding proteins. By virtue of their hydrophobicity, they are able to penetrate readily the lipid portion of the cell membrane. Receptors for these hormones exist intracellularly in the cytoplasm or nucleus and usually act as regulators of gene expression. These hydrophobic signaling molecules exist in plasma bound to protein, so that the concentration of this class of regulators does not fluctuate rapidly in plasma, and their actions are in general slower in onset and more prolonged than those of the water-soluble class.

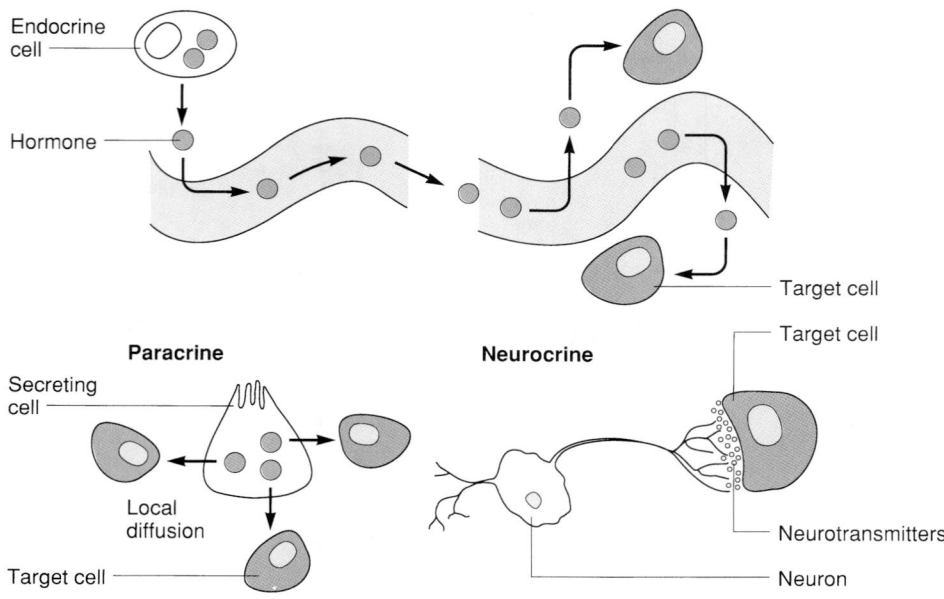

Figure 1.44. Endocrine, paracrine, and neurocrine modes of cell-to-cell communication.

Intracellular Receptors and the Control of Gene Expression

The primary molecular structure of most intracellular receptors is known from molecular cloning. Receptors for steroid hormones, thyroid hormones, vitamin D, and retinoic acid are homologous and form a superfamily of receptors with similar structure and function (42,43). All have two properties in common: they bind DNA, and they also bind a particular ligand (hormone). The DNA-binding region in the center of the molecule is highly homologous within the superfamily. The carboxyl-terminal end binds the ligand, and the amino terminus is a variable region believed to be active in regulating gene transcription (Fig. 1.45). Other receptors of unknown function exist, termed *orphan receptors.*

Most cells contain approximately 10,000 receptors for one or more steroid hormones or other, similar receptors. Some types of steroid receptors, particularly for glucocorticoids, are located in the cytosol in the inactive state; others, including thyroid hormone receptors, are located in the nucleus (42). Once the ligand binds, the receptor undergoes a conformational change, termed *activation.* This allows cytoplasmic receptors to move into the nucleus and bind to DNA. Receptors already in the nucleus increase their affinity for DNA. In the case of glucocorticoid receptors and probably others of this class, the inactive receptor is associated with another protein, the heat-shock protein (molecular weight of 90 kd). Heat-shock proteins block the DNA-binding domain of the receptor. Activation involves the dissociation of the inhibitor protein.

Activated steroid and thyroid receptors bind to specific regions of DNA and influence the synthesis of specific mRNA (43,44), thereby regulating the production of proteins that mediate the cellular response to the hormone (Fig. 1.46). The specific region of DNA occupied by the receptor can be identified because the bound protein makes this region resistant to cleavage by nucleases. Electrophoretic analysis of a mixture of DNA fragments resulting from a nuclease digestion in the presence of a bound receptor is called *DNA footprinting.* The receptor-binding

DNA sequence (called a *response element*) consists of 8 to 10 base pairs. Response elements for glucocorticoids (termed *glucocorticoid response elements*) exhibit homology sufficient that the consensus sequence can be used to identify potential glucocorticoid-regulated genes. Deletion of these sequences abolishes glucocorticoid regulation, and their transfer to another gene confers regulation. Thyroid hormone receptors interact with a different sequence, termed a *thyroid hormone response element.* The interaction of these receptors with DNA is believed to involve a cysteine-rich region of the receptor that forms loops or fingers coordinated by Zn^{2+}. This so-called *zinc finger structure* is also present in other transcription factors that interact with DNA.

Only a small number of genes are immediately influenced by a particular steroid hormone (primary response). Synthesis of other steroid-regulated proteins occurs later. This observation has led to the concept that some of the primary gene products may in turn activate other genes responsible for the later or secondary response (Fig. 1.47). In addition to stimulating gene expression, steroid hormones may also inhibit transcription of genes. Furthermore, steroids do not induce the same gene in all cells, which indicates that the steroid receptor does not work alone but must interact with other transcription factors termed *coactivators,* some of which are cell-type specific.

Transduction by Cell Surface Receptors

All water-soluble regulatory molecules, including peptide and protein hormones and smaller neurotransmitters, bind to cell surface receptor proteins. Binding of the appropriate ligand evokes an intracellular signal, which usually regulates enzyme activity, membrane transport, or, in some cases, gene expression. The notion that the role of the ligand is to generate a conformational change in the receptor is supported by the observation that antibodies directed against the receptor can sometimes mimic the effect of the normal ligand. This is the case in which autoanti-

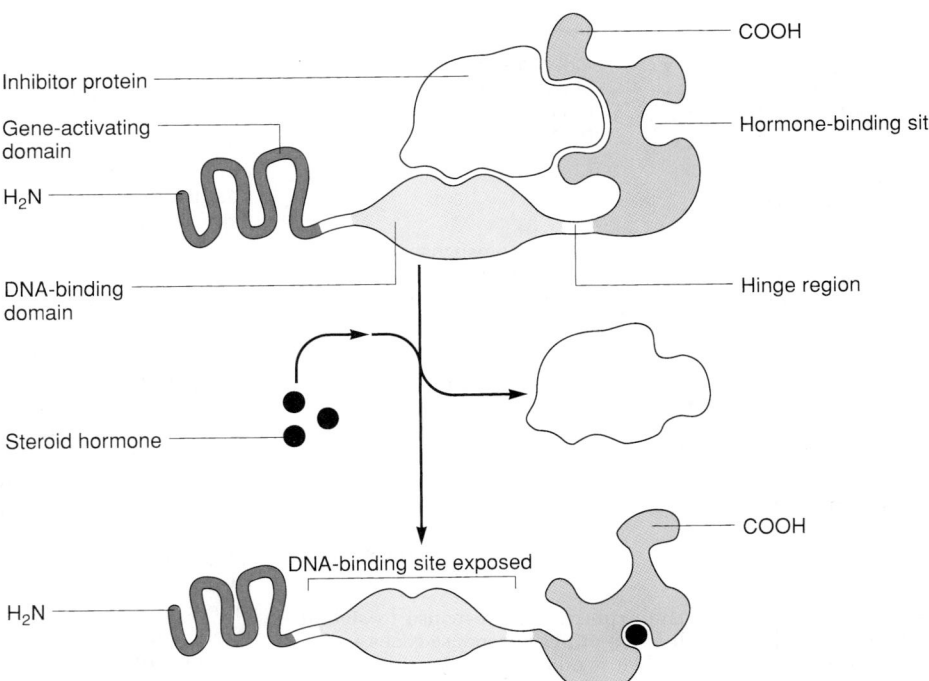

Figure 1.45. Schematic diagram of the domain structure of a steroid hormone receptor and its associated inhibitor protein. After steroid binding, the inhibitor dissociates, exposing the DNA-binding site.

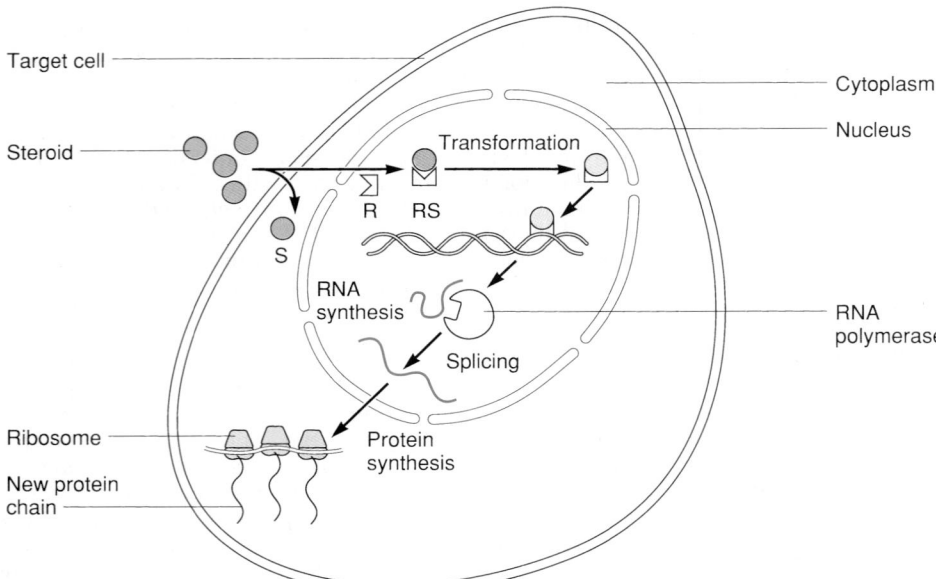

Figure 1.46. Schematic diagram of steroid hormone action. Steroids (S) enter the target cell and bind to a receptor (R), which is then transformed and binds to DNA in the nucleus, where it acts as a transcription factor to regulate the binding of RNA polymerase and the synthesis of new mRNA.

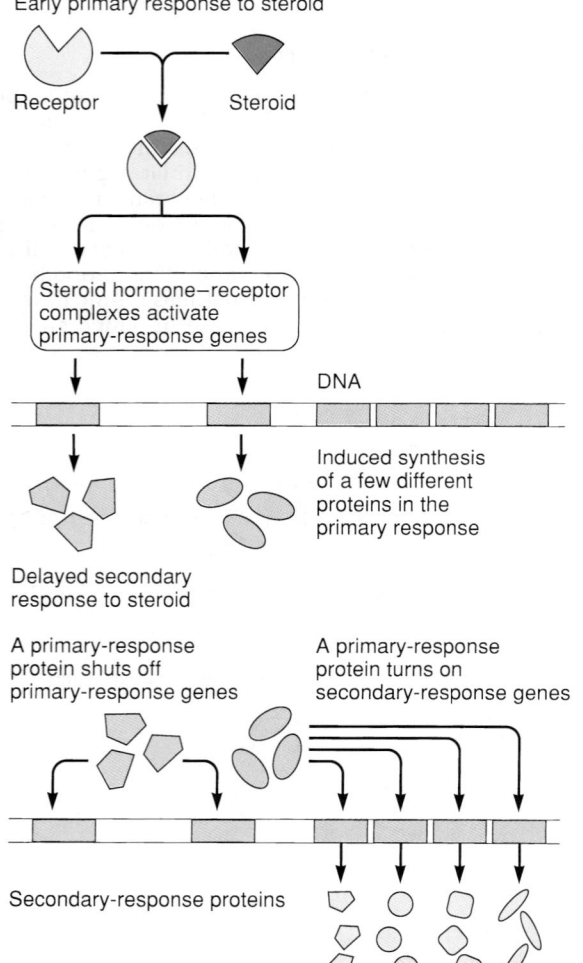

Figure 1.47. Pattern of gene expression in response to steroid hormone, whereby a few different primary-response genes are activated, and their products then regulate the expression of secondary-response genes.

bodies against the thyroid-stimulating hormone receptor overactivate thyroid cells and result in the disease state of hyperthyroidism. The number of receptors can vary from a few hundred to 100,000 or more per cell. In polarized cells, receptors may be limited to a specific membrane domain, usually that which is in closest contact with the blood supply.

Most cell surface receptors belong to one of three functional classes. These are ion channel receptors, catalytic receptors, and G-protein-linked receptors (Fig. 1.48A–C). Ion channel receptors, such as the nicotinic cholinergic receptor, are multisubunit assemblies; each subunit has multiple membrane-spanning segments. Together, these subunits form an ion-selective pore that can be gated (i.e., opened or closed) by a change in the transmembrane electrical potential or by the binding of a ligand to one of the subunits. These channels are in general restricted to nerve, muscle, and some endocrine cells and transduce information either by changing the membrane potential or by allowing entry of Ca^{2+}.

Catalytic receptors are membrane proteins that possess enzymatic activity. They usually consist of three regions—an extracellular ligand-binding domain, a membrane-spanning region, and an intracellular catalytic domain. The best understood receptors of this class are tyrosine kinases (45), which transfer phosphate from ATP to tyrosine residues. Other catalytic receptors possess enzymatic activity as serine kinases, tyrosine phosphatases, and as a form of guanylate cyclase, the enzyme synthesizing cyclic guanosine monophosphate (cGMP) from GTP. Receptors with tyrosine kinase activity include those for EGF, platelet-derived growth factor, and insulin. The insulin receptor contains four disulfide-linked chains, two of which span the membrane and are in proximity. The EGF receptor is a single chain but has been shown to dimerize in the membrane after binding EGF. Interaction between protein subunits may be involved in the signal transduction mechanism by which extracellular ligand binding alters the activity of an intracellular enzyme. In the case of the tyrosine kinase receptors, the kinase initially phosphorylates itself on tyrosine residues (autophosphorylation), a process that may involve the adjacent member of the dimer. Subsequently, the kinase may also phosphorylate

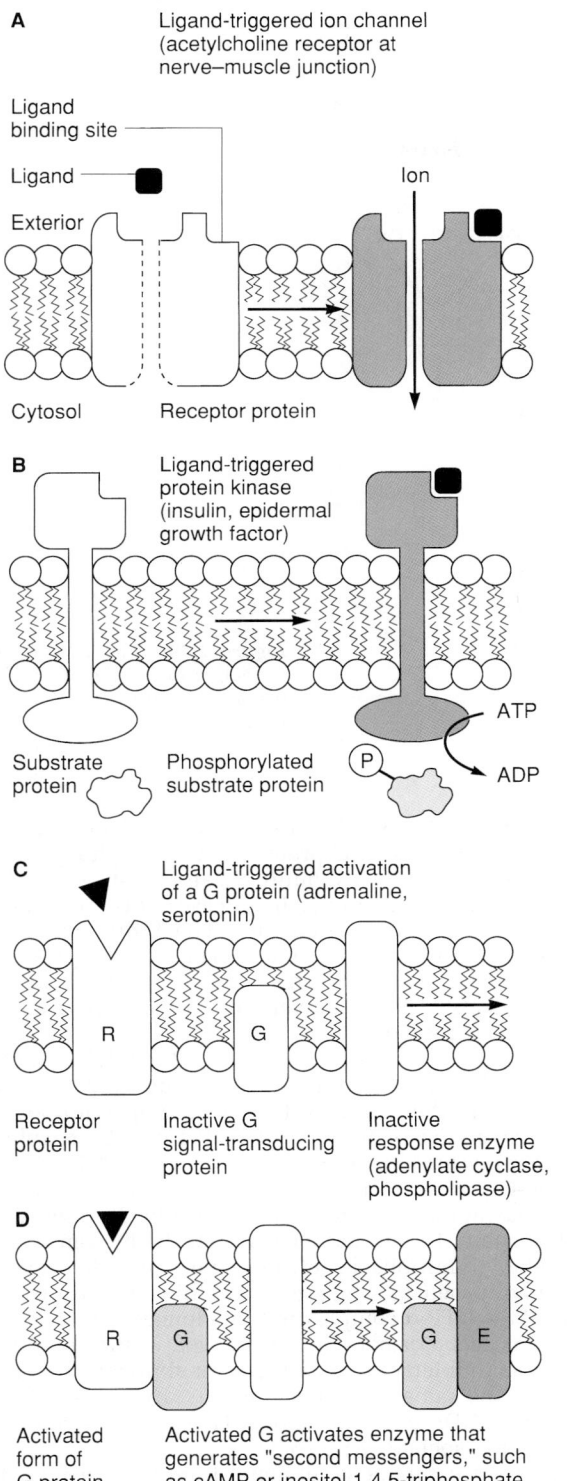

A Ligand-triggered ion channel (acetylcholine receptor at nerve–muscle junction)

Ligand binding site

Ligand

Exterior

Ion

Cytosol   Receptor protein

B Ligand-triggered protein kinase (insulin, epidermal growth factor)

ATP

ADP

Substrate protein   Phosphorylated substrate protein

C Ligand-triggered activation of a G protein (adrenaline, serotonin)

R   G

Receptor protein   Inactive G signal-transducing protein   Inactive response enzyme (adenylate cyclase, phospholipase)

D

R   G   G   E

Activated form of G protein   Activated G activates enzyme that generates "second messengers," such as cAMP or inositol 1,4,5-triphosphate

Figure 1.48. Types of cell surface receptors. *(A)* Ligand-activated ion channel; binding results in a conformational change, opening or activating the channel. *(B)* Ligand-activated protein kinase; binding activates the kinase domain, which phosphorylates substrate proteins. *(C and D)* Ligand activation of a G protein, which then activates an enzyme that generates second, or intracellular, messengers.

tyrosine residues on cytoplasmic proteins such as the insulin-receptor substrate-1 (IRS-1). Multiple signaling pathways are initiated by the binding of intracellular proteins to the phosphotyrosine residues on the receptor or on IRS-1. These proteins include a GTPase-activating protein, phospholipase Cγ, a tyrosine phosphatase, and PI 3-kinase, all of which possess a highly conserved domain called SH2 (for *src* homology), which was first found in the oncogene *src*. A pathway for activation of MAP kinase (46,47) (Fig. 1.49) involves the adaptor protein Grb2, which binds the activated receptor by an SH2 domain and then binds an effector, SOS (named after a gene in *Drosophila*), which promotes the release of GDP from Ras, allowing it to bind GTP and thereby becoming active. Activated Ras binds the protein kinase Raf, causing it to translocate to the plasma membrane, where it is activated. The protein kinase Raf initiates a kinase cascade by phosphorylating a MAP kinase kinase (also called MEK), which phosphorylates and activates a MAP kinase, ERK (*e*xtracellularly *r*egulated *k*inase).

It is now known that mammalian cells possess three parallel kinase cascades, each containing three kinases acting in series and leading to activation of ERKs, JNKs (*J*un *N*-terminal *k*inase), and p38 (48). All three MAP kinases are activated by dual phosphorylation on threonine and tyrosine residues and, when activated, can phosphorylate structural molecules, enzymes, and transcription factors, as shown for ERKs in Fig. 1.49. Whereas ERKs are key enzymes in cell growth, JNKs and p38 are activated by cell stress and are sometimes called *stress kinases.* The balance of the three kinase cascades along with other cell signaling mechanisms, including NF-kB, can lead to apoptosis (programmed cell death).

Other receptors, such as those for growth hormone, erythropoietin, and various cytokines, are not themselves tyrosine kinases, but when activated by a specific ligand, the cytoplasmic portion of the receptor binds a cytoplasmic tyrosine kinase of the janus family such as JAKs, which then phosphorylates the receptor itself, and intracellular targets including members of the Stat family of transcription factors. This promotes dimerization of the Stat and translocation to the nucleus. This JAK-Stat pathway is another major pathway by which these membrane receptors regulate gene transcription (49). In an analogous manner, the transforming growth factor-β receptor, which possesses serine kinase activity, phosphorylates another intracellular protein, Smad, which dimerizes and translocates to the nucleus to regulate transcription.

The largest family of cell surface receptors is the G-protein-linked receptors. These are homologous structurally in that they possess seven membrane-spanning hydrophobic domains, an extracellular amino terminus, three extracellular connecting loops, three intracellular connecting loops, and a carboxyl tail (Fig. 1.50). They are also functionally homologous in that they all interact with guanine nucleotide–binding proteins (G proteins), which both activate the production of the intracellular message and influence the affinity of the receptor.

The transmembrane segments form a binding pocket for small molecules such as acetylcholine and catecholamines. The external segments are more important in the interaction with peptide hormones. The third cytoplasmic loop between the fifth and sixth transmembrane domains is the largest and most variable and is believed to interact with the appropriate G protein. Phosphorylation of serine, threonine, and tyrosine residues in the carboxyl tail are important in desensitization, whereby continued occupancy of the receptors leads to the loss of the cell response.

The G proteins are a family of proteins that bind and hydrolyze GTP (50,51). Those in the plasma membrane were

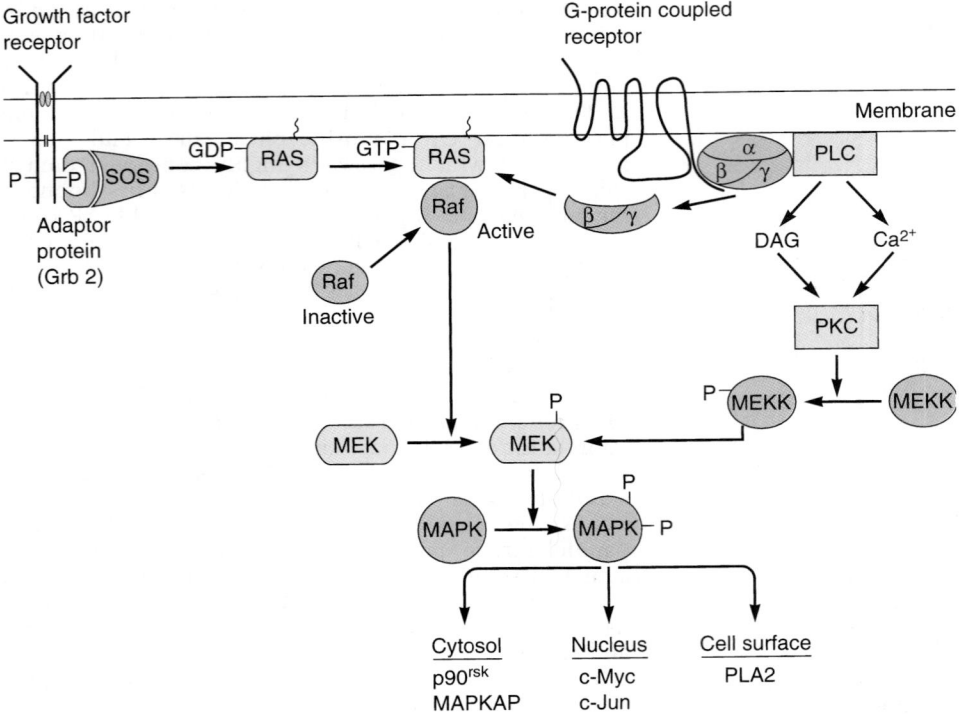

Figure 1.49. Schematic diagram for activation of the MAP kinase cascade, leading to ERK activation.

originally identified as a component in the activation of adenylate cyclase, but are now known also to be involved in the inhibition of adenylate cyclase, the activation of phospholipases C and A_2, the regulation of Ca^{2+} and K^+ channels, and the perception of light and odor. G proteins involved in membrane signal transduction are heterotrimeric proteins with unique α subunits and common or extremely similar β and γ subunits (51). The α subunits for the G-protein-stimulating adenylate cyclase (α_s) and for the G-protein-inhibiting adenylate cyclase (α_i) have been identified and shown to exist in multiple isoforms. Other homologous α subunits have been identified by purification and molecular cloning, which regulate other membrane effectors. One, termed α_o (the G protein is termed

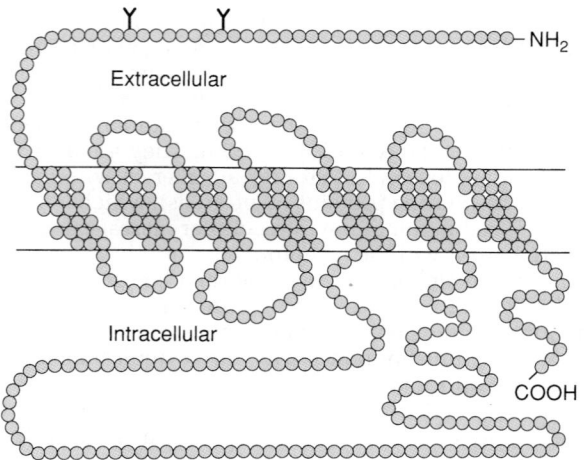

Figure 1.50. Schematic view of a G-protein-coupled receptor, showing the typical seven-transmembrane domain structure. Each sphere represents an amino acid. Y indicates N-linked sugar side chain.

G_o), is especially abundant in brain and is believed to regulate ion channels. A G-protein-activating phospholipase C, termed G_q, and its α subunit, α_q, also exist, as do related α subunits α_{11}, α_{14}, and α_{15}. In all cases, it is the α subunit that binds the guanine nucleotide. The βγ dimer portion of the G protein is involved in anchoring the complex to the membrane but has also been shown to mediate specific biologic effects such as activation of K^+ channels and the MAP kinase cascade.

In a generally accepted model of G-protein function, binding of the ligand to its receptor allows the receptor to interact with the G protein (52). This interaction leads to the dissociation of the bound GDP from the α subunit, which allows it to be replaced by GTP (Fig. 1.51). The receptor–G-protein complex rapidly dissociates, so that each receptor can interact with multiple G proteins. The GTP-α subunit then dissociates from the βγ complex and activates or inhibits its effector (i.e., adenylate cyclase, phospholipase C). The system amplifies because the lifetime of the GTP-α complex is much longer than that of the hormone receptor complex. Moreover, it allows multiple receptors to interact with the same or similar G proteins to regulate the same physiologic events. Eventually, GTP is cleaved to GDP by an intrinsic GTPase activity, and the α subunit reassociates with βγ.

The final component in signal transduction by G-protein-linked cell surface receptors is the effector that generates the intracellular messenger. The two best-understood effectors are adenylate cyclase, which converts ATP to cAMP, and the polyphosphoinositide-specific phospholipase C, which cleaves PI 4,5-bisphosphate (PIP_2), producing 1,4,5-inositol trisphosphate (IP_3) and DAG. Adenylate cyclase has been cloned, and its primary structure is consistent with an integral membrane protein with a molecular size of 150 kd with multiple membrane-spanning domains. The catalytic site is clearly intracellular. The PI-specific phospholipase C has also been purified and cloned and is known to exist in multiple forms (β, γ, and

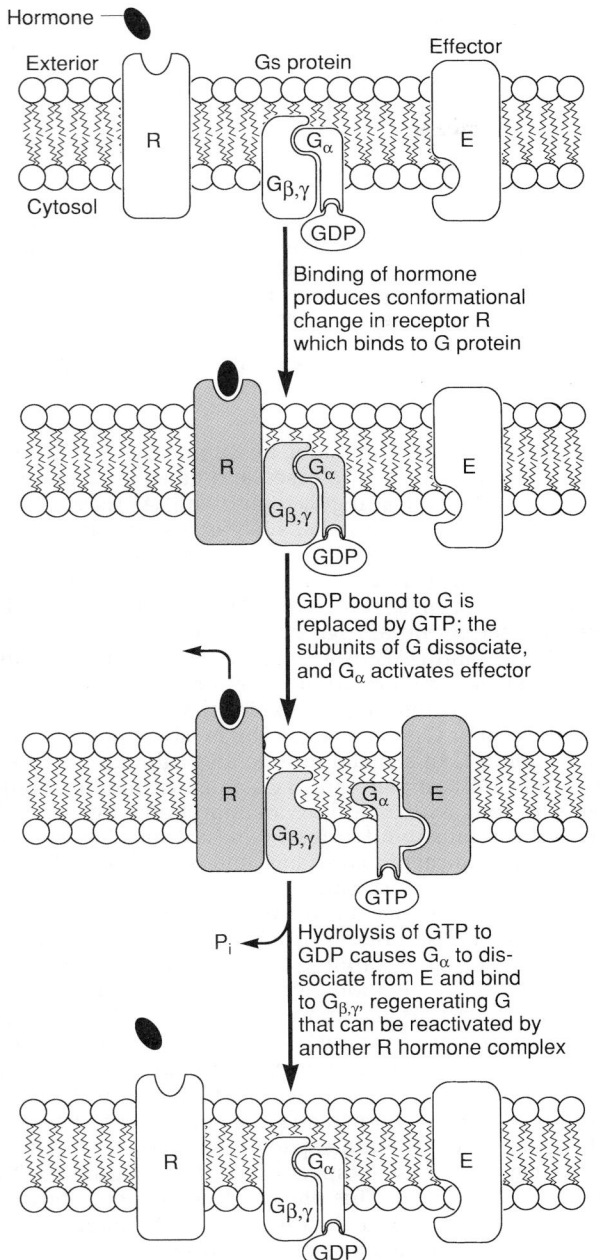

Figure 1.51. Activation of a membrane enzyme such as adenylate cyclase by the binding of hormone to its receptor. The G protein is here shown with its constituent α, β, and γ subunits. Blue units are in the activated state.

δ), which are expressed in different tissues (53). The importance of multiple forms and whether they couple to the same or distinct G proteins remains to be established. The γ isoform, however, can be activated in a different manner, involving tyrosine phosphorylation by the EGF receptor.

Other specific effectors activated by G proteins may include phosphatidylcholine-specific phospholipases C and D, phospholipase A_2, Na^+–H^+ ion exchangers, and various ion channels. Regulation of ion channels is distinct mechanistically from that in which a ligand binds directly to a subunit of the channel. An example of G-protein regulation of ion channels occurs in the heart, where certain types of α_i activate K^+ in response to cholinergic receptor occupancy channels, thereby slowing the heart rate.

Intracellular Messengers

Cyclic Nucleotides

The prototypic intracellular messenger cAMP is produced by the action of the enzyme adenylate cyclase in the plasma membrane. In liver cells, cAMP causes glycogenolysis by activation of the enzyme glycogen phosphorylase. To function as a mediator, the concentration of cAMP must change rapidly. In resting cells, cAMP exists at a concentration of 10^{-8} to 10^{-6} mol/L, and is continually being degraded by a specific enzyme, cAMP phosphodiesterase. cAMP levels can increase 10-fold or more within seconds of receptor binding through activation of adenylate cyclase. The rise is reversed on cessation of stimulation by the phosphodiesterase. The cAMP response system can also be modulated in some cases by regulation of phosphodiesterase activity. The increase in cAMP can also be inhibited by regulators activating the inhibitory G protein (Fig. 1.52).

Cyclic adenosine monophosphate acts as an allosteric regulator, and most if not all of its actions are mediated by activation of cAMP-dependent protein kinase A (PKA), which catalyzes the phosphorylation of proteins. In its inactive form, PKA consists of two regulatory subunits that bind cAMP and two catalytic subunits (Fig. 1.53). cAMP binds to the regulatory subunit, causing it to release the active catalytic subunit. In some cases, cAMP action is localized within a cell by a family of anchoring proteins termed AKAPs that bind the regulatory subunit of PKA. The active kinase then catalyzes the phosphorylation of serine and threonine residues of target proteins, thus effecting a change in their activity. For example, phosphorylation of phosphorylase kinase in liver and muscle activates glycogenolysis. Phosphorylation of hormone-sensitive lipase in fat cells activates lipolysis. A great many other structural and enzymatic proteins are known to be phosphorylated in response to various hormones, but the physiologic significance of the phosphorylation is not always understood. In some cases, cAMP is known to activate gene expression. All genes activated by cAMP contain a DNA sequence termed a *cAMP-response element* (CRE), which functions analogously to steroid response elements. When activated, PKA translocates to the nucleus and phosphorylates the transcription factor CREB (CRE binding protein), which, in conjunction with the coactivator protein CBP/300 (54), stimulates transcription.

Cyclic adenosine monophosphate also inhibits the dephosphorylation by intracellular phosphatases of proteins phosphorylated by PKA. It does so by phosphorylating an inhibitor protein, which allows it to bind to and inhibit certain protein phosphatases.

Cyclic adenosine monophosphate is not the only cyclic nucleotide active as an intracellular messenger. Most animal cells also produce cGMP from GTP, and this cyclic nucleotide is known to activate a specific protein kinase. In most cases, cGMP is produced by a cytoplasmic enzyme, guanylate cyclase, which is activated by NO (55) or oxidative radicals. NO is produced by NO synthase enzymes from arginine and diffuses locally both within and between cells as a gaseous mediator. Membrane-associated forms of guanylate cyclase also exist, and one has been identified as the receptor for atrial natriuretic factor. cGMP also plays a signaling role in rod cells of the retina, although in this situation, the fall in cGMP by a light-induced, G-protein-mediated phosphodiesterase influences Na^+ channels and the receptor potentials of these cells.

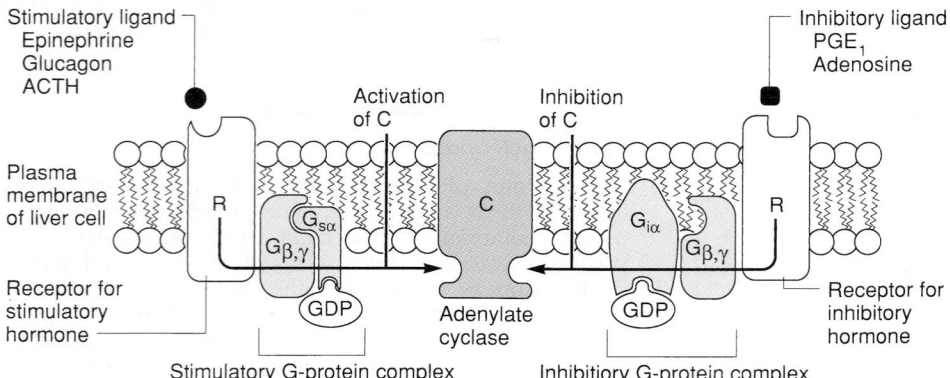

Figure 1.52. Stimulatory and inhibitory regulation of adenylate cyclase (C) by different G proteins. The βγ subunits are the same in both stimulatory and inhibitory G proteins, whereas the α subunits and receptors differ.

Ca²⁺ and Diacylglycerol

Intracellular calcium ions function as second messengers in many cells (56). The intracellular concentration of Ca^{2+} increases as a result of the enzymatic hydrolysis of PIP_2 by a specific phospholipase C enzyme. PIP_2, which accounts for less than 1% of cellular phospholipid, is produced by the ATP-dependent phosphorylation of PI (Fig. 1.54) and is believed to exist primarily in the inner leaflet of the plasma membrane. PIP_2 is cleaved by a phospholipase C that is activated by receptors coupled through a G protein of the G_q or in some cases G_i family. The cleavage of PIP_2 generates two products–IP_3, which is water soluble and diffuses through the cell, and DAG, which remains in the membrane and activates the enzyme protein kinase C (PKC) (57,58).

Inositol trisphosphate in the cytoplasm binds to a receptor on the ER, which as a homotetramer forms a gated Ca^{2+} channel (59); its opening leads to the release of sequestered Ca^{2+}. Normally, cytoplasmic Ca^{2+} $[(Ca^{2+})_i]$ is maintained at a concentration of approximately 100 nmol/L by a system of pumps and leaks in the plasma membrane and by a Ca^{2+}-ATPase, which sequesters Ca^{2+} in intracellular organelles. By releasing sequestered Ca^{2+}, an increase in IP_3 can transiently increase $[Ca^{2+}]_i$ to as much as 1 μmol/L, although this level usually falls within a few minutes (Fig. 1.55). Continued maintenance of an elevated $[Ca^{2+}]_i$ requires additional Ca^{2+} influx from extracellular fluid, which may be controlled by a metabolite of IP_3 or by virtue of depletion of the intracellular stores. This latter mechanism, known as the *capacitative model,* implies an unknown mediator that regulates plasma membrane Ca^{2+} channels. After its production, IP_3 is rapidly hydrolyzed to IP_2 and IP by specific phosphatases or phosphorylated to 1,3,4,5-IP_4 and higher phosphate derivatives by IP_3 kinase (58). 1,3,4,5-IP_4 is hydrolyzed to yield the inactive isomer, 1,3,4-IP_3.

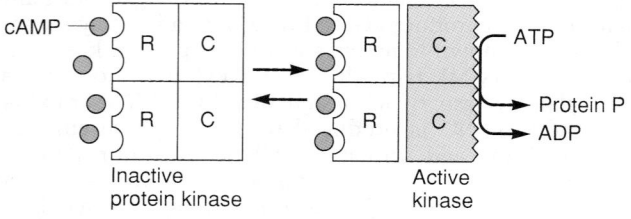

Figure 1.53. Activation of adenosine monophosphate (AMP)-dependent protein kinase by cyclic AMP (cAMP). Binding of cAMP to the regulatory (R) subunits induces dissociation and activation of the catalytic (C) subunits. C is enzymatically active only when dissociated.

When cells are stimulated by submaximal concentrations of agonist, Ca^{2+} is released and taken back up by intracellular stores, leading to repetitive $[Ca^{2+}]_i$ oscillations (57,60). In some larger cells, such as oocytes or neurons, an increase in $[Ca^{2+}]_i$ can be seen to propagate across the cell. This propagation, along with other evidence, has led to the concept of Ca^{2+}-induced Ca^{2+} release as being important after an initial triggering of Ca^{2+} release by IP_3.

Both Ca^{2+} and DAG exert many of their effects by altering protein phosphorylation. Most of the actions of Ca^{2+} are mediated by binding to proteins that can be thought of as intracellular Ca^{2+} receptors. The most common of these are troponin C in skeletal muscle and calmodulin, which is found in all animal and plant cells. Calmodulin binds four Ca^{2+} ions with an affinity of approximately 1 μmol/L. Calmodulin must bind at least two Ca^{2+} ions before it undergoes a conformational change and is able to activate enzymes. In some cases, calmodulin exists as a permanent regulatory subunit of a multisubunit enzyme, as is the case for phosphorylase kinase; in most cases, the calmodulin exists free, and after binding Ca^{2+} can interact with target proteins, which include cyclic nucleotide phosphodiesterase, some Ca^{2+} transport ATPases, and NO synthase (Fig. 1.56). A variety of Ca^{2+}-calmodulin-activated protein kinases exist, including myosin light-chain kinase, which is specific for myosin, and Ca^{2+}-calmodulin-regulated kinase II, which has a broad substrate specificity. These are all serine- and threonine-specific kinases. Ca^{2+}-calmodulin also activates a specific serine–threonine phosphatase, calcineurin. This phosphatase has been shown to be essential for T-cell activation and is the target for immunosuppressants such as cyclosporine (61).

The DAG that is produced by PIP_2 hydrolysis has as its primary function the activation of another kinase, PKC (62), which also requires the presence of Ca^{2+} and acidic phospholipids. The action of DAG is to lower the K_m for Ca^{2+}, such that the enzyme can be activated even at resting $[Ca^{2+}]_i$ concentrations. An increase in $[Ca^{2+}]_i$ probably contributes to activation because Ca^{2+} also promotes binding of the cytoplasmic enzyme to membranes. When activated by DAG and Ca^{2+}, PKC transfers phosphates from ATP to serine and threonine residues on target proteins. PKC can also be activated by phorbol esters, tumor promoters that bind to PKC and are used experimentally to activate this pathway (63). DAG can be produced not only by PIP_2 hydrolysis but by hydrolysis of other membrane phospholipids, particularly phosphatidylcholine, which may be cleaved by either a phospholipase C or phospholipase D enzyme. This means that DAG and Ca^{2+} signals, although initially coordinated, may diverge and that some extracellular signals can increase DAG without an increase in Ca^{2+}. It has also been discovered that PKC is actually a

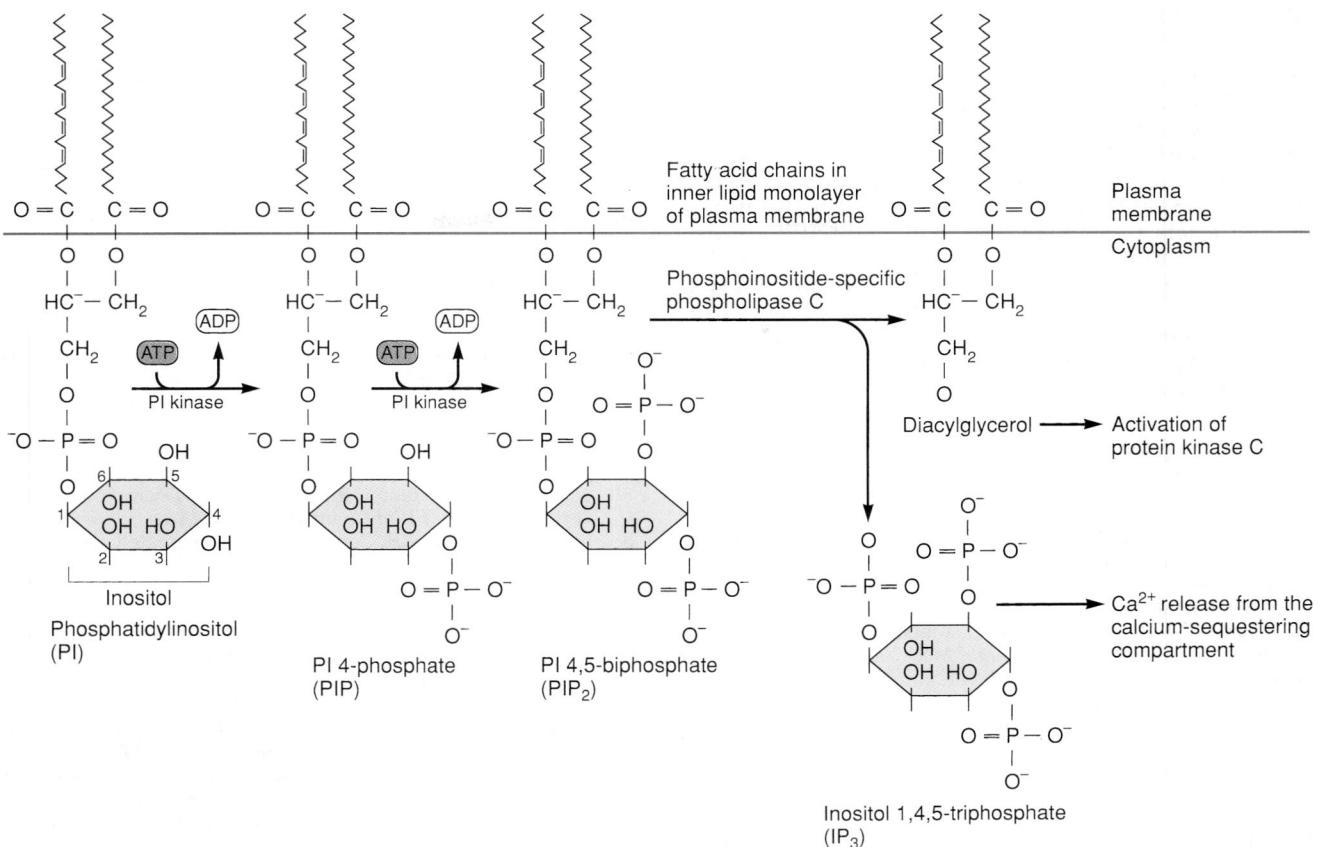

Figure 1.54. Synthesis and hydrolysis of inositol phospholipids. Phosphatidylinositol is phosphorylated in the membrane to produce polyphosphoinositides, PIP and PIP$_2$. PIP$_2$ is the primary target for phosphoinositide-specific phospholipase; the products of this enzymatic cleavage are inositol trisphosphate (IP$_3$), which releases intracellular Ca^{2+}, and diacylglycerol, which activates protein kinase C.

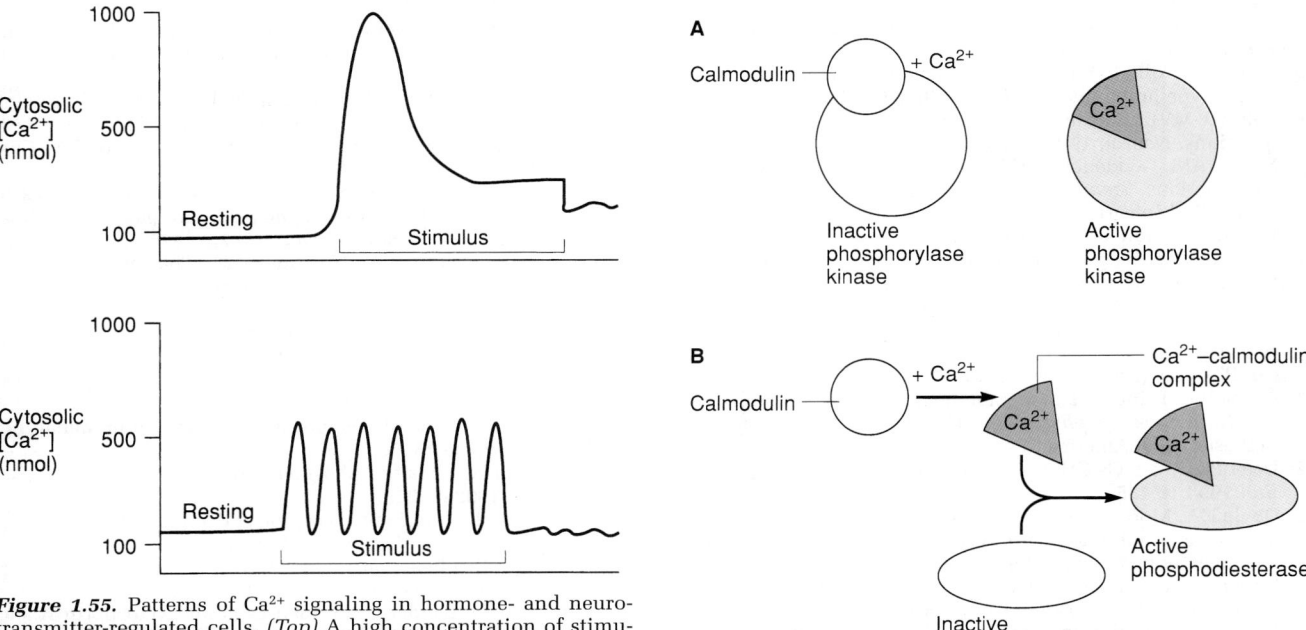

Figure 1.55. Patterns of Ca^{2+} signaling in hormone- and neurotransmitter-regulated cells. *(Top)* A high concentration of stimulant induces a large amount of inositol trisphosphate (IP$_3$), which transiently increases Ca^{2+} to approximately 1 µmol by release of Ca^{2+} from intracellular stores, followed by a much lower sustained increase, which is due to Ca^{2+} influx across the cell membrane. *(Bottom)* Low concentrations of stimulant that induce small increases in IP3 lead to transient release and reuptake of sequestered intracellular Ca^{2+}, leading to oscillations in intracellular free Ca^{2+}.

Figure 1.56. Ca^{2+} binding to the protein calmodulin alters its conformation and thereby activates enzymes. In the case of phosphorylase kinase, calmodulin is an integral subunit of the enzyme, whereas for other enzymes, such as phosphodiesterase, the activated calmodulin binds to the inactive enzyme, thereby activating it.

family of kinases and that some forms possess lipid binding but lack Ca^{2+}-binding domains.

Protein kinase C is believed to phosphorylate a number of important membrane molecules, including the Na^+–H^+ exchanger, ion channels, and certain receptors. Much of the evidence for this is based on the use of phorbol esters to activate PKC artificially. PKC is also able to activate the MAP kinase cascade. In some cases, the activation of PKC increases the transcription of specific genes, which are said to contain a phorbol ester response element. This probably involves activation of a DNA-binding transcription factor after a PKC-mediated phosphorylation.

REFERENCES

1. Lodish H, Berk A, Zipursky SL, et al. *Molecular cell biology,* 4th ed. New York: WH Freeman, 1999.
2. Aberts B, Bray D, Lewis J, et al. *Molecular biology of the cell,* 3rd ed. New York: Garland, 1994.
3. Bretscher MS. The molecules of the cell membrane. *Sci Am* 1985;253:100.
4. Cuervo AM, Dice JF. Lysosomes: a meeting point of proteins, chaperones, and proteases. *J Mol Med* 1998;76:6–12.
5. Masters C, Crane D. Recent developments in peroxisome biology. *Endeavor* 1996;20:68.
6. Schliwa M. *The cytoskeleton.* New York: Springer-Verlag, 1986.
7. Bray D. *Cell movements.* New York: Garland, 1992.
8. Hall A. Rho GTPases and the actin cytoskeleton. *Science* 1998;279:509.
9. Coluccio L. Myosin I. *Am J Physiol* 1997;273:C347.
10. Furukawa R, Fechheimer M. The structure, function, and assembly of actin filament bundles. *Int Rev Cytol* 1997;175:29.
11. Fuchs E, Cleveland DW. A structural scaffolding of intermediate filaments in health and disease. *Science* 1998;279:514.
12. Maccioni RB, Cambiazo V. Role of microtubule associated proteins in the control of microtubule assembly. *Physiol Rev* 1995;75:835.
13. Hirokawa N. Kinesin and dynein superfamily proteins and the mechanism of organelle transport. *Science* 1998;279:519.
14. Mitic L, Anderson J. Molecular architecture of tight junctions. *Annu Rev Physiol* 1998;60:121.
15. Geiger B, Volk T, Volberg T. Molecular heterogeneity of adherins-type junctions. *J Cell Biol* 1985;101:1523.
16. Bennett MVL. Gap junctions: new tools, new answers, new questions. *Neuron* 1991;6:305.
17. Simon AM, Goodenough DA. Diverse functions of vertebrate gap junctions. *Trends Cell Biol* 1998;8:477.
18. Hynes RO. Integrins: versatility, modulation, and signalling in cell adhesion. *Cell* 1992;69:11.
19. Yamada KM, Geiger B. Molecular interactions in cell adhesion complexes. *Curr Opin Cell Biol* 1997;9:76.
20. Finkelstein A, Mauro A. Physical principles and formalisms of electrical excitability. In: Kandel ER, ed. *Handbook of physiology: the nervous system, vol I.* Bethesda, MD: American Physiological Society, 1977:161.
21. Dawson D. Principles of membrane transport. In: Schultz SG, ed. *Handbook of physiology: the gastrointestinal system.* Bethesda, MD: American Physiological Society, 1991:1.
22. Deen PMT, van Os CH. Epithelial aquaporins. *Curr Opin Cell Biol* 1998;10:435.
23. Doyle DA, Morais Cabral J, Pfuetzner RA, et al. The structure of the potassium channel: molecular basis of K^+ conduction and selectivity. *Science* 1998;280:69.
24. Stryer L. *Biochemistry,* 4th ed. New York: WH Freeman, 1995.
25. Frank J. How the ribosome works. *Am Sci* 1998;86:428.
26. Pain VM. Initiation of protein synthesis in eukaryotic cells. *Eur J Biochem* 1996;236:747.
27. Georgopoulous C, Welch WJ. Role of the major heat shock proteins as molecular chaperones. *Annu Rev Cell Biol* 1993;9:601.
28. Walter P, Lingoppa VR. Mechanism of protein translocation across the endoplasmic reticulum membrane. *Annu Rev Cell Biol* 1986;2:499.
29. Matlack K, Mothes W, Rappaport TA. Protein translocation: tunnel vision. *Cell* 1998;92:381.
30. Kornfeld R, Kornfeld S. Assembly of asparagine-linked oligosaccharides. *Annu Rev Biochem* 1985;45:631.
31. Spies M. Heads or tails: what determines the orientation of proteins in the membrane. *FEBS Lett* 1995;369:76.
32. Melchoir F, Gerace L. Two-way trafficking with Ran. *Trends Cell Biol* 1998;8:175.
33. Schatz G. The protein import system of mitochondria. *J Biol Chem* 1996;271:31763.
34. Gilbert H. Protein disulfide isomerase and assisted protein folding. *J Biol Chem* 1997;272:29399.
35. Rothman JE. Mechanisms of intracellular protein transport. *Nature* 1994;372:55.
36. Kornfeld S. Trafficking of lysosomal enzymes. *FASEB J* 1987;1:462.
37. Farquhar MG, Palade GE. The Golgi apparatus: 100 years of progress and controversy. *Trends Cell Biol* 1998;8:2.
38. Schimmöller F, Simon I, Pfeffer SR. Rab GTPases, directors of vesicle docking. *J Biol Chem* 1998;273:22161.
39. Burgess TL, Kelly RB. Constitutive and regulated secretion of proteins. *Annu Rev Cell Biol* 1987;3:243.
40. Pfeffer SR. Transport-vesicle targeting: tethers before SNAREs. *Nature Cell Biol* 1999;1:E17.
41. Riezman H, Woodman PG, vanMeer G, et al. Molecular mechanisms of endocytosis. *Cell* 1997;91:731.
42. Evans RM. The steroid and thyroid hormone receptor superfamily. *Science* 1988;240:889.
43. Mangelsdorf DJ, Thummel C, Beato M, et al. The nuclear receptor superfamily: the second decade. *Cell* 1995;83:835.
44. Johnson PF, McKnight SL. Eukaryotic transcriptional regulatory proteins. *Annu Rev Biochem* 1989;58:799.
45. Fantl WJ, Johnson DE, Williams LT. Signaling by receptor tyrosine kinases. *Annu Rev Biochem* 1993;62:453.
46. Blenis J. Signal transduction via the MAP kinases: proceed at your own RSK. *Proc Natl Acad Sci USA* 1993;90:5889.
47. Seger R, Krebs EG. The MAPK signaling cascade. *FASEB J* 1995;9:726.
48. Cano E, Mahadevan LC. Parallel signal processing among mammalian MAPKs. *Trends Biochem Sci* 1995;20:117.
49. Schindler C, Darnell JE. Transcriptional responses to polypeptide ligands: the JAK-STAT pathway. *Annu Rev Biochem* 1995;64:621.
50. Bourne HR, Saunders DA, McCormick F. The GTPase superfamily: conserved structure and molecular mechanism. *Nature* 1991;349:117.
51. Simon MI, Strathman MP, Gautam N. Diversity of G proteins in signal transduction. *Science* 1991;252:802.
52. Bourne HR. How receptors talk to trimeric G proteins. *Curr Opin Cell Biol* 1997;9:134.
53. Singler WD, Brown HA, Sternweis PC. Regulation of eukaryotic phosphatidylinositol-specific phospholipase C and phospholipase D. *Annu Rev Biochem* 1997;66:475.
54. Goldman PS, Tran UK, Goodman RH. The multifunctional role of the co-activator CBP in transcriptional regulation. *Recent Prog Hormone Res* 1997;52:103.
55. Hobbs AJ. Soluble guanylate cyclase: the forgotten sibling. *Trends Pharmacol Sci* 1997;18:484.
56. Rasmussen H. The cycling of calcium as an intracellular messenger. *Sci Am* 1989;261:66.
57. Berridge MJ. Inositol trisphosphate and calcium signalling. *Nature* 1993;361:315.
58. Majerus PW. Inositol phosphate biochemistry. *Annu Rev Biochem* 1992;61:225.
59. Mikoshiba K. The InsP3 receptor and intracellular Ca^{2+} signaling. *Curr Opin Neurobiol* 1997;7:339.
60. Berridge MJ. Elementary and global aspects of calcium signaling. *J Physiol (Lond)* 1997;499:291.
61. Bierer BE, Holländer G, Fruman D, et al. Cyclosporin A and FK506: molecular mechanisms of immunosuppression and probes for transplantation biology. *Curr Opin Immunol* 1993;5:763.
62. Parker PJ, Kour G, Marais RM, et al. Protein kinase C: a family affair. *Mol Cell Endocrinol* 1989;65:1.
63. Ron D, Kazanietz MG. New insights into the regulation of protein kinase C and novel phorbol ester receptors. *FASEB J* 1999;13:1658.

SURGERY: SCIENTIFIC PRINCIPLES AND PRACTICE, Third Edition, edited by Lazar J. Greenfield, Michael W. Mulholland, Keith T. Oldham, Gerald B. Zelenock, and Keith D. Lillemoe. Lippincott Williams & Wilkins Publishers, Philadelphia, © 2001.

CHAPTER 2

NUTRITION AND METABOLISM

J. STANLEY SMITH, JR., WILLIAM G. AUSTEN, JR., AND WILEY W. SOUBA

The maintenance of adequate nutritional status is paramount to good patient care. Although it is intuitive that the well-nourished patient responds more favorably to surgical intervention than a malnourished patient, little formal nutritional education has been included in the core teaching curriculum at many medical schools. Moreover, because of the lack of well-designed studies, it has been difficult to prove that nutritional intervention favorably affects outcome. Historically, nutrition has been considered the province of physicians treating chronic medical diseases, and the surgeon, before the introduction of total parenteral nutrition (TPN), did not become involved in the care of debilitated, malnourished patients. It is now well established that malnutrition is common in hospitalized surgical patients and that the usual kinds of diets provided to patients may contain inadequate amounts or proportions of certain nutrients. Recent developments have increased our understanding of the relationship between nutrition and metabolism, and it is increasingly clear that the optimum nutritional care for a given patient depends, in large part, on the primary diagnosis and underlying metabolic status. The mediators that regulate the body's metabolic and nutritional response to injury, sepsis, and cancer have now been well described. Today, nearly all hospitalized patients can be fed safely and effectively. As a consequence, surgeons must become familiar with the changes in body metabolism that develop during catabolic illnesses and with the indications for and delivery of perioperative nutritional support.

Although the disease process is usually the major cause of malnutrition, many patients lose additional weight during their hospitalization as a result of withholding of meals for diagnostic tests or procedures. Critically ill patients are frequently anorectic secondary to illness and confinement. Now, however, these patients can be fed, but controlled trials done in patients with normal body composition undergoing elective surgery show that such nutritional support produces little improvement in outcome. Therefore, limited weight loss in selected hospitalized patients is acceptable because short-term undernutrition does not prolong a life-limiting illness, nor does it complicate convalescence after major operation or other therapy. Other patients, such as those sustaining major injury or life-threatening complication such as sepsis, require vigorous nutritional care.

This chapter reviews the field of nutrition and metabolism as it relates to surgical patients. Portions of this review have been previously published (1–5), and it includes sections from the chapter by Watters and colleagues (6) in the first edition of this textbook.

BASIC NUTRITIONAL BIOCHEMISTRY

Body Composition

Total body mass consists of an aqueous component and a nonaqueous component. The nonaqueous portion comprises bone, tendons, and mineral mass as well as adipose tissue. The aqueous phase contains the body cell mass, which is made up of skeletal muscle, intraabdominal and intrathoracic organs, skin, and circulating blood cells. Also contributing to the aqueous portion is the interstitial fluid and the intravascular volume. Total body water in the average-sized (70-kg) adult man makes up approximately 55% to 60% (~40 L) of total body mass. Of this 40 L, approximately 22 L is intracellular, 14 L is interstitial fluid, and the plasma volume is approximately 3 to 3.5 L. Body composition varies as a function of age and sex (Fig. 2.1) and becomes altered after injury or surgery. These changes are characterized by a loss of lean body mass, a loss of body fat, and expansion of the extracellular fluid compartment. Thus, the metabolically active body mass becomes diminished.

Bioelectrical impedance is one way to measure this change in lean body mass, based on the principle that electrical resistance is proportional to the fluid and electrolyte content of tissue. Because the lean body mass or body cell mass has most of the fluid and electrolyte content, passage of an electrical current through the body at the bedside can measure the lean body or "fat-free" mass (7). This appears to work well in both healthy and criti-

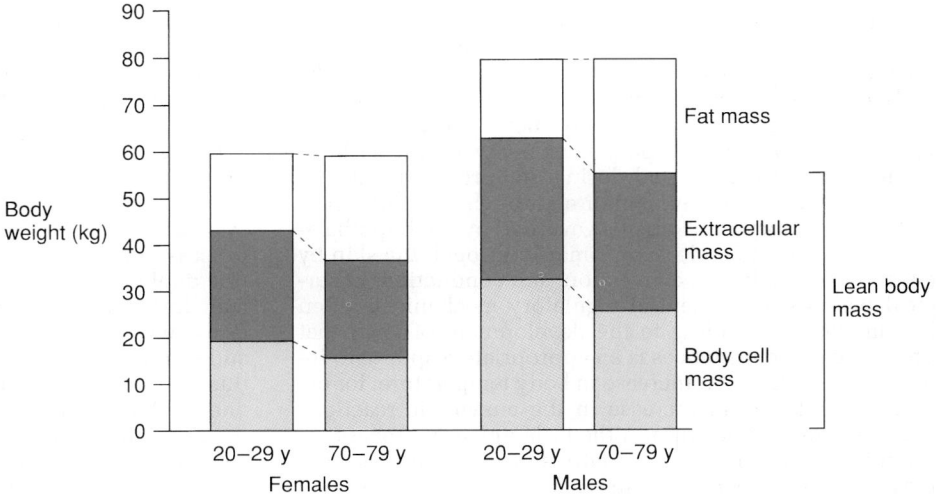

Figure 2.1. Body composition as a function of sex and age. (Data from Cohn SH, Vaartsky D, Yasumura S, et al. Compartmental body composition based on total-body nitrogen, potassium, and calcium. *Am J Physiol* 1980;239:E524–E530.)

Table 2.1. FUEL RESERVES OF A HEALTHY (70-KG) ADULT MAN

Energy source	Weight (kg)	kcal Value
Fat	14	125,000
Protein		
Skeletal muscle	6	24,000
Other	6	24,000
Glycogen		
Muscle	0.15	600
Liver	0.075	300
Free glucose	0.02	80

cally ill patients, and can give the practitioner a guide for accurately gauging nutritional support.

For energy, the body contains fuel reserves that it can mobilize and use during times of starvation or stress (Table 2.1). By far the largest energy component is fat, which is calorically dense, providing approximately 9 kilocalories (kcal) per gram. Body protein comprises the next largest mass of utilizable energy, but amino acids yield only approximately 4 kcal/g. Unlike fat reserves, body protein is not a form of energy storage, but rather a structural and functional component of the body. Loss of body protein, if severe, has functional consequences because after injury, proteolysis is accelerated to generate amino acids to support gluconeogenesis and other key synthetic processes. In the long run, a chronic catabolic state can lead to erosion of body protein stores such that susceptibility to infection is increased, wound healing is impaired, and outcome is unfavorably affected.

Energy Metabolism

From a simplistic mechanical standpoint, the human body is nothing more than an engine. It burns fuel to generate energy that, in turn, is used to perform work. The human body does several kinds of work, including mechanical work (e.g., locomotion, breathing), transport work (e.g., carrier-mediated uptake of nutrients into cells), and synthetic work (biosynthesis of proteins and other complex molecules). Indeed, all of these kinds of work are essential for life. The energy used to do this work comes from the energy present in the chemical bonds of the nutrients we consume. The human body has the capacity to "oxidize" several types of fuels, including glucose (carbohydrates), amino acids (proteins), fatty acids (lipids), ketone bodies, and alcohol. Thus, the human body converts energy stored in the chemical bonds of nutrients into internal (e.g., enzymatic catalysis) and external work (e.g., muscular contraction for locomotion). During starvation or after operative procedures when nutrition is not provided, the body oxidizes stored energy sources to generate work. In humans, this process is relatively inefficient because approximately half of this potential energy is lost as heat. Some of the heat generated during this process is used to help maintain body temperature through carefully controlled regulatory mechanisms governed by the hypothalamus. Excess heat is released primarily through the skin by evaporation, radiation, convection, and conduction. In surgical patients, these central regulatory mechanisms often become "reset," leading to the development of fever that under most circumstances is an appropriate response to injury and infection. An increase in body temperature, for example, results in an increase in the enzymatic reactions that are necessary to support the inflammatory process.

Amino acids, glucose, and fatty acids are the major energy sources the body uses to perform work. Amino acids come from endogenous proteins and the dietary proteins we consume, or are provided as crystalline L-amino acids for intravenous administration. Glucose is produced when carbohydrates are broken down in the gut lumen, or is generated in the liver from other sugars. Fatty acids are derived from the hydrolysis of triglycerides. Glucose provided in TPN solutions is in the form of dextrose, which is a hydrated glucose molecule that provides 3.4 kcal/g. One liter of of 5% dextrose in water (D_5W) contains 50 g of dextrose, or 170 kcal. Therefore, the usual postoperative surgical patient given an intravenous glucose solution at 125 mL/h receives approximately 500 kcal/d, far less than the actual number of kilocalories needed to meet energy requirements. However, this is enough glucose to stimulate pancreatic release of insulin, the primary anabolic hormone that stimulates amino acid uptake and protein synthesis.

Triglycerides are made up of three fatty acids bound to a glycerol molecule. Naturally occurring fatty acids may be saturated (no double bonds) or unsaturated (one or more double bonds). In most tissues, fatty acids are readily oxidized for energy and are especially important energy sources for the heart, liver, and skeletal muscle. In adipose tissue, fatty acids may be reesterified with glycerol and stored as triacylglycerols (triglyceride) in adipocytes. Nearly the entire volume of an adipocyte consists of a large fat droplet. This stored fat is mobilized during starvation and stress, whereas structural lipid usually is preserved. The major lipids in plasma do not circulate in free form. Free fatty acids are bound to albumin, whereas cholesterol, triglycerides, and phospholipids are transported as lipoprotein complexes. Lipoproteins are cleared from the circulation by the action of lipoprotein lipase, an enzyme located on the surface of the capillary endothelium. This enzyme catalyzes the breakdown of triglycerides to free fatty acids and glycerol. The second lipase, which regulates the supply of free fatty acids to tissues, is hormone-sensitive lipase. It is present only in adipose tissue and catalyzes the breakdown of stored triglycerides into glycerol and fatty acids. The fatty acids that are produced are released into the circulation.

Hormone-sensitive lipase is rapidly activated by the counterregulatory hormones, epinephrine, norepinephrine, and glucagon, which bind to a cell membrane receptor. Growth hormone and glucocorticoids also increase the activity of hormone-sensitive lipase, but this process takes time because it involves de novo protein synthesis. Thus, during stress, the activity of hormone-sensitive lipase increases, leading to mobilization of fat, but stress also decreases the activity of lipoprotein lipase on endothelial cells, impairing the clearance of fat from the bloodstream. Nonetheless, fat is an important fuel source for critically ill patients, and as a general rule the amount of fat administered to patients receiving TPN should comprise approximately 15% to 30% of total nonprotein caloric needs.

Free fatty acids must be activated in the cytoplasm by condensation with coenzyme A before they can be oxidized. The resulting fatty acyl coenzyme A molecules are transported into the mitochondria by means of a shuttle system in which L-carnitine acts as an acyl carrier. This process may be rate limiting in severe stress states. Carnitine depletion has been shown to be characteristic of critical illness, and therefore supplementation of TPN solutions with carnitine has been proposed to enhance endogenous utilization of fats as a fuel source. Although this has not proven to be effective, it is another example of one of the attempted nutritional approaches to improve the metabolic care of critically ill patients.

Energy is measured in calories. A calorie is the amount of heat required to raise the temperature of 1 g of water from 14.5°C to 15.5°C at a pressure of 1 standard atmosphere. A kilocalorie (1,000 calories) is the unit of energy measurement used in the United States for reference to body metabolism and nutrition. Basal energy requirements are those measured with normal resting subjects when no external work is being done; basal energy is used mainly for transport work and synthetic work in cells. When energy is measured for patients by indirect calorimetry, this is referred to as the *resting energy expenditure* (REE). A surprisingly small percentage (<5%) of this energy is spent on cardiac output and the work of breathing in normal subjects. In contrast, for people with chronic obstructive lung disease or patients on ventilators, the work of breathing may account for 15% to 20% of caloric expenditure. Thus, the REE measures the basal energy expenditure plus any extra required by the patient's disease process.

Caloric requirements (metabolic rate) are related to oxygen consumption by the formula:

$$\text{Metabolic rate} = 4.83 \times \text{O}_2 \text{ consumption}$$

where metabolic rate is expressed in kilocalories per unit time and O_2 consumption $\dot{V}$ is expressed in liters of oxygen consumed per unit time. For example, the average resting postabsorptive 70-kg man consumes approximately 200 mL of oxygen per minute, or 288 L of oxygen per day. This is equal to approximately 1,450 kcal/d.

In most adult surgical patients, energy requirements can be estimated and complicated formulas usually are not required. Basal metabolic rate (BMR) can be estimated from body weight alone (Table 2.2) except in extremely obese people. Although metabolic rate varies with age and sex, these factors are not major determinants of caloric needs. When caloric requirements for surgical patients are determined, they provide the physician with an estimation of how many kilocalories should be provided to the patient. REE can be measured at the bedside by indirect calorimetry. Patients must be either intubated or able to tolerate a hood placed over their face. Patients should not be receiving O_2 in excess of 70%. Protocols have been developed to measure the REE with just a 5-minute steady state because most patients are rarely quiet for more than that time (8). In general, energy needs increase as the severity of the illness increases (Table 2.3). Interestingly, the expenditure of kilocalories is only minimally increased after elective surgery. The largest increase in energy expenditure occurs in patients with severe multiple trauma or major thermal injury. Thus, the average-sized adult who sustains a major burn rarely requires more than 3,500 kcal/d for maintenance.

Although the provision of enough calories is beneficial, giving too many calories can "overfeed" the patient. Excess calories, especially in the form of sugars, lead to lipogenesis and hepatic steatosis that interferes with hepatic function. Critically ill patients may not fit the factors used to estimate their energy requirements and need indirect calorimetry to measure energy expenditure more accurately.

Table 2.2. APPROXIMATE BASAL METABOLIC RATES IN ADULTS

Weight (kg)	Basal metabolic rate (kcal/d)
50	1,300
60	1,450
70	1,600
80	1,750
90	1,900
100	2,050

Table 2.3. CALORIC REQUIREMENTS FOR THE AVERAGE ADULT (70-KG) MAN

Disease process	Kcal/d
Basal	1,450
Postoperative (uncomplicated)	1,500–1,700
Sepsis	2,000–2,400
Multiple trauma (ventilator)	2,200–2,600
Major burn	2,500–3,000

The only significant source of usable energy in mammalian tissues is the carbon–hydrogen bond in carbohydrates, fats, and amino acids. When the bond is broken by intracellular catalysis, energy is liberated and carbon dioxide and water are formed. The reaction also forms adenosine triphosphate (ATP) by adding a phosphate to adenosine diphosphate (ADP). This requires a pool of phosphate to be available to form the ATP. In those patients with chronic malnutrition or starvation, this pool of phosphate may be depleted and dangerously lower serum phosphate levels as dextrose is reintroduced to the metabolism. This hypophosphatemia can lead to cardiac arrest and is known as the *refeeding syndrome*. Although not usually seen in elective surgical patients, the refeeding syndrome may manifest in patients with cancer or critically injured patients receiving only borderline nutrition.

The general formula for glucose oxidation is:

$$\text{C}_6\text{H}_{12}\text{O}_6 + 6\text{O}_2 \rightarrow 6\text{ CO}_2 + 6\text{H}_2\text{O}$$

The respiratory quotient (RQ) is the ratio between the volume of CO_2 produced to the volume of O_2 used (RQ = $\dot{V}\text{CO}_2/\dot{V}\text{O}_2$). The RQ for the preceding reaction is the ratio of six volumes of CO_2 to six volumes of oxygen, which equals 1.00.

For the oxidation of fats, more oxygen is required to oxidize the multiple carbon–carbon bonds, and thus the RQ is less than 1. The oxidation of triglyceride is as follows:

$$2\text{C}_{51}\text{H}_{98}\text{O}_6 + 145\text{ O}_2 \rightarrow 102\text{ CO}_2 + 98\text{ H}_2\text{O}$$

The RQ is 102/145, which equals 0.703.

The RQ for proteins is more difficult to calculate because the composition of the various amino acids varies from protein to protein. However, on the average, the RQ for protein is 0.8. Can the RQ ever be greater than 1? Yes: the process of lipogenesis, in which fatty acids are synthesized from glucose, has an RQ much greater than 1. For a sample fat ($\text{C}_{55}\text{H}_{104}\text{O}_6$) containing a balanced mixture of fatty acids, the equation is as follows:

$$27\text{ C}_6\text{H}_{12}\text{O}_6 + 6\text{ O}_2 \rightarrow 2\text{ C}_{55}\text{H}_{104}\text{O}_6 + 52\text{ CO}_2 + 58\text{ H}_2\text{O}$$

The RQ for this reaction is 52 divided by 6, which equals 8.67. The clinical significance of this reaction is that when very high carbohydrate loads are given, the patients' RQ may increase to 1.3 or even 1.4, indicating that a portion of the infused glucose is being converted to fat. In this process, considerable quantities of carbon dioxide are produced that must be removed from the body during the process of breathing. On occasion, however, in patients with pulmonary insufficiency, a high PCO_2 may develop during high-glucose feedings, necessitating a decrease in glucose calories to prevent acid–base abnormalities. This is another reason why overfeeding can be dangerous.

Protein/Amino Acid Metabolism

Protein is the building block of life and the most important nutrient for life. Approximately 15% of total body weight consists of proteins, approximately half of which are intracellular and half extracellular. Extracellular proteins include those that circulate in the bloodstream (i.e., albumin, transferrin, hemoglobin); those that comprise the intracellular matrix include collagen and other fibrous proteins. In humans and other mammals, dietary protein is the source of most amino acids. Intestinal absorption is the only physiologic pathway by which the body obtains exogenous amino acids, except when they are provided therapeutically by the intravenous route. Enterocytes are responsible for amino acid absorption and can transport amino acids across the brush border or basolateral membrane. Small peptides may be absorbed passively, but free amino acids are transported actively into the enterocyte cytoplasm by functionally and biochemically distinct amino acid transport systems. These have been defined on the basis of their amino acid selectivities and physicochemical properties. Each transport system relates to an integral cell membrane-associated transporter protein and functions to translocate the amino acid from the intraluminal environment into the cytoplasm.

Many factors, including nutritional status, have been shown specifically or nonspecifically to alter amino acid transport activities. The first is a reversible hyperplasia of the intestinal mucosa after a prolonged period of oral hyperalimentation, resulting in an increase of epithelial cell numbers and of the absorptive surface area. This nonspecific hyperplasia can increase amino acid uptake by a factor of five. The second mechanism is a reversible, severalfold increase of specific amino acid transport activities. Surgery, infection, and cancer also influence intestinal transport activity. Ileus changes the brush border transport activity and may also alter nutrition and absorption in surgical patients.

Digestion of ingested protein provides free amino acids, dipeptides, tripeptides, and polypeptides that are absorbed by the small intestine and delivered to the body where they can be incorporated into new proteins or other biosynthetic products. Excess amino acids are degraded and their carbon skeletons are oxidized to produce energy or are incorporated into glycogen or free fatty acids. In addition to the metabolism of dietary amino acids, the existing proteins in the cell are continuously recycled, such that total protein turnover in the body is approximately 300 g/d (Fig. 2.2). Vertebrates cannot reuse nitrogen with 100% efficiency; therefore, obligatory nitrogen losses occur, mainly in the urine. Most of the nitrogen lost in the urine is in the form of urea (85%), with lesser amounts excreted as creatine and ammonia. Urinary nitrogen losses diminish in people fed a protein-free diet, but never become zero because of the body's inability completely to reuse nitrogen. In stressed patients, this ability to adapt to starvation is compromised such that proteolysis of body proteins continues at a substantial rate (Fig. 2.3). Although it is often assumed that skeletal muscle bears the brunt of this protein wasting, it is now apparent that net proteolysis also occurs in organs such as the gut and liver. If the ability to synthesize proteins is compromised by malnutrition or disease, function is usually correspondingly affected. This may show clinically in patients as impaired wound healing, immunoincompetence, or breakdown of the gut mucosal barrier.

Because of these obligatory nitrogen losses accentuated by catabolic disease states, stressed surgical patients have increased energy and nitrogen needs. The recommended daily allowance for protein in the United States is 0.8 g/kg/d; this requirement may triple in critically ill patients because of their profound catabolism and inefficient protein economy (Table 2.4). One gram of nitrogen, on the average, is equivalent to 6.25 g of protein.

Nitrogen (N) balance can be calculated from the difference between the amount of nitrogen taken in by the patient and the amount of nitrogen lost in the urine, stool, skin, wounds, and fistula drainage. Nitrogen balance is

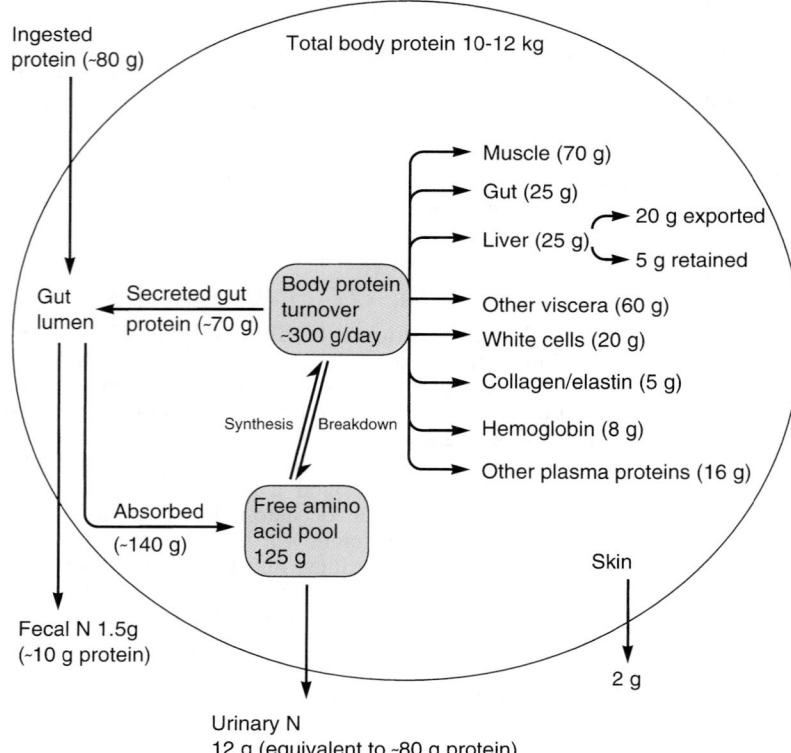

Figure 2.2. Whole-body protein metabolism in a normal, 70-kg man.

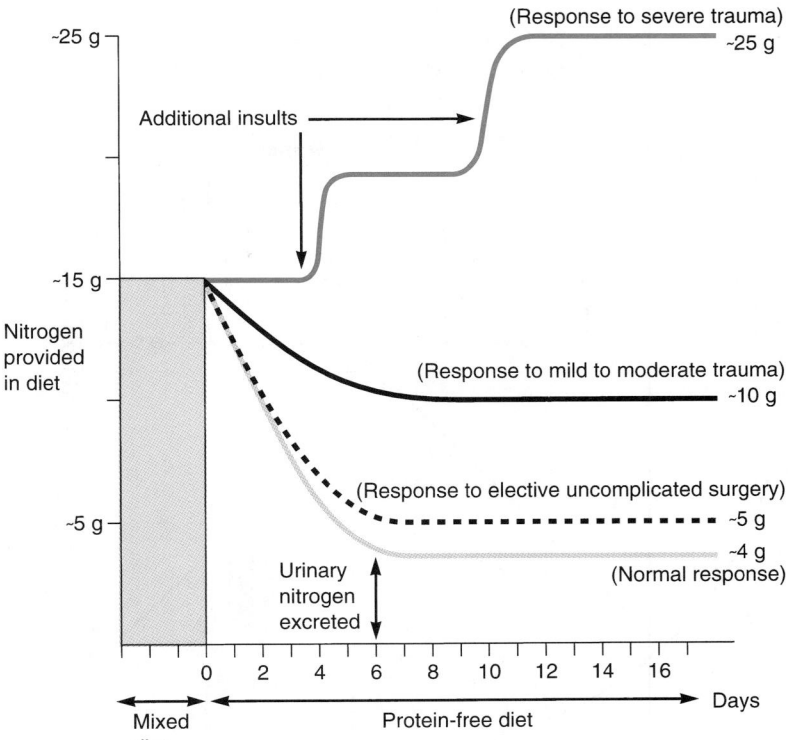

Figure 2.3. The response to starvation in normal subjects and postoperative, septic patients. The normal person adapts to starvation by conserving body protein, which is manifested by a decrease in nitrogen excretion in the urine. Septic patients do not adapt to starvation by using ketones for energy, and therefore urinary nitrogen losses are much greater.

measured from the amount of nitrogen given minus the amount excreted in the urine in a 24-hour sample. Nitrogen loss from a high-output fistula may also be measured, but stool, skin, and wound losses usually cannot be measured and are estimated (e.g., diarrhea) or not calculated.

$$N_{balance} = N_{intake} - N_{out}$$

Positive $N_{balance}$ indicates $N_{in} > N_{out}$
Examples: growth (child), anabolism after surgery

Negative $N_{balance}$ indicates $N_{in} < N_{out}$
Examples: starvation, injury, severe infection

Over relatively long periods, the healthy adult remains in nitrogen equilibrium (zero nitrogen balance). In contrast, surgical patients are prone to development of negative nitrogen balance because of their underlying disease process. This is most often manifested clinically as wasting of skeletal muscle secondary to rates of protein breakdown, which exceeds protein synthesis.

Metabolism of amino acids (from enteral or parenteral feedings) generates ammonia, which is one of the most toxic and reactive compounds in physiologic fluids. Ammonia levels in blood are usually kept at nontoxic concentrations (20 to 40 μmol/L); this is done primarily by hepatic conversion of ammonia to urea, a nontoxic, soluble compound. A large portion of the ammonia used for urea

synthesis arises from nitrogen catabolism in extrahepatic tissues. Excretory or transport amino acids, primarily glutamine and alanine, serve as vehicles for transporting ammonia in a nontoxic form from peripheral tissues to the visceral organs. In these organs, ammonia is reformed and then either excreted (kidneys) or detoxified (liver). From the intestinal tract, the large ammonia load delivered to the liver escapes the systemic circulation because of the biochemical pathways in the liver that detoxify it. Only the liver has all the enzymes of urea synthesis, and these enzymes are located only in periportal hepatocytes. Thus, diseases affecting the periportal areas lead to an increased ammonia load in the systemic circulation.

Urea is a highly soluble (2 mol/L), nontoxic molecule with a high nitrogen content (47%), but little chemical energy is required for its biosynthesis. Normal human subjects that ingest a Western diet excrete approximately 30 g of urea daily. This may increase to over 60 g/d in catabolic surgical patients. Urea accounts for 85% of the total urinary nitrogen, with the remaining 15% contributed by ammonia and creatinine.

The biosynthesis of urea involves four important steps: transamination, oxidative deamination, ammonia transport, and the reactions of the urea cycle. Transamination, catalyzed by enzymes termed transaminases or aminotransferases, exchanges an NH$_2$ and an OH between a pair of amino acids and a pair of ketoacids. Transamination is usually a freely reversible process permitting transaminases to function both in amino acid catabolism and biosynthesis. The most important transamination reaction in the body is catalyzed by glutamate transaminase. This reversible reaction forms glutamate from α-ketoglutarate, using a variety of amino acids as nitrogen donors. Hence, the amino acid groups of most amino acids ultimately are transferred to α-ketoglutarate by transamination with glutamate. This is important because glutamate is the only amino acid in mammalian tissues that undergoes oxidative deamination at an appreciable rate. Release of the ni-

Table 2.4. **AMINO ACID REQUIREMENTS FOR THE AVERAGE ADULT (70-KG) MAN**

Disease process	Amino acids g/kg/d
Postoperative (uncomplicated)	1–15
Sepsis	1.5–2.0
Multiple trauma (ventilator)	1.5–2.0
Major burn	2.0–3.0

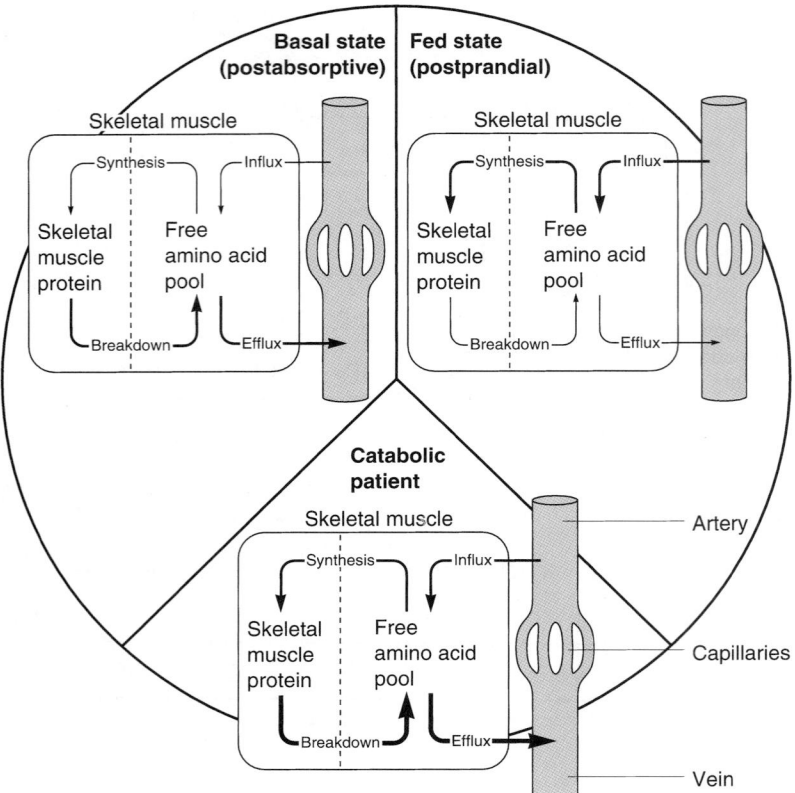

Figure 2.4. Relatives rates of protein synthesis and breakdown in skeletal muscle in postabsorptive, postprandial, and catabolic states. After an overnight fast, muscle releases net amounts of amino acids to help maintain the circulating pool. Breakdown exceeds synthesis, although this may not be measurable using standard techniques. After a meal, muscle amino acid uptake is greater than release and protein synthesis is greater than catabolism. In the catabolic surgical patient, protein synthesis may be increased, but this rate is exceeded by the rate of breakdown. In the absence of nutritional support, profound muscle wasting can occur.

trogen as ammonia is catalyzed by glutamate dehydrogenase, an enzyme with highest activity in the liver. This enzyme plays an important role in the funneling of nitrogen from glutamate to urea.

In the postabsorptive state (after an overnight fast), the gut lumen is empty of ingested proteins. Therefore, absorption of luminal amino acids is relatively low. Circulating amino acid levels are maintained by the release of preformed amino acid pools and the breakdown of cellular proteins. Protein degradation generates amino acids exported directly to the circulation as well as providing amino acid precursors for synthesis of other amino acids subsequently released. In catabolic surgical patients, protein synthesis in skeletal muscle may be increased but protein breakdown is accelerated to a greater extent, such that net proteolysis and depletion of the amino acid pool is observed (Fig. 2.4). This is manifested clinically as loss of lean body mass and negative nitrogen balance.

Thermoregulation

Alterations in the body's central thermostat located in the hypothalamus are almost always observed in patients with systemic infection. Core temperature reflects the balance between heat production and heat loss, both of which can be altered in surgical patients. Most of the heat production in the postabsorptive basal state occurs in the brain and the abdominal organs. Increased heat production occurs after an infectious challenge and is due to a resetting of the hypothalamic setpoint, mediated by proinflammatory cytokines such as interleukin (IL)-1. Such an increase in body temperature is thought to be an adaptive one because rates of cellular reactions increase as a function of temperature. The metabolic rate increases approximately 10% for each degree Celsius increase sin temperature.

Heat loss is regulated by adjustments in skin blood flow and in perspiration. In cooler environments, heat loss is through dissipation of skin heat; in warmer environments, heat loss occurs primarily through sweating. Burn patients exhibit an impaired ability to preserve body heat; for this reason, warmer ambient temperatures in the intensive care unit and the operating room are essential for the maintenance of thermoneutrality in such patients. During surgery, general anesthesia may reduce the capacity for shivering, leading to heat loss, and increased evaporation from the open body cavities may lead to mild hypothermia.

HOMEOSTATIC RESPONSES AND ADJUSTMENTS TO STRESS

Built into the body's defense mechanisms is a complex set of orchestrated responses initiated within moments of injury or insult. These responses are indelible, essential for survival, and designed to maintain body homeostasis at a time when key physiologic processes are threatened. These responses are immediately set into motion by various components of the injury response such as volume loss, tissue damage, fear, and pain. Later factors reinitiating or perpetuating these responses include invasive infection and starvation. These events are in general related to the severity of injury—that is, the greater the insult, the more pronounced the specific response. Incorporated into the human genome are genes encoding the synthesis of key hormones and peptides that allow the body to respond to such insults with remarkable resilience. From an evolutionary standpoint, these biologic responses result from a process favoring survival of the fittest in the struggle to preserve the species. From a teleologic standpoint, these responses are designed to benefit the organism, enhance recovery, and ensure a relatively speedy return to health.

Table 2.5. DIFFERENCES BETWEEN ELECTIVE SURGERY AND ACCIDENTAL INJURY

Insult	Elective operation	Accidental injury (trauma)
Tissue damage	Minimal; tissues are dissected with care and reapproximated	Can be substantial; tissues usually torn or ripped; débridement often necessary
Hypotension	Uncommon: preoperative hydration used and fluid status is carefully monitored intraoperatively	Fluid resuscitation often not immediate; blood loss can be substantial, leading to shock
Pain/fear/anxiety	Usually can be alleviated with preoperative medication	Usually present
Infectious complications	Uncommon: prophylactic antibiotics often administered	More common because of contamination, hypotension, and tissue devitalization
Overall stress response	Controlled and of lesser magnitude; starvation better tolerated	Uncontrolled; proportional to the magnitude of the injury; malnutrition poorly tolerated

Whether the body is injured accidentally or in the carefully monitored confines of an operating room, the responses to such trauma are similar. However, it is apparent to the student of surgery that such settings are also different in ways that influence the extent and magnitude of the stress response (Table 2.5). Accidental injury is unplanned and uncontrolled; tissues are torn, ripped, bruised, and contaminated. The associated volume loss may be substantial, leading to tissue hypoperfusion that, if prolonged, results in cellular deterioration and death in tissues that were not initially traumatized. Pain, excitement, and fear are usually heightened and uncontrolled. As a consequence, the magnitude of the physiologic responses to major accidental injury is considerable.

In contrast, the "elective" tissue trauma that is inflicted in the confines of an operating room is calculated, planned, and monitored. Although elective surgery causes pain, often interrupts food intake, and is usually associated with the removal of an organ or tissue, the perioperative management of elective surgical patients is often designed to attenuate such changes. Patients are seen before surgery by anesthesiologists and surgeons and evaluated to determine the need for preoperative nutritional support or additional medical consultation. Hydration before surgery is common, as is the administration of prophylactic antibiotics and drugs to relieve anxiety and fear. In the operating theater, the surgical site is prepared in a sterile fashion to minimize contamination, and numerous physiologic responses (e.g., blood pressure, pulse, urine output) are continually monitored. Blood and blood products are invariably available. During the operation, tissues are carefully dissected and incised to minimize tissue trauma; tissues are reapproximated with care when possible. Appropriately selected pharmacologic agents are used to block undesirable cardiovascular responses, and specific techniques such as epidural anesthesia or patient-controlled analgesia are effective in minimizing postoperative pain. As a consequence, the physiologic responses to elective surgery are usually of a lesser magnitude than those after major accidental injury. Improvements in surgical and anesthetic care now allow us to perform major elective operations with minimal morbidity and mortality.

SPECIFIC COMPONENTS OF THE STRESS RESPONSE

Volume Loss and Tissue Hypoperfusion

After reduction of the circulating blood volume, the body immediately attempts to compensate to maintain adequate organ perfusion. Pressure receptors in the aortic arch and carotid artery and volume (stretch) receptors in the wall of the left atrium detect the fall in blood volume and immediately respond by signaling the brain. Heart rate and stroke volume, the two determinants of cardiac output, increase. Afferent nerve signals are also initiated that stimulate the release of both antidiuretic hormone (ADH) and aldosterone. ADH is produced by the posterior pituitary gland in response to hypotonicity and increases water reabsorption in the kidney. Aldosterone is produced by the renin–angiotensin system, which is activated when the juxtaglomerular apparatus in the kidney is stimulated by a fall in pulse pressure. Aldosterone increases renal sodium reabsorption, thereby conserving intravascular water. These mechanisms are only partially effective and severe hemorrhage, in the absence of adequate resuscitation, often leads to a prolonged low-flow state. Under these circumstances, oxygen delivery is inadequate to meet tissue demands and the cell is forced to switch to anaerobic metabolism, leading to lactic acidosis.

Tissue Damage

Injury of body tissues appears to be the most important factor setting the stress response into motion. Hypovolemia and malnutrition may act synergistically with tissue destruction, but in and of themselves hypovolemia and starvation do not initiate a hypermetabolic/hypercatabolic response unless they result in infection or tissue injury. For example, prolonged underperfusion may lead to ischemia, cellular death, and the release of toxic products that can initiate the "stress" response. Afferent neural pathways from the wound signal the hypothalamus that injury has occurred; tissue destruction usually is sensed in the conscious patient as pain. Efferent pathways from the brain are immediately triggered and stimulate a number of responses designed to maintain homeostasis.

Pain and Fear

Pain and fear are established components of the stress response. Both lead to excessive production of the catecholamines preparing the body for the "fight-or-flight" response.

Lack of Nutrient Intake and the Consequences of Malnutrition

The metabolic response to injury and surgery brings increased energy expenditure. In many patients undergoing surgery, nutrient intake is inadequate for a period (1 to 5 days) after operation. If energy intake is less than expenditure, oxidation of body fat stores and erosion of lean body mass occur, with the resultant loss of weight. Body glycogen stores are limited and are depleted within 24 to 36 hours. Consequently, glucose, which is required by the central nervous system and white blood cells, must be synthesized de novo. Amino acids, released principally by skeletal muscle, are the major gluconeogenic precursors.

Most injured patients can tolerate a loss of 15% of their preinjury weight without a significant increase in the risk of surgery. When weight loss exceeds 15% of body weight, the complications of undernutrition interact with the stress process, impairing the body's ability to respond appropriately to the injury and to added complications such as infection.

A major goal of nutritional support in the trauma patient is to match the energy and nitrogen expenditure that occurs after injury to aid host defense. In contrast to injured patients, the catabolic and hypermetabolic responses that occur after elective operations are of a lesser magnitude because there is less tissue destruction and the neurohormonal/inflammatory response is less intense. Consequently, well-nourished patients undergoing major operations do not require nutritional support after surgery unless it is anticipated that food intake will be precluded for more than 7 days.

Invasive Infection

The major complication observed in surgical patients is infection. Most patients, particularly those in intensive care units, are exposed to a variety of infectious agents in the hospital. Normal barrier defense mechanisms are disrupted by multiple indwelling pieces of plastic such as intravenous catheters and nasotracheal and nasogastric tubes. Breakdown of skin and mucous membrane allows portals of entry for bacteria. Infection alone may initiate catabolic responses that are similar to (but not the same as) those after injury in noninfected patients. Both processes cause fever, hyperventilation, tachycardia, accelerated gluconeogenesis, increased proteolysis, and lipolysis, with fat used as the principal fuel source. Inflammatory cells release a variety of soluble mediators that aid host resistance and wound repair, but undernutrition may compromise the available host defense mechanisms and thereby increase the likelihood of invasive sepsis, multiple organ system failure, and death.

DETERMINANTS OF HOST RESPONSES TO SURGICAL STRESS

The pattern of physiologic changes elicited in response to surgical stress results from the specific interaction of an individual patient with the stressful stimulus. The host must be capable of transmitting and integrating injury signals, both neural and humoral, and then mounting an appropriate response that requires the interaction of a number of organ systems. The nature, intensity, and duration of the stress are fundamental determinants of both the host mediators activated and the physiologic changes observed. The responses that follow a minor elective operation are similar to those observed during a comparable, brief period of fasting and bed rest. On the other hand, major thermal injury results in a prolonged period of hypermetabolism and a severe drain on the body's energy and protein stores, resolving only with wound closure and resolution of the sepsis that may have developed. Thus, there are profound metabolic differences between the body's response to simple starvation and major stress (Table 2.6).

Body Composition

Body composition is a major determinant of the metabolic responses observed during surgical illness. Posttraumatic nitrogen excretion is directly related to the size of the body protein mass. The balance of nitrogen intake versus output from the body serves as a marker of protein metabolism. The net loss of a certain amount of nitrogen from the body implies the net breakdown of the corresponding amount of protein. In women, the size of the skeletal muscle mass is approximately one half that of age-matched men; thus, it is the muscular young man in whom nitrogen losses are most marked after injury, and it is the elderly, sedentary woman in whom they are least marked.

Nutritional Status

Patients undergoing major elective surgery with preexisting nutritional depletion have diminished nitrogen losses compared with normally nourished patients, although endocrine responses are similar. A strong relation between protein depletion and postoperative complications has been demonstrated in nonseptic, immunocompetent patients undergoing elective major gastrointestinal surgery. Protein-depleted patients had significantly lower preoperative respiratory muscle strength and vital capacity, an increased incidence of postoperative pneumonia, and longer postoperative hospital stays. Impaired wound healing as well as decreased respiratory, hepatic, and muscle function in protein-depleted patients awaiting surgery has also been reported.

Age

Many of the changes in the metabolic responses to surgical illness that occur with aging can be attributed to alterations in body composition and to longstanding patterns of physical activity. Although weight remains more or less stable, fat mass tends to increase with age, whereas muscle mass tends to decrease. The loss of strength that accompanies immobility, starvation, and acute surgical illness may have marked functional consequences. The capacity of muscle to serve as a substrate source may be limited during prolonged illness in the elderly patient, and muscle strength may rapidly become inadequate for respiratory and other vital muscle function.

The changes in REE occurring with aging can be accounted for, in large part, by changes in body composition, specifically decreases in muscle mass. After the limited stress of elective surgery, increases in energy expenditure are independent of age. Endocrine responses to elective operation and to trauma appear intact in older patients in terms of plasma cortisol levels and urinary excretion of epinephrine, norepinephrine, and 17-hydroxycorticosteroids.

The prevalence of cardiovascular and pulmonary diseases increases with age. Diminished arterial compliance, impaired vasoconstriction, altered autonomic function and sensitivity to catecholamines, and decreased barore-

Table 2.6. METABOLIC DIFFERENCES BETWEEN THE RESPONSE TO SIMPLE STARVATION AND TO INJURY

	Simple starvation	Severe injury
Basal metabolic rate	—	++
Presence of mediators	—	+++
Major fuel oxidized	Fat	Mixed
Ketone body production	+++	±
Hepatic ureagenesis	+	+++
Negative nitrogen balance	+	+++
Gluconeogenesis	+	+++
Muscle proteolysis	+	+++
Hepatic protein synthesis	+	+++

flex sensitivity may all impair the maintenance of cardio-vascular homeostasis during acute surgical illness. Thus, the delivery of oxygen to the tissues may be impaired in the elderly at every step of the oxygen transport pathway and may be inadequate when oxygen demands are highest. The physiology of aging, in general terms, is marked by a diminished sensitivity to perturbations of homeostasis and diminished effectiveness of the mechanisms to restore and maintain homeostasis.

Sex

Observed differences between the metabolic responses of men and women in general reflect differences in body composition. Lean body mass, expressed as a proportion of body weight, is lower in women than in men, and this difference is thought to account for the lower net loss of nitrogen after major elective abdominal surgery in women.

MEDIATORS OF THE STRESS RESPONSE

The response to operative stresses (elective injury) or accidental injury (trauma) comprises two components: a neurohormonal arm and an inflammatory arm. These pathways work together to determine the magnitude of the response. The principal counterregulatory hormones involved are the catecholamines, the corticosteroids, and glucagon. The inflammatory component of injury involves the local elaboration of cytokines and the systemic activation of humoral cascades involving complement, eicosanoids, and platelet-activating factor. These mediators promote wound healing by stimulating angiogenesis, white cell migration, and ingrowth of fibroblasts. During elective surgical procedures, the local inflammatory response is confined to the wound, and significant amounts of these mediators do not gain access to the systemic circulation. After accidental injury, where there is massive tissue destruction or prolonged hypotension leading to cell injury, these substances may be produced locally in the wound in excessive amounts, resulting in "spillover" into the systemic circulation. In addition, cells in other tissues (such as Kupffer cells in the liver) may become activated to produce these mediators. Such responses can lead to a systemic response in which these mediators cause detrimental effects such as hypotension and organ dysfunction.

Counterregulatory Hormones

After moderate to severe injury, there is a marked rise in the elaboration of the counterregulatory hormones glucagon, the glucocorticoids, and epinephrine. During the ebb phase of injury, the sympathoadrenal axis helps maintain the pressure–flow relationships necessary for an intact cardiovascular system. With the onset of hypermetabolism, characteristic of the flow phase, these and other hormones exert a variety of metabolic effects. Glucagon has potent glycogenolytic and gluconeogenic effects on the liver that signal the hepatocytes to produce glucose from hepatic glycogen stores and gluconeogenic precursors. Cortisol mobilizes amino acids from skeletal muscle and increases hepatic gluconeogenesis. The catecholamines stimulate hepatic glycolysis and gluconeogenesis and increase lactate production from peripheral tissues (skeletal muscle). Catecholamines also increase the metabolic rate and stimulate lipolysis. The level of growth hormone is elevated, even in the presence of hyperglycemia, and thyroid hormone levels are reduced to low-normal concentrations. Infusion of counterregulatory hormones into normal subjects reproduces many of the metabolic alterations characteristic of injury (9).

Cytokines

Cytokines, which are produced both at the site of injury by endothelial cells and by diverse immune cells throughout the body, also occupy a pivotal position in the stress response (10). Cytokines differ from classic endocrine hormones in that they are produced by a variety of cell types and have the capacity to exert their tissue effects locally through direct cell-to-cell communication ("networking") in a paracrine or autocrine fashion. Cytokines can also stimulate the production of other cytokines, leading to important cascades that amplify and diversify the effects of the proximal cytokine. Occasionally, when produced in excess, cytokines may act as hormones, spilling over into the systemic circulation and becoming detectable in the bloodstream. Under these circumstances, cytokines produce systemic responses through endocrine mechanisms.

The cytokines that appear to play the most important role in regulating the metabolic response to injury are tumor necrosis factor-α (TNF-α, cachectin), IL-1, IL-2, IL-6, and interferon-γ (IFN). These polypeptide signalers, produced by the organism in response to tissue injury, necrosis, bacteremia, or endotoxemia, induce both adaptive (e.g., stimulation of the acute-phase response) and adverse (organ dysfunction) responses after severe injury (Fig. 2.5). The production of cytokines is likely to be greatest when the injury is most severe. Under these circumstances, local cytokine production may gain access to the systemic circulation and trigger detrimental responses such as hypotension and organ dysfunction. Tissue injury and necrosis produced by higher concentrations of TNF-α are

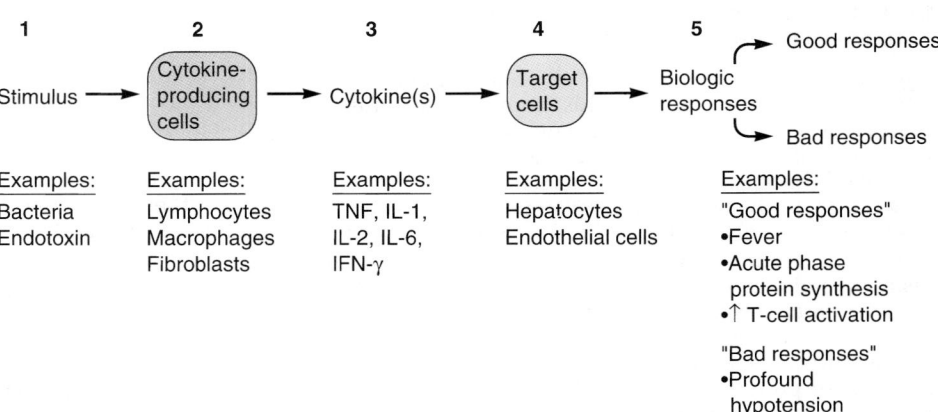

Figure 2.5. Cytokines can elicit both beneficial and deleterious responses.

mediated by effects on the microvasculature that produce an intense inflammatory reaction leading to ischemic and hemorrhagic necrosis.

Tumor necrosis factor-α is considered to be the primary mediator of the systemic effects of endotoxin, producing anorexia, fever, tachypnea, and tachycardia at low doses and hypotension, organ failure, and death at higher doses. TNF-α is produced primarily by macrophages, but lymphocytes, Kupffer cells, and a number of other cell types have been identified as sources of TNF-α. In healthy humans, plasma levels of TNF-α are quite low, usually ranging from 0 to 35 pg/mL. Concentrations in tissues are likely to be higher. In animal models, stimulation of TNF-α-producing cells with endotoxin induces both transcription and translation of the protein within minutes, with detection in serum after 20 minutes. In both humans and animals, TNF-α levels peak between 90 minutes and 2 hours after injection of endotoxin. TNF-α leads to IL-1 release.

Interleukin-1, like TNF-α, has a variety of proinflammatory activities. A single low in vivo dose of IL-1 results in fever, neutrophilia, hypozincemia, increased hepatic acute-phase protein synthesis, decreased albumin synthesis, anorexia, sleep, and release of adrenocorticotropic hormone (ACTH), glucocorticoids, and insulin. At higher doses, IL-1 induces hypotension, leukopenia, tissue injury, and death in a manner characteristic of septic shock. IL-1 induces many of the same biologic effects as TNF-α, and the combined effect of these two cytokines is often greater than the effect of either alone.

Interleukin-6 is now recognized as the primary mediator of altered hepatic protein synthesis, known as the acute-phase protein synthetic response. Glucocorticoid hormones augment the cytokine effects on acute-phase protein synthesis. Elevated levels of IL-6 are found in the circulation of patients with infections, trauma, and cancer.

The IFNs are a family of proteins originally identified for their ability to inhibit viral replication in infected cells. IFN-γ is a type II IFN, totally unrelated in structure and function to the type I IFNs, which have antiviral properties. IFN-γ has the ability to up-regulate the number of TNF-α receptors on various cell types.

If Cytokines Have Detrimental Effects, Why Do They Exist?

The genes that regulate cytokine biosynthesis are highly conserved, indicating that these peptides confer a survival advantage after injury. Although excess production can be dangerous to the host, cytokines exert a number of beneficial effects under most circumstances that appear to outweigh the detrimental effects seen in extreme pathophysiologic states.

Mobilization of Amino Acids and Stimulation of Acute-phase Protein Synthesis

Cytokines act in concert with other mediators to promote mobilization of amino acids from skeletal muscle. This response provides key nutrients to support cellular metabolism at a time when the animal usually cannot acquire food because of the associated immobility and anorexia. The primary metabolic component of the acute-phase response effected by IL-6 is a qualitative alteration in hepatic protein synthesis with a resulting alteration in plasma protein composition. Characteristically, proteins acting as serum transport and binding molecules (albumin, transferrin) are reduced in quantity, and acute-phase proteins (fibrinogen, C-reactive protein) are increased. Acute-phase proteins are elaborated, in part, for the purpose of reducing the systemic effects of tissue damage. Al-

though the true physiologic role of many of the acute-phase proteins remains unclear, many act as antiproteases, opsonins, or coagulation and wound-healing factors, and they likely inhibit the generalized tissue destruction that is associated with the local initiation of inflammation. For example, increases in fibrinogen enhance thrombus formation, whereas antiproteases reduce tissue damage caused by proteases released by dead or dying cells. C-reactive protein has been hypothesized to have a scavenger function. This acute-phase response confers a significant survival advantage after injury and infection.

Elevation in White Blood Cell Count

Leukocytosis is recognized clinically by an elevated circulating white blood cell count, with an increase in the proportion of immature cells. This phenomenon has been attributed, in part, to the release of neutrophils and their precursors into the circulation from the bone marrow. Both TNF-α and IL-1 produce an increase in the number and immaturity of circulating neutrophils because of a direct action on the bone marrow. Locally produced TNF-α and IL-1 are also chemotactic for neutrophils.

Hypoferremia and Hypozincemia

Serum iron and zinc levels are reduced in septic patients, an event that is cytokine mediated. The decrease in serum iron is probably important in protecting the host against various bacteria. The reduction in iron can inhibit the growth rate of microorganisms that have a strict requirement for iron as a growth factor. Both TNF-α and IL-1 have been shown to mediate hypoferremia, hypozincemia, and other alterations in trace element metabolism.

Localization of the Wound/Inflammatory Site

Localization or containment of tissue injury may be an important response designed to minimize systemic effects from the inflammation at the trauma site. This is accomplished by vasodilatation, migration of neutrophils and monocytes to the wound, initiation of the coagulation cascade, and proliferation of endothelial cells and fibroblasts in later stages of wound healing. These effects confine the insult as much as possible, and activate defense mechanisms to minimize adverse systemic effects, such as cardiovascular collapse and subsequent organ failure. Cytokines are involved in all of these functions. The wound becomes an organ of cytokine production in which local metabolism is controlled in part by cytokines.

Fever/Subjective Discomfort

Fever is the systemic response to invading microorganisms and their toxins elicited by changes in the microenvironment of the anterior hypothalamus. These febrile responses are cytokine mediated. Fever has both beneficial and detrimental effects on the host, but it is generally believed that the generation of fever by endogenously produced substances has adaptive value and imparts a survival advantage on the organism. Fever induced by the injection of cytokines in humans is associated with symptoms of malaise, myalgia, headache, and joint pain. These constitutional symptoms are likely to be beneficial because they encourage the "sick" animal to seek shelter, safety, and rest and to avoid additional stressful situations.

Gut Mucosal Barrier Dysfunction as a Mediator of the Stress Response

Under certain circumstances, the gut may become a source of sepsis and serve as the motor of the systemic inflammatory response syndrome. The maintenance of an intact brush border and intercellular tight junctions prevents the movement of toxic substances into the intestinal lymphatics and circulation; these functions may become altered in critically ill patients. Maintenance of a gut mucosal barrier that effectively excludes luminal bacteria and toxins requires normal perfusion, an intact epithelium, and normal mucosal immune mechanisms.

Microbial translocation is the process by which microorganisms migrate across the mucosal barrier and invade the host. Translocation can be promoted in three general ways: (a) altered permeability of the intestinal mucosa, (b) decreased host defense, and (c) an increased number of bacteria in the intestine. Hemorrhagic shock, hypoxemia, sepsis, distant injury, or administration of cell toxins leads to altered permeability. Glucocorticoid administration, immunosuppression, or protein depletion decreases host defense. Bacterial overgrowth, intestinal stasis, or even feeding bacteria to experimental animals increases the luminal bacterial count and may cause translocation. Even if actual migration of whole bacteria does not occur, the gut may absorb their endotoxin into the portal venous system. A number of retrospective and epidemiologic studies have associated infection in specific patient populations with bacterial invasion from the gut. These studies have demonstrated an increase in mucosal permeability both in normal volunteers who received endotoxin as well as infected burn patients. Because many of the factors that facilitate bacterial translocation occur simultaneously in surgical patients, and their effects may be additive or cumulative, patients in an intensive care unit may be extremely vulnerable to the invasion of enteric bacteria or the absorption of their toxins. Such patients usually do not receive enteral feedings, and current parenteral therapy results in gut atrophy. Methods used to support critically ill patients neither facilitate repair of the intestinal mucosa nor maintain gut barrier function.

ELECTIVE SURGERY

Physiologic Responses to Surgery

The physiologic responses to surgical stress are multiple and complex (Fig. 2.6). One of the earliest consequences of a surgical procedure is the rise in levels of circulating cortisol that occurs in response to a sudden outpouring of ACTH from the anterior pituitary gland. The rise in ACTH stimulates the adrenal cortex to elaborate cortisol, which remains elevated for 24 to 48 hours after operation. Cortisol has generalized effects on tissue catabolism and mobilizes amino acids from skeletal muscle that provide substrates for wound healing and serve as precursors for the hepatic synthesis of acute-phase proteins or new glucose. Associated with the activation of the adrenal cortex is stimulation of the adrenal medulla through the sympathetic nervous system, with elaboration of epinephrine and norepinephrine. These circulating neurotransmitters

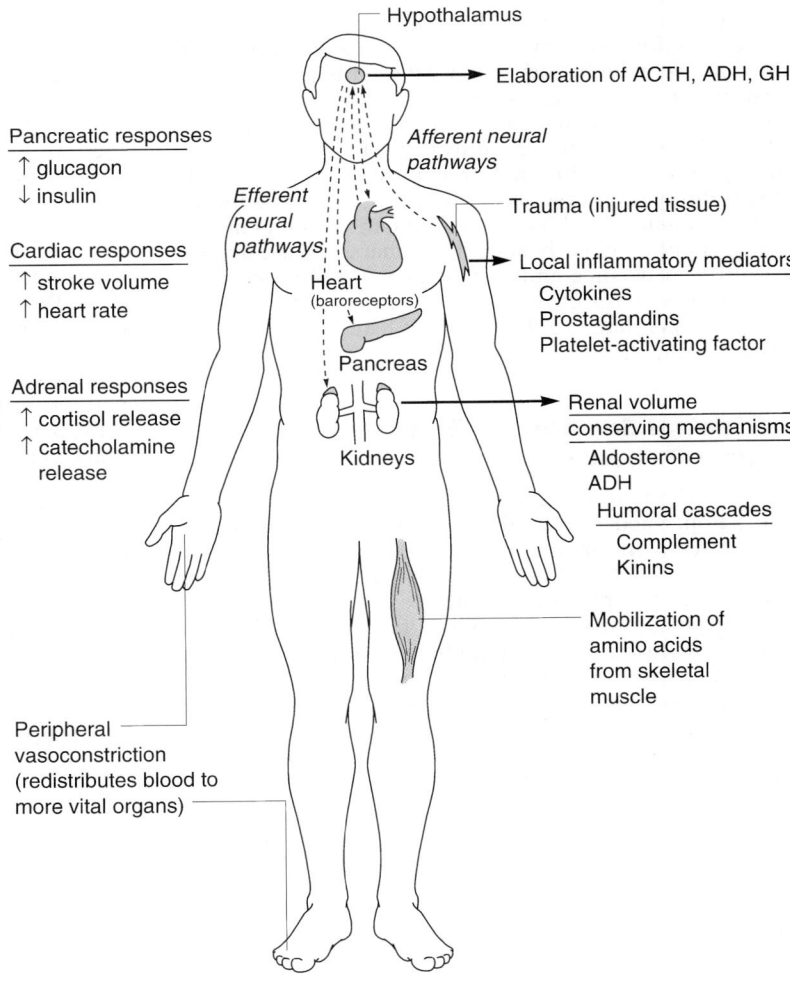

Figure 2.6. Homeostatic adjustments initiated after injury.

play an important role in circulatory adjustment, but may also elicit metabolic responses if the augmented secretion rate continues over a prolonged period.

The neuroendocrine responses to surgery also modify the various mechanisms that regulate salt and water excretion. Alterations in serum osmolarity and tonicity of body fluids secondary to anesthesia and the operative stress stimulate the secretion of aldosterone and ADH. Aldosterone is a potent stimulator of renal sodium retention, whereas ADH stimulates renal tubular water reabsorption. Thus, the ability to excrete a water load after elective surgical procedures is restricted and weight gain secondary to salt and water retention is usual after surgery. Edema occurs to a varying extent in all surgical wounds, and this accumulation is proportional to the extent of tissue dissection and local trauma. This "third-spaced" fluid eventually returns to the circulation as the wound edema subsides and diuresis commences 2 to 4 days after the operation.

Alterations occur in the response of the endocrine pancreas after elective surgery. In general, insulin elaboration is diminished and glucagon concentrations rise. This response may be related to increased sympathetic activity or to the rise in levels of circulating epinephrine known to suppress insulin release. The rise in glucagon and the corresponding fall in insulin is a potent signal to accelerate hepatic glucose production, and, with the help of other hormones (epinephrine and glucocorticoids), gluconeogenesis is maintained.

The period of catabolism initiated by surgery, characterized by a combination of inadequate nutrition and alteration of the hormonal environment, has been termed the *adrenergic–corticoid phase.* This phase usually lasts 1 to 3 days and is followed by the *adrenergic–corticoid withdrawal phase,* which lasts 1 to 3 days. This period is followed by the onset of anabolism, which occurs at a variable time in the patient's convalescence. In general, in the absence of postoperative complications, this phase starts 3 to 6 days after an abdominal procedure of the magnitude of a colectomy or gastrectomy, often concomitant with the commencement of oral feedings. The patient then enters a prolonged period of early anabolism characterized by positive nitrogen balance and weight gain. Protein synthesis is increased as a result of sustained enteral feedings, and this change is related to the return of lean body mass and muscular strength.

Nutritional Support of Elective Surgical Patients

Most patients undergoing elective surgery are adequately nourished. Unless the patient has had significant preoperative malnutrition, characterized by a weight loss greater than 10% to 15%, or has a major intraoperative or postoperative complication, solutions containing 5% dextrose may be administered for 5 to 7 days before the return of feeding with no detrimental effect on outcome. Therefore, the increased cost of feedings and the potential complications associated with intravenous nutrition cannot be justified. The use of jejunal feedings in the postoperative period may be useful in some patients, especially those undergoing extensive upper gastrointestinal surgery.

Nutritional Assessment

The two major objectives of nutritional assessment are (a) to determine the patient's nutritional status; and (b) to determine energy, protein, and other nutrient requirements. Part of the careful medical history and physical examination should be focused to inquire about associated diseases and history of weight loss, and to establish the diagnosis of cachexia, protein–energy malnutrition, or specific nutrient deficiencies. Measurements of skinfold thickness are helpful to determine fat mass, and a 24-hour urine collection with measurement of creatinine allows determination of the creatine-height index, a factor proportional to the size of muscle mass.

Immunologic status also has been used to evaluate nutritional status; total peripheral lymphocyte count, delayed hypersensitivity using a skin test response to common antigens, and lymphocyte transformation have all been used as indicators of immunocompetence in the critically ill patient. The depressed immune function often returns to normal with nutritional repletion, but altered immunologic responses are not specific for nutritional deficiencies and can be observed in patients with advanced malignant disease or in those who have had a severe injury. Serum albumin and transferrin are the most common serum proteins measured, and they correlate well with body protein deficiency in isolated cases of malnutrition.

Determining Nutritional Requirements

Total energy requirements are based on several factors: (a) the BMR, (b) the degree of stress imposed by the disease process, and (c) the amount of energy expended with activity. Standard nomograms relate normal metabolic requirements to a person's age, sex, height, and weight. The principal determinants of nitrogen requirement in surgical patients are total energy intake, nitrogen intake, and the metabolic state of the patient. Malnourished patients with intact protein-conserving mechanisms can achieve nitrogen equilibrium when 7% to 8% of the total caloric needs are provided as protein. This translates into a calorie-to-nitrogen ratio of approximately 350 kcal to 1 g N_2. Hypermetabolic, catabolic patients, on the other hand, have a diminished protein economy and require much more protein.

Routes of Feeding

For patients who can eat and have a functional gastrointestinal tract, adequate nutrition is best provided by the regular hospital diet. The enteral route of feeding is always the preferred route of feeding, and a variety of enteral diets are available for patients with a functional intestinal tract who will not or cannot eat. In these patients, nasogastric or nasojejunal feedings may be indicated. For patients with a diseased or nonfunctional gastrointestinal tract, parenteral nutrition may be necessary. Peripheral venous feedings provide dilute nutrients in a large fluid volume and rely on fat emulsions as a principal calorie source. Central venous feedings consist of hypertonic glucose and amino acid solutions infused through a catheter placed in the superior vena cava. Adequate calories can be administered in a small fluid volume, but this method of feeding requires placement and care of a central venous catheter and possible infectious complications.

TRAUMA

General Overview and Time Course of the Injury Response

In the 1930s, Cuthbertson (11) described the time course for many of the posttraumatic responses, and two distinct periods were identified. The early "ebb" or shock phase was usually brief (12 to 24 hours) and occurred immediately after injury. Blood pressure, cardiac output, body temperature, and oxygen consumption were reduced. These events were often associated with hemorrhage and resulted in hypoperfusion and lactic acidosis. With restoration of blood volume, ebb-phase alterations gave way to more accelerated responses. The "flow" phase was then characterized by hypermetabolism, increased cardiac output, increased urinary nitrogen losses, altered glucose metabolism, and accelerated tissue catabolism. The flow-phase responses to accidental injury are similar to those seen after elective operation. The response to injury, however, is usually much more intensive and extends over a longer time.

Characteristics of the Flow Phase of the Injury Response

Hypermetabolism

Hypermetabolism is defined as an increase in BMR above that predicted on the basis of age, sex, and body size. Metabolic rate is usually determined by measuring the exchange of respiratory gases and by calculating heat production from oxygen consumption and carbon dioxide production. The degree of hypermetabolism (increased oxygen consumption) usually is related to the severity of the injury. Patients with long-bone fractures have a 15% to 25% increase in metabolic rate, whereas the metabolic needs of patients with multiple injuries increase by 50%. Patients with severe burn injury [>50% of body surface area (BSA)] have resting metabolic rates that may reach twice basal levels. These metabolic rates in trauma patients are contrasted to those in postoperative patients, who rarely increase their BMR by more than 10% to 15% after surgery.

Altered Glucose Metabolism

Hyperglycemia commonly occurs after injury, and the elevation of fasting blood sugar levels usually parallels the severity of stress in the ebb phase. During the ebb phase, insulin levels are low and glucose production is only slightly elevated. Later, during the flow phase, insulin concentrations are normal or elevated, yet hyperglycemia persists. This phenomenon suggests an alteration in the relationship between insulin sensitivity and glucose disposal, hence insulin resistance. Hepatic glucose production is increased, and studies show that much of the new glucose generated by the liver arises from three-carbon precursors released from peripheral tissues.

Measurements of substrate exchange across injured and uninjured extremities of severely burned patients indicate that glucose is used in small amounts by the uninjured extremity. In contrast, the injured extremity extracts large amounts of glucose. The wound converts most of the glucose to lactate, which is recycled to the liver in the Cori cycle. Additional studies have shown that uninjured volunteers are able to dispose of an exogenous glucose load much more readily than injured patients. Moreover, the quantity of insulin elaborated by the patients was greater than in control subjects; nonetheless, these rising insulin concentrations failed to increase glucose clearance in these patients. Other studies have demonstrated a failure to suppress hepatic glucose production in trauma patients during glucose loading or insulin infusion. Either of these perturbations usually inhibits hepatic glucose production in normal subjects. Thus, profound insulin resistance occurs in injured patients.

Alterations in Protein Metabolism

Extensive urinary nitrogen loss occurs after major injury. Like other responses, the loss of nitrogen after injury is related to the extent of the trauma, but it also depends on the previous nutritional status, as well as the age and sex of the patient, because these factors determine, in part, the size of the muscle mass. In unfed patients, protein breakdown rates exceed synthesis, and negative balance results. Providing exogenous calories and nitrogen increases protein synthesis, but, even with achievement of energy balance, the nitrogen loss is not attenuated (12). The nitrogen loss can be balanced only by providing enough nitrogen intake.

Skeletal muscle is the major source of the nitrogen that is lost in the urine after extensive injury. Although it is now recognized that amino acids are released by muscle in increased quantities after injury, it has only recently been appreciated that the composition of amino acid efflux does not reflect the composition of muscle protein. The release is skewed toward glutamine and alanine, each of which comprises approximately one third of the total amino acids released by skeletal muscle. The kidney extracts glutamine, which contributes ammonium groups for ammonia generation, a process that excretes acid loads. The gastrointestinal tract also takes up glutamine to serve as an oxidative fuel. The gut enterocytes convert glutamine primarily to ammonia and alanine, and these two substances are released into the portal venous blood. This ammonia is then removed by the liver and converted to urea, and the alanine may be removed by the liver to serve as a gluconeogenic precursor. After elective surgical stress, glutamine consumption by the bowel and kidney is accelerated in a reaction that appears to be regulated by the increased elaboration of glucocorticoids. Although skeletal muscle releases alanine at an accelerated rate, the gastrointestinal tract and kidney also release increased amounts of alanine. The alanine is then extracted by the liver to be used in the synthesis of glucose and acute-phase proteins. Hence, glutamine and alanine are important participants in the transfer of nitrogen from skeletal muscle to visceral organs; however, their metabolic pathways favor the production of urea and ammonia, both of which lose nitrogen from the body.

Alterations in Fat Metabolism

To support hypermetabolism, increased gluconeogenesis, and interorgan substrate flux, stored triglyceride is mobilized and oxidized at an accelerated rate. Glucose administration poorly attenuates this lipolysis, which may be the result of continuous stimulation of the sympathetic nervous system. Although mobilization and use of free fatty acids are accelerated in injured subjects, ketosis during brief starvation is blunted, and the accelerated protein catabolism remains unchecked. If unfed, severely injured patients rapidly deplete their fat and protein stores. Such malnutrition increases their susceptibility to added stresses of hemorrhage, surgery, and infection and may contribute to organ system failure, sepsis, and death.

Nutritional Support of the Injured Patient

Case Example

A 37-year-old, nonobese man (BSA, 2.0 m^2) is admitted to the hospital with blunt abdominal trauma. He is resuscitated and noted to have a positive diagnostic peritoneal lavage. At operation, a liver laceration is repaired and the patient is noted to have a large retroperitoneal hematoma that is nonexpanding. The patient is admitted to the trauma intensive care unit of the hospital, and a nasogastric tube is placed. Over the next 24 hours, his blood volume is restored, and he is given maintenance solutions with 5% dextrose and appropriate electrolytes at the rate of 125 mL/h. Because of a prolonged ileus, the patient is not fed, and he is started on TPN on postoperative day 7. On the 12th day after the accident, the patient starts taking clear liquids and is gradually advanced to regular diet over the next 3 days. He is discharged from the hospital.

Nitrogen balance studies from hospital days 1 through 7 reveal a cumulative 7-day nitrogen loss of 122 g. During this 7-day period, the patient had no nitrogen intake and received 500 calories of glucose per day. When TPN was started, he had lost 9 lb, half of which was lean body mass, and the remainder fat. He gained his weight back over the next 4 weeks.

Consequences of Malnutrition

The metabolic response to injury results in increased energy expenditure. If energy intake is less than expenditure, oxidation of body fat stores and erosion of lean body mass occur, with resultant loss of weight. When body weight loss exceeds 10% to 15%, the complications of undernutrition interact with the disease process, increasing morbidity and mortality rates. Undernutrition to this extent after injury may impair the body's ability to respond appropriately to the injury and inhibit responses to added stress such as infection.

The major impact of nutritional support in the trauma patient is to aid host defense. These patients are exposed to a variety of infectious agents in the hospital, and their injuries and requirements of care increase the risk of infection. Undernutrition may compromise the available host defense mechanisms and thus increase the likelihood of invasive sepsis, multiple organ system failure, and death. Additional consequences of malnutrition include poor wound healing, decreased mobility and activity, occurrence of pressure sores and decubitus ulcers, altered gastrointestinal function, and occurrence of edema secondary to reduced colloid osmotic pressure.

Priorities of Care

Resuscitation, oxygenation, and arrest of hemorrhage are immediate priorities for survival. Wounds should then be repaired or stabilized as expeditiously as possible. Nutritional support is an essential part of the metabolic care of the critically ill trauma patient and should be instituted before significant weight loss occurs. Adequate nutrition supports normal responses that optimize wound healing and recovery.

Goals of Nutritional Support

Most injured people are not malnourished at the time of injury, but the increased metabolic demands after injury quickly lead to a malnourished state if the patient is not nutritionally supported. On stabilization of the patient's condition and development of a care plan, nutritional support can be gradually initiated. The goal of nutritional support is the maintenance of lean body cell mass and the limitation of weight loss to less than 10% of preinjury weight. The nutritional requirements of the trauma patient can be determined as follows:

1. Determine BMR for age, sex, and BSA (BMR in kilocalories per day).
2. Determine the percentage of increase in metabolic rate due to the injury.
3. If active, add 25% × BMR for hospital activity (walking, physical therapy, sitting, treatment).
4. The sum of steps 1 to 3 is an estimated daily caloric requirement for maintenance of body weight.
5. Divide step 4 by 150 to determine nitrogen requirements (convert to protein = 6.25 × nitrogen).
6. Give approximately 70% of caloric requirement as glucose. Give remaining caloric requirement as fat.

Reassess energy and nitrogen needs at least twice weekly.

7. If nutritional support seems inadequate because of progressive weight loss, consider direct measurement of oxygen consumption or measurement of nitrogen balance.

SEPSIS

General Overview and Time Course of the Metabolic Response to Sepsis

The response patterns after major infection are less predictable than those after elective operations and trauma. The invasion of the body by microorganisms initiates many host responses, including mobilization of phagocytes, an inflammatory response at the local site, fever, tachycardia, and other systemic responses. Systemic events during the hyperdynamic phase of sepsis can be categorized into two general types of responses: (a) those related to the host's immunologic defenses, and (b) those related to the body's general metabolic and circulatory adjustments to the infection. The changes in metabolism relate to alterations in glucose, nitrogen, and fat metabolism, as well as the redistribution of trace metals.

Systemic Metabolic Responses

Severe infection is characterized by fever, hypermetabolism, diminished protein economy, altered glucose dynamics, and accelerated lipolysis, much like the injured patient. Anorexia is commonly associated with systemic infection and contributes to the loss of lean body tissue. These effects are compounded in the patient with sepsis by multiorgan system failure, which includes the gastrointestinal tract, liver, heart, and lungs.

Hypermetabolism

Oxygen consumption is usually elevated in the infected patient. The extent of this increase is related to the severity of infection, with peak elevations reaching 50% to 60% above normal. Such responses often occur in the postoperative and postinjury periods secondary to severe pneumonia, intraabdominal infection, or wound invasion. If the patient's metabolic rate is already elevated to a maximal extent because of severe injury, no further increase will be observed. In patients with only slightly accelerated rates of oxygen consumption, the presence of infection causes a rise in metabolic rate that adds to the preexisting state. A portion of the increase in metabolism may be ascribed to the increase in reaction rate associated with fever (Q_{10} effect). Calculations suggest that the metabolic rate increases 10% to 13% for each elevation of 1°C in central temperature. On resolution of the infection, the metabolic rate returns to normal.

Altered Glucose Dynamics

The increased glucose production observed in infected patients appears to be in addition to the augmented gluconeogenesis that occurs after injury. For example, uninfected burn patients have an accelerated glucose production rate approximately 50% above normal; with the onset of bacteremia in similar patients, hepatic glucose production increases to twice basal levels. Glucose dynamics after infection are complex, and profound hypoglycemia and diminished hepatic glucose production have also been described in both animals and human patients. Studies in animals and in human patients show that deterioration in gluconeogenesis is associated with more progressive stages of infection and may be related to alterations in splanchnic blood flow.

Alterations in Protein Metabolism

Accelerated proteolysis, increased nitrogen excretion, and prolonged negative nitrogen balance occur after infection, and the response pattern is similar to that described for injury. Amino acid efflux from skeletal muscle is accelerated in patients with sepsis, and this flux is matched by accelerated visceral amino acid uptake. In infected burn patients, splanchnic uptake of amino acids is increased 50% above rates in uninfected burn patients with injuries of comparable size. These amino acids serve as glucose precursors and are used for synthesis of acute-phase proteins. Studies in animals have demonstrated that an increase in hepatic amino acid uptake during systemic infection is due to an increase in the activities of specific amino acid transporters that reside in the hepatocyte plasma membrane.

Severe infection is often associated with a hypercatabolic state that initiates marked changes in interorgan glutamine metabolism (Fig. 2.7). The cycle may begin with a breakdown in the gut mucosal barrier, resulting in microbial translocation. Bacteria and their endotoxins stimulate macrophages to release cytokines, which activate the pituitary–adrenal axis. The release of cortisol stimulates glutamine synthesis and release by tissues such as the lungs and skeletal muscle. The bulk of the glutamine is taken up by the liver at the expense of the gut. Acidosis frequently occurs in the patient with sepsis, and this stimulus serves as a signal for accelerated glutamine uptake by the kidney. Glutamine liberates an ammonia ion that combines with a hydrogen ion and is excreted in the urine, thus contribut-

ing to acid–base homeostasis. Because the glutamine arises from skeletal muscle proteolysis, this complication of sepsis is yet another sign of heightened skeletal muscle breakdown.

Alterations in Fat Metabolism

Fat is a major fuel oxidized in infected patients, and the increased metabolism of lipids from peripheral fat stores is especially prominent during a period of inadequate nutritional support. Lipolysis is most probably mediated by the heightened sympathetic activity that is a potent stimulus for fat mobilization and accelerated oxidation. Serum triglyceride levels reflect the balance between rates of triglyceride production by the liver and use and storage by peripheral tissues. Marked hypertriglyceridemia has been associated with gram-negative infection on occasion, but plasma triglyceride concentrations are usually normal or low, indicating enhanced clearance by other organs. Infected patients cannot convert fatty acids to ketones efficiently in the liver, and hence do not adapt to starvation like fasted, unstressed people. It has been suggested that the low ketone levels of infection may be a consequence of the hyperinsulinemia associated with catabolic states.

Changes in Trace Mineral Metabolism

Changes in the balance of magnesium, inorganic phosphate, zinc, and potassium usually follow alterations in nitrogen balance. Although the iron-binding capacity of transferrin is usually unchanged in early infection, iron disappears from the plasma, especially during severe pyrogenic infections; similar alterations are observed with serum zinc levels. These decreases cannot be totally ac-

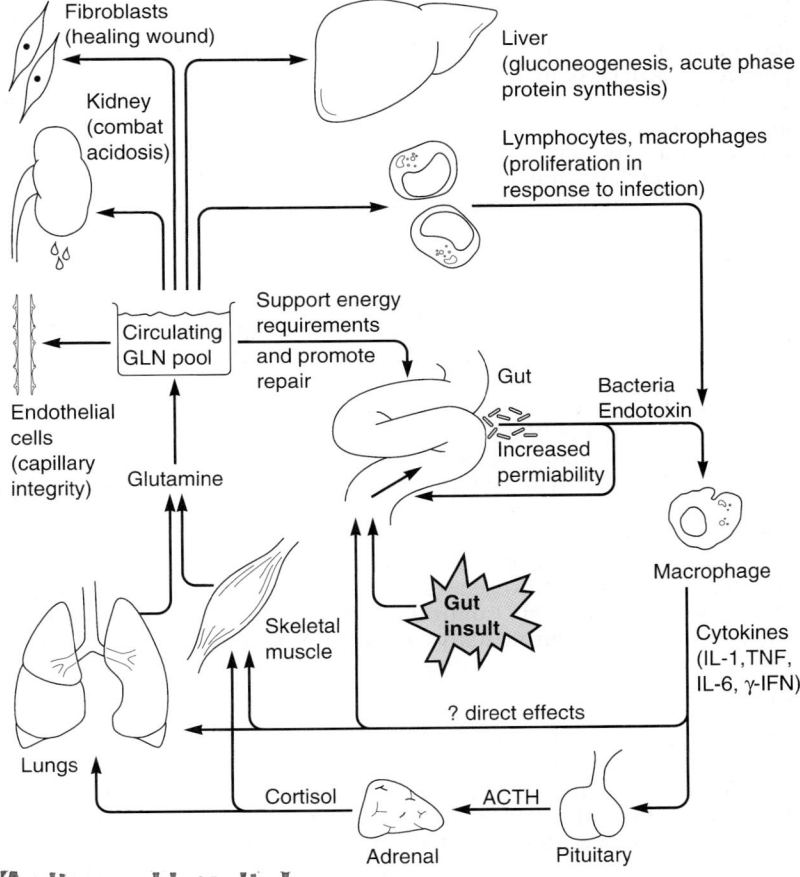

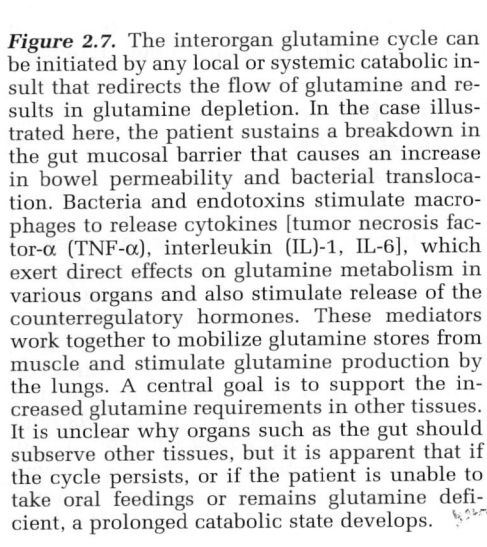

Figure 2.7. The interorgan glutamine cycle can be initiated by any local or systemic catabolic insult that redirects the flow of glutamine and results in glutamine depletion. In the case illustrated here, the patient sustains a breakdown in the gut mucosal barrier that causes an increase in bowel permeability and bacterial translocation. Bacteria and endotoxins stimulate macrophages to release cytokines [tumor necrosis factor-α (TNF-α), interleukin (IL)-1, IL-6], which exert direct effects on glutamine metabolism in various organs and also stimulate release of the counterregulatory hormones. These mediators work together to mobilize glutamine stores from muscle and stimulate glutamine production by the lungs. A central goal is to support the increased glutamine requirements in other tissues. It is unclear why organs such as the gut should subserve other tissues, but it is apparent that if the cycle persists, or if the patient is unable to take oral feedings or remains glutamine deficient, a prolonged catabolic state develops.

counted for by losses of the minerals from the body. Rather, both iron and zinc accumulate in the liver, and this accumulation appears to be another host defense mechanism. The administration of iron to the infected host, especially early in the disease, is contraindicated because increased serum iron concentrations may impair resistance. Unlike iron and zinc, copper levels usually rise, and the increased plasma concentrations can be ascribed almost entirely to the increase in ceruloplasmin produced by the liver.

Nutritional Requirements and Special Feeding Problems

As with all patients, the primary objectives of nutritional assessment are to evaluate the patient's current nutritional status and to determine energy, protein, and macronutrient and micronutrient requirements. Weight gain and anabolism usually are difficult to achieve during the septic process, but they do occur once the disease process has abated. Total energy requirements can be calculated using the stress equation; mild to moderate infections increase energy requirements 20% to 30%, and severe infection increases caloric needs approximately 50% above basal levels. The most severe complication of sepsis is the multiple organ dysfunction syndrome, which may result in death. The current treatment of systemic infection consists of (a) removal or drainage of the septic source; (b) use of appropriate antibiotics; (c) supportive therapy of specific organ failure, whether cardiac, pulmonary, hepatic, renal, or gastrointestinal; and (d) vigorous support of the host through nutritional means.

Respiratory Insufficiency

A common problem associated with systemic infection is oxygenation and elimination of carbon dioxide. Patients often require intubation and vigorous ventilatory support. Most of the enteral and parenteral formulas used to provide nutritional support for critically ill patients contain large amounts of carbohydrate, which generate large quantities of carbon dioxide after oxidation. Such a large carbon dioxide load may worsen pulmonary function or delay weaning from the ventilator. If this factor becomes a problem, the carbohydrate load should be reduced to 50% of metabolic requirements and fat emulsion administered to provide additional calories.

Renal Failure

When renal failure becomes progressive, the early use of hemodialysis minimizes the effects of uremia superimposed on the metabolism of sepsis. Metabolic studies in patients with acute and chronic renal failure have limited the intake of nonessential amino acids in an attempt to lower urea production. Proteins of high biologic value, but in much smaller quantities (<0.5 g/kg/d) than usually given, are administered along with adequate calories, usually in the form of glucose. When enteral feedings are not feasible, a central venous infusion of an essential amino acid solution and hypertonic dextrose provides calories and a small quantity of nitrogen, to reduce protein catabolism while simultaneously controlling the rise in blood urea nitrogen (BUN). During dialysis, protein intake is liberalized, but the BUN is maintained below 100 mg/dL.

Gut Dysfunction

Sepsis causes marked changes in gastrointestinal function. The most common abnormality is ileus, which can result from intraabdominal disease or from the effects of bacteria elsewhere. Breakdown of the gut mucosal barrier with translocation of luminal bacteria and their toxins can initiate a prolonged hypermetabolic state.

Hepatic Failure

Hepatic dysfunction is a common manifestation of septicemia. The degree of dysfunction is variable and may appear early as a slight elevation of liver enzymes, or it may cause severe jaundice and hyperbilirubinemia. Hepatic dysfunction usually resolves on resolution of the sepsis, but if the inflammatory process persists, adjustments in the feeding formulation will be necessary. The carbohydrate load is usually reduced to consist of no more than 50% of metabolic requirements, and the additional calories should be provided as fat emulsion. The patient should be observed for the presence of encephalopathy; if this complication occurs, the protein load should also be reduced.

Cardiac Dysfunction

The myocardial dysfunction that occurs in sepsis may be secondary to the elaboration of cytokines such as TNF-α or IL-1, which have direct myocardial depressant activity, or the heart failure may be secondary to pulmonary insufficiency with an increased pulmonary vascular resistance and right ventricular overload. Malnourished patients with sepsis may be sensitive to volume overload, and use of a concentrated solution of hypertonic dextrose mixed with amino acids may be indicated to maximize calories and minimize volume. In addition, 20% fat emulsion can be administered to provide additional energy.

NUTRITION AND METABOLISM IN THE PATIENT WITH CANCER

Cachexia is especially common in patients with advanced malignant disease, and it has been shown to have a negative impact on outcome. Malnutrition is associated with increases in postoperative complications, including sepsis, ileus, and wound dehiscence, and it has been shown to have adverse effects on immune function and treatment tolerance. The rationale for providing nutritional support is to prevent or reverse host tissue wasting, broaden the spectrum of therapeutic options, improve the clinical course, and ultimately prolong patient survival.

The use of nutritional support in patients with cancer, especially the use of TPN, was initially heralded with enthusiasm. However, conflicting results from numerous subsequent clinical studies was the rule rather than the exception; this discrepancy was due to poor study design and the use of different end points to assess efficacy. Consequently, the enthusiasm has waned, accompanied by a more conservative approach to patient selection. Nonetheless, the role for nutritional support in the patient with cancer remains an important component of overall therapy.

Which Patients with Cancer Should Receive Specialized Nutritional Support?

If the patient has a functional gastrointestinal tract and can consume adequate calories by mouth, a regular hospital diet should be provided and no specialized nutritional support is necessary. In patients with head and neck cancers who have difficulty chewing or swallowing, a blenderized diet can be consumed orally or nutrition can be given through a soft nasogastric tube that is inserted into the stomach by the nasal or oral route. If the cancer obstructs the nasopharyngeal route such that tube passage is contraindicated, placement of a feeding gastrostomy or jejunostomy (in the operating room) is almost always well tolerated. Because it is anticipated that patients with head and neck cancer will continue to lose weight, such a feed-

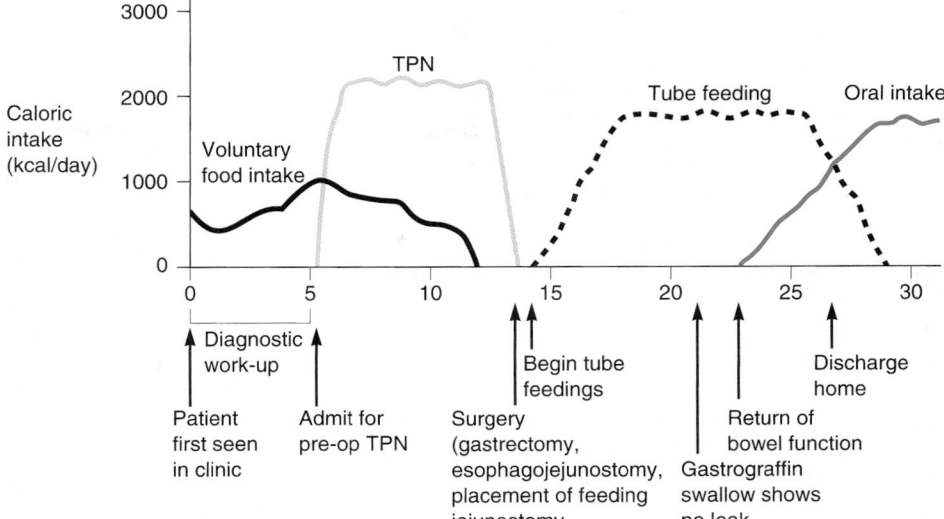

Figure 2.8. The use of total parenteral nutrition in a patient with cancer with an obstructing carcinoma of the stomach in whom preoperative enteral nutrition is contraindicated. The gastrointestinal tract should be used as soon as bowel function returns. Placement of a feeding jejunostomy at the time of surgery may be useful.

ing strategy should be initiated early, especially in those who will have prolonged radiation or chemotherapy.

Preoperative nutritional support should be given only to those patients who do not require an emergency operation and who have severe weight loss (>15% of preillness body weight) and a serum albumin less than 2.9 mg/dL. If the patient can tolerate preoperative tube feedings, this route of feeding is preferred as long as adequate calories and nitrogen can be delivered. For patients in whom this is not feasible (i.e., a patient with profound weight loss from an obstructing carcinoma of the stomach), admission to the hospital for administration of preoperative TPN (Fig. 2.8) has been shown to decrease the rate of postoperative complications. Preoperative nutrition (enteral or parenteral) should not be given for longer than 7 to 10 days. If it is anticipated that oral intake after surgery will be delayed for greater than 7 days, placement of a jejunal feeding tube at the time of surgery should be strongly considered, especially if the patient was malnourished before surgery.

Patients with gastrointestinal side effects from chemotherapy or radiation therapy (e.g., mucositis, crampy pain, nausea, and diarrhea) may feed by the enteral route, although voluntary intake is likely to be diminished. Such patients can tolerate 5 to 7 days of inadequate nutrition, especially if they were previously well nourished. If the side effects are severe, resulting in a longer period of gastrointestinal toxicity, the use of TPN should be considered. The use of TPN for patients receiving bone marrow transplantation has been shown to be a valuable component of overall care.

Enteral Nutrition in Patients with Cancer

Enteral nutrition is always the preferred route of feeding any patient, including those with cancer, if the gastrointestinal tract is functional. This can be accomplished by using between-meal supplements, by inserting soft, comfortable nasogastric feeding tubes, or by inserting gastrostomy or jejunostomy feeding catheters. Infusing nutrients into the gastrointestinal tract (as opposed to intravenously) allows them to be processed and absorbed in a normal physiologic fashion. There are several benefits of using the bowel lumen for nutrient delivery. The trophic effects of enteral feeding on the small bowel mucosa have been well

described. The integrity of the mucosal lining is maintained and may provide an effective barrier to intraluminal enteric organisms that might otherwise be absorbed into the systemic circulation. Atrophic changes may be seen in the intestinal epithelium after several days of bowel rest; this atrophy is not reversed by currently available TPN solutions. Newer enteral diets contain pharmacologic amounts of gut-specific nutrients such as glutamine, a conditionally essential amino acid that is required for intestinal function.

Total Parenteral Nutrition in Patients with Cancer

Numerous clinical trials have failed to yield a consensus with regard to the efficacy of TPN in patients with cancer. However, several prospective studies have helped to clarify both the indications for and contraindications to the use of TPN in the surgical patient with cancer. The 1991 multicenter Veterans Affairs Total Parenteral Nutrition Cooperative Study demonstrated that preoperative TPN is beneficial in surgical patients (many of whom had cancer) with severe preoperative malnutrition (13). However, TPN was not effective in patients who were minimally or moderately malnourished. Brennan and colleagues (14) examined the use of routine postoperative TPN after major pancreatic resection. In patients randomized to receive TPN starting on postoperative day 1, the investigators found a statistically significant increase in the incidence of intraabdominal abscesses as well as a tendency toward an increased incidence of peritonitis and bowel obstruction. The control group received a standard peripheral infusion of dextrose, suggesting that the increase in complications was not due to the absence of luminal nutrients but rather to some toxic effect of the TPN. The authors concluded that routine use of postoperative TPN was not indicated and may in fact have harmful side effects after pancreatic resection. Many surgeons would elect to place a feeding jejunostomy in such patients.

In contrast to the Brennan study, Fan and colleagues (15) studied the use of perioperative (starting 7 days before the planned procedure) TPN for patients undergoing hepatectomy for hepatocellular carcinoma. They found that patients randomized to receive perioperative TPN had a statistically significant reduction in infectious complications and a decreased diuretic requirement compared with similar patients who did not receive TPN. The significance of this study is that it is only one of two studies showing a benefit to the use of routine perioperative TPN for patients who did not have severe malnutrition. In addition, it establishes a select group of patients in whom routine perioperative TPN may be of benefit.

As a general rule, the most important factor to consider when making decisions about the use of TPN for patients with cancer is the response of the tumor to antineoplastic therapy. The following guidelines will undergo future revision as more effective antitumor regimens become clinically available.

TPN for relatively short hospital stays of 7 to 14 days

TPN is not indicated in well-nourished or mildly malnourished patients undergoing chemotherapy, radiation therapy, or surgery. Such patients can usually consume some nutrition enterally and can tolerate short periods (up to 7 days) of inadequate intake.

TPN is not indicated for patients with rapidly progressive malignant disease who fail to respond to treatment. Such patients are terminal and should not receive TPN.

TPN is indicated in severely malnourished patients, or those in whom gastrointestinal or other toxicities preclude adequate enteral intake for 7 days or longer. Available evidence suggests that patients who are candidates for TPN under these circumstances should, when feasible, receive TPN before or in conjunction with the institution of therapy.

Lengthy periods of in-hospital TPN (>2 weeks) or home TPN

TPN is not indicated for patients with rapidly progressive tumor growth unresponsive to therapy. Such patients are terminal.

TPN is indicated in those patients for whom treatment-associated toxicities preclude the use of enteral nutrition and represent the primary impediment to the restoration of performance status. Such patients usually respond to antitumor therapy.

TPN is indicated in selected malnourished patients with cancer where the natural history of the disease can be expected to permit a period of normal or near-normal performance status. Such patients should be receiving antitumor therapy with a reasonable anticipation of response, or the natural history of the untreated tumor should be such that a reasonable quality of life can be expected.

CHOICE OF NUTRITION IN SURGICAL PATIENTS: ENTERAL OR PARENTERAL?

Although the physiologic advantage of enteral nutrition is apparent, preoperative nutritional repletion by the enteral route has not been as extensively studied as preoperative TPN. Although its use can be associated with the development of nausea, diarrhea, and distention, we recommend the use of enteral nutrition (through a feedings tube or as between-meal supplements) in malnourished patients if it is feasible. Candidates must have a functional gastrointestinal tract and must be able to receive adequate amounts of calories and nitrogen. In many critically ill patients, enteral nutrition-related gastrointestinal complications are high and associated with decreased nutrient intake from the ordered levels (16,17).

Total Parenteral Nutrition as Primary Therapy

Patients with Enterocutaneous Fistulae

Patients with gastrointestinal–cutaneous fistulae represent the classic indication for TPN. In such patients, oral intake of food almost invariably results in increased fistula output, which can lead to metabolic disturbances, dehydration, and death. Several comprehensive reviews have concluded that TPN clearly affects the treatment and course of disease for patients with gastrointestinal fistulae. The following conclusions can be drawn from studies evaluating the use of TPN in patients with enterocutaneous fistulae: (a) TPN increases the spontaneous closure rate of enterocutaneous fistulae, but does not markedly decrease the mortality rate in patients with fistulae (improvements in mortality are mainly due to improved surgical and metabolic care); (b) if spontaneous closure of the fistula does not occur, patients are better prepared for operative intervention because of the nutritional support they received; and (c) certain fistulae (radiated bowel) are associated with a higher failure rate of closure than others, and should be treated more aggressively surgically after a defined period of nutritional support (unless closure occurs).

Patients with Short Bowel Syndrome

Prospective, randomized trials designed specifically to examine the impact of TPN on patients with short bowel syndrome have not been initiated, mainly because such patients have no choice but to receive TPN. Most of these patients, who would have certainly died before the availability of TPN, now survive for long periods on home parenteral nutrition. In selected patients with residual small intestine (at least 18 inches), postresectional hyperplasia may develop with time such that they can tolerate enteral feedings. Studies by Wilmore and colleagues (18) have demonstrated that the requirement for TPN could be decreased or even eliminated in patients with short gut syndrome by providing a nutritional regimen consisting of supplemental glutamine, growth hormone, and a modified high-carbohydrate, low-fat diet. There was a marked improvement in the absorption of nutrients with this combination therapy and a decrease in stool output. In addition, TPN requirements were reduced by 50%, as were the costs associated with care of these patients. Discontinuation of the growth hormone did not increase TPN needs in these patients once they had undergone successful gut rehabilitation.

Patients with Hepatic Failure

Patients with liver disease usually are malnourished because of excessive alcohol intake and diminished food intake. These patients are protein depleted yet intolerant of protein because of their tendency to become encephalopathic with a high nitrogen intake. Because of liver damage and portosystemic shunting, derangements in circulating levels of amino acids develop in these patients. The plasma aromatic/branched-chain amino acid ratio is increased, favoring the transport of aromatic amino acids across the blood–brain barrier. These amino acids are precursors of false neurotransmitters that contribute to lethargy and encephalopathy. Treatment of patients with liver failure with solutions enriched in branched-chain amino acids and deficient in aromatic amino acids results in improved tolerance to the administered protein and clinical improvement in the encephalopathic state.

Patients with Major Thermal Injury

Aggressive nutritional support in patients with major burns seems to be associated with improved survival, particularly when increased amounts of dietary protein are provided (19). Burned patients often require ventilatory support or have ileus that prevents using the gastrointestinal tract for feeding. Even if the gastrointestinal tract is usable, such patients are often unable to eat enough because of frequent trips to the operating room combined with the anorexia of severe injury. Most burn authorities believe that aggressive nutritional support in patients with major thermal injury has influenced outcome in a positive manner.

Patients with Acute Renal Failure

Total parenteral nutrition with amino acids of high biologic value may decrease the mortality rate in patients with acute renal failure (20). The use of solutions containing high-quality amino acids can improve nitrogen balance and diminish urea production. It is thought that provision only of essential amino acids allows the body maximally to reuse nitrogen for the synthesis of nonessential amino acids and thereby helps prevent rapid rises in BUN. This translates into a decreased frequency of dialysis. However, there is no advantage and, in fact, there is a cost disadvantage to using essential amino acid solutions if the patient is already being dialyzed every other day. Therefore, a balanced standard amino acid formulation is recommended.

Total Parenteral Nutrition as Secondary Therapy

Prolonged Ileus after Operative Procedure

Occasionally patients have a prolonged ileus after an abdominal procedure that precludes the use of the intestinal tract as a route of feeding. Such an occurrence usually is unpredictable and the cause of the ileus often is not demonstrated. If the patient is unable to eat by the seventh postoperative day, TPN should be started. The ileus may persist for several weeks. Although provision of TPN does not influence the disease process *per se*, it is beneficial because it prevents further erosion of lean body mass.

Acute Radiation and Chemotherapy Enteritis

In malnourished patients who receive abdominal or pelvic radiation or chemotherapy, mucositis and enterocolitis may develop that preclude using the gastrointestinal tract for prolonged periods. In such patients, TPN should be provided until the enteritis resolves and oral feeding can be resumed.

Preoperative Total Parenteral Nutrition in the Perioperative Setting

In general, the use of perioperative nutrition (particularly parenteral feedings) cannot be justified unless a clear benefit to the patient can be demonstrated. The results of prospective, randomized trials evaluating the efficacy of preoperative TPN are conflicting because of the variations in the nutritional status of patients studied, the differences in types of diseases in these malnourished patients, the differences in the type and length of nutritional support administered, and the failure to accrue enough patients to avoid type II statistical error. The following questions are important to consider: Does preoperative nutritional support decrease the morbidity and mortality associated with major operative procedures? How long should nutritional support be administered? What type of nutritional repletion should be administered?

One of the best studies to date evaluating the efficacy of preoperative TPN was published by the Veterans Affairs Total Parenteral Nutrition Cooperative Study Group (13). More than 3,500 patients requiring mainly elective ab-

dominal surgery were entered into this prospective, randomized trial. They were initially screened for evidence of malnutrition using subjective criteria or by determining their Nutritional Risk Index Score, which included objective criteria such as percentage weight loss and serum albumin level. The patients were further divided into categories assigning them to one of four groups: well nourished, borderline malnourished, moderately malnourished, or severely malnourished. Patients in each malnourished category were randomized to receive at least 7 days of preoperative TPN or to proceed with surgery without preoperative TPN. Patients randomized to receive TPN received 1,000 kcal/d in excess of calculated caloric requirements. Lipid was provided on a daily basis. One criticism of this study was that patients were allowed to eat in addition to receiving parenteral feedings.

Analysis of the data from this study indicated that there was no difference in short-term or long-term complications between groups. Infectious complications, including pneumonia, abscess, and line sepsis, were statistically significantly higher for patients receiving TPN. Noninfectious complications (impaired wound healing) were significantly lower only in those patients receiving TPN who were in the severely malnourished group (>15% weight loss and serum albumin <2.9 mg/dL). This study strongly suggests that preoperative TPN should be provided only to severely malnourished patients who cannot be nourished by the enteral route. Contraindications to the use of preoperative TPN include patients requiring emergency surgery and those who are only mildly or moderately malnourished. In such patients, TPN should be continued after surgery only if the gastrointestinal tract cannot be used for tube feedings. Nasojejunal or jejunostomy tubes should also be considered in patients undergoing major upper abdominal procedures in whom it is anticipated that oral feedings may not be resumed for 7 to 10 days after surgery.

Composition of Total Parenteral Nutrition Formulations

Total parenteral nutrition solutions are administered through a central venous catheter usually inserted into the subclavian vein (Fig. 2.9). The composition of a standard TPN solution is shown in Table 2.7. Because of the hyperosmolarity of such solutions, they must be delivered into a high-flow system to prevent venous sclerosis. Patients receiving TPN should be monitored regularly by measuring blood sugar, serum electrolytes, and liver function tests. Elevations in serum glucose are common in surgical patients receiving TPN, especially if the patient is stressed and is relatively glucose intolerant. Hyperglycemia usually can be controlled by adding insulin to the TPN formulation or by decreasing the amount of glucose in the solution. It has been shown that injured humans can maximally oxidize approximately 5 to 6 mg of glucose/kg/min. For a 70-kg man, this is equal to approximately 500 to 600 g/d (2,000 to 2,400 kcal/d). Glucose calories in excess of this amount are converted to fat or result in hyperglycemia and glycosuria. The amounts of the various electrolytes that are provided to patients receiving TPN vary depending on factors such as previous nutritional and hydration status. Careful monitoring is critical because as new cell mass is accrued, the intracellular ions potassium and phosphate may accumulate, leading to severe hypokalemia or hypophosphatemia. These electrolyte disturbances can develop rapidly and are much more life threatening than hyponatremia. Vitamin (Table 2.8) and trace mineral (Table 2.9) requirements must also be taken into consideration.

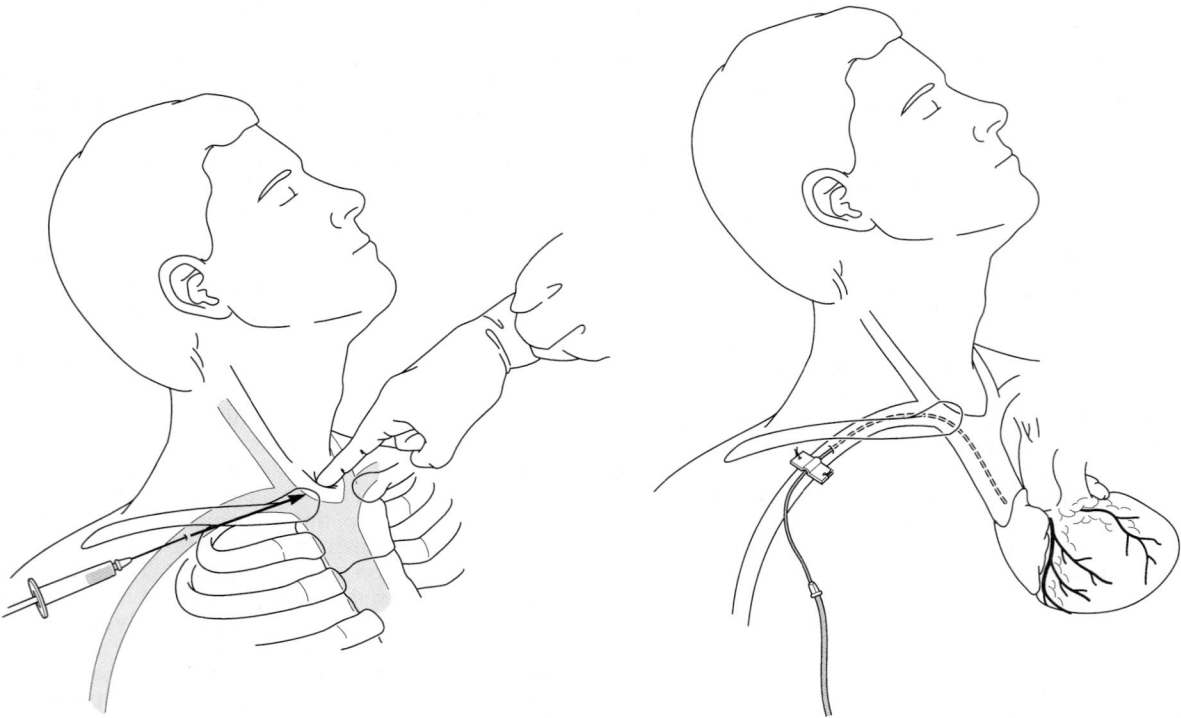

Figure 2.9. Technique for insertion of a subclavian catheter (see text for details).

The use of lipids in TPN was developed to meet the requirement for linoleic acid and the full caloric needs in hypermetabolic patients, in recognition of the complications associated with infusing large amounts of dextrose. Intravenous fat emulsions consist of soy or safflower oils (vegetable fat emulsions) that contain primarily long-chain triglycerides composed of fatty acids with 16- and 18-carbon chain lengths. The provision of fat provides essential linoleic acid, inhibits lipogenesis from carbohy-

drates, and lowers the RQ, which may benefit patients with respiratory compromise. However, the high content of ω-6 polyunsaturated fatty acids (especially linoleic acid) in these emulsions may have harmful effects. Linoleic acid is a precursor for the synthesis of various prostaglandins and leukotrienes, which can cause immunosuppression and suppress cytokine activity. Standard intravenous fat emulsions may alter the cell membrane phospholipid composition of cells of the

Table 2.7. COMPOSITION OF A STANDARD CENTRAL VENOUS SOLUTION

VOLUME

10% Amino acid solution	500 mL
50% Dextrose solution	500 mL
Fat emulsion	—
Electrolytes + vitamins + minerals	~50 mL
Total volume	~1,050 mL

COMPOSITION

Amino acids	50 g
Dextrose	250 g
Total N	50/6.25 = 8 g
Dextrose kcal	250 g × 3.4 kcal/g = 840 kcal
mOsm/L	2000

ELECTROLYTES ADDED TO TPN SOLUTIONS

	Usual concentration	Range of concentrations
Sodium (mEq/L)	60	0–150
Potassium (mEq/L)	40	0–80
Acetate (mEq/L)	50	50–150
Chloride (mEq/L)	50	0–150
Phosphate (mEq/L)	15	0–30
Calcium (mEq/L)[a]	4.5	0–20
Magnesium (mEq/L)	5	5–15

[a]Usually added as calcium gluconate or calcium chloride; one ampule of calcium gluconate = 1 g of calcium = 4.5 mEq.
TPN, total parenteral nutrition.

Table 2.8. VITAMIN REQUIREMENTS

Vitamin	Unit	Recommended dietary allowance for daily oral intake	Daily requirement of the moderately injured	Daily requirement of the severely injured	Amount provided by one vitamin pill	Daily amount provided by standard intravenous preparations
Vitamin A (retinol)	IU	1,760 (women)–3,300 (men)	5,000	5,000	10,000	3,300 (retinol)
Vitamin D (ergocalciferol)	IU	200	400	400	400	200
Vitamin E (tocopherol)	mg TE	8–10	Unknown	Unknown	15	10[a]
Vitamin K (phylloquinone)	µg	20–40[b]	20	20	0	0[c]
Vitamin C (ascorbic acid)	µg	60	75	300	100	100
Thiamine (vitamin B_1)	µg	1.0–1.5	2	10	10	3.0
Riboflavin (vitamin B_2)	µg	1.2–1.7	2	10	10	3.6
Niacin	mg	13–19	20	100	100	40
Pyridoxine (vitamin B_6)	µg	2.0–2.2	2	40	5	4.0
Pantothenic acid	mg	4–7 (adults)[b]	18	40	20	15
Folic acid	mg	0.4	1.5	2.5	0	0.4
Vitamin B_{12}	mg	3.0	2	4	5	5
Biotin	mg	100–200[b]	Unknown	Unknown	0	60

[a]Equivalent to recommended dietary allowance.
[b]Estimated to be safe and adequate in dietary intakes.
[c]Must be supplemented in peripheral venous solutions.
From Rombeau JL, Rolandelli RH. Nutritional support. In: Wilmore DW, Brennan MF, Harken RH, et al., eds. Care of the surgical patient: II. Care in the ICU. New York: Scientific American Medicine, 1989:6.

reticuloendothelial system, resulting in changes in membrane fluidity such that clearance of bacteria and toxins is impaired. In addition, ω-6 polyunsaturated fatty acids may alter the local production of cytokines such that chemotaxis is negatively impacted. Newer nutritional methods of modifying the catabolic response to injury and infection propose the use of the ω-3 fatty acids, which may decrease eicosanoid biosynthesis and thereby diminish the vasoconstriction, platelet aggregation, and immunosuppression that may occur when ω-6 derivatives are administered. Studies suggest that ω-3 fatty acids may be of benefit to the critically ill patient. The ω-3 fatty acids have been added to enteral formulas, but are not in parenteral formulas yet.

Fat is an important fuel source for critically ill patients. The septic and injured human seems preferentially to use endogenous fat as an energy source, which appears to be related in part to the effects of counterregulatory hormones on stimulating fat mobilization. These patients have a relative unresponsiveness to the administration of carbohydrates in that free fatty acid mobilization is only marginally decreased and free fatty acid oxidation is not suppressed as in "pure starvation." Despite glucose infusion above energy expenditure, a hormonal milieu is maintained that favors fat mobilization and oxidation.

Potential Complications of Total Parenteral Nutrition

Advances in technology, monitoring, and catheter care have greatly reduced the incidence of complications associated with the use of TPN. The establishment of a nutrition support team (physician, dietitian, nurse, pharmacist) and the recognition of such a team as an important part of overall patient care has also been a key factor in reducing complications. Complications of TPN occur and can be divided into three types: mechanical, metabolic, and infectious (Table 2.10). The management of the patient who becomes septic while receiving TPN is shown in Fig. 2.10.

Effects of Total Parenteral Nutrition on the Gastrointestinal Tract

Most studies that have examined the effects of TPN on intestinal function and immunity have been done in animals. These studies clearly demonstrate that TPN poses risks related to intestinal disuse. A unique feature of TPN is that subjects can remain on prolonged bowel rest without concomitant malnutrition, thereby facilitating the study of intestinal disuse as an independent variable. In rats, TPN results in significant disruption of the intestinal

Table 2.9. MINERAL AND TRACE ELEMENT REQUIREMENTS

Mineral	Recommended dietary allowance for daily oral intake (mg)	Suggested daily intravenous intake (mg)	Daily amount provided by a commercially available mixture (mg)
Zinc	15	2.5–5.0[a]	5.0
Copper	2–3[b]	0.5–1.5	1.0
Manganese	2.5–5.0[b]	0.15–0.8	0.5
Chromium	0.05–0.2[b]	0.01–0.015	0.1
Iron	8 (women)–10 (men)	3	—

[a]Burn patients require an additional 2 mg.
[b]Estimated to be safe and adequate in dietary intakes.
From Rombeau JL, Rolandelli RH. Nutritional support. In: Wilmore DW, Brennan MF, Harken RH, et al., eds. Care of the surgical patient: II. Care in the ICU. New York: Scientific American Medicine, 1989:6.

TABLE 2.10. COMPLICATIONS ASSOCIATED WITH THE USE OF TOTAL PARENTERAL NUTRITION

Complication	Cause	Treatment
MECHANICAL		
Pneumothorax	Puncture/laceration of lung pleura	Serial chest radiographs; chest tube if indicated
Subclavian artery injury	Penetration of subclavian artery during needle stick	Chest radiographs; serial monitoring of vital signs
Air embolism	Aspiration of air into the subclavian vein and right heart	Place patient in Trendelenburg and left lateral decubitus; aspirate air
Catheter embolization	Shearing off the tip when withdrawing catheter	Retrieve catheter transvenously under fluoroscopic guidance
Venous thrombosis	Clot formation in great vein secondary to catheter	Heparinization if clinically significant
Catheter malposition	Tip of catheter directed into internal jugular or opposite subclavian vein	Reposition under fluoroscopy
METABOLIC		
Hyperglycemia	Excessive glucose calories or glucose intolerance	Decrease glucose calories; administer insulin
Hypoglycemia	Sudden cessation of TPN	Bolus 50% glucose solution; monitor blood glucose
Carbon dioxide retention	Infusion of glucose calories in excess of energy needs	Decrease glucose calories and replace with fat
Hyperglycemic, hyperosmolar nonketotic coma (HHNC)	Dehydration from excessive diuresis	Discontinue TPN immediately; give insulin; monitor glucose/electrolytes
Hyperchloremic metabolic acidosis	Excessive chloride administration	Give Na and K as acetate salts
Azotemia	Excessive amino acid administration with inadequate calories	Decrease amino acids; increase glucose calories
Essential fatty acid deficiency	Inadequate essential fatty acid administration	Administer fat solution
Hypertriglyceridemia	Rapid fat infusion of decreased fat clearance	Slow rate of fat infusion
Hypophosphatemia	Inadequate administration of electrolyte in question	Increase administration
Hypocalcemia		
Hypomagnesemia		
Hypokalemia		
Bleeding	Vitamin K deficiency	Administer vitamin K
INFECTIOUS		
Line sepsis	Cather tip infected	Remove catheter; antibiotics
Infection at skin site	Bacteria at site of catheter entry into skin	Remove catheter; local wound care

TPN, total parenteral nutrition.

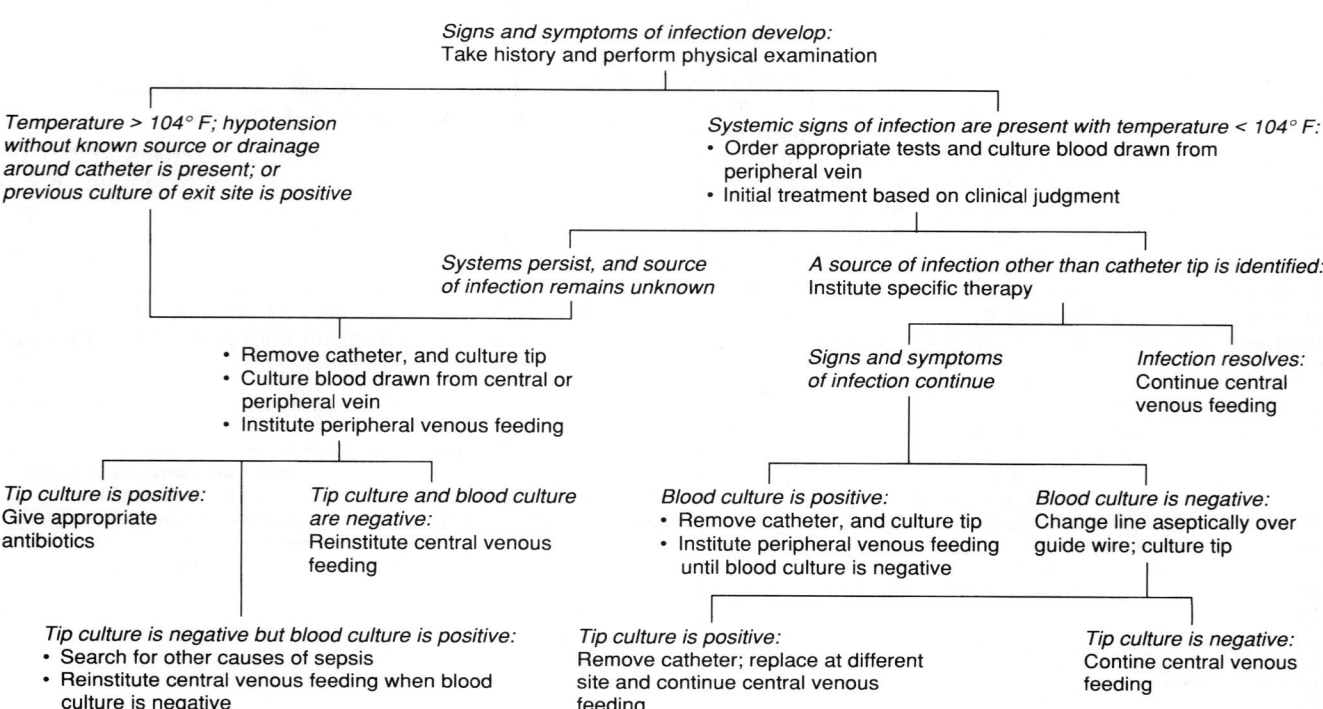

Figure 2.10. Management of the patient on total parenteral nutrition who becomes septic.

microflora, with bacterial translocation from the gut lumen to the mesenteric lymph nodes. In addition, when stresses such as burn injury, chemotherapy, or radiation are introduced in these models, animals on TPN have a much higher mortality rate. This body of literature suggests that TPN, under certain circumstances, may predispose patients to an increase in gut-derived infectious complications (21).

A provocative study in human volunteers demonstrated that people receiving TPN had an accentuated systemic response to endotoxin challenge compared with enterally fed volunteers (22). The study is consistent with an impairment in gut barrier function during parenteral feedings that may promote the release of bacteria or cytokines, leading to pronounced systemic responses and possibly multiple organ failure.

NUTRITIONAL SUPPORT OF THE GUT IN CRITICALLY ILL PATIENTS

The intestinal tract has long been considered an organ of inactivity after operation or injury. Ileus usually is present, nasogastric decompression is often necessary, and the gut is usually unused in the immediate postoperative period. In the past, digestion and absorption was thought to be the only physiologic role of the gut. Disuse of the intestine, either through starvation or nutritional support by TPN, may lead to numerous physiologic derangements as well as changes in gut microflora, impaired gut immune function, and disruption of the integrity of the mucosal barrier. Thus, maintaining gut function in the perioperative period may be essential to minimize septic complications and organ failure.

Treatment strategies designed to support the gut during critical illness should be directed toward the provision of appropriate nutrition and maintenance of mucosal structure and function. Presumably, such efforts assist the gut in its role as a metabolic processing station and as a barrier.

Enteral Feeding

Enteral feedings are probably the best single method of maintaining mucosal structure and function. The trophic effects of luminal nutrition are crucial, and the beneficial effects are well documented even if relatively small amounts of nutrients are provided.

Gut-specific Nutrients

It is now clear that the composition of the diet as well as the route of delivery plays an important role in maintaining gut structure and function. Several gut-specific nutrients have been studied, but glutamine has received the most attention. Glutamine has been classified as a nonessential or nutritionally dispensable amino acid. Because this categorization implies that glutamine can be synthesized in adequate quantities from other amino acids and precursors, it has not been considered necessary to include glutamine in nutritional formulas. It has been eliminated from TPN solutions because of its relative instability and short shelf life compared with other amino acids. With few exceptions, glutamine is present in oral and enteral diets only at the relatively low levels characteristic of its concentration in most animal and plant proteins (approximately 7% of total amino acids).

Several studies, however, have demonstrated that glutamine may be a conditionally essential amino acid during critical illness, particularly as it relates to supporting the metabolic requirements of the intestinal mucosa. In general, these studies demonstrate that dietary glutamine is not required during states of health, but appears to be beneficial when glutamine depletion is severe or when the intestinal mucosa is damaged by insults such as chemotherapy and radiation therapy. Addition of glutamine to enteral diets reduces the incidence of gut translocation, but these improvements depend on the amount of supplemental glutamine and the type of insult studied. Glutamine-enriched TPN partially attenuates the villous atrophy that develops during parenteral nutrition. The use of intravenous glutamine in humans appears to be safe and effective and it has been shown to diminish complications and reduce hospital stay (23,24).

In contrast to glutamine, short-chain fatty acids are the primary energy source for colonocytes. Diets enriched in short-chain fatty acids have been shown to increase colonic DNA content and mucosal morphometrics as well as strengthen colonic anastomoses in rats.

Use of Growth Factors to Support the Gut Mucosa

Specific growth factors that may promote intestinal mucosal growth have been implicated in a number of physiologic processes, including growth, tissue repair, and regeneration. Among these is epidermal growth factor, a polypeptide secreted by submaxillary glands and by Brunner's glands of the small intestine. The most widespread effect of epidermal growth factor on the gastrointestinal mucosa is the overall stimulation of DNA synthesis as evidenced by thymidine incorporation.

OTHER METHODS OF MODIFYING THE CATABOLIC RESPONSE TO SURGERY AND CRITICAL ILLNESS

Besides nutritional intervention, several other methods of modifying the physiologic and biochemical responses to an elective operative procedure have been studied in an effort to reduce the magnitude of the stress of operations and to provide insight into mechanisms in these responses. Studies suggest that regional anesthetic techniques block afferent signals from the wound and interrupt sympathetic nervous efferent signals to the adrenal gland and possibly the liver. The effect of sympathetic blockade is a reduction in the apparent magnitude of the stress response. Others have studied stress responses in sympathectomized animals by blocking the efferent limb of the neuroendocrine reflex response. These reports indicate that central nervous system blockade interrupts afferent signals stimulated by operative procedures.

More recent studies have documented the safety and efficacy of long-term exogenous recombinant growth hormone administration (25). Growth hormone stimulates protein synthesis during hypocaloric feedings and increases retention of sodium and potassium by the kidney. The potential synergistic effects of specialized nutrition in combination with growth hormone require further study. Cyclooxygenase inhibitors such as aspirin and ibuprofen attenuate the symptoms and endocrine responses that occur with critical illness without altering cytokine elaboration. It is anticipated that researchers will eventually be able selectively to block the deleterious effects of excessive cytokines and preserve their beneficial effects.

TECHNIQUES OF NUTRITIONAL SUPPORT

Transnasal (Nasogastric and Nasoduodenal) Feeding Catheters

The use of transnasal feeding catheters for intragastric feeding or for duodenal intubation is a popular adjunct for providing nutritional support by the enteral route. The stomach is easily accessed by the passage of a soft, flexible feeding tube. Intragastric feedings provide several advantages for the patient. The stomach has the capacity and reservoir for bolus feedings. Feeding into the stomach results in the stimulation of biliary/pancreatic axis, which is probably trophic for the small bowel, and gastric secretions has a dilutional effect on the osmolarity of the feedings, reducing the risk of diarrhea. The major risk of intragastric feeding is the regurgitation of gastric contents and their aspiration into the tracheobronchial tree. This risk is highest for patients who have an altered mental sensorium or are paralyzed.

The placement of the feeding tube through the pylorus into the fourth portion of the duodenum reduces the risk of regurgitation and aspiration of feeding formulas. To place a transnasal intraduodenal feeding catheter, the patient should be in the sitting position with the neck slightly flexed. This allows for the passage of a lubricated 8-French polyurethane feeding catheter (with a stylet in place) through the patient's nose in a posterior and inferior direction, bringing the catheter to the level of the pharynx. The head is brought back to a neutral position and the patient is instructed to swallow while the feeding catheter is passed into the esophageal lumen. The advancement of the catheter is continued for a distance of approximately 45 to 50 cm. The stylet is removed and the position of the catheter is confirmed radiographically before the initiation of feedings. Tubes can be positioned fluoroscopically if necessary. The patient who frequently removes the feeding catheter may be a candidate for a feeding tube bridle (Fig. 2.11).

A variety of enteral formulas are commercially available and can be adjusted for calorie, nitrogen, or fiber content.

Technique of Gastrostomy Placement

A feeding gastrostomy should be considered for patients requiring long-term enteral nutrition and in patients with obstruction of the esophagus or locally advanced head and neck cancers that preclude eating. A temporary Stamm gastrostomy is a popular method for access to the gastric lumen and can be performed at the time of any major abdominal procedure. A circular pursestring suture (3-0 silk) with a 1.5-cm diameter is placed in the body of the anterior wall of the stomach. The ideal location is in the midportion of the stomach closer to the greater curvature in a relatively avascular site. A second circular pursestring suture is then placed outside the first one. The feeding catheter is then brought through the abdominal wall (left upper quadrant). Using the electrocautery, a stab wound is made in the anterior portion of the stomach directly in the center of the concentric pursestring sutures. The feeding catheter is introduced into the gastric lumen and the inner concentric suture is secured in place. The second pursestring is then secured, inverting the gastric mucosa completely. The stomach is drawn upward toward the anterior abdominal wall. Placement of Lembert silk sutures in all four quadrants around the catheter secures the stomach to the anterior abdominal wall. The catheter is then secured to the skin by placement of sutures at the base of the catheter exit site.

Technique of Percutaneous Endoscopic Gastrostomy

Percutaneous endoscopic gastrostomy (PEG) to provide access for gastric feedings can be performed without laparotomy or general anesthesia. Using intravenous sedation and topical anesthetic, a gastroscope is passed through the mouth and the esophagus into the stomach, which is inflated. The light from the gastroscope is then transilluminated through the anterior abdominal wall in the epigastrium or left subcostal area. The abdomen is prepared and draped and a wheal of local anesthetic is injected at the area of transillumination. A 1-cm vertical incision is made and an angiocatheter or needle is inserted through the abdominal wall into the stomach under the direct vision of the gastroscope. A wire loop is passed through the catheter into the stomach and grasped with a snare passed through the gastroscope. The gastroscope and wire loop are withdrawn through the mouth and the wire is looped through a corresponding wire on the end of the PEG tube. By pulling the wire out through the abdominal wall, the PEG tube is pulled in through the mouth and out the anterior abdomen while followed through the esophagus by the gastroscope. The gastroscope then visualizes the inner part of the PEG tube to ensure it seats properly against the stomach wall. The tube protruding through the abdominal wall is attached securely at the exit site to prevent accidental dislodgment. The tube can later be removed with just a hard pull.

Technique of Feeding Catheter Jejunostomy Placement and Witzel Jejunostomy

A feeding catheter jejunostomy should be considered after any major upper abdominal procedure if prolonged

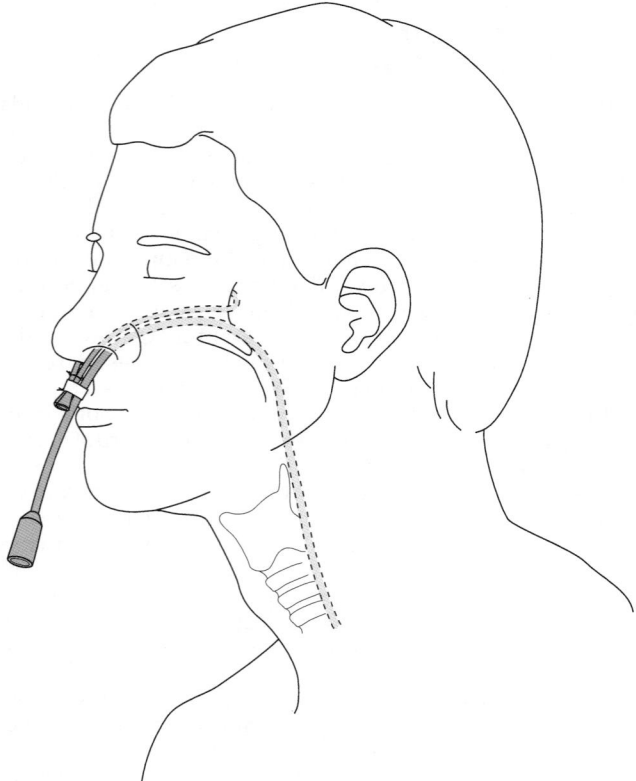

Figure 2.11. Use of a feeding tube bridle for patients who are prone to extubate the feeding catheter.

enteral nutrition support is anticipated. The simplest method is a needle jejunostomy performed fairly quickly at the end of the definitive operation. A 14- or 16-gauge needle is used to create a tunnel subserosally at approximately 30 to 40 cm distal to the ligament of Treitz, and then the needle tip is introduced into the jejunal lumen. A feeding catheter is inserted through the needle and advanced 30 to 40 cm distally into the bowel lumen to the desired location, and the needle is then withdrawn. The loop of jejunum is then anchored to the parietal peritoneum with permanent sutures, and the catheter is secured to the skin with nylon sutures.

A feeding jejunostomy can also be performed using the Witzel technique. A loop of proximal jejunum 20 to 30 cm from the ligament of Treitz is delivered into the wound. A pursestring suture is placed on the antimesenteric border of the bowel and an incision is made with electrocautery in the intestinal wall in the center of the pursestring suture. A red rubber catheter (14 French) is inserted into the lumen of the jejunum and advanced distally. The pursestring suture is secured in place, and a serosal tunnel is then constructed by placing 000 silk sutures from the catheter's exit site extending 5 to 6 cm proximally. The catheter is then delivered through the abdominal wall through a separate stab incision. The adjacent loop of intestine is anchored with two 000 silk sutures spread over 2 to 3 cm to prevent twisting of the loop and possible obstruction. The catheter is secured to the skin with a 3-0 nylon suture. Jejunal feeding catheters can be used immediately for feeding purposes after the operation.

Peripheral Intravenous Feedings

Peripheral veins may be used for infusion of glucose, amino acid solutions, and fat emulsions. However, these solutions must be nearly isotonic to avoid peripheral vein sclerosis. Ten percent glucose solutions may be used to increase the efficacy of amino acid utilization. Fat emulsions can be administered simultaneously with glucose and amino acid solutions because they provide an efficient fuel source and are isotonic. The major disadvantage of these peripherally administered mixtures is limited caloric delivery to meet catabolic demands within tolerated fluid volumes. Indications for peripheral vein feeding include the following: (a) as a supplement when enteral feedings can be only partially tolerated because of gastrointestinal dysfunction; (2) as a method of nutritional support when the gastrointestinal tract must be kept relatively empty for short periods during diagnostic work-up; and (3) as preliminary feedings before subclavian catheter insertion in patients requiring TPN.

Technique of Central Venous Catheter Placement

The preferred method of access to the superior vena cava is by percutaneous cannulation of the subclavian vein (Fig. 2.8). Alternate sites include the jugular approach, but the catheter exiting in the neck region makes it more difficult to secure the dressing site and maintain sterility.

A person who is experienced in the technique should perform the placement of a central venous catheter. To reduce the risk of bleeding complications, patients with a platelet count below 50,000 should receive fresh platelets before catheter insertion. The procedure is performed using aseptic technique; the surgeon should wear a hat, mask, gown, and gloves. The procedure can take place in the operating room or in the patient's room if there is adequate lighting and assistance. An environment should be created to minimize patient anxiety, and informed consent must be obtained. The patient is placed in the Trendelenburg position with both arms at the sides and the head turned away from the site of insertion. The chest is shaved, prepared, and draped in a sterile fashion. Local anesthesia is infiltrated near the insertion site and the underlying tissues along the inferior border of the clavicle. The tip of the needle is inserted into the skin and subcutaneous tissues at the midpoint of the clavicle, aiming for the suprasternal notch.

The needle is directed parallel to the patient's bed, inserting beneath the clavicle and at all times with negative pressure applied to the syringe. The prompt inflow of blood into the syringe indicates entrance into the subclavian vein, and the needle is advanced a few millimeters to ensure the bevel is within the lumen of the vessel. The patient is instructed to perform a Valsalva maneuver to prevent an air embolism, the syringe is disconnected from the needle and the guide wire is passed through the needle lumen, and the needle is then withdrawn over the guide wire. The passage of the wire through the needle should meet with minimal resistance, and the needle should be removed only after 15 cm of the wire has been passed into the vessel. A small incision is made at the guide wire exit site and a dilator is passed over the wire. The dilator is then removed over the wire and is replaced by the catheter, which is fully advanced. The wire is withdrawn and the catheter is flushed with sterile saline. The catheter is then sutured into position, the insertion site cleaned, and a sterile dressing placed. A portable chest radiograph is done to confirm placement of the catheter and rule out pneumothorax.

Complications from long-term central venous catheterization include venous thrombosis and catheter-related infections. Thrombosis of the central vessels is a complication that is often overlooked. The rate of clinical suspicion for subclavian vein thrombosis is only approximately 3%, whereas studies that use phlebography or radionuclide venography indicate that the incidence is as high as 35%. Febrile episodes are not uncommon in the cancer population, particularly in the neutropenic patient. If primary catheter sepsis is confirmed, the catheter must be removed immediately and the tip cultured.

NUTRITION SUPPORT AND HEALTH CARE REFORM

Health care reform is forcing hospitals to begin to scrutinize expensive therapies such as nutrition support and the personnel involved in delivering them (26). Nutrition support teams are now considered a cost center rather than a revenue center. The risk to the nutrition support team is that it will lose its independence, becoming a passive participant in the care of the patient who requires nutritional support. The risk to the patient is that cost issues may override those of quality care.

The evolution of an interdisciplinary nutrition support team approach was seen as a way to maximize efficiency and patient care. Recently, there has been a tendency to diminish the size of these units. At the same time, the challenge to nutrition support professionals is to coordinate efficient and early intervention and to document its efficacy and outcome. In the absence of any documented efficacy, many people argue, there is no need for formal nutrition support or the team in charge of that service. Therefore, it becomes imperative that the team justify its importance to the hospital, pointing out that a formal nutrition support team provides quality control and polices the administration of nutritional support. To do this, the nutrition support team must (a) identify specific patient populations who will benefit from nutrition support, (b) establish clinical pathways (guidelines), and (c) develop and implement measurements of efficacy (outcomes).

Table 2.11. STRATEGIES FOR COST-EFFECTIVE NUTRITION SUPPORT

PROMPTLY IDENTIFY HIGH-RISK PATIENTS

Screen for those who would benefit from nutritional support
To prevent complications associated with poor nutritional status

PROVIDE APPROPRIATE CARE

Use critical pathways and clinical guidelines
Use early postoperative nutrition when indicated
Use total parenteral nutrition only when indicated
Transition to regular diet as soon as feasible
Document use of feeding on length of stay

PROVIDE ECONOMICAL CARE

Oral vs. enteral vs. parenteral
"Shop" for best prices for equipment, solutions, formulas
Centralize compounding
Standardize orders, hang times, and the like

MONITORING

Incorporate patient outcomes and continuous quality
   improvement into daily practice
Proactively justify team costs and savings

Modified from Nelson J. The impact of health care reform on nutrition support: the practitioner's perspective. Nutrition in Clinical Practice 1995;5:22.

In the past, the costs required to pay the members of the nutrition support team have been more than offset by the reimbursements for the services provided, particularly for the delivery of TPN. In a capitated environment, hospitals find themselves in the peculiar situation where less is better. The danger of this approach as it relates to the nutritional support of hospitalized patients, particularly patients with complicated problems and complex diseases, is that the withholding of nutritional support from certain patients may result in serious consequences. Aggressive early feeding may be the best approach if it reduces complications in the long run. Methods of ensuring that nutrition support is cost effective have been suggested (Table 2.11).

Nutrition support may also play a role in quality assurance. In a report from a level 1 trauma center (27), acute nutritional interventions were necessary in 5% of their nutritional support team evaluations. Overfeeding unrecognized by the clinical service prompted most of the interventions. This was especially important because of the severity of illness and mortality rate in the overfed group. Estimation of total caloric need from body weight grossly overestimates basal energy needs, and indirect calorimetry is required to measure true caloric needs (28).

In conclusion, nutrition is extremely important to the surgical patient because of the changes in metabolism brought about by the surgery, trauma, or sepsis they endure. Changes in body composition occur with loss of lean body mass, increase in energy requirements, and decreased resistance to infection. Although we can provide for these changes, we really cannot stop them. Thus, knowledge of the changes and ways we can ameliorate them is essential.

REFERENCES

1. Souba WW, Wilmore DW. Diet and nutrition in the care of the patient with surgery, trauma, and sepsis. In: Shils M, Young V, eds. *Modern nutrition in health and disease,* 8th ed. Philadelphia: Lea & Febiger, 1994:1202–1240.
2. Souba WW. Total parenteral nutrition. In Copeland EM III, Levine BA, Howard RJ, et al., eds. *Current practice of surgery–CD-Rom.* New York: Churchill Livingstone, 1995.
3. Souba WW. Cytokines: key regulators of the nutritional/metabolic response to critical illness. *Current Problems in Surgery* 1994;31:577–652.
4. Hautamaki RD, Souba WW. Principles and techniques of nutritional support in the cancer patient. In: Karakousis CP, Copeland EM, Bland KI, eds. *Atlas of surgical oncology* Philadelphia: WB Saunders, 1995:741–748.
5. Souba WW. Homeostasis: bodily changes in trauma and surgery. In: Sabiston D, ed. *Essentials of surgery,* 2nd ed. Philadelphia: WB Saunders, 1987:10–23.
6. Watters JM, Van Woert JH, Wilmore DW. Metabolism and nutrition. In: Greenfield LJ, Mulholland MW, Oldham KT, et al., eds. *Surgery: scientific principles and practice.* Philadelphia: JB Lippincott, 1993:38–86.
7. Frankenfield DC, Cooney RN, Smith JS, et al. Bioelectrical impedance plethysmographic analysis of body composition in critically injured and healthy subjects. *Am J Clin Nutr* 1999; 69:426.
8. Frankenfield DC, Sarson GY, Blosser SA, et al. Validation of a 5-minute steady state indirect calorimetry protocol for resting energy expenditure in critically ill patients. *J Am Coll Nutr* 1996;15:397.
9. Bessey PQ, Watters JM, Aoki TT, et al. Combined hormonal infusion simulates the metabolic response to injury. *Ann Surg* 1984;200:264.
10. Fong Y, Lowry SF. Cytokines and the cellular response to injury and infection. In: Wilmore DW, Brennam MF, Harker AH, et al., eds. *Care of the surgical patient (critical care): IV. Trauma.* New York: Scientific American Medicine, 1992:1.
11. Cuthbertson DP. Alterations in metabolism following injury: Part 1. Injury. *QJM* 1980;11:175–189.
12. Frankenfield DC, Smith JS, Cooney RN. Accelerated nitrogen loss after traumatic injury is not attenuated by achievement of energy balance. *J Parenter Enteral Nutr* 1997;21:324.
13. Buzby GP, and The Veterans Affairs Total Parenteral Nutrition Cooperative Study Group. Perioperative total parenteral nutrition in surgical patients. *N Engl J Med* 1991;325:525.
14. Brennan MF, Pisters PWT, Posner M, et al. A prospective randomized trial of total parenteral nutrition after major pancreatic resection for malignancy. *Ann Surg* 1994;220:436–444.
15. Fan ST, Lo CM, Lai ECS, et al. Perioperative nutritional support in patients undergoing hepatectomy for hepatocellular carcinoma. *N Engl J Med* 1994;331:1547–1552.
16. McClave SA, Sexton LK, Spain DA, et al. Enteral tube feeding in the intensive care unit: factors impeding adequate delivery. *Crit Care Med* 1999;27:1252.
17. Montejo JC. Enteral nutrition-related gastrointestinal complications in critically ill patients: a multicenter study. *Crit Care Med* 1999;27:1447.
18. Wilmore DW, Byrne TA, Young LS, et al. A new treatment for patients with the short bowel syndrome: growth hormone, glutamine, and a modified diet. *Ann Surg* 1995;222:243–254.
19. Alexander JW, MacMillan BG, Stinnert JD, et al. Beneficial effects of aggressive protein feeding in severely burned children. *Ann Surg* 1980;192:505.
20. Abel RM, Beck CH, Abbott WM, et al. Improved survival from acute renal failure following treatment with intravenous essential L-amino acids and glucose: results of a prospective, double-blind study. *N Engl J Med* 1973;288:695.
21. van der Hulst RRWJ, van Kreel BK, von Meyenfeldt MF, et al. Glutamine and the preservation of gut integrity. *Lancet* 1993; 341:1363–1365.
22. Fong Y, Marano MA, Barber A, et al. Total parenteral nutrition and bowel rest modify the metabolic response to endotoxin in humans. *Ann Surg* 1989;210:449–457.
23. Ziegler TR, Young LS, Benfell K, et al. Clinical and metabolic efficacy of glutamine-enriched parenteral nutrition following bone marrow transplantation: a double-blind randomized controlled trial. *Ann Intern Med* 1992;116:821–828.
24. Scheltinga MR, Young LS, Benfell K, et al. Glutamine-enriched intravenous feedings attenuate extracellular fluid expansion after standard stress. *Ann Surg* 1991;214:385–395.
25. Jiang ZM, He GZ, Zhang SY, et al. Low-dose growth hormone and hypocaloric nutrition attenuates the protein-catabolic response after major operation. *Ann Surg* 1989;210:514.
26. Nelson J. The impact of health care reform on nutrition support: the practitioner's perspective. *Nutr Clin Pract* 1995;5:22.
27. Klein CJ, Henry SM. Acute nutrition interventions help identify indicators of quality in a trauma service. *Nutr Clin Pract* 1999;14:85.
28. Frankenfield DC, Wiles CE, Bagley S, et al. Relationships between resting and total energy expenditure in injured and septic patients. *Crit Care Med* 1994;22:1796.

SURGERY: SCIENTIFIC PRINCIPLES AND PRACTICE, Third Edition, edited by
Lazar J. Greenfield, Michael W. Mulholland, Keith T. Oldham, Gerald B. Zelenock,
and Keith D. Lillemoe. Lippincott Williams & Wilkins Publishers, Philadelphia, © 2001.

CHAPTER 3

WOUND HEALING

NEIL A. FINE AND THOMAS A. MUSTOE

An understanding of wound healing is fundamental to all of surgery and involves a broad range of cellular actions and interactions. Wound healing is a fundamental homeostatic process in response to injury. It involves the activation of basic cellular processes of inflammation, cell proliferation, and growth as well as regulation of these processes once repair is complete. Increased understanding of the cellular and molecular events involving growth factors and cytokines, and the realistic prospects for pharmacologic manipulation, have focused a great deal of research interest from a broad range of disciplines. Although much new knowledge has been gained, there remain many unanswered questions. This chapter outlines a basic set of concepts regarding wound healing, with emphasis on the clinical principles of basic surgical techniques and the care of surgical incisions, and open, acute and chronic wounds.

NORMAL WOUND HEALING

Wound healing is the body's response to injury. Injury can be acute or chronic and involve multiple tissues, but wound healing is most clearly illustrated by examining the response to full-thickness injury (e.g., a cut or an incision) to the epidermis and dermis. This injury sets in motion a sequence of interrelated reparative forces. Although the events overlap in time, it is helpful to consider the process as stages or phases of wound healing; these are presented as separate events. This provides for clear conceptualization of the individual events and conforms with standard conventions. These events, however, do not occur independently, and the degree of temporal overlap is significant (Fig. 3.1).

Every tissue in the body undergoes reparative processes after injury. Bone has the unique ability to heal without scar. Liver has the potential to regenerate parenchyma and is the only organ that has maintained that ability in the adult human. Although liver does regenerate, it often heals with scar (cirrhosis). With these exceptions, all other human tissues heal with scar. This chapter reviews the healing process of human skin with particular emphasis on surgical applications. Delineation of the individual mediators is still evolving, so the emphasis is on the underlying physiologic processes and the patterns of response.

Inflammatory Phase

The inflammatory phase of acute wound healing begins immediately after injury. The initial response to the disruption of blood vessels is bleeding. The homeostatic response to this is clot formation to stop hemorrhage. Platelet plug formation initiates the hemostatic process along with clotting factors activated by collagen and basement membrane proteins exposed by the injury. Fibrin, produced by the clotting cascade, binds the platelet plug and forms a matrix for the cellular responses that follow. After injury, transient vasoconstriction is mediated by catecholamines, thromboxane, and prostaglandin (PG) $F_{2\alpha}$. Platelet degranulation, the evacuation of the granules into the extracellular space, provides the contents of α granules and dense granules, most notably platelet-derived growth factor (PDGF) and transforming growth factor-β (TGF-β). These substances initiate chemotaxis and proliferation of inflammatory cells, beginning the inflammatory response that ultimately heals the wound (Table 3.1). Transient vasoconstriction is necessary to decrease blood loss at the time of the initial wounding and also to allow clot formation. Vasoconstriction lasts for 5 to 10 minutes. Once a clot has been formed and active bleeding has stopped, vasodilation increases local blood flow to the wounded area, supplying cells and substrate necessary for further wound repair. The vascular endothelial cells also deform, increasing vascular permeability. The vasodilation and increased endothelial permeability are mediated by histamine, PGE_2, and PGI_2 (prostacyclin) as well as vascular endothelial cell growth factor. These vasodilatory substances are released by injured endothelial cells, and

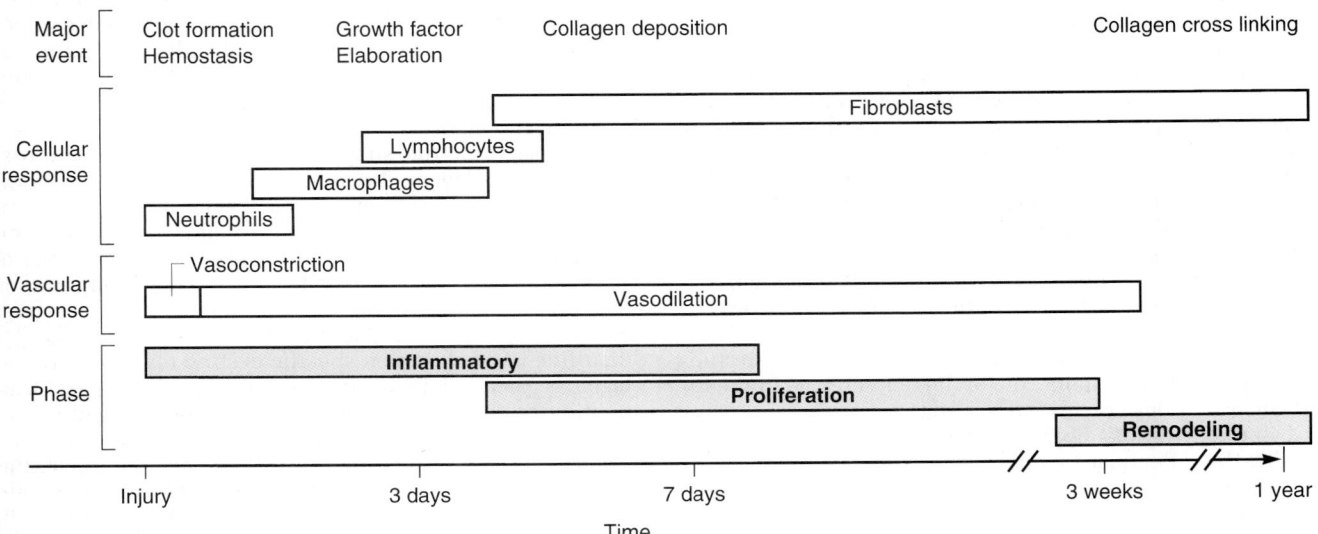

Figure 3.1. Time line of phases of wound healing with dominant cell types and major physiologic events.

Table 3.1. **PLATELET GRANULES AND MEDIATORS OF PLATELET AGGREGATION**

PLATELET GRANULES

α Granules: Contain Platelet-specific Proteins

Platelet factor 4
β-Thromboglobulin
Platelet-derived growth factor
Transforming growth factor-β

Dense Granules

Adenosine diphosphate
Serotonin
Calcium

MEDIATORS OF PLATELET AGGREGATION

Thomboxane A_2
Thrombin
Platelet factor 4

mast cells, and enhance the egress of cells and substrate into the wounded tissue (Fig. 3.2).

At this stage, the wound is full of debris from the initial injury. This material consists of a mixture of injured, and devitalized tissue (fat, muscle, epithelium), clot (platelets, erythrocytes, fibrinogen), bacteria (from the skin surface and external environment), extravasated serum proteins (glycoproteins and mucopolysaccharides), and foreign material introduced at the time of injury (suture, dirt). During the next several days, the wound is cleared of bacteria, devitalized tissue, and foreign material by recruited and activated phagocytic cells. Polymorphonuclear leukocytes (PMNs) begin to arrive immediately, attaining large local numbers within 24 hours. The process of clearing the wound of debris usually takes several days, but the time varies depending on the amount of material to be cleared. The PMN reflex is followed by macrophages, which appear in wounds in significant numbers within 2 or 3 days. These macrophages are mononuclear phagocytic cells derived from circulating monocytes or resident tissue macrophages. They complete the process of removing all material not necessary for the ensuing steps of wound healing.

In the absence of significant bacterial contamination, macrophages promptly replace PMNs as the dominant cell type during the inflammatory phase. The role of the macrophages is not limited to phagocytosis (1). Macrophages are also the sources of more than 30 different growth factors and cytokines. These growth factors induce fibroblast proliferation, endothelial cell proliferation (angiogenesis), and extracellular matrix production. They also recruit and activate additional macrophages. The result is the induction of a wound healing amplification cycle as growth factors recruit macrophages and elicit additional growth factor release. Studies using specific antibodies that destroy PMNs or block certain aspects of the amplification function (such as adhesion) have shown that wounds still heal normally in the absence of bacteria, but that healing is significantly impaired without functional macrophages (even in the absence of bacteria). These studies confirm the dominant role of the macrophage in the inflammatory phase of wound healing.

Lymphocytes also appear in wounds in small numbers during the inflammatory phase. The role of lymphocytes in the wound healing process remains to be clarified, but they are thought to be related more to chronic inflammatory processes than to the initial response to wounding. Because recombinant growth factors are available now in sufficient quantities for clinical use, the prospect of using growth fac-

tors as pharmacologic agents to stimulate wound healing (and potentially modulate abnormal scarring) is the focus of much research. Only one agent, however, has been approved for human use in the United States. After a 7-year process, involving 1,000 patients, becaplermin gel, a PDGF preparation (Regranex; Ortho McNeil Pharmaceuticals, Raritan, NJ), was approved in 1997 by the U.S. Food and Drug Administration (FDA) for use in diabetic foot ulcers (2,3). Studies with PDGF for other indications, as well as trials of other growth factors, are undergoing active clinical investigation. Another product, an artificial skin equivalent made of a dermis-like matrix covered with cultured epithelium from heterologous human foreskins (Apligraf; Novartis Pharmaceuticals, East Hanover, NJ), was FDA approved in 1998 for use in refractory venous ulcers of more than 1 year's duration. The main effect of this product is most likely the delivery of growth factors produced by the neonatal cells. Increased knowledge of the role of growth factors in wound healing has also provoked consideration of strategies using other pharmacologic agents for indirect modulation of growth factor levels in wounds.

Proliferative Phase

The proliferative phase begins with the formation of a provisional matrix of fibrin and fibronectin as part of initial clot formation. The provisional matrix is populated by macrophages initially; however, by 3 days after injury, fibroblasts appear in the fibronectin–fibrin framework and initiate collagen synthesis. Fibroblasts proliferate in response to growth factors to become the dominant cell type during this phase. Growth factors produced by macrophages simultaneously induce angiogenesis, which regulate the ingrowth and proliferation of endothelial cells to form new capillaries. This neovascularity is visible through the epithelium and gives the wound a pink or purple-red appearance. Capillary ingrowth provides the fibroblasts with oxygen and nutrients to sustain cell proliferation and support the production of the permanent wound matrix. This latter material is composed of collagen and proteoglycans or ground substance, replacing the provisional fibronectin–fibrin matrix.

Collagen is the dominant structural molecule in the wound matrix and the final scar. This is not surprising because collagen is the principal structural protein in skin, bone, and indeed all human tissue. Collagen is synthesized into an organized cable-like network in a multistep process with both intracellular and extracellular components (Fig. 3.3). The collagen molecule has abundant quantities of two unique amino acids, hydroxyproline and hydroxylysine. The hydroxylation process that forms these amino acids requires ascorbic acid (vitamin C) and is necessary for the subsequent stabilization and cross-linkage of collagen. Procollagen is formed in the fibroblasts as a long linear amino acid segment with regular repeats of hydroxyproline every third amino acid and with terminal extension peptides. Procollagen molecules aggregate in the case of type 1 collagen (the most common) as three alpha chains to form a triple-helical complex (Fig. 3.3A). The triple helix is maintained by intramolecular disulfide bonds between specific cystine residues. Procollagen is secreted in its triple-helical form; extracellular peptidases cleave the extension peptides at the amino and carboxyl termini, leaving the central collagen molecule. Collagen cross-linking (Fig. 3.3B) then occurs in the extracellular space as the collagen molecules aggregate into larger structures. Lysyl oxidase catalyzes the conversion of lysine and hydroxylysine into aldehyde forms. These aldehydes form intermolecular bonds by undergoing spontaneous condensation. This produces stable, cross-

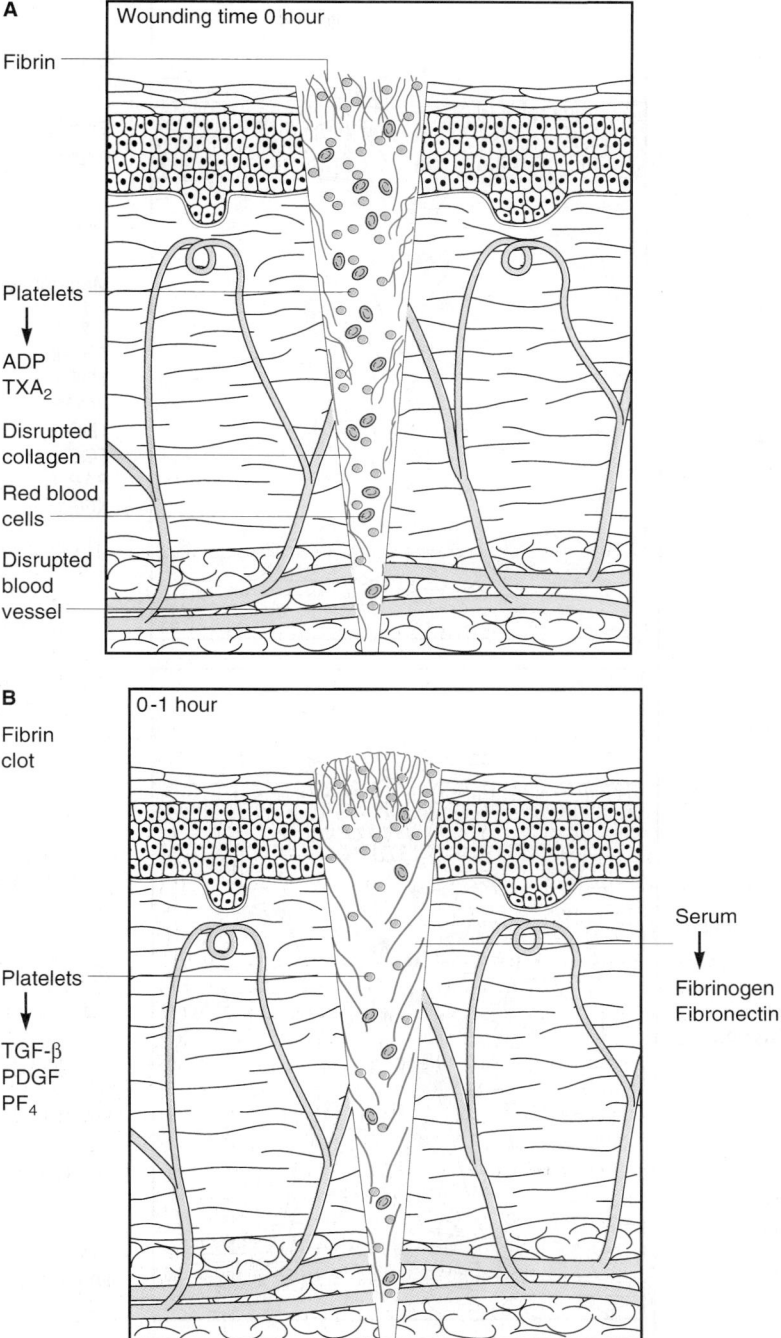

Figure 3.2. Schematic representation of wound healing processes. ADP, adenosine diphosphate; TXA$_2$, thromboxane A$_2$; TGF-β, transforming growth factor-β; PDGF, platelet-derived growth factor; PF$_4$, platelet factor 4; TNF-α, tumor necrosis factor-α; FGF, fibroblast growth factor; PAF, platelet-activating factor; KGF, keratinocyte growth factor. *(continues)*

linked collagen fibrils. These intramolecular and intermolecular bonds provide strength and stability. As the wound matures, fibrils cross-link to form large cables of collagen, providing increased tensile strength (Fig. 3.3C). The wound is now more appropriately considered a scar.

Although there are several types of collagen, type I predominates throughout the body. The principal collagen in scar is type I, with lesser amounts of type III collagen. Other collagen types make important contributions to the basement membrane, cartilage, and other structures (Table 3.2).

Remodeling Phase

The transition from the proliferative phase to the remodeling phase is defined by reaching collagen equilib-

rium. Collagen accumulation in the wound reaches a maximum within 2 to 3 weeks after wounding. Although supranormal rates of synthesis and degradation continue throughout remodeling, there is no further change in total collagen content (4). Tensile strength gradually increases as random collagen fibrils are replaced by organized fibrils with more intermolecular bonds. During the initial phase of wound healing, there is a relative abundance of type III collagen in the wound. With remodeling, the normal adult 4:1 ratio of type I to type III collagen is restored. Under normal wound healing conditions, the capillary density gradually diminishes and the number of fibroblasts is reduced. The wound loses its pink or purple vascular color and becomes progressively pale. The collagen undergoes constant remodeling. New collagen is formed and collagen

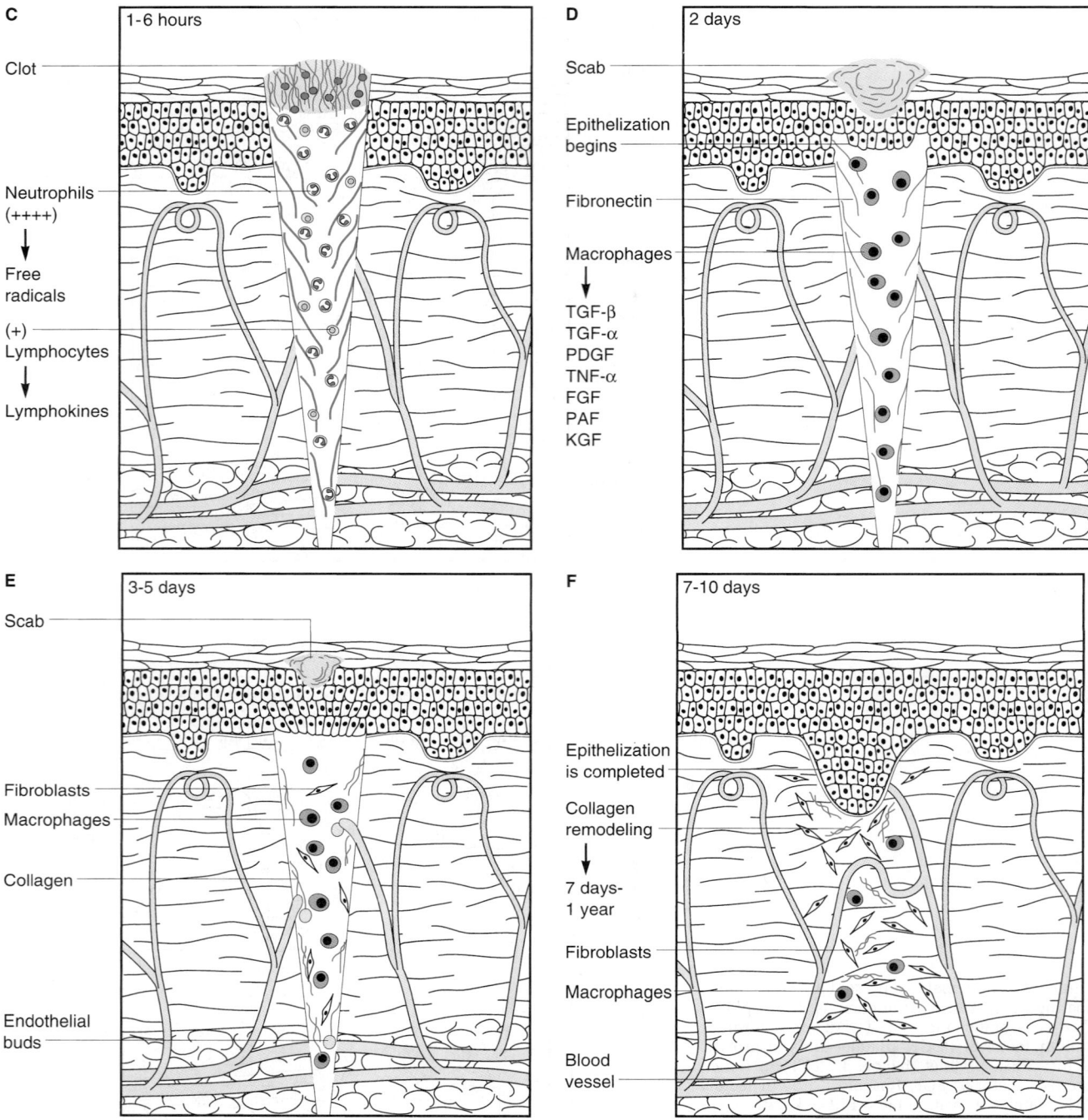

Figure 3.2. *(Continued)*

degradation by specific collagenases continues. Collagenase activity is balanced against new production of collagen to produce a steady state. As equilibrium is achieved, the collagen fibrils align themselves in a longitudinal arrangement as dictated by stress placed on the wound. Scars never achieve the degree of order achieved by collagen in normal skin or tendons, but they do increase in strength for 6 months or longer, eventually reaching 70% of the strength of unwounded skin (Fig. 3.4).

The other important component of the extracellular matrix is the ground substance or proteoglycans. These substances are composed of a protein backbone with long hydrophilic carbohydrate side chains. The hydrophilicity of these molecules accounts for much of the water content of a scar. In the early immature wound, there is a disproportionately large amount of proteoglycans (particularly hyaluronic acid). During the maturation phase, the proteoglycan content returns to a level that closely approximates that of normal skin.

Until recently, the extracellular matrix (predominantly collagen and proteoglycans) was thought to be inert. It is becoming increasingly clear, however, that the extracellular

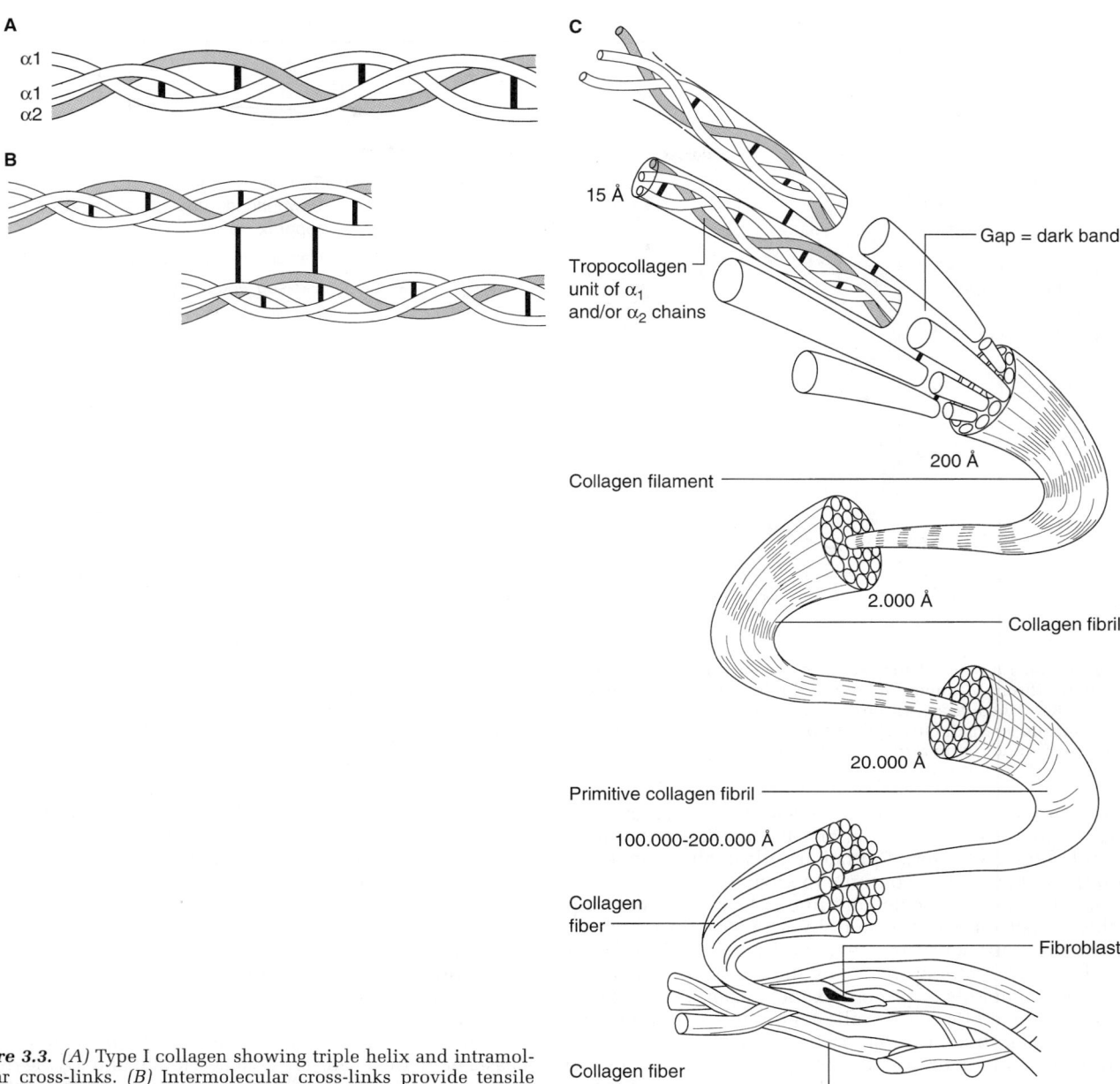

Figure 3.3. *(A)* Type I collagen showing triple helix and intramolecular cross-links. *(B)* Intermolecular cross-links provide tensile strength. *(C)* Assembly of collagen fibrils, fibers, and fiber bundles.

Table 3.2. **COLLAGEN TYPES**

Type	Property of aggregate unit	Tissue distribution
I	Rigid fibrils	All connective tissue except cartilage
II	Rigid fibrils	Cartilage and vitreous
III	Elastic fibrils	Elastic tissue (e.g., fetal skin, blood vessels, uterus)
IV	Sheet	Basement membrane
V	Fibril	Widespread
VI	Beaded filaments	Widespread
VII	Anchoring fibrils	Interface of basement membrane and underlying stroma
VIII	Sheet	Descemet's membrane
IX	Fibril	Hyaline cartilage
X	Sheet	Hypertrophic cartilage
XI	Fibril	Hyaline cartilage
XII	Fibril	Similar to type I

matrix has an important role in transmitting cellular signals through cell attachment receptors (integrins). It also serves as a reservoir for growth factors. No doubt other roles will be defined in the future. The role of proteoglycans as signaling molecules is just beginning to be delineated.

Epithelialization

The skin is composed of two layers, the epidermis and the dermis. The outermost layer, the epidermis, is the protective barrier that forms the external interface between the body and the environment. The epidermis protects against water loss, allowing the other cells of the body to live in a liquid environment, as well forming a barrier to bacteria and other environmental factors. Reconstruction of the epithelial barrier (epithelialization) begins within hours of the initial injury. As a first step, epithelial cells from the basal layer at the wound edge flatten and migrate across the wound, completing wound coverage within 18 to 24 hours in a coapted surgical wound. The cells along

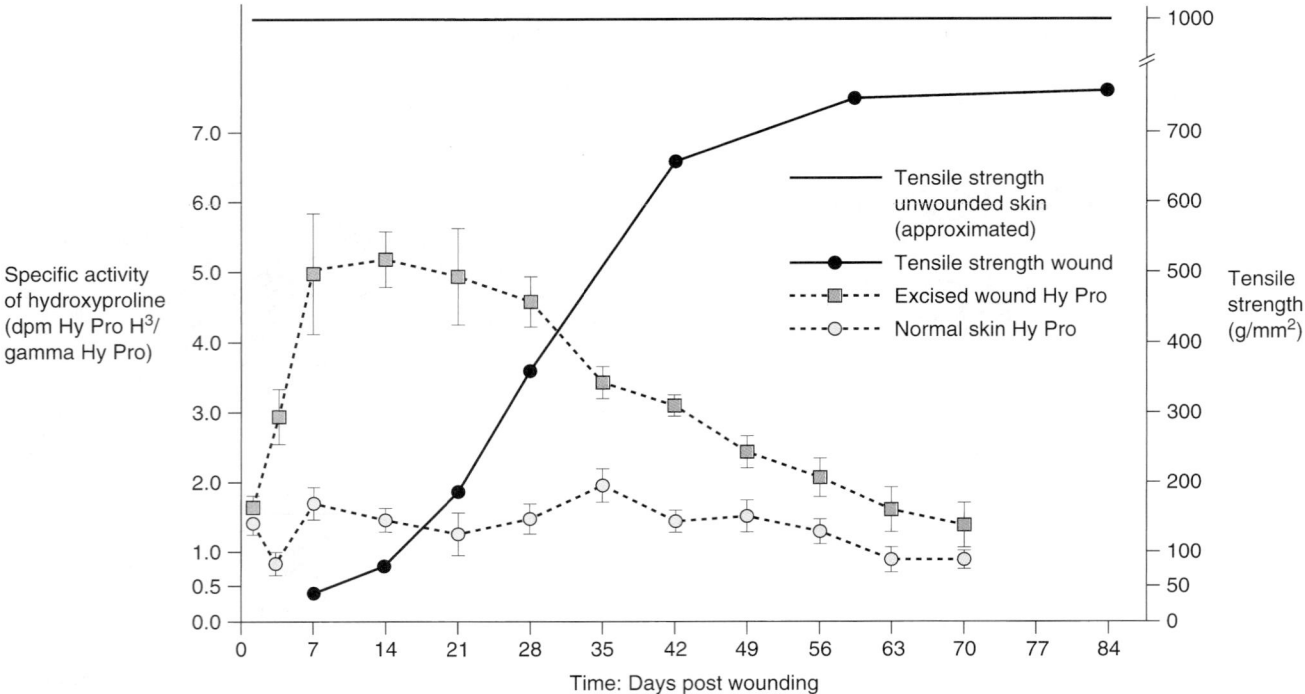

Figure 3.4. Relation of the rate of collagen synthesis to the gain of tensile strength in rat skin wounds. (From Madden JW, Peacock EE Jr. Studies on the biology of collagen during wound healing: 1. Rate of collagen synthesis and deposition in cutaneous wounds of the rat. *Surgery* 1968;64: 288; tensile strength curve taken from Levenson SM, Gever EF, Crowley LV, et al. The healing of rat skin wounds. *Ann Surg* 1965;161:293, with permission.)

the margin are also dividing to reform the characteristic basilar-to-apical differentiation of multilayered mature epithelium (see later). Epithelial cells exhibit contact inhibition; that is, they continue to migrate across an appropriate bed until a single continuous layer is formed. Epithelial cell migration occurs by a process in which the epithelial cells send out pseudopods, attaching to the underlying extracellular matrix by integrin receptors. Bacteria, large amounts of protein exudate from leaky capillaries, and necrotic tissue all compromise this process, delaying epithelialization. Delayed epithelialization results in a more profound and prolonged inflammatory process, thereby contributing to unsatisfactory or hypertrophic scarring.

In superficial, partial-thickness wounds, epithelialization results from migration of epithelial cells from remaining dermal appendages, sweat glands, and hair follicles (Fig. 3.5). This is relatively rapid because the distance between hair follicles and sweat glands is short; epithelialization is usually complete within 7 to 10 days. In more complex injuries, however, such as deep second-degree burns, the combination of increased necrosis and fewer remaining dermal appendages can result in delayed epithelialization with prolongation of the inflammatory process.

A partial-thickness burn or abrasion that requires more than 2 weeks to epithelialize has a high incidence of hypertrophic scarring. The increased scarring is presumably secondary to prolonged inflammation. This can be minimized by achieving a closed wound through skin grafting or other techniques.

With full-thickness injury, the entire dermis is destroyed or removed. Epithelialization occurs only from the margins of the wound, at a maximal rate of 1 to 2 mm/d. In practice, adequate coverage of sizable wounds is rarely

achieved. Thus, lower leg ulcers rarely heal faster than 1 cm/mo; that is, a 2-cm diameter ulcer typically takes 2 months to heal under ideal conditions. In an open wound, the rate of epithelialization is critically dependent on the vascularity and health of the underlying granulation tissue (neodermis) across which it migrates. Thus, although chronic wounds are characterized by a failure of epithelial migration, the cause is most often a problem in the underlying wound bed.

Epithelial cells alone provide little strength when not anchored to dermis. They are therefore prone to injury. The basal epidermal cells are attached to the underlying dermis by hemidesmosomes. These structures attach to keratin filaments in the epithelial cells. The hemidesmosomes connect by a series of intermediate proteins to anchoring filaments, long proteins that intertwine with the collagen network of the dermis. Intact epithelium is resistant to shear forces because of these strong dermal attachments. Without an adequate dermal base, however, epidermis provides unstable wound coverage and is characterized by chronic and recurrent breakdown.

After the first layer of cells restores the epithelial barrier, additional layers develop, restoring the basilar-to-apical order. As the cells mature, they resume keratin formation. This regenerates the stratum corneum of the epidermis and completes the restorative process of epithelialization and provides stable coverage.

Visible scarring occurs only when the injury extends deeper than the superficial dermis. Superficial abrasions and burns usually heal without scarring, but deeper abrasions and burns can scar significantly. Whenever the dermis is incised, a scar forms. The prominence of the scar is variable and can be minimized by location and closure technique. If an incision is made, however, a scar is inevitable.

A

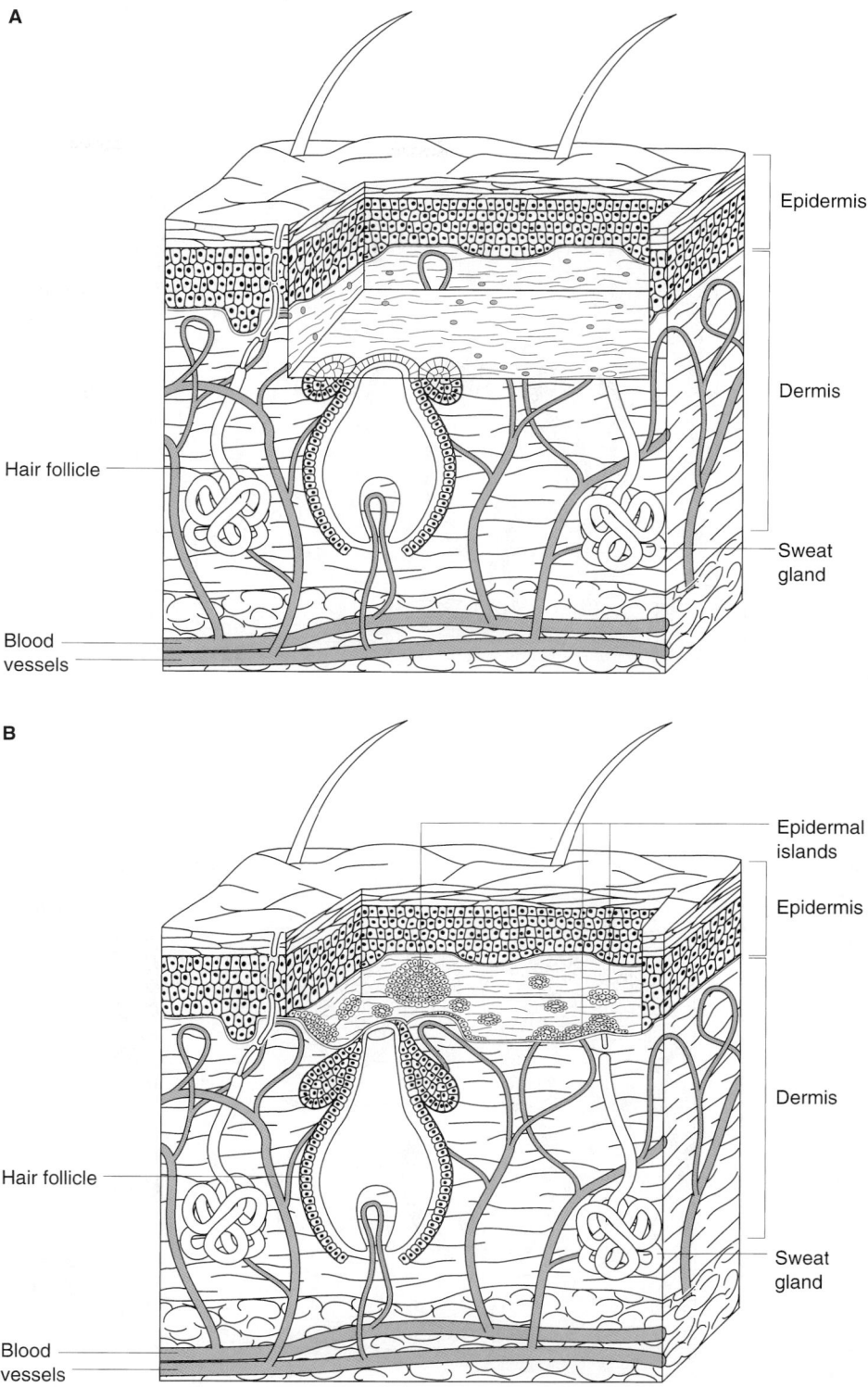

Epidermis

Dermis

Hair follicle

Sweat gland

Blood vessels

B

Epidermal islands

Epidermis

Hair follicle

Dermis

Sweat gland

Figure 3.5. Reepithelialization of a partial-thickness wound. *(continues)*

Blood vessels

Stretch marks are a unique type of scar. Stretch marks occur when the collagen fibers in the dermis are stretched to the point of disruption, but the epidermis is not disrupted. This results in scar formation in the dermis that is visible through an intact, unscarred epidermis.

Clinical Implications

This review of normal wound healing has numerous practical implications for the care of wounds and surgical incisions. Meticulous hemostasis reduces the inflammation and phagocytosis necessary to clear the wound of blood. Atraumatic handling of tissue decreases the load of necrotic or nonviable cells at the wound margin. This is best achieved using fine forceps or skin hooks to retract and assist in coapting the dermis. Crush injury to the epidermis with forceps should be avoided. Deep sutures are best placed only into collagen-laden structures that have the tensile strength to hold sutures under tension, that is, fascia and dermis. Fat does not contain collagen and does

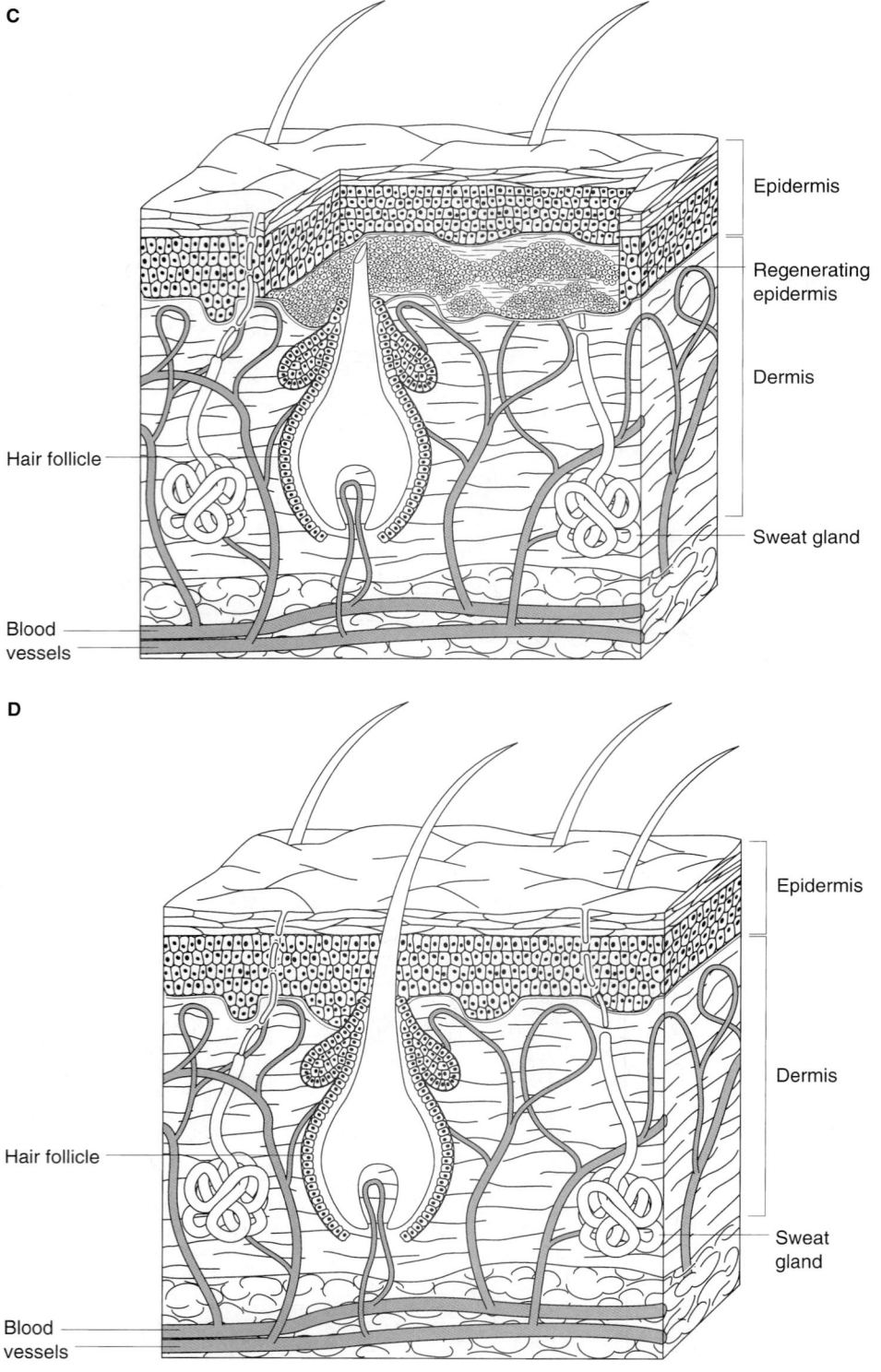

C

Epidermis

Regenerating epidermis

Dermis

Hair follicle

Sweat gland

Blood vessels

D

Epidermis

Dermis

Hair follicle

Sweat gland

Blood vessels

Figure 3.5. *(Continued)*

not hold together tissues under tension. Therefore, fatty tissue should not be sutured as a separate layer. Dead space obliteration and fluid evacuation are best achieved by suction drainage rather than by adding additional foreign material to the wound in the form of suture material. Therefore, in closing a laparotomy incision, even in a morbidly obese patient with a 2-inch panniculus, the closure should be limited to the abdominal fascia, the skin, and rarely Scarpa's fascia.

Under normal circumstances, epithelialization of an incision is complete within 24 to 48 hours, and there is no reason to protect the incision from water after this time. Allowing the patient to wash or shower 1 or 2 days after surgery has significant psychological benefits and gently débrides the incision and keeps it clean by rinsing away surface bacteria and debris. Blood and protein exudate create an excellent culture medium for any skin surface bacteria. Showers reduce the chance of bacterial accumulation in surface crusts along the incision and on the sutures. This decreases inflammation and prevents breakdown of the fragile epithelial layer over the incision, improving the quality of the scar.

OPEN WOUNDS (ACUTE)

Open wounds, whether ulcers or open surgical incisions closing by secondary intention, heal with the same sequence of inflammation, matrix deposition, epithelialization, and scar maturation as previously described. However, there are some important differences. In the closed (sutured) incisional wound, the healing process progresses through an orderly temporal sequence. In an open wound, the healing events are spatially separated. In the open wound, a bed of granulation tissue forms over the exposed subcutaneous tissue. Granulation tissue is composed of new capillaries, proliferating fibroblasts, and an immature matrix of collagen, proteoglycans, substrate adhesion molecules (including fibronectin, laminin, and tenascin), and acute and chronic inflammatory cells. In addition, there are variable amounts of bacteria and protein exudate, depending on the "health" of the wound. At the advancing edge of epithelium, the process of acute inflammation is taking place. Behind the advancing edge, there is a proliferative area; and further behind, the scar is maturing and remodeling. An understanding of the biologic principles of wound healing has direct clinical implications in wound care, particularly in the case of chronic wounds (e.g., pressure sores, lower leg ulcers, diabetic foot ulcers).

The most important clinical factor in the healing of surgical incisions is the gain in tensile strength of the wound. This was discussed previously and depends almost entirely on collagen deposition. The rate of collagen synthesis determines the initial wound strength. Ultimate wound strength is determined by the degree of collagen organization and cross-linking. The healing of open wounds is defined primarily by epithelialization, and successful healing is related more to the maintenance of epithelial integrity than to the tensile strength of the scar. As discussed earlier, the rate of epithelialization in open wounds is limited by the rate of migration of the proliferating epithelial edge. Factors that regulate epithelial migration are an area of active research. There is clear evidence that the extracellular matrix (collagen, fibronectin, basement membrane proteins, glycosaminoglycans) is composed of structural elements that are not inert. They function as an essential substrate, with adhesion molecules regulating intercellular communication. The cellular elements of the matrix express specific receptors that recognize amino acid sequences on the matrix proteins. This allows for cellular attachment at specific sites, cell locomotion, and intracellular signal transduction. Rapid epithelialization therefore depends on an optimal matrix, manufactured by the underlying granulation tissue, as well as on optimal delivery of nutrients and oxygen by an adequate blood supply.

Inflammatory cells in open wounds, especially the macrophages, release growth factors. Growth factors enhance migration and proliferation of fibroblasts and endothelial cells in wounds. In an open wound, this leads to the formation of granulation tissue, the cobblestone-like, pink surface of healthy new tissue. The ability of an open wound to form granulation tissue is governed by the blood supply to the tissue and the relative absence of devitalized tissue and bacteria. Therefore, wounds that form granulation tissue should heal or be amenable to surgical closure with flaps or skin grafts. Wounds that do not form granulation tissue are very likely to be recalcitrant to all treatments except those directed at the underlying cause of the failure to form granulation tissue (i.e., vascular bypass to restore adequate blood flow to an ischemic extremity wound).

Wound Contraction

Wound contraction is an important event that differentiates open wounds and closed incisions. When open wounds contract, the surrounding skin is pulled over the wound to reduce its size. This can occur much faster than epithelialization. In addition to increasing the speed of wound closure, another advantage is that the open wound is resurfaced by the normal sensate skin surrounding the wound. Most animals are loose skinned, meaning that the skin (epithelium, dermis, subcutaneous fat) is only loosely attached to the underlying muscle fascia. Some animal wounds heal almost entirely by contraction; for example, a 2-cm ulcer heals to a 3-mm point in a loose-skinned animal. Humans, however, do not have this degree of skin mobility in most sites because skin is tightly adherent and less elastic, especially in the lower leg. Therefore, although contraction may account for 90% of the reduction in wound size on the perineum, it accounts for at most 30% to 40% of the healing of a lower leg ulcer. This is one important reason why leg ulcers are so slow to heal. All healing wounds generate a strong contractile force (5). When this contractile force is exerted across a joint, or an area of motion, such as the neck, axilla, or elbow, it may result in a scar contracture. A contracture is a scar that limits the functional range of motion of a joint.

At the cellular level, the forces that drive wound contraction come from the fibroblasts. Fibroblasts, like muscle cells, contain actin microfilaments. When these filaments increase in number, the cells take on the morphologic appearance of myofibroblasts. Myofibroblasts are seen in increased numbers in contracting wounds, but their role is unclear. It is unknown whether the fibroblasts that attach to the collagen fibrils by means of integrin receptors move collagen fibers together using a locomotor action or whether the contraction comes from intrinsic cellular contraction.

Unless created and dressed under sterile conditions, all open wounds are contaminated by the bacterial flora on the surrounding skin and from the environment. Bacterial colonization of the wound is routine and is not deleterious to normal healing. Bacterial infection, however, is deleterious and can delay or prevent healing. Cellulitis or invasive bacterial infection of the surrounding tissues is relatively easy to diagnose with experience. Treatment typically requires systemic antibiotic therapy. Distinguishing wound colonization from invasive infection, however, can be difficult. The burn wound experience has demonstrated that bacterial counts of more than 10^5 organisms per gram of tissue on quantitative analysis are associated with failure of surgical wound closure. This is an important diagnostic technique because clinical judgment is inadequate. The failure of wound closure in this circumstance is in part due to bacterial and phagocytic proteases that prevent healing. In a similar fashion, if the bacterial count is above this threshold in the wound granulation tissue, the excessive proteases and endotoxins delay epithelialization.

Any nonepithelialized wound leaks plasma. With more inflammation, capillary permeability is further increased. Increased microvascular permeability results from endothelial cell injury or dysfunction. This is mediated by many components of the inflammatory cascade, including histamine, kinins, complement, PGE_2, PGI_2, and others. This exudate of serum proteins and inflammatory cells serves as a rich culture medium, which may continue the cycle of bacterial proliferation and lead to more exudate formation. In addition, the edema that results from capillary dysfunction increases the distance for diffusion of oxygen and nutrients to their metabolic targets.

The net result of this cycle is delayed or absent wound healing.

Clinical Features

Basic principles of wound care should be tailored to assist the mechanisms elaborated earlier, leading to more rapid healing. Although many approaches to wound care are practiced, Winter and Scales (6) first recorded that epithelialization is more rapid under moist conditions than dry conditions. Without dressings, a superficial wound or one with minimal devitalized tissue forms a scab or crust. The scab forms when blood and serum coagulate, dry, and form a protective moisture barrier over the open wound (Fig. 3.6). Epithelialization occurs with controlled clot proteolysis and migration of the epithelium under the clot. If the wound is kept moist with an occlusive dressing, however, and the exudate does not become infected, then epithelial migration is optimized. A skin graft donor site, for example, epithelializes several days faster under an occlusive dressing than a dry dressing. In addition, the pain of an open wound or skin graft donor site is dramatically reduced under an occlusive dressing.

Moist healing can be achieved by occlusive dressings, occlusive ointments or creams, or continually moistened dressings. The traditional wet-to-dry dressing, however, if truly left to dry, simply produces desiccation and necrosis of the surface layer of the wound, delaying epithelialization. Although wet-to-dry dressings can be effective for débridement of wound exudate, they are usually less desirable than a moist healing environment combined with effective cleaning of the wound (i.e., water irrigation).

Role of Oxygen

Oxygen is necessary for normal metabolic cellular function, but in wounds with actively proliferating and metabolically stimulated cells, it is even more critical. PMNs require ambient PO_2 levels of 25 mm Hg to produce superoxide radicals, which serve an essential role in bacterial killing. The enzyme system that generates superoxide and its derivative oxidant products functions optimally at PO_2 levels greater than 50 mm Hg. Collagen synthesis is also highly dependent on adequate tissue oxygen tension. A fresh wound is initially avascular and is always hypoxic relative to the surrounding tissues. In the center of a new wound, the tissue PO_2 can drop to near zero. After angiogenesis and the delivery of oxygenated blood, the tissue PO_2 quickly rises. In general, the tissue oxygen tension in a wound is lower than that of surrounding normal tissues. Atherosclerosis of major arteries, small vessel disease from other causes, impaired oxygen delivery, local scarring with fibrosis, and other events may reduce local tissue PO_2 levels from normal (approximately 40 mm Hg) to less than 25 mm Hg. If so, tissue hypoxia may result in significantly impaired wound healing. In the postoperative patient, suboptimal skin perfusion due to even modest hypovolemia, smoking-related arteriopathy, or excess circulating epinephrine can result in a low tissue PO_2. Subcutaneous tissue oxygen levels have been correlated clinically with surgical complication rates. Supplemental oxygen, optimal fluid administration, pain control, and arterial reconstruction all have potentially beneficial roles in the effort to enhance the tissue PO_2. Oxygen delivery to tissue is the primary determinant of healing; anemia alone is not specifically detrimental to wound healing (7).

Hyperbaric oxygen therapy (HBO) can achieve high oxygen levels in most wounds for the duration of the treatment, usually 1.5 hours at a time. The patient is placed in

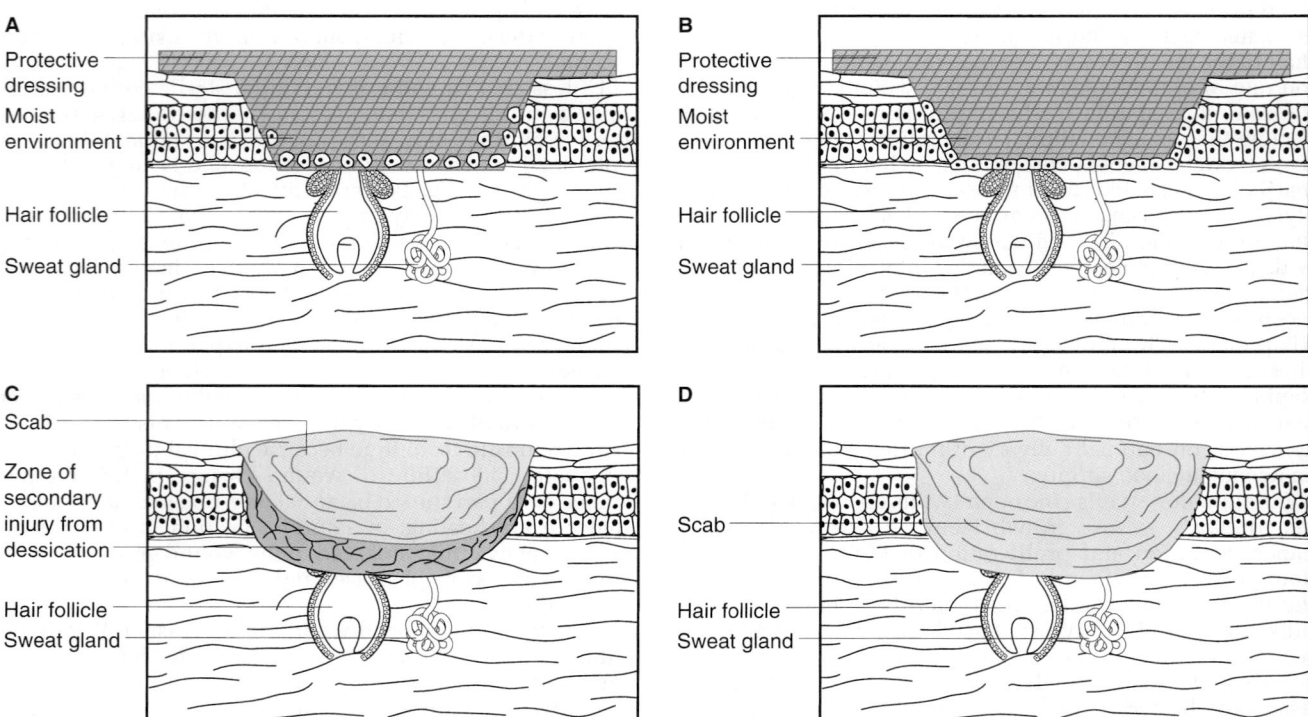

Figure 3.6. Rapid epithelialization occurs in a moist environment. Desiccation delays healing by causing tissue necrosis in the exposed wound. The scab ultimately forms a moisture barrier, and epithelialization occurs from the wound edge and any remaining dermal appendages (see Fig. 3.5).

the hyperbaric chamber and is exposed to 2 to 2.5 atmospheres of pressure and 100% oxygen. Although oxygen is a necessary component in aerobic metabolism, it may also act as a signaling molecule for growth factor production. Clinical experience suggest efficacy of HBO, but conclusive prospective, randomized trials have not been conducted (8). It is clear that HBO can raise the P_{O_2} in ischemic wounds, but the indications, length of treatment, and number of treatments are still empiric. Based on the findings in a number of retrospective studies, use of HBO has become widespread, particularly with diabetic foot ulcers and wounds that have been irradiated.

Role of Edema

In normal tissue, each cell is only a few cell diameters away from the nearest capillary and receives nutrients and oxygen by diffusion. However, with inflammation, venous insufficiency, or other causes of edema formation, the sequestered extracellular and extravascular fluid increases the diffusion distance for oxygen and results in a lower tissue P_{O_2}. In the case of lower extremity venous insufficiency, the chronic protein leak from the capillaries results in pericapillary deposition. This "cuffing" is a further barrier to oxygen and nutrient diffusion, and possibly functions as a site for nonspecific binding of growth factors, making them less available to the wound environment. The importance of edema control is often underestimated. Even in extremities that are not noticeably swollen, elevation and other methods of edema control (elastic wraps, compression stockings, sequential compression machines) can be of substantial benefit. The most important therapeutic maneuver in the healing of leg ulcers associated with venous insufficiency is edema control with leg elevation, compression stockings, or compressive dressings and, in severe cases, intermittent or sequential compression devices.

Role of Tissue Necrosis and Exudate

Open wounds often contain devitalized tissue as a result of injury, and may be complicated by infection or suboptimal tissue perfusion. If the amount of dead tissue is large, the impairment to healing is obvious, but it is often not fully appreciated that smaller amounts of necrotic tissue or fibrinous exudate also delay healing. In addition, any open wound constantly produces an exudate of serum proteins and dead inflammatory cells, which increases devitalized tissue, if present. The net result is that increased exudate, higher bacterial counts, edema, and more proteases and other inflammatory mediators have a deleterious effect on healing. Therefore, devitalized tissue, especially dermis, usually requires surgical excision. If necrotic dermis is left in place, the underlying subcutaneous tissue (fat), which is less vascular, eventually becomes infected. Small amounts of devitalized tissue and exudate can be débrided or removed with dressings, enzyme application, whirlpools, water irrigation, or simple washing. However, the mechanical débriding action must be sufficient and frequent enough to remove the exudate and debris, producing a clean wound before healing is optimal. Because wounds are painful and the dressings or washing insufficient, the exudate often is not removed adequately. This results in delayed healing.

CHRONIC WOUNDS

A practical definition of a chronic wound is one that has failed to heal within 3 months. Although there are a variety of underlying causes, most can be categorized as pressure sores, diabetic foot ulcers, or leg ulcers. An important question is whether chronic wounds are intrinsically different from acute wounds. For instance, does local tissue senescence make healing a chronic wound impossible? Or, do chronic wounds have the inherent potential to heal, but are subject to a combination of factors that lead to delayed healing? Research has begun to address the question of what is different about the environment in a chronic wound.

Clinicians have long recognized that most chronic wounds do indeed have the potential to heal. Healing usually fails because of inadequate attention to the basic principles of open wound care—adequate cleansing, débridement, edema control, avoidance and treatment of ischemia, and achievement of a moist wound healing environment. However, the wound environment in many chronic wounds does differ in important ways from acute wounds. Studies have examined wound fluid and biopsy samples collected from chronic wounds. These reveal significant increases in tissue levels of proteases and collagenases, which are capable of degrading matrix proteins and growth factors. Degradation of growth factors inhibits their crucial functions of proliferation and chemotaxis. When wound fluid from a chronic wound is compared with fluid from an acute surgical wound, there is indeed a lower level of growth factors. It is not clear what influence bacteria have in this process, although the direct release of bacterial proteases and the indirect effect of protease release from phagocytic cells are both relevant. It is unknown whether growth factor levels are depressed because of proteolysis, primary inhibition of release, or secondary phenotypic changes in the cells of the chronic wound.

WOUND MANAGEMENT

Surgical Incisions

It takes at least 3 weeks for collagen to undergo sufficient remodeling and cross-linking to attain moderate strength. Figure 3.4 shows that at 1 to 2 weeks, the time when most sutures are removed, a wound has a small fraction of its eventual strength and may therefore disrupt with even modest stresses. Therefore, deep sutures are placed in collagen-containing structures to hold prolonged tension. Dermis, intestinal submucosa, muscular fascia, tendon, ligament, Scarpa's fascia, and blood vessel wall represent a partial list of tissues with high collagen content. These deep sutures are often absorbable. The most common absorbable materials, polyglycolic acid (Dexon) and polygalactic acid (Vicryl), retain tensile strength for approximately 3 weeks. Sutures used for tendon and abdominal fascia are usually permanent or, if absorbable, should ideally retain their tensile strength for close to 6 weeks. After 6 weeks, wounded tissue has gained approximately 50% of its eventual strength. To prevent hernia formation, heavy lifting is avoided after major abdominal surgery for 6 weeks. Tendon repairs are splinted and activity restricted to avoid full tension for a similar period.

Open Wound Dressings

There are at least 150 dressing products commercially available. These include multiple topical antibiotics, irrigants, and débriding agents. Although becaplermin gel (Regranex) and an artificial skin equivalent made of a dermis-like matrix covered with cultured epithelium from heterologous human foreskins (Apligraf) have been shown to decrease healing times in certain wounds, standard treatment, which adheres to the principles outlined earlier, may be successfully applied to most wounds. There are many good alternative treatments, but to avoid confusion they should be judged according to the following criteria:

1. How effectively is the wound cleaned or débrided?
2. Is moist wound healing achieved?
3. Is edema minimized in the periwound tissue?
4. Are new pressure insults or wound soilage prevented?
5. Is tissue oxygenation (blood flow) adequate?

In some situations, reduction of tissue bacteria is an important additional need; this is most often addressed by adequate cleaning and débridement. In the absence of large amounts of necrotic tissue, wound débridement does not need to be accomplished surgically. Proteinaceous exudate can be tenacious, however, and simple application of moist dressings may not be adequate to remove it. Water irrigation, either in whirlpools or by water from a hand-held shower spray or from dental water cleaning devices, can be gentle and yet generate enough power to débride effectively (9). Frequent moist dressing changes can accomplish this as well, and in some cases, occlusive absorptive dressings can generate enough tissue proteases effectively to degrade proteins that the absorptive dressings remove. This deceptively simple principle is the most frequently overlooked in wound care. The typical open surgical wound often contains deep interstices that packing or other absorptive dressings may not reach. The deeper portions of the wound may then accumulate exudate and bacteria. This is one example where water irrigation may be particularly useful. Commonly used agents such as hydrogen peroxide are actually harmful to normal tissue, and are weak oxidants and thus do a poor job of débriding. These are to be avoided. Enzymatic débriding agents can be effective when properly used.

As discussed, a desiccated wound undergoes delayed healing. Most wounds require an absorptive dressing to remove exudate. This can be gauze, which is inexpensive and effective but requires frequent dressing changes and is not occlusive, so that an ointment or cream must be added. Skin graft donor sites do well with an occlusive polyurethane film dressing. Most of the newer dressing products have been designed to be more absorptive and achieve moist healing without infection from excess exudate. An emphasis has been to decrease the frequency of dressing changes. It must be emphasized that although factors such as convenience, patient acceptance, and cost are good reasons for choosing a product, as long as moist healing is achieved, there is no evidence that one is better than another.

Edema is detrimental to wound healing and is often undertreated, in part because of difficulties in patient education. Edema can be a factor in virtually any ulcer of the lower extremity, although venous insufficiency is the most important. Because patients often have personal habits that are hard to modify, this can be a refractory problem. Patients often object to compression stockings, the most effective method for limiting edema. This leaves intermittent leg elevation, elastic wraps, and elevation of the foot of the bed as alternative measures. The critical factor is getting the patient to realize that leg swelling must be avoided, and so in the course of their day, each patient must modify behavior sufficiently to treat this problem.

Systemic Factors Affecting Wound Healing

Several important systemic factors or conditions influence wound healing. Interestingly, there are no known systemic conditions that lead to more rapid wound healing. The discussion that follows relates to factors that may retard or inhibit wound healing.

Nutrition

Wound healing requires energy and is an anabolic process (10). Patients who are severely malnourished or who are actively catabolic demonstrate impaired healing. Although there is no single measure of nutritional adequacy, the serum albumin level is the most readily available and clinically useful parameter. A serum albumin greater than 3.5 g/dL suggests adequate protein stores and positive nitrogen balance. However, albumin has a serum half-life of 19 days. Therefore, the serum albumin level does not drop early in a catabolic process and is slow to rise when protein stores are repleted and an anabolic state returns. Serum transferrin has a shorter half-life and therefore responds more promptly to nutritional fluctuations, but it is not part of a routine chemistry panel and has not gained widespread clinical use. There is no consensus on nutritional parameters that accurately predict surgical complications. In considering closure of a chronic wound such as a pressure sore, the ability to form granulation tissue and begin wound contraction are clinical indications of acceptable wound healing potential. The presence of a granulating, contracting wound argues strongly that the patient has adequate nutrition to undergo surgery, just as the absence of granulation and contraction argues strongly against. Certainly, an albumin level of less than 3 mg/dL raises concern for potential wound healing problems. Most surgeons avoid trying to close chronic wounds surgically until nutritional levels are considered acceptable.

Vitamins play an important role in wound healing as well. Vitamin A is involved in the stimulation of fibroplasia, collagen cross-linking, and epithelialization. In animal studies, vitamin A reverses the inhibitory effects of glucocorticoids on the inflammatory phase of wound healing (11). Although there is no conclusive evidence in humans, vitamin A may be useful clinically for steroid-dependent patients who have problematic wounds or who are undergoing an extensive surgical procedure. Vitamin A may be used either topically or systemically, but attention should be paid to the dosage and duration of therapy because vitamin A is fat soluble and has a well defined toxicity state. An oral dose of 25,000 IU daily or topical application of 200,000 IU ointment three times a day should be sufficient in adults.

Vitamin C is a necessary cofactor in the hydroxylation of lysine and proline in collagen synthesis and cross-linkage. The deficiency state, scurvy, is rarely seen in the Western world today. The utility of vitamin C supplementation in patients who are taking a normal diet is not established.

Vitamin E is applied to wounds and incisions by many patients. The evidence to support this practice is entirely anecdotal and, in fact, large doses of vitamin E have been found to inhibit wound healing (12). Only, massage, pressure, and silicone sheeting have been shown to flatten and soften scars. Many people perceive a healing benefit from topical creams, but the two main variables that determine how a scar appear are the following: (a) scars improve with the passage of time; and (b) natural variability occurs in scar formation, between different individuals, and in the same individual in different locations and at different ages.

Essential fatty acids are required for all new cell synthesis. Essential fatty acid deficiency is first noted in areas of high cellular turnover, such as healing wounds, skin, and gastrointestinal mucosa. Early experience with total parenteral nutrition in which essential fatty acids were lacking showed that difficult wounds and dramatic skin changes developed in patients. These were rapidly reversed with the addition of fat to the parenteral nutritional program.

Zinc and copper are also cofactors for many enzyme systems that are important to wound healing. Deficiency states have been seen with parenteral nutrition but are rare and now readily recognized and treated with supplements.

Vitamin and mineral deficiency states clearly show the necessity of these agents for wound healing. However, these deficiency states are extremely rare in the absence of parenteral nutrition or other extreme dietary restrictions. There is no evidence to support the concept that supranormal provision of these factors enhances wound healing in normal patients. Significant complications, especially with excessive fat-soluble vitamin supplementation, are reported. However, malnutrition can be a significant problem in the elderly and debilitated patient. These patients require nutritional supplementation and should receive vitamin and mineral supplementation as part of their protein and caloric repletion.

Aging

There are important age-dependent aspects of wound healing. The elderly heal more slowly and with less scarring. There is gradual attenuation of the inflammatory response with age, and decreased wound healing is one of the consequences. In vitro studies have documented an age-dependent decrease in the proliferative potential of fibroblasts and epithelial cells. Clinically, this accounts for the formation of finer scars and an improved cosmetic appearance in the elderly. Hypertrophic scars are rarely seen in the elderly. Sutures should be left in place longer to allow for the slower gain in tensile strength in the aged. This may be done without formation of suture marks because slower epithelialization occurs along the sutures. Although the aged usually heal surgical incisions without complications, the combination of age with other adverse factors can result in severe healing deficits and high surgical complication rates.

Pharmacologic Impairment to Wound Healing

Bone marrow suppression, a common consequence of chemotherapy, is detrimental to wound healing. Quantitative and qualitative lymphocyte and monocyte deficiency impairs cellular proliferation in the inflammatory phase of wound healing. Any chemotherapeutic agent that suppresses the bone marrow impairs healing. Fortunately, this is predictably reversible with cessation of chemotherapy. Glucocorticoids inhibit wound healing based on their antiinflammatory and immunosuppressive effects. The antiinflammatory effect of steroids is in part the result of inhibiting arachidonic acid metabolism through impairment of macrophage migration and altered neutrophil function. Glucocorticoids also inhibit synthesis of procollagen by fibroblasts, delaying wound contraction. Steroid-dependent patients have a persistent decrease in wound tensile strength even after healing is complete. Patients who require chronic systemic steroid therapy have attenuation of the dermis, which therefore is susceptible to injury. Even minor shearing forces may produce tearing of the skin and full-thickness wounds because of the decreased tensile strength.

Ischemia

Adequate tissue oxygenation plays a critical role in wound healing (13). It is needed for aerobic metabolism and also for proper neutrophil function, especially in bacterial killing. It is also a requirement for hydroxylation of proline and lysine to form stable collagen fibrils (Table 3.3).

Table 3.3. **FACTORS THAT CONTRIBUTE TO WOUND ISCHEMIA**

Poor arterial inflow—atherosclerosis
Poor venous flow—venous stasis
Smoking
Radiation
Edema
Diabetes mellitus—accelerates atherosclerosis
Vasculitis
Fibrosis—chronic scarring
Pressure—pressure sores or decubitus ulcer

Smoking. Smoking or use of nicotine patches inhibits oxygen delivery through sympathomimetic vasoconstriction. Also, smoking elevates carboxyhemoglobin levels in the blood. This shifts the oxygen delivery curve to the left because of the high affinity of carboxyhemoglobin for oxygen, resulting in less available oxygen in the wound. Animal studies demonstrate that even moderate decreases in tissue oxygen tension result in severe impairment of wound healing with substantially increased infection rates. Smoking has been shown to increase wound complication rates when skin flaps are elevated with a marginal distal blood supply.

Radiation. Radiation injury leads to arteriolar fibrosis and impaired oxygen delivery. In addition, there is progressive obliteration of blood vessels in the radiated area over time. Radiation also causes intranuclear and cytoplasmic damage to fibroblasts, and this appears to limit their proliferative potential.

Edema. Edema impairs local oxygen delivery, as outlined earlier. Also, edema is often associated with increased venous pressure. This postcapillary obstruction decreases the perfusion pressure in the capillary bed, resulting in ischemia. Increased venous pressure also leads to protein extravasation and pericapillary cuffing. This acts as a diffusion barrier to oxygen, further impairing tissue oxygenation and wound healing.

Diabetes. Diabetes mellitus is often associated with decreased healing of open wounds and increased susceptibility to infection. Many factors contribute to poor healing in diabetic patients, and most of these reflect local wound ischemia. However, healing is not impaired in a normally perfused area in a well controlled diabetic patient. This subject is discussed in detail later.

Other Local Conditions

Peripheral arterial occlusive disease secondary to atherosclerosis can be a primary cause of impaired healing, and may also be a cofactor with other conditions discussed. Also, conditions such as vasculitis, prolonged pressure, lower leg venous insufficiency, and tissue fibrosis affect wound healing through the mechanism of local tissue ischemia.

Chronic Wound Care

As noted, a chronic wound is commonly defined as an open wound that has failed to respond to standard care and remains open at 3 months. Typically, the wound size is static, with no visibly advancing epithelial edge. The etiology of a chronic wound is often multifactorial. One or more factors that impair wound healing, such as advanced age, ischemia, bacterial contamination, edema, and malnutrition or immunosuppression, are often present in patients with chronic wounds. A systematic approach is needed to identify these factors. Once all of the potentially applicable factors have been identified, those amenable to treatment are reversed. Age is, of course, fixed, but most other factors can be modified. Wounds should be débrided and topical as well as systemic antibiotics may be indicated for true bacterial infection. Arterial revascularization can increase oxygenation in the wound and elevation and compression dressings can decrease edema. Skin grafting or other surgical procedures are indicated as long as the underlying processes has been identified and appropriately treated. The underlying causes of some chronic wounds, such as diabetes or venous insufficiency, cannot be corrected.

Specific chronic wounds are discussed in the sections that follow.

Pressure Sores

Pressure sores are sometimes mistakenly referred to as *bed sores* or *decubitus ulcers.* These sores are not always acquired in bed or while lying flat in a decubitus position. All pressure sores, regardless of location, do involve prolonged pressure over a bony prominence. The ability of tissue to withstand pressure is defined by the duration of the pressure, the amount of pressure, and related shear forces. The most frequent locations of pressure sores are overlying the ischium, sacrum, and trochanter. The heel, knee, and ankle are less common locations.

Prolonged pressure produces ischemia in the tissue by occluding the microcirculation. This occurs when the tissue pressure exceeds the capillary filling pressure of 25 mm Hg. Pressure on the tissue overlying the sacrum can reach 80 mm Hg in a recumbent patient, so tissue necrosis can occur within hours if the pressure is not relieved by frequent changes in position.

Skin is more resistant to pressure than the underlying subcutaneous fat or muscle. This accounts for the common finding of a small skin ulceration overlying a large area of subcutaneous necrosis. Efforts to identify and control factors that contribute to impaired wound healing should be made. Nutrition is often a problem, as is bacterial overgrowth. If the patient can avoid pressure on the involved area and other contributing factors are controlled, most pressure sores heal. However, there is a higher incidence of recurrence if pressure sores are allowed to heal by secondary intention rather than by surgical closure. This is explained by the increased scarring that occurs in healing by secondary intention and the fact that this places the scar directly over the pressure point. Because scars are never as strong as intact skin, they are more prone to breakdown than intact skin that has been placed over these pressure points by surgical closure.

Leg Ulcers

Leg ulcers are perhaps the most common type of chronic ulcer. The disease process responsible is most often local tissue ischemia. The underlying cause of this local tissue ischemia should be identified and appropriate treatment initiated.

Approximately 90% of all leg ulcers in the United States are secondary to venous insufficiency (valvular incompetence). Venous insufficiency leads to local tissue ischemia by increased venous pressure, which lowers the transcapillary perfusion pressure, and by leg edema. Initial treatment should be directed to cleansing and débriding the wound of proteinaceous exudate and limiting the edema and protein loss with compression dressings and elevation. A common treatment has been the Unna boot, a paste bandage that is absorptive, limits edema, and can be changed weekly. This allows the physician complete control of treatment with weekly visits. If this dressing is made compressive by adding an elastic wrap, it is highly effective in reducing edema, absorbing the exudate, and providing an occlusive wound environment. Its limitations are that it requires weekly visits and precludes normal showering or bathing. Compression garments or elastic wraps with frequent dressing changes, thorough cleaning, and an occlusive dressing can be equally effective. Surgical treatment of venous insufficiency is addressed elsewhere.

Additional causes of leg ulcers include arterial insufficiency and other vasculitis syndromes. These are treated best by correcting the underlying disease and providing local wound care. If the underlying problem cannot be treated, there is little hope of securing a stable, healed wound.

Diabetic Foot Ulcers

Diabetic foot ulcers are caused by pressure over bony prominences, usually the metatarsal heads, in the setting of neuropathy. However, there is no evidence to support the often-cited concept that these ulcers may result from small vessel disease. This theory originated with a non-blinded study of the microvasculature in amputation specimens by Goldenberg in 1959. Subsequent blinded studies have failed to reveal any architectural differences in small blood vessels of diabetic amputation specimens. The ischemia in diabetic foot ulcers is most likely due to prolonged pressure on insensate toes and feet. This pressure ischemia is enhanced by the increase in blood viscosity related to nondeforming erythrocytes, which develop because of nonenzymatic glycosylation of cell membrane proteins. These rigid red blood cells plug capillary beds and decrease microvascular flow. In addition, the glycosylated hemoglobin has increased affinity for oxygen, thereby making less oxygen available to the tissues. Diabetic patients also have a predilection for infrapopliteal arterial occlusive disease and may therefore benefit from arterial reconstructive surgery. The requirements for successful treatment of diabetic ulcers include pressure relief with non-weight-bearing strategies and aggressive débridement of callus and marginally vascularized wound edges. Preventive measures with appropriate orthotic shoes are essential once healing is achieved. Finally, the clinician should bear in mind that the clinical effectiveness of becaplermin gel has been demonstrated in clean diabetic forefoot wounds.

Agents to Optimize Wound Healing

Dressings

Although becaplermin gel has been shown to speed healing in diabetic forefoot wounds, many types of dressings are commercially available, and none has been demonstrated to be effective if standard care is ignored. Despite marketing claims, standard wound care, keeping wounds clean, moist, and as free of edema and bacteria as possible, is still the most important factor in wound healing.

The ideal dressing should be simple, inexpensive, highly absorptive, and nonadherent. It should achieve moist healing and have antibacterial properties. Other factors to be considered are less frequent dressing changes, an all-in-one dressing that does not require tape or an overlay, and a gentle adhesive that is effective but not injurious to the skin when removed (14).

The simplest dressing is gauze and tape—it is inexpensive, absorptive, and, when used with an ointment, can achieve moist healing. The primary disadvantages are the necessity for frequent dressing changes and the potential for tape irritation and wound desiccation. Other products

Table 3.4. **WOUND DRESSINGS**

Classification	Composition	Indications	Functions	Examples
Films	Semiocclusive (semipermeable)— polyurethane or copolyester	Acute partial- or full-thickness wounds with minimal exudate Nondraining primarily closed wounds	Mimics skin performance Is water vapor permeable Is water and bacterial impermeable Is retention dressing for gel Is retention dressing for tubes Provides moist environment	Op-site Bioclusive Tegaderm Blisterfilm Visulin
Hydrocolloids	Contain hydrophilic colloidal particles (quar, karaya, gelatic, carboxymethl cellulose) in an adhesive mass (usually polysorbutylene)	Acute or chronic partial- or full-thickness wounds Stage I to IV decubitus ulcers	Absorbs fluid Débrides soft necrotic tissue by autolysis Protects wounds Provides good adhesiveness without adherence to wound Encourages granulation Promotes reepithelialization Protects wounds from trauma	Cutinova Hydro Duoderm Comfeel Restore Intrasite Ultec J&J ulcer dressing
Hydrogels	Contain 80%–99% water Cross-linked polymer such as polyethyleneoxide, polyvinyl pyrrolidone, or acrylamide	Acute or chronic partial-thickness wound with minimal exudate	Creates moist environment Usually requires secondary dressing Has low absorbency Débrides minimally Decreases pain Does not adhere to wound	Vigilon Geliperm Elastogel Intrasite gel
Foams	Either hydrophilic or hydrophobic Nonocclusive Usually polyurethane or gel film-coated High absorbency	Acute or chronic partial-thickness wounds that are highly secreting and require mechanical débriding	Débrides Has high absorbancy Water vapor permeable	Cutinova Plus Lyofoam Allevyn
Impregnates	Fine-mesh gauze impregnated with moisturizing, antibacterial, or bactericidal compounds Nonadherent	Acute or chronic partial-thickness wounds with minimal to moderate exudate	Does not adhere to wound Promotes reepithelialization May contain antibacterial or bactericidal agents Requires secondary dressing	Aquaphor-Gauze Adaptic Biobrane Scarlet Red
Absorptive powders and pastes	Consist of starch, copolymers, or colloidal hydrophilic particles Can absorb up to 100 times their weight in fluid	Chronic full-thickness wounds with large amounts of exudate	Has high absorbancy Débrides necrotic and fibrous material from wound	Spand-Gel Geliperm Envisan paste Bard absorption dressing Duoderm granules Hydrogran Hollister Exudate Absorber

Compiled by M.C. Crossland, RN, Wound Healing Center, Medical College of Virginia, Richmond, VA.

are classified into films, foams, hydrocolloids, hydrogels, and absorptive powders (Table 3.4). Films are semipermeable to water, usually made of polyurethane, and nonabsorptive. These are useful to achieve a moist wound healing environment over minimally exudative wounds, such as a split-thickness skin graft donor site.

Other dressing types have been designed for increased absorptive capacity. This requires fewer dressing changes and maintains an environment for moist healing.

The hydrocolloids deserve special mention because they have achieved widespread use. These contain hydrophilic materials, such as quar, karaya, gelatin, or carboxymethylcelluose, with an adhesive material and are covered by a semipermeable polyurethane film. These dressings use material that adheres to the skin surrounding a wound, is highly absorptive, and achieves a moist healing environment. Adhesion is maintained until the absorptive capacity is exhausted, after which atraumatic removal is easily accomplished. Similar materials have been extensively used for peristomal care. These are best used for open wounds that have only moderate exudate.

The increased absorptive capacity of these products allows infrequent, minimally traumatic dressing changes.

This, along with ease of use and achievement of moist healing, is their principal advantage.

Antibiotics

The role of antibiotics in wound care is controversial. All open wounds are colonized with bacteria. Only when the surrounding tissue is invaded (cellulitis) are systemic antibiotics clearly indicated. Antibiotics may be useful in other situations, such as when the granulation tissue has a high bacterial count, or in a case of reduced resistance to bacteria, such as in a diabetic foot ulcer, but these situations are not clearly defined. The routine use of systemic antibiotics for chronic wounds should be avoided to reduce the development of resistant bacterial strains in the wound.

Topical antibiotics are frequently used and can be useful. The ointment vehicle may help keep the wound moist, and the bacterial count in a wound may be lowered as a result. With most antibiotics, however, resistant organisms emerge quickly and allergic, hypersensitivity reactions are common. Most topical antibiotic ointments should be limited to 3 weeks of therapy to avoid development of a rash or other signs of inflammation resulting from the antibiotic ointment, rather than bacteria. The expense is substantial, and the benefits are not well demonstrated. Silver sulfadiazine, frequently used for burn care, is also useful for chronic wounds. Its broad spectrum of activity, the lack of relevant drug-resistant plasmids in bacteria, and its low cost make it a good choice.

Débriding Agents

Collagenases have been used to débride wounds since the late 1970s and can be a highly effective adjunct in the treatment of chronic wounds with necrotic tissue. These agents are used after surgical débridement to help clean a wound and to avoid a painful mechanical débridement. Collagenases combined with antibiotic powder have been proposed as a useful treatment for chronic wounds. A combination of collagenase and a nonenzymatic débriding agent (papain/urea) has also shown promise (15).

Pharmacologic Agents

Growth factors found naturally in wounds have improved healing in both normal and complex animal wounds (Table 3.5). The growth factors with the most evidence for efficacy are PDGF, TGF-β, epidermal growth factor, and members of the fibroblast growth factor family, although insulin-like growth factor-1, interleukin (IL)-1, IL-2, granulocyte–macrophage colony-stimulating factor, and vascular endothelial cell growth factor have also been associated with improved rates of healing in animal models (16,17). Clinical trials are in progress, and only becaplermin (PDGF) has been approved by the FDA. PDGF has shown efficacy in accelerating healing for patients with clean, well vascularized diabetic forefoot ulcers. A limiting factor in these clinical trials has been the variability in patients in terms of both systemic factors that affect healing and the number of variables in the wounds. The clinical studies are therefore difficult to perform and interpret.

Growth hormone deserves brief mention because it has been used successfully in some situations to reverse the catabolic impact of many severe injuries. Wound healing is a fundamentally anabolic event (creating new tissue), and in the setting of a severe burn, growth hormone administration significantly accelerates donor site healing, presumably because it minimizes catabolism.

EXCESSIVE SCARRING

Many factors are involved in the formation of an ideal scar. The most important of these are

- Accurate alignment of sharply incised tissue parallel to the natural lines of resting skin tension
- Closure of the wound without tension on the epidermis and without underlying dead space
- Primary healing without complications such as infection or dehiscence

The patient's genetic makeup and the location of the wound on the body are also important factors. The more negative factors associated with a particular wound, the more likely it will form a scar that is less than ideal. From an evolutionary viewpoint, wound healing has been programmed to be rapid and exuberant to minimize the problems of an open wound. As part of the aging process, the proliferative phase of wound healing becomes less exuberant, and although wound healing is slower, scars are improved.

The distinctions between an unsightly scar, a hypertrophic scar, and a true keloid can be confusing. An accurate diagnosis of most scars can be made by clinical observation and the history of the lesion.

Keloids

True keloids are uncommon and occur predominantly in dark-skinned people with a genetic predisposition for keloid formation (18). In most cases, this trait appears to be transmitted in an autosomal dominant pattern. The primary difference between a keloid and a hypertrophic scar is that a keloid extends beyond the boundary of the original tissue injury. It behaves as a benign tumor and extends into or invades the normal surrounding tissue. This creates a scar that is larger than the original wound.

Table 3.5. **SELECTED GROWTH FACTORS RELEVANT TO WOUND HEALING**

Factor	Source	Target	Function
TGF-β	All cells	All cells	Fibrosis
			Proliferation
TGF-α	Platelets	Epithelial cells	Proliferation
	Keratinocytes	Fibroblasts	
	Macrophages	Endothelial cells	
PDGF	Platelets	Neutrophils	Chemotaxis
	Macrophages	Macrophages	Proliferation
	Fibroblasts	Fibroblasts	Collagenase synthesis
	Endothelial cells	Smooth muscle cells	
	Smooth muscle cells		
FGF	Macrophages	Endothelial cells	Proliferation
	Fibroblasts	Epithelial cells	Chemotaxis
	Endothelial cells	Fibroblasts	Angiogenesis
		Chondroblasts	
EGF	Platelets	Epithelial cells	Proliferation
	Macrophages	Endothelial cells	Chemotaxis
	Keratinocytes	Fibroblasts	
IGF-I/Sm-C	Fibroblasts	Fibroblasts	Cell replication
		Endothelial cells	Collagen synthesis
IL-I	Macrophages	Fibroblasts	Proliferation
		Neutrophils	Collagenase synthesis
			Chemotaxis

TFG-β, transforming growth factor-β; TGF-α, transforming growth factor-α; PDGF, platelet-derived growth factor; FGF, fibroblast growth factor; EGF, epidermal growth factor; IGF-I/Sm-C, insulin-like growth factor I/somatomedin C; IL-I, interleukin-I.

Histologically, keloids contain an overabundance of collagen. The absolute number of fibroblasts is not increased, but the production of collagen continually outpaces the activity of collagenase, resulting in a scar of ever-increasing dimensions. The cause of keloid formation is unknown. Immunoglobulin G levels are increased, which suggests possible autoimmune stimulation resulting in a chronic inflammatory response with continued collagen deposition.

The treatment of keloids is difficult. The cause is unknown and the underlying disorder is not resolved by any specific therapy. Some improvement is usually seen with excision followed by intralesional steroid injection (19). In unresponsive cases, excision followed by a short course of radiation therapy has been successful, but the resulting scar is unpredictable and potentially worse. Keloids typically develop several months after injury and rarely, if ever, subside. Although many therapies have been tried, with anecdotal reports of success, none is ideal (20).

Hypertrophic Scars

Hypertrophic scars are histologically similar to keloids. They contain an overabundance of dermal collagen. Hypertrophic scars, however, respect the boundaries of the original injury and do not extend into normal unwounded tissue. They have less genetic predisposition, but hypertrophic scars also occur more frequently in Asians and blacks. They are often seen on the upper torso and across flexor surfaces. They usually develop within the first month after wounding and often subside gradually.

Improvement of hypertrophic scars may be obtained with pressure garments, topical silicone sheeting applications, or reexcision and closure (21). Reexcision and closure should be considered if conditions of the closure can be improved. This is especially true for wounds that originally healed by secondary intention or were complicated by infection. Simple reexcision and closure is unlikely to improve a scar that was closed with proper alignment and healed primarily without complications (22).

Unsightly Scars

A wound that is closed under tension or without adequate or accurate alignment, or a wound that runs across the lines of natural skin tension, is often unsightly. Surgical excision and closure with attention directed to correcting the underlying cause of the unsightly scar usually results in improvement.

FETAL WOUND HEALING

Much interest and research have focused on the process of fetal wound healing. It has been demonstrated that humans and several other mammalian species undergo fetal skin healing with little or no scar if the injury occurs early enough during gestation (23,24).

The physiologic mechanisms involved in scarless fetal healing are under active investigation. Adult wounds heal with a significant inflammatory response followed by abundant collagen deposition and remodeling into a mature scar. Numerous studies have shown that fetal wounds heal with little or no inflammation and no excess collagen formation. The fetal wound matrix is also higher in hyaluronic acid than the adult wound. This substance is seen only early in adult healing. Amniotic fluid is rich in hyaluronic acid and may provide the hyaluronic acid found in the fetal wound. Experiments that have exposed adult skin to amniotic fluid, however, demonstrate adult-type healing with scar formation.

Clearly, the fetal wound differs from the adult wound in several ways. The scarless healing appears multifactorial. Further research may identify factors (i.e., growth factors) that can be applied to wounds to diminish scar formation. This has potentially important application in virtually all of surgery, but has proved to be an elusive goal despite aggressive research interest.

REFERENCES

1. Leibovich SJ, Ross R. The role of the macrophage in wound repair: a study with hydrocortisone and antimacrophage serum. *Am J Pathol* 1975;78:71.
2. Wieman TJ, Smiell JM, Su Y. Efficacy and safety of a topical gel formulation of recombinant human platelet-derived growth factor BB (becaplermin) in patients with chronic neuropathic diabetic ulcers: a phase III, randomized, placebo-controlled, double-blind study. *Diabetes Care* 1998;21:822.
3. Ladin D, and the Plastic Surgery Educational Foundation DATA Committee. Becaplermin gel (PDGF-BB) as topical wound therapy. *Plast Reconstr Surg* 2000;105:1230.
4. Madden JW, Peacock EE. Studies on the biology of collagen during wound healing: I. Rate of collagen synthesis and deposition in cutaneous wounds of the rat. *Surgery* 1968;64:288.
5. Peacock EE Jr. *Wound repair,* 3rd ed. Philadelphia: WB Saunders, 1984.
6. Winter GD, Scales JT. Effect of air drying and dressings on the surface of a wound. *Nature* 1963;197:91.
7. Jonsson K, Jensen JA, Goodson WH, et al. Tissue oxygenation, anemia, and perfusion in relation to wound healing in surgical patients. *Ann Surg* 1991;214:6.
8. Kindwall EP, Gottlieb LJ, Larson DL. Hyperbaric oxygen therapy in plastic surgery: a review article. *Plast Reconstr Surg* 1991;88:898.
9. Gross A, Cutright DE, Bhaskar SN. Effectiveness of pulsating water jet lavage in treatment of contaminated crushed wounds. *Am J Surg* 1972;124:373.
10. Demling RH, DeSanti L. The stress response to injury and infection: role of nutritional support. *Wounds* 2000;12:3.
11. Seifter E, Rettura G, Padawer J, et al. Impaired wound healing in streptozotocin diabetes: prevention by supplemental vitamin A. *Ann Surg* 1981;194:42.
12. Ehrlich P, Tarver H, Hunt TK. Inhibitory effect of vitamin E on collagen synthesis and wound repair. *Ann Surg* 1972;175:235.
13. LaVan FB, Hunt TK. Oxygen and wound healing. *Clin Plast Surg* 1990;17:463.
14. Carver N, Leigh IM. Synthetic dressings. *Int J Dermatol* 1992;31:10.
15. Alvarez OM, Fernandez-Obregon A, Rogers RS, et al. Chemical débridement of pressure ulcers: a prospective, randomized, comparative trial of collagenase and papain/urea formulations. *Wounds* 2000;12:15.
16. Mustoe TA, Pierce GF, Thomason A, et al. Accelerated healing of incisional wounds in rats induced by transforming growth factor-β. *Science* 1987;237:1333.
17. Brown GL, Nanney LB, Griffen J, et al. Enhancement of wound healing by topical treatment with epidermal growth factor. *N Engl J Med* 1989;321:76.
18. Rockwell WB, Cohen IK, Enrlich HP. Keloids and hypertrophic scars: a comprehensive review. *Plast Reconstr Surg* 1989;84:827.
19. Griffith H. The treatment of keloids with triamcinolone acetonide. *Plast Reconstr Surg* 1966;38:202.
20. Lawrence WT. In search of the optimal treatment of keloids: report of a series and a review of the literature. *Ann Plast Surg* 1991;27:164.
21. Ahn ST, Monafo WW, Mustoe TA. Topical silicone gel: a new treatment for hypertrophic scars. *Surgery* 1989;106:781.
22. Khouri RK, Mustoe TA. Trends in the treatment of hypertrophic scars. *Adv Plast Reconstr Surg* 1991;8:129.
23. Mast BA, Diegelmann RF, Krummel TM, et al. Scarless wound healing in the mammalian fetus. *Surg Gynecol Obstet* 1992;174:441.
24. Siebert JW, Burd AR, McCarthy JG, et al. Fetal wound healing: a biochemical study of scarless healing. *Plast Reconstr Surg* 1990;85:503.

SURGERY: SCIENTIFIC PRINCIPLES AND PRACTICE, Third Edition, edited by
Lazar J. Greenfield, Michael W. Mulholland, Keith T. Oldham, Gerald B. Zelenock,
and Keith D. Lillemoe. Lippincott Williams & Wilkins Publishers, Philadelphia, © 2001.

CHAPTER 4

HEMOSTASIS

THOMAS W. WAKEFIELD

BASIC CONSIDERATIONS

The coagulation mechanism is a dynamic interactive network that relies on the interaction between platelets and coagulation complexes for clot formation. Initiating agents for coagulation include collagen and tissue factor. Tissue factor, released from injured cells, activates the extrinsic pathway of coagulation. Disruption of the endothelium of blood vessels exposes underlying collagen to platelets, activating them. In the blood, tissue factor complexes with activated factor VII, activating factors IX and X to factors IXa and Xa (activated factors IX and X) (1). The enzyme responsible for the initial activation of factor VII is unknown. However, factors Xa and VIIa catalyze activation of factor VII, so there is amplification for the formation of factor VIIa (2). At the same time, activated platelets spread in shape, with their procoagulant phospholipid phosphatidylserine and phosphatidylinositol (termed platelet factor 3) becoming externalized (3). This allows for the coagulation proteins to assemble on the surfaces of platelets, accelerating the coagulation reactions (4) (Fig. 4.1). Platelet membranes contribute critical surfaces for coagulation complex assembly. Activated but not resting platelets express binding sites for coagulation factors. During platelet activation in vitro, microparticles are released that are rich in receptors for factors Va and VIIIa (5,6). Von Willebrand factor (vWF) is responsible for platelet adhesion through binding to glycoprotein (Gp) Ib (7), whereas fibrinogen forms bridges between activated platelets by binding to GpIIb/IIIa on adjacent stimulated platelets (8). Unstimulated platelets attach to immobilized fibrinogen by the same receptor (9).

Once the platelet plug has formed, the stage is set for coagulation protein assembly. Activated factor X (Xa), activated factor V (Va), ionized calcium, and factor II (prothrombin) form on the platelet phospholipid surface to initiate the prothrombinase complex, which catalyzes the formation of thrombin faster than can be achieved with factor Xa alone (4) (Fig. 4.2). When the amount of tissue factor is limited, activation of factor IX rather than factor X is favored (10,11), allowing for tissue factor activation in situations of low tissue factor concentration. The pathway so described up to this point corresponds to the classic extrinsic pathway of coagulation. Thrombin is central to all of coagulation and acts to cleave fibrinopeptide A (FPA) from the α chain of fibrinogen and fibrinopeptide B (FPB) from the β chain (12). This leads to the release of fibrinopeptides and the formation of new fibrin monomers, which then cross-link, resulting in fibrin polymerization. Thrombin also activates factor XIII, which catalyzes the cross-linking of fibrin to make the clot firm (13), activates platelets, and activates factors V and VIII, two nonenzymatic cofactors, to Va and VIIIa (4). This is important because only factors Va and VIIIa are involved in coagulation. Factor XIIIa also cross-links other plasma proteins, such as fibronectin and α_2-antitrypsin, resulting in their incorporation into clot (14).

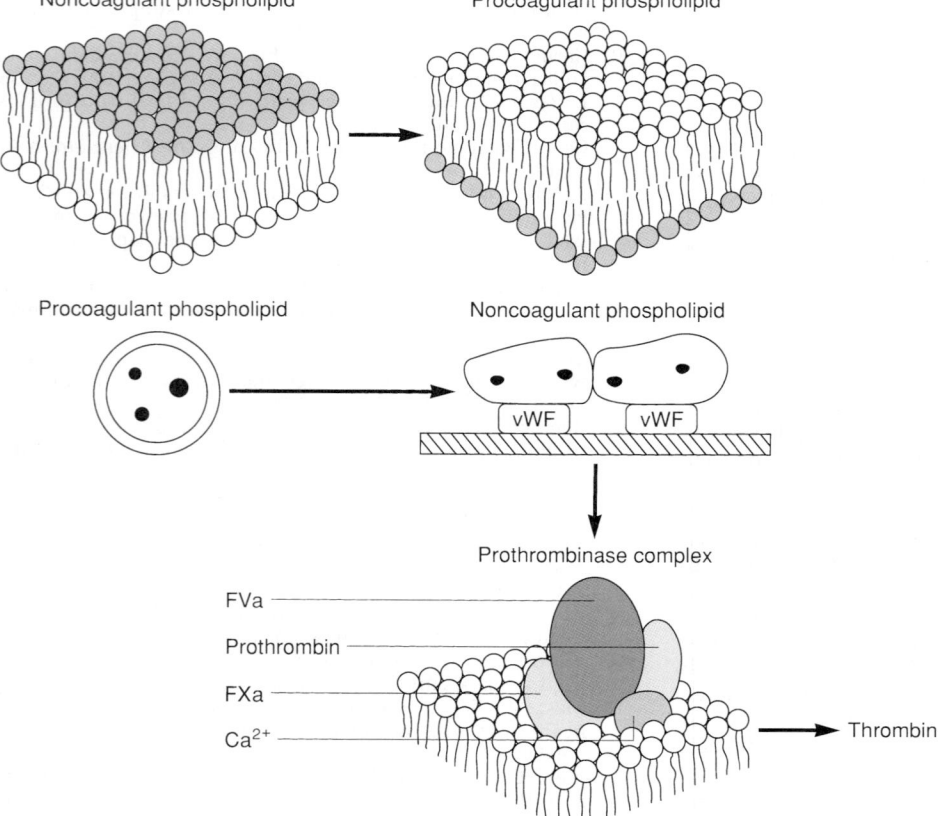

Noncoagulant phospholipid → Procoagulant phospholipid

Procoagulant phospholipid → Noncoagulant phospholipid

vWF   vWF

Prothrombinase complex

FVa
Prothrombin
FXa
Ca^{2+} → Thrombin

Figure 4.1. Formation of coagulation cascade assembly on the platelet phospholipid surface. (After Hassouna HI. Laboratory evaluation of hemostatic disorders. *Hematol Oncol Clin North Am* 1993;7:1188.)

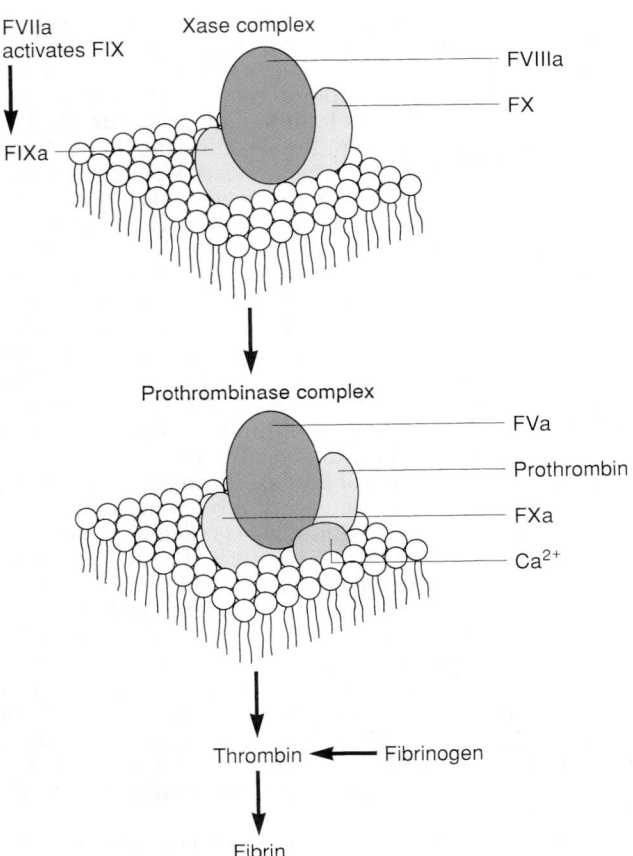

Figure 4.2. Formation of the Xase complex and prothrombinase complex with amplification of thrombin and fibrin formation. (After Hassouna HI. Laboratory evaluation of hemostatic disorders. *Hematol Oncol Clin North Am* 1993;7:1177.)

The intrinsic pathway of blood coagulation requires activation of factor XI to XIa. This may occur by both the contact activation system through activation of factor XII, plasma prekallikrein and high-molecular-weight kininogen, and, more importantly, through thrombin with negatively charged surfaces (15). Factor XIa activates factor XI autocatalytically (15) and also catalyzes the conversion of factor IX to IXa (16). Factor IXa, X, ionized calcium, and thrombin-activated factor VIII (VIIIa) then assemble on the platelet surface in a complex called the *Xase complex* to catalyze the activation of factor X to Xa (4) (Fig. 4.2). Factor Xa then shunts into the prothrombinase complex for further amplification of thrombin formation. The importance of a mechanism of factor XI activation independent of the contact activation system is apparent because patients deficient in those factors of the contact activation system, including factor XI, bleed, whereas patients deficient in factor XII, prekallikrein, and high-molecular-weight kininogen do not usually bleed (14).

NATURAL ANTICOAGULANT MECHANISMS

At the same time that thrombin forms, natural anticoagulant mechanisms oppose further thrombin formation. Just as thrombin generation is key to coagulation, antithrombin III is the central anticoagulant protein. This glycoprotein of 70-kd molecular weight binds to thrombin, preventing the removal of FPA and FPB from fibrinogen (17), preventing the activation of factors V and VIII, and

inhibiting the activation and aggregation of platelets. In addition, antithrombin III inhibits factors IXa (18), Xa, and XIa (19). A second natural anticoagulant is activated protein C, which inactivates factors Va (20,21) and VIIIa (22), thus reducing the Xase and prothrombinase complex acceleration of the rate of thrombin formation. In the circulation, protein C is activated to protein Ca on endothelial cell surfaces by thrombin complexed with one of its receptors, thrombomodulin (23–25) (Fig. 4.3), in a one-to-one complex (26), highlighting another important role for thrombin. The formation of this thrombin–thrombomodulin complex accelerates the activation of protein C compared with thrombin alone. Thrombin, at the same time, by binding to thrombomodulin, loses its platelet-activating activity (27) as well as its enzymatic activity for fibrinogen and factor V (28). Protein S is a cofactor for protein Ca (29) (Fig. 4.4). A third natural anticoagulant is heparin cofactor II (30). Its concentration in plasma is estimated to be significantly less than that of antithrombin III, and its action is implicated primarily in the regulation of thrombin formation in extravascular tissues. Finally,

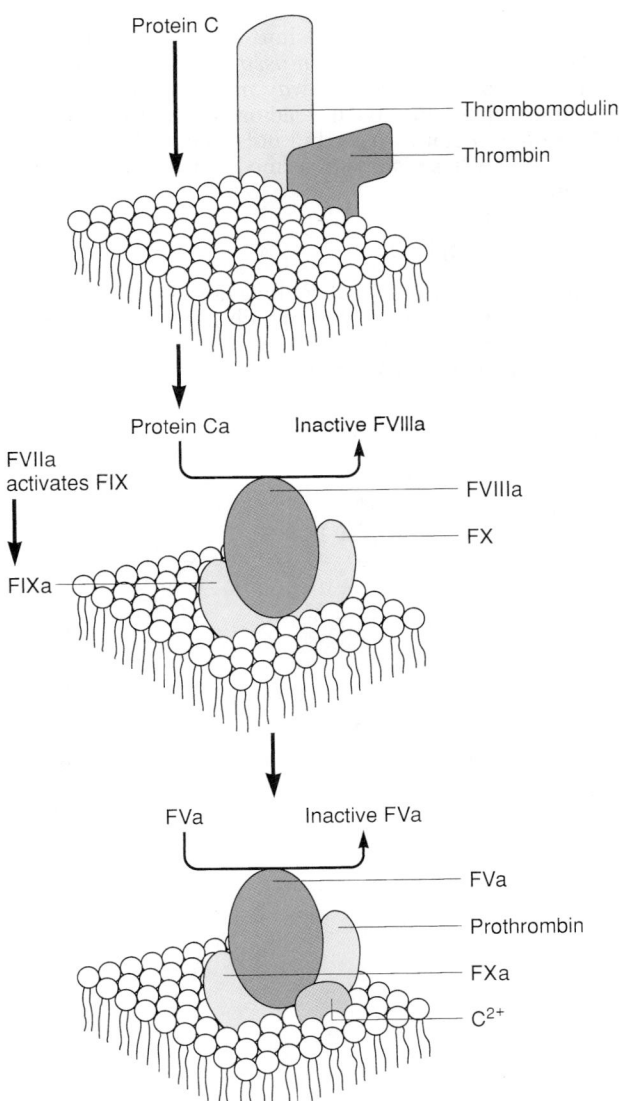

Figure 4.3. Activation of protein C by thrombin–thrombomodulin interaction. (After Hassouna HI. Laboratory evaluation of hemostatic disorders. *Hematol Oncol Clin North Am* 1993;7:1175.)

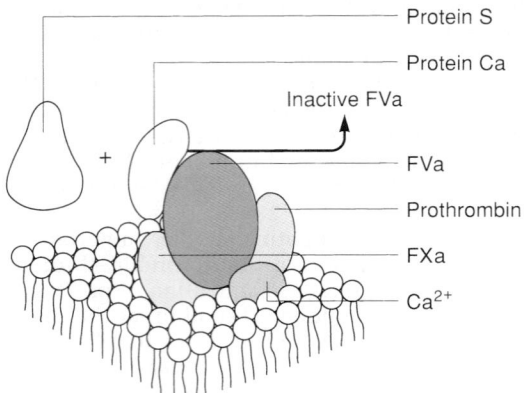

Figure 4.4. Actions of protein S. (After Hassouna HI. Laboratory evaluation of hemostatic disorders. *Hematol Oncol Clin North Am* 1993;7:1176.)

thrombin is inactivated when it becomes incorporated into the clot.

The extrinsic pathway is short lived owing to an inhibitor called the *lipoprotein-associated coagulation inhibitor* (31) or *extrinsic pathway inhibitor* (32). This protein inactivates the tissue factor–factor VIIa complex activation of factor X to Xa, but not of factor IX to IXa (14). This inhibitor has also been termed *tissue factor pathway inhibitor.*

FIBRINOLYSIS

During the process of thrombus formation, there is a constant process of clot lysis, which prevents physiologic thrombus formation from leading to pathologic intravascular thrombosis. Plasminogen, tissue plasminogen acti-

vator (tPA), and α_2-antiplasmin (α_2-AP) become incorporated into the fibrin clot as it forms (4) (Fig. 4.5). In fact, thrombin (both α and γ) promotes tPA release from endothelial cells as well as the production of plasminogen activator inhibitor (PAI-1) from endothelial cells (33,34). tPA converts plasminogen to plasmin, the main fibrinolytic enzyme. This is a serine protease whose main substrates include fibrin, fibrinogen, and other coagulation factors. Plasmin also interferes with platelet adhesion through vWF by proteolysis of GpIb (35). Fibrin, when digested by plasmin, yields one molecule of fragment E and two molecules of fragment D. In physiologic clot formation, fragment D is released in dimeric form (D-dimer) (4). The D-dimer fragment is a marker for ongoing thrombosis and fibrinolysis of formed clot (fibrin). The natural inhibitor of excess plasmin, α_2-AP, is also released by endothelial cells. In physiologic fibrinolysis, α_2-AP is bound to fibrin and excess plasmin is readily inactivated. In fibrinolytic states (fibrinogenolysis), however, and during treatment with fibrinolytic agents, circulating fibrinogen, in addition to clot-bound fibrin, is degraded by circulating plasmin, which is not readily inactivated by α_2-AP. Circulating fibrinogen is degraded by removal of FPB and the carboxyl-terminal portion of the α chain, yielding fragment X, which clots slowly (36). Fragment X is further degraded to one molecule of fragment D and a fragment Y, neither of which clot thrombin; fragment Y is broken down to two molecules of fragment D and one molecule of fragment E (4) (Fig. 4.6). In these fibrinogenolytic states, the D fragments are not cross-linked, and D-dimer is not formed. The Y and D fragments are potent inhibitors of fibrin formation.

The major categories of plasminogen activators include exogenous factors, such as streptokinase; endogenous factors, such as tPA and urokinase; and intrinsic factors (4). Intrinsic factors include factor XII, prekallikrein, and high-molecular-weight kininogen. These factors of the contact system are more important in clot lysis than

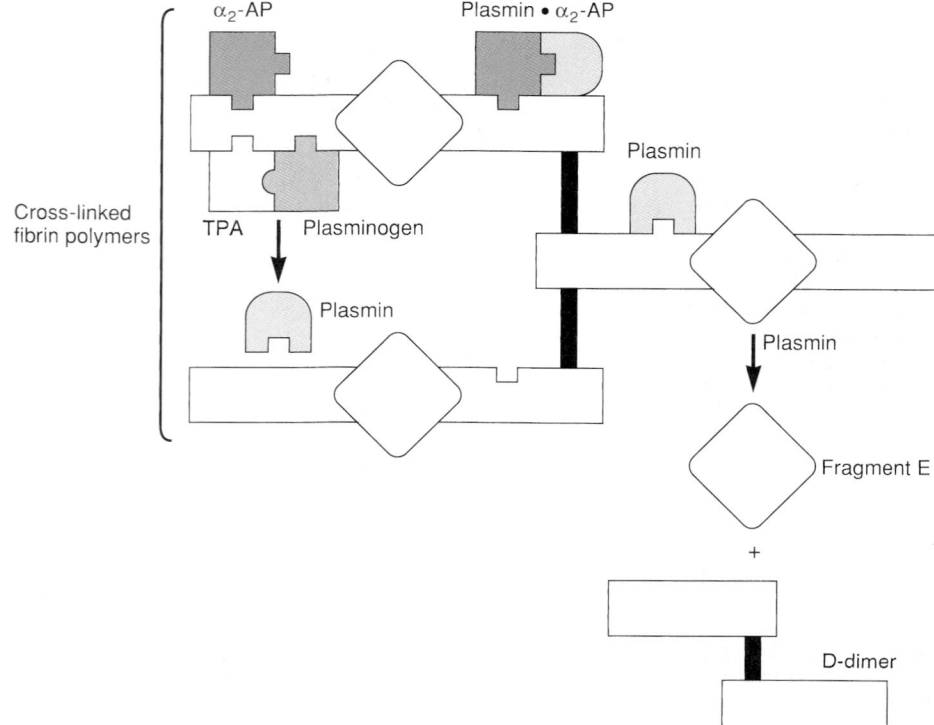

Figure 4.5. Incorporation of plasminogen, tissue plasminogen activator (tPA), and α_2-antiplasmin (α_2-AP) into the fibrin clot as it forms with production of D-dimer fragments. (After Hassouna HI. Laboratory evaluation of hemostatic disorders. *Hematol Oncol Clin North Am* 1993;7:1186.)

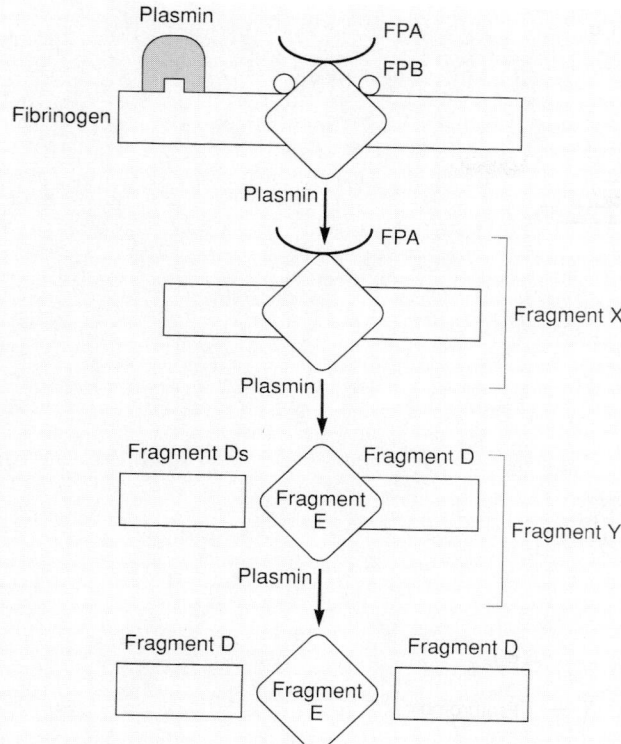

Figure 4.6. Process of fibrinogenolysis and formation of non-cross-linked fragment Ds. (After Hassouna HI. Laboratory evaluation of hemostatic disorders. *Hematol Oncol Clin North Am* 1993; 7:1193.)

thrombus formation. Activated forms of factor XII, kallikrein, and factor XI independently can convert plasminogen to plasmin (37). These enzymes may also liberate bradykinin from high-molecular-weight kininogen, resulting in an increase in vascular permeability, prostacyclin liberation, and tPA secretion. Finally, activated protein C (factor Ca) has been found to inactivate proteolytically the inhibitor to tPA, thus promoting tPA activity and fibrinolysis (26).

The endothelial cell itself appears to be in an excellent position to act as a nonthrombogenic surface (Fig. 4.7). It has three systems for the promotion of a nonthrombotic surface, including thrombin–thrombomodulin interaction, heparin–antithrombin III binding, and a membrane-bound fibrinolytic system. Circulating plasminogen exists in an N-terminal glutamic acid form (Glu-Plg). On the endothelial cell surface, Glu-Plg is converted to its N-terminal ly-

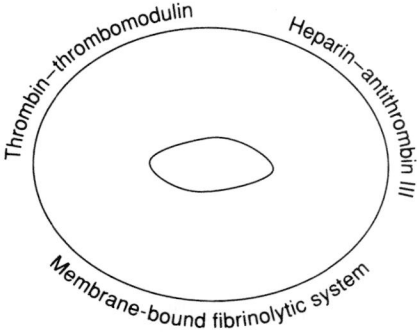

Figure 4.7. Vessel wall endothelial cell antithrombotic properties.

sine form (Lys-Plg) by locally generated plasmin (38). Local cell concentrations of tPA may be great enough to saturate high-affinity receptors, elaborate small amounts of plasmin, and convert Glu-Plg to Lys-Plg. Lys-Plg is then converted to plasmin with improved catalytic efficiency and the generation of a local fibrinolytic response.

In summary, coagulation is an ongoing process of thrombus formation, inhibition of thrombus formation, and thrombus dissolution. The central mediator is thrombin (4) (Fig. 4.8). Abnormalities in coagulation occur when one process—thrombus formation, thrombus inhibition, or fibrinolysis—overcomes the others and dominates the delicate balance that is hemostasis.

THROMBOSIS AND INFLAMMATION

Thrombosis and inflammation are closely linked. Tumor necrosis factor (TNF), a polypeptide cytokine of stimulated macrophages released in response to inflammation and sepsis, down-regulates thrombomodulin expression through endocytosis and degradation of thrombomodulin (39). TNF increases the level of C4b-binding protein, decreasing the amount of free protein S available to function as a cofactor for protein C. In addition, TNF induces tissue factor expression on the surface of endothelial cells. In a study of six normal human volunteers given TNF, factor X was activated to Xa early after administration, followed by prothrombin activation in a more gradual pattern of increase observed hours after maximal concentrations of factor Xa had been reached (40). TNF also inhibits fibrinolysis by suppressing the release of tPA and inducing the expression of tPA inhibitor type I (41–46). In vivo, TNF initially increases plasma plasminogen activator activity, followed by an even greater increase in PAI-1 antigen, leading to an overall inhibition of the fibrinolytic system (47). In addition, by down-regulating thrombomodulin, TNF decreases protein C production. Because protein C inhibits PAI-1, a decrease in protein C decreases the fibrinolytic potential of the blood. Along with its effects on coagulation, TNF facilitates inflammation. TNF and other cytokines stimulate adherence proteins on endothelial cells (48–51) for leukocytes and induce endothelial and vascular wall smooth muscle cell production of interleukin-8 (IL-8) gene expression and monocyte chemotactic protein-1 mRNA expression (52). These cytokines activate neutrophils in vitro and stimulate neutrophil and monocyte movement in vivo. They are also involved in the process of cytokine networking, in which one cytokine activates other cytokines, producing a physiologic response. The association between TNF and activation of both the coagulation and inflammatory pathways has been firmly established.

A model for the possible interactions between thrombosis and inflammation has been proposed (53) (Fig. 4.9). In this model, vascular injury results in the margination of circulating platelets along the vessel wall, probably mediated by vWF binding to GpIb on the platelet surface. The platelets then activate and aggregate in an interaction mediated by fibrinogen, resulting in platelet plug formation. Blood clotting is stimulated by the expression of tissue factor, and the clotting complexes are propagated on the phospholipid surfaces of activated platelets, resulting in the formation of a fibrin clot. Circulating neutrophils and monocytes then interact with the platelets through P-selectin and with the endothelial cells through P-selectin and E-selectin, events that result in the stable interaction between leukocytes and platelets at the thrombus–wall interface. Neutrophils and monocytes participate in this local inflammatory response, and monocytes may specifically contribute to clot formation by further tissue factor

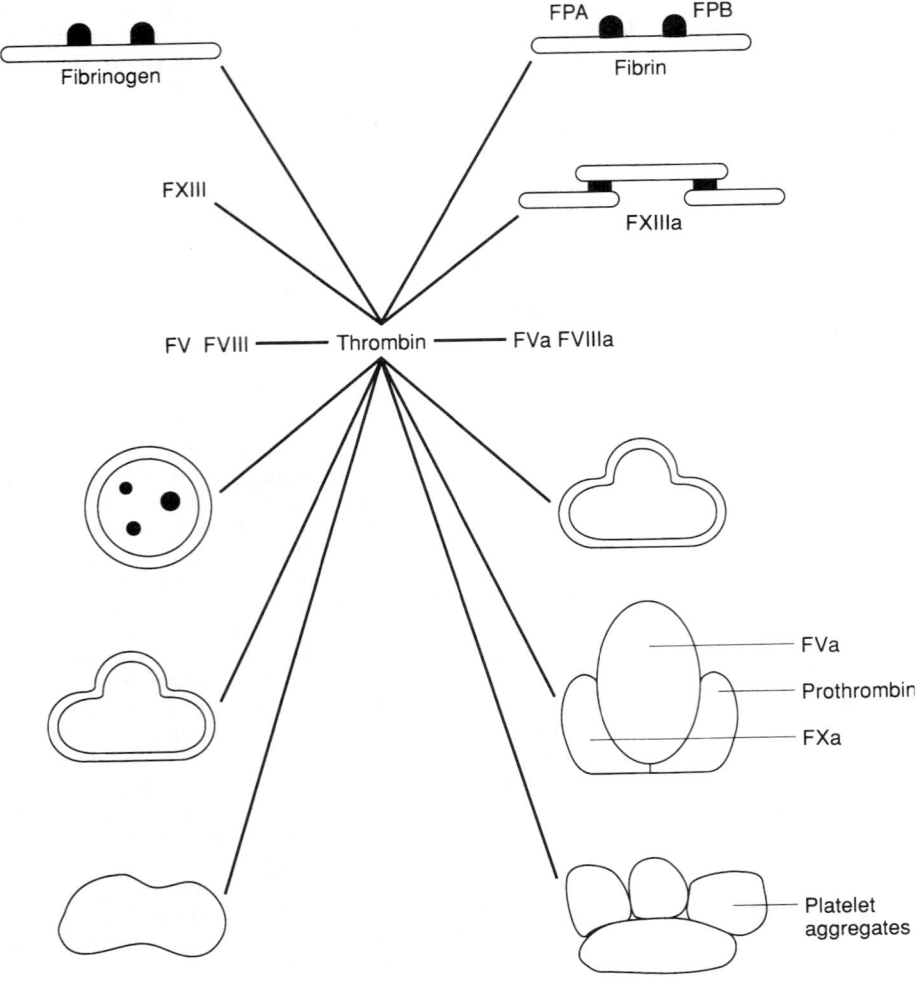

Figure 4.8. Thrombin as the central mediator of coagulation. (After Hassouna HI. Laboratory evaluation of hemostatic disorders. *Hematol Oncol Clin North Am* 1993;7:1177.)

expression on their surface. This has been suggested in a study involving fibrin formation under the influence of a monoclonal antibody to P-selectin in a primate arteriovenous fistula model (54).

In the venous circulation, a series of steps linking thrombosis and inflammation has been suggested (55). In step 1, thrombus formation involving platelets, neutrophils, and monocytes is initiated at venous confluences, saccules, and valve pockets. In step 2, adherent neutrophils and platelets become activated, releasing substances such as adenosine diphosphate (ADP, platelets) and neutrophil-activating peptide-2 (NAP-2, platelets and neutrophils), activating and attracting more platelets and neutrophils. Catepsin G, secreted from activated neutrophils, converts

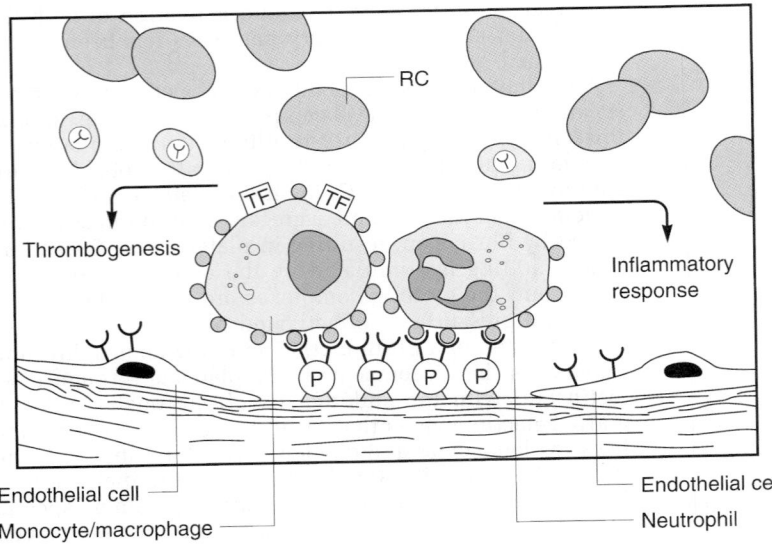

Figure 4.9. Cellular basis for blood coagulation, including platelets (P), neutrophils, monocytes, P-selectin (Y), and red blood cells (RC). (After Furie B, Furie BC. Molecular and cellular biology of blood coagulation. *N Engl J Med* 1992;326:803.)

β-thromboglobulin (secreted from platelets) into NAP-2 by proteolytic cleavage (56). This NAP-2 stimulates more catepsin G secretion, which in turn stimulates more platelet secretion (57,58), providing more substrate for NAP-2 and causing feedback activation for the recruitment of more platelets and neutrophils. In step 3, coagulation is initiated and promoted on the phospholipid surface of the platelets. Finally, in step 4, new layers of neutrophils and platelets form on the surface of fibrin, activate, and begin another round of the clotting process.

Leukocytes extravasate into the vein wall by a chemotactic gradient that develops in the wall in response to the venous thrombosis. In a baboon model of deep vein thrombosis (DVT) induced by stasis, the presence of a venous catheter for a short time, and the administration of the thrombogenic reagents TNF and antibody to protein C, we have observed by enzyme-linked immunosorbent assay (ELISA) protein measurements and immunohistochemical tissue staining the presence of inflammatory cytokines in the vein wall directly beneath the luminal thrombus, including IL-8, IL-6, monocyte chemotactic protein-1 (MCP-1), epithelial neutrophil-activating protein-78 (ENA-78) and macrophage inflammatory protein-1α (MIP-1α) (59). We have similarly observed in a pure stasis model of inferior venal caval thrombosis in both primates and rats a similar occurrence in the vein wall, with the early influx of neutrophils followed by the later extravasation of monocytes, macrophages, and lymphocytes in a typical inflammatory progression. This suggests that the sequence may lead to a complete inflammatory response in the vein wall. Further research to block the inflammatory response and the subsequent effect this interference may have on the detrimental interactions between the thrombus and the vein wall and valves may have significant implications for treatment of venous thrombosis. Approaches to interfere with the inflammatory response include blocking initial leukocyte adhesion, leukocyte activation, or both.

PROCOAGULANT STATES

A number of conditions can lead to a procoagulant state, including heparin-associated thrombocytopenia, antithrombin III deficiency, protein C and S deficiencies, resistance to activated protein C, lupus anticoagulant and the presence of antiphospholipid antibodies, fibrinogen abnormalities, defective fibrinolytic activity, platelet abnormalities, prothrombin 20210 polymorphism, homocystinemia, and disseminated intravascular coagulation (DIC).

Heparin-induced Thrombocytopenia

Heparin-induced thrombocytopenia occurs in 0.6% to 30% of patients who receive heparin, although severe thrombocytopenia (platelet counts <100,000/μL) is seen much less frequently (60). It is caused by a plasma factor, most likely a heparin-dependent immunoglobulin G (IgG) platelet antibody, that causes platelet aggregation when combined with platelet factor IV. The antibody may not be heparin specific, the main contributing mechanism being the degree of sulfonation of the heparin-like compound (61), and the actual platelet aggregation likely depends on the Fc region of the antibody (62). Activation of platelets in this setting can result in thrombocytopenia, thrombosis, and embolic episodes. Morbidity and mortality rates as high as 61% and 23%, respectively, have been reported (63). Both bovine and porcine heparin have been associated with this syndrome, although bovine heparin appears to be more commonly associated. Even low-molecular-weight heparins (LMWH) have been associated with the

syndrome. The syndrome usually begins 3 to 14 days after heparin administration, although it may begin earlier if the patient has been exposed to heparin in the past with preformed antibodies already present. The pathophysiology has been summarized: (a) heparin combines with platelet factor IV; (b) IgG forms to the heparin–platelet factor IV complex; (c) the antibody binds to a platelet FcγRIIA receptor by its Fc receptor; (d) platelet activation occurs; (e) platelet release and aggregation occurs; (f) platelet microparticles are formed; (g) cytokines and catecholamines enhance platelet aggregation; (h) immunoglobulins/complement deposit on the surface of endothelial cells, stimulating tissue factor; and (i) resulting thrombosis may then occur (64). Arterial and venous thromboses have all been noted and are likely to occur in diseased or traumatized vessels. Even small exposure as with heparin coating on pulmonary artery catheters has been reported to cause this problem.

Heparin-induced thrombocytopenia should be suspected in a patient when thrombosis occurs while receiving heparin or when there is a fall in platelet count to less than 100,000/μL. The laboratory diagnosis includes the gold standard serotonin release assay (sensitivity 94%; specificity 100%) (65), a less sensitive platelet aggregation assay, an ELISA assay detecting the antibody in the patient's plasma (66), as well as fluorescence-activated cell sorter analysis for the platelet microparticles (67). Other coagulation tests are usually negative in these patients. Treatment consists of cautious administration of protamine sulfate to reverse the heparin if active thrombosis has occurred, or discontinuation of heparin, allowing its effects to wear off, followed by another anticoagulant while beginning warfarin therapy. Patients with circulating platelet microparticles have a heightened thrombotic risk, and warfarin administration initially can potentiate this hypercoagulable state. Thus, warfarin should be begun under the protection of another anticoagulant (68). Available alternatives recommended include aspirin, which has only limited success. Iloprost, a prostacyclin analogue, although effective (69), is no longer recommended because of its strong vasodilatory and hypotensive effects. LMWHs with greater than 90% cross-reactivity by serotonin assay should not be substituted, although some have suggested that if an LMWH tests negative in vitro, it may be substituted (70). Danaparoid sodium (Orgaran; Organon Teknika, Durham, NC), a heparinoid, has a low (24%) level of cross-reactivity (71) and may be used if there is no cross-reactivity. The GpIIb/IIIa receptor antagonist c7E3 has been used, but it is associated with potential bleeding risks (72). Ancrod, a defibrinating agent, requires 12 hours before anticoagulation is achieved (73). Last, direct thrombin inhibitors have been used (74), and a direct thrombin inhibitor, lepirudin (Refludan; Aventis Pharmaceuticals, Parsippany, NJ) (75), has been approved by the U.S. Food and Drug Administration (FDA) for use in this syndrome. With early diagnosis and appropriate treatment, morbidity and mortality rates as low as 7.4% and 1.1%, respectively, have been reported (76).

Antithrombin III Deficiency

Antithrombin III deficiency accounts for approximately 1% to 2% of venous thrombotic events. Episodes of native arterial and arterial graft thrombosis have been described in antithrombin III deficiency (77). Although uncommon, this hypercoagulable state is a significant risk for recurrent, life-threatening thrombosis. Most cases occur early in life, with most apparent by 50 years of age. Antithrombin III is a serine protease inhibitor (serpin) of thrombin and factors Xa, IXa, VIIa, kallikrein, and XIa and has a half-life of 2.8 days. The diagnosis of antithrombin III deficiency should be suspected in a patient who cannot be adequately anticoagulated on heparin or who has thrombosis while on heparin, because heparin's effect is due to its ability to potentiate the anticoagulant effects of antithrombin III. The diagnosis is made by measuring antithrombin III antigen and activity levels with the patient off anticoagulants. Heparin decreases antithrombin III levels by 30%, and this effect can be noted for up to 10 days after stopping heparin therapy, whereas warfarin increases antithrombin III levels. During significant thrombotic episodes, antithrombin III levels may also become lowered by antithrombin III consumption. The nephrotic syndrome can lead to a relative antithrombin III deficiency because of the loss of intermediate-sized proteins into the urine along with albumin (molecular weight, 68 kd), with subsequent acute thrombosis of renal veins (78). Additional causes of antithrombin III deficiency include liver disease (site of production), malignancy, malnutrition, decreased protein production, and DIC (79). There are also less frequent causes of antithrombin III deficiency, including defective antithrombin III activity with normal quantitative levels and an abnormal interaction between antithrombin III and heparin (80). Homozygous individuals usually die in utero, whereas heterozygous patients usually demonstrate levels less than 70%. Treatment for a patient with antithrombin III deficiency who needs to be anticoagulated with heparin usually requires fresh frozen plasma, 2 units every 8 hours decreasing to 1 unit every 12 hours, followed by oral anticoagulants. Antithrombin III concentrates are also available (81).

Protein C and S Deficiencies

Protein C and S deficiencies lead to a hypercoagulable state. Protein C, with its cofactor protein S, are both synthesized by the liver. Activated protein C inactivates factors Va and VIIIa in the prothrombinase and Xase complexes, respectively (Fig. 4.10). This effect results in less formation of thrombin, the main clotting enzyme, and

therefore down-regulation of the clot-promoting system. In addition, activated protein C inhibits the inhibitor to tPA, thus increasing the fibrinolytic potential of blood. Protein C is activated to activated protein C when thrombin binds to the endothelial cell receptor thrombomodulin (82). Thrombomodulin brings protein C in proximity to thrombin to be activated. The half-life of protein C and protein S is approximately 4 to 6 hours. Although most cases of protein C or protein S deficiency involve venous thrombosis, cases of arterial thrombosis have been reported, especially in young patients (<51 years of age) (83). Both protein C and S deficiency states exhibit congenital and acquired forms and, when present, both lead to significant risk for thrombosis. When the condition is present as a homozygous state at birth, infants usually die from unrestricted clotting and secondary clot lysis, a condition of extreme DIC termed *purpura fulminans*. Patients heterozygous for protein C deficiency usually have protein C levels less than 60% of normal (4). Acquired deficiency states for protein C occur with liver failure, DIC, and nephrotic syndrome, for much the same reasons as for acquired antithrombin III deficiency.

Protein S is a cofactor to activated protein C. Protein S deficiency results in clinical states identical to protein C deficiency. Nephrotic syndrome can also lead to a reduction in free protein S levels and, subsequently, a hypercoagulable state due to protein S loss in the urine. Moreover, inflammatory states such as systemic lupus erythematosus (SLE) can result in an elevation of the protein S binding protein, C4b binding protein, thus reducing free protein S. It is free protein S that serves as a cofactor to activated protein C activity. The diagnosis of protein C or S deficiency is made by measuring protein C and S levels. For protein C, both antigen and activity levels are measured, whereas for protein S, only antigen levels are measured. The clinically important value of protein S is measurement of its free antigen. A condition also exists in which there is an abnormality in the function of the protein C molecule itself, resulting in a decrease in protein C activity without a decline in antigenic protein C levels.

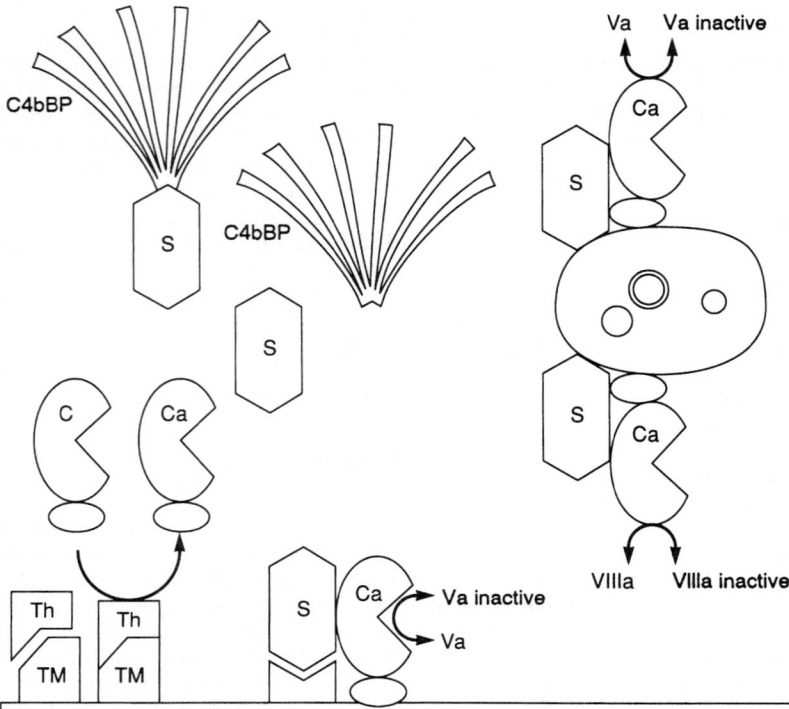

Figure 4.10. Role of proteins C and S. Th, thrombin; TM, thrombomodulin; C4bBP, C4b binding protein. (After Esmon CT. The regulation of natural anticoagulant pathways. *Science* 1987;235:1348.)

Thrombosis usually occurs between 15 and 30 years of age for deficiency of both of these proteins. When the diagnosis has been made with episodes of thrombosis, treatment consists of anticoagulation, initially with heparin, followed by lifelong oral anticoagulation. However, there have been reports that in large populations of asymptomatic blood donors, low protein C levels may be found in asymptomatic people, suggesting that not all patients with low levels of these factors thrombose. Many heterozygous family members of homozygous protein C-deficient infants also are unaffected (84). Thus, anticoagulation therapy in an individual patient should be instituted only after thrombosis.

During the initiation of oral anticoagulation, blood may become transiently hypercoagulable because the vitamin K-dependent factors with short half-lives (proteins C and S, factor VII) are inhibited before the other vitamin K-dependent factors (factors II, IX, and X). In a patient already partially deficient in protein C or S, the levels of these anticoagulant factors diminish even further with the initiation of oral anticoagulation, thus resulting in a temporary hypercoagulable state. This can result in microcirculatory thrombosis and the syndrome of warfarin-induced skin necrosis (85), leading to full-thickness skin loss, especially over fatty areas where blood supply is poor to begin with, such as breasts, buttocks, and abdomen. To prevent this devastating syndrome, warfarin therapy at lower loading doses should be begun under the protection of systemic heparin anticoagulation (standard heparin or LMWH), especially in those patients needing oral anticoagulation for thromboembolic disease.

Resistance to Activated Protein C (Factor V Leiden)

Resistance to activated protein C (factor V Leiden) is a relatively newly described syndrome, reported in 20% to 60% of cases of idiopathic venous thrombosis (86). It is the most common cause for thrombosis, although alone is a relatively low risk factor for thrombosis. A common polymorphism of factor V causing activated protein C resistance is present in 1% to 2% of the general population, and is much more common in whites than in minority Americans (87). The defect is due to a resistance to inactivation of factor Va by activated protein C as a result of the substitution of a glutamine for arginine at position 506 in factor V (88), called factor V Leiden. This single amino acid substitution is due to a single base pair mutation in the factor V gene. Thrombotic manifestations are noted in those either homozygous or heterozygous for this mutation. Patients homozygous for this mutation usually do not die in infancy. The incidence of thrombosis also is correlated to the presence of additional risk factors for thrombosis, especially in women using oral contraceptives (88). Combined defects with other hypercoagulable states, such as protein C and S deficiency (89,90), also result in a markedly increased thrombotic risk. The relative risk for thrombosis in patients heterozygous for factor V Leiden is increased 7-fold, whereas it is increased 80-fold for those homozygous for factor V Leiden (91). In addition to the large number of cases of primary venous thrombosis, recurrent venous thrombosis is also more common in patients with this entity, with an increase in the recurrent venous thrombosis relative risk of 2.4-fold (92). Although venous thrombosis predominates, arterial thrombosis, especially involving lower extremity revascularizations, has also been reported (93). The prevalence is increased in patients with peripheral vascular occlusive disease, measured both by the functional assay (94,95) and by genetic analysis (96).

The diagnosis of activated protein C resistance is made by a clot-based assay with the addition of activated protein C. Over 90% of people with activated protein C resistance have the factor V Leiden mutation (i.e., the arginine-to-glutamine substitution at position 506). Treatment options for activated protein C resistance include anticoagulation, initially heparin, followed by oral anticoagulation. The long-term use of warfarin is controversial because no data exist to suggest that long-term warfarin should be given after a first episode of venous thrombosis in a patient with this syndrome, especially if the patient is heterozygous for the syndrome. The fact that activated protein C resistance carries a relatively low (2.4-fold) increased risk for recurrent thrombosis suggests that not all patients after their first episode of thrombosis need long-term anticoagulant treatment, and that patients must be evaluated in light of their overall risk for thrombosis.

Lupus Anticoagulant

The "lupus anticoagulant" is a misnomer. It is unfortunate that this syndrome is called *anticoagulant* because it is associated with or results in a hypercoagulable state. It is associated with antiphospholipid antibodies, usually IgG, which result in thrombosis (97). The antiphospholipid antibody syndrome consists of the presence of an antiphospholipid antibody in association with episodes of thrombosis, recurrent fetal loss, thrombocytopenia, and livedo reticularis. Strokes, myocardial infarctions, visceral infarctions, and extremity gangrene may occur. The diagnosis is suspected in a patient with a prolonged activated partial thromboplastin time (aPTT) with other coagulation test results normal and a measured antiphospholipid or anticardiolipin antibody. The prolongation in the aPTT is a laboratory artifact; the antiphospholipid antibody interacts with the anionic phospholipids in the aPTT assay, prolonging the assay. The diagnosis may be made with either an abnormal clot-based functional assay with the patient off anticoagulants, or by direct ELISA antibody measurement. There is imperfect agreement between diagnostic tests for this abnormality. Approximately 80% of patients with a positive aPTT test (lupus anticoagulant) have a positive antiphospholipid antibody by ELISA, but only 10% to 50% of patients with a positive antiphospholipid antibody by ELISA have a positive aPTT test. Patients with both tests positive are reported to have the same thrombotic risk as those with either alone (98). The prolonged aPTT appears to be a better predictor for thrombotic events, whereas a high-titer antiphospholipid antibody (especially an IgG anticardiolipin antibody) is more predictive of recurrent fetal loss (99). In fact, up to 10% of women with two or more unexplained abortions are found to have a positive antiphospholipid antibody. Although low-titer antibody occurs in 2% of healthy young women and a high-titer antibody in 0.2% of healthy young women, apparent healthy women with high-titer antibody have an approximately 28% chance of fetal loss (100). The mechanisms responsible for fetal loss are unknown, although new data suggest that levels of annexin V (a phospholipid-binding protein with potent anticoagulant activity) in trophoblasts and endothelial cells are reduced in the presence of antiphospholipid antibodies (101).

Although the lupus anticoagulant has been reported in 5% to 40% of patients with SLE, it can exist in patients without SLE and also can be induced in patients by medications, cancer, and certain infectious diseases. A number of possible thrombotic mechanisms have been suggested. These include inhibition of prostacyclin synthesis or its release from endothelial cells (102), inhibition of protein C activation by thrombin binding to thrombomodulin (103), raised PAI-1 levels (104), direct platelet activation

(105), and endothelial cell activation with antiphospholipid antibodies (106). Increased monocyte tissue factor expression and low free protein S plasma levels also have been noted in patients with the antiphospholipid syndrome and thrombosis (107). Although each of these mechanisms has been supported in the literature, no one dominant mechanism has emerged, suggesting that the cause of thrombosis in these patients is multifactorial.

Thrombosis can involve both the arterial and venous circulations, especially peripheral vessels of the extremities (108). At least one third of patients with lupus anticoagulants have a history of one or more thrombotic events, with over 70% in the venous circulation (97). Arterial graft thrombosis has also been associated with this syndrome. One half of a series of 18 arterial vascular bypass grafts thrombosed in those patients positive for antiphospholipid antibody (109). In a second series, the incidence of graft thrombosis was 27% in the presence of either a lupus anticoagulant or heparin-induced thrombocytopenia, compared with 1.6% when no hypercoagulable state was identified (110). In a third study, anticardiolipin antibodies were associated with an increased risk of vein graft failure over a short, 6-month follow-up (111). The incidence of antiphospholipid antibodies was also elevated (26%) in a group of young white men (<45 years of age) with chronic lower leg ischemia, compared with control patients (13%) (112). However, a recent prospective comparison of patients undergoing elective infrainguinal bypass grafting revealed that even though one third were positive for antiphospholipid antibodies, there was minimal difference in primary or assisted patency rates, limb salvage, or survival rates between positive and negative patients (113).

Treatment of the antiphospholipid antibody syndrome involves anticoagulation in the face of thrombotic events (100). Higher levels of warfarin [international normalized ratio (INR) >3.0] have been recommended for the treatment of the antiphospholipid syndrome (114). For recurrent fetal loss, heparin or LMWH throughout the pregnancy is recommended. Patients with lupus anticoagulants can have heparin monitored successfully with a thrombin time or anti-factor Xa level, whereas warfarin can be monitored by factor X levels.

Other Hypercoagulable States

Defective fibrinolysis is another cause of a hypercoagulable state. Abnormal plasminogens (dysplasminogenemia), although quite rare (<1%), have been noted in spontaneous arterial or venous thrombosis. Other defects in fibrinolysis that are not well defined may affect up to 10% of the otherwise normal population (115). Abnormal fibrinogens (dysfibrinogenemia) also can cause venous thrombosis, and may account for 1% to 3% of patients with thrombosis.

Other pathways for fibrinolysis could contribute to thrombosis if defective. To date, however, no specific defects have been characterized. tPA is released from endothelium in response to thrombin, histamine, and bradykinin. Thrombin binding to thrombomodulin activates protein C, which inactivates the inhibitor to tPA, thus enhancing fibrinolysis (116). Although factors of the contact activation system are direct activators of plasminogen to plasmin, evidence indicates that prekallikrein activation on endothelial cells results in kinetically favorable single-chain urokinase activation and subsequent plasmin formation (117). Corresponding to the fibrinolytic activators, inhibitors include α_2-AP and PAI-1. Elevated levels of PAI-1 have been associated with DVT and myocardial infarction. Defective fibrinolysis may also occur because of a decreased content or release of plasminogen activators, or an increase in their inhibitors (118). A fibrinolytic shutdown in the postoperative period due to increased inhibitors to tPA has been observed. Although the relationship between venous thrombosis and abnormal fibrinolysis is debated, it is clear that there is a relationship between impaired postoperative fibrinolysis and venous thrombosis (119). In addition, PAI-1 release is upregulated by thrombin, endotoxin, and IL-1, explaining the elevated levels of PAI-1 found during certain infections. TNF down-regulates protein C, decreasing the ability of activated protein C to inactivate PAI-1, which is also up-regulated during sepsis (120). Both of these mechanisms result in decreased fibrinolysis.

There are two clinical settings in which *abnormal platelet aggregation* has been associated with thrombosis. The clinical settings include advanced malignancy of the lung and uterus and after carotid endarterectomy. Hyperactive platelets have also been seen during graft thrombosis in peripheral vascular surgical reconstructions (83). Diabetes mellitus, which is known to be associated with hyperactive platelets, may be a contributor to these conditions. Because platelet function testing is not a highly developed quantitative assay, and because the availability of such testing is limited in many laboratories, the importance of abnormal platelet aggregation to the hypercoagulable condition is unknown. Antiplatelet agents alone therefore are not very likely to eliminate such a thrombogenic hypercoagulable potential (121).

Two new syndromes have been described as contributory to the hypercoagulable state. *Prothrombin 20210 polymorphism* involves a genetic polymorphism in the distal 3′ untranslated region of the prothrombin gene (122). This syndrome has been described in patients with venous thrombosis. This base pair polymorphism, G20210A, has been found to increase the risk for venous thrombosis by 5.4-fold. Of 219 patients with confirmed venous thrombosis, 12 or 5.5% were found to be heterozygous carriers of the 20210A allele, whereas in a corresponding group of healthy control subjects, the incidence was only 1.2%. In addition, this genotype, although not increased in frequency in patients with arterial disease, has been found to be associated with venous thrombosis in simple heterozygotes and double heterozygotes for other procoagulant conditions, and to have synergy with factor V Leiden (123). This syndrome also has been seen in younger women exhibiting myocardial infarction.

A second newly described syndrome associated with hypercoagulability is *hyperhomocystinemia*. Hyperhomocystinemia, a risk factor for atherosclerosis and vascular disease, has been found to increase the risk for venous thrombosis in those younger than 40 years of age (124), and to increase the risk for recurrent venous thrombosis in patients between 20 and 70 years of age (125). In addition, an especially strong association in older women has been found (126). The combination of high homocysteine levels with other hypercoagulable markers such as factor V Leiden has been suggested to result in an increased risk of thrombosis. The mechanism of thrombosis is not clear. Suggested mechanisms range from an impairment in endothelium-dependent vasodilation from decreased bioavailability of nitric oxide (127–129), a decreased production of nitric oxide due to lipid peroxidation (130–132), a toxic effect on vascular endothelium (133) and the clotting cascade, to abnormal methionine metabolism affecting the methylation of DNA and cell membranes (134,135). Elevated levels of homocysteine may also reduce the activation of protein C on thrombomodulin (136,137) and increase thromboxane production. Furthermore, elevated homocysteine has been shown to decrease tissue plasminogen binding and plasmin formation (138–139). The association between hyperhomocystinemia and venous thrombosis has been strongly established. Additional evidence suggests that treatment specifically to lower homocysteine levels, such as vitamin B$_6$, vitamin B$_{12}$, or folic acid, is salutary, although there are no data to substantiate that such treatment lowers the thrombotic risk. Evidence suggest that moderate folate ingestion lowers plasma homocysteine levels.

Disseminated Intravascular Coagulation

Disseminated intravascular coagulation is the primary form of acute thrombosis. Causes of DIC include abruptio placentae, gram-positive and gram-negative sepsis, endotoxemia, malignant tumors, pelvic operations, certain snake bites, hematologic malignancies, and hepatic failure (4). Coagulation is activated by the release into the circulation of tissue factor, which activates factor VII to VIIa, leading to massive thrombin production and fibrin generation. Fibrinolysis then becomes activated, leading to bleeding in the later stages of the syndrome because of the consumption of clotting factors, depletion of fibrinogen, and unchecked plasmin activity. Laboratory values in DIC reveal a decline in platelet count and fibrinogen level with a concomitant elevation in fibrin split products. A more chronic form of DIC has been reported, with the release of small amounts of tissue factor into the circulation in conditions such as tumors of the prostate, diabetes mellitus, use of factor IX concentrates, total hip replacement, and abdominal aortic aneurysm (4). In a prospective study of 76 patients with extensive aortic aneurysms, 4% of patients (especially those with thoracoabdominal involvement) exhibited clinically overt DIC before surgery (140). In this more chronic form of DIC, fibrinogen tends to remain within the normal range.

In summary, a number of conditions can lead to a procoagulant state. A procoagulant screen should include routine coagulation tests such as the aPTT and platelet count, antithrombin III activity and antigen assay, protein C antigen and activity levels, protein S antigen level, and mixing studies to identify a lupus anticoagulant (if indicated); activated protein C resistance assay and factor V Leiden gene analysis; prothrombin 20210 genetic analysis; homocysteine level; an antiphospholipid antibody screen that includes anticardiolipin antibody; fibrinogen level; functional plasminogen assay; and platelet aggregation testing, if possible. Although conditions exist that lead to these hypercoagulable states, only 10% to 15% of patients with venous thrombosis have one of the conditions listed here, with the most frequent condition involving abnormalities in protein C and protein S. The incidence increases with the concentration of patients at high risk in specialized coagulation centers (80), and may be even higher with the measurement of new parameters such as resistance to protein C where the incidence may be as high as 20%–40% (87–89). Thus, not every patient with a thrombotic event should be screened. However, patients with strong positive family histories, young patients with arterial and venous thromboses without obvious cause, and patients with multiple episodes of thrombosis without an underlying anatomic abnormality should be investigated and screened.

BLEEDING DISORDERS

Although the surgeon deals more often with procoagulant states than bleeding disorders, it is important to recognize these disorders when they occur.

Coagulation Factor Deficiency

Coagulation factor deficiency states are important causes of bleeding. Factor VIII and IX deficiency states are involved in hemophilia A and B and type I von Willebrand's disease. Hemophilia A (Fig. 4.11) is inherited as a sex-linked recessive deficiency of factor VIII, with fewer cases secondary to spontaneous mutation. The incidence of this abnormality is approximately 1 in 10,000 births. Clinical findings range from bleeding into joints and muscles, epistaxis, hematuria, and bleeding after minor trauma, to prolonged postoperative bleeding, retroperitoneal bleeding, and intramural bowel hemorrhage. Laboratory screening tests usually reveal a prolongation of the aPTT, with other test results being normal. The minimum level of factor VIII required for hemostasis is 30%, and spontaneous bleeding is uncommon with factor VIII levels greater than 5% to 10% of normal (141). Levels less than 2% constitute severe, 2% to 5% moderate, and greater than 5% mild deficiency (142). Severe deficiency with levels less than 1% poses the risk for spontaneous bleeding episodes. Although the half-life of factor VIII is 2.9 days in normal subjects, the half-life of factor VIII concentrates is only 9 to 18 hours (4). Levels between 80% to 100% of normal should be attained for surgical bleeding or life-threatening hemorrhage. Acquired deficiency has been reported to occur with the development of antibodies to factor VIII after therapy. Inhibitor antibodies develop in approximately 10% to 15% of patients with hemophilia A, although the incidence of antibody formation may be much higher in previously untreated patients and in those with severe hemophilia A. A new recombinant factor VIII preparation has been developed and tested in children and infants. Despite the development of low levels of in-

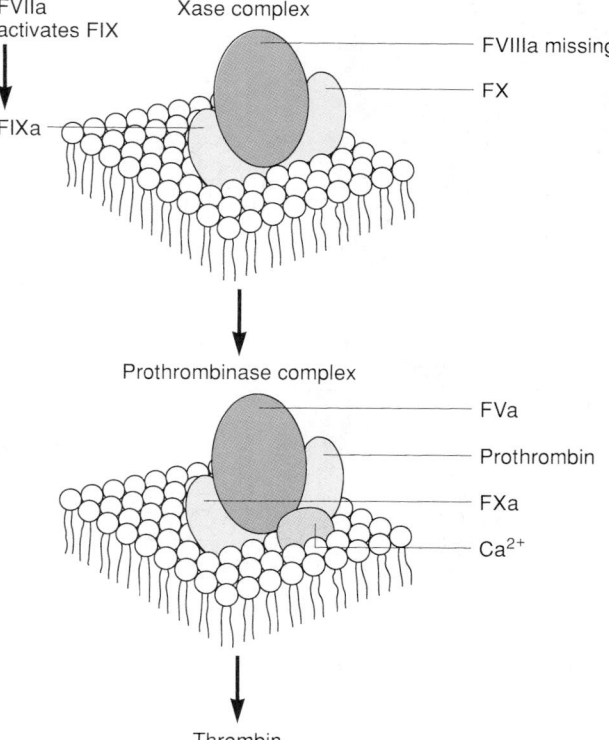

Figure 4.11. Hemophilia A involves a deficiency of factor VIII. (After Hassouna HI. Laboratory evaluation of hemostatic disorders. *Hematol Oncol Clin North Am* 1993;7:1187.)

hibitors in 20% of children at a mean 9 days after first administration, these inhibitors either disappeared or remained at low levels (143). Because this recombinant preparation is virus free, the benefits outweigh the risks of low levels of inhibitor development for the treatment of hemophilia A (especially because in 1992, almost 30% of the entire hemophilic population in the United States had reported AIDS, and more than 22% had died of AIDS) (144).

Factor IX deficiency (Christmas factor), known as hemophilia B (Fig. 4.12), is transmitted as an X-linked recessive trait. It also may be acquired because of enhanced factor IX clearance in states such as the nephrotic syndrome, abnormal protein production in vitamin K deficiency, and acquired specific inhibitors to factor IX in various autoimmune diseases, such as SLE. It is clinically indistinguishable from hemophilia A, and laboratory screening tests reveal a prolonged aPTT, with other test results normal, although a greater proportion of patients have only mild or moderate deficiency (145). Severe deficiency (approximately 30% of cases) is defined as a level of activity less than 4% of normal, whereas moderate deficiency is reported with activity levels between 20% and 40% (4). Treatment consists of plasma or factor IX concentrates and vitamin K. It has been recommended that levels greater than 30% be achieved for hemostasis (141).

Von Willebrand factor causes platelet adhesion to collagen, initiating platelet plug formation. It also forms a complex with factor VIII in the blood. Produced in endothelial cells and megakaryocytes (compared with the liver for factor VIII), it has a circulating half-life of 6 to 20 hours (4). A number of different subtypes have been identified for its deficiency state (Fig. 4.13), and the syndrome is transmit-

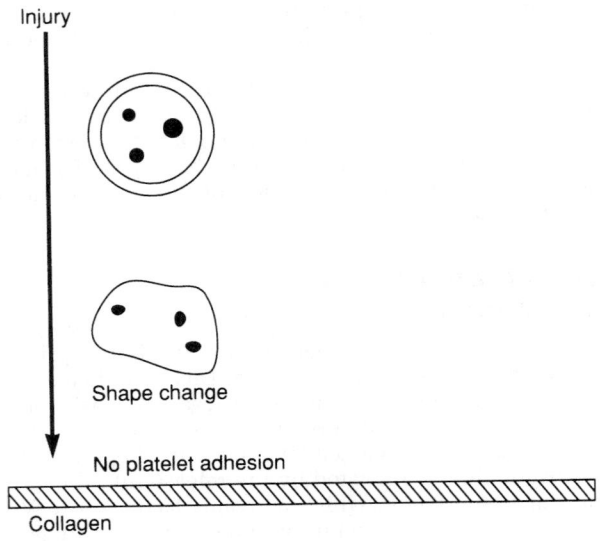

Figure 4.13. Von Willebrand's disease involves an absence of platelet adhesion to collagen. (After Hassouna HI. Laboratory evaluation of hemostatic disorders. *Hematol Oncol Clin North Am* 1993;7:1187.)

ted as both autosomal dominant (heterozygous) and autosomal recessive (homozygous) forms. Variants include types I and III (quantitative decreases in normal-appearing vWF) and type II (qualitative abnormalities in structure and function of vWF) (146). vWF deficiency is probably as common as hemophilia A, although the true incidence may surpass what is generally appreciated because many mild cases probably remain undiagnosed. The classic syndrome is caused by a reduction of factor VIII activity (although not as great as in hemophilia A) and vWF (vWF–factor VIII complex). Clinical manifestations include mild to moderate epistaxis, gingival bleeding, menorrhagia, rare joint or muscle bleeding, and subcutaneous bleeding (4). Spontaneous bleeding is not as common as in hemophilia A. Screening laboratory tests include prolonged aPTT, with other coagulation test results normal; a prolonged bleeding time; a decreased level of factor VIII activity; decreased immunoreactive levels of the vWF; and abnormal platelet aggregation response to ristocetin (4). The most reliable source of vWF is cryoprecipitate, although many concentrates of factor VIII have vWF present and show promise. Desmopressin acetate (DDAVP) is available for the treatment of mild cases; serum levels of 25% to 50% are needed for hemostasis (141).

Other specific factor deficiencies are much less common and receive only a brief overview here. Factor XI (plasma thromboplastin antecedent), complexed to high-molecular-weight kininogen in the plasma, has a half-life of 40 to 80 hours (4). Deficiency of this factor carries an autosomal recessive inheritance. Homozygous patients have levels up to 20% of normal, whereas heterozygous patients typically show levels between 30% and 65% of normal (4). This syndrome is particularly frequent in certain ethnic groups such as Ashkenazi Jews. Screening tests include a prolonged aPTT and whole-blood clotting time, with other coagulation test results normal (4). A factor XI assay is the definitive test for the diagnosis. Treatment includes administration of fresh frozen plasma, and hemostasis requires at least 25% of normal factor XI activity (141).

Factor V (proaccelerin) deficiency is rare. This factor produced in the liver has a half-life of 12 to 36 hours, and its deficiency is inherited as autosomal recessive (4). Severe deficiency (called *parahemophilia*) occurs with 1%

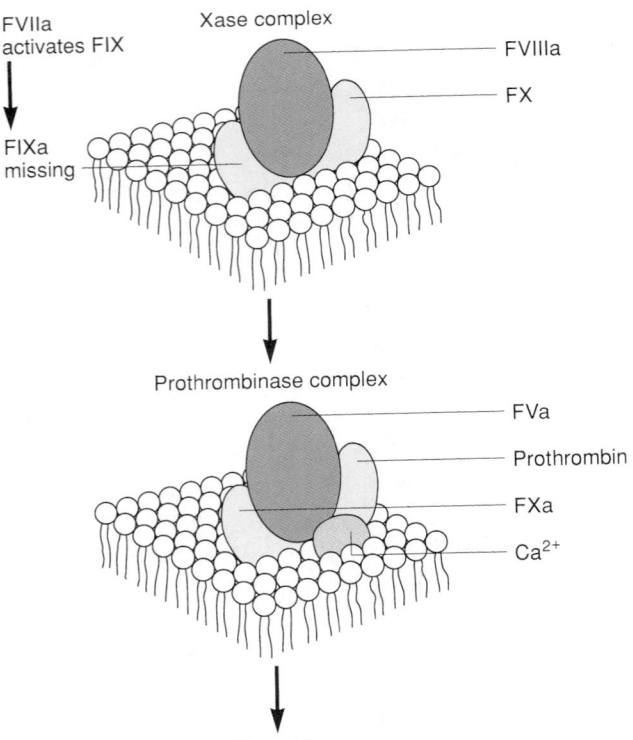

Figure 4.12. Hemophila B involves a deficiency of factor IX. (After Hassouna HI. Laboratory evaluation of hemostatic disorders. *Hematol Oncol Clin North Am* 1993;7:1190.)

plasma activity, whereas moderate deficiency is characterized by 25% plasma activity (4). Deficiency of factor V becomes important in the coagulopathy associated with early liver transplantation. Dysfunctional factor V syndrome has also been described. An acquired syndrome has been seen in patients with acute and chronic liver disease (4). Screening tests include prolonged aPTT, prothrombin time (PT), and whole-blood clotting times; levels of factor V may be measured. Treatment consists of fresh frozen plasma; levels at least 15% of normal are needed for hemostasis (141).

Factor VII (proconvertin) deficiency is inherited as an autosomal recessive trait. Homozygous deficiency is found with levels of 10% of normal, whereas heterozygous patients have levels 40% to 60% of normal (4). A dysfunctional syndrome has also been described with normal levels of factor VII and decreased enzymatic activity. Again, this deficiency state can also be acquired in the presence of liver disease and vitamin K deficiency. Heterozygous patients do not have symptoms, but homozygous patients often display bleeding. Screening tests include a prolonged PT, with other coagulation test results normal (4). A factor VII assay confirms the diagnosis, and treatment involves the administration of fresh frozen plasma. Levels as low as 10% of normal allow for hemostasis (141).

Factor X (Stuart-Power factor) deficiency is transmitted as an autosomal recessive, heterogeneous, incomplete recessive trait (4). Homozygous patients (severe deficiency) have less than 1% of normal plasma activity, whereas those with moderate deficiency demonstrate levels between 10% and 20% of normal plasma activity (4). Acquired deficiency states have been described. Screening tests include a prolonged aPTT, PT, and whole-blood clotting time with a normal thrombin clotting time (TCT), and a specific factor X assay exists (4). Clinical findings include minor or more major bleeding episodes, and treatment involves the use of fresh frozen plasma. Plasma levels should be maintained above 10% of normal to prevent bleeding (141).

The rarest of the inherited disorders of bleeding is factor II deficiency. This deficiency, transmitted as an autosomal recessive trait, can also be related to liver disease, oral anticoagulation, and the newborn period. Screening tests include a prolonged aPTT and PT, with normal TCT and platelet function (4). Factor II has a half-life of 2 to 5 days, and treatment involves the use of fresh frozen plasma and prothrombin concentrates; levels of 40% are needed for hemostasis (141).

Deficiencies of fibrinogen can also lead to bleeding disorders. This is the only factor deficiency state in which the TCT is prolonged. It is generally believed that a fibrinogen level of 100 mg/mL should be achieved to stop bleeding related to fibrinogen abnormalities. Fibrinogen deficiency may also occur from consumption during DIC and from primary fibrinolytic states.

Platelet Disorders

Platelet disorders are another important cause of bleeding. Platelets have three major roles in coagulation: (a) initial adhesion to areas of endothelial denudation; (b) externalization of a phospholipid surface for coagulation complex assembly, accelerating the speed of coagulation; and (c) aggregation for platelet plug formation. Platelet function can be related to three distinct zones. The outer zone contains the glycoprotein receptors responsible for platelet adhesion (GpIb) and platelet aggregation (GpIIb/IIIa); receptors for fibrinogen, vWF, and fibronectin (GpIIb/IIIa); and the receptor for thrombospondin (GpIIIb)

(4). The second zone, the sol-gel zone, contains elements that allow platelet contraction; the third zone, the organelle zone, contains electron-dense bodies that store calcium, serotonin, ADP and adenosine triphosphate, and the nondense α granules that store markers for platelet activation (4). Bleeding associated with platelets includes mucosal bleeding (e.g., epistaxis), easy bruisability, petechiae, purpura, and menorrhagia.

Extracorporeal bypass circuits, such as cardiopulmonary bypass and extracorporeal membrane oxygenation circuits (ECMO), activate platelets regardless of the type of oxygenator used and can produce bleeding. During cardiopulmonary bypass, after fibrinogen and IgG become adsorbed onto the bypass circuit, platelets are immediately activated. These activated platelets change their shape, aggregate, and adhere to the fibrinogen surface through multiple interactions between the GpIIb/IIIa receptor and the exposed binding sites on the carboxyl terminus of the γ chain of fibrinogen and the Fc regions of IgG antibodies. Fibrinogen also can induce both platelet activation and aggregation. Platelets release granule contents, such as platelet factor 4, β-thromboglobulin, serotonin, adenine nucleotides, and thromboxane, and their sensitivity to various platelet agonists decreases. Some adherent platelets break away and leave membrane fragments on the surface of the extracorporeal circuit. Platelet aggregates form; new, larger platelets arrive from the bone marrow; and a heterogeneous mixture of platelet fragments, degranulated platelets, resealed platelets with damaged membranes, reversibly activated platelets, and new platelets results (147). Thus, bleeding time increases are usually recorded. In addition, cardiopulmonary bypass activates factor XII and complement (the contact activation system), leading to neutrophil activation, release of lysosomal enzymes, generation of oxygen free radicals, and the harmful "inflammatory" response noted with extracorporeal circuits along with the direct activation of the fibrinolytic system by plasmin activation. Prosthetic vascular grafts likewise activate platelets, and platelet uptake on both Dacron (Fig. 4.14) and expanded polytetrafluoroethylene grafts has been found in a number of animal models and in patients for up to 6 months to 10 years after graft implantation (148). This platelet uptake appears to be mostly a phenomenon of recruitment with three different mechanisms: the release of ADP from activated platelets, the production of thromboxane from activated platelets, and the generation of thrombin.

Inherited defects of platelet receptors include defects of GpIIb/IIIa (Glanzman's thrombasthenia), characterized by impaired platelet binding to vWF, fibrinogen, and fibronectin. In patients with defects in GpIb (Bernard-Soulier syndrome), the absolute number of platelets is decreased, the platelets are larger, and platelet aggregation and adhesion are abnormal (4). Acquired deficits occur in uremia, with both GpIb and GpIIb/IIIa receptors are defective, resulting in impaired adhesion and aggregation. Acquired deficits also occur in patients who previously received platelet transfusions and then acquire immune-mediated anti-platelet antibodies. Patients with Glanzman's thrombasthenia also show abnormalities in the sol-gel zone, and their platelets lack the ability to contract and retract. A number of platelet disorders associated with abnormalities of the organelle zone have also been described.

Abnormalities in Fibrinolysis

Abnormalities in fibrinolygis may play a role in abnormal bleeding disorders. Genetic or acquired deficiencies in α₂-AP may be associated with bleeding, whereas deficiencies in factor XIII (fibrin stabilizing factor) may lead to

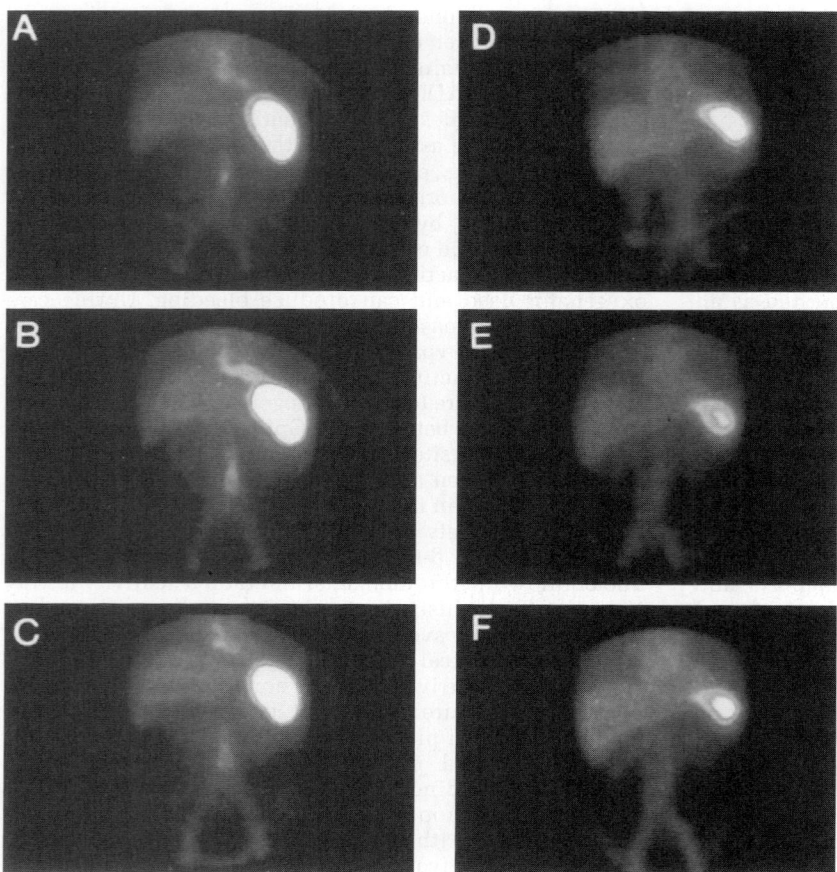

Figure 4.14. Human Dacron aortic graft platelet activity at 1 week *(A)*, 3 months *(B)*, and 6 months *(C)*, versus absence of human expanded polytetrafluoroethylene (ePTFE) aortic graft platelet activity at 1 week *(D)*, 3 months *(E)*, and 6 months *(F)*. (After Wakefield TW, Shulkin BL, Fellows EP, et al. Platelet reactivity in human aortic grafts: a prospective, randomized mid-term study of platelet adherence and release products in Dacron and ePTFE grafts. *J Vasc Surg* 1989;9:238.)

highly lysable clot. α_2-AP deficiency is treated with ε-aminocaproic acid or tranexamic acid. Homozygous patients with factor XIII deficiency and less than 1% of normal plasma activity often show bleeding from the umbilical cord at birth, bleeding after trauma or surgery, and delayed bleeding 24 to 36 hours later (4). Intracranial bleeding also has been noted. Screening test results include a shortened euglobulin lysis time and the presence of clot solubility in 5 mol/L urea, 2% acetic acid, or 1% monochloroacetic acid (4). A specific assay for factor XIII activity exists. Treatment consists of fresh frozen plasma, cryoprecipitate, and factor XIII concentrates. Finally, a deficiency of PAI-1 has been described that may lead to bleeding.

PHARMACOLOGIC/NONPHARMACO-LOGIC INTERVENTIONS

Heparin

Heparin, discovered by Jay McLean in 1916, is a heterogeneous mixture of sulfated polysaccharide molecules of varying molecular weights, ranging from 2 to 40 kd. Heparin is obtained from beef lung or porcine intestine. Heparin accelerates the reaction between thrombin and anti-thrombin III, accelerating the inhibition of thrombin and other serine proteases by antithrombin III. Heparin also directly binds and inhibits coagulation proteases and is important for the selective inhibitor of thrombin, heparin cofactor II. After bolus injection, heparin's half-life is approximately 90 to 120 minutes, although the half-life depends on the amount injected—the more injected, the longer the half-life. Activated factor X and activated factor II are most sensitive to the heparin–antithrombin III com-

plex. Heparin is cleared through the reticuloendothelial system and does not cross the placental barrier. Clinical use of heparin in venous thrombosis and pulmonary embolism and as a prophylactic agent has been established (149). A lower frequency of bleeding complications has been found with continuous infusion rather than bolus injections. In addition, a lesser degree of thrombin accumulation has been found with continuous administration. In monitoring heparin, an aPTT 1.5 times control or a TCT 2 times control reflects adequate anticoagulation. Activated clotting times (ACTs) in a range of 150 to 200 seconds also suggest adequate anticoagulation. In many situations, direct measurements of heparin levels do not correlate with the level of anticoagulation as measured by aPTT. Heparin decreases platelet aggregability while enhancing the generation of thromboxane from platelets (150). Noncoagulant high-molecular-weight heparin fragments may also potentiate platelet aggregation, and heparin-associated thrombocytopenia from an immune mechanism is a potential complication of heparin use. Any patient undergoing heparin therapy should have a platelet count measured every other day after the fourth day of therapy (or earlier if the patient is known to have been exposed to heparin in the past) to evaluate for thrombocytopenia. The most common complication of heparin therapy is bleeding. The risk of hemorrhage is increased in the elderly, postmenopausal women, and in patients with preexisting abnormalities of coagulation, thrombocytopenia, and uremia. Long-term therapy may be associated with alopecia and osteoporosis; osteoporosis has been found in patients receiving large doses of heparin for longer than 6 months.

Use of heparin for venous thrombosis prophylaxis has received considerable attention. Low-dose heparin protects against venous thrombosis through three different mechanisms. First, antithrombin III activity, with its inhibition of factor Xa, is enhanced by trace amounts of heparin; second, there may be a decrease in thrombin availability, preventing its activation and its fibrin-stabilizing effect; and third, small doses of heparin may inhibit the second wave of platelet aggregation and the subsequent platelet release reaction. In a review of 27 clinical trials concerning the use of low-dose heparin for venous thromboembolism prophylaxis, the incidence of venous thrombosis in the nontreated patients averaged 25%, compared with only 7% in those receiving low-dose heparin (151). In addition, thrombi likely to produce major pulmonary embolism were decreased from 6% in the nontreated patients to 0.6% in the group treated with low-dose heparin. Low-dose heparin was found to decrease the incidence of massive pulmonary embolism seen at autopsy. Low-dose heparin does, however, carry an increased risk of wound hematoma, and only higher-risk patients should be treated. The sodium and calcium salts of heparin appear to be equally effective for prophylaxis, and the incidence of wound hematoma is not related to the type of salt in the heparin preparation. In addition, there is only a slight advantage to giving 5,000 units three times a day compared with twice a day.

The use of low-dose heparin therapy has been endorsed for a number of applications by a concensus statement on venous thrombosis prophylaxis (152). In a metaanalysis of 70 randomized trials in 16,000 patients comparing low-dose heparin with standard therapy for venous thrombosis prophylaxis, the odds of development of DVT with low-dose heparin decreased 67% ± 4%, whereas for pulmonary embolism (both fatal and nonfatal), the odds decreased 47% ± 10% (153). For fatal pulmonary embolism, the odds reduction was even greater (64% ± 15%). No increase in mortality from other causes was found in patients treated with low-dose heparin. Importantly, these reductions were seen in urologic, elective orthopedic, and traumatic orthopedic procedures. This is somewhat at variance concerning urologic and orthopedic patients, in whom low-dose heparin is not thought to be efficacious, but it may reflect previous errors in interpretation of studies with small numbers of patients (type II error). Bleeding complications were more frequent in the heparin-treated patients, with no difference between 5,000 units twice a day and 5,000 units three times a day. Low-dose heparin prophylaxis appears to be a good means of preventing venous thromboembolic events during many surgical procedures, but should be confined to those patients known to be at high risk owing to the potential for increased bleeding complications. Other methods of pharmacologic prophylaxis are not reviewed here. Heparin plus other agents, such as dihydroergotamine, sodium warfarin, dextran, and aspirin, and mechanical measures have been evaluated and are reviewed in the consensus statement (152).

Because of the bleeding complications related to low-dose heparin, there is considerable interest in LMWH for venous thrombosis prophylaxis. Standard heparin is a mixture of polysaccharide molecules that vary in size from 2 to 40 kd. The anticoagulant effect is primarily centered over the lower end of the molecular weight spectrum. Standard unfractionated heparin is able to inhibit thrombin because it is large enough to make a ternary complex between itself, thrombin, and antithrombin III. LMWHs are not large enough to make this complex because the minimum chain length necessary for formation of such a ternary complex is 18 saccharide units. Thus, LMWHs demonstrate less antithrombin activity. However, for inhibition of factor Xa, such a ternary complex

is not necessary. Thus, LMWHs are able to inhibit factor Xa. Each LMWH preparation has its own antifactor Xa–to–antifactor IIa (thrombin) ratio, depending on its size and molecular weight. Most commercially available LMWHs have ratios between 4 : 1 and 2 : 1, whereas standard unfractionated heparin has a 1 : 1 ratio (154). Because the bleeding potential of heparin is related largely to its antithrombin activity, LMWHs should have a lower bleeding potential. In addition, LMWHs have less antiplatelet activity and less risk for heparin-induced thrombocytopenia.

The LMWHs have other advantages over standard unfractionated heparin. These include an improved pharmacokinetic profile due to reduced nonspecific binding to plasma proteins, less lipolysis, a half-life that is not dose dependent, more constant antifactor Xa inhibition, less interference with protein C activation, less complement activation and interference with appropriate platelet aggregation, less risk for osteoporosis, and a lower level of fibrin monomer production (154). High and sustained plasma antifactor Xa levels exist for greater than 16 hours after LMWH administration in therapeutic doses, and its excretion is primarily renal. There is no available agent effective for LMWH reversal as measured by antifactor Xa levels (155).

The LMWHs were first used in DVT prophylaxis, and they have become the prophylactic agent of choice in orthopedic hip and knee surgery, and in high-risk general surgery patients (153). More recently, they have been used in the full treatment of DVT and pulmonary embolism. A number of level 1 studies and metaanalyses have compared LMWH with standard unfractionated heparin in the treatment of DVT (156,157). Together, these studies demonstrate a lower risk of major bleeding, a lower risk of recurrent thromboembolic events, and a lower risk of death than with standard unfractionated heparin. Even for pulmonary embolism, LMWH appears at least equivalent if not superior to standard unfractionated heparin, but much more convenient (158). It is not necessary to monitor LMWH with coagulation testing except in specific situations such as renal failure, and most dosage schemes use either fixed-dose or weight-adjusted dosing given subcutaneously. Because there is no need for coagulation testing, outpatient treatment has become a reality. However, a number of different services need to be coordinated for such outpatient treatment to be successful, including home nursing, pharmacy, coagulation (for warfarin monitoring), and physician.

The economic impact of the use of LMWH as opposed to standard unfractionated heparin for the treatment of venous thromboembolism has been investigated. Cost savings have ranged from greater than $300,000 for 125 patients (or approximately $25,000/case) in the United States (159), to approximately $4,000 (U.S. dollars) per case in Canada (160), and to a greater than 60% reduction in costs in a study involving centers in Europe, Australia, and New Zealand (161). In addition, treatment with LMWH (dalteparin) once daily resulted in large cost reductions in a large, multicenter Swedish study (162). Expanded indications have resulted in greater than 80% of patients becoming eligible for outpatient treatment (163). With expanded use, over 90% of patients report high satisfaction with home outpatient treatment (164).

Low-molecular-weight heparin has also been studied in unstable angina (154). LMWH has been found superior to placebo and equivalent or superior to standard unfractionated heparin when evaluating the outcomes death or myocardial infarction, without any increase in major bleeding. The question remains whether one preparation of LMWH will be found superior to another, or whether all preparations are equivalent and share the same advantages for the treatment of DVT, pulmonary embolism, and unstable angina.

Reversal of heparin anticoagulation with protamine sulfate is often associated with adverse hemodynamic and hematologic side effects, including hypotension, bradycardia, pulmonary artery hypertension or hypotension, declines in oxygen consumption, leukopenia, and thrombocytopenia (165,166). Although the pulmonary changes have been observed in up to 3% to 4% of cases, hypotension is more frequent. In addition, deaths have been reported after the use of protamine, with noncardiogenic pulmonary edema and right heart failure accompanying the most severe reactions. In a survey sent to members of the Society for Vascular Surgery and the European Society for Vascular Surgery, the incidence of noteworthy protamine-related side effects was significant at 4% to 5%, as reported by approximately 650 surgeons. The most likely cause of the hypotension appears to involve the elaboration of a vasodilator factor, such as nitric oxide, as well as a direct depression of myocardial function, including the development of bradycardia (167,168). Pulmonary artery hypertension, on the contrary, is thought to result from thromboxane release from nonplatelet sources in the pulmonary circulation (169). Finally, thrombocytopenia and leukopenia are most likely the result of a direct effect of protamine on phospholipid membranes of these blood elements (170). Immunologic reactions also may occur in patients with prior exposure to protamine, especially in diabetic patients taking NPH insulin that contains protamine (to allow for more prolonged absorption) or those previously exposed to protamine. Unfortunately, no other effective and safe agent for heparin neutralization exists, and in those situations when heparin must be reversed, such as at the completion of major aortic reconstructions and cardiopulmonary bypass, protamine must be given.

Although it has been suggested that the rate of administration is the most crucial factor in protamine-related reactions, declines in hemodynamic parameters and oxygen consumption still occur with slow administration (166). Work from our laboratory has demonstrated that total cationic charge appears to be an important determinant for both anticoagulation reversal efficacy and hemodynamic toxicity (171). Effective and less toxic alternatives to protamine for the reversal of both standard unfractionated heparin and LMWH anticoagulation should be available in the future.

Warfarin

Warfarin oral anticoagulant therapy is recommended for chronic treatment of venous thromboembolism. Warfarin interferes with the vitamin K-dependent clotting factors II, VII, IX, and X; protein C; and protein S. In the liver, these factors are γ-carboxylated in a reaction catalyzed by the reduced form of vitamin K. During this reaction, 10 to 12 glutamic acid residues are converted to γ-carboxyglutamic acid residues (Fig. 4.15). When these factors are released from the liver, they are secreted as active proteins (4). The carboxyglutamic acid residues are responsible for these proteins binding to phospholipid membranes and the formation of the Xase and prothrombinase complexes on activated platelet surfaces. Warfarin prevents the reduction of vitamin K once it has functioned as a cofactor for the γ-carboxylation (Fig. 4.16). There are two classes of compounds possessing anticoagulant effects: 4-hydroxycoumarins [of which crystalline warfarin sodium (Coumadin; Du Pont Pharmaceutical, Wilmington, DE) is the most common] and the 2-substituted 1,3-indanediones (4). Bleeding complications are associated with the level of anticoagulation. The level of anticoagulation is monitored with the PT. At levels higher than a one-stage PT of 1.4 ×

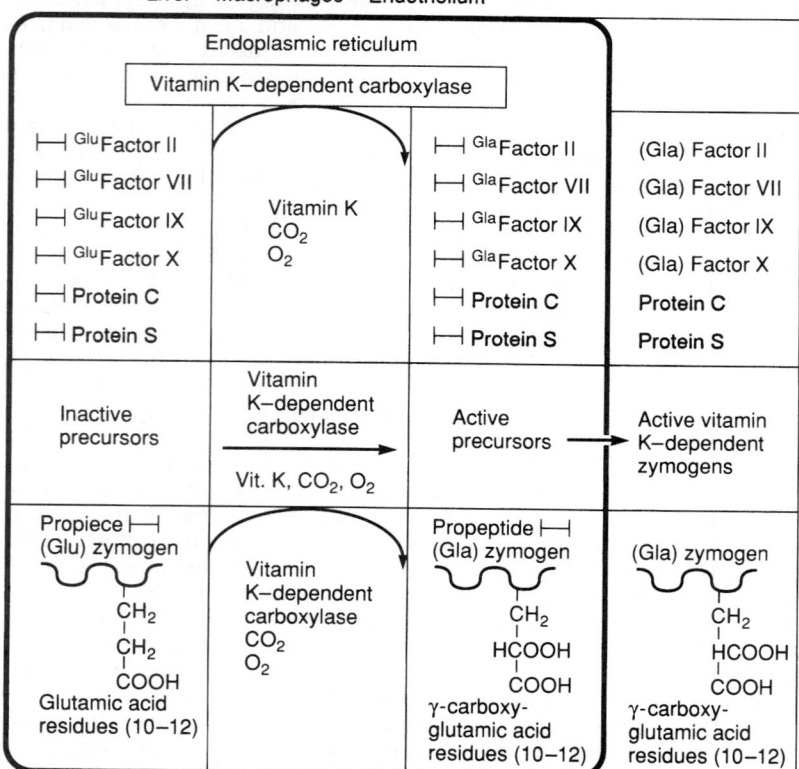

Figure 4.15. Conversion of glutamic acid residue to γ-carboxyglutamic acid residues by vitamin K-dependent carboxylase for factors II, VII, IX, and X, protein C, and protein S. (After Hassouna HI. Laboratory evaluation of hemostatic disorders. *Hematol Oncol Clin North Am* 1993;7:1219.)

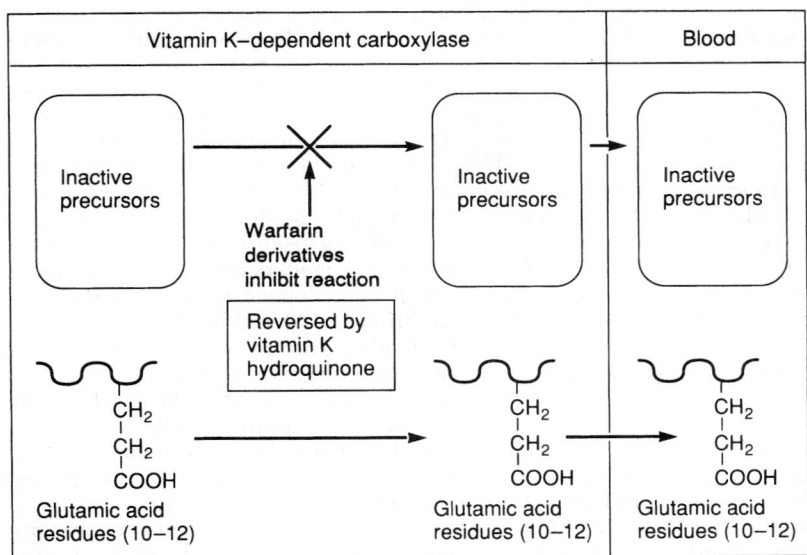

Figure 4.16. Secretion of inactive vitamin K-dependent precursor factors from the liver into the blood after warfarin administration. (After Hassouna HI. Laboratory evaluation of hemostatic disorders. *Hematol Oncol Clin North Am* 1993;7:1220.)

control, there is nearly a fivefold increase in the frequency of bleeding complications (172). Because of variations in the thromboplastins used for the PT determinations in various countries, the INR system, in which the sensitivity of thromboplastins has been standardized, was developed (173). Using this system, the proper range for treatment of venous thrombosis by warfarin is an INR of 2 to 3.

Major complications of sodium warfarin therapy include recurrent thrombosis, bleeding, and skin necrosis. It is recommended that warfarin be continued 4 to 6 months after an initial episode of DVT. Between 10 weeks and 4 months after DVT, the recurrent thrombosis rate is 8.3 episodes per 1,000 patient months. Between 4 months and 3 years, this incidence falls to 4 episodes per 1,000 patient months. At approximately 4 months, the risk of bleeding matches and exceeds the benefit from anticoagulant therapy. With recurrent DVT, the thrombotic risk is greater, and sustained anticoagulation is appropriate. Repeat venous thrombosis has been found in up to 20% of patients with recurrent venous thrombosis who are treated with only a short, 6-month course of warfarin (174). In addition, for idiopathic DVT, a prolonged course greater than 3 months may be appropriate (175). Patients at highest risk for bleeding on warfarin include the elderly, patients with gynecologic or urologic disorders, women after childbirth, and patients given large warfarin loading doses. A final important complication of warfarin is skin necrosis, which occurs more frequently in patients with protein C deficiency. This usually involves full-thickness skin sloughing over fatty areas such as the breasts and buttocks, but can also be seen in other anatomic distributions such as the extremities and digits.

Antiplatelet Agents

Antiplatelet agents are used to prevent cardiovascular events such as coronary thrombosis and neointimal hyperplasia. Platelet aggregation is mediated by receptors that are part of the mammalian integrin family. This family includes the β_1 family, mediating platelet interaction with cells, collagen, fibronectin, and laminin; the β_2 family (LeuCAM), present on leukocytes mediating interactions between leukocytes and other cells important in inflammation; and the β_3 family (cytoadhesion), including the megakaryocyte-specific GpIIb/IIIa receptor and the vitronectin receptor present on platelets and other cells (176).

Platelet aggregation is mediated by GpIIb/IIIa, which binds fibrinogen, vWF, fibronectin, vitronectin, and thrombospondin to activated platelets. These high-density receptors are hidden on unactivated platelets; they become exposed on the surface of activated platelets. Evidence suggests that fibrinogen on the surface of biomaterials can also bind these receptors and itself activate platelets. Fibrinogen's dimeric structure allows for platelet–platelet interactions and platelet aggregation. At high shear rates on biomaterials, however, vWF may mediate platelet aggregation. The GpIIb/IIIa receptor contains a binding site for the tripeptide sequence arginine–glycine–aspartic acid (RGD), which is common to many of the receptor proteins. Agonists for platelets expose this receptor, cause aggregation, and initiate the release of arachidonic acid, leading to thromboxane A_2 release and further platelet aggregation. Arachidonic acid release is not necessary for aggregation, however, because most agonists can directly expose GpIIb/IIIa. In addition, initial platelet adhesion is a stimulus for platelet aggregation and receptor exposure.

Platelet aggregation can be inhibited by the following methods:

1. Blocking cyclooxygenase, the first step converting arachidonic acid to thromboxane and prostacyclin
2. Blocking thromboxane synthase, the enzyme leading to thromboxane A_2
3. Blocking the thromboxane A_2 receptor
4. Increasing intraplatelet levels of cyclic adenosine monophosphate (AMP) or guanosine monophosphate (GMP), which inhibit the exposure of the platelet GpIIb/IIIa receptor
5. Directly blocking the platelet receptor GpIIb/IIIa

Aspirin and indomethacin inhibit cyclooxygenase. Although aspirin inhibits thromboxane, it also inhibits prostacyclin. In clinical situations, the use of lower doses of aspirin in an attempt to inhibit thromboxane generation but preserve prostacyclin generation has not proven successful. Methylxanthines, such as dipyridamole (Persantine; Boehringer Ingelheim, Ridgefield, CT), inhibit phosphodiesterase, the enzyme that normally degrades cyclic AMP, leading to higher levels of cyclic AMP. Endothelium-derived relaxing factor (nitric acid), nitroglycerin, and nitroprusside mediate platelet aggregation through modulation of cyclic GMP. In addition, monoclonal antibodies to GpIIb/IIIa itself or synthetic peptide blockers of this receptor containing the RGD sequence or the fibrinogen γ-chain carboxyl-terminal sequence directly inhibit the function of this receptor. Receptor blockage is the most specific way to inhibit aggregation; when the GpIIb/IIIa receptor is blocked, even high concentrations of agonists cannot stimulate platelets. In models of prosthetic vascular graft–platelet interactions, thromboxane synthase inhibitors appear less effective than aspirin, suggesting that endoperoxide intermediates are proaggregatory and can interact at the platelet thromboxane receptor, thus subverting any potential antiaggregatory effect of thromboxane reduction. Thromboxane receptor antagonists thus should rectify this situation and exhibit a synergistic effect with thromboxane synthase inhibitors. Thromboxane synthase inhibitors, not thromboxane receptor antagonists, are associated with a decreased urinary excretion of thromboxane metabolites and a marked increase in prostacyclin generation. Combined compounds with both thromboxane synthase inhibition and receptor antagonism have been developed with the intent of enhancing prostacyclin production from endoperoxide intermediates (antiaggregatory) while preventing these intermediates from combining with the thromboxane receptor and augmenting platelet aggregation. Ticlopidine, a relatively new antiplatelet agent, inhibits the exposure of the GpIIb/IIIa receptor by unknown mechanisms. This agent, however, takes several days to become effective. Because of ticlopidine-associated neutropenia, an analogue of ticlopidine, clopidogrel, was developed. This thienopyridine compound is not associated with the same degree of neutropenia and has been shown to reduce the composite end points of stroke, myocardial infarction, and death in patients with vascular disease [3].

Direct inhibitors of the GpIIb/IIIa receptor were first developed as murine-derived monoclonal antibodies. The compound C7E3Fab (ReoPro; Eli Lilly, Indianapolis, IN), a chimeric monoclonal antibody directed at GpIIb/IIIa, is the first agent of this class to become clinically available [3]. Its receptor binding is nonspecific and it binds to other cell surface integrins. Agents in development include RGD mimics that are competitive antagonists to the GpIIb/IIIa receptor, including the cyclic peptide eptifibatide (Integrilin; Key Pharmaceutical, Kenilworth, NJ), the parenteral nonpeptide mimetics tirofiban (Aggrastet; Merck & Co., West Point, PA) and lamifiban, the oral nonpeptide mimetics xemilofiban, orbofiban, roxifiban, sibrafiban, lefradafiban, and SB 214857, and the parental and oral nonpeptide mimetic RPR-109891 (Klerval; Aventis Pharmaceuticals) [177]. All studies to date with these agents have involved coronary interventions,

Other Agents

Other agents for anticoagulation include hirudin, aprotinin, desmopressin acetate, and ancrod. Hirudin, obtained from the saliva of leeches, is a single-chain polypeptide composed of 65 amino acids, with three disulfide bonds and a molecular weight of 8,000 to 9,000 daltons. It is highly specific for thrombin inhibition. Hirudin has a short half-life of 15 to 30 minutes and is excreted unchanged in the urine. Hirudin has no natural inhibitors, compared with heparin, which has the natural inhibitors platelet factor 4 and fibrin II-monomer. As an inhibitor of thrombin, hirudin prevents conversion of fibrinogen to fibrin; thrombin-catalyzed activation of factors V, VIII, and XIII; and, importantly, thrombin-induced platelet aggregation [178]. In addition to its small size and high potency for thrombin, hirudin has a dominant antiplatelet effect, even with platelet-rich thrombi. Hirudin has been found to be more effective than heparin in reducing platelet deposition and mural thrombus at similar aPTT levels [179]. aPTT levels two to three times control (0.7 to 1.0 mg/kg hirudin) are effective in limiting arterial thrombosis and platelet deposition. Hirudin prevents thrombus growth at both high and low shear rates of blood flow, and has even been found to stop thrombus growth in severe stenoses. Unlike heparin, which can inhibit only free, circulating, unbound thrombin, hirudin and other thrombin inhibitors act against both circulating and clot-bound thrombin. The high incidence of bleeding from hirudin, however, limits its usefulness clinically [178]. The gene for hirudin was cloned in 1986, leading to the recombinant production of analogues such as Hirulog (The Medicines Co., Cambridge, MA) and lepirudin (Reflodan; Aventis Pharmaceuticals). Hirulog is less potent than hirudin but also demonstrates an apparent lack of toxicity and immunogenicity [178]. Argatroban (a synthetic organic antithrombin) has been found useful for the treatment of patients with heparin-induced thrombocytopenia, and lepirudin has now been approved by the FDA for use in this syndrome, with an acceptable bleeding profile.

One area of interest for all prosthetic surfaces, ranging from cardiopulmonary bypass and ECMO circuits to prosthetic vascular grafts, is the ability to *passivate* the surface, which means to lessen platelet–surface interactions, as well as leukocyte activation. Inhibition of platelet function during cardiopulmonary bypass has been accomplished using iloprost, but at the cost of hypotension because of its vasodilatory properties [180]. A unique finding is that passivation lasts far beyond the time when the drug is present in the circulation. Other compounds that have been suggested for this purpose include a class of reversible platelet–fibrinogen receptor inhibitors, the RGD-containing peptides called *disintegrins* obtained from viper venom that inhibit receptors associated with platelet GpIIb/IIIa receptor complexes [181,182]. In sheep, disintegrins limit thrombocytopenia, preserve platelet responsiveness to ADP, attenuate release of platelet factor IV, and decrease the GpIIIa antigen associated with a 24-hour ECMO circuit surface [182]. Inhibitors of the contact activation portion of extracorporeal systems are less well described. Factor XII is activated by the cardiopulmonary bypass circuit. Corn trypsin inhibitor is a weak inhibitor of factor XII activation [147], whereas aprotinin inhibits prekallikrein, kallikrein, and fibrinolysis, and preserves platelet function (perhaps by inhibiting the deleterious high levels of plasmin) [183]. The inhibition of prekallikrein and kallikrein produces an anticoagulant state, whereas the inhibition of plasmin prevents fibrinolysis. Aprotinin has greater affinity for plasmin than kallikrein, and an anticoagulant effect is noted only at very high doses [184]. This agent has successfully reduced transfusion requirements and blood loss in open heart surgery [185]. Another agent that has been suggested to preserve platelet function is desmopressin acetate, a synthetic analogue of vasopressin, which releases preformed vWF from storage sites (Weibel-Palade bodies) in endothelial cells [186]. vWF then stimulates the production of factor VIII coagulant protein, stabilizes its structure, and forms a circulating noncovalent complex with factor VIII. This vWF–factor VIII complex supports platelet adhesion and improves platelet–platelet interactions. The aPTT shortens and prothrombin consumption increases owing to the increase in factor VIII coagulant protein. In addition, desmopressin elevates the plasma levels of larger vWF multimers, which are more effective than smaller vWF multimers. Finally, tPA secretion is stimulated by desmopressin. Desmopressin corrects the hemorrhagic tendency in mild hemophilia A and von Willebrand's disease, and has been found to reduce blood loss and the need for transfusion by 30% to 40% in complex cardiac operations. Qualitative platelet defects found in uremia and cirrhosis of the liver may be corrected transiently (187), and the platelet lesion caused by small doses of aspirin also may be corrected by desmopressin acetate. Despite the effectiveness of desmopressin acetate, it has not been shown to increase the risk of thrombosis.

Another anticoagulant that has been used in place of heparin is ancrod, a thrombin-like enzyme derived from the Malayan pit viper (188). This enzyme produces a controlled decrease in fibrinogen levels by depleting FPA from fibrinogen but not FPB. The fibrin monomers that result stimulate the local production of tPA. Both of these actions lead to a state of anticoagulation. The amount of fibrinogen depletion must be carefully titrated to prevent bleeding. Other agents under development but not discussed include factor X inhibitors, tissue factor pathway inhibitor, and activated protein C.

Fibrinolytic Agents

Fibrinolytic agents are direct or indirect activators of plasminogen, the inactive proteolytic enzyme of plasma that binds to fibrin during the formation of thrombus. Fibrin-bound plasminogen is more susceptible to activation than is free plasminogen in plasma. Streptokinase isolated from group C β-hemolytic streptococci, and acylated plasminogen–streptokinase (APSAC) act through a streptokinase–plasmin complex; urokinase, single-chain urokinase-type plasminogen activator (SCU-PA), and recombinant tPA act directly on plasmin without an intermediate drug–plasmin complex (189) (Fig. 4.17). tPA (originally isolated from a melanoma cell line and now produced through recombinant DNA technology), APSAC, and SCU-PA are termed *fibrin selective* because of their high ratio of activity for fibrin-bound plasminogen compared with circulating plasminogen.

Acylation of the streptokinase–plasminogen complex on the active serine moiety on the light chain stabilizes the catalytic serine site, making this complex inert to circulating plasminogen. Binding to fibrin occurs through the heavy-chain lysine–plasminogen portions; over time, the acetyl group leaves the complex, resulting in a fibrin-spe-

cific thrombolytic effect. Urokinase, a double-chain polypeptide, is formed by the cleavage of SCU-PA by plasmin to single-chain urokinase (a proenzyme-like substance); this cleavage is fibrin specific and occurs through a mechanism whereby SCU-PA activates plasminogen at the fibrin surface, converting it to plasmin. This activation is 10-fold more active at a fibrin surface than in circulating blood. Thus, only the fibrin-bound plasminogen is converted to plasmin for thrombolysis at the fibrin clot surface. tPA occurs in either a single- or double-polypeptide chain form. tPA has a fibrin-binding site and a catalytic site that are widely separated from each other. This separation allows tPA to be activated to its fibrin target, thus establishing its fibrin-specific nature. The level of the lytic state is greatest with streptokinase and APSAC, intermediate with urokinase, less with SCU-PA, and least with single-chain tPA (189) (Table 4.1). Half-lives also vary among different agents, from 5 minutes for single-chain recombinant tPA to 90 minutes for APSAC (189). Streptokinase and APSAC, produced by group C β-hemolytic streptococci, are antigenic; urokinase and SCU-PA, produced from human fetal kidney cells in tissue culture, are nonantigenic. Because of its antigenicity, allergic reactions to streptokinase have been reported in 2% to 20% of cases. In addition, serum sickness has been reported with streptokinase.

Bleeding complications associated with fibrinolytic agents (reported in up to half of patients receiving systemic fibrinolytic agents for venous thrombosis) are related to the invasive procedures associated with drug therapy. Factors involved in bleeding include hypofibrinogenemia and fibrin degradation products. The latter inhibit fibrin polymerization and, in combination with a decrease in the clotting factors V and VIII (from excess plasmin not neutralized by α_2-AP), inhibit the ability of blood to clot. Although coagulation tests in general do not correlate well with bleeding, a fibrinogen level less than 100 mg/dL is associated with an increased risk and severity of bleeding. In addition, newly formed thrombi are easily lysed as they form. Platelets are both inhibited and stimulated by fibrinolytic agents. Because fibrinogen is a necessary cofactor for ADP-

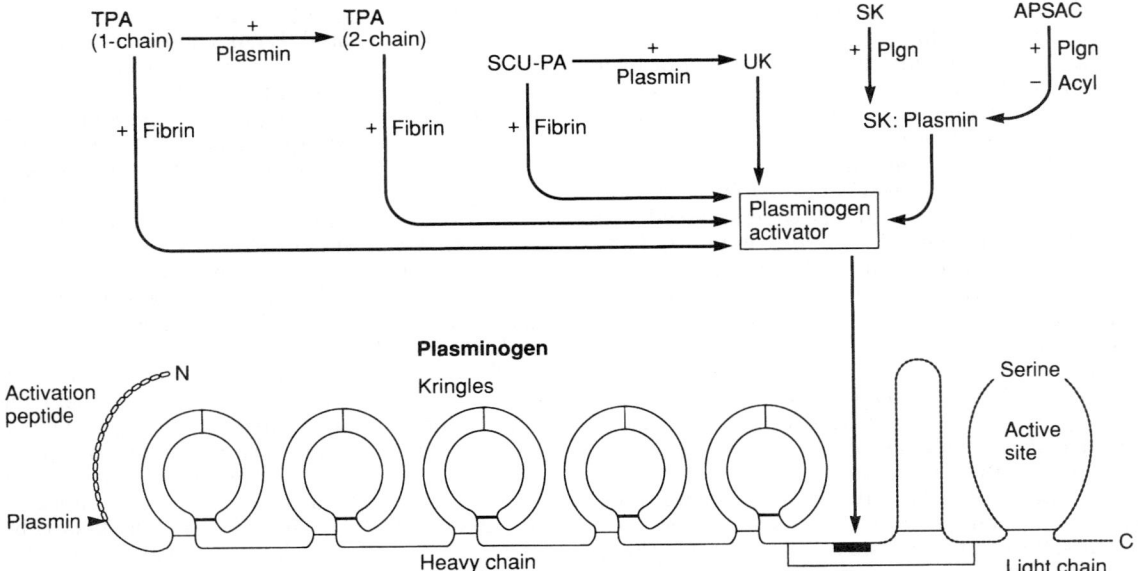

Figure 4.17. Sites of action of plasminogen activators on plasminogen. TPA, tissue plasminogen activator; SCU-PA, single-chain urokinase plasminogen activator; UK, urokinase; SK, streptokinase; Plgn, plasminogen; APSAC, acylated plasminogen–streptokinase. (After Marder VJ, Sherry S. Thrombolytic therapy: current status. *N Engl J Med* 1988;318:1513.)

Table 4.1. CHARACTERISTICS OF FIBRINOLYTIC AGENTS[a]

	SK	APSAC	UK	SCU-PA	rTPA[a] 2-Chain	rTPA[a] 1-Chain
Half-life (min)	23	90	16	7	8	5
Fibrin enhancement	1+	1+	2+	4+	4+	3+
Plasma proteolytic state	4+	4+	3+	2+	2+	1+
Duration of infusion	60 min	2–5 min	5–15 min	Several hours	Several hours	Several hours
Thrombus specificity (vs. hemostatic plug)	0	0	0	0	0	0
Incidence of reperfusion (% within 3 h)	60–70	60–70	60–70	60–70	60–70	60–70
Speed of reperfusion (min)	45	45	45	45	45	45
Frequency of reocclusion (estimated %)	15	10	10	NA	20	20
Simultaneous administration of heparin	No	No	No	Yes	Yes	Yes
Bleeding complications	4+	4+	4+	4+	4+	4+
Allergic side effects	Yes	Yes	No	No	No	No
Antigenicity	Yes	Yes	No	NK	NK	NK
Expense	1+	2+	3+	4+	4+	4+

[a]The clinical data were derived mostly from reported experience with current intravenous dosages in the treatment of acute myocardial infarction.
SK, streptokinase; APSAC, acylated plasminogen–streptokinase activator complex; UK, urokinase; SCU-PA, recombinant single-chain urokinase plasminogen activator; rTPA, recombinant tissue-type plasminogen activator; NA, data not available; NK, not known; 0, none; 4+, highest.
From Marder VJ, Sherry S. Thrombolytic therapy: current status. N Engl J Med 1988;318:1514.

induced platelet aggregation, low fibrinogen levels aggravate a platelet defect. At the same time, plasminogen bound to platelets leads to impaired adhesion and a decrease in their ability to aggregate. Plasmin-induced cleavage of adhesive proteins, such as thrombospondin, fibronectin, and fibrin, also disrupts the bonds that hold platelet aggregates together. In addition, plasmin formed on the endothelial cell surface impairs platelet adhesion to areas of vascular injury during therapy with fibrinolytic agents. Despite these mechanisms that decrease the clotting ability of blood during fibrinolytic therapy, it has been found that these agents promote reocclusion in up to 30% of cases early after thrombolysis through platelet activation, suggesting that platelet activation occurs early after lysis and platelet inhibition occurs later (176). In addition, increased synthesis of endothelial cell PAI-1 has been demonstrated experimentally after treatment with tPA, another mechanism that could potentially contribute to early thrombotic reocclusion (190).

Indications for thrombolytic therapy remain controversial. Clearly, in DVT, fibrinolytic agents allow for greater clot lysis than heparin and help preserve valve function to a greater degree, but at the risk of a higher rate of bleeding complications (191). Thirteen studies of thrombolytic therapy for acute DVT have been compiled from the literature (192). In these studies, patients were assessed with venography. Of those patients treated with anticoagulants, only 4% had complete lysis and 14% revealed partial lysis. In contrast, 45% of patients treated with thrombolytic agents showed significant or complete clot lysis and an additional 18% revealed partial lysis. Two studies evaluated the long-term success of thrombolytic therapy compared with anticoagulation for DVT. In 39 patients with follow-up of 1.6 to 5 years, 21% of patients treated with heparin had no evidence of postthrombotic symptoms, and 64% of patients treated with streptokinase did not have symptoms (193,194). Similarly, significant functional benefit was reported 5 to 10 years after therapy in patients with significant clot lysis as measured by photoplethysmography (PPG) times and foot volumetric studies, although PPG did not completely normalize in the lysis group. In addition, in a large prospective study in patients followed after DVT with either heparin or streptokinase, no major improvement in deep venous valvular compe-

tence was found with lytic agents at 2-year follow-up, and venous functional preservation appeared the same whether clot lysis was complete or incomplete (195). Approximately half of patients who present with their first episode of DVT and who begin lytic therapy within 72 hours of the onset of symptoms achieve significant dissolution of their thrombus. Only approximately 15% of patients who present acutely with lower extremity DVT, however, fit into this category because most patients who have leg swelling or leg pain for the first time do not immediately seek medical attention (196). The use of thrombolytic therapy for DVT thus remains controversial.

The main questions about the use of lytic therapy for DVT are which agent, what dose, and for how long? In a study comparing streptokinase to urokinase in DVT (197), little cost difference was found after considering the longer infusion time and greater bleeding complications associated with streptokinase versus urokinase. Another study (198) compared tPA, 0.5 mg/kg twice over 4 hours or 8 hours, with heparin versus placebo plus heparin for proximal venous thrombosis. Over 50% total clot lysis was found in 58% of a group of patients treated over 4 hours, 23% in a group treated for 8 hours, and only 7% complete clot lysis in the placebo-treated group. Follow-up of patients who achieved greater than 50% clot lysis revealed evidence of chronic venous insufficiency in only 25%, compared with 56% of those with less than 50% clot lysis, a difference that was close to but not statistically significant ($p = .07$). This study suggests that further investigation into the use of the fibrin-specific agents for proximal DVT may be enlightening.

Fibrinolytic therapy has been suggested for use in upper extremity effort venous thrombosis, catheter-induced venous thrombosis, Paget-Schroetter syndrome, and superior vena caval thrombosis. An interesting approach combining thrombolytic therapy and thoracic outlet decompression has been proposed (199). Thrombolytic therapy is initiated locally with urokinase (250,000 IU bolus, then 1,000 to 4,000 IU/min) by a small catheter positioned from a basilic vein approach. After clot lysis, anticoagulation is continued for 3 months, with heparin followed by sodium warfarin to allow for thrombophlebitis (the inflammatory response in the vein that occurs due to the thrombus) to resolve. In approximately 3 months, thoracic outlet decompression is performed. Percutaneous transluminal angioplasty is not successful in the presence of an anatomic defect. Long-term results have been reported to be excellent and correlate well with the initial ability to clear the thrombus. A recent trend to more immediate thoracic outlet decompression has been advocated, avoiding the 3-month interval.

Thrombolytic therapy in pulmonary embolism has been extensively studied. Two carefully designed studies have evaluated the use of either urokinase or streptokinase. Although both agents rapidly lysed clot and improved pulmonary hemodynamics, there was no difference in patient mortality rate or recurrence rate of pulmonary embolism compared with heparin alone (200,201). Urokinase dissolved pulmonary arterial clot within 24 hours of treatment and, in certain instances, reversed shock. By 7 days, both the thrombolytic- and heparin-treated patients revealed equal improvement in pulmonary hemodynamics, and there was no difference in lung scan resolution. In addition, no difference was seen between urokinase and streptokinase. Bleeding complications were more frequent in the thrombolytic-treated patients. Patients who received urokinase responded better if they were younger, if the embolus was less than 48 hours old, or if the embolus was large. As a general guide, thrombolytic therapy for pulmonary embolism should be considered when there is angiographically documented lobar or greater pulmonary embolism causing acute pulmonary hypertension and shock; lesser degrees of pulmonary embolism should be treated with standard heparin anticoagulation.

Tissue plasminogen activator, 0.6 mg/kg over 2 minutes, plus heparin, versus placebo plus heparin for patients with pulmonary embolism has also been reported, with use of lung scans at 24 hours and 7 days to document treatment efficacy (198). No increase in bleeding complications was noted and lysis was significantly improved at 24 hours in the tPA group (34.4%) versus the placebo group (12%, $p = .026$). However, again, the advantage for tPA had disappeared by 7 days (59% lysis compared with 56% lysis). The benefit for tPA thus would be expected only early in the small number of patients who die as a result of massive pulmonary embolism in the first hour after the embolus occurs.

Thrombolytic therapy for peripheral arterial applications is becoming more frequently used, especially when the agents are given intraarterially. The method of McNamara and Fischer (202) has gained the most recognition, involving passage of a guide wire through the thrombus and then infusion of a large dose of urokinase at 4,000 IU/min for 1 to 2 hours, directly into the clot. If progress is made, further thrombolytic therapy is given at 1,000 to 2,000 IU/min for 6 to 12 hours or until complete clot lysis has occurred. Using this method, the mean infusion time was found to be 18 hours, and the incidence of bleeding was significantly lessened. McNamara and Fischer (202) compared these results with those of streptokinase from the literature and found a 13% incidence of severe bleeding with streptokinase versus only a 4% incidence with high-dose intraarterial urokinase therapy. McNamara and Bomberger (203) reported on their first 100 cases of selective intraarterial infusion of urokinase and found complete clot lysis in 77%, with native arterial occlusions responding better than arterial graft occlusions (71% vs. 41% success) at 6-month follow-up. After thrombolytic therapy has reopened an occluded vessel or graft, however, radiologic or surgical correction of the lesion responsible for the thrombosis must be addressed for long-term success. A 1-year graft patency rate of 89% in those grafts in which an underlying lesion was successfully repaired, compared with 23% in grafts without a correctable lesion, has been reported (204). At 2 years, this difference

was even greater (79% compared with 10%). Complications associated with thrombolytic therapy for arterial thrombosis include bleeding, rethrombosis, embolization treated with further thrombolytic therapy, and sepsis from prolonged catheter placement. The most recent innovation in intraarterial thrombolytic therapy involves lacing the entire length of the thrombus with high-dose urokinase before continuous infusion and then using pulse-spray techniques. The application of tPA to peripheral vascular cases has been reported; although promising results were described, 17% of patients still responded with a decrease in systemic fibrinogen levels to less than 100 mg/dL (205). In addition, three patients had groin hematomas, and one had a stroke soon after therapy had been completed. Although fibrin specific, tPA can still cause systemic thrombolytic effects.

The use of intraoperative thrombolytic therapy has been advocated for situations in which complete clot evacuation cannot be accomplished (as may be seen in up to 40% of patients undergoing balloon embolectomy with an embolectomy catheter for acute arterial occlusion), or when the distal vasculature is occluded and precludes appropriate inflow patency (191). One method involves urokinase administration distal to an occluding clamp, infused at 250,000 IU combined with 1,000 IU of heparin in 250 mL saline, and allowed to remain for 30 minutes. If necessary, another 125,000 IU is infused for 30 minutes. Using this technique, 70% of limbs with critical ischemia at the completion of successful balloon embolectomy were spared amputation, with only one bleeding complication (206). For patients with multivessel occlusions or for whom any degree of systemic fibrinolysis would be risky, a new, high-dose isolated limb perfusion technique has been described. This technique involves anticoagulation, limb exsanguination with an Esmarch bandage, application of a proximal tourniquet, and direct arterial infusion of 1,000,000 IU or more of urokinase for 45 to 60 minutes, with direct drainage of the venous effluent below the tourniquet.

Although much work has been carried out on the use of thrombolytic agents in the sphere of acute myocardial infarction, this area is also evolving. In general, the use of streptokinase reduces in-hospital mortality rates by 30%, although prospective comparisons between various thrombolytic agents have not yet been reported (207). The clinical benefits associated with coronary thrombolysis most likely are determined by the rapidity of coronary artery reperfusion. Platelet-mediated thrombotic events may be responsible for the 25% to 30% incidence of reocclusion associated with current protocols and agents. Heparin therapy added to tPA may improve the efficacy of this thrombolytic agent during coronary thrombolysis and helps to prevent reocclusion after thrombolysis is completed.

Contraindications to thrombolytic therapy, whether regional or systemic, are well defined and consist of active internal bleeding, recent surgery or trauma (usually within 10 days of infusion), recent cerebrovascular accident (within 2 months), or documented left heart thrombus (Table 4.2). Relative contraindications include recent surgery, gastrointestinal bleeding or trauma, severe hypertension, mitral valve disease, endocarditis, a history of a defect in hemostasis, or pregnancy. Finally, the recent withdrawal of urokinase from the market needs to be kept in mind when considerations turn to the use of thrombolytic agents.

Dextran

Dextran is a high-molecular-weight polysaccharide produced from sucrose by *Leuconostoc mesenteroides*. Fractionation and hydrolysis produce a product with an average molecular weight of either 40 kd [dextran-40 (Rheomacrodex; Medisan, Parsippany, NJ)] or 70 kd (Dex-

Table 4.2. **CONTRAINDICATIONS TO THROMBOLYTIC THERAPY**

ABSOLUTE

Active internal bleeding
Recent (<2 mo) cerebrovascular accident
Intracranial disease

RELATIVE

Major

Recent (<10 d) major surgery, obstetric delivery, or organ biopsy
Left heart thrombus
Active peptic ulcer or gastrointestinal abnormality
Recent major trauma
Uncontrolled hypertension

Minor

Minor surgery or trauma
Recent cardiopulmonary resuscitation
Atrial fibrillation with mitral valve disease
Bacterial endocarditis
Hemostatic defects (i.e., renal or liver disease)
Diabetic hemorrhagic retinopathy
Pregnancy

CONTRAINDICATIONS TO STREPTOKINASE

Known allergy
Recent streptococcal infection
Previous therapy within 6 mo

Data from NIH Consensus Development Conference. Thrombolytic therapy in treatment. Ann Intern Med 1980;93:141.

tran-70). Dextran-40 has been studied in detail for its ability to augment patency of difficult lower extremity bypass grafts in the early postoperative period. Dextran-40 acts as a volume expander, causing hemodilution, decreasing blood viscosity, decreasing platelet adhesiveness, reducing factor VIII activity, and increasing the lysability of clots (208). In addition, dextran has been found to coat endothelial cell surfaces, decreasing their electronegativity. Two 500-mL bottles on the day of bypass surgery followed by one on each of the succeeding 3 postoperative days at 75 mL/h increase bypass patency 1 day, 1 week, and 1 month after surgery for femorotibial bypasses and all infrainguinal bypasses in which autologous vein could not be used. A number of other applications for dextran-40 have been suggested, including vascular trauma, endarterectomy, arterial and venous thrombectomy, venous reconstruction, and as a prophylactic agent for prevention of the development of venous thrombosis. None of these other indications has been substantiated by a clinical study, such as in the case of difficult lower extremity bypass procedures.

Mechanical Measures

Mechanical measures are used for the prevention of DVT during operative procedures or in patients who cannot be given pharmacologic prophylaxis. These measures include early ambulation, elastic stockings, electrical calf muscle stimulation, and external pneumatic compression, either with uniform-pressure stockings or graded-pressure stockings. In many well controlled studies of venous prophylaxis, intermittent pneumatic compression has been found as effective as low-dose heparin therapy. In addition to augmentation of venous return with these devices, local and systemic fibrinolysis appears to be stimulated, even in areas remote from the application of the compression. The length of time that intermittent pneumatic compression

should be used has not been adequately determined, but most data suggest that at least 5 days or longer in the face of prolonged immobilization may be optimal.

LABORATORY MONITORING OF COAGULATION AND ANTICOAGULATION

Tests of Platelet Function

Platelet tests include peripheral platelet counts, bleeding times, and platelet aggregation. Usually, a platelet count of 50,000/μL or more ensures adequate hemostasis, whereas counts less than 10,000/μL are dangerous and may lead to spontaneous bleeding. Thrombocytosis is considered to exist when the platelet count exceeds 500,000/μL, although in some cases (especially those involving myeloproliferative disorders), counts may be greater than 1,000,000/μL (4). Bleeding time assays assess the ability of platelets to form hemostatic plugs and are usually shorter than 8 minutes. A bleeding time between 8 and 15 minutes most often reflects a low plasma level of vWF, the use of antiplatelet drugs, the presence of lupus-like antibodies, or a factor XI deficiency (4). A bleeding time greater than 15 minutes is clearly prolonged and indicates severe platelet functional impairment, very low levels of vWF, or afibrinogenemia and severe factor V deficiency (4). Platelet aggregation testing involves the use of a number of different agonists, such as ADP, collagen, epinephrine, arachidonic acid, calcium ionophores, platelet-activating factor, thromboxane, and thrombin. Thrombin and collagen appear to be the primary in vivo stimuli, whereas thromboxane, ADP, serotonin, and platelet-activating factor appear to be amplifiers of aggregation after platelet secretion. Although a strong agonist, such as thrombin, can produce irreversible platelet aggregation independent of the arachidonic acid pathway, weak agonists such as epinephrine, ADP, and collagen require an intact cyclooxygenase pathway for the induction of irreversible platelet aggregation. Although a relatively straightforward technique, platelet aggregation is not available in most laboratories, probably because of the observer-dependent nature of the test. Characteristic curves for the various agonists have been reported, such as the presence of a second wave of aggregation for ADP at relatively low concentration (10^{-6} mol/L) versus only a single wave at higher levels (2×10^{-5} mol/L). The first wave is due to ADP, and the second wave arises from products released from the platelets on activation, such as thromboxane. Platelet aggregability has been studied in 685 male and 273 female patients in a prospective study of the role of hemostasis on the development of peripheral vascular occlusive disease (121). Platelet aggregability was found to increase with age, was greater in white than in black patients (especially among men), and tended to decrease with higher levels of habitual alcohol intake. Platelet aggregability was less among smokers, especially among men, but it was increased in the presence of elevated plasma fibrinogen levels.

Coagulation Tests

Coagulation tests include PT (intrinsic and extrinsic pathways and fibrinogen), PTT and aPTT (contact and intrinsic pathway), TCT (fibrinogen conversion to fibrin), and ACT (whole blood and platelets). The only abnormality that causes an isolated elevation in PT with all of the other test results normal is factor VII deficiency, the factor that is activated by tissue factor and then stimulates generation of the extrinsic pathway of coagulation (4). In addition, the PT is sensitive to small decreases in factor V levels. The PT is the most common manner of measuring the level of oral anticoagulant therapy. The aPTT identifies abnormalities of the contact and intrinsic phases of coagulation. The aPTT evolved from the PTT, first described in 1953 and 1954. The PTT uses a phospholipid derived from either brain or lung tissue to mimic the function of platelets in the scheme of coagulation. The aPTT standardizes the activation of factor XII by agents such as cephaloplastin. Because the blood specimen, activator, and phospholipid must be incubated for a period, the blood specimen must be anticoagulated during the activation step; this is usually accomplished with sodium citrate. After incubation, the specimen is recalcified to begin the test. Conditions that cause a prolonged aPTT include the presence of heparin; deficiencies in factors VIII, IX, and XII; and the presence of lupus-like anticoagulants (4). aPTT values have variably been shown to correlate with heparin dosages and serum heparin levels. Heparin levels of 0.2 IU/mL or greater usually correlate with an aPTT of 1.5 times normal or greater. TCT is a measurement of the time it takes for exogenously added thrombin to turn plasma fibrinogen into fibrin clot. As such, it is extremely sensitive to levels of heparin and is an excellent means of measuring the level of heparin-induced anticoagulation. The beauty of the TCT is that it is not specific for any disease condition; thus, it may be used to differentiate factor deficiencies from the presence of heparin or to separate lupus anticoagulant from abnormalities in fibrinogen levels (4). The ACT is a measurement of the ability of whole blood to clot, and as such is an available technique for monitoring intraoperative heparin levels. The ACT responds linearly to increasing heparin dosage and correlates well with observed clinical anticoagulation (thrombus-free surface on cardiopulmonary bypass devices) (209). Adequate anticoagulation for extracorporeal circulation is defined as an ACT of 480 seconds or more, but most cardiovascular surgeons would agree that any value between 300 and 600 seconds is acceptable. For peripheral vascular applications, values of 250 seconds or greater are considered appropriate levels representative of full intraoperative anticoagulation. The ACT may be affected by hemodilution, cardioplegia solutions, hypothermia, platelet dysfunction, hypofibrinogenemia, and other coagulopathies, as well as by certain medications and excess protamine administration.

Test of Fibrinolysis

Tests of fibrinolysis are less well characterized. The euglobulin lysis test time is a crude screening test for problems with fibrinolysis (4). Patients with accelerated fibrinolysis are often found to have a deficiency of α_2-AP (of which the total amount normally is only half of the total plasmin that can be generated) or the fibrin clot-stabilizing factor XIII (4). A deficiency of PAI-1 also may lead to accelerated fibrinolysis. During normal clot formation and breakdown, the D-dimer fragment of fibrinogen is a marker for ongoing thrombosis and physiologic fibrinolysis, whereas for fibrinogenolysis, the two D fragments that are produced are not cross-linked into the D-dimer form (4).

REFERENCES

1. Zur M, Radcliffe RD, Oberdick J, et al. The dual role of factor VII in blood coagulation: initiation and inhibition of a proteolytic system by a zymogen. *J Biol Chem* 1982;257:5623.
2. Radcliffe R, Nemerson Y. Mechanism of activation of bovine factor VII: products of cleavage by factor Xa. *J Biol Chem* 1976;251:4749.
3. Ferguson JJ, Waly HM, Wilson JM. Fundamentals of coagulation and glycoprotein IIb/IIIa receptor inhibition. *Eur Heart J* 1998;19[Suppl D]:D3.
4. Hassouna HI. Laboratory evaluation of hemostatic disorders. *Hematol Oncol Clin North Am* 1993;7:1161.
5. Sims PJ, Faioni EM, Wiedmer T, et al. Complement proteins C5b-9 cause release of membrane vesicles from the platelet surface that are enriched in the membrane receptor for coagulation factor Va and express prothrombinase activity. *J Biol Chem* 1988;263:18205.
6. Gilbert GE, Sims PJ, Wiedmer T, et al. Platelet-derived microparticles express high affinity receptors for factor VIII. *J Biol Chem* 1991;266:17261.
7. Hickey MJ, Williams SA, Roth GA. Human platelet glycoprotein IX: an adhesive prototype of leucine-rich glycoproteins with flank-center-flank structures. *Proc Natl Acad Sci USA* 1989;86:6773.
8. Bennett JS, Vilaire G, Cines DB. Identification of the fibrinogen receptor on human platelets by photoaffinity labeling. *J Biol Chem* 1982;257:8049.
9. Savage B, Ruggeri ZM. Selective recognition of adhesive sites in surface-bound fibrinogen by glycoprotein IIb/IIIa on nonactivated platelets. *J Biol Chem* 1991;266:11277.
10. Osterud B, Rapaport SI. Activation of factor IX by the reaction product of tissue factor and factor VIII: additional pathway for initiating blood coagulation. *Proc Natl Acad Sci USA* 1977;74:5260.
11. Bauer KA, Kass BL, ten Care H, et al. Factor IX is activated in vivo by the tissue factor mechanism. *Blood* 1990;76:731.
12. Blomback, B, Blomback M. The molecular structure of fibrinogen. *Ann NY Acad Sci* 1972;202:77.
13. Folk JE, Finlayson JS. The epsilon-(gamma-glutamyl) lysine crosslink and the catalytic role of transglutamines. *Adv Protein Chem* 1977;31:1.
14. Davie EW, Fujikawa K, Kisiel W. The coagulation cascade: initiation, maintenance, and regulation. *Biochemistry* 1991;30:10363.
15. Naito K, Fujikawa K. Activation of human blood coagulation factor XI independent of factor XII: factor XI is activated by thrombin and factor XIa in the presence of negatively charged surfaces. *J Biol Chem* 1991;266:7353.
16. DiScipio RG, Kurachi K, Davie EW. Activation of human factor IX (Christmas factor). *J Clin Invest* 1978;61:1528.
17. Rosenberg RD, Damus PS. The purification and mechanism of action of human antithrombin-heparin cofactor. *J Biol Chem* 1973;248:6490.
18. Kurachi K, Fujikawa K, Schmer G, et al. Inhibition of bovine factor IXa and factor Xab by antithrombin III. *Biochemistry* 1976;15:373.
19. Kurachi K, Davie EW. Activation of human factor XI (plasma thromboplastin antecedent) by factor XIIa (activated Hageman factor). *Biochemistry* 1977;16:5831.
20. Kisiel W, Canfield WM, Ericsson LH, et al. Anticoagulant properties of bovine plasma protein C following activation by thrombin. *Biochemistry* 1977;16:5824.
21. Marlar RA, Kleiss AJ, Griffin JH. Mechanism of action of human activated protein C, a thrombin dependent anticoagulant enzyme. *Blood* 1982;59:1067.
22. Vehar GA, Davie EW. Preparation and properties of bovine factor VIII (antihemophilic factor). *Biochemistry* 1980;19:401.
23. Esmon CT, Owen WG. Identification of an endothelial cell cofactor for thrombin-catalyzed activation of protein C. *Proc Natl Acad Sci USA* 1981;78:2249.
24. Owen WG, Esmon CT. Functional properties of an endothelial cell cofactor for thrombin-catalyzed activation of protein C. *J Biol Chem* 1981;256:5532.
25. Esmon NL, Owen WG, Esmon CT. Isolation of a membrane-bound cofactor for thrombin-catalyzed activation of protein C. *J Biol Chem* 1982;257:859.
26. Esmon CT. The regulation of natural anticoagulant pathways. *Science* 1987;235:1348.
27. Esmon NL, Carroll RC, Esmon CT. Thrombomodulin blocks the ability of thrombin to activate platelets. *J Biol Chem* 1983;258:12238.
28. Esmon CT, Esmon NL, Harris KW. Complex formation between thrombin and thrombomodulin inhibits both thrombin-catalyzed fibrin formation and factor V activation. *J Biol Chem* 1982;257:7944.

29. Walker FJ. Regulation of activated protein C by a new protein: a possible function for bovine protein S. *J Biol Chem* 1980;255:5521.

30. Tollefsen DM, Majerus PW, Blank MK. Heparin cofactor II: purification and properties of a heparin-dependent inhibitor of thrombin in human plasma. *J Biol Chem* 1982;257:2162.

31. Broze GJ, Girard TJ, Novotny WF. Regulation of coagulation by a multivalent Kunitz-type inhibitor. *Biochemistry* 1990; 29:7539.

32. Rapaport SI. Inhibition of factor VIIa/tissue factor-induced blood coagulation: with particular emphasis upon a factor Xa-dependent inhibitory mechanism. *Blood* 1989;73:359.

33. Gelehrter TD, Sznycer-Laszuk R. Thrombin induction of plasminogen activator inhibitor in cultured human endothelial cells. *J Clin Invest* 1986;77:165.

34. Dichek D, Quertermous T. Thrombin regulation of mRNA levels of tissue plasminogen activator and plasminogen activator inhibitor-1 in cultured human umbilical vein endothelial cells. *Blood* 1989;74:222.

35. Adelman B, Michelson AD, Loscalzo J, et al. Plasmin effect on platelet glycoprotein Ib–von Willebrand factor interactions. *Blood* 1985;65:32.

36. Schmaier AH. Disseminated intravascular coagulation: pathogenesis and management. *J Intensive Care Med* 1991;6:209.

37. Hajjar KA, Nachman RL. Endothelial cell–mediated conversion of Glu-plasminogen to Lys-plasminogen: further evidence for assembly of the fibrinolytic system on the endothelial cell surface. *J Clin Invest* 1988;82:1769.

38. Coleman RW. Activation of plasminogen by human plasma kallikrein. *Biochem Biophys Res Commun* 1969;35:273.

39. Esmon NL, Esmon CT. Protein C and the endothelium. *Semin Thromb Haemost* 1988;14:210.

40. Van der Poll T, Buller HR, ten Cate H, et al. Activation of coagulation after administration of tumor necrosis factor to normal subjects. *N Engl J Med* 1990;322:1622.

41. Nawroth PP, Stern DM. Modulation of endothelial cell hemostatic properties by tumor necrosis factor. *J Exp Med* 1986;163:740.

42. Bevilacqua MP, Pober JS, Majeau GR, et al. Recombinant tumor necrosis factor induces procoagulant activity in cultured human vascular endothelium: characterization and comparison with the actions of interleukin-1. *Proc Natl Acad Sci USA* 1986;83:4533.

43. Conway EM, Bach R, Rosenberg RD, et al. Tumor necrosis factor enhances expression of tissue factor mRNA in endothelial cells. *Thromb Res* 1989;53:231.

44. Schleef RR, Bevilacqua MP, Sawdey M, et al. Cytokine activation of vascular endothelium: effects on tissue-type plasminogen activator and type I plasminogen inhibitor. *J Biol Chem* 1988;263:5797.

45. Van Hinsbergh VW, Kooistra T, van den Berg EA, et al. Tumor necrosis factor increases production of plasminogen activator inhibitor in human endothelial cells in vitro and rats in vivo. *Blood* 1988;72:1467.

46. Medina R, Schocher SH, Han JH. Interleukin-1, endotoxin, or tumor necrosis factor/cachectin enhance the level of plasminogen activator messenger RNA in bovine aortic endothelial cells. *Thromb Res* 1989;54:41.

47. Van der Poll T, Levi M, Buller HR, et al. Fibrinolytic response to tumor necrosis factor in healthy subjects. *J Exp Med* 1991;174:729.

48. Pohlman TH, Stanness KA, Beatty PG, et al. An endothelial cell surface factor(s) induced in vitro by lipopolysaccharide, interleukin-1, and tumor necrosis factor-alpha increases neutrophil adherence by CD18 dependent mechanism. *J Immunol* 1986;136:4548.

49. Schleimer RP, Rutledge BK. Cultured human endothelial cells acquire adhesiveness for neutrophils after stimulation with interleukin-1, endotoxin, and tumor-promoting phorbol diesters. *J Immunol* 1986;136:649.

50. Rothlein R, Dustin ML, Marlin SD, et al. A human intercellular adhesion molecule (ICAM-1) distinct from LFA-1. *J Immunol* 1986;137:1270.

51. Bevilacqua MP, Stengelin S, Gimbrone MA, et al. Endothelial leukocyte adhesion molecule 1: an inducible receptor for neutrophils related to complement regulatory proteins and lectins. *Science* 1989;243:1160.

52. Kunkel SL, Standiford T, Metinko AP, et al. Endothelial cell-derived novel chemotactic cytokines. In: Lefant C, ed. *Lung vascular injury: molecular and cellular response.* New York: Marcel Dekker, 1991:213-226.

53. Furie B, Furie BC. Molecular and cell biology of blood coagulation. *N Engl J Med* 1992;326:800.

54. Palabrica T, Lobb R, Furie BC. Leukocyte accumulation promoting fibrin deposition is mediated in vivo by P-selectin on adherent platelets. *Nature* 1992;359:848.

55. Stewart GJ. Neutrophils and deep venous thrombosis. *Haemostasis* 1993;23:127.

56. Holt JC, Yan Z, Lu W, et al. Isolation, characterization, and immunological detection of neutrophil-activating peptide 2: a proteolytic degradation product of platelet basic protein. *Proc Soc Exp Biol Med* 1992;199:171.

57. Ferrer-Lopez P, Renesto P, Schattner M, et al. Activation of human platelets by C5a-stimulated neutrophils: a role for cathepsin G. *Am J Physiol* 1990;258:C1100.

58. Evangelista V, Rajtar G, de Gaetano G, et al. Platelet activation by fMLP-stimulated polymorphonuclear leukocytes: the activity of cathepsin G is not prevented by antiproteases. *Blood* 1991;77:2379.

59. Wakefield TW, Greenfield LJ, Rolfe MW, et al. Inflammatory and procoagulant mediator interactions in an experimental baboon model of venous thrombosis. *Thromb Haemost* 1993; 69:164.

60. Ansell JE, Price JM, Shah S, et al. Heparin-induced thrombocytopenia: what is its real frequency? *Chest* 1985;88:878.

61. Greinacher A, Michels I, Mueller-Eckhardt. Heparin-associated thrombocytopenia: the antibody is not heparin specific. *Thromb Haemost* 1992;67:545.

62. Adelman B, Sobel M, Fujimura Y, et al. Heparin-associated thrombocytopenia: observations on the mechanism of platelet aggregation. *J Lab Clin Med* 1989;113:204.

63. Silver D, Kapsch DN, Tsoi EK. Heparin-induced thrombocytopenia, thrombosis, and hemorrhage. *Am Surg* 1983;198:301.

64. Cancio LC, Cohen DJ. Heparin-induced thrombocytopenia and thrombosis. *J Am Coll Surg* 1998;186:76.

65. Sheridan D, Carter C, Kelton JG. A diagnostic test for heparin-induced thrombocytopenia. *Blood* 1986;67:27.

66. Jackson MR, Krishnamurti C, Aylesworth CA, et al. Diagnosis of heparin-induced thrombocytopenia in the vascular surgery patient. *Surgery* 1997;121:419.

67. Lee DH, Warkentin TE, Hayward CP, et al. The development and evaluation of a novel test for heparin induced thrombocytopenia. *Blood* 1994;84:188a(abstr).

68. Warkentin TE, Elavathil LJ, Hayward CP, et al. The pathogenesis of venous limb gangrene associated with heparin-induced thrombocytopenia. *Ann Intern Med* 1997;127:804.

69. Gruel Y, Lermusiaux P, Lang M, et al. Usefulness of antiplatelet drugs in the management of heparin-associated thrombocytopenia and thrombosis. *Ann Vasc Surg* 1991;5:552.

70. Slocum MM, Adams JG Jr, Teel R, et al. Use of enoxaparin in patients with heparin-induced thrombocytopenia syndrome. *J Vasc Surg* 1996;23:839.

71. Magnani HN. Heparin-induced thrombocytopenia (HIT): an overview of 230 patients treated with Orgaran (Org 10172). *Thromb Haemost* 1993;70:554.

72. Liem TK, Teel R, Shukla S, et al. The glycoprotein IIb/IIIa antagonist c7E3 inhibits platelet aggregation in the presence of heparin-associated antibodies. *J Vasc Surg* 1997;25:124.

73. Cole CW, Fournier LM, Bormanis J. Heparin-associated thrombocytopenia and thrombosis: optimal therapy with ancrod. *Can J Surg* 1990;22:207.

74. Lewis BE, Iaffaldano R, McKiernan TL, et al. Report of successful use of argatroban as an alternative anticoagulant during coronary stent implantation in a patient with heparin-induced thrombocytopenia and thrombosis syndrome. *Cathet Cardiovasc Diagn* 1996;38:206.

75. Greinacher A, Volpel H, Janssens U, et al. Recombinant hirudin (Lepirudin) provides safe and effective anticoagulation in patients with heparin-induced thrombocytopenia: a prospective study. *Circulation* 1999;99:73.

76. Almeida JI, Coats R, Liem TK, et al. Reduced morbidity and mortality rates of the heparin-induced thrombocytopenia syndrome. *J Vasc Surg* 1998;27:309.

77. Towne JB, Bernhard VM, Hussey C, et al. Antithrombin deficiency: a cause of unexplained thrombosis in vascular surgery. *Surgery* 1981;89:735.

78. Siddiqi FA, Tepler J, Fantini GA. Acquired protein S and antithrombin III deficiency caused by nephrotic syndrome: an unusual cause of graft thrombosis. *J Vasc Surg* 1997;25:576.

79. Flinn WR, McDaniel MD, Yao JS, et al. Antithrombin III deficiency as a reflection of dynamic protein metabolism in patients undergoing vascular reconstruction. *J Vasc Surg* 1984; 1:888.

80. Eby CS. A review of the hypercoagulable state. *Hematol Oncol Clin North Am* 1993;7:1121.

81. Menache D. Antithrombin III concentrates. *Hematol Oncol Clin North Am* 1993;6:1115.

82. Clouse LH, Comp PC. The regulation of hemostasis: the protein C system. *N Engl J Med* 1986;314:1298.

83. Eldrup-Jorgensen J, Flanigan DP, Brace L, et al. Hypercoagulable states and lower limb ischemia in young adults. *J Vasc Surg* 1989;9:334.

84. Esmon CT. The regulation of natural anticoagulant pathways. *Science* 1987;235:1348.

85. Cole MS, Minifee PK, Wolma FJ. Coumadin necrosis: a review of the literature. *Surgery* 1988;103:271.

86. Svensson PJ, Dahlback B. Resistance to activated protein C as a basis for venous thrombosis. *N Engl J Med* 1994;330:517.

87. Ridker PM, Miletich JP, Hennekens CH, et al. Ethnic distribution of factor V Leiden in 4,047 men and women: implications for venous thromboembolism screening. *JAMA* 1997; 277:1305.

88. Kalafatis M, Mann KG. Factor V Leiden and thrombophilia. *Arterioscler Thromb Vasc Biol* 1997;17:620.

89. Koeleman BP, Reitsma PH, Allaart CF, et al. Activated protein C resistance as an additional risk factor for thrombosis in protein C–deficient families. *Blood* 1994;84:1031.

90. Koeleman BP, van Rumpt D, Hamulyak K, et al. Factor V Leiden: an additional risk factor for thrombosis in protein S deficient families? *Thromb Haemost* 1995;74:580.

91. Rosendaal FR, Koster T, Vandenbroucke JP, et al. High risk of thrombosis in patients homozygous for factor V Leiden (activated protein C resistance). *Blood* 1995;85:1504.

92. Simioni P, Prandoni P, Lensing AW, et al. The risk of recurrent venous thromboembolism in patients with an Arg506 Gln mutation in the gene for factor V (factor V Leiden). *N Engl J Med* 1997;336:399.

93. Ouriel K, Green RM, DeWeese JA, et al. Activated protein C resistance: prevalence and implications in peripheral vascular disease. *J Vasc Surg* 1996;23:46.

94. Donaldson MC, Belkin M, Whittemore AD, et al. Impact of activated protein C resistance on general vascular surgical patients. *J Vasc Surg* 1997;25:1054.

95. Foley PW, Irvine CD, Standen GR, et al. Activated protein C resistance, factor V Leiden, and peripheral vascular disease. *Cardiovasc Surg* 1997;5:157.

96. Sampram ES, Lindblad B, Dahlback B. Activated protein C resistance in patients with peripheral vascular disease. *J Vasc Surg* 1998;28:624.

97. Greenfield LJ. Lupus-like anticoagulants and thrombosis. *J Vasc Surg* 1988;7:818.

98. Lockshin MD. Antiphospholipid antibody syndrome. *JAMA* 1992;268:1451.

99. Lynch A, Marlar R, Murphy J, et al. Antiphospholipid antibodies in predicting adverse pregnancy outcome: a prospective study. *Ann Intern Med* 1994;120:470.

100. Lockshin MD. Antiphospholipid antibody: babies, blood clots, biology. *JAMA* 1997;277:1549.

101. Rand JH, Wu XX, Andree HA, et al. Pregnancy loss in the antiphospholipid-antibody syndrome: a possible thrombogenic mechanism. *N Engl J Med* 1997;337:154.

102. Carreras LO, Defreyn G, Machin SJ, et al. Arterial thrombosis, intrauterine death, and "lupus" anticoagulant: detection of immunoglobulin interfering with prostacyclin formation. *Lancet* 1981;1:244.

103. Comp PC, DeBault LE, Esmon NL, et al. Human thrombomodulin is inhibited by IgG from two patients with non-specific anticoagulants. *Blood* 1983;62[Suppl 1]:299a(abstr).

104. Violi F, Ferro D, Valesini G, et al. Tissue plasminogen activator inhibitor in patients with systemic lupus erythematosus and thrombosis. *BMJ* 1990;300:1099.

105. Vermylen J, Blockmans D, Spitz B, et al. Thrombosis and immune disorders. *Clin Haematol* 1986;15:393.

106. Ferro D, Pittoni V, Quintarelli C, et al. Coexistence of antiphospholipid antibodies and endothelial perturbation in systemic lupus erythematosus patients with ongoing prothrombotic state. *Circulation* 1997;95:1425.

107. Reverter JC, Tassies D, Font J, et al. Hypercoagulable state in patients with antiphospholipid syndrome is related to high induced tissue factor expression on monocytes and to low free protein S. *Arterioscler Thromb Vasc Biol* 1996;16:1319.

108. Williams FM, Hunt BJ. The antiphospholipid syndrome and vascular surgery. *Cardiovasc Surg* 1998;6:10.

109. Ahn SS, Kalunian K, Rosove M, et al. Postoperative thrombotic complications in patients with the lupus anticoagulant: increased risk after vascular procedures. *J Vasc Surg* 1988;7:749.

110. Donaldson MC, Weinberg DS, Belkin M, et al. Screening for hypercoagulable states in vascular surgical practice: a preliminary study. *J Vasc Surg* 1990;11:825.

111. Nielsen TG, Nordestgaard BG, von Jessen F, et al. Antibodies to cardiolipin may increase the risk of failure of peripheral vein bypasses. *Eur J Vasc Endovasc Surg* 1997;14:177.

112. Valentine RJ, Kaplan HS, Green R, et al. Lipoprotein (a), homocysteine, and hypercoagulable states in young men with premature peripheral atherosclerosis: a prospective, controlled analysis. *J Vasc Surg* 1996;23:53.

113. Lee RW, Taylor LM Jr, Landry GJ, et al. Prospective comparison of infrainguinal bypass grafting in patients with and without antiphospholipid antibodies. *J Vasc Surg* 1996;24: 524.

114. Khamashta MA, Cuadrado MJ, Mujic F, et al. The management of thrombosis in the antiphospholipid-antibody syndrome. *N Engl J Med* 1995;332:993.

115. Towne JB, Bandyk DF, Hussey CV, et al. Abnormal plasminogen: a genetically determined cause of hypercoagulability. *J Vasc Surg* 1984;1:896.

116. Rodgers GM. Hemostatic properties of normal and perturbed vascular cells. *FASEB J* 1988;2:116.

117. Motta G, Rojkjaer R, Hasan AA, et al. High molecular weight kininogen regulates prekallikrein assembly and activation on endothelial cells: a novel mechanism for contact activation. *Blood* 1998;91:516.

118. Nilsson IM, Ljungner H, Tengborn L. Two different mechanisms in patients with venous thrombosis and defective fibrinolysis: low concentrations of plasminogen activator or increased concentration of plasminogen activator inhibitor. *Br Med J Clin Res Ed* 1985;290:1453.

119. Prins MH, Hirsh J. A clinical review of the evidence supporting a relationship between impaired fibrinolytic activity and venous thromboembolism. *Arch Intern Med* 1991;151: 1721.

120. Paramo JA, Perez JL, Serrano M, et al. Types 1 and 2 plasminogen activator inhibitor and tumor necrosis factor alpha in patients with sepsis. *Thromb Haemost* 1990;64:3.

121. Meade TW, Vickers MV, Thompson SG, et al. Epidemiological characteristics of platelet aggregability. *BMJ* 1985;290:428.

122. Cumming AM, Keeney S, Salden A, et al. The prothrombin gene G20210A variant: prevalence in a U.K. anticoagulant clinic population. *Br J Haematol* 1997;98:353.

123. Ferraresi P, Marchetti G, Legnani C, et al. The heterozygous 20210 G/A prothrombin genotype is associated with early venous thrombosis in inherited thrombophilias and is not increased in frequency in artery disease. *Arterioscler Thromb Vasc Biol* 1997;17:2418.

124. Falcon CR, Cattaneo M, Panzeri D, et al. High prevalence of hyperhomocyst(e)inemia in patients with juvenile venous thrombosis. *Arterioscler Thromb* 1994;14:1080.

125. den Heijer M, Blom HJ, Gerrits WB, et al. Is hyperhomocysteinemia a risk factor for recurrent venous thrombosis? *Lancet* 1995;345:882.

126. den Heijer M, Koster T, Blom HJ, et al. Hyperhomocysteinemia as a risk factor for deep vein thrombosis. *N Engl J Med* 1996;334:759.

127. Loscalzo J. The oxidant stress of hyperhomocyst(e)inemia. *J Clin Invest* 1996;98:5.

128. Tawakol A, Omland T, Gerhard M, et al. Hyperhomocyst(e)inemia is associated with impaired endothelium-dependent vasodilation in humans. *Circulation* 1997;95:1119.

129. Upchurch GR, Welch GN, Randev N, et al. The effect of homocysteine on endothelial nitric oxide production. *FASEB J* 1995;9:A876(abstr).

130. Blom HJ, Kleinveld HA, Boers GH, et al. Lipid peroxidation and susceptibility of low-density lipoprotein to in vitro oxidation in hyperhomocystinemia. *Eur J Clin Invest* 1995;25:149.

131. Chin JH, Azhar S, Hoffman BB. Inactivation of endothelium derived relaxing factor by oxidized lipoproteins. *J Clin Invest* 1992;89:10.

132. Liao JK, Shin WS, Lee WY, et al. Oxidized low-density lipoprotein decreases the expression of endothelial nitric oxide synthase. *J Biol Chem* 1995;270:319.

133. Starkebaum G, Harlan JM. Endothelial cell injury due to copper-catalyzed hydrogen peroxide generation from homocysteine. *J Clin Invest* 1986;77:1370.

134. Rees MM, Rodgers GM. Homocystinemia: association of a metabolic disorder with vascular disease and thrombosis. *Thromb Res* 1993;71:337.

135. Ueland PM, Refsum H, Brattstrom L. Plasma homocysteine and cardiovascular disease. In: Francis RB Jr, ed. *Atherosclerotic cardiovascular disease, hemostasis, and endothelial function.* New York: Marcel Dekker, 1993:183.

136. Hayashi T, Honda G, Suzucki K. An atherogenic stimulus homocysteine inhibits cofactor activity of thrombomodulin and enhances thrombomodulin expression in human umbilical vein endothelial cells. *Blood* 1992;79:2930.

137. Rodgers GM, Conn MT. Homocysteine, an atherogenic stimulus, reduces protein C activation by arterial and venous endothelial cells. *Blood* 1990;75:895.

138. Graeber JE, Slott JH, Ulane RE, et al. Effect of homocysteine and homocystine on platelet and vascular arachidonic acid metabolism. *Pediatr Res* 1982;16:490.

139. Nehler MR, Taylor LM Jr, Porter JM. Homocystinemia as a risk factor for atherosclerosis: a review. *Cardiovasc Surg* 1997;5:559.

140. Fisher DF Jr, Yawn DH, Crawford ES. Preoperative disseminated intravascular coagulation associated with aortic aneurysms: a prospective study of 76 cases. *Arch Surg* 1983;118:1252.

141. Collins JA. Blood transfusion and disorders of surgical bleeding. In: Sabiston DC, ed. *Textbook of surgery,* 14th ed. Philadelphia: WB Saunders, 1991:85.

142. Lusher JM, Warrier I. Hemophila A. *Hematol Oncol Clin North Am* 1993;7:1021.

143. Lusher JM, Arkin S, Abildgaard CF, et al. Recombinant factor VIII for the treatment of previously untreated patients with hemophilia A: safety, efficacy, and development of inhibitors. *N Engl J Med* 1993;328:453.

144. Telfer MC. Clinical spectrum of viral infections in hemophilic patients. *Hematol Oncol Clin North Am* 1993;7:1047.

145. Larson PJ, High KA. Biology of inherited coagulopathies: factor IX. *Hematol Oncol Clin North Am* 1993;7:999.

146. Ginsburg D. Biology of inherited coagulopathies: von Willebrand factor. *Hematol Oncol Clin North Am* 1993;7:1011.

147. Edmunds LH. Blood contact activation during cardiopulmonary bypass. *J Vasc Surg* 1990;12:213.

148. Wakefield TW, Shulkin BL, Fellows EP, et al. Platelet reactivity in human aortic grafts: a prospective randomized midterm study of platelet adherence and release products in Dacron and ePTFE grafts. *J Vasc Surg* 1989;9:234.

149. Hirsh J. Heparin. *N Engl J Med* 1991;324:1565.

150. Saba HI, Saba SR, Morelli GA. Effect of heparin on platelet aggregation. *Am J Hematol* 1984;17:295.

151. Kakkar VV. The current status of low-dose heparin in the prophylaxis of thrombophlebitis and pulmonary embolism. *World J Surg* 1978;2:3.

152. Clagett GP, Anderson FA Jr, Geerts W, et al. Prevention of venous thromboembolism. *Chest* 1998;114:531S.

153. Collins R, Scrigmeour A, Yusuf S, et al. Reduction in fatal pulmonary embolism and venous thrombosis by perioperative administration of subcutaneous heparin: overview of results of randomized trials in general, orthopedic, and urologic surgery. *N Engl J Med* 1988;318:1162.

154. Hirsh J. Low–molecular-weight heparin. *Circulation* 1998;98:1575.

155. Salzman EW. Low–molecular-weight heparin: is small beautiful? [Editorial]. *N Engl J Med* 1986;315:957.

156. Leizorovicz A. Comparison of the efficacy and safety of low molecular weight heparins and unfractionated heparin in the initial treatment of deep venous thrombosis: an updated meta-analysis. *Drugs* 1996;52[Suppl 7]:30.

157. Siragusa S, Cosmi B, Piovella F, et al. Low–molecular-weight heparins and unfractionated heparin in the treatment of patients with acute venous thromboembolism: results of a meta-analysis. *Am J Med* 1996;100:269.

158. Simonneau G, Sers H, Charbonnier B, et al. A comparison of low–molecular-weight heparin with unfractionated heparin for acute pulmonary embolism. *N Engl J Med* 1997;337:663.

159. Groce JB. Patient outcomes and cost analysis associated with an outpatient deep venous thrombosis treatment program. *Pharmacotherapy* 1998;18:175S.

160. Hull RD, Raskob GE, Rosenbloom D, et al. Treatment of proximal vein thrombosis with subcutaneous low–molecular-weight heparin vs. intravenous heparin: an economic perspective. *Arch Intern Med* 1997;157:289.

161. van den Belt AG, Bossuy PM, Prins MH, et al. Replacing inpatient care by outpatient care in the treatment of deep venous thrombosis: an economic evaluation. *Thromb Haemost* 1998;79:259.

162. Lindmarker P, Holmstrom M. Use of low molecular weight heparin (dalteparin), once daily, for the treatment of deep vein thrombosis: a feasibility and health economic study in an outpatient setting. *J Intern Med* 1996;240:395.

163. Wells PS, Kovacs MJ, Bormanis J, et al. Expanding eligibility for outpatient treatment of deep venous thrombosis and pulmonary embolism with low–molecular-weight heparin. *Arch Intern Med* 1998;158:1809.

164. Harrison L, McGinnis J, Crowther M, et al. Assessment of outpatient treatment of deep-vein thrombosis with low–molecular-weight heparin. *Arch Intern Med* 1998;158:2001.

165. Horrow JC. Protamine: a review of its toxicity. *Anesth Analg* 1985;64:348.

166. Wakefield TW, Ucros I, Kresowik TF, et al. Decreased oxygen consumption as a toxic manifestation of protamine sulfate reversal of heparin anticoagulation. *J Vasc Surg* 1989;9:772.

167. Pearson PJ, Evora RR, Ayrancioglu K, et al. Protamine releases endothelium-derived relaxing factor from systemic arteries: a possible mechanism of hypotension during heparin neutralization. *Circulation* 1992;86:289.

168. Wakefield TW, Bies LE, Wrobleski SK, et al. Impaired myocardial function and oxygen utilization due to protamine sulfate in a isolated rabbit heart preparation. *Ann Surg* 1990;212:387.

169. Morel DR, Zapol WM, Thomas SJ, et al. C5a and thromboxane generation associated with pulmonary vaso- and broncho-constriction during protamine reversal of heparin. *Anesthesiology* 1987;66:597.

170. Eika C. On the mechanism of platelet aggregation induced by heparin, protamine, and polybrene. *Scand J Haematol* 1972;9:248.

171. DeLucia A, Wakefield TW, Andrews PC, et al. Efficacy and toxicity of differently charged polycationic protamine-like peptides for heparin anticoagulation reversal. *J Vasc Surg* 1993;18:49.

172. Coon WW. Anticoagulant therapy. *Am J Surg* 1985;150:45.

173. Hirsh J. Oral anticoagulant drugs. *N Engl J Med* 1991;324:1865.

174. Hull R, Carter C, Jay R, et al. The diagnosis of acute, recurrent, deep-vein thrombosis: a diagnostic challenge. *Circulation* 1983;67:901.

175. Kearon C, Gent M, Hirsh J, et al. A comparison of three months of anticoagulation with extended anticoagulation for a first episode of idiopathic venous thromboembolism. *N Engl J Med* 1999;340:901.

176. Coller BS. Platelets and thrombolytic therapy. *N Engl J Med* 1990;322:33.

177. Madan M, Berkowitz SD, Tcheng JE. Glycoprotein IIb/IIIa integrin blockade. *Circulation* 1998;98:2629.

178. Fenton JW, Ofosu FA, Brezniak DV, et al. Thrombin and antithrombotics. *Semin Thromb Haemost* 1998;24:87.

179. Jang IK, Gold HK, Ziskind AA, et al. Prevention of platelet-rich arterial thrombosis by selective thrombin inhibition. *Circulation* 1990;81:219.

180. Addonzio VP Jr, Fisher CA, Jenkin BK, et al. Iloprost (ZK 36 374), a stable analogue of prostacyclin, preserves platelets

during simulated extracorporeal circulation. *J Thorac Cardiovasc Surg* 1985;89:926.

181. Musial J, Niewiarowski S, Rucinski B, et al. Inhibition of platelet adhesion to surfaces of extracorporeal circuits by disintegrins. RGD-containing peptides from viper venoms. *Circulation* 1990;82:261.

182. Shigeta O, Gluszko P, Downing SW, et al. Protection of platelets during long-term extracorporeal membrane oxygenation in sheep with a single dose of a disintegrin. *Circulation* 1992;86[Suppl II]:398.

183. Mohr R, Goor DA, Lusky A, et al. Aprotinin prevents cardiopulmonary bypass-induced platelet dysfunction: a scanning electron microscope study. *Circulation* 1992;86[Suppl II]:405.

184. Quereshi A, Lamont J, Burke P, et al. Aprotinin: the ideal anti-coagulant? *Eur J Vasc Surg* 1992;6:317.

185. Royston D, Bidstrup BP, Taylor KM, et al. Effect of aprotinin on need for blood transfusion after repeat open heart surgery. *Lancet* 1987;2:1289.

186. Salzman EW, Weinstein MJ, Reilly D, et al. Adventures in hemostasis. Desmopressin in cardiac surgery. *Arch Surg* 1993;128:212.

187. Mannucci PM. Desmopressin: a nontransfusional form of treatment for congenital and acquired bleeding disorders. *Blood* 1988;72:1449.

188. Cole CW, Bormanis J, Luna GK, et al. Ancrod versus heparin for anticoagulation during vascular surgical procedures. *J Vasc Surg* 1993;17:288.

189. Marder VJ, Sherry S. Thrombolytic therapy: current status (first of two parts). *N Engl J Med* 1988;318:1512.

190. Fuji S, Sawa H, Saffitz JE, et al. Induction of endothelial cell expression of the plasminogen activator inhibitor type I gene by thrombosis in vivo. *Circulation* 1992;86:2000.

191. Quinones-Baldrich WJ. Principles of thrombolytic therapy. In: Rutherford RB, ed. *Vascular surgery*, 4th ed. Philadelphia: WB Saunders, 1995:334.

192. Comerota AJ, Aldridge SC. Thrombolytic therapy for acute deep vein thrombosis. *Semin Vasc Surg* 1992;5:76.

193. Elliot MS, Immelman EJ, Jeffrey P, et al. A comparative randomized trial of heparin versus streptokinase in the treatment of acute proximal venous thrombosis: an interim report of a prospective trial. *Br J Surg* 1979;66:838.

194. Arnsen H, Hoiseth A, Ly B. Streptokinase or heparin in the treatment of deep vein thrombosis: follow-up results of a prospective study. *Acta Med Scand* 1982;211:65.

195. Kakkar VV, Lawrence D. Hemodynamic and clinical assessment after therapy for acute deep vein thrombosis: a prospective study. *Am J Surg* 1985;150:54.

196. Porter JM, Taylor LM. Current status of thrombolytic therapy. *J Vasc Surg* 1985;2:239.

197. Graor RA, Young JR, Risius B. Comparison of cost effectiveness of streptokinase and urokinase in the treatment of deep vein thrombosis. *Ann Vasc Surg* 1987;1:524.

198. Turpie AGG. Thrombolytic agents in venous thrombosis. *J Vasc Surg* 1990;12:196.

199. Machleder HI. Evaluation of a new treatment strategy for Paget-Schroetter syndrome: spontaneous thrombosis of the axillary-subclavian vein. *J Vasc Surg* 1993;17:305.

200. National Heart and Lung Institute Cooperative Study Group. Urokinase pulmonary embolism trial: phase 1 results. *JAMA* 1970;214:2163.

201. National Heart and Lung Institute Cooperative Study Group. Urokinase-streptokinase embolism trial: phase 2 results. *JAMA* 1974;229:1606.

202. McNamara TO, Fischer JR. Thrombolysis of peripheral arterial and graft occlusions: improved results using high-dose urokinase. *AJR Am J Roentgenol* 1985;144:769.

203. McNamara TO, Bomberger RA. Factors affecting initial and 6 months patency rates after intraarterial thrombolysis with high-dose urokinase. *Am J Surg* 1986;152:709.

204. Gardiner GA, Sullivan KL. Catheter directed thrombolysis for the failed lower extremity bypass graft. *Semin Vasc Surg* 1992;5:99.

205. Graor RA, Risius B, Young JR, et al. Peripheral artery and bypass graft thrombolysis with recombinant tissue-type plasminogen activator. *J Vasc Surg* 1986;3:115.

206. Comerota AJ, White JV. Intraoperative, intra-arterial thrombolytic therapy as an adjunct to revascularization in patients with residual and distal arterial thrombus. *Semin Vasc Surg* 1992;5:110.

207. Doorey AJ, Michelson EL, Topol EJ. Thrombolytic therapy for acute myocardial infarction: keeping the unfulfilled promises. *JAMA* 1992;268:3108.

208. Rutherford RB, Jones DN. The role of Dextran-40 in preventing early graft thrombosis. In: Bergqvist D, Lindblad B, eds. *Pharmacological intervention to increase patency after arterial reconstructions*. Malmo, Sweden: ICM AB, 1989:44.

209. Stenbjerg S, Berg E, Albrechtsen OK. Heparin levels and activated clotting times (ACT) during open heart surgery. *Scand J Haematol* 1981;26:281.

SURGERY: SCIENTIFIC PRINCIPLES AND PRACTICE, Third Edition, edited by Lazar J. Greenfield, Michael W. Mulholland, Keith T. Oldham, Gerald B. Zelenock, and Keith D. Lillemoe. Lippincott Williams & Wilkins Publishers, Philadelphia, © 2001.

CHAPTER 5
CYTOKINES
LISA M. COLLETTI

Cytokines are soluble protein mediators that are secreted by one cell to influence another cell, tissue, or organ in an autocrine, paracrine, or endocrine fashion. A multitude of soluble protein mediators with a wide range of biologic effects have been described. Cytokines play an important role in regulating the immune response and act in various ways on T cells, B cells, cells of the monocyte/macrophage lineage, neutrophils, fibroblasts, smooth muscle cells, endothelial cells, and epithelial cells. Immunologic functions that are influenced by these polypeptides include the host response to both acute and chronic bacterial, viral, fungal, and parasitic infections, trauma, burns, allograft rejection, ischemia/reperfusion injury, and autoimmune diseases. Cytokines also play important roles in tumor biology, in response to the tumor itself and in mediating tumor growth and metastasis. Angiogenesis, as well as cellular growth and differentiation, are also under cytokine-mediated regulation. An excessive cytokine release is responsible for the development of the adult respiratory distress syndrome (ARDS) and multiple organ system failure (MOSF). Cytokines have a multitude of actions and effects, and a complete discussion of all of these areas is beyond the scope of this chapter. Instead, this chapter focuses on some of the actions of cytokines that have particular pertinence to surgery. As such, we focus on their role in tissue injury, inflammation, and wound repair, in addition to discussing some new data pertaining to their role in angiogenesis, as well as tissue growth and repair.

Cytokine production at various tissue sites depends in part on the proximity of the site to a stimulus. It has been suggested that cytokine concentrations increase concomitantly with the magnitude of injury or inciting stimulus. However, in both laboratory and clinical settings, it has been difficult to correlate plasma cytokine concentrations with the extent of tissue damage. The reason appears to be that cytokines typically function in an autocrine and paracrine fashion and are therefore designed to signal the presence of local, rather than systemic, inflammation. Tumor necrosis factor-α (TNF-α) and interleukin (IL)-1 are important early mediators of the inflammatory response and trigger a variety of host responses. These include an increase in neutrophil margination, activation of the antimi-

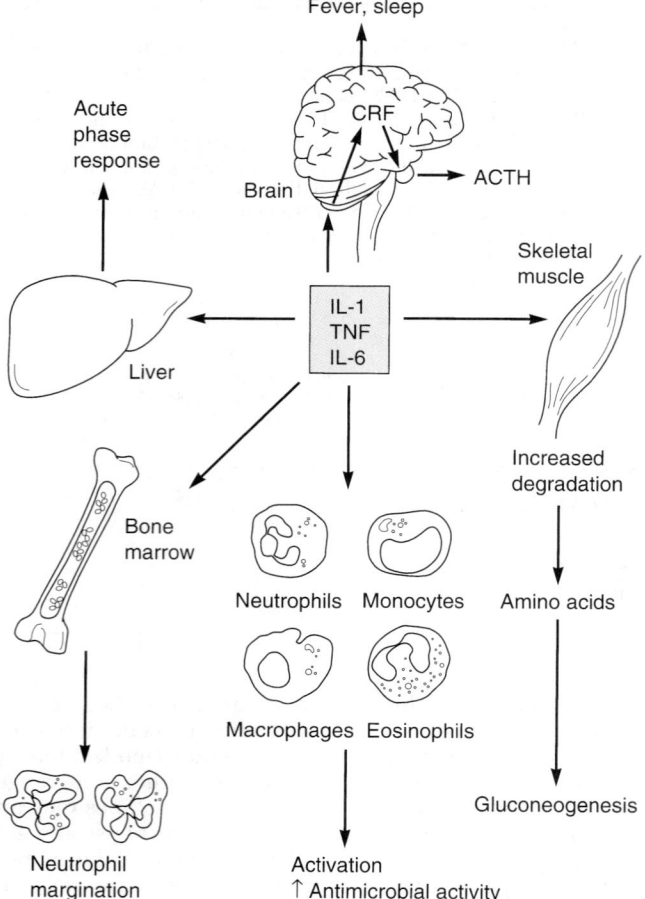

Figure 5.1. Early-response cytokines and the initiation of inflammation. Tumor necrosis factor-α (TNF-α), interleukin (IL)-1, and IL-6 have a multitude of effects in the initiation of the inflammatory response, including the increased breakdown of skeletal muscle to yield amino acids for gluconeogenesis; the activation of monocytes, macrophages, neutrophils, and eosinophils, with an increase in neutrophil margination and an overall increase in leukocyte antimicrobial activity; and the induction of the acute-phase response. In the brain, these molecules cause changes that induce fever and sleep. In addition, they up-regulate corticotropin-releasing factor, which stimulates the production of adrenocorticotropic hormone (ACTH).

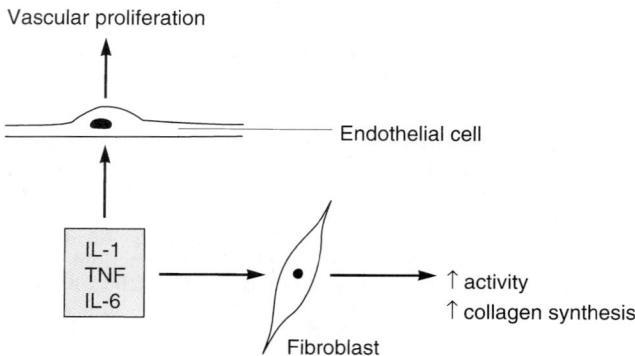

Figure 5.2. Effects of tumor necrosis factor-α (TNF-α), interleukin (IL)-1, and IL-6 on acute tissue injury and wound repair. After injury, TNF-α, IL-1, and IL-6 regulate fibroblast activity and collagen synthesis, as well as vascular proliferation in the initiation of tissue repair

crobial activity of monocytes, macrophages, neutrophils, and eosinophils, induction of the acute-phase response, and increased skeletal muscle degradation to yield amino acids for gluconeogenesis (1) (Fig. 5.1). During wound repair, the same molecules play an important role in regulating vascular proliferation, fibroblast and osteoclast activity, and collagen synthesis (2,3) (Fig. 5.2). Although these activities constitute the normal physiologic response to injury and are directed by relatively low, local concentrations of cytokines, excessive concentrations of these molecules can cause adverse effects (Fig. 5.3). They include tachycardia, hypotension, pulmonary inflammation, edema, vascular congestion and hemorrhage, acute renal tubular necrosis and fibrinous renal thrombi, acute hepatic inflammation, and lactic acidosis, all of which can be associated with sepsis, systemic inflammation, and MOSF (4–7) (Table 5.1). The capacity of the host to generate an acute inflammatory response is necessary to clear offending agents, such as bacteria, viruses, and fungi. Once the inciting agent is removed, the inflammatory reaction resolves and normal tissue repair and remodeling occur, reestablishing normal host function. Although many of the mechanisms responsible for this response have been determined, precise details of all of the pathways have not been fully elucidated. Both immune and nonimmune cells participate in the generation of reactive oxygen metabolites, as well as lipid and protein mediators of inflammation. All of these mediators are essential for the full expression of the inflammatory response.

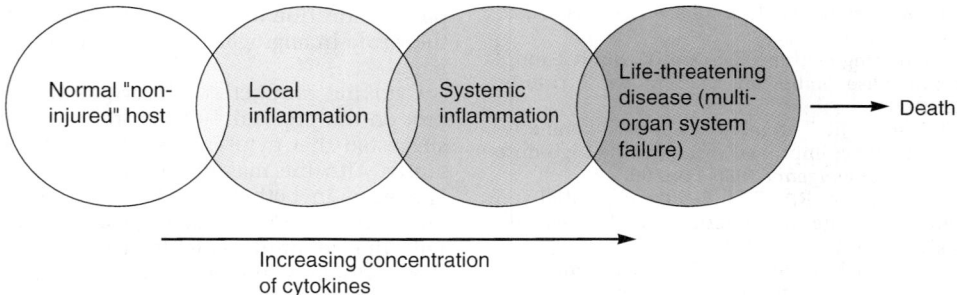

Figure 5.3. Spectrum of normal to pathologic effects of cytokines based on increasing concentrations. Low local concentrations of cytokines represent normal physiology and the normal initial response to injury or infection. Increasing concentrations of cytokines, resulting in systemic cytokine levels, result in severe physiologic derangements, often leading to multiple organ system failure and death of the host.

Table 5.1. ADVERSE PHYSIOLOGIC EFFECTS SEEN WITH SYSTEMIC CYTOKINE LEVELS LEADING TO MULTIPLE ORGAN SYSTEM FAILURE

Organ system	Effect
Cardiovascular	Tachycardia
	Hypotension
Pulmonary	Inflammation
	Edema
	Vascular congestion
	Hemorrhage
Renal	Acute tubular necrosis
	Fibrinous renal thrombi
Hepatic	Acute hepatic inflammation
Musculoskeletal	Skeletal muscle breakdown
	Lactic acidosis

EARLY RESPONSE CYTOKINES

Tumor Necrosis Factor-α

Tumor necrosis factor-α was initially demonstrated to be important in the development of sepsis and MOSF. Septic shock is a pathologic condition characterized by circulatory failure and collapse. It is typically associated with ARDS, MOSF, and death (5–7). The interplay between monocytes, tissue macrophages, neutrophils, and endothelial cells appears to be particularly important in the pathophysiology of this process. At the cellular level, this syndrome is associated with hypermetabolism and an energy deficit, ultimately leading to cellular injury and death. The cascade of inflammatory events that culminates in MOSF is initiated by trauma, microorganisms, microbial by-products, and cytokines (5–7). Although MOSF can also occur in an aseptic state, particularly with multiple trauma, severe burns, or severe pancreatitis, there is always a cytokine-dependent response associated with these acute inflammatory syndromes (Fig. 5.4). The exact agent that initiates MOSF is unknown, particularly in the aseptic state. In the septic state, however, endotoxin triggers the expression of several cytokines, particularly TNF-α and IL-1, which orchestrate the subsequent inflammatory response in a cascade fashion. If unchecked, this cascade can precipitate MOSF and eventual death.

Tumor necrosis factor-α has pleiotropic effects on many cellular functions. At local inflammation sites, this cytokine mediates the normal initiation, maintenance, and repair of tissue injury. In contrast, exaggerated systemic levels of TNF-α can cause MOSF and increase the host morbidity and mortality rate (8–12). Cells of the monocyte–macrophage lineage are the principal cellular sources of TNF-α. However, TNF-α can also be expressed by glial cells in the brain, Kupffer cells in the liver, keratinocytes in the skin, mast cells, natural killer cells, T cells, and B cells (13). A variety of exogenous and endogenous factors produced by bacteria, viruses, parasites, and tumors can induce cells to produce TNF-α; however, endotoxin is the most potent stimulus for TNF-α production and release (13,14). The regulation of TNF-α gene expression is multifactorial, and several molecules, such as interferon-γ (IFN-γ), can increase TNF-α production, whereas others, such as IL-4, IL-10, corticosteroids, and pentoxyfylline, decrease TNF-α production (15). Studies with monoclonal antibodies against TNF-α for sepsis syndromes in humans have shown only modest benefits. TNF-α is a member of a growing family of cytokines, which include TNF-α, TNF-β, Fas ligand, TNF-related apoptosis ligand, nerve growth factor, and CD40 ligand. In

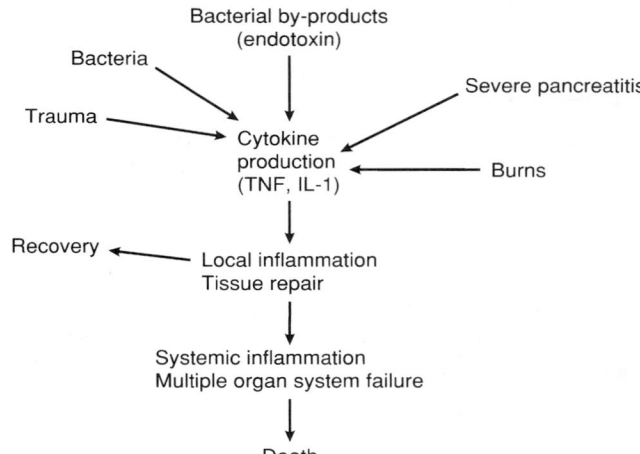

Figure 5.4. Multiple organ system failure (MOSF). A multitude of potential insults to the host can initiate the cascade of events that can ultimately culminate in MOSF and death. Trauma, burns, bacterial infection, or severe pancreatitis are all well known initiating events precipitating MOSF. These events cause expression of tumor necrosis factor-α (TNF-α) and interleukin-1 (IL-1), which initiate the inflammatory cascade. When the cascade proceeds in a controlled, well orchestrated fashion, tissue repair and recovery of the host occurs. However, if the cascade continues in an exaggerated, uncontrolled fashion, with elevated systemic concentrations of a variety of inflammatory cytokines, MOSF ensues with potential death of the host.

contrast to TNF-α, most of the members of this family are involved in the regulation of cellular proliferation and apoptosis. TNF-α is unique in its inflammatory characteristics. The observation that TNF-α has both proinflammatory and apoptosis-inducing properties is perplexing. TNF-α can induce a variety of other proinflammatory cytokines known to antagonize apoptosis, including IL-1, IL-6, and granulocyte–macrophage colony-stimulating factor (GM-CSF). There is experimental evidence that suggests that TNF-α directly stimulates apoptotic cell death, as well as inducing pathways to protect this same cell from apoptotic death (16). The exact mechanisms responsible for the control of these opposing functions remain to be determined.

Tumor necrosis factor-α has a marked procoagulant effect on endothelial cells, precipitating intravascular thrombosis (Fig. 5.5; Table 5.2). TNF-α induces the endothelium to release numerous factors with procoagulant activity, as well as altering the antithrombotic properties of the vascular endothelium itself. Although TNF-α overall tends to facilitate a hypercoagulable state, this molecule can also induce endothelial synthesis of prostacyclin and urokinase-type plasminogen activator, thus facilitating antithrombotic tendencies (Fig. 5.6; Table 5.2). It is clear that this multitude of mediators can exert conflicting effects, and the net effect of TNF-α depends on the location and quantity in which it is produced and the vascular bed with which it interacts.

Tumor Necrosis Factor-α Regulation

Tumor necrosis factor-α biosynthesis is a tightly regulated process, controlled at several levels, including gene transcription, message translation, and protein processing. TNF-α is expressed on the cell membrane as a bioactive 26-kd protein, and is cleaved into its 17-kd soluble form by a specific TNF-α converting enzyme, an adamolysin and member of the matrix metalloproteinase family. Shedding of the extracellular domains of the two TNF-α recep-

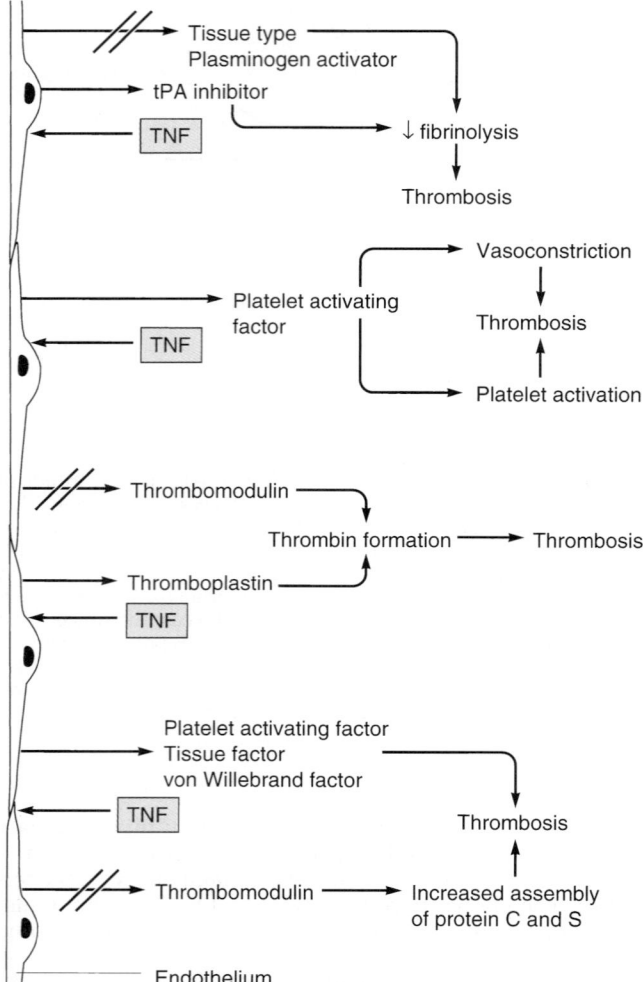

Figure 5.5. Actions of tumor necrosis factor-α (TNF-α) favoring thrombosis. TNF-α has numerous procoagulant effects, favoring intravascular thrombosis. TNF-α causes endothelial cells to release a variety of factors with procoagulant properties, including tissue factor, platelet-activating factor, von Willebrand factor, thromboplastin, and tissue-type plasminogen activator inhibitor. It also inhibits the formation of tissue-type plasminogen activator and thrombomodulin. The inhibition of thrombomodulin increases coagulation through two mechanisms. A decrease in thrombomodulin allows both an increase in the assembly of protein C and S complexes, as well as increasing thrombin formation. In addition, both the decrease in thrombomodulin and the increase in thromboplastin further facilitate thrombin formation. Similarly, the decrease in tissue-type plasminogen activator and the increase in tissue-type plasminogen activator inhibitor decrease overall fibrinolysis, again favoring thrombosis. The TNF-α-mediated increase in platelet-activating factor favors thrombosis through platelet activation and vasoconstriction.

tors, by matrix metalloproteinases, can further alter the biologic activity of TNF-α by decreasing the number of cell signaling sites on target tissues and increasing the amount of circulating inhibitors (17). TNF-α signaling occurs through two different receptors: TNFR1 (p55) and TNFR2 (p75) (17). Their expression is differentially regulated and exhibits some tissue specificity (Fig. 5.7). It is thought that one receptor may be responsible for activing inflammatory pathways, whereas the other receptor activates apoptotic functions (17). Although investigations have suggested

Table 5.2. PRIMARY EFFECTS OF TUMOR NECROSIS FACTOR AND INTERLEUKIN-1 ON THE VASCULAR ENDOTHELIUM

INCREASE LEUKOCYTE ADHESION BY INCREASING THE EXPRESSION OF ENDOTHELIAL ADHESION MOLECULES; FACILITATES EXTRAVASATION OF NEUTROPHILS

Intercellular adhesion molecule-1
Platelet–endothelial cell adhesion molecule-1
Vascular cell adhesion molecule-1
E-selectin
P-selectin

INCREASE THROMBOGENICITY

Increases tissue factor
Decreases thrombomodulin
    Blocks assembly of protein C and S complexes
Increases synthesis of thromboplastin
    Increase in thromboplastin plus a decrease in thrombomodulin results in an increase in thrombin formation at the endothelial surface
Decrease fibrinolysis
    Increases tissue-type plasminogen activator inhibitor
    Decreases tissue-type plasminogen activator
Increases platelet-activating factor
    Potent platelet and leukocyte activator
    Powerful vasoconstrictor
Increases von Willebrand factor

DECREASE THROMBOGENICITY

Increases prostacyclin synthesis
    Powerful vasodilator
    Inhibits platelet aggregation
Increases urokinase-type plasminogen activator
    Activates fibrinolysis
Increases nitric oxide synthesis
    Inhibits platelet aggregation
Causes release of many substances that increase vasodilation
    Prostaglandin E_2
    Prostacyclin
    Thromboxane A_2
    Nitric oxide

STIMULATE CYTOKINE EXPRESSION AND SECRETION THAT RESULT IN LEUKOCYTE RECRUITMENT AND ACTIVATION

IL-1
IL-6
GM-CSF
G-CSF
IL-8
Monocyte chemoattractant protein-1

INCREASE PLATELET-DERIVED GROWTH FACTOR

Cause morphologic change
Stimulate angiogenesis

G(M)-CSF, granulocyte (macrophage) colony-stimulating factor; IL, interleukin.

that each type of receptor activates a distinct signaling pathway, in vitro and in vivo data have yielded conflicting results as to which receptor activates which pathway.

Proinflammatory signals, including TNF-α and IL-1, regulate the shedding of TNF-α receptors and increase the appearance of shed TNF-α receptors in the circulation. TNF-α also directly induces the expression and release of TNF-α inhibitors, including IL-10, corticosteroids, and prostanoids, which act in a negative feedback loop to suppress TNF-α production and processing. TNF-α is the principal inducer of IL-10, and IL-10 effectively suppresses TNF-α release in response to endotoxin. Thus, TNF-α down-regulates its own bioactivity in an autocrine manner by altering the number of cell receptors and by releasing self-acting inhibitors. TNF-α-

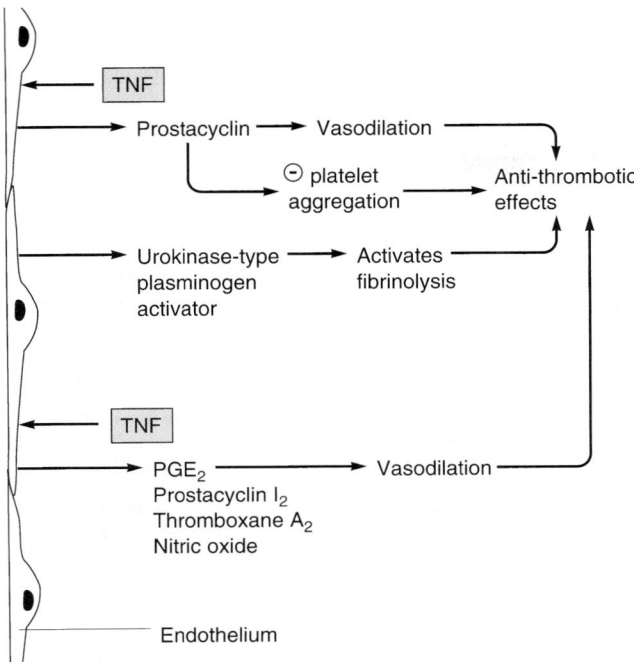

Figure 5.6. Anticoagulant effects of tumor necrosis factor-α (TNF-α). Although most TNF-α -induced effects on the endothelium favor thrombosis, this cytokine also has antithrombotic actions. These include an increase in endothelial synthesis of prostacyclin and urokinase-type plasminogen activator. Prostacyclin inhibits platelet aggregation and is a potent vasodilator. Urokinase-type plasminogen activator induces fibrinolysis. TNF-α also up-regulates endothelial production of prostaglandin E_2, prostacyclin I_2, thromboxane A_2, and nitric oxide, which are all powerful vasodilators.

mediated disease is associated with either excessive initial TNF-α production or inadequate production of its inhibitors. This is the basis for several therapeutic strategies used for sepsis, rheumatoid arthritis, inflammatory bowel disease, and multiple sclerosis.

Figure 5.7. Tumor necrosis factor-α (TNF-α) receptors. The p55 TNF-α receptor has a highly conserved intracellular domain of approximately 70 amino acids that plays an important role in triggering cellular apoptosis. It is termed the *death domain* (DD) and is critically important in intracellular signaling. Binding of the intracellular DDs triggers the intracellular signaling cascade, ultimately leading to the recruitment of Fas-associating protein with DD (FADD), which leads directly to the pathway triggering apoptosis. The p55 receptor requires an additional binding protein, TNFR1-associated DD protein (TRADD) to recruit FADD. TRADD can also interact with two other proteins, TRAF1 and TRAF2 (TNF-α receptor-associated factors). TRAF2 is important in the cascade leading to the activation of NF-KB by TNF-α, which leads to the activation of the inflammatory effects of TNF-α. Thus, TRADD is the branch point for TNF-α activation of apoptosis versus inflammation. The p75 TNF-α receptor also activates an intracellular signaling pathway leading to the binding of TRAF1 and TRAF2, resulting in inflammatory TNF-α effects. It can also induce apoptosis, but it does not share the p55 pathway. Rather, the p75 pathway to apoptosis is through the induction of acid or neutral sphingomyelinases.

Tumor necrosis factor-α and the Fas ligand are mediators of apoptosis in several immune cell populations. TNF-α-mediated apoptosis may be responsible for removal of T-cell populations during sepsis, and neutrophils from inflammatory foci. Studies suggest that there is a delicate balance between and within TNF-α signaling pathways, regulating the balance between ongoing inflammation and apoptosis.

Interleukin-1

Interleukin-1 is a complex, multifunctional molecule that shares many biologic properties with TNF-α and markedly potentiates the lethal effects of TNF-α when given concurrently (18). Overall, IL-1 alone probably has weaker effects than TNF-α in the induction of shock. Many cells can synthesize and release IL-1 in response to a wide variety of stimuli. Cells that are typically involved in the immune response can produce IL-1, most importantly the monocyte–macrophage cell line, including blood monocytes, alveolar and peritoneal macrophages, Kupffer cells, and synovial macrophages. These cells are the major sources of secreted IL-1 (Fig. 5.8). Lymphocytes, including natural killer cells, B cells, and helper T cells, are also sources of IL-1. In addition, a variety of other "nonimmune" cells produce IL-1. In the central nervous system, astrocytes, microglia, and glioma cells produce IL-1, as do vascular smooth muscle cells and endothelial cells. Neutrophils, fibroblasts, chondrocytes, epithelial cells, keratinocytes, Langerhans cells, and renal mesangial cells have also been shown to produce IL-1. IL-2, GM-CSF, transforming growth factor-β (TGF-β), TNF-α, all of the interferons, and IL-1 are all endogenous mediators that can induce IL-1 production. Other endogenous stimuli for IL-1 production include antigen–antibody complexes, the Fc region of immunoglobulin G, and C5a. Other nonspecific exogenous stimuli include silica particles and ultraviolet irradiation. For macrophages to present antigen to T cells, macrophage-derived IL-1 participation and synthesis are required. Exogenous products, such as endotoxins, peptidoglycans, muramyl dipeptide, virus particles, yeast particles, and zymosan, are also IL-1-stimulating agents.

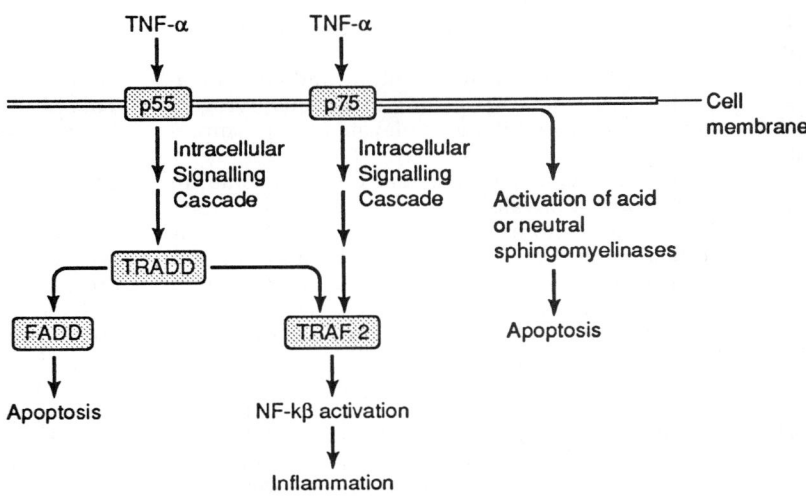

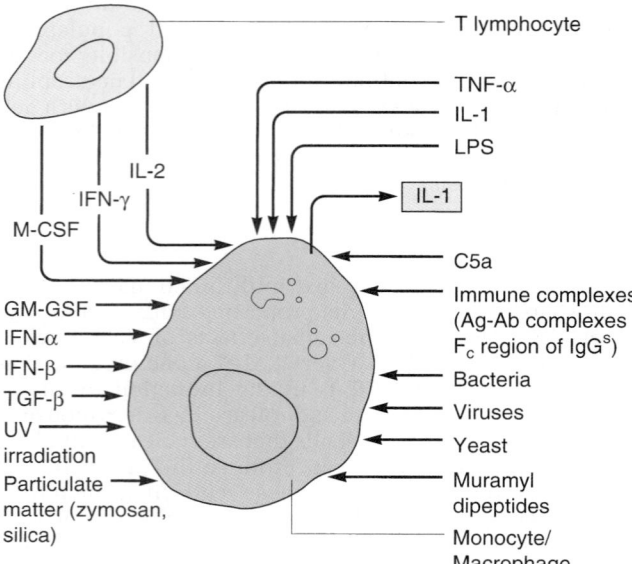

Figure 5.8. Stimuli for interleukin-1 (IL-1) production in cells of the monocyte–macrophage lineage. The macrophage is the most important cellular source of IL-1 in vivo.

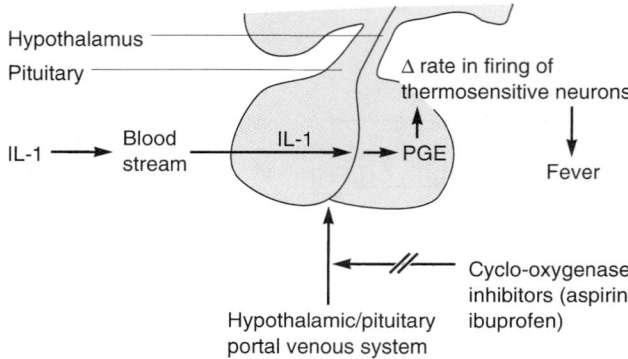

Figure 5.9. Etiology of interleukin-1 (IL-1)-induced fever. Although there is no evidence that IL-1 crosses the blood–brain barrier, IL-1 induces fever when injected into animals. IL-1 interacts with the endothelial cells of the pituitary–hypothalamic–portal venous system, inducing production and release of E-series prostaglandins. These prostaglandins then act on the thermosensitive cells of the hypothalamus, altering their firing rate, resulting in fever. Antipyretic drugs inhibit cyclooxygenase, preventing the generation of prostaglandins from arachidonic acid.

Metabolic and Inflammatory Effects of Interleukin-1

The proinflammatory effects of IL-1 are well documented and include effects on fibroblasts, synovial cells, chondrocytes, endothelial cells, hepatocytes, and osteoclasts. A key feature of IL-1-induced actions is the stimulation of arachidonic acid metabolism and the secretion of a variety of inflammatory proteins, including other cytokines and proteases (18). IL-1 stimulates the release of pituitary stress hormones, increases the synthesis of collagenases, resulting in the destruction of cartilage, and stimulates prostaglandin production (18). IL-1 induces fever when injected into experimental animals (18). There is no evidence that IL-1 crosses the blood–brain barrier, and it is likely that this pyrogenic action occurs by interacting with the endothelial cells of the hypothalamic–pituitary–portal venous system, which generates prostaglandins of the E series (18) (Fig. 5.9). These prostaglandins then act on the hypothalamus to alter the firing rates of the thermosensitive neurons, resulting in fever (18). Antipyretic drugs, such as aspirin, are effective because they inhibit the cyclooxygenase enzyme involved in converting arachidonic acid to prostaglandins. Fever is an evolutionarily conserved, nonspecific reaction to infection and inflammation. Although IL-1 can serve as an endogenous pyrogen, other cytokines can also induce an elevated body temperature.

Experimental evidence suggests that IL-1 has some interesting functions in physiologic homeostasis. For example, somnolence and anorexia are common manifestations of acute infection, and the central administration of IL-1 can induce slow-wave sleep in experimental animals. IL-1 administration has an anorectigenic effect, inhibits lipoprotein lipase activity, and mobilizes neutrophils from the bone marrow with a resultant neutrophilia.

The effects of TNF-α and IL-1 overlap (18). TNF-α can stimulate the production of IL-1, and the effects of the two cytokines together are far greater than the the effects of either molecule alone (Table 5.3). IL-1 is also produced in the sepsis syndrome in concert with TNF-α; however, the mechanism of IL-1-induced shock appears to be related to the release of other small mediator molecules, such as platelet-activating factor, prostaglandins, and nitric oxide, which all potentiate hypotension (19). In animals, a single intravenous dose of IL-1 decreases the mean arterial pressure, lowers systemic vascular resistance, and induces leukopenia and thrombocytopenia (19). One of the most important properties of IL-1 involves its interaction with the vascular endothelium. These particular actions are again redundant, however, and overlap with those of TNF-α (Fig. 5.10). Other manifestations of IL-1–endothelial cell interactions include prostaglandin production, production of platelet-activating factor, and a variety of colony-stimulating factors. These responses facilitate the mobilization and activation of appropriate leukocyte populations for specific localized immune responses. IL-1 also affects the vascular endothelium by shifting the balance toward thrombosis and a procoagulant state by down-regulating the fibrinolytic system and enhancing the activity of plasminogen activator inhibitor and tissue-factor-like procoagulant, as well as thrombomodulin and the protein-C system (20). IL-1 shifts the fibrinolytic properties of the endothelium by increasing plasminogen activator inhibitor-1 production while leaving unchanged or decreasing tissue-type plasminogen activator (20). IL-1 enhances thrombin formation on the endothelial surface by inducing the synthesis of thromboplastin and concomitantly suppressing thrombomodulin gene expression. Furthermore, IL-1 induces platelet-activating factor synthesis. This phospholipid is a potent platelet and leukocyte activator, as well as a powerful vasoconstrictor.

Although most IL-1-induced changes facilitate a hypercoagulable state, this cytokine can also stimulate the endothelial synthesis of prostacyclin and urokinase-type plasminogen activator. This facilitates antithrombotic tendencies. Prostacyclin inhibits platelet aggregation and is a potent vasodilator, whereas urokinase-type plasminogen activator activates the fibrinolytic system. This IL-1-induced increase in prostacyclin facilitates vasodilation at sites of inflammation, as well as the hypotension associated with systemic cytokine release (i.e., septic shock). Cyclooxygenase inhibitors prevent hypotension in this setting (19). It is clear that this multitude of mediators can exert conflicting effects, and the net effect of IL-1 can depend on its location and quantity, as well as the vascular bed with which it interacts.

Table 5.3. **TISSUE SOURCES AND EFFECTS OF EARLY-RESPONSE CYTOKINES**

	Tumor necrosis factor	**Interleukin-1**	**Interleukin-6**
Source	Monocytes/macrophages, keratinocytes, Kupffer cells, fibroblasts, astrocytes, glial cells, mast cells, NK cells, T and B lymphocytes	Monocytes/macrophages, keratinocytes, Kupffer cells, fibroblasts, endothelial cells, astrocytes, microglial cells, epithelial cells, PMNs, vascular smooth muscle cells epithelial cells, NK cells, T and B lymphocytes	Monocytes/macrophage, keratinocytes, Kupffer cells, fibroblasts, endothelial cells, astrocytes, PMNs, microglial cells, T and B lymphocytes, epithelial cells
Introduction of fever	++	+++	+
Induction of shock	+++	++	+/−
Stimulation of acute-phase response	+	++	+++
Endothelial cells activation	+++	++	+/−
Procoagulant activity	+++	++	+/−
Anorexia, weight loss	+++	++	+/−
Fibroblast proliferation	++	++	−

NK, natural killer; PMNs, polymorphonuclear leukocytes.

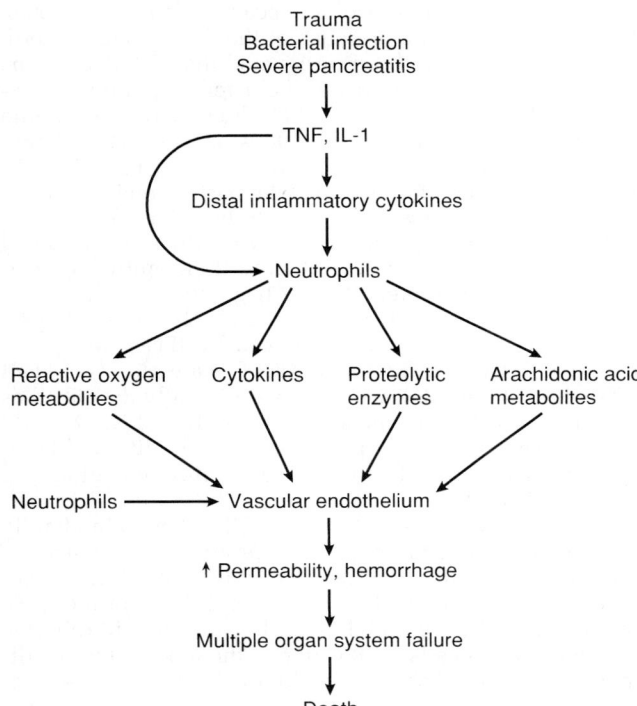

Figure 5.10. Cascade leading to multiple organ system failure (MOSF). A variety of noxious events—including trauma, burns, infection, and pancreatitis—can trigger this cascade of events. Tumor necrosis factor-α (TNF-α) and interleukin-1 (IL-1) are important early mediators, initiating adherence of neutrophils to the vascular endothelium by up-regulating both leukocyte and endothelial adhesion molecules. TNF-α and IL-1 are also responsible for triggering the release of more distal inflammatory cytokines, which are important neutrophil chemotactic and activating agents. These activated neutrophils are recruited into the area of injury or infection, where they elaborate reactive oxygen metabolites, other cytokines, proteolytic enzymes, and arachidonic acid metabolites, all of which injure the surrounding tissues and microvasculature, resulting in increased microvascular permeability, hemorrhage, and accentuated leukocyte migration into these tissues. Neutrophil recruitment and activation is one of the key events in this cascade because the activated neutrophil appears to be one of the most important effector cells in mediating tissue injury in multiple organ system failure, regardless of the precipitating event.

Interleukin-6

Interleukin-6 also is important in host defense because it regulates the hepatic response to inflammation. IL-6 was initially termed *hepatocyte-stimulating factor,* and its most important function appears to be regulating the hepatic acute-phase response (21). The hepatic acute-phase response is a series of homeostatic responses induced by injury or infection. After the injurious or infectious stimulus, several physiologic changes develop within several hours. These changes typically reflect alterations in the set point of a variety of physiologic parameters and include alterations in thermoregulation typically manifested by fever, nitrogen balance manifested by the development of a catabolic state, and changes in circulating levels of a group of particular proteins, classically termed *acute-phase proteins* (Table 5.4). These physiologic changes allow the host to recover from the injury or infection. IL-6 is one of the primary stimuli for the production of these proteins by the liver (22) (Table 5.5). Most of these proteins are glycoproteins, and they play various roles in the homeostatic response to injury and infection (22). IL-6 expression is stimulated by a multitude of cytokines and growth factors, as well as by bacterial endotoxins (23). In monocytes and macrophages, lipopolysaccharide (LPS) is the most potent stimulus for IL-6 production; the most potent stimuli for fibroblast-derived IL-6 are IL-1 and TNF-α (23). Platelet-derived growth factor (PDGF) and fibroblast growth factor (FGF) can also cause significant induction of IL-6 in fibroblasts (23). Steroids inhibit IL-6 induction in

Table 5.4. **MAJOR ACUTE-PHASE REACTANTS**

Protein	Function
C-reactive protein	Opsonin
Serum amyloid A	Apolipoprotein
α_2-Macroglobulin	Antiproteinase
α_1-Acid glycoprotein	Transport
Fibrinogen	Coagulation
α_1-Proteinase inhibitor	Antiproteinase
α_1-Antichymotrypsin	Antiproteinase
Haptoglobin	Binds and removes hemoglobin
Hemopexin	Binds heme
Ceruloplasmin	Oxygen scavenger, transport
Complement C_3	Opsonin
Serum amyloid P	Unknown
Albumin	Unknown
Transferrin	Transport

Table 5.5. **ACUTE-PHASE PROTEINS REGULATED BY CYTOKINES**

INDUCED BY IL-6

C-reactive protein
α_2-Macroglobulin
α_1-Acid glycoprotein
Fibrinogen
α_1-Proteinase inhibitor
α_1-Antichymotrypsin
Haptoglobin
Hemopexin
Ceruloplasmin
Complement C_3
Serum amyloid P
Serum amyloid A

INDUCED BY II-1

C-reactive protein
α_1-Acid glycoprotein
Complement C3
Serum amyloid P
Serum amyloid A
Haptoglobin
Hemopexin

cells of the monocyte–macrophage lineage. Most, if not all nucleated cells have the capacity to express IL-6 in vitro. In vivo, the most prominent source of IL-6 appears to be LPS-stimulated monocytes or macrophages and IL-1- or TNF-α-stimulated stromal cells, particularly fibroblasts, epithelial cells, and endothelial cells (23) (Fig. 5.11). In vitro studies have shown that IL-6 can be expressed by central nervous system cells, particularly astrocytes, microglial cells, and folliculostellate cells. Despite these in vitro data, it appears that only a few cell types in vivo secrete IL-6 in pathologic situations. Plasma levels of IL-6 rise rapidly after an in vivo challenge by LPS. There appears to be a temporal lag between elevations in plasma TNF-α and subsequent elevations in plasma IL-6. Thus, it is likely that macrophage-derived IL-1 and TNF-α are responsible for producing IL-6. These macrophage-derived, early-response cytokines can activate adjacent stromal cells, such as fibroblasts and endothelial cells, to release high levels of IL-6. This cascade increases plasma levels of IL-6 and subsequently stimulates the hepatic acute-phase response.

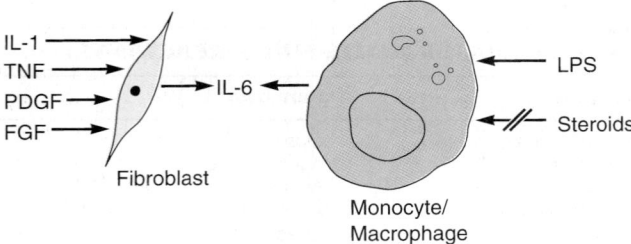

Figure 5.11. Stimuli for interleukin (IL)-6 production in fibroblasts and cells of the monocyte–macrophage lineage. In vivo, tumor necrosis factor-α (TNF-α) and IL-1 are the most potent stimuli for fibroblast IL-6 production, whereas lipopolysaccharide (LPS) is the most potent stimulus for monocyte–macrophage IL-6 production. Steroids inhibit monocyte–macrophage IL-6 production and release. Platelet-derived growth factor (PDGF) and fibroblast growth factor (FGF) are also capable of inducing fibroblast IL-6 production in vivo.

CHEMOTACTIC FACTORS

Several peptide, polypeptide, and lipid mediators have chemotactic properties. Although TNF-α, IL-1, and LPS were initially reported to have direct neutrophil chemotactic activity, more recent studies have shown that these molecules are not directly chemotactic for neutrophils (5). This finding suggests that cytokine networks may be operative in vivo and again depend on the initial expression of early-response cytokines (i.e., TNF-α and IL-1). This initial interaction is followed by the generation of more distal inflammatory mediators that directly influence neutrophil chemotaxis and activation. Because neutrophil chemotaxis and activation is a key component of inflammation, this is clearly an important part of the inflammatory cascade.

There is a particularly important group of chemotactic cytokines that share significant homology, with the presence of four conserved cysteine amino acid residues (24). These cytokines in their monomeric forms are all less than 10 kd, are characteristically basic heparin-binding proteins, have specific neutrophil chemotactic activity, and display four highly conserved cysteine amino acid residues, with the first two cysteines separated by one nonconserved amino acid residue. Because of their chemotactic properties and the presence of the CXC cysteine motif, these cytokines have been designated the *CXC chemokine family*. These chemokines are all clustered on human chromosome 4, and exhibit 20% to 50% homology at the amino acid level (5). Since the mid-1980s, at least 12 different CXC chemokines have been identified. They include NH$_2$-terminal truncated forms of platelet basic protein [connective tissue activating protein-III, β-thromboglobulin, and neutrophil-activating peptide-2 (NAP-2)], growth-related oncogene (GRO)-α, GRO-β, GRO-γ, IL-8, epithelial neutrophil-activating protein (ENA-78), granulocyte chemotactic protein-2, platelet factor-4 (PF-4), IFN-γ-inducible protein (IP-10), and monokine induced by IFN-γ (MIG) (25) (Table 5.6). GRO-α, GRO-β, and GRO-γ are closely related CXC chemokines (25), with GRO-α originally described as a mitogen for human melanoma cells. IL-8, ENA-78, and granulocyte chemotactic protein-2 were all initially identified by their ability to induce neutrophil activation and chemotaxis (25).

Interleukin-8 is the best-studied CXC chemokine family member and has been found to be produced by an array of both immune and nonimmune cells, including monocytes, alveolar macrophages, neutrophils, keratinocytes, mesangial cells, epithelial cells, hepatocytes, fibroblasts, and endothelial cells. IL-8 is one of the most potent mediators of neutrophil chemotaxis in this family of molecules. The early-response cytokines, TNF-α and IL-1, are key molecules for inducing IL-8, which in turn plays an im-

Table 5.6. **CXC CHEMOKINES**

Name	Abbreviation
Connective tissue-activating protein III β-thromboglobulin	CTAP-III
Neutrophil-activating peptide-2	NAP-2
Growth-related oncogene-α	GRO-α
Growth-related oncogene-β	GRO-b
Growth-related oncogene-γ	GRO-γ
Interleukin-8	IL-8
Epithelial neutrophil-activating protein	ENA-78
Granulocyte chemotactic protein-2	GCP-2
Platelet factor-4	PF-4
γ-Interferon-inducible protein	IP-10
Monokine induced by γ-interferon	MIG

portant role in inducing neutrophil recruitment and activation and in continuing the inflammatory response. Similarly, in vitro studies have identified ENA-78 as a potent neutrophil chemotaxin that is produced by endothelial cells stimulated by either TNF-α or IL-1, neutrophils, monocytes, pulmonary epithelial cells, and pulmonary fibroblasts. Both IP-10 and MIG are interferon-inducible CXC chemokines. Although IP-10 induces all three interferons (IFN-α, IFN-β, and IFN-γ), MIG is unique in that it appears to be expressed only in the presence of IFN-γ. IFN-γ also attenuates the expression of both IL-8 and ENA-78. These concepts suggest that both immune and nonimmune cells can produce neutrophil chemotactic cytokines and thus help to propagate the inflammatory response. They also show that members of the CXC chemokine family demonstrate disparate regulation by IFN-γ, and suggest that IFN-γ may be an important molecule with respect to the control and regulation of inflammation.

CXC Chemokine Structure and Function

Studies have demonstrated an important amino acid sequence in the primary CXC chemokine structure that appears to account for the disparate abilities of these molecules to function as promoters or inhibitors of neutrophil chemotaxis (26–28). The three amino acid residues that immediately precede the first cysteine amino acid are critically important in receptor binding and neutrophil activation (26–28). This area has been designated as the ELR motif, and is made up of the amino acid sequence Glu-Leu-Arg (26–28) (Fig. 5.12). The ELR motif appears to be the most critical region in these molecules for CXC receptor interactions (26–28). There are two types of human CXC receptors mediating transmembrane signals: CXC-R1 and CXC-R2 (29). Both CXC-R1 and CXC-R2 bind IL-8 with similar high affinity; however, the receptor affinities are significantly different for other CXC chemokines (29). CXC-R1 binds these other molecules with relatively low affinity (29). In contrast, CXC-R2 binds all ELR-containing

CXC chemokines with high affinity (29). The ELR motif is present in all members of the CXC family that activate neutrophils and bind to CXC-R2 (28,29). The ELR region can be modified so that biologic activity is lost, even though receptor binding is retained (28). These antagonist analogues, including IL-8 (6-72) and (Ala4,5) IL-8 (4-72), have a much lower receptor affinity compared with native IL-8, suggesting that the ELR motif is important for receptor binding as well as activation (28).

The ELR sequence is notably absent in some CXC chemokines, particularly IP-10, MIG, and PF-4 (26–28). These molecules have a significantly decreased ability to induce neutrophil chemotaxis (26–28). When the ELR motif was introduced into PF-4, its neutrophil chemotactic properties increased 1,000-fold (27). Thus, this particular region of the CXC molecules is important for neutrophil chemotactic activity. Further studies have demonstrated that ELR-containing CXC chemokines are angiogenic, whereas CXC chemokines lacking the ELR sequence are angiostatic (30). When non-ELR-containing chemokines are combined with ELR-positive chemokines, the angiogenic properties of the ELR-positive molecules are suppressed, suggesting that the ELR motif is critical for dictating angiogenic activity (27,28,30). The ELR-negative molecules also suppress the angiogenic properties of FGF-β, suggesting that a receptor system other than the CXC receptors is operative in this setting (30). These studies suggest that differing molecules in the CXC family are promoters or suppressors of biologic activity, and that the balance between these promoters and suppressors may regulate these biologic activities in the chemokine family.

CXC Chemokines and Angiogenesis

Interleukin-8 is a potent neutrophil chemotaxin and activator; in addition, IL-8 is a potent angiogenic factor. In vitro, recombinant IL-8 mediates endothelial cell chemotaxis and proliferation. IL-8 also demonstrates potent angiogenic activity in an in vivo angiogenesis model using a corneal micropocket system in rabbits or rats. Endothelial cell chemotaxis occurs in response to recombinant IL-8 at a concentration of 1.25 nmol/L and is comparable with chemotaxis toward recombinant FGF at a concentration of 6 nmol/L (31–33). Similar concentrations of IL-8 are angiogenic in the corneal micropocket model. Because monocytes and macrophages can represent a major source of angiogenic activity in wounds, chronic diseases, and solid tumors (31–33), IL-8 may be an important angiogenic factor liberated by these cells in a variety of pathologic states, as well as during normal wound repair.

In contrast, another member of the CXC chemokine family, PF-4, has angiostatic properties. In vivo, PF-4 was found to attenuate the growth of murine melanoma and human colon cancer, and this appeared to be related to its angiostatic properties (32–35). This angiostatic activity was initially postulated to be secondary to the heparin-binding domain in the carboxyl terminus of the molecule (32–35). This does not appear to be the case, however, because a recently produced PF-4 analogue without the heparin-binding domain was equipotent in vivo to native PF-4 in attenuating tumor growth (32–35). The ELR area appears to be critically important in binding and activating neutrophils (Fig. 5.12). This particular motif is absent in certain members of the CXC chemokine family, notably PF-4, IP-10, and MIG. These particular molecules display a markedly reduced potency in mediating neutrophil chemotaxis. When the ELR motif is introduced into these molecules, they gain significantly in their potency for neutrophil chemotaxis. Thus, this particular structural difference may also explain, at least in part, the disparate an-

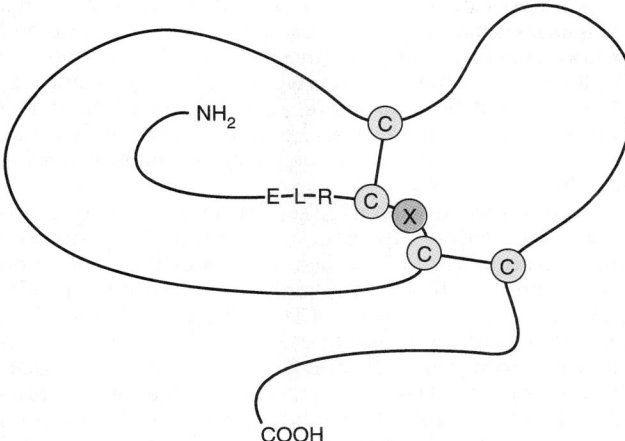

Figure 5.12. Schematic structure of CXC cytokines, demonstrating the four highly conserved cysteine amino acids. The first two cysteines are separated by one nonconserved amino acid. The ELR motif that precedes the first cysteine amino acid is also illustrated. The presence of the ELR motif appears to be important for neutrophil chemotactic activity and possibly also for angiogenic activity. Platelet factor-4 (PF-4), interferon-γ-inducible protein (IP-10), and monokine induced by interferon-γ (MIG) lack the ELR motif and have a significantly reduced ability to induce neutrophil chemotaxis. This property is restored when the ELR motif is added to these molecules.

giogenic activity between members of the CXC chemokine family. This suggests that the CXC chemokines can function as either angiostatic or angiogenic factors, and the biologic balance that is maintained between these factors can govern overall angiogenic potential in a variety of physiologic and pathophysiologic states.

CXC Chemokines and Mitogenesis

Although the best known and studied CXC chemokine effect is neutrophil chemotaxis, the biologic actions of these molecules are more wide ranging, and include mitogenesis and angiogenesis. IL-8 induces keratinocyte proliferation, with this effect being directly attributable to specific IL-8 receptors on the keratinocyte (36,37). Subsequent keratinocyte binding studies showed that the IL-8 receptor–ligand interactions were specific for IL-8, and similar in concentration to those needed for optimal neutrophil chemotaxis and angiogenesis. This suggests that IL-8 may be important in wound healing after tissue injury and inflammation. Further, macrophage inflammatory protein-2 (MIP-2) causes rat alveolar epithelial cell proliferation in vitro and GRO-α, GRO-β, and GRO-γ are mitogenic for melanoma cells, again demonstrating the mitogenic properties of these molecules (36,37). Monocytes and macrophages are likely a major source of mitogenic activity in wounds.

COUNTERREGULATORY CYTOKINES

Interleukin-6, Interleukin-10, and Interleukin-13

At least three counterregulatory interleukins have been identified: IL-6, IL-10, and IL-13. These molecules were initially identified by their ability to inhibit TNF-α generation in macrophages stimulated with LPS (38). Blockade of any of these interleukins increases TNF-α levels and neutrophil recruitment. IL-1 receptor antagonist (IL-1ra) is a product of stimulated macrophages and is also a counterregulatory factor in the inflammatory response (38). When the inflammatory response is triggered, there is a rapid and profound loss of IKB because of its hydrolysis by the 26S proteosome. This allows translocation of NF-KB to the nucleus, where gene activation occurs (38). In the presence of IL-10 or IL-13, activation of NF-KB fails to take place and the generation of inflammatory mediators is accordingly suppressed (38). Although the exact mechanisms are unclear, IL-10 and IL-13 inhibit fundamental processes leading to signal transduction and gene activation in the pathways of the inflammatory response. IL-10 appears to be the most potent antiinflammatory agent in this group.

Interleukin-10 is produced by multiple cell types, specifically types 1 and 2 helper T cells. IL-10 is secreted predominantly by human monocytes and macrophages, as well as by T and B lymphocytes. It specifically is not produced or released by neutrophils. IL-10 production is increased by exposure to LPS, TNF-α, IL-2, IL-4, IL-13, as well as other agents, with TNF-α being a particularly strong stimulus for IL-10 production and release. IL-10 inhibits cytokine production in multiple cell types; in monocytes and macrophages, IL-10 down-regulates synthesis of TNF-α, IL-1, IL-6, and IL-8. A similar pattern was also seen in neutrophils. IL-10 also promotes the release of other antiinflammatory molecules, specifically soluble TNF-α receptors and IL-1ra.

In the setting of injury, burns, sepsis, ARDS, and MOSF, serum IL-10 levels are often increased. In these studies, patients with the highest levels of IL-10 died (38). It is unclear whether this is actually a pathologic response, or a marker of injury severity. The preponderance of the litera-

ture suggests that IL-10 is not a mediator of immunosuppression, but rather important for the control of the inflammatory response. IL-10 may be an important molecule in the development of inflammatory bowel diseases such as ulcerative colitis and Crohn's disease. Recent studies with IL-10 knockout mice demonstrate that chronic enterocolitis develops in these animals, pathologically and clinically resembling ulcerative colitis and Crohn's disease in humans (39). A preliminary clinical trial suggests that there may be a therapeutic benefit with IL-10 treatments in these patients, which in turn suggests that these disease processes may be the result of an imbalance between proinflammatory and antiinflammatory cytokines.

Interferon-γ

Interferon-γ is a macrophage-activating factor and, as such, is usually a proinflammatory cytokine (40). It is known to modulate cellular differentiation, cytotoxicity, cytokine production, cellular adhesion, and oxidative metabolism through its effects on leukocytes and endothelial cells (40). It also regulates numerous macrophage functions, including tumor cell cytotoxicity, antimicrobial activity, increased killing of intracellular pathogens, and antigen processing and presentation to lymphocytes through the induction of major histocompatibility complex (MHC) antigens (40). Other studies have documented antiinflammatory effects for this molecule. Mucosal gene transfer of IFN-γ inhibits pulmonary allergic responses in mice (41). There is also a down-regulatory role for IFN-γ in autoimmune encephalomyelitis (42). More recent investigations suggest a more complex regulatory role for IFN-γ in the cascade of mediators that affect neutrophil recruitment; IFN-γ selectively inhibits LPS-induced expression of CXC chemokines (43). Similarly, there is a selective inhibition of CXC chemokine expression in neutrophils treated with IFN-γ (44). IFN-γ up-regulates macrophage production of IP-10 and MIG, ELR-negative CXC chemokines that are known to inhibit neutrophil chemotaxis and activation. In addition, IFN-γ decreases macrophage secretion of the ELR-positive CXC chemokines IL-8, KC, and ENA-78. The ELR-positive CXC chemokines are potent neutrophil chemotactic agents and are important in the neutrophil-mediated phase of injury. IFN-γ also modulates Kupffer cell production of TNF-α and IL-1, although by different mechanisms. IFN-γ increases Kupffer cell production of TNF-α and prostaglandin E$_2$ (PGE$_2$), but not IL-1; further, PGE$_2$ is a known inhibitor of Kupffer cell TNF-α release, through a negative feedback loop, thus suggesting an autoregulatory feedback mechanism involving IFN-γ.

Interferon-γ is involved in regulation of a variety of adhesion molecules important in neutrophil recruitment and activation (40). IFN-γ also modulates the expression of endothelial cell adhesion molecules. Endothelial cells exposed to IFN-γ express CD54. This facilitates firm neutrophil adhesion by the CD11/CD18 ligand. Neutrophil-endothelial cell adhesion requires the CD54-CD18 complex. CD54 expression is augmented by low-dose IFN-γ, but decreases in the presence of high-dose IFN-γ. IFN-γ has also been shown to inhibit the up-regulation of E- and P-selectin on activated endothelial cells.

INJURY, INFLAMMATION, AND WOUND HEALING: BASICS OF THE INFLAMMATORY RESPONSE

Polypeptide mediators, such as TNF-α and IL-1, are early-response cytokines actively involved in initiating the cascade of events that precipitates acute inflammation. They trigger other cytokines that are important in the in-

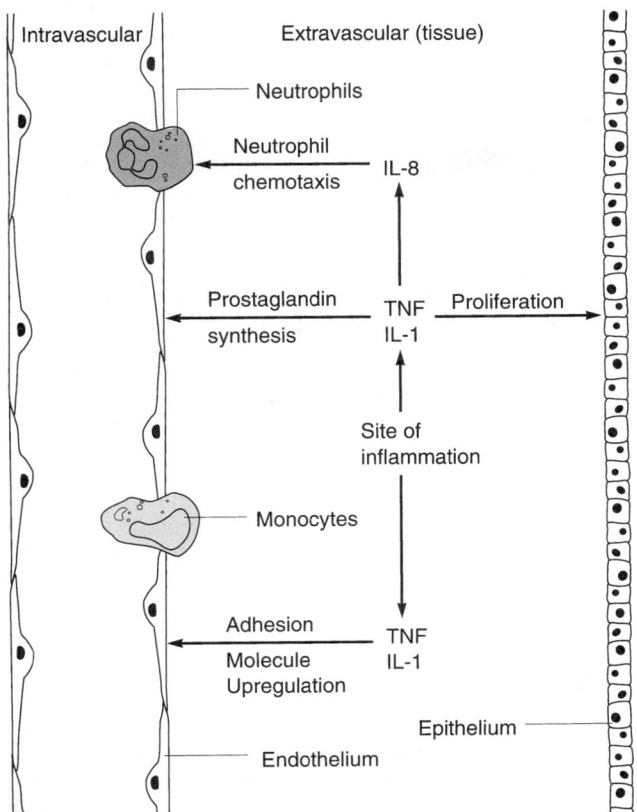

Intravascular	Extravascular (tissue)

Neutrophils

Neutrophil chemotaxis   IL-8

Prostaglandin synthesis   TNF IL-1   Proliferation

Site of inflammation

Monocytes

Adhesion Molecule Upregulation   TNF IL-1

Epithelium

Endothelium

Figure 5.13. Initial interaction between leukocytes and the endothelium. Tumor necrosis factor-α (TNF-α) and interleukin (IL)-1 are important early mediators in the initial interaction between the endothelium and leukocytes. The early adherence of leukocytes to the endothelium is an important first step in the recruitment of leukocytes into an area of injury or inflammation, and TNF-α and IL-1 are critical mediators in this process because they are capable of up-regulating endothelial and leukocyte adhesion molecules. TNF-α and IL-1 can also induce IL-8, a powerful neutrophil chemotactic agent.

flammatory network and also appear to promote the adherence of inflammatory cells to the endothelium, thus enhancing the trafficking of immunologically active cells into an area of injury or infection. The actual physical interaction between the endothelium and neutrophils is a critical event in initiating the inflammatory response and is responsible for localizing inflammatory cells into an

area of injury (Fig. 5.13). Adhesion molecules are grouped according to their protein structures, and three classes of molecules are important for leukocyte–endothelial interactions (Table 5.7): the immunoglobulin gene superfamily, the selectins, and the integrins (45). The major cytokine-induced adherence proteins that are expressed on the surface of endothelial cells include intercellular adhesion molecule-1 (ICAM-1), platelet–endothelial cell adhesion molecule (PECAM), vascular cell adhesion molecule (VCAM), all members of the immunoglobulin gene superfamily, E-selectin, and P-selectin (45). The major groups of cytokine-induced adherence proteins expressed on neutrophils include members of the integrin and selectin families (45). The most important integrins expressed on the neutrophil cell surface that mediate neutrophil–endothelial adherence are the β₂ integrins. These include CD11a/CD18, CD11b/CD18, and CD11c/CD18 (25). The L-selectins and the very late after activation (VLA) antigens are also important leukocyte adhesion molecules.

Tumor necrosis factor-α alters cell surface adhesion molecule expression on neutrophils and endothelial cells, stimulating endothelial cell–neutrophil adhesion and altering chemotaxis and procoagulant and antimicrobial neutrophil activity by up-regulating more distal inflammatory cytokines, particularly IL-8 and other chemokines. TNF-α activates neutrophils directly and indirectly through the release of more distal inflammatory cytokines. This induces the production and release of reactive oxygen metabolites and induces the production of additional cytokines (Fig. 5.10). Neutrophil recruitment and activation is a key process in the development of MOSF because the activated neutrophil appears to be one of the primary effector cells mediating the development of tissue injury in MOSF, regardless of the precipitating event (5). Activated neutrophils release a variety of inflammatory mediators, including proteolytic enzymes, arachidonic acid metabolites, reactive oxygen species, and cytokines, which can all directly affect the microvasculature, leading to increased microvascular permeability, hemorrhage, and accentuated leukocyte migration into the affected tissues (5).

Tissue injury results in a complex cascade of events that initiate the inflammatory response, progress to wound healing and tissue repair, and ultimately restore the host to its preinjury state. Inherent in these events is a unique and precise regulation of cytokine and growth factor release into the circulation, as well as into the wound environment. Cytokines are critical to the regulation of the immune response, cellular growth and differentiation, angiogenesis, and extracellular matrix production that occurs during injury, inflammation, and tissue repair. Lack of proper regulation of these complex events can lead to a

Table 5.7. MAJOR SUBFAMILIES OF ADHESION MOLECULES

Subfamily	Major glycoprotein	Primary distribution
IgG superfamily	Intercellular adhesion molecule-1	Endothelial cells, fibroblasts, epithelial cells, hematopoietic cells
	Vascular cell adhesion molecule-1	Endothelial cells
	Platelet–endothelial cell adhesion molecule-1	Intercellular junction of endothelial cells, platelets
Selectins	L-selectin	All leukocytes
	E-selectin	Activated endothelial cells
	P-selectin	Platelets, Weibel-Palade bodies of endothelial cells
Integrins	β₁: VLA antigens	T lymphocytes (types 1–6)
	β₂: CD₁₁ₐ, LFA-1	All leukocytes
	CD₁₁ᵦ, MAC-1	PMNs, monocytes
	CD₁₁ᵧ, gp150,95	PMNs, monocytes
	β₃, CD₁₁ᵦ, gp11b/111a	Platelets, endothelium

gp, glycoprotein; LFA-1, lymphocyte function-associate antigen-1; PMNs, polymorphonuclear leukocytes; VLA, very late after activation.

destabilization of hemodynamics, metabolism, and the overall process of inflammation, culminating in pathologic processes such as ARDS and MOSF.

Injury and Inflammation

Neutrophil recruitment to a site of inflammation is the hallmark of acute inflammation. This process depends on a complex series of events, which includes the following steps: endothelial cell activation, expression of endothelial cell-derived neutrophil adhesion molecules, neutrophil–endothelial cell adhesion, neutrophil activation and expression of neutrophil-derived adhesion molecules, neutrophil diapedesis, and neutrophil migration beyond the vascular barrier along chemotactic gradients. This initial phase is also characterized by the interaction of platelets, acute inflammatory cells, growth factors, and cytokines. The exposure of connective tissue during the process of wounding initiates the coagulation cascade and platelet degranulation with the release of growth factors. The factors then induce inflammatory cell chemotaxis into the wound site. Neutrophils are the first cells to populate the wound, peaking at 24 to 48 hours; although not essential to wound healing, they are critical in the host defense against infection. Macrophages appear within 48 to 96 hours, and are critical to the overall healing process. They promote the inflammatory process, débridement, and activation of mesenchymal cells to proliferate and produce extracellular matrix. Their influx into the wound and eventual role in the repair process depends largely on the generation of a diverse range of mononuclear phagocyte chemoattractants in the wound site. T lymphocytes appear 4 to 5 days after wounding and are also critical to tissue repair.

Leukocyte–Endothelial Cell Interactions: Role of Adhesion Molecules and Chemotactic Factors

Leukocyte extravasation is a crucial determinant of inflammatory and immunologic reactions. Endothelial cells and leukocytes interact closely in initiating the hemostatic, inflammatory, and immune responses to injury and infection. Although cytokines are an important mechanism of communication between leukocytes and endothelial cells, the expression of a receptor and counterreceptor on the surface of these cells also permits physical interaction and subsequent communication between them. The binding of inflammatory cells to the endothelium is a key proximal event in initiating the inflammatory response that precedes chemotaxis. This event localizes inflammatory cells to an area of inflammation, infection, or injury. The endothelium is another important source of cytokines, which are then responsible for continuing to propagate the inflammatory response. Although this recruitment process is not unique to any particular organ, certain tissues, such as the lung, appear to be particularly susceptible to leukocyte recruitment and subsequent inflammatory injury. Leukocyte–endothelium adherence is unique in that it must both be strong enough to allow significant attachment of the leukocyte to the endothelium and be controlled by one or more mechanisms that allow the adherence process to be transient and reversible. Once the adherence process occurs, a chemotactic signal triggers the inflammatory cells to transmigrate across the basement membrane into the interstitium.

Leukocyte and Endothelial Cell Adhesion Molecules

Although many of the specific mechanisms that recruit neutrophils into tissues during acute inflammation are not fully known, the temporal events that initiate and propagate neutrophil recruitment likely include endothelial cell activation and expression of endothelial-derived neutrophil adhesion molecules, neutrophil activation and expression of neutrophil-derived adhesion molecules, neutrophil–endothelial cell adherence, and neutrophil transendothelial migration by established neutrophil chemotactic gradients. The initial neutrophil–endothelial cell adhesion is a requisite event for successful neutrophil extravasation at sites of inflammation (Table 5.7).

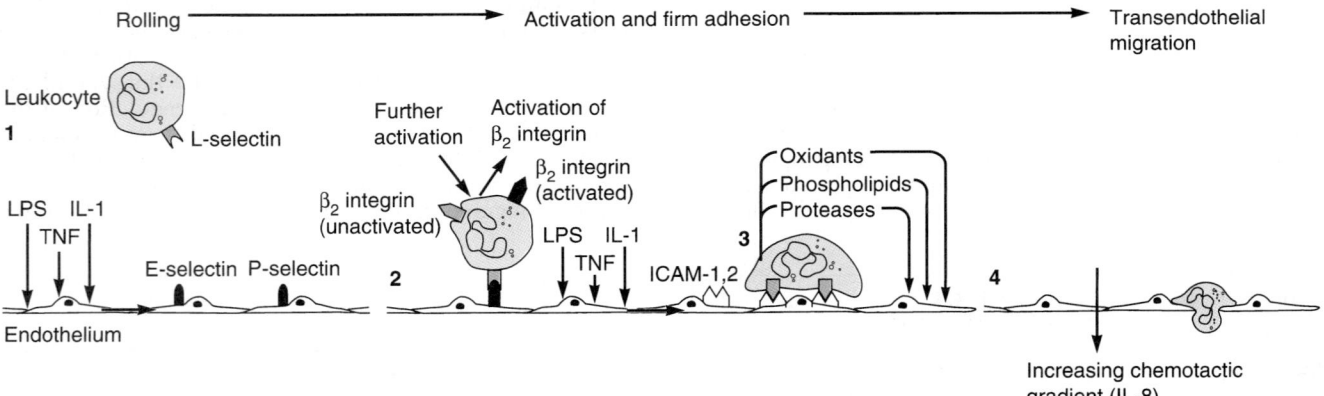

Figure 5.14. Neutrophil recruitment and activation into areas of inflammation. (1) Selectins mediate early loose adhesion or "rolling." This is a low-affinity adherence between constitutively expressed L-selectin on the neutrophil and E-selectin or P-selectin on the activated vascular endothelium. (2) This rolling slows the neutrophil enough to allow it to be activated, with expression and activation of β_2-integrins on the cell surface. Further activation of the endothelium by tumor necrosis factor-α (TNF-α), interleukin-1 (IL-1), or lipopolysaccharide (LPS) leads to increased expression of intercellular adhesion molecule (ICAM)-1 and ICAM-2, with subsequent firm adherence of the neutrophil to the endothelium. This is mediated through ICAM–β_2-integrin interactions. (3) The activated adherent neutrophil can then release proteases, oxidants, and phospholipids, resulting in endothelial cell injury and increased microvascular permeability. (4) Neutrophils then diapedese into the extravascular space along established chemotactic gradients. Platelet–endothelial cell adhesion molecule-1 (PECAM-1) may be important in transendothelial migration.

Three major families of adhesion molecules are expressed on the surface of leukocytes and endothelial cells, and they are important for leukocyte–endothelial cell interactions (45). These include the immunoglobulin supergene family, the selectins, and the integrins. The immunoglobulin supergene family includes ICAM-1, VCAM-1, and PECAM-1, which all can be expressed on endothelial cells and are important for leukocyte adherence (45). E-selectin and P-selectin are members of the selectin family that are expressed on the surface of endothelial cells and are also important for leukocyte adherence (45). L-selectin is also a member of the selectin family, and this molecule is expressed on the cell surface of all leukocytes (45). It is particularly important for the early adherence of neutrophils to the activated endothelium.

The family of integrins is further divided into three subfamilies: β_1, β_2, and β_3 (45). The β_1 subfamily includes the VLA antigens 1 through 6 (45). These molecules are primarily distributed on T lymphocytes. However, the interaction of monocyte-derived VLA-4 with VCAM-1 may be an important mechanism for monocyte adherence to the activated endothelium (45). The β_2 subfamily includes CD11a, CD11b, CD11c, which represent lymphocyte function-associated antigen-1, MAC-1, and glycoprotein (Gp) 150,95 (Fig. 5.14). CD11a, CD11b, and CD11c exist in a heterodimeric form, complexed to CD18. All of these molecules are expressed on the cell surface of a variety of leukocytes and are probably the most important subgroup of this family with respect to leukocyte–endothelium interactions (45). Included in the β_3 subfamily are GpIIb and GpIIb/IIIa, which are expressed on platelets as well as the endothelium (45).

The leukocyte β_2-integrin adhesion molecule family consists of a complex group of heterodimeric glycoproteins that are expressed only on the surface of leukocytes. The three members of the β_2-integrin family display a variable α and a constant β chain with the cluster designations CD11a/CD18, CD11b/CD18, CD11c/CD18.46 The CD11a/CD18 complex is expressed on all leukocytes; CD11b/CD18 is predominantly expressed on neutrophils and monocytes (46). Neutrophils have a substantial pool of CD11b/CD18 in their secondary and tertiary granules, and when the neutrophil is activated, CD11b/CD18 rapidly translocates to the cell surface (46). The ligand/receptor for neutrophil-derived CD11b/CD18 complex is the split product of complement (iC3b) and ICAM-1.

Intercellular adhesion molecule-1 is a member of the immunoglobulin supergene family and is found on the surface of both immune and nonimmune cells (46). Although originally described as the counterreceptor for CD11a/CD18 complex, ICAM-1 is also an important ligand/receptor for CD11b/CD18 complex expressed on neutrophils. ICAM-1 is constitutively expressed on endothelial cells and is up-regulated in response to endotoxin, TNF-α, or IL-1 (46). Neutralizing monoclonal antibodies to either CD11b, CD18, or ICAM-1 in models of acute lung injury have been shown to attenuate neutrophil-dependent lung injury. These findings suggest that neutrophil-derived β_2-integrins and endothelial cell-derived ICAM-1 play a pivotal role in the pathogenesis of acute inflammation and lung injury.

Another group of molecules involved in neutrophil–endothelium adhesion are selectins. These include L-selectin, which is constitutively expressed on leukocyte cell surfaces, E-selectin, which is induced on activated

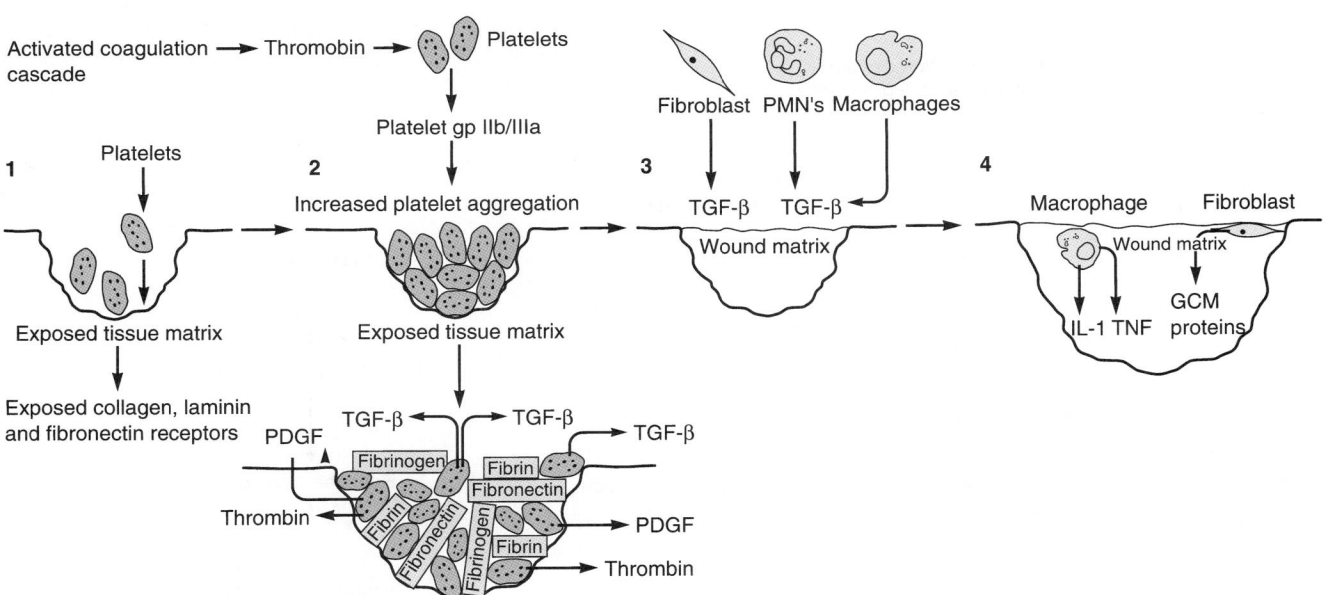

Figure 5.15. Establishment of a provisional wound matrix. (1) Platelets bind to exposed wound matrix through interaction of β_1- and β_3-integrins and collagen, laminin, and fibronectin receptors. (2) After wounding, the coagulation cascade is activated, generating thrombin, which activates platelet glycoprotein (Gp) IIb/IIIa and increases platelet aggregation. A provisional wound matrix is formed and is made up of platelets, fibrin, fibrinogen, and fibronectin. The activated platelets in the wound generate transforming growth factor-β (TGF-β), platelet-derived growth factor (PDGF), and thrombin. (3) TGF-β is strongly chemotactic for neutrophils, macrophages, and fibroblasts, recruiting these cells into the provisional wound matrix, where they are also subsequently activated by TGF-β. (4) Increasing concentrations of TGF-β result in macrophage activation, producing increased amounts of tumor necrosis factor-α (TNF-α) and interleukin-1 (IL-1). TGF-β also stimulates fibroblast production of extracellular matrix proteins. These reactions further enhance migration of macrophages and fibroblasts into the wound, facilitating tissue repair.

endothelial cells by endotoxin, TNF-α, or IL-1, and P-selectin (47) (Fig. 5.14). Both E-selectin and P-selectin facilitate neutrophil–endothelial cell adherence through neutrophil-derived L-selectin (47). Data indicate the importance of the combination of selectins, β₂-integrins, ICAM-1, and chemotaxins for the full development of neutrophil–endothelial cell adhesion and subsequent transendothelial migration.

Adhesion Molecules and Wound Repair

The β₂-integrins are key components for initiating neutrophil–endothelial cell adherence and perpetuating the inflammatory cascade. The β₁- and β₃-integrins are key molecules in generating a wound matrix after tissue injury (45). After tissue damage, platelets bind to the exposed matrix. This requires the interactions of the β₁- and β₃-integrins and the collagen, laminin, and fibronectin receptors (45) (Fig. 5.15). Activation of the coagulation cascade generates thrombin. This activates platelet GpIIb/IIIa, promoting further platelet aggregation (45). A wound matrix is subsequently formed, containing platelets, fibrinogen, fibrin, and fibronectin. The activated platelets in the wound matrix elaborate TGF-β, PDGF, and thrombin (45). TGF-β is strongly chemotactic for neutrophils, macrophages, and fibroblasts. In addition, as these inflammatory cells migrate into the wound, they encounter increasing concentrations of TGF-β, which subsequently activates these inflammatory cells. Macrophages increase their synthesis of TNF-α and IL-1, and fibroblasts increase their synthesis of extracellular matrix proteins. These reactions stimulate the up-regulation of macrophage and fibroblast integrins, which promote further migration of these inflammatory cells into the wound site and increase deposition of provisional matrix. This sets the stage for the tissue repair process.

Other Factors in Neutrophil Recruitment

Although chemotactic signals and adhesion molecules are considered to be the major determinants of leukocyte recruitment, changes in the rheologic properties of blood can also play a role in extravasating leukocytes. In addition, prostaglandins greatly amplify the activity of locally injected chemoattractants, such as IL-8. Cytokine-induced prostaglandin production acts in concert with the expression of adhesion molecules and the production of chemotactic cytokines.

WOUND HEALING

Normal wound repair rapidly restores tissue integrity and function after various insults, such as trauma, burns, and infection. Healing involves a complex interplay between humoral, cellular, and extracellular matrix networks. Nevertheless, it occurs in a controlled, sequential manner that depends on the cells communicating with one another (Fig. 5.16). Although this communication often occurs by direct cell-to-cell contact through specific cellular adhesion molecules, cells can also signal one another through soluble mediators, such as cytokines. The CXC chemokines have been previously discussed as

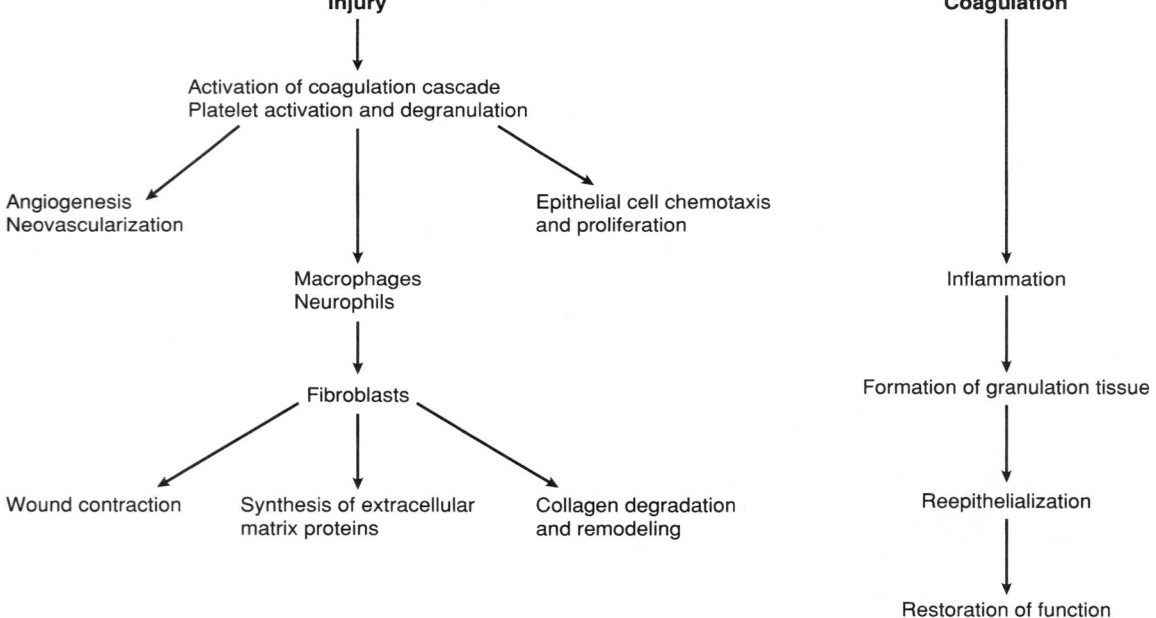

Figure 5.16. Wound healing and tissue repair. Injury initially results in platelet activation and degranulation, as well as activation of the coagulation cascade. The release of a variety of factors, both from the activated platelets and through the coagulation cascade, initiates the process of angiogenesis and neovascularization, activates neutrophils, monocytes, and macrophages, and recruits these cells into the area of injury. In addition, the process of epithelial cell chemotaxis and proliferation begins. These processes represent acute inflammation. Macrophages and neutrophils and the cytokines and mediators they elaborate are then important in the progression from acute inflammation to active tissue repair with the formation of granulation tissue. Recruitment and activation of fibroblasts in the provisional wound matrix is the next key step in tissue repair. Fibroblasts increase their synthesis of extracellular matrix proteins, as well as elaborating proteases and collagenases that are important for tissue remodeling. This progresses to wound contraction, reepithelialization, and restoration of function.

chemotactic factors, but they also appear to have reparative activities. Experimental findings support the importance of these molecules in angiogenesis and mitogenesis,
which are important processes in tissue repair and wound
healing.

After injury, the reparative process immediately begins
with hemorrhage and extravasation of plasma into the
wound (Fig. 5.17). This activates the intrinsic and extrinsic coagulation pathways, leading to fibrin deposition and
establishment of a provisional matrix (48). Platelet activation and degranulation also occur during coagulation,
leading to the deposition of cytokines into the provisional
matrix. These cytokines include TGF-α, TGF-β, PDGF, and
NAP-2, which is a proteolytic cleavage product of platelet

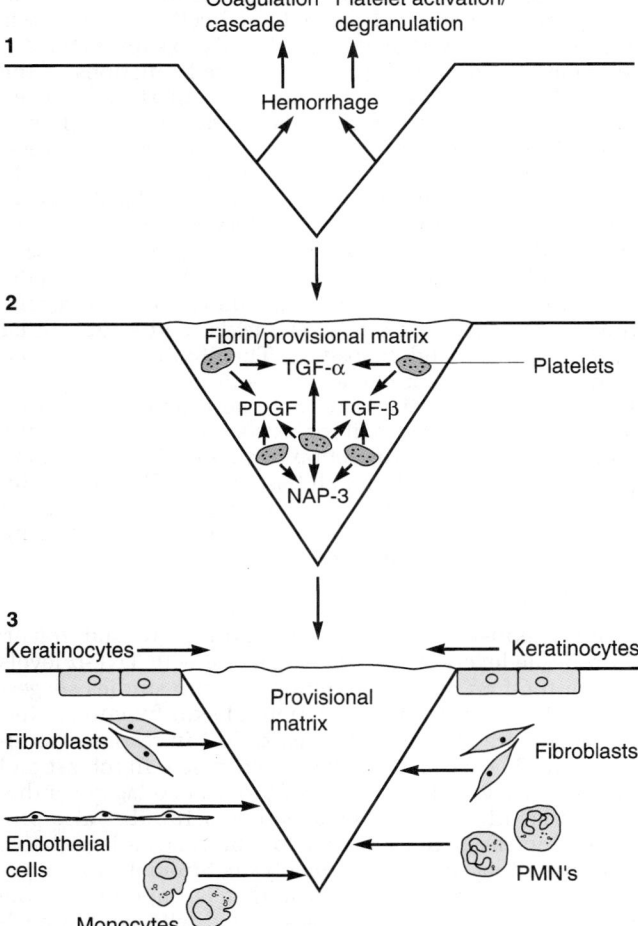

Figure 5.17. The wound matrix. (1) After injury, hemorrhage occurs, with activation of coagulation and deposition of fibrin in the
wound. (2) Concurrently, platelets are activated, resulting in degranulation, with the deposition of transforming growth factor
(TGF)-α, TGF-β, platelet-derived growth factor (PDGF), and neutrophil-activating peptide-2 (NAP-2) in the provisional wound
matrix. (3) TGF-α, TGF-β, PDGF, and NAP-2 are important growth
factors and chemotaxins for recruiting or activating fibroblasts,
endothelial cells, monocytes, and neutrophils into the wound.
Neutrophils are typically the first cells recruited into a site of injury, and produce a number of cytokines that are important for
initiating wound repair. Although neutrophils are important in
initial host defense, the monocyte–macrophage is recruited into
the wound after inflammation is established and is important in
converting the provisional wound matrix into mature granulation
tissue. Thus, coagulation and platelet degranulation are key
processes for the subsequent cellular recruitment and activation
necessary for wound healing.

basic protein (48). These cytokines are either important
growth factors or chemotaxins that elicit leukocytes, endothelial cells, fibroblasts, and keratinocytes, which are
important in tissue repair (48). Thus, coagulation and
platelet activation provide the initial foundation for subsequent cellular recruitment.

Neutrophils are typically the first leukocytes to arrive at
the wound, with their primary function to phagocytize debris. These cells can also produce cytokines that help to
orchestrate the progression of wound repair. Although
neutrophils are important for initial host defense, the second wave of leukocytes consists of mononuclear cells,
with the mononuclear phagocyte representing a pivotal
leukocyte in the progression of wound repair. The mononuclear phagocyte can generate inflammatory mediators
that are important in transforming the provisional matrix
to more mature granulation tissue (3).

Proliferative Phase of Wound Healing

The transition of wound repair from acute inflammation
to granulation tissue is essential because granulation tissue consists of appropriate extracellular matrix constituents, fibroblasts, endothelial cells, leukocytes, and
mediators that form either the connective tissue foundation or stimulus for neovascularization (3,48). This occurs
approximately 3 days after wounding, and continues for at
least 3 weeks. Fibroblasts achieve peak numbers on day 7
after wounding. They are synthetic cells and produce most
of the structural proteins used during tissue reconstruction. The accelerated production of collagen with subsequent cross-linking provides the scaffold on which wound
strength depends. The process of angiogenesis is important because it sustains a continual supply of oxygen and
nutrients to the cellular constituents of the wound and
provides a substructure for the eventual reepithelialization of the wound surface (Table 5.8). It proceeds in parallel with fibroplasia. It is regulated by cytokines released
from activated inflammatory cells and local conditions,
such as hypoxia and lactic acid accumulation. Data suggest that the cytokines of the CXC chemokine family play
an important role in the angiogenic process that occurs
during wound healing (36,37). During the early phases of
granulation tissue formation, the immature connective tissue resembles undifferentiated mesenchyme with persistent fibrin, an embryonic form of fibronectin, a predominance of collagen type I, fibronectin, and
protease-dependent remodeling of the extracellular matrix
(Fig. 5.16). The granulation tissue provides the foundation
for reepithelialization of the wound surface. As basal keratinocytes migrate from the wound edge over the surface
of the mature granulation tissue, keratinocytes at the
wound margin begin to proliferate. This response is
followed by epidermal regeneration and production of

**Table 5.8. KERATINOCYTE-DERIVED CYTOKINES
WITH ACTIVITY IN WOUND HEALING**

Cytokine	Major effect
Tumor necrosis factor	Tissue remodeling
IL-1	Matrix deposition
	Tissue remodeling
IL-6	Inflammation
IL-8	Inflammation
TGF-β	Matrix deposition
TGF-α	Epithelialization
Platelet-derived growth factor	Granulation tissue formation

IL, interleukin; TGF, transforming growth factor.

basement membrane extracellular constituents (i.e., fibronectin, type IV and VII collagen, heparin sulfate proteoglycans, and laminin) that provide the integrity between epidermal and dermal structures (49). The sequential yet overlapping interplay of coagulation, inflammation, and formation of granulation tissue provides the foundation for the subsequent reepithelialization that is necessary to restore tissue function under normal conditions of wound repair. The stimulus for reepithelialization is mediated by a combination of cytokines, loss of contact inhibition, and exposure of constituents of the extracellular matrix, particularly fibronectin.

Cytokines and Angiogenesis in the Healing Wound

Angiogenesis is an important component of tissue repair and wound healing. The ingrowth of new blood vessels is critical for a continued supply of oxygen and nutrients to the regenerating tissues. One of the key features of the normal, physiologic process of angiogenesis is that it is a local, transient event under strict control. Strong evidence suggests that a biologic imbalance in the production of angiogenic and angiostatic factors contributes to the pathogenesis of several angiogenesis-dependent disorders. These disease states are typically associated with an overexpression of angiogenic activity, which may be associated with the maintenance and progression of a chronic disease state. Disorders associated with chronic inflammation, such as rheumatoid arthritis, scleroderma, psoriasis, atherosclerosis, and idiopathic pulmonary fibrosis are examples of nonmalignant diseases with chronic angiogenic activity (50).

Persistent neovascularization in these disorders is a prerequisite for perpetuating fibroproliferation (2,50). For example, in rheumatoid arthritis, the unrestrained proliferation of fibroblasts and neovascularization leads to the formation of persistent granulation tissue, whose degradative enzymes contribute to the profound destruction of joint spaces (51). A subpopulation of macrophages isolated from rheumatoid synovium produce factors that are potentially angiogenic in vivo and chemotactic for capillary endothelial cells in vitro (31,32,52). The inability of macrophages to express appropriate angiogenic activity may also contribute to the pathogenesis of diseases that are associated with defective angiogenesis. Blood monocyte-derived macrophages from patients with scleroderma fail to generate the expected angiogenic activity when exposed to the agonist LPS (53), suggesting that a defect in macrophage responsiveness to activating signals contributes to the attenuated neovascularization encountered in scleroderma. Psoriasis is a well known angiogenesis-

dependent disorder, characterized by marked dermal neovascularization. Keratinocytes derived from psoriatic plaques are angiogenic compared with keratinocytes obtained from normal people. This appears to be at least partly due to an overproduction of the angiogenic cytokine, IL-8, and a deficiency in the production of the angiogenesis inhibitor, thrombospondin-1, with the net result being a proangiogenic environment (54,55). It is well established that angiogenesis is a tightly regulated process that is under complex positive and negative controls. It is also apparent that overexuberant angiogenesis is common with most chronic inflammatory disorders (Table 5.9).

Cytokine–Fibroblast Interactions

The replacement of normal functional organs by nonfunctional scars has long been associated with the exchange of differentiated parenchymal cells for fibroblasts and collagen. By virtue of their inability to express the differentiated and often highly specialized functions of the original parenchymal cells, these fibroblasts have been viewed as passive structural cells and devoid of vital functions. Their unchecked proliferation inhibits the successful repair and regeneration of normal functional tissues. In the past, little attention was paid to the fibroblast's potentially active role in the inflammatory response. Because these cells are the primary source of the connective tissue found in fibrotic lesions, an increasing effort has been devoted to studying the mechanisms underlying the regulation of fibroblast growth, chemotaxis, and extracellular matrix synthesis and deposition. The fibroblast is appreciated as an important element in both normal and pathologic processes, particularly those surrounding tissue injury and repair. Because fibroblasts are present in virtually all tissues, cytokine production by these cells plays an important role in most, if not all tissues. The fibroblast is involved in many functions, including regulation of tissue repair and fibrosis, hematopoiesis, bone metabolism, inflammation, and immune response.

Interleukin-1

Interleukin-1 is important for normal wound repair, with tissue levels of IL-1 peaking along with TNF-α levels within the first day of wounding. In vitro studies suggest that IL-1 is important for a variety of skin functions. Keratinocytes are known to synthesize IL-1 in response to injury, and IL-1 has been shown to stimulate fibroblast and keratinocyte growth as well as fibroblast collagen synthesis and keratinocyte chemotaxis (Fig. 5.18). IL-1 also promotes increased transcription of the matrix-degradative enzymes collagenase and stromelysin. Stromelysin is a potent tissue-degrading proteinase that is important in the tissue remodeling processes associated with wound healing. The up-regulation of stromelysin may also be an important component of many pathologic processes, such as those involved in joint destruction in arthritis and tumor invasion. In addition, IL-1 induces macrophages to produce plasminogen activator inhibitor, which is important for tissue remodeling and repair as well as for fibroblast proliferation. In contrast, other studies have demonstrated that IL-1 inhibits fibroblast growth and matrix synthesis and stimulates collagenase production (Table 5.10). These actions are at least partly due to the ability of IL-1 to up-regulate PGE$_2$ production, which, in an autocrine fashion, results in down-regulation of matrix synthesis and cellular proliferation. The stimulation of prostaglandin production by IL-1 appears to be mediated through the up-regulation of phospholipase A$_2$ and cyclooxygenase activities due at least in part to the increased synthesis of these enzymes. As would be expected, IL-1-induced inhibition of

---

Table 5.9. DISEASE PROCESSES ASSOCIATED WITH ABNORMALITIES IN NEOVASCULARIZATION

DISEASES ASSOCIATED WITH EXCESSIVE NEOVASCULARIZATION
  Rheumatoid arthritis
  Psoriasis

DISEASES ASSOCIATED WITH INSUFFICIENT NEOVASCULARIZATION
  Scleroderma

DISEASES ASSOCIATED WITH CHRONIC INFLAMMATION
  Idiopathic pulmonary fibrosis
  Atherosclerosis

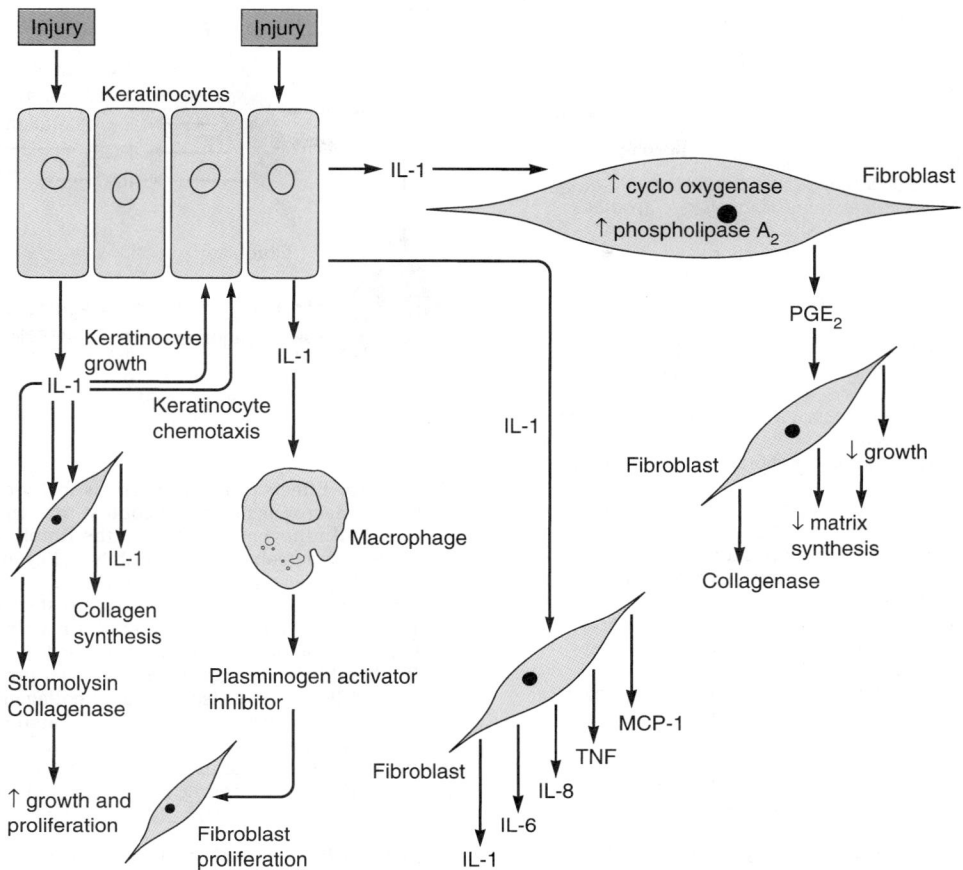

Figure 5.18. Actions of interleukin (IL)-1 on keratinocytes, macrophages, and fibroblasts in the context of wound healing. Keratinocytes produce IL-1 in response to injury. IL-1 then stimulates keratinocyte growth and chemotaxis. In addition, this keratinocyte-derived IL-1 has multiple effects on other cells, particularly fibroblasts and macrophages. IL-1 induces fibroblasts to produce many cytokines that are important for wound healing, including IL-1, IL-6, IL-8, tumor necrosis factor-α (TNF-α), and monocyte chemoattractant protein-1 (MCP-1). IL-1 also induces fibroblast growth and proliferation, collagen synthesis, and the synthesis of collagenase and stromelysin. Collagenase and stromelysin are important in the process of tissue remodeling, which is a vital component of wound healing. In the macrophage, IL-1 induces the synthesis of plasminogen activator inhibitor, which is important for tissue remodeling and also increases fibroblast proliferation. IL-1 also has some inhibitory actions on the fibroblast, which are mediated through the up-regulation of prostaglandin E_2 (PGE$_2$). IL-1 increases cyclooxygenase and phospholipase A_2, increasing the synthesis of PGE$_2$. PGE$_2$ then functions in an autocrine fashion to decrease fibroblast growth and matrix synthesis and further increases collagenase production.

fibroblast proliferation and matrix synthesis is blunted by treatment with cyclooxygenase inhibitors. The effects of IL-1 on fibroblast collagen gene expression are complicated by the inhibitory effects of PGE$_2$ on collagen synthesis, as well as the IL-1-induced up-regulation of the matrix-degradative proteins, particularly stromelysin and collagenase. PGE$_2$ is known to stimulate collagenase secretion and to elevate intracellular cyclic adenosine monophosphate, which inhibits net collagen production. Despite what appears to be multiple IL-1-induced inhibitory effects on net collagen synthesis, there is evidence that IL-1 induces an increase in steady-state levels of procollagen mRNA. The collagen synthesis-promoting properties of IL-1 can be unmasked when the inhibitory effect of PGE$_2$ is blocked with cyclooxygenase inhibitors. Because of both its promoting and inhibiting effects on fibroblast collagen synthesis, the overall activity of IL-1 in this area is somewhat unclear compared with other well-defined fibroblast growth-promoting cytokines.

Although IL-1 appears to have multiple effects on soft-tissue wound healing, it also has important modulating effects on bone and cartilage. IL-1 stimulates bone resorption and the synthesis of PGE$_2$. IL-1 also has degradative effects on cartilage proteoglycans and may be involved in the destructive joint inflammation that occurs in rheumatoid arthritis. In fact, the effects of IL-1 on fibroblasts were initially studied in arthritic joints. Many of the effects of IL-1 on the fibroblast are similar to those induced by TNF-α, and synergistic effects are seen when the two agents are used together.

Tumor Necrosis Factor-α and Interleukin-6

As with other cytokines, the effects of TNF-α on the fibroblast are varied and difficult to separate in vivo from the influence of other cytokines, particularly IL-1. TNF-α appears to be important in the early inflammatory response to wounding and in orchestrating tissue repair. Studies suggest that TNF-α is important for normal wound

Table 5.10. **ACTIONS OF CYTOKINES ON FIBROBLASTS**

Cytokine	Effect
TNF	Stimulates proliferation Stimulates PGE$_2$ production Stimulates collagenase production May stimulate or inhibit collagen synthesis Induces IL-1, IL-6, IL-8, and MCP-1
IL-1	Stimulates PGE$_2$ production Stimulates growth and proliferation Stimulates collagen synthesis Induces IL-1, IL-6, IL-8, TNF, and MCP-1 Induces stromolysin and collagenase May stimulate or inhibit extracellular matrix production

IL-6	Upregulates tissue inhibitor of metalloproteinase
	   production
	Inhibits the proliferation-inducing properties of
	   TNF

PDGF	Potent chemotactic agent for fibroblasts

TGF-β	Induces TGF-β and PDGF
	Stimulates PGE$_2$ production
	Enhances collagen synthesis, deposition, and
	   maturation
	Stimulates extracellular matrix production
	Inhibits matrix degradation by increasing
	   synthesis of protease inhibitors
	May inhibit or promote cellular proliferation

Epidermal
  growth factor
	Stimulates cellular proliferation and
	   collagen synthesis
	Induces PDGF
	Potent chemotactic agent for fibroblasts

IL, interleukin; MCP-1, monocyte chemoattractant protein-1; PGE$_2$, prostaglandin E$_2$; PDGF, platelet-derived growth factor; TGF-β, transforming growth factor-β; TNF, tumor necrosis factor.

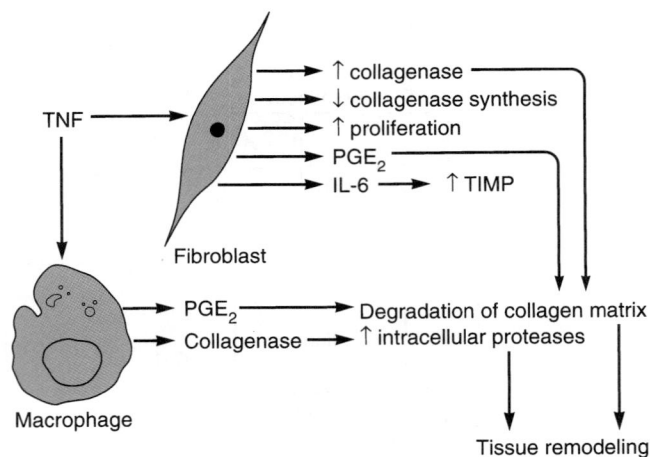

Figure 5.19. Effects of tumor necrosis factor-α (TNF-α) on fibroblasts and macrophages in the context of wound healing. TNF-α has powerful mitogenic actions on the fibroblast, increasing proliferation. Conversely, it also inhibits collagen synthesis and increases collagenase production. TNF-α also increases fibroblast production of interleukin-6 (IL-6) and prostaglandin E$_2$ (PGE$_2$). IL-6 appears to play a role in extracellular matrix metabolism by increasing production of tissue inhibitor of metalloproteinase (TIMP). In addition to increasing fibroblast production of collagenase and PGE$_2$, TNF-α also increases collagenase and PGE$_2$ production by the macrophage. Increased amounts of collagenase and PGE$_2$ facilitate collagen matrix degradation, as well as increase the production of intracellular proteases, which are all important in tissue remodeling, a key aspect of wound healing.

repair, with tissue levels of TNF-α peaking within the first day of wounding (56). Furthermore, TNF-α has potent angiogenic activity in wounds, as demonstrated in an in vivo subcutaneous sponge implant model (57). Other studies suggest that abnormal levels of TNF-α or the continued presence of TNF-α in the wound inhibit healing, demonstrating that TNF-α inhibits the ingrowth of granulation tissue, retards the accumulation of collagen hydroxyproline, and down-regulates collagen synthesis. Although TNF-α inhibits fibroblast collagen synthesis (58), it also has potent mitogenic effects. The mitogenic response correlates well with an increased stimulation of tyrosine phosphorylation and is down-regulated by IFN-γ (58). TNF-α has no chemotactic effect on fibroblasts and does not alter the fibroblast response to other chemoattractants. TNF-α does, however, stimulate the production of fibroblast PGE$_2$ and enhances transcription and translation of IL-6. IL-6 may play a role in fibroblast extracellular matrix metabolism through its ability to enhance the production of tissue inhibitor of metalloproteinase. More recent studies suggest that TNF-α acting locally may block wound healing by inhibiting the expression of the gene for type I collagen. TNF-α also stimulates cartilage resorption and the release of proteoglycans from cartilage by a limited proteolytic degradation, and it inhibits proteoglycan synthesis (Fig. 5.19). These particular phenomena may be mediated and promoted by collagenase and PGE$_2$, because both are up-regulated in fibroblasts and macrophages by TNF-α and are involved in the degradation of collagen matrix and stimulation of the intracellular proteases responsible for tissue remodeling (58). TNF-α may also inhibit fracture healing in experimental animals. The decline in the rate of fracture repair appears to be related to TNF-α-

induced inhibition of cartilage formation early in new bone synthesis. This is due to its inhibition of mesenchymal cell differentiation into chondroblasts. All of these functions may be important in the normal process of wound healing and remodeling, as well as in the pathologic settings of degenerative joint diseases and altered wound healing.

Epidermal Growth Factor

The family of epidermal growth factor (EGF)-like molecules is characterized by high-affinity binding to the EGF receptor, thus inducing mitogenesis in EGF-sensitive cells. EGF stimulation is associated with the activation of a phospholipase C, which is specific for phosphatidylcholine, reflecting cytokine-sensitive phosphatidylcholine pools or selective diacylglycerol metabolism. The extracellular matrix influences fibroblast responses to cytokines. EGF, applied topically in microgram quantities, can enhance soft-tissue wound healing by increasing soft-tissue neovascularization (59). In human clinical trials, EGF has also been shown to accelerate epidermal regeneration in cutaneous wounds (59). Similarly, in vitro studies have shown that recombinant EGF enhances keratinocyte migration when the cells are grown on connective tissue matrices of collagen or fibronectin. The mechanism of this enhanced migration may be related to increased expression of the α$_2$β$_1$-integrin, which is responsible for keratinocyte migration on collagen type I and IV. EGF is also a potent chemoattractant for granulation tissue fibroblasts, and cells at all stages of wound repair are responsive to this factor (60). These chemotactic properties of EGF for fibroblasts and keratinocytes may at least partially explain the ability of EGF to accelerate wound healing in vivo.

Transforming Growth Factor-β

Transforming growth factor-β appears to be one of the key cytokines in controlling tissue repair (Fig. 5.20). Fur-

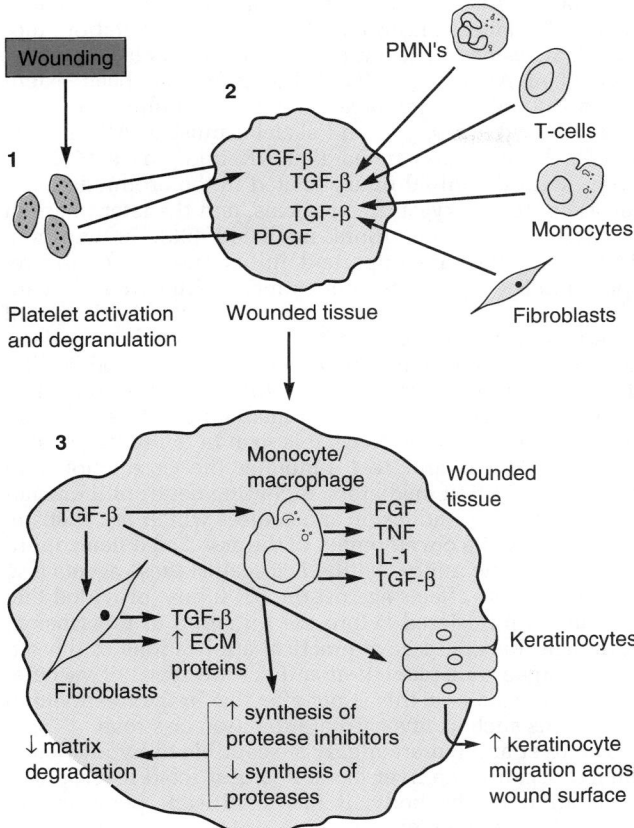

Figure 5.20. Transforming growth factor-β (TGF-β) in wound healing. TGF-β is one of the key cytokines in the orchestration of tissue repair. Immediately after wounding, platelets are activated and degranulated, releasing large amounts of TGF-β and platelet-derived growth factor (PDGF) into the wounded tissue. TGF-β is a powerful chemotactic agent for neutrophils, T lymphocytes, monocytes, and macrophages, which are all recruited into the wound. As these cells encounter increasing concentrations of TGF-β, they become activated and release a variety of other factors that are important for perpetuating wound healing. Monocytes and macrophages release fibroblast growth factor (FGF), tumor necrosis factor-α (TNF-α), interleukin-1 (IL-1), and additional TGF-β. Fibroblasts also generate more TGF-β and increase their synthesis of extracellular matrix proteins. TGF-β inhibits matrix degradation by increasing the synthesis of extracellular matrix proteins, as well as increasing synthesis of protease inhibitors and decreasing protease synthesis. TGF-β also increases keratinocyte migration across the wound surface, facilitating reepithelialization.

thermore, the sustained production of this cytokine has been implicated in the development of tissue fibrosis in various chronic disease states. Wound healing is a complex series of coordinated events. It begins with platelet-induced hemostasis, followed by an influx of inflammatory cells and fibroblasts, the deposition of extracellular matrix and neovascularization, and the proliferation of cells that reconstitute the injured tissue (40). TGF-β plays a role in each of these events (49). Platelets contain high concentrations of TGF-β and PDGF, which are released into the tissue at the site of injury (2). TGF-β is strongly chemotactic for neutrophils, T cells, monocytes, and fibroblasts (2). As these inflammatory cells move into the site of injury, they are activated as they encounter increasing concentrations of TGF-β. Monocytes begin to elaborate FGF, TNF-α, and IL-1, and fibroblasts increase their synthesis of extracellular matrix proteins (49). TGF-β also in-

duces both the infiltrating cells and resident cells to produce more TGF-β. This autoinduction amplifies its biologic effects at the site of injury and may contribute to the development of chronic fibrosis in various pathologic states (61). At physiologic concentrations, TGF-β regulates PDGF production in smooth muscle cells and fibroblasts, FGF production in endothelial cells, and TNF-α and IL-1 production in monocytes (61). TGF-β also modulates macrophage cytotoxicity by suppressing the production of superoxide and nitric oxide (61).

The extracellular matrix is a dynamic superstructure of self-aggregating macromolecules, including fibronectin, collagens, and proteoglycans, to which cells attach by means of surface receptors called integrins (49). TGF-β is a potent inducer of extracellular matrix production, stimulating the synthesis of collagen types I, II, and V, fibronectin, and glycosaminoglycans (61). The matrix surrounding the cells in a wound is continually degraded by proteases. TGF-β inhibits matrix degradation by increasing the synthesis of protease inhibitors, such as metalloproteinase inhibitor and plasminogen activator inhibitor, and by inhibiting gene expression and synthesis of protease, stromelysin, and collagenase. TGF-β simultaneously stimulates cells to increase the synthesis of matrix proteins, decrease the synthesis of matrix-degrading proteases, increase the production of protease inhibitors, and modulate the expression of integrins to increase cellular adhesion to the matrix. TGF-β binds to the proteoglycans in the matrix near the cell surface, and such binding can act as a signal to terminate the production of TGF-β after tissue repair is complete.

Fibrosis represents a pathologic excess of the normal process of tissue repair. The excessive or sustained production of TGF-β is a key molecular event in inducing tissue fibrosis, and this molecule may be an important mediator in a variety of disease states, including pulmonary fibrosis, liver cirrhosis, scleroderma, keloid formation, and rheumatoid arthritis. The topical application of TGF-β accelerates wound healing. In rats, topical or limited intravenous administration of TGF-β normalizes wound healing that is impaired by age or glucocorticoids (62). In contrast, repeated injections of high-dose TGF-β induces serious systemic effects, including marked fibrosis of the kidneys and liver (63). Recombinant TGF-β has been shown to accelerate soft-tissue wound healing in both normal and diabetic animals (64). Normal healing was accelerated by 30% in wounds treated with recombinant TGF-β (64). Further in vivo studies demonstrated that this cytokine enhances collagen synthesis, deposition, and maturation (64). TGF-β also appears to enhance keratinocyte migration across a wound surface by increasing the expression of keratinocyte cell surface integrins that facilitate the migratory component of reepithelialization. Thus, the overall in vivo effects of TGF-β clearly favor its role as an important promoter of tissue repair, wound healing, and reepithelialization. These actions are clearly relevant for many potential clinical applications, including surgical wound healing in debilitated patients or those undergoing chemotherapy, treatment of diabetic, decubitus, and varicose ulcerations, and burns.

Platelet-derived Growth Factor

A heterodimeric protein composed of α and β chains, PDGF is one of the most important mediators of the tissue repair process. This molecule was originally described as the most potent mitogen for cells of mesenchymal origin. In addition, the homodimers of both the α and β chains are also potent growth factors, encoded by separate genes that are independently regulated and expressed. PDGF is synthesized by megakaryocytes, fibroblasts, endothelial cells, macrophages, and smooth muscle cells. It is a potent mitogen for fibroblasts, smooth muscle cells, and endothelial cells. This molecule is also a chemotactic and activating factor for neutrophils, smooth muscle cells, and fibroblasts. PDGF is also a fibroblast chemoattractant, with the chemotactic response inversely related to the rate of cellular proliferation. PDGF has been shown to accelerate the normal wound healing process by as much as 30% (64). This is attributed to a PDGF-dependent increase in early deposition of fibronectin and glycosaminoglycans, which accelerates the deposition of the provisional wound matrix (64). There is a subsequent increase in collagen synthesis (64). Topically applied PDGF accelerates the healing of surgical incisions in both normal and healing-impaired animals (65,66). Enhanced wound-breaking strength was seen for as long as 49 days postwounding after a single topical application of PDGF at the time of wounding (65,66). Other studies have shown that PDGF enhances the healing of dermal ulcers in both porcine and diabetic mouse models (64–66). In one prospective, randomized, double-blind study in humans, topically applied PDGF enhanced the healing of stage 3 and 4 decubitus ulcers (67). It appears that during tissue injury and wound healing, PDGF stimulates a cascade of autocrine and paracrine activities. The accelerated healing responses that are seen in response to PDGF are associated with an enhanced influx and activation of macrophages, followed by the accumulation, activation, and proliferation of fibroblasts. Increases then occur in extracellular matrix deposition, particularly glycosaminoglycans and fibronectin, neovascularization, and the reepithelialization process (64).

ISCHEMIA/REPERFUSION AND INFLAMMATORY CYTOKINE CASCADES

Ischemia/reperfusion (I/R) is involved in the pathophysiologic process of many clinical disorders, including myocardial infarction, stroke, mesenteric ischemia, peripheral vascular disease, organ transplantation, and circulatory shock. The latter condition, followed by resuscitation, represents a systemic I/R injury and often leads to the development of ARDS and MOSF. I/R injury has been extensively studied in many organ systems, including the heart, brain, liver, kidney, gut, and skeletal muscle. All of these studies have demonstrated that I/R injury is a biphasic event, with the initial injury related to the production and release of toxic oxygen free radicals, and the later phase of the injury being neutrophil-mediated (68). In addition, TNF-α and IL-1 are important initial triggers for the response to I/R injury, and pretreatment with anti-TNF-α antibodies or anti-IL-1 antibodies before the initiation of reperfusion can prevent some of the associated tissue damage. Unfortunately, administration of these antibodies after the initiation of reperfusion does little to inhibit the ensuing tissue injury. The cascade of mediators unleashed in response to I/R is similar to what is seen in the setting of sepsis, with TNF-α and IL-1 inducing the production and release of addition mediators, including neutrophil chemotactic agents and adhesion molecules, which are then responsible for the development of the associated neutrophil-mediated tissue injury. Antibodies against these agents also have protective effects against the I/R injury, provided that they are administered before the initiation of reperfusion. Although this could have practical applications in the setting of organ transplantation and certain types of vascular surgical procedures, this is not effective in the treatment of conditions such as myocardial infarction or stroke.

The liver and gut are highly susceptible to hypovolemic shock. Because the liver has the largest fixed macrophage population in the body, it has significant potential for macrophage-dependent cytokine production and release. Cytokines released from the liver or gut during hypovolemic shock and resuscitation (I/R injury) may play a major role in the subsequent pathogenesis of ARDS and MOSF (Fig. 5.21). Further, the translocation of bacteria

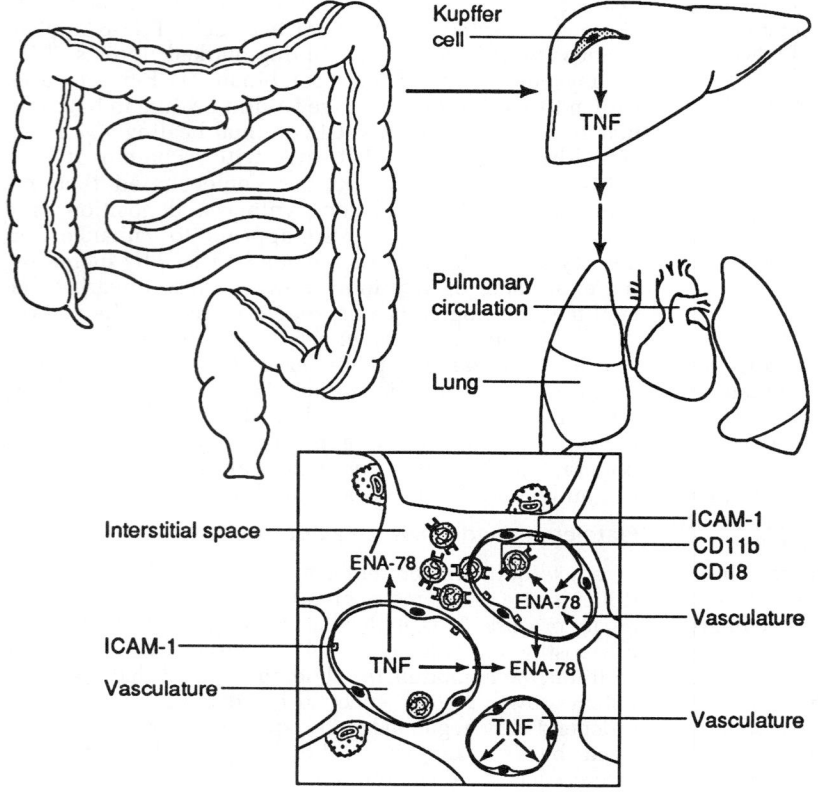

Figure 5.21. Gut, liver, and lung interactions in the development of multiple organ system failure (MOSF). After a severe total body insult, there is often a systemic ischemia/reperfusion injury. For example, hypovolemic shock with resuscitation represents a systemic ischemic event with subsequent reperfusion after resuscitation. In these instances, it is postulated that the development of adult respiratory distress syndrome (ARDS) and MOSF is the result of systemic levels of early-response inflammatory cytokines, such as tumor necrosis factor-α (TNF-α) and interleukin (IL)-1. The major source of these cytokines is the gut and liver. Further, the lung is the next vascular bed to be exposed to high levels of these cytokines, and the lung is particularly sensitive to these molecules. This may precipitate the development of ARDS. High levels of TNF-α and IL-1 trigger the production and release of CXC chemokines, such as IL-8, MIP-2, and epithelial neutrophil-activating protein (ENA-78), as well as up-regulating adhesion molecules on the vasculature, such as intercellular adhesion molecule-1 (ICAM-1). All of these molecules then facilitate the migration of neutrophils into the area, with subsequent neutrophil-mediated tissue damage and the development of ARDS.

and bacterial products from the gut into the mesenteric circulation, with subsequent passage into the portal circulation during the course of hypovolemic shock with resuscitation, may result in significant hepatic cytokine production and release and be important with respect to the potential development of ARDS and MOSF after many forms of shock with resuscitation. In addition, the hepatic reperfusion injury inherent to resectional hepatic surgery, mesenteric vascular surgery, and orthotopic liver transplantation can also be associated with pulmonary and other end-organ dysfunction.

CYTOKINES AND LIVER DISEASE AND REGENERATION

The liver is unique in that it is the only mammalian organ that can regenerate its biologically functional parenchymal mass after resection or injury instead of healing with biologically nonfunctional scar. A patient's ability to restore preoperative hepatic mass after major liver resection is well known (69). A multitude of mediators that are hepatic mitogens, both in vitro and in vivo, have been identified, but the precise mechanisms involved in liver regeneration remain to be defined (70). Some of the well known hepatic mitogens include hepatocyte growth factor, EGF, and TGF-α. More recently, TNF-α and some of the other inflammatory cytokines have been demonstrated to have mitogenic actions on the liver, suggesting a continuum of effects of these molecules from tissue injury and inflammation to repair and regeneration (Table 5.11). Patients with poor hepatic function have a baseline increase in circulating levels of TNF-α, IL-1, IL-6, and other proinflammatory cytokines (71,72). These baseline increases in cytokine production are unrelated to the type or chronicity of liver disease, but are disease stage dependent (71,72). There are several potential explanations for ongoing cytokine production during hepatic disease. First, in liver disease associated with ongoing infection, there may be persistent hepatic macrophage stimulation, with increased cytokine production. Second, there may be impaired Kupffer cell or hepatocyte clearance of circulating mediators secreted in otherwise normal amounts, allowing these substances access to the systemic circulation. Finally, the inflammatory mediators may be important in initiating hepatic regeneration after liver injury, and are therefore chronically up-regulated for ongoing hepatic repair.

Alterations in immune function and cytokine production may be related to the pathophysiologic changes seen in chronic liver diseases. There is increasing evidence that the monocyte–macrophage system is chronically activated in patients with alcoholic liver disease. These patients have enhanced spontaneous monocyte cytokine production, as well as baseline elevations in circulating IL-1, IL-6, and TNF-α (71,73,74). Patients with alcoholic cirrhosis have increased levels of soluble TNF-α receptor type I (sTNFR-55), with serum sTNFR-55 levels paralleling disease severity (72). Increased soluble TNF-α receptors in ascitic fluid and plasma from patients with other forms of liver disease have also been reported (75,76). The increase

in soluble TNF-α receptors is likely a response to increased TNF-α production due to ongoing hepatic injury, and is probably a protective mechanism against increased systemic TNF-α concentrations. These data suggest that TNF-α production is increased in the face of liver disease or injury, and that cytokines may be important in the host response to these insults. It is unclear whether the increases in TNF-α seen with hepatic disease play a detrimental or beneficial role—in other words, are these chronically elevated levels of TNF-α, and possibly other inflammatory cytokines, perpetuating inflammation and injury to the host, or are they important in the reparative processes that are ongoing within the liver?

Injury and inflammation are intimately linked to wound healing and tissue repair. In a healthy adult liver, most hepatocytes are growth arrested and perform various liver-specific functions (70). However, mature hepatocytes undergo DNA synthesis and cell division after liver injury (70,77). Within 24 hours of injury, the resident hepatocytes begin to proliferate, and this continues until the original hepatic mass is reestablished (70). Entry into the proliferative phase of the cell cycle is synchronous, with a sharp peak in hepatocyte DNA synthesis occurring 18 to 24 hours after injury (70). This process is an active area of research, and many growth-stimulatory factors and inhibitors have been identified. However, the exact mechanisms controlling hepatic regeneration remain to be defined. Kupffer cells produce a multitude of mediators and likely play a central role in the regulation of hepatocyte proliferation (77,78). Kupffer cells and hepatic endothelial cells actively produce soluble mediators, including cytokines, which play a pivotal role in maintaining the hepatic microenviroment (78–82). Kupffer cells become activated after partial hepatectomy, with an augmented in vitro production of both TNF-α and IL-1 (83,84). Conditioned media from activated Kupffer cells initiate DNA synthesis in cultured hepatocytes (85). Histologic analysis of the remaining hepatic parenchyma after partial hepatectomy demonstrates a neutrophil infiltrate, an increase in MHC class II antigen expression, and changes in Kupffer cell morphology indicating an activated state, including cellular swelling, numerous vacuoles, and a high number of lysosomes (86).

Studies support a role for TNF-α in hepatic regeneration. Treatment with antibodies to TNF-α immediately before partial hepatectomy inhibits liver regeneration (87). Administration of exogenous TNF-α to normal rats stimulates hepatic DNA synthesis, with an overall increase in hepatic size and weight (88). In similar studies, exogenous TNF-α administered after 70% hepatectomy increased the rate of hepatic regeneration compared with animals receiving a saline control (89). Hepatocyte proliferation can be induced in rats by treatment with lead nitrate, without the need for hepatic resection or injury (90). In this setting, a significant increase in serum TNF-α occurs without a concurrent increase in serum hepatocyte growth factor, and the serum TNF-α increases parallel hepatocyte proliferation (90). In vitro, hepatocytes tolerate TNF-α, and TNF-α elicits hepatocyte DNA synthesis in serum-free media (70). Further studies (91) have shown that relatively brief periods of hepatic ischemia accelerate hepatic regeneration after partial hepatectomy. This study demonstrated that ischemic periods of less than 60 minutes led to an enhanced regenerative capacity in the remaining liver after partial hepatectomy. Hepatic injury and inflammation may be intimately linked to hepatic regeneration and repair through the pluripotent actions of cytokines released in response to hepatic injury. TNF-α, or other TNF-α-inducible cytokines, may act as physiologic stimuli for liver regeneration, particularly in the setting of hepatic in-

---

Table 5.11. **PROTEIN MEDIATORS THAT MAY HAVE PROLIFERATIVE EFFECTS IN THE LIVER**

Hepatocyte growth factor
Epidermal growth factor
Transforming growth factor-α
Tumor necrosis factor
Interleukin-6

jury or inflammation; however, the precise mediators and their mechanisms of action remain to be fully elucidated.

REFERENCES

1. Larrick JW, Kunkel SL. The role of tumor necrosis factor and interleukin-1 in the immunoinflammatory response. *Pharm Res* 1988;5:129.
2. Clark RAF. Basics of cutaneous wound repair. *J Dermatol Surg Oncol* 1993;19:693.
3. Leibovich SJ, Weisman DM. Macrophages, wound repair, and angiogenesis. *Prog Clin Biol Res* 1988;266:131.
4. Tracey KJ, Beutler B, Lowry SF, et al. Shock and tissue injury induced by recombinant human cachectin. *Science* 1986;234:470.
5. Strieter RM, Lynch JP III, Basha MA, et al. Host responses in mediating sepsis and the adult respiratory distress syndrome. *Semin Respir Infect* 1990;5:233.
6. Tracey KJ, Lowry SF, Cerami A. Cachectin/TNF-α in septic shock and septic adult respiratory distress syndrome. *Am Rev Respir Dis* 1988;138:1377.
7. Schlag G, Redl H, Hallstrom S. The cell in shock: the origin of multiple organ failure. *Resuscitation* 1991;21:137.
8. Waage A, Halstensen A, Espevik T. Association between tumor necrosis factor in serum and fatal outcome in patients with meningococcal disease. *Lancet* 1987;11:355.
9. Girardin E, Grau GE, Dayer JM, et al., and the J5 Study Group. Tumor necrosis factor and interleukin-1 in the serum of children with severe infectious purpura. *N Engl J Med* 1988;319:397.
10. Marks JD, Marks CB, Luce JM, et al. Plasma tumor necrosis factor in patients with septic shock: mortality rate, incidence of adult respiratory distress syndrome. *Am Rev Respir Dis* 1990;141:94.
11. Tracey KJ, Fong Y, Hesse DG, et al. Anti-cachectin/TNF monoclonal antibodies prevent septic shock during lethal bacteremia. *Nature* 1987;330:662.
12. Shalaby MR, Halgunset J, Haugen OA, et al. Cytokine-associated tissue injury and lethality in mice: a comparative study. *Clin Immunol Immunopathol* 1991;61:69.
13. Cerami A. Inflammatory cytokines. *Clin Immunol Immunopathol* 1992;62:S3.
14. Bauss F, Droge W, Mannel DN. Tumor necrosis factor mediates endotoxic effects in mice. *Infect Immun* 1987;55:1622.
15. Philip R, Epstein LB. Tumor necrosis factor as immunomodulator and mediator of monocyte cytotoxicity induced by itself, gamma interferon, and interleukin-1. *Nature* 1986;323:86.
16. Tartaglia LA, Ayres TM, Wong GH, et al. A novel domain with the 55kd TNF receptor signals cell death. *Cell* 1993;74:845.
17. Tartaglia LA, Weber RF, Figare IS, et al. The two different receptors for tumor necrosis factor mediate distinctive cellular responses. *Proc Natl Acad Sci USA* 1991;88:9292.
18. Le J, Vilcek J. TNF and IL-1: cytokines with multiple overlapping biological activities. *Lab Invest* 1987;56:234.
19. Okusawa S, Gelfand JA, Ikejima T, et al. Interleukin-1 induces a shock-like state in rabbits: synergism with tumor necrosis factor and the effect of cyclooxygenase inhibition. *J Clin Invest* 1988;81:1162.
20. Bevilacqua MP, Scheel RR, Gimbrone MA Jr, et al. Regulation of the fibrinolytic system of cultured human endothelial cells by interleukin-1. *J Clin Invest* 1986;78:587.
21. Gauldie J, Richards C, Harnish D, et al. Interferon β2/B-cell stimulatory factor type 2 shares identity with monocyte-derived hepatocyte-stimulating factor and regulates the major acute-phase protein response in liver cells. *Proc Natl Acad Sci USA* 1987;84:7251.
22. Gauldie J, Baumann H. Cytokines and acute phase protein expression. In: Kimball EH, ed. *Cytokines in inflammation.* Toronto: Telford Press, 1991:136.
23. Van Snick J. Interleukin-6: an overview. *Annu Rev Immunol* 1990;8:253.
24. Walz A, Burgener R, Car B, et al. Structure and neutrophil-activating properties of a novel inflammatory peptide (ENA-78) with homology to IL-8. *J Exp Med* 1991;174:1355.
25. Baggioloini M, Dewald B, Walz A. Interleukin-8 and related chemotactic cytokines. In: Gallin JI, Goldstein IM, Snyderman R, eds. *Inflammation: basic principles and clinical correlates.* New York: Raven Press, 1992:69.
26. Herbert CA, Vitangcol RV, Baker JB. Scanning mutagenesis of interleukin-8 identifies a cluster of residues required for receptor binding. *J Biol Chem* 1991;266:18989.
27. Clark-Lewis I, Dewald B, Geiser T, et al. Platelet factor-4 binds to interleukin-8 receptors and activates neutrophils when its N-terminus is modified with Glu-Leu-Arg. *Proc Natl Acad Sci USA* 1993;90:3574.
28. Clark-Lewis I, Kim KS, Rajarathnam K, et al. Structure–activity relationships of chemokines. *J Leuk Biol* 1995;57:703.
29. Chuntharapai A, Kim KJ. Regulation of the expression of the IL-8 receptor A/B by IL-8: possible functions of each receptor. *J Immunol* 1995;155:2587.
30. Strieter RM, Polverini PJ, Kunkel SL, et al. The functional role of the ELR motif in CXC chemokine-mediated angiogenesis. *J Biol Chem* 1995;270:27348.
31. Ward PA, Lentsch AB. The acute inflammatory response and its regulation. *Arch Surg* 1999;134:666–669.
32. Koch AE, Polverini PJ, Leibovich SJ. Stimulation of neovascularization by human rheumatoid synovial tissue macrophages. *Arthritis Rheum* 1986;29:471.
33. Polverini PJ. *Cytokines,* vol 1. Basel: S. Karger, 1989:54.
34. Sharpe RJ, Byers HR, Scott CF, et al. Growth inhibition of murine melanoma and human colon carcinoma by recombinant human platelet factor 4. *J Natl Cancer Inst* 1990;82:848.
35. Maione TE, Gray GS, Hunt AJ, et al. Inhibition of tumor growth in mice by an analog of platelet factor 4 that lacks affinity for heparin and retains potent angiogenic activity. *Cancer Res* 1991;51:2077.
36. Driscoll KE, Hassenbein DG, Howard BW, et al. Cloning, expression, and functional characterization of rat MIP-2: a neutrophil chemoattractant and epithelial cell mitogen. *J Leuk Biol* 1995;58:359–364.
37. Michel G, Kemeny L, Peter Ru, et al. Interleukin-8 receptor-mediated chemotaxis of normal human epidermal cells. *FEBS Lett* 1992;305:241.
38. Selzman CH, Shames BD, Miller SA, et al. Therapeutic implications of interleukin-10 in surgical disease. *Shock* 1998;10:309.
39. Neurath MF, Buschenfelde KH. Protective and pathologic roles of cytokines in inflammatory bowel diseases. *J Invest Med* 1996;44:516.
40. Young HA, Hardy KJ. Role of interferon-gamma in immune cell regulation. *J Leuk Biol* 1995;58:373381.
41. Li XM, Chopra RK, Chou TY, et al. Mucosal IFN-γ gene transfer inhibits pulmonary allergic responses in mice. *J Immunol* 1996;157:3216.
42. Willenborg DO, Fordham S, Bernard CA, et al. IFN-γ plays a critical down-regulatory role in the induction and effector phase of myelin oligodendrocyte glycoprotein-induced autoimmune encephalomyelitis. *J Immunol* 1996;157:3223.
43. Ohmori Y, Hamilton TA. IFN-γ selectively inhibits lipopolysaccharide-induced JE/monocyte chemoattractant protein-1 and KC/GRO/melanoma growth stimulating activity gene expression in mouse peritoneal macrophages. *J Immunol* 1994;153:2204.
44. Kasama T, Strieter RM, Lukacs NW, et al. Interferon γ modulates the expression of neutrophil-derived chemokines. *J Invest Med* 1995;43:58.
45. Benton LD, Khan M, Greco RS. Integrins, adhesion molecules surgical research. *Surg Gynecol Obstet* 1993;177:311.
46. Springer TA. Adhesion receptors of the immune system. *Nature* 1990;346:425.
47. Stoolman LM. Adhesion molecules controlling lymphocyte migration. *Cell* 1989;56:907.
48. Thornton FJ, Schaffer MR, Barbul A. Wound healing in sepsis and trauma. *Shock* 1997;8:391.
49. Davidson JM. Wound repair. In: Gallin JI, Goldstein IM, Snyderman R, eds. *Inflammation: basic principles and clinical correlates.* New York: Raven Press, 1992:244.
50. Zetter BR. Angiogenesis: state of the art. *Chest* 1988;93:159S.
51. Harris ED Jr. Recent insight into the pathogenesis of the proliferative lesion in rheumatoid arthritis. *Arthritis Rheum* 1976;19:68.
52. Koch AE, Podlverini PJ, Kunkel SL, et al. Interleukin-8 (IL-8)

as a macrophage-derived mediator of angiogenesis. *Science* 1992;258:1798.

53. Koch AE, Litvak MA, Burrows JC, et al. Decreased monocyte-mediated angiogenesis in scleroderma. *Clin Immunol Immunopathol* 1992;64:153.

54. Rastinejad F, Polverini PJ, Bouck NP. Regulation of the activity of a new inhibitor of angiogenesis by a cancer suppressor gene. *Cell* 1989;56:345.

55. Good DJ, Polverini PJ, Rastinejad F, et al. A tumor suppressor-dependent inhibitor of angiogenesis is immunologically and functionally indistinguishable from a fragment of thrombospondin. *Proc Natl Acad Sci USA* 1990;87:6624.

56. Fahey TJ III, Sherry B, Tracey KJ, et al. Cytokine production in a model of wound healing: the appearance of MIP-1, MIP-2, cachectin/TNF and IL-1. *Cytokine* 1990;2:92.

57. Mahadevan V, Hart IR, Lewis GP. Factors influencing blood supply in wound granuloma quantitated by a new in vivo technique. *Cancer Res* 1989;49:415.

58. Scharffetter K, Heckman M, Hatamochi A, et al. Synergistic effect of tumor necrosis factor alpha and interferon-gamma on collagen synthesis of human skin fibroblasts in vitro. *Exp Cell Res* 1989;181:409.

59. Hom DB, Maisel RH. Angiogenic growth factors: their effects and potential in soft tissue wound healing. *Ann Otol Rhinol Laryngol* 1992;101:349.

60. Buckley-Sturrock A, Woodward SC, Senior RM, et al. Differential stimulation of collagenase and chemotactic activity in fibroblasts derived from rat wound repair tissue and human skin by growth factors. *J Cell Physiol* 1989;138:70.

61. Barnard JA, Russette ML, Moses HL. The biology of transforming growth factor beta. *Biochim Biophys Acta* 1990; 1032:79.

62. Beck LS, DeGuzman L, Lee WP, et al. One systemic administration of transforming growth factor-β1 reverses age- or glucocorticoid-impaired wound healing. *J Clin Invest* 1993;92: 2565.

63. Terrell TG, Working PK, Chow CP, et al. Pathology of recombinant human transforming growth factor-β1 in rats and rabbits. *Int Rev Exp Pathol* 1993;34:43.

64. Lynch SE, Colvin RB, Antoniades NH. Growth factors in wound healing. *J Clin Invest* 1989;84:640.

65. Greenhalgh DG, Sprugel KH, Murray MJ, et al. PDGF and FGF stimulate wound healing in the genetically diabetic mouse. *Am J Pathol* 1990;136:1235.

66. Mustoe TA, Purdy J, Gramates P, et al. Reversal of impaired wound healing in irradiated rats by platelet-derived growth factor BB: requirement for an active bone marrow. *Am J Surg* 1989;158:345.

67. Mustoe TA, Cutler NR, Allman RM, et al. A phase II study to evaluate recombinant platelet-derived growth factor-BB in the treatment of stage 3 and 4 pressure ulcers. *Arch Surg* 1994;150:213.

68. Jaeschke H, Bautista AP, Spolarics Z, et al. Superoxide generation by neutrophil and Kupffer cells during in vivo reperfusion following hepatic ischemia in rats. *J Leuk Biol* 1992; 52:377.

69. Weinbren K, Hadjis NS. Compensatory hyperplasia of the liver. In: Blumgart LH, ed. *Surgery of the liver and biliary tract.* London: Churchill Livingstone, 1990:51–54.

70. Fausto N, Laird AD, Webber EM. Role of growth factors and cytokines in hepatic regeneration. *FASEB J* 1995;9:1527.

71. Khoruts A, Stahnke L, McClain CJ, et al. Circulating tumor necrosis factor, interleukin-1, and interleukin-6 concentrations in chronic alcoholic patients. *Hepatology* 1991;13:267.

72. Diez-Ruiz A, Tilz G, Gutierrez-Gea F, et al. Neopterin and soluble tumor necrosis factor receptor type I in alcohol-induced cirrhosis. *Hepatology* 1995;21:976.

73. Deviere J, Content J, Denys C, et al. Excessive in vitro bacterial lipopolysaccharide-induced production of monokines in cirrhosis. *Hepatology* 1990;11:628.

74. Torre D, Zeroli C, Giola M, et al. Serum levels of interleukin-1-α, interleukin-1-β, interleukin-6, and tumor necrosis factor in patients with acute viral hepatitis. *Clin Infect Dis* 1994;18: 194.

75. Andus T, Gross V, Holstege A, et al. High concentration of soluble tumor necrosis factor receptors in ascites. *Hepatology* 1992;16:749.

76. Tilg H, Vogel W, Wiedermann CJ, et al. Circulating interleukin-1 and tumor necrosis factor antagonists in liver disease. *Hepatology* 1993;18:1132.

77. Grisham JW. A morphologic study of deoxyribonucleic acid synthesis and cell proliferation in regenerating liver: autoradiography with ³H-thymidine. *Cancer Res* 1962;22:842.

78. Billiar TR, Curran RD. Kupffer cell and hepatocyte interactions: a brief overview. *JPEN J Parenter Enteral Nutr* 1990; 14:175.

79. Arii S, Monden K, Itai S. Depressed function of Kupffer cells in rats with CCl₄-induced liver cirrhosis. *Res Exp Med* 1990; 190:173.

80. Higashitsuji H, Arii S, Furutani M, et al. Expression of cytokine genes during liver regeneration after partial hepatectomy in rats. *J Surg Res* 1995;58:267.

81. Mawet E, Shiratori Y, Hikiba Y, et al. Cytokine-induced neutrophil chemoattractant release from hepatocytes is modulated by Kupffer cells. *Hepatology* 1996;23:353.

82. Thornton AJ, Ham J, Kunkel SL. Kupffer cell–derived cytokines induce synthesis of a leukocyte chemotactic peptide, interleukin-8, in human hepatoma and primary hepatocyte cultures. *Hepatology* 1991;14:1.

83. Katsumoto F, Miyazaki K, Nakayama F. Stimulation of DNA synthesis in hepatocytes by Kupffer cells after partial hepatectomy. *Hepatology* 1989;9:405.

84. Goss JA, Mangino MJ, Callery MP, et al. Prostaglandin E₂ down regulates Kupffer cell production of IL-1 and IL-6 during hepatic regeneration. *Am J Physiol* 1992;264:G601.

85. Nagata Y, Tanaka N, Orita K. Endotoxin-induced liver injury after extended hepatectomy and the role of Kupffer cells in the rat. *Surg Today* 1994;24:441.

86. Boermeester MA, Straatsburg IH, Houdijk APJ, et al. Endotoxin and interleukin-1 related hepatic inflammatory response promotes liver failure after partial hepatectomy. *Hepatology* 1995;22:1499.

87. Akerman P, Cote P, Yang SQ, et al. Antibodies to tumor necrosis factor-α inhibit liver regeneration after partial hepatectomy. *Am J Physiol* 1992;263:G579.

88. Feingold KR, Soued M, Grunfeld C. Tumor necrosis factor stimulates DNA synthesis in the liver of intact rats. *Biochem Biophys Res Commun* 1988;153:576.

89. Beyer HS, Stanley M. Tumor necrosis factor-alpha increases hepatic DNA and RNA and hepatocyte mitosis. *Biochem Int* 1990;22:405.

90. Kubo Y, Yasunaga M, Masuhara M, et al. Hepatocyte proliferation induced in rats by lead nitrate is suppressed by several tumor necrosis factor-α inhibitors. *Hepatology* 1996;23: 104.

91. Maruyama H, Harada A, Kurokawa T, et al. Duration of liver ischemia and hepatic regeneration after hepatectomy in rats. *J Surg Res* 1995;58:290.

SURGERY: SCIENTIFIC PRINCIPLES AND PRACTICE, Third Edition, edited by
Lazar J. Greenfield, Michael W. Mulholland, Keith T. Oldham, Gerald B. Zelenock,
and Keith D. Lillemoe. Lippincott Williams & Wilkins Publishers, Philadelphia, © 2001.

CHAPTER 6

INFLAMMATION

VAISHALI DIXIT SCHUCHERT AND TIMOTHY R. BILLIAR

Cornelius Celsus, a Roman writer of the first century A.D., described the four cardinal signs of inflammation: *rubor* (redness), *tumor* (swelling), *calor* (heat), and *dolor* (pain). *Laesio functio* is the loss of function that accompanies any combination of these effects (1). In 1793, the Scottish surgeon John Hunter was the first to postulate that inflammation does not represent a disease state *per se,* but rather a nonspecific response that can produce a "salutary" effect on its host. He also recognized that excessive inflammation can be deleterious to the host. Inflammation thus became known as the "first principle of surgery" (1). Julius Cohnheim (1839–1884) provided one of the first microscopic descriptions of inflammation. While examining the blood vessels of the frog mesentery and tongue, he described in vivid detail the initial vasodilatation and blood flow changes, subsequent edema due to altered vascular permeability, and the associated leukocyte migration pattern seen in acute inflammation (2). The Russian biologist, Elie Metchnikoff, discovered the process of phagocytosis by observing the ingestion of rose thorns by amebocytes of starfish larvae (1882), and of bacteria by mammalian leukocytes (1884). He concluded that the purpose of inflammation was to bring phagocytic cells to the injured area to engulf invading bacteria (3). This theory contradicted the prevailing view of the time that the purpose of inflammation was to bring in factors from the serum to neutralize the infectious agents. It soon became clear that both cellular (phagocytosis) and humoral factors (antibodies) were critical in the defense against microorganisms. For these observations, both Metchnikoff and Paul Ehrlich (who developed the humoral theory) shared the Nobel Prize in 1908 (4). Sir Thomas Lewis was the first to establish the concept that chemical substances, locally induced by injury, mediate the vascular changes of inflammation (5), opening the doors to the discovery of the chemical mediators of inflammation and the potent antiinflammatory agents.

Inflammation represents the body's natural response to injury (e.g., microbial invasion, physical trauma, burns). Although an adequate inflammatory response provides an essential defense mechanism against such insults, an inappropriate or excessive response can cause considerable morbidity and even mortality. Inflammation represents the end product of a complex interplay of cellular and humoral elements. Humoral components are molecules circulating in the blood, including antibodies and the complement system. Cellular components consist of the granulocytes, mononuclear phagocytes, lymphocytes, and a wide variety of nonleukocytes that affect a multitude of processes involved in inflammation. Microscopically, these cellular and humoral elements produce changes in the local vasculature and leukocyte recruitment mediated by kinins, cytokines, chemokines, lipid mediators, neuropeptides, and reactive oxygen and nitrogen species. Within 30 to 60 minutes, neutrophils marginate, extravasate, and accumulate at the site of injury, where they engulf offending pathogens and release oxidants and proteases. Within 4 to 5 hours, mononuclear cells (monocytes and lymphocytes) begin to accumulate at the site of injury (6). Recruited monocytes and activated resident macrophages participate in nonspecific phagocytic activity, whereas lymphocytes orchestrate specific, antibody-dependent lysis of cells. These leukocytes continue to release mediators to regulate the local and sometimes systemic inflammatory responses. Redness and warmth result from local vasodilatation, primarily in the postcapillary venules. Increased vascular permeability leads to accumulation of fluid at the site of injury. The vasodilatation, swelling, and local production of neuropeptides, prostanoids, kinins, and cytokines also produce the sensation of pain and contribute to the loss of function in the affected tissues.

This chapter focuses on the cellular and humoral components of local and systemic inflammatory responses and the complex interplay among the various inflammatory mediators. Although an in-depth discussion of immunology is provided elsewhere, the essential immune effector cells and their roles in inflammation are reviewed.

CELL DEVELOPMENT

During intrauterine development, hematopoiesis occurs initially in the embryonal yolk sac, followed temporally by the liver, spleen, and lymph nodes (7). By the fifth month of gestation, hematopoiesis is initiated in the bone marrow. By birth, it occurs exclusively in the bone marrow, and continues throughout adult life in the flat bones of the skull, ribs, sternum, vertebral column, and pelvis, as well as in the proximal ends of long bones. All of the cellular elements of blood, including the red blood cells that transport oxygen, the platelets that trigger blood clotting in damaged tissues, and the white blood cells of the immune system, derive ultimately from the same progenitor or precursor cells, the hematopoietic stem cells. These pluripotent stem cells, in turn, give rise to cells of more limited potential, which are the immediate progenitors of red blood cells, platelets, and white blood cells. Cells progress to a blast phase, after which they begin to decrease in size and assume the typical characteristics of their fully differentiated and mature forms. The different types of blood cells and their lineage relationships are summarized in Fig. 6.1.

Totipotential hematopoietic stem cells give rise to two principal cellular lineages—lymphoid and myeloid. The common lymphoid progenitor gives rise to B and T lymphocytes, as well as natural killer (NK) cells. Lymphocytes are unique in that they proliferate and mature both within and outside of the bone marrow. When B lymphocytes (or B cells) are activated, they differentiate into plasma cells that secrete antibodies. T lymphocytes (or T cells) develop into CD8+ (cytotoxic) or CD4+ (helper) phenotypes. Cytotoxic lymphocytes and NK cells patrol the tissues and are capable of eliminating infected or transformed cells. Helper T cells assist in the generation of an immune response by promoting the activation of cells such as B cells and macrophages. All other cellular constituents of blood are derived from the myeloid progenitors. These include erythrocytes (red blood cells), thrombocytes (platelets), monocytes, and granulocytes. Erythroblasts develop to reticulocytes before becoming mature erythrocytes. The primary stimulus for erythropoiesis is erythropoietin produced by the kidney. As development progresses, hemoglobin content increases. Fully mature red blood cells lack organelles and nuclei. Megakaryocytes differentiate into platelets.

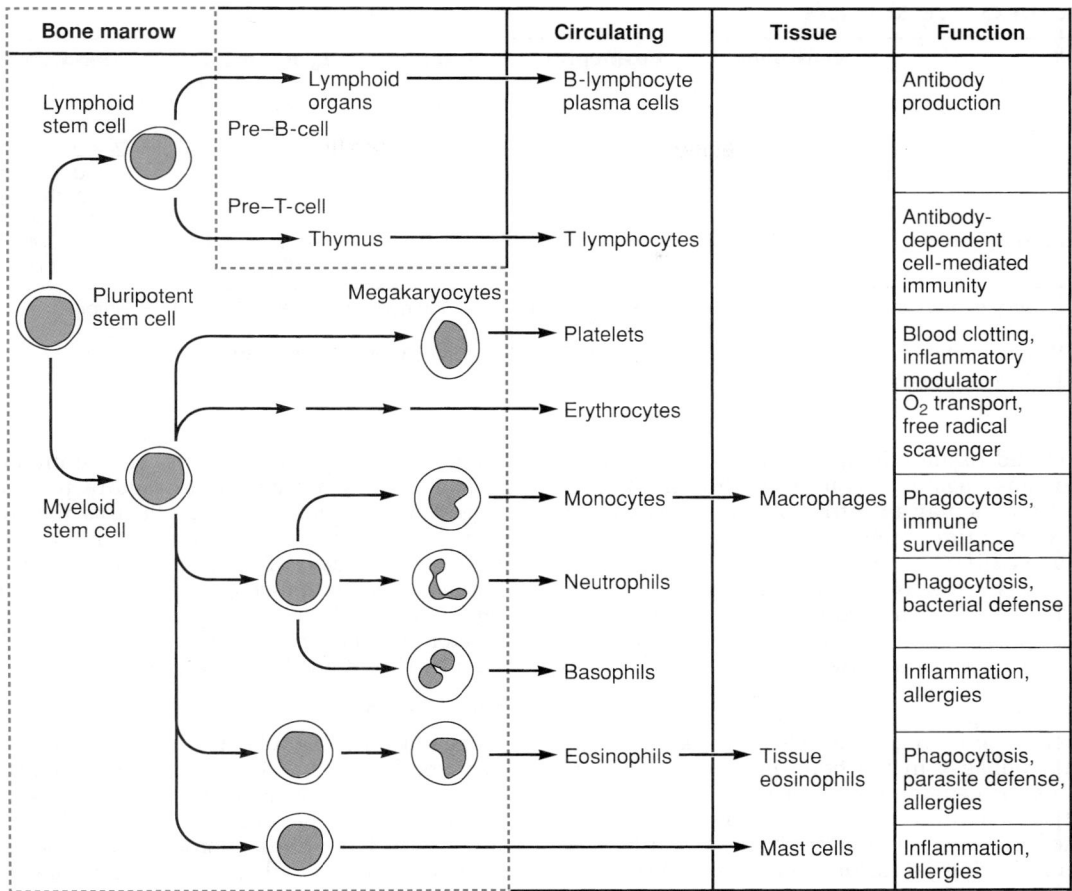

Figure 6.1. Cells of the hematopoietic cell system. Pluripotent stem cells in the bone marrow differentiate into lymphoid or myeloid stem cells. Lymphoid stem cells differentiate into pre-B cells or pre-T cells. In lymphoid organs, pre-B cells differentiate into B cells, which are released into the circulation. B cells further develop in the lymphoid organs into plasma cells, the antibody-producing cells of the immune system. Myeloid stem cells further differentiate in the bone marrow to produce mature cells. These mature cells are released into the circulation, with the exception of mast cells, which are not found in the circulation. Circulating monocytes migrate into tissues, where they develop into macrophages.

Leukocytes are the primary cellular effectors of the inflammatory process. The leukocytes encompass lymphocytes of the lymphoid lineage as well as monocytes and granulocytes of the myeloid lineage. Differentiation and maturation of specific leukocyte subsets is driven by the presence of specific cytokines and growth factors. No factor has absolute lineage specificity. The range for a normal leukocyte count is 5,000 to 10,000/mm³ circulating blood. The relative composition of the leukocyte subsets is shown in Table 6.1.

Monocytes, from the myeloid lineage, are also called *round cells* based on their round to oval nuclei. They do not have cytoplasmic granules visible by light microscopy, and nuclei are round rather than lobulated (7). Monocytes are released into the blood, where they migrate to the tissues of the body and differentiate into macrophages capable of a wide variety of effector functions. Myeloid progenitors can also differentiate into three principal lineages of granulocytes (neutrophils, eosinophils and basophils).

Granulocytes are characterized by conspicuous and abundant cytoplasmic granules containing inflammatory mediators and enzymes (7). The three types of granulocytes are named according to the staining characteristics of their specific granules. Eosinophils stain with acidic dyes such as eosin. Basophils stain positive with basic dyes such as hematoxylin or methylene blue. Neutrophils have little affinity for acidic or basic dyes. Each of the granulocyte lineages develops through myeloblast, promyelocyte, myelocyte, metamyelocyte, and band phases before becoming mature granulocytes. During development, granulocyte nuclei become increasingly segmented, and thus granulocytes are commonly referred to as *polymorphonuclear leukocytes*. Neutrophils are the most numerous and most important cellular component of the innate immune response. Hereditary deficiencies in neutrophil function can lead to overwhelming bacterial infection. Eosinophils are thought to be important chiefly in defense against parasitic infections. Basophils and mast cells elaborate substances affecting vascular tone and permeability, and play important roles in protecting the mucosal surfaces of the body.

Neutrophils

Neutrophils are the principal cellular component of the acute inflammatory response. First to arrive at sites of

Table 6.1. **LEUKOCYTE SUBSETS**

Cell	Neutrophil	Eosinophil	Basophil	Lymphocyte	Monocyte/Macrophage
Size	13 μm	12–16 μm	15 μm	9–16 μm	16–20 μm
Differential in circulating blood	40%–75%	1%–6%	<1%	20%–45%	2%–6%
Development	6–9 d	6–9 d	3–7 d	1–2 d	2–3 d
Life span	6 h to ~5 d	8–12 d in tissue	~1 y	Months to years	1–2 d as monocytes/ months to years as macrophages
Growth factors and activators	G-CSF, IL-8	G-CSF, IL-5	G-CSF, IL-3	IL-2, IL-12 (T_H1), IL-4 (T_H2)	M-CSF, GM-CSF, interferon-γ, tumor necrosis factor

(G, M)-CSF, (granulocyte, monocyte) colony-stimulating factor; IFN, interferon; IL, interleukin; T_H, helper T cell; TNF, tumor necrosis factor.
Modified from Wheater's functional histology: a text and colour atlas, 3rd ed. Burkitt G, Young B, Heath JW, eds. Edinburgh, New York: Churchill Livingstone, 1993.

inflammation and tissue injury, they are essential in the early host defense against invading pathogens. Consequently, neutrophils play a central role in virtually every inflammatory condition, including adult respiratory distress syndrome (ARDS), ischemia/reperfusion injury, inflammatory bowel disease, and rheumatoid arthritis (8–11). The magnitude of neutrophil influx is directly related to the severity of injury. The importance of neutrophils in host defense is underscored by the fact that 55% to 60% of the hematopoietic output of bone marrow is dedicated to the production of neutrophils (12). Granulocyte colony-stimulating factor (G-CSF), elaborated by activated macrophages in the bone marrow, is the primary stimulus for development and maturation of neutrophils (13). On exiting the bone marrow, neutrophils have a limited life span, circulating in the blood for 7 to 10 hours before taking up residence in tissues for a total of 1 or 2 days (14,15).

Neutrophils respond to injury by adhering to the vascular endothelium near the site of injury and then migrating to the inflammatory focus. There they destroy microbes by phagocytosis and release of toxic cellular contents. To accomplish this task, neutrophils express an array of receptors capable of a wide variety of functions. Aggregation, adhesion, and transmigration of neutrophils are mediated by the sequential cell surface expression of selectins and integrins, discussed in detail in the section on Phagocyte–Endothelial Cell Interactions. In addition, neutrophils express receptors for IgG (immunoglobulin G) (FcγR) and for complement component C3b [complement receptor type 1 (CR1)] (12). Binding of IgG to the neutrophil FcγR triggers the respiratory burst, antibody-dependent cellular cytotoxicity (ADCC), and the release of cytokines and prostanoids. C3b acts as a chemotaxin to neutrophils. The most significant consequence of ligand binding to FcγR or C3b is the activation of phagocytosis. IgG and C3b are the most important opsonins, or agents that enhance phagocytosis.

Neutrophils also express receptors that respond to endogenously generated chemoattractants [e.g., leukotriene (LT) B_4, platelet-activating factor (PAF), C5a], and the neutrophil-activating CXC chemokines such as interleukin (IL)-8. The bacterial cell wall constituents N-formylmethionyl-leucyl-phenylalanine (fMLP) and lipopolysaccharide (LPS) are important exogenous chemoattractants. Chemoattractants in low concentrations stimulate migration and priming, whereas higher concentrations stimulate degranulation and release of reactive oxygen species (ROS). Primed neutrophils respond to chemotactic stimuli more vigorously. Inflammatory cytokines [e.g., tumor necrosis factor (TNF), granulocyte–macrophage colony-stimulating factor (GM-CSF), G-CSF] can also act as priming agents. The priming process can be initiated within 1 hour and does not appear to require protein synthesis, suggesting a direct signaling effect as the likely mechanism (6). Receptors specific for each inflammatory mediator trigger a cascade of reactions that culminates in the formation of second messengers by a set of effector enzymes. Signal transduction between cell surface receptors and the effector enzymes in the cell interior is carried out principally by G proteins (discussed later).

Antimicrobial Functions

The antimicrobial effector functions of neutrophils are mediated by a host of intracellular proteins and oxygen derivatives. The major extralysosomal cytosolic protein of neutrophils is calprotectin, a complex of calcium-binding proteins that deprives microorganisms of zinc and performs important regulatory functions. Most microbicidal proteases are found in neutrophil granules (16) (Table 6.2). These proteases not only destroy phagocytosed pathogens, but they can spill out of the cell to damage surrounding host tissues. The initial classification of neutrophil granules was based on peroxidase staining characteristics. Primary, or azurophil granules formed during the promyelocyte stage contain neutral proteases, acid hydrolases, and myeloperoxidase (MPO). The smaller, MPO-negative secondary granules, or specific granules, are formed later during the myelocyte stage and contain metalloproteinases. Later classifications based on immunocytochemical properties divided granules into four categories: azurophil (primary), specific (secondary), gelatinase (tertiary), and secretory.

Azurophil granules release their contents into intracellular phagolysosomes. The major constituents of azurophil granules are MPO, the defensins, lysozyme, serprocidins, and bactericidal/permeability-increasing protein (BPI). MPO participates in the generation of toxic oxygen derivatives such as the superoxide radical, hypohalous acids, and the highly reactive singlet oxygen. The greenish color of pus is due to neutrophil MPO (17). Optimal microbicidal activity in neutrophils requires the generation of MPO and hydrogen peroxide (H_2O_2). This requirement is illustrated in patients with chronic granulomatous disease. Neutrophils from these patients engulf invading pathogens by phagocytosis but are unable to destroy them in the phagolysosomes, resulting in chronic unresolved infections (18).

Defensins and other cationic peptides such as polylysine and protamine interact with the negatively charged plasma membrane to increase the permeability of microbe cell walls (19). The four α defensins (human neutrophil peptides 1 through 4) are also chemotactic to T lymphocytes. Lysozyme, present in both primary and secondary

Table 6.2. **NEUTROPHIL GRANULES AND THEIR CONSTITUENTS**

Azurophil granules	Specific granules
Myeloperoxidase	Lysozyme
Lysozyme	Phospholipase A_2
Cathepsins	Gelatinase
Elastase	Collagenase
Proteinase 3	Lactoferrin
Azurocidin (CAP37/heparin-binding protein)	Tumor necrosis factor
BPI	fMLP-R
Defensins	Mac-1 (CD11b/CD18; CR3)
iNOS	Cytochrome b_{558}
α_1-Antitrypsin	Fibronectin-R
α-Mannosidase	Laminin-R
Sialidase	Vitronectin-R
Ubiquitin protein	Thrombospondin-R
β-Glucuronidase	β_2-microglobulin
Acid mucopolysaccharide	Histaminase
	Heparanse
	Sialidase
	Urokinase-type plasminogen activator
	Urokinase-type plasminogen activator-R

Gelatinase granules	Secretory vesicles
Gelatinase	Mac-1 (CD11b/CD18; CR3)
Mac-1 (CD11b/CD18; CR3)	Alkaline phosphatase
Cytochrome b_{558}	Cytochrome b_{558}
DAG-deacylating enzyme	CR1
fMLP-R	CD14 (lipopolysaccharide receptor)
Lysozyme	fMLP-R
Acetyltransferase	Albumin
β_2-microglobulin	Urokinase-type plasminogen activator-R
Urokinase-type plasminogen activator-R	

"-R" indicates "receptor." BPI, bactericidal/permeability-increasing protein; CAP, cationic antibiotic protein; CR1, complement component C3b; CR3, $\alpha_M\beta_2$ integrin; DAG, diacylglycerol; fMLP, N-formylmethionyl-leucyl-phenylalanine; iNOS, inducible nitric oxide synthase.

granules, attacks the outer surfaces of bacteria or fungi (20). The serprocidins (*serine protease* homologues) are atypical in that they are released extracellularly. Elastase is the best-characterized serprocidin and perhaps the most important oxygen-independent mediator of neutrophil-related microbicidal activity and tissue injury. Elastase cleaves extracellular matrix components, including proteoglycans, collagen types I, III, and IV, and fibronectin in addition to elastin. It can promote cellular detachment from surfaces and kill cells directly (20). The most important plasma inhibitor of neutrophil elastase is α_1-proteinase inhibitor. Elastase itself inactivates most of the other important plasma enzyme inhibitors such as α_2-plasmin inhibitor, C1 inhibitor, and antithrombin III. Other serprocidins include cathepsin G, azurocidin/CAP-37/heparin-binding protein (AZU), and proteinase-3/myeloblastin. Cathepsins play a role in the digestion of proteoglycan. Proteinase-3/myeloblastin induces platelet aggregation and degranulation. AZU is chemotactic for monocytes and stimulates LPS-induced release of IL-6 and TNF from monocytes. BPI increases the permeability of gram-negative bacterial outer membranes and is noted for its high homology with the LPS recognition protein known as LPS binding protein (21,22).

Unlike azurophilic granules, specific granules release their contents extracellularly (16). Cathelicidins have direct cytotoxicity and may act as a neutrophil chemoattractant. These protease inhibitors have also been shown to induce nitric oxide (NO) release from macrophages. Phospholipase A_2 (PLA_2) of specific granules participates in the calcium-dependent degradation of bacterial membrane phospholipids. Lactoferrin, a member of the transferrin family, limits the availability of iron to microbes and in-

hibits proinflammatory cytokine release from monocytes. Secretory vesicles, the fastest of the granules to be mobilized, are unique in that they are of endocytic origin and possess alkaline phosphatase on their luminal surface. Tertiary granules contain the powerful metalloproteinase, gelatinase (23).

Neutrophils are an important source of ROS that have potent antimicrobial activity. As such, they are also capable of effecting nonspecific tissue injury. Superoxide anion generated through activation of the reduced nicotinamide-adenine dinucleotide phosphate (NADPH) oxidase (respiratory burst) system can dismutate to H_2O_2 and can be converted to the highly toxic hydroxyl radical (24). In combination with NO, superoxide can produce the peroxynitrite radical (discussed separately) (25). Neutrophil MPO interacts with H_2O_2 and halides to form hypohalous acids, particularly hypochlorous acid (HOCl). Hypochlorous acid is released extracellularly once generated. In addition to their direct bactericidal effects, these oxygen derivatives can induce bystander tissue injury by inducing DNA strand breaks, triggering membrane lipid peroxidation, and inducing apoptotic pathways (26). Oxygen radicals can also activate signaling pathways leading to nuclear factor-kappa B (NFκB) activation and cytokine release (27).

Eosinophils

Eosinophilic granulocytes share a common bone marrow origin and certain properties with neutrophilic granulocytes. Both eosinophils and neutrophils adhere to inflamed endothelium, migrate through the extracellular matrix to sites of inflammation, and release inflammatory mediators and toxic agents from cytoplasmic granules. They both release superoxide anion and H_2O_2 through a respiratory burst, although eosinophils are less efficient than neutrophils in ingesting and killing microorganisms. The NADPH oxidase (respiratory burst) system is probably similar in eosinophils and neutrophils. There are important differences, however. Whereas tissue recruitment of neutrophils is prominent at sites of bacterial infection, recruitment of eosinophils is pronounced at sites of parasitic infection and allergen challenge. Differential expression of chemokine receptors and their responses to individual chemokines allows selective recruitment of adherent eosinophils and neutrophils to sites of inflammation. In general, neutrophils migrate in response to CXC chemokines (IL-8), whereas eosinophils respond to CC chemokines (eotaxin, MIP-1α, MCP-3, RANTES) (28). The primary eosinophilopoietic cytokines are IL-3, GM-CSF, and IL-5. These cytokines are involved in differentiation, activation of effector functions, and survival by inhibiting apoptosis. Once they leave the bone marrow, eosinophils circulate in the bloodstream for a few hours and then enter tissues of the gastrointestinal tract, lung, and genitourinary tract, where they reside for several days. For every circulating eosinophil, there are 100 tissue eosinophils. Unlike neutrophils, they can reenter the circulation (28).

The visual hallmark of the eosinophil is an electron-dense crystalline core in the specific granules. These bicompartmental granules make up 95% of the total cytoplasmic granules. The crystalline core contains major basic protein (MBP) and the cytokine GM-CSF (29). MBP is cytotoxic to parasites and normal cells and stimulates histamine release from mast cells and basophils. The granule matrix contains eosinophil peroxidase (EPO), eosinophil-derived neurotoxin, lysosomal enzymes, catalase, TNF, transforming growth factor-β (TGF-β), and cationic proteins that stimulate formation of transmembrane pores to increase target cellular permeability (30). EPO is distinct from the MPO found in neutrophils. Eosinophils release EPO extracellularly on target cell surfaces. Hydrogen peroxide is converted to hydrogen halides by EPO. Approximately 30% of oxygen consumed by stimulated eosinophils is accounted for by the formation of halogenating species. Thiocyanate may be the major halide for the EPO–H_2O_2–halide system (31). EPO also stimulates neutrophil aggregation and adhesion to endothelial cells. If ingested by a neighboring phagocyte, EPO can combine with H_2O_2 and halides to form hypohalous acids. The sparse unicompartmental granules contain Charcot-Leyden crystal protein, hydrolytic enzymes (acid phosphatase, arylsulfatase), and EPO. Charcot-Leyden crystals make up approximately 10% of the total eosinophil protein and have lysophospholipase activity (32). Eosinophils contain esterified arachidonic acid in their cytoplasmic lipid bodies that can act as substrate for the formation of inflammatory lipid mediators such as leukotriene C_4 and platelet activatias factor (33,34).

After an allergen or parasitic challenge, resident mucosal mast cells and macrophages secrete cytokines that up-regulate expression of endothelial cell adhesion molecules. Eosinophils have a unique mechanism of adherence to the endothelium. Adhesion involves interactions between the β_1 integrin very late antigen-4 (VLA-4) on eosinophil to vascular cell adhesion molecule-1 (VCAM-1) and fibronectin on endothelial cells. IL-4 can activate both the binding and the up-regulation of endothelial cell VCAM-1. Adhesion to endothelial cells and transmigration also requires mechanisms shared with neutrophils involving selectins and β_2 integrins. Eosinophils are activated by IL-3, GM-CSF, IL-5, PAF, CC chemokines, and the complement-derived anaphylatoxins C3a and C5a. Activated eosinophils produce cytokines and chemokines that recruit and activate more eosinophils and other leukocytes. IL-5, PAF, LTB_4, and fMLP are chemotactic for eosinophils. C5a, the most potent proinflammatory mediator derived from the complement system, is chemotactic for eosinophils. The eosinophil cell membrane expresses G protein-linked chemokine receptors for eotaxin, MIP-1α, MCP-2, MCP-3, RANTES, and other CC chemokines (35).

Although eosinopenia may be indicative of acute inflammation, it is associated with allergic inflammation, asthma, and chronic parasitic infections. The primary targets for eosinophil cytotoxicity are probably extracellular parasites (helminths) (36). Release of EPO and other granule contents confers cytotoxic properties to eosinophils against these parasites. Eosinophils act in conjunction with basophils and mast cells as primary effectors in allergic inflammation and asthma. They express IgE receptors and stimulate histamine release from basophils and mast cells through the actions of MBP (30). Eosinophils can also regulate basophil and mast cell function by releasing enzymes that inactivate histamine and slow-reacting substance of anaphylaxis. Eosinophil-derived prostaglandins inhibit mast cell function. Eosinophil apoptosis has also been shown to be markedly delayed in atopic diseases (37).

Basophils and Mast Cells

Basophils and mast cells are central to the development of allergic inflammation. In addition, they produce cytokines, lipid mediators, vasoactive amines, and proteases that participate in nonallergic inflammatory responses. Mast cells share a common progenitor cell with basophils in the bone marrow but develop as a separate cell type (38). The primary growth factors for basophil development are IL-3 and GM-CSF (39). The primary growth factor for mast cells is stem cell factor, also called KIT ligand (40). Although basophils and mast cells are distinct cell types, they are often grouped together because of their similarity in granule content, activating stimuli, and effector functions.

Mature basophils constitute only 0.5% to 1% of circulating leukocytes. Mast cells do not circulate freely but rather are fixed in the connective tissue. The primary stimulus for basophil and mast cell activation and degranulation is binding of IgE antigen to the high-affinity IgE antibody receptor (FcεR). They are also activated by such diverse agents as contrast media, opiates, anaphylatoxins (C3a and C5a), chemokines, and neuropeptides. Basophils and mast cells elaborate both preformed and newly synthesized inflammatory mediators. The main basophil proteoglycan is chondroitin sulfate A (41). Mast cells contain heparin, chondroitin sulfate A, and chondroitin sulfate E. Mast cell granules also store neutral proteases.

There are two subpopulations of mast cells based on the neutral proteases. The subpopulation designated MC_{TC} produces tryptase, chymase, cathepsin G, and carboxypeptidase, and is found in the skin and small intestinal submucosa. The other subtype, designated MC_T, produces only tryptase and is found in lung and small intestinal mucosa (40). The latter subtype depends on T cells for its generation and maintenance. The lipid mediators LTB_4, LTC_4, and prostaglandin D_2 (PGD_2) are synthesized de novo in response to stimulation. The leukotrienes are powerful vasoconstrictors, bronchoconstrictors, and chemoattractants for neutrophils and eosinophils. PGD_2 inhibits platelet aggregation and is chemotactic for neutrophils. Of all the secretory products, histamine is the one classically associated with basophil and mast cell function.

Histamine

Both basophils and mast cells synthesize and secrete histamine. Histamine, or 2-(4-imidazolyl)ethylamine, is formed by the carboxylation of histidine (42). It is stored in preformed granules at acid pH as a complex with proteins and proteoglycans. Mast cells carry greater quantities of histamine than do basophils. The classic vasoactive properties of arteriolar dilatation, increased vascular permeability, and bronchoconstriction are mediated by the H_1 receptors (the target of most antihistamines). H_2 receptors are involved in modulation of the immune response and stimulating gastric output and mucus secretion. H_3 receptors participate in neuroconduction.

Monocytes and Macrophages

Monocytes and macrophages (the mononuclear phagocytes) are derived from the same stem cell precursor that gives rise to granulocytes. The stem cell differentiates in response to IL-3, GM-CSF, and monocyte colony-stimulating factor (M-CSF) into monoblasts and then into promonocytes that possess phagocytic capabilities (43). Promonocytes further differentiate into monocytes. Mature monocytes are the largest of the leukocytes and are characterized by round, eccentric nuclei and prominent pseudopodia. Blood monocytes have the shortest life span of all circulating leukocytes, circulating in blood only 1 to 2 days before migrating into tissues and differentiating into macrophages (7,14). Monocytes constitutively migrate into different tissues during homeostasis. Once inside the tissues, monocytes undergo transformation into macrophages that reside there for months to years. Macrophages are found in practically every tissue in the body. The phenotype of macrophages varies according to the tissue in which they differentiate and their state of activation. Differentiated macrophages include Kupffer cells of the liver, alveolar macrophages of the lung, and brain microglial cells. Resident macrophages are typically found at interfaces with blood (liver, spleen) and with lymph (lymph nodes and gastrointestinal tract), where they can readily detect, ingest, and destroy invading microorganisms. Interferon-γ (IFN-γ) is the primary activator of macrophages (44). Other important activators include GM-CSF, TNF, IL-1, and LPS. Activated macrophages and monocytes can produce approximately 100 different products, including GM-CSF, M-CSF, and G-CSF. They are also important sources of IL-1, TNF, eicosanoids (arachidonic acid metabolites), and NO (45) (Table 6.3).

Table 6.3. MACROPHAGE PRODUCTS

Product	Functions
Enzymes	
Lysozyme	Antimicrobial
Urokinase	Plasminogen activation and fibrinolysis, neutral proteinase activation
Collagenase	Connective tissue catabolism
Angiotensin-converting enzyme	Vasopressor
Acid hydrolases (many)	Lysosomal digestion
Cytokines	
IL-1	Multiple local and systemic host defense functions
TNF	Multiple local and systemic host defense functions
IFN-α/β	Antiviral, immune modulation
IL-6	Acute-phase response
IL-10	Antiinflammatory cytokine, antigen presentation cell functions
IL-12, IL-18	Stimulate IFN-γ production by NK and helper T cells
FGF	Fibroblast growth
GMN-CSF	Granulocyte, macrophage, and DC growth and differentiation
IL-8	Granulocyte chemoattractant
MIP-1α/β	Chemoattractant, hematopoietic regulator
MCP-1	Monocyte recruitment
RANTES	Recruitment of monocytes and helper T cells
MDC	Chemotactic for DC and NK cells
Complement proteins	Local opsonization and complement activation
Coagulation factors	Local initiation and regulation clotting
Adhesion, matrix molecules	Localization, migration; modulation of cellular interactions and phagocytosis
Fibronectin, thrombospondin, proteoglycan	
Transport proteins	
Transferrin	Iron transport
B_{12}-binding protein	Vitamin transport
Apolipoprotein E	Lipid transport
Bioactive lipids	
Cyclooxygenase, lipooxygenase, products of arachidonate	Inflammatory mediators (e.g., pain, vasodilation, edema)
Platelet-activating factor	Platelet activation
Reactive oxygen intermediates	Killing and stasis of microorganisms and cells by activated macrophages
Superoxide anion, hydrogen peroxide, single oxygen, hydroxyl radicals	
Reactive nitrogen intermediates	Killing of microbial, parasitic, and cellular targets by activated macrophages, inflammatory mediator
Nitric oxide, nitrites, nitrates	
Defensins	Antibacterial

DC, dendritic cell; FGF, fibroblast growth factor; GM-CSF, granulocyte/macrophage colony-stimulating factor; IFN, interferon; IL, interleukin; MCP, membrane cofactor protein; MDC, macrophage-derived chemokine; MIP, macrophage inflammatory protein; NK, natural killer; RANTES, regulated on activation, normally T-cell expressed and secreted; TNF, tumor necrosis factor.

Modified from Gordon S. Development and distribution of mononuclear phagocytes: relevance to inflammation. In: Gallin JI, Snyderman R, eds. Inflammation: basic principles and clinical correlates, 3rd ed. Philadelphia: Lippincott Williams & Wilkins, 1999.

During inflammation, monocytes, like other leukocytes, are mobilized and recruited from the blood by adhesion to the endothelium, followed by transendothelial migration and locomotion to the target tissue. Monocytes are recruited to sites of inflammation in response to chemoattractants such as PAF, C5a, and the CC chemokines (46). RANTES, MIP-1α, and chemokines of the MCP family are important monocyte–macrophage chemotaxins (47). Mononuclear phagocytes in turn elaborate chemoattractants such as IL-8, PAF, and LTB$_4$ that recruit neutrophils and other leukocytes. The adhesion molecule L-selectin mediates the loose reversible tethering of monocytes to endothelial cells. Firm adhesion of monocytes to the endothelium involves the interactions of β_1 and β_2 integrins on monocytes with the cell adhesion molecules intercellular adhesion molecule-1 (ICAM-1) and vascular cell adhesion molecule-1 (VCAM-1) on endothelial cells (48).

A defining feature of monocytes and macrophages is their phagocytic capacity. Monocytes and tissue macrophages phagocytize particulate material through two distinct receptors present in their plasma membrane: the IgG receptor (FcγR) and the receptor for the complement factor C3b. Fc receptors of macrophages recognize pathogens targeted by specific antibodies. Terminal sugar patterns on the surfaces of infectious agents also allow recognition by macrophages for nonspecific phagocytosis (49). The respiratory burst seen in the mononuclear phagocytes is similar to that of neutrophils. Blood monocytes carry MPO in their cytoplasmic granules. MPO is released into phagosomes after particle ingestion and can react with H_2O_2 and halides to produce toxic hypohalous acids, superoxide anion, H_2O_2, and hydroxyl radical. Peroxidase activity diminishes with further differentiation of monocytes to macrophages. On activation, however, macrophages can release H_2O_2, hydroxyl radical, and singlet oxygen. Macrophages can use peroxidase released by adjacent neutrophils, eosinophils, and monocytes and acquired through endocytosis. When phagocytosis occurs, there is some release of cytotoxic lysosomal enzymes to the exterior of the cell. Released serine proteases (plasminogen activator), cysteine proteases (cathepsins B, H, and L), and metalloproteinases (collagenase, gelatinase) can effect injury to the surrounding tissue. Macrophages also play an important immunoregulatory role by scavenging apoptotic neutrophils at sites of inflammation and apoptotic thymocytes during positive and negative selection of T cells (50).

The functions of the mononuclear phagocytes are intimately related to those of T lymphocytes. Mononuclear phagocytes are antigen-presenting cells (APC) (51). Portions of phagocytosed materials are processed and presented on the cell surface to T lymphocytes during the development of specific immunity. The processed antigen is expressed in conjunction with major histocompatibility complex (MHC) molecules on the APC surface that are recognized specifically by T-cell receptors. CD4+ T cells, or helper T cells, recognize MHC class II molecules on the APC surface and stimulate B cells to differentiate into memory B cells or specific antibody-producing plasma cells. The activated helper T cells can also stimulate macrophage production of NO, oxygen intermediates, and other inflammatory mediators. CD8+ cytotoxic T lymphocytes (CTL) recognize MHC class I molecules and can induce target cell lysis. Monocytes and activated macrophages release IL-12, the major activator of the type 1 helper T cell (T$_H$1) subset of T lymphocytes, which themselves produce a host of inflammatory cytokines. Monocytes also elaborate IL-15, whose actions are similar to those of IL-2 (T-cell growth factor) (43). Optimal macrophage activation requires both IFN-γ and an agent to sensitize the macrophage to IFN-γ. Both activators can be provided by activated T lymphocytes. CD40 ligand (CD40L) on T cells can bind CD40 on macrophages to sensitize the macrophage. Alternatively, membrane-associated TNF or lymphotoxin (TNF-β) found on lymphocytes can activate macrophage TNF synthesis and sensitize the macrophage. IL-10 from T cells promotes monocyte maturation and macrophage differentiation (52).

Lymphocytes

The lymphoid division of hematopoiesis gives rise to the lymphocytes. There are three varieties of lymphocytes: B cells, T cells, and NK cells. B and T lymphocytes respond to specific antigens, whereas NK cells do not have antigenic specificity. NK cells, also called *large granular lymphocytes,* make up approximately 15% of the total lymphocyte population and are a part of the innate, or nonspecific immune response. They are the first line of defense against many viral infections. Virus-infected cells lose surface expression of MHC class I molecules. The lack of the normally expressed MHC class I molecules serves as the target for NK cells. NK cells bind cell-bound antibody and participate in antibody-dependent cell cytotoxicity (ADCC). Cells targeted by antibody engagement or by the lack of appropriate MHC class I signal undergo cell death (53).

B and T lymphocytes are central to the adaptive, or specific, immune response. B lymphocytes (B cells) and T lymphocytes (T cells) are unique in that they proliferate in and outside the bone marrow. B cells develop in the bone marrow but reach final maturity in lymph nodes, spleen, and mucosal lymph nodules such as tonsils and Peyer patches. Activated B cells differentiate into antibody-producing plasma cells. Antigen–antibody reactions are involved in the neutralization of viruses and bacterial toxins, opsonization for phagocytosis, and complement activation. Activation of B cells requires antigen binding to cell surface receptors and stimulation by helper T-cell-derived cytokines. Polyclonal B-cell activation can occur in a T-cell-independent manner if the antigen has a large repeating polymeric sequence, as does Epstein-Barr virus or LPS. B cells are activated by free antigen; they do not need the help of APC (discussed in the section on T-Cell-mediated Immune Response) (54).

Development of T lymphocytes progresses from bone marrow to the thymus. Most developing T cells, or thymocytes, undergo apoptosis (programmed cell death) during positive and negative selection (55). Any ubiquitous protein synthesized by normal host cells will be presented in the thymus by APC. Thymocytes reactive to these self-proteins are deleted (negative selection) (56). Positive selection expands cells that respond to nonself antigen. IL-7 stimulates the proliferation and differentiation of developing T cells. There are two types of mature T cells, CD4+ (helper) T cells and CD8+ (cytotoxic) T cells. The mature T cell that leaves the thymus and enters the bloodstream is a committed CD4+ or CD8+ T cell (57).

Lymphocytes, the smallest of the leukocytes, constitute approximately 20% of circulating leukocytes (Table 6.1). Most circulating lymphocytes are T cells. Sixty percent of peripheral T cells are CD4+. The normal ratio of CD4+ to CD8+ T cells is 2 : 1. Lymphocytes continuously recirculate through lymph nodes, spleen, lymphatics, lymph nodules, and blood. A T cell that encounters its particular antigen can be activated to become an effector T cell. Activation of a T cell requires its specific antigen binding plus a costimulatory signal provided by the interaction between designated costimulatory molecules on the APC and their corresponding receptors on the T cell (57). CD4+ and CD8+ T lymphocytes each proliferate and differentiate into effector cells with specific functions.

The CD4+ or helper T cells recognize antigen presented on MHC class II molecules. Cytokines are the mediators of effector helper T cell functions. CD4+ T cells, like CD8+ T cells, produce IL-2 to stimulate growth and activation of T cells. Helper T cells are further divided into T_H1 and T_H2 effector cells (Fig. 6.2). The principal stimulus for differentiation of helper T cells to the T_H1 subtype is IL-12 produced by phagocytes on infection with intracellular bacteria such as *Mycobacteria* and *Listeria*. Interferons stimulate T_H1 development by augmenting IL-12 production from macrophages or by maintaining expression of IL-12 receptors on CD4+ T cells. The principal effector action of T_H1 cells is the activation of macrophages. T_H1 cells regulate production of opsonizing and complement-fixing antibodies and are effectors of phagocyte-dependent responses. T_H1 responses are also referred to as *cell-mediated immunity* (CMI) or *delayed-type hypersensitivity* (DTH) (58,59).

The principal stimulus for differentiation to the T_H2 subset of CD4+ T cells is IL-4. T_H2 cells are the cellular effectors of humoral, or antibody-mediated immunity. They

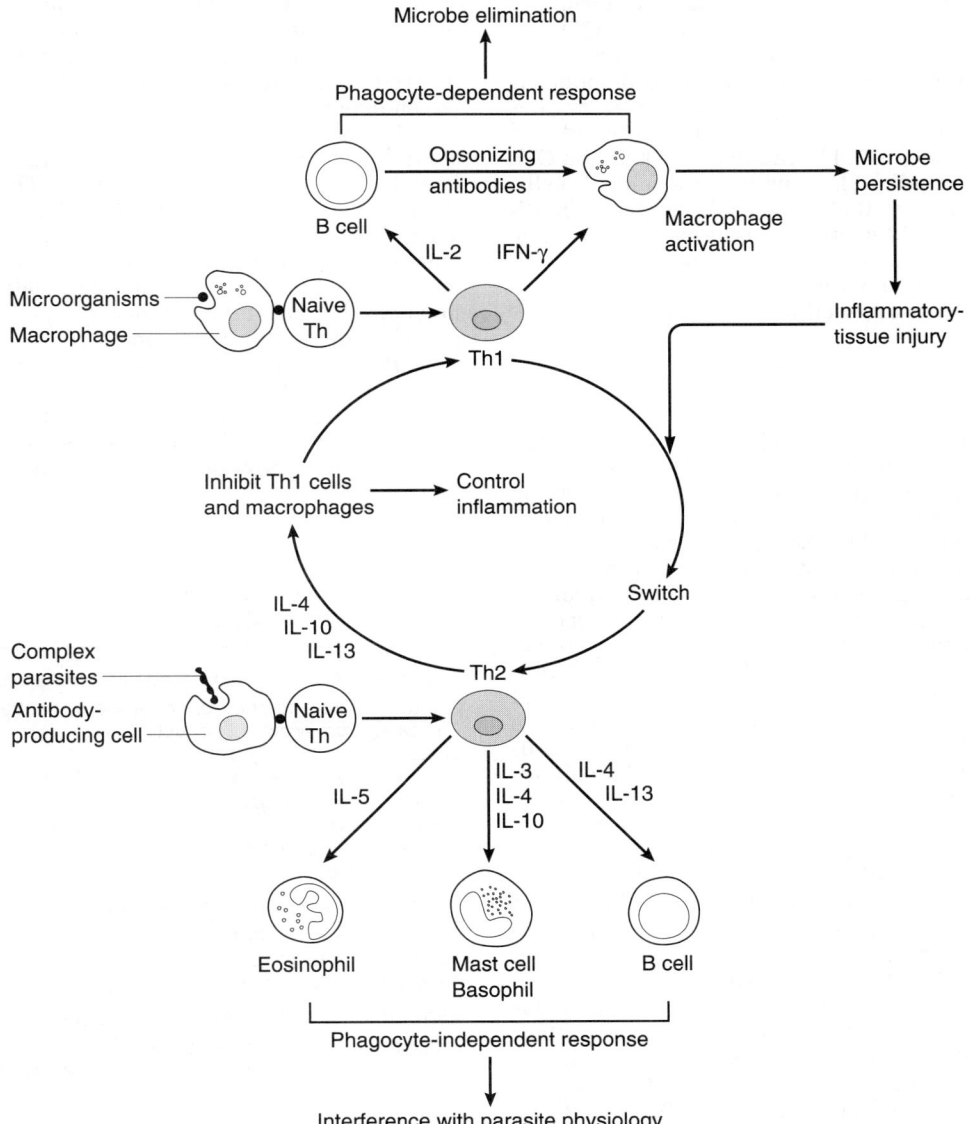

Figure 6.2. The helper T cell (T_H) T_H1/T_H2 paradigm. Microorganisms (especially intracellular parasites) are challenged by T_H1 cells, which are able to promote both the activation of microphages [through the release of interferon-γ (IFN-γ)] and the production of opsonizing antibodies [through the release of interleukin-2 (IL-2) and IFN-γ]. This phagocyte-dependent response usually promotes the elimination of the microorganism. If, despite such responses, the pathogen persists, the inflammatory reaction triggered by T_H1 cells and macrophages can result in tissue injury. Large and complex parasites, such as gastrointestinal nematodes, which cannot be rapidly eliminated by T_H1 cells because of their size, are challenged by T_H2 cells, which do not kill them but instead interfere with their physiology. T_H2 cells inhibit the development and function of T_H1 cells (through IL-4 and IL-10) as well as several macrophage functions (through IL-4, IL-10, and IL-13). Such a phagocyte-independent response may also occur as a result of a switch during infections that are not rapidly cleared by T_H1 cells, thus resulting in the control of dangerous inflammation. (Redrawn from Romagnani S. Understanding the role of T_H1/T_H2 cells in infection. *Trends Microbiol* 1996;4:470–473.)

produce B-cell-activating molecules such as IL-4, IL-5, and CD40L in addition to other proinflammatory and antiinflammatory cytokines. Activation of mast cells and eosinophils by extracellular pathogens is associated with activation of T_H2 cells. T_H2 cells down-regulate the inflammatory response by inhibiting macrophage functions and T_H1 responses. Helper T cells that express both T_H1 and T_H2 patterns of cytokine expression have been called T_H0 cells (60). The expanding population of helper T cell subsets also includes the T_H3 subtype that produces high quantities of TGF-β (61).

CD8+ effector cells are called cytotoxic T lymphocytes (CTL). CTL recognize viruses and other intracellular pathogens presented on MHC class I molecules. CTL kill their targets by inducing apoptosis, or programmed cell death. The primary mechanism of CTL-induced apoptosis is the release of the cytotoxins perforin and granzymes from cytoplasmic granules. Apoptosis can also be induced by the binding of Fas (CD95) ligand (FasL, CD95L) on CTL to Fas on the target cell (62). As with CD4+ helper T cells, early evidence suggests that CD8+ cells may also be divided into T_C1 and T_C2 subtypes based on their cytokine profiles and effector functions. The mechanisms of antigen presentation, costimulation, and effector T-cell functions are reviewed in the section on T-Cell-mediated Immune Response.

Platelets

Platelets (thrombocytes) are anucleated cytoplasmic fragments derived from the bone marrow megakaryocyte whose primary function is in thrombosis and hemostasis. However, it has become clear that thrombotic and inflammatory events are linked as part of the host defense to tissue injury.

Thrombin or abnormal endothelial surfaces in areas of vessel injury induce platelet aggregation and activation. Clot formation triggers platelet release of vasoactive agents and inflammatory mediators (Table 6.4). Vasoactive substances include the vasodilators PGE_2 and prostacyclin (PGI_2), and the vasoconstrictors $PGF_{2\alpha}$ and platelet-derived growth factor (PDGF). Serotonin, PGE_2, PAF, and cationic proteins increase vascular permeability. The adhesion molecule platelet–endothelial cell adhesion molecule (PECAM-1) and the β_3 integrins, or the cytoadhesins, on the surface of platelets are involved in platelet plug formation, endothelial cell adhesion, and leukocyte emigration. Platelet activity is the primary source of chemoattractants for neutrophils in blood and blood clots. Neutral proteinases released from stimulated platelets cleave complement factor C5, liberating the chemoattractant C5a. PDGF binds strongly to the extracellular matrix, providing a long-acting source of chemoattractant. Platelet factor 4 (PF_4) is a cationic protein that penetrates the vascular wall and is a chemoattractant. Thrombospondin released from activated platelets mediates monocyte binding to platelets. Together these substances promote leukocyte margination, activation, and recruitment to sites of injury (6).

Almost every neutrophil response at the site of inflammation is modulated by platelets. Platelets can either augment or attenuate neutrophil-mediated tissue injury by modulating neutrophil adherence to the endothelium, release of proteinases and inflammatory mediators, and oxygen radical generation. Neutrophils and platelets synergize to produce greater amounts of PAF than the sum of their individual production. The influx of platelets to sites of injury parallels that of neutrophils, peaking 1 to 3 hours from the onset of injury.

The vasoactive substances and inflammatory mediators of platelets are either stored in cytoplasmic granules or synthesized de novo. The dense granules contain adenosine diphosphate (ADP), adenosine triphosphate (ATP), serotonin, and calcium. ADP is the most important platelet agonist during platelet plug formation. The more abundant alpha granules contain fibrinogen, thrombospondin, P-selectin, PF_4, PDGF, TGF-β, high-molecular-weight kininogen, and many other biologically active proteins. The lipid mediators, including PAF and thromboxane A_2 (TXA_2), are newly synthesized on stimulation. PAF and TXA_2 are potent constrictors of vascular and bronchial smooth muscle. Among the many functions of PAF are platelet aggregation, increased vascular permeability, enhanced phagocyte free radical formation, and the adhesion of platelets to neutrophils. Platelet activation appears to occur in allergic asthma and may precede the delayed accumulation of eosinophils in the lung after allergen exposure. PF_4 can also stimulate histamine release from basophils (63).

Platelets are an important source of eicosanoids (metabolites of arachidonic acid). Thromboxane synthetase in platelets is responsible for the production of TXA_2. TXA_2 constricts vascular smooth muscle and increases vascular permeability. Its most important effect may be in stimulating platelet aggregation. Aspirin and nonsteroidal antiinflammatory drugs (NSAIDs) inhibit platelet function by inhibiting thromboxane production. The effects of aspirin on platelet function are irreversible. Only the production of sufficient numbers of new platelets, which requires 7 to 10 days, can reverse the effect of aspirin. Platelets participate in transcellular metabolism for lipooxygenase (LO) products. Transcellular

---

Table 6.4. FACTORS DERIVED FROM PLATELET ACTIVATION

CHEMOATTRACTANTS DERIVED FROM PLATELET ACTIVITY

C5a derived from complement cleavage by neutral proteinases released from activated platelets
Lipids
    12-Hydroxy eicosatetraenoic acid (12-HETE)
    Platelet-activating factor
    α-Granule proteins
    Platelet-derived growth factor
    Platelet factor 4

GROWTH FACTORS PRODUCED BY PLATELETS

Transforming growth factors α and β
Fibroblast growth factor
Platelet-derived growth factor

ANTIMICROBIAL ACTIVITY FROM PLATELETS

Cationic bactericidal protein (β lysin)
IgE-mediated oxidant production by platelets directed at schistosomes

VASOACTIVE SUBSTANCES FROM PLATELETS

Vasodilators
    Prostaglandin E_2
    Prostaglandin I_2
Vasoconstrictors
    Prostaglandin $F_{2\alpha}$
    Serotonin
    Platelet-derived growth factor

AGENTS RELEASED BY PLATELETS THAT INCREASE VASCULAR PERMEABILITY

Serotonin
Platelet-activating factor
Prostaglandin E_2
Cationic proteins (e.g., prostaglandin F_4)

metabolism refers to eicosanoid production through the interactions of neighboring cells of different types. Endothelial cells can use platelet-derived endoperoxides to synthesize PGI_2. Platelets interact with neutrophils in several pathways, providing a direct link between thrombosis and inflammation. Released 12-hydroxyeicosatetraenoic acid (12-HETE) from activated platelets can be used by unstimulated neutrophils to produce 12,20-diHETE, a chemoattractant that cannot be produced by either cell alone. 12-HETE from activated platelets and 5-HETE from activated neutrophils can combine in either cell type to form 5,12-diHETE. The diHETEs may have indirect antiinflammatory effects by diverting production away from the proinflammatory leukotrienes. 12-LO from platelets can act on LTA_4 formed by neutrophils to produce the intermediate 5(6)-epoxytetraene. This intermediate produces lipoxin A_4 and lipoxin B_4, vasoactive agents that have primarily counterinflammatory effects (64,65).

Erythrocytes

The primary function of the erythrocyte, or red blood cell, is to transport oxygen to and carbon dioxide from tissues. They may also play important roles in the acute inflammatory response. The enzyme adenosine deaminase may be involved in the acute inflammatory response after ischemia/reperfusion injury by metabolizing adenosine released from ischemic cells, liberating ammonia (NH_3). NH_3 amidates complement factor C3. Amidated C3 can act as an alternative complement pathway convertase, generating membrane attack complex (MAC) formation and stimulating phagocytic oxidative metabolism (66). Amidated C3 also stimulates release of superoxide and MPO from neutrophils. Antioxidant enzymes in erythrocytes may play a role in regulating oxidant-induced tissue injury during ischemia/reperfusion and other acute inflammatory responses in which phagocytes liberate reactive oxygen derivatives. Erythrocytes have large quantities of superoxide dismutase and catalase that function to neutralize superoxide anion and H_2O_2, respectively.

CELLULAR EFFECTOR MECHANISMS IN INFLAMMATION

Phagocyte–Endothelial Cell Interactions

The activity of phagocytic leukocytes against foreign particles is a nonspecific early line of defense in the battle against invading pathogens. Phagocytes are derived from both the granulocyte lineage (neutrophils, eosinophils, basophils) and mononuclear cell lineage (monocytes, macrophages). Circulating phagocytes are actively recruited to the site of injury through a well-orchestrated series of steps. Local resident mast cells and macrophages activate the neighboring endothelium, rapidly altering its surface properties. The activated endothelium is able to attract circulating leukocytes and prepare them for combat. Once localized, the leukocytes can respond more readily to soluble mediators that direct cells to the inflammatory focus. Phagocytic leukocytes engulf the offending pathogens and release toxic proteins and ROS both to propagate and contain the inflammatory response. Neutrophil influx is the most rapid. Mononuclear cell influx is slower but more persistent. Lymphocytes are also actively recruited in a similar manner, but are involved in specific immune responses that are discussed elsewhere. Central to the process of recruitment is the interaction between the circulating phagocytes and endothelial cells.

Vascular Response to Injury

The immediate vascular response to injury is the same regardless of whether the injury is due to physical, chemical, or microbial agents. Mediators of the vascular response include vasoactive amines (histamine, serotonin), kinins, complement factors, eicosanoids (prostaglandins, leukotrienes), PAF, neuropeptides, and NO. Vasodilation of local arterioles and the microvasculature leads to tissue congestion, or an "active hyperemia," to deliver cells to the inflammatory site. Edema fluid begins to accumulate secondary to the increased hydrostatic pressure in the microvasculature and larger intercellular gaps between endothelial cells as they contract. The pattern of vascular permeability changes is related to the intensity of injury. Mild injury causes increased permeability limited to the postcapillary venules, whereas severe injury is associated with increased permeability in postcapillary venules, capillaries, and arterioles (6,17).

Margination

Leakage of plasma out of the local vasculature in combination with the release of vasoactive substances leads to a relative hemoconcentration and stasis in the local microcirculation. Stasis promotes rouleaux formation by erythrocytes in the center of the bloodstream, whereas leukocytes move to the periphery of the vessel. This is referred to as *leukocyte margination*.

Rolling

The peripherally located leukocytes begin "rolling" along the vascular endothelium through a series of loose, reversible attachments. This rolling, or tethering, is mediated by transmembrane glycoproteins that bind sugar groups on other cell surfaces, the selectins. E-selectin and P-selectin are present on the endothelium, and L-selectin is found on leukocytes (Fig. 6.3).

L-selectin is exclusively and constitutively expressed on leukocytes. Cytokines such as TNF, GM-CSF, and G-CSF increase the affinity of leukocyte L-selectin for its counterreceptor. On leukocyte activation, L-selectin is rapidly shed from the cell surface. The endothelial selectins (P- and E-selectin) are up-regulated in response to inflammatory stimuli. P-selectin is stored intracellularly in the membranes of Weibel-Palade bodies of endothelial cells and platelet alpha granules and can therefore be expressed on the cell surface within minutes after activation. Fusion of these granules with the endothelial plasma membrane is stimulated by thrombin, histamine, complement fragments, oxygen species, LPS, and cytokines such as IL-1 and IFN-γ. E-selectin must be synthesized de novo and requires 4 to 6 hours for maximum expression in vivo. Substance P, LPS, TNF, IFN-γ, and IL-1 increase endothelial surface expression of E-selectin. Ligands for P- and E-selectins are polysaccharide structures, such as sialyl Lewis expressed on granulocytes, monocytes, and a small proportion of lymphocytes. P-selectin glycoprotein ligand is a ligand for both P- and E-selectin. Soluble P-selectin may have a role in maintaining the nonadhesiveness of circulating neutrophils and limiting inflammatory reactions or vascular damage (67–69).

Leukocyte Activation

Leukocytes become activated on tethering to the endothelial surface. Binding to endothelial selectins results in the up-regulation of leukocyte integrin expression. Activation of leukocytes requires the association of leukocyte-specific integrins and their endothelial ligands, cell adhesion molecules. PAF released by activated endothelial cells promotes leukocyte activation. Activated leukocytes have

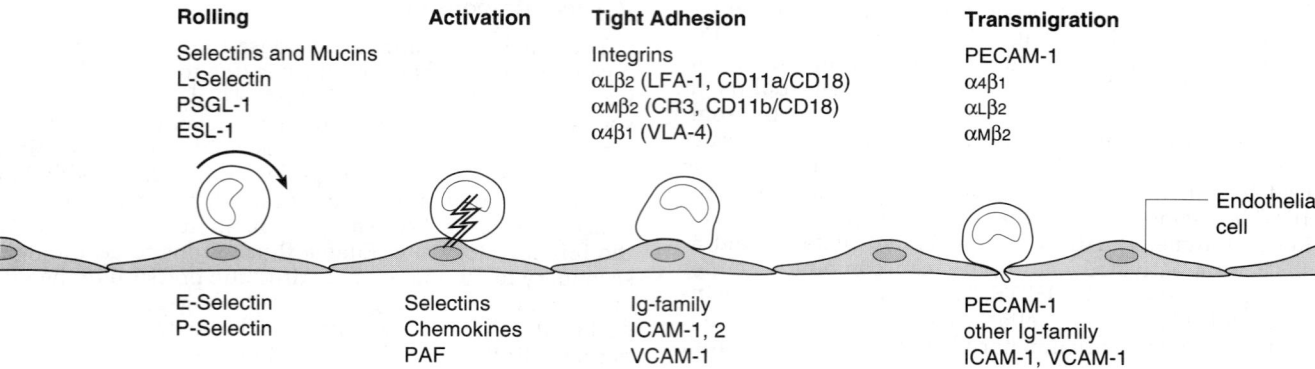

Figure 6.3. Leukocyte emigration is molecularly dissectable into distinct steps involving sequential interactions of different families of adhesion molecules on the leukocyte and endothelial cell. Some of the leukocyte adhesion molecules implicated in these steps are printed above the leukocytes, whereas those involved on the endothelial cells are printed below the endothelial cells *(shaded)*. The rolling step involves interaction between members of the selectin family of adhesion molecules and their sialylated Lewis-bearing ligands, some of which are on defined proteins that have been identified (P-selectin glycoprotein ligand, ESI-1). Leukocytes rolling along the endothelium are in a position to have their integrins activated by a variety of stimuli presented by the endothelial cell. Activation of integrin is followed rapidly by tight adhesion to the apical surface of the endothelial cell. This adhesion depends on leukocyte integrins of the β_2 family as well as $\alpha_4\beta_1$. Where the counterreceptors for this adhesion have been identified, they are members of the immunoglobulin gene superfamily. Adhesion must be reversible because the leukocytes crawl over the endothelium to an intracellular border. Transmigration involves the squeezing of leukocytes in ameboid fashion between tightly apposed endothelial cells. This step is sometimes referred to as *diapedesis*. Platelet–endothelial cell adhesion molecule (PECAM-1) on both leukocytes and endothelium plays a crucial role in this process. There is evidence that the leukocyte integrins and their counterreceptors are involved, as well. (Redrawn from Muller WA. Leukocyte recruitment in inflammatory disease. In: Peltz G, ed. Austin, TX: RG Landers, 1996:5.)

increased receptors for adhesion molecules and chemoattractants to facilitate firm adhesion and transmigration.

Adhesion

After the initial weak attachment, firm adhesion of activated leukocytes to the endothelium occurs through activated integrins of the β_2 family and $\alpha_4\beta_1$. ICAM-1 is the most important endothelial cell counterreceptor for the β_2 integrins. β_2 Integrins (the leukocyte integrins) are essential in the firm adhesion of leukocytes to endothelium. Neutrophils from people who lack the capacity to express functional β_2 integrins are unable to bind stably to the endothelial wall, resulting in a clinical condition known as *leukocyte adhesion deficiency*. These patients have neutrophilia, recurrent soft-tissue infections, and poor wound healing. Each β_2 integrin has a unique function in neutrophil binding. The β_2 integrin, $\alpha_L\beta_2$, also present on T cells, is commonly known as *lymphocyte functional antigen* (LFA-1). Its interaction with ICAM-1 is critical for maximal T-cell function in cell lysis, B-cell help, antigen-induced mitogenesis, and the mixed lymphocyte reaction. $\alpha_M\beta_2$ (CR3) binds the complement factor C3 fragment iC3b. Secretory granules in neutrophils are the major reservoir for $\alpha_M\beta_2$ and $\alpha_X\beta_2$. Translocation of the β_2 integrins from secretory granules occurs during stimulation with inflammatory mediators. α_4 Integrins mediate both rolling and adhesion in recruitment of monocytes independent of selectins and b_2 integrins. $\alpha_4\beta_1$ Integrin, also known as very late antigen (VLA-4), binds VCAM-1 on the endothelial surface to mediate tight adhesion (70–72).

Transmigration

The transmigration, or diapedesis, of adherent leukocytes out of the postcapillary venule also depends on the integrins. The β_1 integrins, or VLAs, are cell surface receptors for the extracellular matrix constituents laminin, fibronectin, and collagens. The β_3 family of integrins consists of glycoprotein (gp) $III\beta III\alpha$ and the vitronectin receptor. Leukocyte PECAM-1 and endothelial PECAM-1 are crucial for transmigration of neutrophils and monocytes (70,71,73,74). PECAM is concentrated along the intercellular junctions of endothelial cells. The cell forces its way across the endothelium by thrusting pseudopods between endothelial cells and then squeezing through by ameboid movement. Locomotion and changes in cell shape are mediated by intracellular actin and myosin microfilaments. Once the leukocyte has crossed the endothelial layer, it must traverse the subendothelial basal lamina. This may involve proteolysis of extracellular matrix components, including collagen type IV, laminin, and fibronectin. Alternatively, it may involve interactions of the basal lamina with a distinct domain of leukocyte PECAM-1. Membrane-bound elastase localizes to the migrating front of neutrophils possibly to facilitate transendothelial migration. Whereas neutrophil transmigration into tissues occurs upon inflammatory stimulation, monocytes emigrate constitutively at low levels and differentiate into tissue macro-phages. On activation by inflammatory mediators, monocytes are actively recruited in higher numbers. T cells constitutively cross venules to lymph nodes.

Chemotaxis

The directed migration of leukocytes through tissue is due to chemotactic factors. These factors are usually water-soluble peptides of either endogenous or exogenous origin that direct leukocyte migration by forming concentration gradients leading to the inflammatory focus. Important neutrophil chemotaxins include complement C5a, IL-8, LTB$_4$, and fMLP. fMLP is the major chemotactic peptide secreted by bacteria. The ability of fMLP and C5a to increase permeability correlates with their activity as leukocyte chemoattractants. Endotoxin activates macrophages to produce IL-8 and macrophage chemotactic peptides. C5a may be involved in the initial recruitment of neutrophils, whereas prolonged recruitment may be due to the production of chemotactic cytokines such as IL-8 by emigrated leukocytes (46,75,76).

Which leukocyte subset will infiltrate a lesion is regulated by the differential expression of chemoattractant receptors and adhesion molecules on various leukocytes. Monocyte extravasation requires endothelial cells to express membrane cofactor protein-1 (MCP-1) at the cell to cell junction to allow diapedesis to occur along a chemoattractant gradient. Once inside the intima, the monocytes amplify the MCP-1 signal by synthesizing and secreting their own MCP-1. Chemotactic factors bind to specific receptors on the leukocyte plasma membrane resulting in an influx of calcium ions. Neutrophils move rapidly along a chemotactic gradient, whereas macrophages move slowly. Recruited leukocytes themselves can release chemotactic factors either as a result of phagocytosis or through other inflammatory mediators.

Phagocytosis

Phagocytosis is triggered when opsonin receptors on the phagocyte cell surface interact with ligands on the surface of a particle to be ingested. Opsonins are substances that enhance phagocytosis. Antibodies and complement factor C3b are the most important opsonins. Once an antibody coats the particle surface, the phagocyte can bind to the Fc fragment of the antibody and ingest the particle. C3b is fixed to the surface of microorganisms during complement activation. Both neutrophils and macrophages have C3b receptors. This receptor acts in conjunction with neutrophil and macrophage receptors for the Fc fragment of IgG. Other complement components such as mannose-binding protein can also act as opsonins. β_1 integrins act as opsonins by promoting the binding and ingestion of invasin-bearing bacteria such as *Yersinia* species. Phagocytosis mediated through Fc receptors leads to a proinflammatory response, whereas complement-mediated uptake does not initiate the same responses. Activation of the phagocyte results in the formation of pseudopods that engulf the particle. The ingested target is encapsulated in a membrane-bound phagolysosome derived from the fusion of lysosomes and phagosomes (77,78).

Pathogen Killing

The destruction of pathogens involves an oxygen-dependent pathway, in which a "respiratory burst" results in production of biologically active oxygen derivatives, and oxygen-independent pathways involving degranulation of toxic proteinases.

Degranulation (Oxygen-independent Killing). Chemotactic factors, chemokines, complement factors, FcγR ligands, proinflammatory cytokines, and possibly adhesion receptors stimulate degranulation in neutrophils. The fusion of cytoplasmic granules with the plasma membrane involves the receptor-triggered activation of PLA_2, phospholipase D (PLD), cytoplasmic protein tyrosine kinases, RHO proteins, and the generation of messengers through hydrolysis of phosphatidylinositol 4,5-bisphosphate (PIP_2) by G protein-coupled receptors. Once formed, the phagocytic vacuole (phagolysosome) fuses with cytoplasmic granules of the neutrophil and the granules discharge their contents into the phagosome. This is termed *degranulation*. During degranulation, lysosomal enzymes may leak out into the extracellular space, resulting in release of plasmin and other proteases that generate anaphylatoxin fragments of complement, release of kallikrein, and release of phospholipase, which can generate arachidonic acid. The neutrophil enzymes that appear to have the greatest potential to act as mediators of tissue destruction are elastase, collagenase, and gelatinase. These enzymes attack components of the extracellular matrix responsible for tissue architecture. Serum and tissue antiproteinases such as α_1-antitrypsin and α_2-macroglobulin limit the activity of these proteolytic enzymes. Hypochlorous acid (HOCl) can inactivate key proteinase inhibitors that are intended to protect the host tissues from injury. Antibacterial factors in neutrophil granules and their functions are listed in Table 6.2 (6,12, 16,79).

Oxygen-dependent Killing of Pathogens. Neutrophils have two oxygen-dependent defenses against microbes, the MPO system and the nonenzymatic respiratory burst. Macrophages produce toxic oxygen metabolites only through the respiratory burst.

The multicomponent NADPH oxidase, or respiratory burst oxidase, is present on the phagocyte plasma membrane. The activated NADPH oxidase consumes molecular oxygen and cytosolic NADPH as a source of electrons to produce superoxide. The active enzyme is assembled from proteins in the cytosolic and membrane compartments of neutrophils. The core components include flavocytochrome b_{558}, the electron transporting apparatus, which consists of gp91(phox) and p22(phox); the cytosolic components p47(phox) and p67(phox); and the oxidase cofactor Rac (Fig. 6.4). In resting neutrophils, most b_{558} is in the secondary granules. On neutrophil activation, b_{558} moves to the plasma membrane and phagolysosomes. Phosphorylation of p47(phox) with protein kinase C induces conformational changes resulting in the appearance of a binding site through which p47(phox) interacts with cytochrome b_{558} during the activation process. The cytochrome subunits gp91 and p22 are tightly bound in the membrane, with Rap1A also bound to the gp91 subunit. p47(phox), p67(phox), and guanosine diphosphate (GDP) dissociation inhibitor (GDI)–Rac2 complex are in the cytosol. On activation, GDI releases Rac2, and p47(phox) becomes phosphorylated. This causes translocation of Rac2, p47(phox), and p67(phox) to the membrane and complexation with the cytochrome components, thus completing assembly of the active oxidase. Phosphorylation of p47(phox) is mediated by protein kinase C, and dissociation of GDI–Rac2 may be mediated by lipid signal, such as arachidonate or phosphatidate (6,80).

Neutrophils of patients with chronic granulomatous disease have a defective NADPH oxidase system and are thus unable to generate superoxide. Although they are able to phagocytose bacteria, they are unable to kill the intracellular microbes, and chronic, unresolved infections result (18).

Digestion

Digestion of the dead microorganisms by lysosomal enzymes degrades any bacterial products that may perpetuate the inflammatory reaction. Lysosomal enzymes are also capable of activating complement, which in turn can promote even more phagocyte chemotaxis. Cells that have successfully ingested pathogens may travel to regional lymph nodes where, in the case of dendritic cells (DC) or macrophages, they may become potent antigen-presenting cells. Apoptosis is a major means of clearing neutrophils from an inflammatory site. In fact, only apoptotic neutrophils are engulfed by macrophages (50).

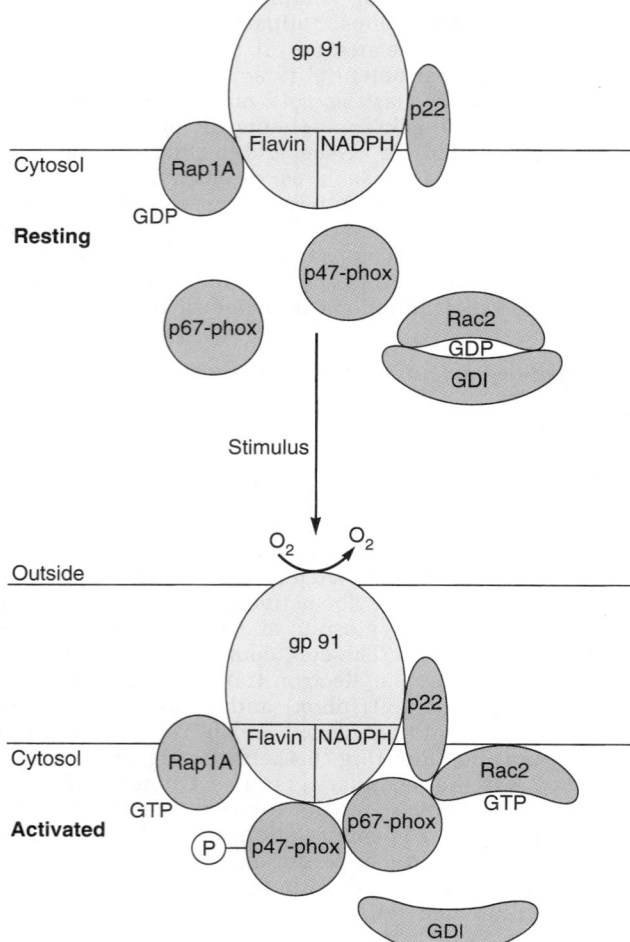

Figure 6.4. Activation of the reduced nicotinamide-adenine dinucleotide phosphate (NADPH) oxidase in human neutrophils. In the resting neutrophil, the cytochrome subunits gp91 and p22 are tightly bound in the membrane, with Rap1A also bound to the gp91 subunit. p47(phox), p67(phox), and guanosine diphosphate (GDP) dissociation inhibitor (GDI)–Rac2 complex are in the cytosol. On activation, GDI releases Rac2, and p47(phox) becomes phosphorylated. This causes translocation of Rac2, p47(phox), and p67(phox) to the membrane and complexation with the cytochrome components, thus completing the assembly of the active oxidase. Phosphorylation of p47(phox) is mediated by protein kinase C, and dissociation of GDI–Rac2 may be mediated by lipid signal, such as arachidonate or phosphatidate. Other components also may be involved.

T-Cell–mediated Immune Response

Many of the microorganisms that invade the body are eliminated by being engulfed and destroyed by phagocytes. Pathogens that can evade elimination by this first line of defense, the innate immune system, must be removed by other means. It is the function of the adaptive, or antigen-specific immune response, to eliminate such pathogens. There are two major types of adaptive immune responses: cell-mediated immunity and humoral immunity. CMI is also called *delayed-type hypersensitivity*. CMI is mediated by the T_H1 subtype of CD4+ helper T lymphocytes, cytotoxic CD8+ lymphocytes, and macrophages. Humoral immunity is mediated by T_H2 CD4+ cells, B cells, plasma cells, and antibodies. The division is an oversimplification as there is considerable overlap between the

two pathways. Antibody formation and the humoral immune system are better addressed in a discussion of immunology. Presented here is a brief review of the T-cell-mediated adaptive immune responses.

Activation of naive T lymphocytes into effector T lymphocytes (CTL, T_H1, or T_H2 cells) requires an antigen-specific signal (signal 1) and a nonspecific costimulatory signal (signal 2). Both signals are provided by specialized APC localized in lymphoid organs.

Antigen-presenting Cells

T cells can recognize only those antigens associated with surface MHC molecules. MHC class I molecules are expressed on all nucleated cells, whereas MHC class II molecules are expressed only on antigen-presenting cells (APC). APC present peptide fragments of antigenic proteins to recirculating T lymphocytes in the form of an antigen–MHC molecule complex. The three professional APC are DC, macrophages, and B cells (54) (Fig. 6.5).

Dendritic cells (DC) are the most potent and specialized APC. DC, named for their appearance when fixed, share a common origin with macrophages, but become specialized to process and present antigen to naive T cells. They develop by one of several pathways. Monocytes stimulated with M-CSF, GM-CSF, and IL-4 are driven toward macrophage maturation, whereas those stimulated with GM-CSF and IL-4 or IL-13 differentiate toward DC. Maturation of DC requires cytokine (TNF) or LPS stimulation. Tissue DC such as the epidermal Langerhans cells are immature DC. They have phagocytic capabilities but lack costimulatory activity. If these tissue DC encounter antigen, they become activated, travel through the lymph to lymphoid organs, and differentiate into mature DC. As mature DC, they have costimulatory function but lose their phagocytic capacity. Monocytes that reverse-transmigrate have the phenotype of immature DC. Monocytes that reverse-transmigrate in the presence of inflammatory stimuli become mature DC (81,82).

Each of the professional APC is specially equipped to present certain types of antigen. DC are particularly effective in presenting viral proteins. Most viral protein is found in the cytosol. Cytosolic viral protein is processed and presented in conjunction with MHC class I molecules on the surface of the APC. MHC class I molecules are recognized by CD8+ T lymphocytes. Viral envelope proteins translocate to the endoplasmic reticulum, where they can be processed in endosomes and presented on MHC class II molecules to stimulate either a CD4+ T_H1 response or a T_H2 response. Therefore, in many viral infections, DC prime both CD8+ and CD4+ T cells. DC can also present antigens derived from apoptotic cells in the context of MHC class I (83).

Macrophages present antigenic peptides from ingested pathogens that persist in the phagosomes. These peptides, usually bacterial in origin, are expressed in conjunction with MHC class II molecules on the macrophage surface. B cells bind specific soluble molecules through their cell surface immunoglobulins. The bound antigen is endocytosed, processed, and presented on surface MHC class II molecules. Insect toxins, venoms, and allergens are examples of such soluble antigens. The importance of B cells as APC in vivo is not fully known (83–85).

A third mechanism of T-cell recognition involves lipid antigens such as cell wall antigens from intracellular bacteria such as *Mycobacterium leprosum*. These antigens bind CD1, an MHC-related cell surface molecule, that presents these antigens to certain subtypes of T cells (86). A superantigen is an unprocessed bacterial or retroviral product that binds the MHC molecule and the T-cell receptor outside the usual antigen-binding sites. Superantigen bind-

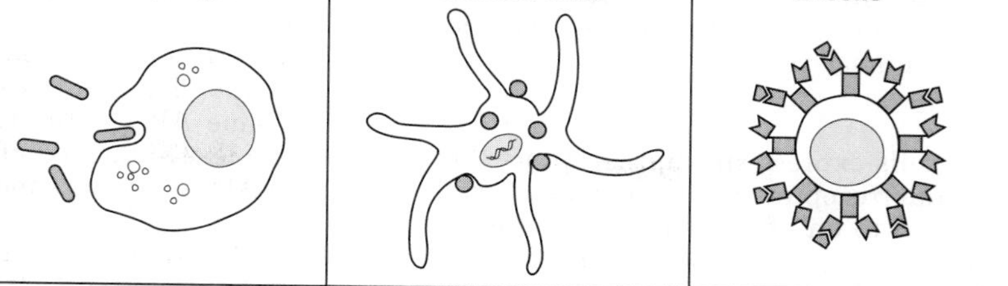

	Macrophages	Dendritic cells	B cells
Antigen uptake	Phagocytosis +++	+++ Phagocytosis by tissue dendritic cells. ++++ Viral infection	Antigen-specific receptor (Ig) ++++
MHC expression	Inducible by bacteria and cytokines - to +++	Constitutive ++++	Constitutive. Increases on activation +++ to ++++
Co-stimulator delivery	Inducible - to +++	Constitutive; by mature non-phagocytic lymphoid dendritic cells. ++++	Inducible - to +++
Antigen presented	Particulate antigens. Intracellular and extracellular pathogens	Peptides. Viral antigens (allergens?)	Soluble antigens. Toxins. Viruses
Location	Lymphoid tissue. Connective tissue. Body cavities	Lymphoid tissue. Connective tissue. Epithelia	Lymphoid tissue. Peripheral blood

Figure 6.5. The properties of professional antigen-presenting cells. Macrophages, dendritic cells, and B cells are the major cell types involved in the initial presentation of exogenous antigens to naïve T cells. These cells vary in their means of antibody uptake, major histocompatibility complex (MHC) class II expression, costimulator expression, the antigens that appear to be crucial for presentation, and their locations in the body. (Redrawn from Janeway CA Jr, Travers P. *Immunobiology: the immune system in health and disease,* 3rd ed. 1997;7:15.)

ing leads to polyclonal stimulation of whole families of T cells and is likely involved in the pathogenesis of toxic shock syndrome and certain autoimmune diseases (87).

Primary Immune Response

The first encounter of naïve T cells with antigen on APC is the primary immune response. The primary immune response results in the formation of effector T cells and memory T cells that respond more vigorously and expeditiously to the same antigen (54). Memory T lymphocytes still require activation by professional APC to regenerate effector T cells.

Pathogens or their products are carried constitutively to the local downstream lymph nodes. Pathogens in the blood travel to the spleen. Those on mucosal surfaces localize to lymphoid nodules such as Peyer patches or tonsils. Professional APC are concentrated in these peripheral lymphoid organs. Some APC circulate and pick up pathogens at sites of infection, then travel to the local lymph nodes. There they wait for the specific T lymphocytes that will recognize their antigen.

Naïve T lymphocytes circulate continuously between blood and lymphoid organs, making contact with many APC and "sampling" their antigens. Lymphocytes enter the cortical region of lymph nodes by migrating across the high endothelial venules (88). The homing of naïve T cells to lymphoid organs requires selectins. L-selectin, found constitutively on all lymphocytes, binds sialyl Lewis carbohydrate on the endothelium. For example, L-selectin on lymphocytes binds GlyCAM-1 on the high en-

dothelial venules in lymph nodes. Another ligand for L-selectin, MAdCAM-1 (mucosal addressin cell adhesion molecule-1) on the endothelium of mucosa, guides the lymphocyte entry into mucosal lymphoid tissues. The migration of lymphocytes across the endothelium requires integrins. Lymphocyte functional antigen-1 (LFA-1), a member of the β_2 integrin family (the leukocyte integrin family), is the most important adhesion molecule for lymphocyte activation (89). Binding of LFA-1 to ICAM-1 and ICAM-2 on endothelial cells facilitates migration. Most lymphocytes are carried back to the blood by the efferent lymphatics. If a T lymphocyte recognizes its specific antigen on the surface of an APC, it remains for several days, then returns to blood as an armed effector T cell ready to home to the site of infection.

Adhesion molecules mediate the transient interactions between T cells and APC required for the T cell to sample each antigen it encounters. Lymphocyte LFA-1 can bind to the APC in a loose, reversible fashion by ICAM-1, ICAM-2, and ICAM-3 on the APC. If a match between T cell and antigen is found, conformational changes in LFA-1 greatly increase its affinity for ICAM-1 and ICAM-2 to stabilize the association between lymphocyte and APC. The T cell can then proliferate and differentiate into armed effector T cells. Effector T cells lose surface expression of L-selectin and no longer recirculate through lymph nodes. Instead, they express VLA-4, a β_1 integrin, which binds vascular endothelium at sites of infection. Effector T cells have increased LFA-1 and CD2 adhesion molecule expression that facilitates tight binding to the target cell (90,91).

Binding of the T-cell receptor to its specific antigen on the MHC molecule is the first signal for activation. The second signal, costimulation, is required for antigen-specific clonal expansion of the T cells.

Costimulation

Antigen-presenting cells express specific receptors that must bind to their counterreceptors on the attached T cell to convert a naïve T cell to an effector T cell. These costimulatory molecules on the APC surface are the B7 molecules, B7.1 (CD80) and B7.2 (CD86). The costimulatory signal must come from the same APC that provides signal 1 (57,92). DC are the most potent APC because they express both classes of MHC molecules and the B7 molecules constitutively. Macrophages and B cells must be activated to express the costimulatory molecules. The only counterreceptor on naïve T cells is CD28. Activated T cells express CTLA-4 (CD152), which binds B7 molecules 20 times more avidly than CD28 does (93). Activated T cells are induced to produce IL-2 (T-cell growth factor) and IL-2 receptor (IL-2R). IL-2 drives further proliferation and differentiation. CTLA-4 regulates the proliferative response by limiting the amount of IL-2 production (94).

The absence of costimulation results in an unresponsive, or anergic T cell. Anergic T cells do not produce IL-2 and therefore cannot proliferate and differentiate into effector cells even when presented with antigen at a later time. A three-signal model of T-cell activation has been proposed. Signal 1 is antigen binding. Signal 2 is the association of B7 molecules with CD28 on T cells. Signal 3 is the association of B7 molecules with CTLA-4. Signal 1 plus signal 3 results in anergy. All three signals could result in either activation or anergy, depending on specific conditions (95–97) (Fig. 6.6).

The differentiation of naïve CD8+ T cells to cytotoxic T lymphocytes (CTL) requires a stronger costimulatory signal. This can be provided by either DC as the APC, as they have the greatest intrinsic co-stimulatory activity, or by a CD4+ helper T lymphocyte. Naive helper T cells attached to the same APC as the CD8+ T cell can be activated to elaborate IL-2. Attached effector helper T cells can stimulate the APC to express more co-stimulatory molecules. In the case of virulent viruses, cytotoxicity substitutes for CD28 costimulation, and so the typical costimulatory signal is not required for activation. For less virulent viruses, costimulation is necessary for CTL induction (95).

The initial encounter between T cells and APC induces expression of CD40 ligand (CD40L). CD40L combines with CD40 on APC to stimulate expression of B7 molecules or result in CD28-independent costimulation. Effector cells do not require a costimulatory signal. When effector T cells encounter their specific antigens at the site of infection, they can immediately attack their target cells.

Effector T-Cell Functions

Cytotoxic lymphocytes, the CD8+ effector cells, target cells expressing viruses and other intracellular pathogens presented on MHC class I molecules. CTL kill their targets by inducing apoptosis, or programmed cell death. The most important mechanism of CTL-induced apoptosis is the calcium-dependent release of cytotoxic granule contents. Perforin and granzymes are the chief cytotoxins elaborated by CTL. Granzymes are serine proteases that trigger DNA fragmentation and apoptosis. Perforin stimulates cell membrane pore formation that facilitates granzyme entrance to cells. Fas ligand (FasL) (CD95L) is a membrane protein expressed on CTL that initiates apoptosis on binding to Fas on the target cell. CTL also release

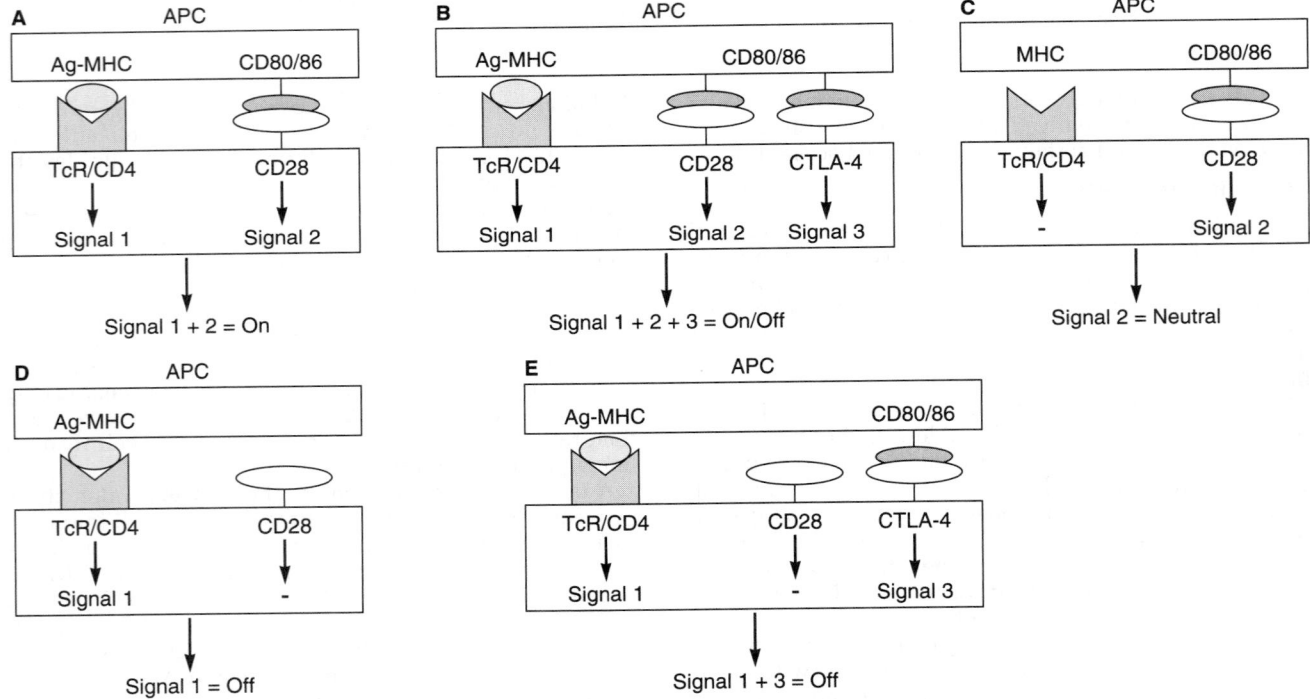

Figure 6.6. The three-signal model of lymphocyte activation. Different types of antigen-presenting cells activate distinct forms of signal transduction in T cells, leading to differential signaling to CD28 and CTLA-4 (CD152), and the balance of signals determines the outcome of activation, anergy, or apoptosis. (Redrawn from Lee KP, Harlan DM, June CH. Role of co-stimulation in the host response to infection. In: Gallin JI, Snyderman R, eds. *Inflammation: basic principles and clinical correlates,* 3rd ed. Philadelphia: Lippincott Williams & Wilkins, 1999:193.)

the cytokines IFN-γ, TNF, and CC chemokines. IFN-γ and certain CC chemokines have antiviral properties, and both IFN-γ and TNF are potent activators of macrophage function. IL-2 produced by CTL and local helper CD4+ lymphocytes expands CTL. IL-12 released by APC also stimulates CTL activity (62).

The CD4+ or helper T cells recognize antigen presented on MHC class II molecules. Effector helper T cells secrete cytokines that promote proliferation, differentiation, and activation of inflammatory cells. The differentiation to either the T_H1 or T_H2 subset is determined at the first encounter between the naïve CD4+ T cell and antigen (58,59). APC produce IL-12, favoring the T_H1 response, or cell-mediated immunity (CMI). IL-12 also stimulates production of IFN-γ, the principal macrophage activator, by NK cells and CD4+ T lymphocytes. The actions of T_H1 responses are macrophage dependent. T_H1 cells produce macrophage-activating molecules including IFN-γ, GM-CSF, TNF, CD40L, and FasL, in addition to other cytokines. T_H1 CMI responses are protective against most invading organisms and usually result in the elimination of the pathogen. If the pathogen persists, the ongoing T_H1 response can result in injury to host tissue.

T cells, mast cells and basophils produce IL-4, which drives T_H2 formation and the humoral, or antibody-mediated response. T_H2 cells inhibit macrophage functions and T_H1 responses, resulting in the down-regulation of the inflammatory response. It is likely that the initial helper T-cell response is T_H1 mediated, followed by a shift to T_H2 responses (58) (Fig. 6.2).

Reactive Oxygen Species

Free radicals and reactive oxygen species (ROS) are implicated in the pathogenesis of practically every inflammatory condition. A free radical is any species capable of independent existence that contains one or more unpaired electrons. Free radicals may be positive, negative, or neutral in charge. The term *reactive oxygen species* includes free radicals as well as molecules such as H_2O_2 that are capable of radical formation in the extracellular and intracellular environments. Activated phagocytes (neutrophils, monocytes, macrophages, and, to a lesser extent, eosinophils) are the primary generators of ROS. ROS have extremely short half-lives (10^{-11} to 10^{-6} seconds) but can cause significant tissue injury by initiating free radical chain reactions. The most important species implicated in inflammatory injuries to tissues are the superoxide anion, the hydroxyl radical, H_2O_2, singlet oxygen, NO, and peroxynitrite. ROS can have direct toxicity to local tissues and can act as the early alarm molecules that activate inflammatory cells and stimulate release of proinflammatory cytokines. There is evidence that ROS can mediate proinflammatory events through indirect mechanisms such as assembly of MAC in complement and inactivation of normal serum leukocyte protease inhibitors. They also have been shown to activate apoptotic pathways (98,99).

Superoxide Anion

Reduction of molecular oxygen by a single electron results in formation of the superoxide anion:

$$O_2 + e^- \rightarrow O_2^{\cdot -} \tag{1}$$

This reaction may occur accidentally because 5% of electrons leak through their carriers in the respiratory chain of mitochondria (100). The most important sources of superoxide, however, are from the activation of NADPH oxidase (or hexose monophosphate) and MPO systems (as in the respiratory burst) in phagocytes. Lymphocytes and fibroblasts produce superoxide to a lesser degree. Other mechanisms of superoxide production in inflammation include uncoupling of the xanthine dehydrogenase system, uncoupling of mitochondrial and endoplasmic reticulum electron transport chains, and nonenzymatic reactions such as autooxidation of hemoglobin and thiol compounds by oxygen. The mechanism for superoxide production in ischemic tissues involves the cell's inability to maintain proper ion gradients as ATP levels fall due to decreased oxidative phosphorylation. The resulting elevated cytosolic calcium concentration activates a protease that catalyzes the conversion of xanthine dehydrogenase to xanthine oxidase. When the ischemic site is reperfused, xanthine oxidase catalyzes the conversion of hypoxanthine and xanthine to uric acid. Superoxide and H_2O_2 are generated as by-products of this reaction (101). Superoxide exists in equilibrium with its protonated form, perhydroxyl radical:

$$O_2^{\cdot -} + H^+ \leftrightarrow HO_2^{\cdot} \tag{2}$$

At neutral or alkaline pH, almost all this is in the form of superoxide. The local acidic environment in phagosomes may drive the equilibrium toward perhydroxyl radical, a stronger oxidant than superoxide anion. Superoxide itself is a relatively weak radical, but can spontaneously dismutate in aqueous solution to form H_2O_2 and singlet oxygen:

$$2H^+ + O_2^{\cdot -} + O_2^{\cdot -} \rightarrow H_2O_2 + O_{2(singlet)} \tag{3}$$
$$\text{spontaneous or via superoxide dismutase (SOD)}$$

Superoxide can also be converted to the more potent hydroxyl radical through the metal-catalyzed Haber-Weiss reaction:

$$H_2O_2 + O_2^{\cdot -} + Fe^{3+} \rightarrow O_2 + OH^- + {\cdot}OH + Fe^{2+} \tag{4}$$

Superoxide can react with nitric oxide (NO) in the vascular endothelium or in activated cells to form the hydroxyl radical through an intermediate peroxynitrite ion ($ONOO^-$):

$$NO^{\cdot} + O_2^{\cdot -} \rightarrow ONOO^- + H^+ \leftrightarrow$$
$$ONOOH \rightarrow {\cdot}OH + NO_2^{\cdot} \tag{5}$$

The roles of NO and peroxynitrite in inflammation are discussed later in a separate section:

Hydrogen Peroxide

Hydrogen peroxide can be produced by bacteria and after dismutation of superoxide in phagocytes (Equation 3). It is a weak oxidant with many physiologic functions, but has high potential to produce damage because of its ability to diffuse freely across cell membranes and undergo Fenton reactions to form hydroxyl radicals (eq. 6). Hydrogen peroxide can combine with MPO in the presence of halides to form hypohalous acids such as hypochlorous acid (HOCl). It can also effect cellular injury by synergizing with proteinases and activating NFκB to trigger proinflammatory cytokine release. ATP levels fall in cells exposed to H_2O_2 because of the oxidation of the glycolytic enzyme glyceraldehyde 3-phosphate dehydrogenase. H_2O_2 release also can stimulate apoptosis (27,98).

Hydroxyl Radical

The hydroxyl anion (${\cdot}OH$) is the most reactive oxidizing radical known to date. It is formed from superoxide through the Haber-Weiss reaction under physiologic conditions (Equation 4), or in increased amounts from H_2O_2 through the Fenton reaction:

$$H_2O_2 + Fe^2 \rightarrow Fe^{3+} OH^- + {\cdot}OH$$

$$Hb\text{-}Fe^{2+} + H_2O_2 \rightarrow Hb\text{-}Fe^{3+} + OH^- +$$
$${\cdot}OH \text{ (in erythrocytes)} \tag{6}$$

In the Haber-Weiss reaction, superoxide anion is the reductant. Other reducing agents such as glutathione (GSH), reduced pyridine nucleotides (NADH, NADPH), or ascorbate can substitute for superoxide as the required reductant for hydroxyl formation. Copper and other metals can also act in place of iron in the Haber-Weiss catalysis. Under physiologic conditions, lactoferrin found in neutrophil specific granules provides the iron catalyst for the Haber-Weiss reaction. Both lactoferrin and transferrin can catalyze hydroxyl radical formation, but only when fully saturated with iron. Partially saturated lactoferrin or transferrin inhibits the catalysis. In the Fenton reaction, superoxide or other biologic reducing agents such as lactate or ascorbate donate electrons to generate the ferrous ions required to react with H_2O_2 to form $\cdot OH$.

Mechanisms of tissue damage mediated by hydroxyl include DNA strand breaks and base hydroxylations leading to ATP depletion and gene mutations. The formation of single-strand breaks in DNA activates the enzyme poly(ADP-ribose) polymerase (PARP) as part of the repair process. ATP levels fall as NAD^+ is depleted by PARP if substantial DNA damage has occurred (25). It can also stimulate lipid peroxidation. When close to membrane phospholipids, the hydroxyl radical can attack lipid side chains to form radical intermediates called *peroxyl radicals,* H_2O_2, and lipid hydroperoxides. Hydroperoxides can disrupt membrane function or can decompose to form cytotoxic aldehydes. Lipid peroxidation end products also uncouple Ca^{2+}-ATPase, which leads to an accumulation of intracellular calcium. The activation of Ca^{2+}-dependent enzymes such as proteases and phospholipase then causes further cell damage.

Hypohalous Acids and the Myeloperoxidase System

Hypohalous acids are formed by neutrophil MPO or lactoperoxidase in the presence of halides such as chloride or bromide. Once formed, hypohalous acids are released extracellularly. The respiratory burst of phagocytes is the primary source of H_2O_2 for MPO-catalyzed reactions. The MPO–H_2O_2–halide system inactivates bacterial toxins and metabolites, while stimulating secretion of vasoactive agents from platelets and mast cells. It can regulate the complement pathway by differential stabilization of C1q, the initiating component of the classical pathway.

Hypochlorous acid (HOCl) is the most important hypohalous acid in vivo. HOCl is a powerful antibacterial agent capable of activating neutrophil collagenase and oxidizing α_1-antitrypsin, the major serum protease inhibitor limiting elastase-induced tissue injury. Cell lysis occurs at higher concentrations. HOCl can contribute to hydroxyl radical and singlet oxygen production. Hypochlorite (OCl^-), the dissociated form of HOCl, can chlorinate amino groups, resulting in monochloramine and dichloramine production. These metabolites are long-lived and can oxidize amino acid residues, heme proteins, membrane lipids, and sulfur-containing moieties. Chloramines can combine with halide anions to release toxic free halides that can halogenate cellular constituents. Combination of HOCl with taurine chloramine can result in the activation of complement C5 to trigger formation of MAC (24,98).

Singlet Oxygen

Singlet oxygen, a highly reactive and extremely short-lived species, is formed by an input of energy to O_2 that reverses the spin direction of one of the outermost unpaired electrons away from a parallel spin. It is produced during reactions of the MPO–H_2O_2–halide system and is a potential product of superoxide dismutation and the Haber-Weiss reaction. It is highly electrophilic and reacts with compounds containing electron-rich double bonds (e.g., unsaturated fatty acids) or unsaturated heterocyclic rings (e.g., some amino acids). Singlet oxygen reacts with membrane lipids to produce peroxides.

Antioxidants and the Defense against Reactive Oxygen Species

A delicate balance exists between prooxidant mechanisms of tissue damage and defense and repair systems. Superoxide is removed from tissues by spontaneous dismutation to H_2O_2, a process that can also be catalyzed by the enzyme superoxide dismutase (Equation 3). The susceptibility of cells to injury by H_2O_2 depends on the level of scavenging enzymes in the target cell. Hydrogen peroxide formed intracellularly is removed by the enzyme catalase:

$$\text{catalse } 2\,H_2O_2 \rightarrow 2\,H_2O + O_2 \qquad (7)$$

The role of catalase in the extracellular environment is performed by GSH peroxidase, a selenium-dependent enzyme that reduces H_2O_2 while oxidizing reduced GSH to its oxidized form. The degradation of H_2O_2 by the GSH cycle is coupled to the activation of the hexose monophosphate shunt (Fig. 6.7). There is evidence that increasing GSH concentrations in monocytes and macrophages block ROS-mediated activation of NFκB and subsequent proinflammatory cytokine production (98). Mechanisms of preventing hydroxyl radical-induced tissue damage include the binding of transition metal ions by albumin, ceruloplasmin, haptoglobin, lactoferrin, and transferrin. Taurine is a scavenger for HOCl.

In addition to the specific antioxidant enzymes listed previously, other endogenous antioxidants play an important role in regulating the oxidant status. Vitamin E (α-tocopherol) is located in cell membrane phospholipids and is a major chain-breaking antioxidant. Vitamin C (ascorbic acid) has many antioxidant properties, including its ability to regenerate α-tocopherol from the tocopherol radical that forms at membrane surfaces. It can prevent activation of neutrophil-derived collagenase and is a powerful scavenger of hypochlorous acid, superoxide, singlet oxygen, and hydroxyl radicals. Carotenoids (vitamin A) have long double bonds to attract and quench radical attack. Uric acid, the major antioxidant in saliva, is a powerful scavenger of water-soluble radicals such as hypochlorous acid and singlet oxygen. It can also bind copper and iron ions to suppress hydroxyl radical formation. The mitochondrial electron transfer chain coenzymes pyrroloquinolinequinone and the reduced form of

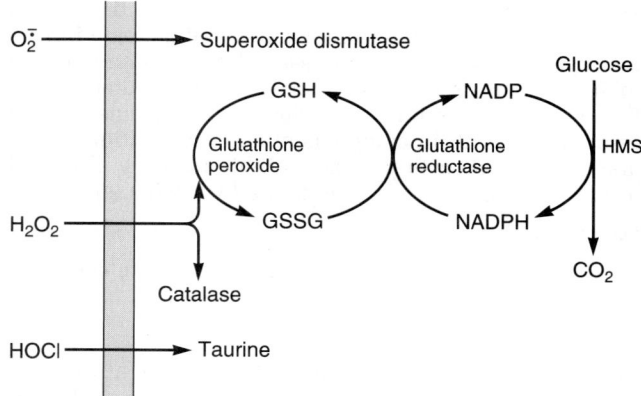

Figure 6.7. Scavengers of reactive oxygen species. HMS, hexose monophosphate shunt. (Redrawn from Klebanoff SJ. In: Gallin JI, Snyderman R, eds. *Inflammation: basic principles and clinical correlates,* 3rd ed. Philadelphia: Lippincott Williams & Wilkins, 1999:723.)

ubiquinone (coenzyme Q) have antioxidant properties. Stress proteins or heat-shock proteins are induced by oxygen radicals and ischemia, and may play a role in the defense against excess oxygen radical production. The major 32-kd stress protein, heme oxygenase-1, catalyzes the cleavage of heme to biliverdin, which is subsequently converted to bilirubin, an efficient free radical scavenger (98).

Nitric Oxide

Since Palmer and colleagues identified endothelium-derived relaxing factor as NO in 1987 (102), investigators have discovered a multitude of roles and functions for NO in almost every aspect of physiology and pathophysiology (103). More recent discoveries into NO's roles in inflammation have opened exciting new avenues of investigation with therapeutic implications. NO is a weakly reactive radical that diffuses short distances from cell to cell independent of membrane channels or receptors. It has an extremely short half-life because of its rapid inactivation by hemoglobin and other endogenous substances. It is thus primarily a paracrine and autocrine mediator. The family of enzymes called NO synthase (NOS) catalyzes the formation of NO and citrulline using the terminal guanido nitrogen of the amino acid L-arginine and oxygen as substrates (104). NOS contains prosthetic groups for flavin-adenine dinucleotide, flavin mononucleotide, tetrahydrobiopterin, iron protoporphyrin IX, and zinc. Three isoforms of NOS have been identified and cloned in humans (Table 6.5). The calcium-dependent constitutive isoforms, neuronal NOS (nNOS or NOS1) and endothelial NOS (eNOS or NOS3) produce small amounts of NO that mediate physiologic processes on a second-to-second basis. The inducible NOS (iNOS or NOS2) produces larger, sustained amounts of NO with both cytoprotective and cytotoxic properties in response to activating stimuli. However, low levels of iNOS may be expressed constitutively in certain cell types, and levels of constitutive NOS transcripts can be elevated by certain stimuli such as shear and hypoxia. Many of the physiologic effects of NO are mediated by the activation of soluble guanylate cyclase. Reductions in calcium concentrations triggered by increased levels of intracellular cyclic guanosine monophosphate promote vascular smooth muscle relaxation and the inhibition of platelet aggregation and adhesion. The cellular response to NO also likely involves multiple signal transduction mechanisms including mitogen-activated protein (MAP) kinase signaling pathways.

Inflammation associated with endotoxemia, hemorrhagic shock, and ischemia/reperfusion is associated with increased NO production by iNOS. iNOS, first described in macrophages, can be expressed in essentially any cell type in response to immunologic stimuli. Important activators of iNOS up-regulation include LPS, IL-1, TNF, and IFN-γ. Unlike nNOS and eNOS, iNOS does not depend on elevations in intracellular calcium levels for its activity. The expression of iNOS is regulated primarily at the level of transcription and at the level of iNOS mRNA stability. IFN-γ may stabilize iNOS mRNA, whereas TGF-β can destabilize it. Transcription of the iNOS gene is controlled by NFκB, IFN-γ-responsive element, and TNF-responsive element. Induction of iNOS can be inhibited by glucocorticoids, thrombin, macrophage deactivation factor, PDGF, IL-4, IL-8, IL-10, and IL-13. Dexamethasone may inhibit iNOS induction by impairing the DNA binding capacity of NFκB and by increasing levels of the inhibitory IκB (105, 106).

The endothelial dysfunction and vascular hyporeactivity seen in septic shock is at least partly mediated by NO produced by iNOS (107). NO has been shown to mediate the negative inotropic effects of TNF, IL-6, and IL-2 on cardiac muscle as well as TNF-induced vasodilation in the systemic and microcirculations (108). NO may indirectly increase prostaglandin production by increasing the catalytic activity of cyclooxygenase (COX) through a process known as S-nitrosylation. NO also has been shown to decrease leukotriene production by inhibiting 5-lipoxygenase (109). NO plays an autoregulatory role in the T_H1 subset of helper T lymphocytes by limiting their own proliferation (110).

Nitric oxide can mediate tissue injury in inflammation by modulating organ perfusion, mediating interactions with neutrophils, contributing to proinflammatory signaling, and possibly by regulating apoptosis (111). Whereas eNOS is a primary regulator of blood flow under physiologic conditions, both eNOS and iNOS modulate organ blood flow in pathophysiologic states. Basal NO release from eNOS prevents the adherence of neutrophils (in addition to lymphocytes and monocytes) to the endothelium and inhibits chemotaxis under physiologic conditions. Animal studies have demonstrated that pharmacologic inhibition of iNOS or genetic deletion of iNOS attenuates neutrophil accumulation in organs after ischemia/reperfusion injury (112). Conversely, similar experiments in endotoxemia implicate an antiadhesive role for iNOS in endotoxemia, indicating that the effect of induced NO on neutrophil accumulation is insult specific (111). Activated neutrophils can be stimulated by receptor-mediated agonists such as fMLP, PAF, and LTB_4 to produce NO. NO produced by neutrophils at sites of inflammation can combine with superoxide to form peroxynitrite as another means of effecting toxicity (113).

The reaction of NO with superoxide is the only reaction that outcompetes the reaction of superoxide with superoxide dismutase. Although small amounts of peroxynitrite are produced under basal conditions from constitutively produced NO and superoxide from mitochondria and other cellular sources, endogenous antioxidants such as GSH, vitamin E, vitamin C, and superoxide dismutase likely limit its toxicity. A low concentration of peroxynitrite has been

Table 6.5. ISOFORMS OF NITRIC OXIDE SYNTHASE

	Constitutive		Inducible
	nNOS (NOS1)	**eNOS (NOS3)**	**iNOS (NOS2)**
Calcium dependence	Yes	Yes	No
Regulation	Constitutive	Constitutive	Transcriptional
Cell types	Neuronal	Endothelial cells	All
NO production	Intermittent	Intermittent	Sustained, 6–10X greater

NOS, nitric oxide synthase; eNOS, endothelial NOS; iNOS, inducible NOS; nNOS, neuronal NOS.

shown to inhibit neutrophil adhesion. Higher concentrations of peroxynitrite can initiate a wide range of toxic oxidative reactions through a peroxynitrous acid intermediate. These include the initiation of tyrosine nitration, lipid peroxidation, and direct inhibition of mitochondrial respiratory chain enzymes. The balance between superoxide and NO determines the reactivity of peroxynitrite: excess NO reduces the oxidation elicited by peroxynitrite. In addition, peroxynitrite may contribute to cytotoxicity by a more indirect pathway. Peroxynitrite-induced single-strand breaks in DNA activate the nuclear enzyme poly(ADP-ribose) synthetase, leading eventually to irreversible energy depletion of the cells and necrotic-type cell death (25).

Inducible NOS plays a key role in host defense, with NO or peroxynitrite exhibiting potent antimicrobial activity against a number of pathogens including virus, fungi, and bacteria. Although microbial susceptibility to NO-mediated killing can vary considerably between species, essential roles have been identified in tuberculosis and bacterial peritonitis (114). Induced NO has been shown to be essential for the up-regulation of the inflammatory response in hemorrhagic shock and is likely to be so in other inflammatory processes. NO produced by iNOS leads to the activation of NFκB (115). This is followed by the induction of proinflammatory cytokines and increased leukocyte recruitment and activation.

Both proapoptotic and antiapoptotic effects have been demonstrated by NO under various conditions. NO derived from eNOS may inhibit apoptosis. Proapoptotic effects appear to be associated with pathophysiologic conditions in which iNOS is up-regulated. However, adenoviral transfer of iNOS has been shown to inhibit endothelial cell apoptosis (116). Low concentrations of peroxynitrite have also been shown to induce apoptosis, whereas higher concentrations promote cell necrosis in vitro (25). The role of NO-mediated apoptosis in the regulation of the inflammatory response is yet to be more clearly defined.

In summary, NO mediates tissue injury both directly through the formation of peroxynitrite, and indirectly through the amplification of the inflammatory response. Like many mediators, however, NO has dual regulatory functions and is therefore difficult to characterize as either proinflammatory or antiinflammatory. In general, basal levels of NO produced by constitutive NOS may confer antiinflammatory effects, whereas induced NO may tend to promote the up-regulation of the inflammatory response. It is likely that an optimal level of NO is necessary in the host defense; too little NO may be as harmful as too much.

The Stress Response

The stress response is an individual cell's reaction to a threat to its microenvironment. Every cell of every organism undergoes a stress response to reestablish homeostasis when the normal equilibrium is disrupted. It is often referred to as the *heat-shock response* after the identification in the 1960s of a group of genes expressed after exposure to heat, the heat-shock proteins (HSP) (117). Later, it became evident that HSP as well as other cellular proteins were expressed in response to a wide variety of insults and are thus probably more accurately referred to as *stress proteins*. Inducers of the stress response include physical stresses (burns, radiation, trauma), chemical agents and mediators (toxins, heavy metals, cytokines, ROS), infectious agents (bacteria, viruses, parasites), and allergens. Clinically, expression of HSP has been observed under conditions in which oxygen delivery is compromised, as in hemorrhage or ischemia. The mechanism by which the stress response is initiated may involve stress-induced alterations in protein structure or the formation of protein aggregates that induce stress protein gene expression (118).

Activation of the stress response is associated with morphologic and metabolic alterations in the cell. Morphologic alterations include the accumulation of unprocessed forms of mRNA in the nucleus, aggregation of protein complexes in the nucleolus, and increased numbers of actin microfilaments in the cytoplasm. Changes in cellular metabolism include a rapid reduction in intracellular ATP levels, most likely correlated with alterations in the integrity of mitochondria. The stress response is characterized by a transient down-regulation of most cellular products and by the up-regulation of stress proteins (119). It is the induction of stress proteins that confers the primary adaptive and protective effects of the stress response. After expression of stress genes, cells become resistant to subsequent stresses. Members of the stress protein family include heme oxygenase, involved in the breakdown of heme into biliverdin; the multiple-drug resistance gene product or P-glycoprotein; ubiquitin, involved in targeting proteins for degradation; scavengers such as superoxide dismutase, ferritin, and metallothioneins; and the glycolytic enzymes enolase and glyceraldehyde 3-phosphate dehydrogenase. It is, however, the HSP that comprise the largest and most intensively studied group of stress proteins.

Heat-shock proteins can be either constitutive or inducible upon heat shock or other stresses. Constitutive HSP are referred to as *molecular chaperones* because of their central role in the synthesis, folding, and translocation of proteins (120). HSP are classified into families according to their molecular mass and degree of homology. The most extensively studied is the Hsp70 family. Their size is on the order of 70 kd and they share greater than 70% homology. Members of the Hsp70 family bind ATP. Under conditions of ATP depletion, the cell perceives a decrease in stress protein levels, leading to activation of the stress response. Hsp70 is essential for the ability of cells to adapt to and survive environmental stresses. Both Hsp72 and Hsp73 are present in the cytosol and nucleus. However, Hsp73 is constitutively expressed, whereas Hsp72 is exclusively induced after stress. In most studies, Hsp72 is used as a marker of HSP induction. The Hsp60 family members are also referred to as *chaperonins*. The glucose-regulated protein group of HSP are induced with glucose starvation, inhibitors of *N*-glycosylation, and calcium ionophores. The decrease in glucose content may affect the pool of sugar donors during protein glycosylation. The low-molecular-weight HSP (molecular masses of 20 to 30 kd) may be important regulatory components of the actin-based cytoskeleton. Transcription of heat-shock genes is mediated by the activation of heat-shock elements in the gene promoters. Two heat-shock transcriptional factors (HSF) have been identified. HSF1 activates transcription of the *Hsp72* gene in response to heat, heavy metals, and other inducers of the stress response. On heat shock, unbound HSF1 oligomerizes, translocates to the nucleus, and binds to the HSP promoter to activate the transcription of the gene. HSF2 is not activated by the classic inducers of heat shock genes but may be important in controlling the activities of *Hsp* gene expression in the normal or unstressed cell (118,121,122).

A number of inflammatory states such as rheumatoid arthritis, ARDS, or asthma have been shown to benefit experimentally from increased HSP expression (117–119, 122). HSP can play multiple roles in modulating the inflammatory response. Functions of HSP during inflammation include enhancement of immune responses, thermotolerance, regulation of apoptosis, hemostasis, and cytoprotection against ROS and other inflammatory mediators. Induced HSP in macrophages contribute to antigen processing and presentation. HSP may shift the balance between T_H1 and T_H2 toward an increase in the more antiinflammatory T_H2 cells. ROS, including H_2O_2, hydroxyl radical, and peroxynitrite, activate HSP synthesis, most likely by altering protein structure or function. In the presence of iron, ROS also induce the oxidation-specific stress protein heme oxygenase or ferritin. These proteins contribute to protection against oxidative stress by binding iron and preventing it from participating in the Fenton reaction (see section on Reactive Oxygen Species). Mechanisms of HSP-mediated cytoprotection from the toxic effects of ROS include the maintenance of cellular GSH levels (Hsp27) and mitochondrial protection (Hsp70). ROS thus induce a cytoprotective response that counteracts their own toxicity. Other inflammatory mediators such as NO have also been shown to induce expression of HSP. HSP may participate in intracellular signaling pathways that modulate the production or function of inflammatory mediators. For example, Hsp90 has been shown to facilitate signaling that leads to NO formation by eNOS (123). Hsp70 has been reported to prevent apoptosis, which may actually serve to promote propagation rather than resolution of inflammation. In addition, the body's immune response to bacterial and parasitic stress proteins likely protects the host from infection. The bacterial homologue of Hsp60, GroEL, is a major target of the mammalian humoral response to bacterial infections. Many activators of HSF1 are potent inhibitors of the proinflammatory transcription factor NFκB. Aspirin and other NSAIDs activate HSF while inhibiting NFκB. Therefore, the antiinflammatory effects associated with the stress response might relate more to the inhibition of NFκB activation (118,124).

Apoptosis

The host response to inflammation must include regulatory mechanisms that limit inflammatory tissue injury. At the cellular level there must be a balance between cellular proliferation/ differentiation, and cell death. Apoptosis, or programmed cell death, is distinguished from necrotic cell death by biochemical and structural differences (125) (Table 6.6). Necrosis is a pathologic form of cell death characterized by cellular swelling and loss of membrane integrity. Although also seen in pathologic states, apoptosis is usually a physiologic process. Apoptosis follows an orderly sequence of events. DNA fragmentation and plasma membrane blebbing is followed by the formation of apoptotic bodies consisting of cytoplasmic and membrane fragments. Cell death by apoptosis does not trigger an inflammatory response because cytoplasmic granule contents do not leak out of the apoptotic cell. On the other hand, cell lysis in necrosis releases intracellular contents, triggering inflammatory reactions. Phagocytosis of necrotic cells and substances released by them activate surrounding macrophages, amplifying the inflammatory re-

sponse. Thus, whether a cell undergoes apoptotic or necrotic death is crucial to the regulation of inflammation.

Apoptosis plays a major role in limiting neutrophil-mediated tissue toxicity. Neutrophils are programmed to undergo apoptosis constitutively. Once a neutrophil becomes apoptotic it is recognized and engulfed by local macrophages. This is the preferred mechanism for clearing neutrophils from inflammatory foci. Similar mechanisms have been implicated in the clearance of eosinophils, monocytes, and lymphocytes. The uptake of apoptotic neutrophils by macrophages does not elicit macrophage secretion of inflammatory mediators. Phagocyte lectins and various scavenger receptors may recognize elements on the surface of apoptotic cells exposed by the loss of normal plasma membrane asymmetry. Neutrophil apoptosis is accelerated by phagocytosis of bacteria and slowed by GM-CSF and other neutrophil growth factors and activators (126,127).

Apoptosis plays a prominent role in the immune system. Most developing T cells undergo apoptosis during the selection process in the thymus (55). Termination of the cellular immune response also involves cytokine-induced apoptosis. Apoptosis can be used by lymphocytes as a means of effecting death in other cells. CTL kill target cells by inducing apoptosis a Fas-induced pathway and a perforin- and granzyme-mediated pathway (62) (see section on T-Cell—mediated Immune Response). Increased apoptosis has been observed in lymphoid tissues of patients dying of sepsis, suggesting that excessive lymphocyte apoptosis may contribute to fatal sepsis (128).

Mechanisms of Apoptosis Activation

Apoptosis occurs constitutively as well as in response to a wide variety of stimuli. Inducers of apoptosis include oxidant stress, radiation, viral infection, trauma, and cytokines. Many of the pathologic agents that induce apoptosis at low concentrations can cause necrosis at higher concentrations. Apoptogenic stimuli activate the cell's "suicide" program through both receptor-dependent and -independent pathways. The sphingomyelin breakdown product, ceramide, is implicated as a transducer of apoptosis (129). DNA damage secondary to radiation or oxygen radical formation results in the accumulation of the tumor suppressor gene *p53*. *p53* promotes non-receptor-mediated modulation of apoptosis (130).

Receptor-mediated pathways involve "death receptors" that belong to the TNF receptor superfamily (131). Ligands shown to induce apoptosis include FasL, TNF, TNF-related apoptosis-inducing ligand (TRAIL), nerve growth factor, and CD40L. The best-characterized death receptors are Fas (CD95, Apo1) bound by FasL (CD95L)) and TNFRI (p55, CD120a) bound by TNF and lymphotoxin α (TNFβ). Although primarily produced by macrophages, TNF is expressed on many cell types, whereas FasL appears to be restricted mainly to the surfaces of CTL, activated macrophages, and neutrophils. TNF and FasL also differ in that whereas FasL directly activates a cell death pathway, TNF does so through a more indirect route and concurrently stimulates pathways that inhibit apoptosis (Fig. 6.8). Independent and divergent proinflammatory signaling pathways by TNF lead to the induction of NFκB, an inhibitor of apoptosis (132). The mechanism by which several cytokines, including IL-1, IL-6, and GM-CSF, inhibit apoptosis is through induction of NFκB. The balance between induction of NFκB and the induction of apoptosis is one of many factors that ultimately determines the cell's fate.

Ligation of death receptors recruits "death domain"-containing adaptor proteins that interact with the receptor's intracellular death domain. This protein–protein in-

Table 6.6. APOPTOSIS VERSUS NECROSIS

	Apoptosis	Necrosis
Inducers	Physiologic/pathologic	Pathologic
Programmed	Yes	No
Cell size	Shrinkage	Swelling
Plasma membrane	Intact	Fragmented
Inflammatory response	No	Yes

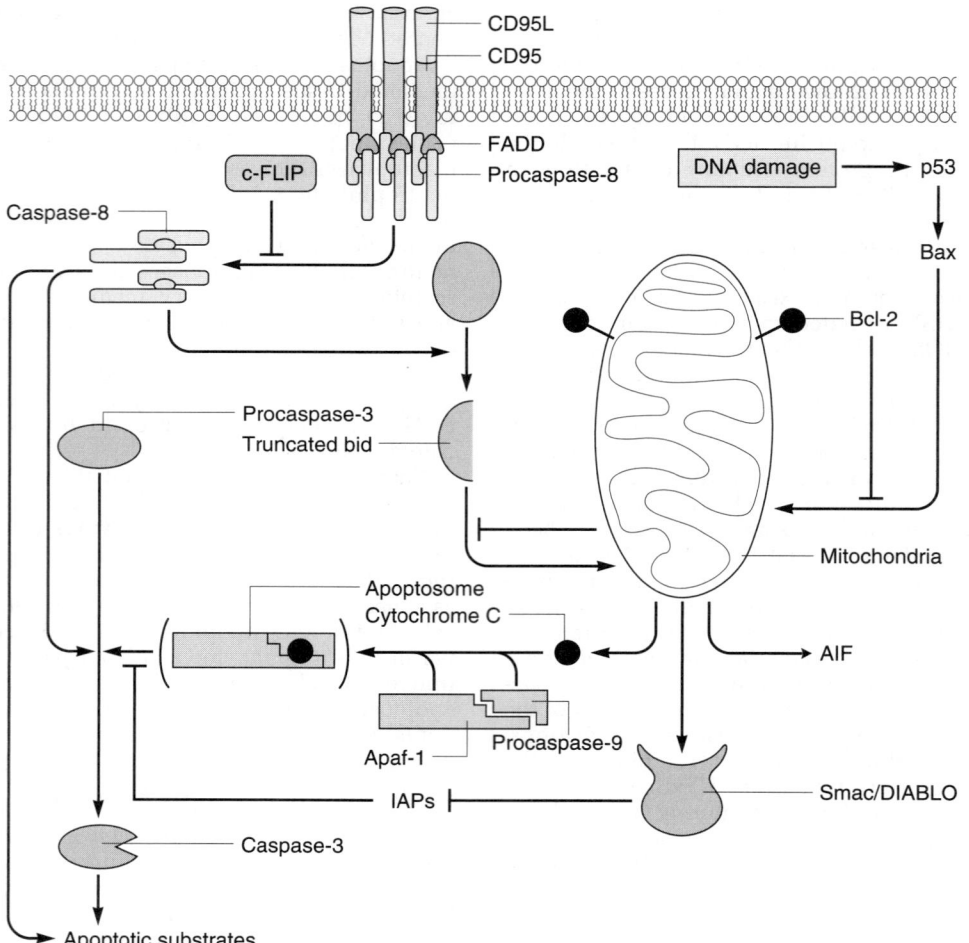

Figure 6.8. The death receptor pathway is triggered by members of the death receptor superfamily such as CD95 (Fas) and TNFRI. Binding of CD95 ligand to CD95 induces receptor clustering and formation of a death-inducing signaling complex. This complex recruits, through the adapter molecule Fas-associated death domain (FADD) protein, multiple procaspase-8 molecules, resulting in caspase-8 activation through induced proximity. Caspase-8 activation can be blocked by recruitment of the degenerate caspase homologue c-FLIP. The mitochondrial pathway is used extensively in response to extracellular cues and internal insults such as DNA damage. These diverse response pathways converge on mitochondria, often through the activation of a proapoptotic member of the Bcl-2 family. Unlike Bcl-2, which seems to spend most if not all of its life attached to intracellular membranes, many other proteins, including Bax, Bad, Bim, and Bid, can shuttle between the cytosol and organelles. The cytosolic forms represent pools of inactive, but battle-ready proteins. Proapoptotic signals redirect these proteins to the mitochondria, where the fight for the cell's fate will take place. Activation of proapoptotic members can occur through proteolysis, dephosphorylation, and probably several other mechanisms. Proapoptotic and antiapoptotic Bcl-2 family members meet at the surface of mitochondria, where they compete to regulate cytochrome c exit. If the proapoptotic camp wins, an array of molecules is released from the mitochondrial compartment. Principal among these is cytochrome c, which associates with Apaf-1 and then procaspase-9 to form the apoptosome. The death receptor and mitochondrial pathways converge at the level of caspase-3 activation. Caspase-3 activation and activity is antagonized by the IAP proteins, which themselves are antagonized by the Smac/DIABLO protein released from mitochondria. Cross-talk and integration between the death receptor and mitochondrial pathways is provided by Bid, a proapoptotic Bcl-2 family member. Caspase-8-mediated cleavage of Bid greatly increases its prodeath activity, and results in its translocation to mitochondria, where it promotes cytochrome c exit. Under most conditions, this cross-talk is minimal, and the two pathways operate largely independently of each other. AIF, apoptosis-inducing factor; Apaf-1, apoptotic protease-activating factor; c-FLIP, c-FLICE inhibitory protein (c-FLICE, caspase-8/FADD-like IL-1β–converting enzyme); DIABLO, direct IAP binding protein with low pI; IAP, inhibitor of apoptosis protein; Smac, second mitochondria-derived activator of caspases.

teraction initiates the enzyme cascade responsible for apoptosis effector mechanisms—the caspases. All signaling pathways, receptor dependent or independent, converge on the activation of cysteine proteases related to IL-1β-converting enzyme (ICE) called *caspases* (133). Cas-

pases propagate apoptotic signaling by cleaving/activating other caspases, and eventually execute the terminal events in apoptosis by cleaving specific target proteins. Caspases 8 and 10 activate apoptosis signaling by linking Fas-associated death domain protein (FADD) with the caspase cascades. Caspases 3 and 7 are the executor molecules in the nucleus that cleave death substrates, including nuclear structural proteins, protein kinases, and proteins involved in cell cycle regulation or DNA fragmentation. Cytochrome C release from mitochondria is a key component in the activation of caspases. Cytochrome C release, and therefore apoptosis, is inhibited by Bcl-2. Bcl-2 is the primary death protection protein that belongs to the Bcl family of proaproptotic and antiapoptotic proteins integrally involved in the regulation of apoptosis (134).

Cell Signaling Mechanisms

G Proteins

Guanine nucleotide-binding proteins [guanosine triphosphatases (GTPases), or G proteins] are cell receptors for lipid mediators (eicosanoids, PAF), kinins, neuropeptides, chemokines, and other inflammatory ligands. G proteins are unique in that they contain both ligand binding domains on the cell exterior and intracellular signaling domains. They are particularly important and classically associated with neutrophil activation. There are two types of G proteins, heterotrimeric and monomeric. Heterotrimeric G proteins are seven-span transmembrane signal transducers composed of α, β, and γ subunits, each with multiple isoforms (Fig. 6.9). In the inactivated form, G proteins are bound tightly by GDP. Binding of an inflammatory ligand to its receptor releases GDP from the α subunit. GTP re-

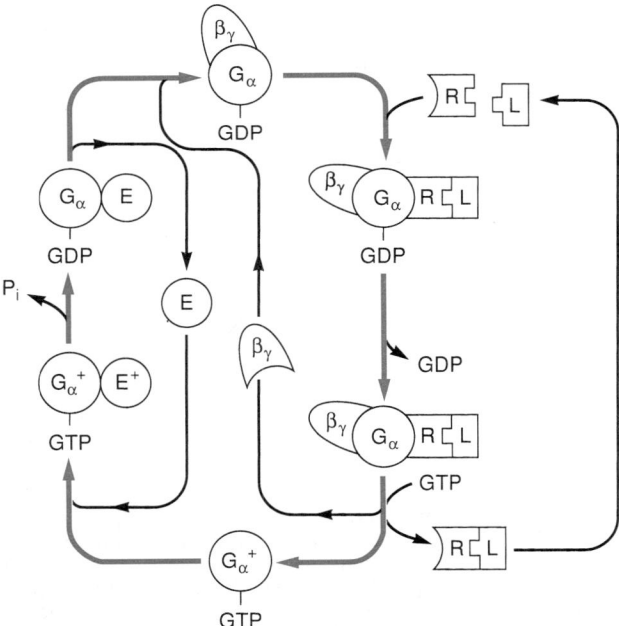

Figure 6.9. The G protein cycle of activation. When a ligand (L) binds to its receptor (R) on the cell surface, this LR complex activates a guanosine triphosphate (GTP)-binding protein located on the cytoplasmic side of the cell membrane. Formation of the LR complex causes the release of guanosine diphosphate (GDP) from the G protein. The vacant guanine nucleotide-binding site is rapidly filled by GTP from the cytosol, causing the release of the G protein from the LR complex and the dissociation of the G$_\alpha$ subunit from the β-γ subunit of the G protein. The GTP–G$_\alpha$ complex represents the activated G protein component that binds and activates an effector (E) in the cell. The catalytic activity of the effector continues until the bound GTP is hydrolyzed by the G$_\alpha$ subunit. The GDP–G$_\alpha$ complex rapidly dissociates from the effector (which is no longer active), associates with a β-γ subunit, and is ready for another cycle of activation. P$_i$, inorganic.

places GDP, followed by dissociation of the GTP–α complex from the $\beta\gamma$ subunits. The activated GTP–α complex then interacts with downstream effector enzymes. Intrinsic GTPase activity results in hydrolysis of GTP to GDP, promoting reassociation of the inactive $\alpha\beta\gamma$ complex, which is then available to begin a new cycle (6,135,136).

The monomeric G proteins are also known as low-molecular-weight G proteins, small G proteins, or the Ras superfamily. Families of small G proteins include Ras, Rho/Rac, and Arf. These small proteins regulate intracellular events within neutrophils such as the respiratory burst, chemotaxis, degranulation, and phospholipid metabolism. They act downstream of the cell surface G proteins. Like the heterotrimeric G proteins, small G proteins carry out cycles of guanine nucleotide exchange and GTP hydrolysis. Their activation is regulated by GTPase-activating proteins that increase GTP hydrolysis, and guanine nucleotide dissociation inhibitors. The small G proteins Arf and Rho mediate activity of phospholipase D stimulated by che-moattractants. Ras is important in the activation of MAP kinases, discussed later (6,137).

Second Messengers

Signal transduction through heterotrimeric G proteins results in the activation of multiple second messenger pathways. The two subclasses of heterotrimeric G proteins are the cholera toxin-sensitive G$_s$ (stimulatory) proteins and the pertussis toxin-sensitive G$_i$ (inhibitory) proteins. G$_s$ proteins are ubiquitously distributed, and are responsible for the activation of adenylate cyclase with subsequent generation of cyclic adenosine monophosphate (cAMP; Fig. 6.10). Stimulation of G$_i$ proteins, conversely, inhibits the activation of adenylate cyclase. Stimuli that increase cytosolic cAMP levels (PGE$_1$, histamine, ATP, epinephrine, adenosine) function in the neutrophil to inhibit chemoattractant-induced responses and play an important regulatory role in neutrophil activation (6,135–137).

G proteins also mediate the activation of phospholipases (Fig. 6.11). Phospholipase C (PLC) hydrolyzes PIP$_2$ to diacylglycerol (DAG) and inositol triphosphate (IP$_3$). IP$_3$ induces calcium release from intracellular stores. Increased concentrations of calcium stimulate neutrophil degranulation and combine with DAG to activate phospholipase-dependent protein kinase C. DAG interacts with phospholipase-dependent protein kinase C, resulting in its translocation to the cell membrane, activation, and subsequent phosphorylation of cellular proteins. DAG is rapidly phosphorylated by a specific kinase to form phosphatidic acid (PA). DAG can also be formed de novo utilizing PA as a precursor. PLD hydrolyzes phosphatidylcholine (PC) to PA and choline. PLA$_2$ hydrolyzes PC or phosphatidylethanolamine (PE) to arachidonic acid and lyso-PC or lyso-PE. Arachidonic acid can then be used as substrate for eicosanoid (prostaglandin, leukotriene) synthesis. Activation of both PLA$_2$ and PLD requires calcium and protein kinase C activation. Protein kinase C is a target for calcium, DAG, PA, and arachidonic acid. It is known to phosphorylate specific components of the NADPH (respiratory burst) oxidase in neutrophils. Several other protein kinases are activated in neutrophils, including the MAP kinases (6,136).

Transcription Factors

The inflammatory response requires the rapid transcription of genes that encode effector proteins. This gene expression is regulated by specific DNA-binding proteins called *transcription factors*. Transcription factors are "instructed" to bind regulatory elements in gene promoters

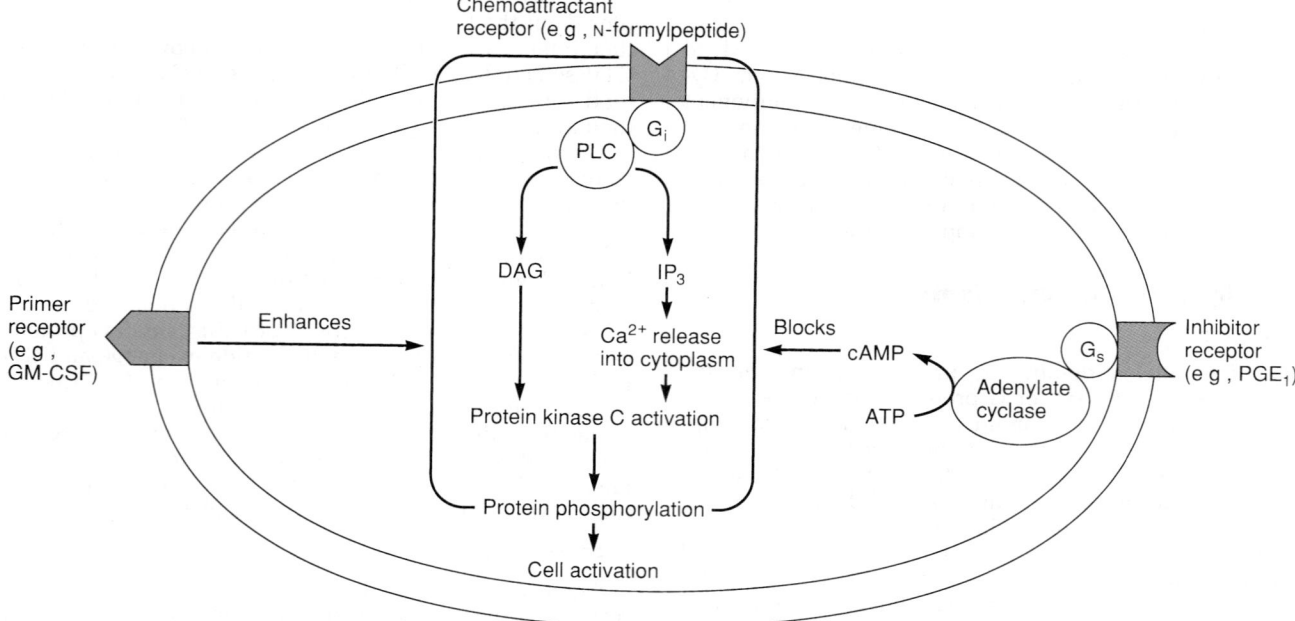

Figure 6.10. Modulation of neutrophil signal transduction pathways. The chemoattractant-mediated signal transduction pathway is enhanced by priming agents, such as granulocyte–macrophage colony-stimulating factor (GM-CSF). The mechanism is not clearly defined, but it may involve an enhanced expression of chemoattractant receptors on the cell surface. The chemoattractant-mediated signal transduction pathway is inhibited by agents such as prostaglandin E_1 (PGE$_1$) and β-adrenergic agonists that cause G_S-mediated activation of adenylyl cyclase. This inhibition is thought to occur by way of cyclic adenosine monophosphate (cAMP)-mediated phosphorylation events. ATP, adenosine triphosphate; G_i, G protein that mediates phospholipase C (PLC) activation by chemoattractants; G_S, G protein that stimulates adenylate cyclase; DAG, diacylglycerol; IP$_3$, inositol 1,4,5-trisphosphate.

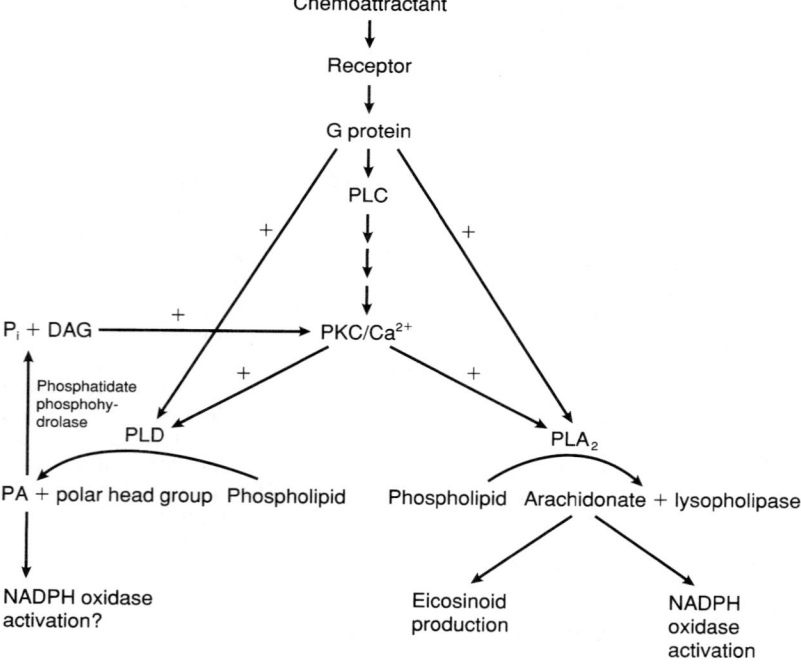

Figure 6.11. The role of phospholipases in neutrophil signal transduction. Ligand binding to its receptor activates G proteins, which activate phospholipase C (PLC). This in turn results in increased cytosolic Ca^{2+} and activation of protein kinase C (PKC). Activated G proteins also activate phospholipases D and A_2 (PLD and PLA$_2$), but elevated Ca^{2+} levels and PKC activation are also required. Thus, PLC activation is required for activation of PLD and PLA$_2$. PLD produces phosphatidate (PA), which can be dephosphorylated to give diacylglycerol (DAG). PLA$_2$ cleaves arachidonate from the *sn*-2 position of glycerophospholipids, leaving a lysophospholipid. NADPH, reduced nicotinamide-adenine dinucleotide phosphate; P$_i$, inorganic phosphate.

by signals transmitted from the cell surface. Cell surface receptor binding by inflammatory ligands such as cytokines triggers intracellular signal transduction pathways that link the cell exterior to the nucleus. Alternately, certain activators such as redox stress and reactive oxygen derivatives may enable intracellular transduction pathways without specific receptor binding. Signal transduction systems can often overlap and modify one another to activate specific transcription factors differentially. Transcription factors of particular importance during inflammation include NFκB, activator protein (AP-1), signal transducer and activator of transcription (STAT) proteins, nuclear factor of activated T cells (NFAT), and nuclear factor-IL6 (NF-IL6; Table 6.7).

Activation of NFκB is critical for maximal expression of many proinflammatory cytokines, including TNF, IL-1, IL-6, and IL-8. In addition, NFκB binding sites are common in genes encoding growth factors, adhesion molecules, and acute-phase proteins. NFκB activation also increases transcription of enzymes such as COX-2 and iNOS that in turn produce inflammatory mediators. The prototype is a heterodimeric protein composed of DNA-binding proteins p50 (NFκB1) and p65 (Rel A). However, it can be composed of dimers of any combination of Rel DNA binding proteins. A group of inhibitory proteins called IκB sequester NFκB in the cytoplasm of immune and inflammatory effector cells. IκB is phosphorylated after activation by ROS, cytokines, NO, hypoxia, redox stress, and bacterial metabolites. A phosphorylation-regulated ubiquitination leads to rapid degradation of IκB to release NFκB. Free NFκB then translocates from the cytoplasm to the nucleus, where it binds to regulatory elements in target gene promoters to induce gene expression and protein synthesis (27,138,139) (Fig. 6.12).

Many of the stress stimuli that trigger NFκB also activate AP-1. AP-1 consists of homodimers or heterodimers of members of the c-*Jun* and c-*Fos* families of protooncogenes. These proteins are exclusively nuclear proteins. The signal for AP-1 activation arises from a group of serine/threonine kinases, the mitogen-activated protein (MAP) kinases. Small G proteins such as Ras activated by cell surface receptor binding trigger MAP kinase kinase kinase (MAP KKK) activity and the MAP kinase cascade. MAP kinases can be grouped into major classes: extracellular signal-regulated kinases (ERKs), c-Jun N-terminal kinases (JNKs), and p38. ERK is activated by mitogens and growth factors. JNK and p38 are also referred to collectively as the *stress-activated protein kinases* (SAPKs).

SAPKs are activated by proinflammatory cytokines (TNF, IL-1) and cellular stress (heat shock, ROS, ultraviolet radiation, osmotic stress) (140). Not surprisingly, there is evidence of cooperative interactions between AP-1 and NFκB activation pathways that can result in functional synergy (141).

The STAT proteins mediate the cellular effects of most cytokines. There are seven STAT proteins identified to date. These proteins are activated by Janus kinase (JAK) proteins that associate with cell surface cytokine receptors. On cytokine binding, the JAKs dimerize and transphosphorylate each other. STAT proteins associate with the phosphorylated JAKs and are themselves phosphorylated. The activated STAT proteins form dimers and translocate to the nucleus, where they bind to recognition sequences in the promoter regions of genes to activate transcription (142,143) (Fig. 6.13).

The NF-IL6 transcription factor is the nuclear factor for the IL-1-responsive element in the IL-6 gene. It is known by many names, such as C/EBP (CCAAT enhancer binding protein) and LAP (liver-activating protein). Activators of NF-IL6 include LPS, cytokines, iNOS, and neutrophil granule enzymes. Phosphorylation of serine or threonine residues of NF-IL6 by calcium/calmodulin-dependent kinases, protein kinase C, and especially the MAP kinases, activates DNA binding and transcription of inflammatory genes. Activation of NF-IL6 leads to transcription of class I (IL-1- and IL-6-induced) acute-phase protein genes. It is also associated with the up-regulation of cytokines, adhesion molecules, iNOS, and COX-2. Like AP-1, many of its effects involve cooperative interactions with NFκB (144).

Nuclear factor of activated T cells (NFAT) is primarily involved in regulating the production of effector proteins of the immune responses. Although first identified in the IL-2 promoter of T cells, it is expressed in a host of cell types, including mast cells, mononuclear phagocytes, eosinophils, and endothelial cells. It is activated by stimulation of receptors coupled to calcium mobilization. Examples of such receptors are antigen receptors on T and B lymphocytes, the Fcε receptor on mast cells and basophils, the Fcγ receptor on macrophages, and G protein-coupled receptors. Receptor binding activates PLC, leading to increased calcium concentrations. Calcineurin, a calcium/calmodulin-dependent phosphatase activated by elevated levels of intracellular calcium, activates NFAT. NFAT participates in multiple cooperative interactions with AP-1 (139).

Table 6.7. SELECTED TRANSCRIPTION FACTORS, THEIR ACTIVATORS, AND GENES REGULATED IN INFLAMMATION

Transcription factor	Examples of activators	Examples of genes regulated
AP-1	TNF, IL-1, UV, H_2O_2, LPS, GFs, stress, ROS/redox stress, antioxidants, hypoxia, T-cell receptor	TNF, IL-1, IL-2, IL-5, IFN-γ, ICAM-1, E-selectin, GM-CSF, MMPs, COX-2
NFκB/REL	TNF, IL-1, UV, H_2O_2, LPS, mitogens, viral proteins, NO, ROS/redox stress	IL-1, IL-2, IL-6, IL-8, IL-12, TNF, E-selectin, VCAM-1, ICAM-1, MIP-1, MCP-1, eotaxin, RANTES, COX-2, iNOS, PLA_2, G-CSF, GM-CSF, IFN-β
STAT	IFNs, CSFs, GFs, IL-1 through IL-15	FOS, E-selectin, MYC, ICAM-1, FcγRI
NF-IL6	IL-1, TNF, IL-6, LPS, IL-8, IL-12, G-CSF, iNOS, elastase, MPO, lysozyme	Acute-phase proteins, IL-7, IL-8, ICAM-1, iNOS, COX-2
NFAT	T-cell receptor, B-cell receptor, Fcε-receptors, Fcγ receptors, histamine and thrombin receptors	IL-2, IL-3, IL-4, IL-5, IL-8, IL-13, TNF, GM-CSF, IFN-γ, CD40L, FASL

AP, activator protein; CSF, colony-stimulating factor; COX, cyclooxygenase; GFs, growth factors; ICAM, intercellular adhesion molecule; IFN, interferon; IL, interleukin; iNOS, inducible nitric oxide synthase; LPS, lipopolysaccharide; MMP, matrix metalloproteinases; MPO, myeloperoxidase; NFAT, nuclear factor of activated T cells; NF-IL6, nuclear factor-IL6; NFκB, nuclear factor kappa-B; PLA_2, phospholipase A_2; ROS, reactive oxygen species; STAT, signal transducer and activator of transcription; TNF, tumor necrosis factor; UV, ultraviolet; VCAM, vascular cell adhesion molecule.
Modified from Gallin JI, Snyderman R, eds. Inflammation: basic principles and clinical correlates, 3rd ed. Philadelphia: Lippincott Williams & Wilkins, 1999.

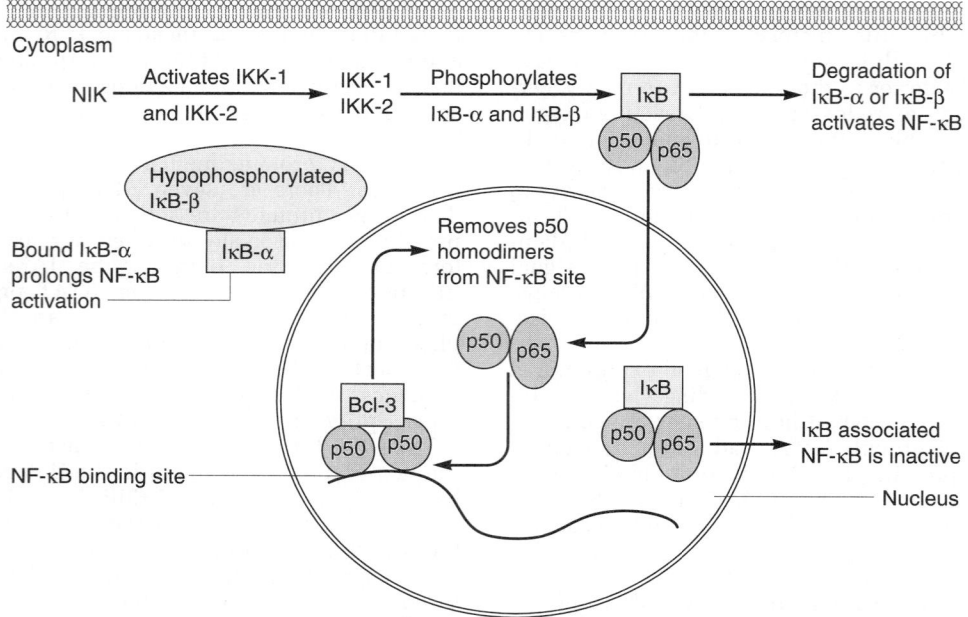

Figure 6.12. Pathways regulating nuclear factor-kappa B (NF-κB) activation and the ability of NF-κB to act as a transcriptor enhancer, NIK, NF-κB-inducing kinase; IκB, inhibitor of κB. (Redrawn from Abraham E. NFκB activation. *Crit Care Med* 2000;28[Suppl 4]:101.)

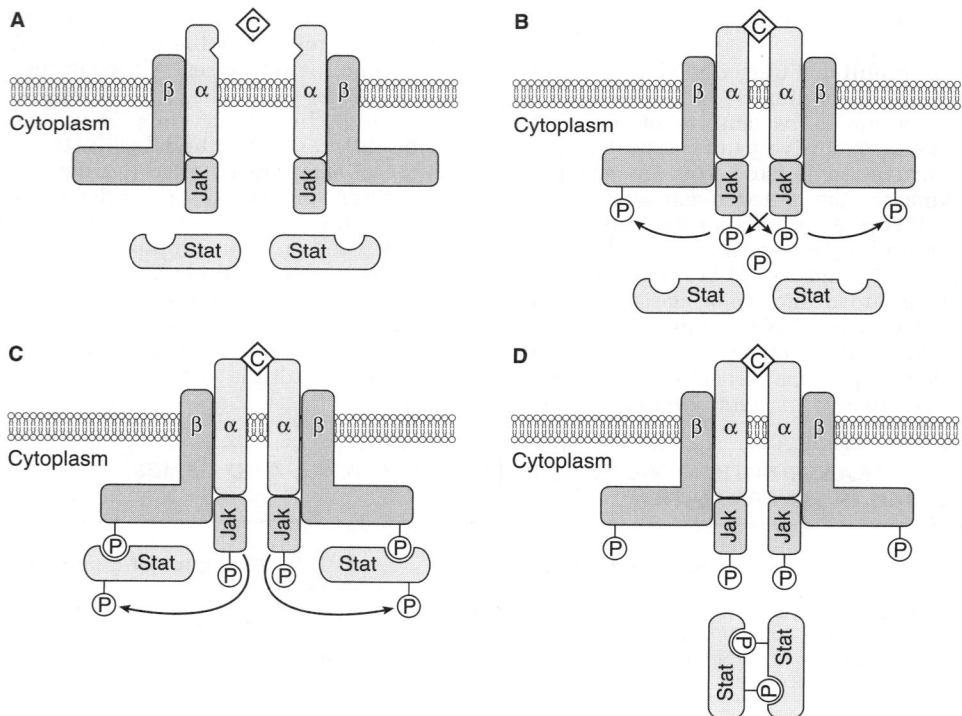

Figure 6.13. JAK-STAT signaling pathway. *(A)* JAK (Janus kinase) components are associated in an inactive form with the cytoplasmic portion of cytokine receptors. *(B)* Cytokine binding leads to cytokine receptor aggregation. Adjacent JAK proteins become activated and phosphorylate each other and phosphorylate tyrosine residues on the cytoplasmic region of the cytokine receptor. *(C)* Through the Src homology 2 (SH2) domain, STAT (signal transducer and activator of transcription) proteins bind phosphotyrosine residues on the cytoplasmic portion of cytokine receptors. Bound STAT proteins are phosphorylated by bound JAK proteins and subsequently dissociate. *(D)* Phosphorylated STAT proteins dimerize and then move to the nucleus, where they activate transcription by binding to specific sequences. (Redrawn from Sundy JS, et al. In: Gallin JI, Snyderman R, eds. *Inflammation: basic principles and clinical correlates,* 3rd ed. Philadelphia: Lippincott Williams & Wilkins, 1999:438.)

HUMORAL COMPONENTS OF INFLAMMATION

The Complement System

The complement system plays an important role in the host response to invading organisms as well as in the pathogenesis of a number of inflammatory diseases such as immune complex diseases, ischemia/reperfusion injury, and ARDS (145–148). Complement has the unique ability to recognize and eliminate pathogens or damaged host cells in the absence of antibody or specific cellular immune mechanisms. Perhaps more important, complement enhances host defenses by marking foreign particles for phagocytosis through opsonization. There are over 30 distinct plasma and cell membrane proteins involved in the initiation, activation, amplification, regulation, and termination of the complement system. Complement components are synthesized mainly by hepatocytes, but also by local mononuclear phagocytes. Initiation occurs by one of three pathways: the classical pathway, the mannose-binding lectin (MBL) pathway, and the alternative pathway. All three pathways lead to sequential activation of inactive precursor molecules, or zymogens, through proteolysis. The cascades culminate in the generation of a C3 convertase enzyme that binds to target cells and activates C3. Subsequent formation of the membrane attack complex (MAC) leads to lysis of target cells or pathogens. The principal components of the complement cascade are outlined in Fig. 6.14 (145–147).

Initiation

Classical Pathway. The classical complement pathway is the primary mediator of adaptive humoral (antibody-mediated) immunity. The initial activation step of the classical pathway is the interaction of C1 with antigen–antibody complexes containing either IgM or IgG. Other substances such as lipid A in endotoxin and mitochondrial membranes have been shown to activate the classical pathway independent of antigen–antibody complexes in vitro. C1 is a calcium-dependent macromolecule composed of three glycoproteins, C1q, C1r, and C1s, as two reversible subunits, C1q and C1r2s2. C1q, the recognition unit of the classical pathway, interacts with the Fc region of the immunoglobulin, leading to a conformational change in C1q that allows autocatalytic activation of C1r. C1r then cleaves C1s. The activated C1s cleaves and activates C4 and C2. C4 is cleaved into the smaller peptide C4a, an anaphylatoxin, and C4b, which can bind immune complexes on the surface of target cells and, more important, can provide a magnesium ion-dependent binding site for C2. The proconvertase C4bC2 is activated by C1s, cleaving C2 into C2a and C2b. The C2a fragment possesses the enzymatic site of the classical pathway C3 convertase C4b2a (147,149).

Control of classical pathway activation occurs at several different levels. Excessive classical pathway C3 convertase activity is prevented by the inherent instability of this enzyme due to the rapid decay of C2a off the complex. C1 inhibitor covently binds C1s and thus gives activated C1 a

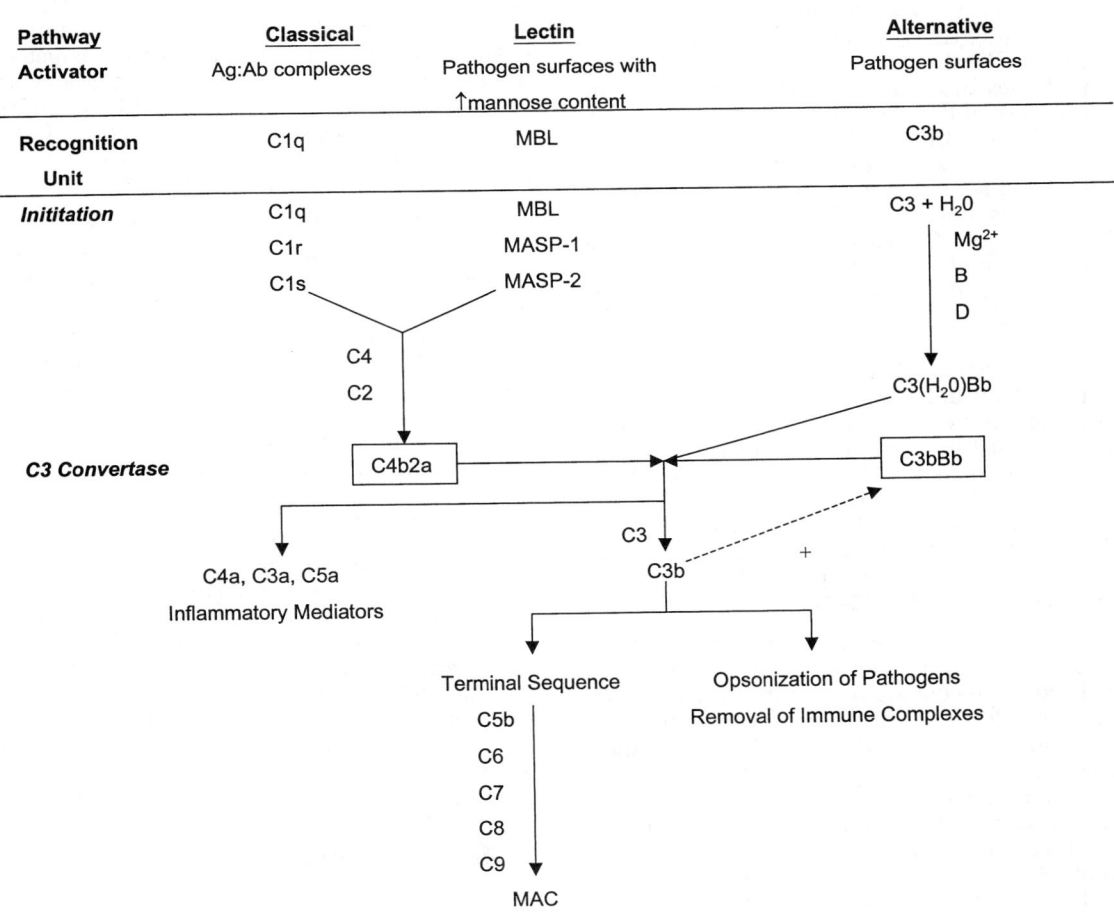

Figure 6.14. Principal components of the complement cascade. All three pathways culminate in the formation of a C3 convertase enzyme that binds to target cells and activates C3. Formation of the membrane attack complex (MAC) leads to lysis of target cells or pathogens. Phagocytes carry membrane receptors for C3b leading to opsonization and phagocytosis. MBL, mannose-binding lectin; MASP, MBL-associated serine protease.

half-life of only 13 seconds. C4 binding protein (C4bp) enhances spontaneous dissociation of C4b2a and also acts as a cofactor for C3b/C4b inactivator (I), which degrades C4b.

Mannose-binding Lectin Pathway. Mannose-binding lectin, a member of the C-type lectin (collectin) family, acts as the recognition unit of the MBL pathway. MBL recognizes polysaccharides with high mannose content and other oligosaccharides with characteristic linkages found exclusively on pathogens and not on normal host components. The calcium-dependent binding of MBL with the pathogenic polysaccharide results in activation of MBL-associated serine proteases (MASP-1 and MASP-2). Activated MASP-2 cleaves and activates C4 and C2 in the same fashion as in the classical pathway. The classical and MBL pathways converge at the activation of C4 and C2 and share a common pathway after that. In fact, MBL, MASP-1, and MASP-2 are so similar to the classical components C1q, C1r, and C1s, that at one time it was thought that these components were interchangeable variants of the same pathway. It has since been demonstrated that they are indeed distinct entities (147,150,151).

Alternative Pathway. The alternative pathway is a major mediator of innate, or nonspecific immunity. Because the alternative pathway activation is independent of antibody, it is able to react very quickly as a line of host defense. The alternative pathway exists in a low-grade activated state and becomes fully activated in the presence of a suitable activating surface. Bacteria, viruses, fungi, and parasites can all activate the alternative pathway. Initiation of the pathway occurs through low-grade spontaneous hydrolysis of C3 to give C3(H$_2$O). C3(H$_2$O) then binds B in the presence of magnesium. D, already present in plasma in its activated form, cleaves B, releasing Ba and C3(H$_2$O)Bb, the initial C3 convertase of the alternative pathway. This convertase cleaves C3 into the anaphylatoxins C3a and C3b, which bind covently by a thiol ester bond to nearby particle surfaces. C3b is the recognition component of the alternative pathway. This binding of C3b is responsible for the opsonization of bacteria. A positive feedback loop then ensues, with each C3b molecule forming a more efficient C3 convertase, C3bBb, in the presence of B, D, and magnesium. Properdin prolongs the half-life of C3 convertase by delaying the decay of Bb from C3bBb.

Excessive amplification of the alternative pathway is checked by β1H globulin factor H and factor I. H accelerates the decay and delays the formation of C3bBb. It also acts as a cofactor for I to degrade C3 into iC3b, which is unable to bind B to generate C3 convertase. The chemokine (MCP) can also act as a cofactor for I in C3 degradation. Decay acceleration factor (DAF) hinders C3 convertase assembly and mediates its dissociation in all three pathways. Complement receptor type 1 (CR1) has activities similar to MCP and DAF (145–147).

Terminal Sequence. All three pathways share a common final pathway to complete complement activation. The terminal sequence consists of 1 molecule each of C5, C6, C7, and C8, in addition to up to 18 molecules of C9, resulting in the formation of the MAC C5b-9. This complex forms a transmembrane channel with a hydrophobic outer layer and hydrophilic core that can lead to water and ion fluxes, osmotic lysis, and ultimately death of target cells or pathogens (145–147,152).

Cleavage of C5 leaves the anaphylatoxins C5a and C5b, which bind C6 and then C7. The C5b67 complex binds to the lipid membrane of the target cell, allowing the new complex to penetrate deeper into the lipid membrane. This initial 30-Å diameter transmembrane channel created by the C5-8 complex can increase in size up to 100 Å with the addition of C9 molecules (C9 polymerization), allowing

significant water and ion fluxes. Antagonists of MAC-induced cell injury include protein S and very low-density lipoprotein, which inhibit C5b67 binding to membranes, and C8 and C9 binding glycoproteins, which inhibit pore formation. Protein S also prevents C9 polymerization.

Functions of Complement

Complement is involved in the destruction of pathogens and altered host cells by mediating inflammation and chemotaxis, through cytolytic actions of MAC, and by enhancing phagocytosis through opsonization of foreign particles. Complement regulates immune complex processing by solubilizing complexes and regulating size of complexes, and through CR1-mediated clearance of immune complexes.

Anaphylatoxins. The anaphylatoxins, C4a, C3a, and especially C5a, play a significant role in increasing blood vessel permeability, vasodilatation, edema formation, neutrophil adhesion and activation, chemotaxis, and the release of toxic oxygen species and lysosomal enzymes from phagocytic cells. In biologic fluids, C5a is rapidly converted to the more physiologically stable form, C5a des-Arg, by plasma carboxypeptidase N. C5a and C5a des-Arg are approximately equipotent in increasing vascular permeability. The mechanism of C5a-induced permeability changes appears to involve an interaction between circulating neutrophils and the endothelium, resulting in an increased permeability to plasma proteins.

Opsonization and Phagocytosis. Opsonization and phagocytosis is the most important mechanism for the destruction of pathogens. Phagocytes (neutrophils, monocytes/macrophages) carry membrane receptors for complement factor C3 components attached to targeted cells and proteins. CR1 is the C3b receptor on phagocytes involved in binding C3b and C4b. CR3 and CR4 are β$_2$-integrins that bind the iC3b processing fragment of C3. C1q and MBL can act as indirect opsonins by enhancing phagocytosis initiated by CR1 or Fcγ receptors.

Membrane Attack Complex-induced Cytolysis

For the *Neisseria* species of bacteria, complement-mediated cell lysis is the primary host defense. Patients with deficiencies in the terminal components C5, C6, C7, and C8 are susceptible to meningococcal and gonococcal infections. MAC formation is also associated with local prostanoid generation in an animal model of complement-induced lung injury as well as release of platelet alpha granules and dense bodies.

Complement Component Deficiencies

Deficiencies in classical or lectin pathway initiators or C3 result in a spectrum of recurrent pyogenic infections. Defects in the MAC components (C5–C9) or in properdin result in susceptibility to *Neisseria* species infection. Deficiencies in the early components of the classical pathway can lead to defective clearance of immune complexes. Patients lacking DAF have paroxysmal nocturnal hemoglobinuria. Deficiency of C1 inhibitor allows uncontrolled cleavage of C2 and generation of the vasoactive fragment C2a. This syndrome, called *hereditary angioneurotic edema,* is associated with fluid accumulation in tissues and risk of suffocation due to epiglottal swelling.

Lipid Mediators

Eicosanoids

Eicosanoids are 20-carbon oxygenation products of eicosatetraenoic acid, also called *arachidonic acid.* These lipid mediators are not stored in tissues, but are synthesized within seconds in response to a variety of stimuli, including tissue injury and chemical mediators. Although most cells are capable of producing eicosanoids, neutrophils and macrophages are particularly important sources during inflammation. The rapid destruction of eicosanoids in the circulation limits their role primarily to that of autocrine and paracrine mediators of local inflammatory changes (153–155).

The liberation of the precursor molecule, arachidonic acid, from membrane phospholipids is the major rate-limiting step in eicosanoid production. PLA_2 is a family of enzymes that is responsible for the formation of arachidonic acid from cell membranes. The 14-kd PLA_2 forms arachidonate from plasma membranes and is transcriptionally regulated by IL-1 and TNF, or is preformed in some cells. The 85-kd PLA_2, regulated by MAP kinase phosphorylation and by calcium-dependent translocation to membranes, acts on nuclear and endoplasmic reticulum membranes rather than the outer plasma membrane. In mast cells, arachidonate may be generated by cleavage of DAG rather than by PLA_2. Once formed, arachidonic acid metabolism proceeds along one of two different pathways: the COX pathway or the LO pathway (Fig. 6.15).

Cyclooxygenase Pathway. Cyclooxygenase catalyzes the first step in a series of reactions that converts arachidonic acid to the prostanoids (prostaglandins and thromboxane). There are two isoforms of COX, the constitutively expressed COX-1 and the inducible COX-2. COX-2 is generally thought to play a more important role in inflammatory processes such as fever, hyperalgesia, and edema formation. COX oxidizes arachidonic acid to the endoperoxidase prostaglandin G_2 (PGG_2), which is converted to PGH_2. PGH_2 is converted to specific prostaglandins or thromboxane by the action of tissue-specific enzymes such as prostacyclin synthetase in endothelial cells and thromboxane synthetase in platelets. PGE_2 synthesis does not require the PGH_2 intermediate. The prostanoids are chemically unstable and are rapidly converted to inactive products by enzymatic pathways.

The effects of prostanoids, like those of all eicosanoids, on target cells are mediated by receptors belonging to the G protein family. The prostanoids possess both opposing and overlapping effects during an inflammatory response (Table 6.8). The major endothelial prostaglandin is PGI_2 (prostacy-

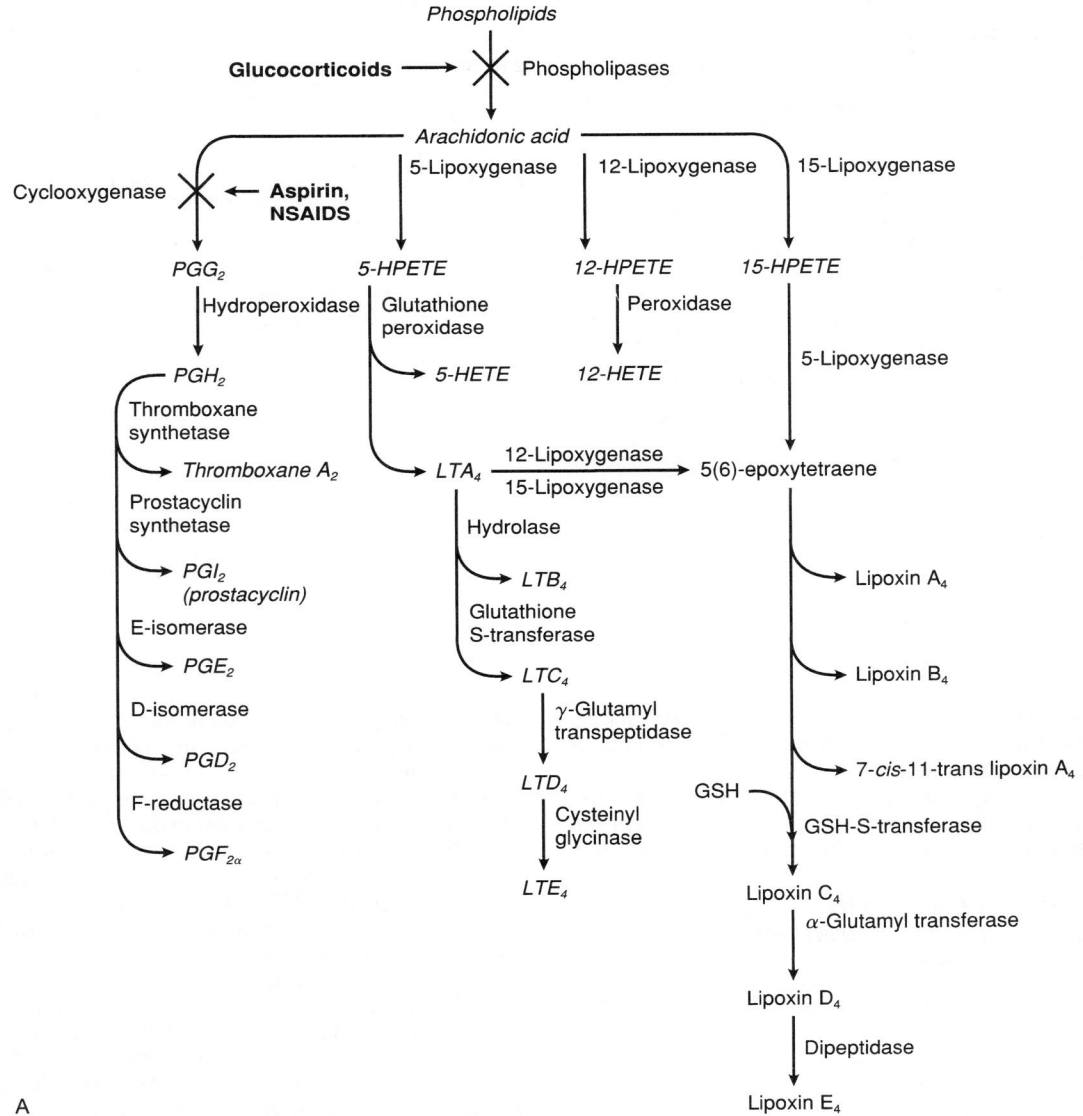

A

Figure 6.15. Pathways of eicosanoid production. Inflammatory mediators derived from arachidonic acid *(A)* and their structures *(B)*. Sites of inhibition by antiinflammatory drugs are shown. NSAIDs, nonsteroidal antiinflammatory drugs (e.g., ibuprofen). *(continues)*

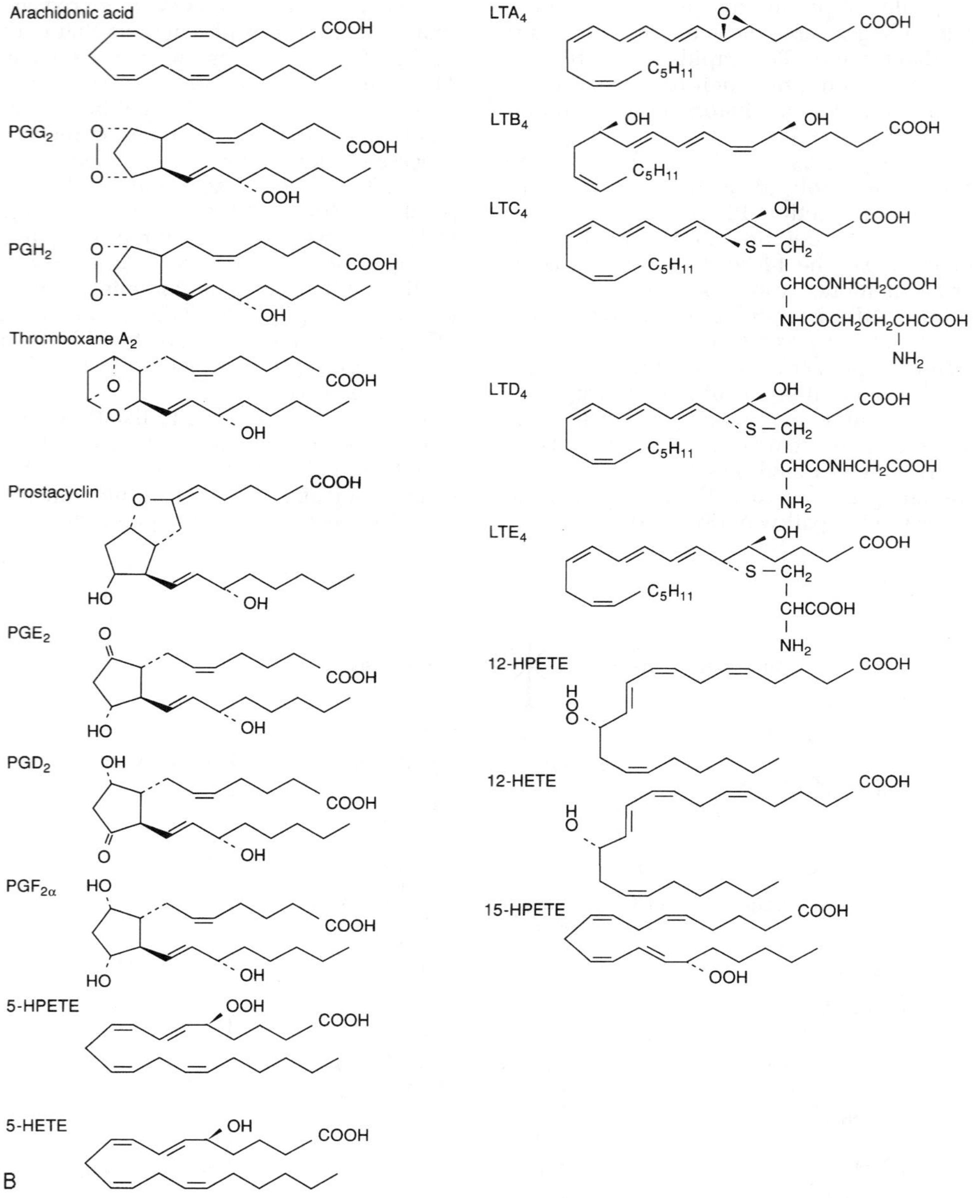

Figure 6.15. *(Continued)*

clin), a potent vasodilator. Prostacyclin inhibits platelet aggregation and adhesion, and inhibits neutrophil chemotaxis and activation. It acts synergistically with PGE$_2$ to increase vascular permeability through the effects of bradykinin. Prostacyclin is a weak bronchodilator of large airways but constricts small airways. The predominantly antiinflamma-

tory PGE$_2$ is generated in large quantities by macrophages, neutrophils, lymphocytes, and eosinophils. PGE$_2$ contributes to the fever response and synergizes with bradykinin and histamine to mediate pain. PGE$_2$ is a bronchodilator, although in low concentrations it may have some bronchoconstrictor action. PGE$_2$ inhibits both IL-1 production and T-cell responsiveness to IL-1. Low concentrations of PGE$_2$ stimulate TNF release, whereas higher concentrations suppress TNF production. Other counterinflammatory properties include the inhibition of neutrophil chemotaxis and activation and inhibition of T$_H$1 lymphocyte proliferation. PGD$_2$ is a potent bronchoconstrictor that inhibits neutrophil chemotaxis and activation. The mast cell is the major source of PGD$_2$ in allergic inflammatory reactions. TXA$_2$, PGG$_2$, and PGH$_2$ oppose the actions of prostacyclin by promoting platelet aggregation and inducing bronchoconstriction. TXA$_2$ produced by platelets and macrophages is a powerful vasoconstrictor that induces neutrophil accumulation and increases vascular permeability (153–156).

Table 6.8. PROINFLAMMATORY AND ANTIINFLAMMATORY EFFECTS OF PROSTANOIDS

	PGG$_2$	PGH$_2$	PGI$_2$	PGE$_2$	TXA$_2$
Chemotaxis	↑	↑	↓	↓	↑
Bronchial tone	↑	↑	↓	↓	↑
Platelet aggregation	↑	↑	↓	↓	↑
Systemic vascular tone			↓	↓	↑↑
Pulmonary vascular tone	↑	↑	↓	↓	↑

PG, prostaglandin; TX, thromboxane.

Lipooxygenase Pathway

Leukotrienes. Leukotrienes are leukocyte-derived molecules with three conjugated double bonds. The initial step in the production of leukotrienes and lipoxins is the oxidation of arachidonic acid by one of three lipooxygenase (LO) enzymes: 5-LO, 12-LO, and 15-LO. Leukotrienes produced by the 5-LO pathway have received the most attention. 5-LO associates with the perinuclear membrane protein 5-LO-activating protein (FLAP) in activated leukocytes to catalyze the formation of 5-hydroperoxyeicosatetraenoic acid (5-HPETE) from arachidonic acid. The subsequent conversion of 5-HPETE to LTA_4 is carried out by a dehydrase and is also catalyzed by 5-LO. LTA_4 can either be transformed to LTB_4 by a hydrolase or to LTC_4 by the addition of GSH by means of GSH-S-transferase. LTC_4 can in turn be successively hydrolyzed to the dipeptide derivative LTD_4 and the single-amino acid derivative LTE_4. Additional LO activity results in the production of 12-HPETE, 12-HETE, and 15-HPETE. These compounds exhibit biologic activity, although they are not as potent as the leukotrienes or COX products. The leukotrienes are inactivated by oxidation followed by dehydrogenation (6,154–157).

The major LO product of neutrophils is LTB_4. It is also produced by macrophages. LTB_4 is an important neutrophil and eosinophil chemotaxin that also promotes adhesion to the endothelium. It increases vascular permeability, either directly or through interaction with neutrophils and endothelial cells. LTB_4 has also been shown to induce hyperalgesia. In addition, LTB_4 serves as an intracellular messenger as a ligand for peroxisome proliferator-activated receptor-α (PPAR), a nuclear receptor that acts as a transcription factor to induce expression of enzymes for fatty acid oxidation and adipogenesis (158).

Slow-reacting substance of anaphylaxis (SRS-A), which is activated in mast cells during anaphylactic reactions, consists of the sulfidopeptide leukotrienes LTC_4, LTD_4, and LTE_4. LTC_4 is the major eicosanoid product of eosinophils and the only mast cell-derived product of LO. These three leukotrienes constrict the vascular and bronchial smooth muscle. In fact, LTC_4 and LTD_4 are probably the most powerful bronchoconstrictors in humans, being more than 1,000 times more potent than histamine in compromising airway function. They also increase capillary permeability to allow plasma exudation and are vasodilatory in skin, causing the classic wheal-and-flare reaction (159).

Lipoxins. Lipoxin biosynthesis can occur by several routes, depending on the tissue. It is unclear which subset of leukocytes is the primary source of lipoxins, but eosinophils have been implicated. Lipoxin synthesis may require cell–cell interactions. A 5(6)-epoxytetraene intermediate can be formed by 5-LO activity on 15-HPETE. This reaction when carried out in blood vessels requires the interaction between platelets and neutrophils. On mucosal surfaces, 12-LO and 5-LO activity on LTA_4 can result in formation of this lipoxin intermediate through leukocyte–epithelial cell interactions. The 5(6)-epoxytetrane intermediate is then converted to lipoxin A_4, lipoxin B_4, or lipoxin C_4. Lipoxin C_4 can be sequentially modified to form lipoxin D_4, then lipoxin E_4 (158,160,161).

The actions of lipoxins are only incompletely understood, but appear to be counterregulatory to the leu-ko-trienes. Lipoxins inhibit the generation of leukotrienes by down-regulating 5-LO as 15-LO is up-regulated. The antiinflammatory cytokines IL-4 and IL-13 contribute further to the down-regulation of inflammatory responses by up-regulating 15-LO. Lipoxins inhibit the actions of LTB_4 and LTD_4. Lipoxin A_4 and B_4 are potent vasoactive compounds. Lipoxin A_4 is a vasodilator, whereas lipoxin B_4 is a vasodilator in some tissues and a vasoconstrictor in other tissues. Vascular and smooth muscle actions of lipoxins include increased NO and prostacyclin production, increased arachidonate release, and reversal of endothelin-induced vasoconstriction. Lipoxin A_4 is also a potent bronchoconstrictor. Counterinflammatory functions of lipoxin A_4 include the inhibition of leukotrienes, $PGF_{2\alpha}$, fMLP, and other chemoattractants. Lipoxin A_4 also down-regulates LTB_4-mediated delayed-type hypersensitivity reactions.

Inhibitors of Eicosanoid Production. A large number of antiinflammatory drugs act by interfering with eicosanoid synthesis. Corticosteroids inhibit inflammation at least in part by inhibiting PLA_2 through the induction of the 30,000-kd protein lipocortin (162). They have been shown selectively to inhibit COX-2 activity without affecting COX-1. NSAIDs block synthesis of prostaglandins and thromboxane by inhibiting COX activity. In contrast to the other NSAIDs, aspirin inhibits COX in an irreversible manner. The effects of aspirin on platelet function can be reversed only by the arrival of new platelets 7 to 10 days later. Aspirin has more recently been shown to stimulate formation of 15-epilipoxin (15R-HETE) from endogenous arachidonic acid in endothelial or epithelial cells through the acetylation of COX-2 or by oxidation of arachidonic acid by cytochrome P_{450} or 5-LO. These aspirin-triggered 15-epilipoxins appear to be more potent in their antiinflammatory effects because of longer half-lives. A potential negative effect of NSAID use is that inhibition of COX can shunt arachidonic acid through the 5-LO pathway, resulting in the synthesis of higher levels of proinflammatory leukotrienes, thus minimizing any benefit achieved from reduction of other eicosanoid levels. More important, NSAIDs act systemically in a nonselective manner, so that inhibition of prostaglandin synthesis can result in dangerous side effects in locations where prostaglandins normally exert cytoprotective effects (e.g., mucosal ulceration in the stomach).

Platelet-activating Factor

Platelet-activating factor was originally described as a substance released from sensitized rabbit basophils that activated rabbit platelets (164). PAF is a heterogeneous mixture of 1-0-alkyl-2-acetyl-*sn*-glycero-3-phosphocholines that plays a prominent role in physiologic and pathologic inflammatory states. Like other lipid mediators, it is not stored in cells but is rapidly produced by activated inflammatory cells. Synthesis of PAF involves either the remodeling of membrane phospholipids by PLA_2, usually more important under inflammatory conditions, or by de novo synthesis usually seen in resting cells (165) (Fig. 6.16). De novo synthesis is regulated by substrate availability and involves a constitutively active enzyme that produces PAF in small basal amounts. The membrane phospholipid precursor of PAF, 1-0-alkyl-2-acyl-*sn*-glycero-3-phosphocholine (ether-PC), is present in high amounts in neutrophils. Other cells that can synthesize PAF include platelets, basophils, monocytes, eosinophils, mast cells, and vascular endothelial cells. Like the eicosanoids, the synthesis of PAF is initiated by calcium-mediated activity of PLA_2, which yields 1-0-alkyl-*sn*-glycerophosphocholine (lyso-PAF). Acetylation of lyso-PAF yields PAF. PAF may be released from the cell, or it may be converted back to lyso-PC by acetylhydrolase and to the precursor ether-PC (6).

Biologic effects of PAF are mediated by the G protein-coupled PAF receptor. Although it induces platelet aggregation and degranulation, PAF has critical functions in the inflammatory response that extend well beyond its actions on platelets. Its vasoactive properties include vasodilatation and increased vascular permeability. PAF is also a potent bronchoconstrictor. The effect of PAF on phagocytes (neutrophils, monocytes/macrophages) is to enhance ara-chidonic acid metabolism, leading to increased motility, de-

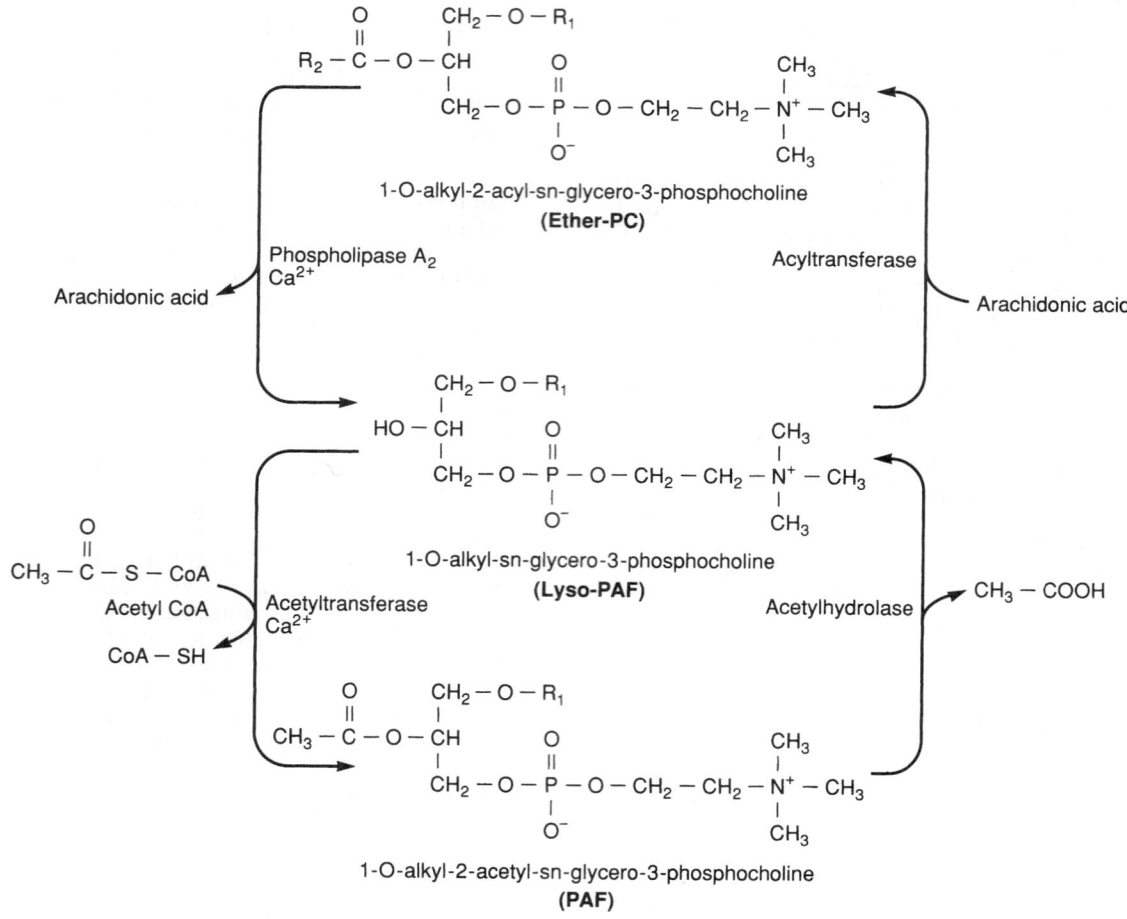

Figure 6.16. Pathways of platelet-activating factor (PAF) biosynthesis and breakdown.

granulation, and free radical formation. PAF plays an integral role in promoting activation and adherence of inflammatory cells to the vascular endothelium (166). During the early leukocyte response, activated endothelial cells synthesize and express PAF on the cell surface. Leukocytes tethered to the endothelium by P-selectin are activated by endothelial PAF. This "signaling," or activation step, results in the induction of tight integrin-dependent adhesion of leukocytes to the vascular endothelium with subsequent emigration and chemotaxis. Acyl-PAF, the major acetylated lipid from mast cells, basophils, and endothelial cells, is a less potent derivative of PAF that likely plays a role in the regulation of neutrophil adhesion to endothelial cells as well. In the case of a persistent pathologic stimulus, PAF may escape into the circulation and activate circulating leukocytes, leading to systemic sequelae of an excessive inflammatory response. PAF also promotes the adhesion of platelets to neutrophils, contributing to the prothrombotic features of the inflammatory process. As a mediator of sepsis, PAF augments endotoxin-induced hypotension and neutrophil and platelet accumulation in lungs. There is evidence that the NO-induced hypotension in experimental models of endotoxemia is mediated by PAF (167). PAF acetylhydrolase, an enzyme regulated by dexamethasone, estrogen, and PAF itself, is the enzyme responsible for the degradation of PAF.

Kinins

Kinins (from the Greek *kineo,* to move) are small vasoactive peptides generated during the inflammatory response, of which bradykinin and lysyl-bradykinin are the most important. Additional kinins (T-kinin, hyp[3]-bradykinin) are usually modifications of the nonapeptide bradykinin. There are three mechanisms of kinin formation during inflammation—one involving plasma proteins, a second involving tissue proteins, and the third involving cellular proteinases. Bradykinin is formed from the sequential cleavage of inactive precursors by serine protease kininogenases. As shown in Fig. 6.17, kinin formation is closely linked to the clotting and complement cascades (6,168,169).

Production of Bradykinin in Plasma

The biosynthetic pathway commences with the activation of Hageman factor (HF), factor XII of the coagulation cascade. HF undergoes autoactivation on binding to negatively charged surfaces such as basement membrane of injured vessel walls, heparin, or lipid A of endotoxin. HF can also be activated by LPS or by proteolytic cleavage by kallikrein. Prekallikrein is found in plasma as a 1 : 1 complex with high-molecular-weight kininogen (HK), a nonenzymatic protein. Kininogen enhances the binding of prekallikrein to negatively charged surfaces. Activated HF converts bound prekallikrein to kallikrein, which in turn activates more HF in a positive feedback cycle. HFf, a cleavage product of activated HF, is also capable of activating prekallikrein. Plasma kallikrein in plasma, tissues, and secretions such as saliva specifically cleaves HK to release the nonapeptide bradykinin. In addition to bradykinin production, kallikrein participates in the activation of plasminogen and C1q of the complement system. The only major plasma inhibitor of activated HF is C1 inhibitor The primary inhibitors of kallikrein in plasma are α_2-macroglobulin and C1 inhibitor.

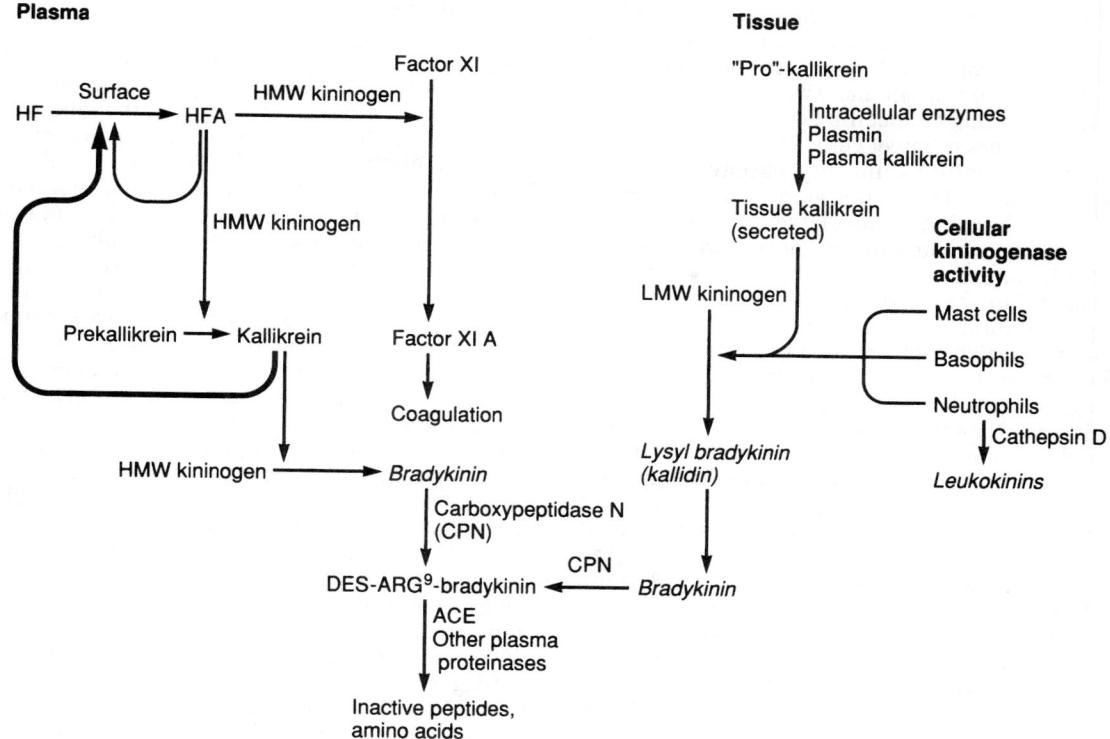

Figure 6.17. Three pathways of kinin formation. ACE, angiotensin-converting enzyme; CPN, carboxypeptidase N; HF, Hageman factor; HFA, activated Hageman factor; HMW, high molecular weight; LMW, low molecular weight. (After Proud D, Kaplan AP. Kinin formation: mechanisms and role in inflammatory disorders. *Annu Rev Immunol* 1988;6:49.)

Kinin Production in Tissue

Lysyl-bradykinin, or kallidin, is the product of cleavage of either HK or low-molecular-weight kininogen (LK) by tissue kallikreins. Tissue kallikreins are distinct proteins, different from their plasma counterparts. LK is present in higher concentrations intracellularly compared with HK. Whereas both HK and LK can be converted to kallidin by tissue kallikrein, only HK is cleaved by plasma kallikrein. Kallidin itself can be converted to bradykinin by a plasma aminopeptidase. Both kallidin and bradykinin use the same receptors and perform similar functions, but kallidin is approximately 85% as potent as bradykinin. Tissue kallikrein is synthesized as a preproenzyme converted intracellularly to tissue prokallikrein by enzymes that are not yet well characterized. The secreted prokallikrein is then converted to tissue kallikrein extracellularly by plasmin or plasma kallikrein. The only significant inhibitor of tissue kallikreins is α_1-proteinase inhibitor.

Cellular Kininogenase Activity

Neutrophils, mast cells, and basophils have been implicated as sources of kininogenase activity. Neutrophils produce leukokinins, distinct 21- to 25-amino acid peptides, by way of cathepsin D. Their role inflammation is unclear. Bradykinin is metabolized sequentially to the partially active eight-amino acid peptide, des-Arg-bradykinin, by carboxypeptidase N (anaphylatoxin inactivator), and then to inactive five-amino acid and three-amino acid fragments by angiotensin-converting enzyme (ACE). ACE is the predominant enzyme to inactivate bradykinin in the pulmonary vasculature. Arginine released as a by-product of the carboxypeptidase N reaction may contribute further to the modulation of inflammation by acting as substrate for the formation of NO (170).

There are two well characterized types of kinin receptors and possibly a third type (168). B1 receptors have a limited distribution and are expressed primarily on the vasculature under pathologic conditions such as tissue injury. Des-Arg-bradykinin and des-Arg-kallidin are the major agonists for B1 receptors. Activated B1 receptors on the vasculature help mediate hypotension in sepsis and are thought to mediate pain (171). Both B1 and the more widely distributed B2 receptors are G protein-coupled receptors. Activation of B2 receptors stimulates IP and phospholipase C (PLC) turnover, resulting in the accumulation of IP_3, DAG, and calcium as second messengers. The B2 receptors are more important in mediating the effects of kinins most closely associated with inflammation. Bradykinin and lysyl-bradykinin, the main ligands for B2 receptors, induce arteriolar dilatation and mediate pain. Like histamine, bradykinin increases gaps between postcapillary venule endothelial cells to cause a transient increase in vascular permeability. It is a potent constrictor of bronchial, uterine, and gastrointestinal smooth muscle, as well as a constrictor of coronary and pulmonary vasculatures (168). Activation of endothelial B2 receptors stimulates production of NO to enhance vasodilatation further. The antihypertensive and cardioprotective effects of ACE inhibitors have been shown to be at least partly mediated by kinins (172). ACE, in addition to catalyzing the formation of angiotensin II from angiotensin I, promotes the hydrolysis of bradykinin to inactive metabolites. In addition, bradykinin can modulate platelet function by stimulating endothelial cell secretion of PGI_2 and thromboxane through activation of PLA_2.

Neuropeptides

Nerves in every tissue carry neuropeptides that can participate in an inflammatory response. Neuropeptides may provide the neuroendocrine link between psychological stress and inflammatory diseases such as psoriasis and inflammatory bowel disease. Like cytokines, neuropeptides may act in a pleiotropic and redundant fashion. Neuropeptides execute their inflammatory and immunomodulatory effects by binding to specific G protein-coupled receptors on the surfaces of target cells. Neuropeptides may be proinflammatory, antiinflammatory, or both. For example, the hypothalamic fever response to PGE$_2$ induced by IL-1 and TNF elaboration is mediated by substance P, whereas it is down-regulated by adrenocorticotropic hormone (ACTH), arginine vasopressin (AVP), and α-melanocyte stimulating hormone (α-MSH). Neuropeptides are also important immunomodulators. The pituitary peptides prolactin, corticotropin-releasing hormone (CRH), and AVP, have been shown to augment immune responses by enhancing T$_H$1 activity (173,174).

Tachykinins are important proinflammatory neuropeptides that mediate pain and promote the classic inflammatory signs of erythema and edema formation through their vasodilatory effects. The tachykinins are derived from two genes: preprotachykinin I, which gives rise to substance P, neurokinin A, neuropeptide K, and neuropeptide γ; and preprotachykinin II, which encodes neurokinin B (175). Substance P stimulates monocyte and neutrophil influx and neutrophil phagocytosis. Its inflammatory effects appear to be mediated by the proinflammatory cytokines TNF and IL-1 from mast cells, monocytes, macrophages, bone marrow, and endothelial cells. During allergic inflammation, substance P stimulates histamine release from mast cells. As an effector of immune function, substance P promotes T-cell proliferation and antibody production. Substance P released locally by nerve terminals is important in mediating the perception of pain.

Corticotropin-releasing hormone stimulates release of IL-1, IL-6, and superoxide from macrophages. Proinflammatory consequences of CRH release are self-regulated, however, through cortisol release. Cortisol down-regulates production of proinflammatory cytokines (IL-1, TNF, IL-2, IL-6), metalloproteinases, and iNOS, and, through negative feedback loops, inhibits the production of CRH as well as ACTH and AVP. AVP, growth hormone, and prolactin are other important proinflammatory neuropeptides (173,174).

Vasoactive intestinal peptide (VIP) and its homologous peptide, pituitary adenylate cyclase-activating polypeptide (PACAP), display both proinflammatory and antiinflammatory effects. VIP, found throughout the central and peripheral nervous systems, is a chemoattractant for macrophages, neutrophils, and T cells, and may play an important role in granulomatous reactions. VIP also stimulates release of histamine and IL-5. Both VIP and PACAP are vasodilators. However, VIP and PACAP are also known as macrophage deactivating factors. They inhibit IL-6, TNF, and IL-12 release and inhibit iNOS expression in activated macrophages. VIP and PACAP have been shown to stimulate production of the antiinflammatory cytokine IL-10 by macrophages (177). VIP also inhibits IL-2 and IFN-γ production by lymphocytes and inhibits T-cell proliferation.

Somatostatin and α-MSH are primarily antiinflammatory in action. Somatostatin, which colocalizes with substance P in sensory nerves, inhibits IgE formation and NK cell activity. α-MSH inhibits chemotaxis and IFN-γ production, and down-regulates T$_H$1 activity. ACTH, calcitonin, and β-endorphin are other neuropeptides with predominantly antiinflammatory properties.

Calcitonin gene-related peptide (CGRP) is primarily an immune modulator, inhibiting activity of T cells and macrophages, partly through the induction of IL-10. It also is an inhibitor of antigen presentation. CGRP promotes vasodilatation and neutrophil influx, and synergizes with bradykinin and histamine to promote edema formation through vasodilatation and increased vascular permeability.

Cytokines

Cytokines are small polypeptides or glycoproteins that interact with high-affinity receptors on their target cells to modulate cell growth, tissue repair, the immune response, and inflammation. Constitutive production of cytokines is usually low, if present at all. Typically, cytokines are synthesized and secreted in response to cellular activation or injury. Although cytokines such as IL-1, IL-6, and TNF can manifest systemic effects in the acute-phase response or in septic shock, cytokines primarily exert their effects as paracrine or autocrine mediators. Target cells respond to cytokine stimulation by altering gene expression. The terminology used in the cytokine literature is often confusing and has evolved over the years. Monokines are cytokines produced by cells of the monocyte lineage. Lymphokines are lymphocyte-derived cytokines. It has become evident, however, that both can be produced by different cell types, so these terms may now be obsolete. Chemokines, the largest family of cytokines, represent a subset chemotactic for leukocytes and are discussed separately (178).

Cytokine secretion requires new protein synthesis. Production of cytokines is regulated mainly at the level of gene transcription. Transcription for cytokine synthesis is rapid and transient after cell activation. Bacterial metabolites, ROS, and cytokines themselves can act as alarm molecules to trigger a cascade of phosphorylations that culminates in the activation and binding of nuclear transcription factors (see section on Transcription Factors, earlier). NFκB is probably the most important activator of cytokine gene expression (138,139). Production of cytokines is a function of the sum of interactions between NFκB and other transcription factors such as AP-1 and NF-IL6. Cytokine synthesis is also regulated at the posttranscriptional and posttranslational levels. Cytokine protein precursors are often processed by specific proteinases before being expressed as biologically active cytokines. Receptors for cytokines on target cells can be classified into families based on their structure. Most cytokine receptors are of the class I family of dimeric (and sometimes trimeric) proteins. Class I cytokine receptors are further divided into subfamilies based on a common receptor chain shared by cytokines. The major means for most cytokine receptors to communicate with the target cell nucleus to activate gene transcription involves the JAK-STAT signal transduction pathway (142, 143) (see section on Transcription Factors).

Cytokines are characterized by pleiotropy (one cytokine has many functions) and redundancy (many cytokines have the same function). IL-1 and TNF, probably the best-characterized cytokines, highlight these features. Both cytokines affect practically every cell type. They are both associated with the development of physical signs and symptoms of the acute-phase response and the systemic inflammatory response syndrome (SIRS). These include the induction of fever, chills, hypotension, altered pituitary hormone secretion, and acute-phase protein synthesis. Cytokines are capable of synergistic interactions. IL-1 and TNF do not synergize because they often share a common signal transduction pathway. On the other hand, synergism between TNF and IFN-γ is possible because they activate distinct signaling pathways that amplify each other. TNF and IFN-γ synergize to increase the cytotoxicity of TNF on tumor cells and to induce NO production in macrophages. Cytokines can act in an antagonistic fashion. One cytokine can also directly or indirectly affect the production of another cytokine. IL-2 production in T cells occurs in response to stimulation with IL-1. IL-12 increases IFN-γ production in T cells and NK cells, and IFN-γ in turn increases IL-12 production in macrophages. Table 6.9 highlights selected cytokines and their sources, targets, and main functions.

Table 6.9. **SELECTED CYTOKINES**

Cytokine	Source	Target cells	Main functions
IL-1	Mo/Mφ, B, EC, epith, fibro	All	Neutrophil and Mo emigration, shock, fever, APP production, ↑ adhesion molecules
IL-2	T	T, B, NK, Mo/Mφ	T activation and proliferation, Mo/Mφ activation
IL-4	T, Ba, MC	T, B, NK, neutrophil, Eo, Mo/Mφ, EC, fibro	T_H2 differentiation and proliferation; T_H1, B, and Mo inhibitor
IL-6	Mo/Mφ, B, fibro, EC, epith	T, B, Mo/Mφ, epith, hepatocytes	APP synthesis, T and B differentiation
IL-8	Mo/Mφ, T, Neutrophils, fibro, EC, epith	Neutrophils, T, Mo/Mφ, EC, Ba	Neutrophil activation, adherence, and migration; Mo and T migration; Ba histamine release
IL-10	Mo/Mφ, T, B, MC	Mo/Mφ, T, B, NK, MC	Inhibits T_H1 differentiation, ↓ Mφ secretion
IL-12	Mφ	T, NK	T_H1 activator
IL-13	T	Mo/Mφ, B, EC	↓ Mφ secretion, ↑ adhesion molecules and CC chemokines on EC
IFN-α/β	All	All	Antiviral; antitumor; activates T, Mφ, NK; ↑ MHC class I antigen
IFN-γ	T, NK	All	Mφ activator, T_H1 differentiation, Ig secretion, ↑ MHC class II antigen, antiviral fever, anorexia, shock, capillary leak, APP synthesis, inflammatory cytokine induction, NK activator
TNF	Mo/Mφ, MC, Ba, Eo, NK, B, T, fibro, epith	All except RBC	
G-CSF	Mo/Mφ, fibro, EC, epith, stromal cells	Myeloid cells, EC	Myelopoiesis, neutrophil function and survival
GM-CSF	T, Mo/Mφ, fibro, EC, epith	Mo/Mφ, neutrophils, Eo, fibro, EC	Myelopoiesis, Mφ and NK activator, dendritic cell maturation
TGF-β	Almost all	Almost all	Inhibits T, Mφ, granulocyte activity; ↑ matrix protein synthesis

APP, acute-phase protein; B, B cell; Ba, basophil; Eo, eosinophils; epith, epithelial cells; fibro, fibroblasts; GM-CSF, granulocyte/macrophage colony-stimulating factor; IFN, interferon; IL, interleukin; MHC, major histocompatibility complex; Mo, monocytes; Mφ, macrophages; NK, natural killer; T, T cell; T_H, helper T cell; TGF, transforming growth factor; TNF, tumor necrosis factor.
Modified from Gallin JI, Snyderman R, eds. Inflammation: basic principles and clinical correlates, 3rd ed. Philadelphia: Lippincott Williams & Wilkins, 1999.

Tumor Necrosis Factor

Tumor necrosis factor (cachectin) was the first monocyte/macrophage-derived cytokine identified. It was originally described as a cytotoxic agent that induces necrosis in tumor cells (179). Today it is recognized as a primary mediator of the immune and inflammatory response produced by many different types of cells. Among the many types of cells that can produce TNF, monocytes and macrophages are the most significant. TNF is produced in response to stimulation with LPS, complement 5a, GM-CSF, hypoxia, IL-1, irradiation, leukotrienes, NO, ROS, viruses, and TNF itself. There are two forms of biologically active TNF: a transmembrane pro-TNF and the secreted TNF. TNF mediates its multitude of effects by binding to receptors that are present on all nucleated cells. There are two types of transmembrane receptors—type I (p60 or p55) and type II (p80 or p75). The type I receptor appears to be more significant in mediating TNF's effects. The type I TNF receptor has three functional domains: a neutral sphingomyelinase activating domain (NSD), an acidic activating domain (ASD), and the death domain (180) (Fig. 6.10). Each of these domains is associated with an adaptor protein. Differential expression of adaptor proteins and downstream proteins determines the net effect of TNF binding. The death domain pathways are associated with either proapoptotic or antiapoptotic activity. Activation of the NSD and ASD pathways is more directly associated with the inflammatory response, but overlap between the death domain pathway and the ASD pathway allows all three pathways to mediate an inflammatory response. Soluble TNF receptors formed by proteolytic processing of both types of receptors bind and neutralize TNF and TNF receptors, and may be an endogenous regulator of TNF activity. For a discussion of death domain signaling, the reader is referred to the section on Apoptosis.

Tumor necrosis factor is central to the pathogenesis of SIRS and septic shock (181–183). The acute overproduction of TNF is associated with capillary leak and hypotension at least partly secondary to induction of NO. TNF induces release of pituitary hormones (ACTH, prolactin, thyroid-stimulating hormone, growth hormone) and other proinflammatory cytokines (IL-1, IL-6, IL-8, GM-CSF). It initiates neutrophil margination by inducing expression of adhesion molecules and stimulates degranulation and superoxide production. TNF activates monocytes, macrophages, and NK cells, resulting in enhanced cytotoxicity. TNF-activated macrophages produce high mobility group-1 protein (HMG-1), which has been shown to act as a late mediator in sepsis (184). The procoagulant state associated with inflammation is partly mediated by TNF activation of the coagulation and complement cascades (185).

Interleukin-1

Interleukin-1 has been known by many names, including lymphocyte-activating factor, mitogenic protein, leukocyte pyrogen, endogenous pyrogen, B-cell activating factor, and leukocyte endogenous mediator. The main producers of IL-1 are monocytes, macrophages, and lymphocytes. IL-1 appears to be released either in parallel with or in response to TNF secretion. There are three members of the IL-1 gene family: IL-1α, IL-1β and IL-1 receptor antagonist (IL-1RA). Most IL-1α remains in the cytosol in a precursor form or is associated with the cell membrane in a biologically active form. Transcription of IL-1β is induced by such variegated stimuli as C5a, hypoxia, or thrombus formation, but translation to the mature form of IL-1β requires cytokine stimulation (may be IL-1) or LPS. Although IL-1β can be cleaved from its precursor by trypsin, plasmin, and other proteases, processing is usually linked to peptide cleavage by

IL-1β–converting enzyme (ICE) (186). ICE has been the object of considerable interest by investigators because it is the first member of the family of intracellular cysteine proteases, or caspases, which are known to participate in apoptosis.

The two IL-1 receptors (IL-1RI and IL-1RII) belong to the immunoglobulin superfamily of proteins (187). Both receptors bind IL-1α, IL-1β, and IL-RA. IL-1RI activates signal transduction, whereas IL-1RII is a decoy receptor that does not transduce a signal (188). The exact mechanisms of signal transduction have yet to be uncovered, although it appears that different target cells use different mechanisms. The nuclear transcription factors NFκB and AP-1 are common to many IL-1- and TNF-inducible genes. Signaling by the IL-1 receptor and TNF receptor appears to converge at the level of NFκB-inducing kinase, although MAP kinase may play a role in the signaling of both receptors as well (189).

Interleukin-1, like TNF, affects nearly every cell type. Unlike TNF, IL-1 is not directly lethal, but reproduces many of the acute hematologic and metabolic phenomena associated with sepsis. The biologic activities of IL-1α and IL-1β are usually indistinguishable. IL-1 mediates many of the systemic manifestations of the acute-phase response, usually in conjunction with TNF and IL-6. These including fever, myalgia, somnolence, and hypotension. IL-1 stimulates the hypothalamic–pituitary axis, increasing thyroid-stimulating hormone, ACTH, and cortisol levels. IL-1 also stimulates acute-phase protein synthesis either directly or by inducing IL-6 release. It promotes neutrophil differentiation and activation by inducing GM-CSF and M-CSF. Overproduction of IL-1 produces excessive margination of activated neutrophils into the vascular wall, stimulates endothelial cell procoagulant activity, and increases leukocyte binding.

Interleukin-1 receptor antagonist modulates the proinflammatory effects of IL-1 by acting as a competitive inhibitor. Binding of IL-1RA to IL-1RI does not result in a signal. A soluble form of the IL-1 receptor (sIL-1R) binds and neutralizes IL-1 as another potential means of self-regulating the proinflammatory effects of IL-1.

Interleukin-2

Interleukin-2 (or T-cell growth factor) produced by activated T cells is the primary stimulator of T-cell proliferation and differentiation (190). Receptors for IL-2 are present only on activated T cells, B cells, a small proportion of NK cells, and mononuclear phagocytes. The heterotrimeric IL-2 receptor belongs to the subfamily of class I receptors that shares a common γ chain. Antigen activation of resting T cells initiates transcription of IL-2 and up-regulates cell surface expression of IL-2 receptors, resulting in clonal expansion of those cells. Antigen binding to the T-cell receptor in the absence of a costimulatory signal results in clonal anergy (unresponsiveness) secondary to the selective inhibition of IL-2 gene expression. IL-2 in conjunction with IFN-γ and IL-12 can trigger a positive feedback cycle of NK cell activation. The net effect of T- and NK cell activation is increased cytolysis and release of proinflammatory cytokines. Local injection of IL-2 produces the classic signs of inflammation—rubor, calor, tumor, and dolor. Continuous intravenous administration of IL-2, as seen when IL-2 is used for cancer immunotherapy, results in SIRS features (fever, rigor, myalgia, capillary leak, vascular collapse) (191).

Interleukin-6

Interleukin-6 is constitutively produced in many cells but induced in infection, trauma, or immune stimulation in almost every cell type. The IL-6 receptor is a heterodimeric protein that shares its gp130 signal transduction component with related cytokines [leukemia inhibitory factor (LIF), IL-11, oncostatin M (OSM), ciliary neurotrophic factor (CNTF), cardiotrophin-1 (CT-1)]. IL-6 is the chief regulator of acute-phase proteins. Together with IL-1 and TNF, IL-6 mediates

the systemic manifestations of the acute-phase response such as fever, somnolence, and altered pituitary hormone secretion (192). IL-6 increases central secretion of vasopressin, which may partly explain the incidence of the syndrome of inappropriate antidiuretic hormone seen with some inflammatory states. It potentiates the immune response by inducing B-cell differentiation and activating T cells. IL-6 interacts with TNF to enhance T-cell proliferation and promotes neutrophil activation and accumulation. IL-6 is also an important regulator of the inflammatory response. Many of its biologic activities, including the induction of acute-phase protein synthesis and the stimulation of corticosteroid release, dampen the inflammatory response. Whereas antecedent TNF and IL-1 production potentiates IL-6 release, IL-6 antagonizes LPS-induced TNF production and TNF-induced IL-1 production (193,194).

Interleukin-12

Interleukin-12 (also called *NK cell stimulatory factor* and *cytotoxic lymphocyte maturation factor*) augments cytotoxicity of NK and T cells. IL-12 is produced primarily by APC (monocytes and DC) by two pathways: a T-cell-independent pathway induced by bacteria or intracellular parasites during the early inflammatory response and a T-cell-dependent pathway induced by the interaction of CD40L on activated T cells with CD40 receptor on IL-12-producing cells (195,196). The class I IL-12 receptor complex includes the gp130 chain of the IL-6 receptor. IL-12 shares a special partnership with IFN-γ. Activated NK cells and T_H1 cells produce IFN-γ that potentiates IL-12 production by macrophages in a positive feedback cycle. Through the induction of IFN-γ production, IL-12 enhances the function of phagocytic cells and promotes antitumor activity. IL-12 is the major cytokine responsible for the differentiation of T_H1 cells and the suppression of T_H2 cells (58). The inhibition of T_H2 and IL-4 activity confers antiallergic properties to IL-12.

Interferons

The interferons are unique in that they possess potent antiviral and antitumor qualities. They are divided into type I (IFN-α, IFN-β) and type II (IFN-γ). Type I interferons do not share molecular homology with type II interferon, but they share important biologic properties.

Type I Interferons (IFN-α, IFN-β). Type I interferons can be produced by practically any cell when properly stimulated. Viruses are the most potent inducers of IFN-α/β, but LPS, double-stranded RNA, IL-1, and TNF can act as inducers as well. Interferons bind to the class II (interferon) family of cytokine receptors that includes receptors for IFN-α/β, IFN-γ, IL-10, and tissue factor. The type I IFNs have greater antiviral and antitumor activity compared with IFN-γ and are an important component of the first line of defense against viral infection. IFN-α and IFN-β regulate the expression of MHC class I molecules and $β_2$-microglobulin that stabilize the MHC class I complex. They can also stimulate B-cell development, proliferation, and immunoglobulin heavy chain switching from IgM to IgG. Type I interferons inhibit cell replication of normal and tumor cells and enhance CTL and NK cell activity. They are used in clinical settings against hepatitis B and C infection, multiple sclerosis, CML, and Kaposi's sarcoma (197–199).

Type II Interferon (IFN-γ). Interferon-γ displays all the signature features of cytokines—pleiotropy, redundancy, synergism, and antagonism. Unlike the type I interferons, IFN-γ is produced only by T cells and activated NK cells. CD8+ T cells and the T_H1 subset of CD4+ T cells produce IFN-γ in response to MHC-bound peptide antigen with a costimulatory signal. Other inducers include mitogens and TNF plus IL-12. NK cells produce IFN-γ independent of MHC-associated antigen. The class II receptors for IFN-γ are found on all cells (pleiotropy). IFN-γ is primarily an immune modulator. In addition to its antiviral and antitumor features shared with type I interferons (redundancy), IFN-γ is the major activating factor for macrophages. It regulates expression of MHC class II as well as MHC class I molecules. IFN-γ is involved in reciprocal stimulation with TNF and IL-12. Stimulated macrophages activate NK cells by releasing TNF and IL-12. These activated NK cells then release IFN-γ, which further stimulates macrophages to secrete more TNF and IL-12. The result is a positive amplification loop. IL-10, by suppressing macrophage release of TNF and IL-12 in the initiation of this loop, is the major negative regulator of IFN-γ production. The IL-12 released from monocytes and macrophages differentially activates T_H1 cells while inhibiting the T_H2 subset. IFN-γ induces macrophage release of IL-1 and IL-6 in addition to TNF and IL-12, and can synergize with these cytokines in mediating cytotoxicity (synergism). IFN-γ promotes inflammatory cell recruitment by enhancing adhesion of lymphocytes to endothelial cells, inducing morphologic changes in endothelial cells, and attracting neutrophils. Microbicidal activity is enhanced in macrophages and neutrophils with IFN-γ stimulation. However, IFN-γ antagonizes the actions of GM-CSF (antagonism) (200,201).

Colony-stimulating Factors

Colony-stimulating factors derive their name from their tendency to promote the formation of granulocyte or mononuclear cell colonies in semisolid media. Receptors for GM-CSF and G-CSF are of the class I family of cytokine receptors. GM-CSF is expressed by T cells, B cells, macrophages, mast cells, fibroblasts, and endothelial cells in response to stimuli such as IL-1, IL-2, LPS, TNF, or oxidized lipoproteins. Its target cells are neutrophils, monocytes, macrophages, and DC. It is a powerful stimulus for hematopoiesis and mobilization of blood progenitors. GM-CSF enhances cytokine release, degranulation, and the phagocytosis of opsonized particles by neutrophils. In monocytes and macrophages, GM-CSF enhances cytotoxicity and cytokine release. It also stimulates differentiation and proliferation of DC and promotes the activity of APC (81,202).

Granulocyte colony-stimulating factor is produced by macrophages, endothelial cells, fibroblasts, and bone marrow stromal cells. It has strict target cell specificity for members of the neutrophil lineage to support proliferation and maturation (203). IL-1 and TNF produced in conjunction with G-CSF in activated macrophages induce fibroblasts and endothelial cells to release G-CSF into the circulation to stimulate granulopoiesis. In 1991, the U.S. Food and Drug Administration approved use of G-CSF in patients with neutropenia induced by chemotherapy or immunosuppressive agents after organ transplantation (204).

Antiinflammatory Cytokines

Although cytokines are usually thought of as proinflammatory, cytokines with antiinflammatory effects are critical in regulating the host response. The principal antiinflammatory cytokines are IL-4, IL-10, IL-13, and TGF-β. The antiinflammatory cytokines inhibit the production of proinflammatory cytokines from mononuclear phagocytes and granulocytes. They further antagonize proinflammatory effects by up-regulating IL-1RA and soluble TNF receptor units. IL-4, IL-10, and IL-13 are produced by the T_H2 subset of helper T cells and share many similar effects. The procoagulant state of inflammation is attenuated by their inhibition of LPS-induced tissue factor activity. IL-4, IL-10, and IL-13 inhibit the induction of COX-2 and iNOS in monocytes and macrophages.

Interleukin-4 and IL-13 share 25% homology, a common receptor chain, and many biologic properties (205). They increase 15-LO activity, leading to increased 15S-HETE and lipoxin A_4, both of which antagonize proinflamma-

tory leukotrienes. They also down-regulate surface expression of Fcγ receptors on monocytes, contributing to decreased antibody-dependent cell cytotoxicity (ADCC) (206). In APC, IL-4 and IL-13 can have immunostimulatory effects by up-regulating expression of MHC class II and costimulatory molecules on monocytes. Either IL-4 or IL-13 can be used in combination with GM-CSF to stimulate differentiation of monocyte precursors into DC in culture (202).

Interleukin-10, once called *cytokine synthesis inhibiting factor,* is perhaps the most powerful anti-inflammatory cytokine. IL-10 is produced by T_H2 cells, B cells, monocytes, and macrophages in response to LPS, immune complexes, and proinflammatory cytokines. Agents that increase cAMP, such as catecholamines and PGE_2, enhance IL-10 release. Receptors for IL-10 are of the class II (interferon) family of cytokine receptors. IL-10 plays a critical role in regulating the systemic inflammatory response. Its chief effects involve the deactivation of APC and granulocytes. In addition to inhibiting proinflammatory cytokine release, IL-10 inhibits the expression of adhesion molecules, MHC class II proteins, and the costimulatory molecules on monocytes. In neutrophils, IL-10 inhibits cytokine release, superoxide generation, migration, and even survival, to limit the duration of the acute inflammatory response (207). IL-10 and IL-4 inhibit IFN-γ and IL-12 production to limit differentiation and function of T_H1 cells and favor differentiation of T_H2 cells (58). Activation of T cells in the presence of IL-10 results in anergy, or nonresponsiveness, of those T cells. IL-10 inhibits TNF and IL-12 production by macrophages. Like IL-4, IL-10 can inhibit macrophage activation after LPS challenge, leading to decreased production of NO and H_2O_2 (208). The addition of IL-10 to GM-CSF and either IL-4 or IL-13 in monocyte cultures inhibits differentiation to DC (209). IL-10 also displays some immunostimulatory effects. By up-regulating surface expression of Fcγ receptors on monocytes, IL-10 enhances ADCC and the phagocytosis of opsonized particles (210).

Transforming growth factor-β received its name owing to the observation that it induced phenotypic transformation of fibroblast cell lines in vitro (211). TGF-β promotes wound healing by increasing extracellular matrix protein synthesis and stimulating mononuclear cell and fibroblast influx (212). It is a powerful immunomodulator that favors differentiation of CD4+ T cells to the T_H2 subset and inhibits MHC class II surface expression. TGF-β can synergize with IL-4, IL-13, and IL-10 to antagonize the production or effects of proinflammatory cytokines. Macrophages exposed to TGF-β have a weakened respiratory burst and decreased production of TNF and NO. Signaling by TGF-β receptors is unique. TGF-β binds to the type II receptor, a constitutive kinase that phosphorylates the type I receptor, activating a serine/threonine kinase. The kinase phosphorylates mothers against decapentaplegic-related protein (MADR), an inactive cytoplasmic element, allowing the phosphorylated MADR to move into the nucleus to activate transcription (213).

Chemokines

Chemokines *(chemo*attractant cyto*kines)* make up the largest family of cytokines (214–217). They consist of small, dimeric, proinflammatory proteins that show 20% to 50% homology at the amino acid level. The primary function of chemokines is leukocyte chemotaxis. Unlike the classic chemoattractants that have little specificity, members of the chemokine family recruit specific subsets of leukocytes. Chemokines have direct chemotactic effects as well as indirect effects through the induction of other mediators (histamine, ROS, defensins, or other neutrophil enzymes). They are produced by resident macrophages, recruited leukocytes, endothelial cells, fibroblasts, and many other cell types on induction by LPS, phagocytosis, and inflammatory cytokines such as IL-1, TNF, IL-6, and IFN-γ. Constitutively produced chemokines such as SDF-1, TARC, MDC, MIP-3β,

SLC, and RANTES, are likely to be involved in leukocyte trafficking under normal conditions. Most chemokines, however, are produced on cell activation. Several of the constitutively expressed chemokines are up-regulated with inflammatory and immunologic stimulation. Four subfamilies of chemokines have been identified to date, based on their arrangement of cysteine residues. The α-chemokines have the first two cysteine residues separated by an amino acid, and are needed more commonly called *CXC chemokines*. The first two cysteine residues of β-chemokines are adjacent to each other, so these are termed *CC chemokines*. The other two cysteine motif subfamilies are represented by lymphotactin (C or γ-chemokine) and fractalkine (CX3C or δ-chemokine). Che-mokine receptors are seven transmembrane receptors that signal by G proteins and the formation of IP$_3$ and DAG as second messengers. To date, there are five CXC chemokine receptors identified, nine CC chemokine receptors, and one receptor each for C and CX3C chemokines. The list of chemokines and their receptors continues to expand and evolve at an explosive rate.

CXC Chemokines and Their Receptors. CXC chemokines chemoattract and activate neutrophils and, to a somewhat lesser degree, lymphocytes. IL-8, also called *neutrophil activating peptide* (NAP), is the prototype CXC chemokine. IL-8 is chemotactic for all granulocytes (neutrophils, eosinophils, and basophils) and activates practically every aspect of neutrophil function. It stimulates neutrophil degranulation, phagocytosis, transendothelial migration, shedding of L-selectin, up-regulation of β$_2$ integrins, and augmented superoxide production in response to bacterial metabolites. In addition to granulocytes, IL-8 attracts T cells directly or indirectly by inducing neutrophil degranulation of the T-cell chemoattractants CAP37/azurocidin and defensins. IL-8 binds two receptors, CXCR1 and CXCR2 (IL-8RA and IL-8RB, respectively). Binding of CXCR1 is responsible for respiratory burst activity and activation of phospholipase D, whereas both receptors promote chemotaxis and degranulation. Other ligands for CXCR1 and CXCR2 (GCP-2; GRO-α, -β, -γ; NAP-2; ENA-78) are neutrophil activating chemokines. Interestingly, G-CSF, an important growth factor for neutrophils, can up-regulate mRNA for CXCR1 and CXCR2.

The interferon-influenced chemokines, IP-10 (IFN-γ-inducible protein) and Mig (monokine induced by IFN-γ), are unique in that they do not target neutrophils. These chemokines may play a more prominent role in mediating inflammatory responses to viral infections and autoimmune disorders. Mig, chemotactic for tumor-infiltrating lymphocytes or activated T cells and monocytes, promotes CTL activity. IP-10 is constitutively expressed in high amounts in thymic and splenic stromal cells. It is chemotactic for monocytes, T cells, and NK cells and promotes T-cell adhesion. IP-10 and Mig bind the CXCR3 receptor found exclusively on IL-2-activated T cells. Stromal cell-derived factor-1 (SDF-1) is the only known ligand for the CXCR4 receptor. SDF-1 is found in almost all organs except in blood cells. It stimulates proliferation of pre-B-cell clones and growth of bone marrow B progenitor cells in the presence of IL-7. This receptor has gained much interest since the discovery that it is a coreceptor for HIV-1. Platelet factor-4 (PF$_4$) and neutrophil-activating protein-2 (NAP-2) are CXC chemokines released from platelets. PF$_4$, from platelet alpha-granules, binds heparin with high affinity to stimulate coagulation.

CC Chemokines and Their Receptors. The β-chemokines recruit monocytes, granulocytes, T cells, NK cells, and DC. RANTES is produced by stimulated T cells, platelets, and endothelial cells, and is constitutively produced by resting T cells, suggesting a physiologic role under normal conditions. MIP-1α and MIP-1β are produced largely by stimulated T lymphocytes. Macrophage-inflammatory protein-1 (MIP-1)

is primarily a chemotactic agent for neutrophils, monocytes, eosinophils, basophils, and T lymphocytes. Other effects include the development of fever, the stimulation of hematopoietic progenitor cells, and the up-regulation of TNF, IL-1, and IL-6. MIP-3α/LARC (liver and activation-regulated chemokine)/exodus is expressed in lymphoid tissues and is chemotactic for peripheral lymphocytes. MIP-3β/ELC (Epstein-Barr virus-induced gene 1 ligand chemokine), the ligand for CCR7, has no relation to MIP-3α.

The membrane cofactor protein (MCP) family of chemokines (MCP 1 through 4) are mainly chemotactic for monocytes and T cells. MCP chemokines promote differential functions by binding to different receptors. Binding to CCR1 enhances chemotaxis, whereas activation of CCR2 increases the release of intracellular substances such as histamine and leukotrienes from basophils on binding by MCP-1. MCP-1 is produced in nonlymphocytic cells (endothelial cells, epithelial cells, fibroblasts, smooth muscle cells, macrophages, and mast cells). Eotaxin and eotaxin-2, chemotactic for eosinophils and basophils, are selective for CCR3. Eotaxin-2/MPIF-2 (myeloid progenitor inhibitory factor)/Ckβ-6 is chemotactic for resting T cells in addition to its actions on eosinophils.

Chemokines may have anti-inflammatory effects as well. MPIF-1/Ckβ-8 is chemotactic for resting T cells, monocytes, and neutrophils. Its inhibitory function is aimed at myeloid progenitors (granulocytes, mononuclear phagocytes), whereas that of MPIF-2 is directed at colony formation of multipotential hematopoietic progenitors in vitro. Macrophage-derived chemokine (MDC), expressed, as its name implies, from monocytes and macrophages, is constitutively expressed in thymus, lung, and spleen. Its chemotactic properties are directed toward DC and activated NK cells.

C and CX3C Chemokines. Lymphotactin (single cysteine motif), the only member of the C chemokine family, is produced by CD8+ lymphocytes, thymocytes, NK cells, and, to a lesser degree, by DC and activated mast cells. As its name implies, it selectively recruits lymphoid cells. Fractalkine, the sole CX3C chemokine, is produced by activated endothelial cells. In its membrane-bound form, fractalkine acts as a solid-phase adhesion molecule. The soluble form is cleaved from the membrane-bound form and can act as a soluble chemoattractant for lymphoid cells and monocytes.

INTEGRATION OF THE INFLAMMATORY COMPONENTS

Acute-phase Response

The acute-phase response that occurs in response to trauma or cellular injury is characterized by alterations in hepatic metabolism and gene regulation; activation of the central nervous system, leading to fever and adaptive behaviors; an altered hematologic profile; activation of complement and the fibrinolytic and clotting cascades; and the release of neuropeptides, kinins, and hormones. Although named the *acute-phase response*, these changes accompany both acute and chronic inflammatory disorders. It is a rapid, nonspecific response that occurs before any specific immune response. Although the acute-phase response is believed to benefit the host defense in the face of altered homeostasis, excessive production of inflammatory mediators could have detrimental and even lethal effects (e.g., systemic amyloidosis, SIRS, septic shock). Cytokines are the chief mediators of the acute-phase response, and of the cytokines, IL-6, IL-1, and TNF play particularly central roles (192,218).

Acute-phase Proteins

An acute-phase protein is defined as a protein whose concentration increases by at least 25% during inflammatory disorders (219,220). Acute-phase proteins begin to rise

Table 6.10. **ACUTE-PHASE PROTEINS**

Acute-phase Protein	Production during acute phase	Function
C-reactive protein	↑ 1,000×	Opsonin
Serum amyloid A	↑ 1,000×	Apolipoprotein
α_1-Acid glycoprotein	↑ 2–5×	Platelet inhibitor
Fibrinogen	↑ 2–5×	Coagulation, tissue repair
α_2-Macroglobulin	↑ 2–5×	Antiproteinase
α_1-Proteinase inhibitor	↑ 2–5×	Antiproteinase
α_1-Antichymotrypsin	↑ 2–5×	Antiproteinase
Haptoglobin	↑ 2–5×	Antioxidant
Hemopexin	↑ 2–5×	Antioxidant
Ceruloplasmin	↑ 0.5×	Antioxidant, transport
C3	↑ 0.5×	Complement
Factor B	↑ 0.5×	Complement
C1 Inhibitor	↑ 0.5×	Complement
C4b-binding protein	↑ 0.5×	Complement
Mannose-binding lectin	↑ 0.5×	Complement
Albumin	↓ 0.1–0.5×	Transport
Transferrin	↓ 0.25–0.5×	Transport

after a delay of approximately 6 hours and serve important functions in restoring homeostasis after infection or inflammation (Table 6.10). These include hemostatic functions (fibrinogen), microbicidal and phagocytic functions [complement components, C-reactive protein (CRP)], antithrombotic properties (α_1-acid glycoprotein, plasminogen, protein S), antioxidant properties (haptoglobin, hemopexin), and antiproteolytic actions (α_2-macroglobulin, α_1-protease inhibitor, and α_1-antichymotrypsin). Negative acute-phase proteins, including albumin, prealbumin, transferrin, retinol-binding protein, α_2-HS glycoprotein, and α- and β-lipoproteins, decrease by at least 25%. Changes in production by hepatocytes are primarily responsible for their changing plasma levels. The magnitude of the response depends on the severity of the stress and varies from patient to patient. Whereas trauma and burns lead to significant increases in acute-phase protein concentrations, exercise and psychiatric illness can lead to more moderate responses.

The two major acute-phase proteins in humans are CRP and serum amyloid A (SAA). CRP, named because of its reaction with pneumococcal C-polysaccharide during pneumococcal pneumonia, appears to have both proinflammatory and antiinflammatory effects. It has been shown to activate complement, recognize foreign pathogens, bind phagocytic cells, and enhance activation of tissue factor, the main initiator of coagulation. Digestion of CRP by neutrophil proteinases releases chemotactic peptides. CRP can also inhibit superoxide production by neutrophils and inhibit neutrophil adhesion by decreasing surface expression of L-selectin. CRP peaks at approximately 48 hours and returns to baseline within 8 days after elective operation. Changes in plasma or serum CRP, although nonspecific, may reflect the magnitude of an inflammatory process, and may help differentiate between inflammatory and noninflammatory conditions. Measurement of CRP is more precise than the erythrocyte sedimentation rate, which largely depends on plasma fibrinogen levels and is influenced by miscellaneous other factors in the circulation. SAA, the other major acute-phase protein in humans, may affect cholesterol metabolism and promote chemotaxis and adhesion of phagocytes during inflammation.

Each component of the acute-phase response is individually and differentially regulated. CRP and SAA are upregulated up to 1,000-fold during the acute-phase reaction. In general, the antiproteinases and antioxidants are upregulated twofold to fivefold, whereas complement components may show a modest 50% rise. Unlike other acute-phase proteins, complement proteins are also synthesized to a small degree in extrahepatic sites, including the spleen and tissues of the reticuloendothelial system. C1 inhibitor is of special interest as an acute-phase protein because of its effects outside of the complement cascade. This antiprotease inhibits the activity of Hageman factor (HF), limiting kinin production and factor XI production. Thus, the up-regulation of a complement inhibitor protein during the acute phase affects clotting, fibrinolysis, and kinin release pathways. Levels of the negative acute-phase proteins albumin and transferrin drop almost immediately after operation and remain depressed for several days. The rapid initial loss of these proteins is likely due to increased vascular permeability and loss to the extravascular space.

Acute-phase proteins can be roughly divided into two groups based on their responses to cytokines. Type I proteins include CRP, SAA, C3, factor B, and α_1-acid glycoprotein, and are induced by IL-1-like cytokines (IL-1α, IL-1β, TNF). Type II proteins include fibrinogen, haptoglobin, α_1-antichymotrypsin, α_2-macroglobin, hemopexin, ceruloplasmin, and α_1-antitrypsin. Type II proteins are induced by IL-6-like cytokines. In general, IL-6-like cytokines (LIF, IL-11, OSM, CNTF, and CT-1) synergize with IL-1-like cytokines in the induction of type I proteins, whereas IL-1-like cytokines have no effect on, or may even inhibit the induction of type II proteins. The categorization of types I and II acute-phase proteins is clearly an oversimplification. Overlap and exceptions follow these general guidelines.

Systemic Manifestations of the Acute-phase Response

In the acute-phase response, the host undergoes a resetting of set-points to combat the altered homeostasis. Systemic manifestations include neuroendocrine changes, changes in the hematologic profile, metabolic and chemical changes, and alterations in plasma trace metal levels. The classic neuroendocrine manifestation is fever. IL-1, IL-6, and TNF mediate the fever response by resetting the hypothalamic temperature set-point through the synthesis of PGE_2. The secretion of neuropeptides such as CRH and AVP, and of hormones such as glucagon, insulin, thyroxine, and aldosterone is also characteristic of the acute-phase response. CRH and AVP released by the hypothalamus increase ACTH and cortisol levels. The rise in plasma cortisol levels occurs rapidly, peaking at 6 hours, and is one of the earliest apparent systemic changes. Cortisol release inhibits the fever response and cytokine gene expression, contributing a potential regulatory function in the acute-phase response. Another means by which glucocorticoids inhibit inflammation is through stimulation of macrocortin synthesis. Macrocortin inhibits synthesis of PLA_2, limiting the availability of arachidonic acid for prostaglandin synthesis. Glucocorticoids increase the rate of synthesis of certain acute-phase proteins involved in connective tissue repair and clotting (e.g., fibrinogen), as well as antioxidants and antiproteinases (haptoglobin and α_2-macroglobin). They also may function to counteract the hypoglycemic response to insulin overproduction during infection or stress. In this way, glucocorticoids may act in conjunction with glucagon and epinephrine to increase blood glucose concentrations in the acute phase. Patients typically display a leukocytosis that peaks at approximately 10 hours after an elective operation, and can later manifest thrombocytosis and "anemia of chronic disease." Metabolic changes include altered lipid metabolism and negative nitrogen balance. Changes in the chemical and enzymatic profile include increased hepatic production of metallothionein, inducible NOS, heme oxygenase, manganese superoxide dismutase, and glutathione (GSH). Plasma levels of zinc and iron are noted to drop, whereas copper levels increase slightly. The initial drop in iron and zinc levels parallels the fall in their plasma binding proteins (transferrin and albumin, respectively). A second phase of reduction persists for the duration of inflammation and is likely due to sequestration induced by IL-6, glucocorticoids, and catecholamines. Low levels of iron and zinc may confer protective antimicrobial effects because they are essential for microbial growth.

Mediators of the Acute-phase Response

Bacterial products such as LPS are probably the most potent activators of tissue macrophages, the initiators of the acute-phase response. LPS, through its interactions with LPS-binding protein, CD14, and Toll-like receptors, induces macrophage synthesis of ROS, including NO; lipid derivatives such as PGE_2, thromboxane A_2, and PAF; and acute-phase cytokines. The primary signals inducing synthesis of acute-phase cytokines in the absence of bacterial infection may be free radicals, prostaglandins, or modified proteins acting as foreign materials.

Acute-phase cytokines can be proinflammatory (IL-1, TNF, INF-γ, IL-8) or antiinflammatory (IL-10, IL-4, IL-13, TGF-β). However, it is IL-6 and IL-6-type cytokines (LIF, IL-11, OSM, CNTF, and CT-1) that are most critical in the acute-phase response. IL-6 is the major inducer of acute-phase protein synthesis and, together with IL-1 and TNF, is responsible for the systemic features classically associated with the acute-phase response (fever, anorexia, leukocytosis, and hormonal changes).

In addition to the aforementioned cytokines, IFN-γ is a potent inducer of complement components. The antiinflammatory cytokine TGF-β stimulates synthesis of antiproteases, urokinase, and negative acute-phase proteins. IL-4 is inhibitory to some acute-phase proteins. Growth factors, including hepatocyte growth factor and TGF-β, are also able to modulate the synthesis of acute-phase proteins. Glucocorticoids augment the response to cytokines, and insulin attenuates the cytokine-induced rise in acute-phase proteins.

Effects of the cytokines are influenced by cytokine receptors, receptor antagonists, and hormones. IL-1RA competes with IL-1 and attenuates the acute-phase response in vivo. Soluble receptors for IL-1 and TNF act as antagonists. In contrast, soluble receptors for IL-6 act as agonists.

Regulation of Acute-phase Cytokines and Proteins

Several major families of transcription factors participate in the up-regulation of acute-phase cytokines and acute-phase proteins, the most important being NF-IL6, AP-1, and NFκB (221). NF-IL6 participates in the induced expression of the cytokines IL-1, TNF, IL-6, and IL-8, among others. Activation of cytokine gene expression by NFκB is probably the most important pathway. The triggering of IL-6 in monocytes in vitro by IFN-γ involves a change in the amount of the phosphorylated transcription factor Sp1, together with the induction and activation of IFN regulatory factor.

All known acute-phase proteins are regulated primarily at the transcriptional level, with the exception of apoferritin, which is translationally controlled. Activation of TNF and IL-1 receptors triggers signaling pathways that activate transcription factors AP-1 and NFκB. Many type I (IL-1-responsive) acute-phase protein genes contain response elements for NFκB, NF-IL6, and AP-1 in their promoters. Acute-phase protein responses to IL-6 are mediated through the JAK-STAT signal transduction pathway. STAT3 is also known as *acute-phase response factor*. In addition, both IL-1 and IL-6 signal transduction mechanisms activate the MAP kinase pathway that activates transcription factor NF-IL6, linking the IL-1 and IL-6 pathways.

Reperfusion Injury

Prolonged tissue ischemia produces irreversible injury and cell death. Tissues subjected to sublethal durations of ischemia can be salvaged with timely restoration of blood flow. A paradoxical situation occurs when reoxygenation actually increases injury. Reperfusion injury is the damage caused by the restoration of blood flow in previously ischemic tissue. Reperfusion injury has classically been associated with myocardial ischemia. However, any tissue or organ deprived of blood flow is subject to reperfusion injury. Reperfusion injury contributes to morbidity and mortality in any situation where ischemic tissues are reperfused, as in organ transplantation and peripheral revascularization procedures. Injury is directly due to activation of the inflammatory response. The principal pathways leading to reperfusion injury are complement activation and neutrophil influx. Components of the complement cascade promote tissue damage through generation of anaphylatoxins and by formation of the MAC. Invading neutrophils injure tissue through the generation of ROS and the release of proteolytic enzymes. The pathogenesis of reperfusion injury begins in the microcirculation.

Microvascular Endothelium

Alterations in the microvascular endothelium are central to the pathophysiologic process of reperfusion injury. Endothelial dysfunction characterized by a loss in constitutive NO production occurs within minutes after reperfusion of ischemic vasculature (222). The loss of endothelial NO contributes to a marked degree of neutrophil adherence and an up-regulation of cell adhesion molecules such as P-selectin. Decreased endothelial NO production also impedes blood flow by inhibiting vasorelaxation. The endothelium can become a target of oxidant injury. In times of low oxygen concentrations, endothelial xanthine dehydrogenase is converted to xanthine oxidase. Reperfusion supplies oxygen, the remaining substrate required for xanthine oxidase activity, resulting in the formation of superoxide anion and H_2O_2 (see section on Reactive Oxygen Species). As neutrophils and other cellular effectors are progressively recruited and activated, released mediators further contribute to increased vascular permeability and oxidant and nonoxidant injury. Capillary plugging by neutrophils and platelets can impair local blood flow and cause the "no-reflow phenomenon." PAF and other factors released by neutrophils activate circulating platelets and promote vascular plugging. Platelets also release factors that enhance platelet–neutrophil adhesion. Both cell types also release vasoconstricting agents that can further exacerbate no-reflow.

Neutrophils and Reperfusion Injury

Neutrophil depletion studies have shown attenuated tissue injury compared with subjects with normal numbers of neutrophils (223). Neutrophil recruitment to sites of inflammation is governed by chemoattractant factors and by the regulated expression of adhesion molecules found on the surface membranes of neutrophils and vascular endothelial cells (Fig. 6.3). Adhesion molecules are expressed soon after reperfusion. Indeed, animal studies using blocking monoclonal antibodies to selectins and β_2 integrins show improved organ function after reperfusion after ischemia (224). The selectins (L-selectin on neutrophils, E-selectin and P-selectin on endothelial cells) mediate the loose reversible contact through interaction with their sialyl Lewis-containing counterreceptors. Cytokines activate these rolling neutrophils to enhance the affinity of neutrophil β_2 integrins (LFA-1, Mo1/Mac-1; p150,95) for their counter-receptor ICAM-1 expressed on activated endothelium. Ischemic tissues elaborate chemoattractant factors such as C5a, IL-8, PAF, and LTB$_4$ that recruit neutrophils and activate them to release toxic agents through the respiratory burst and degranulation. These adhesion molecule- and chemoattractant-mediated events lead to neutrophil infiltration, capillary leak, impairment of blood flow, tissue necrosis with impaired organ function, and death.

Neutrophils affect direct toxicity to the surrounding tissue through the elaboration of ROS and granule contents. Superoxide anion, hydroxyl anion, hypochlorous acid, chloramine, H_2O_2, and singlet oxygen are all produced by the neutrophil respiratory burst and myeloperoxidase systems. Activated local macrophages amplify their effect by releasing oxygen derivatives, inflammatory cytokines, and NO. Peroxynitrite formed by the reaction of NO and superoxide can contribute directly to tissue injury during reperfusion. Neutrophil granule proteases such as elastase, collagenase, and gelatinase alter the vascular permeability and are highly destructive to local tissue.

Complement System in Reperfusion Injury

The mechanisms by which complement is activated on reperfusion are not completely understood. Ischemia may transform cells into complement-activating surfaces by altering the plasma membrane or through the exposure of basement membrane or subcellular organelle components. Reperfusion may result in binding of natural antibody and activation of complement (148). Complement activation has been shown to occur in the setting of therapeutic interventions for the reversal of ischemia. Plasmin-dependent fibrinolytic agents (streptokinase) and plasmin generation after administration of tissue plasminogen activator have been associated with activation of complement (225).

Anaphylatoxins appear to have important functions in the activation and propagation of complement-mediated injury. The anaphylatoxins mediate alterations in vascular permeability, induce smooth muscle cell contraction, and release histamine from mast cells and basophils. C3a and C5a are also potent chemoattractants for cellular constituents of inflammation, including neutrophils. C5 can be converted to an active form by oxygen free radicals, which rapidly appear in the extracellular milieu on reperfusion. The conversion of C5 to a functionally active C5b-like form by hydroxyl radicals results in the formation of the complete MAC.

In addition to its direct lytic effects, the MAC may participate in the recruitment of neutrophils during ischemia/reperfusion. MAC components induce expression of neutrophil activators and other inflammatory mediators, including cytokines (TNF, IL-1, IL-8), ROS, prostaglandins, leukotrienes, and cell surface adhesion molecules (226). MAC deposition provides a mechanism for transmembrane ion fluxes. Increased levels of intracellular calcium may activate calcium-dependent phospholipases. MAC components also regulate inflammatory cytokine and adhesion molecule production through the modulation of NFκB activity (227).

Systemic Inflammatory Response Syndrome

The inability of host defenses to control a localized inflammatory process or an unchecked inflammatory response can result in SIRS. The diagnosis of SIRS requires the presence of two or more defined variables (228) (Table 6.11). Sepsis is defined as SIRS with a documented infection. There is a continuum from the development of SIRS to sepsis, with progression to septic shock and multiple organ dysfunction syndrome (MODS) (229). MODS may be defined as the failure to maintain homeostasis without intervention. The outcome (resolution, MODS, or death) depends on the balance between SIRS and host compensatory mechanisms. In one prospective study, 26% of patients with SIRS went on to development of sepsis, and 7% eventually died (230).

The systemic inflammatory response syndrome may be initiated by infectious or noninfectious causes, such as trauma, autoimmune reactions, or pancreatitis. The development of SIRS has been described to occur in three stages (231). In stage I, local cytokine production recruits inflammatory cells to the injured site. In stage II, an acute-phase response is initiated and small quantities of cytokines are released into the circulation to enhance the local response. Enhanced levels of CRP, the major acute-phase protein in humans, are seen in SIRS/sepsis, and clinical resolution is preceded by a drop in CRP levels. If homeostasis cannot be reestablished, stage III (SIRS) ensues. Cytokines then become mediators of tissue destruction by triggering numerous humoral cascades.

The elaboration of proinflammatory cytokines is central to the pathogenesis of SIRS. The most critical of these are IL-1, TNF, and IL-6. They are the primary mediators that trigger increased expression of adhesion molecules and induce secondary proinflammatory mediators (chemokines). Endotoxin, or LPS, is one of the most powerful triggers of SIRS. LPS activates the complement and coagulation cascades, induces endothelial cell activation, and increases TNF and IL-1 synthesis. LPS, TNF, and IL-1 also induce increased production of NO by iNOS in macrophages and other inflammatory cells. PGI$_2$ (prostacyclin), along with other metabolites of arachidonic acid, together with induced NO contribute to decreased systemic vascular resistance and hypotension. Autocrine and paracrine NO production also results in myocardial depression. Increased vascular permeability promotes extravascular third spacing and edema formation. Activated endothelial cells express tissue factor, PECAM, and TXA$_2$, which promote a procoagulant local environment that predisposes to microthrombi formation. Adherent leukocytes further exacerbate organ injury by me-

---

Table 6.11. SYSTEMIC INFLAMMATORY RESPONSE SYNDROME

Two or more of the following must exist:

Temperature	>38°C or <36°C
Heart rate	>90 beats/min
Respiratory rate	>20 breaths/min or Paco$_2$ <32 mm Hg
White blood cell count	>12,000 cells/mm^3, <4,000 cells/mm^3, or >10% bands

From Muckart DJJ, Bhagwanjee S. American College of Chest Physicians/Society of Critical Care Medicine Consensus Conference definitions of the systemic inflammatory response syndrome and allied disorders in relation to critically injured patients. Crit Care Med 1997;25:1789–1795.

chanically impeding microvascular blood flow and by damaging the endothelial cells and surrounding connective tissue. The results are end-organ hypoperfusion, inadequate oxygen delivery, initiation of anaerobic metabolism, and end-organ failure. The metabolic and nutritional sequelae of an activated cytokine milieu include fever, protein catabolism, cachexia, and altered fat, glucose, and trace mineral metabolism.

The proinflammatory SIRS is counteracted by an antiinflammatory response termed the *compensatory antiinflammatory response syndrome* (CARS) (231). Many of the proinflammatory mediators that participate in SIRS modulate the immune function of lymphocytes and mononuclear cells. Proinflammatory mediators can inhibit their own synthesis or enhance the synthesis of natural antagonists by negative feedback mechanisms. Thus, at any given time, the clinical manifestation is SIRS, CARS, or an intermediate, mixed inflammatory response syndrome. The spectrum of features that characterize these syndromes has been termed CHAOS (*c*ardiovascular shock, *h*omeostasis, *a*poptosis, *o*rgan dysfunction, and immune *s*uppression). No specific therapies exist in the treatment of SIRS. Several antibodies to cytokines and cytokine receptors are under investigation for the management of SIRS. Until specific interventions become available, the mainstay of therapy remains addressing the underlying cause and instilling supportive maneuvers.

Chronic Inflammation

There are no clear boundaries between an acute and chronic inflammatory response. In general, if the source of an acute inflammatory process is incompletely eliminated, a state of chronic inflammation eventually ensues. Chronic lesions usually are not characterized by the signs classically associated with acute responses, such as swelling, heat, or redness. Pain is minimal if not absent. Microscopically, chronic lesions are characterized by mononuclear cell infiltration (lymphocytes, monocytes, plasma cells) and proliferation of fibroblasts and vascular elements.

Etiologic agents for chronic inflammation include persistent infectious agents, remnants of dead organisms, foreign bodies (e.g., silicosis), and metabolic by-products (e.g., gout). However, a chronic inflammatory response can develop in the absence of a preceding acute response. This is also manifested in infections with agents of low toxicity such as *Mycobacteria* and *Treponema* (232). Ultimately, chronicity of inflammation is a result of the immune response to a persistent antigen. CD4+ T lymphocytes and macrophages are the primary cellular orchestrators of a chronic inflammatory response (233). T$_H$1 CMI responses are protective against most microbes and usually results in the elimination of the pathogen. If the microbe persists, the ongoing T$_H$1 response results in inflammatory tissue injury. Cytokines and growth factors released by T lymphocytes and macrophages stimulate proliferative responses. Neutrophils and eosinophils contribute to the release of proteolytic enzymes and oxygen derivatives. Eosinophilia is seen with chronic parasitic infections and hypersensitivity conditions. Fibroblasts are actively recruited by chemoattractants such as fibrin, collagens, and cytokines. Local IL-1 stimulates fibroblast proliferation and collagen production. Irreversible tissue damage can occur through the replacement of normal parenchyma with fibrous connective tissue. Fibroblasts can release metalloproteinases that degrade normal tissue, further contributing to tissue destruction. Mast cells are elevated in chronic conditions and may play a part in cell-mediated immune responses. Inflammatory cyst formation may occur as a result of epithelial hyperplasia.

A special subset of chronic inflammation is granulomatous inflammation. Granulomatous inflammation is characterized by two subtypes of granulomas. Immune, or epithelioid, granulomas are associated with granulomatous diseases (e.g., tuberculosis) (234). Caseous necrosis and aggregations of epithelioid cells surrounded by mononuclear leukocytes and fibroblasts are seen in this type. Chronic granuloma formation results from specific immune responses. Foreign body granulomas are made up of foreign body giant cells that develop from nonspecific phagocytosis by macrophages.

REFERENCES

1. Cotran RS. Inflammation: historical perspectives. In: Gallin JI, Snyderman R, eds. *Inflammation: basic principles and clinical correlates,* 3rd ed. Philadelphia: Lippincott Williams & Wilkins, 1999.
2. Cohnheim J. *Lectures in general pathology* [translated by McKee AD from the German], 2nd ed, vol 1. London: New Sydenham Society, 1889.
3. Heifets L. Centennial of Metchnikoff's discovery. *J Reticuloendothel Soc* 1982;1:381–391.
4. Cotran RS, Kumar V, Collins T, eds. *Robbins pathologic basis of disease,* 6th ed. Philadelphia: WB Saunders, 1999.
5. Lewis T. *The blood vessels of the human skin and their responses.* London: Shaw and Sons, 1927.
6. Omann GM, Hinshaw DB. Inflammation. In: Greenfield LJ, Mulholland MW, Oldham KT, et al., eds. *Surgery: scientific principles and practice,* 2nd ed. Philadelphia: Lippincott–Raven, 1997:130–159.
7. Burkitt HG, Young B, Heath JW, eds. *Wheater's functional histology: a text and colour atlas,* 3rd ed. Edinburgh: Churchill Livingstone, 1993.
8. Wortel CH, Doerschuk CM. Neutrophils and neutrophil–endothelial cell adhesion in adult respiratory distress syndrome. *New Horiz* 1993;1:631–637.
9. Jordan JE, Zhao ZQ, Vinten-Johansen J. The role of neutrophils in myocardial ischemia-reperfusion injury. *Cardiovasc Res* 1999;43:860–878.
10. Pillinger MH, Abramson SB. The neutrophil in rheumatoid arthritis. *Rheum Dis Clin North Am* 1995;21:691–714.
11. Grisham MB, Yamada T. Neutrophils, nitrogen oxides, and inflammatory bowel disease. *Ann NY Acad Sci* 1992;664:103–115.
12. Wheeler JG, Abramson JS. *The neutrophil.* Oxford: IRL Press at Oxford University Press, 1993.
13. Edwards SW. *Biochemistry and physiology of the neutrophil.* Cambridge: Cambridge University Press, 1994.
14. Bainton DF. The cells of inflammation: a general view. In: Weissman G, ed. *The cell biology of inflammation,* vol 2. New York: Elsevier/North-Holland, 1980.
15. Dancey JT, Deubelbeiss KA, Harker LA, et al. Neutrophil kinetics in man. *J Clin Invest* 1976;58:705–715.
16. Borregaard N, Cowland BJ. Granules of the human neutrophilic polymorphonuclear leukocyte. *Blood* 1997;89:3503–3521.
17. Trowbridge HO, Emling RC, eds. *Inflammation: a review of the process,* 5th ed. Chicago: Quintessence, 1997.
18. Quie PG, White JG, Holmes B, et al. In vitro bactericidal capacity of human polymorphonuclear leukocytes: diminished activity in chronic granulomatous disease of childhood. *J Clin Invest* 1967;46:668–679.
19. Lehrer RI, Ganz T, Selsted ME. Defensins: endogenous antibiotic peptides of animal cells. *Cell* 1991;64:229–230.
20. Gabay JE, Scott RW, Campanelli D, et al. Antibiotic proteins of human polymorphonuclear leukocytes. *Proc Natl Acad Sci USA* 1989;86:5610–5614.
21. Elsbach P. The bactericidal/permeability-increasing protein (BPI) in antibacterial host defense. *J Leukoc Biol* 1998;64:14–18.
22. Beamer LD, Carroll SF, Eisenberg D. The BPI/LBP family of proteins: a structural analysis of conserved regions. *Protein Sci* 1998;7:906–914.
23. Dewald B, Bretz U, Baggiolini M. Release of gelatinase from a novel secretory compartment of human neutrophils. *J Clin Invest* 1982;70:518–525.
24. Warren JS, Ward PA, Johnson KJ. Oxygen radicals as mediators of inflammation. In: Henson PM, Murphy RC, eds. *Handbook of inflammation,* vol 6. *Mediators of the inflammatory process.* Elsevier Science Publishers BV, 1989.
25. Szabo C. The role of peroxynitrite in the pathophysiology of

shock, inflammation, and ischemia-reperfusion injury. *Shock* 1996;79–88.

26. Klebanoff SJ. Myeloperoxidase: occurrence and biological function. In: Everse J, Everse KE, Grisham MB, eds. *Peroxidases in chemistry and biology,* vol 1. Boca Raton, FL: CRC Press, 1991.

27. Gius D, Botero A, Shah S, et al. Intracellular oxidation/reduction status in the regulation of transcription factors NFκB and AP-1. *Toxicol Lett* 1999;106:93–106.

28. Broide DH, Hoffman H, Sriramarao P. Insights from model systems: genes that regulate eosinophilic inflammation. *Am J Hum Genet* 1999;65:302–307.

29. Weller PF. Eosinophils: structure and functions. *Curr Opin Immunol* 1994;6:85–90.

30. Giembycz MA, Lindsay MA. Pharmacology of the eosinophil. *Pharmacol Rev* 1999;51:213–340.

31. Slungaard A, Mahoney JR Jr. Thiocyanate is the major substrate for eosinophil peroxidase in physiologic fluids: implications for cytotoxicity. *J Biol Chem* 1991;266:4903–4910.

32. Weller PF, Bach DK, Austen KF. Biochemical characterization of human eosinophil Charcot-Leyden crystal protein (lysophospholipase). *J Biol Chem* 1984;259:15100–15105.

33. Lewis RA, Austen KF. The biologically active leukotrienes: biosynthesis, metabolism, receptors, and pharmacology. *J Clin Invest* 1984;73:889–897.

34. Sugiura T, Mabuchi K, Ojima-Uchiyama A, et al. Synthesis and action of PAF in human eosinophils. *J Lipid Mediat* 1992;5:151–153.

35. Elsner J, Kapp A. Regulation and modulation of eosinophil effector functions. *Allergy* 1999;54:15–26.

36. Wardlaw AJ, Moqbel R, Kay AB. Eosinophils: biology and role in disease. *Adv Immunol* 1995;60:151–266.

37. Wedi B, Raap U, Lewrick H, et al. Delayed eosinophil programmed cell death in vitro: a common feature of inhalant allergy and extrinsic and intrinsic atopic dermatitis. *J Allergy Clin Immunol* 1997;100:536–543.

38. Rodewald H-R, Dessing M, Dvorak AM, et al. Identification of a committed precursor for the mast cell lineage. *Science* 1996;271:818–822.

39. Valent P, Schmidt G, Besemer J, et al. Interleukin-3 is a differentiation factor for human basophils. *Blood* 1989;73:1763–1769.

40. Metcalfe DD, Baram D, Mekori YA. Mast cells. *Physiol Rev* 1997;77:1033–1079.

41. Nilsson G, Costa JJ, Metcalfe DD. Mast cells and basophils. In: Gallin JI, Snyderman R, eds. *Inflammation: basic principles and clinical correlates,* 3rd ed. Philadelphia: Lippincott Williams & Wilkins, 1999.

42. Wood-Baker R. Histamine and its receptors. In: Busse WW, Holgate ST, eds. *Asthma and rhinitis.* Boston: Blackwell Science, 1994.

43. Vignola AM, Gjomarkaj M, Arnoux B, et al. Updates on cells and cytokines: monocytes. *J Allergy Clin Immunol* 1998;101:149–152.

44. Nathan CF, Murray HW, Wiebe ME, et al. Identification of interferon-gamma as the lymphokine that activates human macrophage oxidative metabolism and antimicrobial activity. *J Exp Med* 1983;158:670–689.

45. MacMicking J, Xie Q-W, Nathan C. Nitric oxide and macrophage function. *Annu Rev Immunol* 1997;15:323–350.

46. Kuijpers TW, Hakkert BC, Knol EF, et al. Membrane surface antigen expression on human monocytes: changes during purification, in vitro activation and transmigration across monolayers of endothelial cells. In: van Furth R, ed. *Mononuclear phagocytes: biology of monocytes and macrophages.* Boston: Kluwer Academic, 1992.

47. Ben-Baruch A, Michiel DF, Oppenheim JJ. Signals and receptors involved in recruitment of inflammatory cells. *J Biol Chem* 1995;270:11703–11706.

48. Thornhill MH, Haskard DO. Leukocyte adhesion to endothelium. In: Horton MA, ed. *Blood cell biochemistry,* vol 5. *Macrophages and related cells.* New York: Plenum Press, 1993.

49. Ezekowitz RAB. The mannose receptor and phagocytosis. In: van Furth R, ed. *Mononuclear phagocytes: biology of monocytes and macrophages.* Boston: Kluwer Academic, 1992.

50. Fadok VA, McDonald PP, Bratton DL, et al. Regulation of macrophage cytokine production by phagocytosis of apoptotic and post-apoptotic cells. *Biochem Soc Trans* 1998;26:653–656.

51. Chain BM, Levine TP. Antigen processing. In: Horton MA, ed. *Blood cell biochemistry,* vol 5. *Macrophages and related cells.* New York: Plenum Press, 1993.

52. de Waal Malefyt R, Yssel H, Roncarloo MG, et al. Interleukin-10. *Curr Opin Immunol* 1992;4:314–320.

53. Gumperz JE, Parham P. The enigma of the natural killer cell. *Nature* 1995;378:245–248.

54. Janeway CA Jr, Travers P, eds. *Immunobiology: the immune system in health and disease,* 3rd ed. 1997.

55. Surh CD, Sprent J. T-cell apoptosis detected in situ during positive and negative selection in the thymus. *Nature* 1994;372:100–103.

56. Zal T, Volkmann A, Stockinger B. Mechanisms of tolerance induction in major histocompatibility complex class II-restricted T cell specific for a blood-borne self antigen. *J Exp Med* 1994;180:2089–2099.

57. von Boehmer H. The developmental biology of T lymphocytes. *Annu Rev Immunol* 1993;6:309–326.

58. Romagnani S. Understanding the role of TH1 and TH2 cells in infection. *Trends Microbiol* 1996;4:463–466.

59. Mosmann TR, Coffman RL. TH1 and TH2 cells: different patterns of lymphokine secretion lead to different functional properties. *Annu Rev Immunol* 1989;7:145–173.

60. Mosmann TR, Sad S. The expanding universe of T-cell subsets: TH1, TH2, and more. *Immunol Today* 1996;17:138–146.

61. Chen Y, Kuchroo VK, Inobe J, et al. Regulatory T cell clones induced by oral tolerance: suppression of autoimmune encephalomyelitis. *Science* 1994;265:1237–1240.

62. Griffiths GM. The cell biology of CTL killing. *Curr Opin Immunol* 1995;7:343–348.

63. Marcus AJ. Platelets: their role in hemostasis, thrombosis, and inflammation. In: Gallin JI, Snyderman R, eds. *Inflammation: basic principles and clinical correlates,* 3rd ed. Philadelphia: Lippincott Williams & Wilkins, 1999.

64. Serhan CN, Haeggstrom JZ, Leslie CC. Lipid mediator networks in cell signaling: update and impact of cytokines. *FASEB J* 1996;10:1147–1158.

65. Marcus AJ, Safier LB, Ullman HL, et al. Platelet–neutrophil interactions: (12S)-hydroxyeicosatetraen-1,20-dioic acid, a new eicosanoid synthesized by unstimulated neutrophils from (12S)-20-dihydroxyeicosatetraenoic acid. *J Biol Chem* 1988;263:2223–2229.

66. Hostetter MK, Johnson GM. The erythrocyte as instigator of inflammation: generation of amidated C3 by erythrocyte adenosine deaminase. *J Clin Invest* 1989;84:665–671.

67. Dustin ML, Springer TA. Role of lymphocyte adhesion receptors in transient interactions and cell locomotion. *Annu Rev Immunol* 1991;9:27–66.

68. Kansas GS. Selectins and their ligands: current concepts and controversies. *Blood* 1996;88:3259–3287.

69. Tedder TF, Steeber DA, Chen A, et al. The selectins: vascular adhesion molecules. *FASEB J* 1995;9:866–873.

70. Frenette PS, Wagner DD. Adhesion molecules—part I. *N Engl J Med* 1996;334:1526–1529.

71. Frenette PS, Wagner DD. Adhesion molecules—part II: blood vessels and blood cells. *N Engl J Med* 1996; 335: 43–45.

72. Hynes RO. Integrins: versatility, modulation, and signaling in cell adhesion. *Cell* 1992;69:11–25.

73. Vaporciyan AA, DeLisser HM, Yan HC, et al. Involvement of platelet–endothelial cell adhesion molecule-1 in neutrophil recruitment in vivo. *Science* 1993;262:1580–1582.

74. Muller WA, Weigl SA, Deng X, et al. PECAM-1 is required for transendothelial migration of leukocytes. *J Exp Med* 1993;178:449–460.

75. Rot A. The role of leukocyte chemotaxis in inflammation. In: Whicker JT, Evans SW, eds. *Biochemistry of inflammation.* Boston: Kluwer Academic, 1992.

76. Wagner JG, Roth RA. Neutrophil migration during endotoxemia. *J Leukoc Biol* 1999;66:10–24.

77. Indik ZU, Park JG, Hunter S, et al. Structural/functional relationships of Fcγ receptors in phagocytes. *Semin Immunol* 1995;7:45–54.

78. Ezekowitz RAB, Sim RB, Hill M, et al. Local opsonization by secreted macrophage complement components. *J Exp Med* 1983;159:244–260.

79. Woessner JF Jr. Role of cellular proteinases and their protein inhibitors in inflammation. In: Whicker JT, Evans SW, eds. *Biochemistry of inflammation.* Boston: Kluwer Academic, 1992.

80. Park HS, Kim IS, Park JW. Phosphorylation induces conformational changes in the leukocyte NADPH oxidase subunit p47(phox). *Biochem Biophys Res Commun* 1999;259:38–42.

81. Lane PJL, Brocker T. Developmental regulation of dendritic cell function. *Curr Opin Immunol* 1999;11:308–313.

82. Banchereau J, Steinman RM. Dendritic cells and the control of immunity. *Nature* 1998;392:245–252.

83. Braciale TJ, Morrison LA, Sweetser MT, et al. Antigen presentation pathways to class I and class II MHC-restricted T lymphocytes. *Immunol Rev* 1987;98:95–114.

84. Razi-Wolf Z, Freeman GJ, Galvin F, et al. Expression and function of the murine B7 antigen, the major co-stimulatory molecule expressed by peritoneal exudate cells. *Proc Natl Acad Sci USA* 1992;89:4210–4214.

85. Lanzavecchia A. Receptor-mediated antigen uptake and its effect on antigen presentation to class II-restricted T lymphocytes. *Annu Rev Immunol* 1993;8:773–793.

86. Sieling PA, Chatterjee D, Porcelli SA, et al. CD1-restricted T cell recognition of microbial lipoglycan antigen. *Science* 1995;269:227–230.

87. Huston DP. The biology of the immune system. *JAMA* 1997;278:1804–1814.

88. Picker LJ. Control of lymphocyte homing. *Curr Opin Immunol* 1994;6:394–406.

89. Dustin ML, Springer TA. T-cell receptor crosslinking transiently stimulates adhesiveness through LFA-1. *Nature* 1989;341:619–624.

90. Springer TA. Traffic signals for lymphocyte recirculation and leukocyte emigration: the multistep paradigm. *Cell* 1994;76:301–314.

91. Janeway CA, Bottomly K. Signals and signs for lymphocyte responses. *Cell* 1994;76:275–285.

92. Liu Y, Janeway CA Jr. Cells that present both specific ligand and co-stimulatory activity are the most efficient inducers of clonal expansion of normal CD4 T cells. *Proc Natl Acad Sci USA* 1992;89:3845–3949.

93. Bluestone JA. Is CTLA-4 a master switch for peripheral T cell tolerance? *J Immunol* 1997;158:1989–1993.

94. Blair PJ, Riley JL, Levine BL, et al. CTLA-4 ligation delivers a unique signal to resting human CD4 T cells that inhibits interleukin-2 secretion but allows Bcl-X(L) induction. *J Immunol* 1998;160:12–15.

95. Lee KP, Harlan DM, June CH. Role of co-stimulation in the host response to infection. In: Gallin JI, Snyderman R, eds. *Inflammation: basic principles and clinical correlates,* 3rd ed. Philadelphia: Lippincott Williams & Wilkins, 1999.

96. Perez VL, Van Parijs L, Biuckians A, et al. Induction of peripheral T cell tolerance in vivo requires CTLA-4 engagement. *Immunity* 1997;6:411–417.

97. Johnson JG, Jenkins MK. Accessory cell-derived signals required for T cells. *Immunol Res* 1993;12:48–64.

98. Chapple ILC. Reactive oxygen species and antioxidants in inflammatory diseases. *J Clin Periodontol* 1997;24:287–296.

99. Kasahara Y, Iwai K, Yachie A, et al. Involvement of reactive oxygen intermediates in spontaneous and C95 (Fas/APO-1)-mediated apoptosis of neutrophils. *Blood* 1997;89:1748–1753.

100. Nohl H. Generation of superoxide radicals as byproducts of cellular respiration. *Ann Biol Clin (Paris)* 1994;52:199–204.

101. Winyard PG, Perrett D, Harris G, et al. The role of toxic oxygen species in inflammation with special reference to DNA damage. In: Whicker JT, Evans SW, eds. *Biochemistry of inflammation.* Boston: Kluwer Academic, 1992.

102. Palmer RM, Ferrige AG, Moncada S. Nitric oxide release accounts for the biological activity of endothelium-derived relaxing factor. *Nature* 1987;327:524–526.

103. Moncada S, Palmer RMJ, Higgs EA. Nitric oxide: physiology, pathophysiology, and pharmacology. *Pharmacol Rev* 1991;43:109–141.

104. Nathan C, Xie Q. Nitric oxide synthases: roles, tolls, and controls. *Cell* 1994;78:915–918.

105. Kleinert H, Euchenhofer C, Ihrig-Biedert I, et al. Glucocorticoids inhibit the induction of nitric oxide synthase II by down-regulating cytokine-induced activity of transcription factor nuclear factor-kappa B. *Mol Pharmacol* 1996;49:15–21.

106. DeVera ME, Taylor BS, Wang Q, et al. Dexamethasone suppresses iNOS gene expression by upregulating I-kappa B alpha and inhibiting NF-kappa B. *Am J Physiol* 1997;273:G1290–G1296.

107. Titheradge MA. Nitric oxide in septic shock. *Biochim Biophys Acta* 1999;1411:437–455.

108. Finkel MS, Oddis CV, Jacob TD, et al. Negative inotropic effects of cytokines on the heart mediated by nitric oxide. *Science* 1992;257:387–389.

109. Goodwin DC, Landino LM, Marnett LJ. Effects of nitric oxide and nitric oxide-derived species on prostaglandin endoperoxide synthase and prostaglandin biosynthesis. *FASEB J* 1999;13:1121–1136.

110. Allione A, Bernabei P, Bosticardo M, et al. Nitric oxide suppresses human T lymphocyte proliferation through IFN-gamma-dependent and IFN-gamma-independent induction of apoptosis. *J Immunol* 1999;163:4182–4191.

111. Ou J, Carlos TM, Watkins SC, et al. Differential effects of nonselective nitric oxide synthase (NOS) and selective inducible NOS inhibition on hepatic necrosis, apoptosis, ICAM-1 expression, and neutrophil accumulation during endotoxemia. NO: *Biol Chem* 1997;1:404–416.

112. Isobe M, Katsuramaki T, Hirata K, et al. Beneficial effects of inducible nitric oxide synthase inhibitor on reperfusion injury in the pig liver. *Transplantation* 1999;68:803–813.

113. Xia Y, Zweier JL. Superoxide and peroxynitrite generation from inducible nitric oxide synthase in macrophages. *Proc Natl Acad Sci USA* 1997;94:6954–6958.

114. Szabo C, Billiar TR. Novel roles of nitric oxide in hemorrhagic shock. *Shock* 1999;12:1–9.

115. Hierholzer C, Harbrecht B, Menezes JM, et al. Essential role of induced nitric oxide in the initiation of the inflammatory response after hemorrhagic shock. *J Exp Med* 1998;187:917–928.

116. Tzeng E, Kim YM, Pitt BR, et al. Adenoviral transfer of the inducible nitric oxide gene blocks endothelial cell apoptosis. *Surgery* 1997;122:255–263.

117. Polla BS, Bachelet M, Dall'ava J, et al. Heat shock proteins in inflammation and asthma: Dr. Jekyll or Mr. Hyde? *Clin Exp Allergy* 1998;28:527–529.

118. Polla BS, Bachelet M, Elia G, et al. Stress proteins in inflammation. *Ann NY Acad Sci* 1998;851:75–85.

119. Multhoff G, Botzler C. Heat-shock proteins and the immune response. *Ann NY Acad Sci* 1998;851:87–93.

120. Perdrizet GA. Heat shock and tissue protection. *New Horiz* 1995;3:312–320.

121. Mathew A, Morimoto RI. Role of the heat-shock response in the life and death of proteins. *Ann NY Acad Sci* 1998;851:99–111.

122. Ribeiro SP, Villar J, Slutsky AS. Induction of the stress response to prevent organ injury. *New Horiz* 1995;3:301–311.

123. Garcia-Cardena G, Fan R, Shah V, et al. Dynamic activation of endothelial nitric oxide synthase by Hsp90. *Nature* 1998;392:821–824.

124. Wong HR, Ryan M, Wispe JR. Stress response decreases NF-κB nuclear translocation and increases I-κBa expression in A549 cells. *J Clin Invest* 1997;99:2423–2428.

125. Cummings MC, Winterford CM, Walker NI. Apoptosis. *Am J Surg Pathol* 1997;21:88–101.

126. Newman SL, Henson JE, Henson PM. Phagocytosis of senescent neutrophils by human monocyte-derived macrophages and rabbit inflammatory cells. *J Exp Med* 1982;156:430–432.

127. Savill J. Apoptosis in resolution of inflammation. *J Leukoc Biol* 1997;61:375–380.

128. Mahidhara R, Billiar TR. Apoptosis in sepsis. *Crit Care Med* 2000;28[Suppl]:N105–N113.

129. Hannun YA. Functions of ceramide in coordinating cellular responses to stress. *Science* 1996;274:1855–1859.

130. Vogelstein B, Kinzler KW. p53 function and dysfunction. *Cell* 1992;70:523–526.

131. Ashkenazi A, Dixit VM. Death receptors: signaling and modulation. *Science* 1998;281:1305–1308.

132. Van Antwerp DJ, Martin SJ, Verma IM, et al. Inhibition of TNF-induced apoptosis by NF-kappa B. *Trends Cell Biol* 1998;8:107–111.

133. Thornberry NA, Lazebnik Y. Caspases: enemies within. *Science* 1998;281:1312–1316.

134. Adams JM, Cory S. The Bcl-2 protein family: arbiters of cell survival. *Science* 1998;281:1322–1326.

135. Freissmuth M, Casey PJ, Gilman AG. G-proteins control diverse pathways of transmembrane signaling. *FASEB J* 1989;3:2125–2131.

136. Spiegel AM. Signal transduction by guanine nucleotide binding proteins. *Mol Cell Endocrinol* 1987;49:1–16.

137. Spiegel A, Carter A, Brann M, et al. Signal transduction by guanine nucleotide binding proteins. *Recent Prog Horm Res* 1988;44:337–375.

138. Blackwell TS, Christman JW. The role of nuclear factor-kappa B in cytokine gene regulation. *Am J Respir Cell Mol Biol* 1997;17:3–9.

139. Rahman I, MacNee W. Role of transcription factors in inflammatory lung diseases. *Thorax* 1998;53:601–612.

140. Kyriakis JM, Avruch J. Sounding the alarm: protein kinase cascades activated by stress and inflammation. *J Biol Chem* 1996;271:24313–24316.

141. Schulze-Osthoff K, Ferrari D, Riehemann K, et al. Regulation of NF-κB activation by MAP kinase cascades. *Immunobiology* 1997;198:35–49.

142. Heim MH. The Jak-STAT pathway: specific signal transduction from the cell membrane to the nucleus. *Eur J Clin Invest* 1996;26:1–12.

143. Schindler C, Darnell JE. Transcriptional responses to polypeptide ligands: the JAK-STAT pathway. *Annu Rev Biochem* 1995;64:621–651.

144. Poli V. The role of C/eBP isoforms in the control of inflammatory and native immunity functions. *J Biol Chem* 1998; 273:29279–29282.

145. Frank M, Fries LF. The role of complement in inflammation and phagocytosis. *Immunol Today* 1991;12:322–326.

146. Roitt I, Brostoff J, Male D. Complement. In: Roitt I, Brostoff J, Male D, eds. *Immunobiology,* 3rd ed. St. Louis: Mosby, 1993.

147. Cooper NR. Biology of the complement system. In: Gallin JI, Snyderman R, eds. *Inflammation: basic principles and clinical correlates,* 3rd ed. Philadelphia: Lippincott Williams & Wilkins, 1999.

148. Weiser MR, Williams JP, Moore FD Jr, et al. Reperfusion injury of ischemic skeletal muscle is mediated by natural antibody and complement. *J Exp Med* 1996;183:2343–2348.

149. Cooper NR. The classical complement pathway: activation and regulation of the first complement component. *Adv Immunol* 1985;37:151–207.

150. Sim RB, Malhotra R. Interactions of carbohydrates and lectins with complement. *Biochem Soc Trans* 1993;22:106–111.

151. Matsushita M, Fujita T. Activation of the classical complement pathway by mannose-binding protein in association with a novel C1s-like serine protease. *J Exp Med* 1992;176: 1497–1502.

152. Muller-Eberhard HJ. The membrane attack complex of complement. *Annu Rev Immunol* 1986;4:503–528.

153. Marnett LJ, Rowlinson SW, Goodwin DC, et al. Arachidonic acid oxygenation by COX-1 and COX-2. *J Biol Chem* 1999; 274:22903–22906.

154. Smith WL, Garavito RM, DeWitt DL. Prostaglandin endoperoxide H synthases (cyclooxygenases)-1 and -2. *J Biol Chem* 1996;271:33157–33160.

155. Seeds MC, Bass DA. Regulation and metabolism of arachidonic acid. *Clin Rev Allergy Immunol* 1999;17:5–26.

156. Gerritsen ME. Physiological and pathophysiological roles of eicosanoids in the microcirculation. *Cardiovasc Res* 1996; 32:720–732.

157. Serhan CN. Inflammation: signalling the fat controller. *Nature* 1996;384:23–24.

158. Serhan CN, Haeggstrom JZ, Leslie CC. Lipid mediator networks in cell signaling: update and impact of cytokines. *FASEB J* 1996;10:1147–1158.

159. Vamecq J, Latruffe N. Medical significance of peroxisome proliferator-activated receptors. *Lancet* 1999;354:141–148.

160. Leff JA. Leukotriene modifiers as novel therapeutics in asthma. *Clin Exp Allergy* 1998;28[Suppl 5]:147–153.

161. Marcus AJ. Transcellular metabolism of eicosanoids. *Prog Hemost Thromb* 1986;8:127–142.

162. DeCoterina R, Sicari R, Giannessi D, et al. Macrophage-specific eicosanoid synthesis inhibition and lipocortin-1 induction by glucocorticoids. *J Appl Physiol* 1993;75:2368–2375.

163. Serhan CN. Lipoxins and novel aspirin-triggered 15-epi-lipoxins (ATL): a jungle of cell–cell interactions or a therapeutic opportunity? *Prostaglandins* 1997;53:107–137.

164. Henson PM. Activation and desensitization of platelets by platelet-activating factor (PAF) derived from IgE-sensitized basophils: I. characteristics of the secretory response. *J Exp Med* 1976;143:937–952.

165. Snyder F, Fitzgerald V, Blank ML. Biosynthesis of platelet-activating factor and enzyme inhibitors. *Adv Exp Med Biol* 1996;416:5–10.

166. Snyder F. Metabolic processing of PAF. *Clin Rev Allergy* 1994;12:309–327.

167. Noguchi K, Matsuzaki T, Shiroma N, et al. Involvement of nitric oxide and eicosanoids in platelet-activating factor-induced haemodynamic and haematologic effects in dogs. *Br J Pharmacol* 1996;118:941–950.

168. Hall JM. Bradykinin receptors: pharmacological properties and biological roles. *Pharmacol Ther* 1992;56:131–190.

169. Schreiber AD. Plasma inhibition of the Hageman factor dependent pathways. *Semin Thromb Hemost* 1976;3:32–51.

170. Volpe AR, Giardina B, Preziosi P, et al. Biosynthesis of endothelium-derived nitric oxide by bradykinin as endogenous precursor. *Immunopharmacology* 1996;33:287–290.

171. Dell'Italia LJ, Oparil S. Bradykinin in the heart: friend or foe? *Circulation* 1999;100:2305–2307.

172. Tschope C, Gohlke P, Zhu YZ, et al. Antihypertensive and cardioprotective effects after angiotensin-converting enzyme inhibition: role of kinins. *J Card Fail* 1997;3:133–148.

173. Chikanza IC, Grossman AB. Neuroendocrine immune responses to inflammation: the concept of the neuroendocrine immune loop. *Baillieres Clin Rheumatol* 1996;10:199–225.

174. A role for neuropeptides in inflammation. In: Whicker JT, Evans SW, eds. *Biochemistry of inflammation.* Boston: Kluwer Academic, 1992.

175. Canning BJ. Potential role of tachykinins in inflammatory diseases. *J Allergy Clin Immunol* 1997;99:579–582.

176. Delgado M, Pozo D, Martinez C, et al. Vasoactive intestinal peptide and pituitary adenylate cyclase-activating polypeptide inhibits endotoxin-induced TNF-alpha production by macrophages: in vitro and in vivo studies. *J Immunol* 1999; 162:2358–2367.

177. Delgado M, Munoz-Elias EJ, Gomariz RP, et al. Vasoactive intestinal peptide and pituitary adenylate cyclase-activating polypeptide enhance IL-10 production by murine macrophages: in vitro and in vivo studies. *J Immunol* 1999;162: 1707–1716.

178. Thomson A, ed. *The cytokine handbook,* 3rd ed. New York: Academic Press, 1998.

179. Carswell EA, Old LJ, Kassel RL, et al. An endotoxin-induced serum factor that causes necrosis of tumors. *Proc Natl Acad Sci USA* 1975;72:3666–3670.

180. Adam-Klages S, Schwandner R, Adam D, et al. Distinct adaptor proteins mediate acid versus neutral sphingomyelinase activation through the p55 receptor for tumor necrosis factor. *J Leukoc Biol* 1998;63:678–682.

181. Ksontini R, MacKay SL, Moldawer LL. Revisiting the role of tumor necrosis factor alpha and the response to surgical injury and inflammation. *Arch Surg* 1998;133:558–567.

182. Beutler B, Cerami A. Cachectin and tumor necrosis factor as two sides of the same biological coin. *Nature* 1986;320: 584–588.

183. Tracey KJ, Fong Y, Hesse DG, et al. Anti-cachectin/tumor necrosis factor monoclonal antibodies prevent septic shock during lethal bacteraemia. *Nature* 1987;330:662–664.

184. Wang H, Bloom O, Zhang M, et al. HMG-1 as a late mediator of endotoxin lethality in mice. *Science* 1999;285:248–251.

185. van der Poll T, Buller HR, ten Cate H, et al. Activation of coagulation after administration of tumor necrosis factor to normal subjects. *N Engl J Med* 1990;322:1622–1627.

186. Fantuzzi G, Dinarello CA. Interleukin-18 and interleukin-1 beta: two cytokine substrates for ICE (caspase-1). *J Clin Immunol* 1999;19:1–11.

187. Sims JE, March CJ, Cosman D, et al. cDNA expression clong of the IL-1 receptor, a member of the immunoglobulin superfamily. *Science* 1988;241:585–589.

188. Colotta F, Dower SK, Sims JE, et al. The type II "decoy" receptor: a novel regulatory pathway for interleukin-1. *Immunol Today* 1994;15:562–566.

189. Kuno K, Matsushima K. The IL-1 receptor signaling pathway. *J Leukoc Biol* 1994;56:542–547.

190. Smith KA. Interleukin-2: inception, impact, and implications. *Science* 1988;240:1169–1176.

191. Smith KA. Lowest dose interleukin-2 immunotherapy. *Blood* 1993;18:1414–1423.

192. Moshage H. Cytokines and the hepatic acute phase response. *J Pathol* 1997;181:257–266.

193. LeMay LG, Olterness IG, Vander AJ, et al. In vivo evidence that the rise in plasma IL-6 following injection of a fever-inducing dose of LPS is mediated by IL-1 beta. *Cytokine* 1990;2:199–204.

194. Tilg H, Trehu E, Atkins MB, et al. Interleukin-6 (IL-6) as an anti-inflammatory cytokine: induction of circulating IL-1 receptor antagonist and soluble tumor necrosis factor receptor p55. *Blood* 1994;83:113–118.

195. D'Andrea A, Rengaraju M, Valiante NM, et al. Production of natural killer cell stimulatory factor (NKSF/IL-12) by peripheral blood mononuclear cells. *J Exp Med* 1992;176:1387–1398.

196. Shu U, Kiniwa M, Wu CY, et al. Activated T cells induce interleukin-12 production by monocytes via CD40–CD40 ligand interaction. *Eur J Immunol* 1995;25:1125–1128.

197. Uzé G, Lutfalla G, Mogensen KE. Alpha and beta interferon and their receptor and their friends and relations. *J Interferon Res* 1995;15:3–26.

198. Bogdan C. The function of type I interferons in antimicrobial immunity. *Curr Opin Immunol* 2000;12:419–424.

199. DeMaeyer E, DeMaeyer-Guignard J. Type I interferons. *Int Rev Immunol* 1998;17:53–73.

200. Boehn U, Klamp T, Groot M, et al. Cellular responses to interferon-gamma. *Annu Rev Immunol* 1997;15:749–795.

201. Billiau A, Heremans H, Vermeire K, et al. Immunomodulatory properties of interferon-gamma: an update. *Ann NY Acad Sci* 1998;856:22–32.

202. Romani N, Gruner S, Brang D, et al. Proliferating dendritic cell progenitors in human blood. *J Exp Med* 1994;180:83–93.

203. Metcalf D, Nicola NA. Proliferative effects of purified granulocyte colony-stimulating factor (G-CSF) on normal mouse hematopoietic cells. *J Cell Physiol* 1983;116:198–206.

204. Crawford J, Ozer H, Stoller R, et al. Reduction by granulocyte colony-stimulating factor of fever and neutropenia induced by chemotherapy in patients with small cell lung cancer. *N Engl J Med* 1991;325:164–170.

205. Zurawski SM, Vega F Jr, Huyghe B, et al. Receptors for interleukin-13 and interleukin-4 are complex and share a novel component that functions in signal transduction. *EMBO J* 1993;12:2663–2670.

206. de Waal Malefyt R, Figdor CG, Huijbens R, et al. Effects of IL-13 on phenotype, cytokine production, and cytotoxic function of human monocytes: comparison with IL-4 and modulation by IFN-γ or IL-10. *J Immunol* 1993;151:6370–6381.

207. Cassatella MA, Meda L, Bonora S, et al. Interleukin 10 inhibits the release of proinflammatory cytokines from human polymorphonuclear leukocytes: evidence for an autocrine role of tumor necrosis factor and IL-1 beta in mediating the production of IL-8 triggered by lipopolysaccharide. *J Exp Med* 1993;178:2207–2211.

208. Bogdan C, Vodovotz Y, Nathan C. Macrophage deactivation by interleukin 10. *J Exp Med* 1991;174:1549–1555.

209. Macatonia SE, Doherty TM, Knight SC, et al. Differential effect of IL-10 on dendritic cell-induced T cell proliferation and IFN-gamma production. *J Immunol* 1993;150:3755–3765.

210. te Velde AA, de Waal Malefyt R, Huijbens RJ, et al. IL-10 stimulates monocyte Fc gamma R surface expression and cytotoxic activity: distinct regulation of antibody-dependent cellular cytotoxicity by IFN-gamma, IL-4, and IL-10. *J Immunol* 1992;149:4048–4052.

211. Lawrence DA. Transforming growth factor-β: an overview. *Kidney Int* 1995;47:S19–S23.

212. Wahl SM, Hunt DA, Wakefield L. Transforming growth factor β (TGF-β) induces monocyte chemotaxis and growth factor production. *Proc Natl Acad Sci USA* 1987;84:5788–5792.

213. Macias-Silva M, Abdollah S, Hoodless PA, et al. MADR2 is a substrate of the TGF-beta receptor and its phosphorylation is required for nuclear accumulation and signaling. *Cell* 1996;87:1215–1224.

214. Baggiolini M, Dewald B, Moser B. Human chemokines: an update. *Annu Rev Immunol* 1997;15:675–705.

215. Rollins B. Chemokines. *Blood* 1997;90:909–928.

216. Bacon KB, Greaves DR, Dairaghi DJ, et al. The expanding universe of C, CX3C, and CC chemokines. In: Thomson A, ed. *The cytokine handbook*, 3rd ed. New York: Academic Press, 1998.

217. Schall TJ, Bacon KB. Chemokines, leukocyte trafficking, and inflammation. *Curr Opin Immunol* 1994;6:865–873.

218. Suffredini AF, Fantuzzi G, Badolato R, et al. New insights into the biology of the acute phase response. *J Clin Immunol* 1999;19:203–214.

219. Gabay C, Kushner I. Mechanisms of disease: acute-phase proteins and other systemic responses to inflammation. *N Engl J Med* 1999;340:448–454.

220. Pepys MB, ed. *Acute phase proteins in the acute phase response.* New York: Springer-Verlag, 1989.

221. Koj A. Initiation of acute phase response and synthesis of cytokines. *Biochim Biophys Acta* 1996;1317:84–94.

222. Giraldez RR, Panda A, Xia Y, et al. Decreased nitric oxide synthase activity causes impaired endothelium-dependent relaxation in the postischemic heart. *J Biol Chem* 1997;272:21420–21426.

223. Romson JL, Hook BG, Kunkel SS, et al. Reduction of the extent of ischemic myocardial injury by neutrophil depletion in the dog. *Circulation* 1983;67:1016–1020.

224. Vedder NB, Winn RK, Rice CL, et al. A monoclonal antibody to the adherence-promoting leukocyte glycoprotein, CD18 reduces organ injury and improves survival from hemorrhagic shock and resuscitation in rabbits. *J Clin Invest* 1988;81:939–944.

225. Agostoni A, Gardinali M, Frangi D, et al. Activation of complement and kinin systems after thrombolytic therapy in patients with acute myocardial infarction: a comparison between streptokinase and recombinant tissue-type plasminogen activator. *Circulation* 1994;90:2666–2670.

226. Morgan BP. Complement membrane attack on nucleated cells: resistance, recovery, and non-lethal effects. *Biochem J* 1989;264:1–14.

227. Kilgore KS, Schmid E, Shanley TP, et al. Sublytic concentrations of the membrane attack complex of complement induce endothelial interleukin-8 and monocyte chemoattractant protein-1 through nuclear factor-kappa B activation. *Am J Pathol* 1997;150:2019–2031.

228. Muckart DJ, Bhagwanjee S. American College of Chest Physicians/Society of Critical Care Medicine Consensus Conference definitions of the systemic inflammatory response syndrome and allied disorders in relation to critically injured patients. *Crit Care Med* 1997;25:1789–1795.

229. Bone RC. Sepsis, sepsis syndrome, and the systemic inflammatory response syndrome (SIRS): Gulliver in Laputa. *JAMA* 1995;273:155–156.

230. Rangel-Frausto MS, Pittet D, Costigan M, et al. The natural history of the systemic inflammatory response syndrome (SIRS): a prospective study. *JAMA* 1995;273:117–123.

231. Davies MG, Hagen P-O. Systemic inflammatory response syndrome. *Br J Surg* 1997;84:920–935.

232. Trowbridge HO. Immunological aspects of chronic inflammation and repair. *J Endodont* 1990;16:54–61.

233. Dvorak HF, Galli SJ, Dvorak AM. Cellular and vascular manifestations of cell-mediated immunity. *Hum Pathol* 1986;17:122–137.

234. Williams GT, Williams WJ. Granulomatous inflammation—a review. *J Clin Pathol* 1983;36:723–733.

SURGERY: SCIENTIFIC PRINCIPLES AND PRACTICE, Third Edition, edited by Lazar J. Greenfield, Michael W. Mulholland, Keith T. Oldham, Gerald B. Zelenock, and Keith D. Lillemoe. Lippincott Williams & Wilkins Publishers, Philadelphia, © 2001.

CHAPTER 7

DIAGNOSIS, PREVENTION, AND TREATMENT OF INFECTION IN SURGICAL PATIENTS

DAVID L. DUNN AND ORI D. ROTSTEIN

Although we live in a state of constant exposure to microbial pathogens both within the environment and within ourselves, the occurrence of infection is the exception rather than the rule. This is because potentially invasive microbes are held in check by a series of host defense barriers—physical, chemical, and immunologic—that act to maintain the integrity of the mammalian organism. When these barriers are breached or depressed, however, these omnipresent microorganisms are able to proliferate and invade normal tissues, and they may produce infection. This is of importance to surgeons due to the fact that host barriers are violated routinely in order to obtain access to a particular portion of the body to allow performance of the required procedure. Because this very process predisposes patients to infection, surgeons have studied infectious disease entities and almost invariably have been the investigators who have determined how to reduce the incidence of infection in surgical patients.

Surgical patients may develop infection due to many different types of bacterial, fungal, viral, and parasitic microorganisms. In an attempt to describe the interaction of host and invading microbes, researchers have categorized many organisms in relation to *virulence* and *pathogenicity.* These are relative terms, however, that reflect a composite of both microbial and host factors. Some organisms possess virulence factors that facilitate the development of severe infection in both the normal and the immunosuppressed host, while others that are nonpathogenic and rarely cause infection in a normal individual may produce infection and mortality in the immunocompromised patient. In general, virulence is exaggerated in the immunosuppressed host, and thus virtually any microorganism can become pathogenic in an individual lacking intact host defenses.

HOST DEFENSES

Host defenses act both to prevent microbes from causing infection and to contain and eradicate infection once it occurs. Scientific doctrine for many years has divided host defenses into humoral and cellular components. More recently, it has become clear that host defenses are exceedingly complex and that additional stratification is necessary, primarily because of the intricate interactions that occur among various facets of host defense. Two important points should be emphasized: (a) while individual host defenses act as a series of barriers to infection, many components of host defense also may act in tandem and/or synergistically to prevent and contain infection; and (b) many host defense components are capable of exerting deleterious effects upon the host such that an overexuberant host response may alone produce disease. Host defenses can be classified into the following categories: barrier, microbial flora, humoral, cellular, cytokine, and immune procoagulant. Each of these categories will be discussed in turn.

Barriers

The barrier defenses of the mammalian host are numerous and varied, but all serve to separate our sterile body tissue from either the external environment or those portions of the body (e.g., oropharynx, gut) that possess a resident microbial flora *(vide infra).* Thus the skin, mucous membranes, and epithelial layers of various organs of the body constitute effective physical barriers against microbial invasion. In certain portions of the body these barriers have developed ancillary adaptations to increase the effectiveness of the barrier functions. For example, the skin of those areas of the body that are in direct contact with the environment (hands, feet) is particularly thick and durable. In addition, skin structures such as sebaceous glands secrete chemical compounds that serve to maintain a relatively low pH providing effective bacterial stasis. Mucus secretion by specialized glands within the bronchi and gut provides a

mucus layer that represents a physical and chemical barrier to microbial invasion. Within the respiratory tract, ciliary function serves to extrude microorganisms trapped within this mucus layer. In the alimentary tract, the very low pH within the stomach and gut peristalsis both serve to prevent microbial adherence and invasion. Although traumatic disruption of any of these barriers may immediately produce infection, disease states that affect barriers within a particular organ may also diminish protective function and lead to acute or chronic infections.

Microbial Flora

The terms *commensal, resident, indigenous,* and *autochthonous* have all been used to describe those microorganisms that reside in our bodies. Many of these organisms are indeed symbionts, acting to promote host defense and health, while concomitantly benefiting from sequestration within the host milieu. The importance of this microflora should not be underestimated. Under normal circumstances, it is critical to the developing neonatal immune system and acts in concert with other host defenses to prevent the invasion of nonresident pathogens. Unfortunately, the autochthonous microflora—because of proximity and composition—also can provide the initial inoculum that may lead to established infection once host barrier defenses are breached (1).

The composition of the gut microflora is established in neonates after ingestion of microbes that are acquired during contamination from the birth canal and during initial feeding, and remains relatively constant thereafter. Although this flora acts to promote development of the immune system, the specific interactions that produce this effect have not been elucidated fully. Studies performed with gnotobiotic animals have demonstrated that the absence of the gut microflora leads to poor development of gut-associated lymphoid tissue, and absence of local responses to many antigens. Gnotobiotic rodents possess a huge, distended cecum, and are susceptible to otherwise nonlethal bacterial inoculum via a variety of routes of administration. Hepatic Kupffer cell numbers and responses are markedly diminished, as are a wide variety of systemic cellular and humoral immune responses.

The gut microflora also contributes to physical and chemical barriers at the mucous membrane level, in that many autochthonous microbes possess adhesion proteins by which they bind only to certain areas of the mucosal cell, or to specific types of other bacteria. This serves two purposes: (a) potential binding sites for pathogenic organisms are occupied (organisms that cannot adhere cannot cause infection, a phenomenon termed "colonization resistance"); and (b) a substantial physical "mucobacterial" layer is present. This layer is maintained despite the constant shedding of enterocytes, mucus, and bacteria via the high division rates of both bacterial and mammalian cells within this microenvironment.

The oropharynx contains both aerobic and anaerobic microorganisms, generally consisting of a variety of gram-positive aerobic and anaerobic organisms, lactobacilli, *Branhamella, Bacteroides melaninogenicus* and *oralis,* and other anaerobic forms. Microbial inhabitants of the oropharynx do not usually pass into the intestine, however, because the stomach itself represents a significant barrier to invading microorganisms by virtue of its low pH, which kills most microbes unless very large numbers are present or the organisms are acid resistant (e.g., *Mycobacterium, Candida*). This barrier function, coupled with the rapid transit time within the normal stomach and upper small intestine, probably explains why so few microbes (0 to 10^2 gram-positive facultative aerobes, lacto-

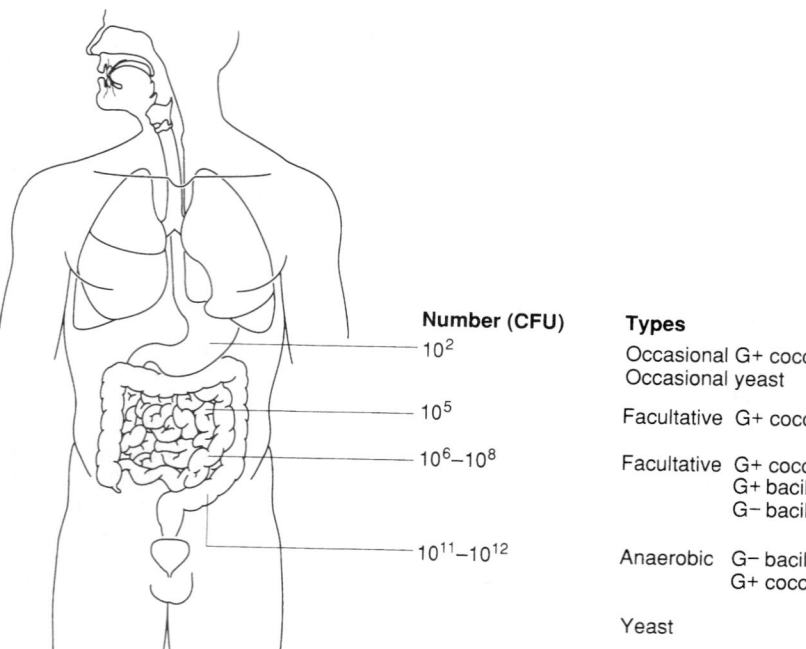

Number (CFU)	Types
10^2	Occasional G+ cocci Occasional yeast
10^5	Facultative G+ cocci
$10^6–10^8$	Facultative G+ cocci G+ bacilli G– bacilli
$10^{11}–10^{12}$	Anaerobic G– bacilli G+ cocci Yeast

Figure 7.1. Autochthonous microflora of the gastrointestinal tract. Large numbers and different types of anaerobic bacteria are present in both the oropharynx and distal gut. The stomach is virtually sterile in normal individuals, but the number of microorganisms increases in an aboral direction. These organisms provide the initial inoculum of microorganisms when perforation of a viscus occurs.

bacilli, and *Candida*) are present in this portion of the gut. Passage of oropharyngeal microflora and ingested microbes into the small intestine can occur during meals, at which time the gastric pH is temporarily elevated, or in patients with diseases that cause alterations in gastric pH or motility. Beyond the stomach, there is an increase in both diversity and number of total organisms and anaerobic flora as the gut microflora is progressively examined in an aboral direction, progressing from the stomach to the colon and rectum (Fig. 7.1).

Similar to the stomach, the upper small intestine contains few organisms, mainly gram-positive aerobes and lactobacilli. The lower small intestine, however, contains large numbers of aerobes and anaerobic forms, especially in patients in whom the ileocecal valve allows free backwash of cecal contents into the terminal ileum. Within the colon, a wide diversity and large number of facultative and strict anaerobic isolates are present. Only a relatively small number of aerobes (*Enterococcus faecalis, Escherichia coli,* and other *Enterobacteriaceae)* are present, these microbes being outnumbered 100 to 300:1 by anaerobes (*Bacteroides fragilis, Bacteroides* sp., *Fusobacterium,* and many others). Microbes compose as much as one third of the dry weight of feces, with as many as 10^{11} to 10^{12} organisms present per gram of feces. Thus, the number of bacteria in the colon approaches 10^{10} to 10^{12} per gram of feces for *Bacteroides* and is typically 10^8 to 10^{10} per gram of feces for *E. coli,* while other microorganisms are present at variable, but often high numbers. Within the lower gastrointestinal (GI) tract, the endogenous anaerobic flora appears to regulate relative bacterial numbers through the process of colonization resistance, wherein their abundance prevents aerobic gram-negative bacilli from achieving overgrowth and host invasion.

Humoral Defenses

Stimulation of the immune system occurs after a variety of antigen-presenting cells (B lymphocytes, macrophages, dendritic cells, Langerhans cells) act to engulf, process, and present antigen to T lymphocytes of the helper lineage. These T lymphocytes, in turn, act to stimulate B lymphocytes to become mature plasmacytes (via secretion of cytokines such as interleukin-4 and -6) dedicated to the production of antibody directed against this specific antigen. An antigen may be defined as any substance that stimulates the host immune response, i.e., that the host immune system recognizes as foreign. Thus an antigen may be an invading microorganism, an inert particle, or any type of chemical compound (protein, lipid, saccharide, complex biomolecule, etc.) that triggers the host immune system. Although some antigens are able to directly stimulate B lymphocytes in and of themselves to produce antibody (many polysaccharides), most antigens require the coordinated efforts of these various components of the immune system (2).

Humoral defenses consist of antibody (immunoglobulin, Ig) and complement (Fig. 7.2). All Ig classes (IgM, IgG, IgA, IgE, and IgD) and IgG subclasses (1 to 4 in humans) are composed of one type (M, G, A, E, D) of heavy (H) and one type

Figure 7.2. Humoral defenses consist of immunoglobulin and complement. (*A, Immunoglobin Structure*) All Ig classes (IgM, IgG, IgA, IgE, and IgD) and IgG subclasses (1 to 4 in humans) are composed of one type (M, G, A, E, D) of heavy (H) and one type (κ or γ) of light (L) protein chains. Each L chain is linked to an H chain, and both H chains are interlinked via disulfide bonds. The H chain of certain Ig types contains domains that activate complement or bind to receptors of either macrophages or polymorphonuclear leukocytes. The amino terminus of the H and L chains together forms the antigen-binding site. (*B, Complement System*) The complement system consists of a series of serum proteins that may become activated via either a classic or alternate (properdin) pathway, both of which eventuate in deposition of terminal complement pathway components on the antigenic cell surface

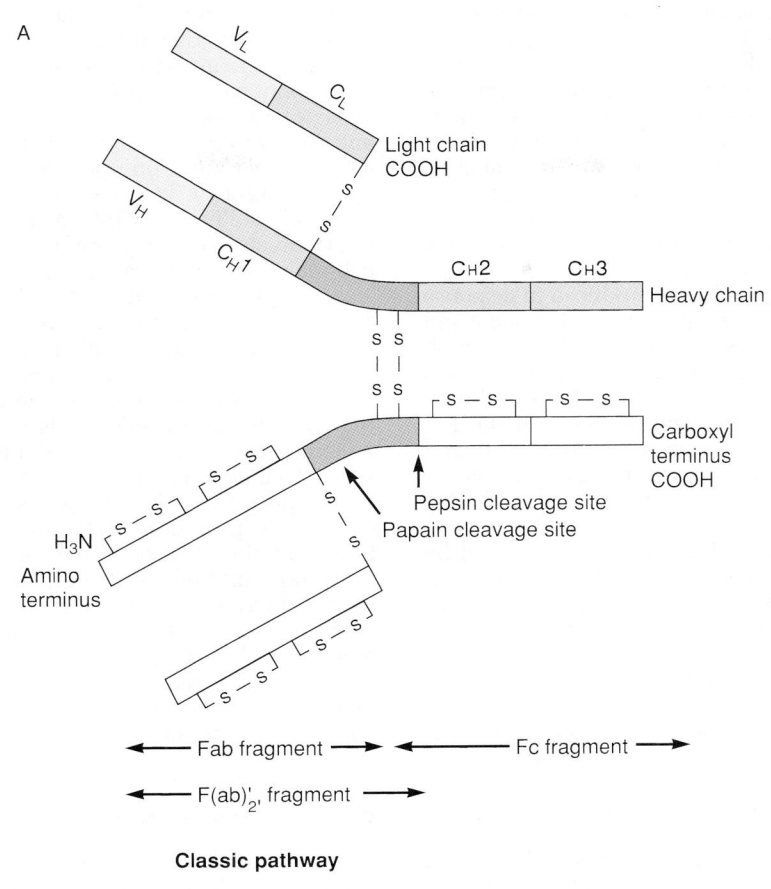

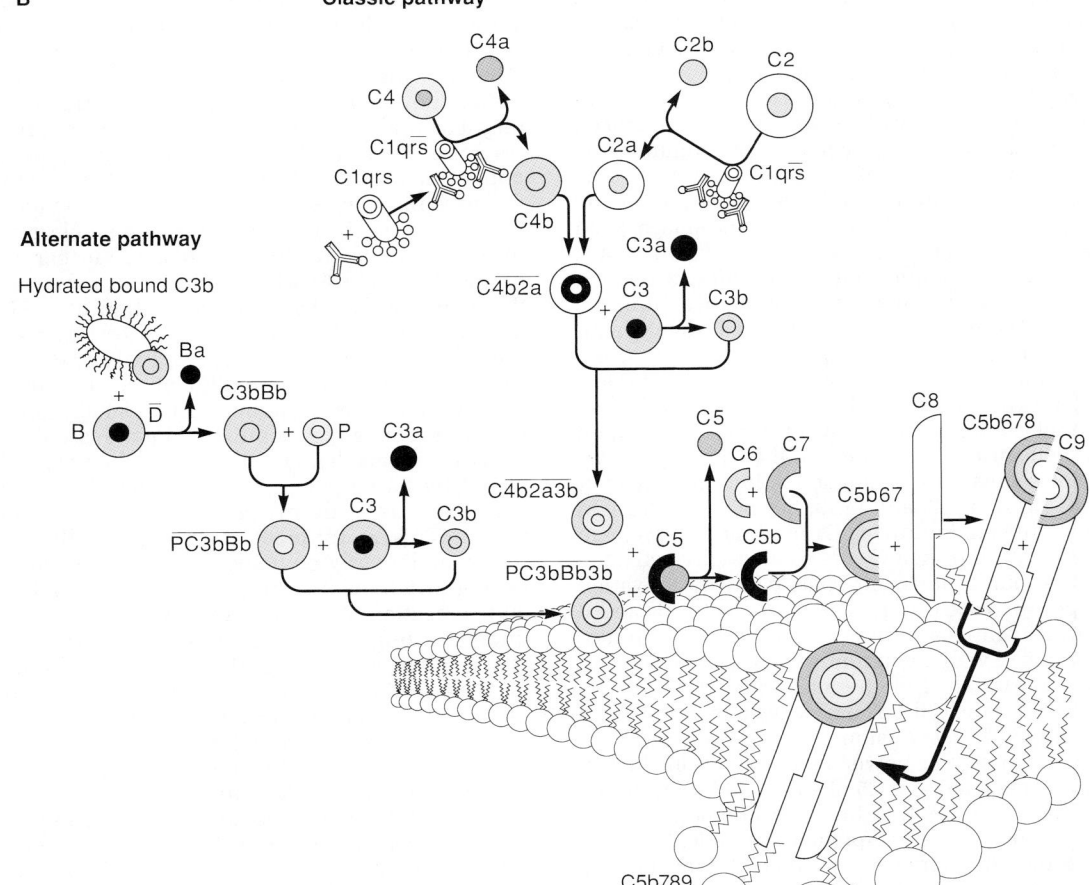

(κ or γ) of light (L) protein chains that consist of several domains both structurally and functionally. Each Ig molecule contains one or more units that consist of two H and two L chains linked by disulfide bonds. The amino terminus of both H and L chains contains several hypervariable regions that fold in three dimensions to produce the antigen-binding site. The carboxy terminus of the H chains contains regions that activate complement and bind Fc receptors by which direct adherence to polymorphonuclear leukocytes (PMNs) and macrophages takes place after antigen binding occurs (Fig. 7.2, upper panel).

Initially, antibody of the IgM class is produced in response to an antigenic challenge. IgM is a pentameric molecule and thus possesses ten binding sites per molecule (i.e., five molecules with two binding sites each). A second exposure to the same antigen, or a cross-reactive antigen, leads to the so-called second set response in which antibody of the IgG class with two binding sites is produced more rapidly and in larger quantity, compared to the initial IgM primary response. Evidence also indicates that antibody of increasing affinity is produced in response to the second antigenic challenge. Immunoglobulin of the IgA class is secreted by gut-associated lymphoid tissue and is combined with a secretory component protein to form a dimer termed secretory IgA. This antibody acts at a variety of epithelial sites to prevent microbial adherence and invasion. IgD and IgE exist in smaller amounts in the circulation and do not appear to play a major role as host defense components, the latter immunoglobulin class being associated with many hypersensitivity reactions and mast cell activation. Membrane bound forms of IgM and IgD serve as antigen receptors on B lymphocytes, and are thus important in antigen recognition and subsequent T- and B-lymphocyte activation.

Ongoing antigenic stimulation enhances plasmacyte replication so that a clone of identical cells develops that secretes the same Ig. Thus, each plasmacyte secretes Ig that is of one class and one specificity and that acts to bind a particular antigen. This binding process may serve to neutralize toxic compounds, as well as to promote enhanced phagocytosis by cellular components of the immune system. The Fc receptor portion of the heavy chain of some subclasses of IgG binds to a specific receptor present on many opsonophagocytic cells (PMNs and macrophages) and acts to markedly enhance phagocytosis. In addition, many, but not all, Igs activate complement after binding to antigen.

The complement system consists of a series of serum proteins that exist in a quiescent or very low level state of activation in the uninfected host (Fig. 7.2, lower panel). Complement activation can occur via either classic or alternate (properdin) pathways, both of which eventuate in deposition of terminal complement pathway components upon the antigenic cell surface. Activation of the classic pathway of complement begins with C1qrs activation, usually after binding to IgG (IgG1, IgG2, and IgG3, but not IgG4) or IgM that has bound antigen. Following C1 binding, complement components C4, C2, and then C3 are sequentially activated via cleavage to subunit forms. Alternate pathway activation occurs in response to activation of alternate factors D and B by IgG4 binding to antigen or directly via contact with fungal and bacterial cell wall compounds such as zymosan and gram-negative bacterial lipopolysaccharide (LPS; endotoxin). The C4b2a or the C3bBb complexes may serve as C3 convertases to amplify conversion of C3 in each pathway, exponentially increase the power of the reaction. Subsequent activation steps include C5 cleavage and then formation of the C5b-9 complex that involves interaction of all the terminal portions of the complement cascade.

Several specific complement components contribute to host defenses, acting to recruit or augment cellular host defenses, or to directly inactivate invading microbes via lytic activity. Primarily, the production of complement component fragments C3a and C5a during activation of this cascade serves to markedly increase vascular permeability, and C5a functions as a PMN and macrophage chemoattractant. This process leads to the recruitment of additional humoral and cellular defenses to a specific area of infection. In addition, C3b deposition upon an antigenic surface enhances opsonophagocytosis via receptors separate from those of the Fc class. Finally, C5b-9 complex deposition upon membrane targets leads to lysis after the formation of gaps in the cell membrane and osmotic fluid shifts.

Although certain types of antibody are extremely effective activators of complement, many foreign substances are able to directly activate either the classic or alternate pathways of complement. For example, many gram-negative microorganisms are able to activate one or both pathways of the complement system, while many yeast cell wall components directly activate the alternative complement pathway. The complement cascade most likely represents a relatively primitive host defense mechanism that is extremely effective in preventing infection, particularly when acting in conjunction with other host defense components.

Overall, antibody and complement act together to neutralize microbial toxins, lyse invading microbial organisms, and/or markedly enhance phagocytosis of those organisms that escape initial neutralization and lysis. Simultaneously, fragments of certain complement components act to recruit additional cellular components of host defenses and direct them toward the area of infection.

Cellular Defenses

A wide variety of cell types serve to provide host defense at several levels. As mentioned above, macrophages can act as initial antigen-processing cells by presenting antigen to T-helper cells, thus initiating the immune response. In addition, however, macrophages are pluripotent cells that play a central role in coordinating the overall inflammatory response. Their resident nature in many tissues affords the opportunity for these cells to represent the first line of host defenses in many areas of the body. In this location, these cells may participate in initial microbial clearance through phagocytosis of invading organisms. Further, this interaction with microbes and their products leads to activation of these cells with subsequent generation of a wide array of mediator molecules capable of orchestrating a number of immune functions. For example, PMNs, cells with a large capacity for microbial engulfment and killing, are present within the bloodstream, but only in small numbers within the tissue. They are mobilized to extravascular sites of infection via diapedesis in response to chemotactic stimuli released by tissue macrophages, bacterial breakdown products such as N-formyl-peptides, and complement activation. This recruitment process generally takes several hours, and clearly coincides with the critical time period during which the interplay between microbial proliferation and abrogation of infection by host defenses occurs. As our understanding of the nature of this process increases, it has also become clear that local activation of host defenses can exert deleterious effects upon the mammalian host. Secretion of lysosomal enzymes (cathepsin, elastase), free radicals (superoxide, hydroxyl), nitric oxide, and cytokines by macrophages and PMNs can directly injure nearby cells, but, in addition, can lead to injury to tissues distant from the site of infection. Specifically, the systemic activation of the inflammatory response may induce overactivation of circulating immune cells as well as those in distant organs resulting in organ injury and the development of the multiple organ dysfunction syndrome (MODS).

Cytokines, Chemokines, and Procoagulant Molecules

Macrophages, endothelial cells, lymphocytes, and other cells secrete and express on their surfaces a large number of different molecules that most probably evolved for the purpose of local intercellular and intracellular signaling. Cytokines are generally low molecular weight polypeptides secreted by cells that exert a wide variety of biologic effects at both the local and systemic levels. The gene for many cytokines has been sequenced, isolated, and cloned and cellular receptors have been identified for many as

well. Cytokines frequently are secreted after initial lymphocyte or macrophage activation, and may act upon the secreting cell itself (autocrine activation) or other cells within the same local environment (paracrine activation) to cause increased secretion of the same cytokine or other cytokines, respectively. For example, interleukin-2 (IL-2) is secreted by T-helper lymphocytes and serves to increase the expression of IL-2 receptors followed by additional IL-2 production by this same cell. Simultaneously, IL-2 secretion activates other cell types. Chemokines are secreted molecules that induce directed migration of cells to sites of inflammation.

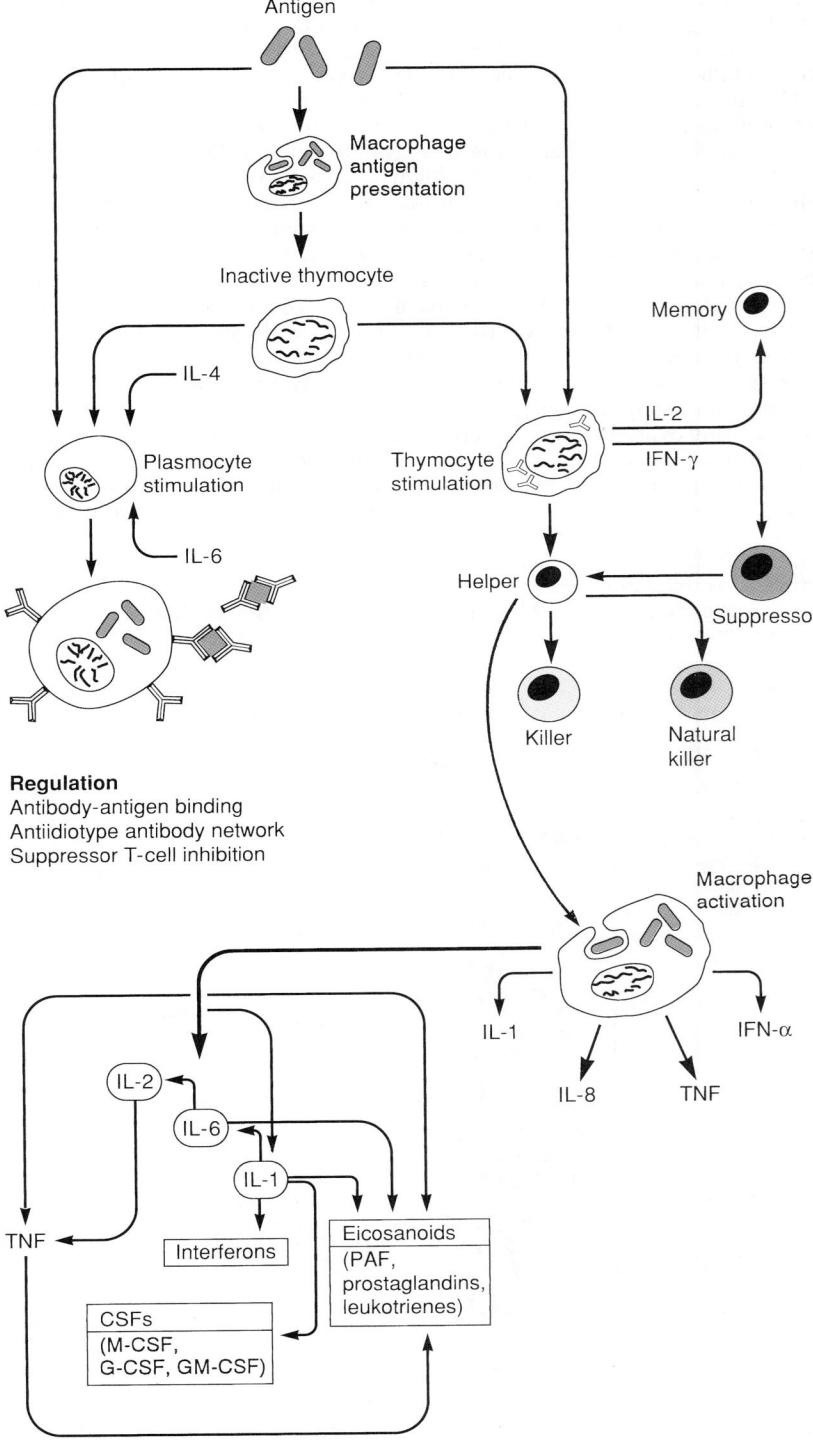

Figure 7.3. Inflammatory and immune response cytokine cascade. After initial antigen processing and presentation by macrophages and other cells, T lymphocytes act to stimulate B lymphocytes to become mature plasmacytes via secretion of cytokines such as interleukin-4 (IL-4) and IL-6 dedicated to the production of antibody directed against a specific antigen. Initial macrophage stimulation in response to bacterial products, interferon-γ (IFN-γ) release by T cells, and IL-1 release by macrophages themselves may be followed by macrophage tumor necrosis factor (TNF) production, and subsequently secretion of IL-6 and other cytokines.

In all probability, a series of activation steps occur in which various cytokines serve to provide regulation of the ensuing cellular response. Thus, during initial macrophage stimulation in response to bacterial products, interferon-γ (IFN-γ) release by T cells and IL-1 release by macrophages may be followed by macrophage tumor necrosis factor (TNF) production, and subsequently secretion of IL-6 and other cytokines takes place (Fig. 7.3) (3). In experimental model systems, IL-1 is capable of producing fever and hypotension, while TNF produces fever, hypotension, gut ischemia, and death. Prior administration of anti-TNF antibody ameliorates these effects. Administration of LPS to human volunteers has provided evidence that IL-1 and TNF are produced approximately 1.5 to 2 hours after LPS challenge, following which IL-6 and IL-8 secretion occurs. Administration of TNF to human volunteers leads to many of the physiologic effects evidenced after LPS challenge (vide infra).

The duality of the effects of the cytokine component of host defenses, exerting both salutary and deleterious effects upon the host, is becoming increasingly evident. For example, experimental models in which TNF or IL-1 is administered have provided evidence that this process actually leads to host defense enhancement and provides protection against a subsequent otherwise lethal TNF or LPS challenge. Initial administration of high doses of TNF, however, produces lethality. Most likely, many cytokines act within the local host defense environment to provide feedback signals and regulate various components of the host defense microenvironment. Thus, cytokines may serve to regulate the "set-point" of host defenses on a continual basis. During overwhelming infection, the body's attempt to contain infection with humoral, cellular, and cytokine defenses after physical barriers are breached may limit infection in some cases. However, as noted above, excessive activation of local defenses may result in egress of cytokines into the systemic circulation with widespread triggering of host defenses throughout the body. This process most probably represents the explanation for the appearance of the "septic state" or systemic inflammatory response syndrome in patients in whom no active infection can be identified.

While the coagulation cascade has classically been associated with the physiologic process of hemostasis, work over the past several decades has suggested that coagulation also plays an important role in the local and systemic inflammatory responses. This process of immune coagulation is mediated by inducible cell surface molecules such as tissue factor as well as plasminogen activator and plasminogen activator inhibitor, whose relative contributions will determine the balance between procoagulant response and anticoagulant/fibrinolytic activity. In general, infection and inflammation induce a net procoagulant response with up-regulation of molecules such as tissue factor and plasminogen activator inhibitor on monocytes/macrophages and endothelial cells and an overall reduction in plasminogen activator activity. The ensuing fibrin deposition promotes local inflammation due to the potent immunomodulatory effects of its degradation products and also may contribute to distant organ injury through the induction of microvascular thrombosis. In studies in experimental models and also in humans, antagonists of coagulation such as antibodies to tissue factor, tissue factor pathway inhibitor, or activated protein C, a molecule with anticoagulant effects, have been shown to impair the procoagulant response and improve outcome. This is, in part, related to the prevention of fibrin deposition but also may be a result of impaired thrombin generation, a downstream product of coagulation with potent proinflammatory capacity.

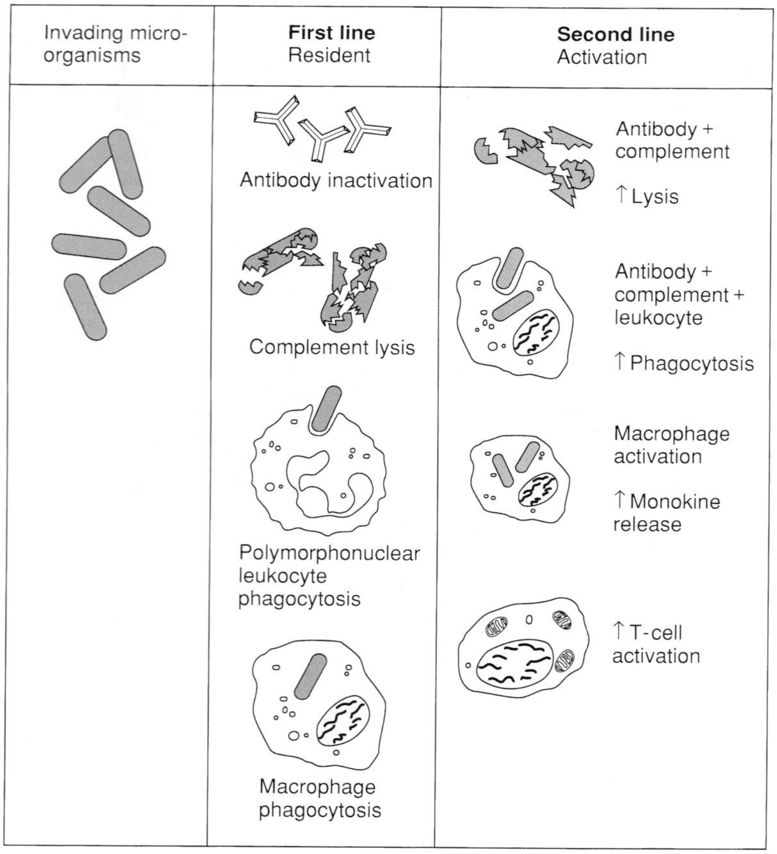

Invading micro-organisms	**First line** Resident	**Second line** Activation
	Antibody inactivation	Antibody + complement ↑ Lysis
	Complement lysis	Antibody + complement + leukocyte ↑ Phagocytosis
	Polymorphonuclear leukocyte phagocytosis	Macrophage activation ↑ Monokine release
	Macrophage phagocytosis	↑ T-cell activation

Figure 7.4. Interactions of various portions of mammalian host defenses. Antibody and complement act in concert to enhance bacteriolysis and phagocytosis, simultaneously recruiting additional humoral and cellular components to the site of infection. Macrophages act as pluripotent cells involved in first-line (resident) host defense, antigen presentation, and T-cell activation, and subsequent activation and cytokine secretion.

Host Defense Component Interactions

Several different components of the immune response are subsequently invoked after the primary initiation steps. A humoral response network exists in which plasmacyte stimulation is markedly enhanced by the presence of IL-4 and IL-6, which are derived from thymocytes and macrophages. Regulation of the humoral immune response network occurs at three different levels: (a) antibody-antigen binding, (b) antiidiotype antibody networks, and (c) inhibition via suppressor T-lymphocyte activation. The initial stages of the immune response are closely linked with the initiation of the host defense response. Invading microorganisms encounter preformed antibody, complement, as well as PMNs and macrophages. These factors represent the first-line or resident host defenses and are able to prevent the development of infection in many cases. These first-line host defenses work closely together as second-line or activation host defenses become operative. For instance, antibody and complement act together through immunoglobulin Fc receptor interactions, C3b deposition, and the lytic effects of terminal complement factors C5b-9 to enhance bacteriolysis as well as phagocytosis of microorganisms. In addition, macrophage stimulation occurs so that enhanced cytokine release and further T-cell activation occurs (Fig. 7.4). T-cell activation is regulated by both positive and negative feedback systems. For instance, initial activation leads to IL-2 secretion, which induces the formation of additional IL-2 receptors on T-cells, which, in turn, causes further stimulation of T-helper and the induction of T-memory cells. On the other hand, T-suppressor cells are activated and these serve to regulate the cellular and humoral immune response. Effector cells (T-killer and natural killer cells) are also stimulated, and additional macrophage stimulation occurs via T-cell–mediated effects. It is noteworthy that the macrophage acts as a key cell in the initiation of the immune response, as well as a first-line resident and as a second-line activated phagocytic and cytokine secreting cell.

MICROBIOLOGIC DIAGNOSTIC TECHNIQUES

The surgeon relies heavily on receiving information from the microbiology laboratory in order to appropriately prevent and treat perioperative infection. Simultaneously, expeditious preparation and transport of specimens and provision of salient clinical information allows the microbiologist to assist the surgeon in interpreting the culture data.

STAINING TECHNIQUES

As a rapid readout of the infecting microbe, a Gram's stain can be performed upon a specimen. This simple technique employs (a) fixation of the specimen with heat, (b) staining with a basic dye such as crystal violet, (c) stain fixation with an iodine-potassium iodide solution, (d) washing with ethanol/acetone, and (e) counterstaining with safranin red. Gram-positive organisms do not decolorize and thus remain dark blue, while gram-negative microorganisms are decolorized during washing and exhibit retention of only the lighter red counterstain. Observation under high-power oil emersion light microscopy may indicate significant infection in a normally sterile body area based on the presence of (a) >2 bacteria (gram-positive, gram-negative, or both) per 1000× magnification high powered field, which is equivalent to 5×10^4 to 10^5 colony-forming units (CFU)/mL within the initial specimen; and (b) white blood cells.

Potassium hydroxide is used to lyse bacteria and other cellular elements within a preparation and allows observation of yeast or mycelial elements. The Gomori methenamine-silver and Giemsa stains are also useful for observing fungal hyphae or spores within tissue, and protozoa may also be observed by this technique. The Ziehl-Neelsen stain is used to identify acid-fast bacteria such as *Mycobacteria*.

Culture Techniques and Sensitivity Determinations

Because most surgical infections are polymicrobial, specimens should be cultured for aerobic and anaerobic bacteria plus fungi. Although aerobic and aerotolerant microorganisms often do not require special transport media, a delay in specimen processing may markedly reduce the yield. Anaerobic transport media have been demonstrated to increase the culture yield of this type of organism. Most specimens are processed by initial growth on a variety of different types of selective media, although blood and catheter specimens are allowed to grow in broth media first, followed by plate growth upon a semisolid agar medium. Catheter specimens may also be directly rolled onto solid agar plates, allowing quantitative determination of the degree of infection. Quantitative cultures are also useful in some cases to determine the degree of infection of burn wounds, and some aggressive soft tissue infections. In all cases, isolation of single colonies on plates allows further growth and identification of a specific organism.

Automated detection systems are available that perform a series of simultaneous biochemical tests that allow precise identification of a specific pathogen. Automated techniques also allow determination of sensitivity patterns to a wide array of antimicrobial agents active against aerobes, anaerobes, fungi, and viruses. Initial culture results may solely indicate that microorganism are growing, but full characterization may require 2 to 3 days, or sometimes longer. An initial report may tentatively indicate the number of different organisms, Gram's stain characteristics, and simple biochemical characteristics such as the presence or absence of lactose fermentation. In some cases, sensitivity reports may be available prior to complete identification of the organism. Once a specific microorganism is identified, a sample of approximately 10^5 CFUs is inoculated during log phase into Mueller-Hinton broth containing varying amounts of an antibiotic. After an 18- to 24-hour period, the tube or well that exhibits no visible growth is then noted, and the reciprocal of this dilution is termed the minimal inhibitory concentration (MIC). This value is compared to either measured or known achievable serum levels for a particular antimicrobial agent, and a designation of sensitive/resistant will be assigned to the particular agent. Based on this information, antibiotics should be adjusted to conform with the known sensitivity of the microbes. Determination of serum bactericidal levels may be of use in some cases, and involves obtaining serum from a patient after antimicrobial agent administration. This antibiotic-containing serum is then used to determine inhibitory concentrations against a specific pathogen or series of pathogens. This test may be especially helpful in patients who are being treated with several antimicrobial agents and who are infected with several different pathogens. In general, antimicrobial agents that achieve in excess of a four- to eightfold increase over the MIC during the peak serum level have been demonstrated to be efficacious in experimental animal models of infection as well as clinical studies. This information may lead the clinician to at least consider a change in the antimicrobial agent regimen, although in some cases this may be premature, especially if the patient is doing well.

Confounding factors that do not allow direct extrapolation of this microbiologic information to a specific surgical patient include evidence that (a) most surgical infections are polymicrobial in nature and may involve synergistic microbial interactions, (b) the initial inoculum size is not known and almost assuredly differs from the inoculum size used to determine the MIC, and (c) the host milieu (pH, blood supply) may affect both the activity as well as penetration of antimicrobial agents (4).

Because the ultimate decision to alter antimicrobial therapy often is based on the initial response of the surgical patient to both the operation and empiric antimicrobial therapy, it is not unreasonable to ask why cultures should be obtained and how the information will be used. The answer revolves around two issues: (a) the patient's response, and (b) the types and antimicrobial resistance patterns of the infecting organisms. For example, although many patients improve, and do not require a change in antimicrobial agent regimen, those patients who exhibit evidence of persistent infection require an assiduous search for the reason. In some cases the cause may be an undrained source of infection or the presence of necrotic tissue, both of which require surgical intervention, while in other cases an organism not normally within the spectrum of activity of the antimicrobial agents selected or resistant to the antimicrobial agent(s) may be present. In the absence of obvious undrained infection, an alteration in antimicrobial agents is indicated when the initial lack of response to therapy is coupled with evidence of microorganisms resistant to the existing antimicrobial agent regimen.

Newer Detection Methods

Classically, the detection of microorganisms has taken place based on the clinical evidence of infection (fever, leukocytosis, etc.) and culture evidence of a specific organism. Increasing reliance, however, is being placed on assays that do not employ culture data. Specifically, the antibody and cytokine host response is being intensely examined, and extremely sensitive amplified assays that rely on antigen, antibody, or microbial DNA detection are being employed in the clinical setting. Routinely, antigen and antibody detection assays have employed hemagglutination, complement fixation, and radioimmunoassay techniques. More recently, enzyme-linked immunosorbent assay (ELISA), immunodot blot, Western immunotransblot, and immunofluorescence are being more frequently employed. Antigen-based assays such as the ELISA typically rely on the nonspecific binding of antigen within the well of a microtiter plate, following which a blocking agent is added to occupy unbound well sites. A specimen that may contain antibody that will bind to the antigen is added and allowed to react with antigen, and then a secondary labeled (e.g., peroxidase) antibody is added that can be used for detection based on colorimetric changes after substrate and an indicator are added. This type of assay represents a very rapid immunologic assay that can be used for both antigen and antibody detection for determination of antibody titer, as well as screening for monoclonal antibody production of a certain specificity by a hybridoma cell line.

Transblot techniques also are being increasingly used in the clinical setting. In most cases, nucleic acid or protein is subjected to electrophoresis so that separation is achieved based on molecular weight. In most cases, sodium dodecyl sulfate-polyacrylamide gel electrophoresis is utilized. Immunoelectrophoretic transfer to nitrocellulose paper then takes place and a probe may be employed to detect the presence of a certain antigen, antibody, or nucleic acid sequence. Direct blotting can take place using dot or slot blots in which DNA or RNA digests are directly layered onto nitrocellulose and then the probe consists of a labeled cDNA

sequence. Similarly, antigen or antibody can be directly blotted onto nitrocellulose and the probe can consist of labeled antibody or antigen. Southern, Northern, and Western immunotransblot techniques are used to detect DNA, RNA, or proteins, respectively.

The polymerase chain reaction (PCR) is being employed in some centers as a very sensitive assay to detect small amounts of microbial DNA. In this assay, nucleic acid is extracted from the test sample that may include the microbial nucleic acid in question. The readout from this test depends on the amplification of microbial nucleic acid present in the sample. In essence, amplification takes place in vitro through repeated nucleic acid denaturing and polymerization of complementary portions of nucleic acid so that the gene copy number increases exponentially. The probe for this assay consists of a copy of a portion of the nucleic acid sequence of the microorganism. Because the probe itself can be copied and used in large quantity, and because the sample nucleic acid has been markedly amplified with regard to gene copy number, the test is extremely sensitive and can detect infection in its very early stages.

These tests are being utilized in the clinical setting to detect a wide variety of infectious agents, including cytomegalovirus (CMV) and human immunodeficiency virus (HIV). Some preliminary observations also indicate that it may be possible to detect fungal pathogens such as *Candida* by using monoclonal antibodies directed against cell wall structures such as mannan, but this test has not found widespread clinical utility.

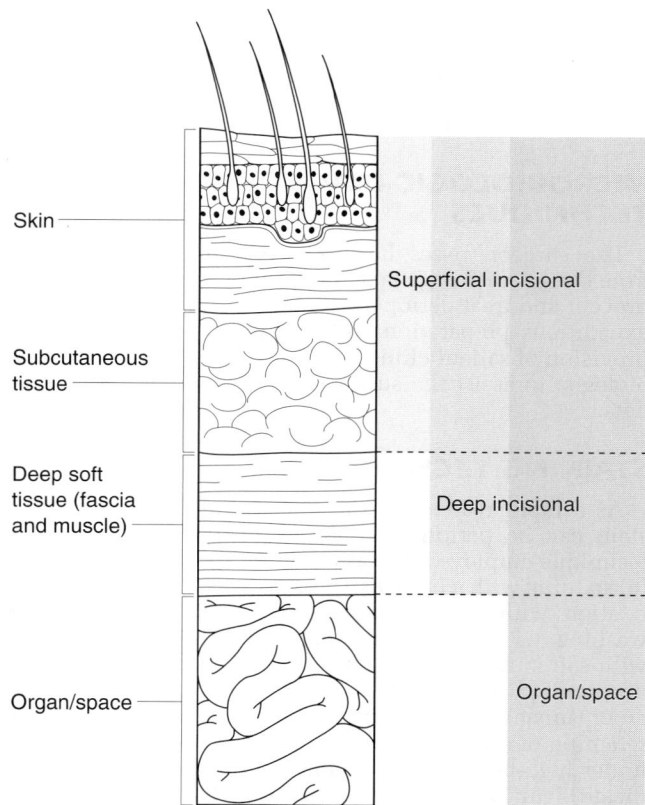

Figure 7.5. Diagrammatic representation of abdominal wall demonstrating the scheme for classification of surgical site infections. (From Mangram AJ, Horan TC, Pearson ML, et al. The Hospital Infection Control Practices Advisory Committee. Guidelines for Prevention of Surgical Site Infection, 1999. *Infect Control Hosp Epidemiol* 1999;20:247, with permission.)

ANTIMICROBIAL AGENTS

Because practicing surgeons are frequently called upon to diagnose and treat infection, they are continually bombarded with persuasive arguments regarding the attributes and potential benefit of an increasingly large number and wide diversity of antimicrobial agents. For this reason, it has become increasingly difficult to choose those agents that are appropriate for a specific indication. Primarily, the surgeon must observe the clinical course of the patient, and interpret the available microbiologic data in this context. In this regard, it must be remembered that (a) antimicrobial agents do not supplant, but are adjunctive to, surgical therapy (débridement of devitalized tissue and drainage of infected material); and (b) there is frequently no requirement to alter antimicrobial therapy in the face of clinical improvement, despite the data obtained from the culture results. The rational use of antimicrobial agents in surgical patients involves the following areas: (a) prophylaxis, (b) empiric therapy, and (c) directed therapy.

Classes of Antimicrobial Agents

Antibacterial agents can be categorized with regard to their structure, mechanism of action, and activity pattern against various types of bacterial pathogens. Penicillins [including several classes of extended spectrum drugs (carboxypenicillins, ureidopenicillins, and penicillins plus β-lactamase inhibitors)] cephalosporins, carbapenems, and monobactams possess a β-lactam ring of some type and act to bind to bacterial division plate proteins, thus inhibiting cell wall peptidoglycan synthesis, resulting in autolytic bacteriolysis. Due to the fact that gram-positive and gram-negative bacteria possess different types of division plate proteins, many of these agents exhibit differential activity between these two types of microorganisms. For example, while first-generation cephalosporins bind avidly to gram-positive division plate proteins, and poorly to those of most gram-negative bacteria, the converse is true for many third-generation cephalosporins, explaining their spectrum of activity.

Tetracyclines, chloramphenicol, and macrolides (e.g., erythromycin) inhibit bacterial ribosomal activity and thus overall protein synthesis via a variety of different mechanisms. Aminoglycosides act to inhibit protein synthesis, but also presumably act on a second target site, a supposition based on the fact that aminoglycosides are bacteriolytic while the other agents are bacteriostatic. Vancomycin inhibits assembly of peptidoglycan polymers, while quinolones bind to DNA helicase proteins and inhibit bacterial DNA synthesis. Sulfonamides inhibit para-aminobenzoic acid incorporation into dihydropteroic acid, thus reducing folinic acid synthesis and thereby purine synthesis. Trimethoprim acts to inhibit dihydrofolate reductase, an enzyme also in the purine synthesis pathway such that these two agents in combination act synergistically. Rifampin binds to bacterial RNA polymerase, acting to directly inhibit bacterial replication. It should be remembered, however, that each agent may possess significant clinical toxicity that may be related to structure and mechanism of action, combined with the degree of differential activity between bacterial and mammalian enzyme systems. The general spectrum of activity of each antimicrobial agent class is shown in Table 7.1.

Prophylactic Antibiotics

Prophylactic antibiotic use is defined as the administration of antibiotics in patients without established infection, with the expectation that prophylaxis will lessen the risk of

Table 7.1. GENERAL SPECTRUM OF ACTIVITY OF COMMONLY USED ANTIMICROBIAL AGENTS[a]

| Antimicrobial Agent | Gram-positive | | | | Gram-negative | Anaerobic | |
	Streptococci	Staphylococci	Enterococci	Enterics	Pseudomonas	Cocci	Bacteroides
Penicillins							
Penicillin G	3	1	1	0	0	2	1
Ampicillin	2	1	3	1	0	1	0
Carboxypenicillins	1	1	1	3	2	1	1
Ureidopenicillins	2	2	2	3	3	1	2
Ampicillin + β-lactamase inhibitor	2	2	3	2	1	2	2
Carboxypenicillins + β-lactamase inhibitor	2	2	2	3	2	2	3
Cephalosporins							
First generation	2	3	0	1	0	2	0
Second generation*	1	2	0	2	1	1	2
Third generation*	0	0	0	3	3	1	1
Monobactams	0	0	0	3	2	0	0
Carbapenems	3	3	0	3	3	2	3
Aminoglycosides	0	1	1	3	3	0	0
Vancomycin	3	3	3	0	0	3	0
Erythromycin	2	2	2	0	0	2	0
Quinolones*	2	1	1	3	2	1	0
Tetracyclines	2	1	1	1	0	1	2
Chloramphenicol	2	2	1	1	0	2	2
Clindamycin	2	1	2	0	0	2	3
metronidazole	0	0	0	0	0	1	3
Trimethoprim-sulfamethoxazole	2	1	0	3	2	1	0

[a]Note: Higher numbers correspond to higher sensitivity of the organism to the antibiotic.
*Different specific agents within the same general class vary markedly with respect to spectrum of activity.

Table 7.2. WOUND INFECTION STRATIFICATION SCHEME

Class I/clean: An uninfected operative wound in which no inflammation is encountered and the respiratory, alimentary, genital, or uninfected urinary tract is not entered. In addition, clean wounds are primarily closed and, if necessary, drained with closed drainage. Operative incisional wounds that follow nonpenetrating (blunt) trauma should be included in this category if they meet the criteria.

Class II/clean-contaminated: An operative wound in which the respiratory, alimentary, genital, or urinary tracts are entered under controlled conditions and without unusual contamination. Specifically, operations involving the biliary tract, appendix, vagina, and oropharynx are included in this category, provided no evidence of infection or major break in technique is encountered.

Class III/contaminated: Open, fresh, accidental wounds. In addition, operations with major breaks in sterile technique (e.g., open cardiac massage) or gross spillage from the gastrointestinal tract, and incisions in which acute, nonpurulent inflammation is encountered are included in this category.

Class IV/dirty-infected: Old traumatic wounds with retained devitalized tissue and those that involve existing clinical infection or perforated viscera. This definition suggests that the organisms causing postoperative infection were present in the operative field before the operation.

Note: As one progresses from class I to class IV, the probability of a wound infection increases.

Adapted from Mangram AJ, Horan TC, Pearson ML, et al., and the Hospital Infection Control Practices Advisory Committee. Guidelines for prevention of surgical site infection—1999. Infect Control Hosp Epidemiol 1999;20:247.

subsequent infection. In the context of surgical patients, this refers primarily to the intravenous administration of antimicrobials in the immediate preoperative period in order to prevent wound infection in skin incisions that are closed at the end of an elective operative procedure. Postoperative wounds may be classified according to their risk of developing infection. One simple stratification system is shown in Table 7.2. Current practice generally dictates that antimicrobial agents should be administered for class II (clean contaminated) and class III (contaminated) types of cases, while patients undergoing clean surgery do not invariably require antimicrobial agents. However, prophylaxis may be indicated for operations under the clean classification, i.e., no organ is entered, when a surgical site infection would represent a catastrophe. This would include cases when prosthetic material is placed, and sternotomy for cardiac surgery and for neurosurgical cases. Some recent studies, however, suggest that a reduction in the wound infection rate can be achieved in clean cases via administration of prophylactic antimicrobial agents and that they may be indicated in high-risk patients.

Experimental studies performed by surgical investigators were the first to find that a finite number of organisms in the initial inoculum to which the wound was exposed determined whether or not infection would result. Studies by Burke (5) and others led to the conclusion that for many organisms this number was 10^5 CFU/g tissue. In an attempt to prevent infection, antimicrobial agents were administered before and at a series of time points after wounding and bacterial contamination of the wound. These studies unequivocally demonstrated that antimicrobial agents reduced infection to the greatest extent when administered prior to contamination, and that the progressive loss of antimicrobial efficacy after contamination was

directly related to growth of microbes within the tissues surrounding and within the wound. Thus a limited period of time existed during which antimicrobial efficacy could be demonstrated. These studies provided the biologic basis for the use of antimicrobial prophylaxis in surgery.

The majority of clinical evidence is derived from studies performed on patients undergoing either biliary or upper GI surgery and receiving first-generation cephalosporin agents. Interestingly, although the combined use of orally administered intraluminal antiaerobic and antianaerobic antimicrobial agents plus mechanical preparation of the bowel significantly reduces the superficial and deep wound infection rates after elective colonic resection (compared to mechanical bowel preparation alone or mechanical bowel preparation plus only an antiaerobic or an antianaerobic intraluminal antimicrobial agent), the addition of an intravenous antimicrobial agent does not significantly further reduce the rate of infection (6). Despite this, the practice of most colorectal surgeons (87%) is to use a combined regimen of oral plus intravenous antibiotics in addition to mechanical preparation in elective colorectal procedures. Thus, in colorectal surgery, while the use of added intravenous prophylactic antimicrobial agent with a spectrum of activity directed against the microflora in that region of the body has not been entirely substantiated, it appears that the conceptual advantage related to lowering the initial inoculum (using oral agents) and plus protecting the wound from contamination with residual organisms (with intravenous agents) seems to dictate the prevailing approach to prophylaxis for colon surgery.

Other important principles related to the use of antimicrobial prophylaxis include the following: (a) The agent selected should be safe, inexpensive, and have a spectrum that includes the likely pathogens contaminating the wound at the time of surgery. (b) The agent should be administered immediately preoperatively, such that bactericidal levels are present in the tissues throughout the procedure. If massive blood loss occurs, the patient is obese, or the operation is prolonged, a second intraoperative dose should be considered. (c) Antibiotics need not be administered postoperatively. This has not been shown to improve effectiveness and may promote adverse drug reactions, the development of resistant microbes in the institution, and the occurrence of superinfections in a given patient.

Empiric Therapy

The surgeon must frequently decide whether or not to institute therapy with antimicrobial agents based on the clinical course of a given patient without the benefit of well-defined microbiologic data. The dilemma thus centers around an attempt to determine whether or not the patient has a source of infection, and at what point does the evidence provide enough support of this diagnosis so that it would be imprudent to withhold antimicrobial therapy. Several tenets should be followed in this setting: (a) an assiduous search for a septic source should be undertaken and continued (cultures, radiographic procedures, et al.), and (b) initial limits should be placed on the course of empiric therapy, and these should be continually reevaluated based on the clinical course of the patient. Should cultures prove negative, discontinuation of antimicrobial therapy would seem appropriate. Care must also be taken to select antimicrobial agents based on known activity patterns in a given institution.

Controversial issues regarding the use of empiric antimicrobial therapy in this setting concern the use of multiple agent regimens in which each agent is specifically targeted against a specific class of pathogens, versus the use of more broad-spectrum agents (many second- and third-generation cephalosporins, carboxypenicillins, urei-dopenicillins, penicillins plus β-lactamase inhibitors, carbapenems) that may suffer slightly from a lack of individual pathogen specificity, but overall are directed against several groups of pathogens. These broad-spectrum agents are being used more and more commonly as empiric therapy, particularly because they often avoid many of the toxic effects such as nephrotoxicity that are present with combined modality regimens. Other broad-spectrum classes of agents remain virtually untested in surgical patients with severe sepsis (e.g., amdinocillin, spectinomycin analogues such as trospectomycin, and newer quinolones). Careful selection among all these agents is required based on known spectra of activity.

Directed Therapy

Simply stated, directed antimicrobial therapy consists of the targeting of specific antibacterial agents against identified pathogens, once sensitivity reports are available. Culture reports from patients with severe, polymicrobial infections may create confusion and lead to administration of three or more antibacterial agents. Because there are no absolute rules, only general guidelines can be provided. Primarily, because experimental and clinical evidence supports the concept of aerobic-anaerobic synergy, therapy should be directed against both potential components of the infection if the body site is such that these microorganisms may be present. This issue is less well defined clinically regarding enterococcal infection. While several experimental studies indicate that this organism can act with other components of the infection to enhance lethality, it has not routinely been included as part of the antimicrobial coverage in all mixed flora infections, e.g., secondary bacterial peritonitis or intraabdominal abscesses. Secondarily, administer agents that exhibit specific activity against various components of the infection, and attempt to balance the effect by selecting those agents that exhibit minimal toxicity, while retaining suitable efficacy. This can often be achieved via administration of extended-spectrum penicillins or second- or third-generation cephalosporins in combination with other agents, or perhaps with carbapenem agents alone. Single-agent therapy has been shown to be equivalent to an aminoglycoside plus an antianaerobic agent (clindamycin or metronidazole) for the treatment of peritoneal contamination due to gangrenous appendicitis or penetrating GI injury and established bacterial peritonitis, as long as the spectrum of activity includes aerobes and anaerobes. Selection of single agent versus combination should be decided based on patient factors, safety profile under the circumstances, and finally cost and ease of administration. As mentioned above, extended-spectrum agents should not be used for prophylaxis, or when less expensive, more routine agents can be directed against a specific pathogen. They are often ideal for treatment of the patient with several pathogenic organisms present, or with a nosocomial infection due to a resistant organism that is within the spectrum of activity of a particular extended-spectrum agent and not other antimicrobials. The duration of therapy for surgical infections has not been well defined, although some guidelines for intraabdominal infections have been established (see Intraabdominal Infection, below).

APPROACHES TO DIAGNOSIS OF INFECTION IN THE SURGICAL PATIENT

Clinical Manifestations of Infection

The interaction of invading microbes and host defenses produces the clinical manifestations of infection. In many cases, the classic local symptoms and signs of pain, swelling, and redness at the infected site and fever as part of the systemic response will all occur, but their absence does not exclude infection, particularly in the immunocompromised host. Systemic leukocytosis with a preponderance of PMNs may be noted, and severe systemic infections may produce confusion, ileus, hypotension, and profound shock. Thus, any of these premonitory signs mandates a thorough diagnostic evaluation to establish or exclude the presence of significant infection.

Initially, a carefully directed review of the patient's previous history, operative procedure(s), and current physical status should be undertaken. Pertinent laboratory and physiologic monitoring data should also be carefully studied. Several diagnostic procedures should be performed in order to collect specimens to obtain concrete microbiologic information. Blood, urine, sputum, and any obviously infected site should be cultured for potential bacterial pathogens as well as fungi and viruses. Although a number of routine studies (e.g., chest radiograph) should be performed, a concentrated effort should be directed toward the superficial and deep components of the surgical wound *(vide infra)*, as this is the area where the vast majority of infections occur. For example, close examination of the wound may reveal a small amount of drainage that will prompt opening the wound to reveal a significant wound infection. Studies such as chest and sinus radiographs in a patient who has undergone prolonged intubation for the purpose of mechanical ventilation may identify diffuse pneumonitis, a discrete infiltrate, or sinusitis and will serve to direct further studies. Subsequent bronchoscopy or sinus aspiration can then be performed to obtain specific site cultures. Catheter sepsis, urinary tract infections, and systemic sepsis must also be considered. The patient in the intensive care unit (ICU) represents a particular challenge to the clinician, as evaluation may be limited by a number of factors including reduced level of consciousness, use of sedation or narcotics, immunosuppressed state, and comorbid disease. Liberal use of computed tomography (CT) scanning in this patient group may aid in detecting pathologic processes in the chest and abdomen. Finally, it bears mention that numerous disease entities not related to infection can cause fever in the immediate postoperative period (atelectasis, thrombophlebitis, pulmonary embolism, drug allergy) and that these must also be included in the differential diagnosis.

Wound Infection

A recent publication entitled *Guideline for the Prevention of Surgical Site Infection—1999* documents the recommendations by the Centers for Disease Control and Prevention (CDC) for prevention of surgical site infection. This document provides an evidence-based approach to the epidemiology of surgical site infections and recommendations for their prevention. This document, available from the CDC Web site (www.cdc.gov) or in various journals (7), represents the most comprehensive guide presently available. Various highlights will be included herein, but the reader is referred to the full Web-based or hardcopy document for details.

The concept of surgical wound infections has been broadened and now includes infections deep to the incision itself. The new terminology is "surgical site infection" and is divided into infections of either the incision or the deeper organs/spaces (Fig. 7.5). The incisional site is further divided into superficial (skin and subcutaneous tissue) and deep (deeper soft tissues of the incision) compartments. Organ/space site infections are defined to involve tissues at the site of surgery other than the incised body wall layers. Surgical site infections, in general, have been shown to in-

Table 7.3. FACTORS INFLUENCING RISK OF SURGICAL SITE INFECTION

Patient factors
  Advanced age
  Smoking
  Obesity
  Coexisting infection at remote site
  Skin or mucous membrane colonization with microorganisms
  Impaired systemic immunity
  Prolonged preoperative stay
  Hypothermia
  Reduced arterial oxygen saturation
Operative factors
  Improper skin antisepsis
  Preoperative shaving
  Blood transfusion
  Duration of operation
  Antimicrobial prophylaxis
  Operating room ventilation
  Inadequate sterilization of instruments
  Foreign material in surgical site
  Surgical technique
    Poor hemostasis
    Tissue trauma
    Skin closure technique
Personnel factors
  Infected or colonized surgical personel
  Duration of surgical scrub inadequate
  Use of fluid resistant surgical drapes and gowns
  Appropriate use of surgical masks, gloves, and caps

Adapted from Mangram AJ, Horan TC, Pearson ML, et al., and the Hospital Infection Control Practices Advisory Committee. Guidelines for prevention of surgical site infection—1999. Infect Control Hosp Epidemiol 1999;20:247.

crease hospital stay, patient morbidity, and costs. Among the different depths of site infection, organ/space infections constitute a greater burden to health care costs overall.

The risk of surgical site infection can be simplistically considered in the form of an equation:

$$\text{Risk of infection} = \frac{\text{Bacterial inoculum} \times \text{bacterial virulence}}{\text{Local host defenses} \times \text{systemic immune competence}}$$

Thus, in defining risk factors for infection and means of minimizing risk, one can consider each of the four components in turn. Factors increasing bacterial inoculum and virulence and decreasing local and systemic host defenses will heighten the risk for the development of surgical site infection. Interventions that lower bacterial inoculum and virulence and increase host defenses will lessen the risk of infection. An individual's risk for infection may be generally predicted based on this equation. For example, systemic immunosuppression and inadequate prophylactic antimicrobial tissue levels or use of antimicrobial agents to which an organism is resistant may foster the development of infection even when low inocula are present. Even the normal host with adequate levels of an appropriate antimicrobial agent may not be able to combat the development of infection, however, if an extremely large bacterial inoculum is introduced.

Many factors influence the occurrence of wound infections. Table 7.3 lists several potential factors that may contribute to the development of surgical site infection by virtue of altering one or more of the factors in the risk equation. Most importantly, these help to define optimal practice aimed at minimizing infection. For each of the factors listed in Table 7.3, there is a variable degree of ex-

perimental, clinical, or epidemiological evidence supporting recommendations regarding implementation of the technique. These are documented in the CDC guidelines and should be referred to for specific details (7).

Intraabdominal Infection

The peritoneal cavity is a mesothelium-lined potential space that under normal circumstances contains only a small amount of serous, sterile fluid. Infection of this potential space can occur after the introduction of microorganisms during peritoneal dialysis or in patients with ascites in whom no viscus perforation has occurred (primary peritonitis) or after perforation of a viscus with spillage of the autochthonous flora takes place (secondary peritonitis). The change in microbial flora in patients with initial secondary bacterial peritonitis so that ongoing infection with normally low-virulence pathogens (e.g., *Staphylococcus epidermidis, Candida albicans*) occurs has been termed tertiary or persistent peritonitis. The introduction of microorganisms into the normally sterile peritoneal environment invokes several potent specialized host antimicrobial defense mechanisms: (a) clearance, (b) phagocytosis and killing, and (c) sequestration (Fig. 7.6) (8).

Bacterial clearance, by translymphatic absorption, occurs via specialized structures found only on the peritoneal mesothelium on the underside of the diaphragm that act as conduits for both fluid and particulate matter. Stomata (10 to 16 μm) between mesothelial cells lead into lymphatic structures (lacunae), that subsequently drain into larger mediastinal lymphatic vessels. These in turn pass material via the thoracic duct into the venous circulation. This efficient means of clearing bacteria from the peritoneal cavity presumably serves as the conduit for the development of bacteremia and the septic host response in patients with intraabdominal infection. Those microbes that are not cleared are rapidly engulfed by resident and recruited phagocytic cells. During the initial stages of infection, resident macrophages and possibly mast cells act as the first line of peritoneal host defense in concert with clearance to diminish bacterial numbers. As noted above, this interaction between bacteria and resident macrophages serves to amplify the local immune response, with release of proinflammatory mediator molecules that both attract and prime other cells such as PMNs. Indeed, after the first several hours, there is an influx of PMNs into the peritoneal cavity. These cells act to engulf those invading microbes that have escaped other defense mechanisms. There are, however, quantitative limitations to the capacity of each of these mechanisms to deal with contamination. In experimental models, only extremely large bacterial inocula (2×10^{10} E. coli) are capable of saturating both clearance and phagocytosis mechanisms simultaneously. The limits of these defenses in humans, however, are not established.

Those microorganisms that evade both clearance and phagocytosis are confronted by a final, primitive host defense mechanism (sequestration) that functions to protect the host from the bacterial inoculum. A fibrinogen-rich inflammatory exudate containing plasma opsonins appears during peritoneal infection, and fibrin polymerization occurs. Acting in conjunction with the omentum and other mobile viscera, perforations are sealed, and as ileus develops, contaminated enteric contents are walled off, thereby preventing continued soilage of the peritoneal cavity and bacteremic spread of bacteria. Fibrin itself has the capacity to trap large numbers of bacteria and also amplify the immune response. Intraabdominal abscess formation is probably promoted both by the fluid influx into the peri-

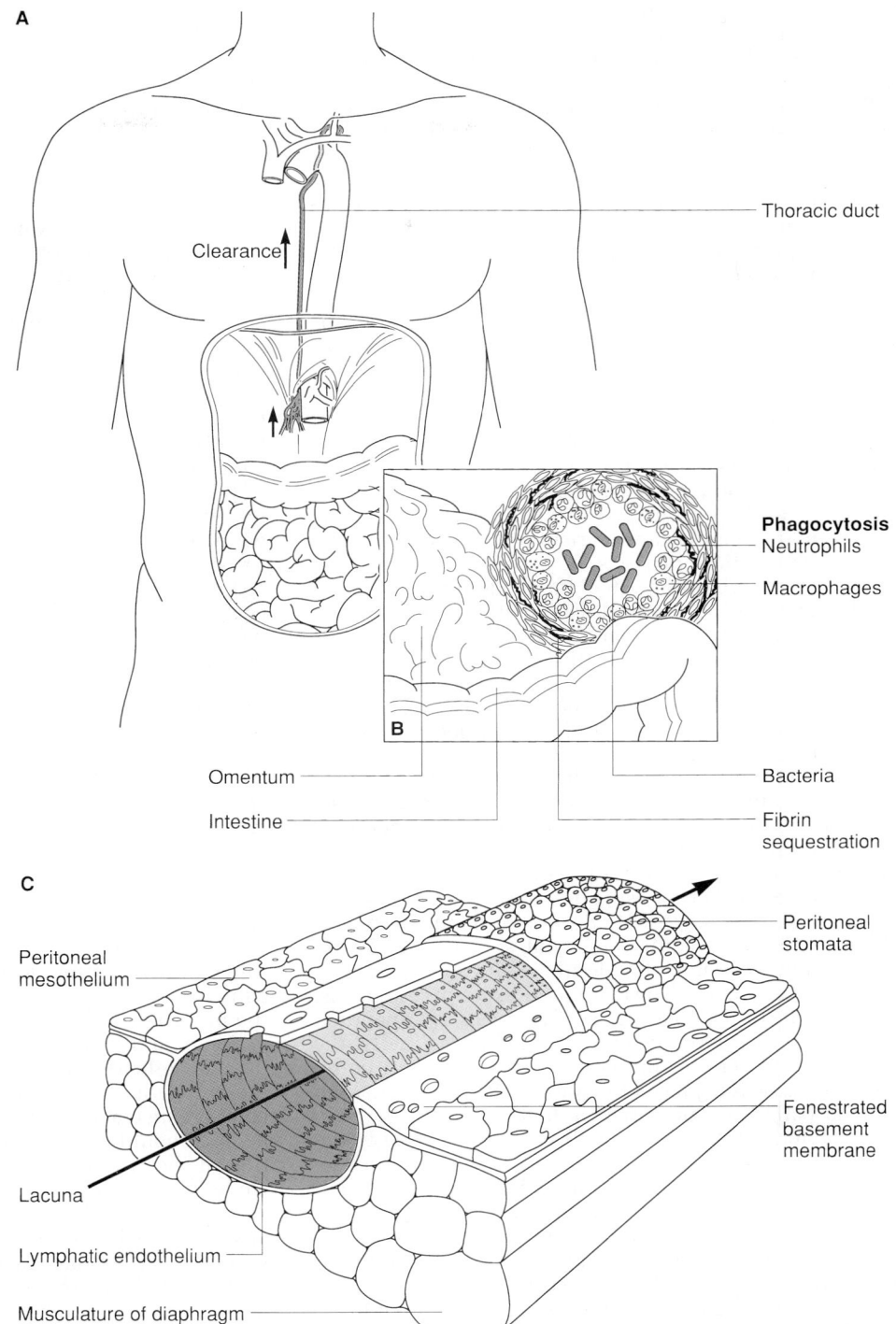

Figure 7.6. Host defenses of the peritoneal cavity consist of clearance, phagocytosis, and sequestration. Clearance occurs via translymphatic absorption, and resident macrophages engulf invading microorganisms. These two components represent the first line of peritoneal host defense, while recruitment of polymorphonuclear leukocytes after 3 to 4 hours and sequestration serve to further limit the development of infection.

toneal cavity, which inhibits opsonization and phagocytosis, and by the fibrin deposition, which isolates the bacteria from the phagocytes, thereby creating a protected microenvironment for bacterial proliferation free from host leukocytes. Typically, intraabdominal infection results from the perforation of a hollow viscus and the ensuing contamination of the normally sterile peritoneal cavity. The normal bacterial flora found in that particular location of the alimentary tract thus determines the initial inoculum.

In parallel with the overall quantity of microorganisms (both aerobes, but predominantly anaerobes), perforations of the lower small bowel and colon produce a higher frequency of infections that contain anaerobic microorganisms, and these patients develop a greater number of infectious complications and exhibit a higher mortality rate. In addition, certain predictable patterns of bacterial isolates are found, and the isolation of these organisms is independent of the site of perforation, indicating that a marked simplification of the numerous microbial forms present in the initial inoculum occurs. This simplification process may be related to synergistic interactions occurring among certain components of the initial inoculum, as well as the selection pressure exerted by host defenses upon certain microbial forms. Overall, an average of four to five isolates have been reported to occur in patients with established intraabdominal infection, more than half of which are anaerobes. Both aerobic and anaerobic isolates are encountered in 80% to 90% of specimens, isolation of either aerobes or anaerobes alone being less common. Commonly encountered aerobic isolates are *E. coli* and other gram-negative enteric bacilli such as *Enterobacter* sp. and *Klebsiella* sp., gram-positive bacteria (various streptococci, staphylococci, and enterococci species), and other gram-negative pathogens (*Proteus* and *Pseudomonas* sp.), and *Candida* sp. Among the anaerobes, *Bacteroides* (especially *Bacteroides fragilis*), *Clostridium,* and the anaerobic cocci are most consistently isolated (9).

From a clinical standpoint, intraabdominal infection may be classified according to whether it is walled off by host peritoneal defenses, i.e., peritonitis versus abscess formation. Peritonitis is subclassified into primary, secondary, or tertiary peritonitis; secondary represents the most common manifestation arising from visceral transmural inflammation, necrosis, or perforation. Evaluation of the patient with suspected intraabdominal infection should begin with a physical examination and an initial flat plate and upright or decubitus roentgenogram of the abdomen. In the acute setting, the presence of peritoneal irritation manifested by local or generalized pain and tenderness with evidence of free intraperitoneal air is diagnostic of visceral perforation and is an indication for surgical intervention. If no obvious viscus perforation is noted, clinical judgment is required to define what course of action should be pursued. The presence of acute-onset diffuse peritonitis with systemic signs of inflammation is usually considered sufficient for recommending surgical therapy. By contrast, the finding of localized peritonitis might suggest further investigation for clarification of the diagnosis and management. Several inflammatory processes that do not require emergent surgery may be revealed though the use of abdominal ultrasound or a CT scan of the abdomen. These include acute diverticulitis, cholecystitis, or pancreatitis. The diagnosis of appendicitis may also be clarified by these methods. Finally, the presence of visceral or nonvisceral abscesses will be revealed by these imaging techniques. The approach to each of these pathologic processes is highlighted in the specific chapter in this text and will not be discussed in detail here.

The diagnosis of intraabdominal infection is particularly challenging in the patient in the ICU setting. These patients are frequently immunosuppressed, have a reduced level of consciousness, have comorbid disease, and may be receiving narcotic analgesics. Together, these factors make history and clinical examination difficult to assess. Several approaches have been advocated in this patient population including diagnostic peritoneal lavage and abdominal CT scanning with GI and rectal contrast. Bedside mini-laparotomy may be helpful in this setting, although there are clearly shortcomings to this approach. Recently, laparoscopy at the bedside has been advocated and has shown promise as a diagnostic tool in experienced hands (10). Further evaluation of this approach appears warranted. The value of empiric laparotomy in this setting is controversial, and in general, does not add to diagnostic accuracy or outcome in this patient population.

Although the primary treatment of a perforated viscus is surgical, antimicrobial therapy is an extremely important adjunct. Empiric antimicrobial therapy for secondary bacterial peritonitis should be directed against both aerobes and anaerobes. Administration of an agent directed against only one component of the infection or the other is inferior to combined therapy. This has been substantiated in carefully stratified groups of patients with perforated or gangrenous appendicitis or who suffer penetrating abdominal trauma that causes perforation of a viscus. As mentioned above, several studies indicate that the results of using several agents in combination is equivalent to the use of single-agent therapy as long as the agents selected possess activity against both components of the infection (11). Selection of inferior single agents with significantly less activity against anaerobes, for example, will most probably produce deleterious results. The availability of newer antibiotics with excellent oral bioavailability has afforded the opportunity to convert from intravenous to oral antibiotics during the course of therapy. In one study, conversion from intravenous therapy to combination oral ciprofloxacin/metronidazole when the patient is tolerating oral nutrition was shown to have equivalent outcome to continued intravenous therapy . The implications for reduced patient morbidity and lower hospital costs are obvious. In patients with straightforward "off the street" peritonitis, the addition of antienterococcal or antifungal agents as initial therapy has not been substantiated by existing data. Their use in more complex patients is better supported by clinical trials. In patients with recurrent GI perforations or anastomotic leakage, prophylaxis with the antifungal agent fluconazole was shown to reduce *Candida* infection and colonization, although overall mortality was not affected in this relatively small study (12). These findings suggest that judicious use of this agent in this selected high-risk group may be beneficial. In a similar fashion, antienterococcal therapy might be considered appropriate for this group of high-risk patients.

Determining the most beneficial duration of antimicrobial therapy in this setting for a specific patient is difficult. Retrospective data suggest that the following criteria should be fulfilled prior to discontinuing antibiotics: (a) The patient is clinically well and afebrile for 48 hours. (b) The leukocyte count has normalized for 48 hours. (c) The band count is <3%. If these three criteria are fulfilled, then the probability of recurrent infection following discontinuation of antibiotics is low (<2%). By contrast, should the patient be febrile or have a persistent leukocytosis, then the probability of residual infection is high (>30%) and a comprehensive search for the cause of persistent inflammation should be initiated. Using these criteria, the duration of therapy ranges from 4 to 7 days postoperatively. Under certain circumstances, the duration of therapy may be shortened such that it resembles "prophylactic" therapy. This includes diseases such as acute appendicitis without perforation, acute cholecystitis, small bowel necrosis with perforation, and acute diverticulitis. Common among these processes is the fact that the pathology is completely extirpated and little infection/inflammation remains in the peritoneal cavity.

During repeated episodes of intraabdominal soilage, patients more frequently develop infections due to gram-positive cocci such as *S. epidermidis, Enterococcus fecalis* and *faecium*, gram-negative organisms such as *Pseudomonas aeruginosa,* and fungi (primarily *Candida*) (13). These organisms are probably selected out by both the failure of host defenses and initial antimicrobial agent therapy. In the setting of tertiary microbial peritonitis, treatment with antimicrobial agents directed against the specific pathogens isolated seems reasonable, although a salutary effect on patient mortality has only been demonstrated with respect to anti-*Candida* therapy.

Necrotizing Soft Tissue Infections

Soft tissue infections may involve any of the individual layers of soft tissues including the skeletal muscles, the deep muscular fascia, the superficial fascia, the skin and subcutaneous tissues, or a combination of all these areas. The nomenclature used to categorize severe soft tissue infections has become progressively more confusing because there have been many eponyms (e.g., Meleney's synergistic gangrene) applied to what is probably the same disease process occurring in different layers or sites. The most common form of progressive necrotizing soft tissue infection seen by a surgeon will be some form of necrotizing fasciitis, an infection of the deep and superficial fascia that is associated with a mortality as high as 40% in many series. Currently, this disease is probably best categorized by (a) site, (b) infecting organism(s), and (c) extent of initial disease and rapidity of progression. Importantly, while this infection primarily involves the fascial layers, the skin may exhibit evidence of necrosis. For example, Fournier's gangrene is a form of necrotizing fasciitis. The pathognomonic presenting sign of necrosis of the scrotal skin is a result of necrosis of the vessels as they traverse the fascial layers into the closely applied overlying skin.

Although many underlying disease processes predispose patients to necrotizing fasciitis, three common factors are almost invariably present: (a) impairment of the immune system (e.g., diabetes mellitus, malignancy, alcoholism), (b) compromise of the fascial blood supply, and (c) the presence of microorganisms that are able to proliferate within this area. Thus, patients who may be immunocompromised and who develop perineal or lower extremity decubitus ulcers, those who undergo closure of heavily contaminated wounds, or those who suffer heavy contamination in the process of traumatic wounding are predisposed to develop this type of infection. Infections of this type are usually polymicrobial in nature with gram-positive organisms such as staphylococci and streptococci (aerobic and anaerobic), gram-negative enteric bacteria, and gram-negative anaerobes being frequently identified. These polymicrobial culture results are assuredly indicative of the occurrence of a synergistic process perhaps, in large part accounting for the severity of these infections. Some microorganisms, however, possess virulence factors that in conjunction with an underlying host predisposition allow this disease process to occur without dependence of other bacteria. Examples of this form of disease include necrotizing fasciitis due to *Clostridium, Pseudomonas,* and *Aeromonas* sp. In these patients, the process is often fulminant and is frequently associated with cellulitis, myositis, fasciitis, and bacteremia with an attendant high mortality probably due to both the soft tissue infection as well as the occurrence of bacteremia with concurrent bacterial exotoxin production. Although rare, tetanus, and toxic shock syndrome due to *Clostridium tetani* and certain toxin-producing strains of streptococci and staphylococci may become established in or about the surgical wound. These unusual infections are associated with few if any of the classic signs of wound infection (e.g., erythema, pain, fluctuance, drainage) but are frequently associated with signs of septic shock, organ failure, and high lethality.

In the vast majority of cases, a high index of suspicion that a necrotizing soft tissue infection is present will exist based solely on clinical signs present within the soft tissues (e.g., skin discoloration or necrosis; blebs; drainage of thin, watery, grayish foul-smelling fluid; subcutaneous crepitus; etc.). Confirmatory evidence can be provided via local exploration of the wound (with direct observation and performance of a Gram stain) and radiologic studies— plain films, CT, or magnetic resonance imaging (MRI) of the involved area. Soft tissue x-rays and/or CT scanning of the area may also help to elucidate the extent of the infection and often the origin, e.g., the presence of a perineal abscess in patients with Fournier's gangrene. However, performance of these studies should not preclude early operative intervention in a clear-cut case or when the diagnosis is highly probable in a patient with evidence of clinical deterioration.

Early recognition based on clinical signs, local site exploration, or CT scanning in selected individuals, in conjunction with prompt, aggressive, and extensive débridement to remove all devitalized and infected tissue, broad-spectrum antibiotics, fluid resuscitation, hemodynamic monitoring, and nutritional support, would appear to afford patients the best chance of survival (14). Often such aggressive surgery is mutilating, requiring the removal of larger amounts of body tissue and one or more extremities. The clearest guidelines to determine the limits of resection involve removal of clearly infected, necrotic tissue so that margins several centimeters into grossly normal, healthy tissue are achieved. Some authors advocate the use of frozen section analysis to determine adequacy of excision, and this may be useful in some cases, particularly those in which the observer is unsure whether infected tissue remains at the margin of resection. More appropriately, planned reexploration should be considered a useful adjunct to initial surgery. The empiric administration of antimicrobial agents active against gram-positive, gram-negative, and anaerobic bacteria should be initiated promptly. In most cases, this will involve the use of several antimicrobial agents in combination. Because of the concern in all such cases of the presence of *Clostridium* infection, high doses of aqueous penicillin G are administered. Gram-positive organisms are treated with vancomycin or a semisynthetic penicillin, while gram-negative organisms are treated with an aminoglycoside or a monobactam. Anaerobic coverage is typically achieved by use of metronidazole or clindamycin. The use of extended-spectrum agents (e.g., carbapenem, ticarcillin-clavulinic acid, piperacillin-tazobactam) to treat gram-negative and anaerobic organisms may be acceptable. As for all infections where empiric therapy is initiated based on likely pathogens, Gram stain and culture data should be used to focus and direct antimicrobial therapy.

Continued areas of controversy concern the efficacy of hyperbaric oxygen therapy, particularly in cases of clostridial gangrene, the need for performing a colostomy in patients with the perineal form of the disease (i.e., Fournier's gangrene), and the continuing high mortality exhibited in patients with all forms of necrotizing fasciitis. Experimental studies using hyperbaric oxygen in models of infection in animals have demonstrated clear benefit to its use. However, while measurement of subcutaneous oxygen tension in patients with necrotizing fasciitis demonstrated a 2.5-fold increase in oxygen tension in patients receiving hyperbaric oxygen (15), controlled clinical trials demonstrating additional benefits derived from hyperbaric oxygen therapy in humans are lacking. At present, therefore, this form of therapy must be considered an adjunct to therapy and should not delay timely and aggressive surgical intervention. Because the entire perineal region and buttocks are frequently involved in patients with perineal necrotizing fasciitis, performance of fecal stream diversion via colostomy often improves wound care and patient management, although it has not invariably improved outcome. Interestingly, several authors have speculated that the mortality rate of necrotizing fasciitis has remained unchanged because improvements in treatment and critical care may have been offset by the occurrence of this disease process in an increasingly high-risk group of older and/or immunocompromised patients.

Gram-negative Bacterial Sepsis, Shock, and Multiple Organ Dysfunction Syndrome (MODS)

Gram-negative bacterial sepsis is a lethal disease process that currently produces substantial morbidity and mortality in both normal and immunocompromised patients (10% to 20% and >30% lethality, respectively), despite therapeutic intervention with antimicrobial agents, aggressive hemodynamic monitoring, fluid resuscitation, and metabolic support. This disease process represents one of the most severe infections that can occur in the surgical patient. Over the last several decades, nosocomial infections due to gram-negative pathogens have increased in frequency; several series report an average incidence of 3 to 13 cases of gram-negative bacteremia per 1,000 hospital admissions. Many factors predispose patients to these infections: (a) underlying host disease processes such as malignancy, renal insufficiency, congestive heart failure, and diabetes mellitus; (b) old age and disability; (c) malnutrition; (d) prior or concurrent antimicrobial therapy; (e) major operations; (f) respiratory or urinary manipulation or intubation; and (g) immunosuppression (acquired or inherited). Fatality in most series has paralleled the presence and severity of the underlying host disease, polymicrobial bacteremia, shock, and lack of early appropriate antimicrobial therapy.

Although many different organisms cause this form of sepsis, *E. coli* predominates in overall frequency. Also common are isolates of *Klebsiella, Enterobacter,* and *Serratia,* while *Pseudomonas* bacteremia is somewhat less common. Sepsis due to *Proteus* sp., *Providencia* sp., *Acinetobacter* sp., *Aeromonas* sp., *Citrobacter* sp., *Achromobacter* sp., *Salmonella* sp., *Shigella* sp., *Bacteroides* sp., and numerous other organisms has also been reported. Some studies have demonstrated that non–E. coli sepsis is more lethal than sepsis caused by E. coli, and that *Pseudomonas* sepsis is associated with the highest lethality, although not all investigators have been able to substantiate this finding. In several series 10% to 20% of patients had polymicrobial sepsis, and most investigators agree that polymicrobial sepsis is more lethal. This appears to be true even when patients are stratified regarding severity of underlying disease and appropriate or inappropriate antimicrobial therapy.

The manner in which gram-negative bacterial infection causes the initial physiologic host septic response (i.e., fever, systemic acidosis, arterial hypoxemia, disordered substrate and oxygen utilization, abnormal metabolism, hyperkalemia, hyperglycemia, decreased systemic vascular resistance, elevated cardiac output, and hypotension), the failure of organs separated spatially from the infected site, and eventual lethality have intrigued investigators for years. Although initially it seemed patent that blood-borne bacteria or bacterial toxins were responsible, it would appear that more complex interactions probably take place. The triggering and amplification of numerous components of several host mediator systems play an important role, and increasing evidence has accumulated that indicates that organ failure and death may occur subsequent to such an overexuberant host response.

Activation of the complement and coagulation cascades occurs and has been associated with leukopenia due to PMN aggregation, macrophage stimulation, and thrombocytopenia. Release of cellular products such as superoxide radicals, lysosomal enzymes (e.g., cathepsin, elastase),

prostaglandins, and monokines appears to follow the initial activation steps. Neither bacteria, bacterial toxins, nor host-mediated events alone can account for all the alterations that occur in host physiology, and thus some composite effect may be responsible. In particular, several groups of investigators have developed experimental models and made clinical observations that provide evidence that cellular mediators are released in response to a variety of stimuli, including bacterial products, and that excessive mediator secretion initiates events that lead to target organ damage and failure. Precise translation of this information to the clinical setting and demonstration of similar pathogenetic mechanisms have been difficult, however, and a unified sequence of events that eventuate in lethality has proven elusive.

Increasing evidence has implicated gram-negative bacterial LPS (endotoxin) as that portion of the gram-negative bacterial cell membrane responsible for many, if not all, of the toxic effects that occur during gram-negative bacterial sepsis. For this reason, LPS has been intensively examined from an immunologic, physiologic, and microbiologic standpoint. The biochemical structure of LPS has been determined for many species of gram-negative microorganisms, and generally consists of repeating O-antigen polysaccharide subunits linked to a polysaccharide core region that, in turn, is attached to membrane bound lipid A (Fig. 7.7). The O-antigen polysaccharide subunits are unique for each organism, and thus largely are responsible for the wide serotypic diversity seen among strains of even a particular gram-negative bacterial species. The core region of LPS

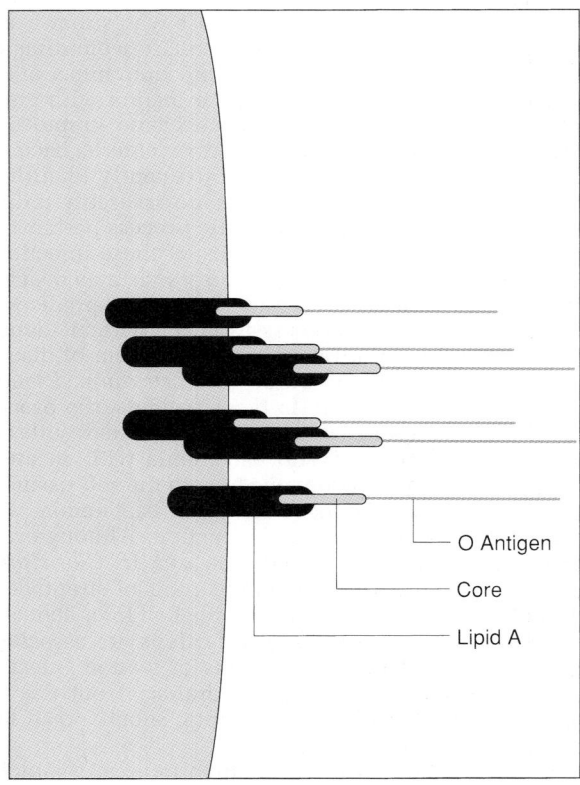

Figure 7.7. Structure of gram-negative bacterial lipopolysaccharide (LPS). LPS consists of three regions: (a) O antigen, a series of repeating polysaccharide units; (b) core LPS, a short series of biochemically and immunologically conserved saccharide residues; and (c) lipid A, which consists of diglucosamine residues associated with nonhydroxylated fatty acids embedded within the outer membrane itself and responsible for the majority of toxicity.

demonstrates a significant degree of structural conservation among genera of gram-negative bacteria and consists of a short series of saccharide residues. The innermost or deep portion of core LPS consists of two to three saccharide residues in most gram-negative bacteria and is the most highly conserved portion of this region. Lipid A is embedded within the outer membrane, and consists of diglucosamine residues associated with nonhydroxylated fatty acids of 12 to 16 carbon atom chain length. Although relatively insoluble in aqueous solutions, injection of isolated lipid A produces toxicity in a variety of animal models, leading to the hypothesis that the hydrophilic O-antigen solubilizes LPS in the mammalian host milieu, while lipid A interacts with lipid components of the host cell membrane.

The LPS molecule exerts diverse effects on the mammalian host. Immunologic responses to LPS include nonspecific polyclonal B-cell proliferation, macrophage activation and monokine secretion, tolerance to a subsequent LPS or bacterial challenge, and production of antibody directed against various portions of the LPS molecule following repeated challenge with either LPS or intact bacteria. Physiologic responses similar to those seen during gram-negative bacterial sepsis occur during LPS administration and include hypotension, hypoxemia, acidosis, bacterial translocation across the gut, complement and coagulation cascade activation, white blood cell and platelet margination, and death.

LPS exerts direct and indirect effects on host tissues to produce the septic response. Indirect, i.e., mediated, effects result from LPS triggering of host macrophages. Activated macrophages secrete a wide array of monokines that include TNF-α, IL-1α,β, IL-6, and IFN-γ. Excessive secretion of cytokines produce substantial systemic effects in the mammalian host. The most compelling evidence supporting this contention is the demonstration in experimental models and humans that administration of TNF by itself produces manifestations nearly identical (fever, leukopenia, hypotension, death) to the administration of LPS. In addition, serum levels of TNF are elevated in patients with gram-negative bacterial sepsis, and administration of LPS to humans and nonhuman primates is associated with elevations of TNF after 1.5 to 2 hours. In several animal models anti-TNF antibody ameliorates the lethal effects of either an LPS challenge or a TNF challenge.

TNF-α and IL-1β appear to be primary mediators within the local host milieu, exerting deleterious effects on the host only after large amounts are secreted and reach the systemic circulation. Macrophage IL-2 and IL-6 (and perhaps IL-8 in humans) appear to be secreted after TNF-α and/or IL-1β stimulation events occur, while IFN-α is secreted at low levels by macrophages during both the initial and subsequent activation and secretion stages. IFN-γ may act to facilitate the continued activation of macrophages, recruitment of additional activated macrophages, and the ongoing output of the above-mentioned monokines. Serum IL-1β levels are increased in humans after exogenous endotoxin administration and are elevated after gram-negative bacterial challenge in nonhuman primates. Protective doses of anti-TNF antibody abrogates this increase in IL-1. IL-1 also has been shown to enhance survival in neutropenic mice after gram-negative bacterial challenge.

Similarly, IL-6 levels are elevated systemically and at the site of infection in animal and clinical studies. In humans, administration of LPS leads to increased serum levels of IL-6, and anti-TNF antibody abrogates the serum increase in IL-6 seen after gram-negative bacterial challenge in animal models. While IL-6 administration does not itself lead to increased mortality, anti-IL-6 antibodies have been shown to improve survival after experimental gram-negative bacterial challenge. Several studies have also indicated that prior administration of low-dose LPS, TNF, or high doses of IL-2 may actually enhance survival during experimental gram-negative bacterial infection, indicating that the level of activation or ability of the host to respond to cytokine secretion may be of critical importance.

Thus, this portion of the host response that normally acts to contain and localize infection may injure the host during systemic infection, leading to the high mortality events of septic shock and MODS. Isolated pulmonary failure (adult respiratory distress syndrome) is common following systemic sepsis, while gut, hepatic, and renal failure may occur subsequently. Many studies have clearly correlated an increase in mortality with an increased evidence of organ dysfunction during sepsis (16).

The diagnosis of systemic sepsis is frequently suspected when the above physiologic alterations occur after a known or suspected source of infection is identified, but the diagnosis is truly confirmed only after blood cultures become positive for a specific microorganism. Identification of the presence of gram-negative LPS is problematic at best, as available assays such as the limulus lysate test are subject to a great deal of variation. Antibody detection tests for LPS, gram-positive, or fungal cell wall components have been examined experimentally and clinically, but most suffer from a lack of specificity when biologic fluids are tested and are not routinely available. During the time in which a diagnosis is being established, clinical deterioration frequently occurs and therapy must be instituted prior to the availability of confirmatory culture data, based on a high index of suspicion that bacteremia may be present.

Many studies have demonstrated a salutary effect when appropriate treatment is begun early in the course of disease. Evidence also exists that empiric antimicrobial therapy directed against gram-negative aerobes may have a salutary effect in febrile, neutropenic patients with hematologic malignancies. The majority of these studies indicate that two agents in combination may provide greater survival than use of a single agent, and this information has been extended to therapy in nonneutropenic individuals (a reasonable but perhaps unwarranted assumption). While systemic sepsis is classically identified with gram-negative bacteremia, other microbes including gram-positive bacteria, occasionally anaerobes, fungi, and viruses can initiate similar host responses. This further underscores the fact that systemic sepsis derives from the host response to microbial infection rather than the infecting microbe per se.

Catheter and Prosthetic Device Infections

Prosthetic catheter and device infections are common among surgical patients. Of these, infection of intravascular devices, particularly central venous catheters, is a significant cause of nosocomial infection and is associated with a significant increase in patient morbidity, hospital stay, and cost (17). Gram-positive organisms such as *S. epidermidis* and *Staphylococcus aureus* are the most frequent pathogens, although infection due to gram-negative bacteria and yeast can also occur, particularly in immunocompromised patients who have received antecedent antibiotic therapy. Microbial factors such as adherence to catheters with formation of biofilm serve to prevent antimicrobial agent penetration as well as the activity of host defenses. A recent meta-analysis reviewed studies examining techniques for preventing central venous catheter–related infections. These included the use of barrier precautions during catheter insertion, no routine replacement of central venous catheters, antiseptics in the hub of the central venous catheters, and use of antiseptic- or antibiotic-impregnated short-term central venous catheters (18). Heparin bonding of catheters and heparin administration also appear to reduce catheter colonization and catheter-related bacteremias.

Treatment consists of device removal and antimicrobial agents directed against the infecting organism. While this is a simple proposition with regard to percutaneously inserted catheters, many types of chronic indwelling catheters and devices require operative removal. Recent studies indicate, however, that a prolonged course of antibiotic therapy will serve to eradicate infection in some cases, although not in overtly bacteremic or fungemic patients. This latter approach may be indicated in patients who experience 1relatively few systemic manifestations due to the infection and who would be adversely affected by removal of the device (e.g., loss of access for intravenous nutrition). Removal should never be delayed, nor should antimicrobial agents be withheld in a patient who has obvious purulence in the region of the catheter and evidence of systemic sepsis.

Urinary Tract Infections

Urinary tract infections are often of concern, particularly in the hospitalized patient because they represent the most common cause of gram-negative bacterial sepsis. The presence of >10^5 CFU/mL in a patient without a Foley catheter in place is diagnostic of infection, while 10^2 to 10^3 CFU/mL is considered significant in a patient who has been catheterized for a short period of time. Prostatitis should also be considered in this setting in the male patient, and usually can be identified based on rectal exam findings, although transrectal ultrasonography may prove useful in selected cases. Because many antimicrobial agents concentrate to a high degree in the urine, it is often possible to quickly eradicate a urinary tract infection. Culture and sensitivity reports should be obtained, and follow-up urine specimens should be sent to the laboratory to ensure the successful treatment of such infections. Gram-negative bacilli are frequent pathogens involved in these infections, but gram-positive organisms such as enterococcus and even staphylococci are not uncommonly identified.

Nosocomial Pneumonia

Nosocomial pneumonia also represents a difficult diagnostic and therapeutic problem, frequently being suspected in the septic patient who requires prolonged intubation and mechanical ventilation. Chest radiographs often are difficult to interpret in these patients, particularly when some component of congestive cardiac failure, intravascular volume overload, or adult respiratory distress syndrome may be present. Although transtracheal aspiration can be performed in some cases, most patients require bronchoscopy in order to obtain appropriate samples for diagnosis. Bacterial, fungal, acid-fast bacterial, viral, and protozoan pathogens should all be considered so that Gram, potassium hydroxide, Ziehl-Neelsen, the Gomori methenamine-silver, Giemsa, and CMV rapid antigen stains, and appropriate cultures should all be performed. Gram-negative bacillary pathogens including *P. aeruginosa* represent commonly isolated organisms in this setting, but gram-positive bacteria and yeast such as *Candida* are also common pathogens.

Other Specific Site Infections

Parotitis can also occur in the surgical patient, particularly in elderly, dehydrated individuals. Therapy should be directed toward rehydration, enhancing salivation, en-suring that no mechanical obstruction of the duct of Stensen is present, obtaining stains and cultures, and administering antibiotics directed against *S. aureus,* which is the most common offending organism. In ICU patients who are often colonized with gram-negative bacteria, the possibility of gram-negative bacterial parotitis should be considered and appropriate empiric therapy used.

Sinusitis can occur in those patients who undergo prolonged nasal intubation. Although routine radiographs may identify this entity, CT scans are often required for diagnosis. Once significant sinus opacification is identified, aspiration and drainage should be performed to obtain material for stain and culture, but this procedure is also therapeutic.

Pseudomembranous colitis is caused by *Clostridium difficile* overgrowth and toxin secretion within the colon, and is associated with alterations in the colonic microflora that occur most frequently during antimicrobial agent administration but also may take place during debilitating illness. Treatment consists of oral metronidazole or vancomycin and it is prudent to discontinue or truncate the intravenous antimicrobial treatment course. Rarely, patients develop fulminant pseudomembranous colitis and become refractory to medical therapy, requiring subtotal colectomy to effect cure.

FUNGAL INFECTIONS

Infections due to fungal pathogens have become increasingly common within the last decade, frequently occurring in patients undergoing prolonged hospitalization in the surgical ICU and in immunocompromised individuals. *Candida* sp. *(C. albicans, C. tropicalis, C. parapsilosis, C. kruseii,* and *C. glabrata)* are the most frequent fungal pathogens isolated, and are common elements of the host microflora. Prophylaxis with oral antifungal agents is warranted, especially during periods of maximal immunosuppression in transplant patients, in patients with uncontrolled diabetes, or during antibacterial antimicrobial therapy.

In general, local, apparently noninvasive *Candida* infections involving the integument and mucous membranes are treated with oral decontamination and topical antifungal therapy using topical agents such as nystatin. *Candida* urinary tract infections can be treated with either an oral antifungal agent or topical amphotericin B as a continuous bladder irrigation. More difficult decisions concern the use of amphotericin B in patients who have fungal pathogens isolated from several sites. Several studies have demonstrated that those patients with three sites positive, or with peritoneal or blood cultures positive for *Candida,* exhibit higher survival rates when amphotericin B therapy is instituted early in the course of infection. Thus, an obvious site of infection such as pneumonitis with a positive fungal culture on bronchoscopy, positive fungal blood cultures, the presence of retinal changes compatible with *Candida* retinitis, or *Candida* present as a monomicrobial isolate within the peritoneal cavity, are generally considered indications for a limited course of amphotericin B therapy (300 to 500 mg). This issue, however, remains controversial, and the role of combination therapy with 5-fluorocytosine or therapy with azole class drugs (e.g., miconazole, ketoconazole, fluconazole, itraconazole) remains to be established.

Infection due to *Aspergillus niger, fumigatus, flavus,* and *terreus* and other less common species can involve the lung, upper respiratory tract, oropharyngeal region, ear, sinuses, skin and soft tissue, and central nervous system. Preexisting pulmonary cavities with subsequent invasion by fungi and formation of an aspergilloma or fungus ball has been the classic description of this disease, but patients more commonly develop a diffuse pneumonia with patchy infiltrates on chest roentgenograms. Central nervous system involvement can also occur as an extremely insidious but lethal process with the development of a fungal brain abscess. Therapy with systemic amphotericin B should be instituted based on even a presumptive diagnosis. Patients with severe infections probably should also receive 5-fluorocytosine and rifampin. Deep fungal infections such as these require long-term systemic amphotericin B therapy with a total dose between 2 and 3 g. The timing of surgical extirpative therapy has not been well defined. In general, however, fungal lesions that do not regress after 1 to 3 weeks of antifungal therapy may require excision following which antifungal therapy is continued. Occasionally, discrete areas of fungal infection are located adjacent to vital structures and should be considered for early excision.

Cryptococcus neoformans is an encapsulated fungus that causes pulmonary, central nervous system, and disseminated cutaneous infection in immunosuppressed patients. Pulmonary disease may be very insidious and produce mild fever, malaise, and a nonproductive cough. Central nervous system disease may present as malaise, fever, or headache either alone or in combination. Any patient with pulmonary cryptococcosis should undergo lumbar puncture. India ink preparations may demonstrate the organism in the cerebrospinal fluid (CSF), but tests for CSF cryptococcal antigen and serum antibody directed against the organism may also be helpful in establishing the diagnosis. Therapy consists of combined amphotericin B and 5-fluorocytosine. The total dose of amphotericin B that should be administered is between 1 and 1.5 g. Azole agents such as fluconazole also may be effective in the treatment of this disease.

Histoplasma capsulatum can cause both pulmonary and disseminated disease in transplant patients. It can produce skin lesions that resemble erythema nodosum, and recognition of these lesions may be a key to the diagnosis. *Coccidioides immitis* may produce disease in healthy or immunosuppressed individuals who inhale the highly infective arthrospores in an endemic region. Treatment of either disease consists of the long-term administration of systemic amphotericin B. Phycomycoses due to *Mucor* and *Rhizopus* spp. can produce locally destructive rhinocerebral or soft tissue infections that are very difficult to eradicate. Central nervous system involvement is common and often fatal. Treatment consists of local aggressive surgical excision and long-term systemic amphotericin B.

Treatment of fungal infection consists of a clinical assessment to determine the severity of disease (superficial versus deep) as well as any laboratory information concerning the sensitivity patterns of the organism. As a general rule, superficial infections and those due to a relatively low virulence organisms (*Candida* esophagitis or sepsis) can be treated with 350 to 500 mg of systemic amphotericin B. Increasing evidence suggests that azole agents such as fluconazole may be highly efficacious in this setting, although further study through well-designed clinical trials are indicated. More aggressive *Candida* infections and organisms with more invasive potential such as *Cryptococcus neoformans* require a more prolonged course of this agent and often the addition of a second agent such as 5-fluorocytosine. Infections due to *Aspergillus* and *Mucor* require very prolonged treatment (2 to 3 g total dose) with amphotericin B and 5-fluorocytosine, and often the addition of a third agent such as rifampin may be beneficial. The use of ketaconazole and more potent azole class agents such as fluconazole and itracona-

zole should also be considered in selected cases. These agents are less toxic, but have not been demonstrated to be of equivalent efficacy to amphotericin B. Lastly, patients receiving exogenous immunosuppressive agents should undergo a marked dosage reduction, and some agents should be discontinued until the infection is adequately controlled or is eradicated. Finally, prophylaxis or empiric antifungal therapy has been evaluated in high-risk patients such as those undergoing bone marrow transplants, those with cancer neutropenia, and patients following liver transplants. In general, treatment with fluconazole or low-dose amphotericin B reduces fungal colonization and invasive infection but has no clear effect on mortality (19).

VIRAL INFECTIONS

Formerly, outside of the field of transplantation, the practicing surgeon was not frequently called upon to treat viral disease. Solid organ transplant patients are prone to develop viral infections by virtue of exogenous immunosuppression. Although this section will emphasize the nature of viral infections in transplant patients, it is being increasingly recognized that viral infections exert a significant impact on other groups of patients that the practicing surgeon may be called upon to treat.

Herpes Virus Infections

The most common posttransplant viral infections are those caused by herpes viruses [CMV, herpes simplex virus (HSV), Epstein-Barr virus (EBV), and varicella-zoster virus (VZV)] and herpes virus type 6 (HV-6). All are most common during the periods of maximal host immunosuppression that occur immediately posttransplant and during treatment of allograft rejection. CMV is a common cause of fever after solid organ transplantation, and evidence of CMV infection occurs in approximately 30% of patients. Incidence factors associated with the occurrence of CMV infection include antirejection therapy, especially with antilymphocyte antibody preparations, advanced age, or receiving an organ from a cadaver. Those individuals who have no serologic evidence of CMV and who receive an organ from a CMV seropositive donor are at highest risk to develop primary CMV infection and disease. Reactivation CMV infection can occur, however, in those CMV seropositive recipients, and superinfection CMV disease (e.g., the occurrence of both primary and reactivation disease due to distinct strains of CMV) has also been reported.

Manifestations of CMV infection range from asymptomatic evidence of infection based on a rise in anti-CMV titers or culture evidence of viral shedding, mild to moderate disease in which systemic signs and symptoms such as fever, leukopenia, malaise, lethargy, and myalgias occur, to severe disease manifestations in which the above-mentioned signs and symptoms are accompanied by profound hypotension, pulmonary failure, hepatitis, pancreatitis, massive GI hemorrhage (upper or lower) due to viral-induced mucosal ulcerations, multiple system organ failure, and death. The most common presentation is that of a febrile, leukopenic patient with a cough, diffuse interstitial infiltrates on a chest radiograph, and hypoxia. Recently, a small subset of patients who develop solely GI manifestations has been recognized.

The diagnosis of CMV can be supported based on the above-mentioned symptoms and signs, and can be confirmed by several tests. Serologic evidence is usually based on evidence of a more than fourfold increase in anti-CMV antibody titer in two specimens obtained at separate times. Culture evidence or the demonstration of typical

CMV inclusion bodies from body fluid or a tissue specimen provides unequivocal evidence of CMV infection. More recently, fluorescein-labeled anti-CMV monoclonal antibodies have been employed in either direct or growth augmented (shell vial) tests to provide a rapid diagnosis in <24 hours. Direct observation of the stained specimen by fluorescence microscopy is performed to detect the presence of CMV. Direct nucleic acid blotting and PCR analysis have also been used to detect the presence of CMV in body fluid samples with high specificity and sensitivity, although these tests are not routinely available.

Previously, the diagnosis of CMV relied heavily on serologic data, while culture data were often not available for several days or several weeks. The above-mentioned tests allow the diagnosis of CMV to be made much more rapidly, and their development has coincided with the availability effective anti-CMV therapy with agents such as ganciclovir. Thus the surgical clinician is able to both diagnose and treat CMV in a very effective fashion.

Although CMV disease continues to be associated with decreased patient and allograft survival, several studies indicate that a reduction in disease incidence is possible by the use of either prophylactic administration of ganciclovir (GCV), acyclovir (ACV), or anti-CMV immune globulin preparations or various combinations. Treatment of CMV disease with GCV, a drug that possesses substantially more in vitro activity against CMV than ACV, is efficacious, and preliminary data indicate that it may be possible to treat patients with mild CMV disease with GCV and concurrently treat rejection as well. Foscarnet is a another drug with considerable activity against CMV that has also been demonstrated to be efficacious in a limited number of patients, although this agent possesses both neuro- and nephrotoxicity.

HSV infection causes painful oropharyngeal ulcerations in most cases, although sporadic cases of disseminated disease (meningoencephalitis, hepatitis, pneumonitis) have been reported. Although HSV alone does not appear to adversely affect patient or allograft survival, combined HSV and CMV infection exerts a deleterious effect on these parameters over and above the effect of CMV alone. EBV causes an occasional case of a mononucleosis-type syndrome, but has also been clearly implicated in the pathogenesis of posttransplant lymphomas. VZV infection can present as disseminated and occasionally life-threatening infection in the nonimmune transplant patient, or as painful herpes zoster in patients who have previously developed chicken pox. HV-6 causes malaise, fever, and lethargy. Primary HSV, EBV, and VZV infections are effectively treated with acyclovir. Evidence of initial life-threatening disease or of rapid disease progression, mandate a concurrent reduction in immunosuppression, intravenous acyclovir, and hospitalization. VZV hyperimmune globulin may also provide benefit as prophylaxis for VZV seronegative patients with clear-cut VZV exposure, or for treatment of severe cases in conjunction with acyclovir, although little data supports this latter recommendation.

Acquired Immunodeficiency Syndrome (AIDS)

A great deal of information has accumulated within the last several years with regard to the etiology and pathogenesis of AIDS. This syndrome is caused by a human retrovirus (HIV-1) that infects T lymphocytes and causes severe immunosuppression. HIV is a member of a family of lymphotrophic viruses, many of which appear to primarily affect other mammalian hosts such as felines or primates. Infection is acquired via parenteral or sexual transmissions. Intravenous drug abuse, homosexuality, and prostitution all represent high-risk types of behavior that predispose to HIV infection. Individuals who live or travel in sub-Saharan Africa where the virus is endemic also represent a potential high-risk group.

HIV detection typically consists of initial ELISA screening. Although sensitive, the 1% to 3% false-positive rate of this test mandates that all positive ELISA individuals be retested by the sensitive and specific Western immunotransblot analysis in which viral capsid antigens are first subjected to electrophoresis followed by immunoelectrophoretic transblotting onto nitrocellulose, and antibody directed against specific antigens can be detected. In particular, the HIV p24 antigen appears to be a sensitive indicator of HIV infection. Current evidence indicates that initial infection with HIV is followed by a latent period that may last several months, following which viremia can be detected by culture data, after which time evidence of anti-HIV antibody is detectable.

Several concerns over HIV disease transmission have arisen with regard to surgical patients. First, transfusion-associated HIV transmission has been documented and this has increased enthusiasm for limiting blood transfusions through the use of cell salvage and autotransfusion devices, as well as autodonation of blood prior to elective operative procedures. Screening of all blood products prior to transfusion and exclusion of blood donors based on a history of high-risk activities has reduced the probability of transfusion-associated AIDS to a very low level. It is possible, however, to transfuse HIV-infected blood or blood products that are ELISA negative, because an occasional individual may donate prior to developing an anti-HIV antibody response. Second, surgeons are concerned about the risk to themselves and other health care workers who are exposed to blood or body fluids from HIV-infected patients. Several cases of HIV transmission due to accidental sticks with hollow-core needles used in patients with AIDS have been reported. These usually involved direct inoculation of several milliliters of blood deep into the soft tissues, rather than a needle-stick exposure with a solid needle, such as that which might occur during suturing. Overall, HIV transmission appears to require a larger inoculum than hepatitis B virus. Third, the concern over possible transmission of HIV from an HIV-infected surgeon to a patient has arisen. For this reason, the highly controversial issues of HIV screening of both patients and surgeons has been the subject of intense discussion.

Many institutions have employed universal blood and body substance precautions that entail treating all invasive procedures as having the potential to transmit disease such as HIV and hepatitis. Arguments in favor of such a policy consist of the above-mentioned fact that HIV-infected patients may not be detected by routine antibody tests even though they are infective, and that stringent precautions to prevent disease transmission to health care workers should be applied to each and every case. Some surgeons, however, believe that all patients should undergo preoperative HIV testing so that additional measures—only one surgeon operating at a time with minimal assistance, use of Kevlar gloves, etc.—could be undertaken, and that the benefits of such a policy may outweigh the potential risk of being unable to maintain the anonymity of a patient identified as being infected with HIV or the occasional initial labeling of a patient as being HIV test positive who subsequently is found to be negative. The issue of HIV transmission from surgeon to patient is a difficult one, and has not been unequivocally documented. Except when performing procedures where the surgeon's blood intermingles with the patient's tissues due to a deep cut or needle stick, transmission seems a remote possibility and the examples (orthopedic procedures, vaginal hysterectomy) of procedures during which this might occur do not really seem concordant with the manner in which these procedures can be performed in order to minimize this risk. These highly controversial issues are being deliberated, but are unlikely to be resolved in the immediate future.

The CDC has provided guidelines regarding needle-stick exposure to health care workers as they relate to HIV. Needle sticks should be reported to occupational health services at the institution and consideration given to the risk of HIV exposure. If the source is known HIV positive or of unknown HIV status, the health care worker should be followed clinically and serologically for 6 months. The initial serology should be performed soon after the exposure, and if the worker is seronegative, it should be repeated at 6 weeks, 12 weeks, and 6 months. The value of prophylactic azidothymidine (AZT) use remains undetermined. This agent shows efficacy in animal models as prophylaxis when started early after exposure, is effective in patients with established disease, and does not induce significant short-term toxicity (nausea, vomiting). However, the low incidence of seroconversion following parenteral exposure (overall 0.4%) has made it virtually impossible to adequately test its effectiveness as a prophylactic agent. Therefore, no specific recommendations exist regarding its use. In deciding, one should consider the risk of transmission (e.g., needle stick versus accidental injection of blood), the interval between exposure and initiation of AZT, and finally the tolerance for side effects.

Individuals who become infected with HIV are prone to a variety of infections and different types of malignancy. Currently, a spectrum exists in which patients progress from asymptomatic infection, to development of the AIDS-related complex (ARC) of diseases, to AIDS itself. Common infections occurring in AIDS patients are *Pneumocystis carinii* pneumonia, CMV pneumonitis, gastroenteritis, hepatitis, meningitis due to *Cryptococcus neoformans,* and pneumonia and disseminated infection due to atypical mycobacteria such as *Mycobacterium avium-intracellulare, M. kansasii,* and *M. chelonei,* as well as gastrointestinal infections due to *Cryptosporidium* and *Campylobacter jejuni.* Predisposition to these infections is due in large part to the lymphotrophic nature of HIV, that markedly reduces the number of T-helper cells as well as the absolute number of T cells.

Treatment of AIDS consists of aggressive antiinfective therapy, once a specific infection occurs, and use of AZT. AZT appears to prolong survival when administered early on in the course of disease and is now considered routine therapy. It is by no means clear, however, that it is possible to eradicate this type of infection. Identification of CD3 antigen as the target molecule on the human T cell for HIV has led to proposals for drugs that will mimic this receptor and prevent binding. This approach holds much promise, but prevention of disease transmission by education and convincing individuals in high-risk groups to use condoms during sexual intercourse and to avoid sharing of needles may have the greatest impact on reducing the incidence of AIDS.

HEPATITIS VIRUSES

Seven distinct hepatitis viruses have been identified: hepatitis A, B, C (formerly non-A, non-B), D (delta), E, F, and G (20). Hepatitis A is usually spread through fecal-oral routes and only occasionally comes to the attention of the surgeon. It is characterized by acute infection rather than the development of chronic liver disease. Hepatitis B is transmitted via the parenteral route in most cases, although oral and sexual transmission has been described. Infection results in symptomatic disease characterized by

jaundice, fever, malaise, and a rise in serum transaminases in 25% of patients. The other 75% remain asymptomatic or experience mild flu-like symptoms during the acute phase of the infection; elevation of IgM antibody directed against surface and subsequently core antigens of the hepatitis B viral particle occurs, and this is followed by the development of IgG antibody production.

Acute infection usually resolves without further sequelae, although antibody titers against surface and core antigens remain elevated. Rarely, acute hepatitis may progress to fulminant hepatic failure, coma, and death. Approximately 5% of patients go on to develop evidence of chronic active or chronic persistent hepatitis. These patients most frequently have few or no symptoms but have mildly abnormal liver function tests with evidence of chronic antigenemia. Over time, this disease may evolve into end-stage liver failure with cirrhosis and its sequelae, and in many patients hepatocellular carcinoma may develop. High-risk groups of patients (e.g., hemodialysis, transplant, hemophiliacs) and health care workers (surgeons, dentists, hemodialysis unit personnel) should receive three vaccinations of the recombinant-DNA hepatitis B vaccine if no previous exposure has been documented. In general, about 95% of individuals will seroconvert by 1 month after the three-dose schedule. Failure to do so mandates a second series of vaccinations. Vaccination is not recommended in individuals who possess anti–hepatitis B antibody. Examination of postvaccination antibody titers indicates that hemodialysis patients do not invariably respond to the initial vaccination series, and this group may require subsequent antibody level determination and booster vaccinations. Administration of antihepatitis B immunoglobulin and subsequent vaccination should occur in nonimmune individuals after exposure to hepatitis B virus.

Hepatitis B is a major risk to health care personnel, with a much higher transmission rate than that observed following a needle-stick exposure to HIV-1. In general, surgeons should be aware of their antibody status, since exposure is not uncommon and the status of patients is not uniformly known. If exposed, those with adequate titers require no further therapy. Those whose titers are absent or low after exposure should receive hepatitis B immunoglobulin and a booster vaccination. Finally, if unvaccinated, the individual should receive the immunoglobulin plus the full three-dose vaccination schedule.

Hepatitis C can cause acute elevations in hepatic enzyme and chronic antigenemia much in the same way as occurs with hepatitis B. Transmission occurs via blood products, and this virus is probably responsible for the majority of transfusion-related hepatitis. Like hepatitis B, significant clinical symptoms occur in only about 30% of patients with acute infection. Identification is currently possible via an ELISA-based technique as well as more sophisticated recombinant immunoblot assays and PCR-based assays. If exposure occurs, antibody titers and PCR-based detection can be performed at baseline and 6 weeks later. Transmission is a function of the mode of injury as well as the status of the patient. The combination of IFN-α plus the antiviral drug ribavirin appears to eradicate the virus in a significant proportion of patients. There is no recommended prophylaxis against infection following exposure to hepatitis C. In individuals developing chronic hepatitis C, treatment with combination IFN plus ribavirin appears to be superior to IFN monotherapy in inducing a sustained virologic response. Hepatitis D is transmitted parenterally. It cannot cause disease alone, but acts as a secondary virus to hepatitis B. The disease caused by both together is more severe than that caused by hepatitis B alone. Immunization against hepatitis B serves to eliminate risk of infection with hepatitis D. Hepatitis E is transmitted by fecal-oral spread and is similar to hepatitis A in terms of symptoms and outcome. The diagnosis is frequently made when patients with symptoms of hepatitis A are seronegative, stimulating investigation for other viral causes. As for hepatitis A, the disease is rarely fatal and is treated with supportive management. The existence of hepatitis G has only recently been reported. At present, little is known about the long-term outcome and no therapy is recommended.

PROTOZOAN AND PARASITIC PATHOGENS

The surgeon will occasionally treat patients with disease due to either protozoan or parasitic organisms, and this is largely dependent upon geographic location because these types of infections are more common in semitropical and tropical habitats. Thus, occasional cases of echinococcal liver disease may require operation, and rare cases of bowel obstruction with or without free peritoneal perforation and widespread dissemination due to various helminths or biliary tract disease due to the oriental liver fluke *Clonorchis sinensis* will be seen. Amebic liver abscesses can be managed medically with metronidazole and do not require percutaneous or operative drainage, unless secondarily infected. Both solid organ transplant and AIDS patients can develop unusual infections due to some more common protozoan pathogens such as *Pneumocystis carinii* and *Toxoplasma gondii.*

P. carinii causes cough, tachypnea, and mild fever, and bilateral diffuse alveolar infiltrates and interstitial pneumonia are seen on the chest roentgenogram. The diagnosis must be rapidly established via bronchoscopy and in some cases open lung biopsy due to the high attendant mortality of untreated disease. Treatment consists of parenteral trimethoprim-sulfamethoxazole, trimethoprim-dapsone, or pentamidine even if the diagnosis is presumptive. This disease rarely occurs in patients receiving trimethoprim-sulfamethoxazole prophylaxis. *T. gondii* can cause a mononucleosis syndrome in healthy patients, while in the immunosuppressed patient necrotizing encephalitis, myocarditis, pneumonitis, and death can occur. *Toxoplasma*-naive solid organ transplant patients are more prone to develop infection if they receive an organ from a donor with evidence of previous infection due to this agent, and this disease is more common in cardiac allograft recipients. Treatment consists of administration of pyrimethamine and sulfadiazine.

NEW TREATMENT MODALITIES

Although the concept of host defense modulation is by no means new, increasing understanding of the host response has led to the accumulation of significant amounts of new information. It must be recognized, however, that the imperfect level of our understanding of the pathophysiology of infection makes the prediction of the ultimate ramifications of even precisely targeted current intervention difficult. Thus, a large number of antiinflammatory and antiinfective agents have been tested experimentally and clinically, with few concrete changes in clinical practice. For instance, although many experimental studies have provided evidence that administration of corticosteroids may reduce septic lethality, in most cases the effect is maximized by steroid treatment prior to the septic insult. Two clinical trials examining the effect of corticosteroid administration during septic shock reached the conclusion that administration of these agents did not reduce septic lethality and may adversely influence outcome in some patients. However, a recent trial that evaluated low-dose corticosteroid therapy in patients according to adrenocortical re-

sponsiveness suggested a clinical advantage to using steroids in individuals with low responsiveness to cosyntropin testing, a group of patients previously shown to have poor outcome from sepsis. These findings suggest that identification of subgroups of patients who may benefit from a given therapy may permit tailoring of therapy that thus enhances its effectiveness.

Endogenous opioids (e.g., beta-endorphin) are released into the cerebral ventricles and systemic circulation in conjunction with endogenous adrenocorticotropic hormone (ACTH), which promotes corticosteroid secretion during various types of stress and shock including LPS administration. Many studies have demonstrated the salutary effects of opioid antagonist administration to animals subjected to shock due to a variety of causes including sepsis. Mortality, however, has not been affected routinely when opioid antagonists are administered without other agents. Those clinical studies performed to date have not uniformly indicated a successful treatment of septic shock. Other opioid antagonists such as thyrotropin-releasing hormone may prove to be more efficacious. Fibronectin has been administered to septic patients in an effort to enhance bacterial clearance, bacteriolysis, and host leukocyte phagocytosis. Despite several clinical trials, administration of cryoprecipitate, which contains high levels of fibronectin, has not been clearly demonstrated to be efficacious.

Since activation of the coagulation cascade occurs during sepsis and the development of microvascular thrombosis contributes to organ ischemia and dysfunction, anticoagulant strategies in the management of sepsis have been investigated in both animal models and in humans. Neutralization of tissue factor with antibodies or with tissue factor pathway inhibitor have demonstrated efficacy in animals and are under study in humans. Similarly, activated protein C (APC) appears promising in this setting and the data suggest its potential efficacy in humans.

Gut Decontamination

The composition of the gut microflora is altered during hospitalization, antimicrobial agent administration, and various disease states. In most cases, the number of facultative aerobic isolates increases throughout the intestine, the number of anaerobic forms decreases, and thus the ability of anaerobic colonization resistance to prevent microbial adherence and invasion is presumably diminished. In addition to providing the initial inoculum when overt intestinal perforation occurs, the altered upper GI microflora has been implicated in the development of nosocomial pneumonia, and the lower GI microflora is implicated in the process of bacterial translocation.

Prolonged intubation for the purpose of mechanical ventilation is associated with initial or oropharyngeal, and subsequent gastric, colonization with facultative gram-negative aerobic organisms such as *E. coli, P. aeruginosa,* and *Klebsiella pneumoniae.* This phenomenon has also been associated with gram-negative respiratory infections due to the identical organisms in a given patient. These same organisms may colonize and proliferate in the distal GI tract despite so-called colonization resistance due to anaerobic organisms.

Bacterial translocation is a process in which bacteria are able to transgress the gut barrier, and are engulfed by local macrophages that reside within mesenteric lymph nodes. Portal and systemic bacteremia and endotoxemia occur in some cases, depending on the severity of the insult. This process has been primarily documented in experimental models via (a) so-called monoassociation of gnotobiotic or conventional antibiotic gut decontaminated animals with specific types of bacteria, or (b) subjecting conventional animals to a variety of insults (e.g., endotoxemia, thermal injury, intestinal ischemia). Although experimental and some clinical evidence exists to support the role of bacterial translocation during sepsis, exact cause and effect has not been clearly established. Of critical importance may be the influence of translocating bacteria and LPS on hepatic metabolism, as hepatic macrophages (Kupffer cells) may be stimulated to produce cytokines such as TNF or IL-1 that act at the local and systemic levels to produce adverse effects on the host.

To reduce the quantity of aerobic gram-negative bacillary organisms present within the intestinal tract, several groups have studied the impact of selective gut decontamination. This technique involves the use of orally administered antimicrobial agents that achieve high intraluminal level directed against gram-negative aerobes and yeast, leaving the host anaerobic intestinal microflora relatively undisrupted. In ICU patients, this technique, combined with a short course of intravenous cephalosporin prophylaxis, appears to be effective in preventing nosocomial infections, particularly pneumonia. One meta-analysis suggests its efficacy in surgical patients in the ICU setting (21). However, at best, the impact on overall mortality is relatively small and thus, in the context of its potential for promoting microbial resistance and its difficulty of administration, the technique has not been embraced with much enthusiasm in North American centers.

LPS Neutralization and Other Sepsis Therapies

Because LPS may be responsible for toxicity both directly and through host mediator systems, the ability of various agents to bind to against this portion of the gram-negative bacterial outer membrane to reduce mortality has been intensively examined. PolymyxinB, a polypeptide antibiotic, binds stoichiometrically to the lipid A region of LPS, but is extremely toxic when administered systemically. Administration of this drug may reduce lethality during experimental gram-negative bacteremia or endotoxemia, but toxicity has largely precluded clinical utility to date. Recent advances in its use including incorporation into extracorporeal hemofiltration devices as well as coupling to dextran to lessen systemic toxicity may make this approach more feasible in the future.

Gram-negative bacterial infection or injection of LPS in experimental models results in the development of antibody primarily directed against O antigen, while very little antibody directed against the core/lipid A region of LPS is produced. Anti-O antigen antibody is serotype specific, and is not cross-reactive. This same phenomenon appears to occur clinically. Because of the wide range of gram-negative bacterial serotypes that cause clinical infection, an intensive effort has been directed toward the identification of cross-reactive components of LPS against which antibody can be directed. This has stimulated the development of a series of so-called rough mutants of both *Salmonella minnesota* and *E. coli* 0111:B4, where the varying portions of the core regions of the LPS are expressed without O antigen. The deep core/lipid A region of LPS may represent a suitable immunogen for the development of cross-reactive antibodies because it is biochemically and immunologically highly conserved among a wide variety of gram-negative microorganisms and it also represents the toxic moiety of LPS. Rough mutants have also been defined for other gram-negative microorganisms including other types of *E. coli*, *Salmonella typhimurium*, and *P. aeruginosa*.

All of the initial studies performed in this field used polyclonal antibody derived from animal or human sources and indicated that type-specific (anti-O antigen) antibody could provide potent non–cross-reactive protection during experimental gram-negative bacterial sepsis. These initial studies were hampered by the fact that monospecific antibody reagents were not available, and thus nonspecific effects could not be excluded. Subsequent studies using monoclonal antibodies have indicated that anti-LPS antibody can provide protection against either an LPS or a bacterial challenge. While some authors have stated that only IgM antibodies will enhance survival, others have provided evidence demonstrating that anti-LPS antibodies of similar but not identical specificity of either IgG or IgM classes provided similar protective capacity. Several groups have developed monoclonal antibodies directed against various portions of the core region of LPS as well as lipid A, and have demonstrated that administration of these cross-reactive anti-core LPS reagents provides protective capacity during experimental endotoxemia and gram-negative bacteremia or peritonitis. In general, however, although anti-core LPS/lipid A monoclonal antibodies are more cross-reactive in vitro, these antibodies provide less potent protective capacity in vivo than anti-O antigen reagents.

That the presence of an anti-core LPS antibody titer occurs naturally and may be protective during clinical gram-negative bacterial infection has been demonstrated in several retrospective clinical studies. In addition, immunization of human volunteers with rough mutant organisms produces an antibody titer, and this serum or plasma is protective in experimental models of sepsis. Using polyclonal anti–*E. coli* J5 human antibody preparations, several authors have demonstrated a reduction in mortality when antiserum was administered to septic patients, although one group could not demonstrate protection when this antiserum was administered as single-dose prophylaxis to neutropenic patients to prevent septic complications. Several recent clinical trials have been performed using anti-core LPS/lipid A monoclonal antibody preparations. Although preliminary evidence suggested that a reduction in lethality could be observed using either HA-1A or E5 anti-lipid A IgM monoclonal antibody, subsequent large multicenter, randomized trials have failed to demonstrate a beneficial effect. Several explanations have been advanced to explain this lack of efficacy: (a) The anti-LPS activity of the reagents tested was low. (b) The patient selection process led to enrollment of patients who had sepsis related to microbes other than gram-negative bacteria. (c) There was significant heterogeneity among patients enrolled in the study, therefore potentially masking a beneficial effect on a specific subgroup. Several other trials using other anti-LPS therapies are in various stages of completion including polymyxin-dextran preparations as well as bactericidal permeability increasing protein, an endogenous leukocyte granular protein with anti-LPS activity.

As an alternative to anti-LPS therapy, other investigators have evaluated strategies aimed at neutralizing more downstream mediator molecules. Trials are also under way to determine the effect of anti-TNF antibody preparations during gram-negative bacterial sepsis, and the concept of combining anti-LPS and anti-TNF antibody preparations may prove fruitful.

Immunostimulants

Although a large number of compounds have been studied experimentally, few have provided clinical efficacy in reducing the rate or severity of infection. Several compounds derived from mycobacterial or yeast cell wall extracts (muramyl dipeptide, zymosan, and glucan) probably act as direct macrophage stimulants, thereby directly enhancing the state of activation of host defenses. Levamisole, an antihelminthic agent, appears to directly stimulate PMNs, and has been shown to possess limited clinical efficacy in a single trial. More recently, thymopentin and several other synthetic compounds have undergone clinical testing. Thymopentin is a peptide that contains the active site of thymopoetin, a thymic hormone that acts to stimulate T-lymphocyte activity. Preliminary trials indicate that this agent ameliorates the host septic response after major operations and trauma, but conclusive evidence of a concurrent reduction in infection-related mortality is not yet available.

REFERENCES

1. Dunn DL. Autochthonous microflora of the gastrointestinal tract. *Perspect Colon Rectal Surg* 1990;2:105.
2. Dunn DL, Meakins JL. Humoral immunity to infection and the complement system. In: Howard RJ, Simmons RL, eds. *Surgical infectious diseases.* Norwalk, CT: Appleton & Lange, 1988:175.
3. Durum SK, Oppenheim JJ. Macrophage-derived mediators: interleukin-1, tumor necrosis factor, interleukin-6, interferon, and related cytokines. In: Paul WE, ed. *Fundamental immunology,* 2nd ed. New York: Raven Press, 1989:639.
4. Dunn DL. The role of infection and use of antimicrobial agents during multiple system organ failure. In: Deitch EA, ed. *Multiple organ failure: pathophysiology and basic concepts of therapy.* New York: Thieme Medical, 1990:150.
5. Burke JF. Preventing bacterial infection by coordinating antibiotic and host activity: a time dependent activity. *South Med J* 1977;1:24.
6. Bartlett JG, Condon RE, Gorbach, et al. Veterans Administration cooperative study on bowel preparation for elective colorectal operations: impact of oral antibiotic regimen on colonic flora, wound irrigation cultures, and bacteriology of septic complications. *Ann Surg* 1978;188:249.
7. Mangram AJ, Horan TC, Pearson ML, et al. The Hospital Infection Control Practices Advisory Committee. Guidelines for Prevention of Surgical Site Infection, 1999. *Infect Control Hosp Epidemiol* 1999;20:247.
8. Dunn DL, Barke RA, Knight NB, et al. The role of resident macrophages, peripheral neutrophils, and translymphatic absorption in bacterial clearance from the peritoneal cavity. *Infect Immun* 1985;49:257.
9. Dunn DL, Simmons RL. The role of anaerobic bacteria in intraabdominal infections. *Rev Infect Dis* 1984;6:S139.
10. Walsh RM, Popovich MJ, Hoadley J. Bedside diagnostic laparoscopy and peritoneal lavage in the intensive care unit. *Surg Endosc* 1998;12:1405.
11. Bohnen JM, Solomkin JS, Dellinger EP, et al. Guidelines for clinical care: anti-infective agents for intra-abdominal infection—a Surgical Infection Society policy statement. *Arch Surg* 1992;127:83.
12. Eggimann P, Francioli P, Bille J, et al. Fluconazole prophylaxis prevents intra-abdominal candidiasis in high-risk surgical patients. *Crit Care Med* 1999;27:1066.
13. Rotstein OD, Pruett TL, Simmons RL. Microbiologic features and treatment of persistent peritonitis in patients in the intensive care unit. *Can J Surg* 1986;29:247.
14. Bilton BD, Zibari GB, McMillan RW, et al. Aggressive surgical management of necrotizing fasciitis serves to decrease mortality: a retrospective study. *Am Surg* 1998;64:397.
15. Korhonen K, Kuttila K, Niinikoski J. Tissue gas tensions in patients with necrotising fasciitis and healthy controls during treatment with hyperbaric oxygen: a clinical study. *Eur J Surg* 2000;166:530.
16. Marshall JC, Cook DJ, Christou NV, et al. Multiple organ dysfunction score: a reliable descriptor of a complex clinical outcome. *Crit Care Med* 1995;23:1638.
17. Rello J, Ochagavia A, Sabanes E, et al. Evaluation of outcome of intravenous catheter-related infections in critically ill patients. *Am J Respir Crit Care Med* 2000;162:1027.
18. Mermel LA. Prevention of intravascular catheter-related infections. *Ann Intern Med* 2000;132:391.
19. Gotzsche PC, Johansen HK. Meta-analysis of prophylactic or empirical antifungal treatment versus placebo or no treatment in patients with cancer complicated by neutropenia. *BMJ* 1997;314:1238.
20. Fry DE. The ABCs of hepatitis. *Advances in surgery,* vol 33. St. Louis: Mosby, 1999:413–437.
21. Nathens AB, Marshall JC. Selective decontamination of the digestive tract in surgical patients: a systematic review of the evidence. *Arch Surg* 1999;134:170.

SURGERY: SCIENTIFIC PRINCIPLES AND PRACTICE, Third Edition, edited by Lazar J. Greenfield, Michael W. Mulholland, Keith T. Oldham, Gerald B. Zelenock, and Keith D. Lillemoe. Lippincott Williams & Wilkins Publishers, Philadelphia, © 2001.

CHAPTER 8

SHOCK

TIMOTHY G. BUCHMAN AND ERIC JACOBSOHN

Shock remains one of the surgeon's most formidable foes. Sixty years after publication of Alfred Blalock's classic textbook, *Principles of Surgical Care: Shock and Other Problems* (1), the diagnosis of shock and the management of shock resuscitation continue to challenge the clinician and investigator. The objective of this chapter is to provide the reader with practical methods for recognizing and resuscitating patients who are in shock. Scientific information is included where helpful to explain or reinforce clinical practice, but this chapter does not attempt a comprehensive review of molecular and cellular events in shock.

As Maier pointed out in the previous edition of this text (2), shock is less a diagnosis than it is a syndrome. Descriptions of the shock syndrome aggregate pathogenesis, manifestation, and physiologic responses in ways that facilitate clinical recognition but conveniently obscure causal relationships. Despite decades of research, the causes of shock (or, more important, the causes of irreversibility and the sequelae of shock) remain enigmatic. The problem with current descriptions, many of which focus on a mismatch between metabolic supply and demand and its consequences, is that they do not capture either the self-sustaining nature of shock or the importance of timeliness in recognition and management. Whereas most authors cite these latter characteristics as "features" of shock and of shock therapy, the self-sustaining characteristic and the effectiveness of early intervention may well be fundamental to the physiologic derangement and rescue, respectively (3).

Because "shock" is commonly described in terms of metabolic shortfall (metabolic demand exceeding supply of essential nutrients), "not shock" or the basal physiologic state must also be examined through the lens of energetics. All life forms, from the prokaryotes to complex mammals, share three imperatives: to extract energy from the environment to hold entropy at bay; to adapt to (the variable) external environment to maintain constant the internal environment; and to replicate. We focus first on energy extraction.

Organisms and their constituent cells are thermodynamically open systems. Ingested carbohydrate, fat, and protein are biochemically degraded into primitive units. The currency of biochemical energy, high-energy phosphates (including adenosine triphosphate, guanosine triphosphate, creatine phosphate, and others), can be generated directly from the primitives or, alternatively, the primitives can be stored. Most humans have several months' worth of stored fat and a day's worth of stored carbohydrate (hepatic and muscle glycogen). There is no storage form of protein: all known proteins are structural or catalytic. The primitives—glucose and fatty acids—generate high-energy phosphates through two biochemical pathways, one that requires molecular oxygen (oxidative phosphorylation) and one that does not (anaerobic glycolysis). The yield of high-energy phosphates through the oxidative pathway is sufficient to sustain life, whereas the yield through the anaerobic pathway is not. Proof of this distinction is clinical: carbon monoxide poisoning (which prevents oxygen transport on hemoglobin) and cyanide poisoning (which uncouples oxidative phosphorylation) are lethal. These represent two unusual causes of shock that the surgeon occasionally encounters.

There is no storage form of oxygen. Arterial hemoglobin is normally 95% to 98% saturated with oxygen, whereas mixed venous blood is normally 70% to 75% saturated, suggesting that approximately one fourth of the available oxygen is removed during each circuit through vital organs and tissues. Human blood volume normally circulates approximately once each minute. These facts suggest that even if every oxygen molecule could be unloaded from hemoglobin to cells, unreplenished oxygen delivery will be exhausted in approximately 4 minutes. This is important for three reasons. It points to oxygen as the critical nutrient; it points to the importance of efficient resuscitation; and it points to restoration of oxygen delivery as the imperative in resuscitation from shock.

If resuscitation is untimely or incomplete, the consequences are predictable and often lethal. Cells initially switch from oxidative phosphorylation to the more anaerobic metabolic pathways. End products of anaerobic metabolism, notably lactic acid, accumulate. More important, the electrochemical gradients across cytoplasmic and subcellular membranes that are normally maintained by a constant supply of high-energy phosphates start failing. As gradients fail, water and salt on either side equilibrate, disrupting the three-dimensional organization of proteins. Disrupted proteins cannot be repaired because the repair mechanisms require high-energy phosphates. Disrupted proteins cannot be recycled because the recycling mechanisms require high-energy phosphates. Beyond a salvage threshold of failed gradients and disrupted proteins, the affected cell becomes necrotic. Unfortunately, clean-up of necrotic tissue also requires energy. The result is a collective, accelerating spiral of deteriorating function of cells, tissues, and organs. Decades of research offer no better therapy than the prompt restoration of oxygen delivery.

The adequacy of oxygen delivery is properly local, but oxygen delivery itself can be estimated from global measures. Thus, oxygen delivery is the geometric product of arterial oxygen saturation, hemoglobin concentration, stroke volume, and heart rate. The product of stroke volume and heart rate is cardiac output, or, equivalently, the amount of venous blood returning to the heart. The focus of shock resuscitation is the optimization of these parameters, and it is therefore worthwhile restating the definition of oxygen delivery in the form of a relation:

$$\dot{D}O_2 \propto S_aO_2 \times [Hgb] \times heart\ rate \times stroke\ volume$$

However, optimization of these four parameters is only the second most important clinical imperative.

The most important task in shock intervention is early recognition of the shock syndrome. The syndrome is composed not only of the metabolic derangements directly attributable to inadequate perfusion but also of the reflex responses teleologically aimed at mitigating the inadequate perfusion. *The reflex responses are clinically appreciable far earlier than the derangements themselves.* These reflex responses are mediated by the neuroendocrine system, which secretes a series of hormones to sustain delivery of nutrients to cells and promote diffusion and transport of nutrients into cells.

Several classes of hormones are released during the initial response to shock, the catecholamines, the renin–angiotensin–aldosterone axis, as well as antidiuretic hormone. The catecholamines, epinephrine and norepinephrine, are full agonists for both α-adrenergic (vasoconstrictor) and β₁-adrenergic (increased heart rate, increased heart contractility, increased heart conduction velocity) receptors. (Each is a partial agonist for β₂-adrenergic receptors, which mediate vasodilatation). The catecholamines cause three early events. First, the heart rate accelerates, second, peripheral arterial beds and splanchnic beds empty into the systemic circulation, and third, potassium is shifted to intracellular compartments. These events are appreciated as tachycardia; as delayed capillary refill and a slight rise in diastolic blood pressure; and as mild hypokalemia. Catecholamine secretion is prominent in all forms of shock and the effects of catecholamines are nearly always the first physical signs of shock. The observed response to catecholamines is less effective when the specific cause of shock renders target cells refractory to catecholamines, namely, septic shock. The response is also less effective when catecholamine responsiveness has been altered with drugs such as β-adrenergic blockers.

Renin is released from the kidneys in response to hypovolemia, and the release is potentiated by epinephrine. The release catalyzes the conversion of angiotensinogen to the angiotensins. The sudden rise in circulating angiotensins contributes substantially to overall splanchnic vasoconstriction. Such constriction can mobilize up to 30% of the total blood volume, compensating for but also masking the loss of blood from the systemic circulation. The combination of catecholamines, renin, and antidiuretic hormone released early in response to shock causes the kidneys to retain water and sodium and decreases splanchnic perfusion. Urine output is therefore modulated relatively early in the response to shock.

Other hormones secreted somewhat later in response to shock include glucagon, cortisol, and growth hormone. Collectively, they alter physiology to create a state similar to diabetes, including mild hyperglycemia and insulin resistance. Both muscle protein and fat stores are mobilized during recovery from shock to augment plasma glucose through gluconeogenesis. Except to correct demonstrable deficiencies, administration of these hormones has not been shown to improve outcome from shock.

THE PATHWAYS TO SHOCK

Once shock is recognized, the surgeon must simultaneously identify and reverse the underlying cause while performing resuscitation. The former is more difficult than the latter. It is helpful to remember that there are three fundamental pathways to shock. These pathways reflect problems with the "three P's": the perfusate (intravascular volume); the pump [problems with the heart or getting blood into the heart (obstruction)]; and the pipes (distributive problems that allow blood to pool into the periphery and to pass by starving tissues without unloading nutrients). This classification is simple enough to commit to memory and can guide decision making for the first several minutes of resuscitation. However, a more detailed classification (Table 8.1) is helpful to refine therapy.

The surgeon most commonly encounters shock through the perfusate pathway. The associated clinical syndromes are hypovolemic shock due to dehydration and hemorrhagic shock due to acute loss of blood volume. Mild perfusate loss

Table 8.1. **A CLASSIFICATION OF SHOCK**

Type	Etiology	Specific causes
1. Hypovolemic shock (perfusate deficit)	Hemorrhagic	Obvious bleeding
		Occult bleeding
	Nonhemorrhagic	Absolute fluid loss (renal, gastrointestinal)
		Relative fluid loss (redistribution secondary to injury, drugs)
2. Cardiac shock (pump failure)	Myocardial failure	Ischemia, infarction
		Cardiomyopathy
		Drug effect
		Metabolic (hypophosphatemia, hypocalcemia, acidosis)
		Excess afterload
		Myocardial rupture
		Myocardial injury (e.g., true contusion)
	Valve failure	Infection
		Proximal aortic dissection
		Injury
		Ruptured papillary muscle
		Obstruction from thrombus, myxoma
		Stenosis
	Conduction	Tachyarrhythmia, bradyarrhythmia
	Tamponade	Acute (injury)
		Chronic (uremia, infection, neoplasm)
3. Distributive shock (pipe failure)	Sepsis	
	Noninfectious systemic inflammatory response syndrome	Burn, pancreatitis, other causes
	Acute adrenal insufficiency	
	Anaphylaxis, drug reactions	
4. Obstructive shock (venous return compromise, outflow blockage)	Pericardial tamponade	
	Increased intrathoracic pressure	Tension pneumothorax
		Excess positive end-expiratory pressure
	IVC obstruction	Gravid uterus on IVC
		Tumor, thrombus
	Pulmonary embolism	
5. Neurogenic shock	Anatomic	Trauma, tumor
	Induced	Spinal or epidural anesthetic
6. Miscellaneous	Toxins	Carbon monoxide, cyanide poisoning
	Metabolic	Myxedema coma
7. Mixed	Combinations	

IVC, inferior vena cava.

is common and does not cause clinical symptoms. For example, voluntary blood donation corresponds to acute loss of approximately 10% of the circulating blood volume. The skin and skeletal muscle vasculature experience a slight decrease in perfusion. However, such a small acute loss is well tolerated because the intravascular volume can be quickly recruited from interstitial and intracellular reserves. Beyond 10% loss, however, the neuroendocrine response to shock becomes clinically apparent. The adrenal medulla increases its blood flow, ensuring both adequate oxygen delivery to its own tissues as well as swift delivery of catecholamines into the systemic circulation. As occupancy of the peripheral adrenergic receptors increases, heart rate and diastolic blood pressure rise, even while blood is squeezed out of the splanchnic bed. This compensatory redistribution fails at approximately 30% volume loss, a failure clinically manifested as the onset of systolic and diastolic hypotension. The decrease in urine flow in the early stages of volume loss is not due to early failure of renal blood flow, but rather to (a) a fall in glomerular filtration rate, (b) the sympathetically induced increases in resorption of sodium from the proximal tubules, and (c) the effects of antidiuretic hormone on retention of free water and that of aldosterone on distal tubular sodium resorption. Once hypotension occurs, further blood flow redistribution occurs in favor of the brain, but at the expense of the heart and the kidneys. A 40% to 50% volume loss exhausts all compensatory mechanisms. The need to restore perfusion and eliminate the cause of shock is evident.

The pump pathway to shock has two important entrances: primary pump failure and inability of the pump to accept the perfusate. The latter is commonly termed *obstructive shock* and is considered separately. The causes of pump failure, or cardiogenic shock, are familiar: acute failure of the cardiac muscle or a cardiac valve, and acute dysrhythmias. Specific diagnoses include myocardial infarction, rupture of a papillary muscle, and fracture of the chordae tendineae (the latter processes, thankfully rare, lead to acute regurgitation and failure of the left heart). The diagnosis and management of acute perioperative myocardial infarction and of arrhythmias are discussed in Chapter 63. The obstructive pathway to shock, the inability of the pump to accept the perfusate, is frequently traversed by injured patients. The specific diagnoses causing obstruction in the acutely injured are tension pneumothorax and pericardial tamponade, both discussed in greater detail in Chapter 65. These diagnoses share a pathophysiologic process that transmits pressure to the external wall of the atria, thereby preventing blood flow into the cardiac chambers. Decompression (of the pleural space or of the pericardial space) is lifesaving. Acute embolism of a blood clot from the systemic veins into the heart (pulmonary embolism) is a common cause of obstructive shock among surgical patients. Therapy is

Table 8.2. CLINICAL PARAMETERS AND MEASURED CORRELATES IN SHOCK

Class	Skin	Right heart filling pressure	Cardiac output	Left heart pressure	Vascular resistance	Myocardial oxygen consumption
Hypovolemic	Cool, pale	↓	↓	↓	↑	↓
Cardiogenic	Cool, pale	↑	↓	↑	↑	↓
Septic (early)	Warm, pink	↔	↑	↓	↓	↑
Septic (late)	Cool, pale	↓	↓	↓	↑	↓
Spinal	Warm, pink below lesion	↓	↓	↓	↓	↔
Obstructive	Cool, pale	↑	↓	↓	↑	↓

focused on relief of the intraluminal obstruction. A less common but deadly cause of obstructive shock is air embolism consequent to underfilled systemic veins brought into contact with the atmosphere, either during surgery or by a central venous catheter. A large air embolus obstructs the right ventricular outflow tract, whereas slow entrainment of air causes distal pulmonary arteries to become obstructed with acute right ventricular dysfunction. Therapy of a large right ventricular air lock requires relief of the obstruction through positioning (placing the patient in the right side down, head down position to try to move the embolus to the apex of the right ventricle), aspirating the right heart through a preexisting central venous catheter, cardiac massage, or direct puncture of the right heart to aspirate the air. These maneuvers are usually performed in the sequence listed until one is successful.

Discrimination between "perfusate" problems and "pump" problems is critical because the therapies are distinct. Unfortunately, the neuroendocrine response to pump shock is clinically indistinguishable to the response to perfusate shock: the skin is poorly perfused, moist, and cool; the pulse is weak; the heartbeat and respiratory rates are rapid; and the urine flow is reduced. Bedside discrimination between pump and perfusate shock is based directly on mechanism: in pump shock, the capacitance (venous) vascular beds are full because the pump cannot or will not accept inflow. Thus, in pump shock, the neck veins are distended, the patient has an elevated central venous pressure, and abnormal heart sounds may be present. In perfusate shock, the neck veins are collapsed and the central venous pressure is low. This difference cannot be overemphasized: given a patient with the classic presentation of shock (ashen facies, diaphoresis, tachycardia, tachypnea, and hypotension), attention should be immediately directed at the neck veins to discriminate pump from perfusate pathways.

"Pipe" shock (formally, distributive shock and neurogenic shock) follows failure of mechanisms that regulate tissue-specific resistance and capacitance. There are two routes to this form of shock. The first is through interruption of the sympathetic nervous system, the consequence of either spinal cord injury or neuraxial instillation of local anesthetic agents (spinal or epidural anesthesia). The second route is through attenuation of the sympathetic effects in the periphery, most commonly in the context of sepsis. Unlike the patient with perfusate or pump shock, patients with pipe shock fail to vasoconstrict in the periphery and therefore usually have warm skin. Tachycardia may be absent and bradycardia is often observed in spinal shock, particularly when the level of the spinal cord injury is at or above T-4. Importantly, the distributive cause of the shock also underlies the early failure of redistributive compensatory mechanisms. Neck veins are typically flat and the central venous pressure remains low.

These observations discriminating among the causes of shock and comparing clinical findings with gross cardiovascular correlates are summarized in Table 8.2.

The physiology underlying these parameters is discussed in detail in the next section.

GUYTON'S MODEL OF THE CIRCULATION AND ITS RELEVANCE TO SHOCK

At the heart of the surgeon's interest in shock are the abilities to recognize and to treat shock. Both require a mechanistic model of the circulation. The most useful for the purposes of understanding and treating shock may well be Guyton's (4,5).

After the work of Harvey, Weber (6), and Bayliss and Starling (7), the next major advance in understanding the driving force of the circulation was the work of Starr and Rawson. They focused on what we today call *preload,* the pressure driving venous return to the heart. Their key experiment was to measure "no-flow" pressure in recently deceased patients. This no-flow pressure in the systemic circulation (P_{ms}, or mean systemic pressure) is the equilibration pressure in the systemic arteries and veins after the heart is stopped. Their studies showed that patients dying of noncardiac causes had a P_{ms} of approximately 10 cm H_2O (approximately 8 mm Hg), whereas those dying of congestive heart failure had a no-flow pressure approximately twice that value (8). Guyton collected several key observations concerning the interrelationships between the venous pressure, cardiac function, and circulation.

1. Sympathetic stimulation of the heart increases cardiac activity to a much greater degree than it increases cardiac output.
2. Replacing the heart by a pump capable of pumping unlimited volumes of blood increases cardiac output only slightly. The pumping is limited by the input volume available.
3. Conversely, even a slight increase in blood volume available on the input side of the pump causes a near-instantaneous increase in cardiac output.
4. Similarly, even a slight decrease in peripheral (arterial) resistance causes a marked increase in cardiac output.

Based on these observations, Guyton reasoned that the normal circulation was at least as dependent on venous pressure driving blood to the heart as on the heart itself for maintaining circulation. The "force from behind" returning blood to the heart had to be balanced with the "force forward" ejecting blood from the heart. Balanced forces represent an equilibrium state for the circulation. To describe the "force from behind," Guyton emphasized the role of the distensible "capacitance" vessels where most of the blood resides and introduced the twin concepts of the venous pressure gradient and the venous return curve. Guyton reasoned that the venous return from the periphery to the heart depended on a pressure gradient, that P_{ms} was the driving pressure, and that the right atrial pressure (P_{ra}) was the upstream pressure. Thus, venous return (or flow) could be described by:

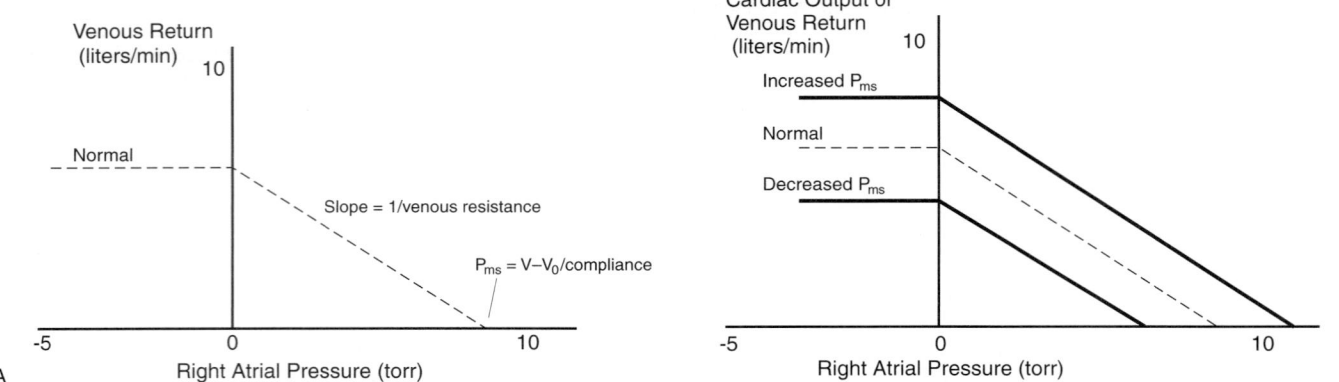

Figure 8.1. *(A)* A schematic venous return curve. Reading from right to left, the intersection of the curve with the abscissa is the mean systemic pressure (P_{ms}), meaning that when the right atrial pressure is equal to the no-flow pressure in the venous circulation, forward flow into the heart ceases. The slope of the curve is the reciprocal of the venous resistance. At all points on the curve, Ohm's law applies: the venous return is equal to the difference between the no-flow and right atrial pressures, divided by the venous resistance. *(B)* Effects of changing the P_{ms} on the venous return curve. The normal venous return curve is reproduced. Because the circulatory system is a closed system, cardiac out put and venous return are equal. Augmenting the P_{ms} (e.g., by a fluid bolus) shifts the oblique portion of the curve to the right, whereas acute diminution of P_{ms} pressure (e.g., during homorrhage) shifts the oblique portion of the curve to the left.

$$\text{Venous return} = \frac{P_{ms} - P_{ra}}{\text{venous resistance}}$$

Figure 8.1 illustrates the concept that a pressure gradient must exist between the capacitance vessels and the right atrium for blood to flow. Reading the figure from right to left, there is no flow if the venous and right atrial pressures are equal. As right atrial pressure falls, flow increases. Both disease and therapy can shift this venous return curve, but only two basic types of shifts occur. If there is a change in blood volume, the curve shifts so that the diagonal portion of the curve moves parallel to its previous position: hypervolemia shifts the curve up and to the right, whereas hy-

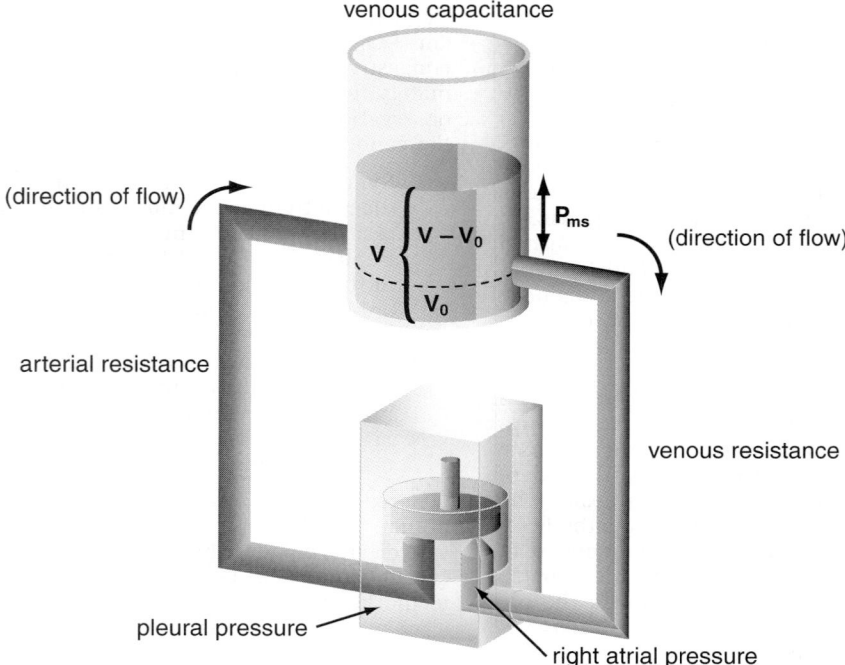

Figure 8.2. Guyton's single-circuit model of the circulation. The capacitance of the venous circulation is represented by the cylinder at the top of the model. The total volume of blood in the capacitance vessels, V, includes the blood required to fill the capacitance vessels, the unstressed volume (V_o) and the blood that exerts pressure (or the stressed volume, $V - V_o$). The pressure exerted by the stressed volume is mean systemic pressure (P_{ms}), or the pressure in the entire circulation as flow ceases and the pressure is permitted to equilibrate. The heart is represented by a cylinder in the pleural space, and the piston causes blood to flow from the venous circuit into the arterial circuit. Venous return is equal to cardiac output.

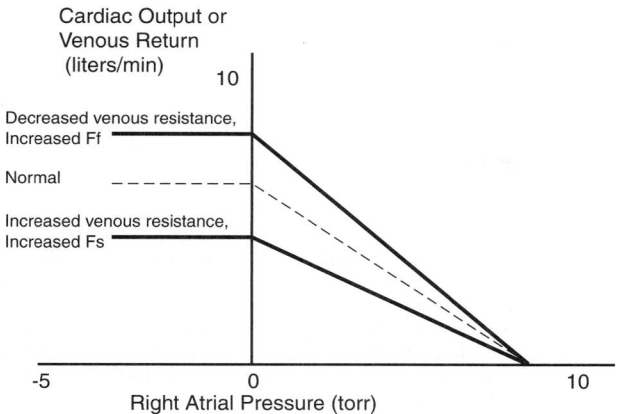

Figure 8.3. The effects of changing venous resistance and of fractional distribution of blood flow across venous beds. The normal venous return curve is reproduced. The no-flow pressure (P_{ms}), and hence the intersection of the curve with the abscissa, is unchanged. A fall in venous resistance or, alternatively, a redistribution of venous blood into beds with fast time constants pivots the oblique portion of the curve up and to the right (clockwise). This happens clinically in neurogenic shock. Conversely, a rise in venous resistance or redistribution of blood into beds with slow time constants causes a pivot of the oblique portion of the curve down and to the left (counterclockwise). Such an increase in venous resistance could follow, for example, compression of the inferior vena cava by the surgeon's hand during an abdominal operation.

povolemia shifts the curve down and to the left. In contrast, changes in vascular tone shift the curve so that it pivots around its intersection with the abscissa. Increases in tone pivot the curve down and to the left, whereas decreases in tone pivot the curve up and to the right. The reasons for these shifts may be inferred from a schematic representation of the circulation (Fig. 8.2).

The reservoir at the top of Fig. 8.2 represents the (large) capacitance of the venous system, and the height of the reservoir is the no-flow pressure, P_{ms}. Note that there is a volume remaining in the reservoir when the pressure of the system is zero. This is the unstressed volume, V_0. This volume is the volume of blood that remains in the circulation when the heart is stopped and the P_{ms} is reduced to zero (i.e., allowing a recently deceased patient to bleed passively until there is no more flow). The P_{ms} is therefore "created" by the incremental volume above V_0 that creates the total blood volume. Increments in total blood volume

obviously increase P_{ms}. What is less obvious, perhaps, is that changes in venous tone change V_0 such that "more" tone diminishes V_0; blood is squeezed from the unstressed volume into the stressed volume. Keep in mind that in the human circulation, changes in arterial blood pressure have no direct effect on venous tone. Thus, either an increase in total vascular volume, a decrease in V_0, or a decrease in the capacitance can cause a right shift of the venous return curve. Changes in the venous resistance, however, change the slope of the venous return curve, causing it to pivot on the abscissa. Three variables affect venous resistance: constriction of the veins themselves, a change in the viscosity of the blood, or redistribution of the blood between venous beds with different time constants. Every vascular bed has a characteristic time constant, τ, which reflects both the volume of blood in that bed and the flow rate of blood through that bed. For example, the skin has a very slow time constant (high volume, very low flow), whereas the kidney has a very fast time constant (low volume but rapid flow). The fractions of blood distributed among slow- and fast-time-constant beds are described as F_s and F_f, respectively. A decrease in F_s and an increase in F_t expedite venous return, changing it in the same direction as decreasing the venous resistance (Fig. 8.3).

The next observation is that right atrial pressure is a surrogate determinant of cardiac function, and that a plot of right atrial pressure versus cardiac output is a valid representation of cardiac function. Frank and Starling recognized that cardiac muscle function was determined by cardiac muscle tension, and right atrial pressure is a valid proxy for that tension in health and in many disease states. Because the venous return and cardiac function curves share the same coordinate space, they can be superimposed on each other (Fig. 8.4). Because (a) the cardiac function curve describes ejection of blood from the heart, (b) the venous return curve describes return of blood to the heart, and (c) the circulation is a closed system, it follows that the equilibrium state of the circulation exists at the unique point where the two curves intersect. It also follows that the only way that circulation can be altered is to "move" the intersection by shifting either one or both function curves. Every individual, whether in health or in a state of shock, has a unique venous return curve and cardiac function curve. In large measure, manipulation of the cardiac output during treatment of shock depends on moving this intersection by simultaneously shifting the venous return and cardiac function curves.

We have already discussed the two ways in which the venous return curve can be shifted. The cardiac function curve

Figure 8.4. Graphic representation of circulatory performance. In this figure, the venous return curve introduced in Fig. 8.1 is superimposed on the familiar Frank-Starling curve that relates a surrogate for left ventricular preload (right atrial pressure) to cardiac output. Because the circulatory system is closed, venous return must equal cardiac output, and the system's performance is described by the intersection of the two curves. The curves can be shifted by disease and further shifted by interventions to counteract disease states. The reason the cardiac function curve extends into the negative range of right atrial pressures is that pleural pressure is normally negative. The net transmural pressure (the pressure across the wall of the right atrium that will cause blood to flow into the right ventricle) remains positive even when right atrial pressure is marginally negative relative to the atmosphere.

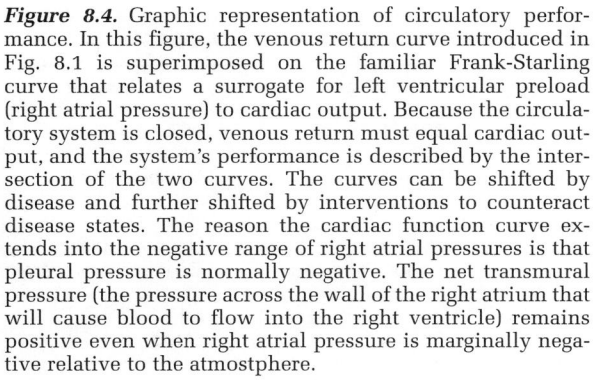

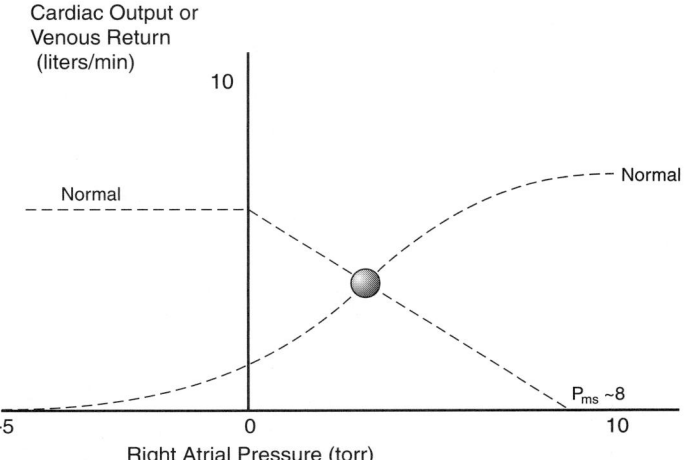

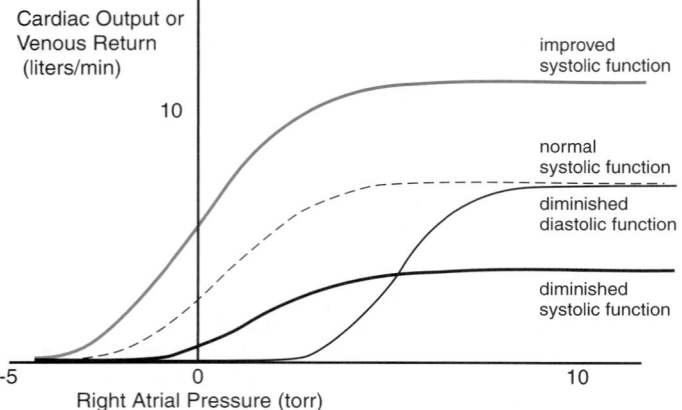

Figure 8.5. Cardiac function illustrated on the Frank-Starling curve. The normal relationship between preload and performance is shown on the *dotted curve*. Systolic deterioration rotates the curve downward, whereas diastolic deterioration shifts it rightward *(black curves)*. Administration of an inotrope rotates the normal curve up and to the left (counterclockwise; *blue curve*).

also has two fundamental shifts (Fig. 8.5). Changes in contractility generally pivot the cardiac function curve around its intersection with the abscissa (x-axis). Improvement in cardiac function pivots the curve up and to the left, whereas cardiac depression pivots it down and to the right. Pure changes is diastolic function shift the curve left and right, with the most common clinical problem—diastolic dysfunction—shifting the cardiac function curve to the right.

TYPES OF SHOCK

Hypovolemic Shock

The most common shock state encountered by the surgeon is hypovolemic shock. Acute hypovolemia causes a parallel left shift of the venous return curve. The intersection with the normal cardiac function curve also shifts down and to the left. The neuroendocrine response, by releasing catecholamines into the circulation, rotates the cardiac function curve up and to the left, increasing cardiac flow, but only marginally. Clinically, tachycardia, tachypnea, and oliguria are reliable guides to the depth of the hypovolemia. The stages of hypovolemia have been classified and are presented in Table 8.3.

A substantial rise in cardiac output can be achieved only by volume resuscitation (starting with crystalloid also causes some hemodilution; Fig. 8.6).

Cardiogenic Shock

Cardiogenic shock causes a pivot, rotating the cardiac function curve down and to the right (Fig. 8.7). The equilibrium intersection between the venous return curve and the depressed cardiac function curve causes the low cardiac output. The physiologic compensatory response is to increase P_{ms}, thus shifting the venous return curve up and to the right in parallel to the original venous return curve. This is a good time to consider and compare the vascular effects of dopamine (which has a predominantly vasoconstrictor effect in high doses) with the effects of dobutamine (which has a more vasodilatory profile). The two drugs have similar inotropic effects, so that administration of either drug partially restores cardiac function, pivoting the cardiac function curve up and to the left. The increase in afterload associated with dopamine may attenuate the left pivot. The effects on the venous return curve are quite different, however. Dopamine further increases P_{ms}, shifting the venous return curve to the right in parallel with the other venous return curves. Dobutamine functions quite differently, keeping P_{ms} roughly constant and pivoting the curve up and to the right as vascular resistance falls. These effects (Fig. 8.7) help to explain why dobutamine is usually preferred over dopamine in cardiogenic shock.

Septic Shock

Septic shock is the most common form of distributive shock encountered by the surgeon. Figure 8.8 illustrates septic shock and resuscitation in terms of venous return and cardiac function curves. Absent medical intervention, the venodilatation of sepsis causes not only a decrease in venous resistance but a fall in P_{ms}. Volume resuscitation restores P_{ms} to its normal value, but now with a markedly decreased venous resistance. The competing cardiac effects of sepsis are readily modeled with appropriate shifts in the cardiac function curves: whereas afterload reduction tends to increase cardiac performance, direct myocardial depression overwhelms the advantage of this after-

Table 8.3. CLASSIFICATION OF HYPOVOLEMIC SHOCK (ASSOCIATED WITH ACUTE BLOOD LOSS)

	Class I	Class II	Class III	Class IV
Estimated blood loss (% blood volume)	≤15%	15%–30%	30%–40%	40%
Typical pulse rate	<100	>100	>120	>140
Typical blood pressure	Normal	Normal mean, with declining systolic and rising systolic pressures	Decreased	Markedly decreased
Pulse pressure	Normal	Narrowed	Narrowed	Unobtainable
Central nervous system/mental status	Normal to slightly anxious	Mildly anxious	Anxious and confused	Confused or lethargic
Urine output	Normal	~0.5 mL/kg/h	<0.5 mL/kg/h	Nil
Volume required	Often none	Crystalloid	Crystalloid and blood	Blood

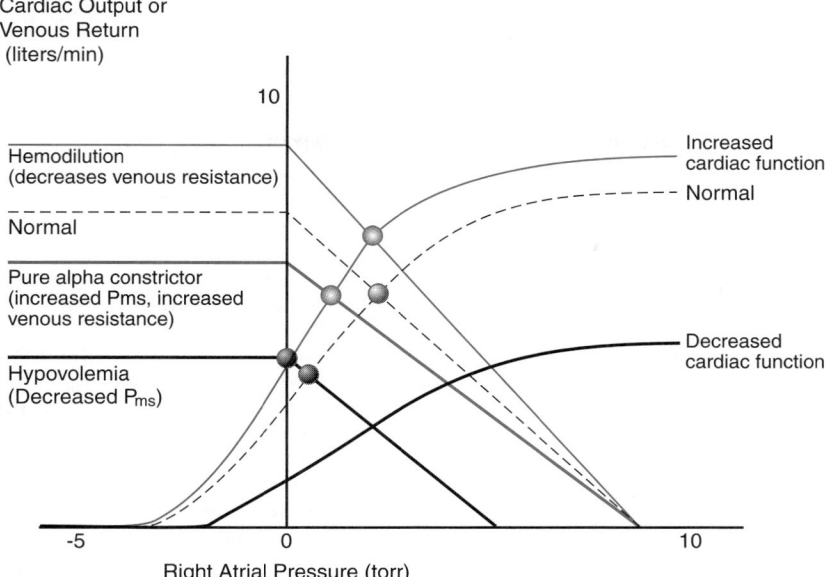

Figure 8.6. Cardiac performance during hypovolemic shock and resuscitation. Beginning with normal performance *(rightmost black dot),* acute hypovolemia shifts the venous return curve down and to the left, reflecting the acute fall in mean systemic pressure (P_{ms}). The intersection of the normal cardiac function curve with the left-shifted hypovolemic venous return curve causes the decrease in cardiac output *(lowermost black dot).* The physiologic "fight-or-flight response" releasing catecholamines from the circulation improves cardiac performance, sliding the cardiac performance curve upward and leftward along the compromised venous return curve *(second black dot).* Administration of a pure vascular constrictor such as phenylephrine would improve P_{ms} but worsen venous resistance, leading to a less favorable slope in the venous return curve *(lowermost blue dot).* The most effective therapy is restoration of circulating volume. Crystalloid resuscitation further diminishes resistance by dilution of the rheologically active erythrocytes, and therefore shifts the venous return curve up and to the right. The new cardiac output is even higher than the original cardiac output *(uppermost dot)* because of these favorable effects on resistance. Also illustrated is a compromised cardiac function curve that can be used to predict the consequences of volume loss in patients with limited cardiac function.

Figure 8.7. *(A, top)* Cardiogenic shock and the effect of dopamine. The normal intersection of the cardiac function and venous return curves is located at the green dot. Cardiac dysfunction causes the typical change in the cardiac output curve, pivoting it down and to the right *(lowermost black dot).* The homeostatic response of the venous circulation—the accumulation of fluid—allows venous pressure to rise, shifting the mean systemic pressure (P_{ms}) to the right while leaving venous resistance (the slope of the venous return curve) unchanged. The new intersection is at the *rightmost black dot.* Dopamine increases not only cardiac performance but P_{ms}, leaving venous resistance more or less unchanged. These combined effects result in a new intersection located at the *blue dot.* Compare with Fig. 8.7B. *(B, bottom)* Cardiogenic shock and the effect of dobutamine. The normal intersection of the cardiac function and venous return curves is illustrated by the *leftmost dot,* and the shift caused by the cardiac dysfunction is illustrated by the *lowermost black dot.* The homeostatic compensation is again illustrated by the *rightmost black dot.* The administration of dobutamine improves cardiac function similar to dopamine. However, the predominantly β-adrenergic stimulation of dobutamine (vs. dopamine) causes a fall in venous resistance. There are two consequences. First, the mean systemic pressure (P_{ms}) may actually fall back to normal when dobutamine is administered, and second, the slope of the venous function curve (the reciprocal of venous resistance) changes, pivoting the curve up and to the right *(blue dot).*

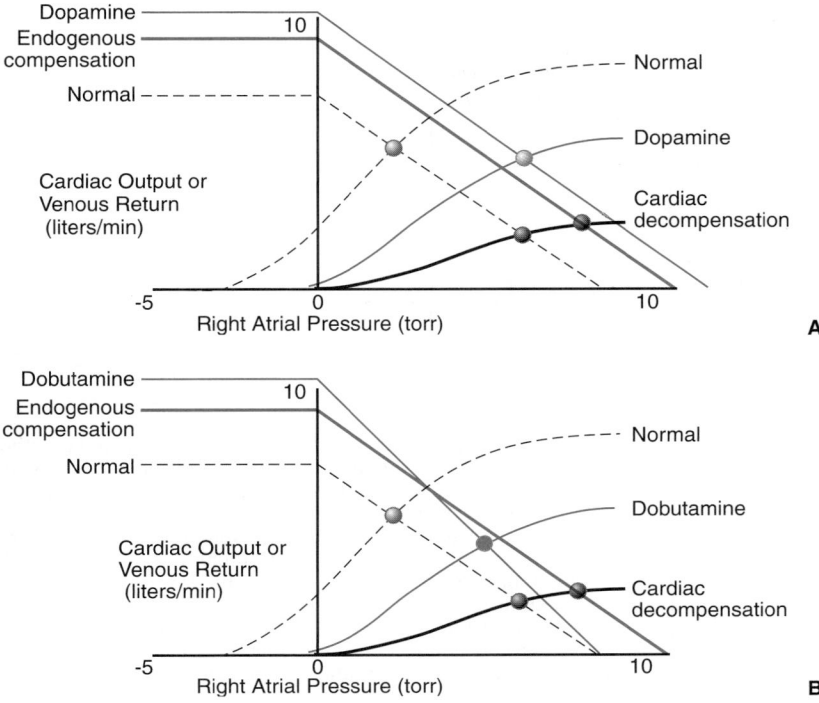

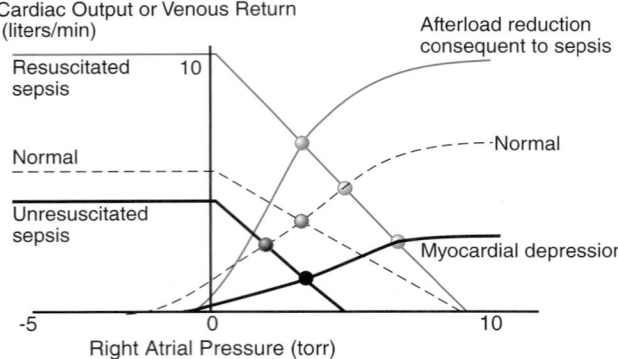

Figure 8.8. Septic shock, resuscitation, and effects on cardiac output. The intersection of the normal curves is located at the *centermost dot*. Early sepsis causes a sudden, marked vasodilation. Mean systemic pressure (P_{ms}) and venous resistance both fall. As a consequence, the oblique portion of the venous return curve shifts to the left (fall in P_{ms}) and also rotates downward and to the left (increase in venous resistance). The intersection of the normal cardiac function curve and the shifted venous return curve is illustrated by the *leftmost dot*. If sepsis is recognized promptly, aggresive volume resuscitation can restore P_{ms} while venous resistance remains constant, creating a resuscitated venous function curve. Cardiac output is defined at the *middle blue dot*. Sepsis can cause both an afterload reduction leading to seemingly increased cardiac performance *(uppermost blue dot)* or severe myocardial dysfunction *(lowermost blue dot)*. If sepsis is unrecognized and myocardial depression supervenes, cardiac function can be inadequate to sustain life *(lowermost dot)*.

load reduction in late, uncompensated sepsis, or in sepsis with preexisting cardiac disease.

Obstructive Shock

Obstruction to venous return is a surgical emergency. The two common causes encountered by general surgeons are pericardial tamponade and tension pneumothorax; ob-

stetricians encounter a similar physiologic effect when the gravid uterus presses on the inferior vena cava. All abdominal surgeons occasionally cause transient obstructive shock by pressing on the inferior vena cava during surgery. Pulmonary embolism and air embolism are the other two major causes of obstructive shock.

Analysis of tension pneumothorax according to Guyton's principles is presented in Fig. 8.9. The venous return curve is markedly distorted because the pleural pressure exceeds the right atrial pressure. Venous return no longer depends on the arithmetic difference between P_{ms} and right atrial pressure, but on the difference between P_{ms} and (the very positive) pleural pressure. The cardiac function curve is also adversely affected by two mechanisms. The rightward shift occurs because the transmural filling pressure is zero when the right atrial pressure falls to the (now positive) value of the pleural pressure. The downward pivot of the cardiac function curve is caused by a reflex increase in pulmonary vascular resistance. Although there is an endogenous catecholamine surge, it is apparent from the analysis that neither a volume load nor administration of exogenous catecholamines will have a significant effect on circulation. The only effective therapy is immediately to reduce pleural pressure by relieving the tension pneumothorax. Pericardial tamponade provides a nearly identical analysis, except that the limitation on transmural pressure is not pleural pressure but pericardial pressure.

Neurogenic Shock

Surgeons encounter neurogenic shock in two arenas: the trauma resuscitation bay and the operating room. Traumatic spinal injury occurs when the cord is severed at a level within or above the sympathetic chain, whereas neurogenic shock encountered in the operating room is the consequence of a neuraxial anesthetic that has extended beyond its intended effect. Bearing in mind that the heart also receives sympathetic input, there is an important functional distinction between an injury above T-4 and one below T-4. The former depresses cardiac function in addi-

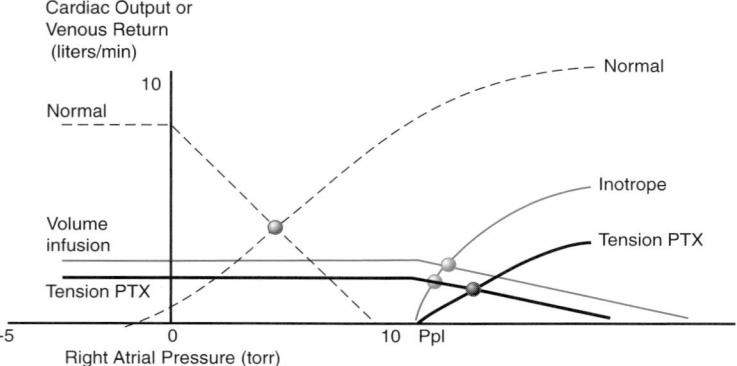

Figure 8.9. Obstructive shock caused by tension pneumothorax. The intersection of the normal curves is located at the *leftmost dot*. The effect of the tension pneumothorax on cardiac function is to shift it far to the right. Note that the intersection of the cardiac function curve with the abscissa is equal to the pleural pressure: at right atrial pressures less than pleural pressures, the atrium cannot fill and therefore no blood can be ejected. Neither endogenous nor exogenous inotropes can shift the cardiac function curve to the left; the intersection with the abscissa is fixed by the pleural pressure. Inspection of the lowermost venous return curve shows that pleural pressure similarly limits venous return. The composite performance is described by the *rightmost dot*. The mean systemic pressure (P_{ms}) is markedly increased owing to blood being squeezed out of the thorax and by endogenous catecholamine release. Neither volume infusion (the middle venous return curve) nor administration of catecholamines (the left-shifted cardiac function curve) creates much improvement in cardiac output *(blue dots)*. The only effective therapy is immediate relief of the excessive pleural pressure by conversion of the tension pneumothorax to an open pneumothorax (needle decompression).

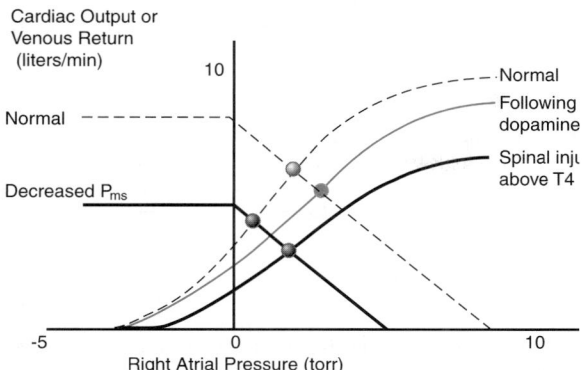

Figure 8.10. Circulation in neurogenic shock. The intersection of the normal curves is marked by the *uppermost dot.* With a spinal injury below T-4, cardiac performance is unchanged, and the major effect is on venous tone. Mean systemic pressure (P_{ms}) falls, with relatively little effect on venous resistance, yielding the performance intersection marked by the *middle black dot.* Sympathetic denervation of the heart, characteristic of spinal cord lesions above T-4, leads to compromised cardiac performance and a circulatory equilibrium *(lowermost black dot).* Volume infusion is required to restore P_{ms}, and the addition of dopamine yields improved venous return and cardiac function curves *(blue dot).*

tion to affecting venous return, whereas the latter leaves cardiac performance unaffected (Fig. 8.10). When cardiac performance is unaffected, limited volume resuscitation and treatment with a pure α–agonist such as phenylephrine is sufficient therapy. However, if the cardiac sympathetic innervation is compromised, vagal parasympathetic innervation may predominate and administration of phenylephrine may aggravate reflex bradycardia. To preclude this undesirable effect of therapy, a mixed inotrope and chronotrope such as dopamine or norepinephrine is used. In extreme cases, temporary cardiac pacing may be lifesaving. Volume restoration is also required.

SHOCK RECOGNITION AND RESUSCITATION: PRACTICAL ASPECTS

Resuscitation from shock must begin immediately on recognition. Restoration of oxygen delivery is the imperative. The simple ABC approach is effective: establish and maintain an airway, ensure breathing with 100% oxygen, and restore the circulation. Supplemental oxygen must be administered by nonrebreather face mask, Ambu-bag, or tracheal intubation. Chronic obstructive airway disease is not a contraindication to the administration of oxygen. Ventilation should be confirmed by auscultation (axillae and stomach) and by demonstration of end-tidal carbon dioxide if the trachea has been intubated. The neck veins should be inspected to discriminate pump shock from perfusate shock. If the neck veins are distended, the axillae should be reauscultated to exclude a tension pneumothorax and consideration should be given to the possibility of pericardial tamponade. The heart should be auscultated to determine whether heart sounds are audible and, if so, whether abnormal heart sounds such as pathologic murmurs and third and fourth heart sounds are present.

A pulse should be sought. The absence of central pulses (femoral, carotid) mandates cardiac life support including cardiopulmonary resuscitation, determination of rhythm, and cardioversion–defibrillation. More commonly, a faint pulse is palpable. The carotid pulse ordinarily is present in adults with systolic blood pressures greater than 60 mm Hg. A short, wide-bore intravenous catheter should be inserted into a peripheral vein and an aliquot of blood taken for analysis. Given the frequency of hypovolemic blood loss in the surgical population, one of the most important steps is an immediate crossmatching of blood. A hemoglobin determination is also desirable. The venous catheter then serves as the conduit for rapid infusion of a balanced salt solution such as lactated Ringer's solution; 20 mL/kg should be administered as rapidly as practicable (within 5 minutes). The fluid bolus serves to increase preload, diminish venous resistance, and possibly decrease arterial afterload, all of which augment cardiac performance. Stroke volume improves by this mechanism even in patients who have sustained an acute myocardial infarction or have pericardial tamponade, as seen in the Guyton diagrams. Fluid bolus should therefore be withheld only when there is incontrovertible evidence that the cause is cardiogenic and associated with frothy pink pulmonary edema. The fluid bolus can be repeated immediately if the shock is not immediately responsive.

While the fluid is being administered, electrophysiologic monitoring should begin. An electrocardiogram (ECG) should be obtained and the rhythm monitored continuously. The systemic blood pressure and heart rate should be determined at regular, frequent (e.g., every 2 to 5 minutes) intervals and recorded on a purpose-specific form. A pulse oximeter should be applied to determine the oxygen saturation of capillary blood. The signal may be difficult to obtain because of intense vasoconstriction, and application of the probe to the earlobe or nose may be helpful. The stomach should be decompressed to prevent the complication of aspiration.

None of the aforementioned methods is especially effective in determining the quality of organ perfusion or the adequacy of shock reversal. The best first proxy for the adequacy of organ perfusion appears to be urine output, which should be measured every 30 minutes by an indwelling bladder (Foley) catheter. The best first proxy for the adequacy of shock reversal is the pH on arterial blood gas analysis. During shock, the pH falls into the acid range as a consequence of anaerobic metabolism with obligatory accumulation of lactic acid. Once resuscitation is adequate, the lactate should be metabolized and the anion gap acidosis should normalize. Persistent anion gap acidosis suggests inadequate resuscitation or frankly nonviable tissue. A non-anion gap acidosis is less worrisome and may follow resuscitation with normal saline. To avoid confusion, Ringer's solution is often used as the balanced salt solution. To reiterate, heart rate and urine output are often the best indicators of the current depth of shock but do not indicate adequacy of resuscitation. Because shock is operationally defined as metabolic shortfall, the adequacy of resuscitation is reflected in tissue perfusion. The most immediately available measures of this perfusion include arterial blood gas analysis for pH and the by-product of anaerobic metabolism, lactate.

Neither of these proxies directly assesses oxygen delivery to tissues most vulnerable to nutrient deprivation, such as neural tissue. However, owing to the sensitivity of the splanchnic bed to even mild shock states, perfusion of abdominal viscera can be used as an intermediate surrogate. The mucosal lumen of the gastrointestinal (GI) tract is accessible though the mouth and the rectum, and there appears to be a tight correlation between the adequacy of mucosal perfusion and outcome. The adequacy of mucosal perfusion can be assessed by tonometry, a technique that indirectly measures the accumulated acids in mucosal cells. However, it is disputed whether titration of care to a predetermined tonometric value improves outcome (9).

Given the metabolic imperatives, it is important frequently to reassess the determinants of oxygen delivery. Oxygen saturation should be maintained above 95%. After resuscitation from shock, metabolic demands can be substantial. The ideal hemoglobin concentration in unstable patients is unknown. Although stable patients can often tolerate hemoglobin levels as low as 7 g/dL, the unstable patient may be better served by targeting a slightly higher level until the shock is fully reversed. The heart rate should be maintained in a physiologic range, usually between 80 to 120 beats/min. (The upper constraint on heart rate is lifted for children, who regulate cardiac output almost exclusively by heart rate.) The stroke volume should be optimized by augmenting preload. If (and usually, only if) there is uncertainty about the magnitude of the cardiac output, it should be measured. This can be done by the thermodilution technique [after insertion of a pulmonary artery catheter (PAC)], by the less invasive dye clearance technique, or by aortic flow assessment with an esophageal ultrasound transducer. Resuscitation from shock states ordinarily requires a minimum indexed cardiac output (cardiac index) of 2.5 L/min/m² of body surface area, and often considerably more, to deliver sufficient oxygen. Although the definition of "sufficient" oxygen delivery is still contested, all agree that a subnormal oxygen delivery is never adequate. Thus "sufficient" is at least "normal" oxygen delivery, which is approximately 500 mL/min/m². Because fully saturated oxyhemoglobin at a normal hemoglobin concentration of 15 g carries approximately 20 mL oxygen per 100 mL blood, the minimum cardiac index of 2.5 L/min/m² is adequate only if there is a normal hemoglobin concentration that is fully saturated with oxygen. Decreases in either hemoglobin concentration or oxygen saturation require compensatory proportionate increments in cardiac output to maintain oxygen delivery at a minimum value of 500 mL/min/m².

ADJUNCTS TO RESUSCITATION

As we have discussed, the compensatory mechanisms and good resuscitation are often effective in previously healthy patients. However, some patients with severe shock and those with preexisting medical diseases often lack sufficient compensatory responses and do not respond to administered oxygen and fluids. Adjunctive therapy is required. There are two major classes of adjuncts, pharmacologic and mechanical.

All patients in shock should be immediately considered possible candidates for one mechanical and two pharmacologic adjuncts. Because severe hypocalcemia and severe acidosis both can thwart shock resuscitation, the ionized calcium and base deficit should be determined early in resuscitation. Calcium should be administered to bring the ionized calcium into the normal range, and consideration should be given to giving sufficient bicarbonate to bring the plasma pH up to 7.2. There is no benefit to administration of calcium or bicarbonate in excess of these targets. Temperature should also be measured, and patients whose temperatures are less than 33° to 34°C should be actively rewarmed because the circulation cannot be readily restored at lower temperatures.

Several classes of drugs serve as adjuncts to resuscitation from shock. Sympathetic and sympathomimetic amines are the most widely used. The selection of one or more of these drugs is based less on the cause of the shock and more on the specific needs of the individual patient. Each drug is titrated to effect, but (with the exception of dopamine) the relative effects of each drug on the different receptor classes are drug specific. The approximate relative effects are listed in Table 8.4.

Table 8.4. RELATIVE EFFECTS OF VASOACTIVE DRUGS

Drug	α	β₁	β₂
Phenylephrine	++/+++	—	—
Norepinephrine	+++	++	+
Epinephrine	+++	+++	+++
Dopamine	+ to +++	++	++
Dobutamine	+	+++	+
Isoproterenol	—	+++	+++

For example, consider a patient with an isolated spinal cord injury at C-6 who has "pipe" failure (distributive shock) with relative bradycardia. Although phenylephrine could be used to stimulate α receptors, there is a possibility of causing further baroreceptor-mediated reflex bradycardia with the rising blood pressure. However, the use of a pressor that also has cardioaccelerator effects is unlikely to cause further bradycardia. Norepinephrine is a drug with strong α and β₁ characteristics and would serve such a patient well, as would dopamine (as discussed previously). In contrast, a patient with an acute myocardial infarction ordinarily requires more efficient myocardial contraction against (a pharmacologically reduced) peripheral resistance. The characteristics of such a drug include low α activity and sufficient β₂ activity to offset the vasoconstriction of β₁ effects. Dobutamine is a typical first choice.

Dopamine differs from the other pressors by having accumulating effects with increasing doses. The receptors occupied first are dopaminergic receptors on the kidney and in splanchnic beds that regionally augment blood flow. Urine output can rise rapidly. Before those receptors are saturated, however, dopamine begins to occupy β receptors. Vasodilation predominates owing to the combined effects on dopaminergic and β receptors, and as a consequence the heart rate increases. As the dose is increased (but before the β receptors are saturated), the α receptors become occupied. Vasoconstriction dominates and the heart rate may slow somewhat. The relationship between infusion rate and receptor occupancy is patient specific. Dopamine must therefore be titrated to desired effect.

The effects of sympathomimetic amines are modulated by several factors. In addition to being most effective in a slightly acid milieu (pH 7.2 to 7.4), the hemodynamic effect depends on receptor number and occupancy, and coupling of the receptor to second messengers: all sympathomimetic amines appear to act through one or more internal cell signaling systems. Receptor number and second messenger coupling appear to be especially important for dobutamine because tachyphylaxis can render the drug ineffective after just a few days' administration. A practical solution is to rotate dobutamine therapy with amrinone or milrinone therapy. Amrinone, although not a sympathomimetic amine, is a steroid-like drug that has cardiac effects indistinguishable from those of dobutamine. Dobutamine acts through a G protein to activate adenyl cyclase and thereby increase the concentration of the second messenger, cyclic adenosine monophosphate (cAMP). Amrinone augments the concentration of cAMP by inhibiting the degrading enzyme, phosphodiesterase. The signal transduction pathways of the adrenergic receptors are given in Table 8.5.

Patients in shock may have preexisting medical conditions that are either compensated by physiologic reserve or have not been diagnosed before the shock episode. Resuscitation from shock is occasionally thwarted by unrecognized endocrinopathies, including hypothyroidism and adrenal cortical insufficiency. Patients who are refractory to resuscitation and those who appear dependent on ex-

Table 8.5. SIGNAL TRANSDUCTION PATHWAYS OF ADRENERGIC RECEPTORS

Receptor type	Action	Second messenger path
α_1	Vasoconstriction	G protein coupled to phospholipase C, cleavage of phosphoinositol, elevation of intracellular calcium
α_2	Decreased central sympathetic outflow, vasoconstriction	G protein to inhibit adenyl cyclase, reduce cAMP
β_1	Increased heart rate, increased contractility, increased conduction velocity	G protein to activate adenyl cyclase, increase cAMP
β_2	Vasodilation	G protein to activate adenyl cyclase, increase cAMP
Dopaminergic	Mixed/vasodilation	G protein to activate adenyl cyclase, increase cAMP

cAMP, cyclic adenosine monophosphate.

ogenous pressor agents in the face of adequate urine output should be evaluated by measurement of thyroid-stimulating hormone (TSH) levels (to evaluate the adequacy of peripheral thyroid activity) and by performance of a cosyntropin test (to evaluate the ability of the adrenal gland to secrete cortisol). Elevated TSH levels in critically ill patients suggest hypothyroidism, which should be treated with levothyroxine. Low basal cortisol levels or cortisol levels that fail to augment after infusion of the adrenocorticotropic hormone analogue suggest adrenal insufficiency. Very rarely, patients with sufficient endogenous vasopressin to prevent diabetes insipidus before shock have hypotension responsive to vasopressin.

Mechanical adjuncts to the management of shock are reserved for patients with true pump failure. The adjuncts include intraaortic balloon counterpulsation and ventricular assist devices. All are bridges to definitive therapy. Intraaortic balloon counterpulsation increases coronary blood flow through critical stenoses by augmenting afterload during diastole. Direct effects on cardiac output are thought to be minimal. In contrast, left and right ventricular assist devices unload the heart directly and can therefore be used when the myocardium itself has failed, not merely its blood supply. The mechanical adjuncts usually require systemic anticoagulation, which may be relatively contraindicated in patients with recent surgery.

RISKS OF RESUSCITATION

Perhaps the most vexing aspect of shock is that resuscitation is not synonymous with reversal, much less a guarantee of recovery. Despite timely intervention and aggressive management, a significant number of patients with shock sustain secondary injuries attributable to reperfusion and inflammation associated with resuscitation. The biology of reperfusion and inflammation is complex, incompletely understood, and far beyond the scope of a practical chapter. A synthesis of existing data that may be clinically useful to the surgeon managing shock includes the following:

- Resuscitation and recovery from shock are medical events that may not have been anticipated during evolution. There is no *a priori* way to discriminate between salutary and harmful physiologic responses to shock or to shock therapies. Even monitoring tools such as the PAC have been cited as contributors to poor outcomes (see later).
- Studies in both animals and humans suggested that the behavior of specific cell populations during shock is influenced by circulating mediators and by direct cell–cell interactions.
- Manipulation of specific cell behavior in animals demonstrated a potential to improve outcome after re-

suscitation from shock. However, manipulation of cell behavior either by manipulation of a particular mediator or of a particular cell–cell interaction has not yet proven to be a helpful therapeutic strategy in humans. Emulation of dozens of manipulations proven helpful in animal models of shock, sepsis, and organ failure have proven ineffective or harmful in humans (10). Why therapies helpful in animal models are harmful to human patients is not known, but the most likely explanation is that the models are inadequate.

- The cell populations that laboratory studies suggest have the greatest influence over the outcome of shock include nucleated blood cells, endothelial cells, and immunocytes (including macrophages and lymphocytes). Each of these cell types is accessible to therapy, but no cell-specific therapy has yet been identified as helpful.
- Endogenous responses and therapeutic interventions trigger secretion of no fewer than 100 mediators, ranging from small gaseous molecules (e.g., nitric oxide) to large, modified polypeptides such as the cytokines tumor necrosis factor and interleukin-1. Each of these mediators is produced by or affects one or more of the cell types listed previously. Although discussion of specific molecules is beyond the scope of this chapter, in general, each mediator appears to have at least one well developed clearance mechanism, ranging from simple diffusion, through autodestruction, to specific molecular antagonists. These clearance mechanisms appear important in the regulation of inflammation, and dysregulation of this complex system is probably important in the adverse sequelae of shock.
- Although the network of mediators contains sophisticated self-limiting mechanisms, the cells affected by the mediators can be activated to secrete additional mediators, thereby amplifying the initial mediator signal. Such amplification appears salutary when the cause of the inflammation is relatively minor and potentially survivable with limited medical intervention.
- A sufficiently large stimulus leads to unbridled inflammation. Nucleated blood cells stick to endothelial walls and the interaction precipitates widespread leakage of fluid and indiscriminate emigration of inflammatory cells into tissues distant from the stimulus. Immunocytes proliferate to mount a further inflammatory response.
- When a further stimulus fails to materialize, an excessive antiinflammatory response ensues. The excessive antiinflammatory response renders the patient immunoincompetent and susceptible to overwhelming infection.

The conclusion that emerges from biologic studies is that the network of mediators and the many affected cells is complex and that mechanisms limiting inflammation are effective as long as the inflammation itself is limited. At present, the safest course appears to include rapid identification and definitive control of inflammatory stimuli before the network of mediators and affected cells is activated. The clinical imperative is to find the cause of the shock, to rectify the cause of the shock, and to do so as rapidly as practical. A common clinical problem serves as an illustration. Restoration of circulating volume remains a cardinal goal of resuscitation from circulatory shock. However, if complete fluid resuscitation is attempted before definitive control of the bleeding, a second occult shock episode may occur. This has been clinically tested: a prospective, randomized study now suggests that severe hemorrhagic shock secondary to penetrating torso injuries is best treated by withholding complete resuscitation until after surgical control of the bleeding is obtained (11).

PULMONARY ARTERY CATHETER IN SHOCK MANAGEMENT: WHETHER AND WHEN

The indications for use of the PAC (Swan-Ganz catheter) are in flux. This device is nontherapeutic and performance depends heavily on the skill of the operator and the expertise of the interpreter. Conclusions regarding its value need to be considered in the context of its use. With this in mind, the PAC appears to be overused. Although several investigators had previously questioned the value of pulmonary artery catheterization, a multicenter trial reported in 1996 that use of a pulmonary artery increased attributable mortality (12). Given the widespread use of PACs, a consensus conference was convened to examine the available evidence. The following questions, answers, and recommendations relevant to PAC use in shock are extracted directly from that report (13):

1. Does Management with the Pulmonary Artery Catheter Improve Outcome in Patients with Myocardial Infarction Complicated by Progressive Hypotension or Cardiogenic Shock? Answer: Yes; Grade: E (weakest support; derived from nonrandomized studies, historical controls and expert opinion). Recommendation: Based on expert opinion, management guided by the PAC may be beneficial for patients with acute myocardial infarction complicated by progressive hypotension or cardiogenic shock. There is, however, no conclusive proof that the PAC improves outcomes in this patient population. Research is needed to determine whether patients with acute myocardial infarction complicated by progressive hypotension or cardiogenic shock managed using the PAC have better outcomes than those patients who are managed using less-invasive diagnostic modalities.

2. Does Management with the Pulmonary Artery Catheter Improve Outcome in Patients with Shock or Hemodynamic Instability? Answer: Uncertain; Grade: E. Recommendation: The PAC may be useful in the management of patients with shock unresponsive to fluid resuscitation and use of vasopressors. Clinical trials are needed to determine whether management of various types of shock with the PAC leads to better outcomes than management using less invasive means of monitoring.

3. Does Pulmonary Artery Catheter-guided Management Improve Outcomes in Patients with Sepsis or Septic Shock? Answer: Uncertain; Grade: D (supported by at least one nonrandomized study employing contemporaneous controls). Recommendation:

The PAC may be useful in patients with septic shock who have not responded to initial aggressive fluid resuscitation and low dose inotropic/vasoconstrictor therapy. Various management strategies for sepsis and septic shock (intravenous fluids, vasoactive medications, inotropic medications, etc.) should be evaluated in prospective, randomized, controlled trials. Patient groups should be carefully defined, by source of sepsis, severity of illness, and organ dysfunction. Investigations should be designed to determine both the effectiveness of the PAC in accurate diagnosis and in monitoring patient response to therapeutic intervention. Management protocols need to be defined for both PAC-guided and non-PAC-guided groups. An independent determination of adequacy of therapeutic intervention (how closely management protocols were followed) should be an integral part of study design.

Acknowledging the paucity of data from randomized, prospective studies, it is suggested that surgeons managing myocardial infarction with progressive cardiogenic shock are justified in prompt placement of a PAC. The value of the PAC in other forms of shock is indeterminate, but in any case its use should follow routine management with fluids and pressors guided by central venous and systemic arterial pressure monitoring. Failure to respond to routine management or uncertainty concerning the response are adequate reasons to use a PAC with its attendant risks.

PROBLEM OF SECONDARY SEPSIS

Once a patient has been resuscitated and moved to the intensive care unit (ICU), the risks of sepsis are increased. The ICU has an indigenous microflora of virulent organisms available to attack immunocompromised, resuscitated patients whose defenses are further weakened by invasive devices. Prevention of secondary sepsis remains an important but very elusive goal for surgical critical care. The nosocomial component of ICU sepsis is widely acknowledged but poorly controlled. Transmission of disease from patient to provider to patient has been documented in many studies, yet compliance with hand washing and barrier (isolation) directives is poor. The indigenous flora is different from the endogenous flora, most likely as a consequence of widespread (ab)use of potent antimicrobials. As in the initial shock, recognition that the resuscitated patient is becoming secondarily septic is difficult. Once the diagnosis is suspected, selection of appropriate antibiotic therapy is relatively simple.

Patients fresh from the street, the operating room, or the surgical ward typically present with a near-classic picture including fever, flushing, and hypotension and perfusion abnormalities. Recognition of the sepsis in such cases is rapid. In sharp contrast, sepsis is extremely difficult to recognize when it occurs in patients who have been in the ICU for several days. The objective clues contributing to that impression include the following:

1. Mental status changes. The brain is exquisitely sensitive to the metabolic derangements of sepsis. Sudden, unexplained deterioration in responsiveness (or, alternatively, diminished dependence on a dose of sedative drug) must always suggest either an oxygen delivery problem (stroke, bleed, myocardial infarction) or sepsis.

2. Increased minute ventilation. Sepsis causes tachypnea. This is difficult to appreciate in the mechanically ventilated patient. Respiratory therapists provide a diagnostic tool in their charting of minute ventilatory

volume. Increasing minute ventilatory volume, particularly when oxygen saturations have been adequate, suggests sepsis or pulmonary embolism.

3. Falling urine output. Patients who have had stable urine output (a proxy for adequate organ perfusion) should continue to have a stable urine output. A falling urine output means there is a problem perfusing the kidneys, there is an acute obstruction, or the kidneys have been poisoned. The nephrotoxins are well known and recognizable on the medication list. Perfusion problems mandate interrogation of the pathways to shock. If the patient is not bleeding and not having a myocardial infarction, then he or she is septic until proven otherwise.

4. Glucose intolerance. Sepsis renders patients resistant to endogenous or administered insulin. New-onset hyperglycemia or glycosuria, or an increase in a previously stable dose of insulin, suggests sepsis.

5. Feed intolerance. Non-ICU patients who contract infections typically become anorectic; they decline food. ICU patients, who are typically fed by tube into the proximal GI tract, become intolerant of those feedings. This intolerance presents either as "residuals," which are evacuated per tube by the nurse, or more dramatically as regurgitation and vomiting.

6. Diarrhea. The administration of narcotics to surgical patients makes constipation more common than normal bowel motions. New-onset diarrhea, especially when the onset is not associated with hyperosmolar tube feedings, suggests that the normal gut mucosal barriers to infection may be failing.

7. Coagulopathy. A new-onset coagulopathy, presenting as a GI bleed or as bleeding from catheterization or surgical sites, is a common presentation of sepsis in the ICU.

8. Falling platelet count. Leukocytosis is a poor indicator of sepsis in surgical patients, for two reasons. First, elective surgery, trauma, and drug reactions cause leukocytosis in many patients. Second, leukopenia is common in advanced sepsis. The progression from leukocytosis to leukopenia traverses the normal range of values, a trajectory that may be erroneously interpreted as improvement. The clue to sepsis in the hemogram of the surgical patient is the platelet count: thrombocytopenia is common owing to the remarkable sensitivity of megakaryocytes to infection. Although thrombocytopenia may be caused by several drugs (heparin and cimetidine are commonly cited as causal), sepsis should always be considered. Occult sepsis-induced thrombocytopenia is more common in many ICUs than drug-induced thrombocytopenia.

Many patients ultimately proven septic often "just don't look right" in the initial stages. The surgeon should always address sepsis as a diagnostic possibility in that situation.

SPECIFIC INTERVENTIONS IN PERIOPERATIVE SEPTIC SHOCK

The approach to septic shock in the perioperative period requires recognition, stabilization of the patient, and identification and reversal of the underlying cause. No matter how often this adage is repeated, one or the other imperative is often neglected. The patient should be moved promptly to an ICU. Stabilization of the septic patient is conveniently organized as a resuscitation. Although the airway is rarely a problem *per se*, sepsis imposes a substantial work of breathing on patients who may be marginal to begin with. The decision to intubate and mechanically ventilate septic patients is based on clinical examination, not laboratory tests or radiographs. The metabolic load of sepsis is enormous, and few septic patients appear to breathe comfortably. The question the surgeon should ask is, "Do I think the patient is going to last 24 hours without an endotracheal tube?" Uncertainty, or any evidence of deterioration on serial examinations (which should be repeated every few minutes), should prompt intubation and mechanical support. Given the frequency of pneumonia as the underlying cause of the sepsis, sampling of tracheal secretions through the newly placed endotracheal tube for Gram's stain and culture is strongly advised. Resuscitation from the shock state should proceed rapidly. An arterial catheter may help guide therapy but is not required for initial resuscitation. It is a common error to focus time and resources on insertion of an arterial catheter before stabilization of the patient. Serial assessment of heart rate, blood pressure, pulse pressure, and central venous pressure, coupled with palpation of central pulses and the extremities, is nearly always sufficient to steer initial fluid and pressor therapy. Once the initial resuscitation is complete and specimens are sent to the laboratory, the next critical steps are to review the medical chart, the medication administration record, and the patient. The medical chart frequently contains information about past infections and medication dependencies. "Sepsis" may be confused with addisonian crisis due to inadvertent omission of corticosteroids from a prescription. The nurses' medication administration record describes the medications the patient is actually receiving as opposed to what is believed to have been ordered. Finally, there is no substitute for performing a head-to-toe examination of the newly septic patient.

If a surgical site infection (other than necrotizing myofascial infection) is identified, it must be drained. Computed tomography (CT) scans are helpful in diagnosis, and percutaneous drainage of CT-identified abscesses is often useful. If there is uncertainty regarding a surgical site infection in a patient who is deteriorating, operative inspection of a surgical site is usually a low-risk procedure in the first postoperative week. Delays for scans and studies that push the exploration clock into the second postoperative week substantially complicate the exploration because surgical inflammation is likely to intensify.

Antimicrobial therapy should be tailored to the patient and to local conditions, including the indigenous flora and resistance patterns. Decision making should consider:

1. The reflex to begin broad-spectrum antimicrobial therapy is ingrained and unlikely to change. To make this strategy useful, guidelines for what constitutes such empiric therapy for perioperative sepsis in a particular hospital should be disseminated and followed. The reason for this is that although empiric therapy often has no discernible effect on a particular patient, it has substantial effect on the flora indigenous to the ICU.

2. "Stop antibiotic" orders are rarely executed owing to confusion regarding the role of antibiotics in the patient's course. The clinician should be prepared to continue the initial selection for a long time. Given the prime directive ("First, Do No Harm"), consideration of antibiotic toxicity should play a role in the initial selection of drugs.

3. Microbiologic culture and toxin data need to be collected before, during, and after the antibiotic course. Data collected before and during the course often pro-

vide the only objective basis for simplifying broad-spectrum regimens. Data collected after the course, particularly screening data from stool specimens, may illuminate unexpected effects. Pseudomembranous colitis confirmed by detection of *Clostridium difficile* toxin is a common consequence of broad-spectrum antibiotic therapy. *Enterococcus faecium* (vancomycin-resistant enterococcus) appears with disquieting frequency.

4. Not all pathogens are bacterial. Yeasts are challenging adversaries; in particular, abdominal and bloodstream sepsis that does not respond promptly to antibacterial therapy should always raise questions regarding the presence of yeast. Immunosuppressed patients such as solid organ transplant recipients are also susceptible to viral infections, especially cytomegalovirus and other herpes viruses.

SPECIFIC PERIOPERATIVE PROBLEMS WITH SHOCK

Shock in the operating room and the perioperative period constitutes a specific problem that surgeons confront in their practice. Although the classifications discussed previously should be applied, certain diagnostic and management sequences also should be considered.

Shock in the Operating Room

Although anesthetics and operations have become progressively safer, most surgeons are eventually confronted with sudden circulatory collapse of a patient in the operating room. Such situations can be salvaged if the surgeon and anesthesiologist work rapidly to analyze and correct the problem. Should the anesthesiologist announce that the patient is *in extremis,* the most important next step is to determine whether there is ventilation and circulation. Presence of carbon dioxide in the end-tidal gas confirms that both are present. Conversely, absence of end-tidal carbon dioxide means that either ventilation or circulation, or both, has failed. Such failure requires immediate confirmation that the endotracheal tube is in the airway, immediate ventilation, and initiation of cardiac compression while the underlying cause of the arrest is sought. Open cardiac massage is more effective than closed massage, and there should be no hesitation in performing a sternotomy or thoracotomy if closed massage is not immediately effective. The cardiac rhythm should be inspected on the monitor, and the anesthesiologist asked about any changes in morphology (suggestive of myocardial ischemia or infarction) before the collapse. If a life-threatening arrhythmia is noted, it should be treated using advanced cardiac life support guidelines. If ventilation and circulation are present but there is circulatory collapse in the context of a reasonably normal cardiac rhythm, the next step is to look at the operative field while asking the anesthesiologist about the airway pressures. The surgeon must look for excessive bleeding and at the shape of the diaphragms. If significant bleeding is observed, isolation and control become the next priority. The reason to inspect the diaphragms while asking about airway pressures is that pneumothoraces are not only common, but quickly become tension pneumothoraces under positive-pressure ventilation. The diaphragm on the affected side billows into the abdomen and remains relatively distended throughout the ventilatory cycle. The airway pressures are higher than previously observed. If such a billowing diaphragm is observed, it should be immediately incised (1 to 2 cm) to convert the tension pneumothorax into an open pneumothorax.

While the surgeon is inspecting the diaphragms, the anesthesiologist should be listening for breath sounds and heart sounds. The reason for listening to the heart sounds is to exclude a rarer cause of obstructive shock, air embolism, a cause that should be suspected in any patient who either has a central venous catheter in place or who has had a large vein open in the operative field. Diagnosis is based entirely on suspicion, but the central venous catheters should be inspected and the heart should be auscultated for a continuous murmur. If air embolism is thought likely, an attempt should be made to aspirate air back through the central catheter while the patient is placed in Trendelenburg position. Management of this complication in the operating room is typically operative, aspirating the right ventricular outflow tract by direct puncture if cardiac massage proves insufficient immediately to break up the air lock. If breath sounds and heart sounds are normal and bleeding is not a problem, it should be ascertained whether there was a drop in end-tidal carbon dioxide just before the circulatory collapse. When such a drop has occurred, it suggests acute pulmonary embolism. Refractory shock caused by acute pulmonary embolism can occasionally be reversed by direct cardiac massage (breaking up the large embolus into smaller pieces) or, if appropriate personnel and equipment are immediately available, surgical retrieval of the clot.

Finally, the possibilities of anaphylaxis to a recently administered drug and of a major transfusion reaction need to be considered. In the operating room and ICU, a view of the heart and aorta in real time can provide helpful information about cardiac performance. Personnel skilled in transesophageal echocardiography who can avail themselves of the necessary equipment can rapidly obtain information about cardiac performance, exclude pericardial tamponade, and make inferences about whether the venous system is sufficiently filled within a minute or two. Resuscitation should not be interrupted while the views are being obtained.

Shock in the Immediate (0- to 4-Hour) Postoperative Period

Shock in the immediate postoperative period is attributed to bleeding until proven otherwise. Plans should be made to return the patient to the operating room while an alternative cause is sought. Alternative causes are common and include acute myocardial dysfunction and delayed presentation of a pneumothorax after positive-pressure ventilation. The value of an immediate ECG and chest radiograph cannot be overemphasized. More often than not, bleeding is either an obvious cause of the shock state or is suggested by a lower-than-expected hematocrit. Although exploration of the surgical site is mandatory, the cause of the bleeding is not always surgical, and appropriate coagulation studies should be ordered along with blood products as soon as immediate postoperative shock is recognized.

Shock in the Intermediate (4- to 24-Hour) Postoperative Period

As anesthetics and pain medications wear off, patients often experience significant pain and respond with a catecholamine surge. The associated increase in heart rate can cause or mask an evolving myocardial infarction in patients at cardiovascular risk. Surgical site pain can extinguish anginal pain, and an ECG along with chemical tests for myocardial damage should be obtained promptly. Bleeding should be no lower than number two on the differential diagnosis of shock, and resuscitation should proceed even while plans are made to return the patient to the operating room. During this interval, serious surgical site infections can cause shock. These site infections, typically streptococcal, cause a brawny cellulitis (sometimes associated with brown edema fluid) that masks a necrotizing myofascial infection. For this reason, shock appearing during the intermediate postoperative period mandates at least an inspection of the wound. If cellulitis is present, the wound should be promptly explored in the operating room, where radical débridement is undertaken. Aggressive antibiotic therapy, an adjunct to surgical débridement (not a substitute), may be lifesaving.

Shock in the Late (>24 Hours) Postoperative Period

There are four common causes of unexplained shock in the late postoperative period. Sepsis is by far the most common, including surgical site infections, bloodstream (catheter-associated) infections, urinary tract infections, and pneumonias. Myocardial infarction is also common and can occur without significant pain during the first few postoperative days. Pulmonary embolism in the setting of occult deep venous thrombosis tends to occur somewhat later because the operation and consequent immobility are usually the cause of the deep venous thrombosis, and pulmonary embolism must follow its formation. Shock and unexplained hypoxemia should suggest pulmonary embolism. Finally, occult GI bleeding causes painless hypovolemic shock that is unexplained until the oral or rectal passage of blood.

Above all, the surgeon should be aware of time. Regardless of the cause of the shock, prompt recognition of the shock state, correction of the underlying problem, and immediate resuscitation appear to be the best guarantors of a favorable outcome.

REFERENCES

1. Blalock A. *Principles of surgical care: shock and other problems.* St. Louis: Mosby, 1940.
2. Maier R. Shock. In: Greenfield LJ, Mulholland M, Oldham KT, et al, eds. *Surgery: scientific principles and practice,* 2nd ed. Philadelphia: Lippincott–Raven, 1997:182–215.
3. Godin PJ, Buchman TG. Uncoupling of biological oscillators: a complementary hypothesis concerning the pathogenesis of multiple organ dysfunction syndrome. *Crit Care Med* 1996;24:1107–1116.
4. Jacobsohn E, Chorn R, O'Connor M. The role of the vasculature in regulating venous return and cardiac output: historical and graphical approach. *Can J Anaesth* 1997;44:849–867.
5. Guyton A, Jones C, Coleman T. *Circulatory physiology: cardiac output and its regulation.* Philadelphia: WB Saunders, 1973.
6. Weber E. The law of pulsatile flow and its application to the circulation: primitive model of the circulation. In: *Berichte über die Verhandlungen der Königlich Sächsische Gessellschaft der Wissenschaften zu Leipzig.* Weidmanische Buchhandlung, 1850;2:164. Cited in Lodato RF. Cardiovascular derangement in septic shock and nitric oxide. *J Crit Care* 1996;11:151–154.
7. Bayliss WM, Starling EH. Observations on venous pressures and their relationship to capillary pressures. *J Physiol (Lond)* 1894;16:159–202.
8. Starr I, Rawson AJ. Role of the "static blood pressure" in abnormal increments of venous pressure, especially in heart failure: I. Theoretical studies on an improved circulation schema whose pumps obey Starling's law of the heart. *Am J Med Sci* 1940;199:27–39.
9. Gomersall CD, Joynt GM, Freebairn RC, et al. Resuscitation of critically ill patients based on the results of gastric tonometry: a prospective, randomized, controlled trial. *Crit Care Med* 2000;28:607–614.
10. Zeni F, Freeman B, Natanson C. Anti-inflammatory therapies to treat sepsis and septic shock: a reassessment. *Crit Care Med* 1997;25:1095–1100.
11. Bickell WH, Wall MJ Jr, Pepe PE, et al. Immediate versus delayed fluid resuscitation for hypotensive patients with penetrating torso injuries. *N Engl J Med* 1994;331:1105–1109.
12. Connors AF Jr, Speroff T, Dawson NV, et al. The effectiveness of right heart catheterization in the initial care of critically ill patients. *JAMA* 1996;18:889–897.
13. Anonymous. Pulmonary Artery Catheter Consensus Conference: consensus statement. *Crit Care Med* 1997;25:910–925.

SURGERY: SCIENTIFIC PRINCIPLES AND PRACTICE, Third Edition, edited by Lazar J. Greenfield, Michael W. Mulholland, Keith T. Oldham, Gerald B. Zelenock, and Keith D. Lillemoe. Lippincott Williams & Wilkins Publishers, Philadelphia, © 2001.

CHAPTER 9

CRITICAL CARE

ROBERT H. BARTLETT

Although critical care has emerged as a distinct discipline, it involves nothing more or less than the care of our sickest patients. Intensive care units (ICUs) originated with the beginnings of cardiac surgery in the early 1960s. Cardiac surgical patients had new and special monitors—continuous electrocardiograms, intraarterial catheters, and central venous pressure catheters. It was often necessary to keep these patients on mechanical ventilators overnight and sometimes for 1 or 2 days. Monitors and devices made it possible to treat patients according to the principles of cardiorespiratory physiology, previously possible only in the laboratory. As surgeons learned these techniques in cardiac surgery, they extended them to the care of other surgical patients—vascular, trauma, and neurologic. Some of the recovery room nurses learned to manage ventilators, amplifiers, oscilloscopes, and the other gadgetry of the extended recovery room. Eventually, care of these patients became a full-time nursing responsibility. Nurses and machinery began to overflow the recovery room, and ICUs were established. Through the 1970s, critical care became a defined nursing specialty, with special training and certification required, and a society and a journal established. Every major hospital developed intensive care nursing units, where these nurses could practice their specialty. The concept spread among medical disciplines, from surgery to medicine to pediatrics to neonatology. By the 1980s, some physicians began to focus their practices on critically ill patients, and some internists and anesthesiologists limited their practices to the critically ill patients of other, primary physicians. "Reanimation" became a subspecialty of anesthesiology throughout Europe.

Surgeons have always been at the forefront of critical care as part of their routine practices. The concept of assigning preoperative or postoperative care to other colleagues runs counter to the training and responsibility of surgeons. Surgical intensive care nursing units, however, required policies, administration, and supervision, and surgeons took on these jobs. Within the past decade, the discipline has become specialized enough to warrant fellowship training, examination, and certification by the American Board of Surgery in surgical critical care. Similar certification is offered by the boards of medicine, anesthesiology, and pediatrics.

Issues of administration and supervision aside, critical care remains simply the business of applying the principles of physiology and pharmacology in the treatment of the sickest patients. This chapter focuses on the basic principles and mechanics of that practice. Although the principles of management and physiology are universal, the examples and numbers in this chapter relate to adult patients. The chapter assumes a thorough knowledge of basic physiology on the part of the reader.

The ICU affords the possibility to monitor a wide variety of physiologic variables continuously and to use that information to prevent and treat organ failure. Central to the intelligent use of this information is an understanding of homeostatic physiology: integrated cardiac, respiratory, and metabolic physiology (oxygen kinetics); respiratory physiology; body fluids and hemodynamics; nutrition and metabolism; and renal pathophysiology.

OXYGEN KINETICS: INTEGRATING HEMODYNAMIC, RESPIRATORY, AND METABOLIC PHYSIOLOGY

Oxygen Consumption

Oxygen consumed in the process of metabolism is expressed as the volume of oxygen per minute ($\dot{V}O_2$). $\dot{V}O_2$ is normally 100 to 120 mL/m^2 per minute, or 200 mL/min for a typical adult. Resting $\dot{V}O_2$ is a function of the metabolizing body cell mass, with fine-tuned control provided by thyroid and catecholamine hormones and a poorly understood metabolic regulator in the hypothalamus. $\dot{V}O_2$ decreases under conditions of hypothermia, paralysis, and hypothyroidism. $\dot{V}O_2$ increases during exercise or other muscular activity, hyperthermia, profound hypothalamic injury, hyperthyroidism, and rises in the levels of catecholamines and inflammatory mediators, particularly the interleukin cytokines. Under steady-state conditions, the amount of O_2 consumed in systemic metabolism is exactly equal to the amount of O_2 taken up in the pulmonary capillaries through the airway. This is true regardless of the status of pulmonary function or dysfunction, so $\dot{V}O_2$ is measured across the lung with the assumption that this is exactly the amount consumed in systemic metabolism.

Oxygen Delivery

The amount of O_2 that is delivered to peripheral tissues is the product of the O_2 content in arterial blood and the cardiac output. Normally, the O_2 content of arterial blood (CaO_2) is about 20 mL/dL, and the normal cardiac index is 3.2 L/m^2 per minute, or 5 L/min for a typical adult. Therefore, the normal systemic delivery of O_2 (DO_2) is 20 mL/dL $\times$ 50 dL/min, or 1,000 mL/min. Although the O_2 content is the most important measure of O_2 in blood, the partial pressure of oxygen (PO_2) and the oxyhemoglobin saturation are more commonly measured in the ICU; hence, it is necessary to convert these measurements. Each gram of hemoglobin can bind 1.36 mL of O_2. If the hemoglobin level of the blood is normal (15 g/dL) and the hemoglobin is 98% saturated, the amount of O_2 bound to hemoglobin is 19.9 mL/dL. In addition, a small amount of O_2 is physically dissolved in the water that makes up plasma and red blood cells. The solubility coefficient for O_2 is 0.0031 mL/mm Hg per deciliter; therefore, the amount of O_2 dissolved in 1 dL of blood at a PO_2 of 100 mm Hg is 0.3 mL, so that the O_2 content of normal arterial blood 19.9 + 0.3 or 20.2 mL/dL, conveniently rounded off to 20 mL/dL. Through the same arithmetic, the O_2 content of venous blood (CvO_2) is 16 mL/dL; hence, the normal arteriovenous difference in O_2 content (avO_2 difference) is 4 mL/dL. The relation between PO_2, saturation, and O_2 content for different concentrations of hemoglobin is shown in Fig. 9.1. Note that the arterial partial pressure of oxygen (PaO_2) and saturation are the same for normal arterial and venous blood, even though the O_2 content is severely decreased in anemia.

Autoregulation to Maintain Oxygen Delivery

The relations between $\dot{V}O_2$ and DO_2 represent one of the most interesting autoregulation systems in homeostasis. First of all, if one of the three components of O_2 delivery is abnormal, endogenous mechanisms regulate the other two until normal O_2 delivery has been restored. In compensation for acute hypoxia or acute anemia, cardiac output increases, but only until normal O_2 delivery is reestablished. In chronic hypoxia, the red cell mass increases until systemic O_2 delivery is normal at normal cardiac output. In chronic anemia, cardiac output increases and remains increased. When cardiac output is decreased, no mechanism induces superoxygenation or polycythemia. In this situation, O_2 consumption generally continues at the normal metabolic rate and relatively more O_2 is extracted from the flowing blood, so that the avO_2 difference is widened. The various combinations of these compensatory mechanisms supply adequate O_2 for systemic metabolism through a wide range of values for O_2 delivery. If the level of O_2 delivery cannot be maintained at the least at twice the level of O_2 consumption, an unstable state results, described later.

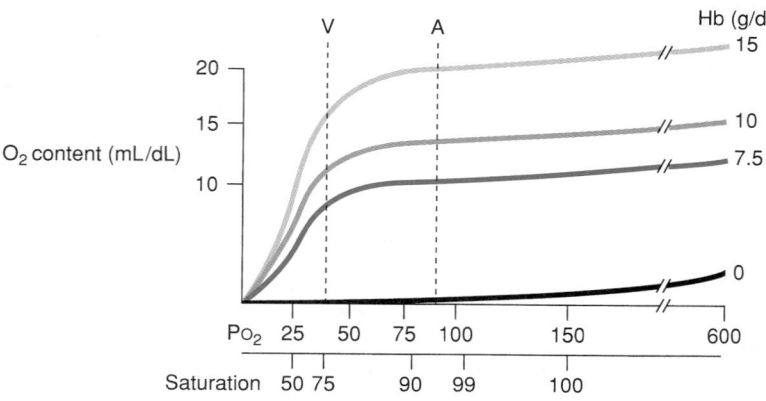

Figure 9.1. The relation of O_2 content, saturation, and PO_2. Typical normal levels in arterial and venous blood are defined at various levels of hemoglobin. (After Bartlett RH. *University of Michigan critical care handbook*. Boston: Little, Brown, 1996, with permission.)

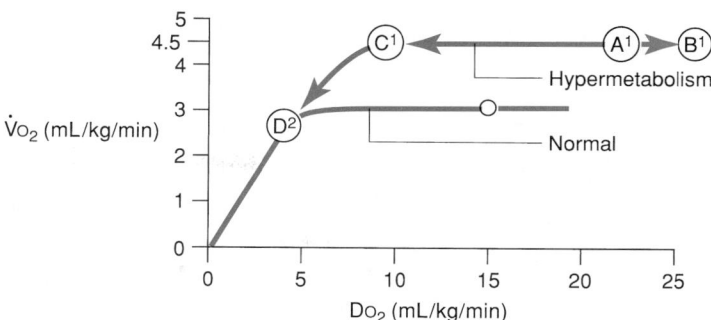

Figure 9.2. The relation of O_2 consumption to a wide range of changes in O_2 delivery. Examples are shown for normal metabolism *(circle)* and hypermetabolic status *(A¹)*. (After Bartlett RH, Anderson HL. Multiorgan failure. In: Zelenock GB, D'Alecy LG, Fantone JC, et al., eds. *Clinical ischemic syndromes: mechanisms and consequences of tissue injury.* St. Louis: Mosby, 1989:565, with permission.)

Autoregulation for Changing Oxygen Consumption

When a change in $\dot{V}O_2$ occurs, a proportional change in DO_2 occurs almost immediately, mediated completely by a change in cardiac output. For example, if a person goes from rest to mild exercise, an increase in $\dot{V}O_2$ occurs, followed promptly by an increase of cardiac output (*A* to *A¹* in Fig. 9.2), which reestablishes the ratio of delivery to consumption at about 5:1. The mechanism that mediates this change in cardiac output is not fully understood but is probably related to a chemoreceptor on the venous side of the circulation. This autoregulation occurs whether the change in $\dot{V}O_2$ is an increase or a decrease and whether it is caused by exercise, sepsis, catecholamines, or other mediators.

Autoregulation for Changing Oxygen Delivery

Conversely, a primary change in O_2 delivery is *not* followed by any change in O_2 consumption, nor would $\dot{V}O_2$ be expected to change; systemic O_2 delivery is not one of the controllers of metabolism. If DO_2 fell below the level of $\dot{V}O_2$, however, $\dot{V}O_2$ would become supply-dependent. In theory, this situation would occur when the ratio of delivery to consumption fell below 1:1. In actuality, this condition of $\dot{V}O_2$ supply dependency occurs when the DO_2 value falls to below twice the $\dot{V}O_2$ value; in other words, supply dependency occurs when the ratio of DO_2 to $\dot{V}O_2$ is less than 2:1. This relation is shown in Fig. 9.3, which demonstrates the biphasic nature of the $\dot{V}O_2$ and DO_2 relationship. When a state of supply dependency exists, anaerobic metabolism occurs, the patient experiences O_2 "debt," and hemodynamic instability eventually results. If the situation lasts long enough, progressive organ failure develops, and the patient can be said to be in a state of circulatory, ischemic,

or hypoxic shock. The same relations exist when $\dot{V}O_2$ is elevated during a hypermetabolic state (Fig. 9.2). Supply dependency occurs during hypermetabolism whenever the $DO_2/\dot{V}O_2$ ratio is less than 2:1, although during hypermetabolism, this happens at a higher level of actual DO_2 than it does during normal metabolism. The primary goals of intensive care and management are to estimate or determine the $\dot{V}O_2$ and DO_2 values, maintain the patient near the normal ratio of 5:1, and, if O_2 delivery fails, intervene before the ratio reaches the critical low level of 2:1.

Monitoring of Venous Saturation

The relation between DO_2 and $\dot{V}O_2$ is reflected in the amount of O_2 in venous blood. Under normal conditions, DO_2 is 1,000 mL/min and $\dot{V}O_2$ is 200 mL/min. The amount of O_2 extracted is 20% of that delivered, with 80% of the O_2 still present in venous blood returning to the heart. Usually, arterial blood is fully saturated, and under normal circumstances, the saturation of mixed venous blood ($S\dot{V}O_2$) is 80%. (This measurement must be made in mixed venous blood because the relative rates of extraction in organs served by the superior and inferior venae cavae and coronary sinus are different.) If an $S\dot{V}O_2$ of 80% corresponds to a 5:1 ratio, then 75% corresponds to 4:1, 60% to 3:1, 50% to 2:1, and so on. As long as the arterial blood is fully saturated, this observation holds true regardless of the absolute level of DO_2 or $\dot{V}O_2$ (Fig. 9.4). If the arterial blood is less than fully saturated, the difference between arterial and venous saturation corresponds to the O_2 extraction and, hence, to the $DO_2/\dot{V}O_2$ ratio. For example, if the arterial blood were 80% saturated and the venous blood were 64% saturated, the ratio would be 5:1.

All these interrelations were originally defined by Fick in 1870. Fick's axiom is that O_2 consumption through the airway is equal to that in peripheral tissues. In his equation, cardiac output equals $\dot{V}O_2$ divided by the avO_2 differ-

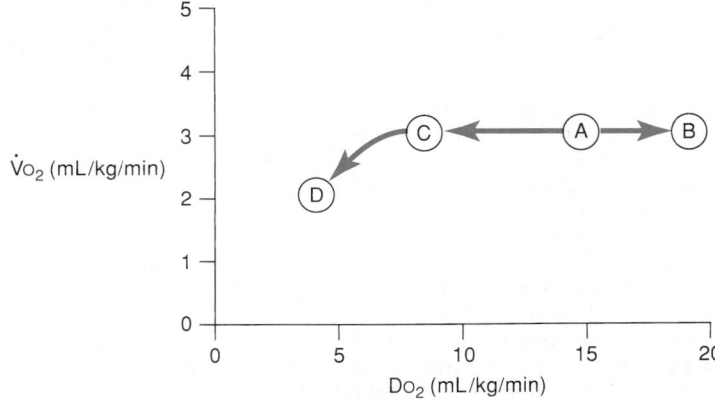

Figure 9.3. Normally *(A),* systemic O_2 delivery is about 15 mL/kg per minute and O_2 consumption is 3 mL/kg per minute. Consumption becomes supply-dependent when delivery is very low *(C to D).* Delivery increases in response to increased metabolism *(A to B).* (After Bartlett RH, Anderson HL. Multiorgan failure. In: Zelenock GB, D'Alecy LG, Fantone JC, et al., eds. *Clinical ischemic syndromes: mechanisms and consequences of tissue injury.* St. Louis: Mosby, 1989:565, with permission.)

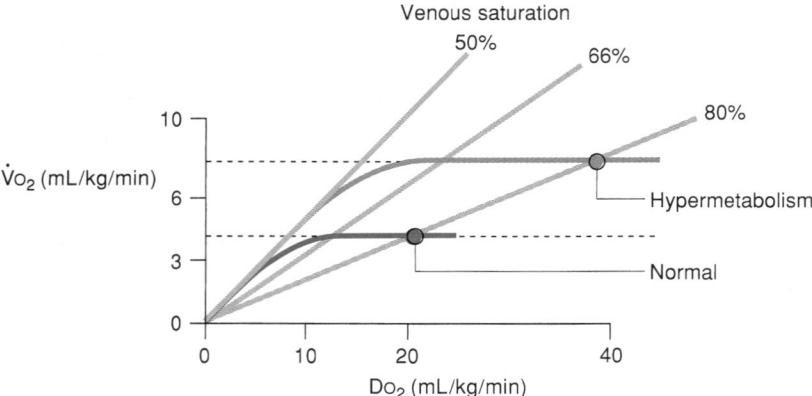

Figure 9.4. Saturation of mixed venous blood for a wide range of ratios between O_2 delivery and consumption. Provided that arterial blood is nearly saturated, venous saturation reflects the ratio between delivery and consumption. (After Bartlett RH. *University of Michigan critical care handbook*. Boston; Little, Brown, 1996, with permission.)

ence, which can also be expressed as avO_2 difference times cardiac output equals $\dot{V}O_2$.

In critically ill patients, $\dot{V}O_2$ may be elevated or depressed, but a slight to moderate elevation in $\dot{V}O_2$ is the most common abnormality in critically ill patients. $\dot{V}O_2$ is elevated in proportion to the degree of inflammation (either bacterial or sterile, as in burns and pancreatitis). A febrile patient with significant signs of septic toxicity typically has a $\dot{V}O_2$ that is 1.5 to 2 times normal. It is unusual for the $\dot{V}O_2$ of a critically ill patient to be more than twice normal. This occurs only in situations of severe muscular exercise, as in seizures or tetanus. $\dot{V}O_2$ is decreased in critically ill patients who are hypothermic.

During hypermetabolism, a change in $\dot{V}O_2$ is followed promptly by a proportional change in DO_2; thus, it is normal for a hypermetabolic patient to have a high cardiac output and pulse rate—that is, to be hyperdynamic. Rarely, the hyperdynamic response exceeds the increase in $\dot{V}O_2$; this situation, reflected in a ratio higher than 5:1 and a venous saturation above 80%, can occur when a large arteriovenous fistula is present, caused either by direct vascular communication or by hyperperfusion of tissues, as in portal hypertension with excessive perfusion of the splanchnic viscera. Some patients cannot mount an increased DO_2 in response to an increased $\dot{V}O_2$ because of any combination of hypoxia, anemia, and myocardial failure. If this occurs, then the $DO_2/\dot{V}O_2$ ratio is less than 5:1, the avO_2 difference widens, the $S\dot{V}O_2$ falls, the amount of O_2 extracted from each deciliter of blood increases, and the patient is using up the systemic O_2 reserves. This increased extraction is perfectly adequate compensation, however, and the patient remains stable as long as the ratio is greater than 2:1. When the various mechanisms of delivery cannot maintain a DO_2 of at least twice the $\dot{V}O_2$, supply dependency and shock occur.

In a series of clinical studies, it has been claimed that the biphasic relation is absent and that a continuous state of $\dot{V}O_2$ supply dependency exists in patients with acute respiratory distress syndrome or sepsis. These studies are marred by artifacts of clinical investigation and are not supported by laboratory studies in which all the variables can be evaluated. It appears, however, that the "knee" of the biphasic curve may be shifted to the right in sepsis, so that the critical ratio is closer to 3:1 than 2:1.

The shape of the oxyhemoglobin dissociation curve, shown in Fig. 9.1, changes in various conditions, moving to the right during acidosis, hypercarbia, and hyperthermia. Although these changes are of physiologic importance (e.g., they facilitate systemic O_2 unloading during ischemia and acidosis), their effects on O_2 content and the relation to PO_2 and saturation are relatively minor compared with the effects of hemoglobin on O_2 content.

RESPIRATORY PHYSIOLOGY AND PATHOPHYSIOLOGY

Carbon Dioxide Kinetics: Ventilation and Metabolism

As mentioned, O_2 uptake across the lung is related to ventilation–perfusion ($\dot{V}/\dot{Q}$) relations and alveolar PO_2. The excretion of carbon dioxide (CO_2), on the other hand, is related to the amount of ventilation. Because CO_2 is much more diffusible than O_2, and because a large amount of CO_2 is excreted during a short period of hyperventilation, the limiting factors controlling oxygenation and CO_2 removal are different.

The total amount of CO_2 produced by systemic metabolism is roughly equivalent to the amount of O_2 consumed (100 to 120 mL/m^2 per minute, or 200 mL/min in a typical adult). The ratio between CO_2 produced and O_2 consumed is referred to as the *respiratory quotient* (RQ) and varies slightly depending on the foodstuff being metabolized.

The production of CO_2 is increased or decreased by each of the factors that causes an increase or decrease in $\dot{V}O_2$. Most of the CO_2 in blood is present as bicarbonate ion, the amount of which cannot change quickly (somewhat analogous to the total blood hemoglobin or red cell mass in relation to O_2). The metabolically produced CO_2, however, is mostly present as dissolved CO_2, added to the blood in the peripheral tissues and excreted in the lung. The relations between CO_2 content, bicarbonate, and dissolved CO_2 are shown in Fig. 9.5. Note that the avO_2 difference for CO_2 is 4 mL/dL, the same as that for O_2. In a steady state, the amount of CO_2 excreted through the lung is exactly equal to the amount of CO_2 produced in peripheral tissues. Because the amount excreted is so easily influenced by minor changes in ventilation, however, the assurance of a steady state is particularly important when $\dot{V}CO_2$ is measured at the airway. The amount of CO_2 excreted is a function of ventilation of perfused alveoli (i.e., alveolar ventilation per minute). The relation between alveolar ventilation and CO_2 excretion is shown in Fig. 9.6.

Pathophysiology of Gas Exchange

Gas transfer in the lung and the causes of hypoxemia are demonstrated in Fig. 9.7. Under normal conditions, red blood cells in the pulmonary capillaries become fully saturated and O_2 dissolves in the plasma; the result is a blood PO_2 of 100 mm Hg (when equilibrium is reached at the end of a resting expiration) and a saturation of 100% (alveolus *A* in Fig. 9.7). This equilibration may be disturbed by hypoventilation in relation to perfusion, or $\dot{V}/\dot{Q}$ mismatch (alveolus *B* in Fig. 9.7); diffusion block caused by intersti-

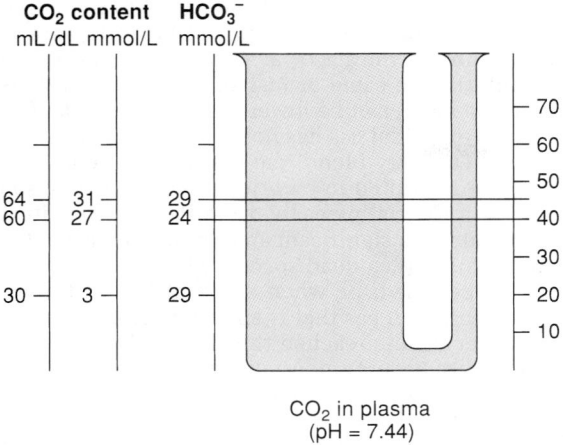

CO₂ content   HCO₃⁻
mL/dL mmol/L   mmol/L

Figure 9.5. A beaker holding CO_2 represents the partitioning of CO_2 between the bicarbonate fraction and the dissolved or carbonic acid fraction in blood. Normal levels for arterial and venous blood are defined. (After Bartlett RH. Post-traumatic pulmonary insufficiency. In: Cooper P, Nyhus L, eds. *Surgery annual, 1971.* New York: Appleton-Century-Crofts, 1971, with permission.)

tial fibrosis (alveolus *C* in Fig. 9.7); or perfusion of non-ventilated alveoli, which is simply the extreme of hypoventilation (alveolus *D* in Fig. 9.7). Diffusion block and $\dot{V}/\dot{Q}$ mismatch can be almost completely overcome by breathing 100% O_2; thus, hypoxemia during exposure to high alveolar PO_2 is caused by total $\dot{V}/\dot{Q}$ mismatch, called *transpulmonary shunting* or *venous admixture.* Under normal conditions, about 5% of the blood entering the left atrium has been shunted away from the pulmonary capillaries, either as a result of bronchial nutritive blood flow or through thebesian veins opening directly into the left side of the heart. This phenomenon, combined with the normal minor $\dot{V}/\dot{Q}$ mismatch associated with breathing at rest and positional effects on pulmonary blood flow, results in a normal arterial PO_2 of 90 to 100 mm Hg and a normal arterial blood oxygen saturation (SaO_2) of 98%. The extent to which various degrees of transpulmonary shunting affect arterial oxygenation is shown in Fig. 9.8. The shunt fraction is actually calculated by assuming that the blood in capillaries in those alveolar units that are functioning normally is fully saturated and oxygenated. In addition, it is assumed that the blood passing through areas of transpulmonary shunt is identical to venous blood. With these assumptions, the fraction of blood passing through the shunt can be calculated as the O_2 content

of blood leaving the capillaries of normal alveoli minus the O_2 content of arterial blood divided by the O_2 content of blood leaving normal alveoli minus the O_2 content of venous blood.

Obviously, the effect of the O_2 content of venous blood in the shunt calculation is considerable; when O_2 delivery is decreased because of low cardiac output or a low hemoglobin concentration, the venous saturation falls and the shunt fraction is increased. The shunt fraction can be calculated at any value for the fraction of inspired oxygen (FIO_2), but such a calculation includes components of diffusion block and $\dot{V}/\dot{Q}$ mismatch when the FIO_2 is less than 1. The level of lung dysfunction can be similarly estimated by calculating the alveolar–arterial (Aa) gradient for O_2 or the PaO_2 divided by the FIO_2. The Aa gradient is calculated as follows:

$$AaO_2 \text{ gradient} = (P_B - P_{H_2O}) \times FIO_2 - PaCO_2 - PaO_2$$
where
$$P_B = \text{barometric pressure}$$
$$P_{H_2O} = 47 \text{ mm Hg at } 37°C$$

and the alveolar PCO_2 is identical to the arterial PCO_2 (not necessarily true).

With these assumptions, the normal Aa gradient is about 10 mm Hg, and an Aa gradient above 500 corresponds to about 30% transpulmonary shunt. Dividing the PaO_2 by the FIO_2 is simply a shortened method to characterize the Aa gradient without all the calculations. The normal value is 500, and a value of 100 corresponds to a 30% shunt. Finally, interruption of the blood flow to alveoli has no effect on oxygenation, except for the diversion of blood flow to all the other areas of lung (alveolus *E* in Fig. 9.7). If the remainder of the lung is basically normal, then occlusion of the pulmonary arteries should have no effect on oxygenation. Patients with pulmonary embolism can become hypoxic, however, because (a) blood flow must increase through areas of $\dot{V}/\dot{Q}$ mismatch and shunting, (b) right atrial pressure increases to the point at which right-to-left shunting occurs through the foramen ovale, or (c) the residence time of red blood cells in pulmonary capillaries becomes so short that the time for oxygenation is inadequate. Of these causes, the latter can be largely corrected with supplemental O_2, which raises the gradient for O_2 diffusion in the pulmonary capillaries.

Carbon Dioxide Transfer in the Lung

The excretion of CO_2 is directly related to the alveolar ventilation, as discussed earlier. Even if 70% to 80% of the alveoli are not inflated, hyperventilation of the remaining 25% can maintain normocarbia in arterial blood, whereas profound hypoxemia results from 70% to 80% shunt re-

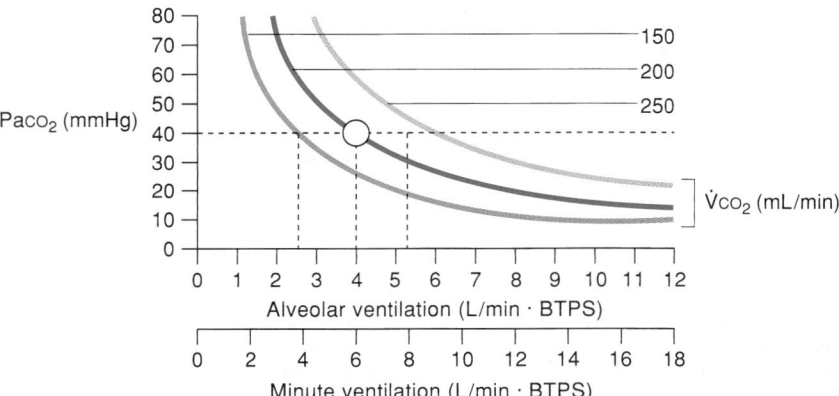

Figure 9.6. Alveolar ventilation required to excrete different levels of metabolically produced CO_2. (Adapted from Nunn JF. *Applied respiratory physiology.* London: Butterworth-Heineman, 1969;2:9, with permission.)

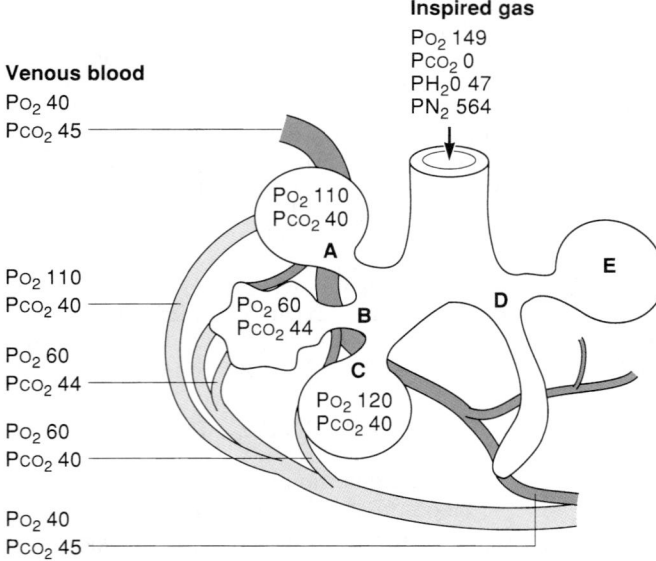

Figure 9.7. Variables affecting pulmonary gas exchange while air is breathed. In alveolus *A,* blood flow and ventilation are equal and normal. The values in the alveolus and the exiting blood represent the end of a normal resting exhalation. Alveolus *B* represents hypoventilation. Alveolus *C* represents diffusion block. Alveolus *D* represents collapse or transpulmonary shunt. Alveolus *E* is ventilated without blood flow. (After Bartlett RH. Posttraumatic pulmonary insufficiency. In: Cooper P, Nyhus L, eds. *Surgery annual, 1971.* New York: Appleton-Century-Crofts, 1971, with permission.)

gardless of the level of FIO_2 or ventilation of the remaining alveoli. These relations are shown in Fig. 9.9, which again illustrates that oxygenation is a function of matching blood flow to alveolar inflation, whereas CO_2 excretion is a function of ventilation or hyperventilation of alveoli with some blood flow. Normally, the end-tidal CO_2 represents mixed alveolar gas that is in equilibrium with pulmonary capillary blood and hence with arterial blood. Therefore, the end-tidal CO_2 and the partial pressure of arterial carbon dioxide ($PaCO_2$) should be almost identical.

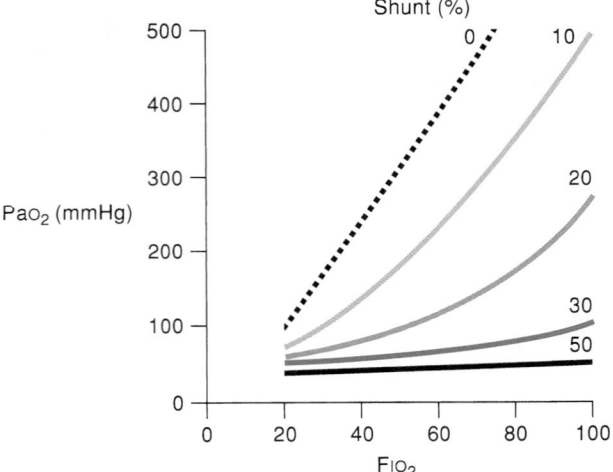

Figure 9.8. The PaO_2 values achieved at variable levels of FIO_2 and variable levels of shunt. These calculations assume normal hemoglobin and a venous saturation of 75%. (After Bartlett RH. *University of Michigan critical care handbook.* Boston; Little, Brown, 1996, with permission.)

The respiratory center is keenly sensitive to the $PaCO_2$, so that the automatic rate and depth of breathing are regulated to maintain the $PaCO_2$ at 40 mm Hg. The end-tidal CO_2 should be the same or just slightly less. There is no way that the $PaCO_2$ can be lower than the end-tidal CO_2. If some of the end-tidal gas has not been in equilibrium with pulmonary capillary blood, the gas does not contain CO_2 and the CO_2 is diluted in end-tidal measurements, so that the end-tidal CO_2 is lower than the $PaCO_2$. This situation occurs whenever a significant amount of lung is ventilated but not perfused (i.e., dead space) or is overventilated and minimally perfused, or when some of the end-tidal gas represents inflation gas that is simply compressed and released, never having reached the alveoli. The latter situation inevitably occurs under any positive-pressure ventilation circumstance but creates a significant end-tidal $PaCO_2$ gradient only when peak airway pressures are very high (> 30 cm H_2O) and when the compression volume is a significant component of each exhaled breath. The end-tidal CO_2 measurement, then, becomes a useful continuous monitor of $PaCO_2$ when the lung is nearly normal, as in ventilator weaning. In addition, the gradient between end-tidal and arterial CO_2, when it is large, serves as an indirect measure of nonperfused alveoli or compression volume, or both.

Pulmonary Mechanics

The interrelations of gas volumes and pressures in ventilation are referred to as *pulmonary mechanics.* The use of a mechanical ventilator is an exercise in pulmonary mechanics, which can be illustrated by comparing the compliance curve for a normal lung with that for an atelectatic or edematous lung. The standard compliance or volume–pressure curve, shown in Fig. 9.10, is drawn by mea-

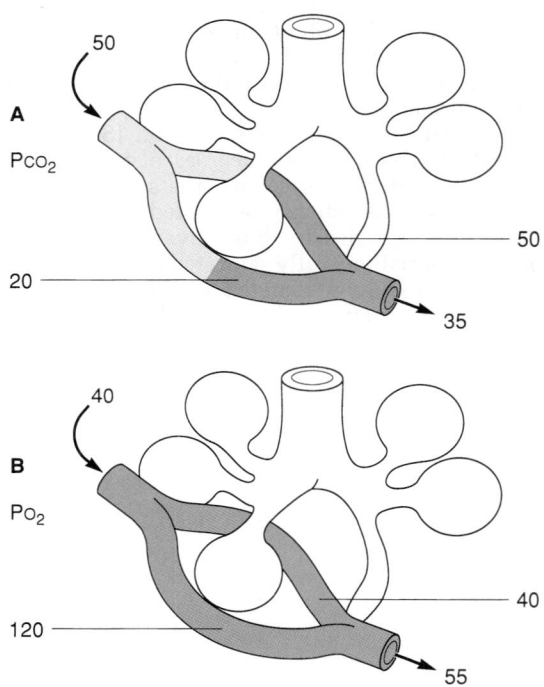

Figure 9.9. The effects of collapsed alveoli (transpulmonary shunt) on the exchange of O_2 and CO_2 in the lung. *(A)* Exchange of CO_2 is limited by ventilation of perfused lung. *(B)* Exchange of O_2 is limited by blood uptake of O_2 in ventilated lung. (After Bartlett RH. Pulmonary pathophysiology in surgical patients. *Surg Clin North Am* 1980;60:1323, with permission.)

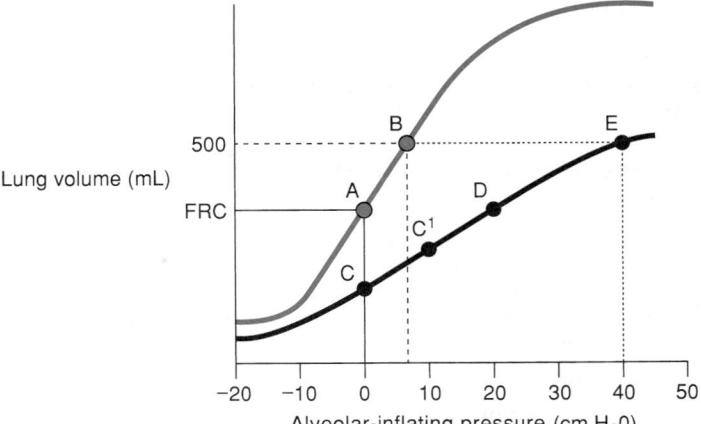

Figure 9.10. Volume–pressure (compliance) curves representing a normal lung *(A and B)* and an atelectatic or edematous lung *(C through E)*. The functional reserve capacity is decreased *(A to C)*, and more pressure is required for inflation *(C to D to E)*. (After Bartlett RH. Use of mechanical ventilation. In: Holcroft J, ed. *Care of the surgical patient,* vol 1. *Critical care.* New York: Scientific American Medicine, 1989;2:9, with permission.)

suring volume and pressure at stages of lung *deflation* after total inflation. (Although the *inflation* volume–pressure curve provides useful information, the literature and this discussion focus on the standard deflation curve.) Volume–pressure curves for normal lungs in three different patients are shown in Fig. 9.11. Notice that the curve for a normal 35-kg child is the same as that for an adult with major atelectasis. (It would be similar after pneumonectomy in an adult.) This emphasizes the point that the functional lung in acute respiratory failure is smaller, but not necessarily "stiffer." In the example shown in Fig. 9.10, inflation of the normal lung with 500 mL of gas requires a pressure of 8 cm H_2O and moves the patient from point *A* to point *B*. When the pressure is released, exhalation occurs passively, and lung volume returns to point *A*. Periodic inflation to 25 or 30 cm H_2O would achieve near-total alveolar inflation without causing overdistension. Each exhaled breath includes gas that is compressed in the ventilator system and compressed in the air space of the lung during ventilation (appearing as additional dead space ventilation), but this compression volume is small at the pressure of 8 cm H_2O required for normal tidal volume when compliance is normal.

In acute respiratory failure, the cause of decreased compliance is almost always associated with a decrease in the functional residual capacity (FRC) (Fig. 9.10). The decreased FRC represents lost alveoli, which are either collapsed or filled with fluid but still perfused with blood. Because the lung is smaller, the compliance curve is shifted to the right, and much higher pressures are required to achieve the same level of inflation. To inflate the lung to point *E,* for example, a pressure of 40 cm H_2O would be necessary. One way of managing ventilation in this circumstance is to maintain positive end-expiratory pressure (PEEP) at 10 cm H_2O *(C¹ in Fig. 9.10)* and ventilate to point *D* with tidal breathing. The PEEP is set at this level to maintain the inflation of alveoli that might close at lower end-expiratory pressures. The elevated peak inspiratory pressure is used to recruit closed alveoli. When that happens, the functional lung is bigger, and the entire compliance curve shifts back toward the left.

Several measurements must be taken to determine whether positive airway pressure is recruiting collapsed alveoli or simply distending normal alveoli (Fig. 9.12). As collapsed alveoli are reinflated, compliance improves, dead space ventilation decreases, cardiac output is unaffected, oxygenation increases at the same ventilator settings as shunt decreases, and the risk of air leak is minimal. These principles and measurements must be kept in mind during the treatment of the patient on a mechanical ventilator.

Lung damage can be caused by high airway pressure, so that the overdistension shown in Fig. 9.12 is not merely inefficient but actually detrimental. Because the most normal areas of lung have the best compliance, they are the

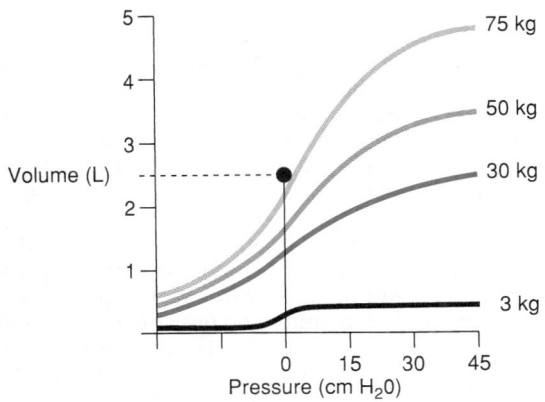

Figure 9.11. Lung volume and pressure in patients of different sizes (or lung volumes of different sizes in an adult patient). The decreased compliance in acute respiratory distress syndrome occurs because the lung is smaller, not because it is stiffer.

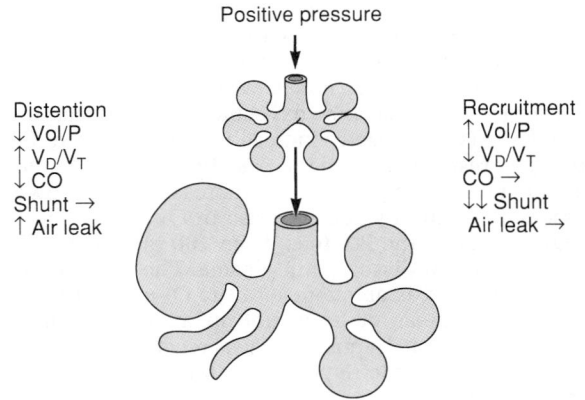

Figure 9.12. During mechanical ventilation, the gas volume may inflate alveoli equally (recruitment) or overdistend selected alveoli (distention). (After Bartlett RH. Pulmonary pathophysiology in surgical patients. *Surg Clin North Am* 1980;60:1323, with permission.)

most vulnerable to overdistention, and this vulnerability contributes to the steady progression of lung dysfunction in patients ventilated at high peak pressure. Every effort should be made to keep the peak inspiratory pressure under 45 cm H_2O, preferably lower.

Pathophysiology of Respiratory Failure

Regardless of the specific cause, pulmonary dysfunction can be classified as (a) *alveolar collapse,* partial or complete (i.e., decreased FRC), or (b) *pulmonary edema,* caused by high hydrostatic pressure, increased capillary permeability, or both.

Alveolar Collapse

A decrease in FRC is caused by incomplete alveolar inflation related to (a) shallow breathing; (b) partial or complete airway occlusion, which can be generalized (as in bronchospasm) or localized (as in gastric aspiration); (c) absorption atelectasis, which occurs when O_2 is substituted for nitrogen in the inspired gas; or (d) conditions in which air or fluid occupies potential alveolar space in the chest, such as pneumothorax, hemothorax, or pulmonary edema. Pulmonary arteriolar spasm in response to local hypoxia autoregulates pulmonary blood flow and maintains adequate gas exchange during alveolar collapse—up to a point. When the loss in ventilation exceeds the decrease in perfusion, $\dot{V}/\dot{Q}$ mismatch occurs, which results in incomplete oxygenation of blood perfusing that area of lung. The resultant hypoxemia stimulates an increased rate and depth of breathing, which may serve to reexpand the partially inflated area of lung. If it does not, the hypoxemia continues, but increased ventilation in other areas of lung results in excess CO_2 excretion, hypocapnia, and respiratory alkalosis. This blood gas picture, hypoxemia with respiratory alkalosis, is the most common abnormality of gas exchange in surgical patients and is the hallmark of $\dot{V}/\dot{Q}$ imbalance.

The oxygenation of blood in the poorly ventilated area of lung can be increased by increasing the concentration of O_2 in the inspired gas. As long as the airways are pinhole patent and the alveoli are inflated at all, the hypoxemia of $\dot{V}/\dot{Q}$ imbalance can be reversed by providing supplemental O_2. Of course, the use of supplemental O_2 treats the symptom rather than the basic cause and may actually make problems worse by exacerbating absorption atelectasis and depriving the poorly ventilated area of nitrogen to hold open the alveoli. This situation can lead to total alveolar collapse. In that circumstance, blood perfusing the nonventilated area (transpulmonary shunt) mixes with blood from other areas of the lung; the result is hypoxemia that is not significantly relieved by the administration of O_2.

The reasons for this are shown in Fig. 9.9. Blood perfusing the atelectatic lung mixes with blood perfusing the more normal lung, so that oxygenation is decreased and blood CO_2 is increased. Increasing the inspired O_2 to 100% may result in a large increase in P_{O_2} in the blood exiting the normal lung. The major increase in P_{O_2}, however, is associated with a small increase in O_2 *content* because the O_2 that raises the P_{O_2} (e.g., from 100 to 500 mm Hg) is the small amount dissolved in plasma. The oxygenation of the arterial blood is an average of the O_2 content of blood from the two areas of lung, not an average of the P_{O_2}. Therefore, systemic hypoxia persists regardless of the F_{IO_2}. When this hypoxemic hypercapnic blood reaches the respiratory center, the rate and depth of breathing are increased. The result is hyperventilation of the normal lung but no change in ventilation of the atelectatic lung. The hyperventilation has a minimal effect on the oxygenation of blood exiting the normal lung for the reasons just out-

lined. It results in excessive excretion of CO_2, however, that leads to respiratory alkalosis, just as in the lesser degrees of $\dot{V}/\dot{Q}$ mismatch, discussed earlier.

Aside from the effects on gas exchange, the loss of alveolar space changes the volume–pressure relations in the lung (e.g., pulmonary mechanics). As shown in Fig. 9.10, a decrease in FRC results in a shift in the volume–pressure relation toward a condition of decreasing compliance. In other words, more pressure is required to achieve the same degree of lung inflation. The pressure specified in this graph is the alveolar-inflating pressure, or transalveolar pressure. It is plotted as positive if it serves to inflate alveoli, whether the relation to atmospheric pressure is positive (as in mechanical ventilation) or negative (as in spontaneous breathing). This method of expressing volume–pressure relations is a standard procedure and appears straightforward. It can become complex, however, when a patient is breathing spontaneously while positive pressure is applied to the airway. Remember that negative pressure applied to the pleural space through the diaphragm and positive pressure applied to the airway with a ventilator are additive when volume–pressure characteristics are considered.

To measure compliance, the intrapleural pressure and the airway pressure must be measured exactly. In studies of pulmonary physiology, esophageal pressure is often substituted for intrapleural pressure. When the airway is intubated, airway pressure can be measured directly, and with some assumptions about pleural pressure, reasonable estimates of volume–pressure relations can be made. The compliance calculated by using such pressures measured in the airway is referred to as *effective compliance.* The normal value is 100 mL/cm H_2O for adults, or 1 to 2 mL/kg per centimeter of H_2O.

Pulmonary Edema

The causes of pulmonary edema are (a) increased hydrostatic pressure (left ventricular failure or gross fluid overload), (b) decreased plasma oncotic pressure (rarely a problem unless the concentration of plasma protein is very low), and (c) increased capillary permeability. When fluid begins to collect in the lung interstitium, it migrates to the loose areolar portions of the lung microanatomy that surround the small bronchioles and pulmonary arteries. Edema in these areas has the effect of narrowing the bronchi and increasing resistance in the pulmonary vasculature. This decreases both ventilation and perfusion in the edematous area; however, ventilation is often affected more than blood flow, which results in a decreased $\dot{V}/\dot{Q}$ ratio, with all of its attendant effects on gas exchange. As more fluid collects in the lung, it may compress alveoli and eventually floods into the alveoli, further decreasing the FRC and ultimately leading to transpulmonary shunting.

The interrelations between lung edema, atelectasis, and gas exchange in postoperative patients are often misunderstood. Significant changes in lung function do not occur until the level of interstitial water is grossly above normal, and at that point, $\dot{V}/\dot{Q}$ mismatch begins. With slightly more transcapillary filtrate, alveolar flooding and shunting occur. With these relations in mind, consider the effect of ventilator treatment; increased airway pressure tends to hold alveoli open, spread out the space available for water accumulation, and overcome the effects of small bronchial occlusion. These effects are observed while edema is minimal, right up to the point at which the lung becomes filled with fluid, which is why positive airway pressure improves gas exchange in pulmonary edema. (Positive pressure does not affect the actual degree of edema in the lung, only its manifestations.) The point is that only extreme edema affects pulmonary function, and even then, minor changes in pulmonary water can lead to major changes in function. This fact, combined with the observation that atelectasis can develop in any patient for reasons unrelated to pulmonary edema, leads to confusion and misunderstanding regarding this aspect of pathophysiology.

The relation of pulmonary edema to infection and fibrosis is more important than the effect of pulmonary edema on lung function. Atelectasis may exist for weeks with no permanent effects on lung structure. Just a few days, however, of pulmonary edema—particularly the protein-rich, capillary-leakage type of edema—sets the stage for pulmonary infection, rapidly developing fibrosis, or both.

Management of Respiratory Failure

The University of Michigan algorithm for the management of severe respiratory failure is shown in Fig. 9.13. For the purposes of this discussion, *severe respiratory failure* is defined as the requirement for intubation, mechanical ventilation, and supplemental inspired O_2. Although routine ventilator patients can be treated without a pulmonary artery catheter, that device provides essential information for the management of severe respiratory failure, and placement of a pulmonary artery catheter is assumed for purposes of this discussion. Whenever a pulmonary artery catheter is placed, we use a fiberoptic oximeter catheter (Oximetrix, Abbott Critical Care Systems, Walnut Creek, CA), which continuously measures mixed venous saturation. We do this because most of the important steps in the management of severe respiratory failure are based on the monitoring of mixed venous saturation.

Although the cause of respiratory failure is usually found in the lung interstitium and parenchyma, it is important not to overlook simple mechanical causes, such as pneumothorax, hydrothorax, plugged endotracheal tubes, occluded airways, or ascites. Bronchoscopy should be performed if there is any question of aspiration or any evidence of mucous plugging or impaction in the airways. Although ventilator management with an indwelling endotracheal tube can be continued for days or weeks, the increased incidence of bacterial pneumonia during long-term intubation, the gas flow resistance of endotracheal tubes, and the obligatory linkage of extubation with ventilator weaning all prompt us to recommend tracheostomy rather than long-term intubation for the treatment of patients with severe respiratory failure. Pulmonary embolism should be considered as a cause of respiratory failure in any patient if the pulmonary artery systolic pressure is above 40 mm Hg.

Optimizing the systemic O_2 delivery in relation to the O_2 requirement is the primary goal of management. In-

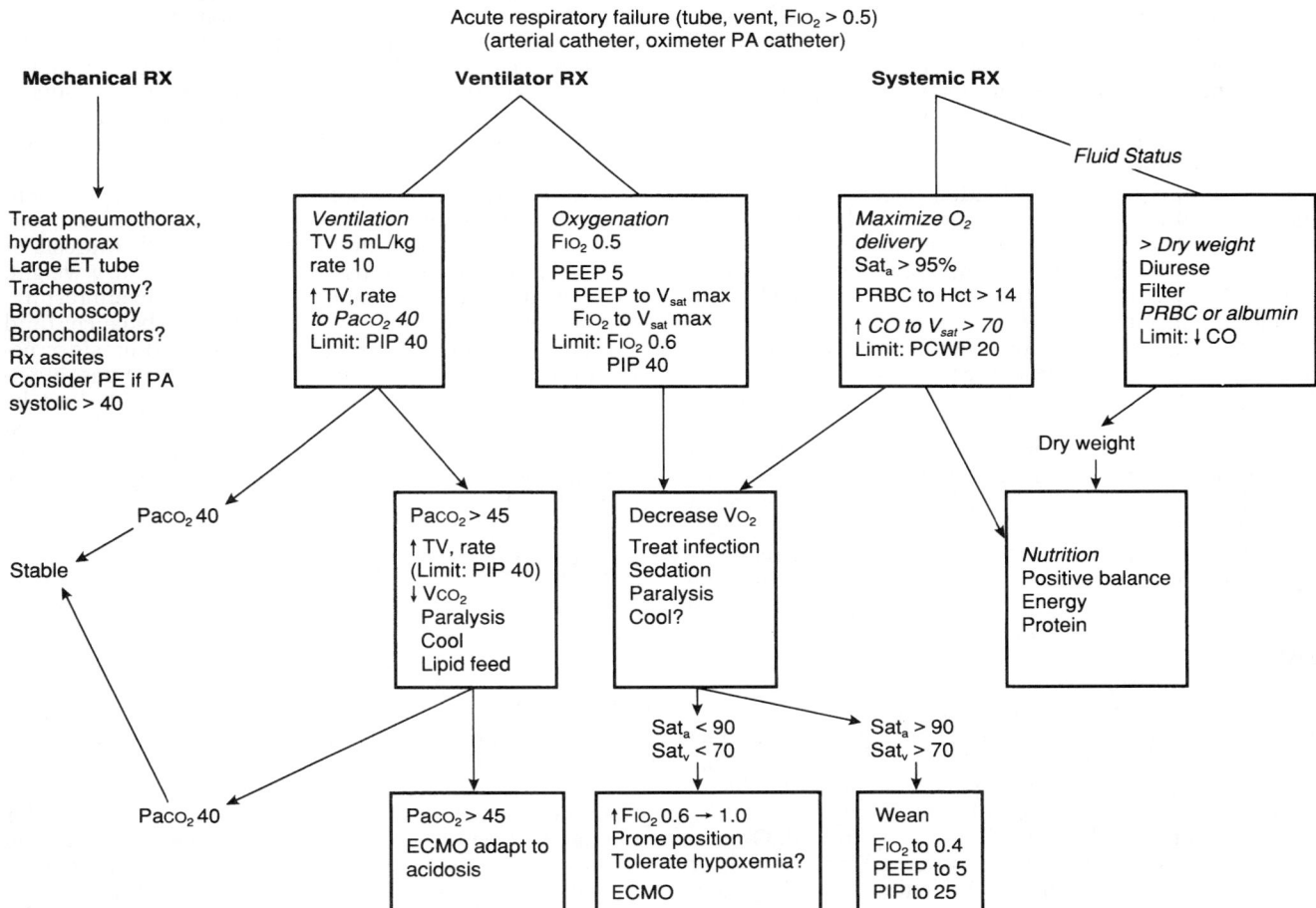

Figure 9.13. Algorithm for the management of respiratory failure. *ET,* endotrachial; *PE,* pulmonary embolism; *PA,* pulmonary artery; *PEEP,* positive end-expiratory pressure; *ECMO,* extracorporeal membrane oxygenation; *PRBC,* packed red blood cells; *PCWP,* pulmonary capillary wedge pressure. (After Bartlett RH. *University of Michigan critical care handbook.* Boston: Little, Brown, 1996, with permission.)

creasing oxygenation of the blood by improving alveolar inflation is only one of the steps involved in optimizing O_2 delivery. Equally or more important are treating anemia and optimizing cardiac output. Most patients in the ICU are anemic, and O_2 delivery is maintained by a compensatory increase in cardiac output. This is an acceptable practice because most patients have an adequate cardiac reserve to compensate for anemia and because blood transfusion is potentially associated with infectious complications. Patients with severe respiratory failure, however, are at risk for death resulting from decreased O_2 delivery (or related multiple-organ failure), so that the risk of transfusion is minor compared with the risk associated with the primary problem. This situation is complicated by the fact that cardiac output may be compromised in these patients, either by the primary disease or by efforts to increase oxygenation with the use of airway pressure. Accordingly, O_2 delivery in these patients should be optimized first by maintaining a normal hematocrit. Second, cardiac output should be optimal (not necessarily maximal) to maintain delivery at four to five times consumption. In general, this means avoiding situations that decrease cardiac output rather than actively trying to increase cardiac output. The airway pressure is kept as low as possible to maximize venous return, abdominal distention is avoided, appropriate blood volume is maintained based on a pulmonary capillary wedge pressure in the range of 15 mm Hg, and blood pressure is kept high enough to maintain coronary perfusion (mean arterial pressure > 50 mm Hg), but not so high as to limit left ventricular function (mean arterial pressure > 90 mm Hg). If all these steps are taken, cardiac output usually autoregulates so that delivery is four to five times consumption. If myocardial contractility is inadequate, then inotropic drugs such as dopamine or dobutamine should be used. These drugs, however, increase O_2 consumption in addition to contractility. Determination of the overall benefit and the titration of inotropic agents should be based on measurements of mixed venous saturation.

Finally, O_2 delivery can be maintained by ensuring adequate saturation of arterial blood. This can be done by supplying supplemental O_2 to the airway and by improving the inflation of collapsed or poorly ventilated alveoli. The FIO_2 is increased to 50% or 60% as the initial step in treating hypoxemia. Alveolar collapse is treated, as outlined earlier, by cleaning the airways, avoiding 100% O_2, removing fluid from the lung or chest, and using the PEEP to hold open those alveoli that have been opened by other measures. The optimal level of PEEP is that at which arterial oxygenation is maintained but venous return or cardiac output is not decreased. The optimal level is best determined by monitoring mixed venous saturation. When the PEEP is varied, the position of the patient on the pressure–volume curve should be noted and the volume should be decreased if the peak airway pressure exceeds 40 cm H_2O. Another step in optimizing lung function is to take advantage of the gravitational effects on pulmonary blood flow by turning the patient to a prone position or to a full lateral position to direct the blood flow to areas of optimal alveolar inflation. (This step often results in the opening of closed posterior alveoli compressed by the weight of fluid in the lung.)

At the same time that O_2 delivery is optimized, O_2 consumption should be decreased to normal, or even below normal if necessary. Treating infection, providing adequate sedation, and establishing muscular paralysis all decrease O_2 consumption and decrease the need for O_2 delivery. Like the other steps used in management, sedation or paralysis is adjusted according to the mixed venous saturation. If the O_2 delivery is still inadequate for metabolic needs despite implementation of these measures (i.e., ve-

nous saturation < 60% to 70%), O_2 consumption can be further decreased by actively cooling the patient, with the understanding that cooling will result in coagulopathy and arrhythmia if the temperature falls below 33°C.

Optimizing CO_2 removal is usually an easier step than optimizing O_2 delivery. The ventilator rate and tidal volume are adjusted to achieve a normal $PaCO_2$, with care taken to avoid a peak airway pressure greater than 40 cm H_2O. If the $PaCO_2$ exceeds 45 mm Hg, the tidal volume, rate, or both are increased until it is normal. The production of CO_2 can be minimized by sedation, paralysis, and treatment of infection. It can be further decreased by avoiding heavy carbohydrate loads in the nutritional regimen and by cooling the patient. If the $PaCO_2$ still exceeds 45 mm Hg despite these measures (and tube or airway occlusion has been ruled out), it is permissible to tolerate hypercarbia and achieve acid–base balance with bicarbonate or Tham buffer solution. This step is preferable to proceeding to extremes of airway pressure, which further injures the lung. Some of the other details of mechanical ventilator management are discussed later.

If O_2 delivery or CO_2 excretion remains inadequate despite all these measures, the likelihood of patient survival is low. In this situation, it is reasonable to consider extracorporeal circulation with gas exchange (extracorporeal membrane oxygenation) as an alternative. In this procedure, catheters are placed into large vessels. Venous blood is removed and oxygenated, CO_2 is removed, and the blood is returned to the arterial or venous circulation to provide mechanical support of pulmonary (or cardiopulmonary) function. This procedure requires systemic heparinization and a well-trained and experienced team. Extracorporeal membrane oxygenation in these patients is often necessary for 1 to 4 weeks. The survival rate for moribund adult patients with severe respiratory failure is 60% to 70%.

General steps are important in patient management throughout the course of severe respiratory failure. In particular, fluid overload should be treated with diuresis or hemofiltration until the patient is returned to dry weight. Successful outcome in the management of severe respiratory failure is correlated with overall fluid balance; fluid overload results in a lower survival rate. As diuresis or hemofiltration is carried out, the patient becomes hypovolemic. As mentioned earlier, cardiac output must be supported, and the combination of diuresis and packed red cell transfusion is usually the best approach to maintaining normal blood volume in the early stages of severe respiratory failure.

Mechanical Ventilation

Mechanical ventilation should be considered when spontaneous breathing is inadequate to maintain gas exchange, or when the effort required to maintain gas exchange is exhausting the patient. Orotracheal intubation is preferred. Nasotracheal intubation is equally uncomfortable and requires the use of a smaller, longer tube. The use of oral or nasal tracheal intubation for as long as 2 to 3 weeks is common practice but is probably not wise. Aside from the obvious damage to the larynx and discomfort for the patient, the tube enters the sterile airway through the grossly contaminated pharynx. Despite the best attempts at oral hygiene, the posterior pharynx harbors a slurry of virulent organisms that inevitably track down along the endotracheal tube to colonize the airway, if not the alveoli. Tracheostomy is much more comfortable for the patient, poses much less airway resistance, and, most importantly, avoids contamination of the lower airway. Having been through a phase of favoring long-term intubation, we now prefer early (in 1 to 2 days) tracheostomy for any patient with major respiratory failure.

The ventilator should be set on the assist–control mode at a low sensitivity. In this fashion, the patient breathes at a rate that maintains the $PaCO_2$ at a normal level, but each breath is mechanically assisted to provide maximal inflation. The volume of each breath is set by limiting the maximal pressure or maximal volume of each breath. Whichever method is used, the peak plateau pressure should generally not exceed 40 cm H_2O. If the patient is comatose or paralyzed, the assist mode cannot be used, and the rate is set in addition to the volume (controlled mechanical ventilation or intermittent mechanical ventilation). The use of the assist mode allows the patient to exercise respiratory muscles while deriving the maximal benefit from the invasive endotracheal tube.

Adequate weaning indices are the following: inspiratory force greater than 20 cm H_2O, vital capacity twice the tidal volume, adequate gas exchange on assisted ventilation at an FiO_2 of 0.3 and PEEP of 5 cm H_2O, and minute ventilation below 10 L/min. Weaning from mechanical ventilation is best accomplished by going straight from the assist–control mode to spontaneous breathing with continuous gas flow (Fig. 9.14). Spontaneous breathing should be associated with adequate gas exchange, adequate tidal volume, a respiratory rate below 20 breaths per minute, and a pulse rate below 120 beats per minute. If the patient is hypermetabolic or is receiving excess carbohydrate as nutritional support, the minute ventilation will be elevated, even during assisted mechanical ventilation. If this is the case, the patient tires rapidly on spontaneous breathing, and the primary problem must be treated before ventilator weaning is attempted.

Treatment of the Interstitial Space

The treatment of edema has two important goals. The first is to increase oxygenation if it is impaired, and the second is to minimize fibrosis and bacterial infection, which often accompany pulmonary edema caused by capillary injury. (Fibrosis and infection are unusual after hydrostatic edema.) The treatment of interstitial edema is to maintain the hydrostatic pressure as low as is compatible with adequate cardiac output and to raise the oncotic pressure selectively in the vascular space. These measures, combined with fluid restriction and diuresis, decrease pulmonary edema. Regulating the hydrostatic pressure and cardiac output requires the use of a pulmonary artery catheter and frequent determinations of cardiac output.

Because it is desirable to keep the filling pressure of the left ventricle as low as possible while good cardiac output is maintained, inotropic drugs to increase left ventricular contractility are helpful. Isoproterenol or dopamine should be used, with serial measurements of cardiac output and filling pressure. A Starling curve can be constructed and the optimal combination of filling pressure and inotropic drug determined.

Simple extracellular fluid (ECF) overload may contribute to interstitial edema in the lung. For example, in some centers, an infusion of 5 to 10 L of salt solution is routinely administered to trauma patients, in addition to blood. This is done in an attempt to replace presumed losses into the "third" extracellular space. (The plasma volume and interstitial fluid are the normal interstitial spaces; the pathophysiologic third space is the transient edema in the area of operation or injury.) The third space expands as long as salt water is poured into the patient, and the difference between what is required and what is actually given is often measured in liters. The fact that most patients tolerate iatrogenic edema does not mean that this is a good practice. If sepsis occurs in an edematous patient, the increased capillary permeability can lead to pulmonary, myocardial, or brain dysfunction.

The first step in decreasing pulmonary edema is to decrease the pulmonary capillary hydrostatic pressure to a level as low as is compatible with adequate cardiac output. This is accomplished through diuresis and fluid restriction. As the patient's blood volume decreases, signs of hypovolemia may appear. Blood volume is then replenished with a fluid that remains in the vascular space. Packed red blood cells are ideal for this application. When the hematocrit is normal, concentrated salt-poor albumin should be used. This hyperoncotic fluid replenishes the blood volume by drawing interstitial fluid from throughout the body into the vascular space and supplementing diuresis. This technique is useful even in the septic patient, whose capillary permeability may be increased and who may lose albumin from the vascular space at a rapid rate. Even when albumin "leaks out" at a rate that is three or four times normal, the short-term effects of expanding blood volume and decreasing edema appear. Experience with infusion of albumin solution into patients who are already hypervolemic has led to the mistaken impression that the use of concentrated albumin in the *hypo*volemic patient may cause problems. On the contrary, it is an efficient way to reexpand blood volume. The use of concentrated globulins would be better yet, but such a preparation is not available. Although furosemide is usually used as the diuretic of choice, mannitol should be mentioned. This drug provides osmotic diuresis in addition to a transient plasma hyperosmolarity, "pulling" fluid into the vascular space.

BLOOD VOLUME AND HEMODYNAMICS

The monitoring and management of systemic perfusion represent one of the easier aspects of intensive care. In

Figure 9.14. Weaning from mechanical ventilation. As mechanical support is decreased, patient effort must increase. If the respiratory rate is high and the tidal volume small, the patient is not ready for extubation. *IMV,* intermittent mechanical ventilation; *CPAP,* continuous positive airway pressure. (After Bartlett RH. Respiratory failure: life support systems. In: Bartlett RH, Whitehouse WM Jr, Turcotte JG, eds. *Life support systems in intensive care.* Chicago: Year Book, 1984:363, with permission.)

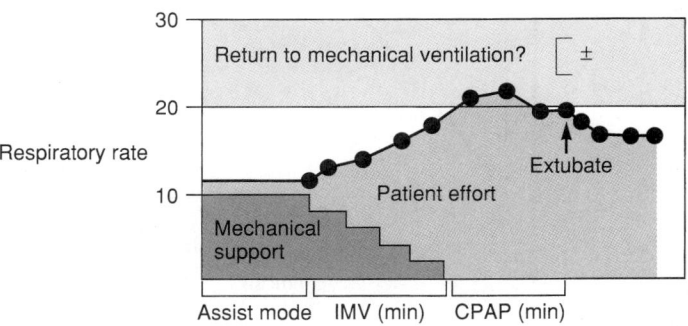

fact, an inordinate amount of attention is given to the monitoring and management of blood pressure, sometimes to the exclusion of other, more important parameters, such as O_2 delivery or metabolic rate. This section reviews cardiac physiology and pathophysiology, cardiac function in relation to blood volume and filling pressure, and systemic vascular physiology in the management of hypotension and inadequate systemic perfusion.

Cardiac Function

Cardiac function is regulated by a complex set of baroreceptors and chemoreceptors that continually adjust the cardiac rate, strength of contractility, and ECF volume (by diuresis or antidiuresis), all of which act to maintain systemic O_2 delivery at four to five times systemic O_2 consumption. Because normal O_2 consumption is 120 mL/m^2 per minute and normal arterial O_2 content is 20 mL/dL, normal cardiac output is autoregulated to a level of 3 L/m^2 per minute. If the rate of metabolism increases or decreases, chemoreceptors readjust the cardiac output proportionally. If the O_2 content of arterial blood falls because of anemia or hypoxemia, the cardiac output increases until normal systemic O_2 delivery is reestablished. If the cardiac output drops because of hypovolemia, increased catecholamine secretion results in an increased cardiac rate and contractility to maintain normal systemic O_2 delivery until transcapillary refilling or exogenous treatment restores the blood volume to normal. Any or all of these complex interactions may be taking place in the same critically ill patient at the same time. To assess these factors in the critically ill patient, we estimate cardiac output, blood volume, and filling pressure based on physical examination findings. Specifically, we examine the quality and numeric values of the pulse pressure, the adequacy of urine output and brain function, the warmth and perfusion of the skin, and the endogenous autoregulation required to maintain perfusion (tachycardia, chest wall cardiac impulse). All these findings make it possible to estimate the cardiac output reasonably well. Examination of the lungs for signs of vascular congestion and of the visible veins in the neck to estimate venous pressure provides some indication of filling pressure. Often, these physical findings are adequate to establish a diagnosis and

institute management. If this level of monitoring is not satisfactory to solve clinical problems, direct measurement of the filling pressure of the right side of the heart (central venous pressure) or the left side of the heart (pulmonary artery pressure) is required. Placement of a pulmonary artery catheter allows the measurement of cardiac output by thermodilution and, more important, the sampling of mixed venous blood to determine saturation. These measurements provide the ratio of systemic O_2 delivery to O_2 consumption.

From all these measurements, one can determine whether the cardiac output is normal for the level of filling pressure of the left ventricle, or whether contractility is decreased. In the latter case, the cardiac output is lower than predicted for a given level of filling pressure. These relations are described in the familiar Frank-Starling curve (Fig. 9.15). If the measurements are within the normal range, then myocardial function can be assumed to be normal. If the values are to the right of the normal range, then cardiac function is compromised because of valvular disease, extrinsic pressure such as pericardial tamponade, or (most commonly) a decrease in contractility.

Cardiac Function, Blood Volume, and Filling Pressure

The filling pressure described earlier and illustrated in Fig. 9.15 reflects the relationship between the cardiac function and the effective blood volume. If the cardiac function and anatomy are normal, then blood volume, filling pressure, and cardiac function are related as shown in the normal area of the Starling curve. The intake and output of fluid and salt are autoregulated to maintain the filling pressure of the left ventricle at about 10 mm Hg. ECF expansion (generalized edema) is usually associated with a normal blood volume. It is important to remember this fact when the critically ill patient with fluid overload is being considered. Gross expansion of the extracellular space, with all the deleterious effects of tissue edema, can and often does coexist with a perfectly normal blood volume. For example, a pulmonary capillary wedge pressure of 5 to 10 mm Hg does not rule out fluid overload as the cause of pulmonary or gastrointestinal dysfunction. Even a minor decrease in ECF volume, however, leads to antidiuresis as soon as hypovolemia is reflected by decreased

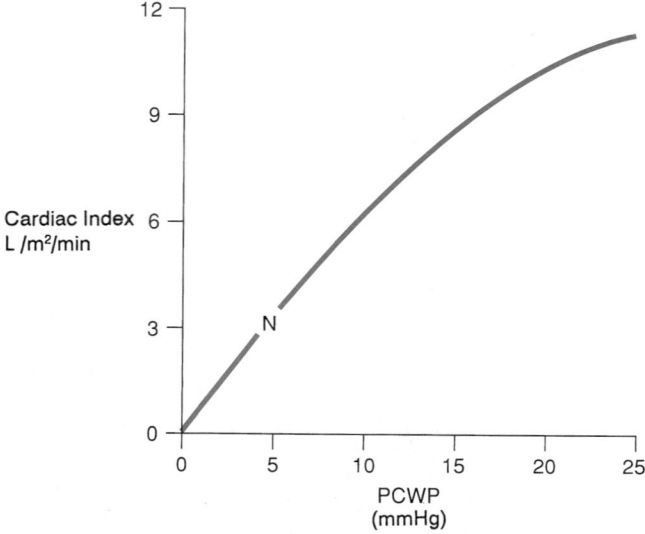

Figure 9.15. Left ventricular function curve (modified from the Frank-Starling curve). *N* is the normal resting status, and the curve represents normal cardiac output response to changes in filling pressure. *PCWP*, pulmonary capillary wedge pressure. (After Bartlett RH. *University of Michigan critical care handbook.* Boston; Little, Brown, 1996, with permission.)

atrial filling pressures. Systemic blood pressure autoregulatory mechanisms increase the cardiac output to compensate. In the case of bleeding, the change in blood volume is immediate and is immediately reflected in these compensatory mechanisms. If the bleeding stops before a critical level of exsanguination is reached, the normal combination of hydrostatic and osmotic forces that control the flow of salt and water at the capillary level results in the net transfer of ECF back into the plasma volume (transcapillary refilling), which restores the normal blood volume, albeit with hemodilution.

The fear that hypotension and ineffective perfusion will develop in a critically ill patient, although it may be appropriate, usually results in the infusion of intravenous salt and water in quantities that exceed losses. Consequently, most patients in the ICU have edema (worse in areas of injury or inflammation), anemia, dilutional hypoproteinemia, and a compensatory increase in cardiac output. In response to anemia, tachycardia develops, even though the blood volume is normal, filling pressures are normal, and total body ECF is excessive. All these factors are reflected in the autoregulatory mechanisms designed to maintain systemic O_2 delivery at four to five times O_2 consumption. If the arterial saturation is close to 100%, then cardiac function is normal for that patient if the venous saturation is in the range of 75% to 80%.

Systemic and Regional Blood Flow

This entire discussion has addressed cardiac output as if blood flow were ideally distributed to each of the various organ systems. In fact, this is usually the case. Even in periods of high cardiac output and low cardiac output, the organs that require increased O_2 delivery (i.e., blood flow) receive the extra blood flow at the expense of other organs that need it less. This autoregulation is based primarily on the maintenance of total systemic vascular resistance as determined by arteriolar tone in all organs throughout the vascular system. Some organs, such as the heart and brain, maintain a constant blood flow over a wide range of inflow pressures. In other organs, such as the kidney, blood flow is more sensitive to arterial inflow pressure. (To state it more accurately, arteriolar resistance regulates organ blood flow in an active fashion.) The management of regional or organ-specific blood flow is rarely possible or even considered in the treatment of critically ill patients. Notable exceptions are the use of vasopressin and glucagon to increase or decrease splanchnic blood flow, and the use of hypocapnic alkalosis to decrease cerebral blood flow. Low doses of dopamine are said to increase renal blood flow selectively, although this phenomenon may be primarily the result of a generalized increase in cardiac output.

In the context of the peripheral circulation, the calculation of resistance is a useful short way to describe the interrelations of cardiac output and systemic or pulmonary blood pressure, but it is no more than that. It is impossible to measure resistance. Resistance is simply a calculation in which blood pressure is divided by blood flow. The results should be expressed as Wood units, or millimeters of mercury per liter per minute per square meter. It is naïve to apply laws of fluid dynamics that are described for the flow of newtonian fluids through rigid tubes, and it is ridiculous to convert resistance units to dynes per second per centimeter to the minus fifth power, as if the resulting number would somehow be more accurate. (Multiplying Wood units times 79.9 to express resistance is common practice but has no rationale.) All cardiovascular measurements should be normalized to body weight or body surface area, and this is particularly true of resistance calculations. The cardiac index rather than the cardiac output should always be used for resistance calculations to compare each patient with the theoretic norm. For example, imagine a 4-year-old with a blood pressure of 90/60 and a well-trained 300-pound adult athlete with a blood pressure of 110/80. Both have a normal cardiac index. The calculated systemic vascular resistance based on the cardiac *index* is the same for both and is normal. The calculated systemic vascular resistance based on cardiac *output* would be pathologically high in the child and pathologically low in the athlete.

Management of Hypotension and Hypoperfusion

The University of Michigan algorithm for hemodynamics is shown in Fig. 9.16. Despite the previous discussion, the first sign that brings hemodynamic problems to the physician's attention is often low blood pressure. If a patient with a low blood pressure or tachycardia, confusion, syncope, or a narrow pulse pressure is identified as possibly having an inadequate systemic O_2 delivery to meet metabolic needs (i.e., shock), the first response is to make some assessment of venous pressure by physical examination. If the venous pressure is high, the problem is presumed to be related to the heart or some mechanical obstruction to blood flow. If the venous pressure is low, the problem is presumed to be attributable to hypovolemia or systemic vasodilation. If the patient does not respond to initial simple management, more detailed monitoring is required in the form of a central venous pressure catheter or perhaps pulmonary artery catheter. If this level of monitoring provides a diagnosis, the physician can proceed to appropriate treatment. If signs of inadequate blood flow persist despite treatment based on venous pressure measurement, then transfer to the ICU and direct monitoring of pulmonary artery pressure, saturation, and cardiac output are required.

With the pulmonary artery catheter in place, the physician can determine whether delivery is adequate to meet metabolic needs (i.e., venous saturation is above 65% provided that arterial saturation is above 95%). If delivery is adequate, then no further acute treatment is needed. If delivery is not adequate, then an appropriate blood volume expander should be given until the wedge pressure is more than 10 mm Hg or the central venous pressure is more than 5 mm Hg. The appropriate blood volume expander may be blood, crystalloid, or plasma, depending on the presumed or proven fluid loss that led to hypovolemia.

If, despite adequate filling pressure, cardiac output is still decreased or venous saturation is less than 65%, then the cause is probably related to cardiac function, and appropriate treatment can be undertaken. If mechanical factors are ruled out and contractility is the limiting factor, then inotropic drugs are the appropriate treatment (Fig. 9.17). If the cardiac output is high and hypotension persists, the cause may be systemic vasodilation (resulting from sepsis, paralysis, or vasodilator drugs), or the problem may be metabolic in origin (hypoglycemia, hypocalcemia, or Addison's disease). If the blood pressure is normal or high and the cardiac output is decreased despite adequate filling pressure, then the problem may be systemic hypertension or systemic hypertension combined with decreased contractility. Only in the latter circumstance is the use of systemic vasodilators appropriate.

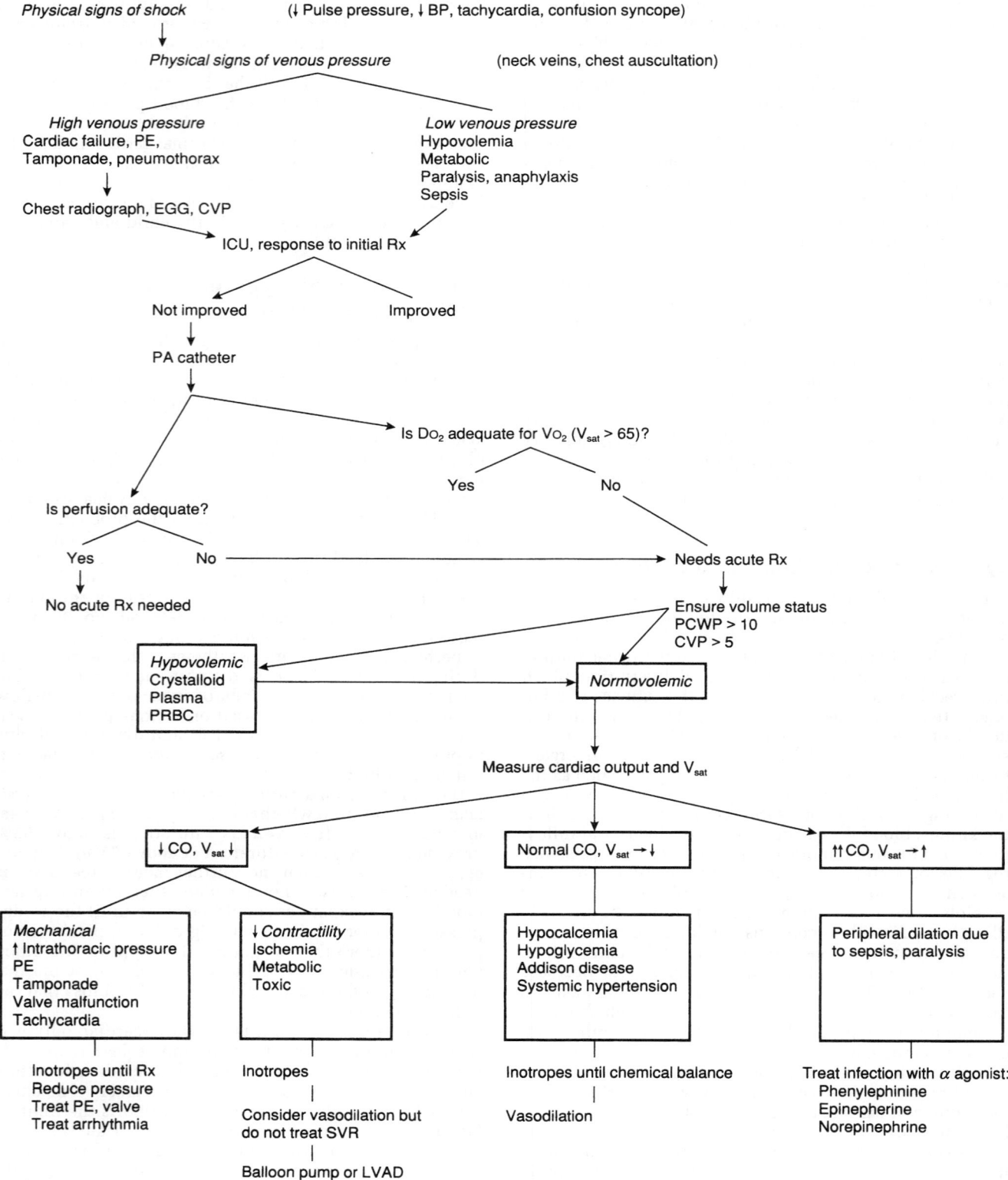

Figure 9.16. Hemodynamic algorithm. (After Bartlett RH. *University of Michigan critical care handbook.* Boston; Little, Brown, 1996, with permission.)

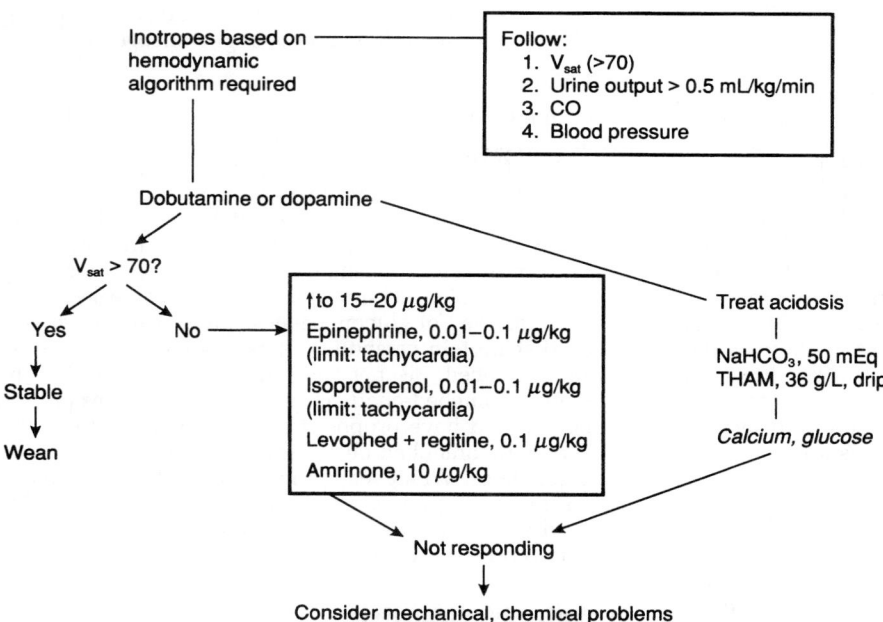

Figure 9.17. Commonly used inotropic drugs.

METABOLISM AND NUTRITION

Metabolic Requirements

The typical expenditures of energy and protein in normal subjects and critically ill patients are shown in Fig. 9.18. Protein and energy requirements are continuous. These are met by endogenous sources during fasting or through exogenous treatment (nutrition). Energy expenditure is referred to as the *basal metabolic rate,* or the *basal energy expenditure*. The basal energy expenditure is properly expressed in joules, the standard unit of energy, but is more commonly and more practically expressed in calories. The basal energy expenditure decreases with advancing age and varies with sex and body size. It is a function of cellular metabolism, and hence of the body cell mass. The basal energy expenditure is usually estimated from a chart combining age, sex, and body size.

Estimating and Measuring Energy Requirements

The actual metabolic rate of any given patient can be estimated by modifying the predicted basal rate according to the clinical condition. For example, the metabolic rate is decreased by 10% in a starving person and increased by 10% with minor activity. This further estimation of metabolic activity in the resting (as opposed to basal) state is referred to as the *resting energy expenditure*. Trauma, stress, sepsis, and surgical operations are all known to increase the metabolic rate. Several authors have proposed tables or formulas for estimating the metabolic rate according to the degree of physiologic stress. This amount of energy is most conveniently expressed in calories per day. The metabolic rate is normalized to body surface area; however, the actively metabolizing tissue is the lean body cell mass. Consequently, reporting "per square meter" underestimates metabolism in a fat person and overestimates it in a lean person.

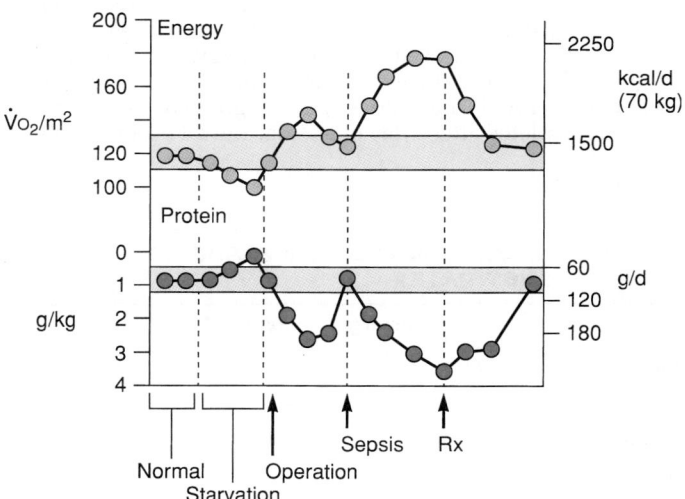

Figure 9.18. Energy and protein metabolism in normal, starving, operative, and septic states. (After Bartlett RH. Nutritional support. In: Dantzker DR, ed. *Cardiopulmonary critical care.* Orlando, FL: Grune & Stratton, 1986:263, with permission.)

Although most of the studies on nutrition in critical illness have been based on estimated energy expenditure, actual measurement is much more accurate and is becoming an important aspect of critical care. The most commonly used method of measurement is indirect calorimetry. In this method, the amount of O_2 absorbed across the lungs into the pulmonary blood is measured during a given period of time. Provided the patient is at a metabolic steady state during this time, the amount of O_2 absorbed across the lungs is equal to the amount of O_2 consumed in metabolic processes. The energy released by the oxidation of various food substrates is known from direct measurements, so that the metabolic rate measured in milliliters of O_2 per minute can be converted to calories per hour or per day if the oxygenated substrates are known. For practical purposes, a conversion factor of 5 kcal of energy per liter of O_2 consumed is a reasonable approximation. It overestimates the metabolic rate slightly, but it is a much more accurate approximation of the actual metabolic rate than a number derived from an arbitrary chart or table.

Energy Sources

The major sources of energy are carbohydrates (including ketones and alcohols) and fats. Protein can be oxidized through gluconeogenesis and is often a significant source of energy in critically ill patients. The goal of nutritional planning is to supply energy from sources other than protein, so that endogenous and exogenous protein can be used for anabolism rather than catabolism. In normal volunteers and surgical patients, the breakdown of protein is decreased by giving the subject exogenous fuel—be it glucose, fat, or xylitol. This is referred to as the *protein-sparing effect*. Small amounts of glucose (400 cal/d) provide some degree of protein sparing, but full caloric support is required for maximal effect.

Carbohydrate is the major source of energy during normal, nonstarving existence. The brain, red cells, and possibly other organs are obligate users of glucose. They require glucose as the primary energy source under normal conditions. Other organs also use glucose preferentially as a source of energy. The brain and red blood cells can develop the capacity to use ketones as an energy source, a process called *starvation adaptation*. When fully oxidized, carbohydrate produces 4 cal of energy per gram of substrate metabolized, 5 cal of energy per liter of O_2 consumed, and one molecule of CO_2 for each molecule of O_2 consumed. The latter ratio is the respiratory quotient (RQ), which is 1 for carbohydrate (Table 9.1).

Fat is the most efficient source of energy. Fat produces 9 cal of energy per gram of substrate metabolized and 4.7 cal of energy per liter of O_2 consumed in this oxidation; its RQ is 0.7. Fat is stored as triglyceride, and for each three molecules of fatty acid oxidized to produce energy, one molecule of glycerol is also oxidized. Endogenous fat is the major source of energy during starvation. The glycogen stores are basically depleted after a day of fasting, and fat becomes the major source of energy, with protein breakdown supplying some glucose through the process of gluconeogenesis.

Mediators

The mediators of the hypermetabolic state are incompletely understood. Elevated catecholamine levels have been identified in burn patients. Corticosteroids, glucagon, growth hormone, and thyroid hormone have all been implicated as mediators of the hypermetabolic state in various critical conditions. Interleukin-2 causes both hypermetabolism and protein catabolism. Certain amino acids may play a modulating role. Alanine, for example, has easy access into the pathway of gluconeogenesis, and it has been suggested that protein catabolism depends on the amount of alanine produced. Fischer and others have shown that the infusion of branched-chain amino acids diminishes protein catabolism and have proposed the administration of solutions rich in branched-chain amino acids to patients in catabolic states. Whatever the mediator of the hypermetabolic state is, it appears preferable to treat the underlying cause while feeding metabolic fuel to the fire rather than to attempt to reverse the hypermetabolic state *per se*.

Protein Metabolism

Estimating and Measuring Protein Requirements

In normal protein metabolism, a continuous excretion of nitrogen (mostly as urea) equivalent to about 50 g of protein each day is matched by a protein intake of 50 g/d. The rate of protein synthesis and breakdown is about 300 g/d, with most endogenous amino acids being recycled into new protein. In starvation, protein catabolism continues (although at a slower rate) without a corresponding protein intake, leaving the patient in a negative protein balance. This protein flux is most conveniently measured as nitrogen flux; consequently, the condition is commonly referred to as *negative nitrogen balance*. During critical illness, the rate of protein catabolism generally increases while intake stops, so that a negative nitrogen balance results. It is convenient to think of this protein breakdown as necessary to produce glucose through gluconeogenesis when other carbohydrate stores have been exhausted.

Protein Sources

The fact that the nitrogen balance is negative does not mean that protein synthesis stops or slows down. On the contrary, the synthesis of new cells, inflammatory cells, collagen, coagulation factors, antibodies, and scores of other proteins occurs at an accelerated rate during critical illness. Amino acids derived from muscle tissue or other somatic and visceral proteins become the building blocks for protein in healing tissue and host defenses. The site of a traumatic or surgical wound or an area of acute inflammation becomes a protein parasite on other body tissues. Eventually, this parasite may overwhelm the host because proteins that would otherwise strengthen the diaphragm or myocardium or participate in host defense processes are thrown to the metabolic flames. A large part of the goal of nutritional management is to provide sources of energy so that endogenous proteins are not required for energy (i.e., protein sparing), and to supply exogenous proteins so that all the needs of protein synthesis can be met without a breakdown of endogenous sources. Although oversimplified, a convenient number to remember for the basal protein requirement is 1 g/kg per day or 40 g/m^2 per day.

Mediators of Protein Catabolism

The mediators of protein catabolism appear to be different from the mediators of the metabolic rate. Although the

---

Table 9.1. CALORIC VALUE OF METABOLIC SUBSTRATES

	kcal/g	kcal/L O_2	RQ
Carbohydrate	4.0	5.0	1.0
Fat	9.5	4.7	0.7
Protein	4.8	4.5	0.8
Carbohydrate → fat	—	—	8.0

RQ, respiratory quotient.

energy requirement and protein breakdown often follow similar patterns, major protein catabolism sometimes occurs in a patient with a normal metabolic rate, and a patient can be hypermetabolic while conserving protein. Tumor necrosis factor is a specific mediator released from monocytes that stimulates the breakdown of endogenous protein. This is in accord with clinical observations that the degree of protein catabolism is generally related to the degree of inflammation and (presumed) neutrophil–monocyte activation.

Vitamins and Minerals

Vitamin stores are plentiful and deficiency states develop slowly, so that vitamin loss is not a concern during the early days of critical illness. A hypermetabolic patient catabolizes vitamins more rapidly than is normal and can reach a deficiency state sooner. A patient who is severely malnourished before entering the ICU may already have a vitamin deficiency. Some evidence suggests that high doses of vitamins A and C may be beneficial to patients with injuries. Because vitamins are inexpensive and safe, we deal with vitamins in the ICU in the same way that we do in the clinic—by prescribing more than enough for the patient who is not eating. Commercial preparations for enteral or parenteral administration provide gross excesses but do not lead to overdose.

Trace metals must be managed more carefully than vitamins because a deficiency can occur sooner and overdose can be deleterious. Calcium, phosphorus, magnesium, and sulfur are more than trace elements. They are lost continuously through the urine, stool, gastric juices, and other drainage. Although large body stores (particularly of calcium and phosphorous) are available, deficiency can develop rapidly. Enteral and parenteral feeding must include these elements. Serum levels of calcium, phosphorus, and magnesium should be measured at regular intervals. Zinc, copper, chromium, selenium, and manganese must be supplied to patients who are supported with enteral or parenteral feeding for more than 2 weeks.

Endogenous Sources of Energy and Protein

In a normal 80-kg man, about 1,000 cal are available as glycogen and other stored carbohydrates. About 140,000 cal are stored as fat. The body contains about 6 kg of protein, which can be consumed as a source of energy or maintained to do work. Nutritional assessment is the process of measuring the amount of these energy and protein reserves.

Energy Reserves

The simplest measurement of nutritional status is body weight in relation to body height. Major changes in weight that are not caused by fluid shifts are related to changes in body fat. Energy reserves are generally estimates of body fat because the amount of carbohydrate held in reserve is negligible. The first approach to measuring energy reserve is an estimation of caloric balance. The daily resting energy expenditure is estimated as described earlier, and the daily energy intake is estimated from the caloric value of nutrients. The latter estimate is easy for critically ill patients because they usually receive nothing by mouth, with all calories supplied through parenteral or tube feeding. A 10,000-cal deficit in a critically ill patient is a severe, acute energy deficit, although this represents only 5 or 6 days of semistarvation. The problem of a 10,000-cal deficit is not the loss of a few pounds of fat but rather the protein catabolism commonly associated with an energy deficit of this size. Fat reserves can be estimated by measuring the thickness of the triceps skin fold or by examining changes in body weight, corrected for fluid balance. Arm circumference includes both fat and muscle mass. Any of these measurements of body fat is at best a gross approximation.

Protein Reserves

Because protein is the functional and structural chemical of the body, most nutritional assessment techniques are estimates of protein reserves. The creatinine–height index is basically a measurement of creatinine excreted (as a measure of muscle breakdown) normalized for body size. Because muscle is a major source of endogenous protein, muscle wasting is characteristic of the malnourished state. This can be detected by testing muscle strength and endurance. Few standardized measures of muscle testing are used for nutritional assessment. One such test is the maximal breathing capacity (also known as the *maximal voluntary ventilation*). In this test, the maximal amount of air that can be moved through rapid breathing during a period of 12 seconds is recorded. The values are expressed as a "percentage of predicted" for a person of a given age, sex, and size (normal is 80% to 120%). In the absence of significant obstructive or restrictive disease, a low value usually indicates a lack of muscular strength and endurance. Inspiratory force is another strength test that is easily and commonly performed in the ICU. The normal range of values is 80 to 100 cm H_2O.

The actual nitrogen balance can be determined by measuring the amount of nitrogen excreted. This is most conveniently done by measuring the amount of urea excreted in the urine, if one assumes that urea constitutes 85% of the total nitrogen excretion. It is better to measure the total nitrogen in urine and other lost fluids because the percentage contained in urea can vary considerably. If the nitrogen excretion is known, the amount of protein catabolized can be estimated and compared with the amount of protein ingested. Indirect assessments of protein reserves are based on the single measurement of body substances that are maintained at normal levels by rapid protein synthesis. Conventional serum proteins, such as albumin and globulin, are not affected by malnutrition until it is severe. Proteins such as prealbumin and transferrin, which turn over more rapidly, are better indicators of protein status. Lymphocytes are rapidly destroyed, and protein is required for the formation of new cells. Consequently, the absolute lymphocyte count is a useful measure of the status of protein reserves. The lymphocyte count, in our experience, is the best single static measurement characterizing nutritional status.

Protein is also required for synthesizing the cells and mediators involved in skin test reactivity. Although skin test reactivity is a manifestation of lymphocyte-mediated immunity, its usefulness in patient assessment is probably as an indicator of the inflammatory response rather than of lymphocyte activity *per se*. Some chronically and acutely malnourished patients convert from a reactive to an anergic state, and reactivity can be restored by nutritional repletion.

These methods are used to classify the nutritional status of patients at the time of injury, operation, or critical illness (Table 9.2). Patients who are depleted of both energy and protein at the time of major physiologic stress have higher morbidity and mortality rates than do patients with normal nutritional status. In an excellent study, Forse and Shizgal measured body cell mass (the gold standard in the measurement of nutritional status) and found that a depleted state could not be reliably detected based on the

Table 9.2. **ASSESSMENT OF ENERGY AND PROTEIN STORES**

	Excess	Normal	Depletion Mild (kcal)	Severe (kcal)
Energy reserves				
Cumulative caloric balance	+	0	−5,000	−10,000
Triceps skinfold	−	Per table	−5%	−40%
Arm circumference	−	Per table	−5%	−30%
Weight change	−	Variable	−	−20%
Protein reserves				
Creatinine/height index	−	Per table	−5%	−30%
Lymphocyte count	>2,000	1,800/μL	1,600	500
Cumulative nitrogen balance	+	0	−30 g	−300 g
Albumin	>3	3 g/dL	2.5	1.5
Total protein	>8	6 g/dL	5.5	4.0
Muscle strength				
Inspiratory force	>100	100 cm H_2O	50	20
Maximal volume ventilation	>120	100% predicted	60	30
Skin test reactivity		Reactive	Anergic	

weight-to-height ratio, triceps skin fold, midarm circumference, albumin level, total protein level, hand strength, or creatinine-to-height ratio. Actual measurements of metabolic rate and nitrogen balance are the best methods of determining nutritional status in critically ill patients.

Energy Balance

Energy expenditure is most conveniently measured through the techniques of respirometry and indirect calorimetry. Respirometry is the process of measuring O_2 consumption and CO_2 production. The consumption of O_2 can be determined by measuring direct volumetric change in a closed-circuit rebreathing spirometer system with a CO_2 absorber, the volume and composition of exhaled gas and inhaled gas, or the O_2 content of arterial and mixed venous blood and multiplying the avO_2 difference by the cardiac output. The latter method requires pulmonary artery catheterization and is complicated by potential errors in the measurements, assumptions, and calculations. The analysis of mixed expired gas is the easiest method to use in normal subjects but is not suitable for patients on supplemental O_2 or mechanical ventilation because of minor variations in the inspired volume and O_2 concentration during the respiratory cycle. Direct volumetric spirometry is the best method for measuring O_2 consumption. This technique also lends itself well to simultaneous measurement of CO_2 production. With measurement of O_2 consumption and CO_2 production, the RQ can be calculated.

With the RQ, the relative amounts of carbohydrate and fat that are oxidized can be determined. The RQ for protein is 0.8. By measuring urinary nitrogen, the amount of protein catabolized can be calculated, and the measured RQ can be corrected for the amount of O_2 and CO_2 involved in protein catabolism. For example, if the urinary nitrogen excretion rate is 0.5 g/h, then protein is being metabolized at a rate of 3 g/h, which accounts for 3,200 mL of O_2 consumed per hour and 2,560 mL of CO_2 produced per hour. This nonprotein RQ is used to define the amount of fat or carbohydrate used as energy sources. Ketones have a low RQ (0.6), so ketone metabolism lowers the overall RQ. Conversely, the conversion of glucose to fat generates CO_2, so the RQ of that reaction is more than 1. Measurement of the RQ is helpful as an internal check on the accuracy of the calorimetry measurements and as a guideline to patient management. For example, if a patient has been receiving only 500 cal/d and has a metabolic rate of 2,500 cal/d, one

would expect that the use of fat would be maximal, and the RQ should be between 0.7 and 0.8. If such a patient is treated with parenteral nutrition and glucose used as the major source of energy, the RQ should be 1 when the caloric replacement matches caloric losses. If the RQ exceeds 1, then some of the infused carbohydrate is being converted to fat and excess CO_2 is being produced, which increases the need for breathing. Hypercaloric feeding with glucose can cause respiratory failure that requires mechanical ventilation simply by increasing the load of CO_2. Energy balance is helpful because it serves to identify the high-risk patient. In our studies, acutely ill patients with caloric deficits greater than 10,000 cal had a much higher mortality rate than patients with positive caloric balances.

Nutrition Supplies

Energy and Protein

The goals of nutritional therapy in critical ill patients are to maintain a positive nitrogen balance and avoid the breakdown of endogenous protein. Exogenous protein can be given through the gastrointestinal tract or parenterally. Parenteral administration is usually in the form of amino acid solutions, although peptide solutions may be adequate for most conditions.

In the steady state, a 70-kg adult typically consumes 1,800 cal and 60 g of protein each day, a ratio of 30 cal/g of protein or 187 cal/g of nitrogen. This would be the appropriate amount of nutrients for a patient who is not nutritionally depleted and is not hypermetabolic—a patient on ventilator support for Guillain-Barré syndrome, for example. If the patient is nutritionally depleted but not hypermetabolic (e.g., a patient with esophageal cancer being prepared for surgery), the maximal amount of protein that can be "loaded into" the active body cell mass should be given. The actual amount depends on the simultaneous caloric support because a greater positive nitrogen balance can be achieved with a given nitrogen supply when a positive caloric balance is achieved at the same time. In such a patient, it would be appropriate to give 150 g of protein and 2,500 cal daily (a ratio of 13 cal/g of protein or 85 cal/g of nitrogen). If most of the calories are given as carbohydrate, some of the carbohydrate will be converted to fat and so produce CO_2 and raise the minute ventilation requirement. A patient who is actively catabolizing protein because of a depletion of carbohydrate energy stores combined with a hypermetabolic state (e.g., a patient with major burns) requires an energy supply to match the hypermetabolic losses (e.g., 3,500 cal in a burn patient who is metabolizing 3,000 cal/d). An exogenous supply of energy may slow down or turn off protein catabolism, but it may not, and it is common practice to provide gross excesses of protein to these patients. Such a patient would typically receive 3,500 mL of a 4% protein formula, hence 140 g of protein with 3,500 cal (a ratio of 25 cal/g of protein or 160 cal/g of nitrogen).

Methods of Supplying Nutrition

Feeding by mouth is the most efficient way of providing energy and protein and is feasible in many critically ill patients. The possibility of oral feeding is one of several reasons why tracheostomy is preferable to endotracheal intubation for the long-term management of patients with acute respiratory failure.

Enteral Feeding. If the patient cannot or will not take food by mouth, liquid food should be administered directly into the stomach or intestine through a feeding tube.

Enteral feeding can be accomplished through a tube passed directly into the duodenum or jejunum at surgery, or through a tube passed into the stomach through the nose or mouth. Soft, small-bore feeding catheters with weighted tips are commercially available, but small-bore nasogastric tubes can serve just as well. It is generally possible to accomplish tube feeding with gastric infusion. Patients with gastric ileus, such as those who have just undergone abdominal operations, can be fed in the jejunum during the period of gastric atony. Formulas for tube feeding range from milk to commercial preparations. The commercial preparations generally contain 1 to 2 cal/mL and include 3% to 7% protein. Most of the calories are supplied as glucose or sucrose, so that the solutions have a high osmolarity. Cramps or diarrhea can result when these high-osmolarity solutions are placed into the stomach or intestine. Diarrhea is the major complication with most tube feeding formulations, and it can usually be controlled by adding pectin to the feedings. A large amount of pectin may be required. Diarrhea can also be minimized by the use of starch or fat as an energy source in tube feedings. This can be supplied as part of the commercial preparation or added in the form of medium-chain triglycerides or other oils. The best results are usually achieved by supplying about half of the calories as carbohydrate and half as fat. Although some of the formulations are advertised to produce little residue, almost all the liquid feeding formulas are completely absorbed in the small intestine. Typical formulas are shown in Table 9.3.

Feedings should be given by continuous infusion into the stomach rather than as large boluses. It is rarely necessary to administer more than 100 mL/h. When possible, the patient should be placed in a sitting position to prevent regurgitation along the tube. Gastric residuals should be checked if the patient feels uncomfortable or appears distended, but it is not necessary to check the residual more than once a day under most circumstances. With continuous tube feeding, a residual of 200 to 300 mL is normal.

It is better to start with a small amount of full-strength formula rather than a large amount of diluted formula. The amount (rather than the concentration) should be gradually increased until the desired volume is reached. Tube feedings can be supplemented by oral intake. Hypernatremia can result if the tube feeding is rich in sodium. This should be managed by the use of low-salt solutions or the administration of free water. A serious problem with tube feeding is complete cessation of feedings by the nursing staff because of diarrhea or a large gastric residual. If the tube feeding needs to be curtailed for any reason, it should be reinstituted the next hour at a smaller volume and gradually increased until the prescribed caloric load is reached.

Parenteral Feeding. Commercial preparations for parenteral feeding are limited to glucose (5% to 45%) and fat (10% to 20%) as energy sources and amino acid or peptide solutions (2% to 10%) as protein sources. Both parenteral and tube feedings are planned so that total energy requirements can be met through fat, carbohydrate, or both. Any protein administered should be available for anabolic processes. Parenteral feeding with carbohydrate is limited by the sclerotic effect of hyperosmolar solutions on veins. Effective parenteral feeding with carbohydrate alone requires solutions of at least 1 cal/mL (25% sugar). This type of solution must be administered into an area of rapid blood flow, generally the superior vena cava. Complications still occur, which are discussed later in this chapter. Fat is a more efficient energy source and can be given through peripheral veins in concentrations of either 10% or 20%. The total daily energy requirement can be given as fat, or a major portion can be given as fat with the rest as carbohydrate. Both fat and carbohydrate are equally effective sources of energy. The fat has the advantage of peripheral administration, and the carbohydrate has the advantage of about 10% less expense. The ratio between fat and carbohydrate energy sources and the ratio between total energy sources and grams of protein vary depending on the clinical state. For example, a patient with cardiac failure may require a solution that is low in volume, low in sodium, but high in calories and protein. A patient with multiple intestinal fistulae may require large volumes, which allow fewer calories and grams of protein per milliliter. Because of the potential problems with central venous cannulation, the administration of 10% glucose, amino acid solutions,

Table 9.3. COMPONENTS OF COMMONLY USED ENTERAL FEEDING FORMULAS

Name	Nonprotein calories			Protein (g)	Osmolarity (mOsm/kg)
	Total	Fat	Carbohydrate		
Milk	565	369	196	33	277
Eggnog	881	297	584	58	480
Isocal	924	396	528	34	300
Ensure	909	333	576	37	450
Vivonex	913	9	904	21	550
Vivonex HN	845	9	844	43	810
Magnacal	1,720	720	1,000	70	590

Table 9.4. COMPONENTS OF COMMONLY USED PARENTERAL FEEDING FORMULAS[a]

	Glucose		Amino acid (g)	mOsm	Calories: gram of nitrogen
	Grams	Calories			
Peripheral vein	100	400	25	880	85:1
Plus 500 mL 10% fat	100	900	25	880	222:1
Standard central	250	1,000	45	1,750	140:1
Concentrated cardiac	350	1,400	45	2,250	200:1

[a]Values per liter of solution.

and fat through peripheral veins has become popular. Two liters of 10% glucose supply 800 cal, and 500 mL of 20% lipid supply 1,000 cal. The total is ample for most patients who are not hypermetabolic.

Any hospital that routinely cares for critically ill patients should have a standardized approach to parenteral nutrition, including vascular access, catheter management, solution preparation, stock solutions, and protocols for the management of risks and complications. The standard solution for total parenteral nutrition is made by mixing equal amounts of 50% glucose and 9% amino acids. This solution contains the equivalent of 1 carbohydrate calorie per milliliter at a ratio of 25 cal/g of protein. The osmolarity of this solution is 1,800 mOsm/L, and it must be administered into an area of rapidly flowing blood. Sterile technique must be followed during insertion and care of the catheter. The standard solution can be modified for individual patients by raising or lowering the concentration of glucose and amino acids and by varying the electrolyte and trace metal composition. Vitamins and trace minerals are added to the solution at regular intervals, according to the general principle of providing more than basal requirements, as discussed earlier. The standard solution is supplemented with intravenous fat to provide at least 100 g of fat emulsion each week to preclude fatty acid deficiency. We favor giving 25% to 50% of the calories each day as fat emulsion. Fat emulsion is usually administered through a peripheral vein, although it can be given through a central catheter at the same time as the hypertonic glucose solution. Typical formulas are shown in Table 9.4.

The most common complication of total parenteral nutrition is infection on or around the intravascular catheter. Of course, infection can occur with any indwelling vascular catheter, but it is more likely in the presence of hypertonic glucose and protein solutions. If catheter infection is suspected, the catheter must be removed and a new catheter placed. The second most common complication is hyperglycemia, which is managed with insulin and the use of fat rather than glucose as the primary calorie source. Other complications are largely those of hyperglycemia—that is, hyperosmolar coma, osmotic diuresis, and localized thrombosis. These complications can be caused by running the solution too rapidly. This is prevented by always using a rate-limiting pump when hypertonic solutions are administered. The presence of systemic infection is an indication for nutritional support, not a contraindication to placing a central catheter. Other complications are related to disease states and specific amino acids. Aromatic amino acids are neurotransmitter precursors. Symptoms of central nervous system disturbances (confusion, seizures, coma) occur in patients receiving total parenteral nutrition, particularly those with liver dysfunction. The symptoms often cease when amino acid infusion is stopped. A solution low in aromatic amino acids has been proposed for patients with liver failure.

Application of Metabolic Economics to the Critically Ill Patient: Assessment of Nutritional Status

Whenever possible, patients who are identified as malnourished through the nutritional assessment process previously described should be returned to normal nutritional status before they undergo a major elective operation. Except in this circumstance, however, patients who require hospitalization because of critical illness cannot be nutritionally prepared ahead of time. The nutritional status of each patient admitted to the ICU should be evaluated. Patients who show evidence of malnutrition should be started on a feeding regimen soon after admission (Fig. 19.19).

During the period of critical illness, the nutritional and metabolic status should be assessed daily. Although estimation from tables or graphs varies considerably from the actual protein and caloric requirements, estimation is better than nothing. Correlation of daily fluid balance with daily weight is an essential step in evaluating nutritional status during critical illness. Along with a daily estimation or measurement of caloric balance, periodic measurement of acute-phase, protein-dependent reactants such as lymphocytes is also helpful. Many patients reach a state of hypoproteinemia in the critical care unit; however, this should never happen if appropriate attention is given to protein and calorie status. The University of Michigan algorithm for management of nutrition in critical illness is shown in Fig. 9.20. In our studies, patients who were in a positive caloric balance at the time of ICU discharge had a higher survival rate than patients in a

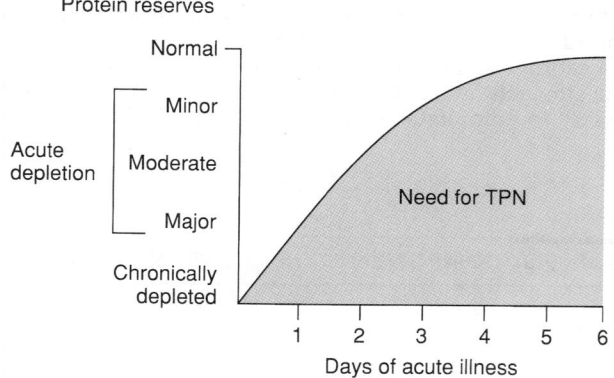

Figure 9.19. General guidelines for determining when to institute parenteral nutrition after acute illness or operation. Patients at risk for multiple-organ failure should be started on total parenteral nutrition within 48 hours. (After Bartlett RH. Nutritional support. In: Dantzker DR, ed. *Cardiopulmonary critical care.* Orlando, FL: Grune & Stratton, 1986:263, with permission.)

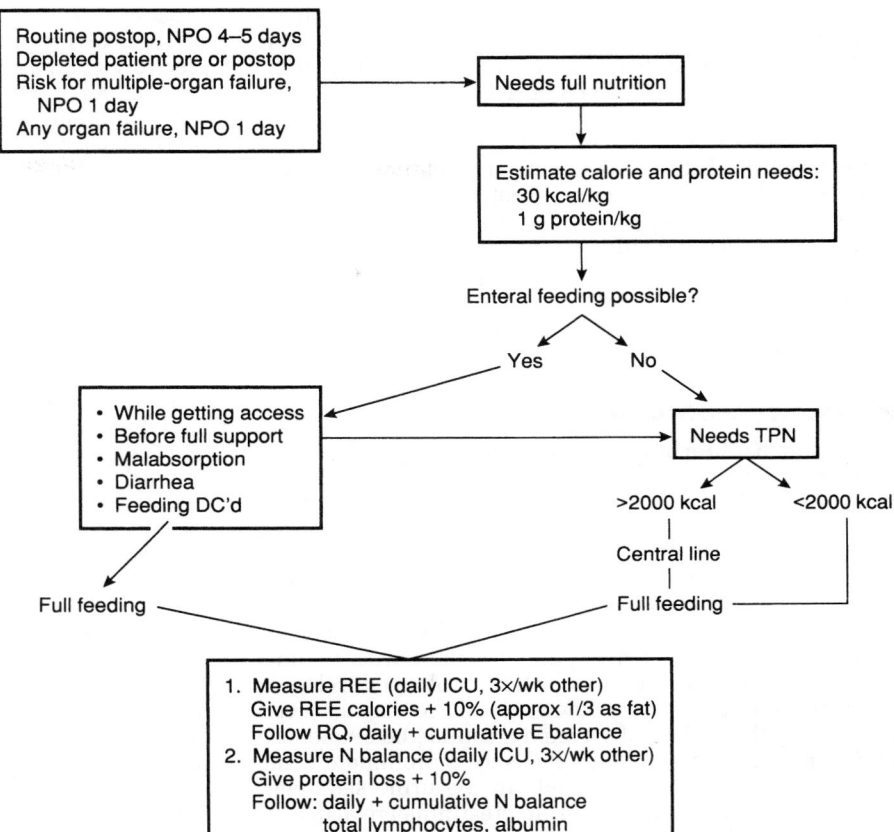

Figure 9.20. Nutritional management algorithm. *TPN,* total parenteral nutrition; *REE,* resting energy expenditure; *RQ,* respiratory quotient. (After Bartlett RH. *University of Michigan critical care handbook.* Boston; Little, Brown, 1996, with permission.)

negative balance. In particular, patients with a 10,000-cal cumulative deficit at the time of discharge from the ICU had a high mortality rate.

Energy requirements should be measured, specifically in patients with respiratory failure, because overfeeding with carbohydrate results in excess CO_2 production through the conversion of carbohydrate to fat. A positive RQ can make it necessary to continue mechanical ventilation in a patient who would otherwise be ready for weaning from the ventilator.

A patient with systemic infection (sepsis) has an elevated metabolic rate and an elevated protein catabolic rate. Such a patient requires an energy and protein supply to meet these needs. The fact that the patient has a systemic infection should not deter the physician from placing a central venous catheter or whatever access is required for enteral or parenteral feeding.

ACUTE RENAL FAILURE

Acute renal failure (ARF), by definition, is an abrupt decrease in kidney function that results in the accumulation of nitrogenous solutes. ARF may be oliguric (urine output < 400 mL/d) or nonoliguric (urine output is normal or increased while solute clearance is markedly decreased) (Table 9.5). The mortality of ARF in the surgical ICU is high (50% to 90%) because ARF is usually just one component of severe multiple-organ failure. The mortality from nonoliguric ARF is significantly less than that from oliguric ARF, although many patients progress to oliguria with its poor outcome. Regardless of urine output, the sequelae of ARF result from the retention of metabolic wastes and are indicated by a progressive rise in blood urea nitrogen (BUN) and serum creatinine concentrations.

Hypervolemia and electrolyte imbalances further complicate the management of oliguric ARF.

The pathogenesis of ARF is commonly classified as prerenal, postrenal, or intrinsic parenchymal disease. This discussion is limited to parenchymal disease.

Parenchymal abnormalities include acute tubular necrosis, pigment nephropathy (secondary to circulating myoglobin and hemoglobin), and those caused by nephrotoxic agents (various drugs and contrast material). Other causes of parenchymal renal disease, such as acute glomerular nephritis and vasculitis, are not typically responsible for ARF in the surgical patient and are not discussed in this chapter.

Acute Tubular Necrosis

Acute tubular necrosis results from ischemia in the renal parenchyma and is the most common pathologic finding of ARF. Under conditions of diminishing renal blood flow, perfusion of the kidneys is first maintained by vasomotor responses, which dilate the afferent arteriole

Table 9.5. **STANDARD MEASUREMENTS IN THE DIAGNOSIS OF RENAL FAILURE**

Test	Prerenal	Parenchymal
Urine osmolarity (mOsm)	>500	250–350
U/P osmolality	>1.5	<1.1
U/P creatinine	>20	<10
Urine sodium	<20	>40
FE_{Na}	<1%	>3%

FE_{Na}, fraction of excreted sodium; U/P, urine-to-plasma ratio.

and constrict the efferent arteriole. As continued hypotension is detected by the juxtaglomerular apparatus, the renin–angiotensin system is activated in concert with the sympathetic release of other vasoactive hormones. These substances produce vasoconstriction of the afferent arteriole and further exacerbate cortical hypoperfusion. Casts of cellular debris obstruct the lumen, and cellular edema occurs. As tubular cells become necrotic and slough off, the leakage of glomerular ultrafiltrate back across the proximal tubular membrane into the interstitium causes edema. Acute tubular necrosis comprises a spectrum of effects of cortical ischemia, ranging from polyuria with tubular dysfunction to temporary anuria to renal cortical necrosis with chronic anuria.

Pigment Nephropathy

Pigment nephropathy is a common cause of ARF and may occur after trauma, burn, operation, or hemodynamic catastrophe. During ischemia or after blunt injury to large muscle masses, myoglobin is released into the circulation. In the kidney, it is filtered from the blood and reabsorbed by the tubule. Although myoglobin is not a direct nephrotoxin, in the presence of aciduria, myoglobin is converted to ferrihemate, which is toxic to renal cells. Rhabdomyolysis should be suspected in patients with burns, trauma, seizures, alcohol or drug intoxication, prolonged ischemia in muscle groups, and extended coma. The diagnosis can be made by the finding of elevated creatine phosphokinase and a urine microscopy study that shows prominent heme pigment without red blood cells in the urine sediment. Hyperkalemia and elevated serum creatinine are also consistent with injury to muscle masses. Prevention of myoglobin-induced ARF may include the use of diuretics and alkalization of urine.

Nephrotoxic Agents

Drug-induced ARF is responsible for about 5% of all cases of ARF. Its pathophysiology differs according to the offending agent. Through normal reabsorption and secretion, the kidney is exposed to high concentrations of drugs and solutes, which may be toxic. This problem is compounded by hypovolemia, which causes an increased reabsorption of water and solutes and exposes the lumen to even higher concentrations of toxins. Although the damage to tubular function can be significant, much drug-induced ARF remains nonoliguric because of the sparing of glomerular function.

Radiographic contrast dye has been documented to cause ARF. The incidence of contrast nephropathy is about 1% to 10% and may be predicted according to a number of risk factors. These include contrast load, age, preexisting renal insufficiency, and diabetes, although some of these factors are disputed. The incidence in patients with normal renal function is a significantly lower, at 1% to 2%. Contrast nephropathy is usually experienced as an asymptomatic, transient rise in creatinine but may progress to oliguric renal failure that requires hemodialysis. Induced diuresis with fluids and diuretics before contrast injection may decrease the incidence and severity of ARF in high-risk patients.

Management of Acute Renal Failure

In surgical patients, ARF rarely occurs in an isolated fashion. Rather, ARF is only one component of a syndrome of multiple-organ failure that is often accompanied by infection. The treatment of these patients, therefore, should be focused on managing the underlying disease processes. The development of ARF complicates the care of surgical patients by introducing difficulties in fluid, electrolyte, and nutritional management. The adverse effects of renal replacement therapies further compound these problems. A favorable outcome can be achieved only through aggressive intervention. This includes surgical drainage of septic foci, excision of necrotic tissue, early implementation of effective renal replacement therapy, and full nutritional support.

General Care

The University of Michigan algorithm for the evaluation and management of renal failure is shown in Fig. 9.21. With nonoliguric ARF, the treatment may differ little from that required for identical patients with normal renal function. The management of fluids, solutes, and nutrition is usually unaffected by nonoliguric ARF, although the BUN may be elevated. The extent of renal dysfunction is limited and almost always reversible. The use of renal replacement therapies (and their inherent complications) is rarely necessary.

Oliguria and anuria pose several management difficulties. In the absence of normal urine output, problems of fluid overload can lead to anasarca, pulmonary edema, and congestive heart failure. The pharmacokinetics of drugs becomes difficult to predict as a result of decreased elimination and increased volume of distribution. In light of these risks, the volume status of patients with ARF must be carefully monitored. Fluid intake and output must be precisely tabulated, and the body weight should be measured daily. Pulmonary artery catheterization may be necessary to monitor the fluid status of these patients more closely. Treatment options for hypervolemia consist of fluid restriction or fluid removal with artificial kidney techniques. Fluid restriction, however, limits the administration of intravenous medications and may preclude adequate nutrition.

Acute renal failure can create severe derangements in electrolyte and acid–base physiology. Serum electrolytes should be measured daily. Of all the electrolyte abnormalities that can occur with ARF, hyperkalemia is the most serious. Under the conditions of hypercatabolism and tissue necrosis that characterize these patients, large amounts of potassium may be generated and accumulate during a short period of time. Acute hyperkalemia causes a decrease in cardiac excitability, which can ultimately result in asystole. The removal of potassium must be accomplished with renal replacement therapy or ion-exchange resins. Other electrolyte abnormalities, such as hyponatremia, hyperphosphatemia, hypocalcemia, and metabolic acidosis, are common in ARF and must be monitored closely. Treatment consists of appropriate additions or restrictions of intravenous solutions and effective use of the artificial kidney.

Platelet dysfunction and coagulopathy are often associated with ARF. A reproducible platelet defect can be demonstrated experimentally with a BUN of 100 mg/dL.

Anemia also accompanies ARF in surgical patients. In addition to the loss of blood during hemorrhage or operation, the production of erythropoietin has been shown to decrease in direct proportion to the decrease in renal function.

Nutrition

The goal of nutritional support in ARF is to provide optimal amounts of calorie and protein substrates to minimize autocatabolism and allow tissue anabolism, wound healing, and sustained immune function. In any discussion of nutrition and renal failure, it is necessary to point out the distinction between acute and chronic renal failure. Patients with chronic renal failure are generally healthy, and their energy requirements differ little from

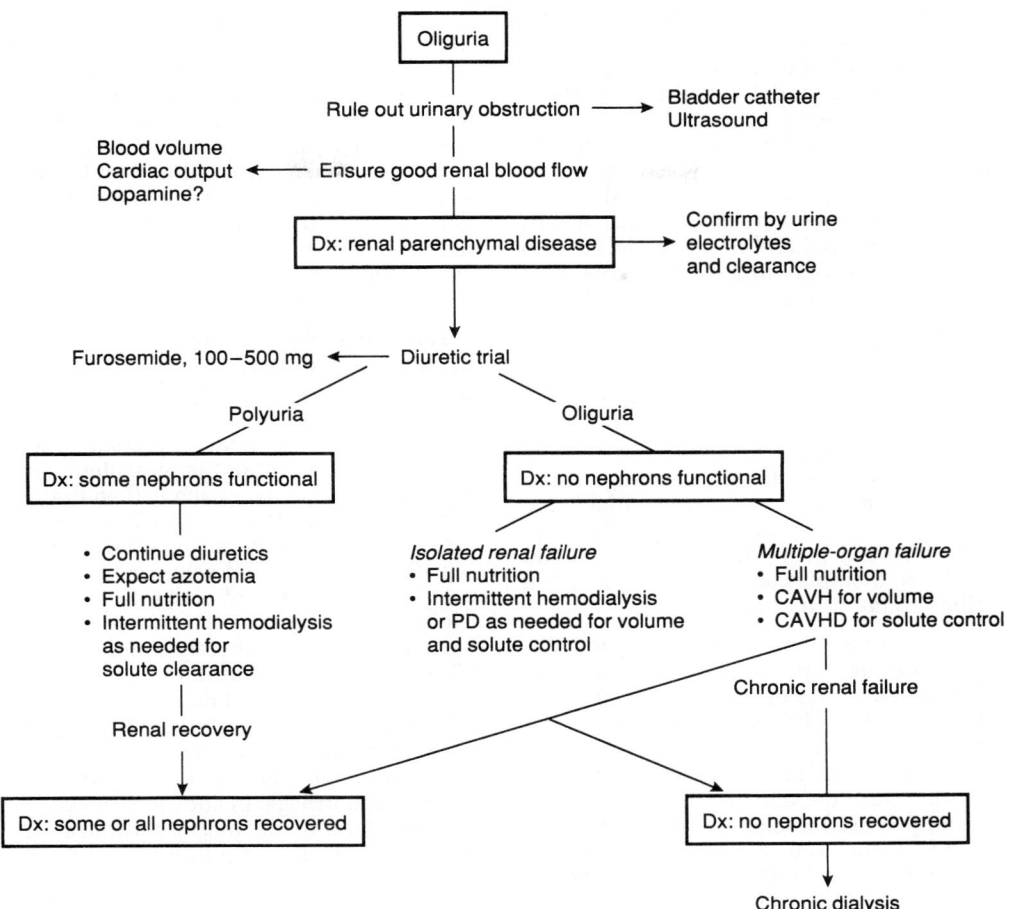

Figure 9.21. Algorithm for the management of acute renal failure. *PD*, peritoneal dialysis; *CAVH*, continuous arteriovenous hemofiltration; *CAVHD*, continuous arteriovenous hemodialysis. (After Mault JR, Bartlett RH. Acute renal failure. In: Greenfield LJ, ed. *Complications in surgery and trauma*, 2nd ed. Philadelphia: JB Lippincott, 1989:149, with permission.)

those of persons without chronic renal failure. Protein intake is required only for metabolic turnover and is restricted to the minimize the generation of urea and other products of protein metabolism.

By contrast, the metabolic requirements of a patient with ARF are those of a critically ill, hospitalized patient. Actual measurement of resting energy expenditure has shown that the caloric requirements of patients with multiple-organ failure and ARF are often 50% above those of normal, healthy subjects. Measured protein requirements may be increased to as much as 2.5 g/kg to provide for anabolic wound healing and sustained immune function. For these patients, protein restriction is counterproductive and potentially detrimental. Urea generation is best minimized by providing enough energy substrates (carbohydrates and lipids) to prevent the cannibalization of endogenous protein as an energy source. Investigations emphasizing energy and protein balance have demonstrated an improved outcome in ARF.

A positive energy balance may also make the management of uremia and hyperkalemia less difficult. When a patient receives fewer calories than those expended, the difference must be made up from endogenous stores. In a well-nourished person, carbohydrate stores rarely exceed 2,500 kcal. After these stores have been depleted, lipid and protein stores are mobilized. In the diseased state, endogenous protein has been shown to be catabolized pref-

erentially as an energy substrate in the absence of readily available glucose. With the catabolism of protein, urea is generated. In addition, catabolic wasting of tissues and cells liberates excess potassium. Maintaining a positive energy balance with glucose and lipids should reduce protein catabolism, urea generation, and hyperkalemia.

Although protein restriction may be advocated in chronic renal failure, the protein requirements in ARF are usually elevated. Abel and colleagues were among the first to suggest that survival is improved with the addition of amino acids to intravenous nutrition. Others have confirmed these findings. The two important concerns regarding protein supplementation in ARF are what type and how much to administer. The rate of protein catabolism reported in various studies ranges from 70 to 200 g/d. In light of this wide range of values for protein catabolism, the actual measurement of protein balance is desirable. In an oliguric patient, the protein catabolic rate can be reasonably approximated by calculating the rate of urea generation. In this calculation, the changes in BUN and fluid balance are recorded for a 24-hour period. The nitrogen content is also determined in collections of dialysate or ultrafiltrate, nasogastric suction fluids, wound drainage, and so on, obtained during the same time interval. If one assumes that the urea produced during protein catabolism is not reused and is contained within the extracellular space, the urea generation rate can be calculated. With this information, the daily protein balance can be monitored. Maintaining a positive protein balance is the goal, although this may be difficult to achieve. Most investigators supplement protein at a rate of 0.5 to 1 g/kg daily, and the effects of providing larger amounts have yet to be studied.

Much effort has been dedicated to determining the best proteins and amino acids to administer to ARF patients. Some contend that a solution of only essential amino acids should be given, whereas others have shown benefit with the use of mixed (essential and nonessential) amino acids. In addition, solutions containing a high proportion of branched-chain amino acids may enhance a positive nitrogen balance.

Renal Replacement Therapy

Indications for the use of renal replacement therapy include fluid overload (pulmonary edema, congestive heart failure), hyperkalemia, metabolic acidosis, uremic encephalopathy, coagulopathy, and acute poisoning. Three modalities of renal replacement therapy are available for the treatment of ARF: hemodialysis, peritoneal dialysis, and continuous arteriovenous hemofiltration (CAVH). The features of each of these therapies are contrasted in Table 9.6 and are described in the next sections.

Hemodialysis. In the contemporary form of hemodialysis, blood is circulated through a porous, hollow-fiber membrane that is permeable to solutes of less than 2,000 d. An isotonic solution surrounding the membrane provides a concentration gradient for the selective removal of solutes such as potassium, urea, and creatinine while plasma concentrations of sodium, chloride, and bicarbonate are unchanged. A roller pump is used to maintain an extracorporeal blood flow of about 300 mL/min through an arteriovenous shunt or a double-lumen venovenous access. The transmembrane pressure gradient created by the pump effects the desired amount of fluid removal. Full systemic anticoagulation is required for this procedure, although less heparin may be used in patients with a baseline coagulopathy. Hemodialysis is typically performed every other day for a 3- to 4-hour period but is required more frequently in catabolic patients with high rates of urea generation. Solute and volume removal with hemodialysis is considered very efficient relative to removal with the other methods of renal replacement. This efficiency is reflected in the clearance of water-soluble drugs such as aminoglycosides, cephalosporins, and penicillins. Plasma concentrations may be decreased by as much as 50% per treatment; accordingly, these drugs should be administered after treatments with close monitoring of serum concentrations. Hemodialysis is also the method of choice for the rapid removal of life-threatening toxins and poisons.

Although the incidence of complications of hemodialysis is insignificant in the treatment of patients with chronic renal failure, frequent and often profound complications may occur when it is used to treat critically ill patients with ARF. In the acute setting, hemodialysis has been shown to cause hypotension, hypoxemia, and hemolysis and to precipitate cardiac arrhythmia. These events limit the application of dialysis in patients with unstable conditions.

Peritoneal Dialysis. Peritoneal dialysis is performed by infusing several liters of a sterile electrolyte solution with hypertonic glucose into the abdominal space. With the peritoneal membrane used as a selective barrier, the dialysate solution creates an osmotic pressure gradient that extracts ECF and solutes out of the mesenteric circulation and into the peritoneal cavity, which is then drained after an equilibration period of 1 to 2 hours. The rate of extracellular volume removal usually ranges from 0.5 to 1 L/h, although a higher rate of fluid and solute clearance can be attained by using larger volumes of dialysate and performing exchange cycles more frequently. The use of automated delivery systems makes this a relatively simple procedure with respect to nursing time and training.

Peritoneal dialysis has several advantages over other methods of renal substitution. The technique does not require vascular access or systemic anticoagulation, so that it is useful in patients with peripheral vascular disease or at risk for hemorrhage. In addition, the slow rate of equilibration and fluid extraction in peritoneal dialysis minimizes the problems of dysequilibrium and hemodynamic compromise experienced with conventional hemodialysis.

Peritoneal dialysis is associated with many risks and complications, particularly in surgical patients. The most frequent and significant of these is catheter infection and peritonitis. Rigid peritoneal catheters inserted percutaneously in the acute setting become predictably colonized after 48 to 72 hours. Subcutaneously placed Silastic catheters are associated with a lower incidence of peritonitis (1.6 episodes per patient-year) and should be implanted in patients undergoing peritoneal dialysis for prolonged periods. Other access-related complications include visceral injury at the time of catheter placement and formation of intraabdominal adhesions. In light of these risks, peritoneal dialysis is generally the last-choice method of renal replacement after abdominal operation or trauma.

Table 9.6. COMPARISON OF RENAL REPLACEMENT THERAPIES

	Hemodialysis	**Peritoneal dialysis**	**CAVH/CAVHD**
Description	Rapid, intermittent	Slow, intermittent	Slow, continuous
Access	Arteriovenous or venovenous	Abdominal catheter	Arteriovenous
Anticoagulation	Required	None required	Required
Solute removal	Excellent	Excellent	Good with standard CAVH; excellent with CAVHD
Fluid removal	Good to excellent	Good	Excellent
Hemodynamic instability	Significant	None	None
Risks of procedure	Hypotension/hypoxemia, dysequilibrium syndrome	Infection or peritonitis, intraabdominal adhesions, respiratory distress	Dehydration, hemorrhage, electrolyte imbalance
Overall appraisal	Useful for urgent removal of solutes or poisons	Contraindicated with abdominal operation	Allows great flexibility with fluid and electrolyte balance
	Hemodynamic instability limits use in intensive care patients	Useful in burn patients and those with poor vascular access	Solute removal enhanced with CAVHD

CAVH, continuous arteriovenous hemofiltration; CAVHD, continuous arteriovenous hemodialysis.

Other complications of peritoneal dialysis include hyperglycemia secondary to the hypertonic glucose of the dialysate and respiratory distress secondary to reduced diaphragmatic compliance resulting from increased intraabdominal pressure. Finally, repeated lavage of the peritoneal cavity causes a daily protein loss of 10 g or more and may exacerbate malnutrition in patients with catabolic ARF.

Continuous Arteriovenous Hemofiltration. CAVH was conceived by Kramer and colleagues in 1977 and is specifically intended for the treatment of ARF. CAVH is an extracorporeal ultrafiltration technique that removes ECF across a synthetic membrane by means of a hydrostatic pressure gradient created between indwelling arterial and venous catheters. When the systolic blood pressure is 80 mm Hg or higher, blood flows through the porous, hollow-fiber capillary membrane at a rate of 50 to 150 mL/min, driving plasma water and solutes of up to 10,000 d out of the hemofilter at a rate of 500 to 700 mL/h. A replacement solution formulated to resemble ECF without toxic solutes is simultaneously infused into the venous access port of the circuit at a rate sufficient to achieve the desired hourly fluid balance. This exchange transfusion of 12 to 17 L of ECF per day provides clearance of about 10 to 14 g of urea per day (if a BUN concentration of 80 mg/dL is assumed). Arteriovenous access is accomplished by percutaneous cannulation of the femoral artery and vein with a low incidence of complications. Although full systemic anticoagulation is not necessary for CAVH, heparinization of the extracorporeal circuit is required, usually at a rate of 500 U/h. CAVH is run continuously for as many days as renal replacement is required. Hemofilter performance (monitored by the ultrafiltration rate) decreases with time, so that replacement with a new hemofilter is required about every 2 days. Continuous hemofiltration can also be accomplished by venous drainage with a pump, with return to the venous system.

Experience with CAVH has shown that it causes little or no hemodynamic instability when unstable, critically ill patients with ARF are treated. The stable nature of this therapy is attributed to the slow and continuous removal of fluid and solutes and to the fact that the membrane (polysulfone) does not induce complement activation when in contact with blood.

With ultrafiltration rates averaging 10 to 12 L/d, CAVH also allows great flexibility in volume management and eliminates the need for fluid restriction in patients with oliguric ARF. Fluid balance and serum electrolyte concentrations can be titrated to any value in a matter of hours by manipulating the composition and rate of flow of the replacement solution. CAVH facilitates the provision of optimal amounts of nutrition to patients with ARF.

Solute clearance with CAVH is limited by the ultrafiltration and replacement fluid exchange rate. In patients with a high rate of urea generation, solute removal by CAVH may be inadequate, and variations of the technique may be used to enhance clearance. The most promising of these variations is continuous arteriovenous hemodialysis (CAVHD), in which the same filter and circuit are used as in CAVH with the addition of a dialysate bath to increase solute clearance to equal that achieved with standard hemodialysis. In CAVHD, ultrafiltration is diminished to about 150 mL/h, so that little replacement fluid is required and the procedure is simplified. With either CAVH or CAVHD, complications of dehydration, electrolyte imbalance, and hemorrhage can occur. Accurate tabulation of fluid balance and frequent measurements of serum electrolytes and coagulation indices are necessary.

Guidelines for Renal Replacement Therapy in Acute Renal Failure. The current recommendations for renal replacement therapy in ARF are as follows:

1. Volume (intravenous fluids, total parenteral nutrition) should be supplemented as the patient requires, regardless of the method of renal replacement.
2. Renal replacement therapy should be instituted early in the course of ARF, before hypervolemia, azotemia, or hyperkalemia occurs.
3. For severely ill patients with ARF, CAVH is the renal replacement therapy of choice.
4. If solute clearance is insufficient with CAVH, conversion to CAVHD or supplementation with standard hemodialysis should be carried out.
5. Peritoneal dialysis may be used when vascular access is unavailable or when the risk for hemorrhage is prohibitive.
6. Hemodynamically stable patients with isolated ARF should be treated with intermittent hemodialysis or peritoneal dialysis.

Prognosis

The survival of patients with ARF depends on the successful treatment of the primary disease causing renal failure. The anephric patient supported with renal replacement therapy survives until disease of some other organ system supervenes. In a study of patients with "pure" acute tubular necrosis after renal transplantation, Mentzer and colleagues reported the mortality rate of ischemic acute tubular necrosis without other organ failure to be 6%. In contrast, the mortality rate of multiple-organ failure complicated by ARF ranges from 50% to 90%.

For patients who survive the acute phase of illness, the recovery of renal function after ARF depends on the type and extent of injury to the renal parenchyma. Renal replacement therapy may be required for several weeks until urine output and solute excretion return to acceptable levels. If renal function has not returned after 6 weeks, recovery is unlikely, and provisions should be made for long-term renal substitution therapy.

MULTIPLE-ORGAN FAILURE

For the purposes of this discussion, multiple-organ failure is defined as dysfunction of two or more of the six vital organ systems: cardiovascular, respiratory, nervous system, renal, hepatic, and host defenses. Failure of other organ systems (e.g., skin, coagulation, digestive system) may occur, but this is of secondary importance in comparison with failure of the major organ systems. A definition of organ system failure appears in Table 9.7. One of the important contributions of the adult extracorporeal membrane oxygenation study sponsored by the National Institutes of Health was to identify multiple-organ failure as a

---

Table 9.7. CRITERIA FOR ORGAN FAILURE[a]

Cardiovascular	Cardiac index <2.5 L/m^2/min with left atrial pressure >10 mm Hg
	Inotropic or vasopressor drugs required to maintain adequate perfusion
Respiratory	Alveolar–arterial O_2 gradient >300 mm Hg
Nervous	Glasgow Coma Score <10
Renal	Creatinine >3 mg/dL
Hepatic	Bilirubin >5 mg/dL
Host defenses	Positive blood culture
	Invasive tissue infection
	Anergic to common antigens

[a]Arbitrary definitions of the University of Michigan Surgical Intensive Care Unit.

syndrome and to define the mortality risk. The 713 patients in that study were selected because they had respiratory failure, and the mortality rate of respiratory failure alone was 40% in patients ages 12 to 65 years. With failure of two organ systems, the mortality rate rose to 55%; it was 75% with failure of three organ systems, and 90% with failure of four or more. In a study of isolated acute postoperative renal failure without failure of other organ systems, the mortality rate was 6%. The mortality rate with multiple-organ failure that included renal failure was 70% to 90%. Failure of the host defense system, defined as locally invasive infection or systemic sepsis, is both a cause and a result of failure of other organ systems and carries a high risk for mortality.

The specific mechanism of organ injury during ischemia is the subject of many other chapters in this book. Understanding the mechanism is of major importance because it may be possible to prevent or delay tissue injury by pharmacologic or mechanical means during periods of ischemia. The pharmacologic prevention of tissue injury associated with ischemia by using enzyme inhibitors, O_2 radical "scavengers," and other agents is a subject of major interest and is discussed in detail in other chapters in this book. The most effective short-term form of protection during ischemia is hypothermia. Cooling organs during the ischemic period of transplantation and cardiac operations has been standard practice for decades. Hypothermia offers protection from ischemic injury for minutes to hours. We rarely take advantage of this phenomenon in the ICU, but the use of moderate hypothermia (with paralysis and anesthesia to prevent shivering) is worthy of investigation as a short-term means of preventing tissue injury. In fact, this is a normal protective mechanism. Any patient in profound circulatory shock rapidly becomes hypothermic.

If a single organ sustains a major ischemic injury and perfusion is then reestablished, other organs may progress through the early phases of tissue injury identified earlier. Specifically, after prolonged ischemia and reperfusion of a leg, for example, generalized capillary leakage is commonly seen. The organs that malfunction when edematous are most obviously affected (lung, brain, heart, and gut). However, the fact that tissue edema also occurs in kidney, muscle, skin, and all other organs suggests that chemical or cellular mediators from the ischemic reperfused tissue act to increase capillary permeability throughout the body. The increased permeability in organs other than the lungs suggests that microemboli are not mediators, as they would be trapped in pulmonary capillaries, but rather that humoral or cellular mediators are at work. A wide variety of substances have been implicated as mediators of increased capillary permeability, including lysosomal enzymes, by-products of coagulation and fibrinolysis, platelets and the products of platelet activation, white cells and the products of white cell activation, arachidonic acid metabolites, activated complement, leukocytic cytokines, and superoxide radicals. In addition to these general factors, tissue-specific agents may cause systemic toxicity, such as myoglobin after muscle ischemia or bacterial endotoxin after gut ischemia. The actual mechanism of systemic capillary injury after local ischemia probably includes many or all of these mediators, so that a single pharmacologic approach to prevention would be naïve.

Clinically, the patient with multiple-organ failure progresses through well-defined phases. Identification of these phases may help shed some light on the mechanisms of tissue injury in systemic ischemia. After an episode of shock and resuscitation, the phases of multiple-organ failure can be described as follows:

Phase I: Generalized increased capillary permeability results in edema, weight gain, intravenous volume requirement, and increased protein concentration in urine and lymph. Although the pulmonary microvasculature has been studied the most thoroughly, it is apparent that the lung is the most obvious end-organ in a generalized permeability defect.

Phase II: A hypermetabolic state is characterized by an increased $\dot{V}O_2$, and a compensatory increase in O_2 delivery is characterized by tachycardia and a high cardiac output. The similarity of this condition after systemic ischemia and reperfusion to hypermetabolism after endotoxemia, localized sterile inflammation, and infusion of stress hormones suggests a common mechanism.

Phase III: Organ malfunction results from localized edema (particularly in the lung and heart) and cellular injury, particularly in the kidney, liver, brain, and host defense system. Hemorrhagic shock predisposes to bacterial translocation and endotoxin absorption from the intestine. The theory that gut bacteria are the cause of systemic hypermetabolism and capillary leakage in shock is an old one that is receiving renewed attention.

Phase IV: In the absence of systemic sepsis, organs may recover to normalcy or may be irreversibly damaged and require long-term support (e.g., the kidney). If the phases of organ failure lead to systemic infection or irreversible tissue damage in the lung or brain, then death of the entire organ is likely.

The management of multiple-organ failure is the business of intensive care and is only briefly summarized here. The important goals are to avoid further episodes of local or systemic ischemia and to keep the brain viable by pharmacologic or mechanical support of the failing organs until they recover.

Respiratory failure is treated by providing mechanical assistance for lung inflation and ventilation and by decreasing lung edema as much as possible. Airway intubation is usually required, with the use of positive end-expiratory pressure and continuous positive airway pressure to achieve and sustain alveolar inflation for the purpose of systemic oxygenation, and the use of mechanical ventilation for the purpose of CO_2 removal. Peak airway pressures greater than 40 cm H_2O are damaging to the lung, and much of the progressive respiratory failure seen in the past decade in the ICU may have been iatrogenic barotrauma. Good evidence now indicates that forced diuresis with a negative fluid balance is associated with improved survival in acute respiratory failure.

Cardiac failure is treated with inotropic drugs and with mechanical devices (usually the intraaortic balloon pump) if inotropes are ineffective. Although inotropic drugs are usually titrated to achieve a desired arterial blood pressure, it is more sensible to titrate inotropes to achieve a normal $\dot{D}O_2/\dot{V}O_2$ ratio. Monitoring of pulmonary artery pressure and mixed venous saturation is essential to the intelligent treatment of patients with severe respiratory or cardiac failure.

Adequate nutrition is important for recovery from multiple-organ failure. Usually, the gut malfunctions early in this syndrome (ileus), and it is necessary to provide nutrients intravenously. Sugar and fat are given to meet requirements according to $\dot{V}O_2$ measurement and the arithmetic of indirect calorimetry. Protein is given to match protein losses, usually in the range of 1 to 2 g/kg per day. Our data indicate that results are improved if nutritional support is begun in critically ill patients within 24 hours of admission to the ICU.

Renal failure is treated by the mechanical substitution of renal function. Although hemodialysis and peritoneal dialysis can serve this purpose, each is associated with significant drawbacks in the critically ill patient with multiple-organ failure. CAVH and CAVHD are the methods of choice for renal replacement therapy and have totally replaced intermittent dialysis for critically ill patients in our hospital. An important change during the last few years in the management of patients with renal failure has been the substitution of full nutritional support for the protein and fluid restriction practiced in the past.

Hepatic failure is often part of this syndrome, for which no specific treatment is available. The effects of hepatic failure (coagulopathy, hypoproteinemia, ascites, ammonia intoxication) are treated symptomatically.

Host defense failure (locally invasive or systemic infection) is treated by local drainage, excision, or both whenever possible, with the addition of systemic antibiotics. Despite an incredible proliferation of synthetic antibiotics, sepsis is the final common pathway in most of these patients.

REFERENCES

General

Preoperative and Postoperative Care Committee of the American College of Surgeons. *Care of the surgical patient*, vol 1. *Critical care*. New York: Scientific American Medicine, 1988.

Bartlett RH. *University of Michigan critical care handbook*. Boston: Little, Brown, 1996.

Oxygen Kinetics

Bartlett RH. A critical carol: being an essay on anemia, suffocation, starvation, and other forms of intensive care, after the manner of Dickens. *Chest* 1984;85:687–693.

Cain SM. Oxygen delivery and uptake in dogs during anemic and hypoxic hypoxia. *J Appl Physiol* 1977;42:228.

Cilley RE, Scharenberg AM, Bongiorno PF, et al. Low oxygen delivery produced by anemia, hypoxia, and low cardiac output. *J Surg Res* 1991;51:425.

Fleming A, Bishop M, Shoemaker W, et al. Prospective trial of supranormal values as goals of resuscitation in severe trauma. *Arch Surg* 1992;127:1175.

Hirschl RB, Heiss KF, Cilley RE, et al. Oxygen kinetics in experimental sepsis. *Surgery* 1992;112:37.

Russel JA, Phang PT. Oxygen delivery/consumption controversy: approaches to management of critically ill. *Am J Respir Crit Care Med* 1994;149:533.

Shoemaker W, Appel PL, Kram HB. Hemodynamic and oxygen transport responses in survivors and nonsurvivors of high-risk surgery. *Crit Care Med* 1993;21:977.

Tremper KK, Barker SJ. Pulse oximetry. *Anesthesiology* 1989;70:98.

Tuchschmidt J, Fried J, Astiz M, et al. Elevation of cardiac output and oxygen delivery improves outcome in septic shock. *Chest* 1992;102:216.

White KM. Completing the hemodynamic picture: S$\dot{V}$O$_2$. *Heart Lung* 1985;14:272.

Hemodynamics

Camm AJ, Garratt CJ. Adenosine and superventricular tachycardia. *N Engl J Med* 1991;325:1261.

Fick A. *On the measurement of the blood quantity in the ventricles of the heart*. Proceedings of the Physiological, Medical Society of Wurzburg, July 9, 1870.

Hansen PD, Coffey SC, Lewis FR. The effects of adrenergic agents on oxygen delivery and oxygen consumption in normal dogs. *J Trauma* 1994;37:283.

Ognibene FP, Parker MM, Natanson C, et al. Depressed left ventricular performance: response to volume infusion in patients with sepsis and septic shock. *Chest* 1988;93:903.

Sarnoff SJ. Myocardial contractility as described by ventricular function curves: observations on Starling's law of the heart. *Physiol Rev* 1955;35:107.

Starling EH. The Linacre lecture on the law of the heart. Given at Cambridge, 1915. London: Longmans, Green, 1918.

Swan HJC, Ganz W, Forrester JS, et al. Catheterization of the heart in man with the use of a flow-directed balloon-tipped catheter. *N Engl J Med* 1970;283:447.

Vincent JL, Preiser JC. Inotropic agents. *New Horizons* 1993;1:137.

Respiration

Arensman R, Cornish JD, eds. *Extracorporeal life support*. Cambridge, MA: Blackwell Science, 1993.

Artigas A, Carlet J, LeGall JR, et al. Clinical presentation, prognostic factors, and outcome of ARDS in the European collaborative study, 1985–1987: a preliminary report. In: Zapol W, Lamare F, eds. *Adult respiratory distress syndrome*. New York: Marcel Dekker Inc., 1991.

Bartlett RH. Use of mechanical ventilation. In: Holcroft J, ed. *Care of the surgical patient*, vol 1. *Critical care*. New York: Scientific American Medicine, 1989;2:9.

Bartlett RH, Morris AH, Fairley HB, et al. A prospective study of acute hypoxic respiratory failure. *Chest* 1986;589:684.

Bernard GR, Artigas A, Brigham KL, et al. The American–European consensus conference on ARDS: definitions, mechanisms, relative outcomes, and clinical trial coordination. *Am J Respir Crit Care Med* 1994;149:818.

Gattinoni L, Bombino M, Pelosi P, et al. Lung structure and function in different stages of severe adult respiratory distress syndrome. *JAMA* 1994;271:1772.

Gattinoni L, D'Andrea L, Pelosi P, et al. Regional effects and mechanism of positive end-expiratory pressure in early adult respiratory distress syndrome. *JAMA* 1993;269:2122.

Hechtman HB, Weisel RD, Vito L, et al. The independence of pulmonary shunting and pulmonary edema. *Surgery* 1973;74:300.

Hickling KG, Walsh J, Henderson S, et al. Low mortality rate in ARDS using low volume, pressure-limited ventilation with permissive hypercapnia: a prospective study. *Crit Care Med* 1994;22:1568.

Kolobow TA, Moretti MP, Fumagali R. Severe impairment of lung function induced by high peak airway pressure during mechanical ventilation: an experimental study. *Am Rev Respir Dis* 1987;135:312.

Pelosi P, D'Andrea L, Vitale G, et al. Vertical gradient of regional lung inflation in adult respiratory distress syndrome. *Am J Respir Crit Care Med* 1994;149:8.

Shanley CJ, Bartlett RH. The management of acute respiratory failure. *Curr Opin Gen Surg* 1994;94:7–16.

Simmons RS, Berdine GG, Seidenfeld JJ, et al. Fluid balance in the adult respiratory distress syndrome. *Am Rev Respir Dis* 1989;135:924.

Vasilyev S, Schaap RN, Mortensen JD. Hospital survival rates of patients with acute respiratory failure in the modern respiratory intensive care unit: an international, multi-center, prospective survey. *Chest* 1995;107:1083.

Nutrition and Metabolism

Bartlett RH, Dechert RE, Mault J, et al. Measurement of metabolism in multiple organ failure. *Surgery* 1982;92:771.

Bessey PQ. Metabolic response to critical illness. In: Wilmore DW, Brennan MF, Harken AF, et al., eds. *Care of the surgical patient*, vol 1. *Critical care*. New York: Scientific American Medicine, 1988.

Cahill G. Starvation in man. *N Engl J Med* 1970;282:668.

Christou NV, MacLean APH, Meakins JL. Host defense in blunt trauma: interrelationships of kinetics of anergy and depressed neutrophil function, nutritional status, and sepsis. *J Trauma* 1980;28:833.

Cook DJ, Laine LA, Guyatt GH, et al. Nosocomial pneumonia and the role of gastric pH: a metaanalysis. *Chest* 1991;100:7.

Dudrick SJ, Wilmore DW, Vars HM, et al. Can intravenous feeding be a sole means of nutrition support growth in the child and restore weight loss in an adult? An affirmative answer. *Ann Surg* 1969;169:974.

Kresowik TF, Dechert RE, Mault JR, et al. Does nutritional support affect survival in critically ill patients? *Surg Forum* 1984;35:108.

Moore FA, Moore EE, Kudsk KA, et al. Clinical benefits of an immune-enhancing diet for early postinjury enteral feeding. *J Trauma* 1994;37:607.

Shizgal HM, Milne CA, Spanier AH. The effect of nitrogen- sparing, intravenously administered fluids on postoperative body composition. *Surgery* 1979;85:496.

Tryba M. Sucralfate vs. antacids or H₂ antagonists for stress ulcer prophylaxis: a metaanalysis on efficacy and pneumonia rate. *Crit Care Med* 1991;19:942.

Renal Failure

Abel RM, Beck CH, Abbot WM, et al. Improved survival from acute renal failure after treatment with intravenous essential L-amino acids and glucose: results of a prospective double-blind study. *N Engl J Med* 1973;208:695.

Bartlett RH, Bosch J, Geronemus R, et al. Continuous arteriovenous hemofiltration for acute renal failure: workshop summary. *Trans Am Soc Artif Intern Organs* 1988;34:67.

Bartlett RH, Mault JR, Dechert RE, et al. Continuous arteriovenous hemofiltration: improved survival in surgical acute renal failure? *Surgery* 1986;100:400.

Geronemus R, Schneider N. Continuous arteriovenous hemodialysis: a new modality for treatment of acute renal failure. *Trans Am Soc Artif Intern Organs* 1984;30:610.

Kolff WJ, Berk HTJ. Artificial kidney: dialyzer with great area. *Acta Med Scand* 1944;117:121.

Mault JR, Bartlett RH, Dechert RE, et al. Starvation: a major contributor to mortality in acute renal failure? *Trans Am Soc Artif Intern Organs* 1983;29:390.

Mault JR, Dechert RE, Lees P, et al. Continuous arteriovenous filtration: an effective treatment for surgical acute renal failure. *Surgery* 1987;101:478.

Mentzer SJ, Fryd DS, Kjellstrand CM. Why do patients with postsurgical acute tubular necrosis die? *Arch Surg* 1985;120:907.

Teschan PE, Post RS, Smith LJ, et al. Post-traumatic renal insufficiency in military casualties. *Am J Med* 1955;18:172.

Fluids and Electrolytes

Brimioulle S, Berre J, Dufaye P, et al. Hydrochloric acid infusion for treatment of metabolic alkalosis associated with respiratory acidosis. *Crit Care Med* 1989;17:232.

Davenport HW, ed. *The ABC of acid–base chemistry*, 4th ed. Chicago: University of Chicago Press, 1958.

Demling RH, Manohar M, Will JA, et al. The effect of plasma oncotic pressure on the pulmonary micro-circulation after hemorrhagic shock. *Surgery* 1979;86:323.

Huckabee WE. Abnormal resting lactate. I. Significance in hospital patients. *Am J Med* 1961;30:838.

Lyons LY, Owns JH, Moore FD. Posttraumatic alkalosis: incidence and pathophysiology of alkalosis in surgery. *Surgery* 1966;60:93.

Moore FD. Determination of total body water and solids with isotopes. *Science* 1946;104:157.

Virgilio RW, Rice CL, Smith DE, et al. Crystalloid vs. colloid resuscitation: is one better? *Surgery* 1979;85:129.

Central Nervous System

Arbit E, Krol G. Coma, seizures, and brain death. In: Wilmore DW, Brennan MF, Harken AF, et al., eds. *Care of the surgical patient*, vol 1. *Critical care*. New York: Scientific American Medicine, 1988.

Griffin D, Fairman N, Coursin D, et al. Acute myopathy during treatment of status asthmaticus with corticosteroids and steroidal muscle relaxant. *Chest* 1992;102:510.

Kaufman HH, Bretaudiere JP, Rowlands BJ, et al. General metabolism in head injury. *J Neurosurg* 1987;20:254.

Marion DW. The Glasgow Coma Scale score: contemporary application. *Intensive Care World* 1994;11:101.

McGillicuddy JE. Cerebral protection: pathophysiology and treatment of increased intracranial pressure. *Chest* 1985;87:85.

Teasdale G, Jennett B. Assessment of coma and impaired consciousness. *Lancet* 1974;2:81.

Watling SM, Dasta JF. Prolonged paralysis in intensive care unit patients after the use of neuromuscular blocking agents: a review of the literature. *Crit Care Med* 1994;22:884.

Host Defenses

Baker JW, Deitch EA, Berg RD, et al. Hemorrhagic shock induces bacterial translocation from the gut. *J Trauma* 1988;28:896.

Bernard GR, Loose JM, Sprung CL, et al. Hydrocorticosteroids in patients with the adult respiratory distress syndrome. *N Engl J Med* 1987;317:1565.

Christou NV, MacLean APH, Meakins JL. Host defense in blunt trauma: interrelationships of kinetics of anergy and depressed neutrophil function, nutritional status, and sepsis. *J Trauma* 1980;20:833.

Clagett P. Hemostasis in surgical patients. In: Miller TA, Rolands BJ, ed. *Physiologic basis of modern surgical care*. St. Louis: Mosby, 1988.

Lacroix J, Infante-Rivard C, Jenicek M, et al. Prophylaxis of upper gastrointestinal bleeding in intensive care units: a meta-analysis. *Crit Care Med* 1989;17:862.

Pugin J, Aukenthler R, Lew D. Oropharyngeal decontamination decreases incidence of ventilator-associated pneumonia: a randomized, placebo-controlled, double-blind clinical trial. *JAMA* 1991;265:2704.

Rock CS, Lowry SF. Tumor necrosis factor. *J Surg Res* 1991;51:434.

Shoemaker WC, Appel PL, Kram HB, et al. Hemodynamic and oxygen transport monitoring to titrate therapy in septic shock. *New Horizons* 1993;1:145–159.

Staab DB, Sorensen VJ, Fath JJ, et al. Coagulation defects resulting from ambient temperature-induced hypothermia. *J Trauma* 1994;36:634.

Weiss SJ. Tissue destruction by neutrophils. *N Engl J Med* 1989;320:365.

SURGERY: SCIENTIFIC PRINCIPLES AND PRACTICE, Third Edition, edited by Lazar J. Greenfield, Michael W. Mulholland, Keith T. Oldham, Gerald B. Zelenock, and Keith D. Lillemoe. Lippincott Williams & Wilkins Publishers, Philadelphia, © 2001.

CHAPTER 10

FLUIDS, ELECTROLYTES, AND ACID–BASE BALANCE

RICHARD B. WAIT, KIM U. KAHNG, AND ISHA A. MUSTAFA

A complete understanding of fluid and electrolyte balance is essential for surgeons and for those caring for surgical and other critically ill patients. Only with a thorough knowledge of normal physiologic control mechanisms can one hope to understand the complex pathophysiology of abnormal or disease states. Similarly, an understanding of the techniques used to evaluate and monitor patients must precede any attempt at treatment. This chapter reviews normal fluid and electrolyte physiology as well as acid–base physiology. In addition, the physiologic changes in fluids and electrolytes that commonly take place in response to disease, injury, and surgical therapy are discussed.

The study of body fluids began centuries ago, but our understanding of the complex interactions between water, electrolytes, and nonelectrolyte components that make up the body fluids has increased substantially in recent decades. With these advances have come more sophisticated studies of the mechanisms regulating the exchange of fluids and electrolytes. To understand how the body's internal milieu is regulated, the basic concepts of fluid compartments, osmotic forces, and oncotic pressure must be addressed.

TOTAL BODY WATER AND THE FLUID COMPARTMENTS

The total volume of water within the body is termed *total body water* (TBW). The relationship between TBW and body weight is relatively constant for any given person and depends on the amount of fat present in the body. Because fat contains little water, TBW as a percentage of body weight decreases with increasing body fat. Using isotopic water dilution techniques (deuterium or tritium), the estimated average TBW in men is 60% of body weight, whereas in women, who typically have more adipose tissue, the estimated average TBW is 50% of body weight (1). The percentage of body weight accounted for by water also varies with age. In infants, water makes up approximately 80% of body weight. This value decreases to approximately 65% by 1 year of age. Throughout adult life, a gradual decrease occurs in TBW because the amount of fat in the body usually increases with age. Estimates of TBW should be adjusted for very thin or obese patients. In obese patients, estimates of TBW should be decreased by 10% to 20%, whereas in lean patients, estimates should be increased by approximately 10%.

Total body water is distributed in intracellular and extracellular compartments (Table 10.1). Intracellular fluid (ICF) makes up approximately two thirds of the TBW, or approximately 40% of body weight. ICF cannot be measured directly but is calculated as the difference between the TBW and the measured extracellular water. Although localized within cells, the ICF is readily exchangeable with the water in the extracellular compartment.

Extracellular fluid (ECF) volume can be measured directly. Methods for these measurements are much less reliable than those used to measure TBW because no substance used for the measurement of extracellular water distributes itself solely into the extracellular compartment. Use of inulin as a measure of extracellular volume yields results that range from 30% to 33% of TBW, or approximately 20% of body weight (Table 10.1).

The ECF compartment may be further subdivided into the intravascular and interstitial spaces. The intravascular space, which accounts for 25% of the ECF, contains the plasma volume, which is approximately 8% of the TBW or 5% of body weight. The interstitial water volume can be calculated as the difference between the total ECF and the intravascular fluid; it constitutes approximately 25% of TBW, or 15% of body weight. The interstitial space extends from the blood vessels to the cells themselves and includes the complex ground substance making up the acellular matrix of tissue. Although the water in this space is thought to be freely exchangeable with intravascular, lymphatic, and intracellular water, this water exists in two phases. The free phase contains water that is generally freely exchangeable and in a constant state of flux. The bound or gel phase is composed of water that is closely associated with glycosaminoglycans, mucopolysaccharides, and other matrix components. This water is much less freely exchangeable. An additional ECF compartment, the transcellular compartment, consists of water that is poorly exchangeable under normal circumstances. This fluid is separated from other compartments by both endothelial and epithelial barriers. Included in this category are cerebrospinal fluid, synovial fluid, water in cartilage and bone, fluids of the eye, and the lubricating fluids of the serous membranes. Together, these fluids constitute approximately 4% of TBW.

In summary, TBW is contained in intracellular, intravascular, and interstitial compartments. These three compartments are in dynamic equilibrium, and alterations in one ultimately lead to compensatory changes in the others.

COMPOSITION OF BODY FLUIDS

Sodium and potassium are the dominant cations in the body. Sodium is primarily restricted to the ECF and potassium to the ICF. Sodium content in the average adult is approximately 60 mEq/kg. Approximately 25% of this sodium is nonexchangeable because it is confined to bone. Of the exchangeable fraction, approximately 85% is in the ECF. Small amounts of potassium, calcium, and magnesium make up the remainder of the cations present in the ECF (Table 10.2).

These extracellular cations are electrochemically balanced, primarily by chloride anions as well as by bicarbonate, phosphate, and sulfate ions. In the plasma, anionic proteins also contribute to ion balance. The interstitial fluid, an ultrafiltrate of plasma, contains little protein. As a result of the Donnan equilibrium, the content of both cations and anions in interstitial fluid is slightly higher than in plasma (Table 10.2). The Donnan equilibrium describes the unique relation between solutions of permeable and impermeable complex anions when these anions are unevenly distributed across a semipermeable membrane. This special type of equilibrium exists between the ICF and ECF because of the high concentration of protein and nondiffusible phosphates in the cell. Interstitial fluid, in contrast, contains little protein. The Donnan equilibrium exists across the capillary endothelial membrane because the concentration of

Table 10.1. BODY FLUID COMPARTMENTS

Total body water	Body weight (%)	Total body water (%)
Total	60	100
Intracellular	40	67
Extracellular	20	33
Intravascular	5	8
Interstitial	15	25

Table 10.2. ELECTROLYTE CONCENTRATIONS OF INTRACELLULAR AND EXTRACELLULAR FLUID COMPARTMENTS

	Extracellular Fluid (mEq/L)		Intracellular fluid
	Plasma	Interstitial fluid	
CATIONS			
Na^+	140	146	12
K^+	4	4	150
Ca^{2+}	5	3	10^{-7}
Mg^{2+}	2	1	7
ANIONS			
Cl^-	103	114	3
HCO_3^-	24	27	10
SO_4^{2-}	1	1	—
HPO_4^{3-}	2	2	116
Protein	16	5	40
Organic anions	5	5	—

protein is higher on the blood side of the capillary than on the interstitial fluid side. The concentrations of diffusible ions are not necessarily equal across these membranes because of the presence of complex anions. As mentioned, potassium is the dominant cation of the ICF. Total body potassium is normally approximately 42 mEq/kg, and most of this potassium is intracellular and freely exchangeable. Magnesium and sodium ions also contribute to the cationic component of the ICF. These cations are balanced by phosphate and sulfate anions as well as bicarbonate and intracellular proteins.

CONCENTRATION OF BODY FLUIDS

Despite the difference in composition between the ECF and ICF, the overall concentration of water in these fluids is identical. When concentration differences of water occur, they are only transient because water freely equilibrates between compartments. The concentration of water in the fluid compartments depends on the osmotic activity generated by the ion species contained in each compartment.

Osmotic Activity of Body Fluids

Body fluids are aqueous solutions composed primarily of water and contained in the different compartments of the body. For the purpose of simplicity, we consider the fluid compartments to be static, although there is a continuous flux of both water and electrolytes among these compartments. The movement of water depends on a number of physical principles, the most important of which is osmosis. According to the principles of osmosis, if two solutions are separated by a semipermeable membrane (i.e., a membrane that is permeable to water but impermeable to electrolytes and nonelectrolyte particles), water moves across the membrane to equalize the concentration of osmotically active particles. In so doing, osmotic equilibrium is achieved.

The osmotic activity across a semipermeable membrane is determined by the concentration of the solutes on each side of the membrane. Traditionally, electrolyte concentrations are expressed as milliequivalents per liter (mEq/L). The concentration of nonelectrolytes is usually expressed in milligrams per deciliter (mg/dL) or grams per deciliter (g/dL). The concentration of multivalent ions such as calcium and magnesium may be expressed as either milliequivalents per liter or milligrams per deciliter. The movement of water across a semipermeable membrane is based primarily on the number of particles rather than on the molar concentration of the solution, so this measurement is made by dividing the molar concentration of the substance by the number of particles into which it can freely dissociate in water. The unit of measurement for these particles is the osmole (osm) or milliosmole (mOsm). Therefore, when 1 mol of NaCl dissociates in water to Na^+ and Cl^-, it produces 2 osm, whereas 1 mol of a nondissociating molecule, such as glucose, produces 1 osm (1,000 mOsm). Osmolarity, measured in milliosmoles per liter (mOsm/L), or osmolality, measured in milliosmoles per kilogram (mOsm/kg) water, defines the osmotic activity of the particles in solution. Osmolality is measured by freezing-point depression techniques; however, the measured osmolality of a solution may not equal the calculated osmolality if the ions do not totally dissociate. This occurs more frequently as ionic solutions increase in concentration. The osmotic coefficient of a solution describes the amount of dissociation of the ions in solution, and it can be calculated by dividing the observed (measured) osmolality by the calculated value:

$$\text{Osmotic coefficient} = \frac{\text{observed (measured) osmolality}}{\text{calculated osmolality}} \quad (1)$$

Because cells are bounded by a semipermeable membrane, adding free water to the fluid surrounding a cell causes water to move across the cell membrane to equalize the osmolality differential between the intracellular and extracellular compartments. On a larger scale, adding free water to the ECF of the body causes an immediate expansion of the extracellular space, followed by a redistribution of water into the intracellular compartment (Fig. 10.1A). Similarly, loss of free water from the extracellular space (contraction of the extracellular compartment) ultimately leads to a shift of water from the intracellular to the extracellular space (Fig. 10.1B). These osmotic forces are not trivial. An osmotic gradient of just 1 mOsm generates a pressure equivalent to 19.3 mm Hg. Thus, changes in the osmotic activity of the ECF determine in part the volume of water in the intracellular space.

Whereas *osmolality* defines the concentration of particles in a fluid solution, *tonicity* refers to the effect of the particles on cell volume. Permeant solutes can freely cross cell membranes, whereas impermeant solutes cannot. Thus, although permeant solutes contribute to the osmolality of a solution, they have no effect on tonicity. This is because freely moving particles do not change the oncotic gradients, which govern movement of fluid. Permeant solutes therefore do not alter cell volume. Sodium is an example of an impermeant solute that is excluded from the intracellular space. As such, sodium affects not only osmolality but fluid movement and cell volume. In contrast, urea is a permeant solute that freely crosses cell membranes. Although urea contributes to the osmolality of a solution, it has no effect on the tonicity because it distributes equally across membranes, and as such does not

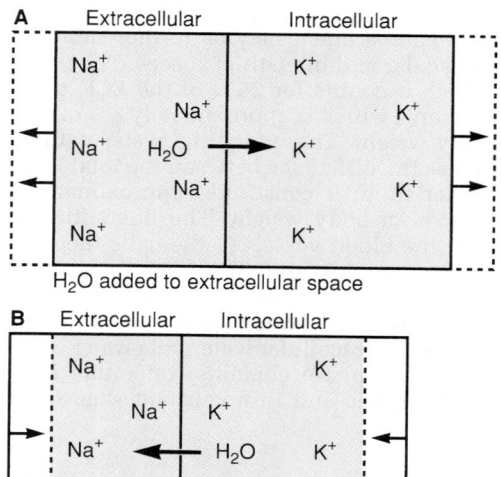

Figure 10.1. *(A)* The equilibration of water from the extracellular to the intracellular space after the addition of free water to the extracellular fluid compartment. Osmolality transiently decreases in the extracellular compartment, causing water to move across the cell membranes into the intracellular space. *(B)* Similar shifts after free water loss from the extracellular compartment. Water moves from the intracellular space to the extracellular space in response to the osmolal gradient that is established.

contribute to the osmoles that effect cell volume. Thus, urea is an "ineffective" osmole.

The term *hyperosmolar* is used to describe concentrations of body fluids that are higher than normal, whereas *hypoosmolar* describes concentrations lower than those considered physiologic. Although hypoosmolar (dilutional) states are always accompanied by hypotonicity, hyperosmolar states are not always associated with hypertonicity. For example, hypertonicity does not occur in the patient with a markedly elevated blood urea nitrogen (BUN) level despite the fact that there may be marked hyperosmolality because urea is a permeable molecule. Glucose, however, does contribute effective osmoles to the ECF, which can result in hyperosmolar fluid with associated hypertonicity. Insulin increases the transport of glucose across cell membranes, rendering these osmoles ineffective. In diabetic patients, hyperglycemia contributes to both hyperosmolality and hypertonicity of the ECF. Water shifts from the intracellular space to the extracellular space, causing expansion of the ECF and a decrease in the concentration of plasma sodium. For every 100 mg/dL elevation in blood glucose measured, serum sodium falls 1.5 mEq/L. When insulin is administered, glucose moves into the cells and no longer contributes to the hypertonic state. Water shifts back into the cells, correcting the apparent hyponatremia.

Plasma osmolality (P_{osm}) is an excellent measure of total body osmolality. Osmolality differentials between fluid compartments are only transient because fluid shifts maintain isosmotic conditions. Sodium is the predominant extracellular cation; thus, estimates of P_{osm} can be made by simply doubling the serum sodium concentration (serum $[Na^+]$):

$$P_{osm} \text{ (mOsm/L)} = 2 \times \text{serum } [Na^+] \qquad (2)$$

Because glucose and BUN may make significant contributions to P_{osm} in certain disease states, this formula is modified for glucose and for BUN:

$$P_{osm} \text{ (mOsm/L)} = 2 \times \text{serum } [Na^+] + \frac{glucose}{18} + \frac{BUN}{2.8} \qquad (3)$$

This simple calculation is clinically useful despite its inherent errors. If there is a discrepancy of greater than 15 mOsm/L between the calculated P_{osm} and that measured by osmometry in the clinical laboratory, an osmolal gap exists. This gap may be the result of the presence of osmotically active particles, such as mannitol, ethanol, or ethylene glycol, or of a reduced fraction of plasma water secondary to myeloma proteins or hypertriglyceridemia.

Colloid Oncotic Pressure (Colloid Osmotic Pressure)

Plasma proteins are confined primarily to the intravascular space and contribute to the osmotic pressure developed between the plasma and the interstitial fluid. Normal plasma protein levels of 7 g/dL contribute approximately 0.8 mOsm/L. The van't Hoff equation can be used to convert osmolality to osmotic pressure:

$$\pi = CRT \qquad (4)$$

where π = osmotic pressure, C = osmolal solute concentration, R = gas constant, and T = absolute temperature. At body temperature, each milliosmole develops a 19.3-mm Hg pressure gradient; thus, normal plasma protein concentrations generate a colloid oncotic pressure of 15.4 mm Hg (19.3 mm Hg × 0.8 mOsm/L). When measured directly, plasma oncotic pressure equals approximately 24 mm Hg. The difference between the calculated and measured pressures is due to the shift in solute particles caused by the pressure of protein anions on one side of a semipermeable membrane (in the intravascular space). This redistribution is explained by the Donnan equilibrium, described previously.

Osmoregulation

The body is capable of fine regulations of solute and water concentrations, so that osmolality remains fairly constant at an average of 289 mOsm/kg H_2O. In response to small changes in cell volume, osmoreceptor cells in the paraventricular and supraoptic nuclei of the hypothalamus send signals to the neuronal centers that control the two primary regulators of water balance, thirst and antidiuretic hormone (ADH, arginine vasopressin) secretion. In the presence of excess free water, ECF osmolality falls. As the osmolality approaches 280 mOsm/kg H_2O, thirst is inhibited, and ADH levels decline (2). In the absence of ADH, the permeability of the renal collecting tubules to water is decreased, and the urine becomes maximally dilute, with urine osmolality (U_{osm}) approaching 100 mOsm/kg H_2O (Fig. 10.2). This causes an increase in free water excretion, and the P_{osm} begins to rise. With water depletion, thirst is stimulated, and ADH secretion is increased as P_{osm} approaches 295 mOsm/kg H_2O. As ADH levels rise to approximately 5 pg/mL, the renal collecting tubules become maximally permeable to water. Water is reabsorbed from the collecting ducts in response to the concentration gradient developed in the renal medullary interstitium. Thus, the final concentration of urine depends on both the permeability of the collecting ducts (controlled by ADH secretion) and the concentration of the medullary interstitium. Maximal U_{osm} may approach 1200 mOsm/kg H_2O. The net effect is to decrease free water excretion dramatically and to return P_{osm} toward normal.

The high sensitivity of the osmoreceptors, combined with the high gain achieved through the ADH feedback system, ensures that even small changes in P_{osm} result in marked alterations in urine concentration. This relation can be expressed as follows:

$$\text{Urine osmolality} = 95 \times \text{plasma osmolality} \qquad (5)$$

A 1-mOsm change in P_{osm}, therefore, results in a 95-fold change in U_{osm}.

In addition to the signals from the hypothalamic osmoreceptors, neural input from baroreceptor regions of the medulla as well as angiotensin II can influence ADH secretion and thirst. Consequently, changes in either osmolality or hemodynamics influence water balance. ADH secretion is exponentially related to changes in pressure, so that relatively small changes in pressure have little effect, but large decreases in pressure can cause tremendous increases in ADH secretion. In general, changes in osmolality have a much greater effect on ADH secretion than do hemodynamic changes. The changes in ADH secretion elicited by changes in P_{osm} can be profoundly affected by large changes in blood pressure (Fig. 10.3).

Sodium Concentration and Water Balance

Changes in TBW content are reflected by changes in the extracellular solute concentration. Because sodium is the primary extracellular cation and potassium is the predominant intracellular cation, the serum $[Na^+]$ approximates the sum of the exchangeable total body sodium (Na_e^+) and exchangeable total body potassium (K_e^+) divided by TBW:

$$\text{Serum } [Na^+] = \frac{Na_e^+ + K_e^+}{TBW} \qquad (6)$$

Because total body solute content ($Na_e^+ + K_e^+$) remains relatively stable over time, changes in TBW content result in inversely proportional changes in serum Na^+ (Fig.

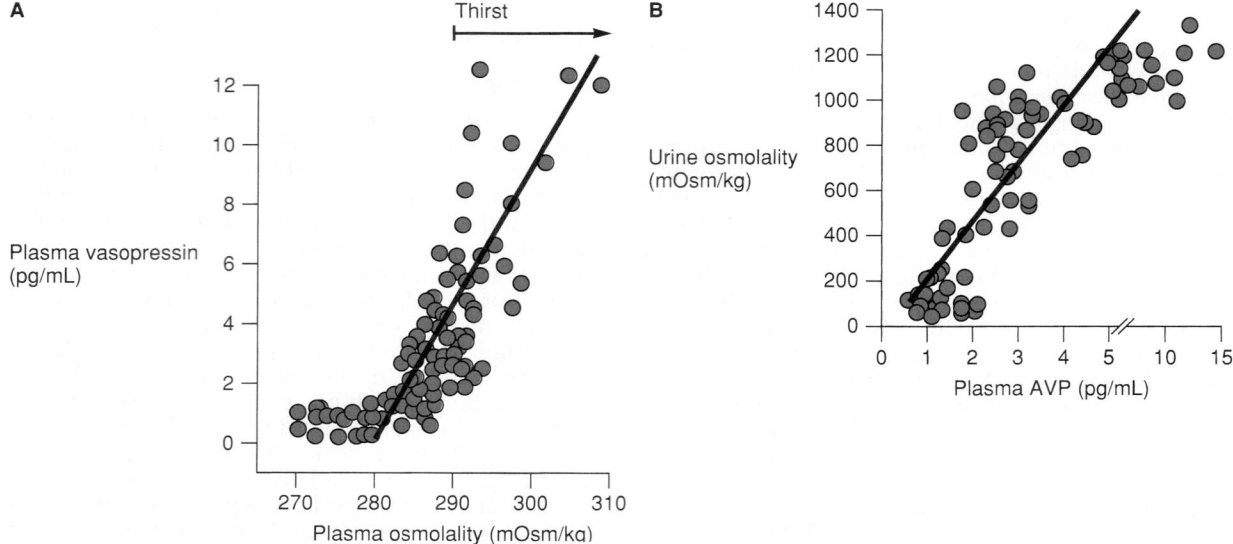

Figure 10.2. The relation of plasma antidiuretic hormone (arginine vasopressin or AVP) secretion to plasma *(A)* and urine *(B)* osmolality in healthy adults in varying states of water balance. (From Robertson GL, Berl T. Water metabolism. In: Brenner BM, Rector FC Jr, eds. *The kidney.* Philadelphia: WB Saunders, 1986:392.)

10.4). Thus, abnormalities in serum sodium are an indication of abnormal TBW content.

Effective Circulating Volume

Effective circulating volume is a term used to describe that portion of the extracellular volume that perfuses the organs of the body and affects the baroreceptors. The effective circulating volume normally corresponds to the intravascular volume, but in certain disease states the two can be substantially different. An example of this is the patient with congestive heart failure in whom the intravascular volume is actually high but the effective circulating volume is low because of cardiac failure. Similarly, patients with arteriovenous fistulae, either surgically created or resulting from trauma or aneurysms, have a deficit in effective circulating volume.

The effective circulating volume is usually in a state of equilibrium with the remainder of the extracellular volume, so that changes in the total extracellular volume are reflected by changes in the effective circulating volume. This relation can be drastically altered in certain disease

states, many of which are familiar to the surgeon. Abnormal shifts of fluid from the intravascular space into the tissues is often termed *third-space* fluid loss. Examples of disorders that cause third-space loss of fluid include bowel obstruction, which causes edema of the bowel wall and transudation of fluid into the bowel lumen, pancreatitis, which causes retroperitoneal fluid extravasation, and *sepsis syndrome,* with resulting capillary leak. Although fluid remains in the extracellular compartment, it is poorly exchangeable while the disease process persists. In these situations, total ECF remains constant or increases, and interstitial water is increased at the expense of intravascular volume.

Volume Control

Changes in volume are detected both by osmoreceptors, which detect changes in P_{osm}, and baroreceptors, which are sensitive to changes in pressure. The osmoreceptors are responsible for the day-to-day fine-tuning of volume, whereas the baroreceptors contribute relatively little to the control of fluid balance under normal conditions (3). As

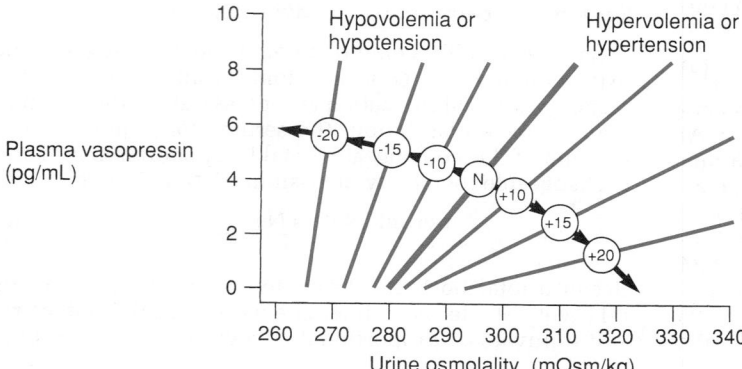

Figure 10.3. Effect of acute changes in blood volume or pressure on the osmoregulation of antidiuretic hormone (vasopressin). The heavy oblique line in the center represents the relation between plasma ADH and osmolality under normovolemic, normotensive conditions. The lines to the left and right show the shift in the relation when blood volume or blood pressure is acutely decreased or increased by the percentage indicated in the circles. [From Robertson GL. Physiology of ADH secretion. *Kidney Int* 1987;32(Suppl 21):520.]

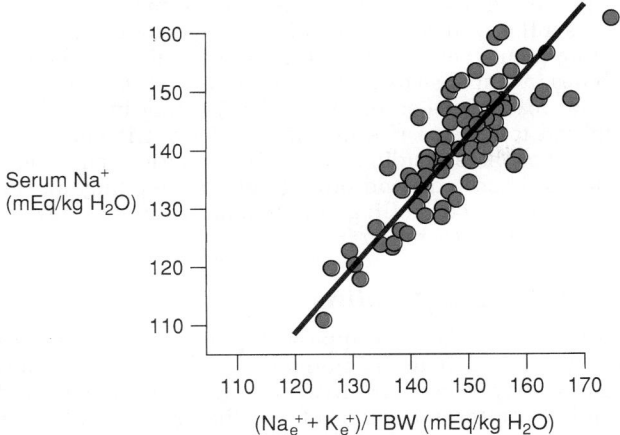

Figure 10.4. Relation between serum [Na$^+$] and the ratio of (Na$_e^+$ + K$_e^+$) to total body water (TBW). (From Edelman IS, Liebman J, O'Meara MP, et al. Interrelationships between serum sodium concentration, serum osmolarity and total exchangeable sodium, total exchangeable potassium and total body water. *J Clin Invest* 1958;37:1236.)

mentioned earlier, large changes in circulating volume can modify the osmoregulation of ADH secretion. These changes must be on the order of a 10% to 20% loss of blood volume. The atria of the heart respond to both volume and pressure. Baroreceptors control volume by means of sympathetic and parasympathetic connections, whereas atrial natriuretic peptide (ANP) released by atrial myocytes in response to atrial wall distention influences sodium-linked volume control. A small rise in right atrial pressure of 1 mm Hg produces a 30-pg/mL rise in the plasma ANP level. ANP may also directly inhibit renal sodium reabsorbtion. Higher, pharmacologic doses also affect renal blood flow and glomerular filtration rate. All of these actions function to control volume through sodium-linked pathways.

Baroreceptor Modulation of Volume Control

Changes in the effective circulating volume are sensed by the volume receptors of the intrathoracic capacitance vessels and atria, the pressure receptors of the aortic arch and carotid arteries, the intrarenal baroreceptors, and, to a lesser extent, the hepatic and cerebrospinal volume receptors. These stretch receptors are sensitive to changes in pressure and also to changes in circulating volume that are manifested by changes in pressure. The responses of these receptors to altered circulating volume are neural, by way of the sympathetic and parasympathetic fibers, and hormonal. The primary hormonal mediators include the renin–angiotensin system, aldosterone, ANP, dopamine, and the renal prostaglandins. The end result of this complex system of receptors and messengers is a change in sodium and water balance mediated by the kidneys. It is through changes in sodium and water reabsorption that volume and pressure are ultimately normalized.

Baroreceptor Function

The low-pressure baroreceptors of the intrathoracic vena cava and atria are located in vessels that are distensible and not affected by sympathetic stimulation; thus, they are ideally situated to detect changes in venous volume (4). These receptors send continuous signals through vagal afferent nerves to the cardiovascular control centers of the medulla and hypothalamus, which, in turn, send signals through parasympathetic and sympathetic fibers to

the heart and kidneys. Changes in stretch of these vessels result in changes in the frequency of signal output from these receptors. Increases in atrial distention cause decreased nerve signal traffic, which ultimately causes increased sympathetic tone to the heart and results in tachycardia and inhibition of sympathetic tone to the kidney. This leads to increased renal blood flow and decreased tubular sodium reabsorption. Conversely, low volume in the intrathoracic vessels results in increased sympathetic tone to the kidneys, decreased renal blood flow, and increased sodium reabsorption.

The kidneys are richly innervated with sympathetic fibers whose terminals are located throughout the vascular tree, especially on afferent and efferent arterioles. In addition, the tubules are directly innervated by sympathetic nerves. The kidneys receive little parasympathetic innervation. Experimental evidence clearly indicates that renal sympathetic nerve stimulation results in decreased renal blood flow and increased tubular sodium reabsorption. The effects of renal sympathetic nerve activity on sodium reabsorption are probably mediated both by direct innervation of the renal tubule and by β–adrenergic stimulation of renin production. The renal sympathetic nervous system may not be crucial to the fine regulation of sodium balance under normal physiologic conditions because experiments in conscious, unstressed animals reveal minimal effects of renal denervation on either blood flow or sodium reabsorption. The effects of renal denervation become much more marked in the presence of anesthesia or hypotension, suggesting that sympathetic effects on renal function may be important during periods of stress.

Arterial baroreceptors are located in the aortic arch and carotid arteries. They respond to changes in heart rate, arterial pressure, and the rate of rise in the arterial pressure. Arterial baroreceptors are important during periods in which there are extremes in the changes in arterial pressure characteristics, as occur during hemorrhage. They are probably not involved in controlling subtle volume or pressure changes. In addition to large-vessel baroreceptors, there are arterial baroreceptors in the afferent arterioles of the kidneys. These baroreceptors modulate renin secretion. Increases in transmural pressure cause suppression of renin release, and decreases in transmural pressure stimulate renin release.

Hormonal Mediators of Volume Control

Renin–Angiotensin System. The key to much of the volume and pressure control exerted by the kidneys is the release of renin from the juxtaglomerular cells of the afferent arterioles. Renin is a 40-kd proteolytic enzyme that is released in response to changes in arterial pressure, changes in sodium delivery to the macula densa of the distal convoluted tubule, increases in β–adrenergic activity, and increases in cellular cyclic adenosine monophosphate. The latter may be stimulated by prostaglandins, histamine, glucagon, and other hormonal influences.

Renin cleaves the decapeptide angiotensin I from circulating angiotensinogen and α$_2$-globulin produced by the liver. Angiotensinogen is abundant, so this reaction is enzyme dependent rather than substrate dependent. Angiotensin I is further cleaved to the octapeptide angiotensin II by angiotensin-converting enzyme, which is produced by vascular endothelial cells. One pass through the pulmonary microvasculature converts most angiotensin I to angiotensin II. Angiotensin II acts both locally and systemically to increase vascular tone. In addition, it stimulates catecholamine release from the adrenal medulla, increases sympathetic tone by acting centrally, and stimulates catecholamine release from sympathetic nerve terminals. Angiotensin II also affects sodium reab-

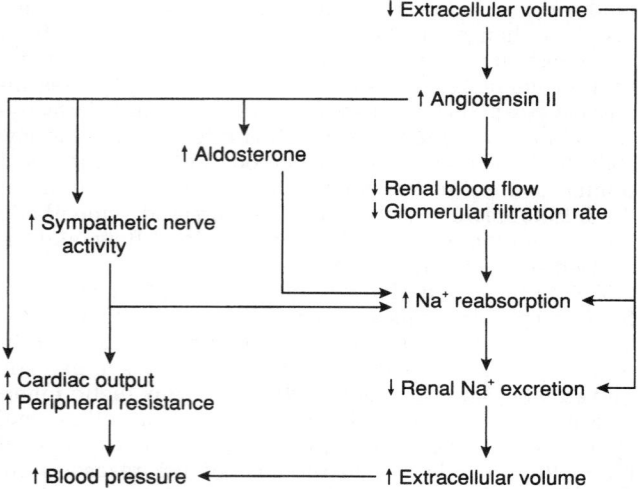

Figure 10.5. Multiple effects of increased angiotensin II release in response to the stimulus of decreased extracellular volume.

sorption by decreasing renal plasma flow and the glomerular filtration coefficient. This results in altered tubuloglomerular feedback, the mechanism by which changes in distal tubular NaCl delivery alter glomerular blood flow. Finally, angiotensin II increases sodium reabsorption by direct tubular action as well as by stimulation of aldosterone release from the adrenal cortex. The multiplicity of actions of angiotensin are depicted in Fig. 10.5. Angiotensin II can be further cleaved by aminopeptidase A to form angiotensin III. This hormone has actions similar to its precursor. Its half-life is short, and its physiologic significance has yet to be fully determined.

Aldosterone. Aldosterone is a mineralocorticoid produced in the zona glomerulosa of the adrenal cortex. This hormone exerts a major influence over sodium balance by increasing renal tubular reabsorption of sodium. Aldosterone acts directly on the distal tubular segments, predominantly on the collecting tubules. By increasing protein production in these tubular cells, aldosterone induces an influx of sodium, which causes an increase in cellular Na^+-K^+-adenosine triphosphatase activity. The net result is increased sodium reabsorption and increased potassium excretion. Although the primary regulator of aldosterone secretion is angiotensin II, aldosterone release is also stimulated by increased potassium levels, adrenocorticotropic hormone, endothelins, and prostaglandins.

ATRIAL AND RENAL NATRIURETIC PEPTIDES

The role of the cardiac atria and renal tubules in sodium and volume control is becoming clearer. ANP is synthesized and released by atrial myocytes in response to atrial wall distention. As mentioned previously, small changes in right atrial pressure produce large increases in plasma levels of ANP (5). There is evidence that ANP has a direct inhibitory effect on renal sodium reabsorption, which is probably maximal at the level of the medullary collecting tubules. Although pharmacologic doses of ANP can cause changes in both renal blood flow and glomerular filtration rate, physiologic levels do not appear to have any major effect on these parameters. Other active fragments of the ANP prohormone have been found to have natriuretic activity. The best described is urodilatin, also known as *renal natriuretic* peptide. Urodilatin is a peptide with

ANP-like activity that was first isolated from human urine. It is synthesized and luminally secreted by cortical-collecting tubule cells. Like ANP, it is released in the kidney tubules in response to atrial distention and saline loading. It is at least twice as potent as ANP, acting in the distal nephron to cause a rise in intracellular cyclic guanosine monophosphate, leading to sodium, chloride, and water diuresis. Urodilatin and other peptides may play an important role in controlling intravascular volume and water and electrolyte secretion (6).

Renal Prostaglandins

Renal prostaglandins appear to play a role in volume control, although under normal physiologic conditions, this role may be minimal. Disease states such as sepsis and jaundice, or the induction of anesthesia, may make the contribution of the prostaglandins more pronounced.

Prostaglandin E_2 (PGE_2) and prostaglandin I_2 (PGI_2) appear to be the predominant prostaglandins produced in the kidney. PGE_2 is produced primarily by the interstitial cells of the renal medulla. The release of PGE_2 has been shown to depend on increases in interstitial pressure, which can be induced by changes in renal perfusion, ureteral obstruction, or alterations in oncotic pressure. Under these conditions, PGE_2 increases sodium excretion in the absence of changes in glomerular filtration rate. PGE_2 antagonizes the action of vasopressin (ADH) and inhibits ADH-induced sodium reabsorption along the medullary collecting duct and thick ascending limb. PGI_2 is produced by the glomeruli and endothelial cells of the kidney and is present in the greatest concentrations in the renal cortex. PGI_2 is a vasodilator, and its effects on renal vascular resistance increase both renal blood flow and glomerular filtration rate. PGI_2 production is augmented by increases in angiotensin, catecholamines, and sympathetic tone, and may act to counterbalance their vasoconstricting effects. Although under normal physiologic conditions, inhibition of prostaglandin production has little effect on renal function, administration of nonsteroidal antiinflammatory agents, which inhibit cyclooxygenase, to patients with conditions known to cause renal dysfunction (e.g., cirrhosis) can precipitate renal failure, presumably because of loss of the protective effects of the renal prostaglandins (7).

Endothelins

Angiotensin was thought to be the most potent vasoconstrictor produced in the body until the discovery of endothelin. Endothelins are peptide vasoconstrictors that are also involved in volume and pressure regulation. Endothelin is produced and released by endothelial and other cells acting in a paracrine fashion on adjacent smooth muscle cells. In addition to increasing peripheral resistance, endothelin infusion has a direct inotropic effect on the myocardium, increasing cardiac output. In contrast to its vasoconstrictive effects, endothelin stimulates the release of other vasoactive mediators, particularly endogenous vasodilators like nitric oxide, which act to limit its intense vasoconstrictor effect.

Endothelin exerts a complex influence on sodium and water exchange through varied interactions with many other hormones that govern fluid and electrolyte balance. One net effect of endothelin is a decrease in the filtered load of sodium in the kidney. This results in inhibition of water reabsorption and decreased sodium excretion. Endothelin increases ANP secretion, activates angiotensin-converting enzyme, and inhibits renin release by the juxtaglomerular apparatus. At low doses, endothelin-1 produces a dose-dependent natriuresis and diuresis. Endothelin also modulates the biosynthesis of aldosterone, thereby inhibiting water reabsorption through aldosterone-controlled mechanisms. Vasopressin-mediated water reabsorption is also inhibited. Endothelin appears to have complex interactions with other regulators of renal perfusion and handling of water and electrolytes, which has stimulated research to evaluate the contribution of endothelin to the pathophysiology of various renal diseases (8).

Nitric Oxide

Nitric oxide is a free radical produced from L-arginine by nitric oxide synthases. Formation of nitric oxide is blocked by a variety of L-arginine analogues, such as L-NG-monomethyl-arginine (L-NMMA). With a half-life of 3 to 5 seconds, nitric oxide is rapidly neutralized by hemoglobin, methylene blue, and superoxide anions.

Nitric oxide has many biologic functions, including regulation of vessel tone and tissue blood flow. In addition to its flow-regulating properties, nitric oxide inhibits platelet aggregation and adhesion and participates in host defenses. Macrophages produce nitric oxide after exposure to cytokines. Nitric oxide production has proved to be cytotoxic to tumor cells as well as bacteria. This bacteria-induced macrophage nitric oxide production contributes to the vasodilatation and low systemic vascular resistance that is characteristic of sepsis. In the gastrointestinal system, nitric oxide functions as a neurotransmitter, participating in the relaxation of the lower esophageal sphincter, sphincter of Oddi, stomach, small intestine, and anus. Nitric oxide is also produced by the gastric mucosa, where it protects mucosal blood flow by dilating vessels to the mucosa (9).

Nitric oxide production occurs throughout the kidney in smooth muscle cells, mesangial cells, tubules, and endothelial cells. In the kidney, nitric oxide participates in the regulation of renal hemodynamics and renal handling of water and electrolytes. Nitric oxide and PGI_2 each independently cause renal vasodilation in response to a variety of stimuli. Nitric oxide is important in the regulation of medullary (vasa recta) blood flow. Pressure-dependent sodium excretion is ablated with inhibitors like L-NMMA and restored with L-arginine. Nitric oxide also contributes to tubuloglomerular feedback, which modulates the delivery and reabsorption of sodium and chloride in the renal tubules. Nitric oxide synthase in macula densa cells is activated by tubular solute reabsorption to release nitric oxide as a vasodilating component of the tubuloglomerular feedback response. Nitric oxide also participates in regulating renin release by the juxtaglomerular apparatus. Finally, nitric oxide produced in the proximal tubule may mediate the effects of angiotensin on tubular reabsorption (10).

NORMAL WATER AND ELECTROLYTE EXCHANGE

Under normal circumstances, the body's homeostatic mechanisms are capable of controlling the volume and composition of the fluid compartments at a remarkably constant level, so that a stable internal milieu is maintained. Surgical patients, however, are particularly prone to fluid and electrolyte abnormalities, not only because of disease but because perioperative fluid replacement may sidestep some of these homeostatic mechanisms. Although it is important to recognize and correct the abnormalities brought about by disease, trauma, and stress, it is equally important to know how to maintain normal fluid and electrolyte balance, thereby avoiding iatrogenic abnormalities.

Normal Water Exchange

Water losses are both sensible (measurable) and insensible (unmeasurable). Sensible losses include losses through urine, stool, and sweat. Table 10.3 summarizes the normal sensible and insensible losses encountered in a 24-hour period. The volumes of these losses may vary considerably. Urinary loss usually varies in proportion to intake plus other losses. The minimal amount of water needed to excrete normal metabolic waste products is approximately 300 mL/d.

Water loss in stool is usually small, on the order of 150 mL/d, but may increase markedly in disease conditions. The gastrointestinal tract has a net secretory action down to the level of the jejunum, and the reabsorptive capacity of the remainder of the small and large intestines keeps water loss by this route to a minimum. Bowel obstruction, severe diarrhea, and enterocolic fistulae are examples of conditions that may increase gastrointestinal losses of water and electrolytes.

Sweat does not usually account for much of the daily water loss. Sweating is an active process involving the secretion of a hypotonic mixture of electrolytes and water, and it should be differentiated from the insensible water loss of evaporation from the skin.

Insensible water loss is the evaporatory loss of water from both the skin and the respiratory tract (Table 10.3). Evaporatory skin losses depend on the body surface area, the temperature of the patient, and the relative humidity of the environment. Evaporation through the skin functions as a mechanism for heat loss and is proportional to calories expended. Approximately 30 mL of water is lost for every 100 kcal expended. Respiratory exchange depends on the ambient temperature and the relative humidity as well as on the rate of air exchange. Respiratory water loss is also energy dependent; thus, at normal respiratory rates, 13 mL of water is lost for every 100 kcal expended. Overall, normal insensible water losses average approximately 8 to 12 mL/kg/d. Insensible water loss increases 10% for each degree of body temperature above 37.2°C (99°F). In addition, patients with tracheostomies who breathe unhumidified air lose additional free water. Conversely, patients who are on respirators or who breathe air that is 100% humidified have no respiratory losses and may gain free water.

A person normally consumes approximately 2,000 mL/d of water, although this quantity is highly variable. Approximately one third of this amount comes from water bound to food, and the remainder originates from free water intake. In addition, water may be gained when carbohydrates and proteins, which are kept in solution by water in the cell, are metabolized. Although this gain is usually minimal, catabolic states may increase the amount

Table 10.3. WATER LOSSES IN A 60- TO 80-KG MAN

	Average daily volume (mL)	Minimal daily volume (mL)
Sensible losses		
Urinary	800–1,500	300
Intestinal	0–250	0
Sweat	0	0
Insensible losses		
Lungs and skin	600–900	600–900

Adapted from Shires GT, Canizaro PC. Fluid and electrolyte management of the surgical patient. In: Sabiston DC, ed. Textbook of surgery. Philadelphia: WB Saunders, 1986:77.

of oxidative free water gain to approximately 500 mL/d. To maintain proper fluid volumes, intake and excretion are well balanced through thirst mechanisms and the changes in renal excretion described earlier.

Normal Salt Exchange

In industrialized nations, daily salt intake averages 100 to 250 mEq/d Na+, or 6 to 15 g/d NaCl. This amount of intake is normally balanced by losses through sweat, stool, and urine. Renal sodium excretion is the mechanism by which fine control of sodium balance can be exerted. In cases of hyponatremia, the kidney can conserve sodium with urinary losses of less than 1 mEq/d. Conversely, urinary excretion can be maximized to rates up to 5,000 mEq/d if necessary to achieve sodium balance. The normal sodium requirement is in the range of 1 to 2 mEq/kg/d.

Potassium balance in the body is also finely controlled. Because most potassium remains in the intracellular compartment, potassium homeostasis is maintained by a balance between intake and gastrointestinal and renal losses, and by a balance between extracellular and intracellular potassium. In a normal diet, approximately 40 to 120 mEq of potassium is ingested daily. Of this potassium, 10% to 15% is excreted in the feces, and the remainder is excreted in the urine. Normal daily potassium requirements are approximately 0.5 to 1 mEq/kg/d. Abnormal renal function markedly changes this figure; consequently, potassium intake must be minimized in patients with renal failure.

FLUID AND ELECTROLYTE THERAPY

Parenteral Solutions

A number of electrolyte solutions are available for parenteral administration. Selection of the appropriate fluid is determined by assessment of the patient's maintenance fluid requirements, existing fluid deficits, and ongoing fluid losses. Table 10.4 lists the commonly available electrolyte solutions and the electrolyte composition of each. Although use of these solutions is convenient, there are occasions when a particular solution does not accurately replace the electrolyte components of the losses or deficits, and more than one type of solution may be indicated. Ions such as potassium, magnesium, or calcium may be necessary and can be added to parenteral solutions to suit the patient's requirements.

Lactated Ringer's solution is a physiologic solution containing many of the electrolytes found in plasma. This solution is commonly used to replace losses of fluid with the ionic composition of plasma, such as edema fluid and small bowel losses. It is ideal for the replacement of existing fluid deficits when the serum electrolyte concentrations are normal. The disadvantage of this solution is the relatively low sodium content (130 mEq/L) compared with plasma. Normal renal function usually ensures that the extra free water in this solution (150 mL/L) is excreted. Hyponatremia can occur with extended use of lactated Ringer's solution, or with use in patients who have impaired renal function, especially dilutional abnormalities such as those secondary to increased ADH secretion. Because lactate anions are readily metabolized to bicarbonate, the lactate ions in lactated Ringer's solution rarely contribute to acidosis if tissue perfusion has been maintained or restored.

Isotonic saline (0.9% or normal saline) contains 154 mEq of both sodium and chloride. Although this solution can be useful in patients with hyponatremia or hypochloremia, the excess of both sodium and chloride can lead to electrolyte and acid–base disturbances. Infusion of large volumes of 0.9% saline can lead to total body sodium overload and hyperchloremia. The added chloride load can result in a hyperchloremic metabolic acidosis or can aggravate preexisting acidosis. In addition, the pH of this solution and of the related solutions (0.45%, 0.33%, and 0.2% saline) is 4.0 to 5.0.

The less-concentrated saline solutions are used to replace ongoing fluid losses, such as nasogastric tube losses, and are also used in maintenance fluid therapy. The solution is determined by the calculated requirements. The 0.45%, 0.33%, and 0.2% saline solutions are hypoosmotic and thus have excess free water. In addition, 0.33% and 0.2% saline solutions are hypotonic with respect to plasma and can result in red blood cell lysis if rapidly infused. For this reason, 5% dextrose (50 g of dextrose per liter) is added to these solutions to increase the tonicity. In addition, when metabolized, 5% dextrose represents 200 kcal for each liter of solution.

Hypertonic saline solutions (3% NaCl and 5% NaCl) are usually reserved for replacement of sodium deficits in patients with symptomatic hyponatremia or those at high risk for development of symptoms. Calculations for replacement of sodium deficits are addressed later in this chapter. Hypertonic saline solutions have been used in the early resuscitation of hypovolemic trauma and burn patients. These solutions appear to increase intravascular volume in these patients more quickly than lactated Ringer's solution, and the total resuscitation volume requirement may be decreased. Patients resuscitated with hypertonic solutions require close monitoring of serum electrolytes to prevent hypernatremia and hyperosmolar coma. Although these experimental findings are of interest, the efficacy of hypertonic saline resuscitation has yet to be determined.

Plasma expanders are also commonly used in surgical patients. Some of these solutions and their contents are given in Table 10.5. These solutions are usually reserved for special clinical situations and are not used routinely in fluid management. Plasma protein solutions, such as 5% and 25% albumin, act initially by increasing plasma oncotic pressures. Exogenously administered protein is retained in the intravascular space, and interstitial water may move into the intravascular space. Abnormalities in microvascular permeability, such as those found in the pulmonary circulation in the adult respiratory distress syndrome, in regional circulatory beds in burns or infections, and in the systemic circulation in sepsis, can result in the extravasation of these proteins into the interstitial space. This, in turn, can lead to increased rather than de-

Table 10.4. ELECTROLYTE CONTENT OF COMMONLY USED INTRAVENOUS ELECTROLYTE SOLUTIONS

Solution	Electrolyte (mEq/L)					
	Na+	K+	Ca2+	Mg2+	Cl-	HCO3-
0.9% NaCl (normal saline)	154	—	—	—	154	—
0.45% NaCl	77	—	—	—	77	—
0.33% NaCl	56	—	—	—	56	—
0.2% NaCl	34	—	—	—	34	—
Lactated Ringer's solution	130	4	4	—	109	28
3.0% NaCl	513	—	—	—	513	—
5.0% NaCl	855	—	—	—	855	—

Table 10.5. PLASMA EXPANDERS

Solution	Concentration (%)
HUMAN ALBUMIN	
Albutein 5% (Alpha Therapeutic)	5
Albutein 25% (Alpha Therapeutic)	25
Albuminar-5 (Armour)	5
Albuminar-25 (Armour)	25
Buminate 5% (Hyland)	5
Buminate 25% (Hyland)	25
PLASMA PROTEIN FRACTIONS: ALBUMIN 4.4%	
Plasmanate (Cutter)	
Plasmatein (Alpha Therapeutic)	
Plasma-Plex (Armour)	
Proteinate (Hyland)	
DEXTRANS AND STARCH	
Dextran 40 (Rheomacrodex)	10
Dextran 70 (Macrodex)	6
Hetastarch (Hespan)	6

Adapted from Carroll HJ, Oh MS. Water, electrolyte, and acid–base metabolism. Philadelphia: JB Lippincott, 1989:82.

creased interstitial edema formation. Approximately half of all exogenously administered albumin eventually ends up in the extravascular space. In addition, the half-life of exogenously administered albumin is approximately 11 days, considerably shorter than endogenously produced protein. Hydroxyethyl starch (hetastarch) and dextran are synthetic plasma expanders. They have half-lives longer than or similar to that of albumin and are less expensive. The usefulness of oxygen-carrying synthetic plasma expanders, including stroma-free hemoglobin and perfluoro chemical compound-containing solutions, is under intense investigation. In the future, these solutions may prove beneficial in selected clinical settings.

Goals of Fluid and Electrolyte Therapy

The goals of fluid therapy are to normalize hemodynamic parameters and body fluid electrolyte concentrations. These goals are accomplished by correction of preexisting volume and electrolyte abnormalities, administration of fluids to replace normal daily losses (maintenance fluid therapy), and replacement of additional ongoing fluid losses. Replacement of fluids is crucial for patients who have sustained traumatic injuries or undergone surgical interventions or dissection, and in the management of postoperative fluid shifts.

Correction of Existing Volume Abnormalities

Volume Deficit. Volume deficits can be either acute or chronic. Chronic volume deficits may manifest as decreased skin turgor, weight loss, sunken eyes, hypothermia, oliguria, orthostatic hypotension, and tachycardia. In addition, serum BUN and creatinine may be elevated, with a high BUN/creatinine ratio (above 15 : 1), and the hematocrit may be elevated as well. Assuming no change in red cell mass, the hematocrit can be expected to increase 6 to 8 points for each liter deficit in intravascular volume. In this situation, urine concentration is usually high, and urine sodium excretion is low (<20 mEq/L Na^+). Unlike urine sodium levels, plasma sodium is not an indicator of intravascular volume. Plasma sodium concentration remains normal when fluid loss is isotonic, despite the volume of fluid lost.

Acute volume losses are usually manifested by changes in vital signs. If organ perfusion is compromised, urine

output may be low. Attempts to quantify volume deficits are usually of little value. The volume of fluid required to restore blood pressure, heart rate, and urine output is the best estimate of what the volume deficit has been. All deficits should be immediately addressed. Volume resuscitation should continue until hemodynamic parameters are normalized.

Fluid resuscitation for hypovolemia is initiated with an isotonic solution such as lactated Ringer's solution. Urine flow in critically ill patients is monitored with an indwelling Foley catheter. In general, urine output of greater than 0.5 mL/kg/h is desirable. After fluid resuscitation has been initiated, a thorough history and physical examination may help to determine the origins of the volume deficits, and the underlying causes can be appropriately addressed. Central venous pressure may be monitored with a central venous catheter or pulmonary artery catheter. Invasive monitoring with a central venous or pulmonary artery catheter should be considered in elderly patients or patients with cardiac disease. Placement of these catheters should occur concurrently with, not in place of, ongoing resuscitation. This type of invasive monitoring can be used to guide fluid resuscitation as well as determine the need for inotropic or vasoactive agents in critically ill patients. As stated earlier, the goal of initial therapy is the normalization of heart rate, blood pressure, and tissue perfusion.

Volume Excess. Surgical patients usually do not present with volume excesses, although it is not uncommon for patients to manifest volume excess during the course of their hospitalization. Large volumes of fluid can be sequestered in extravascular spaces (third-space losses) as a consequence of surgery, trauma, and disease processes. With the resolution of pathologic conditions and normalization of microvascular permeability, these fluid losses stop and eventually reverse. Thus, the sequestered fluid is autotransfused at variable rates. This may lead to volume overload if appropriate adjustments in fluid management are not made. In addition, postoperative patients and traumatized patients may be unable to excrete normal fluid loads secondary to increased ADH secretion. Frequent manifestations of volume overload are weight gain, elevated central venous pressure, pulmonary edema, peripheral edema, and an S_3 gallop. Intravascular volume excess is best treated by appropriate volume restriction and judicial use of loop diuretics if acute symptoms become evident.

Maintenance Fluid Therapy

Maintenance fluid replacement is aimed at replacing fluids normally lost during the course of a day. Calculation of maintenance fluid replacement does not include replacement of either preexisting deficits or ongoing additional losses. Maintenance fluid replacement should begin after the reestablishment of normal hemodynamic status with appropriate resuscitation fluids.

Basal requirements for water and electrolytes are determined by sensible and insensible losses. Insensible water loss averages approximately 8 to 12 mL/kg/d and increases 10% for every degree of body temperature above 37.2°C (99°F). For example, a 70-kg man without a fever has a daily insensible water loss of approximately 840 mL. In addition, urinary and stool losses must be added to this figure. A useful formula for calculating maintenance water requirements is provided in Table 10.6. This formula adjusts for differences in body weight and for changes in body water content. A smaller (or younger) person who has a high percentage of TBW in relation to body weight requires a greater amount of maintenance fluid per kilogram than a larger (or older) person. For example, a 10-kg child requires 100 mL H_2O/kg/d or 1,000 mL/H_2O/d. A 70-

Table 10.6. CALCULATION OF MAINTENANCE FLUID REQUIREMENTS

Body weight	Fluid requirement[a]	
For 0–10 kg	Give 100 mL/kg/d	A
For the next 10–20 kg	Given an additional 50 mL/kg/d	B
For weight >20 kg[b]	Give 20 mL/kg/d	C

[a]Maintenance fluid requirements = sum of A + B + C.
[b]For elderly patients or patients with cardiac disease, this amount should be reduced to 15 mL/kg/d.

Table 10.7. ELECTROLYTE CONCENTRATIONS IN GASTROINTESTINAL SECRETIONS

Secretion	Electrolyte (mEq/L)					Rate (mL/d)
	Na$^+$	K$^+$	Cl$^-$	HCO$_3^-$	H$^+$	
Salivary	50	20	40	30	—	100–1,000
Gastric						
Basal	100	10	140	—	30	1,000
Stimulated	30	10	140	—	100	4,200
Bile	140	5	100	60	—	500–1,000
Pancreatic	140	5	75	100	—	1,000
Duodenum	140	5	80	—	—	100–2,000
Ileum	140	5	70	50	—	100–2,000
Colon	60	70	15	30	—	

kg man requires 1,000 mL/d for the first 10 kg (100 mL/kg × 10 kg), plus 500 mL/d for the second 10 kg (20 mL/kg × 10 kg), plus 1,000 mL/d for the last 50 kg (20 mL/kg × 50 kg). Thus, the total daily water requirement for a 70-kg man is approximately 2,500 mL/d. Because hypervolemia is poorly tolerated in older patients and in patients with cardiac disease, the requirement per kilogram over 20 kg is decreased to 15 mL/kg/d in these patients. Thus, the volume calculated for a 50-kg octogenarian is 1,950 mL/d (1,000 mL + 500 mL + 450 mL). These calculations are estimates only, and each patient must be observed closely for signs of volume depletion or volume overload.

Sodium requirements in patients are variable, and excess sodium administration is usually balanced by increased urinary sodium excretion. As a general estimate, 1 to 2 mEq/kg/d of sodium is required for maintenance therapy. Potassium requirements are approximately half those of sodium; thus, 0.5 to 1 mEq/kg/d is the normal calculated potassium requirement. If sodium is replaced at the rate of 2 mEq/kg/d and potassium is replaced at the rate of 1 mEq/kg/d, then a 70-kg patient requires 2,500 mL of water with 140 mEq of sodium and 70 mEq of potassium added to the solution. One liter of parenteral solution would therefore contain 56 mEq of sodium and 28 mEq of potassium. Of the available crystalloid solutions, 0.33% saline solution (56 mEq/L Na$^+$) is the solution that best fits this patient's daily requirements for maintenance therapy. Potassium chloride can be added to each liter of solution (20 to 30 mEq/L), but this is best done after clinical assessment of the patient's electrolyte, acid–base, and renal functional status.

Normal maintenance therapy requires the administration of sodium and potassium. Replacement of calcium, phosphate, or magnesium usually is not necessary in patients requiring short-term therapy. In critically ill patients, however, critical deficits of these electrolytes may occur and must be replaced. In patients requiring long-term fluid replacement, addition of these electrolytes, as well as trace elements, vitamins, protein, and calories, is essential. For this reason, parenteral nutrition solutions should be considered in all patients not expected to resume full enteral nutrition for more than 1 week.

Replacement of Ongoing Fluid Losses

Surgical patients are likely to have extraordinary fluid losses at some point during their hospitalization, especially if they have undergone operative procedures. Once volume deficits have been replaced and maintenance fluids have been calculated and given, the overall fluid balance of the patient can be maintained by replacement of any fluid losses over and above those considered to be maintenance. Although intraoperative and postoperative losses as well as third-space fluid losses must be estimated, ongoing losses from nasogastric tubes, ileostomies, fistulae, and so forth can be easily measured and quantitated. In addition, the electrolyte contents of

these fluids can often be predicted (Table 10.7), and the exact electrolyte content of the fluids can frequently be measured and replaced with precision. Ongoing losses should be detailed on a flow chart that documents the intake and output of all fluids. Patients needing emergent operation require adequate fluid resuscitation before being taken to the operating room, except in the circumstance of uncontrolled hemorrhage, for which operative intervention is the only means of stabilizing the volume loss. Operative and postoperative fluid management must be carefully controlled and monitored to ensure an optimal patient outcome.

Intraoperative Fluid Therapy

Anesthesia interrupts normal baroreceptor reflexes, so the patient with volume depletion that was compensated preoperatively by increased vascular resistance and heart rate may become acutely hypotensive on induction of anesthesia. For this reason, adequate resuscitation before surgery is mandatory. During operative procedures, fluid losses result from blood loss, third-space sequestration from trauma or manipulation of tissues, and evaporative losses from the wound itself. Although most patients can tolerate an unreplaced blood loss of at least 500 mL, losses above this level may require replacement during the operation. The shifts of fluid from the intravascular space to the extravascular space that occur in response to third-space volume losses from operative manipulation, tissue trauma, and evaporation cannot be measured but should be anticipated. Replacement with isotonic solutions, such as lactated Ringer's solution, is given at a rate of 500 to 1,000 mL/h during the operation. Close intraoperative monitoring of blood pressure and urine output aids the surgeon and anesthesiologist in avoiding periods of hypotension secondary to volume depletion.

Central venous pressure is monitored in those patients undergoing more complex procedures. In critically ill patients or patients at high risk for development of cardiac or fluid balance abnormalities during surgery, cardiac output and pulmonary artery wedge pressures are used to gauge the adequacy of fluid resuscitation. Elderly and high-risk patients may also benefit from preoperative placement of a pulmonary artery catheter to optimize preoperative, operative, and postoperative cardiac function and fluid resuscitation.

Postoperative Fluid Therapy and Monitoring

Fluid therapy during the postoperative period should be tailored to each patient and depends on the adequacy of the patient's volume status at the completion of the operative procedure as well as on the ongoing fluid losses. Maintenance fluid therapy should be supplemented by replacement of the additional fluids needed to replace the ongoing third-space losses as well as losses from various tubes and drains. In general, isotonic solutions should be used for volume resuscitation during the early postoperative period. It is best not to give potassium supplements during this period unless they are specifically required as indicated by serum electrolyte measurements.

Monitoring fluid status during the postoperative period is best accomplished by careful monitoring of vital signs, urinary output, and, if necessary, central venous pressure. Urine output is maintained at a level greater than 0.5 mL/kg/h. Urine specific gravity is usually measured more easily than U_{osm} and serves as an indicator of both volume status and renal ability to concentrate and dilute the urine. Urine specific gravity of greater than 1.010 to 1.012 indicates that the urine is being concentrated (compared with plasma), and a urine specific gravity of less than 1.010 indicates that dilute urine is being produced.

Both volume depletion and cardiac failure are usually accompanied by concentrated urine and low flow rates. Urine specific gravity in the range of plasma (1.010 to 1.012) may indicate either adequate hydration or the inability of the kidneys either to dilute or concentrate the urine. Renal failure in the postoperative period may be accompanied by low urine volumes (oliguric renal failure, <500 mL/d), or normal or high urine volumes (nonoliguric or high-output renal failure). When there is a high risk for renal failure during the postoperative period, urine collections should be obtained for measurement of urine electrolytes as well as creatinine clearance. High-risk patients include those with preexisting renal disease, those who were hypotensive before or during surgery, and those receiving nephrotoxic drugs.

An accurate and direct method of monitoring a patient's fluid status is to measure central pressures. This may be accomplished using a central venous catheter placed in the superior vena cava. Central venous pressures of 5 to 12 mm Hg or 6 to 15 cm H_2O are considered normal. Pressures above this range usually indicate volume overload or cardiac failure, whereas pressures below this range indicate intravascular volume depletion. Serial monitoring of central venous pressure is a valuable indicator of both volume status and adequacy of fluid management.

Because central venous pressure is affected by venomotor tone and cardiac performance as well as by circulating volume, measurements may not accurately define the causes of abnormalities in effective circulating volume, especially in conditions in which central venous pressures are high. Insertion of a pulmonary artery catheter enables much more accurate determinations of both volume status and cardiovascular performance. Pulmonary artery pressure, pulmonary artery wedge pressure, and thermodilution measurement of cardiac output can be easily accomplished using the Swan-Ganz catheter. In addition, venous saturation in the pulmonary artery, which may reflect global adequacy of oxygen delivery, can be continuously measured. Critically ill patients can be closely monitored using serial measurements of wedge pressure and cardiac output, achieving more precise control of fluid management.

Both short- and long-term fluid management are facilitated by daily measurement of body weight and fluid intake and output, which are carefully recorded on the patient's chart. Insensible fluid losses are estimated and added to the total outputs. Balancing daily intake and output with appropriate fluid management is essential. Normally, hospitalized patients with no caloric intake lose weight at a rate dependent on the catabolic state. Weight gain usually indicates increases in TBW rather than in protein or fat content.

CONCENTRATION CHANGES IN BODY FLUIDS

Volume excess or deficits are often isotonic but may be accompanied by changes in extracellular sodium concentration and osmolality. Normal sodium homeostasis has been discussed in previous sections. The mechanisms controlling normal osmoregulation may be affected by the same processes responsible for controlling volume. Volume depletion is the most common disorder of volume status encountered in surgical and trauma patients. These patients usually present with isotonic dehydration (Fig. 10.6A). In this condition, the volume lost is isotonic with plasma. Examples of isotonic volume deficits include blood loss, third-space losses, and gastrointestinal losses. Volume depletion may also be accompanied by hypoosmolar conditions (hypotonic dehydration; see Fig. 10.6B), which is often iatrogenic and the result of incomplete volume resuscitation with hypotonic solutions. Dehydration associated with hyperosmolar states (hypertonic dehydration; see Fig. 10.6C) is infrequent and usually indicates impaired consciousness and thirst mechanisms, or a patient's inability to drink or obtain water. As mentioned previously, volume excesses often occur some time after

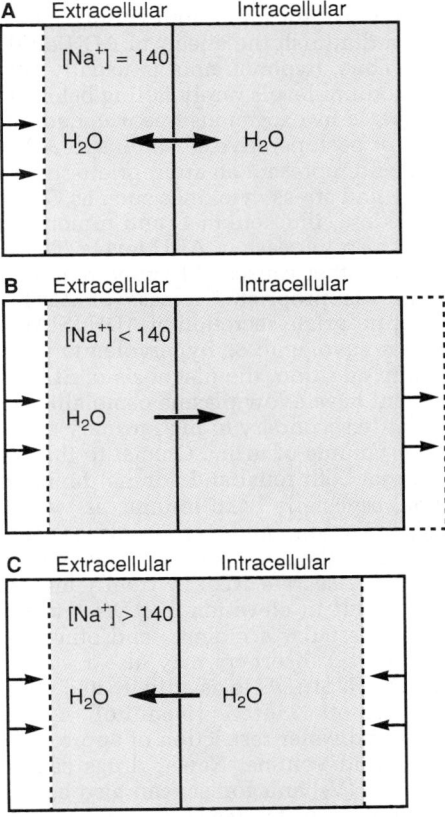

Figure 10.6. *(A)* Isotonic dehydration. Extracellular fluid is lost, but sodium concentration and osmolality remain unchanged. There is no change in intracellular volume. *(B)* Hypotonic dehydration caused by an extracellular fluid deficit with hyponatremia. Water moves into the intracellular space, causing further extracellular depletion and intracellular fluid (ICF) expansion. *(C)* Hypertonic dehydration caused by loss of extracellular free water, resulting in hypernatremia. Water from the ICF shifts to the extracellular space, resulting in contraction of both ICF and extracellular fluid compartments.

hospitalization rather than at presentation. The most frequent concentration defect associated with volume excess is hyponatremia.

Hyponatremia

Causes

Hyponatremia is classified as either primary or secondary. Primary hyponatremia refers to low plasma sodium levels that are the direct result of sodium loss. Secondary hyponatremia is due to excess water in relation to a normal sodium. Gastrointestinal losses, fistula drainage, or the use of diuretics, as well as adrenal insufficiency can all produce primary hyponatremia. Secondary hyponatremia can be caused by infusion of hypotonic solutions, excess ingestion of free water, and increased reabsorption of free water.

The most common cause of hyponatremia is an excess of free water rather than a deficit in total body sodium. Hyponatremia in this situation is associated with a low P_{osm}. Hyponatremia is frequently seen in the postoperative or postinjury period because ADH is elevated as part of the stress response to injury. Increased ADH secretion acts on the collecting tubules of the kidney to increase free water reabsorption. Volume expansion due to increased free water reabsorption may stimulate natriuresis, which may exacerbate the problem. Most instances of increased postoperative or postinjury hyponatremia *per se* result in increased sodium reabsorption. Both volume expansion and hyponatremia diminish the effects of ADH on the collecting tubules. Thus, hyponatremia is usually self-limiting, with serum sodium levels rarely falling below 130 mEq/L unless aggravated by exogenous free water administration.

Postinjury or postoperative elevations in ADH secretion are transient and represent an appropriate stress response. Inflammatory and stress cytokines such as C-reactive protein, interleukin-6, interleukin-1, and tumor necrosis factor all result in an increase in ADH levels. There are however, numerous other causes of hyponatremia that are the result of an "inappropriate" release of ADH. The syndrome of inappropriate secretion of ADH (SIADH) is diagnosed when a euvolemic or hypervolemic patient is hyponatremic. In addition, the diagnosis of SIADH requires that the patient have a low plasma osmolality with a high urine osmolality secondary to high urinary sodium excretion in a low volume of urine. Crucial to the diagnosis is the concept that both renal and adrenal function are normal. Trauma, especially head trauma, as well as alcohol withdrawal, infection, and certain drugs can produce SIADH. Tumors of the lung, pancreas, duodenum, bladder, and prostate may secrete ADH. Virtually any pulmonary disease may result in elevation of ADH levels. Brain tumors, cerebral vascular accidents, and other central nervous system (CNS) disorders may also result in varying degrees of SIADH. SIADH is usually treated with a combination of an osmotic diuretic (mannitol), a loop diuretic (furosemide), and water restriction of approximately 50% maintenance fluid volume. Newer drugs called nonpeptide vasopressin (V_2) antagonists can also be used. These work by inhibiting water reabsorption by competitively blocking the binding of arginine vasopressin to V_2 receptors. The net result is increased water excretion without concomitant electrolyte excretion.

Hyponatremia can also be associated with low effective circulating volume. This most commonly occurs in edematous states or cirrhosis with ascites, but it can also result from dehydration with concomitant volume replacement with hypotonic solutions. Because of the low intravascular volume, renal plasma flow and glomerular filtration rate are low, resulting in increased sodium reabsorption by the kidneys. This renal compensation may not be sufficient to correct the abnormality.

Although hyponatremia most often results from excess free water, it can occur in the presence of excess solute. In this situation, TBW content is either normal or diminished, and P_{osm} is increased. The hyperosmolality shifts water from the intracellular to the extracellular space, resulting in hyponatremia. The most common example of this hyperosmolar/hyponatremic state is untreated hyperglycemia. Excess solute may also be due to the exogenous administration or ingestion of mannitol, ethanol, methanol, or ethylene glycol. In addition to shifts in water, cellular exchange of potassium for sodium as a compensatory mechanism for potassium loss may result in hyponatremia. In both hyperosmolar and hypokalemic conditions, total body sodium remains normal.

Finally, hyperproteinemia and hyperlipidemia can cause falsely low sodium values. This has been termed *pseudohyponatremia*, and is an abnormality in laboratory measurement of sodium that is not accompanied by any symptoms attributable to hyponatremia.

Clinical Features

The development of symptoms depends on both the level of hyponatremia and the rapidity with which serum [Na$^+$] falls. Chronic hyponatremia is often asymptomatic until the serum [Na$^+$] falls below 110 to 120 mEq/L. An acute drop in serum [Na$^+$] to 120 to 130 mEq/L may result in a variety of symptoms. The clinical manifestations of hyponatremia are primarily related to the CNS and are the result of cellular water intoxication, although gastrointestinal and musculoskeletal symptoms are also common. Weakness, fatigue, muscle cramps, mental confusion, anorexia, nausea, and vomiting occur frequently. Headaches, confusion, and delirium may herald frank seizure activity and coma. Permanent CNS damage can occur if hyponatremia is left untreated, but overzealous treatment may also lead to CNS injury. Rapid infusion of hypertonic saline may result in central pontine myelinolysis and the quadriplegia, dysarthria, and dysphasia of the "locked-in" syndrome. Because of the dangers inherent in rapid treatment, the underlying causes and the risks to the patient with hyponatremia must be carefully considered before deciding on the appropriate therapy.

Diagnosis

Differentiating the causes of hyponatremia may be difficult. Once hyperosmolar hyponatremia (caused by hyperglycemia, mannitol administration, or radiologic contrast medium) has been excluded, and pseudohyponatremia has been eliminated from the differential diagnosis, the clinician must determine whether the effective circulating volume is low (hyponatremic dehydration) or normal.

Hyponatremic dehydration may be caused by renal or extrarenal sodium losses. Renal sodium losses are usually the result of diuretic use, chronic renal failure, adrenal insufficiency, or a defect in aldosterone secretion. The hallmark of these disorders is a urine sodium level above 20 mEq/L in the face of hyponatremia. This is in contradistinction to extrarenal sodium loss such as may be secondary to vomiting, diarrhea, or fluid loss through nasogastric tubes, fistulae, or drains. The dehydration resulting from these conditions causes increased renal sodium reabsorption and urine sodium levels below 20 mEq/L. Normal or high effective circulating volume in combination with hyponatremia is almost always caused by SIADH or by increased sensitivity of the renal collecting tubules to the action of normal levels of ADH.

Treatment

Treatment of hyponatremia depends on the severity of the symptoms, the chronicity with which the condition develops, and the hydrational status of the patient. Hypovolemic patients often benefit primarily from rehydration because their symptoms are frequently caused by dehydration rather than hyponatremia. Isotonic saline or lactated Ringer's solution can often be used in these patients to normalize volume. Because rapid normalization of volume may lead to hypernatremia, serial monitoring of serum $[Na^+]$ is performed during judicious volume replacement. Most surgical patients with hyponatremia are euvolemic or hypervolemic. Patients without symptoms in this category are best treated by free water restriction because free water overload is the usual cause of the condition.

Patients who have significant symptoms require aggressive treatment tempered by the duration of the hyponatremia. Because the risk of central pontine myelinolysis is greatest in patients who have been hyponatremic for longer than 48 hours, 5% or 3% saline solution is given relatively slowly to increase serum $[Na^+]$ at a rate not exceeding 0.5 mEq/L/h. The amount of sodium needed to increase the serum $[Na^+]$ to a desired level can be calculated as follows:

$$Na^+ \text{ required (in mEq)} = (\text{desired } [Na^+]_s - \text{actual } [Na^+]_s) \times TBW \quad (7)$$

where $[Na^+]_s$ = serum sodium concentration. For example, a 70-kg patient has been hyponatremic for more than 48 hours and has a serum sodium level of 120 mEq. To avoid central pontine myelinolysis, correction of serum $[Na^+]$ during the first 24 hours is limited to 0.5 mEq/L/h × 24 = 12 mEq/L. Using formula 7,

$$Na^+ \text{ required} = (132-120) \times TBW \quad (8)$$

Because TBW is 60% of body weight,

$$\begin{aligned} Na^+ \text{ required} &= (132 - 120) \times [0.6(70)] \quad (9) \\ &= 12 \times 42 \\ &= 504 \, mEq \end{aligned}$$

Because 5% saline contains 850 mEq/L of sodium,

$$504 \, mEq \times \frac{1L}{850} \, mEq = 0.593 \, L \, 5\% \text{ saline} \quad (10)$$

Administration of this fluid would supply 593 mL of water and expand the TBW by this amount, so that the increase in serum $[Na^+]$ is slightly less than calculated. A high degree of accuracy is rarely needed in the formulation of treatment. Frequent serum electrolytes should be obtained, and increasing symptoms may necessitate more rapid therapy despite the inherent risks.

For acute hyponatremia (<48 hours), more rapid treatment may be used. Symptomatic acute hyponatremia may be treated with hypertonic saline to correct serum $[Na^+]$ at a rate of 1 to 2 mEq/L/h. Hyperacute hyponatremia, which may result from inadvertent infusion of large volumes of water or from dialysis accidents, can be treated to increase serum $[Na^+]$ at rates of 5 mEq/L/h. The treatment goal in any of these settings is to achieve a serum sodium level above 125 mEq/L or to achieve resolution of symptoms. It is unnecessary to increase serum sodium levels rapidly to normal values. Prophylactic anticonvulsant therapy may also be beneficial.

Hypernatremia

Causes

Hypernatremia is a less common problem in surgical patients than hyponatremia and is usually the result of excessive free water loss associated with hypovolemia. Patients with tracheostomies who breathe unhumidified air or patients with high fevers can lose large volumes of free water through increased insensible water losses. Large volumes of free water can also be lost when hypertonic glucose solutions are used for peritoneal dialysis. Head trauma or neurosurgical procedures may be complicated by the development of diabetes insipidus. In this condition, secretion of ADH is depressed, which results in free water diuresis. On occasion, free water losses secondary to diabetes insipidus can be massive.

Hypernatremia can also be caused by increased total body content of sodium, which is usually related to exogenous administration of sodium. Infusion of excessive amounts of sodium bicarbonate during acute resuscitation from cardiopulmonary arrest is frequently associated with subsequent hypernatremia. Administration of solutions containing large amounts of sodium for replacement of free water deficits may also lead to hypernatremia.

Clinical Features

Moderate degrees of hypernatremia are tolerated well, and symptoms rarely develop unless serum $[Na^+]$ levels exceed 160 mEq/L or serum osmolality exceeds 320 to 330 mOsm/kg. The development of symptoms also depends on the rapidity with which the hypernatremia develops. The symptoms of hypernatremia are related to the hyperosmolar state. Cellular dehydration occurs as water passes into the extracellular space. CNS effects predominate. The most common symptoms are restlessness, irritability, ataxia, fever, tonic spasms, and seizures. Subarachnoid hemorrhage may also occur.

Treatment

Once hypernatremia becomes symptomatic, it is associated with significant morbidity and mortality. Prompt treatment of hypernatremia is essential. Rapid correction carries a significant risk of cerebral edema and brain stem herniation. In chronic hypernatremia, the cells in the brain gradually adapt by increasing intracellular osmotic solute content, thereby regaining cellular volume. These cellular changes are not readily reversed. A sudden decrease in extracellular sodium concentration, and therefore osmolality, results in cell swelling. Because chronic hypernatremia is relatively well tolerated, there are few advantages to correcting the free water deficit rapidly. Free water is administered to correct serum $[Na^+]$ at a rate not exceeding 0.7 mEq/L/h. The amount of water required to correct a hypernatremic state depends on the free water deficit, the insensible free water losses, and the urinary free water excretion rate. The water requirement to replace the free water deficit can be calculated using the following formula:

$$\text{water requirement} = \frac{\text{actual } [Na^+]_s}{\text{desired } [Na^+]_s - 1} \times TBW \quad (11)$$

Because

$$\text{desired change in } [Na^+]_s = \text{actual } [Na^+]_s - \text{desired } [Na^+]_s \quad (12)$$

It follows that

$$\frac{\text{desired change in } [Na^+]_s}{\text{desired } [Na^+]_s} = \frac{\text{actual } [Na^+]_s}{\text{desired } [Na^+]_s - 1} \quad (13)$$

Substituting into formula 8,

$$\text{water requirement} = \frac{\text{desired change in } [Na^+]_s}{\text{desired } [Na^+]_s} \times TBW \quad (14)$$

For example, a 70-kg patient with a TBW of 42 L (TBW 60% of body weight) has a serum sodium of 170 mEq/L. The maximum desired change in serum sodium over 1 day would be approximately 16 mEq (0.7 mEq/L/h). Substituting into formula 9,

$$\text{water requirement} \quad = \frac{16 \times 42}{154} \quad (15)$$
$$= 4.3 \text{ L}$$

The desired level of serum sodium would not be achieved unless insensible losses (approximately 8 mL/kg/d) and urinary free water losses were also replaced. Urinary losses of free water can be determined by calculating free water clearance:

$$C_{H_2O} = V - C_{osm} \ V - \frac{U_{osm} \times V}{P_{osm}} \quad (16)$$

where C_{H_2O} = free water clearance, C_{osm} = osmolar clearance rate, V = urine flow rate, and U_{osm} and P_{osm} = urine and plasma osmolalities.

The U_{osm} and P_{osm} can be estimated by the total sodium and potassium concentrations. Therefore,

$$C_{H_2O} = V - \frac{(U_{Na} + U_K) \times V}{[Na^+]_s} \quad (17)$$

where U_{Na} and U_K = urinary sodium and potassium concentrations. A positive number signifies net free water loss and adds to the water requirement, whereas a negative number indicates free water absorption and is subtracted from the water requirement. Thus, the total water requirement to achieve the desired decrease in serum $[Na^+]$ is the sum of the calculated water deficit plus the calculated insensible water loss plus the urinary free water clearance.

COMPOSITIONAL CHANGES IN BODY FLUIDS

Potassium

Potassium is the major intracellular cation and is the major determinant of intracellular osmolality. Normally, intracellular potassium concentration is approximately 150 mEq/L, whereas extracellular potassium levels range from 3.5 to 5 mEq/L. Because of the large difference between intracellular and extracellular potassium concentrations, a transmembrane potential is generated. Alterations in the potassium concentration gradient have profound effects on transmembrane potential and consequently on cellular function. This is especially true for cardiac, skeletal, and smooth muscle. The membrane potential (E_m) developed in cells is described by the Nernst equation:

$$E_m = -\log 60 \frac{[K_I]}{[K_E]} \quad (18)$$

where $[K_I]$ and $[K_E]$ = intracellular and extracellular potassium concentrations, respectively.

Normally, the membrane potential of cells is approximately −90 mV as produced by a $[K_I]/[K_E]$ ratio of 30 : 1. Intracellular potassium levels are relatively stable, but extracellular potassium levels are often altered in pathologic situations. Overall potassium balance is determined by potassium intake and by renal and extrarenal excretion.

Extracellular potassium concentration is primarily determined by renal excretion. Approximately 90% of ingested potassium is excreted in the urine. Most potassium filtered by the glomerulus is reabsorbed in the proximal tubule, so that net excretion of potassium is determined by the amount of potassium secreted by the distal tubule and collecting duct of the nephron. In these nephron segments, movement of potassium into the tubular lumen is determined by the difference between intracellular and luminal fluid potassium concentrations, the permeability of the luminal cell membranes to potassium, and the electrical po-

tential gradient across the luminal cell membrane. Potassium secretion is stimulated by increased urine flow in the distal nephron segments, increased sodium delivery to these segments, high plasma potassium concentrations, and alkalosis. In addition, humoral factors, including aldosterone, vasopressin, and β-adrenergic agonists, stimulate renal excretion of potassium. Because of the central role of the kidneys in potassium excretion, renal failure (either acute or chronic) can easily lead to hyperkalemia.

Sweat accounts for a small amount of daily potassium excretion. Nonrenal excretion of potassium is primarily fecal, and 5 to 10 mEq/d is excreted in the feces. This amount may be greatly increased in hyperkalemic states or in renal failure.

Extracellular potassium levels can be greatly influenced by the acute flux of potassium into or out of the cells. Insulin causes potassium to move into the cell, inducing a change in membrane potential and stimulating glycolysis. Alkalosis causes potassium to shift into cells in exchange for H^+. Conversely, acidemia induces the cellular exchange of intracellular K^+ for extracellular H^+. A redistribution of potassium into the ECF can also occur in hyperosmolar conditions because the movement of water into the extracellular compartment causes "solvent drag" and may increase the flux of potassium in response to its concentration gradient.

Hyperkalemia

Causes. Hyperkalemia rarely develops from excessive potassium intake in the absence of renal insufficiency because the capacity for renal potassium excretion is large. In the surgical patient, diminished renal function is perhaps the most common problem leading to hyperkalemia. Both chronic and acute renal failure result in a defect in potassium excretion. Nonoliguric renal failure, a form of renal failure common in critically ill patients, may lead to potassium intoxication despite apparently adequate urine formation. Serum potassium levels may increase by 0.3 to 0.5 mEq/L/d in noncatabolic patients with acute renal failure, but this level can increase to 0.7 mEq/L/d or more in catabolic patients or those with other sources of potassium intake. Hospitalized patients may have varied sources of potassium intake. Obvious sources include intravenous fluids as well as total parenteral nutrition formulas containing potassium. Less obvious sources include medications that are bound to potassium. For example, β-lactam antibiotics can contain significant amounts of potassium.

In patients with chronic renal disease, potassium balance is normalized by increased colonic potassium excretion, as well as increased potassium excretion per functional nephron. Infusion of cationic amino acid solutions, such as arginine and lysine, can be associated with hyperkalemia because these amino acids are taken up by cells in exchange for potassium. In addition, hyperkalemia has been reported to occur with administration of beta blocking agents and other medications.

Cellular disruption with release of potassium may result in hyperkalemia. The classic example of this is hyperkalemia associated with crush injuries. Reperfusion of ischemic limbs can also lead to substantial elevations in potassium when newly created blood flow washes out the by-products of ischemia-induced cell lysis. Hyperkalemia may also occur when potassium is released from lysed erythrocytes in large hematomas or after massive blood transfusion. Similarly, potassium release from tumor lysis may result in increased serum potassium. Hyperkalemia can also be associated with the depolarizing muscle relaxants (e.g., succinylcholine). Although unusual, hyperkalemia can also result from absorption of potassium after the use of solutions containing high potassium levels, such as cardioplegia solutions or organ preservation solutions (Collin or University of Wisconsin solutions).

Clinical Features. The clinical manifestations of hyperkalemia are primarily related to membrane depolarization caused by a decrease in the $[K_I]/[K_E]$ ratio. The most life-threatening manifestations are related to the cardiac effects of membrane depolarization. Mild hyperkalemia results in peaked T waves on the electrocardiogram (ECG) and can cause paresthesia and weakness. More severe forms of hyperkalemia cause flattened P waves, prolongation of the QRS complex, and deep S waves on the ECG. Ventricular fibrillation and cardiac arrest can result. Neuromuscular manifestations of severe hyperkalemia include weakness progressing to flaccid paralysis.

Treatment. The treatment of hyperkalemia is dictated by the serum level and by ECG changes or symptoms. Severe hyperkalemia with ECG abnormalities requires urgent treatment. The effects of hyperkalemia on membrane potentials can be reduced by increasing calcium levels. Rapid infusion of 10% to 20% calcium gluconate may be lifesaving. The effects are transient and usually last approximately 30 minutes. Administration of sodium bicarbonate is another temporary measure. The increase in serum sodium antagonizes the effects of hyperkalemia on the membrane potential, whereas the increase in extracellular pH shifts potassium into the cells. Movement of potassium into the intracellular compartment can also be achieved by giving 10 to 20 units of regular insulin. Twenty-five to 50 g of glucose (50 to 100 mL of 50% glucose solution) is administered concurrently to avoid insulin-induced hypoglycemia.

Definitive therapy of hyperkalemia requires increasing potassium excretion. This may be accomplished by the administration of K^+/Na^+ exchange resins such as sodium polystyrene sulfonate (Kayexalate; Sanofi Winthrop Pharmaceuticals, New York, NY). The usual oral dose is 40 g dissolved in 20 to 100 mL of sorbitol. Each gram removes approximately 1 mEq of potassium. Kayexalate can also be given as a retention enema in a dose of 50 to 100 g in 200 mL of water. Retention of the enema may be facilitated by inflating the balloon of a Foley catheter in the rectum. Each gram removes approximately 0.5 mEq of potassium. Peritoneal dialysis or hemodialysis is indicated for severe hyperkalemia and for patients with renal failure.

Hypokalemia

Causes. Hypokalemia can be caused by total body potassium depletion secondary to decreased potassium intake, increased extrarenal potassium losses, or increased renal potassium losses. Normally, hypokalemia is not secondary to diminished potassium intake, although intravenous fluid replacement with potassium-free solutions for prolonged periods can result in hypokalemia, especially in patients with increased potassium losses from the gastrointestinal tract.

Decreased serum potassium levels may also be caused by redistribution of potassium into the intracellular space. Acute increases in blood pH secondary to bicarbonate administration during resuscitation can cause acute hypokalemia, as can administration of insulin to hyperglycemic diabetic patients.

Causes of hypokalemia include the following:

- Shift of potassium to the intracellular space
- Acute alkalosis
- Administration of glucose and insulin
- Catecholamines
- Increased gastrointestinal loss
- Diarrhea
- Mucus-secreting colon tumors (villous adenoma)
- Excessive renal loss
- Metabolic alkalosis
- Magnesium deficiency
- Hyperaldosteronism (adrenal adenoma or hyperplasia)

Clinical Features. Symptoms of hypokalemia, like those of hyperkalemia, are manifestations of disturbances in the $[K_I]/[K_E]$ ratio with resultant alterations in membrane potentials. As potassium levels fall below 2.5 mEq/L, muscle weakness is common. Severe hypokalemia can cause paralysis involving the muscles of respiration. Intestinal peristalsis can be impaired and result in intestinal ileus. Cardiac muscle abnormalities are reflected by the predisposition to digitalis intoxication, the development of cardiac arrhythmia, including ventricular fibrillation, and sensitization to epinephrine-induced arrhythmia. ECG abnormalities include flattened T waves, depressed ST segments, prominent U waves, and prolongation of the QT interval. Renal changes include decreased renal blood flow and glomerular filtration rate. These effects may be relatively minor, and they may be accompanied by polyuria, polydipsia, metabolic alkalosis, and sodium retention. Decreased peripheral vascular resistance with ensuing hypotension may be due to a decrease in vascular sensitivity to angiotensin II.

Treatment. The primary treatment of hypokalemia is potassium replacement, although the patient's acid–base balance should be considered before initiating therapy. The route and rate of potassium replacement depends on the presence and severity of symptoms. A reduction in serum potassium of 1 mEq/L represents a total body potassium deficiency of approximately 100 to 200 mEq. Potassium should be administered intravenously if the symptoms are severe, if the serum concentration is below 2 mEq/L, or if the patient is unable to take oral potassium. Intravenous potassium can be administered at a rate of approximately 10 mEq/h, and the concentration of potassium should be 40 mEq/L or less. If less fluid is desired, up to 20 mEq in 100 mL of intravenous solution can be given, although no more than 40 mEq should be administered per hour. Potassium should be given orally if possible. Oral formulations include potassium salts such as potassium chloride, potassium phosphate, and potassium bicarbonate.

Calcium

Calcium is a divalent cation found in abundance in the human body. Approximately 99% of total body calcium is located in bone in the form of hydroxyapatite crystals. Although the bulk of this calcium is not readily exchangeable, the calcium on the surface of bones can be exchanged and serves as the major store of calcium for maintenance of calcium balance. Calcium homeostasis depends on exchange of calcium between bone and ECF, renal excretion, and intestinal absorption. These three processes are controlled to a great extent by parathyroid hormone (PTH).

The total plasma calcium concentration is approximately 10 mg/dL. In ECF, calcium exists in three forms: ionized calcium, nonionized calcium, and protein-bound calcium. Ionized calcium, which makes up approximately 45% of total calcium, is responsible for most physiologic actions of calcium in the body, and its level is tightly controlled by regulatory mechanisms. Normal serum concentration of ionized calcium is approximately 4.5 mg/dL. Because laboratory measurement of the ionized form is more difficult than measurement of total calcium, many laboratories report only total calcium values. Some nonionized calcium is complexed with nonprotein anions, including phosphate and citrate, and does not easily dissociate. These molecular forms make up only 15% of the total calcium present in plasma. Approximately 40% of extracellular nonionized calcium is bound to proteins. Most is bound to albumin, with the remainder bound to α= and β-globulins.

Changes in either plasma protein levels or pH can alter the proportion of calcium in the ionized state. The protein binding of calcium is pH dependent because of competition by H^+ for protein-binding sites. Prompt correction of changes in ionized calcium by various homeostatic mechanisms usually prevents symptoms from occurring, but rapid changes in pH can result in symptoms. The change in ionized calcium can be predicted if the changes in pH and protein concentrations are known. A 0.1 change in pH alters protein-bound calcium by 0.17 mg/dL in the same direction as the pH change. Thus, acidosis decreases protein-bound calcium levels and increases ionized calcium levels. Similarly, a change in albumin concentration of 1 g/dL changes protein-bound calcium by 0.8 mg/dL in the same direction. Because little of the calcium is bound to globulins, changes in globulin concentration of 1 g/dL change protein-bound calcium by only 0.16 mg/dL.

Despite a 10,000-fold concentration gradient with the ECF, the intracellular calcium concentration is normally maintained at extremely low levels, 10^{-7} mol/L. This is accomplished by active transport of calcium out of the cell and by sequestration of calcium in mitochondria and the endoplasmic reticulum. Calcium influx occurs through calcium channels, and cytosolic calcium is often bound to specific calcium-binding proteins such as calmodulin. These control mechanisms are key to the central role of calcium as a second messenger in multiple physiologic cellular functions such as neurovascular transmission, muscle contraction, and enzyme regulation.

Calcium Homeostasis

Calcium homeostasis is maintained through a balance of bone exchange, renal excretion, and intestinal absorption. All of these functions are controlled to a great degree by PTH. Of these three homeostatic mechanisms, calcium exchange with bone is the most important. Although the mechanisms are not clearly understood, it appears that decreased levels of ionized calcium lead to increases in PTH and increases in 1,25-dihydroxyvitamin D_3, both of which stimulate bone absorption by increasing osteoclastic activity. Increased levels of ionized calcium result in decreased PTH and 1,25-dihydroxyvitamin D_3, which decreases bone absorption. In addition, an elevated ionized calcium concentration results in increased calcitonin and 24,25-dihydroxyvitamin D, which increases osteoblastic activity.

Intestinal absorption of calcium depends primarily on 1,25-dihydroxyvitamin D_3, which stimulates calcium absorption from all parts of the small intestine. Renal excretion of calcium is regulated by PTH and vitamin D, which increase distal tubular reabsorption of calcium, and by calcitonin, which inhibits calcium reabsorption. Both metabolic and respiratory alkalosis can increase calcium excretion. Acidosis has the opposite effect. The fundamentals of the regulation of calcium homeostasis are depicted in Fig. 10.7.

Hypercalcemia

Causes. The most common causes of hypercalcemia are hyperparathyroidism and malignancy. Hyperparathyroidism is termed primary when one or more parathyroid glands produce inappropriately elevated amounts of PTH in relation to the serum calcium level. This is the result of

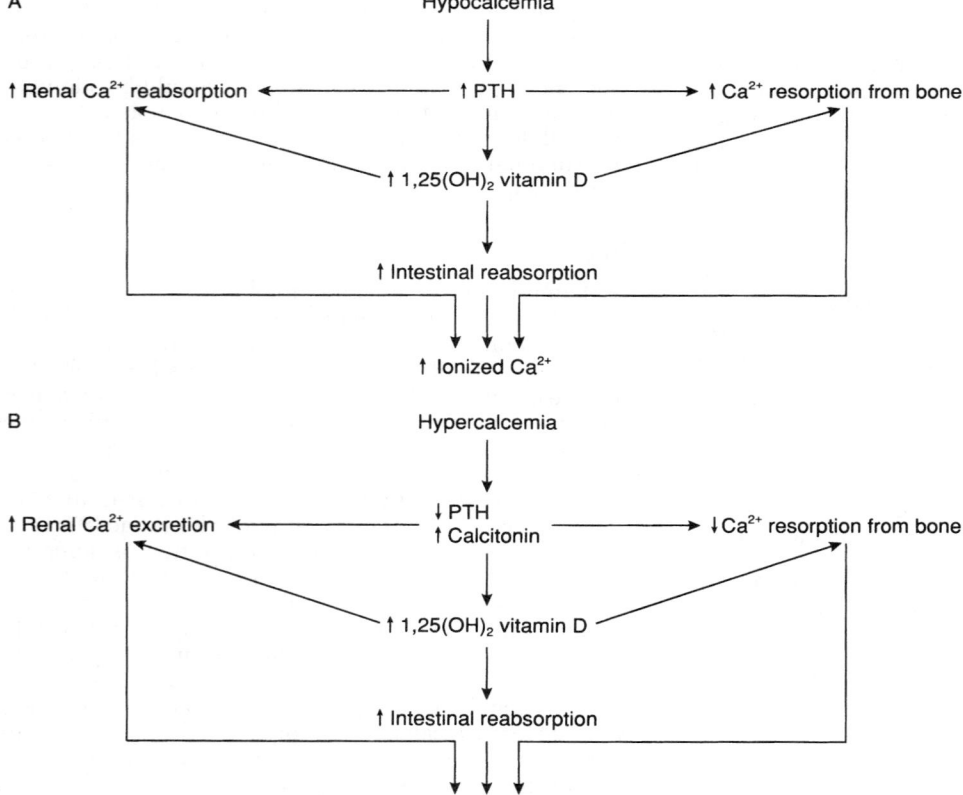

Figure 10.7. Effects of hypocalcemia *(A)* and hypercalcemia *(B)* on the mediators of calcium homeostasis. PTH, parathyroid hormone.

a parathyroid adenoma in approximately 80% to 90% of cases. Chief cell hyperplasia accounts for an additional 15% of cases, whereas parathyroid cancer is responsible for less than 1% of cases. In secondary hyperparathyroidism, elevated PTH secretion occurs because of an abnormality of an organ system other than the parathyroid glands. Usually this is the result of renal failure, though Paget's disease, osteogenesis imperfecta, and multiple myeloma represent other known etiologies of secondary hyperparathyroidism. In renal failure, poor renal excretion of phosphate results in increased serum levels of phosphate that, in turn, result in decreased serum calcium levels. In addition, gut absorption of calcium is decreased because of a deficiency in renal vitamin D metabolism. Finally, diseased kidneys are not capable of clearing the breakdown products of PTH. Tertiary hyperparathyroidism is the development of parathyroid hyperplasia with autonomous PTH production. Up to 30% of patients with pre-renal transplantation hyperparathyroidism have persistent elevations in the PTH and calcium after renal transplantation despite the fact that renal function has returned toward normal.

Hypercalcemia can be caused by malignant disease, either because of bony destruction from metastases or autonomous tumor secretion of PTH-like substances that alter calcium homeostasis. Common causes of hypercalcemia from bone destruction include multiple myeloma, lymphoma, or metastatic breast carcinoma. Interleukin-1, colony-stimulating factor, and tumor necrosis factor have been implicated as local mediators of the osteolytic activity associated with tumor metastases. Tumors that elaborate humoral factors resulting in hypercalcemia are primarily squamous cell carcinomas of the head and neck, esophagus, lung, kidney, and genitourinary tract. Secretion of PTH-like peptides, prostaglandins, transforming growth factor, and vitamin D metabolites has been reported. Humorally mediated hypercalcemia may also occur with metastatic tumors, especially breast carcinoma.

Other causes of hypercalcemia include the use of thiazide diuretics, acute adrenal insufficiency, granulomatous disease, milk-alkali syndrome, hyperthyroidism, and prolonged immobilization in otherwise young and healthy patients.

Clinical Features. The clinical manifestations of hypercalcemia depend on both the severity and duration of the abnormality. Neuromuscular effects may be the earliest manifestations and include muscle fatigue, weakness, personality disorders, psychoses, confusion, depression, and coma. Cardiovascular effects are less prominent, with hypertension being the most frequent problem encountered. ECG changes include shortening of the QT interval. Gastrointestinal side effects, such as nausea, vomiting, and abdominal pain, are not uncommon. Pancreatitis and increased gastric acid secretion with ulcer formation have also been reported.

The renal side effects of chronic hypercalcemia are numerous and can be severe. The combination of increased renal calcium excretion and decreased intestinal calcium reabsorption in response to hypercalcemia results in a new state of equilibrium at a higher serum concentration of calcium. A decrease in glomerular filtration rate, which may be a direct effect of hypercalcemia or secondary to dehydration from vomiting, can exacerbate the hypercalcemia by increasing calcium reabsorption by the kidney. In addition, nephrocalcinosis can occur, ultimately leading to chronic renal failure. Nephrolithiasis, interstitial nephropathy, renal tubular acidosis (RTA), and nephrogenic diabetes insipidus may also accompany prolonged hypercalcemia.

Treatment. Elevation of total serum calcium concentrations to greater than 14 mg/dL requires prompt treatment to prevent the many serious and potentially lethal complications of hypercalcemia. This is even more urgent for hypercalcemia associated with hyperphosphatemia because of the risk of metastatic calcification. Immediate measures are directed toward maximizing renal excretion of calcium. Because these patients are often dehydrated, 0.9% or 0.45% saline solution with 20 to 30 mEq/L of potassium is administered intravenously. Hydration should proceed at rates of 200 to 300 mL/h to promote diuresis. Furosemide may be given to enhance calcium excretion, but adequate hydration must precede diuretic therapy.

Long-term treatment depends on the underlying cause of the hypercalcemia. Primary hyperparathyroidism is usually readily treated by resection of the parathyroid abnormality (adenoma or hyperplasia). Definitive treatment of secondary or tertiary hyperparathyroidism may be either subtotal parathyroidectomy or total parathyroidectomy with autonomous parathyroid transplantation. Hypercalcemia secondary to tumor secretion of hormonal mediators may be controlled by extirpation of the tumor. In the presence of metastatic bone disease, inhibition of bone resorption with mithramycin or calcitonin may yield good results. In addition, hypercalcemia due to metastatic breast carcinoma or hematologic malignancies may respond to steroid therapy. Patients with renal failure benefit from dialysis using a low-calcium dialysate.

Hypocalcemia

Causes. Hypocalcemia secondary to hypoparathyroidism can complicate thyroid or parathyroid surgery by either inadvertent total parathyroidectomy or loss of parathyroid function due to devascularization. This has been reported to occur in as many as 2% to 3% of total thyroidectomies, although this figure appears to be declining. After resection of a parathyroid adenoma, hypocalcemia can occur because of atrophy of the remaining glands. Calcium replacement therapy may be required until the remaining glands resume normal function.

Hypocalcemia can also complicate acute pancreatitis owing to calcium precipitation into the peripancreatic tissues. In addition, pancreatic and small bowel fistulae may result in loss of calcium-rich fluid. Long-standing vitamin D deficiency secondary to malnutrition, malabsorption, or lack of exposure to sunlight can lead to hypocalcemia. Renal failure can lead to a deficiency in 1,25-dihydroxyvitamin D_3 and result in diminished intestinal absorption of calcium. Severe magnesium deficiency can also lead to hypocalcemia because of suppression of PTH levels.

Clinical Features. Serum calcium levels below 8 mg/dL may be associated with symptoms and signs that are primarily manifestations of neuromuscular abnormalities. These include muscle cramps, perioral tingling, paresthesia, laryngeal stridor, tetany, seizures, and psychotic behavior. Classic signs of hypocalcemia include hyperactive deep tendon reflexes. Two well described physical findings occur when a patient becomes hypocalcemic. One of these is Chvostek's sign, which consists of facial muscle spasm when the trunk of the facial nerve is tapped. The other finding is Trousseau's sign, carpal spasms when a blood pressure cuff is inflated to occlude the brachial artery for 3 minutes. This finding indicates latent tetany. ECG changes include a prolonged QT interval caused by prolongation of the ST segment.

Treatment. Asymptomatic hypocalcemia, which may be secondary to low protein or albumin levels with normal ionized calcium levels, need not be treated. Symptomatic hypocalcemia is best treated with intravenous infusion of calcium in the form of calcium gluconate or calcium chloride. Calcium chloride dissociates primarily to the ionized form and is therefore more efficacious in raising ionized calcium levels. Calcium should be administered at a rate not exceeding 50 mg/min (2.5 mEq/min). Prolonged calcium replacement is given orally in the form of calcium lactate, calcium citrate, or calcium carbonate. Vitamin D_3, also known as calcitriol, increases the rate of intestinal absorption and decreases the oral calcium dose requirement.

Magnesium

Total body content of magnesium in the average adult is 2,000 mEq, half of which is confined to bone. Most of the remaining magnesium is distributed in the intracellular space. Less than 1% of total body magnesium is located in the extracellular space, at concentrations of 1.4 to 2 mEq/L (or 1.7 to 2.3 mg/dL). Sixty percent of this magnesium exists in the ionized form, 25% is in the protein-bound state, and the remainder is complexed with nonprotein anionic species.

Magnesium consumed in the diet is primarily absorbed by the small intestine. The amount absorbed depends on the intake, which averages 25 mEq/d. Magnesium absorption may also be influenced by the levels of 1,25-dihydroxyvitamin D_3. Bone stores constitute the other major source of available magnesium, although regulation of magnesium exchange with bone is poorly understood.

Magnesium is excreted primarily by the kidneys. Approximately 40% of the filtered magnesium is reabsorbed in the proximal tubule, predominantly in the ascending limb of Henle. Thus, loop diuretics cause a marked increase in magnesium excretion. Magnesium excretion is also increased by hypermagnesemia, hypercalcemia, metabolic acidosis, and phosphate depletion. Conversely, magnesium excretion is decreased by metabolic alkalosis.

Hypermagnesemia

Causes. Renal failure is the primary cause of hypermagnesemia. Because of the ability of the kidneys to excrete large magnesium loads, hypermagnesemia rarely occurs if renal function remains normal. In patients with chronic or acute renal failure, administration of magnesium-containing antacids or laxatives is often the cause of magnesium excesses. Hypermagnesemia may also be due to the release of magnesium from injured tissues; thus, severe burns, crush injuries, and other causes of rhabdomyolysis may lead to high magnesium levels. Severe metabolic acidosis, extracellular volume depletion, and renal insufficiency with creatinine clearances below 30 mL/min may also cause hypermagnesemia.

Clinical Features. Neuromuscular function is depressed by hypermagnesemia because of the inhibition of synaptic acetylcholine release. Loss of deep tendon reflexes can occur with magnesium levels above 8 mg/dL. Paralysis and eventually coma can develop if levels exceed 12 to 18 mg/dL. Acute hypermagnesemia may be manifested by hypotension or even cardiac arrest if levels exceed 18 mg/dL.

Treatment. Because it is usually associated with renal failure, withholding magnesium-containing drugs in patients with hypermagnesemia usually prevents the development of magnesium excesses. Calcium antagonizes the effects of magnesium, so that infusion of 5 to 10 mEq of calcium by slow intravenous injection may serve as adequate emergency treatment. Volume expansion, correction of acid–base disturbances, administration of loop diuretics, and hemodialysis may also be used to decrease magnesium levels.

Hypomagnesemia

Causes. Because the kidneys are able to conserve magnesium well in states of magnesium depletion, hypomagnesemia rarely occurs from poor intake alone, although malnutrition is a common cause of hypomagnesemia. The combination of low intake and increased gastrointestinal loss can lead to hypomagnesemia. Malabsorptive states, especially steatorrhea, can result in significant losses of magnesium. Other causes of hypomagnesemia include prolonged periods of intravenous fluid replacement without magnesium replacement and chronic use of loop diuretics. Drugs, such as cyclosporine, aminoglycosides, cisplatin, and insulin, can also produce magnesium depletion. Burns, acute pancreatitis, treatment of diabetic ketoacidosis, and the diuretic phase of acute renal failure have been associated with the development of hypomagnesemia.

Clinical Features. Magnesium plays an integral role as a cofactor in many enzyme systems and also affects neuromuscular function. Deficiencies in magnesium may present symptoms and signs similar to hypocalcemia. Muscle fasciculations and weakness, tetany, carpopedal spasm, nausea, vomiting, and personality changes may occur. Electrolyte disturbances may also be caused by hypomagnesemia. Hypocalcemia caused by impaired PTH secretion and PTH resistance may develop. Hypokalemia caused by renal potassium wasting may also occur.

Treatment. Magnesium may be administered orally in mild cases of hypomagnesemia, but large oral doses frequently lead to diarrhea. Correction of major deficits is therefore managed by intravenous administration of magnesium sulfate at a dose of 50 to 100 mEq/d. Treatment of patients who have severe symptoms with up to 3 g of magnesium sulfate may be accomplished by bolus intravenous injection followed by an infusion of 1 to 2 mEq/kg/d.

ACID–BASE BALANCE

Definitions

An acid is defined as a chemical that can donate a hydrogen ion (H^+), for example, HCl and H_2CO_3, and a base is a chemical that can accept a H^+, for example, OH^- and (HCO_3^-). Ampholytes are both acids and bases; an example is $H_2PO_4^-$, which can donate a H^+ to become HPO_4^{2-} but can also accept H^+ to become H_3PO_4. Because HCl is a strong acid that almost completely dissociates, Cl^- is not considered a base. Bases are commonly anions, but neutral substances can also function as bases (e.g., ammonia and creatinine). Some chemicals do not fit the classic definition of an acid, although they retain acidic properties when dissociated in water. For example, when $CaCl_2$ is dissolved in water, the Ca^{2+} accepts OH^- to form $Ca(OH)_2$. Because $[H^+] \times [OH^-]$ in water remains constant at 10 to 14, the consumption of OH^- by Ca^{2+} results in increased dissociation of water. Consequently, the concentration of hydrogen ions increases, and $CaCl_2$ dissolved in water is an acidic solution.

The concentration of hydrogen ions ($[H^+]$) determines the acidity of a solution. The pH is the negative logarithm of $[H^+]$ expressed in moles per liter (mol/L). The concentration of H^+ in biologic systems is in the range of nanomoles (10^{-9} mol) per liter (nmol/L). When

$$[H^+] = 40 \text{ nmol/L} = 4 \times 10^{-10} \text{ mol/L} \qquad (19)$$

then

$$pH = -\log [H^+] = -(-7.4) = 7.4 \qquad (20)$$

When

$$[H^+] = 80 \text{ nmol/L} = 8 \times 10^{-10} \text{ mol/L} \qquad (21)$$

then

$$pH = -\log [H^+] = -(-7.1) = 7.1 \qquad (22)$$

The degree to which an acid dissociates determines its strength. If an acid, HA, dissociates to H^+ and A^-, then

$$[H^+] \times [A^-]/[HA] = K \qquad (23)$$

where K = dissociation constant. The greater the value of K, the greater the ability to dissociate, and therefore the greater the strength of the acid. Because most acids have a K value considerably below 1.0,

$$pK = -\log K \qquad (24)$$

Rearranging,

$$[H^+] = K \times [HA]/[A^-] \qquad (25)$$
$$-\log [H^+] = -\log K \times -\log [HA]/[A^-]$$
$$pH = pK \times \log [A^-]/[HA]$$

This is the derivation for the Henderson-Hasselbalch equation.

Buffer Systems

Buffers are chemicals in solution that tend to minimize changes in pH that would otherwise occur after the addition of acid or alkali. If a strong acid is added to the salt of a weak acid and a strong base, the reaction produces another salt and a weak acid:

$$HCl + NaHCO_3 \rightarrow NaCl + H_2CO_3 \qquad (26)$$

Thus, the decrease in pH that would have occurred in the absence of $NaHCO_3$ is minimized. Conversely, if a strong base is added to a weak acid, the base is neutralized:

$$NaOH + H_2CO_3 \rightarrow NaHCO_3 + H_2O \qquad (27)$$

The elevation in pH after the addition of NaOH is prevented.

One type of buffer is a mixture of a weak acid and its salt, which forms an amount of weak acid or base equivalent to the amount of strong acid or base added to the system. The presence of such buffer systems in the body is crucial to minimizing changes in pH secondary to the daily production of the 70 mEq of acid generated from dietary precursors. There is a relatively narrow range of pH for optimal function of the chemical reactions necessary for cell function.

The principal intracellular buffers are organic phosphates, bicarbonate, and peptides. In addition, hemoglobin functions as a significant buffer in red blood cells. The major extracellular buffer is bicarbonate. An approximation of the total body buffer capacity is 15 mEq/kg. More than half of the total body alkaline buffer content is located outside the ECF and may in large part reside in bone (11). The buffer pair carbonic acid/bicarbonate (H_2CO_3/HCO_3^-) is the focus of the ensuing discussion because it is the primary buffer system of the body and the components of this buffer system are easily measured. Because all body buffer systems are in equilibrium, the state of the H_2CO_3/HCO_3^- system essentially reflects the state of all the body buffers.

From a chemical point of view, the ideal buffer should have a pK that approximates the pH to be preserved. The H_2CO_3/HCO_3^- buffer system has a pK of only 6.1, but this buffer system is efficient because of the presence of large amounts of bicarbonate, the conversion of its acid H_2CO_3 to CO_2 that is rapidly excreted through the lungs, and an inexhaustible supply of CO_2, although at low concentrations.

The H_2CO_3/HCO_3^- buffer system is defined by the Henderson-Hasselbalch equation. This equation (equation 15), when applied to the H_2CO_3/HCO_3^- buffer system, yields the following:

$$pH = pK + \log [HCO_3^-]/[H_2CO_3] \qquad (28)$$

In the clinical use of this equation, $[H_2CO_3]$ is replaced by $[CO_2]$ because measurement of the low concentrations of $[H_2CO_3]$ present in body fluids is difficult, whereas $[CO_2]$, which is in equilibrium with $[H_2CO_3]$ in a fixed ratio, can be readily measured. Making this substitution, the equation becomes

$$pH = pK + \log [HCO_3^-]/[CO_2] \qquad (29)$$

Because the pK for this buffer system is 6.1,

$$pH = 6.1 + \log [HCO_3^-]/[CO_2] \qquad (30)$$

Using normal values for $[HCO_3^-]$ (24 mEq/L) and $[CO_2]$ (1.2 mmol/L),

$$pH = 6.1 + \log 24/1.2 \qquad (31)$$
$$= 6.1 + \log 20 = 7.4$$

A pH of 7.4 is maintained as long as the ratio of $[HCO_3^-]$ to $[CO_2]$ remains 20 : 1. The amount of $[CO_2]$ in solution is estimated from P_{CO_2} and its solubility coefficient (0.03 in plasma). Making these substitutions,

$$pH = 6.1 + \log [HCO_3^-]/(P_{CO_2} \times 0.03) \qquad (32)$$

Anion Gap

The anion gap is defined as follows:

$$\text{Anion gap} = [Na^+] - ([Cl^-] + [HCO_3^-]) \qquad (33)$$

Normally, the difference between the serum $[Na^+]$ and the sum of the chloride and bicarbonate anion concentrations is a reflection of the sum of the serum proteins, sulfate anions, inorganic phosphates, and organic acids present in low concentrations. The anion gap is usually 12 ± 2 mEq/L. Variances from the normal may be caused by a change in unmeasured anions or cations. Calculation of the anion gap may help define both simple and mixed forms of acid-base disturbances. Acidosis associated with a high anion gap is usually secondary to increases in endogenously produced acids (e.g., lactic acidosis or ketoacidosis), decreases in renal excretion of acids (e.g., renal failure), or ingestion of toxins.

ACID–BASE DISTURBANCES

There are four primary acid-base disturbances, each of which are related to changes in either $[HCO_3^-]$ or P_{CO_2}. Metabolic acidosis is a decrease in pH as a result of a primary decrease in $[HCO_3^-]$, whereas metabolic alkalosis is an increase in pH caused by a primary increase in $[HCO_3^-]$. Respiratory acidosis is a decrease in pH secondary to a primary increase in P_{CO_2}. Likewise, respiratory alkalosis is an increase in pH caused by a primary decrease in P_{CO_2}. In each of these disorders, compensatory changes occur to minimize changes in the relative ratio of $[HCO_3^-]$ to P_{CO_2} and thereby blunt the effect of the primary disturbance on pH (Table 10.8).

Metabolic Acidosis

Three mechanisms result in a decrease in extracellular bicarbonate concentration and metabolic acidosis:

1. Dilutional acidosis. Rapid infusion of an alkali-free solution results in dilution of the bicarbonate concentration.

Table 10.8. HCO₃⁻ AND PCO₂ DERANGEMENTS IN PRIMARY AND SECONDARY ACID–BASE DISTURBANCES

Disorder	Primary			Secondary	
	pH	HCO₃⁻	Pco₂	HCO₃⁻	Pco₂
Metabolic acidosis	↓	↓			↓
Metabolic alkalosis	↑	↑			↑
Respiratory acidosis	↓		↑	↑	
Respiratory alkalosis	↑		↓	↓	

2. Cellular retention of K⁺ in exchange for Na⁺ and H⁺. Buffering of the H⁺ may result in a transient decrease in extracellular bicarbonate concentration.
3. Decreased body bicarbonate content. This occurs when net loss of bicarbonate exceeds bicarbonate generation.

The first two mechanisms are relatively infrequent and usually produce only mild, self-limiting metabolic acidosis; however, aggressive "overresuscitation" of surgical or trauma patients with normal saline solution may result in a dilutional acidosis. Most clinically significant metabolic acidosis is related to net loss of bicarbonate, which occurs when consumption due to either loss or titration is greater than bicarbonate generation. Under normal circumstances of ingestion of the average amount of protein in the American diet, approximately 70 mEq of acid is generated daily. The major source of acid production is sulfuric acid from the metabolism of sulfur-containing amino acids. In addition, normal physiologic processes result in the generation of organic acids, the titration of which consumes bicarbonate. Although the resulting organic anions are further metabolized with regeneration of bicarbonate, urinary excretion of some organic anions occurs and results in net loss of bicarbonate.

These sources of acid gain are partially offset by net gastrointestinal absorption of metabolizable anions, such as citrate, which are metabolized to yield bicarbonate. The remainder of the excess acid is balanced by renal excretion of acid with simultaneous generation of bicarbonate. A decrease in body bicarbonate content may therefore be the result of a primary increase in net acid generation, termed *extrarenal acidosis,* or a primary reduction in renal acid excretion, termed *renal acidosis.*

In extrarenal acidosis, the normal compensatory mechanism is increased renal excretion of acid, usually as ammonia, with generation of bicarbonate. This mechanism is sensitive to decreases in bicarbonate concentration and has the capacity to generate large amounts of bicarbonate.

In contrast, renal acidosis is not as readily compensated because the renal abnormality is the primary mechanism. The level to which serum bicarbonate concentration decreases depends on several factors, including the magnitude of the disparity in acid production and acid excretion as well as its duration. In general, the development of renal acidosis is slow but progressive, whereas the development of extrarenal acidosis is rapid but usually self-limiting. Despite persistent net loss of bicarbonate, extracellular bicarbonate concentration may stabilize at a subnormal level rather than continue to decrease. This may be due to bone buffering, which has the capacity to buffer as much as 28 to 37 mEq/d of acid.

Mechanisms Resulting in Decreased Body Bicarbonate Content

Increased Production of Organic Acids. Increased protein intake and tissue catabolism resulting in greater metabolism of sulfur-containing amino acids can lead to generation of increased amounts of sulfuric acid. With normal kidney function, any decline in serum bicarbonate concentration stimulates renal acid excretion, which can compensate nearly completely for the increase in acid production.

Administration of Exogenous Acid. Ingestion of a sufficient quantity of exogenous acid can exceed renal compensatory capacity and result in metabolic acidosis. Examples of acids that may be ingested include ammonium chloride, calcium chloride, nitric acid, sulfuric acid, and hydrochloric acid.

Nonrenal Loss of Bicarbonate. Diarrhea, intestinal or pancreatic fistulae, and burns can cause metabolic acidosis secondary to loss of bicarbonate. In addition, ureterosigmoidostomy and ureteroileostomy result in loss of bicarbonate because of reabsorption of NH₄Cl from the urine. The potential for fistulae to result in metabolic acidosis depends on the concentration of bicarbonate in the fluid and the rate of external drainage. Thus, metabolic acidosis is less common with biliary fistulae than pancreatic fistulae because bicarbonate concentration in bile is usually less than 50 to 60 mEq/L, and the amount of drainage tends to be modest. In pancreatic fistulae, bicarbonate concentration in pancreatic juice approaches 150 mEq/L, and the drainage can be profuse.

Organic Acidosis. The two most common types of organic acidosis are ketoacidosis and lactic acidosis. The abnormality primarily responsible for ketoacidosis is deficiency of insulin, whether primary, as in diabetic ketoacidosis, or secondary to hypoglycemia. Normally, free fatty acids generated from breakdown of triglycerides in adipose tissue are either used as an energy source by various organs such as muscle, or carried to the liver, where they are reesterified to triglycerides and incorporated into very-low-density lipoprotein, or further metabolized. Ketoacids are produced by mitochondrial metabolism of free fatty acids to acetyl-CoA, with subsequent formation of acetoacetate and β-hydroxybutyrate (redox forms of the same compound). Under normal conditions, a small amount of ketoacidosis is produced. During prolonged starvation, production of ketoacids increases to modest levels, providing an important source of energy to nonhepatic tissues, particularly the brain.

In diabetic ketoacidosis, the ketoacid production is excessive because of insulin deficiency, which drives ketoacid production by increasing free fatty acid release from adipose tissue, increasing transport of free fatty acids into hepatic mitochondria, promoting conversion of acetyl-CoA to ketoacids, and impairing extrahepatic use of ketoacids (12). Insulin deficiency also contributes to hyperglycemia by decreasing the metabolism of glucose by extrahepatic tissues and increasing hepatic production of glucose. The resulting osmotic glucose diuresis causes increased renal excretion of sodium and water. Additional losses of sodium and potassium occur as the result of renal excretion of the excess ketoacid anions. Potassium excretion is further enhanced by hyperaldosteronism due to the increased delivery of sodium to the distal tubule that occurs in association with the osmotic diuresis. Despite total body potassium depletion, serum potassium concentration is often increased in diabetic ketoacidosis secondary to metabolic acidosis, renal insufficiency, insulin deficiency, and hyperosmolality. These pathophysiologic changes result in the typical clinical presentation, which includes dehydration, polyuria, polydipsia, hyperglycemia, hyperventilation, and metabolic acidosis with an increased anion gap (normochloremic).

Spontaneous decarboxylation of acetoacetate to acetone occurs with excretion of acetone through the lungs, resulting in the characteristic odor described in diabetic ketoacidosis. Patients may be lucid, although some degree of mental obtundation is common, and coma may occur.

In hyperosmolar, hyperglycemic, and nonketotic coma, moderate acidosis may be observed. The mechanism of the acidosis is not clear. In contrast to the moderate hyperglycemia, averaging 600 mg/dL, seen in diabetic ketoacidosis, the marked hyperglycemia, averaging 1,200 mg/dL, that occurs in hyperosmolar nonketotic hyperglycemia is not associated with ketoacidosis.

Lactic acidosis can be divided into type A, caused by tissue hypoxia, and type B, caused by other mechanisms. Hypoxia, the most common cause of lactic acidosis, impairs the mitochondrial oxidation of the reduced form of nicotinamide-adenine dinucleotide (NADH) to NAD, which is necessary for glycolysis. Under these conditions, NADH is oxidized by the reduction of pyruvate, the end product of glucose metabolism in the Embden-Meyerhof pathway, to lactic acid. Thus, generation of lactic acid is the final step of anaerobic glycolysis. Lactic acid is normally produced by muscle, blood elements, intestine, and skin, and is used by the liver and kidney. Normal serum lactate concentration is below 2 mEq/L. Lactic acidosis secondary to hypoxia is usually due to increased production of lactate as well as decreased use, and serum lactate concentration is greater than 6 mEq/L.

The most common cause of type B lactic acidosis is ethanol intoxication. Lactic acidosis is caused by increased generation of NADH by the metabolism of alcohol, which interferes with hepatic gluconeogenesis and, therefore, lactate use.

In lactic acidosis, the L-isomer is usually elevated because of the specificity of mammalian lactate dehydrogenase. Various bacteria found in colonic flora are capable of generating large amounts of D-lactic acid. D-Lactic acidosis has been reported in humans only in the presence of short-gut syndrome because the small bowel normally absorbs the dietary substrate for bacterial D-lactic acid production. In addition, the colon must be selectively colonized by bacteria that possess D-lactate dehydrogenase. Typically, the patient has short-gut syndrome, and the acidosis is preceded by food ingestion and is accompanied by characteristic neurologic findings, including mental confusion, slurred speech, staggering gait, and nystagmus. These neurologic manifestations are secondary to bacterial neurotoxins. The acidosis is accompanied by an increased anion gap, but L-lactate and ketone levels are normal. Treatment includes oral antibiotics, recolonization of the colon with non-D-lactate dehydrogenase-forming bacteria, and a low-carbohydrate diet.

Metabolic Acidosis Caused by Drugs and Toxins. Acetylsalicylic acid (aspirin) is rapidly metabolized to salicylic acid, which is eventually further metabolized and excreted by the kidney. Ingestion of more than 4 to 6 g/d results in excretion of unmetabolized salicylic acid. Salicylate intoxication causes a respiratory alkalosis secondary to direct stimulation of the respiratory center as well as a metabolic acidosis with an increased anion gap. In addition, acidosis increases the toxicity of salicylate by increasing the concentration of the nonionized form, which results in higher intracellular concentrations. Manifestations of salicylate overdose include tinnitus, asterixis, noncardiogenic pulmonary edema, hypotension, vascular collapse, vomiting, seizures, and coma. Blood levels of salicylate correlate poorly with the severity of the clinical presentation because of the variability in time between ingestion and hospitalization. Treatment is usually required when more than 10 g have been ingested. It includes alkalinization of the urine to prevent reabsorption of salicylate and hemodialysis in patients with severe neurologic symptoms.

Ethylene glycol, the principal component of antifreeze, is converted by alcohol dehydrogenase to glycoaldehyde, then to glycolic acid with production of one NADH at each step. The acidosis produced by ingestion of ethylene glycol is secondary to accumulation of glycolic acid, although lactate also accumulates because of the production of NADH. Bicarbonate is not regenerated when the glycolate is further metabolized, so exogenous alkali is required to replace what was titrated. In addition, 3% to 10% of ethylene glycol is converted to oxalic acid, which may result in hypocalcemia and contribute to acute renal failure. Three stages of toxicity are described. CNS dysfunction characterizes the first stage. This is followed by cardiopulmonary failure and finally by oliguric acute renal failure. Treatment includes the administration of ethanol, which has greater affinity for alcohol dehydrogenase and delays the metabolism of ethylene glycol to its toxic metabolites. Treatment also includes hemodialysis or peritoneal dialysis to remove ethylene glycol and glycolate.

Metabolism of methanol by alcohol dehydrogenase results in the formation of formaldehyde and formic acid, both of which are severely toxic. The acidosis is associated with an increase in anion gap secondary to the accumulation of formate. The clinical presentation includes blurred vision or blindness associated with the funduscopic findings of hyperemic discs and retinal edema, malaise, headache, abdominal pain, vomiting, convulsions, and coma. Treatment includes ethanol infusion to delay the metabolism of methanol by alcohol dehydrogenase, hemodialysis, bicarbonate administration, and intravenous folate to enhance metabolism of formate.

Renal Acidosis: Decreased Net Acid Excretion

The impaired ability of the kidney to excrete acid and hence generate bicarbonate may be secondary to a decrease in the number of functioning nephrons and is termed *uremic acidosis* or *renal tubular acidosis*. Uremic acidosis, which can occur in both acute and chronic renal failure, is primarily caused by a reduction in ammonia excretion secondary to a reduction in the number of functioning proximal tubular cells. In addition, decreased proximal tubular bicarbonate reabsorption contributes to the development of acidosis. Although the onset of uremic acidosis may be related to declining renal function, its appearance can also be influenced by diet-dependent protein and organic anion ingestion, use of diuretic therapy that stimulates acid excretion, and the extent of tubular versus glomerular injury.

Renal tubular acidosis can be classified as distal (classic, type I) or proximal (type II), depending on the primary site of the renal tubular defect leading to acidosis. Distal RTA is characterized by a defect in urinary acidification. It is associated with either hypokalemia or hyperkalemia, depending on the underlying pathophysiologic mechanisms. Proposed mechanisms of distal RTA with hypokalemia include reduced H+ pump activity and increased tubular permeability with back-leak of secreted H+ into the tubular cell. In RTA with hyperkalemia, the mechanism is decreased luminal negativity secondary to impaired sodium reabsorption. The major defect in proximal RTA is proximal tubular dysfunction resulting in diminished reabsorption of filtered bicarbonate. Urinary excretion greater than 15% of the filtered load of bicarbonate at normal serum bicarbonate levels is pathognomonic for proximal RTA. Other indicators of proximal tubular dysfunction include glycosuria, aminoaciduria, uricosuria, and phosphaturia.

Clinical Features of Acute Metabolic Acidosis

The major cardiovascular effects of acute metabolic acidosis are peripheral arteriolar dilatation, decreased cardiac contractility, and central venous constriction. These can lead to cardiovascular collapse and pulmonary edema. Catecholamine secretion is stimulated by metabolic acidosis, and in mild cases (pH >7.1), heart rate may be increased. In more severe metabolic acidosis (pH <7.1), the direct effects of acidosis override the catecholamine effects and result in bradycardia and decreased contractility. These depressive effects are magnified by beta blockers. In addition to these cardiovascular effects, metabolic acidosis can affect oxygen delivery by shifting the oxygen–hemoglobin dissociation curve to the right. In more prolonged metabolic acidosis, this may be partially offset by decreased production of 2,3-diphosphoglycerate in red blood cells because of a slower rate of glycolysis. Metabolic acidosis can also cause gastric distention, abdominal pain, nausea, and vomiting.

Compensatory Mechanisms

Renal Compensation. The kidney is extremely sensitive to changes in serum bicarbonate concentration and responds by increasing net acid excretion primarily by increasing ammonia excretion. Maximal renal compensation requires 2 to 4 days. In addition, the maximal amount of ammonia excreted during acidosis depends on factors that include the rate of glutamine delivery, effects on glomerular filtration rate by associated conditions such as dehydration, and the type of anion that accompanies the acid because renal acid secretion is stimulated to varying degrees by different anions. Although renal compensation is effective in achieving normal net acid excretion with extrarenal causes of metabolic acid, variable results are seen with renal acidosis. Compensation at times is complete for proximal RTA, whereas compensation usually is incomplete for distal RTA.

Respiratory Compensation. Delay in achieving maximal renal response to an increased acid load causes blood pH to decline, which stimulates hyperventilation. Although effective in promptly raising blood pH, ventilatory compensation is only partial, and full respiratory compensation requires 12 to 24 hours. The mechanism behind this delay remains unclear. The magnitude of the decrease in Pco_2 in response to a given degree of metabolic acidosis can be used to determine whether the metabolic acidosis is complicated by coexisting respiratory acidosis or respiratory alkalosis. Although a number of sophisticated mathematic models relating Pco_2 to serum bicarbonate, serum hydrogen ion, and pH have been described, the following is a simple equation that is readily applicable to the clinical situation (12):

$$d Pco_2 = 1.2 \times d[HCO_3^-] \pm 2.0 \qquad (34)$$

where $dPco_2$ = expected decrease in Pco_2 given the measured decrease in serum bicarbonate concentration. For example, if serum bicarbonate is 18, $d[HCO_3^-]$ is 6 (24 − 18). The expected $dPco_2$ is 7.2 ± 2, or Pco_2 = 32.8 (40 − 7.2) ± 2 mm Hg. This equation is applicable in mild to moderate metabolic acidosis because pulmonary edema complicating severe metabolic acidosis interferes with maximal ventilatory compensation.

Treatment

Acute Metabolic Acidosis. The major principle of treatment for mild to moderate acute metabolic acidosis is correction of the underlying cause. In surgical and trauma patients, metabolic acidosis is often the result of hypoxia secondary to inadequate tissue perfusion and subsequent lactic acidosis. Volume and blood resuscitation alone may be enough to correct the acidosis. Attempts to correct acidosis with exogenous bicarbonate without correction of inadequate tissue perfusion are usually unsuccessful. Likewise, attempts to treat hypotension in volume-depleted patients with vasopressor agents increase tissue hypoxia and acidosis and may exacerbate the problem. The immediate goals are volume replenishment and correction of acidosis, and the long-term goal is to identify and treat definitively the underlying disease process.

The use of bicarbonate for the treatment of lactic acidosis is controversial. In several studies, the use of bicarbonate in patients with lactic acidosis has not improved clinical parameters or outcome. In addition, bicarbonate administration does not change the clinical course or outcome of patients with diabetic ketoacidosis. Bicarbonate is best reserved for patients with other, not easily reversible causes of metabolic acidosis to prevent cardiovascular collapse, and usually is not used until the pH falls to 7.1 to 7.2. Because older patients and those with cardiovascular disease have decreased tolerance for acidosis, bicarbonate may be given before the pH has fallen to such low levels. The amount of bicarbonate required to increase its serum concentration to any given level cannot be calculated. The goal is to increase the pH to 7.2 to 7.3 by administering one or two ampules of bicarbonate (44.5 to 50 mEq/amp) initially, basing the need for additional bicarbonate on repeated arterial blood gas results. Rapid correction to achieve normal serum bicarbonate concentration may be harmful because organic anions are precursors of bicarbonate, and their eventual metabolism combined with administered bicarbonate may result in metabolic alkalosis. This may be further complicated by persistent hyperventilation in the face of rapidly normalized serum bicarbonate concentration, resulting in the superimposition of a respiratory alkalosis. In addition, rapid correction of serum bicarbonate concentration may not allow reversal of 2,3-diphosphoglycerate depletion in red blood cells. The resulting shift of the oxygen–hemoglobin dissociation curve to the left may result in tissue hypoxia.

Chronic Acidosis. Most cases of distal RTA require treatment with daily doses of alkali to correct acidosis and prevent nephrocalcinosis and nephrolithiasis. Patients with distal RTA and hypokalemia require potassium supplementation as well. In proximal RTA in adults, mild cases do not require specific therapy. Severe cases ($[HCO_3^-]$ <18) are treated with thiazide diuretics and a low-salt diet to achieve a modest degree of volume depletion, which reduces the requirement for bicarbonate supplementation. Children are particularly susceptible to the growth-retarding effects of even mild acidosis, and the threshold for treatment should be low.

Diabetic Ketoacidosis. The correction of both acidosis and hyperglycemia is best achieved by the administration of insulin. Metabolism of the anions of the ketoacids begins promptly with insulin therapy and results in the generation of bicarbonate. In addition, insulin inhibits ketone formation and gluconeogenesis and stimulates peripheral use of ketones and glucose. A general recommendation is to administer a loading dose of 20 IU of regular insulin intravenously, followed by a continuous intravenous infusion of 5 to 10 IU/h. Infusion of small amounts of insulin (1 to 3 IU/h) should be continued until acidosis clears. Volume resuscitation is also required; the average amount is 4 or 5 L in the first 24 hours. Alternating liters of normal and half-normal saline is recommended, despite increased extracellular osmolality, to minimize the risk of cerebral edema. Potassium replacement is essential, even in the face of normal or high serum potassium, because hypokalemia develops as acidosis and hyperglycemia are corrected. Unrecognized hypokalemia is a major cause of death from diabetic ketoacidosis.

Hyperosmolar Nonketotic Acidosis. The key to successful treatment is to seek, recognize, and treat any underlying cause for the hyperosmolar nonketotic hyperglycemia, such as gram-negative sepsis. Hyperglycemia is corrected by the administration of insulin, as described previously. Volume depletion can be more severe than that seen with diabetic ketoacidosis. Potassium supplementation must be given as well.

Metabolic Alkalosis

Causes

Sustained metabolic alkalosis occurs only if extracellular bicarbonate concentration is increased and renal excretion of excess bicarbonate is inhibited. Alone, neither is sufficient to result in metabolic alkalosis. Extracellular bicarbonate concentration is increased by numerous mechanisms. Loss of HCl is a leading cause of metabolic alkalosis in surgical patients. The most common example of this cause of metabolic alkalosis is loss of pure gastric secretion due to vomiting or nasogastric drainage in the face of gastric outlet obstruction. The gastric secretion of HCl generates equal amounts of bicarbonate in the blood. External loss of gastric acid results in a net gain in bicarbonate, which causes metabolic alkalosis. Although the kidney can excrete excess bicarbonate, this must be accompanied by excretion of sodium. Renal excretion of sodium is limited in the face of the volume depletion, which also occurs with external losses of gastric secretion. As volume depletion progresses, sodium is conserved in exchange for hydrogen. Thus, in metabolic alkalosis secondary to gastric outlet obstruction, the urine initially is alkalotic but becomes paradoxically acidotic in prolonged or uncorrected cases.

Increased extracellular bicarbonate concentration can occur with administration of either bicarbonate or precursors of bicarbonate, such as lactate, citrate, or calcium carbonate, or as a result of increased renal production of bicarbonate. Conditions in which acid excretion exceeds endogenous acid production and in which the renal threshold for bicarbonate reabsorption is increased can result in metabolic alkalosis. Such conditions include moderate potassium depletion, excess mineralocorticoids, and high P_{CO_2}.

Hypokalemia and cellular exchange of potassium for hydrogen can also lead to metabolic alkalosis. Hypokalemia results in enhanced proximal tubular bicarbonate reabsorption and distal tubular acid excretion. When potassium leaves the cell, it is exchanged for either sodium or hydrogen to maintain electrical neutrality. Loss of potassium from the body then results in a net gain in bicarbonate in the ECF.

Maintenance of elevated extracellular bicarbonate concentration can occur by a number of mechanisms. Volume contraction leads to decreases in renal blood flow and glomerular filtration rate that reduce the filtered load of bicarbonate. This, in addition to decreased proximal tubular reabsorption of bicarbonate, maintains high extracellular concentrations of bicarbonate. High P_{CO_2} causes an increase in renal threshold for bicarbonate secondary to decreased intracellular pH of the renal tubular cell. The net result is increased bicarbonate reabsorption.

Hypercalcemia and low PTH levels both result in increased proximal tubular reabsorption of bicarbonate, which may be enhanced by a decrease in glomerular filtration rate. Renal failure also leads to an inability of the

kidney to excrete excess bicarbonate. Diuretics can cause or exacerbate metabolic alkalosis by both causing rapid contraction of intravascular volume and increasing renal excretion of acid. Chloride deficiency is another common factor that maintains an alkalotic state. In some instances of metabolic alkalosis, urinary excretion of chloride is markedly reduced. Reversal of metabolic alkalosis in these cases can be readily achieved by administration of chloride-containing solutions. Although chloride deficiency *per se* can result in an increased renal threshold for bicarbonate and in increased renal reabsorption of bicarbonate, this apparent association may also be related to volume contraction. Metabolic alkalosis can be divided into chloride-responsive and chloride-resistant types.

Respiratory Compensation

The major compensatory mechanism in metabolic alkalosis is respiratory because the presence of the metabolic alkalosis implies renal dysfunction in either generating or failing to excrete increased amounts of bicarbonate. Hypoventilation is limited by the development of hypoxemia, which stimulates ventilation, and P_{CO_2} rarely exceeds 60 mm Hg (Table 10.9). Among the four major types of acid–base disorders, this compensatory mechanism is the least effective. For a given degree of metabolic alkalosis, the following equation can be used to predict the compensatory increase in P_{CO_2}:

$$dP_{CO_2} = 0.7 \times d[HCO_3^-] \pm 5 \qquad (35)$$

where dP_{CO_2} = expected increase in P_{CO_2} given the measured increase in serum bicarbonate concentration.

Clinical Features

Clinical signs of metabolic alkalosis may not be prominent because the condition usually develops relatively slowly. If acute, CNS manifestations of confusion, obtundation, stupor, and coma may be present as well as tetany and neuromuscular irritability.

Treatment

Correction of the underlying cause is the mainstay of treatment in this disorder. In general, correction of potassium depletion and volume depletion corrects the metabolic alkalosis. Renal excretion of bicarbonate cannot occur in the face of persistent volume depletion. Volume depletion should be corrected with chloride-containing solutions. In patients without intravascular volume deficits, renal excretion of bicarbonate can be enhanced by administration of the carbonic acid anhydrase inhibitor

Table 10.9. CALCULATIONS FOR ESTIMATING THE COMPENSATORY RESPONSES TO PRIMARY ACID–BASE DISTURBANCES

Type of Disorder	Degree of Compensation	Time Required
Metabolic acidosis	$dP_{CO_2} = d[HCO_3^-] \times 1.2 \pm 2$	12–24 h
Metabolic alkalosis	$dP_{CO_2} = d[HCO_3^-] \times 0.7 \pm 5$	12–24 h
Acute respiratory acidosis	$d[HCO_3^-] = dP_{CO_2} \times 0.07 \pm 1.5$	Minutes
Chronic respiratory acidosis	$d[HCO_3^-] = dP_{CO_2} \times 0.4 \pm 3$	3–5 d
Acute respiratory alkalosis	$d[HCO_3^-] = dP_{CO_2} \times 0.2 \pm 2.5$	Minutes
Chronic respiratory alkalosis	$d[HCO_3^-] = dP_{CO_2} \times 0.5 \pm 2.5$	2–3 d

diuretic acetazolamide. If renal excretion of bicarbonate cannot be increased because of underlying renal insufficiency, or if the metabolic alkalosis is severe, acid may be administered to titrate directly the excess extracellular bicarbonate. Acids that can be used include ammonium chloride, arginine hydrochloride, lysine hydrochloride, or dilute hydrochloric acid (0.1 N). Partial correction of the alkalosis is the initial goal. A general guide is that 2.2 mEq/kg decreases serum bicarbonate by approximately 5 mEq/L. In the face of renal failure, dialysis may be necessary to remove excess bicarbonate.

Respiratory Alkalosis

A primary decrease in P_{CO_2} resulting in increased extracellular pH is referred to as *respiratory alkalosis*. Hyperventilation and the ensuing fall in P_{CO_2} may be secondary to hypoxia, reflex stimulation from decreased pulmonary compliance, drugs, mechanical ventilation, and other causes.

Hypoxia stimulates ventilation through peripheral chemoreceptors in the carotid and aortic body. Decrease in arterial P_{O_2}, rather than in oxygen content, is the main stimulus. Acute drops in arterial P_{O_2} result in sustained hyperventilation only when the P_{CO_2} decreases below 60 mm Hg. Although hyperventilation occurs with even slight degrees of hypoxia, the resulting increase in brain pH suppresses the stimulus for hyperventilation unless severe hypoxia is present. In contrast, chronic hypoxia results in hyperventilation even with mildly decreased P_{CO_2} because brain pH is lowered by metabolic compensation. The two most common causes of hypoxia resulting in respiratory alkalosis are pulmonary disease and exposure to high altitudes.

Compensatory Mechanisms

Tissue buffering is the initial response to a decrease in P_{CO_2}. Red blood cells provide one third of the buffering. Consumption of bicarbonate results from cellular liberation of H^+. Although immediate, the magnitude of tissue buffering is slight and can be predicted by the following formula:

$$d[HCO_3^-] = dP_{CO_2} \times 0.2 \pm 2.5 \qquad (36)$$

Renal compensation is achieved, not by increasing excretion of bicarbonate, but by decreasing net acid excretion, primarily through reductions in ammonia excretion and increases in organic anion excretion. These organic anions are excreted as sodium and potassium salts. As a result, potassium excretion is increased, resulting in hypokalemia. Complete renal compensation requires 2 or 3 days.

Clinical Features

Chronic respiratory alkalosis is usually asymptomatic because compensatory mechanisms are successful in maintaining pH close to normal. Acute respiratory alkalosis may cause sensations of breathlessness, dizziness, and nervousness and can result in circumoral and extremity paresthesias, altered levels of consciousness, and tetany. These signs are related to decreased cerebral blood flow secondary to decreased P_{CO_2}, and decreased ionized calcium concentration secondary to the increased blood pH.

Treatment

The underlying stimulus for the hyperventilation should be addressed. The cause of hypoxemia should be determined and corrected. In acute symptomatic respiratory alkalosis, rebreathing or breathing 5% CO_2 temporar-

ily relieves the symptoms. If the condition is secondary to mechanical ventilation, adjustment of tidal volume or respiratory rate should result in resolution of the respiratory alkalosis.

Respiratory Acidosis

Respiratory acidosis, the decrease in extracellular pH from a primary increase in P_{CO_2}, is due to inadequate ventilation. Although pulmonary disease commonly causes hypoxemia, respiratory acidosis is far less common because diffusion of O_2 is more readily impaired than diffusion of CO_2. The main causes of hypoventilation include depression of the respiratory center, impaired respiratory excursion of the thorax, airway obstruction, and chronic obstructive pulmonary disease. In addition, inappropriate ventilatory settings in the mechanically ventilated patient may result in respiratory acidosis.

Compensatory Mechanisms

Increased P_{CO_2} results in increased H_2CO_3, which dissociates into H^+ and HCO_3^-. Cellular exchange of Na^+ and K^+ for H^+ allows the reaction to continue in this direction with increased extracellular bicarbonate. This tissue buffering is accomplished within minutes. Persistently elevated P_{CO_2} also stimulates increased renal acid excretion, primarily the chloride salt of ammonia, and results in increased renal generation of HCO_3^-. Full renal compensation occurs over 3 to 5 days. The following formula describes chronic respiratory acidosis:

$$d[HCO_3^-] = dP_{CO_2} \times 0.4 \pm 3 \qquad (37)$$

Clinical Features

The magnitude of clinical manifestations depends on the chronicity and rate of development of respiratory acidosis. Acute changes in P_{CO_2} result in acute cerebral acidosis, which may cause drowsiness, restlessness, and the development of a flapping tremor, or, if more severe, stupor or coma. The response of the cerebral vasculature to acidosis is dilation. The consequent increase in cerebral blood flow may result in increased intracranial blood pressure, headache, and papilledema. Systemic acidosis results in peripheral vasodilatation, depressed cardiac contractility, and insensitivity to catecholamines.

Treatment

Treatment should be directed to the underlying cause of the hypoventilation. Endotracheal intubation to achieve adequate ventilation is key to the treatment of acute respiratory acidosis of any cause. The treatment of chronic, compensated respiratory acidosis may be complicated by the accompanying hypoxemia. In chronic hypercapnia, the central chemoreceptors may be insensitive, and the accompanying hypoxemia may supply the main respiratory drive through stimulation of peripheral chemoreceptors. In such patients, complete correction of the hypoxemia may further suppress respiration and worsen the respiratory acidosis. In addition, P_{CO_2} should not be normalized rapidly. Reequilibration of cerebral bicarbonate concentration lags behind systemic changes. Thus, even if P_{CO_2} is normal, cellular and cerebral metabolic alkalosis may develop.

Mixed Acid–Base Disorders

Combinations of two or more of the four primary acid–base disorders may occur and should be suspected when blood pH approaches normal despite abnormal P_{CO_2} and $[HCO_3^-]$, or when compensatory changes appear to be either excessive or inadequate (Fig. 10.8). The com-

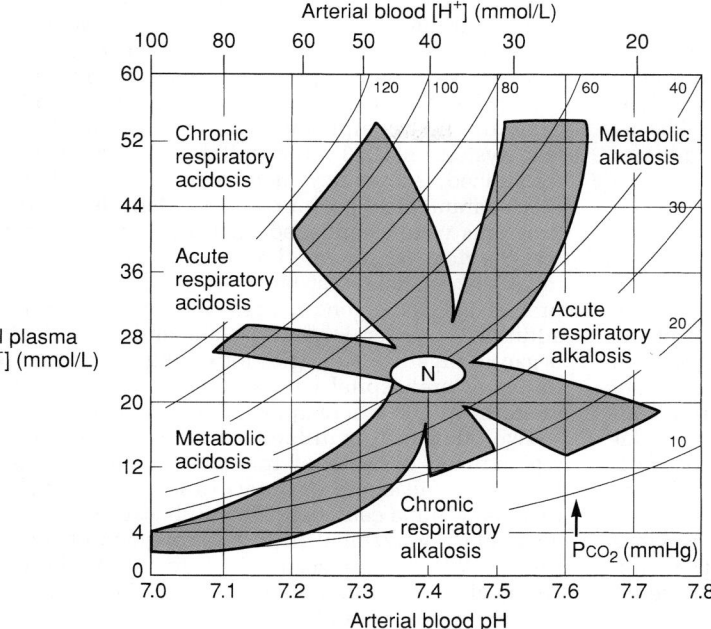

Figure 10.8. Acid–base nomogram. Shown are the 95% confidence limits of the normal respiratory and metabolic compensations for primary acid–base disturbances. (From Cogan MG, Rector FC Jr. Acid–base disturbances. In: Brenner BM, Rector FC Jr, eds. *The kidney*. Philadelphia: WB Saunders, 1986:473.)

bination of respiratory acidosis and respiratory alkalosis is impossible, but any other combination is possible. Familiarity with the acid–base disorders associated with various clinical situations and the expectation of mixed abnormalities allows appropriate interpretation of arterial blood gases and serum electrolyte determinations. A summary of the calculations for estimating the compensatory responses and timing of these responses is presented in Table 10.9 (13).

REFERENCES

1. Edelman IS, Leibman J. Anatomy of body water and electrolytes. *Am J Med* 1959;27:256.
2. Robertson GL. Physiopathology of ADH secretion. In: Tolis G, Labrie F, Martin JB, et al., eds. *Clinical neuroendocrinology: a pathophysiological approach.* New York: Raven Press, 1979:247.
3. Briggs JP, Sawaya BE, Schnerman J. Disorders of salt balance. In: Kokko JP, Tannen RL, eds. *Fluid and electrolytes.* Philadelphia: WB Saunders, 1990:70.
4. Gauer OH, Henry JP. Neurohumoral control of plasma volume. *Int Rev Physiol* 1976;9:145.
5. Salazar FJ, Granger JP, Joyce MLM, et al. Effects of hypertonic saline infusion and water drinking on atrial peptides. *Am J Physiol* 1986;251:R1091.
6. Goetz KL. Renal natriuretic peptide (urodilatin?) and atriopeptin: evolving concepts. *Am J Physiol* 1991;261:F921.
7. Wait RB, Kahng KU. Renal failure complicating obstructive jaundice. *Am J Surg* 1989;157:256.
8. Reuzzi G, Benigni A. Endothelins in the control of cardiovascular and renal function. *Nature* 1993;342:589.
9. Rodeberg DA, Chaet MS, Bass RC, et al. Nitric oxide: an overview. *Am J Surg* 1995;170:292.
10. Bachman S, Mundel P. Nitric oxide and the kidney: synthesis, localization, and function. *Am J Kidney Dis* 1994;24:112.
11. Lemann JJR, Lennon EJ. Role of diet, gastrointestinal tract, and bone in acid–base homeostasis. *Kidney Int* 1972;1:275.
12. Foster DW, McGarry JD. The metabolic derangements and treatment of diabetic ketoacidosis. *N Engl J Med* 1983; 309:159.
13. Carroll HJ, Oh MS. *Water, electrolyte and acid–base metabolism.* Philadelphia: JB Lippincott, 1989:206.

SURGERY: SCIENTIFIC PRINCIPLES AND PRACTICE, Third Edition, edited by Lazar J. Greenfield, Michael W. Mulholland, Keith T. Oldham, Gerald B. Zelenock, and Keith D. Lillemoe. Lippincott Williams & Wilkins Publishers, Philadelphia, © 2001.

CHAPTER 11

TRAUMA

DAVID B. HOYT, RAUL COIMBRA, HENRY MAGILL CRYER III, JAMES W. DAVIS, RANDALL M. CHESNUT, LISA A. ORLOFF, GREGORY J. JURKOVICH, ROBERT J. WINCHELL, DAVID H. WISNER, ROBERT C. MACKERSIE, SANDRA L. ENGELHARDT, MICHAEL J. SISE, STEVEN R. SHACKFORD, M. MARGARET KNUDSON, RICHARD K. SIMONS, AND GRACE S. ROZYCKI

Introduction

DAVID B. HOYT AND RAUL COIMBRA

The beginnings of surgery can be linked closely with trauma care and casualty management during war. Today, trauma is a principal public health problem in every country, regardless of the level of socioeconomic development. In the United States, trauma is the leading cause of death among people between 1 and 44 years of age. The number of annual deaths in the United States due to trauma is over 150,000, more than three times the number of combat casualties that occurred during the entire Vietnam conflict. In 1995, 59 million people were accidentally injured in the United States; this represents an annual injury incidence of approximately one in four people and accounts for one third of all hospital admissions. During the same period, the number of trauma-related deaths was 147,691, which represents a rate of 55.93 deaths per 100,000 people (1). Individual loss, pain, suffering, incapacitation, and disability are difficult to quantify. Although injuries occur to people of all ages and both sexes, young men are most often affected. Because many severe injuries result in long-term disability, consideration of the lifetime cost of injury should take into account acute and chronic care as well as the cost of lost economic productivity. Recent calculations have estimated the total cost of injury in the United States to be approximately $260 billion per year (1).

HISTORICAL DEVELOPMENT OF TRAUMA CARE

The approach to modern trauma has grown out of the care of wounds and casualty management resulting from war. Advances in rapid transport, volume resuscitation, wound management (both débridement and infection control), blood banking, enteric injury management, vascular surgery, surgical critical care, and the need for early nutritional management have all grown out of military experience. Salient historical events are shown in Table 11.1. Although by no means complete, this table provides examples of the many and significant contributions derived from the large military experience with multiple injuries.

Civilian progress has in general followed the evolution of military systems with regard to trauma care. In 1922, the importance of orthopedic trauma was first recognized in the United States with the establishment of the Committee on the Treatment of Fractures. This evolved into the Committee on Trauma of the American College of Surgeons in 1949. Increased awareness of traffic injuries and fatalities during the 1950s and 1960s began to raise surgical awareness and public concerns. A specific trauma unit was opened in 1961 at the University of Maryland, and the concept of the "golden hour" was established. In 1966, the National Academy of Sciences and the National Research Council published an important white paper entitled *Accidental Death and Disability: The Neglected Disease of Modern Society*. This publication increased public awareness and led to a federal agenda for the general improvement of trauma care. Coupled with leadership from key academic centers and often by surgeons with recent military experience, the spread of advanced trauma systems began. The Maryland Institute of Emergency Medicine became the first completely organized, statewide, regionalized system in 1973. Prehospital provider programs were formalized, emergency medical technicians (EMTs) and other paramedical personnel were identified, and training programs were established. In 1973, the Emergency Medical Service Act became law, providing specific endorsement and financial assistance for the development of comprehensive emergency medical service systems. In addition to federal efforts, state and local legislatures began to organize strategies for caring for injured patients by using prehospital care systems to deliver patients to major hospitals where appropriate care could be given.

Two other factors influenced the rapid development of regionalized systems of trauma care in the late 1970s. First, major teaching hospitals in large cities had become regional trauma centers by default because of their experience and involvement in the trauma care of indigent patients. With strong academic leadership, these centers were able to develop regionalization of systems of trauma care by setting examples.

Of at least equal importance, the American College of Surgeons Committee on Trauma developed a task force to publish *Optimal Hospital Resources for the Care of the Seriously Injured* in 1976, thus establishing a standard for evaluation of care. The current version was published in 1999, and is the most comprehensive of these reports (2). It establishes criteria for prehospital and trauma care personnel and establishes the importance of ongoing quality assessment. In addition, the American College of Surgeons Committee on Trauma developed the Advanced Trauma Life Support course in 1980, which has contributed to uniformity of initial care and the development of a common language for all care providers (3).

In summary, the current awareness of trauma is the result of many historical factors, both military and civilian

Table 11.1. **SIGNIFICANT HISTORICAL DEVELOPMENTS RELATES TO TRAUMA CARE**

Period or person	Contribution
Greek medicine	Wound care and fracture management
Roman Empire	Realization that laudable pus was undesirable
	Healing by second intention
16th-century, Paré	Use of dressing and ligature in wound management
French and Indian War, John Hunter	Differentiation between primary and secondary wound healing
Early 1800s, Dominique Jean Larrey	Developed the principle of the ambulance and the concept of triage
Crimean War, 1853–1856	Demonstrated value of nursing care (Florence Nightingale)
Samuel Gross, 1862	Described shock as the root unhinging of the machinery of life
Civil War	Rediscovery of importance of field ambulance, nonsuppurative wound care
	Initial use of antiseptics
	Further development of nursing care by Clara Barton, American Red Cross founder
World War I	Principle of débridement and delayed closure for wounds more than 8 hours old
	Established primary closure for wounds less than 8 hours old only
	Field ambulance mechanized with automobile availability
	Recognition that shock was due to blood or fluid loss and use of seawater to replace blood volume
	Introduction of Dakin solution
World War II	Débridement and delayed closure practiced
	Diverting colostomies standard care
	Blood transfusion, rapid evacuation, specialized surgical units close to the front
Korean conflict	Development of Mobile Army Surgical Headquarters (MASH) units, use of helicopters, development of vascular surgery, field research leading to better understanding of posttraumatic renal failure
Vietnam conflict	Development of an airbase regional emergency medical system with transport from injury to intervention in 1 hour
	Better fluid resuscitation
	Understanding of adult respiratory distress syndrome

in origin. The prevalence and economic impact of trauma and the commitment required to provide optimal care make it a significant challenge for the surgeon.

MORTALITY PEAKS AFTER TRAUMA INJURY

Trauma deaths occur at three traditionally recognized times after injury (Fig. 11.1). Approximately half of all trauma-related deaths occur within seconds or minutes of injury and are related to lacerations of the aorta, heart, brain stem, brain, and spinal cord. Few of these patients are saved by health care systems, regardless of efficacy. In general, these injuries are best addressed using prevention strategies, either devices that prevent injury or laws that limit certain behavior patterns (4).

The second mortality peak occurs within hours of injury and accounts for approximately 30% of deaths, half of which are due to hemorrhage and half to central nervous system (CNS) injuries. Important reductions in mortality rates during this period have resulted from the development of trauma and rapid transport systems. Overall trauma mortality rates have been reduced from approximately 30% to 2% to 9% where well organized trauma care systems exist (5,6). Only approximately 25% of the United States is served by such systems. Further development of trauma systems, organized care protocols, and expansion of these systems to rural areas will undoubtedly result in further reductions in mortality rates during this period.

The third mortality peak includes deaths that occur from 1 day after trauma to weeks later. This late mortality usually is attributed to infection and multiple organ failure (7). Ten percent to 20% of trauma deaths occur during this period. The development of efficient trauma systems, however, has changed the epidemiology of these deaths. During the first week after trauma, refractory intracranial hypertension after severe head injury now accounts for a significant number of these deaths. The incidence of sepsis and multiple organ failure has diminished as a result of aggressive and better early resuscitation and care. Sepsis and multiple organ failure now account for approximately 5% of overall mortality and only 30% of late mortality where organized trauma systems exist. Finally, fatal pulmonary embolism accounts for a significant number of these late deaths (8).

Efforts to reduce the morbidity and mortality of trauma must include specific programs for each of the three different mortality peaks. Early deaths can best be reduced with accident prevention programs or legislated protective devices. Focus on the regional planning of trauma system development will affect the number of avoidable deaths during the second mortality peak. Finally, late deaths will be diminished as research generates better understanding of the processes related to sepsis, multiple organ failure, and CNS injury (9).

General Considerations
DAVID B. HOYT AND RAUL COIMBRA

EPIDEMIOLOGY

In the United States, approximately 2.6 million people are hospitalized annually as a result of accidental injury, and approximately 35 to 40 million emergency department visits occur for the evaluation and treatment of injuries (1). Over 40% of these patients are between 25 and 44 years of age, and 20% are between 15 and 24 years. People younger than 45 years of age sustain almost 80% of all injuries and account for 75% of the total lifetime costs. Young men are the highest risk group, not because of physiologic distinctions but because of the propensity to engage in high-risk activities.

According to data provided by the National Center for Injury and Prevention Control, during 1997, considering all injury-related deaths (total of 149,691), 56.6% occurred in the age group of 15 to 49 years, predominantly in the male population. Overall, the risk of dying after injury for the male population is seven times higher than that for the female population (10).

Although morbidity and mortality figures are important, another important variable related to injury cost for the society is measured in years of productive life lost (YPLL), which reflects the potential productivity that is lost as a result of premature death. Traumatic deaths result in a higher number of YPLL compared with deaths associated with cancer and cardiovascular diseases. This is because injuries are more prevalent in the younger population. In 1996, the age-adjusted YPLL before age 75 years (per 100,000 population) was 1,919, 1,554, and 1,223 for in-

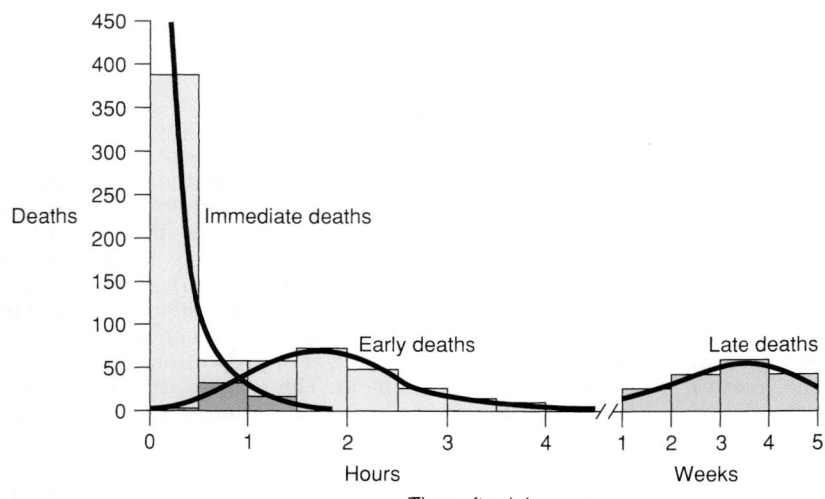

Figure 11.1. Three periods of peak mortality after injury.

jury, cancer, and heart diseases, respectively (1). For each traumatic death there are, on average, 36 YPLL, compared with 16 for cancer and 12 for cardiovascular diseases (11).

The leading causes of injury include motor vehicle accidents, falls, firearms, injuries due to cutting or piercing instruments, and burns. Fatalities after injury are mainly due to motor vehicle accidents (32%), gunshot wounds (22%), and falls (9%) (12).

There are several important differences among the various ethnic groups in the United States in terms of the epidemiology of injury. The three leading causes of traumatic death for people younger than 35 years of age are the same in all groups: motor vehicle accidents, homicide, and suicide. In the African-American population, the leading cause of death in this age group is homicide. The mortality rate from motor vehicle accidents is approximately 42 per 100,000 among Native Americans, 20 per 100,000 among the white population, and 11 per 100,000 in the Asian population (11). Suicide rates are higher for Native Americans than for any other group (1).

The impact of injury in children is also significant. The leading causes of injury in this group are motor vehicle accidents, burns, drowning, falls, and poisoning. Injury in this age group leads to a significant number of deaths, disabilities, days of missed school, medical costs, and missed work days for parents.

Adolescents are also at increased risk for injury. In fact, more adolescents die from injuries than from all other diseases combined (13). Forty percent of all deaths in this age group are caused by intentional injuries, such as homicide and suicide (14). Considering adolescents 15 to 19 years of age, one fourth of the deaths are caused by firearms (15).

Unfortunately, alcohol ingestion is a major cause of fatal vehicular accidents. Although significant progress has been made in the prevention of drinking and driving, 39% of all traffic fatalities in 1997 were alcohol related (National Highway Traffic Safety Administration) (16). More important, it has been determined that that 60% of the time that a child passenger dies in a car crash, it is the driver of the child's car who was intoxicated (17). Other drugs, such as marijuana and cocaine, have been implicated in 18% of motor vehicle accident-related fatalities (18).

Those who plan injury research and prevention must take into account the characteristics of the specific target population, as well as other important epidemiologic factors such as alcohol and drug use.

BIOMECHANICS OF INJURY

All traumatic injury occurs as a result of deformation of tissues beyond a threshold that results in structural damage. Understanding the biomechanics of specific injuries is important in guiding initial evaluation. In general, injury is categorized as either penetrating or nonpenetrating (blunt) trauma. After blunt trauma, the injury is produced as the tissues are compressed or as deceleration occurs. In penetrating trauma, the injury is produced by crushing and separation of tissues along the path of the penetrating object.

Energy Transfer

The severity of any injury is directly proportional to the amount of kinetic energy transferred to the tissues, whether by a projectile or by blunt impact. Kinetic energy (KE) is a function of the mass (M) of an object and its velocity (V):

$$KE = \frac{M \times V^2}{2} \qquad (1)$$

It is clear from this equation that changes in velocity alter the kinetic energy transfer more significantly than changes in mass. This fact becomes critical in the assessment of high- and low-velocity gunshot wounds. Likewise, a small child and a large adult, although significantly different in size and weight, are subjected to similar levels of energy transfer in a high-speed vehicular collision, the primary determinant being velocity rather than mass.

Cavitation

Cavitation occurs as tissue struck by a moving body recoils from the point of impact, away from the object. After blunt trauma, this may result in a cavity from temporary deformation of the tissues by a lap belt or steering wheel. The resulting transient tissue cavity may be caused by rapid acceleration or deceleration. Extreme strain occurs at points of anatomic fixation during the formation of these temporary cavities. Forces can be produced both along the longitudinal axis (tensile or compression strain) and across the transverse axis (shear strain). These types of forces cause deformity, tearing, and tissue failure or fracture.

With penetrating trauma, transient cavitation is caused by the transfer of kinetic energy from the projectile. A permanent cavity is produced by tissue displacement.

The tolerance of biologic tissue to traumatic injury is directly proportional to the elasticity of the organ—that is, its ability to return to its original shape and position. This characteristic is directly affected by the rate of loading or the rate at which strain is applied to the tissues. More rapid application of force increases the likelihood of exceeding the tolerance of the tissue. Tissue injury occurs when a lower strain or shear force is applied at a higher rate of loading.

BIOMECHANICS OF BLUNT TRAUMA

Blunt trauma results in two types of forces during impact. First, changes in speed (acceleration or deceleration) create shear strain, and second, deformity changes (stretch or compression) create tensile strain. Analyses of injuries associated with changes in speed have facilitated the understanding of specific injuries to the head, thorax, and abdomen. For example, shear stress to the head secondary to deceleration leads to brain stem stretching, and injury to the spinal cord occurs from shear stress at points of attachment. Contrecoup brain injuries include stretch forces placed on bridging veins, which may lead to hemorrhage and a subdural hematoma. Understanding the biomechanics of blunt injuries allows us to predict patterns for specific types of trauma.

Shear Strain Injuries

Differential acceleration in the thorax makes the aorta the most common site of shear injuries, the most frequent point of injury being the ligamentum arteriosum. Here, the descending aorta is tightly fixed to the thoracic spine, whereas more proximally it is relatively mobile. Shear stress in this area allows the proximal aorta to move in relation to the fixed distal aorta and, therefore, to tear. Abdominal injuries can result as a consequence of acceleration of the viscera at a rate out of proportion to movement of the points of attachment. The kidneys, small intestine, large intestine, and spleen are all vulnerable to this type of shear injury. Similarly, with deceleration, the liver may continue to travel relative to the ligamentum teres, generating shear forces that transect or lacerate the hepatic parenchyma.

Rapid deceleration can place sudden flexion and extension forces on the cervical spine, which can cause cervical fractures, subluxation, or ligamentous injury.

Tensile Strain Injuries

Tensile strain creates injury by directly compressing the tissue. For the head, tensile strain results in fractures of the skull, which in turn may cause intracranial bleeding or contusions of the underlying brain parenchyma. In the thorax, external chest compression can lead to cardiac contusion, pulmonary contusion, pneumothorax, and fractured ribs or a flail chest. In the abdomen, the pancreas, liver, spleen, and occasionally the kidneys are subject to tensile strain injuries, particularly after a frontal impact. In addition, direct compression of the abdomen may increase intraabdominal pressure, rupturing the diaphragm. Similarly, external compression of the pelvis is associated with bladder rupture and other pelvic injuries.

Understanding how these shear and tensile (compression) injuries occur allows us to predict certain injury patterns for specific types of trauma.

Motor Vehicle Collisions

Patterns of injury are recognized for several specific types of motor vehicle collisions. These include (a) head-on or frontal impact, (b) rear impact, (c) lateral or side impact, (d) rotational impact, and (e) rollover. Some estimate of injury pattern is possible by analysis of damage to the vehicle, but the presumption is usually that any or all of these forces may have been involved. In general, a vehicle's occupant receives a kinetic energy transfer similar to that of the vehicle itself. In this regard, description of vehicular damage may be useful for general categorization of patients. As an automobile collides with an object, passengers collide with the interior of the automobile, and the internal organs collide with the body wall or are sheared from anatomic attachment.

It has been shown that better automotive design has greatly improved the outcome for occupants if the safety features of the vehicle are in use at the time of the accident. Active safety restraint systems include shoulder and lap seat belts, air bags (frontal and lateral), and door locks; passive restraint systems include front and rear energy-absorbing collapsible chassis, lateral bars, and improved lateral wall design.

Frontal and Rear Impact

With a frontal impact, the vehicle stops abruptly, and unrestrained front-seat occupants move in one of two predictable pathways—down and under the dashboard or up and over the steering wheel.

With the former movement, the knees strike the dashboard, and the upper legs absorb the primary energy transfer. Dislocated knees, fractured femurs, and posterior fracture–dislocations of the hips are expected. After the knees strike, the upper body flexes forward, moving up and over the steering wheel. The chest or abdomen strikes the steering wheel and the head strikes the windshield. The head stops the forward momentum of the torso and kinetic energy is absorbed by the cervical spine (Fig. 11.2).

Predictable injury patterns resulting from the up-and-over component of a frontal impact include the following:

- Rib fractures, pulmonary contusion, flail chest, and myocardial contusion may occur after the anterior chest wall is compressed by the steering wheel.
- Hollow abdominal viscera and solid organs are compressed, resulting in intestinal perforation and lacerations of the mesentery and solid organs with accompanying hemorrhage.
- After the anterior chest stops, intrathoracic organs continue to move, and shear injuries such as lacerations of the aorta or liver result.
- Shear injuries also may occur to the kidneys and other solid viscera.
- Injury to the brain can occur from direct compression with scalp lacerations, skull fractures, and cerebral contusions, or from deceleration and shear stress, which cause diffuse axonal injury and cerebral contusion or subdural hematoma.
- Acute neck flexion, hyperextension, or both can occur, causing cervical spine injury.

Rear impact collisions occur when stationary objects or slow-moving vehicles are struck from behind. The amount of kinetic energy generated depends on the difference between the velocities of the two vehicles, rather than the sum, as with forward collisions. After a rear impact, the vehicle and its occupants accelerate forward, during which time cervical spine hyperextension with injury may occur. If the vehicle slows to a stop spontaneously, often the occupants are not severely injured. If the car strikes another object, the occupants are thrown forward, with injury potential similar to that seen with a frontal impact. Thus, rear impact collision can potentially cause two types of injury: those caused by the primary rear impact and those resulting from the secondary frontal impact.

Lateral and Rotational Impact and Rollover

Two patterns of injury result from lateral impact, depending on whether energy is transferred to the vehicle directly or imparts motion to the vehicle. If the target vehicle remains in place or there is significant passenger compartment intrusion, typical injuries include lateral crushing compression injuries to the torso, pelvis, and spine. Energy delivered to the chest with lateral compression can cause a flail chest, pulmonary contusion, and ruptured liver or spleen. Depending on the location of the occupant's arm, humeral and clavicular fractures may occur. The pelvis and femur are often struck by the door, forcing the femoral head medially, causing an acetabular fracture. Head injuries range from simple lacerations to cerebral contusions with intracranial hemorrhage.

If the vehicle does not move away from the point of lateral impact, an occupant who is restrained remains fixed in place and is more vulnerable to the intruding vehicle. More commonly, the vehicle is moved by the force of the impact, and passenger restraints markedly reduce injury. In this case, the occupant begins lateral motion with the car and is pulled away from the impact point by the restraint. As the torso is pushed laterally, the head stays in its original position, producing lateral flexion and rotation to the cervical spine, which leads to fractures. Passengers sustaining lateral impact also should be considered for injuries resulting from secondary collisions with other passengers.

Rotational impact injuries occur when the car strikes a moving vehicle laterally. The moving vehicle rotates around the point of impact, resulting in combinations of the injuries seen in head-on and lateral impacts.

During rollover accidents, the automobile may sustain impacts many times from many different angles, and as a result, the occupant may have virtually any injury. All potential injury mechanisms should be considered. Rollover accidents with passenger ejection are associated with a profound increase in fatality rates, in part because the second impact can cause injuries that compound or exceed those resulting from the initial impact. Rollover accidents

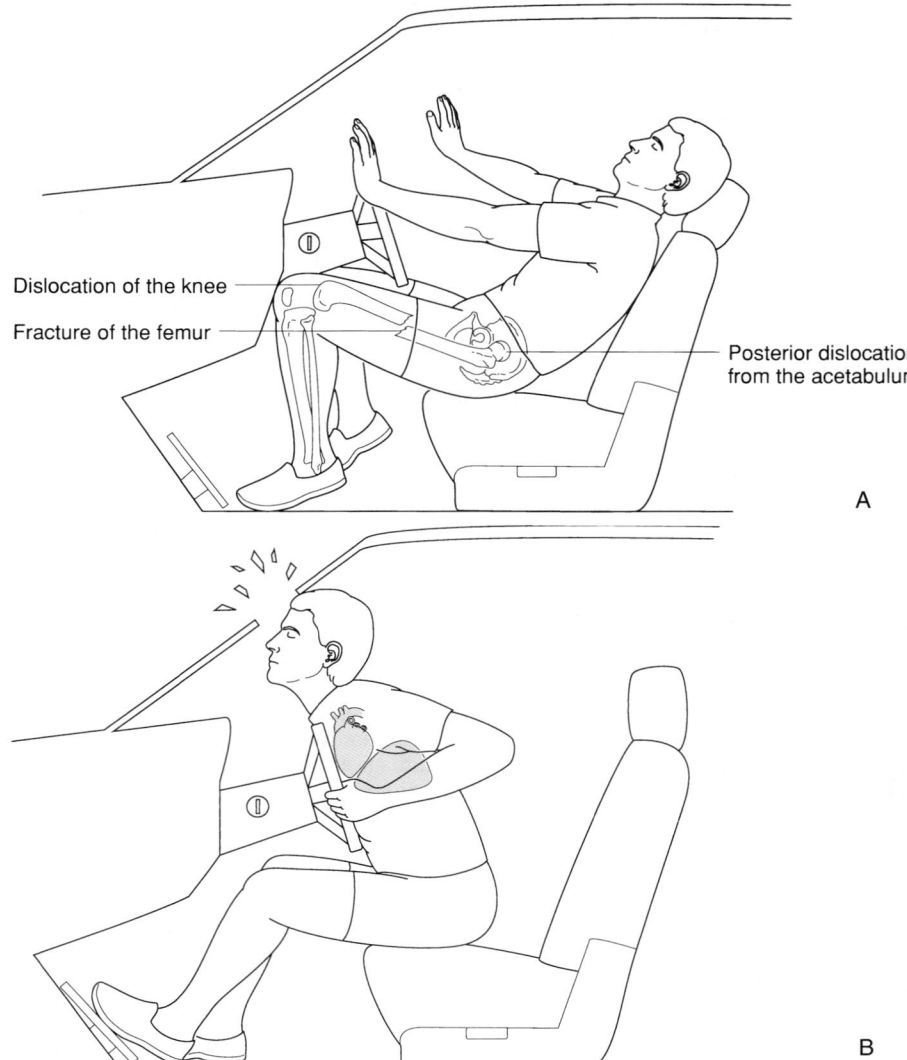

Dislocation of the knee

Fracture of the femur

Posterior dislocation from the acetabulum

A

B

Figure 11.2. Down-and-under *(A)* and up-and lower *(B)* mechanisms of injury after frontal deceleration impact.

with passenger ejection are considered to have the greatest injury potential.

Restraint Device Injury

Theoretically, three-point passenger restraints, when used properly, allow the kinetic energy transferred by the impact to be absorbed by the bony pelvis and chest. If improperly positioned, however, lap belts may rise above the pelvis, delivering the compression force to the soft tissues of the abdominal cavity or retroperitoneum. The number of injuries related to restraint devices is increasing, probably reflecting the broader general use of these systems. Although there is no question of the overall efficacy of these devices, specific related injuries must be recognized by the clinician.

Common injuries when lap belts are incorrectly strapped above the anterior iliac crest include compression injuries of the intraabdominal organs (liver, pancreas, spleen, small bowel, large bowel), increased intraabdominal pressure and diaphragmatic rupture, and anterior compression of the lumbar spine. Diagonal shoulder straps should be worn in combination with lap belts to prevent forward motion of the trunk. Diagonal shoulder straps should not be worn alone because this can be associated with chest and neck injuries if the pelvis is not secured by the lap belt. Injuries associated with shoulder straps in-

clude carotid artery contusion with or without thrombosis and clavicle and rib fractures.

Air bags have enormous potential for injury prevention because they prevent the initial collision of passenger and automobile interior that occurs with frontal impacts. To be effective, air bags must be used in combination with seat belts because they deflate immediately and therefore do not prevent secondary collisions. Lateral air bags have been recently incorporated in some, but not all vehicles. Injuries such as lateral collisions of the head with the middle column and lateral compression of the chest wall may be, at least in part, prevented by these new devices. Airbags are not effective in rear impact collisions. Given the predominance of frontal impact accidents, however, public health considerations in favor of air bags should be strongly emphasized.

Motorcycles

Motorcycle injuries involve four types of impacts: frontal, angular, ejection, and rear end collision. In a frontal impact, the center of gravity is above and behind the front axle as the motorcycle tips forward and the rider travels over the handlebars. Injuries to the head, chest, or abdomen may occur, depending on which part of the anatomy strikes the handlebars. If the rider's feet are placed on the pegs, the upper leg strikes the handlebars in forward motion, causing bilateral midshaft femur fractures. Angular or lateral impact usually results in crush injuries of the lower extremities. With ejection, the rider is thrown into the air until the head, chest, or extremities strike another object. Injury occurs at the point of impact and, just as with the ejected occupant from an automobile, the potential for severe injury is high. This mechanism of injury is frequent and contributes importantly to the extraordinary injury potential for motorcycle passengers. In rear end collisions, the motorcycle is usually at a stop when it is hit by a second vehicle from behind. The injury pattern is that of rapid acceleration with hyperextension and crush.

Pedestrians

Two general patterns are seen in motor vehicle pedestrian accidents, depending on whether the patient is an adult or a child. In adults, the initial impact is often by the car bumper, producing fractures to the tibia and fibula. As the victim falls over the moving vehicle, the pelvis and upper femur are struck by the front of the vehicle's hood, and the abdomen and thorax continue onto the top of the hood. The secondary strike can result in fractures of the femur or pelvis and produce serious intraabdominal or intrathoracic injury. Injury to the head depends on whether the patient's head strikes the car hood or is protected with the arms. A third impact occurs as the victim falls away, striking the ground. This impact commonly leads to head injury as well.

In children, the initial impact is predictably higher and may produce injury to the pelvis or upper femur. The second impact occurs when the front of the hood strikes the thorax. The final impact may not occur on top of the hood but rather as the child is dragged underneath the vehicle. As the child falls backward, multiple impacts with the ground, underside of the vehicle, and wheels are possible, so virtually any injury may occur. Because of the potential for forceful impact and the direct blow to the middle torso, any child struck by a vehicle must be considered to have potentially severe injuries.

Falls

Falls result in multiple impacts. Energy transfer is a result of the velocity that develops during the fall, so the height of the fall usually determines the magnitude of injury. Falls from more than three times the height of the victim, or from more than 20 feet are considered severe. The surface on which the victim lands and its degree of compressibility (e.g., water vs. concrete) also have an effect on the energy transfer and the types of shear and tensile strain that occur. A typical injury pattern after falls in which the victim lands on the feet includes bilateral calcaneal fractures and multiple compression fractures of the thoracic and lumbar spine (Fig. 11.3).

If the victim falls forward with the arms extended, frequent associated fractures include bilateral Colles wrist fractures. Hip dislocation and pelvic fractures are common if these structures sustain impact, and significant head and torso injuries are always possible, depending on the orientation of the victim at the time of impact.

GENERAL ANATOMIC CONSIDERATIONS IN BLUNT INJURY

The first and second ribs, sternum, scapula, and femur are considered to be some of the strongest and least vulnerable bones in the body. Therefore, fractures of these bones are indicators of severe trauma. Clear association exists between first and second rib fractures and injuries to the head, chest, and abdomen. Similarly, fractures to the sternum, although unusual, have a relatively high frequency of associated myocardial contusion. Fractures to the scapula indicate significant thoracic trauma. The presence of a femur fracture in a frontal impact injury should raise the concerns of acetabular fractures or dislocation of the knee. An inventory of specific orthopedic injuries and their common associated findings is provided in Table 11.2. These associations should be routinely considered during initial evaluation after major blunt trauma.

The anatomic orientation of certain structures also leads to predictable injury patterns. For example, the right ventricle is the most anterior portion of the heart and therefore is the most commonly contused area. The association of splenic injury with rib fractures on the left side and liver injuries with rib fractures on the right side is also frequently seen after blunt trauma.

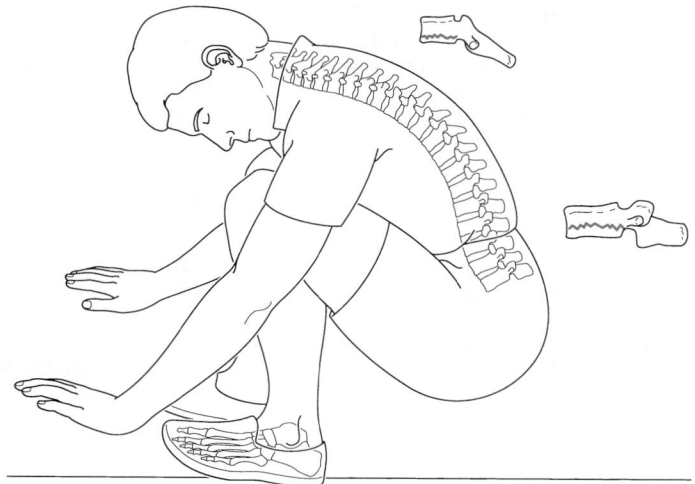

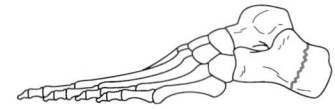

Figure 11.3. Hyperflexion injury after a fall.

TABLE 11.2. PATTERNS OF INJURY TO THE HEAD, NECK, TRUNK, AND EXTREMITIES ASSOCIATED WITH ORTHOPEDIC INJURIES

Diagnosed injury	Associated injury
Fracture—temporal, parietal bone	Epidural hematoma
Maxillofacial fracture	Cervical spine fracture
Sternal fracture	Cardiac contusion
First and second rib fracture	Descending thoracic aorta, intraabdominal bleeding
Fractured scapula	Pulmonary contusion
Fractured ribs 8–12, right	Lacerated liver
Fractured ribs 8–12, left	Lacerated spleen
Fractured pelvis	Ruptured bladder, urethral transection
Fractured humerus	Radial nerve injury
Supracondylar humerus fracture	Brachial artery injury
Distal radius fracture	Median nerve compression
Supracondylar femur fracture	Popliteal artery thrombosis
Anterior dislocation shoulder	Axillary nerve injury
Posterior dislocation of hip	Sciatic nerve injury
Posterior dislocation of knee	Popliteal artery thrombosis

BIOMECHANICS OF PENETRATING INJURIES

Penetrating trauma involves the transfer of energy to a relatively small tissue area. The velocity of a gunshot wound is exceedingly high compared with any type of blunt trauma. The kinetic energy of a bullet disrupts and fragments cells and tissues, moving them away from the path of the bullet. The actual size of the frontal area of impact is determined by three factors: profile, tumble (spin and yaw), and fragmentation.

The profile, or frontal area, of a knife, screwdriver, or smooth bullet is that of a pointed missile. If the missile is crushed or deformed as a result of impact, the frontal area changes shape and disperses the impact over a wider tissue area, producing greater energy exchange and therefore greater injury. A knife or jacketed bullet does not deform significantly during impact, whereas a hollow-point bullet flattens, spreads, and fragments on impact, enlarging the area of injury.

Tumble results when the center of gravity of a bullet is eccentric, usually because it is located near the base rather than the apex of the bullet. Spin and axial movement (yaw) are bullet movements that occur after a gun is fired. At impact, spin and yaw continue to carry the base of the bullet forward, resulting in end-over-end motion, or tumble. This increases the area of energy exchange and results

in greater tissue damage. Gunshot wounds are an example of the effect of fragmentation injury. The frontal impact damage can be estimated by classifying penetrating injuries into low-, medium-, and high-energy capacities.

Low-energy Stab Wounds

Low-energy missiles include knives and other objects that produce damage only by their sharp cutting edges. Cavitation is minimal, and injury can be predicted simply by tracing the pathway of the weapon in the body. Knowledge of the type of weapon and the sex of the attacker is sometimes helpful. Men tend to stab with the blade on the thumb side of the hand in an upward thrust. Conversely, women tend to stab downward holding the blade to the outside of the hand. The attacker may stab and move the knife or weapon inside the body, which can lead to more injury than that perceived from the cutaneous wound. Judgment of the potential scope of injury by examination of the entrance wound is not reliable.

Low- and Medium-velocity Gunshot Wounds

Low-velocity gunshot wounds are defined as those with an initial muzzle velocity of less than 1,200 ft/s. Medium-velocity projectiles have muzzle velocities between 1,200 and 2,000 ft/s. Most handguns and some rifles are low- or medium-energy weapons. Table 11.3 provides a comparison of bullets and initial muzzle velocity for firearms frequently associated with penetrating civilian trauma. The primary point of classification is that these weapons not only damage the tissue directly in the path of the missile but produce cavitation injury to tissues close to the impact. The size of the cavitation injury is directly proportional to the velocity of the bullet. With low- and medium-velocity gunshot wounds, the cavity is usually three to six times the area of the bullet frontal surface. The amount of tumble, fragmentation, and profile change also influence the extent of injury.

High-energy Weapons

High-velocity projectiles are those with a muzzle velocity of more than 2,000 ft/s. The essential difference in these weapons is that their projectiles produce a much larger cavity or pressure cone than low- and medium-velocity missiles. The temporary cavity extends well beyond the actual bullet tract, producing a wider injury. The vacuum created by the cavitation pulls clothing, bacteria, and other debris from the surrounding areas into the wound, creating the additional risk of contamination. The proliferation of semiautomatic weapons also has resulted in an

Table 11.3. MUZZLE VELOCITY, KINETIC WEIGHT OF PROJECTILE, AND APPROXIMATE MAXIMUM KINETIC ENERGY OF FREQUENTLY USED FIREARMS

Description (caliber)	Projectile weight (g)	Muzzle velocity (ft/s)	Kinetic energy (ft/lb)
Pistols			
.22 Short	29	1,000	72
.38 Special	158	870	263
9-mm Luger	125	1,150	440
.45	250	860	410
.357 Magnum	158	1,430	695
.44 Magnum	240	1,470	1,150
Rifles			
.22 Long	40	1,150	150
.56-mm M-16	55	3,200	1,248
.30-30 Winchester	170	2,200	1,830

increased number of wounds a victim may experience. Instead of a single gunshot wound, the surgeon may be faced with multiple wounds in multiple body locations.

Blast Injuries

Blast injuries caused by close-range shotgun fire constitute devastating injuries comprising extensive tissue destruction. Besides specific organ injury, blast injuries have the highest potential for secondary infection. These injuries, in general, should be surgically explored, devitalized tissue should be extensively débrided, and the wounds should be left open and packed with sterile dressing that should be changed and reviewed in the operating room (19).

GENERAL ANATOMIC CONSIDERATIONS OF PENETRATING INJURIES

Evaluation of entrance and exit wounds is essential to assess the number of projectiles, their courses, and which organs are at risk of injury. Entrance wounds for bullets typically cause tattooing, burning, and abrasion as a result of the spin. Depending on the range, there may be direct burning of skin. Weapons fired within 2 to 3 inches of the skin cause burns. Tattooing occurs if the muzzle is within 12 inches of the skin at the time of firing. The range from which a gun is fired is also significant in that the air resistance that slows bullet velocity and reduces kinetic energy is directly proportional to the distance traveled.

Once a missile penetrates tissue, the energy is distributed predictably within a closed space and, depending on the organs struck and the types of tissue traversed, certain injuries can be anticipated. For example, a bullet penetrating the skull may have insufficient residual energy to traverse and exit the opposite side of the skull. It may instead follow the curvature of the interior of the skull, generating a more severe brain injury than would result from a simple linear passage.

In the thorax, lung parenchyma has low mass and therefore sustains less damage from penetrating injury than any other thoracic tissue. Similarly, blood vessels that are not fixed may be pushed aside without significant damage. Large, fixed vessels, however, such as the aorta and vena cava, are particularly susceptible to fatal injury. If bones are penetrated, fragments may become secondary missiles and can lacerate the surrounding tissues. Muscles may expand out of the path of a missile, but this can result in stretching and hemorrhage. Injury to adjacent blood vessels can result in intimal damage with subsequent thrombosis even if the vessel as a whole remains intact. Low-velocity bullets may not follow a straight path but rather ricochet through the body cavity, injuring other organs.

Penetrating injuries also should be evaluated with regard to topography. For example, penetrating wounds of the neck are commonly associated with injury to the jugular veins, trachea, and carotid artery. Injuries to the trachea are commonly associated with injuries to the esophagus, and injuries to the carotid artery are commonly associated with injuries to the internal jugular vein. In penetrating wounds to the thorax, the clinician must consider the possibilities of injury to the heart, lung, and diaphragm. The anterior location of the right ventricle makes it particularly vulnerable to penetrating trauma. All penetrating wounds below the nipple line or inframammary groove must be considered for potential intraabdominal injury (Fig. 11.4). Similarly, wounds that cross the midline, so-called axial traverse wounds, are important to recognize.

In the thorax, this indicates that every mediastinal structure is at risk, and in the abdomen, the possibility of major vascular injury, particularly to the aorta and vena cava, must be considered. Associated abdominal injuries often include hepatic and splenic injuries, as well as diaphragmatic, pulmonary, and gastric injuries. Duodenal and pancreatic injuries are commonly seen with injuries of the liver, inferior vena cava, stomach, and colon. Examples of injuries associated with specific vascular trauma include the following:

- Superior mesenteric artery or superior mesenteric vein injury with pancreas and liver
- Renal artery injury with liver, kidney, and colon
- Inferior vena cava injury with liver, small bowel, colon, pancreas, and duodenum
- Portal vein injury with inferior vena cava, liver, pancreas, and duodenum
- Axillary artery injury with brachial plexus trauma

SCORING SYSTEMS AND INJURY ASSESSMENT

Many systems have been developed in an effort to allow comparison of injuries and trauma patients among institutions. Some provide considerable help, although none is perfect. The impetus for injury severity scoring systems is provided by the need to identify and classify severely injured patients in the prehospital phase, to predict mortality, to assess results, and to improve communication.

One simple way to classify trauma patients is to place them into three groups according to severity of injury: (a) those patients with injuries that are rapidly fatal, (b) those with injuries that are potentially fatal, and (c) those with injuries that are not fatal. The first group includes patients who have exsanguinating injuries, massive head injuries, cervical spinal cord transection, or major airway disruption producing death in less than 10 minutes. Five percent of traumatic injuries and half of all deaths fall in this category. The third group, which accounts for 80% of trauma patients, includes patients with injuries that are minor or confined to soft tissue and isolated extremity fractures. This group seldom has major injury, and urgent treatment is not essential. These patients survive without significant disability even if prolonged delays occur before definitive therapy. The real impact of improved prehospital care and organized trauma systems is on the second category of patients (approximately 15% of the total), those who can be saved if effective medical care is provided quickly. It is for this group that scoring systems have been developed.

Revised Trauma Score and Triage

The trauma score developed by Champion and Sacco (20) in 1981 has been the most widely applied as well as the most useful scoring system for the initial evaluation of trauma victims. It mathematically combines the physiologic parameters of blood pressure, respiratory rate, and Glasgow Coma Score to assess injury severity and predict which patients need the most timely and sophisticated medical care. Table 11.4 shows the components of the Revised Trauma Score (RTS).

In addition to physiologic scores, specific anatomic aspects of injury are correlated with high injury potential. Penetrating injuries to the head, neck, torso, and extremities; the presence of multiple broken ribs and flail chest; the presence of two or more proximal long-bone fractures; pelvic fractures; limb paralysis; and amputation proximal to the wrist have been identified as anatomic indicators of severe injury. Finally, the mecha-

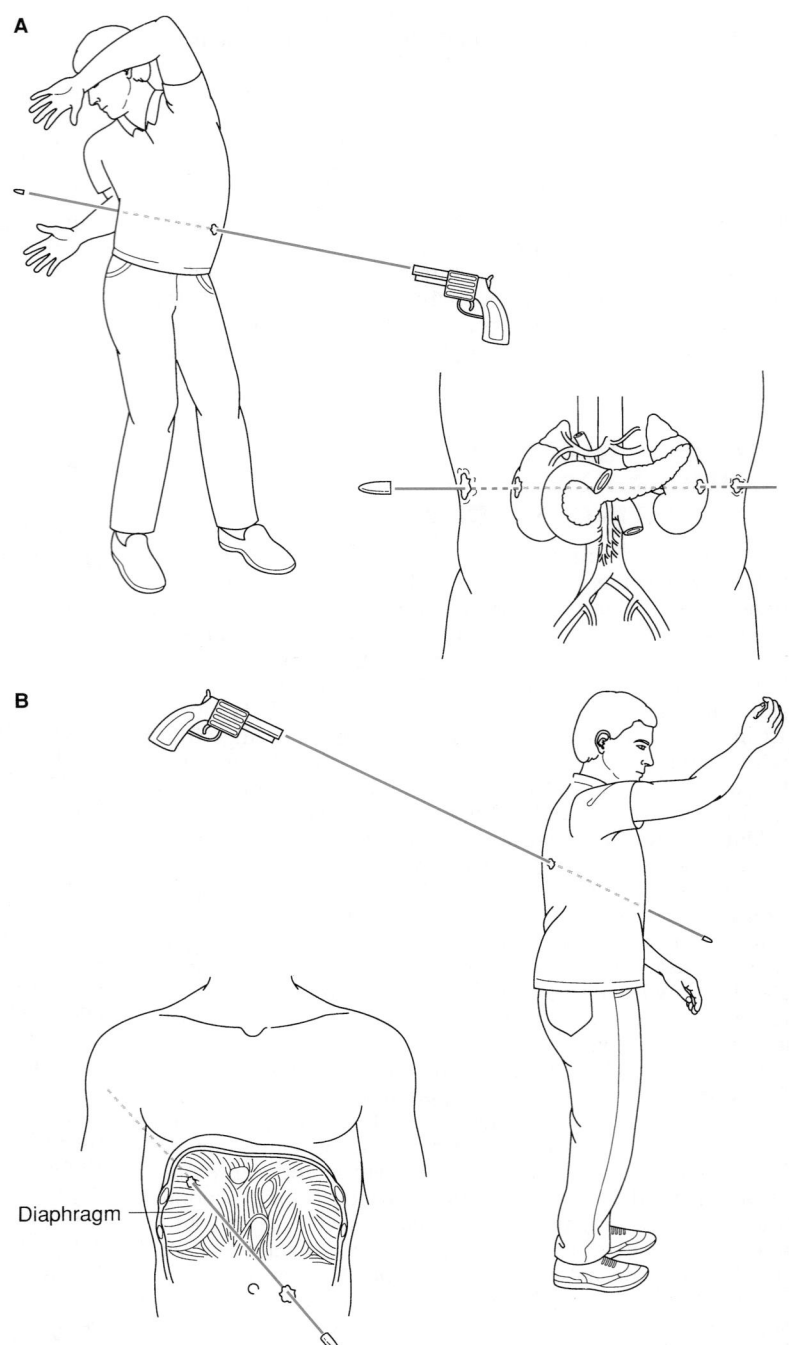

Figure 11.4. Axial traverse *(A)* and transdiaphragmatic *(B)* wounding mechanisms with associated injury potential for combined thoracic and abdominal injuries.

nism of injury is used to identify patients who are at high risk for significant injuries and are best evaluated at a trauma center. These data have been integrated with factors of age and comorbid disease into a triage decision scheme that is recommended by the American College of Surgeons (Fig. 11.5).

The major criticism of this triage scheme is that it leads to the frequent triage of patients to trauma centers (overtriage), which may not be necessary in all cases. On the other hand, it diminishes the number of patients with severe injury who are overlooked, and overtriage is the inherent cost of a sufficiently sensitive scoring system.

Table 11.4. **REVISED TRAUMA SCORE COMPONENTS**

Glasgow Coma Scale	Systolic blood pressure (mm Hg)	Respiratory rate (breaths/min)	Coded value
13–15	>89	10–29	4
9–12	76–89	>29	3
6–8	50–75	6–9	2
4–5	1–49	1–5	1
3	0	0	0

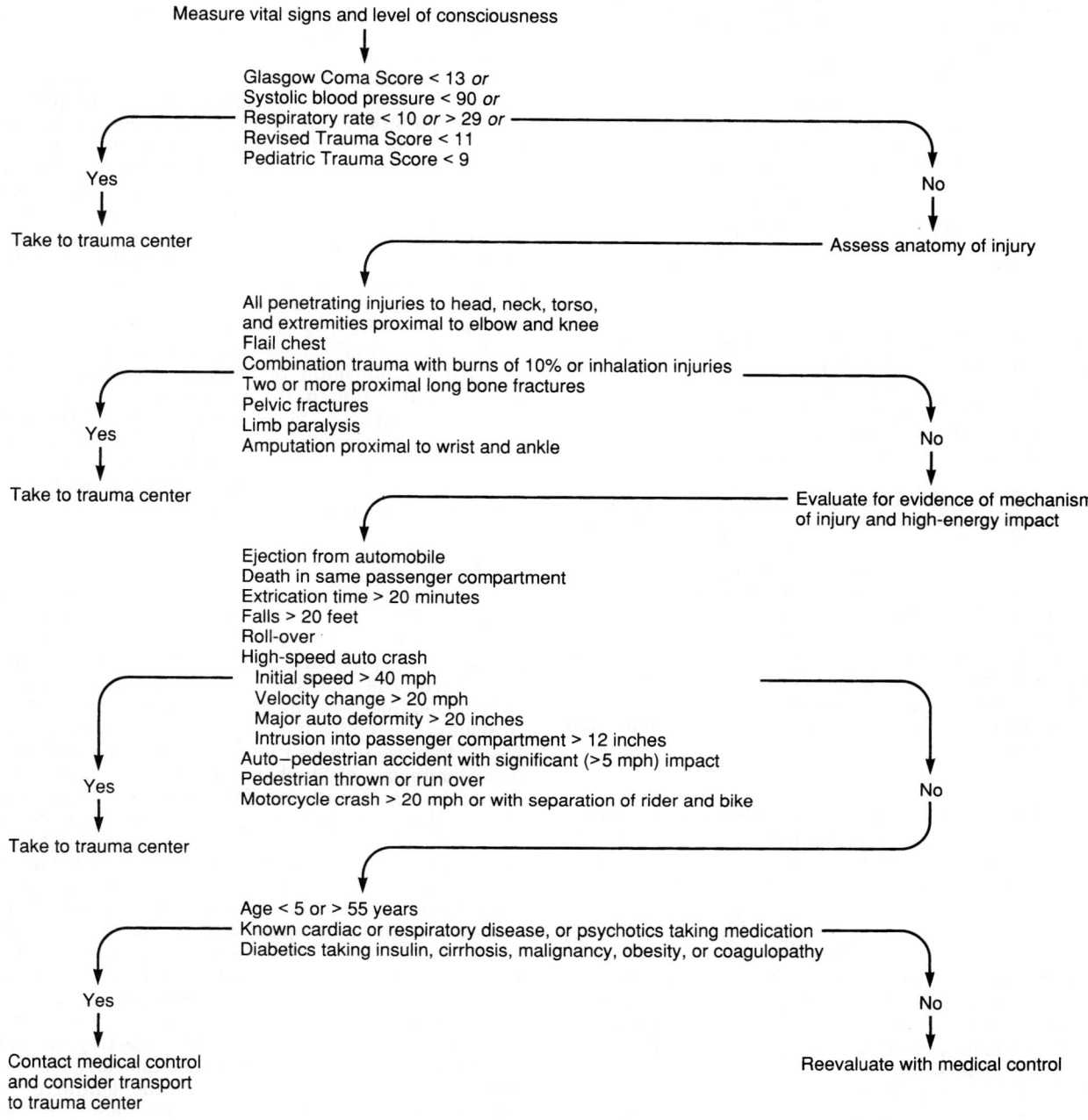

Measure vital signs and level of consciousness

Glasgow Coma Score < 13 *or*
Systolic blood pressure < 90 *or*
Respiratory rate < 10 *or* > 29 *or*
Revised Trauma Score < 11
Pediatric Trauma Score < 9

Yes   No

Take to trauma center   Assess anatomy of injury

All penetrating injuries to head, neck, torso,
and extremities proximal to elbow and knee
Flail chest
Combination trauma with burns of 10% or inhalation injuries
Two or more proximal long bone fractures
Pelvic fractures
Limb paralysis
Amputation proximal to wrist and ankle

Yes   No

Take to trauma center   Evaluate for evidence of mechanism
of injury and high-energy impact

Ejection from automobile
Death in same passenger compartment
Extrication time > 20 minutes
Falls > 20 feet
Roll-over
High-speed auto crash
    Initial speed > 40 mph
    Velocity change > 20 mph
    Major auto deformity > 20 inches
    Intrusion into passenger compartment > 12 inches
Auto–pedestrian accident with significant (>5 mph) impact
Pedestrian thrown or run over
Motorcycle crash > 20 mph or with separation of rider and bike

Yes   No

Take to trauma center

Age < 5 or > 55 years
Known cardiac or respiratory disease, or psychotics taking medication
Diabetics taking insulin, cirrhosis, malignancy, obesity, or coagulopathy

Yes   No

Contact medical control
and consider transport
to trauma center   Reevaluate with medical control

When in doubt take to a trauma center

Figure 11.5. Field triage decision scheme as recommended by the American College of Surgeons.

Outcome Assessment

Also important are the needs to compare specific injuries accurately and develop a scale for rating severity of tissue damage. Outcome analysis based on the parameters developed is a major objective of these types of scoring systems (21).

Abbreviated Injury Scale

The Abbreviated Injury Scale (AIS) (22) was developed in 1971 for use in blunt trauma and has subsequently been updated on a periodic basis. The 1990 revision of the AIS includes descriptors for penetrating trauma. Injury severity is determined in six different body areas on a scale of

0 to 6, where 0 indicates no injury, 5 indicates critical injury, and 6 indicates a nonsurvivable injury. The AIS evaluates individual injuries but does not account for multiple injuries. Thus, it is a specific anatomic index (7). Table 11.5 shows an example of the AIS for abdominal injuries. The shortcoming of the AIS is that it evaluates only the most severe injury in each body area and fails to account for multiple serious injuries in the same body compartment, thereby underscoring the true severity of injury.

Injury Severity Score

In 1974, Baker developed the Injury Severity Score (ISS), which is calculated by assigning AIS values to each

Table 11.5. ABBREVIATED INJURY SCALE SCORING SYSTEM FOR ABDOMINAL INJURIES

Score	Injury examples
1	Abdominal wall abrasion
2	Liver, stomach, colon, mesentery contusion
3	Minor liver or spleen laceration
	Bowel laceration without perforation
4	Major liver or spleen laceration
	Bowel laceration with perforation
5	Major liver or spleen laceration with tissue loss
	Bowel laceration with tissue loss

injury in six body areas: (a) head and neck, (b) face, (c) chest, (d) abdomen and pelvic contents, (e) extremities and pelvis, and (f) general and cutaneous. To derive the ISS, the scores for the three most severely injured areas are squared and added. ISS values vary from 3 to 75. If the value of the AIS is 6 in any body area, the ISS automatically is 75.

The result is that substantial quadratic correlation between injury severity based on ISS and death can be developed. The ISS is extremely helpful and has been widely used. However, it does not adjust for patient age or patient-related comorbid risk factors, such as chronic disease. Further, the severity of head injury is disproportionately underscored in that combinations of injuries in other areas can result in a higher ISS score than a fatal head injury. Despite this drawback, the ISS is an excellent tool for the study of groups of patients with multiple injuries from blunt trauma and allows comparison of outcomes and quality assurance.

TRISS

The TRISS methodology (23) is of great importance because it attempts to combine the trauma score, or physiologic component, and the ISS, or anatomic component. It also incorporates the patient's age. The equation used is as follows:

$$P_s = \frac{1}{(1+e^{-b})} \qquad (2)$$

where P_s = the probability of survival, and b = b_0 + b_1 (RTS) + b_2 (ISS) + b_3 (patient age); b_0, b_1, b_2, and b_3 are coefficients derived from a regression analysis applied to data from thousands of patients analyzed in the Major Trauma Outcome Study.

The TRISS method yields a specific probability of survival. Adjustments are made for age and mechanism of injury sustained (blunt or penetrating). The methodology allows patient groups to be compared. Individuals with an unexpected outcome can be specifically identified.

The TRISS method can be used for quality assurance evaluations both within and between institutions. Typically, a cutoff point (e.g., P_s = 50%) is chosen, and records of the deaths of patients with a probability of survival greater than the cutoff value are submitted for peer review. TRISS also can be used to examine cases in which the survivors exceeded the cutoff value. In addition, TRISS has been used to compare trauma outcomes between different institutions. To achieve this goal, a Z factor is calculated: the Z factor is equal to the number of observed deaths minus the expected number of deaths, divided by a population variation factor specific for the institution. A positive Z statistic indicates more survivors than expected, and a negative Z statistic indicates fewer than the expected number of survivors. Another factor that is added to the comparison is the W statistic. This methodology attempts to compare the average increase or decrease in the number of survivors per 100 patients with the normal population. In theory, then, comparisons can be made (24).

Other potentially relevant scoring systems are in various stages of development and validation. These include evaluation of specific mechanisms of injury, comparison of penetrating and blunt injuries, and provision of patient outcome indices in the intensive care unit. A specific Organ Injury Scaling system has been developed in an attempt to standardize the description of anatomic injuries. Another system, A Scoring Characterization of Trauma (ASCOT), uses descriptors of anatomic injury, patient physiology, age, and type of injury (25). Like TRISS, the ASCOT system uses logistic modeling and multivariate analysis to calculate a probability of survival.

Finally, to simplify the coding of trauma scores, a method that uses discharge diagnoses based on the International Classification of Diseases has been described (26,27). In this system, the first and second discharge diagnoses as well as the first operative code and the injury E code are used to calculate a Mortality Risk Ratio, which can be used in quality assurance. The validity and applicability of this system for intrainstitutional quality assurance remains to be documented.

SUMMARY

Trauma is a major national health care problem that affects one of four U.S. citizens annually. The cost of trauma injury and treatment to the U.S. society is greater than $200 billion dollars per year when loss of future productivity is considered. The causes of traumatic death vary considerably depending on demographics. Urban and politically unstable areas typically have a higher incidence of penetrating trauma, whereas rural and stable communities have a predominance of blunt injuries, usually vehicular accidents. Nonetheless, causes of death after injury are remarkably similar. Central nervous system injury accounts for approximately half of all fatalities, hemorrhage for 35%, and sepsis, multiple organ failure, and pulmonary embolism for approximately 15%. With the introduction of trauma systems during the last three decades, the incidence of preventable death has dropped from approximately 25% to less than 5%. This is the result of improvements in care both for acute head injuries and for control of hemorrhage. In addition, the incidence of late death attributable to sepsis and multiple organ failure has diminished, possibly as a result of better and early resuscitation. The responsibility of the surgeon for trauma encompasses the early recognition of injury, the resuscitation, and then the definitive care of the patient. As we improve the operative and intensive care rendered to trauma patients, we are beginning to reach the flat portion of the outcome curve (24,28). The area of injury prevention is still open to substantial improvement. To reduce the morbidity and mortality from trauma, surgeons must take a more active role in the prevention of trauma at the community level.

Trauma Systems

DAVID B. HOYT AND RAUL COIMBRA

The development of civilian regional trauma systems has provided the single most significant improvement in the care of injured patients in the last three decades. However, data show that only 23 states in the United States have functional, statewide trauma systems, and 8 states have no trauma system at all (29). The necessary elements of a trauma system have been defined. These include four primary patient needs—access to care, prehospital care, hospital care, and rehabilitation. In addition, five issues require social and political solutions to supplement medical efforts: prevention, disaster medical planning, patient education, research, and rational financial planning. Recent federal legislation (The Trauma Care Systems Planning and Development Act) authorized planning, implementation, and development of statewide trauma care systems (28).

COMPONENTS OF A TRAUMA CARE SYSTEM

Access

A first step in providing broad access to trauma care is to establish adequate emergency communication systems. Although many urban centers have capitalized on modern electronic technology to establish emergency systems, most rural communities in the United States have not. This type of access includes emergency telephone numbers (e.g., 911), emergency telephones located along major freeways, and a host of individualized radio and telephone networks. Access also requires that all users know how to enter the system. Public safety and information programs and school educational programs are used to inform health care providers and the public about emergency medical access.

Prehospital Care

Prehospital care encompasses many components. The primary focus is on education of paramedical personnel to provide initial resuscitation, triage, and treatment of injured patients. The development of coordinated response systems for ground ambulances, fixed-wing aircraft, and helicopters is an essential part of a modern trauma system. Effective prehospital care requires coordination between various public safety agencies and hospitals to maximize efficiency, minimize duplication of services, and provide care at a reasonable cost.

Hospital Care

Hospital care of the injured patient requires commitments from specific facilities to provide administrative support, medical staff, nursing staff, and other support personnel. The unpredictable nature of trauma care may generate demands for diagnostic services, operating rooms, laboratory services, and critical care beds, which may disrupt other programs in a hospital. Ultimately, the responsibility for a decision to commit to becoming a trauma center rests with the Board of Trustees and the medical staff of a hospital. This decision must be made within a complex social, financial, and ethical framework that is beyond the scope of this review.

Rehabilitation

Rehabilitation, the long-term component of trauma patient care, is as important as prehospital and hospital care, although it is traditionally underdeveloped. Only 1 of 10 trauma patients in the United States has access to adequate rehabilitation programs. The long-term functional recovery of patients after injury is also poorly understood (30). It makes little sense to develop sophisticated prehos-

pital and hospital care systems only to have patients obtain posttraumatic rehabilitation in inadequate facilities.

Other Essential Components

Effective trauma programs must focus on injury prevention. As noted, more than half of deaths occur within minutes of injury. Identification of risk factors and high-risk groups, development of strategies to alter personal behavior through education or legislation, and other preventive efforts are the only rational approach to these types of injuries. Education is the second component of a trauma system, with the goal being both public and professional understanding of the available regional resources and how to access them. Disaster planning for a region is another responsibility of a trauma system, and emergency services in a community must be coordinated prospectively. Finally, societal commitment to support effective research and fund the financial operations of trauma systems is necessary. Most of the industrialized world has begun to approach this complex problem. Fitting trauma care systems into the changing managed health care environment remains a challenge.

PRIMARY ROLE OF SURGEONS IN A TRAUMA SYSTEM

The key individual participants in the development of a system of trauma care are the general surgeons. Surgeons have political responsibilities that include interaction with local police, fire, and emergency medical service authorities; with the individual hospitals; and with any other institutions that participate in the system of care. Planning with the recognized verification authorities at a state or local level is necessary. Implied is a fiscal responsibility to optimize the use of resources and to maintain cost containment so that the system can be successful.

Surgeons should be involved in needs assessment for both ground and air prehospital care services and should assume an active role in the training of emergency medical technicians (EMTs) and paramedics. This includes responsibility for prehospital management protocols and for direct input to EMTs for treatment of injured patients before hospital admission. The final responsibility in the prehospital arena is to monitor and analyze prehospital care outcome and correct deficiencies as they occur.

During the resuscitation phase, surgeons should maintain a vital involvement in initial management of injured patients. Advanced Trauma Life Support protocols for initial management have been established and provide a basis for initial care. Many models have worked well, including surgeons resuscitating patients initially and surgeons working together with emergency department physicians and other members of the resuscitation team. It is essential, however, for the surgeon to maintain active involvement in initial resuscitation and to prioritize and orchestrate the sequence of evaluation and management of complex injuries. The greatest source of preventable deaths and morbidity occurs during the initial phase of care and is related to the need for rapid operative intervention. The central role of surgeons in this capacity is obvious. Establishing protocols for evaluation of life-threatening injuries becomes the responsibility of the surgeon so that operative care can be provided in a timely fashion. Modern trauma care requires the ability to move rapidly, to prioritize multiple injuries, and to accomplish several tasks simultaneously. No training other than that of the general surgeon allows a single person to function effectively in such a capacity.

Postinjury care is ongoing and does not end after operation. Critical care includes mechanical ventilatory support, hemodynamic support, and management of renal, hepatic, and gastrointestinal dysfunction, important postoperative surgical requirements that contribute to prevention of death (31). In addition, nutritional support in the treatment of multiple organ failure is an important domain of the general surgeon.

The quality of surgical leadership is of fundamental importance in the development of trauma systems. Successful trauma systems cannot develop without the commitment of the surgical department and the surgeons themselves within a hospital or community.

TRAUMA SYSTEM DEVELOPMENT

Trauma system development involves the redistribution of patients and medical and economic resources. It therefore requires public and legislative support and community-wide education. The first step in the development of such a system is to determine the need. In general, this has been done in communities by a quality assurance program that reviews the outcome of trauma cases in that region. This review traditionally has been focused on trauma deaths and their potential preventability. It is at least as important, however, to demonstrate whether there is potential for preventing permanent disability. The involvement of local physicians in such an audit usually leads to unambiguous conclusion, and, coupled with increased public awareness, the need for change becomes a community issue. The role of the surgeon is critical in both leadership and commitment to establish a better standard of care.

The second phase of the review is to establish legal authority for the development of a system. This usually requires legislation at a state or local level that provides public agency authority. Recent federal and state legislative efforts continue to define this relationship (28). The designated agency then works with trauma surgeons to develop criteria for the trauma system, design facilities to care for the patients, and establish a registry for tracking all injured patients and maintaining a quality assurance program.

Specific aspects of the system that are required include developing a prehospital communications and transport system, training personnel, and specifying qualifications for trauma care personnel for every phase of hospital care, including resuscitation, surgery, critical care, and rehabilitation. With criteria established, the process is democratized. The authoritative body requests proposals from major hospitals and appropriate local health care professionals. These proposals demonstrate the commitment of the hospital and medical staff and their ability to comply with established standards. The standard criteria were developed by the American College of Surgeons Committee on Trauma and appear in their 1993 report entitled *Resources for the Optimal Care of the Injured Patient* (2). External peer review usually is used to critique proposals and verify a specific hospital's capabilities. The purpose of peer review is not to certify a hospital within a region but to verify that the hospital and medical personnel can in fact deliver the appropriate level of care. The verification process can be accomplished through the American College of Surgeons Committee on Trauma or by inviting outside reviewers who are expert in the field of trauma.

After verification, formal designation is carried out by the authoritative body established at the outset. Designation is contractual and generally binding on prehospital providers. The designation process sets standards of care for the trauma system that can be monitored on an ongoing basis and implies a specific commitment from the providers.

The final component of program development involves design of the mechanisms for ongoing monitoring of needs assessment and quality assurance for the system. The trauma registry allows accurate documentation of epidemiologic data and monitoring of standards of care (32). Clinical indicator cases in which care is questioned are selected for review, and care is improved over time. The use of the Injury Severity Score using the TRISS methodology previously discussed allows for the identification of patients who die and for analysis of the predicted mortality rate. This methodology also allows for unanticipated deaths to be automatically reviewed.

Analysis of Trauma System Performance

Trauma system effectiveness has been measured by several scientific approaches and study designs. The most common include panel, trauma registry, and population-based studies, all with positive and negative aspects.

Panel review studies usually are conducted by a panel of experts (variable number) that reviews trauma-related deaths to determine preventability. Although this method has evolved in recent years by including well defined criteria and standardized definitions, significant methodologic problems are still in place that cause a great deal of inconsistency in the interpretation of the data.

Registry studies usually are used to compare data on outcome from a trauma center or a trauma system with a national reference norm. The Major Trauma Outcome Study (MTOS) has been used for this purpose; however, several limitations merit mention. The MTOS data are outdated; it is not population based; it includes a disproportionate number of patients with blunt trauma (79%); it includes patients from trauma centers with different levels of care; and autopsy data were not reported in 15% of the cohort. These issues compromise the reliability of the comparison with data from other systems or centers.

Trauma registries are advantageous because they include a detailed description of injury severity and contain physiologic data.

Population-based studies include information on all injured patients in a region using death certificates, hospital discharge claim data, and fatal accident reporting system. Although these databases have limited information regarding physiologic data, injury severity, and treatment provided to an individual, they are useful to evaluate changes in outcome before and after, or at different times after the implementation of trauma systems in a defined region.

An "Academic Symposium to Evaluate Evidence Regarding the Effectiveness of Trauma Systems" was recently carried out (33). Participants in this symposium agreed that the available data, although not always consistent, show that trauma systems implementation improves patient care. They also concluded that functional outcomes, financial outcomes, patient satisfaction, and cost effectiveness should be evaluated in addition to mortality in future prospective, well controlled studies.

SUMMARY

The development of a trauma system in a geographic area (city, county, or state) provides for access to trauma care and rapid transport of major trauma victims to specific hospitals in that region. The development of trauma systems has resulted in a significant reduction in patient mortality rates within the first hours after injury. These specific hospitals, called *trauma centers,* have concentrated resources and expertise to treat severely injured patients immediately and effectively throughout their care. Experience gained from the development of trauma systems has demonstrated the importance of the commitment required from surgeons to meet the specific problems encountered in the process.

Patient Care Phase: Prehospital and Resuscitation Care

HENRY MAGILL CRYER III

Care of the injured patient begins in the prehospital setting with a tightly integrated multidisciplinary Emergency Medical Service (EMS) System. The goal of the EMS System is to provide immediate access to lifesaving medical care. This usually entails the use of a first-response team, such as the fire department or other public safety personnel, with the capability of providing basic life support (BLS) within minutes of an accident. When available, a rapid transport team capable of providing advanced life support (ALS) moves the injured patient to a trauma center, where a multidisciplinary team meets the patient to continue resuscitation, identify injuries, and provide expeditious therapy, with the aim of completing all of these processes within 1 hour (the so-called golden hour). The goal of the EMS System is to assess for life-threatening injuries, initiate emergency care, and transport the injured patient as expeditiously and safely as possible to a trauma center.

PREHOSPITAL CARE

Personnel

The initial goal of any EMS System is to provide a rapid response by personnel trained in BLS skills to the scene of the injured patient. In most cases, this function is preformed by Emergency Medical Technician Basics (EMT-B). The EMT-B's responsibility is rapidly to assess the patient's airway, breathing, and circulation and look for evidence of obvious external hemorrhage. The EMT-B's skills include extrication, spinal protection, immobilization, splinting, and control of external hemorrhage. In most EMS Systems, BLS is followed by ALS. ALS personnel are usually paramedics (EMT-P) with some type of transportation. In some systems, ALS personnel are specially trained nurses or physicians and may have air transportation capabilities. ALS personnel carry an assortment of equipment and supplies, such as endotracheal tubes, cricothroidotomy kits, needles for chest decompression, intravenous fluids, and an assortment of medications for initial treatment of the critical trauma patient.

The controversy between rapid transport ("scoop and run") and field stabilization philosophies continues to appear in the literature. The choice of procedure for the individual patient often requires complex judgments. Decisions made by experienced on-scene EMTs communicating with the trauma center that will receive the patient provide the best patient outcome (34,35). The procedures performed and the time invested depend on factors such as the patient's hemodynamic stability, level of consciousness, complexity of extrication, distance from the receiving trauma center, and experience of the personnel at the scene and in the transport vehicle.

Injured patients who are at risk for progressive deterioration from continued bleeding, which requires rapid transport to a trauma center, may be better served with stabilization procedures done en route rather than at the scene (34).

Nationally standardized training programs for EMTs, both BLS and ALS, have become popular. These programs, Basic Trauma Life Support (BTLS) and Prehospital Trauma Life Support (PHTLS) provide EMS personnel a curriculum to assist them in making these complex decisions (36).

Assessment and Management Priorities

Airway Assessment

Because the most immediately life-threatening problem to the injured patient is loss of airway patency, this is the first priority of the first-response team on arrival at the injury site. Patients who are awake, alert, and talking obviously have a patent airway, but patients who are unconscious or have evidence of respiratory insufficiency require immediate attention. Typical BTLS skills, such as suctioning, the placement of oropharyngeal airways, and the use of bag–mask devices, are usually sufficient at least temporarily to restore oxygenation at the injury scene. On the other hand, approximately 10% of patients require endotracheal intubation (37), and up to 20% of patients would benefit from field intubation. Endotracheal intubation is the best procedure for airway control for patients who are in shock, have abnormal breathing patterns, or are unable to protect the airway because they are unconscious. Endotracheal intubation is a skill that requires proper training and regular use of the technique. In addition, ongoing quality assurance and reeducation are needed to maintain skills over time.

Training of paramedical personnel almost always includes endotracheal intubation, but the indications for intubation vary. Most trauma systems underuse prehospital endotracheal intubation. Endotracheal intubation is far superior to bag–valve–mask systems because it provides larger tidal volumes and less risk of aspiration (37). Unconscious or obtunded patients with absent or diminished gag reflexes have a high risk of aspiration of gastric contents. Positive-pressure ventilatory assistance by bag–valve–mask or mechanical ventilation device can cause gastric distention and increase the risk of aspiration. Some indications for endotracheal intubation in the field should include respiratory distress, unconsciousness, hypovolemic shock, significant head injury, severe chest injury, and facial burns. Reported rates of successful intubation by paramedical personnel vary between 90% and 98%, and complications are rare (38). More liberal indications for endotracheal intubation include all patients in major injury cases with unstable vital signs or altered mental status. On the other hand, intubation in an uncontrolled environment like the prehospital setting can be difficult at times. Patients with head injuries may have cervical spine injuries, so in-line mobilization techniques are necessary to ensure intubation without further injury to the cervical spinal cord. In cases where intubation is not successful, the use of a pharyngeal lumen airway may be an option. Patients often clench their teeth, in which case either nasotracheal intubation or the use of neuromuscular blocking agents such as succinylcholine may be necessary for successful intubation. Nasotracheal intubation is an effective technique if practiced frequently, but most paramedical personnel lack training in this technique. The use of neuromuscular blocking agents in the field is becoming more popular (38).

Needle and surgical cricothyroidotomy in the field are currently controversial, but are growing in popularity. Occasionally, cricothyroidotomy may be the only way to establish an airway. Reasonable results have been obtained in the prehospital setting using cricothyroidotomy (39,40).

Breathing

After establishment of a patent and controlled airway, the next priority is to ensure that air exchange is taking place. Immediately life-threatening injuries that preclude air exchange include tension pneumothorax, massive open chest wounds, sucking chest wounds, and tracheal disruption. There are no maneuvers likely to correct tracheal disruption in the field. Both open chest wounds and sucking chest wounds respond to endotracheal intubation and positive-pressure ventilation. Tension pneumothorax occasionally requires field decompression. Field techniques to deal with tension pneumothorax include needle thoracostomy and chest tube thoracostomy.

Some trauma systems allow paramedical personnel to place chest tubes in the field or en route under medical control (41). Chest tube placement probably is not necessary in urban trauma systems with short response times but can be of value in rural areas, where transport times can exceed 1 hour.

Circulation

The most common cause of death during the first hour after injury is hemorrhage. Therefore, after establishment of a patent airway and adequate air exchange, the next priority is support of the circulation. Direct pressure controls obvious external hemorrhage. The placement of one or two large-bore intravenous lines in the upper extremities en route to the trauma center facilitates resuscitation. However, placement of lines must not delay transport unless the patient is undergoing a complex extrication or is more than 30 minutes from a trauma center (36). The standard of care in the prehospital setting for hypotensive patients has been volume replacement and application of the pneumatic antishock garment (PASG). However, recent data raise questions about both therapies.

In a large, prospective, randomized study, Mattox and colleagues (42) found that in an urban setting with predominantly penetrating trauma, the PASG offers no survival advantage and actually increases the mortality rate if it is used in patients with thoracic injuries. On the other hand, there was a suggestion of benefit for patients who had a field blood pressure lower than 50 mm Hg. Cayten and colleagues (43) also found that patients with a field blood pressure lower than 50 mm Hg had increased survival with PASG use. Taken together, these studies suggest that PASG use is beneficial if the field blood pressure is less than 50 mm Hg. It is also possible that the PASG is of value in other settings, particularly those involving lengthy transport times or patients with blunt trauma, or if the PASG is used as a splint. These situations have not been adequately studied in prospective clinical trials.

The controversy between the "scoop and run" philosophy and the field resuscitation philosophy in seriously injured patients has more or less been resolved by common sense (34). Patients who are a short distance from a trauma center should not undergo field placement of intravenous lines. Instead, they should be expeditiously transported to the trauma center with attempts made during transport to obtain intravenous access. This facilitates initiation of resuscitation on arrival at the trauma center. On the other hand, patients who are a long distance from a trauma center or who require long extrication times benefit from the placement of intravenous lines and administration of intravenous fluids. However, a new controversy has arisen regarding the use of intravenous fluids in the prehospital setting for injured patients.

Experimental and clinical evidence raises the possibility that internal hemorrhage from major vascular injuries should not be treated with intravenous fluid infusion until the bleeding can be controlled in the operating room (44). In the hypotensive state, such major vascular injuries have a chance to clot and temporarily stop hemorrhage. But if intravenous volume restores normal blood pressure, the clot can dislodge and the rate of bleeding can increase significantly. This can lead to loss of both oxygen-carrying capacity and clotting factors and, ultimately, to exsanguination. If this theory is correct, it would be particularly relevant to the use of such agents as hypertonic saline. Hypertonic saline restores intravascular volume and blood pressure to almost normal levels very rapidly, albeit transiently. A prospective, randomized trial of normal saline versus hypertonic saline administration (45) demonstrated a significant improvement in survival when the data were compared with Major Trauma Outcome Study data for patients who had a probability of survival of 25% or less, patients who had nontamponaded injuries, and patients who had an entry Glasgow Coma Scale (GCS) score of 8 or less. There was no evidence that nontamponaded bleeding was exacerbated by the use of hypertonic saline, despite the fact that blood pressure and intravascular volume increased. This study included patients in an urban trauma setting in which the median time from injury to arrival at the trauma center was 54 minutes. The median time from the beginning of infusion to arrival at the trauma center was 15 minutes. These data were confirmed by similar results obtained in a multiinstitution trial (46) in urban trauma systems. In this setting, it appears that the most severely injured patients can benefit from the use of hypertonic saline resuscitation. It is not known whether similar results would be obtained in settings with longer prehospital times.

With some prehospital field interventions being controversial in the critical trauma patient, and with prolonged prehospital scene times being potentially harmful, the standardized trauma training programs (BTLS, PHTLS) for EMS personnel suggest that a single trauma patient who does not require extrication should be assessed, treated, and packaged for transportation in less than 8 to 10 minutes. Any additional assessment and treatment interventions should be done en route to the trauma center.

RESUSCITATION PHASE

Adoption of the trauma center concept increased dramatically and has produced documented improvement in survival of multiply injured patients in numerous reports. Trauma centers are hospitals committed to the total care of the trauma patient 24 hours a day. Multidisciplinary trauma teams consist of emergency physicians, general and orthopedic surgeons and neurosurgeons, critical care nurses, and diagnostic technicians. After notification of a major injury from the scene, the trauma team assembles in a specially equipped resuscitation room and waits for the patient to arrive. On arrival, care is immediately transferred from the prehospital team to the trauma team, and the trauma team rapidly initiates the resuscitation phase without a delay or lapse. Seriously injured patients should bypass hospitals without these resources and be taken to the nearest trauma center.

Many patients have relatively minor injuries that do not require mobilization of this expensive team and resources. Therefore, an important function of a trauma system is to allow communication between prehospital personnel and the trauma center to identify those patients who can benefit from trauma hospital and trauma team care. In addition to communication between the prehospital care team and the trauma team, a written report briefly describing the mechanism and extent of injury, vital signs, and significant treatment started by the prehospital personnel should be provided. These details identify high-risk patients to alert the trauma center team to look for injury patterns of high probability and to guide further work-up. Assessment and treatment then follow a logical sequence based on nationally standardized protocols through the Advanced Trauma Life Support format.

Team Composition

The trauma team consists of members from different disciplines, each of whom sees the patient from a particular point of view. By necessity, the team must have a single captain whose responsibility it is to organize and prioritize treatment efforts while the team is performing the primary and secondary survey to identify and treat life-threatening conditions. In a well orchestrated team, the team leader integrates and coordinates several tasks simultaneously. In most level I and II trauma centers, the team captain is a general surgeon trained in trauma care. In the ideal situation, the trauma surgeon should be present when the patient arrives. Although this is true in every level I and II trauma center, this may not be practical in many areas where the incidence of trauma is too low to justify the expense of an in-house trauma surgeon 24 hours a day, 365 days a year. In many rural and nonacademic level III trauma centers, the initial team captain is an emergency physician, with a general surgeon assuming the role on arrival. Academic institutions with both emergency medicine and surgical residency programs have the obligation of training both specialties to assume the role of trauma team leadership.

Although responsibilities vary between institutions, anyone involved in the resuscitation of trauma patients must master several procedures: all types of airway management, including cricothyroidotomy; establishment of vascular access through both percutaneous and open approaches; decompression of the pleural space using needle or tube thoracostomy; and decompression of the pericardial space by pericardiocentesis, subxiphoid window, or emergency thoracotomy.

Primary Survey: Initial Assessment

The multidisciplinary trauma team receives the patient from the transport team in a specially equipped resuscitation room. The team's first priority is simultaneously to assess the airway, blood pressure, and level of consciousness of the patient. This examination begins with observation of the patient's ability to talk and breathe as well as palpation of the wrist for a pulse. Although in reality the primary survey is performed in a simultaneous fashion, for descriptive purposes it is broken down here into its individual components and their appropriate priorities.

The first priority is reassessment of the airway. Airway obstruction often responds to simple maneuvers such as suctioning, the chin lift, jaw thrust, or placement of an oropharyngeal airway. Protection of the cervical spine with in-line immobilization is imperative during these maneuvers. Persistence of respiratory insufficiency requires endotracheal intubation. Unsuccessful intubation necessitates cricothyroidotomy. Occasionally, the anatomy does not allow cricothyroidotomy, as can occur with laryngeal fracture. In these cases, a formal tracheotomy must be performed. After an airway is established, a physician auscultates the chest to confirm air exchange and obtains a chest radiograph to ensure proper tube position.

The next priority is to ensure adequate ventilatory exchange by rapid auscultation of both lung fields and assessment for mechanical factors that may interfere with breathing. These include compression of the lung from hemothorax, pneumothorax, or visceral herniation; loss of chest wall stability from flail chest; lung damage from pulmonary contusion; and airway obstruction from aspiration. A dramatic presentation with cyanosis, intense respiratory effort without air movement, distended neck veins, and lack of breath sounds on chest auscultation indicates that a tension pneumothorax is present. Clinical diagnosis of tension pneumothorax requires immediate needle thoracostomy followed by chest tube thoracostomy. Sucking chest wounds should be sealed with an occlusive dressing secured on three sides to function as a flap valve. Most other problems become evident on the initial chest radiograph and are relieved by chest tube insertion, suctioning, or repositioning of the endotracheal tube. The optimal position for chest tube insertion is the mid-axillary line at the fifth or sixth interspace, avoiding the axilla, the large muscles of the back and chest, and the breast. Insertion of a finger into the chest before chest tube placement ensures entry into the pleural space and provides the opportunity to search digitally for defects in the diaphragm.

After establishment of an airway, ventilation, and appropriate pleural drainage, the next priority is an assessment of the patient's circulatory status. This includes estimation of blood volume and cardiac function. Blood pressure, pulse, skin perfusion and capillary refill, mental status, presence of breath sounds, and neck vein distention are all useful clinical indicators of hemodynamic status. The first issue is to establish whether the patient is in hypovolemic shock and, if so, the magnitude of this shock. The initial survey evaluates blood pressure, pulse, and skin perfusion. Circulatory collapse in the injured patient is almost always caused by hypovolemia secondary to hemorrhage. Occasionally, concurrent heart disease, spinal cord injury, and massive soft tissue swelling or cardiac tamponade also contribute. The mainstay of treatment for hypotension in the injured patient is volume resuscitation with crystalloid solution and packed red blood cells (RBCs). A lack of response to intravenous infusion of 2 L of lactated Ringer's solution indicates significant, ongoing hemorrhage and necessitates immediate blood transfusion.

Effective resuscitation from hemorrhagic shock requires both restoration of intravascular volume and control of hemorrhage. Most hypotensive patients are compensating maximally on arrival in the emergency department (ED) and many have ongoing hemorrhage. The less responsive a patient is to initial volume resuscitation, the more urgent is the need for hemorrhage control. One need not wait for a response to resuscitation before taking the patient to the operating room. Another situation that requires vigilance is the cool, pale patient with relatively normal vital signs. These patients are compensating maximally and have a normal blood pressure because of intensive peripheral vasoconstriction. However, this compensatory mechanism is of only limited duration, and such patients require immediate rapid volume transfusion, blood transfusion, and operative control of bleeding. A similar trap exists for patients with the mangled extremity syndrome or multiple open fractures. Patients may have lost significant blood volume at the injury scene. Before resuscitation, there may be relatively little hemorrhage from the open wounds. However, the patient may exsanguinate after initiation of intravenous fluids that increase blood pressure and cause vasodilation of previously vasoconstricted extremities.

These patients also require immediate volume resuscitation and operative control of their wounds.

The final priority in the primary survey is a brief neurologic evaluation using components of the GCS. The GCS is scored by assessing eye opening, verbal responses, and motor responses. In addition, pupillary size and reactivity and the presence of other lateralizing signs are assessed. Mental status may improve in response to volume resuscitation; however, a patient with a GCS score of 8 or less is assumed to have a significant brain injury. In this case, aggressive brain resuscitation, including appropriate ventilation, restoration of circulating volume, and the provision of adequate oxygenation, are important considerations.

Emergency department resuscitative thoracotomy is an aggressive, desperate attempt to save a dying patient. The dramatic return to full consciousness of a clinically dead patient after release of a pericardial tamponade from a stab wound to the heart provides complete justification for ED thoracotomy to those who have witnessed it. However, the widespread use of the technique in all patients arriving without vital signs has resulted in an extremely low survival rate at a very high cost. At first glance, the cost of an unsuccessful ED thoracotomy would seem to be nothing more than the cost of sterilizing the instruments and the physician's time. Many times, however, vital signs are temporarily restored, and the patient dies in the operating room or in the intensive care unit after massive blood transfusion and the use of considerable resources. Even worse from the resource management perspective is the rare patient who survives in a permanent vegetative state. The cost of the care for these patients must be included in any cost/benefit analysis.

Boyd and colleagues (47) performed a metaanalysis on 24 reports concerning the outcome of ED thoracotomy. They found that the overall survival rate after ED thoracotomy was 11% (264 of 2,294 patients). There were no survivors among patients with no signs of life at the trauma scene. Signs of life were defined as supraventricular electrical activity, pupillary reaction, and agonal respirations. In addition, there were no neurologically intact survivors among blunt trauma patients who were without signs of life on arrival in the ED. Considering these findings, the researchers proposed an algorithm that would indicate ED thoracotomy for penetrating trauma only if the patient had signs of life at the scene and had lost signs of life less than 5 minutes before arrival in the ED. Blunt trauma patients would be allowed ED thoracotomy only if the patient had signs of life on arrival in the ED. For patients who meet these criteria and lose cardiac function, airway placement and fluid resuscitation are initiated simultaneously with, or are immediately followed by, left anterior thoracotomy, pericardiotomy, and internal cardiac massage.

Secondary Survey

The secondary survey is directed at specific identification of suspected and unsuspected injuries. It consists of a thorough physical examination that includes observation and palpation of the entire body for evidence and characterization of injury. However, the priorities of the secondary survey depend on the results of the primary survey and the patient's response to initial resuscitative efforts. The secondary survey for a patient in hemorrhagic shock unresponsive to initial resuscitative efforts during the primary survey consists only of rapid identification of the bleeding site and rapid transport to the operating room for definitive control of hemorrhage. At the other end of the spectrum, a completely stable patient with relatively minor injuries undergoes a complete physical examination with confirmatory laboratory and radiographic tests before initiation of the treatment phase. The secondary survey can be interrupted at any time if a patient's status deteriorates. Many aspects of the secondary survey, such as physical examination, radiographic examination, and blood drawing for laboratory tests and crossmatching of blood, are performed simultaneously. For the purposes of description, the secondary survey is broken down into its individual components.

Head and Face

The head-to-toe examination usually begins with palpation of the skull and the head to identify hematomas, lacerations, and fractures. Scalp lacerations can cause significant blood loss and should be closed with a full-thickness running suture to provide hemostasis. Potential ocular injuries are assessed by testing visual acuity, pupillary function, and ocular range of motion. A funduscopic examination is important to identify increased intracranial pressure, vitreal hemorrhage, or retinal detachment. The findings of ecchymosis over the mastoid process, hemotympanum, otorrhea, rhinorrhea, and periorbital ecchymosis often indicate basilar skull fracture. Thorough palpation of the facial bones identifies step-offs or instability associated with facial fractures. Reassessment of the airway and a careful bimanual examination of the oral cavity identify loose teeth as well as mandibular and maxillary fractures. Bleeding from nasal fractures may require posterior and anterior packing for hemostasis.

Neck

Examination of the cervical region is conducted while axial immobilization of the cervical spine is maintained. The cervical collar is removed and the neck is examined for tracheal deviation, subcutaneous emphysema, hematomas, or distended jugular veins. The posterior cervical spine is palpated to elicit tenderness or other signs of obvious fracture. Cranial nerve function should be determined and recorded. Evidence of laryngeal fracture includes subcutaneous emphysema, tenderness or distortion of the thyroid and cricoid cartilage, and voice change. The presence of a fractured larynx is a relative contraindication to endotracheal intubation because of the possibility of extending the injury or creating a false passage leading to loss of the airway. Patients with suspected laryngeal fractures should be taken to the operating room immediately for formal tracheotomy. Carotid pulses are assessed, and bruits or expanding hematomas that may be suggestive of carotid artery injury are identified.

Penetrating injuries should not be probed, cannulated, or explored past the platysma because uncontrollable hemorrhage may ensue if a clot is dislodged from a major vascular injury. Wounds that have penetrated the platysma are evaluated either by formal operative exploration of the neck or by some combination of angiography, triple endoscopy (pharyngoscopy, laryngoscopy, and esophagoscopy), radiographic contrast study, computed tomography (CT) scan, and observation. If a water-soluble contrast swallow does not show a pharyngeal or esophageal leak, a subsequent barium swallow is indicated. Injuries encompassing the area from the cricoid cartilage to the angle of the mandible are usually explored. Angiography is mandatory for injuries between the cricoid cartilage and the clavicle and for injuries between the angle of the mandible and the base of the skull. Radiographic evaluation of the cervical spine should include anteroposterior, lateral, and odontoid views. A CT scan is often used further to evaluate suspect bony injuries, and careful flexion and extension films may be necessary to rule out potentially unstable ligamentous injuries of the cervical spine.

Chest

The chest wall is inspected for evidence of instability (flail chest) and for lacerations, including sucking chest wounds, abrasions, and contusions. Auscultation is performed to identify hemothorax or pneumothorax, and palpation is used to elicit tenderness that may be associated with rib fractures. As has been mentioned, tension pneumothorax can be identified by cyanosis, tracheal deviation, distended neck veins, lack of breath sounds, and inability to move air. Tension pneumothorax causing cardiopulmonary collapse is a clinical diagnosis that requires immediate treatment by needle thoracostomy followed by chest tube insertion.

Virtually all other life-threatening and potentially life-threatening chest injuries are diagnosed or suspected on chest radiography. Hemothorax is identified by opacification of a hemithorax and is treated by chest tube thoracostomy. Most pulmonary parenchymal bleeding stops with reexpansion of the lung and evacuation of the pleural space. However, thoracotomy is indicated if the initial blood loss exceeds 1,500 mL or if the rate of ongoing blood loss exceeds 200 to 300 mL/h in an adult. Blood evacuated from the pleural space can be autotransfused with appropriate chest tube drainage systems. Pneumothorax is usually treated by chest tube thoracostomy. Occasionally, small, stable pneumothoraces can be treated successfully by needle aspiration or close observation.

Pulmonary contusion is identified by radiographic findings of an irregular interstitial pattern or frank consolidation in the lung parenchyma. The clinical manifestations of pulmonary contusion vary from mild dyspnea to overt pulmonary failure with development of adult respiratory distress syndrome. The magnitude of the injury is rarely appreciated during the initial evaluation, and it is important to follow up with serial blood gas determinations and a repeat chest radiograph at 6 hours.

All patients with chest trauma should have an electrocardiographic evaluation and continuous monitoring during the first hour in the ED. Patients with electrocardiographic changes during the initial hour may have myocardial contusions and should be monitored for at least 24 hours. If there is any sign of myocardial failure, the patient should undergo echocardiography. Most myocardial contusions are self-limited and require only careful monitoring and treatment of significant dysrhythmias during the first 24 to 48 hours. Rarely, patients have all of the manifestations of overt myocardial failure and require full support, including aortic balloon pump.

Patients with rapid deceleration blunt injuries to the chest may sustain a transection of the thoracic aorta. The chest radiograph should be evaluated for widening of the mediastinum (more than 8 cm on a 40-inch anteroposterior chest radiograph), apical capping of the lung with blood, tracheal displacement, depression of the left main-stem bronchus, loss of the aortic window, deviation of the nasogastric tube, and loss of the parispinous stripe. Each of these findings suggests the presence of a mediastinal hematoma, which is often associated with a transection of the aorta. Additional radiographic findings that indicate a substantial force to the mediastinum include fractures of the sternum, first or second ribs, or scapula. Patients with a significant mechanism of injury and suspicion of mediastinal hematoma on chest radiography should undergo arch aortography to rule out transection of the aorta. Recent use of spiral dynamic CT and transesophageal echocardiography (48) is encouraging,

and these techniques also have a place in the identification of aortic injury in patients with severe blunt chest trauma.

Evidence of a ruptured diaphragm on chest radiograph includes the presence of the nasogastric tube or bowel above the normal plane of the diaphragm. If the patient has a diagnosis of ruptured diaphragm and respiratory distress, consideration should be given to careful placement of a chest tube. Placement of the chest tube to water seal instead of suction decreases intrathoracic pressure and prevents further herniation. These patients should undergo expeditious exploratory laparotomy to repair the defect.

Major bronchial injuries typically present with massive subcutaneous mediastinal emphysema and pneumothorax. Chest tube placement results in a vigorous air leak.

Management of penetrating injuries to the chest depends on the trajectory of the missile. Wounds confined to one lung or pleural cavity are usually treated by chest tube placement alone, with reexpansion of the lung. If the missile may have traversed the mediastinum, further evaluation is necessary, potentially including bronchoscopy, esophagoscopy, and aortography. Echocardiography is used to rule out pericardial blood and heart injury. False-negative studies have occurred when blood in the pericardium decompresses into the pleural space. However, echocardiography may be a sufficient screening tool if there are no clinical signs or symptoms and no hemothorax.

Abdomen

The abdominal examination should attempt to determine whether there is a significant injury requiring surgical intervention. Although physical examination is often accurate and reliable, it can be misleading in 20% to 30% of patients (49). This is particularly true in patients who are obtunded from head injury, alcohol, drug use, or shock. If patients are hemodynamically unstable, it is important to determine rapidly whether free intraperitoneal hemorrhage is responsible for the hypotension. Diagnostic peritoneal lavage (DPL) accomplishes this goal rapidly and safely and is extremely reliable in the hemodynamically unstable patient.

Diagnostic peritoneal lavage is considered grossly positive if more than 10 mL of blood is aspirated after catheter insertion. If less than 10 mL of blood or no blood is aspirated, 1 L of normal saline solution is infused into the peritoneum and then drained. A sample of the drained fluid is sent to the laboratory for RBC count; DPL is considered microscopically positive if the RBC count is higher than 100,000/mL. If the goal is to find the source of hemorrhage in a hypotensive patient, a grossly positive DPL pinpoints the abdomen as at least one source, and the patient should undergo immediate laparotomy. On the other hand, a microscopically positive DPL indicates intraabdominal injury that will eventually require laparotomy, but the major source of hemorrhage causing the hypotension may be elsewhere (chest or pelvis) (50).

In the hemodynamically stable patient, the lack of specificity of the DPL often leads to nontherapeutic and therefore unnecessary laparotomies. For this reason, CT has become routine for the evaluation of the abdomen in hemodynamically stable patients. Sequential CT scans may be necessary. Injuries that often have subtle findings during the first several hours after injury but may be found on a delayed CT scan include duodenal rupture, pancreatic transection, and blunt rupture of the intestine. Laboratory evaluations that may be helpful include liver enzyme levels and, to a lesser extent, serum amylase levels.

The use of ultrasound is popular in some institutions, replacing DPL for the diagnosis of free intraperitoneal fluid.

The work-up for patients with penetrating abdominal injuries depends on the missile. Gunshot wounds to the abdomen are an indication for exploratory laparotomy because 90% to 95% of these patients have intraabdominal injuries. The occasionally encountered patient with a tangential subcutaneous wound can be evaluated by laparoscopy (51) to determine whether peritoneal penetration injury has occurred. Stab wounds to the abdomen are often evaluated initially by local exploration of the wound. If the wound traverses the anterior fascia, then the patient can be evaluated by DPL or laparoscopy and should undergo exploratory laparotomy if the results are positive. Stab wounds to the flank and back are best evaluated by CT scan and serial observation (52). CT scan findings that mandate exploratory laparotomy include retroperitoneal hematoma, free air, extravasation of contrast material, and free intraperitoneal fluid.

Pelvis

After evaluation of the abdomen, the pelvis is assessed by physical examination. The bones of the pelvis are palpated gently to elicit tenderness that could indicate fracture. The genitalia should be inspected for scrotal hematoma or blood at the urethral meatus, which indicates probable urethral transection. A bimanual pelvic examination in women identifies evidence of vaginal laceration, indicating an open pelvic fracture. A rectal examination is performed to identify blood indicative of bowel injury and, occasionally, a mobile prostate, which indicates urethral transection. Evidence of a free-floating prostate, blood at the urethra, or scrotal hematoma should prompt a retrograde urethrogram before placement of a bladder catheter is attempted. All patients sustaining blunt trauma should undergo plain radiography of the pelvis to diagnose potential pelvic fracture. If a pelvic fracture is present, the patient should be assessed for retroperitoneal pelvic bleeding.

If the patient is hemodynamically unstable, the pelvic fracture must be considered a potential source of hemorrhage. This is important because pelvic fracture bleeding is retroperitoneal and rarely controllable at exploratory laparotomy. Potential pelvic fracture bleeding should be evaluated and treated by early angiography. If the patient is hemodynamically stable, the pelvic fracture should be evaluated further with additional plain radiographs and CT scans.

Extremities

Finally, the extremities are evaluated for open wounds with potential sources of hemorrhage or occult open fractures. Evaluation of pulses may indicate vascular injury. Palpation and passive range of motion tests diagnose potential long-bone fractures, dislocations, and ligamentous injuries. Dislocations require prompt reduction, especially if there is any evidence of neurovascular compromise. Penetrating wounds to the extremities necessitate evaluation for potential vascular injury by palpation of pulses, auscultation for bruits, and recognition of expanding hematomas. Proximity wounds can be evaluated by duplex ultrasound scan or arteriography.

The ideal trauma system consists of a prehospital care team that quickly and safely transports an injured patient to a trauma center, where a multidisciplinary trauma team immediately begins resuscitation of the patient. Treatment of immediately life-threatening injuries begins during transport and continues after arrival at the trauma center.

Rapid initial evaluation, followed by a more detailed secondary survey, allows identification of injuries while therapy is simultaneously begun. The management priorities are to identify and treat airway obstruction, hemorrhage, epidural or subdural hematoma, retroperitoneal or mediastinal hematoma, peripheral vascular injury, nonbleeding visceral injury, and long-bone fracture, in that order. The secondary survey is interrupted as necessary to treat life-threatening and limb-threatening injuries as they are identified according to this priority list. If interruption occurs, the secondary survey is completed at a later time.

Patient Care Phase: Shock
JAMES W. DAVIS

Shock can result from a variety of insults, including hypovolemic, septic, cardiac, or neurologic compromise. It is a condition caused by blood flow that is insufficient to meet the metabolic demands of organs and tissues. This section describes the hemorrhagic and hypovolemic causes of shock; other causes of shock are covered elsewhere.

PATHOPHYSIOLOGY

Hemorrhage initiates both rapid and slower, more sustained compensatory responses. Rapid responses, which occur within 1 minute of injury, are primarily increased adrenergic output, reflex tachycardia, and vasoconstriction. More sustained responses include resorption of fluid into the intravascular space and renal conservation of water and electrolytes.

Rapid Response

The body responds to maintain homeostasis almost immediately after the onset of hemorrhage. Decreased activation of the arterial baroreceptors through a decrease in blood pressure or, even more subtly, through a decrease in pulse pressure, causes an increased sympathetic discharge, which results in reflex tachycardia and vasoconstriction.

Increased adrenergic output with increased secretion of catecholamines also leads to vasoconstriction, increased heart rate, and increased myocardial contractility. Constriction of the systemic capacitance of small veins and venules shifts blood back to the central venous circulation, increasing right-sided cardiac filling pressures. Left-sided filling and pressure are augmented by pulmonary vasoconstriction. Concomitantly, vasoconstriction occurs in the skin, kidneys, and viscera, effectively shunting blood to those tissues with locally dominant blood flow regulatory mechanisms (e.g., heart and brain). Adrenergically mediated vasoconstriction increases cardiac filling and causes increased contractility and reflex tachycardia, all of which combine to increase stroke volume and cardiac output.

Sustained Response

Sustained compensatory responses include the release of vasoactive hormones and fluid shifts from the interstitium and the intracellular space. Decreased renal blood flow and increased adrenergic activity lead to the secretion of renin from the juxtaglomerular complex. Renin stimulates the release of adrenocorticotropic hormone (ACTH) and also stimulates the formation and release of angiotensin I by the liver. Circulating angiotensin I is converted in the lungs to angiotensin II, which is probably the most potent known vasoconstrictor. The increased concentrations of angiotensin and ACTH also increase aldosterone secretion. Aldosterone acts to increase resorption of sodium (Na^+) in the renal tubules. The release of vasopressin is increased because of reduced stimulation from the arterial baroreceptors, and this hormone causes increased resorption of water from the renal ultrafiltrate. After hemorrhage, vasopressin is sufficiently elevated also to function as a vasoconstrictor.

Adrenergically mediated vasoconstriction affects arterioles, precapillary and postcapillary sphincters, and small veins and venules. The decrease in intravascular hydrostatic pressure distal to the precapillary sphincter leads to resorption of interstitial fluid [water, Na^+, and chloride (Cl^-)] into the vascular space and thereby functions to restore circulating volume. This is known as *transcapillary refill.*

The increased release of the stress hormones (epinephrine, ACTH, cortisol, and glucagon), coupled with relative insulin resistance after shock, leads to high extracellular concentrations of glucose. In addition to glucose, products of anaerobic metabolism (i.e., lactate) from hypoperfused cells accumulate in the extracellular compartment, inducing hyperosmolarity. This extracellular hyperosmolarity draws water from the intracellular space, increasing interstitial osmotic pressure, which in turn drives water, Na^+, and Cl^- across the capillary endothelium into the vascular space (53).

Loss of Compensation

If the shock state continues, the postcapillary sphincter remains in spasm, but the arteriolar and precapillary sphincters cannot maintain the tension, and they become relaxed. As the sphincters relax, the capillary hydrostatic pressure increases, and Na^+, Cl^-, and water are moved into the interstitium by Starling forces, leading to further depletion of intravascular volume.

Cellular membrane function is also impaired in hemorrhagic shock. The normal, negative membrane potential approaches neutrality, leading to increased permeability and interstitial concentration of potassium (K^+). This is caused at least in part by a decrease in the normal function of the adenosine triphosphate-dependent Na^+-K^+ membrane pump that is induced by cellular hypoxia. The loss of the membrane potential difference and the Na^+-K^+ pump also leads to an intracellular influx of fluid, with concomitant cellular swelling. Some experimental evidence indicates that the decrease in membrane potential may be partly mediated by endorphins and that the decrease is partially reversible with naloxone.

EVALUATION OF SHOCK

Shock is easily recognized by even the most inexperienced caregiver after the compensatory mechanisms have been overcome by the severity of the injury. It is more difficult to recognize the patient in compensated shock, who presents with vital signs that are almost normal. It is critically important to the patient's ultimate outcome that recognition and treatment of shock occur before decom-

pensation. The clinical assessment must be guided by the knowledge that the severity of the symptoms and signs of shock varies from patient to patient and also in relation to the volume of blood lost. The patient is evaluated based on clinical appearance, hemodynamic measurements, and biochemical analysis.

The initial vasoconstriction described earlier causes the skin to be cool, with poor capillary refill. Patients in shock hyperventilate to compensate for metabolic acidosis. As the shock state progresses, mental status changes also occur; decreased cerebral perfusion pressure and increased catecholamine stimulation of the reticular activating formation may lead to anxiety and restlessness. With increasing blood loss, stupor or coma may result.

The hemodynamic assessment should include evaluation of the rate and character of the pulse, the blood pressure, and, in some cases, the central venous pressure (CVP) and pulmonary artery pressure. Tachycardia is a normal response to volume loss but also to pain, anxiety, and fear, all of which are commonly present in the trauma patient. Assessment of the pulse (full and strong or weak and thready) may be helpful in determining the proper diagnosis. Because of the body's ability to compensate for hypovolemia, changes in blood pressure do not occur reliably until 20% to 30% of blood volume has been lost. In patients for whom there is no concern of spinal injuries, postural vital signs can be assessed. A drop of more than 10 mm Hg in the systolic blood pressure or an increase of 20 beats/min in the heart rate with upright posture suggests volume loss. In addition, the pulse pressure usually narrows, even in compensated shock, because of the effects of vasoconstriction on the diastolic blood pressure. In patients with multisystem injuries or significant premorbid medical conditions, more invasive cardiovascular monitoring may be necessary. The CVP reflects the efficiency of the cardiac pump, the adequacy of the blood volume, and the state of the venous tone. Changes in CVP in response to treatment or from continuing hemorrhage are more revealing than a solitary measurement.

An indirect but extremely valuable measure of perfusion and volume status is urine output. A urinary catheter should be inserted in every trauma patient evaluated for shock. Hourly urine output should be 0.5 to 1 mL/kg for adult patients, at least 1 mL/kg for most pediatric patients, and 1 to 2 mL/kg for patients younger than 2 years of age.

Biochemical analysis of shock is based on the shift from aerobic to anaerobic metabolism in underperfused tissues. Increased lactate production is associated with tissue hypoperfusion (54). Broder and Weil (55) reported increased lactate levels in patients with shock. Subsequently, Vitek and Cowley (56) demonstrated higher lactate levels in survivors than in nonsurvivors (8.1 vs. 4.5 mEq/L) and that the median lethal level for lactate in hemorrhagic shock was 7.3 mEq/L. In addition, a decrease in serum lactate levels occurs in hypovolemic patients with resuscitation (57). The time required to normalize serum lactate levels through resuscitation is an important prognostic factor for survival (58).

Another biochemical marker of shock and resuscitation is the base deficit. This is defined as the amount of a fixed base (or acid) that must be added to an aliquot of blood to restore the pH to 7.40. The base deficit can be obtained as part of the arterial blood gas analysis and is reflective of metabolic acidosis, oxygen debt, and the changes in lactate (59) (Fig. 11.6). Base deficit values have been categorized as normal (2 to −2), mild (−3 to −5), moderate (−6 to −9), and severe (< −10) (60). Progressive worsening of base deficit values, by categories,

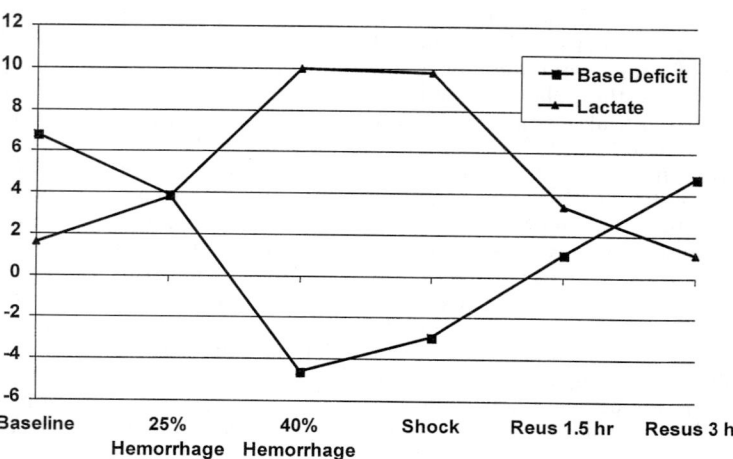

Figure 11.6. The relationship of base deficit to lactate in porcine hemorrhagic shock and resuscitation. The animals were subjected to incremental hemorrhage of 25% and 40% of calculated blood volume. The "shock" measurement was obtained 30 minutes after completion of hemorrhage, but before resuscitation. Resuscitation was performed with crystalloid (Resus 1.5 hours) and return of shed blood (Resus 3 hours). There was a statistically significant correlation between base deficit and lactate at each interval ($p < .01$) as well as the overall regression coefficient (R = -0.794, $p < .001$). (Modified from Davis JW. The relationship of base deficit to lactate in hemorrhagic shock. *J Trauma* 1994;36:168, with permission.)

has been shown to correspond to increased injury severity (by anatomic and physiologic scoring systems), and decreased survival. Base deficit is a useful guide to the fluid and blood volume required for resuscitation (61) (Fig. 11.7).

Changes in the base deficit with volume infusion can be used to judge the efficacy of resuscitation (61). Further, base deficit has been shown to be superior to pH values in assessing the normalization of acidosis after shock resuscitation, and the time required for normalization of base deficit has perhaps even greater prognostic significance than that for lactate (62).

The biochemical changes associated with the hypoperfusion of shock (i.e., increased lactate concentration and base deficit) occur even with compensation. Because of the potential difficulties in diagnosing compensated shock, an arterial blood gas analysis including base deficit should be obtained for every major trauma patient, and any patient with a base deficit of 6 mEq/L or less should be considered to be in shock until proven otherwise.

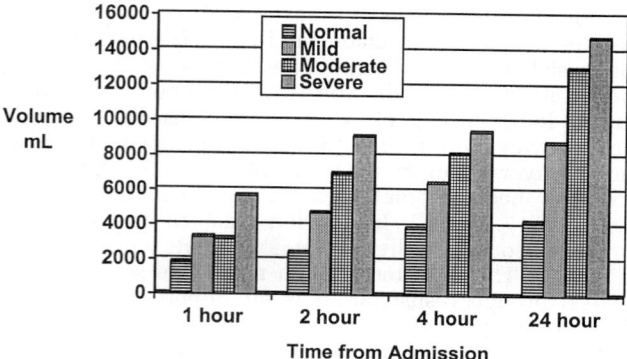

Figure 11.7. Resuscitation fluid requirements and admission base deficit. The amount of fluid (crystalloid and blood) infused at each time interval by base deficit category is shown. Base deficit categories are: normal (2 to -2), mild (-3 to -5), moderate (-6 to -9), and severe (< -10). The differences in volume between groups and time intervals are statistically significant. (Modified from Davis JW, Shackford SR, Mackersie RC, et al. Base deficit as a guide to volume resuscitation. *J Trauma* 1988;28:1464, with permission.)

CLASSIFICATION OF HEMORRHAGE

The signs and symptoms of shock vary with both the severity and duration of blood loss. A review of the Advanced Trauma Life Support classification system of the American College of Surgeons is useful to comprehend the manifestations and physiologic changes associated with hemorrhagic shock in adults (63). Blood volume is estimated at 7% of ideal body weight, or approximately 4,900 mL in a 70-kg patient.

Class I: Mild hemorrhage, up to 15% of total blood volume. This condition is exemplified by voluntary blood donation. In the supine position, there are no measurable changes in heart or respiratory rates, blood pressure, or pulse pressure. Capillary refill is normal. This degree of hemorrhage requires little or no treatment, and blood volume is restored within 24 hours by transcapillary refill and the other compensatory methods.

Class II: Loss of 15% to 30% of blood volume (800 to 1,500 mL). Clinical symptoms include tachycardia and tachypnea. The systolic blood pressure may be only slightly decreased, especially in the supine position, but the pulse pressure is narrowed (because of the diastolic increase from adrenergic discharge). Urine output is reduced only slightly (20 to 30 mL/h). Mental status changes (e.g., anxiety) are frequently present. Capillary refill is usually delayed. Patients with class II hemorrhage usually can be resuscitated with crystalloid solutions, but some may require blood transfusion.

Class III: Loss of 30% to 40% of blood volume (up to 2,000 mL). Patients with class III hemorrhage present with inadequate perfusion that is obvious; marked tachycardia and tachypnea; cool, clammy extremities with significantly delayed capillary refill; hypotension; and significant changes in mental status (e.g., confusion, combativeness). Class III hemorrhage represents the smallest volume of blood loss that consistently produces a decrease in systolic blood pressure. The resuscitation of these patients frequently requires blood transfusion in addition to administration of crystalloids.

Class IV: Loss of more than 40% of blood volume (more than 2,000 mL), representing life-threatening hemorrhage. Symptoms include marked tachycardia, a significantly depressed systolic blood pressure, and narrowed pulse pressure or unobtainable diastolic pressure. The mental status is depressed (e.g., lethargy, stupor) and the skin is cold and pale. Urine output is negligible. These patients require immediate transfusion for resuscitation and frequently require immediate surgical intervention.

TREATMENT OF HEMORRHAGIC SHOCK

The treatment of hemorrhagic shock requires control and arrest of hemorrhage as well as restitution of the circulating blood volume. The search for the source of hemorrhage should occur simultaneously with the institution of volume infusion (Fig. 11.7).

A minimum of two large-bore (14- to 16-gauge) intravenous catheters should be established in adults (63). Lactated Ringer's solution is then infused at the same time as blood is obtained for arterial blood gas analysis, typing, and screening. Fluid can be infused up to 175 to 200 mL/min through a 14-gauge catheter and up to 220 mL/min through intravenous tubing placed into a vein through a cutdown. A fluid challenge of 1 to 2 L is administered to the hypotensive patient and the response is assessed. If the blood pressure returns to normal and is stabilized, the blood loss was relatively small, and the only treatment required may be infusion of a balanced saline solution.

If the increase in blood pressure is transient after fluid bolus, the hemorrhage was severe or may be ongoing. Additional crystalloid is administered, and the need for blood transfusion is assessed. Patients who continue to require large amounts of fluid and blood to support perfusion usually have ongoing hemorrhage and require surgical intervention. No response or a minimal response to apparently adequate infusions of crystalloid solution and blood indicates exsanguinating hemorrhage and the need for urgent surgery.

Some controversy has developed over how much resuscitation should be attempted before definitive control of hemorrhage. Animal studies have demonstrated increased blood loss and increased mortality rates after infusion of isotonic and hypertonic solutions in models with uncontrolled hemorrhage (64). In a similar study of uncontrolled hemorrhage, improved survival rates and decreased hemorrhage were achieved by infusion of only enough fluid to maintain a mean arterial pressure of 40 mm Hg (instead of 80 mm Hg) (65). It seems logical that restoration of normal blood volume would lead to increased hemorrhage if the sites of bleeding were not controlled. However, this approach to resuscitation (i.e., withholding of intravenous fluids) in patients at high risk for ongoing hemorrhage, such as those with penetrating truncal trauma, remains controversial (66).

The same clinical indicators used to evaluate shock are used to evaluate the patient's response to resuscitative efforts. The commonly considered end points of resuscitation include a normal blood pressure, decreased heart rate, adequate urine output, and normal CVP. The same compensatory mechanisms that can allow shock to go unrecognized, however, also can lead to underresuscitation. This is particularly true of blood pressure. CVP depends on intravascular volume and the state of venous tone. Assessment of the adequacy of volume replacement by CVP can be improved by observing the changes in CVP after rapid administration of small volumes (250 mL) of Ringer's solution. A CVP that does not change after administration of a bolus may indicate that normovolemia is still not restored.

Metabolic parameters also should be used to assess the end points of resuscitation. With adequate restoration of volume, the metabolic acidosis should resolve, and the base deficit and serum lactate level should normalize. A base deficit that persists despite an apparently adequate volume of resuscitation necessitates a diligent search for ongoing hemorrhage (61).

Monitoring changes in cellular perfusion by measurement of tissue oxygen tension (tissue PO_2) has significant appeal as an end point of resuscitation. The measurement of tissue PO_2 during inspired oxygen challenges is both sensitive and specific in determining flow-dependent oxygen consumption (67). Although this technology has significant potential, it is not widely available at present, and the confounding variables of vasoconstriction from hypothermia and catecholamine release have not been resolved.

Because blood flow is not uniformly distributed to all tissue beds, assessment of regional blood flow may indicate tissue beds with hypoperfusion even when the more global indices (base deficit, lactate) are normalizing. Because the splanchnic circulation is one of the first to be compromised and one of the last to be restored, assessing gut perfusion, specifically gastric mucosal perfusion, has been suggested as an appropriate and accessible regional circulatory bed to be monitored. Low gastric mucosal pH (pHi < 7.32) has been associated with increased organ failure and a higher mortality rate (68). Another approach to assessment of regional perfusion is the measurement of mitochondrial cytochrome a,a_3 redox shifts using near-infrared spectroscopy. Early investigational efforts suggest that this technique may be useful in identifying regional hypoperfusion (69).

Resuscitative Fluids

Crystalloids

Balanced salt solutions are the most commonly used resuscitative fluids, and their use to restore extracellular volume significantly decreases the transfusion requirement after hemorrhagic shock. Lactated Ringer's solution is isotonic, readily available, and inexpensive. It rapidly replaces the depleted interstitial fluid compartment and does not aggravate any preexisting electrolyte abnormalities. Previous investigations have shown that administration of lactated Ringer's solution does not lead to aggravation of the lactic acidosis that is present in shock (57). As volume and perfusion are restored, lactate is mobilized and metabolized to bicarbonate in the liver. Mild metabolic alkalosis may occur 1 or 2 days after large-volume resuscitations with lactated Ringer's solution. Normal saline solution is also effective for resuscitation of hypovolemic patients. Previous concerns about inducing hypernatremic, hyperchloremic metabolic acidosis with massive resuscitation volumes have not been borne out by further investigation with normal saline and the hypertonic saline solutions. Resuscitation with crystalloid solutions requires a volume administration ratio of 3 : 1 to 4 : 1 over volume lost. Investigations have raised concerns about the proinflammatory effects of resuscitation with lactated Ringer's solution. Increased apoptosis in both the small intestine and the liver was seen after resuscitation from hemorrhage with lactated Ringer's solution, but not with hypertonic solutions or blood resuscitation (70). In addition, increased leukocyte adhesion and neutrophil activation have been shown after resuscitation with lactated Ringer's solution, changes not seen with hypertonic or colloidal resuscitation (71,72).

Colloids

Although colloids do not replete the interstitial space, they have a volume-expanding effect somewhat greater than the amount infused. Colloids have the theoretic advantages of increasing the colloid oncotic pressure and requiring smaller volumes for resuscitation than crystalloids (73). Colloids commonly used for volume expansion in hypovolemia include albumin, dextran 70, dextran 40, and hydroxyethyl starch.

Albumin solutions have been used during resuscitation to increase colloid oncotic pressure and, hypothetically, to protect the lung from interstitial edema; however, there is a relatively rapid flux of albumin across the pulmonary capillary membranes and relatively rapid clearance through the pulmonary lymphatics. In addition, it has been estimated that albumin passage from the intravascular to the extravascular space occurs at a rate of up to 500 mL/h.

Dextran 70 and dextran 40 are polysaccharides with molecular weights of 70,000 and 40,000, respectively. Dextran 40 (10%) is hyperoncotic and initially exerts a volume-expanding effect that is almost twice the volume infused. However, because of its lower molecular weight, it is more rapidly excreted than the other colloids. The gain in intravascular volume is roughly equal to the amount of dextran 40 infused within the first 3 or 4 hours of administration. Dextran 40 is more commonly used in cases of peripheral vascular disease and hyperviscosity syndromes. Dextran 70 is provided as a 6% solution and does not exert the hyperoncotic effect produced by dextran 40. The volume expansion is somewhat greater than the amount infused, but because of its larger molecular size, its volume-expanding effect may be maintained for 24 to 48 hours. The dextran preparations also cause decreased platelet adhesiveness and decreased factor VIII activity. They carry an incidence of allergic reaction of up to 5%, and anaphylaxis of 0.6% (73). In addition, because of the rheologic properties of dextran, blood incompatibility can be simulated, making identification of compatible blood more difficult.

Hydroxyethyl starch [hetastarch, Hespan (DuPont Merck Pharmaceuticals, Wilmington, DE)] is an amylopectin. It exerts a volume-expanding effect similar to that of dextran 70. The duration of expansion is approximately 36 hours. Hetastarch is reported to have side effects similar to those of dextran, but with less frequency. The incidence of anaphylaxis is 0.006%. A new hydroxyethyl starch, pentastarch, has a lower molecular weight and fewer hydroxyethyl groups. Pentastarch has a shorter duration of action (2.5 hours) than hetastarch and has been reported to have less effect than other colloids on coagulation in burn resuscitation and in postoperative cardiac surgery patients (74,75).

The controversy regarding use of crystalloids versus colloids in resuscitation has not been resolved. Both types of solutions can restore circulating volume. The effects of the solutions on pulmonary function are at issue and are summarized as follows: (a) the use of crystalloid solutions decreases plasma oncotic pressure, thereby leading to lung edema at lower microvascular pressures; and (b) colloids given in the face of pulmonary injury (contusion) can extravasate, promoting edema because of the reduced plasma interstitial oncotic gradient. Several studies have indicated an advantage to crystalloids in resuscitation. It has been demonstrated that saline and dextran are cleared from the alveolar space more rapidly than either starch or plasma (76). In addition, a metaanalysis of colloid versus crystalloid resuscitation after hemorrhagic shock demonstrated a higher mortality rate among the colloid-resuscitated patients, partly because of pulmonary complications (77).

Blood

Most patients with class I or II hemorrhage can be resuscitated with balanced salt solutions only. Patients who lose more than 25% to 30% of total blood volume need blood for resuscitation. Blood administered within 24 hours of its collection is probably ideal for resuscitation of trauma patients. The availability of whole blood, however, has progressively decreased with the increasing separation of donated blood into components such as packed red blood cells (RBCs), plasma, and platelets. There remains some controversy about whether fresh whole blood therapy is superior to component therapy in the treatment of hemorrhage and resuscitation-induced coagulopathy. The failure of component therapy to resolve nonsurgical bleeding in some trauma patients has led to recommendations that whole blood be used more often (78), but there is no scientific evidence to indicate that whole blood has additional benefits.

The decision about the composition of blood to be transfused is determined in part by the urgency of the situation. Blood that has been fully typed and crossmatched carries the least risk of transfusion reactions, but it also takes the most time to obtain (usually 45 minutes or longer). Other transfusion options include the use of type O, Rh-negative or type-specific blood (Table 11.6).

Type O, Rh-Negative Blood

Type O, Rh-negative (universal donor) blood is immediately available without a crossmatch. Because type O blood contains no AB cellular antigens, administration of packed RBCs is relatively safe for patients of any blood type, with little risk of hemolytic reaction. The administration of more than 4 units of type O, Rh-negative blood to a non-O blood type patient, however, theoretically can result in an admixture of blood type. Rarely, administration of a high-titered anti-A or anti-B unit of type O blood to a non-O blood type patient results in a positive direct Coombs' test or, even more rarely, a hemolytic reaction.

A pretransfusion blood specimen should be sent to the blood bank when the patient is admitted, and type-specific blood should be transfused as soon as it is available. Previous concerns that administration of type O blood to patients with non-O blood types would lead to hemolytic reactions after the transfusion is changed to appropriate type-specific blood are probably unwarranted.

Table 11.6. COMPARISON OF BLOOD AVAILABILITY

Blood	Typing	Antibody screen	Crossmatch	Time
Type O negative	No	No	No	Now
Type specific	Yes	No	No	<10 min
Type and screen (gel technique)	Yes	Yes	Yes	30 min
Type and crossmatch	Yes	Yes	Yes	45–60 min

Type-specific Blood

Type-specific blood is available from most blood banks within 5 to 10 minutes of receipt of the blood specimen, while the patient is being resuscitated with balanced salt solutions. Although not crossmatched, this blood can be administered safely, as demonstrated in both military (79) and civilian (80) experiences. The rapid availability and safety of type-specific blood makes it the blood of choice for resuscitation in trauma.

Autotransfusion

Autotransfusion involves collection of the shed blood and its reinfusion through a filter back into the patient. Autotransfusion can be as simple as aspiration of the blood into a citrate-containing collection chamber, followed by reinfusion through a 40-μm filter. A more elaborate system, the Haemonetics autotransfuser (Haemonetics Corp., Braintree, MA), centrifuges the collected blood and delivers washed, packed RBCs for reinfusion. The advantages of autotransfusion include transfusion with warm, compatible blood without delays and with no risk of transmission of hepatitis, human immunodeficiency virus, or other blood-borne pathogens.

Autotransfused blood can produce disseminated intravascular coagulation and activation of fibrinolysis. In addition, collection of blood from the peritoneal cavity after hollow viscus injury, even with cell washing, can lead to bacterial contamination of the autotransfused blood (81). Successful autotransfusion of contaminated blood has been demonstrated (82), but blood obtained from enteric-contaminated cavities probably should not be used, except perhaps in extreme circumstances, until its safety is better determined. Inadequate scavenging of shed blood has been a problem because suction power is limited to 30 to 60 mm Hg to avoid hemolysis. It appears, however, that this level could be increased to 100 mm Hg with little effect on hemolysis and some improvement in blood scavenging (83). Despite that improvement, investigators have found that the autotransfuser was used in only 22% of the trauma patients for whom it was prepared. The precise role of autotransfusion in trauma is not well defined, but, with increasing concerns about homologous blood transfusion, its use is likely to increase.

Experimental Resuscitation Fluids

Hypertonic Saline

Hypertonic saline solutions have been used in resuscitation of patients after burn shock, elective vascular surgery, and trauma. Hypertonic fluid resuscitation expands intravascular volume both from the fluid infused and from an osmotically induced shift of intracellular fluid into the intravascular compartment. In addition to expanding volume, hypertonic saline solutions have been shown to increase left ventricular performance (84), decrease peripheral resistance from arteriolar dilatation (85), and redistribute cardiac output to the kidneys and viscera (85,86).

The optimal osmolarity of hypertonic saline solutions for resuscitation from hypovolemia has not been determined. Investigations with 2,400-mOsm saline solutions administered in boluses of 4 mL/kg have shown that this concentration rapidly restores blood pressure to baseline levels after hemorrhagic loss of 40% to 50% of blood volume (87). However, the response to bolus administration was not sustained. The addition of colloid to the hypertonic saline solution led to sustained increases in arterial pressure, cardiac output, and measured plasma volumes, with the colloid acting to hold the water drawn into the intravascular space by the hypertonic saline solution. Other reports have described more effective volume replacement with smaller-volume infusions of 500-mOsm solutions than with lactated Ringer's solution (88), and suggest a mortality advantage in head-injured patients (89,90). Excessively hypertonic solutions (3,600 to 4,800 mOsm) can be associated with seizure activity.

Studies of hypertonic saline resuscitation in models of uncontrolled hemorrhage have demonstrated increased hemorrhage and increased mortality rates after administration of hypertonic saline solutions compared with resuscitation with normal saline solution (91). The increased hemorrhage is thought to be caused in part by the peripheral vasodilatation produced by administration of hypertonic saline solutions. Other investigations of hypertonic saline have demonstrated improved survival with small-volume administration and no real increase in hemorrhage. In addition, hypertonic solutions may have some advantages over lactated Ringer's solution. More recent investigations have demonstrated increased leukocyte adherence and neutrophil activation (71,72) as well as increased apoptosis in liver and small intestine with lactated Ringer's resuscitation, but not with resuscitation with hypertonic saline solutions (70).

Blood Substitutes

Readily available oxygen-carrying solutions have tremendous potential for trauma patient resuscitation. The "ideal blood substitute" would be nonantigenic, free of transmissible disease, and have normal or near-normal oxygen-carrying capacity. Efforts to produce this "ideal" solution have included perfluorocarbon preparations and stroma-free hemoglobins from human, bovine, and recombinant sources.

Perfluorocarbons

Perfluorocarbon preparations were stabilized with emulsifiers, and added to solutions of hetastarch and balanced salt solutions as one of the first clinically used blood substitutes. These compounds did improve oxygen delivery and restore volume but had significant side effects, including depression of platelet counts, fibrinogen levels, and the immune system (92–94). These compounds have been withdrawn from clinical use.

Stroma-free Hemoglobin

After removal from an erythrocyte, hemoglobin retains its oxygen-carrying capacity. Hemoglobin solutions prepared from lysis of RBCs have been shown to be effective oxygen-carrying resuscitative fluids in animal models (95). The side effects from the use of hemolyzed blood (e.g., renal dysfunction, coagulopathy) are caused by stromal elements of the erythrocyte. Removal of these stromal elements by lysis decreases the incidence of such problems. However, isolated preparations of stroma-free hemoglobin as a blood substitute have a short half-life and a marked affinity for the oxygen molecule, becoming half-saturated at a Po_2 of 14 mm Hg instead of the normal 27 mm Hg (76,77).

Efforts to produce a clinically useful stroma-free hemoglobin have included diaspirin cross-linking of the hemoglobin tetramer, glutaraldehyde or pyridoxylated polymerization of human and bovine hemoglobins, and recombinantly cross-linked hemoglobin (98,99).

The diaspirin cross-linked hemoglobin successfully completed phase I and II trials. However, this blood substitute was found to increase blood pressure from increased vasomotor tone through its role as a nitric oxide scavenger (99). Pulmonary hypertension and increased mortality rates in phase III trials led to the withdrawal of this agent (100–103).

Polymerized, pyridoxylated, stroma-free hemoglobin (PolyHeme; Northfield, Evanston, IL) is a different formulation. This substance has been shown to have essentially the same oxygen-carrying capacity and P_{50} as whole blood (104,105). Clinical phase I and II studies with this substance have demonstrated safety and efficacy in restoration of blood volume and oxygen-carrying capacity in severely injured hypovolemic patients (105). There have been no adverse consequences from this blood substitute with infusion of volumes up to the equivalent of 10 units of blood (98,106).

COMPLICATIONS OF SHOCK

Hemorrhagic shock can lead to a cascade of related complications, each requiring its own intervention if the clinician is to achieve the goal of resuscitating the patient from the shock state. The most commonly encountered of these complications are metabolic acidosis, hypothermia, and coagulopathy. Other complications of shock and resuscitation, such as ischemia–reperfusion, multiorgan system dysfunction or failure, adult respiratory distress syndrome, and others are covered elsewhere in this text.

Metabolic Acidosis

The acidosis of hemorrhagic shock results from tissue hypoperfusion, anaerobic metabolism, and lactate accumulation. The treatment for acidosis from shock is restoration of adequate tissue perfusion. Acidosis can lead to cardiac compromise, however, and some therapeutic drugs (e.g., lidocaine) are inactive if the pH is less than 7.2. Severe acidosis therefore should be treated with judicious administration of bicarbonate, with frequent monitoring of the pH and base deficit by arterial blood gases, to achieve a pH of 7.2 or higher. Overadministration of bicarbonate should be avoided because it shifts the oxyhemoglobin dissociation curve to the left, resulting in greater oxygen affinity for the hemoglobin molecule and less oxygen release into the tissues.

Hypothermia

Hypothermia (core temperature < 35°C) is common after severe injury. Heat loss is increased in the trauma patient. In addition to immobilization, both prehospital and postadmission exposure can lead to conductive, convective, and evaporative heat loss. The administration of room-temperature intravenous fluids and of cold stored blood also contributes to hypothermia (107). Hypothermia increases fluid requirements and independently increases acute mortality rates after major trauma (108).

As the core temperature decreases, the rate of oxygen consumption also decreases, to approximately 50% of normal at 28°C. The decrease in oxygen consumption is accompanied by increased production of acid metabolites. A leftward shift in the oxyhemoglobin dissociation curve also occurs with hypothermia but is partially compensated by the acidosis. Central nervous system effects progress from confusion and loss of manual dexterity to obtundation and frank coma as the core temperature decreases from 35° to 26.5°C. The heart rate decreases to approximately half of baseline at 28°C, with a concomitant decrease in cardiac output. All cardiac electrical conduction intervals are prolonged, consistent with the changes in heart rate, and both atrioventricular dissociation and refractory ventricular fibrillation occur at 28°C. Other physiologic effects include ileus and pancreatitis (from cold enzyme activation) at temperatures lower than 35°C.

Compensatory responses to hypothermia include increased excretion of catecholamines, with potential doubling of the basal metabolic rate, and increased production of thyroid hormones, with potential increases in the basal metabolic rate to five times baseline. Shivering can increase heat production as well, but it represents a significant energy expenditure, and has been shown to be inhibited during episodes of hypotension or hypoxemia (109). Compensatory responses to hypothermia are lost at temperatures below 30° or 31°C, and a state of complete poikilothermy is reached.

The treatment for hypothermia is rewarming. The core temperature (rectal or bladder) should be obtained on admission of the trauma patient. Patients whose core temperatures are 33° to 35°C can be treated with passive rewarming, warm blankets, and hot packs. Patients with core temperatures lower than 33°C require active rewarming. If the patient is unconscious, airway control should first be obtained. Because severe hypothermia causes vasoconstriction, noninvasive blood pressure measurements may not be feasible or accurate, and an arterial line should be placed for monitoring and blood gas sampling. The inspired gas through the ventilator should be heated to 41°C and fully saturated with water vapor to increase heat conductance into the capillary beds of the lung.

The intravenous fluids should also be warmed. Commercially available rapid infusion systems with heating elements should be used. Continuous arteriovenous rewarming is a method of rewarming that uses femoral artery and venous catheters, and the patient's own systolic blood pressure to create an extracorporeal circulatory "fistula" through a counter-current fluid warmer (107). In patients in extremis, extracorporeal pump systems can be used for both circulatory support and rewarming.

Other warming methods include lavage of heated saline through nasogastric and thoracostomy tubes as well as peritoneal lavage, but are not as effective.

Coagulopathy

Coagulopathy is a frequent problem in the trauma patient who has received large volumes of crystalloid solution and blood for resuscitation. Although this problem is incompletely understood, it is clear that posttraumatic coagulation defects are multifactorial. The presence of shock, the fluid volume required for resuscitation, the presence of hypothermia (110), and preexisting diseases (e.g., liver, renal, or congenital coagulation disorders) all influence the likelihood and severity of coagulopathy.

The major factor in coagulopathy has been postulated to be the dilutional thrombocytopenia that occurs after massive volume resuscitation. Although bleeding times can be prolonged with platelet counts less than 100,000 cells/mL, platelet counts of 50,000 cells/mL or greater are usually adequate for surgical hemostasis. Dilutional thrombocytopenia becomes more likely with infusions of more than one blood volume. Each unit of platelets administered increases the platelet count by 10,000 to 15,000 cells/mL. Control of surgically remediable hemorrhage is prudent before platelet transfusion to prevent the loss of the transfused platelets into the surgical field.

Dilution of other coagulation factors also plays a role in development of coagulopathy. Factors V and VIII are the most labile in banked blood, but levels of less than 10% of normal for factors VII, X, XI, XII, and XIII are associated with abnormalities in hemostasis, as demonstrated by prolonged partial thromboplastin time and prothrombin time. Fresh frozen plasma can be administered as a source of all the soluble coagulation factors. The administration of cryoprecipitate may be necessary as a concentrated source of factor VIII and fibrinogen, particularly if adequate hemostasis is not obtained with the use of fresh frozen plasma.

Definitive Care Phase: Head Injuries

RANDALL M. CHESNUT

EPIDEMIOLOGY

Brain injury is the most common cause of death in trauma victims, accounting for approximately half of deaths at the accident site. The injuries usually are blunt, and motor vehicle accidents are the most frequent mechanism of injury. Of particular significance are motorcycle accidents involving unhelmeted passengers, which produce severe injuries. As many as two thirds of all motor vehicle accident victims sustain some head injury. Complications from closed head injuries are the single largest cause of morbidity and mortality in patients who reach the hospital alive. Of patients who require long-term rehabilitation, head trauma is usually the primary injury. These data are generally applicable to children as well. Although the mechanisms vary, head injuries are the major cause of morbidity and mortality in childhood trauma victims, accounting for an annual mortality rate of 1 per 1,000 in this age group.

PATHOPHYSIOLOGY

Traumatic injury to the brain involves a primary brain injury that occurs at impact and leads to disruption of brain substance and blood vessels. In addition, secondary brain injury may result from hypoxia, hypotension, the effects of increased intracranial pressure (ICP) and altered cellular biochemical processes.

Primary Injury

Energy transfer to the head causes direct disruption of neurons, glial cells, and microvasculature localized at the area of impact. As the brain accelerates within the skull, it is also vulnerable to impact with the opposite inner table. Therefore, contrecoup injury to the opposite underlying brain is relatively common. Diffuse axonal injury from brain distortion may lead to damage and disruption of deep brain structures. The brain is also subject to torsion injury resulting from rotation around the fixed brain stem. This type of injury can damage the reticular activating system, leading to unconsciousness. Intracranial hemorrhage results from disruption of bridging subdural veins and bleeding from cortical tissue damage (subdural hematoma), direct laceration of epidural arteries from impact fractures (epidural hematoma), or intraparenchymal bleeding (intracerebral contusion and hematoma). Bleeding and brain laceration from penetrating injuries are due to direct energy transfer. Whether direct impact causes contusion, subdural hematoma, epidural hematoma, or diffuse axonal injury, little can be done therapeutically to change the magnitude or location of the primary injury once it has occurred.

Secondary Injury

Secondary brain injuries result from events occurring after the primary insult, due either to the direct consequences of the process initiated by the primary injury or to deleterious outside influences. The occurrence and magnitude of secondary insults is often the determining factor in outcome from brain injury. Because, in contrast to primary injuries, secondary insults are amenable to medical management, they are the focus toward which the medical treatment of brain injury is directed.

Primary tissue injury initiates a variety of biochemical processes, including free radical-mediated lipid peroxidation, excitotoxic "superactivation" of glutamate–aspartate neurotransmitter systems, alterations in membrane receptor and ionic channel characteristics, and others. These events can proceed for significant periods after primary injury and often are self-sustaining. It is the goal of the numerous clinical trials involving treatment of brain trauma patients with various pharmacologic agents to determine means by which these processes may be attenuated or reversed.

The major external secondary injury processes after brain injury are hypotension and hypoxia. Hypotension is the number one treatable determinant of severe head injury. A single episode of systolic blood pressure less than 90 mm Hg during the period from injury through resuscitation doubles the mortality rate and significantly increases the morbidity of any given brain injury (111). Furthermore, an early hypotensive episode strongly increases the probability of later intracranial hypertension. It is for these reasons that rapid and complete restoration of blood pressure is the most important goal in the resuscitation of the brain-injured patient. This has led to the somewhat unconventional suggestion of using pressors as temporizing agents during volume resuscitation (111).

Hypoxia (apnea or cyanosis in the field or a $PaO_2 < 60$ mm Hg) is also an independent predictor of poor outcome. The frequency and magnitude of hypoxia have been notably decreased by modern airway management techniques, particularly early endotracheal intubation and assisted ventilation.

Intracranial Pressure

Intracranial pressure results from the aggregate volumes of brain, cerebrospinal fluid (CSF), and blood in the fixed intracranial compartment. Mild or slow expansion of one or two of these compartments can be buffered by compensatory decreases in either the CSF or blood compartments (into the spinal subarachnoid space or the venous sinuses, respectively). When this buffering capacity is exceeded, the compliance of the brain is compromised and small additional increases in intracranial volume produce marked elevations in ICP.

Intracranial hypertension may be considered deleterious through two somewhat separable mechanisms: herniation and ischemia. Herniation occurs when a pressure gradient exists across an incomplete barrier such as the tentorium or the falx cerebri. It is deleterious because of the tissue damage that obtains when herniation occurs. Transtentorial herniation is the most important of these and is manifest by anisocoria, motor posturing, autonomic disturbances, and death. The specter of herniation is the major determinant of the absolute threshold for ICP treatment, generally accepted as 20 to 25 mm Hg, although this has not been well defined scientifically. A major unanswered question is how ICP should be managed when considered independently from perfusion. The issues involve both risk of herniation and also whether there are detrimental effects of elevated pressure *per se*. It is the goal of ongoing research in the area of cerebral compliance that clinically useful information regarding these issues will result.

The second deleterious aspect of intracranial hypertension is that the resulting increase in resistance to cerebral blood flow (CBF) results in or exacerbates ischemia. This resistance can be roughly approximated by cerebral perfusion pressure (CPP), which is defined as the difference between arterial blood pressure and ICP:

CPP = mean arterial pressure – ICP

Under normal circumstances, cerebral vascular autoregulation maintains stable CBF over a wide range of CPP (approximately 50 to 150 mm Hg; Fig. 11.8). After injury to the brain, this autoregulation is usually disrupted. This disruption can be complete, resulting in a pressure-passive system (*straight dashed line* in Fig. 11.8). More frequently, the disruption is incomplete, characterized by a normal sigmoid shape but with abnormal elevation of the lower breakpoint above the normal value of 50 mm Hg *(sigmoid dashed line)*. A possible consequence of this disruption is that a CPP that is satisfactory for uninjured patients may be insufficient after head trauma (range of hypoperfusion).

In a pressure-passive system, cerebral blood volume (CBV) increases in proportion to CPP. In such an instance, the goal is to keep the CPP just above the level of cerebral ischemia, thereby minimizing iatrogenic intracranial hypertension caused by increased CBV. In the situation of incomplete disruption, the goal is to keep CPP within the range of autoregulation because this not only avoids ischemia but may decrease ICP if autoregulatory vasoconstriction in response to increased CPP decreases CBV.

Confounding this situation is the recent information that CBF may be significantly depressed during the early postinjury period. Therefore, it is particularly critical that CPP be supported assiduously from the first point of patient contact. Because hyperventilation causes vasoconstriction, thereby decreasing CBF, the use of hyperventilation during this early period is somewhat more hazardous than after the first 24 to 48 hours.

The preceding physiologic reasoning has given rise to "cerebral perfusion pressure therapy" wherein CPP is elevated to 70 mm Hg throughout the course of intracranial hypertension. The efficacy of CPP therapy has been suggested by studies without internal control subjects reporting decreased morbidity and mortality with CPP therapy compared with historical control subjects. The result of such reports has been that CPP-based therapy has become widely accepted as standard practice. Unfortunately, more recent reports suggest that such acceptance may have been premature. It appears that errors in selecting historical control groups for comparison with CPP-based therapy groups may prevent the ability to differentiate the impact of increasing CPP from simply avoiding in-hospital hypotensive episodes. When proper control groups are selected to address this deficiency, it appears that CPP-based therapy may be simply a proxy for avoidance of transient ischemia (112). Such a possibility is further supported by preliminary analysis of data from the National Institutes of Health-sponsored North American Brain Injury Study on Hypothermia, which suggests that episodes in which CPP falls below 50 mm Hg are much more highly correlated with outcome than maintaining CPP above 70 mm Hg (Guy Clifton, M.D., personal communication).

In addition, it appears that elevating CPP may increase the duration of intracranial hypertension (113,114). This might be due to the elevation of hydrostatic forces that favor formation of vasogenic edema, thereby prolonging brain swelling and ICP elevation. Finally, the results of a prospective, randomized investigation of CPP-based versus ICP-based management have suggested that there is no overall difference in outcome between the two strategies. The major effect of CPP-based therapy is the alteration in the mode of death, with ICP-related deaths being replaced by later mortality from systemic complications (especially respiratory distress syndrome) (Claudia Robertson, M.D., and Alex Valadka, M.D., personal communication). Such considerations imply that, although attention to CPP (and, thus, cerebral perfusion) is important, the proper method of managing CPP remains to be determined.

Ultimately, the goal of managing blood pressure and CBF is to maintain a level of perfusion that meets the metabolic cellular demands of the brain. The major problem with managing traumatic brain injury (TBI) based on pressure measurements is that relevant alterations in cerebral metabolism are missed. This is significant because the usual course after injury is for cerebral metabolism to decrease drastically, slowly returning toward normal in patients who improve. One implication of such a metabolic course is that CBF values that would be dangerous under

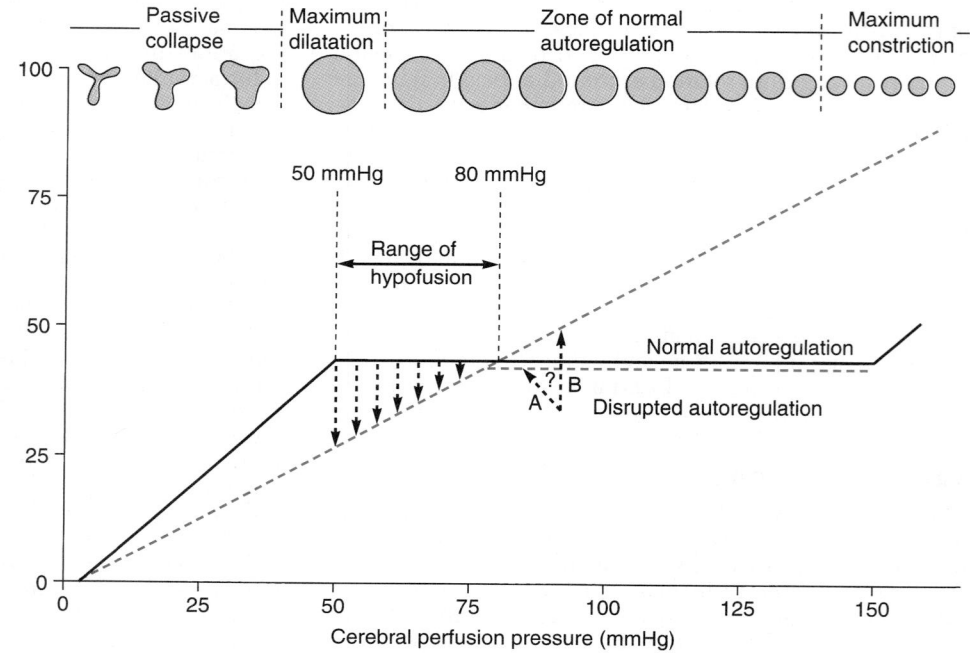

Figure 11.8. Cerebral pressure autoregulation. The normal relationship is indicated by the solid line with autoregulatory breakpoints at 50 and 150 mm Hg. Two disrupted states are also diagrammed. Complete loss of autoregulation *(line B)* results in a pressure-passive system wherein cerebral blood flow and cerebral blood volume (CBV) increase linearly with cerebral perfusion pressure. The more common form of disruption is indicated by the *sigmoid dashed line (line A),* where the major alteration is a right shift in the lower breakpoint. The circles at the top of the figure represent the diameters of the resistance vessels in the normal situation. The area of the circles represent CBV. Shifting this relationship to the right by 30 mm Hg represents the partially disrupted state. (© R.M. Chesnut, M.D., FCCM, reproduced with permission.)

normal metabolic conditions might be quite satisfactory when cerebral metabolism is depressed. Indeed, because metabolic autoregulation is usually preserved after TBI, low values of CBF might reflect flow–metabolism matching. One result of such a course of metabolic change might be that CPP elevation is reasonable during the early (i.e., first 12 to 24 hours) posttraumatic period when metabolism is near normal and ischemia is both probable and extremely devastating. Subsequently, when metabolic demands fall, CPP elevation may not be necessary and, indeed, may be counterproductive.

Unfortunately, metabolic information is not readily available in the clinical setting. The balance between metabolic needs and substrate delivery, however, often can be estimated by monitoring the oxygen saturation in the internal jugular vein ($JVSO_2$). Although limited by technical problems of averaging, incomplete sampling of the total cerebral tissue volume, and accuracy, the monitoring of $JVSO_2$ is a clinically useful method of detecting some otherwise occult episodes of ischemia as well as tailoring therapy to individual patient needs as they evolve (115). By monitoring arteriojugular lactate difference, occult areas of ischemia or anaerobic metabolism also can be detected and treatment changes made. We have found that combined monitoring of ICP, CPP, $JVSO_2$, arteriojugular lactate difference, and quantitative regional CBF [with cold xenon computed tomography (CT) CBF studies] has allowed individualized management of cerebral needs, thereby avoiding over- and undertreatment, minimizing the likelihood of iatrogenic injury, and shortening the intensive care unit (ICU) stay.

Treatment of hypertension is rarely indicated in the head-injured patient. There is no evidence that hypertension promotes continued intracranial hemorrhage, and hypertension related to brain injury usually resolves when the intracranial hypertension is controlled. When profound hypertension requires treatment, short-acting, selective β-adrenergic antagonists should be used. Vasodilators such as sodium nitroprusside should be avoided because they increase CBV.

As noted previously, metabolic autoregulation is the other and more fundamental type of intrinsic CBF control. Vasoconstriction is nonlinearly proportional to pH and, therefore, subject to manipulation of $PaCO_2$. As a result, hyperventilation-induced alkalosis produces vasoconstriction, resulting in a decrease of both CBF and CBV. Although the latter is beneficial in controlling ICP, the former is potentially deleterious and mandates caution when using hyperventilation. For reasons outlined earlier, hyperventilation is best avoided whenever possible during the early postinjury course when the risk of ischemia is extremely high.

Cerebral Edema and Osmolar Therapy (Mannitol)

Cerebral edema during the early postinjury period is usually cytotoxic (intracellular). Later, vasogenic (extracellular) edema may play a role in brain swelling. Although resulting from different mechanisms (cellular membrane dysfunction and blood–brain barrier breakdown), present treatment for cerebral edema is limited to the administration of osmotic agents, most commonly mannitol. Mannitol increases the osmotic gradient, drawing fluid from the interstitial compartment into plasma, thereby reducing brain volume. In regions where the blood–brain barrier has been disrupted, however, mannitol is minimally effective and may actually leak into tissues (116). Fortunately, the area of blood–brain barrier breakdown is usually much smaller than the area of edema that it creates, and mannitol is usually quite effective in lowering ICP.

Mannitol also has other mechanisms of action. It creates an acute increase in intravascular volume, which may transiently improve cardiac output and CBF. It also appears to cause acute and transient vasoconstriction as a result of its ability to decrease blood viscosity and improve flow. Both effects are more immediate than the osmotic effects and may be responsible for its early effects on ICP. They also may explain why mannitol is more effective in lowering ICP when administered as a bolus rather than as a slow infusion.

Unfortunately, mannitol can produce significant diuresis. The resulting hypovolemia can result in hypotension, not only producing secondary insult to the brain but causing intracranial hypertension due to autoregulatory vasodilatation. Evidence has suggested that the apparent relationship between early mannitol use and hypotensive episodes correlates with increased morbidity and mortality rates (117). Therefore, mannitol should be used only for proven or strongly suspected intracranial hypertension and should be avoided under conditions of hypovolemia, and fluid losses should be diligently replaced. Because lower doses of mannitol (0.25 g/kg) are just as efficacious as larger doses (1 g/kg) in lowering ICP, the lower doses should be used.

CLINICAL ASSESSMENT

The objectives during early clinical assessment of the head-injured patient are multiple and must be accomplished simultaneously. These include the establishment of adequate oxygenation, appropriate ventilation, and circulatory stability and evaluation of the extent of brain injury while treating ICP elevations. Although there is now some evidence that systemic hypotension may infrequently be the result of a head injury, the clinician must always presume initially that hypotension in a trauma patient is the result of hypovolemia. It is a significant error to withhold volume resuscitation in a misdirected effort to control cerebral edema. During initial assessment, mental status changes cannot be presumed to be the result of drugs or alcohol, although routine toxicology screening is appropriate. It should be presumed that any change in mental status or the neurologic examination, or any evidence of herniation (such as anisocoria) suggests an expanding intracranial mass lesion.

Table 11.7. GLASGOW COMA SCALE

Component	Score
Eye score	
Never open	1
Open to pain	2
Open to command	3
Open spontaneously	4
Verbal score	
No verbalizations	1
Garbled	2
Inappropriate	3
Confused	4
Oriented	5
Motor score	
No movement	1
Decerebrate posturing	2
Decorticate posturing	3
Withdraws to pain	4
Localizes pain	5
Obeys commands	6
Total score	3–15

From Teasdale G, Jennett B. Assessment of coma and impaired consciousness: a practical scale. Lancet 1974;2:81–84.

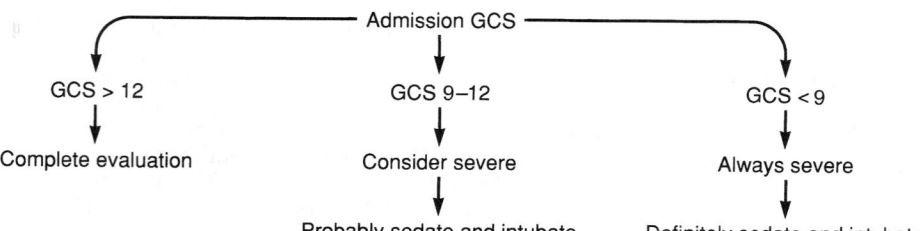

Figure 11.9. Glasgow Coma Scale (GCS) triage guide for initial evaluation of head injury. For the motor scale, the best response for any limb is recorded.

Under such circumstances, therapeutic ICP reduction becomes the first priority and emergency imaging or surgical decompression must be accomplished immediately.

Noxious stimuli such as urinary catheter, nasogastric tube, or vascular cannula placement can precipitate ICP peaks during resuscitation. These procedures, therefore, should be done quickly and efficiently, optimally after sedation.

With regard to the brain injury, several critical assessments are necessary and should be precisely recorded because trends are at least as important as any single observation. The three key parameters are level of consciousness, pupillary reflexes and size, and the motor examination.

Glasgow Coma Scale

The single most useful assessment for a head-injured patient is to evaluate the level of consciousness. In this regard, the Glasgow Coma Scale (GCS) has become an international standard that is easily, rapidly, and reliably obtained (Table 11.7). It is not, and was never intended to be, a neurologic examination and should not be substituted for this.

Glasgow Coma Scale components include assessment of eye opening, verbal response, and motor response. The routine use of GCS provides a useful measure of initial injury severity and allows stratification for initial therapy as well as for outcome analysis.

Patients can be stratified for triage purposes into those with severe injuries (GCS score of 8 or less), moderate injuries (GCS score of 8 to 12), or mild injuries (GCS score of more than 12; Fig. 11.9). Patients with severe head injuries require immediate endotracheal intubation, mechanical ventilation, and complete resuscitation, and any clinical evidence of intracranial hypertension (such as signs of herniation) mandates maximal therapy to decrease ICP.

Many significant injuries occur in patients with GCS scores between 8 and 12. Although this is defined as the moderate injury group, all these patients require maximal brain resuscitation until a definitive diagnosis can be made. A patient with a GCS of 12 or more tends to be confused but responsive to verbal stimulation. These patients need serial neurologic evaluations because this is the group who can "talk and die" because of missed or delayed intracranial pathologic processes. In general, however, whenever expedient, attention to other major injuries can take priority over cerebral imaging or management.

Pupils

Pupillary asymmetry, dilation, or loss of light reflex in an unconscious patient usually reflects herniation due to mass effect from intracranial hemorrhage ipsilateral to the dilated pupil. The probability of an intracranial mass lesion can be roughly approximated given the degree of anisocoria (1 or 3 mm), the mechanism of injury (± motor vehicle accident), and age (118) (Fig. 11.10). Occasionally, pupillary signs may indicate direct second or third nerve injury or trauma to the globe, but this must always be a diagnosis of exclusion. An unequal and nonreactive pupil is the cardinal sign that herniation is occurring and rapid lowering of ICP is essential. An ovoid pupil is also ominous and is associated with injuries that result in herniation in approximately 15% to 20% of patients.

Motor Examination

The motor system is examined for asymmetry, abnormal posturing, or lack of movement. Hemiparesis, paraparesis, or quadriparesis suggests a cervical or thoracolumbar spine fracture with spinal cord injury. Hemiparesis secondary to brain stem herniation due to mass effect may be either ipsilateral or contralateral to the side of the dilated pupil. Hemiparesis also may result from significant brain contusion. In the unconscious patient, a painful stimulus should be used to evaluate motor function. All four extremities should be examined and the results noted because only the response of the best limb is reflected in the GCS score.

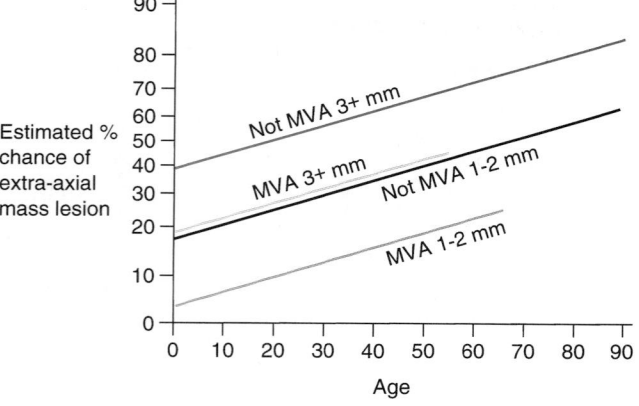

Figure 11.10. Estimated percentage chance of an extraaxial intracranial mass lesion greater than 25 cm³ as a function of degree of anisocoria, age, and mechanism of injury. Mechanism of injury was defined as motor vehicle accident (MVA) or other mechanism (Not MVA). (Reproduced from Chesnut RM, Gautille T, Blunt BA, et al. The localizing value of asymmetry in pupillary size in severe head injury: relation to lesion type and location. *Neurosurgery* 1994;34:840–845, with permission.)

INITIAL TREATMENT

Evidence-based Medicine and the Management of Traumatic Brain Injury

The recent publication of the Guidelines for the Management of Severe Brain Injury represents a significant step in standardizing the management of TBI based on published, peer-reviewed literature (119). This document represents the application of a strict evidence-based process to 14 topics relevant to TBI care. After an exhaustive, explicitly defined literature search covering each topic, the recovered literature was carefully classified along a three-point continuum. Each report was ranked as Class I, Class II, or Class III, depending on whether the data resulted from a randomized, prospective trail, well done retrospective analysis, or lesser but still valuable line of evidence. This process produced a set of Standards, Guidelines, and Options for treatment, where Standards (based on Class I evidence) represent principles with a high degree of clinical certainty, Guidelines (based on Class II evidence) reflect principles with a moderate degree of clinical certainty, and Options (based on Class III evidence) reflect principles for which there is unclear clinical certainty. By specifically defining the scientific foundation of 14 TBI management issues, the Guidelines for the Management of Severe Brain Injury provide an unbiased reference focused on facilitating scientific management of TBI. For details of this document, the reader is referred to the source document (119). Wherever applicable, the findings contained in the Guidelines for the Management of Severe Brain Injury have been incorporated into this text.

Early intracranial hypertension may certainly exert a detrimental influence on clinical outcome. At present, there is no technology for ICP measurement before the insertion of an ICP monitoring device. Unfortunately, all treatment modalities for intracranial hypertension have potentially serious complications, and many of them directly interfere with resuscitation procedures (e.g., use of diuretics). The efficacy of systemic resuscitation in improving the likelihood of survival from trauma is well accepted. In addition, the acknowledged negative influence of secondary insults such as hypotension and hypoxia on outcome from severe head injury render systemic resuscitation a *sine qua non* that provides a vital infrastructure on which treatment of intracranial hypertension must be based. Therefore, all treatment must be consistent with optimal systemic resuscitation. When signs of transtentorial herniation develop, they should be interpreted as definitive evidence of intracranial hypertension and prompt rapid and definitive treatment specifically focused on lowering ICP but maintaining physiologic resuscitation.

The composition and volume of the intravenous fluids used to resuscitate patients with head injuries should be selected with the purpose of restoring intravascular blood volume. Although the widely disseminated but scientifically unsupported adage of "keeping TBI patients dry" has been discarded, the concept of restricting free water remains desirable. Isotonic crystalloid solution in the form of 0.9% normal saline is preferable to lactated Ringer's solution as a resuscitation fluid for TBI. Furthermore, there is a growing body of scientific support for initiating the use of 250 mL of 7.5% normal saline as the initial resuscitation fluid in TBI victims (120–122).

The objectives of resuscitation do not depend on the presence or absence of a head injury. Blood volume should be normal, with an appropriate blood pressure, a normal central venous pressure, adequate urine output, good peripheral perfusion, and progressive improvement of any base deficit. The systolic blood pressure should not be allowed to drop below 90 mm Hg in adults. There is some evidence that there may be an advantage to targeting a mean arterial pressure of 90 to 100 mm Hg during resuscitation until ICP monitoring can be initiated. Once ICP data are available, a minimal CPP of 70 mm Hg should be the initial goal.

Resuscitation in the Absence of Clinical Signs of Herniation

An algorithm developed by the Oregon Health Sciences University based on the Guidelines for the Management of Severe Brain Injury for use by prehospital care providers and emergency physicians in Oregon is illustrated in Fig. 11.11. The algorithm is meant to guide decision making in resuscitating TBI victims and determining the necessity for ICP-lowering therapy. In addition, individual care providers can optimize their ability to accomplish eucapnea or mild hypocapnea by determining their individual Ambu-bag tidal volumes, calculating the ventilatory rate necessary for that tidal volume to deliver the proper minute ventilation (see later), and writing these values for infants, children, and adults of various weights on the pocket card.

Elevating the head of the bed (reverse Trendelenburg position in the absence of clearance of the axial skeleton) has been shown generally to lower the CPP in the absence of adequate volume resuscitation (123). Because this may elevate the ICP *per se,* it is not advised until complete resuscitation has been accomplished. The confusion and agitation often attendant to head injury render sedation desirable and can contribute to intracranial hypertension. Therefore, patients with suspected head injury usually should be sedated. Neuromuscular relaxation, however, has the notable effect of limiting the neurologic examination to the pupils and the CT scan. Therefore, in the absence of evidence of herniation, its use should be limited to situations where sedation alone is not sufficient for safe and efficient patient transport and resuscitation. When used, short-acting agents are strongly preferred. The prophylactic administration of mannitol is not recommended because of its volume-depleting diuretic effect. In addition, although it is desirable to achieve a low normal $PaCO_2$ during transport of a patient with suspected brain injury, the risk of exacerbating early ischemia by vigorous hyperventilation outweighs the questionable benefit to the patient without evidence of herniation. Therefore, ventilatory parameters consistent with optimal oxygenation and normal ventilation are recommended. The minute ventilation should be targeted at 100 mL/kg/min unless quantitative measurement of $ETCO_2$ or $PaCO_2$ is available. In the absence of signs of intracranial hypertension, ventilation should be adjusted to accomplish a $PaCO_2$ of 35 mm Hg when arterial gas values become available.

Resuscitation in the Presence of Clinical Signs of Herniation

Signs of intracranial hypertension consist of evidence of transtentorial herniation (pupillary dilation or loss of reactivity, motor posturing or flaccidity) or progressive neurologic deterioration not attributable to other causes (e.g., sedation). When such signs are present, aggressive treatment of intracranial hypertension is indicated. Hyperventilation should be accomplished by increasing the minute ventilation to 120 to 140 mL/kg/min. This does not depend on or interfere with successful volume resuscitation. Because hypotension can produce both neurologic deterioration and intracranial hypertension, the use of mannitol is less desirable unless adequate volume resuscitation has been accomplished. If such is the case, however, mannitol should be administered by bolus infusion. Under such circumstances, it is obviously critical that the diagnosis and treatment of the neurologic injury be accomplished with utmost haste.

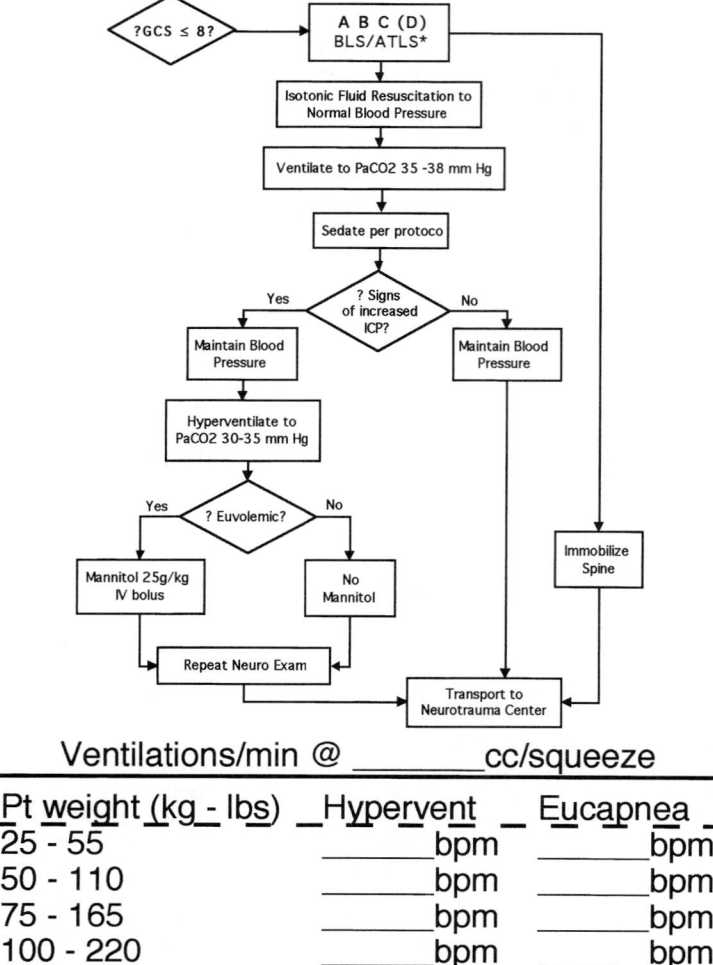

Figure 11.11. An algorithm developed for a pocket card to guide decision making in resuscitating traumatic brain injury (TBI) victims and determining the necessity of intracranial pressure (ICP)-lowering therapy. In addition, individual care providers can optimize their ability to accomplish eucapnea (100 mL/kg/min) or mild hypocapnea (120 to 140 mL/kg/min) by determining their individual Ambu-bag tidal volumes, calculating the ventilatory rate necessary for that tidal volume to deliver the proper minute ventilation, and writing these values for infants, children, and adults of various weights on the pocket card. (© R.M. Chesnut, M.D., FCCM, reproduced with permission.)

Ventilations/min @ _____cc/squeeze		
Pt weight (kg - lbs)	Hypervent	Eucapnea
25 - 55	_____bpm	_____bpm
50 - 110	_____bpm	_____bpm
75 - 165	_____bpm	_____bpm
100 - 220	_____bpm	_____bpm

Radiographic Priorities

Neurosurgical evaluation and assessment is initiated as soon as the potential for significant head injury is realized. Prompt radiographic evaluation is essential and CT scan is the imaging modality of choice for virtually all acute neurologic conditions. Patients with mild head injuries usually can be observed with sequential examinations, and radiographic evaluation may be unnecessary unless the results determine whether the patient can be discharged from the hospital. A very cogent argument, however, has been made for liberal application of CT scan, even to patients with minimal evidence of TBI, as a method of making safe, efficient, and economic triage decisions (124). In any instance, evidence of neurologic deterioration or the occurrence of a situation wherein the neurologic examination cannot be followed (e.g., the need for general anesthesia) mandates CT scan or intraoperative ICP monitoring.

In general, indications for neurologic imaging (usually CT scan) include the following:

- Suspected skull penetration by a foreign body
- Discharge of CSF, blood, or both from the nose
- Hemotympanum or discharge of blood or CSF from the ear
- Protracted unconsciousness
- Altered state of consciousness at the time of examination
- Focal neurologic signs or symptoms

- Any situation precluding proper surveillance
- Head injury plus additional trauma
- Possible head injury in the presence of additional pathologic findings, such as stroke
- Head injury with alcohol intoxication

Patients with moderate or severe injuries require prompt neurosurgical consultation and rapid radiographic evaluation using the CT scan. Hemodynamically stable patients with significant neurologic deterioration should go to the CT scanner immediately after Advanced Trauma Life Support resuscitation. In hemodynamically unstable patients who require immediate surgical intervention to sustain intravascular volume, exploratory thoracotomy or laparotomy must take precedence and measurement of ICP or air ventriculography can be performed concurrent with life-saving surgery. Treatment of significant intracranial mass lesions is initiated immediately on diagnosis.

The spine should be cleared radiographically or immobilized and protected in every patient with a severe head injury. Although only 13% of patients with severe head injuries have spinal cord injuries, the potentially devastating consequences of an overlooked spinal injury require constant vigilance.

Plain Skull Radiographs

With the routine availability of the CT scan, the use of plain skull radiography has diminished. Several authors have concluded that the presence of a fracture on a skull radiograph rarely influences treatment, does not reflect the severity of injury or predict outcome, and has seldom been a legal concern. On the other hand, the likelihood of an intracranial hematoma requiring surgical treatment is strongly correlated with the presence or absence of a skull fracture and a negative neurologic examination (125). Therefore, the value of skull films in head injury remains controversial.

In general, any patient meeting one of the aforementioned criteria should undergo CT imaging. Skull radiographs should be reserved for the patient with a mild head injury who has a negative neurologic examination, where the results of the skull radiographic study will alter the care plan (i.e., allow discharge from the hospital without a CT scan or determine the necessity for a CT scan). As noted previously, there is a growing body of evidence supporting more liberal use of CT imaging, which will obviate the use of plain skull radiographs except under circumstances where a CT scan is unobtainable.

If a CT scan is unavailable, lateral displacement of the calcified pineal gland of more than 2 mm from midline on a skull radiograph suggests a mass lesion. However, if there is suspicion of an intracranial pathologic process, more definitive diagnostic maneuvers are indicated.

Linear skull fractures appear as two radiolucent lines with sharp, well demarcated edges typically coursing from the point of impact on the calvarium toward the base of the skull. Significant depressed skull fractures are easily seen on plain frontal and lateral skull films. The mechanism of injury is usually a direct blow to the skull by a blunt object. Closed depressed skull fractures that are comminuted and those with a fragmented outer margin displaced beneath the inner table usually have been treated surgically, although there is growing evidence that many may be treated nonoperatively if there is no neurologic dysfunction or CT scan evidence of underlying tissue injury. Open fractures are also usually treated surgically, although, again, there is growing evidence that fresh, noncomminuted fractures without neurologic deficit, CSF or brain extrusion, gross contamination, or underlying tissue injury can be closed and treated with prophylactic antibiotics.

Basilar skull fractures are usually diagnosed from clinical evidence because they are poorly visualized on plain films. Only approximately 20% of patients with clinical evidence of basilar skull fractures have discernible injury on plain skull radiographs. These clinical signs include otorrhea or rhinorrhea, subcutaneous ecchymoses overlying the mastoid region (Battle's sign), bilateral periorbital ecchymoses (raccoon eyes), or hematotympanum. A basilar skull fracture may involve the paranasal sinuses, piriform sinus, petrous bone, sphenoid sinus, or sella turcica. Injury to adjacent structures, such as the seventh or eighth cranial nerves, brain stem, and carotid or basilar artery, are not uncommon. Basilar skull fractures are usually visualized on CT scan, although special protocols may be required. In the acute situation, no specific therapy is indicated. A CSF leak should not be tamponaded unless associated bleeding is brisk, and antibiotics should not be administered for the purpose of prophylaxis of meningitis.

Computed Tomography

The CT scan finding that correlates most with intracranial hypertension is compression or obliteration of the basilar cisterns (Fig. 11.12). Not only does this finding portend a stormy ICP course, but the primary predictor of outcome in patients with this CT picture is the peak level of intracranial hypertension occurring during the first 72 hours (126,127). When cisternal compression is coincident with a midline shift of greater than 5 mm, the prognosis is even more ominous. ICP monitoring should be im-

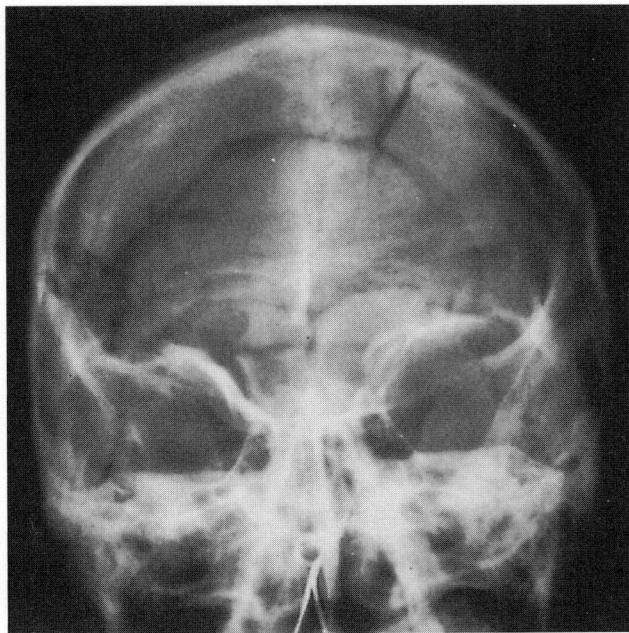

Figure 11.12. A computed tomography scan that is highly predictive of intracranial hypertension. The basilar cisterns are obliterated and the sulci are flattened.

mediately initiated in any patient with cisternal compression, and intracranial hypertension vigorously treated. These patients, particularly those with minimal evidence of parenchymal contusion, die primarily from secondary insults, suggesting that they are potentially salvageable.

Acute epidural hematomas correlate well with skull fractures. The most common association is a linear, nondisplaced fracture in the temporoparietal region, crossing the middle meningeal artery. The classic clinical course involves a lucid interval after a brief loss of consciousness with subsequent neurologic deterioration. However, such a course occurs in fewer than 50% of patients with epidural hematoma, so clinical suspicions must remain high. The typical CT scan appearance of an epidural hematoma is a high- or mixed-density concave extraaxial mass with smooth borders (Fig. 11.13).

Acute subdural hematomas occur over the convexity of the brain. The hematoma may evolve because of rupture of bridging cortical veins or bleeding from the underlying parenchymal injury, which is common. It is this subjacent tissue damage that usually determines the neurologic outcome of patients not succumbing to intracranial hypertension. On CT scan, a subdural hematoma appears as an extraaxial, high- or mixed-density crescentic mass that spreads out over the hemisphere, following the cortical irregularities (Fig. 11.14). The midline shift may be out of proportion to the size of the hematoma because of the contributing mass effect from an underlying brain contusion or hemispheric swelling.

Intracerebral hemorrhage and cerebral contusion are common after trauma and are readily visualized on CT scan. Brain contusion appears as a focal, heterogeneous density with hemorrhage interspersed with injured tissue (Fig. 11.15). Intracerebral hematomas are usually more homogeneous in their high-density appearance. These lesions tend to "blossom" over time because of continued hemorrhage and the development of edema. Therefore, it is important closely to observe and monitor the ICP of such patients because significant and hazardous mass effect may evolve, requiring surgical treatment.

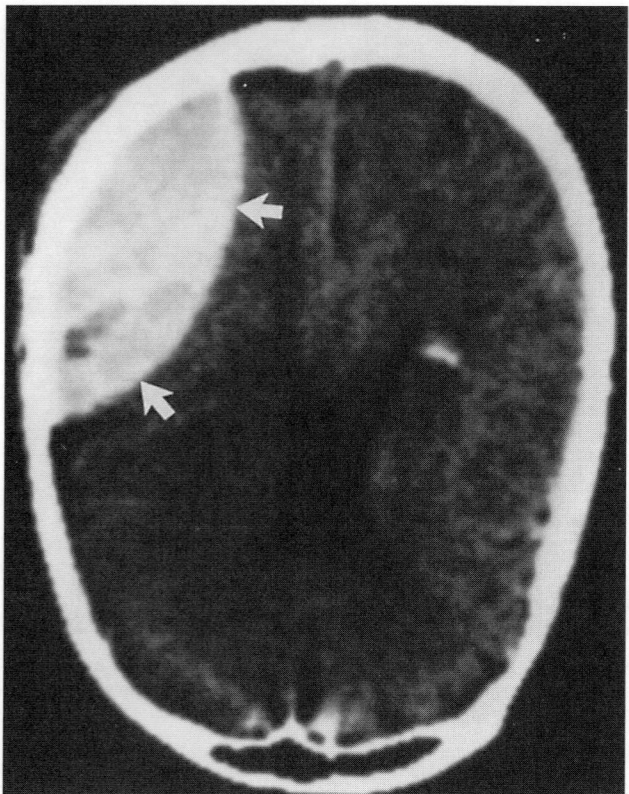

Figure 11.13. Typical computed tomography scan appearance of mixed-density, lens-shaped, acute epidural hematoma with mass effect.

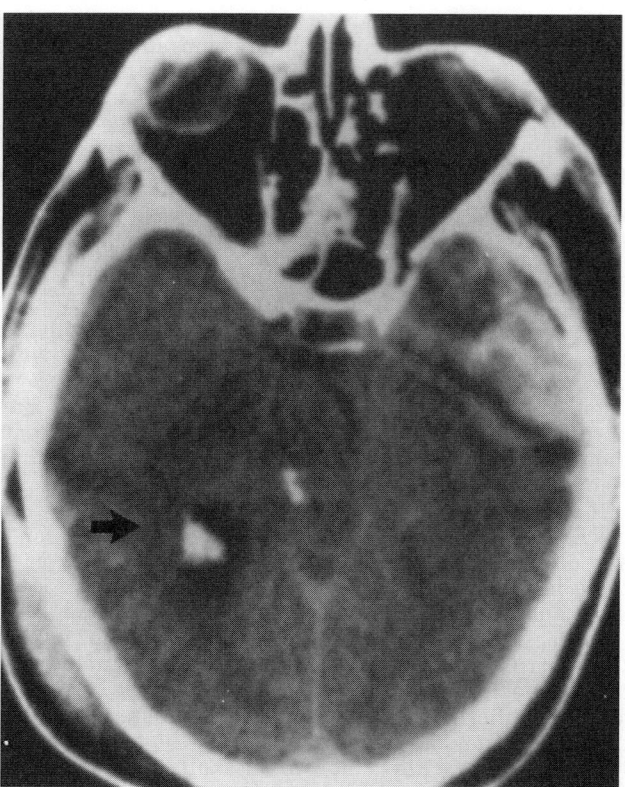

Figure 11.15. Contusion and associated intracerebral hematoma in the frontotemporal area.

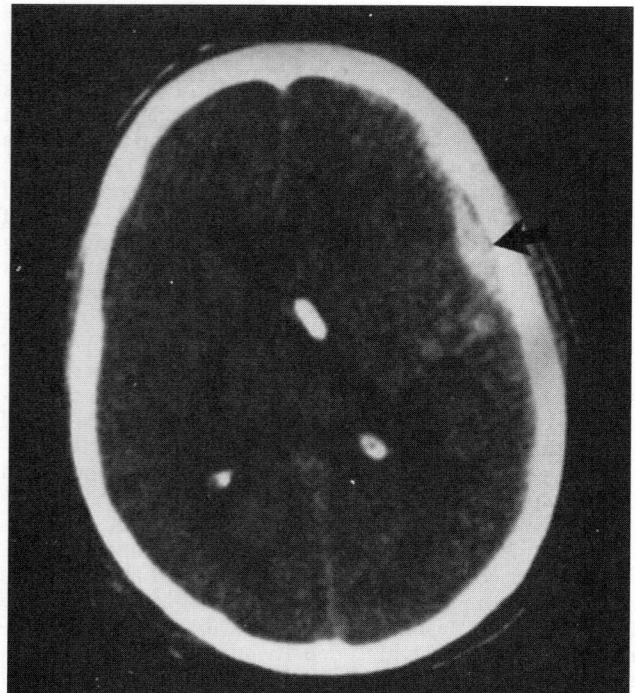

Figure 11.14. Usual computed tomography scan appearance of a crescent-shaped, high-density blood collection conforming to the contour of the cerebral hemisphere in a subdural hematoma.

The typical CT scan appearance of subarachnoid hemorrhage is a layer of blood over the cerebral cortex, layering over the tentorium and commonly filling the basal cisterns. Cerebral edema appears as areas of decreased density that may be either focal or diffuse. Posttraumatic edema formation usually takes hours to days to develop unless compounded by hypoxia or hypotension. The "swollen brain" commonly seen in the setting of trauma may be due to edema or increased CBV (unclotted, intravascular blood is low density). Diffuse axonal injury, typical of acute acceleration–deceleration injury, appears on CT scan as cerebral swelling and small areas of focal hemorrhage in the brain stem, thalamus, deep nuclear region, or corpus callosum, as well as in the hemispheric white matter. Finally, gunshot wounds or other penetrating injuries can be evaluated with CT scan to allow accurate preoperative assessment of the anatomic injury for prognostic and therapeutic planning purposes.

One significant issue of recent origin is the "blossoming" or appearance of new lesions subsequent to CT images obtained at very short intervals after injury. Reports as recent as the early to mid-1990s often presented initial CT scan data from studies done hours after trauma. With improved prehospital transport and the ready availability of CT imaging, many initial studies are now performed 15 to 30 minutes after injury. As a result of such "ultra-early" CT scans, there is now a risk of missing significant intracranial lesions because imaging is completed before their appearance or during an early phase of their evolution. For this reason, any patient with an intracranial lesion or intracranial hypertension should routinely have an early follow-up CT scan 4 to 6 hours after admission. At this time, CT imaging of the cervical spine also can be done in an effort to facilitate its clearance.

DEFINITIVE MANAGEMENT

Surgical Decompression and Outcome

The objective of management for acute subdural or epidural hematomas is emergent surgical decompression. The timing of decompression is critical; delay of more than 4 hours is associated with a poorer outcome (128). The possibility of a mass lesion must be entertained in any patient who shows evidence of herniation. Under optimal circumstances, this herniation can be reversed medically (with hyperventilation and mannitol), allowing an emergent CT scan that will demonstrate not only the location and size of any intracranial mass lesions, but which patients are herniating because of diffuse, nonsurgical processes.

When CT scan is not immediately available or herniation is refractory to medical management, emergency trephination is a useful and life-saving option. The first bur hole is placed in the ipsilateral temporal region and the dural mater is opened if an epidural hematoma is not in evidence (Fig. 11.16). If this exploration is negative, a second hole is placed in the opposite temporal region. If this is unrewarding, serial trephines are performed in the region of the parietal boss and the frontal convexity, first on the ipsilateral side, then contralaterally. A bur hole exploration is not negative until six holes have been drilled. A positive trephine is turned into a craniotomy and the hematoma is thoroughly evacuated.

Epidural hematomas are frequently of arterial origin and have a tendency to expand. Prognosis varies directly with level of consciousness at time of surgery, ranging from 0% for patients conscious throughout, to 27% with the classic lucid interval, to over 50% if the patient never regains consciousness. Given these data, epidural hematomas should almost uniformly undergo immediate surgical evacuation. Such an approach has resulted in an overall mortality rate of approximately 9% (127).

Subdural hematomas are more common, particularly in non-motor vehicle trauma. For subdural hematomas, the prognosis is less optimistic, with mortality rates of approximately 50%. To a great extent, this is related to the often significant injury to the underlying brain. Subdural hematomas with mass effect (i.e., midline shift > 5 mm) usually should be evacuated. Some smaller lesions may be managed medically and often disappear over a relatively short time.

Cerebral contusions and intracerebral hematomas are usually treated operatively when mass effect results in intracranial hypertension or signs of herniation. When such lesions are located in the temporal lobe, however, there is a risk of precipitous herniation without impressive ICP elevation because of the confining nature of the middle cranial fossa and the direct apposition of the temporal lobe to the brain stem and tentorial incisura. For this reason, many trauma neurosurgeons are much more aggressive with surgical débridement of temporal contusions than similar lesions in other locations.

Diffuse brain injury has a mortality rate that is directly related to the significance of the associated intracranial hypertension. As such, the mortality rate of diffuse injury with open basilar cisterns is approximately 13%, whereas compression or absence of cisterns has an associated mortality rate of approximately 38%. Diffuse injuries are not amenable to surgical therapy unless decompressive craniectomy is indicated for control of intractable intracranial hypertension.

Intracranial Pressure Monitoring

All patients with severe brain injuries and a significant percentage of those with moderate injuries should have continuous monitoring of ICP. The Guidelines for the Management of Severe Brain Injury indicate that Class II evidence supports monitoring of all patients with a postresuscitation GCS score of 8 who either have any CT scan evidence of intracranial lesions or who have a negative CT scan but two or three of the following: (a) age greater than 40 years, (b) any history of hypotension, or (c) abnormal motor posturing. The use of ICP monitoring in other patients is considered discretionary. ICP monitoring should be considered in any patient with a GCS score of 12 who cannot be closely monitored clinically or whose CT scan demonstrates evidence of intracranial hypertension (i.e., mass lesion, obscured or absent basal cisterns, or midline shift).

Although many ICP monitoring techniques are available, the most common involve small fiberoptic or strain-gauge catheter tip pressure sensors placed millimeters into the brain. Fluid-coupled catheters are also placed into the lateral ventricles. The minimally invasive catheters are reliable and have a very low complication rate, making them an ideal choice in instances where a minimum-risk ICP monitoring technique is desired (e.g., in a moderate head injury in a patient who needs general anesthesia). They are also useful when the ventricles are too small to cannulate or there is an uncorrected coagulopathy. Ventriculostomy catheters have the added capability of allowing CSF drainage for ICP control. However, they are technically more difficult to place and the complication rate is somewhat higher. In any case, there is a monitoring technology available for any instance in which ICP monitoring is desired. Monitoring ICP not only provides early warning of herniation but, by allowing calculation of CPP, offers the possibility of more precisely optimizing CBF and preventing ischemic secondary brain injury.

Medical Management

Aggressive restoration of intravascular volume, maintenance of adequate CPP, and avoidance of hypoxia are fundamental to the medical treatment for intracranial hypertension. In addition, control of pain and the response to noxious stimuli, detection and treatment of seizures, and management of hypermetabolism (e.g., fever) are necessary. Venous drainage of the brain should be facilitated by

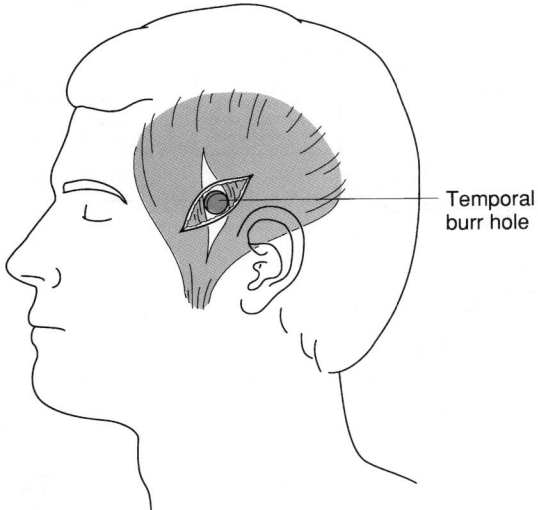

Figure 11.16. Location for placement of initial exploratory bur hole in the temporal region for emergency diagnosis and decompression.

Temporal burr hole

avoiding constriction of the jugular system in the neck and elevating the head of the bed in euvolemic patients. In addition, attention should be paid to intrathoracic pressures, particularly when the use of positive end-expiratory pressure or continuous positive airway pressure is entertained. Finally, meticulous systemic critical care is vital because the ICU stay and the associated needs of endotracheal intubation, mechanical ventilation, and other artificial support significantly increase the risk of nosocomial and iatrogenic complications.

Cerebrospinal fluid drainage, hyperventilation, and the administration of mannitol and barbiturates are the mainstays of therapy to control documented intracranial hypertension. However, each has significant potential complications that can obviate the beneficial effects. Therefore, they should not be used unless intracranial hypertension is demonstrated by monitoring. Caution and vigilance must attend their use. Although the treatment of intracranial hypertension is not the primary focus of this chapter, some brief comments are useful.

The algorithm contained in the Guidelines for the Management of Severe Brain Injury for treating intracranial hypertension is shown in Fig. 11.17. When consulting this algorithm, it should be remembered that it represents a consensus opinion (Class III evidence).

The initial treatment of intracranial hypertension should include adequate sedation and analgesia, control of fever, and optimization of systemic physiologic conditions that might exacerbate ICP elevation (e.g., intrathoracic pressure).

Neuromuscular blockade should be considered if these treatments are not effective. However, the value of interruption of paralysis to recheck the neurologic examination must be kept in mind when neuromuscular blockade is initiated.

When available through ventriculostomy, CSF external drainage should be the first method of managing intracranial hypertension. There is no consensus on what pattern of drainage is most effective. ICP measurement cannot be performed when the ventricular catheter is open to drain. For this reason, we usually drain against approximately 10 cm H_2O resistance for 2-minute intervals, then reclamp the catheter and measure the ICP.

As discussed previously, mannitol is a useful tool for treating intracranial hypertension. There are no specific physiologic indications for the use of mannitol over other agents. Mannitol should be avoided under conditions of hypovolemia or increased serum osmolarity (>320 mOsm/L). When administered, mannitol should be given as a bolus. It appears that lower doses (e.g., 0.25 g/kg) are just as effective in lowering ICP as larger doses (e.g., 1 g/kg) (119).

Hyperventilation is usually effective at lowering ICP. As noted, however, it works by vasoconstriction-induced decreases in CBV, which allows the possibility of inducing ischemia by diminishing CBF. At present, there is no clinically applicable method for measuring CBV, and it is unclear how often elevated CBV *per se* is a primary physiologic abnormality in intracranial hypertension. Therefore, lowering CBV to treat intracranial hypertension includes risks that need be minimized. In general, hyperventilation

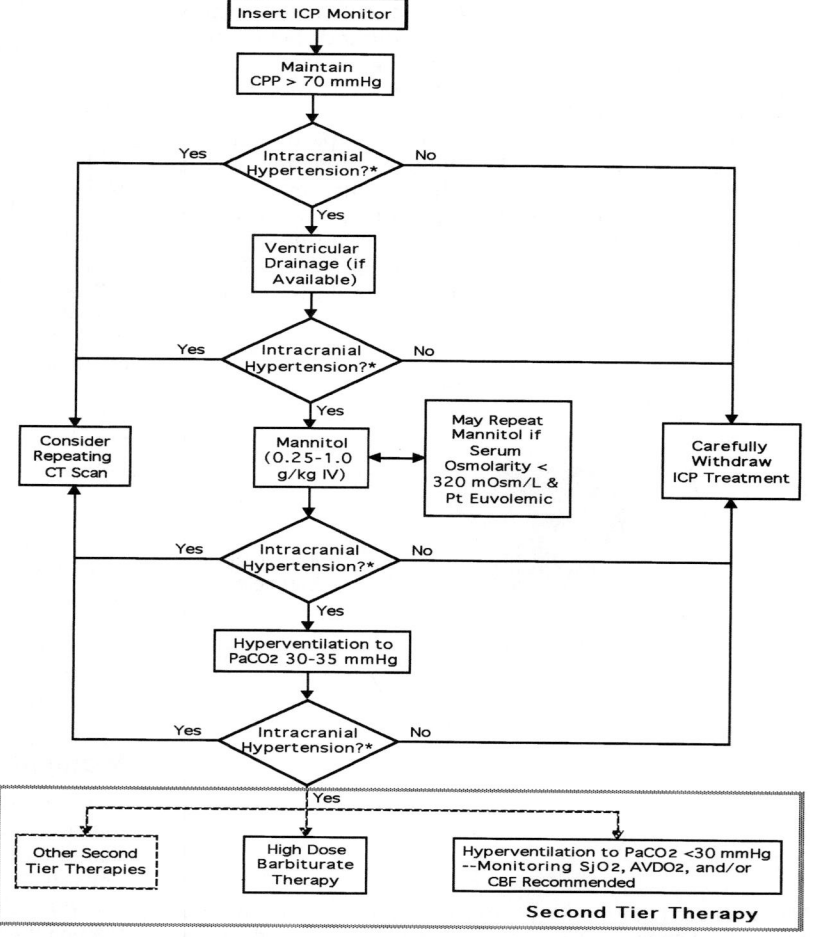

Figure 11.17. The algorithm from the Guidelines for the Management of Severe Brain Injury illustrating an approach to the early care of the patient with severe traumatic brain injury (TBI), developed by consensus. The necessity of ensuring the ABCs (airway, breathing, and circulation) is stressed, emphasizing the establishment of a satisfactory cerebral perfusion pressure. The decision tree for administering mannitol or using hyperventilation is also illustrated. The importance of safely and quickly obtaining a computed tomography (CT) scan of the brain in directing the choice between surgery or intracranial pressure (ICP) monitoring should be noted. (From Bullock R, Chesnut RM, Clifton G, et al. *J Neurotrauma* 1996;13:639–734, with permission.)

* Threshold of 20-25 mmHg may be used. Other values may be substituted in individual conditions.

Table 11.8. MODIFIED THERAPEUTIC INTENSITY LEVEL

Treatment	Score
Sedation/neuromuscular blockade	1
Ventricular drainage	1
Mannitol (1 g/kg/h)	2
Mannitol (>1 g/kg/h)	4
Pressors/inotropes for cerebral perfusion pressure management	2
Hyperventilation ($PaCO_2$ 30–35 mm Hg)	4
Vigorous hyperventilation ($PaCO_2$ <30 mm Hg)	6
Barbiturate/propofol coma	15
Hypothermia	15
Surgical decompression	15

($PaCO_2$ <35 mm Hg) should be avoided during the first 24 hours after TBI (119). Thereafter, if intracranial hypertension continues, hyperventilation to $PaCO_2$ values between 30 and 35 mm Hg may be considered. Whenever hyperventilation is used, and certainly when $PaCO_2$ values of less than 30 mm Hg are targeted, methods of monitoring the effects on CBF or flow–perfusion matching should be considered. These include quantitative CBF measurement, jugular venous saturation monitoring, and following cerebral tissue oxygen saturation.

Although controversial, decompressive craniotomy appears to be useful in achieving survival in patients without devastating primary brain injury who are succumbing to secondary brain injury related to intracranial hypertension. Decompressive craniotomy should be considered in patients when ICP elevations become refractory to medical management, when the rate of rise of the hourly therapeutic intensity level (Table 11.8) presages refractory ICP, or the risk–benefit ratio of ongoing therapy for intracranial hypertension appears unfavorable. The latter is a difficult clinical judgment, but a very important issue because putting the patient through a very complex ICP management course through the use of extreme medical maneuvers (e.g., barbiturate coma), only to lose the patient to respiratory distress syndrome, is not a satisfactory outcome.

Although we are just beginning to understand the pathophysiologic mechanisms involved in TBI and the optimal way to manipulate them, the burgeoning number of systems now amenable to monitoring various aspects of cerebral physiology present a very encouraging picture for the future. It appears that through the application of excellent critical care and unified trauma management approaches from the field through hospital discharge, we can minimize the effects of the primary brain injury, avoid secondary injuries, and achieve substantial improvements in recovery from severe TBI.

Definitive Care Phase: Maxillofacial Injuries

LISA A. ORLOFF

The major causes of maxillofacial trauma are motor vehicle accidents, direct assault, industrial injuries, sports-related injuries, and low- and high-velocity gunshot injuries. Maxillofacial injuries are present in one third of se-

riously injured patients with multisystem trauma (129), and such injuries can be life threatening. Airway compromise and hemorrhage are immediate concerns in patients with maxillofacial trauma; associated brain and cervical spine injuries must be sought and recognized, and appropriate timing of treatment must be coordinated with care of trunk and extremity injuries. An awareness of maxillofacial anatomy and dynamics is essential to effect survival from acute injuries and to restore normal form and function.

ANATOMY

Maxillofacial trauma constitutes most extracranial head injuries. Facial skeletal fractures and soft-tissue damage in the frontal, orbital, nasal, zygomatic, maxillary, and mandibular regions are included. Ocular trauma, a specific form of maxillofacial injury that is the province of the ophthalmologic surgeon, is not discussed here.

The frontal bone, which houses the frontal sinuses, is particularly strong because of its arched configuration and its thick, hard bone. Up to 2,200 lb. of force is necessary to fracture the frontal sinus; this force is two to three times greater than that required to fracture other facial bones (130). The frontal sinus is fully developed by approximately 19 years of age, but its size and degree of pneumatization are variable. The thick anterior wall makes up the central inferior portion of the forehead. The inferior wall or floor of the sinus is the roof of the orbit. The thin posterior wall abuts the frontal lobe of the brain. The frontonasal duct communicates with the nasal cavity.

The nasoethmoid complex, located at the junction of the frontal, nasal, lacrimal, and ethmoid bones and sinuses, is susceptible to compression and collapse during blunt facial trauma. The medial canthal tendons and the nasolacrimal drainage system are also vulnerable. Injury to these structures can result in telecanthus (widening of the intercanthal distance) and lacrimal dysfunction. Cerebrospinal fluid (CSF) rhinorrhea and anosmia secondary to cribriform plate or ethmoidal roof disruption with olfactory tract damage should be suspected.

The orbit comprises seven bones: frontal, zygoma, maxilla, lacrimal, ethmoid, sphenoid, and palatine. The four walls of the orbit form a pyramid, with its base anteriorly at the level of the eyelids and its apex posteriorly at the optic foramen. The lateral and superior walls are strong and are not easily fractured. On the other hand, the orbital floor (or roof of the maxillary sinus) and medial wall (mostly lamina papyracea) are thin and easily fractured. The orbital rims themselves are sturdy and protect the globe. Bony fragments of the orbit can impinge on the optic nerve or on the ophthalmic and retinal arteries and veins, especially at the orbital apex. Extraocular muscles, especially the inferior rectus, can become entrapped between bone fragments, limiting ocular movement.

The nasal bones are the most commonly fractured bones in the body. If injury to the nose is not detected and corrected, nasal obstruction and deformity can result. Traumatic epistaxis or nose bleeding can occur with blunt midface trauma with or without fracture of the nose. The thin, paired nasal bones project like a tent on the frontal process of the maxilla. The internal nasal septum provides tenuous support and is frequently injured.

The blood supply to the nose derives from the internal and external carotid arteries. The external carotid gives off the maxillary artery, whose sphenopalatine and descending pharyngeal branches supply the nose and ethmoid and maxillary sinuses, and the facial artery, whose superior labial branch supplies the anterior inferior nasal cavity. The internal carotid artery gives off the ophthalmic artery, which in turn sends anterior and posterior ethmoidal arteries to the nose. The most common sites of epistaxis are along the anterior septum (the Kiesselbach or Little area) and behind the middle turbinate. However, any midface fractures and associated mucosal lacerations can present with epistaxis.

The zygoma is divided into the zygomatic arch and the malar bone. The zygoma articulates with the frontal, maxillary, temporal, and sphenoid bones. Predictable fracture patterns result from specific forces on the zygoma. Posterolateral blows cause zygomatic arch fractures. More anterior blows to the zygoma cause tripod (or trimalar) fractures, so called because of the three main fracture sites: the frontozygomatic suture line, the maxilla along the infraorbital rim, and the zygomatic arch.

The maxilla serves as a shock absorber for the skull and the cranial cavity. It is connected to the skull by the palatine bone, the zygoma, and the nasal processes. Consistent fracture patterns from blows to the maxilla, first classified by LeFort in 1901 (131), occur in and along the maxilla at its junction with the weaker and aerated bone of the paranasal sinuses and nasal cavity. Significant force is required to produce such fractures, and they are most often the result of motor vehicle accidents. With increased survival from automobile accidents, mainly as a result of increased seat belt use, has come an increased frequency of maxillofacial or LeFort fractures, perhaps because the upper torso and face are not completely restrained. The more recent addition of airbags to automobiles may result in a decrease in the incidence of facial fractures, although cases of facial trauma have been reported that have been the direct result of airbag deployment. The classic LeFort fractures are defined as follows (Fig. 11.18):

LeFort I: The fracture line runs along the floor of the maxillary sinus and posteriorly along the maxillary tubercle and into the pterygoid plates. A mid-palatal split fracture, running anteroposteriorly, may be present.

LeFort II: Also called a *pyramidal fracture,* the apex of the fracture runs across the nasofrontal suture line; the fracture lines then run down the lamina papyracea of the ethmoid bone, across the orbital floor, and around the zygoma to the pterygoid plates.

LeFort III: Also known as *craniofacial dysjunction,* this fracture runs through all buttresses connecting the maxilla to the skull. Separation occurs across the root of the nose near the cribriform plate, across the frontoethmoidal suture and superior orbit to the region of the frontozygomatic suture, across the temporal fossa

to the pterygomaxillary space, and usually across the base of the pterygoid plates. The cribriform plate, ethmoidal arteries, optic nerve, and internal maxillary artery are all vulnerable in such fractures. The patient has a characteristic "mule" face, but initially this may not be obvious because of facial edema.

In practice, LeFort fractures are frequently asymmetric, mixed, or impure. For instance, there may be a "hemi-LeFort II" fracture, or a mixed LeFort I fracture on one side and a LeFort II fracture on the other side of the face.

The mandible is the second most frequently fractured facial bone, after the nasal bones. The configuration of an open arch, the position on the face, and the tendency to atrophy with age and the edentulous state make the mandible especially vulnerable to trauma. The most common cause of mandible fractures is interpersonal violence, especially among men. Mandible fractures are uncommon in children and are usually caused by child abuse or falls. Motor vehicle accidents account for most of the remaining mandible fractures. Sports injuries (even boxing) account for only 2% of mandible fractures (132). The sites of fracture, in decreasing order of frequency, are the body, angle, condylar neck, symphysis and parasymphysis, ramus, and alveolar ridge. Multiple fractures occur in 53% of cases (133). Although discussion of dental injuries is beyond the scope of this chapter, knowledge of dental anatomy is essential in the management of mandible injuries. The universal numbering system of permanent dentition and the Angle classification of occlusion facilitate description of injuries, planning of repair, and prediction of outcome.

Soft-tissue injuries of the face are encountered even more often than facial fractures. Such injuries can be devastating, both functionally and cosmetically. Surgical management of soft-tissue injuries requires attention to details of superficial anatomy in addition to awareness of subcutaneous structures.

The facial nerve is the most important underlying structure at risk because blunt or penetrating trauma to the facial nerve trunk or branches can cause complete or partial ipsilateral facial paralysis. The most common cause of facial nerve injury is fracture of the temporal bone (134), but injury can occur anywhere from the intracranial to the external facial course of the nerve. After exiting the stylomastoid foramen, the facial nerve trunk enters the parotid gland and divides into temporal, zygomatic, buccal, marginal mandibular, and cervical branches. Injuries to the middle branches distal to the parotid rarely result in significant deficit, but the temporal and marginal mandibular branches have the least cross-innervation with other branches, so they are vulnerable throughout their course.

In general, nonpenetrating trauma to the extracranial facial nerve is managed conservatively by expectant observation. Penetrating injuries are best repaired at the time of wound débridement and closure. If primary neurorrhaphy is not feasible, interposition grafts (usually from the greater auricular nerve or sural nerve) may be necessary.

EARLY CONSIDERATIONS

Initial priority in the patient with maxillofacial trauma, as in any trauma victim, must be directed at performing an efficient and orderly physical examination and stabilizing life-threatening problems. Because the airway is in the midst of the maxillofacial region, confirming and securing airway support may immediately lead to identification of maxillofacial injuries. Facial skeletal instability, soft-tissue edema, and hemorrhage can hinder airway access. Teeth and blood may be aspirated, contributing to respiratory distress. If a patient cannot be safely intubated by ei-

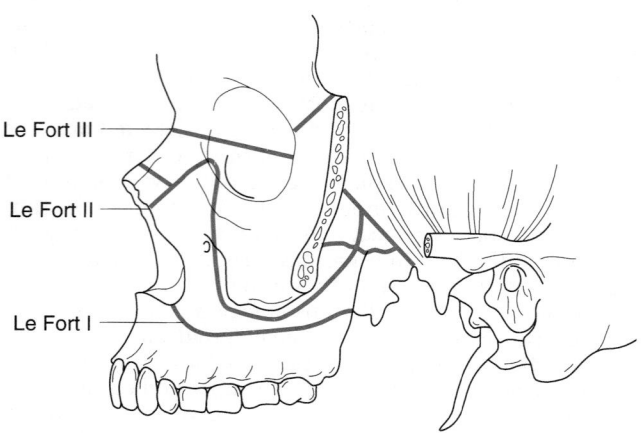

Figure 11.18. LeFort classification system of maxillofacial fractures.

ther the orotracheal or the nasotracheal route, a tracheotomy or cricothyrotomy may be necessary. Although initial airway control should be obtained by the simplest and most direct route, management of midface and mandibular injuries may necessitate subsequent tracheotomy in the definitive phase of management.

Two percent to 4% of patients with maxillofacial injuries have concomitant cervical spine fractures (135). Throughout the initial resuscitation and until proven otherwise, the patient with maxillofacial injuries should be treated as if the cervical spine is unstable. Any airway access maneuvers must be performed with attention toward maintaining in-line traction on the cervical spine.

Bleeding from facial injuries, especially in conjunction with blood loss from additional injuries, can be life threatening and warrants immediate attention. Direct pressure can be applied to external sites of bleeding, but intranasal and pharyngeal hemorrhage are usually best treated initially by packing. However, packing of nasoethmoid or cribriform plate fractures can lead to direct intracranial injury. In this situation, a combined craniofacial approach to fracture reduction, dural repair, and control of epistaxis and rhinorrhea may be required.

Most nosebleeds come from anterior intranasal vessels. These can be controlled with anterior nasal packs consisting of 0.5- or 1-inch wide gauze impregnated with antibiotic ointment. In the conscious patient, the nasal mucosa is vasoconstricted and anesthetized topically with oxymetazoline (Neo-Synephrine; Sanofi Winthrop Pharmaceuticals, New York, NY) and tetracaine (Pontocaine; Sanofi Winthrop Pharmaceuticals) or 4% cocaine. Gauze is then layered into the nose, starting inferiorly along the floor and packing superiorly. The tail of gauze is brought out anteriorly to facilitate pack removal in 3 to 5 days. Various prefabricated nasal packs are often available in emergency departments.

Posterior nasal bleeding requires posterior packing for control. A no. 16 or 18 Foley catheter can be inserted through the nose into the nasopharynx; the balloon is then inflated with 10 to 15 mL of saline solution, and the catheter is pulled anteriorly against the vomer and sphenoid rostrum in the posterior naris. An anterior pack is then inserted to abut the Foley balloon. The catheter is secured anteriorly with a clamp, dental roll, or piece of plastic tubing, with care taken to avoid pressure on the nasal ala or columella. The packs are removed in 3 to 5 days. Whenever a posterior pack is in place, the patient must be monitored for potential airway obstruction and hypoxemia.

Epistaxis that fails to respond to nasal packing requires more invasive management. Endoscopic cauterization may successfully control superficial bleeding. Surgical ligation of the anterior and posterior ethmoidal arteries may be necessary to control anterior bleeding. These vessels are approached through a standard external ethmoid incision between the medial canthus and the nasal root. If bleeding persists, a more posterior source should be suspected, and the internal maxillary artery is then ligated as well. This vessel is usually exposed through a transantral approach. The maxillary sinus is opened through a Caldwell-Luc (gingivobuccal sulcus) incision, and the posterior wall of the sinus is then opened to reach the pterygomaxillary space. In some cases of severely comminuted midface fractures, this approach is not feasible, and an intraoral approach is preferred.

An alternative but less specific means of controlling posterior epistaxis is by ligation of the external carotid artery. Because this vessel is somewhat removed from the actual site of bleeding, there is frequently collateral blood flow into the maxillary artery system distal to the point of ligation. Nevertheless, the external carotid artery can be accessed easily through the neck, even under local anes-

thesia. It is essential to identify at least two branches of the external carotid artery before ligating it to avoid accidental ligation of the internal carotid artery. Care must be taken to avoid injury to the vagus nerve, superior laryngeal nerve, hypoglossal nerve, sympathetic chain, and marginal mandibular nerve.

Patients with epistaxis and maxillofacial fractures who can be taken to surgery immediately and given a general anesthetic may have their bleeding controlled most effectively by fracture reduction. Early fracture treatment can obviate the need for formal nasal packing or vessel ligation.

Finally, a nonsurgical technique is that of selective arterial catheterization and embolization for control of epistaxis. The bleeding sites are identified angiographically and then occluded with embolization materials (such as polyvinyl alcohol foam, polymerizing fluids, or even microballoons). This procedure is performed by interventional radiologists at specialized centers (136).

Pharyngeal bleeding can occur as a result of mucosal laceration or penetrating injury to the internal carotid artery. Initial management after airway stabilization consists of packing the throat with layers of gauze wrap. The end of the gauze roll should be brought out through the mouth to facilitate pack retrieval after more definitive management is implemented.

EVALUATION

Physical Examination

After the airway has been secured and life-threatening hemorrhage controlled, the secondary survey can be performed. An efficient but systematic physical examination of the entire body should be carried out. The maxillofacial examination is part of the evaluation of the head and neck, including the neurologic system.

The scalp and face should be inspected for any lacerations or bruises. All loose soft tissue and bone fragments should be saved.

The eyes are checked for pupil size and reactivity to light and accommodation. Pupil asymmetry can indicate an elevation of intracranial pressure but also may be a sign of trauma to the globe. Extraocular movements are tested, and diplopia and unequal pupillary levels are assessed. Limitation suggests orbital injury with entrapment of periorbital tissues (Fig. 11.19). Visual acuity is evaluated (e.g., by tests of light perception, ability to count fingers, ability to read print). Proptosis and enophthalmos suggest hemorrhage within and fracture of the orbital walls, respectively. Periorbital swelling frequently accompanies fracture of the zygoma or maxilla. Subconjunctival hemorrhage suggests a fractured zygoma or direct trauma to the globe. Pooling and leakage of tears may indicate disruption of the lacrimal system.

The nose is inspected for deformity, pain, mobility, septal hematoma, and obstruction. Bleeding should be managed immediately, as previously discussed. Leakage of CSF suggests a cribriform plate or ethmoid roof fracture and, if present, should warn against insertion of any nasal tubes or packing. Any watery nasal discharge should be tested on filter paper: CSF forms a ring around blood or mucus. Intercanthal distance is measured; if it is more than 3.5 cm, a nasoethmoid fracture should be suspected.

The ears are examined for bleeding, CSF leakage, tympanic membrane perforation, and hemotympanum. Lacerations of the external auditory canal usually indicate the presence of a mandible fracture.

The facial soft tissues are examined for sensory and motor deficits. Peripheral or central injury to cranial nerves V and VII must be sought in relation to other in-

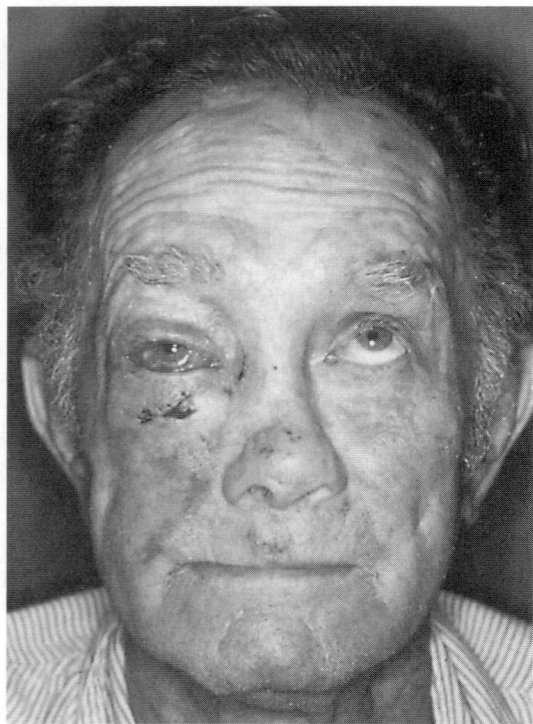

Figure 11.19. Orbital blow-out fracture with entrapment of inferior rectus muscle and limitation of upward gaze on the patient's right side.

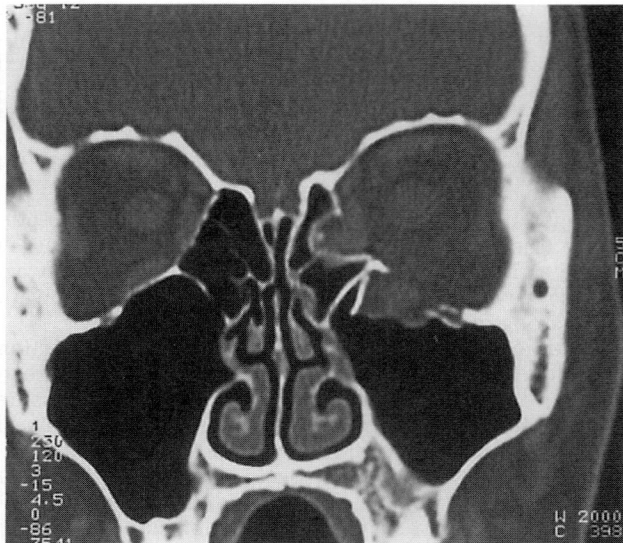

Figure 11.20. Coronal computed tomography scan showing orbital floor fracture.

juries. Subcutaneous emphysema in the middle and upper face suggests paranasal sinus fracture, and in the lower face and neck implies injury to the larynx, trachea, or lungs. Venous engorgement of the face suggests trauma to the major vessels of the neck or thorax. Leakage of clear or pink fluid from a facial wound may be a sign of parotid duct or gland injury.

The face as a whole is examined for asymmetry and deformity. Elongation with bilateral swelling suggests bilateral maxillary fracture. Step-off defects, tenderness, and ecchymoses around the orbit suggest maxilla and zygoma fractures. The midface is palpated for mobility. Bimanual palpation (with one hand grasping the maxilla and palate intraorally while the other hand stabilizes the forehead) may reveal palate, cheek, or nose mobility, indicating a LeFort I, II, or III fracture of the maxilla. Eye injuries occur in 60% of patients with mid-facial trauma, and blindness is a particular risk in LeFort III fractures (133). Therefore, any patient with suspected orbital fractures should have a formal ophthalmologic examination.

The mandible is palpated externally from one temporomandibular joint to the other. Tenderness, step-off defects, and crepitus are external signs of fracture. Intraoral hematoma (especially involving the sublingual and gingival mucosa), lacerations, bleeding, loose or broken teeth, mobile jaw segments, malocclusion, and decreased bite strength (i.e., inability to grip a tongue blade between the maxillary and mandibular molars) are internal signs of mandible fracture.

Radiographic Examination

In the conscious and cooperative patient with maxillofacial trauma, plain facial films and panoramic mandible radiographs can be obtained initially to assess bony injury.

The cervical spine must be confirmed as uninjured before any manipulation of the head is done. Plain films are entirely adequate for isolated zygoma and orbit fractures. More detailed and definitive radiographic assessment is obtained with computed tomography (CT).

Computed tomography is part of the standard management of the head-injured patient, and sections through the facial skeleton can be obtained simultaneously, providing information on the extent of facial fractures in addition to the status of the brain. Axial and coronal sections are complementary; only axial views can be obtained in patients with cervical spine injury, although coronal reconstructions can be made. The coronal CT scan images (obtained with the patient's head hanging with the neck extended) are especially helpful in delineating the cribriform plate and ethmoid roof region, the orbital rims, and the overall vertical facial height (Fig. 11.20). Newer, three-dimensional CT scanning is neither necessary nor particularly advantageous in evaluating most cases of maxillofacial trauma.

DEFINITIVE CARE

Timing of Repair

Most maxillofacial injuries do not require immediate definitive repair. Although soft-tissue injuries usually are best treated as early as possible for optimum healing with minimum infection, treatment of facial fractures can be delayed while attention is directed toward more life-threatening injuries. Fracture reduction is difficult to perform and results are difficult to assess early after injury because of edema. If surgery can be performed within 3 to 6 hours of trauma and is planned for treatment of brain injury acutely, maxillofacial repair can be carried out simultaneously or serially. Otherwise, it is preferable to wait for edema to subside and to perform elective repair at 3 to 7 days after injury. After 10 days, fracture reduction become increasingly difficult as fibrosis develops. For mandible fractures, definitive repair should be performed within 24 hours to minimize fracture contamination and risk of osteomyelitis, as well as to alleviate pain.

Infection Prophylaxis

Contaminated wounds usually should be treated with prophylactic antibiotics until definitive treatment has been delivered. Coverage against *Staphylococcus* and *Streptococcus* species usually suffices. The rich vascularity of the facial soft tissues helps to minimize infection and optimize wound healing. Even animal bites, a particularly common cause of facial soft-tissue injuries in children, can be repaired primarily and successfully treated with antibiotics, unlike animal bites elsewhere on the body.

Facial fractures involving the paranasal sinuses usually cause bleeding into the sinuses, which, if stagnant, may lead to sinusitis. Nasal packing for epistaxis control always should be accompanied by antibiotic therapy to avoid inducing sinusitis or toxic shock syndrome.

Open reduction and fixation of facial fractures with alloplastic hardware carries a risk of prosthetic implant contamination and infection; therefore, perioperative antibiotic use is appropriate.

In addition to antibiotic therapy, oral hygiene is extremely important in patients with maxillary or mandibular fractures who have altered oral function. Oral rinses with saline and dilute hydrogen peroxide or commercial mouthwash are effective.

The use of antibiotic prophylaxis in the presence of CSF fistulae is controversial. Antibiotics in this setting have not been shown to reduce the incidence of meningitis, and they can encourage the growth of resistant organisms (137).

Management of Soft-tissue Injuries

The outcome of soft-tissue injuries can be greatly influenced by the surgeon. Although secondary reconstruction and scar revision are frequently necessary, the primary wound management should incorporate the principles of wound healing and aesthetic soft-tissue surgery.

Wound cleansing is an extremely important preliminary step. Foreign bodies, gross debris, and bacterial contamination should be scrubbed and then rinsed from the wound. Application of antiseptic solutions such as chlorhexidine gluconate, hexachlorophene, or povidone–iodine is followed by copious irrigation with sterile saline solution. Tissues should be kept moist with saline until they are actually closed.

Adequate anesthesia is essential to ensure patient comfort and cooperation. Even with general anesthesia, infiltration of local anesthetic can help with vasoconstriction during surgery and with pain relief after surgery. Common anesthetic solutions include 1% or 2% lidocaine with epinephrine 1 : 100,000, mixed with the longer-acting 0.5% bupivacaine. Doses up to 300 mg lidocaine or 120 mg bupivacaine are usually safe for the average adult; the addition of epinephrine counteracts the vasodilatory effect of lidocaine and prolongs its duration of action. Local infiltration and regional nerve blocks are usually sufficient for repair of facial wounds, but general anesthesia is often required for repair of significant facial injuries in children, large wounds in adults, and lacrimal and facial nerve lacerations, as well as for prolonged cases and for multiply injured patients with concurrent repair of other sites.

The surgical instruments needed may not be available in the emergency department, and the surgeon should specifically request or bring a set of facial plastic surgery instruments. Choice of suture material depends on the location and dimensions of the wounds and the age and reliability of the patient. Absorbable suture is usually used for closure of subcutaneous layers. Chromic catgut is absorbed in tissues by macrophage activity and retains its tensile strength for 7 to 10 days. A fast-absorbing catgut can be used for skin closure in cases in which it is preferable not to have to remove skin sutures (e.g., in young children or noncompliant patients). The longer-acting absorbable sutures derived from polyglycolic acid maintain their tensile strength for 30 to 45 days. They are absorbed by acid hydrolysis with less associated inflammatory reaction than chromic catgut. These are the preferred sutures for closure of wounds with considerable tension or inflammation. Nonabsorbable monofilament suture is the preferred material for skin closure because it incites very little tissue reaction and can be used for running intradermal or epidermal suturing.

Hemostasis is achieved with direct pressure, cautery, or ligation of identified vessels. Before wound closure, tissue should be assessed for damage and loss. Abraded skin heals with an abnormal texture and color; if small amounts of tissue are abraded or crushed, they should be excised. Larger areas should be allowed to heal acutely and undergo scar revision later. Jagged wound edges should be reapproximated without being trimmed; their closure often resembles running W-plasties or geometric broken-line closures, which are preferable to linear scars. Avulsion wounds and defects with tissue loss should be closed. If the loss is small, the local tissue can be undermined and advanced to close the wound primarily. Larger defects can be closed with local skin flaps, skin grafts, or regional flaps. If in doubt, the surgeon can close the wound with a skin graft and perform a revision later under more elective conditions.

Avulsed tissue that has been saved can be cleaned and reimplanted. Avulsed ears are best reattached with microvascular repair of nutrient arteries and veins. Simple suturing of the ear itself is less successful but can be enhanced by multiple cutaneous incisions on both sides of the ear and by treatment of the patient with hyperbaric oxygen for 2 weeks. Avulsed cheek or lip defects are better treated by rearranging surrounding tissue to achieve closure.

Skin closure consists of deep stitches to approximate the dermis and remove tension from the wound edge, followed by skin approximation. Deep stitches of absorbable suture are placed with knots buried and wound edges everted. Cutaneous stitches also should be placed so as to evert the approximated wound edges; interrupted vertical mattress sutures, simple interrupted stitches, a running subcuticular suture, a simple running stitch, or a running locking stitch can be used.

Drains should be used for large wounds with oozing or with high potential for infection. A small rubber drain usually suffices; latex should be avoided in allergic patients. Antibiotic ointment or an occlusive dressing should be applied. Skin sutures are removed from the face after 4 or 5 days. Sutures left in longer are likely to cause permanent marks where epithelium grows down the suture track.

Facial scars, like those elsewhere on the body, mature over months and years. Even aesthetically unacceptable scars improve with maturation. Nevertheless, any scar that is larger than 2 cm, is wider than 2 mm, distorts normal anatomy, or does not lie in a favorable skin tension line can be improved by scar revision. Revision should be performed no sooner than 6 months after initial injury, and preferably approximately 1 year later.

Facial nerve lacerations are best repaired primarily at the time of soft-tissue repair. If primary repair is not feasible because of other, life-threatening injuries, the severed nerve endings should be tagged with metal microvascular clips or nonabsorbable suture, if possible. The optimal technique of neurorrhaphy is debatable, but epineural, perineural, and interfascicular repair are all effective. The most important variables are the atraumatic handling of the nerve, the use of microsuture (e.g., 8-0 to 10-0 monofilament nylon) in end-to-end anastomosis, and the absence of tension. If tension is present or a segment of facial nerve is missing, an interposition graft should be inserted. The greater auricular nerve in the neck and the sural nerve from the leg are the most common donor nerves.

Duct injuries (mainly the lacrimal ducts and the parotid ducts) should be repaired primarily. The duct is cannulated with fine silicone tubing and then, if possible, sutured over the cannula. The parotid duct can be marsupialized into the oral cavity, and the lacrimal duct can be diverted into the nasal cavity by dacryocystorhinostomy if primary repair fails. Medial and lateral canthal tendon injuries should be repaired with permanent suture that is passed through periosteum or even bone.

Management of Bony Injuries

Facial fractures are treated by closed or open reduction, with or without wire or rigid fixation. Hardware for rigid internal fixation consists of plates and screws made of titanium, stainless steel, or, more recently, absorbable polymers such as polylactide. Nondisplaced fractures, such as those involving the nasal bones, zygoma, and maxilla, may require no treatment at all. On the other hand, displaced fractures require not only reduction and stabilization but also treatment of associated injuries to the facial soft tissues and intracranial structures.

Treatment of frontal sinus fractures is a function of fracture complexity. Nondisplaced anterior wall fractures can be left alone. Displaced anterior wall fractures should be opened and repaired to avoid later mucocele formation and a residual depressed area over the fracture site. The frontal sinus mucosa adjacent to the fracture line is removed, and the anterior wall fragments are reduced and stabilized with either stainless steel wire (26 or 28 gauge) or microplates and screws.

Posterior wall fractures should be explored, preferably using an osteoplastic flap (138) or craniotomy approach. Any dural defects are repaired first. The sinus mucosa is then either removed from all fracture lines or stripped from the sinus completely and replaced by autologous fat packing within the sinus. The frontonasal duct is also obliterated with a fat or muscle plug. The bony fragments are then reduced and stabilized. If posterior wall fractures are severely comminuted or bone is missing, the frontal sinus is best cranialized by removing the entire posterior wall and the sinus mucosa while preserving the anterior wall. The cranialization procedure (139) eliminates the sinus altogether and makes room for edematous brain to expand. The normal forehead contour is preserved, and the frontal lobes of the brain are still protected by bone.

Nasoethmoid fractures are rarely amenable to closed reduction because of the frequent disruption of the medial canthal tendons and nasolacrimal system. Open reduction is often performed with the help of an ophthalmologic surgeon. The bone fragments of the nasal, lacrimal, and ethmoid bones are restored to their correct anatomic positions and stabilized with stainless steel wires or microplates. The medial canthal tendons are realigned and stabilized with transnasal wires. Lacrimal injuries are repaired with a dacryocystorhinostomy, with the use of silicone catheters to reestablish routes for tear flow.

Orbital floor blow-out fractures are best exposed through a subciliary or transconjunctival lower eyelid incision. Herniated orbital contents, such as inferior rectus and inferior oblique muscles and orbital fat, are replaced within the periosteum of the orbit. Exposure of the fracture extent should be made with great caution, especially to avoid injury to the infraorbital nerve, the optic nerve, and the globe itself. The fractured orbital floor should be reduced if possible, or reconstituted with an implant if support is inadequate. Implants of silicone sheeting [0.04 inch (0.1 cm) thick], Gelfilm, autogenous bone and cartilage, titanium mesh, polylactide mesh, or hydroxyapatite all have been used successfully.

Medial blow-out fractures also should be explored to reduce herniated fat and muscle and to assess the lacrimal system and ethmoid vessels. Implants are usually not necessary, but larger defects can be reconstituted with the same implant materials used for inferior wall blow-out fractures.

Superior and lateral orbital blow-out fractures are quite rare. Orbital contents should be reduced, associated frontal sinus injuries addressed, and the fractures stabilized.

Orbital apex fractures are perhaps the most serious type of orbital fractures. The approach for exploration and decompression depends on the fracture site. Options include a lateral orbitotomy, an extended external sphenoethmoidectomy, a frontal craniotomy, or an endoscopic intranasal approach. The surgeon must be familiar with the entire three-dimensional anatomy of the orbit and its surrounding structures to achieve safe decompression of the optic nerve and the ophthalmic neurovascular bundle.

Reduction of nasal fractures often must await resolution of local swelling. Isolated nasal fractures identified within hours of their onset can be reduced early; otherwise, closed reduction is best carried out within 4 to 10 days. Most nasal fractures can be managed with closed techniques. Open reduction is used for early correction of nasal fractures that cannot be reduced adequately in a closed fashion and for correction of previously existing nasal deformity or malunion. Unsuccessful attempts at closed reduction and open wounds of skin and mucosa are indications for open reduction. Only surgeons experienced in rhinoplasty should perform open repair.

Topical intranasal anesthesia with regional local anesthetic blocks to the nasal dorsum, anterior maxilla, base of the septum, infraorbital nerve, greater palatine nerve, and superior alveolar nerve enable closed reduction of nasal fractures in the emergency department or clinic setting. General anesthesia may be necessary, but it still should be supplemented with topical and local anesthetics to enhance visualization and reduce bleeding. Depressed and displaced fractures are reduced with the use of an intranasal elevator and manual pressure or with special forceps. The septum can also be realigned with the use of these instruments. Internal packing and external splinting help to stabilize the reduction.

Most isolated zygomatic arch fractures cause purely cosmetic deformities. Reduction can be performed through a Gillies (temporal scalp), lateral brow, or intraoral incision. Fixation is usually unnecessary. Zygomatic arch fractures are particularly difficult to treat secondarily if they heal in a displaced position.

Malar complex and tripod fractures usually require reduction and fixation at a minimum of two points to maintain stability. The lateral brow and subciliary or transconjunctival lower lid incisions yield access to zygomaticofrontal and inferior orbital rim fractures. The malar complex can be reduced and then wired or plated to these locations.

Maxillary fractures are some of the most challenging facial fractures to manage. The main goal is reestablishment of adequate dental occlusion, and secondary goals are reunion of the bony fractures and cosmetic facial restoration. The mainstay of treatment is open reduction and internal fixation of the maxillary fragments. Intermaxillary fixation (IMF), also known as *maxillomandibular fixation*, usually plays a role in the realignment and stabilization of the occlusion. IMF traditionally is achieved by wiring arch bars to the maxillary and mandibular teeth and then binding the arch bars and maxillae to one another with wires or rubber bands. An alternative and safer method (for the surgeon handling the wires) for achieving IMF is the four-screw technique, whereby self-tapping 2.7-mm bone screws are placed into the maxilla and mandible bilaterally, and wires are secured between the screws above and below (140).

Most LeFort I fractures are adequately reduced and stabilized by IMF with or without circumzygomatic and orbital rim suspension wires. LeFort II fractures are handled similarly. Miniplates or microplates are also used to stabilize individual maxillary fractures. Associated nasoethmoid and orbital fractures are managed concomitantly, as previously described. LeFort III fractures often require suspension wiring to the stable frontal bone. External fixation devices must be considered for severely comminuted maxillary fractures. Alveolar and palatal fractures associated with any LeFort-type injury are best managed with intraoral acrylic splints that are wired into place.

The general approach to proper midface reduction and stabilization is to establish the mandible as a solid base and to rebuild the facial skeleton vertically after centric occlusion has been restored. The upper midface is secured to the cranial base, and mid-facial height is preserved. If mandible fractures are also present, these should be reduced first, if possible.

Successful management of mandible fractures requires not only restoration of premorbid occlusion but complete immobilization of the fragments during healing. Infections must be prevented to avoid malunion or nonunion and osteomyelitis. In general, teeth in the line of fractures can and should be preserved, because they actually improve the likelihood of successful mandible fracture repair (141). Exceptions include teeth that are grossly mobile in the bony mandible fragment, those with root fractures or periapical radiolucency, those with extensive caries, and those that interfere with fracture reduction.

Intermaxillary fixation is the fundamental therapy for maxillary and mandibular arch fractures, as previously described. IMF is usually left in place for 4 to 6 weeks, although less time is necessary in pediatric patients and in patients with subcondylar fractures. Displaced and "unfavorable" fractures (i.e., those whose fragments are distracted by the pull of the muscles of mastication) require open exposure of the fracture line and direct reduction and fixation. Unfavorable fractures occur most commonly in the angle, body, and symphyseal regions. Exposure is achieved through an extraoral, intraoral, or transbuccal approach. IMF is used at least intraoperatively to establish proper occlusion. Fixation with wires does not provide rigid fixation, whereas miniplate or reconstruction plate osteosynthesis does have this primary advantage. Unless rigid fixation is obtained, IMF should be maintained for 4 to 6 weeks after surgery. Dynamic compression plates have the ability to apply compressive forces to the fracture site that facilitate the primary bone healing process. Lag screws and even plates that use hollow screws that encourage osseointegration are also useful.

Mandible fractures in edentulous patients pose special problems. Although occlusion is no longer a primary issue of concern, edentulous mandibles are typically atrophic and less able to accept hardware. Occasionally, open reduction and internal fixation is possible. Otherwise, if dentures are available, they can be wired circumferentially to the maxilla and mandible and then placed in IMF. Gunning splints can be placed intraorally to bridge the fracture, or external fixation can be achieved with percutaneous pins inserted into the mandible on either side of the fracture and connected by an acrylic bar that maintains reduction and immobilization. Elderly patients require immobilization for 6 to 10 weeks because of their slower rate of healing.

Nonunion is more likely to occur with mandible fractures than with fractures of other facial bones. Débridement, rewiring, and restabilization may not be adequate; bone grafts and external fixation are usually required. Hyperbaric oxygen therapy can be helpful in preparation for bone grafting.

Definitive Care Phase: Neck Injuries

GREGORY J. JURKOVICH

The vital structures of the neck are concentrated in a small anatomic area, generally unprotected by bone or dense muscular covering. Yet, because of its relatively small size, only 5% to 10% of traumatic injuries involve the neck. Although infrequent in occurrence, neck injuries often require prompt surgical management. Disruption of the airway or carotid circulation is an immediate life-threatening problem, and esophageal or peripheral nerve injury can cause chronic morbidity. Penetrating injuries are most common and most severe, with fatality rates ranging from 1% to 2% for stab wounds, from 5% to 12% for gunshot wounds, and up to 50% for rifle or shotgun blasts (142–144). Up to 50% of these deaths are preventable with appropriate early care. Significant blunt neck trauma is less common but can be particularly difficult to manage because it often involves the airway. Carotid or vertebral artery injury can also occur as a consequence of acute cervical spine hyperextension, even in the absence of bony injury. The initial diagnosis of these injuries can be difficult, and the consequences of missing an injury are severe.

As a general guideline, all patients with penetrating neck wounds that traverse the platysma muscle should be admitted to the hospital for evaluation, observation, and treatment. Likewise, all patients with blunt traumatic injuries of the neck should be admitted. This section of the text focuses on the preferred and available diagnostic and treatment options for patients with blunt or penetrating neck trauma.

ANATOMY

The neck is classically divided into a number of anatomic triangles (Fig. 11.21). The two large anterior and posterior triangles are particularly important in neck trauma. Wounds to the posterior triangle rarely involve the esophagus, airway, or major vascular structures, although if the blow is directed inferiorly, intrathoracic injury can occur. In contrast, penetrating wounds that enter through either the sternocleidomastoid muscle or the anterior triangle carry a high likelihood of vascular, airway, or esophageal injury (Fig. 11.22).

The anterior neck is further divided into three zones defined by horizontal planes. Zone I represents the base of the neck and is variably defined. In the Roon and Christensen classification (145), zone I is defined as extending from the sternal notch to the lower border of the cricoid cartilage (Fig. 11.23). Injuries here carry the highest mortality rate because of the risk of major vascular and intrathoracic injury. Zone II is the central and largest portion of the neck. It extends from the top of zone I to the angle of the mandible. Zone II injuries are most common but

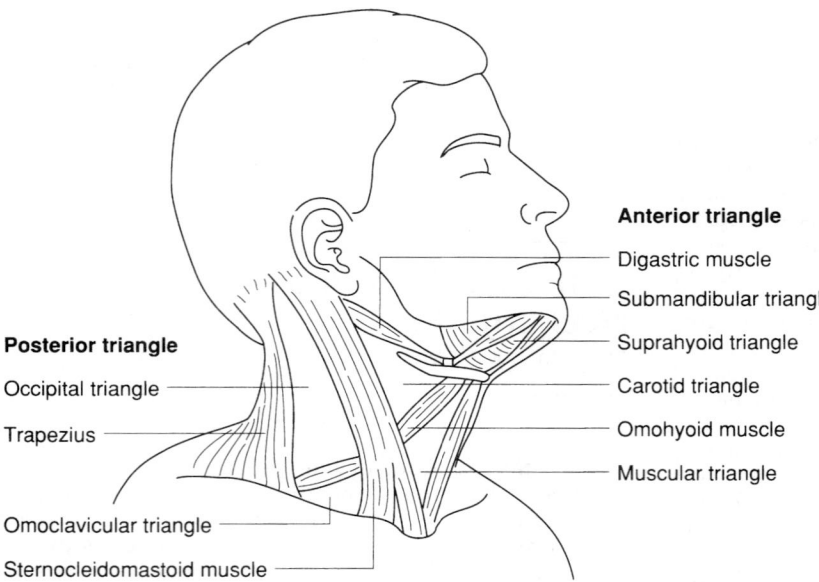

Posterior triangle

Occipital triangle

Trapezius

Omoclavicular triangle

Sternocleidomastoid muscle

Anterior triangle

Digastric muscle

Submandibular triangle

Suprahyoid triangle

Carotid triangle

Omohyoid muscle

Muscular triangle

Figure 11.21. Anatomic triangles of the neck. The posterior triangle is composed of the smaller occipital and omoclavicular triangles. The anterior triangle has as smaller divisions the carotid, muscular, submandibular, and suprahyoid triangles.

carry a lower mortality rate than either zone I or III injuries because injury is usually apparent and exposure of vital structures is readily accomplished. Zone III is that part of the neck above the angle of mandible. The risk of injury to the distal carotid artery, salivary glands, and pharynx is greatest in this zone. Exposure in this region can be particularly difficult.

The other major anatomic landmark in the neck is the platysma muscle. This thin, broad muscle lies just beneath the skin and covers the entire anterior triangle and anteroinferior aspect of the posterior triangle. Wounds that fail to penetrate the platysma are considered superficial and do not warrant extensive evaluation. A wound that penetrates the platysma must be considered a serious sur-

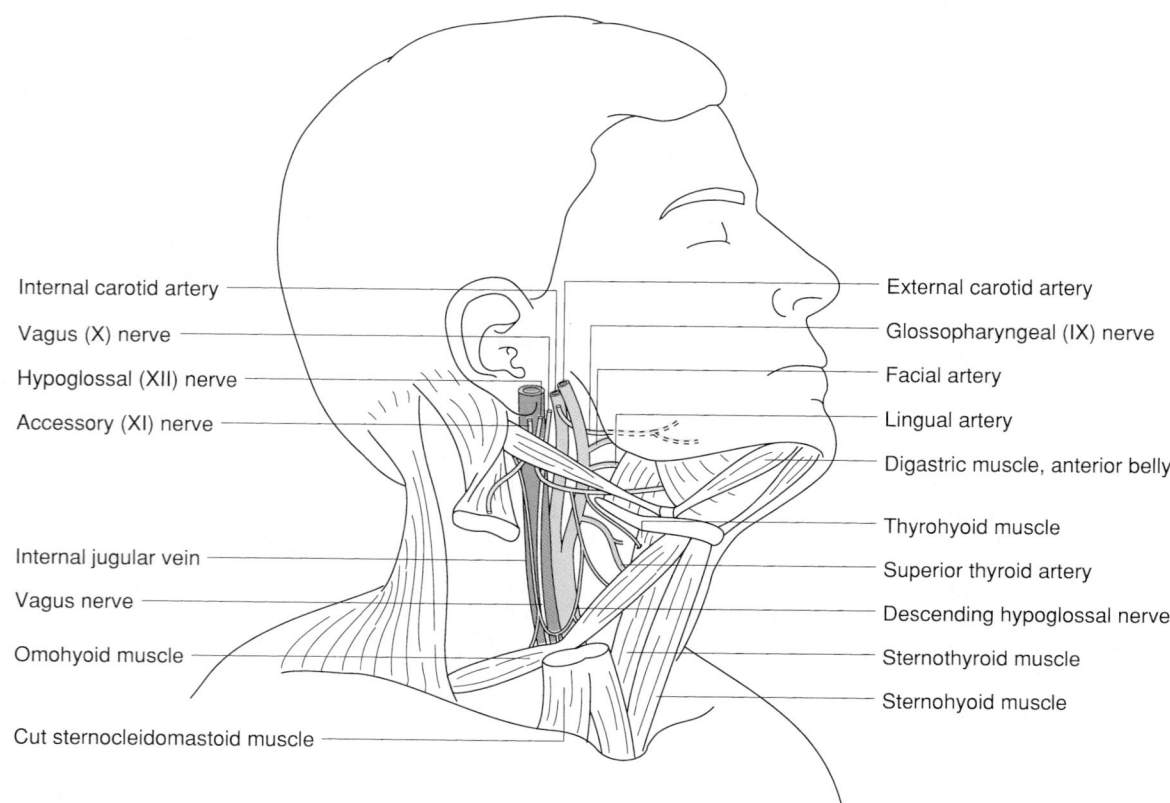

Internal carotid artery

Vagus (X) nerve

Hypoglossal (XII) nerve

Accessory (XI) nerve

Internal jugular vein

Vagus nerve

Omohyoid muscle

Cut sternocleidomastoid muscle

External carotid artery

Glossopharyngeal (IX) nerve

Facial artery

Lingual artery

Digastric muscle, anterior belly

Thyrohyoid muscle

Superior thyroid artery

Descending hypoglossal nerve

Sternothyroid muscle

Sternohyoid muscle

Figure 11.22. Proximity of cranial nerves to the carotid arteries of the neck. Trauma resulting in cranial nerve deficits in this region is often associated with vascular injury.

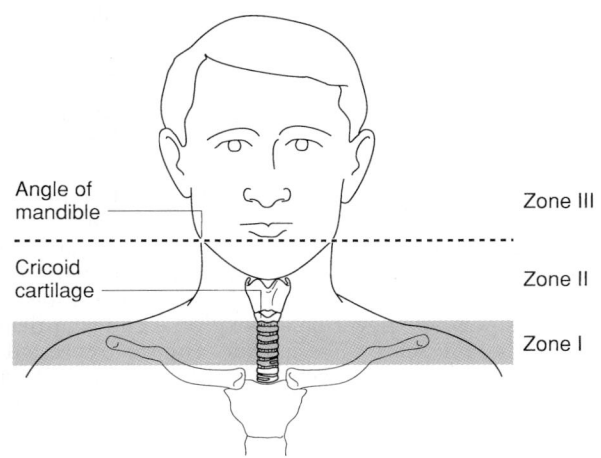

Figure 11.23. Zones of the neck. The junction of zones I and II is variously described as being at the cricoid cartilage or at the top of the clavicles. The important implication of a zone I injury is the greater potential for intrathoracic great vessel injury.

gical problem that mandates hospital admission and further evaluation.

INITIAL MANAGEMENT

The same priorities for initial care of the multiply injured patient apply to the management of isolated neck trauma. Airway control remains the primary tenet of initial trauma care, and it takes precedence over all other aspects of the evaluation and resuscitation. If injury involves the airway itself or surrounding structures, this management task takes on special significance. Rapid inspection for air movement, crepitus, hoarseness, and subcutaneous emphysema is the first step. Supplemental oxygen always should be administered, and adequate lighting and suction are essential. If spontaneous ventilation appears adequate, close observation and pulse oximetry monitoring are suggested because acute decompensation can occur with little warning. If spontaneous respirations are inadequate, if blood or other material obstructs the airway, or if progressive cervical swelling from hemorrhage threatens to occlude the airway, emergency intubation is necessary. Procrastination converts a simple intubation into a difficult and bloody emergency tracheostomy. Direct visualization of the vocal cords and oral endotracheal intubation are usually preferred. If cervical spine injury has not been excluded, hyperextension of the neck must be avoided. Two-man intubation with in-line cervical traction is an alternative to nasotracheal intubation.

Massive pharyngeal or neck hematoma can totally occlude the airway, making direct intubation impossible. Attempts at blind nasotracheal intubation cause further mucosal or laryngeal injury, and an emergency surgical airway (cricothyroidotomy or tracheostomy) is required. Occasionally, blunt laryngeal trauma is so severe as to disrupt and occlude the airway. The preferred method of controlling the airway in this setting is controversial (see Trachea and Larynx), but provisions for a surgical airway must be at hand. Options include primary tracheostomy or a single attempt at endoscopically assisted endotracheal intubation. Temporization with transtracheal needle-jet insufflation can be a valuable adjunct in these settings.

Concurrent with airway control is awareness of potential cervical spine injury, particularly in unconscious patients who have sustained blunt head and neck trauma.

The head and neck should be supported in the neutral position until this possibility is excluded radiographically and by physical examination. In the emergency department, support of the head and neck is best accomplished by a strong, steady assistant rather than by collars, sandbags, or tape. The lateral cervical spine film is an essential component of the initial evaluation of patients with either blunt or penetrating neck trauma, both to assess the bony cervical spine and to evaluate soft tissues for edema or misplaced air.

The initial management continues to follow the ABC guidelines of trauma care advocated by the Advanced Trauma Life Support course of the American College of Surgeons, with particular attention directed at adequacy of ventilation, treatment of shock, and baseline neurologic examination. Patients with blunt neck trauma often have concomitant thoracic injuries, and penetrating neck wounds may follow a caudal trajectory, injuring lung or intrathoracic great vessels, particularly if the entrance is in zone I (146). Rapid physical examination of the thorax is therefore part of the initial evaluation of neck trauma patients and should include inspection, palpation, and auscultation. Pneumothorax must be treated rapidly by needle decompression or tube thoracostomy, or both, and treatment should not necessarily be delayed for radiographic confirmation. Major neck hemorrhage is treated with direct pressure. Blind clamping of vessels is discouraged to avoid inadvertent injury to nerve or esophagus. Adequate peripheral intravenous access is required in all patients with neck trauma and usually requires at least two peripheral intravenous catheters lines of 16 gauge or larger. Blood is drawn for typing and crossmatching and routine laboratory evaluations, and fluid resuscitation is initiated based on the degree of shock and anticipated hemorrhage. A rapid yet thorough neurologic examination is also part of the initial management, with particular attention to the patient's level of consciousness and the status of cranial and brachial plexus nerves. Changes in the results of neurologic examination are key indicators of ongoing injury.

After the initial resuscitation, a complete physical examination is performed to detect associated injuries and better define the extent of neck trauma. Close visual inspection of the neck alerts the physician to the possibility of underlying injuries and the mechanism of injury. For example, an oblique 4- to 6-cm bruise on the neck of a restrained passenger in a motor vehicle accident should alert the physician to the possibility of blunt cervical vascular trauma from a seat belt injury. Neck wounds should not be probed for fear of dislodging a clot and reinstituting hemorrhage. The neck should be palpated with attention to normal anatomic landmarks and areas of tenderness. Crepitus or subcutaneous emphysema indicates injury to the trachea, esophagus, or lung until proven otherwise. It should never be assumed that a penetrating skin wound itself is responsible for subcutaneous air. If the patient is able to talk, the presence of hoarseness, dysphagia, or dysphonia should be determined. Hemoptysis and hematemesis are also signs of tracheal and esophageal injury. Table 11.9 lists the clinical signs of significant injury that usually mandate neck exploration to exclude or treat vascular, airway, esophageal, and nerve injuries.

All patients with blunt or penetrating neck trauma should have a chest radiograph to rule out thoracic trauma. Stable patients should have soft-tissue neck films to look for retropharyngeal hematoma, tracheal narrowing or deviation, retained missile fragments and pathways, and subcutaneous or retropharyngeal air. Computed tomography (CT) scan of the neck is particularly helpful in blunt trauma to evaluate laryngeal structures. Patients who have sustained blunt neck trauma and whose neuro-

Table 11.9. CLINICAL SIGNS OF SIGNIFICANT INJURY IN PENETRATING NECK TRAUMA

Vascular
  Shock
  Active bleeding
  Large or expanding hematoma
  Pulse deficit
Airway
  Dyspnea
  Stridor
  Hoarseness
  Dysphonia or voice change
  Subcutaneous emphysema

Digestive tract
  Hemoptysis
  Dysphagia or odynophagia
  Hematemesis
  Subcutaneous emphysema
Neurologic
  Focal or lateralized neurologic
    deficit

logic examination is inconsistent with findings on head CT scan should undergo four-vessel cerebral angiography.

SELECTIVE VERSUS MANDATORY EXPLORATION

There is uniform agreement that all unstable patients and all patients with clinical signs of significant neck injury require prompt exploration. All other patients with wounds that penetrate the platysma should at least be admitted to the hospital and observed. Controversy exists, however, in the management of asymptomatic, stable patients with penetrating neck injury. Two distinct schools of thought exist, one advocating mandatory surgical exploration of all wounds that penetrate the platysma (143,147,148) and the other favoring a more selective approach (149–153). A comprehensive review of selective versus mandatory operative management published in 1991 documents similar rates for injury incidence, overall mortality rate, and delayed complications, as well as similar hospital costs, but with a significant reduction of negative neck explorations in the selective management group (154) (Table 11.10). Most recent studies have advocated some type of selective management in a clinical setting with explicit guidelines and expertise in the appropriate use of various diagnostic modalities (155–160).

Advocates of a mandatory exploration policy cite the low morbidity and negligible mortality rate after negative neck exploration as justification for the high rate of nega-

tive findings (40%–60%). The disastrous complications of missed injuries further support this stance. A 67% mortality rate is reported after delayed operations for neck vascular injuries, and a 44% mortality rate for delayed operations for esophageal injuries (144). A 1986 literature review reported an overall mortality rate of 16.7% for patients initially observed after penetrating neck trauma who subsequently required surgical exploration (161). In addition, a few reports have documented major structural injury in a small percentage of patients who undergo exploration despite a clinically silent physical examination; in one report, 5.5% of patients with wounds that appeared innocuous but were nevertheless explored had significant injuries (148). Transcervical gunshot injuries represent a special category of neck wounds, with one report documenting the high likelihood of injuries to cervical structures (83%) and supporting aggressive surgical exploration in all cases (162).

Supporters of a more selective approach berate the high incidence of negative explorations, the cost of a surgical exploration, and the fact that some injuries are missed in spite of a surgical exploration. They also argue that the original data supporting mandatory neck exploration are based on World War II and Vietnam War experience with large-caliber, high-velocity projectiles, unlike the typical knife or handgun injury observed in civilian trauma. The wide availability and diagnostic accuracy of angiography, endoscopy, and esophagography further support a selective management plan. Merion and colleagues (151), as part of a review of the cost of managing penetrating neck trauma, analyzed 27 reported series in which the clinical courses of more than 4,000 patients with penetrating neck trauma were documented. Fifty-two percent of patients treated by surgeons advocating selective exploration underwent immediate operation, compared with almost 90% of patients treated by those advocating mandatory exploration. Reexamination of these series revealed that the mortality rate was no different in the two groups, and only 2.4% of initially observed patients required subsequent operation (161).

No uniform policy has been accepted for selective management of patients with penetrating neck injury in the absence of positive clinical findings. There is a general agreement that zone I and III injuries require diagnostic studies such as angiography, endoscopy, and esophageal contrast studies (163). The management of the zone II injury, however, is variable and subject to the experience

Table 11.10. MANDATORY OPERATION COMPARED WITH SELECTIVE MANAGEMENT OF PENETRATING NECK TRAUMA

	Mandatory	Selective
Patients		
Number of series	11	24
Number of patients	1,653	2,540
Outcome		
Mortality rate (range)	5.85% (0.3%–11.0%)	3.75% (0%–9.8%)
Cases explored	1,492 (90.2%)	1,596 (62.8%)
Positive explorations	803 (53.8%)	1,117 (70.0%)
Cases observed	161 (9.8%)	944 (37.2%)
Delayed exploration	3 (1.9%)	20 (2.1%)
System injured		
Arterial injuries	213 (12.9%)	303 (11.9%)
Venous injuries	310 (18.8%)	459 (18.0%)
Esophagus or pharynx	163 (9.9%)	191 (7.5%)
Larynx or trachea	150 (9.1%)	181 (7.1%)

Modified from Asensio J, Valenziano C, Falcone R, et al. Management of penetrating neck injuries: the controversy surrounding zone III injuries. Surg Clin North Am 1991;71:267.

and preference of individual surgeons and trauma centers (155–160). The disagreement concerns whether patients should routinely undergo surgical neck exploration, undergo extensive diagnostic evaluation similar to that performed in zone I and III injuries, or simply be observed. Because a number of clinical reviews demonstrate similar patient outcomes, each institution or surgeon should adopt a management plan most consistent with local resources and experience.

At Harborview Medical Center in Seattle, all patients with neck wounds who are in hypovolemic shock or who have evolving stroke are immediately explored for vascular control. Most of those with neck wounds that penetrate the platysma in zone II undergo exploration, as do all patients with clinical signs of tracheal, esophageal, or major vascular injury. Preoperative angiography is not usually required for zone II injuries because of the relative ease of exposure and control of critical vascular structures. The track of the offending agent is followed throughout its course to exclude any possible vascular, tracheal, esophageal, or neurologic injury. Intraoperative endoscopy is usually performed if pharyngeal, esophageal, or tracheal injury is suspected but cannot be readily identified.

Zone I and III penetrating injuries are selectively managed based on clinical presentation and the results of diagnostic studies. Hemodynamically unstable patients undergo immediate exploration, with operative incision based on the most likely source of vascular injury. Zone I injuries are managed like mediastinal traversing wounds (162,164). Angiography is performed in hemodynamically stable patients with penetrating wounds to zone I to identify potential injuries to the thoracic outlet vessels or to facilitate planning the operative approach. Cinefluoroesophagography, first with water-soluble contrast material and then with barium, is performed after angiography for zone I injuries. Endoscopy is considered a complementary procedure to the esophagography, and should follow if there is any question of an abnormality. Angiography is also performed for zone III injuries because of the possible inaccessibility of internal carotid artery lesions or to demonstrate a need for systemic anticoagulation. In addition, most of the vascular lesions identified at the base of the skull are best managed by interventional angiography techniques. Esophageal studies are not done for zone III injuries.

OPERATIVE EXPLORATION

Twenty-five percent to 50% of patients with penetrating neck trauma (depending on mechanism) present with obvious signs of injury requiring prompt operation. An additional 10% to 20% of patients without clinical signs of injury are discovered to have significant vascular, esophageal, or airway injury on further diagnostic testing. A physician treating patients with neck trauma must be capable of performing a complete neck exploration and repair of vascular and aerodigestive injuries. Neck exploration should be performed in the operating room under general endotracheal anesthesia. In the hemodynamically stable patient with a patent airway, intubation can be deferred until laryngoscopy and bronchoscopy have been performed. A nasogastric tube is usually passed to ensure an empty stomach. Preparation and draping of the patient before induction of anesthesia allows control of hemorrhage if the patient starts to gag at the time of placement of the endotracheal tube. The chest is also auscultated before surgery, and a chest radiograph is routinely obtained because penetrating injuries may follow a downward path with pleural penetration. A pneumothorax may not develop until positive-pressure ventilation is applied, and it may initially present as unexplained hypotension during anesthesia.

The incision is planned to allow full exposure of the tract of the injury (Fig. 11.24). The oblique incision along the anterior border of the sternocleidomastoid muscle is preferred for unilateral and high (zone III) injuries, whereas the transverse collar incision is preferable for bilateral or neck-traversing wounds. Extension of either neck incision into a median sternotomy affords excellent exposure of the thoracic great vessels. Proximal and distal control of the major vessels also must be considered in the length and position of the incision, and the patient is always surgically prepared for a possible median sternotomy. The tract of the injury is followed to its depth, systematically examining each structure in or near the tract.

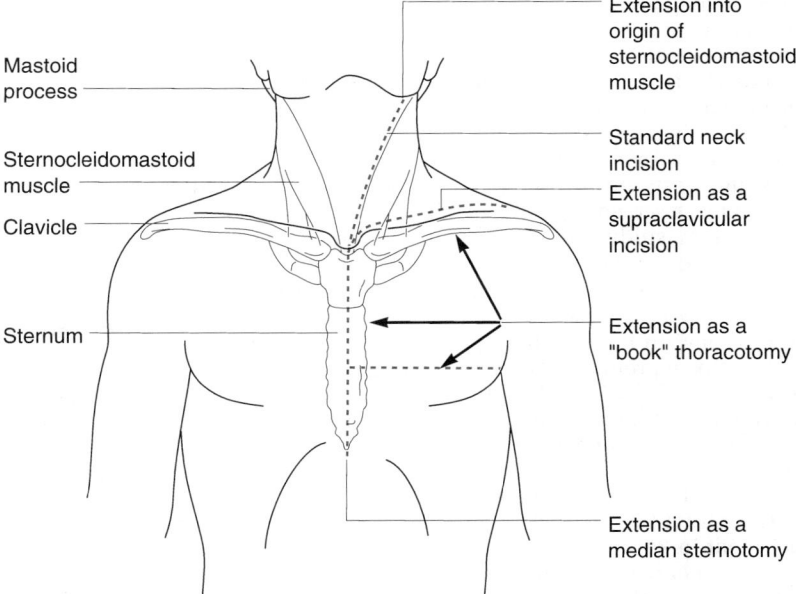

Figure 11.24. Neck exploration incisions. Extension of oblique or collar incision into a median sternotomy affords excellent exposure of the great vessels.

Mastoid process

Sternocleidomastoid muscle

Clavicle

Sternum

Extension into origin of sternocleidomastoid muscle

Standard neck incision

Extension as a supraclavicular incision

Extension as a "book" thoracotomy

Extension as a median sternotomy

MANAGEMENT OF SPECIFIC INJURIES

Blood Vessels

Blood vessels are the most commonly injured structures in the neck. Major arterial and venous injuries occur in 18% and 26% of penetrating neck wounds, respectively (160). Blunt vascular injury accounts for perhaps only 3% of all carotid injuries (165). There has been an increase in reported blunt carotid injuries, perhaps because of better recognition (166,167). However, the initial diagnosis remains a difficult one and must be suspected based on the mechanism of injury.

Carotid Artery

In the largest series reported in the English literature, 85 blunt carotid injuries were recognized in 67 patients over 11 years in a level I trauma center (166). Automobile crashes were the most common injury mechanism (82%), followed by motorcycle crashes (7%) and assaults (6%). All but two of the patients had associated injuries, and combinations of blunt carotid injury with closed head and cervical spine injuries occurred in 48% and 6% of patients, respectively. The initial physical examination demonstrated neurologic findings that were not compatible with brain CT scan findings in 34%, and soft-tissue injury in the anterior neck in 14% of the patients. A neurologic deficit developed subsequent to hospital admission in 43% of the patients. The average interval from injury to definitive diagnosis was 53 hours, highlighting the point that, although its recognition is often delayed, blunt carotid trauma must be suspected in patients who begin to have focal neurologic signs or symptoms after a latent interval. In a multicenter review, significant neurologic deficits developed in 29% of patients more than 12 hours after admission (168). Other physical findings—expanding hematoma, audible bruit, pulsatile neck mass, palpable thrill, Horner's syndrome, or any neurologic symptom not explained by other injuries—may be absent at the initial examination. Because there is some evidence to suggest improved outcome with early diagnosis (166–168), there must be a high index of suspicion if the mechanism of injury involves a direct blow to or compression of the neck, basilar skull fracture, cervical hyperextension and rotation, or blunt intraoral trauma (165). Cerebral angiography remains the gold standard for diagnosis. However, angiography is invasive and time consuming, and therefore not a suitable screening test. There is encouraging evidence regarding the use of duplex ultrasound, magnetic resonance, and helical CT angiography (HCTA) as screening diagnostic tools (169–172). However, these modalities still lack sufficient evidence to demonstrate their accuracy, require the presence of around-the-clock expertise, and possess high costs, all of which may make them impractical to use as mass screening tools for blunt trauma patients. In a multicenter study, duplex ultrasound demonstrated 86% (12 of 14) of the arterial injuries but was unable to discern dissection of the internal carotid artery at the base of the skull in two patients; proximal flow characteristics were also normal in both of these patients (168,169). HCTA appears to be a promising future screening tool (170,171); the advantage of HCTA is that it can be incorporated in the work-up of a blunt trauma patient who is having a head CT scan because of concomitant head injury, and it can evaluate the intracranial vessels.

The mortality rate remains high with blunt carotid injury, ranging from 20% to 40%, with permanent neurologic impairment in 25% to 80% of survivors (166–168,173). There is a reasonably good neurologic outcome, better than 55%, for an uncomplicated arterial dissection, and a uniformly poor outcome, with close to a 100% mortality rate, for complete arterial disruption and bilateral arterial occlusion (166–168). Treatment is highly variable and the efficacy has not been proven in a prospective study (166,167,174). Therapy depends on the type and location of the vascular lesion, concomitant injuries, availability of the interventional techniques, and preference of the treating surgeon. Arterial dissections can be managed best by systemic anticoagulation (166). For patients with contraindication to anticoagulation, antiplatelet therapy also has been suggested (167). The anticoagulation is to prevent propagation, embolization, and thrombosis. Stenting and primary surgical therapy, in anatomically favorable locations, also has been used in the management of arterial dissection in small studies (166–168, 175). If it is anatomically feasible, pseudoaneurysms may be resected. Larger inaccessible pseudoaneurysms are a difficult management challenge; the treatment includes anticoagulation, balloon occlusion, stenting, ligation, or extracranial–intracranial bypass (174,176,177). Patients with carotid–cavernous fistulae have been treated with balloon occlusion with variable results (166,168). The outcome of an arterial injury with complete vascular thrombosis depends more on the neurologic status than on any treatment regime. Nonsurgical management seems appropriate for most of these patients (173). The rare and fortunate patient with complete carotid thrombosis without neurologic deficits is best treated with anticoagulation to prevent further or contralateral damage (166,178).

Patients with penetrating carotid artery injury most commonly present with exsanguinating hemorrhage. The principles of operative repair of vascular structures in the neck are the same as those for other major vessels. What makes neck vascular trauma unique is the intolerance of the perfused end organ (brain) to even short periods of ischemia. The indication for repair versus ligation of a carotid injury depends in part on the neurologic presentation. Patients without a neurologic deficit should have restoration of vascular continuity, with a good neurologic outcome anticipated. Also, patients with all grades of neurologic deficits short of coma also should have primary vascular repair (179). Although the experience with revascularization of patients sustaining acute stroke from arteriosclerotic occlusive disease suggests that hemorrhagic infarction and death can result from revascularization, several reviews of acute revascularization in the trauma patient note that the combined morbidity and mortality rate is significantly lower in patients undergoing primary repair (15%) compared with those treated with arterial ligation (50%) (180–182). In comatose patients, neither repair nor ligation appears to influence what is a uniformly poor prognosis. Ligation of the carotid artery is indicated in the comatose patient with no prograde flow, in the presence of uncontrollable hemorrhage, or if technical reasons prohibit repair. There is little experience or evidence to favor extracranial–intracranial bypass in the patient requiring carotid artery ligation for trauma, although it has been used selectively in patients requiring selective carotid occlusion (178,183).

Vertebral Artery

Traumatic injury to the vertebral artery, once only rarely diagnosed, is now more commonly identified, certainly because of the liberal application of neck angiography after both penetrating and blunt neck injuries. Blunt vertebral artery injuries occur more commonly than blunt carotid injuries, probably because of the close association of bony and ligamentous structures. Mechanisms reported to cause vertebral artery injury are remarkably diverse, including hyperextension and rotation, direct blows, chiropractic manipulation, yoga exercises, volleyball, and even "head banging" to heavy metal rock music (184,185). Unilateral vertebral artery occlusion seldom results in a neurologic deficit, despite a 15% incidence of congenital unilateral hypoplastic vertebral arteries (186). Treatment of blunt vertebral artery injury with thrombosis usually is nonoperative: systemic anticoagulation (if possible) is recommended to avoid further propagation of existing thrombus. More often with penetrating wounds, acute hemorrhage, pseudoaneurysm, or formation of an arteriovenous fistula are reasons for surgically addressing a known vertebral artery injury. Operative exposure and exploration can be difficult. The extraosseous first portion of the vertebral artery can be exposed by a supraclavicular incision with transection of the sternal head of the sternocleidomastoid muscle (Fig. 11.25). More distal exposure (second or third portion) is best obtained by an anterior approach (187,188). An incision is made along the anterior border of the sternocleidomastoid muscle, and the carotid sheath is identified and retracted either anterosuperiorly or posteroinferiorly to expose the prevertebral space (Fig. 11.26). Hemoclips are blindly applied where the vertebral artery is free of the osseous vertebral canal between the transverse processes, behind the longus cervicis (colli) muscle. High ligation of the vertebral artery at the C-1 to C-2 level (fourth portion) is a satisfactory method of obtaining distal control without unroofing the bony canal of the vertebral artery (186). Percutaneous embolization both distal and proximal to the site of arterial injury simplifies the management, but it requires a skilled and experienced interventional angiographer to cross the site of injury without causing further, uncorrectable damage. Contralateral vertebral angiography is recommended to determine accurately the extent of injury or the adequacy of embolization.

Trachea and Larynx

Blunt laryngeal trauma typically results from an anterior impact force (e.g., dashboard, steering wheel) that drives the larynx posteriorly against the rigid cervical spine. The impact can produce a simple or comminuted fracture of laryngeal cartilage, disruption of the mucosa of the endolarynx, or perforation and tears of the hypopharynx. Figure 11.27 depicts the critical laryngeal anatomy and the most common blunt injury pattern. These injuries are frequently occult and are often initially overlooked as attention is directed to injuries of the head, face, and thorax. Delayed recognition of blunt laryngeal trauma is the single greatest contributor to mortality, followed by aspiration of blood, missed esophageal injury, and overlooked concomitant intraabdominal injury. Subtle clinical signs and symptoms of laryngeal injury cannot be ignored. One report identifies hoarseness as the most common symptom, followed by shortness of breath, inability to tolerate the supine position, pain, dysphagia, and aphonia. Tenderness was identified as the most common clinical sign, followed by subcutaneous emphysema, neck contusion, tracheal deviation, and hemoptysis (189). Liberal use of fiberoptic endoscopy and neck CT aids in the diagnosis (190).

Unlike blunt laryngeal trauma, penetrating injuries to the trachea and larynx are usually readily apparent and dramatic in their clinical presentation. Subcutaneous emphysema (occasionally massive), pain, hoarseness, and respiratory distress are hallmarks of tracheal injury. However, rapid endotracheal intubation by field paramedics can mask a high tracheal injury. Concomitant esophageal, vascular, and thoracic injuries are frequent. A 20-year review of 106 tracheobronchial injuries documented a 22% incidence of concomitant esophageal injuries, a 16% incidence of major vessel injury, and a 40% incidence of hemopneumothorax (191).

As with any trauma victim, the first treatment priority for those with laryngotracheal injuries is to secure an adequate airway. With a laryngeal injury, this usually straightforward task can be extremely challenging. If an emergency airway is required, direct endotracheal intubation can be attempted initially if the laryngeal structures are well visualized and the endotracheal tube is passed over a flexible endoscope. However, this risks further damage to

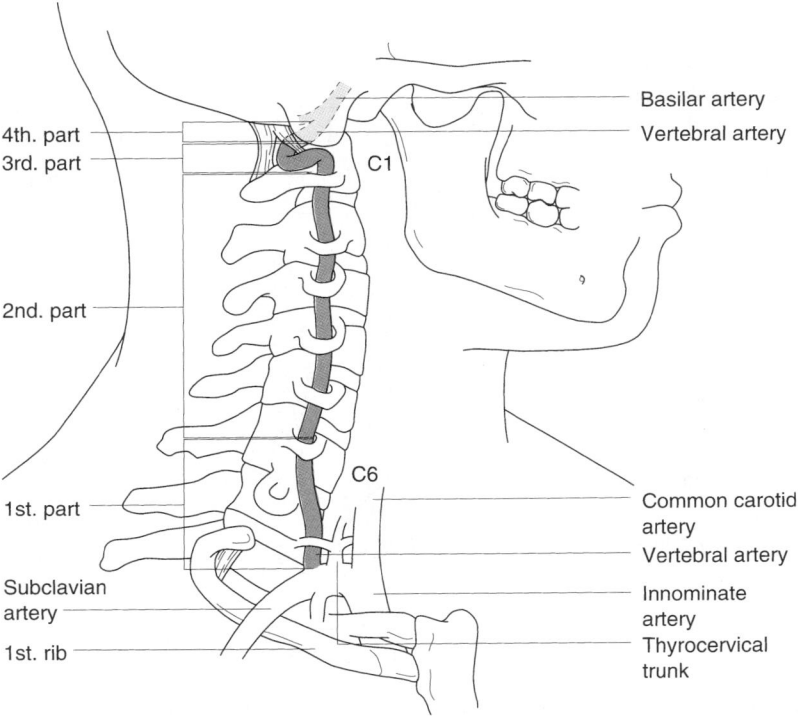

Figure 11.25. Normal anatomy of the vertebral artery, showing its division into four parts.

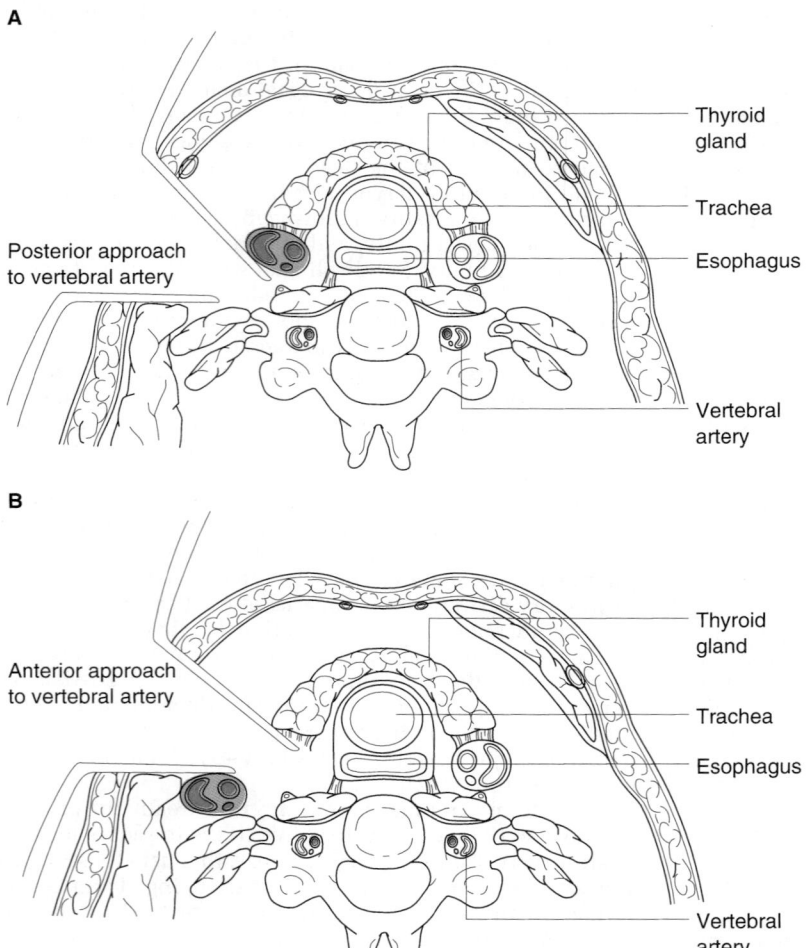

A

Posterior approach
to vertebral artery

Thyroid
gland

Trachea

Esophagus

Vertebral
artery

B

Anterior approach
to vertebral artery

Thyroid
gland

Trachea

Esophagus

Vertebral
artery

Figure 11.26. Operative approach to the vertebral artery. *(A)* Carotid artery and sheath retracted anteriorly. *(B)* Carotid artery and sheath retracted posteriorly.

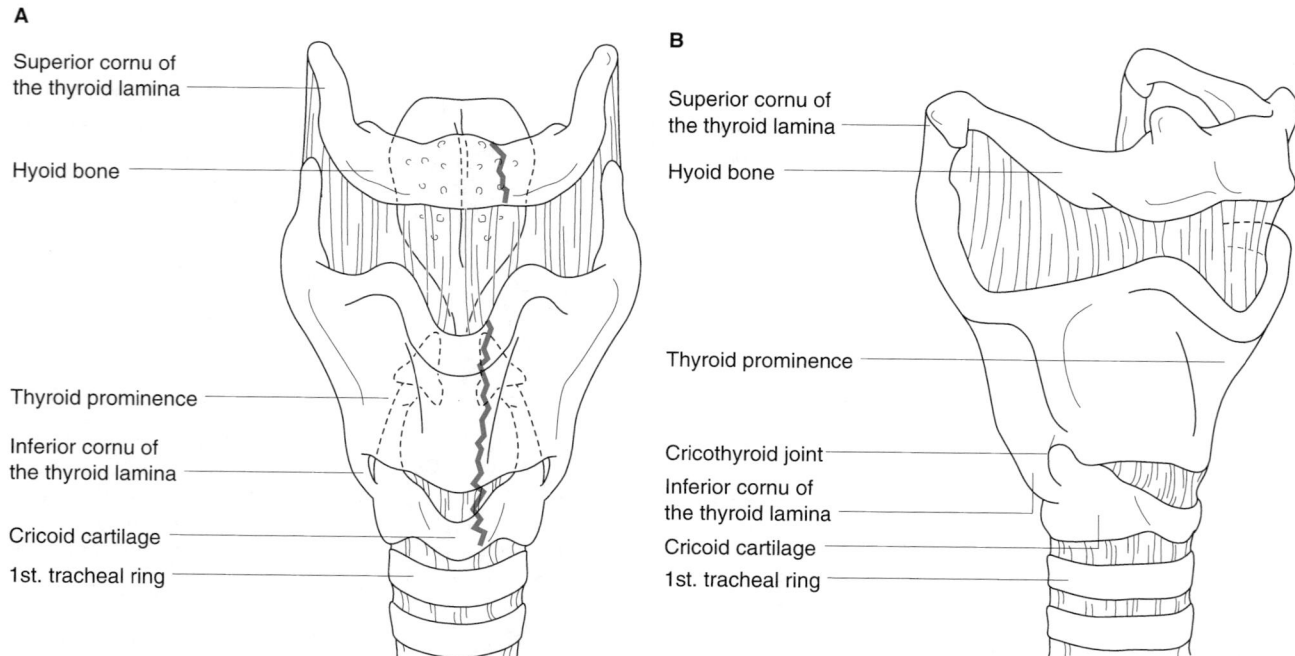

A

Superior cornu of
the thyroid lamina

Hyoid bone

Thyroid prominence

Inferior cornu of
the thyroid lamina

Cricoid cartilage

1st. tracheal ring

B

Superior cornu of
the thyroid lamina

Hyoid bone

Thyroid prominence

Cricothyroid joint

Inferior cornu of
the thyroid lamina

Cricoid cartilage

1st. tracheal ring

Figure 11.27. Frontal view *(A)* and three-quarters view *(B)* of larynx.

the trachea even in the most experienced hands. Equipment and preparation for emergency tracheostomy should always be at hand, and tracheostomy is usually recommended if an emergency airway is required, even though it also carries some risk of further injury (192). Pulse oximetry monitoring is essential, and care must be taken to prevent episodes of hypoxia while alternative airway access techniques are attempted. Transtracheal needle-jet insufflation can temporize a critical situation and allow a more controlled tracheostomy.

Operative repair is not usually required for patients with simple laryngeal edema, hematomas without mucosal disruption, small lacerations of the endolarynx not involving the anterior commissure or the free margin of the vocal fold, and small lacerations of the supraglottic larynx that do not disrupt the integrity of this site (192). Indications for primary open repair of the larynx include virtually all penetrating tracheal or laryngeal wounds, vocal cord disruption, mucosal tears with exposed cartilage, thyrohyoid separation, thyroid or cricoid cartilage fractures, and hypopharyngeal perforations. The basic tenets of operative care are débridement of devitalized cartilage, reduction of cartilaginous fractures, mucosal coverage of exposed cartilage, and closure of tracheal defects. Tracheostomy is not always required, but it is useful if extensive edema or prolonged airway compression is anticipated. Controversial areas in the surgical care of laryngotracheal trauma patients include the timing of operation, the role of laryngeal stents, the use of steroids, indications for skin grafting, and the techniques of operative exposure of the larynx (193).

Pharynx and Esophagus

Esophageal injuries occur in only 5% of patients with penetrating neck wounds. Esophageal perforation from external blunt trauma is rare and accounts for less than 10% of all esophageal perforations (194,195). Most blunt injuries are due to a direct blow to the neck with a hard object, such as a steering wheel in high-speed motor vehicle crashes, but it can occur from minor trauma. The diagnosis of an esophageal injury can be difficult. The clinical signs of esophageal injury, such as hematemesis, odynophagia, neck pain, crepitus, and air in the soft tissues on chest and neck radiographs, are often absent or obscured by concomitant laryngotracheal injury (196). In one study, the blunt cervicothoracic esophageal injury had a 56% incidence of associated tracheolaryngeal injury (195). In a review of 77 patients with penetrating esophageal injuries, 45 had cervical esophageal wounds (197). Overall, physical findings were diagnostic in only 26% of patients. Furthermore, the morbidity of a missed esophageal injury is catastrophic. One review of penetrating neck wounds contained 109 cases of esophageal injuries; the mortality rate was 2% if operation was performed immediately but increased to 44% if operation was delayed because of an initially missed injury, and to 100% if no operation was performed (144). This information is widely used as support for a mandatory neck exploration policy. However, other authors have documented a small but significant incidence of missed esophageal injury even after neck exploration. In one report, cervical esophageal injury was initially missed at neck exploration in three patients, and all three died (197). As a result, an aggressive effort at excluding esophageal injury is warranted, and some authors recommend routine esophagography or esophagoscopy, or both, to aid in the diagnosis of isolated esophageal injuries. However, the sensitivity of esophagography in detecting esophageal injury varies from approximately 50% to 90%, and the sensitivity of endoscopy varies from 29% to 100% (161). These modalities should be considered complementary; when combined, they have an accuracy of almost 100% (198). The choice of rigid or flexible esophagoscopy is largely a matter of individual preference.

Careful evaluation of the entire tract of the offending penetrating agent or region of blunt hematoma is required to document esophageal integrity. This can be technically challenging and time consuming, but it is a crucial component of the neck exploration. Concomitant intraoperative endoscopy, esophageal air insufflation, or even vital dye instillation can be helpful in excluding injury. Because almost all reported deaths from cervical esophageal injuries are the result of a delayed or missed diagnosis, a particularly thorough search is warranted. The key to successful management of cervical esophageal and pharyngeal injury is early adequate drainage (199). All such wounds should be drained to avoid deep neck infection or development of a salivary fistula, which occurs in 9% to 18% of these patients (196,200). Esophagography before drain removal is also recommended, because approximately half of postrepair fistulae are initially clinically silent. The injured esophagus should be meticulously débrided and repaired primarily, in two layers, with absorbable and nonabsorbable suture. Single-layer closure may be adequate (200). A sternocleidomastoid or strap muscle always should be placed between the trachea and esophagus in a combined repair. If primary closure is not realistic or safe because of an extensive loss of tissue as with shotgun blast, it may be necessary to perform a cutaneous esophagostomy for feeding purposes and a cutaneous pharyngostomy for salivary drainage. A secondary reconstructive procedure is then required after the initial healing is complete. There have been reports of nonoperative management of small injuries confined to the upper hypopharynx, above the arytenoid cartilage, if there are no other associated injuries (199). The treatment includes close observation, intravenous antibiotics, and restricted oral intake. Most surgeons advocate primary repair of all esophageal injuries, if it can be accomplished early. Delays of longer than 12 hours significantly increase the risk of repair dehiscence, wound abscess, and death. Neck esophageal injuries diagnosed more than 24 to 48 hours after injury are best managed initially by diversion and drainage.

Nerves

The preoperative determination of level of consciousness and lateralizing gross motor or sensory deficits is required in all patients; a more detailed neurologic examination of the brachial plexus, deep cervical plexus, phrenic nerve, and cranial nerves should be performed in all but the most unstable patients. A hypoglossal or spinal accessory nerve injury is particularly easy to miss unless a preoperative neurologic examination is performed. The vagus nerve can be evaluated by examination of the vocal cords. Primary débridement and repair of all severed or lacerated "named" nerves is preferred, with the use of fine interrupted nonabsorbable suture on the perineurium. Repair of a *single* recurrent nerve injury is controversial. An avulsed recurrent laryngeal nerve (blunt laryngotracheal disruption) should be implanted into the posterior cricoarytenoid muscle (201). If a motor nerve deficit is apparent, an expendable sensory nerve such as the great auricular can be interposed as a nerve graft to allow anastomosis without tension. If the patient's condition precludes primary repair, the nerve ends should be marked with silver clips or nonabsorbable colored suture. Secondary repair 3 weeks after injury is advised.

Definitive Care Phase: Chest Injuries

ROBERT J. WINCHELL

Chest injuries are common after trauma and are frequently severe. Approximately half of all accident fatalities include some element of chest injury, and approximately one fourth of these deaths can be directly attributed to thoracic injuries. Blunt injuries to the chest, such as from motor vehicle crashes or falls, are more common than those from penetrating trauma, except in some urban areas where penetrating injuries predominate. Among penetrating injuries, stab wounds are in general more common than gunshot wounds.

Most chest injuries can be treated with relatively simple methods, such as tube thoracostomy, appropriate analgesic management, and good pulmonary care (202). However, delay in diagnosis and treatment of severe chest injuries (e.g., tension pneumothorax, aortic transection, rib fractures with pulmonary contusion) is a common cause of preventable death after trauma. An organized structure for understanding chest injuries and their pathophysiology is necessary to guide diagnostic and therapeutic decisions.

ANATOMIC CONSIDERATIONS

For purposes of injury classification, the thorax can be divided into four anatomic zones: (a) the chest wall, (b) the pleural space, (c) the pulmonary parenchyma, and (d) mediastinal structures. Injuries to the chest wall include injuries to the bony thorax and shoulder girdle, as well as soft-tissue injuries. Pleural space injuries include the pneumothorax and hemothorax, in which the potential space between the visceral and parietal pleurae is occupied by either blood or air. Pulmonary parenchymal injuries include contusion, laceration, hematoma, and pneumatocele. Mediastinal injuries involve major vascular structures and the aerodigestive tract. Mediastinal vascular injuries include injuries to the heart, aorta, and great vessels. Aerodigestive injuries include tracheal and bronchial disruptions, traumatic asphyxia, and esophageal injuries.

DIAGNOSIS

Initial Evaluation

The initial evaluation and treatment of a patient with chest injuries is the same as for any trauma victim. An effective airway is secured, adequacy of breathing is ensured, and circulation is assessed and supported with control of external hemorrhage and establishment of large-bore peripheral venous access. Therapy for potentially life-threatening problems should be initiated immediately.

Whenever possible, a careful history relevant to the chest should be obtained, including details of the mechanism of injury. The speed and direction of impact and the degree of frontal deceleration are important factors in motor vehicle crashes. Aortic transection is associated with severe deceleration injury. Patients not using restraint systems are likely to contact the steering wheel or the dashboard of the car, placing them at an increased risk for chest injuries, such as rib fractures, flail chest, and pulmonary contusion, as well as tracheal or laryngeal injuries.

In patients who sustain penetrating trauma, the characteristics of the wounding instrument are important, but accurate information often is not available. External wounds can be misleading. All information from the patient should be carefully considered, even if the complaints are distant from the perceived trajectory of the injury. Patients with complaints of hoarse voice, dyspnea, throat pain, and dysphagia should be carefully evaluated for injuries to the larynx and the cervical portion of the esophagus. Complaints of dyspnea or pressure in the chest with or without chest wall pain may be indicative of pneumothorax or hemothorax.

The patient's past medical history is also important. A history of pulmonary disease, heart disease, or prior thoracic surgery can alter interpretation of diagnostic studies and affect therapeutic decisions. In addition, a history of medications, allergies, smoking, and the recent ingestion of drugs and alcohol should be obtained.

The physical examination begins with complete exposure of the chest and inspection for signs of contusions, lacerations, or penetrating wounds. These visible signs may give clues to the mechanism of injury. The breathing pattern, its effectiveness in ventilation, and any abnormal motion of the chest wall should be observed. Chest wall splinting and shallow respiration may be noted in patients with rib fractures. Asymmetric chest wall expansion with hyperinflation of one hemithorax is suggestive of tension pneumothorax. Paradoxical motion of a segment of chest wall is diagnostic of flail chest.

The presence of penetrating wounds should be noted, both anteriorly and posteriorly, and marked with metal clips for radiographic reference. In general, these wounds should not be probed. Little if any valuable information is obtained from probing chest wounds, and the maneuver can turn a minor laceration injury into a pneumothorax, requiring a chest tube and longer hospitalization. The location of penetrating injuries, and the likely trajectory of missiles, should modulate the physician's search for mediastinal and pulmonary parenchymal injuries. Penetrating injuries below the nipple line must be presumed to involve the abdominal cavity as well.

The examination of the chest continues with auscultation. The breath sounds should be compared bilaterally for quality and symmetry. Absence of breath sounds on one side is highly suggestive of hemothorax or pneumothorax. Asymmetric hypoventilation may be secondary to splinting from rib fractures, pulmonary contusion, hemothorax or pneumothorax, or main-stem intubation. The presence of rales and rhonchi should alert the clinician to possible intercurrent problems, such as pneumonia or cardiogenic shock from a myocardial infarction.

Gentle but firm palpation of the chest wall demonstrates areas of point tenderness that may be associated with fractures of the ribs, sternum, or clavicles. Areas of referred pain or tenderness should be noted, such as sternal compression causing lateral rib pain in the case of lateral rib fractures. Shoulder pain may be associated with the diaphragmatic irritation of splenic injury (Kehr's sign). The presence of crepitus over the manubrium or in the neck may be an early sign of tracheobronchial injury. Crepitus over the chest wall may be caused by rib fractures or by air in the subcutaneous tissues from a pneumothorax.

Percussion of the chest can also provide valuable information. Hyperresonance should raise suspicion of pneumothorax. This finding is most dramatic with tension pneumothorax, and it may be the most reliable physical sign of tension pneumothorax. Dullness to percussion is suggestive of hemothorax.

Adjunctive Diagnostic Modalities

The chest radiograph is by far the most important diagnostic study, and it should be obtained early in all patients with significant chest trauma. Standard posteroanterior and lateral chest films provide the most accurate information and should be obtained whenever possible. However, because of urgency, concerns about unstable spinal or pelvic injuries, and conflicting priorities, this is rarely possible in the trauma patient. In most patients, 100-cm supine anteroposterior chest radiographs are obtained during the initial evaluation.

Most thoracic injuries can be diagnosed simply from the plain films, making evaluation of chest films a vital skill for the trauma surgeon. A systematic approach to reading chest radiographs is important to ensure that all available information is considered. All chest films should be evaluated for abnormalities of the bony thorax, the soft tissues of the mediastinum, the diaphragm, the pleural space, and the pulmonary parenchyma.

In addition to rib fractures, injuries to the clavicle, scapula, and thoracic spine should be apparent on direct examination of the chest film. A lateral chest film may be necessary to make the diagnosis of sternal fracture, and specific oblique views may increase the diagnostic yield for rib fractures. These special studies are not essential because both rib fracture and sternal fracture are frequently clinical rather than radiographic diagnoses. Presence of significant bony injuries is indicative of major energy transfer to the chest and should raise suspicion of other underlying injuries.

Evaluation of the mediastinum is performed next, looking not only for abnormal widening of the superior mediastinum but for more subtle changes in mediastinal contour. Abnormalities of the aortic contour should raise the suspicion of vascular injury. The presence of air in the mediastinum is suggestive of injury to the esophagus or tracheobronchial tree. The diaphragmatic contours should be sharp and located in normal anatomic position. Poor visualization of a hemidiaphragm may result from traumatic rupture of the diaphragm or from hemothorax. A depressed hemidiaphragm associated with hyperexpansion of the hemithorax suggests tension pneumothorax.

Haziness over one hemithorax on the supine chest radiograph can indicate a hemothorax. Conversely, lucency of one hemithorax should raise suspicion of pneumothorax. Pneumothorax is often confirmed by identification of lung parenchyma collapsed away from the chest wall, but this finding is not always present, especially in patients on positive-pressure ventilation. The radiograph also should be carefully evaluated for lucency in the region of the diaphragm and deepening of the costophrenic sulcus, which are indicative of subpulmonic pneumothorax. The diagnostic accuracy for a suspected pneumothorax may be increased by upright inhalation and exhalation radiographic views.

In patients with potential esophageal injuries, contrast studies should be obtained. The use of a water-soluble contrast agent instead of barium in esophageal evaluation is controversial. The water-soluble medium causes less reaction in the mediastinum if there is an esophageal injury, but it can cause significant pneumonitis if there is a tracheoesophageal fistula. Barium contrast studies give superior mucosal detail in esophageal injuries. It is prudent to begin with water-soluble contrast and proceed with a larger volume of barium for better mucosal detail if no extravasation occurs. In patients who are conscious and alert, the oral contrast should be swallowed under fluoroscopic visualization. In unconscious adult patients, a nasogastric tube is placed just below the pharynx and a 30- to 50-mL bolus of contrast material is injected with enough pressure gently to distend the esophagus while obtaining a plain radiograph.

Angiography is the best study to rule out major injury to the great vessels in the chest in most circumstances, and angiography remains mandatory in most patients at risk for aortic disruption who have abnormal findings on the chest radiograph. Advances in computed tomography (CT) technology have greatly improved the diagnostic accuracy of this modality, and studies suggest that dynamic CT scan of the chest may rival angiography in diagnostic accuracy (203,204) in centers experienced in its use. Dynamic CT scan of the chest is a very useful modality to assess the mediastinum and aortic arch in patients with a negative chest film, where the concern for aortic injury is based on mechanism of injury alone. Transesophageal echocardiography for the evaluation of the aortic arch has been used successfully in some centers (205,206). It is a potential alternative for patients who cannot be transported to the angiography suite because of hemodynamic instability or immediate need for other surgery.

Angiography should be obtained whenever the diagnosis of occult vascular injury in the thoracic cavity is considered. Accurate knowledge of the anatomy of an injury may be essential to planning the correct surgical approach. Patients with penetrating injuries to the thoracic inlet, wounds that cross the midline, or penetrating injuries with trajectories that suggest vascular involvement should undergo angiography if they are hemodynamically stable. Such injuries may present with subtle angiographic findings, and biplanar views are mandatory. Patients with occult vascular injury are at risk for development of massive bleeding during or after angiography, and they must be monitored with great care throughout the procedure.

Video-assisted thoracoscopy is emerging as a potential diagnostic tool for the evaluation of chest trauma. It provides good visualization of mediastinal structures as well as the pleural cavity. The procedure requires general anesthesia and intubation with a double-lumen endotracheal tube to facilitate complete examination, which may limit its usefulness as a screening tool. Video-assisted thoracoscopy is not yet widely used as a diagnostic modality, and experience remains concentrated primarily in centers with an interest in its use.

TREATMENT

General Considerations

Most injuries to the chest can be successfully managed without surgical intervention. The routine use of tube thoracostomy for treatment of hemothorax and pneumothorax is a cornerstone of therapy. Thoracotomy is most often needed for the control of massive bleeding or bleeding that persists despite tube thoracostomy. Approximately 80% to 85% of patients with hemorrhage in the chest can be treated by tube thoracostomy alone.

Most bleeding in the chest is the result of injuries to the low-pressure pulmonary circulation. Partial or complete collapse of the lung associated with pneumothorax or hemothorax allows small tears or lacerations in the pulmonary parenchyma to continue to bleed. The insertion of a chest tube with subsequent evacuation of the air, blood, and clot allows for reexpansion of the lung and restoration of the normal negative intrathoracic pressure. The reexpanded parenchyma is then apposed against the relatively nondeformable chest wall, leading to tamponade of the low-pressure bleeding. For larger and deeper lacerations, still with relatively low-pressure bleeding from the pulmonary circulation, bleeding can be controlled by the reinflated parenchyma and by the edema in the injured tissue. Tube thoracostomy with full expansion of the lung results in adequate hemostasis in most cases. Persistent bleeding is most commonly a result of injuries to major proximal branches of the pulmonary circulation or to systemic arteries, including the intercostal and internal mammary arteries.

The key to successful closed drainage is complete evacuation of blood and clot with full reexpansion of the lung. Patients with ongoing bleeding can form significant clots and are at risk for occlusion of the thoracostomy tube. Therefore, it is vital to use a relatively large tube in patients with hemothorax and to monitor the tube to ensure its continued patency. In most adults, a 36F chest tube is a reasonable choice.

Insertion of a chest tube should be performed as a sterile procedure. After appropriate skin preparation with povidone–iodine solution, local anesthetic is injected, and the chest tube is placed through a skin incision in the fifth or sixth intercostal space, slightly anterior to the mid-axillary line. This relatively cephalad location for the chest tube is chosen to ensure intrathoracic placement of the tube and to avoid injury due to a potentially elevated or ruptured hemidiaphragm. Slightly anterior placement, just behind the body of the pectoralis muscle, is important to minimize risk of injury to the long thoracic nerve. The tube is directed posteriorly to facilitate evacuation of blood from the thorax when the patient is supine. A finger should be inserted through the incision into the thorax before placement of the thoracostomy tube. This digital exploration allows the physician to confirm the thoracic location, assess for the presence of pleural adhesions, feel for viscera (suggesting a ruptured diaphragm), and, possibly, palpate injuries in the diaphragm and pericardium before inserting the chest tube. After insertion, the thoracostomy tube should be placed to closed suction drainage until the air leak is resolved and the output is less than 2 mL/kg (or approximately 150 mL) in a 24-hour period.

The use of prophylactic antibiotics has been shown to decrease infectious complications after tube thoracostomy (207,208). Other data suggest that the risk of major infectious complications, such as empyema, after tube thoracostomy under appropriate sterile technique is low, leading to the conclusion that prophylactic antibiotics are unnecessary (209). The use of prophylactic antibiotics after tube thoracostomy is reasonable, but has not been uniformly adopted.

Indications for Surgery

Chest Wall Injuries

Most chest wall injuries do not require surgical repair; however, these patients frequently have associated abdominal, orthopedic, or other injuries that do require operative management (210). The open pneumothorax, or sucking chest wound, requires operative débridement and closure. Sternal fractures with significant posterior displacement also require operative repair.

Injuries Manifesting in the Pleural Space

Thoracotomy is indicated for control of ongoing hemorrhage. Pleural space injuries that require operative repair include massive hemothorax with ongoing bleeding, and clotted or caked hemothorax.

Parenchymal Injuries

The cause of hemothorax requiring surgery occasionally is ongoing hemorrhage from lung parenchymal injuries. Deep parenchymal injuries can also produce severe hemoptysis that necessitates thoracotomy. In addition, operative repair is required for injuries to the trachea or major bronchi that exceed approximately one-half the circumference of the airway, or if there are large continuing air leaks that cannot be controlled by insertion of chest tubes.

Mediastinal Injuries

Mediastinal injuries that require surgery include blunt or penetrating cardiac trauma with associated exsanguination, cardiac tamponade, or great vessel injury. Injuries to the thoracic esophagus require thoracotomy and repair.

Other Injuries

Thoracotomy can be of value in resuscitation of trauma patients with hypovolemia unresponsive to massive volume infusion. Resuscitative thoracotomy also may be indicated in patients with cardiac arrest after penetrating chest trauma, but rarely after blunt trauma.

General Conduct of Surgery

The choice of position and surgical approach is dictated by the nature of the patient's thoracic injuries, the certainty of diagnosis, and the potential for associated injuries involving other body sites. The standard posterolateral thoracotomy provides optimal exposure to the contents of a particular hemithorax, but the lateral position of the patient makes access to the other side of the chest or the abdomen difficult if not impossible. Therefore, although posterolateral thoracotomy provides the best access, it can be used only in patients who have injuries isolated to a given hemithorax. This determination usually can be made in patients with clearly defined injury and in those who have been under observation for a period before thoracotomy.

In most patients undergoing emergency thoracotomy for chest trauma, an anterolateral approach must be used. The patient remains supine to allow for access to the abdomen and contralateral chest cavity. Exposure through an anterolateral thoracotomy is considerably more difficult but is adequate with proper technique. The ipsilateral side of the body should be elevated to facilitate posterior exposure. The posterior aspect of the incision must extend as far as possible, at least to the border of the latissimus dorsi, and particular care must be taken to follow the curvature of the underlying rib. The mobility of the ribs is limited in the anterolateral approach, and it may be necessary to divide the one or more costal cartilages at the sternum to gain sufficient access. The medial portion of the incision should curve superiorly to facilitate this maneuver (Fig. 11.28A).

The anterolateral thoracotomy incision can be carried transversely across the sternum into the opposite hemithorax to allow exposure to the heart, mediastinum, and structures in the opposite pleural cavity. The sternum can be divided with a sternal saw, a Lebsche knife, or heavy scissors. This bilateral, or clamshell, thoracotomy provides excellent exposure to the heart, mediastinum, and bilateral pulmonary hila (Fig. 11.28B). It is necessary to divide both internal mammary arteries in making this incision, and they must be carefully ligated at the time of closure to prevent recurrent bleeding.

The median sternotomy incision provides excellent exposure to the heart and the great vessels in the anterior mediastinum, but it provides difficult exposure for repair of injuries of the lungs, descending aorta, chest wall, diaphragm, or esophagus. Therefore, like the posterolateral thoracotomy, it can be used only if the patient's injuries can be determined with relative certainty. This is not often the case, and most penetrating injuries to the heart are best approached through a left anterolateral thoracotomy, with extension across the sternum transversely if necessary.

The median sternotomy can be extended into the neck or over the clavicle for exposure of the aortic arch and innominate vessels (Fig. 11.29A). This approach may pro-

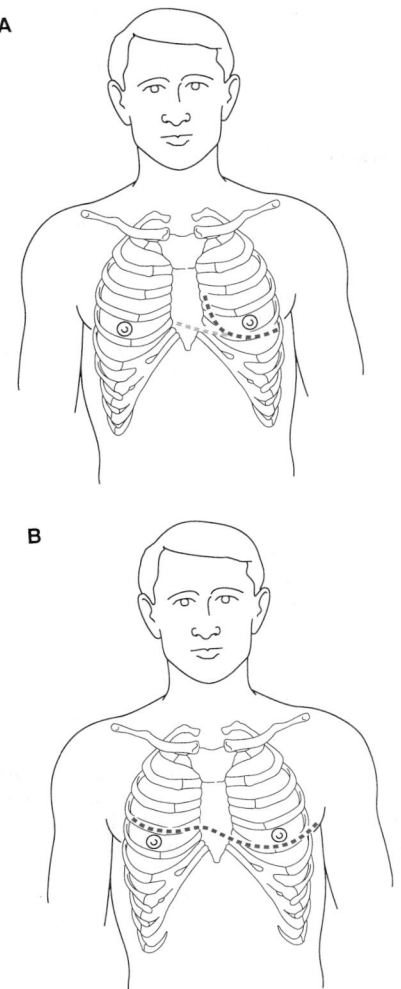

Figure 11.28. *(A)* Anterolateral thoracotomy showing correct (dark) and too-transverse (light) incisions. *(B)* A clamshell, or bilateral thoracotomy incision.

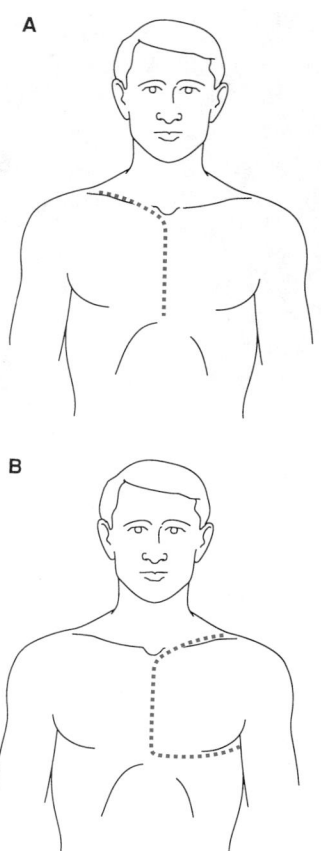

Figure 11.29. Median sternotomy with clavicular extension *(A)* and trapdoor incision *(B)* for exposure of the intrathoracic great vessels.

vide the best access to vascular injuries at the thoracic inlet. The median sternotomy combined with the clavicular extension and left anterolateral thoracotomy, the so-called trapdoor incision, can be used for exposure to the entire left thoracic inlet (Fig. 11.29B). Such an incision may be the only way to approach proximal injuries in this difficult area. This exposure should be used only if it is absolutely necessary for control of hemorrhage because it can lead to traction injury of the brachial plexus and disabling long-term sequelae. Care also must be taken to avoid injury to the phrenic nerve on the anterior border of scalenus anterior muscle.

Specific Injuries

Injuries to the Chest Wall

Rib Fractures. Rib fractures are the most common injury associated with blunt chest trauma. They can occur directly at the site of force or laterally as a result of significant anteroposterior compression of the chest. The location and area of rib fracture may be indicative of associated injuries. The first rib is protected by the shoulder girdle and clavicle, so fractures of the first rib indicate a significant amount of energy transferred to the torso. First rib fractures have been

associated with severe chest and abdominal injuries and with aortic injuries. Posterior rib fractures are also associated with significant energy transfer to the thorax. Fractures of the lower ribs may be associated with intraabdominal injury. A 20% incidence of splenic injury is associated with fractures of ribs 9, 10, and 11 on the left side (211). There is similar association between right lower rib fractures and hepatic parenchymal injuries.

The diagnosis of rib fracture is primarily clinical, and fractures often cannot be seen on routine radiographs. Rib tenderness (either directly or on anteroposterior compression), crepitus over the possible area of fracture, and decreased breath sounds on the side of injury are all suggestive of rib fracture or injury. Specific rib detail films increase the diagnostic yield of chest radiographs, but radiologic confirmation of the diagnosis is not essential (Fig. 11.30). Chest radiographs may demonstrate associated injuries, such as pneumothorax, pulmonary contusion, or hemothorax.

The treatment of rib fractures is directed primarily at control of their adverse effect on ventilation. Because of the pain associated with chest wall injury, poor inspiratory effort, splinting, and an ineffective cough commonly result. If these are not prevented or appropriately treated, atelectasis and pneumonia ensue. Elderly patients, especially those with preexisting pulmonary disease, are particularly prone to these complications. An assessment of the patient's ventilatory compromise from pain can be made by bedside pulmonary function tests, with primary

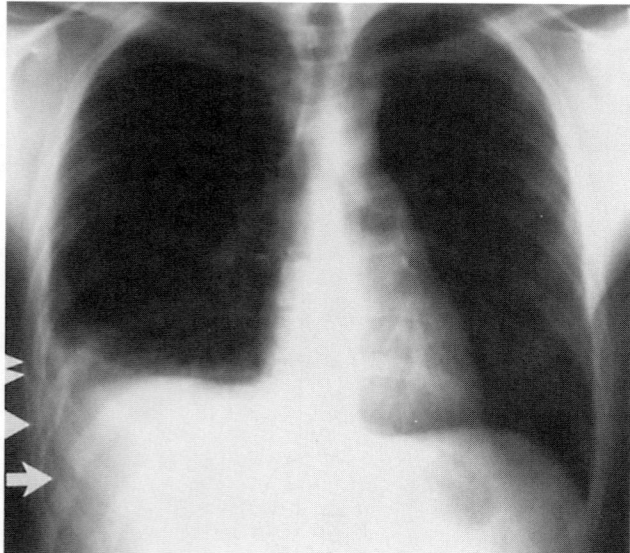

Figure 11.30. Chest radiograph showing multiple rib fractures (ribs 7 to 10). The costophrenic angle is blunted, representing a 400-mL hemothorax.

attention to the forced vital capacity and tidal volume. A forced vital capacity of less than 10 mL/kg or a tidal volume of less than 5 to 7 mL/kg is indicative of significant respiratory compromise.

Adequate pain relief and pulmonary care are the primary therapeutic goals. Good analgesia and careful pulmonary care can markedly improve the patient's ventilatory function. The use of intercostal nerve blocks is effective but has been largely supplanted by newer techniques such as patient-controlled analgesia, continuous opioid infusion, and epidural analgesia. Careful use of parenteral opioids, either on a routine basis or through patient-controlled analgesia, suffices in most cases. Epidural techniques are of particular value in elderly patients and in those with underlying pulmonary disease, in whom parenteral opioid use may be limited by respiratory side effects. One study showed that use of epidural opioid produces improvement in pulmonary function superior to that obtained from continuous intravenous administration of narcotic (212). Ventilatory function should be measured both before and after analgesic treatment is begun, and the narcotic dose should be titrated to ventilatory response. The practice of taping fractured ribs is not only ineffective but counterproductive because it can increase the pain from the rib fractures and may further restrict an already compromised ventilatory ability.

Although epidural and continuous intravenous analgesia appear to be the most effective methods for pain control from rib fractures, not all patients with fractured ribs require hospitalization. Patients who are generally healthy with no underlying medical problems, and who demonstrate good ventilatory function with oral analgesics, may be treated on an outpatient basis with careful follow-up. Patients with a history of smoking, chronic obstructive pulmonary disease, or other pulmonary problems who sustain rib fractures are at increased risk for complications. These patients usually benefit from hospital admission to ensure adequate analgesia and to monitor pulmonary function.

Sternal Fractures. Sternal fractures are frequently associated with a significant blow to the anterior chest. The incidence of sternal fractures historically is low, occurring in approximately 5% of patients with severe chest injuries. Sternal fracture has been reported to occur in unrestrained motor vehicle accident victims who strike the steering wheel. The mortality rate associated with sternal fractures in older series has been as high as 25% to 30%, mainly because of other injuries to the chest, such as aortic transection, cardiac contusion or tamponade, or tracheobronchial rupture. More recent studies have suggested a change in the pattern and severity of injuries associated with sternal fracture (213). Major improvements in automobile safety, including collapsible steering columns, interior padding, and passive restraints, have probably contributed to this change. Isolated sternal fracture may result from shoulder belt use, and it does not necessitate hospital admission in the stable patient (214–216).

Sternal fractures are usually transverse but can be longitudinal, especially if they are associated with sternal flail chest. Posterior displacement of the fractured sternum can impinge on the heart. The diagnosis of sternal fracture is made by palpation of the sternum if an obvious step-off is present. A lateral chest radiograph can reveal sternal fractures and the degree of posterior displacement (Fig. 11.31). The treatment of sternal fracture is primarily adequate pain relief and pulmonary care, as for rib fractures. If severe displacement is present, operative reduction with fixation of the fracture may be required.

Flail Chest. A flail chest occurs when consecutive ribs are fractured in more than one place, creating a free-floating segment of the chest wall. The free-floating segment can involve the sternum, with separation of the costochondral junction on either side (Fig. 11.32). Flail chest occurs in up to 20% of patients with severe blunt chest injuries.

Flail chest may result in paradoxical chest wall motion, as the free-floating segment responds to pressure gradients, not to the organized motion of the chest wall during

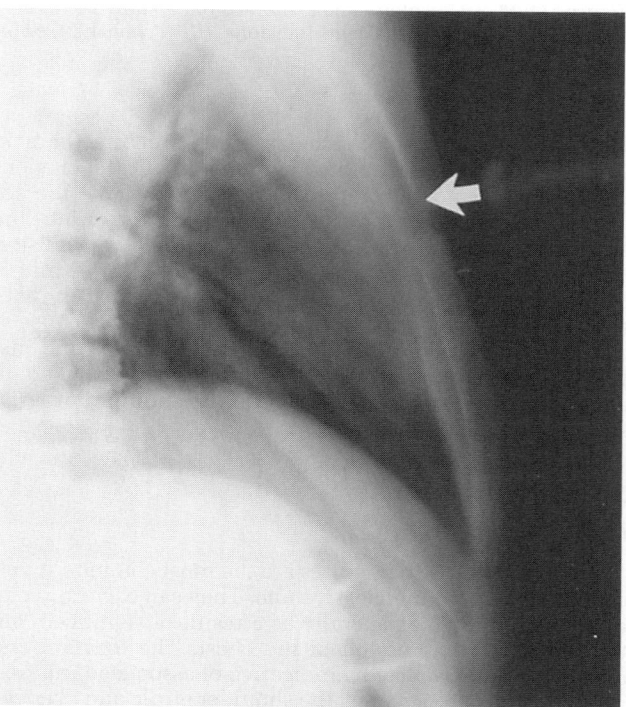

Figure 11.31. Posterior displacement of a sternal fracture *(arrow),* as demonstrated on a lateral chest radiograph.

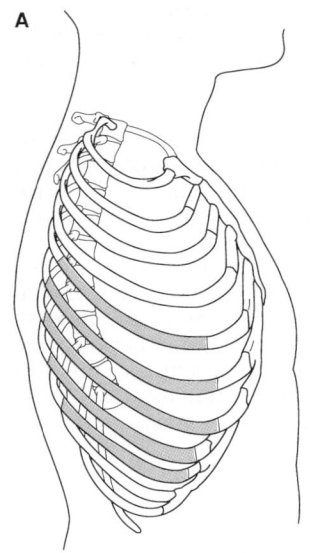
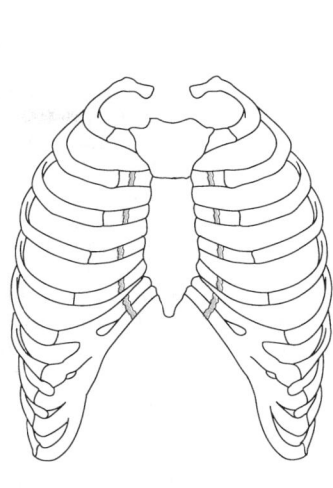

A   **B**

Figure 11.32. *(A)* Right lateral flail chest. *(B)* Sternal flail chest.

breathing. The intact chest wall expands during inspiration, but the negative intrathoracic pressure generated causes the flail segment to move inappropriately inward. On expiration, the flail segment moves outward as the rest of the chest wall moves inward. Historically, it was believed that this paradoxical motion was the cause of the severe ventilatory insufficiency associated with flail chest, and therapeutic efforts were focused on stabilization of the flail segment. Stabilization was attempted with dressings, sandbags, surgical fracture fixation, even towel clips through the chest wall into the rib, attached to the frame of the bed. Mortality rates with these modes of treatment were between 30% and 40% (217).

Our understanding of the pathophysiologic consequences of the flail chest has evolved. The ventilatory impairment is not caused simply by the paradoxical motion of the chest wall but rather by the underlying pulmonary parenchymal injury in combination with the hypoventilation and splinting that result from the pain of multiple contiguous rib fractures. The weak and ineffective ventilatory effort frequently leads to progressive atelectasis and pneumonia. Improved understanding of the pathophysiology of flail chest also has altered the therapeutic focus, with dramatic improvements in survival. The current approach to the patient with flail chest stresses adequate analgesia to prevent the cycle of pain, splinting, and hypoventilation, and early ventilatory support. The need for mechanical ventilation is determined by the degree of pulmonary parenchymal injury and by the inability to achieve adequate pain relief. Using such methods, the mortality rate for flail chest has decreased to approximately 2% in nonventilated patients and approximately 20% in patients requiring mechanical ventilation. Mortality is usually related to severe head injuries, or other associated injuries (218–220).

The patient's ventilatory status is assessed at the time of initial presentation. Mechanical problems contributing to respiratory compromise, such as airway obstruction, pneumothorax, or hemothorax, should be treated rapidly. Patients with a flail chest who present with respiratory distress and hypoxemia require immediate endotracheal intubation and mechanical ventilation. If the patient's ventilatory function is initially adequate, aggressive measures to ensure analgesia are undertaken. Epidural techniques are often required, and they should be considered early.

The patient is carefully monitored, because the pulmonary injuries commonly progress over the first several hours. Mechanical ventilation should be initiated at the first early signs of impending ventilatory failure, not after the patient is in an advanced state of respiratory compromise.

Vigorous chest physiotherapy and pulmonary care are an integral part of the treatment protocol. Usually, the amount of pain experienced by the patient decreases within 72 hours, and the amount of analgesia required is concomitantly less. These patients are continued on aggressive chest physiotherapy and pulmonary care under careful observation until their pain is well controlled, tidal volume is adequate, and cough has improved. Then they can be weaned gradually from systemic to oral analgesia.

Open Pneumothorax. The open pneumothorax, or sucking chest wound, is an uncommon injury that produces a large chest wall defect and is usually caused by impalement, high-speed motor vehicle accident, or shotgun blast. These injuries can also occur from large lacerations in the chest wall after an assault. The defect in the chest wall allows equilibration of intrathoracic and ambient pressures, leading to collapse of the lung. If the defect is large enough, air flows through the chest wall defect rather than through the trachea and into the lungs with each inspiratory effort. This can result in rapid and profound ventilatory compromise, an immediately life-threatening situation. The diagnosis of a sucking chest wound can be made on simple inspection of the chest wall and hearing the flow of air through the wound. The defect should be occluded with an impermeable dressing, such as petrolatum gauze, essentially converting the situation to a closed pneumothorax. Tube thoracostomy is then performed to reexpand the lung. The chest wall defect usually requires operative débridement and formal chest wall closure. In most cases, closure can be accomplished primarily, although large soft-tissue defects may require tissue transfer techniques.

Pleural Space Injuries

Simple Pneumothorax. Pneumothorax, defined as air in the potential space between the visceral and parietal pleurae, is a common occurrence. The loss of negative intrapleural pressure allows the lung to collapse from elastic recoil. Pneumothorax ordinarily results from ruptured alveoli or from small lacerations in the pulmonary parenchyma and is frequently associated with rib fractures. Pneumothorax also can result from lacerations through the chest wall (e.g., stab or gunshot wounds) and from iatrogenic injuries (e.g., as a complication of placement of a central venous catheter). The diagnosis of pneumothorax is suggested on physical examination by decreased ipsilateral breath sounds; decreased expansion of the affected hemithorax; hyperresonance to percussion; crepitus; or subcutaneous emphysema. The chest radiograph is usually diagnostic (Fig. 11.33). In patients on positive-pressure ventilation, the radiologic diagnosis can be somewhat more difficult because the lung does not always collapse away from the chest wall. The diaphragmatic contour should be carefully evaluated for evidence of subpulmonic air, the deep sulcus sign.

In patients with penetrating trauma to the chest but no pneumothorax apparent on supine chest film, upright posteroanterior and inhalation–exhalation views may improve the diagnostic yield. Patients who manifest no evidence of pneumothorax on upright chest radiography after 6 hours of observation may be discharged safely (221).

Traumatic pneumothorax is treated by placement of a tube thoracostomy, as previously described. A large (36F) chest tube should be inserted to evacuate the air and any blood and blood clots that may be present. Patients with only subcutaneous emphysema who are to undergo general anesthesia with positive-pressure ventilation should be considered for prophylactic tube thoracostomy to prevent the potentially lethal complication of tension pneumothorax. A chest radiograph should be obtained after insertion of the chest tube to confirm that proper tube positioning and reexpansion of the lung have occurred.

Patients with small, asymptomatic pneumothoraces who do not require general endotracheal anesthesia or positive-pressure ventilation may be observed carefully without placement of a tube thoracostomy. If the air leak from the lung has sealed, the air in the pleural cavity will be reabsorbed, with subsequent complete reexpansion of the lung. Serial chest films should be obtained to ensure that the pneumothorax is progressively decreasing and that the lung is not collapsed. Small pneumothoraces, par-

ticularly those from spontaneous bleb rupture or iatrogenic injury, can be drained effectively with smaller thoracostomy tubes, causing less patient discomfort and shortening hospital stay (222,223).

Tension Pneumothorax. A tension pneumothorax occurs if the pressure of accumulated air in the pleural space exceeds the ambient pressure, resulting in a net positive intrathoracic pressure. Although tension pneumothorax can occur in patients who are breathing spontaneously, it is most commonly associated with positive-pressure ventilation. Positive-pressure ventilation increases the air leak into the ipsilateral pleural space and can convert a simple pneumothorax to a tension pneumothorax. Mediastinal shift leads to decreased venous return to the heart and compression of the opposite functional lung. Tension pneumothorax often causes severe respiratory distress and hemodynamic compromise.

Patients with tension pneumothorax can have tachypnea, dyspnea, absent breath sounds on the affected side, and hyperresonance to percussion. As the situation progresses, central cyanosis, tracheal deviation, jugular venous distention, and arterial hypotension occur. The chest radiograph may reveal a collapsed lung, a depressed ipsilateral hemidiaphragm, widened intercostal spaces, and a mediastinal shift away from the hemithorax with positive intrathoracic pressure (Fig. 11.34).

Immediate decompression of the affected hemithorax is required in patients with respiratory and hemodynamic compromise from tension pneumothorax. Decompression is most rapidly accomplished by needle thoracostomy, which involves placing a large-bore (14- or 16-gauge) needle through the chest wall to relieve the positive intrathoracic pressure. Historically, the second intercostal space in the mid-clavicular line was suggested as the site for this procedure, but the anatomic landmarks are rather difficult, and the potential for mediastinal vascular injuries is significant. The author recommends that the needle thoracostomy be done in the fifth or sixth intercostal space at the mid-axillary line, in the same position as the tube thoracostomy. The body wall is thinnest at this site, and the anatomy is much less complex. Placement of a tube thoracostomy after needle decompression constitutes definitive therapy.

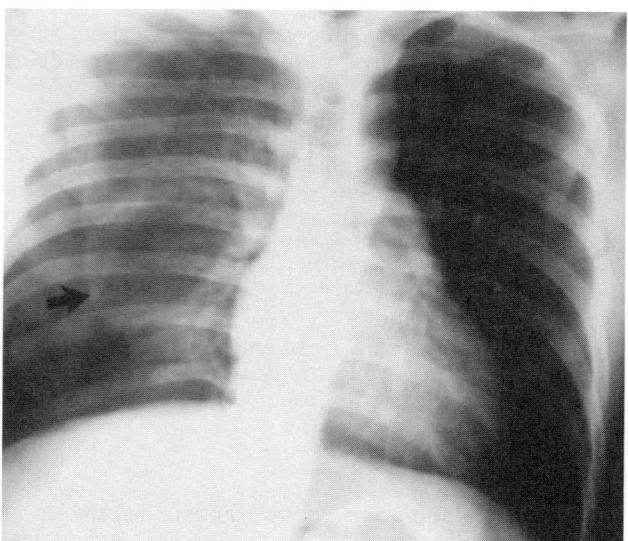

Figure 11.33. Right-sided simple pneumothorax with no significant mediastinal shift (*arrow* indicates lung margin).

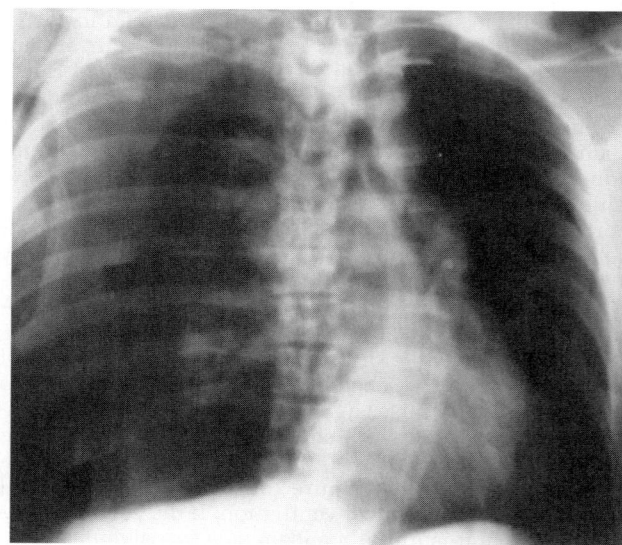

Figure 11.34. Right-sided tension pneumothorax with tracheobronchial and mediastinal shifts.

Hemothorax. A hemothorax is the accumulation of blood in the pleural space, and it occurs in 50% to 75% of patients with severe blunt or penetrating chest trauma. Though the amount of bleeding is often minimal with small lung lacerations or puncture wounds, there is potential for massive bleeding from injuries to larger branches of pulmonary arteries and veins, major rents in the pulmonary parenchyma, or lacerations of systemic arteries. Patients may be relatively asymptomatic or in frank hypovolemic shock at the time of presentation, and may complain of dyspnea or shortness of breath. Physical examination usually reveals decreased breath sounds and dullness to percussion on the injured side. Supine chest films usually show haziness of the affected lung field or, with massive hemothorax, complete opacification (Fig. 11.35).

The treatment of hemothorax begins with tube thoracostomy to evacuate the blood and reexpand the lung. The pressure of the pulmonary parenchymal circulation is relatively low, and reexpansion of the lung compresses the areas of injury against the interior of the relatively rigid chest wall. This acts to tamponade low-pressure bleeding. In addition, the pulmonary parenchyma has a high concentration of tissue thromboplastin, which probably contributes to hemostasis and sealing of air leaks. Simple tube thoracostomy is adequate treatment for up to 85% of patients with hemothorax.

Massive hemothorax (i.e., more than 1,000 to 1,500 mL) may require thoracotomy for evacuation of clot and control of bleeding. Efforts should be made to evacuate all of the blood from the chest and to reexpand the lung, which leads to tamponade of the injured lung parenchyma. If reexpansion fails or if the patient continues to bleed rapidly, thoracotomy is required for control of bleeding. Persistent bleeding, at a rate greater than 200 mL/h for 4 hours, or greater than 100 mL/h for 8 hours, is also an indication for thoracotomy in adults. If the patient manifests any hemodynamic instability during this period of observation, urgent thoracotomy is mandatory.

Caked or Clotted Hemothorax. In some cases, a clot remains around the lung despite the presence of a well placed large-bore tube thoracostomy. This clot keeps the lung from completely reexpanding and can cause pulmonary entrapment or an eventual fibrothorax (Fig. 11.36). The incidence of infected, clotted, or caked hemothorax after tube thoracostomy is 5% to 15% in major

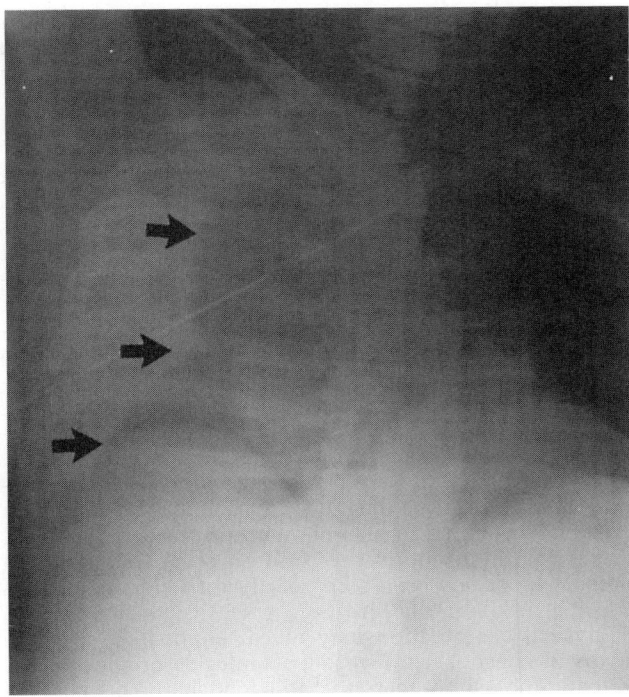

Figure 11.36. Large accumulation of intrapleural blood or clotted hemothorax with compression of right lung *(arrows).*

trauma patients. Although a small hemothorax is spontaneously absorbed over time, a large hemothorax does not resolve without mechanical drainage. The magnitude of the residual hemothorax that necessitates thoracotomy has not been clearly defined.

Surgical therapy for a clotted hemothorax consists of evacuation of retained clot and decortication of the lung if a thick fibrinous peel is present. If done relatively early, before the clot has become organized, evacuation often can be accomplished using thoracoscopy, with or without the addition of a limited thoracotomy (224–226). This procedure is usually well tolerated, with full reexpansion of the

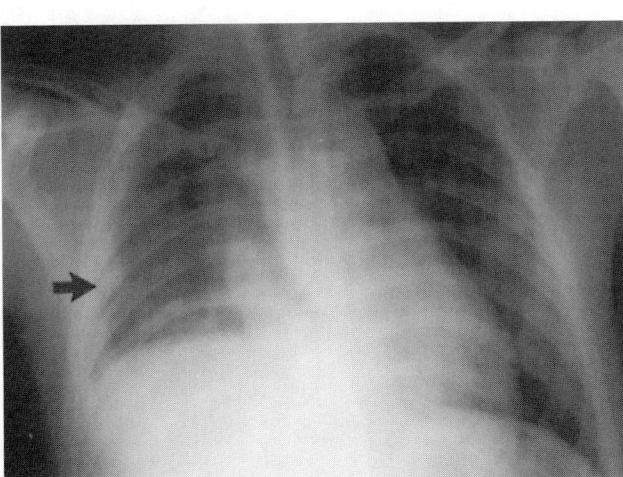

Figure 11.35. Right-sided hemothorax with diffuse unilateral haziness and pleural-based density *(arrow),* indicating intrapleural blood.

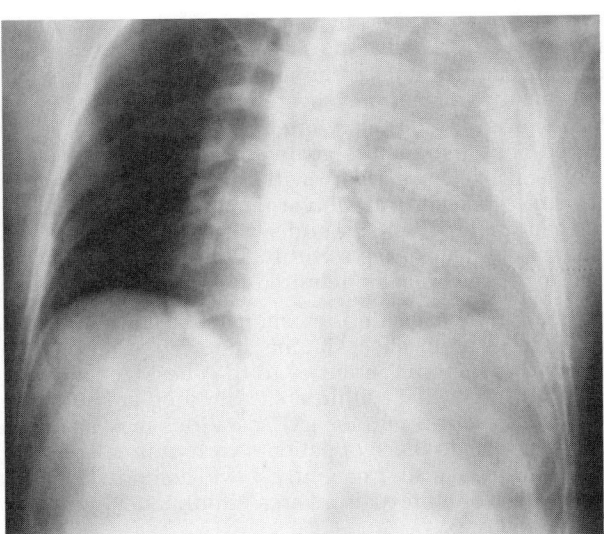

Figure 11.37. Hemothorax and associated massive left pulmonary contusion after blunt chest trauma.

lung and discharge from the hospital within a week. After the first 7 to 10 days, removal of the clot is more likely to require full thoracotomy and decortication, which has a significantly greater physiologic impact.

Parenchymal Injuries

Pulmonary Contusion. Pulmonary contusion occurs in up to 70% of patients with severe blunt chest trauma. It is associated with rib fractures, flail chest, and sternal fractures. Pulmonary contusion involves extensive interstitial hemorrhage within the parenchyma, with alveolar collapse and extravasation of blood and plasma into the alveoli. As a result, a ventilation–perfusion mismatch develops, which leads to arterial hypoxemia. Under these circumstances, the hypoxemia is usually refractory to increases in inspired oxygen concentration. In addition, pulmonary compliance decreases, and work of breathing increases. These effects tend to worsen over the first several hours after injury and can combine to produce severe respiratory failure. The diagnosis of pulmonary contusion must be considered in patients with rib fractures and flail chest or with any other severe blunt chest trauma. Such patients must be observed carefully for evidence of progressive ventilatory failure.

Physical examination may reveal contusions over the involved chest as well as the rib injuries previously described. The patient who is unable to meet the demands of increased work of breathing may present with significant ventilatory distress. The classic radiographic appearance is that of a poorly defined infiltrate consistent with both alveolar and interstitial edema (Fig. 11.37). These findings on the chest radiograph are present within 1 hour of injury in 70% of patients. The remainder, however, have a delay of 4 to 6 hours before the contusion becomes visible on the chest film. Hypoxemia and significant alveolar–arterial gradient may be evident on arterial blood gas examination.

Treatment of patients with pulmonary contusion is primarily supportive. Patients who can maintain satisfactory arterial blood gases (i.e., partial pressure of oxygen >60 mm Hg with inspired oxygen concentration of 50%) and adequate ventilatory mechanics (i.e., a respiratory rate <24 breaths/min, a tidal volume >5 to 7 mL/kg, and a forced vital capacity >10 mL/kg) may not require intubation. These patients should be carefully monitored, and care should be taken to provide adequate analgesia for rib fractures.

Patients who cannot sustain adequate pulmonary function require mechanical ventilation. Gas exchange can be improved in most cases by use of a moderate level of continuous positive airway pressure. Careful optimization of intravascular volume status and cardiac performance is often required in more severely injured patients, and placement of a pulmonary artery catheter should be considered. The therapeutic goals are to maintain adequate peripheral oxygen delivery with airway pressure and inspired oxygen concentration at the lowest possible levels.

Depending on their size and severity, pulmonary contusions may start to resolve within 48 to 72 hours of injury, but 2 to 3 weeks may be required for complete resolution.

Pulmonary Laceration. Pulmonary lacerations can be the result of blunt chest trauma, but they are more common with penetrating injuries to the chest. A pulmonary laceration may exist within a surrounding area of contusion. Patients with pulmonary lacerations may have complaints similar to those of patients with pulmonary contusion, but they also frequently have hemoptysis. Chest radiography often reveals an area of pulmonary contusion and hemothorax.

The hemorrhage from pulmonary lacerations is usually from the low-pressure pulmonary system and can be treated with tube thoracostomy and reexpansion of the lung. If the air leak from the tube thoracostomy is large and the lung is not completely reexpanded, the placement of a second tube may be necessary. Bronchoscopy should be performed in patients with large air leaks or hemoptysis to rule out a bronchial injury.

Patients who have a pulmonary laceration and require positive-pressure ventilation are at risk for development of significant bronchopleural fistulae. If the air leak is very large, conventional modes of volume ventilation may not provide adequate alveolar ventilation. Strategies to improve alveolar ventilation include pressure-limited ventilatory modes, higher-frequency low-volume ventilation, and, in rare circumstances, independent lung ventilation. Bronchoscopic procedures to occlude the distal airway leading to the fistula also have been reported (227,228). In most circumstances, the air leak eventually closes, especially if the patient can be weaned from positive-pressure ventilation. If a significant leak persists, if the lung fails to expand, or if hemorrhage from the pulmonary laceration continues at a significant rate, thoracotomy may be necessary.

Pulmonary Hematoma. Pulmonary hematoma occurs when bleeding from a laceration is contained within the surrounding parenchyma. The mechanisms of injury and presenting complaints are similar to those for contusion, but hemoptysis is more likely with intraparenchymal hematoma. On the chest radiograph, the margins of a pulmonary hematoma are more clearly defined and spherical, in contrast to the diffuse, ill-defined borders of a contusion (Fig. 11.38). The degree of ventilatory compromise is usually less severe than in patients with pulmonary contusion because the hematoma displaces rather than infiltrates the lung tissue.

Conservative treatment with good pulmonary care and chest physiotherapy is the rule, and these lesions usually resolve without specific therapy in 2 to 3 weeks. During this time, the patient may have intermittent low-grade fever; however, if the fever remains high or increases, the

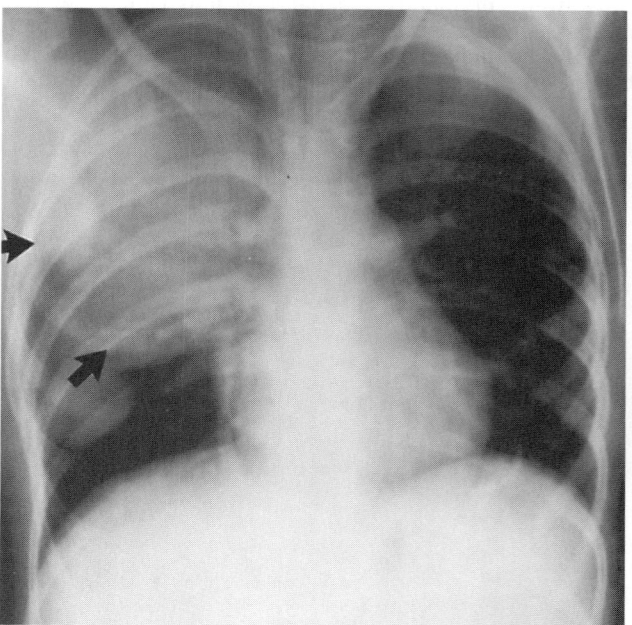

Figure 11.38. Right-sided pulmonary hematoma with well-defined spherical margins *(arrows),* in contrast to the ill-defined borders of a contusion.

possibility of an infected pulmonary hematoma should be entertained. Bronchoscopy should be performed to rule out a retained foreign body or clot in the airway. Antibiotics should be started, and vigorous chest physiotherapy should be initiated. A CT scan of the chest may reveal an air–fluid level in the hematoma. Percutaneous placement of a drainage catheter can be effective in resolving infected pulmonary hematomas. If this is unsuccessful, surgical resection may be needed.

Pneumatocele. A traumatic pulmonary pneumatocele occurs if there has been sufficient force to rupture a small airway without causing major hemorrhage, forming an air-filled pulmonary cavity. Pneumatocele is usually well tolerated, but the patient may complain of mild chest pain, dyspnea, or hemoptysis. A chest radiograph reveals a spherical, air-filled cavity that may show a fluid level on upright chest film. Preexisting disease, such as pulmonary abscess, tuberculosis, or other cavitary lesion in the lung, should be ruled out. A CT scan of the chest is helpful in establishing the diagnosis. Because infections occur in fewer than 10% of patients with these injuries, prophylactic antibiotics are not indicated. Conservative management with good pulmonary care and observation is the treatment of choice. Resolution of these lesions is slow, taking up to 4 months.

Mediastinal Injuries

Tracheobronchial Injuries. Tracheobronchial injuries from blunt trauma are relatively uncommon, occurring in fewer than 1% of patients with severe trauma. These injuries can result from blunt trauma (e.g., high-speed motor vehicle accidents) or from crushing injuries. If significant anteroposterior compressive force is applied to the chest, it causes rapid lateral deformation of the thoracic cavity and results in traction injury of the trachea or main-stem bronchi, usually within 2 cm of the carina. Penetrating injuries to the tracheobronchial tree are most common in the cervical area but can occur anywhere. Clothesline-type injuries can occur in bicyclists, motorcyclists, or drivers of other recreational vehicles. These blunt injuries can cause transection of the cervical trachea, resulting in airway obstruction.

Most patients with severe airway injuries die at the scene of the accident as a result of airway obstruction. Patients who survive to reach the hospital may complain of dyspnea, cough, or hemoptysis. Physical examination may reveal stridor, and subcutaneous emphysema is almost always found. Chest radiographs may reveal pneumothorax, extensive pneumomediastinum, and air in the soft tissues of the neck and chest wall. Placement of a tube thoracostomy may result in a continued massive air leak from the chest tube with no expansion of the lung (Fig. 11.39). If so, a second chest tube should be placed, and bronchoscopy should be undertaken to confirm the diagnosis.

Most bronchial injuries, including complete disruptions, heal spontaneously; however, stricture formation is common with more extensive injuries. If the injury involves less than one third of the circumference of the bronchus and the lung can be reexpanded with chest tube placement, nonoperative management probably will be successful. If the injury involves more than one third to one half of the circumference of the airway, early surgical repair is indicated to prevent late stricture (229). Persistent large air leak and inability to reexpand the lung also may necessitate surgical repair of bronchial injuries.

A right posterolateral thoracotomy gives excellent exposure to the thoracic trachea and right main-stem bronchus. Proximal left main-stem bronchial injuries also can be reached through this incision. Complete transection of the

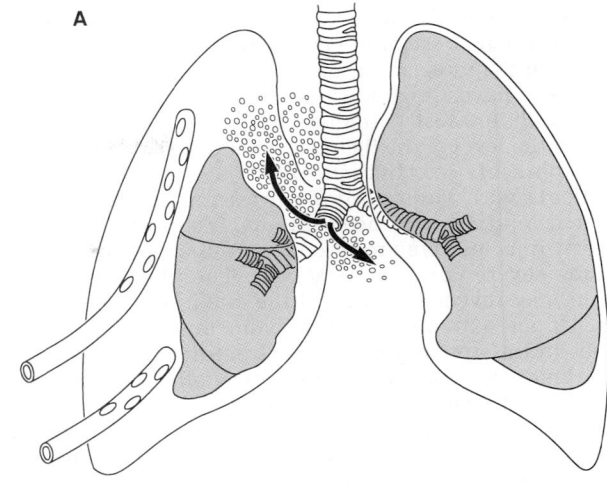

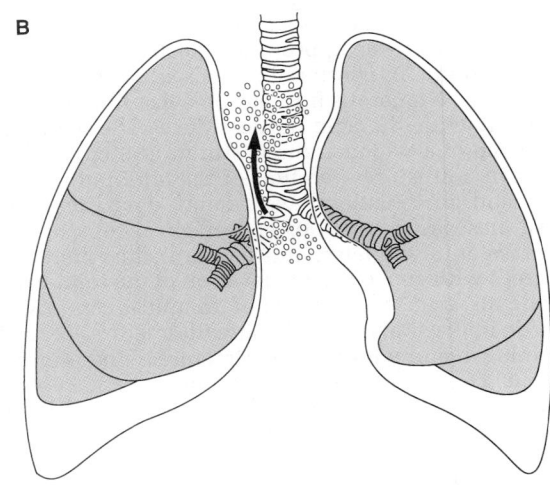

Figure 11.39. *(A)* Ruptured bronchus demonstrating pneumothorax with intrapleural rupture. *(B)* Pneumomediastinum with extrapleural rupture.

left main-stem bronchus requires left posterolateral thoracotomy, especially if the transection is more than 1 cm distal to the carina. Primary repair is the goal in most cases, although severe injuries may require sleeve resection of the bronchus or even lung resection. The repair should establish a mucosal closure with an absorbable suture material to decrease the incidence of suture-line granuloma formation or anastomotic stenosis. Bronchoscopic stent placement also has been used successfully in the repair of isolated bronchial injuries (230).

Transection of the trachea in the low cervical area may be associated with retraction of the tracheal stump into the mediastinum. Preparations should therefore be made for extension of the cervical incision into a median sternotomy if necessary. The repair of cervical tracheal injuries is discussed in greater detail in the section on neck trauma.

Aortic Injuries. Blunt aortic disruption is associated with the mechanism of abrupt deceleration. Shear forces act on the vessel at points of anatomic fixation, resulting in transection of the vessel. In patients who survive the initial injury, the hemorrhage is contained by the adventitia and tissues of the mediastinum, forming a pseudoaneurysm. The most common sites are the proximal aortic arch near the aortic valve; just distal to the origin of the left subclavian artery origin at the ligamentum arteriosum; and at the diaphragmatic hiatus. Patients with ascending aortic tears have a high mortality rate and rarely reach the hospital alive. Most patients who present alive have injuries at the level of the ligamentum arteriosum. Injuries at the diaphragm occur infrequently.

Patients with blunt aortic injuries frequently have associated injuries, with head trauma, fractures, and major visceral injuries being most common. Specific symptoms include severe chest or back pain. The physical examination may reveal fractures of the clavicles, sternum, or ribs. Upper extremity hypertension and asymmetry of pulses in the upper and lower extremities (pseudocoarctation) may be diagnostic. This presentation occurs if the ends of the transected aorta are not in perfect alignment. A careful neurologic evaluation is important because patients may have paraplegia or paraparesis from loss of blood flow through the intercostal arteries that supply the spinal cord.

The timely diagnosis of blunt injury of the thoracic aorta depends on a thorough search for it, which should be triggered initially by an appropriate mechanism of injury (i.e., deceleration). A chest radiograph is a useful screening procedure. Numerous findings on chest film have been associated with thoracic aortic injury. These include the presence of a widened mediastinum (>8 cm at the aortic knob in adults); obliteration of the aortopulmonary window and an indistinct aortic knob; deviation of the trachea, nasogastric tube, or endotracheal tube to the right; depression of the left main-stem bronchus more than 140 degrees with concomitant elevation of the right main-stem bronchus; and the presence of an apical cap (Fig. 11.40). Aortic injury is also associated with fractures of the first or second rib and with scapular fractures. The finding of abnormal contour of the mediastinum or aortic knob is probably the most reliable early finding on chest film and demands further work-up. An anteroposterior chest film taken with the patient in the supine position tends to magnify the size of the mediastinum to some extent. It is often helpful to obtain an upright chest film, if it is not contraindicated.

Abnormal findings on the chest film—or any suspicion of the injury—must be aggressively investigated. Because of the high morbidity associated with missed injuries, angiography has been the diagnostic study of choice in patients at significant risk. It is important to obtain full arch aortography, four-vessel run-off, and a full aortogram to avoid missing injuries at the aortic root, the diaphragmatic hiatus, or the origins of the great vessels. As discussed earlier in this section, dynamic helical CT scan of the chest may be equivalent to angiography in experienced hands. Chest CT scan is certainly a useful screening procedure in patients who have a negative chest film but significant mechanism of injury (231). Transesophageal echocardiography, also described earlier in the section, has been used with success. Transesophageal echocardiography is especially promising for use in unstable patients who cannot be transported to the angiography suite or the CT scanner.

Most blunt injuries of the aorta require immediate surgical repair. The literature suggests that a subset of patients have stable pseudoaneurysms that may be safely managed with delayed operation if necessary in the presence of other life-threatening injuries (204). In most cases, rapid surgical repair is vital to the survival of patients with blunt aortic injury (232,233). If the pseudoaneurysm ruptures before definitive repair, the mortality rate is extremely high. The preoperative treatment of patients with aortic disruption involves careful control of blood pressure and avoidance of hypertension. A short-acting β-antagonist such as esmolol or labetalol is probably the best choice if blood pressure control is needed. These agents are easy to titrate and they decrease both blood pressure and myocardial contractility, which results in lower shear stress in the arterial wall. Pure arteriolar vasodilation, such as that achieved using sodium nitroprusside, may actually lead to increased wall shear stress because pulse pressure often increases as systolic blood pressure decreases. The use of sodium nitroprusside also should be avoided in patients with head injuries.

An intraarterial catheter should be placed for direct arterial pressure monitoring, and a central venous or pulmonary artery catheter should be placed by an internal jugular or femoral route. The subclavian approach should be avoided because of the danger of entering the mediastinal hematoma.

Injuries of the ascending aorta often require full cardiopulmonary bypass for repair, and median sternotomy provides the best exposure (234). The repair of aortic injuries at or below the level of the ligamentum arteriosum is accomplished through a left posterolateral thoracotomy. Relatively simple injures can be repaired primarily. In young patients, it is often prudent to use pledgetted sutures for the repair. The thoracic aorta has relatively limited mobility, and intercostal vessels should not be sacrificed to facilitate primary repair owing to concerns about spinal cord perfusion. More extensive injuries require placement of a prosthetic graft.

The technique of aortic repair has been the subject of some controversy, primarily because of the risk of spinal cord ischemia with cross-clamping of the thoracic aorta. One review (235) showed no difference in the rate of paraplegia (8%) with or without placement of a heparin-bonded shunt to maintain distal flow during repair. The use of complete cardiopulmonary bypass with full heparinization has been shown to increase the mortality rate in patients who have other cerebral and vascular injuries, and it is probably contraindicated in blunt trauma. However, more recent advances in pump technology allow left

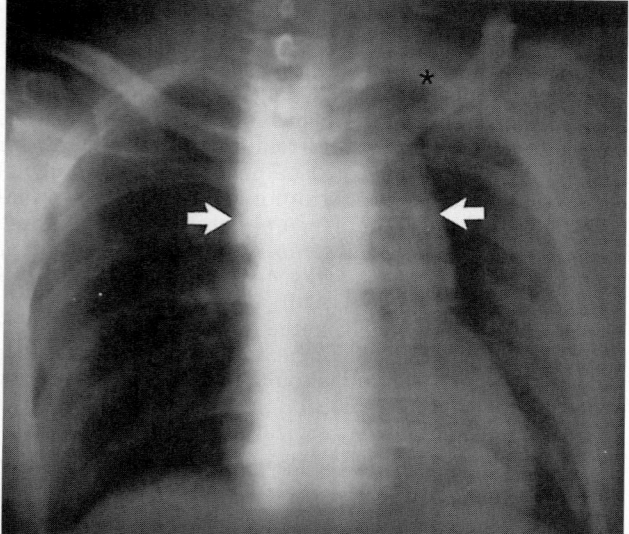

Figure 11.40. Chest radiograph demonstrating wide mediastinum *(arrows),* a left pleural cap *(asterisk),* and obliteration of the aortic notch, all consistent with an aortic transection.

heart bypass with much lower levels of systemic anticoagulation, and this technique can be safely used in multiply injured patients (233). Although definitive data are lacking, left heart bypass techniques probably decrease the rate of paraplegia, and should be used whenever possible.

Penetrating injuries to the aorta can occur anywhere along its length. Some penetrating injuries, especially from low-velocity projectiles, may result in the formation of a contained pseudoaneurysm, and have limited hemorrhage in the early postinjury phase. It is essential to investigate fully all injuries with a trajectory in proximity to the aorta, especially those traversing the posterior mediastinum. Aortography is essential in stable patients with evidence of mediastinal hematoma, but other modalities, including helical CT, are useful in low-risk patients (236).

Penetrating injuries are often amenable to primary repair, although prosthetic graft placement may be required in larger wounds. As in the case of blunt injuries, left heart bypass techniques are probably beneficial, and should be used in complex cases when circumstances allow.

Myocardial Contusion. The incidence of myocardial contusion is difficult to determine because there is no consensus with regard to its definition and diagnostic criteria. It has been suggested that as many as 75% of patients with major blunt chest injury sustain myocardial contusion, although the incidence of clinically significant findings or complications is clearly much lower. Clinically significant dysrhythmia or pump failure probably occurs in fewer than 5% of patients admitted to a trauma center. The mechanisms of injury associated with myocardial contusion include deceleration or crush injuries to the anterior thorax. There are no classic signs or symptoms, although the patient may complain of chest pain and sometimes of palpitations. Physical examination may reveal bruising and tenderness over the anterior chest. Findings of pericardial rubs or murmurs are rare.

The sensitivity and specificity of diagnostic tests for myocardial contusion cannot be determined because there are no universally accepted diagnostic criteria. Findings on electrocardiogram (ECG) that have been associated with myocardial contusion include ST-T-wave alterations, supraventricular and ventricular dysrhythmia, and sinus and atrioventricular nodal dysfunction. Right and left bundle-branch blocks also have been observed. None of these, however, is specific. For example, the ST-T-wave alterations also may be associated with pain, anxiety, hypoxia, and hypovolemia, all of which are common after severe trauma. Determination of creatine kinase (CK) isoenzymes, specifically the myocardial band (MB) fraction, also has been used to aid in the diagnosis of myocardial contusion. Elevation of the CK-MB fraction to greater than 5% of the total, or a total plasma CK concentration greater than 50 to 100 IU/mL, is considered diagnostic of myocardial contusion at some trauma centers, but the clinical significance of this finding is unclear. Elevation of the CK-MB fraction is neither sensitive nor specific for clinically significant injury leading to complications.

Two-dimensional echocardiography also has been used in an effort to diagnose myocardial contusion. This is a sensitive and specific method to assess global cardiac performance, wall motion defects, intramural hematomas, valvular dysfunction, and pericardial effusion. Positive findings are uncommon in patients presenting with trauma, and none of these tests is specific for myocardial contusion (237).

The need for treatment is based on clinical presentation. Dysrhythmias should be treated aggressively, but there are no data to support the use of prophylactic antidysrhythmics. Patients in whom dysrhythmias are likely to develop usually present with dysrhythmia or other ECG abnormalities. It is uncommon for significant dysrhythmia to develop in patients with a normal admitting ECG. Patients with suspected myocardial contusion and clinical evidence of poor myocardial performance should undergo echocardiography. Patients at risk for myocardial contusion who require surgery for other problems should be carefully monitored, but emergency surgery can be accomplished without significant additional morbidity or mortality. Myocardial pump failure is rare, and its treatment is not specifically altered in the posttraumatic patient should it occur.

Some controversy has surrounded the asymptomatic patient. A typical scenario involves the patient with some chest wall pain after a motor vehicle accident but without dysrhythmia. Stable patients with no evidence of dysrhythmia or other injury that would mandate hospitalization can be monitored for as little as 8 hours and discharged safely (238).

Cardiac Tamponade. Injuries to the heart resulting in cardiac tamponade can occur from either blunt or penetrating trauma, although penetrating injuries are much more common. The incidence of pericardial tamponade from blunt mechanisms is difficult to assess. Blunt cardiac injuries with tamponade can result from motor vehicle accidents, crush injuries, falls, construction injuries, and explosions. According to autopsy series, approximately 10% of motor vehicle accident fatalities show evidence of some cardiac damage, and 5% of deaths are from cardiac injuries, but patients presenting alive with tamponade from blunt injury are rare.

Pericardial tamponade occurs after blunt trauma from rupture of a chamber of the heart. This occurs with a severe blow to the chest at the moment when the heart is at end-diastole and maximally distended with blood. The part of the heart most likely to rupture in this scenario is the portion with the thinnest, least muscular wall, usually the right atrial appendage. Rupture of other chambers and disruption of the inferior vena cava from the right atrium also can occur, but these lesions are usually associated with death at the scene. A small atrial injury may allow the patient to survive to be transported to the hospital.

Penetrating trauma is the usual cause of pericardial tamponade, and the outcome is directly related to the character of the weapon. High-velocity, large-caliber weapons or shotguns are predictably lethal. Large stab wounds with free chamber perforation larger than 2 cm are also frequently fatal. Smaller stab wounds and iatrogenic cardiac injuries from central venous catheterization or percutaneous transcoronary angioplasty are more likely to have a good outcome (239).

The diagnosis of pericardial tamponade should be considered in any patient with penetrating chest trauma, particularly to the central portion of the chest. Tamponade also should be considered in patients with severe blunt chest trauma who remain hypotensive and have no evidence of external blood loss or hemorrhage into the thorax, abdomen, or pelvis. The classic Beck's triad, consisting of muffled heart sounds, decreased pulse pressure, and jugular venous distention, occurs in a minority of patients. If the patient is hypovolemic, jugular venous distention may not develop until late in the presentation. Chest radiography may reveal a pneumothorax or hemothorax, or be entirely negative. The pericardium is not acutely distensible, and an enlarged cardiac silhouette is not reliably seen in acute tamponade.

Two-dimensional echocardiography is highly sensitive for the presence of pericardial fluid and wall motion abnormalities. If available in a timely fashion, echocardiography is the best diagnostic study to rule out tamponade in the stable patient. Placement of a central venous catheter to measure central venous pressure has been advocated as a diagnostic test in the hemodynamically stable patient. A very high central venous pressure (>20 to 25 cm H_2O) is probably diagnostic, although elevations of this magnitude are usually associated with visible venous distention. Moderately elevated pressures, in the range of 14 to 16 cm H_2O, require further evaluation. Measurements of central venous pressure are neither sensitive nor specific for the diagnosis of pericardial tamponade, and they depend on the patient's volume status and level of agitation. Such tests may be of value, but they must be interpreted with extreme care. Under most circumstances, there is little role for diagnostic pericardiocentesis.

In hemodynamically stable patients with high likelihood of cardiac tamponade, the preferred approach is to perform a subxiphoid pericardial window incision with the patient under general anesthesia, unless echocardiography is immediately available in the resuscitation area or operating room. An extraperitoneal approach is made through a midline incision, or a transperitoneal approach is used at the time of concurrent laparotomy. The xiphoid is retracted superiorly or resected, and an incision is made through the diaphragm into the pericardium. This test is highly accurate for the presence of blood in the pericardial sac, and it allows for decompression of the tamponade. Decompression of tamponade through a subxiphoid window may result in significant hemorrhage that cannot be well controlled. Necessary preparations for immediate median sternotomy must be made before a window incision is performed.

Patients with hemodynamic instability and a penetrating wound in the left chest or parasternal region should undergo immediate left anterolateral thoracotomy with a wide, longitudinal opening of the pericardium. Cardiac lacerations should be digitally controlled until adequate blood volume is restored and the patient is relatively stable. The use of staples also has been advocated to close cardiac lacerations rapidly but temporarily for immediate hemostasis. Small lacerations in the beating heart can be then repaired using nonabsorbable sutures placed through Teflon pledgets. Larger lacerations may require cardiopulmonary bypass for adequate decompression and repair. The left thoracotomy incision can be carried transversely across the sternum into the right chest to facilitate exposure of the entire heart and great vessels if necessary.

Reported survival rates for small injuries to a single chamber are between 60% and 87%, although patients who arrive moribund do poorly regardless of care. The postpericardiotomy syndrome occurs commonly after repair of traumatic cardiac injury. It can occur in mild form in up to half of patients. The more severe form includes pericarditis with fever, malaise, and a friction rub. Pericarditis is usually treated with nonsteroidal antiinflammatory drugs. Symptomatic pericardial effusions should be treated with percutaneous drainage. Recurrent symptomatic pericardial effusions may require complete anterior pericardiectomy.

Esophageal Injury. Injury to the thoracic esophagus from external force or compression is a rare event and occurs in fewer than 0.01% of patients who sustain multiple blunt injuries (240). If it does occur, the site of blunt rupture is most often in the distal third of the esophagus, just above the gastroesophageal junction. This injury probably results from an abrupt increase in intraabdominal pressure while the glottis is closed during impact. The resultant rapid rise in pressure causes rupture at the weakest point of the esophagus, similar to that seen in Boerhaave's syndrome. Penetrating trauma to the thoracic esophagus is also uncommon and is usually associated with injuries to the adjacent structures. Symptoms include chest pain and dysphagia, and a Hamman crunch may be noted on auscultation of the mediastinum. A nasogastric tube should be carefully passed for gastric decompression and may return blood. Late findings with missed esophageal rupture include subcutaneous emphysema, fever, and shock. The chest film may reveal air in the retroesophageal space, pneumomediastinum, pneumothorax, or left pleural effusion, but it also may be negative.

Esophagography should be performed in every patient with suspected esophageal injury. This is best begun with water-soluble contrast rather than barium because of the problems associated with barium contamination of the mediastinum (Fig. 11.41). Patients who are conscious and alert can swallow the contrast material under fluoroscopy. In unconscious and intubated patients, a nasogastric tube is carefully placed into the proximal esophagus, and 30 to 50 mL of water-soluble contrast medium is injected with sufficient pressure to distend the esophagus. If the initial study is negative, a barium study is then performed.

Esophagoscopy is also of value in the diagnostic work-up. Both flexible and rigid techniques have been advocated, and the choice is probably best made based on operator experience. Visualization of an esophageal laceration is diagnostic, but a negative esophagoscopy must be accompanied by a contrast study of the esophagus to achieve sufficient diagnostic certainty. Esophagoscopy should be used to follow up suspect or technically imperfect contrast studies

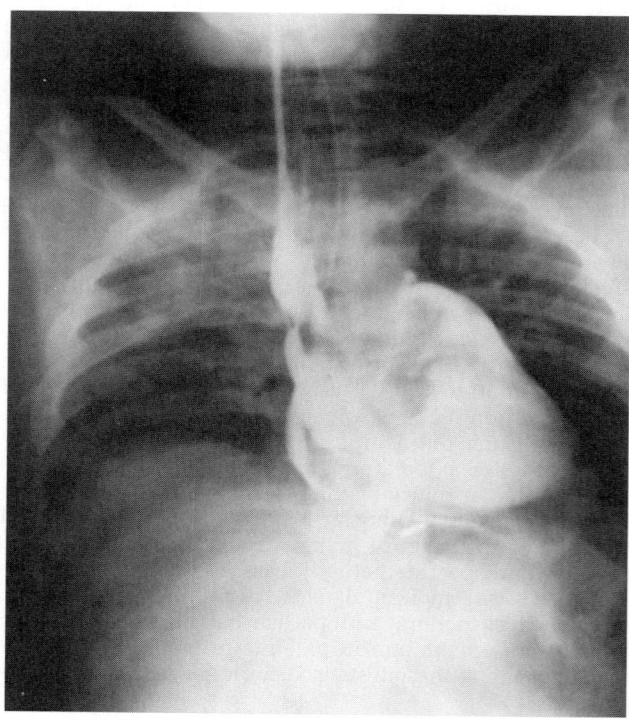

Figure 11.41. Water-soluble contrast esophagogram demonstrating leak from the esophagus into the pericardial sac consistent with a distal esophageal injury.

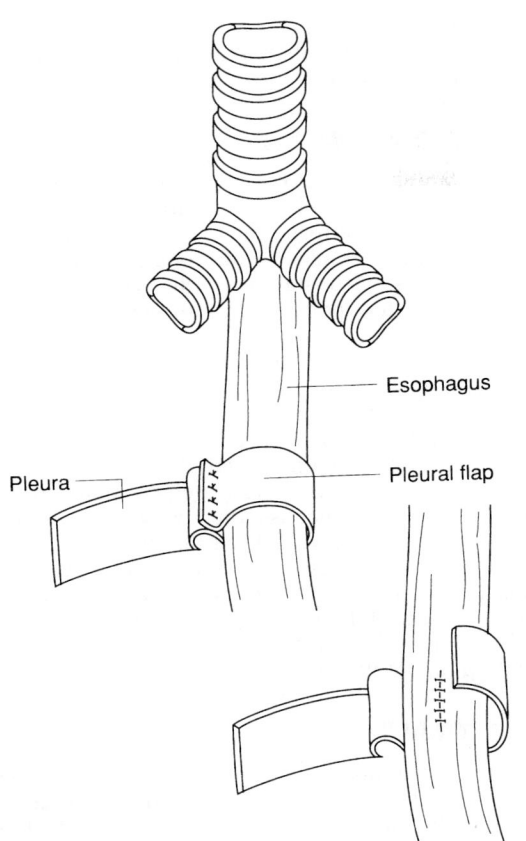

Figure 11.42. Pleural patch reinforcement of primary closure of the esophagus after penetrating injury.

and as a security measure in patients with a high likelihood of esophageal injury. If an esophageal injury is identified, immediate exploration is undertaken.

The surgical approach is dictated by the location of the injury. Cervical esophageal lesions can usually be approached through a collar incision, repaired primarily, and drained widely. This topic is covered more fully in the section on neck injuries. Most injuries of the proximal thoracic esophagus can be approached through a right posterolateral thoracotomy. Injuries near the diaphragmatic hiatus may be more accessible through a left posterolateral thoracotomy. If the diagnosis is made rapidly, most lacerations of the esophagus can be repaired primarily and the mediastinum drained widely. Reinforcement of the repair with a pleural flap or other tissue is recommended for complex injuries (Fig. 11.42). If an adequate pleural flap cannot be obtained, an intercostal muscle pedicle flap can be used to buttress the esophageal repair in a similar fashion. Esophageal injuries at the diaphragmatic hiatus may be repaired primarily and reinforced with a circumferential (Nissen) or partial (Thal) fundoplication.

If the diagnosis of esophageal injury has been delayed, simple repair usually is not feasible because of established mediastinitis. In cases of severe mediastinal contamination, repair of the injury, wide mediastinal drainage, and esophageal exclusion with cervical esophagostomy and temporary closure of the gastroesophageal junction is recommended. A proximal gastrostomy is performed for decompression, and a feeding jejunostomy is performed for nutritional support (Fig. 11.43). Such an approach often allows primary healing of the esophageal injury, avoiding later reconstruction (241). In cases of extensive injury, late reconstruction is required and may be complex (see Chapter 20) (242).

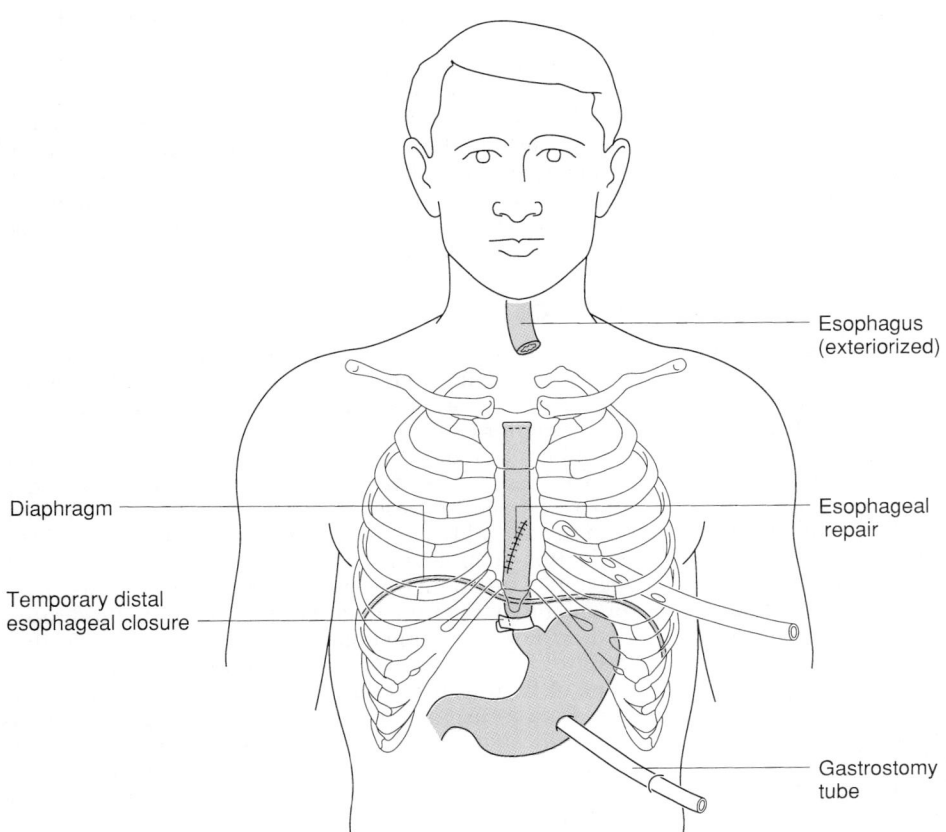

Figure 11.43. Esophageal exclusion including transection and proximal esophagostomy with temporary closure of the distal esophagus to prevent reflux and ongoing leak.

Definitive Care Phase: Abdominal Injuries

DAVID H. WISNER AND DAVID B. HOYT

Most civilian abdominal injuries are caused by blunt trauma secondary to high-speed automobile crashes, although penetrating injuries are common in urban environments. The failure successfully to manage abdominal injuries accounts for most of the preventable deaths that follow multiple trauma. Failure to recognize occult abdominal hemorrhage and to control bleeding from intraabdominal organs leads to significant morbidity, and such injuries account for approximately 10% of the traumatic deaths that occur annually in the United States.

ANATOMIC CONSIDERATIONS

The abdomen is defined by the diaphragm at its superior aspect and by the infragluteal fold at its caudal aspect; it includes the entire circumference of the torso. Abdominal injury is often accompanied by trauma to other sites, such as the central nervous system, the chest, and the musculoskeletal system. To simplify the initial trauma evaluation, the abdomen can be divided into four areas: (a) intrathoracic abdomen, (b) true abdomen, (c) pelvic abdomen, and (d) retroperitoneal abdomen (Fig. 11.44). With the exception of the true abdomen, all of these areas are difficult to assess by physical examination alone.

The intrathoracic abdomen is the portion of the upper abdomen that lies beneath the rib cage (Fig. 11.44A). Bony and cartilaginous structures make this area essentially inaccessible to palpation. Its contents include the diaphragm, liver, spleen, and stomach. Each of these organs can be injured when blunt or penetrating impact is delivered to the rib cage. Diagnostic peritoneal lavage (DPL) is useful in evaluating this anatomic area.

The pelvic abdomen is defined by the bony pelvis (Fig. 11.44B). Its contents include the rectum, bladder, urethra, small intestine, and, in female patients, the uterus, fallopian tubes, and ovaries. Trauma to the pelvis, particularly pelvic fractures, can damage the organs within, and penetrating injuries of the buttocks can injure any or all of the pelvic organs. Injury to these structures may be extraperitoneal and therefore difficult to diagnose. For this reason, suspected injuries may require adjunctive procedures such as bladder catheterization, urethrocystography, and sigmoidoscopy for diagnosis.

The retroperitoneal abdomen contains the kidneys, ureters, pancreas, second and third portions of the duodenum, great vessels, aorta, and vena cava (Fig. 11.44C). Injury to these structures can also occur secondary to penetrating or blunt trauma. The kidneys can be damaged by injury to the lower ribs posteriorly, and any of these structures can be damaged by crushing injuries to the front or side of the torso. Again, injury to these structures may result in few physical findings, and physical examination and DPL are of little use. Evaluation of the retroperitoneal abdomen requires use of radiographic imaging procedures, including computed tomography (CT), angiography, ultrasound, and intravenous pyelography.

The true abdomen contains the small and large intestines, the bladder when distended, and the uterus when gravid. Perforation of these organs is usually manifested by pain from peritonitis and is associated with significant abdominal physical findings. DPL is a useful adjunct if injury is suspected, and a plain abdominal film can be helpful if free air is present.

PENETRATING INJURY

Handguns are the most common cause of serious penetrating injury to the abdomen. Significant intraabdominal injury occurs in approximately 80% of patients who sustain abdominal gunshot wounds but in only 20% to 30% of patients with stab wounds. The frequency of organ injury after penetrating abdominal trauma is shown in Table 11.11.

Injuries to both thoracic and abdominal cavities occur in 25% of patients with penetrating wounds of the abdomen. Patients with penetrating wounds of the thorax also may have significant intraabdominal injury because the bullet can readily traverse the diaphragm. Patients with gunshot wounds to the abdomen and lower chest should routinely undergo laparotomy because the probability of intraabdominal injury is high. Whether selective management or mandatory laparotomy is the best method for treating stab wounds is a controversy discussed later. The difference in injury potential between gunshot wounds and stab wounds is a function of the higher kinetic energy associated with gunshot wounds.

BLUNT TRAUMA

Automobile accidents are the cause of at least 60% of all traumatic injuries. Table 11.12 shows the frequency with which specific organs are injured by blunt abdominal trauma. Some series list the liver rather than the spleen as the most commonly injured intraabdominal organ; this difference probably reflects the means of diagnosis. Small liver injuries are often detected in patients who undergo CT scan of the abdomen, whereas splenic injuries in adults are more likely to be clinically significant and to require surgical intervention.

Solid organs are most frequently injured from blunt trauma. The sudden application of pressure to the abdomen is more likely to rupture a solid organ than a hollow viscus, and this accounts for the greater incidence of solid organ injury. The more elastic tissues of young people tolerate trauma better than those of older people, and this accounts in part for the differences in injuries between children and adults with blunt abdominal trauma.

PREHOSPITAL CARE

Little can be done outside of a hospital for patients with abdominal injuries. For penetrating wounds, sterile dressings should be applied, and the patient should be carefully monitored. Foreign bodies embedded in the trunk should not be removed because major bleeding can follow. Evisceration is best left undisturbed except for application of a moist sterile dressing and protection of the patient from further injury. General principles of stabilization and evaluation should be followed, including ensuring an adequately functioning airway, inserting intravenous lines (preferably in the upper extremity), beginning fluid resuscitation, and providing rapid transport to a trauma facility. Despite recent controversy surrounding the issue of the value of fluid resuscitation in the early posttraumatic period, fluid resuscitation in the prehospital phase of care is still indicated. Preoccupation with fluid resuscitation should not, however, delay rapid transport to a trauma center. The prehospital application of the pneumatic antishock garment is usually not indicated for severe abdomi-

A

Intrathoracic abdomen
    Diaphragm
    Liver
    Spleen
    Stomach

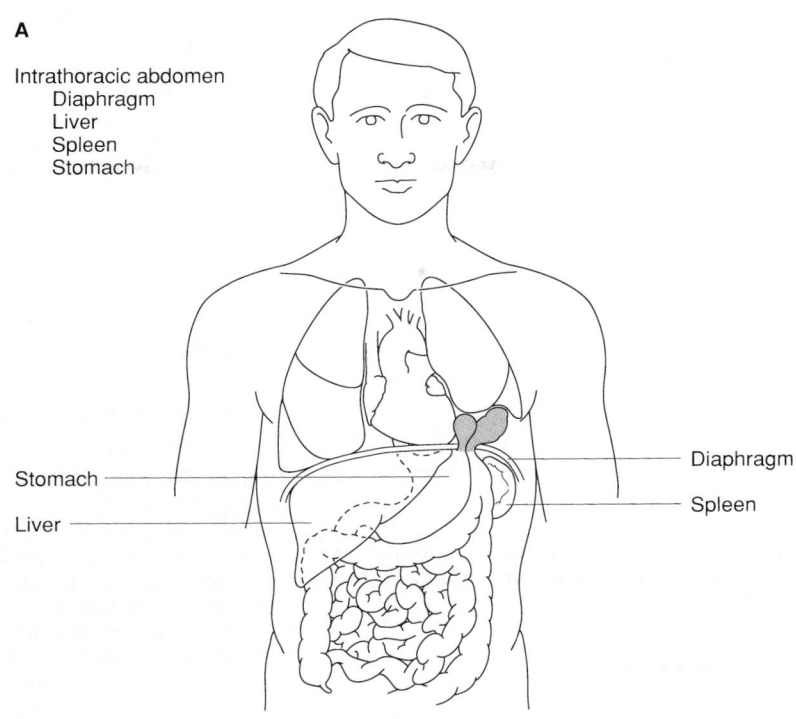

Stomach

Liver

Diaphragm

Spleen

B

Pelvic abdomen
    Urinary bladder
    Urethra
    Rectum
    Small intestine
In addition
    Uterus, fallopian tubes,
    ovaries (female)

Bladder

Urethra

Rectum

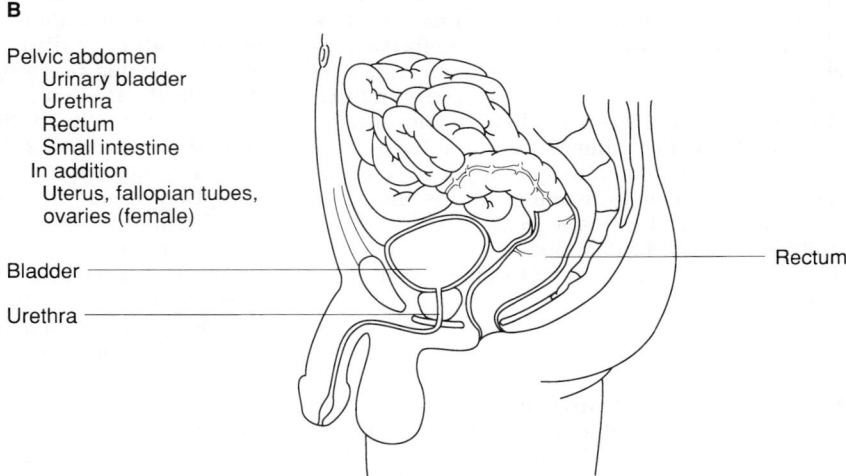

Figure 11.44. Four traditional anatomic divisions of the abdomen. *(A)* Intrathoracic abdomen. Contents of this area are subdiaphragmatic but cephalad to the costal margin. With respiration, the diaphragm is presumed to ascend to the level of the nipples (fourth intercostal space anteriorly). A ruptured left hemidiaphragm is illustrated with herniation of the stomach and distal transverse colon into the left hemithorax. *(B)* Similarly, the contents of the pelvic abdomen are within the bony pelvis. *(C)* The structures in the retroperitoneal abdomen. The true (intraperitoneal) abdomen contains the remainder of the viscera, and the inventory of its contents is dynamic, depending on body position and respiration (not shown).

C

Retroperitoneal abdomen
    Kidneys
    Ureters
    Pancreas
    Great vessels
    Duodenum (2nd
    and 3rd parts)

Duodenum

Inferior vena cava

Right kidney

Aorta

Pancreas

Spleen

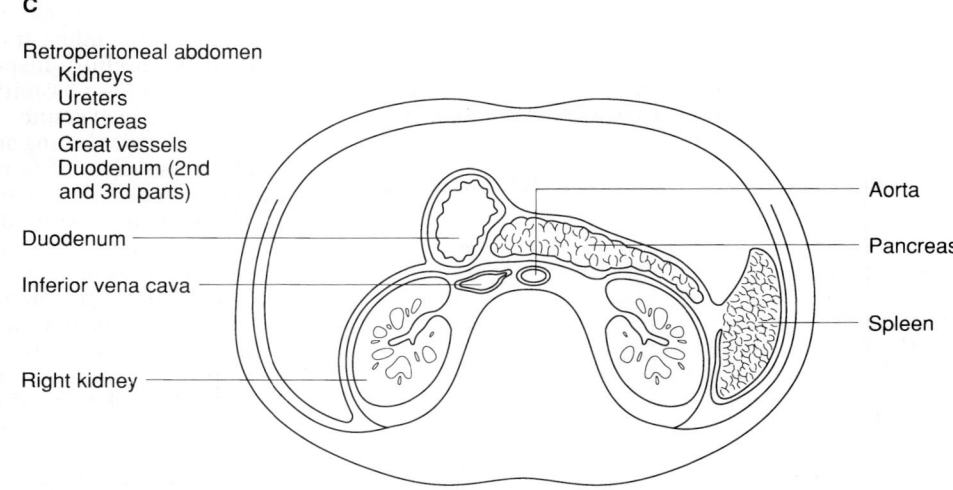

Table 11.11. FREQUENCY OF ORGAN INJURY IN PENETRATING ABDOMINAL TRAUMA

Organ	Occurrence (%)
Liver	37
Small bowel	26
Stomach	19
Colon	17
Major vascular	13
Retroperitoneal	10
Mesentery and omentum	10
Spleen	7
Diaphragm	5
Kidney	4
Pancreas	4
Duodenum	2
Biliary system	1
Other	1

nal hemorrhage but may play a role in the temporary stabilization of severe pelvic fractures, particularly if prolonged transport times are anticipated.

HOSPITAL RESUSCITATION AND DIAGNOSIS

Diagnosis and treatment should proceed concurrently after established protocols, many of which have been reviewed previously. A functioning airway must be established, particularly in the comatose patient, before evaluation of the abdomen. If necessary, an endotracheal tube is placed and assisted ventilation is begun. Upper extremity, large-bore intravenous catheters are initiated, and resuscitation is begun with lactated Ringer's solution. Early crystalloid resuscitation is indicated despite theoretic considerations that instillation of intravenous fluids increases bleeding and causes a dilutional coagulopathy (243). When operative intervention is necessary, however, it should not be delayed by overly zealous attempts at fluid resuscitation.

History

Penetrating injuries present little diagnostic challenge other than the question of whether to explore the abdomen operatively. An attempt should be made to establish details of the trauma event and the weapon used. The blunt trauma assessment can be aided considerably by an accu-

Table 11.12. FREQUENCY OF ORGAN INJURY IN BLUNT ABDOMINAL TRAUMA IN ADULTS

Organ	Occurrence (%)
Liver	30
Spleen	25
Retroperitoneal hematoma	13
Kidney	7
Urinary bladder	6
Intestine	5
Mesentery	5
Pancreas	3
Diaphragm	2
Urethra	2
Vascular	2

rate history. If the patient was involved in an automobile accident in which the steering wheel was struck or if there was no seat belt used, specific thoracic and epigastric abdominal trauma should be suspected. If the patient was restrained, it can be helpful to determine whether the restraint was a two-point lap belt or a three-point shoulder belt. The patient who sustains rib fractures involving the lower left chest has a 20% chance of associated splenic injury; the patient with rib fractures on the right has a 10% chance of liver injury. A compression fracture of the lumbosacral region carries a 20% risk of significant renal parenchymal injury. A relevant history combined with a directed physical examination guides the initial assessment of patients with abdominal trauma.

Physical Examination

The objective of the physical examination in abdominal trauma is rapidly to identify the patient who needs laparotomy. Precise definition of specific organ injury is unnecessary because immediate operative indications are usually applicable to any specific organ. These fundamentally consist of significant hemorrhage or perforation of a hollow viscus. Unfortunately, the specificity and sensitivity of physical examination are not adequate to make these determinations. Associated injuries often cause tenderness and spasm in the abdominal wall and make diagnosis difficult. Lower rib fractures, pelvic fractures, or abdominal wall contusions can mimic the signs of peritonitis.

In patients with gunshot wounds, no presumptions should be made about entrance and exit wounds. Their determination is difficult in the emergency department, and unfounded presumptions can lead to inaccurate estimations about the number of times a patient was shot and the course of the bullets. If time permits, radiographs should be obtained to determine the location of any bullets or bullet fragments that remain in the patient. Presumptions about entrance and exit wounds can also lead to subsequent legal difficulties.

Because the primary manifestation of blunt solid organ injury is hemorrhage, the patient should be monitored closely during the initial assessment, and continuing or refractory shock is presumed to result from continuing or massive hemorrhage. A hemodynamically stable patient can undergo complete evaluation, including physical examination, DPL, and adjunctive radiographic and laboratory studies.

The patient should be examined from head to toe for signs of blunt trauma and for penetrating wounds. Small abrasions or areas of ecchymosis suggest significant local intraabdominal injury. Penetrating wounds should be marked with radiopaque clips to allow radiographic delineation of the injury tract. The abdominal wall and back should be carefully inspected, and posterior ecchymosis should raise the possibility of retroperitoneal injury. The absence of bowel sounds is consistent with an ileus, but it is a nonspecific finding and, in the context of a busy emergency department, it is insensitive for discriminating between patients who do and do not need laparotomy.

The patient's respiratory pattern should be evaluated. Halting, labored breathing may be caused by diaphragmatic irritation or may accompany significant upper abdominal injury. Inspiratory left shoulder pain correlates with irritation of the left hemidiaphragm from bleeding, which is often the result of a splenic laceration.

Palpation can reveal localized tenderness, spasm, or rigidity of the abdominal wall. These findings and the finding of rebound tenderness are consistent with peritonitis and perforation of hollow viscera. Exploratory laparotomy is required for this presumed diagnosis. Suprapubic tenderness and pelvic lateral wall tenderness, which can indicate a pelvic fracture, are assessed in the conscious patient. Inspection of the perineum and urethral meatus for blood is routine to look for signs of pelvic fracture.

As assessment continues, a urinary catheter is placed, and a urine sample is sent for analysis for microscopic hematuria. If there is suspicion of injury to the lower urinary tract, the bladder, or the urethra because of an associated pelvic fracture, retrograde urethrography is performed before catheterization. Rectal examination is performed, and sphincter tone is evaluated. The integrity of the rectal wall and the position and mobility of the prostate are evaluated. The stool should be tested for the presence of gross or occult blood. A nasogastric tube is passed, and gastric contents are aspirated and tested for blood.

The physical findings for injuries to these different structures are often a function of the time between injury and examination. Hollow viscus perforations may require several hours before peritonitis becomes apparent. Colon or gastric perforations produce peritonitis more rapidly, small bowel perforations less so. Because of the wide spectrum of injury, frequent reevaluation becomes an essential strategy in the treatment of patients with blunt abdominal trauma.

Laboratory Studies

Blood studies of value in the initial evaluation of a patient with abdominal trauma include the hematocrit and serum amylase or lipase. Plasma aminotransferase levels may be of some value in the diagnosis of liver injury, particularly in children. Leukocyte counts, serum creatinine, glucose, and serum electrolyte determinations are often obtained for reference but ordinarily have little value in the early management period.

The diagnosis of massive hemorrhage is usually obvious from hemodynamic parameters, and the hematocrit merely confirms the diagnosis. Iatrogenic dilutional anemia is common and, in the presence of hemodynamic stability, is well tolerated. Urinalysis confirms the presence of microscopic hematuria. For blunt trauma, radiographic evaluation of the kidneys and bladder should be initiated if the patient has gross hematuria or microscopic hematuria and shock (systolic blood pressure <90 mm Hg in an adult) at any point during the prehospital or emergency department course. The serum amylase is insensitive and nonspecific as a marker for major pancreatic or enteric injury. Injuries to the head and face commonly cause increased plasma amylase concentrations. Persistent or symptomatic hyperamylasemia, however, should raise the concern of significant intraabdominal injury and is an indication for aggressive radiographic or surgical investigation. Pancreatic or duodenal injury is best assessed with intraluminal gastrointestinal and intravenous contrast media with dynamic CT scan.

Radiographic Evaluation

Radiologic studies of potential value in the evaluation of abdominal trauma include a chest radiograph, abdominal plain films, retrograde urethrography and cystography, excretory urography, CT scans, ultrasound, and angiography. All injuries from penetrating trauma should be evaluated with a plain radiograph with the use of radiodense markers on the wound sites to allow evaluation of the missile trajectory. With blunt trauma, an anteroposterior film of the pelvis can delineate pelvic fractures not detectable on physical examination. The initial pelvic film or chest radiograph can also demonstrate fractures of the thoracic or lumbar spine. A transverse fracture of the vertebral bodies, or Chance fracture, should increase the search for serious blunt intestinal injury. In addition, free intraperitoneal air,

trapped retroperitoneal air from duodenal perforation, or loss of the psoas shadow from retroperitoneal bleeding all may be seen. The overall value of plain abdominal films after blunt trauma is limited.

Of greater value are CT scans, ultrasound, and angiography. CT has real value in the accurate assessment of solid organ injuries, particularly the liver, kidney, and spleen; contrast-enhanced CT has great accuracy in the delineation of intraabdominal bleeding. The accuracy of CT scan in evaluation of hollow viscus injury is limited, but this is not an obstacle because this limitation is well known. CT is specific in the evaluation of retroperitoneal injuries and is the single most useful and informative diagnostic study for patients with abdominal trauma. Ultrasound has become increasingly popular in the initial diagnostic management of abdominal trauma (244). There is a learning curve for the use of ultrasonography in the emergency department, but in the hands of experienced personnel it is effective in determining the presence or absence of intraperitoneal blood. Emergency department ultrasound is not very sensitive for the detection of specific organ injuries and, like CT, is relatively insensitive to diagnose bowel injuries. It has proved much better for the evaluation of blunt trauma than for penetrating trauma, although interrogation of the pericardial space with an ultrasound probe placed in the subxiphoid position is quite sensitive to the presence of pericardial blood in patients with penetrating cardiac injuries.

Angiography is reserved for specific situations, such as suspected aortic or renal arterial injuries, and is not considered an initial screening investigation.

Laparoscopy also has been used for both diagnosis and treatment of trauma patients (245). It has not proven useful in the management of blunt trauma patients. After penetrating trauma, it has a role in the diagnosis of a selected group of patients. Laparoscopy is helpful in patients in whom it is unclear whether the peritoneum has been penetrated. In these circumstances, laparoscopy can rapidly and relatively noninvasively determine if there is a hole in the peritoneum. In patients in whom peritoneal penetration is seen, the use of laparoscopy subsequently to explore the peritoneal cavity and repair injuries is more controversial. The adequacy of abdominal exploration, particularly examination of the bowel and retroperitoneum, has been questioned, and repair of large injuries through the laparoscope can be tedious. Patients with a left lower chest wound are also potential candidates for laparoscopy. In these patients, both peritoneal penetration and diaphragmatic injury can be diagnosed. Diaphragmatic injury in such circumstances is one area in which repair through the laparoscope has proven feasible. When laparoscopy is used in patients with potential diaphragmatic injury, positive pressure in the peritoneal cavity can lead to tension pneumothorax if the chest is not adequately vented.

Abdominal Paracentesis and Peritoneal Lavage

Diagnostic peritoneal lavage is a standard technique to detect significant intraabdominal hemorrhage after blunt trauma. Its applicability after low-velocity gunshot or stab wounds is less clear, and it has no place in the evaluation of high-velocity gunshot wounds. Abdominal paracentesis can be used in place of DPL if the suspicion of intraabdominal hemorrhage is high and time is critical. A negative result on abdominal paracentesis is of no definitive diagnostic significance, however, and it is usually preferable to perform formal DPL to establish whether a hemoperitoneum is present. DPL, like paracentesis, is of greatest value in patients whose physical findings do not clearly establish whether intraperitoneal injury is present.

Table 11.13. COMPARISON OF DIAGNOSTIC PERITONEAL LAVAGE AND COMPUTED TOMOGRAPHY IN THE DIAGNOSIS OF VISCERAL INJURY AFTER BLUNT ABDOMINAL TRAUMA

	Diagnostic peritoneal lavage	Computed tomography
False-negative result	<1%	5%–20%
False-positive result	5%–12%	5%
Time to complete	5 min	55 min
Cost	$125	$900

The specific indications for DPL in blunt trauma include the following:

- Unconscious patient with question of potential abdominal injury
- Patient with a high-energy injury, suspected intraabdominal injury, and equivocal physical findings
- Patient with multiple injuries and unexplained shock
- Patient with major noncontiguous or thoracoabdominal injuries
- Patient with spinal cord injury
- Intoxicated patient in whom abdominal injury is suspected
- Patient who has a suspected intraabdominal injury with equivocal diagnostic findings and who will be undergoing prolonged general anesthesia for another injury, making continued reevaluation impossible

Relative contraindications include patients with previous abdominal operations, pregnancy, morbid obesity, obvious peritonitis, and exsanguinating hemorrhage. If the patient is hemodynamically stable, CT scan is prudent and, if the patient is unstable, immediate exploratory laparotomy is indicated. Children have somewhat different indications, and this is discussed separately.

Diagnostic peritoneal lavage is not useful for patients with abdominal gunshot wounds, all of whom require immediate laparotomy (246). If local exploration of a stab wound suggests penetration of the anterior fascia and peritoneum, DPL can help distinguish those with significant and insignificant injuries. It is most sensitive in the diagnosis of hemoperitoneum, but significant hemoperitoneum does not necessarily accompany hollow viscus lacerations.

In blunt trauma, DPL is considered positive if 10 mL of grossly bloody aspirate is obtained before instillation of lavage fluid, or if the siphoned lavage fluid has more than 100,000 red blood cells (RBCs) per milliliter. Evaluation of lavage fluid in stab wounds should be based on a different protocol. In general, more than 1,000 RBCs/mL is considered a positive DPL result, and laparotomy should follow.

Diagnostic peritoneal lavage and CT scan are both satisfactory tests for the diagnosis of visceral injury after blunt abdominal trauma. DPL has distinct advantages, including higher sensitivity, lower cost, immediate interpretation, and rapidity (Table 11.13). The major disadvantages are a 1% to 3% risk of iatrogenic intraperitoneal injury and the high sensitivity of the test. The high sensitivity can lead to nontherapeutic laparotomies (i.e., when there are no injuries requiring repair). False-positive DPL results are relatively common if an infraumbilical approach is used in a patient with a pelvic fracture. A pelvic radiograph should be obtained before DPL if a pelvic fracture is suspected, so that the incision is placed cephalad to the umbilicus. This avoids a false-positive result from traversing a pelvic hematoma that has dissected into the anterior infraumbilical abdominal wall. Finally, an important related issue is whether every patient with hemoperitoneum from abdominal trauma requires laparotomy.

Before DPL, the bladder should be emptied by drainage with a catheter. The abdomen is prepared with povidone–iodine solution and draped with sterile towels. The lower abdominal midline is infiltrated by lidocaine with epinephrine, and a 3-cm incision is carried down to the linea alba. This is opened, and a peritoneal dialysis catheter is placed through the peritoneum under direct vision. After peritoneal entry, the catheter is directed at a 45-degree angle into the pelvis and aspirated. If the aspirate returns 5 to 10 mL of bloody fluid, the study is considered positive and is terminated. If little or no blood is aspirated, 1,000 mL of normal saline or lactated Ringer's solution (or 10 mL/kg in a child) is rapidly infused into the peritoneal cavity. After the infusion is complete, the empty intravenous bottle is placed on the floor, allowing the intraperitoneal fluid to be siphoned into the bottle for analysis.

The general approaches to the diagnosis of blunt and penetrating trauma are outlined in Figs. 11.45 and 11.46.

Indications for Surgery

It is the unique job of the general surgeon directing a trauma team to integrate the various specialties involved in the care of the multiply injured patient. In this regard, judgments about specialized procedures for problems that are not life threatening need to be made with an overall view of the patient's physiologic status. This requires both important managerial skills and technical skills. With specific regard to abdominal injuries, indications for laparot-

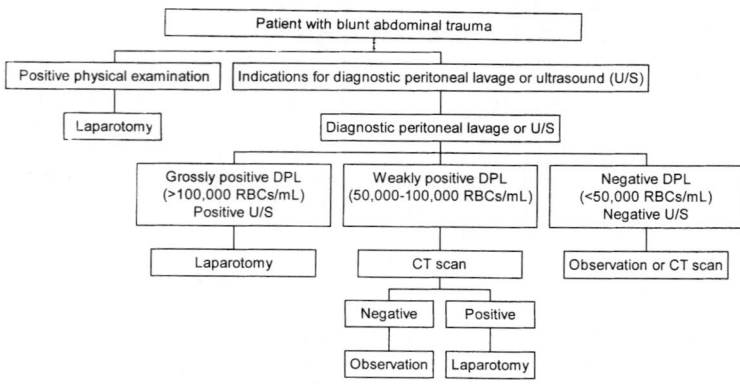

Figure 11.45. Diagnostic algorithm for blunt abdominal trauma.

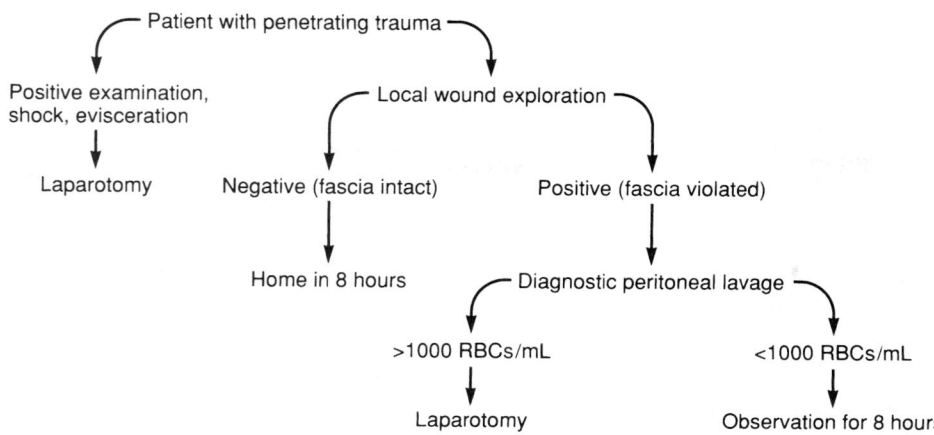

Figure 11.46. Diagnostic algorithm for low-velocity penetrating abdominal trauma.

omy include signs of peritonitis, unexplained shock, evisceration, uncontrolled hemorrhage, clinical deterioration during observation, and, in general, a DPL consistent with hemoperitoneum.

In preparation for laparotomy, certain issues must be considered to protect the patient against hypotension during the early stages of surgical exploration. Vascular access must be secure. Femoral venous lines and large-bore catheters placed by saphenous cutdown at the ankle are options for the rapid infusion of large volumes of fluid. If the patient has lost a large amount of blood, central venous catheterization should be done prospectively if at all possible. Arterial cannulae should be placed to allow perioperative blood pressure monitoring and sequential blood gas determinations.

Broad-spectrum antibiotics are given as soon as the decision to perform a laparotomy is made. The postoperative use of antibiotics is dictated by the operative findings. The spectrum of coverage should include anaerobic and aerobic organisms. Several large studies have compared the efficacy of a second-generation cephalosporin (cefoxitin) with clindamycin plus an aminoglycoside (gentamicin or tobramycin) in abdominal trauma. Cefoxitin as a single agent is as effective as any combined treatment. The ideal length of coverage is uncertain. In general, if patients have gross enteric contamination with established peritonitis, treatment should last 5 to 7 days. Patients with minimal contamination can be treated with prophylaxis for 24 hours or less.

Tetanus prophylaxis should be administered, particularly with transenteric gunshot wounds. If fully immunized as a child, a patient is adequately treated with a booster immunization. If adequate childhood immunization is absent, unlikely, or unknown, then passive immunization should be provided with hyperimmune globulin (Hyper-Tet; Bayer Corporation, West Haven, CT).

Operative Approach

The patient should be placed supine on the operating room table and the entire anterior torso from the sternal notch to the groins should be prepared and draped to allow for maximum exposure. The initial operative approach for abdominal trauma is straightforward. A midline incision is preferred, and there are few reasons to deviate from this choice. In addition, the patient should be routinely prepared from the sternal notch to the middle thigh to allow harvesting of the saphenous vein for any vascular injury encountered. This also allows extension into a median sternotomy in the event that more proximal control of the vena cava or aorta is needed or if the patient is found to have a cardiac injury.

After the abdomen is opened, obvious blood and clot is sequentially removed, first from the lower abdomen and then from the upper abdomen, by packing of all four quadrants of the abdomen. If the peritoneal cavity is full of blood, the location of clot is often a clue to the site of bleeding. Any area that is found to be the source of hemorrhage can be repacked. Inflow occlusion can be accomplished, if needed, by clamping of the aorta at the diaphragmatic hiatus. Obvious hollow viscus wounds should be rapidly sutured. This initial closure does not need to be definitive and is done primarily to minimize contamination during the course of the operation. Retroperitoneal hematomas may be the source of exsanguinating hemorrhage if rupture into the free peritoneal cavity has occurred. If not, these can be left for investigation at a later time, depending on the location. Hematomas of the pelvis that are associated with pelvic fractures should not be disturbed. Stable hematomas in the perinephric space lateral to the midline are also best left undisturbed. Central hematomas that can involve injury to the major vascular structures, pancreas, or duodenum are noted and explored after control of injuries within the peritoneal cavity.

After packing has controlled hemorrhage and ongoing contamination has been stopped, time is taken to allow resuscitation of the patient's circulating blood volume. Warming is also appropriate at this time if massive blood loss has occurred. Sustained periods of hypotension should be avoided at all costs, and usually this can be accomplished with packing. After the intraabdominal injuries have been repaired, a complete and thorough exploratory laparotomy is performed methodically to investigate the entire contents of the abdomen.

In some patients, a temporizing approach to intraabdominal injuries is appropriate. This approach has been dubbed *damage control laparotomy* (247). Minimizing operative time is emphasized and the definitive management of all injuries is not necessary. Appropriate candidates for damage control laparotomy are patients with profound coagulopathy, hypothermia, massive intraabdominal injuries, or severe associated nonabdominal injuries. Hollow viscus injuries should be temporarily controlled so that there is no ongoing contamination, but restoration of gastrointestinal continuity is not done. The abdominal wall is either left open or closed temporarily, and resuscitative efforts are continued with particular emphasis on correcting coagulopathy and hypothermia. A planned reoperation is then undertaken when the patient's condition permits. Definitive injury repair management is undertaken at that time.

SPECIFIC INJURIES

Diaphragm

Injuries to the diaphragm occur in approximately 4% of patients with blunt abdominal or thoracic trauma; these injuries involve the left hemidiaphragm most of the time. All diaphragmatic injuries must be repaired to avoid the long-term potential for herniation, incarceration, and strangulation of abdominal viscera. The diagnosis of diaphragm injury should be suspected if respiratory distress and radiologic evidence of pleural effusion are not relieved by tube thoracostomy or if an upright radiograph demonstrates obvious visceral herniation into the thorax (Fig. 11.47). Chest radiograph findings in patients with blunt diaphragmatic rupture are sometimes subtle and may appear only as a blurring of the costophrenic angle or the line of the hemidiaphragm.

Epigastric and low-thoracic penetrating injuries should be presumed to have traversed the diaphragm. During exploratory laparotomy, the entire diaphragmatic surface should be exposed and directly visualized. Linear lacerations can be repaired with a simple running suture or interrupted horizontal mattress sutures, whereas larger lacerations and tissue deficits occasionally require repair with prosthetic material. Frequently, the left side of the medial portion of the defect is directly adjacent to the pericardium, and care must be taken to avoid iatrogenic injury to the pericardium or heart. Exploration of acute traumatic diaphragmatic rupture is usually accomplished through the abdomen because of the high potential for associated intraperitoneal injury. Defects discovered at a later date can be addressed satisfactorily by a transthoracic approach, which facilitates lysis of adhesions. The principal complication of diaphragmatic rupture is visceral incarceration

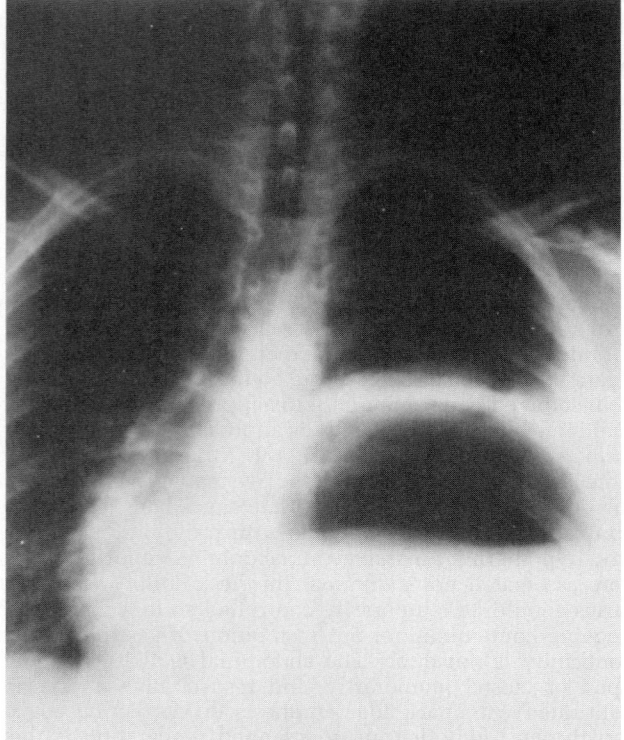

Figure 11.47. Chest radiograph showing gastric bubble in the left chest consistent with a rupture of the left hemidiaphragm.

and possible strangulation associated with an unrecognized injury. After surgical repair, specific problems are rare.

Spleen

The spleen is the intraabdominal organ most frequently injured in blunt trauma. Splenic injury is often accompanied by rib fractures on the left because the spleen lies in the left upper quadrant of the abdomen just to the left and slightly posterior to the stomach. Blunt injury is usually the result of compression of the spleen between the anterior body wall and the posterior thorax. The history is helpful if the patient can describe a specific fall or direct blow to the left chest, flank, or abdomen. For penetrating trauma, a wound entry or exit in this area should raise the suspicion of splenic injury. The clinical signs may be few and subtle; a high level of suspicion must be maintained simply on the basis of mechanism of injury. Clinical evidence of splenic injury includes signs of blood loss, left upper quadrant abdominal pain or tenderness, and pain referred to the left shoulder (Kehr's sign).

In general, laboratory studies are of limited help. Leukocytosis and decreased hematocrit are present, but neither is specific for splenic injury. CT scan is useful in hemodynamically stable patients for demonstrating splenic injury. Ultrasound confirms hemoperitoneum, if present, with splenic injury.

Historically, splenic injury was routinely treated with splenectomy. During the last few decades, several factors have contributed to a change in this management strategy. Postsplenectomy sepsis, with its high attendant mortality rate, has been characterized. In addition, the relative success rates for splenic salvage techniques and nonoperative management have become particularly important in the treatment of children with splenic injury. Initial nonoperative approaches emphasized the importance of the CT scan appearance of the splenic injury. More recent algorithms focus more on the clinical presentation of the patient rather than the CT scan appearance, although the presence of a "blush" on the CT scan is indicative of potential ongoing bleeding and an increased likelihood of operative intervention (248) (Fig. 11.48). Although increasingly practiced, nonoperative management is not without dangers and limitations. Potential disadvantages include prolonged hospitalization and possibly more exposure to transfused blood, but the principal risks of the nonoperative approach are ongoing hemorrhage and missed associated intraabdominal injuries, particularly to the pancreas or bowel.

The spleen is evaluated for hemorrhage during the course of laparotomy. If hemorrhage is noted, a decision must be made regarding splenic salvage. This assessment requires complete mobilization of the spleen from its attachments (see Pancreas, later), and care must be taken to prevent further injury. After the spleen is mobilized, the tail of the pancreas is released from the posterior retroperitoneum, and the spleen is delivered into the abdominal incision. The spleen and tail of the pancreas must be mobilized together to evaluate adequately the extent of splenic injury. Ongoing bleeding can be controlled during mobilization by manual compression.

Topical hemostatic agents usually can control capsular tears of the spleen. Lacerations of the splenic substance can be controlled with interlocking absorbable sutures. Major lacerations of the splenic substance involving less than half of the splenic tissue can be treated with segmental splenic resection. Splenic salvage should not be attempted if the patient has protracted hypotension or other severe injuries or if undue delays are encountered in the attempt to repair the spleen. With penetrating injury, dam-

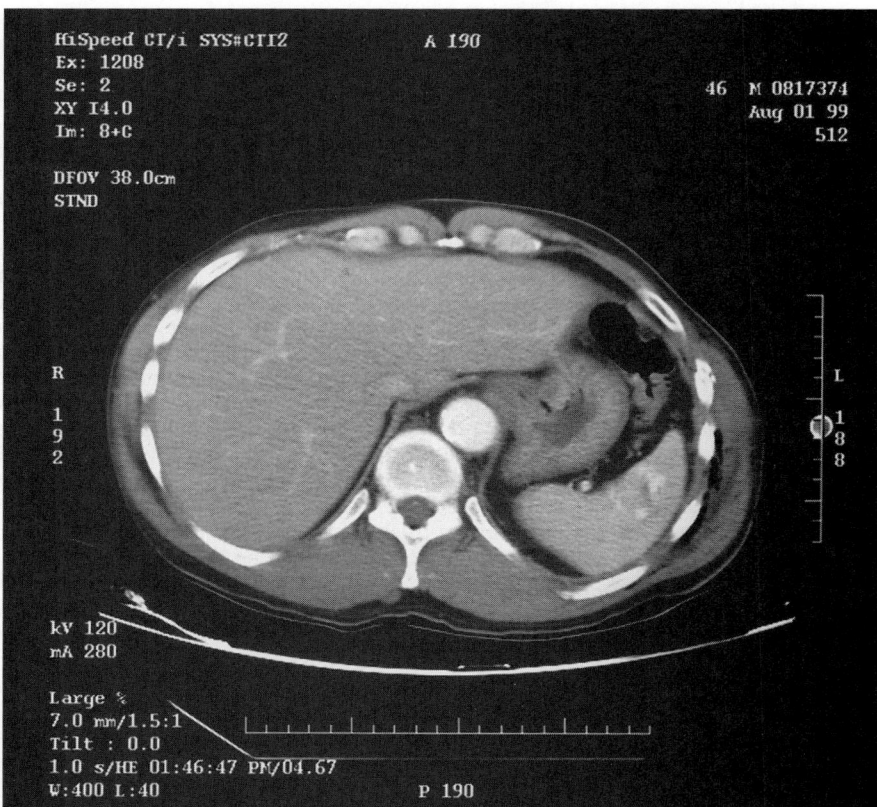

Figure 11.48. A cut from a computed tomography scan through the upper abdomen of a patient with a splenic injury. The spleen has evidence of several areas of contrast "blush."

age to adjacent structures, such as the stomach, pancreas, colon, and diaphragm, must be anticipated and investigated. The nonoperative management of splenic trauma in adults is most attractive if the diagnosis has been made with an abdominal CT scan, the patient is hemodynamically stable, and there are no other signs of abdominal injury. Nonoperative management is successful in such circumstances approximately 90% of the time in adults, and even more often in children. Follow-up CT scans are routinely obtained by some surgeons, but they are probably not necessary if the patient is doing well clinically (249). In general, nonoperative management should be carried out for the initial 24 to 48 hours in an intensive care unit, and patients should remain hospitalized for 1 week postinjury because of the risk of delayed bleeding.

Complications after splenectomy include early transient thrombocytosis, which usually resolves spontaneously within 2 or 3 months. Anticoagulation is neither necessary nor helpful. Delayed hemorrhage, pancreatitis, and subphrenic abscess also may occur. Subphrenic abscess is primarily related to associated hollow viscus injuries and is uncommon after blunt trauma. Routine drainage of the subphrenic space should not be done; it is associated with an increased rather than a decreased incidence of abscess.

Postsplenectomy Sepsis

Fatal pneumococcal septicemia after splenectomy was first noted in the mid-1950s in children. This postsplenectomy sepsis syndrome is caused by failure to clear one of several encapsulated bacteria in the absence of the spleen. The incidence varies from 0.5% to as much as 12% or 15%, depending on age and the underlying disease. The incidence is inversely related to age and is higher with underlying hematologic disorders such as lymphoma or thalassemia. The incidence of life-threaten-

ing sepsis in adult trauma patients is low, but it is higher than in the normal population. The overall clinical significance is not easily defined. Concern about the possibility of postsplenectomy sepsis should not obscure the fact that the initial priority is to arrest hemorrhage and deal with the patient's immediate life-threatening injuries.

Certainly in children, and possibly in adults, efforts at splenic salvage are appropriate. If splenectomy is performed, postoperative follow-up is essential. Immunization with the polyvalent pneumococcal vaccine is required, and booster immunization should be done every 3 years. In addition, prophylactic antibiotics, usually oral penicillin, should be given any time the patient is undergoing instrumentation, such as during dental repair or surgery, and probably should be given prophylactically as well. Such patients should be advised of their increased potential for postsplenectomy sepsis and should carry an identification card to alert health care workers of this possibility if they have an infection. All infections should be considered emergencies and treated aggressively with intravenous antibiotics in the hospital.

Liver

The liver is the largest organ in the abdominal cavity and is commonly damaged in blunt and penetrating abdominal trauma as well as in thoracoabdominal injuries. Some series have found that the incidence of liver injuries exceeds that of injuries to the spleen. In any case, the two together account for approximately 75% of all blunt intraabdominal injuries. Trauma sufficient to lacerate the liver is often associated with injuries to other organs. Spontaneous hemostatic mechanisms are sufficiently effective that approximately 85% of patients with liver injuries are not actively bleeding at the time of laparotomy, and these injuries are predictably well tolerated. At laparotomy, most liver injuries require no specific therapy, and drainage is usually unnecessary. Those injuries that do require definitive surgical care present a complex and life-threatening series of problems.

Patients with significant liver injuries usually have a history of major blunt energy transfer to the right thorax or upper abdomen. Physical findings may be minimal because early bleeding may not cause peritoneal irritation or abdominal distention. Any patient with unexplained hypotension after blunt abdominal trauma must be considered at risk for a severe liver injury. Likewise, major liver injury should be suspected if a patient has a history of shock at the scene after blunt trauma. DPL is most helpful in establishing the diagnosis of hemoperitoneum, and if DPL results are positive, laparotomy is appropriate. In hemodynamically stable patients and in those with a contraindication to DPL, CT scan is precise in evaluating subcapsular hematomas, lacerations, and other hepatic parenchymal injuries. Liver injuries seen on CT scan in hemodynamically stable patients can be treated nonoperatively as long as the patient is followed closely and the possibility of associated hollow viscus or pancreatic injury is borne in mind (250).

Injuries vary from simple capsular tears and nonbleeding lacerations, to complex fractures with lobar destruction and extensive parenchymal disruption, to bile duct disruption, to hepatic artery and venous injuries. The type of injury dictates the character of the surgical therapy required. The principles of liver injury management are the same regardless of the severity of injury. They involve control of bleeding, removal of devitalized tissue, and establishment of adequate drainage.

Simple lacerations that have stopped bleeding at the time of surgery do not require drainage unless they are deep into the parenchyma, in which case they have a high probability of postoperative biliary leakage. Subcapsular hematomas can be simply evacuated or left intact if there is no associated parenchymal injury. Lacerations that continue to bleed despite attempts at local control require exploration of the liver wound. The depths of the liver wound are explored and specific vessels and biliary radicals are individually ligated.

In the event that bleeding continues despite segmental ligation of parenchymal vessels, the structures of the porta hepatis should be compressed as a diagnostic maneuver (Pringle maneuver; Fig. 11.49). If the bleeding stops as a result of this maneuver, it is presumed to originate from the portal veins or the hepatic artery. If the bleeding continues, it is presumed to arise principally from the hepatic veins or inferior vena cava, although this distinction is seldom clear-cut in the operating room. The portal triad also can be intermittently occluded with this maneuver to allow improved visualization during placement of sutures as parenchymal vessels are ligated. If selective parenchymal ligation fails, ligation of the hepatic artery is an alternative if the trial Pringle occlusion has had a salutary effect. This is rarely necessary but can occasionally produce dramatic hemostasis without subsequent liver failure. The vessel is usually occluded as close to the liver injury as possible, and after initial efforts at hemostasis have failed.

An alternative for deep lacerations with persistent bleeding is resectional débridement of the involved segment of the liver. This is accomplished by the finger fracture technique, removing devitalized liver or an appropriate portion of the liver up to and including formal lobectomy. This is required in approximately 5% to 8% of all patients with liver injuries. Subsegmental resection is usually adequate; if segmentectomy or lobectomy is required, a knowledge of the anatomy is imperative so as not to compromise inflow or outflow of the remaining segments. This decision should be made early in the exploration, the blood bank notified,

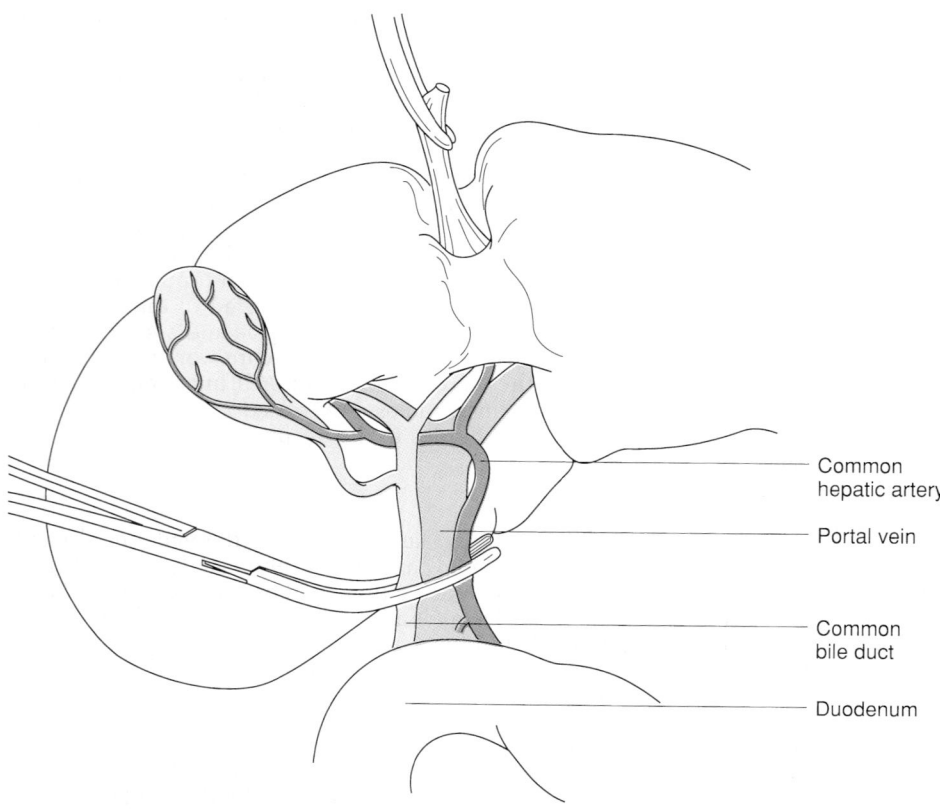

Common hepatic artery

Portal vein

Common bile duct

Duodenum

Figure 11.49. Pringle maneuver compression of the portal triad structures with a noncrushing vascular clamp for hepatic inflow control. If possible, clamp times should be limited to 15- to 20-minute intervals.

adequate help procured, and exposure obtained. Exposure is best accomplished by complete division of the capsular attachments of the liver. Parenchymal débridement and division is done after formal dissection of the porta hepatis. This is an alternative associated with operative mortality rates usually in the range of 10%.

In the event that parenchymal or hepatic vein bleeding cannot be controlled and the patient remains difficult to resuscitate, is hypothermic, and has a coagulopathy from massive transfusion, packing of the injury and further resuscitation after the abdomen is closed are appropriate. Subsequent operative removal of the packs 24 to 72 hours later can be accompanied by resection and suture ligation in a stable, resuscitated patient. After hemostasis has been achieved, the area should be drained. Either sump drainage or wide-open drainage can be used. The packing is done with laparotomy pads placed either directly onto the bleeding liver surface or on top of a plastic drape. For packing to be successful, it should be used early, before coagulopathy has become too severe.

Inability to control bleeding by any of the previously described techniques suggests significant retrohepatic vena caval bleeding or bleeding from the hepatic veins. If bleeding is unilobar, débridement and resection may be sufficient. With bilobar involvement or uncontrollable hemorrhage from a single lobe, early consideration should be given to the placement of an intracaval shunt or complete vascular isolation. This approach is rarely necessary and should be undertaken only if packing has not controlled hemorrhage from the liver (Fig. 11.50). To accomplish this, the midline laparotomy incision is extended into the chest, either by a right anterior thoracotomy or, preferably, by a median sternotomy. Infrahepatic (cephalad to the renal veins) and suprahepatic (usually intrapericardial) control of the vena cava is obtained. A shunt or other large conduit is then inserted through a right atrial pursestring into the vena cava, and vascular occlusion around the conduit at these sites is obtained. The resultant vascular isolation is always imperfect but may allow better visualization of hepatic vein and vena cava lacerations for direct suture ligation or repair. Total venous occlusion may be equally effective and serves the same general purpose. The risk of hypotension is significant with either approach. With the former, significant blood loss is inevitable during a trial cannulation. With the

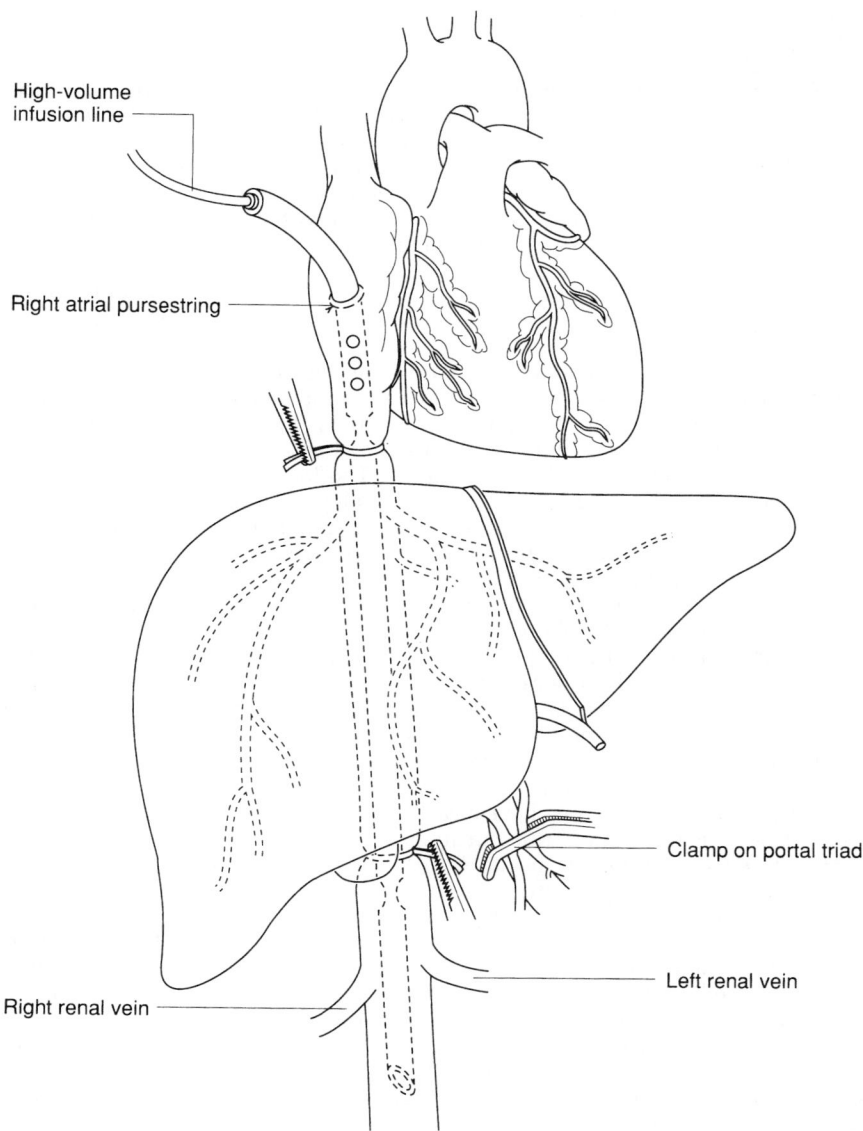

Figure 11.50. Intracaval shunt used for retrohepatic venous injuries, combined with a Pringle maneuver for isolation of the retrohepatic vena cava for operative repair.

High-volume infusion line

Right atrial pursestring

Clamp on portal triad

Left renal vein

Right renal vein

latter, diminished venous return to the right atrium is always a result. This is such an unusual injury that personal preference dictates the approach.

The major complications after liver injury include hemorrhage, respiratory insufficiency, coagulopathy, hypoglycemia, biliary fistula or other bile duct injury, hemobilia, and subdiaphragmatic or intraparenchymal abscess formation. The coagulopathy after liver resection is usually the result of hypothermia and inadequate replacement of blood components. Patients undergoing major hepatic resection after trauma need continuous glucose infusion, often 10% dextrose, during the early postoperative period. Hypoalbuminemia is not common and does not usually require albumin administration. It should be treated simply with aggressive nutritional support unless hemodynamic consequences arise. Hyperbilirubinemia is transient and usually peaks in 2 to 3 weeks after major resection; it usually does not exceed 10 mg/dL. Intrahepatic and subphrenic abscesses can develop, particularly if significant débridement has been necessary. These are diagnosed by clinical evidence of sepsis combined with ultrasound or CT scan and often can be treated with percutaneous drainage. When percutaneous drainage is unsuccessful or not available, drainage can be effected surgically either transperitoneally or posteriorly through the bed of the 12th rib. Biliary fistulae usually close spontaneously, and major extrahepatic ductal injuries are rare. For the rare biliary leak or fistula that does not close spontaneously, placement of a temporary intrabiliary stent either at the site of injury or through the sphincter of Oddi (to decrease intrabiliary pressure) is a possibility. Experience to date with such stents is limited. A T-tube placed in an otherwise normal common bile duct is inappropriate unless the extrahepatic biliary tree is injured. Hemobilia is a rare complication presenting with intrahepatic bleeding into the bile ducts and is best diagnosed with angiography or endoscopy. Angiographic embolization is the treatment of choice.

Stomach

The stomach is vulnerable to penetrating injuries of the upper abdomen and lower chest. The upper abdominal viscera underlie the lower ribs to a level as high as the fourth intercostal space. The stomach is injured in 5% to 10% of patients with penetrating abdominal trauma. The location of external wounds should lead to the initial suspicion of gastric injury. As with injuries to other intraabdominal viscera, physical examination of the abdomen often points to the presence of injury. It is difficult to differentiate between gastric injuries and injuries to other intraabdominal viscera based on palpation of the abdomen alone, but a physical examination that is positive for peritoneal signs mandates expeditious abdominal exploration. Precise preoperative characterization of injuries is not necessary. Hematemesis or blood found on aspiration of the stomach with a nasogastric tube is another finding suggestive of gastric injury. Although many patients with blood in the stomach after penetrating abdominal trauma have a gastric injury, the absence of these signs does not rule out such an injury.

Abdominal exploration is begun by a standard upper midline incision. Adequate diagnosis requires mobilization and visualization of the entire stomach. Most of the anterior surface of the stomach can be adequately visualized without extensive mobilization. Visualization is facilitated if the edge of the greater curve of the stomach is grasped, either with the fingers or with several Babcock clamps, and the stomach is pulled down into the operative field. For greater traction, the Babcock clamps can be used to grasp the nasogastric tube through the stomach wall. If the clamps are placed far apart, this maneuver also can be used to spread out the stomach so that the entire surface can be seen. It is also helpful to place a nasogastric tube and empty the stomach with suction.

Exposure of the anterior surface of the gastroesophageal junction can be difficult if the flare of the costal margin is narrow or if the left lobe of the liver is in the way. Improved exposure is accomplished with extension of the midline incision as high as possible by creating a paraxiphoid extension. The left hepatic lobe is retracted to the right after division of the left triangular ligament, as would be done for exposure of the gastroesophageal junction for performance of a vagotomy or antireflux procedure. Finally, mobilization of the gastroesophageal junction, encirclement with a tape or drain, and caudal traction into the operative field allow for improved visualization and the performance of any necessary repairs.

The posterior wall of the stomach should be examined for the presence of injuries. This is especially true if there is an injury on the anterior surface. The posterior stomach is exposed by opening the gastrocolic ligament. This can be done bluntly if the hole is made to the left of the midline approximately halfway between the stomach and the transverse colon in a relatively avascular area. The lesser sac is entered, and the posterior wall of the stomach can then be seen.

As with exposure of the anterior surface, the greater curve of the stomach should be grasped. By lifting the greater curve superiorly and out into the wound, the posterior wall of the stomach can be displayed and visualized. If necessary, the attachments of the gastrohepatic and gastrocolic ligaments to the lesser and greater curvature, respectively, should be cleared to rule out an underlying injury. The excellent blood supply of the stomach allows this to be done with minimal risk of devascularization.

Injuries to the stomach are usually easy to repair. Most can be repaired primarily in two layers, with an inner running layer of 3-0 or 4-0 absorbable sutures followed by an outer layer of 3-0 or 4-0 permanent Lembert sutures. Because of the ample blood supply and large lumen of the stomach in all areas except the gastroesophageal junction and pylorus, there is minimal concern for excessive inversion and luminal compromise. Good blood supply also leads to excellent healing in most cases. On rare occasions, especially after shotgun wounds, large injuries of the stomach may require resection. Injuries to the pylorus are rare. If they do occur, they should be closed with a Heineke-Mikulicz pyloroplasty if possible; a concomitant vagotomy is not necessary.

Because of the stomach's position high in the abdomen, injuries to the stomach are frequently associated with lacerations of the diaphragm. This is especially true for gunshot wounds. During spontaneous ventilation, there is negative pressure in the pleural cavity and positive pressure in the abdomen. The resultant pressure gradient causes movement of gastric fluid and particulate matter from the abdomen into the chest if both the stomach and diaphragm have been injured. The degree to which movement of such debris into the chest has occurred can be deceptive in the operating room because most of the movement occurs before the institution of positive-pressure ventilation and laparotomy. Small holes in the hemidiaphragm may appear innocuous when in fact significant pleural contamination has occurred.

Even small amounts of contamination with gastric contents can result in the development of an empyema. It is difficult to drain particulate matter with a chest tube, especially if there is associated clotted blood. In the presence of combined injuries to the stomach and diaphragm, therefore, the pleural cavity should be lavaged before closure of the diaphragmatic hole. The diaphragmatic laceration should be enlarged enough to allow lavage from the abdomen. The course of the phrenic nerve in the diaphragm should be borne in mind, and enlargement of the diaphragmatic laceration should be done either radially or as peripherally as possible (Fig. 11.51).

Occasionally, adequate lavage of the pleural cavity using an abdominal approach is difficult. This occurs if the amount of pleural contamination is massive or if enlargement of the diaphragmatic laceration cannot be done without risk of denervation of the diaphragm. In such instances, the abdomen should be closed and a limited anterolateral thoracotomy should be performed for removal of contaminating particulate debris and saline lavage fluid. Although this seemingly drastic strategy rarely proves necessary, it significantly reduces the risk of empyema development. An alternative approach to this problem is the use of thoracoscopy to lavage the hemithorax. Experience with thoracoscopy in this setting is minimal, but it is an attractive alternative to thoracotomy.

Blunt injuries to the stomach are rarer than penetrating injuries and account for only 1% of blunt hollow viscus injuries. The stomach is large, distensible, and mobile. A great deal of force is necessary to cause a blowout of the gastric wall. As a consequence, the mortality rate from associated injuries is high in patients with blunt stomach injuries. Blowout injuries of the stomach also tend to be large. The stomach may be more likely to be injured from blunt trauma if it is full at the time of the injury, and blunt trauma injuries are therefore often associated with significant intraperitoneal contamination. Associated injuries usually make the need for abdominal exploration obvious. Principles of operative exposure and repair are the same as for penetrating injuries.

Duodenum

Penetrating Injuries

Because of the retroperitoneal location of the duodenum close to a number of other viscera and major vascular structures, isolated penetrating injuries to the duodenum are rare. The need for abdominal exploration is usually dictated by associated injuries, and the diagnosis of duodenal injury is usually made in the operating room. Associated injuries lead to a mortality rate of 15% to 20% in patients with duodenal injury. The duodenum is also susceptible to complications of repair (251).

In the rare instances in which isolated penetrating injury to the duodenum occurs, the most reliable means of making the diagnosis is with serial abdominal examinations. Although theoretically appealing as a means of diagnosis, the use of serum amylase concentrations in the diagnosis of penetrating duodenal injury is neither sensitive nor specific. The sensitivity of DPL in the diagnosis of penetrating duodenal injury is also poor because of the retroperitoneal location of the duodenum.

As with the stomach, diagnosis of duodenal injuries in the operating room depends on adequate exposure. The lateral and posterior portions of the duodenum cannot be visualized without mobilization. This mobilization is done by incising the lateral peritoneal reflection of the duodenum and mobilizing the duodenum from right to left with a combination of blunt and sharp dissection. This technique is known as the Kocher maneuver, and it can be carried well across the midline to the level of the abdominal aorta, providing exposure of the underlying vena cava and aorta.

Entry into the lesser sac by way of the gastrocolic ligament provides exposure of the posterior aspect of the proximal part of the first portion of the duodenum and the medial aspect of the second portion. Exposure of the third and fourth portions of the duodenum, if necessary, is carried out by incising the ligament of Treitz and mobilizing the right colon from right to left so that the right colon and small intestine can be elevated. This is sometimes referred to as the Cattell maneuver. With this combination of maneuvers, the entire duodenum can be mobilized and exposed for identification and thorough evaluation of any injury. It is critical to identify all injuries at the time of the initial abdominal exploration, because overlooked injuries

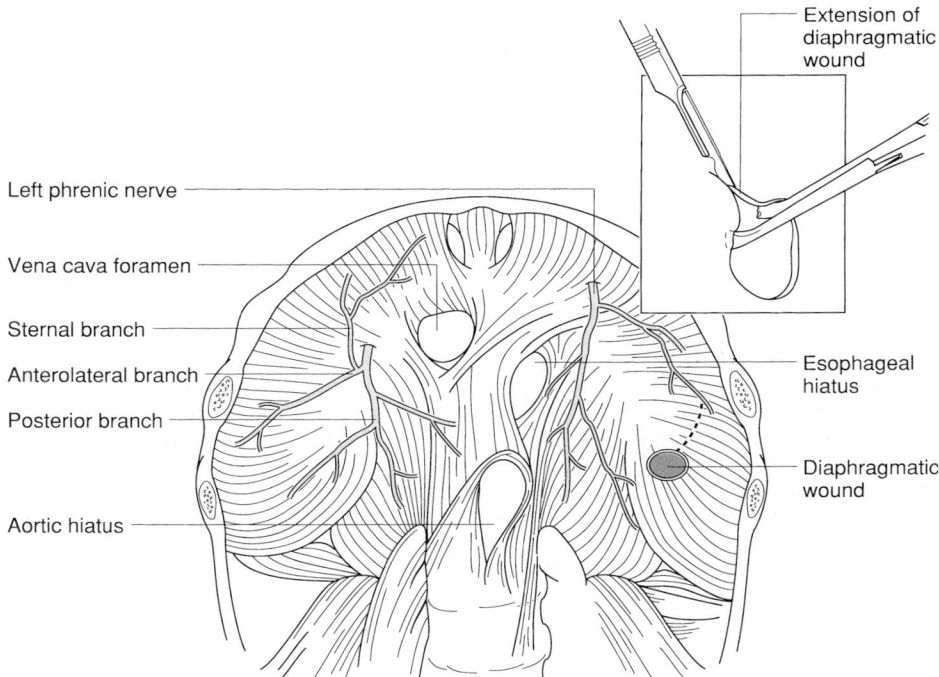

Figure 11.51. Phrenic nerve distribution of the diaphragm. Enlarging diaphragmatic wounds to carry out pleural lavage should be done with this innervation in mind. Either radial incision (as shown) or circumferential incisions should be used.

Left phrenic nerve

Vena cava foramen

Sternal branch

Anterolateral branch

Posterior branch

Aortic hiatus

Extension of diaphragmatic wound

Esophageal hiatus

Diaphragmatic wound

are associated with a significant increase in subsequent morbidity.

Grading systems have been devised to characterize duodenal injuries. Although useful for research purposes, the specifics of the grading systems are less important than several simple aspects of the duodenal injury: (a) the anatomic relation to the ampulla of Vater; (b) the character of the injury (i.e., a simple laceration versus destruction of the duodenal wall); (c) the involved circumference of the duodenum; and (d) associated injuries to the biliary tract, pancreas, or major vascular structures.

Most penetrating injuries to the duodenum are simple lacerations that can be repaired primarily. Such repairs should be done in two layers, with an inner absorbable layer of 3-0 or 4-0 running sutures followed by an outer layer of 3-0 or 4-0 permanent Lembert sutures. The closure should be oriented transversely, if possible, to avoid luminal compromise, but transverse orientation is not as critical in the duodenum as it is in the rest of the small intestine. Excessive inversion should be avoided. The biliary tract does not require drainage in such cases unless there is a primary biliary tract injury, and the duodenum does not require tube decompression, although both of these maneuvers have been advocated in the past. The periduodenal area should be drained with either closed suction drainage or passive rubber drains.

Large injuries to the duodenum are more difficult to repair. Injuries that encompass as much as 40% or 50% of the duodenal wall can be successfully closed primarily. Primary repair of injuries larger than that, however, can lead to luminal compromise. If the duodenum has been transected or almost transected, the edges should be débrided and a two-layer primary anastomosis done without tension after mobilization of the duodenum, provided that the transection is not close to the ampulla of Vater. Large injuries of the duodenum also can be treated with a jejunal patch by bringing up a loop of jejunum and laying it onto the area of injury so that the serosa of the jejunum buttresses the duodenal repair (Fig. 11.52). Alternatively, a duodenojejunostomy can be done to drain a large defect internally.

Destruction of a portion of the duodenum is rarely so complete as to preclude either primary closure or jejunal patch repair. If the duodenum alone has been injured, a rare occurrence, the patient should undergo a duodenojejunostomy to the defunctionalized Roux-en-Y limb of jejunum. If there are severe associated injuries to the pancreas or biliary tract, pancreaticoduodenectomy may be necessary. The morbidity associated with pancreaticoduodenectomy is substantial, and this operation is indicated only if the extent of injury is so great that the necessary resection has, in essence, been done by the injury. If débridement of devitalized tissue results in a pancreaticoduodenectomy, the necessary pancreatic, gastric, and biliary anastomoses should be made.

Some duodenal repairs are tenuous. This is a particular problem if there is associated pancreatic injury, raising concern about the digestive action of activated pancreatic enzymes on the repair. Pyloric exclusion is a technique devised to defunctionalize the duodenum and protect the repair from activated pancreatic enzymes until it has had time to heal. The original procedure devised to accomplish these objectives was called *pyloric diverticulization,* and it consisted of antrectomy, oversewing of the duodenal stump, tube decompression of the duodenum and biliary tract, and gastrojejunostomy to restore gastrointestinal continuity. Pyloric exclusion was devised as an alternative to this extensive procedure to shorten operating time and make the procedure reversible.

Pyloric exclusion is started with a gastrotomy along the greater curvature of the stomach. The pylorus is closed

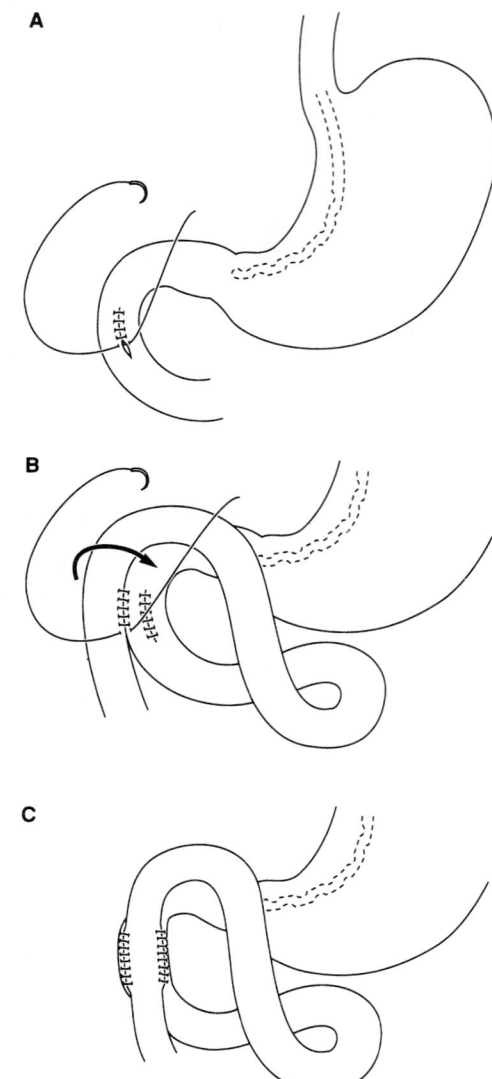

Figure 11.52. A jejunoileal patch can be used to reinforce repairs of the duodenum. *(A)* The duodenum is first repaired. *(B)* The retrocolic loop of jejunum is brought up to the area of repair. *(C)* The serosa is sewn over the repair.

with a large running suture placed through the gastrotomy or, alternatively, the pylorus is stapled closed. Gastrointestinal continuity is then restored by a gastrojejunostomy (Fig. 11.53). Tube decompression of the duodenum should be performed in severe duodenal injuries, but the biliary tract does not require decompression unless there has been an associated biliary tract injury. As with all duodenal injuries, the periduodenal area should be externally drained to ensure that a postoperative leak becomes a controlled fistula.

If patients who undergo pyloric exclusion are studied a number of weeks after the exclusion procedure with upper gastrointestinal contrast series, most are found to have normal reconstituted gastrointestinal continuity. The closure of the pylorus breaks down, and the normal gastrointestinal route is reestablished. This occurs regardless of whether the pylorus was closed with absorbable or nonabsorbable suture. As the pylorus reopens, the gastrojejunostomy may gradually close of its own accord. It is for this reason that

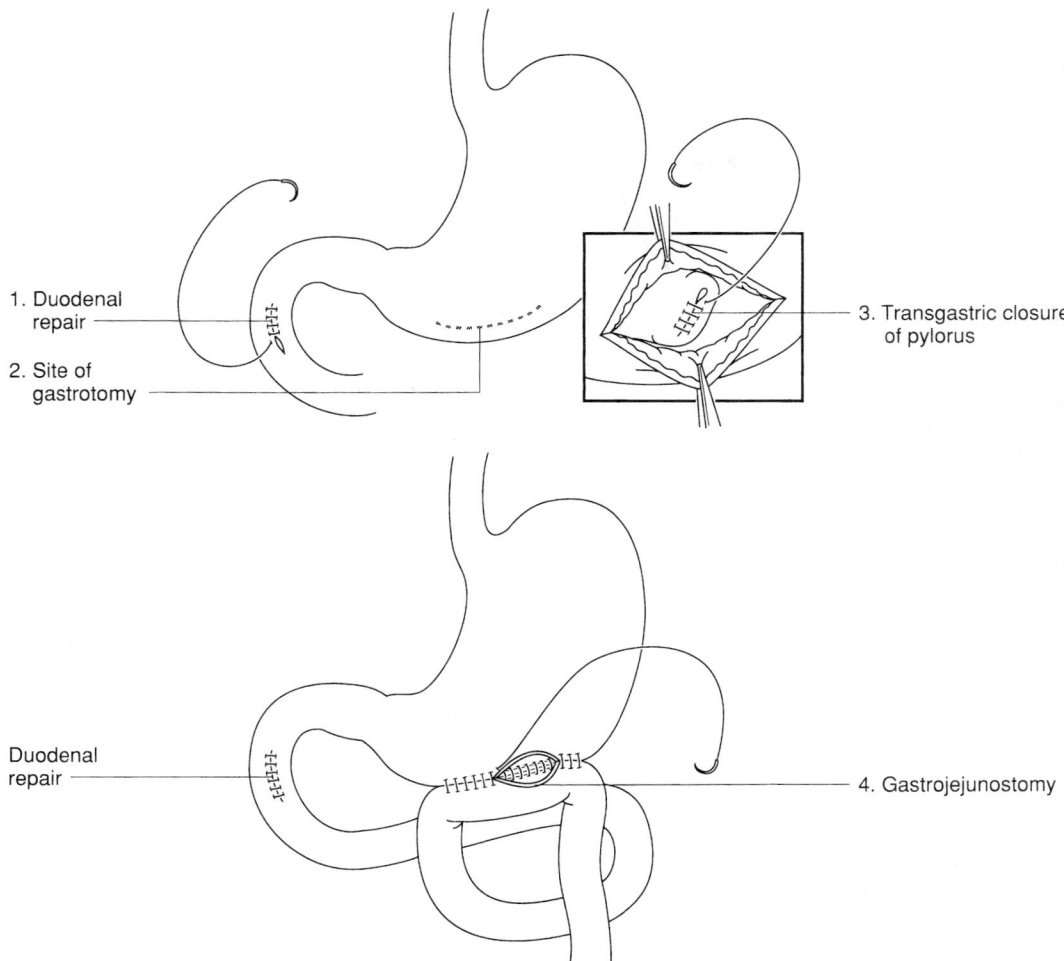

1. Duodenal repair
2. Site of gastrotomy
3. Transgastric closure of pylorus
Duodenal repair
4. Gastrojejunostomy

Figure 11.53. Technique of pyloric exclusion for complex duodenal injury.

pyloric exclusion, although an inherently ulcerogenic procedure, does not require a concomitant vagotomy.

Blunt Injuries

Blunt injuries to the duodenum are both less common and more difficult to diagnose than penetrating injuries. They can occur in isolation or with pancreatic injury. These are instances in which the need for immediate abdominal exploration is not obvious. Because the duodenum is located in the retroperitoneum, findings on physical examination of the abdomen may be subtle unless there are associated intraabdominal injuries. Nonetheless, the physical examination is still one of the best methods for determining the presence of a duodenal injury. This is true even if the admission examination is indeterminate, emphasizing the need for serial abdominal examinations.

In theory, perforations of the duodenum should be associated with leak of amylase and other digestive enzymes, and it has been suggested that determination of the serum amylase concentration may be helpful in the diagnosis of blunt duodenal injuries. However, the test lacks sensitivity. The duodenum is retroperitoneal, the concentration of amylase in the fluid that leaks is variable, and amylase concentrations often take hours to days to increase after injury. Although serial determinations of serum amylase are better than a single, isolated determination on admission, sensitivity is still poor, and necessary delays are inherent in serial determinations.

Plain abdominal radiographs have been advocated for the diagnosis of blunt duodenal injuries. The characteristic finding is that of extraluminal retroperitoneal air in the area of the duodenum. If present, this finding on plain film is often indicative of duodenal injury and should prompt operative exploration. Because many blunt injuries to the duodenum do not demonstrate this finding, however, it is not a reliable way to rule out injury.

Upper gastrointestinal series and CT scans of the abdomen are more sensitive than plain abdominal radiographs for the presence of duodenal contusion or perforation after blunt trauma. Performance of these tests requires a stable patient without any other obvious indications for abdominal exploration. Upper gastrointestinal series are less expensive to perform than CT scans, are widely available, and may have slightly increased sensitivity for subtle injuries of the duodenum. An advantage of CT, conversely, is that the rest of the retroperitoneum and peritoneal viscera are also visualized. With either study, extravasation of contrast material from the duodenum constitutes an indication for surgical intervention and repair.

Operative exposure and repair of the duodenum after blunt trauma are the same as for penetrating injuries. Crush injuries are more common after blunt trauma and occasionally require extensive resection, but the injuries can be treated by simple techniques of repair if they are diagnosed in a timely fashion.

Intramural hematoma of the duodenum is a rare injury specific to patients with blunt trauma. It is most common in children after isolated localized force to the upper abdomen, possibly because of the relatively flexible and pliable musculature of the child's abdominal wall. Intramural hematoma occur when the duodenum is crushed and there is bleeding in the submucosal or subserosal layers of the duodenum. The duodenum is not perforated. Such hematomas can lead to obstruction of the lumen. If the diagnosis is not made at the time of the initial injury, the obstruction usually takes several days to develop, presumably because of increased accumulation of intramural water as the hemoglobin in the hematoma begins to break down and osmotic forces increase absorption of water. This mechanism is similar to that proposed to explain the increase in size of subdural hematomas with time.

If exploration takes place shortly after injury, intramural hematomas of the duodenum are seen as periduodenal hematomas through the abdominal incision. At the time of initial operative evaluation, all hematomas in the area of the duodenum should be explored to rule out the possibility of perforation. Such exploration includes a Kocher maneuver and mobilization of the duodenum, which in most instances successfully drains subserosal hematomas. Submucosal hematomas may require drainage with deeper, separate incisions. If surgery does not occur shortly after injury, obstructive symptoms become manifest after a number of days. An upper gastrointestinal series or CT scan should be performed to demonstrate obstruction. The obstruction is usually in the second portion of the duodenum and, in the classic picture, demonstrates a coiled-spring appearance.

Some debate surrounds the treatment of intramural hematomas of the duodenum if the diagnosis is delayed, but the weight of opinion argues for initial nonoperative treatment. This strategy is usually successful because the hematoma gradually resolves and the obstructive symptoms subside without long-term residual sequelae. If obstructive symptoms persist beyond 10 to 14 days from the time of diagnosis, abdominal exploration should be undertaken to rule out the presence of a duodenal perforation or injury to the head of the pancreas that may be an alternative cause of duodenal obstruction.

Complications

Both penetrating and blunt injuries of the duodenum can lead to complications associated with leak of the duodenal repair. The duodenum is particularly susceptible to leak of repairs because of the presence of intraluminal digestive enzymes. Adequate drainage of the periduodenal area ensures that such leaks are controlled and do not result in an intraabdominal abscess. Placement of a decompressive duodenal tube to protect duodenal repairs is controversial and has been abandoned by many surgeons. In theory, a decompressive tube protects the duodenal repair and lessens the incidence of repair failure. If a duodenal repair breaks down and the duodenum is adequately drained, a duodenal fistula results. In the absence of distal obstruction, foreign body, or persistent infection (the chances of which are minimized by adequate drainage), many of these controlled fistulae ultimately close. They may be slow to resolve, and a wait of several months is advised to allow them to resolve spontaneously. Trials of total parenteral nutrition may increase the rate of spontaneous closure. If a fistula fails to close after an appropriate waiting period, further surgical intervention is warranted. It consists of reexploration of the abdomen and construction of a duodenojejunostomy as a form of internal drainage. The duodenojejunostomy should be constructed with the use of a defunctionalized Roux-en-Y limb of jejunum.

Pancreas

Penetrating Injuries

Penetrating injuries to the pancreas are usually diagnosed in the operating room (252). Like the duodenum, the pancreas is located in the retroperitoneum, surrounded by a number of other viscera and major vascular structures. As a result, an isolated injury to the pancreas is unusual, and patients with penetrating pancreatic trauma usually have obvious indications for abdominal exploration. Major vascular injuries are seen in 40% to 50% of patients with penetrating pancreatic injuries, in 50% of those with injuries to the liver, and in 25% of those with injuries to the duodenum. Preoperative serum amylase concentrations are not helpful; they are elevated only in approximately 30% of patients with penetrating pancreatic injuries.

On abdominal exploration, signs of pancreatic injury include a projectile path that passes near the pancreas, a central hematoma in the upper abdomen, and injuries to the duodenum, vena cava, suprarenal aorta, or mesenteric vessels. In all these instances, the pancreas should be thoroughly explored.

The anterior surface of the pancreas is visualized by entry into the lesser sac of the peritoneal cavity. This is done in the same fashion as outlined previously for exposure of the posterior aspect of the stomach, with division of the gastrocolic ligament in a relatively avascular area to the left of the midline. A thin layer of peritoneum overlies the anterior surface of the pancreas at this point, and complete visualization of the surface sometimes requires incision of this layer.

The tail of the pancreas can be more fully visualized, especially in its posterior aspect, by mobilization of the spleen and the tail of the pancreas as a unit. This is accomplished by incision of any lateral attachments of the spleen to the abdominal wall and mobilization of the spleen with blunt dissection laterally to medially by development of the plane between the anterior surface of the left kidney and the posterior aspect of the spleen. This brings the spleen into the abdominal wound and elevates the posterior aspect of the pancreatic tail for inspection.

The posterior aspect of the body of the pancreas is visualized by development of the avascular area at the inferior margin of the body and tail of the pancreas with a combination of sharp and blunt dissection. The pancreas can then be mobilized inferiorly to superiorly. This maneuver is also important for mobilization of the pancreas in preparation for distal pancreatic resection.

The posterior aspect of the head of the pancreas can be exposed by an extensive Kocher maneuver. In combination with entry into the lesser sac, this also allows for bimanual palpation of the pancreatic head, with one hand placed on the anterior surface of the pancreas through the hole in the lesser sac and the other hand placed behind the pancreas in the plane developed by the Kocher maneuver.

In the evaluation of penetrating pancreatic injuries, the key to operative management is the determination of whether a ductal injury is present. Transduodenal intraoperative pancreatography has been recommended, but the use of this technique in the identification of ductal injuries is controversial. The advantage of this maneuver is that it allows for more definitive determination of the type of operative intervention that should be undertaken. The major disadvantage is that it necessitates entry into the duodenum when there is no associated duodenal injury, which turns simple pancreatic injuries into combined pancreaticoduodenal injuries, with an attendant increase in potential postoperative morbidity. A further argument against intraoperative pancreatography is that most injuries to the pancreas can be adequately evaluated and decisions made about appropriate operative treatment without radiographic examination of ductal anatomy. In certain circumstances, the use of intraoperative endoscopic retrograde cholangiopancreatography (ERCP) eliminates this problem.

The operative management of penetrating pancreatic injuries is somewhat controversial. Injuries can be classified according to both location and severity. With respect to location, injuries can be subdivided into those of the head, body, and tail of the pancreas. With respect to severity, classification systems have been devised that not only have comparative and research applications but can be used in the determination of the best treatment. Class I injuries are simple contusions of the pancreas; class II injuries are lacerations of the parenchyma in the body or tail of the pancreas; class III injuries are those with severe disruption of the head or body; and class IV injuries are those in which there is an associated injury to the duodenum.

Class I injuries should be observed or simply drained externally. The optimal type of drainage is a matter of some debate, and a variety of different drainage methods have been espoused. For many years, passive rubber drains were routinely used. Several reports published in the 1970s and early 1980s sought to demonstrate the superiority of sump drainage for pancreatic injuries, although other reports published since that time have not demonstrated superiority for any particular form of drainage. A report on a randomized series of patients seemed to demonstrate an advantage of closed suction drainage over sump drainage, but the data were inconclusive. The type of drain used after pancreatic injury is probably not important as long as adequate drainage is effected. This can be accomplished with passive, sump, or closed suction systems.

If drains are used, they should be left in place for at least 5 to 7 days to ensure that a drain tract develops. Pancreatic fistulae can develop on a delayed basis 3 to 7 days after injury, and if the drains are removed before that time, drainage may be inadequate. The morbidity rate for patients with undrained pancreatic secretions is much greater than for those with drained pancreatic secretions.

The timing of drain removal should be based on both the amount and character of the pancreatic drainage. Drain outputs in excess of 150 to 200 mL/d are suggestive of pancreatic fistulae. Determinations of drain amylase concentration are moderately helpful, but amylase concentrations in the drainage are of little benefit if patients are tested within a few days of injury because even high levels (>50,000 IU/L) do not correlate with the development of a pancreatic fistula or other complications. Determinations done at 7 days after injury correlate with the presence of a pancreatic fistula or other pancreatic complication only if the level is higher than 100,000 IU/L. The negative predictive value of a concentration below 100,000 IU/L is poor, however, and does not rule out the presence or subsequent development of a pancreatic complication.

The treatment of class II injuries depends on the presence or absence of a ductal injury, a determination that can be difficult to make. The argument for intraoperative pancreatography is made for class II injuries. The presence of a ductal injury in the head of the pancreas does not usually make a difference with respect to treatment because most of these injuries should be drained regardless. On the other hand, if a ductal injury is present or suspected in the body or tail of the pancreas, the appropriate treatment is resection of the distal pancreas. If no ductal injury is present, simple drainage is adequate. Although this reasoning is clear, the difficulty lies in determining whether injuries to the body or tail of the pancreas do, in fact, include ductal injury.

Class III injuries of the body or tail of the pancreas, as mentioned previously, should be treated with a distal pancreatectomy. Distal resection can include up to 80% of the gland, if necessary. Subsequent endocrine or exocrine insufficiency is rare if the pancreas is normal. Class III injuries of the head of the pancreas should be drained. Resection of these injuries requires internal drainage, near-total pancreatectomy, or pancreaticoduodenectomy procedures that are associated with a high rate of morbidity and mortality. If a pancreatic fistula develops, the drains can control the fistula. If the fistula does not resolve with time, the pancreas can be drained internally at a later date.

Class IV injuries of the pancreas involve injuries to the duodenum as well as to the pancreas. If the injuries to the duodenum and pancreas are simple, the duodenum can be repaired primarily and the pancreas can be drained, or a distal resection can be carried out if the pancreatic injury is in the body or tail. For more complicated, combined injuries, pyloric exclusion can be done to minimize pancreatic stimulation and protect the duodenal repair (see Duodenum, earlier). For massive injuries to the duodenum and head of the pancreas, pancreaticoduodenectomy with reconstruction should be reserved for cases in which débridement of devitalized tissue results in a de facto removal of the duodenum and head of the pancreas. Penetrating injuries to the ampulla of Vater also may require formal pancreaticoduodenectomy.

Internal drainage of the pancreas has been suggested as a means of treating ductal injuries without the need for resection of viable and functional pancreatic tissue. Although in theory this approach preserves pancreatic function and minimizes the risk of postoperative pancreatic insufficiency, it is not without risks. The risk of postoperative pancreatic insufficiency after pancreatic resection is minimal if the remaining pancreas is normal. The pancreaticojejunal anastomosis is prone to break down and leak, especially if suboptimal conditions of associated injury and hemodynamic instability exist. The construction of a Roux-en-Y jejunal limb requires the opening of the intestine and the creation of a small bowel anastomosis. If the intestine has not been injured, this procedure increases the amount of contamination associated with the injury and also increases the likelihood of postoperative morbidity. For these reasons, most major trauma centers rarely carry out internal drainage procedures in the early postinjury period, relying instead on either resection or drainage. Internal drainage is usually reserved for cases in which persistent pancreatic fistulae or pseudocysts develop late (253), and is done on a delayed basis.

Distal pancreatectomy for traumatic injuries should be performed only after the pancreas has been thoroughly mobilized and exposed. In some cases, the pancreas has already been transected, and the site of resection has therefore already been determined for the surgeon. If this is not the case, the pancreas should be transected just proximal to the site of known or presumed ductal injury. If associated splenectomy is planned, elaborate dissection is unnecessary. The splenic artery can be identified near the superior margin of the pancreas and ligated. The splenic vein also can be individually ligated at this point. Commonly, the splenic vein lies behind the body and tail of the pancreas, and its isolation requires more dissection. As an alternative to extensive dissection to isolate the splenic vein behind the pancreas, the vein can be transected along with the pancreatic parenchyma. Individual ligation of the splenic vein stump can be done after the distal pancreas and spleen have been removed.

It is helpful first to mobilize the spleen and tail of the pancreas.

The pancreas should be mobilized at the site of transection and can be encircled with a rubber drain. Mobilization and encirclement are best done by an approach to the pancreas along its inferior margin and mobilization inferiorly to superiorly. The pancreas can be divided either distal to a bowel clamp or with a stapler. There are some indications that a sutured closure is less likely to break down and lead to fistula formation than a stapled closure. If a bowel clamp is used, the pancreatic stump should be oversewn with a running suture. Typically, nonabsorbable suture has been recommended for this purpose, but the type of suture used is probably not of major consequence with respect to the subsequent development of complications. It is also recommended that an individual figure-of-eight suture be placed in the cut end of the pancreatic duct. This proves exceedingly difficult in patients with normal pancreatic ductal systems because the duct is small and not easily identified in the cut edge of the pancreatic stump. A pancreatic duct that can be seen easily may indicate preexisting proximal ductal obstruction. In this case, the duct should be individually ligated. If the cut end of the duct is not immediately apparent, time and effort should not be taken to locate and individually ligate it.

It is possible to perform a distal pancreatectomy without a concomitant splenectomy. Splenic salvage involves individual ligation and division of the branches of the splenic artery and vein that supply the body and tail of the pancreas. This adds to operative time and can increase the risk of bleeding, particularly if there is an associated injury to the spleen treated with splenorrhaphy. Splenic salvage should be attempted, therefore, only in hemodynamically stable patients with minimal or no associated intraabdominal or extraabdominal injuries.

Pancreatic injuries can lead to a number of complications, including pancreatic fistulae, pseudocysts, bleeding in the area of the pancreatic bed, and pancreatitis. Pancreatic fistulae after trauma are characterized by persistent drainage of pancreatic enzymes and secretions from the pancreatic injury for a number of weeks after injury. Most of these fistulae close spontaneously, especially if there is no proximal obstruction of the pancreatic ductal system. A trial of total parenteral nutrition may improve the rate and incidence of spontaneous closure. Experience with the use of somatostatin in patients with posttraumatic pancreatic fistulae is limited. Somatostatin given to patients with pancreatic fistulae after elective pancreatic resections seems to decrease the amount of fistula drainage but has not consistently decreased the time to fistula closure.

Pseudocysts that develop after pancreatic trauma often resolve on their own or with percutaneous aspiration. If, after 4 to 6 weeks of observation with serial ultrasound or CT scans, the pseudocyst does not show signs of resolution, it should be drained internally with a defunctionalized limb of jejunum.

Bleeding in the area of the pancreatic bed is usually an early complication that is caused by inadequate drainage with resultant autodigestion of the pancreas and surrounding tissue. Bleeding can be avoided by identifying all injuries at the time of exploration and ensuring adequate drainage. If massive bleeding does occur, it should be dealt with through operative intervention.

Pancreatitis, another complication of pancreatic injury, is also related to inadequate drainage of pancreatic secretions. Treatment consists of provision of adequate drainage and supportive care. If the pancreatitis is localized to the distal pancreas and a trial of conservative management fails, distal pancreatectomy should be considered.

Blunt Injuries

The major difference between penetrating and blunt injuries of the pancreas concerns diagnosis. Penetrating injuries are usually discovered on abdominal exploration for associated injuries, but blunt injuries may occur in isolation and the preoperative diagnosis can be difficult. Blunt pancreatic injuries are relatively rare, which increases the difficulty of diagnosis. In one series of pancreatic injuries, delays in diagnosis of blunt injuries ranged up to several days. Making the diagnosis as quickly as possible is important because delays in diagnosis are associated with increased morbidity.

The body of the pancreas lies directly anterior to the vertebral column and is vulnerable to crush injuries when the anterior abdominal wall is forcibly compressed, as can occur from a seat belt or a sharp blow to the epigastrium. In such instances, the pancreas may be the only intraabdominal organ injured.

A variety of different means are available to make the diagnosis of blunt pancreatic injury. Physical examination of the abdomen is useful, but because of the retroperitoneal location of the pancreas, the results can be misleadingly benign until a number of hours after injury. This emphasizes the importance of serial examinations. In most cases, the abdomen becomes progressively more tender to palpation during the first 24 to 48 hours after injury and the need for abdominal exploration becomes more obvious. The physical examination of the abdomen is much less reliable in young children and in patients with head injuries.

The serum amylase concentration is elevated on admission in approximately 70% of patients with blunt pancreatic injury. However, elevated serum amylase has a poor positive predictive value and also occurs in many patients without pancreatic injury. The amylase concentration can be elevated because of trauma to other organs, including the salivary glands and the ovaries. In addition, the remaining 30% of patients with normal admission serum amylase concentrations must be considered. Serum lipase concentrations and serial determinations of serum amylase are occasionally helpful in monitoring the courses of patients with normal or only mildly elevated admission values, but reliance on these methods of diagnosis results in delays in diagnosis, and a percentage of diagnoses are missed for a considerable period.

Diagnostic peritoneal lavage and emergency department ultrasound are of little help in the early diagnosis of pancreatic injury unless there have been associated intraperitoneal injuries. The retroperitoneal location of the pancreas results in minimal findings in the lavage fluid, and obtaining amylase concentrations in the lavage fluid is not helpful.

Computed tomography scan of the abdomen allows for visualization of the retroperitoneum, including the pancreas. In the case of isolated injury to the pancreas, the sensitivity of the CT scan is at its lowest shortly after injury. Although it may be a good test for the diagnosis of pancreatic injury after a number of hours have passed, immediate CT scan of the abdomen misses some pancreatic injuries, particularly if expert interpretation is not available.

Finally, ERCP is a means of diagnosing pancreatic injury. ERCP is an attractive diagnostic method because it is less invasive than abdominal exploration and also provides information about the status of the ductal system, but there are several practical disadvantages to the technique. Most of the studies that have reported successful use of ERCP have involved stable patients studied hours to days after injury and sent to a referral center specifically because of suspicion of a pancreatic injury. These patients are a selected group, quite different from patients who are freshly injured. ERCP is not universally available and, even in large centers, is often unavailable at the odd hours necessary for early diagnosis in acutely injured patients. Many endoscopists are fearful of inducing an exacerbation of pancreatitis in patients with mild pancreatic injuries lacking ductal involvement. The logic of using ERCP dictates that in the absence of a ductal injury on the study, the patient should be treated conservatively; worsening of traumatic pancreatitis in some of these patients is an undesirable side effect.

To summarize, the early diagnosis of blunt pancreatic injuries, particularly if they occur in isolation, can be extremely difficult, and no single test allows for an easy and reliable diagnosis. A combination of serial abdominal examinations and serum amylase determinations, CT scan, and ERCP in selected patients is the best diagnostic strategy available. These studies should be combined, with a low threshold for operative intervention if a pancreatic injury is suspected.

Basic principles of exposure and operative management of blunt injuries of the pancreas are the same as for penetrating injuries. In many instances of severe injury, the pancreas already has been transected by the trauma, making the pancreatic resection somewhat simpler to carry out. Isolated injuries of the pancreas from blunt trauma also lend themselves to distal pancreatectomy with splenic preservation. As in penetrating injury, splenic salvage should be attempted only in stable patients without associated splenic rupture or severe associated intraabdominal or extraabdominal injuries. Complications of blunt pancreatic injury are similar to those outlined for penetrating injuries.

Small Intestine

Because the small intestine occupies more volume in the peritoneal cavity than any other organ, it is the intraabdominal viscus most frequently injured by penetrating abdominal trauma. The severity of injury ranges from trivial rents in the bowel serosa or mesentery to massive perforation or devascularization injuries requiring extensive resection.

Diagnosis of small bowel injury can be made by a number of methods. Physical examination of the abdomen reveals peritoneal signs in many patients with penetrating small bowel injuries. Patients with gunshot wounds routinely undergo laparotomy. Routine exploration of all other penetrating anterior abdominal injuries that violate the abdominal wall fascia can be performed. An alternative to this is to use serial abdominal examinations, hematocrits, and leukocyte counts. If the patient shows increasing signs of intraperitoneal injury, abdominal exploration is performed. In stable patients with penetrating injuries to the anterior abdomen, a third approach is DPL. A variety of criteria for positivity in patients who undergo DPL for blunt trauma have been proposed, ranging from 1,000 RBCs/mL of lavage fluid as a threshold for positivity, up to the conventional 100,000 RBCs/mL used in blunt trauma patients. Use of the more stringent criteria naturally decreases the rate of false-negative results for small penetrating injuries to the small intestine and other subtle intraperitoneal injuries, but it does so at the cost of an increased rate of false-positive results.

Regardless of the approach taken for the preoperative diagnosis of penetrating injuries of the small intestine, the operative approach is the same. The abdomen should be explored through a standard upper midline incision, and initial attention should be directed toward bleeding from associated injuries or from the small bowel mesentery. Bleeding from the mesentery usually can be controlled with suture ligation or with a rapid running closure of the mesenteric rent. This closure does not need to constitute definitive repair, but it temporarily controls bleeding until definitive treatment is delineated.

After bleeding has been controlled, steps to prevent ongoing leakage of intestinal contents from the injured small bowel should be taken. This is done by rapid examination of the small intestine and by either application of Babcock or Allis clamps or a temporizing running single-layer closure of the injured areas. After initial control of the leak, the intestine should be examined more carefully. Definitive repair or resection should not be done until the entire length of the intestine has been carefully examined because a thorough knowledge of the extent of injury is necessary for a logical and rational approach to operative management. It makes no sense, for example, to repair a segment of small intestine, only to determine after further exploration that injuries to adjacent segments of the bowel dictate resection of the entire segment.

The entire length of the small intestine should be carefully examined, starting at the ligament of Treitz and moving sequentially, proximally to distally, to each successive loop. This should be done in a systematic manner and should include inspection of the small bowel mesentery by fanning out the mesentery and examining each new loop. If there is a suspect area along the mesenteric border of the intestine, the mesentery should be cleared away to allow for adequate visualization. The small intestine has a good blood supply and easily tolerates this maneuver. Any blood or other debris found on the serosa of the bowel should be wiped away. Sometimes, such debris overlies an otherwise unsuspected area of injury.

In theory, the number of holes found in the small intestine should add up to an even number because there should be an identical number of entrance and exit wounds. This rule is sometimes violated in practice, however, because the intestine is extensively coiled in the peritoneal cavity and tangential wounds of the bowel are common. Rather than focusing on the number of holes in the bowel, attention should be directed to a close inspection of the entire length of the intestine. After all areas of injury have been identified, a decision about repair or resection is made. Areas of massive destruction of the bowel or the mesentery, with associated ischemia, should be treated with resection. If after débridement, more than 40% to 50% of a portion of the wall of the small intestine is missing, that segment also should be resected. Increasing experience with stapled anastomoses in trauma patients has shown them to be a safe and practical alternative to sutured anastomoses. Stapled anastomoses are particularly useful when time is of the essence and should be constructed in a side-to-side, functional end-to-end fashion.

Knife wounds to the small intestine are usually easy to manage and rarely require extensive débridement or resection. On rare occasions, a large rent in the small bowel mesentery results in enough devascularization to require resection of a segment of intestine. Gunshot wounds require more débridement. However, because the small bowel is filled largely with air and is pliable and mobile, it is resistant to the effects of a bullet. Débridement of gunshot wounds does not need to be done beyond obviously devitalized areas, regardless of the type of gun used and the velocity of the bullet.

Minor mesenteric lacerations should be treated with suture ligation of bleeding points and closure of the rent. Major lacerations with devascularization should be treated with resection and primary anastomosis. Small bowel anastomoses, if properly done and after adequate débridement of devitalized tissue, have an excellent rate of healing even with severe associated injuries, shock, and peritonitis.

Shotgun wounds to the abdomen from close range are often associated with massive tissue destruction and should be treated in a manner similar to that described previously. At medium or long range, they sometimes result in a diffuse pattern of shot injury, creating multiple small perforations of the small intestine. In such instances, the general principles outlined previously should be followed and obvious areas of injury repaired. It is sometimes impossible to ensure closure of all the numerous areas of perforation. In such cases, obvious areas of injury should be closed; smaller areas of perforation often do not require surgical closure because they rarely leak and are of minimal consequence.

On rare occasions, injuries to the small intestine occur in patients who are hemodynamically unstable as a result of associated injuries. In such instances, the small intestine can be treated most expeditiously by application of the gastrointestinal anastomosis stapler as necessary to remove the injured areas of bowel. If a second operation is planned because of associated injuries, definitive anastomosis can be deferred and the stapled ends of the intestine simply returned to the abdomen until the second procedure is performed.

Blunt injuries to the small intestine are much less common than penetrating injuries. As with other blunt intraabdominal injuries, they are more difficult to diagnose because the need for urgent intraabdominal intervention is not always obvious. Blunt perforations and devascularizations of the small intestine often occur in isolation, either as the only injury or as the only intraabdominal injury present. This makes early diagnosis even more difficult (254).

Seat belts have been implicated in the pathogenesis of blunt injuries of the small intestine. The intestine is compressed between the seat belt and the vertebral column and can be distended to the point of rupture or torn violently on its mesentery, resulting in either perforation or devascularization. Because of the severe degree of force necessary to produce a blunt intestinal injury, there is a frequent association with transverse fractures of a lumbar vertebral body (Chance fracture).

Diagnosis is made primarily by physical examination of the abdomen. Abdominal examination is usually positive shortly after injury, but initial findings in some cases can be subtle, resulting in delays in diagnosis. If head injury or intoxication makes physical examination of the abdomen unreliable, DPL should be performed. The false-negative rate of DPL for this injury is 5%. CT and ultrasound, particularly if done early after injury, are not reliable in ruling out blunt intestinal injury. The injury itself may not be obvious, and small amounts of intraperitoneal fluid from the injury may not be detectable.

Blunt injuries to the small intestine are most common in either the proximal jejunum or the distal ileum, probably because the intestine is fixed at these two points and more vulnerable to compression and stretch injuries. Multiple injuries to the small intestine from blunt trauma occur in approximately 25% of cases. Second or even third areas of injury should be carefully sought if a blunt intestinal injury is discovered on abdominal exploration.

After the suspicion of blunt intestinal or other intraabdominal injury has been raised and the decision to explore the abdomen has been made, the basic principles of abdominal exploration and operative management of blunt small bowel injuries are the same as for penetrating injuries. Because of the nature of the mechanism of injury, the perforations are usually amenable to primary repair. Mesenteric rents that cause devascularization and require

resection are relatively more common after blunt injury than after penetrating injury.

Colon and Rectum

Most injuries to the colon and rectum are the result of penetrating or perforating trauma. Blunt trauma accounts for only approximately 5% of colonic injuries. Rectal injuries can occur in association with pelvic fractures, and the possibility of rectal injury must be considered in any patient with a significant pelvic fracture in addition to evaluation of other pelvic viscera such as the bladder, distal ureters, uterus, and vagina.

Signs and symptoms of peritonitis result from injury to the colon and rectum but are not specific. Injury to the extraperitoneal rectum is particularly difficult to recognize because peritonitis does not result. Conventional laboratory studies usually are not helpful. Plain radiographs may show free air in the peritoneal cavity, but this finding is relatively uncommon; when it is not present, the patient cannot be assumed to be free of bowel perforation. DPL may be of value if intraperitoneal colonic injury is present, yielding lavage fluid with blood, bacteria, or fecal material. If the injury is confined to the extraperitoneal colon and rectum, however, DPL is of no value. Extraperitoneal colonic or rectal injury is extremely difficult to diagnose. The possibility of rectal injury must be considered in any patient with penetrating trauma to the lower abdomen or buttocks. Digital examination is essential. The presence of blood on examination is strong evidence for colon or rectal injury, and proctoscopic and sigmoidoscopic examinations should be performed. Water-soluble contrast studies also may be useful, but direct bowel examination usually is preferable. Approximately 95% of colon injuries are caused by gunshot, shotgun, or stab wounds, and, whenever the possibility of colonic injury is entertained, broadspectrum intravenous prophylactic antibiotics should be started immediately. The number of doses continued after surgery is determined by the degree of colon injury, but it is prudent to treat most patients for 7 to 10 days, as for established peritonitis.

The central issue in the operative management of colonic injuries is the controversy between primary repair of low-risk colonic injuries and repair or resection with exteriorization (255). Primary repair may be selected after additional risk factors have been excluded. Complications increase with primary repair in the presence of preoperative hypotension, intraperitoneal hemorrhage exceeding 1 L, more than two additional injured organs (hepatic, pancreatic, and splenic injuries have the highest morbidity rates), significant fecal spillage, or an elapsed time since injury of more than 6 hours. Many patients with low-risk penetrating colon can be treated with primary closure in the absence of these risk factors. High-risk colonic injuries or those associated with severe injuries, as indicated previously, should be treated with resection and colostomy. This is a relatively conservative approach, and recent series indicate that primary repair may be safe even in the presence of some of the circumstances listed. When resection is necessary, primary anastomosis usually is not advised. The colon is unprepared in this setting and experience with primary anastomosis after trauma is not yet sufficient to allow its recommendation.

A compromise between colostomy and primary repair has been advocated, with exteriorization of the repaired segment. The success of this technique is low, and it probably has little benefit over diverting colostomy alone. Postoperative complications include abscess formation, anastomotic leak, peristomal hernia, and the morbidity and mortality associated with colostomy closure.

The morbidity and mortality from rectal injuries is primarily a result of inadequate initial therapy and the complications associated with delayed sepsis. Rectal injury must be suspected if there is any penetrating injury or if there is a sacral fracture that produces a pelvic ring disruption. Sigmoidoscopic examination is essential.

The principles of operative management include the following:

- Placement of the patient in the lithotomy position to provide simultaneous exposure of both the perineum and abdomen.
- Wide débridement of all dead and devitalized tissue.
- A totally defunctioning colostomy (simple loop colostomy may be inadequate).
- Rectal wall closure, if the injury is easily accessible from a peritoneal approach.
- Retrorectal drainage only in highly selected severe injuries, with coccygectomy, if necessary, to attain adequate rectal drainage.
- Distal rectal stump washout.
- Broad-spectrum intravenous antibiotics, nutritional support, and serial débridement.

Complete rectal destruction is a rare injury for which primary abdominoperineal resection with packing may be necessary. If done, the packing should be removed operatively in approximately 48 hours. Complications of rectal injuries include pelvic abscesses, urinary or rectal fistulae, rectal incontinence and stricture, urinary incontinence, and loss of sexual function.

Retroperitoneal Hematoma

The optimal management of retroperitoneal hematoma depends on a number of factors, including its cause, its location, and the presence of associated injuries.

The retroperitoneum can be divided into anatomic zones for purposes of decision making (Fig. 11.54). Central retroperitoneal hematomas (zone 1) are associated with pancreaticoduodenal injuries or major abdominal vascular injury. Flank or perinephric hematomas (zone 2) may be associated with injuries to the genitourinary tract or, in the case of penetrating trauma, with injuries to the colon. Zone 3 injuries, which are confined to or originate from the pelvis, are most often associated with pelvic fractures.

Retroperitoneal hematomas in zone 1, regardless of cause or size, are formally explored with inspection of each of the relevant structures. This is required because of the high incidence of associated major vascular, pancreatic, or duodenal injuries and the high morbidity and mortality rates if these are overlooked.

Zone 2 hematomas caused by penetrating injuries should be routinely explored. Whether proximal control of the renal pedicle should be obtained before exploration of a perinephric hematoma is controversial. If there is severe ongoing hemorrhage, time should not be taken to obtain proximal control, and the kidney should be mobilized directly. If time and the degree of hemorrhage permit, however, it is acceptable to obtain vascular control before mobilization of the kidney. Zone 2 hematomas caused by blunt trauma can be left alone if they are not expanding and the intravenous urogram is normal.

Zone 3 retroperitoneal hematomas in patients with penetrating injuries should be explored to exclude major vascular injuries. Local bleeding encountered at exploration under these circumstances usually is easy to control, and the associated injuries can be identified. Patients with zone 3 hematomas secondary to blunt trauma usually have associated pelvic fractures. Exploration of the hematoma can be hazardous and is usually avoided. There is often

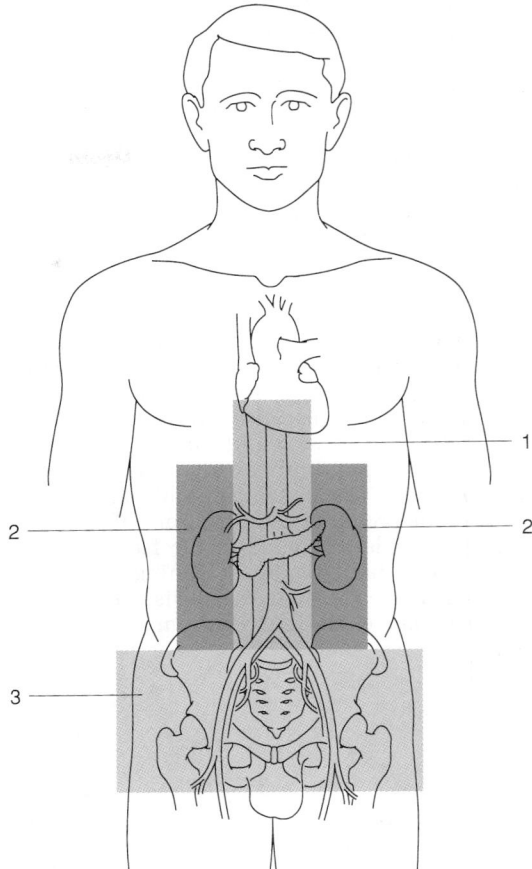

Figure 11.54. Zones of the retroperitoneum.

extensive injury to the rich presacral venous and arterial circulation. Incision of the peritoneum releases the tamponade, and dissection within the hematoma can produce catastrophic bleeding. Discrete bleeding points rarely can be identified. Exploration of these hematomas is associated with an increased requirement for transfusion and a higher mortality rate.

Definitive Care Phase: Retroperitoneal Injuries

ROBERT C. MACKERSIE

The process of identifying and controlling sources of major hemorrhage after injury is of primary importance early in the resuscitation of multiply injured patients. This should be undertaken as a logical, stepwise process that includes evaluation of external, thoracic, abdominal, retroperitoneal, and fracture sites of hemorrhage. The initial diagnoses of fracture site hemorrhage and external hemorrhage usually can be made on the basis of the physical examination. The diagnoses of thoracic and abdominal hemorrhage are reliably made using chest radiography and diagnostic peritoneal lavage (DPL), abdominal ultrasound, or abdominal computed tomography (CT), as discussed earlier in this chapter. The diagnosis of retroperitoneal hemorrhage, however, cannot be made reliably with DPL, plain radiographs, or abdominal ultrasound, and requires a separate set of screening and diagnostic studies. Two of the most common causes of major hemorrhage in the retroperitoneum after blunt trauma are pelvic fractures and injuries to the kidney. With appropriate screening and evaluation performed early in the resuscitation, timely therapeutic intervention can be instituted, resulting in decreased morbidity and mortality rates.

PELVIC FRACTURES

Most pelvic fractures occur as a result of high-energy blunt trauma, such as occurs in motor vehicle crashes or falls. The spectrum of pelvic fracture injuries ranges from minor, isolated, nondisplaced fractures of the pubic rami to severe crush injuries with multiple fractures that can be rapidly lethal. The proximity of adjacent organs results in a high incidence of associated genitourinary and abdominal injuries. The potential complications of pelvic fracture injury may be underestimated in the face of other, more obvious injuries. Radiographic screening, early control of associated hemorrhage, and diagnosis and treatment of other injuries are essential to minimize morbidity and mortality.

Unlike most long-bone fractures, only approximately 25% of pelvic fractures are apparent on the basis of physical examination. The practice of forced bimanual manipulation of the iliac crests to elicit pelvic instability is to be condemned because it is neither a sensitive nor specific finding. The so-called pelvic rock test is also painful at best and may exacerbate hemorrhage with more severe fractures. Screening radiographs of the pelvis, although not universally required in examinable patients, should be obtained on most patients with a major mechanism whose examination is at all impaired, and on all blunt trauma patients with hypotension or other evidence of shock.

A number of classification schemes have been proposed for pelvic fractures (256–258). One of the simpler schemes is shown in Fig. 11.55. Pelvic fractures are divided into fractures that are comminuted and unstable (type 1); fractures involving two separate breaks in the pelvic ring, which are also unstable (type 2); and stable fractures involving either single breaks in the ring or fractures of the pubic rami or iliac crest (type 3) (259). As a general rule, anterior arch fractures are more commonly associated with injury to the urethra in male patients or to the bladder, whereas posterior arch fractures are more commonly associated with major hemorrhage. Although an approximate relationship exists between the number of breaks in the pelvic ring and the blood transfusion requirement, the

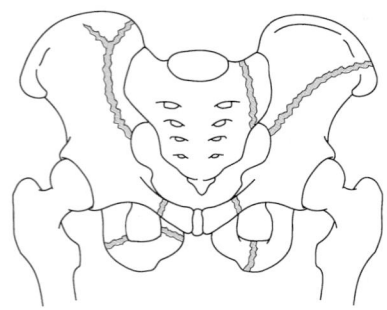

Type I: Unstable (crush)
Mortality: 20%–30%
Blood loss: >10 units
Complications: 60%–75%

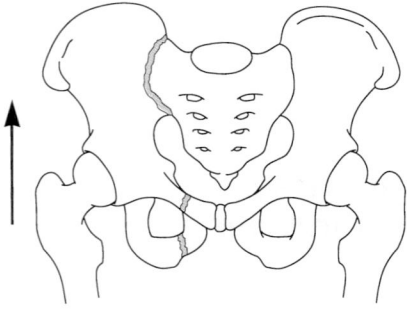

Type II: Unstable
Mortality: 8%–12%
Blood loss: 2–10 units
Complications: 30%–50%

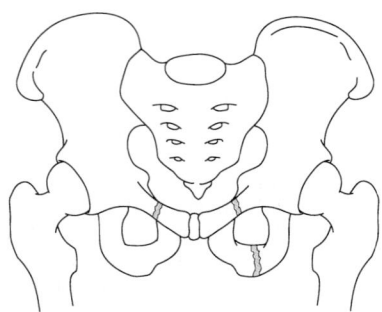

Type III: Stable
Mortality: <5%
Blood loss: 1–4 units
Complications: 10%–20%

Figure 11.55. Classification of pelvic fractures with relative stability.

precision with which the pelvic radiograph alone can predict massive transfusions is limited. This is particularly true of complex, crush-type injuries.

Hemorrhage resulting from injury to the sacral venous plexus, laceration of multiple arterial branches of the hypogastric vessels, or fractured cancellous bone presents a formidable challenge to the trauma surgeon. Massive hemorrhage is the principal cause of early death in patients with pelvic fracture, and survival depends primarily on rapid identification and control. The presence of hemorrhage from associated intraperitoneal injuries should be considered first. The presence of a major pelvic fracture, independent of other injuries, increases the probability of a significant intraabdominal injury by approximately 10%. For this reason, an objective evaluation of the abdomen (DPL, CT, ultrasound) is indicated for most patients with pelvic fractures. Hypotensive patients should undergo a supraumbilical lavage as soon as possible. This method is preferable because of the possibility of catheter penetration of a large retroperitoneal hematoma dissecting into the preperitoneal space. DPL performed incorrectly in the infraumbilical site with a major pelvic fracture can yield an incidence of false-positive results as high as 45% (Fig. 11.56). If DPL is performed soon after injury using proper position and technique, however, the incidence of false-positive results caused by pelvic fracture hemorrhage may be as low as 1% (260).

Grossly positive findings on DPL should prompt an expeditious exploratory laparotomy because more than 90% of these patients have significant intraabdominal injuries. Patients with major pelvic fractures whose DPL results are positive only by cell count criteria have a lower incidence of major intraabdominal injuries, and primary control of pelvic fracture hemorrhage may be considered first in these patients (261).

At laparotomy, after a thorough abdominal exploration has been performed and injuries repaired, the size of the pelvic hematoma can be assessed. Exploration of retroperitoneal pelvic fracture hematomas is contraindicated under almost all circumstances. Pelvic fracture hemorrhage rarely can be controlled surgically, and decompression of the hematoma can further exacerbate bleeding. Ligation of the internal iliac arteries is ineffective in controlling bleeding because of the rich collateral blood supply and frequency of venous bleeding. Rarely, actual disruption of the iliac vessels requires operative control. For rapidly expanding pelvic hematomas, placement of laparotomy packs in the pelvis to aid tamponade can provide effective temporary control. Rapid closure of the abdominal wound under these circumstances should be followed immediately by pelvic angiography and embolization of active arterial bleeding. Patients with large pelvic fracture hematomas should be observed carefully for the development of intraabdominal compartment syndrome, discussed elsewhere in this chapter.

In patients with negative DPL results and evidence of major pelvic fracture hemorrhage, three modalities are available to help reduce blood loss: application of external counterpressure for venous tamponade, arteriography and embolization of arterial pelvic bleeding sites, and placement of an external pelvic fixator (262).

The early identification of patients requiring specific pelvic fracture hemorrhage control is essential in reducing transfusion requirements and morbidity and mortality. The combination of hemodynamic status and fluid and blood requirements during the first 30 to 45 minutes of resuscitation identifies patients who require immediate arteriography and embolization. As a general rule, adults requiring more than 2 to 3 units of blood in the first hour attributable to pelvic fracture hemorrhage benefit from some form of specific hemorrhage control. In patients who are eligible for pelvic and abdominal CT scan (those without clinical evidence of shock), dynamic CT scan of the pelvis, particularly with newer helical CT scanners, can discern even less severe active pelvic fracture arterial bleeding with good sensitivity. Patients with evidence of active CT contrast extravasation or a large, inhomogeneous fracture hematoma suggesting major recent hemor-

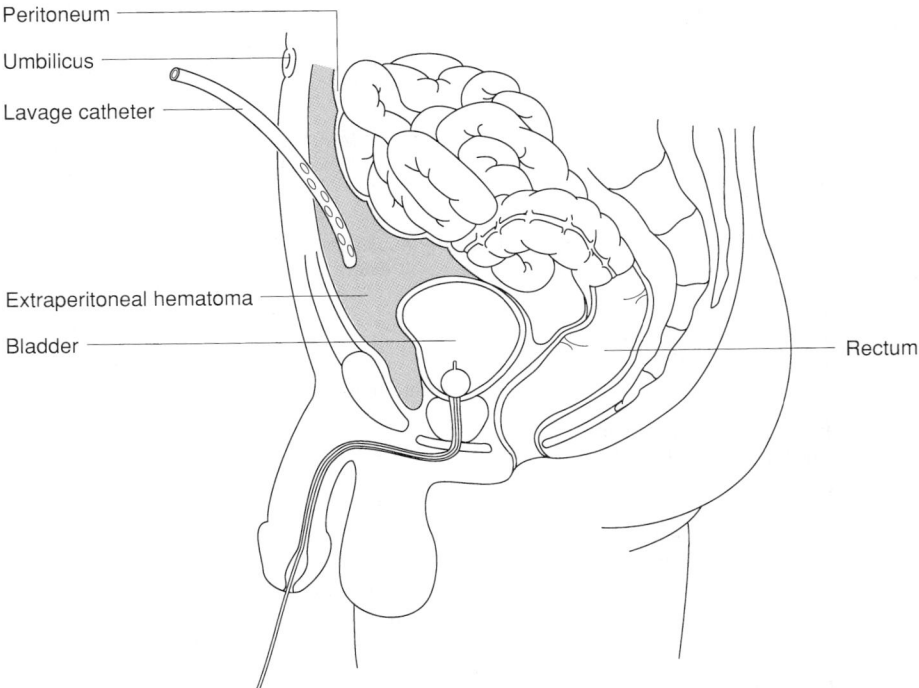

Peritoneum

Umbilicus

Lavage catheter

Extraperitoneal hematoma

Bladder

Rectum

Figure 11.56. Peritoneal lavage performed through the infraumbilical site with pelvic fracture can be complicated by placement of the catheter into the extraperitoneal hematoma. Supraumbilical lavage is therefore indicated in the presence of a pelvic fracture.

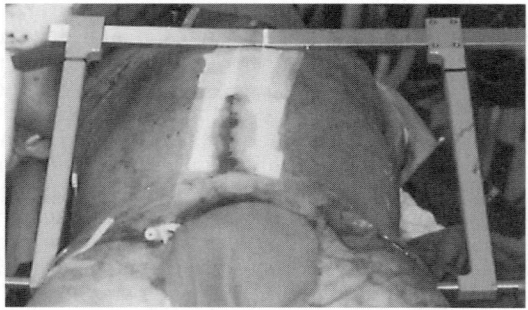

Figure 11.57. C-clamp external fixator allows rapid application of posterior fixation. External pelvic fixation should precede arteriography only if it is immediately available. PASG, pneumatic antishock garment.

rhage also should be strongly considered for arteriography and embolization.

The application of external counterpressure (i.e., the pneumatic or military antishock garment) has been shown in several adult series to be effective in lowering transfusion requirements, presumably by producing tamponade of venous hemorrhage. Because of its inability definitively to control arterial hemorrhage and its adverse effects on ventilation and lower extremity perfusion, this type of garment should be used only for the short-term stabilization of patients with more profound shock as a bridge to embolization or pelvic external fixation. The role in children is even more limited because of limitations inherent in obtaining a proper fit of the garment.

Definitive control of major arterial pelvic fracture bleeding is best accomplished by pelvic arteriography. Internal iliac arteriography with selective embolization of bleeding branches is associated with minimal morbidity and results in complete control of arterial bleeding in more than 85% of patients (263,264).

In selected patients with unstable fractures involving the sacrum or pubic diastasis injuries, the application of pelvic external fixation can further reduce hemorrhage from cancellous bone and the sacral venous plexus. More recently, the use of the C-clamp fixator has decreased application time and may reduce posterior fracture hemorrhage in patients with associated ligamentous disruption (Fig. 11.57). The ease of placement and the rotational mobility of the clamp arm allow immediate placement without interference with subsequent arteriographic embolization for combined treatment of severe pelvic fracture hemorrhage.

In many patients, particularly those with unstable (type 1) injuries, both embolization for arterial hemorrhage control and pelvic fixation for venous tamponade and control of bone bleeding are required for optimal early control of hemorrhage. The precise sequence of these interventions varies according to institutional resources, depending on the relative availability and time requirements for both arteriography and pelvic fixation, which vary considerably from institution to institution. Many centers have developed institutional protocols for pelvic fracture management that take these variables into account. One such algorithm is shown in Fig. 11.58.

After control of pelvic fracture hemorrhage has been achieved, pelvic fracture management may require orthopedic stabilization of the fracture sites. In patients with open

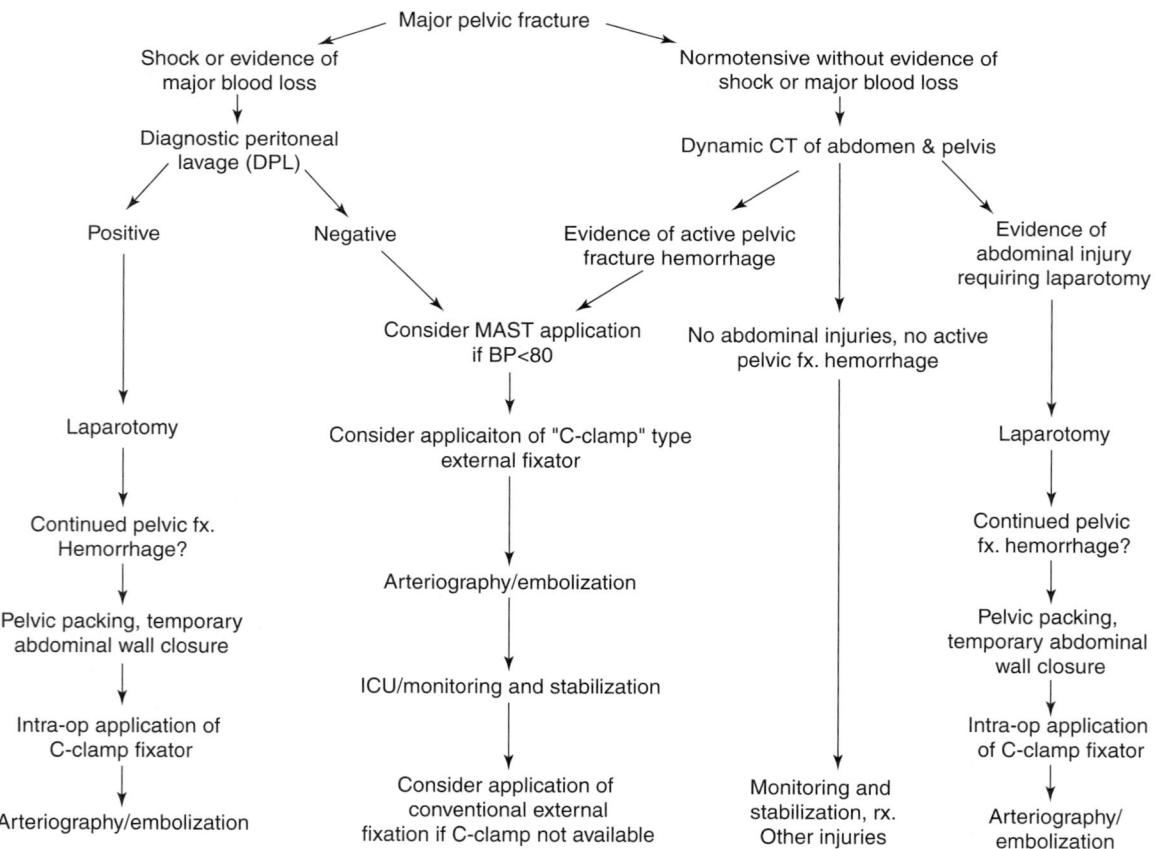

Figure 11.58. Algorithm for the initial management of abdominal and pelvic hemorrhage.

pelvic fractures involving rectal or extensive perineal (perirectal) injuries, fecal contamination and secondary infection of the fracture site and surrounding hematoma result in a high incidence of sepsis and septic mortality unless the fecal stream is diverted. Complete proximal fecal division (no loop colostomies) has been shown to reduce the mortality rate by approximately 50% in patients with these injuries. The performance of a diverting colostomy should be undertaken only after definitive control of pelvic fracture hemorrhage has been obtained and the patient has been fully resuscitated from a metabolic standpoint, including correction of hypothermia, coagulopathy, and acidosis.

RENAL INJURIES

Renal injuries constitute the greatest proportion of genitourinary tract injuries. The kidneys are relatively well protected from blunt injury in adults, but less so in children. Mild contusions manifested clinically by hematuria are common, occurring in 6% to 15% of patients with major blunt trauma. The critical decisions with respect to renal trauma involve the need for and extent of radiologic evaluation, and the indications, based on clinical or radiographic findings, for operative intervention.

The presence of hematuria remains the most sensitive clinical indicator of renal trauma. The specificity of hematuria is low, however, and the practice of performing intravenous pyelography (IVP) on all patients with blunt trauma and microscopic hematuria is both time consuming and unnecessary. Although many patients sustaining blunt trauma have microscopic hematuria, in most cases it results from clinically insignificant renal contusions. In studies examining clinical features associated with significant renal trauma, three factors have been identified: shock, gross hematuria, and major associated injuries (i.e., pelvic fractures, spinal or other abdominal injuries). The incidence of renal trauma requiring operation in the absence of these factors was zero in several combined series. Although major renal injuries can occur in patients without shock or gross hematuria, the incidence is less than 1%, and this fact has prompted some investigators to suggest that specific radiographic evaluation is unnecessary in the absence of one of these two findings.

The indications for radiographic assessment of renal injury in the face of penetrating trauma should be far more liberal because there are conflicting reports on the degree of correlation between the injury severity and the degree of hematuria (265). Penetrating renal injuries can occasionally present without any hematuria whatsoever. For this reason, renal imaging should be considered in all patients with stab wounds and selected gunshot wounds to the flank or upper abdomen if the clinical status allows time to complete the study, recognizing that most patients with gunshot wounds go directly to the operating room.

Radiographic options for the diagnosis of renal trauma include single- or multiple-film IVP, formal nephrotomography, and CT scan. Because of the insensitivity of IVP for both blunt and penetrating renal injuries, and the excellent specificity and sensitivity of CT, the use of IVP should be confined to the occasional intraoperative study, as indicated by clinical findings at general laparotomy (266). Even the single-film ("one-shot") IVP, which has been used extensively in the past as a means for documenting the presence of two functioning kidneys, probably has little place in most resuscitations, and there is little evidence to suggest that it affects clinical decision making, particularly given the option of intraoperative IVP (267). Patients needing immediate operative exploration should not be delayed by the performance of a one-shot IVP. Patients whose clinical condition allows additional diagnostic studies and who, on the basis of proximity (penetrating) or hematuria (for blunt trauma, as previously discussed), need renal imaging, should undergo CT scan as the procedure of choice. Renal arteriography, which is highly sensitive and specific for vascular injuries, is infrequently required because renal CT provides sufficient information to allow exploration and repair of renal vascular injuries.

The decision to perform renal exploration as an independent procedure should be based on both radiographic and clinical evaluation. CT allows more precise assessment of the degree of perinephric hemorrhage and the degree of collecting system disruption than operative inspection (268) (Figs. 11.59 and 11.60). Most blunt renal injuries diagnosed with preoperative CT scan are contusions and minor lacerations, and can be treated nonoperatively with close monitoring and follow-up CT scan. Renal

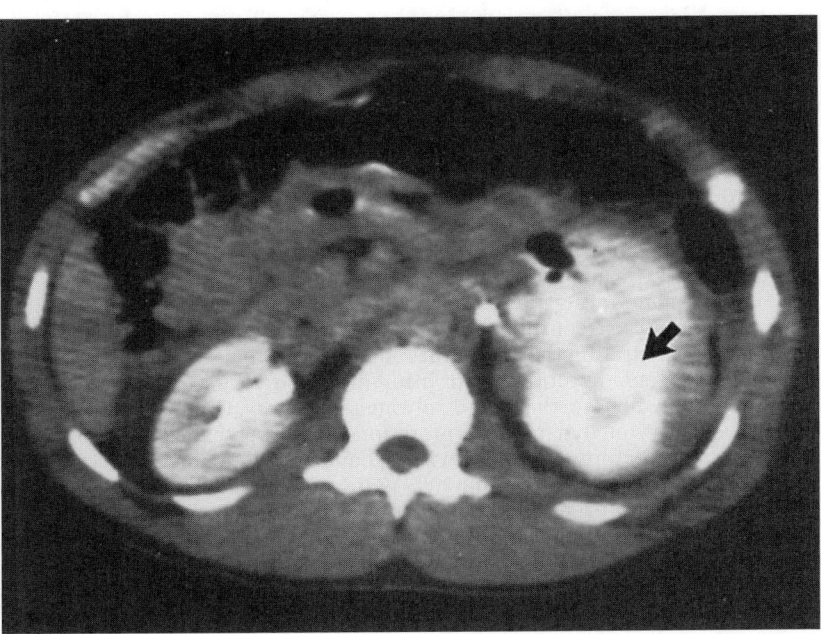

Figure 11.59. Ruptured kidney *(arrow)* requiring operation for intractable pain and continued hemorrhage.

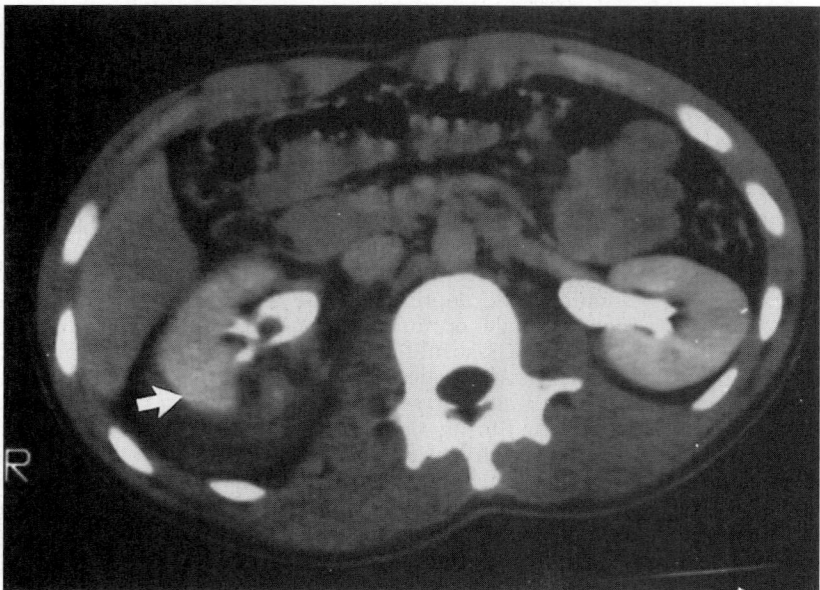

Figure 11.60. Ruptured kidney *(arrow)* treated nonoperatively.

parenchymal injuries and even minor lacerations of the collecting system caused by blunt trauma usually heal without complications. Patients with clinical evidence of ongoing hemorrhage, larger or expanding perinephric hematomas, major collecting system disruptions, or persistent hemorrhage into the collecting system usually benefit from early operation.

Penetrating injuries, particularly gunshot wounds, routinely require exploratory laparotomy because of the high incidence of associated intraabdominal injuries and the likelihood of complex renal injury. The overall incidence of renal injuries in penetrating torso trauma is 6% to 8%. Stab wounds occasionally produce only minor, isolated renal lacerations, without hilar or collecting system involvement, and minimal hematomas. Selected patients have been successfully treated nonoperatively with close clinical examination and follow-up (269).

A number of major renal injuries are diagnosed at the time of initial laparotomy, often in hemodynamically unstable patients. Most commonly, a perinephric hematoma is encountered in association with blunt hepatic or splenic injuries. Indications for renal exploration at laparotomy after blunt trauma include an expanding or pulsatile perinephric hematoma and suspected renal vascular injury. In patients with blunt injuries, it is preferable to defer exploration of nonexpanding, nonpulsatile perinephric hematomas until treatment of intraabdominal and other associated life-threatening injuries is completed. Postoperative CT scan can be performed for formal staging of these injuries. In many instances, injuries can be better defined and treated nonoperatively. Perinephric hematomas found during laparotomy for penetrating trauma should be explored carefully. Continued or recurrent hemorrhage is more often a problem in penetrating than in blunt renal injuries.

The goal of renal exploration for blunt or penetrating injury is to control hemorrhage and salvage the kidney. Contrary to the notion that renal exploration often creates a need for nephrectomy, recent reviews have reported an overall salvage rate approaching 90% (270).

The operative approach to renal trauma should include proximal control of both the renal artery and renal vein. After control of the renal hilum is obtained, the kidney can be explored by mobilization of either the right or left colon centrally and dissection through the Gerota fascia, with elevation of the kidney from the retroperitoneum. Although initial proximal renal vascular control can potentially result in a lower overall nephrectomy rate, it may not be appropriate in patients who are hemodynamically compromised as a result of their renal injury. Under these circumstances, rapid mobilization of the kidney with digital control of the hilum is necessary to stem what can be exsanguinating hemorrhage. Many of these patients ultimately require nephrectomy.

The specific operative approach depends on the injury. The general objectives are to control hemorrhage, repair any injury to the collecting system, and revascularize or remove nonperfused renal tissue. Options include simple suture repair of lacerations with or without pedicle flap coverage, partial nephrectomy with oversewing of vessels and repair of the collecting system, and total nephrectomy. Although some enthusiasm exists for revascularization of arterial injuries involving intimal tears and complete occlusion of the renal artery, this is rarely successful in patients with blunt trauma. To be successful, repair should be performed within 6 to 8 hours of injury.

Postoperative complications from renal trauma include recurrent or ongoing hemorrhage, arteriovenous fistula, and urinary extravasation with fistula or urinoma. Late hypertension also may occur in a small number of patients as a result of either central renal vascular injuries or severely injured kidneys treated nonoperatively. The outcome of complications from renal trauma depends on the extent and timeliness of postinjury evaluation.

BLADDER INJURIES

Injury to the urinary bladder, because of its relatively protected position, is often associated with other serious injuries. Diagnostic methods are straightforward and effective and should be undertaken in every patient with suspected bladder injury. Outcome is directly related to early diagnosis and treatment.

Most blunt bladder injuries (>95% in some series) occur in association with pelvic fractures. The most common mechanism is laceration of the extraperitoneal bladder. Severe deceleration can also result in a bursting rupture at the dome of the bladder. Penetrating injuries to the bladder may occur in isolation but are more commonly associ-

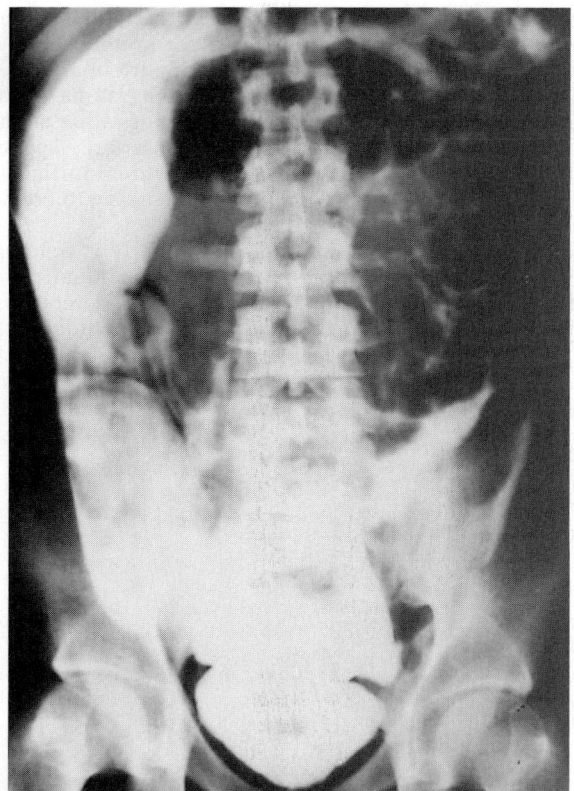

Figure 11.61. Intraperitoneal rupture of the bladder as demonstrated on cystogram.

ated with other intraabdominal injuries. The absence of peritoneal signs on physical examination is not a reliable means of excluding bladder rupture, because intraperitoneal rupture occurs less frequently, and urine, if present in the peritoneum, produces little inflammatory reaction. The classic diagnostic method of choice for suspected rupture of the urinary bladder is a static cystogram followed by a postvoid film. More recently, CT cystography has begun to replace conventional cystography in some centers. Cystography should be performed in any patient with visible blood in the urine in association with a pelvic fracture. Static cystography can be conducted easily in the trauma resuscitation area and involves the placement of a

urinary catheter and the performance of low-volume contrast (100 to 150 mL), high-volume contrast (350 to 400 mL), and postvoid radiographs.

Prior experience with CT in the diagnosis of bladder injuries suggested that injuries may be missed using this technique. More recent experience with higher-resolution scanners and deliberate contrast distention of the bladder (typically with retrograde filling of the bladder) suggests results comparable with those obtained by conventional static cystography. The variation in reported results may be a function of the technical conduct of the CT study (with and without active retrograde contrast filling of the bladder) (271,272).

Urethral injury in men is frequently associated with bladder rupture, and all male patients should be carefully examined for the presence of scrotal or urethral hematoma, free-floating prostate, or blood at the meatus. Retrograde urethrography should be performed before placement of urinary catheters in these patients.

Bladder ruptures are classified into those that rupture freely into the peritoneal cavity (Fig. 11.61) and those with extravasation limited to the retroperitoneum (Fig. 11.62). Intraperitoneal bladder ruptures, often involving burst injuries of the dome, are characteristically large injuries, and they require early operative repair. Occasionally, this form of bladder rupture is discovered at the time of laparotomy for other immediately life-threatening problems. Bladder repair is accomplished by a layered closure using absorbable sutures. Although many urologists prefer to place a suprapubic cystostomy tube at the time of bladder repair, patients also can be managed with simple urethral catheter drainage alone.

In the past, extraperitoneal bladder ruptures were treated primarily by operative repair. It has since become evident that most extraperitoneal bladder injuries can be treated nonoperatively by urethral catheter drainage alone (273). This method obviates bladder exploration with manipulation of the extraperitoneal hematoma. The early and late complications after nonoperative management of extraperitoneal bladder injuries are minimal. Follow-up cystography, performed after approximately 10 days, demonstrates healing of the bladder injury in approximately 85% of patients (274). Occasionally, a patient requires prolonged catheter drainage, and consideration should be given to performing a suprapubic cystostomy under these circumstances. With this management regimen, even large extraperitoneal bladder injuries heal without the need for operative repair.

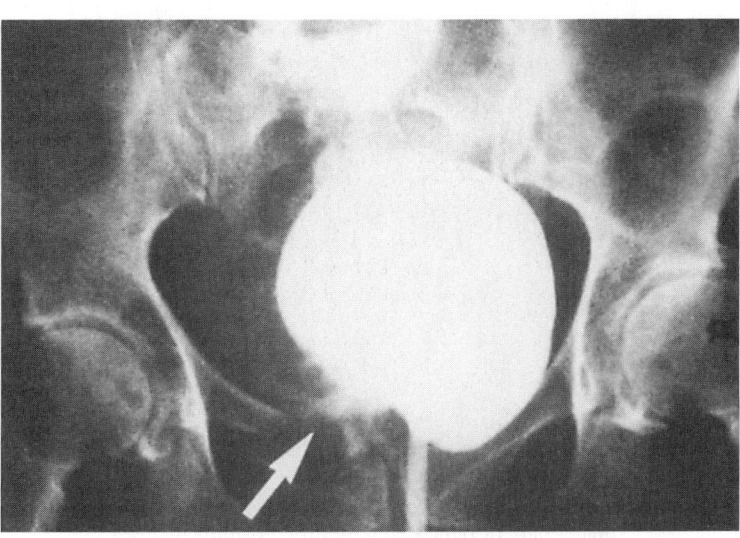

Figure 11.62. Cystogram demonstrating contained retroperitoneal bladder rupture.

Most complications of bladder rupture involve delay or error in diagnosis. Contamination of the large pelvic hematoma with infected urine is reported rarely. Patients with extraperitoneal bladder rupture usually should be given antibiotics for the duration of urinary catheter placement.

URETERAL INJURIES

Ureteral injuries occur less frequently than injuries to either the bladder or the kidney. They are most often caused by gunshot wounds and stab wounds but in rare cases are secondary to blunt external trauma. Because iso-

lated ureteral injuries can present without even microscopic hematuria, a vigorous search for ureteral injury is required for any patient with penetrating trauma.

The diagnosis of a ureteral injury after trauma usually can be made on the basis of an IVP showing either a cutoff in ureteral drainage or contrast extravasation. Approximately 15% of ureteral injuries are not evident initially on IVP, and retrograde ureterography is necessary to confirm the diagnosis.

The luxury of preoperative IVP frequently is not available in patients with life-threatening intraabdominal injuries who require immediate laparotomy. Ureteral injuries under these circumstances must be excluded at the

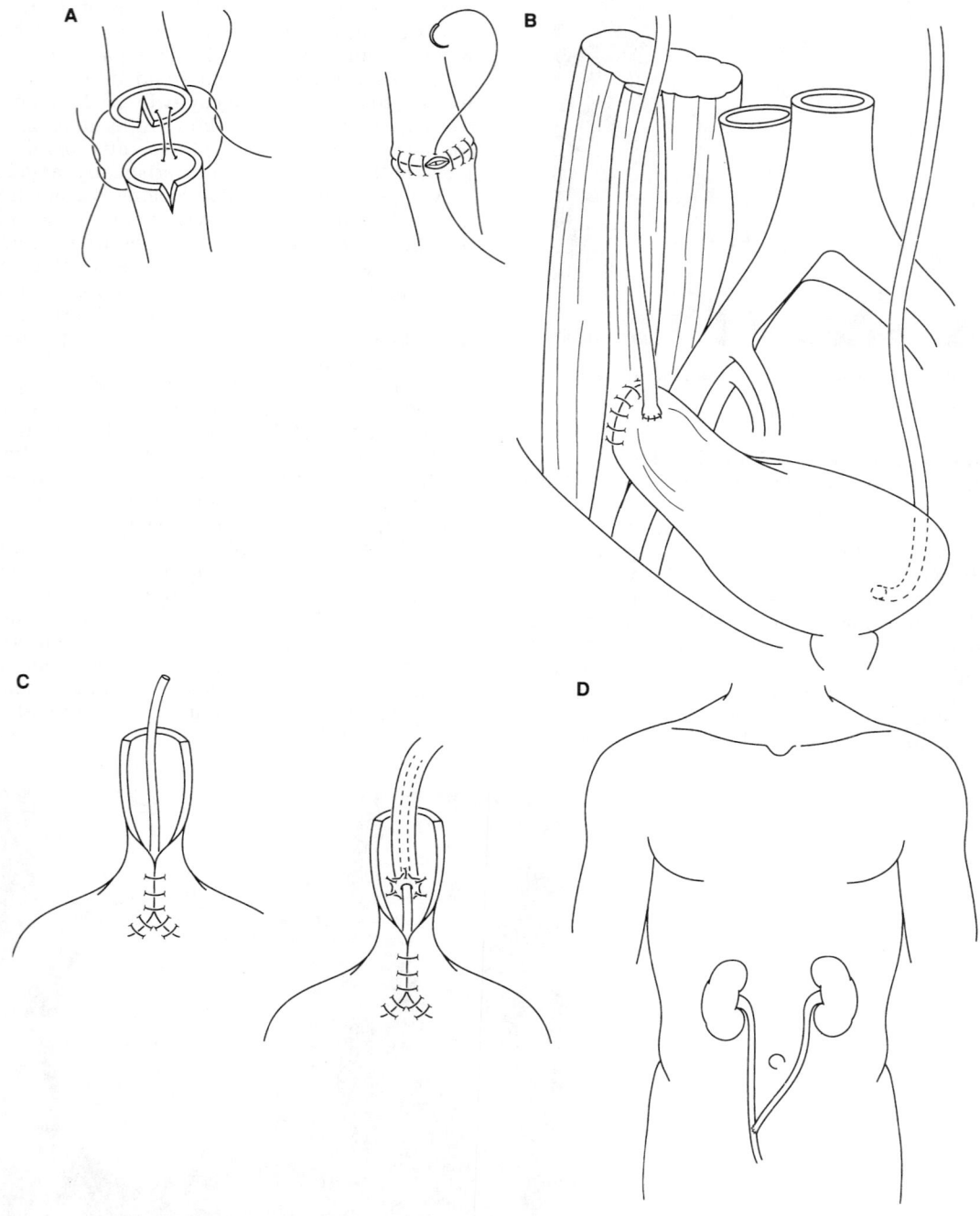

Figure 11.63. Options for repair of the ureter: *(A)* primary ureteroureterostomy; *(B)* psoas hitch; *(C)* (Boari) flap; or *(D)* transureteroureterostomy.

time of surgery. In most cases, exploration of the bullet or stab wound tract is sufficient to exclude or confirm ureteral injury. With massive retroperitoneal hematomas or the presence of multiple penetrating injuries, direct inspection of the entire ureter is not feasible, and extensive dissection should be avoided because of the danger of devascularization. Under these circumstances, an intraoperative IVP can be performed. An alternative is intraoperative chromopyelography using intravenous methylene blue to color the urine and better delineate any extravasation.

Treatment of ureteral injuries is best performed at the time of initial exploration. Specific treatment depends primarily on the location and extent of injury. In most cases with penetrating trauma, short segments of ureter are involved, and there is little if any loss of length. Under these circumstances, primary ureteroureterostomy with stenting or reimplantation of the distal ureter into the bladder is the preferred technique (Fig. 11.63A). For ureteral injuries involving long segment loss, such as those that occur with shotgun injuries, the problem is more complex. Lower ureteral injuries can be repaired by reimplantation of the distal ureter into the bladder, combined with either a psoas hitch (Fig. 11.63B) or a bladder pedicle (Boari) flap (Fig. 11.63C) to reduce tension. Transureteroureterostomy is an option for both lower and middle ureteral injuries (Fig. 11.63D). For long segment loss in the upper ureter, autotransplantation of the kidney to the iliac fossa has been described, as has small bowel interposition.

Missed ureteral injuries can present as urinoma, characterized by nausea, vomiting, fever, and lower quadrant pain. Urinary fistulae with drainage through either a surgical wound or the original penetrating injury can also occur. Screening for these missed ureteral injuries is best done with IVP, ultrasound, or CT scan to look for urinomas. A definitive diagnosis is best obtained by retrograde ureterography.

URETHRAL INJURIES

The occurrence of urethral injuries after trauma is limited almost entirely to the male population because of the length and exposure of the membranous urethra (275) (Fig. 11.64). Pelvic fractures and straddle-type injuries are the most common mechanisms. Injuries above the urogenital diaphragm (posterior urethra) occur most commonly in association with pelvic fractures. Injuries to the anterior urethra (below the urogenital diaphragm) usually occur as the result of a fall or straddle-type injury. Most posterior urethral injuries involve complete disruption, as opposed to anterior injuries that result in partial tears in approximately half of patients.

A urethral tear should be suspected in any male patient with pelvic fracture. These patients should be examined carefully for signs of urethral injury, including scrotal or perineal hematomas, blood at the urethral meatus, or anterior displacement of the prostate gland on rectal examination. The presence of any of these clinical findings constitutes a contraindication to immediate placement of a urethral catheter. A retrograde urethrogram should be obtained in these cases by the placement of a small balloon catheter in the fossa navicularis and gravity infusion of 10 to 15 mL of contrast material. This is a rapid, simple, and reliable means of diagnosing urethral injuries (Fig. 11.65). Contrast material should never be injected under pressure for this examination.

Urethral injuries, particularly partial tears that are not associated with prostate displacement, can occur in the

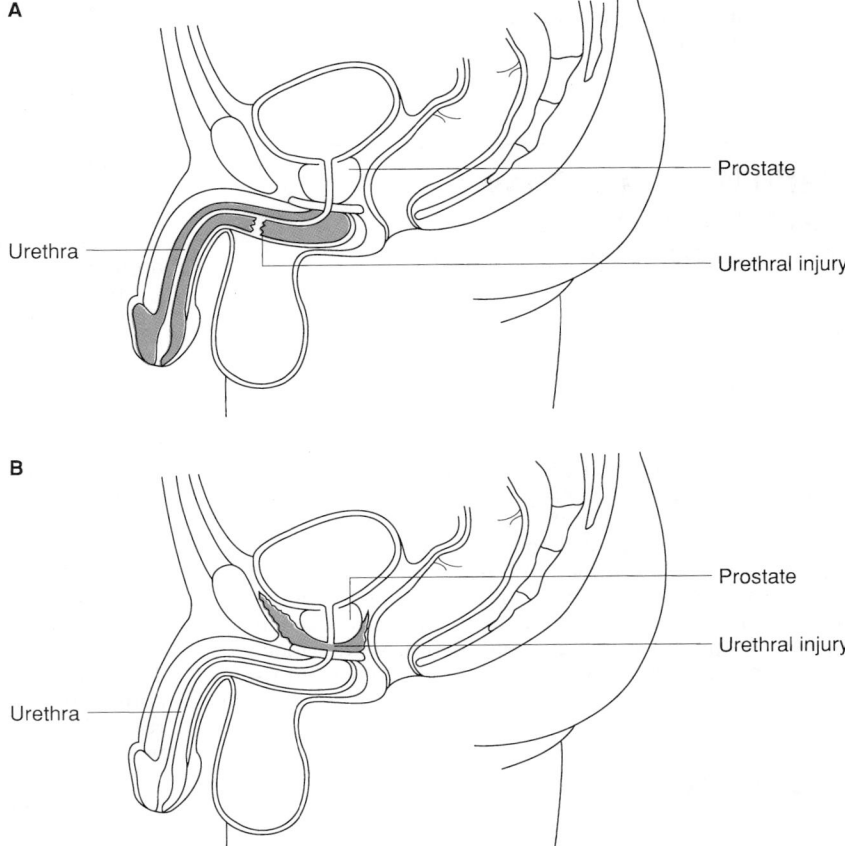

Figure 11.64. *(A)* Anterior tear of the urethra with the Buck fascia intact. *(B)* Posterior tear with prostate displacement.

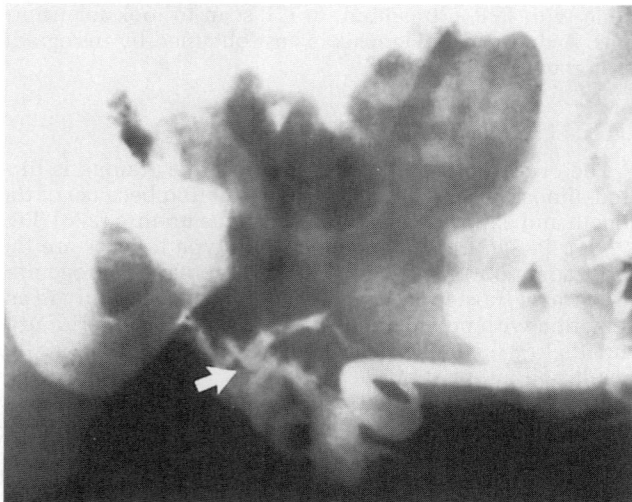

Figure 11.65. Retrograde urethrogram showing tear of the membranous urethra (posterior) with contrast extravasation *(arrow).*

absence of any clinical findings. Urinary catheters should be placed with great care in any patient with a pelvic fracture, and any difficulty in catheter placement should be an indication for a retrograde urethrogram.

Initial management of urethral tears consists of suprapubic cystostomy for urinary drainage. Because of the increased incidence of impotence and urinary stricture, immediate repair or reconstruction of the injured urethra usually is not attempted. Formal reconstruction of urethral tears can be undertaken after several months and usually involves a perineal urethroplasty. Impotence, which occurs in approximately 20% of late repairs, is the major complication, and its severity is related to the degree of initial injury.

Definitive Care Phase: Vascular Injuries

MICHAEL J. SISE AND STEVEN R. SHACKFORD

Vascular injuries have become increasingly common because of the epidemic of urban violence as well as the widespread application of invasive diagnostic and therapeutic techniques that use vascular access. The development of regional trauma systems with rapid transport has also contributed to the increased incidence of vascular injuries by delivering patients with previously fatal injuries to the trauma center in a timely fashion. Injuries range from isolated penetrating extremity trauma with minimal signs to major vessel injury with blunt mechanism, multiple-system trauma. Early diagnosis and successful management require a thorough examination with a focus on both mechanism and location of injury, an efficient use of diagnostic modalities, and a timely application of operative management.

EPIDEMIOLOGY

Vascular trauma typically affects men between the ages of 20 and 40 years and is primarily a result of a penetrat-

ing injury (276). In urban environments, gunshot wound is the most frequent cause. Because many vascular injuries of the head, neck, and torso are immediately lethal, most patients with vascular injury surviving transport and initial resuscitation have extremity trauma. However, trauma centers in urban environments with brief prehospital transport times are seeing an increase in patients arriving with major vascular injuries that were previously fatal (277). The increase in the use of endovascular therapies has also increased the number of iatrogenic injuries, which now account for approximately one third of the vascular trauma seen in many centers.

PATHOPHYSIOLOGY

The principal physiologic consequences of vascular injury result from either hemorrhage or inadequate distal perfusion. Great vessel injury is more likely to result in the former, whereas peripheral arterial injuries are usually associated with the latter (278). Exsanguinating hemorrhage is most often the result of intrathoracic or intraabdominal great vessel injury, which is usually lethal before medical treatment is available. Noncavitary hemorrhage can also result in exsanguination if there is unopposed flow, although this is a slower process and is usually treated easily at both the prehospital and definitive care levels. Blunt extremity trauma can result in extensive local hemorrhage, which can produce life-threatening hypovolemia in combination with other injuries. Hypovolemic shock is the important systemic consequence of all these injuries; it is discussed in detail elsewhere in this text.

Local consequences of vascular injuries are usually related to acute arterial occlusion from thrombosis after injury. This results in ischemia distal to the injury site and can lead to limb or organ loss. The degree of tissue loss is related to the adequacy of collateral flow, the sensitivity of the distal tissue to ischemia, and the delay involved in repairing the injury and restoring blood flow. The variability in these factors is great. The brain is most sensitive to ischemia because of high basal energy requirements and the absence of glycogen stores. Brain ischemia for longer than 4 minutes results in irreversible injury. Peripheral nerves and muscles are much more resilient, tolerating periods of ischemia of up to 4 hours without permanent injury. An important principle of vascular repairs, however, is that outcome is time dependent, necessitating an aggressive approach and a high priority.

Protracted arterial ischemia produces anoxic cell death. The restoration of arterial flow after complete ischemia often results in a reperfusion injury. This phenomenon is initiated by biochemical events that occur during ischemia. Xanthine dehydrogenase is converted to xanthine oxidase under anoxic or ischemic conditions, allowing hypoxanthine to accumulate. When oxygen is reintroduced, as a result of reperfusion, the accumulated hypoxanthine is converted to xanthine with the generation of superoxide anion, a highly reactive oxygen free radical. Because skeletal muscle contains little xanthine oxidase, the major source of free radicals in reperfusion injury is the polymorphonuclear leukocyte (279). The free radicals initiate lipid peroxidation, which injures the microvascular endothelium, resulting in interstitial edema formation (280). The interstitial edema increases the interstitial fluid pressure, which compresses capillaries and venules and interrupts flow, ultimately leading to a "no reflow" phenomenon and muscle necrosis.

If the severity of ischemia is significant enough to cause skeletal muscle necrosis, rhabdomyolysis, with the release of potassium and myoglobin into the systemic circulation, follows. Acute acidosis, hyperkalemia, and myoglobin-induced renal failure can occur. Beyond the immediate threat of limb loss, the systemic effects of extremity ischemia with muscle necrosis can ultimately prove fatal.

The type of vascular injury is related to both the mechanism of trauma and the location of the target vessel. Simple lacerations are the most common penetrating injuries to both arteries and veins. Incomplete lacerations often cause more hemorrhage than complete transections because of the inability of a partially transected vessel to undergo retraction, vasoconstriction, and thrombosis as it would if completely transected. Complex associated soft-tissue injuries also exacerbate local hemorrhage. Intimal flap occlusion, arterial contusion with thrombosis, and arteriovenous fistulae are all common outcomes of acute penetrating vascular injury. Chronic problems include pseudoaneurysm formation, thrombosis, and distal embolization.

Blunt trauma usually is caused by the deceleration injuries associated with motor vehicle crashes or falls from heights, and it commonly results in complete or partial disruption of the vessel wall. As the arterial wall is deformed, the elastic adventitia and muscular layers remain intact while the intima fractures. Blood dissects beneath the fractured intima, causing protrusion into the lumen and thrombosis. In the aorta and its major branches, this process can result in an acute pseudoaneurysm with only the adventitial layer remaining intact; delayed rupture, occurring minutes to days later, can cause exsanguinating hemorrhage.

The increasing incidence of high-velocity wounds in the setting of urban violence has led to the appearance of "shock-wave" vessel injuries. The high-velocity projectile produces a shock wave that displaces tissues in a 90-degree direction away from the path of the bullet. A temporary cavity is created that significantly distorts adjacent tissue several centimeters away from the actual bullet tract. The shock wave can stretch and disrupt blood vessels and create intimal tears with localized dissection, thrombosis, or embolization. Although these injuries are usually immediately apparent, partial intimal disruption can lead to a delayed onset of thrombosis or embolization with resultant ischemia.

DIAGNOSIS

Vascular trauma may be immediately apparent on initial presentation or remain occult. The assessment of blood loss during the prehospital phase of care is frequently unreliable. However, a history of pulsatile arterial bleeding or a large amount of hemorrhage surrounding the site of injury is an important finding suggestive of vascular injury. Hypotension in the prehospital phase of care or on initial presentation also deserves particular attention because an occult vascular injury may be present.

Intraabdominal or intrathoracic vascular injuries should be suspected in hypotensive victims of penetrating injury. Blunt great vessel injury in the chest should be considered whenever there is external evidence of major thoracic trauma or a history of rapid deceleration. The physical signs that raise the index of suspicion include sternal fracture, flail chest, thoracic spine fracture, and first rib fracture. Other signs associated with intrathoracic vascular trauma include differential arm blood pressures or differential arm to lower extremity blood pressures; radiographic evidence of a widened mediastinum (>8 cm on an anteroposterior exposure) or loss of normal aortic contour; and thoracic outlet hematoma.

For victims of blunt trauma, the mechanism and force of injury should be carefully considered. Motor vehicle accidents that cause fatalities are often associated with signif-

icant energy transfer. A history of altered mental status or intermittent paralysis also should alert the examiner to the possibility of a carotid or aortic injury.

Complete occlusion or arterial disruption results in distal ischemia and produces the classic physical findings of pain, pallor, pulse deficit, paresthesia, and diminished perfusion (Table 11.14). Partial occlusions produce lesser signs and symptoms and are therefore more likely to be missed. The course of a penetrating injury should be estimated both visually and radiographically, using plain films with radiopaque markers for entrance and exit wounds. Patients with blunt injuries require a complete evaluation with emphasis on examination of the pulses. This can be difficult in a hypovolemic and hypotensive patient with multiple fractures and splints. After adequate fluid resuscitation has been completed, peripheral pulses should be palpable. Segmental arterial pressure determination by Doppler technique is a valuable adjunct in the examination of extremity vascular trauma. However, the presence of audible Doppler signals over an artery in the extremity does not rule out an arterial injury or indicate adequate perfusion.

The use of a Doppler device for extremity evaluation should include determination of distal blood pressure. This is accomplished by placing the probe over the selected artery in the foot or at the wrist and slowly inflating the blood pressure cuff at the ankle or the forearm. The pressure at which Doppler signals cease indicates the perfusion pressure at the level of the blood pressure cuff. This pressure should be compared with the other extremity in upper extremity evaluation or with the highest upper extremity pressure in lower extremity evaluation. In a healthy and normovolemic person, the ankle–brachial index is 1.1. A ratio of less than 0.9 or a 20-mm Hg difference between extremities should arouse suspicion of significant arterial trauma. However, in hypovolemic patients, frequently both lower extremity ankle–brachial indices are diminished to as low as 0.75. Reevaluation after resuscitation is essential if both lower extremity indices are diminished. Doppler examination for acute venous disruption has not been evaluated and is likely to be unreliable.

Duplex scanning is increasingly used in the evaluation of acutely injured extremities and the proximal extracranial carotid arteries. This technique, if performed by an experienced technician, is both sensitive and specific for detecting vascular injuries in areas that can be directly examined. It is particularly effective as a screening technique when patients do not have classic signs of vascular trauma. For instance, patients with blunt force trauma to the neck are ideal candidates for evaluation with Duplex scan of the carotid arteries. In vessels that are easy to image, this technique can rule out the presence of thrombosis, pseudoaneurysm, intimal flap, and arteriovenous fistula. When thoughtfully applied, this technique has al-

---

Table 11.14. PHYSICAL FINDINGS ASSOCIATED WITH EXTREMITY VASCULAR INJURY

Classic signs	Signs of occult injury
Pulsatile bleeding	History of significant hemorrhage
Thrill or bruit	Proximity wounds
Pain	Peripheral nerve deficit
Pulselessness	Diminished pulse
Pallor	Fracture–dislocation (knee, elbow)
Paresthesias	Unexplained shock
Paralysis	
Poikilothermia	

lowed the more selective use of arteriography and has become a valuable tool in the initial work-up of the acutely injured patient.

Arteriography is indicated in patients with suspected vascular trauma unless there is a clear indication for immediate operative therapy, such as exsanguinating hemorrhage or clear signs of arterial occlusion in which the operative approach is straightforward. For example, patients with posterior knee dislocation and loss of distal pulses with signs of ischemia require an immediate operative repair of the popliteal artery. In this instance, arteriography is both unnecessary and time consuming. In contrast, a hemodynamically stable patient with penetrating trauma to the thoracic inlet cannot be successfully managed without arteriography if aortic arch or great vessel injury is suspected.

The indications for arteriography include a history of moderate hemorrhage at the penetrating injury site, injury near major arterial structures, diminished pulses, and peripheral nerve injury in the distribution of a nerve that is near a major vessel. Proximity as the sole indication for arteriography, in the absence of a diminished ankle–brachial ratio or other signs of major injury, has proved to be an unreliable indicator of the need for arteriography (281). In the absence of the classic signs of major vascular injury, patients with penetrating wounds near major vessels can be observed closely without arteriography.

Formal arteriography using the Seldinger technique is preferred in stable patients. In unstable patients with other major injuries and suspected occult extremity arterial trauma, arteriography can be performed in the emergency department or on the operating table. In these cases, rapid bolus injection of sufficient contrast material without inflow occlusion is sufficient to produce adequate visualization of extremity vessels.

Arteriography for vascular trauma must be performed with attention to several essential details:

1. Entrance and exit wounds should be marked with radiopaque markers.
2. The contrast agent should be injected well above the suspected site of injury.
3. Biplanar views of at least 15 cm of artery above and below the site of injury should be obtained.
4. Early and late views should be taken to rule out the presence of early venous filling from an arteriovenous fistula or late filling of a pseudoaneurysm.
5. Any abnormality should be attributed to vessel injury unless there is unequivocal evidence of underlying chronic vascular disease in the contralateral noninjured extremity.

The appropriate use of arteriography can significantly reduce the rate of unnecessary explorations for suspected vascular trauma. If routine surgical exploration is performed whenever vascular injury is suspected, a negative exploration rate of approximately 60% or more can be expected. Selective use of arteriography reduces the negative exploration rate to approximately 35%. With experience, arteriography is an extremely reliable method of excluding vascular trauma. In this context, the sensitivity is 97% to 100%, and the specificity is 90% to 98%, with overall accuracy between 92% and 98% (281). Arteriography has an associated minor complication rate of 2% to 4% and a major complication rate of 0.6%.

NONOPERATIVE MANAGEMENT

The aggressive application of arteriography for suspected occult vascular trauma results in the detection of clinically insignificant lesions that can be treated nonoperatively. These include intimal irregularity, focal spasm with minimal narrowing, and small pseudoaneurysms. Although these lesions have been aggressively managed with operative therapy in the past, considerable evidence suggests that nonoperative therapy of some asymptomatic lesions is safe and effective. Ongoing surveillance for subsequent occlusion or hemorrhage is mandatory, however. Duplex scanning offers an accurate, noninvasive method to follow these lesions in the extremities. Operative therapy is indicated for thrombosis, for chronic symptoms of occlusive disease, and for failure of small pseudoaneurysms to undergo thrombosis. Nonoperative therapy also may be indicated for clinically insignificant lesions in patients with multiple injuries for whom vascular repair presents a prohibitive risk.

Endovascular Management

Interventional radiologic management of vascular injuries is rapidly evolving. Effective use of this new modality requires special training and expertise on the part of the radiologist or surgeon and an integration of these skills into the overall flow of management of the injured patient. Nowhere is the "captain of the ship" function of the trauma surgeon more important. A clear understanding of the importance of timely restoration of blood flow is essential for the appropriate and successful use of endovascular techniques. Endovascular procedures that are successful in patients with chronic vascular disease are not necessarily effective in patients with acute vascular injury. When in doubt, conventional operative techniques should be the standard in the care of these injuries.

The indications for endovascular techniques include hemorrhage from branch vessels that may be occluded without producing significant ischemia, acute pseudoaneurysms with a small lateral wall arterial injury, intimal flap without significant underlying thrombosis, and acute arteriovenous fistulae. Complete arterial disruption or thrombosis, particularly in the presence of multiple other injuries, is not appropriately managed with endovascular techniques. Endovascular placement of stents and stent grafts for noniatrogenic vascular trauma remains largely experimental and should be limited to centers with extensive experience in the use of these technologies.

Endovascular embolization is particularly effective in branch vessel hemorrhage. A pelvic fracture with hemorrhage from the hypogastric arterial distribution responds well to this technique. Extremity trauma with significant hemorrhage from branch vessels also can be successfully managed by embolization. Coils may be placed with or without thrombotic protein foam material. Biologic glues also have been used effectively. Balloon catheter occlusion of the underlying artery distal to branch vessels is an important adjunct and is frequently effective in preventing distal embolization. Stent grafts are a relatively new technology that involves placement of collapsible stents covered with graft material. These are somewhat limited in their application to larger vessels because of the risk of precipitating thrombosis or distal embolization. Long-term results are not yet available, and their application remains limited to specialized centers with training, expertise, and the appropriate equipment.

Ultrasound-guided Therapy

Reports have documented the success of color flow duplex-guided compression of iatrogenic pseudoaneurysms of the femoral artery (282,283). This has been used in pseudoaneurysms that are greater than 3 cm in diameter. Pseudoaneurysm of less than 3 cm spontaneously close from thrombosis within 4 weeks and require simple follow-up with ultrasound rather than treatment. Complete occlusion of large pseudoaneurysms can require probe compression of up to 3 hours and is often associated with moderate patient discomfort and occasional skin necrosis over the pseudoaneurysm, ultimately leading to surgical therapy. An alternative to compressive therapy of pseudoaneurysms is ultrasound-guided thrombin injection (284). Large (>3 cm in diameter) pseudoaneurysms and those associated with arteriovenous fistulae have been effectively thrombosed in a matter of seconds with the injection of 0.5 to 1.0 mL of thrombin solution (1,000 U/mL).

OPERATIVE MANAGEMENT

The initial step in the management of all vascular injuries is the adequate restoration of circulating blood volume. External bleeding should be controlled by direct pressure. Blind clamp placement is to be condemned. Tourniquets also are to be avoided unless there is extensive soft-tissue loss with extensive hemorrhage. If the use of a tourniquet is unavoidable, a pneumatic cuff of the type used for distal extremity orthopedic procedures is preferred. Tourniquets occlude collaterals, making distal ischemia significantly worse. If applied improperly, they allow arterial inflow, occlude venous outflow, and increase bleeding.

The operative management of vascular injuries must be orchestrated with the overall care of the patient's other injuries. Although life-threatening abdominal or thoracic injuries take priority over limb-threatening arterial injuries, every attempt should be made to begin simultaneous vascular repair by an additional team of surgeons while the abdominal or chest injury is being treated.

The goal of operative management of vascular injuries is the rapid control of hemorrhage and the restoration of perfusion, with salvage of the extremity or organ in jeopardy. Intravenous broad-spectrum antibiotics should be administered as preparations for surgery are being made. In isolated extremity vascular injury with arterial occlusion, systemic heparin also should be administered to avoid the propagation of thrombus in vessels distal to the occlusion. In multiply injured patients, especially those with central nervous system trauma, heparin is inappropriate. Tetanus prophylaxis should be included, as in the treatment of any penetrating wound. A wide sterile operative field should be prepared to allow for adequate exposure of vessels with both proximal and distal control. A lower extremity always should be prepared as a potential site for saphenous vein harvest. In patients with lower extremity injury, the contralateral limb should be made ready for vein harvest. For patients with suspected neck or abdominal sites of vascular trauma, the chest should be prepared to allow access to the aorta and its branches.

The early involvement of an orthopedic surgeon is an essential part of the surgical management of extremity vascular trauma associated with skeletal injury. The surgical procedure should be a combined effort. In general, the vascular repair is performed first, followed by stabilization of the skeletal injury, but the vascular surgeon's role does not end after perfusion is restored. Careful surveillance to ensure that orthopedic appliances do not obstruct the arterial repair and reexamination to confirm patency before wound closure are essential to successful limb salvage. A similar approach should be taken to vascular injuries associated with large soft-tissue defects. The early involvement of a surgeon experienced with plastic and reconstructive surgery is essential to the successful management of these wounds.

A few patients have extensive soft-tissue loss in an extremity associated with neurologic deficit, extensive fractures, and vascular injuries, with limbs that appear mangled. Usually, there is little hope for functional recovery, and careful consideration should be given to primary amputation. An objective scoring system has been developed to aid with this difficult problem (285) (Table 11.15). A score of 7 or greater has been found to predict eventual amputation in 100% of patients. This decision must be made in consultation with orthopedic and reconstructive surgical colleagues and should take into account the patient's overall status. In cases of extensive skeletal damage and severe hemorrhage, primary amputation can be lifesaving. The decision to take this course is complex and difficult.

Vascular reconstruction for trauma should be performed with attention to proper technique. The use of fine monofilament sutures on the appropriately sized needles, vascular instruments, and loupe magnification are all appropriate. It is in the best interest of the patient that surgeons unfamiliar with techniques of vascular reconstruction obtain assistance from experienced colleagues.

The initial step in the surgical management of vascular injuries is to obtain proximal and distal control of the injured vessel. This is most easily accomplished through uninjured areas adjacent to the injury, using incisions normally used for elective exposure of these vessels. Direct approach through the site of injury is fraught with the hazards of severe hemorrhage and iatrogenic trauma to the vessel itself or to adjacent nerves. Balloon-tipped catheters can be valuable in obtaining proximal and distal control if they are inserted carefully through the site of injury and inflated. Subsequent dissection then establishes proximal and distal control.

After control has been established, careful thrombectomy of the proximal and distal arteries is carried out until there is no evidence of thrombus. Heparinized saline, 10 IU/mL, is then flushed proximally and distally into the lumen of the artery. The technique for arterial repair should not be selected until the entire extent of the injury is known and the injured vessel has been débrided. The injured arterial segment is inevitably longer than appreciated at first inspection. End-to-end anastomosis can be used in the repair of many larger arteries if there is sufficient length to perform the repair without undue tension.

Table 11.15. COMPONENTS OF THE MANGLED EXTREMITY SEVERITY SCORE

	Points
Skeletal or soft tissue injury	
Low energy: stabs, simple fractures, low-velocity gunshot wounds	1
Medium energy: open or multiple fractures, dislocations	2
High energy: close-range shotgun wounds, high-velocity gunshot wounds; crush injuries	3
Very high energy: high-energy plus gross contamination, major soft-tissue loss	4
Limb ischemia	
Pulses reduced or absent, perfusion normal	1
Pulseless, with paresthesia, delayed capillary refill	2
Cool, paralyzed insensate, numb	3
(All ischemia scores are doubled if ischemia time >6h)	
Shock	
Systolic blood pressure always >90 mm Hg	0
Transient hypotension	1
Persistent hypotension	2
Age	
<30 y	0
30–50 y	1
>50 y	2

Although 2 cm frequently has been cited, there is no definitive length of artery for safe resection and primary repair.

In the repair of more extensive arterial injuries, reversed saphenous vein from an uninjured lower extremity is the first choice for interposition graft. Although PTFE grafts have been used with success at many centers, saphenous vein remains the usual choice for interposition grafting (286). Care must be taken to avoid either kinking from a redundant graft or stenosis from undue tension. A spatulated anastomosis should be performed between artery and graft to avoid stenosis. Intraoperative completion angiography is mandatory to determine the adequacy of repair, confirm patency, and visualize the distal arterial runoff.

The repair of concomitant venous injuries is controversial. The priority of venous repair in combined arterial and venous injuries has not been firmly established. Proximal extremity veins and the great veins are repaired whenever technically possible to avoid the sequela of venous occlusion. Techniques of repair vary from simple suture closure to saphenous vein patch or graft interposition. Venous repair should not be attempted in a hemodynamically unstable patient; rather, ligation should be performed to expedite the operation.

The use of intraluminal shunts provides a valuable adjunct for patients in need of complex arterial reconstructive procedures (287). Standard shunts used in elective carotid operation function well in the early restoration of arterial and venous flow if extensive grafting or limb reimplantation is required. Limb ischemia time is significantly reduced when shunts are used properly. Interposition grafting can be performed by placing the interposition graft over the shunt. Shunts effectively restore flow to injured extremities in patients who are too unstable to undergo completion of peripheral arterial repair. Shunts have been left in place for extended periods with ultimate salvage of the extremity (287).

Extraanatomic bypass plays a limited but important role in arterial trauma. Penetrating abdominal trauma with aortic or iliac artery disruption associated with extensive bowel injury and contamination by enteric contents can make in situ arterial repair highly susceptible to infection and disruption. In this situation, arterial ligation and extraanatomic bypass through the axillofemoral or femorofemoral route may be the only acceptable means to restore distal perfusion. The long-term patency rate of such grafts is inferior to in situ reconstruction, but these grafts do provide an excellent means to maintain perfusion and avoid life-threatening complications. Patients must be observed closely for graft occlusion and the need for subsequent reconstructive procedures.

The development of an extremity compartment syndrome is a devastating complication after arterial trauma.

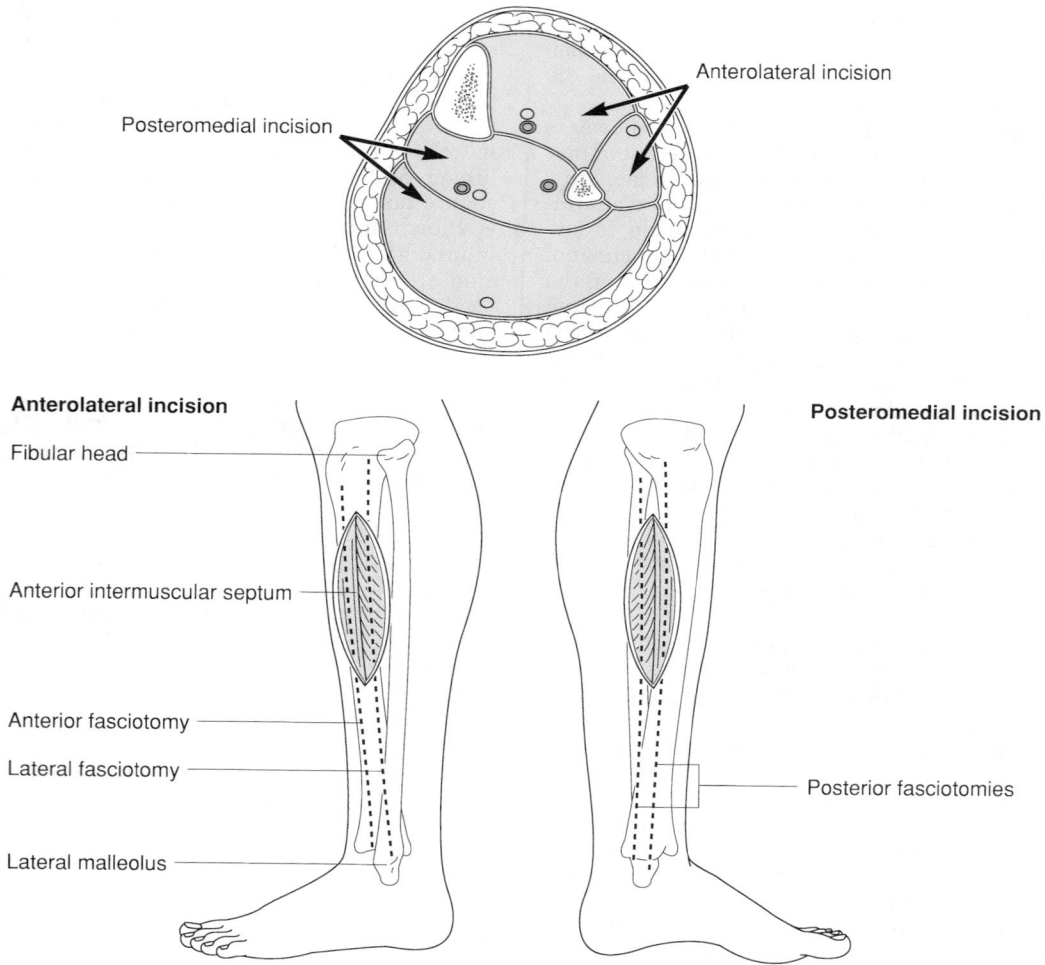

Figure 11.66. Surgical approach for four compartment fasciotomies through incisions on the medial and lateral aspects of the calf.

The syndrome is uncommon in the thigh and forearm but is frequently seen in the calf. The most sensitive sign of compartment syndrome is pain on passive stretch of the involved muscle. Although many devices are available to measure compartment pressures in the calf, many trauma surgeons are aggressive in the application of four-compartment fasciotomy whenever there is extensive soft-tissue injury or skeletal trauma in the lower leg combined with vascular trauma or the history of prolonged ischemia (Fig. 11.66). In any patient with lower extremity trauma who exhibits signs of pain or distal ischemia, the compartment pressure should be measured and fasciotomy performed as needed. An untreated or unrecognized compartment syndrome produces nerve and muscle damage and prevents good functional recovery despite the patency of the vascular repair. Factors that suggest the need for fasciotomy are as follows:

- Prolonged period (≥6 hours) between injury and restoration of perfusion
- Associated crush injury
- Preoperative calf swelling
- Combined arterial and venous injuries
- Extensive venous ligation
- Postoperative signs or disproportionate muscle pain, pain on passive stretch, or tender and firm muscles
- Elevated compartment pressures

Proper wound management is essential to successful limb salvage after vascular trauma in the extremities. Aggressive wound débridement and pulse irrigation with copious amounts of antibiotic solution should be performed routinely. Coverage of the vascular repair with viable muscle or fascia and subcutaneous tissue is essential to prevent desiccation and infection. The assistance of a plastic and reconstructive surgeon is essential in the management of injuries that involve extensive tissue loss. Flap rotation and, in the case of extreme tissue loss, myocutaneous free flap transfer may be required. Delayed primary skin closure also should be considered in all injuries except those involving minimal trauma and surgical dissection.

The use of low-molecular-weight dextran can prevent early thrombosis and improve microvascular circulation in patients with prolonged ischemia. Dextran 40 at 40–50 mL/h for 24 hours does not cause significant bleeding complications and can improve patency rates of arterial reconstructions, especially in small arteries. The routine use of a postoperative heparin infusion, however, significantly increases the incidence of wound hematoma. Heparin should be reserved for patients with documented thrombotic complications, including deep venous thrombosis and definable hypercoagulable states. Vasodilators are of limited value in the perioperative management of vascular injuries.

Postoperative monitoring for early failure of the vascular reconstruction is essential to ensure limb salvage. Monitoring in the intensive care unit with frequent peripheral vascular examination should be used. The immediate challenges after operation are restoration of adequate intravascular volume and rewarming of the patient. Evaluation of distal circulation is difficult until the patient is normovolemic and normothermic. In the early postoperative period, pulses are frequently absent and Doppler ratios decreased, despite a patent repair; however, there should be audible Doppler signals over the distal arteries. Normal pulses and a normal pulse ratio may not return for 6 to 8 hours after reconstruction. Early reoperation should be performed if Doppler signals become inaudible or if pulses and a normal ratio do not return. The salvage rate for reoperation after initially successful reconstruction is more than 90% if performed in a timely fashion. Delay in reoperation dooms the reconstruction to almost certain failure.

COMPLICATIONS

Early thrombosis of the vascular reconstruction is the most immediate postoperative complication. Careful surveillance, as outlined previously, allows for prompt recognition and reoperation. Significant swelling in the early postoperative period suggests venous thrombosis. A duplex scan should be obtained to confirm the presence of venous thrombus. If the popliteal vein or more proximal veins are involved, heparin should be started and continued until the patient has been therapeutically anticoagulated with warfarin. Elevation of the extremity decreases the swelling and discomfort.

Infection in the area of a vascular reconstruction is a potentially devastating complication. Disruption of the suture line and hemorrhage usually follow. Suture repair of the disrupted anastomosis is doomed to failure. The safest course is ligation in an area of the artery not involved in the infection, combined with extraanatomic bypass in uninvolved tissue to restore the distal perfusion.

Late complications include stenosis or occlusion of the arterial repair, aneurysmal changes in vein grafts, and the postthrombotic syndrome after venous thrombosis or ligation. All patients who require surgical treatment of vascular trauma should be monitored regularly on a long-term basis because of the potential for late complications. Early detection allows for timely treatment and a reduction in morbidity.

MANAGEMENT OF SPECIFIC VASCULAR INJURIES

Most patients presenting to trauma centers with vascular trauma have injuries of the extremities. Vascular injuries of the head, neck, chest, and abdomen are often immediately fatal. In contrast to the military experience, in which many of the wounds are from high-velocity missiles, civilian penetrating injuries tend to result from low-velocity weapons. As a result, more patients with torso and head and neck injuries survive to reach the trauma center. Table 11.16 compares the civilian experience with

Table 11.16. COMPARISON OF VASCULAR INJURIES FROM THE VIETNAM EXPERIENCE WITH TWO MODERN URBAN EXPERIENCES

Site	Vietnam	Houston	San Diego	Total
Neck	50 (5%)	17 (8%)	53 (8%)	120 (6%)
Chest	11 (1%)	40 (18%)	194 (29%)	245 (13%)
Abdomen	29 (3%)	41 (18%)	154 (23%)	197 (11%)
Upper extremity	342 (34%)	64 (29%)	102 (16%)	508 (28%)
Lower extremity	568 (57%)	59 (27%)	161 (24%)	788 (42%)
Total	1,000	221	664	1,858

military experience with regard to the distribution of vascular injuries. Most military vascular injuries occur in the lower extremity and are inflicted by antipersonnel weapons. In contrast, civilian trauma most frequently involves the torso and upper extremity. Penetrating trauma is the predominant mechanism of injury in the military experience, whereas in the civilian experience the mechanisms of injury are related to the environment in which the trauma center is located. In suburban areas, motor vehicular trauma with blunt vascular injuries predominates. In the inner city, penetrating injuries are more common. Cervical vascular injuries are discussed elsewhere in this chapter.

Injury to the Thoracic Great Vessels

Both penetrating and blunt injuries of the great vessels in the chest can occur. They are predictably life threatening because of the associated hemorrhage and the high frequency of concomitant injury to major adjacent structures (288). These injuries are discussed in the broader context of complex thoracic trauma elsewhere in this chapter. This review is undertaken with specific attention to the management of injuries to the aorta and its main branches.

Penetrating injuries of the great vessels usually are associated with hemothorax and evidence of hypovolemia. Tube thoracostomy reveals severe ongoing hemorrhage, and either emergency department thoracotomy or an urgent transfer to the operating room is required. In patients with penetrating trauma who remain stable and do not have significant ongoing hemorrhage after tube thoracostomy, there are a number of signs that suggest the need for arteriography to rule out great vessel injury. These include missile emboli to peripheral vessels, the presence of missiles or missile trajectories near great vessels, and a mediastinal hematoma on chest radiography. Confirmation of the diagnosis is obtained at angiography, if possible, but the magnitude of hemorrhage may well preclude any maneuver other than immediate thoracotomy.

Penetrating wounds to the ascending aorta, innominate artery, and right subclavian artery are best approached by a median sternotomy. Extrathoracic extensions may be necessary to obtain proximal and distal vascular control. The approach to a penetrating wound of the innominate

vein and left common carotid artery is shown in Figs. 11.67 and 11.68. In general, venous ligation is well tolerated, and arterial repair is performed. Left subclavian and descending thoracic aortic injuries require a left thoracotomy for exposure. If an emergency department thoracotomy is required, exposure of all but the apex of the mediastinum can be obtained by carrying the incision across the sternum into the right chest (Fig. 11.29). Almost all survivable blunt great vessel injuries result in acute pseudoaneurysms of the aortic isthmus or the proximal arch vessels (Figs. 11.69 to 11.71). The aortic isthmus (the area of the descending aorta between the ligamentum arteriosum and the origin of the left subclavian artery) is susceptible to shear injury in deceleration accidents. These typically involve transection of the intima and media with containment of hemorrhage by the elastic adventitia. The mortality rate from delayed rupture of this lesion approaches 50% in the first 24 hours if left untreated.

The initial results of stent graft placement in stable patients with aortic or great vessel injuries have been promising. Patients who are hemodynamically stable with either intimal flap or small acute pseudoaneurysms have been successfully treated with the placement of these devices. These successes, however, have been limited to centers with special training and expertise and carefully developed preexisting protocols. Stent graft placement for acute thoracic aortic pseudoaneurysm at the aortic isthmus is particularly promising in view of the morbidity of the operative approach. However, these techniques must be carefully planned, thoughtfully applied, and orchestrated with the overall care of the injured patient. Whenever stent grafts are placed, immediate access to the operating room in the case of failure or complications is required.

Conventional surgical management of the aortic injuries consists of direct suture repair or synthetic graft interposition. If possible, cardiopulmonary bypass capability should be available in the event that aortic occlusion proves necessary for repair. For patients who arrive at a trauma center without severe hypotension, the results of surgical therapy are encouraging. Paraplegia is an important complication because the anterior spinal artery originates from branches of the thoracic intercostal arteries. Cross-clamping of the aorta in the chest for arterial repair

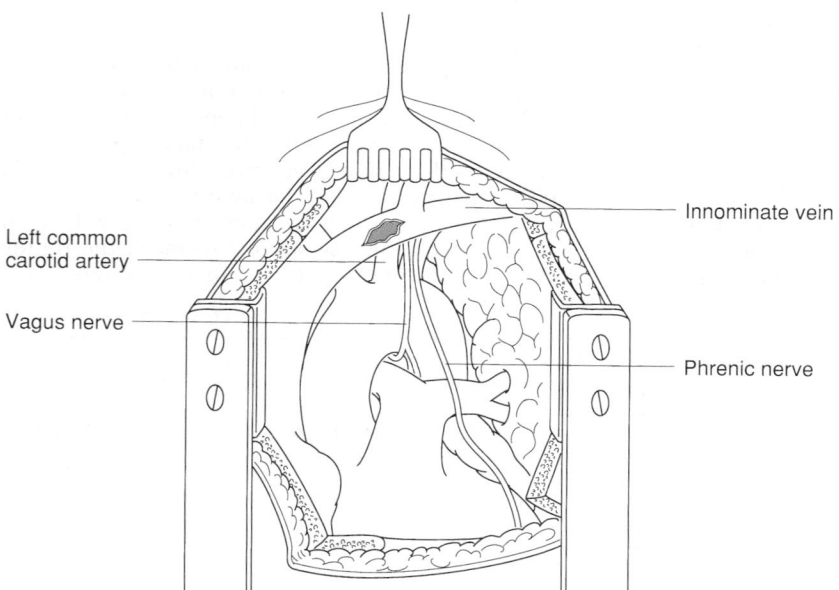

Left common carotid artery

Vagus nerve

Innominate vein

Phrenic nerve

Figure 11.67. Proximal and distal control of both venous and arterial injuries must be obtained without injury to the adjacent structures, such as the phrenic, vagus, or recurrent laryngeal nerves.

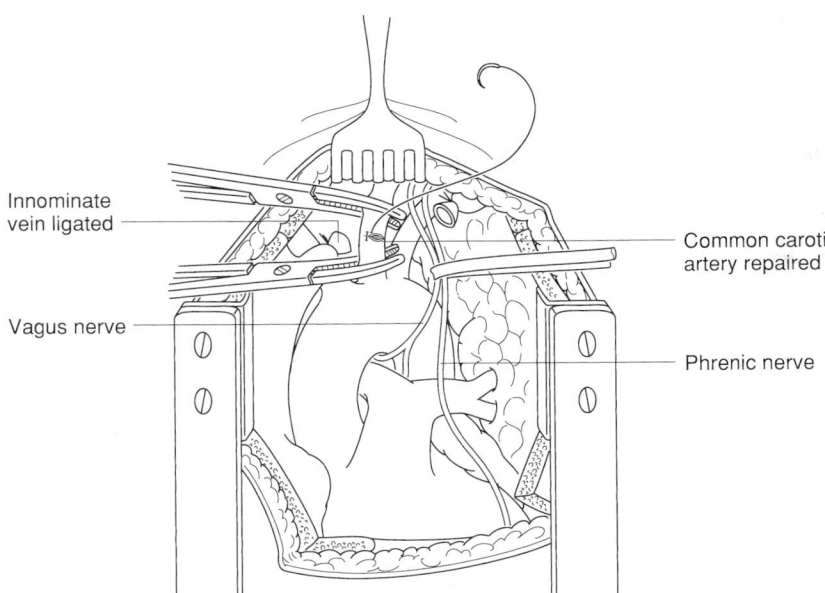

Innominate
vein ligated

Common carotid
artery repaired

Vagus nerve

Phrenic nerve

Figure 11.68. Combined arterial and venous injuries often are best treated with ligation of the vein, whereas isolated venous injuries may be safely repaired. Common carotid arterial repair is shown.

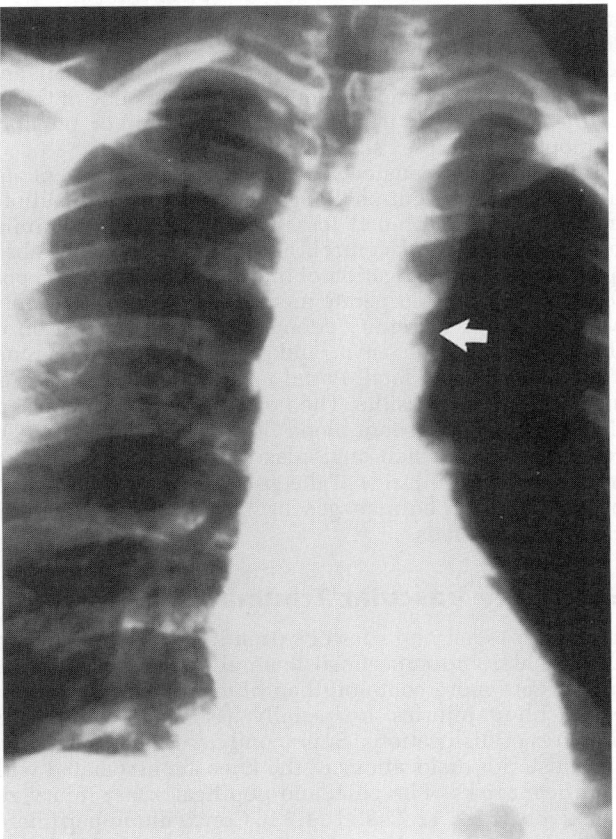

Figure 11.69. Portable chest radiograph demonstrating an indistinct aortic knob *(arrow)* and left apical pleural cap in a 21-year-old man who sustained a significant deceleration injury to the chest.

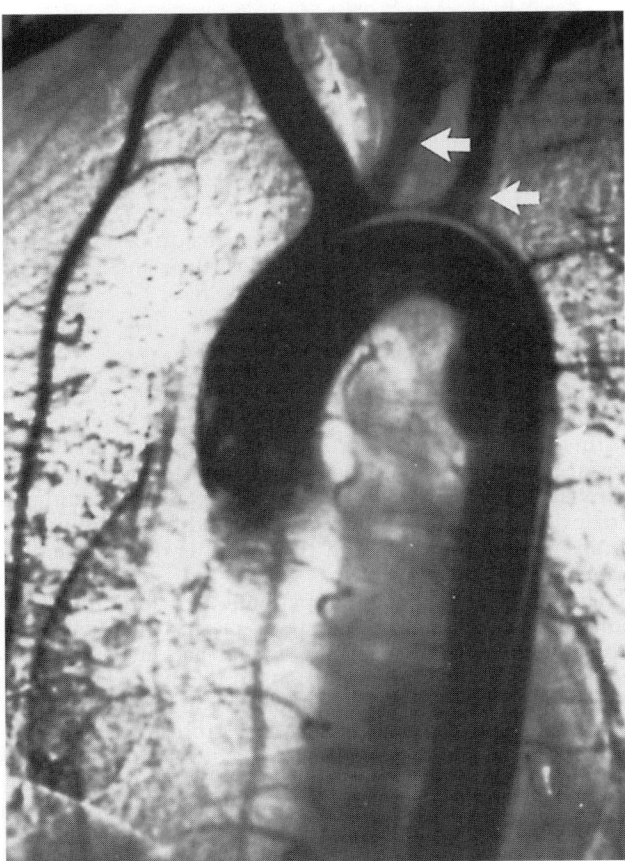

Figure 11.70. Thoracic aortogram revealing traumatic pseudoaneurysm of the aortic isthmus, the left common carotid artery, and the left subclavian artery *(arrows)* in the same patient shown in Fig. 11.69.

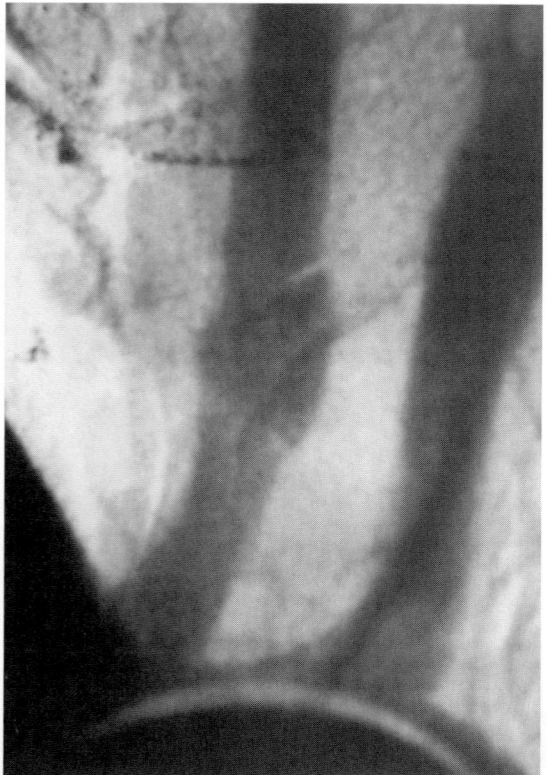

Figure 11.71. Enlarged view of the carotid and subclavian injury in the same patient shown in Fig. 11.69.

results in paraplegia in approximately 8% of these patients despite modern techniques to maximize distal perfusion. The best approach includes avoidance of hypovolemia and rapid vascular repair.

Abdominal Vascular Injury

The diagnosis of major intraabdominal vascular injury is most often made at celiotomy. The common exception to this is blunt disruption of the renal artery with thrombosis, which is typically detected on arteriography after nonvisualization of the involved kidney. Rarely, blunt aortic or iliac artery disruption is suspected from diminished or absent distal pulses, and the injury is documented by arteriography.

The initial management of patients with abdominal vascular trauma is dictated by the severity of hemorrhage from the site of injury. In the agonal patient, emergency department thoracotomy and aortic occlusion above the diaphragm must be performed to control hemorrhage during transport to the operating room. Rapid fluid resuscitation and expeditious celiotomy are required in all patients with abdominal vascular injury.

The priorities in the management of abdominal vascular trauma are similar to those in other areas. If active bleeding is encountered at celiotomy, it is controlled by direct pressure. If contained retroperitoneal hemorrhage is encountered, proximal and distal vascular control is obtained before the hematoma is opened. Associated bowel injury should be closed expeditiously to avoid ongoing contamination from enteric contents. The most common finding at celiotomy in patients with blunt abdominal trauma is either retroperitoneal or intramesenteric hematoma. Less commonly, intestinal ischemia may be present as a result of thrombosis or avulsion of mesenteric vessels.

Exposure of the great vessels of the posterior abdomen is essential in the management of significant abdominal vascular trauma. If active hemorrhage is encountered, precise identification of the source of bleeding can be difficult. If it is necessary, exposure of the aorta at the diaphragmatic hiatus for clamp placement is best performed by entering the lesser sac and longitudinally splitting the crural fibers.

The infrarenal aorta and its bifurcation are best approached by mobilization of the small intestine to the right upper quadrant and opening of the retroperitoneum in the midline or lateral to either the ascending or descending colon. The superior and inferior mesenteric arteries, the left renal hilum, and the left iliac artery can be exposed by reflection of the spleen and entire left colon for entry into the retroperitoneum. Similarly, the vena cava, right renal hilum, and right iliac artery can be exposed by a Kocher maneuver combined with mobilization of the right colon. The portal area is best exposed by the combination of a Kocher maneuver and mobilization of the hepatic flexure of the colon from the underlying duodenum and head of the pancreas.

Arterial and venous repair in the abdomen follow the same general principles of vascular technique used elsewhere. Primary suture repair, patch angioplasty, and saphenous vein interposition are used selectively to restore adequate flow. The use of synthetic graft material should be avoided if there is associated bowel or pancreatic injury. All mesenteric arterial repairs should include a careful inspection of the intestine for evidence of ischemia. Completion angiography after abdominal vascular repair is difficult and suboptimal. Therefore, documentation of patency of the repair is best achieved using Doppler ultrasound or, possibly, intraoperative duplex scanning.

Injuries to the vena cava or the portal vein present significant management challenges because of the insidious nature of ongoing blood loss, the difficulty of obtaining proximal and distal control, and the high risk of subsequent thrombosis. Ligation of these vessels should be performed only as a desperate measure in unstable patients. Massive lower extremity edema accompanies ligation of the infrarenal vena cava, and ligation above the renal veins is uniformly fatal. Portal venous ligation should be avoided if at all possible. The portal vein provides 80% of the oxygen and nutrient blood flow to the liver (289). Direct suture and patch angioplasty are the most effective means to repair injuries of the great veins. Mesenteric venous injury can be managed by ligation without significant complications.

Extremity Vascular Trauma

The most common sites of extremity arterial trauma are the brachial and superficial femoral arteries. Penetrating injuries are more common than blunt injuries. If they do occur, blunt injuries are usually associated with major fractures or dislocations. Supracondylar humeral fractures and posterior dislocations of the knee are associated with significant risks of brachial and popliteal artery injury, respectively (Figs. 11.72 and 11.73). Concomitant peripheral nerve injuries occur in 60% of patients with vascular injuries in the extremities.

The extensive collateral circulation and the smaller muscle mass in the arm make acute arterial occlusion in the arm less likely to cause limb-threatening ischemia than in the leg. The priorities of prompt diagnosis and timely restoration of perfusion, however, remain applicable to upper extremity arterial trauma. A potentially limb-threatening situation is caused by injury to the brachial artery proximal to the origin of the profunda brachii artery

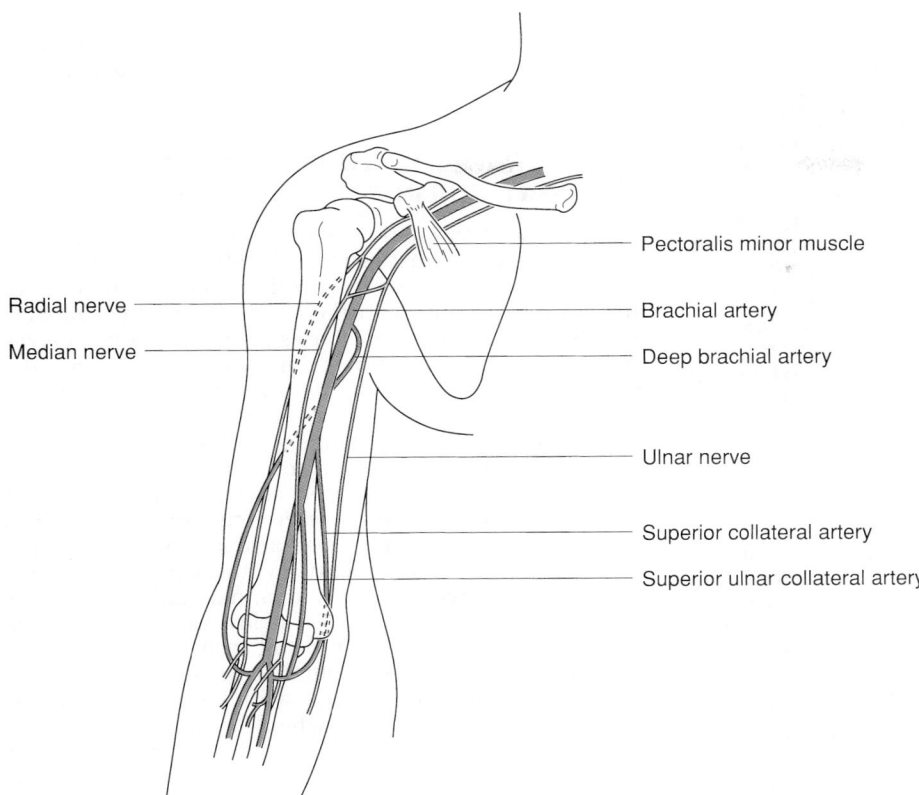

Figure 11.72. The proximity of the distal brachial artery to the humerus leads to a predisposition to arterial injury with supracondylar fractures.

or by occlusion of both the ulnar and radial arteries in the forearm; prompt arterial repair should be undertaken. In contrast, if isolated radial or ulnar artery occlusion occurs, reconstruction is not required provided adequate flow into the hand through the remaining vessel can be documented. Fasciotomy in the forearm is rarely required and

is necessary only after prolonged delays in restoration of flow or if there is extensive soft-tissue injury.

In the lower extremity, vascular trauma is a significant management challenge. The large muscle mass of the leg and the lack of significant arterial collaterals increase the risk of limb loss whenever arterial occlusion occurs. Early

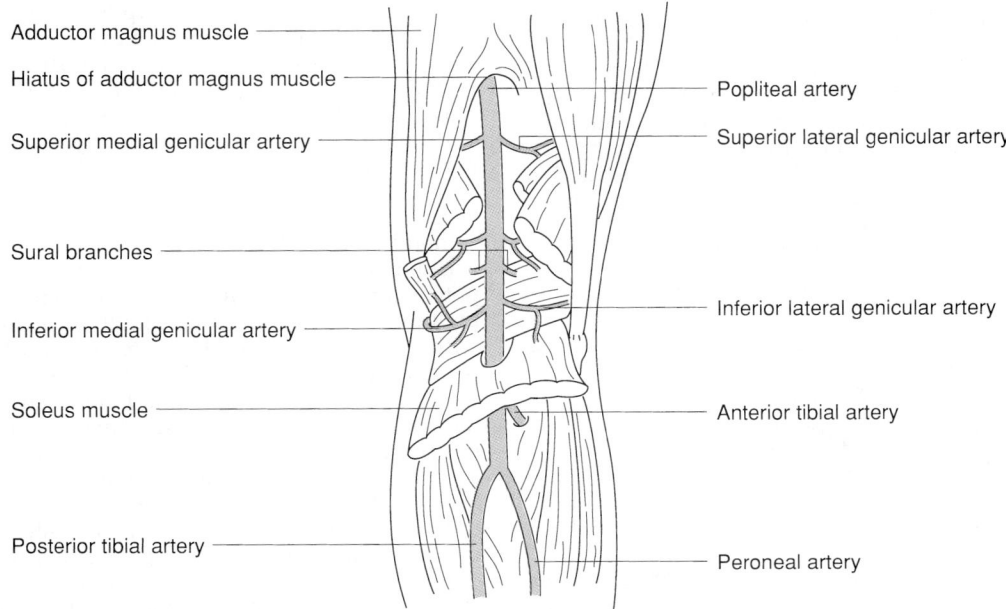

Figure 11.73. The popliteal artery is bound above and below the knee joint by the muscles of the thigh and calf and is immobile. Posterior knee dislocation frequently results in injury to the popliteal artery.

diagnosis, timely operation, and proper vascular technique are therefore essential. Injuries to the femoral arteries, whether blunt or penetrating, often can be successfully managed by direct repair. Popliteal artery injuries usually require interposition grafting (286). Isolated tibial vessel injury does not require treatment if one of the other leg arteries is patent. As outlined previously, the liberal use of fasciotomy in the lower leg is necessary to avoid compartment syndrome. After reconstruction, intraoperative completion arteriography and close postoperative monitoring are essential to detect and successfully treat early occlusion of the arterial reconstruction. The management of lower extremity venous injuries remains controversial, as has been discussed briefly. Whenever possible, veins should be repaired, but never at the expense of physiologic stability. Rarely, if soft-tissue and skeletal injury are extensive and significant vascular injury has occurred, primary amputation is required.

OUTCOME

The results of properly diagnosed and expeditiously treated vascular trauma are encouraging. The mortality rate after isolated peripheral vascular trauma is low, with no mortalities reported in many series. The mortality rate for suprarenal aortic injuries remains approximately 50% to 70%. Infrarenal aortic injuries have mortality rates of 20% to 40%. The amputation rate after peripheral vascular trauma continues to decrease, with several series reporting amputation rates of less than 2%. The recent improvement in limb salvage is a result of a combination of factors, most of which decrease the warm ischemia time. Early amputation, if necessary, appears to be related to prolonged ischemia but is clearly multifactorial. Late amputation is done primarily for disability or infection.

The initial success rate of vascular repair for traumatic injury approaches 100%. However, initial technical success implies neither limb salvage nor satisfactory functional outcome. The early results depend on the extent of the soft-tissue and bone injury. If successful soft-tissue healing occurs without infection, there is usually long-term vascular patency. The functional outcome, however, is directly related to the severity of orthopedic injury and can be particularly dependent on the extent of neurologic recovery. It is not uncommon to have a successful vascular repair result in a limb that is, for all intents and purposes, totally nonfunctional because of the underlying neurologic injury or the severity of disruption of muscle, bone, and ligament. A multidisciplinary approach with input from orthopedic surgery, plastic and reconstructive surgery, and, when needed, neurosurgery, in addition to comprehensive rehabilitation services is the best way to ensure the most successful long-term outcome.

Definitive Care Phase:
Orthopedic and Spinal Injuries

SANDRA L. ENGELHARDT AND ROBERT J. WINCHELL

Clinically significant orthopedic injuries occur in over 70% of multiply injured patients and are more than twice as common as serious intrathoracic or intraabdominal trauma (290). Orthopedic injuries are rarely immediately life threatening, but they can contribute greatly to morbid-

ity and are one of the principal determinants of functional recovery. For these reasons, it is imperative that the clinician caring for injured patients has a thorough understanding of basic orthopedic principles.

ORTHOPEDIC INJURIES AND THE PRIMARY SURVEY

The initial resuscitation of the trauma patient is directed at identifying and treating immediately life-threatening injuries that affect the airway, breathing, and circulation. Although major injuries to the head, chest, and abdomen usually take precedence, injuries to the axial spine, pelvis, or multiple long bones can significantly affect hemodynamic stability and the ability to assess other injuries.

Cervical spine fractures can cause varying degrees of respiratory compromise, ranging from loss of intercostal, abdominal wall, and cervical accessory muscles to apnea if the spinal cord is damaged above the phrenic nerve roots (C-3 to C-5). Patients with ventilatory failure from acute cord injury exhibit a paradoxical breathing pattern in which the abdomen seesaws with respiration. This is caused by paralysis of the abdominal wall musculature and may be seen with injuries as low as T-11. Decreased abdominal muscle tone can result in marked ventilatory insufficiency that is compounded by loss of intercostal and accessory muscles. Patients with high cervical lesions are even more seriously disabled because their muscle weakness is potentially exacerbated by loss of diaphragmatic function. Intubation and mechanical ventilation must be considered early, even in patients who initially appear well compensated. There is a tendency for respiratory failure to develop in such patients several hours after injury secondary to fatigue. With or without intubation, they are at high risk for pulmonary complications related to atelectasis and inadequate clearance of secretions.

In addition to pulmonary compromise, high spinal cord injuries can lead to significant hypotension. Most of the arteriolar tone is mediated through the sympathetic nervous system. Sympathetic nerves arise from the ventral roots of the thoracic spinal segments and are controlled by descending pathways from the brain stem. These controlling pathways may be interrupted in high thoracic and cervical cord injuries, resulting in loss of vasomotor tone. Lack of sympathetic drive to the sinoatrial node causes a predominance of vagal tone and bradycardia. This produces the classic clinical picture of spinal cord injury with hypotension and relative bradycardia. In contrast to patients with hypovolemic shock, the extremities of patients with high cord lesions are warm and well perfused because the injury ablates sympathetically mediated peripheral vasoconstriction.

Hypovolemia must be presumed to be the cause of hypotension in the initial evaluation of any trauma patient, including the patient with spinal cord injury. A patient with spinal shock should be managed with volume expansion until sources of significant blood loss have been ruled out and volume deficits have been replaced. Once the circulating volume has been restored and hemorrhage has been controlled, persistent hypotension is best managed with a pure α-adrenergic agonist like phenylephrine. Volume status should be optimized with the use of a central venous or pulmonary artery catheter to avoid fluid overload and exacerbation of pulmonary problems.

Hemorrhage from fracture sites is a potential cause of instability in the blunt trauma patient. Although hypovolemic shock *always should* prompt a search for intracavitary hemorrhage, bleeding from fractures and lacerations frequently contributes to hypotension and may be its sole cause. It is important, therefore, to assess the degree of bleeding caused by fractures. The fractured pelvis can be a source of life-threatening hemorrhage and must be identified early in the evaluation of the injured patient. Blood loss at a closed fracture site is frequently underestimated (291), and the amount of bleeding in the field from open fractures is often unknown. A closed femoral fracture may result in 1 to 2 units of blood loss (292). Closed tibial fractures typically cause loss of less than 1 unit of blood. Although multiple fractures can cause shock, hypotension is unusual in the setting of a single long-bone fracture. An additional source of bleeding is likely in such a patient.

Pain from orthopedic trauma can complicate the assessment of other injuries. Physical examination of the spine, chest, and abdomen relies on the patient's ability to report tenderness to palpation. Intense competitive pain from fractures may alter the perception of visceral pain or pain from spinal fractures. Therefore, in multiply injured patients, especially those with significant long-bone fractures, strong emphasis must be placed on the objective evaluation of all potential injuries. This equates to routine use of diagnostic peritoneal lavage, computed tomography, or ultrasonography to screen for intraabdominal injuries, and liberal use of radiographs to screen for fractures in these multiply injured patients.

TRUE ORTHOPEDIC EMERGENCIES

Most orthopedic injuries do not require truly emergent treatment. Fixation of skeletal injuries usually can be deferred until the patient is stable. Certain circumstances, however, dictate immediate therapy to preserve life and limb.

Pelvic Fracture

Many reports in the literature underscore the importance of hemorrhage associated with pelvic fractures (293,294). Fifteen percent to 20% of patients present with hypotension, and the mortality rate in this subgroup often exceeds 40% (295). High-energy mechanisms, such as those involved in motor vehicle crashes and falls from height, subject the patient to enormous forces. Therefore, there is a high incidence of serious associated injury, especially to the central nervous system and the abdominal viscera. Associated injuries contribute significantly to the 5% to 20% overall mortality rate for pelvic fractures. Equally important is the hemorrhage related to the broken pelvis itself. The severity of blood loss is usually related to the fracture's location. Anterior ring disruptions, located anterior to the acetabula and involving the superior and inferior rami, typically bleed 1 to 2 units. They are more commonly associated with urogenital injury than with massive hemorrhage. Fractures posterior to or involving the acetabula, especially vertical disruption of the sacroiliac joint, can produce life-threatening blood loss. Bone fragments can lacerate branches of the internal iliac artery, and the sacral venous plexus, intimately associated with the sacrum's anterior aspect, can be torn. There can also be significant bleeding from the fracture itself. Successful management of these patients requires an aggressive multidisciplinary approach, possibly involving early use of the pneumatic antishock garment (PASG) and selective use of external fixation devices and angiography with therapeutic embolization of bleeding vessels. The methods used to treat the patient with a pelvic fracture are institution dependent and should reflect the approach with which the orthopedic, interventional radiology, and trauma teams are most comfortable and familiar.

Spinal Cord Injury with Neurologic Compromise

After the critical problems with acute respiratory and circulatory embarrassment after spinal cord injury have been addressed, the approach to the patient is driven primarily by the stability of the neurologic condition. The nature of the fracture and the presence or absence of canal compromise are also important in determining initial therapy. Patients with over 50% effacement of the spinal canal and those with deteriorating neurologic examinations are candidates for emergency surgical decompression.

Careful neurologic assessment should be performed to determine the level of motor and sensory function, evaluate the presence of spinal shock, and assess whether the lesion is complete. Patients with a complete lesion have no sensory or motor function below the level of injury. Once spinal shock has resolved, a patient with an incomplete lesion demonstrates some sensory or motor function and sacral sparing of sensation. Patients with incomplete lesions and improving examination results are followed with serial neurologic testing. Stabilization is performed once the neurologic examination results have plateaued. Patients with significant canal compromise and a worsening examination may benefit from early surgery to decompress the spinal cord. Those with complete injuries, especially in the cervical spine, should be observed for a time before surgery to minimize the risk of further injury to the compromised spinal cord. The loss of even a single level of function during a prematurely performed operation can have a profound effect on the patient's ultimate rehabilitation status. Patients with a stable examination and an incomplete lesion represent difficult management decisions and must have their care individualized.

Clinical trials involving several pharmacologic interventions for patients with acute spinal cord injury are ongoing. In the Second National Acute Spinal Cord Injury Study, patients with spinal cord injury who received high doses of methylprednisolone sodium succinate within 8 hours of injury had improved neurologic recovery. At 6 weeks postinjury, treated patients demonstrated modest but statistically significant improvements in motor and sensory function. This benefit continued to be observed 6 months and 1 year after injury. Accepted treatment for patients with spinal cord injury consists of an initial bolus of 30 mg/kg of methylprednisolone followed by an infusion of 5.4 mg/kg/h for 23 hours. Steroid treatment begun more than 8 hours after injury has resulted in increased complications and worsened neurologic outcome, and should be avoided (296,297).

Patients with either complete or incomplete injuries should have definitive spinal stabilization at the earliest practical opportunity. Evidence from a variety of centers demonstrates prevention of early complications and significant acceleration of the rehabilitation process in patients undergoing early spinal stabilization.

Open Fracture

The importance of open fractures relates to the greatly increased risk of infection when a broken bone is associated with overlying soft-tissue injury. Aggressive management protocols for open fractures are designed to reduce the incidence of early infection, as well as the subsequent development of osteomyelitis and nonunion. The Gustilo classification (Table 11.17), initially applied to tibial fractures, offers a useful framework within which to classify these injuries (298,299).

All open fractures require thorough irrigation and débridement of devitalized tissues within 8 hours of injury.

Table 11.17. CLASSIFICATION OF OPEN FRACTURES

Type I	Wound <1 cm; low-energy mechanism, minimal crush damage or contamination
Type II	Wound 1–10 cm; high-energy mechanism, moderate soft-tissue damage
Type III	Wound >10 cm; high-energy mechanism, extensive soft-tissue damage; fracture often highly comminuted; automatically includes high-velocity gunshot wounds, displaced segmental fractures, extensive crush injuries, concomitant vascular injuries, and extensive contamination of soft tissues
Type IIIA	Limited periosteal stripping; no major soft-tissue defects; complex reconstruction usually not required
Type IIIB	Extensive periosteal stripping; major soft-tissue loss; complex reconstruction required
Type IIIC	Type IIIA or IIIB injury associated with major vascular injury

This should be performed using sterile technique in the operating room or resuscitation area. Patients should be treated with broad-spectrum parenteral antibiotics, usually a cephalosporin, with the addition of an aminoglycoside for grade III fractures.

Early stabilization is an important component of open fracture management. Challenges arise when local soft-tissue injury limits the options available for skeletal fixation. External fixation is often the best choice for fractures associated with large soft-tissue defects. In wounds involving less soft-tissue destruction, internal fixation is safe and may offer significant advantages in selected cases (300).

Bones broken by projectiles should be managed like other open fractures. With low-velocity gunshot wounds, débridement of the wound with immediate internal fixation of the fracture is well tolerated and associated with a low risk of infection. High-velocity wounds require extensive débridement and individualized management. Regardless of the mechanism of injury or the treatment method chosen, patients who undergo early fixation of open fractures fare better in both the short and long term.

Dislocations with Potential Neurovascular Compromise

Joint dislocations present with pain and deformity and may or may not be found in conjunction with fractures. The immediate importance of dislocations relates to the possibility of concomitant neurovascular injury (Table 11.18). Such injuries can be overlooked unless each joint and pulse is evaluated systematically. Vascular injuries

Table 11.18. ARTERIAL INJURIES ASSOCIATED WITH FRACTURES AND DISLOCATIONS

Orthopedic injury	Artery injured
Clavicle or first rib fracture	Subclavian artery
Anterior shoulder dislocation	Axillary artery
Humeral neck fracture	Axillary artery
Supracondylar humerus fracture	Brachial artery
Elbow dislocation	Brachial artery
Middle third femur fracture	Superficial femoral artery
Supracondylar femur fracture	Popliteal artery
Posterior knee dislocation	Popliteal artery
Proximal tibia/fibula dislocation	Popliteal artery, tibioperoneal trunk, anterior tibial artery

occur with 1% to 2% of most dislocations (301). An important exception is the posterior knee dislocation, which is associated with popliteal artery injury in one third of cases. There is a high incidence of limb loss if this injury is missed and not repaired (302). As a rule, any dislocation with neurovascular compromise must be reduced immediately. Angiography should be obtained in any patient with signs of vascular injury, with severe ligamentous disruption or multiple fractures around the knee, or in whom the pulse was absent before reduction.

Avascular necrosis of the femoral head is a disabling condition sometimes caused by acute dislocation of the hip. The femoral head's blood supply through the central artery is tenuous and is compromised by dislocation. In addition, tension on the joint capsule can greatly impede collateral flow. It is imperative to reduce hip dislocations as soon as possible to minimize the incidence of this complication.

Reduction of dislocations, particularly those involving large joints, may require considerable force to overcome muscular spasm and reestablish anatomic relations. Although reduction dramatically relieves pain, the process itself can be difficult for the surgeon and the patient. Dislocations of smaller joints can be reduced with analgesia alone, but those involving larger joints, especially the hip and knee, are often best reduced under general anesthesia. The absence of pain and profound muscle relaxation provide optimal conditions for anatomic reduction.

COMPARTMENT SYNDROME

When bleeding and edema occur in a closed fascial compartment, the pressure in the compartment may become high enough to impair capillary blood flow, impede oxygen delivery, and ultimately result in cellular death. This so-called compartment syndrome can occur after crush injury of an extremity, severe fractures, or after a period of ischemia followed by reperfusion. The ischemia–reperfusion mechanism typically follows repair of a vascular injury or, less frequently, occurs after use of the PASG or improper positioning of an extremity during surgery. Compartment syndrome may be present during the patient's initial evaluation, or it may not appear until the postoperative or postresuscitative period. It must be diagnosed expeditiously to avoid further damage to the extremity. In the patient with multiple injuries, this requires a thorough evaluation of all extremities and measurement of compartment pressures in any suspect limb. The clinical presentation and treatment of this syndrome are described in the segment of this chapter addressing vascular trauma.

SYSTEMATIC IMPACT OF ORTHOPEDIC INJURIES

Although rarely lethal in their own right, orthopedic injuries are often a source of major morbidity in trauma patients. The immobility imposed by fractures places the patient at increased risk for a variety of problems. Pulmonary complications are the most common of these. Several studies have demonstrated a decreased incidence in all types of pulmonary complications when early fixation of spine, long-bone, and pelvic fractures is used (303,304). Although early fixation allows prompt mobilization and improved pulmonary toilet, and is thought to contribute to improved outcomes for the multiply injured patient, a potential exception to this beneficial effect is discussed later.

One of the most catastrophic postinjury complications is pulmonary embolism (PE). Among patients who survive their initial injuries, it is one of the leading causes of death. All patients with orthopedic injury, particularly those with lower extremity, spine, and pelvic fractures, are at high risk for deep venous thrombosis (DVT) and subsequent PE. A randomized study of DVT and PE in trauma patients revealed an incidence of 8.8%, which could be reduced to 2.9% with the use of sequential compression devices or low-dose heparin. Among patients with spinal cord injury, this incidence was reduced from 27% to 10% (305). Prophylactic measures are therefore helpful, but imperfect, and DVT develops in a subset of patients despite maximal therapy. Aggressive prophylaxis and surveillance therefore are necessary for the multiply injured patient. This should include sequential compression devices, subcutaneous heparin if possible, and weekly venous duplex examinations of the lower extremities. It usually is possible to initiate low-dose heparin therapy in most trauma patients within the first 48 hours after injury (305). Patients who have contraindications to anticoagulation or who are immobilized secondary to multiple orthopedic injuries should be considered for placement of an inferior vena cava filter. Prophylactic vena cava filter placement has been shown to decrease the incidence of PE in high-risk trauma patients from 17% to 2.5% (306). The use of vena cava filters, although not risk free, is associated with a fairly low incidence of early complications (307). Collection of data regarding the truly long-term effects of filter placement is ongoing.

The classic triad of acute respiratory failure, altered mental status, and petechiae of the head, torso, and sclera suggests the fat embolism syndrome. The syndrome is to be distinguished from fat embolism, which is simply the presence of fat globules in the peripheral circulation and lung parenchyma after long-bone fracture or multiple trauma. This can be detected by various techniques in greater than 90% of patients with long-bone fractures. Fat embolism syndrome is less common and has an incidence of 0.5% to 2.0% in patients with isolated long-bone fractures and of 5% to 10% in patients with multiple long-bone or concomitant pelvic fractures (308,309). A high index of suspicion is necessary when looking for this syndrome because most patients do not present with the typical fulminant course (310). There are no reliable tests to confirm the diagnosis. The presence of lipiduria or of fat globules in alveolar macrophages on bronchoalveolar lavage, previously thought to be diagnostic of the syndrome, has been shown to be nonspecific (310).

The pathophysiologic process of fat embolism syndrome has been the subject of much debate. Recent work suggests that an interaction of fat, platelets and the clotting cascade results in intravascular coagulation and leukocyte activation. The inflammatory response causes endothelial damage, increased capillary permeability, and decreased levels of functional surfactant in the lung. These changes produce hypoxemia and pulmonary edema, which may progress to the adult respiratory distress syndrome (ARDS).

The only current therapy for fat embolism syndrome is supportive care with mechanical ventilation and intensive care unit monitoring as needed. Although the use of corticosteroid therapy has been shown to attenuate the pulmonary injury induced by intravascular infusion of free fatty acids in animals (311), human trials merely suggest a benefit from their use (312). Concerns about increased infection risk and the inability to predict who will be affected by fat embolism syndrome limit the usefulness of steroid therapy.

Early fracture fixation has been advocated as a means of reducing the incidence of fat embolism syndrome. Some researchers have challenged this concept, and have reported that a subset of patients with femoral fractures and pulmonary contusion had a higher incidence of ARDS if fractures were repaired early rather than late (313). Avoidance of reaming of the femoral canal may prevent this effect (314). Further analysis of this subgroup is needed to define the optimal management scheme for these patients.

Patients with spinal fractures associated with cord injuries are vulnerable to a myriad of immediate and delayed morbidities. Although these complications are not unique to patients with spinal cord injuries, their clinical presentation may be dramatically altered, leading to serious delays in diagnosis. Extra surveillance and prophylactic measures for gastrointestinal, genitourinary, and integumentary complications are warranted in patients with spine fractures and neurologic compromise.

OTHER ISSUES IN ORTHOPEDIC TRAUMA

General Principles of Fracture Fixation

During the initial phase of treatment, immobilization is sufficient management for most extremity fractures. Definitive treatment ranges from simple anatomic reduction and casting to complex open reduction and internal fixation. The choice of therapy involves a number of variables and is aimed at optimizing functional recovery.

Fractures of the lower extremity can be classified roughly by anatomic site. Hip fractures, including those of the proximal femur, almost always require rigid fixation to maintain anatomic relations and hip function. Although midshaft femoral fractures can be treated with skeletal traction and bed rest, most are managed with intramedullary rods that allow early ambulation. Simple fractures of the lower leg are well managed with cast application and crutch mobilization. Complex fractures usually call for internal fixation to obtain adequate anatomic realignment. Ankle fractures almost always require open reduction and internal fixation to achieve good functional recovery.

Upper extremity fractures often can be managed with closed techniques. Breaks of the proximal and middle third of the humerus rarely need rigid fixation because accurate anatomic reduction is not critical. Fractures around the elbow are more likely to require open reduction and internal fixation to preserve function. In the lower arm, fractures involving only one bone (ulna or radius) are most commonly managed by casting. Involvement of both bones almost always necessitates internal fixation to preserve rotational function of the forearm. Wrist fractures commonly demand rigid fixation to maintain anatomic reduction. Similarly, fractures of the small bones of the hand often require rigid fixation because accurate alignment is vital to function.

Fixation can be achieved by a variety of methods, including intramedullary instrumentation, various plates, screws and wires, and external fixators. Completely implantable instrumentation is preferred. In open fractures, however, especially those with soft-tissue loss, risk of infection often necessitates use of the external technique. External fixators are usually rapidly applied and obviate the need for long operations with potentially significant blood loss in critically ill, multiply injured patients.

Mangled Extremities

The badly damaged extremity with significant skeletal, soft-tissue, and neurovascular injury presents a difficult management problem. Complex open fractures with degloving, near-amputation, or extensive nerve and vessel injuries may be technically repairable, but the salvage of a painful and functionally useless limb serves little purpose. Reconstructive efforts often require multiple operations and may continue for years. By comparison, young patients who undergo primary amputation usually return to productive lives within a year of injury. The decision to proceed with the primary amputation of a mangled extremity can be exceedingly difficult, but it is of vital importance. A variety of scoring systems, including the Mangled Extremity Severity Score (MESS), Mangled Extremity Severity Index (MESI), Limb Salvage Index (LSI), and Predictive Salvage Index (PSI), have been designed to facilitate the prediction of patients who will require amputation (315–318). Although all of the scoring systems are able to identify most of the patients who require amputation, none is able to predict functional outcome (319). Decisions regarding a mangled extremity require a multidisciplinary approach, and it is the responsibility of the general trauma surgeon to consider the impact of attempts at limb salvage on the overall care of the patient.

Timing of Fracture Fixation

An important advance in trauma care has been the recognition that early treatment of orthopedic injuries (i.e., within 24 hours) is associated with decreased hospital stay, shortened intensive care unit stay, and diminished morbidity and mortality rates. Early fixation of orthopedic injuries must be incorporated into the overall resuscitation of the patient and must be individualized. Previously accepted contraindications to early orthopedic surgery, such as burns (320) or head injury (321,322), have been challenged. Some contraindications still exist (323), including hemodynamic instability, significant hypothermia, or coagulopathy. In these situations, it is likely that prolonged surgery or additional blood loss will jeopardize the patient's survival or potential for meaningful neurologic recovery. When such problems are encountered, surgery should not be postponed indefinitely. Rather, aggressive correction of the abnormality should be undertaken, with frequent reappraisal of the patient's readiness for orthopedic repair at the earliest possible opportunity.

Early orthopedic intervention must be efficient and expert. Long operations by inexperienced personnel not only negate the benefit of early intervention, but can cause increased morbidity and mortality. There are occasions in which the care of orthopedic injuries is compromised by patient instability. This may necessitate washout of open fractures or fasciotomy at the bedside in the intensive care unit. More rarely, it may mean that the patient's life is preserved at the expense of the viability or function of an injured limb. Because such patients require the expertise of multiple subspecialties, the general trauma surgeon must be familiar with diagnostic and therapeutic options and use this knowledge to coordinate the optimal care of these challenging patients.

Definitive Care Phase: Pediatric Trauma

M. MARGARET KNUDSON

EPIDEMIOLOGY

Injury remains the single most important health problem for children and adolescents. An estimated 22 million children are injured each year in the United States, and the death and disabilities resulting from trauma surpass all other major diseases in the pediatric population. The best available data on pediatric trauma are maintained in the National Pediatric Trauma Registry (324). To date, data have been collected on over 27,000 pediatric trauma patients cared for at the 85 participating trauma centers. Over 90% of the injuries in this population resulted from blunt mechanisms, and were unintentional. Only 3% of these children died, but 40% were left with functional limitations. Most of those who died did so before they ever reached the hospital; thus, *the most effective method of reducing deaths in children and adolescents is injury prevention.*

Figure 11.74 summarizes the data from the National Pediatric Trauma Registry by mechanism of injury. As can be seen, protective measures (e.g., child restraint devices, helmets) were seldom used. When examining these data by age of the child, it becomes apparent that falls are the major mechanism of injury in children younger than 10 years of age, but carry a mortality rate of less than 1%. On the other hand, pedestrian injuries are the next most common in frequency, with an associated mortality rate of 5%. Among adolescents, motor vehicular trauma is the major mechanism of injury, with an associated mortality rate of 4%; gunshot wounds are fourth in order of frequency, but carry the highest mortality rate (10%). Mortality rates for all types of trauma are greater in rural parts of the country than in cities and suburbs, presumably because of longer times from injury to definitive care (325,326).

A striking difference between injured children and adults is that the "trimodal" mortality curve described in

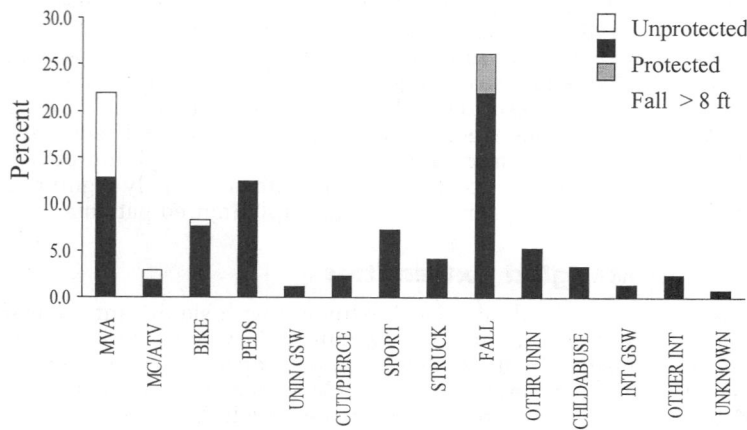

Figure 11.74. Mechanism of injury in pediatric trauma from the National Pediatric Trauma Registry data. Note the large incidence of unrestrained passengers and unhelmeted bicycle riders.

adult patients is not seen in children. Those pediatric patients who die do so either at the scene or within a few hours of hospital admission. Late deaths due to sepsis or organ failure are decidedly rare in young children. Next to injury control, then, the most important method of saving lives and preventing disability after pediatric trauma is prompt recognition and emergent treatment of all life-threatening injuries.

PREHOSPITAL CARE

Pediatric patients represent only 10% of all paramedic calls in this country, and some have questioned whether prehospital providers are capable of maintaining the skills necessary to resuscitate severely injured children. Some authors have reported fatalities in the prehospital arena that were associated with inadequate airway management in children, whereas others have found similar success rates with intubation in children as in adults (327,328). Clearly, it is the responsibility of physicians involved in training prehospital providers to ensure continued practice in airway management and fluid resuscitation techniques for all patients, regardless of age. Similarly, all ambulances must be equipped with pediatric equipment in various sizes, including blood pressure cuffs, masks, endotracheal tubes, and intravenous (IV) access devices.

As with all injured patients, prehospital care of pediatric patients should be limited to maintaining spinal precautions, assurance of an adequate airway, administration of oxygen, and rapid transport to definitive care. Establishment of IV access is unnecessary unless the transport time is longer than 20 minutes. For very young children in shock, we have been particularly pleased with the use of intraosseous infusions in the prehospital setting. These devices can be rapidly established in an emergency vehicle during transport, thus avoiding delays. Preventing secondary brain insults associated with hypoxia or hypotension in the prehospital arena by providing fluid and controlling the airway has the potential to significantly affect the outcome after major head trauma in children.

The inclusive trauma system must provide for the needs of injured children as well as adults. Prehospital providers must be instructed to deliver the injured child to the closest appropriate facility with the capabilities of caring for major trauma. This may be a pediatric trauma center or a regional trauma center with pediatric commitment. The receiving center must have the necessary personnel and equipment to care for the injured child, as outlined in *Resources for Optimal Care of the Injured Patient: 1999* by the Committee on Trauma, American College of Surgeons. Thus, when *primary* prevention methods have failed, the goal shifts to minimizing the trauma once it has occurred *(secondary prevention)* and to preventing postinjury complications *(tertiary prevention)*.

INITIAL RESUSCITATION AND EVALUATION

Preparation is the key to a successful pediatric trauma resuscitation. In addition to having the proper equipment in the room, the room itself must be warmed in advance so that heat loss can be prevented. Small children are especially prone to hypothermia, which in turn may render the child unresponsive to resuscitation efforts. Use of convective air blankets can be helpful, if the blankets are left in place. All IV fluids should be warmed and the head wrapped, if possible, because small children lose substantial amounts of heat through their relatively large heads.

As with all trauma resuscitations, the initial focus is on the airway. The best protection for the airway in the child who is breathing spontaneously is to maintain a superior and anterior position of the middle face (sniffing position), while keeping the cervical spine immobilized. If the airway is inadequate, it can be opened with a gentle chin lift or jaw thrust. Because infants are obligate nose breathers, clearing of the nasal passages may be required. The mouth is cleared of blood and foreign material and supplemental oxygen is applied in all cases. In a young child, respiratory compromise can result from gastric dilatation or from compression of the diaphragm by intraabdominal blood or air. The use of nasogastric or orogastric tubes is therefore necessary in pediatric trauma patients.

Children with obvious respiratory distress, with major head injury, or those who arrive in shock must have endotracheal intubation immediately. The proper-sized endotracheal tube can be estimated by choosing one that corresponds to the diameter of the child's small finger or the nares (Table 11.19). One good approach is the use of color-coded drawers with all the equipment necessary for a certain size child, using the Broselow Pediatric Resuscitation Measuring Tape to estimate the child's weight. (Fig. 11.75). In children younger than 12 years of age, nasotracheal intubation is avoided because of the small size of the tube and the potentially serious complications associated with blind passage. Compared with an adult, the child's airway is more cephalad and anterior, and the trachea is soft and short (7 cm by 18 months). These anatomic changes must be kept in mind during intubation. After preoxygenation, a rapid-sequence intubation is performed as outlined in Fig. 11.76. A chest radiograph should be obtained to confirm proper position of the endotracheal tube. If the airway cannot be secured by the most senior person in the resuscitation room, a temporizing needle cricothyroidotomy is placed and jet insufflation initiated, until an airway can be established in the operating room. There should be no attempt at emergency department tracheostomy in young children. This is reserved for experienced surgeons under operating room conditions only.

After assurance of an adequate airway, attention is directed toward establishment of IV access. Preferred sites for percutaneous access are the back of the hand, the antecubital fossa, and the saphenous vein at the ankle. If the child is in shock, and no IV line can be established after two attempts, an intraosseous nail is placed in an uninjured proximal tibia (in children 6 years or younger). Alternatively, percutaneous femoral vein lines can be placed by an experienced physician. It is important to follow a protocol so that time is not wasted by too many attempts at percutaneous IV access before resuscitation can begin.

Table 11.20 outlines the normal vital signs for children of various ages. A child's systolic blood pressure should

---

Table 11.19. EXAMPLES OF APPROPRIATELY SIZED ENDOTRACHEAL AND THOROCOSTOMY TUBES[a]

Age	Endotracheal tube	Thoracostomy tube
Premature	2.5 mm	12F
Newborn	3.0 mm	14F
Toddler	4.5 mm	20F
6 y	5.5 mm	24F
10 y	6.5 mm	28F
Adolescent	7.0 mm	32F

[a]The Broselow Pediatric Resuscitation Tape can also be used to estimate weight based on the height of the child to select appropriate drug doses.
From Lubitz DS, Siedel JS, Chameides L, et al. A rapid method for estimating weight and resuscitation drug dosages from length in the pediatric age group. Ann Emerg Med 1988;17:567, with permission.

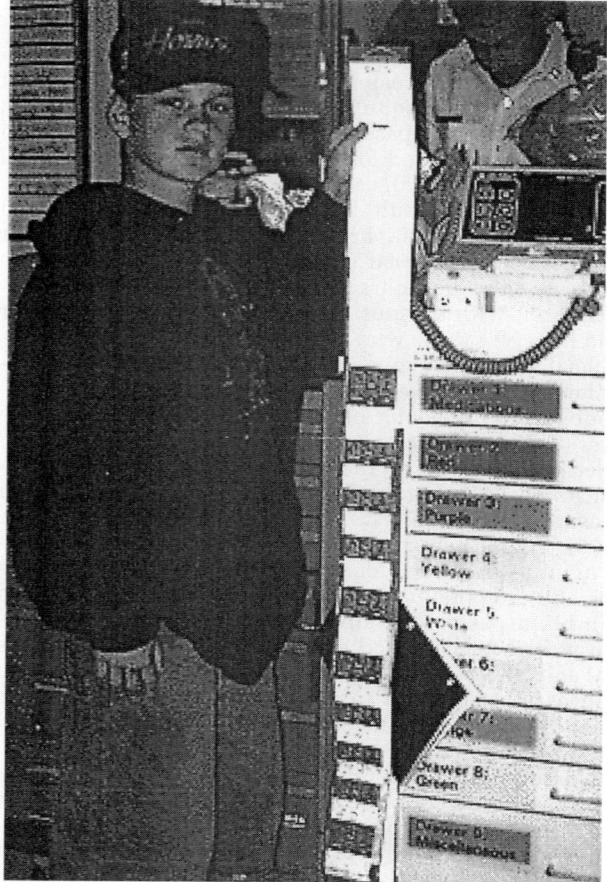

Figure 11.75. The Broselow Resuscitation Measuring Tape and the corresponding cart with drawers to match the colors/sizes on the tape. Each drawer contains the appropriately sized equipment for each size of child.

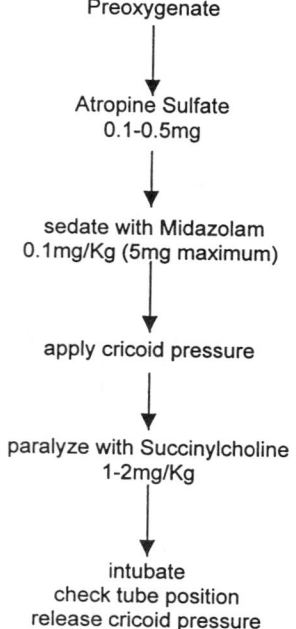

Figure 11.76. Rapid-sequence intubation for the pediatric patient.

Table 11.20. NORMAL VITAL SIGNS BY AGE

	Pulse	Systolic blood pressure (mm Hg)	Respiratory rate
Infant (<1 y)	160	80	40
Preschool (<5 y)	140	90	30
Adolescent (>10 y)	120	100	20

be 80 mm Hg plus twice the age in years. In general, a blood pressure of less than 80 mm Hg systolic is considered to be shock in a child, with the exception of small infants. Hypotension, however, is a late sign of shock in a child because of the child's increased physiologic reserve compared with an adult. The initial signs of shock can be very subtle in a child, and may be manifested by only a slight tachycardia or lethargy. Once hypotension has developed, the child has already lost approximately 45% of the circulating blood volume and death is imminent if treatment is delayed.

Resuscitation begins with 20 mL/kg of warmed lactated Ringer's solution given as a push (Fig. 11.77). This can be repeated twice, but if the child remains in shock, the source of bleeding should be quickly addressed. Transfusions of packed cells are given at a dose of 10 mL/kg. In addition to reestablishment of normal blood pressure, a proper response to resuscitation includes a slowing of the heart rate, return of skin color and warmth to the extremities, clearing of the sensorium, and a urinary output of 1 to 2 mL/kg/h.

During the resuscitation, radiographic studies of the chest and pelvis are performed and cervical spine protection is maintained until at least three views can be obtained (anteroposterior, lateral, and odontoid). Clearing of the cervical spine is relatively elective; time should not be wasted on these films if other injuries take priority. In the unstable child, a quick sonographic evaluation of the pericardium and the peritoneum (the FAST examination, or *f*ocused *s*onographic *a*ssessment for *t*rauma) for blood can be helpful in establishing the priorities of treatment (Fig. 11.78). Blood in the pericardial or peritoneal cavity in the persistently unstable child demands surgical intervention. In the stable child, a computed tomography (CT) scan of the abdomen with contrast is indicated when one of the following conditions is met:

- History of shock but now stable
- Unexplained drop in hematocrit
- Presence of hematuria
- Presence of lower rib or pelvic fractures
- Unreliable abdominal examination because of head injury
- Presence of abdominal pain/ecchymosis
- Uncorrected base deficit

Although ultrasound is reasonably sensitive in detecting the presence of fluid in the abdomen, its accuracy is highly dependent on the operator. Although limited, initial experience with the FAST examination in pediatric trauma patients has been favorable, and some data suggest that hospital resources are conserved when the FAST examination is incorporated into the algorithm in the evaluation of the pediatric abdomen after blunt trauma (329). Ultrasound, however, may not detect the presence of solid organ injuries without free blood, may miss small amounts of blood early in the resuscitation, cannot be used to stage the degree of injury to a solid organ, and cannot exclude pancreatic injury. In addition, the finding of blood in the peritoneum in a stable child does not dictate laparotomy. For

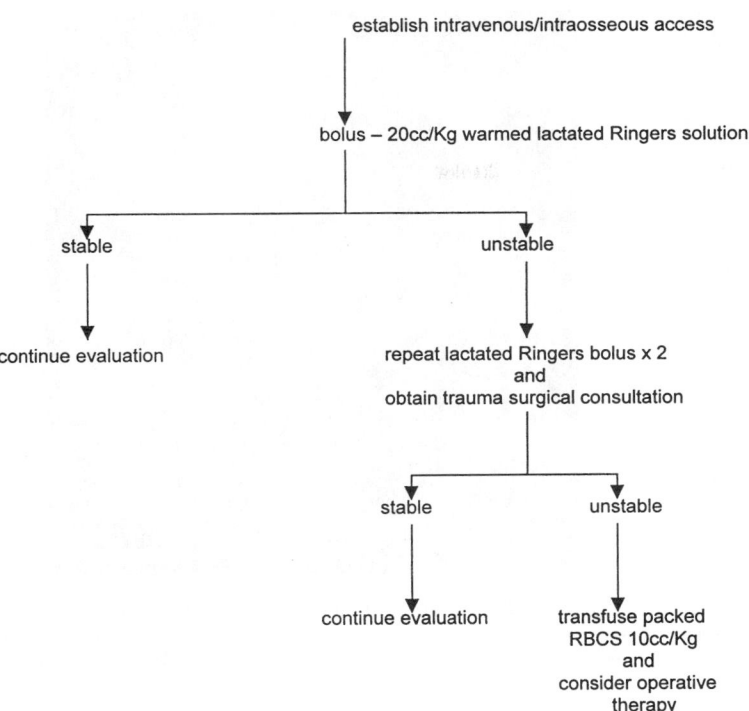

establish intravenous/intraosseous access

bolus – 20cc/Kg warmed lactated Ringers solution

stable

continue evaluation

unstable

repeat lactated Ringers bolus x 2
and
obtain trauma surgical consultation

stable

continue evaluation

unstable

transfuse packed
RBCS 10cc/Kg
and
consider operative
therapy

Figure 11.77. Pediatric resuscitation algorithm.

all of these reasons, the role of FAST in pediatric trauma patients remain controversial. Neither ultrasound nor CT reliably detects the presence of a bowel injury (see later).

Throughout this critical period of resuscitation and evaluation, the emotional needs of the child must be kept constantly in mind. The frightened child is emotionally labile and may regress to infantile behavior. A calm and reassuring approach with attempted explanation of procedures gains the most cooperation. There is evidence that the psychological effects surrounding a traumatic event are long lasting, even if the trauma is relatively minor (see later). The needs of the "injured" family must also be met by providing a continual flow of information to the distressed parents during the resuscitation.

MANAGEMENT OF SPECIFIC INJURIES

Neurologic Trauma

Head injury is the leading cause of death in children who have sustained trauma. According to the National Pediatric Trauma Registry, 26% of all injured children have sustained central nervous system trauma (330). In those children who survive, the long-term disabilities have a major impact on the quality of life for them and for their families. Unique to infants is the large number of head injuries resulting from child abuse. Although children in general have a higher survival rate after head injury, they

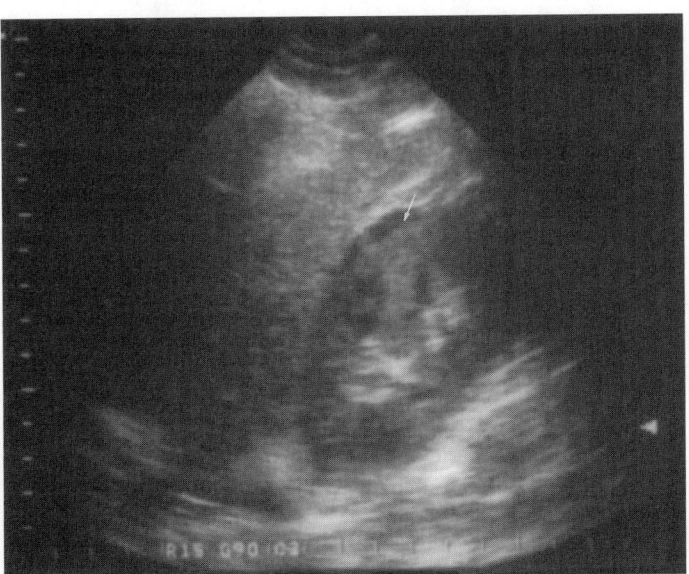

Figure 11.78. Positive FAST (*f*ocused *s*onographic *a*ssessment for *t*rauma) examination showing a small amount of fluid in Morison's pouch (right hepatorenal space).

actually may be more vulnerable to long-term disability than adults. In addition, in children who have the combination of head injury and hypotension, the age advantage generally associated with childhood is eliminated.

Evaluation of the child with head injury begins with assurance of adequate airway, breathing, and circulation to avoid secondary brain insults. A thorough neurologic examination is performed and documented, including the Glasgow Coma Scale (GCS) score. The verbal portion of the score has been adapted for application in children (Table 11.21), but it is the motor score that correlates best with outcome. Except for the most minor cases, a head CT scan is performed in all children with evidence of neurologic injury. Although mass lesions from hemorrhage requiring surgical intervention are relatively uncommon in children, cerebral edema is very common, and such a finding on CT scan dictates the treatment (Fig. 11.79).

Children with a GCS score of 8 or less and those with evidence of cerebral edema on CT scan require sedation, paralysis, endotracheal intubation, and mechanical ventilation to keep the $PaCO_2$ at approximately 35 mm Hg. An intracranial pressure monitor (or ventriculostomy catheter) is placed so that cerebral perfusion pressure can be maintained at at least 70 mm Hg. Brain metabolism is minimized by treating fever and avoiding seizures. Despite aggressive treatment, the overall mortality rate from severe head injury in pediatric patients is 6%, and the coexistence of extracranial injury significantly reduces recovery potential.

Fortunately, only 5% of all spinal cord injuries occur in children. Certain anatomic features predispose younger children (age ≤8 years) to injury of the upper cervical spine, from the occiput to the base of C-2 (331,332). These characteristics include a proportionately heavier head and weak ligaments that permit greater mobility in C-1 to C-2 compared with the lower spine; horizontally inclined articulating facets and immature vertebral joints that facilitate sliding; growth centers that are susceptible to shear forces during rapid deceleration or hyperflexion–extension; and a higher fulcrum of flexion. In children older than 8 years, cervical spine fractures are seen primarily at C-5 to C-6, resulting from motor vehicular trauma or from diving mishaps.

Some normal anatomic variables make interpretation of cervical spine films in children somewhat challenging. Pseudosubluxation occurs normally in approximately 40% of children, most commonly seen as anterior displacement of C-2 on C-3. An increased distance between the dens and the anterior arch of C-1 also may occur without any pathologic consequences. Skeletal growth centers may resemble fractures, especially at the odontoid and the spinous processes. If there is doubt over whether an abnormality exists, it is wise to protect the spine until expert consultation can be arranged.

Another abnormality seen more commonly in children is spinal cord injury without radiologic abnormality (SCI-

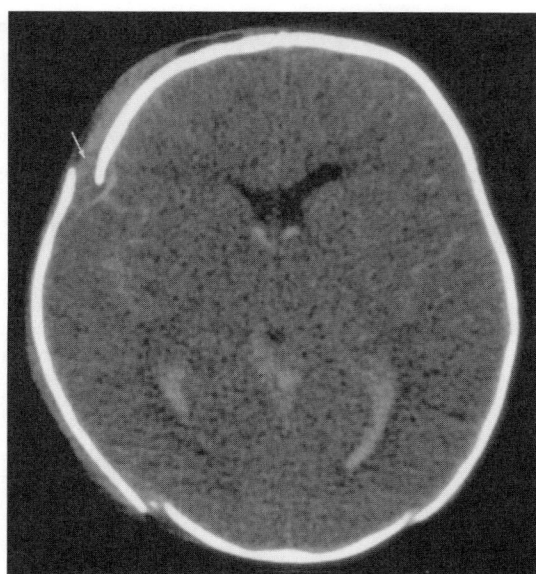

Figure 11.79. Computed tomography scan of the head in a child with massive head trauma. Note the skull fracture with underlying brain edema and compression of the underlying ventricle.

WORA). Some authors have suggested that SCIWORA represents more than 50% of spinal cord injuries in children, especially for those younger than 8 years of age (333). This phenomenon is attributed to the elastic nature of the child's spine and may result from longitudinal distraction, hyperflexion, hyperextension, or spinal cord ischemia. SCIWORA may present with a central cord syndrome (i.e., upper limbs weaker than the lower limbs). The diagnosis is established by magnetic resonance imaging, and high-dose steroid therapy should be initiated immediately.

Thoracic Trauma

Blunt thoracic trauma may result in pulmonary contusion, hemothorax, pneumothorax, and rib fractures. Although rib fractures are less common in children than in adults because of the elastic nature of the chest wall, when they do occur, they represent a high-energy transfer to the chest. Some authors have reported mortality rates of 25% to 50% in children with major chest injuries. Pulmonary contusion may not be obvious on the initial chest radiograph, but can produce hypoxia after several hours. Hemothoraces and pneumothoraces are managed as in adults (see Table 11.23 for chest tube sizes). Tracheobronchial disruption should be suspected in a child with a tension pneumothorax, massive subcutaneous emphysema, and a continuing air leak or persistent collapse of the lung despite a functioning chest tube. The diagnosis is confirmed by bronchoscopy.

Although initially thought to be rare, blunt cardiac injuries do occur in children and range from mild to lethal. One multicenter review from 16 institutions over 10 years identified 184 cases of blunt cardiac injury (334). The primary mechanisms of injury associated with this diagnosis were motor vehicle and pedestrian crashes. Although no hemodynamically stable patient with a normal sinus rhythm subsequently had a cardiac dysrhythmia or cardiac failure, there were three deaths attributed to pump failure after blunt cardiac trauma, and 5% of the survivors had significant valvular dysfunction. In another study, 14% of 282 children who died after trauma had evidence of cardiac injuries, and rupture of a cardiac chamber was

Table 11.21. PEDIATRIC VERBAL SCORE

Verbal response	V-score
Appropriate words or social smile, fixes and follows	5
Cries, but consolable	4
Persistently irritable	3
Restless, agitated	2
None	1

Adapted from American College of Surgeons Committee on Trauma. Advanced trauma life support course: instructor manual. Chicago: American College of Surgeons, 1997.

identified as the major cause of death from blunt cardiac trauma (335). Although it is obvious that significant cardiac injuries rarely occur in isolation, and that most of these children die at the scene, a few survive and are transported to trauma centers. Use of the FAST examination can readily identify these children and allow for prompt treatment.

Thoracic aortic rupture is also a rare injury in children but is highly lethal if undiagnosed. A report from the National Pediatric Trauma Registry describes 29 patients (from a total of 53,000) with traumatic aortic disruptions and a mortality rate of 51% (336). Multisystem trauma from motor vehicle crashes or pedestrian collisions are the most common scenarios in these children. The mechanism of injury and a chest radiograph demonstrating a widened mediastinum should raise suspicion and prompt investigation. Dynamic spiral CT scan of the chest may be used as a screening test, but arch angiography remains the most definitive method of diagnosis. Good outcomes can be expected from early diagnosis, antihypertensive therapy, and definitive operative management.

Abdominal Trauma

Twenty-five percent of children who sustain trauma have abdominal injuries because the protruding pediatric abdomen receives little protection from the short rib cage and small pelvis. The kidney is relatively large and anterior, and a significant abdominal blow often manifests with hematuria. Hematuria, however, is associated with a liver or splenic injury more often than with a significant renal injury; therefore, the presence of hematuria demands an objective evaluation of the abdomen. Because of the limitations of physical examination of the abdomen in young children, most stable pediatric trauma patients with major injury mechanisms or abdominal tenderness are best evaluated with abdominal CT scans (see earlier for the indications for CT scans in the pediatric patient). Although some authors advise against the use of gastrointestinal contrast in pediatric patients, citing the potential for aspiration, most pediatric institutions administer both IV and oral contrast for abdominal CT. We have not seen complications with this approach, and the presence of oral or gastrointestinal contrast greatly enhances the specificity of the examination. On the other hand, persistently unstable patients should undergo a FAST examination in the trauma room, and those with positive findings should be taken straight to surgery (Fig. 11.80).

The approach to solid organ injuries (liver, spleen, kidney) discovered on CT scan is primarily observational. Most (>90%) of these injuries heal without operation (Fig. 11.81). The indications for surgery in children with solid organ injuries include evidence of ongoing bleeding, uncorrected base deficit, hemodynamic instability, the development of peritoneal signs or other signs and symptoms of an associated gastrointestinal injury, or major urinary extravasation or necrosis in the presence of renal injuries (Fig. 11.82). In one study, the need for operation in pediatric patients with liver injury was predicted by a low Trauma Score on arrival, a 25% or greater lobar disruption with pelvic blood collections seen on CT scan, and the need for transfusion within the first 2 hours of admission (337). Thus, although most pediatric patients with blunt abdominal trauma do not require operation, the need for surgical judgment in determining those children who fail nonoperative therapy is critical.

Although there is general agreement that the initial approach to the pediatric trauma patient with solid organ injury is nonoperative, until recently there has been little consensus on the need for intensive care, the amount of transfusion considered acceptable, the need for and timing of follow-up imaging procedures, and the activities allowed after discharge. One review of the practice patterns of pediatric surgeons caring for stable patients with traumatic solid organ injuries revealed a very low incidence of nonoperative failures (zero in some centers), a general agreement that transfusions were not required unless the hemoglobin fell to 7 to 8 g/dL, and that most children should be observed in an intensive care unit (ICU) setting for 24 to 48 hours (338). Children were allowed out of bed when the hematocrit had stabilized, the pain had resolved, and hematuria was no longer present (renal injuries). Most surgeons agreed that stabilization of hematocrit was the most important factor in determining the timing of discharge. However, there was general lack of agreement on the need for follow-up imaging and the recommendations on activity level after discharge. Although the liver usually does not rebleed once it has stopped, delayed rupture of the spleen is a recognized complication of nonoperative management. Fortunately, these delayed ruptures occur most commonly in the first few days after injury, while the child is still in the hospital. Delayed rupture is associated with continued bleeding under the splenic capsule that eventually bursts, or is due to the presence of a splenic arterial injury that ruptures (pseudoaneurysm). These complications of splenic injury are readily apparent on a follow-up CT scan.

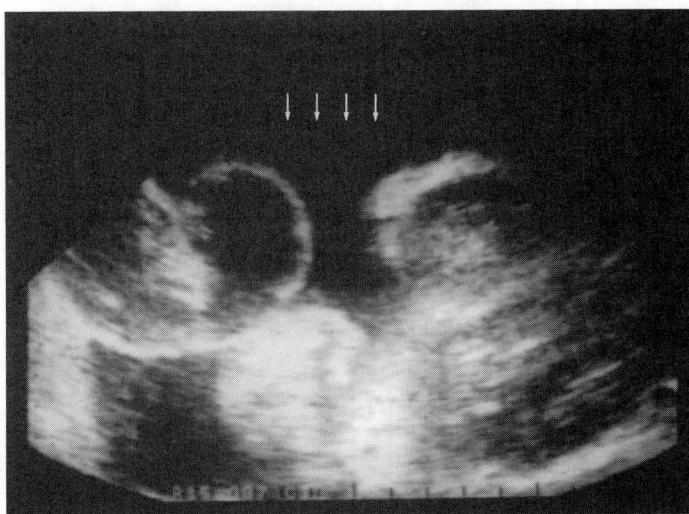

Figure 11.80. Pelvic ultrasound in a child with a ruptured spleen demonstrating a large amount of blood with floating loops of small intestine. The child, who also had a major head injury, was unstable and treated with immediate splenectomy.

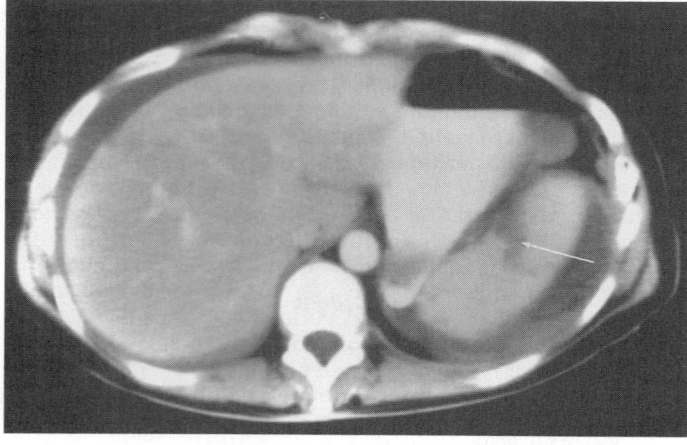

Figure 11.81. Computed tomography scan of the abdomen in a child who was hemodynamically stable. Note the grade III laceration of the spleen with blood around the liver. This child was managed successfully without surgery.

Other authors have documented complete resolution of these injuries by CT imaging 6 weeks after injury and concluded that outpatient CT imaging seldom changed clinical management unless a return to contact sports before 6 weeks postinjury was being considered (339). Thus, a reasonable approach to the stable child with a solid organ injury can be outlined as follows:

- Documentation of the degree of injury by CT scan
- A short ICU stay until the hematocrit has stabilized
- Allow ambulation when out of the ICU
- Allow oral intake when the ileus resolves
- Discharge when eating and ambulating without pain
- CT scan before discharge for all splenic and renal injuries
- Selectively repeat CT scan for those with liver injuries
- Documentation of injury resolution before contact sports
- Continued investigation into the use of ultrasound in follow-up

Pancreatic injuries occur in less than 1% of pediatric trauma patients, but carry a high morbidity and mortality rate if overlooked. The mechanism of injury is usually a blow to the epigastrium, as with the handlebars of a bicycle, or, in some cases, child abuse. Abdominal tenderness frequently is absent initially. The most sensitive diagnostic study is an abdominal CT scan with contrast, but this injury can be missed on the initial scan. The approach to a blunt pancreatic injury is conservative unless major ductal disruption is present (340). Postinjury complications include pancreatic fistula, but even this complication may resolve with drainage alone (Fig. 11.83).

With abdominal CT scan as the cornerstone of diagnosis after blunt abdominal trauma in children, and with the general nonoperative approach to solid organ injuries, much attention has been directed toward the diagnosis of small intestinal injuries in these patients (341–343). Blunt intestinal injuries occur in 1% to 5% of pediatric patients with abdominal trauma, and the initial findings on physical examination may be subtle. Findings on CT scan may be equally subtle; rarely is extravasation of contrast material seen. However, the presence of free fluid in the pelvis that is not associated with a solid organ injury should raise the question of intestinal injury. Other signs of these injuries on CT scan include blood or streaking in the mesentery and thickening of the bowel wall (Fig. 11.84). The presence of a small intestinal injury also should be suspected when there are associated spinal fractures caused by the use of a lap belt (lap belt complex or "Chance" fractures) without a shoulder harness, as shown in Fig. 11.85 (344). Occasionally, a blunt injury to the ab-

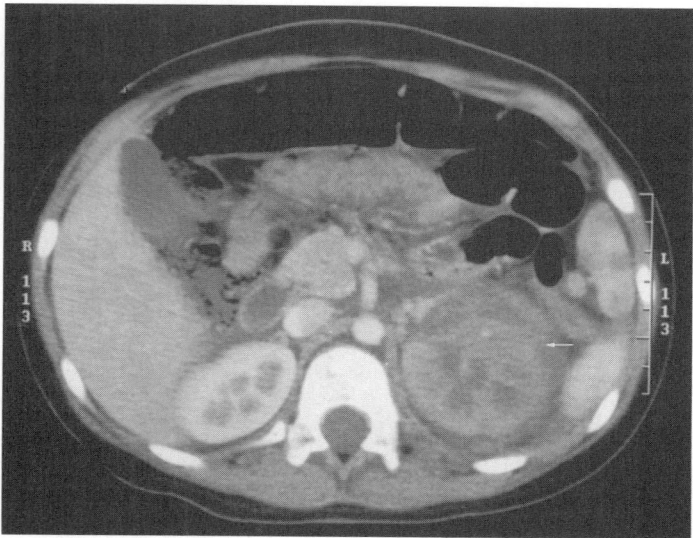

Figure 11.82. Major left renal injury in a young child. Note the lack of renal perfusion, but no extravasation is seen.

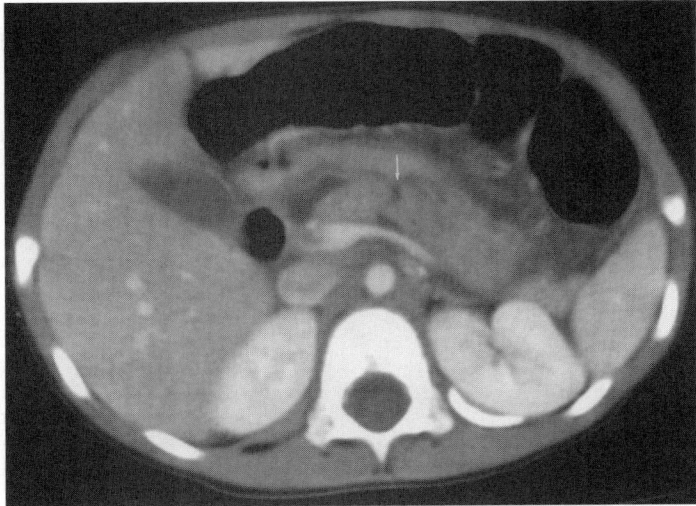

A

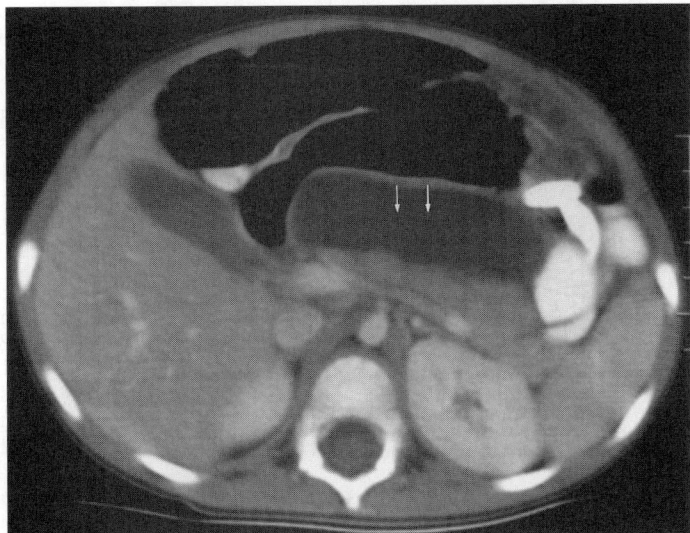

B

Figure 11.83. *(A)* Pancreatic injury after child abuse. Head and body of pancreas appear nearly completely transected (at *arrow*). *(B)* Large pancreatic pseudocyst that developed despite operative drainage in the same child. This fistula was managed with interventional radiologic drainage procedures.

domen results in a hematoma that causes obstruction but not full-thickness injury. This is most common in the duodenum and usually resolves with conservative treatment (Fig. 11.86). Although there is considerable debate as to whether a delayed diagnosis of intestinal injury affects outcome, there certainly are children in whom a missed injury causes significant complications. Signs and symptoms in children whose injuries are initially missed include fever, peritoneal irritation, increasing white blood cell count, and vomiting.

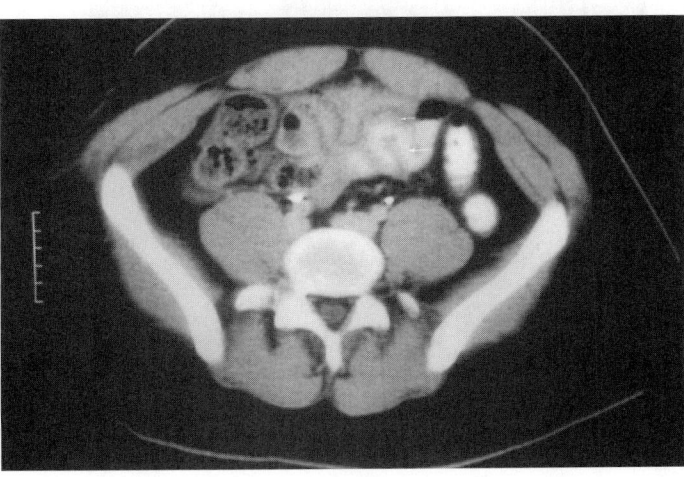

Figure 11.84. Computed tomography scan showing thickened bowel was in a child with a small intestinal injury.

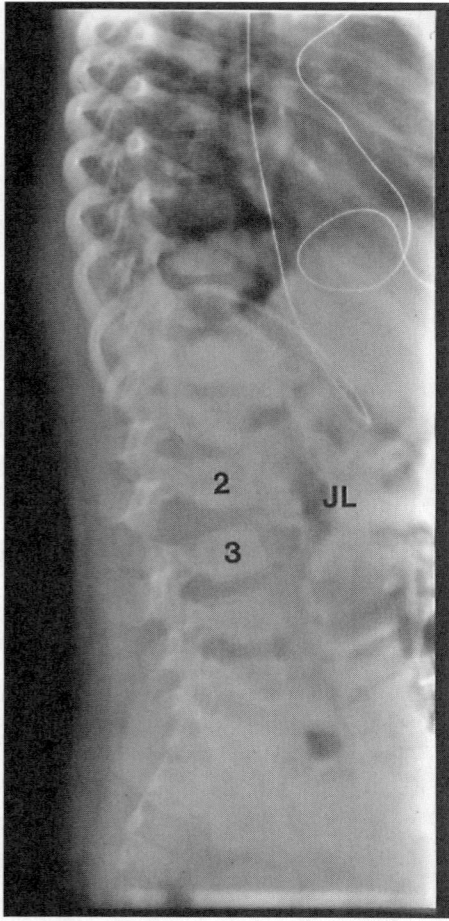

Figure 11.85. Lumbar Chance fractures in a child secondary to a lap belt injury.

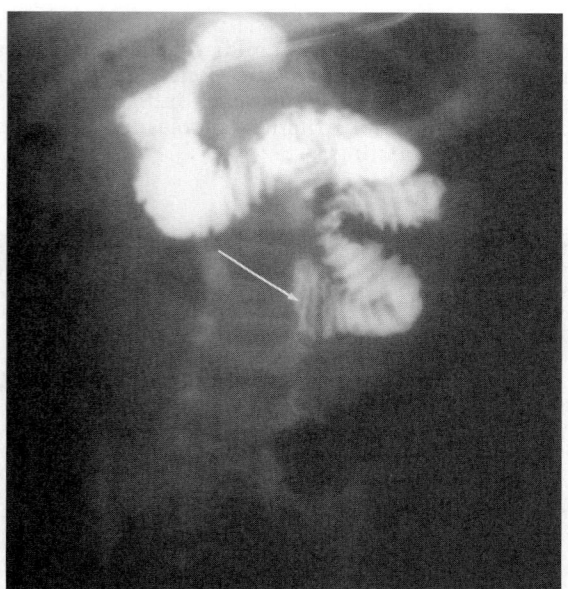

Figure 11.86. Mesenteric hematoma of the proximal jejunum after blunt trauma. This injury responded to conservative measures.

Pelvic Fractures and Extremity Trauma

Trauma to the growing extremity of a child can cause a bend without actual fracture of the bone (greenstick fracture). If the epiphysis of a long bone is involved, there may be long-term consequences in terms of growth and development. On the other hand, many fracture deformities in young children correct themselves spontaneously, a process termed *remodeling*. The blood loss associated with bony injuries, especially in the pelvis, is proportionately greater in the child than in the adult, and this must be considered during the resuscitation phase. Supracondylar fractures at the elbow are relatively common in children and always should raise the concern of an accompanying vascular injury. All injured extremities must be monitored carefully with frequent neurovascular examinations for possible development of a compartment syndrome.

Children with pelvic fractures are at risk for life-threatening hemorrhage as well as associated abdominal injuries (345). Patients at significant risk for hemorrhage are those with bilateral anterior and posterior fractures (346). The presence of multiple pelvic fractures also predicts the presence of associated genitourinary and abdominal injuries. Because pelvic fractures in children rarely occur in isolation, associated injuries to the head, abdomen, chest, and extremities must be suspected.

CHILD ABUSE

All physicians caring for injured children have an ethical and legal responsibility to recognize and report the possibility of child abuse. Centers for Disease Control and Prevention estimates suggest that abuse and neglect kill 4.5 of every 10,000 children 4 years of age and younger. Sadly, most children who die or sustain serious injury from child abuse have been injured previously. These deaths and injuries are potentially preventable if the abusive behavior is recognized. The initial hint of abuse may be a discrepancy between the history offered and the apparent degree of injury. In addition, the history may be inconsistent among the adults involved. Frequently, the child has been taken to several different emergency departments to avoid raising suspicion. Physical signs of child abuse include perioral injuries, retinal hemorrhages, multiple subdural hematomas without a fresh skull fracture, genital or perianal injuries, burns in unusual areas (including burns caused by cigarettes), and radiographic evidence of multiple old or healed fractures. If abuse is suspected, hospital admission is mandatory and a formal report is required by law in most states.

PERFORMANCE INDICATORS

The pediatric trauma system requires constant reevaluation. Because death after trauma is relatively less common in those children who are brought to the hospital alive (compared with adults), pediatric performance filters are aimed at reducing the morbidity after injury. Participation in system-wide reviews and a commitment to correction of identified problems is required of all professionals caring for injured children to ensure the best possible outcomes.

FUNCTIONAL RECOVERY

Children who survive their trauma may still experience long-term problems related to both physical and psychological impairment. Findings from a study of disabilities related to bicycle injuries found that whereas one third of children had persistent disability noted at the time of hospital discharge, only 11% received appropriate physical therapy treatments (347). Cognitive or behavioral changes were noted in one third of children, including changes in school performance and sleep disorders. It is clear that when protocols for the rehabilitative care of injured children are lacking, full recovery from injury is limited. In a related prospective study, 92 injured children with injuries were compared with a matched control group of 59 children who were admitted for acute appendicitis (348). Fifty-four percent of children with minor injuries and 71% of those with major injury had persistent physical limitations at 12 months. The incidence of behavioral disturbances among major trauma patients rose to 41% at 12 months, and many exhibited a decrease in academic performance. Mothers of injured children showed significant psychological trauma compared with mothers of children with appendicitis, and these symptoms were most common when their children had persistent physical limitations. Only 73% of families of major trauma patients had returned to normal family life, compared with 87% of the minor injury group families and 100% of the control subjects. It is clear from these data that severe injuries cause a great deal of morbidity among children and their families, and that programs designed to address these issues must be instituted before discharge and be continued during the first year after trauma.

Posttraumatic stress disorder (PTSD) also may develop after a traumatic event. Symptoms of this disorder in young children include sleep disturbances and nightmares, separation anxiety, difficulties in concentration, intrusive thoughts, difficulties in talking with parents and friends, mood disturbance, deterioration in academic performance, specific fears, and accident-related play. PTSD was reported in 35% of children involved in road traffic accidents compared with only 3% of children injured while playing sports (349). Unfortunately, none of the children had received any psychological help at the time of assessment. Research conducted at our own center found the PTSD symptoms of reexperiencing, avoidance and numbing, and increased arousal were present in 52% of children discharged from a pediatric trauma center. Their symptoms were not recognized by most of the personnel caring for the children, nor were they appreciated by their families. Interventional programs that are aimed at both recognition and treatment of PTSD symptoms have the ability to improve functional recovery after injury in children.

INJURY PREVENTION

The overwhelming majority of pediatric injuries are preventable using available methods of injury prevention. A national survey addressing parental attitudes and knowledge of child safety revealed that parents worried more about kidnapping and drug abuse than about childhood injury (350). These parents were relatively well informed about automobile safety, but knew little about pedestrian and bicycle injuries, burns, and drowning. Physicians were cited as the parent's first choice for information on injury control and child safety, but most physicians know little about injury prevention. It is clear that major educational programs aimed at all caregivers would have a significant impact on pediatric trauma mortality rates.

Methods aimed at reducing childhood injury can be described as active or passive. Active intervention requires a behavioral change to be effective, such as securing a child in a safety seat. On the other hand, passive intervention requires little action from the individual. The most effective injury prevention programs incorporate the four "E"s:

> *Engineering* of products and environments
> *Enactment* of legislation to promote safety
> *Education* of children, caregivers, health care professionals, legislators
> *Evaluation* of the efficacy of specific interventions

Successful injury prevention programs have resulted in a significant reduction in the number of burn injuries in children. Contributing to this reduction is the use of fire-retardant sleepwear and working smoke detectors. There has been less success in reducing injuries to pediatric pedestrians: risk factors for pedestrian injuries in children include an age of 5 to 9 years, male sex, poverty, household crowding, inadequate parental supervision, family stress, and minority race or ethnic group (351). Environmental contributions include living on streets with high traffic, lack of pedestrian-control devices, absence of alternatives to the street for play, and a high density of curbside parking. Successful environmental modifications, termed *traffic calming,* have been pioneered in Europe and include diversion of high-speed traffic away from the core of the city and residential areas and decreasing the speed limit to 10 to 20 mph. These changes reduce the risk of injury for all pedestrians, but especially for children. Bicycle helmets are effective in reducing the risk of head injuries by 85% and the risk of brain injuries by 88%. There is evidence that educating pediatricians improves the use of car seats for children in the short run. Although the rate of use of car seats for newborns and infants is approximately 75%, their use in toddlers is estimated at only 29%, and as many as half of car seats for children are not used correctly.

Preventing penetrating trauma is more complicated but still can be done effectively. Laws that make gun owners responsible for storing firearms in a manner that makes them inaccessible to children have resulted in a 23% reduction in unintentional shooting deaths among children where they are in effect (352). An injury prevention program in Harlem that included improving the safety of the environment, supporting the development of the community, providing safe and supervised activities for children and adolescents, and providing effective health education resulted in a 50% reduction in assault and gun injuries in the intervention community, whereas these same injuries increased in a neighboring community (353). Thus, there is hope for curbing the epidemic of pediatric injuries, but it will require a combination of legislative efforts, education of all child care providers, enforcement of existing safety laws, and use of widespread, community-based prevention programs using methods that have proven effective.

Definitive Care Phase: Geriatric Trauma
SANDRA L. ENGELHARDT

For a variety of reasons, geriatric trauma is becoming one of the major challenges to health care providers in the 21st century. The population of the United States is aging. In 1997, 34.1 million Americans were 65 years of age or older. By the year 2030, it is projected that more than 20% of the populace, or 70 million people, will be older than

65 years. Life expectancy is increasing in the United States. Babies born in 1997 have a life expectancy of 76.5 years, and a person reaching age 65 in 1997 could expect to live an additional 17.6 years (354). The more active lifestyle many older people are enjoying, in conjunction with increasing life expectancy, is producing a larger geriatric population that is more prone to injury than at any time in the past.

Trauma was the seventh leading cause of death among those older than 65 years of age in 1997. Despite being less frequently injured than their younger counterparts, elderly patients are more likely to have fatal outcomes after trauma. Although they constitute 12% of the populace, the elderly account for 33% of trauma deaths (355). Geriatric patients who survive injury are more likely to experience complications and permanent loss of independent function than are younger patients. One third of trauma care dollars are spent on the elderly, and their hospital length of stay averages twice as long as that of similarly injured, nongeriatric patients (356).

Having lost the physiologic flexibility of youth, the elderly trauma patient requires special attention and care. A favorable outcome is best ensured by an aggressive approach to resuscitation, evaluation, and management. Avoidance of complications and careful attention to previously existing medical conditions help optimize the functional recovery of the geriatric trauma patient.

MECHANISMS OF INJURY

Falls

Falls are the most frequent cause of accidental injury and death among the elderly (Fig. 11.87). In 1997, 12,000 geriatric deaths were due to falls. Eighty-three percent of these deaths occurred in people 75 years of age or older (357). Falls in the elderly are rarely from great heights, as they are in younger patients. They usually occur at the home, on steps or level ground. Although trauma due to falls is usually orthopedic, serious injury has been reported in 17.5% to 47% of cases (358). The economic consequences of falls are staggering. Five percent of hospital admissions for older adults are due to fall-related injuries, and charges total more than $50 million a year. Adding to overall expenditures, patients who have fallen are discharged to nursing homes more frequently than other elderly patients (359).

Risk factors for geriatric falls include sensory impairments, neuromuscular disorders, unstable gait, dementia, lower extremity weakness, postural hypotension, and the effects of medications or alcohol (360). Approximately 25% of falls in the elderly are caused by an underlying medical problem; therefore, in addition to treating the injuries sustained in the fall, a cause for it should be sought (358). Environmental factors contribute to many potentially preventable falls. In the home, falls can be caused by poor lighting, obstacles on the floor, or lack of hand rails on stairways. Identification of people at risk for falling, modification of their surroundings, aiding their vision and hearing, and improving their lower extremity and truncal strength may decrease the incidence of falls. A postfall assessment, which includes laboratory studies, electrocardiogram, 24-hour Holter monitoring, and environmental evaluation by a nurse practitioner, has been documented to result in 26% fewer hospitalizations, a 52% reduction in hospital days, 9% fewer falls, and 17% fewer deaths (361).

The mortality rate from geriatric falls is improving; this has been ascribed to better trauma care rather than improved injury prevention. From 1962 to 1988, mortality rates per 100,000 declined from 165 to 60 (63%) for falls in men in their 80s and from 86 to 20 (76%) for women in their late 70s (362).

Motor Vehicle Crashes

Trauma from motor vehicle crashes is the second leading cause of accidental death in the elderly, resulting in 8,300 deaths in 1997 (357). There are approximately 21.8 million (13%) licensed drivers older than 65 years of age in the United States, 6.6 million of whom are older than 75 years. Although older drivers log fewer miles on the road, they are involved in a disproportionately high number of crashes. The elderly have the second highest accident rate of any age group, behind those "new drivers" aged 16 to 25 years (363).

In contrast to younger drivers, older adults are less likely to be involved in crashes in which alcohol plays a role. Only 6.6% of fatally injured drivers older than 65 years have blood alcohol levels greater than 0.10%, compared with 23% for all other age categories (364). On the other hand, the elderly are more likely to be involved in crashes during daylight hours, good weather, and closer to home (364). Their crashes are more likely to involve intersections, right-of-way judgments, traffic sign violations, and two-car incidents than are crashes involving younger drivers (365). Crash patterns in the geriatric population probably relate in some measure to preexisting medical conditions, diminution of cognitive and motor skills, and potentially to side effects of medications. These statistics have fueled ethical debates regarding stricter control of driving privileges for senior citizens.

Pedestrian Injuries

In 1997, 1,300 geriatric pedestrians were struck and killed by automobiles in the United States (357). The aged are involved in crashes as pedestrians more frequently than any other group, including children (360). Elderly patients have a significantly higher death rate than younger pedestrian victims with comparable Injury Severity Scores (ISS) (366). Even in supposedly safe areas like crosswalks, those older than age 65 account for 46% of fatalities. A number of factors contribute to these findings. The elderly are hindered by decreased visual and auditory acuity,

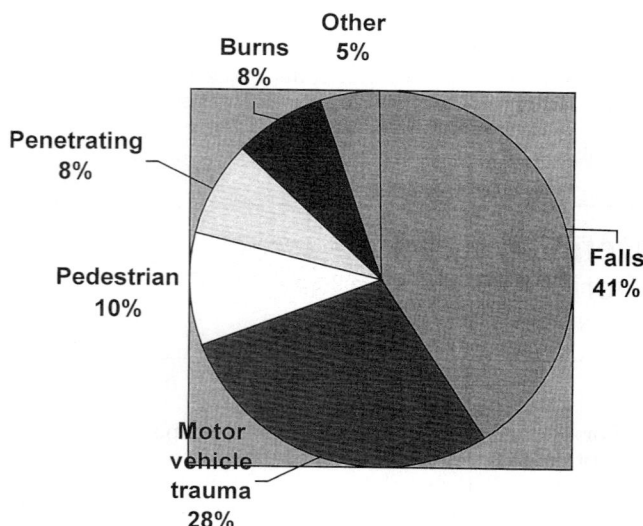

Figure 11.87. Causes of death among the elderly.

slowed gait (less than the United States' standard of 4 feet per second crossing time allotment), and kyphoscoliosis (restricting the ability to gaze upward at traffic signals).

Burns

Burns are responsible for 8% of traumatic deaths among the elderly. Geriatric patients are more likely to sustain deeper, larger burns than are younger patients. This may be related to difficulty in removing themselves from a burning environment. Most burns in the elderly occur in their place of residence. Fatal burns often involve alcohol, smoking in bed, or being trapped in a burning building. The elderly have a higher mortality rate for the same extent of burn than do younger patients (367). Burns over 50% to 70% of total body surface area are almost uniformly fatal in those older than 65 years. The presence of inhalation injury increases this mortality rate. Among survivors, more than half of elderly burn patients are less independent after injury and many require placement in extended care facilities.

Nonaccidental Trauma

Penetrating trauma accounts for another 8% of traumatic elderly deaths. Perhaps because of their poor vision, decreased balance and strength, and cognitive changes leading to poor judgment, the elderly are especially vulnerable to violent crime. Although the literature addressing this issue is sparse, 4% to 14% of trauma admissions among the elderly are due to assault (368). Although attacks with blunt instruments are most frequently reported, the incidence of penetrating injuries is increasing. Geriatric patients have a higher mortality rate in this arena as well. In a case-controlled study, the mortality rate for stab wounds was 4.7% for those younger than 65 and 17.3% for those older than 65 years. Similarly, the gunshot wound mortality rate was 19.5% in the young and 52.1% in the old (369).

The problem of elder abuse is receiving more attention than it has in the past. Up to 10% of geriatric trauma may be nonaccidental, with 4% of patients being victims of moderate to severe abuse. Elder abuse has been linked to changes in family structure, longer life expectancy, financial difficulties, lack of community support, and increasing violence in our society (370). As with potential victims of child abuse, suspicions should be raised when a geriatric patient appears bruised, malnourished, or unkempt. Health care providers must take steps to initiate investigation of any such suspect circumstances.

ANATOMIC AND PHYSIOLOGIC CHARACTERISTICS OF AGING

Table 11.22 summarizes some of the major physiologic changes associated with aging.

Cardiovascular System

With aging, the myocardium and arterial system undergo a progressive loss of compliance, resulting in a less effective pumping mechanism. This is accompanied by a decreased sensitivity of the cardiovascular system to catecholamines. The adequacy of the geriatric patient's stress response is compromised further by diminution in contractility, stroke volume, and ability to increase heart rate. These changes may be exacerbated by the use of prescribed beta blocking and calcium channel blocking drugs. Age-associated changes in the cardiac conduction system result in frequent dysrhythmias, including atrial fibrilla-

Table 11.22. ANATOMIC AND PHYSIOLOGIC CHANGES OF AGING

Organ system	Changes
Cardiovascular	Decreased cardiac output
	Decreased catecholamine response
	Decreased compliance
Respiratory	Increased functional residual capacity
	Decreased vital capacity
	Decreased compliance
	Decreased oxygen tension
Renal	Decreased glomerular filtration rate
	Decreased concentrating ability
Metabolic	Decreased lean body mass
	Protein, calorie, and vitamin deficiencies
Immunologic	Decreased cellular and humoral immunity
Skeletal	Decreased bone density

tion, premature ventricular contractions, supraventricular beats, and a variety of heart blocks. Atherosclerotic heart disease limits oxygen delivery to the myocytes, impairing the ability of the aged myocardium to respond to stress. In light of these physiologic aberrations, it is not uncommon for dysrhythmias, congestive heart failure, myocardial ischemia, or even sudden death to occur after major trauma in the elderly.

Pulmonary System

Changes in the respiratory system that accompany aging include decreased vital capacity and forced expiratory volume, increased functional residual capacity, decreased compliance, and decreased diffusion capacity. Although arterial oxygen tension diminishes, arterial carbon dioxide tension remains unchanged. Increased anteroposterior diameter of the chest contributes to diminished diaphragmatic excursion, altering pulmonary mechanics and decreasing the strength of the cough. Age-related changes in the lungs' defense mechanisms, such as mucosal atrophy and diminished mucociliary clearance, also occur. Elderly patients' oropharynxes have a high rate of colonization with gram-negative organisms, further increasing their risk for development of pneumonia (371). These alterations in pulmonary function make the elderly trauma patient highly susceptible to pulmonary complications.

Renal System

The kidneys are not immune to changes with aging, and demonstrate a decreased glomerular filtration rate and decreased excretory capacity due to loss of functional glomeruli. Diminished muscle mass makes serum creatinine an insensitive measure of renal function. In the elderly patient, measurement of creatinine clearance is a more reliable way to gauge function, and should be used to guide dosing of renally excreted drugs.

Osteoporosis

Osteoporosis is virtually endemic among the elderly and accounts for the frequent observation of fractures following seemingly minor trauma. The etiology of osteoporosis is multifactorial, and includes increased bone resorption, loss of estrogenic hormones, diminished physical activity, and impaired calcium absorption by the gut. An increased risk of fracture in the elderly trauma patient mandates a careful history and physical examination to avoid missed injuries.

Nutrition and Metabolism

Body composition changes profoundly with aging, with increased fat mass and decreased lean muscle mass, total body water, and bone density. The elderly have lower caloric requirements than when they were younger. Their protein, vitamin, and mineral requirements are largely unchanged. Geriatric patients frequently have preexisting protein-calorie malnutrition. After trauma, nutritional support must address underlying deficiencies as well as provide adequate protein and calories to sustain the stressed patient. Early institution of aggressive feeding protocols ought to have a salutary effect on such complications as pneumonia, sepsis, and poor wound healing.

Immune System

Aging adversely affects the immune system through a variety of mechanisms. The best studied of these are the consequences of aging on T-cell function. Although the number of T cells is unchanged (372), their activation, proliferation, and ability to produce cytokines are impaired (373). T-helper cell impairment decreases the humoral immune response (374). Delayed hypersensitivity is also diminished in the elderly (375). The results of these immunologic changes are an increased susceptibility to infection and a higher incidence of multiple organ system failure after trauma.

Neurologic System

The dura becomes more tightly adherent to the skull as the brain ages, making the development of an epidural hematoma more uncommon in the elderly patient. Progressive loss of cerebral volume creates more space around the brain. Although this may protect the brain from contusion in some settings, it also elongates bridging veins, and makes them more prone to tearing. These factors increase the likelihood of a subdural hematoma in the elderly trauma patient (376). The enlarged space around the brain can accommodate a relatively large volume of blood and may mask significant intracranial hemorrhage. A heightened index of suspicion for a significant intracranial lesion must be present during the neurologic evaluation of the older patient.

INITIAL EVALUATION AND RESUSCITATION

Prehospital triage decisions for elderly patients need not deviate from established routines. Patients with significant mechanism of injury, obvious head or thoracoabdominal injuries, or who demonstrate physiologic impairment as measured by the Trauma Score at the scene of injury should be triaged to a trauma center.

The initial resuscitation of the elderly patient should follow basic tenets of trauma care, with attention paid to the details of geriatric physiology. General principles of establishing adequate airway and breathing are unchanged. The older patient with altered mental status is at high risk for aspiration, and definitive airway control should be obtained early. Hypoxia must be recognized and addressed to prevent the sequelae of systemically inadequate oxygen delivery. An arterial blood gas should be obtained promptly on admission and oxygen saturation monitored continuously with pulse oximetry.

As the circulatory status is assessed, blood should be obtained for laboratory studies and type and crossmatch. Intravenous access should be established with two large-bore peripheral intravenous catheters. When evaluating the vital signs, the clinician should remember that elderly patients are often accustomed to higher-than-normal blood pressures. As such, a blood pressure of 100 mm Hg in a 70-year-old patient with a usual blood pressure of 150 mm Hg may represent hypovolemic shock. Volume loading should begin with crystalloid and be followed by packed red blood cells as needed. Aggressive monitoring of volume status should be instituted early because it has been shown to benefit elderly patients (377,378).

Various criteria have been suggested to guide the use of arterial line monitoring and pulmonary artery catheterization in the elderly trauma patient, including an ISS greater than 9, evidence of shock as demonstrated by metabolic acidosis, or the presence of comorbid conditions. Volume loading should be used to achieve a pulmonary capillary wedge pressure of 15 mm Hg. Once adequate filling pressures have been established, inotropic support should be initiated as needed to support oxygen delivery and cellular metabolism. Oxygen transport variables, mixed venous oxygen saturation monitoring, and lactate levels can be used to assess the adequacy of resuscitation. Scalea et al. have shown that early invasive monitoring of these variables in the elderly trauma patients improved survival rates from 7% to 53% (377).

The aged trauma patient's limited reserve should prompt a rapid but thorough evaluation for injury. Computed tomography (CT) scan of the brain should be obtained for any history of loss of consciousness, amnesia, or lateralizing signs on neurologic examination. Intracavitary hemorrhage can be rapidly assessed with a chest radiograph and objective evaluation of the abdomen with ultrasound, CT scan, or diagnostic peritoneal lavage. To avoid missed injuries, the secondary survey should be done with careful attention to detail. Immediately after resuscitation and evaluation are complete, the patient should be admitted to a setting in which close, invasive monitoring can be continued.

Routine radiographic evaluation of the elderly patient should include cervical spine, chest, and pelvic films. Radiographs should be obtained liberally in areas of obvious deformity or pain. Degenerative changes are frequent in the aged skeleton, and additional views or CT scans may be necessary for further assessment of areas in question, particularly in the cervical spine.

A careful history regarding the circumstances surrounding the trauma can be helpful in determining contributing factors. It is not uncommon for a myocardial infarction or stroke to precipitate an automobile crash. A fall may have been caused by a dysrhythmia or by orthostatic hypotension. A careful medication history is crucial. β-Adrenergic blockade obviously blunts the chronotropic response to hypovolemia. Hypoglycemic agents can precipitate coma, mimicking closed head injury. Diuretic use can lead to fluid and electrolyte abnormalities that exacerbate hypovolemia. Many elderly patients are also taking anticoagulants; therefore, coagulation abnormalities must be recognized and addressed early in this group.

MANAGEMENT OF SPECIFIC INJURIES

Head Injuries

The initial management of the elderly patient with a closed head injury is similar to that of the head-injured younger patient. A thorough search for intracranial lesions must be undertaken. Support of airway, breathing, and circulation and prompt diagnosis of the specific neurologic injury are of paramount importance. Twenty percent of elderly patients who present with a Glasgow Coma Scale

(GCS) score of greater than 13 have an intracranial hematoma, and 12% of these patients die (379). The early, aggressive use of invasive monitors is essential in maintaining adequate oxygen delivery to the injured brain.

Outcome after geriatric closed head injury is much worse than in younger cohorts. In a comparison of patients with closed head injury older than 60 years with patients aged 20 to 40 years, the mortality rate in the elderly was 79% compared with 36% in the younger patients. This was despite having similar admission GCS, Revised Trauma Score (RTS), ISS, Abbreviated Injury Score (AIS), resuscitation, nutritional support, and neurosurgical intervention. Of the nine older patients who left the hospital, six were persistently vegetative and two were severely disabled (380). Another study demonstrated that patients older than 51 years of age in whom coma persisted more than 5.5 days had zero chance of mental restitution, compared with patients aged 22 to 50 years, who had a 50% chance of recovery even if coma lasted 7 days or longer (381).

Thoracic Trauma

A less compliant chest wall and osteoporotic bones result in a high incidence of rib fractures among older blunt trauma victims. These fractures can be complicated by pneumothorax or hemothorax, which should be treated as in younger patients. Aggressive pain control is especially beneficial in the elderly and may minimize the development of pneumonia and the need for mechanical ventilation. A thoracic epidural catheter should be used if enteral or parenteral narcotics offer inadequate analgesia.

Myocardial contusion should be suspected when dysrhythmias follow blunt chest trauma. Continuous electrocardiographic monitoring is indicated when cardiac rhythm abnormalities are present. Echocardiography can confirm the diagnosis of myocardial contusion by demonstrating cardiac wall motion abnormalities.

Because of atherosclerotic changes, the thoracic aorta of older patients may be at higher risk for disruption after deceleration injury. Angiography remains the gold standard for diagnosis of aortic injury and should be used liberally when there is a history of significant deceleration. Unfortunately, even with prompt recognition and treatment, thoracic aortic injury carries a grim prognosis for the elderly patient. A comparison of patients older than 55 years of age with blunt thoracic aortic injury demonstrated a mortality rate of 82%, versus 12% in patients with similar injury who were younger than 55 years (382).

Several papers have analyzed outcomes in elderly victims of blunt thoracic trauma. Allen and Schwab reviewed 48 patients older than 60 years of age who sustained blunt chest injury. Almost half were injured in motor vehicle crashes, and the other half in falls. Only 15% of patients required mechanical ventilation. Among those who did not, 89% survived and 81% returned to independent living. Only 8% required discharge to a skilled nursing facility (371). With aggressive pulmonary toilet, excellent pain control, avoidance of complications, and good nutrition, the outlook for elderly victims of thoracic trauma may be excellent.

Abdominal Trauma

Higher pain tolerance, dementia, closed head injury, or intoxication may affect the geriatric patient's abdominal examination. Occult injuries must be diligently sought. Initial evaluation of the stable patient with focused abdominal ultrasound or CT scan is appropriate. The elderly should be well hydrated before receiving intravenous contrast because they are at higher risk for development of acute tubular necrosis after its administration (367).

Avoidance of missed injuries is crucial. Although geriatric patients usually are able to tolerate operative intervention for abdominal trauma, they are less able to handle shock or sepsis due to delays in diagnosis.

When operative therapy is required in the elderly patient, several principles should be remembered. Careful monitoring of fluid status with an arterial line, central line, or pulmonary artery catheter is essential in cases in which large fluid shifts are expected. Older patients have compromised thermoregulation, and careful attention must be paid to maintaining intraoperative normothermia. Every effort must be made to avoid the development of the lethal triad of hypothermia, acidosis, and coagulopathy.

Critical Care Considerations

Mortality in elderly trauma patients has been correlated with the development of cardiac complications and sepsis (377). It has been postulated that aggressive intensive care unit monitoring can improve outcomes in this population by decreasing the frequency of such events. Sepsis and subsequent multiple organ system failure cause most late deaths after trauma in the elderly. Urosepsis is common in older patients, as is the development of pneumonia. When these conditions develop, they should be promptly diagnosed and aggressively treated. Acalculous cholecystitis should be suspected in the setting of abdominal pain, tube feeding intolerance, and hyperbilirubinemia. Catheter-related sepsis should be avoided because it prolongs hospital stay and increases costs. The complication rate in the elderly can be diminished by careful attention to nutritional requirements, with institution of enteral nutrition as soon as it can be tolerated. In addition, prompt mobilization out of bed and strength training by physical therapists help the patient mobilize secretions and maintain strength and muscle mass.

Geriatric patients are at increased risk for thromboembolic complications after trauma. Patients with hip and pelvic fractures, neurologic trauma, prolonged immobilization, or a previous history of thromboembolic events are at especially high risk for deep venous thrombosis (DVT) or pulmonary embolism. All trauma patients should have some form of prophylaxis, such as sequential compression devices or low-dose heparin. Systemic anticoagulation or inferior vena cava filter placement should be considered for high-risk patients. Most DVTs are clinically inapparent; therefore, screening high-risk patients with serial duplex venous ultrasound can result in earlier diagnosis and treatment. A low threshold for obtaining ventilation–perfusion scanning and pulmonary angiography should be used in patients with unexpected cardiopulmonary deterioration.

Ethical decision making is an important aspect of geriatric patient care. In most instances, aggressive care is indicated. There are, however, increasing numbers of patients who have made their wishes regarding potentially futile care known in the form of a living will. The competent patient's autonomy to make such decisions must be protected. In other cases, the family may have a clear idea of the patient's wishes regarding quality of life and the use of life support measures after devastating injury. Early and frank communication between the trauma surgeon and the family regarding these issues is required so goals of treatment can be established and unwanted supportive measures can be avoided.

OUTCOME AFTER GERIATRIC TRAUMA

It is undeniable that geriatric patients tolerate injury less well than younger patients and are more likely to die after major trauma (383,384). As previously discussed, several factors may contribute to the higher mortality rate in the elderly. Older trauma patients have a higher rate of preexisting disease and a higher complication rate (385). A review of the Multiple Trauma Outcome Study database by Sacco et al. demonstrated that preexisting diabetes and hepatic, cardiovascular, respiratory, and renal disease were all associated with higher mortality rates. This finding, as well as a higher rate of complications in the elderly, was confirmed by Perdue et al. and others (385–387). The combination of advanced age, premorbid illness, and the development of complications often results in fatal outcome for the elderly patient. The increased mortality rate in this population suggests that geriatric patients should be aggressively triaged to designated trauma centers where resources exist to optimize their care.

Although the mortality rate after trauma is higher in the elderly than in younger patients, there is a significant potential for meaningful recovery among those who survive the acute phase of injury. Rates of independent living from 57% to 81% have been documented (378,383,388). These studies are in contrast to a report by Oreskovich et al. indicating only an 8% return to independent living 1 year after traumatic injury in geriatric patients (386). The potential for significant independent recovery in the elderly, despite their initially higher mortality rate, justifies aggressive triage and initial treatment of these patients.

INJURY PREVENTION

Injury prevention has the potential to benefit most of the geriatric population. The cost of prevention programs is minimal compared with the cost of caring for an elderly trauma patient for weeks in the intensive care unit. Significant impact can be demonstrated by "pre-event" interventions such as home safety inspections, modification of pharmacologic regimens, and treatment of any sensory disturbances that affect the elderly patient's ability fully to perceive and safely navigate the environment.

Drivers with visual and hearing impairments, dementia, and musculoskeletal disorders and those taking certain medications are at higher risk for automobile crashes (360). Driver education courses specifically addressing the needs of the aging driver have been developed by the American Association of Retired Persons and the National Teachers Association. Decreased rates of injury and death have followed implementation of these programs (389). Public safety programs also can reduce the frequency of severe injury and death from pedestrian versus automobile collisions (390). Identification of particularly dangerous intersections can result in crosswalk modification to provide better visibility, longer crossing times, and other improvements.

Definitive Care Phase: Trauma in Pregnancy

GRACE S. ROZYCKI

Although injured pregnant patients comprise approximately 1% of all trauma admissions (391–396), the magnitude of the problem is much greater because two patients are being cared for simultaneously. The overall maternal mortality rate continues to decline in the United States, but trauma accounts for a significant number of deaths in these women (392,397). In fact, this problem may be underestimated because the gravid status may not be routinely recorded on death certificates (398).

In several series (393,399,400), the rate of fetal death parallels the extent of maternal injury, yet it also has been reported to be three to four times greater than the maternal death rate, implying that the survival of the mother is not always sufficient to ensure fetal well-being (391,392,395, 401). Although most trauma involving pregnant patients occurs during the second or third trimester (391,399, 401–403), some reports of domestic abuse show this occurs frequently before 18 weeks' gestation, and then diminishes between 20 and 30 weeks' gestation. Motor vehicle crashes occur with equal frequency throughout the gestational period (403). Fetal demise is directly related to birth weight and gestational age. Fifty percent of fetuses die after serious maternal trauma if they are no older than 26 weeks' gestational age. Ninety percent of fetuses die after significant maternal trauma if their weight is less than 750 g, compared with a 40% mortality rate when the weight is greater than 750 g (404).

An understanding of the anatomic and physiologic changes unique to pregnancy as well as the principles of resuscitation and treatment after trauma are important to provide the best care for both the injured mother and her unborn child.

ANATOMY AND PHYSIOLOGY UNIQUE TO THE GRAVID PATIENT

Anatomic and physiologic changes of pregnancy can alter the injury response, necessitating a modified approach to resuscitation and therapy (Table 11.23). Knowledge of these changes should be kept in mind as the evaluation and resuscitation of the pregnant trauma patient proceeds.

Anatomic Changes

By the 12th week of gestation, the gravid uterus is considered an intraabdominal organ. With the ascent of the enlarged uterus out of the pelvis, it undergoes dextrorotation because of the presence of the rectosigmoid colon (405). Important marks for estimating gestational age include the umbilicus (20 weeks' gestation) and the costal margins (34 to 36 weeks' gestation). During the final 2 weeks of normal gestation, the fetal head descends into the pelvis, accounting for the fetal skull fractures or traumatic brain injuries that are often associated with maternal pelvic fractures. With increasing gestational age, the uterus also becomes relatively thin (1.5 cm at term) and the amount of amniotic fluid decreases (405). As a result, the fetus is more vulnerable to injury, especially when the mother receives a direct blow to the abdomen. Although the myometrium is relatively elastic, the placenta is not, predisposing it to shear forces at the uteroplacental interface, which may lead to abruptio placentae.

Placental perfusion depends on the blood flow through the uterus and ovarian arteries. It is estimated to be approximately 500 mL/min (406), but varies with position and hormonal changes (407). In early pregnancy, there is a softening and cyanosis of the cervix with an eversion of the proliferating columnar endocervical glands (405). These changes make the cervix friable and prone to bleed even with minor trauma. There is also enlargement of ovarian veins and increased vascularity of the maternal vagina with advancing gestational age.

Table 11.23. PHYSIOLOGIC ALTERATIONS IN PREGNANCY

System	Change	Implication
Neurologic	Eclampsia may mimic traumatic brain injury (headache, seizures, hypertension)	Exclude traumatic brain injury (head computed tomography scan) May mask shock
Cardiovascular	Cardiac output increased by 1.0 to 1.5 L/min	Delayed signs of shock
	Heart rate ↑ 10–15 bpm	
	Blood pressure ↓ 5–15 mm Hg in second trimester but returns to normal in third trimester	
	Plasma volume increased by 50%	
	Vena cavalcompression	Supine hypotension syndrome
Respiratory	Residual lung volume decreased	Decreased buffering capacity
	Decreased P_{O_2}	
	Chronic respiratory alkalosis	
Gastrointestinal	Decreased gastrointestinal motility	Increased propensity toward aspiration and vomiting Urinary stasis
	Dilatation of renal system	
Genitourinary		Physiologic hydronephrosis and urinary stasis
	Dilatation of renal system	
Laboratory values	Increased white blood cell count	Difficulty interpreting clinical picture regarding hemorrhage
	Decreased hematocrit	
	Increased fibrinogen and factors VII, VIII, X, XII	Hypercoagulable state

Cardiovascular

Maternal blood volume (plasma and erythrocytes) begins to increase during the first trimester, but expands most rapidly during the second trimester, reaching approximately 45% above nonpregnant levels (408–410). The increase in plasma volume is proportionally greater than the enlarged erythrocyte volume and results in the anemia of pregnancy. Near term, the plasma volume continues to expand, but the red cell mass begins to increase, resulting in a near-normal hematocrit. Pregnancy-induced hypervolemia supplies the extraordinary demands of the enlarged uterus, allows for fewer red blood cells to be lost during parturition, minimizes the loss of oxygen-carrying capacity associated with hemoglobin, and protects the mother from the hypotensive effects of impaired venous return (411). This physiologic hypervolemia masks volume loss after trauma and may give the clinician an unfounded sense of security about the patient's hemodynamic stability. Almost 35% of the mother's blood volume may be lost before clinical signs of shock are noted (412).

As pregnancy progresses, cardiac output increases up to 50% above normal until the 24th week of gestation, after which it plateaus (Table 11.24). This increase in cardiac output is a result of a modest rise in heart rate and stroke volume that relates to the expanded blood volume and the direct inotropic effect of estrogen (413).

If the pregnant patient is in the supine position, the inferior vena cava is partially obstructed by the gravid uterus, which decreases venous blood return to the heart, lowers cardiac output, and causes supine hypotension. The enlarged uterus also compresses the abdominal aorta, reducing blood flow to the fetus through diminished uterine arterial flow. Turning the pregnant patient onto her left side improves venous return and increases cardiac output by approximately 30% (414).

Overall, cardiac work is increased with pregnancy because of the volume load and estrogen effect, despite a decrease in systemic vascular resistance mediated by prostaglandin, progestin, intracellular calcium flux, and endothelial-derived factors (415). Early in pregnancy, the blood pressure, especially the diastolic level, decreases, but then slowly returns to normal by term. Mean normal values for the first trimester are 105 mm Hg systolic and 60 mm Hg diastolic; for the second trimester, 102 and 55 mm Hg, and for the third trimester, 108 and 67 mm Hg. Significant elevation from these levels may indicate pregnancy-induced hypertension (416).

Table 11.24. CENTRAL HEMODYNAMIC CHANGES IN 10 NORMAL NULLIPARIOUS WOMEN BETWEEN 35 WEEKS' GESTATION AND AGAIN WHEN 11 TO 13 WEEKS' POSTPARTUM

	Pregnant[a]	Postpartum	Change
Mean arterial pressure (mm Hg)	90 ± 6	86 ± 8	No change
Pulmonary capillary wedge pressure (mm Hg)	8 ± 2	6 ± 2	No change
Central venous pressure	4 ± 3	4 ± 3	No change
Heart rate (beats/min)	83 ± 10	71 ± 10	+17%
Cardiac output (L/min)	6.2 ± 1.0	4.3 ± 0.9	+43%
Systemic vascular resistance (dyne/s/cm^{-5})	1,210 ± 266	1,530 ± 520	−21%
Pulmonary vascular resistance (dyne/s/cm^{-5})	78 ± 22	119 ± 47	−34%
Serum colloid osmotic pressure (mm Hg)	18.0 ± 1.5	20.8 ± 1.0	−14%
COP–PCWP gradient (mm Hg)	10.5 ± 2.7	14.5 ± 2.5	−28%
Left ventricular stroke work index (g/m/m^2)	48 ± 6	41 ± 8	No change

[a]Made in lateral recumbent position.
COP, colloid osmotic pressure; PCWP, pulmonary capillary wedge pressure.
Adapted from Maternal adaptions to pregnancy. In: Cunningham FG, MacDonald PC, Gant NF, et al., eds. Williams obstetrics, 20th ed. Norwalk, CT: Appleton & Lange, 1997:191–225, with permission.
Adapted from Jurkovich GJ. Hypothermia in the trauma patient. Adv Trauma 1989;4:111, with permission.

Finally, the enlarged uterus causes the heart to be displaced upward and to the left. This change, along with the common development of a serous pericardial effusion (417), results in an enlarged cardiac silhouette and increased pulmonary vascular markings on the chest radiograph (418).

Pulmonary Changes

As the uterus enlarges during pregnancy, the diaphragm rises approximately 4 cm, which results in a lower residual lung volume, diminished ventilatory reserve, and decreased resting arterial oxygen tension. Both diaphragmatic excursion and thoracic circumference increase, resulting in larger tidal volumes (Table 11.25). A chronic respiratory alkalosis shifts the oxyhemoglobin dissociation curve to the left, therefore increasing the affinity of maternal hemoglobin for oxygen. Simultaneously, however, this slight increase in pH stimulates an increase in 2,3-diphosphoglycerate that shifts the curve to the right, facilitating oxygen release to the fetus (405,419). Pulmonary artery pressures remain normal, but pulmonary vascular resistance decreases to accommodate the incremental change in blood volume and cardiac output (413,420).

Gastrointestinal

As pregnancy progresses, the enlarged uterus stretches the abdominal wall and compresses the viscera. This results in a diminished response to peritoneal irritation and altered or referred pain perception, making the clinical examination unreliable. An increased propensity toward aspiration occurs because of compression of the intraabdominal organs, which decreases gastrointestinal motility. Also, the relaxant effect of progesterone and estrogen on smooth muscle diminishes lower esophageal sphincter competency. Alkaline phosphatase levels are almost doubled, most likely from placental alkaline phosphatase enzymes. Progesterone inhibits gallbladder contractility by inhibition of cholecystokinin, leading to bile stasis and a propensity for the development of gallstones (421). Finally, gastrin is produced by the placenta, which lowers gastric pH during pregnancy.

Nutrient changes during pregnancy include decreased nitrogen use (demanding more protein intake) and a diabetogenic state characterized by a mild fasting hyperglycemia, postprandial hyperglycemia, and hyperinsulinemia (409). Progesterone and estrogen may contribute to a peripheral resistance to insulin (409). Also noted are increased plasma lipid levels that may correlate with estradiol, progesterone, and human placental lactogen levels.

Renal

Throughout pregnancy, the renal collection system enlarges to meet the demands of the increased blood volume and urine formation. The renal pelvis and ureter dilate early in the first trimester, resulting in a mild hydronephrosis (1.5 cm longer) and hydroureter (422). Urinary stasis in the collecting system predisposes the pregnant woman to pyelonephritis. In the first trimester, the renal blood flow and the glomerular filtration rate increase by up to 50%; consequently, the levels of creatinine and blood urea nitrogen decrease (423). This event precedes significant increases in cardiac output or blood volume. The clinical significance is that normal or slightly elevated levels of creatinine or blood urea nitrogen may signify renal dysfunction. Davison and Hytten noted the presence of glucosuria in the gravid patient due to the increase in glomerular filtration rate and the decrease in reabsorptive capacity for filtered glucose (424). Because of hormonal and osmoreceptor alterations, the normal serum sodium concentration for a pregnant woman is approximately 132 mEq/L. Increased clearance of uric acid occurs in the first and second trimester, but reabsorption becomes normal later. An elevated serum uric acid level in the first or second trimester may portend toxemia even in the normotensive gravida (425) (Table 11.26).

Musculoskeletal

The relaxation of the interosseous ligaments during pregnancy causes increased mobility of the sacroiliac and sacrococcygeal joints and widening of the symphysis pubis. These changes, coupled with an enlarged uterus, result in lordosis, disrupt the maternal center of gravity, and increase the risk for falls.

Laboratory Values

The peripheral blood leukocyte count increases to approximately 12,000 cells/mL during gestation and may be as high as 25,000 cells/mL during labor (426). The platelet count may appear falsely low because of dilution from increases in plasma volume. Fibrinogen (factor I) and factors VII, VIII, IX, and X are increased considerably during pregnancy, but prothrombin (factor II) is increased only slightly. Although there is a slight decrease in the protein S level and its activity (427), levels of antithrombin III and protein C show no significant change during the pregnancy. The level of plasminogen (profibrinolysin) in plasma increases significantly, most likely induced by estrogen.

Table 11.25. VENTILATORY FUNCTION IN PREGNANT WOMEN COMPARED WITH NONPREGNANT WOMEN

Function	Nonpregnant	Pregnant	Change (%)
Respiratory rate	15	16	
Tidal volume (mL)	485	680	+39[a]
Minute ventilation (mL)	7,270	10,340	+42[a]
Vital capacity (mL)	3,260	3,310	+1
Residual volume (mL)	965	770	20[a]

[a]Significant differences.

Adapted from Maternal adaptions to pregnancy. In: Cunningham FG, MacDonald PC, Gant NF, et al., eds. Williams obstetrics, 20th ed. Norwalk, CT: Appleton & Lange, 1997, with permission.

Table 11.26. RENAL CHANGES IN NORMAL PREGNANCY

Alteration	Manifestation	Clinical relevance
Increased renal size	Approximately 1 cm greater on radiographs	Postpartum decreases in size should not be mistaken for parenchymal loss
Dilation of pelvis, calyces, and ureters	Resembles hydronephrosis on ultrasound or intravenous pyelography (more marked on right)	
Increased renal hemodynamics	Glomerular filtration rate and renal plasma flow increase ~50%	Serum creatinine and urea nitrogen values decrease during normal gestation; an increase >0.8 mg/dL creatinine may be sign of renal insufficiency; protein, amino acid, and glucose excretion all increase
Changes in acid–base metabolism	Renal bicarbonate threshold decreases; progesterone stimulates respiratory center	Serum bicarbonate is 4 to 5 mEq/L lower; Pco_2 is 10 mm Hg lower, (a Pco_2 of 40 mm Hg already represents CO_2 retention)
Renal	Osmoregulation altered: osmotic thresholds for vasoporessin release and thirst decrease	Serum osmolarity decreases ~10 mOsm/L (serum Na ~5 mEq/L) during normal gestations

Adapted from Maternal adaptations to pregnancy. In: Cunningham FG, MacDonald PC, Gant NF, et al., eds. Williams obstetrics, 20th ed. Norwalk, CT: Appleton & Lange, 1997, with permission.

INITIAL ASSESSMENT AND MANAGEMENT

Priorities for the resuscitation of the injured pregnant patient are the same as for any other trauma patient. Patient care, however, is altered to accommodate the unique anatomic and physiologic characteristics of the gravid woman (428).

The best therapy for the unborn child is expedient maternal resuscitation. An adequate airway with supplemental oxygenation is essential to prevent fetal hypoxemia. The release of maternal catecholamines causes uteroplacental vasoconstriction, compromising fetal circulation (429,430). Because fetal blood functions on a different oxyhemoglobin dissociation curve, small positive increments in oxygen concentration improve oxygen content and physiologic reserve for the fetus, even if maternal arterial oxygen content does not change appreciably. Maternal hemorrhagic shock, with its resultant release of catecholamines, causes uterine artery vasoconstriction, reducing uterine perfusion and compromising fetal viability. Hence, vigorous crystalloid resuscitation is encouraged, even for patients who appear normotensive. In late pregnancy, compromised cardiac output and blood pressure secondary to vena cava compression can be relieved by placing the patient in the left lateral decubitus or right hip-flexed position. A nasogastric tube should be inserted because of the pregnant patient's increased propensity toward vomiting and aspiration. Urinary volume per hour should be monitored to provide some indication of perfusion status.

History and Physical Examination

The secondary survey consists of a thorough history (including obstetric history), physical examination, and fetal monitoring (431). Maternal prenatal history is crucial and may alter management decisions if medical problems such as preeclampsia, diabetes, essential hypertension, or congenital heart disease are present. Obstetric history includes the date of the last menstrual period, the expected date of confinement, the perception of fetal movement, and the status of the current and previous pregnancies. Gestational age (fetal maturity) can be estimated from the fundal height, as measured by palpation. (Fundal height at the umbilicus represents approximately 20 weeks' gestation.) These factors help in the decision matrix if emergent delivery is necessary. For example, a 26-week-old fetus is considered viable and has a good chance of survival if

given neonatal intensive care support. Pelvic and rectal examinations are performed with special attention to vaginal discharge (amniotic fluid or blood), effacement, dilation, and fetal station (432).

Fetomaternal hemorrhage occurs in 6% of all pregnancies, but in 20% of injured pregnant patients. Although 0.01 mL of fetal blood (1 to 3 fetal cells per 500,000 maternal red blood cells) sensitizes 70% of Rh-negative patients, the remainder require up to 40 mL, or one third of fetal blood volume. The Kleihauer-Betke test detects fetal cells in the maternal circulation, indicating fetomaternal hemorrhage (433,434). Because this test can determine the risk of isosensitization in Rh-negative gravid women, it is recommended for injured Rh-negative pregnant patients in the second or third trimester to detect impending fetal exsanguination. If positive, the Kleihauer-Betke test should be repeated 24 hours later to identify ongoing fetomaternal hemorrhage. Treatment consists of an initial dose of Rh immune globulin with an additional dose administered for every 30 mL of fetomaternal transfusion estimated by this test.

Fetal Assessment and Monitoring

Fetal evaluation consists of uterine assessment, fundal height measurement, and recording of heart tones, heart rate, and movement. A heart rate of 100 beats/min or less is considered bradycardia. Uterine tenderness and contraction may be related to abruptio placentae, which can occur in the absence of vaginal bleeding. Auscultation for a complete minute determines regularity (acceleration and deceleration) of the fetal heartbeat. However, continuous fetal monitoring is the best predictor of a healthy or distressed fetus (404). There is still no consensus on the indications for fetal monitoring in trauma patients. A guideline for patients with major injuries, including shock, is to provide continuous fetal monitoring for at least 24 hours.

Fetal heart rate and uterine activity can be monitored by either external (indirect) or internal (direct) methods. The external method is noninvasive and has wider clinical application. Internal monitoring requires insertion of an intrauterine catheter and application of a fetal scalp electrode. The normal fetal heart rate ranges between 120 and 160 beats/min. Abnormalities in variability may signal hypoxia or dysrhythmia in the fetus. Early decelerations of fetal heart rate, which conform closely to uterine contractions, are vaguely mediated and not of significance. Similarly, variable decelerations, secondary to transient umbilical cord compression, are not of great concern. The presence of late deceleration of fetal heart rate after uterine contractions is thought to be related to uteroplacental insufficiency and may warrant routine monitoring after injury (404).

Ultrasonography is a valuable adjunct in determining fetal viability. It detects the changes of pregnancy 3 to 4 weeks after ovulation and is therefore useful in the gestational period, especially because it involves no radiation exposure. During the first trimester, an endovaginal ultrasound probe provides close approximation of the transducer to the uterus through cervical tissue. This method does not require bladder catheterization or filling and thus allows for a rapid examination (435–437). Real-time B-mode ultrasound demonstrates fetal cardiac movement and determines fetal size and placental location. Abruptio placentae may be identified as a retroplacental lucency (blood clot) or an echogenic structure in the amniotic fluid.

Diagnostic Modalities

After patient stabilization, several diagnostic modalities are used to define the extent and type of injury for the mother and her unborn child. Initially, laboratory studies are obtained. If blood is urgently needed, type O, Rh-negative blood is chosen. Evaluation of the abdomen may be performed by diagnostic peritoneal lavage, computed tomography (CT) scan, or ultrasound (438). There is an increasing role for ultrasound in the diagnosis of hemoperitoneum secondary to blunt abdominal trauma. Diagnostic peritoneal lavage may be performed in the pregnant patient, but the open, supraumbilical technique is recommended. Reliance on ultrasound to evaluate both the mother and the fetus obviate the need to perform a CT scan or diagnostic peritoneal lavage and can provide valuable information on fetal motion, heart tones, location, and placement.

Liberal but judicious use of radiographic studies is advised for the evaluation of the pregnant trauma patient. A diagnostic modality deemed necessary should not be withheld for fear of potential hazard to the fetus. Factors contributing to the sequelae of prenatal exposure to ionizing radiation are the stage of development, the exposure time, the dose delivered, and the dose absorbed. The absorbed radiation dose varies according to many factors, including instrument model, desired image quality, and distance from the radioactive source. The developmental stages are the preimplantation phase (0 to 8 days after conception), major organogenesis (9 to 60 days), and the fetal period (61 to 270 days). The roentgen (R) is the unit of exposure, and the centigray (cGy) or rad is the unit of absorbed dose. Exposure and absorbed fetal doses for radiographic tests are presented in Table 11.27. No estimates have been made of radiation risk during the first few days of human development. Because the natural prevalence of congenital anomalies is approximately 6%, any effects of such tests are undetectable at low radiologic doses. There is no medical justification for terminating pregnancy in women exposed to 5 cGy or less (439). A 0.1% increase in the rate of spontaneous abortion during the first 2 weeks of development follows a dose of 10 cGy, and there is a 1% increase in congenital abnormalities at the same dose (440). Another concern is the potential for late neoplasia development. The risks for radiation-induced cancer after in utero exposure (during the second and third trimesters) are estimated to be 1 in 15,000 children if exposed to 1 mGy x-radiation (441). If the fetus receives 50 mGy, the risk is increased to 1 in approximately 300 children. Combined studies, such as CT scan of the abdomen with oral and intravenous contrast, obviate the need for multiple

Table 11.27. REPRESENTATIVE ENTRANCE EXPOSURES AND FETAL DOSES FOR FREQUENTLY PERFORMED RADIOGRAPHIC EXAMINATIONS WITH A 200-SPEED IMAGE RECEPTOR

Examination	Entrance exposure (mrad)	Fetal dose (mrad)
Skull (lateral)	70	0
Cervical spine (AP)	110	0
Shoulder	90	0
Chest (PA)	10	0
Thoracic spine (AP)	180	1
Lumbosacral spine (AP)[a]	250	80
Intravenous pyelogram[a]	210	60
Hip[a]	220	50
Wrist or foot	5	0

[a]Abdominal/gonadal shields should be used if possible.
AP, anteroposterior; PA, posteroanterior.
From Bushong SC. Radiologic science for technologists: physics, biology, and protection. St. Louis: CV Mosby, 1988:550, with permission.
Adapted from Jurkovich GJ. Hypothermia in the trauma patient. Adv Trauma 1989;4:111, with permission.

studies such as an intravenous pyelography. Prudent judgment and foresight by the physician should ensure that specific radiographic studies are ordered and accurately performed to avoid repetition.

Blunt Trauma

Motor vehicle crashes remain the chief cause of blunt trauma in the pregnant patient. As pregnancy progresses, the uterus becomes more vulnerable, rising out of the protective bony pelvis, and it absorbs most of the impact of blunt abdominal trauma. These factors often result in direct fetal injury, usually skull fracture or intracerebral hemorrhage. Pelvic fractures in the gravid patient may cause extensive maternal retroperitoneal hemorrhage as a result of engorged pelvic veins.

Uterine rupture from blunt trauma occurs most often at the site of prior cesarean section or at the posterior fundus. It can present with massive hemorrhage or more insidiously with minimal vaginal bleeding if rupture occurs at the fundus, far from the uterine vessels. Repair can be either primary in two layers or with a polytetrafluoroethylene patch (442). Avulsion of the uterus has been reported, with bladder rupture being an associated finding.

Abruptio placentae is the most common cause of fetal death after maternal injury. This carries a 30% to 70% rate of fetal death and a 1% maternal mortality rate. Over 50% placental separation invariably results in fetal demise. Abruptio placentae can occur in the absence of obvious abdominal injury because maternal shock is a far greater stimulus for abruption than are the mechanical forces of trauma disrupting the placenta (432). Abruptio placentae is more common in the presence of hypertension, diabetes mellitus, advanced age, multiparity, and maternal use of tobacco or cocaine. Abruptio placentae presents with vaginal bleeding (in 80% of cases), abdominal pain, disseminated intravascular coagulation due to thromboplastin release, and inexplicable maternal hypovolemia. It invariably occurs within 48 hours after trauma, and pregnant patients who are at risk should be monitored accordingly.

The pregnant patient with minor injury should be observed for several hours. Most patients with insignificant trauma do not require admission unless specific signs and symptoms, such as vaginal bleeding, abdominal cramps, or leakage of amniotic fluid, are present. In one series (396), only 1 of 11 patients had symptoms after minor trauma, and pregnancy outcome was successful. Occult abruptio placentae has been reported after motor vehicle accidents in which the patient displayed only subtle clinical signs and symptoms. Because placental separation can occur with rapid deceleration injuries, a three-point restraint system appropriately applied is recommended for pregnant automobile passengers (444–446). The mechanism of injury may provide invaluable information regarding potential injuries in even a healthy-appearing patient. At a minimum, a prompt and thorough maternal assessment, fetal assessment, and a comprehensive search for injuries are necessary for evaluating the pregnant patient with minor trauma.

Penetrating Trauma

The perinatal mortality rate from penetrating injury to the mother has been reported to range from 47% to 71% (447). In general, pregnant women with gunshot wounds to the abdomen should undergo celiotomy. For those who sustain stab wounds to the abdomen, management is based on the likelihood of intraabdominal injury. The abdominal examination may be unreliable because of a diminished response to peritoneal irritation and altered or referred pain perception. If the clinical presentation is unclear (e.g., absence of peritonitis or evisceration), then a diagnostic peritoneal lavage performed with the open technique in the supraumbilical area may be diagnostic.

Operative Management

General anesthesia is preferred for the gravid patient with multisystem injury. The risks of anesthesia are related to the physiologic changes that accompany pregnancy. For example, because aspiration is more likely, rapid-sequence induction is preferred. The effects of anesthetics are related to the stage of fetal development and the dose of the agent administered. Because premature labor has been shown to be associated with surgery and with various anesthetic regimens, intraoperative fetal monitoring is recommended. One study reported an increase in fetal demise after celiotomy, especially if the operation was performed in the first trimester or in the presence of peritonitis (448). In a multicenter study, fetal death occurred in 35% of cases in which the pregnant women underwent general anesthesia and surgery, compared with 11% of cases in which general anesthesia was not used. However, the mean Injury Severity Score in the surgery group was 18.0, compared with 5.5 in the nonsurgery group.

The standard vertical midline incision is used for maternal celiotomy. Adequate visualization of viscera is mandatory, and the pregnant uterus should not interfere with abdominal exploration or repair of an injury. If labor ensues, vaginal delivery is almost always encouraged. Even early in the postoperative period, vaginal delivery is still preferred and does not appear harmful to the mother or the neonate. Cesarean section prolongs the operative time and increases blood loss, generally by approximately 1 L. Figure 11.88 provides a suggested algorithm for the management of the uterus during a celiotomy (449). During celiotomy for trauma, indications for cesarean section are as follows:

- Maternal shock, pregnancy near term
- Threat to life from exsanguination (injury or disseminated intravascular coagulation)
- Mechanical limitation of maternal treatment
- Risk of fetal distress exceeding risk of prematurity
- Unstable thoracolumbar spinal injury

If fetal delivery is vaginal the uterus is incised longitudinally. After the amniotic membranes are ruptured, the fetus is delivered, and the placenta is removed. The uterus is closed in a running-locking fashion using large absorbable suture. Once the uterus is evacuated, postpartum hemostasis begins. In cases of uterine atony, bimanual compression of the uterus and the intravenous administration of oxytocin are begun. In addition, the surgeon should examine the uterus and cervix for any lacerations and ensure that the uterus is thoroughly evacuated. Other measures to control severe hemorrhage include intravenous methyl ergonovine, or intramyometrial injection of 15-methyl prostaglandin $F_{2\alpha}$. For the most part, massive hemorrhage associated with emergent cesarean section in the injured women is associated with a pelvic fracture. Packing of the pelvis or embolization of the internal iliac arteries may be needed as well.

Successful outcome of a postmortem cesarean section depends on the duration of the gestation and the time interval between maternal death and delivery. Under optimal conditions, at 26 to 28 weeks' gestation, the estimated fetal survival rate is approximately 50%. Therefore, postmortem cesarean section is justified if the estimated gestational age is approximately 26 to 28 weeks. If the time between maternal death and delivery is less than 5 minutes, the fetal prognosis is considered excellent. If the time since maternal death is prolonged to approximately 20 minutes, fetal prognosis is poor. Uncertainty about maternal death time is not a contraindication for this procedure (450).

Burns

Fewer than 0.1% of pregnant patients sustain severe burns. The successful approach to the management of the burn victim relies on maintaining a normal intravascular volume and avoiding hypoxia. In these patients, inadequate initial resuscitation is often responsible for the loss of the pregnancy. In a review of 15 pregnant victims of electric shock, 4 fetuses were viable and only 1 was nor-

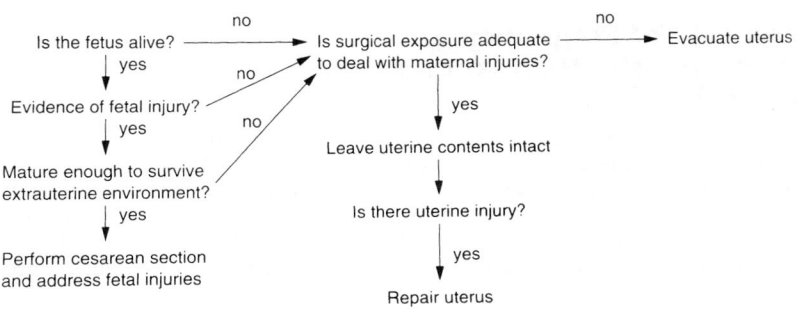

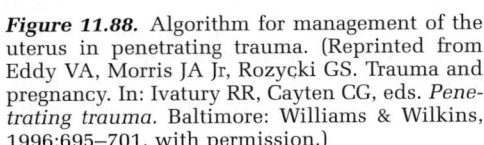

Figure 11.88. Algorithm for management of the uterus in penetrating trauma. (Reprinted from Eddy VA, Morris JA Jr, Rozycki GS. Trauma and pregnancy. In: Ivatury RR, Cayten CG, eds. *Penetrating trauma.* Baltimore: Williams & Wilkins, 1996:695–701, with permission.)

Table 11.28. *CRUDE MORTALITY RATES AFTER MATERNAL BURN INJURIES*

Body surface injured (%)	Maternal mortality rate (%)	Fetal mortality rate (%)
<40	3	22
50	25	53
>80	100	100

From Taylor JW, Plunkett GD, McManus WF, et al. *Thermal injury during pregnancy. Obstet Gynecol* 1976;47:434–438, with permission.

mal (451). Because the fetus is much less resistant to electrical shock, fetal monitoring is strongly recommended after this type of injury. Table 11.28 delineates the estimates of body surface area burned and associated mortality rates in pregnant patients.

Critical Care Management

Critical care management of the traumatized pregnant patient covers a wide range of topics. The basic principles of hemodynamic monitoring, adequate ventilatory support, nutrition, and careful assessment of volume status apply to the injured pregnant patient and are covered in more detail in other chapters. Knowledge of the disease processes that can arise in the pregnant patient within the first 24 hours after injury allows the physician to render high-quality critical care to the traumatized patient and her unborn child.

When administrating medication to the gravid patient, potential risk versus therapeutic benefit must be considered especially carefully. Prophylactic tetanus immunization should be given appropriately, with anti-D globulin for patients who are Rh negative and at risk for isoimmunization. Prophylactic antibiotics are administered if needed, but tetracycline and most sulfa drugs should be avoided.

Cardiopulmonary Resuscitation

The enlarged uterus compresses the vena cava, resulting in a 25% decrease in cardiac output as a result of decreased venous return. To improve the effects of CPR, patients before 24 weeks' gestation can be maintained in the supine position but with manual displacement of the uterus laterally. After 24 weeks' gestation, a procedure table with a 30-degree left lateral tilt is helpful, although cardiopulmonary resuscitation (CPR) is only 80% effective when performed with the patient in this position. Emergent cesarean section may be needed if the patient does not respond to CPR within approximately 5 minutes (452,453). Morris and colleagues found that if the fetus is viable (presence of fetal heart tones) and is at least 26 weeks' gestation, emergent cesarean section is justified (454); they found that infants who met those criteria had a survival rate of 75%.

Toxemia of Pregnancy or Preeclampsia (Pregnancy-induced Hypertension)

Any traumatized pregnant patient presenting with seizures or coma should have head injury excluded, and then the diagnosis of eclampsia should be considered. In the severe state, eclampsia is manifested by hypertension, pulmonary edema, proteinuria, and seizure activity. The pathophysiologic event is vasospasm, which affects he-

patic, renal, cerebral, and placental blood flow. Despite the presence of pulmonary edema, intravascular volume depletion is often present, and a fluid challenge may be appropriate. Rapid control of the hypertension is achieved with hydralazine (455). However, elevated maternal oxygen consumption disrupts uterine vascular oxygen supply and maternal equilibrium, resulting in fetal distress. Smoother control of reduction in blood pressure and myocardial oxygen consumption is accomplished by achieving volume expansion before vasodilation. Inotropic support, in combination with vasodilator treatment, maximizes oxygen delivery and affects afterload reduction. Magnesium sulfate has a slight hypotensive effect but does not decrease systemic vascular resistance. The hemodynamic parameters illustrated in Table 11.24 are guidelines for optimizing maternal hemodynamics, uteroplacental perfusion, and, ultimately, fetal well-being.

Thromboembolism

Pregnant patients are at increased risk of thromboembolism from all three components of Virchow's triad: stasis, intimal damage, and hypercoagulability. Increased venous capacitance, vena cava compression, and weight gain promote venous stasis. Labor and trauma cause intimal damage, and hypercoagulability results from elevated levels of fibrinogen and intrinsic coagulation factors with the gravid state. Advanced age and multiparity further increase these risks. No method of prophylaxis has been demonstrated to be both safe and universally effective in preventing thromboembolism, either in the patient with multiple injuries or in the pregnant patient. In general, warfarin is avoided and heparin is considered the anticoagulant of choice during pregnancy (456).

Amniotic Fluid Embolism

Amniotic fluid embolism after trauma in pregnancy or parturition is characterized by hypotension, hypoxemia, and coagulopathy. The diagnosis is often difficult, and an 80% mortality rate has been reported. Amniotic fluid debris enters the maternal venous circulation, causing sudden dyspnea and hypotension. A mixed metabolic acidosis and respiratory alkalosis ensue. The chest radiograph shows characteristic pulmonary edema or an acute respiratory distress pattern. Hemodynamically, the patient has an elevated pulmonary capillary wedge pressure and a low systemic vascular resistance. Disseminated intravascular coagulation develops in approximately 30% of these patients. Although most cases of amniotic fluid embolism occur during labor, it has been reported to occur after abdominal trauma (457) and abruptio placentae. This diagnosis is established on clinical findings, and the treatment consists of supportive care (i.e., oxygenation, maximization of hemodynamic parameters, and correction of coagulopathy).

Interpersonal Violence

Although motor vehicle crashes and falls are the most common etiologies of trauma during pregnancy, reports indicate that 4% to 17% of pregnant women are victims of interpersonal violence (392–394). In fact, this number may be underestimated because population-based prevalence estimates are often unavailable, pregnancy is not consistently recorded on death certificates (398), and, as with many abuse crimes, it is not always reported.

Poole and colleagues reported that 64 (31.5%) of 203 injured pregnant patients experienced interpersonal violence (401). Of the eight fetal deaths in this series, three occurred 7 days after injury and five occurred in women with an Injury Severity Score of zero. These findings indicate that severe trauma to the fetus may occur without obvious injury to the mother, emphasizing the need for the physician to question the patient directly about abuse. Furthermore, physicians should be encouraged to take measures for early intervention, such as establishing a link with agencies that deal with battered women, so that physical protection, emotional support, and information about legal rights are readily available.

SUMMARY

The pregnant trauma victim presents a unique challenge to the resuscitating physician. Two patients are being treated, and a high degree of expertise is needed to treat both. Initially, evaluation should involve the cooperative efforts of the emergency physician, trauma surgeon, obstetrician, and obstetric nurse. If the pregnancy is near term or delivery is anticipated, a pediatrician and pediatric surgeon should be consulted. The pregnancy should not distract the surgeon from initiating basic resuscitation. Equally important, the injury should not confound the obstetrician. The expertise of the obstetric nurse is useful in coordinating the overall care plan of the mother and her unborn child. Expedient, accurate resuscitation of the mother takes priority because the best chance for fetal survival is maternal survival.

Definitive Care Phase: Critical Care and Postinjury Management

RICHARD K. SIMONS

Trauma systems implementation, wide dissemination of Advanced Trauma Life Support resuscitation protocols, and early definitive care provided by trauma centers have dramatically reduced early mortality rates after injury. Late mortality due to complications, missed injuries, or errors during the postinjury or critical care phases of management are assuming increasing importance in the quest to eliminate preventable death. Studies have indicated that death after injury in a level 1 trauma center was attributed to acute inflammatory processes in over 10% of cases (458), and that provider-related complications are particularly lethal in the intensive care unit (ICU) setting (459).

Trauma patients represent a unique group among the ICU population by virtue of their age (approximate mean, 33 years) and general lack of chronic underlying disease. For these reasons, the prospects for functional recovery are good but dependent on sophisticated and skillful critical care and postinjury management. This care, which is frequently complex and multisystem, requires a high level of expertise, coordination, and prioritization. Integrated care models led by specialty-trained trauma surgeons, delivered in a trauma center setting, and following national guidelines for optimal care appear to have superior outcomes compared with fragmented care models depending on multiple subspecialists to provide care at various stages of the care process (460).

This section reviews those critical care issues that are pertinent or unique to the major trauma patient.

FACTORS RELATED TO POSTINJURY COMPLICATIONS

Local Effects of Tissue Injury

Traumatic injury involves the transfer of kinetic energy to tissue, resulting in the primary possibilities of tissue damage and disruption, with loss of function, local hemorrhage, contamination, and embolization of air, tissue, or particulate matter. These occur immediately but may be exacerbated by inappropriate or poorly timed postinjury management. Secondary effects of tissue injury may occur from minutes to days later, and include inadequate débridement of dead tissue such as burn eschar, further hemorrhage and edema resulting in elevated compartment pressures, inadequate fracture stabilization, persistent local tissue ischemia, high-level contamination or infection with resultant inflammation, and immunosuppression. These secondary effects are major determinants of the subsequent activation of the systemic inflammatory response syndrome (SIRS) and multiple-organ dysfunction syndrome, and are an important focus of early postinjury care.

Shock, Ischemia, and Reperfusion Injury

Tissue ischemia after trauma may be either local or global. The related derangement in cellular metabolism and changes in ion transport across cell membranes have been a major focus of shock research for many years. Although the direct effects of ischemic tissue injury are well documented, it is increasingly recognized that an important component of posttraumatic tissue injury occurs after resuscitation with reperfusion and reoxygenation. Oxygen free radicals (hydroxyl radical, superoxide anion, and others) generated from tissue-derived xanthine oxidase and phagocyte-derived NADPH (nicotinamide-adenine dinucleotide phosphate, reduced form) oxidase systems are thought to be important mediators. This reperfusion injury may be responsible for such diverse events as compartment syndromes and SIRS.

Recognition and aggressive resuscitation of occult shock states prevalent in the postinjury and ICU setting may ameliorate reperfusion injury. Rapid correction of acidosis and tissue hypoperfusion along with reoperation for continuing hemorrhage all have a significant role in blunting this response. Invasive hemodynamic monitoring is required in the more severely injured patients, particularly the elderly or in the presence of significant comorbidity. The use of the pulmonary artery catheter has been recommended in trauma as a means of directing hemodynamic support, particularly when used as an aid to clarify diagnosis and improve functional outcome (461). Definitive markers of adequate resuscitation remain elusive, and goal-directed therapy aimed at achieving arbitrary hemodynamic profiles has not been proven. Restoration of end-organ function, correction of metabolic indicators, and adequate hemodynamic parameters suffice to guide resuscitative end points in most patients. Other therapeutic strategies aimed at ameliorating reperfusion injury remain experimental. They include xanthine oxidase inhibitors, inhibition of neutrophil adherence, and exogenous antioxidant administration. Several of these approaches have shown promise in animal studies, but have yet to enter the clinical arena.

Alterations in Other Homeostatic Mechanisms

Tissue injury, mechanical ventilation, traumatic or chemically induced coma, and massive fluid resuscitation all pose major challenges to the body's homeostatic mechanisms. Thermoregulation is particularly compromised by these events and strict attention to limiting ongoing heat loss and restoring normothermia is required to minimize the devastating consequences of hypothermia. Physiologic collapse and refractory coagulopathy are seen once core temperatures approach 32°C and demand active core rewarming (462). This issue is discussed in detail later in the chapter. For the euthermic patient, maintenance of a warm ambient temperature ensures minimizing metabolic demands and risk of heat loss. Massive transfusion rapidly leads to failure of normal coagulation unless blood product replacement therapy directed by coagulation tests is instituted. Severe head injury, uterine rupture, or unevacuated blood clots may result in disseminated intravascular coagulation, requiring blood product support and treatment of the underlying cause.

Metabolic Response to Injury

The metabolic response to trauma is phasic. The initial period of hypovolemia, shock, hypoperfusion, and hypothermia is associated with increasing oxygen debt, anaerobic metabolism, and alterations in enzymatic function characterized by elevated catecholamine levels, diminished insulin levels, and elevated blood glucose and free fatty acid levels. This is the so-called ebb phase in the metabolic response. Once perfusion has been restored, the normal response is one of a hyperdynamic circulation with elevated cardiac output and increased oxygen consumption with correction of oxygen debt and lactate levels. This is associated with hypermetabolism characterized by elevated insulin levels and glucose production, increased energy expenditure, and normalization of free fatty acid and catecholamine levels. This is the so-called flow phase. Minimization of the ebb phase by early and complete resuscitation limits the magnitude and duration of the flow phase. An unduly prolonged or exaggerated flow phase merges imperceptibly with SIRS and is an indication of either a massive initial physiologic insult or a second or ongoing inflammatory challenge. The increased metabolic demands of the flow phase require adequate substrate support in the form of supplemental oxygen therapy, increased minute ventilation, and adequate nutrition. The more seriously injured patients require caloric intake of 1.5 to 2 times that of basal energy expenditures along with adequate protein intake. Nutritional support should be initiated early in the critical care phase of postinjury management, using the enteral route if at all possible to avoid the infectious and immunosuppressive complications of parenteral nutrition. Early use of the gut also preserves mucosal integrity, minimizes feeding intolerance, and limits the potential for immunologic complications.

Alterations in the Immune and Inflammatory Response

Major perturbations in the immune system occur in patients after injury, contributing to the early inflammatory response and subsequent late mortality from sepsis or organ failure. The changes in the immune system are significant and global, affecting both humoral and cellular components of the system (463). Changes in humoral mediators after trauma include increased levels of proinflammatory cytokines, including tumor necrosis factor, interleukin-1, and interleukin-6, along with decreased levels of interleukin-2, interleukin-3, and interferon-γ. Immunosuppressive complement activation products and other immunosuppressive peptides are present in the serum of trauma patients along with decreased serum fibronectin and opsonic activity.

Cellular immune function is also modified. Polymorphonuclear neutrophil (PMN) function is acutely altered with demargination, with activation resulting in expression of cellular adhesion molecules, increased production of oxygen radicals, and degranulation with sequestration in organ capillary beds. The trauma patient is thought to be vulnerable to secondary insults during this period when PMNs are "primed" (464). Surgical interventions and development of complications during this period may result in an exaggerated response triggering SIRS or organ dysfunction. Subsequently, many PMN antimicrobial functions are suppressed after trauma, including chemotaxis, phagocytosis, respiratory burst, and intracellular killing. Macrophage activation plays a central role in the proinflammatory cytokine milieu that develops after injury. However, macrophage receptor expression and subsequent antigen presentation are subsequently impaired along with the shift toward an immunosuppressive phenotype. Similar defects appear in lymphocyte function, including shifts in T-cell populations with decreased CD3 and CD4 subpopulations, depression of B-cell and immunoglobulin production, and loss of antigen recall. The overall effect of these global changes after trauma may result in the development of SIRS and multiple-organ dysfunction syndrome along with immunosuppression, resulting in the potential for septic complications and death.

The mechanisms by which this immunosuppression develops after trauma are multiple, and include the direct effects of tissue injury itself, the release of multiple immunosuppressive mediators, and immunosuppressive effects of the neuroendocrine response to trauma. In addition, the gastrointestinal tract may play an important role in the development of posttraumatic immunosuppression. Shock, trauma, endotoxemia, and starvation all have been shown to have a negative impact on the functional integrity of the intestine. This could potentially result in translocation of bacteria or endotoxin to the portal circulation or mesenteric lymph nodes (465). Alternatively, activation of gut-associated immune cells may lead to systemic release of gut-derived cytokines. The net result of this process appears to be a generalized cytokine-mediated immunosuppression, although the clinical relevance of this remains to be fully demonstrated.

Immunomodulation

The importance of these immunosuppressive effects is becoming more apparent as our ability to modify this response improves. Potential strategies to reduce the immune consequences of trauma include the early definitive care of wounds, restoration of gastrointestinal tract function and integrity, and initiation of nutritional support, selected immunologic stimulation using biologic response modifiers or specific metabolic or nutritional immunostimulants, and selected immunologic blockade of the more harmful aspects of the immune response. Many of these potential interventions remain experimental, although some are now moving into mainstream critical care. Examples include rapid restoration of organ dysfunction using global and regional indicators of resuscitation and early establishment of enteral nutrition with high-calorie, high-protein products (463).

CLASSIFICATION OF COMPLICATIONS

Disease-related Complications

Careful analysis and classification of complications after traumatic injury show that most complications are directly related to the patient's injuries or the metabolic and immune responses to injury. These disease-related complications are discussed in further detail in the last section of the chapter. Other adverse outcomes, however, can be termed *provider related* and are the focus of quality assurance and continuous quality improvement programs designed to limit unnecessary morbidity and mortality (466–468).

Provider-related Complications

Provider-related complications include errors in diagnosis resulting in delays of treatment, technical errors, errors in communication, or errors of judgment. Some specific examples have been discussed previously. Missed injuries or unrecognized severity of injury during the initial work-up of a trauma patient places the burden of subsequent diagnosis on the critical care phase of trauma management. These missed injuries or unexpected physiologic deterioration after recognized injuries should be anticipated, and frequent monitoring of vital signs and follow-up physical examinations are a required part of the management of the multiply injured patient. Sudden neurologic deterioration may signify a worsening of an intracerebral bleed, and deteriorating vital signs may signify ongoing hemorrhage from an apparently trivial splenic injury or pelvic fracture. A full physical examination, sometimes termed a *tertiary survey,* performed on the second hospital day frequently picks up new minor injuries not appreciated by the patient or physician at the time of admission. Minor orthopedic injuries are a particularly frequent example.

In addition to these early errors, one report demonstrated that 23% of provider-related complications occur during the critical care phase of trauma care. These errors were associated with a disproportionate percentage of preventable deaths (459). Critical care errors included management errors, monitoring errors, errors in electrolyte management or drug administration, and technical and procedural errors. Collectively, these studies demonstrate the importance of continued vigilance in identifying and correcting these provider-related complications, particularly recurrent process errors, to minimize preventable mortality and morbidity. Development of evidence-based and consensus-driven care guidelines help standardize care, limit variation, and reduce error. This process should be an essential component of critical care unit management.

COMPLICATIONS IN MAJOR ORGAN SYSTEMS

Systemic Inflammatory Response Syndrome

Persistence or exaggeration of the hyperdynamic and hypermetabolic state after injury is thought to be detrimental and result in organ injury. Persistent inflammatory response after injury and in the absence of proven infection has been termed *SIRS*. It is defined by manifestation of two or more of the following conditions: (a) temperature greater than 38°C or less than 36°C; (b) heart rate over 90 beats/min; (c) respiratory rate greater than 20 breaths/min or $Paco_2$ less than 32 mm Hg; and (d) white blood cell count greater than 12,000/mm^3, less than 4,000/mm^3, or more than 10% immature (band) forms (469). Development of SIRS should elicit a diligent search for an underlying inflammatory focus, although frequently none is found. Treatment remains supportive in the absence of a reversible inflammatory stimulus.

Sepsis and Organ Dysfunction

Proven infection in the presence of SIRS is termed *sepsis.* If evidence of global or organ-specific hypoperfusion develops, then the term *severe sepsis* applies. Septic shock refers to sepsis associated with hypotension (systolic blood pressure <90 mm Hg) refractory to volume or requiring inotropes (469). Both sustained SIRS and sepsis lead ultimately to organ dysfunction, which is both progressive and sequential if the inflammatory process persists. Typically, the respiratory system is the first to be affected, with other organ system functions deteriorating subsequently. The presence of multiple organ system dysfunction secondary to SIRS or sepsis is termed *multiple organ dysfunction syndrome* and carries a poor prognosis, particularly if dysfunction is severe, prolonged, and involves multiple systems. Organ dysfunction grading has been proposed to aid with prognosis and research, although consensus has yet to be reached on the criteria. Individual organ failure is discussed under each system heading.

Pulmonary System

Pulmonary complications account for a full third of disease-related complications after trauma. Age greater than 55 years, shock at time of admission, and severe head injury are all significant risk factors for the development of the more serious of the pulmonary complications, including pneumonia, atelectasis, pulmonary embolus, and adult respiratory distress syndrome (ARDS) (470).

The general reasons for endotracheal intubation and mechanical ventilation in the trauma patient include (a) the need for a secure airway, (b) augmentation of the work of breathing for patients with acutely increased ventilatory workloads or decreased ventilatory capacity, (c) maintenance of arterial oxygen tension by increasing functional residual capacity and alveolar Po_2, and (d) the temporary need for induced hyperventilation for treatment of acute intracranial hypertension. The most common clinical scenario for intubation and mechanical ventilation involves patients with neurologic injuries. Common indications for posttraumatic mechanical ventilation are shown in Table 11.29.

The presence of thoracoabdominal injuries, the degree of shock, and the patient's age and underlying disease also play a role in the decisions regarding intubation and mechanical ventilation. The rapidly changing physiologic status of many trauma patients often requires that intubation be performed in anticipation of developing indications. Under these circumstances, physiologic trends, including those that may occur over short periods, are often an appropriate indication for intubation and mechanical ventilation. In the trauma setting, it is always prudent to err on the side of aggressive airway and ventilatory control.

Patients who have high peak airway pressures as a result of severe thoracic injury, pulmonary edema, or ARDS are at greatly increased risk for the development of mechanical complications. Prolonged intubation dramatically increases the risk of both infectious and mechanical complications (Table 11.30). Many mechanical complications of the endotracheal tube can be avoided by close monitoring of tube position. Proximal displacement of the endotracheal tube may occur suddenly (usually iatrogenic) or more gradually, usually in association with increased peak airway pressures. An endotracheal cuff leak is often the first clinical manifestation of proximal balloon

Table 11.29. COMMON INDICATIONS FOR MECHANICAL VENTILATION WITH SPECIFIC INJURIES

Airway Compromise
   Massive facial fractures
   Arterial injury in neck
   Aspiration (blood, debris)
   Severe head injury
Inadequate ventilation
   Cervical spine injury (high)
   Shock
   Ruptured diaphragm
   Crushed chest or flail chest
Inadequate oxygenation
   Pulmonary contusion or flail chest
   Massive aspiration
   Shock
   Air or fat embolus
   Adult respiratory distress syndrome
Need for hypocapneic vasoconstriction
   Acutely elevated intracranial pressure

displacement and mandates careful determination of tube position. The blind installation of more air into the endotracheal tube cuff may result in its expulsion proximal to the vocal cords and may precipitate loss of the airway.

Endotracheal tube obstruction may result from mucous plugs, kinking, and balloon herniation over the distal orifice, or the gradual accumulation of proteinaceous debris. Failure to pass a suction catheter easily should prompt close examination of tube position and balloon volume. Bronchoscopy occasionally is required to confirm endotracheal tube position and patency.

Modern endotracheal tubes with high-volume, low-pressure cuffs have greatly reduced the incidence of laryngeal and subglottic injuries previously associated with prolonged endotracheal intubation. Patients who require prolonged intubation or have laryngeal injuries may be candidates for tracheostomy, although the exact timing of this procedure remains a controversial issue. Certainly, patients with profound and persistent neurologic deficits, patients with significant airway injury or edema, or patients with severe respiratory failure requiring mechanical ventilation for more than 2 to 3 weeks are all candidates for early tracheostomy, which may help reduce the incidence of iatrogenic airway injuries. Tracheostomy can be performed by standard surgical techniques or percutaneously at the bedside.

Mechanical ventilation in patients with normal lungs requires positive airway pressures, which rarely cause mechanical problems. In many trauma patients, however, lung abnormalities develop that result in diminished compliance with the risk of high airway pressure generation. The lung pathologic process is usually inhomogeneous, and high pressures result in overdistention (volutrauma) of relatively normal airspaces while the atelectatic areas remain collapsed. Airway pressures must be monitored and ventilator settings adjusted to minimize the risk of ventilator-associated lung injury. Smaller tidal volumes, decreased flow rates, or pressure-controlled modes of ventilation may be required (see Chapter 8).

Bronchopleural fistulae may follow penetrating injury to the chest. Most air leaks are uncomplicated, usually closing spontaneously within 2 to 5 days. Positive-pressure ventilation, particularly in patients with more severe lung injury or disease and diminished lung compliance, potentiates tidal volume loss from a larger bronchopleural fistula. A reduction in tidal volume with an appropriate

Table 11.30. COMPLICATIONS OF MECHANICAL VENTILATION

Complication	Cause	Common conditions
Mechanical		
Tube displacement	High airway pressure	ARDS or infection
	Iatrogenic	Any
Cuff leak	Tube displacement	Any
	Balloon perforation	Any
	Tracheal malacia or dilation	Prolonged ETT intubation
Balloon herniation	Overinflation, obstruction of ETT tip	Any
Main-stem intubation	Iatrogenic	Any
ETT stenosis or kink	Secretions or malposition	Any
Spontaneous pneumothorax	Parenchymal degeneration	ARDS
	High airway pressure	
Bronchopleural fistula	Barotrauma or lung laceration	Infection or ARDS
Nasal erosion	Iatrogenic	Any
Tracheoinominate fistula	Pressure necrosis	Tracheostomy—high pressure
Tracheosophageal fistula		High pressure plus nasogastric tube
Vocal cord granulomas	Pressure necrosis	Prolonged ETT intubation
Aretynoid stenosis	Pressure necrosis	Prolonged ETT intubation
Tracheal stenosis	Pressure necrosis	Tracheostomy
Depressed cardiac output	Impaired venous return	High PEEP or PIP
Increased intracranial pressure	Impaired venous return	High PEEP or PIP
Metabolic		
Hypoxia	Pulmonary edema, $\dot{V}/\dot{Q}$ mismatch	Pneumonia, ARDS, PE
Hypercapnea	$\dot{V}/\dot{Q}$ mismatch	ARDS
Infectious or inflammatory		
Tracheobronchitis	Oropharyngeal colonization	Prolonged ETT intubation
Pneumonia	Gastric and orophyaryngeal colonization	Prolonged ETT intubation
	Variable	Severe injury
ARDS		
Empyema	Iatrogenic pneumonia or gastrointestinal contamination	Variable
Pleural effusion	Reactive or fluid overload	Variable

ARDS, adult respiratory distress syndrome; ETT, endotracheal tube; PE, pulmonary embolus; PEEP, positive end-expiratory pressure; PIP, peak inspiratory pressure; $\dot{V}/\dot{Q}$, ventilation/perfusion.

increase in ventilatory rate usually reduces the volume loss to tolerable levels. Occasionally, more complex ventilatory patterns are required to reduce airway pressures (time-cycle, pressure-controlled, high-frequency, or double-lung ventilation). Elevated airway pressures may be secondary to intraabdominal complications, and abdominal compartment syndrome should be ruled out in any patient with climbing ventilator pressures.

Pneumonia and empyema constitute most posttraumatic thoracic infections. Penetrating trauma that results in pleural contamination sufficient to cause an empyema occurs infrequently. The more common causes are severe chest wall injuries or gastrointestinal contamination through a diaphragmatic defect. *Staphylococcus aureus* is the causative organism in most posttraumatic empyema unless there has been contamination from the abdomen. Iatrogenic contamination and failure or delay in adequately evacuating a hemothorax are contributing factors. The prophylactic use of antibiotics, although possibly of benefit, should not be considered a substitute for aseptic technique, proper chest tube positioning, complete evacuation of a hemothorax or pneumothorax, and complete reexpansion of the lung.

Pneumonia is one of the most prevalent and troublesome infections after trauma. Most postinjury pneumonias occur in patients who require prolonged endotracheal intubation and mechanical ventilation. In patients with severe head injuries who require prolonged muscular paralysis, the incidence of pneumonia approaches 80% to 90%. Causative factors include reduced cough, impaired mucociliary clearance, immunosuppression, aspiration, and oropharyngeal and gastric bacterial colonization (Table 11.31).

Posttraumatic nosocomial pneumonia characteristically is caused by gram-negative enteric organisms such as *Escherichia coli, Klebsiella* species, and *Pseudomonas* species. These organisms are typically found in the gastrointestinal tract and are frequently found colonizing the normally sterile upper gastrointestinal tract and oropharynx in critically ill patients admitted to the ICU. Contamination of the upper respiratory tract by microaspiration of these oropharyngeal or gastric organisms has been implicated in the pathogenesis of nosocomial pneumonia. Consequently, therapeutic strategies have evolved that try to minimize this process. These have included prophylaxis of stress ulceration with the use of cytoprotective agents that preserve gastric acidity rather than acid-neutralizing strategies in the hope that this may reduce gastric colonization and subsequent inoculation of the respiratory tract; and the use of topical antimicrobial agents in the oropharynx and intragastrically to decontaminate these sites selectively by reducing the levels of pathogenic gram-negative organisms. To date, the data comparing different stress ulceration strategies with the incidence of nosocomial pneumonia have yet to demonstrate any consistent benefit of cytoprotective over acid-neutralizing strategies (471,472). The data on selective decontamination of the digestive tract suggest a decreased incidence of nosocomial pneumonia in patients given topical antibiotics, but this has yet to be translated into decreased length of stay in the ICU or improved survival (473,474).

The diagnosis of pulmonary infection in trauma patients with prolonged endotracheal intubation is complicated by the certainty that colonization is present and by the fact that concurrent noninfectious problems are common (atelectasis, pulmonary edema, acute respiratory distress). The use of conventional findings on sputum Gram's stain, evidence of systemic infection, and radiographic findings is problematic. Clinical reports suggest that quantitative cultures of central respiratory secretions also may be inaccurate (475,476). Bronchoscopy with either protected catheter brush sampling or bronchoalveolar lavage promises a higher degree of diagnostic accuracy in patients with recurrent or resistant respiratory infections, but has not entered mainstream ICU care (477,478).

Nosocomial pneumonia requires appropriate and adequate antibiotic therapy. Treatment is often empiric, at least initially, and choice of antibiotic depends on Gram's stain identification of predominant organisms and the knowledge of prevailing antibiotic sensitivities or organisms specific to the unit or hospital. Once the organism and specific antibiotic sensitivities are identified, treatment can be modified accordingly for the purposes of simplicity, consistency, and cost effectiveness. Use of antibiotics, empiric and specific for nosocomial pneumonia, should be standardized by formal protocols, revised on a regular basis in the light of unit or institutional changes in prevailing organisms or sensitivities.

Deep venous thrombosis and its lethal counterpart, pulmonary embolus, are not infrequent complications after traumatic injury. Deaths from pulmonary embolus contribute significantly to delayed mortality after trauma. Patients at high risk for this complication should be prospectively identified and receive adequate prophylaxis using a combination of mechanical calf compression stockings and low-dose anticoagulation. Low-molecular-weight heparins have proven to be more efficacious than unfractionated heparin for the prophylaxis of trauma patients. In high-risk patients in whom standard prophylaxis is not possible, placement of a prophylactic inferior vena cava filter should be considered. Patients with multiple long-bone fractures, pelvic fractures, spinal cord injury, or severe head injury all should be considered at high risk, and because pulmonary embolus is a frequently unheralded but lethal complication, prophylaxis should be initiated at the earliest opportunity (479).

Relief of thoracic pain after blunt chest injury is an important but often neglected adjunct to the maintenance of good pulmonary toilet. Patients with multiple rib fractures derive substantial benefit from adequate analgesia. To this end, patient-controlled narcotic analgesia or the lumbar or thoracic epidural administration of opiate analgesics or local anesthetics may be particularly helpful in appropriately selected trauma patients (480). Adequacy of analgesia can be determined by intermittent assessment of objective parameters such as maximal inspiratory force and vital capacity.

Most trauma patients require mechanical ventilation only for short-term management, and guidelines for ventilator weaning and extubation are similar to those for other surgical patients. Increases in ventilatory work associated

---

Table 11.31. POTENTIAL FACTORS PREDISPOSING TO THE DEVELOPMENT OF POSTINJURY PNEUMONIA

Aspiration at the time of injury (blood, gastric contents)
Muscular paralysis (head injury)
Enforced immobilization (elevated head of bed, head injuries)
Orthopedic injuries (soft-tissue emboli, immobilization)
Sinus infection (bacterial reservoir)
Infected pneumatocele (bacterial reservoir)
Endotracheal intubation (conduit for microaspiration)
Nasogastric intubation (wick for gastric contents)
Neutralization of gastric pH (bacterial overgrowth with aspiration)
Pulmonary contusion or laceration
Oropharyngeal colonization (increased bacterial adherence)
Tracheobronchial bacterial colonization
   (decreased mucociliary clearance)
Postinjury immunosuppression
Pain and reduced ventilatory capacity

with massive volume resuscitation and chest wall or pulmonary edema usually resolve within the first 48 to 72 hours after trauma and rarely require formal weaning in the absence of additional lung disease.

Patients requiring prolonged mechanical ventilation frequently require a formal program of stepwise reduction in ventilator support. This weaning process is discussed in detail in Chapter 8.

Cardiovascular System

Because most trauma patients are young and in good health, the frequency of major cardiovascular complications after injury is usually low. Complications occur most often in three major groups of patients: (a) the elderly, particularly those with preexisting coronary artery or myocardial disease; (b) patients who have sustained direct myocardial injury; and (c) patients in whom sepsis or multiple organ failure develops later in their hospital course.

Preinjury myocardial disease, particularly coronary artery disease, is clearly associated with decreased survival after major injury (481). Indications for hemodynamic monitoring in high-risk or elderly patients after major trauma should be adjusted appropriately. Patients sustaining major thoracoabdominal or orthopedic injuries are usually monitored with central venous pressure and arterial lines. In addition, a flow-directed pulmonary artery catheter should be placed in patients with evidence of inadequate myocardial function, a history of coronary artery or heart disease, or impairment of gas exchange.

Survivors of penetrating cardiac injuries usually have an uncomplicated postoperative course. Lacerations involving the conduction system or coronary artery are exceptions. Blunt cardiac injury does not often lead to clinical complications. Rhythm disturbances usually are transient, easily treated, and occur within the first several hours of injury (482). For the occasional patient exhibiting cardiac insufficiency after myocardial contusion, the recovery time is usually shorter (48 to 72 hours) than that for myocardial infarction, probably related to the lack of underlying coronary artery disease. Inotropic support is considered safe, if required. Patients with evidence of significant cardiac injury also should be screened for pericardial effusion or tamponade, papillary muscle defects, and ventricular wall contractility using echocardiography.

Cardiac failure unrelated to direct injury may occur after global ischemia and profound hemorrhagic shock or in the presence of sepsis. A variety of small polypeptides, myocardial depressant factors, have been isolated in experimental models of hemorrhagic and endotoxic shock. These appear to exert their effects by a negative inotropic action, but their relevance is uncertain. Care of these patients is simply supportive.

Central Nervous System

The principal challenge in the management of head injury resides in postinjury critical care and involves management of increased intracranial pressure (ICP), cerebral perfusion pressure (CPP), as well as multisystem dysfunction. Failure to control ICP and maintain CPP are the most common and serious complications after severe head injury (483). These issues are discussed in detail in a previous section of this chapter. Management of severely head-injured patients requires the sequential introduction of various monitoring and therapeutic strategies based on clinical course, computed tomography (CT) scan findings, and response to treatment. Significant deterioration in clinical course or ICP should be considered an absolute indication for repeat CT scan. This is the only practical method for the prompt identification of patients in whom surgically correctable mass lesions develop during the initial phase of care.

Intracranial pressure monitors include intraventricular catheters, subarachnoid or subdural bolts, and intraparenchymal or extradural fiberoptic sensors. Complications associated with these catheters are predictable and include malfunction, hemorrhage, and infection. CPP can be determined from the difference between mean arterial pressure and ICP. However, cerebral blood flow may not correlate reliably with CPP, particularly if autoregulation of cerebral blood flow is compromised, and adequacy of cerebral perfusion may be difficult to predict on the basis of a given value of CPP. Jugular venous bulb blood gas determination and the calculation of cerebral oxygen extraction ratios may be a more sensitive predictor of occult cerebral ischemia. Optimal care of seriously head-injured patients requires the close collaboration of the neurosurgeon and surgical intensivist to monitor and coordinate necessary therapeutic interventions while maintaining general supportive care. Hypoxia and hypotension must be avoided at all costs and may affect the timing of nonneurosurgical operative procedures or the decision to manage abdominal injuries nonoperatively.

A unique set of issues arises in patients with lethal head injuries who are identified as potential organ donors. The combined use of CT, clinical examination, and ICP monitoring usually allows prompt identification of these patients. The expansion of transplantation programs has increased the need for donor organs, and the effort to solicit this donation is now a legal requirement in many states in the United States. Physiologic support must be continued until the wishes of the patient or family regarding organ donation can be ascertained. Centrally mediated hypotension, pulmonary edema, massive diuresis from diabetes insipidus, hypothermia, and coagulopathy are all predictable problems that require aggressive support until either death or organ donation. The burden of this support is best minimized by prompt solicitation and expeditious organ donation.

Renal System

Despite the frequency of profound hypovolemic shock that occurs after major trauma, the incidence of renal failure in these patients is declining. A multicenter study of 72,757 trauma patients found an incidence of only 0.11% for renal failure requiring dialysis (484). The combined effects of rapid transportation and appropriate fluid resuscitation are responsible for this remarkably low incidence. Inadequate renal perfusion caused by a variety of shock states remains the primary cause of prerenal dysfunction (485). Hypovolemic shock may be produced by ongoing hemorrhage, inadequate fluid resuscitation, and excessive diuresis combined with volume restriction, as is done in head-injured patients. Causes of inadequate renal perfusion not related to hypovolemia include cardiogenic problems such as myocardial contusion, tamponade, and infarction. Intraabdominal hypertension also precipitates decreased renal blood flow and, left uncorrected, results in progressive renal dysfunction.

Direct renal injury in the posttraumatic patient is most commonly associated with prolonged shock or ischemia and is termed *acute tubular necrosis*. Pharmacologic agents, such as the aminoglycosides, amphotericin, and the radiographic dyes used for contrast studies, are all associated with primary nephrotoxicity. Extremity compartment syndromes or crush injuries producing rhabdomyolysis also may precipitate renal failure on the basis of renal tubular precipitation of pigment compounds. Preexisting renal disease often exacerbates any of these insults.

The outcome for patients with posttraumatic renal failure is determined principally by their underlying disease, the cause of the renal failure, and any associated injuries. Previous reports have suggested that the mortality rate from oliguric renal failure is substantially greater (70% to 80%) than for nonoliguric renal failure (20% to 30%). Supportive treatment for posttraumatic renal failure includes correction of the underlying cause, nutritional support, and dialysis.

Most centers rely on hemodialysis performed using percutaneously placed venous access lines. These methods are more suitable for acute, short-term hemodialysis, and they avoid the complications of infection and thrombosis associated with surgically placed arteriovenous shunts. Peritoneal dialysis is often impractical because of associated abdominal and pelvic injuries, but it can be done if necessary.

Continuous arteriovenous hemodialysis or venovenous hemodialysis has been applied to patients with posttraumatic renal failure. Advantages include its ease of use, absence of systemic anticoagulation, and avoidance of the rapid fluid and electrolyte shifts that occur with intermittent dialysis.

Gastrointestinal System

Missed Injuries

Missed injuries along with postoperative intraabdominal infections are important causes of abdominal complications after trauma. Missed injuries with the use of diagnostic peritoneal lavage occur in approximately 0.5% to 3% of patients. These usually consist of diaphragmatic or retroperitoneal injuries of the duodenum, pancreas, colon, or genitourinary tract. Similarly, bowel and pancreatic injuries are difficult to identify with CT scan and ultrasound and may be missed. A high index of suspicion must be maintained with frequent clinical examination of patients at risk for occult abdominal trauma. The onset of new abdominal signs mandates further work-up or exploration.

Fever, leukocytosis, tachycardia, the development of paralytic ileus, increased fluid requirements, and failure to wean from mechanical ventilation may all represent warning signs of the development of intraabdominal infection. Infection is usually the result of either missed injury or a postoperative complication in the trauma setting. CT scan is the single most useful diagnostic tool in this clinical setting because it yields considerable information with regard to organ injury and the presence of intraabdominal abscesses or fluid collections. Ultrasonography may be useful as well. Its major advantages are portability and low cost, but it is less sensitive, less specific, and may well be more operator dependent in an ICU environment. Localized fluid collections, suspect for intraabdominal abscesses, may be treated by interventional drainage procedures using either modality.

No method of noninvasive imaging is completely accurate, and none should be relied on definitively to exclude intraabdominal injury or infection in the face of contrary clinical data. Bowel perforations, mesenteric or segmental ischemia, and diaphragmatic injuries may be impossible to diagnose reliably using CT scan. Diagnostic peritoneal lavage for the evaluation of acute abdominal problems appears effective in several small series. Laparotomy as a diagnostic test for unexplained sepsis has a low yield in critically ill trauma patients and should not be used routinely. It is the rare patient with progressive sepsis, but no identifiable source on imaging, who benefits from laparotomy.

Intraabdominal Infections

Posttraumatic intraabdominal infection is almost always the result of gastrointestinal tract contamination.

Penetrating trauma accounts for the largest proportion of these infections. Intestinal injuries accompany 40% to 50% of gunshot wounds and 15% to 30% of stab wounds, usually resulting in significant intraabdominal contamination. Because of its higher bacterial counts, the colon is consistently associated with a higher incidence of infectious complications than isolated gastric, duodenal, or small bowel injuries. The precise incidence of intraabdominal or incisional wound infection after colonic injuries depends on factors present at the time of injury (blood loss, degree of contamination, and other associated injuries) and on whether the wound is closed or left open.

The use of perioperative antibiotics for trauma has been investigated extensively. Most of these studies compared single-agent, second- or third-generation cephalosporins with combinations of antibiotics effective against anaerobic and coliform bacteria. Most have demonstrated that single-agent cephalosporins are at least as effective as multiagent regimens in retarding intraabdominal abscesses or wound infections resulting from a variety of contaminated traumatic wounds. Single-agent cephalosporins continue to be the first choice of prophylactic and perioperative antibiotics in the treatment of most abdominal trauma.

The optimal duration of administration of postinjury antibiotics has not been determined, but a number of studies suggest that there is no advantage in administering these agents for more than 2 days.

Open Abdomen and Abdominal Compartment Syndrome

Limited or "damage control" surgery is increasingly popular in the multiply injured patient in whom gross physiologic deterioration has occurred to the point that further surgery would be dangerous. Patients are being returned to the ICU with temporary abdominal closures in anticipation of returning to the operating room once physiologic homeostasis has been achieved. These patients need to be monitored for persistent hemorrhage in the face of corrected coagulopathy and hypothermia, mandating early return to the operating room. Abdominal compartment syndrome is also becoming increasingly recognized in the postoperative period after trauma laparotomy. Extensive retroperitoneal hematoma, bowel edema, and the need for intraabdominal packing all place the patient at risk for development of this syndrome. The trauma surgeon should be aware of this possibility not only at the time of abdominal wall closure, but in the postoperative period. Increasingly tense abdominal distention, increasing airway pressures, difficulty in ventilating, and decreasing urine output in the face of normal vascular filling pressures should strongly suggest the diagnosis. Elevated intraabdominal pressures (intraabdominal hypertension) can be confirmed by transducing the bladder after installation of saline. Pressures greater than 25 cm H_2O, indicating the need for decompressive surgery. Patients with abdominal compartment syndrome need to be returned to the operating room for expeditious reexploration and prosthetic closure. As packs are removed, hematomas and edema resolve, prosthetic material can be gradually imbricated, and abdominal contents eventually reduce below the level of the fascia. Once this has been achieved, final definitive closure of fascia should be possible.

Miscellaneous Abdominal Complications

Stress ulceration of the gastric mucosa causing hemorrhage or perforation has been described after trauma. The incidence of this complication has greatly diminished, however, and this has been temporally related with the introduction of routine prophylactic pharmacotherapy aimed at either reducing gastric pH or providing gastric mucosal cytoprotection. Other factors that may have led to this decreasing incidence are the earlier and more aggressive use of intragastric tube feedings and the development of resuscitation end points that more clearly signal restoration of adequate organ perfusion. However, certain patients still appear to be at high risk for development of stress ulceration, including patients who have septic complications, organ dysfunction, severe multisystem injury (Injury Severity Score >20), a high spinal cord injury with neurologic deficit, or a significant burn injury. These patients should receive aggressive prophylaxis and be monitored for evidence of gastrointestinal bleeding (486). Omeprazole may be useful in those patients with clinically significant bleeding and may be preferable to surgical options except in the exsanguinating patient.

A small number of patients have acute surgical problems unrelated to direct injury, such as acalculous cholecystitis, acute appendicitis, acute diverticulitis, and perforated duodenal ulcer. Diminished pain responses in patients with head or spinal cord injuries and the frequent need for endotracheal intubation and ventilatory support complicate accurate diagnosis. With the exception of acalculous cholecystitis, which can be evaluated using ultrasound and biliary scintigraphy, the diagnosis of nontraumatic intraabdominal infection after trauma is frequently delayed.

Orthopedic and Soft-tissue Complications

Major orthopedic injuries to the pelvis, thoracolumbar spine, or long bones occur in approximately 24% of blunt trauma patients. Related morbidity and mortality usually result from hemorrhage, immobilization, or sepsis. Primary failure of fracture healing is relatively uncommon. Hemorrhage is the major source of mortality and has been discussed. Pelvic fractures are clearly the most problematic. Less dramatic but far more common are the pulmonary and septic complications related to prolonged immobilization and enforced bed rest. As has been discussed, early fixation of these injuries is associated with much lower morbidity rates (487).

Open fractures, particularly those associated with significant soft-tissue loss, are often heavily contaminated and prone to local infection, necrosis, and progressive tissue loss. Long-term disability up to and including amputation can result. Aggressive and frequent operative débridement, dressing changes, and systemic antibiotics maximize the probability of a good outcome.

The potential for development of compartment syndrome exists in any patient with prolonged ischemia, particularly when coupled with associated soft-tissue trauma. Reperfusion edema may take several hours to develop, and compartment pressure should be monitored continuously or frequently for high-risk patients. Prophylactic fasciotomy, performed at the time of initial surgery, is often indicated for prolonged (>4 to 6 hours) ischemia or severe crush injuries. Urinary monitoring for presence of myoglobin and monitoring of serum creatine phosphokinase enzyme levels may be useful in detecting any progressive or ongoing rhabdomyolysis. Evidence of progressive muscle necrosis should prompt a complete inspection of the involved muscle groups, usually in the operating room.

Other Infections

Wound Infection

The incidence of incisional wound infection depends on the method of wound treatment and the degree of contam-

ination. One study of wound infections in trauma patients found an incidence of 3.2%, 8.1%, and 24.6% for clean, clean contaminated, and contaminated wounds, respectively (488). The liberal use of delayed primary closure or secondary closure in heavily contaminated wounds, such as colonic injuries, substantially reduces the incidence of wound infection in the latter group.

Wounds heavily contaminated at the time of injury require extensive débridement and washout. Shotgun wounds, degloving injuries, and crush injuries are at high risk. Obviously, the degree and source of contamination are critical. It may be appropriate to return patients to the operating room daily for débridement and washout of major wounds.

Virtually all contaminated wounds, assuming adequate nutritional repletion, respond to this regimen of repeated débridement and conscientious dressing care. Failure to respond initially to this regimen should prompt a thorough investigation, including quantitative wound cultures and examination for invasive fungal infection. Patients with progressive tissue destruction in the absence of identifiable pathogens often benefit from an empiric course of an antifungal agent. Delays in recognizing invasive fungal infections under these circumstances are frequently lethal.

Large degloving injuries or areas of extensive skin loss usually require thorough débridement and eventual skin grafting. Attempts at creative closures of large contaminated or devascularized flaps over drains are usually futile and increase the risk of serious infection and sepsis. The application of fresh cadaver autografts can provide an ideal interim dressing over débrided wounds and reduces the incidence of secondary infection, pain, and fluid loss.

Catheter Infection

Central venous pulmonary artery and arterial catheters continue to be a major source of nosocomial infections. Infection rates for central venous catheters vary depending on catheter type (single lumen or multilumen), insertion site, duration of use, type of use, dressing type, and the patient's underlying condition. The placement of catheters during initial resuscitation may be less than optimal with respect to aseptic technique. In general, emergency lines are best removed routinely within 24 hours. Failure to do so has been associated with an increased risk of infection. Cutdown catheters are particularly prone to infection and should not be used any longer than is absolutely necessary.

Catheter hub colonization with internal migration of bacteria and external catheter contamination with migration of skin wound bacteria are the two principal sources of catheter infections. The incidence of infection at each of these sites varies and is probably a function of placement technique and the frequency of catheter hub manipulation. The duration of catheter placement and the patient's condition (septic vs. nonseptic) are additional risk factors for catheter infections.

Multilumen catheters have been associated with an increased incidence of contamination and infection compared with single-lumen catheters. Causes for this have not been precisely determined but are probably related to the increased frequency of catheter manipulation and the infusion of multiple agents.

Studies using a silver-impregnated antimicrobial subcutaneous cuff attached to central venous catheters or antibiotic-impregnated catheters have reported a decreased incidence of associated line infections (489,490). Such devices may offer the advantages of reduced infections and the need for less frequent line changes. The usefulness of these devices in trauma patients and their efficacy have yet to be determined.

In general, the treatment of the complication of catheter sepsis is removal with replacement at an alternative site if the line is necessary. Systemic antibiotic therapy may be unnecessary, but if given, the duration of treatment should be brief.

Sinusitis

Sinus infections are important both as primary infections and as a potential reservoir for secondary pulmonary infections. Sinusitis is most commonly associated with obstruction caused by indwelling nasotracheal or nasogastric tubes. Surveillance sinus films should be obtained routinely as part of the fever evaluation in patients with nasal tubes. Tube removal or alternative placement, sinus aspiration or drainage, and antibiotics usually provide adequate therapy.

Envenomation and Environmental Injuries

GREGORY J. JURKOVICH

ENVENOMATION INJURIES

Snakebites

More than 375 species of venomous snakes can be found worldwide, and they are responsible for approximately 300,000 bites and 30,000 deaths each year. In the United States, it is estimated that 45,000 snakebites occur annually, resulting in 14 to 20 deaths each year (491–493). However, in 1991, only 3,805 snakebites were reported to the American Association of Poison Control Centers, and 1,039 of these were from snakes generally considered to be nonpoisonous (494). Occasionally a bite by a garter snake (*Thamnophis* species) can be confused early with the bite of a poisonous snake of the Crotalidae family. Progressive local effects (edema, erythema) can be produced by toxic salivary secretions of a parotid-like gland (Duvernoy's glands) if the skin has been broken (495). However, systemic signs fail to develop, and the local signs resolve spontaneously within a few days.

The five main families of poisonous snakes are the Colubridae, Elapidae, Hydrophidae, Viperidae, and Crotalidae. The Colubridae family consists primarily of the boomslang and the bird snake, which are mainly found in Africa. The Elapidae family includes the cobras, the coral snakes, and the adders, which are found throughout Asia, Africa, the Americas, and Australia. The Hydrophidae family consists of the sea snakes, which are found throughout the Pacific and along the west coast of South America. The Viperidae family consists of old world vipers, which are found throughout Africa, Europe, and the Middle East. The Crotalidae are the true pit vipers and are found worldwide.

The native venomous snakes of North America are members of the phylum Chordata, class Reptilia, order Squamata, suborder Serpentes, and of the families Crotalidae and Elapidae (Table 11.32).

Rattlesnakes are members of the family Crotalidae and the genus *Crotalus* or *Sistrurus*. Water moccasins (or cottonmouths) and copperheads are also members of the Crotalidae family, but of the genus *Agkistrodon*. The coral snake is the major representative of the Elapidae family, and of the genus *Micrurus* or *Micruroides*. Other well known members of the Elapidae family not indigenous to North America are the cobras and mambas. The distribution of venomous snakes in the United States is extensive, with at least one native species found in every state except Maine, Alaska, and Hawaii. Rattlesnakes are particularly widely distributed, whereas the water moccasin is found in the southeastern United States, Mississippi Valley, Illinois, and Indiana. The copperhead's range is primarily from central Massachusetts to northern Florida and west to Illinois and Texas.

The Crotalidae, or pit vipers, have a number of characteristics that help distinguish them from benign snakes (Fig. 11.89). Their unique and characteristic thermoreceptor "pit" is an infrared sensor located between the nostril and the eye that helps the snake localize its prey. Pit vipers also have a vertical elliptical pupil, a triangular head, and retractable fangs. Venomous snakes have a single row of plates distal to the anal plate on their ventral surface, whereas harmless snakes have a double row of caudal plates.

Coloration is so variable as to be nearly useless as a distinguishing characteristic. An exception is the coloration of the Elapidae coral snake, which can be identified by the simple rhyme, "red on yellow kill a fellow; red on black venom lack." This refers to the fact that a coral snake has circular bands of colors with red adjacent to yellow, whereas the nonvenomous but similar-looking king snake has red on black bands that do not completely encircle it. It has been noted that the Eastern coral snake has a completely black nose, whereas the king snake usually does not.

Most snakebites in the United States occur in the Sunbelt region between April and October, with the peak occurring in the summer months of July and August. Prehibernation and posthibernation snakes appear to be more aggressive. The victims of snakebites are typically men between 18 and 50 years of age, and up to 60% of victims are deliberately handling snakes (496). In one report (496), the ingestion of alcohol was associated with 56.5% of snakebites incurred while intentionally handling or

---

Table 11.32. SNAKES OF THE FAMILY CROTALIDAE

Genus	Common name	Characteristics	Range
Agkistrodon	Water moccasin and copperhead	No rattles; large plates on crown	North America, southeastern Europe, Asia
Bothrops	New World pit vipers	No rattles; small scales on crown; large scales on ventral tail	Mexico to South America
Crotalus	Rattlesnakes	Rattles; small scales on crown	North, Central, and South America
Lachesis	Bushmaster	No rattles; small scales on crown; small scales on ventral tail	Central and South America
Sistrurus	Massasaugas and pygmy rattlesnakes	Rattles; large plates on crown	North America
Trimeresurus		No rattles; small scales on crown	Asia

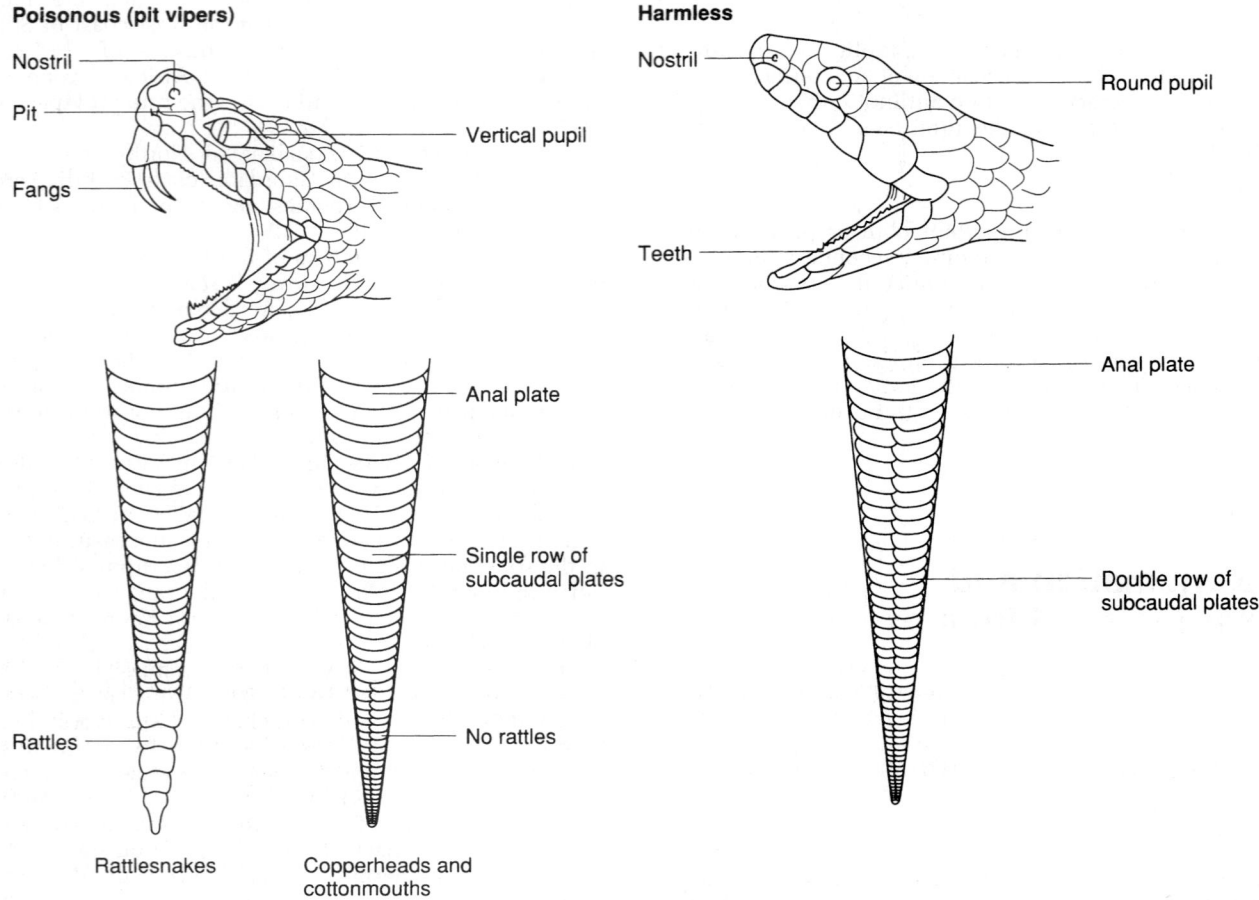

Poisonous (pit vipers)

Nostril

Pit

Fangs

Vertical pupil

Anal plate

Single row of subcaudal plates

Rattles

No rattles

Rattlesnakes

Copperheads and cottonmouths

Harmless

Nostril

Teeth

Round pupil

Anal plate

Double row of subcaudal plates

Figure 11.89. Characteristics of snakes that differentiate poisonous pit vipers from harmless snakes.

knowingly not avoiding a snake. Others suggest that approximately 30% of all snakebite victims are intoxicated (497).

Not every poisonous snakebite results in envenomation, and even the presence of fang marks does not necessarily correlate with envenomation. Venom is produced in large glands located on the dorsal sides of the head, corresponding to the parotid glands, giving the head its characteristic triangular shape. During the bite, the venom is forced through the hollow fangs by the palatine muscles and extruded out the orifices, which are located just proximal to the tip. Therefore, small amounts of clothing or foot gear may significantly diminish the depth of penetration and limit the amount of envenomation.

The severity of envenomation is related to the amount of venom injected, the concentration of the venom, and the size of the snake. Direct intravenous envenomation is unusual but particularly severe (498). Snakebites with a distance between the fangs of more than 15 mm are representative of a large snake and therefore suggest a potentially more significant envenomation. Hibernation also seems to play a role in severity. After hibernation, snakes are relatively dehydrated because they have been in a prolonged fasting state, and therefore they produce a more potent, concentrated venom. The degree of envenomation also varies because even with fang marks, 10% to 25% of bites have no significant envenomation. With each strike, the snake may discharge between 25% and 75% of its venom, so that successive or repetitive strikes tend to diminish the amount of venom available. It has also been observed that

snakes that are angered or fearful may discharge greater amounts of venom.

Venom

The function of venom is to kill or immobilize prey and to aid in digestion. Venom consists of a complex array of proteins and enzymes that are characterized in general as neurotoxins, hemotoxins, and cardiotoxins. More than 26 different proteins and nonenzymatic peptides have been isolated from various venoms (493). The Crotalidae venom consists of approximately 90% water, 5 to 15 enzymes, 3 to 12 nonenzymatic proteins and peptides, and more than 6 other unidentified substances. A partial list of these enzymes is shown in Table 11.33 and includes several proteolytic enzymes, phospholipase, nucleotidase, acetylcholinesterase, and amino acid oxidase.

The low-molecular-weight peptides and polypeptides appear to act by damaging vascular endothelial cells. Electron microscopic analysis of tissue from humans has demonstrated disruption of the vascular endothelium and other plasma membranes. Microangiopathic vascular injury leads to increased permeability, peripheral edema, pulmonary edema and hemorrhage, significant interstitial fluid sequestration, and hypotension. Other venom proteins appear to induce a neuromuscular blockade or coagulopathy. Procoagulant venom factors seem to dominate, primarily exerting their effect late in the clotting cascade by activating factor X or prothrombin or directly converting fibrinogen to fibrin (499). Tissue destruction is aided

Table 11.33. ENZYMES OF SNAKE VENOMS

Proteolytic enzymes
Arginine ester hydrolase
Thrombin-like enzyme
Collagenase
Hyaluronidase
Phospholipase A_2 (A)
Phospholipase C
Lactate dehydrogenase
Phosphomonoesterase
Phosphodiesterase
Acetylcholinesterase
RNase
DNase
5'-Nucleotidase
L-Amino acid oxidase

by several different proteins. L-Amino acid oxidase causes extensive tissue destruction and splits fibrinogen, leading to platelet trapping and unstable clot formation, thus contributing to the genesis of disseminated intravascular coagulation (DIC). Phospholipase A_2 causes hydrolysis of lecithin at the C-2 position, resulting in the formation of lysolecithin. This alters the permeability of erythrocyte membranes and muscle cell plasma membranes, leading to hemolysis and tissue edema. Hyaluronidase induces the lysis of ground substance and thereby aids in the distribution of the venom throughout body tissues.

The Elapidae snakes also have specific neurotoxins and cardiotoxins, which have a more direct effect on the neuroactivity of the prey. Coral snake venom exhibits a direct blocking action on the acetylcholine receptor sites that does not appear to be responsive to neostigmine. This causes ptosis, dysphagia, and slurred speech and can lead to seizures, coma, and death within 8 to 72 hours.

Signs and Symptoms

The important signs and symptoms of snakebites include both local and systemic effects. Immediate pain and progressive edema and erythema at the site of the bite are the norm. Local signs and symptoms progressing at a rate of greater than 30 cm/h, along with microscopic hematuria and bleeding from the puncture sites, indicate significant envenomation (500). Occasionally delayed toxicity has been observed, and rarely severe toxicity has followed after resolution of initial local symptoms (501).

Myonecrosis at or near the bite site is affected by both the direct toxic effects of the venom and the added ischemia of edema and increased compartment pressures. The development of a frank compartment syndrome after a snakebite of the extremity is an unusual occurrence. Studies using purified venom injected into the anterolateral leg compartment of mongrel dogs determined that only intramuscular injection leads to an increase in compartmental pressure (502). Because most snakebites do not penetrate through the superficial fascia, compartment syndromes are unusual and the principal cause of myonecrosis is probably direct toxicity of the venom rather than ischemia from elevated compartment pressure. Nonetheless, in one report of 36 rattlesnake bites, three definitive diagnoses of compartment syndrome were made on the basis of elevated compartment pressures (503). The indication for fasciotomy remains controversial, with some authors recommending fasciotomy in nearly all cases (504), but others believing that aggressive use of antivenin precludes the need for fasciotomy in most instances. In one of those reports, only 1 fasciotomy was required in the treatment of 272 Eastern diamondback and water moccasin bites (505).

Shock is a common finding with significant systemic envenomation, resulting from increased microvascular permeability and the loss of plasma volume. Bradycardia and arrhythmia result from the cardiotoxins. Renal failure may occur from hypoperfusion and shock, DIC with renal tubular necrosis, or as a direct toxic effect of the venom. Sixteen cases of Sheehan's syndrome of pituitary necrosis have also been reported after a Russell viper bite and were thought to be due to the procoagulant activity of the viper's venom (506).

The hematologic effects of venom cause both local and systemic problems. Venom appears to activate factor X as well as factors V and IX, or directly converts fibrinogen to fibrin, leading to activation of the coagulation cascade and a consumptive coagulopathy (499). The prothrombin time (PT) and partial thromboplastin time (PTT) are commonly increased. This may result in persistent bleeding, ecchymosis, or petechia at the puncture site or affected extremity. Microscopic hematuria and bleeding from any preexisting condition, such as peptic ulcer or menstrual bleeding, may aggravate the situation. Venom also causes a mild defibrinogenation state, with unstable clot formation using fibrinogen but sparing platelets. This may contribute to DIC.

Venom also appears to cause myriad neurologic effects, especially the venom from the Elapidae family. The venom of coral snakes, cobras, and sea snakes contains an acetylcholinesterase receptor antagonist that causes ptosis, slurred speech, and impaired swallowing leading to hypersalivation. This venom also has central nervous system activity that results in progressive weakness, paresthesia, and eventually respiratory muscle failure and respiratory arrest. Seizures and psychotic behavior may develop that can lead to coma or death in 8 to 72 hours. The toxins responsible include neurotoxin A, which appears to act on the central nervous system, and neurotoxin B, which acts at the myoneural junction.

Clinical Evaluation

Initial laboratory testing should include electrolytes, complete blood count with platelet count, PT, PTT, fibrinogen level, and urinalysis (500). Frequent clinical examinations should focus on neurologic, hematologic, and hemodynamic profiles. Special immunodiagnostic studies have been developed to help identify the species of snake, but these tests are not yet clinically applicable in the United States (507). Radioimmunoassay is extremely sensitive, with some venoms being detected to levels of 0.4 μg/L. The limited applicability of this assay is due to its expense and the fact that it may take 24 hours to produce a definitive result. The enzyme-linked immunosorbent assay (ELISA) has been widely used and is sensitive to 5 mg/L of venom. ELISA may be run on serum, urine, blister fluid, or aspiration fluid. This test is helpful when attempting to determine the specific snake to direct monovalent antivenin therapy. In the United States, however, there is only one Crotalidae antivenin and only one coral snake antivenin; therefore, this more detailed identification usually is unnecessary (508).

Treatment

First aid begins with immobilization and splinting of the infected part at the level of the heart or at a slightly dependent position, much as a fracture of the extremity would be treated. The utility of incision and suction at the puncture site has been debated for years. In dogs, up to half of the venom can be removed if incision and suction are begun within 3 minutes of the bite (509), but these results have not been verified in humans. Russell has indicated that if immediate incision and suction is started and continued for 1 hour, at best, 11% of the venom may be removed (493,510). Most authorities do not recommend incision and suction therapy (511).

The use of a proximal tourniquet should also be discouraged because it may lead to venous congestion and increased ischemia without demonstrated benefit. Cryotherapy (ice pack) is discouraged universally because it increases tissue ischemia. The effects of cryotherapy and steroids were studied in envenomated mongrel dogs, and it was found that no added benefit could be demonstrated by using corticosteroids or cryotherapy as adjuvants to antivenin alone (512).

Tetanus prophylaxis and the prevention of secondary infections are important objectives of snakebite treatment. Species of the gram-negative bacteria *Aerobacter, Proteus,* and *Pseudomonas* are particularly common causes of bacterial infection, and appropriate systemic antibiotics are given routinely. Cholinergic agonists may be of benefit after an elapid bite because this venom has a significant effect on acetylcholine receptors. Calcium gluconate may also be of benefit after an Elapidae bite to control the onset of seizures. Some snake venoms have been shown to contain metallopeptides, and for this reason, ethylenediaminetetraacetic acid (EDTA) has been tried experimentally in animals as a chelator to inactivate these proteins. The use of EDTA is to be discouraged, however, because it appears to hasten death in laboratory animals for unknown reasons (506). Systemic steroids have no effect in the initial treatment of snakebites, but they play a significant role in treatment of serum sickness that often follows antivenin therapy (513).

Although there is debate over the efficacy and utility of antivenin therapy (514), antivenin remains the mainstay of treatment of significant envenomation throughout the world (515). More than 100 antivenin products are available worldwide, with most recent attention focused on the development and testing of sheep (ovine)-produced antivenin, containing only the venom-binding portion of immunoglobulin G (IgG), termed Fab. (Crotab; Therapeutic Antibodies, Inc., Nashville, TN). This fraction of the antibody is isolated from the ovine serum by sodium sulfate precipitation, followed by papain digestion, which dissociates the venom-binding portion of the IgG, or the Fab component, from the remainder of the antibody, termed Fc (516). Encouraging initial experience suggests that this new ovine antivenin is more potent that the Wyeth-Ayerst (Philadelphia, PA) equine antivenin against all North American crotalids, with fewer allergic reactions (517).

While the newer ovine Fab antivenin is tested and subjected to trials, the two most commonly available antivenins in the United States remain horse serum-based products. The Crotalidae antivenin by Wyeth-Ayerst is a polyvalent, hyperimmune equine serum produced by horse envenomation with the Eastern diamondback, Western diamondback, tropical rattlesnake, and fer-de-lance. The horse serum, before being administered to humans, is partially purified using ammonium sulfate precipitation followed by freeze drying. The other available antivenin is the Eastern coral snake antivenin, also manufactured by Wyeth-Ayerst.

Before administration of antivenin, the patient must be tested for sensitivity to equine serum. Intradermal testing with 0.2 mL of a 1 : 10 or 1 : 100 serum dilution should be performed in all patients, with a positive test consisting of a wheal or erythema within the first 15 to 30 minutes. Similarly, two drops in the conjunctiva with a 1 : 1,000 dilution serum give a positive result with the production of itching and erythema in the conjunctiva. These sensitivity tests have a false-positive rate of approximately 50% and a false-negative rate of 8% to 10%. Anaphylaxis is reported in 3% to 54% of patients treated with antivenin. The latter event is a type I IgE-mediated anaphylactic reaction to the horse serum, which results in mast cell degranulation.

The occurrence of anaphylaxis during or after administration of antivenin mandates immediate cessation of therapy and countermeasures, including antihistamines [diphenhydramine HCl (Benadryl; Parke-Davis, Morris Plains, NJ)], epinephrine infusion, or corticosteroids. The adequacy of the airway and volume status must be ensured. The risk of continuing antivenin must be weighed against the potentially fatal consequences of severe envenomation. The Wyeth-Ayerst antivenin product brochure describes a lengthy desensitization schedule. Concomitant administration of intravenous antihistamine and epinephrine in small, titrated microdrip doses to prevent the most severe manifestations of systemic anaphylaxis has been described in an allergic patient in whom antivenin therapy was deemed essential. This technique requires close physician observation because there are risks from both anaphylaxis and the treatment itself (508).

The other major complication of antivenin therapy is serum sickness. Serum sickness occurs in approximately 50% to 75% of all patients treated with antivenin. It is a type III hypersensitivity reaction in which soluble antigen–antibody complexes are deposited diffusely in the presence of antigen access. In 26 patients who were treated with a total of 507 vials of Crotalidae antivenin, there was a 23% incidence of immediate hypersensitivity reaction and a 50% incidence of serum sickness (513). Eighty-three percent of patients who received more than 8 vials of antivenin had serum sickness, compared with 38% of those receiving fewer than 8 vials. Serum sickness symptoms of urticaria, itching, nephritis, and arthralgia can occur any time up to 3 weeks after antivenin therapy. The exact number of vials of antivenin required to induce serum sickness is not known, but it appears that increasing amounts of antivenin lead to a higher incidence of serum sickness, with almost universal occurrence after the administration of 7 to 10 vials of antivenin. The treatment for serum sickness is systemic corticosteroids in decreasing doses over a 7- to 14-day period.

Pit viper bites may be graded by the following scale (513,518,519):

Grade 0—visible bite but no envenomation
Grade I—minimal pain and edema of less than 25 cm
Grade II—moderate pain, edema of 25 to 40 cm, systemic weakness, and emesis
Grade III—severe pain, edema of 40 to 50 cm, petechia, and systemic vertigo
Grade IV—lethal envenomation with widespread edema, shock, seizures, coma, and renal failure

The estimated initial amount of Crotalidae antivenin needed should correlate with the presenting clinical grade of envenomation. The package insert for Wyeth-Ayerst Crotalidae Antivenin Polyvalent suggests the following dosing estimations:

Grade 0—none
Grade I—none
Grade II—2 to 4 vials
Grade III—5 to 9 vials
Grade IV—more than 10 vials

Each vial is diluted in 50 mL of saline and given intravenously over 15 to 20 minutes. Antivenin therapy is continued until the entire estimated dose is administered or progression of symptoms has stopped. Repeated dosing may be necessary. Children and small adults appear particularly susceptible to envenomation and may require a larger dose than initially anticipated.

Although early surgical excision of the bite wound has been advocated by some, most authorities regard antivenin as the primary therapy and reserve surgery for the occasional compartment syndrome or débridement of necrotic tissue at the site of the bite several days after envenomation. Unless deep intramuscular envenomation has occurred and antivenin therapy has been delayed, fasciotomy is rarely required. Because the musculature and deep compartments of the hand are relatively superficial, however, intramuscular penetration may occur at these sites. Myonecrosis and interstitial edema may cause enough compartmental hypertension in these upper extremity sites that linear finger fasciotomy and digital release are helpful. Fasciotomy may help reduce the ischemic tissue damage caused by increased pressure, but does not alleviate the myonecrosis caused by the direct toxic effect of the venom (502,520). Noninvasive arterial studies may help select patients who require special surgical intervention for ischemia (521).

VENOMOUS LIZARDS

Two species of venomous lizards exist, *Heloderma suspectum* and *Heloderma horridum*. *H. suspectum,* or the Gila monster, is found in the southwestern United States, and *H. horridum,* or the Mexican beaded lizard, is found in central and southern Mexico (522). Physicians may, however, encounter a bite victim anywhere in the world because these colorful animals are common in zoos and often are kept illegally as pets. Nonetheless, human envenomation is very unusual, with only 13 case reports of Gila monster envenomation in the medical literature since 1956, and most from captive animals (523).

Gila monsters grow up to 55 cm in length. They characteristically have slow, lingering movements, but they also have surprisingly quick reflexes and incredibly powerful jaws. Although usually docile, the medical literature reports suggest they can strike without warning or provocation. The mechanism of envenomation is fairly inefficient. The lizard has eight pairs of inferior labial glands located on either side of the lower jaw that secrete venom into the floor of the mouth. By capillary action alone, the venom travels out of the glands and into grooves of the posteriorly curved lower canines (teeth 4 through 7, counting from

the central incisor). Only approximately 60% of bites have significant envenomation because prolonged chewing is required to disperse the venom adequately into the prey. Dislodging the animal from its prey, however, may be difficult because of its extremely powerful jaws. It may be necessary to cut the powerful masseter muscles to pry open the lizard's mouth. More ill-advised techniques of grabbing the tail or igniting the lizard (flame under the lower jaw) have also been attempted. The teeth of the Gila monster are poorly anchored, and periodically shed. Wounds must be thoroughly explored for the teeth because soft-tissue radiographs often fail to demonstrate these foreign bodies (523).

In general, Gila monster bites have local effects, with direct tissue destruction and capillary membrane injury by serotonin, amine oxidases, phospholipase A, hyaluronidase, and a variety of proteases. Pain is the most common clinical symptom, usually subsiding in 8 to 10 hours, although it may persist for several days. Generalized weakness, dizziness, perspiration, and anxiety are other common symptoms. Hypotension is a common clinical finding with envenomation, usually responding to fluid resuscitation alone. There has been one reported case of significant systemic hypotension and myocardial infarction in a 23-year-old after a Gila monster bite (524). Other common signs include erythema, edema, and even lymphangitis, probably from pathogens injected at the time of the bite because injection of sterile venom produces none of these clinical signs. Rather severe nausea and vomiting can also be seen. Laboratory abnormalities are rare. The treatment of Gila monster bites is largely local wound care and systemic support of the patient (fluids, pain relief, antibiotics, antiemetics). No antivenin is available. Tetanus immunization should be current. A period of observation after the bite to assess the potential for systemic toxicity is warranted.

SPIDER BITES

More than six genera of spiders in the United States can inflict painful bites and necrotic ulceration, but most widely known and ones of medical significance are *Loxosceles reclusa* (brown recluse spider), *Tengenaria agrestis* (hobo spider), and *Latrodectus mactans* (black widow spider). In the United States, the brown recluse spider is native to the central South, whereas other *Loxosceles* species exist in the southwestern border state regions (Fig. 11.90).

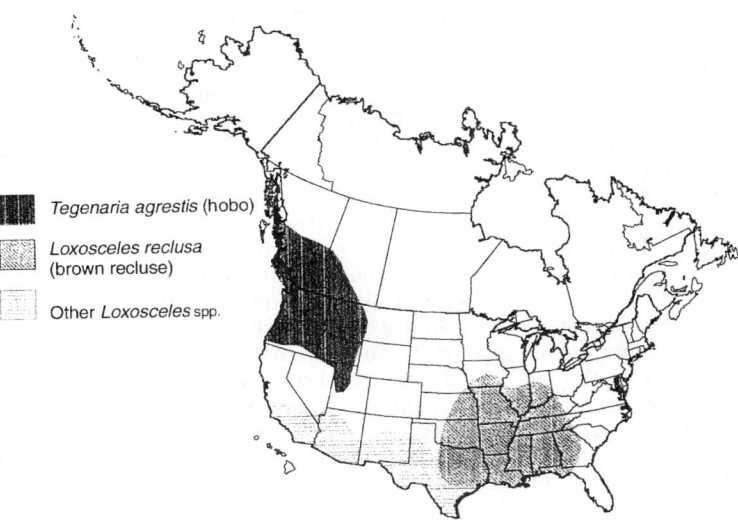

- ■ *Tegenaria agrestis* (hobo)
- ▨ *Loxosceles reclusa* (brown recluse)
- ▢ Other *Loxosceles* spp.

Figure 11.90. The geographic distribution of medically relevant spiders is shown for North America.

Sighting of the brown recluse outside of its native region is rare, and usually attributed to shipping of the spider in boxes of possessions or commerce. On the rare occasion when the brown recluse spider is found outside of its native region, it is a single specimen only, not the typical large populations of spiders that exist when the habitat is conducive to their survival. The hobo spider is indigenous to the Northwest, whereas the black widow spider resides throughout the United States, except for Alaska (525).

All three of these spiders can cause a painful, slow-healing, necrotic ulceration, but not all painful ulcerations should be attributed to spider bites. When a spider has not been positively identified as the offending agent, consideration should be given to other possible causes of necrotic ulceration (526–528). Lyme disease *(Borrelia burgdorferi)* in particular can present with the classic "bull's-eye" patterning characteristic of the brown recluse bite (529). Lyme disease is caused by an *Ixodes* tick-borne spirochete and is most common in the Northeast, Middle Atlantic area and the upper Midwest. Lyme disease is important to distinguish because early treatment with antibiotics (doxycycline) is usually curative, whereas unrecognized infections can cause late arthritic and neurologic symptoms that may not respond to antibiotics.

Tengenaria agrestis was introduced to the Pacific Northwest in the early 1900s from Europe. It was first reported from Seattle in the 1930s, and had become common by the 1960s. It is long-legged (40 mm resting length) and hairy, ranging from light tan to dark brown. Its cephalothorax (10 to 12 mm) is distinguished by two stripes and "butterfly" markings on the dorsal surface, and two stripes marking the ventral surface. It is a poor climber, and hence is usually found in low places. Sometimes referred to as an aggressive house spider, the hobo builds a funnel-shaped web that can be found in woodpiles, crawl spaces, barns, haystacks, and objects that have not been moved in a long time. The hobo spiders are active from spring through fall, and although not overtly aggressive, the most dangerous time to encounter the hobo spider is during the fall mating season; the nests should be avoided and not probed with a finger.

The brown recluse spider is so named because it lives in dark, dry places, emerging only at night. It does not spin a web but catches prey by pursuit. It is small (0.5 to 1 cm wide body; leg span of 3 to 4 cm) and recognizable by the characteristic violin-shaped mark on the cephalothorax. When viewed under a microscope, it has three pairs of eyes rather than the two pairs of eyes most spiders have. Like most biting spiders, they bite humans only when trapped or crushed against the skin. Brown recluse spider bites cause a complex and chronic soft-tissue ulcer. Clinical signs begin first with an erythematous papule (2 to 8 hours), followed by white vasoconstriction (8 to 72 hours), ecchymosis (24 to 72 hours), and a hemorrhagic vesicle (48 to 96 hours) (526). Two to 7 days after the bite, an eschar develops over a characteristic crateriform ulcer, with surrounding soft-tissue induration (530). The eschar may conceal a progressive undermining necrosis that can persist for months. These wounds are most severe in the fatty parts of the body, such as the thighs and buttocks, perhaps because of the relatively poor blood supply to these tissues. There may also be a particular dermonecrotic factor in brown recluse venom. Sphingomyelinase D is present in the venom and appears to interact with the sphingomyelin of the red blood cell membrane, and perhaps capillary endothelial cell membranes, causing cell destruction (531). Histologically, the site of the bite is said to resemble a cutaneous Arthus reaction, with the mechanism involving interactions between complement, neutrophils, and the clotting system (532). Investigations sug-

gest the necrosis is completely dependent on the victim's neutrophils, yet these neutrophils are not activated by the venom. *Loxosceles* venom appears to be a novel yet potent endothelial cell agonist, stimulating the release of interleukin-8 and granulocyte–macrophage colony-stimulating factor, and E-selectin expression (533).

Significant systemic symptoms after a brown recluse bite occur infrequently, perhaps in less than 10% of cutaneous manifestations. The clinical spectrum includes fever, chills, malaise, arthralgia, nausea and vomiting, and a scarlatiniform rash, but can progress to hemolytic anemia, renal failure, and DIC in rare cases, perhaps more commonly in children than adults (534).

Treatment of brown recluse spider bites includes analgesics, wound care, antitetanus therapy, avoidance of early surgical débridement, and perhaps oral dapsone. Antibiotics are reserved for true associated cellulitis. Dapsone if thought to work as an inhibitor of polymorphonuclear leukocyte chemotaxis, but it can cause hemolysis in glucose-6-phosphate dehydrogenase-deficient patients and can produce methemoglobinemia. Some studies show dapsone effective in reducing the size of the skin lesion and limiting the need for surgical débridement (535,536), whereas others demonstrate no benefit in animal models (537). The most common dose is 50 to 100 mg (0.7 mg/kg) twice daily for 3 days to 2 weeks, although it is not approved for this use by the U.S. Food and Drug Administration. One controlled trial of dapsone, electric shock therapy, or no therapy in guinea pigs injected with 30 μg spider venom demonstrated efficacy of dapsone in reducing lesion induration and necrosis area 72 hours after envenomation (538). Electric shock therapy had no benefit. Hyperbaric oxygen treatment of model envenomation in rabbits and pigs also failed to demonstrate any effect on lesion healing time or superficial appearance, although hyperbaric treatments seemed to have decreased the amount of undermining necrosis visualized histologically on day 24 after envenomation (537,539). A trial of hyperbaric oxygen, dapsone, and cyproheptadine in rabbits also failed to demonstrate any significant difference in lesion size, ulcer size, or histopathologic ranking up to 10 days after injection of toxin (540). Local injections of lidocaine, phentolamine, and systemic steroids and antihistamines have been widely used in the past but have no demonstrable benefit. Systemic corticosteroids probably have a role only in the rare case of systemic loxoscelism, which has minimal skin changes but produces massive hemolysis (530). Surgical excision of the lesion itself has no clear benefit (541).

Few living creatures invite such poetic fascination and fear as the black widow spider. Its name, coloring, carnivore diet, and the disconcerting habit of the female eating her sexual partner invite such fascination. And although both the male and female spider possess potent venom, only the female is dangerous to humans because the male is smaller, and its bite cannot penetrate human skin. The mature female has a black body, approximately 6 mm in diameter, with a characteristic red hourglass mark on the ventral aspect of the thorax. This mark is not always present and may consist only of two red dots. The black widow prefers a dry, protected, dimly lit area with access to flies and other insects, such as the outdoor privy. During the period in which the female *L. mactans* is guarding an egg sac, she is particularly aggressive and will attack the male if he disturbs the web, hence earning the particularly dark and descriptive common name (535). The diet most commonly consists of insects of any size, but reportedly includes mice, toads, and tarantulas that wander into the dense web and succumb to the poisonous bite and organ liquefaction.

Black widow venom has a systemic neurotoxin, the primary effect of which is chest pain and abdominal pain. The abdominal pain may mimic an abdominal crisis, with marked cramping and a rigid abdomen. The neurologic signs of hyperreflexia, paresthesia, and cutaneous hyperesthesia help distinguish this from a true intraabdominal catastrophe. Profuse sweating, hypertension, and tachycardia are also common (542). The primary treatment is supportive care and narcotics and muscle relaxants (methocarbamol or benzodiazepam) for pain control, although antivenin therapy also provides effective pain relief in patients with severe envenomations (543). Antivenin is a horse serum-derived immunoglobulin therapy, usually suggested for use in young (<6 years of age), the very infirm, and patients with a severe reaction. The usual dose is 1 ampule in 50 mL of normal saline. Calcium gluconate, 10 mL of a 10% solution given intravenously over 15 to 20 minutes, has usually been considered the first-line treatment of severe envenomations, although one report disputes its efficacy at pain relief (543). Most black widow spider bite symptoms resolve within 1 day, but recurrent symptoms may persist for 2 to 3 days. Antivenin has been reported to be effective up to 30 hours after a bite (544). The reported mortality rate is 2% to 6%, usually as a result of severe acute or delayed hypersensitivity reactions with paralysis, hemolysis, renal failure, and coma.

HYMENOPTERA

The more than 100,000 species of Hymenoptera consist of the well known families of bees, wasps, and hornets, but also include the fire ants, a nonwinged Hymenoptera present in the southeastern United States (545). More envenomations and more deaths (approximately 40 annually) in the United States are caused by Hymenoptera stings than snakebites, emphasizing the fact that the venom of most Hymenoptera is as toxic as the rattlesnake's venom, the difference being the volume administered. The venom is primarily a hemolysin and neurotoxin, known for triggering anaphylactic reactions. Bee venom also contains melittin, phospholipase A_2, and hyaluronidase, which when given in adequate volume can cause endothelial disruption, cell breakdown, and tissue necrosis. It is estimated that approximately 0.4% of the human population is at risk for anaphylaxis from Hymenoptera stings (546). Fortunately, most sting reactions are mild, involving dermal manifestations (hives, edema) only. The clinical effects are related both to the local toxic effects and the anaphylactic systemic effects. The local toxic effects include significant pain, swelling, and pruritus. If a significant amount of toxin is injected, the patient may experience nausea, emesis, and muscle spasms.

Most deaths from Hymenoptera stings are a result of severe anaphylactic reaction, which can occur at any age, but is relatively more common in adults. In this reaction, a preformed IgE antibody activates mast cells, leading to degranulation with massive histamine release and prompting laryngeal and pulmonary edema, vasodilation, and vascular collapse. The treatment for Hymenoptera bites and stings is to remove the stinger, treat the local wound with ice and possibly an enzymatic meat tenderizer, and treat the anaphylactic reactions aggressively with antihistamines (diphenylhydramine HCl, 50 to 100 mg intramuscularly or intravenously) or epinephrine (1 : 1,000 dilution, 0.3 to 0.5 mL intramuscularly or subcutaneously). Patients also require supplemental oxygen and intravenous fluids.

After sting anaphylaxis, approximately 50% of patients remain allergic to subsequent stings, in part determined by the severity of the initial anaphylactic symptoms. Children with benign dermal reactions only are unlikely to have recurrent reactions. Patients with more severe reactions are at risk for repeat anaphylaxis. Patients with a history of insect sting anaphylaxis and positive venom skin tests should have epinephrine available and are candidates for subsequent venom immunotherapy, which provides almost 100% protection against subsequent sting reactions. Such desensitization can take over 3 years (546).

Africanized bees *(Apis mellifera scutellata)* are a more aggressive subspecies than the native European bees of North and South America. Initially imported to Brazil in 1956 in the hope that they would hybridize with the better honey-producing European bee, some escaped and began interbreeding with domestic bees, proliferated, and migrated through Central America, reaching the United States around 1990 (547). Currently located primarily in the arid southwestern United States, these bees now pose a significant threat because massive envenomations (>50 bites) have occurred, resulting in nausea, vomiting, shock, hemolysis, rhabdomyolysis, and DIC; coma and renal failure can follow. Rarely, in patients initially complaining only of pain after multiple bee stings, a delayed (6 to 48 hours) toxic reaction has been reported, and some poison centers now recommend a 24-hour hospitalization for pediatric patients, older patients, and patients with underlying medical problems after an envenomation of 50 or more stings because such patients have an increased risk of delayed severe systemic reaction (548). Laboratory studies on patients sustaining massive envenomations should be performed on presentation and 6 hours later to rule out hemolysis, thrombocytopenia, liver function abnormalities, and rhabdomyolysis.

Two species of imported fire ants now infest large areas of the Gulf Coast states (549). The most aggressive species, *Solenopsis invicta,* has adapted well to environmental conditions in the South, where it has become a considerable agricultural pest and a significant public health problem. Sting reactions typically include a dermal wheal-and-flare reaction followed by sterile pustules at sting sites. Occasionally, large local dermal reactions and pyoderma, or even life-threatening anaphylaxis can occur. Four venom allergens have been isolated and characterized. Clinical studies under way are designed to compare the safety and efficacy of fire ant venom with whole-body extract for diagnosis and treatment of fire ant allergy (545).

SCORPIONS

More than 650 types of scorpions can be found worldwide. In the United States, most are not lethal, and the sting results primarily in local effects. In parts of Brazil, Mexico, North Africa, India, and Israel, however, the scorpion sting may be lethal. The venom toxicity depends greatly on species, season, and the age of the scorpion. In a fatal response, the venom induces a sympathetic storm, resulting in hypertension, tachycardia, and high-output cardiac failure (550). Serum biochemistry reveals increased potassium and glucose, decreased sodium, and markedly elevated catecholamine levels. The treatment is specific antivenin therapy and systemic support directed at controlling hypertension and acute pulmonary edema. The outcome in the United States is usually excellent, with complete resolution of local effects, but in some parts of Brazil, the mortality rates for a scorpion sting have been reported to be as high as 12% in adults and 60% in children (551). In India, of 34 children admitted to hospital after scorpion sting, 14 had hypertension, 9 had acute pulmonary edema, 5 had myocardial failure, and 4 died (550). In one report from Israel, respiratory distress was the main feature in 17 of 54 children with scorpion stings, but only 3 required mechanical ventilation. Two patients died, but both failed to receive antivenin (552). However, another report from Israel evaluated the treatment of 104 children with scorpion envenomation, noting that since 1989 they had discontinued using antivenin, with similar, if not better results in the no-antivenin group (553). The antivenin in this report, however, is prepared from donkeys treated with the venom of the yellow scorpion *(Leiurus quinquestriatus)*, which is not the same as the North American bark scorpion *(Centuroides exilicauda)* antivenin.

HYPOTHERMIA

Because humans are homeotherms, we attempt to maintain a constant body temperature despite changes in environmental temperature. Normal body temperature depends on the site of measurement and is 37°C sublingually, 38°C in the rectum, 32°C at the skin, and 38.5°C deep in the liver. Even minor deviation from normal leads to important symptoms and disability (554). Humans have a remarkable capacity to dissipate heat by evaporating body water; however, our tropical evolutionary heritage has provided us with far less ability to cope with cold conditions. As a result, hypothermia can occur in a variety of clinical settings, and from a number of causes (Table 11.34).

To allow for the normal circadian temperature variation of 0.5° to 1°C, hypothermia is considered to be present in humans if the core temperature drops below 35°C (95°F). Hypothermia is usually classified by temperature zones as mild (32° to 35°C), moderate (28° to 32°C), or severe (<28°C) (555). Primary accidental hypothermia is defined as a decrease in core temperature that occurs as a result of overwhelming environmental cold stress. It most often occurs as a result of recreational misadventures that lead to cold-water immersion or prolonged environmental exposure. Secondary accidental hypothermia occurs in patients with abnormal heat production or thermoregulation, who become cold despite only mild cold stress (e.g., hypothyroidism, stroke, hypoadrenalism, trauma, hypoglycemia, drug overdose). The term *urban hypothermia* sometimes describes the hypothermia of the homeless, typically found in those predisposed to cooling by drugs, alcoholism, age, debilitating diseases, poverty, or some combination of these factors. Chronic hypothermia develops in patients with impaired heat generation (i.e., elderly and infirm) who live in nonheated apartments, are under continual cold stress, and after a time are found always to have a low temperature, as if they have autoregulated to a new set temperature. A multicenter review of 428 cases of accidental hypothermia reported an overall mortality rate of 17% (556), although other reports document mortality rates as high as 80%, primarily due to infection and underlying illness.

The physiologic response to hypothermia is one of transitional changes, with few exact temperature-dependent responses (Fig. 11.91). Broadly speaking, the transition from a "safe zone" of hypothermia (in which physiologic adaptations to heat loss are working) to a "danger zone" of hypothermia (in which shivering is abolished, metabolism decreases, and heat loss is passively accepted) occurs between 33° and 30°C. The initial effects of hypothermia mimic intense sympathetic stimulation, with tremulousness, profound vasoconstriction, tremendous increases in oxygen consumption, and acceleration of heart rate and minute ventilation (557).

The cardiovascular response includes tachycardia, followed by progressive bradycardia, which starts at approximately 34°C and results in a 50% heart rate decrease at 28°C. Cardiac output initially increases with the tachycardia, then progressively decreases, with a concomitant fall in blood pressure. The conduction system is particularly sensitive to hypothermia: the PR, then the QRS, and finally the QT interval become progressively prolonged (558). As temperature falls below 30°C, atrial fibrillation, bradycardia, and ventricular dysrhythmia become common, with asystole occurring at temperatures below 25°C (559). Because palpating pulses or measuring blood pressure in cold, stiff, hypothermic patients is difficult, the presence of an organized cardiac electrical rhythm should be taken as a sign of life that contraindicates cardiopulmonary resuscitation chest compressions, despite the absence of a palpable pulse. Such a rhythm may provide diminished but sufficient circulation in patients with severely reduced metabolism, and it is likely that vigorous chest compressions will convert this perfusing rhythm to fibrillation. Rewarming with close monitoring of rhythm, pulse, and blood pressure are indicated. If cardiac arrest should occur, extracorporeal cardiopulmonary bypass for perfusion and rewarming is indicated (560). One report noted excellent long-term functional outcomes in 15 of 32 young patients successfully rewarmed in this manner (561). All patients were intubated and ventilated and had received ongoing cardiac massage during transportation, and all 15 survivors had documented circulatory arrest (ventricular fibrillation or asystole) and fixed, dilated pupils. The mean interval from discovery of the patient to rewarming with cardiopulmonary bypass was 141 ± 50 minutes; the mean temperature was 21.8° ± 2.5°C.

Respiratory drive is increased during the early stages of hypothermia, but below 33°C progressive respiratory depression occurs, resulting in a decrease in minute ventilation. This usually is not a significant problem until temperatures below 29°C are reached. Occasionally, hypothermia results in the production of a large amount of mucus (cold bronchorrhea) (562). Because ciliary action and the cough reflex are also depressed, this predisposes to atelectasis and

---

Table 11.34. CLINICAL DEFINITIONS OF HYPOTHERMIA AND EXAMPLES OF SETTINGS IN WHICH THEY OCCUR

Type	Settings
Accidental	Recreational environmental exposure, cold water immersion
Therapeutic	Treatment of Reye's syndrome cardiopulmonary bypass, organ preservation
Drug induced	Alcohol, anesthetics, barbiturates, phenothiazines, morphine, others
Central nervous system dysfunction	Transection of spinal cord, hypopituitarism, cerebrovascular accidents
Hypothalamic dysfunction	Wernicke's encephalopathy, anorexia nervosa, head trauma, pinealoma, other tumors
Metabolic	Hypoglycemia, hypothyroidism, hypoadrenalism, malnutrition
Dermal dysfunction	Burns, erythrodermas
Traumatic	Occurs after any major injury

Adapted from Jurkovich GJ. Hypothermia in the trauma patient. Adv Trauma 1989;4:111, with permission.

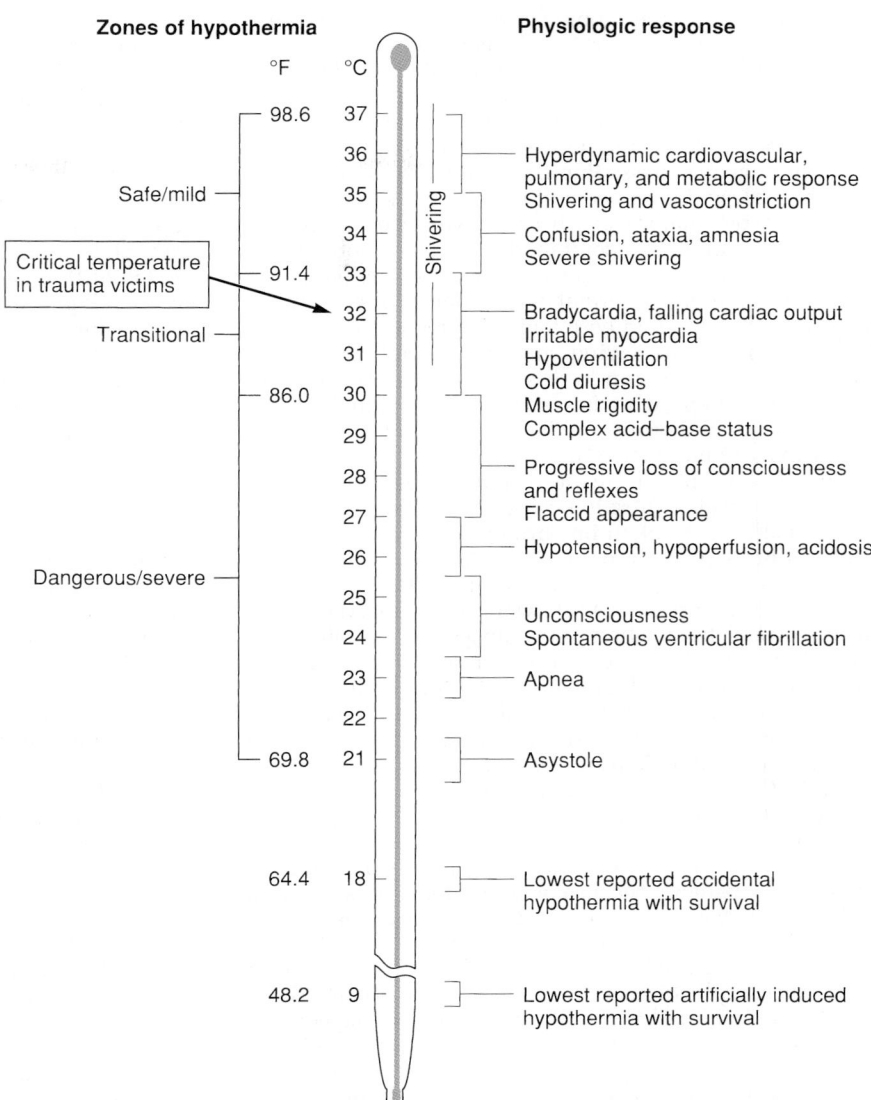

Zones of hypothermia

°F   °C

— 98.6   37

36

Safe/mild   35

34

— 91.4   33

Transitional   32

31

— 86.0   30

29

28

27

26

Dangerous/severe   25

24

23

22

— 69.8   21

64.4   18

48.2   9

Critical temperature in trauma victims

Physiologic response

Shivering

Hyperdynamic cardiovascular, pulmonary, and metabolic response
Shivering and vasoconstriction

Confusion, ataxia, amnesia
Severe shivering

Bradycardia, falling cardiac output
Irritable myocardia
Hypoventilation
Cold diuresis
Muscle rigidity
Complex acid–base status

Progressive loss of consciousness and reflexes
Flaccid appearance

Hypotension, hypoperfusion, acidosis

Unconsciousness
Spontaneous ventricular fibrillation

Apnea

Asystole

Lowest reported accidental hypothermia with survival

Lowest reported artificially induced hypothermia with survival

Figure 11.91. Zones of hypothermia and corresponding physiologic response. Wide biologic variability accounts for physiologic changes rarely occurring at exact temperatures noted. (From Jurkovich GJ. Hypothermia in the trauma patient. *Adv Trauma* 1989;4:111, with permission.)

aspiration. Noncardiogenic pulmonary edema is also occasionally reported, especially in elderly patients, and especially after prolonged periods of hypothermia (563).

Perhaps the greatest controversy regarding the pulmonary effects of hypothermia revolves around the need to correct blood gases to the patient's hypothermic body temperature. Arterial blood gas samples are always warmed to 37°C before measurement. A nomogram of Severinghaus mathematical corrections is then used to estimate the blood gas values at the patient's actual body temperature. With each 1°C temperature reduction, the P_{CO_2} decreases by 4.4% and the P_{O_2} decreases by 7.2%. Thus, a blood gas measured at 37°C with a P_{CO_2} of 40 mm Hg and a P_{O_2} of 70 mm Hg in a 32°C patient is reported as having a P_{CO_2} of 32 mm Hg and a P_{O_2} of 48 mm Hg after temperature correction.

The decrease in partial pressure is related to the increased solubility of gases in cold fluids, and is not a result of a change in carbon dioxide content, oxygen content, or serum bicarbonate level. Clinicians often assume that the normal P_{CO_2} and P_{O_2} at 37°C are the values that should be attained at all temperatures. However, if normothermic end points for P_{CO_2} are attained in a hypothermic patient, they would have increased total body CO_2 stores, which would manifest by a rising P_{CO_2} and a falling

pH during rewarming. Likewise, attempts at increasing a P_{O_2} that reflects normal oxygen content at a lower temperature are also inappropriate. A far simpler strategy is to assess the blood gases at 37°C without temperature correction. Values that are normal and acceptable when reported at 37°C correspond to normal values and contents when "corrected" for hypothermic temperatures.

Temperature correction of blood gases for pH management is also unnecessary. A pH of 7.40 at 37°C would be temperature corrected to 7.47 in a 32°C patient. At 37°C, the acid–base balance of water is neutral (pH = pOH) when the pH is 6.8, and the body functions optimally when its pH is offset 0.6 pH units above the neutral point of water, and has a relatively alkaline pH of 7.40. The pH of water rises with cooling, causing the pH of blood to rise by 0.015 pH units/°C, without a change in bicarbonate content (564,565). Managing a 30°C patient with a pH of 7.40 instead of 7.47 fails to maintain the normal pH offset above the neutral point of water (relative alkalinity), and results in a acidotic cellular and chemical environment that has a multiplicity of effects on enzyme systems. Because blood with a pH of 7.40 assessed at 37°C is reported as having a pH of 7.47 when temperature corrected to 32°C, the simplest strategy when confronted with a 32°C patient is to assess the blood gas at 37°C only, and to use the 37°C uncorrected pH value for management (566,567).

The neurologic response to hypothermia is heralded by progressive loss of lucidity and deep tendon reflexes, and, eventually, by flaccid muscular tone. Patients are often amnestic below 32°C, and between 31° and 27°C they usually lose consciousness. Pupillary dilatation and loss of cerebral autoregulation occur at temperatures below 26°C, and electroencephalography becomes silent at 19° to 20°C (568). These findings, combined with an unobtainable pulse and apparent rigor mortis, may cause the patient to appear dead. It is important to remember that patients have been revived from core temperatures as low as 14°C (569), and hence the saying "no one is dead until warm and dead." An exception to this admonition probably includes the patient who has sustained an anoxic event while still normothermic and has a serum potassium level greater than 10 mmol/L (570).

Reduction in blood pressure and cardiac output decreases glomerular filtration rate, but urinary output is maintained because of an impairment in renal tubular Na^+ reabsorption (cold diuresis) (571,572). Vasoconstriction also results in an initial increase in central blood volume that prompts a diuresis. Ileus, bowel wall edema, depressed hepatic drug detoxification, punctate gastric erosions (Wischnevsky's ulcers), hyperamylasemia, and, rarely, hemorrhagic pancreatitis are hallmarks of the intestinal response to hypothermia. Hypothermia inhibits insulin release and insulin uptake at receptor sites, making hyperglycemia a relatively common finding, especially at temperatures below 30°C (573). Exogenous insulin administration is unwarranted because it may result in rebound hypoglycemia during rewarming. Serum electrolyte changes are unpredictable, but serum potassium is often slightly increased in hypothermic patients because of renal tubular dysfunction, acidosis, and the breakdown of liver glycogen (574). Hypothermia also appears to affect endothelial cell adhesion molecule function, which may partially explain increased infectious complications in hypothermic patients (575).

Body temperature has a significant effect on oxygen uptake. Oxygen consumption ($\dot{V}O_2$) increases dramatically with any fall in body temperature. When involuntary muscle contractions in the form of shivering occur, oxygen consumption increases by as much as three- to fivefold (576,577). This is inefficient because shivering produces heat near the surface of the body, causing most of it to be lost to the environment, with less than 45% being retained by the patient (576).

The thermoregulatory drive is such a powerful one that it takes precedence over many other homeostatic functions. The resultant increase in oxygen utilization may result in anaerobic metabolism, acidosis, and significant cardiopulmonary stress (578). One study noted a 35% increase in oxygen consumption and a 65% increase in CO_2 production in postoperative patients after resolution of anesthesia, when the thermostatic drive reappeared (579). In another study, a core temperature decrease of as little as 0.3°C in postoperative patients was associated with a 7% increase in $\dot{V}O_2$, and temperature reductions between 0.3° and 1.2°C were associated with a 92% increase in $\dot{V}O_2$, with proportional increases in minute ventilation (580). Further details of the specific organ system responses to hypothermia are beyond the scope of this section, but the interested reader is referred to several excellent in-depth monographs (555,564,581–583).

Hypothermia in Trauma Patients

Mild hypothermia is very common after traumatic injury. When ambient temperature falls below the thermoneutral temperature (i.e., the temperature at which no thermogenesis or heat dissipation is necessary), which is 28°C (82.5°F) for humans, an increase in heat production is required to maintain a normal body temperature. Combustion is the only source of endogenous heat production, and this requires an increase in oxygen utilization. However, after shock or injury oxygen supplies are often limited, and further heat loss occurs owing to cold emergency department and operating room environments, cold fluid resuscitation, and open thoracic and abdominal cavities. This is further aggravated by anesthetic and neuromuscular blocking agents that prevent the heat-producing shivering response. Thus, the occurrence of hypothermia in surgical or critically injured patients is most often a form of secondary accidental hypothermia.

In one study, 57% of trauma patients admitted to a level I trauma center were hypothermic at some time, and that temperature loss was most significant in the emergency department (584). Another study reported that the average initial temperature for 94 intubated major trauma victims was 35°C, with no seasonal variation (585). Sixty-six percent of all patients in this study were hypothermic on admission: 43% were mildly hypothermic (34° to 36°C) and 23% had temperatures below 34°C. Likewise, Jurkovich et al. reported that 42% of 71 adult trauma victims with an Injury Severity Score (ISS) of 25 or higher had core temperatures below 34°C, and in 13% the core temperature fell below 32°C (586). Importantly, there were no survivors if core body temperature was below 32°C. Both mortality rate and the incidence of hypothermia increase with higher ISS, massive fluid resuscitation, and the presence of shock, but controlling for these variables still demonstrates that the mortality rate of the hypothermic trauma patient is greater than that of the warm trauma patient (586,587).

Hypothermia in the critically ill surgical patient is also an ominous sign. Although the mortality rate for moderate (28° to 32°C) degrees of primary accidental hypothermia is approximately 20% (556), moderate levels of hypothermia in trauma and critically ill patients are associated with a much higher mortality rate. Rutherford and colleagues have reported that 9.4% of surgical intensive care unit patients had a core body temperature less than 35°C; the mortality rate of the hypothermic trauma patients was 53% (588). Compared with other patient populations, the mortality rate associated with hypothermia in the trauma victim is so high that some have proposed classifying it as a distinct form of hypothermia (589). The following zones of severity for injury hypothermia have been proposed:

Mild hypothermia—36° to 34°C (<96.8° to 93.2°F)
Moderate hypothermia—34° to 32°C (<93.2° to 89.6°F)
Severe hypothermia—less than 32°C (<89.6°F)

Hypothermia appears to occur only in victims of relatively severe trauma. Little and Stoner, reporting on a heterogeneous group of 82 trauma patients, observed that hypothermia occurred only in those patients with an ISS greater than 12 (590). Skin temperature fell from 32.0°C to 31.7°C, whereas core temperature fell from 37.3°C to 36.5°C. Hypothermia did not occur in less severely injured patients, and shivering, which could have been expected, was noted in only one of the hypothermic patients. Mild degrees of injury have, in fact, been associated with small elevations in core body temperature, particularly when the shivering response mechanism has not been ablated (554,591).

The detrimental effect of hypothermia in the human trauma victim is contrasted by a large body of animal experimental evidence suggesting that hypothermia has a protective role in shock. This extensive body of literature is reviewed elsewhere (554), but in general, animals subjected to combined hypothermia and shock (hemorrhage, burn, blunt trauma) usually survive longer than similarly injured but actively warmed animals. Blalock and Mason (1941) were among the first in modern times to recognize the ability of hypothermia to prolong survival times after shock, but they emphasized that the overall survival rate was unchanged (592). However, increases in both survival times and survival rates have been shown in a rat model of induced hypothermia after hemorrhagic shock (593). The protective effects of hypothermia in preventing ischemia–reperfusion injury have been described in a number of models, including muscle, intestine, and rabbit ear (594–596).

Hypothermia has also been suggested to protect the traumatically injured brain. The use of therapeutic hypothermia in a patient with traumatic brain injury was first reported in 1943, and sporadically over the ensuing two decades (597,598). More recently, a randomized, multicenter, controlled trail of core body hypothermia in trauma patients with severe closed head injury [Glasgow Coma Scale (GCS) scores of 3 to 7] has been conducted (599). Select trauma patients with severe head injury were intentionally cooled to 32° to 33°C for 24 hours after injury, and then rewarmed. Early reports suggest an improved or hastened neurologic recovery at 3 and 6 months after injury for those with moderately severe head injury (GCS score of 5 to 7), but there was no difference in functional outcome in any subgroup at 12 months. In addition, the overall patient mortality rate may be higher in the entire cohort of hypothermic patients, although the final report of this study is not yet published. Other authors have reported higher rates of pneumonia and diabetes insipidus in a small study of induced hypothermia in severely head-injured patients (GCS score <8), with no effect on neurologic outcome (600).

Evidence further supporting the harmful effect of hypothermia in the trauma patient is provided by a prospective, randomized trial of rapid rewarming versus conventional rewarming of 57 multiple trauma patients (601). In this study, trauma patients who were rapidly rewarmed with continuous arteriovenous rewarming (CAVR; see later) from less than 34.5°C to greater than 36°C required less resuscitation fluid volume and had a lower early mortality rate than those rewarmed more slowly. Failure to rewarm in either group was uniformly fatal. The survival rate at 3 days after injury was 82% in the rapid rewarm group versus 62% in those conventionally managed. Approximately 50% of the patients in both groups had a severe head injury, defined as a head Abbreviated Injury Severity score of 3 or greater. In this well controlled study, maintenance of hypothermia not only failed to confer an advantage but was detrimental to early survival.

The role of hypothermia in the injured patient remains unresolved. It is apparent that the physiologic consequence of severe trauma is a drop in core body temperature. It remains unclear, however, if this response is an intentional, protective response to shock, or the result of diminished heat production due to failing metabolism. The frequent presence of lactic acid accumulation in cold, seriously injured patients supports the latter hypothesis. Clinical studies indicate that even mild hypothermia in the trauma patient is predictive of a poor outcome. Hypothermia does diminish metabolic demands and oxygen consumption in anesthetized patients, but the price appears to be malfunction of enzymes and physiologic systems necessary to recover from injury.

Perhaps the systems most affected in patients sustaining major trauma are those involved in clotting. Reports of coagulation abnormalities in patients with apparently normal clotting factor levels surfaced shortly after the introduction of hypothermic cardioplegia for cardiac surgery (602,603). Although hemodilution with volume expanders deficient in clotting factors and platelets is usually the primary cause of nonsurgical bleeding, cold platelets are known to undergo morphologic changes that affect adherence, including loss of shape, cytoplasmic swelling, and dissolution of cytoplasmic microtubules necessary for normal motility (604). Platelet activation is also associated with activation of cell membrane phospholipases that hydrolyze phospholipids to arachidonic acid, a precursor to prostaglandin endoperoxides (PGE_2) and thromboxane A_2, a potent vasoconstrictor necessary for normal platelet aggregation (605). Valeri and associates induced systemic hypothermia to 32°C in baboons, but kept one forearm warm using heating lamps and a warming blanket (606). Simultaneous bleeding time measurements in the warm and cold arm were 2.4 and 5.8 minutes, respectively. This effect, which was reversible with rewarming, appeared to be mediated by cold-induced slowing of the enzymatic reaction rate of thromboxane synthetase, which resulted in decreased production of thromboxane A_2.

As with blood gases, clinical tests of coagulation are temperature standardized to 37°C. Fibrometers contain a thermal block that heats the plasma and reagents to 37°C before initiating the assay. Thus, tests of coagulation reflect clotting factor deficiencies but are corrected for any potential effect of hypothermia on clotting factor function. A detailed study of the kinetic effects of hypothermia on clotting factor function has been undertaken by Reed et al., who performed clotting tests (PT, PTT, and thrombin time) on reference human plasma containing normal clotting factor levels at temperatures ranging from 25° to 37°C. The results showed a significant slowing of all coagulation tests at temperatures below 35°C that was proportional to the degree of hypothermia (607). The prolongation of clot formation occurred at clinically relevant levels of hypothermia and was equivalent to that seen in normothermic patients with significant clotting factor depletion. For example, assays conducted at 35°, 33°, and 31°C prolonged the PTT to the same extent as would occur in a euthermic patient with reductions in factor IX levels to 66%, 32%, and 7% of normal, respectively.

Clotting factor supplementation is not the answer to a hypothermia-induced coagulopathy; rewarming is. However, in many seriously injured patients, clotting factor depletion exists in conjunction with hypothermia. A potentiating effect of hypothermia on coagulation dysfunction occurs in plasma of patients with deficient clotting factor levels, although there does not appear to be synergy between the two conditions (608). Hypothermic, coagulopathic trauma patients still benefit from coagulation profile testing. If prolongation of PT and PTT are evident in plasma warmed to 37°C, clotting factor replacement is indicated. If PT and PTT are near normal, rewarming alone reverses the clinically apparent coagulopathy.

Treatment

Rewarming techniques are usually classified as passive external rewarming, active external rewarming, or active core rewarming (555,609). Passive external rewarming simply implies allowing spontaneous rewarming to occur with the patient removed from a hypothermic environment, and is usually used only for the mildly hypothermic patient. Active external rewarming techniques include surrounding the patient with warm blankets or heating pads, infrared heating lights, and immersion in warm water. Active core rewarming includes heated intravenous fluids, as well as heated peritoneal or thoracic lavage, heated gastric, bladder, or colonic lavage, heated and water-saturated inhaled air, and extracorporeal circulatory rewarming. Blood rewarming is currently limited to a maximum temperature of 42°C by the American Association of Blood Banks, but rewarming to 49°C with inline microwave blood rewarmers has been reported as safe, as has intravenous fluid rewarming to 65°C (610,611).

The advantages and disadvantages of each technique are regularly debated, particularly regarding the role of external versus core rewarming. However, it is clear that the rate of heat transfer to the hypothermic patient is greatest using active core rewarming, particularly extracorporeal circulation rewarming. This may be a critical factor in surgical patients for whom rapid restoration of clotting and cardiac function is necessary.

The technique of rewarming the hypothermic victim by extracorporeal circulation has been described by numerous authors, based primarily on small personal experiences (612,613). This technique has limited applicability in surgical patients, but has appeal in cases of primary accidental hypothermia, where maintenance of circulation, correction of hypoxia, and replenishment of intravascular volume may play a role as large as correcting the temperature change itself. Improvements in heparin-bonded circuitry and the use of atraumatic centrifugal pumps may eventually remove the restriction systemic anticoagulation places on extracorporeal bypass.

A simplified technique of extracorporeal active core rewarming is CAVR (614). This technique makes use of the patient's own blood pressure to drive an extracorporeal circuit through an efficient, but small counter-current heat exchange device. Systemic anticoagulation is not necessary because the tubing is heparin bonded and trauma patients are relatively anticoagulated. The relative ease of use may make this device widely applicable in rewarming severely hypothermic patients with an intact circulation. As noted earlier, this device has been used in a prospective, randomized trial of rewarming trauma patients, demonstrating its efficacy (601).

The use of body cavity lavage with warm solutions is a simple, less invasive method of accomplishing active core rewarming. However, rewarming rates with body cavity lavage vary greatly based on initial core temperature, dialysate temperature, infusion rate, and dwell time. Several studies support the notion that active core rewarming by peritoneal lavage is preferable to active external rewarming (555,615). Moss et al. examined three techniques of rewarming hypothermic and cardiac-arrested dogs, concluding that both peritoneal lavage (55°C dialysate) and partial extracorporeal circulation were faster than active external rewarming with a heating blanket (555). A frequently stated disadvantage of external rewarming is that the peripheral tissues are rewarmed in advance of the still cool "core," resulting in peripheral vasodilation. In the presence of inadequate volume resuscitation, this may result in vascular collapse ("rewarming shock") and a subsequent fall in central temperature ("afterdrop") as the cold peripheral blood returns to the core. Whether this is the mechanism of the core afterdrop is debatable because a core afterdrop has been noted to occur in animal models even during complete circulatory arrest. Volume contraction due to vasoconstriction, cold diuresis, and cellular swelling coupled with inadequate fluid resuscitation may be a more appropriate explanation for circulatory collapse during rewarming.

The thermodynamic principles of heat transfer to the hypothermic patient are reviewed in greater detail elsewhere, but a sense of rewarming rates and quantity of heat transferred by various techniques is instructional (609, 616,617). Ventilating a patient with a core temperature of 32°C with water-saturated air at 41°C results in a maximum heat transfer rate of 9 kcal/h. For comparison, basal metabolic heat generation produces approximately 70 kcal/h, and shivering produces up to 250 kcal/h. Given the specific heat of the body (0.083 kcal/kg/°C), 58 kcal is required to raise the temperature of a 70-kg patient by 1°C. Thus, more than 6 hours would be required to warm a 32°C patient using 41°C humidified inspired air.

Heat transfer rates using body cavity lavage can be similarly calculated based on the specific heat of water (1 kcal/kg/°C). If 1 L of 44°C water infused into a body cavity dwells long enough to exit at 40°C, 4 kcal of heat will have been transferred to the patient. Thus, over 14 L of fluid is needed to increase core temperature by 1°C. However, warming becomes less efficient as the patient rewarms because a longer dwell time is required to reduce the temperature of the infusate to 40°C.

Warming by cardiopulmonary bypass or CAVR is the most efficient method of core heating. With flow rates of 15 to 30 L/h, it is possible to deliver 120 to 240 kcal/h if the reinfused blood is heated to 40°C, a rate of heat transfer over 10 times that of the other methods. In any case, the urgency with which rewarming must be accomplished depends on how adversely the hypothermia is affecting the patient. With the exception of extracorporeal circulatory methods, most rewarming techniques serve primarily to prevent loss of endogenously generated heat, and are ineffective in circumstances during which rapid rewarming is indicated. Early and discrete attention to the mechanisms of heat loss is necessary to prevent the metabolic and hemorrhagic complications associated with hypothermia in surgical patients.

COLD INJURY AND FROSTBITE

Cold injuries limited to digits, extremities, or exposed surfaces are the result of either direct tissue freezing (frostbite) or more chronic exposure to an environment just above freezing (chilblain or pernio; trenchfoot). Cold injury has been a major cause of morbidity during war experiences. It resulted in over 7 million lost soldier fighting days by Allied forces in World War II, and was reportedly the most common major injury sustained by British soldiers in the Falklands expedition (618).

Chilblain and *pernio* are descriptive terms for a form of local cold injury characterized by pruritic, red-purple papules, macules, plaques, or nodules on the skin. The lesions are often associated with edema or blistering and are caused by a chronic vasculitis of the dermis (619); this entity does not appear to be related to hereditary protein C or S deficiency (620). This pathologic process is provoked by repeated exposure to cold, but not freezing, temperatures. This injury typically occurs on the face, the anterior surface of the tibia, or the dorsum of the hands and feet, areas poorly protected or chronically exposed to the environment. With continued exposure, ulcerative or hemorrhagic lesions may appear and progress to scarring, fibrosis, and atrophy. Treatment consists of sheltering the patient, elevating the affected part on sheepskin, and allowing gradual rewarming at room temperature. Rubbing and massage are contraindicated because they can cause further damage and secondary infection.

Trenchfoot or cold immersion foot (or hand) describes a nonfreezing injury of the hands or feet, typically in sailors, fishermen, or soldiers, that is caused by chronic exposure to wet conditions and temperatures just above freezing (621). It appears to involve an alternating arterial vasospasm and vasodilatation, with the affected tissue first cold and anesthetic and then hyperemic after 24 to 48 hours of exposure. With the hyperemia comes an intense, painful burning and dysesthesia, and tissue damage is characterized by edema, blistering, redness, ecchymosis, and ulceration. Complications of local infection or cellulitis, lymphangitis, and gangrene may occur. A posthyperemic phase occurs 2 to 6 weeks later and is characterized by tissue cyanosis with increased sensitivity to cold. Treatment is best started during or before the reactive hyperemia state, and consists of immediate removal of the extremity from the cold, wet environment with exposure of the feet (or hands) to warm, dry air. Elevation to minimize edema, protection of pressure spots, and local and systemic measures to combat infection are indicated. Massage, soaking of the feet, or rapid rewarming are not indicated. Demyelination of nerves, muscle atrophy, fallen arches, and osteoporosis may all present long-term complications, and a tendency toward marked vasospasm during subsequent exposure to cold develops in some patients (622).

Frostnip is the mildest form of cold injury. It is characterized by initial pain and pallor, with subsequent numbness of the affected body part. Skiers and other winter outdoor enthusiasts are most likely to experience this cold injury to the nose, ears, or tips of digits. The injury is reversible and warming of the cold tissue results in return of sensation and function with no tissue loss.

Frostbite is a more severe and common form of cold injury. Frostbite damage is caused by direct ice crystal formation at the cellular level with cellular dehydration and microvascular occlusion. Frostbite is traditionally classified into four grades of injury severity:

First degree—tissue freezing with hyperemia and edema, but without blistering
Second degree—tissue freezing with hyperemia, edema, and characteristic large, clear blisters
Third degree—tissue freezing with death of subcutaneous tissues and skin, resulting in hemorrhagic vesicles that are in general smaller than second-degree blisters
Fourth degree—tissue necrosis, gangrene, and eventual full-thickness tissue loss

The affected body part nearly always initially appears hard, cold, white, and anesthetic, regardless of the depth of injury. Because the appearance of the lesion changes frequently during the course of treatment, and because the initial treatment regimen is applicable for all degrees of insult (623), some authorities suggest discarding this classification as a prognostic impossibility, and simply classifying frostbite as either superficial or deep (624).

Weather conditions, altitude, degree of protective clothing, duration of exposure, and degree of tissue wetness are all contributing external factors to the development of frostbite injury. Because sensory nerve activity is abolished at 7° to 9°C, the disappearance of pain is an early warning sign of cold injury. Acclimation to cold may be protective, whereas a previous history of frostbite probably predisposes to another cold tissue injury. Smoking and a history of arterial disease also are contributing factors. In urban environments, over 50% of frostbite injuries are alcohol related, and a significant portion of these patients (16%) have an underlying psychiatric illness (625).

Evidence suggests that frostbite injury has two components—the initial freeze injury and a reperfusion injury that occurs during rewarming. The initial response to tissue cooling is vasoconstriction and arteriovenous shunting, intermittently relieved (every 5 to 7 minutes) by vasodilation, the so-called hunting response (626). With prolonged exposure, this response fails, and the temperature of the freezing tissue approximates ambient temperature until −2°C. At this point, extracellular ice crystals form, and as these crystals enlarge, the osmotic pressure of the interstitium increases, resulting in movement of intracellular water into the interstitium. Cells begin to shrink and become hyperosmolar, disrupting cellular enzyme function. If freezing is rapid (>10°C/min), intracellular ice crystal formation occurs, resulting in immediate cell death (618). Intravascularly, endothelial cell disruption and red cell sludging result in cessation of circulation.

During rewarming, red cell, platelet, and leukocyte aggregation is known to occur and results in patchy thrombosis of the microcirculation. These accumulated blood elements are thought to release, among other products, the toxic oxygen free radicals and the arachidonic acid metabolites $PGF_{2\alpha}$ and thromboxane A_2, which further aggravate vasoconstriction and platelet and leukocyte aggregation (627,628). However, the exact mechanism of tissue destruction and death after freeze injury remains poorly defined. Animal studies suggest that vascular injury in the form of endothelial cell damage and subsequent interstitial edema, but not vessel thrombosis, predominate as initial events in rewarming injury (629). A substantial component of severe cold injury may be neutrophil mediated, as suggested by the observation that a monoclonal antibody to neutrophil–endothelial and neutrophil–neutrophil adherence can markedly ameliorate the pathologic process of a severe cold injury (630). In this rabbit model, animals treated with anti-CD11/CD18 adhesion molecule after cold injury (30 minutes at −15°C) but before rewarming (39°C water bath) had significantly less tissue loss and edema. The implication of these observations is that much of the injury of severe frostbite occurs during rewarming or reperfusion. Clinical application of these experimental observations remains untested.

Treatment

Prehospital or field care of the victim of cold injury should focus on removing the patient from the hostile environment and protecting the injured body part from further damage. Rubbing or exercising the affected tissue does not augment blood flow and risks further cold injury or mechanical trauma. Because repeated bouts of freezing and thawing worsen the injury, it is preferable for the patient with frostbite of the hands or feet immediately to seek definitive shelter and care rather than rewarm the tissue in the field and risk refreezing. Although the initial symptoms may be mild and overlooked by the patient, severe pain, burning, edema, and even necrosis and gangrene may appear with rewarming. With severe injury there is a progressive decrease in range of motion, and edema becomes prominent. The injury may progress to numbness and, eventually, to loss of all sensation in the affected tissue.

The emergency room treatment of a frostbite victim should first focus on the basic ABCs (airway, breathing, and circulation) of trauma resuscitation, and systemic hypothermia should be identified and corrected. Most patients are dehydrated, and resuscitation with warm fluids is an important part of early management. Fractures are often accompanied by frostbite in mountaineers, and although manipulation may be required to treat vascular compromise, open reduction is hazardous, and application of traction should be delayed until after postthawing edema has been assessed.

Rapid rewarming is the goal. Gradual, spontaneous rewarming is inadequate, particularly for deeper injuries, and rubbing the injured part in ice or snow often delays warming and results in marked tissue loss (631). Rapid rewarming should be achieved by immersing the tissue in a large water bath of 40° to 42°C (104° to 108°F). The water should feel warm, but not hot, to the normal hand. The bath should be large enough to prevent rapid loss of heat and the water temperature maintained. Dry heat is not advocated because it is difficult to regulate, and the result of using excessive heat is often disastrous. The rewarming process should take approximately 30 to 45 minutes for digits, with the affected area appearing flushed when rewarming is complete and good circulation has been reestablished. Narcotics are required because the rewarming process can be quite painful.

The skin should be gently but meticulously cleansed, air dried, and the affected area elevated to minimize edema. A tetanus toxoid booster should be administered as indicated by immunization history. Sterile cotton is placed between toes or fingers to prevent skin maceration, and extreme care taken to prevent infection and avoid even the slightest abrasion. The affected tissue should be protected by a tent or cradle, and pressure spots must be prevented. In one review, infection developed in 13% of urban frostbite victims, but one half of these infections were present at time of admission (625). Most clinicians reserve antibiotics for identified infections (632).

After rewarming, the treatment goals are to prevent further injury while awaiting the demarcation of irreversible tissue destruction. All patients should be hospitalized, and affected tissue gently cleansed once or twice a day in warm (38°C) whirlpool baths, with some clinicians adding an antiseptic such as chlorhexidine or an iodophor to the bath (632). Based on the findings of arachidonic acid metabolites in the blisters of frostbite victims, some authors advocate the use of topical aloe vera (thromboxane inhibitor) and systemic ibuprofen or aspirin. Heggers et al. report on a nonrandomized trial in which 56 patients treated with these agents, plus prophylactic penicillin, had less tissue loss, a lower amputation rate, and a shorter hospital stay than 98 patients treated with warm saline, silver sulfadiazine, or Sulfamylon dressings (Bertek Pharmaceuticals, Sugar Land, TX) (627). Another report on frostbite treatment in rabbits demonstrated improved tissue viability if systemic pentoxifylline and topical aloe vera cream were used (633). Uninfected blebs should be left intact because they provide a sterile biologic dressing for 7 to 10 days, and protect underlying epithelialization. After resolution of edema, digits should be exercised during the whirlpool bath and physical therapy begun. Tobacco, nicotine, and other vasoconstrictive agents must be withheld. Weight bearing is prohibited until complete resolution of edema.

Numerous adjuvants have been suggested and tried in an effort to restore blood supply to frostbitten areas. The intense vasoconstrictive effect of cold injury has focused attention on increased sympathetic tone. Sympathetic blockade and even surgical sympathectomy continues to be advocated by some authors, under the theory that it releases the vasospasm that precipitates thrombosis in the affected tissue (633,634). This method of treatment has produced inconsistent results and is difficult to evaluate clinically, with no prospective, randomized trials available. Although sympathectomy appears to mollify the pain, hyperhidrosis, and vasospasm of cold injuries, it may increase vascular shunting and adversely affect healing. In one series, a more proximal demarcation of injury in sympathectomized limbs was noted than in nonsympathectomized ones, despite apparently equal bilateral injury (631).

Experience with intraarterial vasodilating drugs such as reserpine and tolazoline has also been unrewarding. Bouwman and colleagues demonstrated in a controlled clinical study that immediate (mean, 3 hours) ipsilateral intraarterial reserpine infusion coupled with early (mean, 3 days) ipsilateral operative sympathectomy failed to alter the natural history of acute frostbite injury compared with the contralateral limb (635). Heparin, thrombolytic agents, and hyperbaric oxygen have also failed to demonstrated any substantial treatment benefit, whereas low-molecular-weight dextran alleviated postthawing circulatory obstruction as late as 2 hours after thawing, and markedly reduced tissue loss in rabbit feet (636,637).

The difficulty in determining the depth of tissue destruction in cold injury has led to a conservative approach to the care of frostbite injuries (638,639). As a general rule, amputation and surgical débridement are delayed for 2 to 3 months unless infection with sepsis intervenes. The natural history of a full-thickness frostbite injury is the gradual demarcation of the injured area with dry gangrene or mummification clearly delineating nonviable tissue. Often the permanent tissue loss is much less than originally suspected. In an Alaskan series, only 10.5% of patients required amputation, usually involving only phalanges or portions of phalanges (640). The need for emergency surgery is unusual, but vigilance should be maintained during the rewarming phase for the development of a compartment syndrome requiring fasciotomy. Open amputations are indicated in patients with persistent infection and sepsis that is refractory to débridement and antibiotics. Mills and colleagues convincingly demonstrated that of all the factors in the treatment of frostbite that may influence outcome, premature surgical intervention by any means, in any amount, was by far the greatest contributor to poor results (631).

The use of technetium 99m methylene diphosphonate bone scanning has shown some promise in the early detection of eventual bone and soft-tissue viability (641), as has the use of magnetic resonance imaging (642). Technetium 99m "triple-phase" scanning (1 minute, 2 hours, 7 hours) performed 48 hours after admission has been used to assess early tissue perfusion and viability, in an attempt to define the extent of fatally damaged tissues and to allow for early débridement and wound closure (643).

Frostbitten tissues seldom recover completely. Some degree of cold insensitivity invariably remains. Hyperhidrosis (in up to 72% of patients), neuropathy, decreased nail and hair growth, and a persistent Raynaud's phenomenon in the affected part are frequent sequelae to cold injury (636). The affected tissue remains at risk for reinjury and should be carefully protected during any cold exposure. As mentioned previously, chilblain (or chronic pernio) is a specific form of a dermopathy secondary to cold-induced skin vasculitis. Treatment with antiadrenergics (prazosin hydrochloride, 1 to 2 mg/day) or calcium channel blockers (nifedipine, 30 to 60 mg/day) and careful protection from further exposure is often helpful (619,644). However, few therapies afford significant relief to the chronic symptoms after tissue freeze injury, although β- and α-adrenergic blocking agents, calcium channel blockers, topical and systemic steroids, and a host of home remedies have been tried with occasional individual success.

REFERENCES

1. Bonnie RJ, Fulco CE, Liverman CT. Magnitude and costs. In: Bonnie RJ, Fulco CE, Liverman CT, eds. *Reducing the burden of injury, advancing prevention, and treatment.* Washington, DC: National Academy Press, 1999:41–59.
2. American College Of Surgeons Committee on Trauma. *Resources for optimal care of the injured patient: 1999.* Chicago: American College of Surgeons, 1999.
3. American College of Surgeons Committee on Trauma. *Advanced trauma life support course: instructor manual.* Chicago: American College of Surgeons, 1997.
4. Kraus JF, Peek C, McArthur DL, et al. The effect of the 1992 California motorcycle helmet use law on motorcycle crash fatalities and injuries. *JAMA* 1994;272:1506.
5. Lowe DK, Gately HL, Goss JR, et al. Patterns of death, com-

plication, and error in management of motor vehicle accident victims: implications for a regional system of trauma care. *J Trauma* 1983;23:50.

6. Shackford SR, Hollingsworth-Fridlund P, Cooper G, et al. The effect of regionalization upon the quality of trauma care assessed by concurrent audit before and after institution of a trauma system: a preliminary report. *J Trauma* 1986;26:812.

7. Baker CC, Oppenheiner L, Stephens B, et al. Epidemiology of trauma deaths. *Am J Surg* 1980;140:144.

8. Shackford SR, Mackersie RC, Hollingsworth-Fridlund P, et al. The epidemiology and pathology of traumatic death: a population-based analysis. *Arch Surg* 1993;128:571.

9. Grossblatt N, ed. *Injury in America: a continuing public health problem*. Washington, DC: National Academy Press, 1985.

10. National Center for Injury and Prevention Control. Overall injury and averse-event-related deaths and rate per 100,000. E800–E999. www.cdc.gov/ncipc. National Center for Injury and Prevention Control, Centers for Disease Control and Prevention, 1995.

11. Baker S. *The injury fact book*. New York: Oxford University Press, 1992.

12. Rice DP, MacKenzie EJ, and associates, eds. *Cost of injury in the United States: a report to Congress*. San Francisco: Institute for Health & Aging, University of California and Injury Prevention Center, Johns Hopkins University, 1989.

13. Centers for Disease Control and Prevention. *Injury mortality: national summary of injury mortality data 1984–1990*. Atlanta: Centers for Disease Control and Prevention, 1993.

14. Runyan CW, Gerken EA. Epidemiology and prevention of adolescent injury: a review and research agenda. *JAMA* 1989;262:2273–2278.

15. Fingerhut LA. *Firearm mortality among children, youth, and young adults 1–34 years of age, trends and current status: U.S., 1985–1990*. Advance data No. 231. Hyattsville, MD: National Center for Heath Statistics, Centers for Disease Control and Prevention, 1993.

16. National Highway Traffic Safety Administration (NHTSA). *Traffic safety facts 1997: Alcohol*. Washington, DC: NHTSA, 1998.

17. Alcohol-related traffic fatalities involving children—United States 1985–1996. Centers for Disease Control and Prevention. *MMWR Morb Mortal Wkly Rep* 1997;46:1130–1133.

18. National Highway Traffic Safety Administration (NHTSA). *The incidence and role of drugs in fatally injured drivers*. Traffic Tech. Washington, DC: NHTSA, 1993.

19. Hoekstra SM, Bender JS, Levison MA. The management of large soft-tissue defects following close-range shotgun injury. *J Trauma* 1990;30:1489–1493.

20. Champion HR, Fallen WF, Golocovsk M. The trauma score. *Crit Care Med* 1981;9:672.

21. Champion HR, Gainer PS, Yackee E. A progress report on the trauma score in predicting a fatal outcome. *J Trauma* 1986;26:927.

22. American Association for Automotive Medicine. *The Abbreviated Injury Scale (AIS), revised ed*. Des Plaines, IL: American Association for Automotive Medicine, 1990.

23. Boyd CR, Tolson MA, Copes WS. Evaluating trauma care: the TRISS method. *J Trauma* 1987;27:370.

24. Hoyt DB, Hollingsworth-Fridlund P, Winchell RJ, et al. An analysis of recurrent process errors leading to provider-related complications on an organized trauma service: directions for care improvement. *J Trauma* 1994;36;377.

25. Wisner DH. History and current status of trauma scoring systems. *Arch Surg* 1990;127:115.

26. Rutledge R. Injury severity scoring in trauma patients. *Adv Trauma Crit Care* 1993;8:117.

27. Rutledge R. Injury severity grading in trauma patients: simplified technique based upon ICD-9 coding. *J Trauma* 1993; 35:497.

28. U.S. Department of Health and Human Services (DHHS). *Model trauma care system plan*. Washington, DC: U.S. DHHS, September 30, 1992.

29. Bass RR, Gainer PS, Carlini AR. Update on trauma system development in the United States. *J Trauma* 1999;47: S15–S21.

30. Holbrook TL, Hoyt DB, Anderson JP, et al. Functional limitation after major trauma: a more sensitive assessment using the quality of well-being scale—the trauma recovery pilot project. *J Trauma* 1994;36:74.

31. Davis JW, Hoyt DB, McArdle MS, et al. The significance of critical care errors in causing preventable death in trauma patients in a trauma system. *J Trauma* 1991;31;813.

32. Davis JW, Hoyt DB, McArdle MS, et al. An analysis of errors causing morbidity and mortality in a trauma system: a guide for quality improvement. *J Trauma* 1992;32:660.

33. Mullins RJ, Mann NC. Introduction to the Academic Symposium to Evaluate Evidence Regarding the Efficacy of Trauma Systems. *J Trauma* 1999;47:S3–S5.

34. Pepe PE, Maio RF. Evolving challenges in pre-hospital trauma services: current issues in suggested evaluation tools. *Prehosp Disast Med* 1993;8:S25.

35. Sampalis JS, Lovoie A, Williams JI. Impact of on-site care, pre-hospital time, and level of in-hospital care on survival in severely injured patients. *J Trauma* 1993;34:252.

36. Cayten CG, Murphy JG, Stahl WN. Basic life support versus advanced life support for injured patients with an injury severity score of 10 or more. *J Trauma* 1993;35:460.

37. Pepe PE, Copass MK, Joyce TH. Pre-hospital endotracheal intubation: rationale for training emergency medical personnel. *Ann Emerg Med* 1985;14:1085.

38. Vilke GM, Hoyt DB, Epperson M, et al. Intubation techniques in the helicopter. *J Emerg Med* 1994;12:217.

39. Salvino CK, Dries D, Gamelli R, et al. Emergency cricothyroidotomy in trauma victims. *J Trauma* 1993;34:503.

40. Xeropotamos NS, Coats T, Wilson AW. Pre-hospital surgical airway management: one year's experience from the Helicopter Emergency Medical Service. *Injury* 1993;24:222.

41. York D, Dudek L, Larson R, et al. A comparison study of chest tube thoracostomy: air medical crew and in-hospital trauma service. *Air Med J* 1993;12:227.

42. Mattox KL, Bickel LW, Pepe PE, et al. Prospective MAST study in 911 patients. *J Trauma* 1989;29:1104.

43. Cayton CG, Berendt BM, Byrne DW, et al. A study of pneumatic anti-shock garments in severely hypotensive patients. *J Trauma* 1993;34:728.

44. Bickwell WH, Wall MJ, Pepe PE, et al. Immediate versus delayed fluid resuscitation for hypotensive patients with penetrating torso injuries. *N Engl J Med* 1994;331:1105.

45. Vassar MJ, Perry CA, Holcraft JW. Pre-hospital resuscitation of hypotensive trauma patients with 7.5% NaCl versus 7.5% NaCl with added dextran: a controlled trail. *J Trauma* 1993; 34:622.

46. Vassar MJ, Fischer RP, O'Brien PE, et al. A multicenter trial for resuscitation of injured patients with 7.5% sodium chloride: the effect of added dextran—the Multicenter Group for the Study of Hypertonic Saline in Trauma Patients. *Arch Surg* 1993;128:1003.

47. Boyd MV, Vanek VW, Bourguet CC. Emergency room resuscitation thoracotomy: when is it indicated? *J Trauma* 1992; 33:714.

48. Buckmaster MS, Kearney PA, Johnson SB. Further experience with transesophageal echocardiography in the evaluation of thoracic aortic injury. *J Trauma* 1994;30:989.

49. Miller FB, Cryer HM, Chilikuris S, et al. Negative findings on laparotomy for trauma. *South Med J* 1989;82:1231.

50. Evers BM, Cryer HM, Miller FB. Pelvic fracture hemorrhage: priorities in management. *Arch Surg* 1989;124:422.

51. Fabian TC, Croce MA, Stewart RM, et al. A prospective analysis of diagnostic laparoscopy in trauma. *Ann Surg* 1993;217:557.

52. Meyer DM, Thal ER, Wegelt JA. The role of abdominal CT in the evaluation of stab wounds to the back. *J Trauma* 1989; 29:1226.

53. Gann DS, Carlson DE, Byrnes GJ, et al. Impaired restitution of blood volume after large hemorrhage. *J Trauma* 1981;12: 598.

54. Huckabee WE. Relationships of pyruvate and lactate during anaerobic metabolism: II. exercise and formation of O_2 debt. *J Clin Invest* 1958;37:255–263.

55. Broder G, Weil MH. Excess lactate: an index of reversibility of shock in human patients. *Science* 1964;143:1457.

56. Vitek V, Cowley RA. Blood lactate in the prognosis of various forms of shock. *Ann Surg* 1971;173:308–313.

57. Canizarro PC, Prager MD, Shires GT. The infusion of Ringer's lactate solution during shock. *Am J Surg* 1971;122:494–501.

58. Abramson DA, Scalea TM, Hitchcock R, et al. Lactate clearance and survival following injury. *J Trauma* 1993;35: 584–589.
59. Davis JW. The relationship of base deficit to lactate in porcine hemorrhagic shock and resuscitation. *J Trauma* 1994;36:168–172.
60. Davis JW, Parks SN, Kaups KL, et al. Admission base deficit predicts transfusion requirements and risk of complications. *J Trauma* 1996;41:769–774.
61. Davis JW, Shackford SR, Mackersie RC, et al. Base deficit as a guide to volume resuscitation. *J Trauma* 1988;28: 1464–1467.
62. Davis JW, Kaups KL, Parks SN. Base deficit is superior to pH in evaluating clearance of acidosis after traumatic shock. *J Trauma* 1998;44:114–118.
63. American College of Surgeons Committee on Trauma. *Advanced trauma life support: shock.* Chicago: American College of Surgeons, 1988:59–73.
64. Krausz MM, Bar-Ziv M, Rabinovici R, et al. "Scoop and run" or stabilize hemorrhagic shock with normal saline or small-volume hypertonic saline? *J Trauma* 1992;33:6–10.
65. Kowalenko T, Stern S, Dronen S, et al. Improved outcome with hypotensive resuscitation of uncontrolled hemorrhagic shock in a swine model. *J Trauma* 1992;33:349–353.
66. Bickell WH, Wall MJ Jr, Pepe PE, et al. Immediate versus delayed fluid resuscitation for hypotensive patients with penetrating torso trauma. *N Engl J Med* 1994;331:1105–1109.
67. Waxman K, Annas C, Daughters K, et al. A method to determine the adequacy of resuscitation using tissue oxygen monitoring. *J Trauma* 1994;36:852–858.
68. Chang MC, Cheatham MC, Nelson LD, et al. Gastric tonometry supplements information provided by systemic indicators of oxygen transport. *J Trauma* 1994;37:488.
69. Rhee P, Langdale L, Mock C, et al. Near-infrared spectroscopy: continuous measurement of cytochrome oxidation during hemorrhagic shock. *Crit Care Med* 1997;25:166.
70. Deb S, Martin B, Sun L, et al. Resuscitation with lactated Ringer's solution in rats with hemorrhagic shock induces immediate apoptosis. *J Trauma* 1999;46:582–589.
71. Corso CO, Okamoto S, Ruttinger D, et al. Hypertonic saline dextran attenuates leukocyte accumulation in the liver after hemorrhagic shock and resuscitation. *J Trauma* 1999;46: 417–423.
72. Rhee P, Burris D, Pikoulis M, et al. Lactated Ringer's solution resuscitation causes neutrophil activation after hemorrhagic shock. *J Trauma* 1998;44:313–319.
73. Ross AD, Angaran DM. Colloids vs. crystalloids: a continuing controversy. *Drug Intell Clin Pharmacol* 1984;18:202–212.
74. Waxman K, Holness R, Tominaga G, et al. Hemodynamic and oxygen transport effects of pentastarch in burn resuscitation. *Ann Surg* 1989;209:341–345.
75. London MJ, Ho JS, Triedman JK, et al. A randomized clinical trial of 10% pentastarch (low molecular weight hydroxy ethyl starch) vs. 5% albumin for plasma volume expansion after cardiac operations. *J Thorac Cardiovasc Surg* 1989;97:785–797.
76. Mackersie RC, Durelle J. Differential clearance of colloid and crystalloid solutions from the lung. *J Trauma* 1993;35: 448–453.
77. Moss GS, Rice CL, Sehgal LR, et al. Management of traumatic and hemorrhagic shock. *Anesth Rev* 1990;17:25–29.
78. Gervin AS. Transfusion, autotransfusion, and blood substitutes. In: Mattox KL, Moore EE, Feliciano DV, eds. *Trauma.* Norwalk, CT: Appleton & Lange, 1988:161.
79. Whelan TJ, Burkhalter WE, Gomez A. Management of war wounds. In: Welch CE, ed. *Advances in surgery,* vol 3. Chicago: Year Book Medical, 1968:251.
80. Gervin AS, Fisher RP. Resuscitation of trauma patients with type-specific, uncrossmatched whole blood. *J Trauma* 1984; 24:327.
81. Boudreaux JP, Bornside GH, Cohn I. Emergency autotransfusion: partial cleansing of bacteria-laden blood. *J Trauma* 1983;23:31.
82. Glover JL, Smith R, Yaw PB, et al. Autotransfusion of blood contaminated by intestinal contents. *J Am Coll Emerg Physicians* 1978;7:142.
83. Jurkovich GJ, Moore EE, Medina G. Autotransfusion in trauma: a pragmatic analysis. *Am J Surg* 1984;148:782–785.
84. Widenthal K, Mierzwial DS, Mitchell JH. Acute effects of increased serum osmolality on left ventricular performance. *Am J Physiol* 1969;216:898–904.
85. Kramer GC, Walsh JC. Future trends in emergency fluid resuscitation. In: Tuma RF, White JV, Messmer K, eds. *The role of hemodilution in optimal patient care.* Munich: Zuckschwerdt-Verlag, 1989:89–99.
86. Roche T, Silva M Jr, et al. Hypertonic resuscitation from severe hemorrhagic shock: patterns of regional circulation. *Circ Shock* 1986;19:165–176.
87. Smith GJ, et al. A comparison of several hypertonic solutions for resuscitation of bled sheep. *J Surg Res* 1985;39: 517–528.
88. Shackford SR, Fortlage DA, Peters RM, et al. Serum osmolar and electrolyte changes associated with large infusions of hypertonic sodium lactate for intravascular volume expansion of patients undergoing aortic reconstruction. *Surg Gynecol Obstet* 1987;164:127–136.
89. Vassar MJ, Perry CA, Gannaway WL, et al. 7.5% Sodium chloride/dextran for resuscitation of trauma patients undergoing helicopter transport. *Arch Surg* 1991;126:1065–1072.
90. Holcroft JW, Vassar MJ, O'Brien PE, et al. Hypertonic/hyperoncotic resuscitation of trauma patients undergoing helicopter transport: a multicenter trial. *Arch Surg* 1993;128:1003.
91. Gross D, Landau EH, Klin B, et al. Quantitative measurement of bleeding following hypertonic saline therapy in "uncontrolled" hemorrhagic shock. *J Trauma* 1989;29:79–83.
92. Tremper KK, Friedman AE, Levine EM, et al. The preoperative treatment of severely anemic patient with a perfluorochemical oxygen transport fluid: Fluosol-DA 20%. *N Engl J Med* 1982;307:277.
93. Elliot LA, Ledgerwood AM, Lucas CE, et al. Role of Fluosol DA 20% in prehospital resuscitation. *Crit Care Med* 1989; 17:575.
94. McCoy LE, Elliot LA, Lucas CE, et al. Regenerative responses to exchange transfusion. *Biomater Artif Cells Artif Organs* 1988;16:575–583.
95. Greenburg AG, Hayashi R, Siefert I, et al. Intravascular persistence and oxygen delivery of pyridoxalated stroma-free hemoglobin during gradations of hypotension. *Surgery* 1979; 86:13–16.
96. Moss GS, Gould SA, Sehgal LR, et al. Hemoglobin solution: from tetramer to polymer. *Surgery* 1984;95:249.
97. Hoyt DB, Greenburg AG, Perskin GW, et al. Hemorrhagic shock and resuscitation: improved survival with pyridoxalated stroma-free hemoglobin. *Surg Forum* 1980;31:15.
98. Cohn S. Is blood obsolete? *J Trauma* 1996;42:730–732.
99. Cohn S. The current status of hemoglobin substitutes. *Ann Med* 1997;29:371–376.
100. Kelley JS, Prielipp RC. Letter to the editor. *N Engl J Med* 1999;341:126.
101. Sharma AC, Singh G, Gulati A. The role of NO mechanism in cardiovascular effects of diaspirin cross linked hemoglobin in anesthetized rats. *Am J Physiol* 1995;38:H1379–H1388.
102. Dietz NM, Martin CM, Beltran-del-Rio AG, et al. The effects of cross-linked hemoglobin on regional vascular conductance in dogs. *Anesth Analg* 1997;85:265–273.
103. Hess JR, MacDonald VW, Brinkley WW. Systemic and pulmonary hypertension after resuscitation with cell-free hemoglobin. *J Appl Physiol* 1993;74:1769–1778.
104. Gould SA, Moss GS. Clinical development of of human polymerized hemoglobin as a blood substitute. *World J Surg* 1996;20:1200–1207.
105. Gould SA, Moore EE, Hoyt DB, et al. The first randomized trial of human polymerized hemoglobin as a blood substitute in acute trauma and emergent surgery. *J Am Coll Surg* 1998;187:113–122 .
106. Johnson JL, Moore EE, Offner PJ, et al. Resuscitation of the injured patient with polymerized stroma-free hemoglobin does not produce systemic or pulmonary hypertension. *Am J Surg* 1998;176:612–617.
107. Gentilello LM. Advances in the management of hypothermia. *Surg Clin North Am* 1995; 75:243–256.
108. Gentilello LM, Jurkovich GJ, Stark MS, et al. Is hypothermia in the victim of major trauma helpful or harmful? *Ann Surg* 1997;226:439.

109. Stoner HB. Studies on the mechanism of shock: the impairment of thermoregulation by trauma. *Br J Exp Pathol* 1969; 50:125.

110. Gubler KD, Gentilello LM, Hassantash SA, et al. The impact of hypothermia on dilutional coagulopathy. *J Trauma* 1994; 36:847.

111. Chesnut RM, Marshall LF, Klauber MR, et al. The role of secondary brain injury in determining outcome from severe head injury. *J Trauma* 1993;34:216–222.

112. Chesnut RM. Avoidance of hypotension: conditio sine qua non of successful severe head-injury management. *J Trauma* 1997;42:S4–S9.

113. Chesnut RM. Hyperventilation versus cerebral perfusion pressure management: time to change the question. *Crit Care Med* 1998;26:210–212.

114. Cruz J. The first decade of continuous monitoring of jugular bulb oxyhemoglobin saturation: management strategies and clinical outcome. *Crit Care Med* 1998;26:344–351.

115. Robertson CS, Cormio M. Cerebral metabolic management. *New Horiz* 1995;3:410–422.

116. Kaufmann AM, Cardoso ER. Aggravation of vasogenic cerebral edema by multiple-dose mannitol. *J Neurosurg* 1992; 77:584–589.

117. Chesnut RM, Gautille T, Blunt BA, et al. Neurogenic hypotension in patients with severe head injuries. *J Trauma* 1998;44:958–963; discussion 963–964.

118. Chesnut RM, Gautille T, Blunt BA, et al. The localizing value of asymmetry in pupillary size in severe head injury: relation to lesion type and location. *Neurosurgery* 1994;34: 840–845; discussion 845–846.

119. Bullock R, Chesnut R, Clifton G, et al. Guidelines for the management of severe head Injury. *J Neurotrauma* 1996; 13:639–734.

120. Vassar MJ, Perry CA, Gannaway WL, et al. 7.5% Sodium chloride/dextran for resuscitation of trauma patients undergoing helicopter transport. *Arch Surg* 1991;126: 1065–1072.

121. Vassar MJ, Fischer RP, O'Brien PE, et al. A multicenter trial for resuscitation of injured patients with 7.5% sodium chloride: the effect of added dextran 70—the Multicenter Group for the Study of Hypertonic Saline in Trauma Patients. *Arch Surg* 1993;128:1003–1011; discussion 1011–1013.

122. Vassar MJ, Perry CA, Holcroft JW. Pre-hospital resuscitation of hypotensive trauma patients with 7.5% NaCl versus 7.5% NaCl with added dextran: a controlled trial. *J Trauma* 1993;34:622–632; discussion 632–633.

123. Rosner MJ, Coley IB. Cerebral perfusion pressure, intracranial pressure, and head elevation. *J Neurosurg* 1986;65: 636–641.

124. Stein SC, Ross SE. Mild head injury: a plea for routine early CT scanning. *J Trauma* 1992;33:11–13.

125. Mendelow AD, Teasdale G, Jennett B, et al. Risks of intracranial hematoma in head injured adults. *BMJ* 1983;287: 1173–1176.

126. Marmarou A, Anderson RL, Ward JD, et al. Impact of ICP instability and hypotension on outcome in patients with severe head trauma. *J Neurosurg* 1991;75:S159–S166.

127. Marshall LF, Gautille T, Klauber MR, et al. The outcome of severe head injury. *J Neurosurg* 1991;75:S28–S36.

128. Seelig JM, Becker DP, Miller JD, et al. Traumatic acute subdural hematoma: major mortality reduction in comatose patients treated within four hours. *N Engl J Med* 1981;304: 1511–1518.

129. Hayter JP, Ward AJ, Smith EJ. Maxillofacial trauma in severely injured patients. *Br J Oral Maxillofac Surg* 1991;29:370.

130. Nahum AM. The biomechanics of maxillofacial trauma. *Clin Plast Surg* 1975;2:59.

131. LeFort R. Étude experimentale sur les fractures de la machoire siperieuve. *Riv Chir de Paris* 1901;23:208.

132. Stanley RB. Pathogenesis and evaluation of mandible fractures. In: Mathog RH, ed. *Maxillofacial trauma.* Baltimore: Williams & Wilkins, 1984:136–147.

133. Holt GR. Maxillofacial trauma. In: Cummings CW, ed. *Otolaryngology: head and neck surgery.* St Louis: Mosby, 1986:313–344.

134. Coker NJ. Management of traumatic injuries to the facial nerve. *Otolaryngol Clin North Am* 1991;24:215.

135. Haug RH. Cervical spine fractures and maxillofacial trauma. *J Oral Maxillofac Surg* 1991;49:727.

136. Valavanis A. Interventional neuroradiology for head and neck surgery. In: Cummings CW, ed. *Otolaryngology: head and neck surgery, update II.* St Louis: Mosby, 1990.

137. Marentette LJ, Valentino J. Traumatic anterior fossa cerebrospinal fluid fistulae and craniofacial considerations. *Otolaryngol Clin North Am* 1991;24:152.

138. Goodale RL, Montgomery WW. Anterior osteoplastic frontal sinus operation. *Ann Otol Rhinol Laryngol* 1961;70:860.

139. Nadell J, Cline DG. Primary reconstruction of depressed frontal skull fractures including those involving the sinus, orbit, and cribriform plate. *J Neurosurg* 1974;41:200.

140. Busch RF, Prunes F. Intermaxillary fixation with intraoral cortical bone screws. *Laryngoscope* 1991;101:1336.

141. Dierks EJ. Management of associated dental injuries in maxillofacial trauma. *Otolaryngol Clin North Am* 1991;24: 177.

142. Ordog G. Penetrating neck trauma. *J Trauma* 1987;27:543.

143. Saletta J, Lowe R, Lim L, et al. Penetrating neck trauma. *J Trauma* 1976;16:579.

144. Sankaran S, Walt A. Penetrating wounds of the neck: principles and some controversies. *Surg Clin North Am* 1977; 57:139.

145. Roon AJ, Christensen N. Evaluation and treatment of penetrating cervical injuries. *J Trauma* 1979;19:391.

146. Flint L, Snyder W, Perry M, et al. Management of major vascular injuries in the base of the neck: an 11-year experience with 146 cases. *Arch Surg* 1973;106:407.

147. Bishara R, Pasch A, Douglas D, et al. The necessity of mandatory exploration of penetrating zone II neck injuries. *Surgery* 1986;100:655.

148. Jones R, Terrell J, Salyer K. Penetrating wounds of the neck: an analysis of 274 cases. *J Trauma* 1967;7:228.

149. Jurkovich G, Zingarelli W, Wallace J, et al. Penetrating neck trauma: diagnostic studies in the asymptomatic patient. *J Trauma* 1985;25:819.

150. Mansour MA, Moore EE, Moore FA, et al. Validating the selective management of penetrating neck wounds. *Am J Surg* 1991;162:517.

151. Merion RM, Harness JK, Ramsburgh SR. Selective management of penetrating neck trauma: cost implications. *Arch Surg* 1981;116:691.

152. Adolfo A, Kaledzi Y, Parsa M, et al. Penetrating neck wounds: mandatory versus selective exploration. *Ann Surg* 1985;202:563.

153. Demetriades D, Charalambides D, Lakhoo M. Physical examination and selective conservative management in patients with penetrating injuries of the neck. *Br J Surg* 1993; 80:1534.

154. Asensio J, Valenziano C, Falcone R, et al. Management of penetrating neck injuries: the controversy surrounding zone II injuries. *Surg Clin North Am* 1991;71:267.

155. Klyachkin ML, Rohmiller M, Charash WE, et al. Penetrating injuries of the neck: selective management evolving. *Am Surg* 1997;63:189.

156. Irish JC, Hekkenberg R, Gullane PJ, et al. Penetrating and blunt neck trauma: 10-year review of a Canadian experience. *Can J Surg* 1997;40:33.

157. Sofianos C, Degiannis E, Van den Aardweg MS, et al. Selective surgical management of zone II gunshot injury of the neck: a prospective study. *Surgery* 1996;120:785.

158. Biffl WL, Moore EE, Rehse DH, et al. Selective management of penetrating neck trauma based on cervical level of injury. *Am J Surg* 1997;174:678.

159. Roden D, Pomerantz R. Penetrating injuries to the neck: a safe, selective approach to management. *Am Surg* 1993;59: 750.

160. Beitsch P, Weigelt JA, Flynn E, et al. Physical examination and arteriography in patients with penetrating zone II neck wounds. *Arch Surg* 1994;129:577.

161. Carducci B, Lowe R, Dalsey W. Penetrating neck trauma: consensus and controversies. *Ann Emerg Med* 1986;15:208.

162. Hirshberg A, Wall MJ, Johnston RH Jr, et al. Transcervical gunshot injuries. *Am J Surg* 1994;167:309.

163. Sclafani SJ, Cavaliere G, Atweh N, et al. The role of angiography in penetrating neck trauma. *J Trauma* 1991;31:557.

164. Richardson J, Simpson C, Miller F. Management of transmediastinal gunshot wounds. *Surgery* 1981;90:671.

165. Welling R, Saul T, Tew J, et al. Management of blunt injury to the internal carotid artery. *J Trauma* 1987;27:1221.

166. Fabian TC, Patton JH, Croce MA, et al. Blunt carotid injury: importance of early diagnosis and anticoagulant therapy. *Ann Surg* 1996;223:513.

167. Eachempati SR, Vaslef SN, Sebastian MW, et al. Blunt vascular injuries of the head and neck: is heparinization necessary? *J Trauma* 1998;45:997.

168. Cogbill TH, Moore EE, Meissner M, et al. The spectrum of blunt injury to the carotid artery: a multicenter perspective. *J Trauma* 1994;37:473.

169. Davis J, Holbrook T, Hoyt D, et al. Blunt carotid artery dissection: incidence, associated injuries, screening, and treatment. *J Trauma* 1990;30:1514.

170. LeBlang SD, Nunez DB. Helical CT of cervical spine and soft tissue injuries of the neck. *Radiol Clin North Am* 1999; 37:515.

171. Rogers FB, Baker EF, Osler TM, et al. Computed tomographic angiography as a screening modality for blunt cervical arterial injuries: preliminary results. 1999;46:380.

172. James CA. Magnetic resonance angiography in trauma. *Clin Neurosci* 1997;4:137.

173. Fakhry S, Jacques PF, Proctor H. Cervical vessel injury after blunt trauma. *J Vasc Surg* 1988;8:501.

174. Pretre R, Reverdin A, Kalonji T, et al. Blunt carotid artery injury: difficult therapeutic approaches for an underrecognized entity. *Surgery* 1994;115:375.

175. Okada Y, Shima T, Nishida M, et al. Traumatic dissection of the common carotid artery after blunt injury to the neck. *Surg Neurol* 1998;51:513.

176. Sundt T, Pearson B, Piepgras D, et al. Surgical management of aneurysms of the distal extracranial internal carotid artery. *J Neurosurg* 1986;64:169.

177. Gewertz B, Samson D, Ditmore QM, et al. Management of penetrating injuries of the internal carotid artery at the base of the skull utilizing extracranial–intracranial bypass. *J Trauma* 1980;20:365.

178. Martin WSG-GS. Pediatric penetrating head and neck trauma. *Laryngoscope* 1990;100:1288.

179. Brown MF, Graham JM, Feliciano DV, et al. Carotid artery injuries. *Am J Surg* 1982;144:748.

180. Weaver F, Yellin A, Wagner W, et al. The role of arterial reconstruction in penetrating carotid injuries. *Arch Surg* 1988; 123:1106.

181. Unger S, Tucker W, Mrdeza M, et al. Carotid arterial trauma. *Surgery* 1980;87:477.

182. Liekweg W, Greenfield L. Management of penetrating carotid arterial trauma. *Ann Surg* 1978;188:587.

183. Vazquez Anon V, Aymard A, Gobin YP, et al. Balloon occlusion of the internal carotid artery in 40 cases of giant intracavernous aneurysm: technical aspects, cerebral monitoring, and results. *Neuroradiology* 1992;34:245.

184. DeBehnke DJ, Brady W. Vertebral artery dissection due to minor neck trauma. *J Emerg Med* 1994;12:27.

185. Egnor MR, Page LK, David C. Vertebral artery aneurysm: a unique hazard of head banging by heavy metal rockers [Case report]. *Pediatr Neurosurg* 1991;17:135.

186. Golueke P, Scalfani S, Phillips T, et al. Vertebral artery injury: diagnosis and management. *J Trauma* 1987;27:856.

187. Hatzitheofilou C, Strahlendorf C, Kakoyiannis S, et al. Penetrating external injuries of the oesophagus and pharynx. *Br J Surg* 1993;80:1147.

188. Meier D, Brink B, Fry W. Vertebral artery trauma: acute recognition and treatment. *Arch Surg* 1981;116:236.

189. Myers E, Iko B. The management of acute laryngeal trauma. *J Trauma* 1987;27:448.

190. Fuhrman G, Stieg F, Buerk C. Blunt laryngeal trauma: classification and management protocol. *J Trauma* 1990;30:87.

191. Kelly J, Webb W, Moulder P, et al. Management of airway trauma: I. tracheobronchial injuries. *Ann Thorac Surg* 1985; 40:551.

192. Schaefer SD. The acute management of external laryngeal trauma: a 27-year experience. *Arch Otolaryngol Head Neck Surg* 1992;118:598.

193. Gussack G, Jurkovich G. Treatment dilemmas in laryngotracheal trauma. *J Trauma* 1988;28:1439.

194. Beal SL, Pottmeyer EW, Spisso JM. Esophegeal perforation following external blunt trauma. *J Trauma* 1988;28:1425.

195. Jacobs I, Ghassem N, Keely K, et al. Hypopharyngeal perforation after blunt neck trauma: case report and review of literature. *J Trauma* 1999;46:957.

196. Glatterer M, Toon R, Ellestad C, et al. Management of blunt and penetrating external esophageal trauma. *J Trauma* 1985; 25:784.

197. Defore W, Mattox K, Hansen H, et al. Surgical management of penetrating injuries of the esophagus. *Am J Surg* 1977; 134:734.

198. Weigelt J, Thal E, Snyder W, et al. Diagnosis of penetrating cervical esophageal injuries. *Am J Surg* 1987;154:619.

199. Stanley RB, Armstrong WB, Fetterman BL, et al. Management of external penetrating Injuries into the hypopharyngeal–cervical esophagus. *J Trauma* 1997;42:675.

200. Winter RP, Weigelt JA. Cervical esophageal trauma: incidence and cause of esophageal fistulas. *Arch Surg* 1990;125:849.

201. Snow J. Diagnosis and therapy for acute laryngeal and tracheal trauma. *Otolaryngol Clin North Am* 1984;17:101.

202. Shackford SR. Blunt chest trauma: the intensivist's perspective. *J Intensive Care Med* 1986;1:125.

203. Fabian TC, Davis KA, Gavant ML, et al. Prospective study of blunt aortic injury: helical CT is diagnostic and antihypertensive therapy reduces rupture. *Ann Surg* 1998;227:666.

204. Pate JW, Gavant ML, Weiman DS, et al. Traumatic rupture of the aortic isthmus: program of selective management. *World J Surg* 1999;23:59.

205. Vignon P, Rambaud G, Francois B, et al. Quantification of traumatic hemomediastinum using transesophageal echocardiography: impact on patient management. *Chest* 1998; 113:1475.

206. Berenfeld A, Barraud P, Lusson JR, et al. Traumatic aortic ruptures diagnosed by transesophageal echocardiography. *J Am Soc Echocardiogr* 1996;9:657.

207. Gonzalez RP, Holevar MR. Role of prophylactic antibiotics for tube thoracostomy in chest trauma. *Am Surg* 1998;64: 617.

208. Nichols RL, Smith JW, Muzik AC, et al. Preventive antibiotic usage in traumatic thoracic injuries requiring closed tube thoracostomy. *Chest* 1994;106:1493.

209. Mandal AK, Thadepalli H, Mandal AK, et al. Posttraumatic empyema thoracis: a 24-year experience at a major trauma center. *J Trauma* 1997;43:764.

210. Mattox KL. Thoracic injury requiring surgery. *World J Surg* 1983;7:49.

211. Trunkey DD. Spleen.

212. Mackersie RC, Karagianes T, Hoyt DB, et al. Prospective evaluation of epidural and intravenous opiates for pain control and restoration of ventilatory function following multiple rib fractures. *J Trauma* 1991;31:443.

213. Roy-Shapira A, Levi I, Khoda J. Sternal fractures: a red flag or a red herring? *J Trauma* 1994;37:59.

214. Peek GJ, Firmin RK. Isolated sternal fracture: an audit of 10 years' experience. *Injury* 1995;26:385.

215. Chiu WC, D'Amelio LF, Hammond JS. Sternal fractures in blunt chest trauma: a practical algorithm for management. *Am J Emerg Med* 1997;15:252.

216. Gouldman JW, Miller RS. Sternal fracture: a benign entity? *Am Surg* 1997;63:17.

217. Thomas AN, Blaisdell FW, Lewis FR, et al. Operative stabilization for flail chest after blunt trauma. *J Thorac Cardiovasc Surg* 1978;75:793.

218. Richardson JD, Adams L, Flint LM. Selective management of flail chest and pulmonary contusion. *Ann Surg* 1982;196: 481.

219. Shorr RM, Crittenden M, Indeck M, et al. Blunt thoracic trauma: analysis of 515 patients. *Ann Surg* 1987;206:200.

220. Freedland M, Wilson RF, Bender JS, et al. The management of flail chest injury: factors affecting outcome. *J Trauma* 1990;30:1460.

221. Weigelt J, Aubaken R, Meir D, et al. Management of asymptomatic patients following stab wounds to the chest. *J Trauma* 1982;22:291.

222. Roggla M, Wagner A, Brunner C, et al. The management of pneumothorax with the thoracic vent versus conventional intercostal tube drainage. *Wien Klin Wochenschr* 1996;108: 330.

223. Martin T, Fontana G, Olak J, et al. Use of pleural catheter for the management of simple pneumothorax. *Chest* 1996;110: 1169.

224. Sosa JL, Pombo H, Puente I, et al. Thoracoscopy in the evaluation and management of thoracic trauma. *Int Surg* 1998; 83:187.

225. Meyer DM, Jessen ME, Wait MA, et al. Early evacuation of traumatic retained hemothoraces using thoracoscopy: a prospective, randomized trial. *Ann Thorac Surg* 1997;64: 1396.

226. Liu DW, Liu HP, Lin PJ, et al. Video-assisted thoracic surgery in treatment of chest trauma. *J Trauma* 1997;42:670.

227. Ponn RB, D'Agostino RS, Stern H, et al. Treatment of peripheral bronchopleural fistulas with endobronchial occlusion coils. *Ann Thorac Surg* 1993;56:1343.

228. York EL, Lewall DB, Hirji M, et al. Endoscopic diagnosis and treatment of postoperative bronchopleural fistula. *Chest* 1990;97:1390.

229. Jones WS, Mavroudis C, Richardson JD, et al. Management of tracheobronchial disruption resulting from blunt trauma. *Surgery* 1984;95:319.

230. Sim EK, Liam BL, Lee KH, et al. Treatment of delayed partial bronchial rupture with expandable metallic stent. *Singapore Med J* 1999;40:428.

231. Demetriades D, Gomez H, Velmahos GC, et al. Routine helical computed tomographic evaluation of the mediastinum in high-risk blunt trauma patients. *Arch Surg* 1998;133:1084.

232. Fabian TC, Richardson JD, Croce MA, et al. Prospective study of blunt aortic injury: Multicenter Trial of the American Association for the Surgery of Trauma. *J Trauma* 1997; 42:374.

233. Gammie JS, Shah AS, Hattler BG, et al. Traumatic aortic rupture: diagnosis and management. *Ann Thorac Surg* 1998;66: 1295.

234. Symbas PJ, Horsley WS, Symbas PN. Rupture of the ascending aorta caused by blunt trauma. *Ann Thorac Surg* 1998; 66:113.

235. Mattox KL, Holtzman M, Pickard LR, et al. Clamp/repair: a safe technique for the treatment of blunt injury to the descending thoracic aorta. *Ann Thorac Surg* 1985;40:456.

236. Feliciano DV. Trauma to the aorta and major vessels. *Chest Surg Clin North Am* 1997;7:305.

237. Karalis DG, Victor MF, Davis GA, et al. The role of echocardiography in blunt chest trauma: a transthoracic and transesophageal echocardiographic study. *J Trauma* 1994;36:53.

238. Foil MB, Mackersie RC, et al. The asymptomatic patient with suspected myocardial contusion: is hospital admission really necessary? *Am J Surg* 1990;160:638.

239. Moreno C, Moore EE, Majure JA, et al. Pericardial tamponade: a critical determinant for survival following penetrating cardiac wounds. *J Trauma* 1986;26:821.

240. Kemmerer WT, Eckert WG, Gathright JB, et al. Patterns of thoracic injuries in fatal traffic accidents. *J Trauma* 1961; 1:595.

241. Chang CH, Lin PJ, Chang JP, et al. One-stage operation for treatment after delayed diagnosis of thoracic esophageal perforation. *Ann Thorac Surg* 1992;53:617.

242. Urschel HC Jr, Razzuk MA, Wood RE, et al. Improved management of esophageal perforation: exclusion and diversion in continuity. *Ann Surg* 1974;175:587.

243. Bickell WH, Wall MJ Jr, Pepe PE, et al. Immediate versus delayed fluid resuscitation for hypotensive patients with penetrating torso injuries. *N Engl J Med* 1994;331:1105–1109.

244. Rozycki GS, Ballard RB, Feliciano DV, et al. Surgeon-performed ultrasound for the assessment of truncal injuries: lessons learned from 1,540 patients. *Ann Surg* 1998;228: 557–567.

245. Villavicencio RT, Aucar JA. Analysis of laparoscopy in trauma. *J Am Coll Surg* 1999;189:11–20.

246. Moore E, Moore J, Van Duzer-Moore S, et al. Mandatory laparotomy for gunshot wounds penetrating the abdomen. *Am J Surg* 1980;140:847–851.

247. Rotondo MF, Schwab CW, McGonigal MD, et al. "Damage control": an approach for improved survival in exsanguinating penetrating abdominal injury. *J Trauma* 1993;35: 375–382.

248. Schurr MJ, Fabian TC, Gavant M, et al. Management of blunt splenic trauma: computed tomographic contrast blush predicts failure of nonoperative management. *J Trauma* 1995; 39:507–512.

249. Thaemert BC, Cogbill TH, Lambert PJ. Nonoperative management of splenic injury: are follow-up computed tomographic scans of any value? *J Trauma* 1997;43:748–751.

250. Croce MA, Fabian TC, Menke PG, et al. Nonoperative management of blunt hepatic trauma is the treatment of choice for hemodynamically stable patients: results of a prospective trial. *Ann Surg* 1995;221:744–753.

251. Levison MA, Peterson SR, Sheldon GF, et al. Duodenal trauma: experience of a trauma center. *J Trauma* 1984;24: 475–480.

252. Wisner DH, Wold RL, Frey CF. Diagnosis and treatment of pancreatic injuries: an analysis of management principles. *Arch Surg* 1990;125:1109–1113.

253. Lucas CE. Diagnosis and treatment of pancreatic and duodenal injury. *Surg Clin North Am* 1977;57:49–65.

254. Wisner DH, Chun Y, Blaisdell FW. Blunt intestinal injury: keys to diagnosis and management. *Arch Surg* 1990;125: 1319–1322.

255. Stone HH, Fabian TC. Management of perforating colon trauma: randomization between primary closure and exteriorization. *Ann Surg* 1979;190:430–436.

256. Looser KG, Crombie HD Jr. Pelvic fractures: an anatomic guide to severity of injury—review of 100 cases. *Am J Surg* 1976;132:638–642.

257. Cryer HM, Miller FB, Evers BM, et al. Pelvic fracture classification: correlation with hemorrhage. *J Trauma* 1988;28: 973.

258. Burgess AR, Eastridge BJ, Young JWR, et al. Pelvic ring disruptions: effective classification system and treatment protocols. *J Trauma* 1990;30:848–856.

259. Trunkey DD, Chapman MW, Lin RC Jr, et al. Management of pelvic fractures in blunt trauma injury. *J Trauma* 1974;14: 912–923.

260. Mendez C, Gubler KD, Maier RV. Diagnostic accuracy of peritoneal lavage in patients with pelvic fractures. *Arch Surg* 1994;129:477–481.

261. Evers BM, Cryer HM, Miller FB. Pelvic fracture hemorrhage: priorities in management. *Arch Surg* 1989;124:422–424.

262. Flint L, Babikian G, Anders M, et al. Definitive control of mortality from severe pelvic fracture. *Ann Surg* 1990;211: 703–806.

263. Panetta T, Sclafani SJ, Goldstein AS, et al. Percutaneous transcatheter embolization for massive bleeding from pelvic fractures. *J Trauma* 1985;25:1021–1029.

264. Ben-Menachem Y, Coldwell DM, Young JW, et al. Hemorrhage associated with pelvic fractures: causes, diagnosis, and emergent management. *AJR Am J Roentgenol* 1991;157: 1005–1014.

265. Nicolaisen GS, McAninch JW, Marshall GA, et al. Renal trauma: reevaluation of the indications for radiologic assessment. *J Urol* 1985;133:183.

266. Morey AF, McAninch JW, Tiller BK, et al. Single shot intraoperative excretory urography for the immediate evaluation of renal trauma. *J Urol* 1999;161:1088–1092.

267. Stevenson J, Battistella FD. The "one-shot" intravenous pyelogram: is it indicated in unstable trauma patients before celiotomy? *J Trauma* 1994;36:828–833.

268. Carroll PR, McAninch JW. Staging of renal trauma. *Urol Clin North Am* 1989;16:193–201.

269. Wessells H, McAninch JW, Meyer A, et al. Criteria for nonoperative treatment of significant penetrating renal lacerations. *J Urol* 1997;157:24–27.

270. McAninch JW, Carroll PR, Klosterman PW, et al. Renal reconstruction after injury. *J Urol* 1991;145:932–937.

271. Horstman WG, McClennan BL, Heiken JP. Comparison of computed tomography and conventional cystography for detection of traumatic bladder rupture. *Urol Radiol* 1991;12: 188–193.

272. Haas CA, Brown SL, Spirnak JP. Limitations of routine spiral computerized tomography in the evaluation of bladder trauma. *J Urol* 1999;162:51–52.

273. Cass AS, Luxenberg M. Management of extraperitoneal ruptures of bladder caused by external trauma. *Urology* 1989;3: 179–183.

274. Corriere JN Jr, Sandler CM. Management of the ruptured bladder: seven years' experience with 111 cases. *J Trauma* 1986;26:830–833.

275. Cass AS. Urethral injury in the multiple-injury patient. *J Trauma* 1984;24:901–906.

276. Mattox KL, Feliciano DV, Burch J, et al. 5,760 Cardiovascular injuries in 4,459 patients: epidemiologic evolution 1958–1987. *Ann Surg* 1989;209:698.

277. Shackford SR, Baxt WG, Hoyt DB, et al. Impact of a trauma system on the outcome of severely injured patients. *Arch Surg* 1987;122:523.

278. Shackford SR, Rich NM. Peripheral vascular injury. In: Feliciano DV, Moore EE, Mattox KL, eds. *Trauma,* 3rd ed. Norwalk, CT: Appleton & Lange, 1996.

279. Cambria RA, Anderson RJ, Dikdan G, et al. Leukocyte activation in ischemia-reperfusion injury of skeletal muscle. *J Surg Res* 1991;51:13.

280. McCord JM. Oxygen-derived free radicals in postischemic tissue injury. *N Engl J Med* 1985;312:159.

281. Snyder WH, Thal ER, Bredges RA, et al. The validity of normal arteriography in penetrating trauma. *Arch Surg* 1978; 113:424.

282. Fellmeth BD, Buckner NK, Ferreira JA, et al. Postcatheterization femoral artery injuries: repair with color flow US guidance and C-clamp assistance. *Radiology* 1992;182:570.

283. Fellmeth BD, Roberts AC, Bookstein JJ, et al. Postangiographic femoral artery injuries: nonsurgical repair with US-guided compression. *Radiology* 1991;178:671.

284. Kang SS, Labropoulos N, Mansour MA, et al. Percutaneous ultrasound guided thrombin injections: a new method for treating postcatheterization femoral pseudoaneurysms. *J Vasc Surg* 1998;27:1032.

285. Johansen K, Davies M, Howie T, et al. Objective criteria accurately predicting amputation following lower extremity trauma. *J Trauma* 1990;30:568.

286. Feliciano DV, Mattox KL, Graham JM, et al. Five-year experience with PTFE in vascular wounds. *J Trauma* 1985;25:75.

287. Johansen K, Bandyk D, Thiele B, et al. Use of temporary intraluminal shunts: resolution of management dilemma in complex vascular injuries. *J Trauma* 1982;22:395.

288. Mattox KL, Wall MJ. Injury to the thoracic great vessels. In: Feliciano DV, Moore EE, Mattox KL, eds. *Trauma,* 3rd ed. Norwalk, CT: Appleton & Lange, 1996.

289. Graham JM, Mattox KL, Beall AC. Portal venous injuries. *J Trauma* 1978;18:843.

290. Court-Brown CM. Care of accident victims. *BMJ* 1989;298: 115.

291. Perry JF, McClellan RJ. Autopsy findings in 127 patients following fatal traffic accidents. *Surg Gynecol Obstet* 1964;119: 586.

292. Lieurance R, Benjamin JB, Rappaport WD. Blood loss and transfusion in patients with isolated femur fractures. *J Orthop Trauma* 1992;6:175.

293. Burgess AR, Eastridge BJ, Young JWR, et al. Pelvis ring disruptions: effective classification system and treatment protocols. *J Trauma* 1990;30:848.

294. Mucha P Jr, Farnell MB. Analysis of pelvic fracture management. *J Trauma* 1984;24:379.

295. Pedowitz RA, Shackford SR. Non-cavitary hemorrhage producing shock in trauma patients: incidence and severity. *J Trauma* 1989;29:219.

296. Bracken MB, Shepard MJ, Collins WF, et al. A randomized controlled trial of methylprednisolone or naloxone in the treatment of acute spinal cord injury. *N Engl J Med* 1990; 322:1405.

297. Bracken MB, Shepard MJ, Collins WF, et al. Methylprednisolone or naloxone treatment after acute spinal cord injury: 1-year follow-up data—results of the Second National Acute Spinal Cord Injury Study. *J Neurosurg* 1992;76:23.

298. Gustilo RB, Anderson JT. Prevention of infection in the treatment of 1,025 open fractures of long bones: retrospective and prospective analysis. *J Bone Joint Surg Am* 1976;58:453.

299. Gustilo JB, Mendoza RM, Williams DN. Problems in the management of type III (severe) open fractures: a new classification of type III open fractures. *J Trauma* 1984;24:742.

300. Delong WG, Born CT, Wei SY, et al. Aggressive treatment of 119 open fracture wounds. *J Trauma* 1999;46:1049.

301. Bunt TJ, Malone JM, Moody M, et al. Frequency of vascular injury with blunt-trauma induced extremity injury. *Am J Surg* 1990;160:226.

302. Gable DR, Allen JW, Richardson JD. Blunt popliteal artery injury: is physical examination alone enough for evaluation? *J Trauma* 1997;43:541.

303. Lozman J, Deno DC, Feustel PJ, et al. Pulmonary and cardiovascular consequences of immediate fixation or conservative management of long-bone fractures. *Arch Surg* 1986; 121:992.

304. Latenser BA, Gentilello LM, Tarver AA, et al. Improved outcome with early fixation of skeletally unstable pelvic fractures. *J Trauma* 1991;31:28.

305. Dennis JW, Menawat S, Von Thron J, et al. Efficacy of deep venous thrombosis prophylaxis in trauma patients and identification of high-risk groups. *J Trauma* 1993;35:132.

306. Rodriguez JL, Lopez JM, Proctor MC, et al. Early placement of prophylactic vena caval filters in injured patients at high risk for pulmonary embolism. *J Trauma* 1996;40:797.

307. Patton JH, Fabian TC, Croce MA, et al. Prophylactic Greenfield filters: acute complications and long-term follow-up. *J Trauma* 1996;41:231.

308. Levy D. The fat embolism syndrome. *Clin Orthop* 1990;261: 281.

309. Eddy A, Rice C, Carrico C. Fat embolism syndrome: monitoring and management. *J Crit Illness* 1987;2:24.

310. Bulger EM, Smith DG, Maier RV, et al. Fat embolism syndrome: a 10-year review. *Arch Surg* 1997;132:534.

311. Broe P, Toung T, Margolis S, et al. Pulmonary injury caused by free fatty acid: evaluation of steroid and albumin therapy. *Surgery* 1981;89:582.

312. Alho A, Saikku K, Eerola P, et al. Corticosteroids in patients with a high risk of fat embolism syndrome. *Surg Gynecol Obstet* 1978;147:358.

313. Pape H, Regel G, Dwenger A, et al. Primary intramedullary femur fixation in multiple trauma patients with associated lung contusion: a cause of post-traumatic ARDS? *J Trauma* 1993;34:540.

314. Pape H, Regel G, Dwenger A, et al. Influences of different methods of intramedullary femoral nailing on lung function in patients with multiple trauma. *J Trauma* 1993;35:709.

315. Johansen K, Daines M, Howey T, et al. Objective criteria accurately predict amputation following lower extremity trauma. *J Trauma* 1990;30:568.

316. Gregory RT, Gould RJ, Peclet M, et al. The mangled extremity syndrome (M.E.S.): a severity grading system for multisystem injury of the extremity. *J Trauma* 1985;25:1147.

317. Russell WL, Sailors DM, Whittle TB, et al. Limb salvage versus traumatic amputation. *Ann Surg* 1991;213:473.

318. Howe HR Jr, Poole GV Jr, Hansen KJ, et al. Salvage of lower extremities following combined orthopedic and vascular trauma. *Am Surg* 1987;53:205.

319. Durham RM, Mistry BM, Mazuski JE, et al. Outcome and utility of scoring systems in the management of the mangled extremity. *Am J Surg* 1996;172:569.

320. Dossett AB, Hunt JL, Purdue GF, et al. Early orthopedic intervention in burn patients with major fractures. *J Trauma* 1991;31:888.

321. Kalb DC, Ney AL, Rodriguez JL, et al. Assessment of the relationship between timing of fixation of the fracture and secondary brain injury in patients with multiple trauma. *Surg* 1998;124:739.

322. Scalea TM, Scott JD, Brumback RJ, et al. Early fracture fixation may be "just fine" after head injury: no difference in central nervous system outcomes. *J Trauma* 1999;46:839.

323. Phillips TF, Contreras DM. Current concepts review: timing of operative treatment of fractures inpatients who have multiple fractures. *J Bone Joint Surg Am* 1990;72:784.

324. Tepas JJ. Resuscitation of the injured child. In: Trunkey DD,

Lewis FR, eds. *Current therapy of trauma*, 4th ed. St. Louis: Mosby, 1999:81–88.

325. Svenson JE, Spurlock C, Nypaver M. Factors associated with the higher traumatic death rate among rural children. *Ann Emerg Med* 1996;27:625–632.

326. Esposito TJ, Sanddal ND, Dean JM, et al. Analysis of preventable pediatric trauma deaths and inappropriate trauma care in Montana. *J Trauma* 1999;47:243–253.

327. Nakayama DK, Gardner MJ, Rowe MI. Emergency endotracheal intubation in pediatric trauma. *Ann Surg* 1990; 218–223.

328. Paul TR, Marias M, Pons PT, et al. Adult versus pediatric prehospital trauma care: is there a difference? *J Trauma* 1999;47:455–459.

329. Partrick DA, Bensard DD, Moore EE, et al. Ultrasound in an effective triage tool to evaluate blunt abdominal trauma in the pediatric population. *J Trauma* 1998;45:57–63.

330. Tepas JJ, DiScala C, Ramenofsky MLO, et al. Mortality and head injury: the pediatric perspective. *J Pediatr Surg* 1990; 25:92–95.

331. Orenstein JB, Klein BL, Gotschall CS, et al. Age and outcome in pediatric cervical spine injury: 11-year experience. *Pediatr Emerg Care* 1994;10:132–137.

332. Givens TG, Polley KA, Smieth GR, et al. Pediatric cervical spine injury: a three-year experience. *J Trauma* 1996;41: 310–314.

333. Kriss VM, Kriss TC. SCIWORA (spinal cord injury without radiographic abnormality) in infants and children. *Clin Pediatr* 1996;35:119–124.

334. Dowd MD, Krug S. Pediatric blunt cardiac injury: epidemiology, clinical features, and diagnosis. *J Trauma* 1996;40: 61–87.

335. Scorpio RJ, Wesson DE, Smith CR, et al. Blunt cardiac injuries in children: a postmortem study. *J Trauma* 1996;41: 306–309.

336. Cooper A, Barlow B, DiScala C, et al. Mortality and truncal injury: the pediatric perspective. *J Pediatr Surg* 1994;29:33–38.

337. Moulton SL, Lynch FP, Hoyt DB, et al. Operative intervention for pediatric liver injuries: avoiding delay in treatment. *J Pediatr Surg* 1992;27:958–963.

338. Fallat ME, Casale AJ. Practice patterns of pediatric surgeons caring for stable patients with traumatic solid organ injury. *J Trauma* 1997;43:820–824.

339. Prankikoff T, Hirschl R, Schlesinger AE, et al. Resolution of splenic injury after nonoperative management. *J Pediatr Surg* 1994;29:1366–1369.

340. Keller MS, Stafford PW, Vane DW. Conservative management of pancreatic trauma in children. *J Trauma* 1997;42: 1097–1100.

341. Canty TG, Canty TC Jr, Brown C. Injuries of the gastrointestinal tract from blunt trauma in children: a 12-year experience at a designated pediatric trauma center. *J Trauma* 1999;46:234–240.

342. Kurkschubasche AG, Fendya DG, Tracy TF, et al. Blunt intestinal injury in children: diagnostic and therapeutic considerations. *Arch Surg* 1997;132:652–658.

343. Benard DD, Beaver BL, Besner GE, et al. Small bowel injury in children after blunt abdominal trauma: is diagnostic delay important? *J Trauma* 1996;41:476–483.

344. Newman KD, Bowman LM, Eichelberger MR, et al. The lap belt complex: intestinal and lumbar spine injury in children. *J Trauma* 1990;30:1133–1140.

345. Bond SJ, Gotshall CS, Eichelberger MR. Predictors of abdominal injury in children with pelvic fracture. *J Trauma* 1991;31:1169–1173.

346. McIntyre RC, Bensard DD, Moore EE, et al. Pelvic fracture geometry predicts risk of life-threatening hemorrhage in children. *J Trauma* 1993;35:423–429.

347. Nakayama DK, Gardner MJ, Rogers KD. Disability from bicycle-related injuries in children. *J Trauma* 1990;30:1390–1394.

348. Wesson DE, Scorpio RJ, Spence LJ, et al. The physical, psychological, and socioeconomic costs of pediatric trauma. *J Trauma* 1992;33:252–257.

349. Stallard P, Velleman R, Baldwin S. Prospective study of post-traumatic stress disorder in children involved in road traffic accidents. *BMJ* 1998;317:1619–1623.

350. Eichelberger MR, Gotschall CS, Feely HB, et al. Parental attitudes and knowledge of child safety: a national survey. *Am J Dis Child* 1990;144:714–720.

351. Rivara FP, Grossman DC, Cummings P. Injury prevention (part 1). *N Engl J Med* 1997;337:543–548; (part 2) *N Engl J Med* 1997;337:613–618.

352. Cummings P, Gorssman DC, Rivara FP, et al. State gun safe storage laws and child mortality due to firearms. *JAMA* 1997;278:1084–1086.

353. Durkin MS, Kuhn L, Davidson LL, et al. Epidemiology and prevention of severe assault and gun injuries to children in an urban community. *J Trauma* 1996;41:667–673.

354. National Estimates: Annual Population Estimates by Age Group and Sex, selected years from 1990 to 2000. Population Estimates Program, Population Division, U.S. Bureau of the Census, Washington, DC 20233.

355. U.S. Department of Health and Human Services. National Vital Statistics Report. Births and Deaths: Preliminary Data for 1997. Vol 47, No. 4. October 7, 1998. Hyattsville, MD.

356. DeMaria EJ. Evaluation and treatment of the elderly trauma victim. *Clin Geriatr Med* 1993;9:461.

357. National Safety Council. *Accident facts: deaths due to unintentional injury*. Chicago: National Safety Council, 1998.

358. Duthie EH. Falls. *Med Clin North Am* 1989;73:1321.

359. Alexander BH, Rivera FP, Wolf ME. The cost and frequency of hospitalization for fall-related injuries in older adults. *Am J Public Health* 1992;83:1020.

360. Santora TA, Schinco MA, Trooskin SZ. Management of trauma in the elderly patient. *Surg Clin North Am* 1994;74:163.

361. Rubinstein LZ, Robbins AS, Josephson KR, et al. The value of assessing falls in an elderly population: a randomized clinical trial. *Ann Intern Med* 1990;15:113:308–316.

362. Riggs JE. Mortality from accidental falls among the elderly in the United States, 1962–1988: demonstrating the impact of improved trauma management. *J Trauma* 1993;35:212.

363. National Safety Council. *Accident facts*. Chicago: National Safety Council, 1991.

364. National Highway Traffic Safety Administration (NHTSA). *A decade of progress: fatal accident reporting system, 1989*. U.S. Department of Transportation publication HS807071. Washington, DC: NHTSA, 1992.

365. Scalea TM, Kohl L. Geriatric trauma. In: Feliciano DV, Moore EM, Mattox KL, eds. *Trauma*, 3rd ed. Norwalk, CT: Appleton & Lange, 1996:899.

366. Sklar DP, Demarest GB, McFeeley P. Increased pedestrian mortality among the elderly. *Am J Emerg Med* 1989;7:387.

367. Schwab CW, Kauder DR. Trauma in the geriatric patient. *Arch Surg* 1992;127:701.

368. Osler T, Hales K, Baack B, et al. Trauma in the elderly. *Am J Surg* 1988;156:537.

369. Finelli FC, Jonsson J, Champion HR, et al. A case controlled study of major trauma in geriatric patients. *J Trauma* 1989; 29:541.

370. Appleton W. Elder abuse: diagnose, treat, cure. *Ann Emerg Med* 1988;17:1006.

371. Allen JE, Schwab CW. Blunt chest trauma in the elderly. *Am Surg* 1985;51:697.

372. Bender BS, Nagel JE, Adler WH, et al. Absolute peripheral blood lymphocyte count and subsequent mortality in elderly men: the Baltimore Longitudinal Study of Aging. *J Am Geriatr Soc* 1986;34:649.

373. Nagel JE, Chopra RK, Chrest FJ, et al. Decreased proliferation, interleukin 2 synthesis, and interleukin 2 receptor expression is accompanied by decreased mRNA expression in phytohemagglutinin-stimulated cells from elderly donors. *J Clin Invest* 1988;81:1096.

374. Adler WH. Immune function in the elderly. *Geriatrics* 1989; 44[Suppl A]:7.

375. Stead WW, Lofgren JP, Warren E, et al. Tuberculosis as an endemic and nosocomial infection among the elderly in nursing homes. *N Engl J Med* 1985;312:1483.

376. Gennarelli TA, Thibalut LB. Biomechanics of acute subdural hematoma. *J Trauma* 1982;22:680.

377. Scalea TM, Simon HM, Duncan AO, et al. Geriatric blunt multiple trauma: improved survival with early invasive monitoring. *J Trauma* 1990;30:129.

378. DeMaria EJ, Kenney PR, Merriam MA, et al. Aggressive trauma care benefits the elderly. *J Trauma* 1987;27:1200.

379. Bybee DE. Toleration of head injury by the elderly. *Neurosurgery* 1987;20:954.

380. Pennings JL, Bachulis BL, Simons CR, et al. Survival after severe brain injury in the aged. *Arch Surg* 1993;128:787.

381. Carlsson CA, Essen CV, Lofgren J. Factors affecting the clinical course of patients with severe head injuries. *J Neurosurg* 1968;29:242.

382. Camp PC, Rogers FB, Shackford SR, et al. Blunt traumatic thoracic aortic lacerations in the elderly: an analysis of outcome. *J Trauma* 1994;37:418.

383. Van der Sluis CK, Klasen HJ, Eisma WH, et al. Major trauma in young and old: what is the difference? *J Trauma* 1996;40: 78–82.

384. Finelli FC, Jonsson J, Champion HR, et al. A case control study for major trauma in geriatric patients. *J Trauma* 1989; 29:541–548.

385. Perdue PW, Watts DD, Kaufmann CR, et al. Differences in mortality between elderly and younger adult trauma patients: geriatric status increases risk of delayed death. *J Trauma* 1998;45:805–810.

386. Oreskovich MR, Howard JD, Copas MK, et al. Geriatric trauma: injury patterns and outcome. *J Trauma* 1984;24: 565–572.

387. Sacco WJ, Copes WS, Bain LW, et al. Effect of preinjury illness on trauma patient survival outcome. *J Trauma* 1993;35: 538–542.

388. Day RJ, Vinen J, Hewitt-Falls E. Major trauma outcomes in the elderly. *Med J Aust* 1994;160:675–678.

389. State of California Department of Motor Vehicles. Stylos L, Janke MK. *Annual tabulations of mature driving program driving record comparisons.* CAL-DMV-RSS-89-119. Sacramento, CA: State of California Department of Motor Vehicles, 1989.

390. Retting R, Schwartz SI, Kulewiicz M, et al. Queens Boulevard Pedestrian Safety Project, New York City. *MMWR Morb Mortal Wkly Rep* 1989;38:61.

391. Rogers FB, Rozycki GS, Osler TM, et al. A multi-institutional study of factors associated with fetal death in injured pregnant patients. *Arch Surg* 1999;134:1274–1277.

392. Kissinger DP, Rozycki GS, Morris JA, et al. Trauma in pregnancy: predicting pregnancy outcome. *Arch Surg* 1991;126: 1079–1086.

393. Drost TF, Rosemurgy AS, Sherman HF, et al. Major trauma in pregnant women: maternal/fetal outcome. *J Trauma* 1990;30: 574–578.

394. Hoff WS, D'Amelio LF, Tinkoff GH, et al. Maternal predictors of fetal demise in trauma during pregnancy. *Surg Gynecol Obstet* 1991;172:175–180.

395. Esposito TJ, Gens DR, Smith LG, et al. Trauma during pregnancy: a review of 79 cases. *Arch Surg* 1991;126:1073–1078.

396. Pearlman MD, Tintinalli JE, Lorenz RP. A prospective controlled study of outcome after trauma during pregnancy. *Am J Obstet Gynecol* 1990;162:1502–1510.

397. Fildes J, Reed L, Jones N, et al. Trauma: the leading cause of maternal death. *J Trauma* 1992;32:643–645.

398. Dietz P, Rochat R, Goldner T, et al. Osewe PL, ed. Pregnancy status poorly reported on death certificates. In: *Georgia epidemiology report.* Atlanta: Department of Human Resources, 1995:Report #11–6, pp. 1–4.

399. Shah KH, Simons RK, Holbrook T, et al. Trauma in pregnancy: maternal and fetal outcomes. *J Trauma* 1998;45: 83–86.

400. Scorpio RJ, Esposito TJ, Smith LG, et al. Blunt trauma during pregnancy: factors affecting fetal outcome. *J Trauma* 1992;32:213–216.

401. Poole GV, Martin JN Jr, Perry KG Jr, et al. Trauma in pregnancy: the role of interpersonal violence. *Am J Obstet Gynecol* 1996;174:1873–1878.

402. Biester EM, Tomich PG, Esposito TJ, et al. Trauma in pregnancy: normal revised trauma score in relation to other markers of maternofetal status—a preliminary study. *Am J Obstet Gynecol* 1997;176:1206–1212.

403. Connolly A, Katz VL, Bash KL, et al. Trauma and pregnancy. *Am J Perinatol* 1997;14:331–336.

404. Depp R. Clinical evaluation of fetal status. In: Scott JR, DiSaia PJ, Hammond CB, et al., eds. *Danforth's obstetrics and gynecology,* 6th ed. Philadelphia: JB Lippincott, 1990: 315–334.

405. Cunningham FG, MacDonald PC. Maternal adaptations to pregnancy. In: Gant NF, et al., eds. *Williams obstetrics,* 20th ed. Norwalk, CT: Appleton & Lange, 1997:191–225.

406. Edman CD, Toofanian A, MacDonald PC, et al. Placental clearance rate of maternal plasma androstenedione through placental estradiol formation: an indirect method of assessing uteroplacental blood flow. *Am J Obstet Gynecol* 1981; 69:851.

407. Kauppila A, Koskinen M, Puolakka J, et al. Decreased intervillous and unchanged myometrial blood flow in supine recumbency. *Obstet Gynecol* 1980;55:203.

408. Pritchard JA. Changes in blood during pregnancy and delivery. *Anesthesiology* 1965;26:393.

409. Whittaker PG, MacPhail S, Lind T. Serial hematologic changes and pregnancy outcome. *Obstet Gynecol* 1996;88: 33.

410. Scott DE. Anemia during pregnancy. *Obstet Gynecol Ann* 1972;48:638.

411. Smith CV, Phelan JP. Trauma in pregnancy. In: Clark SL, Cotton DB, Hankins GDV, et al., eds. *Critical care obstetrics,* 2nd ed. Boston: Blackwell, 1991:498.

412. Brinkman CRI, Mofid M, Assali NS. Circulatory shock in pregnant sheep: effects of hemorrhage on uteroplacental and fetal circulation and oxygenation. *Am J Obstet Gynecol* 1974;118:77–90.

413. Gonick B. Intensive care monitoring of the critically ill pregnant patient. In: Creasy RK, Resnick R, eds. *Maternal–fetal medicine: principles and practice,* 2nd ed. Philadelphia: WB Saunders, 1989:845.

414. Bieniarz J, Branda LA, Maqueda E. Aortocaval compression by the uterus in late pregnancy: III. unreliability of the sphygmomanometric method in estimating uterine artery pressure. *Am J Obstet Gynecol* 1968;102:1106.

415. Greiss FC, Anderson SG. Effect of ovarian hormones on the uterine vascular bed. *Am J Obstet Gynecol* 1970;107:829.

416. Clark SL, Cotton DB, Lee W. Central hemodynamic assessment of normal term pregnancy. *Am J Obstet Gynecol* 1989; 161:1439.

417. Enein M, Zina AAA, Kassem M, et al. Echocardiography of the pericardium in pregnancy. *Obstet Gynecol* 1987;69:851.

418. Lee W, Cotton DB. Cardiorespiratory changes during pregnancy. In: Clark SL, Cotton DB, Hankins GDV, et al., eds. *Critical care obstetrics,* 2nd ed. Boston: Blackwell, 1991:2.

419. Tsia CH, deLeeuw NKM. Changes in 2,3-diphosphoglycerate during pregnancy and puerperium in normal women and in B-thalassemia heterozygous women. *Am J Obstet Gynecol* 1982;142:520.

420. Hume RF, Killam AP. Maternal physiology. In: Scott JR, DiSaia J, Hammon DB, et al., eds. *Obstetrics and gynecology.* Philadelphia: JB Lippincott, 1990:93.

421. Braverman DZ, Johnson ML, Kern F Jr. Effects of pregnancy and contraceptive steroids on gallbladder function. *N Engl J Med* 1980;302:362.

422. Bailey RR, Rollerston GL. Kidney length and ureteric dilatation in the puerperium. *Br J Obstet Gynaecol* 1971;78:55.

423. Chesley LC. Renal function during pregnancy. In: Carey HM, ed. *Modern trends in human reproductive physiology* 1963;1:205–214.

424. Davison JM, Hytten FF. The effects of pregnancy on the renal handling of glucose. *Br J Obstet Gynaecol* 1975;82:374.

425. Lindheimer MD, Grunfeld JP, Davison JM. Renal disorders. In: Barron WM, Lindheimer MD, ed. *Medical disorders during pregnancy,* 2nd ed. St. Louis: Mosby, 1995:37.

426. Taylor DJ, Phillips P, Lind T. Puerperal hematological indices. *Br J Obstet Gynaecol* 1981;88:601.

427. Bremme K, Ostlund E, Almqvist I, et al. Enhanced thrombin generation and fibrinolytic activity in normal pregnancy and the puerperium. *Obstet Gynecol* 1992;80:132.

428. Advanced trauma life support. American College of Surgeons Committee on Trauma. *Trauma in women,* 6th ed. Chicago: American College of Surgeons, 1997:313–324.

429. Rosenfeld CR, Barton MD, Meschia G. Effects of epinephrine on distribution of blood flow in the pregnant ewe. *Am J Obstet Gynecol* 1976;124:156.

430. Rosenfeld CR, West J. Circulatory response to systemic infusion of nor-epinephrine in the pregnant ewe. *Am J Obstet Gynecol* 1977;127:376.

431. Higgins SD. Perinatal protocol: trauma in pregnancy. *J Perinatol* 1988;8:288–292.

432. Neufeld JDG, Moore EE, Marx JA, et al. Trauma in pregnancy. *Emerg Med Clin North Am* 1987;5:623–640.

433. Kleihauer E, Braun H, Betke K. Demonstration von fetalem hamoglobin in den erythrocyten eines blutausstrichs. *Klin Wochenschr* 1957;35:637.

434. Scott JR, Beer AE, Guy LR. Pathogenesis of Rh immunization in primigravidas: fetomaternal versus maternal-fetal bleeding. *Obstet Gynecol* 1977;49:9.

435. Thorsen MK, Lawson TL, Aiman EJ, et al. Diagnosis of ectopic pregnancy: endovaginal vs. transabdominal sonography. *AJR Am J Roentgenol* 1990;155:307–310.

436. Timor-Tritsch I, Greenidge S, Admon D, et al. Emergency room use of transvaginal ultrasonography by obstetrics and gynecology residents. *Am J Obstet Gynecol* 1992;166:866–872.

437. Mateer JR, Valley VT, Aiman EJ, et al. Outcome analysis of a protocol including bedside endovaginal sonography inpatients at risk of ectopic pregnancy. *Ann Emerg Med* 1996;27:283–289.

438. Reed KL. Ultrasound in obstetrics. In: Scott JR, DiSaia PJ, Hammond CB, et al., eds. *Danforth's obstetrics and gynecology,* 6th ed. Philadelphia: JB Lippincott, 1990:297–314.

439. Brent RL. The effect of embryonic and fetal exposure to x-ray, microwaves, and ultrasound: counseling the pregnant and nonpregnant patient about these risks. *Semin Oncol* 1989;16:347–368.

440. Bushong SC. *Radiologic science for technologists.* Washington, DC: Mosby, 1983:550.

441. Stovall M, Blackwell CR, Novada DH, et al. Fetal dose from radiotherapy with photon beams: report of AAPM Radiation Therapy Committee Task Group No. 36. *Med Phys* 1995;22:63–82.

442. Martin JN, Brewer DW. Successful pregnancy outcome following mid-gestational uterine rupture and repair using Gore-Tex soft tissue patch. *Obstet Gynecol* 1990;75:518.

443. Higgins SD, Garite TJ. Late abruptio placentae in trauma patients: implications for monitoring. *Obstet Gynecol* 1984;63(3)[Suppl]:10S–12S.

444. Crosby WM. Automobile trauma in pregnancy: prevention and treatment. *Prim Care Update Ob/Gyn* 1996;3:6.

445. Crosby WM, Costiloe J. Safety of lap-belt restraint for pregnant victims of automobile collisions. *N Engl J Med* 1971;284:632.

446. Pearlman MD, Viano D. Automobile crash simulation with the first pregnant crash test dummy. *Am J Obstet Gynecol* 1996;175:977–981.

447. Franger AL, Buchsbaum HJ, Peaceman AM. Abdominal gunshot wounds in pregnancy. *Am J Obstet Gynecol* 1989;160:1124–1128.

448. Saunders P, Milton PJ. Laparotomy during pregnancy: an assessment of diagnostic accuracy and fetal wastage. *BMJ* 1973;3:165–167.

449. Eddy VA, Morris JA Jr, Rozycki GS. Trauma and pregnancy. In: Ivatury RR, Cayten CG, eds. *Penetrating trauma.* Baltimore: Williams & Wilkins, 1996:695–701.

450. Rothenberger D, Quattlebaum FW, Perry JF. Blunt maternal trauma: a review of 103 cases. *J Trauma* 1978;18:173.

451. Fatovich DM. Electric shock in pregnancy. *J Emerg Med* 1993;11:175.

452. Marx GF. Cardiopulmonary resuscitation of late-pregnant women. *Anesthesiology* 1982;56:156.

453. Oates S, Williams GL, Rees GA. Cardiopulmonary resuscitation in late pregnancy. *BMJ* 1988;297:40.

454. Morris JA, Rosenbower TJ, Jurkovich GJ, et al. Infant survival after cesarean section for trauma. *Ann Surg* 1996;223:481–449.

455. Common complications of pregnancy: hypertensive disorders in pregnancy. In: Cunningham FG, MacDonald PC, Gant NF, et al., eds. *Williams obstetrics,* 20th ed. Norwalk, CT: Appleton & Lange, 1997:693–744.

456. Ginsberg JS, Hirsch J. Use of antithrombotic agents during pregnancy. *Chest* 1998;114:524S–530S.

457. Judich A, Kuriansky J, Engelberg I, et al. Amniotic fluid embolism following blunt abdominal trauma in pregnancy. *Injury* 1998;29:475–477.

458. Acosta JA, Yang JC, Winchell RJ, et al. Lethal injuries and time to death in a level 1 trauma center. *J Am Coll Surg* 1998;186:528.

459. Davis JW, Hoyt DB, Mackersie RC, et al. The significance of critical care errors in causing preventable deaths in trauma patients in a trauma system. *J Trauma* 1991;31:813–819.

460. Simons RK, Eliopoulos V, Laflamme D, et al. Impact on process of trauma care delivery 1 year after the introduction of a trauma program in a provincial trauma center. *J Trauma* 1999;46:811.

461. Pulmonary artery catheter consensus conference: consensus statement. *New Horiz* 1997;5:175.

462. Kirkpatrick AW, Chun R, Brown DR, et al. Hypothermia and the trauma patient. *Can J Surg* 1999;42:333.

463. Simons RK, Hoyt DB. Immunomodulation. In: *Advances in trauma and critical care,* vol 9. St. Louis: Mosby, 1994:135–167.

464. Botha AJ, Moore FA, Moore EE, et al. Postinjury neutrophil priming and activation: an early vulnerable window. *Surgery* 1995;118:358.

465. Deitch EA. The role of intestinal barrier failure and bacterial translocation in the development of systemic infection and multiple organ failure. *Arch Surg* 1990;125:403–404.

466. Cales RH, Trunkey DD. Preventable trauma deaths: a review of trauma care systems development. *JAMA* 1985;254:1059–1063.

467. Hoyt DB, Hollingsworth-Fridlund P, Fortlage D, et al. An evaluation of provider-related and disease-related morbidity in a level 1 university trauma service: directions for quality improvement. *J Trauma* 1992;33:586–601.

468. Hoyt DB, Hollingsworth-Fridlund P, Winchell RJ, et al. Analysis of recurrent process errors leading to provider-related complications on an organized trauma service: directions for care improvement. *J Trauma* 1994;36:377–384.

469. American College of Chest Physicians—Society of Critical Care Medicine Consensus Conference. Definitions for sepsis and organ failure for the use of innovative therapies in sepsis. *Crit Care Med* 1992;20:864.

470. Hoyt DB, Simons RK, Winchell RJ, et al. A risk analysis of pulmonary complications following major trauma. *J Trauma* 1993;35:524–531.

471. Driks MR, Craven DE, Celli BR, et al. Nosocomial pneumonia in intubated patients given sucralfate as compared with antacids or histamine type 2 blockers: the role of gastric colonization. *N Engl J Med* 1987;317:1376–1382.

472. Simms HH, DeMaria E, McDonald L, et al. Role of gastric colonization in the development of pneumonia in critically ill trauma patients: results of a prospective randomized trial. *J Trauma* 1991;31:531–537.

473. Stoutenbeek CP, van Saene HK, Miranda DR, et al. The effect of oropharyngeal decontamination using topical nonabsorbable antibiotics on the incidence of nosocomial respiratory tract infections in multiple trauma patients. *J Trauma* 1987;27:357–364.

474. Johanson WG Jr, Seidenfeld JJ, de los Santos R, et al. Prevention of nosocomial pneumonia using topical and parenteral antimicrobial agents. *Am Rev Respir Dis* 1988;137:265–272.

475. Johanson WG Jr, Pierce AK, Sanford JP, et al. Nosocomial respiratory infections with gram-negative bacilli: the significance of colonization of the respiratory tract. *Ann Intern Med* 1972;77:701–706.

476. Berger R, Arango L. Etiologic diagnosis of bacterial nosocomial pneumonia in seriously ill patients. *Crit Care Med* 1985;13:833–836.

477. Villers D, Derriennic M, Raffi F, et al. Reliability of the bronchoscopic-protected catheter brush in intubated and ventilated patients. *Chest* 1985;88:527–530.

478. Kahn FW, Jones JM. Diagnosis in bacterial respiratory infection by bronchoalveolar lavage. *J Infect Dis* 1987;155:862–869.

479. Winchell RJ, Hoyt DB, Walsh J, et al. Risk factors associated with pulmonary embolism despite routine prophylaxis: implications for improved protection. *J Trauma* 1994 *(in press).*

480. Rabinovici R, Rudolph AS, Feuerstein G. Characterization of hemodynamic, hematologic, and biochemical responses to administration of liposome-encapsulated hemoglobin in the conscious, freely moving rat. *Circ Shock* 1989;29:115.

481. Morris JA Jr, MacKenzie EJ, Edelstein SL. The effect of pre-existing conditions on mortality in trauma patients. *JAMA* 1990;263:1942–1946.

482. Foil MB, Mackersie RC, Furst S, et al. The asymptomatic patient with suspected myocardial contusion. *Am J Surg* 1990; 160:638–643.

483. Rosner MJ. Pathophysiology and management of increased intracranial pressure. In: Andrews BT, ed. *Neurosurgical intensive care.* New York: McGraw-HIll, 1993:57–112.

484. Morris JA, Much P, Ross S, et al. Acute posttraumatic renal failure: a multicenter perspective. *J Trauma* 1991;31: 1584–1590.

485. Stene JK. Renal failure in the trauma patient. *Crit Care Clin* 1990;6:111–119.

486. Simons RK, Hoyt DB, Winchell RJ, et al. A risk analysis of stress ulceration following trauma. *J Trauma* 1994;36:165.

487. Seibel R, LaDuca J, Hassett JM, et al. Blunt multiple trauma (ISS 36), femur traction, and the pulmonary failure-septic state. *Ann Surg* 1985;202:2283–2295.

488. Weigelt JA. Risk of wound infections in trauma patients. *Am J Surg* 1985;150:782–784.

489. Maki DG, Cobb L, Garman JK, et al. An attachable silver-impregnated cuff for prevention of infection with central venous catheters: a prospective randomized multicenter trial. *Am J Med* 1988;85:307–314.

490. Flowers RH III, Schwenzer KJ, Kopel RF, et al. Efficacy of the attachable subcutaneous cuff for the prevention of intravascular catheter-related infection: a randomized, controlled trial. *JAMA* 1989;261:878–883.

491. Minton S. Poisonous snakes: part 1 and 2. *Clin Med* 1978; 85:13.

492. Parrish H. Incidence of treated snakebites in the United States. *Public Health Rep* 1966;81:269–276.

493. Russell F. Medical problems of snakebite: epidemiology. In: Russell F, ed. *Snake venom poisoning.* Great Neck, NY: Scholium International, 1983:250–258.

494. Litovitz T, Holm K, Bailey K, et al. Annual report of the American Association of Poison Control Centers national data collection system. *Am J Emerg Med* 1992;10:454–505.

495. Gomez H, Davis M, Phillips S, et al. Human envenomation from a wandering garter snake. *Ann Emerg Med* 1994;23: 1119–1122.

496. Curry S, Horning D, Brady P, et al. The legitimacy of rattlesnake bites in central Arizona. *Ann Emerg Med* 1989;18: 658–663.

497. Wingert W, Chan L. Rattlesnake bites in southern California and rationale for recommended treatment. *West J Med* 1988; 148:37–44.

498. Davidson T. Intravenous rattlesnake envenomation. *West J Med* 1988;148:37–44.

499. Hutton RA, Warrell DA. Action of snake venom components on the haemostatic system. *Blood Rev* 1993;7:176–189.

500. Arnold R. Treatment of venomous snakebites in the Western Hemisphere. *Mil Med* 1984;149:361–365.

501. Guisto J. Severe toxicity from crotalid envenomation after early resolution of symptoms. *Ann Emerg Med* 1995;26: 387–388.

502. Garfin S. Rattlesnake bites and surgical decompression: results using a laboratory model. *Toxicon* 1984;22:177–184.

503. Downey D, Omer G, Moneim M. New Mexico rattlesnake bites: demographic review and guidelines for treatment. *J Trauma* 1991;31:1380–1386.

504. Glass T. Early débridement in pit viper bites. *JAMA* 1976; 235:2513–2516.

505. White RR, Weber RA. Discussion of poisonous snakebite in central Texas: possible indicators for antivenin treatment. *Ann Surg* 1991;213:466–471; discussion 471–472.

506. Nelson B. Snake envenomation: incidence, clinical presentation, and management. *Med Toxicol* 1989;4:17–31.

507. Minton S. Present tests for detection of snake venom: clinical applications. *Ann Emerg Med* 1987;16:932–937.

508. Wingert W, Wainschel J. Diagnosis and management of envenomation of poisonous snakes. *South Med J* 1975;68: 1015–1026.

509. McCullough N, Gennaro J. Evaluation of venomous snake bite in southern United States. *J Fla Med Assoc* 1963;40: 959–967.

510. Kunkel D. Bites of venomous reptiles. *Emerg Med Clin North Am* 1984;2:563–577.

511. Treatment of snakebite in the United States. *Med Lett* 1982: 87–90.

512. Clark R. Cryotherapy and corticosteroids in the treatment of rattlesnake bite. *Mil Med* 1971;136:42–44.

513. Jurkovich GJ, Luterman A, McCullar K, et al. Complications of Crotalidae antivenin therapy. *J Trauma* 1988;28:1032–1037.

514. Lindsey D. Controversy in snake bite: time for a controlled appraisal. *J Trauma* 1985;25:462–463.

515. Christopher DG, Rodning CB. Crotalidae envenomation. *South Med J* 1986;79:159–162.

516. Chippaux JP, Goyffon M. Venoms, antivenoms, and immunotherapy. *Toxicon* 1998;36:823–846.

517. Consroe P, Egen NB, Russell FE, et al. Comparison of a new ovine antigen binding fragment (Fab) antivenin for United States Crotalidae with the commercial antivenin for protection against venom-induced lethality in mice. *Am J Trop Med Hyg* 1995;53:507–510.

518. McCullough N, Gennaro J Jr. Treatment of venomous snake bites in the United States. *Clin Toxicol* 1970;3:483–500.

519. Wood J, Hoback W, Green T. Treatment of snake venom poisoning with ACTH and cortisone. *Va Med Monthly* 1955;82: 130–135.

520. Garfin SR, Castilonia RR, Mubarak SJ, et al. The effect of antivenin on intramuscular pressure elevations induced by rattlesnake venom. *Toxicon* 1985;23:677–680.

521. Curry S, Kraner J, Kunkel D, et al. Noninvasive vascular studies in management of rattlesnake envenomations to extremities. *Ann Emerg Med* 1985;14:1081–1084.

522. Russell F. Gila monster. In: Russell F, ed. *Snake venom poisoning.* Great Neck, NY: Scholium International, 1983: 395–419.

523. Hooker K, Caravati E, Hartsell S. Gila monster envenomation. *Ann Emerg Med* 1994;24:731–735.

524. Preston C. Hypotension, myocardial infarction, and coagulopathy following Gila monster bite. *J Emerg Med* 1989;7: 37–40.

525. Necrotic arachnidism—Pacific Northwest, 1988–1996. *MMWR Morb Mortal Wkly Rep* 1996;45:433–436.

526. Walker J, Hogan D. Bite to the left leg: clinical pearls. *Acad Emerg Med* 1995;2:223–237.

527. Russell F. A confusion of spiders. *Emerg Med* 1986;18:8–13.

528. Vetter R. Wounds other than brown recluse spider bites [Online]. December 1, 1998. Department of Entomology, UC Riverside. http://cnas.ucr.edu/enot/Spiders/necrotic.html.

529. Edlow J. Lyme disease and related tick-borne illnesses. *Ann Emerg Med* 1999;33:680–693.

530. Wilson DC, King LE Jr. Spiders and spider bites. *Dermatol Clin* 1990;8:277–286.

531. Wasserman G. Wound care of spider and snake envenomations. *Ann Emerg Med* 1988;17:1331–1335.

532. Futrell JM. Loxoscelism. *Am J Med Sci* 1992;304:261–267.

533. Patel KD, Modur V, Zimmerman GA, et al. The necrotic venom of the brown recluse spider induces dysregulated endothelial cell-dependent neutrophil activation: differential induction of GM-CSF, IL-8, and E-selectin expression. *J Clin Invest* 1994;94:631–642.

534. Ginsberg C, Weinberg A. Hemolytic anemia and mulitorgan failure associated with localized cutaneous lesion. *J Pediatr* 1988;112:496–499.

535. Pennell T, Babu S, Meredith J. The management of snake and spider bites in the southeastern United States. *Am Surg* 1987;53:198–204.

536. DeLozier J, Reaves L, King L, et al. Brown recluse spider bites of the upper extremity. *South Med J* 1988;81:181–184.

537. Hobbs G, Anderson A, Greene T, et al. Comparison of hyperbaric oxygen and dapsone therapy for *Loxosceles* envenomation. *Acad Emerg Med* 1996;3:758–761.

538. Barrett SM, Romine-Jenkins M, Fisher DE. Dapsone or electric shock therapy of brown recluse spider envenomation? *Ann Emerg Med* 1994;24:21–25.

539. Strain GM, Snider TG, Tedford BL, et al. Hyperbaric oxygen effects on brown recluse spider *(Loxosceles reclusa)* envenomation in rabbits. *Toxicon* 1991;29:989–996.

540. Phillips S, Kohn M, Baker D, et al. Therapy of brown spider envenomation: a controlled trial of hyperbaric oxygen, dapsone, and cyproheptadine. *Ann Emerg Med* 1995;25: 363–368.

541. Rees R, Altenbern D, Lynch J, et al. Brown recluse spider bites: a comparison of early surgical excision versus dapsone and delayed surgical excision. *Ann Surg* 1985;202:659–663.

542. Muller GJ. Black and brown widow spider bites in South Africa: a series of 45 cases. *S Afr Med J* 1993;83:399–405.

543. Clark RF, Wethern-Kestner S, Vance MV, et al. Clinical presentation and treatment of black widow spider envenomation: a review of 163 cases. *Ann Emerg Med* 1992;21:782–787.

544. Suntorntham S, Roberts J, Nilsen G. Dramatic clinical response to the delayed administration of black widow spider antivenin [Letter]. *Ann Emerg Med* 1994;24:1198–1199.

545. Freeman TM. Imported fire ants: the ants from hell! *Allergy Proc* 1994;15:11–15.

546. Reisman RE. Stinging insect allergy. *Med Clin North Am* 1992;76:883–894.

547. Schumacher M. Significance of Africanized bees for public health: a review. *Arch Intern Med* 1995;155:2038–2043.

548. Kolecki P. Delayed toxic reaction following massive bee envenomation. *Ann Emerg Med* 1999;33:114–116.

549. Stafford CT. Fire ant allergy. *Allergy Proc* 1992;13:11–16.

550. Bawaskar HS, Bawaskar PH. Cardiovascular manifestations of severe scorpion sting in India (review of 34 children). *Ann Trop Paediatr* 1991;11:381–387.

551. Yarom R. Scorpion venom: a tutorial review of its effects in man and experimental animals. *Clin Toxicol* 1970;3:561–569.

552. Dudin AA, Rambaud-Cousson A, Thalji A, et al. Scorpion sting in children in the Jerusalem area: a review of 54 cases. *Ann Trop Paediatr* 1991;11:217–223.

553. Sofer S, Shahak E, Gueron M. Scorpion envenomation and antivenom therapy. *J Pediatr* 1994;124:973–978.

554. Jurkovich G. Hypothermia in the trauma patient. *Adv Trauma* 1989;4:111–140.

555. Moss J. Accidental severe hypothermia. *Surg Gynecol Obstet* 1986;162:501–513.

556. Danzl D, Pozos R, Auerbach P, et al. Multicenter hypothermia survey. *Ann Emerg Med* 1987;16:1042–1055.

557. Brantigan C, Patton B. Clinical hypothermia, accidental hypothermia, and frostbite. In: Goldsmith H, ed. *Lewis' practice of surgery.*. New York: Harper & Row, 1978.

558. Trevino A, Razi B, Beller B. The characteristic electrocardiogram of accidental hypothermia. *Arch Intern Med* 1971;127: 470–473.

559. Ferguson N. Urban hypothermia. *Anaesthesia* 1985;40: 651–654.

560. Hauty MG, Esrig BC, Hill JG, et al. Prognostic factors in severe accidental hypothermia: experience from the Mt. Hood tragedy. *J Trauma* 1987;27:1107–1112.

561. Walpoth B, Walpoth-Aslan B, Mattle H, et al. Outcome of survivors of accidental deep hypothermia and circulatory arrest treated with extracorporeal blood warming. *N Engl J Med* 1997;337:1500–1505.

562. Cohen D, Cline J, Lepinski S, et al. Resuscitation of the hypothermic patient. *Am J Emerg Med* 1988;6:475–478.

563. Ledingham I, Mone J. Treatment of accidental hypothermia: a prospective clinical study. *BMJ* 1980;1:1102–1105.

564. Rahn H, Reeves R, Howell B. Hydrogen ion regulation, temperature, and evolution. *Am Rev Respir Dis* 1975;112:165–172.

565. Ream A, Reitz R, Silverberg G. Temperature correction of $PaCO_2$ and pH in estimating acid-base status: an example of emperor's new clothes? *Anesthesiology* 1982;56:41.

566. White F. A comparative physiologic approach to hypothermia. *J Thorac Cardiovasc Surg* 1982;82:821–831.

567. Hansen J, Sue D. Should blood gas measurements be corrected for the patient's temperature? [Letter]. *N Engl J Med* 1980;303:341.

568. Orlowski J, Erenberg G, Lüders H, et al. Hypothermia and barbiturate coma for refractory status epilepticus. *Crit Care Med* 1984;12:367–372.

569. Dobson JA, Burgess JJ. Resuscitation of severe hypothermia by extracorporeal rewarming in a child. *J Trauma* 1996;40: 483–485.

570. Schaller M, Fischer A, Perret C. Hyperkalemia: a prognostic factor during acute severe hypothermia. *JAMA* 1990;264: 1842–1845.

571. Moyer J, Morris GJ, DeBakey M. Effect on renal hemodynamics and excretion of water and electrolytes in dog and man. *Ann Surg* 1957;145:26.

572. Anderson M, Nielsen K. Renal function under experimental hypothermia in rabbits. *Acta Med Scand* 1955;151:191.

573. Curry D, Curry K. Hypothermia and insulin secretion. *Endocrinology* 1970;87:750–755.

574. Axelrod D, Bass D. Electrolytes and acid base balance in hypothermia. *Am J Physiol* 1956;186:31.

575. Haddix T, Pohlman T, Noel R, et al. Hypothermia inhibits human E-selectin transcription. *J Surg Res* 1996;64:176–182.

576. Iampietro P, Vaughan J, Goldman R, et al. Heat production from shivering. *J Appl Physiol* 1960;15:632–634.

577. Pozos R, Wittmers L. *The nature and treatment of hypothermia.* Minneapolis: University of Minnesota Press, 1983.

578. Flacke J, Flacke W. Frequent, insidious, and often serious. *Semin Anesth* 1983;2:183–196.

579. Zwischenberger J, Kirsh M, Dechert R, et al. Suppression of shivering decreases oxygen consumption and improves hemodynamic stability during postoperative rewarming. *Ann Thorac Surg* 1987;43:428–431.

580. Roe C, Goldberg M, Blair C, et al. The influence of body temperature on early postoperative oxygen consumption. *Surgery* 1966;60:85–92.

581. Gentilello L. Practical approaches to hypothermia. *Adv Trauma Crit Care* 1994:39–79.

582. Paton B. Accidental hypothermia. *Pharmacol Ther* 1983;22: 331–337.

583. Reuler J. Hypothermia: pathophysiology, clinical settings, and management. *Ann Intern Med* 1978;89:519–527.

584. Gregory J, Townsend M, Cloutier C, et al. Timing and incidence of hypothermia (T<36°C) in operated trauma patients. Presented at the AAST 50th Annual Meeting, 1990, Tucson, AZ.

585. Luna G, Maier R, Pavlin E, et al. Incidence and effect of hypothermia in seriously injured patients. *J Trauma* 1987;27: 1014–1018.

586. Jurkovich G, Greiser W, Luterman A, et al. Hypothermia in trauma victims: an ominous predictor of survival. *J Trauma* 1987;27:1019–1024.

587. Psarras P, Ivatury R, Rohman M, et al. Hypothermia in trauma: incidence and prognostic significance. Presented at the meeting of the Eastern Association Surg. Trauma, 1988, Longboat Key, FL.

588. Rutherford EJ, Fusco MA, Nunn CR, et al. Hypothermia in critically ill trauma patients. *Injury* 1998;29:605–608.

589. Gentilello L, Jurkovich G. Hypothermia in the penetrating trauma victim. In: Ivatury R, Cayten G, eds. *Textbook of penetrating trauma.* Baltimore: Williams & Wilkins, 1996: 995–1006.

590. Little R, Stoner H. Body temperature after accidental injury. *Br J Surg* 1981;68:221–224.

591. Hardy J, Randini I. Some physiologic aspects of surgical trauma. *Am Surg* 1952;136:345.

592. Blalock A, Mason M. A comparison of the effects of heat and those of cold in the prevention and treatment of shock. *Arch Surg* 1945;42:1054–1059.

593. Sori A, El-Assuooty A, Rush B, et al. The effect of temperature on survival in hemorrhagic shock. *Am Surg* 1987;53: 706–710.

594. Cornejo CJ, Kierney PC, Vedder NB, et al. Mild hypothermia during reperfusion reduces injury following ischemia of the rabbit ear. *Shock* 1998;9:116–120.

595. Jurkovich G, Pitt R, Curreri P, et al. Hypothermia prevents increased capillary permeability following ischemia-reperfusion injury. *J Surg Res* 1988;44:514–521.

596. Wright J, Kerr J, Valeri C, et al. Regional hypothermia protects against ischemia-reperfusion injury in isolated canine gracilis muscle. *J Trauma* 1988;28:1027–1031.

597. Fay T. Observations on generalized refrigeration in cases of severe cerebral trauma. *Assoc Res Nerv Ment Dis Proc* 1943; 24:611–619.

598. Milde LN. Clinical use of mild hypothermia for brain protection: a dream revisited. *J Neurosurg Anesthesiol* 1992;4: 211–215.

599. Marion DW, Penrod LE, Kelsey SF, et al. Treatment of traumatic brain injury with moderate hypothermia. *N Engl J Med* 1997;336:540–546.

600. Shiozaki T, Kato A, Taneda M, et al. Little benefit from mild hypothermia therapy for severely head injured patients with low intracranial pressure. *J Neurosurg* 1999;91:185–191.

601. Gentilello LM, Jurkovich GJ, Stark MS, et al. Is hypothermia in the victim of major trauma protective or harmful? A randomized, prospective study. *Ann Surg* 1997;226:439–447; discussion 447–449.

602. Bachmann F, McKenna, Cole E, et al. The hemostatic mechanism after open heart surgery: I. studies on plasma coagulation factors and fibrinolysis in 512 patients after extracorporeal circulation. *J Thorac Cardiovasc Surg* 1975;79:76–85.

603. Harker L, Malpass T, Branson H, et al. Mechanism of abnormal bleeding in patients undergoing cardiopulmonary bypass: acquired transient platelet dysfunction associated with selective alpha-granule release. *Blood* 1980;56:824–834.

604. Kattlove H, Alexander B. The effect of cold on platelets: 1. cold-induced platelet aggregation. *Blood* 1971;38:39–47.

605. Patt A, McCroskey B, Moore E. Hypothermia-induced coagulopathies in trauma. *Surg Clin North Am* 1988;68:775–789.

606. Valeri C, Feingold H, Cassidy G, et al. Hypothermia induced reversible platelet dysfunction. *Ann Surg* 1987;205:175–181.

607. Reed R, Bracey A, Hudson J, et al. Hypothermia and blood coagulation: dissociation between enzyme activity and clotting factor levels. *Circ Shock* 1990;32:141–152.

608. Gubler K, Gentilello L, Hassantash S, et al. The impact of hypothermia on dilutional coagulopathy. *J Trauma* 1994;36: 847–851.

609. Gentilello L, Jurkovich G, Moujaes S. Hypothermia and injury: thermodynamic principles of prevention and treatment. In: Levine B, ed. *Perspectives in surgery.* St. Louis: Quality Medical, 1991.

610. Sheaff C, Fildes J, Keogh P, et al. Safety of 65°C intravenous fluid for the treatment of hypothermia. *Am J Surg* 1996; 172:52–55.

611. Herron D, Grabowy R, Connolly R, et al. The limits of blood-warming: maximally heating blood with an inline microwave bloodwarmer. *J Trauma* 1997;43:219–228.

612. Fruehan A. Accidental hypothermia. *Arch Intern Med* 1960; 105:218–229.

613. Kugelberg J, Schuller H, Berg B. Treatment of accidental hypothermia. *Scand J Thorac Cardiovasc Surg* 1967;1:142–146.

614. Gentilello L, Cortes V, Moujaes S, et al. Continuous arteriovenous rewarming: experimental results and thermodynamic model simulation of treatment for hypothermia. *J Trauma* 1990;30:1436–1449.

615. Patton J, Doolittle W. Core rewarming by peritoneal dialysis following induced hypothermia in the dog. *J Appl Physiol* 1972;33:800–804.

616. Myers R, Britten J, Cowley R. Hypothermia: quantitative aspects of therapy. *J Am Coll Emerg Physicians* 1979;8:523–527.

617. Gentilello L, Moujaes S. Treatment of hypothermia in trauma victims: thermodynamic considerations. *J Intensive Care Med* 1995;10:5–13.

618. Britt LD, Dascombe WH, Rodriguez A. New horizons in management of hypothermia and frostbite injury. *Surg Clin North Am* 1991;71:345–370.

619. Jacob J, Weisman M, Rosenblatt S, et al. Chronic pernio: a historical perspective of cold-induced vascular disease. *Arch Intern Med* 1986;146:1589–1592.

620. Benchikhi H, Roujeau JC, Levent M, et al. Chilblains and Raynaud phenomenon are usually not a sign of hereditary protein C and S deficiencies. *Acta Derm Venereol* 1998;78: 351–352.

621. Auerbach P. Disorders due to physical and environmental agents. In: Mills J, et al., eds. *Current emergency diagnosis and treatment.* Los Altos, CA: Lange Medical, 1985.

622. Francis T, Golden FSC. Non-freezing cold injury: the pathogenesis. *J R Nav Med Serv* 1985;71:3–8.

623. Lloyd E. *Hypothermia and cold stress.* Rockville, MD: Aspen Publications, 1986:84–85.

624. Mills WJ Jr. Frostbite: a discussion of the problem and a review of the Alaskan experience. [1973 classical article.] *Alaska Med* 1993;35:28–49.

625. Urschel JD. Frostbite: predisposing factors and predictors of poor outcome. *J Trauma* 1990;30:340–342.

626. Dana H, Rex I, Samitz M. The hunting reaction. *Arch Dermatol* 1969;99:441.

627. Heggers J, Robson M, Weingarten M, et al. Experimental and clinical observations on frostbite. *Ann Emerg Med* 1987;16: 1056–1062.

628. Ozyazgan I, Tercan M, Melli M, et al. Eicosanoids and inflammatory cells in frostbitten tissue: prostacyclin, thromboxane, polymorphonuclear leukocytes, and mast cells. *Plast Reconstr Surg* 1998;101:1881–1886.

629. Bourne M, Piepkorn M, Clayton F, et al. Analysis of microvascular changes in frostbite injury. *J Surg Res* 1986;40: 26–35.

630. Mileski W, Raymond J, Winn R, et al. Inhibition of leukocyte adherence and aggregation for treatment of severe cold injury in rabbits. *J Appl Physiol* 1993;74:1432–1436.

631. Mills WJ Jr, Whaley R. Frostbite: experience with rapid rewarming and ultrasonic therapy: part I and II. [1960 classical article.] *Alaska Med* 1993;35:6–18.

632. Treatment of frostbite. *Med Lett* 1980;22:112–114.

633. Miller MB, Koltai PJ. Treatment of experimental frostbite with pentoxifylline and aloe vera cream. *Arch Otolaryngol Head Neck Surg* 1995;121:678–680.

634. Rakower S, Shahgoli S, Wong SL. Doppler ultrasound and digital plethysmography to determine the need for sympathetic blockade after frostbite. *J Trauma* 1978;18:713–718.

635. Bouwman D, Morrison S, Lucas C, et al. Early sympathetic blockade for frostbite—is it of value? *J Trauma* 1980;20: 744–749.

636. Purdue G, Hunt J. Cold injury: a collective review. *J Burn Care Rehabil* 1986;7:331–342.

637. Mundth E. Frostbite symposium. Presented at the Arctic Aero Medical Laboratory, 1964, Ft. Wainwright Laboratory, AK.

638. Edlich R, Chang D, Birk K, et al. Cold injuries: comprehensive therapy. 1989;15(9):13–21.

639. Mills W Jr. Comment and recapitulation. *Alaska Med* 1993; 35:69–87.

640. Mills W Jr. Summary of treatment of the cold injured patient: hypothermia. [1980 classical article.] *Alaska Med* 1993;35: 50–53.

641. Mehta RC, Wilson MA. Frostbite injury: prediction of tissue viability with triple-phase bone scanning. *Radiology* 1989; 170:511–514.

642. Barker JR, Haws MJ, Brown RE, et al. Magnetic resonance imaging of severe frostbite injuries. *Ann Plast Surg* 1997;38: 275–279.

643. Greenwald D, Cooper B, Gottlieb L. An algorithm for early aggressive treatment of frostbite with limb salvage directed by triple-phase scanning. *Plast Reconstr Surg* 1998;102: 1069–1074.

644. Rustin M, Newton J, Smith N, et al. The treatment of chilblains with nifedipine: the results of a pilot study, a double-blind placebo-controlled randomized study and a long-term open trial. *Br J Dermatol* 1989;120:267–275.

SURGERY: SCIENTIFIC PRINCIPLES AND PRACTICE, Third Edition, edited by
Lazar J. Greenfield, Michael W. Mulholland, Keith T. Oldham, Gerald B. Zelenock,
and Keith D. Lillemoe. Lippincott Williams & Wilkins Publishers, Philadelphia, © 2001.

CHAPTER 12

BURNS

ROBERT L. SHERIDAN AND RONALD G. TOMPKINS

Management of burn patients is a multifaceted challenge, requiring surgical, critical care, rehabilitative, and psychosocial skills. The prognosis of such patients has improved dramatically since the early 1980s, with most not only surviving but enjoying excellent functional and cosmetic outcomes. This chapter reviews the clinical management of serious burns and relates progress in this management to the growing understanding of the pathophysiology of burn injury.

MANAGEMENT PHILOSOPHY

The management philosophy provides a systematic approach to patients that includes the following:

Individualized resuscitation of virtually all patients regardless of injury severity (the exception being elderly patients with massive injuries for whom survival is highly unlikely and in whom the quality of survival is likely to be inconsistent with their own desires as expressed by health care proxy or close family members)
Early excision and biologic closure of deep wounds
Continuous rehabilitation
Judicious use of broad-spectrum antibiotics with early detection and specific treatment of septic foci
Intensive patient and family psychosocial support
Long-term follow-up with ongoing rehabilitative and reconstructive support

The acute hospitalization is organized into four phases: (a) initial evaluation and resuscitation, (b) initial wound excision and biologic closure, (c) definitive wound closure, and (d) intensification of the continuous rehabilitation effort. With this approach, regardless of injury size, survival with good quality of life can be expected for most burn patients who present without anoxic brain injury.

EPIDEMIOLOGY

Approximately 2 million Americans require medical attention each year for burn injuries. Children 6 months to 2 years of age (1) and elderly people (2) are at particular risk of sustaining burns in domestic cooking and bathing accidents. Young adults are more often injured in the workplace. Structural fires spare no age group. As in motor vehicle trauma, alcohol use frequently contributes to these injuries. Although the life-threatening nature of large injuries is often emphasized, the potentially devastating impact of poorly managed smaller burns should not be neglected (Fig. 12.1) (see color insert following page 1190). Extensive efforts have been made to diminish the incidence of pediatric burn injury through public education, but the effect is variable. For example, legislation that mandates lower temperatures for water heaters has been successful, leading to a decreased incidence of hot water injuries in children (3). Inconsistent application of these laws remains a problem. Approximately 15% of pediatric burn injuries

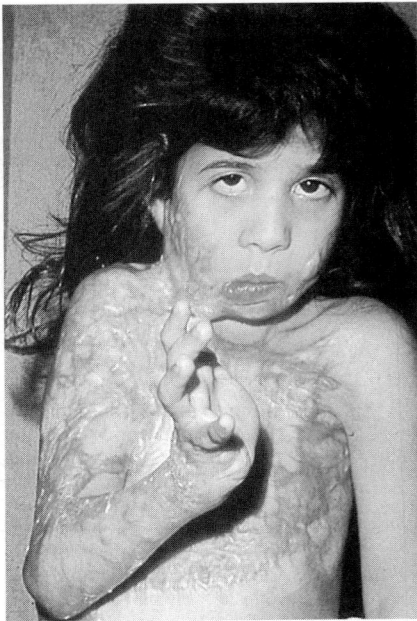

Figure 12.1. Suboptimal management of small burns can have major adverse functional and cosmetic implications.

are attributed to abuse or neglect, and an awareness of this important issue facilitates the prevention of repeated injuries (4).

Predicting mortality is difficult in burned patients. In one statistical evaluation, age over 60 years, full-thickness burn size over 40% of the total body surface area (TBSA), and the presence of inhalation injury were found to be important prognostic factors (5). In the past, age younger than 4 years was reported to be a negative predictor of survival (6,7). However, in a more recent report of over 1,000 children managed over a 7-year period, there was no mortality in any child younger than 4 years of age and no mortality in any child with a burn covering less than 60% of TBSA (8).

NATURAL HISTORY

A skin envelope played a crucial role in allowing aquatic sea animals to adapt to the land environment. Our survival as individuals continues to depend on the vapor and bacterial barriers provided by normal skin. The epidermal layer provides these two essential functions, and the dermis provides flexibility and strength (Fig. 12.2). In addition, dermal appendages prevent desiccation of the skin by producing oils, and the reactive dermal microvasculature is responsible for heat dissipation and conservation, allowing humans to adapt to changes in environmental temperature. These important functions are compromised or lost when substantial areas of the skin are burned. An understanding of the natural history of any disease process facilitates an understanding of the success of intervention. This natural history is examined here at the level of the local tissue and the whole organism.

Local Response to Burn Injury

The local response to thermal injury is principally related to destruction and thrombosis of blood vessels in the dermis. Of particular interest are the microvascular reactions in the surrounding dermis, where progressive vaso-

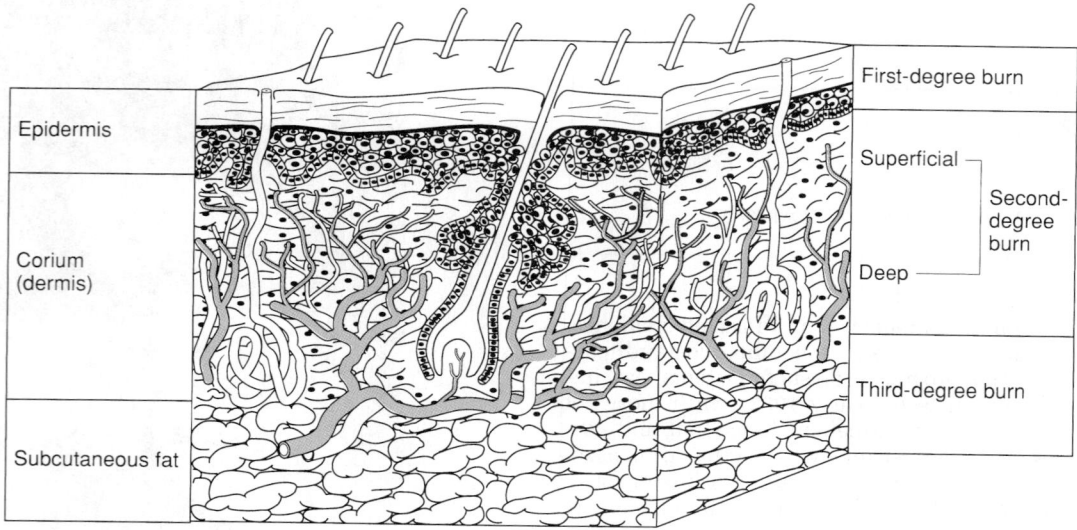

Figure 12.2. Schematic depiction of skin.

constriction and thrombosis are seen to a degree that varies in accordance with the severity of the primary injury (9). In animal models, the secondary injury that follows these microvascular changes is truncated by cyclooxygenase inhibitors (10), lazaroids (11), and fibrinogen depletion (12). These observations suggest possible future therapeutic interventions to minimize secondary injury.

Systemic Response to Burn Injury

The systemic response to cutaneous thermal injury is driven by the loss of the skin's barrier functions. This results in accelerated fluid losses, decreased host resistance to infection, release of mediators from the injured tissue with microvascular and end-organ dysfunction, and bacterial overgrowth in the eschar, resulting in systemic infection. Edema in tissue immediately surrounding the burn occurs secondary to local release of vasoactive mediators, such as prostaglandins, thromboxane A_2, and reactive oxygen radicals. When burn size exceeds 20% or 30% of TBSA, clinically significant interstitial edema is seen in distant soft tissues secondary to a combination of mediators generated in the wound and hypoproteinemia. Distant microvascular injury may interfere with the function of organ systems not directly injured by the burning process (13), thus explaining the frequent occurrence of pulmonary and other end-organ dysfunction in patients with large burns (14). Although exciting work is underway that may ultimately lead to clinically useful modifications of these mediator effects (15), our understanding of these processes is as yet inadequate to allow intelligent intervention.

A burn wound is initially clean but is rapidly colonized by endogenous bacteria. As these bacteria multiply in the avascular eschar over succeeding days, proteases liquefy the eschar, which then separates, leaving a bed of granulation tissue or healing burn, depending on the depth of the original injury. If wounds are small, less than 20% of TBSA, this local infectious challenge is usually well tolerated. When injuries are larger, however, systemic infection frequently results, explaining the rare survival of patients with burns in excess of 40% of TBSA when the wound is managed in this expectant fashion (16).

The physiologic challenge of a burn in excess of 20% of TBSA frequently results in an initial decrease in cardiac output and metabolic rate. Subsequently, a hypermetabolic response is seen, with a near doubling of cardiac output and resting energy expenditure over the next 24 to 48 hours in those who are successfully resuscitated. The magnitude of this response peaks with injuries of 60% or more of TBSA when the metabolic rate is more than double resting values. Enhanced gluconeogenesis, relative insulin resistance, and increased protein catabolism associated with this response have major clinical implications for the support of burn patients. The etiology of the hypermetabolic response is not entirely understood but is assumed to involve a combination of the following and perhaps other factors:

- Change in hypothalamic function with coincident increases in glucagon, cortisol, and catecholamine secretion (17)
- Deficient gastrointestinal barrier function with translocation of bacteria and their by-products (18)
- Bacterial contamination of the burn wound with systemic release of similar products from this source (19,20)
- Some element of enhanced heat loss through evaporation of fluid across the eschar (21)

The hypermetabolic response probably has survival value because it is conserved so broadly over numerous species. An important element of successful treatment of patients who have sustained large injuries is to support this response through the provision of adequate quantity and quality of substrate.

Although limited modifications of the hypermetabolic response in the form of antipyretics have been widely practiced, elimination of this response is of unknown value and may be harmful. The growing number of recombinant protein products capable of affecting the cascade of inflammatory mediators, along with our fledgling understanding to the process, has led to a plethora of laboratory and clinical projects aimed at determining whether seemingly adverse facets of the hypermetabolic response, such as the excessive protein catabolism, can be obviated without harming the patient. Data are still inadequate to support such therapies outside of clinical trials.

INITIAL EVALUATION

Meaningful survival can be expected even in the most severe injuries, so the approach to burn patients is aggressive. An organized approach to serious injuries facilitates the achievement of optimal outcome and begins with a systematic initial evaluation that includes a primary survey, effective vascular and airway access, and a systematic secondary survey (22,23).

Systematic Initial Evaluation

Many burn patients sustain concurrent injuries, and the initial evaluation should therefore be approached as for any victim of multiple trauma. After the airway is evaluated and secured while the cervical spine is controlled, breathing mechanics are assessed, a rough estimate is made of the circulating blood volume, the level of consciousness is documented, and the patient is completely exposed. This should be done in a warm environment to avoid hypothermia. Secure airway and vascular access is crucial and should be obtained early during the evaluation. A badly burned face precludes tape in securing the endotracheal tube; an umbilical tie harness should be used instead (Fig. 12.3) (see color insert following page 1190). Secure venous access is best obtained centrally, although two peripheral intravenous lines are a reasonable option. In hypovolemic children, intraosseous resuscitation can be lifesaving (Fig. 12.4) (see color insert following page 1190), but it should be promptly replaced with venous cannulae as soon as practical. All patients should have a nasogastric tube placed, particularly if they are to be transported by air, because a gas-filled stomach can lead to emesis and aspiration (Fig. 12.5). A bladder catheter facilitates smooth fluid resuscitation. Continuous temperature monitoring with rectal or esophageal probes and arterial access is helpful in selected patients.

The burn-specific secondary survey (Table 12.1) includes a complete history, vital signs, a detailed physical examination, and laboratory and radiographic studies appropriate for the mechanism of injury. The history, particularly details about the mechanism of injury, is important and is ideally obtained from witnesses, rescue personnel, and family members. The mechanism of injury often determines the need for special studies, such as computed tomography (CT) of the head and abdomen or radiography of the cervical spine. Other important historical points include medical and surgical history, time of the last meal, tetanus status, medications and allergies, water temperature in hot-liquid injuries, and extrication time in closed-space injuries. Vital signs are determined during the secondary survey, and age-specific norms should be known (Table 12.2). A complete physical examination should proceed in an organized fashion; the presence of the burn should not distract the examiner from performing a complete assessment.

The patient's neurologic status should be carefully documented early in the evaluation because many patients become progressively obtunded secondary to the administration of analgesics and sedatives and as the result of intravascular volume depletion. If injury mechanism is consistent with a head injury, CT should be performed.

Trauma to the head, face, and neck is determined by inspection and palpation. The corneal epithelium and globes should be examined before the development of adnexal edema, which makes examination more difficult. Major corneal epithelial burns are obvious by the resulting opaque appearance of the cornea. More subtle defects are apparent after staining with topical fluorescein. Upper airway injuries are suspected in the presence of a hoarse voice, burns of the lips or tongue, singed facial hair and nasal vibrissae, or carbonaceous sputum. Hot liquid aspiration may complicate facial scald burns in small children and should be suspected if there is blistering in or around the mouth. If upper airway compromise is imminent, endotracheal intubation is mandatory, particularly before the initiation of long transports. Verification of endotracheal tube security is an important part of the head and neck examination.

The torso should be assessed for compliance, and if ventilation is restricted by overlying circumferential eschar, torso escharotomies should be performed promptly with coagulating electrocautery to minimize blood loss. Incisions are typically made axially along the flanks and are connected by one or more horizontal incisions (Fig. 12.6). The abdomen should be assessed for tenderness or distention. If the mechanism of injury suggests an abdominal injury, CT or peritoneal lavage is appropriate, particularly in the presence of an inappropriately high resuscitative volume requirement. Gastric distention is particularly common in distressed children, and nasogastric decompression is routinely recommended during the initial evaluation and transport. Proper nasogastric tube function should be verified regularly. All burned patients should receive immediate stress ulcer prophylaxis with intraluminal antacids and intravenous histamine receptor blockers because the incidence of stress ulceration is unacceptably high if this precaution is not taken. The presence of genital burns should be noted. If the patient is not circumcised, the foreskin should be reduced after placement of the bladder catheter to avoid paraphimosis secondary to progressive edema.

Regular assessment and documentation of peripheral perfusion is crucial during the first days after injury. Blood flow can be compromised by constricting circumferential eschar as subeschar tissues become progressively edematous or by progressive intracompartmental edema in patients with electrical or deep thermal burns. Both are detected by the development of a progressive increase in the

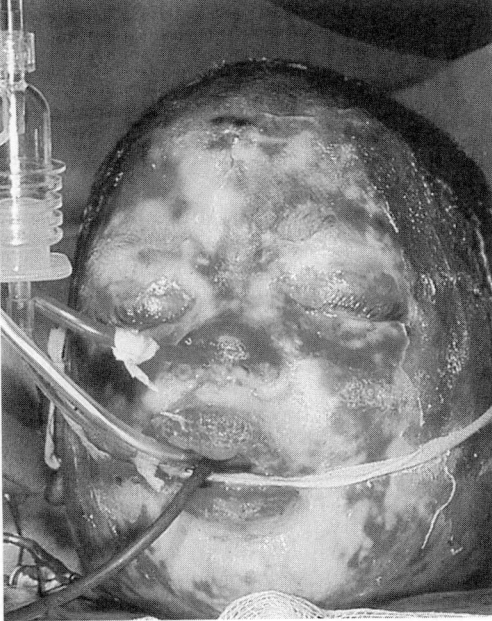

Figure 12.3. Endotracheal tube security is of the utmost importance during the first few postburn days, because airway edema can result in significant difficulty when one is attempting to reinsert displaced endotracheal tubes. Secure airway control is facilitated by the use of umbilical ties, rather than adhesive tape, to anchor endotracheal tubes.

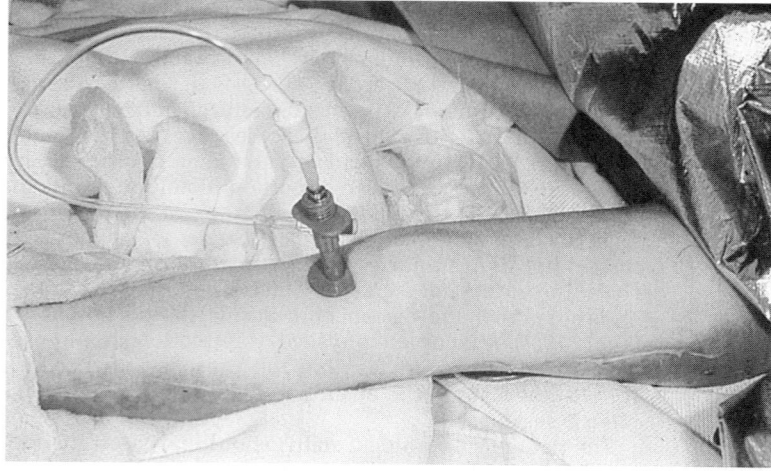

Figure 12.4. Intraosseous infusion can be life-saving in children in whom vascular access cannot be promptly achieved.

extremity's consistency and a decrease in its distal temperature. Pulsatile Doppler signals in the lower pressure distal vasculature, such as the palmar arch and digital vessels, should be documented hourly; their loss is consistent with increasing tissue pressure if intravascular volume is adequate. Constricting circumferential eschar can be opened at the bedside using coagulating electrocautery. This is most commonly done using medial and lateral axial incisions with the patient lightly sedated. It is im-

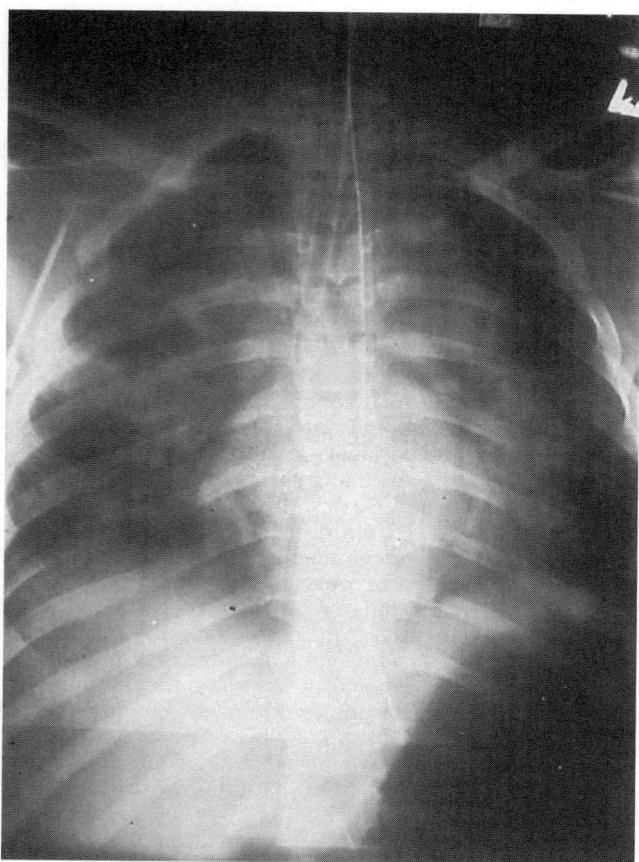

Figure 12.5. Nasogastric tube function, as well as physical presence, must be regularly verified to minimize the possibility of gastric distention and subsequent aspiration during burn resuscitation. Both of these potential problems are shown in this radiograph of a burn patient.

portant to maintain hemostasis during the procedure and to verify that distal blood flow has been enhanced. Particularly in young children, hand escharotomies often are not required once the proximal upper extremity has been adequately decompressed (24). If decompression of the arm to the level of the metacarpophalangeal joints has not resulted in adequate digital blood flow, axial digital incisions are made between the extensor tendons and the neurovascular bundles. Ideally, a single incision on the radial aspect of the thumb and the ulnar aspect of the digits suffices. The incisions on the central digits of the hand can be extended proximally between the extensors.

Weakness of intracompartmental muscle groups or pain with their passive stretch supports the suspicion of elevated intracompartmental pressures, although such signs can be obscured in many burn patients. It can be exceptionally difficult to diagnose an evolving compartment syndrome in acutely burned patients, and the clinician should decompress such extremities based on clinical suspicion (25). Compartment pressure measurements can be a useful adjunct in equivocal situations, but clinical judgment suffices in most cases. If missed, compartment syndromes lead to intracompartmental sepsis or functional deficits later in the patient's course.

Evaluation of the wound is deferred until higher-priority evaluations are complete. Important to the initial evaluation is an assessment of the wound depth, size, and circumferential components. Early burn depth estimates are accurate in very deep or very superficial wounds. Many burns, however, particularly scald injuries, are of indeterminate depth on initial examination. Significant effort has been applied to develop technical aids that accurately gauge burn wound depth during the initial evaluation (26), but none of these aids has had routine clinical success. Fortunately, an accurate determination of depth is not necessary to proceed with initial wound management or fluid resuscitation. In contrast, an accurate assessment of burn size can be made early and is important to initial management because resuscitative fluid administration is determined primarily by overall burn size. Burn size in children is best estimated with an age-specific chart (Fig. 12.7) because the body's proportions change with growth. The major anthropometric change involves the head and legs. The infant head represents 18% and the legs 14% of TBSA. In older adolescents and adults, the head represents 9% and the legs 18% of TBSA. Scattered wounds can be estimated knowing that the palm of the hand represents 0.5% of TBSA over a broad range of ages (27). It is important to identify circumferential components of the

Table 12.1. IMPORTANT ASPECTS OF THE BURN-SPECIFIC SECONDARY SURVEY

History
Closed-space exposure
Extrication time
Delay in seeking attention
Fluid given during transport
Previous illnesses and injuries

Head, eyes, ears, nose, and throat
The globes should be examined and corneal epithelium stained with fluorescein before adnexal swelling makes examination difficult. Adnexal swelling provides excellent coverage and protection during the first days after injury. Tarsorrhaphy is virtually never indicated acutely.
Corneal epithelial loss can be overt, giving a clouded appearance to the cornea, but it is more often subtle, requiring fluorescein staining for documentation. Topical ophthalmic antibiotics constitute optimal initial treatment.
Signs of airway involvement include perioral and intraoral burns or carbonaceous material and progressive hoarseness.
Hot liquid can be aspirated with a facial scald injury and result in acute airway compromise requiring urgent intubation.
Endotracheal tube security is crucial and is best maintained with an umbilical tape harness, rather than adhesive tape, on the burned face.

Neck
The radiographic evaluation is driven by the mechanism of injury.
Neck escharotomies are rarely needed to facilitate venous drainage of the head.

Cardiac
Cardiac rhythm should be monitored for 24 to 72 h in electrical injury.
Elderly patients may experience transient atrial fibrillation if modestly overresuscitated.
Significant arrhythmias are unusual if intravascular volume and oxygenation are adequately supported.
History of myocardial infarction increases the risk of new infarct with the stress of burn injury, and appropriate monitoring is necessary.

Pulmonary
Inflating pressures should be kept below 40 cm H_2O by the performance of chest escharotomies when needed.
Severe inhalation injury may lead to slough of endobronchial mucosa and thick endobronchial secretions. Sudden endotracheal tube occlusions may occur.

Vascular
Burned extremities should be vigilantly monitored by serial examinations. Indications for escharotomy include decreasing temperature, increasing consistency, slowed capillary refill, and diminished Doppler flow in the digital vessels. The clinician should not wait until flow in named vessels is compromised to decompress the extremity.
Fasciotomy is indicated after electrical or deep thermal injury when distal flow is compromised.
Compartment pressure measurement can be helpful, but clinical examination is an indication for decompression regardless of compartment pressure readings.

Abdomen
Nasogastric tubes should be placed and their function verified, particularly, before air transport in unpressurized helicopters.
An inappropriate resuscitative volume requirement may be a sign of an occult intraabdominal injury.
Torso escharotomies may be required to facilitate ventilation of deep circumferential abdominal wall burns.
Immediate stress ulcer prophylaxis with histamine receptor blockers and antacids is indicated with serious burns.

Genitourinary
Bladder catheterization is appropriate in all who require fluid resuscitation and urine output monitoring.
The foreskin should be reduced over the bladder catheter after insertion because progressive swelling may otherwise result in paraphimosis.

Neurologic
Early neurologic evaluation is important because the sensorium is altered by medication or hemodynamic instability during the hours after injury. Computed tomographic scanning is appropriate, if possible, for head trauma.
Patients who require neuromuscular blockade for transport should also receive adequate sedation and analgesia.

Extremities
Extremities with circumferential thermal burns or electrical injury should be promptly decompressed by escharotomy or fasciotomy when clinical examination reveals diminished distal perfusion. Limbs at risk should be dressed so they can be frequently examined.
The need for escharotomy usually becomes evident during the early resuscitation. Most escharotomies can be delayed until transport has been effected if this is less than 6 h.
Burned extremities should be elevated and splinted in a position of function.

Wounds
Wounds are often underestimated in depth and overestimated in size on initial examination.
Size, depth, and the presence of circumferential components are important issues.

Laboratory tests
Arterial blood gas analysis is important when airway compromise or inhalation injury is present.
Normal carboxyhemoglobin concentration on admission does not eliminate the possibility of a significant exposure because the half-life of carboxyhemoglobin is 30 to 40 min in those effectively ventilated with 100% oxygen.
Baseline hemoglobin and electroytes can be helpful later during resuscitation.
Urinalysis for occult blood should be performed with deep thermal or electrical injuries.

Radiographic evaluations
Radiographic evaluation is driven by the mechanism of injury and the need to document placement of supportive cannulae.

Electrical burns
Cardiac rhythm should be monitored in high- (>1,000 V) or intermediate- (>220 V) voltage exposures for 24 to 72 h.
Low- and intermediate-voltage exposures can cause locally destructive injuries but uncommonly result in systemic sequelae.
After high-voltage exposures, delayed neurologic and ocular sequelae can occur, so a carefully documented admission examination is important.
Injured extremities should be serially evaluated for intracompartmental edema and promptly decompressed when necessary.
Bladder catheters are required for high-voltage exposure to assess the possibility of pigmenturia.
This is treated adequately with volume loading in most patients.

Chemical burns
Wounds should be irrigated with tap water for at least 30 minutes. The globe is irrigated with isotonic crystalloid solution.
Blepharospasm may require ocular anesthetic administration.
Exposure to hydrofluoric acid may be complicated by life-threatening hypocalcemia, particularly after exposures to concentrated or anhydrous solutions. Close monitoring and supplementation of serum calcium is necessary. Subeschar injection of 10% calcium gluconate solution is appropriate after exposure to highly concentrated or anhydrous solutions.

Tar burns
Tar should be initially cooled with tap water irrigation, then removed with a lipophilic solvent.

Table 12.2. AGE-SPECIFIC RESUSCITATION END POINTS

Evaluation	Target
Sensorium	Comfortable, arousable
Urine output	
Infants	1–2 mL/kg/h
Children	0.5–1 mL/kg/h
All others	0.5 mL/kg/h
Base deficit	<2 mEq/dL
Systolic blood pressure	
Infants	60–70 mm Hg
Children	70–90 + (twice age in years) mm Hg
Adolescents and adults	90–120 mm Hg

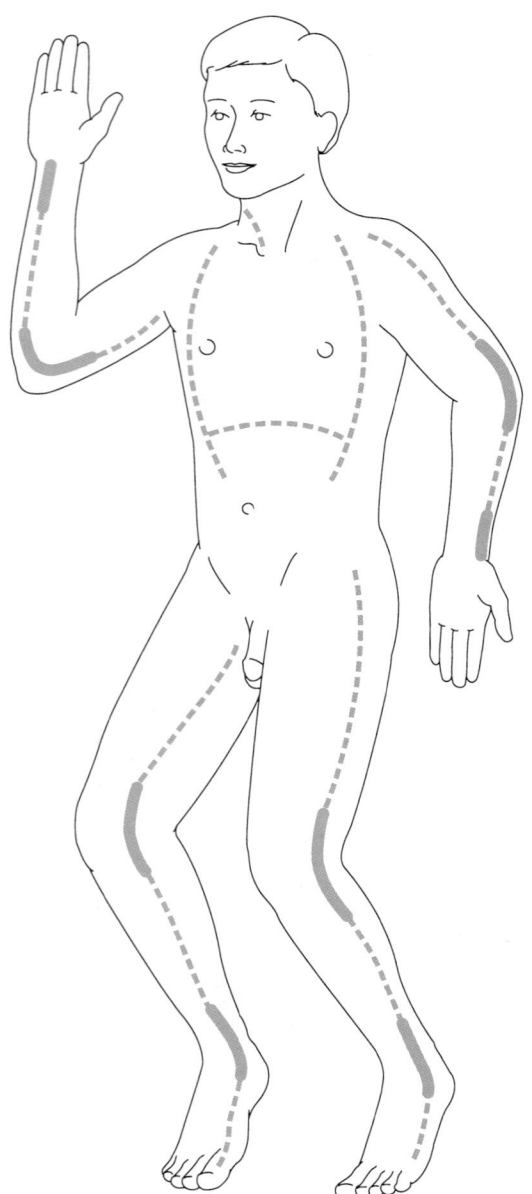

Figure 12.6. Preferred sites of escharotomy. Connecting lateral axial incisions across the midline facilitates ventilation with low inflating pressures. Extremity escharotomies are performed using medial and lateral axial incisions.

wound because these areas need to be closely monitored for compromise of peripheral perfusion in extremity or neck burns and ventilation in torso injuries. It is worthwhile to calculate both burned and unburned areas. Because the sum must equal 100%, mistaken estimates of burn wound size can be avoided easily.

Relatively few laboratory studies are essential during the initial evaluation. Patients with a history of exposure to noxious fumes should have the arterial PaO_2, $PaCO_2$, pH, and carboxyhemoglobin percentage determined. Because the half-life of carboxyhemoglobin is 30 to 45 minutes when patients are ventilated with high concentrations of oxygen, however, a normal carboxyhemoglobin of less than 5% does not preclude significant exposure when patients have been appropriately ventilated during transport. Patients with electrical or deep thermal injuries often require blood products during the initial resuscitation; a blood bank specimen should be sent routinely in such patients. Routine hematology and chemistry profiles are of limited usefulness initially, but a baseline should be established. Urinalysis for occult blood is helpful in patients with electrical or deep thermal burns if gross pigmenturia has been cleared with crystalloid administration. Radiographic evaluation during the initial evaluation is determined largely by the mechanism of injury and the need to evaluate placement of resuscitative cannulae.

The initial evaluation of patients with electrical, chemical, tar, or abuse-related injuries is generally the same as for patients with thermal injuries; a few unique aspects require emphasis, however. Burn units are often called on to manage nonburn diagnoses that require complex wound and critical care resources, such as purpura fulminans, toxic epidermal necrolysis, staphylococcal scalded skin syndrome, or major soft tissue avulsions. Such patients benefit from the unique combination of critical care and surgical resources available in burn units (28). Special aspects of evaluation of patients with purpura fulminans, toxic epidermal necrolysis, and staphylococcal scalded skin syndrome are presented in Table 12.3 and Fig. 12.8 (see color insert following page 1190).

Electrical Injuries

Although lesser voltages can cause locally destructive injuries without systemic sequelae (Fig. 12.9) (see color insert following page 1190), high voltage (>1,000 V) can cause a combination of deep-tissue injury secondary to the passage of current, locally destructive entrance and exit wounds, deep wounds where current arches across flexed joints, flame burns secondary to clothing ignition, flash burns, axial spine fractures secondary to tetanic contraction of paravertebral muscles, and other injuries related to the fall or blast that so commonly accompanies high-voltage injury. Patients with burns caused by exposure to high-voltage electricity require a complete trauma evaluation, cardiac monitoring, bladder catheterization to evaluate the urine for pigment, serial monitoring of compartments at risk for pressure elevation, and spine immobilization pending radiographic examination of the axial spine. Compartment pressure elevation, secondary to edema of injured muscle, can result in additional ischemic injury if compartments are not promptly released (Fig. 12.10) (see color insert following page 1190).

Chemical Injuries

Patients who sustain chemical burns (Fig. 12.11) (see color insert following page 1190) are first treated with at least 30 minutes of copious tap water irrigation. Ocular injuries are irrigated with saline. Topical ophthalmic anes-

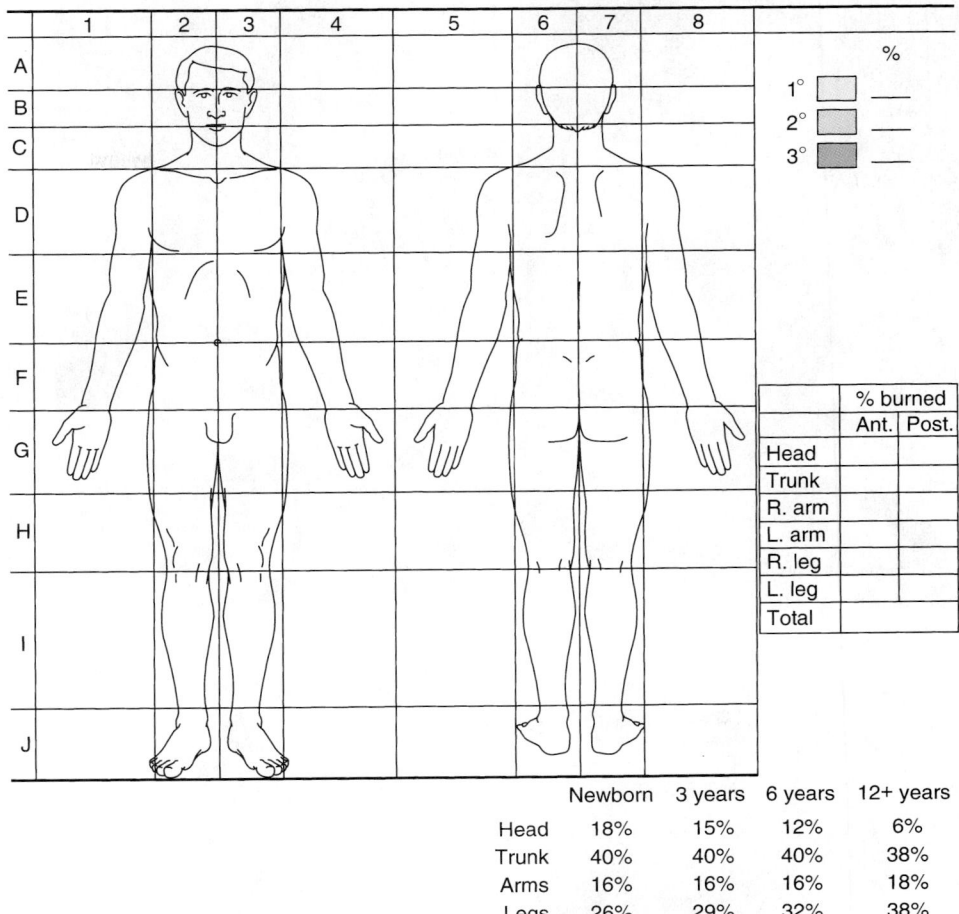

		Newborn	3 years	6 years	12+ years
	Head	18%	15%	12%	6%
	Trunk	40%	40%	40%	38%
	Arms	16%	16%	16%	18%
	Legs	26%	29%	32%	38%

	% burned	
	Ant.	Post.
Head		
Trunk		
R. arm		
L. arm		
R. leg		
L. leg		
Total		

Figure 12.7. An age-specific chart facilitates accurate estimation of burn size over a broad range of ages.

thetics facilitate relief of the blepharospasm that often interferes with effective irrigation of the globe. Patients exposed to concentrated hydrofluoric acid may experience life-threatening hypocalcemia (29). This should be anticipated and managed with subeschar injection of 10% calcium gluconate with monitoring and support of the serum ionized calcium before urgent excision of selected extensive wounds. The more common limited exposures to dilute hydrofluoric acid are managed with irrigation and topical calcium gluconate gel.

Tar Injuries

Tar is often heated to more than 300°F, and contact commonly causes a deep burn. Adherent tar is initially cooled by tap water irrigation to limit the progression of the injury and is later removed with a lipophilic solvent (Fig. 12.12) (see color insert following page 1190). After initial irrigation, chemical and tar burns are managed surgically as indicated by depth, which is frequently underestimated on initial examination.

Table 12.3. KEY ASPECTS OF THE DIAGNOSIS OF PURPURA FULMINANS, TOXIC EPIDERMAL NECROLYSIS, AND STAPHYLOCOCCAL SCALDED SKIN SYNDROME

Purpura fulminans
It is typically a complication of meningococcal sepsis.
It is likely a consequence of transient protein C deficiency; therefore, fresh frozen plasma should be considered as a resuscitative colloid.
It is frequently accompanied by organ failure.
Treatment involves management of organ failures and excision and grafting of wounds.

Toxic epidermal necrolysis
A variant of erythema multiforme major, toxic epidermal necrolysis is an epidermal slough at the dermal–epidermal junction.
The degree of mucous membrane and conjunctival involvement varies, and when severe is usually called Stevens-Johnson syndrome.
Differentiation from staphylococcal scalded skin syndrome can be difficult on clinical grounds, and in such cases, skin biopsy is diagnostic. Treatment involves prevention of wound desiccation

and superinfection with topical antimicrobials and xenografting of confluent areas of slough while awaiting healing.
Ophthalmologic evaluation is important to prevent synechiae. Those with severe oropharyngeal involvement may require intubation for airway protection and enteral tube feeding for nutritional support.

Staphylococcal scalded skin syndrome
Staphylococcal scalded skin syndrome is a reaction to a staphylococcal toxin that causes a separation at the granular layer of the epidermis. This superficial wound usually heals quickly if superinfection and desiccation are prevented.
Involvement of the mucous membrane and conjunctiva is not seen, which is a helpful diagnostic point for separating staphylococcal scalded skin syndrome from toxic epidermal necrolysis.
A detailed search for a focus of staphylococcal infection is warranted while empiric antistaphylococcal antibiotics are administered.

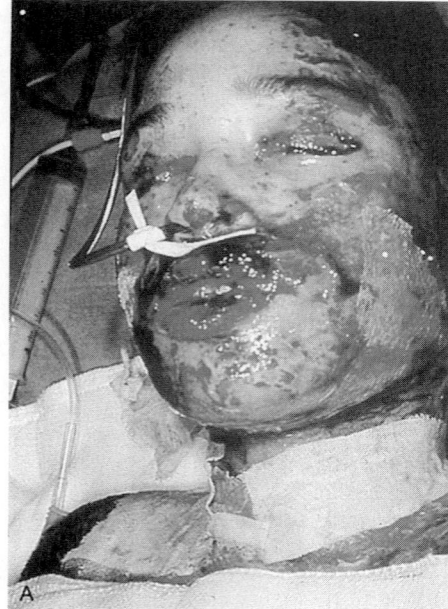
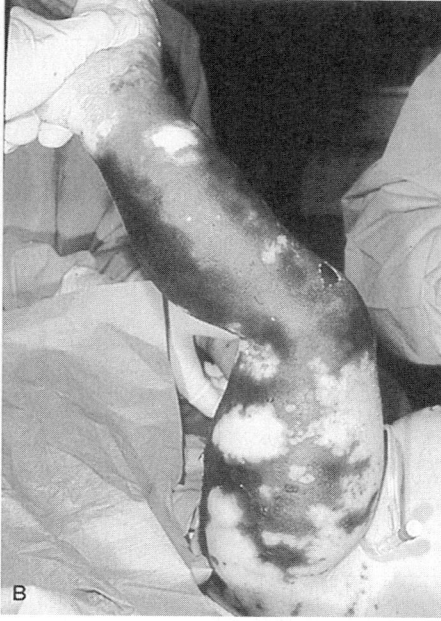

Figure. 12.8. *(A)* Toxic epidermal necrolysis is a severe variant of erythema multiform. When there is major mucous membrane involvement, as in this patient, it is described as Stevens-Johnson syndrome. *(B)* Purpura fulminans describes a syndrome in which extensive soft tissue necrosis results from transient protein C or protein S deficiency complicating meningococcal sepsis.

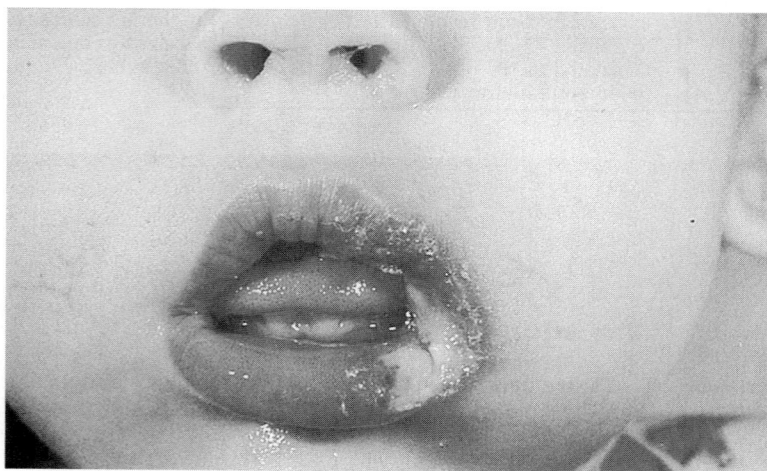

Figure 12.9. Low- and intermediate-voltage injuries can be locally destructive, as in this child who suffered a 110-volt commissure burn to the mouth by biting the cord of an electrical appliance. These injuries are rarely associated with serious systemic sequelae.

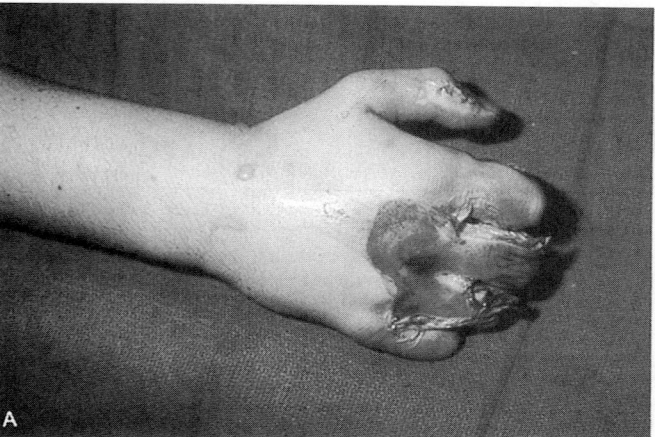
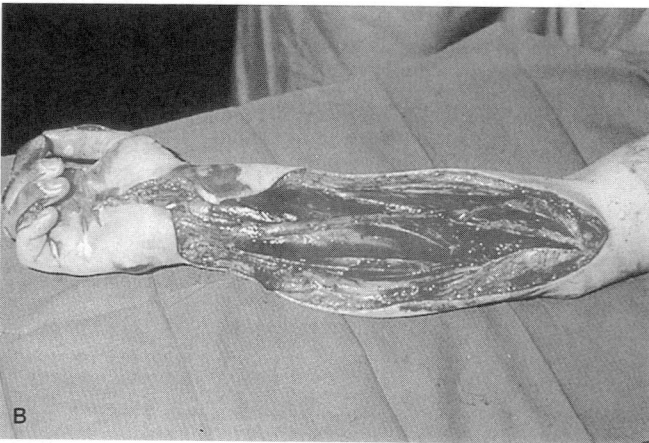

Figure 12.10. *(A)* This patient made contact with a 20,000-volt power line, resulting in a locally destructive entrance wound and occult muscle injury in the proximal extremity, leading to a compartment syndrome. *(B)* Prompt fasciotomy of the forearm and hand prevented the development of an additional ischemic injury secondary to high intracompartmental pressures.

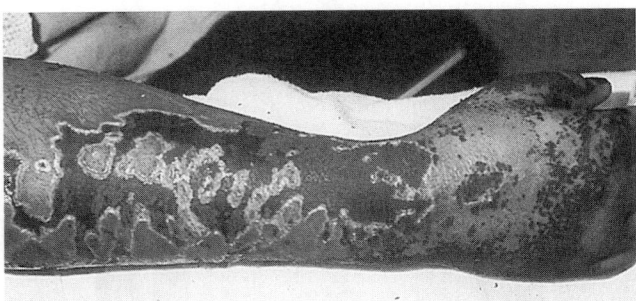

Figure 12.11. Chemical burns are often deeper than they appear on initial examination, as in this patient who suffered a sulfuric acid splash injury. Copious irrigation remains the mainstay of initial therapy.

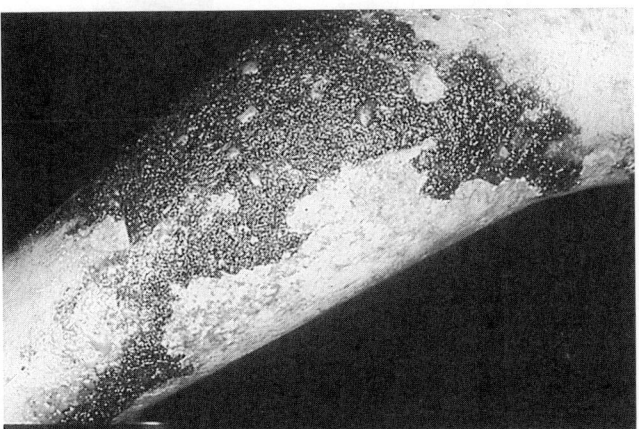

Figure 12.12. Tar burns are managed with initial cooling irrigation followed by later tar removal. In this patient, residual tar is being removed after softening in a lipophyllic solvent. Such burns are usually deep and generally require resurfacing.

Injuries of Abuse

All burned children should be evaluated for abuse or neglect. It is an ethical and legal mandate that suspect injuries be filed with the appropriate local agency (30). Table 12.4 lists important historical points and characteristics of the burn wound that can indicate the burn was caused by abuse, and Fig. 12.13 (see color insert following page 1190) is an example of this type of injury. All such children should be admitted to the hospital regardless of burn size.

Table 12.4. IMPORTANT POINTS OF HISTORY AND PHYSICAL EXAMINATION THAT SUGGEST ABUSE OR NEGLECT

History
Delayed presentation for medical care
Conflicting histories
Previous injuries

Suspect burn patterns
Sharply demarcated margins
Uniform depth
Absence of splash marks
Stocking or glove patterns
Flexor sparing
Porcelain contact sparing
Dorsal location of contact injury of the hands
Very deep localized contact injury

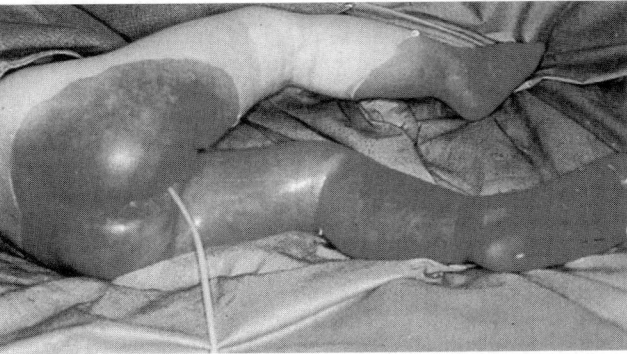

Figure 12.13. This child's wound is consistent with an intentional immersion in scalding water, demonstrating both flexor sparing and sharply defined margins around a deep burn of uniform depth.

Radiographic screening of the head and long bones should be considered for further documentation of possible abuse.

FLUID RESUSCITATION

The large number of fluid resuscitation formulas in common use is a tribute to the fact that no one formula accurately predicts fluid requirements in every patient. No formula can replace a physician at the bedside repeatedly evaluating the patient's physiologic response throughout the resuscitative period. Common controversies in fluid resuscitation relate to the role of colloid, the differences between children and adults, and the influence of inhalation injury and delayed resuscitation on fluid requirements. A reasonable consensus is represented by the Modified Brooke formula (Table 12.5), which serves as the basis for this discussion. Regardless of the formula chosen to initiate resuscitation, subsequent fluid administration is best guided by regular reassessment of resuscitation end points rather than by a formulaic prediction.

Vasoactive mediators released from injured tissue result in a diffuse capillary leak seen shortly after a major burn injury. This loss of microvascular integrity results in the extravasation of crystalloid and colloid solutions for the

Table 12.5. MODIFIED BROOKE FORMULA

First 24 hours
Adults and children >10 kg
   Lactated Ringer's solution: 2–4 mL/kg/% burn/24 h
    (first half in first 8 h)
   Colloid: none

Children <10 kg
   Lactated Ringer's solution: 2–3 mL/kg/% burn/24 h
    (first half in first 8 h)
   Lactated Ringer's solution with 5% dextrose: 4 mL/kg/h
   Colloid: none

Second 24 hours
All patients
   Crystalloid: to maintain urine output. If silver nitrate is used, sodium leeching mandates continued isotonic crystalloid. If a nonaqueous topical solution is used, free water requirement is significant. Serum sodium should be monitored closely. Nutritional support should begin, ideally by the enteral route.
   Colloid (5% albumin in lactated Ringer's solution)
   • 0%–30% burn: none
   • 30%–50% burn: 0.3 mL/kg/% burn/24 h
   • 50%–70% burn: 0.4 mL/kg/% burn/24 h
   • >70% burn: 0.5 mL/kg/% burn/24 h

first 18 to 24 hours after burn injury. This pathophysiology explains the enormous volume requirement in these patients and is the reason that most resuscitative formulas withhold colloid until 24 hours after injury. Despite controlled data to support this common clinical practice (31), controversy over this point remains. Children commonly require intravenous fluid in excess of that predicted by several formulas (32). A urine output of 1 to 2 mL/kg/h is one important resuscitation end point in small children. Infants and very young children have renal concentrating abilities that are not completely mature. In toddlers and older children, however, whose concentrating abilities are adult, targeting a urine flow of 0.5 to 1 mL/kg/h results in lower overall fluid requirements that are closer to those of an adult. Patients with inhalation injury have overall volume requirements greater than predicted by standard formulas (33), possibly because of the release of vasoactive mediators from injured pulmonary parenchyma.

During the first 24 hours, lactated Ringer's solution, 2 to 4 mL/kg/% burn/24 h, is the primary resuscitative fluid. Because hypoglycemia can develop in children who weigh less than 10 kg if glucose is not administered, lactated Ringer's solution or half-normal saline with 5% dextrose at a maintenance rate (4 mL/kg/h) is given along with a reduced amount of the former (3 mL/kg/% burn/24 h). Dextrose-containing fluid should not be given as the primary resuscitative fluid because hyperglycemia and osmotic diuresis may result. Half of the calculated 24-hour total should be administered during the first 8 hours after injury. These calculations should be based on the time of injury, not on the time that vascular access is achieved. During this first 24-hour period, the resuscitative infusion of lactated Ringer's solution should be adjusted up or down in 10% increments every hour based on age-specific resuscitation end points, such as urine output, sensorium, base deficit, cardiac filling pressures, pulse, and blood pressure (Table 12.2). The importance of an hourly bedside evaluation during this period cannot be overemphasized.

It is important to recognize a failing resuscitation as early as possible because this facilitates salvage of these patients. At any point during a resuscitation, the estimated total fluid administration can be calculated based on the known administered volume and the current rate of infusion. This figure is divided by the patient's weight and burn size, resulting in a number that describes the number of milliliters of fluid per kilogram of body weight per percentage of burn that the patient is targeted to receive during the first 24 hours. A failing resuscitation is one in which the patient is likely to receive at least 6 mL/kg/% burn during the first 24 hours after injury. Larger resuscitation fluid volumes are commonly required by patients for whom resuscitation is delayed, who have sustained inhalation injury, or who have extensive and deep burns. These patients often benefit from the early infusion of low-dose dopamine, 3 to 5 μg/kg/min, and placement of a pulmonary artery catheter, or the early administration of colloid (Table 12.5).

Patients with gross pigmenturia are at risk for myoglobin-induced acute tubular necrosis (Fig. 12.14) (see color insert following page 1190). This situation is most common in patients who have sustained high-voltage electrical injury or deep thermal burns. In these patients, pigment must be cleared from the urine promptly. This is ideally accomplished with crystalloid loading, maintaining a brisk urine output of 2 mL/kg/h or more. Also helpful is alkalinization of the urine. This is best accomplished by administration of 0.12 to 0.5 mEq/kg/h of sodium bicarbonate intravenously as a part of the resuscitative fluid, with careful observation of the serum pH. Occasionally, osmotic diuresis using mannitol is required; however, the

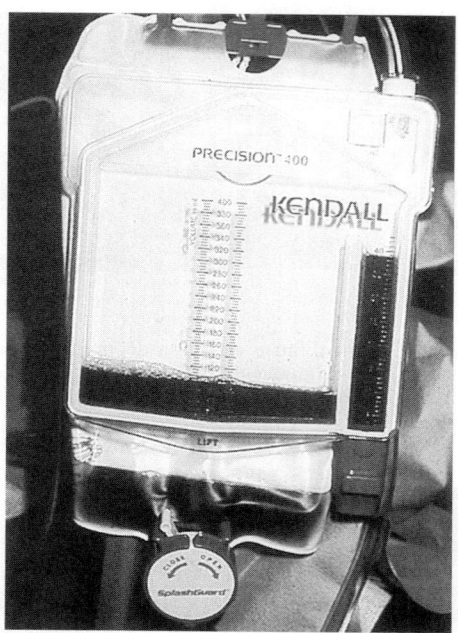

Figure 12.14. Heavily pigmented urine must be cleared of hemochromogens to avoid acute tubular necrosis.

administration of osmotic diuretics obscures the urine output as a measure of intravascular volume status. Therefore, a pulmonary artery or central venous catheter should be placed when mannitol must be used so that cardiac filling pressures can be used to judge the adequacy of fluid administration.

Beginning 24 hours after injury, colloid administration is appropriate, as the diffuse microvascular injury abates and endothelial cell integrity returns. At this time, colloid remains largely in the intravascular compartment. Colloid, usually 5% albumin in lactated Ringer's solution, is infused at a dose based on burn size (Table 12.5). During this second 24-hour period, crystalloid requirements markedly diminish and transeschar free water loss dominates the electrolyte picture unless an aqueous topical antimicrobial such as 0.5% silver nitrate solution is used. In the former situation, free water administration is required; in the latter case, transeschar leeching of sodium (approximately 350 mEq/m^2/24 h) mandates continued administration of isotonic crystalloid. Major morbidity is associated with aberrations of serum sodium concentrations at this time, so diligent electrolyte monitoring is important. Nutritional support, ideally enterally, should commence during the first 48 hours after injury.

INITIAL WOUND EXCISION AND BIOLOGIC CLOSURE

Early removal of extensive areas of devitalized tissue with immediate biologic closure of resulting wounds is the core surgical objective during the first postburn week. This policy of early excision is now widely practiced in the United States. It is accomplished as excision of the entire wound coincident with fluid resuscitation (34) or, more commonly, by staged excision of all deep partial- and full-thickness components of the wound during the first 3 to 7 days after injury (35). Wounds of the face, palms, soles, and genitals usually are not excised early. The emphasis on early excision is based on several documented and perceived advantages over the traditional approach of allowing eschar to liquefy until separation occurs, leaving a bed of granulation tissue that is subsequently autografted. Documented advantages include an improved survival rate in patients with injuries involving more than 30% to 40% of TBSA (36,37), truncated hospital stays (38), lower costs, and fewer painful dressing changes. Although not proved, it appears that a decrease in the duration and intensity of the hypermetabolic response, improved immunologic function, and less hypertrophic scarring may result from early excision.

Estimation of Burn Depth

In practical terms, only deep partial- or full-thickness burns undergo early excision. Such an approach assumes an ability accurately to determine burn depth during the initial examination. Although numerous technical aids, such as laser Doppler flow meters, intravenous fluorescein, burn wound biopsy, thermography, light reflectance, and fluorescence of intravenous dyes, have been proposed (26), none has yet equaled in accuracy or practicality the eye of an experienced examiner. The differentiation of superficial burns that will heal within 3 weeks with topical antimicrobial treatment from deeper injuries that will require excision can usually be made on clinical examination during the first days after injury. Certain patients have a component of their wound for which it is difficult to judge depth on initial examination. If overall wound size is not large (i.e., <15% of TBSA), such indeterminate-depth wounds can be treated with topical antimicrobials initially until the portion that requires grafting becomes evident. This situation is common in patients with small injuries caused by hot liquid. In this case, it is prudent to apply topical antimicrobials for 5 to 7 days and limit excision and grafting to full-thickness and deep dermal wounds.

Topical Antimicrobials

Topical antimicrobials play an important supportive role to excision and grafting because they delay the process of wound colonization and infection. Three topical agents are commonly used in the United States (Table 12.6). Silver sulfadiazine is perhaps the most common because it has a broad spectrum of activity, is painless and simple to apply, and has no metabolic or electrolyte implications. Mafenide acetate is an important element of the topical formulary because it alone reliably penetrates eschar. The major disadvantages are that it is a carbonic anhydrase inhibitor that causes a moderate metabolic acidosis and that it is painful on application. It is typically applied to eschar at risk for infection and to all deep burns

Table 12.6. **THREE COMMON TOPICAL MEDICATIONS USED IN THE UNITED STATES**

Agent	Characteristics
Silver sulfadiazine	Painless on application
	Fair to poor eschar penetration
	No metabolic side effects
	Broad-spectrum antibacterial
Mafenide acetate	Painful on application
	Excellent eschar penetration
	Carbonic anhydrase inhibitor
	Broad-spectrum antibacterial
0.5% Silver nitrate	Painless on application
	Poor eschar penetration
	Leeches electrolytes
	Broad-spectrum antibacterial and antifungal

of the external ear. The latter practice has markedly diminished the incidence of auricular chondritis. Silver nitrate is applied to heavy gauze dressings every 2 hours as an aqueous 0.5% solution. Although it penetrates eschar poorly and can leech large quantities of sodium and potassium from the wounds, its broad antibacterial and antifungal activity, as well as its flexible use on burn wounds, donor sites, and fresh grafts, makes it a valuable topical agent.

Techniques of Excision

A common argument against early burn wound excision is the prodigious blood loss associated with these procedures. Modern blood-conserving practices and the selection of earlier timing for excision of wounds have diminished this concern, however. Tangential wound excisions of the torso, neck, and head are performed after subeschar injection of dilute epinephrine solutions. Tangential wound excisions of the extremities are done after exsanguination and inflation of a pneumatic tourniquet. Although substantial experience is required to differentiate marginal areas of wound, tissue viability is readily accessed by color and texture, rather than the presence of diffuse bleeding. The principle is simply to excise nonviable tissue and conserve that which is viable. Instruments used in tangential excision of burned tissue include hand-operated, compressed gas-powered, and electric dermatomes. When required, excisions to the underlying fascia are performed with coagulating electrocautery, further diminishing blood loss. Although such procedures have traditionally been limited to 2 hours or 20% of TBSA, far larger procedures can be done safely if blood-conserving practices are rigorously followed and patients are kept warm by maintaining operating room temperatures above 90°F or 100°F (39).

Temporary Wound Closure Alternatives

Once necrotic eschar is excised to a bed of viable tissue, immediate biologic closure is mandatory. Ideally, immediate autografting is performed. When donor sites are insufficient for this purpose, a temporary biologic cover must be chosen while donor sites heal. Such covers should prevent desiccation and provide a vapor and bacterial barrier over the excised wound (40). Fresh or cryopreserved human allograft is most appropriate for this purpose. It is placed in a meshed but unexpanded fashion exactly as autograft would be placed. When placed on a viable wound bed, it vascularizes and provides physiologic wound closure until rejected 2 to 4 weeks later; at this time or before, it is replaced with reharvested autograft. Other temporary covers in common use are porcine xenograft, both fresh and reconstituted, and the synthetic bilaminate Biobrane (Dow-Hickman, Sugar Land, TX), which has a porous nylon inner layer and a semipermeable outer layer. Only human allograft will vascularize, however, and it therefore remains the optimal temporary wound closure material. Although application of biologic covers to wounds with residual eschar is dangerous and should not be practiced, a second common use for biologic dressings is to cover selected clean superficial wounds as they epithelialize. This minimizes the pain associated with an open partial-thickness burn. Allograft, screened for malignant and infectious diseases, is a precious resource and is not commonly used as a biologic dressing in these circumstances. Rather, reconstituted porcine xenograft is preferred.

DEFINITIVE WOUND CLOSURE

During the phase of definitive wound closure, allograft is replaced with reharvested autograft, and burns of certain specialized areas are addressed. This phase usually begins 1 week after injury and lasts for several weeks, depending on the extent of burn and the availability of suitable donor sites. Prompt definitive wound closure in patients with large injuries remains an elusive goal. At present, for most patients, split-thickness autograft provides the most practical and durable definitive wound closure material.

Burns of the Face, Ocular Adnexa, and Ears

Because of the thickness and deep appendages of the skin of the central face, relatively deep burns in these areas frequently heal. This is fortunate because it is difficult to achieve a favorable result with primary excision and grafting of the central face. Unless burns in these areas are of extraordinary depth, they are commonly treated with topical antimicrobial agents for 2 weeks. Areas that remain unhealed are excised and closed with thick sheet autograft. The face can be considered to consist of cosmetic units (Fig. 12.15), and it is ideal if full-thickness facial burns can be autografted in cosmetic units if this does not require sacrifice of significant areas of healed burn or unburned skin (41).

Burns of the ocular adnexa are common and potentially difficult management problems. During the first week after injury, lid edema usually ensures that the underlying globe is adequately protected and lubricated. As wound contracture occurs, exposure and desiccation of the globe can ensue (Fig. 12.16) (see color insert following page 1190), with resulting keratitis and corneal ulceration. If this is unresponsive to ocular lubrication, prompt surgical release of the lid is mandatory. Tarsorrhaphy is an ineffective alternative because the forces of wound contraction routinely disrupt the tarsorrhaphy and damage the underlying tarsal plate.

Burns of the external ear are treated with twice-daily cleansing and application of mafenide acetate. It is essen-

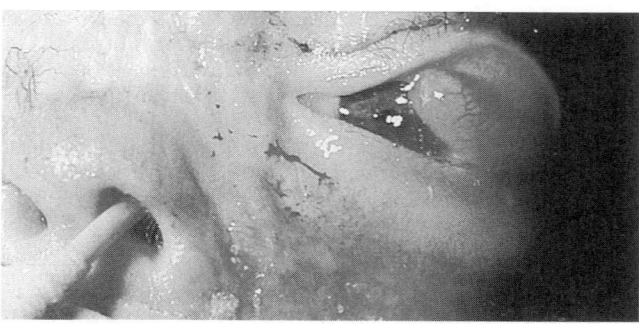

Figure 12.16. Contracture of burned ocular adnexae results in exposure and desiccation of the globe. When ocular lubrication is inadequate, lid release is mandatory.

tial to avoid pressure on the burned auricle from objects such as pillows. Simple devices such as foam ear protectors are effective preventive measures. Deep burns of the external ear are commonly complicated by acute suppurative chondritis if topical mafenide acetate is not applied (42). This complication is recognized by progressive auricular edema, erythema, and pain; it requires that the infected cartilage be immediately débrided to avoid complete loss of the cartilaginous support of the auricle.

Burns of the Hands and Feet

The increasing survival rates of patients with large burns have brought into greater focus the importance of the quality of life after such injuries. A crucial element of postinjury quality of life is hand function. Optimal functional outcome of hand burns is facilitated by an organized, multidisciplinary approach to the injuries.

The initial evaluation of the burned hand should begin with screening for other trauma. A complete hand examination is necessary, with particular attention being paid to perfusion by evaluation of capillary refill, temperature, consistency, and Doppler signals in the palmar arch, digital vessels, and distal pulp. It is not enough simply to demonstrate that there is blood flow in the radial or ulnar arteries. If the hands are cool and firm with distal circulation impaired, prompt escharotomies of the proximal upper extremity and hand are performed as previously described. In cases of high-voltage electrical injury or deep thermal burns, the need for urgent fasciotomy is indicated by progressive firmness of the compartments of the hand and forearm, or progressive neurologic impairment or pain. In equivocal cases, it is most prudent to proceed to decompression promptly rather than wait until ischemia has advanced.

Subsequent management of the burned hand is dictated by the depth of the injury. Superficial burns are managed with elevation, topical antimicrobials, and full passive range of motion twice daily for each joint. Splinting the hand in a functional position, with the metacarpophalangeal joints at 70 to 90 degrees, the interphalangeal joints in extension, the thumb in neutral position with the first web space open, and the wrist in 20 to 30 degrees of extension, is indicated if there is significant edema. Healing can be expected within 2 to 3 weeks if injuries are superficial. Deep partial- and full-thickness injuries are best managed with excision and sheet grafting as soon as practical (Fig. 12.17) (see color insert following page 1190). Hands are immobilized in a functional position for 7 days after surgery before passive and active therapy is resumed. Fourth-degree hand burns, which involve the underlying extensor mechanism, joint capsules, or bone, are significantly more difficult problems and are managed by staged

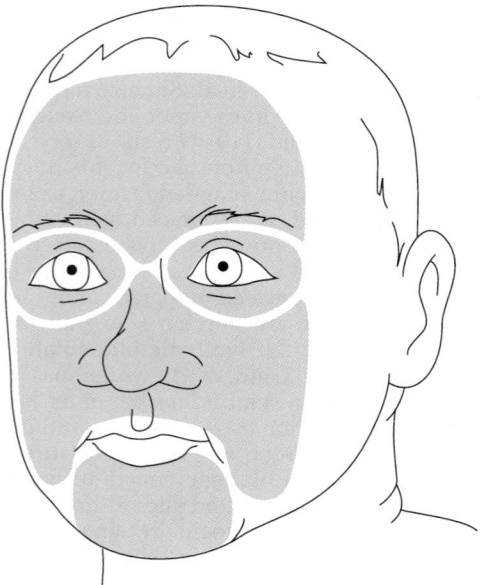

Figure 12.15. The cosmetic units of the face. It is ideal to autograft the face in cosmetic units if this does not require the sacrifice of significant areas of healed burn or unburned skin.

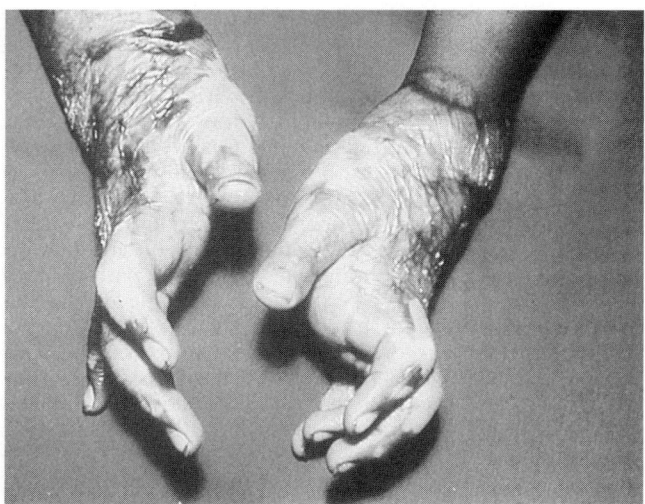

Figure 12.17. Spontaneous healing of deep dermal hand burns can result in a poor functional result.

sheet autografting. They also often benefit from temporary axial Kirschner wire fixation of open and unstable interphalangeal or metacarpophalangeal joints. Patients with smaller overall burn sizes in association with fourth-degree hand burns are often well served by débridement and groin or abdominal flap coverage. When hand burns are addressed in an organized fashion that stresses continuous hand therapy, most patients with deep partial- and full-thickness burns have normal or near-normal long-term function (24,43). Even patients with fourth-degree injuries, although rarely enjoying normal function, can expect to be able to function independently in activities of daily living.

The palmar skin is remarkably thick, so only approximately 20% of palmar burns require resurfacing. Therefore, a conservative approach facilitates preservation of the specialized attachment of the palmar skin to the underlying fascia. Full-thickness injuries are grafted with full-thickness or thick split-thickness sheet grafts and splinted in extension to maintain the palm in an open position.

Burns of the feet are managed in a similar fashion. Prompt excision and grafting of deep dermal and full-thickness injuries of the dorsum of the foot usually results in normal function. Fourth-degree injuries, although more difficult management problems, are entirely consistent with a normal functional result. Burns of the plantar surface of the feet are grafted with full- or thick split-thickness sheet grafts if they fail to heal within 3 weeks.

Genital Burns

On initial presentation, it is important to ensure that the burned foreskin is reduced into a normal position because progressive edema may result in paraphimosis. Bladder catheter drainage is not required to limit contamination of perineal wounds with urine. Bladder catheters should be used only to facilitate resuscitation and should be promptly removed when genital edema is resolved and close monitoring of the urine output is no longer required. Likewise, diversion of the intestinal tract is not required in the management of perineal burns. On occasion, contraction of the deeply burned and desiccated foreskin may render the placement of bladder catheters in the acute setting impossible. In these cases, dorsal or ventral incisions through the contracted foreskin permit catheter placement. When a deeply burned foreskin is being débrided,

any viable remnant should be preserved because such tissue may be useful in later reconstruction. Although there is some enthusiasm for early excision of deep genital burns, these limited surface area injuries can be managed with topical therapy for 2 to 3 weeks unless the wounds are remarkably deep. Unhealed injuries are débrided and grafted with sheet autograft at this time, with generally excellent cosmetic and functional results (44).

SELECTED CRITICAL CARE ISSUES

The enhanced survival of patients with large burns has been facilitated by increasing sophistication of the critical care techniques used to support an aggressive surgical approach to wounds, manage failing organ systems, and support the hypermetabolic response to injury. This section reviews some of the important points relevant to the management of inhalation injury and respiratory failure, techniques of arterial and venous access, nutritional support of the hypermetabolic response, and the recognition and management of multiorgan failure.

Inhalation Injury and Respiratory Failure

The pathophysiology of inhalation injury is complex and varies with the aerosolized toxins particular to the circumstances of individual injuries (45). However, these injuries routinely demonstrate the following:

Upper airway obstruction secondary to progressive edema
Reactive bronchospasm from aerosolized irritants
Small airway occlusion initially from edema and subsequently from sloughed endobronchial debris and loss of the ciliary clearance mechanism
Microatelectasis from loss of surfactant and alveolar edema
Interstitial and alveolar edema secondary to loss of capillary integrity

The physiologic consequences of these aberrations are upper and lower airway obstruction, increased airway resistance, decreased compliance, an increase in the dead space/tidal volume ratio, and intrapulmonary shunting.

Determination of the severity of inhalation injury is surprisingly difficult because the components of the smoke to which a patient has been exposed usually are unknown. Because current treatment is exclusively supportive, diagnosis provides only prognostic information. Suggestive points in the patient's history include entrapment in a closed space or prolonged extrication time. Physical signs that support the diagnosis include singed nasal vibrissae and facial hair, burns of the central face, intraoral burns, carbonaceous debris in the oropharynx, and diffuse wheezing. Bronchoscopy frequently reveals carbonaceous endobronchial debris and mucosal pallor, erythema, or ulceration. Xenon scanning may reveal delayed or asymmetric clearance of the radiotracer secondary to small airway obstruction. Unfortunately, findings at the time of initial evaluation frequently do not correlate with the subsequent clinical course.

The earliest consequence of inhalation injury is upper airway edema, which is commonly seen during the first 6 to 24 hours after injury. It is more prominent in small children and patients with large surface area injuries who experience more significant aberrations of capillary integrity and therefore more soft-tissue edema. Upper airway obstruction is best managed with prompt endotracheal intubation and elevation of the head maintained for 48 to 72 hours. In equivocal cases, diagnostic bronchoscopy is performed and patients with significant upper airway edema are intubated using the bronchoscope as a stylet. Endotracheal tubes are removed when facial edema has largely resolved and there is an audible air leak around the tubes at 30 cm H_2O of inflation with the cuff deflated.

Although severe steam inhalation can result in direct heat injury to the distal tracheobronchial tree, more distal airway injuries are usually caused by aerosolized toxins rather than thermal energy, the upper airway being a highly effective heat sink. The physiologic consequences of small airway injury are obstruction and intrapulmonary shunting with progressive respiratory failure. Small airway occlusion secondary to sloughed endobronchial debris and the loss of the ciliary clearance mechanism results in a high rate (up to 50%) of pneumonia (46). Successful treatment of patients with inhalation injury requires aggressive pulmonary toilet aided by frequent chest physiotherapy and bronchoscopic suctioning and lavage. Positive-pressure ventilation facilitates the treatment of patients with large shunts or compliance sufficiently poor to result in an excessive work of breathing. Positive end-expiratory pressure helps optimize functional residual capacity, minimizing intrapulmonary shunt and enhancing compliance. Although moderate inflating pressures help to expand recruitable segments, peak inspiratory pressures in excess of 40 cm H_2O should be avoided because they are associated with both overt barotrauma and more subtle overpressure injuries to the pulmonary microvasculature and alveoli. The combined effects of barotrauma and oxygen exacerbate respiratory failure (47). High inflating pressures are also ineffective in recruiting additional respiratory units because the compliance decrements are not homogeneous and high pressures simply overdistend more compliant segments. When ventilating patients with respiratory failure, one approach is to use low-volume ventilation and tolerate moderate hypercapnia and respiratory acidosis to facilitate control of inflating pressures (Table 12.7). This is associated with a low incidence of barotrauma and a high rate of survival (48).

Carbon Monoxide and Cyanide Exposure

Both carbon monoxide and cyanide are commonly inhaled by victims of closed-space fires (49). Carbon monoxide is a colorless and odorless gas with a high affinity for hemoglobin. Patients with significant amounts of carboxyhemoglobin have a marked reduction in their ability to deliver oxygen to peripheral tissues despite a normal arterial partial pressure of oxygen. The 2.5-hour half-life of carboxyhemoglobin is reduced by a factor of five by ventilation with 100% oxygen. Fire victims who are well ventilated with high concentrations of oxygen by emergency response personnel from the time of extrication commonly have normal carboxyhemoglobin values (<5%) on initial evaluation despite significant exposures to carbon monoxide at the time of injury. Carboxyhemoglobin is not sensed by standard transmission pulse oximetry, so a normal saturation on such a monitor does not preclude the possibility of significant carboxyhemoglobinemia. In conjunction with a severe carbon monoxide exposure, patients frequently also sustain a hypoxic cerebral insult and on occasion experience late neurologic sequelae. Hyperbaric oxygen can reduce the half-life of carboxyhemoglobin more rapidly than 100% oxygen and may possibly reduce further the incidence of late neurologic sequelae. The latter contention is debated, however, and the obvious danger associated with the loss of patient access during treatment in a monoplace hyperbaric chamber must temper the use of this modality in unstable patients undergoing resuscitation (50).

Hydrogen cyanide, which is commonly present in the smoke of structural fires, interferes with oxidative metabolism at the cellular level and causes lactic acidosis. With proper ventilation and fluid resuscitation, the cyanide-induced acidosis corrects rapidly in most patients, and specific treatment with sodium thiosulfate usually is not required (51).

Vascular Access Techniques

The successful management of large burns, particularly in the presence of respiratory or other organ failures, depends critically on reliable venous and arterial access despite the high rates of catheter sepsis traditionally associated with these patients. Peripheral access is often impractical in burn patients and is associated with unacceptable rates of suppurative thrombophlebitis. For these reasons, central venous access is routine except in patients with small injuries who require venous access for only a few days.

Arterial access, when required, can be safely maintained through the percutaneous radial, pedal, or femoral route (52). The importance of proper technique cannot be overemphasized if complications are to be avoided. The risk of central nervous system emboli associated with axillary arterial lines and the difficulty of maintaining catheters in the radial position for prolonged periods have led to a preference for the femoral position in children (53). Patients intubated for airway protection only, who

---

Table 12.7. **VENTILATOR MANAGEMENT OF RESPIRATORY FAILURE**

1. Treat bronchospasm with nebulized β-adrenergic agonist agents.
2. Treat inadequate chest wall compliance secondary to overlying eschar with escharotomy.
3. Ensure ventilator synchrony with adequate opiate and benzodiazepine infusions. Neuromuscular blockade may be necessary in some situations.
4. Reset end point of ventilation to a physiologic pH (≥7.2). Allow gradual-onset hypercapnia as long as there is no head injury.
5. Reset end point of oxygenation to an arterial saturation of at least 90%, typically associated with an arterial oxygen content of 60 mm Hg or greater.
6. Optimize inflating pressures.
   A. Choose optimal PEEP. This is best done by creating a pressure–volume curve with a graduated inflation and setting PEEP just above the inflection point. This can be

done by evaluating the clinical response (blood gases and hemodynamics) to increasing levels of PEEP.
   B. Choose optimal PIP. This is best done by using pressure-controlled ventilation and targeting a tidal volume of 10–15 mL/kg, as long as total inflating pressures (PIP + PEEP) can be kept under 40 cm H_2O. If this is inconsistent with meeting the reset end points of oxygenation and ventilation, then the pressure cap should be violated.
   C. Choose optimal mean airway pressure (P_{maw}). Lengthen expiratory time to a target of 20 to 25 cm H_2O, as long as auto-PEEP is not detectable.
7. In those rare patients in whom these measures remain insufficient, consider the use of innovative adjuncts, such as nitric oxide, partial liquid ventilation, or extracorporeal support.

PEEP, positive end-expiratory pressure; PIP, peak inflating pressure.

have no significant intrapulmonary shunt or dead space abnormalities, can be well treated with a transmission oximetry probe and central venous blood gasses.

Because most catheter infections arise from the central venous line tract rather than the hub, strict line care, including a nonocclusive insertion site cleansing every 4 hours, minimizes the risk of both arterial and central venous catheter sepsis. Catheters should be changed at least weekly and are inserted through unburned tissue whenever possible. Using this approach, central venous and arterial catheter sepsis rates are not significantly higher than in unburned critically ill patients (54).

Nutritional Support

The hypermetabolic response to burn injury is intense until wound closure is complete. This physiologic response is considered by some to be detrimental to the patient. This assumption must be accepted with caution, however, because this response to injury has been retained by numerous species for millions of years and presumably plays a role in recovery from injury. Conventional wisdom indicates that bacteria and their products that translocate from an incompetent gut barrier, the burn wound itself, and infectious foci are the forces driving the hypermetabolic and inflammatory responses. Accurate nutritional therapy for this response is crucial to achieving a favorable outcome.

Accurate support is essential because overfeeding is associated with hepatic steatosis, hepatic dysfunction, and increased carbon dioxide production that exacerbates respiratory insufficiency. Underfeeding results in inanition and poor wound healing. These factors have led to a plethora of formulas by which nutritional support has been administered to burn patients. Patients treated with prompt wound excision and biologic closure have a reduced energy expenditure compared with historic control subjects (55), and multiple studies have revealed that standard formulas are poorly predictive of actual energy requirements in individual burn patients. For these reasons, indirect calorimetry is commonly used to guide nutritional support of critically burned patients (56). Total energy expenditure can be roughly estimated by using expired gas indirect calorimetry to determine a resting energy expenditure and then multiplying the resting energy expenditure by a factor of 1.3 to 1.7.

Protein loads of 2.5 to 3 g/kg/d are recommended to support the requirements of seriously burned patients (57). Reports have proposed that use of recombinant human growth hormone can accelerate donor site healing and produce an earlier positive nitrogen balance (58). Prompt donor site healing and reliable positive nitrogen balance can be achieved without this expensive therapy, however. In addition, the long-term effects of pharmacologic doses of growth hormone remain undetermined, so the routine use of recombinant human growth hormone in burn patients should be approached with caution.

Multiple Organ Failure and Other Complications of Thermal Injury

It has been said that treatment of patients with large burns requires identification and management of a series of complications while the wound is progressively closed. Successful clinicians interpret any subtle deterioration as a manifestation of an occult complication, usually septic, until it is proved otherwise. Repetitive septic episodes can trigger multiple organ dysfunction in burn patients. Common complications of thermal injury are presented in Table 12.8.

Multisystem organ failure is the leading cause of late death in burn patients (59,60). The etiology of the multisystem organ failure syndrome involves complex cellular and subcellular biologic factors that are only now beginning to be unraveled by investigators using increasing numbers of recombinant products and receptor blocking antibodies. Our fragmentary understanding of this biology makes it clear that we must use caution when considering therapeutic use of these products outside the laboratory. It is widely assumed that the hypermetabolic response is driven by several inciting events, including repeated infections, translocation of bacteria and their products from an incompetent gut barrier, and the burn wound itself, and that these underlying processes cause multiorgan failure through similar mediator cascades after an overly exuberant response.

A deteriorating burn patient commonly has early evidence of multiple organ dysfunction in a predictable cascade: increasing obtundation is followed by progressive intrapulmonary shunting with hypoxia, ileus, nonoliguric renal failure, rising cholestasis, and thrombocytopenia (59). The most common initiating event is one of the many infections to which burn patients are prone. Certainly, wound sepsis is an obvious potential source. This should be infrequently seen now, however, because deep wounds are promptly removed before the onset of infection. The clinical team should search thoroughly for an occult infectious focus when multiorgan dysfunction first becomes evident because addressing such processes promptly can prevent the full development of the syndrome. When an underlying infectious focus can be identified and addressed, organ function improves. If not, failures progress with a predictably fatal outcome. The occult infections that should be considered in such situations (Table 12.8) include nosocomial sinusitis, which is particularly common in those with nasotracheal tubes; intravascular infections, such as endocarditis and suppurative thrombophlebitis, which typically present with fever and bacteremia without localized signs of infection; pneumonia or empyema; intraabdominal infections, such as acute cholecystitis and intestinal infarction; osteomyelitis; and infected intravascular devices.

REHABILITATION AND RECONSTRUCTION

With survival after large burns becoming more the rule than the exception, more attention has been focused on the quality rather than the simple fact of survival. Maximizing physical and psychosocial functional recovery is the key to optimizing the overall quality of life after serious burn injury.

Physical function is best optimized by the continuous involvement of dedicated burn occupational and physical therapists, beginning during the acute resuscitation. At this time, their involvement may be limited to antideformity positioning and splinting of the hands and extremities with twice-daily full range-of-motion exercises of all joints. In more stable patients, and in those with large injuries nearing wound closure, therapy sessions may take many hours each day and involve strengthening, ambulation, active and passive range of motion, development of adaptive skills with modified utensils, performance of activities of daily living, and, in older adolescents and adults, development of work-related skills. These important activities are continued after discharge.

Psychosocial adaptation after severe burns can be difficult, particularly if serious injury involves the hands or face. Preburn psychiatric disorders or family dysfunction may further complicate recovery. The coordinated in-

Table 12.8. COMMON COMPLICATIONS AFTER BURN INJURY

Neurologic

Transient delirium occurs in up to 30% of patients and usually resolves with supportive therapy. Evaluation is for anoxia, metabolic disturbance, and structural lesions.

Seizures most commonly result from hyponatremia or abrupt benzodiazepine withdrawal. Peripheral nerve injuries occur from direct thermal injury, compression from compartment syndrome or overlying nonelastic eschar, major metabolic disturbances, or improper splinting techniques.

Delayed peripheral nerve and spinal cord deficits develop weeks or months after high-voltage injury secondary to small vessel injury and demyelinization.

Renal

Early acute renal failure follows inadequate perfusion during resuscitation or myoglobinuria.

Late renal failure complicates sepsis and multiple organ failure or the use of nephrotoxic agents.

Adrenal

Acute adrenal insufficiency secondary to adrenal hemorrhage presents with hypotension, fever, hyponatremia, and hyperkalemia.

Cardiovascular

Endocarditis and suppurative thrombophlebitis typically present with fever and bacteremia without signs of local infection.

Hypertension occurs in up to 20% of children and is best managed with β-adrenergic blockers.

Venous thromboembolic complications are infrequent in patients with large burns.

Iatrogenic catheter insertion complications are minimized by meticulous technique.

Pulmonary

Pneumonia may occur with or without inhalation injury and is treated with pulmonary toilet and antibiotics.

Early respiratory failure may occur secondary to inhalation of noxious chemicals. Later respiratory failure may occur secondary to sepsis or pneumonia.

Hematologic

Neutropenia and thrombocytopenia, as well as disseminated intravascular coagulation, are common indicators of impending sepsis.

Systemic immunologic deficits contribute to a high rate of infectious complications.

Otologic

Auricular chrondritis secondary to bacterial infection results in rapid loss of viable cartilage. It is preventable by the routine use of topical mafenide acetate on all burned ears.

Sinusitis and otitis media can be caused by transnasal instrumentation and are treated by relocation of tubes, antibiotics, and judicious surgical drainage.

Complications of endotracheal intubation include nasal alar and septal necrosis, vocal cord erosions and ulcerations, tracheal stenosis, and tracheoesophageal and tracheoinnominate artery fistulae. Complications are minimized by compulsive attention to tube position, avoidance of oversized tubes, and attention to cuff pressures.

Enteric

Hepatic dysfunction, secondary to transient hepatic blood flow deficits and manifested as hepatocellular enzyme (aspartate and alanine aminotransferase) elevations, is extremely common. Late hepatic failure begins with elevations of cholestatic enzymes and may progress through coagulopathy and hepatic failure. It is associated with sepsis and multiple organ failure.

Pancreatitis is usually coincident with splanchnic flow deficits early and sepsis-induced organ failures later.

Acalculous cholecystitis can present as sepsis without localized symptoms or signs.

Radiographic evaluation can be followed by bedside percutaneous cholecystostomy in unstable patients.

Gastroduodenal ulceration, secondary to splanchnic flow deficits that degrade mucosal defenses, is common and potentially life threatening if routine histamine receptor blockers antacids are not administered.

Intestinal ischemia is possible if it is secondary to inadequate resuscitation and splanchnic flow deficits.

Ophthalmic

Ectropion, from progressive contraction of burned ocular adnexae, results in exposure of the globe. This requires acute eyelid release. Tarsorrhaphy is rarely helpful, more often resulting in injury to the tarsal plate as contraction forces pull out tarsorrhaphy sutures.

Corneal ulceration can progress to full-thickness corneal destruction if secondary infection. This is prevented by careful globe lubrication with topical antibiotics and possibly acute lid release for ectropion.

Symblepharon, or scarring of the lid to the denuded conjunctiva, occurs after chemical burns or corneal epithelial defects complicating toxic epidermal necrolysis. It is prevented by daily examination and adhesion disruption with a fine glass rod.

Genitourinary

Urinary tract infections are minimized by maintaining bladder catheters only when required.

Neither bladder catheterization nor colonic diversion is required for management of perineal and genital burns.

Candidal cystitis occurs with bladder cathers and broad-spectrum antibiotics. Catheter change and amphotericin B irrigation for 5 days is usually therapeutic. If infections are recurrent, the upper tracts should be screened ultrasonographically.

Muskuloskeletal

Burned exposed bone is usually débrided with a drill until viable cortical bone is reached. This is allowed to granulate and is autografted. Patients whose overall condition and wounds are appropriate are treated with local or distant flaps.

Fractured and burned extremities are best immobilized with external fixators while overlying burns are grafted. Burn patients with coincident fractures in unburned extremities benefit from prompt internal fixation.

Heterotopic ossification develops weeks after injury and is seen most commonly around deeply burned major joints such as the triceps tendon. It presents with pain and decreased range of motion. Most patients respond to physical therapy, but some require excision of heterotopic bone to achieve full function.

Soft tissue

Hypertrophic scar formation is a major cause of long-term functional and cosmetic deformities. It is heralded by a secondary increase in neovascularity 9 to 13 weeks after epithelialization.

Management options include grafting of deep dermal and full-thickness wounds, compression garments, judicious steroid injections, topical silicone products, and scar release and resurfacing procedures.

---

volvement of psychiatric, psychological, and social work staff facilitates maximum psychological recovery and social reintegration. These staff should be actively involved with the patient, family, and local outpatient support services throughout the hospitalization. Planning for discharge and arrangements and funding for needed outpatient services begins at the time of admission. The expectation for every burn patient should be a return to family and mainstream community life.

Hypertrophic Scarring and Reconstructive Surgery

Hypertrophic scar formation is a major source of long-term morbidity after burns (Fig. 12.18) (see color insert following page 1190). All healed and grafted burns become hypervascular shortly after successful epithelialization. Wounds destined to become hypertrophic go through a second surge of neovascularization at 9 to 13 weeks (61).

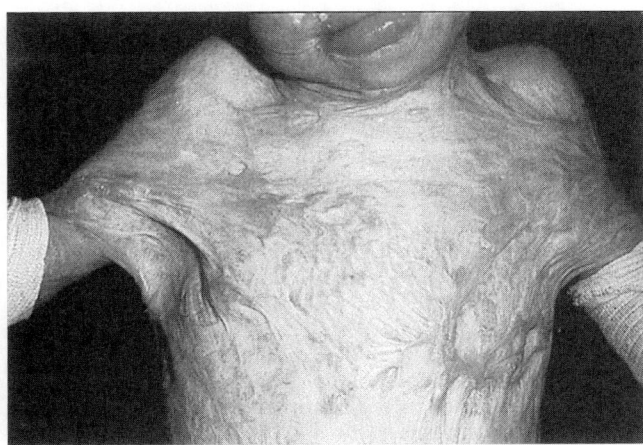

Figure 12.18. Hypertrophic scar formation has major adverse functional and cosmetic implications.

Additional collagen is formed and contraction occurs during the next 4 to 6 months, at which time the hypervascular tissue involutes, becoming less erythematous and raised over the subsequent 8 to 12 months. Despite the importance of hypertrophic scar formation, our basic understanding of the process remains poor (62). This lack of understanding is exacerbated by the absence of an animal model of scar hypertrophy.

Wounds that are associated most commonly with hypertrophy are deep dermal burns that heal in 3 or more weeks and full-thickness wounds that heal by contraction and epithelial spread from wound edges. Wounds across flexor surfaces and across the anterior neck and submental area, where there is much tension across the healed wounds, are also subject to scar hypertrophy with increased frequency. Any wound has the potential to become hypertrophic, however, and it is often difficult to predict accurately the probability that any individual patient will have hypertrophic scar formation.

The ability to influence the development of hypertrophic scars is limited. Current tools include compression garments, topical silicone sheets, steroid injections, and release or excision and autografting. Compression garments are individually measured and worn beginning within 2 weeks of grafting or wound epithelialization. They are not advised for use on the head of a child younger than 1 year of age because they can mold the calvarium. Topical silicone has been advocated by some for hypertrophic scar treatment, although the mechanism of action is not clear and the use of topical silicone sheeting is accompanied by frequent skin irritation and rashes. Judicious intradermal steroid injection has been of value in the management of limited areas of hypertrophic scarring, usually in cosmetically important areas of small size. Intradermal steroid injections can be painful, and the dose must be limited to avoid systemic effects. Patients with recalcitrant areas of hypertrophic scarring often are best served by release or excision. Resultant wounds are covered with sheet autograft or flaps. Tissue expanders can be of great value, particularly in the closure of defects of hair-bearing scalp. When function is not limited, it is ideal to wait 2 years for full scar maturation before embarking on reconstructive procedures. When function is threatened, however, prompt surgery is indicated (Fig. 12.19) (see color insert following page 1190). Patients with large burn wounds commonly require a series of reconstructive procedures during the first few years after injury to attain the best possible cosmetic and functional results.

FUTURE OF BURN MANAGEMENT

Potential innovations likely to be seen in the next decade fall into five broad groups: those intended to support or modify the hypermetabolic response, growth factors, innovations in wound management, new critical care technology, and permanent skin substitutes.

Recent work has shown that although the factors driving the hypermetabolic response may vary from patient to patient, a common web of mediators effects the response. The adverse aspects of the hypermetabolic response are best obviated by minimizing release of inflammatory mediators from the wound by prompt excision and biologic closure. Support of gastrointestinal barrier function is en-

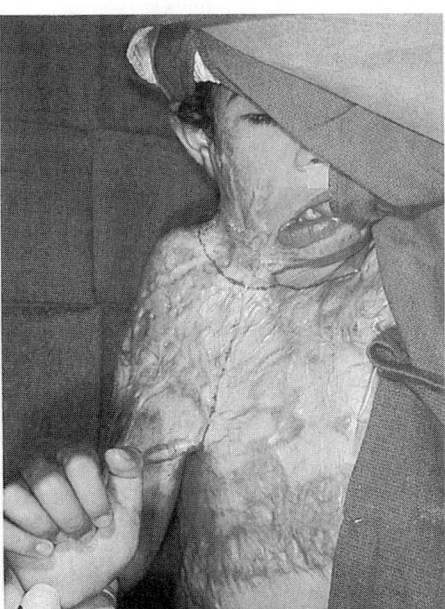

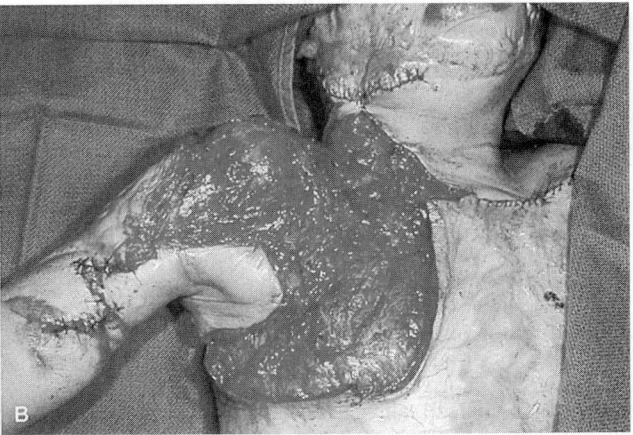

Figure 12.19. Prompt release and autografting is indicated when hypertrophic scar formation threatens to limit function.

sured through establishment of adequate splanchnic blood flow by normalizing hemodynamics and providing enteral nutritional support as soon as possible after injury. Early detection and elimination of infectious foci are fundamental also. These measures are likely to be more effective than attempts to modify the complex cascade of mediators that effect the hypermetabolic response. Support, rather than major modification, of the hypermetabolic response seems most appropriate at present because our understanding of the basic biology is quite fragmentary. Ongoing work with blocking antibodies and recombinant mediators in animal models and humans promises to enhance our understanding of the hypermetabolic response to injury and facilitate treatment of such patients.

Use of topical epidermal growth factor or systemic human growth hormone has been associated with shortened donor site healing times in burn patients. The differences between control and treated patients have been limited, however, and any potential benefit should be weighed against the financial and still undefined long-term physiologic costs of these therapies. Ongoing animal and clinical work with transforming growth factors, platelet-derived growth factors, fibroblast growth factors, and colony-stimulating factors promises to enhance our understanding of the biology of wound healing and may lead to improvements in clinical care in the future.

The ability accurately to determine the depth of wounds on initial presentation has the potential to shorten hospital stays by eliminating the period of observation that is commonly used to facilitate accurate predictions of wound healing in patients with small burns of indeterminate depth. Although several such technical adjuncts, such as laser Doppler flow meters and high-resolution ultrasound, have been developed, none has proved of practical clinical utility. The ability of low-power lasers to cause intravenously administered indocyanine green dye to fluoresce is under evaluation and may prove valuable (63). Bloodless wound débridement using a scanning carbon dioxide laser has been effective in a porcine model and holds potential promise as a means to decrease the blood loss associated with wound excision (64,65). Débriding enzymes have previously been associated with injury to normal tissue, bleeding, pain, infection, and inadequate débridement. New formulations of these enzymes, designed to liquefy necrotic tissue without injuring healthy tissue, may prove of limited value in burn care. If efficacious, these substances may also facilitate both wound depth evaluation and blood-conserving removal of eschar.

Critical care technologies under development that may affect burn care include newer modes of ventilation that stress avoidance of high inflating pressures and techniques of extracorporeal support. Nitric oxide, delivered into the ventilator circuit, has been shown to decrease intrapulmonary shunting by increasing pulmonary blood flow to well ventilated lung segments and decrease pulmonary vascular resistance in patients with respiratory failure. It may prove of value in burn patients with inhalation injury and severe respiratory failure (66).

Definitive wound closure using materials other than autograft is the goal of several ongoing research projects and, if realized, will have an enormous impact on the acute and reconstructive management of burn patients. Substitutes being developed include epidermal analogues, dermal analogues, and composite substitutes. Of the epidermal analogues, sheets of cultured autologous epithelium are in clinical use. Although expensive and associated with low engraftment rates and extreme graft fragility, this technology is of value in the treatment of patients with massive injuries (67). Patients with smaller injuries are better served by a split-thickness autograft. If cultured epidermis becomes fully in-

tegrated with a functional dermal analogue, its value may increase substantially. Dermal substitutes, designed to be combined with ultrathin autograft or cultured epithelium, are best represented by a synthetic bilaminate artificial skin (68), which was successful in a large multicenter trial and is now marketed as Integra artificial skin (Integra Lifesciences, Plainsboro, NJ). This material is approved for use in patients with life-threatening burns, and postmarketing trials are in progress. It has been associated with gratifying long-term cosmetic and functional results and will likely play an important role in wound closure in patients with massive burns (69). Another dermal substitute in early clinical use is AlloDerm (LifeCell, The Woodlands, TX), a cryopreserved human dermal product (70). Experience with these substitutes is limited, but encouraging.

Enormous strides have been made in burn patient management since the early 1980s. Although burn injuries remain a tremendous challenge to the patient, family, and burn unit team, the prognosis for those sustaining such injuries continues to improve. Ongoing progress in the evolution of our ability to modify the hypermetabolic response, fully understand the potential roles of growth factors, develop more effective ways to evaluate and excise wounds, mature critical care technologies, and develop durable permanent skin substitutes will further enhance our patients' quality of survival.

REFERENCES

1. Simon PA, Baron RC. Age as a risk factor for burn injury requiring hospitalization during early childhood. *Arch Pediatr Adolesc Med* 1994;148:394–397.
2. Lindblad BE, Terkelsen CJ, Christensen H. Epidemiology of domestic burns related to products. *Burns* 1990;16:89–91.
3. Erdmann TC, Feldman KW, Rivara FP, et al. Tap water burn prevention: the effect of legislation. *Pediatrics* 1991;88: 572–577.
4. Sheridan RL, Ryan CM, Petras LM, et al. Burns in children younger than two years of age: an experience with 200 consecutive admissions. *Pediatrics* 1997;100:721–723.
5. Ryan CM, Schoenfeld DA, Thorpe WP, et al. Objective estimates of the probability of death from burn injuries. *N Engl J Med* 1998;338:362–366.
6. Erickson EJ, Merrell SW, Saffle JR, et al. Differences in mortality from thermal injury between pediatric and adult patients. *J Pediatr Surg* 1991;26:821–825.
7. Morrow SE, Smith DL, Cairns BA, et al. Etiology and outcome of pediatric burns. *J Pediatr Surg* 1996;31:329–333.
8. Sheridan RL, Remensnyder JP, Schnitzer JJ, et al. Current expectations for survival in pediatric burns. *Arch Pediatr Adolesc Med* 2000;154:245–249.
9. Aggarwal SJ, Diller KR, Blake GK, et al. Burn-induced alterations in vasoactive function of the peripheral cutaneous microcirculation. *J Burn Care Rehabil* 1994;15:1–12.
10. Ehrlich HP. Promotion of vascular patency in dermal burns with ibuprofen. *Am J Med* 1984;77:107–113.
11. Choi M, Ehrlich HP. U75412E, a lazaroid, prevents progressive burn ischemia in a rat burn model. *Am J Pathol* 1993; 142:519–528.
12. Ehrlich HP, McGrane WL, Rajaratnam JB. Ancrod prevents vascular occlusion in thermally injured rats. *J Trauma* 1987; 27:420–424.
13. Katz A, Ryan P, LaLonde C, et al. Topical ibuprofen decreases thromboxane release from the endotoxin-stimulated burn wound. *J Trauma* 1986;26:157–162.
14. Demling R, Picard L, Campbell C, et al. Relationship of burn-induced lung lipid peroxidation on the degree of injury after smoke inhalation and a body burn. *Crit Care Med* 1993;21: 1935–1943.
15. LaLonde C, Knox J, Daryani R, et al. Topical flurbiprofen decreases burn wound-induced hypermetabolism and systemic lipid peroxidation. *Surgery* 1991;109:645–651.
16. Gupta M, Gupta OK, Yaduvanshi RK, et al. Burn epidemiology: the Pink City scene. *Burns* 1993;19:47–51.

17. Youn YK, LaLonde C, Demling R. The role of mediators in the response to thermal injury. *World J Surg* 1992;16:30–36.
18. Deitch EA. Multiple organ failure. *Adv Surg* 1993;26: 333–356.
19. Sasaki TM, Welch GW, Herndon DN, et al. Burn wound manipulation-induced bacteremia. *J Trauma* 1979;19:46–48.
20. Demling RH, LaLonde C, Liu YP, et al. The lung inflammatory response to thermal injury: relationship between physiologic and histologic changes. *Surgery* 1989;106:52–59.
21. Wilmore DW, Mason AD Jr, Johnson DW, et al. Effect of ambient temperature on heat production and heat loss in burn patients. *J Appl Physiol* 1975;38:593–597.
22. Sheridan RL. The seriously burned child: resuscitation through reintegration–1. *Curr Probl Pediatr* 1998;28:105–127.
23. Sheridan RL. The seriously burned child: resuscitation through reintegration–2. *Curr Probl Pediatr* 1998;28:139–167.
24. Sheridan RL, Baryza MJ, Pessina MA, et al. Acute hand burns in children: management and long-term outcome based on a 10-year experience with 698 injured hands. *Ann Surg* 1999; 229:558–564.
25. Sheridan RL, Tompkins RG, McManus WF, et al. Intracompartmental sepsis in burn patients. *J Trauma* 1994;36: 301–305.
26. Heimbach D, Engrav L, Grube B, et al. Burn depth: a review. *World J Surg* 1992;16:10–15.
27. Sheridan RL, Petras L, Basha G, et al. Planimetry study of the percent of body surface represented by the hand and palm: sizing irregular burns is more accurately done with the palm. *J Burn Care Rehabil* 1995;16:605–606.
28. Sheridan RL, Briggs SE, Remensnyder JP, et al. The burn unit as a resource for the management of acute nonburn conditions in children. *J Burn Care Rehabil* 1995;16:62–64.
29. Sheridan RL, Ryan CM, Quinby WC Jr, et al. Emergency management of major hydrofluoric acid exposures. *Burns* 1995; 21:62–64.
30. Montrey JS, Barcia PJ. Nonaccidental burns in child abuse. *South Med J* 1985;78:1324–1326.
31. Goodwin CW, Dorethy J, Lam V, et al. Randomized trial of efficacy of crystalloid and colloid resuscitation on hemodynamic response and lung water following thermal injury. *Ann Surg* 1983;197:520–531.
32. Graves TA, Cioffi WG, McManus WF, et al. Fluid resuscitation of infants and children with massive thermal injury. *J Trauma* 1988;28:1656–1659.
33. Navar PD, Saffle JR, Warden GD. Effect of inhalation injury on fluid resuscitation requirements after thermal injury. *Am J Surg* 1985;150:716–720.
34. Desai MH, Herndon DN, Broemeling L, et al. Early burn wound excision significantly reduces blood loss. *Ann Surg* 1990;211:753–759; discussion 759–762.
35. Sheridan RL, Tompkins RG, Burke JF. Management of burn wounds with prompt excision and immediate closure. *J Intensive Care Med* 1994;9:6–19.
36. Herndon DN, Gore D, Cole M, et al. Determinants of mortality in pediatric patients with greater than 70% full-thickness total body surface area thermal injury treated by early total excision and grafting. *J Trauma* 1987;27:208–212.
37. Merrell SW, Saffle JR, Sullivan JJ, et al. Increased survival after major thermal injury: a nine-year review. *Am J Surg* 1987;154:623–627.
38. Herndon DN, Barrow RE, Rutan RL, et al. A comparison of conservative versus early excision: therapies in severely burned patients. *Ann Surg* 1989;209:547–552.
39. Sheridan RL, Szyfelbein SK. Staged high dose epinephrine clysis in pediatric burn excisions. *Burns* 2000;25:745–748.
40. Sheridan RL, Tompkins RG. Skin substitutes in burns. *Burns* 1999;25:97–103.
41. Gonzalez-Ulloa M. Restoration of the face covering by means of selected skin in regional aesthetic units. *Br J Plast Surg* 1956;9:212–221.
42. Mills DC Jr, Roberts LW, Mason AD Jr, et al. Suppurative chondritis: its incidence, prevention, and treatment in burn patients. *Plast Reconstr Surg* 1988;82:267–276.
43. Sheridan RL, Hurley J, Smith MA, et al. The acutely burned hand: management and outcome based on a ten-year experience with 1,047 acute hand burns. *J Trauma* 1995;38: 406–411.
44. Peck MD, Boileau MA, Grube BJ, et al. The management of burns to the perineum and genitals. *J Burn Care Rehabil* 1990; 11:54–56.
45. Heimbach DM, Waeckerle JF. Inhalation injuries. *Ann Emerg Med* 1988;17:1316–1320.
46. Rue LW III, Cioffi WG, Mason AD, et al. Improved survival of burned patients with inhalation injury. *Arch Surg* 1993;128: 772–778.
47. Slutsky AS. Mechanical ventilation. American College of Chest Physicians' Consensus Conference. *Chest* 1993;104: 1833–1859.
48. Sheridan RL, Kacmarek RM, McEttrick MM, et al. Permissive hypercapnia as a ventilatory strategy in burned children: effect on barotrauma, pneumonia, and mortality. *J Trauma* 1995;39:854–859.
49. Sheridan RL, Shank E. Hyperbaric oxygen treatments: a brief overview of a controversial topic. *J Trauma* 1999;47:426–435.
50. Grube BJ. Therapeutic hyperbaric oxygen: help or hindrance in burn patients with carbon monoxide poisoning? *J Burn Care Rehabil* 1989;10:285.
51. Barillo DJ, Goode R, Esch V. Cyanide poisoning in victims of fire: analysis of 364 cases and review of the literature. *J Burn Care Rehabil* 1994;15:46–57.
52. Sheridan RL, Weber JM, Tompkins RG. Femoral arterial catheterization in paediatric burn patients. *Burns* 1994;20: 451–452.
53. Sheridan RL, Weber JM, Peterson HF, et al. Central venous catheter sepsis with weekly catheter change in paediatric burn patients: an analysis of 221 catheters. *Burns* 1995;21: 127–129.
54. Goldstein AM, Weber JM, Sheridan RL. Femoral venous access is safe in burned children: an analysis of 224 catheters. *J Pediatr* 1997;130:442–446.
55. Carlson DE, Cioffi WG Jr, Mason AD Jr, et al. Resting energy expenditure in patients with thermal injuries. *Surg Gynecol Obstet* 1992;174:270–276.
56. Sheridan RL, Yu YM, Prelack K, et al. Maximal parenteral glucose oxidation in hypermetabolic young children: a stable isotope study. *JPEN J Parenter Enteral Nutr* 1998;22:212–216.
57. Prelack K, Cunningham JJ, Sheridan RL, et al. Energy and protein provisions for thermally injured children revisited: an outcome-based approach for determining requirements. *J Burn Care Rehabil* 1997;18:177–181; discussion 176.
58. Gilpin DA, Barrow RE, Rutan RL, et al. Recombinant human growth hormone accelerates wound healing in children with large cutaneous burns. *Ann Surg* 1994;220:19–24.
59. Sheridan RL, Ryan CM, Yin LM, et al. Death in the burn unit: sterile multiple organ failure. *Burns* 1998;24:307–311.
60. Saffle JR, Sullivan JJ, Tuohig GM, et al. Multiple organ failure in patients with thermal injury. *Crit Care Med* 1993;21:1673–1683.
61. Kischer CW. The microvessels is hypertrophic scars, keloids, and related lesions. *J Submicrosc Cytol Pathol* 1992;24: 281–296.
62. Rockwell WB, Cohen IK, Ehrlich HP. Keloids and hypertrophic scars: a comprehensive review. *Plast Reconstr Surg* 1989;84:827–837.
63. Sheridan RL, Schomaker KT, Lucchina LC, et al. Burn depth estimation by use of indocyanine green fluorescence: initial human trial. *J Burn Care Rehabil* 1995;16:602–604.
64. Glatter RD, Goldberg JS, Schomacker KT, et al. Carbon dioxide laser ablation with immediate autografting in a full-thickness porcine burn model. *Ann Surg* 1998;228:257–265.
65. Sheridan RL, Lydon MM, Petras LM, et al. Laser ablation of burns: initial clinical trial. *Surgery* 1999;125:92–95.
66. Sheridan RL, Hurford WE, Kacmorek RM, et al. Inhaled nitric oxide in burn patients with respiratory failure. *J Trauma* 1997;42:641–646.
67. Sheridan RL, Tompkins RG. Cultured autologous epithelium in patients with burns of ninety percent or more of the body surface. *J Trauma* 1995;38:48–50.
68. Heimbach D, Luterman A, Burke J, et al. Artificial dermis for major burns: a multi-center randomized clinical trial. *Ann Surg* 1988;208:313–320.
69. Sheridan RL, Heggerty M, Tompkins RG, et al. Artificial skin in massive burns: results at ten years. *Eur J Plast Surg* 1994;17:91–93.
70. Sheridan R, Choucair R, Donelan M, et al. Acellular allodermis in burns surgery: 1-year results of a pilot trial. *J Burn Care Rehabil* 1998;19:528–530.

SURGERY: SCIENTIFIC PRINCIPLES AND PRACTICE, Third Edition, edited by
Lazar J. Greenfield, Michael W. Mulholland, Keith T. Oldham, Gerald B. Zelenock,
and Keith D. Lillemoe. Lippincott Williams & Wilkins Publishers, Philadelphia © 2001.

CHAPTER 13

ANESTHESIOLOGY AND PAIN MANAGEMENT

TIMOTHY W. RUTTER AND KEVIN K. TREMPER

Anesthesia is a combination of amnesia, analgesia, and muscle relaxation. This state can be achieved by inhaling various vapors that produce each of these conditions in proportion to the concentration achieved in the central nervous system. Anesthesia can also be achieved by using one of three pharmacologic agents that are each targeted to produce a specific effect. These are the amnesics, analgesics, and neuromuscular blocking agents. As the concentration of inhalation anesthetics increases, cardiovascular and respiratory function are progressively depressed. Because of the surgical procedure's requirements or the patient's preexisting cardiac disease, the concentration of inhalation agent that is required to produce sufficient muscle relaxation may be a relative overdose with respect to its effect on the cardiovascular system. For this reason, modern anesthetics usually require titration to optimize conditions for the surgery while maintaining cardiovascular stability.

The goals of modern anesthesia are (a) to achieve this state quickly and safely by choosing the appropriate techniques and agents for the patient's medical condition; (b) to maintain this state throughout the surgical procedure while compensating for the effects of varying degrees of painful stimuli and blood and fluid loss; and (c) to reverse the muscle relaxation and amnesia, bringing the patient back to physiologic control while maintaining sufficient analgesia to minimize postoperative pain. This process is

accomplished with a high degree of safety 30 to 40 million times a year in the United States, in spite of the serious potential complications of technical or judgment errors. The high degree of success of both surgical and anesthetic outcomes is due to the efforts of thousands of surgeons and anesthesiologists who have advanced the art and science of their fields (1). Although modern techniques and analgesics have made it possible nearly to eliminate all perioperative pain, judgmental feelings about patients who complain of pain still remain. Pain is not only unpleasant; it has significant adverse physiologic effects, and physicians should encourage patients to alert health care personnel when pain is felt.

ANESTHETIC AGENTS AND THEIR PHYSIOLOGIC EFFECTS

Inhalation Agents

Anesthetics are generalized depressants of consciousness, pain, cardiopulmonary function, motor function, and recall. The potent inhalation agents (e.g., halothane, enflurane, isoflurane) produce these effects in a dose-dependent fashion with approximately 1% inhaled concentration. The measurement used to compare the potency of inhalation agents is the minimum alveolar concentration (MAC; measured as a percentage) that prevents movement on painful stimulation (incision) in half of the subjects. There is significant patient-to-patient variability even when patients possess a similar degree of health. Compounding this variability are the effects of age, weight, preexisting heart disease or liver disease, and medications other than the anesthetics. Table 13.1 lists the commonly used inhalation agents and their MACs and side effects. In general, all agents depress blood pressure by myocardial depression and vasodilation. There is a generalized depression of cerebral function and cerebral metabolic rate of oxygen consumption, although cerebral blood flow may increase because of vascular dilatation and a loss of autoregulation. Renal blood flow and glomerular filtration

Table 13.1. COMMON INHALATION AGENTS: MINIMUM ALVEOLAR CONCENTRATIONS AND EFFECTS

Agent	Minimum alveolar concentration (%)	Strengths	Weaknesses
Nitrous oxide	105	Analgesia Rapid uptake and elimination Little cardiac or respiratory depression	Sympathetic stimulation Expansion of closed air spaces Interference with vitamin B_{12} metabolism Limitation of FiO_2
Halothane	0.75	Low cost Effectiveness in low concentrations Little airway irritability Uterine relaxation	Less chemical stability Slow uptake and elimination Biodegradability Hepatic necrosis Cardiac depression and arrhythmias
Enflurane	1.68	Good muscle relaxation Stable cardiac rate and rhythm	Pungent odor Seizure activity on electroencephalography
Isoflurane	1.15	Good muscle relaxation Stable cardiac rate and rhythm Usability in neurosurgery	Pungent odor
Desflurane	6	Rapid induction and emergence	Pungent odor Causes coughing High vaper pressure (Boiling point 23.5°C) Requires special pressurized vaporizer High cost
Sevoflurane	1.71	Rapid induction and emergence Less pungent Good for mask induction	High cost Metabolized in liver, producing increased plasma fluoride

Adapted from Miller FL, Marshall BE. The inhaled anesthetics. In: Longnecker DE, Murphy FL, eds. Introduction to anesthesia, 8th ed. Philadelphia: WB Saunders, 1992:77.

rate are reduced by 20% to 50%. Blood flow to the skin increases and cutaneous autoregulation is reduced, impairing the body's ability to conserve heat. The combination of these effects, the cold environment of the operating room, and open body cavities make the patient extremely vulnerable to hypothermia.

Muscle Relaxants

To prevent movement and to facilitate surgical exposure, neuromuscular blocking agents usually are used. These drugs are competitive or noncompetitive inhibitors of the neurotransmitter acetylcholine at the neuromuscular junction. The only noncompetitive inhibitor used clinically is succinylcholine. This drug rapidly binds to the neuromuscular junction and produces depolarization, clinically obvious as fine muscle fasciculations occurring approximately 60 seconds after injection. Succinylcholine cannot be reversed, but its effects are short acting because it is quickly hydrolyzed in the plasma by cholinesterase. Because of rapid onset, succinylcholine is frequently used to facilitate endotracheal intubation when it must be accomplished quickly.

All other clinically useful muscle relaxants are termed *competitive inhibitors* and do not cause depolarization when they attach at the neuromuscular junction. Because these agents compete with acetylcholine, the block produced is in direct proportion to the concentration of the agent relative to the concentration of acetylcholine. If the concentration ratio is low enough, competitive relaxants can be reversed if the concentration of acetylcholine is artificially elevated. Acetylcholine concentration can be increased by giving a drug that blocks its metabolism, an anticholinesterase (e.g., neostigmine). The neuromuscular blocking agent is still present, but motor function returns if the acetylcholine concentration is high enough to outcompete the blocking agent. There is a ceiling beyond which anticholinesterase drugs cannot elevate acetylcholine; therefore, high levels of nondepolarizing relaxants cannot be reversed. Reversing neuromuscular relaxants is not analogous to using naloxone to reverse the effects of opioids; the reversal agent neostigmine does not compete or combine with the relaxant.

Unfortunately, there are systemic consequences to increasing the plasma concentration of acetylcholine. Acetylcholine is the predominant neurotransmitter in the preganglionic sympathetic and parasympathetic nervous systems and in the postganglionic parasympathetic nervous system. For this reason, an anticholinergic drug (atropine or glycopyrrolate) must be given with an anticholinesterase to prevent the undesirable effects of a generalized acetylcholine overdose. The common neuromuscular blocking drugs and their doses, durations, and side effects are listed in Table 13.2; common regimens of reversal agents are given in Table 13.3.

Nondepolarizing relaxants are frequently used in critically ill patients who are difficult to manage otherwise, such as head-injured patients who require hyperventilation or patients with adult respiratory distress syndrome who require complex modes of ventilation. It is imperative that these drugs be given in conjunction with analgesics and amnesic agents. Neuromuscular blocking agents have no analgesic or amnesic properties and only prevent motion of voluntary muscles. Patients can be totally aware and in pain, but unable to communicate. When prolonged muscle relaxation is required, it is best to administer the relaxant by continuous infusion and then monitor the effect with a nerve stimulator. For these settings, relaxants should be administered only to achieve the degree of relaxation necessary and in a dose that allows reversal at any time. Table 13.2 includes the recommended ranges of infusion rates. There have been reports of patients who have prolonged residual motor weakness after the muscle relaxant is cleared (2). These problems have been primarily noted with the drug pancuronium bromide (Pavulon; Organon Teknika, Durham, NC), especially when the patients are also being treated with steroids. It is therefore recommended that pancuronium bromide not be used for longer than 2 days.

All muscles in the body are not equally sensitive to muscle relaxants. The diaphragm is most resistant to neuromuscular blockade, whereas the neck and pharyngeal muscles that support the airway are most sensitive. It is possible for an intubated patient to ventilate spontaneously and even to produce a large negative inspiratory effort, and yet experience complete airway obstruction

---

Table 13.2. COMMON NEUROMUSCULAR BLOCKING DRUGS AND REVERSAL AGENTS

Muscle relaxant	Intubating dose (mg/kg)	Infusion dose (μg/kg/min)	Strengths	Weaknesses
Depolarizing				
Succinylcholine	1.0	100[a]	Fastest onset (30–60 s) Short duration[b] (5 min)	Associated with malignant hyperthermia, dysrhythmias, bradycardia, and hyperkalemia, especially in patients with burns or neurologic injury
Nondepolarizing				
Long-acting (>1 h) pancuronium	0.1	0.3	No histamine release	Tachycardia Slow onset Long duration
Pipecuronium	0.08	—	Similar to pancuronium, no cardiovascular effects	—
Doxacurium	0.07	—	Similar to pancuronium, minimal cardiovascular effects	—
Intermediate-acting (1 h) atracurium	0.5	10	Spontaneous breakdown in plasma	Histamine release
Vecuronium	0.1	1	No cardiovascular effects	
Rocuronium	0.8	10	Fast onset, no cardiovascular effects	
Mivacurium	0.2	10	Fast onset, short duration	Histamine release

[a]This should not be used for longer than 1 h.
[b]Duration is dramatically increased in patients with abnormal plasma pseudocholinesterase.

Table 13.3. DRUGS FOR ANTAGONIZING NONDEPOLARIZING NEUROMUSCULAR BLOCKADE[a]

Name	Time to peak effect (min)	Dose	Use with
Anticholinesterases			
Edrophonium	1–2	0.5–1.0 mg/kg	—
Neostigmine	3–5	0.04–0.07 mg/kg	—
Pyridostigmine	10–12	0.2–0.3 mg/kg	—
Anticholinergics			
Glycopyrrolate	—	0.008 mg/kg (0.5–0.6 mg/70 kg)	Neostigmine Pyridostigmine
Atropine	—	0.007–0.02 mg/kg8 (0.05–1.5 mg/70 kg)	Edrophonium Neostigmine

[a]For reliable results in reversing the effects of nondepolarizing muscle relaxants, administration of anticholinesterases is delayed until spontaneous recovery permits three of four responses to a train-of-four stimulus. For patients with more profound blockade, larger amounts of anticholinesterases may be required, but doses of neostigmine higher than 0.14 mg/kg are unlikely to produce additional improvement.
Adapted from Watling SM, Dasta JF. Prolonged paralysis in intensive care unit patients after the use of neuromuscular blocking agents: a review of the literature. Crit Care Med 1994;22:884.

when extubated because of the effects of residual muscle relaxant on the upper airway muscles. The definitive clinical test for complete reversal of neuromuscular blockage is the patient's ability to sustain a head lift from the bed for 5 seconds.

Narcotics and Other Intravenous Analgesics

Narcotics and synthetic analogues belong to the class of drugs called *opioids*. The most commonly used drugs in this family are morphine, meperidine, and codeine. Since the mid-1980s, a series of synthetic narcotics have been developed, with fentanyl as the prototype. More recently developed synthetics (sufentanil, alfentanil, and remifentanil) are more potent and of shorter duration (Table 13.4). Narcotics produce profound analgesia and respiratory depression. They have no amnesic properties, no direct myocardial depressive effects, and no muscle-relaxant properties. Narcotics can produce significant hemodynamic effects indirectly by releasing histamine or blunting the patient's sympathetic vascular tone because of analgesic properties. The latter effect depends on the degree of sympathetic tone that is present. Acutely injured patients may be hypovolemic and in pain, with high sympathetic tone and peripheral vascular resistance. Patients in this condition can experience dramatic drops in systemic blood pressure with minimal doses of opioids. For this reason, it is important to titrate narcotics in small incremental doses. Because of the lack of direct myocardial depression and the absence of histamine release with the synthetic opioids, they are frequently used as the primary anesthetic in combination with an amnesic agent and a muscle relaxant in patients with significant myocardial dysfunction.

When opioids are titrated intravenously, patients first become apneic because of the respiratory depressive effect (shifting the CO_2 response curve), but they still breathe on command. As the dose increases, patients become apneic and unresponsive. An unusual side effect of high-dose intravenous opioids is chest wall muscle rigidity, which can make it extremely difficult to ventilate a patient without the assistance of a muscle relaxant.

Opioids are primarily analgesic and not amnesic. Patients can be totally aware and have substantial recall of conversations in spite of appearing completely anesthetized. All opioids can be reversed with naloxone. The duration of action of naloxone can be shorter than that of the narcotic, and patients must be observed carefully after they have been treated with naloxone. Naloxone reversal of opioids can be dangerous because the agent acutely reverses the analgesic effects not only of the opioid, but of native endorphins. Naloxone treatment has been associated with acute pulmonary edema and myocardial ischemia and should not be used electively to reverse the effects of a narcotic. It is appropriately used in an emergency situation when the airway is not controlled and the patient is not ventilating because of a narcotic overdose.

Table 13.4. ANALGESICS

Name	Potency	Sedation dose	Duration	Infusion dose
Opioids				
Morphine	1	0.02–0.1 mg/kg IV	2–7 h	—
Meperidine	0.1	0.2–1 mg/kg IV	2–4 h	—
Fentanyl	100	0.5–1 mg/kg IV	30–60 min	—
Sufentanil	1,000	Not recommended		
Alfentanil	25	10–20 mg/kg IV	10–15 min	
Remifentanil[a]	—	Not recommended	10 min	0.1 mg/kg/min 0.2
Other analgesics and anesthetics				
Propofol		0.1–0.5 mg/kg IV[b,c]	25–50 mg/kg/min	
Ketamine		0.1–0.5 mg/kg IV[b]	80 mg/kg/min	

[a]Produced apnea.
[b]May produce apnea.
[c]Produces pain on injection that can be reduced by treatment with 20 mg of lidocaine.
IV, intravenous.

Propofol

Propofol is a lipid-soluble substituted isopropyl phenol that produces a rapid induction of anesthesia in 30 seconds followed by awakening in 4 to 8 minutes. Intravenous propofol can effectively produce total anesthesia, including amnesia, analgesia, and some degree of muscle relaxation. This agent is unique because it is rapidly cleared through hepatic metabolism to inactive metabolites in such a way that the patient becomes alert very quickly after cessation of infusion. Propofol causes a lower incidence of nausea and vomiting compared with opioid or inhalation anesthetics. Propofol has important roles in intensive care units when used as a continuous-infusion sedative at dosages of 25 to 50 μg/kg/min. When the infusion is discontinued, the patient becomes alert within minutes. Propofol can produce significant hypotension when intravenous induction doses are administered. It also produces significant pain on injection. Pain can be diminished or eliminated by pretreatment with intravenous lidocaine, 0.5 mg/kg. Propofol is insoluble in aqueous solution and therefore comes dissolved in a lipid emulsion.

Ketamine

Ketamine is a phencyclidine derivative that produces anesthesia characterized by dissociation between the thalamus and limbic system. Induction of anesthesia is achieved within 60 seconds after intravenous injection of 1 to 2 mg/kg or within 2 to 4 minutes of intramuscular injection of 5 to 10 mg/kg.

Patients appear to be in a cataleptic state in which their eyes remain open with a slow nystagmic gaze. The drug produces intense amnesia and analgesia, but has been associated with unpleasant visual and auditory hallucinations that can progress to delirium. The incidence of these problems can be significantly reduced if benzodiazepines are also administered with the drug. At low doses, patients continue to ventilate spontaneously but cannot be expected to protect the airway should vomiting occur. At higher doses, ketamine acts as a respiratory depressant and produces complete apnea. Ketamine also has direct and indirect sympathetic nervous system stimulatory effects, which can be useful in hypovolemic patients. These effects are diminished or absent in patients who are catecholamine depleted. The sympathetic stimulatory effect increases myocardial oxygen consumption and intracranial pressure, and ketamine is relatively contraindicated in patients with ischemic heart disease or space-occupy-

ing intracerebral lesions. Ketamine is frequently used as an intravenous analgesic during débridement procedures, at doses listed in Table 13.4.

Amnesics and Anxiolytics

Benzodiazepines are the primary class of agents used as amnesics and anxiolytics. The prototype drug, diazepam, has been largely replaced by its water-soluble analogue of shorter duration, midazolam. Lorazepam also belongs in this family of agents, but because it has a very long duration of action, it is not routinely used during surgery. Lorazepam has intensive care unit applications (Table 13.5). Benzodiazepines produce anxiolysis and some degree of amnesia, but have no analgesic properties. During surgery, midazolam is always used in conjunction with an opioid or inhalation agent. Midazolam can be used in combination with the short-acting opioid, fentanyl, to produce conscious sedation for minor procedures. Benzodiazepines can produce apnea and have synergistic effects with narcotics. Very small doses of midazolam and fentanyl can quickly produce an unconscious, apneic patient. As with all anesthetics, benzodiazepines used as intravenous agents for sedation should be given in small, incremental doses to achieve the desired effect. A reversal agent, flumazenil, is also available for benzodiazepines. The recommended dosages of these drugs and their reversal agent appear in Table 13.5.

Local Anesthetics

Local anesthetics constitute a class of drugs that temporarily block nerve conduction by binding to neuronal sodium channels. As the concentration of the local anesthetic increases around the nerve, autonomic transmission is blocked first, followed by sensory transmission and then motor nerve transmission. These drugs can be injected locally into tissue to produce a field block, around peripheral nerves to produce a specific dermatome block, or into the spinal or epidural space to produce a major conduction block.

Adverse consequences associated with the use of local anesthetics fall into three categories: acute central nervous system toxicity due to excessive plasma concentration, hemodynamic and respiratory consequences due to excessive conduction block of the sympathetic or motor nerves, and allergic reactions. Whenever a local anesthetic is injected, there can be inadvertent intravascular injection or an overdose of the drug because of rapid uptake from the tissues. All can produce seizures. Complications can be minimized

---

Table 13.5. ANXIOLYTICS AND AMNESICS (BENZODIAZEPINES)

Name	Dose (mg/kg)	Duration (h)	Strengths	Weaknesses
Midazolam (Versed)	0.05 (infusion dose 0.25 mg/kg/min)	0.5	Water soluble Short duration Good for sedation for short procedures	Acute respiratory depression
Diazepam (Valium)	0.1	1	Intermediate duration	Irritation on IV injection Phlebitis Acute respiratory depression after IV overdose
Lorazepam (Ativan)	0.02–0.08	6–8	Long duration	—
Benzodiazepine reversal Flumazenil (Romazicon)	4–20 mg/kg (0.2 mg repeated every 2–10 min until reversal is achieved) Maximum dose 1 mg	45–90 min	—	May produce seizures, panic, arrhythmias

IV, intravenous.

TABLE 13.6. LOCAL ANESTHETICS

Name	Maximum single dose (mg)	Duration (h)	Comments
Amides			
Lidocaine	500	1[a]	Fast onset
Ropivacaine	200	4–12[a]	Less cardiac toxicity than bupivacaine
Bupivacaine intravenous injection	200	4–12[a]	Exaggerated cardiotoxicity with
			Slow onset
			Long duration
Esters[b]			
2-Chloroprocaine	1,000	0.5–1[a]	Fast onset
			Lowest toxicity
Tetracaine	80	0.5–1	Slow onset

[a]Addition of 100 mg of epinephrine (0.1 mL of 1:1,000) lowers the toxicity and increases the duration of the local anesthetic.
[b]Metabolism to para-aminobenzoic acid may cause allergic reactions.

by withdrawing before injection to avoid an intravascular injection and limiting dosages to the safe range (Table 13.6).

When local anesthetics are administered for a spinal or epidural block, they produce a progressive blockade of the sympathetic nervous system, which produces systemic vasodilatation. Sympathetic nerves travel along the thoracolumbar region with the first four thoracic branches, including the cardiac sympathetic accelerators. A sympathetic blockade of this entire region produces profound systemic vasodilatation and bradycardia. This condition is referred to as *total sympathectomy*, and the hypotension that ensues is usually below the minimal cerebral perfusion pressure required to maintain consciousness. Affected patients are bradycardic, hypotensive, unconscious, and usually apneic. This disastrous situation is easily remedied if treated quickly with a vasopressor (phenylephrine or ephedrine) and atropine. If not treated promptly, the situation proceeds to cardiac arrest. Because the level of sympathetic block is two to six dermatomal levels higher than the sensory block, it is often difficult to obtain a high spinal sensory level without approaching a total sympathectomy.

Local anesthetics are chemically divided into two groups, esters and amides. The esters (2-chloroprocaine and tetracaine) produce metabolites that are related to *p*-aminobenzoic acid and have been associated with allergic reactions. Amides (lidocaine and bupivacaine) are rarely associated with allergic reactions.

SEDATION ANALGESIA FOR MINOR SURGICAL PROCEDURES

There are a variety of minor surgical procedures that can be accomplished safely and comfortably with anesthesia provided by infiltration of local anesthetics (most commonly 1% lidocaine) and mild sedation/anxiolysis provided by intravenous benzodiazepines. All intravenous benzodiazepines, narcotics, and other intravenous anesthetics produce apnea if given in a high enough dose. Because there is substantial patient-to-patient variability in response to a given dose, it is important that intravenous anxiolytics be given in small, incremental doses slowly to achieve a safe sedated state. Another important factor to remember is that the anesthesia is provided by infiltration of the local anesthetic and not by the intravenous sedative. Intravenous agents, including narcotics, cannot overcome the pain associated with a surgical incision. If large doses of narcotics are given for this purpose, once the surgical stimulus ends, the patient may quickly become apneic. The duration of the respiratory depression for even short-acting narcotics is much longer than the painful stimulus of the incision. Because of the potentially serious consequences of an apneic episode, the regulatory agencies have required that all patients undergoing sedation for minor surgical or medical procedures have the following (3):

1. A preprocedure evaluation, including an airway examination
2. Appropriate monitoring: pulse oximetry as a minimum
3. Documentation of the patient's vital signs and arterial oxygen saturation as well as the dose and timing of sedatives provided during the procedure
4. Documentation of a recovery period and a return to a safe recovered state

The preprocedure evaluation should include current medications, coexisting disease, and a brief physical ex-

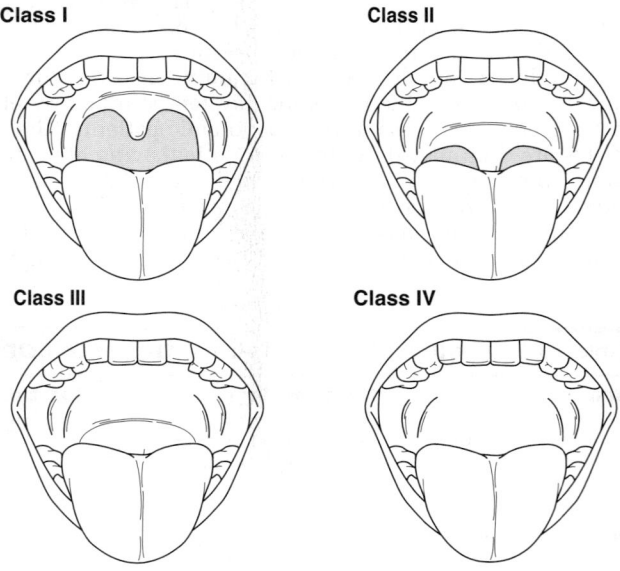

Figure 13.1. Classification of the patient's upper airway based on the size of the tongue and the pharyngeal structures visible on mouth opening. Class I, soft palate, anterior–posterior tonsillar pillars, and uvula visible; class II, tonsillar pillars and part of uvula hidden by base of tongue; class III, soft and hard palate visible; class IV, soft palate not visible, only hard palate visible. (Adapted from Stoelting RK, Miller RD, eds. *Basics of anesthesia,* 3rd ed. New York: Churchill Livingston, 1994:146, with permission.)

Table 13.7. SEDATION SCALE

Sedation scale	Description
1	Awake and alert
2	Awake and sedated
3	Asleep but arousable to touch or verbal stimuli
4	Asleep but arousable to painful stimulus
5	Asleep and not arousable to painful stimulus

amination that includes an evaluation of the airway. It is important to determine how difficult it may be to obtain control of the airway if a patient should become apneic. Although there is no absolute standard to predict a difficult intubation, a simple four-step examination helps to determine the likelihood. First, the patient should have a normal mouth opening. Second, the patient should have normal neck flexion and extension. Third, the physician should be able to fit three fingerwidths under the patient's chin between the thyroid cartilage and the mentum. Finally, when the patient opens his or her mouth and is asked to stick out the tongue, the airway can be classified depending on whether the uvula can be completely seen (class 1), only partly seen (class 2), or not seen, with only the hard and soft palate visible (class 3), or if only the hard palate visible (class 4; Fig. 13.1.). This classification roughly predicts progressive difficulty in intubating because of difficulty in visualizing the larynx (4).

The most common drug used to provide sedation is midazolam. This agent is a fast-onset, relatively short-acting benzodiazepine that can be easily titrated to produce a sedated, yet cooperative arousable state. It is usually given to adults in incremental doses of 1 mg (0.01 mg/kg in children). Adding narcotics, such as fentanyl, even in small doses acts synergistically with benzodiazepines to cause a more sedated state with a much higher incidence of apnea. To assess the effect of the drug, a sedation scale can be of value. The scale used at the University of Michigan is presented in Table 13.7.

RISKS ASSOCIATED WITH ANESTHESIA

Because the anesthetic agents effectively obtund or completely block nearly all physiologic protective mechanisms, there is an associated risk even without a surgical procedure. Fortunately, with the advent of newer agents and monitoring techniques, it is estimated that the mortality rate due to anesthesia alone has decreased from approximately 1 in 10,000 patients in the 1950s to as low as 1 in 100,000 or less for healthy patients today (5). Although a 1 in 100,000 risk of death or serious neurologic impairment may appear small, when these events occur in a young patient undergoing a purely elective procedure, the consequences are devastating for everyone involved. When patients are placed in a condition in which they cannot breathe, there is always the possibility of a technical or judgmental error resulting in hypoxia and brain damage or death. It has been estimated that between 50% and 75% of anesthetic-related deaths are due to human error and are preventable. Because the consequences of an anesthetic mishap are usually severe, the emotional and financial costs are high.

The most common problems associated with adverse outcomes are related to the airway and include inadequate ventilation, unrecognized esophageal intubation, unrecog-

nized extubation, and unrecognized disconnection from the ventilator. The incidence of these problems has been significantly reduced by including capnometry and pulse oximetry in addition to other noninvasive monitors, although a cause-and-effect relation has been difficult to prove. Efforts to improve outcome can be approached at three levels: (a) reduction of the incidence of rare but catastrophic anesthetic-related problems, (b) improvement of the care and experience of every patient undergoing anesthesia and surgery, and (c) improvement of the preparation and management of patients with preexisting medical conditions who have higher morbidity and mortality rates. The first goal has been addressed in part with improved monitoring techniques and anesthesia training. Others have been advanced by the addition of comprehensive pain management, as discussed later in this chapter. Issues of preexisting medical disease and how they affect the anesthetic plan are also briefly discussed later in this chapter.

Cardiovascular Diseases

Hypertension

Hypertension is the most common preexisting medical disease in patients presenting for surgery. Hypertensive patients should be treated medically to render them normotensive before elective surgery. These medications should be continued throughout the perioperative period. The incidence of intraoperative hypotension and myocardial ischemia is higher in untreated hypertensive patients than in adequately treated hypertensive patients if the preoperative diastolic pressure is 110 mm Hg or higher (6). Inadequately treated hypertensive patients undergoing carotid endarterectomies have an increased incidence of neurologic deficits, and those with a history of prior myocardial infarctions have an increased incidence of reinfarction. Patients commonly have an elevated blood pressure on admission to the hospital. Hypertensive patients can have exaggerated responses to painful stimuli and have a higher incidence of perioperative ischemia.

Coronary Artery Disease

Much of the anesthetic preoperative evaluation is directed toward detecting the presence and determining the degree of ischemic heart disease. Coronary artery disease is present in approximately 25% of patients who undergo surgery each year (6). Coronary artery disease is the leading cause of death in the United States and continues to be a major cause of postoperative morbidity and mortality. The goal of the preoperative cardiac evaluation is to identify patients who are at increased risk of perioperative cardiac morbidity.

Although perioperative cardiac events are the leading cause of death after anesthesia and surgery, it has been difficult to define patient characteristics that accurately predict a high risk of adverse outcome (7). Preoperative congestive heart failure (CHF) is clearly a significant risk factor, as is recent myocardial infarction or unstable angina. Diabetes mellitus, atherosclerotic vascular disease, and hypertension also appear to confer risk, although less than CHF or unstable angina. Perioperative risk in patients with valvular heart disease varies with the severity of the disease as represented by CHF, pulmonary hypertension, and dysrhythmias. Dysrhythmias are also a concern in the presence of coronary artery disease. Age and stable angina remain controversial as predictors of perioperative risk, with equal numbers of supporting and refuting studies. Previous coronary artery bypass grafting appears to confer protection against perioperative cardiac events. Because of the incidence of silent ischemia, especially in patients with diabetes mellitus, patients in high-risk groups (i.e., men older than 40, women older than 50 years of age) should be evaluated with preoperative electrocardiography (ECG). In patients without significant pulmonary disease, the ability to climb two flights of stairs without stopping or experiencing symptoms of angina or shortness of breath is considered a good practical test of cardiac reserve. Unfortunately, many patients with ischemic heart disease have concomitant pulmonary disease or other medical problems that limit their activity. The resting 12-lead ECG remains the most cost-effective screening test for ischemic heart disease. The ECG may be normal in patients with extensive ischemic heart disease and does not detect the presence of prior subendocardial myocardial infarction. For patients in high-risk groups, further stress evaluations may be required.

A history of myocardial infarction is important information. Large retrospective studies have found that the incidence of reinfarction is related to the time elapsed since the previous myocardial infarction (7–9). The incidence of reinfarction appears to stabilize at approximately 6% after 6 months. The highest rate of reinfarction occurs in the 0- to 3-month period. The mortality rate from reinfarction for patients undergoing noncardiac surgery has been reported to be between 20% and 50%, and the event usually occurs within the first 48 hours after surgery. Invasive hemodynamic monitoring with a pulmonary artery catheter and aggressive pharmacologic intervention have been shown to reduce reinfarction rates (Table 13.8). The incidence of reinfarction is also increased in patients undergoing intrathoracic or intraabdominal procedures lasting longer than 3 hours (7). The site of surgery and anesthetic technique have not been shown to change the incidence of reinfarction if the procedure is shorter than 3 hours (6). Patients with known three-vessel or left main coronary artery disease are at increased risk, whereas those who have undergone prior coronary artery bypass grafting are at a substantially decreased risk of reinfarction. Although prophylactic therapy with beta blockers, calcium channel blockers, and nitrates has not been proven beneficial, withdrawal of these agents has been associated with perioperative ischemia, myocardial infarction, and death (7).

All patients in high-risk groups or with a history of ischemic heart disease must be evaluated and properly treated before elective surgery. All elective surgery should be delayed for 6 months after myocardial infarction. If this is not feasible, invasive monitoring should be considered in the perioperative period and intensive postoperative observation should continue for at least 48 hours.

Congestive Heart Failure

Congestive heart failure has been described as the single most important factor predicting postoperative cardiac morbidity (10) (Table 13.9). All elective surgical procedures should be deferred until CHF is treated. If surgery cannot be deferred, aggressive perioperative management is warranted with a goal of optimizing cardiac output. In contrast to isolated ischemic heart disease, CHF is more easily diagnosed by history, physical examination, and basic preoperative laboratory work-up, including ECG and chest radiography. Because patients with left, right, or both left and right ventricular dysfunction are less tolerant of the fluid shifts associated with surgery and the myocardial depression associated with the anesthetic, they constitute the highest-risk group for postoperative cardiac complications.

Pulmonary Disease

Pulmonary disease is divided into acute and chronic restrictive and obstructive disease. Restrictive disease is defined by processes that reduce lung volumes, and obstructive disease is characterized by reduced flow rates on pulmonary function tests. Restrictive diseases are further subdivided into intrinsic and extrinsic forms. Intrinsic disease includes adult respiratory distress syndrome, and extrinsic disease is usually due to external restriction of lung volume by chest wall deformities or the patient's excessive weight. Although restrictive diseases can produce significant pulmonary dysfunction, less anesthetic preparation is necessary for these patients. A more sophisticated ventilator may be needed in the perioperative period.

Obstructive diseases are present in patients with ratios of the 1-second forced expiratory volume to forced vital capacity of less than 50%. Obstructive pulmonary disease can be either chronic or acute (e.g., asthma). In either case, the reversible component of obstruction should be reversed before elective surgery. Patients are maintained on bronchodilator medications, and those with chronic secretions are appropriately hydrated and receive therapy to mobilize secretions. In patients with reactive airway disease, the endotracheal tube can induce severe bronchospasm. Even in patients who are well treated before surgery, reactive bronchospasm can complicate anesthetic induction and the emergence from anesthesia. The principal method used to prevent or diminish this foreign body-induced bronchospasm is intubation of the patient at a deep level of anesthesia when reflexes are blunted. The classic way to manage a patient with severe asthma is to induce with an agent that produces bronchodilation and to ventilate the patient with an inhalation agent until the patient is deeply anesthetized before laryngoscopy and intubation. The patient should be extubated while spontaneously ventilating, but with the inhalation agent still in effect. The patient is brought back to consciousness while ventilating by mask. Unfortunately, this technique may not be feasible in patients who have a full stomach because of the risk of aspiration, or in those who are difficult to intubate or ventilate.

For elective surgery, patients should not be wheezing, and chronic patients should have no signs of bacterial infection, such as purulent sputum. Chest physiotherapy combined with hydration helps to remove secretions from the airways. The preoperative use of intermittent positive-

---

Table 13.8. RISK OF MYOCARDIAL REINFARCTION AFTER SURGERY WITH AGGRESSIVE HEMODYNAMIC MONITORING AND INTERVENTIONS AND POSTOPERATIVE INTENSIVE CARE UNIT ADMISSION

Age of previous infarction (mo)	Reinfarction rate (%)
7–12	1.0
3–6	2.3
0–3	5.8

From Rao TKL, Jacobs KH, El Etr AA. Reinfarction following anesthesia in patients with myocardial infarction. Anesthesiology 1983;59:499.

Table 13.9. **CLINICAL FACTORS INDEPENDENTLY RELATED TO PERIOPERATIVE CARDIAC COMPLICATIONS**

Criteria	Points
S_3 gallop or jugular venous distention on preoperative physical examination	11
Transmural or subendocardial myocardial infarction in the previous 6 mo	10
Premature ventricular beats, more than 5 beats/min documented at any time	7
Rhythm other than sinus or presence of premature atrial contractions on last preoperative electrocardiogram	5
Age over 70 y	4
Emergency operations	3
Intrathoracic, intraperitoneal, or aortic site of surgery	3
Evidence for important valvular aortic stenosis	3
Poor general medical condition[a]	3

Total points	Risks of cardiac complication (%)	Risk of death (%)
0–5	0.7	0.2
6–12	5	2
13–25	11	2
≥26	22	5

[a]As evidenced by electrolyte abnormalities, renal insufficiency, abnormal blood gases, abnormal liver status, or any condition that has caused the patient to become chronically bedridden.
From Goldman L, Caldera DC, Nussbaum SR, et al. Multifactorial index of cardiac risk in noncardiac surgical procedures. N Engl J Med 1977;297:845.

pressure breathing has not been shown to decrease the incidence of postoperative pulmonary complications.

Regional anesthetics can be useful in these patients for peripheral surgery or for procedures that require an anesthetic sensory level below T6. As the sensory and motor levels rise to T6 and above, patients lose significant accessory motor function that can decrease expiratory reserve volume and the ability to cough and clear secretions. Because of tenuous pulmonary status and the high incidence of postoperative pulmonary complications, pulmonary patients should be extubated with caution only when they meet adequate extubation criteria relative to preoperative test data. Changes in pulmonary mechanics and frequency of postoperative pulmonary complications are greatest after upper abdominal surgery. Both vital capacity and functional residual capacity are reduced, reaching lowest levels in the first 24 hours after surgery. In high-risk groups, therapy should be directed toward restoring functional residual capacity to preoperative levels. Such therapy improves compliance and gas exchange. Because of the potential adverse effects of systemic narcotics on respiratory drive, the use of epidural narcotics and local anesthetics for postoperative pain control is very popular. These techniques allow the patients to be extubated earlier and, in patients with intrathoracic and upper abdominal surgery, help restore pulmonary function toward preoperative values (11).

Obesity

Obesity causes a host of problems on both sides of the surgical drapes. Obesity is defined as being 20% over ideal body weight. Ideal body weight can be easily estimated as height (cm) − 100 = ideal body weight (kg). The pathophysiologic changes associated with morbid obesity (twice the ideal body weight) affect the respiratory, cardiovascular, and gastrointestinal systems. Patients have an external restrictive disease that reduces functional residual capacity and worsens with the supine position. Breathing effort increases and ventilation becomes diaphragmatic and position dependent. Obese patients frequently desaturate at night and have a high incidence of sleep apnea. Because of increased blood volume and fre-

quent desaturations, pulmonary hypertension and right-sided heart failure can develop in obese patients. Obese people have a high incidence of coronary artery disease. Because of size alone, they have increased cardiovascular demands with limited cardiac reserve and exercise tolerance. Obese patients have a high incidence of hiatal hernia and gastroesophageal reflux, increasing the risk for aspiration on induction and emergence from anesthesia. Because of fatty liver infiltration and fat deposits elsewhere, these patients may experience prolonged effects of anesthetics and other analgesics. Issues as mundane as venous access can cause significant problems in this patient group.

The primary concern of the anesthesiologist is gaining adequate control of the airway. The combined problems of aspiration risk, rapid desaturation caused by reduced functional residual capacity and increased oxygen demand, and the technical difficulties associated with intubation due to anatomic fat deposits make intubation a high-risk procedure. If problems occur, there can be significant technical difficulties in obtaining a rapid cricothyrotomy. For these reasons, a nasal or oral awake intubation can be useful. All patients should receive prophylactic administration of histamine (H_2) receptor antagonists and metoclopramide to decrease the volume of gastric contents. If intubations are to be done after induction of anesthesia, they should be performed in a rapid sequence using cricoid pressure. To prevent aspiration on emergence, obese patients should be extubated when fully awake, preferably in the sitting position. Regional anesthetics can be very useful when peripheral procedures are planned. Unfortunately, morbidly obese patients can experience pulmonary failure just by laying flat, making it difficult to use epidural or spinal anesthetics for abdominal procedures. Epidural analgesics for postoperative pain management allow earlier extubation and ambulation of these patients (11).

Overall hospital mortality rates increase when several chronic diseases are present. Investigators have found that renal failure and CHF are associated with the highest increases in hospital mortality rates, especially in the elderly undergoing emergency procedures (12) (Table 13.10).

Table 13.10. HOSPITAL MORTALITY RATES IN RELATION TO AGE, PREOPERATIVE DISEASE, AND SURGERY

Preoperative disease and surgery	Age (y)[a]		
	<50	**50–69**	**>70**
Chronic heart failure	0.1%/0.5%	0.4%/2%	0.8%/4%
Renal failure	0.2%/1%	0.9%/2%	2%/9%
Abdominal surgery	0.3%/2%	1%/6%	3%/12%
Chronic heart failure and renal failure	0.7%/3%	3%/13%	6%/24%
Chronic heart failure and abdominal surgery	0.9%/4%	4%/17%	7%/30%
Renal failure and abdominal surgery	2%/8%	2%/32%	16%/50%
Chronic heart failure, renal failure, and abdominal surgery	6%/26%	22%/60%	37%/76%

[a]Figures are for elective surgery (first number) and emergency surgery (second number).
From Pederson T, Eliasen K, Henriksen E. A prospective study of mortality associated with anesthesia and surgery: risk indicators of mortality in hospitals. Acta Anaesthesiol Scand 1990;34:176.

RISKS IN PATIENTS RECEIVING LOW-MOLECULAR-WEIGHT HEPARIN

Low-molecular-weight heparin (LMWH) has become a routine method of prophylactically treating patients who are at risk for deep venous thrombosis. LMWH has several advantages over traditional heparin and has been widely adopted in Europe and the United States. Unfortunately, there has been an increased number of reported cases of epidural hematoma formation when regional anesthetics are provided in patients who are being treated with LMWH (13). For that reason, the Society of Regional Anesthesia has published the following guidelines for central conduction block (spinal and epidural anesthesia) to minimize the incidence of this devastating complication:

1. The presence of blood during needle and catheter placement requires delay of 24 hours after surgery before initiation of LMWH therapy.
2. For patients on LMWH (once-daily dosing), needle placement should occur at least 12 hours after last LMWH dose. For patients receiving higher dosing (e.g., enoxaparin 1 mg/kg twice a day), placement should occur at least 24 hours after last LMWH dose.
3. It is recommended that patients who have an indwelling epidural catheter receive LMWH only when there is an extreme risk of deep venous thrombosis, there is frequent monitoring of the patient's neurologic status (every hour), and the catheter is not removed within 12 hours of last dose.
4. After removal of the epidural catheter, LMWH dosing should not occur for at least 2 hours (13).

PREOPERATIVE EVALUATION

The three goals of the preoperative evaluation are (a) to develop an anesthetic plan that considers the patient's medical condition, the requirements of the surgical procedure, and the patient's preferences; (b) to ensure that the patient's chronic disease is under appropriate medical therapy before an elective procedure; and (c) to gain rapport with and the confidence of the patient, answer any questions, and allay fears.

Optimally, to complete this task, an anesthesiologist would meet every patient before the planned surgical procedure to review the medical history, complete a physical examination, discuss the options and associated anesthetic risks, and develop an anesthetic plan. The anesthesiologist prefers to have a comprehensive evaluation of the medical status by the patient's family practitioner or internist, including the results of pertinent laboratory studies. In the past, this was accomplished when the anesthesiologist visited the patient in the hospital the night before surgery. Currently, it is rare to have patients admitted the night before surgery, even before the most comprehensive and complex surgical procedures. The evaluation must still be accomplished, but it must be done on an ambulatory basis, which creates associated logistical problems.

A patient's medical condition should be optimized before an elective surgical procedure. This optimization is best performed by the primary care physician, with medical specialty consultation if necessary. If the procedure is deemed a surgical emergency, the anesthesiologist is responsible for assessing the patient quickly, developing the appropriate anesthetic plan, and proceeding to the operating room as soon as possible. In an emergency situation, the anesthesiologist is not obligated to seek medical consultation to evaluate chronic medical problems because time is essential. The following questions must be answered when evaluating a patient undergoing an elective surgical procedure: What must be included in the preoperative evaluation? Who is involved in this process? When and where are all the steps in this process to be conducted? How should all the information be coordinated so that it is available to the appropriate personnel at the appropriate time?

The following steps must be completed before moving the patient into the operating room:

1. A history and physical examination
2. Appropriate laboratory studies and medical consultations
3. An anesthesiologist preoperative evaluation with assignment of an American Society of Anesthesiologists (ASA) physical status (PS)
4. Discussion with the patient of the options and risks
5. Development of an anesthetic plan

The history and physical examination have repeatedly been shown to be the most valuable parts of the preoperative assessment. It is primarily the surgeon's responsibility to obtain a history that includes current medical conditions, current medication, and previous surgical and anesthetic history. Questions that are of unique interest to the anesthesiologist are those that involve previous anesthetic problems experienced by the patient or blood relatives, and the patient's exercise tolerance. This evaluation not only determines the laboratory tests that may be required, but allows for the assignment of ASA physical status (Table 13.11). The classification serves as a general measure of the patient's state of well-being, taking into account all problems the patient brings to the operating

Table 13.11. PHYSICAL STATUS CLASSIFICATION OF THE AMERICAN SOCIETY OF ANESTHESIOLOGISTS

Physical status classification	Description
PS-1	A normal, healthy patient
PS-2	A patient with mild systemic disease that results in no functional limitation
	Examples: Hypertension, diabetes mellitus, chronic bronchitis, morbid obesity, extremes of age
PS-3	A patient with severe systemic disease that results in functional limitation
	Examples: Poorly controlled hypertension, diabetes mellitus with vascular complications, angina pectoris, prior myocardial infarction, pulmonary disease that limits activity
PS-4	A patient with severe systemic disease that is a constant threat to life
	Examples: Congestive heart failure, unstable angina pectoris, advanced pulmonary, renal, or hepatic dysfunction
PS-5	A moribund patient who is not expected to survive without the operation
	Examples: Ruptured abdominal aneurysm, pulmonary embolus, head injury with increased intracranial pressure
PS-6	A declared brain-dead patient whose organs are being removed for donor purposes
Emergency operation (E)	Any patient in whom an emergency operation is required
	Example: An otherwise healthy 30-year-old woman who requires dilation and curettage for moderate but persistent vaginal bleeding (PS-1E)

room, including systemic disturbances caused by the surgical illness. Although studies of anesthetic mortality show a correlation with the physical status classification, this categorization does not describe the risk directly. The risk of any operation is determined not only by patient-related factors, but by procedure-specific ones. For patients with complex medical problems, it is frequently helpful to supplement the surgical history and physical examination with a recent assessment by the patient's primary physician.

The value of preoperative laboratory studies has undergone substantial reevaluation since the mid-1980s. In the past, a surgical procedure was an opportunity to obtain a battery of baseline laboratory tests, even for ASA PS-I patients. The current thinking is that a laboratory test should not be ordered unless a change in the surgical or anesthetic plan is anticipated. The only preoperative screening test required at the University of Michigan, for example, is an ECG within a year of the planned surgical procedure for men older than 40 and women older than 50 years of age. Pregnancy tests should be obtained only for women who state that they could be pregnant. For procedures with significant anticipated blood loss, a type and crossmatch is ordered, and a preoperative hematocrit is also required. All other tests should have an indication based on history and physical examination. A current strategy for selecting tests indicated by patient history is presented in Table 13.12. Electronic patient questionnaires have also been developed, allowing the appropriate laboratories to be selected based on the patient's response to questions (14).

There has been significant controversy regarding the minimum level for serum potassium for elective surgical procedures. In the mid-1980s, several studies noted that patients undergoing procedures with lower-than-normal potassium levels did not show an increased incidence of cardiac rhythm disturbances (15,16). Although these studies were relatively small (150 patients and 447 patients, respectively), they did conclude that potassium levels of less than 3.5 mmol/L did not appear to increase the intraoperative risk of arrhythmias. More recently, a large study of 2,402 patients undergoing elective coronary artery bypass surgery noted significantly different results (17). Wahr et al. found that perioperative arrhythmia and the need for cardiopulmonary resuscitation increased as the preoperative serum potassium level

decreased below 3.5 mmol/L (17). Although the ischemic myocardium is more prone to dysrhythmias, this is the first time that increased morbidity has clearly been demonstrated (17). It is not known if these results should be extrapolated to patients without ischemic heart disease, but it does open the question of the advisability of proceeding with elective surgery with a potassium level below 3.5 mEq/dL.

The options for anesthetic techniques and the attendant anesthetic risks are best discussed by the anesthesiologist who will provide the anesthetic. If the surgeon prefers a specific anesthetic technique, this is best communicated directly to the anesthesiologist rather than recommended to the patient. The development of the anesthetic plan must be determined by the anesthesiologist.

The history and physical examination and laboratory studies should be performed by the surgeon as soon as the surgical procedure is scheduled. The results of the laboratory studies must be evaluated well in advance of the day of surgery so that positive findings can be attended to in a timely manner. For healthy patients (ASA PS-I and PS-II), the preoperative anesthetic assessment can be conducted by the anesthesiologist on the day of the procedure. If patients have complex medical problems (ASA PS-III or greater) or have significant concerns they want to discuss with an anesthesiologist, they should be evaluated before the day of surgery. Because of the logistical problems of scheduling, most institutions have developed preoperative anesthesia clinics where this process can take place. When specialty medical consultation is considered, the following questions should be answered: Does this patient have ischemic heart disease that requires further medical management or workup? What is the degree of functional improvement of the organ system in question? Is medical treatment of these problems optimized? If not, what needs to be done, and how long will it take?

An obvious problem that concerns anesthesiologists is the potential for a difficult intubation. This can be quickly assessed, as discussed earlier (Fig. 13.1). Even if a patient has no medical problem, the possibility of a difficult airway warrants that the patient be seen before surgery and evaluated. These patients can always be approached by an awake fiberoptic technique, but this takes planning and can cause a significant delay if there is no prior warning.

Table 13.12. **SIMPLIFIED STRATEGY FOR PREOPERATIVE TESTING**[a]

Preoperative condition	Hgb Male	Hgb Female	WBC	PT/PTT	PTL/BT	Electrolytes	Creatinine/ BUN	Blood glucose	AST/Alk PTase	X-ray	ECG	Pregnancy test	T/S
Procedure with blood loss	O	O	—	—	—	—	—	—	—	—	—	—	O
Procedure without blood loss	O	—	—	—	—	—	—	—	—	—	—	—	—
Neonates	—	O	—	—	—	—	—	—	—	—	—	—	—
<40 d	—	O	—	—	—	—	—	—	—	—	—	—	—
40–49 d	—	O	—	—	—	—	—	—	—	—	M	—	—
50–64 d	—	O	—	—	—	—	—	—	—	—	O	—	—
≥65–74 d	O	O	—	—	—	—	O	O	—	?	O	—	—
≥75 d	O	O	—	—	—	—	O	O	—	?	O	—	—
Cardiovascular disease	—	—	—	—	—	—	O	O	—	O	O	—	—
Pulmonary disease	O	—	—	—	—	—	—	—	—	O	O	—	—
Malignancy	O	O	L	L	—	—	—	—	—	O	—	—	—
Radiation therapy	—	—	O	—	—	—	—	—	—	O	O	—	—
Hepatic disease	—	—	—	O	—	—	—	—	O	—	—	—	—
Exposure to hepatitis	—	—	—	—	—	—	—	—	O	—	—	—	—
Renal disease	O	O	—	—	—	O	O	—	—	—	—	—	—
Bleeding disorder	—	—	—	O	O	—	—	—	—	—	—	—	—
Diabetes	O	O	—	—	—	O	O	O	—	—	O	—	—
Smoking	O	O	—	—	—	—	—	—	—	—	—	—	—
Possible pregnancy	—	—	—	—	—	—	—	—	—	—	—	O	—
Drug use	—	—	—	—	—	—	—	—	—	—	—	—	—
Diuretics	—	—	—	—	—	O	O	—	—	—	—	—	—
Digoxin	—	—	—	—	—	O	O	—	—	—	O	—	—
Steroids	—	—	—	—	—	O	—	O	—	—	—	—	—
Anticoagulants	O	O	—	O	—	—	—	—	—	—	—	—	—
CNS disease	—	—	O	—	—	O	O	O	—	—	O	—	—

[a]Not all diseases are included in this table. The physician's own judgment is needed regarding patients with diseases not listed.

?, perhaps obtain; L, obtain for leukemia only; O, obtain; M, obtain for men only; Hgb, hemoglobin; WBC, white blood cell count; PT, prothrombin time; PTT, partial thromboplastin time; PLT, platelet count; BT, bleeding time; BUN, blood urea nitrogen; AST, aspartate aminotransferase; Alk PTase, alkaline phosphatase; ECG, electrocardiogram; TT/S, blood typing and screening for unexpected antibodies; CNS, central nervous system.

MONITORING THE SURGICAL PATIENT

One of the more obvious changes in anesthesia care has been the routine use of an array of electronic monitoring devices to provide continuous surveillance of physiologic status. Because the art and science of anesthesiology involves titrating pharmacologic agents to produce desired physiologic effects, there must be a measured parameter to which drug dosages are titrated. Depending on the severity of preexisting disease and the extent and duration of the surgical procedure, invasive techniques can be used to provide comprehensive, continuous data to guide the titration of fluid therapy and cardiovascular agents.

Monitors of Oxygenation

Pulse oximetry has been called the most significant advance in patient monitoring to date. This device continuously, noninvasively, and inexpensively provides arterial hemoglobin saturation (SaO_2) and peripheral pulse by measuring light absorption in a manner similar to a laboratory cooximeter. A cooximeter shines light through a cuvette filled with a blood sample. Each hemoglobin species absorbs light in direct proportion to its concentration (Beer-Lambert law). A cooximeter requires one wavelength of light for each hemoglobin species to be measured, that is, one wavelength for oxyhemoglobin and one for reduced hemoglobin. To measure other hemoglobins, such as carboxyhemoglobin or methemoglobin, the device requires four wavelengths of light.

The pulse oximeter uses two wavelengths of light, one red and one infrared, that shine through a tissue bed, usually a finger. Opposite the light sources is a photodiode that measures the transmitted light intensity. A large proportion of the light absorbed as it passes through the tissues is not associated with arterial blood but with other components of the tissue, such as skin, muscle, bone, and venous blood. Therefore, the device analyzes only the pulsatile component of absorption and assumes that anything that pulses in the tissue bed is arterial blood, hence the name *pulse oximeter*. Actually, the pulse oximeter measures the ratio of the pulsatile component of red light absorbed to the pulsatile component of the infrared light absorbed. This ratio changes with SaO_2. The exact relation between this ratio and SaO_2 has been empirically determined from volunteer studies and is programmed into the electronics of the oximeter. If any artifacts of a pulsatile nature occur, they may be erroneously integrated into the equation, causing erroneous SaO_2 estimates.

Several things should be remembered when using the pulse oximeter. First, the device measures SaO_2 and not arterial oxygen tension (PaO_2). The PaO_2 must drop below 80 mm Hg before any significant change in SaO_2 occurs. As the PaO_2 drops below 60 mm Hg, the SaO_2 rapidly falls as the inflection point of the sigmoid oxyhemoglobin dissociation curve is approached. As a rough rule of thumb, as SaO_2 drops below 90%, the PaO_2 can be estimated by subtracting 30 points from the SaO_2. For example, an SaO_2 of 85% corresponds to a PaO_2 of 55 mm Hg. Second, the pulse oximeter measures oxygen saturation (milliliters oxygen/deciliter blood) and not arterial oxygen content (CaO_2). Although the dissolved oxygen is ignored because of its small contribution, the oxygen content is directly proportional to the SaO_2 and the hemoglobin concentration. Because the hemoglobin concentration is approximately one third of the hematocrit, the following equation can be used to estimate CaO_2:

$$CaO_2 = 0.45 \, Hct \times SaO_2 \tag{1}$$

or, if SaO_2 is 100%:

$$CaO_2 \times \tfrac{1}{2} \, Hct \tag{2}$$

The oxygen-carrying capacity of blood can be quickly assessed by spinning a hematocrit and measuring the arterial saturation with a pulse oximeter.

Because the pulse oximeter uses only two wavelengths of light, it cannot detect the presence of carboxyhemoglobin (carbon monoxide poisoning) or methemoglobin. Because the absorption characteristics of carboxyhemoglobin are similar to those of oxyhemoglobin, the pulse oximeter registers approximately the sum of both these gases. A pulse oximeter reading of 100% saturation for a patient with smoke inhalation injury may actually indicate severe carbon monoxide poisoning. The only method of determining carbon monoxide poisoning is to send an arterial blood sample for laboratory cooximeter measurement of carboxyhemoglobin. The only clinically accepted device for invasive monitoring of oxygen saturation is the pulmonary arterial oximeter catheter.

Despite the potential drawbacks, the pulse oximeter has been shown to be impressively accurate in a wide variety of patients with a tremendous variation in pulse amplitude (18).

Ventilation Monitors

By definition, a patient is appropriately ventilated when the arterial carbon dioxide tension ($PaCO_2$) is 40 mm Hg. Measuring the respiratory rate can document only the presence of ventilation, not its adequacy. Capnography, or end-tidal CO_2 monitoring, is the visual display of the CO_2 concentration at the airway. To understand the utility of capnography, it is necessary to understand dead space components and how they affect CO_2 removal from the body (19). Dead space (DS) is defined as the portion of the tidal volume (V_T) that does not participate in gas exchange.

$$V_T = DS + V_A \tag{3}$$

The alveolar volume (V_A) is the volume of the inspired gas that reaches well perfused alveoli. The remainder of the V_T, which equals the DS, can be divided into three subcomponents—apparatus dead space (DS_{ap}), anatomic dead space (DS_{an}), and alveolar dead space (DS_{al}).

$$DS = DS_{ap} + DS_{an} + DS_{al} \tag{4}$$

At the end of inspiration, the respiratory apparatus (e.g., endotracheal tube) is filled with inspired gas that should not contain CO_2. Similarly, all the anatomic airways (trachea, bronchi, and all conducting airways down to the alveoli) should be filled with inspired gas and should therefore contain no CO_2. In this model, there are two types of alveoli, those that are well perfused (alveolar gas) and those that are not perfused (DS_{al} gas). At the end of inspiration, the DS_{al} gas, because it is not perfused, does not pick up CO_2, and again contains inspired gas and no CO_2. The alveolar gas should completely equilibrate with the arterial blood and contain CO_2 at the same tension as the arterial blood; ideally, $PaCO_2$ should equal 40 mm Hg. As the patient expires, the CO_2 detected at the patient's mouth first reflects the DS_{ap} gas, which has no CO_2, followed by the DS_{an} gas, again with no CO_2, and finally the alveolar gases, containing both dead space and well perfused alveolar gas. When mixed alveolar gas reaches the airway, it produces a rapid rise in the CO_2 concentration to a level somewhere between the concentration in the alveolar gas (40 mm Hg) and the DS_{al} (0 mm Hg), depending on each component's proportionate volume. For example, if half of the alveoli are DS_{al} and $Paco_2$ equals 40 mm Hg, then the plateau value of the capnogram should be 20 mm Hg, implying that half of the alveoli are not being perfused. With inspiration, the CO_2 value again drops to 0 until another expiration, and a square wave appears again as the alveolar gas is detected at the mouth. With each breath, there should be a square wave whose height approaches the $Paco_2$ value as the amount of the DS_{al} gas approaches 0.

In a healthy young adult, there is no significant DS_{al} gas, and the end-tidal CO_2 value equals the $Paco_2$. Therefore, the difference between these values indicates the proportion of DS_{al} in the patient. The presence of a capnogram itself implies there is metabolism (the production of CO_2), circulation (blood flow to the lungs), and ventilation (respiratory rate and an intact ventilator circuit).

Providing this information on a breath-to-breath basis, the continuous capnogram is extremely useful in many critical situations. It can be used as a surveillance monitor of both the respiratory circuit and the cardiovascular system. Any acute decrease in cardiac output decreases blood flow to the lungs and increases the DS_{al}, causing an acute drop in end-tidal CO_2. For this reason, the device was originally used during neurosurgical procedures with the patient in the sitting position to detect the presence of air emboli. This principle also allows the detection of pulmonary emboli or any acute drop in cardiac output. In fact, the only acute catastrophic cardiopulmonary problem that is not detected by the capnometer is arterial desaturation. Therefore, the combination of the capnometer and the pulse oximeter is an indispensable pairing for beat-to-beat and breath-to-breath surveillance of metabolism, circulation, ventilation, and oxygenation.

Circulation Monitors

Hemodynamic stability can be monitored by a variety of methods, the most basic of which is systemic arterial blood pressure. Intermittent, noninvasive measurement of systemic blood pressure with an oscillometric blood pressure cuff is the standard in the operating room, and its accuracy equals that of clinical measurements by auscultation. Circulation monitors can be cycled as quickly as once per minute, but when used for an extended duration, they should be cycled no more than once every 3 to 5 minutes. When tighter control is required in patients with significant hypertension or serious heart disease, or in those who may sustain acute blood loss, invasive arterial monitoring is used. Although pressure measurements provided by invasive techniques differ from those of noninvasive techniques, they usually coincide closely. A continuous invasive arterial tracing can also be used to assess the adequacy of fluid resuscitation by following the systolic pressure variation with positive-pressure ventilation. A variation greater than 10 mm Hg in the systolic pressure between peak inspiration and end expiration implies inadequate preload and the need for more aggressive fluid resuscitation (20). In patients without left ventricular dysfunction who are undergoing extended surgical procedures with significant fluid shifts and potential blood loss, central venous pressure monitoring is frequently used, with pulmonary arterial catheter monitoring reserved for more critically ill pa-

tients and those with significant left ventricular dysfunction. The adequacy of circulation can be objectively documented by thermodilution cardiac output measurements and mixed venous oxygen saturation monitoring. Transesophageal echocardiography is now commonly used to assess cardiac function. This technique is easily used in the anesthetized, intubated patient and can quickly assess systolic and diastolic function as well as valvular dysfunction.

COMMON PROBLEMS IN THE POSTOPERATIVE PERIOD

Postanesthesia care units are required in any setting where surgical procedures are conducted. The increased scope of surgery and the invasive technology used to monitor sicker patients has increased the service at and training required to operate these facilities. In 1994, the ASA revised the 1988 Standards for Postanesthesia Care (Table 13.13).

The scoring systems used to assess the postoperative patient direct attention to the primary areas of concern. The postanesthesia recovery score is an attempt to evaluate postanesthesia patient status (21) (Table 13.14). This basic information should be incorporated in a record that provides clear documentation of postoperative events. Documentation should also include details of postoperative outpatient care, with a note indicating postoperative telephone contact made to elucidate problems. Problems should receive appropriate follow-up, and written postoperative discharge instructions should be provided for the patient.

Investigators have reported that 24% of patients experience a postanesthesia care unit complication. Nausea, vomiting, and the need for airway support constitute 70% of these complications (22) (Fig. 13.2). The need to maintain airway support was by far the most common respiratory complication. The duration of the procedure as well as ASA classification and type of procedure had a significant bearing on the incidence of complications in this study. Hypothermia was also a common problem that prolonged postoperative postanesthesia care unit stay (Fig. 13.3). Hypothermia has the deleterious effects of altering drug metabolism and delaying recovery. Furthermore, it causes shivering, which increases the metabolic demand for oxygen.

Among cardiovascular complications in the postoperative period, none is more important or more difficult to diagnose than myocardial ischemia. The association of perioperative myocardial ischemia with cardiac morbidity has been clearly documented (23). In a series of high-risk patients undergoing noncardiac surgery, researchers noted that "early postoperative myocardial ischemia is an important correlate of adverse cardiac outcomes" (23). Diagnosis is complicated by the facts that only 10% to 30% of patients with documented myocardial infarction have pain, and that postoperative ECG T-wave changes are often nonspecific (24). Instead, the clinician must seek secondary indications of ongoing ischemia or "angina equivalents," such as hypotension, arrhythmias, elevated filling pressures, or postoperative oliguria. Arrhythmias are common and are significant primarily because of the association with myocardial ischemia or hypoxemia.

Nausea and vomiting are rarely unifactorial and cause considerable discomfort to the patient. There is little evidence to favor one anesthetic or anesthetic technique over

Table 13.13. STANDARDS FOR POSTANESTHESIA CARE[a]

Standards		Criteria to be fulfilled
Standard I[b]	All patients who have received general, regional, or monitored anesthesia care shall receive appropriate postanesthesia management.	1. A PACU or an area that provides equivalent postanesthesia care shall be available to receive patients after anesthesia care. All patients who receive anesthesia care shall be admitted to the PACU or its equivalent except by specific order of the anesthesiologist responsible for the patient's care. 2. The medical aspects of care in the PACU shall be governed by policies and procedures that have been reviewed and approved by the department of anesthesiology. 3. The design, equipment, and staffing of the PACU shall meet requirements of the facility's accrediting and licensing bodies.
Standard II	A patient transported to the PACU shall be accompanied by a member of the anesthesia care team who is knowledgeable about the patient's condition. The patient shall be continually evaluated and treated during transport with monitoring and support appropriate to the patient's condition.	
Standard III	On arrival in the PACU, the patient shall be reevaluated and a verbal report provided to the responsible PACU nurse by the member of the anesthesia care team who accompanies the patient	1. The patient's status on arrival in the PACU shall be documented. 2. Information concerning the preoperative condition and the surgical/anesthetic course shall be transmitted to the PACU nurse. 3. The member of the anesthesia care team shall remain in the PACU until the PCAU nurse accepts responsibility for the nursing care of the patient.
Standard IV	The patient's condition shall be evaluated continually in the PACU	1. The patient shall be observed and monitored by the methods appropriate to the patient's medical condition. Particular attention shall be given to monitoring oxygenation, ventilation, circulation, and temperature. During recovery from all anesthetics, a quantitative method of assessing oxygenation such as pulse oximetry shall be employed in the initial phase of recovery. This is not intended for application during the recovery of the obstetric patient in whom regional anesthesia was used for labor and vaginal delivery. 2. An accurate written report of PACU period shall be maintained. Use of an appropriate PACU scoring system is encouraged for each patient on admission, at appropriate intervals prior to discharge, and at the time of discharge. 3. General medical supervision and coordination of patient care in the PACU should be the responsibility of an anesthesiologist. 4. There shall be a policy to ensure the availability in the facility of a physician capable of managing complications and providing cardiopulmonary resuscitation for patients in the PACU.
Standard V	A physician is responsible for discharging the patient from the PACU.	1. When discharge criteria are used, they must be approved by the department of anesthesiology and the medical staff. They may vary depending on whether the patient is discharged to a hospital room, to the ICU, to a short stay unit, or home. 2. In the absence of the physician responsible for the discharge, the PACU nurse shall determine that the patient meets the discharge criteria. The name of the physician accepting responsibility for discharge shall be noted on the record.

[a]Based on the American Society of Anesthesiologists (ASA) Standards for Postanesthesia Care. A copy of the full text can be obtained from ASA, 520 N. Northwest Highway, Park Ridge, IL 60068-2573.
[b]For nursing care issues, refer to Standards of Postanesthesia Nursing Practice, published by the American Society of Postanesthesia Nurses.
PACU, postanesthesia care unit.

Table 13.14. POSTANESTHESIA RECOVERY SCORE[a]

Parameter	Score
Activity	
Voluntary movement of all limbs to command	2
Voluntary movement of two extremities to command	1
Unable to move	0
Respiration	
Breathes deeply and coughs	2
Dyspnea, hypoventilation	1
Apneic	0
Circulation	
Blood pressure equals 80% of preanesthetic level	2
Blood pressure equals 50%–80% of preanesthetic level	1
Blood pressure equals <50% of preanesthetic level	0
Consciousness	
Fully awake	2
Arousable	1
Unresponsive	0
Color	
Pink	2
Pale, blotchy	1
Cyanotic	0

[a]Patients should score at least 7 before discharge from the postanesthesia care unit.

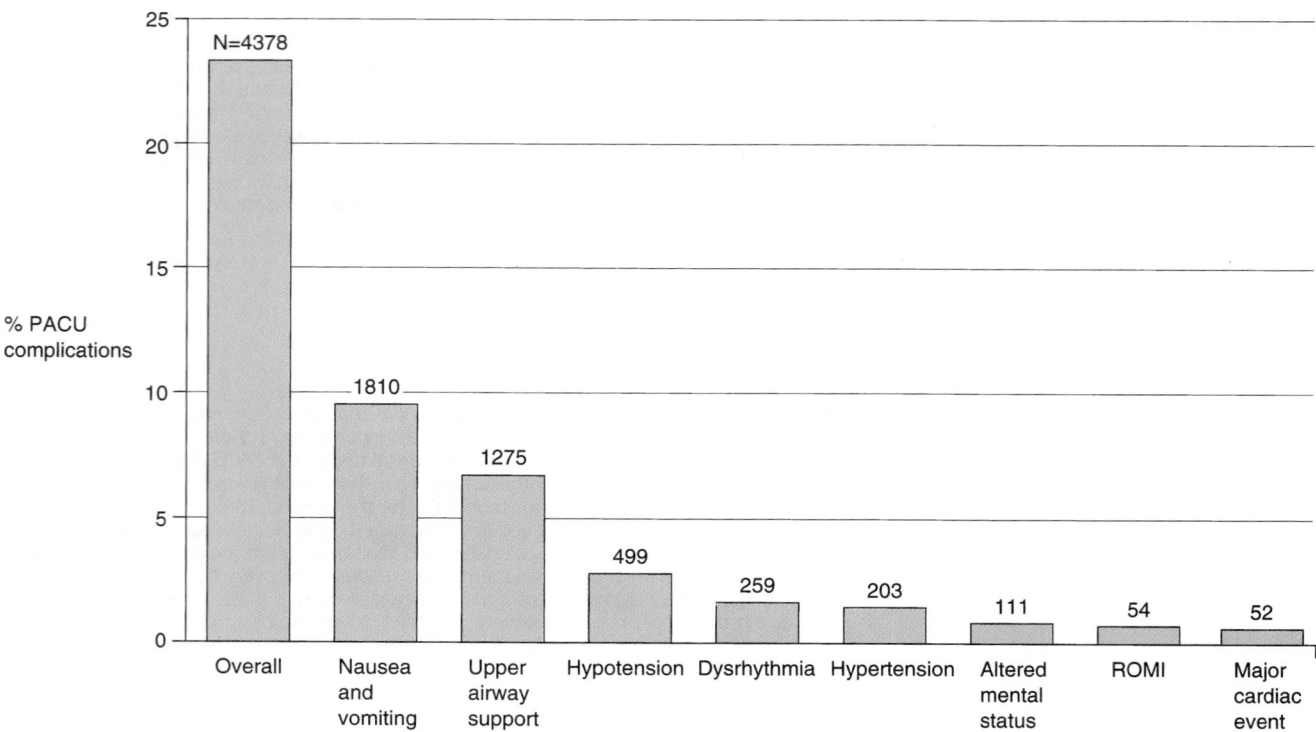

Figure 13.2. Major postanesthesia care unit complications by percentage of occurrence and number of patients experiencing each complication. Nausea and vomiting were the most frequently observed complications. ROMI, rule out myocardial infarction. (After Hines R, Barash PG, Watrous G, et al. Complications occurring in the postanesthesia care unit: a survey. *Anesth Analg* 1992;74:505.)

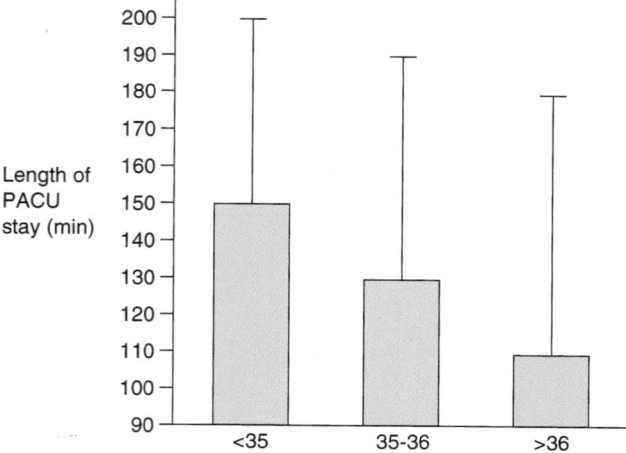

Figure 13.3. Patient body temperature at admission also affects the development of postanesthesia care unit (PACU) complications. The duration of PACU stay as a function of temperature at admission is shown. Stay was significantly reduced in patients whose temperature at admission was 36°C or higher ($p < .01$). (After Hines R, Barash PG, Watrous G, et al. Complications occurring in the postanesthesia care unit: a survey. *Anesth Analg* 1992;74:506.)

another, although propofol appears to have an antiemetic effect. Nitrous oxide, often considered causative, does not appear to increase the incidence of nausea, according to well documented studies. It is not unusual for an antiemetic agent to be included before surgery or as part of the anesthetic technique, especially in patients with a positive history or those deemed to be at risk, such as menstruating young women undergoing laparoscopy. Standard use includes phenothiazines, butyrophenones, metoclopramide, and scopolamine. The U.S. Food and Drug Administration has approved the use of the serotonin antagonist ondansetron, which was shown in several studies to be superior to other agents (25). An algorithm for the treatment of postoperative nausea and vomiting is illustrated in Fig. 13.4.

The most common cause of delayed emergence is the residual effects of anesthesia. A differential diagnosis of delayed anesthetic emergence is presented in Table 13.15. There should be little confusion about the implication of muscle relaxants because physical indications of ventilatory distress, combined with the readings of the blockade monitor, should clearly indicate the role of these drugs. Where appropriate, opioids can be reversed using titrated doses of naloxone. Flumazenil can be used for reversal of benzodiazepines.

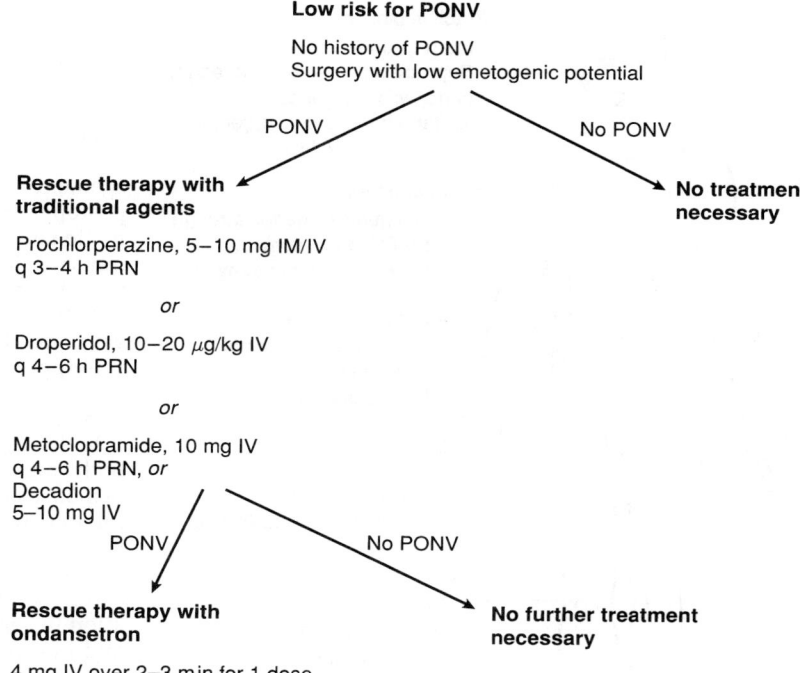

Figure 13.4. Algorithm for preventing and treating postoperative nausea and vomiting (PONV) in adults.

Table 13.15. DIFFERENTIAL DIAGNOSIS OF DELAYED EMERGENCE

Neurologic injury
  Ischemia
  Mass lesions
  Seizure disorders
Metabolic abnormalities
  Hypoglycemia
  Diabetic ketoacidosis
  Nonketotic hyperosmolar hyperglycemic coma
  Hepatic dysfunction
  Electrolyte disturbances
  Renal dysfunction
  Thyroid dysfunction
  Adrenocortical dysfunction
  Cardiorespiratory failure
  Hypothermia
  Malignant hyperthermia
Drug effects
  Inhalational anesthetics
  Opioids
  Barbiturates
  Benzodiazepines
  Ketamine
  Anticholinergics
  Muscle relaxants

POSTOPERATIVE ACUTE PAIN MANAGEMENT

Postoperative pain is an inevitable consequence of surgery. Its severity is site dependent (Table 13.16), but the magnitude of the pain experienced by individual patients after similar surgical procedures is influenced by a multitude of factors. Variation in patient experience has been clearly demonstrated by several authors and is reflected in deficiencies in postoperative pain control (26). The recognition of this clinical problem has prompted interest in underlying pain mechanisms and in innovative ways to alleviate postoperative suffering.

In 1965, the crucial role of nociceptive C-fiber feedback behavior and its modulation by cells in the substantia gelatinosa of the dorsal horn was recognized (27). Repetitive stimulation of these fibers by cellular mediators, such as kinins and catecholamines, promotes neural excitation, prolongs repetitive firing, and lowers the threshold to further excitation. As a result, C fibers do not show fatigue, and the stage is set for continuous pain. Counterirritation of large afferent activity has been shown empirically to have beneficial effects. The gate control theory provides an explanation for the inhibition of C fiber-mediated pain. Serotonergic and enkephalinergic descending inhibitory pathways modulate activity in the dorsal horn before information is relayed to the somatosensory cortex through the spinothalamic tract. The common observation that pain is worse at night, when less sensory information is processed, and that it decreases with daytime activity is

Table 13.16. PERCENTAGE OF PATIENTS WHO REQUIRE ANALGESIC INJECTIONS

Operation	No analgesic needed (%)	Three or more analgesic injections (%)
Minor chest wall	82	0
Inguinal hernia	52	0
Appendectomy	25	10
Lower abdominal surgery	18	40
Upper abdominal surgery	10	45–65

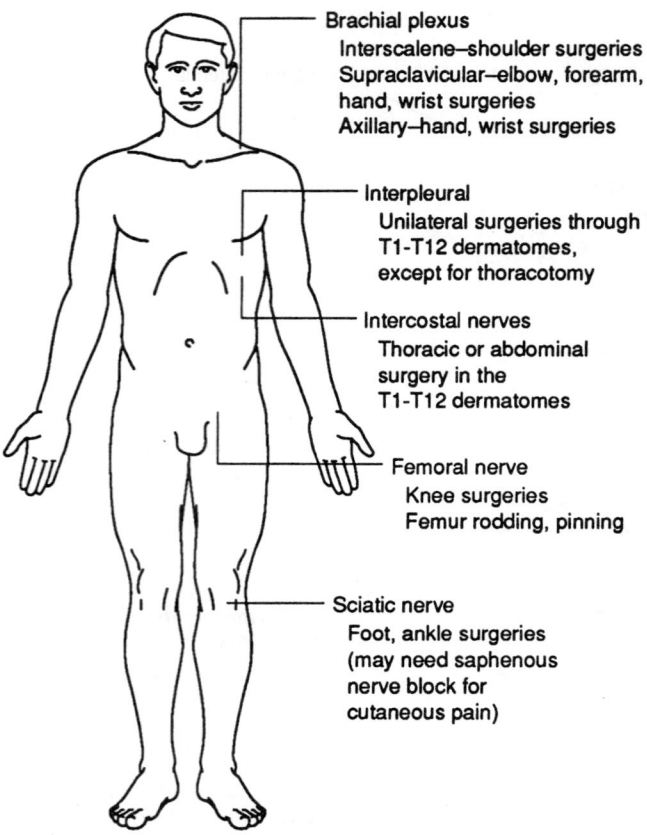

Brachial plexus
Interscalene–shoulder surgeries
Supraclavicular–elbow, forearm,
hand, wrist surgeries
Axillary–hand, wrist surgeries

Interpleural
Unilateral surgeries through
T1-T12 dermatomes,
except for thoracotomy

Intercostal nerves
Thoracic or abdominal
surgery in the
T1-T12 dermatomes

Femoral nerve
Knee surgeries
Femur rodding, pinning

Sciatic nerve
Foot, ankle surgeries
(may need saphenous
nerve block for
cutaneous pain)

Figure **13.5.** Surgical procedures in which peripheral nerve blockade can provide postoperative pain relief.

an example of how this complex neural system functions. Transcutaneous nerve stimulation is a technical attempt to use this principle.

Superficial somatic pain is well localized, has a protective function, and is readily treated by common analgesic techniques. Deep somatic pain may not be well localized, may have some protective function, as in joint immobilization, and is fairly responsive to a variety of analgesics. Visceral pain, served almost entirely by C-fiber activity, is poorly localized, often referred, and difficult to treat. In major operations, all modes can be activated, compounding the clinical challenge of providing adequate pain management. These clinical observations direct the focus of postoperative pain management to the treatment of somatic pain by attacking the nociceptor and the subsequent transmission of the painful impulse by the nerve fiber. The use of nonsteroidal antiinflammatory drugs with or without the injection of local anesthetics into the wound is very effective. If done preemptively at the time of surgery, this approach can significantly improve the patient's postoperative experience (28). Examples of nerve blocks for various procedures are shown in Fig. 13.5.

Including potent opioids in the treatment of deep pain, both somatic and visceral, has been routine. However, the responses to standard regimens have been notoriously unreliable, from inadequate pain relief to narcosis, with complications at both ends of the scale. It was not until the 1980s that variations in response were linked to variable serum concentrations of analgesic drugs. Interpatient variation in serum levels to any standard dose can be fivefold, and interpatient therapeutic concentrations can vary on a similar scale. When these are factored together, there is the potential for a 25-fold variation in patient response to a standard drug prescription. Each patient has an individual therapeutic window (Fig. 13.6), and the clinical implications of this are enormous.

In 1968, investigators demonstrated the virtue of small intravenous doses given on demand (29). As a result, the patient experienced greater pain relief, yet used the same or less total narcotic. Although there was significant patient variation, the demand from any individual patient, although cyclic, was constant. Patient-controlled analgesia (PCA) and the technologic and administrative systems to provide it have developed to a point of some sophistication, requiring servicing and a support structure with its own set of problems (Table 13.17). PCA administration requires a receptive environment, education of all personnel, and ade-

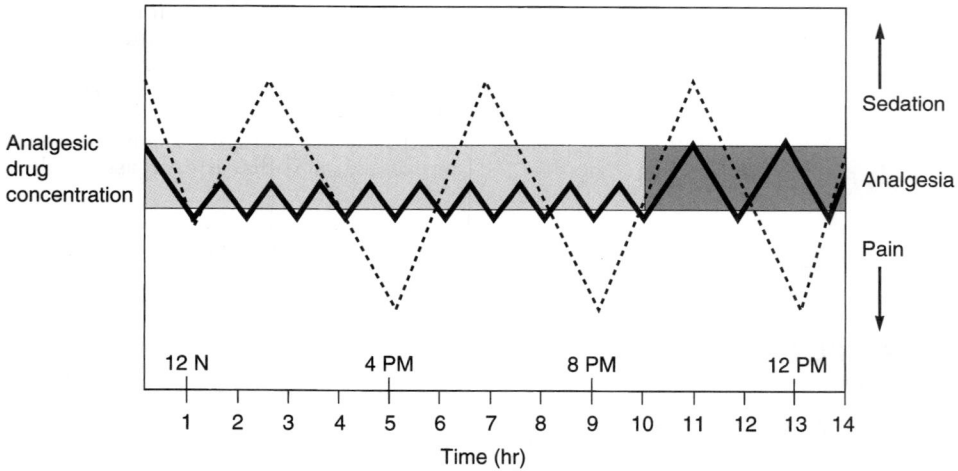

Figure **13.6.** Theoretic relation between dosing interval, analgesic drug concentration, and clinical effects when comparing a patient-controlled analgesia system *(solid line)* with conventional intramuscular therapy *(dashed line)*. (After White PF. Patient-controlled analgesia: a new approach to the management of postoperative pain. *Semin Anesth* 1985;4:261.)

Table 13.17. PROBLEMS THAT CAN OCCUR DURING PATIENT-CONTROLLED ANALGESIA THERAPY

Operator errors
  Misprogramming PCA device
  Failure to clamp or unclamp tubing
  Improperly loading syringe or cartridge
  Inability to respond to safety alarms
  Misplacing PCA pump key
Patient errors
  Failure to understand PCA therapy
  Misunderstanding PCA pump device
  Intentional analgesic abuse
Mechanical errors
  Failure to deliver on demand
  Defective one-way valve at Y-connector
  Faulty alarm system
  Device malfunctions

PCA, patient-controlled analgesia.

quate patient instruction. PCA has received widespread acceptance by patients, nursing staff, and physicians because it provides more prompt and painless analgesia that more closely matches the patient's need over time. PCA is as safe as conventional intramuscular medication. Morphine and meperidine are commonly used drugs, and an example of orders is shown in Table 13.18.

Transdermal narcotic delivery is receiving attention and may become available for postoperative pain. The method is both practical and inexpensive and aims to maintain continuous delivery and constant blood levels. Fentanyl has been the drug of choice and has been well received by patients. The method appears to be safe, but there is a significant lag time between application and the attainment of therapeutic blood levels.

The discovery of endorphins in the 1970s and recognition of their importance in modulating pain at spinal sites led to the supposition that it would be possible selectively to apply opioids directly to receptors. This led to the development of epidural opiate analgesia, in which opioids are applied directly to the receptors at spinal sites. The goal of epidural opiate analgesia is to obtain maximal analgesia while minimizing systemic side effects. For severe acute postoperative pain caused by major surgery, epidural opiate analgesia has proved to be a superior modality for pain control. In high-risk cases, there is evidence that it has an overall beneficial effect on morbidity (11). The effective use of this sophisticated modality requires education and the establishment of protocols with rigorous attention to detail. The potential for respiratory depression demands adherence to monitoring standards. Morphine and fentanyl, often in combination with a dilute local anesthetic solution, are most often prescribed. A typical order form with monitored parameters is shown in Table 13.19.

A comprehensive postoperative pain management service demands resources and must use the physical and pharmacologic modalities available, while recognizing the significant subjective component of any individual's pain problem. The ability to recognize the impact of acute pain or an underlying chronic pain disorder requires that experience be brought to bear on difficult problems. The active involvement of nursing staff and surgeons is essential for the patient to achieve maximal benefit. It is incumbent on the pain management service to render efficient, continuous, and cost-effective care.

Table 13.18. EXAMPLE OF ORDERS FOR PATIENT-CONTROLLED ANALGESIA

1. Patient is to be initiated on PCA with standard monitoring protocol.
2. Drug selection

	Morphine	Meperidine	Dilaudid	
	1 mg/mL	10 mg/mL	0.2 mg/mL	_____ mg/mL
3. Loading → Initial dose (start prn for pain)	2–4 mg	20–40 mg	0.2–0.4 mg	_____ mg
Incremental dose, q5–10 min prn	1–2 mg	10–20 mg	0.1–0.2 mg	_____ mg
Maximum total loading dose	10 mg	100 mg	1 mg	_____ mg
Other	_____ mg	_____ mg	_____ mg	_____ mg
4. Pump setting PCA dose	_____ mg	_____ mg	_____ mg	_____ mg
Lockout interval	_____ min	_____ mg	_____ mg	_____ mg
4-hour limit	_____ mg	_____ mg	_____ mg	_____ mg

PCA, patient-controlled analgesia.
From University of Michigan Hospitals form RP-2044330/982, Rev. 7/93, Acute Pain Service, Patient Controlled Analgesia Standard Orders. Ann Arbor, MI.

Table 13.19. OPIOID PROTOCOLS IN EPIDURAL OPIATE ANALGESIA

	Morphine[a]	Fentanyl[b]
Length of onset	Longer (30–60 min)	Shorter (15–30 min)
Duration	Longer (6–24 h for single bolus)	Shorter (1–2 h for single bolus)
Cephalad spread and side Effects	More prone	Less prone
Indication	Favored for lumbar administration after abdominal surgery	Favored for thoracic administration after chest surgery
Dose	Typically 3–5 mg, q6–8 h	Typically 50–75 mg/h (± dilute bupivacaine)

[a]Hydrophilic: slow in, slow out.
[b]Lipophilic: fast in, fast out.

REFERENCES

1. Calverly RK. Anesthesia as a specialty: past, present, and future. In: Barash PG, Cullen BF, Stoelting RK, eds. *Clinical anesthesia*. Philadelphia: JB Lippincott, 1992.
2. Watling SM, Dasta JF. Prolonged paralysis in intensive care unit patients after the use of neuromuscular blocking agents: a review of the literature. *Crit Care Med* 1994;22:884.
3. Joint Committee on the Accreditation of Healthcare Organizations. *Comprehensive accreditation manual for hospitals: the official handbook: conscious sedation*. Oakbrook Terrace, IL: JCAHO, 1999:73–77.
4. Mallampati SR, Gatt SP, Guigino LD, et al. A clinical sign to predict difficult tracheal intubation: a prospective study. *Can J Anaesth* 1985;32:429.
5. Miller RD. *Anesthesia*, 3rd ed. New York: Churchill Livingstone, 1990.
6. Stoelting RK, Dierdorf SF. *Anesthesia and co-existing disease*, 3rd ed. New York: Churchill Livingstone, 1993.
7. Mangano DT. Perioperative cardiac morbidity. *Anesthesiology* 1990;72:153.
8. Rao T, Jacobs K, El Etr A. Reinfarction following anesthesia in patients with myocardial infarction. *Anesthesiology* 1983;59:499.
9. Tarhan S, Moffitt EA. Myocardial infarction after general anesthesia. *JAMA* 1972;220:1451.
10. Goldman L, Caldera DC, Nussbaum SR, et al. Multi-factorial index of cardiac risk in noncardiac surgical procedures. *N Engl J Med* 1977;297:845.
11. Yaeger M, Glass D, Neff R, et al. Epidural anesthesia and analgesia in high risk surgical patients. *Anesthesiology* 1987;66:729.
12. Pedersen T, Eliasen K, Henriksen E. A prospective study of mortality associated with anaesthesia and surgery: risk indicators of mortality in hospitals. *Acta Anaesthesiol Scand* 1990;34:176.
13. Horlocker TT, Wedel DJ. Neuraxial block and low molecular weight heparin: balancing perioperative analgesia and thromboprophylaxis. *Reg Anesth Pain Med* 1998;23[Suppl 2]:164–177.
14. www.healthquiz.com.
15. Vitez TS, Soper LE, Wong KC, et al. Chronic hypokalemia and intraoperative dysrhythmias. *Anesthesiology* 1985;63:130–133.
16. Hirsch IA, Tomlinson DL, Slogoff S, et al. The overstated risk of preoperative hypokalemia. *Anesth Analg* 1988;67:131–136.
17. Wahr JA, Parks R, Boisvert D, et al. Preoperative serum potassium levels and perioperative outcomes in cardiac surgery patients. *JAMA* 1999;281:2203–2210.
18. Wahr JA, Tremper KK. Pulse oximetry. In: Blitt CD, Hines RL, eds. *Monitoring in anesthesia and critical care medicine,* 3rd ed. New York: Churchill Livingstone, 1994:385.
19. Nunn JF. Respiratory dead space and distribution of inspired gases. In: *Applied respiratory physiology*, 2nd ed. London: Butterworths, 1977:213.
20. Coriat P, Vrillon M, Perel A, et al. A comparison of systolic pressure variations and echo cardiographic estimates of end diastolic left ventricular size in patients after aortic surgery. *Anesth Analg* 1994;78:46.
21. Bonner S. Admission and discharge criteria. In: *Post anesthesia care*. CT: Prentice-Hall International, 1990.
22. Hines R, Barash PG, Waltons G, et al. Complications occurring in the postanesthesia care unit: a survey. *Anesth Analg* 1992;74:503.
23. Mangao DT, Browner WS, Hollenberg M. Association of perioperative myocardial ischemia with cardiac morbidity and mortality in men undergoing noncardiac surgery. *N Engl J Med* 1990;323:1781.
24. Breslow MJ, Miller CF, Parker SD. Changes in T-wave morphology following anesthesia and surgery: a common recovery-room phenomenon. *Anesthesiology* 1986;64:398.
25. Alou E, Himmelseher S. Ondansetron in the treatment of postoperative vomiting. *Anesth Analg* 1992;75:561.
26. Marks RM, Sacher EJ. Undertreatment of medical inpatients with narcotic analgesics. *Ann Intern Med* 1973;78:173.
27. Melzack R, Wall P. Pain mechanisms: a new theory. *Science* 1965;150:97.
28. Tverskoy M, Cozacov C, Ayache M. Post-operative pain after inguinal herniorrhaphy with different types of anesthesia. *Anesth Analg* 1990;70:29.
29. Sechzer PH. Studies in pain with the analgesic demand system. *Anesth Analg* 1971;50:1.

SURGERY: SCIENTIFIC PRINCIPLES AND PRACTICE, Third Edition, edited by Lazar J. Greenfield, Michael W. Mulholland, Keith T. Oldham, Gerald B. Zelenock, and Keith D. Lillemoe. Lippincott Williams & Wilkins Publishers, Philadelphia, © 2001.

CHAPTER 14

TUMOR BIOLOGY

STEVEN D. LEACH, A. SCOTT PEARSON, AND R. DANIEL BEAUCHAMP

Benign and malignant neoplasms represent a common cause of morbidity and mortality in the United States and around the world. Approximately 2.2 million new cases of invasive cancer are diagnosed in the U.S. each year. Among these, approximately 1 million involve either basal cell or squamous cell cancer of the skin, generally posing no risk in terms of systemic spread or cancer-related mortality. The remaining 1.2 million cases of invasive cancer exert a tremendous personal, social, and economic toll in terms of pain and suffering, shortened life, and lost productivity. While the worst of these losses remain impossible to quantify, the economic cost of cancer was estimated to be $107 billion in 1999. These costs include $37 billion for direct health care costs, $11 billion in lost productivity due to illness, and $59 billion in lost productivity due to premature death.

Thirty years ago, President Richard Nixon proclaimed a "War on Cancer" in his 1971 State of the Union Address. The tangible results of this campaign are only now being realized. In 1998, the American Cancer Society reported for the first time a reduction in both the total number of new cancer cases as well as the overall cancer death rate in the U.S. Between 1991 and 1995, the nation's cancer rate fell 2.6%. This drop was the first reported decline in this figure since record keeping was first initiated in the 1930s. While the basis for this decline in cancer deaths remains unknown, several factors are felt to contribute, including public awareness of screening and early detection programs, changes in smoking behavior, and, in some cases, the development of novel effective therapies.

During the past 25 years, tremendous strides have also been made in understanding tumor biology and the molecular basis of neoplasia. The final decades of the 20th century will likely be remembered for the birth of molecular tumor biology. During this period, gain-of-function and loss-of-function mutations were identified in human and animal cancer cells, thereby establishing the principle that tumors are generated by accumulation of mutations in oncogenes and tumor suppressor genes. Moreover, these events have now been ordered into predictable sequences that appear to underlie progression from premalignant precursors to invasive and metastatic cancer. This progress now provides a foundation for development of novel therapies directed against the specific molecular machinery of the tumor cell.

The penetrance of molecular biology into cancer therapeutics now demands that all physicians involved in the care of cancer patients become conversant in molecular oncology. To the extent that tumor biology can be defined by molecular events, so too must the cancer physician be able to understand the molecular basis for the malignant phenotype, and participate in the development of novel molecular therapeutics.

CARCINOGENESIS AND THE SPECTRUM OF NEOPLASIA

For solid tumors, most neoplasms undergo some form of progression from early premalignant lesions to fully invasive and potentially metastatic tumors. The term *neoplasm* implies a "new growth" formed by accelerated and autonomous tissue proliferation. Under this definition, neoplastic growth persists even after the stimuli that initiated the new growth are removed. Neoplasms therefore represent a distinct subset of the broader class of tumors, which includes nonneoplastic "growths" induced by inflammation, suppuration, and/or edema. For any given location, neoplasms may be characterized as benign or malignant based on the propensity for invasive growth and/or metastasis. Among malignant lesions, a neoplasm may be primary, indicating origination in the local tissue, or metastatic, implying origination from a separate regional or distant site.

For many malignant neoplasms, an orderly sequence of events characterizes the progression from premalignant precursor lesions to the fully malignant phenotype. While many of these events may occur on a molecular level without correlative changes in tissue histology, specific histologic precursors have been defined in many tissues. For many neoplasms, the initial histologic manifestation may be in the form of hyperplasia. Hyperplastic lesions are strictly defined as an increase in the number of cells in a tissue or organ. Implicit in the diagnosis of hyperplasia is the notion that the expanded cell number consists of a cell type normally found in that tissue. In many tissues, hyperplasia is felt to represent a premalignant condition that is directly responsible for generating malignant neoplasia, but hyperplasia does not imply the capacity for fully autonomous neoplastic growth, as hyperplasia may regress following withdrawal of initiating stimuli. Examples of processes in which hyperplasia has been implicated in neoplastic progression include atypical ductal hyperplasia in the breast, leukoplakia in the upper aerodigestive tract, endometrial hyperplasia in the uterus, and atypical melanocytic hyperplasia in skin.

In contrast to hyperplasia, metaplasia involves the abnormal transformation of one fully differentiated, adult tissue into another kind of differentiated tissue. Metaplasia involves an acquired transformation, rather than an abnormality in initial development, which is more accurately described as heterotypia or heteroplasia. Metaplastic transformation may involve a reprogramming of epithelial stem cells to a new differentiation pathway, and in some circumstances may also be considered a premalignant condition. Examples of metaplastic conditions associated with an increased risk of future neoplasia include glandular metaplasia of the esophagus (Barrett's esophagus), intestinal metaplasia of the stomach, and ductal metaplasia of the exocrine pancreas.

While the term *dysplasia* is broadly defined as any abnormal tissue development, in the context of tumor biology this term refers to the acquisition of nuclear features characteristic of malignancy. These include nuclear pleomorphism, an increase in nuclear-to-cytoplasmic ratio, prominent nucleoli, and either frequent or aberrant mitotic figures. Dysplastic epithelium may be considered not only a precursor of future malignancy, but also a marker of occult synchronous malignancy. For example, the pres-

ence of high-grade dysplasia documented by endoscopic biopsy of Barrett's esophagus is associated with a 50% risk for invasive carcinoma identified by examination of esophagectomy specimens. Similarly, severe dysplasia in patients with ulcerative colitis is often associated with invasive colonic adenocarcinoma if colectomy is performed. In certain tumor types, the onset of dysplasia has been clearly correlated with the development of tetraploid and/or aneuploid cell populations, as well as the loss of specific tumor suppressor genes. These events may imply an already established autonomous tendency to neoplastic progression.

When dysplastic cells extend to involve the full thickness of involved epithelium, it is commonly referred to as carcinoma in situ, also known as intraepithelial carcinoma. In contrast to invasive carcinoma, these lesions do not invade through the epithelial basement membrane. Carcinoma in situ has no potential for regional or distant spread, as tumor cells have not yet gained access to submucosal lymphatic or vascular channels. When regional lymph node involvement or distant metastases are identified in conjunction with carcinoma in situ, it is generally felt that histologic sampling errors have failed to identify an occult invasive component within the primary neoplasm.

The terms *cancer* and *carcinoma* are often applied in a generic manner to all forms of malignancy. In this generic sense, cancer can be considered a group of diseases characterized by uncontrolled growth and spread of abnormal cells. However, these terms are most accurately applied to neoplasms originating from epithelial tissues. In contrast, a sarcoma is a neoplasm arising from nonepithelial connective tissues, usually of mesodermal origin. These distinctions may also be applied to conditions of widespread metastatic disease, in which the terms *carcinomatosis* or *sarcomatosis* may be applied.

Characteristics of the Transformed Cell

Malignant transformation represents the process by which cells progressively acquire characteristics of the malignant phenotype. The entire malignant phenotype may be characterized by six essential acquired traits: (a) autonomous generation of growth signals, (b) insensitivity to antigrowth signals, (c) evasion of apoptosis (programmed cell death), (d) limitless replicative potential (immortalization), (e) induction of sustained angiogenesis, and (f) capacity for tissue invasion and metastasis.

On a practical level, laboratory assessment of the transformed phenotype involves assays that measure the capacity for cells to exhibit these traits, either as individual components or as an integrated phenotype. As a marker of limitless replicative potential, transformed cells are typically refractory to cellular senescence, allowing for virtually unlimited passage in tissue culture. As an example, the HeLa human cervical cancer cell line has been continuously propagated through countless passages in tissue culture since its initiation in 1951. Other assays of the malignant phenotype include anchorage-independent growth in soft agar, tumorigenesis in athymic mice, and specific assays of angiogenesis, motility, and invasion. In the case of anchorage-independent growth in soft agar, the assay evaluates a number of transformed traits, including the ability of individual cells to generate autonomous growth signals and avoid apoptosis when deprived of substratum attachment. In the case of tumorigenesis in athymic mice, an additional ability to sustain angiogenesis is required.

Multistep Models of Carcinogenesis

A large body of evidence suggests that malignant transformation is a multistep process, now recognized as the stepwise accumulation of genetic and epigenetic events required for neoplastic growth. This process likely explains the age-dependent nature of human tumor incidence, as well as the sequential appearance of histologic intermediates prior to the development of frank malignancy. An early expression of this concept of multistep progression was the "two-hit" model proposed by Knudson in 1971. He noted two distinct patterns of retinoblastoma formation. The first involved the appearance of multiple tumors affecting both eyes in young infants, with an average age of onset of 14 months. Infants in this group frequently had other affected family members, suggesting an inherited predisposition. A second group was characterized by unilateral tumor formation, absence of a family history, and later age of onset. These findings led Knudson to propose the required inactivation of two separate alleles of what later came to be known as the Rb (retinoblastoma) gene. In patients with early bilateral tumors, the first "hit" is provided by the heritable passage of one defective Rb allele in the germline, followed by a second "hit" involving somatic inactivation of the single functioning allele. In patients with unilateral tumors, two independent somatic mutations are required, explaining the longer latency and lower multiplicity of tumors in this group. A similar sequence of events has now been defined for several other tumor suppressor genes, and is frequently referred to as "loss of heterozygosity." This term is generated by the fact that the inherited presence of one mutant and one wild-type allele is initially manifested by the appearance of heterozygosity when DNA is analyzed by restriction fragment length polymorphism. A "second hit" involving loss of the wild-type allele eliminates this heterozygous condition, effectively resulting in a reduction to homozygosity with only the mutated form of the gene remaining (Fig. 14.1).

With the analysis of additional gain-of-function and loss-of-function mutations required for generation of malignant tumors in many tissues, these concepts have been extended to more elaborate models of multistep carcinogenesis, as proposed by Vogelstein and colleagues in the case of colorectal carcinoma. By analyzing the molecular events associated with various stages in the adenoma-carcinoma sequence, the requirement for various genetic mutations during the different stages of tumor progression can be clarified (Fig. 14.2). The earliest histologic event in colorectal carcinogenesis involves the formation of small, benign adenomas consisting primarily of hyperplastic epithelium. This process is accelerated in patients with inherited inactivation of the adenomatous polyposis coli (APC) gene, implying that loss of APC function influences early events in this multistep pathway. While small adenomas frequently harbor only wild-type copies of the K-*ras* proto-oncogene, 50% of adenomas exceeding 1 cm in size will demonstrate activating K-*ras* mutations, implying that this genetic event may be required for adenoma progression. Later events observed during the conversion to carcinoma in situ and fully invasive cancer include allelic loss at the 18q21 chromosome locus, containing the DCC (deleted in colon cancer) gene, and loss of heterozygosity at 17p13, the site of the *p53* tumor suppressor gene. The requirement for multiple rate-limiting molecular events in the process of malignant transformation explains why sporadic neoplasia typically occurs with increasing age, while individuals who inherit mutations in these genes tend to develop early-onset neoplasia.

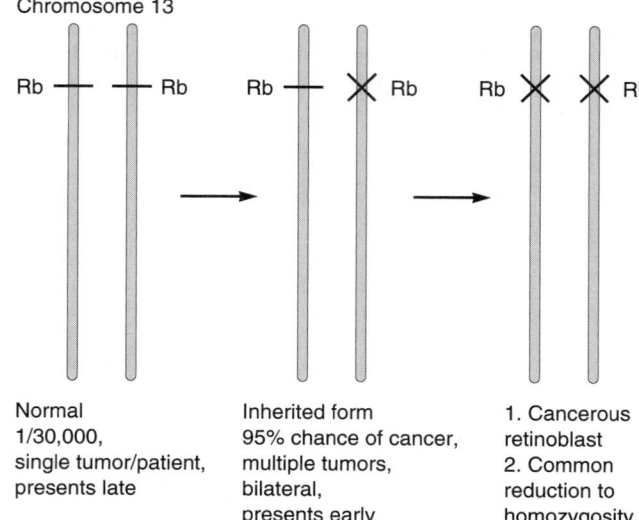

Chromosome 13

Normal
1/30,000,
single tumor/patient,
presents late

Inherited form
95% chance of cancer,
multiple tumors,
bilateral,
presents early

1. Cancerous retinoblast
2. Common reduction to homozygosity

Figure 14.1. The retinoblastoma locus in normal, inherited predisposition, and cancerous cells. Normal individuals have the wild-type Rb gene in all cells and rarely (1/30,000) acquire two somatic mutations, which leads to a single tumor presenting at a late time after birth. An inherited mutation in one Rb allele has a very high (95%) probability of resulting cancer via a reduction to homozygosity at this locus. This results in an early presentation of multiple tumors in the infant. (Redrawn from Mendelsohn J, Howley PM, Israel MA, et al., eds. *The molecular basis of cancer.* Philadelphia: WB Saunders, 1995, with permission.)

The multistep pathway in malignant tumorigenesis is also apparent during attempts to transform primary cells in vitro as well as for in vivo animal models. For primary rodent cells, two cooperative genetic events are required for malignant transformation, often in the form of one growth-promoting gene and one gene that confers resistance to induction of apoptosis. For human cells, a third element involving enhanced telomerase activity is required, conferring a limitless replicative potential. In animal models of chemical carcinogenesis, three distinct phases involving tumor initiation, tumor promotion, and tumor progression have long been noted. In mouse skin, both tumor initiation and promotion are required for the formation of benign papillomas. Tumor initiation appears to involve irreversible DNA damage, while tumor promotion involves reversible epigenetic events often mediated by signaling via membrane growth factor receptors. The factors regulating tumor progression in this system remain less well understood, but may involve repetitive combinations of initiation and promotion with the ultimate selection of malignant clones capable of tissue invasion, angiogenesis, and metastatic spread.

Oncogenes and Tumor Suppressor Genes

The multiple steps required for malignant transformation are primarily accomplished by mutations in oncogenes and tumor suppressor genes. On the simplest level, oncogenes may be considered as genes for which gain-of-function mutations confer a growth advantage during tumorigenesis, while tumor suppressor genes are genes in which loss-of-function mutations confer a selective advantage. The identification of these two classes of tumor-regulating genes emerged from studies of RNA and DNA tumor viruses performed during the 1960s and 1970s.

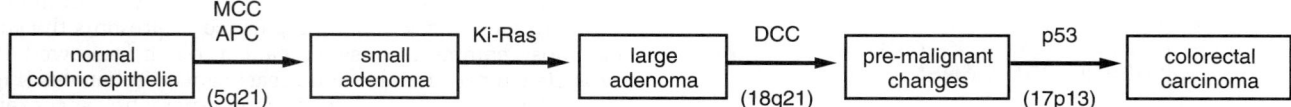

Figure 14.2. The multistep pathway to colorectal cancer. The accumulation of five to ten mutations in several tumor suppressor genes or oncogenes over a lifetime results in cancer. In some cases, an inherited mutation (APC) produces thousands of adenomas, which results in cancer at a younger age. MCC, mutated in colorectal cancer; APC, adenomatous polyposis coli, Ki-*ras*, the Kirsten *ras* oncogene; DCC, deleted in colorectal cancer; *p53*, the *p53* gene. (From Fearon ER. Genetic alterations underlying colorectal tumorigenesis. *Cancer Surv* 1992;12:119, with permission.)

In the case of oncogenes, early studies conducted using tumor retroviruses suggested that, in many instances, a single gene was capable of conferring malignant transformation. However, the significance of these findings was uncertain with respect to human tumorigenesis in which viral etiologies are often not apparent. During the 1970s and 1980s, however, it became clear that many retroviral oncogenes were actually homologous to DNA sequences in uninfected, nonmalignant cells. The oncogene responsible for the transforming capabilities of the Rous sarcoma virus has homologous sequences in the normal chicken genome, thus identifying *src* as a vertebrate oncogene. A human oncogene from a human bladder cancer cell line has proven highly homologous to the Harvey *ras* viral oncogene. Viral and cellular oncogenes have come to be distinguished by the prefixes v- and c-, as in v-*src*, v-*ras*, and c-*src*.

Additional isolation of viral oncogene homologues from normal nontransformed vertebrate cells demonstrated that while viral and human oncogenes were capable of transforming NIH3T3 cells, their normal cellular homologues did not share this transforming capability. Thus the concept of vertebrate proto-oncogenes was established and used to describe genes that required an activation event in order to achieve transforming capability. Multiple mechanisms have now been established for proto-oncogene activation. In the case of cellular *ras* genes, activating point mutations at codons 12, 13, 59, or 61 eliminate guanosine triphosphatase (GTPase) activity, rendering the ras protein constitutively active as a signaling molecule. In other cases, proto-oncogene activation occurs through chromosomal translocations, as in the case of the *bcr/abl* fusion gene produced by the 9:22 translocation (Philadelphia chromosome) observed in chronic myelogenous leukemia (CML). In some cases, cellular oncogenes may also be activated by insertional events occurring during viral integration. Proto-oncogene activation may also occur through overexpression and/or gene amplification, as in the case of c-*myc* and the epidermal growth factor receptor family members HER2-neu and EGFR.

Initial identification of tumor suppressor genes was also achieved by study of tumor viruses, especially the SV40 simian tumor virus, the human papilloma virus (HPV), and various strains of human adenovirus. For each of these viruses, specific viral proteins have been identified that are required for cellular transformation. Examination of the cellular proteins that interact with these viral oncogenes has provided remarkable insight into important tumor suppressor genes whose inactivation is required for malignant transformation. Thus the SV40 large T antigen has been shown to interact with both the *p53* tumor suppressor gene product as well as the retinoblastoma (Rb) protein. In the case of type 5 human adenovirus, the E1A product is responsible for Rb inactivation, while the 55-kd E1B gene product inactivates *p53*. Similarly, HPV E6 pro-

tein binds *p53*, while E7 targets Rb (Fig. 14.3). The fact that three distinct families of DNA tumor viruses all target both *p53* and Rb for inactivation underscores the critical role that these tumor suppressor genes play in preventing malignant transformation.

For both *p53* and *Rb*, additional observations support their identity as tumor suppressor genes. For both of these tumor suppressors, inherited (germline) mutations are associated with a familial predisposition toward neoplasia. In the case of Rb, this is manifested by an inherited predisposition both for retinoblastoma and also for osteogenic sarcoma. In the case of *p53*, germline mutations are associated with the Li-Fraumeni syndrome, in which an increased incidence of sarcomas, breast cancer, leukemia, and central nervous system (CNS) tumors are observed. In addition, inactivating mutations in *Rb* and/or *p53* are observed with significant frequency in sporadic tumors. Finally, rigorous classification as a tumor suppressor gene requires documentation that reintroduction of a wild-type allele into transformed cells lacking a tumor suppressor gene effectively eliminates the tumorigenic ability of transformed cells. While *Rb* and *p53* remain the best characterized tumor suppressor genes in this regard, a growing list of genes have been identified that fulfill at least some of these criteria. These include the APC and DCC genes, the Wilms' tumor WT-1 gene, the neurofibromatosis gene NF-1, BRCA-1 and -2, and the p16 multiple tumor sup-

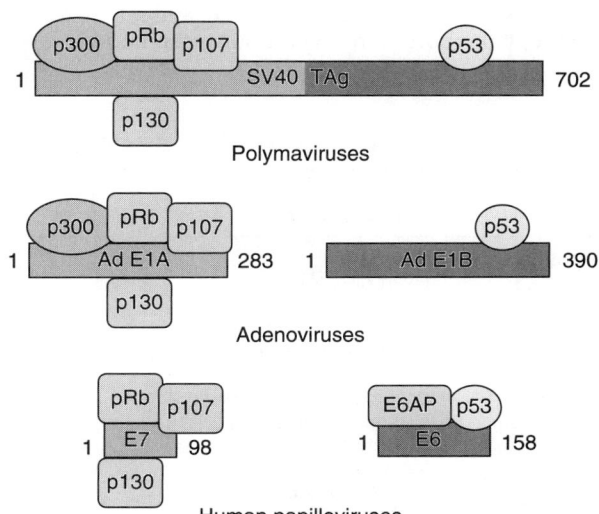

Figure 14.3. The transforming proteins encoded by three distinct groups of DNA tumor viruses target similar cellular proteins. The binding of HPV E6 oncoproteins to p53 mediated by a cellular protein called E6-Ap. (Redrawn from DeVita VT, Hellman S, Rosenberg SA, eds. Cancer: principles and practice. Philadelphia: Lippincott–Raven, 1997:176, with permission.)

Table 14.1. **A PARTIAL LIST OF CELLULAR ONCOGENES AND TUMOR SUPPRESSOR GENES**

Oncogenes
  Ras
  Src
  ErbB
  Myc
  Raf
  Cyclin D1
  Bcl-2
  Fos
  Jun
Tumor suppressor genes
  p53
  RB
  WT-1
  NF-1
  APC
  DCC
  p16INK4/MTS1
  BRCA1
  BRCA2

pressor gene. A partial list of cellular oncogenes and tumor suppressor genes and their functions is provided in Table 14.1.

Cancer Epidemiology

In the U.S., one in every two males and one in every three females will develop an invasive cancer during their lifetime. Cancer represents the second leading cause of death for all ages, exceeded only by heart disease. Over 500,000 deaths per year are attributable to cancer, accounting for 23% of all deaths (Table 14.2). For females between the ages of 35 and 74, cancer is the single leading cause of death. The overall cancer-specific death rate in the U.S. is approximately 170 deaths per 100,000 total population. According to data from the World Health Organization, this places the U.S. in an intermediate position in terms of worldwide cancer death rates, with rates as low as 80/100,000 reported in Mexico, and rates exceeding 200/100,000 reported in several European nations.

In the U.S., 52.4% of all cancer deaths occur in males. For both men and women, lung cancer represents the single most common cause of cancer death, followed by prostate cancer in males and breast cancer in females (Fig. 14.4). For both sexes, colorectal and pancreatic cancer represent the third and fourth most common causes of cancer death, respectively. These common neoplasms account for a sizable fraction of all cancer deaths. For men, lung cancer, prostate cancer, and colorectal cancer account for 54% of all cancer deaths, while cancers of the lung, breast, colon, and rectum account for half of all female cancer deaths.

During the 20th century, dramatic shifts in relative mortality rates have been observed for different cancer sites (Figs. 14.5 and 14.6). In 1930s, carcinoma of the stomach represented the single most common cause of cancer death, while now stomach cancer causes less than 14,000 deaths per year. The factors responsible for this dramatic decline remain uncertain, but are likely related to changes in food storage and processing. Similarly, deaths from lung cancer have risen dramatically as a direct effect of epidemic tobacco use beginning among men in the 1940s and among women later in the 20th century. More recently, tremendous increases in the incidence of melanoma and esophageal adenocarcinoma have been noted.

Cancer Etiology

Cancer epidemiologic data represent integrated effects of countless known and unknown causative agents. In certain situations, tumor causation is straightforward, as in the case of tobacco smoking and lung cancer, chronic hepatitis and hepatocellular cancer, or sun exposure and melanoma. Even among these tumor types, however, dramatic variation in incidence is observed among patients with identical known risk factors, suggesting a complex interplay of positive and negative influences. In general, cancer causation can be categorized according to etiology. Established causes include hereditary factors, viral and other biologic agents, physical agents, chemical agents, hormonal factors, and other lifestyle issues. Estimates of cancer mortality attributable to specific factors suggest that tobacco and dietary factors may account for up to 60% of all cancer deaths in developed countries (Table 14.3).

Table 14.2. **FIFTEEN LEADING CAUSES OF DEATH, UNITED STATES, 1995**

Rank	Cause of death	Number of deaths	Death rate per 100,000 population*	Percent of total deaths
All causes	2,312,132	678.7	100.0	
1	Heart diseases	737,563	205.4	31.9
2	Cancer	538,455	169.1	23.3
3	Cerebrovascular diseases	157,991	42.0	8.8
4	Chronic obstructive pulmonary disease	102,899	30.0	4.5
5	Accidents	93,320	31.6	4.0
6	Pneumonia and influenza	82,923	21.2	3.6
7	Diabetes mellitus	59,254	17.9	2.6
8	HIV infection	43,115	13.1	1.9
9	Suicide	31,284	10.7	1.4
10	Diseases of arteries	26,646	7.7	1.2
11	Cirrhosis of liver	25,222	8.5	1.1
12	Nephritis	23,676	6.5	1.0
13	Homicide	22,895	8.5	1.0
14	Septicemia	20,965	5.9	0.9
15	Alzheimer's disease	20,606	5.0	0.9
	Other and ill-defined	325,318		14.1

*Age-adjusted to the 1970 U.S. standard population. Data source: Vital Statistics of the United States, 1998.

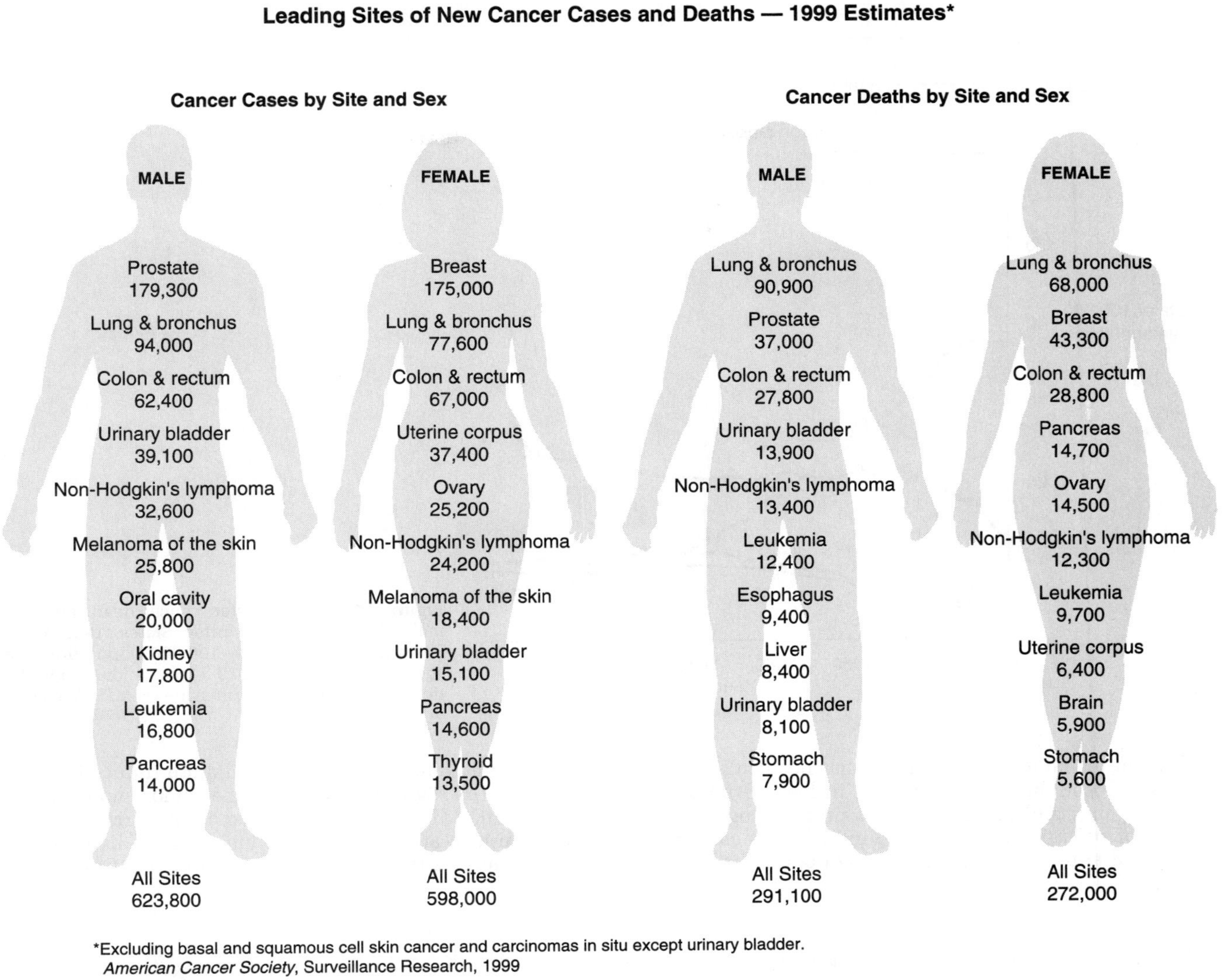

Leading Sites of New Cancer Cases and Deaths — 1999 Estimates*

Cancer Cases by Site and Sex

MALE

Prostate
179,300

Lung & bronchus
94,000

Colon & rectum
62,400

Urinary bladder
39,100

Non-Hodgkin's lymphoma
32,600

Melanoma of the skin
25,800

Oral cavity
20,000

Kidney
17,800

Leukemia
16,800

Pancreas
14,000

All Sites
623,800

FEMALE

Breast
175,000

Lung & bronchus
77,600

Colon & rectum
67,000

Uterine corpus
37,400

Ovary
25,200

Non-Hodgkin's lymphoma
24,200

Melanoma of the skin
18,400

Urinary bladder
15,100

Pancreas
14,600

Thyroid
13,500

All Sites
598,000

Cancer Deaths by Site and Sex

MALE

Lung & bronchus
90,900

Prostate
37,000

Colon & rectum
27,800

Urinary bladder
13,900

Non-Hodgkin's lymphoma
13,400

Leukemia
12,400

Esophagus
9,400

Liver
8,400

Urinary bladder
8,100

Stomach
7,900

All Sites
291,100

FEMALE

Lung & bronchus
68,000

Breast
43,300

Colon & rectum
28,800

Pancreas
14,700

Ovary
14,500

Non-Hodgkin's lymphoma
12,300

Leukemia
9,700

Uterine corpus
6,400

Brain
5,900

Stomach
5,600

All Sites
272,000

*Excluding basal and squamous cell skin cancer and carcinomas in situ except urinary bladder.
American Cancer Society, Surveillance Research, 1999

Figure 14.4. Leading sites of new cancer cases and deaths—1999 estimates. (From http://www.cancer.org/statistics, with permission.)

A large number of hereditary syndromes have been identified that appear to directly increase cancer risk. In many cases, these syndromes are characterized by an autosomal-dominant mode of transmission reflecting inherited mutation of an inactive tumor suppressor gene followed by loss of heterozygosity as described above. For an increasing number of syndromes, the genetic basis has been elucidated. For many of these syndromes, a common theme has emerged in which the genetic lesion causing an inherited predisposition to a given malignancy is observed as a somatic mutation in sporadic, nonfamilial neoplasms involving that site. Thus APC mutations are observed both in familial polyposis and sporadic cases of colon cancer, while germline BRCA-1 mutations are responsible for some forms of familial breast cancer, and somatic BRCA-1 mutations are frequently observed in breast cancers arising in patients with no family history.

Among biologic agents, several human DNA tumor viruses have been causally implicated in human neoplasia. The hepatitis B and hepatitis C viruses have been strongly linked to the development of hepatocellular can-

cer, primarily by indirectly provoking cellular proliferation in response to immune-mediated injury. Similarly, infection with specific high-risk types of human papilloma viruses (e.g., HPV-16, HPV-18, HPV-33) is associated with squamous cell carcinoma of the anogenital tract, including carcinoma or the uterine cervix, carcinoma of the anus, and vulvar carcinoma. In the case of Epstein-Barr virus, latent infection is associated with multiple malignancies, including Burkitt's lymphoma, Hodgkin's disease, T-cell malignancies, and squamous tumors of the oropharynx. More recently, significant attention has been placed on the ability of bacterial pathogens to act as cancer-causing agents. Primary among these, *Helicobacter pylori* infection has been implicated not only in the causation of gastric mucosa-associated lymphoid tissue (MALT) lymphoma, but also in initiating the sequence of events that may result in intestinal-type gastric adenocarcinoma.

Various physical agents are known to be effective carcinogens. Both ionizing and ultraviolet radiation can initiate damage to genomic DNA, which ultimately becomes manifest in the form of neoplasia. In this regard, radiation

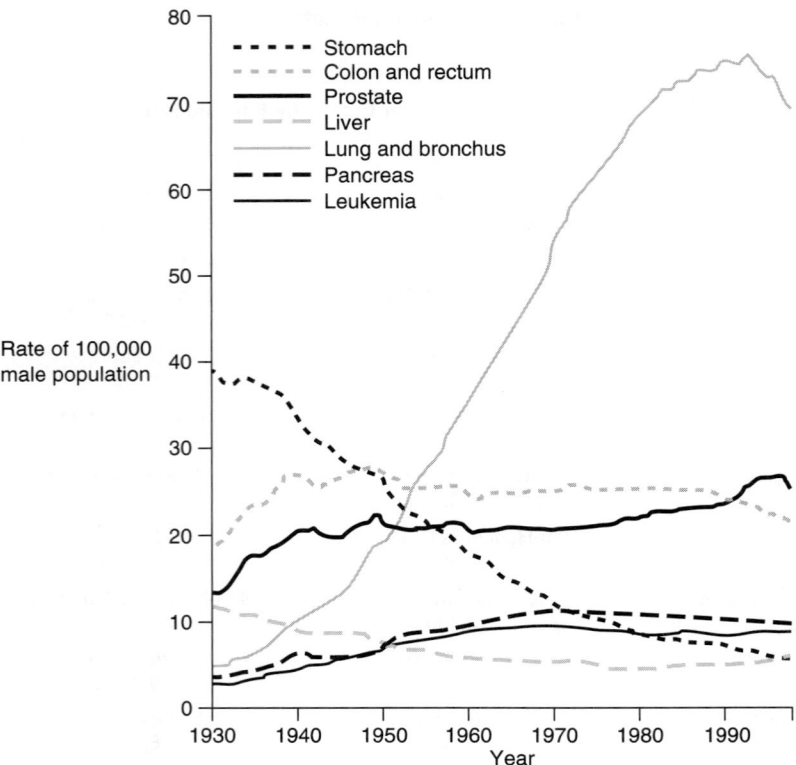

Figure 14.5. Age-adjusted cancer death rates for males by tumor site, United States, 1930–1995. Rates are calculated per 100,000 population and age-adjusted to the 1970 U.S. standard population. (Redrawn with permission of ACS Web site.)

is known to induce high rates of chromosomal deletions and translocations, likely resulting in loss of tumor suppressor genes and/or activation of proto-oncogenes. The ability of superficial radiation to induce skin cancer was suspected almost immediately following the discovery of x-rays. Subsequent examples of radiation-induced cancer included the high incidence of bone tumors noted in radium watch dial painters, lung cancer occurring in uranium miners, and an increased incidence of liver cancer among patients receiving the radiographic contrast mater-

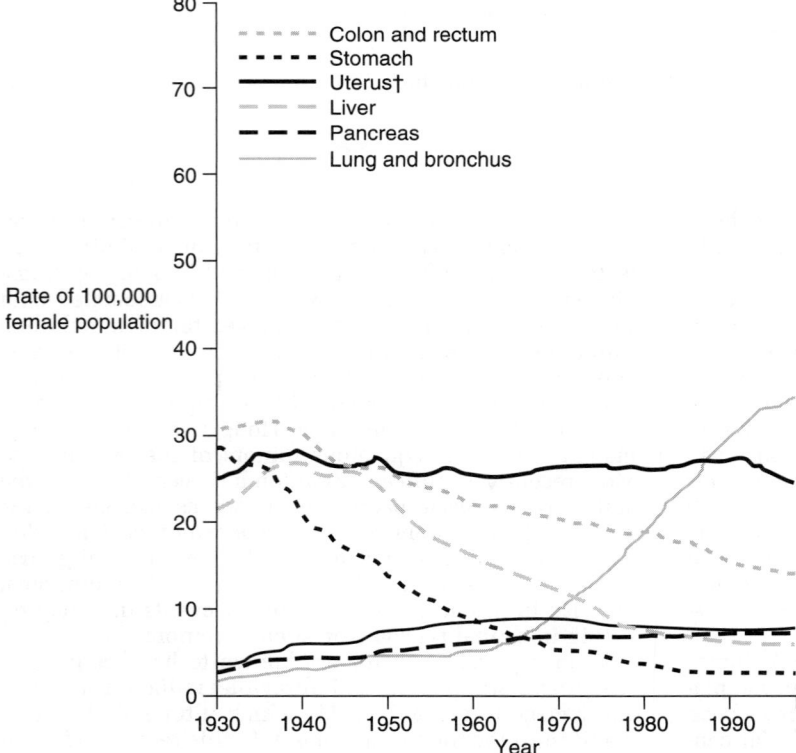

Figure 14.6. Age-adjusted cancer death rates for females by tumor site, United States, 1930–1995. Rates are calculated per 100,000 population and age-adjusted to the 1970 U.S. standard population. (Redrawn with permission of ACS Web site.)

Table 14.3. CANCER MORTALITY ATTRIBUTABLE TO SPECIFIC FACTORS OR GROUPS OF FACTORS IN DEVELOPED COUNTRIES

Factor or group of factors	Percentage
Tobacco	30
Alcohol	3
Diet in adult life (including obesity)	30
Perinatal effects and excessive growth	5
Food additives and contaminants (including salt)	1
Sedentary life	3
Infectious agents	5
Reproductive factors	2
Ionizing and ultraviolet radiation	2
Occupational factors	5
Environmental pollution	2
Medical products and procedures	1
High-penetrance genes	2

ial Thorotrast, which contained the radioactive compound thorium. Widespread examples of ionizing radiation-induced neoplasia were observed among the survivors of Hiroshima and Nagasaki, in whom a high incidence of leukemia and a wide spectrum of solid tumors were reported. Study of these populations suggests both short-term and latent effects of radiation on tumorigenesis. While an increased incidence of leukemia among survivors was noted within 5 to 7 years, an increased incidence of solid tumors continues to be noted even 40 years following radiation exposure. Increased risks for neoplasia may also be noted following therapeutic radiation, as in the case of radiotherapy for cervical cancer, or the historic use of radiation for an enlarged thymus, in which an increased incidence of papillary thyroid cancer is observed. In some instances, the induction of neoplasia following radiation may be due to changes in tissue physiology rather than the direct induction of DNA damage. For instance, patients with Stewart-Treves syndrome develop lymphangiosarcoma in upper extremities affected by chronic lymphedema, often induced by a combination of radical mastectomy and axillary radiation in the treatment of breast cancer.

With respect to ultraviolet radiation, similar mechanisms of carcinogenesis have been observed. Solar ultraviolet radiation represents a potent inducer of DNA damage, often in the form of pyrimidine dimers. These DNA lesions appear to directly lead to mutations in a number of cancer-related genes, including *ras* oncogenes and the *p53* tumor suppressor gene. Inherited syndromes associated with deficiencies in pyrimidine dimer repair such as xeroderma pigmentosum are associated with an increased risk for skin cancer. Acute and chronic ultraviolet injury may also lead to recognition of altered skin antigens by suppressor T lymphocytes, perhaps leading to decreased immune surveillance of malignant cells. Unequivocal evidence confirms ultraviolet radiation as a primary cause of basal cell and squamous cell skin cancer, the two most common forms of human malignancy. While the relationship between melanoma and ultraviolet light is more complex, a large body of evidence suggests that while chronic low-level sun exposure may predispose to squamous and basal cell carcinoma, melanoma risk is specifically enhanced by acute episodes of sunburn, especially early in life. In contrast to the known contribution of ionizing and ultraviolet radiation to cancer risk, the role of other forms of physical energy, including low-frequency electric and magnetic fields, remains uncertain.

Significant attention has been placed on the role of hormonal factors in cancer etiology. Especially as it relates to possible increases in cancer incidence associated with postmenopausal replacement estrogen therapy, this issue has remained an area of significant controversy. In this regard, any adverse effects of hormone therapy on cancer risk must be considered in light of the apparent beneficial effect of estrogen in reducing cardiovascular morbidity and mortality. The importance of understanding the contribution of hormonal factors in cancer etiology is underscored by the fact that approximately 35% of all newly diagnosed male cancers and more than 40% of all newly diagnosed female cancers involve hormone-responsive tissues.

Multiple studies have demonstrated apparent hormone-related risk factors for female breast cancer. In general, factors that increase cumulative estrogen exposure also increase breast cancer risk. These factors include early menarche, late menopause, obesity, and nulliparity or late age of initial pregnancy. In the case of obesity, adipose tissue serves as a rich source of aromatase enzyme activity, leading to increased peripheral conversion of androstenedione to estrone and estradiol. While data are somewhat conflicting, several studies have also suggested that prolonged treatment with higher dose postmenopausal replacement estrogen is associated with moderate increases in breast cancer risk. Together, these factors have generated considerable interest in the role of hormonal manipulation as a means of chemoprevention in high-risk patients. The incidence of several other tumor types may be similarly influenced by hormonal factors, including endometrial cancer, ovarian cancer, and prostate cancer.

Chemical carcinogens appear to represent the most frequent etiologic agents for many common human tumors. Chemical carcinogenesis may be initiated by dietary carcinogens, pharmaceutical carcinogens, occupational exposures, or by lifestyle factors such as tobacco use or betel nut chewing. Chemical carcinogenesis may be mediated by both genotoxic and nongenotoxic mechanisms. Genotoxic mechanisms often involve the formation of covalent adducts involving genomic DNA. Adduct-forming carcinogens include alkylating and arylaminating agents, which transfer alkyl or aryl groups to specific sites on DNA bases. Among these classes of compounds are tobacco-specific nitrosamines, aflatoxins, polycyclic aromatic hydrocarbons, and heterocyclic aromatic amines produced by overcooking meat.

While DNA adduct formation frequently results in inactivating missense and nonsense mutations, evidence suggests that this mechanism may also be involved in carcinogen-induced oncogene activation. For example, methylating N-nitroso compounds are capable of inducing methylation of deoxyguanosine at the O6 position, leading to mispairing with thymine during DNA synthesis and subsequent G:C-to-A:T substitution. This mechanism has been shown to be associated with G-to-A mutations in *ras* proto-oncogenes, with resulting loss of GTPase activity and constitutive activation. In the case of aflatoxins, the most common generated adduct involves the N7 position of deoxyguanosine, causing G:C to T:A transversions. This specific mutation is frequently found at codon 249 in the *p53* tumor suppressor gene within aflatoxin-exposed cells as well as in human liver tumors from patients living in areas of high aflatoxin exposure. Other carcinogens, including some pesticides and herbicides, may act through nongenotoxic means and exert their effects through either toxic cell death with resulting regenerative proliferation or through generation of oxygen radicals. A partial list of chemical carcinogens known or suspected to cause cancer in humans is provided in Table 14.4.

Table 14.4. **KNOWN OR SUSPECTED CHEMICAL CARCINOGENS IN HUMANS***

Target organ	Agents	Industries	Tumor type
Lung	Tobacco smoke, arsenic, asbestos, crystalline silica, benzo(a)pyrene, beryllium, bis(chloro)methyl ether, 1,3-butadiene, chromium V1 compounds, coal tar and pitch, nickel compounds, soots, mustard gas	Aluminum production, coal gasification, coke production, hematite mining, painters	Squamous, large cell, and small cell cancer and adenocarcinoma
Pleura	Asbestos	—	Mesothelioma
Oral cavity	Tobacco smoke, alcoholic beverages, nickel compounds	Boot and shoe production, furniture manufacturer, isopropyl alcohol production	Squamous cell cancer
Esophagus	Tobacco smoke, alcoholic beverages	—	Squamous cell cancer
Gastric	Smoked, salted, and pickled foods	Rubber industry	Adenocarcinoma
Colon	Heterocyclic amines, asbestos	Pattern makers	Adenocarcinoma
Liver	Aflatoxin, vinyl chloride, tobacco smoke, alcoholic beverages	—	Hepatocellular carcinoma, hemangiosarcoma
Kidney	Tobacco smoke	—	Renal cell cancer
Bladder	Tobacco smoke, 4-aminobiphenyl, benzidine, 2-napthylamine	Magenta manufacture, auramine manufacture	Transitional cell cancer
Prostate	Cadmium	—	Adenocarcinoma
Skin	Arsenic, benzo(a)pyrene, coal tar and pitch, mineral oils, soots	Coal gasification, coke production	Squamous cell cancer, basal cell cancer
Bone marrow	Benzene, tobacco smoke, ethylene oxide, antineoplastic agents	Rubber workers	Leukemia

*These carcinogen designations are determined by regulatory or review agencies based on public health needs. They do not imply proof of carcinogenicity in individuals. This table is not all-inclusive. For additional information, the reader is referred to agency documents and publications (95,255–260).

REGULATION OF NORMAL CELL GROWTH

Among the core elements of the transformed phenotype, accelerated proliferation remains a central feature of neoplastic growth. The regulation of normal cell growth is carried out by a number of membrane growth factor receptors initiating signal transduction pathways that ultimately impact on cell cycle regulation. Ultimately, cellular proliferation signals are integrated with cell cycle checkpoints that act to maximize the fidelity of genomic replication, and also with signals governing differentiation, senescence, and programmed cell death (apoptosis).

Growth Factors and Receptors

Under normal circumstances, cellular proliferation is strongly influenced by external signals provided by individual cells, neighboring cells, and the extracellular environment. In many circumstances, this signaling is provided by soluble growth factors that bind to transmembrane receptors on the cell surface. In mammalian cells, a large number of soluble growth factors have been identified that regulate both normal and neoplastic cell growth. These factors may be classified based on structural homology as well as receptor specificity. Among the growth factor systems known to regulate cell proliferation, the epidermal growth factor (EGF), insulin-like growth factor (IGF), hepatocyte growth factor (HGF), fibroblast growth factor (FGF), and transforming growth factor-β (TGF-β) families are known to play critical roles in human malignancy.

Epidermal Growth Factor Family

The actions of EGF and transforming growth factor-α (TGF-α) are mediated by binding to the EGF receptor. The EGF receptor (EGFr) subfamily is a member of the larger family of receptor tyrosine kinases, and contains four closely related receptors. These include EGFr, also known as ErbB1; HER2, also known as ErbB2, neu; HER3, also known as ErbB3; and HER4, or ErbB4. Among these, no activating ligand has yet been described for HER2, and the HER3 receptor exhibits impaired kinase function. Each receptor consists of a cysteine-rich extracellular domain, a single pass transmembrane domain, and a cytoplasmic domain with tyrosine kinase activity and several tyrosine residues that become phosphorylated following receptor activation. Following ligand binding, receptors form either homo- or heterodimers and undergo tyrosine phosphorylation at several sites, with resulting docking of effector proteins (see Signal Transduction, below).

Among EGF receptor ligands, at least eight different growth factors have been identified. These include EGF itself, TGF-α, heparin-binding epidermal growth factor (HB-EGF), amphiregulin, epiregulin, betacellulin, and the neuregulins-1 and -2. These different ligands show preferential binding for different EGF receptor subtypes (Table 14.5). As is evident, a single EGF receptor ligand can bind

Table 14.5. **BINDING OF EGF RECEPTOR LIGANDS TO EGF RECEPTORS**

Ligand	Receptor			
	ErbB1	ErbB2	ErbB3	ErbB4
EGF	X			
TGF-α	X			
Amphiregulin	X			
Neuregulin			X*	X
Neuregulin-2			X*	X
Betacellulin	X			X
Epiregulin	X			X
HB-EGF	X			X

*Ligand binds but does not activate.
EGF; epidermal growth factor; TGF, transforming growth factor.
Note absence of known ligands binding ErbB2. In many cases, receptor heterodimerization can result in ligand-induced phosphorylation (activation) of a nonbinding receptor.

multiple receptors, and a single EGF receptor can bind multiple different ligands. In addition to the complexity implied by four receptors and eight different ligands in the EGF family, additional opportunity for signal diversity is generated by the formation of heterodimers between the different receptor subtypes. Thus receptor subtypes that do not bind a specific EGF receptor ligand when expressed alone can become tyrosine phosphorylated in the presence of a receptor that does interact with that ligand. For example, HER2/neu represents an orphan receptor without known ligands. However, EGF induces tyrosine phosphorylation of HER2 in cells coexpressing EGFr, accompanied by the formation of EGF-stimulated EGFr/HER2 heterodimers. In cells expressing different types of EGF receptor, stimulation by an EGF receptor ligand capable of binding to only one type of receptor often leads to activation of each of the other receptor subtypes.

Recently, EGF receptor activation has been shown to play a role in mediating signals from diverse signaling pathways, suggesting an expanded role of this receptor pathway in regulating cellular events (Fig. 14.7). The critical role of EGF receptor signaling in human malignancy is underscored by upregulated expression of EGF receptors and ligands in many human tumors, by the ability of EGF receptor ligands to promote and accelerate tumorigenesis in several different mouse models, and by the emerging therapeutic role of anti-EGF receptor antibodies in treatment of breast cancer and other malignancies.

Insulin-like Growth Factor Family

Insulin-like growth factor (IGF) receptors are also known to play important roles in tumor biology and malignant cell growth. Among these receptors, there are three known subtypes: the insulin receptor, the IGF-I receptor, and the IGF-II receptor (Fig. 14.8). The insulin receptor and the IGF-I receptor are both heterotetrameric receptor tyrosine kinases. In contrast, the IGF-II receptor is also known as the mannose-6-phosphate receptor and represents a single pass transmembrane protein devoid of intrinsic kinase activity. Upon activation of either the insulin receptor or the IGF-I receptor, tyrosine kinase activation results in phosphorylation of insulin receptor substrate-1 (IRS-1). This signaling molecule then induces docking of signal transduction molecules resulting in activation of mitogenic and cell survival signals. Additional studies have identified a family of insulin growth factor binding proteins (IGFBPs) The IGFBP family includes six proteins with high affinity for insulin-like growth factors, as well as several related proteins with lower binding affinities. Numerous studies have demonstrated that IGF-BPs modulate the mitogenic effects of IGFs. IGFs are present at the cell surface present at levels far in excess of that required for maximal receptor stimulation, and the IGF-BPs provide critical regulation of IGF availability. For IGF-I, the major binding protein appears to be IGFBP-3. This binding protein is capable of inhibiting the growth of

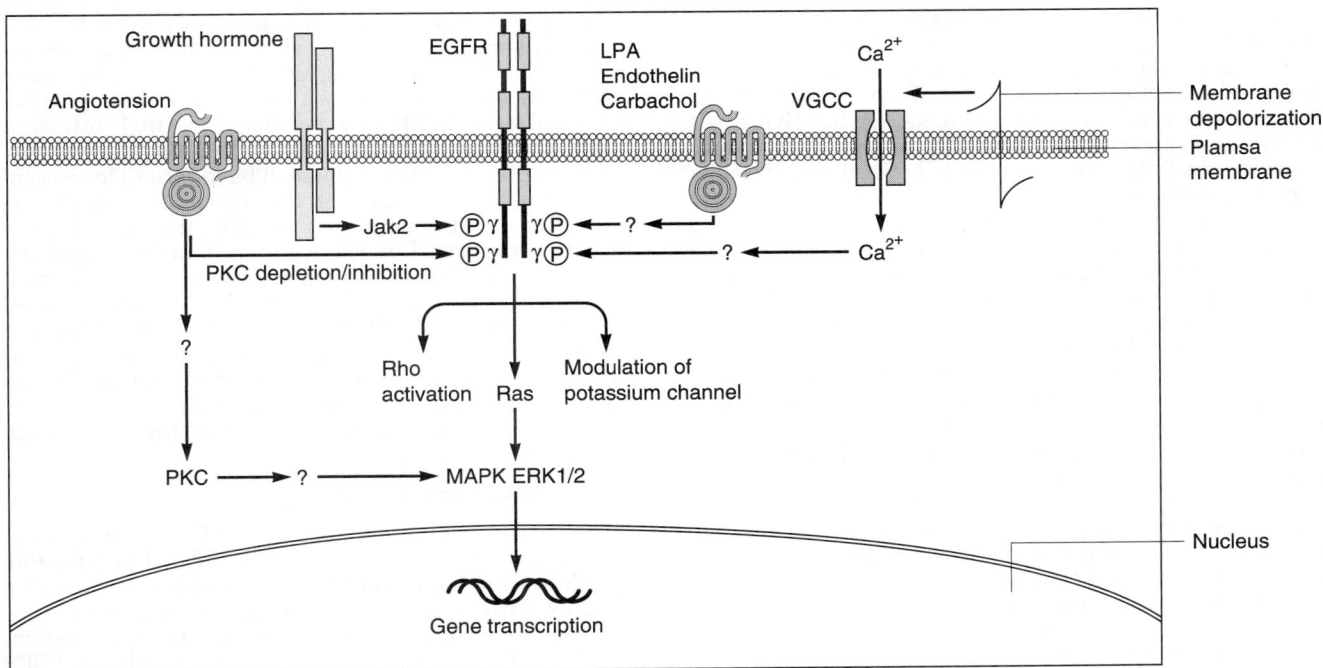

Figure 14.7. Models of EGFR transactivation. In addition to its function as a receptor for its own ligands, the EGFR is used by different signaling pathways as signal transducer for the ativation of downstream targets. LPA, carbachol, and endothelin stimulation of GPCRs or calcium influx as a result of membrane depolarization induce tyrosine phosphorylation of EGFR, which is essential for the activation of the MAP kinase pathway. Carbachol stimulation modulates the activity of a potassium channel in an EGFR-dependent manner and LPA activated RHo and induces stress fibers via the EGFR. In contrast, the activation of the MAP kinase pathway by growth hormone stimulation does not require the kinase activity of the EGFR but does require its tyrosine phosphorylation by Jak2. Angiotensin II uses two different pathways to activate MAP kinase: a PCK-dependent but EGFR- and Ras-independent pathway in naïve control cells and an EGFR- and Ras-dependent pathway when PKC is depleted or inhibited. VGCC, voltage-gated calcium channel. (Redrawn from Hackel PO, Zqick E, Prenzel N, et al. Epidermal growth factor receptors: critical mediators of multiple receptor pathways. *Curr Opin Cell Biol* 1999;11:184–189, with permission.)

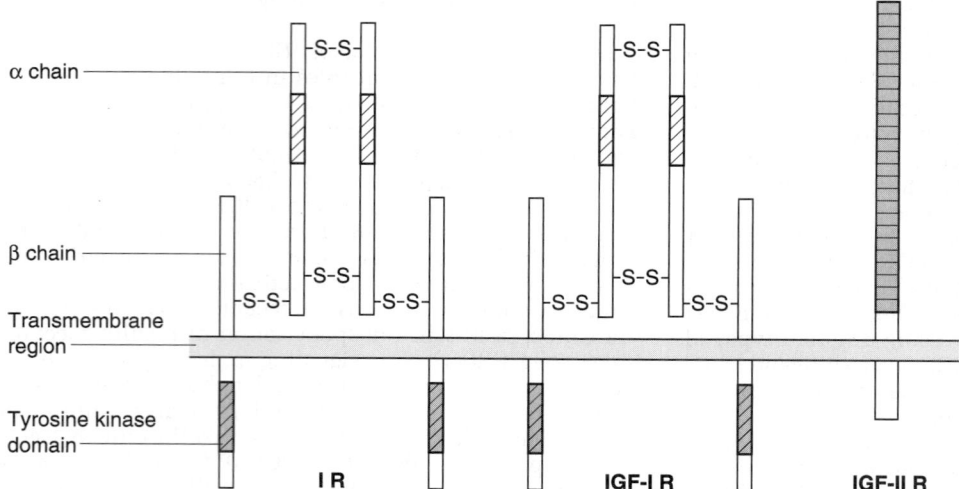

α chain

β chain

Transmembrane region

Tyrosine kinase domain

I R   IGF-I R   IGF-II R

Figure 14.8. The insulin receptor family. The insulin (IR) and insulin-like growth factor-I (IGF-IR) receptors consist of heterotetrameric proteins held together by the indicated disulfide bonds. The two alpha chains are completed extracellular and contain the ligand binding domains (stippled rectangles). The two beta chains cross the transmembrane region and contain the intracellular tyrosine kinase domains (indicated by the shaded rectangles). The insulin-like growth factor II receptor (IGF-IIR) is a single transmembrane protein that is devoid of any kinase activity. (Redrawn from Korc M. Role of growth factors in pancreatic cancer. *Surg Onc Clin North Am* 1998;7:31, with permission.)

breast cancer cells in vitro, and may also play an important role in modulating cancer risk in vivo. Recent epidemiologic studies have demonstrated that high plasma IGF-I and low IGFBP-3 levels are associated with increased risks for prostate, breast, and colorectal cancer.

Hepatocyte Growth Factor

Another receptor tyrosine kinase signaling system known to function in tumor cells is the c-*met* proto-oncogene and its ligand, hepatocyte growth factor (HGF), also known as scatter factor. HGF is a polypeptide that shares structural homology with enzymes of the coagulation cascade. HGF is synthesized as a biologically inactive single chain that is cleaved by the urokinase-type plasminogen activator to a fully active alpha-beta heterodimer. The biologic responses induced by HGF are elicited by binding to its receptor, a transmembrane tyrosine kinase encoded by the c-*met* proto-oncogene. The signaling cascade triggered by HGF induces autophosphorylation of c-*met,* with concomitant activation of different cytoplasmic effectors that bind to a multifunctional docking site. In various tissue culture systems, HGF is capable of inducing tubulogenesis, a complex program of proliferation and cell migration. Activation of c-*met* signaling in papillary thyroid carcinoma and colorectal cancer cells similarly appears to enhance cell migration and invasion. Increased expression of HGF and/or c-*met* has been reported in multiple human tumors including synovial sarcoma, pancreatic carcinoma, and ovarian carcinoma. In several instances, c-*met* expression has been correlated with poor prognosis. Activating mutations in the c-*met* proto-oncogene that result in constitutive tyrosine kinase activity have been reported in papillary carcinomas of the kidney and squamous cell carcinomas of the head and neck.

Fibroblast Growth Factor

Fibroblast growth factors (FGFs) represent a large family of signaling molecules felt to play important roles in cell proliferation, epithelial-mesenchymal interactions during development, cellular differentiation, and angiogenesis. At least 19 different FGFs and four different FGF receptors have been identified. All FGF family members are characterized by a highly conserved 28 amino acid core region as well as a high affinity for heparan sulfate and glycosaminoglcyans. The presence of heparan sulfate proteoglycans (HSPGs) on the cell surface as well as in extracellular matrix allows for significant functional complexity in FGF signaling. Under certain conditions, HSPGs act as co-

receptors, promoting interactions between FGFs and their receptors. Under different circumstances, HSPGs may act to sequester FGFs away from functional receptors, thereby preventing active signaling.

Among the 19 different FGF family members, the two best characterized ligands are FGF1 (acidic FGF), and FGF2 (basic FGF). FGF3 is also known as int3, identified as an integrations locus for the mouse mammary tumor virus. FGF7 is also known as keratinocyte growth factor (KGF). Other FGFs carrying alternate nomenclature include FGF8, known as androgen-induced growth factor, and FGF9, sometimes referred to as glia activating factor. These different FGF family members exert their influence by binding with different affinities to four different FGF receptors (FGFR), several of which have variant forms generated by alternative splicing. FGF receptors are members of the tyrosine kinase receptor superfamily, and are structurally characterized by extracellular domains containing three immunoglobulin-like regions (designated as loops I, II, and III). Among these, ligand binding specificity is determined by the C-terminal portion of loop III. Alternative splice variants involving these immunoglobulin regions further contribute to the functional complexity of FGF signaling, in some cases generating secreted receptor variants that may act to sequester ligand away from functional transmembrane forms of FGFR.

Transforming Growth Factor-β

The transforming growth factor-β (TGF-β) family comprises a large number of structurally related polypeptide growth factors, and each of these is capable of regulating a complex array of cellular processes. These processes include cell proliferation, differentiation, motility, adhesion, and death. Because of the complexity of its actions, TGFB plays an important role in the development, homeostasis, and repair of most tissues. The cellular responses to TGF-β are contextual. In normal epithelial cells, including intestinal epithelium, TGF-β has a predominant growth inhibitory effect, and a substantial body of evidence suggests a role as tumor suppressor.

Neoplastic transformation results in loss of normal growth inhibitory responses to TGF-β. Emerging evidence points toward the involvement of the TGF-β signaling pathway in several malignancies. Reports of the mutational inactivation of genes involved in the TGF-β growth inhibitory signaling in some colorectal cancers and in pancreatic carcinomas have generated considerable excitement. Smad proteins are components of the TGF-β signaling pathway. Recent evidence suggests a significant contribution of *Smad4* gene inactivation in progression to advanced stages of colorectal cancer, such as distant metastasis. Similarly, loss of TGF-β growth inhibitory responses have been observed in several other malignancies such as esophageal cancer and breast cancer. These and other studies provide substantial support for the hypothesis that TGF-β plays a central role in tumor suppression in several organ systems.

The TGF-β ligands bind to and signal through a heteromeric complex of type I and type II receptors that are serine/threonine kinases (Fig. 14.9). The TGF-β type II receptor (TβRII) is necessary for specific ligand binding. Following binding of ligand to type II receptors, the ligand-bound type II receptor forms an oligomeric complex with the type I receptor (TβRI), resulting in type I receptor phosphorylation.

The cloning of the deleted-in-pancreatic-cancer *(DPC4)* gene, and the recognition that *DPC4* had significant homology to the *Drosophila* mothers against decapentaplegic *(Mad)* gene led to the identification and characterization

of the so-called *SMAD* genes in humans and other vertebrates. Mutations in *DPC4* (now also known as *Smad4*) have been identified in 50% of pancreatic cancers. Nine members of the vertebrate TGF-β family intracellular signaling pathways have been identified, and by consensus are now referred to as Smad1 through Smad9. Smads1, 5, 8, and 9 probably function to transduce signals from the TGF-β–related bone morphogenetic proteins (BMPs).

Smads2 and 3 are important substrates of the TGF-β type I receptor that may be activated by either activin or TGF-β selective type II receptors. When phosphorylated by TβRI, Smad2 and Smad3 associate with Smad4, translocate to the nucleus, associate with a DNA-binding partner and activate transcription of specific target genes (Fig. 14.9). Interference with the functions of Smad2, Smad3, or Smad4 alone is sufficient to abrogate Smad-dependent transcriptional activation of selected TGF-β responsive genes. Smads 6 and 7 inhibit the signaling function of the receptor-activated Smads. Smad6 preferentially inhibits BMP signaling, whereas Smad7 can inhibit both TGF-β and BMP signaling by preventing receptor-mediated phosphorylation of the receptor-activated Smad proteins.

There is increasing evidence that the TGF-β serine threonine/kinase receptors may also activate selected members of the mitogen activated protein kinase (MAPK) family of proteins. A rapid increase in p44^{mapk} activity has been observed in response to TGF-β treatment, although the mechanism for this activation remains unclear. Many TGF-β–regulated gene promoters contain AP-1 or CRE response elements, both of which may be direct or indirect targets for activated MAPKs.

TGF-β receptor activation also activates the Jun kinase (JNK) pathway. Jun kinase catalyzes phosphorylation of the c-Jun transactivation domain, and thereby, the function of the AP-1 transcription complex. TGF-β–dependent induction of fibronectin occurs through activation of the JNK pathway in several cell lines (MDA-MB-468 breast cancer, BXPC3 pancreatic cancer, and SW480.7 colon cancer) known to have inactivating mutations of Smad4. Thus, there appears to be TGF-β signaling that may occur independent of the Smad signaling cascade. Furthermore, dominant inhibitory components of the JNK signaling cascade, (including RhoA, Rac1, MEKK1, MKK4/SEK1, c-Jun, and JNK), have been found to inhibit the TGF-β–dependent induction of *3TP-Lux,* a reporter gene that contains elements of the plasminogen activator inhibitor (PAI-1) promoter.

Signal Transduction: A Central Role for Ras

Ultimately, the activation of transmembrane receptor tyrosine kinases by soluble growth factors are coupled to changes in the activity of nuclear transcription factors through a complex system of signal transduction (Fig. 14.10). A number of molecules become physically associated and/or phosphorylated by activated growth factor receptors, including phospholipase C, phosphatidylinositol-3′-kinase, ras GTPase-activating protein (GAP), and the src family of tyrosine kinases. These molecules all contain the src homology regions SH2 and SH3, which are known to be important in regulating interactions among tyrosine-phosphorylated proteins. Through a series of adapter proteins and additional phosphorylation events, growth factor activation ultimately leads to activation of ras proteins, as manifested by an increase in guanosine triphosphate (GTP) binding. The three ras proteins (H-, K-, and N-ras) are members of a large superfamily of ras-related proteins that share significant struc-

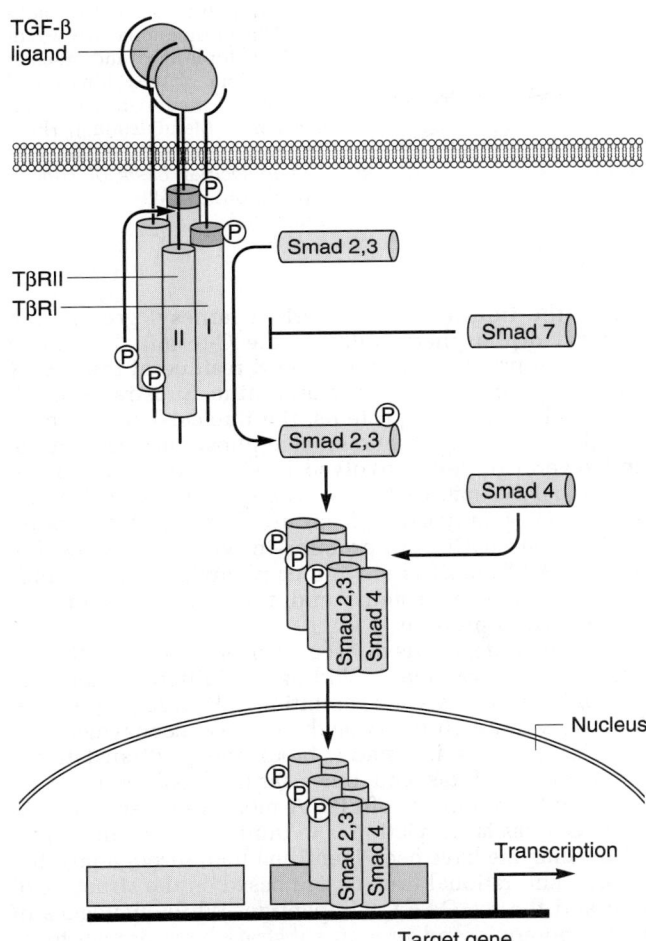

Figure 14.9. TGF-β signal transduction pathways. TGF-β binds to TβRII, causing recruitment, phosphorylation, and activation of TβRI. Substrates of TβRI include the pathway-restricted Smad2 and Smad3. The phosphorylated Smad2 and Smad3 form a heterohexameric complex with Smad4. This complex is transported to the nucleus, where it interacts with other transcription factors and specific cis-acting DNA elements. This pathway has been most closely linked with growth inhibition and tumor suppression in response to TGF-β but is also likely to be involved in other TGF-β responses, such as extracellular matrix production.

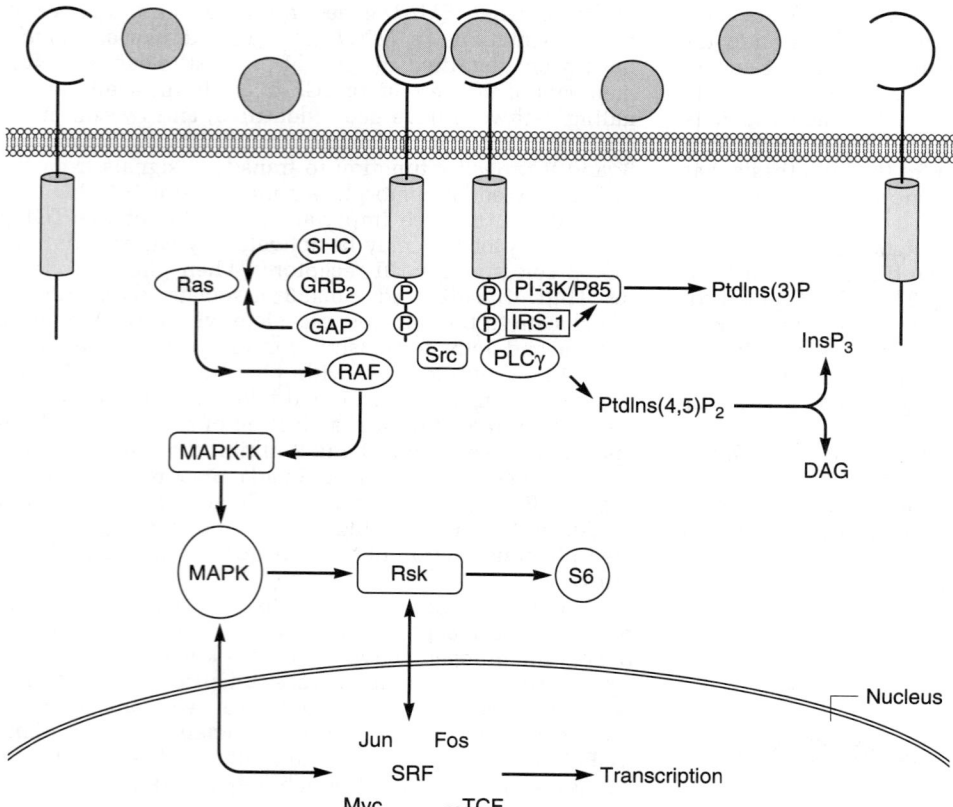

Figure 14.10. Summary of molecules involved in mitogenic signaling through RPTKs. This figure shows a dimerized and activated (tyrosine-phosphorylated) prototypical RPTK and illustrates some of the signaling molecules that associated (unshaded polygons) with receptors or reside further downstream (shaded polygons) in the pathway. The bidirectional arrows indicate cytoplasmic and nuclear localizations of MAP kinase and S6 kinase. (Redrawn with permission of Mendelsohn J, Howley PM, Israel MA, et al., eds. *The molecular basis of cancer.* Philadelphia: WB Saunders, 1995:126.)

tural homology as well as GTPase activity. All known *ras* genes encode an identical nine amino acid domain in the N-terminal half of the protein, which undergoes a major conformational shift when ras binds GTP. Ras-related proteins function as regulated guanosine diphosphate (GDP)/GTP molecular switches involved in the control of diverse cellular functions including growth (ras family), cytoskeletal organization (rho family), or vesicular transport (rab family). The biological activity of ras is controlled by the opposing effects of guanine nucleotide exchange factors (e.g., SOS), which promote formation of the active, GTP-bound state, and GTPase activating proteins (e.g., NF1-GAP), which promote formation of the inactive, GDP-bound state. Structural mutations involving codons 12, 13, and 61 result in mutant ras proteins that lack GTPase activity; these oncogenic ras proteins are locked in the active, GTP-bound state, leading to constitutive activation of downstream targets.

In addition to guanine nucleotide binding, a second critical component of ras function involves a requisite affiliation with the plasma membrane. This membrane affiliation requires posttranslational processing of ras proteins. In order for Ras members to transduce either normal or oncogenic signals, a series of posttranslational modifications must occur. Prenylation on the cysteine residue of the C-terminal CAAX box is followed by peptidase removal of the "AAX" tripeptide and methylation of the resulting cysteine carboxylate. These modifications appear to be required for membrane association and downstream signaling, including recruitment of Raf kinase to the plasma membrane.

Prenylation is a form of posttranslational protein modification that may be mediated by two different enzymes, farnesyl-protein transferase (FPTase) and geranylgeranyl-protein transferase type I (GGPTase I). FPTase cat-alyzes the transfer of a 15-carbon farnesyl group from farnesyl diphosphate (FPP) to the C-terminal cysteine residue of proteins in which the X residue of the CAAX motif is typically serine or methionine. Substrates of FPTase include the ras proteins, the nuclear lamins, the α and β subunits of skeletal muscle phosphorylase kinase, and several proteins involved in signal transduction in the visual system. GGPTase I catalyzes the transfer of a 20-carbon geranylgeranyl group from geranylgeranyl diphosphate (GGPP) to proteins in which the X residue of the CAAX motif is leucine or phenylalanine, including rac and rho proteins and the γ subunits of heterotrimeric G proteins.

Several strategies have been utilized to inhibit the ras farnesylation reaction including inhibition of the isoprenoid biosynthesis and inhibition of FPTase (Fig. 14.11). Inhibitors of 3-hydroxy-3-methylglutaryl coenzyme A reductase, such as lovastatin, block the posttranslational modification of ras and other farnesylated proteins by blocking the synthesis of FPP. A more direct approach to inhibiting ras farnesylation is to inhibit FPTase. Inhibitors of this enzyme have been identified both through targeted screens and rational drug design based on the structure of FPP and the ras CAAX tetrapeptide. While analogues of both isoprenoid and protein substrate have proven to be potent inhibitors of FPTase, the most significant advances have been made with CAAX peptidomimetics. These agents prevent the affiliation of either wild-type or mutant ras with the plasma membrane, interrupting the transduction of growth factor signals to the nuclear transcriptional machinery (Fig. 14.12). Farnesyl transferase inhibitors have proven effective in reversing the malignant phenotype in a large number of preclinical studies; clinical trials are now under way to test the efficacy of these agents in a variety of human tumors.

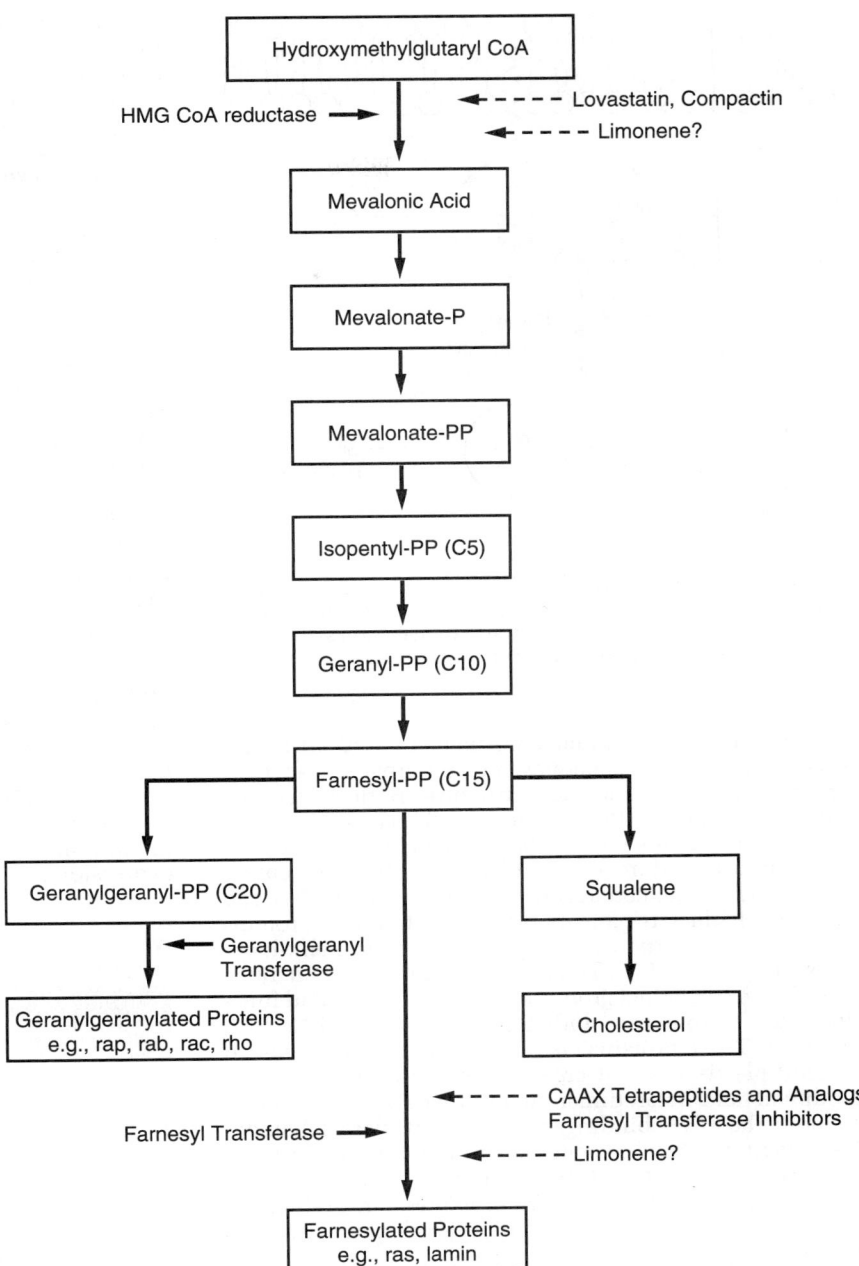

Figure 14.11. Biosynthesis of mevalonic acid derivatives required for posttranslational modification of ras and related proteins.

Differentiation/Senescence

It has long been noted that many aggressive neoplasms lack either morphologic or biochemical markers of a differentiated phenotype. In the case of certain neoplasms, dedifferentiation is documented over time. Thus initially low-grade, well-differentiated myxoid liposarcomas may lose myxoid features at the time of first recurrence, and ultimately exhibit a high-grade, undifferentiated phenotype. While the precise mechanisms of dedifferentiation during tumor formation and propagation remain unknown, several important pathways have been identified to play important roles in both normal and abnormal cellular differentiation.

Helix-Loop-Helix Transcription Factors

For many differentiated cell lineages, the expression of lineage-specific genes is regulated by members of the helix-loop-helix (HLH) family of transcription factors. Over 200 HLH proteins have now been identified, and these proteins appear to play a critical role in regulating cellular differentiation and lineage commitment in all multicellular organisms. In mammals, HLH transcription factors bind to E-box sites on target genes to mediate cell-type–specific gene transcription. For example, the HLH proteins E12 and E47 were originally identified by binding to specific domains in the immunoglobulin kappa light chain enhancer. These E-box sites are specifically identified in DNAase protection assays using B cell nuclear extracts. No protection of these sites is identified in nuclear extracts from nonlymphoid cells, indicating the importance of these HLH binding regions in regulating cell-specific gene activation. Similar E-box sites can be identified in enhancer regions from other genes demonstrating cell-specific patterns of expression, including muscle-specific genes (e.g., myosin light chain kinase, muscle creatine kinase), pancreas-specific genes (e.g., insulin, somatostatin,), and neuron-specific genes.

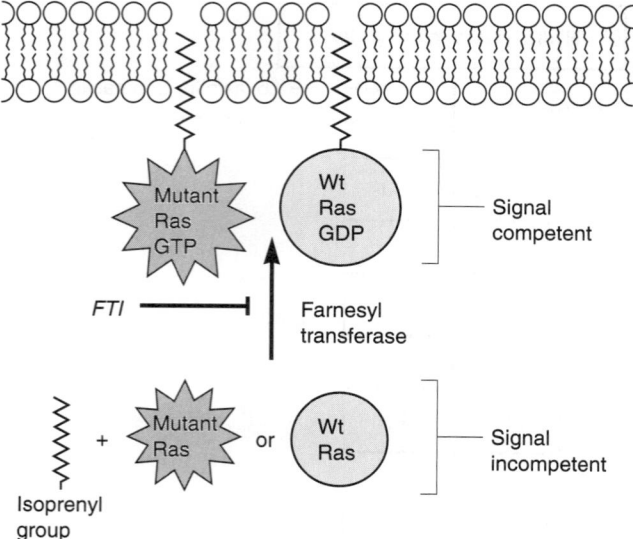

Figure 14.12. Posttranslational farnesylation of ras is required for membrane affiliation and signal compentency. Farnesyl transferase inhibitors (FTI) block posttranslational farnesylation required for activity of either mutant or wild-type ras.

Structurally, HLH proteins are named based on a conserved sequence that generates two amphipathic α-helices separated by a flexible loop structure. Both mutational studies as well as three-dimensional crystal structure analysis have demonstrated that the HLH motif functions as a dimerization domain. Most HLH proteins also contain a basic region that contacts the major groove of DNA and contains residues responsible for E box binding. Proteins containing this structure are known as basic helix-loop-helix proteins (bHLH). HLH transcription factors may be classified into distinct groups based on structure and function. Class I proteins include E proteins such as E12, E47, and HEB. These proteins are often ubiquitously expressed in multiple tissues and are capable of forming both homodimers and heterodimers with other HLH proteins. In general, the DNA binding specificity of class I homodimers is limited to E-box sites containing the core hexanucleotide sequence, CANNTG. In contrast, class II proteins show a tissue-restricted pattern of expression in different cell types and preferentially form heterodimers with class I proteins.

Members of this family play critical roles in regulating lineage-specific gene expression, and include MyoD, myogenin, NeuroD/Beta2, and the achaete-scute family. Class III HLH proteins include the Myc family of transcription factors, and are characterized by an additional leucine zipper domain adjacent to the HLH region. Class IV proteins are composed of proteins able to dimerize with Myc proteins. Class V proteins lack the DNA-binding basic region, and include the Id family of transcriptional repressors. These proteins heterodimerize with class I and class II HLH transcription factors, resulting in transcriptionally inactive complexes. Class VI HLH proteins are characterized by a proline residue in the basic region, and include the the *Drosophila* proteins Hairy and Enhancer of Split, and the mammalian HES proteins. Finally, class VII proteins are characterized by a PAS domain in addition to the bHLH motif.

Myc Regulation of Cellular Differentiation

In human neoplasia, many components of the dedifferentiated phenotype appear to involve regulation by HLH proteins. At least three major pathways have been identified that impact on HLH-regulated cellular differentiation. These include amplification/overexpression of the c-*myc* proto-oncogene, overexpression of Id transcriptional repressors, and activation of Notch signaling. With respect to Myc, the c-*myc* proto-oncogene is amplified in many human tumors, including lung cancer, breast cancer, cervical cancer, and ovarian cancer. In addition, increased expression of c-*myc* is noted in up to one third of breast and colon carcinomas. C-*myc* appears to represent a central switch through which a number of oncogenic pathways including BCR-ABL, β-catenin, and c-*src* converge to stimulate neoplasia (Fig. 14.13). C-*myc* impacts many cellular events relevant to neoplasia including proliferation, apoptosis, adhesion, immortalization, and differentiation. These effects appear to be mediated primarily through formation of heterodimers with the class IV HLH factor Max, leading to activation of Myc target genes (Fig. 14.14). Both during normal development as well as during neoplastic transformation, Myc/Max heterodimers appear to inhibit expression of differentiation-related genes.

Inhibition of Differentiation by Class V HLH Proteins

Another mechanism by which HLH proteins inhibit cellular differentiation involves the Id family of class V HLH proteins. These transcriptional repressors form heterodimers with class I and class II bHLH transcription factors, preventing expression of lineage-specific genes. In addition, Id proteins may directly enhance S-phase entry and cellular proliferation by binding to and inactivating the retinoblastoma gene product. In humans, four members of the Id transcription factor family have been identified. Id expression is normally down-regulated during differentia-

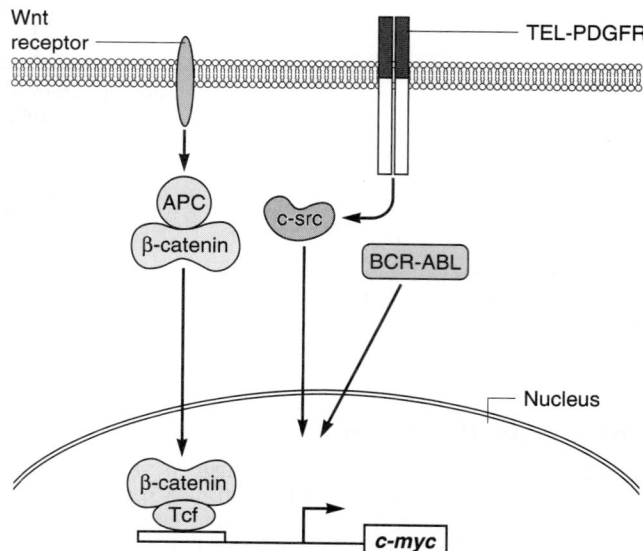

Figure 14.13. The c-myc gene is a central oncogenic switch for oncogenes and the tumor suppressor APC. The APC tumor suppressor protein mediates the degradation of B-catenin. The Wnt oncoprotein is shown activating its receptor, which results in the stabilization of free B-catenin, which sustains activating mutations in human cancers, is a co-factor for the transcription factor Tef. Tef activates c-myc expression through specific DNA binding sites. The oncogenic fusion protein TEL-PDGFR hypothetically activates c-src, as does native PDGFR, resulting in the activation of c-myc. The BRC-ABL oncoprotein likewise requires c-myc for its activity. (Redrawn from Dang CV. c-Myc target genes involved in cell growth, apoptosis, and metabolism. *Mol Cell Biol* 1999;19: 1–11, with permission.)

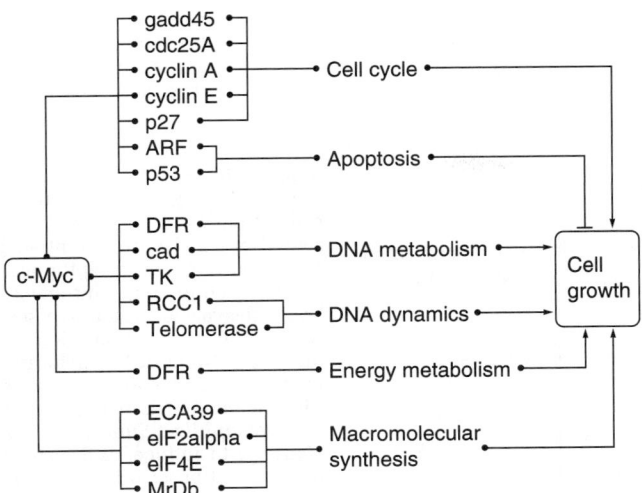

Figure 14.14. Links between c-Myc, selected putative target genes, cellular functions, and cell growth. The diagram illustrates the complexity of the connections between c-Myc and its putative target genes, which are shown clustered according to their functions. The various cellular functions cooperate to promote cell growth. It should be noted that this diagram does not reflect the controversies over the authentication of the various target genes. (Redrawn from Dang CV. c-Myc target genes involved in cell growth, apoptosis, and metabolism. *Mol Cell Biol* 1999;19:1–11, with permission.)

tion of normal cell lineages, while Id overexpression is observed in certain conditions of neoplastic growth. Direct evidence for a role of Id-mediated inhibition of differentiation during neoplastic transformation is provided by the observation that cotransfection of Id3 and bcl-2 results in immortalization of primary rat embryo fibroblasts, while down-regulation of Id2 expression inhibits the growth of pancreatic cancer cells.

Inhibition of Differentiation by Notch Signaling

A third major pathway influencing bHLH-regulated cellular differentiation involves the Notch signaling pathway. Notch signaling appears to play a critical role in regulating

cellular differentiation during both normal development and during malignant transformation. The pathway is highly conserved, with homologous components in *Caenorhabditis elegans, Drosophila,* zebrafish, mice, and humans (Table 14.6). Four human Notch family members have been identified. Notch proteins represent transmembrane receptors containing extracellular tandem EGF-like repeats as well as three Lin/Notch repeats that function in ligand binding and Notch activation. As transmembrane receptors, Notch proteins are unique in apparently lacking any enzymatic activity. Instead, Notch proteins undergo proteolytic cleavage upon activation by binding to DSL ligands (e.g., Delta, Serrate, Lag-2). Recent data suggest that proteolytic cleavage of Notch may be accomplished by γ-secretase, an enzyme also responsible for proteolytic production of β-amyloid from amyloid precursor protein. Following proteolytic cleavage, the Notch intracellular domain (Notch-IC) is released to interact with a number of cytoplasmic and nuclear proteins, including CSL proteins such as *Drosophila Suppressor of Hairless* and mammalian CBF-1. Interactions between Notch-IC and CSL proteins results in transcriptional activation of Hairy/Enhancer of Split (HES) class VI HLH protein. Once bound to DNA, HES proteins recruit a co-repressor known as Groucho, thereby preventing expression of a number of cell lineage–specific class II bHLH proteins, including MyoD, neurogenin 3, and achaete-scute homologues (Fig. 14.15).

Notch signaling therefore represents a mechanism to prevent lineage-specific cellular differentiation. During development, this function appears to play a critical role in lateral inhibition as well as in boundary formation. Notably, Notch signaling has also been implicated in various forms of neoplasia. Notch-IC is capable of transforming rat kidney cells in cooperation with adenoviral E1A, and substitutes for activated ras in this assay. Notch receptors and ligands are upregulated in human cervical cancer, and activating translocations involving Notch family members have been identified in acute T-cell leukemia. Notch also appears to be required for immortalization of B lymphocytes by Epstein-Barr virus, and represents a site for activating integration by the mouse mammary tumor virus. Additional studies have identified an important role of the Notch target gene HES-1 in regulating differentiation status in non–small cell lung cancer.

Table 14.6. CONSERVED COMPONENTS OF THE NOTCH SIGNALING PATHWAY

	Caenorhabditis elegans	*Drosophila*	*Mammals*
Notch receptors	Lin-12 Glp-1	Notch	Notch1 Notch3 Notch2 Notch4
Extracellular ligands (DSL proteins)	Lag-2 Apx-1	Delta	Delta-1 Delta-1 Delta-like 1 (Dll-1) Delta-like 3 (Dll-3)
		Serrate	Jagged1 (Serrate1) Jagged2 (Serrate2)
Intracellular effectors	Lag-1	Suppressor of hairless [Su(H)] Deltex	CBF-1/RBP-J$_\kappa$ Deltex NF$_\kappa$B

Target genes		Enhancer of split [E(spl)]
		  bHLH
		  Groucho
			HES (Hairy/enhancer of split)
			  bHLH
			  TLE

Processing molecules Modifiers	SUP-17	Kuzbanian Fringe	Kuzbanian Lunatic fringe Manic fringe Radical fringe
		Numb	Numb Numb like
		Disheveled	Disheveled 1,2,3

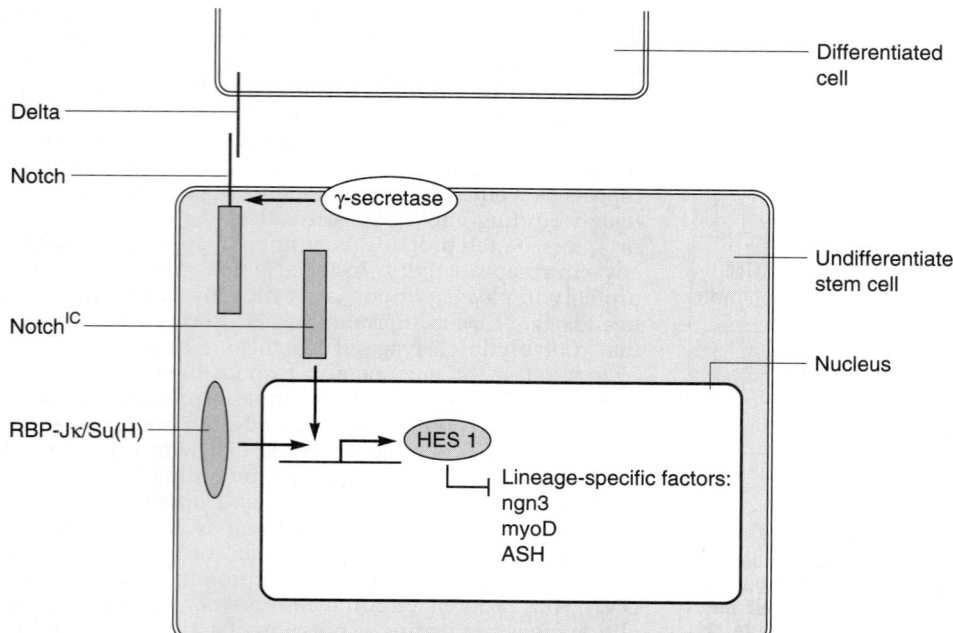

Figure 14.15. Notch signaling inhibits lineage-specific cellular differentiation. Ligands presented by adjacent differentiated cells lead to Notch receptor activation. Following intramembrane cleavage of Notch by γ-secretase, the intracellular domain of Notch (Notch-IC) translocates to nucleus and cooperates with RBP-Jκ- (mammalian homologue of *Drosophila Suppressor of Hairless*) to induce HES1. HES1 represses transcription of lineage-specific transcription factors, including neurogenin3, myoD, and the achaete-scute homologue (ASH). Activation of Notch signaling thereby maintains cells in an undifferentiated, stem cell–like state.

Pharmacologic Regulation of Differentiation

Differentiation is the process by which a cell develops specialized structure and function. Normally, a fully differentiated cell is not capable of further cell division. For example, in the intestinal tract, the pluripotent enterocyte differentiates into either a goblet cell that secretes mucus or an absorptive cell complete with a brush border. Due to alterations in internal or external signaling, the cancer cell is able to continue proliferation and does not undergo terminal differentiation. In this state, the cell is considered to have undergone malignant transformation.

There are a number of agents that can induce cellular differentiation. This can be advantageous in the treatment of cancer because cells committed to terminal differentiation ultimately undergo either senescence or programmed cell death, thus limiting tumor cell proliferation. Examples of differentiation agents that are being used in both the preclinical and clinical setting include retinoids, vitamin D, and butyrate. Retinoids are compounds metabolized from retinol that enter the body through the gastrointestinal tract. Retinoic acid induces transcription by binding to receptors in the cell nucleus, thereby altering transcriptional events that ultimately induce cellular differentiation. Certain forms of retinoic acid have been shown to reverse oral leukoplakia, which is a precursor to squamous carcinoma in heavy smokers. Another differentiating agent is the active form of vitamin D_3 or 1,25-dihydroxyvitamin D_3. Vitamin D receptors are located on breast and colon epithelial cells and vitamin D analogues have been shown to inhibit growth of breast and colon cancer cell lines.

Butyrate compounds also exhibit cytodifferentiating properties. In animal studies, the ability to obtain high levels of butyrate in the colon has stimulated interest in these compounds for chemoprevention in colon cancer.

Telomerase and Cell Immortalization/Senescence

Senescence refers to the process during which a normal cell ages and dies. This process is controlled, in part, by specialized heterochromatic structures at the ends of eukaryotic chromosomes called telomeres that function to stabilize and protect the chromosome. During normal somatic cell replication, telomeres become progressively shorter with each cell division, resulting in chromosome instability. It has been postulated that the shortening of telomeres represents a checkpoint mechanism by which cellular senescence is signaled in normal replicating cell populations.

Telomerase is an RNA-dependent DNA polymerase that stabilizes telomeres by synthesizing the six oligonucleotide repeat TTAGGG. This stabilization can allow indefinite replication and thus "cell immortalization." While inactive in most somatic cells, telomerase remains activated in germ cells and lymphocytes. A unique characteristic of the cancer cell is immortality with the ability to divide repeatedly without undergoing normal cellular senescence. A correlation between telomerase and cancer has recently been documented by the detection of telomerase activity in a high percentage of primary human malignancies including cancer of the lung, colon, breast, and prostate. By remaining in the activated state, telomerase may contribute to the uncontrolled replicative capacity of the cancer cell. This finding has stimulated much discussion of the potential diagnostic, prognostic, and therapeutic implications of telomerase in the management of cancer.

Cell Survival/Programmed Cell Death

Virtually all cell populations are controlled through a balance of survival and death. Under certain conditions such as terminal differentiation, growth factor deprivation, or DNA damage, survival signals to the cell are replaced by death signals. Cell death can occur in a variety of forms, but the most common cause of cell death is either necrosis or apoptosis. Necrotic cell death takes place primarily from noxious stimuli to the cell in the form of chemicals, burns, ischemia, or other insults. In contrast, apoptosis, or programmed cell death, occurs via a complex, genetically determined process. Apoptosis is a continual process in many normal as well as altered cell populations. For instance, during embryogenesis, organ formation undergoes a series of remolding events that are governed by apoptosis. Apoptosis is also an active process in many disease states. Following myocardial infarction, induction of apoptosis occurs in the damaged cardiac muscle cells.

The process of apoptosis is described as a cascade of events, each mediated by intracellular proteins, ultimately leading to apoptotic cell death. After receiving a cell death stimulus, induction of genes that promote apoptosis occurs, thereby shifting the intercellular balance toward proteins with proapoptotic activity. Two of the best studied apoptotic genes are *Bcl-2* and *Bax.* Normally, the levels of antiapoptotic *Bcl-2* allow for continued cell survival. During the apoptotic state, *Bcl-2* levels are down-regulated shifting the balance toward proapoptotic proteins such as Bax. Downstream regulators of the apoptotic cascade are recruited including endonucleases, which cleave chromatin, resulting in nuclear fragmentation. This results in the formation of apoptotic bodies and other morphologic characteristics of apoptosis such as cell shrinkage and loss of contact with adjacent cells. In contrast, necrotic cell death is characterized by cellular swelling and ultimate rupture of the cell membrane. Just as apoptosis is active in embryogenesis and the molding of organ structure and function, it is also recognized to be important in disease states such as cancer. In general, cancer cells that are resistant to cell death have altered their balance of apoptotic regulators. For instance, cancer cells that are resistant to conventional therapies such as radiation and chemotherapy often have increased levels of antiapoptotic proteins such as Bcl-2. To change the balance toward apoptotic cell death, some newer therapies attempt to up-regulate proapoptotic proteins such as Bax, or conversely down-regulate antiapoptotic proteins such as Bcl-2.

In addition to the induction of apoptosis by the above-mentioned proteins, programmed cell death can also occur via recognition events of the immune system. Specifically, the Fas antigen (CD-95, APO-1) is a cell surface protein of the tumor necrosis factor (TNF) family. When stimulated by its ligand (FasL), Fas-bearing cells undergo apoptotic cell death. This is a possible mechanism of cytotoxic T-cell– and natural killer cell–mediated death as well as other autoimmune responses.

ABNORMAL GROWTH REGULATION IN CANCER

Transformation from the normal phenotype to invasive malignancy appears to involve a loss of normal tumor suppressive and growth inhibitory responses as well as the ac-quisition of inappropriate proliferative signals. The presence of inappropriate proliferative signals has been well documented in most malignancies, and includes overexpression of peptide growth factors (TGF-β, amphiregulin, heparin-binding EGF) and of growth factor receptors (e.g., HER2/neu). Alternatively, there may be mutational activation of the signal transduction pathways for the growth factors (e.g., *ras* and *src* oncogenes), activation of oncogenes that are directly involved in stimulating progression of the cell cycle regulation (e.g., *myc, cyclin D1,* etc.), or inactivation of genes that provide checkpoint control on cell cycle progression (e.g., the retinoblastoma gene *p53,* etc.).

Cell Cycle Regulation in Cancer

The cell cycle involves cellular events concerned with replication of chromosomal DNA during the S phase and the separation of replicated chromosomes during cell division (mitosis or meiosis, M phase). The cell cycle is an indispensable process for survival of an organism and is highly conserved throughout evolution. The S phase and M phase are separated by gap periods, or G phases, with the G1 phase preceding the S phase and the G2 phase preceding the M phase (Fig. 14.16). G0 describes cells that are in a quiescent state with regard to cell replication. G0 cells are often differentiated cells that may be metabolically active, but are not involved in the process of cellular replication. The cell has mechanisms for responding to extracellular signals in order that cells in G0 may be recruited into the cell cycle.

The process of cell cycle progression is tightly regulated. The factors responsible for advancing cell cycle progression were initially discovered in yeast and in amphibian eggs. Cyclins were discovered as proteins that oscillated during specific periods of the cell cycle. Subsequent work led to the identification of the catalytic partners of the cyclins, called cyclin-dependent kinases (CDKs). Specific sets of cyclins with their partner CDKs drive progression through specific periods of the cell cycle (Fig. 14.17). It is also critical that mistakes in DNA replication or in chromosomal segregation are monitored and not allowed to propagate. This regulatory function has been called cell cycle checkpoint control. The mechanisms of checkpoint control involve regulation of the levels and activities of the cyclins and CDKs, and also involve the regulation of programmed cell death (apoptosis).

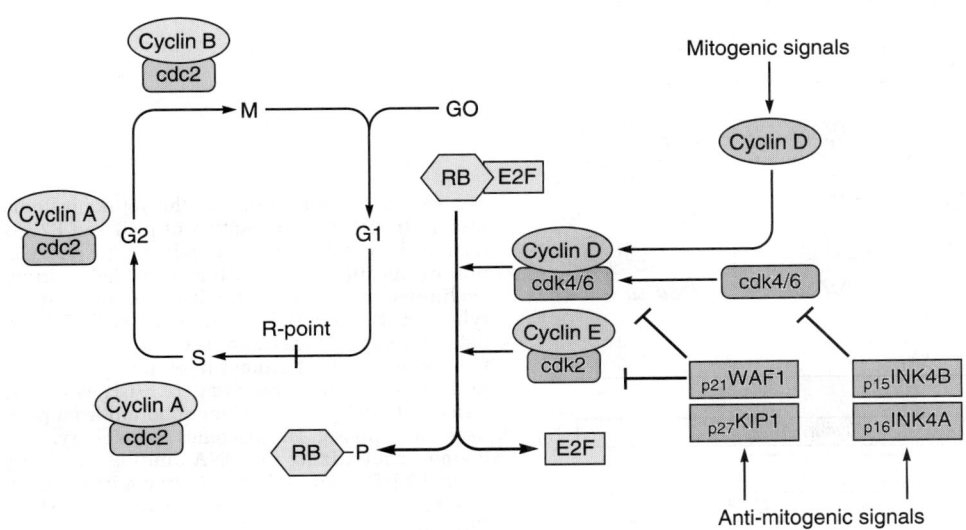

Figure 14.16. The cell cycle clock machinery. G0, M, G1, S, and G2 refer to the quiescence, mitosis, first gap, DNA synthesis, and second gap phases of the cell cycle, respectively. The restriction point (R-point) is shown preceding S phase entry. RB and RB-p represent unphosphorylated and hyperphosphorylated forms of the retinoblastoma protein. (Redrawn from Lundberg AS, Weinberg RA. Control of the cell cycle and apoptosis. *Eur J Cancer* 1999;35:531–539, with permission.)

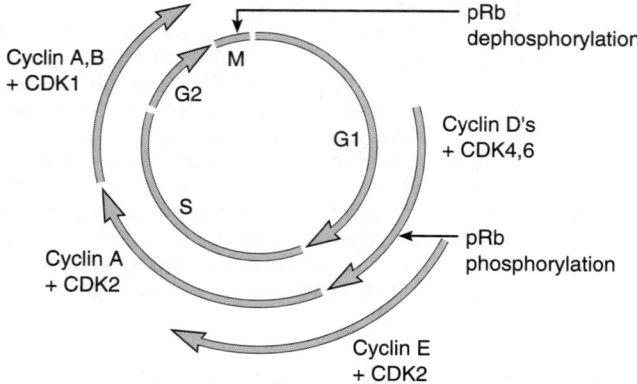

Figure 14.17. The cell cycle clock. This version of the cell cycle shows where the RB (pRB) protein is either phosphorylated or dephosphorylated to regulate cell cycle transit.

Quiescent cells may be recruited to the cell cycle by mitogenic stimulation (e.g., growth factor exposure). Normal cells depend on exogenous mitogenic stimulation only during the first two thirds of the G1 phase. At this two-thirds point, also called the restriction (R) point, the cell may commit itself to advance into the S phase and subsequent phases of the cell cycle (Fig. 14.18). The retinoblastoma protein (pRB) is the molecular switch that controls passage through the R point. Unphosphorylated or hypophosphorylated pRB blocks R point transition, whereas phosphorylation of pRB prevents it from blocking cell cycle progression.

Expression of a specific subset of the cyclins called D-type cyclins (D1, D2, and D3) is increased in early to mid-G1 in response to mitogenic signals. The D-type cyclins assemble with their catalytic partners, CDK4 and CDK6, and the cyclin D/CDK complex enters the cell nucleus where it becomes phosphorylated by a CDK-activating kinase (CAK). A critical function of the cyclin D–dependent kinases is the phosphorylation of the Rb protein. Growth factor activation of Ras signaling and the MAPK cascade induces transcription of the cyclin D1 gene, decreases the turnover of the cyclin D1 protein, and regulates cyclin D-CDK assembly. Expression of the D-type cyclins is dependent on continuous mitogenic stimulation. Progression

through the mid- to late G1 phase of the mammalian cell cycle is dependent on the cyclin D–dependent protein kinases.

Cyclin D–dependent kinases initiate the phosphorylation of Rb in mid-G1, then subsequent activation of the cyclin E/CDK2 complex leads to further phosphorylation of Rb on additional sites. Cyclin A–dependent CDK (CDK2) becomes activated during the S phase and cyclin B–dependent CDK (CDC2) becomes activated during G2 and M. These cyclin–dependent kinases help to maintain Rb in a hyperphosphorylated state until mitosis has been completed and Rb is returned to its hypophosphorylated state at the beginning of G1. Hypophosphorylated Rb inhibits the transcriptional activity of E2F protein family members. Hyperphosphorylation of Rb in late G1 phase disrupts its association with E2F family members, thereby enabling them to express their activity as transcription factors. The activation of the E2F transcription factor complex is required for the expression of a set of genes whose activities are required for S phase progression. These include gene products that regulate nucleotide metabolism and DNA synthesis, as well as cyclins E and A.

The activities of CDKs are governed by other proteins called CDK inhibitors (CKIs). There are two families of CKIs based on structure and their CDK targets. One class includes the INK4 proteins (inhibitors of CDK4), which specifically bind and inhibit the activities of CDK4 and CDK6. This family is composed of four such proteins (p16[INK4a], p15[INK4b], p18[INK4c], and p19[INK4d]). The Cip/Kip family comprises the other family of CKIs. This family includes the proteins p21[Cip1], p27[Kip1], and p57[Kip2]. The CKIs of the Cip/Kip family were originally thought to interfere with the activities of cyclin D–, cyclin E–, and cyclin A–dependent kinases. This view has now evolved with further data confirming that the Cip/Kip proteins are potent inhibitors of cyclin E– and cyclin A–dependent CDK2 activity; however, this family of CKIs appears to act as positive regulators of cyclin D–dependent kinases. Increased levels of cyclin D-CDK4 during the G1 phase results in sequestration of the Cip/Kip CKIs, thereby preventing them from associating with and inhibiting cyclin E– and cyclin A–dependent CDK2. Interestingly, activated CDK2 catalyzes hyperphosphorylation of Rb and also triggers the proteolytic destruction of p27[Kip1].

In addition to transcriptional activation and induction of cyclin gene expression, proteolysis is a critical function

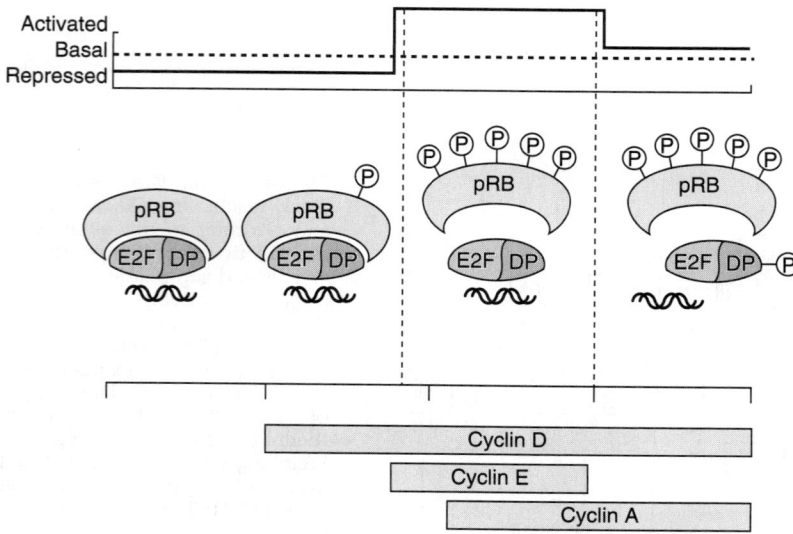

Figure 14.18. Interactions of the retinoblastoma protein (pRB). The interaction of pRB and E2F is regulated by cell cycle–dependent phosphorylation by specific cyclins acting with their partner cyclin-dependent kinases (cdks). Underphosphorylated pRB forms stable complexes with E2F/DP heterodimers and this complex actively represses transcription. pRB becomes hyperphosphorylated in late G1, thereby releasing E2F/DP, which is transcriptionally active when unbound from pRB. Late in S-phase, DP becomes phosphorylated, thereby neutralizing the DNA-binding capability of the E2F/DP heterodimer. (Redrawn from Kaelin WG Jr. Functions of the retinoblastoma protein. *Bioessays* 1999;21:950–958.)

in the regulation of the cell cycle. As mentioned above, proteolytic destruction of p27^{Kip1} is triggered during the S phase. Once the S phase has been initiated, the cell is no longer reliant on mitogenic signals or the D-dependent cyclins for progression through the remainder of the cell cycle. Cyclin E is degraded as cells progress through the S phase, cyclin A is degraded during G2, and cyclin B is degraded by the completion of the M phase in order to reset the system and thereby reestablish a period of mitogen dependence in the next G1 phase (Fig. 14.19).

Disruption of the growth suppressive function of Rb is a common event in cancer. This may occur as the result of mutational inactivation of Rb itself, or because of the disruption of p16 function. Increased expression and activation of cyclin D and CDK4 (via amplification or transcriptional activation) are also common events in human cancer and result in the same type of inactivation of growth inhibitory function of Rb. Interestingly, complete loss of Cip/Kip function has not been observed in cancer, nor have cyclin E gene amplification or mutations resulting in increased cyclin E dependent CDK activity.

The CKIs appear to function as checkpoint controls to ensure that cell cycle progression occurs under the proper environmental conditions and that the proper intracellular signaling has been completed prior to the initiation of DNA synthesis. Further checkpoints are the DNA damage and replication controls that block mitosis when DNA is damaged or DNA replication is incomplete. These checkpoint controls are essential for maintaining genomic stability, the failure of which allows cells to divide when DNA is damaged, DNA synthesis is incomplete, or in the presence of faulty chromosomal segregation.

All cancer cells have abnormalities in one or more of the components of cell cycle control involved in G1 to S phase transition. In some cases loss of Rb function itself is the event that releases the cells from extracellular signaling constraints. Mutational loss of Rb function occurs in the vast majority of retinoblastomas, and less frequently in other tumor types such as lung cancers, soft tissue sarcomas, lung cancers, etc. In the absence of functional Rb protein, E2F is active and there is no requirement for activation of cyclin D/Cdk4 to initiate DNA synthesis. Amplification of the cyclin D1 gene is common in several types of human tumors such as breast, head and neck, esophageal, and hepatic malignancies. Increased expression of cyclin D1 without gene amplification is common in colorectal cancer. Deletion of the p16^{INK4a} gene is also common in human cancers, particularly in melanomas and in a subset of pancreatic cancers. Hereditary loss of p16^{INK4a} function is associated with increased risk for melanoma and pancreatic cancer. All of the above defects in cell cycle regulators result in loss of the same G1/S checkpoint control and it is rare for more than one of the above defects to be identified in the same tumor.

Genomic Instability in Cancer

Genomic instability with a high frequency of chromosomal loss and gain, genome doubling, and subtler genetic mutations are some of the major characteristics of cancer cells. Genomic instability increases the chance of specific gene mutations that are ultimately responsible for the various phenotypes of cancer cells. Cancer cells acquire defects in the checkpoints that control normal mitosis, with its equal distribution of chromosomes into daughter cells and cytokinesis. Failure of this checkpoint may result in unequal distribution of chromosomes or failure to undergo cytokinesis, and either polyploidy (4N, 8N, etc.) or aneuploidy.

The tumor suppressor protein p53 plays a critical role in maintaining genomic stability (Fig. 14.20). p53 function is required to initiate checkpoint-activated cell cycle arrest and programmed cell death in response to DNA damage. This function of p53 is necessary to ensure the integrity of the cellular genome by protecting it from the adverse effects of DNA damage. The p53 protein functions as an important transcription factor mediating expression of a variety of genes whose products may directly regulate growth arrest or apoptosis. Growth arrest induced by p53 may enable a cell to repair DNA that has been damaged. Alternatively, p53 also functions to induce apoptosis in order to prevent propagation of a cell lineage containing mutated DNA sequences.

Expression of p53 may be induced by either DNA damage or by inappropriate mitogenic signaling. An example of an important p53-responsive gene product involved in cell cycle arrest is the cyclin kinase inhibitor protein p21^{Cip1}. Several p53-responsive gene products appear to be involved in the apoptotic response. These include Bax, Fas/Apo, Killer/Dr5, and the redox regulator gene products known as PIGs (p53-induced genes). The expression of Mdm2 is also induced upon activation of the p53 gene. Mdm2 is a negative feedback regulator of p53 whose function is to target p53 for rapid degradation (Fig. 14.20B,C). Interestingly, one of the two products of the *INK4a/ARF* locus, p14^{ARF} inhibits the function of Mdm2, thereby stabilizing and activating p53 and promoting cell cycle arrest and apoptosis in response to inappropriate mitogenic signals. The other product of the *INK4a/ARF* locus is p16^{Ink4a}, the important inhibitor of cyclin dependent kinases 4 and 6, and a mediator of G1 cell cycle.

The protein product of the *Myc* proto-oncogene also regulates both cell proliferation and apoptosis in cell culture systems. *Myc* expression is capable of preventing cells from exiting the cell cycle and of promoting continuous cell cycle progression. Expression of *Myc* also inhibits differentiation in certain cell types. Similar to the situation in which inappropriately increased E2F triggers apoptosis, inappropriate *Myc* expression can also trigger apoptosis.

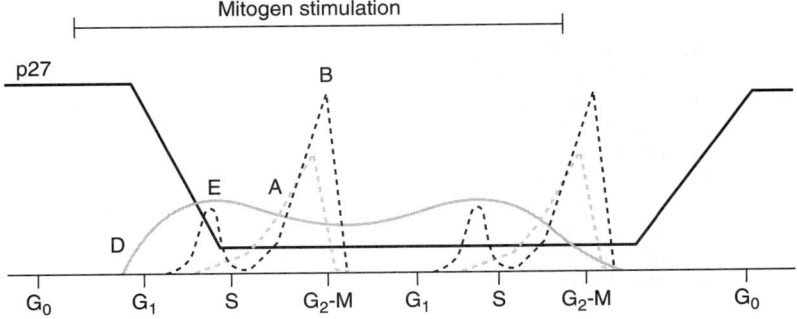

Figure 14.19. Fluctuations of cyclins and cyclin kinase inhibitors during the cell cycle. Cyclins E, A, and B undergo periodic oscillation during each cell cycle. In contrast, the D-type cyclins tend to remain elevated in cycling cells under the influence of growth stimuli. Levels of the inhibitor p27^{Kip1} tend to remain high in quiescent cells, but are decreased in proliferating cells. (Redrawn from Sherr CJ. Cancer cell cycles. *Science* 1996;274:1672–1677, with permission.)

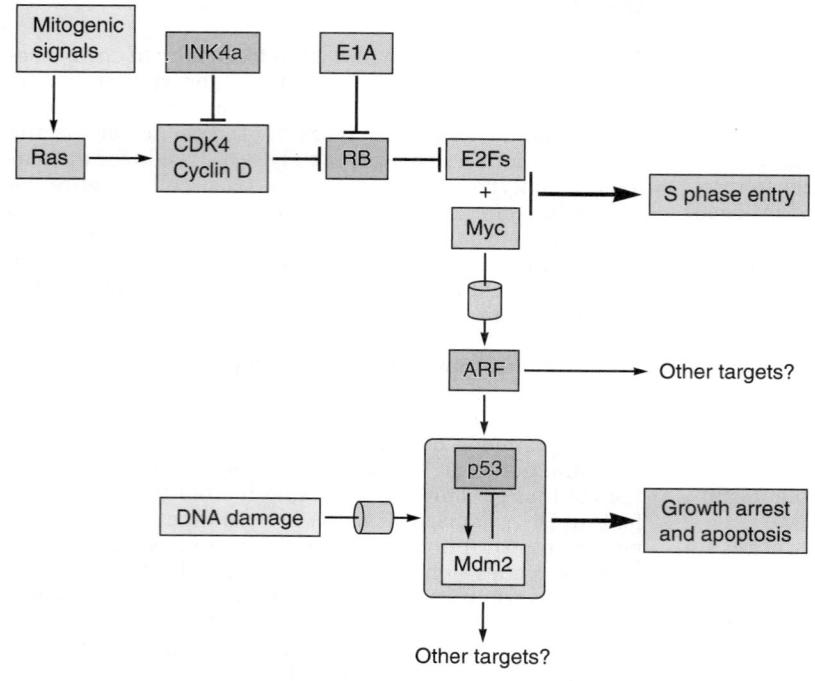

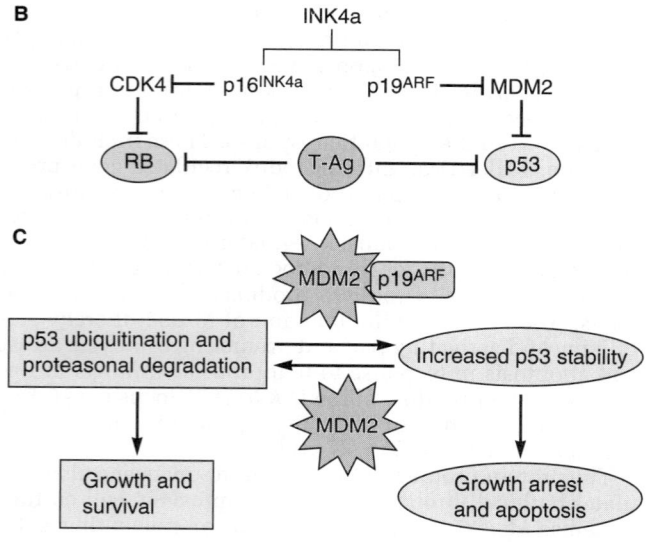

Figure 14.20. The pRB and p53 pathways are connected via an ARF-regulated checkpoint. Mitogenic or oncogene activation of cell cycle entry results in increased E2F and Myc activity and leads to ARF expression. Mdm2 binds to and destabilizes p53, thereby inhibiting its function. ARF binds to Mdm2 and prevents it from destabilizing p53, thereby promoting growth arrest and apoptosis. Loss of ARF can lead to more efficient Mdm2 degradation of p53. Some oncogenic protein products from DNA tumor viruses (e.g., T-antigen [T-Ag]) can interfere with these pathways. The T-Ag inhibits the functions of both pRB and p53. (*A*: redrawn from Sherr CJ, Weber JD. The ARF/p53 pathway. *Curr Opin Genet Dev* 2000;10:94–99, with permission. *B,C*: redrawn from Pomerantz J, Schreiber-Agus N, Liegeois NJ, et al. The INK4a tumor suppressor gene product, p18ARF, interacts with MDM2 and neutralizes MDM2's inhibition of p53. *Cell* 1998;92:713–723, with permission.)

Both increased E2F and *Myc* increase the expression of the ARF protein (p14 and p19), and as described above, increased expression of ARF stabilizes p53, leading to both growth arrest and apoptosis.

There is a growing list of additional proteins that are involved in sensing and repairing DNA damage, or in assuring correct chromosomal segregation during mitosis. Loss of function of these important genomic "caretaker" systems appears to be common in cancer cells, and this loss facilitates genomic instability with the accumulation of additional genetic lesions. The cumulative genetic mutations lead to tumor cells with selective advantages for aggressive biologic behavior including invasiveness and metastatic capacity, resistance to immunosurveillance, resistance to apoptosis, and the ability to resist cancer therapeutic interventions.

Tumor Initiation and Progression in Colorectal Cancer

The Adenoma-Carcinoma Sequence

The development of cancer is a multistep process involving a series of genetic changes that lead sequentially to hyperplasia, adenoma, carcinoma, and finally metastasis (Fig. 14.2). The multistep carcinogenesis process is probably best described and understood for colorectal cancer, but the principles probably apply to all other cancers. The initiating event may be different for cancers arising in different tissues, but the principle of progressive mutational events leading to an accumulation of genetic lesions remains consistent. These genetic lesions consist of loss of critical tumor suppressor functions and mutations that result in gain of function for dominant oncogenes. The current understanding of the development of colon cancer is based on a paradigm developed by Fearon and Vogelstein. Utilizing results from epidemiologic, clinical, and genetic studies they observed that more than 90% of colorectal adenocarcinomas arise from adenomatous polyps. The progression from normal mucosa to adenoma and then to subsequent carcinoma probably occurs over a 10- to 20-year period. Progression of colorectal tumors results from a series of mutations affecting multiple genes involving the regulation of epithelial cell growth, differentiation, and programmed cell death.

This multistep process is developed over the decades and requires several genetic events for completion. Even so, inheritance of a single altered gene can result in a marked predisposition to colorectal cancer in two distinct syndromes, familial adenomatous polyposis (FAP) and hereditary nonpolyposis colorectal cancer (HNPCC). FAP is a syndrome in which an inherited defect in the adenomatous polyposis coli *(APC)* gene leads to the development of multiple benign polyps throughout the colon, some of which slowly progress to invasive lesions. In contrast to FAP, HNPCC is a syndrome characterized by rapid progression of colorectal tumors due to inherited defects in DNA mismatch repair (MMR) genes.

One of the earliest steps in the development of colorectal cancer is the loss of function of the tumor suppressor gene, *APC,* considered a gatekeeper gene in colorectal cancer. This gene was first identified as the gene responsible for FAP by demonstrating co-segregation of mutant alleles in affected kindreds. In fact, over 70% of the sporadic colorectal cancers are believed to involve somatic mutations in *APC.* Further support for the role of *APC* in the development of polyps and colorectal cancer stems from the studies of a mouse genetic model for FAP known as *Min* (multiple intestinal neoplasia). The mutations in *Min* mice, like those in many FAP patients, causes premature truncation of APC protein, and *Min* mice develop multiple adenomatous polyps and cancers of the intestine. The exact mechanism by which *APC* mutations cause abnormal growth of colorectal epithelial cells is still not clear, but several important clues have been uncovered.

Greater than 95% of *APC* mutations in both FAP and sporadic colorectal cancers are C-terminal truncations. Several proteins that interact with the C-terminus of the 2,843 amino acid APC protein may prove to be important in colorectal neoplasia. The majority of somatic and germline mutations in *APC* result in a protein that is truncated in the region containing seven copies of a 20-amino acid repeat that has been shown to both bind and trigger the degradation of β-catenin (Fig. 14.21). β-catenin was initially identified as one of a small group of proteins that colocalizes with the cell adhesion molecule E-cadherin.

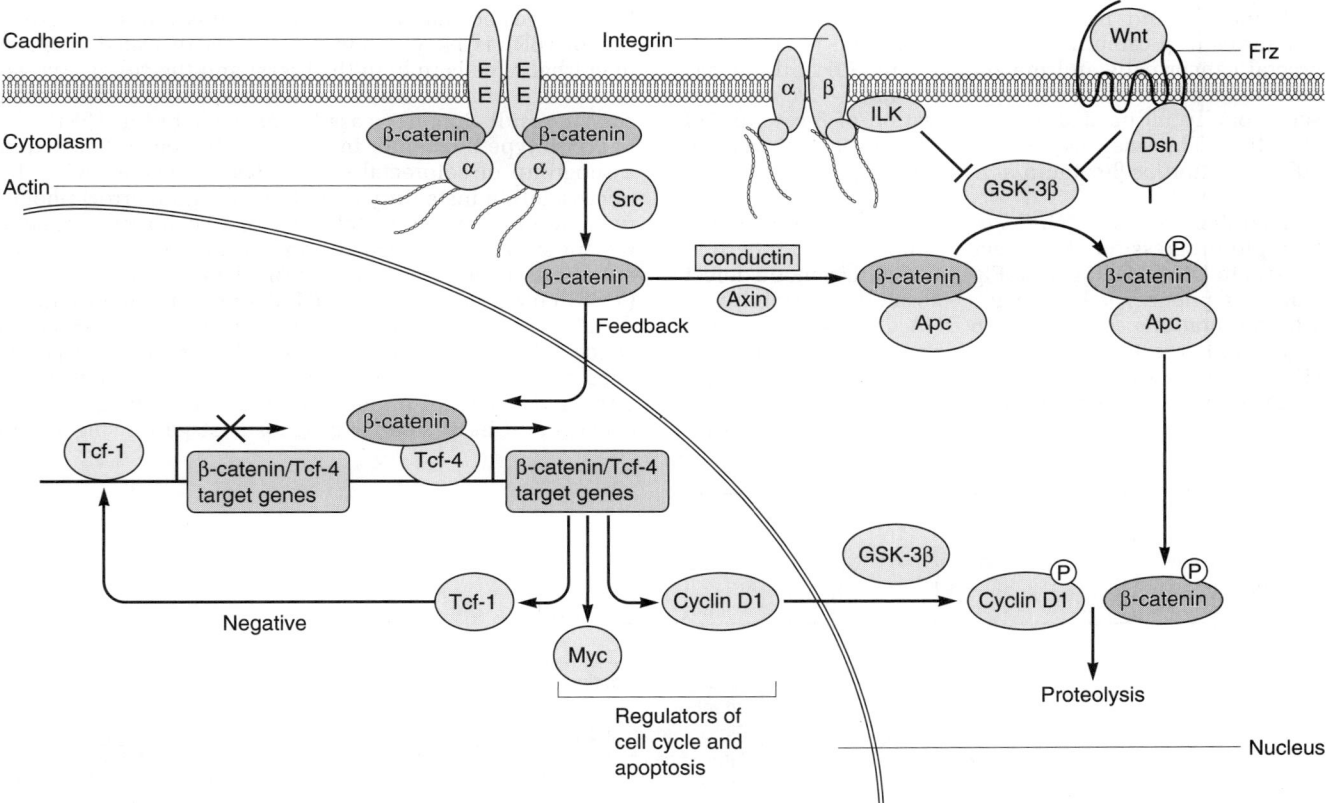

Figure 14.21. The β-catenin/APC/GSK-3b pathway. Signals from cell membrane receptors, adhesion molecules, and levels of E-cadherin regulate the cellular balance of β-catenin. Cytosolic levels of β-catenin are tightly regulated through proteolysis. GSK-3b phosphorylates β-catenin in cooperation with APC, thereby targeting β-catenin for ubiquitin-mediated proteolysis. E-cadherin avidly binds β-catenin to the cell membrane in the adherins junction complex. Inactivation of GSK-3b, loss of APC, or loss of E-cadherin function can result in the cytoplasmic accumulation of β-catenin, enabling it to translocate to the nucleus. In cooperation with the Tcf/Lef transcription factors, β-catenin positively regulates the expression of the c-*myc* and *cyclin D1* proto-oncogenes. Active GSK-3b also targets *cyclin D1* for proteolysis. (Redrawn from MacLeod K. Tumor suppressor genes. *Curr Opin Genet Dev* 2000;1:81–93, with permission.)

β-catenin binds to the cytoplasmic domain of E-cadherin and α-catenin binds to β-catenin, linking this complex with the actin cytoskeleton. Wild-type APC binds to and dramatically reduces the levels of β-catenin by causing increased degradation of the β-catenin protein, whereas *APC* mutants lacking the central region lack this activity and are unable to down-regulate β-catenin.

While β-catenin interacts with cadherins and is necessary for cadherin-mediated cell adhesion, recent evidence has strongly implicated β-catenin as a signal transducer in the *WNT* oncogene pathway. *WNT1* promotes the accumulation of β-catenin in vertebrate cells, and in *Drosophila* the expression of the *WNT* homologue, wingless (Wg), promotes the accumulation of armadillo, the β-catenin homologue. Both *Drosophila* and vertebrate cells down-regulate free cytosolic β-catenin levels through the constitutive activity of the homologous serine/threonine kinases *zeste white* 3 (zw3, *Drosophila*) and glycogen synthase kinase-3 (GSK3, vertebrates), and the functions of these proteins are inhibited by activation of the *WNT1* and *Wg* pathways, respectively. Activation of GSK-3 results in destabilization of β-catenin through phosphorylation. Wnt signaling involves binding of β-catenin with members of the Tcf/Lef family of high mobility group (HMG) transcription factors, cotranslocation to the nucleus, and regulation of selected genes with Tcf/Lef-1 promoter elements. Mutant forms of β-catenin lacking the GSK-3 phosphorylation sites result in accumulation of the β-catenin in the cell nucleus and neoplastic transformation. Stabilizing mutations of β-catenin have been identified in some colorectal cancer cells and melanoma cells. Recently, it has been determined that both *cyclin D1* and c-*Myc* are transcriptionally induced through activation of β-catenin-Tcf signaling. This may explain how the initiating event of *APC* mutation or β-catenin activation may lead to hyperproliferation.

In contrast to FAP, HNPCC is a syndrome characterized by rapid progression of colorectal tumors due to inherited defects in DNA MMR genes (Fig. 14.8). This genetic defect leads to a phenotype known as microsatellite instability in which mutations accumulate in DNA dinucleotide repeat regions. Microsatellite instability is an invariant feature of HNPCC and is also observed in another 5% to 10% of sporadic human colorectal cancers. The DNA repair defect leads to mutations in genes serving important tumor sup-

pressor functions. An example of this is the finding of a high frequency of type II TGF-β receptor mutations among tumors exhibiting microsatellite instability, which is discussed in more detail below.

Loss of Growth Inhibitory Effects of TGF-β in Cancer

TGF-β regulation of epithelial cell proliferation is altered by transformation. Loss of responsiveness to the growth-inhibitory effects of TGF-β occurs in many cancer cell types, including pancreatic, breast and colorectal carcinoma cells. Thus, loss of growth-inhibitory responses to TGF-β appears to be a common and important event that attends malignant transformation of epithelial cells (Fig. 14.22).

TGF-β Signaling Abnormalities in Cancer

The association of colorectal cancers, pancreatic carcinomas, and breast cancers with genetic lesions in the TGF-β signal transduction pathway underscores the importance of TGF-β in maintaining homeostasis in the digestive tract and in the breast. One of the mechanisms by which tumor cells become resistant to the growth inhibitory actions of TGF-β may be through down-regulation or mutation of TβRII. Loss of TGF-β receptor function causes cellular loss of negative growth regulation by TGF-β. Several studies have suggested that a decrease in expression or inactivation of TβRII is a key step for the neoplastic transformation of epithelial cells in both the breast and the colon. Activation of Ras protein, which occurs frequently in colorectal cancer, results in a decreased expression of the TβRII.

TGF-β type II receptor inactivation has been detected in a subgroup of colorectal carcinomas associated with the microsatellite instability or RER (replication error) phenotype found in approximately 13% of all colorectal cancers. Recent studies have also confirmed the presence of TβRII mutations in an additional 15% of microsatellite stable (MSS) colon cancers, and TGF-β signaling abnormalities distal to TβRII in an additional 55% of these MSS colon cancers. It is of interest and seemingly paradoxical that the subset of colorectal cancers that exhibit microsatellite instability (and TβRII mutations) tend to be proximal colon cancers and have a better prognosis (stage for stage) than

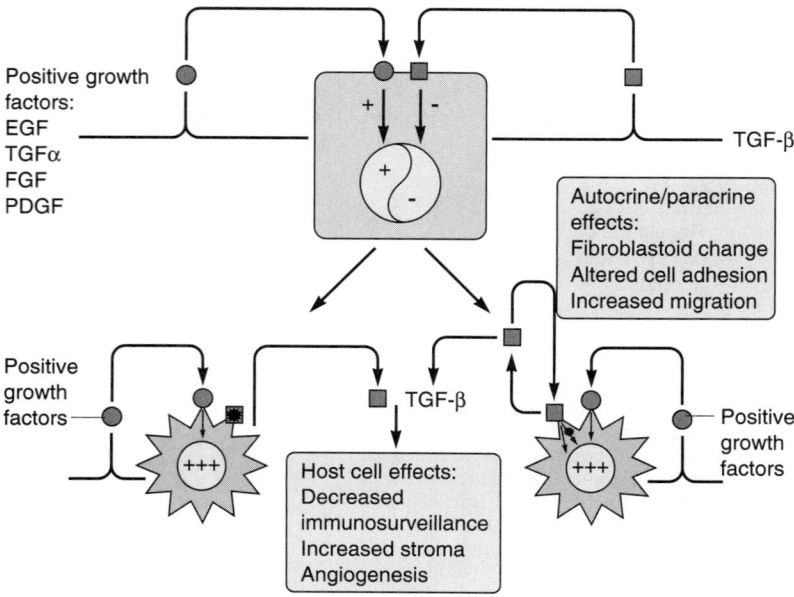

Figure 14.22. The effect of the TGF-β signaling pathway on cells is context-dependent. Normal cells respond to TGF-β with growth inhibition and TGF-β appears to function as a tumor suppressor under normal conditions. While complete loss of the TGF-β receptors is expected to eliminate all autocrine (but not paracrine) effects of tumor-derived TGF-β, postreceptor mutations should not. Tumor cells often lose the ability to undergo growth arrest in response to TGF-β. Despite this loss of growth inhibitory effect, TGF-β autocrine effects on cell morphologic change, and cell adhesion and cell migration (all likely to be advantageous for tumor cells) appear to be retained along with the paracrine effects.

the majority of sporadic colorectal cancers that do not share these genetic defects.

Mutational loss of function of TGF-β signal transduction proteins has been observed in human colorectal cancer. Madr2 (Smad2) mutation was observed in 4%, and DPC4 (Smad4) mutation has been reported in up to 30% of human colorectal cancers. Also, LOH (loss of heterozygosity) of Smad3 has been detected in two (one sporadic and one HNPCC) of 17 cancers examined. These types of mutations may have a significantly different phenotypic outcome as compared with that resulting from loss of the TβRII. Smad4 mutation has also been identified in familial juvenile polyposis, a syndrome characterized by a predisposition to hamartomatous polyps and gastrointestinal cancer. These studies suggest that disruption of Smad signaling may be involved in either the initiation or progression of certain cancers.

TGF-β as a Tumor Promoting Factor

There are several lines of evidence that TGF-β may actually promote malignant transformation and tumor progression for several different cell types and under selected circumstances. TGF-β expression tends to be increased in a wide variety of cancers (including colon cancer) relative to adjacent normal tissues. Transformation of cells with dominant oncogenes (e.g., Ha-*ras* or v-*src*) activates transcription of the TGF-β1 gene. Studies of human colorectal cancers have demonstrated that high-level expression of TGF-β in the primary tumor is associated with advanced stages and is an independent predictor of risk for recurrence and decreased survival.

There are several potential mechanisms for this tumor-promoting effect. For example, TGF-β may suppress tumor immunosurveillance. TGF-β exhibits growth-inhibitory effects on moderate to well-differentiated primary colon carcinomas, but stimulates the proliferation and invasion of poorly differentiated and metastatic colonic carcinomas. Treatment with TGF-β can induce estrogen-independent tumorigenicity of human breast cancer cells. TGF-β treatment can also substitute for wounding as a promoter of fibrosarcomas in chickens infected with the Rous sarcoma virus.

Transformation of preinvasive epithelial neoplasm to the invasive phenotype with metastatic potential is characterized by several profound changes in gene expression and in cellular and tissue morphology. The changes in cellular morphology and tissue architecture can be observed histologically and are accompanied by dramatic changes in the behavior of the transformed cells. The metastatic phenotype is associated with the acquisition of fibroblastoid features and the ability of the cells to invade stroma and blood vessels. There is mounting evidence that autocrine TGF-β expression by tumor cells plays a major role in the epithelial-to-fibroblastoid conversion that accompanies malignant transformation in mammary cells and in keratinocytes. TGF-β1 overexpression enhanced progression of carcinogen-induced skin cancers toward the malignant spindle-cell phenotype in transgenic mice expressing high levels of TGF-β in the skin. The TGF-β–induced epithelial to mesenchymal transition in Ha-*ras* transformed mammary epithelial cells involves disrupted cell-cell adhesion and the loss of epithelial cell polarity in addition to causing the cells to become more spindle-shaped and invasive. The loss of cell polarity in response to TGF-β appears to be the result of a disruption of ZO-1 and F-actin proteins comprising the tight junctions in mammary epithelial cells.

There also appears to be an important regulatory interaction between the TGF-β and cyclooxygenase-2 (COX-2) pathways. Forced overexpression of COX-2 in the non-transformed RIE-1 cells results in down-regulation of the TβRII, and forced overexpression of COX-2 in a human colon cancer cell line results in increased secretion of TGF-β1 from those cells. TGF-β synergistically enhances the expression of COX-2 in conditionally Ha-*ras* transformed RIE-1 cells, and the increase in COX-2 expression by TGF-β in the context of *ras* transformation occurs primarily through a marked increase in the stability of the COX-2 mRNA.

The predominant effect of TGF-β appears to be dependent on the context of the responding cell. Thus, the divergent effects of TGF-β in carcinogenesis may depend on the proliferative capacity and state of differentiation of the epithelial cell, both of which may be altered during the process of neoplastic transformation. Clearly, TGF-β signaling has an important tumor suppressive role; however, after transformation has occurred, TGF-β effects may be detrimental and may actually promote tumor cell survival, invasion, and metastasis (Fig. 14.22). Recent work suggests that these effects may involve TGF-β regulation of COX-2 and other pathways that may contribute to tumor cell aggressiveness.

Cyclooxygenases and Carcinogenesis

Cyclooxygenases are key enzymes in the production of prostaglandins and other eicosanoids that have important roles in the modulation of cell adhesion, growth, differentiation, and apoptosis. Two isoforms of cyclooxygenase (COX) have been identified, and are referred to as COX-1 and COX-2. COX-1 is constitutively expressed in a number of cell types, whereas COX-2 is inducible by a variety of factors, including cytokines, growth factors, and tumor promoters.

Epidemiologic data suggest that prostaglandin synthesis is contributory to the development and progression of intestinal tumors. A number of studies have reported a 40% to 50% decrease in the relative risk of colorectal cancer in persons who are continuous users of aspirin or other nonsteroidal antiinflammatory drugs (NSAIDs). Similarly, experimentally induced colorectal adenomas and cancers are markedly reduced in rodents treated with NSAIDs.

There is now considerable evidence from several different systems that COX-2 is the more important of the two cyclooxygenases with regard to the genesis of colorectal cancer. COX-2 overexpression has been found in 85% of human colorectal cancers. Intestinal adenomas from multiple intestinal neoplasia *(Min)* mice express high levels of COX-2 messenger RNA (mRNA) and protein, and increased COX-2 levels have been reported in azoxymethane-induced rat colon tumors. Similar to the *Min* mice, *Apc*[.716] knockout mice develop multiple intestinal adenomas due to truncating mutations in the *Apc* gene. When the *Apc*[.716] knockout mice were crossbred with mice that were null for the *COX-2* gene, there was a marked reduction in tumor multiplicity and a selective COX-2 inhibitor was more effective than the nonselective NSAID sulindac in reducing polyp number in *Apc*[.716] knockout mice.

Cyclooxygenases may contribute to tumor initiation by catalyzing the oxidation of arachidonic acid to ultimately yield mutagenic metabolites such as malondialdehyde. The cyclooxygenases and their prostanoid products are likely to contribute importantly to carcinogenesis in several other ways. Prostaglandins may impair host immunosurveillance mechanisms to favor tumor progression. COX-2 overexpression may contribute to the tumorigenic potential of dysplastic intestinal epithelial cells by enhancing adhesion to extracellular matrix and by inhibition of apoptosis. Furthermore, forced COX-2 expression in human colon cancer cells resulted in the induction of vascular endothelial tubular morphogenesis when these cells were cocultured with human vascular endothelial cells. This angiogenic induction is abrogated by treatment of the colon cancer cells with NSAIDs. Thus, induction of angiogenesis may be another important tumor-promoting action of COX-2.

PPARδ: A New Target of NSAIDs

Recently, it was reported that PPARδ (peroxisome proliferator-activated receptor-δ) might be a potential target of NSAIDs. PPARδ belongs to the nuclear receptor superfamily that includes steroid hormones, thyroid hormone, and retinoids. PPARδ appears to be down-regulated in the presence of functional APC protein and its expression is elevated in colorectal cancer cells. Eicosanoid products of cyclooxygenase enzymes (including prostaglandins) function as ligands for the PPAR receptors. Genes containing PPARδ-responsive elements are repressed by the NSAID sulindac. Sulindac interferes with the ability of PPARδ to bind to its recognition sequences. These findings suggest that NSAIDs may inhibit tumorigenesis not only through inhibition of COX-2 activity, but also through direct inhibition of PPARδ. The possibility of PPARδ serving as a target of NSAIDs may explain how NSAID-related drugs such as sulindac sulfone that do not inhibit cyclooxygenase activity may induce apoptosis in colon cancer cells.

Tumor Cell Invasiveness and Metastasis

With the exception of inflammatory cells and conditions of wound healing, normal adult cells are constrained in their behavior by intimate contact with neighboring cells and with normal extracellular matrix including that within the basement membrane. Hallmarks of cancer cells include the acquired capacity to invade adjacent tissues and to metastasize. This process involves a change in the types of cell membrane proteins that are responsible for cell-cell and cell-matrix adhesion and communication. Another requirement for tumor cell invasiveness and metastatic behavior is the acquired ability to degrade extracellular matrix. This occurs through up-regulation of extracellular proteases in invasive tumor cells.

The invasive phenotype is characterized by altered expression of proteins known as cell-cell adhesion molecules (CAMS). The altered CAMs include members of the immunoglobulin, the calcium-dependent cadherin, and the integrin families. Both the immunoglobulin and the calcium-dependent cadherins mediate cell to cell interactions, and integrins mediate interactions between cells and extracellular matrix (Fig. 14.21).

An immunoglobulin-related protein that appears to be important in invasion and metastasis is N-CAM. N-CAM switches from a highly adhesive to a poorly adhesive form in Wilms' tumors, neuroblastomas, and small cell lung cancers. Overall expression of N-CAM is decreased in both colorectal cancer and in pancreatic cancer.

Another CAM called E-cadherin is involved in adherens junction complex formation in epithelial cells, and coupling of E-cadherin molecules between adjacent cells functions to constrain growth. One of the proteins bound to E-cadherin is β-catenin, and abundant levels of E-cadherin prevent cytoplasmic accumulation and nuclear translocation of β-catenin. Loss of E-cadherin function is common in epithelial cancers, whereas forced expression of E-cadherin in cultured cancer cells and in transgenic mice inhibits both tumor cell invasion and metastasis. E-cadherin function may be lost in tumor cells by mutational inactivation, transcriptional repression, or increased proteolysis of the extracellular domain.

Cellular adhesion to extracellular matrix and basement membrane proteins is largely mediated by heterodimers of α and β subunits of transmembrane proteins called integrins. There are at least 22 different combinations of the integrin α and β subunits that confer distinct substrate binding preferences to cells. Carcinoma cells facilitate invasion and metastasis by shifting their integrin complement from those that favor binding to extracellular matrix of the normal epithelial basement membrane to other integrin combinations that preferentially bind to partially degraded stromal components produced by extracellular proteases secreted by the tumor cells. Signaling through the integrin receptors can also activate intracellular signal transduction pathways such as the MAPKs and can result in cytoskeletal reorganization to favor the invasive phenotype. These extracellular proteases are also necessary for migration of normal cells such as vascular endothelial cells, fibroblasts, and inflammatory cells.

Two types of extracellular proteases appear to be necessary for tumor cell migration, invasion, and metastasis. These include the urokinase plasminogen activator (uPA) system and the matrix metalloproteinases (MMPs) (Fig. 14.23). The plasmin cascade is regulated by uPA interact-

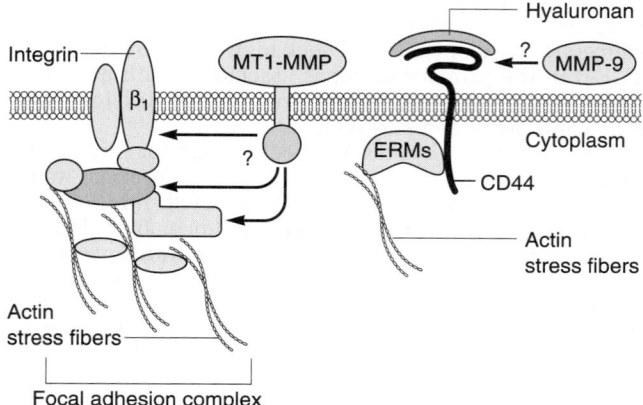

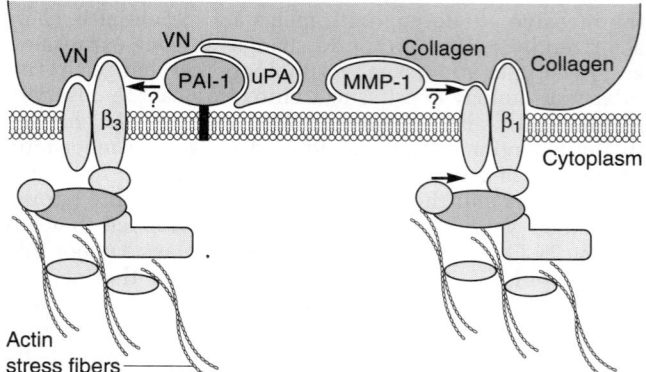

Figure 14.23. Potential interactions of proteinases with the cell surface. The localization of urokinase plasminogen activator (uPA) and uPA receptor (uPAR) at focal adhesion sites may be due to binding to vitronectin (VN) or to selected integrins. Plasminogen activator inhibitor-1 (PAI-1) is the uPA inhibitor and interferes with vitronectin binding to both integrins and uPAR. The matrix metalloproteinases (MMPs) bind to specific components in the extracellular matrix such as collagens, hyaluronan, and heparan sulfate to regulate the interaction of matrix with integrins and the focal adhesion complex. (Redrawn from Hackel PO, Zqick E, Prenzel N, et al. Epidermal growth factor receptors: critical mediators of multiple receptor pathways. *Curr Opin Cell Biol* 1999;11:184–189, with permission.)

ing with the uPA receptor (uPAR) in order to convert the proenzyme substrate plasminogen to the active protease plasmin. Plasminogen activation is also negatively regulated by the plasminogen activator inhibitor (PAI-1). The activation of plasminogen appears to occur in the vicinity of integrins at focal contacts and at the leading edge of migrating cells. Interestingly, uPAR also functions as an adhesion receptor for the extracellular matrix protein vitronectin, and PAI-1 appears to block interaction between vitronectin and uPAR-uPA. There is compelling evidence that uPA expression is necessary for tumor cell invasion of extracellular matrix.

The actions of MMPs are normally regulated by tissue inhibitors of MMPs (TIMPs). The MMPs such as plasmin are involved in regulating cell-matrix interactions through their degradation of matrix protein substrates. Activation of MMPs appears to be focused at the cell surface, and the levels of specific MMPs are increased in tumor cells. At the same time, levels of TIMPs may also be decreased in tumor cells. The actions of MMPs in tumor cells appear to be important for tumor cell invasion, metastasis, tumor angiogenesis, and for release and activation of growth factors such as TGFα.

Tumor Angiogenesis

Cells within tissues must reside within ~100 μm of a capillary blood vessel in order to receive sufficient oxygen and nutrients to sustain survival. New blood vessel growth, angiogenesis, is a carefully regulated process in normal organogenesis. Under normal conditions, once an organ or tissue structure has reached the adult size, little or no further new blood vessel growth occurs. An exception exists in the adult uterus during the normal menstrual cycle. Angiogenesis is also stimulated as part of the normal reparative process in injured tissues. Neovascularization may also be induced under some pathologic conditions such as tissue ischemia, diabetic retinopathy, and neoplasia. Angiogenesis is an essential requirement for tumor growth beyond 2 to 3 mm³. Tumors that continue to grow beyond this early stage must acquire the capacity to induce and sustain angiogenesis. The activation of this "angiogenic switch" appears to be necessary for the rapid growth that is often characteristic of malignant tumors.

The angiogenic switch may be activated via different mechanisms in different tumor types, but its activation results in disruption of the normal balance between proangiogenic and antiangiogenic signals. Importantly, better understanding of the signals that regulate angiogenesis may lead to effective antitumor therapies (Fig. 14.24).

Positive and negative growth signals contribute to the homeostasis of the vascular system. Positive growth signals may be provided by peptide growth factors that interact with specific tyrosine kinase receptors located on the surface of endothelial cells. Examples of these endothelial cell growth factors are vascular endothelial growth factor (VEGF), platelet-derived growth factor (PDGF), and basic and acidic fibroblast growth factors (FGF1 and FGF2). Factors that have inhibitory effects on endothelial cell growth include peptides such as thrombospondin, angiostatin (a proteolytic product of plasminogen), and endostatin (a proteolytic product of collagen XVIII).

Adhesion of endothelial cells to the extracellular matrix and basement membrane is another process that is critical to the development and maintenance of new capillaries. Endothelial cell adhesion is largely mediated by heterodimers of α and β subunits of transmembrane proteins called integrins. Integrins function as receptors for binding to extracellular matrix and basement membrane proteins. Different integrins are expressed on the surfaces of endothelial cells in sprouting capillaries as compared with quiescent vessels. Expression of integrins is modulated by soluble peptide growth factors such as VEGF, FGFs, and TGF-β. Both VEGF and PDGF induce the association of their own receptors with the integrin $\alpha_v\beta_3$, and increase the expression and promigratory effects of $\alpha_v\beta_3$. Association of these growth factor receptors with $\alpha_v\beta_3$ also facilitates the mitogenic response to the growth factors. Integrin $\alpha_v\beta_3$ is also an important survival factor for endothelial cells, and antibodies to $\alpha_v\beta_3$ integrin cause apoptosis of endothelial cells in new blood vessels in experimental animal models.

For endothelial cells to migrate toward a tumor and to form new blood vessels, the tissues must be remodeled to create the space for these new vessels. This remodeling requires the degradation of basement membrane and extracellular matrix by enzymes called matrix metalloproteases (MMPs). Within a tumor, MMPs are expressed by tumor

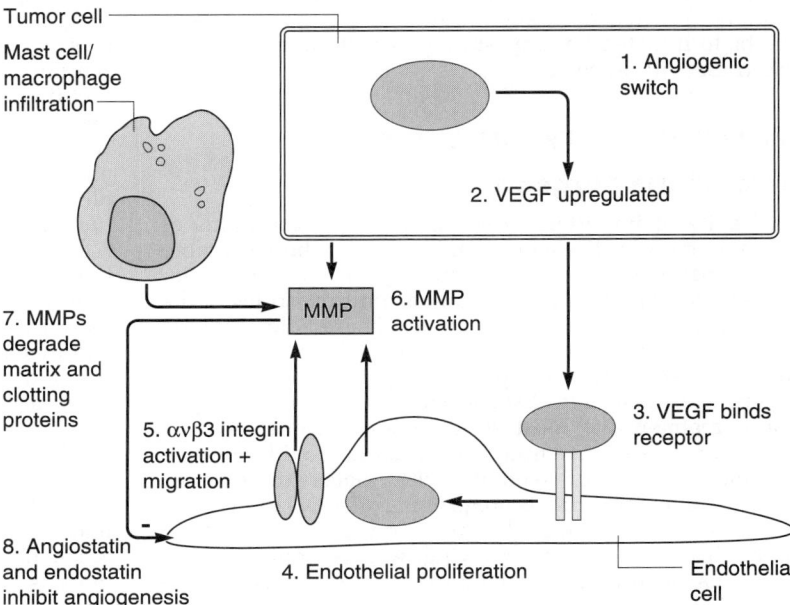

Figure 14.24. Potential targets for antiangiogenic drugs. (Redrawn from Jones PH, Harris AL. The current status of clinical trials in anti-angiogenesis. *Principles Pract Oncol Updates* 2000;14(1): 1–7, with permission.)

Table 14.7. EXAMPLES OF NOVEL CLASSES OF ANTIANGIOGENIC DRUGS IN CLINICAL DEVELOPMENT

Class of drug	Examples	Mode of action	Stage of clinical development
Matrix metalloprotease (MMP) inhibitors	Marimastat, AG-3340 Bay 12-9566	Inhibit MMPs, especially MMP-2 and MMP-9	Randomized phase II studies completed
Vascular endothelial growth factor (VEGF) receptor inhibitors	SU-5416	Inhibits	Phase I trials completed, phase II open
Anti-VEGF antibody	Humanized anti-VEGF antibody	Blocks VEGF activating receptor	Phase II studies
Antiintegrin antibodies	Humanized $\alpha_v\beta_3$ integrin antibody, vitaxin	Cause endothelial apoptosis by blocking $\alpha_v\beta_3$ integrin	Phase I studies completed
Endogenous protein inhibitors	Angiostatin, endostatin	Unknown, generated by MMP and other proteases	Awaiting formulation before phase I studies
Vascular targeting agents	CM101	Fixes complement, causing vasculitis in new vessels	Completed phase I studies

cells, fibroblasts, macrophages, and endothelial cells. MMP2 and MMP9 appear to be particularly important for tumor angiogenesis. They are expressed in several different types of tumors and degrade basement membrane collagens. Inhibition of the functions of MMP2 and MMP9 interferes with angiogenesis in experimental tumor models and inhibits tumor growth. In addition, the matrix metalloproteinase inhibitors also appear to prevent tumor cell invasion of blood vessels and thereby block metastasis in experimental tumor models.

Tumor angiogenesis offers a potentially attractive therapeutic target that may be widely applicable in human cancers (Table 14.7). In fact, there are several classes of antiangiogenic agents that are currently under development for clinical antitumor application. Targeting of the VEGF pathway with humanized anti-VEGF antibody and a VEGF receptor antagonist, SU-5416, are both being applied in phase II clinical trials. At least three different matrix metalloproteinase inhibitors that specifically target MMP2 and MMP9 are being examined in clinical cancer treatment trials. Some MMPIs have progressed to phase III randomized studies for selected cancers. Phase I studies with humanized antibodies to $\beta_v\beta_3$ integrin have been completed, and phase II trials are under way. Vascular targeting agents such as the streptococcal toxin CM-101 with selective toxicity for endothelial cells have also been evaluated in phase I clinical trials and are awaiting further evaluation in phase II trials. If endogenous protein inhibitors of angiogenesis such as angiostatin and endostatin can be formulated for large-scale production, phase I clinical trials will proceed.

MULTIMODALITY CANCER CARE

Role of the Surgeon

In spite of important advances made in the fields of chemotherapy, radiotherapy, and molecular biology, more cancer patients are cured by surgery than by any other treatment modality. The surgeon has multiple roles in the management of the cancer patient. These roles include cancer screening, establishing a diagnosis, initiating primary disease control, and providing palliative care. In the absence of metastatic disease, surgery is the initial primary treatment for most solid tumor malignancies. As such, surgeons are in a unique position to provide curative treatment. Even for patients with metastatic disease, newer surgical treatments are proving effective in decreasing tumor burden and prolonging survival. Thus, the field of surgical oncology is a growing, well-recognized discipline that focuses on the surgical care of the cancer patient. Surgical decision making in oncology requires that

the surgeon understand the natural history of the specific tumor as well as the potential for and pattern of metastatic spread. It is always necessary to balance the oncologic benefit of the surgery with the potential morbidity as stratified by the patient's risk factors.

In general, the treatment of cancer involves a multidisciplinary approach in conjunction with surgical oncology, medical oncology, and radiation oncology. The combination of treatment options can be additive or synergistic in providing more effective care. Therefore, the surgical oncologist must be aware not only of potential surgical treatments but also of how chemotherapy and radiation can be used to augment the successful treatment of cancer patients. This may be in the form of neoadjuvant therapy prior to surgery or in the adjuvant setting following surgical treatment.

The general surgical oncologist provides primary surgical treatment for cancer of the breast, esophagus, thyroid, stomach, liver, pancreas, colon, and rectum, as well as melanoma and sarcoma. Recently, surgical techniques developed by surgical oncologists have substantially altered the diagnosis and treatment of solid tumor malignancies. For example, the technique for determining the presence of lymph node metastasis in breast cancer and melanoma has changed with the development of the sentinel lymph node biopsy. The rationale for this technique is the tenet that spread of malignant cells from the primary tumor to the lymphatic basin follows an orderly progression, that lymphatic flow reaches a sentinel node first prior to progression to secondary nodes. Therefore, removal of the sentinel node followed by careful examination should predict if lymphatic spread has occurred. For patients with a negative sentinel node, the attendant morbidity of further lymphatic dissection may often be eliminated. The technique is accomplished by injecting a blue dye and/or radiopharmaceutical tracer in and around the primary tumor. This injection is followed by identification of the blue node, which can be facilitated further by detection of the radioactive tracer using a hand-held gamma detector. The sentinel node(s) is removed and examined by histologic staining, serial sectioning, immunohistochemistry, and in some cases reverse-transcriptase polymerase chain reaction (RT-PCR) for tumor-specific gene expression. In most cases, if the sentinel node is negative for tumor cells, then further lymphatic dissection is not performed. If the sentinel node does contain tumor cells, then a standard lymphatic dissection is completed. Multiple clinical trials using the technique of sentinel node biopsy have shown that the procedure is accurate in greater than 90% of cases.

The use of ablative therapy for the treatment of liver tumors is being increasingly utilized. Ablative therapy includes cryotherapy (freezing) or radiofrequency ablation (heating). Both techniques use a probe directed by ultrasound guidance into the hepatic tumor that delivers the ablative modality, either freezing with ice ball formation or heating with radiofrequency current. The therapy is performed in situ without removal of tissue. This therapy is limited to patients in whom resection of the tumor is not an option either due to numerous lesions or to the likelihood of inadequate hepatic reserve following hepatic resection.

A treatment modality that combines the expertise of surgical oncology, medical oncology, and radiation oncology is neoadjuvant therapy. Preoperative chemoradiation therapy has several potential advantages. These include (a) shrinkage of the primary tumor, which can facilitate complete resection with less morbidity; (b) well-oxygenated cancer cells respond better to chemoradiation than devascularized cells after surgery; and (c) this therapy provides an in situ assay of chemoresponsiveness that may direct the choice of adjuvant chemotherapeutic agents after the completion of surgical resection. One widely accepted example of this treatment involves preoperative 5-fluorouracil (5-FU)-based chemoradiation in the treatment of rectal cancer when the tumor is staged as T3 or greater by endorectal ultrasound. In addition to increased local tumor control, tumor down-staging may allow for sphincter-saving procedures in select cases. In esophageal carcinoma, neoadjuvant therapy produces a complete response (no remaining viable tumor in the surgical specimen) in up to 25% of cases. In locally advanced breast cancer, neoadjuvant therapy can decrease the extent of surgery that is required and may allow for breast conservation surgery in some cases.

In an attempt to increase the efficacy of adjuvant therapy, these modalities are also being utilized as primary treatment intraoperatively. In patients with extremity melanoma with in-transit metastases, limb perfusion with both cytotoxic and immune stimulating agents can provide high local concentration of the agents compared with typical systemic administration. The active agents, such as melphalan and TNF, are administered intraarterially under hyperthermic conditions and can result in dramatic local tumor response. Similarly, hepatic arterial infusion through implantable subcutaneous ports provides high concentrations of chemotherapy within the liver of patients with unresectable liver metastases from colorectal cancer. Intraoperative radiotherapy (IORT) can be used in patients with microscopically positive margins of resection or other factors that impart a high risk of local recurrence. This technique requires a dedicated operating suite equipped with a machine capable of delivering external beam radiation. IORT has been evaluated predominantly in the treatment of pancreatic cancer and soft tissue sarcoma.

The complexity of intraoperative treatment techniques has necessitated that surgical oncologists develop sophisticated intraoperative skills. This may include the use of ultrasound to image nonpalpable breast masses during surgical biopsy or direct ultrasound of the liver, pancreas, or other organs to detect occult tumors in the operative suite. While the role of laparoscopic resection of malignancy is being evaluated by clinical trials, laparoscopy for staging of disease and placement of enteral feeding tubes is being increasingly used.

Introduction to Clinical Trials

Today, there are a rapidly expanding number of new agents and treatment modalities that are potentially available to treat cancer patients. The key issue is to determine the safety and efficacy of these newer agents compared to more standard treatment. This determination is best evaluated through carefully controlled clinical trials. Clinical trials can be separated into nonexperimental and experimental categories. The nonexperimental category includes (a) case reports; (b) case series, which state what is probable; (c) case control studies, in which there is often difficulty in controlling confounding variables; and (d) patient databases, which can be very useful but have the problem of selection bias. Experimental trials include (a) translational or laboratory studies, which provide preclinical data on a potential treatment; (b) feasibility studies, which assess the feasibility of performing a clinical trial before enrolling large number of patients; and (c) traditional phase I, II, and III studies, in which the treatment modality is taken into the clinical setting. Phase I studies evaluate the safety of the agent and primarily by determining toxicity. The end point of phase II trials is efficacy, which is usually evaluated by measurable tumor response. For agents that are found to be safe and show some efficacy, phase III trials are then performed, which directly compare the new agent to the standard therapy for patients with a particular malignancy. The essentials of any good clinical trial design are (a) hypotheses, (b) clear objectives, and (c) sound statistics. Hypothesis testing is crucial in clinical trial design. The null hypothesis (HO) states there is no difference in the agents being tested. The alternative hypothesis (H1) states there is a difference (i.e., drug A is better than drug B). A type 1 error occurs if the null hypothesis is in fact true (no difference) but the alternative hypothesis is accepted. This could lead to use of an ineffective drug. Type II errors occur when the alternative hypothesis is true (there is a difference) but the null hypothesis is accepted. In this scenario, the opportunity to use an effective drug is missed. There are other problems with the outcome of clinical trials that can result from errors in trial design and analysis. A false-negative outcome can result from small sample size (not enough patients) to detect a difference in treatment. A false-positive outcome can result from multiple significance testing such as unplanned subgroup analysis.

Traditional agents that are evaluated in phase I trials are those with cytotoxic activity such as chemotherapy drugs. Newer agents include those that are cytostatic, antiangiogenic, biologic, as well as gene therapy approaches. The activity of these agents may be to halt tumor growth or be synergistic with other therapies. As the intended mechanism of action of these agents may not cause a decrease in tumor size, standard end points of tumor regression may not be the best method to evaluate their efficacy. Measuring the time to tumor progression is an alternative end point in trials using cytotoxic versus cytostatic agents.

Clinical trials can result in significant changes in surgical practice. The National Surgical Adjuvant Breast and Bowel Project (NSABP) conducted a large trail comparing standard modified radical mastectomy to breast lumpectomy followed by radiation. This trial confirmed the safety of breast conservation therapy and radically changed the surgical treatment of breast cancer.

Surgeons have increasingly recognized the need to conduct large clinical trials to evaluate surgical procedures in cancer patients. However, it is difficult to conduct these large trials within a single institution. In response to this need, the American College of Surgeons Oncology Group (ACOSOG) has recently been formed. This organization accrues patients with the assistance of members throughout the American College of Surgeons.

Chemoprevention

Even though a tremendous amount of effort and research has been given to the treatment of malignant disease, the morbidity from recurrent disease and subsequent mortality remains high. Therefore, a focus on earlier detection and chemoprevention of certain malignancies is being developed. The basis of chemoprevention is targeting specific pathways that are thought to be active in early initiation of solid tumor malignancies. To date, most of the research in chemopreventive strategies has been conducted in malignancies of the breast, colon, and head and neck.

Breast cancer is an endocrine responsive tumor. To block the stimulatory properties of estrogen, the antiestrogen tamoxifen has been used in patients with a diagnosis of breast cancer. The use of tamoxifen not only decreased the risk of recurrence but also decreased the risk of developing cancer in the contralateral breast. In further study by the Breast Cancer Prevention Trial, tamoxifen was shown to markedly reduce the risk of breast cancer in women at high risk of developing breast cancer. This is an example of the efficacy of chemoprevention strategies and has strengthened the focus to develop strategies in other malignancies. Current research is focusing on development of new generation antiestrogens that retain the capacity to enhance cardiovascular and bone health. For example, the Study of Tamoxifen and Raloxifene (STAR) trial is being conducted in postmenopausal women at increased risk of breast cancer to compare the chemopreventive effects as well as the potential reduction in risk of developing osteoporosis.

Studies of large numbers of patients taking aspirin or NSAIDs for various indications have revealed a decrease in the incidence of colorectal cancer compared to patients not taking these agents. It is known that NSAIDs block activity of the enzyme cyclooxygenase (COX) that is involved in the production of prostaglandins. Further investigation has revealed two forms of this enzyme. COX-1 is constitutively expressed and thought to be involved in decreasing inflammation. COX-2, however, is an inducible form of the enzyme and has been found to be elevated in colorectal adenomas and carcinoma. The mechanism of reduction of colorectal cancer risk by NSAIDs is thought to be primarily from inhibition of COX-2. Therefore, selective COX-2 inhibitors have been developed. In addition to their most frequent use in reducing the inflammatory state, these agents are also being used in clinical trials for patients with increased risk for colorectal cancer from familial adenomatous polyposis (FAP). The recommendation for more widespread use of COX-2 inhibitors in the chemoprevention of colorectal cancer will depend on the results of these trials.

BIBLIOGRAPHY

Artavanis-Tsakonas S, Rand MD, Lake RJ. Notch signaling: cell fate control and signal integration in development. *Science* 1999;284:770–776.

Bazzoni G, Gejana E, Lampugnani MG, et al. Endothelial adhesion molecules in the development of the vascular tree: the garden of forking paths. *Curr Opin Cell Biol* 1999;11:573–581.

Boguski MS, McCormick F. Proteins regulating ras and its relatives. *Nature* 1993;366:643–654.

Dang CV, Resar LMS, Emison E, et al. Function of the c-Myc oncogenic transcription factor. *Exp Cell Res* 1999;253:63–77.

Dang CV. c-Myc target genes involved in cell growth, apoptosis, and metabolism. *Mol Cell Biol* 1999;19:1–11.

DeVita VT, Hellman S, Rosenberg SA, eds. *Cancer: principles and practice.* Philadelphia: Lippincott-Raven, 1997:176.

Fearon ER. Genetic alterations underlying colorectal tumorigenesis. *Cancer Surv* 1992;12:119.

Giancotti FG, Ruoslahti E. Integrin signaling. *Science* 1999;285:1028–1032.

Hackel PO, Zqick E, Prenzel N, et al. Epidermal growth factor receptors: critical mediators of multiple receptor pathways. *Curr Opin Cell Biol* 1999;11:184–189.

Hanahan D, Weinberg RA. The hallmarks of cancer. *Cell* 2000;100:57–70.

Jones PH, Harris AL. The current status of clinical trials in antiangiogenesis. *Principles Pract Oncol Updates* 2000;14(1):1–7.

Kaelin WG Jr. Functions of the retinoblastoma protein. *Bioessays* 1999;21:950–958.

Kinzler KW, Vogelstein B. Lessons from hereditary colorectal cancer. *Cell* 1996;87:159–170.

Korc M. Role of growth factors in pancreatic cancer. *Surg Onc Clin North Am* 1998;7:31.

Landis SH, Murray T, Bolden S, et al. Cancer statistics, 1999. *CA Cancer J Clin* 1999;49:8–31.

Levine AJ. Tumor suppressor genes. In: Mendelsohn J, Howley PM, Israel MA, et al., eds. *The molecular basis of cancer.* Philadelphia: WB Saunders, 1995:86–104.

Lundberg AS, Weinberg RA. Control of the cell cycle and apoptosis. *Eur J Cancer* 1999;35:531–539.

Macleod K. Tumor suppressor genes. *Curr Opin Genet Dev* 2000;10:81–93.

Massari ME, Murre C. Helix-loop-helix proteins: regulators of transcription in eucaryotic organism. *Mol Cell Biol* 2000;20:429–440.

Mendelsohn J, Howley PM, Israel MA, et al., eds. *The molecular basis of cancer.* Philadelphia: WB Saunders, 1995:126.

Pomerantz J, Schreiber-Agus N, Liegeois NJ, et al. The INK4a tumor suppressor gene product, p18ARF, interacts with MDM2 and neutralizes MDM2's inhibition of p53. *Cell* 1998;92:713–723.

Riese DJ, Stern DF. Specificity within the EGF family/ErbB receptor family signaling network. *Bioessays* 1998;20;41–48.

Rosen N. Oncogenes. In: Mendelsohn J, Howley PM, Israel MA, et al., eds. *The molecular basis of cancer.* Philadelphia: WB Saunders, 1995:105–116.

Sherr CJ. Cancer cell cycles. *Science* 1996;274:1672–1677.

Sherr CJ, Weber JD. The ARF/p53 pathway. *Curr Opin Genet Dev* 2000;10:94–99.

SURGERY: SCIENTIFIC PRINCIPLES AND PRACTICE, Third Edition, edited by Lazar J. Greenfield, Michael W. Mulholland, Keith T. Oldham, Gerald B. Zelenock, and Keith D. Lillemoe. Lippincott Williams & Wilkins Publishers, Philadelphia, © 2001.

CHAPTER 15

HUMAN GENE THERAPY

BRYCE D. BESETH, ROBERT B. CAMERON, AND JAMES J. MULÉ

Gene therapy is defined as the therapeutic transfer of functional nucleic acids into targeted groups of living cells. As techniques for cloning genes and manipulating genetic material have become both more standardized and refined, gene therapy has rapidly evolved. The completion of the human genome sequence, the development of an increasingly dense single-nucleotide polymorphism map of the genome, and the development of new technologies for functional genomics will deepen our understanding of the molecular basis of disease and further broaden the scope of diseases for which gene therapy strategies can be formulated. Gene therapy has potential applications in the treatment of both heritable and acquired disease as well as their prevention. It is therefore important for all clinicians to have an understanding of the underlying principles and current techniques of gene therapy.

Genetic material can be transferred by an ex vivo or an in vivo approach. In ex vivo transfer, cells are removed from an organism, genetically modified, and then reimplanted. Most early gene therapy investigations used an ex vivo approach. Some of the advantages of such an approach are the ability to isolate and purify target cell populations before treatment and the opportunity to assess the degree of ge-

Table 15.1. GENE THERAPY VECTORS

Vector	Genome	Maximum insert size	Efficiency of transduction	Requires Replication for transduction	Location of vector genome in host	Expression	Immunogenicity	Advantages	Disadvantages	Clinical trials
Viral vectors										
Adeno-associated virus	Single-stranded DNA	4.5 kb	Moderate	No	In the absence of rep protein: episomal or randomly integrated into host genome in the presence of rep protein: preferential site-specific integration into chromosome 19	Stable	No	Stable expression, nonimmunogenic	Small transgene capacity	Cystic fibrosis, Canavan's disease
Adenovirus	Double-stranded DNA	8 kb	High	No	Episomal	Transient	Yes	High transduction efficiency	Immunogenicity leads to elimination of transduced cells and loss of transgene expression	Over 65 trials in a wide range of applications
Gutted adenovirus	Double-stranded DNA	37 kb	High	No	Episomal	Variable, depending on immunogenicity of transgene	Low	High transduction efficiency, low immunogenicity compared with earlier adenoviral vectors	Elimination of transduced cells after expression of immunogenic construct	No
Retrovirus	Single-stranded RNA	7 kb	Moderate	Yes	Random integration into host genome	Stable	No	Integration, long-term expression	Requirement for cell division, labile in vivo, insertional mutagenesis	Over 150 trials in a wide variety of applications, especially for ex vivo manipulation of hematopoietic cells
Lentivirus	Single-stranded RNA	8.8 kb	High	No	Random integration into host genome	Stable	No	Ability to infect nondividing and quiescent cells, integration, long-term expression	Biosafety issues regarding parental virus, insertional mutagenesis	No
Herpes simplex	Double-stranded DNA	30 kb	Moderate	No	Episomal	Transient	No	Neuronal tropism, ability to establish latency, large transgene capacity	Transient transgene expression, viral toxicity in some cell types	One trial for treatment of malignant glioma
Poxviruses	Double-stranded DNA	25 kb	Moderate	No	Cytoplasm	Transient	Yes	Large transgene capacity, wide tropism	Immunogenicity	Cancer immunotherapy and vaccination
Nonviral vectors										
Liposomes	DNA or RNA	50 kb	Low	No	Episomal	Transient	No	Large transgene capacity, nonimmunogenic, ease of manufacture	Low transduction efficiency and transient expression	Over 70 trials in a wide range of applications
Naked DNA	DNA	50 kb	Low	No	Episomal	Transient	No	Large transgene capacity, nonimmunogenic, ease of manufacture	Low transduction efficiency	Several trials in various applications including myocardial angiogenesis, cancer, and hemophilia A
DNA–protein conjugate	DNA	48 kb	Low	No	Episomal	Transient	No	Large transgene capacity, nonimmunogenic, ability to target specific cell types through surface receptors	Low transduction efficiency, degradation within lysosomes	Few

netic transfer before reimplantation. The major drawback of ex vivo techniques is that many potential targets are not amenable to ex vivo manipulation. For such targets, in vivo techniques are required. In an in vivo approach, the vector is introduced directly into the organism. Because of the limitations of current techniques for targeted gene transfer, most in vivo protocols have either injected the vector into a local area of interest or administered it to an area in which exposure of the vector to irrelevant cell populations was minimized. As the ability to target vectors to specific cell populations improves, a greater number of tissues will be accessible for in vivo approaches.

In this chapter, we first review vectorology and the salient characteristics of both viral and nonviral gene therapy vectors (Table 15.1). We then discuss the development of clinical gene therapy approaches for treatment of cancer, acquired diseases, human immunodeficiency virus (HIV) infection, and heritable disorders. Within each of these broad categories, encompassing nearly 400 gene therapy protocols, we discuss gene therapy strategies that are representative of the types of efforts being undertaken. Gene therapy approaches for some diseases such as arthritis, chronic granulomatous disease, and others are not discussed in detail, and for a more complete list of protocols and applications, the reader is directed to the journal *Human Gene Therapy*.

VIRAL VECTORS

To date, five types of viruses have been used as gene therapy vectors in clinical trials: oncoretroviruses, adenoviruses, adeno-associated viruses (AAV), poxviruses, and herpesviruses. Other viruses that are being explored as potential vectors in animal models include alphaviruses, baculoviruses, lentiviruses, and Epstein-Barr virus. All viruses share certain common elements. The viral genome is enclosed in a protein coat termed a *capsid* and, depending on the type of virus, may be surrounded by an outer lipoprotein membrane termed an *envelope*. In enveloped viruses, the envelope and its glycoproteins mediate attachment and entry to the host cell, whereas in nonenveloped viruses, the capsid proteins adopt these functions. The tropism of a virus can therefore be altered by changing its envelope or its capsid proteins, and both of these techniques are commonly used in the development of gene therapy vectors. One of the most common manipulations is termed *pseudotyping* and refers to the replacement of a virus's envelope gene with that of another virus to change its tropism and infectivity.

Viral vectors are designed to be infective but replication defective. The vector genome is therefore deleted of some or all of the genes required for replication. Consequently, viral vectors must be propagated in packaging cell lines that constitutively express these deleted viral proteins. Viral particles manufactured by the packaging cell line are therefore infectious, but are unable to replicate outside of the packaging cell line. In place of the deleted viral genes, a therapeutic gene, termed a *transgene* or *expression cassette,* is inserted. The size of the parent viral genome is therefore an important determinant in the size of the transgene that a viral vector can deliver.

Although much of a viral genome can usually be deleted, it must contain at least two groups of functional elements, the packaging sequence and the *cis*-required elements for infection and gene expression. The packaging sequence is the part of the genome that is required for its incorporation into the protein capsid. The *cis*-required elements, such as promoters, are DNA sequences that must be present on the DNA strand in question to be active. *Trans*-required sequences, on the other hand, need not be physically present on the vector genome, but their gene products such as capsid proteins must have access to the vector genome to carry out their function. For purposes of viral manufacture, *trans*-required elements can be supplied by the packaging cell line. For some types of viral vectors, packaging cell lines are not available. These viral vectors are produced by cotransduction of the vector genome with either another virus or a plasmid that codes for the deleted viral sequences required in *trans.*

One of the risks of viral vector manufacture is the possible generation of replication-competent virus. This can occur through homologous recombination between the vector and the packaging cell line or cotransduced virus. New techniques have minimized this risk by reducing the amount of homologous sequence between vectors and packaging cell lines and by separating the coding sequences for *trans*-required elements such that multiple recombinations are required to generate replication competent virus. In vitro techniques have also been developed to manufacture certain types of viral vectors (1,2).

Retroviral Vectors

Retroviruses are enveloped RNA viruses belonging to the family Retroviridae (Fig. 15.1). The two subfamilies of retroviruses that have received the most attention as gene therapy vectors are the oncoretroviruses and the lentiviruses. A retroviral genome consists of two identical molecules of positive-stranded RNA containing at least three genes: *gag, pol,* and *env*. The *gag* gene codes for group-specific antigens such as capsid proteins, *pol* codes for the reverse transcriptase required to transcribe the RNA genome into DNA, and *env* codes for the envelope glycoproteins that coat the virus. Retroviruses target cells through interactions between the envelope glycoproteins and various cell surface receptors. HIV, for example, targets T cells through an interaction between its glycoprotein (gp)-120 type-specific glycoprotein and the CD4 molecule present on the T-cell surface. After attachment to the target cell, the virus is internalized and uncoated, delivering the virus preintegration complex into the cell cytoplasm. The preintegration complex contains the reverse transcriptase required for transcribing the single-stranded RNA genome into a double-stranded DNA provirus that is then integrated into the host cell genome. The integration of the DNA provirus is random and not site specific. There is therefore a risk of mutagenesis with administration of retroviral vectors.

The retroviruses in use in clinical trials are all members of the oncoretrovirus subfamily. Of the almost 400 clinical trials approved to date, over 40% have used an oncoretrovirus vector. Oncoretroviruses or RNA tumor viruses are so named because most members of this subfamily contain a *src* gene that codes for a protein kinase that imbues them with transforming activity. Most retroviral vectors are derived from an amphotropic strain of the Moloney leukemia virus. The strain is termed *amphotropic* because it can infect both mouse and human cells through the retrovirus amphotropic murine-1 (RAM-1) receptor (3). The only *cis* elements required for viral infection, replication, and integration are the 5′ and 3′ long terminal repeats (LTRs) of the viral genome. All other coding sequences save the packaging sequence can be deleted, yielding a transgene capacity of approximately 7 kb. The feature of retroviruses that has made them most attractive as gene therapy vectors is that they stably integrate into the host cell genome. An integrated retrovirus can therefore express its transgene for the life of the cell, and if a transduced cell population is expanded ex vivo, all progeny of the transduced cell will contain the integrated retrovirus and its transgene. In

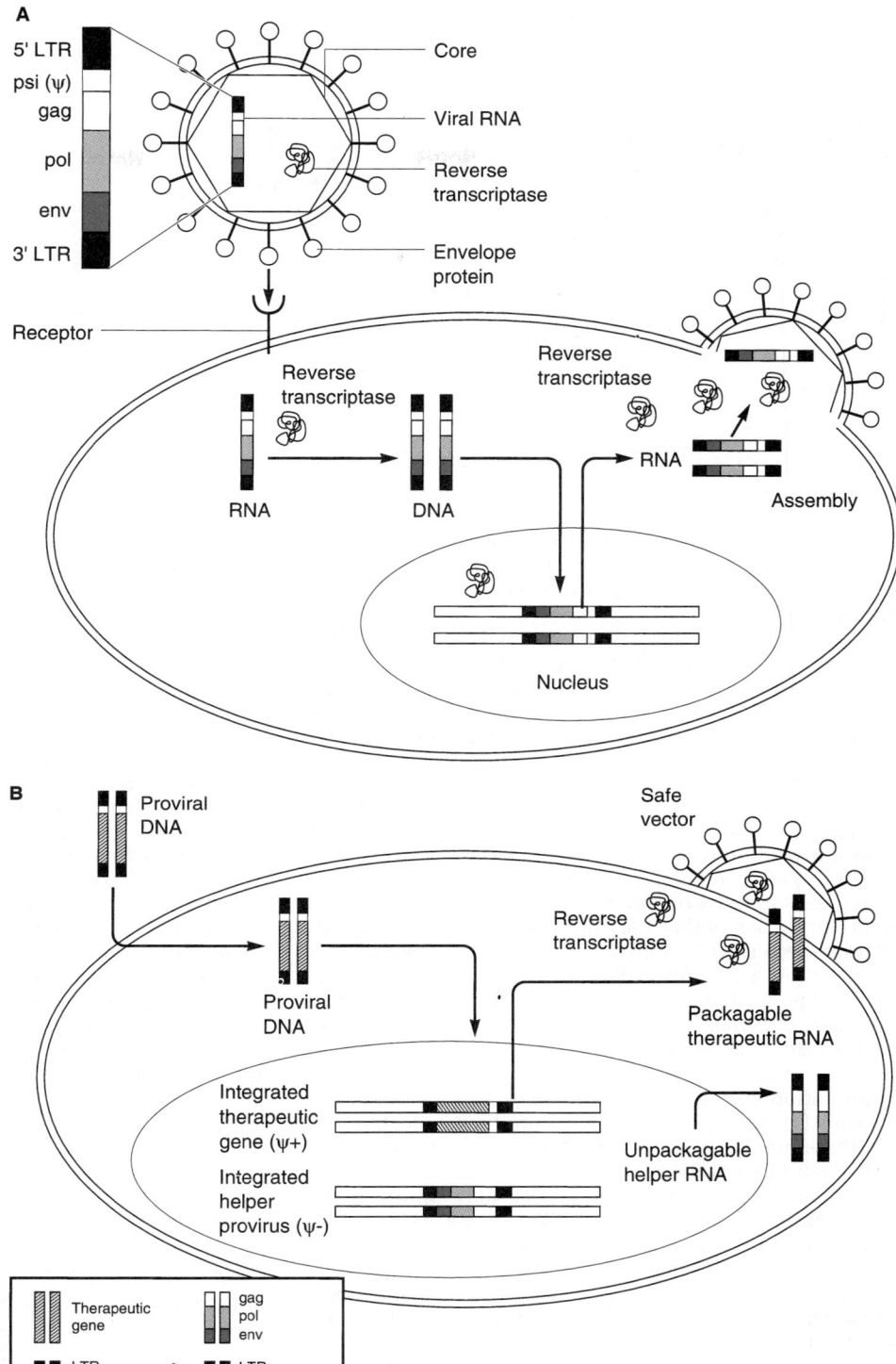

Figure 15.1. *(A)* Processes used in the construction of a retroviral vector. The schematic drawing represents the key features of a retroviral particle. Envelope (env) proteins are important in binding and uptake of the virus by the host cell. Viral reverse transcriptase allows conversion of viral RNA to a DNA provirus. Long terminal repeats (LTRs) are essential for viral integration into the host chromosome. The ψ sequence is necessary for packaging of RNA molecules into virions before budding from the host cell membrane. pol, reverse transcriptase; gag, core proteins. *(B)* Steps in the life cycle of a retrovirus. The envelope glycoproteins bind to specific cell surface proteins and allow fusion of the virus with the cell membrane, permitting entry of virion particles. Once in the cell, molecules of viral reverse transcriptase convert RNA to DNA. Proviral DNA integrates randomly into the genome of the proliferating host cell. Retroviral progeny are synthesized using host cell mechanisms. Packaging of infectious RNA requires ψ sequences. *(Continued on next page.)*

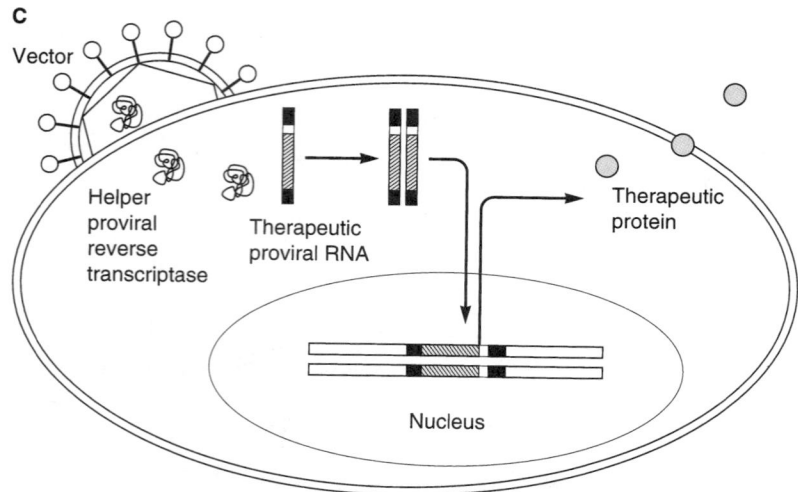

Figure 15.1. *(Continued.) (C)* Steps in construction of therapeutic proviral DNA. Using standard DNA cloning techniques, a therapeutic gene, along with desired promoters, enhancers, and selectable markers, may be substituted for endogenous retroviral structural sequences, such as *gag, pol,* and *env.* By making the therapeutic DNA provirus ψ positive, subsequent therapeutic RNA molecules can be selectively packaged.

addition, because retroviral vectors can be deleted of all viral open reading frames, they do not express any immunogenic viral peptides, minimizing recognition by the immune system.

The major shortcoming of oncoretroviruses is that they can transduce only cells that are actively dividing. This is because the oncoretrovirus preintegration complex cannot transverse nuclear membrane except when the membrane is fragmented during mitosis. Oncoretroviruses are therefore suitable for transducing only those cells that can be grown ex vivo in culture or dividing cells in vivo. This significantly limits the range of applications for which oncoretroviruses are suitable. Cytokines and other techniques, including partial hepatectomy, have been used to make otherwise nondividing cell types more susceptible to transformation by oncoretroviruses. Another liability of oncoretroviruses is that they are labile in the human circulation because of rapid inactivation by complement. This imposes a significant limitation on their use in vivo. It now appears, however, that retroviral vectors packaged in human cell lines have significantly longer half-lives in the primate circulation than do retroviral vectors packaged in nonhuman cell lines. This may be due in part to glycosylation epitopes present in some species but not in primates (4). Changes in retroviral production techniques may therefore increase the utility of retroviruses in vivo.

The lentivirus subfamily of Retroviridae includes HIV, feline immunodeficiency virus (FIV), and equine infectious anemia virus. Lentiviruses, like oncoretroviruses, integrate stably into the host cell genome, but lentiviral vectors have a major advantage in that they can also transduce nonreplicating cells such as neurons and quiescent hematopoietic progenitors. This is because the lentiviral preintegration complex can be efficiently transported through nucleopores and into the nucleus during interphase (5).

Human immunodeficiency virus has been the lentivirus most widely investigated for use in gene therapy applications. The major disadvantage of HIV for use in gene therapy is concern about its biosafety. This has led to the development of progressively attenuated lentiviral vectors based on HIV. In addition to the *gag, pol,* and *env* genes, HIV contains six other genes: *tat, rev, vif, vpr, vpu,* and *nef. Tat* and *rev* are regulatory genes that are required for viral replication, and *vif, vpr, vpu,* and *nef* are accessory genes that are involved in replication and pathogenesis (6). First-generation HIV-based lentiviral vectors were produced using a three-plasmid expression system (7). One plasmid

expressed the *trans*-required elements, a second plasmid coded for a heterologous envelope, and the third plasmid coded for the vector genome and contained the packaging sequence, transgene, and *cis*-required elements. Second-generation HIV-based vectors were created by removing all accessory genes from the construct and demonstrating that these virulence determinants were not required for infectivity in most types of cells (8). The current generation of HIV-based lentiviral vectors combines deletions for *tat, env, vif, vpu, vpr,* and *nef* with a deletion in the 3' LTR, eliminating the transcriptional activity of the LTR. These attenuated lentiviral vectors have been shown stably to transduce both terminally differentiated neurons and quiescent hematopoietic progenitor cells (6,8,9). A lentiviral vector based on FIV has also been developed (10). This FIV-based vector is also able stably to transduce terminally differentiated neurons and other nonreplicating cells. Use of a nonhuman lentivirus avoids some of the concerns raised by HIV-based lentiviruses but introduces new unknowns because the behavior of nonhuman lentiviruses is not well understood in primate hosts. It is likely that lentiviral vectors will be incorporated into gene therapy clinical trials in the near future.

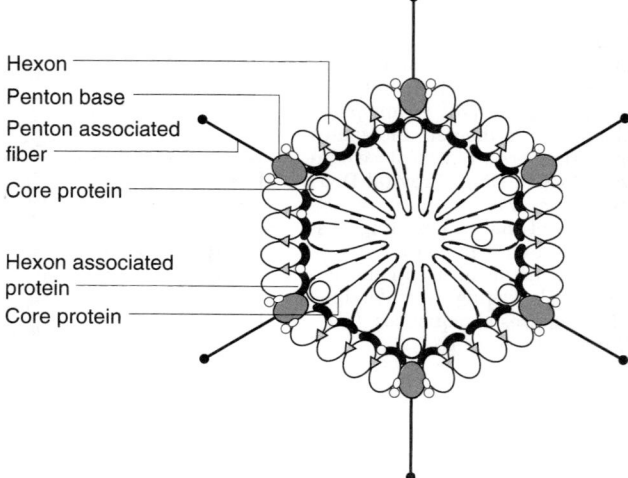

Figure 15.2. Schematic representation of adenovirus structure. Six distinct proteins are subunits of the viral capsid. The core contains two subunit proteins and a terminal protein covalently linked at each of the 5' ends of the linear DNA.

Adenovirus

Adenoviruses are nonenveloped viruses that have a double-stranded DNA genome of between 30 and 35 kb (Fig. 15.2). Currently used adenoviral vectors are derived from viral serotypes 2 and 5, which are endemic in the human population. The adenovirus genome is housed in an icosahedral protein capsid. Projecting from each vertex of the icosahedron is the fiber protein. The fiber protein initiates endocytosis of the virus into the host cell by interacting with one of at least two different cell surface receptors (11,12). Endocytosis of adenoviral vectors depends on the presence of these cell surface receptors as well as α-containing integrins that interact with the capsid proteins. Cells with decreased expression of virus receptors demonstrate resistance to adenovirus infection (13). Importantly, the tropism of adenoviral vectors can be manipulated through modification of the fiber protein (14, 15). Anti-fiber monoclonal antibodies whose Fab fragment is conjugated to a cell receptor ligand have been used to mediate adenoviral vector binding to the folate receptor, present in an up-regulated form on various cancer cells, and to the fibroblast growth factor (FGF)-2 receptor of Kaposi's sarcoma cells (16,17). A bispecific antibody, with specificities for human CD3 and a protein epitope engineered into an adenoviral vector, has been shown to mediate efficient adenoviral transduction of T cells that are otherwise resistant to adenovirus (18).

In the cell, adenovirus disrupts the membrane of the endocytic vesicle to enter the cytoplasm, an important property that has prompted its inclusion into hybrid gene delivery systems. Adenovirus then enters the nucleus through nuclear pore complexes. Once in the nucleus, the adenovirus expresses the early genes, *E1* through *E4*, which code for the nonstructural proteins that direct DNA replication and down-regulation of host cell major histocompatibility complex (MHC) expression. After replication of viral DNA in the nucleus, the mRNA is transcribed and translated into structural viral proteins, followed by viral assembly and lysis of the host cell.

Adenoviruses can infect a broad range of cell types and can transduce both replicating and nonreplicating cells. Most of the adenoviral vectors in clinical trials are *E1*-deleted vectors. These vectors carry a transgene in the deleted *E1* gene region of the viral genome and can be grown to high titers in packaging cell lines that express the adenoviral *E1a* and *E1b* genes. These first-generation vectors are able to transduce cells effectively and can achieve high initial levels of expression. Because they produce low levels of viral proteins from the other early and late gene regions, however, they elicit a cellular immune response, limiting the duration of transgene expression and resulting in destruction of the transduced cells. Immunogenicity is the primary disadvantage of adenoviral vectors, and it both limits the duration of transgene expression and precludes readministration of the vector. Although this does not prevent the use of adenoviral vectors in protocols designed to kill transduced cells, it is problematic for many other types of gene therapy in which prolonged expression of a transgene is desired.

Adenoviral vectors with more expansive deletions in the viral genome have been created in an attempt to reduce leaky viral gene expression and therefore reduce antigenicity. This has culminated in the development of "gutless" adenoviral vectors, which are deleted of all sequences except the packaging sequence and the inverted terminal repeats (19–22). The larger deletion of viral coding sequences in gutless vectors increases the transgene insert capacity to approximately 37 kb, larger than the genome of the parent virus. Studies have shown that gutless adenoviral vectors demonstrate more stable transgene expression and decreased inflammation compared with first-generation *E1*-deleted adenoviral vectors. In mouse strains that do not recognize the gutless adenoviral transgene as foreign, gutless adenoviral vectors can mediate prolonged stable expression of the transgene (23). However, when the transgene is recognized as foreign, a cell-mediated immune response results in diminished levels of transgene expression (24,25). The importance of transgene immunogenicity has been shown in two studies that demonstrated that adenoviral vectors can mediate long-term stable expression of a self-antigen, but that expression of an alloantigen predicts the development of a host immune response and subsequent elimination of transgene expression (26,27). This appears to be because adenovirus vectors effectively transduce dendritic cells, resulting in dendritic cell presentation of transgene peptides (28).

Adeno-associated Virus

Adeno-associated virus is a nonpathogenic, defective human parvovirus with a 4,680-base pair, single-stranded DNA genome housed in a nonenveloped icosahedral capsid. AAV is termed a *defective human parvovirus* because it requires adenovirus or herpesvirus for replication. In the absence of helper virus for replication, AAV establishes latency by integrating into the host genome. AAV preferentially integrates into a site on chromosome 19 designated AAVS1 (29). Membrane-associated heparan sulfate proteoglycan acts as a viral receptor for AAV; however, as for adenovirus, the development of bispecific antibodies to AAV and to other cell surface components enables redirection of the infectious particle (30,31).

The AAV genome consists of the *cap* and *rep* genes flanked by inverted terminal repeats on both ends of the genome. The inverted terminal repeats are the only *cis*-acting elements required for the integration of AAV, although it is now known that *rep* gene products are required in *trans* to make integration site specific. In the absence of *rep*, AAV has been shown both to persist episomally and to integrate into the host genome at sites other than AAVS1 (32). Advantages of recombinant AAV vectors include the ability to be grown to high titers, the capability of transducing both replicating and nonreplicating cells, and the mediation of stable transgene expression in a variety of cell types and animal hosts. Recombinant AAV (rAAV) has been shown in vivo stably to transduce neurons, hepatocytes, skeletal muscle, vascular smooth muscle, hematopoietic progenitor cells, and epithelial cells (33–43).

Adeno-associated virus has also demonstrated the ability to express neoantigens in vivo without generating a cellular immune response. This appears to be because rAAV, unlike adenovirus, does not effectively transduce dendritic cells and does not therefore elicit cell-mediated immunity (28). In animal studies, humoral immune responses to rAAV-encoded transgenes have not prevented stable transgene expression.

The major disadvantage of rAAV vectors is that the size of the transgene is limited to less than 5 kb because of packaging constraints. Although this limits the use of rAAV for some diseases, rAAV has been used successfully to treat a variety of common conditions in animal models. In animal models, several groups have shown long-term correction of factor IX deficiency after transduction of rAAV vectors containing human factor IX into both liver and muscle (39,44,45). Intramuscular administration of rAAV vectors has also been used in murine models to mediate stable rapamycin-regulated secretion of human growth hormone, to mediate stable doxycycline-regulated expression of erythropoietin, and to correct the metabolic abnormalities associated with leptin deficiency (46–48). rAAV vectors are being used clinically in trials for cystic fibrosis and Canavan's disease.

Herpes Simplex Virus Type 1

Herpes simplex virus type 1 (HSV-1) is an enveloped virus belonging to the Herpesvirus family. HSV-1 has a large, double-stranded genome of approximately 150 kb and encodes over 70 viral proteins. HSV-1 attaches to cells by an interaction between glycoproteins on the viral envelope and heparan sulfate moieties of the cell surface. After entry into the cell, the genome circularizes and the early genes for viral replication are transcribed. HSV-1 can then either remain latent, or it can activate the late genes that code for packaging proteins and release daughter virions by cell lysis. HSV-1 vectors have been made by creating deletions in the early gene regions and replacing the early genes with therapeutic genes of interest. Advantages of HSV-1 for use as a gene therapy vector include the ability to carry a transgene of up to 30 kb in size, the ability to establish latency, and the ability to infect nonreplicating cells, particularly neurons. In animal models, HSV-1-based vectors have been able to effect changes in neural physiology after injection into the brain, but the expression of transgene product has been short lived.

There is one ongoing clinical trial using an attenuated, replication-competent HSV vector treatment of malignant glioma. The antitumor activity of this virus is mediated by viral toxicity itself and not by the introduction of an exogenous transgene. Replication of the recombinant is limited to dividing tumor cells in vivo and it has not been shown to infect surrounding brain tissue. Although success in animal models has been shown, the results of human trials are not yet known (49).

Poxviruses

Poxviruses are large, enveloped viruses with a linear, double-stranded DNA genome. Both human and nonhuman poxviruses have been used in clinical trials for gene therapy, although most trials have used the vaccinia virus. Vaccinia is a large virus and can carry up to 25 kb of foreign DNA without loss of infectivity. Importantly, vaccinia virus replicates in the cell cytoplasm using a virally encoded DNA-dependent RNA polymerase, precluding the use of tissue-specific transgene promoters. All steps of the virus life cycle take place in the cytoplasm. Although vaccinia is a cytopathic virus, its pathogenicity in humans is low, as demonstrated by its long record of use as a smallpox vaccine. Advantages of vaccinia include its ability to infect a wide range of cell types as well as a large insert capacity for the expression of multiple genes. The primary disadvantage of poxviruses is immunogenicity, and therefore they are most suited to approaches in which long-term transgene expression is not required. These properties make vaccinia an excellent vehicle for recombinant vaccines. In animal models, recombinant poxviruses have been used effectively as tumor vaccines and in the transfer of immunomodulatory or cytotoxic compounds to neoplastic cells. There are currently 25 gene therapy trials using poxvirus vectors, and most of these involve poxviruses that have been modified to express a tumor antigen such as carcinoembryonic antigen (CEA), prostate-specific antigen (PSA), the MUC-1 mucin antigen (MUC-1), and the melanoma antigen recognized by T cells-1 (MART-1) and gp-100 melanoma antigens.

Chimeric Viral Vectors

Chimeric viral vectors incorporate genetic elements from two or more viral vectors with the goal of creating a vector that is both highly infective and has persistent expression. Chimeric vectors usually combine a highly infective virus, such as adenovirus or herpesvirus, with a viral vector characterized by a high level of stable transgene expression, such as AAV or retrovirus. In adenoviral/retroviral chimeras, retroviral activity in vivo is greatly increased when the retrovirus is protected from complement by an adenovirus capsid and envelope during its delivery to the target cell. In one described adenoviral/retroviral chimera, the chimeric vector directs initially infected cells to produce replication-defective retroviruses that then stably transduce neighboring cells. An example of one of the potential advantages of an rAAV chimera over an rAAV vector is that the chimeric genome can be engineered to code for rep protein in addition to the rAAV vector DNA, allowing for site-specific integration of the rAAV and eliminating the problem of insertional mutagenesis. Although chimeric vectors are now in the beginning stages of development, it is likely that future gene therapy protocols will use vectors that combine favorable aspects of different viral systems (50–54).

NONVIRAL VECTORS

Nonviral systems include liposomes, naked DNA, and DNA–protein complexes and have several advantages over viral vector systems. Nonviral vectors are theoretically safer than viral vectors because there is no danger of replication-competent virus contamination. Nonviral systems are also largely nonimmunogenic, and can therefore be readministered if needed (55). Furthermore, nonviral vectors can carry a larger transgene than most viral vectors. Oncoretroviruses and *E1*-substituted adenoviruses, the two most commonly used viral vectors in clinical trials, have a transgene capacity of no greater than 8 kb, whereas liposomes and DNA–protein complexes can deliver DNA cosmids of up to 50 kb. Finally, production of nonviral vectors is easier than production of viral vectors, largely because they are prepared in vitro, eliminating the need for packaging cell lines. The primary disadvantage of nonviral vectors is low efficiency of gene transfer, which limits their utility for many applications.

Liposomes

Liposomes are a heterogeneous group of compounds composed primarily of phospholipid molecules containing a hydrophobic fatty acid tail and a hydrophilic head group. The charge of the hydrophilic head groups determines whether the liposome is cationic or anionic. Liposomes complexed with DNA can enter a wide variety of cells by endocytosis, and for both types of liposomes, lipid composition can be manipulated to alter the half-life of the liposome in the circulation and help promote lysosomal disruption after endocytosis. After endocytosis, the liposomal DNA must escape from the lysosome before it is degraded by host cell enzymes. This is a critical step in gene transfer, and expression levels depend on preservation of the DNA construct after endocytosis. One approach that has been taken to circumvent the destructive endosomal pathway of liposome uptake has been the incorporation of fusion proteins from the hemagglutinating virus of Japan. These proteins mediate fusion of the liposome with the plasma cell membrane, resulting in direct transfer of DNA into the cytoplasm of the cell and increased efficiency of gene transfer (56).

Because of their negative charge, anionic liposomes do not bind DNA. In an anionic liposome, therefore, the transgene rests in the aqueous compartment in the core of the liposome. This limits the size of the DNA transgene that can be transferred with anionic liposomes. However, the negative charge of anionic liposomes reduces nonspecific binding to cells and therefore enables a greater degree of targeted transfection through glycoproteins incorporated into the liposomal complex (57).

Most animal models and clinical trials have used cationic liposomes. In cationic liposomes, the positively charged head group binds tightly to the negatively charged phosphate groups of the DNA molecule (58). Although the mechanism of cationic liposome entry into the cell is not well understood, it has been shown that cell surface proteoglycans can mediate cationic liposome uptake (59). A disadvantage of cationic liposomes is the tendency to accumulate in the reticuloendothelial system. One approach to evade the cells of the reticuloendothelial system has been to coat the liposome with sialic acid residues (60). The inclusion of various polyethylene glycol-lipids has also been used to decrease the reticuloendothelial cell uptake of liposomes by inhibiting complement-mediated opsonization of the particles (61). Liposomes have been used in a wide variety of animal models and are in use in clinical trials for diseases such as cystic fibrosis and cancer. The major advantages of liposomes are large transgene capacity, low immunogenicity, ease of manufacture, and biosafety. The major shortcoming is the low level and transient nature of expression compared with viral vectors. A newly developed class of synthetic compounds termed *starburst polyamidoamine dendrimers,* however, has a much higher transfection efficiency. Starburst dendrimers are highly branched, spherical polymers that contain large numbers of positively charged surface amino acid groups on their surface. Dendrimers can form stable complexes with polyanions such as plasmid DNA and have been shown dramatically to increase transfection efficiency into a variety of cell types both in vitro and in vivo (62–64). The development of such compounds will likely broaden the scope of applications for which liposomal gene transfer can be considered.

Naked DNA

Naked DNA has been used for gene transfer into a variety of tissues, including skin, respiratory epithelium, skeletal muscle, cardiac muscle, liver, cornea, and various types of cancer. DNA constructs have several advantages over viral vectors: they are easier to produce in quantity than viral vectors, they do not elicit anti-DNA antibodies and can therefore be readministered, and they avoid the biosafety risk of replication-competent virus. At this time, the main disadvantages of naked DNA transfection is the low level of gene expression. New techniques of implantation combined with electrical stimulation, however, have resulted in increased levels of in vivo transgene expression after naked DNA administration (65). By improving the efficiency of naked DNA transfection, electroporation should expand the scope of naked DNA for use in gene therapy.

Naked DNA constructs have proven quite effective as vehicles for vaccination and can be administered by intramuscular injection, intradermal injection, inhalation, oral administration, and also by application of plasmid/liposome complexes onto the skin (66). DNA vaccines can be directed against infectious diseases or tumor antigens and have also demonstrated the ability to break tolerance in a transgenic mouse model of chronic hepatitis B infection (67). Because the level of transgene expression necessary to elicit immunity is much less than that required in other gene therapy applications, low-level expression of plasmid-encoded transgenes has not compromised the effectiveness of naked DNA for use in vaccines. Transfection of skeletal muscle cells alone has been shown to be effective in eliciting cellular immunity (68). A major advantage of DNA vaccines over traditional protein antigen-based vaccines is the elicitation of both humoral and cellular immunity. This is due to the efficient processing of the naked DNA transgene product by host antigen-presenting cells (69). Because traditional antigen vaccines are usually processed as circulating antigen, they elicit only a humoral immunity. Live, attenuated viral vaccines that are processed both as circulating and endogenous antigen can elicit both humoral and cell-mediated immunity, but these attenuated vaccines have the significant disadvantages of increased cost, possible reversion to a more pathogenic strain, and the need for refrigeration, which limits their use in certain parts of the world.

DNA–Protein Complexes

Complexes of DNA and protein consist of DNA associated with a polycation, usually polylysine, which is cova-

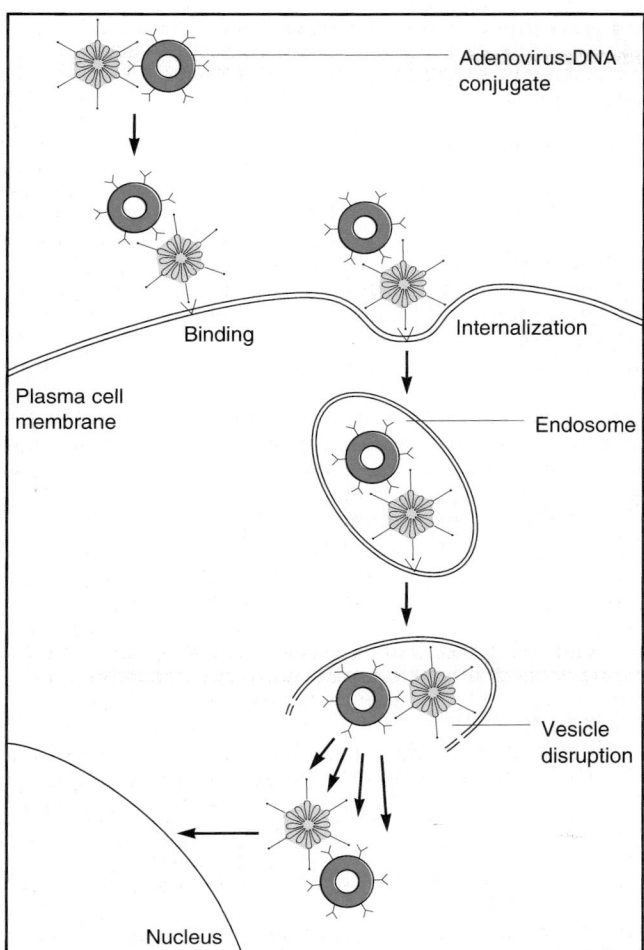

Figure 15.3. Entry pathway of adenovirus–molecular component conjugate into targeted cells. After binding to the target cells, the adenoviral complex is internalized by receptor-mediated endocytosis. Escape from the cellular endosome is accompanied by adenovirus-mediated disruption of the vesicle. This disruption allows the complex to enter the cytosol, where it has access to nuclear pores. The adenovirus may pass the nuclear pores to an intranuclear position.

lently bonded to a ligand moiety specific for a cellular receptor of interest. Because polylysine can be conjugated to a wide variety of ligands, including hormones, antibodies, glycoproteins, mannose, folate, and viral particles, the range of cell types that can be transfected is quite broad (70–76). The first step of gene transfer with DNA–protein complexes is uptake by the receptor-mediated endocytosis pathway. The DNA–protein complex must then escape the lysosomal compartment to avoid degradation (Fig. 15.3). The incorporation of agents that promote lysosomal disruption is important to increase expression (77). Because lysosomal escape is a feature of the adenovirus life cycle, the adenoviral capsid proteins are effective agents for lysosomal disruption and have been incorporated into DNA–protein complexes for this purpose (78–80). DNA complexes have a large transgene capacity and have been used to transfer DNA molecules of up to 48 kb in size (81). Other advantages of this system include the ability to target a specific cell population, the lack of a requirement for cell division, and the opportunity for repeated administration of the complex. The major disadvantage of DNA–protein complexes is that they generate relatively low levels of expression compared with viral vectors, in part because of degradation in lysosomes after endocytosis.

CLINICAL APPLICATIONS OF GENE THERAPY

Cancer

Cell-marking Protocols

The first approved gene therapy protocol was a marker study of tumor-infiltrating lymphocytes in patients with melanoma (82). Tumor-infiltrating lymphocytes were harvested from patients and marked by retroviral-mediated transfer of a neomycin resistance gene. After reinfusion, patient tumors and blood samples were analyzed for the presence of marked lymphocytes. This study provided the first information about the in vivo distribution and trafficking of tumor-infiltrating lymphocytes. Most subsequent gene therapy marker studies have investigated the role of stem cells in hematopoietic reconstitution after bone marrow transplantation for a variety of cancers. Early gene-marking studies provided valuable information by demonstrating that reinfused bone marrow cells contributed to relapse in patients receiving bone marrow transplants for acute myelogenous leukemia, neuroblastoma, and chronic myelogenous leukemia (83–85). Such information is critical for the design of more effective strategies to purge hematopoietic stem cells of contaminating tumor cells before bone marrow transplantation.

Prodrug Treatments

Transfer of "suicide" genes into tumor cells is an approach that has been used in the treatment of many differ-

Table 15.2. **CANCERS TREATED BY GENE TRANSFER OF HSVtk IN CLINICAL TRIALS**

Glioma
Mesothelioma
Ovarian cancer
Prostate cancer
Head and neck squamous cell cancer
Non-small cell lung cancer
Melanoma
Metastatic colon cancer

HSVtk, herpes simplex virus thymidine kinase.

ent types of cancers (Table 15.2). The construct used most often is an adenovirus coding for the HSV thymidine kinase *(HSVtk)* gene. After cell transduction, cells expressing *HSVtk* can then be killed by ganciclovir administration (86). Because ganciclovir must be modified in the transduced target cell to generate the therapeutically active moieties, this type of gene therapy is also termed an *enzyme/prodrug approach.* One of the benefits of the HSVtk system is that not all of the cells in a tumor need to be transduced to ablate the tumor completely. This is due to the bystander effect, which refers to the fact that neighboring cells, although not harboring the *HSVtk* gene, also are killed by ganciclovir administration (87). The bystander effect substantially lowers the transduction efficiency required for therapeutic efficacy. The bystander effect is believed to be due to the presence of gap junctions connecting neighboring cells and consequent passage of the toxic compound, ganciclovir triphosphate, between them (88). HSVtk has also been used to prevent graft-versus-host disease after allogeneic bone marrow transplantation. By transducing donor cells with HSVtk, graft-versus-host reactions can be effectively controlled by administration of ganciclovir (89).

Other enzyme/prodrug systems that have been developed include cytosine deaminase/5-fluorocytosine (5-FC) and cytochrome P-450 2B1/cyclophosphamide (90). Cytosine deaminase is a bacterial enzyme that converts the relatively nontoxic 5-FC into the highly toxic 5-fluorouracil. Use of this system has been shown to eliminate colon cancer tumors in which only 4% of the tumor cells were transduced with cytosine deaminase (91). An adenovirus vector carrying the cytosine deaminase gene is in phase I clinical trials for treatment of colon cancer metastatic to the liver. The cytochrome P-450 2B1/cyclophosphamide system has also proven effective in animal studies and is also characterized by a substantial bystander effect (92). The coexpression of P-450 reductase with cytochrome P-450 has resulted in an increase in tumor kill of up to two orders of magnitude (93). Future directions in the development of cytochrome P-450 vectors include the investigation of other P-450 substrates that have potential as chemotherapeutic prodrugs.

A new approach to increasing the efficacy of drug sensitivity genes has been the development of double suicide gene therapy using a fusion protein composed of cytosine deaminase and HSVtk. The combination of these two systems generates a synergistic antitumor response that is further potentiated when combined with radiation therapy (94). An alternate approach is to increase the catalytic activity of the transferred drug sensitivity gene. A fungal species of cytosine deaminase has been cloned whose catalytic activity for metabolizing 5-FC is approximately 280 times that of the previously developed bacterial cytosine deaminase. Compared with the bacterial enzyme, transfer of fungal cytosine deaminase has been shown to reduce the dose of 5-FC required for in vitro inhibition of tumor growth by approximately 30 times and to increase antitumor efficacy in vivo (95).

Restoration of Tumor Suppressor Function

Restoration of tumor suppressor gene function can be used to treat cancers characterized by loss of a specific regulatory protein. To date, the *p53* tumor suppressor gene has been the most widely used in gene therapy applications. The *p53* tumor suppressor plays a key role in the cell's response to DNA damage and to other stressors such as hypoxia. In response to DNA damage, *p53* expression is up-regulated, and wild-type p53 protein accumulates in the nucleus, causing cell cycle arrest. Mutations in *p53* are found in a wide range of human cancers and are most commonly missense mutations in the DNA binding do-

Table 15.3. CLINICAL TRIALS FOR GENE TRANSFER OF TUMOR SUPPRESSOR GENES INTO HUMAN CANCERS

Tumor suppressor gene	Cancer type
Retinoblastoma gene	Bladder cancer
BRCA-1 gene	Ovarian cancer
	Breast cancer
	Prostate cancer
p53 gene	Lung cancer
	Head and neck squamous cell cancer
	Metastatic colon cancer
	Prostate cancer
	Breast cancer
	Ovarian cancer
	Malignant glioma

main (96,97). Mutations to *p53* may act as dominant negative mutations or loss-of-function mutations, or may actually result in a mutant allele that potentiates the transactivation potential of the wild-type protein (98). In a variety of animal tumor models, introduction of wild-type *p53* into *p53*-deficient tumor cells causes apoptosis and tumor regression. Transfer of *p53* can be combined with other therapies as well. In a murine model, *p53*-mediated tumor regression can be potentiated by concurrent cytokine gene transfer (99). Clinical trials are underway using adenoviral vectors to transduce wild-type *p53* into non-small cell lung cancer, head and neck squamous cell carcinoma, metastatic colon cancer, hepatocellular cancer, prostate cancer, breast cancer, ovarian cancer, and malignant gliomas. Other tumor suppressor genes such as cyclin kinase inhibitors, the *BRCA-1* breast cancer gene, and the retinoblastoma gene have also been shown to mediate apoptosis of cancer cells in vitro and inhibition of tumorigenicity in vivo (100). *BRCA-1, p53,* and the retinoblastoma gene are the three tumor suppressors under evaluation in clinical trials (Table 15.3).

Oncogene Inhibition

To treat cancers that depend on oncogene expression, gene therapy vectors can be designed to eliminate the oncogene mRNA transcript or produce inhibitors of the oncogene protein product. Methods used to prevent oncogene mRNA translation include ribozymes and antisense RNA messages. Ribozymes are small, catalytic RNA molecules that possess sequence-specific RNA cleavage activity (Fig. 15.4). They can be used specifically to target and destroy mRNA transcripts. Ribozymes have been designed

to destroy a large number of different oncogene mRNA species, including those coding for fos, HER-2/neu, H-ras, and bcl-2 (101–104). Ribozymes can also effect RNA repair by cleaving a specified mRNA sequence and then splicing the wild-type sequence in its place, offering the potential for allelic correction in a variety of autosomal dominant disorders (105). The introduction of antisense RNA messages is another technique used to eliminate translation of target mRNA molecules. An antisense RNA message is an RNA molecule whose base pair sequence is complementary to that of a target mRNA message. The antisense RNA molecule anneals to the target RNA to form nontranslatable, double-stranded RNA molecules. Consequently, no protein product can be produced. Antisense strategies targeted at oncogenes are being tested in phase I clinical trials for gliomas, prostate cancer, and breast cancer.

Gene therapy vectors can also be used to produce inhibitors of oncogene products. The bcl-2 family of apoptosis inhibitors is overexpressed in various cancers, including breast cancer, gastric cancer, neuroblastoma, and bladder cancer. Transduction of these types of tumor cells with an adenovirus expressing a bcl-2 inhibitor, bcl-xs, has been shown effectively to mediate apoptosis (106). Hematopoietic stem cells are refractory to the apoptotic effects of the bcl-2 inhibitor, however. Transduction of marrow cells with *bcl-xs* may therefore prove to be a useful method for purging tumor cells before bone marrow transplantation.

Killing by Viral Proliferation

For biosafety, most gene therapy vectors are designed to be replication defective. There are two replication-competent viruses in clinical trials for treatment of cancer whose therapeutic mode of action is selective replication and resultant cytotoxicity in cancerous tissues.

G207 is an attenuated, replication-competent mutant HSV-1 that has replication competence only in dividing cells (49). G207 has been shown to have selective cytotoxicity for neoplastic cells in animal models of intracerebral glioma, breast cancer, subdural malignant meningioma, melanoma, colorectal carcinoma, and squamous cell carcinoma, and is in a phase I study of the treatment of malignant glioma (49,107–111).

CN706 is an attenuated, replication-competent adenovirus that replicates preferentially in cells producing PSA (112). Selectivity is conferred by the presence of a composite prostate-specific promoter/enhancer element placed upstream of the viral *E1a* gene. In vitro, CN706 has been shown selectively to replicate in prostate cancer cells and, in vivo, a single injection of CN706 has been shown

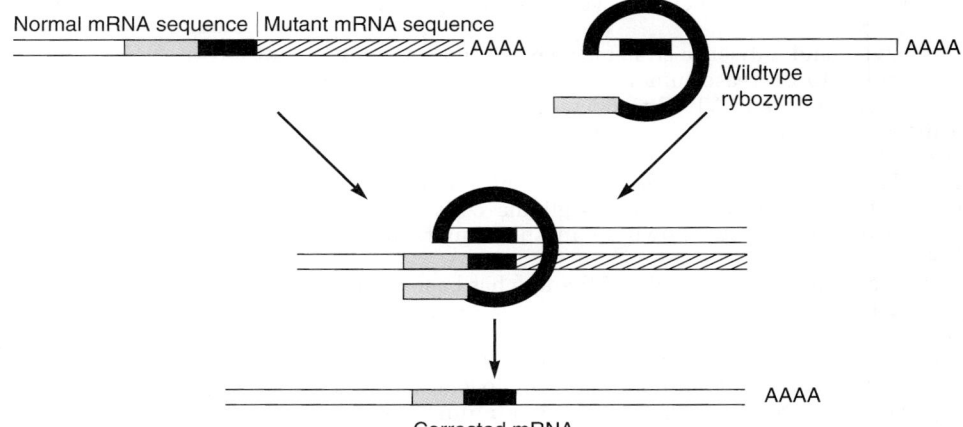

Figure 15.4. Use of ribozymes to correct mutant mRNA. The ribozyme binds to the mutant strand of mRNA, as does an antisense mRNA molecule, but the ribozyme is also capable of editing the mRNA strand and correcting the mutant sequences.

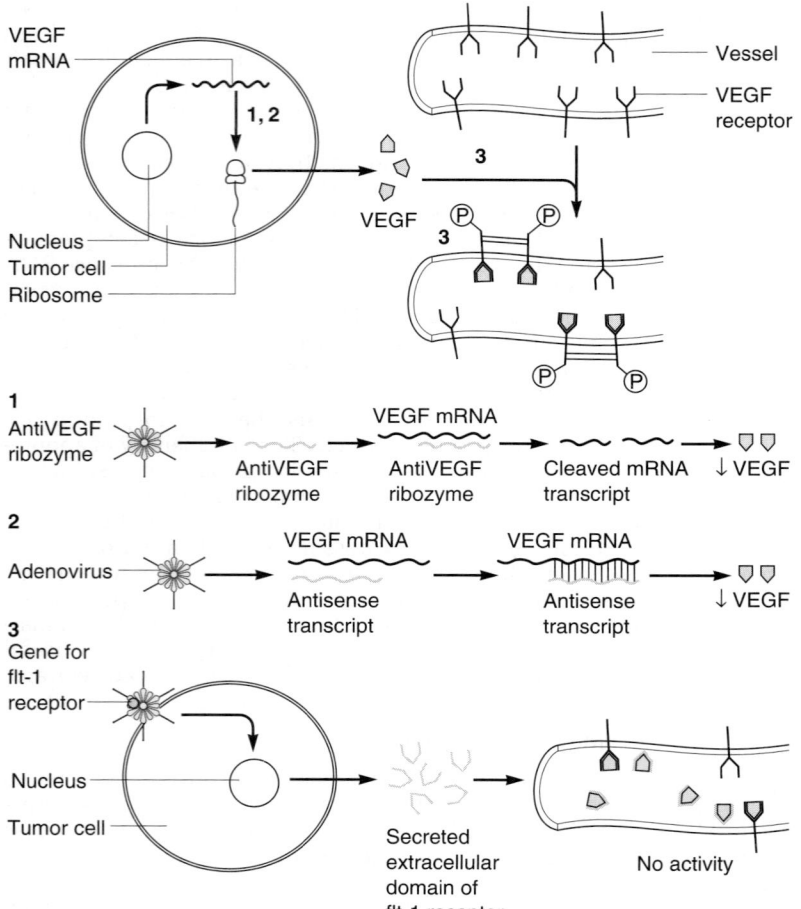

Figure 15.5. Antiangiogenic strategies as a new cancer gene therapy. Binding of vascular endothelial growth factor (VEGF) to the flt-1 receptor results in dimerization, autophosphorylation (P), and activation of intracellular tyrosine kinase domains. The approaches shown are targeted in various ways to block VEGF–VEGF receptor interaction, and include (1) ribozyme, (2) antisense, and (3) the soluble extracellular domain of the VEGF (flt-1) receptor. The latter approach both sequesters available VEGF and acts in a dominant-negative fashion by dimerizing with native flt-1 receptors, preventing autophosphorylation of the intracellular kinase domains.

to kill prostate cancer tumors in nude mice. CN706 is being used in one phase I clinical trial for the treatment of prostate cancer.

Angiostatic Therapies

Antiangiogenic strategies have emerged as a new approach for cancer therapy (Fig. 15.5). The observation that angiogenesis is required for tumor growth and metastasis and that vascular endothelial growth factor (VEGF), a potent angiogenic mediator, is overexpressed in many tumors has prompted the development of anti-VEGF therapies for the treatment of cancer. Although there has been much progress in the development of animal models, angiostatic gene therapies have not yet been incorporated in any clinical trials.

Ribozyme and antisense strategies have both been studied as ways to decrease tumor cell VEGF expression. In glioma cell lines, anti-VEGF ribozymes have been shown to digest from 65% to 95% of VEGF mRNA, causing a greater than 70% decrease in VEGF protein expression (113). In a nude mouse model, transfer of a VEGF antisense construct into subcutaneous glioma cells with an adenovirus vector was shown to inhibit tumor growth (114).

Another approach to anti-VEGF therapy has been the regional delivery of the secreted form of the extracellular domain of the flt-1 VEGF receptor. An abundance of this truncated receptor is capable of binding most of the VEGF present, preventing the initiation of angiogenesis. In a mouse model of colon cancer metastasis, administration of an adenoviral vector coding for this VEGF ligand to the re-

gion of metastasis resulted in regression of metastatic disease (115). In a similar strategy, blockade of the endothelial-specific Tie2 angiogenic signaling pathway with an adenoviral vector coding for a mutant dominant-negative Tie2 receptor has also been shown to mediate the inhibition of tumor growth (116).

Angiostatin and endostatin, two naturally occurring antiangiogenic proteins, are also being investigated for use in

Table 15.4. **CYTOKINES, ALLOANTIGENS, AND COSTIMULATORY MOLECULE GENES TRANSFERRED FOR CANCER IMMUNOTHERAPY**

Cytokines
  IL-2
  IL-4
  IL-7
  IL-12
  Granulocyte–macrophage colony-stimulating factor
  Tumor necrosis factor-α
  IFN-γ
  IL-2/IFN-γ
Costimulatory molecules
  B7-1 (CD80)
Alloantigens
  HLA-B7
Combination therapies
  IL-12/B7-1(CD80)
  IL-2/HLA-B7

HLA, human leukocyte antigen; IL, interleukin.

cancer gene therapy. The angiostatin and endostatin peptides have been shown to inhibit the growth of endothelial cells in vitro, and both have been shown to inhibit tumor growth in animal models (117–119). In a murine model, liposomal administration of angiostatin or endostatin caused a reduction in breast cancer tumor size (120). In a murine metastatic tumor model, intramuscular administration of the endostatin gene inhibited tumor metastasis (121).

Immunotherapeutic Vaccines

Numerous clinical trials of "immunogene therapy" in patients with cancer are underway (Table 15.4). A large percentage of current gene therapy clinical trials for cancer are designed to stimulate the immune system to mount an effective antitumor response. Failure of the immune system to eliminate tumor cells from the body can be viewed as either a defect in the recognition of tumor cell antigens (afferent immune response) or a defect in the cytotoxic or killer cells designed to eliminate tumor cells (effector immune response). Figure 15.6 depicts the breakdown of these clinical efforts by histologic type of the tumors targeted by the various strategies described in this section.

Strategies targeting the efferent limb of the immune system have used delivery of cytokines into the local area of the tumor or into T lymphocytes to stimulate cytotoxic T-cell responses. Interleukin (IL)-2, IL-6, interferon-γ, and tumor necrosis factor-α are all being used in clinical trials to stimulate immune effector mechanisms. Transfer of genes coding for T-cell costimulatory molecules into tumor cells is another strategy for increasing the cytotoxic T-cell response. B7-1 (CD80) is one of the best characterized costimulatory molecules. It is a membrane glycoprotein that binds to the T-cell CD28 receptor and stimulates IL-2 production and T-cell proliferation (122). Not only does B7-1 play an important role in activating T cells, but lack of its costimulatory signal during antigen presentation to the T-cell receptor has been shown to induce T-cell clonal anergy (123). In a number of animal models, transduction of tumor cells with B7-1 has been shown to mediate tumor cell killing and elicit protective immunity (124,125). Gene transfer of B7-1 into tumor cells is being evaluated in clinical trials for treatment of ovarian cancer, colorectal cancer, small cell lung cancer, breast cancer, and melanoma. Animal models have also demonstrated a synergistic antitumor response when tumor cells are transduced with B7-1 in combination with various cytokines such as IL-12 (126). The combination of B-7 and IL-12 is being tested in clinical trials for treatment of melanoma, ovarian, and colorectal cancer.

Gene therapy strategies have also been developed to improve immune recognition of tumor-specific antigens.

Gene transfer of cytokines such as IL-4 and granulocyte–macrophage colony-stimulating factor into tumor cells has been used to generate effective antitumor responses in a large number of murine models and is the most common approach taken to stimulate the afferent limb of the immune system (127,128). Variations on the theme of autologous tumor cell transduction include the inoculation of cytokine-expressing allogeneic tumor cells and fibroblasts. All of these therapies are designed to increase tumor antigen immunoreactivity by delivering cytokine stimuli to antigen-presenting cells and T lymphocytes during the presentation of tumor antigens.

Another approach to stimulating recognition of tumor antigens by the immune system is the development of dendritic cell-based tumor vaccines. Dendritic cells are antigen-presenting cells that are critically important for antigen-specific T-cell activation and can be enriched from the peripheral blood stream after short-term culture with IL-4, granulocyte–macrophage colony-stimulating factor, and tumor necrosis factor-α. Dendritic cells pulsed with tumor antigens or tumor cell mRNA have been shown to elicit T-cell immunity in vivo (129,130). Dendritic cells can also be transduced with vectors coding for specific tumor antigens to elicit potent cell-mediated immunity in vivo (131,132). Systemic IL-2 has been shown to potentiate the antitumor immune response in murine models (133). Clinical trials are underway to assess dendritic cell-based immunotherapies directed against the MART-1 melanoma antigen and CEA.

Poxviruses engineered to express various tumor-specific antigens have also been used successfully to elicit cell-mediated immunity in animal models (134,135). As with dendritic cell-based immunotherapy, the combination of IL-2 with vaccinia inoculation produces greater therapeutic efficacy (136). Clinical trials are assessing poxviruses engineered to express PSA, CEA, MUC-1, the gp100 melanoma antigen, and the MART-1 melanoma antigen.

Alloantigens can also be introduced into tumor cells to increase tumor immunoreactivity. In a murine model, introduction of a foreign MHC protein into poorly immunogenic tumors has have been shown to induce a cytotoxic T-cell response to both the allogeneic MHC protein and to other, unrelated tumor antigens (137). In patients who do not express the MHC class I molecule human leukocyte antigen (HLA)-B7, transfer of HLA-B7 into autologous tumor cells can been used to stimulate immune recognition of both transduced and nontransduced tumor cells. This is believed to occur through alloantigen stimulation of T-cell proliferation and differentiation. Evidence supporting this hypothesis comes from a clinical trial for melanoma in which HLA-B7 gene transfer was shown to

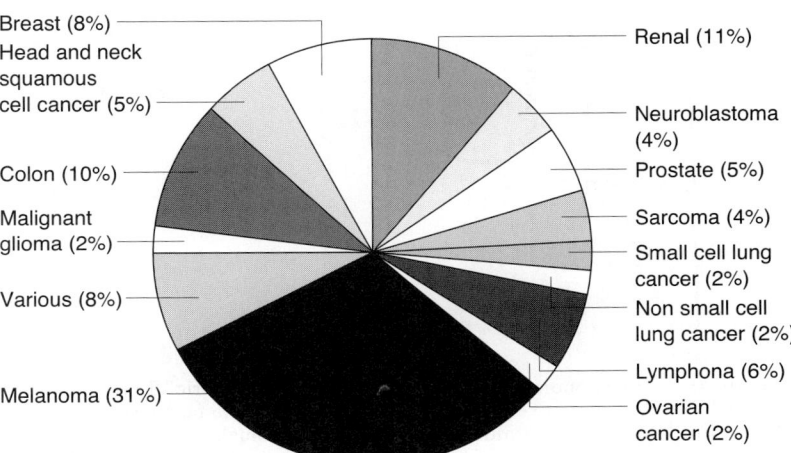

Figure 15.6. Tumor types treated by cytokine, costimulatory molecule, and alloantigen gene transfer in clinical trials of cancer immunotherapy.

Breast (8%)
Head and neck squamous cell cancer (5%)
Colon (10%)
Malignant glioma (2%)
Various (8%)
Melanoma (31%)
Renal (11%)
Neuroblastoma (4%)
Prostate (5%)
Sarcoma (4%)
Small cell lung cancer (2%)
Non small cell lung cancer (2%)
Lymphona (6%)
Ovarian cancer (2%)

alter the T-cell repertoire of tumor-infiltrating lymphocytes located both in the treated lesion and in uninjected nodules (138). Transfer of the HLA-B7 gene into HLA-B7-negative patients is being used in clinical trials for breast cancer, renal cell cancer, melanoma, colon cancer, squamous cell cancer, and non-Hodgkin's lymphoma.

Drug Resistance in Hematopoietic Stem Cells

Transfer of drug resistance genes into hematopoietic stem cells is a strategy designed to permit higher dosing of chemotherapeutic agents by limiting their myelosuppressive side effects. There are three enzymes being used in clinical trials: the human multiple-drug resistance gene (MDR-1), O6-methylguanine-DNA methyltransferase (MGMT), and dihydrofolate reductase (DHFR). MDR1 codes for P-glycoprotein, a transmembrane protein involved in the active transport of various structurally unrelated anticancer drugs out of cells. Overexpression of P-glycoprotein in cancer cells confers resistance to multiple drugs, including vinca alkaloids, anthracyclines, podophyllins, and paclitaxel. Transfer of MDR-1 to imbue hematopoietic stem cells with chemotherapy resistance has been demonstrated in animal models, and MDR-1-transduced hematopoietic stem cells are now being studied in clinical trials for treatment of ovarian cancer, breast cancer, and germ cell tumors (139). MGMT is a DNA repair protein that repairs the promutagenic DNA base lesion in O6-methylguanine introduced by alkylating agents. MGMT is in two clinical trials for treatment of brain tumors (140). DHFR is the primary target of the chemotherapeutic agent methotrexate. Increased expression of DHFR and decreased DHFR binding are both known mechanisms of methotrexate resistance in tumors. A methotrexate-resistant DHFR is in clinical trials for use in chronic myelogenous leukemia, both as part of a bone marrow-purging protocol and as a mechanism to provide transplanted cells with methotrexate resistance.

Chimeric Receptors

An alternative approach that can be taken when tumor cells have a well characterized surface antigen is to engineer mature cytotoxic T cells with chimeric receptors specific to a tumor-associated antigen (141). This approach has been shown to be successful in mediating total tumor regression in mouse models, and cytotoxic T cells expressing recombinant chimeric receptors targeting folate binding protein, CEA, and HER-2/neu are currently in clinical trials (141).

A next step toward applying this technology to the therapy of human cancer involves transduction of human hematopoietic stem/progenitor cells with a chimeric receptor. Figure 15.7 depicts a model therapeutic strategy for patients receiving a chimeric receptor gene-modified hematopoietic stem cell transplant. The progeny lymphocytes and myeloid cells (monocytes and neutrophils) derived from the in vitro transduced hematopoietic stem cells on transplantation and hematolymphoid reconstitution in the recipient would potentially have the ability to recognize and kill in a non-MHC-restricted fashion those cells expressing the specific tumor antigen recognized by the chimeric receptor encoded by the introduced transgene. Because of concern that recognition of "normal" levels of the targeted antigen on normal cells, as opposed to "overexpressed" levels on tumor might lead to toxicity (i.e., by killing normal tissues), vector constructs could also contain suicide cytosine deaminase or thymidine kinase genes to eliminate chimeric receptor-expressing progeny cells if adverse targeting occurs. Because hematopoietic stem cells are self-renewing and pluripotent, they would offer the patient with cancer receiving a bone marrow transplant a long-term immune system with antitumor function.

Another strategy based on redirecting the immune response to recognize tumor-associated antigens after bone

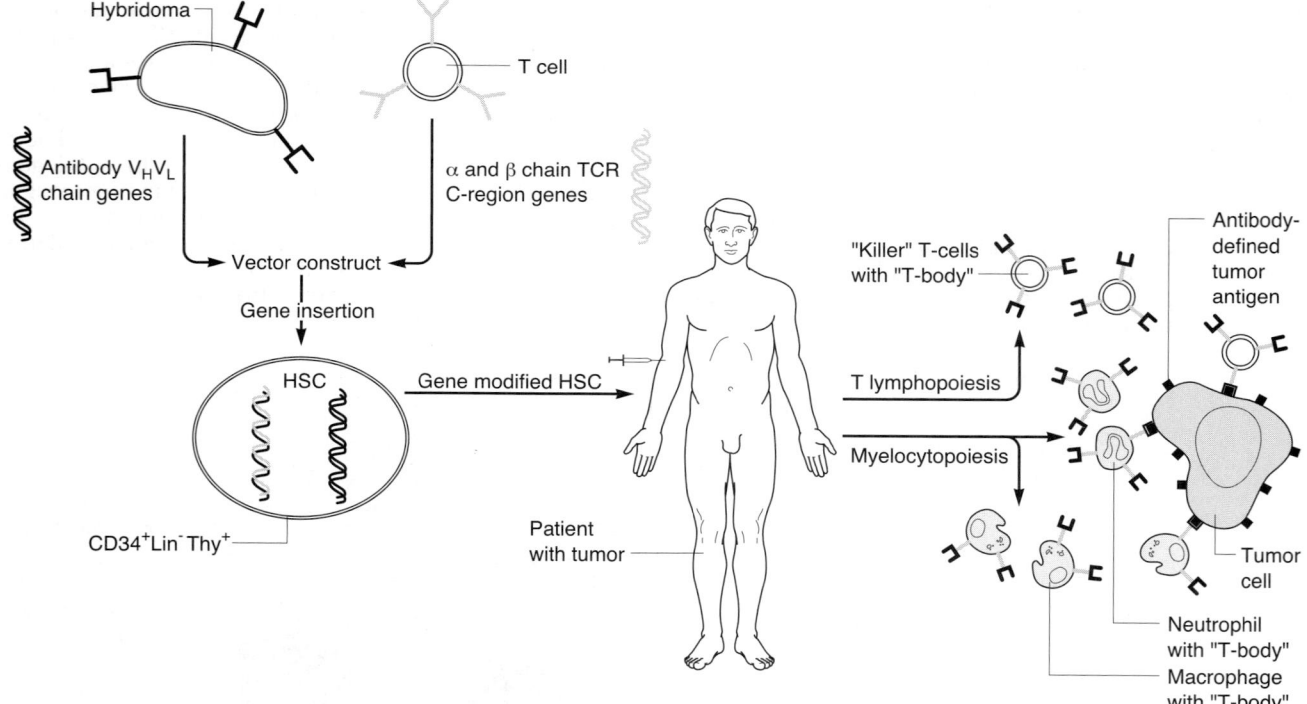

Figure 15.7. Hematopoietic stem cell gene transfer: "chimeric" T-cell receptor approach. The purpose of this strategy is to engineer the antitumor immune response after bone marrow transplantation by producing large numbers of progeny or daughter hematolymphoid cells expressing a transgene encoded receptor ("T-body") directed against tumor-associated antigens.

marrow transplantation is the introduction of genes encoding "classic" T-cell receptors. Unlike the chimeric receptor approach, this strategy would be limited to progeny T cells only, would require coexpression and assembly of two separate chains (α and β), would be MHC restricted, and would be more specific to tumor cells (as opposed to normal tissue). The gene encoding for a T-cell receptor for a cytotoxic T-cell-defined peptide expressed by HLA-A2 on melanoma has been molecularly cloned, which could serve as an initial proof of concept. The prohibitive limitation of this potentially exciting approach, however, may be the difficulty in expressing two independent genes that encode the separate α and β chains of the T-cell receptor in hematopoietic stem cells and their progeny T cells by the currently available vectors.

Acquired Disease

Vascular Disease

Angiogenic gene therapies have been initiated for the treatment of both myocardial ischemia and peripheral vascular disease. All but one of the current clinical trials for therapeutic angiogenesis use an isoform of VEGF as the vector transgene. VEGF is an endothelial cell-specific mitogen and vascular permeability factor that is a prime regulator of angiogenesis and vasculogenesis. In a rabbit model of chronic limb ischemia, intramuscular administration of a plasmid construct coding for VEGF increased collateral circulation and improved perfusion in the treated limb (142). There are three approved protocols for the treatment of peripheral vascular disease studying intramuscular administration of adenoviral and naked DNA VEGF constructs. In a porcine ischemic heart model, intracoronary and intramuscular administration of VEGF have both demonstrated increased collateral vessel development and improved myocardial blood flow (143,144). Two clinical trials are now investigating VEGF intramyocardial gene transfer to the heart (145,146).

Fibroblast growth factor is another angiogenic growth factor that has been investigated for therapeutic myocardial angiogenesis. Administration of FGF in a canine model of cardiac ischemia demonstrated improved collateral blood flow in treated animals (147). In a human clinical trial of patients undergoing cardiac bypass, intramyocardial injection of purified FGF-1 stimulated new capillary development in the area of injection (148). There is one ongoing gene therapy protocol studying the effects of adenovirus-mediated human FGF-4 transfer in patients with stable exertional angina.

Restenosis continues to be a common complication after coronary and peripheral vascular angioplasty procedures, occurring in 30% to 50% of all patients (149,150). Gene therapy approaches to treating restenosis have concentrated on limiting neointima formation by inhibiting the vascular smooth muscle cell proliferation that occurs after balloon dilatation. Animal models have shown inhibition of neointima formation using both cytotoxic approaches, such as the transfer of the *HSVtk* gene or fas ligand into vascular smooth muscle cells, and therapies directed at transduction pathways involved with vascular smooth muscle cell proliferation (151–156). By promoting reendothelialization after injury, VEGF has also been shown to decrease restenosis in some animal models, and is the only gene therapy under study in clinical trials for treatment of restenosis (157,158).

Tissue Regeneration

Gene therapeutic approaches are also being developed for local delivery of growth factors for tissue regeneration.

One of the advantages of using gene transfer for the delivery of growth factors is that it offers the potential for steady, site-specific production of these factors, lowering their systemic levels and therefore limiting their potential toxicities. The feasibility of gene therapy strategies for wound healing has been demonstrated in a canine bone defect model (159). In this model, plasmid vectors encoding a peptide fragment of human parathyroid hormone are encased in a polymer matrix that is implanted at the site of a surgically created bone defect. As a part of the healing process, the matrix is invaded by host fibroblasts that are transfected with the plasmid DNA as they enter the matrix. Thus, the gene-activated matrix provides a mechanism for passive in vivo transfection of host fibroblasts. The fibroblasts then express the parathyroid hormone transgene, resulting in accelerated bone growth and remodeling. Levels of expression are dose dependent and vary proportionally with the titer of plasmid DNA originally present in the polymer matrix. This type of bone healing strategy could find application in the treatment of hip fractures in the elderly.

Parkinson's Disease

Parkinson's disease is a neurodegenerative disorder characterized by a loss of the dopaminergic neurons of the nigrostriatal system. This is manifested clinically by weakness and slowness of movement, fixed facial expression, and resting tremor. Although ex vivo approaches have been successfully used to treat Parkinson's disease, in vivo approaches are preferred because they do not disrupt the neural circuitry of the brain. One gene therapy strategy for treatment of Parkinson's disease is to increase dopaminergic transmission by transduction of tyrosine hydroxylase, the enzyme that produces the dopamine precursor L-dopa, into neurons. An rAAV vector injected into mice has demonstrated tyrosine hydroxlase expression for up to 4 months accompanied by behavioral recovery in treated rats (36). An HSV-1-based vector has also demonstrated long-term tyrosine hydroxylase expression with behavioral improvement in a rat model, although use of this vector also resulted in treatment deaths due to herpes encephalitis (160). The biosafety of HSV-1, despite continuing improvement, does not approach that of rAAV. Cotransduction of tyrosine hydroxlase with aromatic L-amino acid decarboxylase (AADC), the enzyme that converts L-dopa to dopamine, has been shown to potentiate dopamine production and behavioral recovery in a rat Parkinson's model (161). A bicistronic AAV vector coding for both tyrosine hydroxylase and AADC has been used to transduce the striatal cells of dopamine-depleted monkeys treated with the neurotoxin 1-methyl-4-phenyl-1,2,3,6-tetrahydropyridine, a primate model for Parkinson's disease (162). Elevated dopamine levels were observed for a period of up to 2.5 months, although no statistically significant behavioral change was found. Administration of glial-derived neurotropic factor to prevent degeneration of dopaminergic neurons has also been studied for use in Parkinson's disease. In vivo transduction with an rAAV expressing glial-derived neurotropic factor has been successful in the treatment of a progressive-degeneration Parkinson's disease model in rats (163). It is likely that future approaches to gene therapy for Parkinson's disease will combine neuroprotective strategies with techniques to increase dopaminergic transmission.

Human Immunodeficiency Virus

Human immunodeficiency virus is a retrovirus in the lentivirus subfamily and is the etiologic agent responsible for AIDS. There are two types of HIV virus, HIV-1 and HIV-

2, which have approximately 40% sequence homology with one another. HIV-1 is the most common cause of AIDS worldwide and is the target of all current gene therapy protocols. HIV-2 is found predominantly in West Africa. Over 20 clinical trials are investigating the transduction of hematopoietic stem cells and lymphocytes for the treatment of HIV infection. In addition to the *gag, pol,* and *env* genes found in all retroviruses, HIV contains six other genes: *tat, rev, vif, vpr, vpu,* and *nef.* The first step in the HIV life cycle is infection of CD4+ cells mediated by an interaction between the HIV gp120 envelope glycoprotein and a cell surface CD4 molecule in association with other cell surface coreceptors. Once within the cell, karyophilic elements in the HIV preintegration complex direct its transport into the nucleus, where the HIV RNA genome is reverse transcribed into a double-stranded DNA provirus that then integrates into the host genome. Tat and Rev are the two key HIV regulatory proteins. Tat binds to the transactivation response (TAR) element and is a powerful transactivator of HIV gene expression. Rev plays a critical role in the transition from early to late HIV gene expression. By binding to the Rev-responsive element (RRE), a short RNA sequence in the envelope gene, Rev mediates the nuclear export of mRNA species encoding structural proteins, enabling the subsequent production of infectious virus particles (164). Although gene therapy strategies have been formulated to target many of the various HIV gene products, the therapies now in clinical trials are directed toward inhibiting the function of the gp120, Tat, and Rev proteins and eliciting a cytotoxic T-cell response to the envelope glycoproteins on the surface of HIV-infected cells.

The initiation of a cytotoxic T-cell response is an important mechanism for limiting viral pathogenesis, and there are two different gene therapy strategies being tested in clinical trials to elicit a cytotoxic T-cell response against HIV-infected cells. One approach is the ex vivo retroviral transduction of autologous fibroblasts with a portion of the HIV envelope gene. After lethal irradiation, the fibroblasts are then reimplanted into the patient. In animal studies, this technique has been successful in eliciting strong cytotoxic T-lymphocyte and antibody responses directed toward the HIV envelope (165). Another approach is to manipulate autologous T cells by transducing them with chimeric T-cell receptors specific for the HIV gp120 envelope glycoprotein. These chimeric receptors are fusion proteins consisting of human CD4 linked to the intracellular signaling domain of the T-cell receptor ζ chain (166). Cytotoxic T lymphocytes bearing these chimeric receptors are activated to lyse HIV-infected cells after binding of the T-cell receptor to the HIV gp120 envelope protein on the surface of infected cells. One of the strengths of this approach is the fact that the gp120 recognition is not MHC restricted and therefore does not require endogenous processing and presentation in combination with MHC class I surface molecules for recognition and elimination of the infected cell.

In clinical trials, attempts to inhibit the function of the Tat, Rev, and gp120 proteins have included the transduction of transdominant-negative mutant proteins, antisense constructs, decoy genes to prevent regulatory protein binding, intracellular antibodies, and ribozyme constructs. Transdominant-negative mutant proteins lack wild-type activity and also inhibit activity of the wild-type protein. A transdominant negative mutant form of Rev has been used in several protocols to confer T-cell and hematopoietic stem cell resistance to HIV infection. Initial results from a clinical trial studying retroviral transduction of CD4+ cells with a transdominant-negative Rev mutant, Rev M10, have demonstrated long-term engraftment of T cells with an associated survival advantage (167). A fusion construct that combines a transdominant-negative Rev with a transdominant-negative Tat has been shown to inhibit both Tat and Rev activity and is in clinical trials for treatment of HIV. Transduction of an antisense construct to the TAR element in combination with a transdominant-negative Rev construct is another technique being used simultaneously to inhibit both Tat and Rev activity. Alternatively, decoy genes can be used to inhibit regulatory proteins by expressing an oversupply of alternate substrate. In one approach, vector constructs produce RNA species containing multiple RRE elements, binding available Rev protein and limiting HIV replication. Transduction of a RRE decoy gene into hematopoietic progenitor cells is being evaluated in one clinical trial for the treatment of pediatric HIV infection (168).

Intracellular antibodies, also known as *intrabodies,* have also been developed for the inhibition of HIV infection. Intracellular antibodies are single-chain proteins that consist of a variable heavy chain and a variable light chain joined by a polypeptide linker. These antibody constructs are created through the modification of monoclonal antibodies and preserve the specificity of the antigen-binding fragment from which they are derived. Intrabodies also incorporate various peptide motifs that target them to specific subcellular compartments such as the nucleus, cytoplasm, or endoplasmic reticulum. They can be designed specifically to bind and neutralize a variety of proteins, and there are two ongoing clinical protocols studying the use of intracellular antibodies in the treatment of HIV. In one protocol, an intrabody localized in the endoplasmic reticulum binds specifically to the HIV gp160 envelope protein. This prevents the cleavage of gp160 into the gp120 and gp41 proteins, with the effect of limiting expression of gp120 on the cell surface. In animal models, this significantly reduces the infectivity of HIV virions produced by infected cells (169). A second protocol uses a cytoplasmic intrabody to bind Rev protein, inhibiting Rev-mediated nuclear export of structural protein mRNAs (170). Ribozymes are small, catalytic RNA molecules that possess sequence-specific RNA cleavage activity, and although they are being developed for use in a variety of gene therapy applications, at present ribozymes are being used only in protocols for the treatment of HIV. Ribozymes inhibit the function of HIV regulatory proteins by cleaving their RNA transcripts and thereby preventing translation. Ribozymes targeting Tat and Rev as well as the 58-transcribed leader sequence of HIV are being investigated in clinical trials (171,172).

Heritable Disease

There are ongoing gene therapy clinical trials for a variety of hereditary diseases, including adenosine deaminase severe combined immunodeficiency (ADA⁻ SCID), α_1-antitrypsin deficiency, Canavan's disease, chronic granulomatous disease, cystic fibrosis, Fanconi's anemia type C, Gaucher's disease type I, hemophilia A, mucopolysaccharidosis type II (Hunter's syndrome), familial hypercholesterolemia (FH), leukocyte adherence deficiency, ornithine transcarbamylase deficiency, purine nucleoside phosphorylase deficiency, and X-linked SCID. All of these disorders are recessive with the exception of FH, which is caused by loss-of-function mutations of the low-density lipoprotein (LDL) receptor. FH is characterized by a dose dependence in which FH homozygotes have more severe disease than heterozygotes.

Most of the current trials for treating heritable disorders involve gene transfer to the defective cell type. For disorders in which the protein of interest is present in the circulation, however, other target cells capable of transgene expression and secretion, such as fibroblasts or myocytes,

Table 15.5. **CURRENT GENE THERAPY CLINICAL TRIALS FOR HEREDITARY DISORDERS**

Disorder	Gene defect	Phenotype	Incidence	Inheritance	Treatment
Adenosine deaminase SCID	Adenosine deaminase gene	Severe lymphopenia and opportunistic infections	Very rare	Autosomal recessive	Ex vivo retroviral transduction of autologous T cells with the adenosine deaminase gene
α_1-Antitrypsin deficiency	α_1-Antitrypsin gene	Emphysema, cirrhosis	1 in 3,500	Autosomal recessive	Liposomal delivery of plasmid DNA expressing α_1-antitrypsin to the airways
Canavan's disease	Aspartoacylase gene	Severe psychomotor delay, retardation, premature death	1 in 3,500 in the Ashkenazi Jewish population, otherwise very rare	Autosomal recessive	Liposomal delivery of plasmid DNA expressing aspartoacylase to the cerebrospinal fluid
Chronic granulomatous disease[a]	p47-phox gene coding for the p47-phox subunit of the phagocytic NADPH oxidase	Recurrent bacterial and fungal infections	1 per 1,000,000	Autosomal recessive	Retroviral transduction hematopoietic progenitor cells with p47-phox gene
Chronic granulomatous disease[a]	gp91-phox gene coding for the gp91-phox subunit of the NADPH oxidase	Recurrent bacterial and fungal infections	3 per 1,000,000 men	X-linked recessive	Retroviral transduction of hematopoietic progenitor cells with the gp91-phox gene
Cystic fibrosis	Cystic fibrosis transmembrane conductance regulator (CFTR) gene	Bronchitis and pulmonary fibrosis, pancreatic insufficiency, chronic cholestasis, meconium ileus, atresia of the vas deferens	1 in 2,500	Autosomal recessive	Transduction of airway epithelium with adenovirus, liposomes, or recombinant adeno-associated virus carrying the CFTR gene
Fanconi's anemia type C	Fanconi's anemia C complementing gene	Progressive pancytopenia, predisposition to malignancy, hyperpigmentation	1 in 10,000 in the Ashkenazi Jewish population, otherwise very rare	Autosomal recessive	Retroviral transduction of hematopoietic progenitor cells with the Fanconi's anemia C complementing gene
Gaucher's disease type I	Glucocerebrosidase gene	Accumulation of glucocerebroside in the macrophages of the reticuloendothelial system, causing hepatosplenomegaly, splenic sequestration, lytic bone lesions	1 in 9,000; 1 in 1,400 in Ashkenazi Jewish population	Autosomal recessive	Retroviral transduction of hematopoietic progenitor cells with the glucocerebrosidase gene
Hemophilia A (factor VIII deficiency)	Clotting factor VIII gene	Bleeding into soft tissues, muscles, weight-bearing joints	1 in 10,000 men	X-linked recessive	Transfection of plasmid DNA encoding human factor VIII into autologous fibroblast using electroporation
Hunter's syndrome (mucopolysaccharidosis type II)	Iduronate-2-sulfatase gene	Accumulation of heparan sulfate and dermatan sulfate, resulting in hepatosplenomegaly, cardiopulmonary failure, death at age 30–40 y; in severe cases, progressive mental retardation and death in childhood	1 in 100,000 to 1 in 200,000 men	X-linked recessive	Retroviral transduction of peripheral blood lymphocytes with gene for iduronate-2-sulfatase
Hypercholesterolemia	Low-density lipoprotein receptor gene	In heterozygotes, premature coronary artery disease, xanthomata; in homozygotes, coronary artery disease in childhood, planar cutaneous xanthoma	Heterozygotes, 1 in 500	Autosomal dominant	Ex vivo retroviral transduction of autologous hepatocytes with the low-density lipoprotein receptor gene
Leukocyte adherence deficiency	Mutation in the CD18 leukocyte integrin subunit gene	Recurrent bacterial infections	Very rare	Autosomal recessive	Ex vivo retroviral transduction of hematopoietic progenitor cells with the CD18 gene
Ornithine transcarbamylase deficiency	Ornithine transcarbamylase gene	Hyperammonemia causing acute encephalopathy	Very rare	X-linked recessive	In vivo adenoviral transduction of hepatocytes with the ornithine transcarbamylase gene
Purine nucleoside phosphorylase deficiency	Purine nucleoside phosphorylase gene	SCID	Very rare, approximately 40 patients reported	Autosomal recessive	Ex vivo retroviral transduction of peripheral blood lymphocytes with the purine nucleoside phosphorylase gene
X-linked SCID	Common γ-chain of cytokine receptors	SCID marked by severe T-cell lymphopenia, variable B-cell lymphopenia, defective immunoglobulin class switching	1 in 50,000 to 1 in 100,000	X-linked recessive	Ex vivo retroviral transduction of hematopoietic progenitor cells with the γ-chain gene

[a]Chronic granulomatous disease can be caused by two gene defects. Both are listed.
NADPH, nicotinamide–adenine dinucleotide phosphate hydrogenase; SCID, severe combined immunodeficiency.

may be used. In animal models, stable and therapeutic secretion of coagulation factor IX, α_1-antitrypsin, and erythropoietin have all been achieved (43,45,173). In human clinical trials, however, only one trial investigating transduction of fibroblasts with the gene for factor VIII uses such a strategy. Examples of the types of approaches taken in different organ systems with different gene therapy vectors are given in the following sections. For a complete listing of the heritable diseases being treated in gene therapy protocols, refer to Table 15.5.

Adenosine Deaminase Severe Combined Immunodeficiency

Adenosine deaminase SCID was the first disease to be entered into a gene therapy clinical trial. ADA⁻ SCID is caused by an inherited deficiency of ADA, and is associated with the buildup of deoxyadenosine, an ADA substrate, which in T cells is preferentially converted into the toxic compound deoxyadenosine triphosphate. ADA⁻ SCID is characterized by severe lymphopenia, opportunistic infections, and death in early childhood. Enzyme replacement with polyethylene glycol-conjugated ADA enzyme (PEG-ADA) has been developed for treatment of ADA⁻ SCID, but it does not result in full immune reconstitution and costs approximately $250,000 per year. The first gene therapy trials for ADA⁻ SCID, performed concurrently in the United States and Europe, found that retroviral transfer of the ADA gene into peripheral lymphocytes was successful in providing immune reconstitution as measured by improvement of both humoral and cellular immune responses (174,175). In the European trial, both bone marrow and peripheral blood lymphocytes were transduced, and the two different retroviral vectors used to transduce these two cell populations, although both carrying the ADA gene, could be distinguished by digestion with restriction endonucleases. The origin of circulating T lymphocytes could therefore be assessed. This trial demonstrated that although transduced peripheral blood lymphocytes initially constituted most of the circulating T cells, approximately 1 year after treatment T lymphocytes derived from transduced bone marrow precursors began to predominate. Current efforts to treat ADA⁻ SCID have therefore been directed toward transduction of hematopoietic stem cells to provide long-lasting immune reconstitution without the requirement for repeated infusions of modified peripheral blood lymphocytes (176,177). Retroviral gene transfer to hematopoietic stem cells has proven successful in achieving long-term engraftment. However, patients still require supplemental infusions of PEG-ADA for optimal immune function. Further advances in increasing the efficiency of gene transfer will be required before gene therapy alone proves curative for ADA⁻ SCID.

Cystic Fibrosis

Cystic fibrosis is a lethal autosomal recessive disorder caused by mutations of the cystic fibrosis transmembrane conductance regulator gene *(CFTR)* that encodes a cyclic adenosine monophosphate-regulated chloride channel present on the apical surface of epithelial cells. Clinical manifestations of cystic fibrosis affect the lungs, pancreas, small bowel, hepatic bile ducts, and male reproductive tract. Pulmonary disease is the major source of morbidity. Sixteen phase I trials of gene therapy dosing of the lung and airway epithelium have been completed in cystic fibrosis. Adenovirus, AAV, and liposomal delivery systems have been studied in these clinical trials. In general, all of the vectors have been shown to be relatively safe, and there has been no recovery of replication-competent virus after vector administration. In the first trial using adenoviral delivery of *CFTR,* however, the highest dose of viral vector did cause a transient syndrome of hypotension (not requiring vasopressors), tachycardia, dyspnea, fever, fatigue, and headache (178). This is certainly cause for concern, and although the reasons for this constellation of symptoms are not entirely clear, it emphasizes the need for careful titration of gene therapy vectors in clinical use. Although there have been no reported long-term adverse sequelae from vector administration for treatment of cystic fibrosis, neither has there been molecular evidence of significant gene transfer in studies to date. One of the most significant stumbling blocks to gene transfer appears to be the lack of appropriate viral receptors on the apical surface of the airway epithelium (179–181). Although these receptors are present on the basal surface of the epithelial cells, tight junctions between the cells prevent penetration by gene therapy vectors, which are administered in the airway lumen. Further refinements in vector design to overcome this difficulty will be required for future trials.

Hemophilia

Hemophilia A and hemophilia B are X-linked bleeding diatheses that account for most of the congenital coagulation disorders. Hemophilia A, the more common of the two, occurs in 1 in 10,000 male births and is caused by a deficiency of factor VIII, which is a large, 265-kd single-chain protein. Hemophilia B has an incidence of 1 per 25,000 male births and is characterized by a deficiency of factor IX, a single-chain 55-kd protein. Both factors VIII and IX are normally synthesized in the liver. Hemophilia A and hemophilia B are clinically indistinguishable. The phenotype in individual patients varies, depending on the percentage activity of the deficient factor. Clinical manifestations range from episodes of infrequent bleeding, usually associated with trauma, to frequent, severe bleeding episodes unassociated with any stressor. Current therapy for patients with hemophilia is replacement with exogenous clotting factors.

Although the liver is responsible for clotting factor production in the normal person, any tissue capable of secreting factors VIII and IX into the circulation can potentially be targeted for corrective gene transfer. In animal models, gene transfer to both the liver and the skeletal muscle has been successful in mediating long-term correction of hemophilia A and hemophilia B (43,44,182, 183). One phase I clinical trial is studying the safety of peritoneal implantation of autologous fibroblasts transfected with plasmid DNA encoding factor VIII in patients with severe hemophilia A.

Duchenne's Muscular Dystrophy

Duchenne's muscular dystrophy (DMD) is the type of muscular dystrophy that has been most intensively studied for gene therapy. DMD is an X-linked disorder caused by mutations in the 427-kd dystrophin protein. DMD is characterized by the progressive destruction of most skeletal muscles, and most patients with DMD are unable to walk by 12 years of age and die in the second or third decade of life from respiratory failure. Gene therapeutic approaches to treatment of muscular dystrophy have been hindered by poor transduction of terminally differentiated muscle cells by most gene therapy vectors and by the 13.9-kb size of the dystrophin cDNA transcript. Most of the approaches used in mouse models thus far have used a truncated dystrophin cDNA transcript that can mediate partial correction of the DMD phenotype. The development of gutless adenoviral vectors with a large transgene capacity has enabled expression of the entire dystrophin protein in mouse models. Treated animals have, however, generated an immune response to the allogenic dystrophin protein (184). This has led to the investigation of other, less antigenic proteins such as utrophin, a close dystrophin analogue that might be transduced into muscle cells to mitigate the DMD phenotype (185). There are plans to initiate a clinical trial for DMD using a gutless adenovirus vector capable of expressing full-length dystrophin.

Familial Hypercholesterolemia

Familial hypercholesterolemia is an autosomal dominant disorder caused by a variety of mutations in the gene for the LDL receptor. Approximately 1 in 500 people in the United States is heterozygous for a LDL receptor mutation. FH heterozygotes have an elevated plasma cholesterol, manifested by premature coronary artery disease and xanthomas, and constitute approximately 5% of all patients younger than 45 years of age who sustain a myocardial infarction. By 60 years of age, approximately 85% have had a myocardial infarction. FH homozygotes have extremely high elevations of plasma cholesterol and experience life-threatening coronary artery disease in childhood. The Watanabe heritable hyperlipidemic (WHHL) rabbit has been used as an animal model for FH. The WHHL rabbit bears nonfunctional LDL receptors, resulting in accelerated atherosclerosis and premature cardiovascular death (186).

Adenoviral and retroviral vectors have both been investigated for use in gene transfer of the LDL receptor gene to hepatocytes. Although adenoviral vectors have the ability to infect quiescent hepatocytes in vivo, transient expression of the LDL receptor due to leaky viral protein expression and subsequent immune-mediated elimination has limited their utility. Gutless adenoviral vectors demonstrate long-term expression and exhibit less toxicity than first-generation adenoviral vectors, but they have not been studied for LDL receptor gene delivery. Because treatment of FH requires long-term, stable expression of the LDL receptor, research efforts have largely focused on the use of retroviral vectors. Investigation of retroviral transfer of the LDL receptor has as its major challenge the transduction of a cell population that is in a quiescent state. Initial animal models used a strategy of ex vivo hepatocyte culture to induce cell division and render the hepatocytes susceptible to retroviral transduction (187). Stimulation of hepatic regeneration by partial hepatectomy and thymidine kinase/ganciclovir treatment has been used to improve in vivo retroviral gene transfer to the liver (188).

There has been one gene therapy trial for ex vivo treatment of homozygous FH. Hepatocytes were first harvested by partial hepatectomy and cultured ex vivo. After retroviral transduction of the wild-type LDL receptor, the hepatocytes were then infused through an indwelling catheter in the portal vein. Biopsies taken 4 months posttreatment demonstrated evidence of gene-corrected hepatocytes in all patients, although the total cholesterol reduction varied widely from 1% to 20%.

A novel approach under development uses a secretable LDL receptor–transferrin fusion protein that binds to LDL through the amino terminus and provides for receptor-mediated uptake of the lipid–protein complex using the transferrin carboxy-terminal domain (189). This strategy bypasses the LDL receptor for LDL delivery by using hepatic transferrin receptors. Although experiments have been performed only with the protein product and not the vector construct, the strategy of targeting compounds for uptake by heterologous receptors may prove useful in a variety of contexts.

THE FUTURE OF GENE THERAPY AND THE SURGEON

Since the initial trial of gene-based therapy was conducted, surgeons have been intimately involved in the initiation and development of many gene therapy protocols. In the future, it is likely that surgical applications of gene therapy will be developed as some of the first applications of this type of therapy. For instance, it may not be long before cardiothoracic surgeons are asked to administer angiogenic genes in cardioplegia solutions to increase blood vessel development and growth in patients with coronary artery disease. Vascular surgeons may soon be introducing genes to inhibit vascular smooth muscle to decrease postoperative stenoses in patients with severe peripheral vascular disease. Orthopedic surgeons might introduce osteogenic genes into patients with bony defects or fractures to increase bone growth and healing. Surgical oncologists likely will be injecting a variety of genes directly into tumors or introducing them into local circulations in attempts to cure cancer. From these examples, it is clear that surgeons in the future need to continue to play an active role in the development of gene therapy applications. For surgeons, gene therapy represents a unique and powerful tool that can be used to increase the success of surgical interventions, thereby substantially improving the lives of surgical patients.

REFERENCES

1. Ding L, Lu S, Munshi NC. In vitro packaging of an infectious recombinant adeno-associated virus 2. *Gene Ther* 1997;4:1167–1172.
2. Zhou X, Muzyczka N. In vitro packaging of adeno-associated virus DNA. *J Virol* 1998;72:3241–3247.
3. van Zeijl M, Johann SV, Closs E, et al. A human amphotropic retrovirus receptor is a second member of the gibbon ape leukemia virus receptor family. *Proc Natl Acad Sci USA* 1994;91:1168–1172.
4. DePolo NJ, Harkleroad CE, Bodner M, et al. The resistance of retroviral vectors produced from human cells to serum inactivation in vivo and in vitro is primate species dependent. *J Virol* 1999;73:6708–6714.
5. Buckrinsky MI, Haggerty S, Dempsey MP, et al. A nuclear localization signal within HIV-1 matrix protein that governs infection of non-dividing cells. *Nature* 1993;14:666–669.
6. Dull T, Zufferey R, Kelly M, et al. A third-generation lentivirus vector with a conditional packaging system. *J Virol* 1998;72:8463–8471.
7. Naldini L, Blomer U, Gallay P, et al. In vivo gene delivery and stable transduction of nondividing cells by a lentiviral vector. *Science* 1996;272:263–267.
8. Zufferey R, Nagy D, Mandel RJ, et al. Multiply attenuated lentiviral vector achieves efficient gene delivery in vivo. *Nat Biotechnol* 1997;15:871–875.
9. Case SS, Price MA, Jordan CT, et al. Stable transduction of quiescent CD34+CD38– human hematopoietic cells by HIV-1 based lentiviral vectors. *Proc Natl Acad Sci USA* 1999;96:2988–2993.
10. Poeschla EM, Wong-Staal F, Looney DJ. Efficient transduction of nondividing human cells by feline immunodeficiency virus lentiviral vectors. *Nat Med* 1998;4:354–357.
11. Bergelson JM, Cunningham JA, Droguett G, et al. Isolation of a common receptor for coxsackie B viruses and adenoviruses 2 and 5. *Science* 1997;275:1320–1323.
12. Hong SS, Karayan L, Tournier J, et al. Adenovirus type 5 fiber knob binds to MHC class I a2 domain at the surface of human epithelial and B lymphoblastoid cells. *EMBO J* 1997;16:2294–2306.
13. Freimuth P. A human cell line selected for resistance to adenovirus infection has reduced levels of the virus receptor. *J Virol* 1996;70:4081–4085.
14. Dmitriev I, Krasnykh V, Miller C, et al. An adenovirus vector with genetically modified fibers demonstrates expanded tropism via utilization of a coxsackievirus and adenovirus receptor-independent cell entry mechanism. *J Virol* 1998;72:9706–9713.
15. Stevenson SC, Rollence M, Marshall-Neff J, et al. Selective targeting of human cells by a chimeric adenovirus containing a modified fiber protein. *J Virol* 1997;71:4782–4790.
16. Douglas JT, Rogers BE, Rosenfeld ME, et al. Targeted gene delivery by tropism-modified adenoviral vectors. *Nat Biotechnol* 1996;14:1574–1578.
17. Goldman CK, Rogers BE, Douglas JT, et al. Targeted gene delivery to Kaposi's sarcoma cells via the fibroblast growth factor receptor. *Cancer Res* 1997;57:1447–1451.

18. Wickham TJ, Lee GM, Titus JA, et al. Targeted adenovirus-mediated gene delivery to T cells via CD3. *J Virol* 1997;71:7663–7669.

19. Fisher KJ, Choi H, Burda J, et al. Recombinant adenovirus deleted of all viral genes for gene therapy of cystic fibrosis. *Virology* 1996;217:11–22.

20. Kochanek S, Clemens PR, Mitani K, et al. A new adenoviral vector: replacement of all viral coding sequences with 28 kb of DNA independently expressing both full-length dystrophin and beta-galactosidase. *Proc Natl Acad Sci USA* 1996;93:5731–5736.

21. Kumar-Singh R, Farber DB. Encapsulated adenovirus mini-chromosome-mediated delivery of genes to the retina: application to the rescue of photoreceptor generation. *Hum Mol Genet* 1998;7:1893–1900.

22. Parks RJ, Chen L, Anton M, et al. A helper-dependent adenovirus vector system: removal of helper virus by Cre-mediated excision of the viral packaging signal. *Proc Natl Acad Sci USA* 1996;93:13565–13570.

23. Schiedner G, Morral N, Parks RJ, et al. Genomic DNA transfer with a high-capacity adenovirus vector results in improved in vivo gene expression and decreased toxicity. *Nat Genet* 1998;18:180–183.

24. Floyd SS Jr, Clemens PR, Ontell MR, et al. Ex vivo gene transfer using adenovirus-mediated full length dystrophin delivery to dystrophic muscles. *Gene Ther* 1998;5:19–30.

25. Morsy MA, Gu M, Motzel S, et al. An adenoviral vector deleted for all viral coding sequences results in enhanced safety and extended expression of a leptin transgene. *Proc Natl Acad Sci USA* 1998;95:7866–7871.

26. Chen HH, Mack LM, Kelly R, et al. Persistence in muscle of an adenoviral vector that lacks all viral genes. *Proc Natl Acad Sci USA* 1997;94:1645–1650.

27. Tripathy SK, Black HB, Goldwasser E, et al. Immune responses to transgene-encoded proteins limit the stability of gene expression after injection of replication-defective adenovirus vectors. *Nat Med* 1996;2:545–550.

28. Jooss K, Yang Y, Fisher KJ, et al. Transduction of dendritic cells by DNA viral vectors directs the immune response to transgene products in muscle fibers. *J Virol* 1998;72:4212–4223.

29. Kotin RM, Siniscalco M, Samulski RJ, et al. Site-specific integration by adeno-associated virus. *Proc Natl Acad Sci USA* 1990;87:2211–2215.

30. Bartlett JS, Kleinschmidt J, Boucher RC, et al. Targeted adeno-associated virus vector transduction of nonpermissive cells mediated by a bispecific F(ab'gamma)2 antibody. *Nat Biotechnol* 1999;17:181–186.

31. Summerford C, Samulski RJ. Membrane-associated heparan sulfate proteoglycan is a receptor for adeno-associated virus type 2 virions. *J Virol* 1998;72:1438–1445.

32. Kearns WG, Afione SA, Fulmer SB, et al. Recombinant adeno-associated virus (AAV-CFTR) vectors do no integrate in a site specific fashion in an immortalized epithelial cell line. *Gene Ther* 1996;3:748–755.

33. Dudus L, Anand V, Acland GM, et al. Persistent transgene product in retina, optic nerve, and brain after intraocular injection of rAAV. *Vision Res* 1999;39:2545–2553.

34. Fisher KJ, Jooss K, Alston J, et al. Recombinant adeno-associated virus for muscle directed gene therapy. *Nat Med* 1997;3:306–312.

35. Fisher-Adams G, Wong KK Jr, Podsakoff G, et al. Integration of adeno-associated virus vectors in CD34+ human hematopoietic progenitor cells after transduction. *Blood* 1996;88:492–504.

36. Haberman RP, McCown TJ, Samulski RJ. Inducible long-term expression in brain with adeno-associated virus gene transfer. *Gene Ther* 1998;5:1604–1611.

37. Kaplitt MG, Leone P, Samulski RJ, et al. Long-term gene expression and phenotypic correction using adeno-associated virus vectors in the mammalian brain. *Nat Genet* 1994;8:148–154.

38. Kessler PD, Podsakoff GM, Chen X, et al. Gene delivery to skeletal muscle results in sustained expression and systemic delivery of a therapeutic protein. *Proc Natl Acad Sci USA* 1996;93:14082–14087.

39. Osborne WR, Ramesh N, Lau S, et al. Gene therapy for long-term expression of erythropoietin in rats. *Proc Natl Acad Sci USA* 1995;92:8055–8058.

40. Snyder RO, Miao CH, Patijn GA, et al. Persistent and therapeutic concentrations of human factor IX in mice after hepatic gene transfer of recombinant AAV vectors. *Nat Genet* 1997;16:270–276.

41. Song S, Morgan M, Ellis T, et al. Sustained secretion of human alpha-1-antitrypsin from murine muscle transduced with adeno-associated virus vectors. *Proc Natl Acad Sci USA* 1998;95:14384–14388.

42. Xiao X, Li J, Samulski RJ. Efficient long-term gene transfer into muscle tissue of immunocompetent mice by adeno-associated virus vector. *J Virol* 1996;70:8098–8108.

43. Zhang L, Wang D, Fischer H, et al. Efficient expression of CFTR function with adeno-associated virus vectors that carry shortened CFTR genes. *Proc Natl Acad Sci USA* 1998;95:10158–10163.

44. Herzog RW, Hagstrom JN, Kung SH, et al. Stable gene transfer and expression of human blood coagulation factor IX after intramuscular injection of recombinant adeno-associated virus. *Proc Natl Acad Sci USA* 1997;94:5804–5809.

45. Wang L, Takabe K, Bidlingmaier SM, et al. Sustained correction of bleeding disorder in hemophilia B mice by gene therapy. *Proc Natl Acad Sci USA* 1999;96:3906–3910.

46. Bohl D, Naffakh N, Heard JM. Long-term control of erythropoietin secretion by doxycycline in mice transplanted with engineered primary myoblasts. *Nat Med* 1997;3:299–305.

47. Murphy JE, Zhou S, Giese K, et al. Long-term correction of obesity and diabetes in genetically obese mice by a single intramuscular injection of recombinant adeno-associated virus encoding mouse leptin. *Proc Natl Acad Sci USA* 1997;94:13921–13926.

48. Rivera VM, Ye X, Courage NL, et al. Long-term regulated expression of growth hormone in mice after intramuscular gene transfer. *Proc Natl Acad Sci USA* 1999;96:8657–8662.

49. Mineta T, Rabkin SD, Yazaki T, et al. Attenuated multi-mutated herpes simplex virus-1 for the treatment of malignant gliomas. *Nat Med* 1995;1:938–943.

50. Feng M, Jackson WH Jr, Goldman CK, et al. Stable in vivo gene transduction via a novel adenoviral/retroviral chimeric vector. *Nat Biotechnol* 1997;15:866–870.

51. Fisher KJ, Kelley WM, Burda JF, et al. A novel adenovirus-adeno-associated virus hybrid vector that displays efficient rescue and delivery of the AAV genome. *Hum Gene Ther* 1996;7:2079–2087.

52. Holzer GW, Mayrhofer JA, Gritschenberger W, et al. Poxviral/retroviral chimeric vectors allow cytoplasmic production of transducing defective retroviral particles. *Virology* 1999;253:107–114.

53. Johnston KM, Jacoby D, Pechan PA, et al. HSVAAV hybrid amplicon vectors extend transgene expression in human glioma cells. *Hum Gene Ther* 1997;8:359–370.

54. Recchia A, Parks RJ, Lamartina S, et al. Site-specific integration mediated by a hybrid adenovirus-adeno-associated virus vector. *Proc Natl Acad Sci USA* 1999;96:2615–2620.

55. Liu Y, Liggitt D, Zhong W, et al. Cationic liposome-mediated intravenous gene delivery. *J Biol Chem* 1995;270:24864–24870.

56. Saeki Y, Matsumoto N, Nakano Y, et al. Development and characterization of cationic liposomes conjugated with HVJ (Sendai virus): reciprocal effect of cationic lipid for in vitro and in vivo gene transfer. *Hum Gene Ther* 1997;8:2133–2141.

57. Lee RJ, Huang L. Folate-targeted, anionic liposome-entrapped polylysine-condensed DNA for tumor cell-specific gene transfer. *J Biol Chem* 1996;271:8481–8487.

58. Felgner JH, Kumar R, Sridhar CN, et al. Enhanced gene delivery and mechanism studies with a novel series of cationic lipid formulations. *J Biol Chem* 1994;269:2550–2561.

59. Mounkes LC, Zhong W, Cipres-Palacin G, et al. Proteoglycans mediate cationic liposome-DNA complex-based gene delivery in vitro and in vivo. *J Biol Chem* 1998;273:26164–26170.

60. Lasic DD, Martin FJ, Gabizon A, et al. Sterically stabilized liposomes: a hypothesis on the molecular origin of the extended circulation times. *Biochim Biophys Acta* 1991;1070:187–192.

61. Bradley AJ, Devine DV, Ansell SM, et al. Inhibition of liposome-induced complement activation by incorporated poly(ethylene glycol)-lipids. *Arch Biochem Biophys* 1998;357:185–194.

62. Bielinksa AU, Kukowska-Latallo JF, Johnson J, et al. Regulation of in vitro gene expression using antisense oligonucleotides or antisense expression plasmids transfected using starburst PAMAM dendrimers. *Nucleic Acids Res* 1996;24:2176–2182.

63. Kukowska-Latallo JF, Bielinska AU, Johnson J, et al. Efficient transfer of genetic material into mammalian cells using starburst polyamidoamine dendrimers. *Proc Natl Acad Sci USA* 1996;92:4897.

64. Qin L, Pahud DR, Ding Y, et al. Efficient transfer of genes into murine cardiac grafts by starburst polyamidoamine dendrimers. *Hum Gene Ther* 1998;9:553.

65. Rizzuto G, Cappelletti M, Maione D, et al. Efficient and regulated erythropoietin production by naked DNA injection and muscle electroporation. *Proc Natl Acad Sci USA* 1999; 96:6417–6422.

66. Shi Z, Curiel DT, Tang D. DNA-based non-invasive vaccination onto the skin. *Vaccine* 1999;17:2136–2141.

67. Mancini M, Hadchouel M, Tiollais P, et al. Regulation of hepatitis virus mRNA expression in hepatitis B surface antigen transgenic mouse model by IFN-gamma-secreting T cells after DNA-based immunization. *J Immunol* 1998;161:5564–5570.

68. Ulmer JB, Deck RR, DeWitt CM, et al. Expression of a viral protein by muscle cells in vivo induces protective cell-mediated immunity. *Vaccine* 1997;15:839–841.

69. Doe B, Selby M, Barnett S, et al. Induction of cytotoxic T lymphocytes by intramuscular immunization with plasmid DNA is facilitated by bone marrow derived cells. *Proc Natl Acad Sci USA* 1996;6:8578–8583.

70. Chen J, Gamou S, Takayanagi A, et al. Receptor-mediated gene delivery using the Fab fragments of anti-epidermal growth factor receptor antibodies: improved immunogene approach. *Cancer Gene Ther* 1998;5:357–364.

71. Ferkol T, Perales JC, Eckman E, et al. Gene transfer into the airway epithelium of animals by targeting the polymeric immunoglobulin receptor. *J Clin Invest* 1995;95:493–502.

72. Ferkol T, Perales JC, Mularo F, et al. Receptor-mediated gene transfer into macrophages. *Proc Natl Acad Sci USA* 1996;93: 101–105.

73. Martinez-Fong D, Navarro-Quiroga I, Ochoa I, et al. Neurotensin-SPDP-poly-L-lysine conjugate: a nonviral vector for targeted gene delivery to neural cells. *Brain Res Mol Brain Res* 1999;69:249–262.

74. Mulders P, Pang S, Dannull J, et al. Highly efficient and consistent gene transfer into dendritic cells utilizing a combination of ultraviolet-irradiated adenovirus and poly(L-lysine) conjugates. *Cancer Res* 1998;58:956–961.

75. Sosnowski BA, Gonzalez AM, Chandler LA, et al. Targeting DNA to cells with fibroblast growth factor (FGF2). *J Biol Chem* 1996;271:33647–33653.

76. Wu GY, Wu CH. Receptor-mediated in vitro gene transformation by a soluble DNA carrier system. *J Biol Chem* 1987; 262:4429–4432.

77. Perales JC, Ferkol T, Beegen H, et al. Gene transfer in vivo: sustained expression and regulation of genes introduced into the liver by receptor-targeted uptake. *Proc Natl Acad Sci USA* 1994;91:4086–4090.

78. Curiel DT, Agarwal S, Wagner E, et al. Adenovirus enhancement of transferrin-polylysine-mediated gene delivery. *Proc Natl Acad Sci USA* 1991;88:8850–8854.

79. Gottschalk S, Cristiano RJ, Smith LC, et al. Folate receptor mediated DNA delivery into tumor cells: protosomal disruption results in enhanced gene expression. *Gene Ther* 1994;1:185–191.

80. Seth P, Fitzgerald D, Ginsberg H, et al. Evidence that the penton base of adenovirus is involved in potentiation of toxicity of *Pseudomonas* exotoxin conjugated to epidermal growth factor. *Mol Cell Biol* 1984;4:1528–1533.

81. Cotten M, Wagner E, Zatloukal K, et al. High-efficiency receptor-mediated delivery of small and large (48 kilobase) gene constructs using the endosome-disruption activity of defective or chemically inactivated adenovirus particles. *Proc Natl Acad Sci USA* 1992;89:6094–6098.

82. Kasid A, Morecki S, Aebersold P, et al. Human gene transfer: characterization of human tumor-infiltrating lymphocytes as vehicles for retroviral-mediated gene transfer in man. *Proc Natl Acad Sci USA* 1990;87:473–477.

83. Brenner MK, Rill DR, Moen RC, et al. Gene-marking to trace origin of relapse after autologous bone-marrow transplantation. *Lancet* 1993;341:85–86.

84. Deisseroth AB, Zu Z, Claxton D, et al. Genetic marking shows that PH+ cells present in autologous transplants of chronic myelogenous leukemia (CML) contribute to relapse after autologous bone marrow in CML. *Blood* 1994;83:3068–3076.

85. Rill DR, Santana VM, Roberts WM, et al. Direct demonstration that autologous bone marrow transplantation for solid tumors can return a multiplicity of tumorigenic cells. *Blood* 1994;84:380–383.

86. Elion G, Furman P, Fyfe JA, et al. Selectivity of action of an antiherpetic agent 9-(2-hydroxyethoxymethyl) guanine. *Proc Natl Acad Sci USA* 1977;74:5716–5720.

87. Freeman SM, Abboud CN, Whartenby KA, et al. The "bystander effect": tumor regression when a fraction of the tumor mass is genetically modified. *Cancer Res* 1993;53:5274–5283.

88. Fick J, Barker FG Jr, Dazin P, et al. The extent of heterocellular communication mediated by gap junctions is predictive of bystander tumor cytotoxicity in vitro. *Proc Natl Acad Sci USA* 1995;92:11071–11075.

89. Bonini C, Ferrari G, Verzeletti S, et al. HSV-TK gene transfer into donor lymphocytes for control of allogeneic graft-versus-leukemia. *Science* 1997;276:1719–1724.

90. Huber BE, Austin EA, Good SS, et al. In vivo antitumor activity of 5-fluorocytosine on human colorectal carcinoma cells genetically modified to express cytosine deaminase. *Cancer Res* 1993;53:4619–4626.

91. Trinh QT, Austin EA, Murray DM, et al. Enzyme/prodrug gene therapy: comparison of cytosine deaminase/5-fluorocytosine versus thymidine kinase/ganciclovir enzyme/prodrug systems in a human colorectal carcinoma cell line. *Cancer Res* 1995;55:4808–4812.

92. Wei MX, Tamiya T, Chase M, et al. Experimental tumor therapy in mice using the cyclophosphamide-activating cytochrome P450 2B1 gene. *Hum Gene Ther* 1994;5:969–978.

93. Chen L, Yu LJ, Waxman DJ. Potentiation of cytochrome P450/cyclophosphamide-based cancer gene therapy by coexpression of the P450 reductase gene. *Cancer Res* 1997;57: 4830–4837.

94. Rogulski KR, Zhang K, Kolozsvary A, et al. Pronounced antitumor effects and tumor radiosensitization of double suicide gene therapy. *Clin Cancer Res* 1997;3:2081–2088.

95. Hamstra DA, Rice DJ, Fahmy S, et al. Enzyme/prodrug therapy for head and neck cancer using a catalytically superior cytosine deaminase. *Hum Gene Ther* 1999;10:1993–2003.

96. Greenblatt MS, Bennett WP, Hollstein M, et al. Mutations in the p53 tumor suppressor gene: clues to cancer etiology and molecular pathogenesis. *Cancer Res* 1994;54:4855–4878.

97. Wang XW, Harris CC. TP53 tumor suppressor gene: clues to molecular carcinogenesis and cancer therapy. *Cancer Surv* 1996;28:169–196.

98. Forrester K, Lupold SE, Ott VL, et al. Effects of p53 mutants on wild-type p53-mediated transactivation are cell type dependent. *Oncogene* 1995;10:2103–2111.

99. Putzer BM, Bramson JL, Addison CL, et al. Combination therapy with interleukin-2 and wild-type p53 expressed by adenoviral vectors potentiates tumor regression in a murine model of breast cancer. *Hum Gene Ther* 1998;9:707–718.

100. Schreiber M, Muller WJ, Singh G, et al. Comparison of the effectiveness of adenovirus vectors expressing cyclin kinase inhibitors p16INK4A, p18INK4C, p19INK4D, P21WAF1CIP1, and p27KIP1 in inducing cell cycle arrest, apoptosis, and inhibition of tumorigenicity. *Oncogene* 1999;18:16630–16676.

101. Chang MY, Won SJ, Liu HS. A ribozyme specifically suppresses transformation and tumorigenicity of Ha-ras-oncogene-transformed NIH3T3 cell lines. *J Cancer Res Clin Oncol* 1997;123:91–99.

102. Dorai T, Goluboff ET, Olsson CA, et al. Development of a hammerhead ribozyme against BCL-2: II. ribozyme treatment sensitizes hormone-resistant prostate cancer cells to apoptotic agents. *Anticancer Res* 1997;17:3307–3312.

103. Funato T, Ishii T, Kanbe M, et al. Reversal of cisplatin resistance in vivo by an anti-fos ribozyme. *In Vivo* 1997;11: 217–220.

104. Juhl H, Downing SG, Wellstein A, et al. HER-2neu is rate-limiting for ovarian cancer growth: conditional depletion of HER-2neu by ribozyme targeting. *J Biol Chem* 1997;272: 29482–29486.

105. Jones JT, Sullenger BA. Evaluating and enhancing ribozyme reaction efficiency in mammalian cells. *Nat Biotechnol* 1997;15:902–905.

106. Clarke MF, Apel IJ, Benedict MA, et al. A recombinant bcl-xs adenovirus selectively induces apoptosis in cancer cells but not in normal bone marrow cells. *Proc Natl Acad Sci USA* 1995;92:11024–11028.

107. Carew JF, Kooby DA, Halterman MW, et al. Selective infection and cytolysis of human head and neck squamous cell carcinoma with sparing of normal mucosa by a cytotoxic herpes simplex virus type 1. *Hum Gene Ther* 1999;10:1599–1606.

108. Kooby DA, Carew JF, Halterman MW, et al. Oncolytic viral therapy for human colorectal cancer and liver metastases using a multi-mutated herpes simplex virus type-1. *FASEB J* 1999;13:1325–1334.

109. Toda M, Rabkin SD, Martuza RL. Treatment of human breast cancer in a brain metastatic model by G207, a replication-competent multimutated herpes simplex virus 1. *Hum Gene Ther* 1998;9:2177–2185.

110. Toda M, Rabkin SD, Kojima H, et al. Herpes simplex virus as an in situ cancer vaccine for the induction of specific anti-tumor immunity. *Hum Gene Ther* 1999;10:385–393.

111. Yazaki T, Manz HJ, Rabkin SD, et al. Treatment of human malignant meningiomas by G207, a replication-competent multimutated herpes simplex virus 1. *Cancer Res* 1995;55:4752–4756.

112. Rodriguez R, Schuur ER, Lim HY, et al. Prostate attenuated replication competent adenovirus (ARCA) CN706: a selective cytotoxic for prostate-specific antigen-positive prostate cancer cells. *Cancer Res* 1997;57:2559–2563.

113. Ke LD, Fueyo J, Chen X, et al. A novel approach to glioma gene therapy: down-regulation of the vascular endothelial growth factor in glioma cells using ribozymes. *Int J Oncol* 1998;12:1391–1396.

114. Im SA, Gomez-Manzano C, Fueyo J, et al. Antiangiogenesis treatment for gliomas: transfer of antisense-vascular endothelial growth factor inhibits tumor growth in vivo. *Cancer Res* 1999;59:895–900.

115. Kong HL, Hecht D, Song W, et al. Regional suppression of tumor growth by in vivo transfer of a cDNA encoding a secreted form of the extracellular domain of the flt-1 vascular endothelial growth factor receptor. *Hum Gene Ther* 1998;9:823–833.

116. Lin P, Buxton JA, Acheson A, et al. Antiangiogenic gene therapy targeting the endothelium-specific receptor tyrosine kinase Tie2. *Proc Natl Acad Sci USA* 1998;95:8829–8834.

117. O'Reilly MS, Holmgren L, Shing Y, et al. Angiostatin: a novel angiogenesis inhibitor that mediates the suppression of metastases by a Lewis lung carcinoma. *Cell* 1994;79:315–328.

118. O'Reilly MS, Holmgren L, Chen C, et al. Angiostatin induces and sustains dormancy of human primary tumors in mice. *Nat Med* 1996;2:689–692.

119. O'Reilly MS, Boehm T, Shing Y, et al. Endostatin: an endogenous inhibitor of angiogenesis and tumor growth. *Cell* 1997;88:277–285.

120. Chen QR, Kumar D, Stass SA, et al. Liposomes complexed to plasmids encoding angiostatin and endostatin inhibit breast cancer in nude mice. *Cancer Res* 1999;59:3308–3312.

121. Blezinger P, Wang J, Gondo M, et al. Systemic inhibition of tumor growth and tumor metastases by intramuscular administration of the endostatin gene. *Nat Biotechnol* 1999;17:343–348.

122. Gimmi CD, Freeman GJ, Gribben JG, et al. B-cell surface antigen B7 provides a costimulatory signal that induces T cells to proliferate and secrete IL-2. *Proc Natl Acad Sci USA* 1991;88:6575–6579.

123. Gimmi CD, Freeeman GJ, Cribben JG, et al. Human T cell clonal anergy is induced by antigen presentation in the absence of B7 costimulation. *Proc Natl Acad Sci USA* 1993;90:6586–6590.

124. Hodge JW, Abrams S, Schlom J, et al. Induction of antitumor immunity by recombinant vaccinia viruses expressing B7-1 or B7-2 costimulatory molecules. *Cancer Res* 1994;54:5552–5555.

125. Baskar S, Ostrand-Rosenberg S, Nabavi N, et al. Constitutive expression of B7 restores immunogenicity of tumor cells expressing truncated major histocompatibility complex class II molecules. *Proc Natl Acad Sci USA* 1993;90:5687–5690.

126. Putzer BM, Hitt M, Muller WJ, et al. Interleukin 12 and B7-1 costimulatory molecule expressed by an adenovirus vector act synergistically to facilitate tumor regression. *Proc Natl Acad Sci USA* 1997;94:10889–10894.

127. Dranoff G, Jaffee E, Lazenby A, et al. Vaccination with irradiated tumor cells engineered to secrete murine granulocyte-macrophage colony-stimulating factor stimulates potent, specific, and long-lasting anti-tumor immunity. *Proc Natl Acad Sci USA* 1993;90:3539–3543.

128. Wakimoto H, Abe J, Tsunoda R, et al. Intensified antitumor immunity by a cancer vaccine that produces granulocyte-macrophage colony-stimulating factor plus interleukin 4. *Cancer Res* 1996;56:1828–1833.

129. Boczkowski D, Nair SK, Snyder D, et al. Dendritic cells pulsed with RNA are potent antigen-presenting cells in vitro and in vivo. *J Exp Med* 1996;184:465–472.

130. Fields RC, Shimizu K, Mulé JJ. Murine dendritic cells pulsed with whole tumor lysates mediate potent antitumor immune responses in vitro and in vivo. *Proc Natl Acad Sci USA* 1998;95:9482–9487.

131. Kaplan JM, Yu Q, Piraino ST, et al. Induction of antitumor immunity with dendritic cells transduced with adenovirus vector-encoding endogenous tumor-associated antigens. *J Immunol* 1999;163:699–707.

132. Ribas A, Butterfield LH, McBride WH, et al. Genetic immunization for the melanoma antigen MART-1/melan-A using recombinant adenovirus-transduced murine dendritic cells. *Cancer Res* 1997;57:2865–2869.

133. Shimizu K, Fields RC, Giedlin M, et al. Systemic administration of interleukin 2 enhances the therapeutic efficacy of dendritic cell-based tumor vaccines. *Proc Natl Acad Sci USA* 1999;96:2268–2273.

134. Kantor J, Irvine K, Abrams S, et al. Antitumor activity and immune responses induced by a recombinant carcinoembryonic antigen–vaccinia virus vaccine. *J Natl Cancer Inst* 1992;84:1084–1091.

135. Wei C, Storozynsky E, McAdam AJ, et al. Expression of human prostate-specific antigen (PSA) in a mouse tumor cell line reduces tumorigenicity and elicits PSA-specific cytotoxic T lymphocytes. *Cancer Immunol Immunother* 1996;42:362–368.

136. McLaughlin JP, Schlom J, Kantor JA, et al. Improved immunotherapy of a recombinant carcinoembryonic antigen vaccinia vaccine when given in combination with interleukin-2. *Cancer Res* 1996;56:2361–2367.

137. Plautz GE, Yang ZY, Wu BY, et al. Immunotherapy of malignancy by in vivo gene transfer into tumors. *Proc Natl Acad Sci USA* 1993;90:4645–4649.

138. DeBruyne LA, Chang AE, Cameron MJ, et al. Direct transfer of a foreign MHC gene into human melanoma alters T cell receptor V-beta usage by tumor infiltrating lymphocytes. *Cancer Immunol Immunother* 1996;43:49–58.

139. Sorrentino BP, Brandt SJ, Bodine D, et al. Selection of drug-resistant bone marrow cells in vivo after retroviral transfer of human MDR1. *Science* 1992;257:99–103.

140. Allay JA, Dumenco LL, Koc ON, et al. Retroviral transduction and expression of the human alkyltransferase cDNA provides nitrosurea resistance to hematopoietic cells. *Blood* 1995;85:3342–3351.

141. Hwu P. Gene therapy using lymphocyte modification. In: Rosenberg SA, ed. *Principles and practice of the biologic therapy of cancer*, 3rd ed. Philadelphia: Lippincott Williams & Wilkins, 2000:759–769.

142. Tsurumi Y, Takeshita S, Chen D, et al. Direct intramuscular gene transfer of naked DNA encoding vascular endothelial growth factor augments collateral development and tissue perfusion. *Circulation* 1996;94:3281–3290.

143. Lopez JJ, Laham RJ, Stamler A, et al. VEGF administration in chronic myocardial ischemia in pigs. *Cardiovasc Res* 1998;40:272–281.

144. Mack CA, Patel SR, Schwarz EZ, et al. Biologic bypass with the use of a adenovirus-mediated gene transfer of the complementary deoxyribonucleic acid for vascular endothelial growth factor 121 improves myocardial perfusion and function in the ischemic porcine heart. *J Thorac Cardiovasc Surg* 1998;115:168–177.

145. Losordo DW, Vale PR, Symes JF, et al. Gene therapy for myocardial angiogenesis: initial clinical results with direct myocardial injection of phVEGF165 as sole therapy for myocardial ischemia. *Circulation* 1998;98:2800–2804.

146. Rosengart TK, Lee LY, Patel SR, et al. Angiogenesis gene therapy: phase I assessment of intramyocardial administration of an adenovirus vector expressing VEGF121 cDNA to individuals with clinically significant coronary artery disease. *Circulation* 1999;100:468–474.

147. Unger EF, Banai S, Shou M, et al. Basic fibroblast growth factor enhances myocardial collateral flow in a canine model. *Am J Physiol* 1994;266:H1588–H1595.

148. Schumacher B, Pecher P, von Specht BU, et al. Induction of

neoangiogenesis in ischemic myocardium by human growth factors: first clinical results of a new treatment of coronary heart disease. *Circulation* 1998;97:645–650.

149. Bosch JL, Hunink MG. Meta-analysis of the results of percutaneous transluminal angioplasty and stent placement for aortoiliac occlusive disease. *Radiology* 1997;204:87–96.

150. Casterella PJ, Teirstein PS. Prevention of coronary restenosis. *Cardiol Rev* 1999;7:219–231.

151. Chang MW, Barr E, Lu MM, et al. Adenovirus-mediated overexpression of the cyclin/cyclin-dependent kinase inhibitor, p21 inhibits vascular smooth muscle cell proliferation and neointima formation in the rat carotid artery model of balloon angioplasty. *J Clin Invest* 1995;96:2260–2268.

152. Luo Z, Sata M, Nguyen T, et al. Adenovirus-mediated delivery of fas ligand inhibits intimal hyperplasia after balloon injury in immunologically primed animals. *Circulation* 1999;99:1776–1779.

153. Simari RD, San H, Rekhter M, et al. Regulation of cellular proliferation and intimal formation following balloon injury in atherosclerotic rabbit arteries. *J Clin Invest* 1996;98:225–235.

154. Smith RC, Wills KN, Antelman D, et al. Adenoviral constructs encoding phosphorylation-competent full-length and truncated forms of the human retinoblastoma protein inhibit myocyte proliferation and neointima formation. *Circulation* 1997;96:1899–1905.

155. Steg PG, Tahlil O, Aubailly N, et al. Reduction of restenosis after angioplasty in an atheromatous rabbit model by suicide gene therapy. *Circulation* 1997;96:408–411.

156. Ueno H, Yamamoto H, Ito S, et al. Adenovirus-mediated transfer of a dominant-negative H-ras suppresses neointimal formation in balloon-injured arteries in vivo. *Arterioscler Thromb Vasc Biol* 1997;17:898–904.

157. Asahara T, Bauters C, Pastore C, et al. Local delivery of vascular endothelial growth factor accelerates reendothelialization and attenuates intimal hyperplasia in balloon-injured rat carotid artery. *Circulation* 1995;91:2793–2801.

158. Isner JM, Walsh K, Rosenfield K, et al. Arterial gene therapy for restenosis. *Hum Gene Ther* 1996;7:989–1011.

159. Bonadio J, Smiley E, Patil P, et al. Localized, direct plasmid gene delivery in vivo: prolonged therapy results in reproducible tissue regeneration. *Nat Med* 1999;5:753–759.

160. During MJ, Naegele JR, O'Malley KL, et al. Long-term behavioral recovery in parkinsonian rats by an HSV vector expressing tyrosine hydroxylase. *Science* 1994;266:1399–1403.

161. Fan DS, Ogawa M, Fujimoto KI, et al. Behavioral recovery in 6-hydroxydopamine-lesioned rats by cotransduction of striatum with tyrosine hydroxylase and aromatic L-amino acid decarboxylase genes using two separate adeno-associated virus vectors. *Hum Gene Ther* 1998;9:2527–2535.

162. During MJ, Samulski RJ, Elsworth JD, et al. In vivo expression of therapeutic human genes for dopamine production in the caudates of MPTP-treated monkeys using an AAV vector. *Gene Ther* 1998;5:820–827.

163. Mandel RJ, Spratt SK, Snyder RO, et al. Midbrain injection of recombinant adeno-associated virus encoding rat glial cell line-derived neurotrophic factor protects nigral neurons in a progressive 6-hydroxydopamine-induced degeneration model of Parkinson's disease in rats. *Proc Natl Acad Sci USA* 1997;94:14083–14088.

164. Malim MH, Tiley LS, McCarn DF, et al. HIV-1 structural gene expression requires binding of the Rev trans-activator to its RNA target sequence. *Cell* 1990;60:675–683.

165. Galpin JE, Casciato DA, Richards SB. A phase I clinical trial to evaluate the safety and biological activity of HIV-IT (TAF) (HIV-1IIIBenv-transduced, autologous fibroblasts) in asymptomatic HIV-1 infected subjects. *Hum Gene Ther* 1994;5:997–1017.

166. Roberts MR, Qin L, Zhang D, et al. Targeting of human immunodeficiency virus-infected cells by CD8+ T lymphocytes armed with universal T cell receptors. *Blood* 1994;84:2878–2889.

167. Ranga U, Woffendin C, Verma S, et al. Enhanced T cell engraftment after retroviral delivery of an antiviral gene in HIV-infected individuals. *Proc Natl Acad Sci USA* 1998;95:1201–1206.

168. Kohn DB, Bauer G, Rice CR, et al. A clinical trial of retroviral-mediated transfer of a rev-responsive element decoy gene into CD34(+) cells from the bone marrow of human immunodeficiency virus-1 infected children. *Blood* 1999;94:368–371.

169. Marasco WA, Chen S, Richardson JH, et al. Intracellular antibodies against HIV-1 envelope protein for AIDS gene therapy. *Hum Gene Ther* 1998;9:1627–1642.

170. Duan L, Bagasra O, Laughlin MA, et al. Potent inhibition of human immunodeficiency virus type 1 replication by an intracellular anti-Rev single-chain antibody. *Proc Natl Acad Sci USA* 1994;91:5075–5079.

171. Wong-Staal F, Poeschla EM, Looney DJ. A controlled, phase 1 clinical trial to evaluate the safety and effects in HIV-1 infected humans of autologous lymphocytes transduced with a ribozyme that cleaves HIV-1 RNA. *Hum Gene Ther* 1998;9:2407–2425.

172. Yamada O, Yu M, Yee JK, et al. Intracellular immunization of human T cells with a hairpin ribozyme against human immunodeficiency virus type 1. *Gene Ther* 1994;1:38–45.

173. Song S, Morgan M, Ellis T, et al. Sustained secretion of human alpha-1-antitrypsin from murine muscle transduced with adeno-associated virus vectors. *Proc Natl Acad Sci USA* 1998;95:14384–14388.

174. Blaese RM, Culver KW, Miller D, et al. T-lymphocyte-directed gene therapy for ADA-SCID: initial trial results after 4 years. *Science* 1995;270:475–480.

175. Bordignon C, Notarangelo LD, Nobili N, et al. Gene therapy in peripheral blood lymphocytes and bone marrow for ADA-immunodeficient patients. *Science* 1995;270:470–475.

176. Dunbar C, Chang L, Mullen C, et al. Amendment to clinical research project. Project 90-C-195. April 1, 1993. Treatment of severe combined immunodeficiency disease (SCID) due to adenosine deaminase deficiency with autologous lymphocytes transduced with a human ADA gene. *Hum Gene Ther* 1999;10:477–488.

177. Kohn DB, Hershfield MS, Carbonaro D, et al. T lymphocytes with a normal ADA gene accumulate after transplantation of transduced autologous umbilical cord CD34+ cells in ADA-deficient SCID neonates. *Nat Med* 1998;4:775–780.

178. Crystal RG, McElvaney NG, Rosenfeld MA, et al. Administration of an adenovirus containing the human CFTR cDNA to the respiratory tract of individuals with cystic fibrosis. *Nat Genet* 1994;8:42–51.

179. Goldman MJ, Lee PS, Yang JS, et al. Lentiviral vectors for gene therapy of cystic fibrosis. *Hum Gene Ther* 1997;8:2261–2268.

180. Pickles RJ, McCarty D, Matsui H, et al. Limited entry of adenovirus vectors into well-differentiated airway epithelium is responsible for inefficient gene transfer. *J Virol* 1998;72:6014–6023.

181. Walters RW, Grunst T, Bergelson JM, et al. Basolateral localization of fiber receptors limits adenovirus infection from the apical surface of airway epithelia. *J Biol Chem* 1999;274:10219–10226.

182. Snyder RO, Miao C, Meuse L, et al. Correction of hemophilia B in canine and murine models using recombinant adeno-associated viral vectors. *Nat Med* 1999;5:64–70.

183. VandenDriessche T, Vanslembrouck V, Goovaerts I, et al. Long-term expression of human coagulation factor VIII and correction of hemophilia A after in vivo retroviral gene transfer in factor VIII-deficient mice. *Proc Natl Acad Sci USA* 1999;96:10379–10384.

184. Floyd SS Jr, Clemens PR, Ontell MR, et al. Ex vivo gene transfer using adenovirus-mediated full-length dystrophin delivery to dystrophic muscles. *Gene Ther* 1998;5:19–30.

185. Gilbert R, Nalbantoglu J, Petro BJ, et al. Adenovirus-mediated utrophin gene transfer mitigates the dystrophic phenotype of mdx mouse muscles. *Hum Gene Ther* 1999;20:1299–1310.

186. Watanabe Y. Serial inbreeding of rabbits with hereditary hyperlipidemia (WHHL-rabbit). *Atherosclerosis* 1980;36:261–268.

187. Chowdhury JR, Grossman M, Gupta S, et al. Long-term improvement of hypercholesterolemia after ex vivo gene therapy in LDLR-deficient rabbits. *Science* 1991;254:1802.

188. Pakkanen TM, Laitinen M, Hippelainen M, et al. Enhanced plasma cholesterol lowering effect of retrovirus-mediated LDL receptor gene transfer to WHHL rabbit liver after improved surgical technique and stimulation of hepatocyte proliferation by combined partial liver resection and thymidine kinase-ganciclovir treatment. *Gene Ther* 1999;6:34–41.

189. Parise F, Simone L, Antonietta M, et al. Construction and in vitro functional evaluation of a low-density lipoprotein receptor/transferrin fusion protein as a therapeutic tool for familial hypercholesterolemia. *Hum Gene Ther* 1999;10:1219–1228.

SURGERY: SCIENTIFIC PRINCIPLES AND PRACTICE, Third Edition, edited by
Lazar J. Greenfield, Michael W. Mulholland, Keith T. Oldham, Gerald B. Zelenock,
and Keith D. Lillemoe. Lippincott Williams & Wilkins Publishers, Philadelphia, © 2001.

CHAPTER 16

TRANSPLANTATION AND IMMUNOLOGY

JONATHAN S. BROMBERG, JOHN C. MAGEE, JEFFREY D. PUNCH,
ROBERT M. MERION, DARRELL A. CAMPBELL, JR.,
STEVEN RUDICH, RICHARD N. PIERSON III, LARRY R. KAISER,
ROBERT C. GORMAN, AND STEPHEN T. BARTLETT

Transplant Immunology

JONATHAN S. BROMBERG AND JOHN C. MAGEE

The major impediment to universal, long-term allograft function in transplant recipients is the host immune response. Various manifestations of host antidonor immune reactivity result in allograft dysfunction and loss. To prevent these adverse outcomes, systemic immunosuppression is required. Current immunosuppression, however, is not completely reliable in preventing or reversing rejection, and immunosuppression itself results in several undesirable complications. To control the events that occur during clinical organ allografting, it is important to understand the processes of antigen recognition, the effector mechanisms of immune reactivity, and the cellular and molecular interactions that control and regulate the fate of antigen.

INITIATION OF THE IMMUNE RESPONSE

Recognition of Antigen

For allografts to be recognized as foreign and subsequently rejected, or as self and therefore accepted, the potential antigenic determinants of the graft must come into contact with a variety of specific receptors of the immune system. Antigen–receptor interactions are the first steps in a series that ultimately determines the fate of an antigen or an organ. The molecular and cellular participants in these processes are the immunoglobulin receptors of B cells, the antigen or T-cell receptors (TCRs) of T cells, and major histocompatibility complex (MHC) antigens of antigen-presenting cells (APCs).

Direct Recognition of Antigen by Immunoglobulin

Conceptually, the easiest interaction to understand is the direct binding of antigen to immunoglobulin. In this case, antigen can be any cellular constituent (e.g., protein, carbohydrate, lipid, nucleic acid) that is bound by high affinity to a specific immunoglobulin, or antibody. Antibody molecules usually comprise two heavy (H) chains and two light (L) chains. Each chain has an amino-terminal variable (V) region domain, which differs from antibody to antibody. Each chain also has a few to several carboxy-terminal constant (C) region domains, which different antibody molecules may share. There are several different classes of immunoglobulins. The typical IgG dimer, comprising two L chains and two H chains, is shown in Fig. 16.1. Other classes of anti-

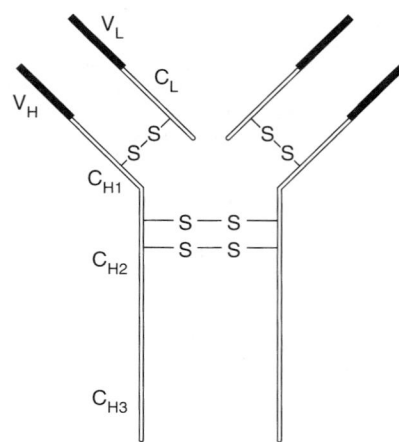

Figure 16.1. Structure of immunoglobulin (IgG). Variable (V) and constant (C) regions of heavy (H) and light (L) chains are joined by disulfide bonds.

bodies differ from IgG in their polymeric structure, number of H-chain constant region domains, and soluble or cell membrane location of the molecules. These features are listed in Table 16.1. Membrane-bound immunoglobulin usually serves as an antigen-specific receptor for stimulating naive or memory B cells, whereas soluble antibodies usually perform effector functions of antigen recognition, opsonization, complement-mediated lysis, or activation of effector cells through Fc receptor interactions. The generation of membrane versus soluble forms of immunoglobulin is usually the result of alternative splicing of messenger (mRNA).

Genetic analysis of immunoglobulin gene structure reveals several features that demonstrate how antibody diversity is generated and maintained. The H-chain gene complex is encoded on chromosome 14 in humans; κ L chains are encoded by chromosome 2 and λ L chains by chromosome 22. A single B cell can produce only a single type of L chain from only one of its chromosomes, a process termed *allelic exclusion*. The molecular determinants of allelic exclusion are just beginning to be elucidated. There appears to be a complex interaction between positive and negative regulatory transcription factors at the level of chromatin structure, and these factors are in turn regulated by membrane-initiated signaling events in response to specific antigens (1).

Heavy- and light-chain loci have a common structural motif of the V regions located upstream, or 5', of the C region. Furthermore, there are many V regions. These have been sequenced and further subdivided into unique or related classes and subclasses. Presumably, these multiple V region families arose by an evolutionary process of gene duplication followed by mutation of individual family members. Further analysis has shown that between the V and C regions are multiple additional genetic elements that provide further structural variation. These elements are termed *joining* (J) and *diversity* (D) regions. J regions are present in both H- and L-chain genes, whereas D regions are present only in H-chain genes. During the process of B-cell maturation, these separate regions are physically brought together in a stochastic process that excises the intervening DNA sequences, including other V, D, and J genes (Fig. 16.2). Because there are many different V-, D-, and J-region genes for each H- and L-chain locus, which all may independently associate, the combinatorial possibilities are extremely large, showing why the immune system is able to generate antibodies for virtually all known antigenic determinants. The general process of gene rearrangement in B cells involves the complex inter-

Table 16.1. STRUCTURAL PROPERTIES OF IMMUNOGLOBULIN CLASSES AND SUBCLASSES

IMMUNOGLOBULIN	IgD	IgM	IgG	IgA	IgE
SUBCLASSES	—	—	G1, G2, G3, G4	A1, A2	—
MOLECULAR WEIGHT (kd)	184	970	146–170	160	188
POLYMERIC STRUCTURE	Dimer	Pentamer	Dimer	Monomer, dimer, or trimer	Dimer
ADDITIONAL CHAINS	—	J chain	—	J chain	—
FUNCTIONAL ASSOCIATIONS	Membrane-bound receptor	Primary antibody, membrane receptor	Secondary antibody	Mucosal antibody	Immediate hypersensitivity

action of membrane-initiated differentiating signals, cytoplasmic transcriptional factors, and nucleic acid excisional machinery at the level of chromatin structure (1–5).

Further diversity is also generated by the nucleic acid template-independent addition of nucleotides (N regions) at the V-D, V-J, and D-J junctions. N regions increase the diversity of immunoglobulin sequences and antibody specificity by another few orders of magnitude. Thus, what is known about the immunoglobulin gene structure explains the presence of diversity at the protein level. Importantly, the regions of greatest nucleotide diversity correspond to the three hypervariable regions of the antibody molecule, which are the amino acid contact residues responsible for direct antigen– antibody or receptor–ligand interactions.

It was previously concluded that a single B cell expresses only a single isotype, or H chain. However, molecular analysis shows that alternative mRNA splicing may allow a single B cell to express different H chains. It was also previously considered that membrane-bound forms of immunoglobulin functioned independently as antigen receptors. However, biochemical analysis demonstrates that at least three invariant chains, Ig-α, Ig-β, and Ig-γ, must as-

sociate with surface immunoglobulin for efficient expression and signal transduction (6,7).

Recognition of Antigen by the T-Cell Receptor in the Context of the Major Histocompatibility Complex

T cells do not bind and recognize antigen directly. T cells recognize a complex composed of a peptide fragment of antigen bound to an MHC molecule. In other words, T cells recognize antigen in the context of MHC, a process termed *MHC restriction*. Structural and genetic analysis of the TCR reveals that it shares many principles with B-cell immunoglobulin receptors. The TCR is composed of separate α and β chains encoded by loci on chromosomes 14 and 7, respectively. Each locus comprises a series of V, D, J, and C segments (Fig. 16.3). The α-chain locus has only V and J genes, whereas the β locus has D regions. These loci undergo rearrangements during T-cell development, maturation, and differentiation, following the principles of gene rearrangement and allelic exclusion. This results in the generation of enormous receptor diversity and the potential to recognize the entire universe of antigens. Diversity is further increased by the insertion of N regions at V-D-J junctions.

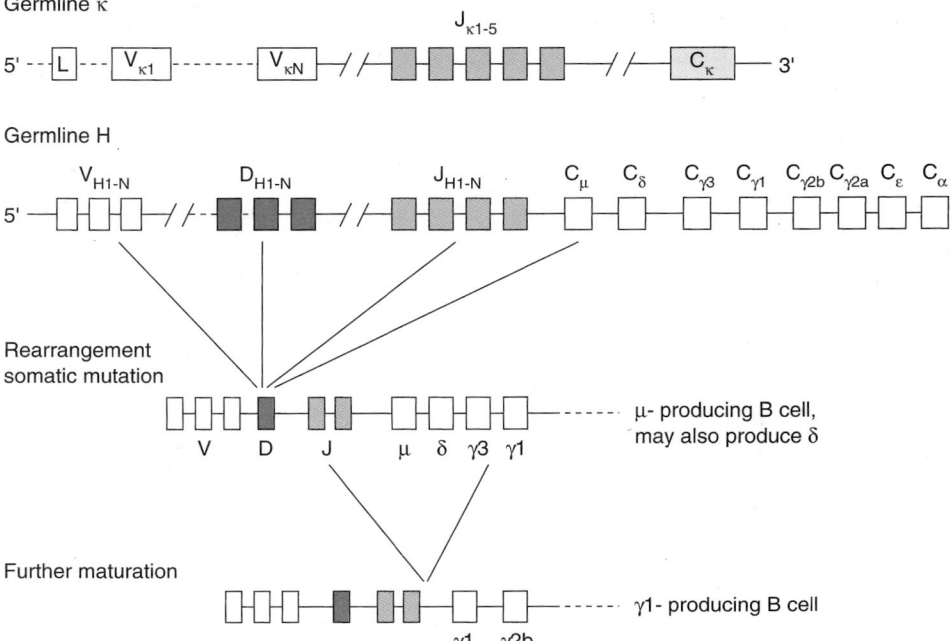

Figure 16.2. Structure of germline immunoglobulin heavy- and light-chain loci showing V, D, J, and C region genes. Maturation results in approximation of specific genes.

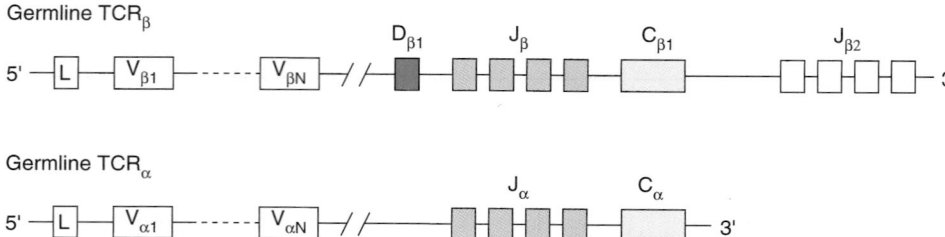

Figure 16.3. Structure of T-cell receptor (TCR) β- and α-chain loci.

T cells may also express alternative TCR γ and δ chains encoded on chromosomes 7 and 14, respectively. These chains are similar to α and β but show somewhat less diversity and are structurally more similar to immunoglobulins than αβ TCRs. Further, γδ T cells recognize not only peptide but nonpeptide antigens (8), and they may play unique roles in recognizing certain intracellular pathogens (e.g., *Mycobacteria, Listeria*) (9,10). γδ TCR T cells are particularly concentrated among intraepithelial lymphocytes of the gastrointestinal tract, further reinforcing the notion that γδ T cells perform functions related to surveillance of certain pathogens. Soluble forms of the TCR exist, resulting from alternative mRNA splicing or from proteolytic cleavage of surface receptors. The function of soluble TCR is not understood; studies show these molecules behave as suppressor factors or proinflammatory mediators.

Similar to surface immunoglobulin, the TCR is not expressed alone in the membrane. The TCR requires the coexpression of a complex of invariant chains termed *cluster determinant 3* (CD3). CD3 is a complex of five transmembrane proteins (γ, δ, ε, ζ, η), as shown in Fig. 16.4, which are important for the assembly of the TCR and its transport and insertion into the cell membrane. The CD3 complex plays an essential role in signal transduction by the TCR, particularly the cytoplasmic domains of the ζ and η chains (11). Additional molecules also function in tandem with the αβ TCR. In particular, the CD4 and CD8 molecules,

transmembrane proteins that are likewise members of the immunoglobulin gene superfamily, physically associate with the αβ TCR and bind to the same MHC molecules as the TCR. This association increases the affinity and avidity of TCR and T cells for antigen. CD4 binds to class II MHC [i.e., human leukocyte antigen (HLA)-DR, DP, and DQ] and is generally considered a cell surface marker for helper T cells (T_H). This explains why T_H are MHC class II restricted. CD8 binds to class I MHC (i.e., HLA-A, B, and C) and is generally considered a cell surface marker for cytotoxic (T_C) or suppressor (T_S) T cells. This explains why T_C are generally MHC class I restricted.

There are two major classes of MHC molecules encoded by linked loci on chromosome 6 and defined by structural and functional associations (Table 16.2). Class I MHC molecules result from the noncovalent association between a polymorphic, transmembrane α chain and a nonpolymorphic soluble β chain, termed b2-microglobulin. Thus, α chains encoded by diverse HLA-A, B, or C alleles each associate with β_2-microglobulin on the cell surface (Fig. 16.5). Class II molecules result from the noncovalent association of polymorphic transmembrane α and β chains encoded by HLA-DP, DQ, or DR (Fig. 16.6). There are separate α and β chains encoded within each separate class II subregion. Despite some structural differences, these class I and II dimers all have four major extracellular domains, with two of the domains contributing the major amino

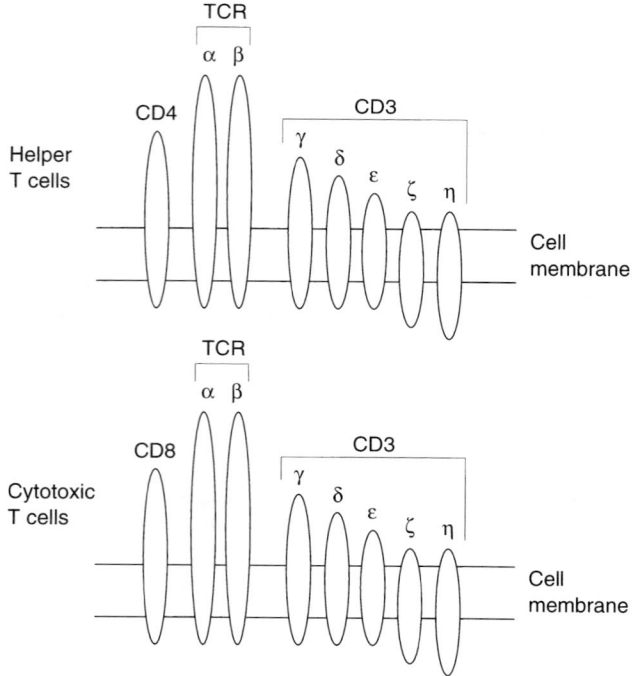

Figure 16.4. T-cell receptor (TCR) complex in the cell membrane composed of TCR αβ, CD3, CD4, and CD8 chains.

Table 16.2. CLASS I AND CLASS II ANTIGENS: STRUCTURE AND FUNCTION

Class I Antigens	Class II Antigens
STRUCTURE	
Encoded by HLA-A, -B, -C loci in humans	Encoded by HLA-D locus (DR, DP, DO)
Single polymorphic heavy chain (45 kd)	Two chains α (29 kd) β (34 kd)
Associated with β_2-microglobulin (12 kd)	—
Five domains α_1, α_2, α_3 extracellular Transmembrane Cystoplasmic	Four domains α_1, α_2 or β_1, β_2 extracellular Transmembrane Cytoplasmic
Expressed on all nucleated cells	Expressed on B cells, antigen-presenting cells, and vascular endothelium
MAJOR FUNCTIONS	
Activator and target for cytotoxic T (CD8+) lymphocytes	Activator of helper T cells (CD4+) and stimulator in mixed lymphocyte reaction
Target for antibody-mediated rejection	Possible target for antibody-mediated rejection
Stimulate antibody response	Stimulator of antibody response (unknown significance)

HLA, human leukocyte antigen.

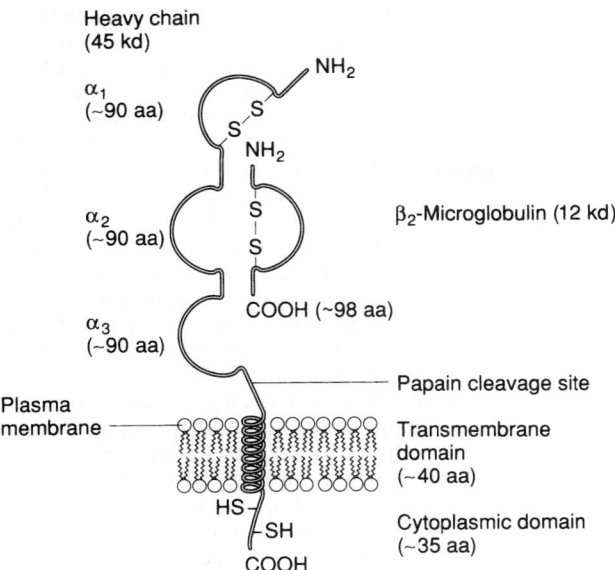

Figure 16.5. Human leukocyte antigen (HLA) class I molecule. The polymorphic heavy chain (45 kd) of the class I polypeptide is noncovalently bound to the invariant light chain, β_2-microglobulin (12 kd). The heavy chain consists of five domains—three extracellular domains (α_1, α_2, and α_3), a transmembrane domain, and a cytoplasmic domain. The α_1 and α_2 domains contain the most polymorphic residues responsible for antigen binding and form the side walls of the peptide binding groove; the transmembrane portion anchors the molecule to the plasma membrane; and the β_2-microglobulin stabilizes the conformation of the extracellular domains.

acid side chains to the walls of the peptide binding groove.

The TCR binds to a complex of MHC plus antigen. X-ray crystallography has determined the three-dimensional structure of these complexes and provided a firm structural and biochemical basis for understanding the cellular

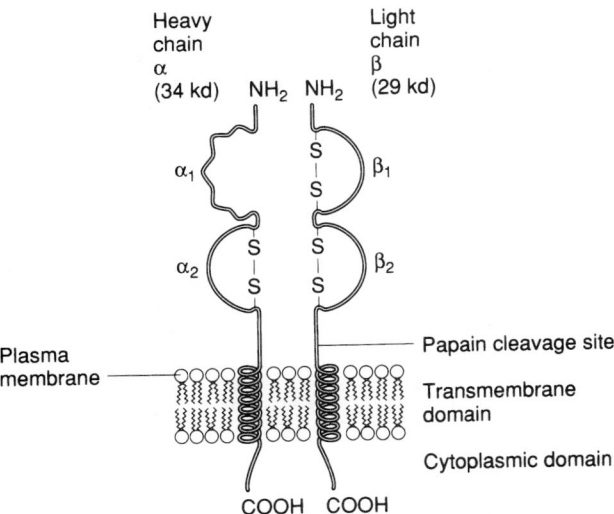

Figure 16.6. Human leukocyte antigen (HLA) class II molecule. The two chains, α (29 kd) and β (34 kd), are noncovalently associated and are made up of four domains—two extracellular domains, a transmembrane domain, and a cytoplasmic domain. Most of the allelic variance is contained in the β chain. The peptide binding site is believed to be in the groove between the α_1 and β_1 domains.

process of MHC restriction (12,13). Figure 16.7 shows that the α_1 and α_2 domains of an MHC class I molecule form a groove on the surface of the MHC molecule. Peptide antigens are loaded into this groove when the functions of antigen processing and presentation are performed. The α_1 and β_1 domains of class II MHC perform a similar function. The TCR residues come in contact with residues of both antigen and MHC. Therefore, polymorphisms of the TCR

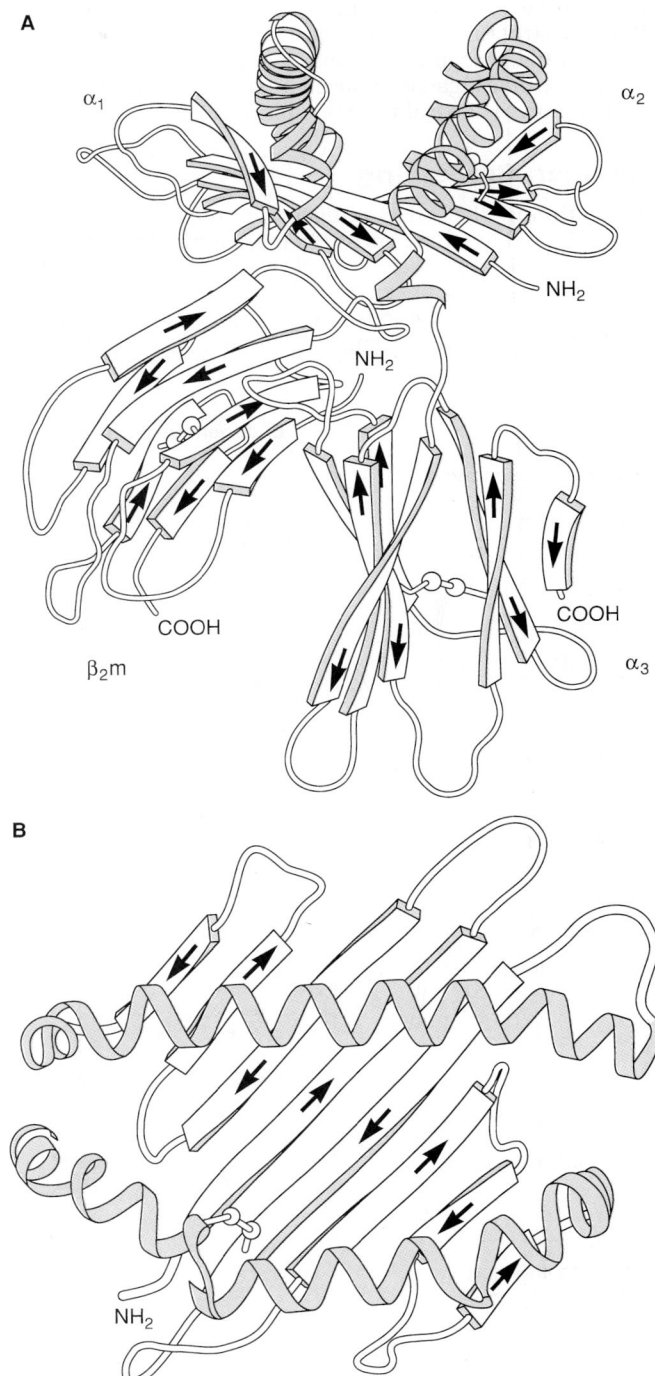

Figure 16.7. Human leukocyte antigen (HLA)-A2 class I molecule. *(A)* There are four domains with the polymorphic α_1 and α_2 on top presenting themselves to the T-cell receptor and α_3 and β_2 below close to the cell membrane. *(B)* Looking at the top of the molecule, the peptide binding groove is shown as made up of the α_1 and α_2 domains forming the side walls and the β pleated sheet forming the floor.

generated by gene arrangement, and polymorphisms of MHC resulting from allelic variation within the population and the expression of several different class I or II molecules, provide the structural variation required to accommodate the potential universe of antigenic determinants. Some of the most important recent advances in immunology have been the determination of the three-dimensional structure of the MHC, peptide binding groove, and TCR and the unequivocal demonstration of the loading of peptide antigen into the MHC molecules. Precise, structurally based approaches to altering the T cell's initial recognition of antigen are now possible and are being investigated experimentally to determine their application to clinical transplantation.

Antigen Processing

Identifying the MHC–antigen complex structure has also initiated much recent study toward defining the pathways by which antigen is loaded onto MHC molecules. The pathways of antigen processing encompass a wide variety of cellular functions, including the receptor-mediated endocytosis of antigen, transfer of cytoplasmic or endosomal antigen to proteolytic organelles, translocation of proteolyzed peptide into the endoplastic reticulum to nascent "naked" MHC molecules, correct folding of new MHC molecules around antigen, transport of antigen–MHC by the *cis-* and *trans-*Golgi apparatus to the cell surface, and recycling of cell surface MHC molecules to endosomal and Golgi compartments to exchange one antigenic peptide for another (Fig. 16.8). This brief list of some of the defined steps of antigen processing and presentation reveals that many of the normal cellular housekeeping processes are coopted during the handling of antigen. These processes include vesicle transport and fusion, microtubule and microfilament function, correct folding and localization of nascent polypeptides coming off the ribosome by chaperonins, and control of intracellular proteolysis. Therefore, the study and eventual understanding of antigen processing and presentation requires knowledge of most normal cellular functions. Immunosuppression may eventually be directed not at T cells or B cells, as is currently the case, but may alter the functions of chaperones, Golgi apparatus, or proteolytic controls.

Figure 16.8 provides a general picture of the major processes, which include antigen uptake, proteolysis,

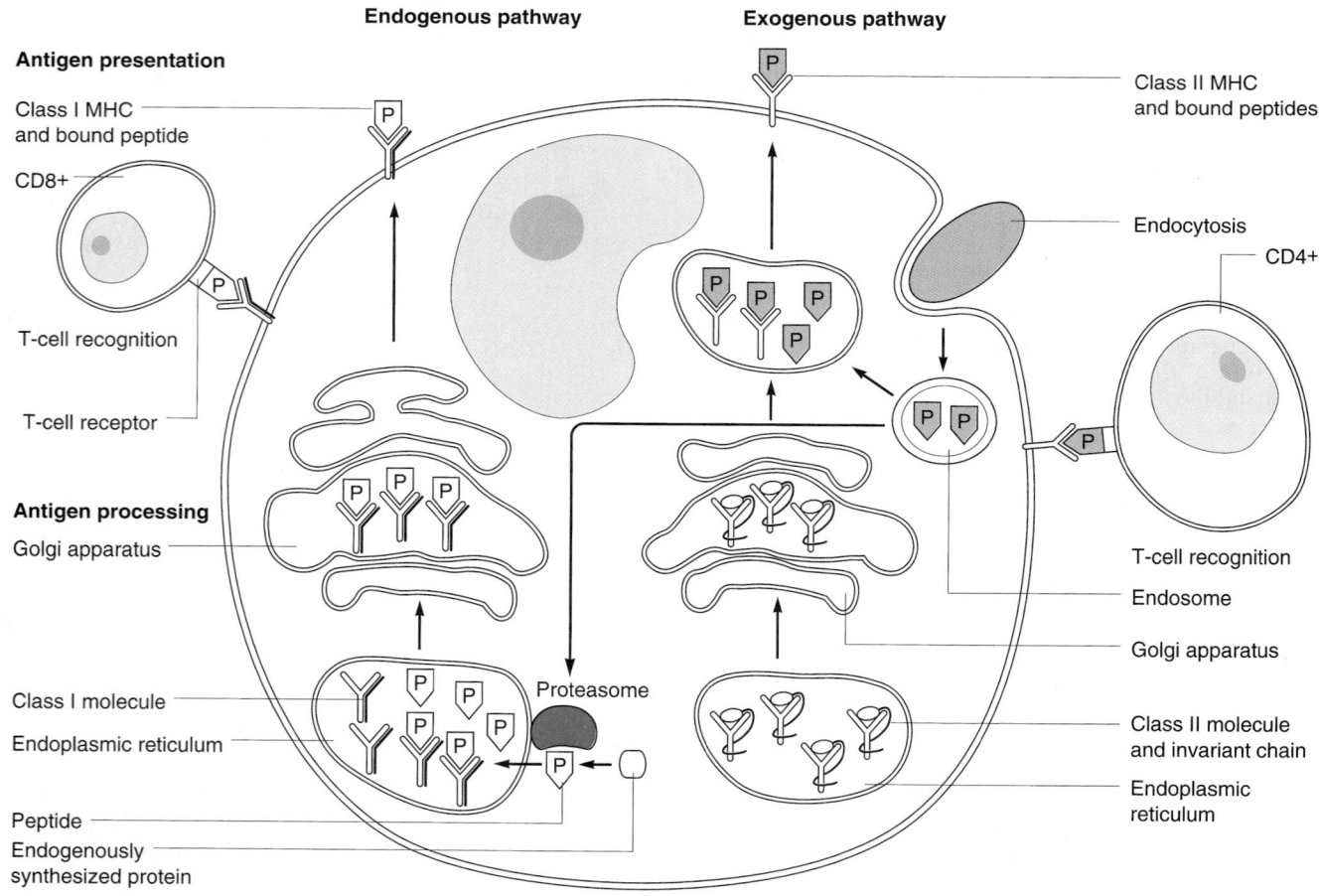

Figure 16.8. Antigen processing and presentation. Endogenously synthesized or intracellular proteins (e.g., viral gene products) are degraded into peptides that are transported to the endoplasmic reticulum. These peptides bind to class I major histocompatibility complex (MHC) molecules and are transported to the surface of the antigen-presenting cell. CD8+ T cells recognize the foreign peptide bound to class I MHC by way of the T-cell receptor complex. Exogenous antigen (e.g., bacterial) is endocytosed and broken down into peptide fragments in endosomes. Class II molecules are transported to the endosome in association with the invariant chain, bound to the peptide, and delivered to the surface of the antigen-presenting cell, where they are recognized by CD4+ cells.

translocation to the endoplasmic reticulum or Golgi, and presentation on the cell surface (14–37). A number of important features should be mentioned. The source of antigen determines how and where it comes into contact with the processing machinery and onto which MHC molecules it is loaded. Thus, endogenously synthesized proteins, such as self-proteins or viral antigens in the cytoplasm, are degraded in the cytoplasm, transported to the endoplasmic reticulum, and loaded onto nascent class I MHC (38). Conversely, exogenously synthesized antigens are taken up in endosomes through receptor-mediated processes, degraded in an endosomal compartment (e.g., lysosome, Golgi apparatus, or a unique structure), transported to the Golgi, and loaded onto nascent class II MHC (39). Although this general scheme for the processing and presentation of endogenous versus exogenous antigens will likely remain intact, there are numerous exceptions where endogenous antigens may be presented by class II MHC or exogenous antigens presented by class I MHC. This undoubtedly reflects the incomplete understanding of vesicle transport, proteolytic control, partitioning of molecules to various endosomal compartments, and the molecular control of MHC folding and peptide loading.

Proteolytic degradation of antigens may be accomplished either in endosomal compartments, probably through fusion with lysosomes, or in the cytoplasm. The latter process seems to be accomplished by a large multiprotein complex called the *proteasome* (40,41). In addition, some of the proteasome subunits are encoded in the MHC region. Thus, the MHC provides the information to degrade antigen and to determine the carrier onto which antigenic peptides are loaded. The control of proteolysis is poorly understood; it is not clear if all cellular constituents have equal access to proteolytic components or if antigens are somehow preferentially shunted into the system. Proteolytic enzymes have specificity for particular peptide bonds; therefore, not all proteins should be equally susceptible to the processing apparatus and some should make "better" antigens than others. This has been confirmed experimentally using amino acid-substituted antigens. In addition, there is allelic variation among the MHC-encoded proteasome subunits so that antigen is processed into different peptides by different alleles. Allelic variation in MHC class I and II peptide binding grooves also determines what set of peptides can be bound by MHC molecules. Thus, heterogeneity of antigens, proteolytic enzymes, and MHC molecules all determine the nature of the peptide ultimately presented to the TCR.

Further molecular analysis demonstrates that the MHC class I peptide binding groove is a fairly closed structure and can accommodate peptides of a relatively restricted size, ranging from 8 to 10 amino acids in length. Conversely, the class II groove is larger and more open ended. It can tolerate more length heterogeneity in the peptide that it binds so that a modal distribution of 12 to 24 amino acids is found loaded onto these molecules. These structural constraints suggest that certain types of antigens may be presented only by certain MHC molecules. Indeed, there is evidence that certain microbial antigens are preferentially presented by class I MHC (42,43). This example also represents one exception where exogenously synthesized antigens are presented by class I. Although the discussion to this point has focused on protein antigens, it is not known if or how nonprotein antigens are loaded into the antigen-binding groove of MHC molecules.

Another important issue is how antigen is transported into the endoplasmic reticulum or Golgi apparatus. The determinants of endosomal transport and its specificity are not defined. The determinants of cytoplasmic transport seem dependent on a transporter complex that phys-

ically links the proteasome to the endoplasmic reticulum. Furthermore, this transporter complex is at least partly MHC encoded. Current models suggest that as a peptide antigen is degraded, it is immediately transported from the proteasome to the lumen of the endoplasmic reticulum, where it is loaded onto class I MHC. The facts that the MHC encodes the transporter and that allelic variation is also present in these molecules provide another level of variation in the ability ultimately to recognize any antigen.

Another noteworthy issue is how peptide is loaded into the binding groove of MHC molecules. Experimental evidence suggests that class I and II dimers are incompletely assembled in the endoplasmic reticulum and are also bound by chaperone proteins. In the case of class II MHC, this chaperone is called the *invariant chain*. Failure to load peptide results in retention of MHC molecules within the endoplasmic reticulum and markedly decreases cell surface MHC expression. Loading of peptide causes the release of MHC by chaperones, completion of folding and assembly, and transport to the cell surface. A related issue is the fate and recycling of cell surface antigen–MHC complexes. There is evidence of endocytosis and reloading of both class I and II molecules with new peptide antigens. The molecular determinants of these processes are still poorly defined.

Antigen Presentation and Antigen-presenting Cells

Based on the previous discussion, it is apparent that antigen processing and presentation depend on a large number of coordinated intracellular events. Many of these events, however, seem to depend on normal cellular processes of transport, proteolysis, and posttranslational modification of proteins. Antigen presentation also depends on the expression of MHC-encoded class I, class II, proteasome, and transporter molecules. All nucleated cells express MHC class I, and many cell types can also express the other loci. This suggests that many different cell types are capable of presenting antigens. In fact, this has been proved in a number of experimental and clinical analyses. Nonetheless, certain cell types are more efficient at processing and presenting antigen and are localized to certain tissues or organs that increase the likelihood that they will participate in antigen presentation. These so-called *professional APCs* are generally considered to be monocytes and macrophages. In addition, closely related interstitial dendritic cells and Langerhans cells of the dermis are extremely efficient APCs. These cells constitutively express class I and II MHC and the other MHC-encoded components. All these products can be up-regulated in response to proinflammatory cytokines, such as interferon-γ (IFN-γ). These cells are also localized to regions, such as the lymph nodes, spleen, and skin, where they are most likely to encounter antigen. Other cell types, such as vascular endothelium, organ parenchymal cells, and tumor cells, can act as APCs under many conditions. The nature of the responding T cell, the cytokine milieu, and the expression of other cell surface adhesion receptors determine APC function.

Alloreactivity

The discussion to this point has centered on general considerations of antigenic recognition. In transplantation, the response to alloantigens is most germane. The immune response to alloantigens is extraordinarily strong and the immune system seems obsessed by allelic variation in MHC antigens. Thus, in a culture of human T lymphocytes stimulated with a purified protein antigen (e.g., murine cytochrome C), far less than 1% of the T cells respond to the antigen. Conversely, if the same culture is stimulated with human allogenic cells expressing different MHC alleles, up to 10% of the T cells respond to the antigenic stimulation. In terms of clinical transplantation, this suggests that the immune system is specifically directed against foreign MHC and that any attempts to improve immunosuppression, prevent rejection, and prolong allograft survival depend on a detailed understanding of alloreactivity.

Current cellular and molecular models of alloreactivity rely on the understanding of TCR and MHC structural interactions. The TCR does not recognize MHC alone but as a complex of antigen plus MHC. During T-cell maturation, autoreactive T cells are eliminated or tolerized (see Development of Lymphocytes). Thus, T cells that recognize self-peptides loaded into self-MHC are no longer present or able to respond to antigen. The remaining T cells have TCR specificities that enable them to recognize foreign peptides loaded onto self-MHC molecules, a concept termed *recognition of altered self.* These same T cells may also fortuitously recognize foreign peptides loaded onto allo-MHC or even self-peptides loaded onto allo-MHC. The reason for these other types of recognition is that TCR–antigen–MHC interactions ultimately rely on the three-dimensional interaction of amino acid side chains of the molecules.

Figure 16.9 shows these potential TCR–MHC interactions, including recognition of self-peptides on self-MHC, or an autoimmune response, and various types of alloantigenic responses. The recognition of foreign or self-peptides loaded onto allo-MHC is termed *direct recognition* because intact allo-MHC is being recognized. The response to foreign MHC peptides loaded onto self-MHC is termed *indirect* recognition because intact allo-MHC is not being recognized. These terms and concepts apply to both class I and class II MHC as well as CD4+ and CD8+ T cells. Most alloreactivity is due to allogenic cells of the donor organ acting as APCs and presenting endogenous peptides in the context of allogenic class I MHC to host CD8+ T cells. However, all permutations of self- and foreign peptides and MHC, and class I and II MHC, have been demonstrated to occur experimentally or clinically. A single T cell may be capable of recognizing one peptide in the context of self-MHC and another peptide in the context of allo-MHC.

Antigenicity

The structural and cellular information in the previous section provides a foundation for considering what determines whether a molecule is perceived as an antigen and how strong an immune response it elicits. In the case of a protein antigen, it must be correctly transported, proteolyzed, loaded onto MHC molecules, and interact with the TCR. Failure to achieve any one of these steps may prevent an appropriate immune response. Immunosuppressive strategies based on this new information are being experimentally evaluated and are discussed later in this chapter. There are many other determinants of antigenicity, such as antigen quaternary structure (44), location of cell types involved in presenting antigen (45), the types of T cells present, and the types of cytokines present during the response. These issues are also discussed later in this chapter. The molecular pathways for antigen processing and presentation are defined for *peptide* antigens. Pathways for carbohydrates, lipids, nucleic acids, or derivatives of these are undefined and may have novel interactions with APC pathways or be incapable of eliciting T-cell immunity. The complexity of the response to antigen demonstrates that many potential loci for immunosuppression exist and that to achieve timely, effective immunosuppression, many of these loci may have to be simultaneously disrupted.

Sites of Antigen Recognition

Anatomic Organization of the Immune Response

In vitro experimental studies of immune function often juxtapose stimulator and responder cells in an environment where all possible cellular interactions may take place more or less equally. In vivo, the situation is quite different because cells and antigen are sequestered or compartmentalized. Thus, interactions among cells are more restricted, resulting in a channeling of immune responses in certain directions. There are several intersecting levels of anatomic organization of the immune system. First, immature T cells, B cells, and APCs arise centrally in the bone marrow. The initial interaction of T and B cells with the bone marrow microenvironment may determine if these cells are tolerized to self-antigens expressed in the bone marrow. T cells undergo further maturation and selection in the thymus (see Development of Lymphocytes). Interactions with thymic medullary and cortical tissues determine that self-reactive cells are tolerized, whereas altered-self–reactive cells remain fully functional.

Second, mature cells circulate in the periphery through the lymphatic and vascular systems, passing through lymph nodes. Lymph nodes are highly organized juxtapositions of T cells, B cells, and APCs, which concentrate antigen in the vicinity of responding lymphocytes. For example, a wound infection or a skin graft introduces bacte-

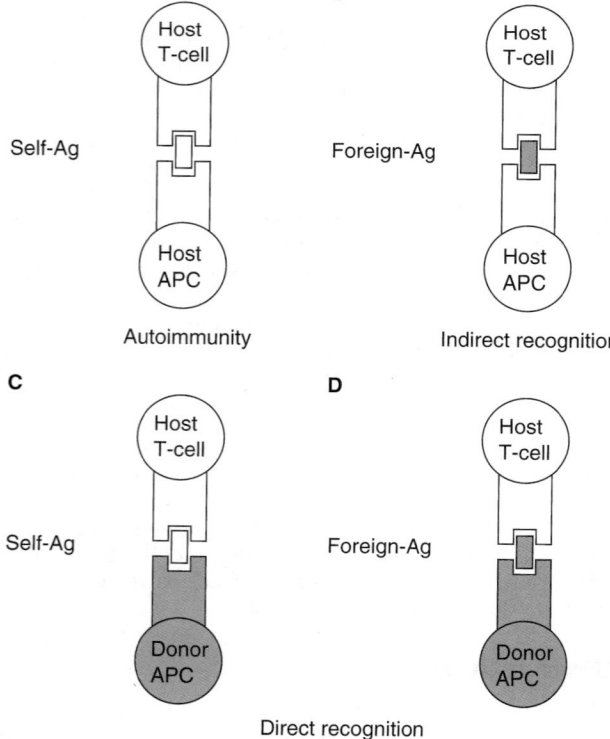

Figure 16.9. T-cell receptor recognition of self- and foreign peptide antigen (Ag) in the context of self- or foreign major histocompatibility complex molecules. *A* represents autoimmunity; *B, C,* and *D* are aspects of alloimmunity. APC, antigen-presenting cell.

rial antigens or alloantigens, respectively, into the dermis. Antigen is taken up by APCs and transported to regional lymph nodes by lymphatic channels. APCs present antigen to T and B cells, which either reside in the node or recirculate through it. This highly organized and stereotyped sequence of events results in antibody production by B cells and priming of T cells to antigen.

Third, regional collections of lymphoid tissue serve specialized functions. The gut-associated lymphoid tissue (GALT) and bronchial-associated lymphoid tissue (BALT) are collections of lymph nodes (e.g., Peyer's patches) and specialized T and B cells, localized to the gut lumen and tracheobronchial tree, areas expected to have a very high burden of antigen and microbial contamination. Most B cells can secrete IgA in these tissues. IgA, or secretory immunoglobulin, is structurally capable of retaining its functions of opsonization and antimicrobial activity within gut and bronchial secretions. There are also intraepithelial γδ TCR T cells of the gut. As mentioned earlier, these cells may have specialized roles in responding to certain microorganisms by virtue of TCR specificity for evolutionarily conserved microbial antigens. The signals that localize IgA+ B cells or γδ+ T cells or that induce cells already present in these regions to express the relevant receptors are not understood.

Fourth, there is a division between the function of central and peripheral lymphoid tissue. Antigen presented peripherally (i.e., subcutaneously or intradermally) localizes to regional lymph nodes and induces long-lived T- and B-cell immunity. Antigen presented centrally (i.e., orally, intrabronchially, or intravenously) may induce transient or local immunity (e.g., intestinal IgA secretion) but also tends to induce systemic unresponsiveness or tolerance to the antigen. This may be an adaptive response to prevent severe, debilitating inflammatory responses to what we ingest or breathe. From the standpoint of transplantation, it may be possible to take advantage of this central versus peripheral difference in antigen presentation to help induce tolerance. What determines this difference is unknown. The possibility that the nature of the APCs in central compartments (e.g., liver, spleen, BALT, GALT) is different than in the peripheral lymph node has been considered. No such differences, however, have been unequivocally demonstrated. More recent inquiries suggest that the microenvironments (e.g., cytokine levels) differ between central and peripheral compartments, and that these differences interact with APCs to channel immune responses in various directions.

Homing and Trafficking

It has long been known that lymphocytes traffic between the vascular and lymphatic compartments and localize to sites of inflammation, and that specialized subsets can home to specific anatomic sites (e.g., IgA+ B cells to the gut). Many of the determinants of lymphocyte homing and trafficking have been defined by molecular and cellular techniques, and determining the physiologic roles of these components is now a much more tractable problem. The major issue to understand in homing and trafficking is leukocyte–vascular endothelial cell interactions. This is the initial interaction required in any immune or inflammatory response. It is not possible for a lymphocyte to home, localize, or circulate without first passing through the vascular endothelial layer. Studies using videomicroscopy and blocking specific molecules with antibodies or genetic techniques have shown that this initial interaction can be divided into several steps (46). Many of these studies have examined neutrophils and monocytes in addition to lymphocytes. In the first step, leukocytes come in contact with the vascular endothelium and adhere to the surface. The cell attaches to and then rolls over the endothelial surface as a result of hemodynamic shear forces. In the second step, the leukocyte is activated to express other receptors and secretes cytokines. The endothelial cell may also become activated and alter receptor expression and cytokine production. In the third step, the leukocyte stops on the endothelial surface, and the adhesive interaction between the cells increases. The final step is transendothelial cell migration.

Each step is associated with several specific interactions between receptors on the leukocyte cell surface and ligands on the endothelial surface or soluble cytokine ligands. Because so many cytokines and surface receptors or ligands have been identified, with many more reported regularly in the literature, the current challenge is to understand how all these signals are integrated in a coherent and specific fashion. Modeling suggests that specific classes of molecules are associated with each of the first three steps of the trafficking process and that these molecules are restricted by cell type (46). The result is a three-digit "zip code," which may specifically direct neutrophils, monocytes, or lymphocytes to the correct anatomic location. This model is illustrated in Fig. 16.10. Different subsets of lymphocytes or other leukocytes can express different receptor and cytokine arrays. Likewise, different subsets of endothelial cells also express different molecular arrays. These differences could account for fine tuning and further specificity of the system.

Cells and Molecules that Participate in Antigen Recognition

T Cells

The central paradigm for the initiation of an immune response is that antigen is taken up by an APC, processed, and then presented to a T cell (Fig. 16.11). The T cell is activated in response to appropriately processed and presented antigen. The activated T cell may become an effector T cell and may also provide help to B cells, other T cells, or even macrophages, which then proceed to act as immune effectors. In this paradigm, the T cell plays a central and indispensable role. For this reason, much of transplantation immunology is directed toward understanding and manipulating T-cell responses.

T cells are divided into two main subclasses: CD4+ and CD8+. CD4+8+ double-positive cells are usually immature T cells or thymocytes, whereas the fully differentiated T cell is usually single positive. Because of the molecular interactions described earlier (47,48), CD4+ T cells are restricted to recognizing antigen in the context of class II MHC and usually perform roles related to B-cell help, T-cell help, and inflammatory responses, such as delayed and contact hypersensitivity. CD8+ T cells are restricted to class I MHC and often perform cytotoxic functions. Under certain circumstances, particularly experimental conditions with transgenic or knockout-derived cells, CD4+ cells can be class I restricted or perform cytotoxic functions. Conversely, CD8+ cells can be class II restricted or perform helper or inflammatory functions. These findings suggest there is sufficient plasticity in TCR structure and cellular programming that a single T-cell subset can perform the functions of other subsets. This may also imply that blocking or ablating the function of a single T-cell subset may not provide reliable immunosuppression from the standpoint of clinical transplantation. However, the complexity of immunoregulatory systems might permit the manipulation of a single T-cell subset to determine the responses of other T-cell subsets.

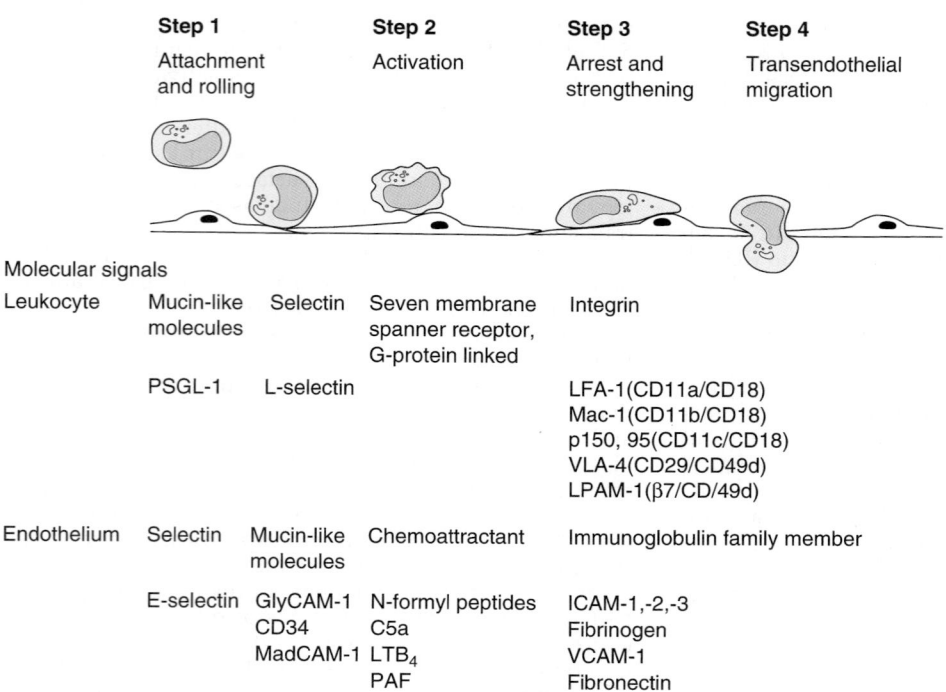

Figure 16.10. Model of leukocyte–vascular endothelial cell interactions important for specific trafficking and homing. The three major classes of cellular adhesion receptors—selectins, integrins, immunoglobulin gene superfamily members—play distinct temporal and functional roles. See Table 16.4 for abbreviations.

The CD4+ T cells fall into one of two major subsets, termed *T helper type 1* (T$_H$1) and *type 2* (T$_H$2) (Table 16.3). T$_H$1 cells are characterized by proinflammatory, delayed-type hypersensitivity effector functions and the release of IFN-γ. T$_H$2 cells are characterized by providing B-cell help, suppressing T-cell responses, and releasing interleukin (IL)-4, IL-5, and IL-10. IL-4 and IL-5 promote B-cell differentiation, maturation, and immunoglobulin production, and IL-4 may act as a feedback cytokine to promote further T$_H$2 proliferation and inhibit T$_H$1 and IFN-γ. IL-10 may also inhibit IFN-γ production. Conversely, IFN-g may promote T$_H$1 and inhibit T$_H$2 production. Furthermore, the potent macrophage-derived T-cell-stimulatory cytokine, IL-12, also promotes T$_H$1 production. Current models suggest that T$_H$1 and T$_H$2 form a regulatory circuit in which one subset inhibits the activity of the other (Fig. 16.12). These models imply that the channeling of an immune response occurs early and is determined by the relative balance of T$_H$ subsets and their cytokines.

Several uncertainties about the T$_H$1/T$_H$2 model remain (49,50). Although these subsets have been repeatedly demonstrated in murine experimental systems, it is not clear if the human subsets are so well defined and compartmentalized. There may be more overlap in humans. Second, it is not clear if T$_H$1 and T$_H$2 interconvert or if their phenotype represents terminal differentiation. A related issue is whether T$_H$1 and T$_H$2 are derived from a common T$_H$0 precursor or if they represent more distant and distinct lineages. Third, the amount and ratio of IL-12, IL-4, IL-2, and IFN-γ at the initiation of an immune response determine whether T$_H$1 or T$_H$2 predominate, yet the initial determinants of these cytokine levels are not well known. Nonetheless, the recognition that distinct cytokines can channel immunity has led to much current experimental and clinical work in which these cytokines are used to drive responses. IL-12 is being considered as a way to boost tumor immunity, and IL-10 is being used to suppress allograft responses.

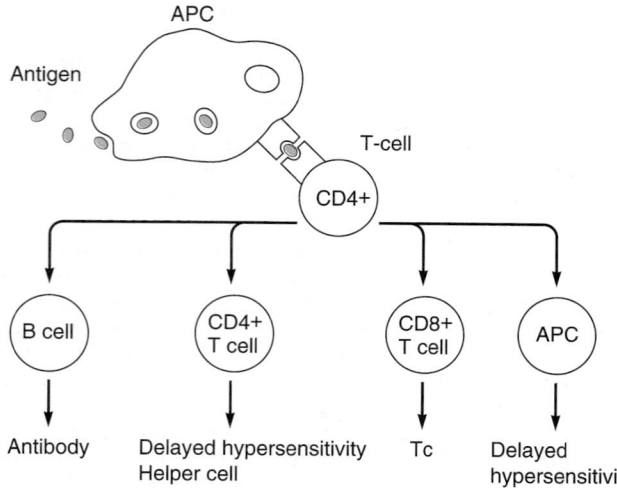

Figure 16.11. Central paradigm for cellular initiation of an immune response. CD4+ T cells respond to appropriately presented antigen on antigen-presenting cells (APCs) and in turn help other T cells, B cells, and APCs.

Table 16.3. T$_H$1 AND T$_H$2 SUBCLASSES

Subclass	Function	Cytokines produced
T$_H$1	Effect delayed-type hypersensitivity	IL-2
	Effect contact sensitivity	IFN-τ
	Provide T$_c$ help	(Respond to IL-12)
T$_H$2	Provide B-cell help	IL-2
	Suppress T-cell responses	IL-4
		IL-5
		IL-10

IFN, interferon; IL, interleukin.

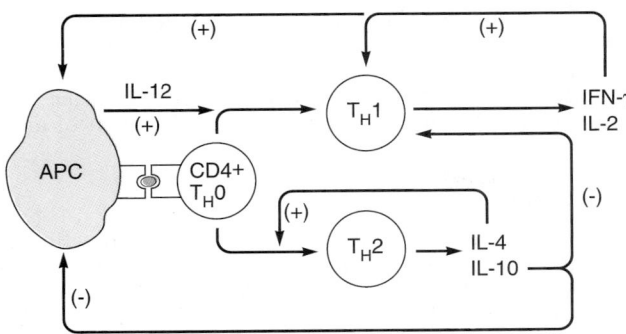

Figure 16.12. T helper type 1 (T_H1)/T_H2 paradigm of CD4+ T-cell subsets. APC, antigen-presenting cell; IFN-γ, interferon-γ; IL, interleukin.

In many texts, CD8+ T cells are also said to perform suppressor functions. The situation is more complicated than this. Experimental results demonstrate that both CD4+ and CD8+ T cells can act as T_S (51–55). In addition, non-T cells may also act as suppressor cells in some circumstances (56). The major problem with most descriptions of suppressor cells is that a phenotypically well-defined population has not been isolated. Thus, only vague descriptions of suppressor cells and their phenotypes have been available. The notion of T_H1 and T_H2 subsets has provided a new context in which to view T_S. Instead of supposing that T_S down-regulate all responses, it is now considered more likely that T_S channel immunity in one direction or another. Thus, T_H2 cells suppress T_H1 and T_C function while supporting B-cell responses. Current models suggest that T_H2 cells are the relevant T_S of cell-mediated immunity, and attempts to boost T_H2 responses during organ allografting are seen as a way to promote graft survival (52).

B Cells

B cells develop initially in the bone marrow, recirculate throughout the vascular and lymphatic systems, and initiate primary and secondary antibody responses, particularly in the germinal centers of lymph nodes. B cells, T cells, and APC-type dendritic cells are brought into close juxtaposition in germinal centers, concentrating antigen to the relevant cells and receptors of the immune system. B cells primarily produce IgM antibody for primary responses and other isotypes for secondary responses. Antibody then performs effector functions of complement fixation, opsonization, clearance, or feedback immune regulation through idiotype–antiidiotype interactions. B-cell responses may be *T independent*, in which B cells respond to antigen in the absence of T_H. These are usually, but not exclusively, IgM responses to polymeric antigens bearing multiple identical epitopes, such as bacterial cell wall polysaccharides. T-independent responses may occur after transplantation and result in graft damage or loss. T-independent responses are also responsible for much of the natural antibody found in graft recipients. Natural antibody is preformed immunoglobulin directed toward alloantigens, despite no previous exposure of the individual to the alloantigen. The antibody putatively arises from exposure to cross-reactive environmental antigens.

T-dependent responses require the T-cell–APC–B-cell interaction. This interaction requires coordinated signaling among these cells of numerous cell surface and soluble ligands. The specificity of the interaction is ensured by the specificity of the T- and B-cell receptors for antigen. Thereafter, a series of nonclonally distributed receptors and ligands interact to amplify and modulate these signals. Figure 16.13 shows some of the important cell sur-

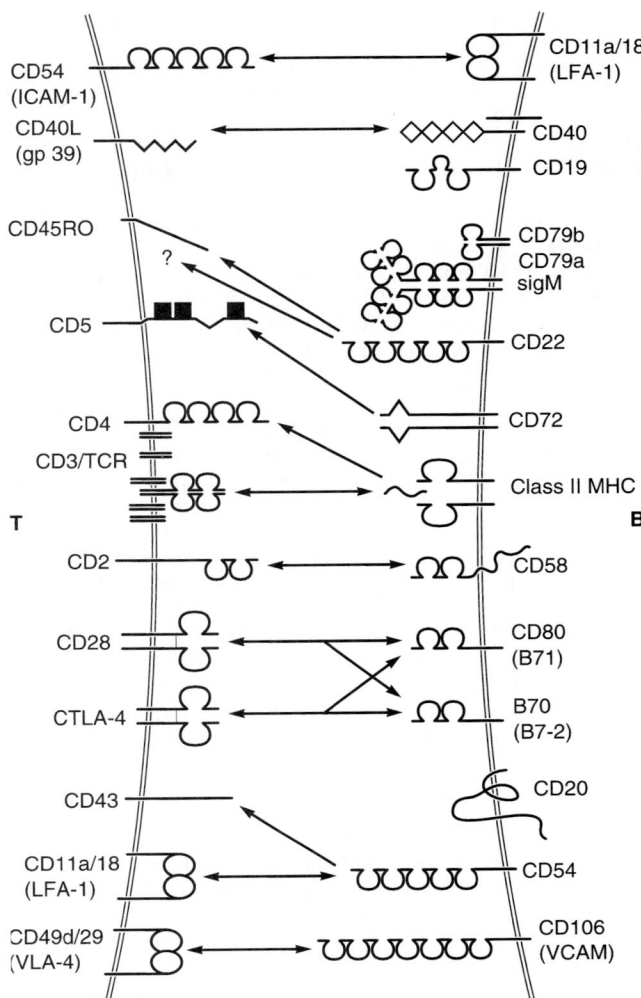

Figure 16.13. Adhesion receptors that may mediate interactions between CD4+ T cells and B cells. ICAM-1, intercellular adhesion molecule-1; LFA-1, leukocyte functional antigen-1; MHC, major histocompatibility complex; TCR, T-cell receptor; VCAM, vascular cell adhesion molecule; VLA-4, very late antigen-4.

face receptor interactions that take place during T-cell stimulation of B cells. Because so many potential interactions may occur, it is unclear which signals are absolutely required or how any one receptor or group of receptors may alter the function of other receptors. Nonetheless, current models (57–61) suggest that the interactions of primary importance are as follows:

- TCR–antigen–class II MHC–CD4
- Antigen–sIgM (B-cell antigen receptor)
- CD28–CD80 (B7-1)/CD86 (B7-2)
- CD40–CD40L

Failure to engage these receptors severely or completely inhibits appropriate responses. Secondary receptor–ligand interactions of importance include CD11a/18 [leukocyte functional antigen-1 (LFA-1)]–CD54 [intercellular adhesion molecule-1 (ICAM-1)], CD2–CD58 (LFA-3), and CD19–(unknown ligand). Failure to achieve these interactions, however, does not necessarily inhibit the B-cell response. Cytokines also required for T and B interactions include IL-4 and IL-5, which promote immunoglobulin class switching to IgE and IgG4 production, and IL-10 and IL-12, which promote switching to IgG1, IgG2, IgG3, and IgA.

The molecular signaling between T and B cells demonstrates that the B cell is not a passive member of the pair that merely receives T-cell-derived signals and then secretes immunoglobulin. As T cells become activated, they express CD40 ligand (CD40L), which binds to CD40 on B cells and activates B cells. B cells in turn then express more CD80 (B7/BB1), which binds to the T cell CD28 receptor. CD28 ligation provides a potent costimulatory signal to T cells, which synergizes with TCR/CD3-derived activational signals. Therefore, there is important bidirectional T and B communication. B-cell-derived immunoglobulins may also regulate T and B immunity through idiotype–antiidiotype interactions. In this case, an antibody recognizes and binds to the polymorphic antigen-binding region of B- or T-cell antigen receptors. The interaction can positively or negatively regulate immunity. Last, the B cell itself may act as an APC. The ability of surface immunoglobulin to bind low concentrations of antigen with high affinity makes B cells particularly efficient APCs. As Fig. 16.13 shows, B cells express the relevant ligands and receptors for direct T-cell interactions. Thus, the T–APC–B ternary complex may really be a T–B binary complex. This is probably the major interaction during secondary responses, when T and B cells are already partially activated and express many of the relevant receptors. For primary responses, CD40L, CD80, CD86, and other receptors are not yet up-regulated, and direct T–B interactions are less efficient. In this case, professional APCs are likely required to initiate appropriate immunity.

Antigen-presenting Cells

It has already been mentioned that virtually any cell type may perform the functions of an APC because many of the steps of processing and presentation take advantage of ubiquitous, constitutive cellular pathways. Most frequently, the term *APC* is applied to monocyte/macrophage or dendritic cells because both express class I and class II MHC, the cells are specialized to take up extracellular components and catabolize them, and these cells are histologically and anatomically located at sites most relevant for antigen entry and recognition. Based on these criteria, B cells are also efficient APCs and are usually most relevant for secondary responses when T cells are already primed or partially activated.

Another cell type of major importance for APC function, particularly in organ allografting, is the vascular endothelial cell (62–71). As discussed earlier, this is the cell that the immune system first comes in contact with and that directs the homing, trafficking, and egress of lymphocytes into regions of inflammation. Vascular endothelial cells are dynamic in their ability to process and present antigen and direct lymphocyte function. Quiescent endothelial cells are far less efficient and active with these processes than activated cells. Activation usually occurs as a result of antigen nonspecific signals during inflammation. Trauma, burns, ischemia, infection, allografting, or any other proinflammatory condition can activate endothelial cells. The signals most relevant for endothelial activation are the cytokines IL-1 and IL-4, tumor necrosis factor (TNF), and bacterial lipopolysaccharide. In turn, activated endothelial cells produce cytokines [IL-1, IL-6, IL-8, IFN-γ, and transforming growth factor (TGF-β)] and display cell surface receptors important for presentation or trafficking [class II MHC, increased class I MHC, vascular cell adhesion molecule-1 (VCAM-1), ELAM-1, and P-selectin]. From the standpoint of transplantation, nonimmunologic events, such as prolonged cold ischemic time or the type of preservation solution, can profoundly affect endothelial cell function and integrity and subsequent lymphocyte–endothelial cell interactions. Despite close tissue matching and good immunosuppression, these nonimmunologic events can activate endothelium, which in turn activates lymphocytes and other leukocytes and facilitates the development of antigen-dependent, immunologic organ rejection.

Adhesion Receptors

An essential feature of lymphocyte communication is the interaction of cell surface receptors with specific ligands (72–78). As shown in Figs. 16.10 and 16.13, a large number of potential interactions among T cells, B cells, APCs, and vascular endothelial cells can occur. Several features are important. First, although these molecules have often been called *adhesion molecules,* most are transmembrane proteins linked to cytoplasmic second messengers. Therefore, receptor engagement is likely to lead to a series of second signals that may alter the transcriptional activation of a wide array of genes and subsequently cellular function. Adhesion is only one function of these molecules.

Although it is possible to describe in detail the individual function of any single receptor–ligand pair, the issue of understanding the integration of many different signals has been a less tractable problem. Figure 16.10 shows current models that assign these receptors to a few related molecular groups and to a few functionally separate steps. Clearly, the immune system has an extraordinary amount of redundancy, so that if a single pathway or receptor–ligand pair is compromised, it is likely other processes circumvent the block.

Adhesion receptors are classified into three major groups based on structural similarities. The *selectins* are transmembrane glycoproteins. The amino-terminal domain is lectin-like in structure. Lectins are molecules that bind carbohydrates. The amino-terminal domain is followed by a domain with homology to epidermal growth factor. This domain is followed by two to nine repeated domains with homology to complement-binding proteins. The ligands for selectins are mucin-like molecules containing large amounts of carbohydrate presumably bound by the lectin domain. Distinct selectins are recognized on leukocytes, platelets, and endothelial cells and termed L-selectins, P-selectins, and E-selectins (Table 16.4). *Integrins* are heterodimeric transmembrane proteins. There are at least eight known integrin β chains that can associate with a wide variety of α chains, generating a large number of possible combinations. The ligands for integrins include many basement membrane components and immunoglobulin gene superfamily members. *Immunoglobulin gene superfamily* members share structural similarities to antibody, particularly tandem extracellular domains each containing a disulfide bond. The ligands for these molecules are often integrin family members. Many cells express both members of the receptor and ligand pair simultaneously. For example, both T and B cells express the selectin LFA-1 (CD11a/CD18) and the immunoglobulin family member ICAM-1 (CD54). How receptor function is regulated such that a cell does not bind to its own surface is not known. Adhesion receptors do not play passive adhesive roles, merely binding ligands that are presented to them. They are involved in more active regulatory processes.

Cytokines and Cytokine Receptors

Immune cells communicate not only by direct cell–cell contact but by soluble factors called *cytokines.* The problem with understanding cytokine action is similar to the problem of defining receptor function. There are so many

Table 16.4. ADHESION RECEPTORS

Molecule	Primary expression	Ligand
SELECTINS		
L-selectin (CD62L)	PMN, lymphocytes	CD34, GlyCAM-1, MAdCAM-1
P-selectin (CD62P)	EC, platelets	P-selectin glycoprotein ligand (PSGL-1)
		Sialyl Lewis^x and others
E-selectin (CD62E)	EC	Sialyl Lewis^x and others
INTEGRINS		
LFA-1 (CD11a/CD18) (β_2, αL)	PMN, lymphocytes	ICAM-1, ICAM-2
Mac-1 (CD11b/CD18) (β_2/αM)	PMN	ICAM-1, IC3b, Fibrinogen, LPS
VLA-4 ($\alpha_4\beta_1$ integrin)	Eosinophils, lymphocytes	VCAM-1, FN

Integrin	Subunits	Ligands and Counterreceptors	Integrin Name
β_1	α_1	Collagens, laminin	VLA-1
	α_2	Collagens, laminin	VLA-2
	α_3	Fibronectin, laminin, collagens	VLA-3
	α_4	Fibronectin, VCAM-1	VLA-4
	α_5	Fibronectin	VLA-5
	α_6	Laminin	VLA-6
	α_7	Laminin	VLA-7
	α_8	?	
	α_V	Vitronectin, fibronectin	
β_2	α_L	ICAM-1, ICAM-2, ICAM-3	LFA-1
	α_M	IC3b, fibrinogen, factor X, ICAM-1	Mac-1
	α_X	Fibrinogen	p150, 95
β_3	α_{IIb}	Fibrinogen, fibronectin, von Willebrand factor, vitronectin, thrombospondin	
	α_V	Vitronectin, fibrinogen, von Willebrand factor, thrombospondin, fibronectin, osteopontin, collagen	
β_4	α_6	?	
β_5	α_V	Vitronectin	
β_6	α_V	Fibronectin	
β_7 (=β_p?)	α_4	Fibronectin, VCAM-1, MAdCAM-1	LPAM-1
	α_{IEL}	?	
β_8	α_V	?	

Molecule	Primary expression	Ligand
IMMUNOGLOBULIN SUPERFAMILY		
ICAM-1 (CD 54)	Lymphocytes, EC	LFA-1, Mac-1
ICAM-2 (CD102)	Lymphocytes, EC	LFA-1
VCAM-1 (CD106)	EC	VLA-4
PECAM-1	EC, PMN, lymphocytes, platelets	?
MAdCAM-1	EC	LPAM-1
CD28	T	CD80 (B7/BB1)
CTLA4	T	CD80, B70/B7-2, B7-3
CD2	T, NK, some B	CD58 (LFA-3), possibly CD59

PMN, polymorphonuclear cell; EC, endothelial cells; T, T cells; NK, natural killer cells; B, B cells; ICAM, intercellular adhesion molecule; PECAM, platelet–endothelial cell adhesion molecule; VCAM, vascular cell adhesion molecule.

known cytokines (Table 16.5) that although individual detailed actions are defined, many of these actions overlap and it is not yet possible to integrate these signals into a unified model (79–102). Furthermore, many different cell types are capable of expressing each cytokine or cytokine receptor. This makes it difficult to define any specificity of cytokine function. Nonetheless, several generalizations have practical implications.

First, the chemoattractant cytokines are important for leukocyte homing and trafficking (Fig. 16.10). Table 16.5 shows that these molecules are categorized according to structural criteria.

Second, the central paradigm of T-cell–APC–B-cell interaction (Fig. 16.11) relies on the production of a few cytokines (Fig. 16.14). The initial CD4+ T-cell–APC interaction results in IL-1 production by APCs, which stimulates CD4+ T cells. These cells then produce IL-2, IL-4, and IL-5. IL-2 and IL-4 help stimulate CD8+ T cells and B cells or even self-stimulate CD4+ T cells by a mechanism termed *autocrine stimulation*. IL-5 primarily helps B cells. Many

other cytokines, however, are involved even in this central paradigm (Fig. 16.12). Blockade of any single cytokine rarely impairs the stimulatory process because other cytokines tend to be redundant.

Third, the distinction between receptors and cytokines is often blurred. Alternative mRNA splicing, posttranslational modifications, or cell surface endopeptidases can convert cell bond receptors into soluble mediators or vice versa. For example, TNF-α can be found as a soluble or cell surface molecule. Cytokine receptors can be processed into soluble fragments that still bind the relevant cytokine. In this case, the soluble receptor may act as an inhibitor of cytokine function because it prevents the interaction of the cytokine with its specific cell surface receptor. Alternatively, these same soluble receptors may prolong the serum half-life of cytokines by preventing proteolytic degradation and may transport the active cytokine to regions of inflammation or antigen presentation. In this case, the soluble receptor potentiates rather than inhibits cytokine function. This situation occurs with a soluble TNF

Table 16.5. **CYTOKINE AND CYTOKINE RECEPTORS**

	Origin	Responding cells
CYTOKINE		
IL-1α or -β	Monocytes, EC	T, B, EC
IL-2	T, B	T, B, monocytes, EC
IL-3	T	T
IL-4	T	T, B, monocytes, mast cells, EC, eosinophils
IL-5	T	T, B, eosinophils
IL-6	T, B, monocytes, EC	T, B, EC
IL-7	T	T, B, monocytes
IL-8	T, EC, monocytes	T, EC, neutrophils
IL-9	T	T, mast cells
IL-10	T	T, B, monocytes
IL-11	Fibroblasts	B, megakaryocytes
IL-12	Monocytes	T, B, NK
IL-13	?	B, monocytes
IL-14	?	B
IFN-α or -β	EC	T, B, EC
IFN-t	T, B	T, B, EC
TNF-a	T, B, EC	T, B, EC
TNF-β	T	T, B, EC
G-CSF	Fibroblasts, osteoblasts	Granulocytes
GM-CSF	T	Granulocytes, monocytes
M-CSF	Fibroblasts, monocytes	Monocytes
Classic Chemoattractants		
N-formyl peptide	Bacterial	Monocytes, granulocytes
C5a	Complement activation	Monocytes, granulocytes
LTB4	Arachidonate metabolism	Monocytes, neutrophils
PAF	Phosphotidylcholine metabolism	Monocytes, granulocytes
C-X-C Chemokines		
IL-8	T, EC, monocytes	T, EC, neutrophils
β-Thromboglobulin	Platelets	T, granulocytes
C-C Chemokines		
MCP-1	T, EC, monocytes	Monocytes
MIP-1a, β	T, monocytes	T, monocytes, granulocytes
RANTES	T, platelets	Monocytes

CYTOKINE RECEPTORS

Type 1 Cytokine Receptors (Hematopoietin Receptors)

IL-2, -4, -7, -9, -13, -15 receptors (share γ-chain)
IL-3, -5, GM-CSF receptors (share KH97 subunit)
LIF, OSM, CNTF, IL-6, IL-1 l receptors (share gp130 subunit)
GH, PRL
EPO, G-CSF

Type II Cytokine Receptors

IFN-α, -β, -γ

TNF-Like Receptors

TNF-α, TNF-β receptors
gp39 (CD30-L)
CD27-L, CD30-L
NGF, 4-1BB
Fas

TGF-β Receptor Family

TGF-β1, TGF-βII receptors (share common TSR-I subunit)
Activin receptor-II, -IIβ

IL-8 Receptor Family (Seven-Membrane Spanner, G-Linked Proteins)

IL-8R
C5a-R
PAF-R
fMLP-R

EC, endothelial cells; T, T cells; B, B cells; (G, GM, M)-CSF, (granulocyte, granulocyte–monocyte, macrophage) colony-stimulating factor; IL, interleukin; IFN, interferon; TNF, tumor necrosis factor; NGF, nerve growth factor; PAF, platelplet activating factor; GH, growth hormone; PRL, prolactin; EPO, erythropoietin; LIF, leukocyte inhibitory factors; OSM, oncostatin M; CNTF, ciliary neutrophic factor.

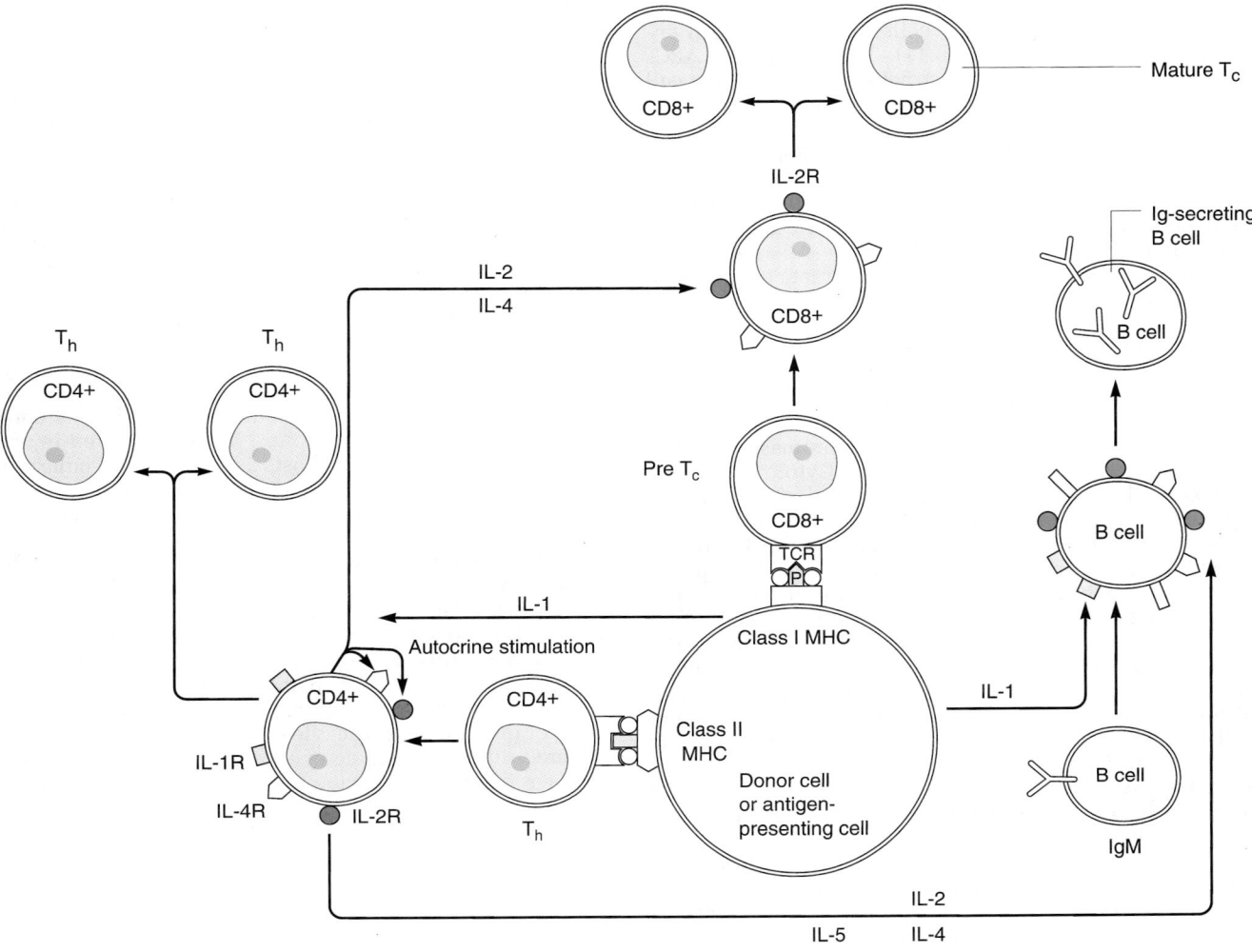

Figure 16.14. T- and B-cell activation. Two signals are required. First, alloantigen binds to antigen-specific receptors–the T-cell receptor (TCR; T cells) or surface immunoglobulin M (IgM; B cells). The second, or costimulatory, signal is provided by interleukin (IL)-1 released by the antigen-presenting cell. CD4+ helper T cells (T_H) release IL-2, IL-4, and IL-5, which provide help for CD8+ cytotoxic T cells (T_C) and for B-cell activation. MHC, major histocompatibility complex.

receptor. Soluble forms of the TCR and class I MHC molecules have also been described. Although their physiologic roles are uncertain, both suppressor and activator functions have been ascribed to these molecules. Likewise, B-cell immunoglobulin may be cell bound and act as the B-cell antigen-specific receptor, or circulate freely as soluble antibody performing a variety of immune regulatory or effector functions.

Fourth, cytokine receptors are often heteromeric complexes sharing common subunits with other cytokine receptors and possessing unique, but related, subunits that confer specificity for an individual cytokine. Genetic or pharmacologic interference with receptor function may therefore impair the effects of only one or of several cytokines. For example, the IL-2, IL-4, IL-7, IL-9, IL-13, and IL-15 receptors all have related cytokine-specific subunits and share a common γ subunit. The same is true for the IL-6, IL-11, leukemia inhibitory factor (LIF), oncostatin M (OSM), and ciliary neurotrophic factor (CNTF) receptors; and the IL-3, IL-5, and granulocyte–monocyte colony-stimulating factor (GM-CSF) receptors.

EFFECTOR MECHANISMS OF THE IMMUNE RESPONSE

Cellular Effectors

Once primed and activated, T cells, B cells, and APCs perform the effector functions of graft rejection (103–110). B cells secrete specific antibody that binds to the allograft cell surface and can kill cells by complement-mediated lysis. Antibody may also alter graft cell function by binding to and cross-linking important cell surface receptors, causing receptor blockade, receptor activation, or inappropriate cellular responses. Antibody may also direct other cells, which possess receptors for the constant region of the immunoglobulin molecule, termed *Fc receptors* (FcRs), to the allogenic cells. Many cell types express FcRs, including T cells, APCs, natural killer (NK) cells, and granulocytes. These FcR+ cells may damage or kill cells with antibody bound to the cell surface by a process called *antibody-dependent cellular cytotoxicity.*

Monocytes and macrophages, the prototypical APCs, become activated by CD4+ T cells during the initial encounter with antigen (Fig. 16.11). These activated APCs can then cause local tissue destruction through direct cell lysis and phagocytosis or indirectly through release of cytotoxic cytokines (e.g., TNF and lymphotoxin). CD4+ T cells can also generate local tissue destruction through inflammatory processes similar to delayed-type hypersensitivity. Cytotoxic lymphokines are released, and other inflammatory cells, such as APCs, are recruited to the local environment.

Cytotoxic CD8+ T lymphocytes kill target cells through direct cell contact. Killer T cells have cytoplasmic granules containing a series of cytotoxic proteins. Contact with a target cell causes the release of these granules onto or into the target. Granule contents include perforins, which assemble to form pores in the target cell membrane, making the cells leaky and susceptible to osmotic death. Granzymes are a series of serine proteases that can disrupt normal intracellular proteins. Cytotoxic T cells also kill cells by engaging a target cell surface receptor called *Fas,* a member of the TNF receptor family (Table 16.5). The interaction of the Fas ligand on the T-cell surface with Fas on the target cell surface leads to apoptotic target cell death. Fas and Fas ligand are distributed not only throughout the immune system but on many other cell types. Fas is probably a general mechanism for determining cellular responses to development, immune activation, and oncogenesis. The regulation and control of the cellular response to engagement of Fas by its ligand involves a poorly understood series of cytoplasmic events comprising second messenger pathways and transcriptional regulators. Delineation of these events will probably lead to important methods for controlling cytotoxic responses.

In addition to the aforementioned cells, a number of other cell types probably also participate in the process of graft destruction and rejection, although their precise roles are not well understood. NK cells are large granular lymphocytes lacking immunoglobulin and most T-cell surface markers (111,112). They do, however, express CD2 (characteristic of T cells) and a subclass of FcR known as CD16, which is characteristic of some B cells. NK cells also express the IL-2 receptor, secrete numerous cytokines (IL-1, IL-2, IL-3, IL-4, IL-6, GM-CSF, TNF, IFN-α, IFN-γ), and produce cytotoxic granzymes and phospholipases. NK cells function by lysing target cells that lack MHC class I. The mechanism by which NK cells recognize targets is through a series of nonclonally distributed receptors that inhibit NK cells if MHC class I is bound, while permitting NK mediated lysis if the receptor is unoccupied. The precise role of NK cells in allograft rejection is not understood, but these cells may be found infiltrating rejecting grafts, and it is presumed they are recruited to the inflammatory site.

Eosinophils are classically found throughout acutely rejecting allografts. Their role and function in graft rejection is also not understood, but they do perform potent cytotoxic effector functions. IL-5, which is secreted by CD4+ T$_H$2 cells, is a potent trophic cytokine for eosinophils. The process of T-cell activation may therefore recruit eosinophils to rejecting grafts (113).

Other cell types, including neutrophils, basophils, and mast cells, can also be found in rejecting grafts or other inflammatory processes (114,115). These cells are presumably recruited to regions of inflammation by cytokines and changes in vascular endothelium. These cells have direct cytotoxic effects, produce cytotoxic cytokines, and recruit additional cells to their locality.

Soluble Effectors

The soluble cytokines have been discussed thus far in terms of promoting homing and trafficking, inducing antigen-specific immunity, and amplifying immune responses. Cytokines also participate directly in the process of inflammation or graft destruction (116–124). TNF-α and TNF-β have direct cytotoxic effects on parenchymal cells and may help mediate the final effector pathway. Many other cytokines (e.g., IL-2, IL-4, IL-5, IL-6, IL-10, and IFN-γ) can be found in rejecting allografts. These cytokines are probably not directly cytotoxic, but recruit additional cells and amplify those already present.

Many other soluble mediators are probably also involved in allograft destruction. Antibody-directed, complement-mediated lysis is an important mechanism in hyperacute and some forms of acute rejection (125). Clotting factors are activated when vascular endothelium is compromised by antibody, cytokines, or cell-mediated injury. Obviously, vascular thrombosis is lethal to vascularized organ allografts. Injured vessels may also release the potent vasoconstricting peptide endothelin, further decreasing blood flow to injured grafts (126). Kinins, prostaglandins, and prostacyclins may all participate in the effector stage of the inflammatory response, serving to potentiate cellular injury or recruit more proinflammatory cells (127). Oxygen intermediates, such as nitric oxide and oxygen free radicals, are also likely important mediators of tissue destruction in transplantation (128–131). So many potential mediators of cellular death make it difficult to control the process at the effector stage. Strategies that interfere with only a single cytotoxic pathway are unlikely to have major therapeutic effects. It will be necessary to subvert many effector pathways or to block initiation processes further upstream of effector mechanisms.

Clinical Syndromes

The wide variety of immune effector mechanisms results in a limited number of defined presentations in clinical transplantation (Figs. 16.15 to 16.18). The pathologic definition of these presentations is defined by the Banff classification system. *Hyperacute rejection* is the result of preformed antibody binding to the allograft at the time of revascularization in the operating room. Complement is activated, resulting in endothelial cell activation, vascular leak, recruitment of platelets and neutrophils, thrombosis of vessels, and destruction of the graft within minutes to hours. Hyperacute rejection can occur if transplantations are performed across an ABO incompatibility or if the recipient possesses high-titer antidonor class I HLA antibodies (132). Because current clinical protocols test for the presence of such incompatibilities or antibodies (see Important Aspects of Antigenicity and Immunity for Clinical Transplantation), hyperacute rejection should not occur. Kidney, heart, pancreas, and lung allografts are all susceptible to hyperacute rejection; however, liver grafts are relatively resistant to this process and are often transplanted across antibody differences (termed a *positive crossmatch*) and even across an ABO difference. The reason for this resistance is not understood but may relate to the large mass of hepatic parenchyma and its ability to absorb antibody and complement, or to the way antibody and complement interact with hepatic endothelium and its dual blood supply. In addition, hyperacute rejection is responsible for the major barrier to xenotransplantation (across-species barrier) (133). Most mammals have high-titer, preformed antibodies directed against cell surface antigens of other species. The current challenge in experimental xenotrans-

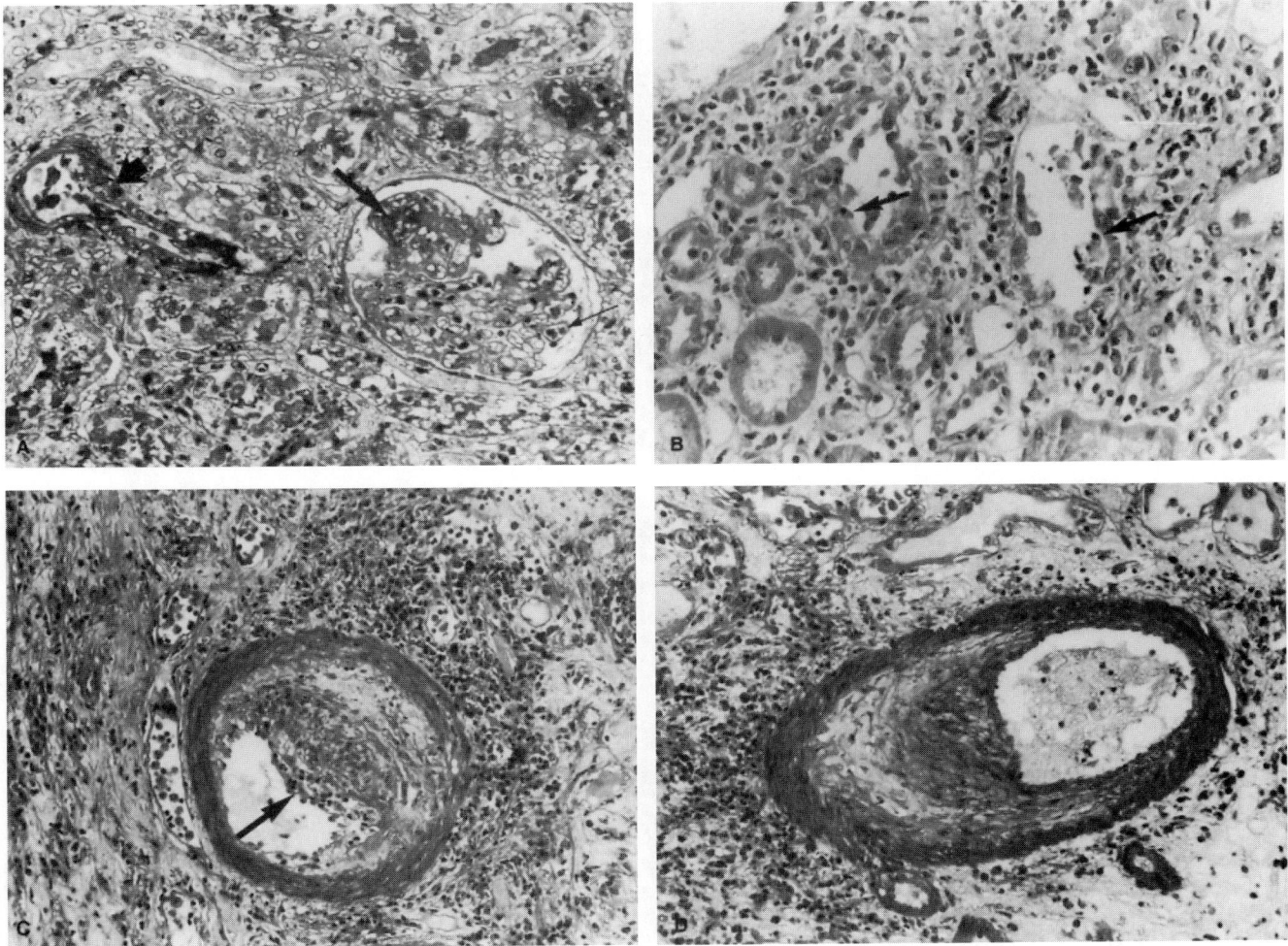

Figure 16.15. Kidney rejection. *(A)* Hyperacute rejection characterized by microthrombi in the glomerular capillaries *(large arrow)*, infiltration with neutrophils *(small thin arrow)*, and endothelial destruction *(thick arrow)*. *(B)* Acute tubulointerstitial rejection showing an interstitial lymphocytic infiltrate, interstitial edema, and infiltration of lymphocytes into the epithelium of the tubules (tubulitis; *arrow*). *(C)* Acute vascular rejection with a subendothelial lymphocytic infiltrate *(arrow)*, along with some evidence of chronic vascular rejection. *(D)* Chronic rejection with severe proliferative endarteritis. (Courtesy of Roger D. Smith, M.D.).

plantation is to control antibody and complement function and prevent hyperacute rejection.

Acute rejection usually occurs days to weeks after transplantation; it rarely occurs months or years later. Acute rejection is initiated by T-cell-dependent immunity and is characterized microscopically by a lymphocytic infiltrate accompanied by plasma cells, eosinophils, and a few mast cells or neutrophils. In the kidney, the infiltrate is in the tubular interstitium, causing a tubulitis. Particularly severe forms also cause a vasculitis or vascular rejection. Hepatic acute cellular rejection is typically a mixed cellular infiltrate in the portal triad with eosinophils, disruption of biliary endothelium, and portal venous endothelialitis. The heart demonstrates an interstitial lymphocytic myositis, whereas the lung shows varying degrees of peribronchiolar and perivascular lymphocytic infiltration. Most clinical immunosuppressive agents are directed toward T cells and preventing or treating acute rejections.

Chronic rejection usually occurs months to years after transplantation. It is characterized by loss of normal histologic structure, fibrosis, and atherosclerosis. Renal chronic rejection demonstrates interstitial fibrosis, tubular and glomerular loss, and vascular obliteration. Hepatic chronic rejection is characterized by portal fibrosis and the disappearance of bile ducts (ductopenia or vanishing bile duct syndrome). Accelerated graft atherosclerosis is the cardinal manifestation with hearts, and bronchiolitis obliterans indicates chronic pulmonary rejection. Chronic rejection is a major cause of graft failure and patient loss with all organs (134). The problem with understanding and eventually treating and preventing chronic rejection is that it undoubtedly represents the final common pathologic pathway of a variety of insults. Thus, repeated bouts of rejection, drug toxicity, recurrent infections (e.g., pneumonias in lung transplants or cholangitis in liver transplants), chronic obstruction (ureter, bile ducts, pancreatic duct), severe ischemic damage to donor organs at the time of transplantation, use of older or suboptimal organ donors, or patient noncompliance with the immunosuppressive regimen can all contribute to a pathologic diagnosis of chronic rejection. Preventing chronic rejection requires attention to each of these problems. Nonetheless, a feature common to all types of chronic rejection is vascular atherosclerosis and obliteration with intragraft expres-

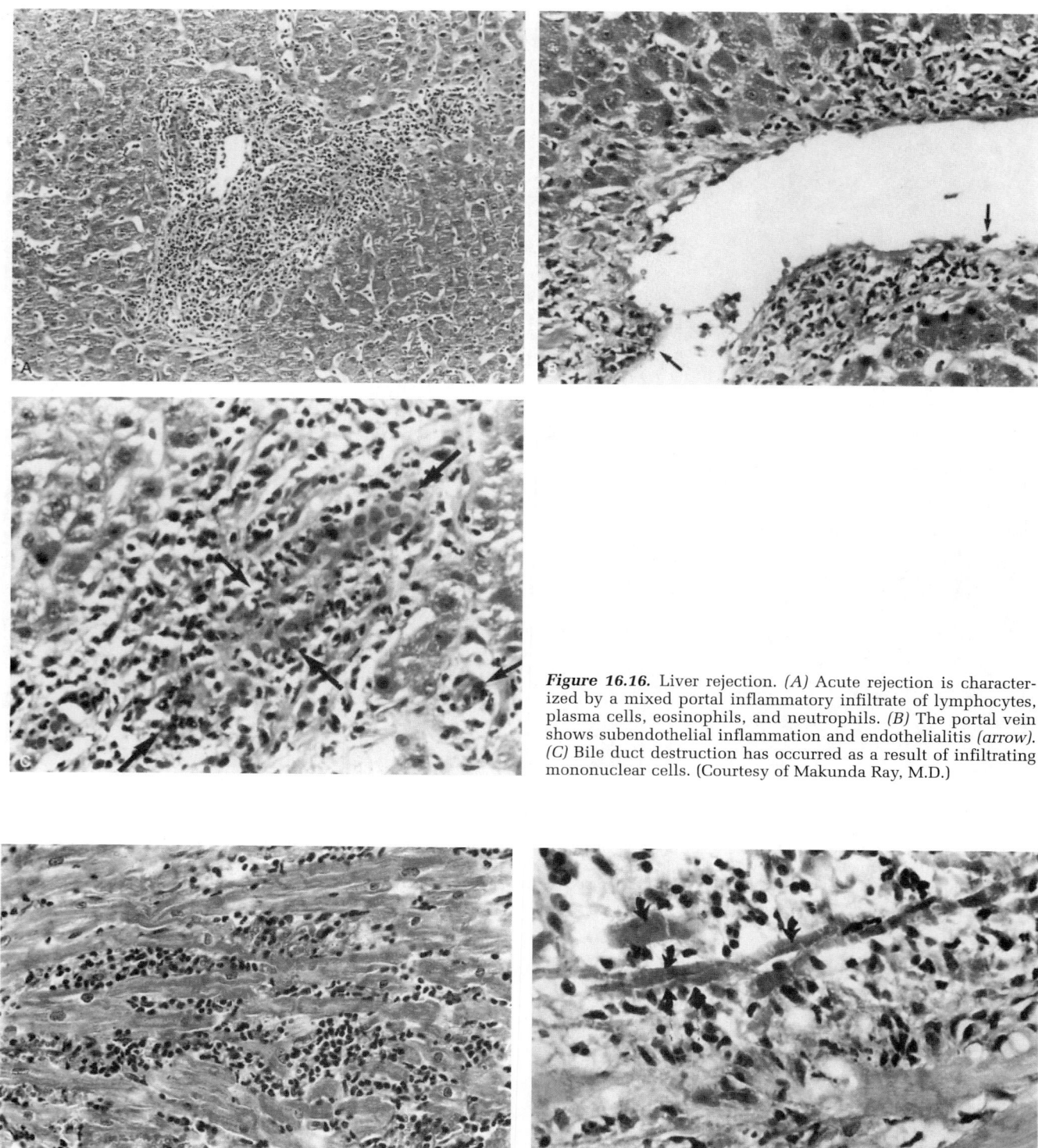

Figure 16.16. Liver rejection. *(A)* Acute rejection is character-ized by a mixed portal inflammatory infiltrate of lymphocytes, plasma cells, eosinophils, and neutrophils. *(B)* The portal vein shows subendothelial inflammation and endothelialitis *(arrow)*. *(C)* Bile duct destruction has occurred as a result of infiltrating mononuclear cells. (Courtesy of Makunda Ray, M.D.)

Figure 16.17. Heart rejection. Severe rejection manifests as a diffuse lymphocytic infiltrate with neutrophils and hemorrhage in the interstitium and myocyte necrosis *(arrows)*. (Courtesy of Jeff Safitz, M.D.)

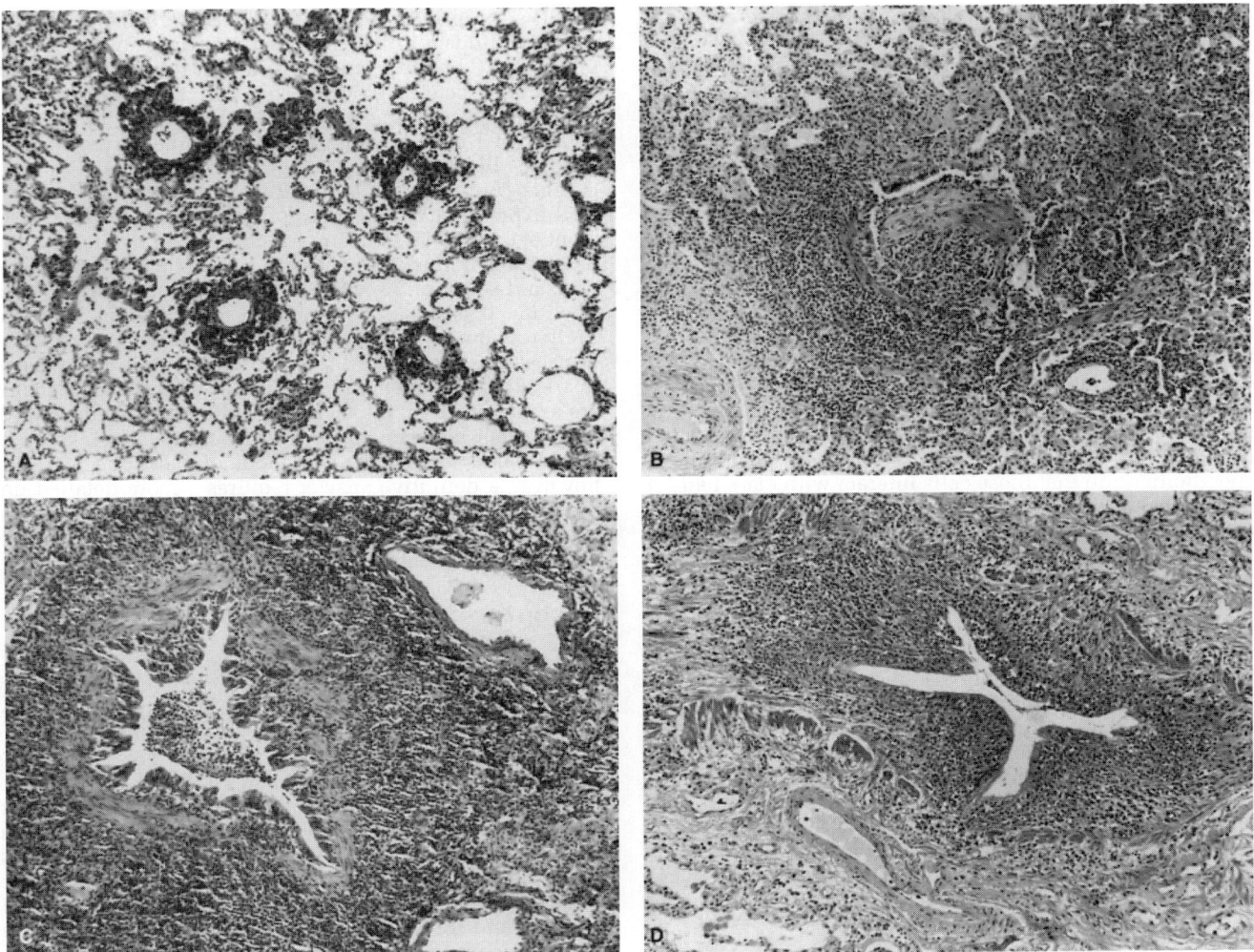

Figure 16.18. Lung rejection. *(A)* Mild acute rejection with a perivascular mononuclear infiltrate around small venules and arterioles. *(B)* With progression to moderate rejection, extension of the infiltrate into the alveolar septa occurs. *(C)* In severe rejection, there is a diffuse perivascular, interstitial, and peribronchiolar infiltrate with abundant fibrin, red blood cells, and neutrophils in the air spaces. *(D)* Bronchiolitis obliterans is the result of chronic rejection and is characterized by narrowing of the bronchioles from scarring. A mild mononuclear infiltrate is still present. (Courtesy of Samuel A. Yousem, M.D., University of Pittsburgh, Pittsburgh, PA.)

sion of certain cytokines and adhesion molecules, such as IL-1, IL-6, TNF-α, and ICAM-1 (135). Methods to prevent chronic rejection may come from a better understanding of vascular biology and how cytokines affect the process of atherosclerosis (136).

REGULATION OF THE IMMUNE RESPONSE

Development of Lymphocytes

The preceding sections have outlined the major molecular and cellular interactions that occur on primary antigenic stimulation and show that different responses, cell types, and molecular entities may be involved. Superimposed on these pathways, however, are several layers of complex immune regulation that result from a variety of cellular interactions. It is important not only that the immune system respond to antigen but that the response is of the appropriate magnitude, type, and duration and that responses to self (i.e., autoimmunity) are avoided (137). The

regulatory processes that control these parameters have important implications for transplantation tolerance and immunosuppression.

The primary determinants of T- and B-cell receptor specificity occur during early lymphocyte development in the bone marrow and thymus (138–144). When developing, immature T or B cells come in contact with self-antigen in these compartments, antigen binds to those cells that possess receptors for self, and the cells are tolerized. The next problem to consider is what happens to cells that are not exposed to self-antigens in these central lymphoid compartments because the antigen is expressed only in the periphery. When lymphocytes mature, migrate to the periphery, and come in contact with these antigens, what prevents subsequent autoimmune responses? There are several levels of control of this process. First, newly emerging lymphocytes are susceptible to tolerizing signals in the periphery, so contact with self-antigen shortly after egress from the bone marrow or thymus can also lead to appropriate nonresponsiveness. Second, because B-cell responses are T-cell dependent, if the T cell is tolerant, the B cell does not respond to the autoantigen. Third, many autoantigens are not expressed on, and therefore not presented by, professional APCs. This results in a failure of appropriate presentation so that T cells cannot "see" the antigen; TCRs may be engaged but tolerance, instead of immunity, ensues.

The problem of T-cell maturation is actually more complex than what was discussed earlier in this chapter. As noted, the TCR is selected to recognize altered self or a foreign peptide loaded into the antigen-binding groove of class I or II self-MHC. The cellular and molecular processes by which this occurs are the subject of intense current investigations and represent one of the major intellectual challenges in immunology. As T cells mature in the thymus, they sequentially acquire β TCR, α TCR, and CD4 and CD8 cell surface receptors. This is accompanied by migration from medullary to cortical regions of the thymus and by extensive proliferation and *loss* of most thymocytes. Numerous experimental studies have revealed that the maturing T cell expresses TCRs of multitudinous specificities and that these cells interact with class I and II molecules on the thymic epithelium. A very strong interaction between a developing T cell and the thymic epithelium indicates autoimmunity and leads to negative selection of those T cells by a process called *programmed cell death,* or *apoptosis.* This is probably responsible for the massive thymocyte loss seen in the normal thymus. Alternatively, complete failure of the T cell to interact with the thymic epithelium probably also results in negative selection by failure to stimulate these developing T cells.

However, a low-affinity interaction between the T cell and the thymic epithelium results in T-cell stimulation, positive selection, and proliferative expansion of those T cells. Thus, these regulatory processes select T cells that have a low affinity for self-peptides and self-MHC (Fig. 16.19). Presumably then, these cells have a higher affinity for allogenic peptides and self-MHC and are able to respond appropriately to antigen. These same cells are also able fortuitously to recognize self-peptides in the context of allo-MHC and allogenic peptides in the context of allo-MHC. This focuses attention again on the fact that T cells are obsessed with the MHC and on why such a high percentage of T cells in an unselected population responds to a single allogenic MHC.

A major unresolved issue in thymic selection of T cells is TCR expression. The process of assortment and rearrangement of α and β V-D-J regions, accompanied by the addition of N regions, must interact with the maturation, proliferation, and selection processes at the level of the thymic epithelium. It is unclear whether TCR expression is an entirely random, stochastic process with subsequent positive or negative selection of T cells or whether there may be an instructional component such that as TCR β and α chains are expressed, they interact with epithelial ligands and direct further assortment and rearrangement of receptor genes. There is evidence for both of these mechanisms; however, a definitive answer requires a more detailed understanding of the precise regulatory and transcriptional mechanisms that connect cell surface TCR receptors to TCR gene rearrangements and expression in the nucleus.

Receptor-driven Stimulation of T and B Responses

The ultimate control of all antigen- and developmentally driven responses depends on a series of receptor–ligand interactions at the cell surface. For B cells, this comprises antigen and cell surface immunoglobulin. For T cells, this includes antigen, TCR, MHC, and CD4 and CD8 interactions. However, these signals usually are not enough completely to stimulate T- and B-cell proliferation, maturation, and effector function. B cells require additional ligands, such as the soluble cytokines IL-2, IL-4, and IL-5. Likewise, T cells also require cytokines, such as IL-1, IL-2, IL-4, IFN-γ, IL-10, and IL-12 (Figs. 16.12 and 16.14). T cells also require the simultaneous or sequential engagement of multiple coreceptors (Fig. 16.13) to become fully activated. CD4 and CD8 are the primary coreceptors, and their engagement is usually absolutely required for T-cell responses. Another major coreceptor is CD28 and the closely related receptor CTLA4 (145,146). The ligands for these receptors are CD80 (B7-1) and CD86 (B7-2). Both receptors can bind both ligands. Blockade of these particular receptor–ligand interactions can prevent T-cell stimulation and cause tolerance to antigen. These pathways are being investigated as a way to produce clinical transplantation tolerance. Additional coreceptors that are important for activation include CD2, CD29/CD49d [very late antigen-4 (VLA-4)] and CD11a/CD18 (LFA-1). Their ligands are CD58 (LFA-3), VCAM-1, and CD54 (ICAM-1), respectively. Despite the description of a large number of important receptor–ligand interactions, there is no unified view of hierarchy among the receptors or of combinations of stimulated receptors that may eventuate a given type of response.

Understanding receptor-driven stimulation and engagement of multiple coreceptors is ultimately the biochemical problem of elucidating the cytoplasmic second messenger pathways and transcriptional transactivators and repressors activated by each receptor or receptor combination. Numerous second messenger pathways, including G proteins, phospholipid and inositol phosphate metabolism, calcium currents, protein phosphorylation, and cyclic adenosine monophosphate (cAMP) metabolism have been described, and many of these are dealt with in other chapters in this text.

For T cells, recent investigations have outlined major signaling pathways important for cellular activation

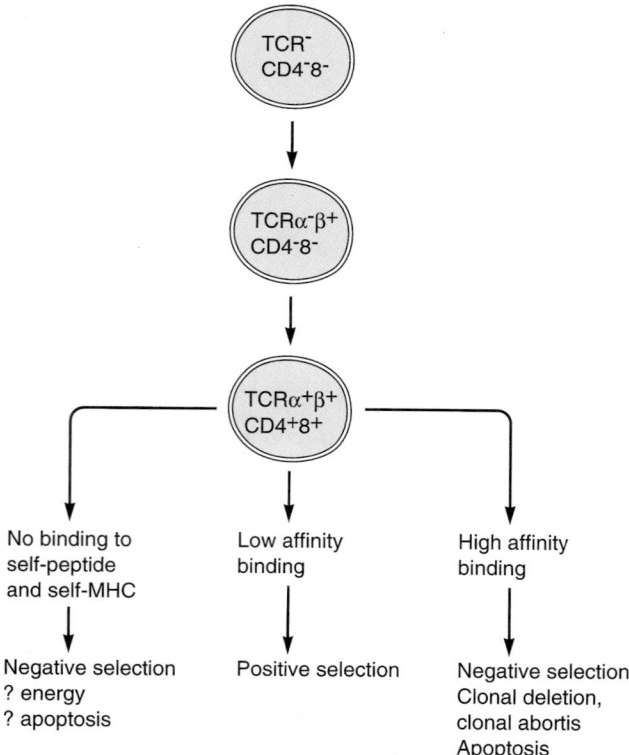

Figure 16.19. Thymic selection of developing T cells. MHC, major histocompatibility complex; TCR, T-cell receptor.

(147–150) (Fig. 16.20). Engagement of TCR/CD3–CD4/8 by antigen–MHC results in the activation and phosphorylation of TCR/CD3 by associated protein tyrosine kinases (PTKs) called p56^{lck}, p59^{fyn}, and ZAP-70. ZAP-70 is a member of the Syk family of PTKs, whereas p56^{lck} and p59^{fyn} are members of the Src family. Phosphorylation of specific cytoplasmic tyrosines of the TCR/CD3 complex enables the receptor to bind an adapter protein, Grb2. Grb2 binds specific phosphorylated tyrosine residues by its Src-homology two (SH2) domain. Grb2 then binds to another protein, Sos, by its SH3 domain. The Grb2 SH3 domain recognizes a proline-rich region on Sos. This complex in turn activates the Ras–guanosine diphosphate complex, causing nucleotide exchange to the activated Ras–guanosine triphosphate (GTP) form. Ras–GTP then activates the Raf-1 serine-threonine kinase. Raf-1 then activates a series of downstream serine-threonine kinases termed MAPKKK, MAPKK (or MEK), and MAPK (for microtubule-associated protein kinase). These downstream kinases serve effector functions by modifying cytoplasmic structural or enzymatic proteins or modifying cytoplasmic transcriptional factors that subsequently translocate to the nucleus. Several levels of control of this cascade are beginning to be elucidated; in particular, cAMP negatively regulates Raf-1 kinase. Thus, two major signaling systems are linked by this recently described interaction. Once an understanding is achieved about what signaling pathways are activated by each T-cell coreceptor, a hierarchy or classification scheme may be possible in which blockade or activation of particular receptors or combinations of receptors will reliably produce specific gene activation or inactivation and tolerance.

The PTKs activate phospholipase Cγ1 (PLC-γ1), which catalyzes the hydrolysis of phosphatidylinositol biphosphate (PIP$_2$) to inositol triphosphate (IP$_3$) and diacylglycerol (DG). IP$_3$ increases intracellular calcium and activates the cytoplasmic protein tyrosine phosphatase, calcineurin. Calcineurin dephosphorylates tyrosines on the inactive cytoplasmic nuclear factor of activated T cells (NF-AT$_c$). The now activated, dephosphorylated NF-AT$_c$ is translocated to the nucleus, where it complexes with nuclear subunits (NF-AT$_n$) and acts as a transcriptional regu-

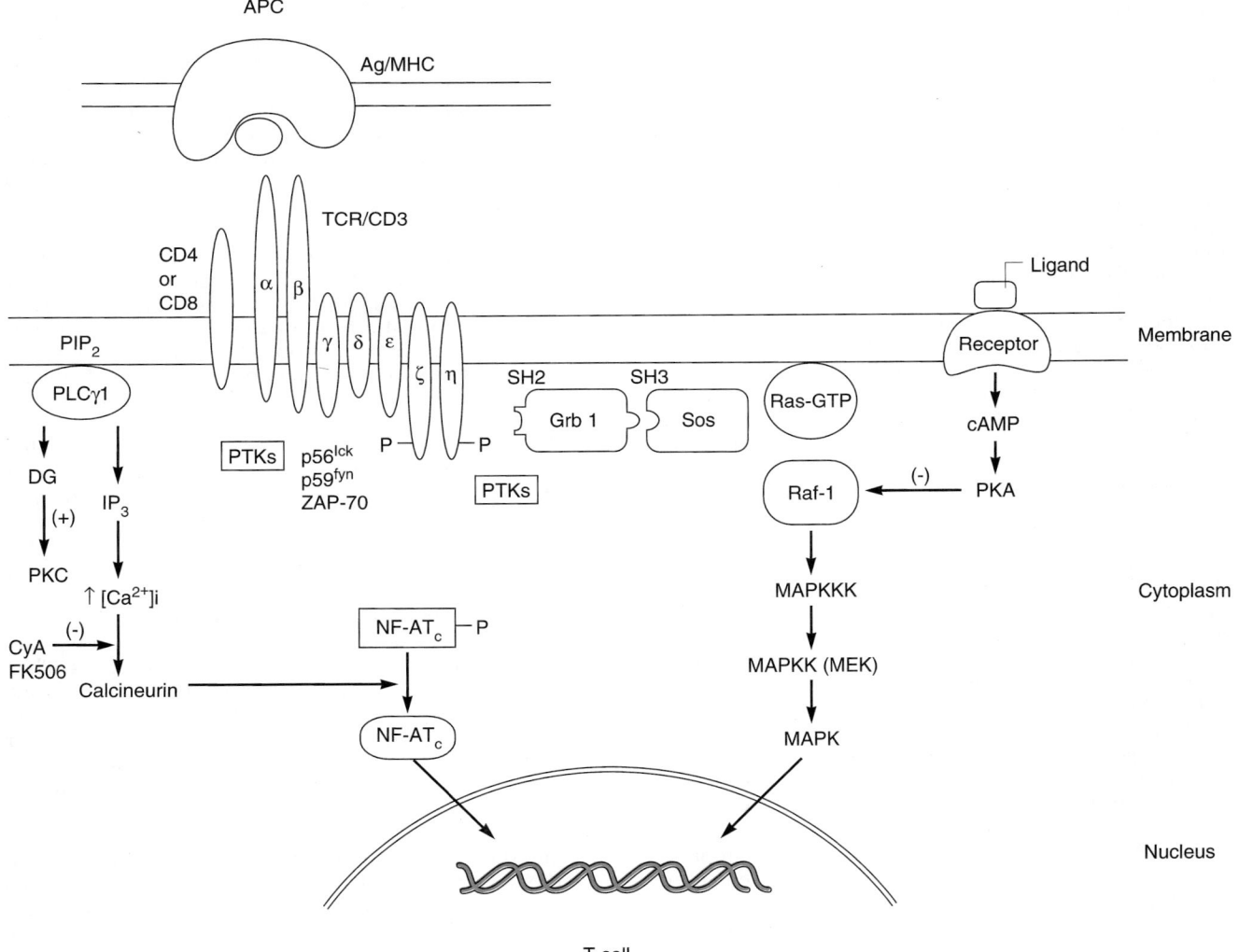

Figure 16.20. Signaling pathways of activated T cells. Ag, antigen; APC, antigen-presenting cell; cAMP, cyclic adenosine monophosphate; CyA, cyclosporine; DG, diacylglycerol; FK506, tacrolimus; IP$_3$, inositol triphosphate; MAPK, microtubule-associated protein kinase; MHC, major histocompatibility complex; NF-AT$_c$, inactive cytoplasmic nuclear factor of activated T cells; PIP$_2$, phosphatidylinositol biphosphate; PKA, protein kinase A; PKC, protein kinase C; PLCγ1, phospholipase Cγ1; PTK, protein tyrosine kinase; SH, Src-homology domain; TCR, T-cell receptor.

lator. This pathway is not only linked to the other important pathways but is blocked by the immunosuppressive agents cyclosporine and tacrolimus.

Tolerance

The term *tolerance* is applied to a variety of different circumstances and therefore presents a semantic problem depending on context. Tolerance usually refers to whole-animal or -organism responses observed experimentally or clinically. It is a functional and not a mechanistic observation. The usual criteria for tolerance include long-term graft acceptance without the need for chronic immunosuppression. In addition, a second donor-specific allograft (i.e., of the same MHC type as the original donor) should also be accepted without the need for additional immunosuppression. The most desirable end point from a clinical view would be true tolerance; however, this is virtually never achieved clinically and achieved only with difficulty experimentally. From a practical standpoint, long-term graft acceptance with minimal chronic immunosuppression, regardless of responses to subsequent second grafts, would be highly desirable and of enormous clinical benefit.

When the term *tolerance* is applied to cellular analyses of lymphocytes, it is again a functional and not a mechanistic description. T and B lymphocytes can be tolerant or nonresponsive to antigen in a variety of specific ways (150–157). *Clonal abortion* refers to the developmental process whereby nascent T- and B-cell clones that recognize autoantigen with high affinity are eliminated. Evidence suggests that at this developmental stage, high-affinity engagement of the antigen-specific receptor and coreceptors leads to second messenger events resulting in apoptosis. In the case of T cells, the complete failure to engage the TCR/CD3 complex may likewise lead to apoptotic clonal elimination.

Clonal deletion can encompass the process of clonal abortion, but it also refers to the elimination of mature T and B cell clones. There are probably several specific cellular and molecular mechanisms responsible for this process. Prolonged or excessive stimulation of the antigen receptor can eventually cause lymphocyte death. Antiidiotype antibodies can eliminate idiotype-positive clones. Suppressor cells may kill or deliver cytotoxic signals to certain antigen-reactive clones. Costimulatory blockade may also result in clonal deletion.

Clonal anergy is a state in which potentially reactive clones and their receptors are physically present but fail to respond to antigen. Anergy may also be the result of several distinct mechanisms, including prolonged receptor stimulation, receptor down-modulation, idiotype–antiidiotype interactions, suppressor cells, and inappropriate APC function in which coreceptor or cytokine function is blocked.

Suppression usually refers to an active process in which a leukocyte or its soluble products inhibit the development or effector function of immune lymphocytes. CD8+ and CD4+ T cells, B cells, macrophages, NK cells, and other cell types have all been shown to act as suppressor cells in certain experimental systems. Given the cellular interactions that can take place during lymphocyte recruitment (Figs. 16.11 and 16.14), it could be anticipated that each interactive site could be a locus for suppression. Given the number of mechanistic possibilities for clonal deletion and clonal anergy, it is also likely that numerous cells could be involved in suppression. Current models of immune regulation suggest that the T_H1/T_H2 dichotomy (Fig. 16.12) may explain much of suppression and be used in practical clinical settings. Thus, IL-10 can be used to suppress allograft responses, and IL-12 can be used to boost anticancer responses.

The term *split tolerance* is used to describe a state in which some responses to alloantigen are suppressed or deleted while other responses remain intact. This is likely a reflection of more detailed cellular analyses of tolerant states where anergy or suppression are dominant mechanisms. Likewise, T cells may proliferate or produce some cytokines, such as IL-2, in response to specific alloantigen but may be unable to generate cytotoxic effector cells because of anergy.

The major problem in clinical transplantation is that despite the detailed description of a large number of potential molecular and cellular mechanisms for inducing and maintaining tolerance, or some type of relative nonresponsiveness, it is not yet possible reliably and reproducibly to control any of these mechanisms in clinical settings. Our ability to induce tolerance will likely rely on a complete understanding of intracellular activational pathways (Fig. 16.20).

Potential Loci for Inducing Nonresponsiveness

The molecular, cellular, and tissue-specific organization of immune development and responses suggests there are a number of discrete steps suitable for interventions designed to promote tolerance or immunosuppression. The thymus is the primary site for T-cell development and for positive and negative selection of specific T-cell clones, depending on the clonotypic expression of the TCR. If specific alloantigen could be placed in the thymus, this could redirect TCR selection and produce tolerance. This has been achieved in experimental models by injecting the recipient thymus with donor-derived cells (158–160). The problem with applying this to humans is the relatively involuted characteristic of the adult thymus. This may be approachable with thymotropic hormones. Nonetheless, the principle remains that thymic presentation of alloantigen "teaches" developing T cells to recognize that alloantigen as self.

The bone marrow is the primary site for B-cell development, and there is some evidence that precursor T cells can be tolerized to some antigens at this stage. In addition, bone marrow precursors populate the thymus. Protocols that attempt to replace part or all of the bone marrow stem cell and precursor population with donor-derived cells should induce tolerance to donor alloantigen (161). In addition, partial replacement of the stem cell compartment results in chimerism, or a state in which both donor- and recipient-derived cells coexist in lymphoid organs. There is much interest in protocols that combine parenchymal organ grafting with bone marrow or stem cell transplantation (162–164). Although these approaches are still experimental, there is evidence that some patients with very long-surviving allografts, who receive minimal or no immunosuppression, have stable low-level chimerism of lymphoid cells (165).

The APC is an absolute requirement for proper T-cell activation. Techniques that alter APC function may induce T_H2 suppressor cells, anergy, or tolerance rather than T_H1 helper cells, CD8+ cytotoxic T cells, or graft rejection. One approach to this is the isolation of specialized APC subpopulations that channel T-cell responses in one direction or another (166). Another approach is the use of ultraviolet B irradiation, which can disrupt APC function and produce suppression or anergy. The problem with both of these methods is that it is not possible to replace, or expose to physical agents, all the APCs in an individual. A more rational approach will be the use of APC receptor–ligand-disrupting agents.

The major intellectual and scientific directions in immunology have been the understanding of the molecular events of receptor–ligand interactions, second messenger pathways, and transcriptional regulation. New immunosuppressive drugs will likely be designed to interact with these pathways. For example, it is now known that cyclosporine and tacrolimus act primarily by inhibiting the NF-AT transcriptional activator. Other potentially promising agents under development are molecules that block the major CD28/CTLA4–CD80/CD86 and CD40–CD40L costimulatory pathways of T cells (167–171). Approaches to support the preferential production of the T_H2 immunosuppressive cytokine IL-10 or disrupt the TCR–antigen–MHC interaction are also under investigation.

Clinical Immunosuppression

Despite the tremendous knowledge of immune regulation, current immunosuppressive regimens used for clinical transplantation are based on empirically derived protocols, using agents such as azathioprine and corticosteroids developed in the 1960s, cyclosporine A developed in the 1970s, and mycophenolate and tacrolimus developed in the 1980s and 1990s (Table 16.6). Newer, more rationally designed drugs are being subjected to clinical trials and several may soon receive approval. Protocols for immunosuppression vary widely from one transplantation center to another and even within a center from one organ to another. The major principle of immunosuppression is to *induce* the patient with high doses of drugs at the time of allografting to prevent rejection. The drugs are then reduced rapidly, within days to weeks, to less toxic *maintenance* levels. Patients are examined frequently, and multiple laboratory tests are obtained to detect rejection or organ dysfunction early for effective treatment. Induction regimens rely on three or four drugs (mycophenolate, corticosteroids, cyclosporine or tacrolimus, antibodies), whereas maintenance regimens rely on two or three of these drugs. Treatment of first or mild rejections is usually accomplished with high-dose "pulse" steroids, whereas steroid-unresponsive, very severe, or secondary rejections are often treated with antibodies, especially OKT3.

The antimetabolites include azathioprine, cyclophosphamide (Cytoxan), and mycophenolate. By interfering with nucleic acid metabolism, these agents inhibit proliferation and clonal expansion of activated lymphocytes, limiting alloantigen-specific immune responses. Many immunosuppressive regimens use these drugs during induction immunosuppression at the time of allografting or for maintenance immunosuppression. They are most useful for preventing rejection but have little role for treating an acute, ongoing rejection. A more recent pharmaceutical, the morpholinoethyl ester of mycophenolic acid, also called CellCept (Roche Laboratories, Nutley, NJ), inhibits de novo purine synthesis. It is more lymphocyte selective than azathioprine. Current data suggest it has important roles in inducing and maintaining immunosuppression and treating ongoing, particularly resistant rejections (172,173).

Glucocorticoids are mainstays of virtually all immunosuppressive regimens and are used for induction and maintenance and for treating rejections. Glucocorticoids are primarily transcriptional regulators, binding to cytoplasmic steroid receptors, which are then translocated to the nucleus, where the complex binds specific gene promoters and other regulatory regions. The glucocorticoids all have similar immunosuppressive actions, and none is more effective than any other at equipotent doses. The relative potency on a milligram basis for the most commonly used drugs are hydrocortisone and cortisol, 1 mg; prednisone, 4 mg; and prednisolone and methylprednisolone, 5 mg. Steroid use is associated with several significant complications and side effects (Table 16.6), and at equipotent doses all have equivalent toxicities. Although the use of multiple-drug regimens has decreased the overall dosing of glucocorticoids, the goal of steroid-free regimens for inducing and maintaining immunosuppression and for treating rejection in all patients has not been achieved.

Cyclosporine is a hydrophobic, cyclic undecapeptide that binds to a cytoplasmic protein, cyclophilin. The major immunosuppressive activity of cyclosporine appears to be related to the ability of the cyclosporine–cyclophilin complex to bind and inhibit the cytoplasmic protein tyrosine phosphatase calcineurin (Fig. 16.20). This in turn inhibits activation of the NF-AT$_c$ transcriptional factor. In essence, cyclosporine is a transcriptional regulator. Cyclosporine is an integral part of all immunosuppressive regimens for induction and maintenance therapy, but seems to have little role in reversing an ongoing acute rejection. The addition of cyclosporine to routine immunosuppressive regimens in 1983 allowed for the exponential growth of transplantation over the following decade. The 1-year graft and patient survival rates for the various organs increased from the 30% to 60% range to the 70% to 90% range. Cyclosporine has several significant toxicities (Table 16.6), but attempts to design congeners with less toxicity but equal immunosuppression have not been successful.

The search for additional immunosuppressive agents led to the discovery of tacrolimus, or FK 506, approved by the U.S. Food and Drug Administration (FDA) in 1994. This macrolide antibiotic binds to a series of related cytoplasmic receptors termed *FK-binding protein* (FKBP). The tacrolimus–FKBP complex inhibits calcineurin. Thus, cyclosporine and tacrolimus have similar mechanisms of action. Tacrolimus is 10 to 100 times more potent than cyclosporine on a molar basis, but it too is associated with a number of significant and similar toxicities (Table 16.6). Tacrolimus has roles in inducing and maintaining immunosuppression and may also be particularly useful for treating resistant rejections. A structurally similar compound, called rapamycin or sirolimus, has recently completed clinical trials and is currently approved (174,175). This macrolide binds to and inhibits FKBP; however, it does not complex to calcineurin. Its molecular mechanism is under investigation. The existence of compounds such as cyclosporine, tacrolimus, and sirolimus suggests that there must be normal cellular constituents that regulate calcineurin function. These regulatory factors are unknown; their purification and isolation will presumably lead to more rational drug design for immunosuppression.

Antimetabolites, glucocorticoids, and calcineurin inhibitors are universally applied both to induction and to maintenance immunosuppression, and any of these agents may be administered chronically to patients. The fourth major group of reagents is antibodies. These may be given for only short periods because of their extreme potency and because of host antiimmunoglobulin responses that limit their efficacy. Antibodies are used for induction to prevent rejection and for treatment of acute, ongoing rejections. There are two major types of antibody preparations (Table 16.7). Polyclonal antibodies, such as antilymphocyte globulin, thymoglobulin, and antithymoctye globulin, are prepared by immunizing animals with human lymphocytes or lymphoid lines, bleeding the animals to obtain serum, and purifying whole immunoglobulin from serum. These preparations are directed against

Table 16.6. CURRENTLY APPROVED IMMUNOSUPPRESSIVE AGENTS

Agent (Brand name)	Mechanism of action	Dosage	Monitoring	Clinical uses	Adverse effects
Azathioprine (Imuran)	Inhibits purine synthesis by active metabolites 6-thioinocinic acid (by conversion to 6-mercaptopurine) and 6-thioguanine nucleotides; inhibits DNA and RNA synthesis; has greater effect on T cells than B cells	1–3 mg/kg/d IV or PO	Maintain WBCs >3,000/µl	Part of regimens to lower doses of cyclosporine or prednisone	Myelosuppression (leukopenia, occasionally thrombocytopenia and megaloblastic anemia), hepatitis, cholestatis, hepatic vein thrombosis, pancreatitis dermatitis, alopecia, increased susceptibility to infection
Cytoxan	Alkylates DNA	0.5–1.5 mg/kg/d	Maintain WBCs >3,000/µL	Substitution for azathioprine if adverse effects occur	Leukopenia, thrombocytopenia, hemorrhagic cystitis, nausea, vomiting, increased susceptibility to infections
Glucocorticoids	Complex; affects T cells and macrophages; has little effect on antibody production by B cells. Steroid–receptor complex binds to DNA; alters transcription of genes responsible for cytokine synthesis; blocks MLR and development of CTL; inhibits IL-1 and IL-6 synthesis	Prednisolone, 1–2 mg/kg/d induction; 0.1–0.2 mg/kg/d maintenance bid, qd, or qod dosing Prednisolone, 2 mg/kg/d for rejection; tapering schedule Solu-Medrol 5–15 mg/kg/d IV for rejection	No objective means to monitor; adjustment done by protocol; adverse effects	Foundation of most multidrug protocols; treatment of rejection	Cushingoid features (moon facies, acne, centripetal obesity, striae), hypertension, weight gain, (increased appetite), hyperglycemia, osteoporosis, type II diabetes, poor wound healing, pancreatitis, peptic ulcer, colonic perforation, psychosis, increased susceptibility to infection
Cyclosporine (Sandimmune)	Binds to cyclophilin; blocks transcription of several early T-cell activation genes, including IL-2, Il-3, IL-4, and interferon-γ; inhibits IL-1 production by macrophages	8–10 mg/kg/d PO qd, bid, or tid or 2.5–3 mg/kg/d IV	Trough levels (usually 12 h); serum creatinine; mg/kg dose (protocol); biopsy (histologic evidence of cyclosporine toxicity)	Induction therapy with prednisolone or azathioprine in most multidrug regimens	Nephrotoxicity, hypertension, hyperkalemia, hyperuricemia and gout, gingival hypertrophy, hepatotoxicity, hirsutism, tremors, seizures, hyperglycemia; hemolytic uremic syndrome increased susceptibility to infection
FK 506, Tacrolimus (Prograf)	Similar to cyclosporine (10–100 times more potent); binds to FK-binding protein; blocks expression of IL-2 receptors on allostimulated T cells	0.15 mg/kg/d PO qd or bid or 0.075 mg/kg IV q 12 h	Trough levels; serum creatinine; dose mg/kg dose (protocol); adverse effects (neurologic)	Induction therapy with prednisone; treatment of rejection; maintenance without prednisolone	Nephrotoxicity, headache weight loss, tremors, paresthesia, increased sensitivity to light insomnia and mood changes, increased susceptibility to infections

MLR, mixed lymphocyte response; CTL, cytotoxic T lymphocytes; IL, interleukin; WBCs, white blood cells.

Table 16.7. POLYCLONAL AND MONOCLONAL ANTIBODIES

Antibody	Source	Mechanism of action	Dosage	Monitoring	Clinical uses	Adverse effects
ALG or ATG	Horse, goat, rabbit	Depletes T cells more than B cells as a result of complement-dependent lysis and opsonization	10–30 mg/kg/d IV qd over 6 h; must be given in central line	Peripheral T-cell levels; monitor for antihorse or antigoat antibody development; platelets; white blood cell count	Induction with azathioprine or prednisone as part of triple or quadruple therapy protocols; treatment of rejection with or without steroids	Fever, chills, leukopenia, thrombocytopenia, nausea, vomiting, diarrhea, arthralgia, headache, myalgia, rash, pruritus, urticaria, chest pain, phlebitis, rarely anaphylaxis or serum sickness
OKT3	Mouse	Reacts with CD3 recognition complex on T cells; blocks recognition of class I or II antigens; inhibits generation and function of effector T cells; opsonizes CD3+ cells; modulates CD3 antigen-recognition complex; renders T cells anergetic or kills them by apoptosis	2.5–10 mg/d IV over 30 min; can be given in peripheral vein	Peripheral CD3 levels; monitor for antimouse antibody development	Same as ALG, ATG	Usually with first dose: fever, chills, diarrhea, headache, nausea, vomiting, dyspnea, wheezing, pulmonary edema, tachycardia, hypotension, aseptic meningitis, seizures, coma; markedly reduced with pretreatment with steroids, acetaminophen, indomethacin, and diphenhydramine hydrochloride

ALG, antilymphocyte globulin; ALT, antithymocyte globulin.

many different antigens present on T cells (e.g., CD2, CD3, CD4, CD8) but also recognize B-cell, monocyte, platelet, and granulocyte antigens. Polyclonal antibodies are very useful for induction (176) but tend to be less effective for treatment of acute rejection. They are associated with a number of side effects related either to their depleting effect on cell populations (leukopenia, thrombocytopenia) or allergic reactions related to host antiimmunoglobulin responses (urticaria, rash, pruritus).

The second type of antibody preparation is monoclonal antibody, derived from cloned hybridoma cells of a single specificity. OKT3, approved by the FDA in 1985, is a mouse monoclonal directed against the nonpolymorphic ε chain of the CD3 complex of the TCR. OKT3 therefore recognizes all T cells (both αβ TCR and γδ TCR) and interferes with their antigen recognition functions in the context of either class I or II MHC. OKT3 is used for both induction and the treatment of rejection. The antibody is used either as first-line treatment for rejection or as treatment for rejections unresponsive to high-dose steroids or polyclonal antibodies. Anti-IL-2 receptor (IL-2R) monoclonal antibodies, basiliximab (Simulect; Novartis, East Hanover, NJ) (177) and daclizumab (Zenapax; Roche Laboratories) (178), were FDA approved in 1998 and are used for induction immunosuppression.

It has previously been considered that polyclonal or monoclonal antibodies function by inhibiting T-cell function either through opsonization, complement-mediated lysis, or steric hindrance of the TCR. Although these mechanisms certainly do occur, it is now clear that other effects may be even more important for immunosuppression. When OKT3 is first administered to a patient, a significant clinical response often occurs within 30 minutes to 4 hours, consisting of fevers, chills, rigors, myalgias, arthralgias, and vascular leak. This has been called the *cytokine syndrome* and is due to OKT3 binding to and crosslinking T-cell CD3, which activates all T cells, thereby causing massive release of IL-2. The IL-2 in turn causes other cells to release IL-1, IL-6, IFN-γ, and TNF-α. These cytokines can be found at very high concentrations throughout the serum, and blocking cytokine production or action can ameliorate the cytokine syndrome. When T cells are stimulated, they lose cell surface CD3, CD4, and CD8 as a result of the antibody. This process is termed *antigenic modulation* and results in naked T cells that are refractory to antigenic stimulation because they lack receptors. Because OKT3 binds CD3 in the absence of other T-cell costimulatory signals (e.g., CD28, CD2, CD29/49d, CD11a/18), this is the equivalent of inappropriate antigen presentation, which experimentally can result in anergy or apoptosis. There is now evidence that because of OKT3, these T cells may also be rendered anergic or even killed by apoptotic mechanisms. The effects of cytokine stimulation, antigenic modulation, anergy, and apoptosis may be separable, and experimental work to produce a form of OKT3 that lacks the clinically deleterious cytokine-inducing properties while preserving the other immunosuppressive characteristics is of significant interest. Polyclonal antibodies also have anti-CD3 specificities and may therefore have a similar mechanism of action. In addition, because polyclonals have many other antireceptor specificities, they may produce a variety of other effects related to receptor cross-linking, antigenic modulation, anergy, and apoptosis.

Other monoclonal antibodies are undergoing clinical evaluation, including anti-CD4, anti-CD8, and anti-CD3. All seem to have some efficacy, but none has yet proved superior to OKT3. Consideration has also been given to toxin-conjugated monoclonal antibodies, but none has reached phase II or III clinical transplantation trials.

Several dozen other compounds of diverse structure and mechanistic activity have been or are being evaluated in experimental and clinical allografting protocols. Several, discussed here briefly, may find a role in clinical transplantation during the next decade. The bacterial product 15-deoxyspergualin is a potent immunosuppressive with mild side effects, including neurotoxicity, anorexia, and bone marrow depression (179). Its mechanism may be related to binding to cytoplasmic members of the heat-shock protein 70 (Hsp 70) family (180) Hsp members are often involved as chaperones in protein folding and transport; therefore, 15-deoxyspergualin may interfere with antigen presentation or the translocation of transcription factors into the nucleus (181). Leflunomide, an isoxazol derivative, has potent immunosuppressive activities and synergizes with cyclosporine (182,183). Its mechanism may be related to inhibiting intracellular messengers and second signals generated by IL-2 and costimulatory receptors such as CD28. Studies suggests that leflunomide may inhibit protein kinases and de novo pyrimidine biosynthesis (184). Molecules aimed at effector mechanisms of cellular destruction have also had some activity in experimental analyses. Thus, inhibitors of complement, platelet-activating factor, nitric oxide synthesis, superoxide synthesis, granzymes, perforins, and interleukins can all prolong graft survival. These latter agents will probably have only adjunctive roles because the most important processes to regulate are probably the initiation of immune responses, immunologic priming, and immunologic memory.

Recent investigations have focused on the design of soluble molecules that mimic various parts of the TCR–antigen–MHC–CD4/CD8 complex. A molecule with high enough affinity for the recognition complex could inhibit T-cell activation and immunity. Analogues of CD4 can perform such a function (185). Likewise, analogues of peptide antigen seem to complete with antigen at the level of binding to the peptide groove of MHC. Furthermore, antigen analogues may induce a negative regulatory signal in T cells and actually anergize T cells as a result of altered receptor affinities and kinetics (186–188). This form of immunosuppression also has the advantage of being strictly antigen specific. One envisions transplanting a patient and then injecting the patient with mimics of the immunodominant peptides corresponding to the mismatched MHC molecules of donor origin to promote selective anergy.

A variety of physical methods have been considered for immunosuppression. Total lymphoid irradiation is successful in experimental transplantation (189). Total lymphoid irradiation ablates much of the immune system and also seems to generate suppressor cells. There is concern that total lymphoid irradiation markedly increases the risk of systemic infection and lymphoid malignancies. It has been known since the early 1970s that prior blood transfusions are associated with a decreased risk of renal allograft rejection and increased graft survival (190). Furthermore, donor-specific transfusions have an antigen-specific protective effect. The cellular and molecular consequences of transfusion or donor-specific transfusion are not certain; however, the presentation of antigen to central lymphoid compartments (e.g., intravenous injection of cells) can generate suppression, anergy, and tolerance (see Sites of Antigen Recognition). Problems with transfusion include the fact that high-titer anti-HLA antibodies develop in 10% to 30% of transfused recipients. These highly sensitized recipients cannot be transplanted. In this respect, transfusions may merely be "selecting" potential high- versus low-reacting recipients. Transfusions and donor-specific transfusions were widely used until the

1980s. The advent of cyclosporine erased much of the benefit that transfusions conferred; they are now only rarely used. Oral feeding of antigen or peptide can also produce suppression, anergy, and tolerance (191,192). A trial of oral peptides in patients with multiple sclerosis suggested they conferred some clinically beneficial immunosuppressive effect (191). It remains to be seen if the same can be accomplished with clinical allografting.

Complications of Immunosuppression

The therapeutic index for immunosuppressives is very low. As a result, numerous toxicities and adverse effects occur, and they are an integral part of treating transplant recipients (Tables 16.6 and 16.7). The most obvious complication is infection. As immunosuppression becomes stronger and more effective, the recipient's ability to resist infection diminishes. Allograft recipients are susceptible both to typical bacterial infections (e.g., urinary tract infection, pneumonia, wound infections) and to infections with unusual organisms (e.g., fungus, virus, atypical bacteria). Immunosuppressives also blunt the inflammatory response to infection so that patients present with very subtle signs and symptoms or very late in the infectious process. The tenets of patient care are the judicious management of immunosuppression to prevent infectious complications, the use of prophylactic antibiotics (i.e., acyclovir or ganciclovir for herpesviruses; sulfamethoxazole for *Pneumocystis;* and nystatin, clotrimazole, or fluconazole for candidiasis), and a low threshold of suspicion for examining, culturing, and treating patients with suspected infections.

Figure 16.21 diagrams the typical transplant-related infections and when they occur. Of particular concern is cytomegalovirus (CMV). CMV, a member of the herpes family, can infect any cell in the body and produce cytopathic effects. CMV infection in immunocompetent people is often clinically inapparent and results in the viral genome persisting in the patient's lymphocytes for life. As a result, organ transplantation almost invariably results in the transfer of viral genomes to the recipient. Evidence of past infection is indicated by elevated serum IgG anti-CMV titers; approximately 70% of the population is CMV seropositive. When seropositive (i.e., previously infected) patients are transplanted and immunosuppressed, CMV virus from their own lymphocytes may be reexpressed and reactivate disease. Reactivation disease is usually mild and self-limited and presents approximately 6 weeks after transplantation as fevers, myalgias, arthralgias, leukopenia, mild elevation of liver enzymes, and mild, nonspecific abdominal complaints. A more serious situation occurs when a previously uninfected, CMV-seronegative patient receives an organ from a CMV-seropositive donor. This situation occurs in 10% to 30% of transplant recipients. The recipient has almost a 100% chance of contracting CMV infection and greater than a 70% chance of having clinically significant or even life-threatening disease, including CMV encephalitis, pneumonitis, hepatitis, and necrotizing gastroenteropathy with perforation and bleeding. Effective prophylactic regimens now include the following: acyclovir, 800 mg four times a day orally for 3 months; ganciclovir, 2.5 mg/kg twice a day intravenously for 2 weeks; and CMV hyperimmune globulin, 150 mg/kg for five doses over 6 to 8 weeks. Therapeutic regimens for established disease include ganciclovir and CMV IgG.

Another complication in allograft recipients is malignancy. There is an increased incidence for only a few histologic types of tumors. The immunosuppressive drugs do

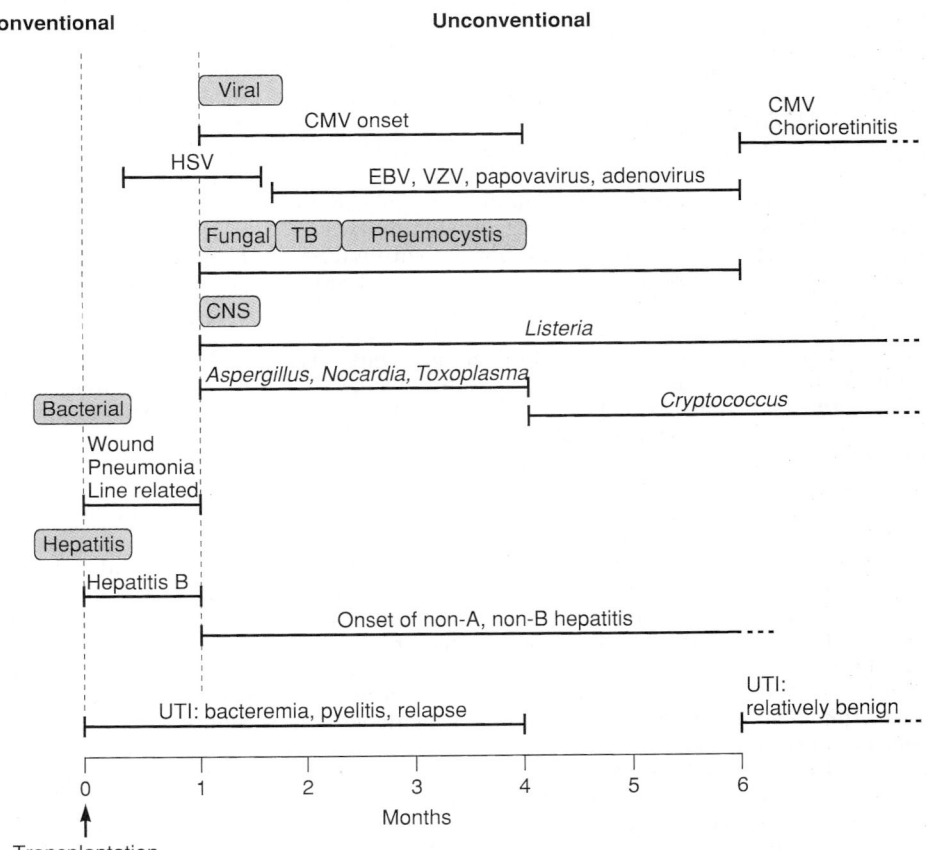

Figure 16.21. Timing of post-transplantation infections. CMV, cytomegalovirus; EBV, CNS, central nervous system; Epstein-Barr virus; HSV, herpes simplex virus; UTI, urinary tract infection; VZV, varicella-zoster virus. (After Rubin RH, Wolfson JS, Cosimi AB, et al. Infection in the renal transplant patient. *Am J Med* 1981;70:405.)

not appear to be directly mitogenic or transforming, but rather suppress immune mechanisms that keep transformed cells in check. Squamous cell carcinomas of the exposed areas of the skin are by far the most common. These usually are not aggressive or invasive tumors and can be cured with simple local excision. Avoiding ultraviolet exposure from the sun is the best preventive measure.

Lymphomas are the next most common tumor and are 10 to 100 times more common in transplant recipients than in the general population. These are usually non-Hodgkin's B-cell lymphomas and are often related to malignant transformation by Epstein-Barr virus (EBV) (193). In immunocompetent people, EBV normally infects B cells and causes polyclonal proliferation of infected cells. The infection is eventually controlled by cytotoxic CD8+ T cells, which recognize and kill viral antigens on the surface of infected B cells. In immunosuppressed patients, T-cell-mediated immunity is impaired, allowing EBV-directed polyclonal B-cell proliferation to continue. Some of the B-cell clones eventually acquire additional mutations, and a benign polyclonal expansion of B cells becomes a more aggressive oligoclonal proliferation. One of these clones can accumulate even more mutations and become an autonomous, monoclonal lymphoma. At this stage, the lymphoma may even lose viral antigens and become insusceptible to immune control. The incidence of lymphoma is directly related to the amount of immunosuppression received over time. Thus, avoiding over-immunosuppression prevents this malignancy. Management of established disease consists primarily of reducing or withdrawing immunosuppression, even to the point of allograft rejection and loss. Although the latter maneuver is possible with renal and pancreatic transplants, where the patient may return to dialysis or insulin, it is not possible with hepatic or cardiac grafts. High-dose intravenous ganciclovir is sometimes effective for treatment and may have a role in prophylaxis. Conventional chemotherapy for lymphoma usually is ineffective for these tumors.

Other tumors with a higher incidence in transplant recipients include Kaposi's sarcoma and a slight increase in cervical carcinoma. The causative agent of Kaposi's sarcoma is human herpesvirus 8, also now called Kaposi's sarcoma herpesvirus. Cervical carcinomas are related to papilloma viruses. This association suggests that immunosuppression primarily interferes with normal antiviral responses in the case of some tumors. Common neoplasms, such as breast, lung, and colon cancer, are *not* more common in transplant recipients than in the general population, suggesting that immune mechanisms are generally irrelevant for these tumors. The effect of immunosuppression on the recurrence of a preexisting or a previously treated cancer is controversial. Data suggest that immunosuppression either has no effect or may slightly increase the incidence of recurrent carcinoma. Current clinical recommendations suggest that after a curative resection, patients should wait at least 2 years before undergoing transplantation (194). It is also possible to transplant a tumor to a recipient from a donor with metastatic disease. Therefore, a history of malignancy excludes potential organ donors. The one exception to this rule is malignant central nervous system tumors that usually do not metastasize. Unfortunately, even these tumors have been transferred by organ transplantation despite no clinical evidence of metastatic disease (195).

Tables 16.6 and 16.7 also show a large number of drug-specific toxicities, many of which are clinically common. This again stresses the point that the therapeutic index for immunosuppression is very narrow and that frequent monitoring of laboratory tests is required for patients re-

ceiving these agents. Of particular concern is atherosclerotic vascular disease. Since the late 1970s, organ failure and infection have become less significant causes of morbidity and mortality while various manifestations of vascular disease have become more important. In fact, coronary artery disease is the primary cause of mortality in the renal transplant population. Many factors related to immunosuppression contribute to vascular disease. Glucocorticoids alter serum lipid components and ratios to unfavorable varieties. They also promote glucose intolerance and insulin resistance. Cyclosporine unfavorably alters serum lipids and contributes to insulin resistance. Cyclosporine also causes hypertension by mechanisms related to vascular endothelial cell-induced release of endothelin and interferes with renal function by altering glomerular hemodynamics and renal prostaglandin production. Prolonged cyclosporine administration may lead to permanent renal damage and eventually the need for dialysis. Sirolimus and tacrolimus share the same toxicities as cyclosporine, causing hypercholesterolemia, insulin resistance, hypertension, and renal insufficiency. Renal insufficiency itself further contributes to hypertension and dyslipidemia. All these variables contribute to atherosclerosis of cerebral, coronary, renal, and peripheral vascular beds. The care of transplant recipients now requires careful monitoring of individual drug doses and levels to reduce their toxicities. Close attention to serum lipid profiles, hypertension, weight, diet, and exercise are also major factors in the long-term treatment of these patients.

Another complication of organ allografting is graft-versus-host disease (GVHD). All vascularized allografts contain lymph nodes and mature lymphocytes. These donor-derived T and B cells can be stimulated by host alloantigen and transiently repopulate the host. The anti-host reactive cells can cause T-cell-mediated lesions, such as hepatitis, dermatitis, or gastrointestinal mucosal lesions, as seen in bone marrow transplant recipients with GVHD. The B cells can produce antihost antibodies; if there is an ABO incompatibility this can even result in a hemolytic anemia. GVHD is usually self-limited as the donor cells are eliminated either by immunosuppression or host antidonor responses.

Important Aspects of Antigenicity and Immunity for Clinical Transplantation

Current clinical protocols determine a limited number of variables and parameters for matching and allocating donor organs to potential recipients. ABO compatibility is obviously required for successful transplantation. Placing an A donor organ in an O recipient results in hyperacute rejection because of the presence of preformed anti-A antibodies. It is possible to transplant A2 donor organs into O recipients because most anti-A antibodies do not bind to the A2 ligand. It is also possible to place O organs into A or B recipients; however, because of the severe organ shortage and long waiting lists, this is not usually performed.

The central position of MHC in immune regulation suggests that HLA matching is very important for allografting. Significant data prove that HLA matching is important for kidney and pancreas transplantation. A well-matched organ has up to a 10% long-term survival advantage over a poorly matched graft. However, as the overall success rate for renal allografting approaches 90%, there is debate over the magnitude of this advantage and what defines poor versus good matching. Good data show that HLA matching is *not* important for liver transplantation and does not affect graft survival. The immunologic reasons for this are not known. The data for cardiac grafting are more controversial; there is probably a small advantage for HLA matching with this organ.

Most laboratories use serologic-based, or antibody-based, techniques to type potential donors and recipients for HLA. The main loci typed are HLA-A, HLA-B, and HLA-DR. For a normal, completely heterozygous person, this results in six antigens typed, and a complete donor–recipient match is referred to as a *six-antigen match* or a *zero-antigen mismatch*. Newer nucleic acid- and polymerase chain reaction-based techniques are being used by an increasing number of HLA laboratories. This technology is more accurate than serologic-based techniques and types for additional loci, including HLA-DP and HLA-DQ and separate α and β chains. Typing for more loci may allow for better matching. However, because HLA heterogeneity is so enormous and because there is such a severe shortage of donor organs, technical advances in typing may confer no benefit on clinical results.

An important test for graft compatibility is the crossmatch. This assay determines if there are preformed antibodies in the potential recipient's serum that react with antigens on the cell surface of the potential donor's lymphocytes (Fig. 16.22). A positive crossmatch means that such antibodies are present and that hyperacute rejection will ensue if the transplantation is performed. Appropriate controls are always performed to exclude autoantibodies. Crossmatching is important for kidney, pancreas, lung, and heart allografting, whereas hepatic allografts resist hyperacute rejection. The reasons for this resistance are not known but may relate to the large mass of hepatic tissue that can absorb antibody and complement and still preserve sufficient functioning cellular mass.

Figure 16.22 shows that the standard crossmatch detects high-titer complement-fixing antibodies. If the recipient has antidonor antibodies that inefficiently fix complement, a positive crossmatch could be missed. Some laboratories use enhancing techniques, such as secondary antibodies or fluorescent flow cytometry, to increase the sensitivity of the crossmatch. The problem with these modifications is that increased sensitivity is accompanied by decreased specificity; therefore, some positive crossmatches could be clinically acceptable. Clinical experience has shown that positive crossmatches from IgG antibodies are the most significant, whereas positive testing from IgM antibodies is not clinically relevant. IgM antibodies can be eliminated from serum specimens by adding a reducing agent such as dithiothreitol.

Figure 16.22 also shows that the standard crossmatch tests donor-derived lymphocytes for the presence of antigen. Because the most relevant antibodies are anti-HLA and because HLA is expressed by essentially all cell types, the experimental design is appropriate. However, if the recipient has antibodies that are cell or organ specific, these antibodies may be missed by the standard crossmatch. Some recipients do occasionally possess cell- or organ-specific antibodies, and hyperacute or severe accelerated acute rejection can ensue in these situations. Experimental studies have also demonstrated a distinct vascular endothelial cell-specific antigen system, which can be a target for hyperacute rejection. This endothelial cell system is, however, still poorly defined and reagents are not available for widespread clinical use. The practical consequence of all these limitations is that hyperacute rejections rarely occur due to noncomplement fixation or antibodies with unusual specificities. Conversely, some positive crossmatches, which have precluded a transplantation, may have been determined by too sensitive a technique.

Another important test that also reflects the presence of host antidonor antibodies is the panel-reactive antibody (PRA). Most recipients on transplant waiting lists send serum samples to the transplantation center on a regular basis. These sera are then periodically tested against a panel of typing cells of known HLA specificities using techniques identical to those for the crossmatch (Fig. 16.22). The percentage of cells with which recipient serum reacts is determined, and this number is the PRA. Most normal people have no anti-HLA antibodies and a low PRA (0% to 5%). Patients who have been transfused, pregnant, previously transplanted, or have an autoimmune disorder that induces a lot of antibodies may have a high PRA (50% to 99%). The presence of a very high PRA suggests a patient is likely to have a positive crossmatch. This information is useful for determining the logistics of organ allocation when cadaveric donor organs become available and have to be transplanted within a short time frame.

A matching technique used in living-related transplantation is the mixed lymphocyte culture or mixed lymphocyte reaction. Lymphocytes are isolated from peripheral blood specimens from both donor and recipient. The donor cells are gamma-irradiated to prevent mitosis, and the two cell populations are placed in culture together. Recipient cells recognize donor antigen in culture, are acti-

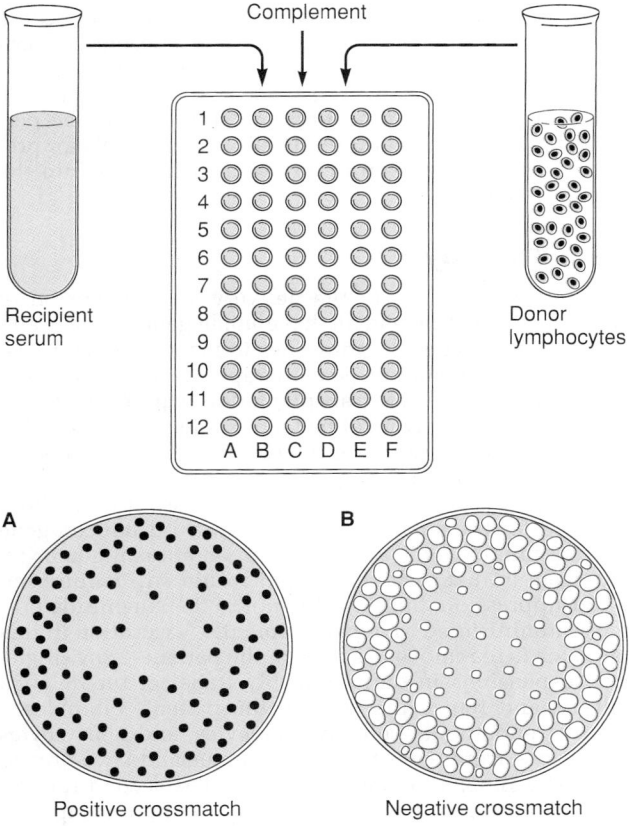

Figure 16.22. Lymphocytotoxicity crossmatch. Recipient serum is incubated with donor lymphocytes and complement in microtiter plates. If donor-specific lymphocytotoxic antibodies are present in the recipient serum, antibody binding results in complement fixation and lysis of the donor lymphocytes. This is detected by the addition of a dye that is taken up through the damaged cell membrane, and a positive crossmatch is noted *(A)*. If no antibodies are present, cells remain viable and do not take up the dye *(B)*. This is a negative crossmatch.

vated, and proliferate rapidly. After a few days of culture, the amount of proliferation is measured by incorporating radiolabeled nucleic acids into the cells. The amount or degree of proliferation compared with appropriate positive and negative controls is assumed to represent the potential for a host antidonor response and the chance of allograft rejection. Unfortunately, the correlation between the mixed lymphocyte reaction and clinical outcome is poor and most centers no longer use this test. Further, because this assay requires several days to complete, it is not useful for cadaveric grafting.

FUTURE DIRECTIONS

Xenotransplantation

One of the most critical problems in clinical transplantation is a shortage of donor organs. There has been continued liberalization of criteria for acceptable cadaveric donors and improvements in operative techniques and preservation solutions. Despite this, only 20% to 30% of potentially suitable donors are ever used. In addition, societal enforcement of mandatory seat belt and helmet laws as well as reduced tolerance for drunk driving have substantially reduced the number of donors available from trauma. At the same time, the increasing success of organ transplantation has increased the indications for transplantation and subsequently the demands for organs. As a result, the number of people waiting for organs in the United States alone is currently more than 70,000 and growing by approximately 10% to 15% each year. One approach to this shortage of organs is xenotransplantation, or the use of organs from different species (196). The successful application of this modality could potentially provide an unlimited supply of organs and make all transplantation operations elective procedures. Unfortunately, there are a number of significant issues that impede the clinical application of xenotransplantation.

The choice of donor species is limited. Primate donors, although phylogenetically similar to humans, are difficult to breed in captivity, and many species are even endangered. In addition, there are significant ethical ramifications of using such closely related species. Furthermore, the transmission of viruses from primates, such as simian retroviruses, could be potentially life threatening. Because of these concerns, attention has been focused on the pig as a suitable donor. The pig is viewed as a good donor because of its size, physiology, acceptance by the public, an extensive knowledge of porcine genetics, and the ability to make inbred and transgenic swine.

The first major hurdle to xenotransplantation between such widely disparate species such as human and pig is hyperacute rejection (197). Humans and many primates have high-titer natural antibodies directed against cell surface determinants present on other species. In the case of pig-to-human xenotransplantation, these antibodies appear to be primarily IgM and are directed against galactose α1-3 galactose present on the porcine cells (198). These natural antibodies are present because humans do not have the enzyme a-galactosyl transferase and do not put these terminal sugar residues on their cell surface. Because of these natural antibodies, pig-to-human transplantation results in hyperacute rejection after these antibodies bind to the endothelium of the porcine organ and activate complement. Several approaches to solving this problem have proven successful in the laboratory. One approach is to deplete serum antibody levels by either plasmapheresis or immunoabsorption while concurrently suppressing B-cell function. Another approach is to eliminate the primary antigenic determinant on the porcine cells by either

creating pigs "knocked out" for α-galactosyl transferase or enzymatically removing the sugar moieties from the graft before transplantation. An alternative tactic is to regulate complement activation (199), which also prevents hyperacute rejection. One such approach is the use of soluble inhibitors of complement activation, such as soluble complement receptor-1. Other approaches have focused on the construction of transgenic pigs that express human complement regulatory proteins on the cell surface (200).

Although the hyperacute rejection barrier to discordant xenotransplantation is relatively severe, it can be overcome (201). Unfortunately, none of these current approaches produces long-term graft survival. This most likely reflects return of humoral immunity and complement function to the recipient as well as generation of a specific cellular immune responses. The relative importance of these processes, and strategies to avert them, is the subject of ongoing investigation.

Another problem with xenotransplantation is the physiologic incompatibility between proteins synthesized by the graft and the recipient. For example, the inability of inhibitors of thrombosis to function adequately on the endothelium surface may predispose a xenograft to thrombosis in the absence of any immune response. In addition, organs such as the liver secrete many serum proteins that might be unable to function in their new host environment. For other organs, such as the heart, this might be less of a barrier.

The final and perhaps most daunting hurdle in xenotransplantation is the transmission of unusual pathogenic organisms to humans, or zoonoses (202). Recent concern has focused on the transmission of porcine retroviruses (203). The subject of zoonoses and xenotransplantation is still in its infancy and appropriate studies must be performed to devise the appropriate clinical protocols for preventing the introduction of any such pathogens into the human population.

Gene Therapy

Technical advances in the delivery and expression of exogenous genetic elements have made gene transfer and gene therapy practical approaches to managing many diseases. In transplantation, gene therapy has at least two potential roles. First, liver transplantation is performed for a number of inborn errors of metabolism (e.g., Wilson's disease). If these diseases are diagnosed before irreversible liver damage, the missing enzyme could be transfected into the patient's own liver and the disease cured without the need for transplantation. The newly introduced gene may be immunogenic and represent an autoantigen or alloantigen. In that case, the patient would still require immunosuppression, but probably not of the magnitude normally administered to organ recipients. A variation in this approach is to remove tissue from the patient, grow single-cell suspensions in culture, stably transfect the cells in culture, and return the cells to the patient. Fibroblasts, vascular endothelial cells, lymphocytes, and hepatocytes are all good candidates for this technique and have proved successful in experimental protocols. The second role for gene therapy is in the actual delivery of immunosuppression. Cytokines, receptors, antisense RNA, or transcriptional regulators could all be engineered into appropriate delivery vectors and introduced directly into the graft. Experimental protocols have successfully demonstrated the utility of these approaches in animals (204–206).

Gene transfer and gene therapy are such new modalities that it is not yet clear how they will eventually be used. A number of difficult technical problems remain to be solved (207). Current transfer vectors result in only transient, low-level expression of the transferred gene within a few cells in the target organ. Sustained, high-level gene expression throughout the graft has not yet been reliably achieved in any system. The transfer vectors and the transferred gene may be highly immunogenic. Additional immunosuppressive strategies are therefore required to circumvent those responses that would limit gene transfer efficacy. The transfer vectors also have potential pathogenic effects that may limit their utility. For example, adenoviral vectors can induce direct cytopathic effects by disrupting lysosomal membranes. Retroviral vectors can incorporate into genomic DNA and therefore have the potential for malignant transformation. Candidate genes for gene therapy have been evaluated in experimental systems, but it is not certain which will be most useful. For example, transforming growth factor-β is a soluble immunosuppressive cytokine; however, it can also induce exuberant fibrosis of the vasculature. IL-10, another immunosuppressive cytokine, can also activate T and B cells in some circumstances. Cytoplasmic or membrane-bound gene transfer products may be better candidates, but unless they can be expressed uniformly throughout the graft, their utility is doubtful. Some of the problems with gene transfer may make it particularly suited to transplantation. The transient expression of an immunosuppressive molecule in a graft at the time of transplantation may be the immunoregulatory signal that would permit the induction of tolerance without the need for long-term, systemic administration of conventional immunosuppression. Low-level expression of gene transfer products may also limit the immunosuppressive effect solely to the target organ, preventing systemic immunosuppression and its deleterious side effects.

Cellular Transplants

There are several situations in which cellular transplantation would better serve the potential recipient than whole-organ transplantation. As mentioned earlier, liver transplantation for certain inborn errors of metabolism could be supplanted by providing a specific gene product. This could be accomplished by infusing liver cells from a normal donor into the portal vein of the recipient and allowing them to populate the recipient liver. Such protocols have been successful clinically but require conventional immunosuppression (208). In addition, the ability to detect rejection would be difficult by either biochemical or histologic means. An alternative is to obtain recipient hepatocytes by partial liver resection, grow them in culture, stably transfect them with the appropriate gene or genes, and reinfuse them into the recipient's portal circulation. Immunosuppression may be required because the new gene product would be recognized as foreign. Similar approaches with fibroblasts, smooth muscle, skeletal muscle, lymphocytes, and vascular endothelial cells have been demonstrated in experimental models.

Pancreas transplantation is performed for type 1 diabetes mellitus, so only the endocrine tissue is required by the recipient. The exocrine tissue in conventional whole-organ pancreas transplantation is often the source of a variety of complications related to the exocrine secretions. Therefore, pancreatic islet transplantation would be preferable. Some islet transplantations have been performed in humans, and the overall success rate for this highly experimental process is still poor, although there are a few notable exceptions. There are two major barriers to islet cell transplantation. First, the physical and mechanical means to separate islets from the whole organ are expensive and inefficient. With current technology, it may be necessary to use several donors for each recipient. With the current donor shortage, this is not a long-term solution to the problem. Xenotransplantation, with the use of porcine islets, may circumvent this problem but introduces the immunologic difficulties of xenoantigens. The second major barrier is immunosuppression and rejection. The success of any organ or cell transplant relies on the ability to detect rejections at an early stage with a simple biochemical or histologic test. None is known for islet transplants, and this is hampering current attempts to provide appropriate immunosuppression for these patients. These issues will likely yield to further experimental endeavors, and islet transplantation will likely supplant whole-organ pancreas transplantation.

REFERENCES

1. Eckhardt LA. Immunoglobulin gene expression only in the right cells at the right time. *FASEB J* 1992;6:2553.
2. Komori T, Okada A, Stewart V, et al. Lack of N regions in antigen receptor variable region genes of TdT-deficient lymphocytes. *Science* 1993;261:1171.
3. Gilfillan S, Dierich A, Lemeur M, et al. Mice lacking TdT: mature animals with an immature lymphocyte repertoire. *Science* 1993;261:1175.
4. Aldhouse P. Transgenic mice display a class (switching) act. *Science* 1993;262:1212.
5. Papavasiliou F, Jankovic M, Gong S, et al. Control of immunoglobulin gene rearrangements in developing B cells. *Curr Opin Immunol* 1997;9:233.
6. Cambier JC, Campbell KS. Membrane immunoglobulin and its accomplices: new lessons from an old receptor. *FASEB J* 1992;6:3207.
7. Clark MR, Campbell KS, Kazalauskas A, et al. The B cell antigen receptor complex: association of Ig-a and Ig-b with distinct cytoplasmic effectors. *Science* 1992;258:123.
8. Constant P, Davodeau F, Peyrat M, et al. Stimulation of human gdT cells by nonpeptidic mycobacterial ligands. *Science* 1994;264:267.
9. Momvaerts P, Arnoldi J, Russ, F, et al. Different roles of and T cells in immunity against an intracellular bacterial pathogen. *Nature* 1993;365:53.
10. Schild H, Mavaddat N, Litzenberger C, et al. The nature of major histocompatibility complex recognition by gd T cells. *Cell* 1994;76:29–37.
11. Weiss A. T cell antigen receptor signal transduction: a tale of tails and cytoplasmic protein-tyrosine kinases. *Cell* 1993;73:209.
12. Williams AF, Beyers AD. At grips with interactions. *Nature* 1992;356:746.
13. Barinage M. Getting some "backbone": how MHC binds peptides. *Science* 1992;257:880.
14. Germain RN. MHC-dependent antigen processing and peptide presentation: providing ligands for T lymphocyte activation. *Cell* 1994;76:287.
15. Townsend A. A new presentation pathway? *Nature* 1992;356:386.
16. Schmid SL, Jackson MR. Making class II presentable. *Nature* 1994;368:103.
17. Howard JC, Seelig A. Peptides and the proteasome. *Nature* 1993;365:211.
18. Powis SJ, Deverson EV, Coadwell WJ, et al. Effect of polymorphism of an MHC-linked transporter on the peptides assembled in a class I molecule. *Nature* 1992;357:211.
19. Lanzavecchia A, Reid PA, Watts C. Irreversible association of peptides with class II MHC molecules in living cells. *Nature* 1992;357:249.
20. Peterson M, Miller J. Antigen presentation enhanced by the alternatively spliced invariant chain gene product p41. *Nature* 1992;357:596.
21. Malnati MS, Marti M, LaVaute T, et al. Processing pathways for presentation of cytosolic antigen to MHC class II-restricted T cells. *Nature* 1992;357:702.
22. Riberdy JM, Newcomb JR, Surman MJ, et al. HLA-DR molecules from an antigen-processing mutant cell line are associated with invariant chain peptides. *Nature* 1992;360:474.
23. Eisenlohr LC, Bacik I, Bennink JR, et al. Expression of a

membrane protease enhances presentation of endogenous antigens to MHC class IB restricted T lymphocytes. *Cell* 1992;71:963.

24. Kaer LV, Ashton-Rickardt PG, Ploegh HL, et al. TAP-1 mutant mice are deficient in antigen presentation, surface class I molecules, and CD4⁻8⁺ T cells. *Cell* 1992;71:1205.

25. Pfeifer JD, Wick MJ, Roberts RL, et al. Phagocytic processing of bacterial antigens for class I MHC presentation to T cells. *Nature* 1993; 361:359.

26. Michalek MT, Grant EP, Gramm C, et al. A role for the ubiquitin-dependent proteolytic pathway in MHC class I-restricted antigen presentation. *Nature* 1993;363:552.

27. Germain RN, Rinker AG. Peptide binding inhibits protein aggregation of invariant-chain free class II dimers and promotes surface expression of occupied molecules. *Nature* 1993;373:725.

28. Driscoll J, Brown MG, Finley D. MHC-linked LMP gene products specifically alter peptidase activities of the proteasome. *Nature* 1993;365:262.

29. Gaczynska M, Rock KL, Goldberg AL. g-Interferon and expression of MHC genes regulate peptide hydrolysis by proteasomes. *Nature* 1993;365:264.

30. Heemels MT, Schumacher TN, Wonigeit K, et al. Peptide translocation by variants of the transporter associated with antigen processing. *Science* 1993;262:2059.

31. Jackson MR, Cohen-Doyle MF, Peterson PA, et al. Regulation of MHC class I transport by the molecular chaperone, calnexin (p88, IP90). *Science* 1994;263:384.

32. Chicz RM, Urban RG, Lane WS, et al. Predominant naturally processed peptides bound to HLA-DR1 are derived from MHC-related molecules and are heterogeneous in size. *Nature* 1992;358:764.

33. Momburg F, Roelse J, Howard JC, et al. Selectivity of MHC-encoded peptide transporters from human, mouse and rat. *Nature* 1994;367:648.

34. Bodmer H, Viville S, Benoist C, et al. Diversity of endogenous epitopes bound to MHC class II molecules limited by invariant chain. *Science* 1994;263:1284.

35. Ortmann B, Androlewicz MJ, Cresswell P. MHC class I/b₂-microglobulin complexes associate with TAP transporters before peptide binding. *Nature* 1994;368:864.

36. Suh WK, Cohen-Doyle MF, Fruh K, et al. Interaction of MHC class I molecules with the transporter associated with antigen processing. *Science* 1994;264:1322.

37. Hunt DF, Michel H, Dickinson TA. Peptides presented to the immune system by the murine class II major histocompatibility complex molecule I-Aᵈ. *Science* 1992;256:1817.

38. Pamer E, Cresswell P. Mechanisms of MHC class I-restricted antigen processing. *Annu Rev Immunol* 1998;16:323.

39. Wolf PR, Ploegh HL. How MHC class II molecules acquire peptide cargo: biosynthesis and trafficking through the endocytic pathway. *Annu Rev Cell Dev Biol* 1995;11:267.

40. Groettrup M, Soza A, Kuckelkorn U, et al. Peptide antigen production by the proteasome: complexity provides efficiency. *Immunol Today* 1996;17:429.

41. Rock KL, Goldberg AL. Degradation of cell proteins and the generation of MHC class I-presented peptides. *Annu Rev Immunol* 1999;17:739.

42. Kurlander RJ, Shawar SM, Brown ML, et al. Specialized role for a murine class I-b MHC molecule in prokaryotic host defenses. *Science* 1992;257:678.

43. Rotzschke O, Falk K, Stevanovic S, et al. Qa-2 molecules are peptide receptors of higher stringency than ordinary class I molecules. *Nature* 1993;361:642.

44. Bachmann MF, Rohrer UH, Kundig TM, et al. The influence of antigen organization on B cell responsiveness. *Science* 1993;262:1448.

45. Guymer RH, Mandel TE. A comparison of corneal, pancreas, and skin grafts in mice. *Transplantation* 1994;57:1251.

46. Springer TA. Traffic signals for lymphocyte recirculation and leukocyte emigration: the multistep paradigm. *Cell* 1994;76:301.

47. Parham P. The box and the rod. *Nature* 1992;357:538.

48. Konig R, Huang L, Germain RN. MHC class II interaction with CD4 mediated by a region analogous to the MHC class I binding site for CD8. *Nature* 1992;356:796.

49. Kelso A. Th1 and Th2 subsets: paradigms lost? *Immunol Today* 1995;16:374.

50. Piccotti JR, Chan SY, VanBuskirk AM, et al. Are Th2 helper T lymphocytes beneficial, deleterious, or irrelevant in promoting allograft survival? *Transplantation* 1997;63:619.

51. Reiner SL, Wang Z, Hatam F, et al. T_H1 and T_H2 cell antigen receptors in experimental leishmaniasis. *Science* 1993;259:1457.

52. Takeuchi T, Lowry RP, Konieczny B. Heart allografts in murine systems. *Transplantation* 1992;53:1281.

53. Gaur A, Haspel R, Mayer J, et al. Requirement for CD8+ cells in T cell receptor peptide-induced clonal unresponsiveness. *Science* 1993;259:91.

54. LaRosa FG, Smilek D, Talmage DW, et al. Evidence that tolerance to cultured thyroid allografts is an active immunological process. *Transplantation* 1992;53:903.

55. Qin S, Cobbold SP, Pope H, et al. "Infectious" transplantation tolerance. *Science* 1993;259:974.

56. Halwani F, Guttmann RD, Ste. Croix H, et al. Identification of natural suppressor cells in long-term renal allograft recipients. *Transplantation* 1992;54:973.

57. Clark EA, Ledbetter JA. How B and T cells talk to each other. *Nature* 1994;367:425.

58. Marx J. Cell communication failure leads to immune disorder. *Science* 1993;259:896.

59. Hill A, Chapel H. The fruits of cooperation. *Nature* 1993; 361:494.

60. Tsubata T, Wu J, Honjo T. B-cell apoptosis induced by antigen receptor crosslinking is blocked by a T-cell signal through CD40. *Nature* 1993;364:645.

61. Carter RH, Fearon DT. CD19: lowering the threshold for antigen receptor simulation of B lymphocytes. *Science* 1992; 256:105.

62. Mantovani A, Bussolino F, Dejana E. Cytokine regulation of endothelial cell function. *FASEB J* 1992;6:2591.

63. Gerritsen ME, Bloor CM. Endothelial cell gene expression in response to injury. *FASEB J* 1993;7:523.

64. Willebrand E, Salmela K, Isoniemi H, et al. Induction of HLA class II antigen and interleukin-2 receptor expression in acute vascular rejection of human kidney allografts. *Transplantation* 1992;53:1077.

65. Fuggle SV, Sanderson JB, Gray DW, et al. Variation in expression of endothelial adhesion molecules in pretransplant and transplanted kidneys: correlation with intragraft events. *Transplantation* 1993;55:1170.

66. Wuthrich RP, Jenkins TA, Snyder TL. Regulation of cytokine-stimulated vascular cell adhesion molecule-1 expression in renal tubular epithelial cells. *Transplantation* 1993; 55:172.

67. Pelletier RP, Morgan CJ, Sedmak DD, et al. Analysis of inflammatory endothelial changes, including VCAM-1 expression, in murine cardiac grafts. *Transplantation* 1993;55:315.

68. Hoffmann MW, Wonigeit K, Steinhoff G, et al. Production of cytokines (TNFα, IL-1β) and endothelial cell activation in human liver allograft rejection. *Transplantation* 1993;55: 329.

69. Morgan CJ, Pelletier RP, Hernandez CJ, et al. Alloantigen-dependent endothelial phenotype and lymphokine mRNA expression in rejecting murine cardiac allografts. *Transplantation* 1993;55:919.

70. Pober JS, Orosz CG, Rose ML, et al. Can graft endothelial cells initiate a host anti-graft immune response? *Transplantation* 1996;61:343.

71. Briscoe DM, Alexander SI, Lichtman AH. Interactions between T lymphocytes and endothelial cells in allograft rejection. *Curr Opin Immunol* 1998;10:525.

72. Albelda SM, Smith CM, Ward PA. Adhesion molecules and inflammatory injury. *FASEB J* 1994;8:504.

73. Hynes RO. Integrins: versatility, modulation, and signaling in cell adhesion. *Cell* 1992;69:11.

74. Lasky LA. Selectins: interpreters of cell-specific carbohydrate information during inflammation. *Science* 1992;258:964.

75. Shimizu Y, Shaw S. Mucins in the mainstream. *Nature* 1993;366:630.

76. Baumhueter S, Singer MS, Henzel W, et al. Binding of L-selectin to the vascular sialomucin CD34. *Science* 1993;262: 436.

77. Berg EL, McEvoy LM, Berlin C, et al. L-selectin–mediated lymphocyte rolling on MAdCAM-1. *Nature* 1993;366:695.

78. Taylor PM, Rose ML, Yacoub MH, et al. Induction of vascular adhesion molecules during rejection of human cardiac allografts. *Transplantation* 1992; 54:451.

79. Paul WE, Seder RA. Lymphocyte responses and cytokines. *Cell* 1994;76:241.

80. Nowak R. Bubble boy paradox resolved. *Science* 1993; 262:1818.

81. Kondo M, Takeshita T, Higuchi M, et al. Functional participation of the IL-2 receptor γ chain in IL-7 receptor complexes. *Science* 1994; 263:1453.

82. Kishimoto T, Akira S, Taga T. Interleukin-6 and its receptor: a paradigm for cytokines. *Science* 1992;258:593.

83. Kishimoto T, Taga T, Akira S. Cytokine signal transduction. *Cell* 1994;76:253.

84. Taga T, Kishimoto T. Cytokine receptors and signal transduction. *FASEB J* 1993;7:3387.

85. Stahl N, Yancopoulos GD. The alphas, betas, and kinases of cytokine receptor complexes. *Cell* 1993;74:587.

86. Hunter T. Cytokine connections. *Nature* 1993;366:114.

87. Stahl N, Boulton TG, Farruggella T, et al. Association and activation of Jak-Tyk kinases by CNTF-LIF-OSM-IL-6 b receptor components. *Science* 1994; 263:92.

88. Ramsay AJ, Husband AJ, Ramshaw IA, et al. The role of interleukin-6 in mucosal IgA antibody responses in vivo. *Science* 1994;264:561.

89. Scott, P. IL-12: initiation cytokine for cell-mediated immunity. *Science* 1993;260:496.

90. Afonso LC, Scharton TM, Vieira LQ, et al. The adjuvant effect of interleukin-12 in a vaccine against leishmania major. *Science* 1994;263:235.

91. Massague J. Receptors for the TGFβ family. *Cell* 1992;69:1067.

92. Wrana JL, Attisano L, Carcamo J, et al. TGFβ signals through a heteromeric protein kinase receptor complex. *Cell* 1992;71:1003.

93. Barral-Netto M, Barral A, Brownell CE, et al. Transforming growth factor-β in leishmanial infection: a parasite escape mechanism. *Science* 1992; 257:545.

94. Attisano L, Carcamo J, Ventura F, et al. Identification of human activin and TGFβ type I receptors that form heteromeric kinase complexes with type II receptors. *Cell* 1993;75:671.

95. Smith CA, Farrah T, Goodwin RG. The TNF receptor superfamily of cellular and viral proteins: activation, constimulation, and death. *Cell* 1994;76:959.

96. Cohen J. New protein steals the show as "costimulator" of T cells. *Science* 1993;262:844.

97. Beutler B, van Huffel C. Unraveling function in the TNF ligand and receptor families. *Science* 1994;264:667.

98. Suda T, Takahashi T, Golstein P, et al. Molecular cloning and expression of the Fas ligand, a novel member of the tumor necrosis factor family. *Cell* 1993;75:1169.

99. Barinaga M. Interfering with interferon. *Science* 1993;259:1693.

100. Huang S, Hendriks W, Althage A, et al. Immune response in mice that lack the interferon-γ receptor. *Science* 1993;259:1742.

101. Darnell JE, Kerr IM, Stark GR. Jak-STAT pathways and transcriptional activation in response to IFNs and other extracellular signaling proteins. *Science* 1994;264:1415.

102. Wu CJ, Lovett M, Wong-Lee J, et al. Cytokine gene expression in rejecting cardiac allografts. *Transplantation* 1992;54:326.

103. Halloran PF, Broski AP, Batiuk TD, et al. The molecular immunology of acute rejection: an overview. *Transplant Immunol* 1993;1:3.

104. Bishop DK, Shelby J, Eichwald E. Mobilization of T lymphocytes following cardiac transplantation. *Transplantation* 1992;53:849.

105. Doherty PC. Cell-mediated cytotoxicity. *Cell* 1993;75:607.

106. Kagi D, Vignaux F, Ledermann B, et al. Fas and perforin pathways as major mechanisms of T cell–mediated cytotoxicity. *Science* 1994; 265:528.

107. Mueller C, Shao Y, Altermatt HJ, et al. The effect of cyclosporine treatment on the expression of genes encoding granzyme A and perforin in the infiltrate of mouse heart transplants. *Transplantation* 1993;55:139.

108. Clement MV, Legros-Maida S, Isreal-Bib D, et al. Perforin and granzyme B expression is associated with severe acute rejection. *Transplantation* 1994;57:322.

109. Clark WR. The hole truth about perforin. *Nature* 1994;369:16–17.

110. Kagi D, Ledermann B, Burki K, et al. Cytotoxicity mediated by T cells and natural killer cells is greatly impaired in perforin-deficient mice. *Nature* 1994;369:31.

111. Whiteside TL, Herberman RB. Role of human natural killer cells in health and disease. *Clin Diagn Lab Immunol* 1994;1:125.

112. Raulet DH. A sense of something missing. *Nature* 1992;358:21.

113. Martinez OM, Ascher NL, Ferrell L, et al. Evidence for a nonclassical pathway of graft rejection involving interleukin 5 and eosinophils. *Transplantation* 1993;55:909.

114. Zhang Y, Ramos BF, Jakschik BA. Neutrophil recruitment by tumor necrosis factor from mast cells in immune complex peritonitis. *Science* 1992;258:1957.

115. Baggiolini M, Boulay F, Badwey JA, et al. Activation of neutrophil leukocytes: chemoattractant receptors and respiratory burst. *FASEB J* 1993;7:1004.

116. Morel D, Norman E, Lemoine C, et al. Tumor necrosis factor alpha in human kidney transplant rejection: analysis by in situ hybridization. *Transplantation* 1993;55:773.

117. Pizarro TT, Malinowska K, Kovacs E, et al. Induction of TNFα and TNFβ gene expression in rat cardiac transplants during allograft rejection. *Transplantation* 1993;56:399.

118. Saito R, Prehn J, Zuo X, et al. The participation of tumor necrosis factor in the pathogenesis of lung allograft rejection in the rat. *Transplantation* 1993;55:967.

119. Martinez OM, Villanueva JC, Lake J, et al. IL-2 and IL-5 gene expression in response to alloantigen in liver allograft recipients and in vitro. *Transplantation* 1993;55:1159.

120. Merville P, Pouteil-Noble C, Wijdenes J, et al. Detection of single cells secreting IFN-gamma, IL-6, and IL-10 in irreversibly rejected human kidney allografts, and their modulation by IL-2 and IL-4. *Transplantation* 1993; 55:639.

121. Kopf M, Baumann H, Freer G, et al. Impaired immune and acute-phase responses in interleukin-6–deficient mice. *Nature* 1994;368:339.

122. Blancho G, Moreau JF, Chabannes D, et al. HILDA/LIF, G-CSF, IL-1β, and TNFα production during acute rejection of human kidney allografts. *Transplantation* 1993;56:597.

123. Bentouimou N, Moreau JF, Peyrat MA, et al. The effects of cyclosporine on HILDA/LIF gene expression in human T cells. *Transplantation* 1993;55:163.

124. Blotnick S, Peoples GE, Freeman MR, et al. T lymphocytes synthesize and export heparin-binding epidermal growth factor-like growth factor and basic fibroblast growth factor, mitogens for vascular cells and fibroblasts: differential production and release by CD4+ and CD8+ T cells. *Proc Natl Acad Sci USA* 1994;91:2890.

125. Johnston PS, Wang MW, Lim SM, et al. Discordant xenograft rejection in an antibody-free model. *Transplantation* 1992;54:573.

126. Stansby G, Fuller B, Jeremy J, et al. Endothelin release: a facet of reperfusion injury in clinical liver transplantation? *Transplantation* 1993;56:239.

127. Spurney RF, Ibrahim S, Butterly D, et al. Leukotrienes in renal transplant rejection in rats. *J Immunol* 1994;152:867.

128. Langreher JM, Hoffman RA, Lancaster JR, et al. Nitric oxide: a new endogenous immunomodulator. *Transplantation* 1993;55:1205.

129. Xenos ES, Stevens RB, Sutherland DE, et al. The role of nitric oxide in IL-1β–mediated dysfunction of rodent islets of Langerhans. *Transplantation* 1994;57:1208.

130. Connor HD, Gao W, Nukina S, et al. Evidence that free radicals are involved in graft failure following orthotopic liver transplantation in the rat: an electron paramagnetic resonance spin trapping study. *Transplantation* 1992;54:199.

131. Land W, Schneeberg H, Schleibner S, et al. The beneficial effect of human recombinant superoxide dismutase on acute and chronic rejection events in recipients of cadaveric renal transplants. *Transplantation* 1994;57:211.

132. Alexandre GP, Latinne D, Gianello P, et al. Preformed cytotoxic antibodies and ABO-incompatible grafts. *Clin Transpl* 1991;5:583.

133. Bach FH. Xenotransplantation: problems for consideration. *Clin Transpl* 1991;5:595.

134. Paul LC, Fellstrom B. Chronic vascular rejection of the heart

and the kidney: have rational treatment options emerged? *Transplantation* 1992;53:1169.

135. Hancock WH, Whitely WD, Tullius SG, et al. Cytokines, adhesion molecules, and the pathogenesis of chronic rejection of rat renal allografts. *Transplantation* 1993;56:643.

136. Hajar DP, Pomerantz KB. Signal transduction in atherosclerosis: integration of cytokines and the eicosanoid network. *FASEB J* 1992;6:2933.

137. Van Parijs L, Abbas AK. Homeostasis and self-tolerance in the immune system: turning lymphocytes off. *Science* 1998; 280:243.

138. Weissman IL. Developmental switches in the immune system. *Cell* 1994;76:207.

139. vonBoehmer H. Positive selection of lymphocytes. *Cell* 1994;76:219.

140. Nossal GJ. Negative selection of lymphocytes. *Cell* 1994;76:229.

141. Allen PM. Peptides in positive and negative selection: a delicate balance. *Cell* 1994;76:593.

142. Marrack P, Parker DC. A little of what you fancy. *Nature* 1994;368:397.

143. Janeway CA. Thymic selection: two pathways to life and two to death. *Immunity* 1994;1:3.

144. vonBoehmer H, Kisielow P. Lymphocyte lineage commitment: instruction versus selection. *Cell* 1993;73:207.

145. Schwartz RH. Costimulation of T lymphocytes: the role of CD28, CTLA-4, and B7/BB1 in interleukin-2 production and immunotherapy. *Cell* 1992;71:1065.

146. Harding FA, McArthur JG, Gross JA, et al. CD28-mediated signaling co-stimulates murine T cells and prevents induction of anergy in T-cell clones. *Nature* 1992;356:607.

147. McCormick F. How receptors turn Ras on. *Nature* 1993;363:15.

148. Marx J. Two major signal pathways linked. *Science* 1993; 262:988.

149. Clements JL. and Koretzky GA. Recent developments in lymphocyte activation: linking kinases to downstream signaling events. *J Clin Invest* 1999;103:925.

150. Schillance RV, Scott JD. Organization of kinases, phosphatases and receptor signaling complexes. *J Clin Invest* 1999;106:761.

151. Jenkins MK, Miller RA. Memory and anergy: challenges to traditional models of T lymphocyte differentiation. *FASEB J* 1992;6:2428.

152. Sprent J. T and B memory cells. *Cell* 1994;76:315.

153. vonBoehmer H. Tolerance by exhaustion. *Nature* 1993;362: 696.

154. Ferber I, Schonrich G, Schenkel J, et al. Levels of peripheral T cell tolerance by different doses of tolerogen. *Science* 1994;263:674.

155. Critchfield JM, Racke MK, Zuniga-Pflucker J, et al. T cell deletion in high antigen dose therapy of autoimmune encephalomyelitis. *Science* 1994;263:1139.

156. Ramsdell F, Fowlkes BJ. Maintenance of in vivo tolerance by persistence of antigen. *Science* 1992;257:1130.

157. Lombardi G, Sidhu S, Batchelor R, et al. Anergic T cells as suppressor cells in vitro. *Science* 1994;264:1587.

158. Araten DJ, Lawton T, Ferrara J, et al. In vitro alloreactivity against host antigens in an adult HLA-mismatched bone marrow transplant recipient despite in vivo host tolerance. *Transplantation* 1993;55:76.

159. Posselt AM, Barker CF, Friedman AL, et al. Prevention of autoimmune diabetes in the BB rat by intrathymic islet transplantation at birth. *Science* 1992;256:1321.

160. Campos L, Alfrey EJ, Posselt AM, et al. Prolonged survival of rat orthotopic liver allografts after intrathymic inoculation of donor-strain cells. *Transplantation* 1993;55:866.

161. Markmann JF, Odorico JS, Bassiri H, et al. Deletion of donor-reactive T lymphocytes in adult mice after intrathymic inoculation with lymphoid cells. *Transplantation* 1993;55:871.

162. Spitzer TR, Delmonico F, Tolkoff-Rubin N, et al. Combined histocompatibility leukocyte antigen matched donor bone marrow and renal transplantation for multiple myeloma with end stage renal disease: the induction of allograft tolerance through mixed lymphohematopoietic chimerism. *Transplantation* 1999;68:480.

163. Wekerle T, Sykes M. Mixed chimerism as an approach for the induction of transplantation tolerance. *Transplantation* 1999;68:459.

164. Miller J, Mathew J, Garcia-Morales R, et al. The human bone marrow as an immunoregulatory organ. *Transplantation* 1999;68:1079.

165. Starzl TE, Demetris AJ, Trucco M, et al. Chimerism and donor-specific nonreactivity 27 to 2 years after kidney allotransplantation. *Transplantation* 1993;55:1272.

166. Fuchs EJ, Matzingert P. B cells turn off virgin but not memory T cells. *Science* 1992;258:1156.

167. Larsen CP, Elwood ET, Alexander DZ, et al. Long-term acceptance of skin and cardiac allografts after blocking CD40 and CD28 pathways. *Nature* 1996;381:434.

168. Kirk AD, Harlan DM, et al. CTLA4-Ig and anti-CD40 ligand prevent renal allograft rejection in primates. *Proc Natl Acad Sci USA* 1997;94:8789.

169. Sayegh MH, Turka LA. The role of T-cell costimulatory activation pathways in transplant rejection. *N Engl J Med* 1998; 338:1813.

170. Kirk AD, Burkly LC, Batty DS, et al. Treatment with humanized monoclonal antibody against CD154 prevents acute renal allograft rejection in nonhuman primates. *Nat Med* 1999;5:686.

171. Harlan DM, Kirk AD. The future of organ and tissue transplantation: can T-cell costimulatory pathway modifiers revolutionize the prevention of graft rejection? *JAMA* 1999;282: 1076.

172. Halloran P, Mathew T, Tomlanovich S, et al. Mycophenolate mofetil in renal allograft recipients. *Transplantation* 1997; 63:39.

173. The Mycophenolate mofetil acute renal rejection study group. Mycophenolate mofetil for the treatment of a first acute renal allograft rejection. *Transplantation* 1998;65:235.

174. Groth CG, Backman L, Morales JM, et al. Sirolimus (Rapamycin)-based therapy in human renal transplantation. *Transplantation* 1999;67:1036.

175. Kahan BD, Julian BA, Pescovitz MD, et al. Sirolimus reduces the incidence of acute rejection episodes despite lower cyclosporin doses in Caucasian recipients of mismatched primary renal allografts: a phase II trial. *Transplantation* 1999; 68:1526.

176. Brennan DC, Flavin K, Lowell JA, et al. A randomized, double-blinded comparison of Thymoglobulin versus Atgam for induction immunosuppressive therapy in adult renal transplant recipients [published erratum appears in *Transplantation* 1999;67:1386] *Transplantation* 1999;67:1011.

177. Kahan BD, Rajagopalan PR, Hall M, et al. Reduction of the occurrence of acute cellular rejection among renal allograft recipients treated with basiliximab, a chimeric anti-interleukin-2 receptor monoclonal antibody. *Transplantation* 1999;67:276.

178. Vincenti F, Kirkman R, Light S, et al. Interleukin-2-receptor blockade with daclizumab to prevent acute rejection in renal transplantation. *N Engl J Med* 1998;338:161.

179. Morris RE. ±15-Deoxyspergualin: a mystery wrapped within an enigma. *Clin Transpl* 1991; 5:530.

180. Nadler SG, Tepper MA, Schacter B, et al. Interaction of the immunosuppressant deoxyspergualin with a member of the Hsp70 family of heat shock proteins. *Science* 1992;258:484.

181. Ramos EL, Nadler SG, Grasela DM, et al. Deoxyspergualin: mechanism of action and pharmacokinetics. *Transplant Proc* 1996;28:873.

182. Chong AS, Finnegan A, Jiang X, et al. Leflunomide, a novel immunosuppressive agent. *Transplantation* 1993;55:1361.

183. Williams JW, Xiao F, Foster P, et al. Leflunomide in experimental transplantation. *Transplantation* 1994;57:1223.

184. Chong AS, Huang W, Liu W, et al. In vivo activity of leflunomide: pharmacokinetic analyses and mechanism of immunosuppression. *Transplantation* 1999;68:100.

185. Jameson BA, McDonnell JM, Marini JC, et al. A rationally designed CD4 analogue inhibits experimental allergic encephalomyelitis. *Nature* 1994;368:744.

186. Travers P. Immunological agnosia. *Nature* 1993;363:117.

187. Weber S, Traunecker A, Oliveri F, et al. Specific low-affinity recognition of major histocompatibility complex plus peptide by soluble T-cell receptor. *Nature* 1992;356:793.

188. Sloan-Lancaster J, Evavold BD, Allen PM. Induction of T-cell anergy by altered T cell-receptor ligand on live antigen-presenting cells. *Nature* 1993;363:156.

189. Roslin MS, Tranbaugh RE, Panza A, et al. One-year monkey heart xenograft survival in cyclosporine-treated baboons. *Transplantation* 1992;54:949.

190. Hardy MA, Reed E, Suciu-Foca N. Antiidiotypic antibodies and pretreatment with blood transfusions in organ transplantation. *Clin Transpl* 1991;5:501.

191. Weiner HL, Mackin GA, Matsui M, et al. Double-blind pilot trial of oral tolerization with myelin antigens in multiple sclerosis. *Science* 1993;259:1321.

192. Hancock WW, Sayegh MH, Kwok CA, et al. Oral, but not intravenous, alloantigen prevents accelerated allograft rejection by selective intragraft T$_H$2 cell activation. *Transplantation* 1993;55:1112.

193. Paya CV, Fung JJ, Nalesnik MA, et al. Epstein-Barr virus-induced posttransplant lymphoproliferative disorders. ASTS/ASTP EBV-PTLD Task Force and The Mayo Clinic Organized International Consensus Development Meeting. *Transplantation* 1999;68:1517.

194. Penn I. The effect of immunosuppression on pre-existing cancers. *Transplantation* 1993;55:742.

195. Colquhoun SD, Robert ME, Shaked A, et al. Transmission of CNS malignancy by organ transplantation. *Transplantation* 1994;57:970.

196. Auchincloss H, Sachs DH. Xenogeneic transplantation. *Annu Rev Immunol* 1998;16:433.

197. Leventhal JR, Matas AJ. Xenotransplantation in rodents: a review and reclassification. *Transplant Rev* 1994;8:80.

198. Gorski A, Grieb P, Makula J, et al. Human xenoreactive natural antibodies: avidity and targets on porcine endothelial cells. *Transplantation* 1993;56:1251.

199. Dalmasso AP, Platt JL. Prevention of complement-mediated activation of xenogeneic endothelial cells in an in vitro model of xenograft hyperacute rejection by C1 inhibitor. *Transplantation* 1993;56:1171.

200. McCurry KR, Kooyman DL, Alvarado CG, et al. Human complement regulatory proteins protect swine-to-primate cardiac xenografts from humoral injury. *Nat Med* 1995;1:423.

201. Lambrigts D, Sachs DH, Cooper DK. Discordant organ xenotransplantation in primates: world experience and current status. *Transplantation* 1998;66:547.

202. Michaels MG, Simmons RL. Xenotransplant-associated zoonoses. *Transplantation* 1994;57:1.

203. Patience C, Takeuchi Y, Weiss RA. Infection of human cells by an endogenous retrovirus of pigs. *Nat Med* 1997;3:282.

204. Shaked A, Csete ME, Shiraishi M, et al. Retroviral-mediated gene transfer into rat experimental liver transplant. *Transplantation* 1994;57:32.

205. Fedoseyeva EV, Li Y, Huey B, et al. Inhibition of interferon-γ mediated immune functions by oligonucleotides. *Transplantation* 1994;57:606.

206. Ramanathan M, Lantz M, MacGregor RD, et al. Inhibition of interferon-γ induced major histocompatibility complex class I expression by certain oligodeoxynucleotides. *Transplantation* 1994;57:612.

207. Magee JC, Sung RS, Bromberg JS. Gene therapy in organ transplantation: applicabilities and shortcomings. In: Sayegh MH, Remuzzi G, eds. *Current and future immunosuppression therapies following transplantation.* Dordrecht, The Netherlands: Kluwer Academic (in press).

208. Fox JJ, Chowdhury JR, Kaufmann SS, et al. Treatment of the Crigler-Najjar syndrome type I with hepatocyte transplantation. *N Engl J Med* 1998;338:1422.

Organ Preservation

JEFRREY D. PUNCH AND ROBERT M. MERION

PATHOPHYSIOLOGY OF ORGAN PRESERVATION INJURY

The removal, storage, and transplantation of a solid organ from a cadaveric donor results in profound alterations in homeostatic control of the organ's interior milieu. These effects manifest themselves in the degree to which the return of normal organ function is delayed or prevented once the transplantation procedure is completed. The injury sustained by an organ during the processes of procurement, preservation, and transplantation occurs primarily as a result of ischemia and hypothermia, ischemic injury being customarily divided into warm and cold ischemia. Warm ischemia and its consequences are associated with normothermic events that occur before removal of the organ from the body. Cold ischemia refers to events occurring during the interval between initial organ cooling and revascularization in the recipient.

The principles of modern organ preservation are to provide for hypothermia, prevention of cellular swelling, and avoidance of biochemical injury (1). These principles are based on known physiologic events that occur during organ storage and result in loss of cellular integrity, changes in ionic composition, and disruption of cellular energy systems. The following sections describe these phenomena. Finally, the effects of oxygen-derived free radicals, cytokines, and nitric oxide at the time of reperfusion are discussed.

Structural Integrity

The cell membrane plays a crucial physical protective role for the cell in addition to providing an active interface with the extracellular environment. Receptors, ion regulation, and enzyme systems linked to the cell membrane complex contain extracellular, transmembrane, and intracellular components essential to their function. The interrelation of such systems with the membrane itself is highly dependent on a stable configuration of the lipid bilayer and on tight control of temperature, pH, and osmolarity. Organ ischemia and preservation disrupt all these relations. Lowering the temperature through the phase transition of lipids results in profound changes in conformation and stability of the membrane in addition to drastically altering the function of membrane-bound enzymes. Physicochemical membrane changes induced by hypothermia result in increased permeability, which in turn adds to the burden of maintaining a stable intracellular environment and contributes to cell swelling. Organ preservation solutions are therefore hypertonic to minimize these alterations.

Ionic Composition

The foregoing membrane changes are compounded by crippling of the Na$^+$-K$^+$-adenosine triphosphatase (ATPase) pump because of the lack of ATP production and by production of excess hydrogen ion because of anaerobic metabolism during ischemia. When the Na$^+$-K$^+$-ATPase pump is paralyzed, potassium is allowed out of the cell and diffuses down its concentration gradient to the extracellular environment, whereas sodium, which is normally kept at a low concentration in the cell, pours in. Current preservation solutions have electrolyte compositions similar to that inside the cell, with high potassium and low sodium concentrations. Osmotic gradients are therefore minimized and the cellular ionic charge remains relatively constant.

Hydrogen ion production continues in ischemic organs and may result in cellular damage. Intracellular pH gradually falls without replenishment of buffering capabilities, and under conditions requiring a switch from aerobic to anaerobic glycolysis, the production of lactic acid also increases. The liver appears to be especially susceptible to this type of injury. A plausible mechanism has been described whereby glucokinase in the liver phosphorylates glucose (endogenous or provided in preservation solution) to glucose-6-phosphate (2). The normal metabolic pathway for glucose-6-phosphate results in production of pyruvate and ultimately lactate by lactate dehydrogenase (Fig. 16.23). Unlike in the kidney, the hepatic isozyme of lactate dehydrogenase, M4, functions particularly well under acidotic conditions in the presence of high concentrations of lactic acid. These biochemical differences underlie the differences in organ "shelf life," that is, the fact that different organs remain functional after different degrees of cold ischemia.

Calcium ion permeability is increased with ischemia, and a rapid influx of calcium may overwhelm intracellular buffering capacity. There is increased activity of calmodulin, a cytoplasmic calcium-binding protein; and a cascade of enzyme activation events, including the up-regulation of phospholipases and subsequent production of prostaglandin derivatives, results in mitochondrial and cell membrane injury. Vascular smooth muscle myofibrillar contraction may be initiated by increased cellular calcium concentrations, with the resulting vasospasm contributing to ischemic damage. Endothelin, a 21-amino acid peptide with potent vasoconstrictor properties, has been recognized as another factor that plays a major role in ischemia by inducing vasospasm, which causes delayed organ function after revascularization (3,4).

Cellular Energy

The energy requirements of aerobic cells are provided by a combination of the enzymatic breakdown of glucose (glycolysis) and by the process of cellular respiration, encompassing the transfer of electrons from organic molecules to molecular oxygen (electron transport and oxidative phosphorylation; Fig. 16.24). Hypothermia results in decreased metabolic rate and slows the rate at which enzymes degrade cellular components, but metabolism is not completely suppressed. It has been calculated that cooling from 37° to 0°C results in a 12-fold reduction in cellular metabolism (1). Although metabolism and utilization of cellular energy stores are slowed, ATP and adenosine diphosphate (ADP), the major sources of cellular metabolic energy, are gradually depleted during hypothermia. This depletion is presumably due to residual energy requirements that exceed the capacity of the cell to produce ATP.

During ischemia and organ preservation, the glycolytic pathway is side-tracked to lactate production as the Krebs tricarboxylic acid cycle and mitochondrial respiration are impaired. Although some of the enzymes of the Krebs cycle may be found in the extramitochondrial cytoplasm, the inner compartment of the mitochondrion is where the enzymatic reactions of the cycle occur. Mitochondrial dysfunction, therefore, is responsible for most of the changes in cellular energy associated with ischemia and organ preservation.

Hypothermic preservation results in reduced activity of mitochondrial enzymes. Cellular respiration, which requires adenine nucleotide substrates, is reduced. For ADP to be transported into the mitochondrion as a substrate for conversion to the high-energy ATP, a membrane adenine nucleotide translocase is required. Hypothermia unfavorably alters the relation between the enzyme and the inner mitochondrial membrane within which it resides, reduc-

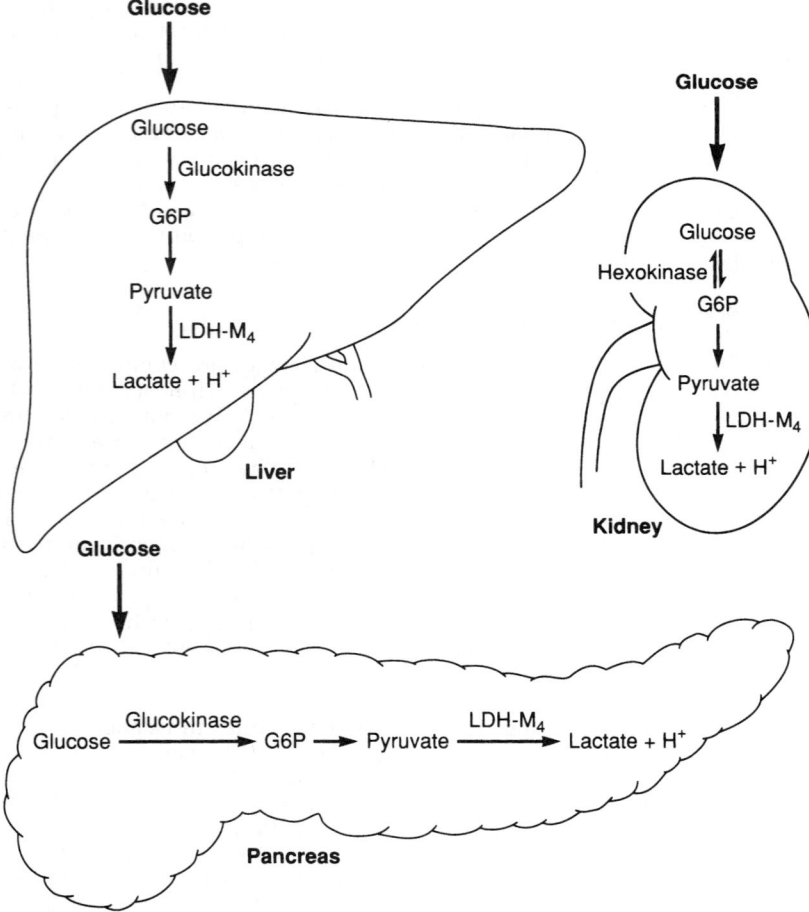

Figure 16.23. The effects of acidosis on glucose metabolism are organ specific. For example, the M4 isozyme of lactate dehydrogenase (LDH) functions well in an acidotic environment in the presence of high concentrations of lactic acid. G6P, glucose-6-phosphate. (After Belzer FO, Southard JH. Principles of solid-organ preservation by cold storage. *Transplantation* 1988;45:673.)

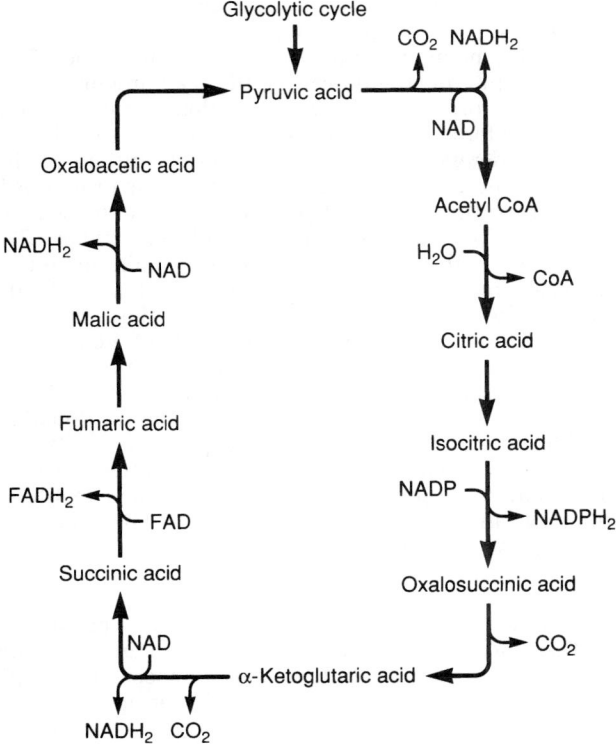

Figure 16.24. Cellular energy requirements are met largely through the processes of glycolysis, the Krebs tricarboxylic acid cycle, and oxidative phosphorylation. CoA, coenzyme A; FAD, flavin adenine dinucleotide; $FADH_2$, reduced form of FAD; NAD, nicotinamide adenine dinucleotide; $NADH_2$, reduced form of NAD.

ing substrate delivery (5). Phospholipid hydrolysis by phospholipases increases levels of free fatty acids, acyl derivatives of which may also affect membrane structure and the function of the translocase. Cannibalization of ADP sequestered in the extramitochondrial cytoplasm by adenylate kinase for conversion to ATP results in accumulation of adenosine monophosphate as a by-product. This reduces purine synthesis and results in the loss of ATP precursors from the cell.

Reperfusion Injury

It is now apparent that much of the injury to transplanted organs actually occurs not during the ischemia *per se,* but on organ reperfusion. This realization has led to many advances in organ preservation aimed at preventing this type of injury. Furthermore, some of the events that occur during reperfusion may result in enhanced immunogenicity of the graft. A better understanding of these events will, it is hoped, lead to the development of preservation methods that decrease the propensity for allograft rejection at a later date.

Oxygen Free Radical-mediated Effects

Fundamental work during the 1970s and 1980s established the mechanisms by which reactive species of oxygen are produced in biologic systems and documented the effects of these molecules on various cells and tissues (6). The best-studied model involves the production of superoxide anion (O_2^-) as a by-product of the enzymatic catabolism of the purine metabolites hypoxanthine and xanthine

to uric acid by xanthine oxidase (Fig. 16.25). During ischemic states, cytosolic enzymes are activated by increased intracellular calcium, resulting in the conversion of xanthine dehydrogenase to xanthine oxidase. Both xanthine dehydrogenase and xanthine oxidase catabolize hypoxanthine and xanthine to uric acid, and xanthine oxidase uses molecular oxygen as an electron acceptor, forming O_2^- as a result. Superoxide anion rapidly reacts with itself to form hydrogen peroxide, a potent oxidant capable of injuring the cell by oxidizing lipid membranes and cellular proteins. Hydrogen peroxide then produces a cascade of oxygen free radicals that are even more potent oxidants, including hydroxyl radical ($OH\cdot$) and singlet oxygen. The damaging effects of oxygen free radicals begin on reperfusion of the organ. During ischemic conditions, tissue oxygen levels fall below the threshold needed to allow xanthine oxidase to metabolize xanthine and hypoxanthine. This allows the intracellular concentration of these metabolites to rise. On reperfusion, oxygen is suddenly available and metabolism proceeds rapidly, resulting in a dramatic and sudden production of reactive oxygen intermediates. The cellular defenses against peroxidation are overwhelmed and injury occurs (7).

Agents that reduce oxygen free radical generation, or scavenge them once they are formed, have been used to determine the contribution of these molecular species to preservation-related reperfusion injury and have the ability to decrease peroxidation due to oxygen free radicals during reperfusion. Allopurinol, an inhibitor of xanthine oxidase, has been shown to have protective effects when used before the ischemic insult in a variety of experimental systems. Unfortunately, allopurinol has other effects, such as vasodilatation and preservation of the purine nucleotide pool, making it a less-than-ideal agent for defining oxygen free radical effects. Other, more specific studies using superoxide dismutase have clearly demonstrated a role for oxygen radicals in reperfusion injury in transplantation (8). Similarly, desferroxamine, an iron chelator, removes an essential metal cofactor for the generation of the extremely reactive hydroxyl radical, resulting in decreased oxidative injury.

Indirect evidence of oxygen free radical effects rests on the documentation of lipid peroxidation. In this process, interaction of highly reactive oxygen species with polyunsaturated fatty acids in the cell membrane starts a chain reaction that may ultimately destroy cellular integrity and result in cell death. The products of this reaction can be measured by several different assays. The magnitude of lipid peroxidation appears to be inversely related to levels of glutathione, which functions as an endogenous free rad-

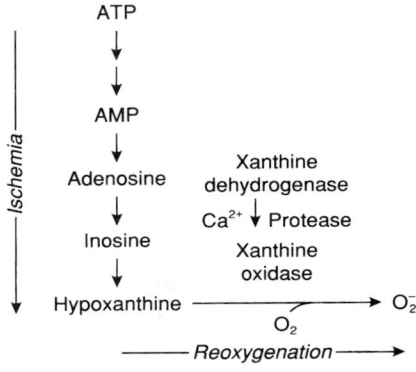

Figure 16.25. The classic pathway of superoxide anion generation by the metabolism of purines by xanthine oxidase. AMP, adenosine monophosphate; ATP, adenosine triphosphate.

ical scavenger. Glutathione and other agents that protect against peroxidation are therefore useful in organ preservation solutions to attenuate reperfusion injury.

Production of oxygen free radicals also initiates production of prostaglandins, including leukotriene B$_4$ by direct activation of phospholipase A$_2$. This chemoattractant causes leukocyte adherence to vascular endothelium. These neutrophils may contribute to local injury by plugging the microcirculation and by degranulation with resulting proteolytic damage to the organ.

Cytokine-mediated Effects

Cytokines are a group of intercellular messenger molecules that may be produced in a variety of normal and pathophysiologic states. Ischemia and reperfusion are known to be associated with marked release of tumor necrosis factor-α, a cytokine with profound systemic effects (9). Other cytokines, including interferon-γ, interleukin-1, and interleukin-8 (neutrophil chemotactic factor), may also be released during organ reperfusion and cause up-regulation of adhesion molecule expression on vascular endothelium. These changes, in addition to adhesion molecule up-regulation, may lead to leukocyte adherence and platelet plugging after revascularization, resulting in graft failure and an increased risk of later rejection.

Nitric Oxide-mediated Effects

Nitric oxide is an extremely labile autocoid generated by nitric oxide synthase from L-arginine. Nitric oxide has potent vasodilatory effects on microvasculature and is responsible for a wide variety of physiologic effects. Evidence is appearing that NO production is induced by inflammatory cytokines, including tumor necrosis factor-α, interferon-γ, and interleukin-1. In the setting of ischemia–reperfusion, NO may therefore mediate injury to organs directly as a result of cytokine release. Inhaled nitric oxide has been demonstrated to attenuate reperfusion injury in transplanted lungs (10). Increased NO synthesis also correlates with acute rejection (11).

CONTEMPORARY CLINICAL PRACTICE

The science of transplantation has developed rapidly since the mid-1970s. Improved understanding of the immune response to allografts and better appreciation of the complexity of organ ischemia- and preservation-related injury have contributed to greatly improved graft and patient survival results. Most solid organ transplantations are now performed as the therapeutic option of choice, and in many cases transplantation offers the only definitive treatment for a given disease entity. As a result, an ever-widening list of indications for solid organ transplantation has emerged, placing increasing pressure on an already limited supply of donor organs. As of November, 1999, there were 66,436 patients awaiting cadaveric organ transplantation in the United States, compared with half that many 4 years earlier (12). Each year, more patients are placed on the waiting lists than are transplanted, causing the waiting time to increase continually.

Determination of Suitability for Cadaveric Organ Donation

General Considerations

The characteristics of a suitable cadaveric organ donor can be divided into those that are general and those that are organ specific. Broadly stated, the general attributes of an acceptable organ donor include the establishment of a diagnosis of brain death, previously good general health, and relative hemodynamic stability from the time of the event precipitating brain death until organ procurement is complete. Informed consent from the donor's next of kin is required before organ procurement. Brain death is discussed in detail later. A detailed understanding of this condition and its associated pathophysiologic processes is essential for the successful procurement and subsequent transplantation of solid organs from cadaveric donors. The circumstances that lead to a diagnosis of brain death usually occur in a setting not conducive to the taking of a detailed medical history. Nevertheless, an effort should be made to contact family members or friends of the potential donor. In this way, the presence of any contraindications to donation can be identified early, and the next of kin can be spared the difficulties of a decision about donation. Cardiorespiratory arrest *per se* should not preclude consideration for organ donation, particularly if the arrest was witnessed, cardiopulmonary resuscitation was instituted promptly, and restoration of effective cardiac hemodynamics was successful.

Age

As experience has been gained with donors considered less than ideal, it has become apparent that arbitrarily defined age limits for organ donors are unnecessary. Ample evidence supports the relaxation of upper age limits for most abdominal organs. For example, renal procurement from cadaveric donors up to 65 years of age is now routinely considered, and successful renal transplantation has been reported from a cadaveric donor 84 years of age (13). Donor age has been similarly deemphasized in some hepatic transplantation programs, in which donors up to 70 years of age have been used, and almost 10% are over 50 years of age. The acceptable upper age limit for cardiac transplant donors has been cautiously but steadily increased, and occasional heart donors older than 45 years of age have been used after careful screening.

Transplantation of organs from donors at the younger extreme of life is usually successful, particularly if the recipient is also a child. Examples include pediatric hepatic and cardiac transplantation. Although the former case is amenable to a reduced-size allograft from an adult as an alternative, no such option exists for the child requiring cardiac replacement. Considerable controversy exists with regard to the advisability of transplanting kidneys from infants and children younger than 5 years of age (14,15) (Fig. 16.26). Lower graft survival rates have been reported when kidneys from very young donors have been transplanted, especially when the recipients are adults (15). However, some centers have reported extremely good short-term results using *en bloc* transplantation of both kidneys from pediatric donors to adults (16).

Overall Premorbid Health

Because most cadaveric organ donors have acute cerebral trauma or intracerebral catastrophe as the cause of brain death, serious associated systemic diseases are relatively uncommon in this population. Nevertheless, careful screening to ascertain that the donor was previously in good health is mandatory. Common disorders, such as hypertension and diabetes mellitus, do not automatically disqualify a person from organ donation, but the duration, severity, and treatment of such conditions should be evaluated for their potential effects on individual organs.

Hemodynamic Stability

Cardiovascular instability and eventual cardiopulmonary collapse occur in all brain-dead patients. Thus,

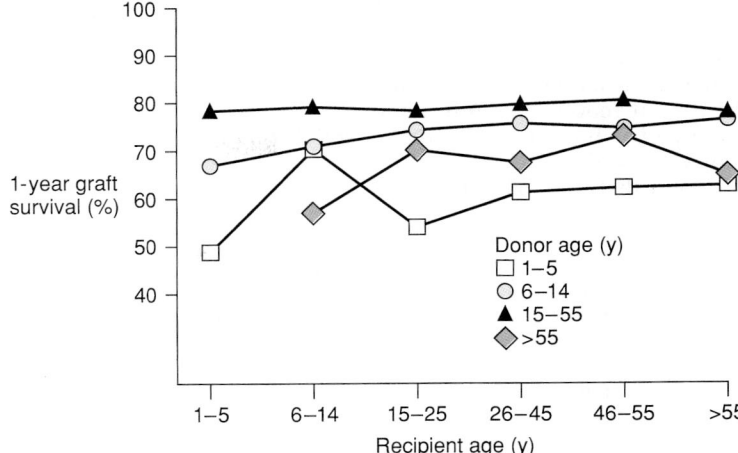

1-year graft survival (%)

Donor age (y)
□ 1–5
○ 6–14
▲ 15–55
◆ >55

Recipient age (y)

Figure 16.26. Relation between donor and recipient age and 1-year kidney graft survival. (After Zhou YC, Cecka JM. Effect of age on kidney transplants. In: Terasaki PI, ed. *Clinical transplantation 1989.* Los Angeles: UCLA Tissue Typing Laboratory, 1989:369.)

hemodynamic management is one of the most important aspects of donor management once brain death has been established and consent for organ donation obtained. As stated previously, however, many potential organ donors sustain significant hypotension or even cardiac arrest during the initial stages of their illness or as the presenting signs of intracerebral catastrophe. Knowledge of the course and management of these episodes is helpful in predicting damage to the various organs and in guiding the work-up of the donor for suitability of the organs for transplantation. In terms of specific organs, the kidneys appear to tolerate transient hypotension best, whereas the liver and pancreas may be more severely damaged by such episodes. The cardiac response to hypotension or actual cardiac arrest depends on the cause of the hemodynamic instability and the magnitude of direct cardiac injury sustained as a result of cardiac compressions during cardiopulmonary resuscitation.

Contraindications

Sepsis. Active systemic infection has traditionally been an absolute contraindication to organ donation. However, because of the current organ shortage, these tenets are being reexamined. A history of diseases such as tuberculosis or HIV infection clearly render a person unsuitable for donation. Pneumonia and urinary tract infection are no longer considered to be problematic in the absence of systemic sepsis. Even in the presence of bacteremia, the risk of transmission of infectious agents by organ transplantation appears to be small (17). In all cases, appropriate antibiotic therapy should be initiated before the procurement procedure.

Viral Infection. All potential organ donors, regardless of whether they are considered high risk, should be tested for evidence of infection with HIV. Under most circumstances, this test is carried out using an enzyme-linked immunosorbent assay. Although the incidence of false-positive results is somewhat of a problem, the high sensitivity of the test ensures that the risk of transmission of this virus is minimized. Testing is also routinely done for evidence of hepatitis B and C. History of viral hepatitis or serologic evidence of past infection has previously been considered an absolute contraindication to organ donation. Many centers are now reconsidering this issue, however, in selected situations. A percentage of organs from donors who have evidence of past infection with the hepatitis B virus are able to transmit the virus, even organs from donors in whom the sole evidence of infection is a positive antibody for hepatitis B core. However, these or-

gans may be considered for recipients who have long-standing infection with this virus or have received the recombinant hepatitis B vaccine and have demonstrated serologic immunity. Similarly, organs from donors with evidence of past infection with the hepatitis C virus are possible sources of infectious virus. The risk of infection is small, however, and these organs are now being considered for patients with known preexisting exposure to the hepatitis C virus (18).

Other viral titers that are frequently determined during work-up of a donor include members of the herpesvirus family, such as cytomegalovirus, Epstein-Barr virus, and herpes simplex virus. Evidence of previous infection with these viruses does not ordinarily preclude organ donation, but may require additional therapy in the recipient, such as hyperimmune globulin administration in the case of cytomegalovirus because this agent can be transmitted with the donor organ.

Cancer. Cancer, regardless of whether treated, has long been considered to contravene organ donation. This tenet of organ transplantation is based on the knowledge that tumor cells may circulate widely throughout the body even in patients with malignant lesions thought to be localized. The transplantation of even a small number of malignant cells into a recipient who is heavily immunosuppressed carries the threat of dissemination of malignancy and a disastrous outcome. The only exception to this rule has been the donor with a primary malignancy of the central nervous system. It has long been thought that as long as the blood–brain barrier is intact, these tumors are rarely capable of systemic spread. Although transmission of a central nervous system tumor of donor origin to a liver transplant recipient has been reported, the rate of transmission depends on the organ transplanted and the type of malignancy involved (19). These cases must be considered on an individual basis.

Specific Organ Dysfunction

The condition of particular organs of interest in great measure dictates their individual suitability for transplantation. With appropriate emphasis on the overall maintenance of donor homeostasis, however, most, if not all, transplantable organs should be procured from most donors. A history of long-standing hypertension may result in fixed damage to the kidneys as a result of hypertensive scarring and secondary to the effects of aortic and renal atherosclerosis. Similarly, insulin-dependent diabetes mellitus produces a well-known renal lesion. These changes may be reversible, however, after transplantation into a nondiabetic recipient (20). The kidneys are relatively resilient organs, and simple measures usually suffice to identify serious renal dysfunction. Measurements of hourly urinary output, coupled with determinations of the central venous pressure, are useful monitors of the adequacy of volume repletion in potential donors. Significant volume depletion occurs during the course of many disorders that lead to brain death. This is the combined result of intentional volume contraction to treat cerebral edema and the effects of diabetes insipidus accompanying lethal brain injury. Serum creatinine should be measured as a global, if imperfect, measure of renal function. Significant elevation of the serum creatinine level during the course of the donor hospitalization may be a sign of renal injury, predisposing to delayed graft function after transplantation. If necessary, an abbreviated form of a creatinine clearance measurement can be made on a 4-hour urine sample.

Preexisting hepatic disease usually can be identified before organ procurement. A history of hepatitis or cirrhosis of any kind precludes donation. Although calculous biliary tract disease would appear to be a contraindication to hepatic procurement, prior cholecystectomy for uncomplicated cholelithiasis is not an absolute contraindication to liver donation. Standard liver function tests, such as serum alanine aminotransferase, aspartate aminotransferase, alkaline phosphatase, and bilirubin, may be helpful in identifying gross injury to the donor liver resulting from traumatic, metabolic, or hemodynamic causes, but the absolute levels of these test results are poor indicators of the likelihood of immediate, life-sustaining graft function in the recipient. Hepatic synthetic function as assessed by prothrombin time may also be deceiving because of the effects of severe brain injury on the coagulation cascade (21).

The pancreas may be difficult to assess until the time of organ procurement. Hyperglycemia and hyperamylasemia are common in patients who sustain brain death, particularly if the cause is traumatic. A careful history establishing the absence of preexisting diabetes mellitus and pancreatitis provides the most useful information. A history of alcohol abuse alone does not correlate well with the finding of chronic pancreatitis at laparotomy. Computed tomographic examination of the abdomen may be indicated if the donor sustained any abdominal injury, but the decision to exclude a potential donor should not be made lightly because of the critical shortage of organs. It is more appropriate to examine the organ at the time of multiple organ harvesting to determine if it is suitable for transplantation rather than making a decision on the basis of historical or laboratory information alone.

Cardiac dysfunction resulting in arrhythmia or the need for inotropic support suggests that the heart is unsuitable for transplantation. Transient supraventricular tachycardia, ventricular arrhythmia associated with severe hemodynamic instability, or cardiac arrest require thorough investigation before acceptance as a cardiac donor. Significant valvular disease and wall motion abnormalities can be readily identified by bedside echocardiographic examination, a study that is routinely obtained by many transplantation centers. In many cases, the fluid management of the donor radically affects the apparent cardiac function because overhydration or underhydration markedly reduce effective cardiac output. Urine output can be extremely misleading because of the loss of antidiuretic hormone secretion from the hypothalamus. Measurements of central venous pressure or pulmonary artery wedge pressure may allow for more accurate management of fluid replacement. Determination of cardiac output using a flow-directed balloon-tipped pulmonary artery catheter is also helpful and complements echocar-

diographic findings. In questionable cases, cardiac catheterization may be required to exclude significant coronary artery disease.

Brain Death

Definition

The concept of brain death was crystallized in the 1968 Report of the Ad Hoc Committee of Harvard Medical School developed to examine the definition of brain death (22). This document established the following clearly defined criteria that were reliably predictive of irreversibility: (a) unreceptivity and unresponsivity, (b) absence of spontaneous muscular movement, (c) absence of reflexes, and (d) silent electroencephalogram. Since the publication of the so-called Harvard Criteria, the prerequisites for the diagnosis of brain death have been refined. Most hospitals have constituted a Brain Death Committee that is responsible for making uniform determinations of brain death according to locally established specific criteria, while conforming generally to the Harvard Criteria. At the University of Michigan Medical Center, the following requirements must be met to make a firm diagnosis of brain death:

1. The presence of reversible causes of coma should be excluded.
2. Clinical criteria establishing the loss of all functions of the entire brain must be met:
   Deep coma
   Absence of brain stem function
   Absence of spontaneous respiration
3. A confirmatory diagnostic test must be carried out.

Reversible causes of coma include sedation, hypothermia below 32.2°C, neuromuscular blockade, and shock. Coma should be deep and fixed, without perception or response to external stimuli, including deep pain. Decerebrate and decorticate responses should not be present. Occasionally, spinal reflexes may be present. Absence of brain stem function can be documented by confirming the absence of pupillary light response, corneal reflex, oculocephalic reflex, oculovestibular reflex, and spontaneous respiration.

An apnea test can be performed to assess spontaneous respiration. Ventilation of the patient with 100% oxygen for 10 minutes before the test reduces the risk of hypoxemia and subsequent cardiovascular collapse. After the period of preoxygenation, passive flow of oxygen into the endotracheal tube is continued, and the patient is monitored for evidence of respiratory effort. During this interval, hypercarbia with a $PaCO_2$ greater than 60 mm Hg should be documented by arterial blood gas testing.

The confirmatory test of choice is an electroencephalogram documenting electrocerebral silence. This may be done 6 hours after the initial clinical determination of brain death and, when accompanied by a second clinical determination, is diagnostic of brain death. Alternatively, four-vessel cerebral arteriography demonstrating cessation of blood flow to the brain may be used within an hour of the clinical brain death declaration. Nuclear scintigraphic determination of brain blood flow has been recognized as a satisfactory method to provide definitive confirmation of brain death. This test has the advantage that it can be done as a portable examination at the patient's bedside in the intensive care unit or emergency department, avoiding the risk of unnecessarily transporting a potentially unstable patient.

Etiology

Any condition that results in an overwhelming cerebral insult may be sufficient to cause brain death. In general, these conditions fall into the broad categories of subarachnoid hemorrhage, direct cerebral trauma, primary malignancy of the central nervous system, and other rare and miscellaneous entities. Subarachnoid hemorrhage may result from rupture of an intracranial aneurysm or other cerebrovascular accident leading to lethal intracerebral hemorrhage. This entity is responsible for most cases of brain death that lead to organ donation. Brain injury after trauma, either vehicular or related to firearms, is also common.

Pathophysiology

Cardiovascular Instability. During the events that lead to brain death, there is usually progressive intracranial hypertension. Important pathophysiologic responses are evident before the actual occurrence of brain death, including the development of marked systemic hypertension associated with vastly increased sympathetic activity and the massive release of catecholamines. Arrhythmia may become manifest at any time during the process of tentorial herniation. Bradyarrhythmia may be associated with the systemic hypertensive response to intracranial hypertension (Cushing's reflex), but ventricular and supraventricular tachyarrhythmia may also be seen in the presence of high levels of catecholamines.

Once herniation is complete and brain death has occurred, a high proportion of donors manifest a hypotensive response related to the loss of sympathetic tone and the failure to maintain circulating catecholamine levels. It has been reported that 62% of brain-dead patients sustain cardiac arrest within 24 hours and 87% by 72 hours in the absence of specific donor maintenance measures (23). Even with aggressive donor support, approximately 10% of donors manifest cardiopulmonary arrest during the interval between the determination of brain death and the procurement of organs (24).

Central Hormonal Failure. As the brain and brain stem cease to function, failure of the central hormonal axis occurs. Pituitary hormones cease to be produced, and diabetes insipidus ensues. Without antidiuretic hormone, urinary output may increase to astonishing rates, sometimes well in excess of 1 L/h. The urine becomes extremely dilute, resulting in increasing serum osmolarity and hypernatremia. The resultant hypovolemia may contribute to cardiovascular collapse if untreated.

The influence of other aspects of central hormonal function are less well understood. There is experimental evidence of reduced circulating levels of triiodothyronine, cortisol, and insulin after brain death in pigs and baboons (25,26). These factors may contribute to the hemodynamic instability, cardiovascular collapse, and hyperglycemia so often seen in association with brain death and have led some to advocate using combinations of these compounds before organ procurement. Confirmatory studies in humans have not shown these hormonal systems to play major roles in the pathophysiology of the hypotensive state after brain death.

Request for Permission from Next of Kin

Most states, as well as the federal government, have passed legislation requiring that relatives of deceased patients be asked whether they are willing to permit organ or tissue donation. Unfortunately, the contribution of such laws to an increase in the actual supply of donor organs is less than clear. What is far more important than required request is the careful training, uniform deployment, and empathetic demeanor of the people who actually approach the family. In many hospitals, trained donor coordinators are on call to discuss the option of organ donation with bereaved families. Such people may come from a variety of fields, including medicine, nursing, social work, or pastoral care. Increasingly, it appears that refusal by the family is one of the biggest stumbling blocks to increasing the supply of organs actually donated. It has also become clear that any discussion of possible organ donation should occur at a time subsequent to and separate from informing the family of the patient's death.

The use of the term *brain death* may be confusing to lay people and professionals alike, implying as it may that brain death is different from other kinds of death. Obviously, the distinction is intended to differentiate this modality of dying from cardiac death, but not to indicate that the person is any less dead. Phrases such as "keeping the organs alive so they can be transplanted" are as misleading and confusing as they are incorrect.

According to the Uniform Anatomical Gift Act, a signed and witnessed organ donor card is a legally binding indication of the decedent's wishes, but throughout North America and most European countries, the family's consent is routinely obtained before organ procurement. Although it is desirable that the entire family be in agreement about donating, the legal next of kin is required to agree to the donation and grant signed permission. The hierarchy for permission from next of kin is as follows:

1. Spouse
2. Adult son or daughter
3. Either parent
4. Adult brother or sister
5. Guardian
6. Any other person authorized to dispose of the body

Non-heartbeating Organ Donors

The profound shortage of organs has led some transplantation centers to initiate efforts aimed at using the organs from patients who are declared dead in the emergency department and do not have effective cardiac function. Once declared dead, the organ procurement team is notified and the organs are rapidly cooled by infusing ice-cold preservation fluids into percutaneously placed cannulae in the aorta and peritoneal cavity. This usually occurs within minutes of arriving in the emergency department, before the next of kin have been notified of the patient's death. Before procuring the organs for transplantation, permission is obtained from the patient's next of kin. In some instances the family refuses donation, in which case the cannulae are removed and the organs are left in place. The rationale behind this approach is based on the realization that many patients die in the emergency department before organ donation can be undertaken. The Institute of Medicine has studied the issues surrounding the use non-heartbeating donors and reached the conclusion that "the recovery of organs from non-heartbeating donors is an important, medically effective, and ethically acceptable approach to reducing the gap that exists now and will continue to exist in the future between the demand for and available supply of organs for transplantation" (27). Growing experience with these techniques demonstrates that when organs are transplanted from non-heartbeating donors, the results are only slightly inferior to those from conventional donors (28).

Donor Maintenance

Tissue Perfusion

Because most donors have been maintained with a minimum of fluids to prevent increased cerebral edema, one of the first priorities in donor maintenance should be the prompt restoration of intravascular volume. Depending on the duration of the donor's underlying illness, this may require from 3 to 10 L of volume resuscitation. In general, the dosage of pressor agents required to support blood pressure can be progressively decreased as the central venous pressure is raised to 10 to 12 cm H_2O. Crystalloid may be used, and lactated Ringer's solution is often given because its slightly lower sodium concentration counteracts the sodium-concentrating effects of diabetes insipidus. If the latter condition has resulted in severe hypernatremia, the addition of free water may be necessary. Colloid and blood should be used to restore and maintain osmotic pressure and normovolemia. The hematocrit should be kept at approximately 35 volume percent to replace traumatic losses and maintain oxygen-carrying capacity. Enough volume should be administered to achieve a urine output of at least 100 mL/h and a systolic arterial pressure of 90 to 120 mm Hg. Higher levels of arterial blood pressure usually are unnecessary because of the loss of sympathetic tone accompanying brain death.

If diabetes insipidus is severe, exogenous vasopressin must be given. Available in a variety of forms, desmopressin acetate (DDAVP), a synthetic analog of 8-arginine vasopressin, appears to have the least splanchnic vasoconstrictive effect compared with its antidiuretic action. This agent can be given by a variety of routes, including intranasally, subcutaneously, or intravenously. The usual dosage is 20 µg intranasally or 2 to 4 µg intravenously or subcutaneously.

Oxygenation and Ventilation

Arterial blood gases should be checked regularly and appropriate adjustments of the ventilator made to optimize gas exchange and acid–base balance. Oxygen supply should be adequate to maintain an arterial oxygen saturation of greater than 95% and, if available, a mixed venous oxygen saturation above 70%. Low levels of positive endexpiratory pressure may facilitate achieving a balanced oxygen supply and demand.

Inotropic Support

Most donors are hypovolemic at the time of brain death and are receiving inotropic support in lieu of volume to support their blood pressure. Dopamine hydrochloride is the most commonly used agent. The need for dosages of this drug in excess of 10 µg/kg/min usually indicates persistent hypovolemia, and the restoration of normovolemia is almost always accompanied by a reduction in dopamine requirements. High doses of dopamine maintained for long periods before organ procurement may be associated with increased rates of acute tubular necrosis and hepatic allograft failure. Cardiac procurement is often abandoned if high doses of inotropic support are required despite adequate volume status.

Other inotropic agents, such as isoproterenol, epinephrine, norepinephrine, and phenylephrine, are occasionally used, but the use of these agents should be discouraged because of their peripheral vasoconstrictive effects. Dobutamine is occasionally used in conjunction with low doses of dopamine.

Prevention of Hypothermia

Thermoregulatory homeostatic mechanisms are destroyed with the occurrence of brain death, and the development of severe hypothermia may lead to ventricular arrhythmia and cardiac arrest. Warming blankets should be used above and below the donor to keep body temperature above 35°C, and exposure for the purposes of examination or intervention should be kept to a minimum. If maintenance of normal body temperature is problematic, intravenous fluids may be prewarmed before administration, and a heated humidifier circuit can be added to the ventilator.

Multiple Organ Procurement

United Network for Organ Sharing and the Coordination of Teams

When brain death has been declared, the person has been identified as a suitable organ donor, and permission has been given by the next of kin, the logistics of organ procurement must be arranged. Since passage of the National Organ Transplantation Act, a national organ procurement and transplantation network has been organized. The federal contract for this important function has been awarded to the United Network for Organ Sharing (UNOS). UNOS is responsible for the fair and equitable distribution of cadaveric donor organs throughout the United States. The 50 states are divided into 11 regions of approximately equal population (Fig. 16.27). Within each region, UNOS-certified local organ procurement organizations (OPOs) are responsible for maintaining the list of potential recipients for their catchment area. All potential recipients in the United States are entered into the UNOS computer system, and a point allocation system is used to determine, in any given OPO, the appropriate recipient for a given donor organ. If a particular organ cannot be used by a recipient in the OPO, the next suitable recipient in the region is offered the organ. Finally, if no recipients in the OPO region can be found, the organ is offered to any recipient in the nation. In each case, recipient priority is ordered by the existing point allocation system. The only exception to these general rules relates to renal transplant recipients who share six antigens with the donor. These kidneys are automatically shared nationwide even if suitable local recipients are available.

Recipients of the various organs may reside in geographically distant locations. Because the recipient transplantation teams must be given considerable detailed information about the donor to decide whether to use a particular organ for a particular recipient, a finite period of time is required to assemble the necessary donor retrieval teams. When all teams are on site at the donor hospital, the donor is transferred to the operating room for the actual procurement procedure.

Surgical Technique for Multiple Organ Procurement

Techniques of multiple organ procurement allow for the removal of the heart, lungs, kidneys, liver, and pancreas from a single donor for transplantation into six or more recipients. The following discussion details the methods used to remove all these organs from a donor.

The heartbeating donor is brought to the operating room from the intensive care unit or emergency department with appropriate hemodynamic and electrocardiographic monitoring. Oxygen is delivered by hand bagging at 100% inspired concentration. Inotropic drug infusions are continued during transport and procurement. The anesthesiologist should maintain close communication with the procurement teams to avoid the development of cardiac arrhythmia, hypotension, and hypoxemia.

The steps in the procedure can be categorized as follows: (a) incision, (b) exploration and inspection, (c) individual organ mobilization, (d) in situ perfusion, (e) removal of organs, and (f) closure of the incision. Postprocurement processing, packaging, and transport to the recipient centers are the final steps.

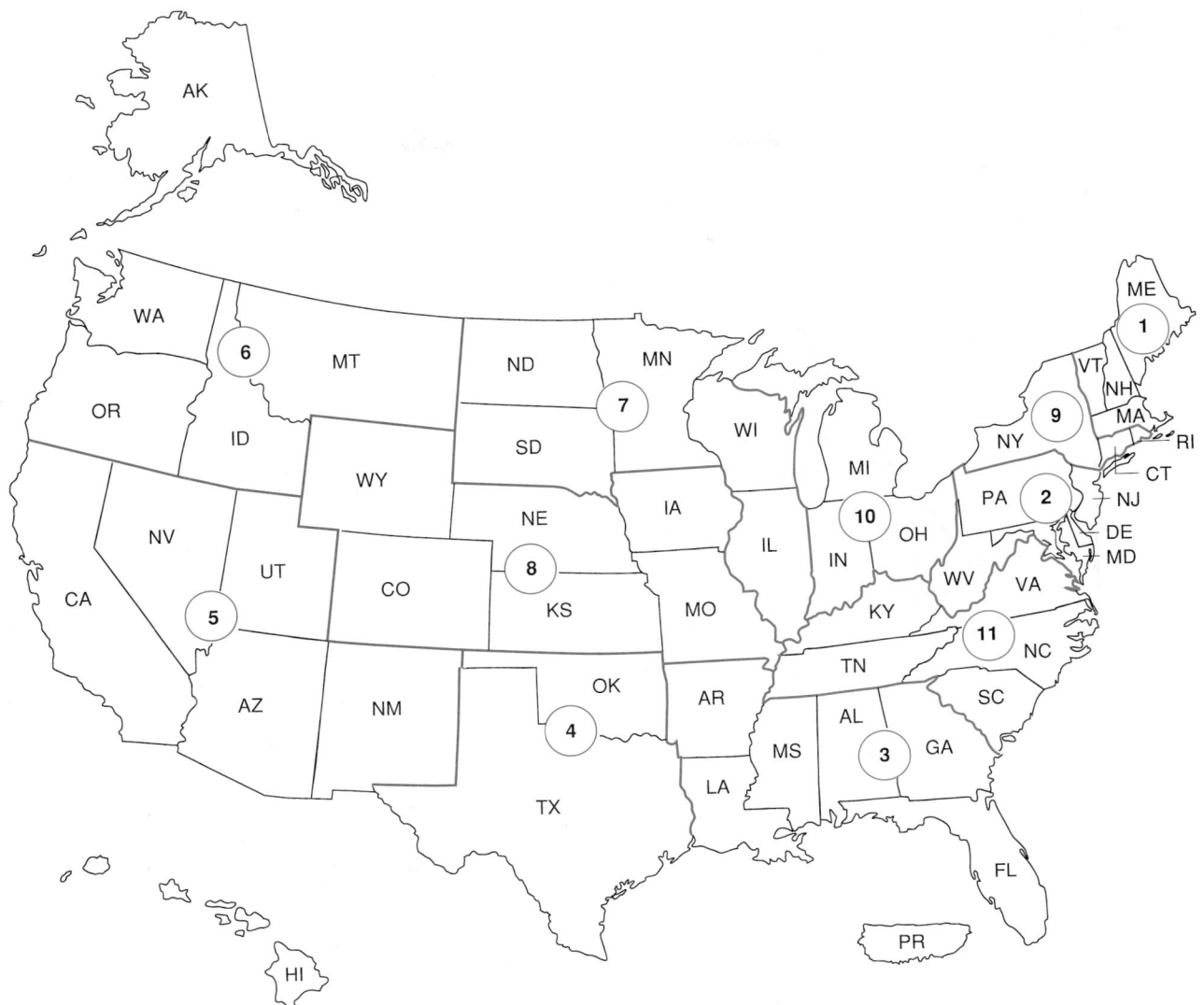

Figure 16.27. The United Network for Organ Sharing has divided the 50 United States into 11 regions of approximately equal populations for purposes of administration of organ procurement, distribution, and educational objectives.

The entire torso is prepared with an iodine-containing solution, and a field is draped from the neck to the pubis. A long, midline incision is made from the suprasternal notch to the pubis. The sternum is split with an electrical or air-powered saw if available, although manual methods using a Lebsche knife or Gigli saw work perfectly well. Exposure of the abdominal organs may be facilitated by the addition of cruciate incisions (Fig. 16.28). A general exploration is carried out to ascertain that no unexpected conditions are present that would preclude donation, such as tumor, infection, or specific organ damage. In general, a "no-touch" technique is used to minimize trauma to the organs during the procurement procedure.

For the so-called rapid technique of organ procurement, little in the way of mobilization of individual organs is necessary. Preparation for in situ perfusion consists of a complete Kocher maneuver, with mobilization of the right colon, duodenum, and small bowel in a cephalad direction to the patient's left (Fig. 16.29). The aorta is exposed from the bifurcation distally to the level of the left renal vein proximally. The inferior mesenteric artery is divided.

Lumbar branches may be ligated and divided at this point. The inferior vena cava is similarly exposed. Next, the left triangular ligament of the liver is taken down, exposing the crural muscle at the aortic hiatus. The aorta is encircled with a tape at the diaphragm (Fig. 16.30A). These maneuvers can be accomplished in approximately 15 minutes and allow in situ perfusion through the distal aorta and crossclamping of the proximal aorta to begin immediately in the event that the donor becomes hemodynamically unstable or sustains cardiac arrest. Warm ischemia is completely prevented by in situ perfusion.

Stable donors afford the luxury of further preparation before in situ flushing. The inferior mesenteric vein is isolated as it enters the retroperitoneum behind the pancreas. This vein provides convenient access for in situ portal flushing by means of a small catheter, such as a Javid shunt. The pars flaccida of the lesser omentum should be inspected for evidence of a replaced left hepatic artery arising from the left gastric artery, and minimal dissection of the hepatic artery is necessary (Fig. 16.30B). The portal triad should be palpated for evidence of a replaced right

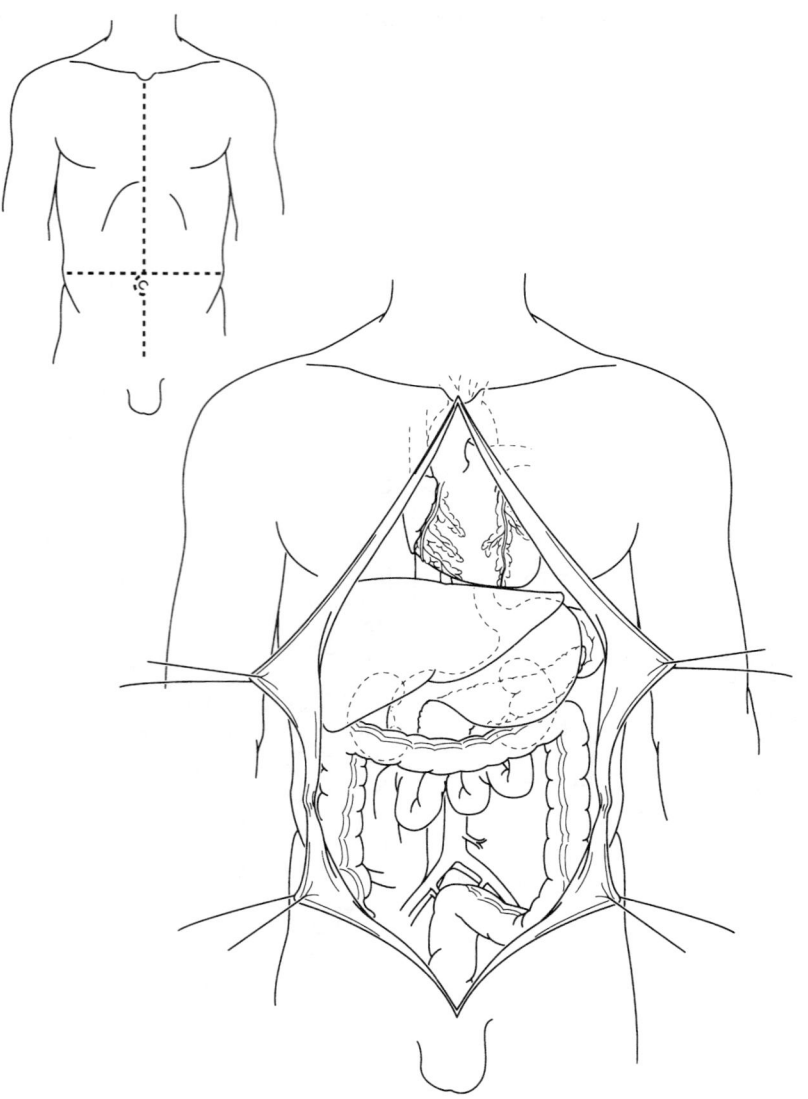

Figure 16.28. A complete midline incision from suprasternal notch to pubis is made for multiple organ procurement. The sternum is split. If necessary, cruciate abdominal incisions are added to facilitate exposure of the intraabdominal organs.

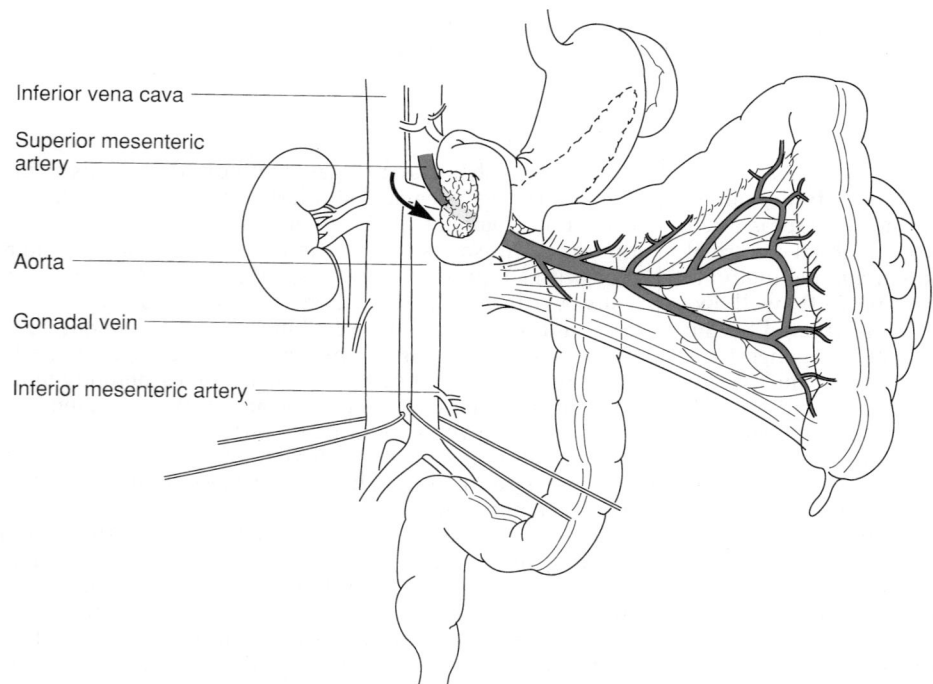

Inferior vena cava

Superior mesenteric artery

Aorta

Gonadal vein

Inferior mesenteric artery

Figure 16.29. The Kocher maneuver is used to mobilize completely the right colon and duodenum, exposing the retroperitoneum, including the aorta, from the level of the superior mesenteric artery to the bifurcation and the inferior vena cava from the iliac veins to the edge of the liver.

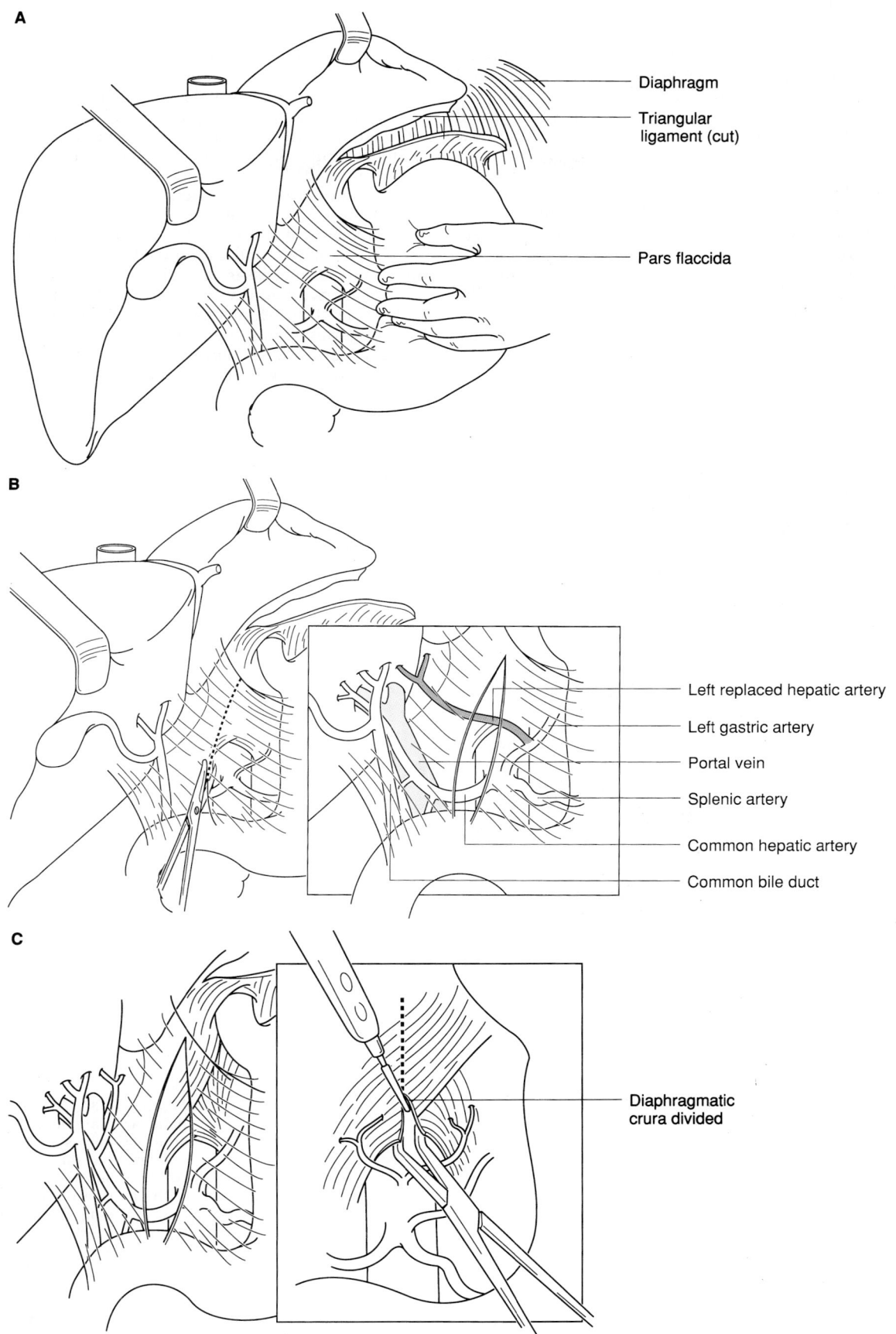

A

Diaphragm

Triangular
ligament (cut)

Pars flaccida

B

Left replaced hepatic artery

Left gastric artery

Portal vein

Splenic artery

Common hepatic artery

Common bile duct

C

Diaphragmatic
crura divided

Figure 16.30. *(A)* The left triangular ligament is divided and the left lateral segment of the liver is retracted to expose the esophagus and aortic hiatus. *(B)* The pars flaccida of the lesser omentum is widely opened after checking for the presence of a replaced left hepatic artery arising from the left gastric artery. *(C)* After division of the diaphragmatic crura, the supraceliac aorta is encircled at the level of the diaphragm.

hepatic artery arising from the superior mesenteric artery. This vessel, when present, can be felt as it courses toward the liver posterior to the common bile duct and along the right side of the portal vein as it emerges from its origin off the superior mesenteric artery posterior to the pancreas (Fig. 16.31).

If the pancreas is to be donated, a total gastrectomy greatly facilitates atraumatic mobilization of the gland. After administration of 250 mL of an iodine-containing solution, followed by a similar volume of amphotericin B solution (50 mg/L), the nasogastric tube is removed and the gastroesophageal junction is divided with a stapling device. After the gastrocolic omental tissue is divided, the short gastric vessels are carefully divided between ligatures or hemostatic clips. The left and right gastric branches to the stomach are then divided. Finally, a stapling device is applied just beyond the pylorus and the

stomach is removed (Fig. 16.32). The spleen is delivered anteriorly, dividing its attachments to the body wall and diaphragm. Using the spleen as a handle, the retroperitoneal attachments of the pancreas are divided from lateral to medial, until the major superior mesenteric vessels are reached (Fig. 16.33). The distal duodenum is likewise divided near the Treitz ligament.

The course of the ureters should be identified. The Gerota fascia is widely incised to allow topical cooling with iced slush solution to supplement the in situ perfusion. Complete mobilization of the kidneys before in situ flushing is unnecessary and risks damage to the renal vessels or inadvertent division of accessory renal arteries.

The heart and lungs can be readied for removal by a team working simultaneously with the abdominal retrieval team. The superior and inferior venae cavae are mobilized, and the aortic arch is dissected sufficiently for

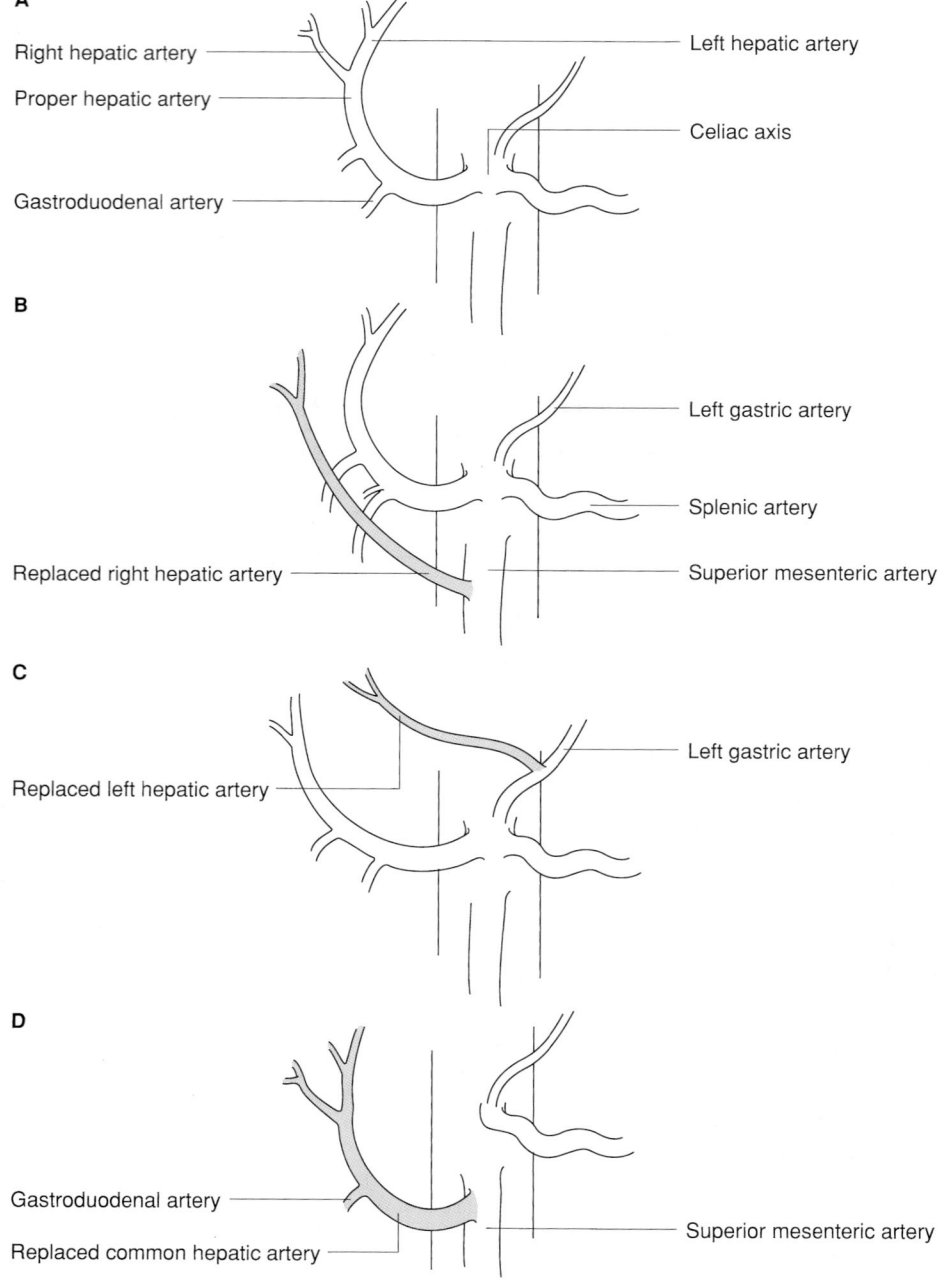

A
Right hepatic artery
Proper hepatic artery
Gastroduodenal artery
Left hepatic artery
Celiac axis

B
Replaced right hepatic artery
Left gastric artery
Splenic artery
Superior mesenteric artery

C
Replaced left hepatic artery
Left gastric artery

D
Gastroduodenal artery
Replaced common hepatic artery
Superior mesenteric artery

Figure 16.31. (A) Standard hepatic arterial anatomy, with the artery arising as a single vessel as a branch of the celiac axis. (B) Aberrant hepatic arterial anatomy, with a replaced right hepatic artery arising from the superior mesenteric artery and ascending posterior to the common bile duct and anterolateral to the portal vein. (C) A replaced left hepatic artery arising from the left gastric artery is usually visible and palpable crossing the pars flaccida of the lesser omentum from the lesser curvature of the stomach. (D) A completely replaced common hepatic artery arising from the superior mesenteric artery.

A

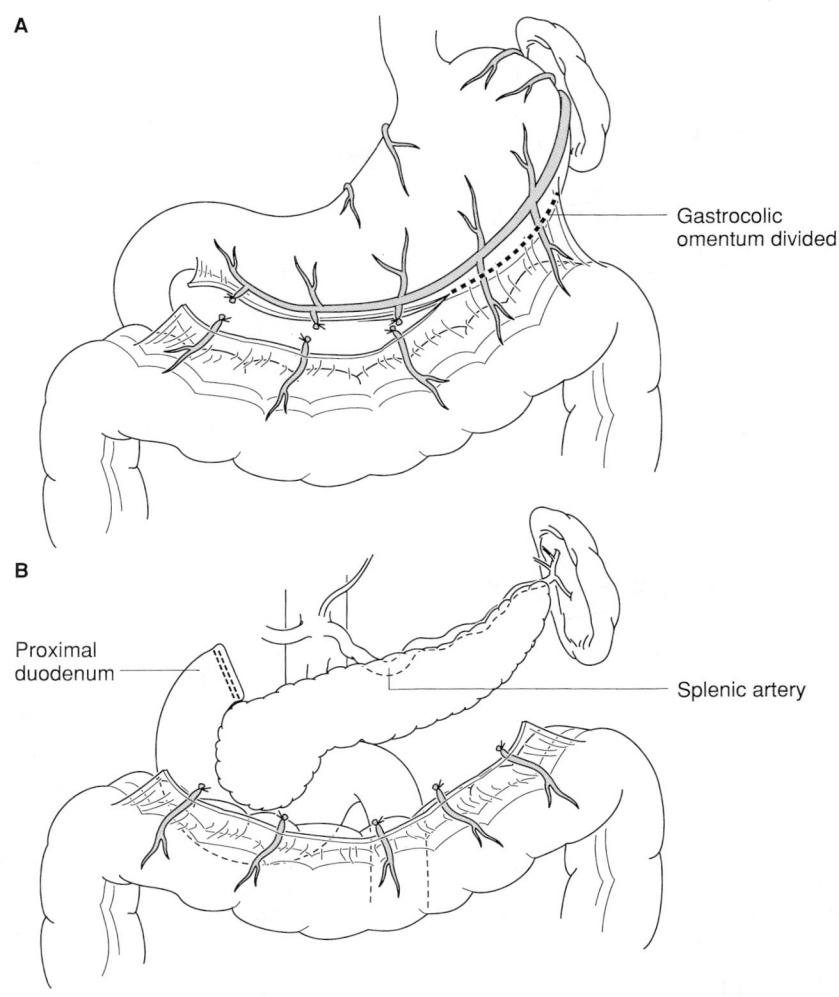

Gastrocolic
omentum divided

B

Proximal
duodenum

Splenic artery

Figure 16.32. *(A)* Division of the gastrocolic omentum exposes the pancreas. The short gastric vessels are ligated and divided, separating the spleen from the stomach. *(B)* After completion of devascularization, the stomach is stapled proximally and distally and removed to facilitate exposure and mobilization of the pancreas.

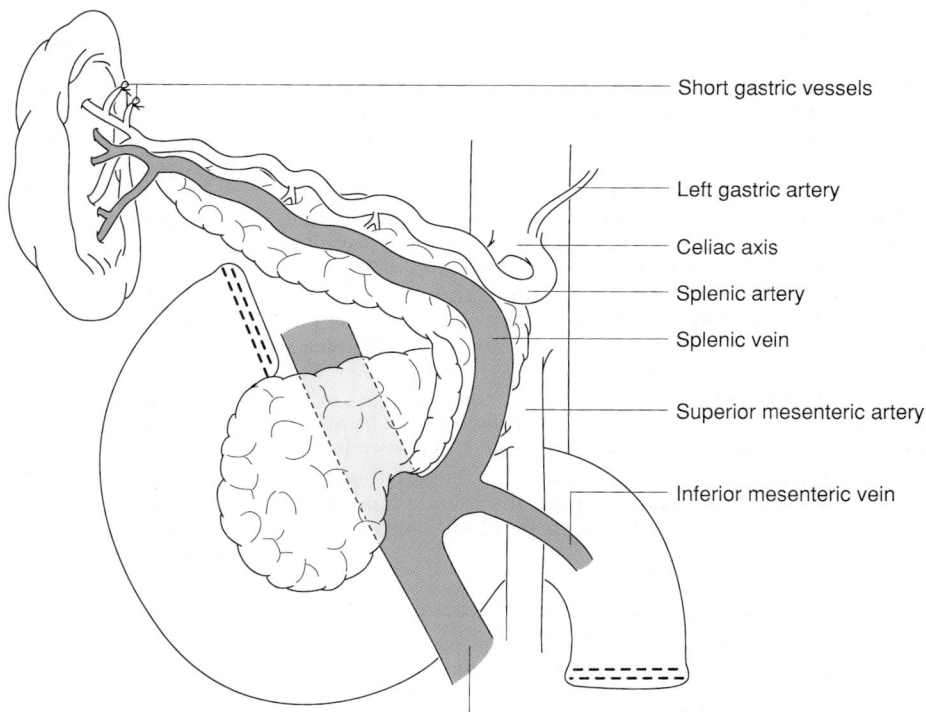

Short gastric vessels

Left gastric artery

Celiac axis

Splenic artery

Splenic vein

Superior mesenteric artery

Inferior mesenteric vein

Superior mesenteric vein

Figure 16.33. The pancreas is reflected anteriorly and to the right to the level of the superior mesenteric vein near the confluence with the splenic vein. The aortic origins of the celiac axis and superior mesenteric arteries are identified.

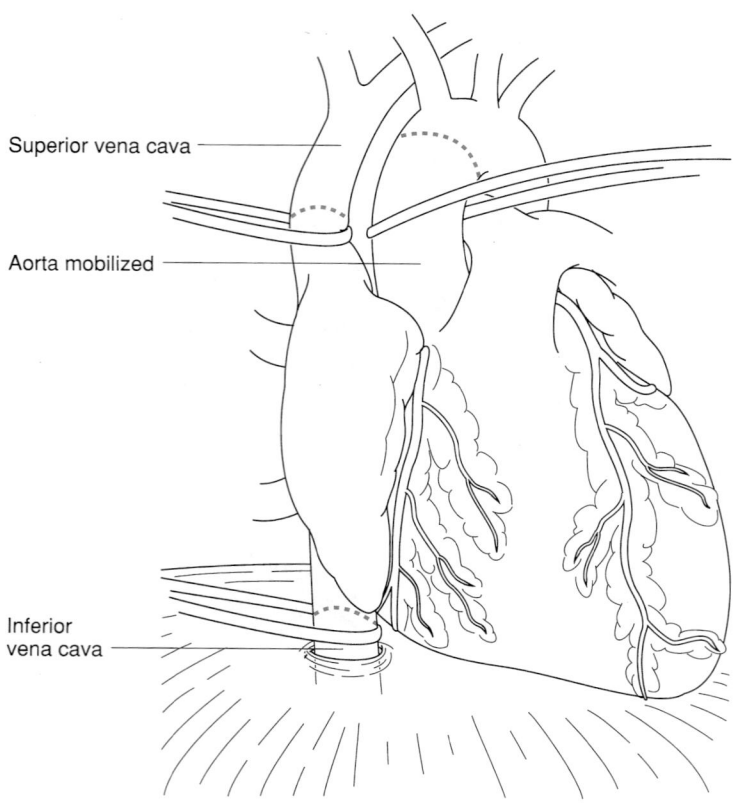

Superior vena cava

Aorta mobilized

Inferior
vena cava

Figure 16.34. Preparation of the heart for cardioplegia. Minimal dissection is necessary. The venae cavae are encircled, and the aorta is separated from the pulmonary artery.

the placement of a crossclamp at the time of infusion of aortic root cardioplegia (Fig. 16.34). Preliminary mobilization of the lungs is usually performed, and access to the pulmonary artery is necessary for pulmonary preservation.

When all teams are ready, a coordinated sequence of events ensures that all organs are simultaneously cooled and protected. The donor is systemically heparinized. A Javid shunt is advanced through the inferior mesenteric vein near the pancreas and advanced into the portal vein (Fig. 16.35A). A cardioplegia needle is positioned in the aortic arch (Fig. 16.35B). The distal abdominal aorta is cannulated for in situ perfusion of the kidneys, liver, and pancreas, and an exsanguination cannula is placed in the distal inferior vena cava (see Fig. 16.35C). Alternatively, the inferior vena caval–right atrial junction may be divided in the chest with suction catheters placed in the caval lumen and right thoracic cavity to decompress the venous circulation at the moment of aortic crossclamping.

The aortic arch and the abdominal aorta at the diaphragm are simultaneously crossclamped. Cardioplegia solution is infused under pressure into the aortic root, perfusing the coronary arteries and arresting the heart. Ventilation is ceased. Portal and distal aortic perfusion is initiated with ice-cold preservation solution. Topical iced slush is placed in the abdomen and chest to assist the cooling process. The heart and lungs are then removed. The clamp is removed from the distal vena caval cannula for exsanguination and to preclude venous congestion.

The liver and pancreas are removed *en bloc.* The diaphragm surrounding the suprahepatic inferior vena cava and adjacent to the bare area of the liver is divided. The infrahepatic inferior vena cava is divided just cephalad to the left renal vein. The liver and pancreas unit is now attached only by the distal superior mesenteric vessels coursing to the small bowel and by the aortic origins of the superior mesenteric artery and celiac axis. The superior mesenteric branches emerging from the uncinate process are ligated and divided, and a cylinder of aorta is removed encompassing the superior mesenteric artery and celiac axis. The liver and pancreas are separated as a bench procedure, retaining the celiac axis with the liver (Fig. 16.36). The splenic artery is divided at its origin. This vessel and the superior mesenteric artery are reconstructed with a bifurcated donor iliac artery graft. The portal vein is divided approximately 1 cm from the pancreas. The common bile duct is divided at the superior edge of the pancreas.

The kidneys are also removed *en bloc.* The ureters are given wide berth to avoid devascularization and are divided near their entrance into the bladder. Dissection is carried out posterior to the aorta and vena cava in the plane of the prevertebral fascia. Once removed, the left renal vein is divided flush with the vena cava (Fig. 16.37). The aorta is opened in the midline to identify the orifices of the renal arteries from within the lumen. In this way, multiple renal arteries can be readily identified and kept on a single aortic Carrel patch. Once the abdominal and thoracic organs have been removed, a sampling of lymph nodes and spleen is taken for tissue typing and crossmatch

Figure 16.36. The liver and pancreas are removed *en bloc.* Separation of the two organs is accomplished as a bench procedure. The celiac axis is retained with the liver, dividing the splenic artery just beyond its origin. The gastroduodenal artery is ligated and divided. The portal vein is divided approximately 1 cm from the superior edge of the pancreas, and the common bile duct is divided just superior to its entrance into the pancreas.

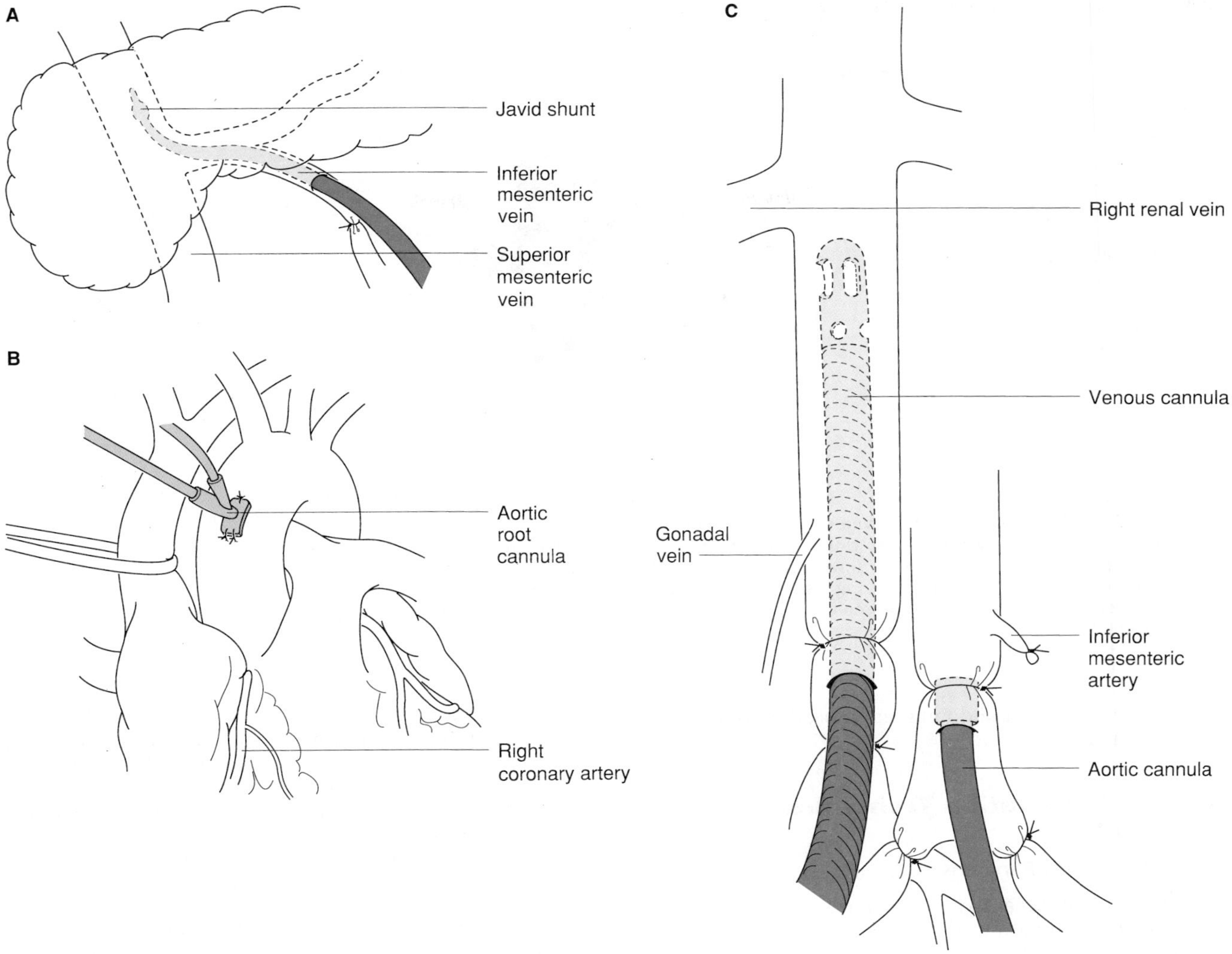

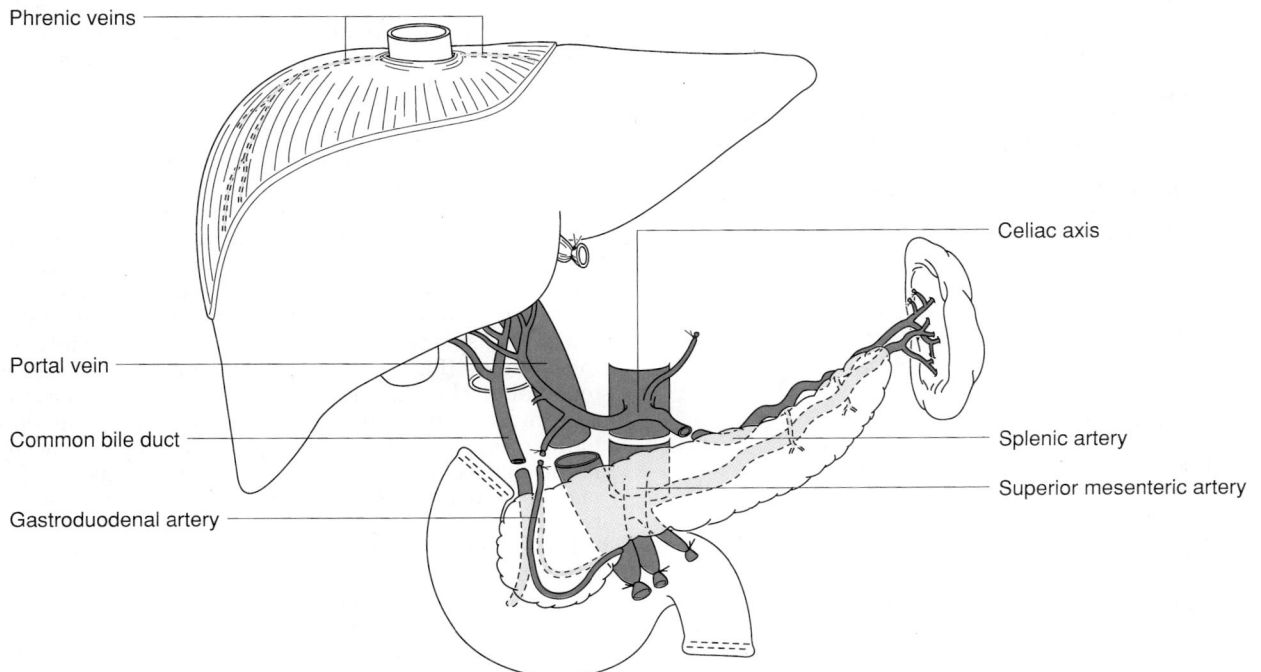

A

Javid shunt

Inferior mesenteric vein

Superior mesenteric vein

B

Aortic root cannula

Right coronary artery

C

Right renal vein

Venous cannula

Gonadal vein

Inferior mesenteric artery

Aortic cannula

Figure 16.35. In situ perfusion set-up. *(A)* A cannula is placed into the portal vein through the inferior mesenteric vein for portal venous perfusion. *(B)* A needle is placed in the aortic root for perfusion of the coronary arteries with cardioplegia solution. *(C)* A cannula is placed in the distal aorta for retrograde perfusion with cold preservation solution. Another cannula is placed in the distal vena cava for venous decompression and exsanguination.

Phrenic veins

Celiac axis

Portal vein

Common bile duct

Splenic artery

Superior mesenteric artery

Gastroduodenal artery

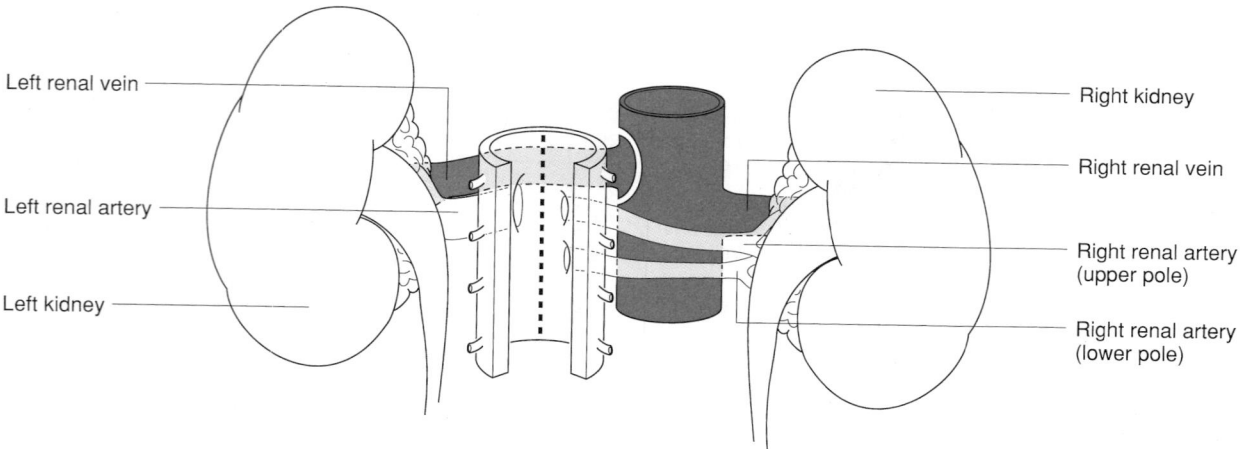

Figure 16.37. The kidneys are removed en bloc and separated on the back bench. Safe division is ensured by viewing the kidneys posteriorly. The aorta is divided between the paired lumbar arteries, and renal arterial orifices can be viewed directly from within the aortic lumen. This avoids any hilar dissection with the accompanying risk of injury to renal arteries. The left renal vein is divided at its entrance to the inferior vena cava, leaving the entire vena cava with the shorter right renal vein.

testing. The chest and abdomen are closed, and standard postmortem care is given.

Current Preservation Techniques and Results

Kidney, Liver, and Pancreas

Until relatively recently, the primary solution used for cold storage preservation of the kidneys was Euro-Collins solution (Table 16.8). This formulation provides a hyperosmolar environment with intracellular electrolyte composition that is intended to reduce cellular swelling. In combination with hypothermia, kidneys can be safely stored in this solution for 36 to 48 hours before transplantation.

In the 1980s, the advent of new immunosuppressive agents, such as cyclosporine, meant that for the first time extrarenal organs could be transplanted with good success rates, and the need for more effective preservation became apparent. Cold ischemia limitations of approximately 8 hours for the liver and pancreas meant that donor and recipient teams had to be exquisitely coordinated; complex recipient operations requiring a multitude of ancillary support services had to be organized in the middle of the night; and all personnel involved in the procedure, including the surgeons, were starting the operation in a fatigued condition.

At the University of Wisconsin, a solution was developed that has totally transformed the practice of hepatic and pancreatic transplantation at most centers in North America and Europe. The new solution, termed UW cold storage solution, is based on the use of lactobionate, raffinose, hydroxyethyl starch, and a host of other ingredients designed to provide high-energy phosphate precursors, hydrogen ion buffering capacity, and antioxidant properties. It is unclear how many of these components are truly necessary. Lactobionate, an impermeant anion to prevent cellular swelling, is used in place of the glucose that is contained in Euro-Collins solution; raffinose, a naturally occurring trisaccharide of fructose, glucose, and galactose, which is found in abundance in sugar beets, provides additional osmotic activity; and hydroxyethyl starch is a colloid intended to prevent an increase in the extracellular space (1). UW solution is used as the preservation method of choice by most programs performing hepatic and pancreatic transplantations. Both organs can be reliably stored for 24 hours (Fig. 16.38), and isolated clinical cases with total cold ischemia times in excess of 30 hours have been reported (29,30). Although these livers will function in terms of hepatocellular metabolism, evidence is accumulating that cold ischemia times of greater than 12 hours may be associated with a higher incidence of biliary strictures.

It is not clear whether the UW cold storage solution has any significant advantages over Euro-Collins solution for the preservation of kidneys. In a large, randomized, multicenter European trial, patient and graft survival rates were similar among recipients of the two solutions, but the in-

Table 16.8. COMPOSITION OF HYPOTHERMIC ORGAN PRESERVATION SOLUTIONS

Component	Amount per liter
EURO-COLLINS SOLUTION	
KH_2PO_4	2.05 g
K_2HPO_4	7.4 g
KCl	1.12 g
$NaHCO_3$	0.84 g
Glucose	35 g
UW SOLUTION	
K^+-lactobionate	100 mmol
KH_2PO_4	25 mmol
$MgSO_4$	5 mmol
Raffinose	30 mmol
Adenosine	5 mmol
Glutathione	3 mmol
Insulin	100 IU
Penicillin	40 IU
Dexamethasone	8 mg
Allopurinol	1 mmol

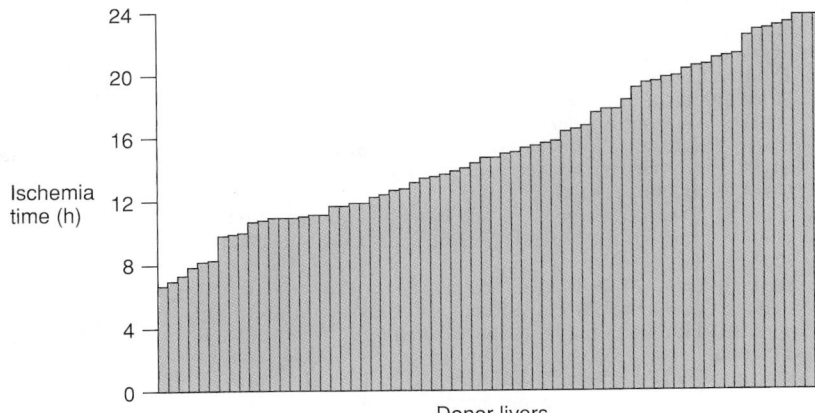

Figure 16.38. Distribution of ischemia times using UW solution for liver transplant preservation at the University of Michigan. Each vertical bar represents the preservation time for an individual donor liver.

cidence of delayed graft function requiring dialysis was reduced by approximately one third in the UW group. The results of other ongoing trials are needed before a definitive statement can be made about the relative merits of the two solutions in renal preservation. Newer preservative solutions, including Celsior (SangStat, Menlo Park, CA), are appearing and may have advantages over UW (31).

Heart and Lungs

Cardiac preservation has changed relatively little in recent years. Hyperkalemic, crystalloid cardioplegia solution is used at 4°C, and 4 hours is the generally accepted limit of cold ischemia. For this reason, donor and recipient operations must be finely coordinated.

A comprehensive review of pulmonary preservation has been published (32). Hypothermia is used along with intracellular-type solutions. Pulmonary inflation also appears to be important. The optimal vascular perfusate for the lungs remains unknown, however, and results with pulmonary transplantation are still limited by deficiencies in the quality and duration of preservation.

Small Bowel

The transplantation of small bowel segments with or without concomitant liver transplantation is being performed with greater regularity as the treatment of choice for short-gut syndrome. Preservation of the bowel is usually done with UW solution, although experimental evidence does not indicate that this solution offers any advantage over simple hypothermia (33). Most small bowel procurements, however, are from donors who have multiple useful organs, hence the use of standard intraaortic preservation techniques. The current limit of cold ischemia time for small bowel is approximately 12 hours (34).

REFERENCES

1. Belzer FO. Evaluation of preservation of the intra-abdominal organs. *Transplant Proc* 1993;25:2527–2531.
2. Belzer FO, Southard JH. Principles of solid-organ preservation by cold storage. *Transplantation* 1988;45:673–676.
3. Simonson MS, Dunn MJ. Endothelins: a family of regulator peptides. *Hypertension* 1991;17:856.
4. Wilhelm SM, Simonson MS, Robinson AV, et al. Cold ischemia induces endothelin gene upregulation in the preserved kidney. *J Surg Res* 1999;85:101–108.
5. Southard JH, Senzig KA, Belzer FO. Effects of hypothermia on canine kidney mitochondria. *Cryobiology* 1980;17:148–153.
6. McCord JM. Oxygen-derived free radicals in postischemic tissue injury. *N Engl J Med* 1985;312:159–163.
7. Clavien PA, Harvey RP, Strasberg SM. Preservation and reperfusion injuries in liver allografts. *Transplantation* 1992;53:957–978.
8. Koyama I, Bulkley GB, Williams GM, et al. The role of oxygen free radicals in mediating the reperfusion injury of cold preserved ischemic kidneys. *Transplantation* 1985;40:590–595.
9. Colletti LM, Burtch GD, Remick DG, et al. The production of tumor necrosis factor alpha and the development of a pulmonary capillary injury following hepatic ischemia/reperfusion. *Transplantation* 1990;49:268–272.
10. Sturber M, Harringer W, Ernst M, et al. Inhaled nitric oxide as a prophylactic treatment against reperfusion injury. *Thorac Cardiovasc Surg* 1999;47:179–182.
11. Devlin J, Palmer RMJ, Gonde CE, et al. Nitric oxide generation. *Transplantation* 1994;58:592–595.
12. United Network for Organ Sharing. On-line: http://www.unos.org (accessed 11/19/99).
13. The 11th report of the human renal transplant registry. *JAMA* 1973;226:1197–1204.
14. Zhou YC, Cecka JM. Effect of age on kidney transplants. In: Terasaki PI, ed. *Clinical transplants 1989*. Los Angeles: UCLA Tissue Typing Laboratory, 1989:369–378.
15. Wengerter K, Tellis VA, Soberman R, et al. Transplantation of pediatric donor kidneys to adult recipients: is there a critical donor age? *Ann Surg* 1986;204:172–175.
16. Bergmeijer JH, Cransberg K, Nijman JM, et al. Functional adaptation of en bloc-transplanted pediatric kidneys into pediatric recipients. *Transplantation* 1994;58:623–624.
17. Freeman RB, Giatras I, Falagas ME, et al. Outcome of transplantation of organs procured from bacteremic donors. *Transplantation* 1999;68:1107–1111.
18. Roth D, Fernandez JA, Babischkin S, et al. Detection of hepatitis C virus among cadaver organ donors: evidence for low transmission of disease. *Ann Intern Med* 1992;117:470–475.
19. Morse JH, Turcotte JG, Merion RM, et al. Development of a malignant tumor in a liver transplant graft procured from a donor with a cerebral neoplasm. *Transplantation* 1990;50:875–877.
20. Abouna GM, Al-Adnani MS, Kremer GD. Reversal of diabetic nephropathy in human cadaveric kidneys after transplantation into non-diabetic recipients. *Lancet* 1983;2:1274–1276.
21. Kaufman HH, Hui KS, Mattson JC, et al. Clinicopathologic correlations of disseminated intravascular coagulation in patients with head injury. *Neurosurgery* 1984;15:34–42.
22. Ad Hoc Committee of Harvard Medical School. A definition of irreversible coma: report of the Ad Hoc Committee of Harvard Medical School to examine the definition of brain death. *JAMA* 1968;205:337–340.
23. Jorgensen EO. Spinal man after brain death. *Acta Neurochir (Wien)* 1973;28:259–273.
24. Emery RW, Cork RC, Levinson MM, et al. The cardiac donor: a six-year experience. *Ann Thorac Surg* 1986;41:356–362.
25. Novitzky D, Wicomb WN, Cooper DKC, et al. Electrocardiographic, hemodynamic, and endocrine changes occurring during experimental brain death in the Chacma baboon. *Heart Transplant* 1984;4:63–69.

26. Novitzky D, Wicomb WN, Cooper DKC, et al. Improved cardiac function following hormonal therapy in brain dead pigs: relevance to organ donation. *Cryobiology* 1987;24:1–10.

27. The Institute of Medicine. *Non-heartbeating organ transplantation: medical and ethical issues in procurement.* Washington, DC: National Academy Press, 1997:1.

28. Sho YW, Terasaki PI, Cecka JM, et al. Transplantation of kidneys from donors whose hearts have stopped beating. *N Engl J Med* 1999;338:221–225.

29. Todo S, Nery J, Yanaga K, et al. Extended preservation of human liver grafts with UW solution. *JAMA* 1989;261: 711–714.

30. D'Alessandro AM, Sollinger HW, Hoffmann RM, et al. Experience with Belzer UW cold storage solution in simultaneous pancreas-kidney transplantation. *Transplant Proc* 1990;22: 532–534.

31. Wieselthaler GM, Chevtchik O, Konetschny R, et al. Improved graft function using a new myocardial preservation solution: Celsior—preliminary data from a randomized prospective study. *Transplant Proc* 1999;31:2067–2068.

32. Haverich A, Scott WC, Jamieson SW. Twenty years of lung preservation: a review. *Heart Transplant* 1985;4:234–240.

33. Kokudo Y, Furuya T, Takeyochi I, et al. Comparison of University of Wisconsin, Euro-Collins, and lactated Ringer's solutions in rat small bowel preservation for orthotopic small bowel transplantation. *Transplant Proc* 1994;26:1492–1493.

34. Furukawa H, Casavilla A, Abu-Elmagd K, et al. Basic considerations for the procurement of intestinal grafts. *Transplant Proc* 1994;26:1470.

Renal Transplantation

ROBERT M. MERION AND JOHN C. MAGEE

HISTORY

Renal transplantation is one of the great success stories of 20th century medicine. First performed successfully in humans by Nobel laureate Joseph Murray in the late 1950s between identical twins, renal transplantation is now the therapy of choice for patients with end-stage renal disease of all etiologies. Compared with chronic dialysis treatments, renal transplant recipients have improved survival, better quality of life, and an enhanced body image and sense of health. In addition, successful transplantation is significantly less expensive than any form of dialytic therapy, the break-even point occurring within 18 months of the procedure.

The biggest challenge facing the field of renal transplantation today is the imbalance between the numbers of suitable recipients and the nearly stagnant number of organ donors (Fig. 16.39). Living renal donation has increased the total number of available organs, but the disparity between donors and recipients continues to increase at an alarming rate.

The procedural aspects of kidney transplantation have become almost completely standardized. Major variables in the clinical application of this modality of treatment include recipient and donor candidate selection criteria, posttransplantation immunosuppressive regimens and follow-up schedules, and the long-term management of immunosuppression-related morbidity, especially neoplasia and opportunistic infection.

RECIPIENT ASSESSMENT

Current indications for renal transplantation are justifiably broad. Any patient with end-stage renal disease should be evaluated as a potential recipient candidate. Patients at the extremes of age can be successfully transplanted provided any associated extrarenal conditions are carefully evaluated. The most frequent categories of end-stage renal disease for which kidney transplantation is performed are shown in Table 16.9. Renal failure from diabetes mellitus and glomerulonephritis remain the most common indications for transplantation in the United States.

For patients who have not yet reached dialysis dependence at the time of referral, a careful assessment of potential reversibility of chronic renal failure should be undertaken. Barring such a situation, most recipients are evaluated with a view toward identification of potential contraindications, rather than by identifying a particular indication. Key factors in the history that preclude transplantation are the presence of uneradicated infection that would complicate the postoperative course or a malignancy other than nonmelanoma skin cancer, unless treatment was for cure and a suitable time has elapsed. Sometimes, pretransplantation treatment of infection can allow for the transplantation to proceed, such as in the case of osteomyelitis complicating diabetes mellitus. An overview of the evaluation of a potential recipient is shown in Table 16.10.

Careful consideration of cardiac reserve is an important element in the evaluation. Diabetic recipients in particular may harbor occult fixed coronary artery lesions amenable to medical, percutaneous, or operative therapy. A stress test evaluating functional cardiac reserve performed either on a treadmill or pharmacologically (e.g., dobutamine

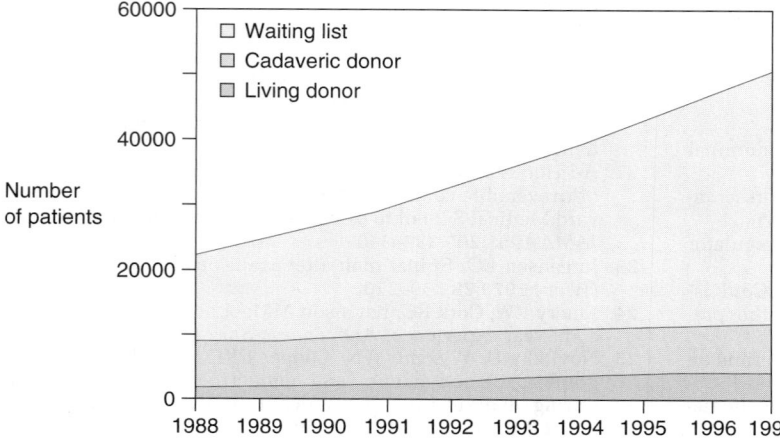

Figure 16.39. Growth of the cadaveric renal transplant waiting list in comparison to modest increases in the numbers of cadaveric and living donor renal transplants performed between 1988 and 1997. Source: UNOS Scientific Registry Data as of September 8, 1998.

Table 16.9. ETIOLOGIES OF END-STAGE RENAL DISEASE AS INDICATIONS FOR RENAL TRANSPLANTATION 1988–1997

Disease	Number of cases	Percent of total
Glomerular diseases	32,330	32%
Diabetes	19,401	19%
Hypertension	13,036	13%
Tubular and interstitial diseases	9,152	9%
Polycystic kidneys	6,183	6%
Congenital, rare familial, and metabolic diseases	3,736	4%
Renovascular and other vascular diseases	2,305	2%
Other	9,787	15%

Data from Cecka JM. The UNOS Scientific Renal Transplant Registry. In: Cecka JM, Terasaki PI, eds. Clinical transplants 1998. Los Angeles: UCLA Press, 1999:1–16.

echocardiography) provides a useful screening tool to determine whether more invasive evaluation with cardiac catheterization is necessary (1).

LIVING DONORS

Since the early 1990s, an increasing proportion of kidney transplantations have been performed using organs procured from volunteer living donors. Considered a selfless, altruistic gift, living kidney donation is a safe and highly successful form of renal replacement therapy. Risks to the donor are minimal, recovery is usually swift and uneventful, and long-lasting psychological benefits have been demonstrated. Results for the recipient are notably better than those achieved with cadaveric grafts.

The evaluation of a potential living kidney donor who has come forward begins with assessment of ABO blood type, histocompatibility testing, and determination of a

Table 16.10. EVALUATION SCHEME FOR WORK-UP OF RENAL ALLOGRAFT RECIPIENTS

SCREENING EVALUATION

History and physical examination
Laboratory analysis
  Biochemistry screen (renal function, electrolytes, liver function)
  Complete blood count; platelet count
  Viral serologies (hepatitis B and C, herpes, cytomegalovirus, HIV)
  ABO blood typing
  Histocompatibility determination
  Cytotoxic antibody screen (panel reactive antibody)
  Prostate-specific antigen (men >50 y)
Chest radiograph
Electrocardiogram
Psychosocial assessment

STANDARD EXAMINATIONS

Dental clearance
Flexible sigmoidoscopy (>50 y)
Gynecologic examination and Pap smear
Mammography (per standard guidelines)

AS-NEEDED EVALUATIONS

Cardiac (all diabetic patients and those >50 y, others by history)
Gastrointestinal (endoscopy as indicated for symptoms, liver biopsy for positive hepatitis serology)
Genitourinary (voiding cystourethrogram, cystoscopy for symptoms)
Pulmonary (arterial blood gases, pulmonary function tests, bronchoscopy as needed)

cytotoxic crossmatch result. The latter tests for preformed antidonor antibody directed toward relevant human leukocyte antigen (HLA)-A, B, and DR gene products. This test must be negative for the transplantation to proceed. A careful medical and psychosocial screening then ensues, looking particularly for inherited renal disease (such as polycystic kidney disease), which would preclude donation, or any other evidence of renal dysfunction. A history of passage of a renal stone is not necessarily a contraindication to donation. General good health is a prerequisite, and, assuming normal results of physical examination, screening with a chest radiograph, electrocardiogram, survey blood work, and urinalysis is completed.

Psychosocial evaluation is directed toward evaluation of the donor's motivation and to the unearthing of any potential secondary gain. Unrelated living donors are increasingly accepted as donors, provided there is a bona fide emotional relationship between donor and recipient.

A detailed recitation of the advantages and disadvantages of renal donation is conveyed to the donor, as well as information on the surgical procedure, hospitalization, postoperative recovery, and long-term outcome. Opportunity should always be afforded to the potential donor to speak to the transplantation team in the absence of the recipient so that any reluctance or issues of coercion can be explored unambiguously.

CADAVERIC DONORS

The most common form of renal transplantation entails the use of an organ from a brain-dead cadaveric donor. The etiology, pathophysiology, and diagnosis of brain death is discussed elsewhere in this chapter, as is consideration of non-heartbeating donors.

Once a suitable cadaveric kidney donor is identified, a series of steps must be completed before the actual transplantation. Pairing of donor kidneys with prospective recipients is coordinated under guidelines promulgated by the United Network for Organ Sharing. Factors related to recipient waiting time, histocompatibility matching, sensitization, and geographic proximity of donor and recipient (a surrogate for reducing ischemia time and improving organ viability) are incorporated into a point system for allocation by a nationwide computer algorithm (2). Donor kidneys are always offered to ABO blood type-identical recipients. National sharing is mandatory for donor–recipient pairs with no HLA mismatches. This occurs in approximately 10% of cases. If no perfectly matched recipients are available, the kidneys are allocated locally to crossmatch-negative recipients according to the point system. If no local recipients are identified, the kidney is offered to a larger region and then nationally, as discussed in the section on organ preservation.

DONOR NEPHRECTOMY

Cadaveric nephrectomy is discussed in an earlier portion of this chapter and is not further considered here. Living donor nephrectomy is traditionally accomplished using an open procedure through a flank incision with the patient in the decubitus position (Fig. 16.40). Dissection is carried down through the muscular layers to the retroperitoneum, taking care to avoid entry into either the abdominal cavity or thorax. Gerota's fascia is opened widely. The renal vein is followed toward the vena cava and the renal artery is dissected to the aorta. The ureter is followed down to the pelvic brim. After disconnection of the ureter, the renal vasculature is divided and the kidney is immediately plunged into iced saline solution and perfused through the artery with a cold preservative solution. The

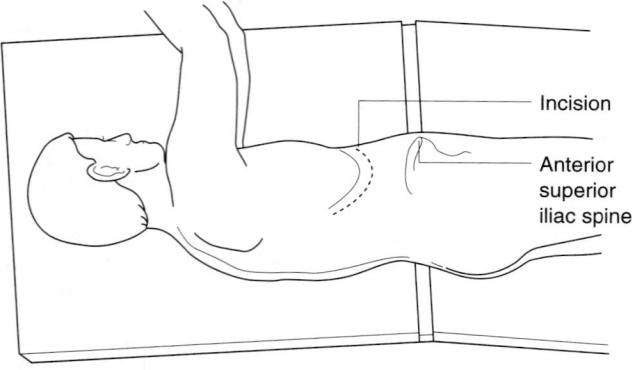

Figure 16.40. Diagram illustrating patient positioning and location of flank incision for open living donor nephrectomy.

remaining stumps of the renal artery and vein in the donor are carefully oversewn and the distal ureter is ligated.

Laparoscopic techniques for living donor nephrectomy have been reported (3). With this technique, the flank incision is avoided. Several technical variations have been described, including a hand-assisted technique in which the incision used ultimately to remove the donor kidney is made at the beginning of the procedure. One hand is passed through this incision, offering the advantage of its use throughout the procedure by the laparoscopic surgeon (Fig. 16.41). Although no prospective, randomized, clini-

cal trials have yet been reported, there are suggestions that laparoscopic donor nephrectomy may be associated with a shorter period of convalescence, earlier return to work, and less pain. No significant adverse effects on renal allograft function have been attributed to the laparoscopic technique, although the shorter right renal vein has led some authors to suggest restricting the procedure to donors with an acceptable left kidney for donation.

Mortality and morbidity related to volunteer renal donation are minimal. It has been estimated that the risk of death is approximately 4 in 10,000. The most common postoperative complications are atelectasis, urinary tract infection, and wound infection. Each of these occurs rarely. The open, flank technique is infrequently associated with hernia formation. The life expectancy of living kidney donors is at least as good as sex- and age-matched control subjects (4).

RECIPIENT OPERATIVE PROCEDURE

The essential features of the recipient operative procedure for renal transplantation include (a) curvilinear iliac fossa incision and dissection of the iliac vessels; (b) siting and anastomosis of the renal artery and vein to the external iliac artery and vein, respectively; (c) revascularization of the kidney; (d) siting and anastomosis of the donor ureter to the recipient bladder; and (e) closure of the incision. The customary incision for renal transplantation follows a curvilinear or "hockey stick" course in the iliac fossa, starting approximately 2 cm medial to the anterior superior iliac spine and proceeding inferomedially to a point just cephalad to the symphysis pubis (Fig. 16.42A).

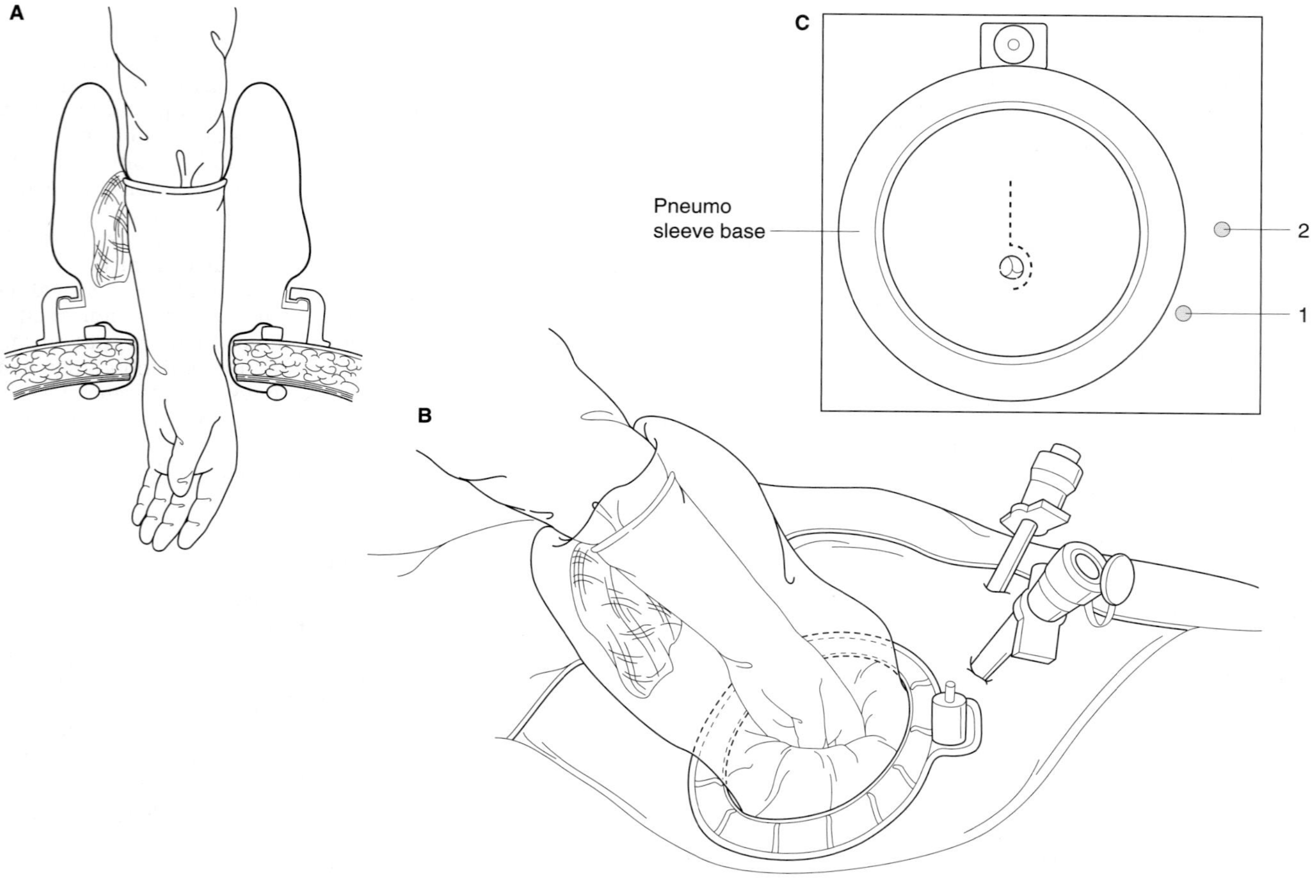

Figure 16.41. *(A)* Laparoscopic port and incision placement for living donor nephrectomy; *(B)* hand-assisted technique facilitates mobilization and reduces operative time.

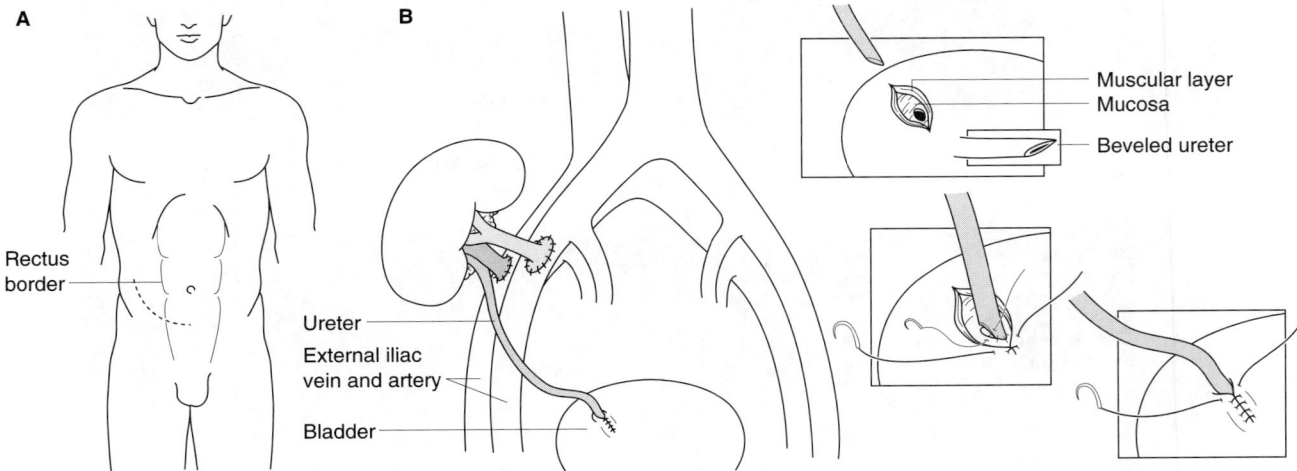

Figure 16.42. *(A)* Curvilinear iliac fossa incision used for kidney transplant recipient operation. *(B)* Vascular anastomoses completed between the external iliac artery and vein and donor renal artery and vein, respectively. *Insets:* ureteral anastomosis performed using the external ureteroneocystostomy technique.

The incision is carried through the abdominal musculature and the peritoneum is carefully reflected medially to expose the external iliac artery and vein. In women, the round ligament is usually taken, whereas the spermatic cord and contents can almost invariably be retracted medially in men. A mechanical retractor aids in exposure, but extreme care must be taken to avoid compression of the femoral nerve and resultant neurologic defect. The artery and vein are dissected free from surrounding retroperitoneal tissues and lymphatic vessels are ligated to avoid postoperative lymphocele formation.

The donor kidney is brought to the surgical field and inspected. Multiple or anomalous vessels, duplication of part or the entirety of the collecting system, and parenchymal abnormalities are identified. The artery and vein are trimmed to appropriate length and any untied tributaries are ligated. Once suitable sites on the external iliac artery and vein have been chosen, an atraumatic vascular clamp is used to occlude the external iliac vein (Fig. 16.42B). Systemic anticoagulation is optionally administered, although the uremic state does not routinely require it. An end-to-side venous anastomosis is carried out, taking care to avoid any kinking or twisting of the renal vein. A similar approach is used for construction of the arterial anastomosis. In the case of a cadaveric donor, a Carrel patch of donor aorta is retained, whereas in living donor transplantation the end of the renal artery is spatulated before anastomosis. After completion of the vascular anastomoses, the donor kidney is revascularized.

Hypothermic storage of donor kidneys is essential to maintain viability, so that once the donor kidney is removed from its 4°C environment, the anastomosis time is important. The donor organ warms at a rate of approximately 1°C per minute, and prolongation of ischemic time is associated with a significantly higher incidence of delayed graft function (5). Additional factors associated with an improved likelihood of immediate graft function include monitoring of intravascular fluid volume to ensure adequate preload at the time of revascularization and administration of osmotic or loop diuretics.

The most commonly used technique for ureteral reconstruction is the external ureteroneocystostomy (6). The bladder is filled with an antibiotic-containing solution. A site is chosen on the dome of the bladder for reconstruction of the lower urinary tract. The muscular coat of the bladder is dissected, allowing the bladder mucosa to herniate. An ellipse of bladder mucosa is excised. The donor ureter should be trimmed to a length sufficient to allow for a tension-free anastomosis to the bladder, but excessive length should be avoided to minimize the risk of ureteral obstruction or stricture formation due to inadequate vascularity, because the donor ureter depends on lower pole branches of the renal artery. The end of the donor ureter is spatulated and a mucosa-to-mucosa anastomosis is constructed using fine absorbable suture (Fig. 16.42, inset). To prevent vesicoureteral reflux, the bladder musculature is closed over the tangential course of the ureter through the bladder wall, so that during micturition the transvesical portion of the ureter is compressed. After completion of the ureteral reconstruction, the wound is inspected for hemostasis, irrigated, and closed in layers.

EARLY GRAFT DYSFUNCTION

The determinants and predictors of graft function start with the organ donor. Living donor grafts nearly all function immediately because of meticulous attention to the evaluation and screening of the potential donor, ideal physiologic and anatomic conditions under which the organ is removed, and the short warm and cold ischemic times that are typical of living donor kidney transplantation. Factors affecting the probability of immediate function in recipients of cadaveric grafts include the occurrence and duration of donor cardiac arrest, need for high-dose vasopressors, and duration of preservation time. In the recipient, adequate volume status and administration of osmotic or loop diuretics are associated with improved function.

Much of the subsequent course of renal transplantation is determined in the minutes and hours after revascularization. Intraoperative assessment of the graft immediately after revascularization should include determination of the adequacy of arterial and venous anastomoses and evaluation of the color and turgor of the graft. A soft, pale kidney suggests inadequate arterial inflow, whereas a tense, distended kidney suggests the possibility of venous obstruction. The typical description of hyperacute rejection is that of a soft, blue graft with a palpable arterial pulse.

Assuming that the graft appearance is satisfactory at the conclusion of the procedure, volume loading should be

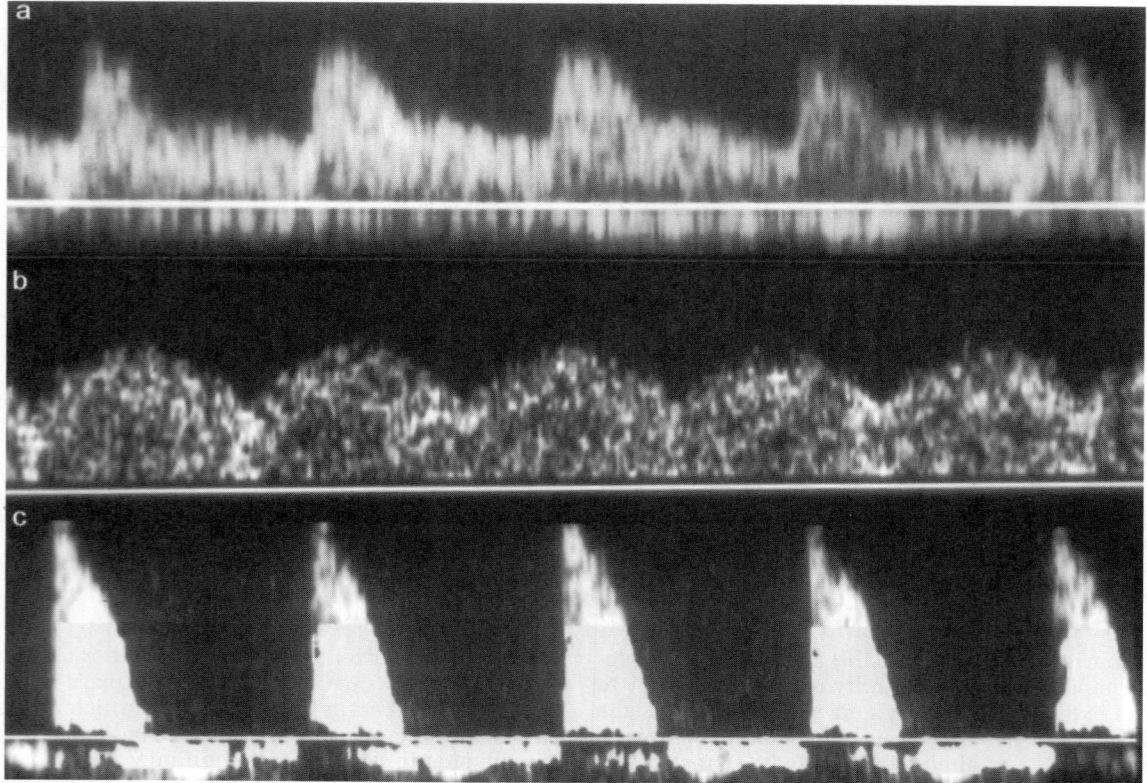

Figure 16.43. *(A)* Normal Doppler ultrasound tracing from a transplanted kidney. *(B)* Transplant renal artery stenosis showing a tardus waveform. *(C)* Doppler ultrasound appearance of reversed diastolic flow associated with allograft rejection of venous obstruction.

continued in the immediate posttransplantation period to encourage diuresis. Loop diuretics may be helpful in this setting. Failure to produce urine should prompt evaluation with bedside color Doppler ultrasonography. Figure 16.43 shows several ultrasound patterns. Absence of the arterial or venous signal should initiate a prompt return to the operating room. A negative examination or one demonstrating only modest reduction in flow with or without reversal of diastolic flow is reassuring, as long as the venous signal is normal, and suggests that the dysfunction is due to an intrarenal problem such as acute tubular necrosis.

Other diagnostic studies are infrequently used and less frequently helpful. Renal allograft arteriography is rarely indicated. Radionuclide scans are used by some to assess function more directly, but the combination of ultrasound and early renal allograft biopsy is simpler, less expensive, and more reliable.

IMMUNOSUPPRESSION

The unmodified immune response to a renal allograft entails a complex series of cellular events that are initiated immediately on revascularization of the transplanted organ. In the absence of immunosuppressive agents, rejection proceeds unabated and can result in complete destruction of the graft within days.

The major objective of immunosuppressive therapy is thus to prevent acute allograft rejection. This goal must be balanced by the risks of immunosuppression, especially opportunistic infection and neoplasia. Both of these are considered in more depth later. Because the immune system recognizes foreign alloantigen so quickly, clinical immunosuppression is started before surgery. Large doses of

corticosteroids are usually given at this stage. The use of induction therapy with polyclonal or monoclonal antibody preparations is still debated, but appears to have advantages for pediatric recipients (7) as well as for patients deemed to be at higher immunologic risk, such as African-Americans, retransplant recipients, and those with high levels of cytotoxic antibody.

Maintenance therapy is typically accomplished using two or three drugs. Corticosteroids are continued indefinitely in most programs. A calcineurin antagonist (cyclosporine or tacrolimus) is the cornerstone of immunosuppression. These agents selectively block T lymphocytes and are critical for the prevention of allograft rejection. The regimen is often rounded out with the addition of a third agent such as mycophenolate mofetil or azathioprine. The former affects T-cell proliferation by blocking purine synthesis through competitive inhibition of inosine monophosphate dehydrogenase. Because T lymphocytes are among the few cells that lack the salvage pathway for purine synthesis, blockade of this step results in significant selective effects on T cells. Azathioprine, long a mainstay of immunosuppressive therapy, also acts as an antimetabolite, but in a much less selective manner, accounting for its major toxicities on rapidly dividing cell populations such as bone marrow.

COMPLICATIONS

Surgical complications occur infrequently after renal transplantation. Vascular compromise in the first hours or days after implantation can be associated with failure of the allograft unless immediately corrected. Renal arterial thrombosis, arterial dissection, pseudoaneurysm formation, and renal vein thrombosis are all fortunately unusual occurrences. Postoperative hemorrhage may result from disruption of the vascular anastomoses, inadequate attention to small tributaries during the retroperitoneal dissection, infection, or renal capsular rupture. The latter is distinctly uncommon with modern methods of organ preservation and pretransplantation immunologic testing to avoid hyperacute rejection.

Transplant renal artery stenosis may present with alteration in renal function, increasing serum creatinine levels, and hypertension. Typically, this complication occurs months to years after transplantation. Doppler ultrasonography provides a very sensitive method to detect this problem and differentiate it from other abnormalities (Fig. 43B).

Morbidity related to the genitourinary system can be broadly divided into leaks and obstruction. Leaks at the ureteroneocystostomy occur infrequently, and can usually be managed nonoperatively by placing a percutaneous nephrostomy tube under ultrasonic guidance (Fig. 16.44). This can be later advanced across the anastomosis into the bladder and converted to a universal stent until healing occurs. If a retroperitoneal urinoma is present, separate drainage of the perinephric space may be indicated.

Obstruction of the urinary system may occur at any time. Early obstruction is usually related to technical imperfection in the anastomosis of the donor ureter to the bladder or other mechanical difficulties such as torsion of the ureter. The donor ureter can be twisted almost 180 degrees before a corkscrew effect is generated as a result of ureteral peristalsis that eventually causes obstruction at the fixed point of the anastomosis. Occasionally, a hematoma or postoperative edema may impede the flow of urine. As pressure increases in the collecting system, urine flow may resume temporarily and the resulting transient decline in serum creatinine may provide false reassurance. Thus, an erratically fluctuating serum creatinine without alternative explanation should be considered a diagnostic clue that partial intermittent ureteral obstruction may be present.

Late obstruction may be due to ischemia of the donor ureter. Because the ureter relies on small arterial branches of the lower pole renal artery for its vascular integrity, it is wise to trim the ureter and avoid leaving excessive length. Multiple episodes of rejection may also adversely affect the microvasculature of the ureter, resulting in long, dense stricture formation requiring reoperation. Reoperation and reconstruction of the ureterovesical anastomosis may be required. In cases where there is inadequate ureteral length once the stenotic segment is resected, a Boari flap procedure may be used (Fig. 16.45).

During the course of the retroperitoneal dissection, care should be taken to ligate lymphatic vessels. Collections of lymph in the perinephric space (lymphocele) may result in urinary obstruction or pain and may become secondarily infected. Diagnosis is straightforward with conventional ultrasound. Percutaneous drainage is associated with a high incidence of recurrence and secondary infection, so the more definitive method of laparoscopic creation of a peritoneal "window" is preferred.

Infection and neoplasia are the two primary categories of posttransplantation complication specifically attributable to the need for maintenance of an immunosuppressed state. Virtually all renal transplant recipients acquire an infection at some point in their course. Early infections tend to be those associated with the surgical procedure, involving the wound, perinephric space, or bladder. Pneumonia may be related to the period of intraoperative intubation and mechanical ventilation. Approximately 4 to 6 weeks posttransplantation, viral infections first start to appear. Cytomegalovirus infection is quite common, especially if a seronegative recipient receives an organ from a seropositive donor. Prophylactic antiviral regimens have been devised for such high-risk combinations, but cytomegalovirus disease may still occur. This herpesvirus infection may become manifest with fever, malaise, and anorexia, along with diminished renal allograft function. Extrarenal manifestations include interstitial pneumonitis, myocarditis, gastrointestinal involvement, and cerebritis. Antiviral therapy with ganciclovir usually is effective, although treatment must be given for 3 to 4 weeks and recurrences may occur, particularly in children.

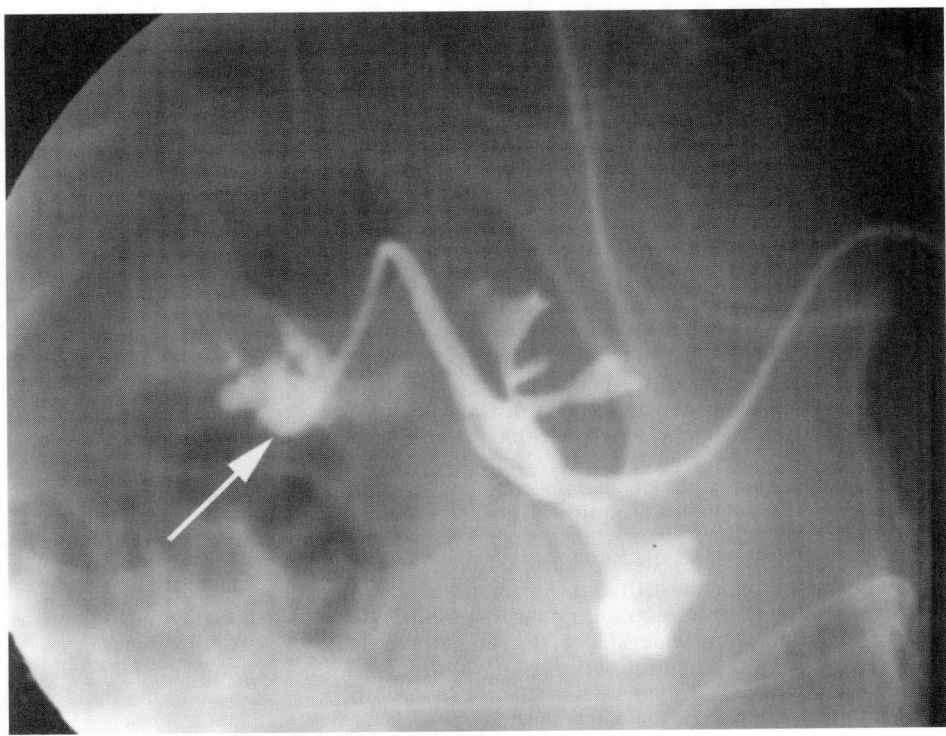

Figure 16.44. Percutaneous nephrostogram showing leak from ureterovesical anastomosis.

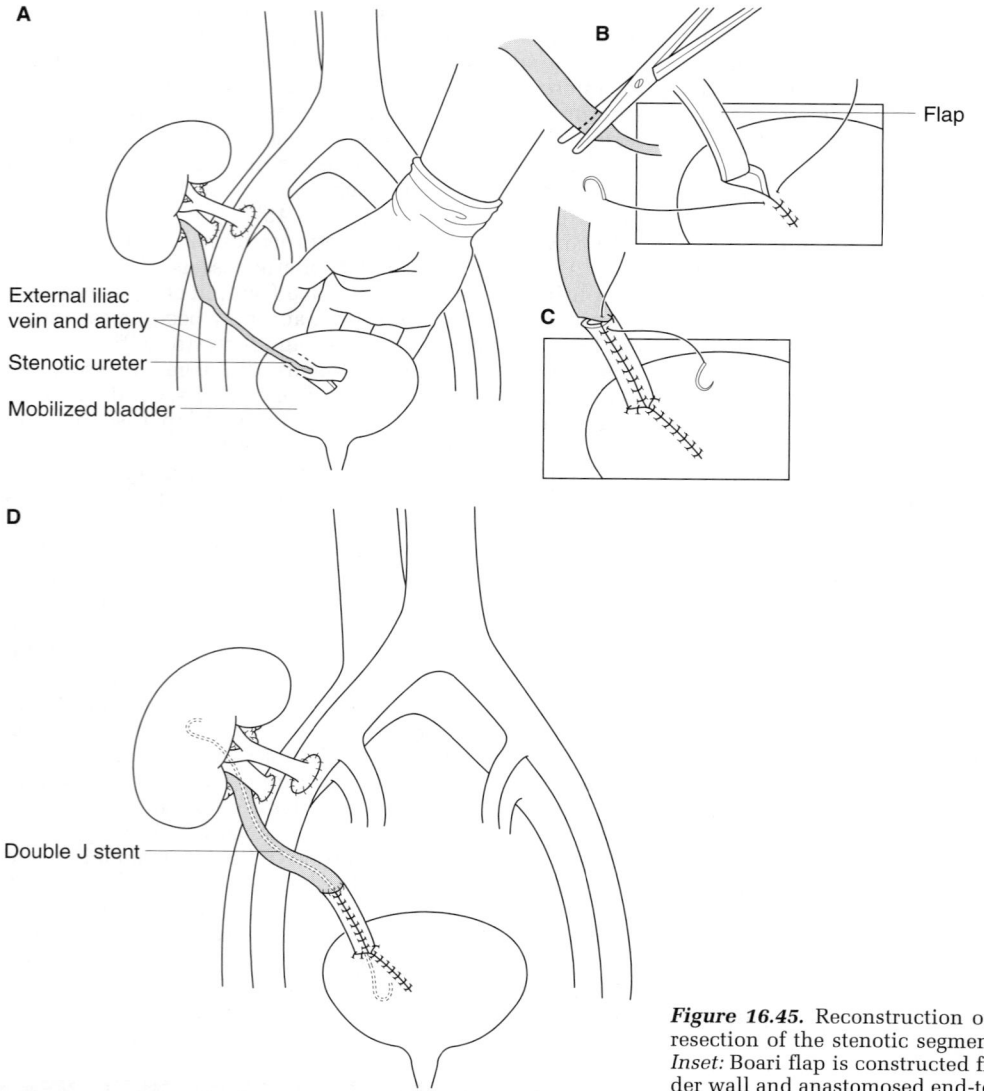

A

External iliac
vein and artery

Stenotic ureter

Mobilized bladder

B

Flap

C

D

Double J stent

Figure 16.45. Reconstruction of a stenotic donor ureter, showing resection of the stenotic segment and mobilization of the bladder. *Inset:* Boari flap is constructed from a tubularized segment of bladder wall and anastomosed end-to-end to the proximal donor ureter.

Other viruses of importance in the renal transplant recipient include herpesvirus (type 1 and 2), Epstein-Barr virus (considered later), and the hepatitis viruses. Varicella can be particularly dangerous in children, and previous infection before transplantation does not guarantee lifelong immune protection in the transplant recipient. The severity of any viral infection may be magnified in the immunosuppressed host. Prophylaxis against herpesvirus is usually given for at least several months after transplantation and at the first indication of mucocutaneous or genital disease. Severe viral infection may necessitate reduction or even temporary cessation of immunosuppressive therapy. Finally, polyomavirus infection has been recently recognized as a cause of renal allograft dysfunction. Histologic demonstration of characteristic viral particles on biopsy material may be required to make a definitive diagnosis.

Bacterial, fungal, and other opportunistic infections are fairly common. A partial listing of the organisms that may affect renal allograft recipients include *Aspergillus, Cryptococcus, Listeria, Pneumocystis carinii,* and *Nocardia,* as well as multisystem infection with *Candida albicans* and non-*albicans* species. Tuberculosis is being seen with in-

creasing frequency as the incidence of infection with this mycobacterium has risen in urban settings.

The incidence of neoplasia is significantly higher in renal transplant recipients than in the general population, and it has been estimated that cancer develops in approximately 4% of recipients. This figure underestimates the true incidence because longer graft and patient survival seem to be associated with a continuing cumulative risk. The most common malignancy seen after renal transplantation is skin cancer, primarily squamous cell carcinoma. Unlike nonimmunosuppressed people, transplant recipients are at a higher risk for nodal spread and multiple tumors.

Posttransplantation lymphoproliferative disease may develop in association with Epstein-Barr virus infection. It is thought that B-cell transformation occurs under the influence of this virus. Initially, polyclonal proliferation occurs, but full-fledged B-cell lymphoma may develop if the condition is not arrested by reduction or cessation of immunosuppression. Progression to oligoclonal or monoclonal disease requires institution of chemotherapy.

Cervical carcinoma in situ occurs at a rate 14-fold higher than in the general population, and there is a 100-fold increase in the incidences of vulvar and anal carcinoma. Unfortunately, the progression of epithelial carcinomas does not appear to be affected by reduction or even cessation of immunosuppressive drugs.

REJECTION

Under cover of modern immunosuppression, only a minority of renal transplant recipients experience one or more episodes of acute allograft rejection. Hyperacute rejection, the most feared manifestation of humorally mediated immune injury, is also fortunately the least common. Hyperacute rejection occurs within minutes to hours of the transplantation procedure when cytotoxic antidonor antibody (presumably undetected by the preoperative crossmatch) binds to vascular endothelium of the graft. This results in activation of the complement cascade and produces destruction of microvascular integrity. The features of hyperacute rejection include the gross intraoperative appearance of a soft, blue kidney despite adequate large vessel arterial inflow and venous outflow. Biopsy at this stage may demonstrate the classic triad of polymorphonuclear leukocytes in the glomerular capillary loops, fibrin deposition, and platelet thrombi. This condition is usually irreversible and removal of the kidney graft is advised to avoid systemic toxicity from a large volume of necrotic tissue and to abort the complement activation engendered by the graft. A less dramatic form of rejection may occur within a few days when memory cells of B-lymphocyte lineage are stimulated to produce an anamnestic antibody response. Histologically, this entity appears as injury primarily focused on the vascular endothelium, although lymphocytic cellular elements are often present as well. Plasmapheresis and substitution of the antiproliferative agent with cyclophosphamide may be helpful in these cases.

Acute rejection typically occurs between 1 week and 3 months after transplantation. Decreased allograft function with rising serum creatinine values and diminished urine output are hallmarks of rejection. Additional signs and symptoms, such as low-grade fever, allograft tenderness, and hypertension may suggest the diagnosis. It is important to confirm the suspicion of allograft rejection with a percutaneous biopsy whenever possible because several other diagnoses can present with similar findings. These include cyclosporine or tacrolimus nephrotoxicity, ureteral obstruction, infection, transplant renal artery stenosis, and recurrence of the underlying renal disease.

Acute allograft rejection is usually treated first by increasing immunosuppression. Pulse corticosteroids (4 to 8 mg/kg of methylprednisolone daily for 3 days) reverses one half to two thirds of first rejection episodes. Those with a more prominent vascular component and those episodes unresponsive to steroids are treated with anti-T-cell antibody. The most common agent is murine monoclonal antibody directed against the CD3 receptor. A 7- to 10-day course of treatment reverses up to 94% of steroid-resistant rejection episodes. Alternatives include equine or rabbit polyclonal antilymphocyte preparations.

Once an acute rejection episode has occurred, the stage is set for a series of events even if the acute process is successfully aborted with enhanced immunosuppression as described previously. The final result of allograft injury is fibrosis with interstitial scarring and proliferative changes in the vascular compartment. These are the features of chronic rejection or chronic allograft nephropathy, a poorly characterized entity that is usually the harbinger of progressive deterioration of graft function and eventual return to dialysis. The course of chronic rejection may extend to months or even several years. No effective treatment has yet been devised and the underlying pathophysiologic process remains unclear.

LONG-TERM COMPLICATIONS AND OUTCOME

Results of renal transplantation continue to improve. More than in any other field of medicine, outcomes of organ transplantation have been collected and studied at the national level for more than 10 years. As the Organ Procurement and Transplantation Network contractor, the Scientific Registry of the United Network for Organ Sharing has carefully assessed results. Similarly, the United States Renal Data System, under contract to the U.S. Department of Health and Human Services, has done similar analyses for all patients with end-stage renal disease. As shown in Fig. 16.46, the overall 1-year actuarial patient survival rate after renal transplantation has risen over the 10-year period from 1987 to 1996 from 91% to 96% for recipients of cadaveric kidneys and from 97% to 98% for living related recipients (8). Patient deaths fall into three main categories. Infection accounts for the plurality of patient deaths, followed closely by complications of atherosclerosis and cardiovascular disease. Malignancy is responsible for a small but important number of deaths.

Despite remarkable improvements in immunosuppressive therapy and corresponding decreases in the incidence of acute allograft rejection in the first weeks and months

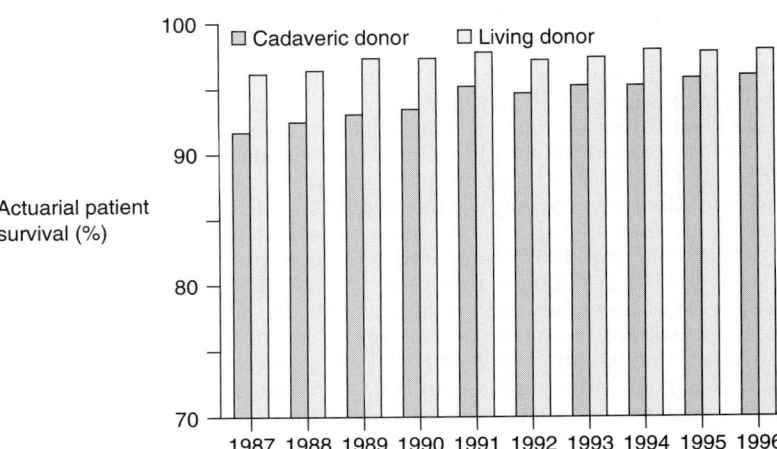

Figure 16.46. Improvements in one year actuarial patient survival after cadaveric and living donor renal transplantation. Source: United States Renal Data System (8).

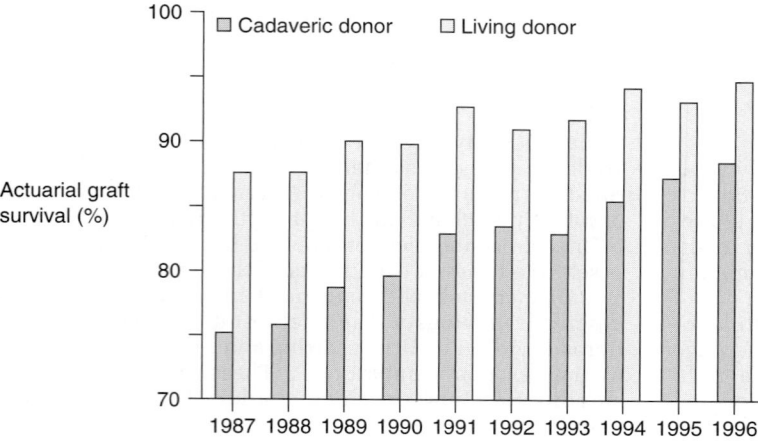

Figure 16.47. Improvements in one-year actuarial graft survival after cadaveric and living donor renal transplantation. Source: United Stated Renal Data System (8).

after transplantation, graft loss continues to exact its inexorable toll. Graft losses due to acute rejection now only barely exceed those from chronic rejection, and medication noncompliance has become the second leading cause of graft loss among patients whose grafts function for at least 5 years. Increasingly, the effects of underlying risk factors for atherosclerosis and the additive effects of immunosuppressive drugs are becoming manifest as more patients die with a functioning graft. Recurrent disease occurs with some regularity in patients with glomerulonephritis, diabetes mellitus, and several other etiologies of end-stage renal disease, but only in unusual circumstances does the recurrent disease lead to allograft failure.

Like patient survival, overall graft survival rates have improved over the 1990s, with 1-year actuarial results of 87.7% and 93.9% reported for first-time recipients of cadaveric and living related grafts, respectively, performed in 1996 (Fig. 16.47). Unfortunately, examination of results on a longer posttransplantation time scale paints a less encouraging picture. Among patients who received their first cadaveric graft in 1987, only 32% were still alive with graft function 10 years later. Clearly, the challenge remains to overcome these continuing graft losses.

Quality of life after kidney transplantation is an important but incompletely studied area. Recent data suggest that patients who receive successful renal transplants have significantly better general and health-related quality of life compared with patients on dialysis (9).

COST EFFECTIVENESS

The federal government has had a long-standing interest in the cost of renal replacement therapy. Since the 1970s, Medicare has covered the costs of such care under the End Stage Renal Disease Program. Annual government outlays for 1997 exceeded $10.7 billion, and it is estimated that the total national direct cost, including patient obligations and non-Medicare coverage, exceeded $15.6 billion (8). Dialysis costs averaged over $51,000 per patient per year between 1993 and 1997, compared with transplantation costs averaging $18,000 per patient per year. Although the initial cost of transplantation is higher than that of dialysis, the break-even point occurs before the end of the second posttransplantation year (8,10,11). Because the typical half-life of a kidney transplant is now in excess of 8 to 10 years, it follows that renal transplantation is significantly less expensive in the long run.

CONCLUSION

Kidney transplantation has established itself as the best form of renal replacement therapy for most patients with end-stage renal disease. Clinical results continue to improve and improved understanding of the immune response to the allograft has led to advances in the efficacy and safety of immunosuppressive therapy. The desperate donor organ shortage continues to stymie more widespread application of this preferred, cost-effective treatment. The growth of living donation is gratifying, but will still fall far short of the demonstrated need.

REFERENCES

1. Reis G, Marcovitz PA, Leichtman AB, et al. Usefulness of dobutamine stress echocardiography for detecting coronary artery disease in end-stage renal disease. *Am J Cardiol* 1995; 75:707–710.
2. United Network for Organ Sharing. On-line: http://www.unos.org (accessed November 25, 1999).
3. Ratner LE, Ciseck LJ, Moore RG, et al. Laparoscopic live donor nephrectomy. *Transplantation* 1995;60:1047–1049.
4. Najarian JS, Chavers BM, McHugh LE, et al. Twenty years or more of follow-up of living kidney donors. *Lancet* 1992;340: 807–810.
5. Cecka JM. The UNOS Scientific Renal Transplant Registry. In: Cecka JM, Terasaki PI, eds. *Clinical transplants 1998.* Los Angeles: UCLA Press, 1999:1–16.
6. Ohl DA, Konnak JW, Campbell DA, et al. Extravesical ureteroneocystostomy in renal transplantation. *J Urol* 1988;139: 499–502.
7. Singh A, Stablein D, Tejani A. Risk factors for vascular thrombosis in pediatric renal transplantation: a special report of the North American Pediatric Renal Transplant Cooperative Study. *Transplantation* 1997;63:1263–1267.
8. U.S. Renal Data System. *USRDS 1999 annual data report.* Bethesda, MD: National Institutes of Health, National Institute of Diabetes and Digestive and Kidney Diseases, April, 1999.
9. Shield CF, McGrath MM, Goss RF, for the FK506 Kidney Transplant Study Group. Assessment of health-related quality of life in kidney transplant patients receiving tacrolimus (FK506)-based versus cyclosporine-based immunosuppression. *Transplantation* 1997;64:1738–1743.
10. Hutton J. The economics of immunosuppression in renal transplantation: a review of recent literature. *Transplant Proc* 1999;31:1328–1332.
11. Schweitzer EJ, Wiland A, Evans D, et al. The shrinking renal replacement therapy "break-even" point. *Transplantation* 1998;66:1702–1708.

Hepatic Transplantation

DARRELL A. CAMPBELL, JR., JOHN C. MAGEE, STEVEN M. RUDICH, AND JEFFREY D. PUNCH

The evolution of hepatic transplantation has been remarkably rapid. Among the many pioneers in this area, Thomas Starzl from the University of Pittsburgh and Roy Calne from Cambridge University stand out. Starzl developed the modern transplantation technique and its clinical application, and Calne was responsible for introducing cyclosporine into clinical practice with parallel development of operative technique. The information presented here derives directly or indirectly from information originally contributed by these two people.

Only since the mid-1980s have technical and immunologic problems been surmounted to the extent that a high level of success with this procedure is now achieved. Advances in donor and recipient selection, organ preservation, anesthetic management, surgical technique, and immunosuppressive protocols have also contributed to improved outcomes. A problem that has not yet been solved is the limitation of donor organ relative to demand. Substantial numbers of patients die each year on the waiting list for lack of a suitable organ. Many strategies have been used to address this problem, the most important of which is the widespread appeal to the public about the need for organ donation. Other strategies have included a relaxation of the previously strict criterion for donor suitability, the development of surgical techniques to split one liver into two segments, each capable of sustaining life, and the development of safe surgical techniques allowing for living volunteers to donate a segment of liver to a recipient.

INDICATIONS FOR HEPATIC TRANSPLANTATION

General Considerations

The most common indication for hepatic transplantation is end-stage liver disease (ESLD), which typically results in the demise of the patient within 1 year and for which no other therapy is effective or suitable. Considering hepatic transplantation thus entails making two determinations. First, it must be determined that the patient actually has ESLD, and second, it must be determined when, in the course of the end-stage disease, transplantation should be done. In practice, the first determination is considerably easier than the second.

The term *end-stage* refers to the culmination of a variety of pathologic processes that leave the damaged liver with minimal function and no potential for recovery. This important assessment is made primarily on a clinical basis, and occasionally supplemented by histologic and serologic information. Instances where histologic information is particularly relevant include the patient presenting with liver failure and a history of alcoholism who might have ESLD or might instead have acute alcoholic hepatitis, a reversible disorder. The distinction could be made by biopsy and would be confirmed by improvement in the absence of alcohol. Histology and serology are also occasionally helpful in other clinical situations when ESLD must be accurately distinguished from acute liver failure with a reversible component, particularly acute viral hepatitis, autoimmune hepatitis, hemochromatosis, or drug toxicity.

The rate of progression of liver disease from a functional state to invalidism to death is variable, and the process may take several years. Previously, patients were placed on a waiting list for transplantation when it was thought that they were unlikely to survive for 1 to 2 years in the absence of a transplant. This was usually a rather subjective determination. In recent years, more standardization has been introduced into the process by the United Network for Organ Sharing (UNOS). According to universally accepted UNOS guidelines, adult patients may be "listed" for transplantation when they have met "minimal listing criteria," meaning seven points on the Child-Turcotte-Pugh (CTP) scale (Table 16.11). Such patients are typically stable outpatients with ESLD and are referred to as status 3 patients. Patients in the 2B category are more ill and have at least 7 CTP points and 1 modifier (active variceal bleed, hepatorenal syndrome, prior history of spontaneous bacterial peritonitis, or ongoing refractory ascites) or at least 10 CTP points without a modifier. Patients in the 2A category are hospitalized in an intensive care unit, have one modifier, and have a life expectancy of less than 7 days. Status 1 patients have either fulminant hepatic failure, primary nonfunction of a liver transplant, or hepatic artery thrombosis occurring within 7 days of liver transplantation.

Referral of a patient with chronic liver disease to a liver transplantation center should be done early in the course of disease rather than later because it may take up to 2 years to receive a transplant after being placed on the transplantation list. Results are significantly improved if the surgery can be done on a semiselective basis rather than urgently. The CTP score can be a useful guide in making the decision for referral. A patient with documented ESLD and seven points (minimal listing criteria) would be an appropriate referral. This means that a liver patient with any two of the following should be referred; grade 1 to 2 encephalopathy, slight ascites, bilirubin greater then 2 mg/dL, international normalized ratio above 1.7, or albumin greater than 3.5 mg/dL. Although severe fatigue and intractable pruritus are often very troublesome symptoms for patients with ESLD, they are not specifically considered indications for transplantation. Usually, patients with these symptoms also have sufficient CTP points to merit listing.

Although these considerations apply to the more chronic forms of liver failure, important emergency decisions about transplantation must be made when the patient presents with fulminant hepatic failure, defined as the progression from good health to liver failure with hepatic encephalopathy within 8 weeks. A certain percentage of these patients recover spontaneously, but most do not. The decision to perform transplantation is based on clinical grounds. The most important consideration is the rate of neurologic deterioration. Surgery is indicated if the

---

Table 16.11. CHILD-TURCOTTE-PUGH SCORE

Points	1	2	3
Encephalopathy	None	1–2	3–4
Ascites	None	Slight	Moderate
Bilirubin[a] (mg/dL)	≤2	2–3	>3
Prothrombin time (seconds prolonged)	≤4	4–6	>6
(INR)	(≤1.7)	(1.7–2.3)	(>2.3)
Albumin	>3.5	2.8–3.5	<2.8

[a]Different values from serum bilirubin are substituted when patients have cholestatic liver disease, such as primary sclerosing cholangitis or primary biliary cirrhosis. These values are ≤4, 4–10, and >10 for 1, 2 and 3 points, respectively.

INR, international normalized ratio.

patient progresses to stage III (stuporous) or IV (unresponsive) coma with documentation of severe hepatic insufficiency, the most reliable indicator being a factor V level of less than 20%.

The number of absolute contraindications to hepatic transplantation has decreased as experience with the procedure has increased. The absolute contraindications for transplantation are inability to withstand the operative procedure, usually for cardiovascular or pulmonary reasons, recent intracranial hemorrhage or irreversible neurologic impairment, active substance abuse, intractable hypotension requiring pressor support, evidence of systemic infection, extrahepatic malignancy, and inability to comply with the posttransplantation regimen.

A number of medical conditions are no longer considered absolute contraindications to hepatic transplantation. For instance, a thrombosed portal vein is no longer a contraindication to transplantation because techniques have been devised to bypass or disobliterate the obstructed segment. The associated comorbidity of juvenile-onset diabetes mellitus formerly precluded transplantation. In current practice, this contraindication is not absolute, depending on the patient's physiologic status at the time of evaluation. Renal insufficiency clearly increases the morbidity of the hepatic transplantation but is not a contraindication. Renal transplantation can be done at the time of hepatic transplantation, and some degree of preoperative renal insufficiency often is reversible after successful hepatic transplantation. Advanced age (>70 years) is a relative contraindication to surgery, but in most centers, the physiologic state of the patient is a more important consideration than the chronologic age.

Specific Diseases for Which Transplantation Is Appropriate

In the absence of contraindications, virtually any disease resulting in liver failure is amenable to treatment (1). Noncholestatic cirrhosis, most frequently caused by alcoholism or chronic viral hepatitis, accounts for over half of the transplantations performed annually in the United States, whereas cholestatic cirrhosis, most commonly caused by primary biliary cirrhosis and primary sclerosing cholangitis, accounts for 10% to 15% (2). Causes of liver failure in 464 patients undergoing primary hepatic transplantation are shown in Table 16.12. A brief description of some of the more common diseases follows.

Alcoholic Liver Disease

Alcoholic liver disease is one of the most common indications for transplantation, and frequently coexists with hepatitis C infection, making the relative contribution of each disease to the potential candidate's condition difficult to ascertain. In some centers, there is a great reluctance to transplant patients who have a long history of alcoholism. On a clinical level, the concern has been that these patients may relapse into alcoholism after transplantation, with medical noncompliance and consequent graft failure. On a broader level, concern has been expressed that society should not pay for expensive treatments for diseases caused by self-destructive behavior. With more experience in this area, it has been recognized that the incidence of alcoholic recidivism after transplantation is low, and results in this category are as good as for non-alcohol-related categories (3). With regard to social policy, firm guidelines have not yet been established, but two points seem relevant. First, society already supports the concept of medical care for other types of self-destructive behavior, such as for the complications of cigarette

Table 16.12. CAUSES OF LIVER FAILURE IN 464 PATIENTS UNDERGOING PRIMARY HEPATIC TRANSPLANTATION SINCE 1993

Primary diagnosis	Number	Percentage
Noncholestatic cirrhosis		
Laennec	82	17.7
Hepatitis C	90	19.4
Hepatitis B	22	4.7
Cryptogenic cirrhosis	55	11.9
Autoimmune hepatitis	22	4.7
Cholestatic liver disease/cirrhosis		
Primary biliary cirrhosis	39	8.4
Primary sclerosing cholangitis	35	7.5
Biliary atresia	40	8.6
Fulminant	30	6.5
Inborns errors of metabolism	26	5.6
Neoplasm	11	2.4
Other	12	2.6
Budd-Chiari syndrome		
Polycystic liver disease		
Sarcoidosis		
Cystic fibrosis		
Caroli's disease		
Congenital hepatic fibrosis		
Neonatal hepatitis		
Hepatic trauma		

smoking. Second, transplantation costs for treating alcoholics do not seem as expensive when viewed in the context of obligatory costs for other treatments for the same disorder, such as portocaval shunting. The decision to perform liver transplantation for an alcoholic patient should be made only after careful examination by an experienced substance abuse specialist, including documentation of adequate patient insight and family support.

In addition to evaluating the risk for recidivism, a careful screening for other comorbid conditions, particularly alcoholic cardiomyopathy, is vital in these patients. A significant number of patients who are actively using alcohol at time of referral also clinically improve with abstinence, frequently improving their liver dysfunction to a point where transplantation can be deferred.

Hepatitis C

Hepatitis C is the major indication for liver transplantation in adults at most centers. It has been estimated that of the over 4 million Americans with hepatitis C, approximately 25% to 30% will progress to cirrhosis (4). Chronic alcohol use appears to promote progression to cirrhosis (5), and patients with hepatitis C are also at risk for development of hepatocellular carcinoma. Results of transplantation for this disease are comparable with those for noninfectious conditions. Hepatitis C invariably recurs in the transplanted liver, but usually follows an indolent course. Additional studies are necessary to evaluate the natural history of recurrent hepatitis C after transplantation and the potential role for antiviral therapy.

Hepatitis B

All patients with hepatitis B who undergo transplantation are at risk for reinfection. Early results after transplantation were poor because of severe recurrent disease, often progressing to early cirrhosis and death. The introduction of long-term hepatitis B immune globulin administration has dramatically diminished the incidence and severity of reinfection. Studies examining the role of nucleoside analogues, both as adjunctive therapy after transplantation and as a means to decrease viral load before transplantation, are underway. It is hoped that in the United States the introduction of universal vaccination against hepatitis B, and the use of potent antiviral agents for patients with chronic hepatitis B, will lead to a reduction in the number of patients requiring liver transplantation for hepatitis B.

Primary Biliary Cirrhosis

Primary biliary cirrhosis is thought to be caused by autoimmune mechanisms and is histologically characterized by portal tract inflammation with destruction of the intrahepatic biliary tract. The disease has a relatively predictable clinical course, characterized by gradually increasing serum bilirubin levels and progressive fatigue. Early stages of the disease are usually asymptomatic, and disease progression may evolve over 20 years. Severe pruritus and hepatic osteodystrophy often develop in these patients and can be quite incapacitating. Transplantation is commonly considered appropriate when the serum bilirubin reaches 10 mg/dL.

Primary Sclerosing Cholangitis

Primary sclerosing cholangitis is a chronic inflammatory process that generates intrahepatic and extrahepatic biliary strictures, and is a common indication for transplantation because there is no other effective long-term treatment. Primary sclerosing cholangitis is often associated with, and indistinguishable from, cholangiocarcinoma. Any doubt about the diagnosis warrants earlier consideration of transplantation. In most cases, colectomy for associated inflammatory bowel disease is done after successful transplantation because the failing liver would make the patient a poor candidate for a large abdominal procedure. Because transplantation is successful treatment, preoperative management should be limited to percutaneous methods of biliary decompression and stricture dilatation. Operative biliary decompression is usually no more effective than percutaneous techniques, and increases the risk of subsequent transplantation by producing adhesions in the right upper quadrant.

Biliary Atresia

Biliary atresia is by far the most common indication for hepatic transplantation in pediatric patients. Recommended treatment includes creation of a portoenterostomy (Kasai procedure), if this can be done before 3 months of age. After this point, success rates diminish markedly. After a successful Kasai procedure, most infants can survive at least to early childhood. Growth and nutritional failure, the development of portal hypertension with variceal hemorrhage, and recurrent cholangitis are indications for hepatic transplantation. In patients with an unsatisfactory course, multiple revisions of the portoenterostomy should be avoided to facilitate subsequent transplantation.

Inherited Metabolic Disorders

Among the more interesting indications for transplantation are the inherited metabolic disorders. Some enzymatic deficiencies in this group result in destruction of the liver; in these conditions, transplantation may resolve the liver failure as well as supply the missing enzyme. Disorders in this category include Wilson's disease, α_1-antitrypsin deficiency, tyrosinemia, and type I glycogen storage disease. In other cases, the liver is not affected by the disease, and transplantation is undertaken solely as enzyme replacement therapy. Diseases that have been cured by hepatic transplantation in this category are hemophilia A or B, homozygous familial hypercholesterolemia, Niemann-Pick disease, and oxalosis.

Fulminant Hepatic Failure

The most common causes of fulminant hepatic failure are viral hepatis, particularly hepatitis B and C, and various drug toxicities. In the latter group, acetaminophen toxicity is particularly prominent. In a significant percentage of cases, the exact etiology is never precisely determined.

Budd-Chiari Syndrome

Budd-Chiari syndrome is characterized by obliteration of the hepatic veins and presents as the triad of right upper quadrant pain, hepatomegaly, and ascites. A side-to-side portocaval shunt, in which the portal vein serves as an outflow tract for the congested liver, is the preferred therapy for cases not yet complicated by the development of cirrhosis. Transjugular intrahepatic portosystemic shunt (TIPS) is another alternative to achieve portal decompression. Transplantation is reserved for cases that present as liver cell failure, cases in which preoperative studies document no significant pressure gradient between portal vein and the inferior vena cava, and cases in which there is associated portal vein or inferior vena caval thrombosis.

Primary Liver Tumors

Transplantation for primary hepatic malignancies was initially plagued by a high frequency of recurrence and poor patient survival. As experience has developed, subsets of patients who might benefit from transplantation have been identified. Hepatocellular carcinoma, either arising de novo or more frequently in the setting of cirrhosis, is the most common malignancy encountered. Most centers consider patients for transplantation if they have a single lesion less than 5 cm or up to three lesions with no lesion greater than 3 cm in size, and there is no evidence of extrahepatic disease after exhaustive evaluation. Because these patients usually need to wait months before a liver is allocated to them, temporizing measures, including chemoembolization, cryotherapy, and radiofrequency ablation, are usually used to arrest tumor progression before transplantation.

Results for transplantation for cholangiocarcinoma have been substantially worse than in most other conditions, and transplantation is not usually an option outside of controlled clinical trials.

PREOPERATIVE ASSESSMENT AND MANAGEMENT

Urgent Transplantation

The patient with an acutely failing liver presents with varying degrees of hemodynamic instability and multiorgan failure. Good results with transplantation can be achieved if the process has not progressed too far before admission and if aggressive treatment strategies are used.

On first assessment, a careful neurologic examination must be done, and the coma grade should be determined. Patients in grade IV coma (unresponsive) benefit from constant monitoring of intracranial pressure (ICP). An ICP monitor may be placed in the subdural space in the operating room. An epidural location is chosen if bleeding is excessive. An attempt is made to keep cerebral perfusion pressure (mean arterial blood pressure minus ICP) above 60 mm Hg. A low mean arterial blood pressure is treated with pressors, and elevation of ICP is treated with hyperventilation and mannitol. Severe elevations of ICP may result in brain death. Hemodynamic stability is maintained by monitoring intravascular volume. Expansion of the intravascular volume may be limited by considerations about ICP, in which case temporary inotropic support is required. Acute renal failure is managed with continuous arteriovenous hemofiltration with or without dialysis, which may be continued during surgery. Because the acutely failing liver produces an acutely failing reticuloendothelial system, florid sepsis often ensues, and broad-spectrum antibiotics are required. Pulmonary insufficiency is a common accompaniment of liver failure and is managed with intubation, high concentration of inspired oxygen, and, if necessary, positive end-expiratory pressure.

Elective Transplantation

Under elective conditions, the potential candidate for hepatic transplantation is usually presented to a multidisciplinary committee for evaluation. Assuming an acceptable indication and no contraindications, attention is directed to the patient's psychological profile and family support resources. These factors are of immense importance because the transplantation process requires a lifelong commitment to a complex medical regimen that involves daily immunosuppression and follow-up care. A history of substance abuse requires careful evaluation by specialists. Demonstrated noncompliance with other types of medical therapy, lack of insight and willingness to confront the issue of substance abuse, and lack of a satisfactory support structure are factors that may make transplantation a poor choice for a patient.

After a decision for hepatic transplantation is made, it is common to wait for several months for a suitable donor organ to become available. During this interval, surveillance of the patient is required so that rapid deterioration is recognized and treated. Encephalopathy is treated with lactulose and protein restriction, variceal hemorrhage with sclerotherapy or TIPS, and refractory ascites with large-volume paracentesis or TIPS. Spontaneous bacterial peritonitis requires hospital admission and antibiotic therapy. For patients awaiting transplantation with a history of substance abuse, any documented relapse warrants removal from the waiting list.

HEPATIC TRANSPLANTATION PROCEDURE

Anesthetic Management

Because most patients report for hepatic transplantation procedures without an opportunity for extensive preoperative preparation, induction of anesthesia is conducted, assuming that the patient has a full stomach, with rapid-sequence technique and cricoid pressure. After intubation, anesthesia is maintained with a combination of inhalation agent and intravenous infusions of paralytic and analgesic drugs. Patients at high risk for cardiovascular problems are often treated with high-dose narcotic technique. Multiple vascular access lines are then placed for monitoring and administration of blood and blood products. Two 8.5-French cannulae are placed in the central venous system by internal jugular or subclavian puncture for transfusion through a rapid infusion device. A balloon-tipped flow-directed pulmonary artery catheter is also inserted. Two arterial lines are placed, one in the radial artery for continuous arterial blood pressure monitoring and a second in the right femoral artery for periodic blood sampling.

Intraoperative Management of Coagulopathy

Bleeding during hepatic transplantation ranges from trivial to torrential. For the most part, administration of blood and blood products during the procedure is dictated more by the central filling pressures, as indicated by the pulmonary artery diastolic pressure, than by estimated blood loss on the operative field. The latter is notoriously inaccurate, and updated estimates lag behind the patient's needs. Early in the operation, preexisting coagulopathy may dictate the use of fresh frozen plasma, cryoprecipitate, and platelet transfusions, but usually these components are reserved for use later in the procedure.

Evaluating the patient's coagulation status during the transplantation procedure requires frequent determinations of standard parameters, such as prothrombin time, partial thromboplastin time, factor levels, and platelet count, as well as clinical assessment of hemostasis in the operative field.

Starting with the anhepatic phase, when the recipient liver is devascularized, a period of fibrinolysis and coagulation failure occurs. This failure is due to the complete cessation of production of hepatic coagulation proteins and fibrinolysis inhibitors and to the inability of the liver to metabolize profibrinolytic compounds. Replacing coagulation factors with fresh frozen plasma and cryoprecipitate is important during this phase.

After revascularization of the donor liver, surgical bleeding may occur. Once this is controlled, a second period of coagulopathy, also characterized by fibrinolysis, may occur. This second fibrinolytic phase results from products of the ischemia and reperfusion injury sustained by the donor organ. This phase usually develops within 1 or 2 hours after revascularization and may be severe, although spontaneous resolution is the rule rather than the exception. When fibrinolysis is unusually severe or persistent, antifibrinolytic therapy with ε-aminocaproic acid is helpful. A loading dose of 5 g is given intravenously, and further doses of 1 g/h may be given if necessary until the period of fibrinolysis has passed. It is important to discontinue e-aminocaproic acid therapy as soon as possible to avoid the potential complications of intravascular thrombus formation or complete thrombosis of major vessels.

Surgical Technique

Transplantation of the liver is one of the most technically demanding surgical procedures. Conceptually, hepatic transplantation may be thought of as comprising three distinct sequential phases. The first phase involves the preliminary dissection and skeletonization of the recipient's diseased liver. The second phase, known as the *anhepatic phase,* refers to the period starting with devascularization of the recipient's liver and ending with revascularization of the newly implanted organ. The third phase is the period after revascularization that includes biliary reconstruction and abdominal closure.

The following sections describe the surgical technique of hepatic transplantation, emphasizing the potential pitfalls and detailing various strategies for circumventing the many technical challenges during this formidable procedure.

Dissection of Recipient Liver

After the anesthetic preparation, the patient's chest, abdomen, left axilla, and left groin are prepared with a povidone-iodine solution and draped as a single large surgical field. The most commonly used incision is a bilateral subcostal incision with an upper midline extension to the xiphoid process (Fig. 16.48). The incision is carried into

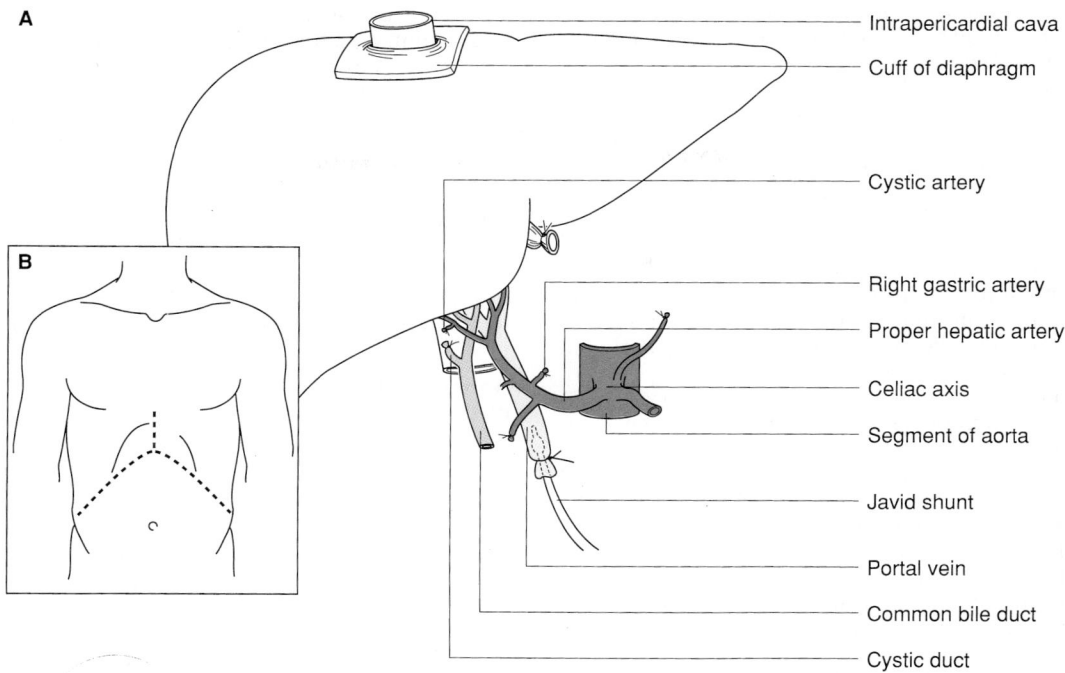

A

B

- Intrapericardial cava
- Cuff of diaphragm
- Cystic artery
- Right gastric artery
- Proper hepatic artery
- Celiac axis
- Segment of aorta
- Javid shunt
- Portal vein
- Common bile duct
- Cystic duct

Figure 16.48. *(A)* The donor liver after excision and before transplantation. *(B)* Bilateral subcostal incision with a subxiphoid extension.

the peritoneal cavity and is held open with a mechanical retractor, providing excellent exposure of the entire upper abdomen.

After inspection of the liver for unforeseen abnormalities, such as an unsuspected hepatoma in a cirrhotic liver, attention is directed to dissecting and skeletonizing the structures of the portal triad. The hepatic artery can be palpated in the anteromedial aspect of the portal triad. Palpation posterior to the common bile duct and lateral to the portal vein reveals the presence of a replaced right hepatic artery. Inspection of the pars flaccida of the lesser omentum along the lesser curvature of the stomach demonstrates a replaced left hepatic artery arising from

the left gastric artery (Fig. 16.49). The proper hepatic artery is freed from the gastroduodenal artery to its bifurcation into the left and right hepatic arterial branches. Because most of the hepatic blood flow in patients with cirrhosis is from the hepatic artery, early division of the hepatic artery can decrease bleeding from the liver during the dissection, but this maneuver may also render the patient functionally anhepatic from that point forward.

The common bile duct is identified and the cystic duct and proximal common hepatic duct are divided. Frequently, collateral venous channels are present running along the course of the bile duct. Care must be exercised during dissection in this area, or significant hemorrhage

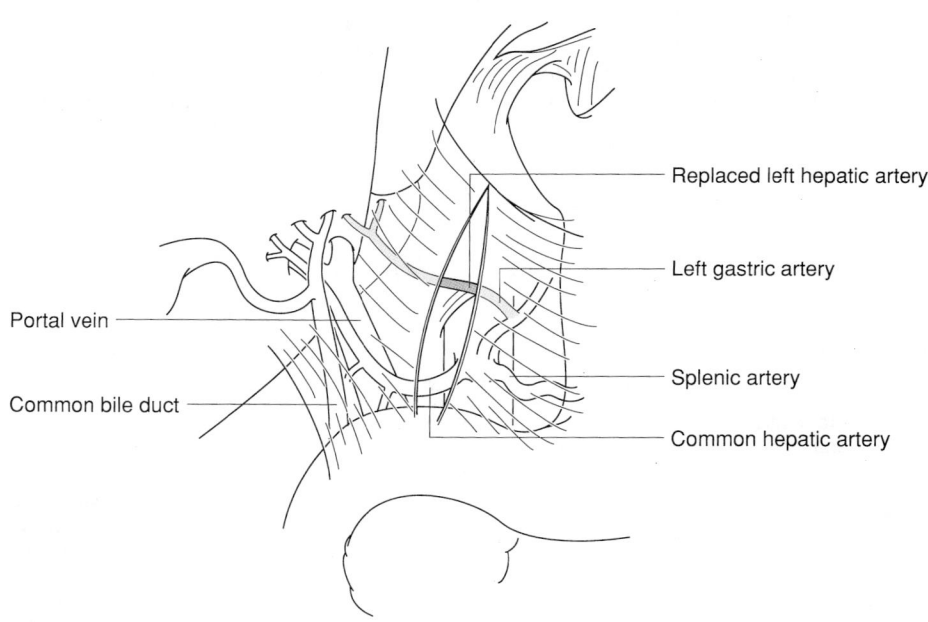

- Replaced left hepatic artery
- Left gastric artery
- Splenic artery
- Common hepatic artery

Portal vein

Common bile duct

Figure 16.49. A replaced left hepatic artery usually arises as a branch of the left gastric artery, traversing the pars flaccida of the lesser omentum from left to right toward the left lobe of the liver.

may occur. In addition, the major blood supply to the distal recipient common bile duct comes from branches of the hepatic artery, so extensive skeletonization of the distal duct should be avoided.

Once the bile duct and the hepatic artery are freed from surrounding tissues, the portal vein can be easily approached from its anterior, medial, and lateral aspects. Anterior branches are rarely found in the portal vein, even in the presence of severe portal hypertension. Thus, dissection is commenced anteriorly between the bile duct and the hepatic artery. The portal vein should be freed over most of its length to the bifurcation in the hepatic hilum. Dissection to the confluence of the superior mesenteric and splenic veins may be necessary if the main portal vein is thrombosed and cannot be disobliterated.

Conventional orthotopic liver transplantation as originally developed included resection of the recipient's intrahepatic vena cava with the diseased liver. This requires occlusion of the inferior vena cava as well as the portal vein for the entire anhepatic period, which can generate significant hemodynamic instability because of decreased venous return, as well as potential difficulties with splanchnic congestion and postoperative renal dysfunction. Venovenous bypass was developed to help restore venous return during this period and was used routinely by many centers. More recently, improvements in anesthetic management and surgical technique have led to the selective use of venovenous bypass only in patients who demonstrate hemodynamic instability after a trial of clamping (6). Alternatively, many are moving to the "piggyback" technique described later, in which the recipient's vena cava is left intact (7). With this technique, the vena cava can either be clamped for a short time, or commonly not at all, and venovenous bypass is rarely necessary.

If the transplantation is to be performed in the conventional manner, the infrahepatic inferior vena cava is mobilized in the retroperitoneum. Large collateral veins may be encountered, and care must be exercised to prevent injury to the renal veins as they enter the vena cava. An avascular plane usually is present behind the vena cava in the segment between the renal veins and the right adrenal vein where it enters the retrohepatic vena cava. Patients with cirrhosis, and especially those with Budd-Chiari syndrome, may have a greatly enlarged caudate lobe, increasing the difficulty of surrounding the vena cava below the liver. Individual hepatic veins draining the caudate lobe may need to be divided to increase the length of infrahepatic vena cava. The remaining ligamentous attachments of the liver are then divided. The falciform and left triangular ligaments are divided. The coronary ligaments and

bare area of the liver are dissected, with care taken to avoid injury to the phrenic or hepatic veins, eventually freeing the suprahepatic inferior vena cava where it traverses the diaphragm. During mobilization of the bare area, the right lobe of the liver is displaced medially to expose, ligate, and divide the right adrenal vein as it enters the retrohepatic vena cava. In some cases, most commonly with Budd-Chiari syndrome, the bare area of the liver and the area around the suprahepatic vena cava may be so densely fibrotic and filled with collaterals that safe dissection is impossible. Transdiaphragmatic exposure of the intrapericardial portion of the inferior vena cava is recommended under these circumstances (Fig. 16.50).

Anhepatic Phase and Implantation of the Donor Liver

At this stage, the liver has been skeletonized sufficiently to permit its rapid removal, and consideration is given to the potential need for venovenous bypass. Proponents of venovenous bypass argue that maintenance of venous return from the kidneys and lower extremities during the anhepatic phase results in a smoother hemodynamic course for most patients, allowing time for a more deliberate approach to hemostasis of the right upper quadrant after recipient hepatectomy and before implantation of the hepatic allograft.

If venovenous bypass is to be used, it is accomplished from the portal vein and inferior vena cava (Fig. 16.51). Cannulae are placed percutaneously in the femoral and internal jugular veins and advanced into the inferior and superior vena cava, respectively. Inferior vena caval blood is delivered to the superior vena cava by a centrifugal pump. The cannulae, tubing, and centrifugal pump head undergo a heparin-bonding process to reduce the chances of thrombus formation and subsequent embolism. Once venovenous bypass has been established, the recipient hepatectomy is completed. After division of the left and right hepatic arteries, the portal vein is divided, and the splanchnic side of the portal vein is added to the venovenous bypass circuit using a Y-connector. This results in total bypass flow rates of 2 to 3 L/min.

The recipient hepatectomy is continued by dividing the infrahepatic inferior vena cava between vascular clamps. Hepatectomy is completed by placing a sturdy clamp on the suprahepatic inferior vena cava as it passes through the diaphragm and excising the diseased liver. The hepatic veins are divided within the substance of the liver to allow the creation of a large suprahepatic cuff comprising the left, middle, and right hepatic veins (Fig. 16.52).

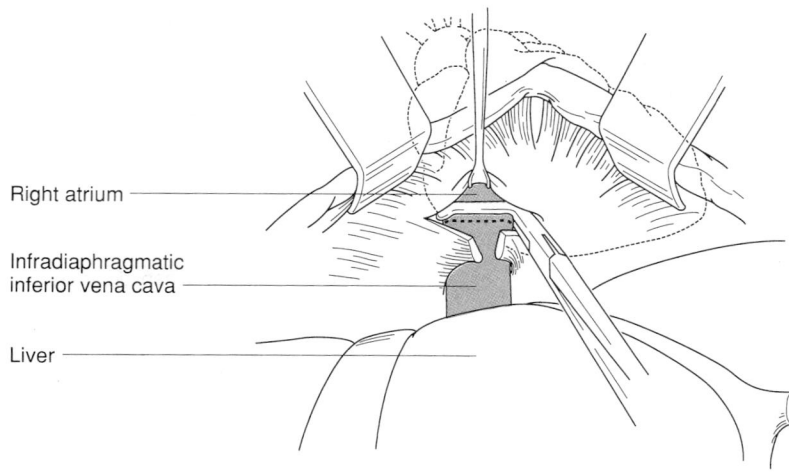

Right atrium

Infradiaphragmatic inferior vena cava

Liver

Figure 16.50. If the suprahepatic vena cava cannot be safely dissected, the intrapericardial segment of the inferior vena cava can be easily exposed by incising the diaphragm. A clamp is placed at the junction between the right atrium and inferior vena cava.

When the piggyback technique is used, the retroperitoneal vena cava is not fully mobilized. The native liver is dissected off the vena cava by ligating the small retrohepatic venous branches draining directly into the vena cava up to the level of the hepatic veins (Fig. 16.53). The hepatic veins may then be clamped at the junction of the hepatic veins and the vena cava, leaving venous return from the lower body intact.

After removal of the recipient liver, the right upper quadrant is carefully inspected, and hemostasis is obtained. Complete hemostasis in the bare area is essential because this region is relatively inaccessible once the donor liver is implanted. Reperitonealization of the bare area can be accomplished using the posterior peritoneum, and it tamponades venous oozing that may occur after transplantation.

The donor liver is brought to the operative field. Bench preparation performed previously includes removal of the gallbladder as well as meticulous ligation of tributaries of the vena cava (right adrenal and phrenic veins), portal vein, and hepatic artery. A Carrel patch of donor aorta is used for the arterial anastomotic site (Fig. 16.54). The vascular anastomoses are carried out using monofilament polypropylene suture. The suprahepatic vena caval anastomosis is performed first by suturing the posterior wall from within the lumen using an imbricating technique (Fig. 16.52). The anterior aspect of the anastomosis is then completed. The infrahepatic vena caval anastomosis is performed next, but the completion of the anastomosis is left until the time of hepatic revascularization to provide a vent for air, for acidotic, hyperkalemic blood, and for residual preservation solution.

With the piggyback technique, the recipient's hepatic veins are divided and fashioned into a common orifice. The donor suprahepatic vena cava is sewn to this hepatic vein orifice. With the piggyback technique, the infrahepatic vena cava of the donor is oversewn or stapled, eliminating one anastomosis (Fig. 16.55).

The arterial anastomosis is completed using a branch-patch technique (Fig. 16.54). In cases were the recipient's arterial inflow is inadequate, a segment of donor iliac vessels can be anastomosed to the supraceliac or infrarenal aorta and used as a conduit to the donor arterial patch. The portal limb of the venovenous bypass circuit is then removed, and the portal venous anastomosis is completed end to end. If portal bypass is not used, many favor performing the portal anastomosis before arterial reconstruction and reperfusing the graft on the portal vein alone to minimize splanchnic congestion. In recipients in whom the portal vein cannot be successfully used, a jump graft of donor iliac vein can be used between the recipient's superior mesenteric vein, or other large portal venous tributary, and the donor portal vein.

During the anastomoses of the venae cavae and the hepatic artery, the donor liver is perfused with saline solution at 4°C by a cannula in the donor portal vein to wash out the preservation solution and keep the organ at a cryoprotective temperature. At the time of revascularization, inflow is restored to the liver through the portal vein. The first 200 to 300 mL of blood is vented through the infrahepatic vena cava. The final suture is then tied, and the suprahepatic caval clamp is removed. Finally, hepatic arterial flow is restored and revascularization is complete.

Postrevascularization Phase and Biliary Reconstruction

After revascularization, the donor liver usually assumes a normal color and consistency within minutes. Identify-

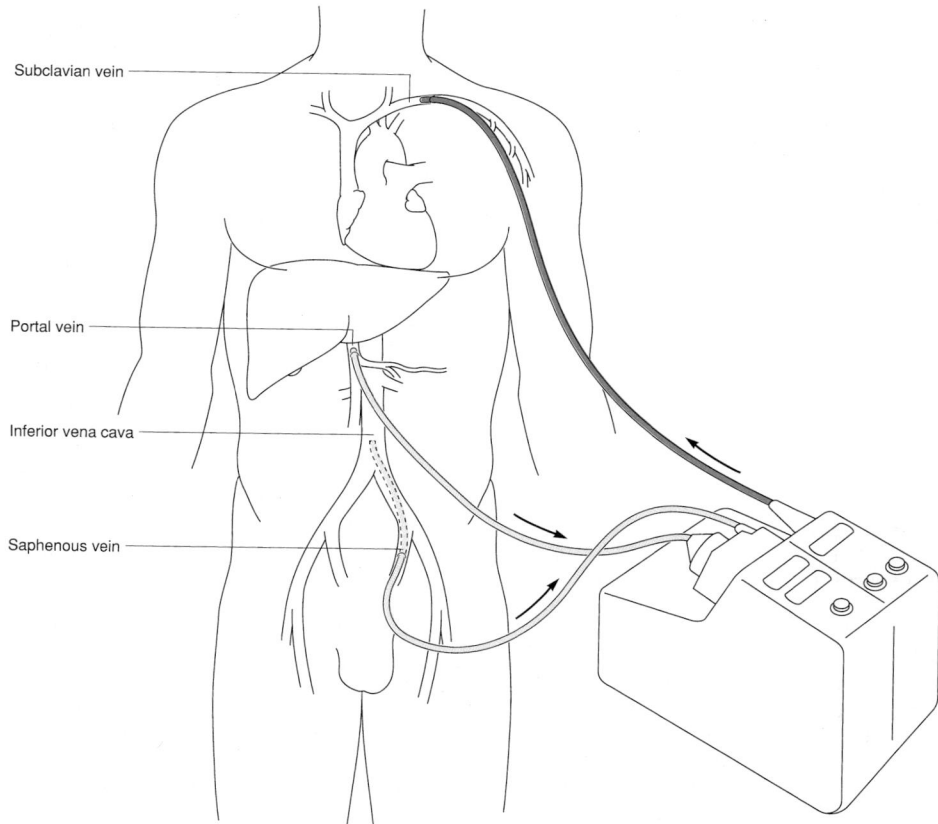

Figure 16.51. Set-up for venovenous bypass during hepatic transplantation. Cannulae are placed into the portal vein to decompress the splanchnic bed and inferior vena cava (through the greater saphenous vein) to decompress the lower extremities and kidneys during the anhepatic phase of the transplantation. A centrifugal pump is used to deliver bypassed blood to the central circulation by means of a cannula passed into the axillary vein.

Subclavian vein

Portal vein

Inferior vena cava

Saphenous vein

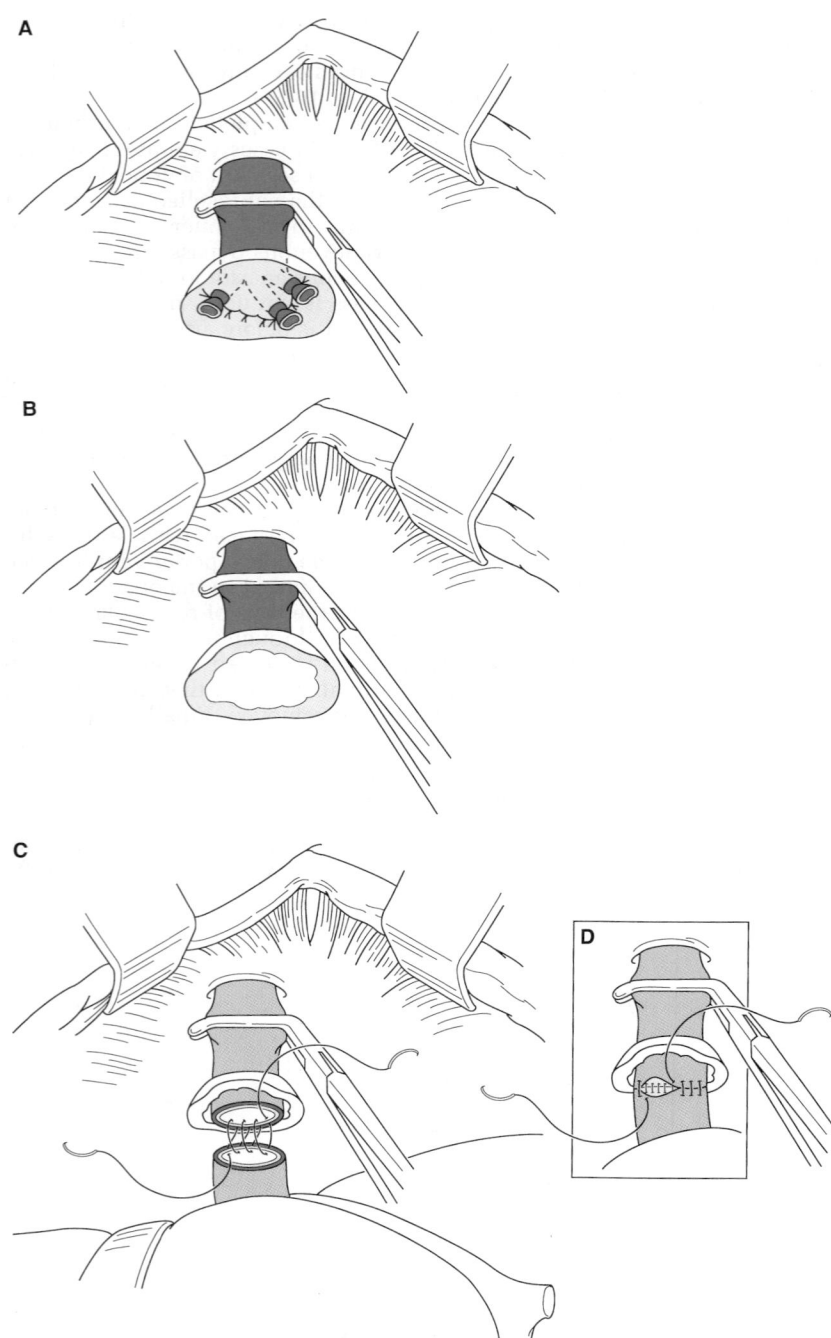

Figure 16.52. *(A)* The diseased recipient liver is removed by incising the liver below the level of the hepatic veins. *(B)* The hepatic veins are then opened to form a large suprahepatic cuff for anastomosis. The suprahepatic vena caval anastomosis: *(C)* posterior suture line; *(D)* anterior suture line.

ing and controlling surgical bleeding entails a meticulous examination of each of the vascular anastomoses as well as a search for unligated branches of the major vessels.

Biliary reconstruction can use any of several options. The most common biliary anastomosis is a choledochocholedochostomy which is a direct end-to-end anastomosis of donor and recipient bile ducts. This anastomosis is carried out using interrupted absorbable monofilament suture. The anastomosis may be stented with a T-tube that exits through the recipient common bile duct or with a smaller straight tube introduced through the donor cystic duct and advanced across the anastomosis (Fig. 16.56), although many centers do not routinely stent the biliary

anastomosis. Patients with a diseased biliary tract, such as those with biliary atresia, primary sclerosing cholangitis, or a recipient duct of inadequate size or quality, require reconstruction with a choledochoenteric anastomosis. Most commonly, a standard Roux-en-Y choledochojejunostomy is carried out and, if possible, a retrocolic loop is used. Under ordinary circumstances, bile is produced immediately (Fig. 16.57).

Abdominal closure is accomplished with nonabsorbable fascial suture in these immunosuppressed patients to reduce the likelihood of dehiscence. Closed-suction peritoneal drains are used only if a bilioenteric anastomosis was performed (Fig. 16.58).

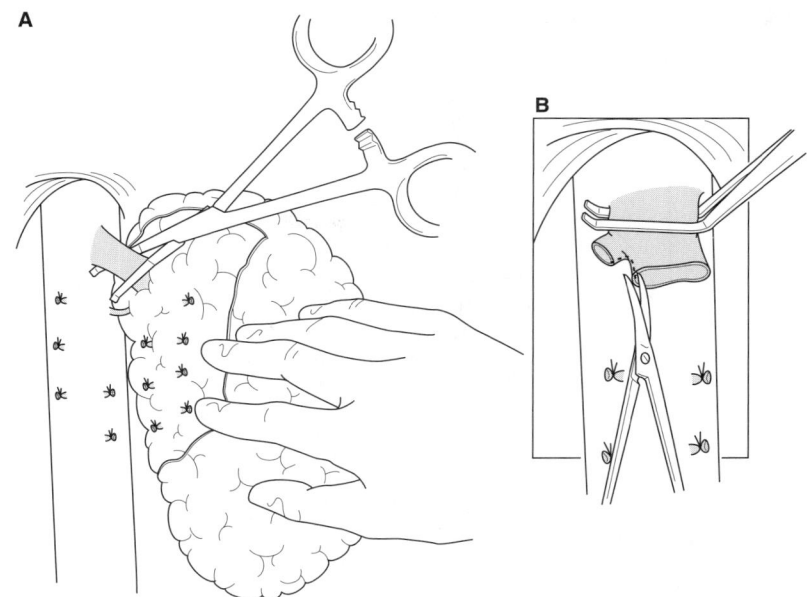

Figure 16.53. *(A)* Recipient liver is dissected off native inferior vena cava by dividing veins draining directly into the inferior vena cava up to the level of the hepatic veins. *(B)* Clamp placed on recipient hepatic veins in preparation of excision of the recipient's native liver.

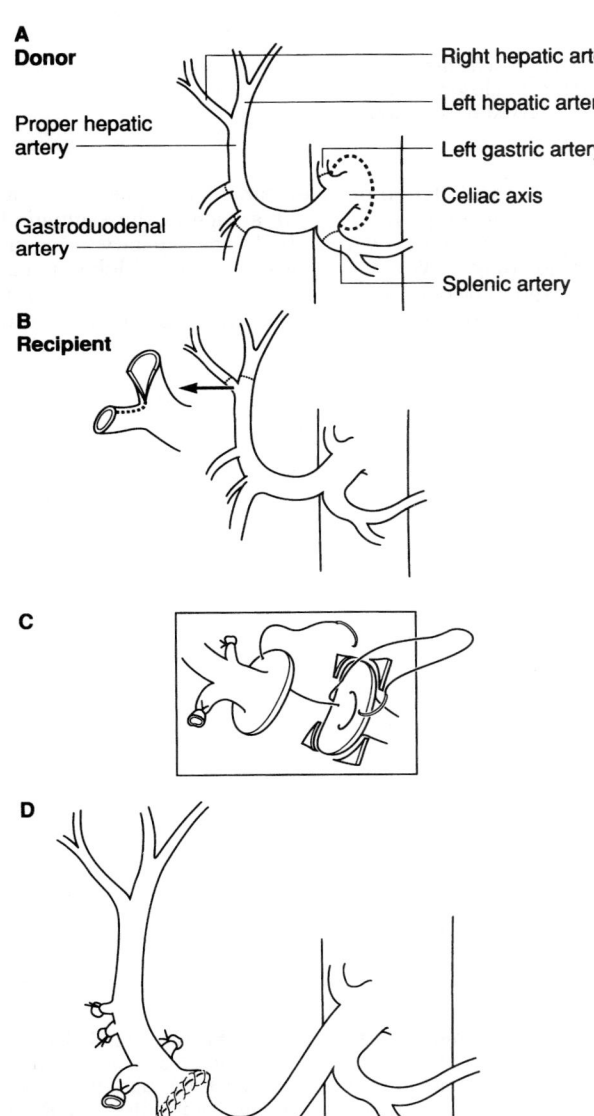

A
Donor

Proper hepatic artery

Gastroduodenal artery

Right hepatic artery

Left hepatic artery

Left gastric artery

Celiac axis

Splenic artery

B
Recipient

C

D

Figure 16.54. *(A)* The donor hepatic artery is procured with a Carrel patch of aorta. *(B)* The recipient hepatic artery bifurcation is used to fashion a branch patch for a larger anastomosis. *(C)* The anastomosis is carried out using continuous monofilament suture material. *(D)* The completed anastomosis.

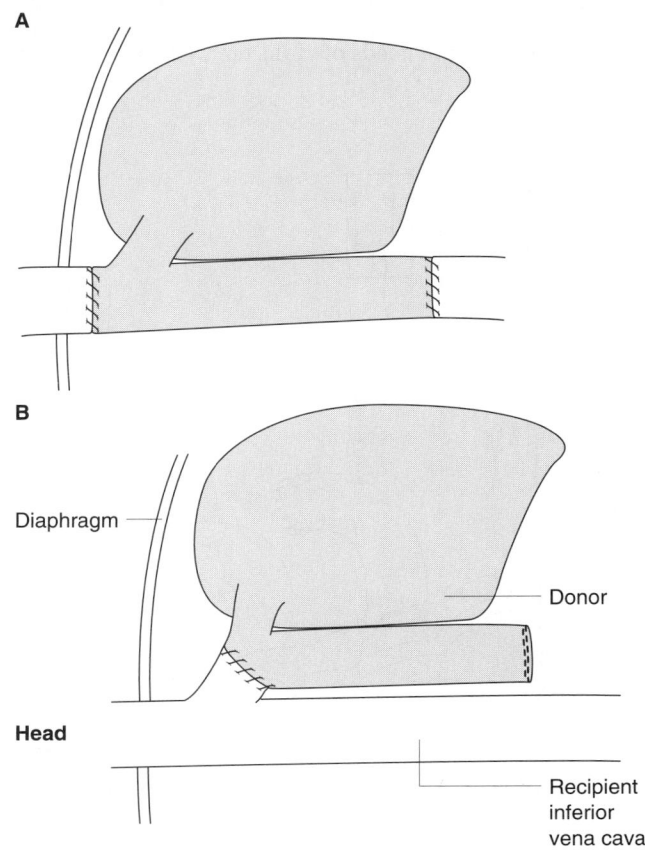

A

B

Diaphragm

Donor

Head

Recipient inferior vena cava

Figure 16.55. Lateral view after completion of caval anastomosis. *(A)* Conventional technique. *(B)* Piggyback technique.

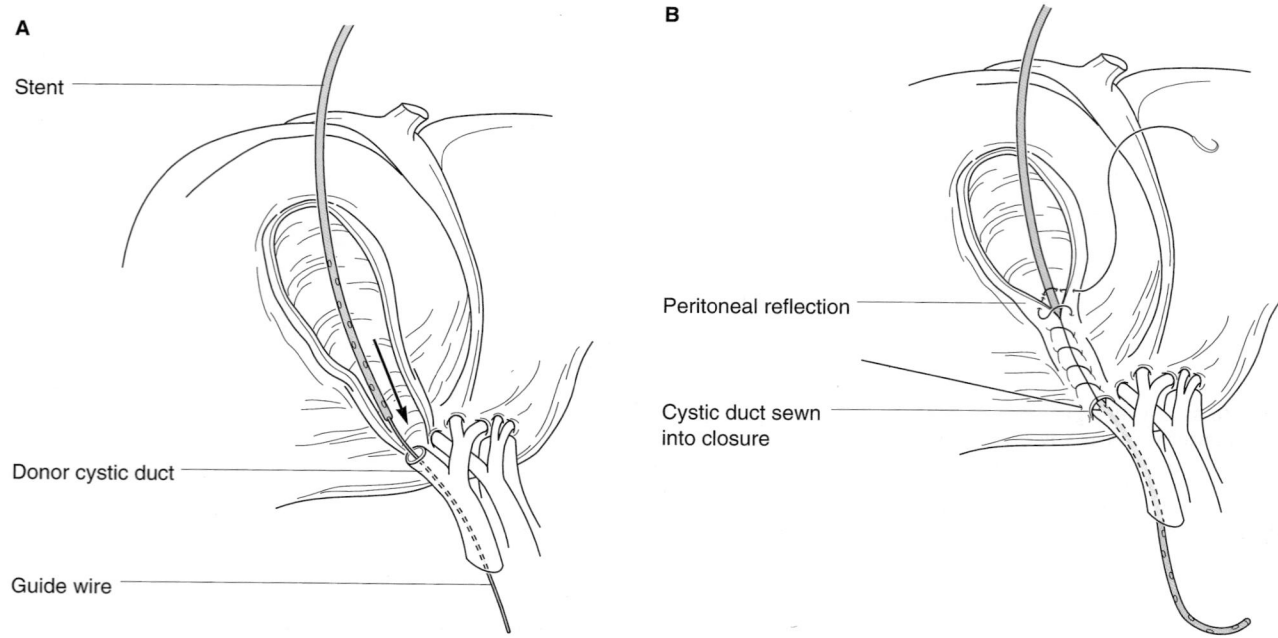

Figure 16.56. Catheter in biliary tree of liver transplant. *(A)* The catheter is passed through the donor cystic duct into the common bile duct. *(B)* The peritoneal reflection is closed over the catheter. The catheter is brought out through the anterior abdominal wall and fixed to the skin.

Techniques for Reduced-size and Split-liver Transplantation

Early in the development of liver transplantation, it was apparent that the number of suitably sized donors was inadequate to meet the needs of children awaiting transplantation. As a result, techniques for transplanting less than the entire liver developed, taking advantage of the segmental anatomy of the liver as well as the liver's capacity to regenerate (Fig. 16.59). With this approach, a single lobe or segment of the liver may be used from a donor who has a body weight up to 10 times greater than the recipient. Careful

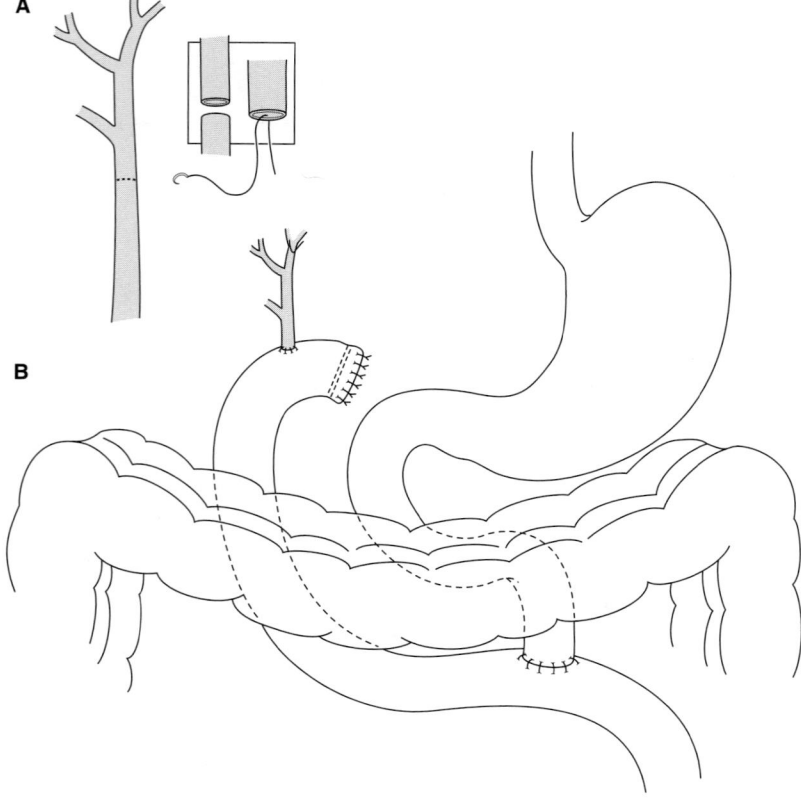

Figure 16.57. *(A)* In most cases, a choledochocholedochostomy is performed over a small drainage tube introduced through the donor cystic duct. *(B)* Patients with a diseased or unsuitable common bile duct require biliary reconstruction with a Roux-en-Y choledochoenterostomy.

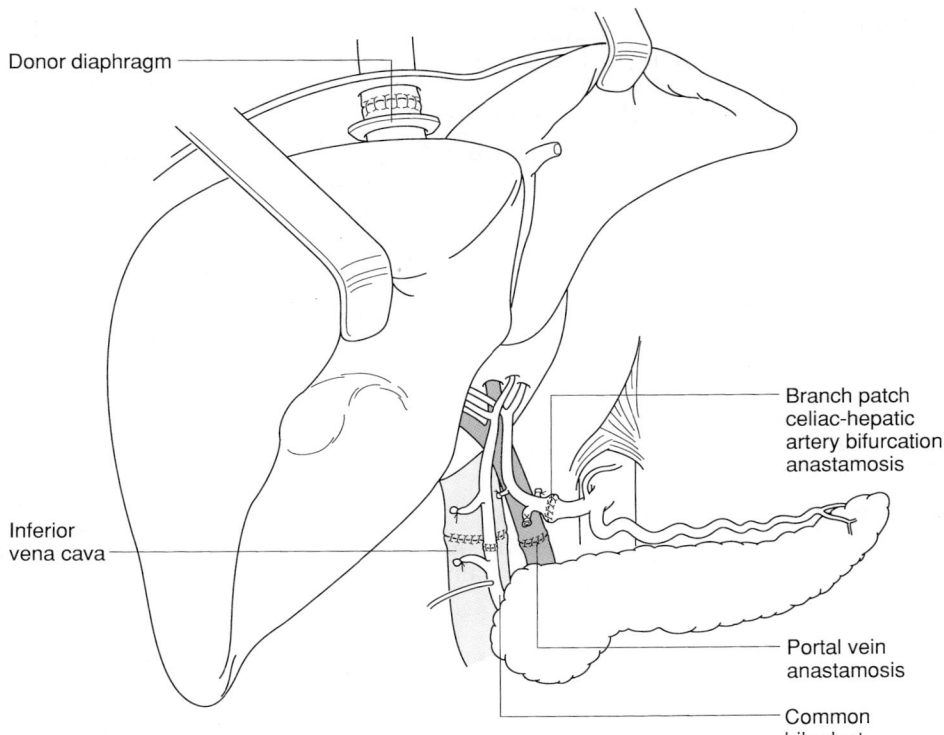

Figure 16.58. The completed hepatic transplantation procedure, showing the liver in the normal orthotopic position and all anastomoses completed.

comparison of donor and recipient dictates the segment or lobe that is chosen so that an adequate mass of liver parenchyma is provided. Typically, donors weighing more than 5 but less than 10 times the recipient could provide a left lateral segment (segments II and III) graft, and donors who were more than 3 but less than 6 times the recipient's weight could provide a left lobe (segments II, III, and IV) graft. Originally, the use of reduced-size segmental grafts in children was performed as a "cutdown" because the unused portion of the liver was discarded.

Although reduced-size liver transplantation permitted livers from adult donors to be used in small children, it did not increase the total number of livers available. A more rational approach is to split the cadaveric liver, whereby the left lateral segment can be used for a child and the remaining liver used for an adult recipient. Unfortunately, analysis of the initial experience with this approach revealed that the outcomes for recipients of split-liver grafts were inferior to those seen in recipients of full-size grafts, and split-liver transplantation fell into relative disfavor. More recently, advances in living donor liver transplantation, discussed later, combined with better donor and recipient selection, have helped resuscitate interest in cadaveric split-liver transplantation, with success rates comparable with those of conventional cadaveric transplantation (8).

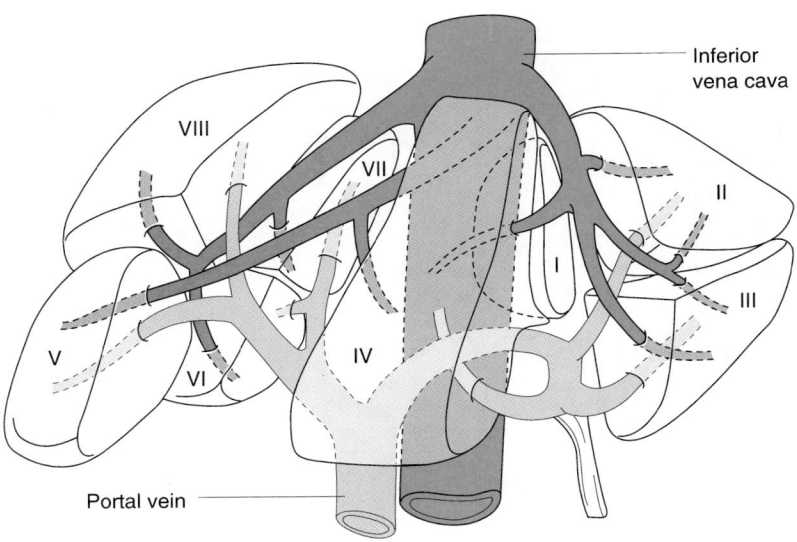

Figure 16.59. Segmental anatomy of the liver as based on Couinaud's nomenclature.

Most of the differences between standard orthotopic hepatic transplantation and segmental transplantation relate to the preparation of the donor organ. In situ splitting of the cadaveric liver can be performed ex vivo, although most groups favor in situ splitting of the cadaveric liver in the same manner as used in procurement of the left lateral segment in living donor procurement. The hepatic parenchyma is divided along anatomic planes, and vascular and biliary structures along the cut surface are meticulously ligated. Biologic glues are not necessary if this step is assiduously completed. In the case of a left lateral segment graft, the recipient retrohepatic vena cava is left in place, and the left hepatic vein of the segmental graft is anastomosed to a cuff fashioned from the recipient's hepatic veins (Fig. 16.60B). Orientation of the graft lobe or segment is important to avoid torsion of the graft and obstruction of venous outflow. Right-lobe grafts can be placed in the usual anatomic position.

Living Donor Liver Transplantation

Despite aggressive application of cadaveric split-liver transplantation and the progressive liberalization of cadaveric donor criteria, including the use of non-heart-beating donors, organ donor shortage is still a significant limitation. As the disciplines of liver surgery and liver transplantation have matured, careful consideration has been given to the possibility that a healthy living donor could donate segments of liver to a potential recipient. Fueled by the success in reduced-size grafts in children and by growing experience in hepatic resections, adult-to-pediatric living liver transplantation using the left lateral segment was pioneered early in the 1990s (9) (Fig. 16.60). This procedure is now routinely performed at many pediatric transplantation programs with an acceptable risk to the donor and graft and recipient survival rates comparable with results for cadaveric liver transplantation.

Living donor liver transplantation has many potential advantages. Preservation time is minimal and primary nonfunction appears rare. Furthermore, the procedure may be performed on an elective basis before severe decompensation of the recipient occurs. Unfortunately, the size of the left lateral segment in the average adult is such that donation of this segment is not an option in children larger than 15 kg. The donor operation appears to have a

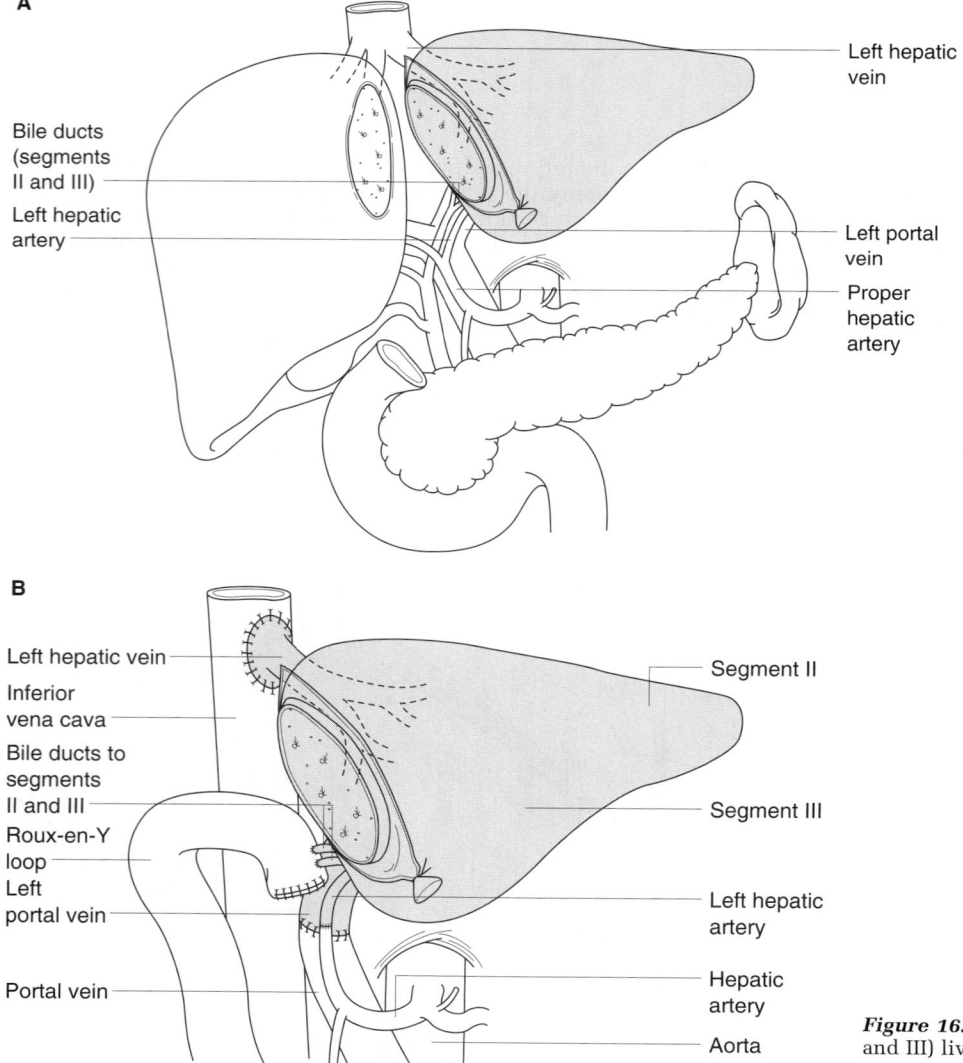

A

Left hepatic vein

Bile ducts (segments II and III)

Left hepatic artery

Left portal vein

Proper hepatic artery

B

Left hepatic vein

Inferior vena cava

Bile ducts to segments II and III

Roux-en-Y loop

Left portal vein

Portal vein

Segment II

Segment III

Left hepatic artery

Hepatic artery

Aorta

Figure 16.60. Left lateral segment (segments II and III) living donor transplantation. *(A)* Donor operation. *(B)* Recipient operation completed.

low and acceptable risk of complications, but donor deaths have been reported.

As experience with adult-to-pediatric living donor liver transplantation has developed, several centers are pursuing adult-to-adult living donor liver transplantation. Because of the size of the average adult recipient, a significant volume of liver must be donated. Both right and left lobes have been donated, but most centers are focusing on right lobe donation for adult recipients (Fig. 16.61).

For any potential living liver donor candidate, the evaluation begins with a thorough medical and psychosocial evaluation. As in living kidney donation, a complete discussion of the risks and benefits to the donor is especially vital because the risks of the donor surgery are not insignificant. A preoperative volumetric assessment of the portion of liver to be donated is performed with computed tomography or magnetic resonance imaging. An estimation of graft size is calculated, with a graft-to-recipient body weight ratio of at least 1% appearing to be a safe minimum. The arterial anatomy is determined before surgery by angiography. A liver biopsy is obtained to rule out occult steatosis, which may affect graft quality. An intraoperative cholangiogram is performed and ultrasound is used to help guide the plane of transection.

The results for both adult-to-pediatric and adult-to-adult living donor liver transplantation have been compa-rable with those observed for recipients of cadaveric transplants. Significant efforts are underway to understand more fully the physiology associated with this undertaking. Small-for-size grafts appear prone to poor function initially, potentially representing inadequate hepatic mass or reflecting an injury caused by portal hyperperfusion. Ensuring adequate venous drainage of the graft to avoid congestion appears vital. Evidence suggests donor liver regeneration to baseline volume is nearly complete in 3 weeks and strategies to promote this process might help provide more graft volume to the recipient in a shorter time.

Living donor liver transplantation has the potential significantly to increase the donor pool, although it is becoming apparent that many recipients will not have a potential donor and many donors will be excluded for medical or psychosocial reasons. Application of this treatment modality must continually ensure that donor safety is paramount.

Auxiliary Liver Transplantation

Under some circumstances, there is a good rationale for placing the donor allograft in a heterotopic rather than orthotopic position, leaving the diseased liver in place. This procedure is referred to as an *auxiliary liver transplantation*. It is used occasionally for cases in which transplantation is indicated for enzymatic defi-

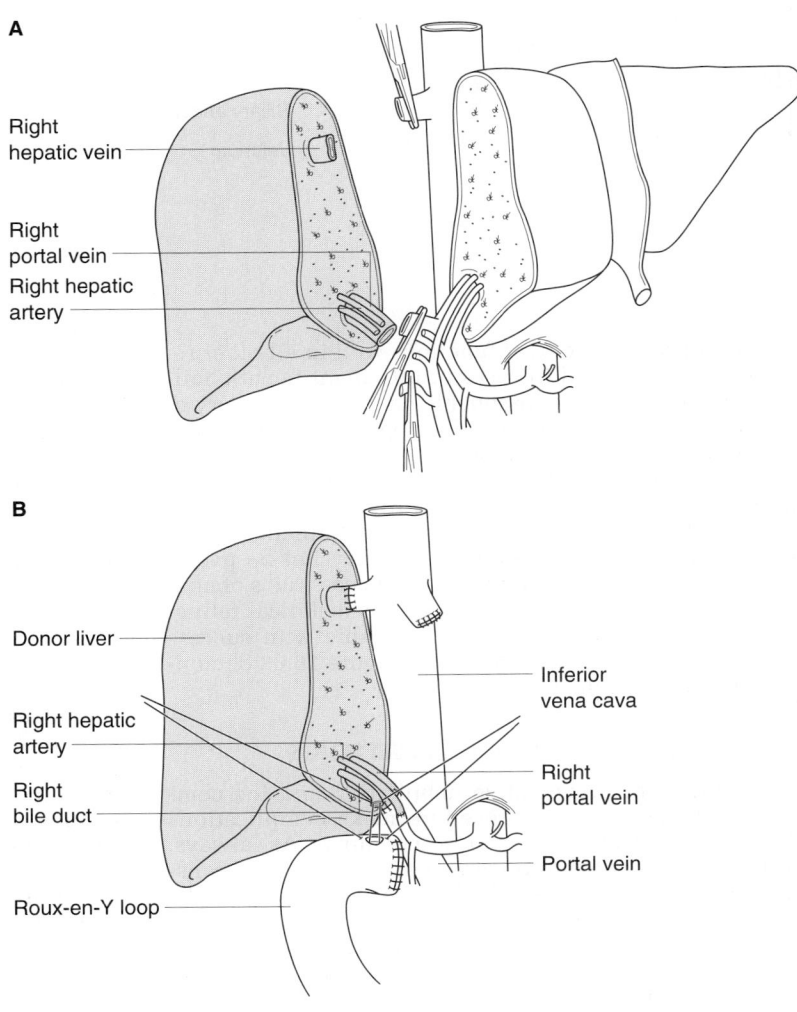

A

Right hepatic vein

Right portal vein

Right hepatic artery

B

Donor liver

Right hepatic artery

Right bile duct

Roux-en-Y loop

Inferior vena cava

Right portal vein

Portal vein

Figure 16.61. Right lobe (segments V to VIII) living donor transplantation. *(A)* Donor operation. *(B)* Recipient operation completed.

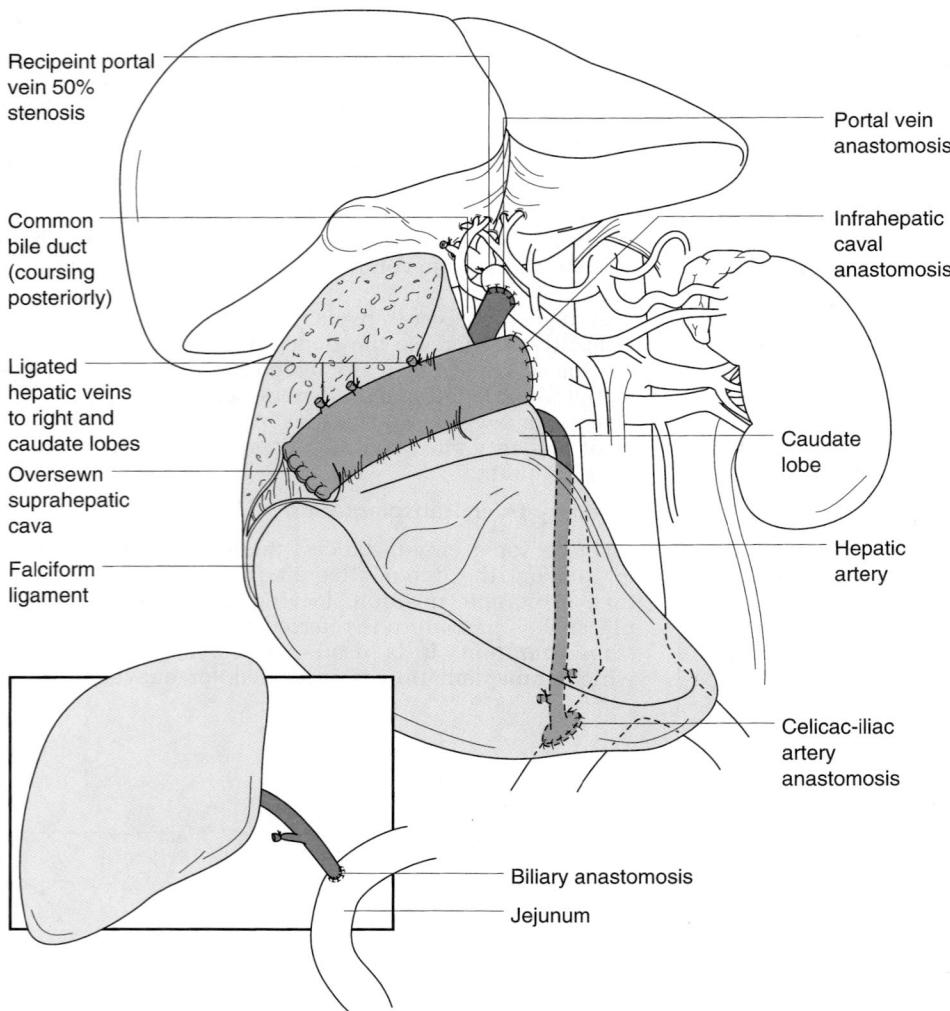

Recipeint portal vein 50% stenosis

Common bile duct (coursing posteriorly)

Ligated hepatic veins to right and caudate lobes

Oversewn suprahepatic cava

Falciform ligament

Portal vein anastomosis

Infrahepatic caval anastomosis

Caudate lobe

Hepatic artery

Celicac-iliac artery anastomosis

Biliary anastomosis

Jejunum

Figure 16.62. Heterotopic auxiliary liver transplantation using a reduced-size allograft.

ciency, but the native liver functions well in all other respects. It is also used in cases of fulminant hepatic failure in which there is a reasonable chance for recovery of the native liver. The major advantages of the auxiliary procedure is that it is a procedure of lesser magnitude than the orthotopic procedure. For patients with enzymatic deficiencies, loss of the graft does not usually result in patient death, and in cases of fulminant hepatic failure, lifelong immunosuppression may not be necessary if native liver function returns. Success rates of auxiliary transplantation have improved as technical refinements have occurred and are comparable with success rates for orthotopic transplantation. Figure 16.62 demonstrates one technique used.

POSTOPERATIVE COMPLICATIONS

The degree of preoperative debilitation and the complexity of the operative procedure make complications after hepatic transplantation a certainty. As always, prompt recognition and treatment are essential. In transplantation, however, the additional burden of early, heavy immunosuppression predisposes to problems not usually encountered in other areas of surgery. Complications associated with immunosuppression, which are predominantly infectious, were detailed earlier. In the following sections, some of the major surgical complica-

tions that occur after hepatic transplantation are described.

Primary Nonfunction

For reasons that are poorly understood, approximately 5% to 10% of transplanted livers function so poorly in the immediate postoperative period that death is likely in the absence of retransplantation. This is referred to as *primary nonfunction* of the allograft. Clearly, most cases of nonfunction are related to inadequate tissue preservation in ice storage or to occult organ dysfunction in the donor, but a sizable percentage of cases may arise from immunologic mechanisms, probably humoral. In the worst cases, the patient does not regain consciousness, a coagulopathy ensues, and multiple organ failure develops. Typically, liver enzyme studies show hepatocellular injury, with aspartate aminotransferase and alanine aminotransferase determinations in the 5,000 to 10,000 IU/dl range, and little bile production. In these cases, urgent retransplantation is required. Because of the tenuous condition of the recipient under these circumstances, however, the morbidity rate is high, usually approximately 50%. Even when the patient survives retransplantation, neurologic injury is common. When the removed hepatic transplant is examined, major arterial and venous blood vessels are patent; histologically, there is complete disruption of the normal lobular architecture, with obliteration of sinusoids by red blood cells, fibrin, and neutrophils. The clinical definition of primary nonfunction of hepatic allografts follows:

Essential Characteristics

Occurrence within 96 hours after the operation
Patent portal vein and hepatic artery

Three of Four Characteristics Required

Bile output <20 mL in 12 hours
Bilirubin level >10 or rising ≥5 mg/d
Prothrombin time/partial thromboplastin time ratio ≥1.5
Factors V and VIII <25% of normal

Early Allograft Dysfunction

In an additional 20% of liver transplant recipients, an entity referred to as *early allograft dysfunction* (EAD) develops (10). EAD is defined as the occurrence of any one of the following between days 2 and 7 posttransplantation: serum bilirubin greater than 10 ng/dL, prothrombin time 17 seconds or more, and hepatic encephalopathy. This syndrome is the result of ischemic injury to the liver sustained before or during the harvesting procedure, as the result of storage for various periods in ice, or damage at the time of transplantation itself. In this regard, EAD is analogous to the development of acute tubular necrosis after renal transplantation.

Patients with EAD experience worse overall survival rates than those without EAD. The 3-year patient survival rate for patients with EAD was 68%, whereas in the absence of EAD, the survival rate at the same interval was 83%. Likewise, the cost of transplantation is significantly higher for patients with EAD.

A number of factors have been identified that are associated with EAD: donor age (>50 years), duration of graft storage in ice, length of donor hospital stay, elevations in recipient prothrombin time and total bilirubin, and UNOS status (degree of urgency of transplantation). Graft steatosis (when percentage of donor hepatocytes with macroscopic fat globules exceeds 40%) is also an important variable predicting both primary nonfunction and EAD.

Biliary Leak or Obstruction

Biliary leak or obstruction is a common surgical complication encountered after hepatic transplantation, accounting for approximately 20% of postoperative surgical problems (11).

Biliary obstruction presents as an unexplained rise in bilirubin and alkaline phosphatase determinations and is confirmed by T-tube cholangiography or by a percutaneous transhepatic cholangiogram. Early strictures do not cause biliary dilatation and usually are not identified by abdominal ultrasound examinations. The most common site of obstruction is at the level of the choledochocholedochostomy, resulting from ischemia, kinking, or technical factors. Because the blood supply of the terminal portion of the donor bile duct derives solely from the hepatic artery, any stricture of the bile duct should prompt an investigation into the patency of the hepatic artery. Strictures of the biliary tree after hepatic transplantation are first treated by balloon dilation using percutaneous techniques. This is successful in 50% of cases, and if not, operative revision is necessary.

Biliary leakage is a feared complication, with a high (50%) mortality rate (12). Most frequently, leakage develops in the third or fourth postoperative week. The high mortality rate may be the result of concomitant hepatic arterial thrombosis, infection of the leaked bile, or the difficulty of bile duct repair in an area of inflamed

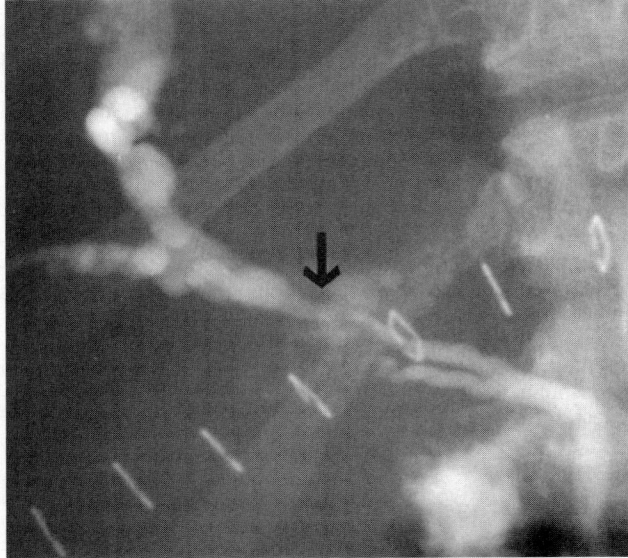

Figure 16.63. Bile leak *(arrow)* from the choledochocholedochostomy after hepatic transplantation.

tissue. Biliary leaks may also occur when an operatively placed T-tube is removed 3 to 6 months after surgery. In these cases, immunosuppression prevents host mechanisms from isolating the T-tube tract with scar tissue. Removal of the T-tube leads to free spill of bile into the peritoneal cavity, an occurrence that is rare in the nontransplantation setting (Fig. 16.63). Late bile leakage from the T-tube site in a transplant recipient is less dangerous than leakage in the immediate postoperative period and is usually treated by hospitalization and intravenous antibiotics, or by placement of a nasobiliary stent inserted retrograde into the common duct by endoscopy. For these reasons, many transplant surgeons avoid using a standard T-tube and place either a smaller-caliber tube through the cystic duct or avoid intubation of the bile duct entirely.

Hemorrhage

Laparotomy to control postoperative bleeding is required in 15% of cases (12). In approximately half of reoperations, a specific bleeding point is identified. The survival rate is higher in these cases, in contrast to those in which diffuse bleeding is encountered, presumably because the latter circumstance is usually associated with poor allograft function and resultant coagulopathy. If significant bleeding occurs after hepatic transplantation, a common and sensible policy is to transfuse the patient until hypothermia and coagulopathy are corrected, with subsequent (1 to 3 days) evacuation of blood from the peritoneal cavity. Evacuation of clot is done to relieve intraabdominal pressure and reduce the chance of intraabdominal infection.

Hepatic Artery Thrombosis

Hepatic artery thrombosis occurs in 5% of adult hepatic transplantation cases and in up to 25% of pediatric cases (13). Technical factors, the flow rate of arterial blood past the anastomosis, and factors causing hypercoagulability all appear to contribute to the overall incidence of this complication.

As in any type of arterial surgery, meticulous technique is essential, and small imperfections may result in catastrophe. The requirement for a complex interposition graft between donor and recipient vessel and the intraoperative revision of the arterial anastomosis are both associated with an increased incidence of thrombosis. In most cases of hepatic artery thrombosis, no obvious technical flaw is detected.

The rate of arterial blood flow in the reconstructed hepatic artery is an important determinant of long-term patency with reduced flow. Children are predisposed to hepatic artery thrombosis because they have smaller vessels and lower mean arterial blood pressure than adults. In pediatric cases, an arterial diameter of less than 3 mm is associated with a doubling in the incidence of hepatic artery thrombosis (14). Rejection is also associated with decreased flow because when it occurs, endothelial cells swell. Hepatic artery thrombosis occurs more commonly in association with rejection.

A postoperative hypercoagulable state associated with hepatic transplantation may predispose to hepatic artery thrombosis. Evidence indicates that relatively poor hepatic production of natural regulatory anticoagulants, such as proteins C and S and antithrombin III, immediately after transplantation promotes coagulation because production of procoagulant factors, such as factor V and VII, occurs more rapidly after revascularization (11). This observation has prompted some centers to administer fresh frozen plasma as a source of antithrombin III and proteins C and S in the postoperative period. Most centers recommend prophylactic aspirin to prevent hepatic artery thrombosis in children. Other factors associated with hepatic artery thrombosis are increased hematocrit, prolonged cold ischemic time, and AB0 incompatibility.

The nature of the clinical problems associated with hepatic artery thrombosis depends on when in the posttransplantation course it occurs. If thrombosis occurs in the early postoperative period, massive hepatocellular necrosis may result. If the diagnosis is made promptly, thrombectomy with or without revision of the arterial anastomosis may obviate the need for repeat transplantation. Late thrombosis (>1 month posttransplantation) may occasionally be asymptomatic, but usually results in recurrent biliary problems such as leak or stenosis. These problems may be treated conservatively, but in most cases retransplantation is required.

Technical factors, size of artery, and coagulation status are not the only variables influencing the development of hepatic artery thrombosis. A twisted or otherwise obstructed hepatic vein outflow produces sluggish flow through the portal vein and hepatic artery and may predispose to thrombosis of either of these vessels. Likewise, preservation injury produces a swollen liver with severe endothelial cell injury, which predisposes to thrombosis. One study suggests that cytomegalovirus (CMV) infection may play a role in arterial thrombosis as well (15). Hepatic artery thrombosis was identified in 12.5% of patients whose donor showed evidence for CMV infection but who themselves had not previously experienced CMV infection, whereas the incidence of thrombosis was 0% in donor–recipient combinations in which neither had experienced CMV infection. The observation is thought to relate to the propensity of CMV to infect endothelial cells and produce a procoagulant effect.

Portal Vein Thrombosis

Postoperative portal vein thrombosis is much less common than hepatic artery thrombosis, occurring in 2% to 3% of cases (13). As for hepatic artery thrombosis, the most important predisposing factors relate to the size of the native portal vein and the rate of blood flow through the native portal vein. The size of the portal vein is influenced by the patient's age and by the presence of previous thrombus, which results in a reduced luminal diameter. Blood flow through the portal vein may be low as a result of the preoperative development of retroperitoneal collaterals from the portal venous system to the renal vein and inferior vena cava. A previous surgically created splenorenal shunt must be disconnected at the time of transplantation because it usually is associated with reduced flow through the portal vein.

Portal vein thrombosis typically presents with marked elevation of enzyme and prothrombin time determinations and progressive liver failure. Occasionally, liver failure does not develop. In this case, the clinical course is one of recurrent variceal hemorrhage, which can be treated by a distal splenorenal shunt.

Vena Caval Thrombosis

Because of the large luminal diameter of the vena cava and its high flow rate, thrombosis of the vena cava rarely occurs after hepatic transplantation and is reported in less than 1% of cases (13).

Intraabdominal Sepsis

Intraabdominal sepsis presents as diffuse peritonitis or localized abscess and occurs in approximately 5% of cases (12). Peritonitis is the result of infection of ascitic fluid, the leakage of infected bile, or leakage of enteric contents into the peritoneum from gastrointestinal perforation. Abscesses develop most commonly in the peritransplant area, but they also develop between loops of small bowel. As would be expected in a frail patient population treated with immunosuppression, the mortality rate from this complication is high (60%). Percutaneous techniques used in association with detailed imaging are useful in making the diagnosis, but are less helpful as treatment. Surgical drainage is usually preferred.

Neurologic Complications

A number of preoperative and postoperative factors predispose to impaired consciousness and seizure activity after transplantation. In one large series, neurologic complications occurred in 30% of patients after liver transplantation (16). Of the neurologic complications encountered, 80% involved altered mental status, whereas 20% involved seizure activity. Preoperative encephalopathy and intraoperative hypotension or anoxia result in cerebral edema, which is worsened by massive resuscitation with administration of intravenous fluids after transplantation. Occasionally, air embolism occurs at the time of revascularization of the transplant, causing neurologic dysfunction. If the patient fails to awaken promptly after transplantation, and particularly if the transplant is functioning well, an urgent computed tomographic scan of the head should be obtained to rule out intracranial hemorrhage and to assess the degree of cerebral edema.

Seizures are common after transplantation and result from any of the factors listed previously as well as from drugs administered, particularly cyclosporine and trimethoprim-sulfamethoxazole. A history of seizures or preoperative encephalopathy greatly predisposes to postoperative seizure activity. Seizures are treated with diazepam and phenytoin and careful monitoring of cyclosporine levels. Rarely, a syndrome similar to progressive multifocal leukoencephalopathy develops, with progressive mental deterioration and death. This is thought to be due in part to the pronounced central nervous system toxicity of cyclosporine (17).

REJECTION AND IMMUNOSUPPRESSION

Rejection can be broadly defined as an immune-mediated host response to graft antigens that leads to allograft damage and may, if not brought under rapid control, cause total destruction of the donor organ. Rejection of the liver allograft is described in several forms: massive hemorrhagic necrosis or acute and chronic rejection. Recognizing rejection in many of its guises, distinguishing it from recurrent hepatic disease, and choosing from an increasing storehouse of ever more potent immunosuppressives is one of the most pressing challenges facing transplantation professionals.

Antibody-mediated Rejection

Hepatic graft injury as a result of massive hemorrhagic necrosis from preexisting host antibodies directed at donor ABO or human leukocyte antigen (HLA) determinants does occur, but in a much less pronounced fashion than in the context of renal transplantation. Large series have documented that overall results of ABO-incompatible donor–recipient transplantations are inferior to ABO-compatible transplantations, with an approximately 20% decrease in 1-year graft survival rates for ABO-incompatible grafts. A substantial percentage of ABO-incompatible grafts function long term, however, and many centers perform ABO-incompatible transplantation in life-threatening situations in which no ABO-compatible donor liver is available (18). It is assumed that the deterioration in graft function relates to isoantibody recognition of foreign ABO antigens on liver tissue.

Hepatic graft loss resulting from recipient antibodies that recognize donor HLA antigens is difficult to document, but most observers believe that it does occur, albeit in a much less predictable fashion than with renal transplantation. It is a rare event, however, and most transplantation programs do not insist on a negative crossmatch between recipient serum and donor cells before transplantation, as is the case in renal transplantation. In one large series, a retrospective evaluation of crossmatch information failed to show any deleterious effect of a positive crossmatch on ultimate hepatic graft survival. When it does occur, antibody-mediated rejection manifests as deterioration of allograft function, usually in the first weeks after surgery (19). Biopsy reveals infiltration by neutrophils, endothelial cell hypertrophy, and focal deposits of fibrin. Immunofluorescence studies may show antibody and complement in the vessel wall. This is similar to an accelerated acute vascular rejection sometimes seen in renal transplant recipients. Treatment usually consists of plasma exchange combined with increased immunosuppression.

Why the liver is less susceptible to antibody-mediated destruction than the kidney is not clearly understood, but probably relates to several factors. First, the liver has a vastly different microcirculation than does the kidney, with a preponderance of sinusoidal channels and a smaller capillary network. It is probable that antibody-mediated injury affects blood flow through the delicate capillary network of the kidney more than it does liver sinusoids. In addition, each hepatocyte is exposed to two sinusoidal channels, presumably permitting survival if only one sinusoid is occluded. Third, the resident macrophages of the liver, Kupffer cells, process antigens for presentation and this may have an effect on the internal immunologic milieu of the organ, quite distinct from that of the kidney. Finally, differences in HLA expression are known to exist in the two organs, with the kidney the more antigenic of the two.

Although humoral (antibody-mediated) rejection has classically been thought of as pertaining to the immediate time frame after transplantation, the role that antibody plays in the initiation and prolongation of chronic rejection has been receiving increased attention. Antibodies have been identified to graft parenchyma cells, HLA molecules on biliary epithelium, vascular endothelium, as well as to other blood cell elements, all implicating a significant role for antibody in chronic allograft rejection.

Cell-mediated Rejection

Acute, or cell-mediated, rejection occurs frequently and the reported incidence depends on multiple factors, including the manner in which rejection is defined, donor factors, the immunosuppression regimen used, and the extent to which the allograft is surveyed for rejection. Acute rejection occurs most commonly in the first 1 to 2 postoperative months, with nearly 70% of early rejection episodes becoming manifest between 5 and 14 days after engraftment. In modern practice, cell-mediated rejection is a less common cause of graft loss than primary nonfunction, hepatic artery thrombosis, or recurrent hepatic parenchymal disease. Still, the effectiveness of antirejection treatment assumes a relatively early diagnosis, which is in turn the result of careful monitoring by the transplantation physician. Prognosis is much worse when rejection is diagnosed later after transplantation (>28 days) or allowed to fester without treatment, as when the diagnosis is in doubt.

The diagnosis of cell-mediated rejection is made on clinical as well as histologic grounds (Table 16.13). Clinical features may include fever and a decrease in bile output or a change in consistency and color of bile from deep green to a watery, light green. Increasingly, with ever more potent immunopharmaceuticals, rejection does not manifest such overt symptoms and is often first diagnosed based on abnormalities in liver function studies. Laboratory evaluation of peripheral blood demonstrates leukocytosis and occasionally eosinophilia. Biochemical changes include elevated levels of serum aminotransferases and alkaline phosphatase, serum prothrombin time, and serum bilirubin. Any of these findings should prompt a biopsy either to confirm rejection as a cause of dysfunction or to lead to other studies to evaluate for recurrent hepatic dis-

---

Table 16.13. DIAGNOSIS OF HEPATIC ALLOGRAFT REJECTION

CLINICAL

Fever
Malaise
Jaundice
Decrease in bile production
Change in color/consistency of bile

LABORATORY

Elevation of serum bilirubin
Elevation of aminotransferases
Increased prothrombin time

BIOPSY

Portal inflammation
Venous endothelial inflammation
Lymphocytic infiltration of bile ducts

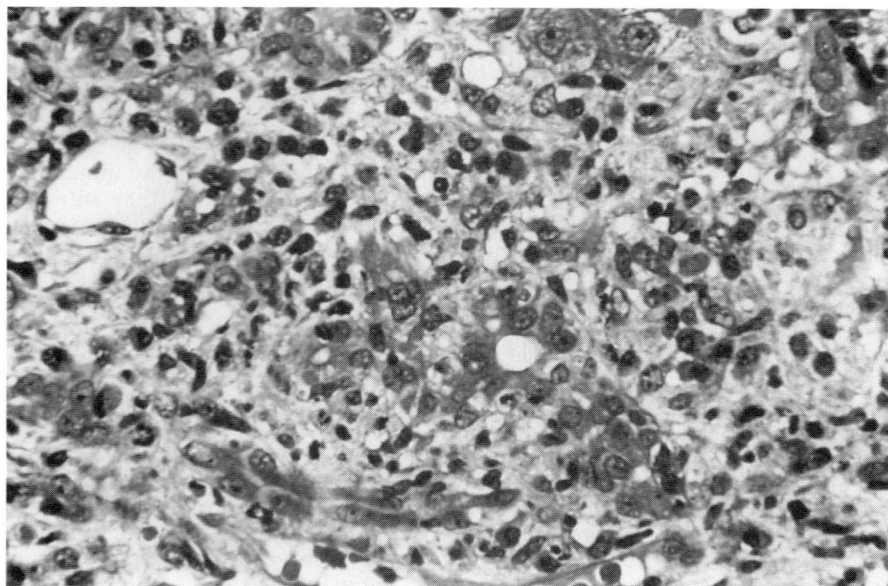

Figure 16.64. Histologic findings in hepatic transplant rejection—bile duct injury. The bile duct *(center)* is infiltrated by lymphocytes.

ease, infection, or malignancy as possible etiologies. Typical biopsy findings in cases of cell-mediated rejection are a triad of portal lymphocytosis, venous endotheliitis (subendothelial deposits of mononuclear cells), and bile duct inflammation and damage (Figs. 16.64 and 16.65). Various classification schemes have been devised to grade the severity of the rejection process based on the degree of cellular involvement or injury in these areas. There is no universally accepted grading system for liver allograft rejection, in contrast to that in renal transplantation. In 1997, a consensus document was published by an international panel that met in Banff, Canada, grading rejections as indeterminate, mild, moderate, or severe, using histologic criteria mentioned previously. Cell characterization analyses have shown that the inflammatory cells appearing in the portal triads during acute rejection episodes are primarily T cells, with fewer macrophages and neutrophils. Bile duct epithelial cells appear to be a prime tar-

get of immune attack, and they are known to express large amounts of class II HLA antigen.

The main risk factors for acute liver allograft rejection are primary immunosuppressive regimen, etiology for liver replacement, donor factors, and other relatively undefined variables, such as preservation time and donor–recipient sex, age, and race mismatch (20). Interestingly, some indications for transplantation are associated with a greater risk for acute cell-mediated rejection than others. Autoimmune diseases, including primary biliary cirrhosis and autoimmune hepatitis, along with hepatitis C, show the highest rates of rejection, whereas hepatitis B infection, in addition to alcoholic liver disease and fulminant hepatic failure, show the lowest rates of rejection (21). The reasons for these differences are far from clear, but the observations have been reproducible.

Occasionally, a biopsy done on a routine or protocol basis shows histologic evidence of rejection in the absence

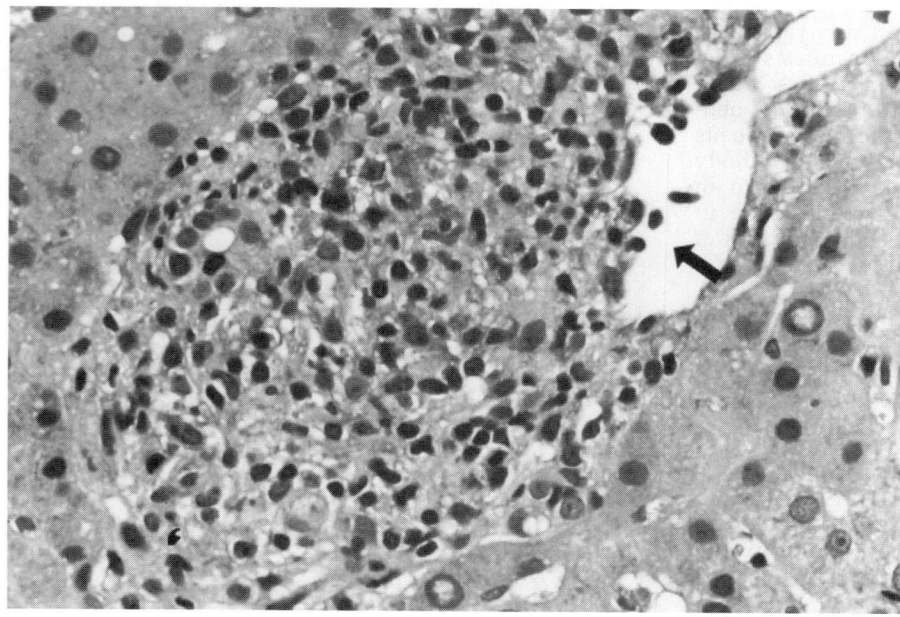

Figure 16.65. Histologic findings in hepatic transplant rejection—portal tract tract lymphocytosis and endotheliitis. The portal triad *(center)* shows a dense cellular infiltrate. The *arrow* indicates endotheliitis.

of clinical or biochemical evidence of rejection. Treatment of this finding is controversial and ranges from full antirejection therapy to no therapy. Spontaneous disappearance of such findings has been reported. Most transplantation specialists would at least perform frequent follow-up biopsies in such cases.

Chronic Rejection

Chronic rejection is characterized by relentless immune attack on small bile ducts and vascular endothelium (22). Clinically, the pattern is one of gradual biliary obstruction, with elevation of alkaline phosphatase and bilirubin, in the absence of abnormalities in large bile ducts. Histologically, small bile ducts are obliterated or completely absent, with a less pronounced cellular infiltrate than is seen with acute rejection. In addition to ductopenia, portal fibrosis, central lobular degeneration, and foam cell arteriopathy are other microscopic hallmarks of chronic rejection. The loss of small bile ducts is partly the result of direct immune-mediated attack on biliary epithelium, comprising both a cellular and humoral component. Relative to other cells in the liver, biliary epithelium tends to express more class I antigen. Class II antigen expression is induced as the result of an episode of acute rejection. Thus, biliary epithelial cells are vulnerable targets for host attack because of their antigenicity. Loss of bile ducts also occurs as the result of ischemia secondary to immune-mediated obliteration of small to medium arteries. Vanishing bile duct syndrome, defined as absence of bile ducts in 15 of 20 portal triads examined, is produced by chronic rejection, but can also be the result of ischemic or other mechanisms; therefore, chronic rejection and vanishing bile duct syndrome are not always synonymous. This syndrome is commonly encountered after transplantation of the liver into a patient with antidonor lymphocytotoxic antibodies. Vanishing bile duct syndrome also has been seen with increasing frequency in patients recovering from CMV infection. Disappointingly, few available agents are effective for treatment of recipients with chronic rejection. As in the case of renal transplantations, chronic rejection responds poorly to increases in immunosuppressive medication, and retransplantation is usually required. Tacrolimus has been shown to be the most effective agent in treating this problem. One multicenter study of the treatment of chronic rejection showed a 70% response rate when patients were converted to tacrolimus (23).

The rate of chronic hepatic allograft rejection is declining, the reason for which is mostly unknown. Between 2% to 5% of liver recipients experience chronic rejection, in marked contradistinction to renal transplant recipients, in which chronic rejection is the major long-term risk factor for graft survival. This decline may be due to improved immunosuppression protocols, particularly the increased use of tacrolimus as primary immunosuppressant in liver transplantation. Many groups have attempted to define risk factors for the development of chronic allograft rejection, yielding conflicting results (24). Factors associated with chronic rejection include multiple or late episodes of acute rejection, immune-mediated etiologies of liver failure (autoimmune hepatitis and cholestatic liver disorders), previous transplantation with development of chronic rejection, and CMV infection.

Immunosuppression Induction and Maintenance

A universal immunosuppressive protocol does not exist for hepatic transplantation. Immunosuppressive protocols are very parochial, based on many factors, not the least of which are a center's past experiences, individual physicians' recent and past experiences, organ recipient variables (etiology of liver failure, prior transplantation, renal dysfunction), donor factors (ischemic time, risk of delayed graft function), difficulty of the recipient surgery (risk of renal dysfunction, hepatic delayed function), and economic factors (25). It is the hope of many that immunosuppressive regimens will become very individualized, based on variables outlined previously. As new agents are developed, the ability to treat each particular transplantation and clinical scenario has greatly increased the complexity of immunosuppression management (Table 16.14). One common immunosuppressive protocol used in hepatic transplantation for a "routine" primary adult liver transplantation consists of placing the recipient on tacrolimus as the primary immunosuppressive agent, in combination with corticosteroids and mycophenolate mofetil as an antiproliferative agent. After 6 to 12 months of excellent graft function (and assuming no acute rejection episodes), the steroids are tapered off and the mycophenolate discontinued, allowing the recipient to be maintained on tacrolimus monotherapy (26). Since the late 1990s, tacrolimus has overtaken cyclosporine as the primary immunosuppressive in nearly 70% of all liver transplant recipients (27). Neoral, a microemulsion formulation of cyclosporine, is an alternative primary immunosuppressive agent with similar efficacy in randomized trials.

This type of multidrug regimen has evolved for several reasons, the most important of which is that more drugs in smaller doses are safer and more effective than larger doses of fewer drugs. Increased efficacy probably relates to the different mechanisms of actions of the drugs involved, which have synergistic effects, in addition to the notion that fewer and less severe side effects result from taking lower doses of most of these pharmaceuticals. For transplant recipients with preexisting renal dysfunction, one of the goals of initial therapy is to avoid potentially nephrotoxic medications. Because this is a well-known side effect of all calcineurin inhibitors, a cyclosporine- (or tacrolimus)-sparing protocol would be followed. In such a regimen, induction therapy with antithymocyte globulin [Thymoglobulin (SangStat, Fremont, CA)] or an interleukin-2 receptor antagonist is used, delaying the introduction of the calcineurin inhibitor for as long as possible, sometimes up to 2 to 3 weeks. After this time,

Table 16.14. IMMUNE MODULATORS USED IN LIVER

ANTIMETABOLITES
Azathioprine
Mycophenolate mofetil

ANTIBODIES
Monoclonal
   Anti-CD3
   Interleukin-2 receptor antagonist
Polyclonal
   Atgam[a]
   Thymoglobulin

CYTOKINE INHIBITORS
Corticosteroids
Calcineurin inhibitors
Cyclosporine
Tacrolimus

CELL CYCLE INHIBITOR
Sirolimus

[a]Atgam (Pharmacia & Upjohn, Kalamazoo, MI): lymphocyte immune globulin plus antithymocyte globulin.

and with improving renal function, tacrolimus or cyclosporine could be introduced into the immunosuppression regimen. Some transplantation centers routinely use induction therapy, not waiting for the development of renal dysfunction, as a kidney-sparing measure.

Both tacrolimus and cyclosporine are monitored by measuring their level in serum. This is a very important element in patient management, especially early after engraftment. Interactions with other medications, especially those that activate or inhibit the cytochrome P-450 system, are relatively commonplace and dose adjustments are not infrequent. Common side effects of this class of drugs include worsening or new-onset diabetes mellitus, renal dysfunction with decreased glomerular filtration, hypertension, headaches, and an increased incidence of skin carcinomas and some types of lymphomas. The goal of long-term immunosuppression management is to decrease the dosages of the mainstay immunosuppressants to as low a level as feasible, balancing between underimmunosuppression (rejection) and overimmunosuppression (infection, increased side effects).

Treatment of Acute Rejection

Despite the overall effectiveness of current immunosuppressive protocols, acute rejection does occur and must be treated promptly (see algorithm Table 16.15). On establishment of the diagnosis, high doses of methylpred-

nisolone (usually 500 mg to 1 g) are administered intravenously on a daily basis for 3 days, followed by a taper. This treatment is usually effective in reversing 50% to 75% of acute rejection episodes. Patients who experience another rejection episode within a short time frame (usually within 1 month) are said to have steroid-resistant rejection. Classically, the treatment for steroid-resistant rejection was either repeat high-dose corticosteroids, or, more frequently, use of Orthoclone OKT3 (Ortho McNeil Pharmaceutical, Raritan, NJ), a murine monoclonal antibody directed to the CD3 determinant of the T-cell receptor complex. OKT3 is administered daily for 7 to 14 days. Treatment is highly effective, and it is unusual to lose an allograft secondary to acute rejection. However, the use of OKT3 for steroid-resistant rejections is not as prevalent as it once was because of (a) significant deleterious adverse effects of this pharmaceutical, including increased incidence of posttransplantation lymphoproliferative disorders, and worsening of posttransplantation hepatitis C; and (b) availability of a wider variety of equally useful immunopharmaceuticals (Table 16.15). Tacrolimus is commonly used as primary immunosuppressant after acute rejection, as well as conversion from an azathioprine-based regimen to one based on mycophenolate mofetil. Other agents finding use to treat acute rejection include antithymocyte globulin and the interleukin-2 receptor antagonists. Because these agents are so new, there have not been any substantive, large, controlled clinical trials showing their efficacy to treat acute rejection.

Table 16.15. MANAGEMENT ALGORITHM OF ACUTE LIVER ALLOGRAFT REJECTION

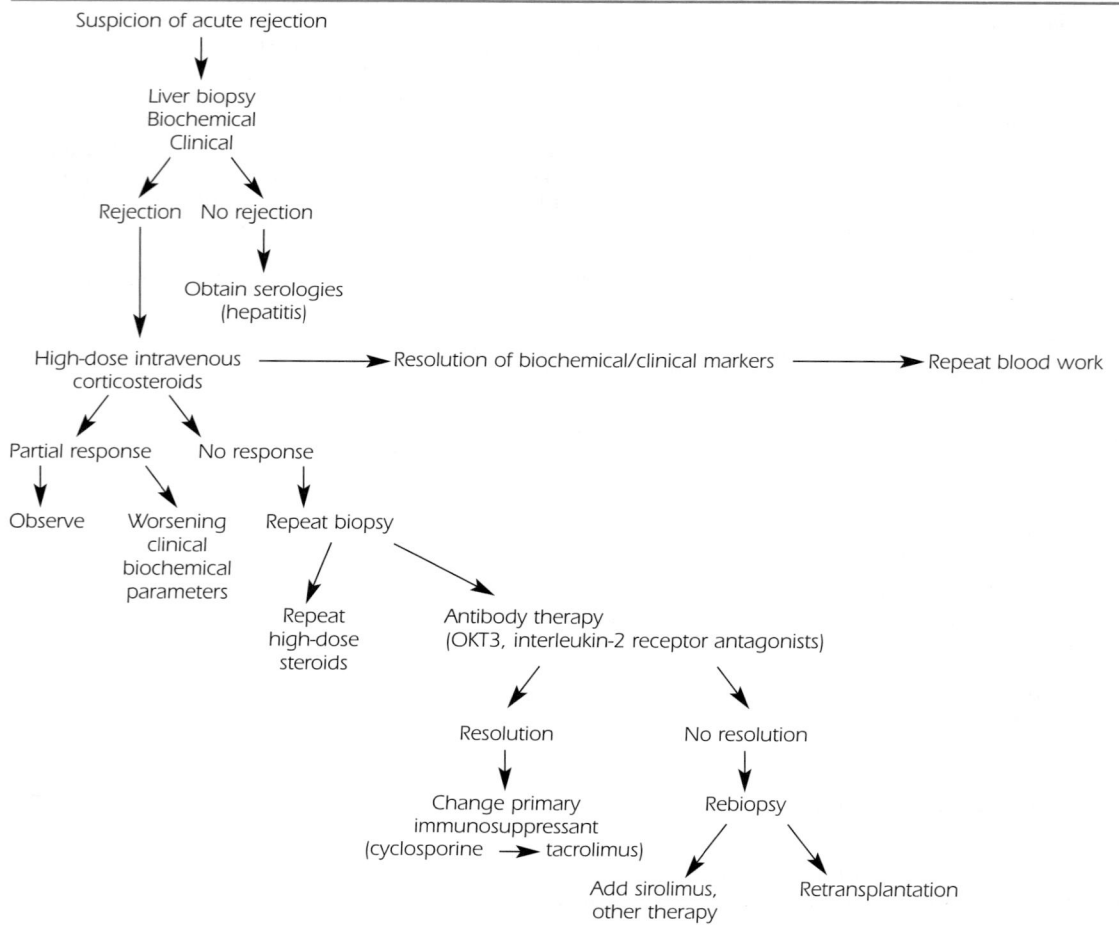

RESULTS

The survival rate after hepatic transplantation has increased gradually. Current 1- and 5-year survival rates are 88% and 74%, respectively (2). Multiple factors affect the likelihood of survival. Registry data from UNOS indicate that the single most significant determinant of survival is whether the patient has had a previous transplantation. Although 88% of patients undergoing their first hepatic transplantation survive, only 67% of patients that have previously undergone hepatic transplantation survive (2). Another important determinant of success is the health status of the patient at the time of transplantation. The patient survival rate after transplantation is 91% for patients not in a hospital before transplantation, 86% for hospitalized patients, and 74% for patients on life support at the time of transplantation (2). Comorbidities such as renal failure and donor factors, particularly donor age, also have a significant impact on posttransplantation survival (28,29). These same factors play a major role in the cost of liver transplantation (30). The cause of liver failure is also an important factor, in that 1-year survival is most likely for patients with cholestatic liver disease (92%), followed by patients with metabolic disorders (92%), noncholestatic cirrhosis (87%), malignancy (87%), biliary atresia (86%), and fulminant hepatic failure (81%) (2). Despite these differences in survival rates, liver transplantation is the only successful therapy for all of these conditions. For example, although patients with fulminant hepatic failure have one of the worst survival rates, most of these patients die if not transplanted. In this context, a survival rate of 81% is excellent.

REFERENCES

1. Carithers RL Jr. Liver transplantation. *Liver Transpl* 2000;6:122.
2. 1999 Annual Report of the U.S. Scientific Registry for Transplant Recipients and the Organ Procurement and Transplantation Network. Transplant Data: 1989–1998. U.S. Department of Health and Human Services, Health Resources and Services Administration, Office of Special Programs, Division of Transplantation, Rockville MD; UNOS, Richmond, VA, p. 89.
3. Campbell DA Jr, Magee JC, Punch JD, et al. One center's experience with liver transplantation: alcohol use relapse over the long term. *Liver Transpl Surg* 1998;4:558.
4. Imperial J. Natural history of chronic hepatitis B and C. *J Gastroenterol Hepatol* 1999;14[Suppl]:S1.
5. Poynard T, Bedosa P, Opolon P. Natural history of liver fibrosis progression in patients with chronic hepatitis C. *Lancet* 1997;349:825.
6. Chari RS, Gan TJ, Robertson KM, et al. Venovenous bypass in adult orthotopic liver transplantation: routine or selective use. *J Am Coll Surg* 1998;186:683.
7. Tzakis A, Todo S, Starzl TE. Orthotopic liver transplantation with preservation of the inferior vena cava. *Ann Surg* 1989;210:649.
8. Busitill RW, Goss JA. Split liver transplantation. *Ann Surg* 1999;229:313.
9. Marcos A, Fisher RA, Ham JH, et al. Right lobe living donor liver transplantation. *Transplantation* 1999;68:798.
10. Deschenes M, Belle S, Krom R, et al. Early allograft dysfunction after liver transplantation. *Transplantation* 1998;66:302.
11. Stahl R, Duncan A, Hooks M, et al. A hypercoagulable state follows orthotopic liver transplantation. *Hepatology* 1990;12:553.
12. Lebeau G, Yanaga K, Marsh J, et al. Analysis of surgical complications after 397 hepatic transplantations. *Surg Gynecol Obstet* 1990;3:317.
13. Lerut J, Tzakis A, Boon K. Complications of venous reconstruction in human orthotopic liver transplantation. *Ann Surg* 1987;205:404.
14. Mazzaferro V, Esquivel C, Makowka L. Hepatic artery thrombosis after pediatric liver transplantation: a medical or surgical event? *Transplantation* 1989;47:971.
15. Madalosso C, deSouza N, Ilstrop P, et al. Cytomegalovirus and its association with hepatic artery thrombosis after liver transplantation. *Transplantation* 1998;66:294.
16. Sterzi R, Santills M, Donato F, et al. Neurologic complications following orthotopic liver transplantation. *Transplant Proc* 1994;26:3679.
17. DeGroen P, Aksamit A, Rakela J. Central nervous system toxicity after liver transplantation. *N Engl J Med* 1986;317:861.
18. Fargos O, Kalil AN, Samuel D, et al. The use of ABO-incompatible grafts in liver transplantation: a life-saving procedure in highly selected patients. *Transplantation* 1995;59:1124.
19. Donaldson PT, Williams R. Cross-matching in liver transplantation. *Transplantation* 1997;63:789.
20. Wiesner RH, Demetris AJ, Belle S, et al. Acute hepatic allograft rejection: Incidence, risk factors, and impact on outcome. *Hepatology* 1998;28:638.
21. Seiler CA, Dufour JF, Renner EL, et al. Primary liver disease as a determinant for acute rejection after liver transplantation. *Langenbecks Arch Surg* 1999;384:259.
22. Wiesner RH, Batts KP, Krom RA. Evolving concepts in the diagnosis, pathogenesis, and treatment of chronic hepatic allograft rejection. *Liver Transpl Surg* 1999;5:388.
23. Sher LS, Cosenza CA, Michel J, et al. Efficacy of tacrolimus as rescue therapy for chronic rejection in orthotopic liver transplantation: a report of the U.S. Multicenter Liver Study Group. *Transplantation* 1997;64:258.
24. Van Hoek B, Weisner RH, Krom RA, et al. Severe ductopenic rejection following liver transplantation: incidence, time of onset, risk factors, treatment, and outcome. *Semin Liver Dis* 1992;12:41.
25. Fisher RA, Ham JM, Marcos A, et al. A prospective randomized trial of mycophenolate mofetil with Neoral or tacrolimus after orthotopic liver transplantation. *Transplantation* 1999;66:1616.
26. Stegall MD, Everson GT, Schroter G, et al. Prednisone withdrawal late after adult liver transplantation reduces diabetes, hypertension, and hypercholesterolemia without causing graft loss. *Hepatology* 1997;25:173.
27. The U.S. Multicenter FK506 Liver Study Group. A comparison of tacrolimus (FK506) and cyclosporine for immunosuppression in liver transplantation. *N Engl J Med* 1994;331:1110.
28. Baliga P, Merion RM, Turcotte JG, et al. Preoperative risk factor assessment in liver transplantation. *Surgery* 1992;112:704.
29. Detre KM, Lombardero M, Belle S, et al. Influence of donor age on graft survival after liver transplantation: United Network for Organ Sharing Registry. *Liver Transpl Surg* 1995;1:311.
30. Brown RS Jr, Lake JR, Ascher NL, et al. Predictors of the cost of liver transplantation. *Liver Transpl Surg* 1998;4:170.

Cardiac Transplantation

RICHARD N. PIERSON III

Since 1964, cardiac transplantation has evolved from a sensational, perilous experiment to become conventional therapy for end-stage heart disease, the paradigm of successful but expensive "high-tech" medicine. This remarkable transformation stemmed from fundamental surgical innovations supported by incremental improvements in the diagnosis and management of common problems. Current challenges revolve around donor supply and allocation, improving long-term outcomes, developing alternative therapies, and related ethical issues.

HISTORICAL PERSPECTIVE

Based on significant contributions by many surgical pioneers (1–8), the first clinical heart transplantation was performed in 1964 by Hardy and colleagues, who attempted to salvage a man dying from cardiogenic shock by replacing his heart with one from a chimpanzee (9). Then, before the concept of brain death achieved wide social or legal acceptance, in 1967 Christian Barnard and his colleagues captured the imagination of the world with the first operative survival, using the heart of a resuscitated cadaveric donor (10). This case, and many others that were performed shortly thereafter, demonstrated the physiologic capacity of the transplanted human heart allograft to support the recipient's circulation, but also the difficulty of managing subsequent immunologic and infectious complications. After a worldwide flurry of activity, generally dismal outcomes at many prominent cardiac surgery centers made clear the need for more thoughtful approaches to what was clearly a difficult constellation of problems beyond that of effective circulatory support.

A few pioneering programs persisted in cautious clinical application supported by parallel laboratory investigation. Recognizing the need for a more sensitive and specific diagnostic technique to diagnose rejection, Phillip Caves, working with Shumway and colleagues at Stanford, developed the technique of transvenous endomyocardial biopsy (11). Frequent, representative surveillance sampling of the graft allowed early detection of pathogenic host immune responses. Perivascular lymphocytic infiltrates were found accurately to diagnose acute cellular rejection in its presymptomatic phase; when detected early, it usually responded to enhanced immunosuppression. Equally important, when rejection was not seen, immunosuppression could be tapered to minimize drug toxicities and reduce the incidence of opportunistic infection. Coupled with important advances in the diagnosis, prevention, and treatment of infectious pathogens in immunosuppressed patients, and in selection and management of patients with end-stage heart failure, patient survival rates at 1 year improved gradually, from approximately 20% in the 1960s to approximately 70% by 1980 (12).

However, even as recently as the early 1980s, when rejection persisted or recurred despite high-dose steroids, alternative treatments (total lymphoid irradiation, intramuscular antilymphocyte preparations, thoracic duct ligation, splenectomy) were often toxic or invasive, and accompanied by a high incidence of major short- and long-term complications. In this context, the discovery and clinical development of cyclosporine (13,14) catalyzed the next major improvement in outcomes. Because its primary mechanism of action (inhibition of calcineurin-dependent cellular activation events) and toxicity profile were fundamentally different from those of azathioprine, an antimitotic agent, or antiinflammatory steroids, combination "triple" therapy allowed each agent to be used more safely. Meanwhile, antithymocyte and antilymphocyte preparations were adapted for safe intravenous use, either as prophylactic induction therapy (quadruple therapy) or as treatment for steroid-resistant rejection. Based primarily on these pharmacologic innovations in the regulation of the immune response, expected 1-year survival rates after heart transplantation gradually rose from approximately 70% to almost 90% between 1980 and 2000 (15) in older and sicker recipients (16,17).

CANDIDATE EVALUATION

End-stage heart failure is the primary indication for heart transplantation in adults, with coronary artery occlusive disease and myopathy of various etiologies each accounting for approximately 45% of cases. Congenital heart disease is the primary indication for infants, whereas myopathy predominates in older children.

The heart transplantation evaluation process seeks to identify patients for whom no other reasonable treatment

---

Table 16.16. INDICATIONS FOR HEART TRANSPLANTATION

GENERAL INDICATIONS

1. End-stage heart disease without lower-risk alternative
2. Absence of any noncardiac condition likely to:
   a. Limit survival independent of cardiac function
   b. Preclude safe administration of adequate immunosuppression
   c. Predispose to life-threatening infection with immunosuppression

SPECIFIC INDICATIONS

1. Heart failure of various etiologies
   a. Myopathy (e.g., ischemic, idiopathic, viral, familial, restrictive)
   b. Valvular
   c. Congenital
   d. Failed transplant
      Early (e.g., primary nonfunction, acute rejection)
      Late (e.g., cardiac allograft vasculopathy)
2. Other indications
   a. Angina not amenable to revascularization
   b. Arrhythmia, failed conventional therapy
   c. Hypertrophic cardiomyopathy
   d. Restrictive cardiomyopathy
   e. Primary cardiac tumor (completely resectable)

---

options exist, and who are at higher risk of death without transplantation than with it, while excluding those whose comorbid conditions are likely significantly to limit length or quality of life. In 1993, a National Institutes of Health consensus conference developed recipient selection guidelines for cardiac transplantation, based on objective criteria known to predict poor outcome without transplantation (18); these guidelines are summarized in Tables 16.16 to 16.18. Among patients with heart failure symptoms, maximal oxygen consumption (MVO_2) is more sensitive and specific than ejection fraction in gauging prognosis, and blunted cardiac output response to exercise may further stratify patients into high- and low-risk groups (19).

When no clear survival advantage is apparent for transplantation or an alternative management strategy, quality of life and other subjective factors are weighed. Contemporary studies defining relative risks, along with basic considerations in the medical management of end-stage heart failure, are well summarized in recent reviews (20–22).

Table 16.17. SELECTION CRITERIA FOR STRATIFYING RISK AND SURVIVAL

SURVIVAL BENEFIT ESTABLISHED

MVO_2 <10 mL/kg/min
Class IV CHF symptoms despite maximal medical therapy
Requiring mechanical circulatory support
Refractory angina without therapeutic alternative
Refractory ventricular arrhythmia without alternative

SURVIVAL BENEFIT LIKELY

MVO_2 10–14 mL/kg/min
Blunted CO response to exercise
Instability of fluid balance or renal function despite documented compliance
Intermittent angina
EF <20% without therapeutic alternative

SURVIVAL BENEFIT NOT ESTABLISHED

MVO_2 10–14 mL/kg/min, preserved CO response to exercise
MVO_2 >14, EF <20% without other indication
History of CHF arrhythmia, controlled with medical therapy

Quality-of-life considerations may influence selection of recipients for whom survival benefit is not established.
CHF, congestive heart failure; CO, cardiac output; EF, ejection fraction; MVO_2, maximal oxygen consumption.

Table 16.18. CONTRAINDICATIONS TO CARDIAC TRANSPLANTATION

ABSOLUTE CONTRAINDICATIONS

High pulmonary vascular resistance[a]
  Transpulmonary gradient >15, fixed
  Pulmonary vascular resistance index >5–6 Woods units
Irreversible renal insufficiency (creatinine clearance <40)[a]
Active infection (viral or bacterial)
Active peptic ulcer disease
Diabetes with end-organ damage (renal insufficiency, neuropathy, retinopathy)
Symptomatic extracardiac vascular disease
  Cerebrovascular obstructive disease with recent transient ischemic attack, cerebrovascular accident
  Pulmonary vascular obstructive disease with claudication, rest pain, or tissue loss
Current malignancy, or recent treatment (<2 y) for life-threatening malignancy
Disease of another organ system that would probably limit survival (established cirrhosis, cardiac or other etiology)
Symptomatic COPD; chronic bronchitis
High risk for inability to comply with complex medical regimen
  Not firmly committed to transplantation
  Inadequate cognitive capacity to comply with postoperative regimen, coupled with inadequate compensatory social support
  Documented psychiatric instability
  Recurrent drug or alcohol abuse
  Demonstrated noncompliance with therapeutic recommendations

RELATIVE CONTRAINDICATIONS

Age >65 y
Established renal failure
Diabetes without end-organ disease
Asymptomatic or previously treated extracardiac vascular disease
COPD with FEV_1 <60% predicted without referable symptoms
Remote malignancy, in remission (>2–4 y with no evidence of disease)
High pulmonary vascular resistance, reversible
Disease of another organ system that would limit quality of life
Difficulty complying with complex medical regimen

---

[a]On optimal medical therapy.
COPD, chronic obstructive pulmonary disease; FEV_1, forced expiratory volume in 1 second.

DONOR SELECTION AND MANAGEMENT

The ideal donor is a young, previously healthy person without cardiac disease or hypertension, who is well matched in size to the intended recipient, and whose hemodynamics have been carefully managed during the evolution of his or her lethal central nervous system injury. Some programs have advocated use of older donors, donors who may transmit infection or malignancy to the recipient, and grafts with hypertensive myocardial hypertrophy for particular recipients (23). Some aggressive programs have even proposed that hemodynamically significant coronary stenoses can be bypassed at the time of transplantation (24). These approaches to donor selection are associated with less favorable short- and long-term outcomes (15,25), but the increased risk may be considered acceptable for patients in whom the short-term prognosis is poor without transplantation.

Donor management requires skill and experience to address successfully the complex physiologic perturbations associated with brain death. Reflex hypertensive and hypotensive responses to intracranial pressure changes, fluid and electrolyte imbalances consequent to the diabetes insipidus from pituitary death, and additional stresses related to hemorrhage, trauma, and surgery often cause hemodynamic and metabolic instability, which may injure a previously healthy heart. The neurohumoral milieu of central nervous system catastrophe may also adversely affect other fundamental cell regulatory functions, such as those dependent on thyroid hormone. Despite controversy regarding the mechanisms involved, thyroid hormone is often administered to the donor as a continuous infusion in the hopes of correcting a "sick euthyroid" syndrome and optimizing cardiac metabolism before explant. Although evidence to date is largely anecdotal, inotrope requirements can often be reduced after thyroid infusion is begun, and donor hemodynamic lability is less common, suggesting improved cardiac and vasoregulatory function (26,27).

Cardiac echocardiography has become a standard component of donor assessment to measure ejection fraction and exclude structural abnormalities or hypertrophy suggestive of hypertensive myopathy. Cardiac catheterization may be requested for donors older than 45 years of age, especially for those with a strong family history of coronary artery disease, for smokers, or when regional wall motion abnormalities are appreciated on echocardiography.

MATCHING DONOR TO RECIPIENT

Once a potential donor is identified, priority among blood type-compatible recipients is determined first by relative severity of illness ("status"), and then by length of time on the waiting list among those at each status in the donor's geographic area. This information is currently tracked and collated by a central, national registry operated by the United Network for Organ Sharing. The heart is first offered to the program whose candidate has seniority on the list and whose registered height and weight range include the potential donor. Donor inotrope requirements and functional assessment, recipient pulmonary vascular resistance, possible infection transmission risks (known hepatitis or potential HIV exposure in the donor), and other logistical considerations (expected graft ischemic time) influence the recipient team's decision regarding acceptance of an organ for an individual patient. If the first program declines the offer for the first patient, the process is repeated for the patient next on the list until the heart is accepted.

Tissue typing, the time-consuming process by which donor and recipient are matched for shared transplant antigens, is not currently used for hearts. The probability is low of identifying a "close" match among the relatively small number of blood type-compatible potential recipients within the geographic radius (usually 1,500 miles) defined by a 4-hour projected ischemic time. In addition, the demonstrated benefit of partial human leukocyte antigen matching is small relative to the added risk of prolonged graft ischemia, a risk augmented by increasing donor age (28).

RECIPIENT MANAGEMENT BEFORE TRANSPLANTATION

The medical therapy of patients awaiting transplantation has improved significantly since the early 1990s, centered around aggressive afterload reduction and diuresis, anticoagulation, and beta blockade (18–20). This trend, coupled with improved mechanical support, has reduced the mortality rate for patients awaiting for transplantation. Because waiting lists have grown faster than the donor pool, and average time waiting has similarly escalated, cardiac decompensation among patients on the waiting list is frequent. In most areas of the country, most hearts go to patients who are sick enough to require hospitalization for intensive diuresis and intravenous inotrope administration.

When inotropic therapy proves inadequate, as gauged by progressive deterioration in renal and other end-organ function, temporary intraaortic balloon pump counterpulsation and mechanical ventilation can stabilize some patients. These interventions are associated with important risks; the relative risk of death is increased threefold in patients who are ventilator dependent at the time of transplantation (15).

In contrast, mechanical circulatory support using ventricular assist devices has emerged as an effective bridging strategy. Although some bridged patients incur serious complications (stroke, renal or hepatic failure, systemic infection) that preclude transplantation, approximately two thirds are successfully transplanted, with excellent outcomes relative to patients not requiring this intervention. Patients with biventricular failure can be supported with either implanted or paracorporeal pulsatile left ventricular support, with or without addition of temporary right heart support (29). Various total artificial heart devices can be implanted in place of the native heart, and have been applied successfully in small numbers (29). This approach is most likely to find a niche as an alternative to heart transplantation in patients not supportable with a left ventricular assist device, such as those with fixed pulmonary hypertension. Intravascular axial flow devices and other nonpulsatile assist systems are also in development.

HEART PROCUREMENT

Cardiac allograft protection depends primarily on hypothermia, which reduces myocardial energy requirements while the heart graft has no nutritive coronary blood flow. Other important principles include avoidance of distention and warm ischemia in both the donor and the recipient, and induction of diastolic (flaccid) cardiac arrest. These goals are accomplished by interrupting of systemic venous return for decompression, placing a clamp across the distal ascending aorta, and infusing a hyperkalemic preservation solution proximal to the clamp, and thus selectively into the coronary arteries. Both the inferior vena cava and left atrium are incised (vented) to prevent distention of either ventricle. Some preservation solutions incorporating free radical scavenging molecules or other cytoprotective agents are associated with improved early graft function (30,31).

Every effort is made to limit the ischemic interval, the time between initial interruption of coronary flow by aortic crossclamping in the donor and removal of the crossclamp in the recipient, to less than 4 hours. Although laboratory studies and isolated clinical reports suggest that good results may be expected with storage times of 8 hours or more using various preservation solutions, increased ischemic time remains a strong and important independent risk factor for poor recipient outcome (15).

OPERATIVE RECIPIENT MANAGEMENT

Timing of the recipient operation requires careful coordination with the procurement team. Anesthesia is induced after the donor heart is visually inspected and

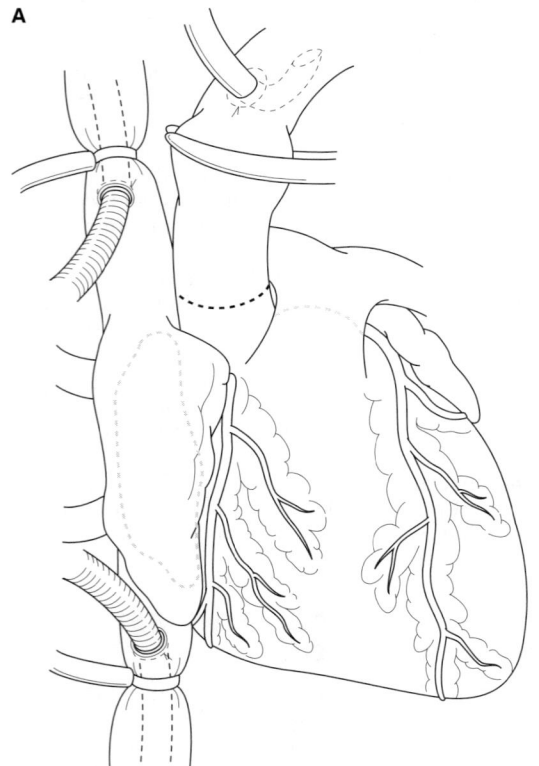

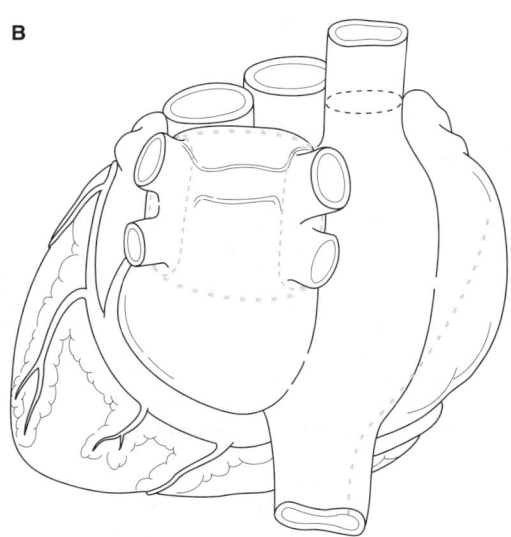

Figure 16.66. Native cardiectomy and donor graft preparation. *(A)* Recipient pericardium after institution of cardiopulmonary bypass and ascending aortic occlusion, with caval snares secured. The diseased native heart can then be safely excised by transecting the recipient aorta and pulmonary artery, and the atria divided as appropriate for the intended implant technique. Shown is the right artial incision for the traditional Lowe/Shumway right atrial cuff. *(B)* Posterior view of the explanted donor heart, indicating various insicions used for artial cuff preparation. Donor atrial cuff incisions made in preparation for traditional Lower/Shumway biatrial implant. The SVC is ligated or oversewn. Right and left pulmonary veins and cavae prepared for the total artioventricular implant technique. For the bicaval technique, the donor SVC and IVC are retained, and the donor left atrial cuff trimmed as for the traditional biatrial approach.

found suitable. Venous access is obtained that permits rapid volume resuscitation and invasive cardiac monitoring after the new heart is implanted. Prior cardiac surgery may complicate coordination of operative timing, and is associated with increased risk of bleeding.

If appropriate, warfarin effect is reversed with fresh frozen plasma and vitamin K. Aprotinin or ε-aminocaproic acid is often used to inhibit fibrinolysis and prevent coagulopathic bleeding associated with hepatic congestion and adhesions from prior cardiac surgery. Increased inotropic infusion, antiarrhythmic agents, or mechanical circulatory support may be required to maintain adequate systemic perfusion before institution of cardiopulmonary bypass.

Vascular access for bypass is accomplished by cannulation of the superior and inferior venae cavae so as completely to divert systemic venous blood to the cardiopulmonary bypass circuit. The ascending aorta or common femoral artery is used for arterial return from the circuit to the patient. Technical misadventures, such as entry into the heart or great vessels before bypass is established, or induction of ventricular arrhythmias, are more common with reoperative procedures, and can greatly complicate the intraoperative course and postoperative management.

Once the proximate arrival of the donor heart is ensured, the recipient is placed on bypass and cooled. Snares are secured around the caval cannulae, the ascending aorta clamped, and the native heart excised (Fig. 16.66) Vascular cuffs are preserved that are appropriate for implantation of the donor heart (Figs. 16.67, 16.68, and 16.69). The donor heart is then prepared according to the implant technique to be used (Fig. 16.66B).

Implant techniques and the sequence of vascular anastomosis vary widely between surgeons, as do strategies used to protect the ischemic organ during implantation. The biatrial orthotopic heart transplantation technique is simple, easy to teach, and still used by many surgeons (8) (Fig. 16.67). The donor atria are spatulated open, trimmed if necessary, and laid over the recipient's atrial remnants. The left atrial suture line is everted to achieve endothelial apposition and to avoid leaving epicardial fat or muscle exposed in the lumen as a potential nidus for thromboemboli. Sinoatrial node dysfunction can usually be prevented by keeping the donor right atriotomy anterior to the sinoatrial node and its blood supply (Fig. 16.67A) and by optimizing graft preservation (31). Even if most of the dilated native atrium is excised, atrioventricular (AV) valve annular geometry may be distorted, causing regurgitation, or the area around the sinus node may be placed under tension, leading to atrial arrhythmias or sinus node dysfunction.

During the 1990s, these considerations led to evaluation of alternate atrial anastomotic techniques, including bicaval

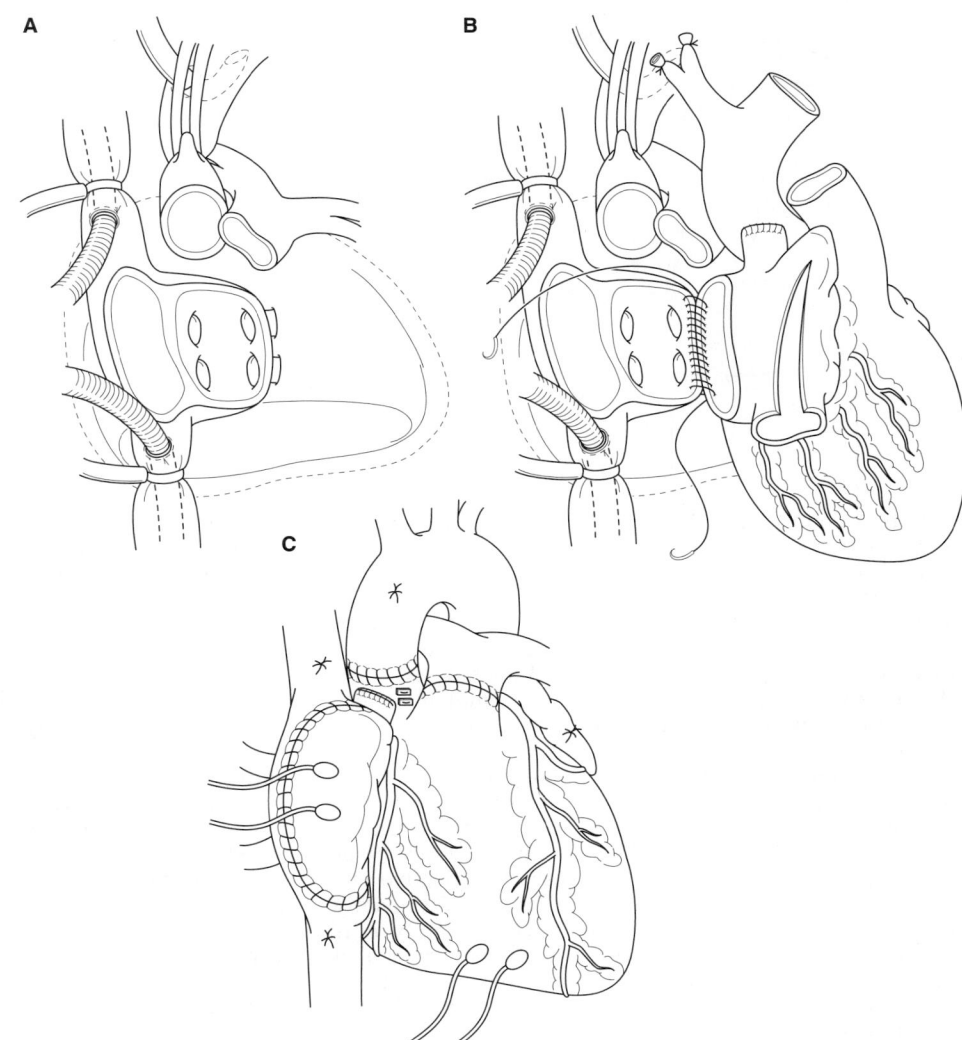

Figure 16.67. Traditional Lower/Shumway biatrial technique. *(A)* Recipient cuffs, prepared for bicaval atrial implant technique. After completion of the left atrial anastamosis *(B)*, the right atrial cuffs are joined. Care is taken to avoid carrying the right atrial incision or suture line close to the donor sinoatrial node, at the SVC/RA junction. *(C)* Appearance of the operative field after completion of great vessel anastomoses, weaning from cardiopulmonary bypass, and decannulation.

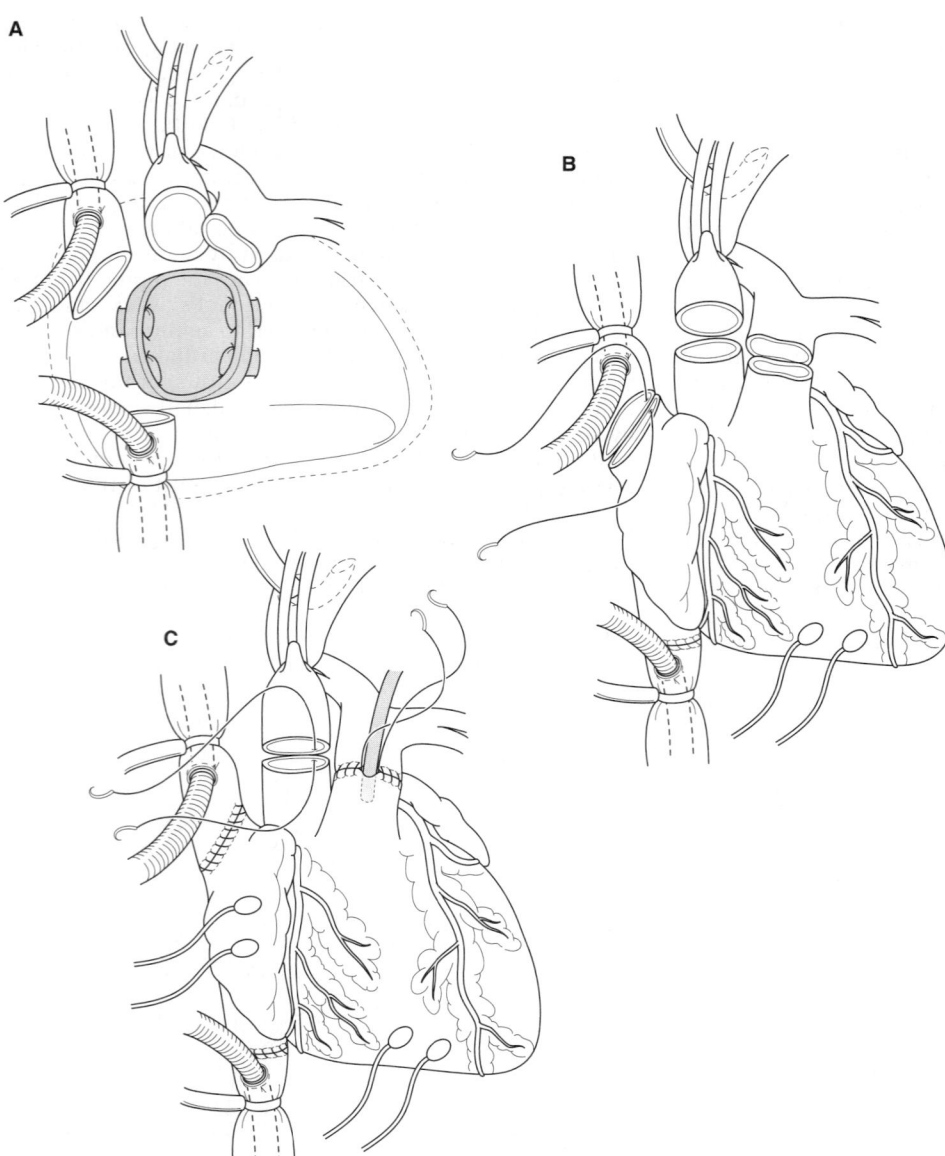

Figure 16.68. Bicaval right atrial implant technique. *(A)* During explanation of the native heart, the interatrial septum may be excised, for end-to-end anastamosis of the cavae *(B)*, or left in place (as in Fig. 16.2A), allowing the back walls of the donor cavae to be laid into those of the recipient. *(C)* Technique for pulmonary artery venting through an opening in the anterior aspect of this anastamosis, which is useful for de-airing and decompressing the right heart. Alternatively, the aorta may be anastamosed earlier in the operation, to minimized graft ischemic time.

right atrial connections (Fig. 16.68) and total AV replacement (two caval and two pulmonary vein anastomoses; Fig. 16.69). In a prospective, randomized trial (bicaval) (32) and several retrospective analyses (33,34), the incidence of atrial arrhythmias and AV valve regurgitation was reduced, and hemodynamic results and survival rates were improved with either the bicaval or total AV technique.

Independent of whether the aorta or pulmonary artery connection is performed first, the anterior aspect of the pulmonary artery anastomosis is usually left open or vented, to allow decompression of the right heart after reperfusion (Fig. 16.68C). The size mismatch between donor and recipient aortas is often dramatic, but can usually be accommodated by beveling the smaller vessel (usually the more pliable donor) to increase its effective circumference, and by distributing the discrepancy evenly over the length of each anastomosis. Occasionally it is necessary to tailor down the larger vessel or to replace an aneurysmal ascending aorta with donor tissue or a prosthetic graft. Functional pulmonary stenosis is avoided by trimming back both donor and recipient sufficiently to prevent redundancy.

An alternate "heterotopic" implantation technique places a second heart in the circulation, in parallel with the retained native heart (35). In principle, leaving the native heart affords protection in the event that the graft fails. The operation is technically demanding, usually produces compressive atelectasis in the right lung, and is associated with a high risk of stroke, perhaps because of stasis of blood in the native heart (36). Notwithstanding, this surgical approach may be considered for patients with high pulmonary vascular resistance unresponsive to vasodilators, and may in the future also find a role in the initial application of cardiac xenografts.

After completion of the anastomoses, the heart is reperfused and allowed to resume contracting without being required to function as a pump ("rested") as the recipient is rewarmed. Atrial and ventricular pacing wires are placed. Cardiac output of the denervated transplant is highly dependent on rate. In addition, the shorter cardiac filling time associated with higher heart rates prevents graft distention. Isoproterenol is initiated before weaning from bypass at a dosage of 0.005 to 0.02 µg/kg/min, and titrated to achieve a heart rate of approximately 110 beats per minute.

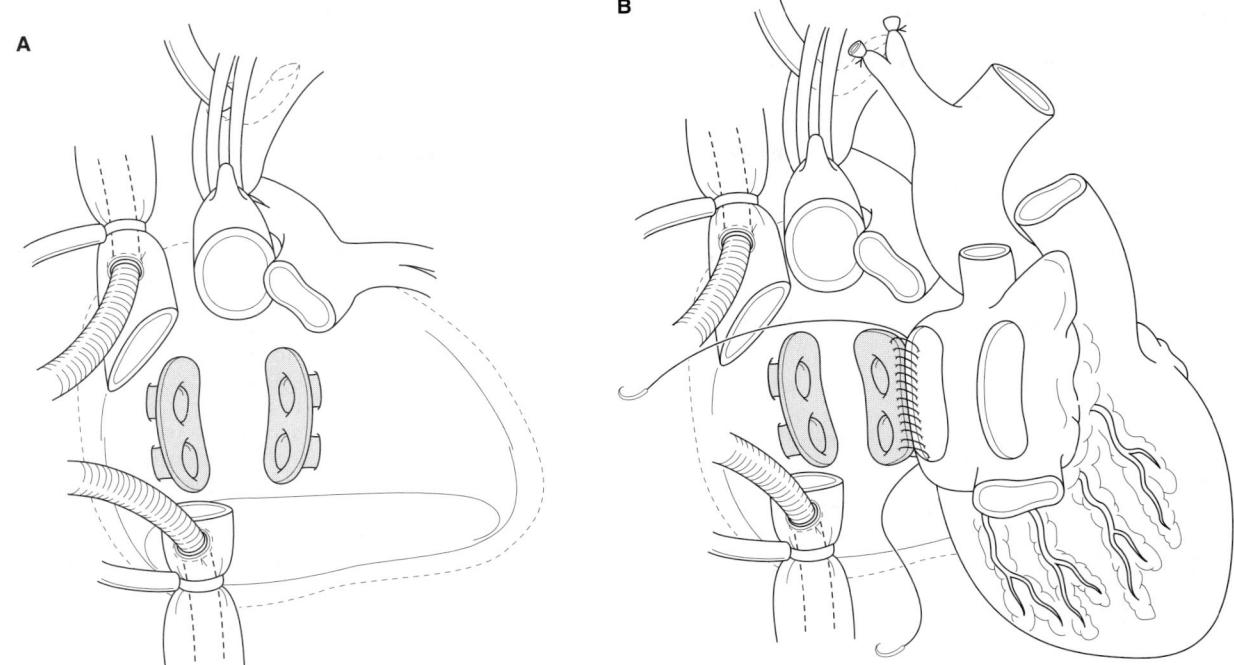

Figure 16.69. Total atrioventricular transplant technique. *(A)* Recipient pericardial well after preparation of bilateral pulmonary vein pedicles and caval cuffs, for total atrioventricular heart transplant. *(B)* Construction of left pulmonary vein anastamosis. As with other left atrial anastamotic approaches, atrial walls or vein cuffs are everted to minimize exposure of thrombogenic fat or muscle to the blood.

Patients with high preoperative pulmonary vascular resistance may be particularly difficult to wean from cardiopulmonary bypass, even with excellent function of the donor heart, because the "normal" donor right ventricle may acutely dilate and fail when confronted by a high-resistance pulmonary vascular bed. Resting the recently ischemic heart on cardiopulmonary bypass, establishing a stable sinus or AV sequentially paced rhythm, instituting inotropic support, and providing intraaortic balloon counterpulsation are useful in managing this problem. Traditional pharmacologic approaches to reducing pulmonary vascular resistance, such as prostaglandins E_1 and I_2 and sodium nitroprusside, may cause transpulmonary shunting of deoxygenated blood; these agents also reduce systemic vascular resistance and thus coronary perfusion pressure. Inhaled nitric oxide selectively dilates the pulmonary vascular bed before being rapidly inactivated by hemoglobin in the blood. We and others have found this very helpful to reduce pulmonary vascular resistance selectively without adverse effects on oxygenation or heart function, and this drug has been approved by the U.S. Food and Drug Administration for clinical use. Poor function of either or both ventricles may necessitate institution of mechanical support as a bridge to graft recovery or to retransplantation.

After surgery, ventilator and inotropic support is weaned, immunosuppression instituted, and diuretic and antihypertensive agents initiated as necessary. Isoproterenol is continued for approximately 5 days, and replaced with theophylline if needed to sustain a resting heart rate over 70. The first surveillance endomyocardial biopsy is performed 7 to 10 days after surgery, and repeated as an outpatient procedure approximately every 2 weeks for the first 3 months. Patient and caregiver education with regard to medication schedules and physiologic monitoring facilitate early discharge for patients without complications.

IMMUNOSUPPRESSION

The goal of immunosuppressive therapy is to prevent immune-mediated injury to the graft while minimizing associated complications, including opportunistic infection. Most programs use a triple-drug regimen, including a calcineurin inhibitor, an antimitotic agent, and steroids. This approach allows each individual drug to be used within its therapeutic window (Table 16.19).

Calcineurin inhibitors block NFkB activation, a cellular activation step critical to T-cell proliferation. Release of cytokines such as interleukin-2 is inhibited, along with activation of other T-cell-dependent pathogenic responses, such as maturation of cytotoxic T cells and provision of T-helper function to B cells. These drugs are not myelosuppressive, and have little direct effect on antigen-presenting cells or macrophages. They are usually dosed orally twice daily, with dose adjustments based on trough blood levels. Antimitotic agents cause an error in DNA replication in dividing cells that lack the purine (guanine and adenosine) salvage pathway, including T and B lymphocytes activated by donor antigens. Their primary toxicity is to other rapidly dividing cells in the surgical wound, bone marrow, and gastrointestinal tract. Dosing is adjusted for depressed white blood cell or platelet counts. Glucocorticoids dampen graft antigen-driven and other inflammatory events in endothelium, parenchyma, and neutrophils, and promote apoptosis of activated lymphocytes. Particularly at high doses or when recurrent rejection prohibits rapid weaning, side effects are multiple and are among those most troubling for patients (Table 16.19). For each class of immunosuppressants, intravenous preparations are available for patients unable to absorb enteral medications; substantial dose adjustments are required when calcineurin inhibitors are given by this route.

Some centers add antibody induction to triple therapy, using one of several available antilymphocyte antibody

Table 16.19. TYPICAL IMMUNOSUPPRESSIVE PROTOCOL AND ASSOCIATED MEDICAL THERAPY AFTER HEART TRANSPLANTATION

Calcineurin inhibitors
    Cyclosporine (2–4 mg/kg PO bid or 1–4 mg/h IV)
    FK506 (0.025–0.15 mg/kg PO bid)
        Side effects: Hypertension, renal insufficiency, tremor, hirsutism (cyclosporine only), gingival hyperplasia, diabetes (FK only)
Anti-mitotic agents
    Azathioprine (1–2 mg/kg/d qd)
    Mycophenylate mofetil (500–1500 mg/d bid)
        Side effects: Marrow suppression, nausea, abdominal cramps, diarrhea
Glucocorticoids
    Methylprednisolone IV, then
    Prednisone PO
        Side effects: Hypertension, insulin resistance, osteoporosis, mood swings, central obesity, cushingoid habitus
Antiprotozoal
    Trimethoprim–sulfamethoxazole (Pneumocystis, toxoplasmosis)
Antiviral
    Acyclovir (herpes)
    Gancyclovir (cytomegalovirus)
Antihypertensives
    ACE inhibitor or ACE receptor blocker
    Diltiazem (retards cyclosporine metabolism, reducing drug requirement)
    Alpha-receptor blockers
Antilipid agents
    Statin class agent

ACE, angiotensin-converting enzyme.

preparations. Monoclonal anti-CD3 or anti-interleukin-2 receptor antibodies selectively disable T-cell populations bearing one of the several receptors critical to the rejection response. These agents tend to delay the onset of the first rejection episode, but not to decrease the overall incidence of acute rejection (37,38). Polyclonal antibody preparations are made by immunizing animals with human lymphocytes or thymocytes; these agents inhibit a broader array of lymphocyte receptors, and may reduce the incidence of acute rejection (39). Induction therapy allows more gradual or delayed introduction of the calcineurin inhibitors, which can help prevent renal insufficiency in patients with marginal preoperative renal function, or when perioperative hemodynamic instability causes additional renal insult. The ability of induction therapy to improve long-term survival has been suggested but not proven for cardiac transplantation; some regimens are associated with a high incidence of "vascular" rejection, viral infection, and lymphoid malignancy (40–42).

Medical management after heart transplantation is focused on anticipation and prevention of common complications. Hypertension and hyperlipidemia are prevalent because of predisposition in the recipient patient population, and as side effects of various immunosuppressive agents. Prophylaxis against opportunistic infections includes agents targeted at common protozoal and viral pathogens (Table 16.19). Surveillance biopsies are performed according to a scheduled routine, and additional biopsies are performed to exclude rejection in the event of hemodynamic instability or unexplained fever. Typically, patients are able to leave the hospital within 10 days of uncomplicated operation, to be followed regularly in outpatient clinic. Monitored physical rehabilitation facilitates optimal cardiovascular and musculoskeletal recuperation (43), and occupational rehabilitation may offer important psychological and social benefits.

COMPLICATIONS

Complications of antirejection therapy relate primarily to the side effects of the specific immunosuppressive agents used. Infections tend to occur in patients with the greatest degree of preoperative debility and malnutrition, or in conjunction with additional stressors such as perioperative bleeding or hepatorenal dysfunction. Bacterial pathogens are common in the first several weeks, particularly in the lung and related to surgical or vascular access sites. Opportunistic viral and fungal infections usually predominate later. Increasingly effective prophylaxis for cytomegalovirus and herpesvirus infections have markedly reduced the morbidity associated with these common pathogens. When infection occurs, immunosuppression is tapered as aggressively as possible based on myocardial biopsy results.

Acute rejection occurs in most patients and is graded histologically according to standardized criteria developed by the International Society for Heart and Lung Transplantation (ISHLT). When detected at an early histologic stage (ISHLT grade 1; Fig. 16.70) in an asymptomatic patient on surveillance biopsy, rejection often responds to augmented oral steroids or an increased dose of calcineurin inhibitor. When a higher grade of rejection is found (Fig. 16.71) when the infiltrate fails to resolve in response to initial interventions, or in the setting of depressed cardiac function or shock, high-dose intravenous steroids are administered and antilymphocyte therapy often added. Inotropic or mechanical support is instituted as needed in hopes of rescuing graft and patient. Anti-

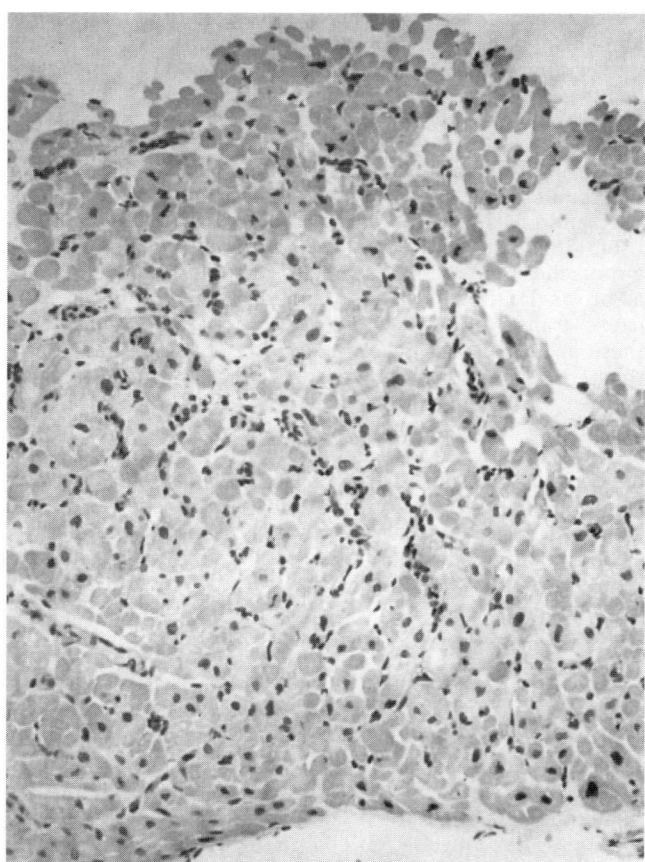

Figure 16.70.   Grade 1B—diffuse, mild acute rejection.

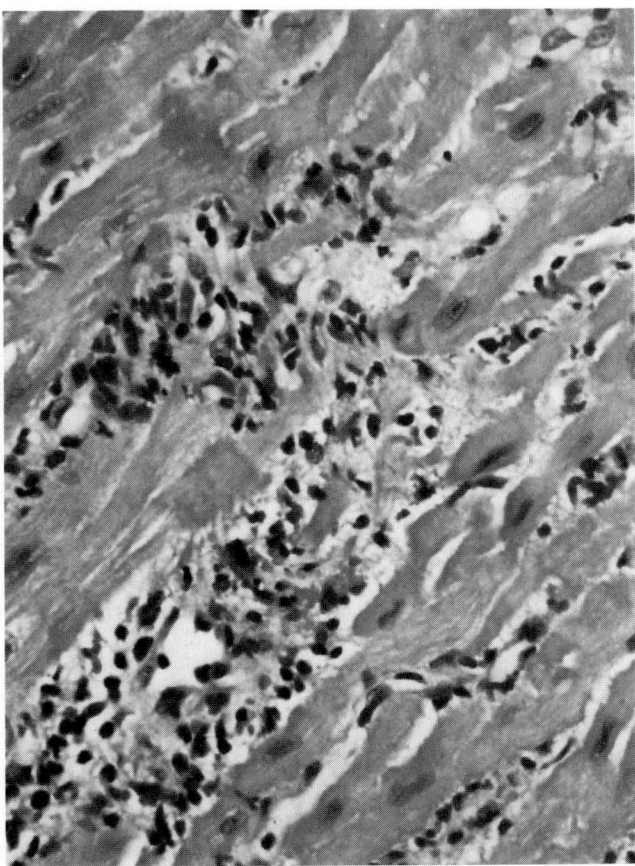

Figure 16.71. Grade 3A—multifocal, moderate acute rejection.

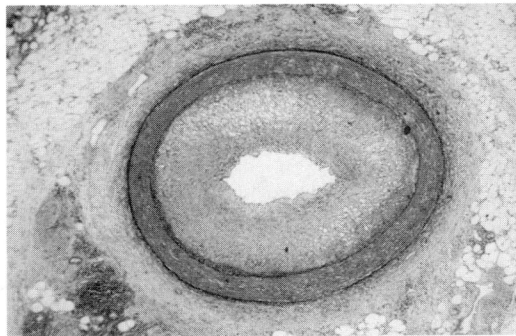

Figure 16.72. Autopsy specimen demonstrating moderately severe concentric fibroproliferative intimal lesion characteristic of cardiac allograft vasculopathy. (Courtesy of Dr. James Atkinson, Vanderbilt University Medical School, Nashville, TN.)

body-mediated vascular rejection is a controversial entity that, when documented by immunohistochemical techniques, may warrant introduction of cyclophosphamide or other agents with increased activity against B cells.

Bradycardia is prevalent in the denervated heart for the first weeks after transplantation, but a resting heart rate of over 70 beats per minute can usually be achieved by initiating a β-adrenergic agonist such as theophylline. Persistent bradycardia may be caused by ischemic, surgical, or immunologic injury to the sinus or AV nodes, or by amiodarone leaching from stores accumulated preoperatively in body fat; pacemaker implantation may be necessary. Atrial flutter or fibrillation may occur spontaneously, or herald acute rejection. This dysrhythmia can be difficult to manage because vagal denervation attenuates digoxin's modulation of the typical rapid ventricular response. Most other agents traditionally used to treat atrial arrhythmias depress AV node conduction or myocardial contractility, particularly undesirable side effects in a recent heart recipient. Amiodarone is in general better tolerated, controls heart rate and promotes conversion to sinus rhythm, and has been used widely in Europe in this circumstance.

Among patients who survive beyond the first year, the primary limit to long-term survival is cardiac allograft vasculopathy (CAV). (Fig. 16.72). Current understanding of the pathogenesis of CAV is incomplete (44). Widely presumed to be a consequence of "chronic rejection," this process has an incidence of approximately 5% per year. CAV may cause progressive insufficiency of coronary flow, myocardial infarction, and ultimately death. Research has drawn attention to the importance of donor stress associated with brain death and ischemia/reperfusion injury in the incidence and severity of CAV in animal models (45). In contrast to the usual pattern of focal proximal lesions in conventional atherosclerosis, coronary arteries are diffusely involved, and conventional revascularization techniques usually are not feasible. In the future, new immunosuppressive or antiproliferative agents may prevent this process or delay its progression (46).

RESULTS

The number of heart transplantations performed worldwide has declined, from a peak of approximately 4,070 in 1995 to fewer than 3,000 in 1999. This decline has occurred despite a steady increase in average donor age (15).

The operative survival rate in adults is over 90%, and both patient and graft 1-year survival rates exceed 80% (15) (Fig. 16.73). The most important risk factors for death in the first year include previous transplantation, increased donor age (with age >60 years conferring greater risk than age >45 years), need for ventilator or left ventricular assist device support before transplantation, and recipient age over 60 years. Rejection and infection together account for most of the mortality during the first year, and contribute approximately equally. Beyond the first year, malignancy, including posttransplantation lymphoproliferative disease, and chronic rejection emerge as prominent additional factors limiting long-term survival. Extrapolating from current early results, more than 50% of recent recipients can expect to be alive 10 years after transplantation, with an actuarial graft half-life of 12.3 years (28).

Repeat heart transplantation accounts for less than 2% of all heart transplantations done. When performed within the first 6 months, typically for early failure of the first graft, the 1-year survival rate is less than 40%. When performed later, usually for CAV, the 1-year survival rate is approximately 60%.

Adolescent (11 to 17 years of age) heart transplantation recipients fare better (>80% 1-year survival rate) than do younger children (1 to 10 years of age; ~77%) or infants (<1 year of age; ~68%). Less favorable short-term outcomes may be ascribed to pulmonary hypertension and anatomic challenges posed by congenital heart disease, and to monitoring and compliance challenges characteristic of these age groups. Nonetheless, the graft half-life for pediatric patients is similar to that for adults, ranging from 11.3 to 13 years of age (15,28).

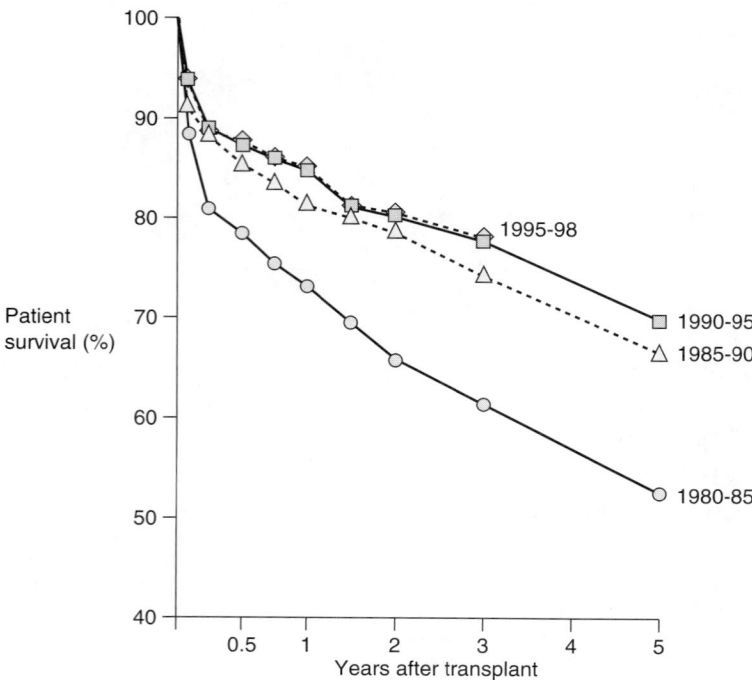

Figure 16.73. Heart transplant survival in adults, 1980–1998. Survival following heart transplantation in adult recipients (≥ 18 years), grouped by era of operation, analyzed by Kaplan-Meier method. After improving steadily during the 1980s, one- and three-year results have plateaued in the 1990s.

ETHICS

Ethical considerations are important to every aspect of heart transplantation. The donor pool is limited and appears to be shrinking despite extended donor acceptance criteria, restricting the number of patients who can undergo transplantation. This shortage forces consideration of ways to limit recipient candidacy (age limits), to increase the donor pool (presumed consent, advertising initiatives, community outreach), and to develop alternatives (mechanical devices; xenografts).

The heart transplantation community has taken the lead in standardizing patient selection and management guidelines, and has established policies for equitable organ allocation. Those given an opportunity to receive the "gift of life" are chosen from a much larger population who might benefit. Recipient candidacy decisions are made by a multidisciplinary group based on objective and subjective input from many people who come to know the patient and family in depth. Some recipient selection criteria are fundamentally arbitrary: age is retained as a criterion because of the limited supply of donor organs and based on the consensus view that younger patients deserve preferred access. Recipient selection criteria become unfair only if they are applied unequally or inconsistently at different programs or between various regions of the country.

Some of the most difficult decisions made by the heart transplantation team involve medically marginal candidates with outstanding and effective social support, or medically suitable candidates with marginal social support. Although most such patients will do well, outcomes in either case can, on average, be expected to fall below outcome benchmarks. For every marginal patient transplanted, a candidate who meets all the criteria may die. Thus, the "right" decision for an individual patient is difficult or impossible to know in advance, and may conflict with the best interests of the population of potential recipients.

CURRENT ISSUES

Quantifiable, objective measures of efficacy beyond survival, such as improvement in exercise capacity, freedom from complications, and reduced costs, are becoming the standards by which individual heart transplantation programs are judged. Most important to the patient are subjective factors such as quality of life and productivity, for which standardized measurement tools are being developed. Meanwhile, the efficacy of any proposed alternative to transplantation must be measured against survival, cost, and quality-of-life benchmarks established by this once-experimental procedure (47).

The most important factor currently restricting the application of heart transplantation is the limited supply of donor organs. Consent is obtained from the donor's legal representatives in only approximately 25% to 50% of cases where hearts are appropriate based on acceptable physiologic parameters. Various proactive approaches, such as institution of presumed consent, have been associated with high per capita donation rates in some countries. However, presumed consent is ethically dubious, and may violate basic cultural or religious precepts of individuals or ethnic groups. An adverse societal response to imposition of this unpopular approach as national policy might paradoxically cripple efforts to maintain organ donation even at current levels. Well-conceived efforts to increase the rate of consent, by passing laws requiring hospitals to facilitate and document the request, by allowing trained people to manage the request process, and by educating the public about "the gift of life," have boosted per capita donation in several U.S. organ procurement regions.

Efforts to develop improved immunosuppressive drugs are important and likely to yield incremental near-term improvements in the incidence of chronic rejection. Ideally, tolerance-permanent graft acceptance could be induced without a requirement for indefinite immunosuppressive therapy. Modulation, rather than suppression, of host responses to donor antigens may allow achievement of this goal (48).

Even if every physiologically suitable donor heart were available, only a minority of patients for whom transplantation would offer a survival advantage could be cared for using this modality. As technical issues related to transcutaneous power delivery, thromboembolism, infection risk, and reliability are addressed, mechanical assist devices are likely to emerge as definitive therapy for some patients. Progress has also been made toward use of porcine xenografts in humans, and the initial immunologic barrier, hyperacute rejection, appears surmountable using organs from pigs genetically modified to express human complement regulatory proteins (49). Control of subsequent cellular and antibody responses has proven difficult in animals models, but life-supporting function of renal xenografts for 3 months and heart xenografts for 1 month have been demonstrated in primates using an intensive regimen of conventional immunosuppressive agents (50–52).

Heart transplantation is one of the most resource-intensive modalities in modern medicine when assessed as cost per year of life saved. The procedure itself, the in-hospital care before transplantation, and maintenance of program infrastructure are very expensive. Ongoing pharmacy charges and surveillance procedure costs are also substantial. Paradoxically, patients physically able to return to work often cannot because they rely on medical disability benefits to pay for medications and follow-up care. Whether heart transplantation will continue to receive wide support is a function of societal acceptance of these costs, as currently reflected by coverage policies established by public and private health care insurers (47). In the future, the application of heart transplantation and related technologies may be limited more by what society chooses to afford, rather than what is medically possible.

REFERENCES

1. Carrel A, Guthrie CC. The transplantation of veins and organs. *Am Med* 1905;10:1101.
2. Carrel A. The surgery of blood vessels. *Bull Johns Hopkins Hosp* 1907;18:18.
3. Neptune WB, Cookson BA, Bailey CP, et al. Complete homologous heart transplantation. *Arch Surg* 1953;66:174.
4. Webb WR, Howard HS, Neely WA. Practical methods of homologous cardiac transplantation. *J Thorac Surg* 1959;37:361.
5. Goldberg M, Berman EF, Akman LC. Homologous transplantation of the canine heart. *J Int Coll Surg* 1958;30:575.
6. Cass MH, Brock R. Heart excision and replacement. *Guys Hosp Rep* 1959;108:285.
7. Demikhov VP. *Experimental transplantation of vital organs* [authorized translation from the Russian by Haigh B]. New York: New York Consultant's Bureau, 1962.
8. Lower RR, Stofer RC, Shumway NE. Homovital transplantation of the heart. *J Thorac Cardiovasc Surg* 1961;41:196.
9. Hardy JD, Chavez CM, Kurrus FE, et al. Heart transplantation in man: developmental studies and report of a case. *JAMA* 1964;188:1132.
10. Barnard CN. The operation: a human cardiac transplant. Interim report of a successful operation performed at Groote Schuur Hospital, Cape Town. *S Afr Med J* 1967;41:1271.
11. Caves PK, Stinson EB, Braham AF, et al. Percutaneous transvenous endomyocardial biopsy. *JAMA* 1973;225:288.
12. Kaye MP, Elcombe SA, O'Fallon WM. The International Heart Transplantation Registry: the 1984 report. *J Heart Transplant* 1985;4:290–292.
13. Calne RY, White DJ, Rolles K, et al. Prolonged survival of pig orthotopic heart grafts treated with Cyclosporin A. *Lancet* 1978;1:1183.
14. Reitz BA, Bieber CP, Raney AA, et al. Orthotopic heart and combined heart and lung transplantation with Cyclosporin-A immune suppression. *Transplant Proc* 1981;13:393.
15. Hosenpud JD, Bennet LE, Keck BM, et al. The Registry of the International Society for Heart and Lung Transplantation: sixteenth official report. *J Heart Lung Transplant* 1999;18:611–626.
16. Everett JE, Djalilian AR, Kubo SH, et al. Heart transplantation for patients over age 60. *Clin Transplant* 1996;10:478–481.
17. Blanche C, Takkenberg JJ, Nessim S, et al. Heart transplantation in patients 65 years of age and older: a comparative analysis of 40 patients. *Ann Thorac Surg* 1996;62:1442–1446.
18. O'Connell JB, Gunnar RM, Evans RW, et al. Task force 1: organization of heart transplantation in the U.S. *J Am Coll Cardiol* 1993;22:8.
19. Chomsky DB, Lang CC, Rayos GH, et al. Hemodynamic exercise testing: a valuable tool in the selection of cardiac transplantation candidates. *Circulation* 1996;94:3176–3183.
20. Stevenson LW. Selection and management of the potential candidate for cardiac transplantation. In: Cooper DKC, Miller LW, Patterson GA, eds. *Transplantation and replacement of thoracic organs,* 2nd ed. Lancaster, UK: Kluwer Academic Press, 1996:161–176.
21. Massie BM. 15 years of heart-failure trials: what have we learned? *Lancet* 1998;352[Suppl 1]:SI29–SI33.
22. Sackner-Bernstein JD. Use of carvedilol in chronic heart failure: challenges in therapeutic management. *Prog Cardiovasc Dis* 1998;41[Suppl 1]:53–58.
23. Jeevanandam V, Furukawa S, Prendergast TW, et al. Standard criteria for an acceptable donor heart are restricting heart transplantation. *Ann Thorac Surg* 1996;62:1268–1275.
24. Drinkwater DC, Laks H, Blitz A, et al. Outcomes of patients undergoing transplantation with older donor hearts. *J Heart Lung Transplant* 1996;15:684–691.
25. Tenderich G, Koerner MM, Stuettgen B, et al. Extended donor criteria: hemodynamic follow-up of heart transplant recipients receiving a cardiac allograft from donors > or = 60 years of age. *Transplantation* 1998;66:1109–1113.
26. Novitsky D, Cooper DKC, Reichart B. Hemodynamic and metabolic responses to hormonal therapy in brain-dead potential organ donors. *Transplantation* 1987;43:852–854.
27. Rosengard BR. Donor management initiative. *Chimera* 1999;10(3):12–13.
28. Opelz G. Results of cardiac transplantation and factors influencing survival based on the collaborative heart transplant study. In: Cooper DKC, Miller LW, Patterson GA, eds. *Transplantation and replacement of thoracic organs,* 2nd ed. Lancaster, UK: Kluwer Academic Press, 1996:417–427.
29. Sapirstein JS, Pae WE Jr. Mechanical circulatory support before heart transplantation. In: Cooper DKC, Miller LW, Patterson GA, eds. *Transplantation and replacement of thoracic organs,* 2nd ed. Lancaster, UK: Kluwer Academic Press, 1996:185–194.
30. Wieselthaler GM, Chevtchik O, Konetschny R, et al. Improved graft function using a new myocardial preservation solution: Celsior. Preliminary data from a randomized prospective study. *Transplant Proc* 1999;31:2067–2068.
31. Jeevanandam V, Barr ML, Auteri JS, et al. University of Wisconsin solution versus crystalloid cardioplegia for human donor heart preservation: a randomized blinded prospective clinical trial. *J Thorac Cardiovasc Surg* 1992;103:194–198.
32. el Gamel A, Yonan NA, Grant S, et al. Orthotopic cardiac transplantation: a comparison of standard and bicaval Wythenshawe techniques. *J Thorac Cardiovasc Surg* 1995;109:721–729.
33. Aziz T, Burgess M, Khafagy R, et al. Bicaval and standard techniques in orthotopic heart transplantation: medium-term experience in cardiac performance and survival. *J Thorac Cardiovasc Surg* 1999;118:115–122.
34. Trento A, Takkenberg JM, Czer LS, et al. Clinical experience with one hundred consecutive patients undergoing orthotopic heart transplantation with bicaval and pulmonary venous anastomoses. *J Thorac Cardiovasc Surg* 1996;112:1496–1502.
35. Cooper DKC, Taniguchi S. Heterotopic heart transplantation: indications, surgical techniques, and special considerations. In: Cooper DKC, Miller LW, Patterson GA, eds. *Transplantation and replacement of thoracic organs,* 2nd ed. Lancaster, UK: Kluwer Academic Press, 1996:353–365.
36. Tagusari O, Kormos RL, Kawai A, et al. Native heart complications after heterotopic heart transplantation: insight into the potential risk of left ventricular assist device. *J Heart Lung Transplant* 1999;18:1111–1119.
37. Starnes VA, Oyer PE, Stinson EB, et al. Prophylactic OKT3 used as induction therapy for heart transplantation. *Circulation* 1989;80[Suppl III]:79–83.
38. van Gelder T, Baan CC, Balk AH, et al. Blockade of the interleukin (IL)-2/IL-2 receptor pathway with a monoclonal anti-IL-2 receptor antibody (BT563) does not prevent the development of acute heart allograft rejection in humans. *Transplantation* 1998;65:405–410.

39. Carey JA, Frist WH. Use of polyclonal antilymphocytic preparations for prophylaxis in heart transplantation. *J Heart Transplant* 1990;9:297–300.

40. Miller LW, Naftel DC, Bourge RC, et al. Infection after heart transplantation: a multiinstitutional study: Cardiac Transplant Research Database Group. *J Heart Lung Transplant* 1994;13:381–392.

41. Swinnen LJ, Costanzo-Nordin MR, Fisher SG, et al. Increased incidence of lymphoproliferative disorder after immunosuppression with the monoclonal antibody OKT3 in cardiac-transplant recipients. *N Engl J Med* 1990;323:1723–1728.

42. Hammond EH, Wittwer CT, Greenwood J, et al. Relationship of OKT3 sensitization and vascular rejection in cardiac transplant patients receiving OKT3 rejection prophylaxis. *Transplantation* 1990;50:776–782.

43. Kobashigawa JA, Leaf DA, Lee N, et al. A controlled trial of exercise rehabilitation after heart transplantation. *N Engl J Med* 1999;340:272–277.

44. Pierson RN III, Miller GM. Late graft failure: lessons from clinical and experimental thoracic organ transplantation. *Graft* 2000;3:88–93.

45. Schmid C, Heemann U, Tilney NL. Factors contributing to the development of chronic rejection in heterotopic rat heart transplantation. *Transplantation* 1997;64:222–228.

46. Hausen B, Morris RE. Review of immunosuppression for lung transplantation: novel drugs, new uses for conventional immunosuppressants, and alternative strategies. *Clin Chest Med* 1997;16:353–366.

47. Evans RW. Socioeconomic aspects of heart transplantation. *Curr Opin Cardiol* 1995;10:169–179.

48. Harlan DM, Kirk AD. The future of organ and tissue transplantation: can T-cell costimulatory pathway modifiers revolutionize the prevention of graft rejection? *JAMA* 1999;282:1076–1082.

49. Cozzi E, White DJ. The generation of transgenic pigs as potential organ donors for humans. *Nat Med* 1995;1:964–966.

50. Zaidi A, Schmoeckel M, Bhatti F, et al. Life-supporting pig-to-primate renal xenotransplantation using genetically modified donors. *Transplantation* 1998;65:1584–1590.

51. Schmoeckel M, Bhatti FN, Zaidi A, et al. Orthotopic heart transplantation in a transgenic pig-to-primate model. *Transplantation* 1998;65:1570–1577; and data presented in abstract form, 5th International Congress of the International Xenotransplantation Association, Nagoya, Japan, October 25, 1999.

52. Vial CM, Bhatti FNK, Ostlie DJ, et al. Enhanced survival of orthotopic cardiac xenografts in an hDAF transgenic pig-to-primate baboon model. Abstract book, 5th International Congress of the Xenotransplantation Association, Nagoya, Japan, October 1999, 49.

Pulmonary Transplantation

LARRY R. KAISER AND ROBERT C. GORMAN

Transplantation of the lung represents one of the last horizons in solid-organ transplantation. After an initial effort at human pulmonary transplantation in 1963, there was considerable excitement but little activity in this area until 1967, when a flurry of pulmonary transplantations followed the first successful human cardiac transplantation. The longest lung transplantation survivor during this early period lived 10 months, most of that time spent in the hospital. The major problems preventing successful pulmonary transplantation have been failure of the airway anastomosis to heal, infection, and rejection (1).

Unlike other solid organs, the lung has no systemic arterial supply that can be reconnected. Bronchial arterial anatomy varies greatly, and the size of bronchial arteries, even when they can be identified, precludes direct anastomosis. Therefore, the bronchial anastomosis is ischemic after the operation, and airway dehiscence may occur ap-

proximately 3 weeks after transplantation. The combination of anastomotic ischemia and other factors, including the susceptibility of the lung to infection because of its direct contact with the outside environment by the airway, prevented successful transplantation despite the efforts of many investigators (2).

The first combined heart and lung transplantation was performed successfully in 1981, but the procedure sometimes required removal of an otherwise normal heart from the recipient. Combined cardiac and pulmonary transplantation introduced a series of new problems related to transplanting two organs, including those associated with heart transplantation and especially accelerated coronary artery atherosclerosis. With combined cardiac and pulmonary transplantation, however, healing of the tracheal anastomosis presents less of a problem, probably because the bronchial artery collaterals in the subcarinal space are preserved.

Recognizing the potential advantage of single-lung transplantation, investigators experimentally defined the factors contributing to failure in pulmonary transplantation (3). They demonstrated the significant detrimental effect that corticosteroids exert on airway healing and showed that cyclosporine did not have this adverse effect. Delaying the administration of maintenance corticosteroids proved advantageous. The investigators also demonstrated that wrapping the bronchial anastomosis with a pedicle of gastrocolic omentum resulted in early capillary ingrowth and revascularization of the airway, promoting healing.

Another significant factor contributing to the improved success of single-lung transplantation was the recognition that careful recipient selection is crucial. Initially, it was felt that the ideal candidate for single-lung transplantation was a patient with end-stage restrictive disease (pulmonary fibrosis), a situation that would lead to preferential ventilation and perfusion of the graft because of the increased compliance and relatively decreased pulmonary vascular resistance of the transplanted lung. In addition, although almost all previous attempts at pulmonary transplantation involved desperately ill, ventilator-dependent patients, lung replacement in a moribund patient who has already experienced significant nutritional depletion and muscle wasting is likely to fail. It is important to select patients who are ambulatory and to place potential recipients in an intense pretransplantation pulmonary rehabilitation program to increase the likelihood of a successful outcome. Improvement in patient selection may indeed be the single most important factor responsible for the success of pulmonary transplantation, even though indications for pulmonary transplantation have broadened considerably.

INDICATIONS

A patient should be referred for transplantation at a point in the course of the disease at which death is considered likely within several years, so that transplantation would be expected to confer a survival advantage. The patient's perception of an unacceptably poor quality of life is an important additional consideration, but the prognosis must be the overriding impetus for referral. Integrated into the decision must be an anticipated waiting time of up to 2 years, during which the candidate's condition must remain functionally suitable for transplantation (4). Patients usually have either predominantly obstructive or restrictive disease, although occasionally they may have a mixed defect. Those with end-stage obstructive physiology may demonstrate changes of emphysema, either nonbullous or bullous, or changes secondary to chronic infection (bronchitic). Patients with cystic fibrosis fall into the latter category, their lung disease resulting from the ravages of chronic, persistent infection (bronchiectasis). Patients

Table 16.20. GENERAL INDICATIONS FOR PULMONARY TRANSPLANTATION

Advanced obstructive, fibrotic, or pulmonary vascular disease with a high risk of death within 2 to 3

Lack of success or availability of alternative therapies

Severe functional limitation, but preserved ability to walk

Less than 60 years old

Less than 60 years old

with cystic fibrosis may also present with a mixed obstructive–restrictive picture. Those with idiopathic pulmonary fibrosis have restrictive physiology. Patients with a congenital deficiency of the α_1-antitrypsin protease commonly present with bullous emphysema, most noticeable at the lung bases. A number of patients also have radiographic and physiologic changes that are similar to those seen in α_1-antitrypsin deficiency, but with levels of α_1-antitrypsin that are normal, suggesting the absence of other, as yet undescribed, proteases.

Patients with pulmonary vascular disease are a distinct group. Those with end-stage disease have either primary pulmonary hypertension, a disease of unknown cause, or secondary pulmonary hypertension, resulting from increased pulmonary perfusion caused by a shunt at the cardiac or supracardiac level. When pulmonary vascular resistance increases sufficiently, the resultant increase in pulmonary artery pressure reverses shunt flow from right to left. This condition is known as *Eisenmenger syndrome.* When shunt reversal occurs, patients are typically considered inoperable because the mortality rate associated with

primary cardiac operations is prohibitive. Theoretically, it is feasible to close the cardiac shunt with insertion of a new lung or lungs, thus unloading the right ventricle with a subsequent decrease in pulmonary vascular resistance to normal levels and improvement of right ventricular function.

Because of problems with donor availability, lung transplantation is limited to patients 60 to 65 years of age or younger who have no other systemic disease and who have no significant coronary artery disease. The criteria used in selecting pulmonary transplant recipients are outlined in Table 16.20.

Candidates for pulmonary transplantation ordinarily have significant functional impairment that interferes with activities of daily living. In patients with restrictive or obstructive disease, abnormal gas exchange is the major problem, and essentially all require supplemental oxygen 24 hours a day. In patients with pulmonary vascular disease, the manifestations of right ventricular failure predominate. These patients may or may not require oxygen.

Disease-specific guidelines for timely referral, which are based on available prognostic indexes, have recently been published (Table 16.21). Of all patients referred for transplantation evaluation, approximately 30% are ultimately accepted.

Potential candidates need to be extremely well motivated to cope with the stresses associated with both the pretransplantation and posttransplantation periods and with the lifelong care they require after transplantation. Transplantation trades one chronic disease for another–the posttransplantation state. Patients require daily medication to maintain their transplanted organ and are constantly at risk for infection.

CONTRAINDICATIONS

Absolute and relative contraindications to lung transplantation are listed in Table 16.22 (5). Relative contraindications include chronic medical conditions such as

Table 16.21. DISEASE-SPECIFIC INDICATIONS FOR PULMONARY TRANSPLANTATION

CHRONIC OBSTRUCTIVE PULMONARY DISEASE
- FEV_1 <25% of predicted value after bronchodilator therapy
- Clinically significant hypoxemia, hypercapnia, or pulmonary hypertension; rapid decline in lung function; or frequent severe exacerbations

IDIOPATHIC PULMONARY FIBROSIS
- Symptomatic disease unresponsive to medical therapy
- Vital capacity <60%–70% of predicted value
- Evidence of resting or exercise-induced hypoxemia

CYSTIC FIBROSIS
- FEV_1 ≤30% of predicted value
- FEV_1 >30% with rapidly declining lung function, frequent severe exacerbations, or progressive weight loss
- Female sex and age <18 y with FEV1 30%[a]

PRIMARY PULMONARY HYPERTENSION
- NYHA functional class III or IV
- Mean pulmonary artery pressure >55 mm Hg
- Mean right atrial pressure >15 mm Hg
- Cardiac index <2 L/min/m²
- Failure of medical therapy, especially intravenous epoprostenol, to improve NYHA functional class or hemodynamic indices.

EISENMENGER'S SYNDROME
- NYHA functional class III or IV despite optimal medical management

[a]These factors are associated with a poorer prognosis; therefore, early referral may be indicated.

FEV_1, forced expiratory volume in 1 second; NYHA, New York Heart Association.

Adapted from Arcasoy SM, Kotloff RM. Lung transplantation. N Engl J Med 1999;340:1081–1091.

Table 16.22. CONTRAINDICATIONS TO PULMONARY TRANSPLANTATION

ABSOLUTE CONTRAINDICATIONS
Severe extrapulmonary organ dysfunction, including renal insufficiency with a creatinine clearance below 50 mL/min, hepatic dysfunction with coagulopathy or portal hypertension, and left ventricular dysfunction or severe coronary artery disease (consider heart–lung transplantation)

Acute, critical illness

Active cancer or recent history of cancer with substantial likelihood of recurrence (except for basal cell and squamous cell carcinoma of the skin)

Active extrapulmonary infection (including infection with HIV; hepatitis B, indicated by the presence of hepatitis B surface antigen; and hepatitis C with evidence of liver disease on biopsy)

Severe psychiatric illness, noncompliance with therapy, and drug or alcohol dependence

Active or recent (preceding 3–6 mo) cigarette smoking

Severe malnutrition (<70% of ideal body weight) or marked obesity (>130% of ideal body weight)

Inability to walk, with poor rehabilitation potential

RELATIVE CONTRAINDICATIONS
Chronic medical conditions that are poorly controlled or associated with target-organ damage

Daily requirement for more than 20 mg of prednisone (or equivalent)

Mechanical ventilation (excluding noninvasive ventilation)

Extensive pleural thickening from prior thoracic surgery or infection

Adapted from Arcasoy SM, Kotloff RM. Lung transplantation. N Engl J Med 1999;340:1081–1091.

osteoporosis, hypertension, diabetes mellitus, and coronary artery disease, which may worsen after transplantation and are acceptable in a candidate only if they have not resulted in end-organ damage and are well controlled with standard therapy. Perioperative corticosteroid therapy was once considered an absolute contraindication because it was thought to be associated with impaired bronchial anastomotic healing (6). Because of improved surgical techniques, transplantation can now be performed safely in patients who receive moderate doses of corticosteroids (7). Although patients receiving mechanical ventilation have undergone successful transplantation, as a group they have a higher mortality rate (4,8).

DONOR CONSIDERATIONS

Plain chest radiographs are used to assess potential donor lungs. In addition, bronchoscopy provides a way to examine directly the potential donor organs and to collect material for culture and Gram stain, the results of which may influence later treatment of the recipient. No other organ has the same risk of infection; a pulmonary infiltrate may preclude the use of a lung. A small infiltrate in one lung without evidence of purulent secretions may still allow this lung to be used in a double-lung transplantation. Likewise, a pulmonary infiltrate does not necessarily preclude use of the contralateral lung for single-lung transplantation. Unfortunately, the lungs of a particular donor may not be suitable when all other organs are acceptable. Because all brain-dead patients have endotracheal tubes and are on mechanical ventilation, there is a high likelihood that the airway is either colonized with bacteria or that there is ongoing invasive infection. With pulmonary infection, an infiltrate is often present on chest radiography. Even with a clear chest radiograph, purulent secretions preclude using the lungs for transplantation.

Problems with the lungs may begin when the insult that results in brain death occurs because the patient may aspirate gastric contents. Signs of aspiration may not be evident on the chest radiograph for 24 to 48 hours, underscoring the importance of bronchoscopy before accepting lungs for transplantation. Characteristic early bronchoscopic evidence of aspiration includes erythematous tracheobronchial mucosa, purulent secretions, and occasionally the presence of food particles.

Major pulmonary contusion resulting from blunt chest trauma also may eliminate lungs from donor consideration, but minor to moderate contusion unilaterally may still allow use of the lungs in a bilateral lung recipient. Evaluating the full extent of contusion at the time of donor retrieval is often difficult because the interval from injury to determination of brain death and donation may be short. Although the detrimental effect on gas exchange caused by a pulmonary contusion is usually transient, further bleeding into the lung parenchyma could occur if cardiopulmonary bypass is required to perform the transplantation, as would be the case in a recipient with pulmonary hypertension.

Pulmonary edema may occur as a result of massive head injury and may be further complicated by certain donor management protocols, which include the following:

- Maintenance of mean arterial blood pressure above 70 mm Hg
- Preference of inotropic support over massive volumes of crystalloid solution to maintain blood pressure (dopamine, 2.5 to 10 mg/kg/min)
- Replacement of fluid at the rate of the previous hour's urine output plus 100 mL
- Maintenance of normothermia

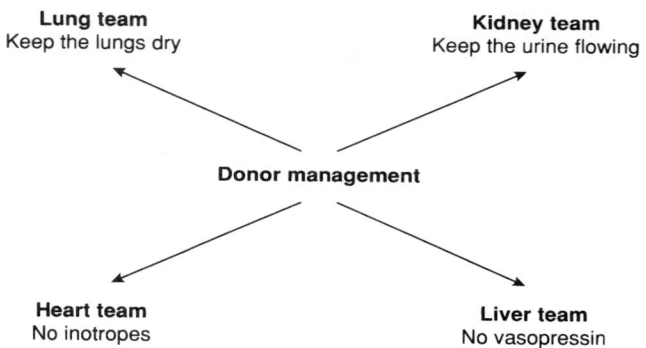

Figure 16.74. Each organ retrieval team has its own set of donor management protocols that often conflict.

- Maintenance of positive end-expiratory pressure at 5 cm H_2O
- Frequent endotracheal suctioning
- Gram staining of sputum
- Monitoring of arterial blood gases every 2 hours

Traditionally, renal transplantation teams have tried to ensure that adequate urine output is preserved; therefore, they preferentially infuse large volumes of crystalloid solutions. Cardiac transplantation teams prefer to avoid using high doses of inotropic agents to maintain blood pressure and also tend to administer large amounts of crystalloid solutions (Fig. 16.74). The importance of coordinating donor management to prevent "flooding" of the lungs, which are much more susceptible to the development of edema after significant cerebral insult, cannot be overstated if lungs are to be available for transplantation. Whether such edematous lungs may be "dried out" when in place in the recipient remains to be determined. The contribution of pulmonary lymphatics, of necessity severed during the donor retrieval at the time of bronchus division, to the clearing of edema in the pulmonary parenchyma is unknown.

Most commonly, lungs are refused after an initial acceptance because the results of bronchoscopy are abnormal or because arterial blood gases deteriorate significantly between the time of acceptance and the time the retrieval team reaches the donor hospital. Size of the donor lungs is less important when the recipient has emphysema, in which each hemithorax is very large, compared with pulmonary fibrosis, in which the hemithorax is contracted. The most important size consideration is a reasonable match between donor and recipient height.

LUNG PRESERVATION

An important area of investigation involves the optimal preservation technique for the ischemic lung. The donor lung must not only remain viable, it must participate actively in gas exchange immediately after implantation. A protocol is employed that uses both a flush technique with cold crystalloid solution and topical cooling to 4°C by immersion. At the time of donor lung retrieval, just before crossclamping of the aorta, prostaglandin E_1 is injected directly into the pulmonary artery to vasodilate the pulmonary vascular bed. Vasodilatation allows for more uniform distribution of the flush solution and for more uniform and rapid cooling. Prostaglandin E_1 may also serve a cytoprotective role by a mechanism yet to be determined. Crystalloid solution (Euro-Collins) at 4°C is rapidly flushed into the pulmonary artery. After removal of the donor heart, leaving a cuff of left atrium around the pulmonary veins, the lungs are removed by dividing the trachea above the carina and the pulmonary artery just proximal to the bifurcation.

The maximal safe interval for the lung to remain ischemic even when cooled has not been defined. Based on empiric observation, 6 hours has been selected as the limit. This time constraint places limits on the distance that may be traveled to procure lungs. The limits of donor lung ischemia have been expanded because of efforts to develop bilateral, sequential lung replacement. The second lung to be implanted perforce is ischemic for a longer time because the lungs are not implanted simultaneously. The longest cold ischemic time has been in the range of 9 to 10 hours, and the lung functioned well within 24 hours after implantation. Although donor lung dysfunction occasionally occurs (5% to 10% incidence), it is usually reversible. Also, the development of this problem has not correlated with prolonged donor lung ischemic time.

Whether one type of preservation solution is superior remains to be determined. A low-potassium dextran solution may be better for early lung function than the standard Euro-Collins solution. One clinical study demonstrated less reperfusion injury, better immediate and intermediate function, as well as better early and long-term survival for donor lungs preserved with low-potassium dextran compared with Euro-Collins (9). Other methods of preservation have also been used experimentally. Core cooling of the donor with an extracorporeal circuit has been used extensively in the United Kingdom for cardiopulmonary transplantation. Others have used an immersion technique without flushing the pulmonary artery.

It is believed that lung injury results not only from the ischemic insult but from reperfusion of the ischemic organ. Several experimental models of acute lung injury implicate oxygen free radicals as a factor in the genesis of reperfusion injury. A significant early increase in lung permeability is seen after an ischemic period followed by reperfusion. Permeability improves within several hours. Changes in the contralateral, nonischemic lung are presumably due to substances released during reperfusion of the ischemic lung. Efforts are directed at identifying techniques to attenuate the reperfusion injury.

Most experimental studies in lung preservation to date have been empiric, evaluating the effects of various techniques on subsequent lung function. Further progress requires a more detailed understanding of events at the cellular level during ischemia and reperfusion so that a rational approach to reduce or eliminate these changes may evolve. Satisfactory preservation techniques must protect not only cell structure and metabolism, but functional integrity of the lung as a whole to maintain normal gas exchange. Methods of preservation that allow for a prolonged ischemic time must also preserve the viability and microcirculation of the airway to prevent subsequent complications of airway healing. It would serve no useful purpose to extend the ischemic time, only to have the airway fail to heal because of thrombosis in small vessels. Given the ability safely to preserve livers and kidneys for 24 hours or longer, it seems likely that donor lung preservation times will be extended in the near future.

TRANSPLANTATION OPERATION

Whether one lung or both lungs are replaced depends on recipient factors, including the cause of the end-stage pulmonary disease as well as donor lung availability. Patients with chronic infection, such as those with cystic fibrosis, require replacement of both lungs. Patients with restrictive physiology (pulmonary fibrosis) do well with single-lung replacement. The situation in patients with end-stage obstructive disease, specifically emphysema, offers considerably more variability. Early in the pulmonary transplantation experience, it became evident that problems resulted from leaving the native emphysematous lung in situ. Air trapping in the remaining native lung, with resultant mediastinal shift, significantly crowded the transplanted lung, resulting in poor expansion and minimal function. Ventilation ($\dot{V}$) preferentially went to the overly compliant native lung, whereas most of the perfusion ($\dot{Q}$) went to the newly transplanted lung, creating a significant $\dot{V}/\dot{Q}$ mismatch that further worsened an already precarious situation.

Despite these concerns, single-lung transplantation not only is an acceptable operation for patients with emphysema, it may be the operation of choice for patients older than 50 years of age (10). Data demonstrate improved forced expiratory volume in 1 second (FEV1) and 6-minute walk results in patients with emphysema undergoing single- versus double-lung transplantation at 1 year. Whether this result will translate into improved long-term survival or functional level is unknown. From a donor standpoint, single-lung transplantation, when acceptable, is a more efficient use of donor organs. The decision to use single-lung transplantation for emphysema evolved mainly from experience with the original *en bloc* double-lung operation, which involved a tracheal anastomosis and routine cardiopulmonary bypass and resulted in significant perioperative cardiac morbidity and mortality.

Replacement of both lungs was greatly simplified by the development and refinement of the bilateral, sequential lung transplantation procedure. A bilateral thoracosternotomy incision ("clamshell" procedure) permits easier completion of the recipient pneumonectomies than is achieved using median sternotomy, and replacing the lungs sequentially usually avoids the need for cardiopulmonary bypass. Even previous chest operations are not contraindications to this procedure. This operation has replaced *en bloc* double-lung procedures and heart–lung transplantation as the operation of choice for patients with end-stage pulmonary disease who need both lungs and for those with pulmonary vascular disease.

In patients with pulmonary hypertension, it has not been determined whether it is preferable to replace one or both lungs. Originally, single-lung transplantation was chosen because replacing one lung allowed adequate unloading of the right ventricle with immediate improvement in right ventricular function and normalization of pulmonary artery pressures (Table 16.23). However, replacing both lungs in this patient population offers a better margin of safety in the perioperative period and results in better hemodynamics in the long term. Whether replacement of both lungs is absolutely required remains to be determined, but currently it is the preferred method in most transplantation centers for patients with pulmonary hypertension, despite donor limitations.

Table 16.23. HEMODYNAMICS DATA FOR SINGLE-LUNG TRANSPLANTATION IN PATIENTS WITH PULMONARY HYPERTENSION

Measurement	Pretransplantation	Posttransplantation
Pulmonary artery pressure		
Mean	58 mm Hg	16 mm Hg
Systolic	94 mm Hg	28 mm Hg
Right ventricular ejection fraction	25%	52%
Cardiac output	4 L/min	7 L/min
Pulmonary vascular resistance	1,302 dyne/cm^5/s	161 dyne/cm^5/s

OPERATIVE TECHNIQUE

Single-lung Transplantation

The performance of the donor operation does not vary because the attempt is always made to use both lungs, either for single-lung replacement on two recipients or for distribution to another transplantation medical center. This practice provides the most efficient use of limited donor organs. In the recipient operation, a standard posterolateral or muscle-sparing axillary thoracotomy is performed, with dissection of the hilar structures as usual for a pneumonectomy (Fig. 16.75). The dissection mobilizes the main pulmonary artery, both superior and inferior pulmonary veins, and the mainstem bronchus. When the donor lung arrives in the operating room, the recipient pneumonectomy is performed by dividing the hilar vessels as far *distally* as possible and the bronchus at the level of the upper lobe take-off.

The implantation operation begins with construction of an anastomosis between the donor and recipient bronchus done in a telescoping fashion with one end brought up inside the other by placing horizontal mattress sutures of nonabsorbable material. This anastomosis is followed by left atrial cuff anastomosis. The pulmonary artery anastomosis is usually performed last. The bronchial anastomosis, formerly wrapped with a pedicle of gastrocolic omentum, now is either wrapped with a piece of pericardial fat or left unwrapped because the telescoping anastomosis offers an added margin of safety for bronchial healing. Once the vascular anastomoses are constructed, clamps are removed and blood flow is reestablished as the lung is inflated. The chest is closed in standard fashion. Either the right or left lung may be transplanted. The decision about which side to transplant is based on both donor lung availability and recipient perfusion lung scan data. If one lung receives most of the perfusion, the opposite lung is transplanted.

Double-lung Transplantation

The technique of double-lung transplantation has evolved considerably since the late 1980s. The favored approach is essentially bilateral, sequential lung replacement (11). With the patient in the supine position, this operation is performed through a bilateral thoracosternotomy incision that includes anterolateral thoracotomies and a transverse sternotomy (Fig. 16.76), or bilateral anterior thoracotomies without sternal division. The bilateral thoracosternotomy incision provides excellent access to both hemithoraces, facilitating dissection and mobilization of hilar structures. This exposure is particularly important in recipients with diffuse or dense adhesions between the visceral and parietal pleural surfaces, as is often seen in patients with cystic fibrosis.

Although both lungs are replaced, the operation can usually be performed without cardiopulmonary bypass. By first replacing the lung with the least function, oxygenation and ventilation are maintained by the lung that receives the major fraction of perfusion. If the patient is unable to tolerate single-lung ventilation because of inadequate gas exchange or rising pulmonary artery pressures with right ventricular dysfunction, then cardiopulmonary bypass is instituted. The donor lungs are separated as for single-lung transplantation, leaving a cuff of left atrium around the pulmonary veins on each side. The recipient pneumonectomy is carried out with the patient maintained on one-lung ventilation. Each donor lung is implanted using essentially the same technique as described for single-lung transplantation. The bronchial anastomosis is completed first, followed by the left atrial and then the pulmonary arterial anastomoses. Flow and ventilation are restored to the newly implanted lung, and this lung then supports the patient while the opposite lung is removed and the second lung is implanted. Although all cardiac output is going through the newly implanted lung once the opposite pulmonary artery is ligated, clinically significant pulmonary edema has not been a problem. Both thoracotomies are then closed, and the sternum is approximated with wire sutures.

Other than procedures performed in patients with pulmonary hypertension, essentially all of these procedures are done without the need for cardiopulmonary bypass. The operation has afforded the opportunity to compare function between lungs with different ischemic times. Lungs may remain ischemic from 7 to 9 hours and still actively participate in gas exchange. Immediate postoperative perfusion scans usually show that the lung with the

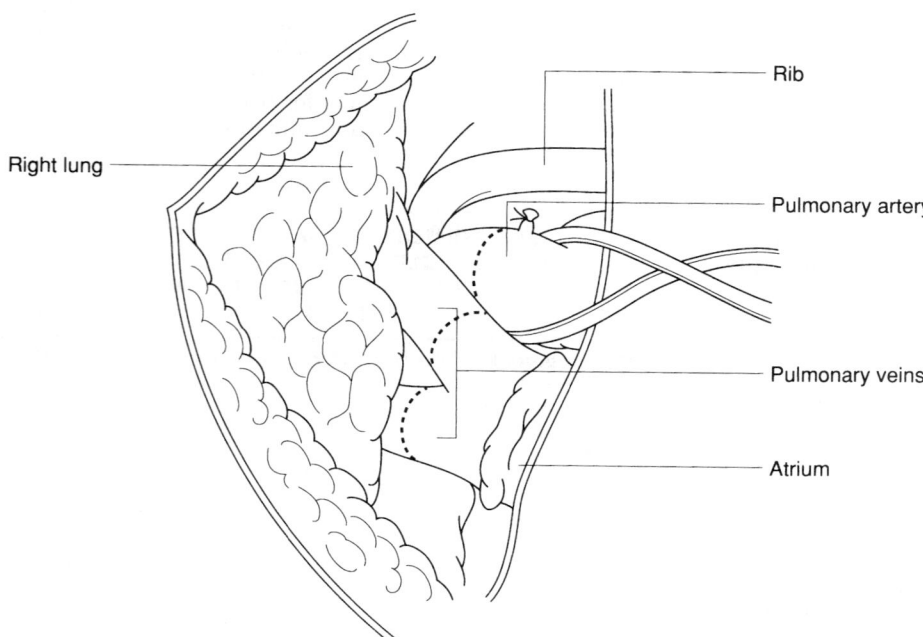

Right lung

Rib

Pulmonary artery

Pulmonary veins

Atrium

Figure 16.75. Mobilization of the hilum of the right lung demonstrating the encircled pulmonary artery with the first branch ligated and divided. The superior and inferior pulmonary veins have been exposed. Both the artery and veins are taken as close to the lung as possible. The bronchus is divided at the level of the take-off of the upper lobe.

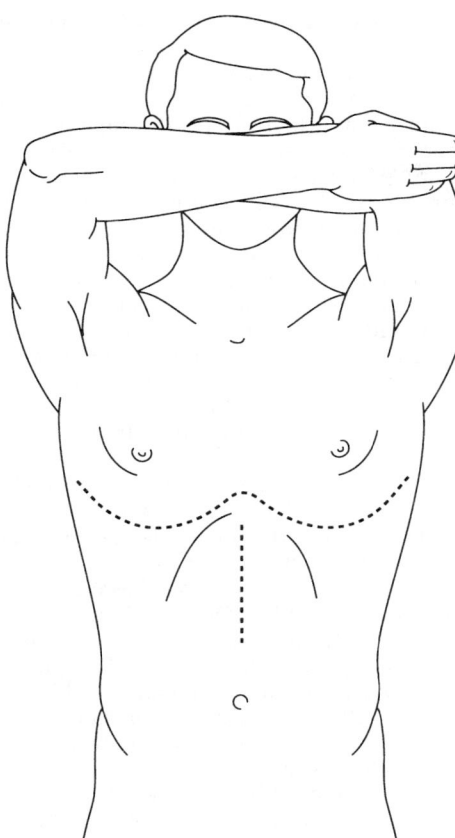

Table 16.24. INDICATIONS FOR PULMONARY TRANSPLANTATION

	Single lung (%)	Double lung (%)
Emphysema	45.1	19.4
α_1-Antitrypsin deficiency	10.7	10.7
Cystic fibrosis	2.1	32.8
Idiopathic pulmonary fibrosis	21.9	7.3
Primary pulmonary hypertension	4.7	9.9
Retransplantation	2.8	2.2

Data from Hosenpud JD, Bennett LE, Keck BM, et al. The Registry of the International Society for Heart and Lung Transplantation: fifteenth official report—1999. J Heart Lung Transplant 1999;18: 611–626.

Figure 16.76. The position of the patient on the operating table before the start of the bilateral, sequential pulmonary transplantation operation. The chest incision, a bilateral thoracosternotomy, is seen, as is the separate midline incision used to expose the omentum. The sternum is divided transversely, and the fifth intercostal space on each side is entered.

longer ischemic time receives less of the perfusion initially, although perfusion normalizes between the two lungs by 24 to 48 hours.

RESULTS

The Registry of the International Society of Heart and Lung Transplantation has recorded 8,598 lung transplantations over a 16-year period. These procedures were performed at 153 centers. Of these, 5,347 were single-lung transplantations. The single most common indication for transplantation was emphysema, either as a result of α_1-antitrypsin deficiency (860 cases) or idiopathy (3,157 cases). Most of the so-called idiopathic cases of emphysema are related to cigarette smoking. Pulmonary fibrosis accounted for 1,438 transplantations (12). Other indications are summarized in Table 16.24.

The overall 1-year actuarial survival rate after lung transplantation is 70%. At 2 years, the survival rate drops to 63%. The 5-year survival is 43% (50% for bilateral and 40% for single). Survival curves for single- and double-lung transplantations diverge after 3 years. Patients with emphysema have the best survival rate, whereas those with pulmonary hypertension have the worst (relative risk of death, 0.52 vs. 1.5). Patients with cystic fibrosis do almost as well as those with emphysema. In a given single institution, survival data may be somewhat better than those observed in the Registry Data. At Barnes Hospital in St. Louis, Missouri, 1- and 2-year survival rates were 87% for patients undergo-

ing single-lung transplantation between 1988 and 1992. For bilateral lung transplantation, the figures were 76% and 73%, respectively (13). Only a small number of lung transplant recipients have survived as long as 7 years, but it should be remembered that it was only in 1988 that significant numbers of transplantations began to be performed. Improved results occurred through 1992, but have plateaued since. The long-term outlook for patients undergoing lung transplantation remains unknown, but some insight can be gained by examining the factors responsible for long-term morbidity and mortality in this patient population.

IMMUNOSUPPRESSION

Immunosuppression is initiated in the immediate perioperative period and continued for the rest of the recipient's life. Standard regimens consist of cyclosporine or tacrolimus, azathioprine or mycophenolate mofetil, and prednisone. Some centers also use antilymphocyte antibody preparations during the induction phase, but there is no convincing evidence that this approach diminishes the incidence of acute or chronic rejection. Two important issues regarding standard immunosuppressive therapy are the myriad side effects associated with these agents and the numerous interactions with other commonly prescribed medications (4).

COMPLICATIONS

Complications resulting from pulmonary transplantation occur frequently, may be severe, and occasionally result in death. Intraoperative complications include technical problems with the vascular or bronchial anastomoses, injury to the phrenic or recurrent laryngeal nerves, and myocardial infarction. Postoperative complications include primary graft dysfunction, infection, and problems with airway healing, rejection, and bronchiolitis obliterans. Intraabdominal complications are not uncommon. Wound infection is noted rarely, although overriding of the sternal edges after double-lung transplantation is not uncommon.

Causes of recipient death can be categorized according to the time frame in which they occur. Early deaths (<90 days posttransplantation) most commonly result from bacterial infection. Primary donor organ failure accounts for the next largest group of deaths, followed by heart failure. Rejection accounts for only 6% of deaths in the early posttransplantation period. Hemorrhage and airway dehiscence each are responsible for 6% of early postoperative deaths. Infection accounts for approximately one third of late deaths (>90 days) posttransplantation. A similar percentage results from manifestations of chronic rejection and bronchiolitis obliterans. Respiratory failure and malignancy are the next most common causes of late mortality, each accounting for approximately 6% of deaths. Despite major strides made in operative and early postoperative care, the complications resulting from chronic immunosuppression continue to plague the transplant recipient.

Primary Graft Dysfunction

Mild, transient pulmonary edema is a common feature of the freshly transplanted allograft. In approximately 15% of cases, the injury is sufficiently severe to cause a form of acute respiratory distress syndrome termed *primary graft failure.* Primary graft failure is presumed to reflect ischemia–reperfusion injury, but surgical trauma and lymphatic disruption may be contributing factors. The diagnosis rests on the presence of widespread infiltrates on chest radiographs and severe hypoxemia within 72 hours after the transplantation and the exclusion of other causes of graft dysfunction, such as volume overload, pneumonia, rejection, occlusion of the venous anastomosis, and aspiration. Treatment is supportive, relying principally on conventional mechanical ventilation. Independent lung ventilation, inhaled nitric oxide, and extracorporeal membrane oxygenation have been used as adjunctive measures. Mortality rates of up to 60% have been reported, and among those who survive, the recovery period is often protracted, but achievement of normal allograft function is possible. The results of emergency retransplantation in such cases have been poor (4,14,15).

Rejection

With few exceptions, acute rejection episodes occur soon after transplantation, usually between posttransplantation days 5 and 7. Usually, two or three rejection episodes occur within the first month. Mild temperature elevation, perihilar fluffy infiltrates, or a minimal decrease in blood oxygenation as measured by arterial oxygen tension may herald rejection. Because rejection occurs so frequently during this period, the distinction between infection and rejection may be difficult. Often, the distinguishing factor between these two entities is that rejection responds positively to the administration of corticosteroids. Treatment of early rejection episodes involves the use of bolus corticosteroid administration given on three consecutive days. Within 12 to 18 hours after the first corticosteroid dose, symptoms relating to rejection usually resolve, including clearing of infiltrates on chest radiograph.

The utility of transbronchial biopsy to diagnose and monitor rejection after cardiopulmonary transplantation is substantial, but the number of biopsies required to maximize specificity is large. One group recommends obtaining 18 separate transbronchial biopsy specimens to achieve 95% specificity. The risks and potential complications of transbronchial lung biopsy do not justify their routine performance because suspected rejection episodes respond so well to corticosteroids. Transbronchial lung biopsy can be used when the issue of rejection versus infection is not resolved after steroid administration. Flexible bronchoscopy can be performed at the bedside, and 6 to 10 separate biopsies can be obtained under fluoroscopic guidance. When symptoms or signs of rejection persist despite adequate treatment, open lung biopsy may be considered.

Infection

Infection in the posttransplantation period continues to be a significant cause of morbidity as well as mortality. Bacterial pneumonia usually responds to appropriate antibiotic therapy, and patients are maintained on specific antibiotics as dictated by sputum culture and results of bronchial washings obtained at bronchoscopy. Antibiotic administration is particularly important if one predominant organism is grown from the donor lung cultures obtained at organ harvest. If a specific organism is grown from donor bronchial washings, the recipient is maintained on an appropriate antibiotic or combination of antibiotics for at least 1 week. The most common organism recovered from donor bronchial washings is *Staphylococcus aureus.* In a series of 32 transplantations, this organism was recovered from donors 11 times and subsequently from 4 transplant recipients. Other commonly recovered pathogens include *Enterobacter* species and *Candida albicans.* The presence of organisms cultured from donor bronchial washings, however, does not absolutely predict the development of invasive infection in recipients. Invasive infection develops in less than half of recipients from whom organisms are recovered.

The second most significant pathogen is cytomegalovirus (CMV). The diagnosis of CMV is usually made from culture of bronchoalveolar lavage fluid or tissue obtained from transbronchial lung biopsy. In the pulmonary transplantation population, CMV pneumonitis is the predominant form of CMV infection, although CMV enteritis and retinitis also occur. Approximately half of lung recipients acquire documented CMV infection. Ganciclovir has proved particularly effective and is the drug of choice for CMV infection in this circumstance. The drug is well tolerated in most patients, with neutropenia accounting for most of the toxicity.

The mortality rate from life-threatening CMV infections treated with ganciclovir has been reported at 10% (16), far better than the 40% or greater mortality rate reported before this agent was available. Major difficulties with life-threatening CMV infection have occurred in CMV-negative recipients who have received a lung from a CMV-positive donor (primary infection) or in recipients already CMV positive (secondary infection). Current practice is to attempt to place only a CMV-negative donor lung in a CMV-negative recipient, but this often proves to be unrealistic given the shortage of donor organs. Despite initial concerns, data from the St. Louis International Lung Transplant Registry fail to demonstrate any survival advantage at 1 or 2 years posttransplantation by avoiding donor–recipient CMV mismatching. Cytolytic therapy, especially with OKT3, is associated with an increased risk and severity of CMV infection. CMV prophylaxis with ganciclovir is used for CMV-positive recipients or for recipients who receive a lung from a CMV-positive donor.

Airway Complications

A major concern after pulmonary transplantation is airway anastomotic healing. During the early pulmonary transplantation experience, problems with airway healing resulted in a significant percentage of deaths. Patients often did well for the first 3 weeks after transplantation, and then the bronchial anastomosis split, often with erosion into the pulmonary artery. Bronchial anastomotic healing initially was facilitated by withholding maintenance corticosteroids until after the first posttransplantation week and using an omental pedicle wrapped around the anastomosis. Historically, most problems with airway healing occurred after the *en bloc* double-lung operation, which involves a tracheal anastomosis. Double-lung transplantation required extensive dissection in the subcarinal space, resulting in the disruption of a number of bronchial collateral vessels. Since this operation was modified to one involving bilateral, sequential lung replacement using two bronchial anastomoses, airway problems have been infrequent and now are rarely implicated in recipient deaths. Partial bronchial dehiscences often heal without sequelae. The use of a telescoping bronchial anastomosis, in which the donor bronchus is intussuscepted into the recipient bronchus, or vice versa, obviates the need for the omental pedicle wrap, allows for immediate use of corticosteroids, and has essentially eliminated anastomotic healing problems.

Bronchiolitis Obliterans

Approximately 20% of pulmonary transplant recipients develop progressive deterioration in pulmonary function because of bronchiolitis obliterans. The incidence of this complication reportedly approaches 50% after heart–lung transplantation. The lesion is characterized histologically by progressive small airway destruction, filling of these small airways with an inflammatory exudate, and, finally, fibrosis. Bronchiolitis obliterans is first manifested clinically by a subtle decrease in pulmonary function reflected in a decreased FEV_1. This complication is likely a form of chronic rejection, although its exact etiology remains unknown. A good animal model of bronchiolitis obliterans does not exist, making study of this entity difficult. If diagnosed early, enhancing immunosuppression may either halt the process or slow progression. It has been hypothesized that the development of bronchiolitis obliterans in cardiopulmonary transplant recipients is related to an A2 antigen mismatch. Others postulate that CMV infection may be implicated. Once diagnosed, it is imperative to increase immunosuppression to prevent what is usually an insidiously progressive disorder. In patients who have bronchiolitis obliterans and then undergo retransplantation, the lesion redevelops in the newly transplanted lungs. The disorder remains a major problem for patients surviving for greater than 2 years posttransplantation. Overall, long-term survival rates for lung transplantation are not likely to change until this problem is solved.

POSTTRANSPLANTATION PHYSIOLOGY

Pulmonary transplantation has afforded an opportunity to observe changes in pulmonary physiology that are not seen under ordinary circumstances. These changes should be viewed relative to the type of transplantation operation.

The development of bilateral, sequential lung replacement provides the opportunity indirectly to assess lung function by perfusion lung scan. Because the newly implanted lungs have different ischemic times, the immediate posttransplantation perfusion scan would be expected to demonstrate less perfusion to the side with the longer ischemic time. Indeed, this situation does occur, especially when ischemic times exceed 6 hours; the relative perfusion to each side usually equalizes within 24 to 48 hours.

Performing single-lung transplantations in patients with pulmonary hypertension has been particularly illustrative in demonstrating the potential for reversing right ventricular dysfunction. As soon as the lung is implanted, the morphology of the right ventricle changes significantly, as assessed by transesophageal echocardiography. The intraventricular septum, previously bulging into the left ventricle, immediately assumes a normal position. An increase in contractility of the right ventricle occurs with a significant decrease in dilatation. The pulmonary artery pressure immediately decreases and is essentially normal by the time the patient leaves the operating room (Table

16.23). Late catheterization studies (2 years posttransplantation) in patients undergoing this operation show continued normal hemodynamics.

The situation after single-lung transplantation in patients with emphysema is also illustrative. A significant $\dot{V}/\dot{Q}$ mismatch would be expected to occur, with ventilation to the native lung occurring preferentially because the native lung is significantly more compliant. Conversely, perfusion should preferentially go to the newly transplanted lung because of lower pulmonary vascular resistance. Despite this occurrence, patients undergoing this operation do well from a functional standpoint (Fig. 16.77). Early data show that physiologic dead space (V_D/V_T) decreases with work, with a shift in ventilation toward the transplanted side. By 3 months posttransplantation, the $\dot{V}/\dot{Q}$ mismatch narrows (Fig. 16.78). Despite the mismatch, no patient has demonstrated carbon dioxide retention.

From a clinical standpoint, improvement in pulmonary function is seen almost immediately after transplantation. The measurement most often used is FEV_1, and marked improvement is seen within 2 weeks. The FEV_1 essentially triples and then remains fairly stable (Fig. 16.79). This observation holds true for both single- and double-lung replacement in patients with obstructive disease. Improvement after bilateral lung replacement is slightly better.

Likewise, exercise studies show significant improvement after lung transplantation. Although patients who receive two lungs may do better on pulmonary function studies, this benefit is not translated into significantly better exercise capability. Maximum oxygen consumption, maximum work, peak ventilation, and anaerobic threshold are increased after lung transplantation but remain well below normal values. This restriction may be due to an accompanying abnormal cardiovascular response to exercise.

When exercise testing is performed, no difference is noted between patients with emphysema who receive one lung or two lungs. The shift in the mediastinum toward the transplanted side results in a relative "volume reduction" on the contralateral side with repositioning of the contralateral hemidiaphragm to a more normal location and to a normal concave configuration. This reconfiguration of the hemidiaphragm allows for significantly better diaphragm excursion and improved lung mechanics and gas exchange. Exercise capacity improves sufficiently to allow most transplant recipients to resume an active and

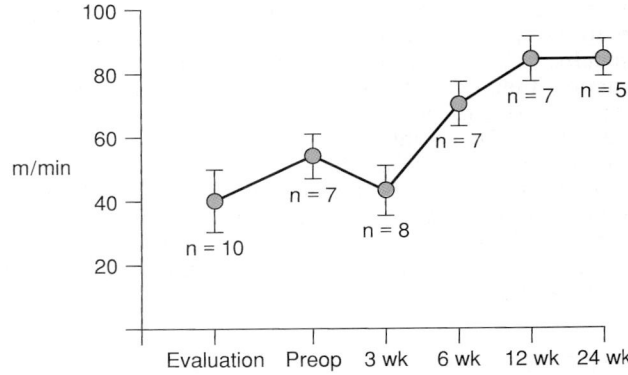

Figure 16.77. Mean 6-minute walk data for a group of patients undergoing single-lung transplantations for emphysema. Marked improvement is seen at the 6-week level, with continued improvement at 12 weeks.

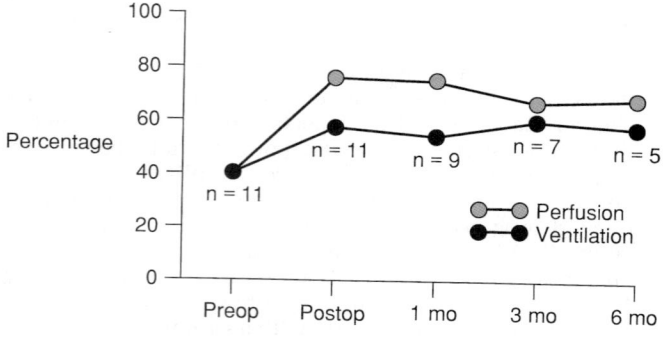

Figure 16.78. Mean values for ventilation and perfusion for patients undergoing single-lung transplantation for emphysema. Note the ventilation–perfusion mismatch that occurs, as expected, after transplantation.

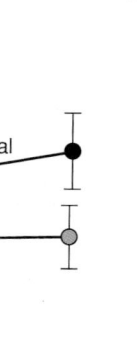

Figure 16.79. Comparison of percentage of predicted forced expiratory volume in 1 second (FEV_1) in 14 patients undergoing single and 10 patients undergoing bilateral sequential pulmonary transplantation for chronic obstructive pulmonary disease.

unencumbered lifestyle. By the end of the first year after transplantation, approximately 80% of recipients report no limitations in activity (4). At the other extreme, only 4% require total assistance. On average, after transplantation the distance a patient can cover during a standard 6-minute walk test is double that achieved before transplantation. Recipients of bilateral lung transplants can walk farther in 6 minutes than recipients of single-lung transplants (4,17), but this difference may reflect the younger age of the bilateral transplant recipients.

FUTURE CONSIDERATIONS

Pulmonary transplantation has slowly evolved from an experimental therapy. The number of these operations performed is still small compared with other solid-organ replacements. Donor availability is still a major issue and will likely continue to be an obstacle. The role of lung volume reduction surgery, as an alternative to transplantation or to delay transplantation in patients with emphysema, remains to be determined. Definition of a role for lung reduction therapy is an important consideration because emphysema is the most common indication for lung transplantation. Questions about long-term follow-up and preservation of lung function also remain to be answered. Pulmonary transplantation has joined other solid-organ transplantations as a viable alternative in patients with end-stage disease. Cost considerations and managed care will likely have a significant impact on transplantation as we enter the 21st century.

REFERENCES

1. Egan TM, Kaiser LR, Cooper JD. Lung transplantation. *Curr Probl Surg* 1989;10:681.
2. Wildevuur CR, Benfield JR. A review of 23 human lung transplants done by 20 surgeons. *Ann Thorac Surg* 1970;9:489.
3. Lima O, Goldberg M, Peters WS, et al. Effects of methylprednisolone and azathioprine on bronchial healing following lung transplantation. *J Thorac Cardiovasc Surg* 1981;83:211.
4. Arcasoy SM, Kotloff RM. Lung transplantation. *N Engl J Med* 1999;340:1081–1091.
5. Maurer JR, Frost AE, Estenne M, et al. International guidelines for the selection of lung transplant candidates. *J Heart Lung Transplant* 1998;17:703–709.
6. Goldberg M, Lima O, Morgan E, et al. A comparison between Cyclosporin A and methylprednisolone plus azathioprine on bronchial healing following canine lung autotransplantation. *J Thorac Cardiovasc Surg* 1983;85:821–826.
7. Schafers HJ, Wagner TOF, Demertzis S, et al. Preoperative corticosteroids: a contraindication to lung transplantation? *Chest* 1992;102:1522–1525.
8. Low DE, Trulock EP, Kaiser LR, et al. Lung transplantation of ventilator-dependent patients. *Chest* 1992;101:8–11.
9. Muller C, Furst H, Reichenspurner H, et al. Lung procurement by low-potassium dextran and the effect on preservation injury. *Transplantation* 1999;68:1139–1143.
10. Kaiser LR, Cooper JD, Trulock EP, et al. The evolution of single lung transplantation for emphysema. *J Thorac Cardiovasc Surg* 1991;102:333.
11. Pasque MK, Cooper JD, Kaiser LR, et al. Improved technique for bilateral lung transplantation: rationale and initial clinical experience. *Ann Thorac Surg* 1990;49:785.
12. Hosenpud JD, Bennett LE, Keck BM, et al. The Registry of the International Society for Heart and Lung Transplantation: fifteenth official report—1999. *J Heart Lung Transplant* 1999; 18:611–626.
13. Davis RD, Pasque MK. Pulmonary transplantation. *Ann Surg* 1995;221:14.
14. Christie JD, Bavaria JE, Palevsky HI, et al. Primary graft failure following lung transplantation. *Chest* 1998;114:51–60.
15. Novick RJ, Kaye MP, Patterson GA, et al. Redo lung transplantation: a North American-European experience. *J Heart Lung Transplant* 1993;12:5–16.
16. Keay S, Peterson E, Icenogle T, et al. Ganciclovir treatment of serious cytomegalovirus infection in heart and heart—lung transplant recipients. *Rev Infect Dis* 1988;10:5563.
17. Bavaria JE, Kotloff RM, Palevsky H, et al. Bilateral versus single lung transplantation for chronic obstructive pulmonary disease. *J Thorac Cardiovasc Surg* 1997;113:520–528.

Pancreas and Islet Transplantation

STEPHEN T. BARTLETT

Diabetes mellitus (DM) is a heterogeneous set of syndromes of impaired glucose tolerance that range from glucose intolerance during stress or pregnancy to severe hyperglycemia and ketoacidosis characteristic of juvenile (type 1) DM. The diagnosis of DM is not difficult to make in most cases. The most common presenting complaints are polyuria, polydipsia, weight loss, and fatigue. In some cases, type 1 DM presents with frank diabetic ketoacidosis. Difficulty can be encountered in the diagnosis of DM when it is based on the results of an oral glucose tolerance test. This test tends to overdiagnose impaired glucose tolerance and DM, in part because the anxiety and pain from phlebotomy may produce a catecholamine response sufficient to elevate the blood glucose in otherwise normal people. Observation of patients 5 years after an abnormal glucose tolerance test result demonstrates that many do not progress to frank DM. The recommendation of the American Diabetes Association, therefore, is that the diagnosis of DM be based on two separate venous plasma glucose values. For the fasting plasma glucose test, normal values should be less than 110 mg/dL. Fasting plasma glucose levels of more than 126 mg/dL on two or more tests on different days indicate DM. When an oral glucose tolerance test is used, a person has DM when two diagnostic tests done on different days show that the blood glucose level exceeds 200 mg/dL 2 hours after ingestion of 75 g of glucose. If the 2-hour value is between 140 and 200 mg/dL and there is one other value greater than 200 mg/dL, then the person is given the diagnosis of impaired glucose tolerance. These people require continued observation because they are at increased risk of progression to symptomatic DM. Progression to frank DM in any given patient with impaired glucose tolerance cannot be predicted (1).

CLASSIFICATION AND PATHOPHYSIOLOGY

Diabetes can be classified into two major groups. Type 2 DM, also referred to as noninsulin-dependent DM, or adult-onset DM, typically presents in obese patients older than 40 years of age. Type 2 DM is a very common disease affecting 1% to 2% of the U.S. population, with wide variation in presentation. If diagnosis is based on an abnormal glucose tolerance test result, the incidences of overt DM and impaired glucose tolerance in Americans are 6.6% and 11.2%, respectively. The genetics of type 2 DM have not been fully elucidated because more than 250 candidate genes have been screened for relevance to DM. It is likely that more than one gene controls the development of type 2 DM. Eighty percent of identical twins are concordant for type 2 DM and 40% of siblings and 30% of offspring of an index case will acquire type 2 DM.

The precise pathophysiologic process of type 2 DM is still a matter of scientific uncertainty. Patients with type 2 DM have two physiologic defects: beta cell hypersecretion and peripheral insulin receptor insensitivity. Both defects must be present for expression of disease, but it remains unclear which defect is primary. Experimentally, insulin hypersecretion can lead to insulin receptor desensitization. Similarly, receptor desensitization can lead to hypersecretion of insulin. From a clinical standpoint, in many cases, the capacity for beta cell hypersecretion is inadequate and exogenous insulin is required. Thus, many patients with type 2 DM require insulin in amounts that can sometimes exceed 100 U/d.

Type 1 DM, or insulin-dependent DM, is an autoimmune disorder that leads to the eventual complete loss of all beta cells in the pancreatic islets. The mean age of onset is 14 years; however, onset may be as early as the first year of life or, rarely, in the seventh decade. Typically, the disease presents in a lean patient complaining of excessive thirst, appetite, and urination with weight loss. Often the disease presents at the time of a concurrent illness such as a viral infection or at the time of major surgery. Occasionally, after the initial stress that exposes the illness abates, there is a brief "honeymoon" period lasting weeks to months during which exogenous insulin is not needed. Eventually the beta cell mass of the patient is completely destroyed by the autoimmune process and exogenous insulin is needed to prevent ketoacidosis, coma, and death. The prevalence of type 1 DM is estimated at 0.26% by age 26 years, with 30,000 new cases annually in the United States.

The pathogenesis of type 1 DM has important implications for transplantation of the pancreas or islets of Langerhans. Genetic susceptibility combined with an unknown environmental event triggers autoimmune islet destruction. That an environmental event is required to trigger the disease is suggested by the observation that although only 30% of identical twins are initially concordant, within two decades of further observation, the concordance rate rises to 50%. This observation and the presence of the honeymoon period demonstrate that the disease is an indolent process of beta cell destruction that may last as long as 7 years. Proof that type 1 DM has an autoimmune pathogenesis also comes from the observation that DM recurred after an initial period of normoglycemia within 6 to 8 weeks after transplantation of a pancreatic segment from a nondiabetic identical twin to the diabetic twin without the benefit of immunosuppression (2). DM has also been transferred in humans from a diabetic sibling to a nondiabetic sibling with bone marrow transplantation (3).

Genetic susceptibility to type 1 DM is strongly related to the human leukocyte antigen (HLA) class II genotype. Ninety-five percent of white people with type 1 DM carry either the DR3 or DR4 HLA antigen. DNA-based typing has shown a strong association between type 1 DM and the HLA DQ β-chain genes $DQ\beta_1{*}0201$ (which segregates with DR3) and $DQ\beta_1{*}0302$ (which segregates with DR4). Conversely, the $DQ\beta_1{*}0602$ gene (which segregates with DR2) is protective. The importance of the HLA genes in disease pathogenesis is not fully understood but may relate to different binding affinities of HLA antigens for oligopeptides from foreign antigens that mimic sequences from normal tissue (molecular mimicry). According to this pathogenetic theory, a chance homology between a viral protein, such as the oligopeptide sequence found in the coxsackievirus, and the beta cell antigen glutamic acid decarboxylase, could result in the activation of an autoimmune response. Diabetic people have a high incidence of antibody to glutamic acid decarboxylase and to epitopes on the coxsackievirus.

Another theory suggests that the disease results from failure to eliminate autoreactive T-cell clones in the thymus during fetal life, possibly because the class I antigens of diabetic patients are poor peptide binders, resulting in the failure to present adequate self-antigen during fetal life. The primary autoantigen that initiates the autoimmune process has not been unequivocally determined, but evidence is accumulating that it is an oligopeptide sequence of the insulin β chain (4). Once the initial autoimmune attack has begun, a variety of previously immunologically silent beta cell antigens are released from dying or injured cells, leading to augmentation of the immune response. At various stages of the autoimmune disease, antibodies to insulin; proinsulin; two forms of glutamic acid decarboxylase; carboxypeptidase A; ganglioside antigens; and the islet cell antigens, ICA 69 and ICA 512, may appear. The appearance of combinations of these antigens has some predictive value in prone populations such as siblings of affected patients or those with a genetic predisposition.

Histologically, the initial lesion of type 1 DM is insulitis or isletitis, an infiltration of the periphery of the islet with macrophages, followed by both CD4+ and CD8+ T lymphocytes. The initial infiltration is nondestructive. Undefined events lead to a switching on of an immunologic attack with beta cell destruction. This event is associated with recruitment of other cells associated with an inflammatory response. Beta cell destruction may be partially mediated by tumor necrosis factor-α (TNF-α), interleukin (IL)-1, and interferon-γ (IFN-γ). Superoxide and nitric oxide also play a role in beta cell destruction. At the conclusion of the process, the beta cell mass, initially estimated at 850 mg, has been reduced to zero.

Secondary Complications of Diabetes

No single pathogenetic sequence can explain all secondary complications of DM. The enzyme aldose reductase converts excess glucose to sorbitol. In experimental animals, sorbitol accumulation in peripheral nerves leads to a loss of myoinositol, abnormal phosphoinositide metabolism, and a decrease in Na^+-K^+-adenosine triphosphatase activity. Aldose reductase inhibitors prevent diabetic neuropathy, cataracts, and retinopathy in experimental animals. Nonenzymatic glycosylation of proteins may also play an important role in the pathogenesis of secondary diabetic complications. Glycosylated low-density lipoprotein cholesterol is not recognized by its receptor and thus the molecule has a prolonged half-life. Formation of cross-links between glycosylated proteins can form advanced glycosylation end-products (AGE). AGE ligation of endothelial cell receptors can activate the release or synthesis of cytokines, endothelin-1, and tissue factor. Activation of the coagulation cascade, in turn, may lead to vascular complications. Prevention of the formation of AGE with aminoguanidine prevents retinopathy, nephropathy, and neuropathy in experimental animals.

Clinical complications of DM include end-stage renal disease (ESRD), retinopathy, peripheral vascular disease, coronary artery disease, and neuropathy. Half of all cases of ESRD are the result of diabetic nephropathy. Approximately 35% of patients with type 1 DM eventually acquire ESRD, which is the most common cause of death and disability in people with DM. DM is also the leading cause of blindness and lower extremity amputations in the United States. Diabetic patients are twice as likely to sustain myocardial infarction or stroke. If secondary complications could be eliminated, DM could be reduced to an inconvenience.

The Diabetes Control and Complication Trial clearly demonstrated that meticulous control of blood glucose prevents and delays the progression of secondary complications. Before this trial, it was uncertain whether blood glucose, elevated insulin levels, or an unknown factor was responsible for progression of secondary complications. In this study, patients with type 1 DM were randomized to conventional treatment with one or two doses of insulin daily versus three or more injections or continuous delivery with an insulin pump. After a mean of 6.5 years, the groups were compared for the degree of progression or prevention of secondary complications. In the primary prevention group, the risk of development of retinopathy was reduced by 76%. Intensive therapy slowed the development of retinopathy by 54%. The occurrence of microalbuminuria was reduced by 39%, and clinical (dipstick positive) albuminuria by 54%. The occurrence of neuropathy was reduced by 60%.

The major side effect of intensive therapy was a threefold increase in the incidence of severe hypoglycemic episodes. Ten percent of patients in the intensive insulin therapy cohort experienced five or more episodes of seizure or coma during the study period and 30% experienced five or more episodes of hypoglycemia severe enough to require third-party assistance but not severe enough to lead to loss of consciousness (5). Thus, there is a trade-off between the prevention of progression of secondary complications and the risk of severe hypoglycemia.

Whether severe hypoglycemia leads to permanent brain injury is uncertain. Diabetic patients who report frequent hypoglycemic episodes have larger cerebral perfusion abnormalities on positron emission scanning than those without a history of hypoglycemia, and school-age children perform worse on neuropsychiatric testing if there is a history of hypoglycemia. People with frequent hypoglycemia are at greater risk of injury during industrial and automobile accidents. Frequent hypoglycemia can lead to a syndrome of hypoglycemic unawareness in which the typical symptoms of tremulousness, anxiety, and hunger resulting from hypoglycemic catecholamine release are lost. These patients may manifest neurologic symptoms of hypoglycemia without the usual adrenergic premonitory symptoms. Management of DM is directed at maintenance of the blood glucose as close to the normal range as possible without incurring undue hypoglycemic morbidity. Unfortunately, for many patients there is no therapeutic window for insulin therapy. They are faced with choosing between freedom from hypoglycemic symptoms and poor overall glycemic control, or tight glycemic control and intolerable episodes of hypoglycemia. For these patients, pancreas transplantation can alleviate these symptoms and the progression of secondary complications.

PANCREAS TRANSPLANTATION

Background

The only reliable cure for DM is pancreas transplantation. The initial experience with pancreas transplantation from the first case in 1966 until the 1980s was marked by a low success rate and very high mortality rates. Before the release of cyclosporine for general use, the results of pancreas transplantation were so poor that there was little interest in the procedure. The first 12 cases used enteric drainage of the duodenum, and only one graft functioned beyond 1 year (6). In 1980, the International Pancreas Transplant Registry (IPTR) reported a 1-year graft survival rate of 21% and a patient survival rate of 67%. Therefore, in the precyclosporine era, fewer than 100 cases were performed in any given year. Subsequent technical and immunosuppressive advances have rendered the operation significantly more successful. In 1983, the technique of bladder drainage was introduced, a technique that became rapidly accepted because of the marked reduction of the risk of posttransplantation sepsis (Fig. 16.80). The release of cyclosporine in the same year led to a significant reduction in the risk of graft loss due to rejection.

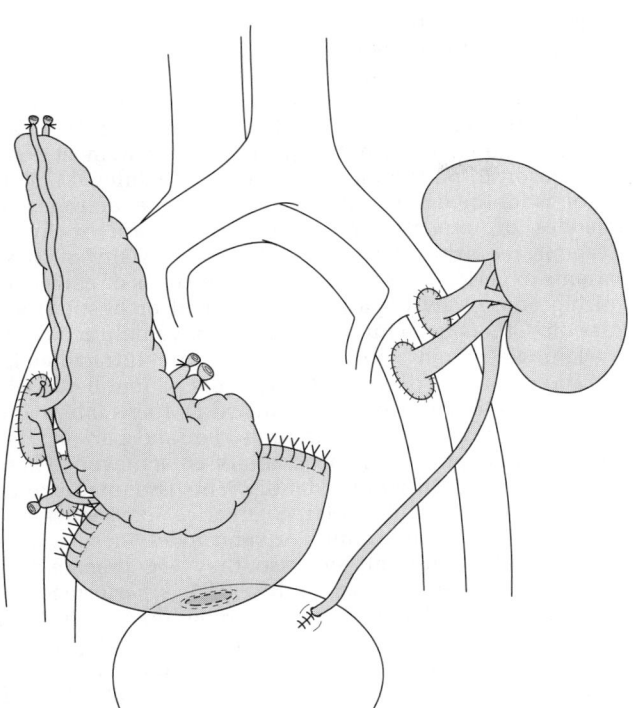

Figure 16.80. Simultaneous pancreas kidney (SPK) transplantation performed with drainage of the pancreatic exocrine secretions into the ruinary bladder (bladder drainage, DB). This has been the predominant technique until recently. Note that a segment of the second portion of the duodenum is left attached to the pancreas. Despite its heterotopic isolation, the transplanted pancreas responds to gastrointestinal hormones with a marked increase in secretion of pancreatic juice that has a very high bicarbonate content. With bladder drainage, recipients must consume as many as forty tablets of sodium bicarbonate daily. Also note that the portal vein drains into the iliac vein, i.e., systemic venous (SV) drainage. In normal individuals 50% of the secreted insulin is extracted from the circulation in the first pass through the liver. Transplant recipients with SV have peripheral insulin levels two- to two-and-a-half times higher than normal.

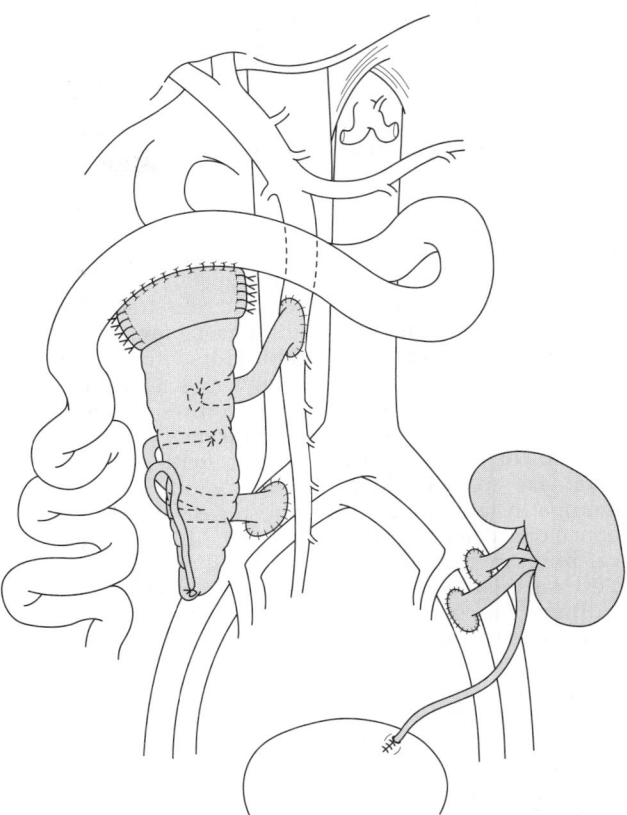

Figure 16.81. Simultaneous pancreas kidney (SPK) transplantation performed with drainage of the pancreatic exocrine secretions into the proximal jejunum (enteric drainage, ED). This technique has been adopted by most transplant centers in the United States for SPK cases. For solitary pancreas transplantation, most centers still utilize BD to allow monitoring of the urinary amylase. Note that the donor portal vein drains into the recipient superior mesenteric vein (portal venous drainage, PV), preventing peripheral hyperinsulinemia. This technique appears to be associated with a lower incidence of rejection. Many centers continue to place the pancreas in the pelvis combining ED and SV. This requires enteric anastomosis to a more distal segment of jejunum or ileum.

More recently, enteric duct drainage has been readopted by many pancreas transplantation centers. According to the IPTR (1), the proportion of enteric-drained cases has continuously increased, as well as the number of centers performing this procedure. In 1993, one group reported a large series of enteric-drained pancreas transplants with success equivalent to a comparable group receiving bladder drainage. This modification was prompted by the identification of the long-term complications of bladder drainage. The current trend is to perform pancreas transplantation with enteric exocrine drainage and systemic venous drainage. However, systemic venous drainage of pancreas transplants has been associated with hyperinsulinemia, which results in dyslipidemia and accelerated atherosclerosis.

To circumvent this problem, investigators have described a more physiologic technique of draining the transplanted pancreas into the recipient's portal circulation (6). Systemic venous drainage is gradually being replaced with the more physiologic portal venous drainage, thus making pancreas transplants totally physiologic (Fig. 16.81). Until July 1999, the operation was still considered experimental by the Health Care Finance Administration. However, as of July 1999, simultaneous pancreas–kidney (SPK) transplantations and pancreas after kidney (PAK) transplantations (a pancreas transplantation performed after a successful kidney transplantation) were awarded Medicare coverage, a step that is generally followed by most insurance carriers and health maintenance organizations.

Patient Selection

Pancreas transplantation has been reserved for patients with type 1 DM. In most cases, there is unequivocal information to confirm the diagnosis of type 1 DM. A history of juvenile onset (the mean age is 14 years), past ketoacidosis, lean body habitus, and a requirement for 20 to 80 U of insulin daily are consistent with this diagnosis. Adult onset, obesity, absence of a history of ketoacidosis, and periods of insulin independence or extraordinary insulin requirements may suggest a diagnosis of type 2 DM. Diagnostic uncertainty should be resolved by the administration of a 100-g oral glucose challenge, followed 1 hour later by simultaneous measurement of a blood C-peptide and glucose. A type 1 diabetic person will have undetectable C-peptide levels despite maximal stimulation of the pancreas with a simultaneously elevated blood glucose. Conversely, a person with type 2 DM will have blood insulin levels that are normal or elevated as a result of insulin resistance. Although some patients with type 2 DM achieve insulin independence with pancreas transplantation, there is no peer-reviewed report of the long-term efficacy of pancreas transplantation in this setting. With only 5,000 cadaver donors in the United States yearly, extension of pancreas transplantation to type 2 diabetic patients should not be widely applied before demonstrable benefits of transplantation and before resolution of the organ donor shortage.

Most patients evaluated for pancreas transplantation have ESRD. Patients are on dialysis or are approaching dialysis, or have had a successful kidney transplantation. Placement on the the United Network for Organ Sharing waiting list for an SPK transplant requires that the potential recipient have a creatinine clearance of less than 25 mL/min. In addition to ESRD, most patients have other secondary complications of DM, including retinopathy, neuropathy, autonomic neuropathy, gastroparesis, and evidence of accelerated atherosclerosis. Although these clinical findings strongly support the indications for SPK or PAK transplantation, they are not required to justify the addition of a pancreas to a kidney transplant. As detailed later, the evidence is overwhelming that pancreas transplantation prevents recurrent diabetic nephropathy in transplanted kidneys. This fact alone, combined with the marked improvement in quality of life achieved with a successful pancreas transplant, strongly supports pancreas transplantation, either simultaneously or after a kidney transplant, in the type 1 diabetic patient with renal failure. It is rare to have ESRD as an isolated secondary complication of DM. Thus, most candidates have varying degrees of other secondary complications that will be arrested or reversed with pancreas transplantation.

Evaluation

All candidates should have noninvasive cardiac stress testing such as dobutamine stress echocardiography or adenosine thallium stress scintigraphy. Potential candidates with reversible myocardial defects should undergo coronary angiography. In many cases, the decision to pursue myocardial revascularization before transplantation is unclear. Patients with ESRD are typically deconditioned, a factor exacerbated if significant diabetic neuropathy is present. Moreover, diabetic neuropathy may prevent patients from experiencing typical angina. Diabetic patients may experience anginal equivalents such as exercise-induced pulmonary edema or paroxysmal nocturnal pulmonary edema. Therefore, the indications for myocardial revascularization are different in this population and should be addressed accordingly. The decision to perform pretransplantation coronary revascularization must be made after considering both perioperative as well as long-term survival (7).

Signs of peripheral arterial occlusive disease should be carefully elicited. The presence of aortoiliac occlusive disease that can compromise arterial inflow to the transplants may require pretransplantation intervention. Correction of aortoiliac disease with angioplasty, placement of an iliac artery endoluminal stent, or aortofemoral bypass should precede transplantation. Similarly, all candidates should be screened for hemodynamically significant carotid occlusive disease that may warrant pretransplantation carotid endarterectomy.

Contraindications to pancreas transplantation include the presence of a recent malignancy, chronic active hepatitis, cirrhosis, psychiatric disease, and social attributes such as active alcoholism and drug dependency that would impair the patient's ability to cooperate with post-transplantation management.

The indications for a pancreas transplant alone (PTA) performed before the development of clinically significant renal insufficiency are obviously different than for those patients who have current or prior ESRD. The most common reason to perform a PTA is severely labile DM. This entity is defined clinically as a syndrome of repeated episodes of hypoglycemic coma or seizure, or hypoglycemia requiring third-party assistance. Many of these patients experience frequent seizure episodes or comas requiring emergency department treatment or hospital admission. Others have industrial or motor vehicle accidents or accidentally injure children in their care. Intractable labile DM should be diagnosed only if the patient has established a relationship with a qualified DM specialist, and despite the best efforts of the physician and patient, reasonably stable glucose control cannot be achieved. These patients are not difficult to identify. They are unable to be alone because they do not recognize or experience the symptoms of hypoglycemia. Advancement in school or employment is difficult because they are preoccupied with their self-care. Occasionally a PTA is performed because the patient has had an inexorable decline in their functional status because of a combination of progressive neuropathy, retinopathy, gastroparesis, and proteinuria secondary to early diabetic nephropathy. Except for a lack of proven effect on retinopathy, successful pancreas transplantation leads to a reversal of all other secondary complications over time.

ORGAN PROCUREMENT AND PRESERVATION

Selection of an appropriate cadaver pancreas donor is integral to the success of pancreas transplantation. The ideal donor is a young, nonalcoholic nonsmoker. Elevation of donor blood glucose in the absence of a history of DM is of no consequence. High-dose catecholamine infusion for donor blood pressure support, rapid dextrose-in-saline infusion for resuscitation, and administration of corticosteroids as a treatment of cerebral edema all contribute to donor hyperglycemia. Successful transplantation of pancreases from donors with a blood glucose in excess of 1,000 mg/dL is not unusual. Elevation of donor serum amylase is not unusual, and commonly is the result of parotitis from craniofacial trauma. Provided that the pancreas is normal in appearance, elevation in amylase and lipase is inconsequential. Ethanol abuse, which is not always revealed by the donor family, can lead to fatty change or fibrosis in the pancreas. Cigarette smoking has been found to produce minor deterioration in glucose-stimulated insulin secretion. The major effect of tobacco abuse on pancreas donors is the development of atherosclerosis in the iliac artery Y-graft needed for the backtable arterial reconstruction of the pancreas (8). Trauma to the pancreas itself is a contraindication to procurement, but a history of donor splenectomy is not usually problematic.

Data from the IPTR demonstrate that the success rate declines if the donor is older than 45 years of age. This controversial report is supported by a single-center study from the University of Minnesota, but disputed by data from the Universities of Pittsburgh and Maryland (9,10). Similarly, there is no difference between donors who have sustained a cardiovascular versus a traumatic death. The critical factor in determining outcome is the selection of pancreases for transplantation that appear phenotypically normal. A normal pancreas is pliable, free of fat in the interlobular

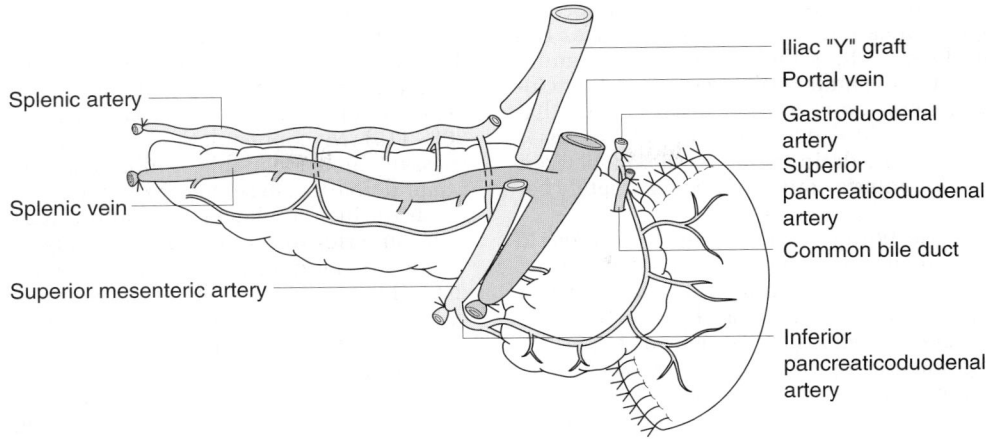

Figure 16.82. Back-table preparation of the pancreas. Prior to transplantation, the pancreas must be prepared in a slush-filled basin to maintain cryopreservation. Preparation includes unifying the arterial blood supply of the pancreas by anastomosis of the donor external iliac artery to the superior mesenteric artery and the donor internal iliac artery to the splenic artery. The donor common iliac artery is used for anastomosis to the recipient iliac artery. During back-table preparation, donor splenectomy is performed and both ends of the duodenum are inverted.

septa, shows no evidence of fibrosis from past pancreatitis, and is salmon-pink. Although preprocurement characteristics associated with a poor outcome may be present, the only certain way to determine the adequacy of a pancreas is to visualize the organ directly at the time of procurement. Some centers have set 55 years of age as the upper limit for pancreas donors because there is evidence that the beta cell mass begins to decrease after this age. Some investigators have also limited donation to people older than 8 years of age or those above a minimum weight of 30 kg. Below this size, vascular reconstruction of the pancreas is very difficult and the risk of thrombosis is unacceptably high.

Procurement Technique

The pancreas is carefully dissected to avoid injury to the capsule of the pancreas. The spleen is used as a handle to dissect the tail from the pancreatic bed. Only a few small vessels are encountered in the region of the tail that require formal division. The tail is lifted from the bed with the electrocautery. The portal triad is dissected in cooperation with the liver transplantation team. Typically, the portal vein is shared by dividing it at the level of the coronary (left gastric) vein. Use of both the liver and pancreas from the same donor should not be problematic even in the presence of a replaced right hepatic artery. The duodenum should be immobilized using electrocautery, and the middle colic vein divided formally. This allows the mesentery of the superior mesenteric artery below the pancreas to be divided with a 60-mm vascular stapler. The duodenum is divided with a stapler just distal to the pylorus and the jejunum is derotated, pulled to the right of the superior mesenteric artery, and divided just distal to the fourth part of the duodenum. Donor arterial perfusion with approximately 3 L of University of Wisconsin perfusate is performed while the abdominal organs are packed in saline slush.

After the pancreas is removed, the distal duodenal staples are removed and the interior of the duodenum is cleansed with bacitracin and kanamycin in saline and amphotericin in sterile water. After the duodenum is cleansed, the interior is filled with perfusate. The entire common iliac artery and its two main branches, the internal and external iliac arteries, are packaged with the pancreas. An iliac venous graft is also included with the pancreas, but extension of the portal vein is rarely needed. Although transplantation should be performed as soon as possible, up to 30 hours of cold ischemia time (time between perfusate infusion and organ reperfusion) has not been associated with reduced graft survival, according to IPTR data.

Back-table Preparation of the Pancreas

The spleen is removed by dividing all vessels in continuity with the pancreatic parenchyma. The distal duodenum is shortened to the point at which the pancreas becomes intimate with the duodenum. Both ends of the duodenum are stapled and inverted with interrupted polypropylene sutures. The iliac artery Y-graft is attached by anastomosis of the internal iliac artery to the splenic artery stump and anastomosis of the external iliac artery to the superior mesenteric artery (Fig. 16.82). The portal vein is lengthened by freeing it from the surrounding adventitial tissue to a point where the splenic vein and superior mesenteric vein meet. Finally, the stumps of the common bile duct and the gastroduodenal artery are suture ligated.

TECHNIQUE OF TRANSPLANTATION

The preferred technique is a fully physiologic transplantation that drains the pancreatic ductal secretions into the recipient jejunum. This technique avoids late complications of drainage into the urinary bladder (11). These include an increased risk of repeated urinary tract infection, episodic hematuria, chemical urethritis and perineal excoriation, and severe bicarbonate wasting that requires daily oral bicarbonate replacement. The major utility of bladder drainage is the ability to monitor urinary amylase. A persistent 25% drop in urinary amylase concentration is associated with pancreatic rejection. This finding can be particularly helpful for solitary transplantation (PAK and PTA) cases. Diagnosis of rejection in SPK cases is facilitated by monitoring serum creatinine.

Many centers use enteric ductal drainage for SPK cases and some centers use enteric drainage in all cases (12). The shift to enteric drainage has been hastened by the realization that approximately 22% of patients with bladder drainage have required late enteric conversion for the aforementioned complications of bladder drainage. Enteric conversion, during which the transplant duodenum is disconnected from the bladder, followed by bladder closure and duodenoenterostomy, is a morbid procedure that required reoperation (a third operation) in 25% of cases (13). As primary enteric drainage is replacing bladder drainage, the need for enteric conversion is fortunately becoming rare.

The decision to use portal venous instead of systemic venous drainage is related to a desire to achieve normal peripheral insulin levels in the recipient. Because 50% of insulin is removed with the first pass through the liver physiologically, systemic venous drainage leads to peripheral insulin levels that are approximately 2.5 times normal (14). If the recipient has had multiple upper abdominal operations or a thick, foreshortened mesentery, systemic venous drainage may be preferred. Conversely, if both the left and right iliac sites have been used, particularly with a prior failed SPK, the portal venous site can be remarkably easy.

The recipient should receive broad-spectrum pretransplantation intravenous antibiotics. If time permits, the recipient should be thoroughly prepared with oral gavage, and oral neomycin and erythromycin, particularly if enteric drainage is planned. Recipients with severe gastrointestinal neuropathy may have marked chronic fecal retention; intraoperative and postoperative management is greatly facilitated if this can be resolved with a preoperative bowel preparation similar to that used for colonic surgery.

The transplantation is performed though a midline incision. The superior mesenteric vein just below the transverse mesocolon is dissected for a length of approximately 3 cm. The right common iliac artery is also completely dissected. The transplantation is accomplished by end-to-side anastomosis of the donor portal vein to the recipient superior mesenteric vein. The iliac artery is passed through a small hole in the jejunal mesentery and the proximal end of the Y-graft is anastomosed to the recipient common iliac artery (Fig. 16.81). If systemic venous drainage is chosen, the recipient right external and common iliac vein is dissected completely, with ligation and division of all the hypogastric vein branches to increase the mobility of the recipient venous system. Arterial inflow is either from the proximal external iliac artery or distal common iliac artery. The transplantation is completed by side-to-side anastomosis of the donor duodenum to the recipient jejunum (Figs. 16.80, 16.81). If the case is an SPK, kidney transplantation is usually performed in the left iliac fossa. Some groups prefer to raise a retroperitoneal flap to place the kidney in a retroperitoneal pocket. This technique has the advantage of preventing torsion of the kidney that is on a long vascular pedicle. Moreover, percutaneous biopsy of a retroperitoneal kidney is somewhat safer because the kidney is enveloped in a pericapsular fibrous rind that prevents postbiopsy hemorrhage. Before it is closed, the abdomen should be thoroughly irrigated.

IMMUNOSUPPRESSION

The pancreas is among the most immunogenic of the solid organ transplants because of the large lymphoid component of the gland. IPTR data show that 75% of pancreas transplantation centers use antilymphocyte induction therapy. Choices include monoclonal or polyclonal antibodies. The value of newer monoclonal antibodies to the IL-2 receptor is not fully proven, but many centers have elected to use them because of low short-term toxicity. Avoidance of antilymphocyte induction appears to lead to an equal one-year graft survival rate, but the incidence of rejection requiring treatment is extremely high at 80% (15). Mycophenolate mofetil, a newer immunosuppressant, is a reversible inhibitor of inosine monophosphate dehydrogenase, an enzyme critical for purine synthesis during lymphocyte activation. This drug has proven to be superior to azathioprine, thereby replacing it in virtually all solid organ transplantations. Mycophenolate mofetil is combined with one of the calcineurin inhibitors, either tacrolimus or cyclosporine. Although there is no clear advantage of one calcineurin inhibitor for SPK transplantation, the results for PTA with cyclosporine have been poor, resulting in the preferential use of tacrolimus-based immunosuppression (16). PAK transplants and PTA are usually immunosuppressed with tacrolimus and mycophenolate mofetil. Most immunosuppressive regimens also include tapering doses of prednisone.

The role of the newer cell cycle inhibitor sirolimus has not been established in pancreas transplantation, but its success in kidney transplantation predicts that it will have a significant role in pancreas transplant management, at least as a replacement for patients experiencing unacceptable toxicity with standard agents.

The major problem with current immunosuppression regimens, beyond known toxicities, is impairment of glucose tolerance. Prednisone leads to peripheral insulin resistance, and both calcineurin inhibitors impair transcription of preproinsulin mRNA. Occasionally this effect leads to hyperglycemia and beta cell degranulation (17). This finding is reversible, responding to calcineurin inhibitor dose reduction and temporary insulin support. Because of peripheral insulin resistance induced by prednisone, the newly transplanted pancreas must secrete approximately twice as much insulin to maintain euglycemia. Despite these limitations, the deleterious effect of immunosuppression rarely affects the overall success of pancreas transplantation.

RESULTS

The increasing success of pancreas transplantation has led to a steady increase in the number of operations performed each year (Fig. 16.83). Although most transplantations are SPK (Fig. 16.84), the number of solitary pancreas transplantations performed is increasing rapidly, particularly since Medicare approval of PAK transplantation. Many patients who were previously excluded for financial reasons can now be transplanted. The national 1-year patient, pancreas, and kidney survival rates for SPK transplantations are 94%, 90%, and 83%, respectively (Fig. 16.85). The 1-year success of PAK and PTA transplantations is 71% and 64%, respectively (Figs. 16.86 and 16.87). Difficulty in the diagnosis of rejection in the solitary pancreas transplantation cases leads to a diminished success rate relative to SPK transplantations. Recent experience has shown that portal venous drainage may be an important factor in improving the success of pancreas transplantation (Fig. 16.88). Regardless of the pancreas transplant type, portal venous drainage leads to reduction in the incidence and severity of rejection, independent of other identifiable factors (18).

Data from both The Netherlands and Sweden strongly suggest that long-term survival is superior for patients with ESRD and type 1 DM who receive an SPK transplant compared with those who receive a kidney transplant

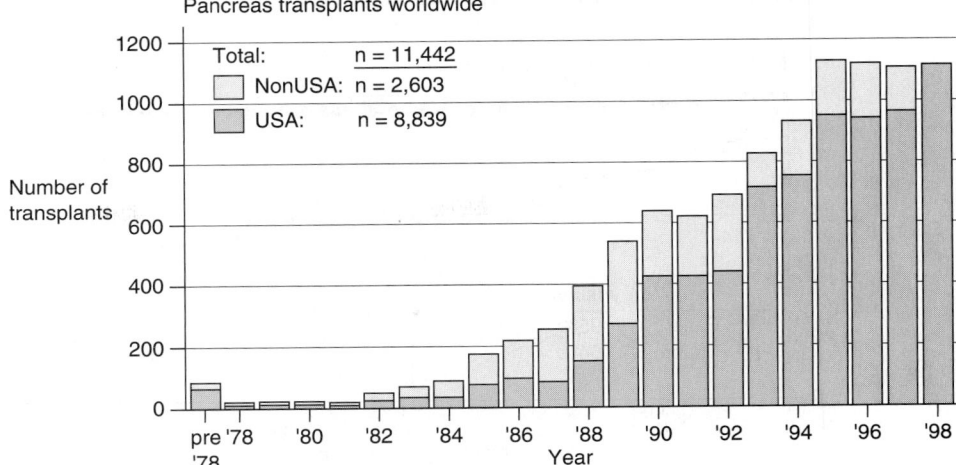

Figure 16.83. Exponential growth of pancreas transplantation, particularly in the United States, has occurred since 1983 as a result of improved immunosuppression and technical improvements that markedly improved the overall success rate.

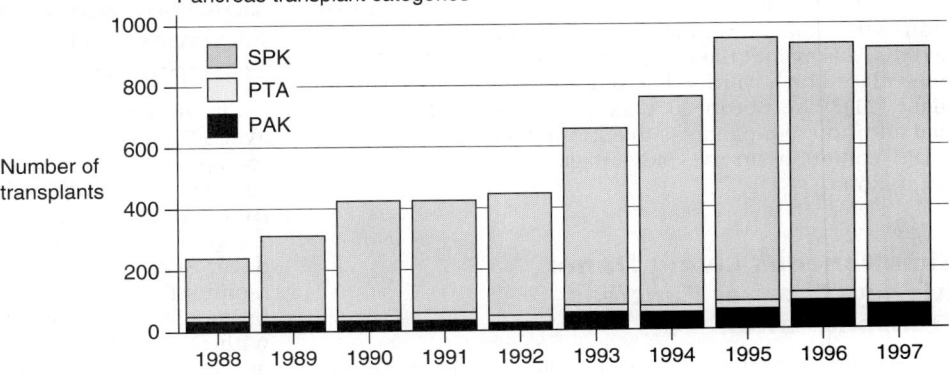

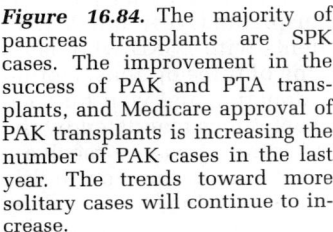

Figure 16.84. The majority of pancreas transplants are SPK cases. The improvement in the success of PAK and PTA transplants, and Medicare approval of PAK transplants is increasing the number of PAK cases in the last year. The trends toward more solitary cases will continue to increase.

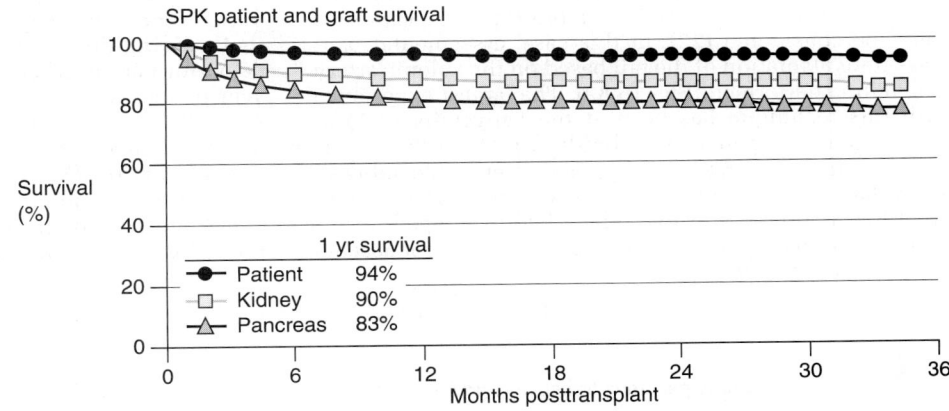

Figure 16.85. The patient, kidney, and pancreas graft survivals are depicted for SPK cases. Addition of a cadaver pancreas simultaneous to transplantation of a cadaver kidney does not jeopardize patient survival or kidney graft survival (data not shown).

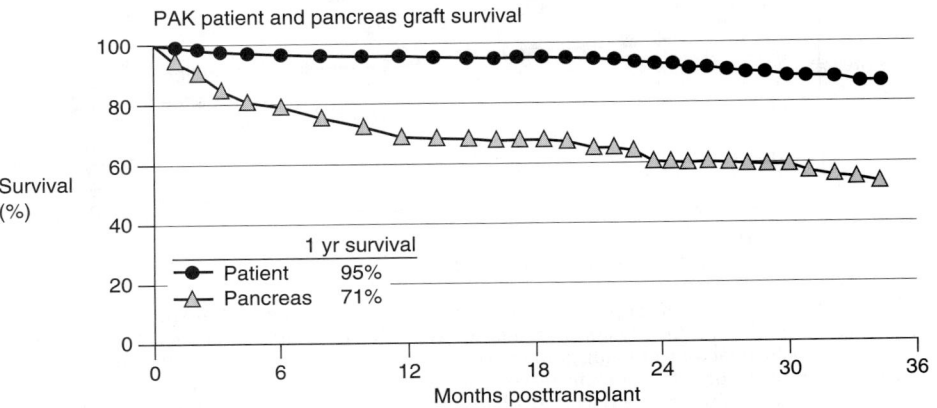

Figure 16.86. Patient and pancreas graft survival for pancreas after kidney cases (PAK). The difference in success between SPK and PAK cases is shrinking in the last four years with the availability of mycophenolate mofetil and tacrolimus immunosuppression combined with biopsy diagnosis of rejection.

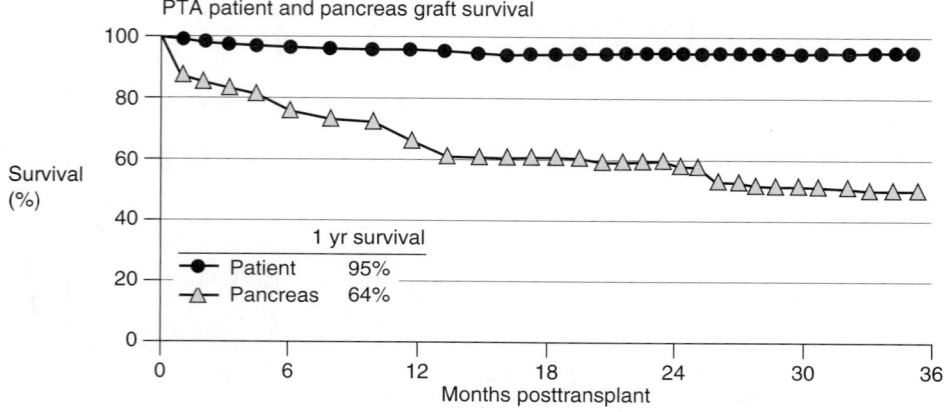

Figure 16.87. Patient and pancreas graft survival for pancreas transplant alone (PTA) cases performed in non-uremic Type 1 diabetics.

alone (19,20). Risk-adjusted data have documented that kidney transplantation for all causes is superior to continued dialysis even if the potential patient is healthy enough to be placed on a waiting list, but does not receive a transplant (21). The European data cited previously confirm that addition of a pancreas to a kidney transplant for type 1 DM confers a survival advantage over a kidney transplant alone.

Simultaneous Living Donor Kidney–Cadaver Pancreas Transplantation

In some circumstances it is justifiable to allow a living donor to donate both a kidney and pancreas segment at the same time. Certainly, with an identical twin donor who has been discordant for DM for more than 20 years, this could be considered (22). In this case, a segmental pancreas transplantation of the tail based on the splenic artery and vein is performed (Fig. 16.89). The largest experience with this technique has been at the University of Minnesota. One-year pancreas and kidney graft survival rates of 78% and 100%, respectively, have been achieved (23). There have been no donor deaths. Gastric varices developed in one donor, and two others had prolonged hospitalization, one for persistent ileus and the other for abscess in the lesser omental sac.

Simultaneous Cadaver Pancreas–Living Donor Kidney Transplantation

There is currently an excess of cadaver pancreases available for transplantation. Potential solitary pancreas transplant recipients are transplanted very quickly. In the past, type 1 diabetic patients with ESRD who had a living donor chose between one of three options. Option 1 was to reject living kidney donation and wait for a cadaver SPK. This choice was sometimes mandated by the recipient's insurance carrier. Option 2 was to receive a living donor kidney transplant alone and accept life with DM. Option 3 was to have a living donor kidney transplantation and then have a PAK procedure, usually 3 to 6 months later. Because of low intrinsic rejection rates in solitary pancreas transplants performed with portal venous drainage, investigators have hypothesized that a living donor kidney and cadaver pancreas could be performed together safely. In one report of 38 cases, 1-year pancreas and kidney graft survival rates were 92% and 97%, respectively (24). Moreover, the waiting time for simultaneous cadaver pancreas–living donor kidney transplantation (SPLK) was substantially less than for cadaver SPK. The cost of SPLK has been less than the combined cost of living donor kidney and PAK transplantation as separate procedures.

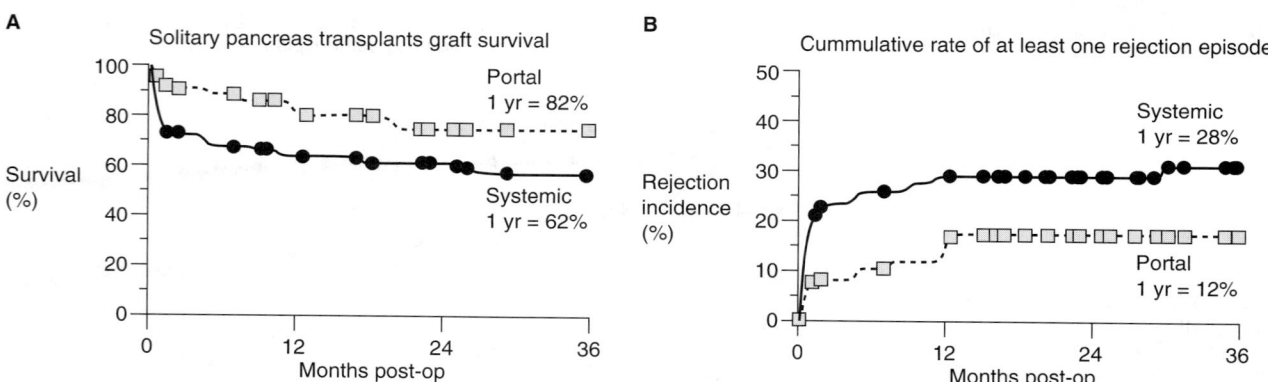

Figure 16.88. (A) Survival of portal venous drained solitary pancreas transplants at the UMMS is significantly higher at three years than that for systemically drained pancreas transplants. Multivariate analysis of factors effecting graft survival demonstrates that portal venous drainage emerges as a significant factor. (B) The main reason for the difference in survival is the markedly reduced incidence of rejection for pancreas transplants performed with portal venous drainage.

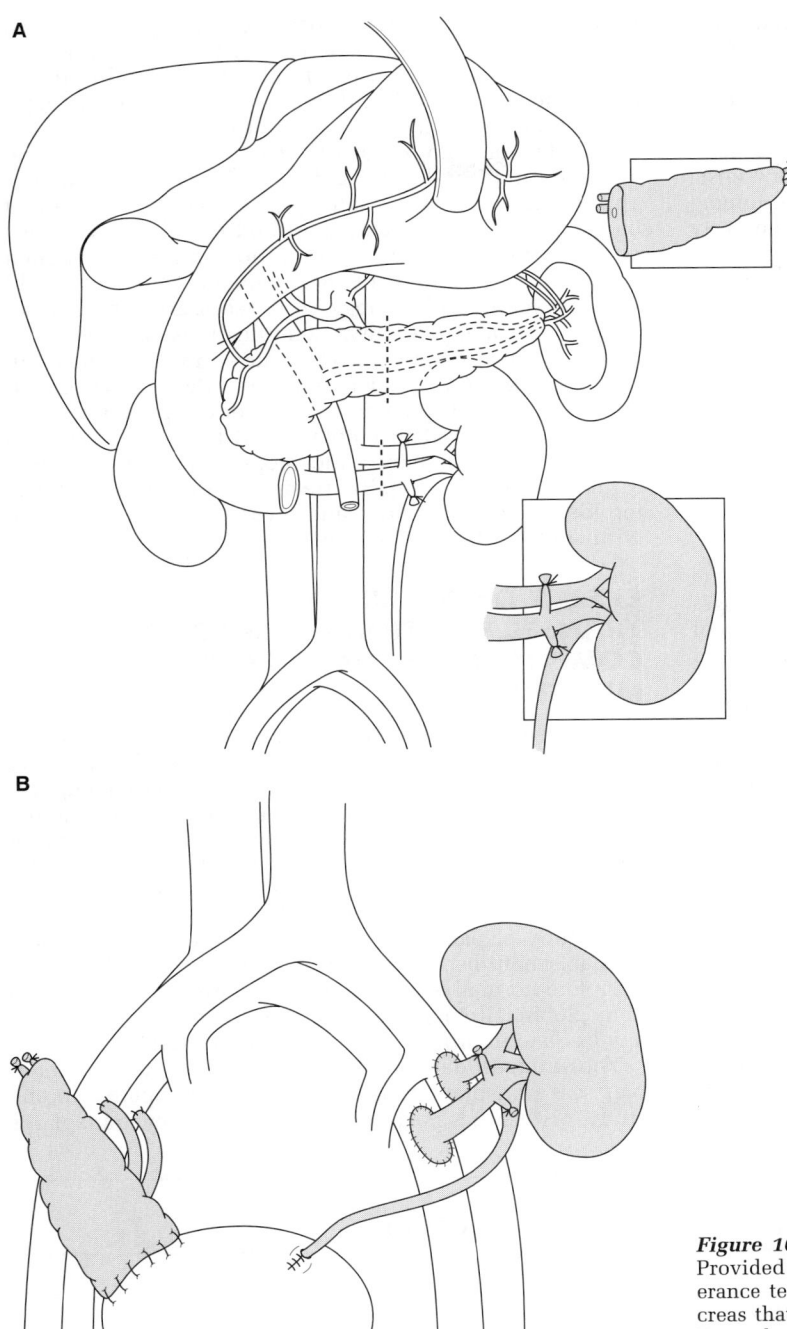

Figure 16.89. Live donor pancreas and kidney transplantation. Provided that the donor has a normal or supra-normal glucose tolerance test, a living donor may donate the segment of the pancreas that is to the left of the superior mesenteric vessels (10a). Transplantation of tail of the pancreas is based on the splenic artery and vein (10b).

COMPLICATIONS

Early thrombosis, usually within 48 hours of surgery, is the most common cause of nonimmunologic graft loss in the first year. Thrombosis is heralded by a sudden rise in blood glucose. Confirmation is usually obtained with duplex ultrasound. Treatment is the immediate removal of the transplant pancreas. Diabetic patients have a relative hypercoagulable state, in part because of defective fibrinolysis. Because SPK transplant recipients have uremic platelet dysfunction, they have only a 2% risk of early pancreatic thrombosis. In contrast, recipients of solitary pancreas transplants are nonuremic and consequently

have an 8% incidence of early thrombosis. To avoid this complication, some centers treat recipients with a continuous low-dose heparin infusion, followed by warfarin anticoagulation. Although this practice has been associated with an increased incidence of reexploration for bleeding, the incidence of early thrombosis has largely been eliminated.

The other major early complication is peripancreatic sepsis, caused by growth of organisms inoculated into the peritoneal cavity on opening the transplant duodenum. The diagnosis should be suspected if the patient has persistent ileus, fever, abdominal pain, leukocytosis, and tenderness between 7 and 14 days after surgery. Treatment includes abdominal lavage, débridement of necrotic peripancreatic fat, and antibiotics (25). There is evidence that prolonged attempts to treat peripancreatic sepsis with antibiotics lead to fungal peritonitis. Peripancreatic sepsis is rarely due to leakage from the duodenum–bladder or duodenoenteric anastomosis. If leakage occurs, one attempt at anastomotic revision can be attempted, but further leaks or sepsis should prompt removal of the pancreas. Computed tomography (CT)-guided drainage is unsuccessful in the early posttransplantation period because the infection is not confined to a discrete collection or cavity. Occasionally a very late (>30 days) presentation of an infected, discrete fluid collection can be resolved with catheter drainage. Although removal of a newly transplanted pancreas is demoralizing for the patient and surgeon, there is no excuse for a patient's death as a result of futile attempts to salvage a pancreas with repeated anastomotic leaks and sepsis. Most patients elect to attempt a second transplantation.

DIAGNOSIS AND TREATMENT OF REJECTION

The most crucial aspect of posttransplantation management is the timely diagnosis of rejection. The diagnosis of rejection is best confirmed with percutaneously obtained biopsy material that demonstrates the classic findings of renal or pancreatic rejection. With SPK transplants, monitoring the serum creatinine can prompt detection of rejection episodes with renal biopsy. Indications for pancreatic biopsy included hyperamylasemia, hyperlipasemia, hyperglycemia, or unexplained fever. Hyperglycemia is usually due to immunosuppression toxicity, but dose reduction without confirming the absence of rejection is hazardous. Moreover, the histologic picture of calcineurin inhibitor toxicity is distinguishable only by biopsy.

Unexplained fever may be the result of posttransplantation lymphoproliferative disorder or cytomegalovirus pancreatitis. In these settings, biopsy may be lifesaving. In SPK cases, both the pancreas and kidney should be sampled when technically feasible because nonsynchronous rejection can occur. If the indication for biopsy is hyperamylasemia, in 14% of cases a pancreatic biopsy is positive and the kidney negative. For bladder-drained solitary pancreas transplants, the appearance of hypoamylasuria, defined as a consistent 25% drop in urinary amylase excretion, or the aforementioned indications should prompt percutaneous biopsy. Blind treatment of rejection without a confirmatory biopsy is rarely appropriate.

Percutaneous biopsy is performed under local anesthesia with ultrasound or CT guidance. Tissue is obtained in approximately 85% of attempts. Usually the cause of biopsy failure is overlying gas-filled bowel loops. A second attempt after a bowel preparation and fasting is often successful. A failure of percutaneous biopsy should prompt laparoscopic biopsy or, if necessary, a biopsy obtained with a laparotomy. Complications from percutaneous pancreatic biopsy have occurred in fewer than 1 in 400 attempts (26). A major advance in the success of solitary pancreas transplantation is the development of a histologic grading system (Table 16.25) for determining the rejection grade in pancreatic biopsies (27) (Fig. 16.90). Mild rejection is usually treated with pulse corticosteroids, whereas moderate and severe rejection are treated with OKT3 or thymoglobulin.

EFFECT OF PANCREAS TRANSPLANTATION ON SECONDARY COMPLICATIONS OF DIABETES MELLITUS

The accumulated data clearly demonstrate that pancreas transplantation decreases mortality, improves the quality of life, and gradually reverses all of the secondary complications of DM except retinopathy. Failure clearly to demonstrate an effect on retinopathy relates to a lack of appropriate long-term studies. A benefit can be inferred because there is a significant effect of intensive insulin therapy on diabetic retinopathy. It is reasonable to assume that a long-term study of pancreas transplant recipients would show similar benefit because pancreas transplantation leads to a complete normalization of blood glucose and glycosylated hemoglobin ($HbA1_c$) levels, whereas intensive insulin therapy leads to improved but still abnormal $HbA1_c$ levels.

The strongest data have related to the dramatic effect of pancreas transplantation on diabetic nephropathy. In one study, within 2.5 years of operation, kidney transplants

---

Table 16.25. GRADING SYSTEM FOR THE DIAGNOSIS OF ACUTE AND CHRONIC REJECTION IN PANCREAS ALLOGRAFT BIOPSIES

Classification	Description
GRADING OF PANCREAS ACUTE ALLOGRAFT REJECTION[a]	
Grade A-0	No rejection (no inflammation)
Grade A-1	No definite rejection (nonspecific septal inflammation)
Grades A-II–III	Minimal–mild acute rejection (mixed inflammation in fibrous septa involving veins and ducts, acinar inflammation)
Grade A-IV	Moderate acute rejection (arterial involvement essential for diagnosis; features of grades II and III are often also present
Grade A-V	Severe rejection (additional severe parenchymal damage—necrosis, secondary to vascular rejection)
GRADING OF PANCREAS CHRONIC ALLOGRAFT REJECTION[b]	
Grade C-0	No fibrosis
Grade C-I	Mild chronic rejection (mild expansion of fibrous septa with very focal acinar loss)
Grade C-II	Moderate chronic rejection (septal fibrosis with 30%–40% parenchymal loss/atrophy)
Grade C-III	Severe chronic rejection (septal fibrosis with 50% parenchymal loss/atrophy)

Note: Ischemia, pancreatitis, viral infections (cytomegalovirus, Epstein-Barr virus), peripancreatic abscess should be excluded before applying the Acute Allograft Rejection Grading Scheme.
[a]Modified from Drachenberg CB, Steinberger E, Hoehn-Saric EW, et al. Evaluation of pancreas transplant needle biopsy: reproducibility and revision of histologic grading system. Transplantation 1997;63:1579–1586.
[b]Modified from Drachenberg CB, Papadimitriou JC, Klassen DK, et al. Chronic pancreas allograft rejection: morphological evidence of progression in needle biopsies and proposal of a grading scheme. Transplantation Proc 1999;31:614.

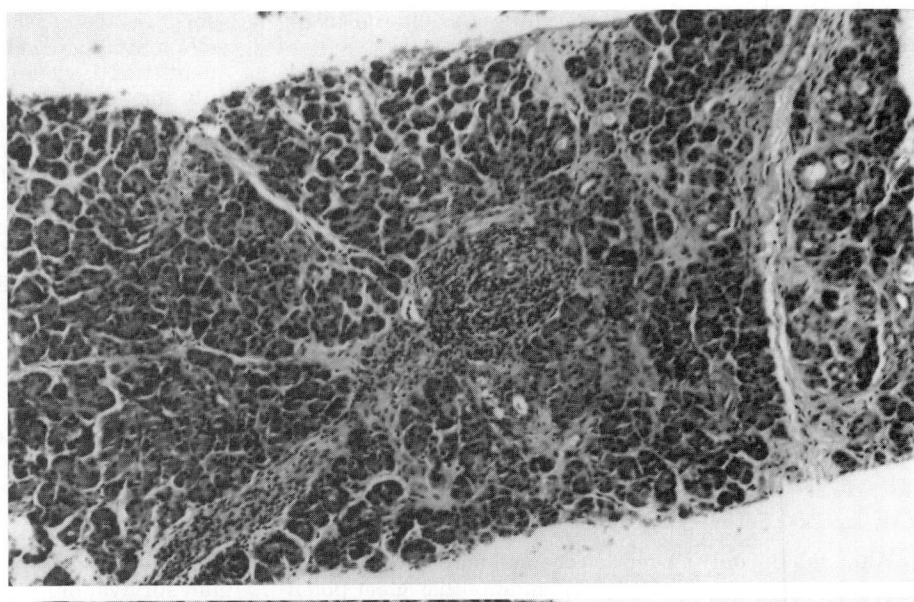

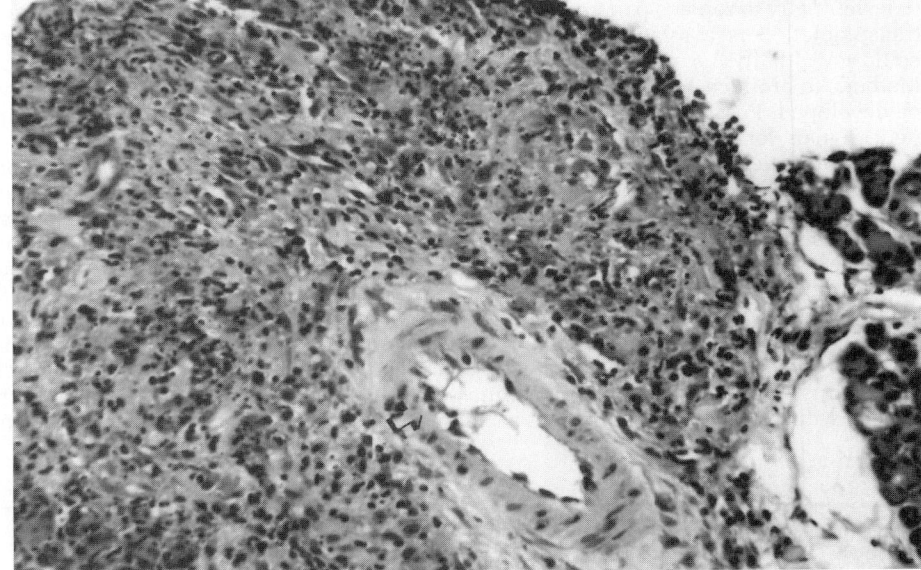

Figure 16.90. *(A)* Percutaneous pancreas biopsy specimen stained with hematoxylin and eosin. Note the predominant mononuclear septal and focal acinar inflammation. The veins are cuffed by the inflammatory infiltrate and the venous endothelium is damaged. Grade A-III rejection. *(B)* Severe acute allograft rejection. An artery shows early endothelitis *(arrow).* The surrounding perenchyma shows extensive necrosis and mixed inflammation. Viable parenchyma is seen to the far right (Grade A-V).

alone in patients with type 1 DM developed thickening of the glomerular basement membrane and mesangial thickening, findings typical of early diabetic nephropathy. In a comparable group of SPK transplant recipients, none of these findings was present on renal biopsy. More surprising was the report that showed a gradual reversal of native diabetic nephropathy in the 10 years after successful pancreas transplantation. These reports clearly show that pancreas transplantation can prevent recurrent diabetic nephropathy in transplanted kidneys. If applied early enough in the course of diabetic nephropathy, renal function may be preserved by pancreas transplantation.

The effect of pancreas transplantation on diabetic neuropathy has been clearly documented using tests of nerve conduction velocity and action potential amplitude. Nerve conduction velocity shows rapid early improvement, and action potential amplitude, a more sensitive indicator of actual axonal recovery, shows gradual recovery over time. No study has shown a significant difference in neurologic recovery by clinical examination. These studies demonstrate continued deterioration of nontransplanted control subjects relative to stable examination findings in patients with successful transplants. Similar to the findings on the effects on nephropathy, the beneficial effect of a pancreas transplantation in arresting progressive neuropathy is immediate, whereas the effect on reversal of clinical and histologic changes is as gradual as the original injury.

Patients with type 1 DM have a 40% 7-year mortality rate from sudden death if there is objective evidence of abnormal cardiorespiratory reflexes, compared with a 14% rate mortality in a cohort of patients with type 1 DM without autonomic neuropathy (28). Consistent with the findings on peripheral neuropathy, successful pancreas transplantation has been shown to lead to gradual improvement in cardiorespiratory reflexes, including improvement in the electrocardiographic RR interval after a Valsalva maneuver. Successful pancreas transplantation can reduce mortality from sudden death. As noted previously, diabetic patients with frequent episodes of hypoglycemia eventually acquire blunted epinephrine responses to hypoglycemia and hypoglycemic symptom unawareness. Successful pancreas transplantation restores both deficits (29).

There are no studies demonstrating a reduction in the incidence or progression of atherosclerosis as result of successful pancreas transplantation. There is evidence that, compared with appropriate control subjects, pancreas transplantation leads to an improvement in serum lipoprotein profiles (30). As might be expected, quality-of-life studies demonstrate improvement in patient sense of well-being as well as psychological health.

In summary, pancreas transplantation has taken a place among the other four solid organ transplantations as a procedure with accepted benefits. The severe shortage of suitable pancreases for transplantation (currently no more than 5,000 per year in the United States) dictates that only patients experiencing diabetic complications are considered as candidates. The development of xenogeneic donors will be necessary to expand the indications for pancreas transplantation.

TRANSPLANTATION OF THE ISLETS OF LANGERHANS

Although the only currently accepted cure for DM is pancreas transplantation, islet transplantation has great potential eventually to replace pancreas transplantation. Islet cell transplantation is a relatively nonmorbid procedure that could eventually be performed on an outpatient basis. Methods to produce an unlimited supply of islets may soon be developed. Possibilities include manipulation of the genetic signals for the differentiation of islets of Langerhans from pancreatic embryonic stem cells, or by clonal expansion of beta cells in vitro under the influence of growth factors. It was initially hoped that the simple transfection of the proinsulin gene into non-beta cells such as hepatocytes might be a solution to the shortage of transplantable islet tissue. Although in vitro insulin secretion can be demonstrated from transfected cells, it is now clear that the cellular mechanisms for stimulus–secretion coupling are highly complex and still incompletely characterized. The possibility that this complex intracellular machinery could be transfected is uncertain. Development of a "humanized" xenogeneic source of islet tissue or development of islets from embryonic stem cells may eventually lead to expanded quantity of tissue for cellular transplantation. Currently, the only source for islet tissue is cadaver pancreases that have been refused for use as solid organ transplants. This arrangement is a practical necessity because the success of pancreas transplantation relative to the developmental status of islet transplantation gives the whole pancreas priority in the current pancreas allocation scheme used by the United Network for Organ Sharing. Despite this allocation scheme, there are regions of the United States with undeveloped interest in pancreas transplantation that allow the use of pancreases for research and clinical application.

Islet Isolation

Techniques for the isolation of intact islets from the whole pancreas were initially developed to facilitate rodent research on islet physiology and transplantation (31). The first report of successful complete reversal of DM in rodents led to general enthusiasm that clinical application was at hand because numerous strategies leading to indefinite graft survival of rodent islets without continuous immunosuppression had been identified (32). These strategies include islet cell culture, treatment with anti-class II antibody and complement, intrathymic transplantation, transfection of immunosuppressive genes into islets or cotransplanted cells, and use of immunoprivileged sites such as the testicle (Table 16.26). In sharp contrast to the rodent experience, in which a large array of strategies leads to indefinite islet acceptance, these same techniques applied to larger mammalian models have virtually no effect. The relative ease of islet isolation in rodents has not been observed for porcine, primate, or human pancreas (Fig. 16.91). Little progress in the development of human clinical islet transplantation was made until the development of a reproducible technique for the mass isolation of human and large animal islets (33). This development was coupled with the commercial availability of highly purified, endotoxin-free collagenase specifically designed for human islet isolation.

Table 16.26. ANTIREJECTION METHODS IN THE ABSENCE OF CONTINUOUS IMMUNOSUPPRESSION IN RODENTS THAT LEAD TO INDEFINITE SURVIVAL

Method	Species	Reference
24°C culture pretreatment of donor islets combined with single injection of antilymphocyte serum	Rat	Lacy PE, et al. Science 1979;204:312–313.
95% O_2 pretreatment of donor islets	Mouse	Bowen KM, et al. Aust J Exp Biol Med Sci 1980;58:441–447.
Microencapsulation of islets	Rat	Lim F, Sun AM. Science 1980;210:908–910.
Donor-specific blood transfusions treated with ultraviolet irradiation	Rat	Lau H, et al. Science 1984;221:754–756.
Ultraviolet irradiation of donor islets combined with a 3-day course of cyclosporine	Rat	Lau H, et al. Science 1984;223:607–609.
Transplantation of islets into the intraabdominally placed testis	Rat	Selawry HJ, Whittington K. Diabetes 1984;33:405–406.
Gamma irradiation pretreatment of donor islets combined with a 3-day course of cyclosporine	Rat	James R, et al. Transplantation 1989;47:929–933.
Intrathymic islet transplantation combined with a single injection of antilymphocyte serum	Rat	Posselt A, et al. Science 1990;249:1293–1295.
Selective costimulatory blockade by anti-CD154 treatment combined with pretransplantation infusion of donor lymphocytes	Mouse	Parker, et al. Proc Nat Acad Sci USA 1995;96:9560–9564.
Cotransplantation of syngeneic myoblasts engineered to express the Fas liquid	Mouse	Lau H, et al. Science 1996;273:109–112.
Cotransplantation of allogeneic testicular cell aggregates	Rat	Korbutt GS, et al. Diabetes 1997;46:317–322.
Antibody-mediated targeting of CD45 isoforms	Mouse	Basadonna GP, et al. Proc Natl Acad Sci USA 1998;95:3821–3826.

Reproduced from Herring BJ, Ricordi C. Islet transplantation for patients with type I diabetes. Graft 1999;2:23, with permission.

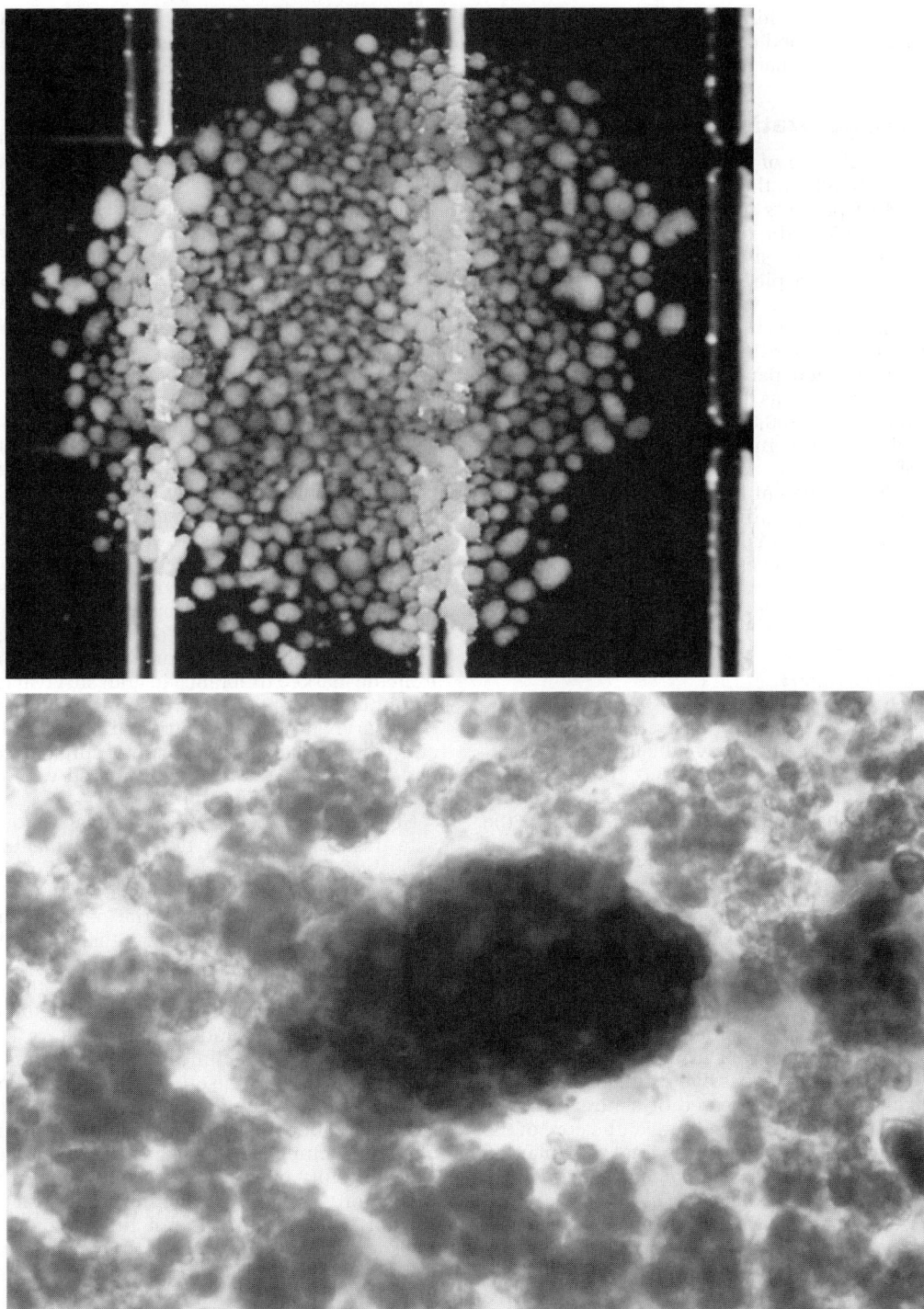

Figure 16.91. *(A)* Five hundred murine islets that have been prepared for transplantation. This number of islets will successfully reverse diabetes in a mouse if transplanted intraportally or under the renal capsule. This usually requires 4–6 mouse donors. (Photograph courtesy of Teruo Okitsu, M.D., University of Maryland.) *(B)* Human islet stained with dithizone. (Photograph courtesy of Alan Farney, M.D., University of Maryland.)

Islet Transplant Technique in Humans

The most common site of islet implantation has been intrahepatic. The portal vein was accessed, in the past, by cannulation of one of major branches of the inferior mesenteric vein during laparotomy. In the case of islet autotransplantations performed on patients undergoing total pancreatectomy for intractable chronic pancreatitis, this is still the usual method for gaining access to the portal circulation. Interventional radiology techniques now allow access to the portal circulation percutaneously by direct needle cannulation of a portal radical, followed by introduction of a temporary Silastic catheter through which islets can by infused. Barring the need for hospitalization due to the administration of antibody immunosuppression, or the surgery necessary to perform simultaneous islet–kidney

(SIK) transplantation, by avoiding laparotomy, islet transplantation could be performed on an outpatient basis, as is commonly done with bone marrow transplantation.

Islet Autotransplantation

The most successful form of islet transplant is the autotransplant, a setting in which there is no immunologic barrier to success. Most patients undergoing this procedure have severe, intractable pain from chronic pancreatitis, have had a previous unsuccessful duct drainage procedure such as the Puestow-Gillespie operation, and have preserved insulin secretion and independence from exogenous insulin requirements. The major limitation to this technique is the increased difficulty in isolating islets from a fibrotic or calcified pancreas. The largest experience with this technique has been at the University of Minnesota. If more than 300,000 islets are successfully isolated, the recipients are insulin independent after 1 year in 74% of cases (34). Approximately 5,000 islet equivalents (an islet equivalent is a 150-μm islet) per kilogram is needed to achieve insulin independence in the autograft setting. The success of islet autotransplants reveals that the major obstacle to successful islet allotransplantation is immunologic.

Barriers to Successful Islet Transplantation

Nonspecific Immunity

Although several world centers have the technical expertise to obtain isolated islets, the combined effects of nonspecific immunity, alloimmunity, and recurrent autoimmunity necessitate a much larger islet cell mass than in the autograft setting. Successful allotransplants have required an average of 12,000 islet equivalents per kilogram. The first barrier to successful allotransplantation is the ability consistently to obtain this increased yield. Some of the early successful cases relied on the combined yield from as many as four pancreases. With the increased success of pancreas transplantation, there is increased pressure to use a single donor pancreas. After transplantation, islets require approximately 10 days to revascularize by capillary ingrowth from the hepatic sinusoid. During the avascular period, the islet must depend on passive diffusion for nutrition. Islets typically undergo a degree of central necrosis during this time. Because the beta cells are at the core of the islet, this process inordinately affects the total transplanted beta cell mass. The nonspecific inflammatory reaction at the site of islet embolization leads to local synthesis of inflammatory cytokines such TNF-α, IFN-γ, and IL-1. Each of these cytokines has been shown to be toxic to the beta cell or to impair insulin secretion. In addition, activation of hepatic macrophages leads to local liberation of oxygen free radicals, to which islets are particularly sensitive because of a constitutive lack of intrinsic antioxidant activity. Inflammatory injury of the islet may sensitize the islet to traditional T-cell alloimmunity and autoimmunity (35,36).

Increased Metabolic Demand

The combined effects of immunosuppression lead to a state of peripheral insulin resistance. Moreover, both calcineurin inhibitors (cyclosporine and tacrolimus) depress transcription of the proinsulin mRNA and lead to abnormal stimulus–secretion coupling of insulin secretion (37). To maintain a euglycemic state, a kidney transplant recipient must increase insulin secretion to 2.5 times normal. This may not be deleterious to a pancreas transplant recipient because the whole beta cell mass is engrafted;

however, because islet cell transplants are often marginal, the effect of immunosuppression can be decisive.

Alloimmunity

There is no experimental or clinical evidence that islet transplants are more sensitive to the effector mechanism of rejection than the whole pancreas (38). This concept has been established by comparing the rapidity of rejection of allogeneic whole-pancreas transplants with that of islet transplants in the Brown Norway to Lewis rodent strain combination. Clinically, the chance of renal rejection in SPK transplants is the same as for SIK transplants, suggesting that islets elicit no greater an alloimmune response than the whole pancreas.

Autoimmunity

Several lines of evidence suggest that islets are particularly sensitive to recurrent autoimmunity. Clinically, recurrent disease in whole-pancreas transplants has been conclusively observed in identical twin pancreas transplantations performed without immunosuppression. In sharp contrast, immunosuppressed pancreatic allografts have had only 2 documented cases of recurrent autoimmunity in more than 10,000 transplantations. Analysis of 300 percutaneous biopsy specimens performed at various times posttransplantation for the diagnosis of rejection did not reveal any histologic evidence of recurrent autoimmunity (39). The clinical evidence for recurrent autoimmunity in islet allografts stems from the marked difference in graft survival in relation to the autoimmune status of the recipient. For instance, the 1-year graft survival of islet allografts in nonautoimmune recipients who are diabetic as a result of surgical extirpation of the pancreas is 45% at 1 year, compared with only 8% in patients with type 1 (autoimmune) DM.

Similarly, whole-pancreas transplants from isogeneic diabetes-resistant (BB-DR) donors transplanted into spontaneously diabetic BB rats leads to indefinite graft survival. Transplantation of isolated islets from the same donors leads to recurrent disease after a brief period of normoglycemia. Investigators have hypothesized that the protective factor in the whole pancreas is the pancreatic lymph node cells, which were demonstrated to engraft in the recipient, creating donor chimerism and ablating the autoimmune state through action of included autoregulatory T cells. Although this concept fits the clinical data well, it has not been conclusively proven in the other animal model of DM, the NOD mouse, or in the human. Nevertheless, the sharply differing results of clinical islet transplantations in autoimmune and nonautoimmune recipients makes it apparent that recurrent autoimmunity plays an important role in human islet transplantation. The ability of immunosuppression to control recurrent autoimmunity is not fully known. The long-term goal of achieving tolerance to human islet transplants will require that the mechanism of recurrent autoimmunity be fully elucidated, and autoimmune as well as alloimmune tolerance will have to be achieved.

Technique of Human Islet Isolation

Islets are isolated from the whole pancreas by enzymatic digestion. The enzyme preparation contains a mixture of collagenase, neutral protease, and thermolysin that permits "liberation" of islets from the acinar and connective tissue elements without disrupting the intraislet cellular connections. Typically, the enzymatic solution is infused through the pancreatic duct, distending the lobules of the pancreas. After a period of digestion at 37°C, the dispersed tissue is separated into a relatively pure fraction of islets using a cell separator. Most islet autotransplantations are performed as a transplantation of a cruder digest to prevent reduction in the marginal yield obtained from the abnormal pancreases used in this procedure. Islet allotransplantations are performed with more highly purified islets.

Immunosuppression

The optimal regimen to achieve permanent islet engraftment has not been established. Two areas have received research emphasis. Protocols must have minimal diabetogenic side effects. Thus, protocols emphasize induction with antibodies that do not induce cytokine release such as anti-IL-2R monoclonal antibodies. Maintenance protocols that avoid or minimize the use of prednisone and the calcineurin inhibitors, cyclosporine and tacrolimus, are desirable. Elimination of the calcineurin inhibitors has been difficult because they have been the most effective class of agents. Newer agents such as sirolimus and mycophenolate mofetil promise to move us closer to a goal of nondiabetogenic immunosuppression.

The second goal of immunosuppression is to achieve true tolerance to transplanted islets. The primate preclinical trials of anti-CD40L (anti-CD154) suggest that this is a realistic possibility (40,41). Investigators have demonstrated 200-day islet allograft survival without immunosuppression in various species of nonhuman primate. Similarly, others have achieved prolonged primate kidney allograft survival without continuous immunosuppression. Many endocrinologists believe that for the stable diabetic patient who is free of secondary complications, the substitution of full-dose immunosuppression for insulin is not a favorable trade. The goal of achieving tolerance to transplanted islets has been the thrust of an enormous amount of grant funding and research activity by transplantation surgeons and immunologists since the first successful rodent islet transplant in 1973. The successful completion of this project will undoubtedly be recognized as one of the greatest achievements in surgery.

Results of Clinical Islet Transplantation

Before 1990, the success of even a single case resulted in case reports in the peer-reviewed literature. With methodical application of strategies to improve early islet function, the success of clinical islet transplantation has markedly improved. The most recent report of the Islet Transplant Registry reveals a rate of insulin independence for at least 1 week of 13% in patients with type 1 DM. The rate of insulin independence after 1 year is only 8% in cases performed between 1990 and 1998. The possibility should be recognized that there is underreporting of unsuccessful cases. Despite the overall disappointing results, some centers are obtaining more promising results. A report from the University of Giessen in Germany revealed that 75% of cases of SIK transplants performed since 1996 retain significant insulin secretion after 1 year, with mean C-peptide levels of 1.8 ng/mL. Although not completely insulin independent in all cases, the patients experienced significant benefit through the elimination of severe hypoglycemic episodes and marked improvement in HbA1$_c$ values. Although only 13% of patients remain insulin independent after 1 year, 33% retain C-peptide levels greater than 0.5 ng/mL and 26% have levels greater than 1.0 ng/mL. On the other hand, 33% lost all function within 1 month, indicating that both immunologic and nonimmunologic attacks take a significant toll in the early posttransplantation period. Using a novel corticosteroid free immunosuppression protocol consisting of daclizamab induction combined with low maintenance doses of sirolimus and tacrolimus, Shapiro has reported a break-through in the success of islet transplantation alone in Type I diabetics. Although islets from two donor pancreas were required, seven

of seven recipients of islet transplants became insulin independent for 4 to 15 months (42). These findings will be reevaluated in an NIH sponsored international, multi-center trial. With the release of several new immunosuppressive agents, these results may improve. Major funding from the Juvenile Diabetes Foundation and the National Institutes of Health to support the establishment of core facilities to perform mass isolation and cryopreservation of human islets have been awarded. This support will accelerate progress by allowing many centers access to large-scale quantities of viable islets for research and clinical trials.

REFERENCES

1. Foster D. Diabetes mellitus. In: Fauci AS, Braunwald E, Isselbucher K, et al., eds. *Harrison's principles of internal medicine.* New York: McGraw-Hill, 1998:2060–2080.
2. Sibley RK, Sutherland DR, Goetz F, et al. Recurrent diabetes mellitus in the pancreas iso- and allograft: a light and electron microscopic and immunohistochemical analysis of four cases. *Lab Invest* 1985;53:132.
3. Lampeter EF, Homberg M, Quabeck K, et al. Transfer of insulin-dependent diabetes between HLA-identical siblings by bone marrow transplantation. *Lancet* 1993;341:1245.
4. Wong FS, Karttunen J, Dumont C, et al. Identification of an MHC class I-restricted autoantigen in type I diabetes by screening an organ-specific cDNA library. *Nat Med* 1999;5: 1026–1031.
5. The Diabetes Control and Complications Trial Research Group. The effect of intensive treatment of diabetes on the development and progression of long-term complications in insulin-dependent diabetes mellitus. *N Engl J Med* 1993;329: 977–986.
6. Kelly WD, Lillehei R, Merkel F, et al. Allotransplantation of the pancreas and duodenum along with the kidney in diabetic nephropathy. *Surgery* 1967;61:827.
7. Schweitzer E, Anderson L, Kuo P, et al. Safe pancreas transplantation in patients with coronary artery disease. *Transplantation* 1997;63:1294–1299.
8. Troppmann C, Gruessner A, Benedetti E, et al. Vascular graft thrombosis after pancreatic transplantation: univariate and multivariate operative and nonoperative risk factor analysis. *J Am Coll Surg* 1996;182:285–316.
9. Kapur S, Bonham C, Dodson S, et al. Strategies to expand the donor pool for pancreas transplantation. *Transplantation* 1999;67:284–290.
10. Bartlett S, Kuo P, Johnson L, et al. Pancreas transplantation at the University of Maryland. *Clin Transpl* 1996;23:271–280.
11. Del Pizzo JJ, Jacobs S, Bartlett ST, et al. Urologic complications of bladder-drained pancreatic allografts. *Br J Urol* 1998; 81:543–547.
12. Bartlett ST. Techniques of pancreatic duct implantation. *Curr Opin Organ Transpl* 1998;3:248–252.
13. Sollinger HW, Odorico JS, Knechtle S, et al. Experience with 500 simultaneous pancreas-kidney transplants. *Ann Surg* 1998;228:284–296.
14. Gaber A, Shokouh-Amiri M, Hathaway D, et al. Results of pancreas transplantation with portal venous and enteric drainage. *Ann Surg* 1995;221:613–624.
15. Jordan M, Shapiro R, Gritsch H, et al. Long-term results of pancreas transplantation under tacrolimus immunosuppression. *Transplantation* 1999;67:266–272.
16. Bartlett ST, Schweitzer EJ, Johnson L, et al. Equivalent success of simultaneous pancreas kidney and solitary pancreas transplantation: a prospective trial of tacrolimus immunosuppression with percutaneous biopsy. *Ann Surg* 1996:224:440–452.
17. Drachenberg CB, Klassen DK, Weir MR, et al. Islet cell damage associated with tacrolimus and cyclosporine: morphological features in pancreas allograft biopsies and clinical correlation. *Transplantation* 1999;68:396–402.
18. Philosophe B, Farnay AC, Schweitzer EJ, et al. The superiority of portal venous drainage over systemic venous drainage in pancreas transplantation. *Annals of Surgery*, 2001 (in press).
19. Smets YF, Westendrop RG, can der Pijl JW, et al. Effect of simultaneous pancreas-kidney transplantation on the mortality

of patients with type-1 diabetes mellitus and end-stage renal failure. *Lancet* 1999;353:1915–1919.

20. Tyden G, Bolinder J, Solders G, et al. Improved survival in patients with insulin-dependent diabetes mellitus and end-stage diabetic nephropathy 10 years after combined pancreas and kidney transplantation. *Transplantation* 1999;67:645–648.

21. Wolfe RA, Ashby VB, Milford EL, et al. Comparison of mortality in all patients on dialysis, patient on dialysis awaiting transplant, and recipients of first cadaveric transplantation. *N Engl J Med* 1999;341(23):1725–1730.

22. Benedetti E, Dunn T, Massad MG, et al. Successful living related simultaneous pancreas-kidney transplant between identical twins. *Transplantation* 1999;67:915–918.

23. Gruessner R, Kendall D, Drangsstveit M, et al. Simultaneous pancreas-kidney transplantation from live donors. *Ann Surg* 1997;226:471–482.

24. Farney A, Cho E, Schweitzer E, et al. Simultaneous cadaver pancreas living donor kidney transplantation (SPLK): a new approach for the type I diabetic uremic patient. *Ann Surg* 2000;232:696–703.

25. Bartlett ST. Pancreas transplantation after thirty years: still room for improvement [editorial]. *J Am Coll Surg* 1996;183:408–410.

26. Klassen DK, Hoehn-Saric EW, Weir MR, et al. Isolate pancreas rejection in combined kidney-pancreas transplantation: results of percutaneous biopsy. *Transplantation* 1996;61:974–977.

27. Drachenberg CB, Steinberger E, Hoehn-Saric EW, et al. Evaluation of pancreas transplant needle biopsy: reproducibility and revision of histologic grading system. *Transplantation* 1997;63:1579–1586.

28. Navarro X, Kennedy WR, Lowenson RB, et al. Influence of pancreas transplantation on cardiorespiratory reflexes, nerve conduction, and mortality in diabetes mellitus. *Diabetes* 1990;39:818–822.

29. Kendall DM, Rooney DP, Smets YF, et al. Pancreas transplantation restores epinephrine response and symptom recognition during hypoglycemia in patients with long-standing type I diabetes and autonomic neuropathy. *Diabetes* 1997;46:249–257.

30. Hughes T, Gaber O, Amiri H, et al. Kidney-pancreas transplantation: the effect of portal versus systemic venous drainage of the pancreas on the lipoprotein composition. *Transplantation* 1995;60:1406–1412.

31. Lacy PE, Kostianovsky M. Method for the isolation of intact islets from the rat pancreas. *Diabetes* 1967;16:35–39.

32. Reekard CR, Ziegler MM, Barker CF. Physiological and immunological consequences of transplanting isolated pancreatic islets. *Surgery* 1973;74:91–99.

33. Ricordi C, Lacy PE, Finke EH, et al. Automated method for isolation of human pancreatic islets. *Diabetes* 1988;37:413–420.

34. Wahoff DC, Papalois BE, Najarian JS, et al. Autologous islet transplantation to prevent diabetes after pancreatic resection. *Ann Surg* 1995;222:562–575.

35. Kaufman DB, Platt JL, Rabe FL, et al. Differential roles of Mac-1+ cells, and CD4+ and CD8+ T lymphocytes in primary nonfunction and classic rejection of islet allografts. *J Exp Med* 1990;172:291–302.

36. Halloran PF, Homik J, Goes N, et al. The "injury response": a concept linking nonspecific injury, acute rejection, and long-term transplant outcomes. *Transplant Proc* 1997;29:79–81.

37. Gillison SL, Bartlett ST, Curry DL. Synthesis–secretion coupling insulin: effect of cyclosporine. *Diabetes* 1989;38:465–470.

38. Bartlett ST, Schweitzer EJ, Kuo PC, et al. Prevention of autoimmune islet allograft destruction by engraftment of donor T cells. *Transplantation* 1997;63:299–303.

39. Drachenberg CB, Papadimitriou JC, Weir MR, et al. Histologic findings in islets of whole pancreas allografts: lack of evidence for recurrent cell-medicated diabetes mellitus. *Transplantation* 1996;62:170–72.

40. Kenyon NS, Fernandez L, Masetti M, et al. Humanized anti-CD154 enhances islet allograft survival in non human primates. Abstract presented at the XVII World Congress of the Transplantation Society, July 12–17, 1998, Montreal, Quebec, Canada.

41. Kirk AD, Harlan DM, Armstrong NN, et al. CTLA4-Ig and anti-CD40 ligand prevent renal allograft rejection in primates. *Proc Natl Acad Sci USA* 1997;94:8789–8794.

42. Shapiro AMJ, Lakey JRT, Ryan EA. Islet transplantation in seven patients with type I diabetes mellitus using a glucocorticoid free immunosuppressive regimen. *N Eng J Med* 2000;343:230–238.

SURGERY: SCIENTIFIC PRINCIPLES AND PRACTICE, Third Edition, edited by Lazar J. Greenfield, Michael W. Mulholland, Keith T. Oldham, Gerald B. Zelenock, and Keith D. Lillemoe. Lippincott Williams & Wilkins Publishers, Philadelphia, © 2001.

CHAPTER 17

EVIDENCE-BASED SURGERY

TOBY GORDON

The principles of evidence-based medicine have been increasingly integrated into the contemporary practice of surgery. The continuous striving of the surgical profession to improve the delivery of health care, the rising demand for surgical services, the close scrutiny by government and managed care of health care costs, and the increasingly knowledgeable health care consumer have all contributed to this trend. Evidence-based surgery draws from the disciplines of medicine and public health, and is centered on the acquisition, evaluation, and application of evidence for the care of the individual patient. More broadly defined beyond the care of the single patient, evidence-based surgery also encompasses population-based outcomes research focused on clinical, economic, and patient-reported data. This chapter was written to assist surgeons in producing and understanding "evidence" related to surgical practice, so they can interpret such information in educational and patient care forums alike.

SURGICAL EVIDENCE: A HISTORICAL PERSPECTIVE

Over the history of surgery, surgical evidence has progressed from anecdote and observations, case studies and reports of patient series, to sophisticated laboratory, clinical, and epidemiologic research. The modern surgical era began in the mid-19th century when major obstacles to the progress of surgery—pain, infection, and hemorrhage—were eliminated. The introduction of anesthesia by Morton in 1846 and the development and acceptance of Lister's principles of antisepsis and aseptic surgery in 1867 led to the development of totally new surgical procedures and the rising use of hospitals as places to care for patients. The formulation of Halsted's conservative surgical principles, the discovery of x-rays, and new principles of hemostasis brought about considerable advances in surgery from the middle to the end of the 19th century. The advent of abdominal, vascular, and orthopedic surgery and increasingly invasive and curative procedures were hallmarks of this era. The increasing professionalism of surgery brought about the promulgation of surgical texts, articles, and journals, the rise of specialty surgical societies, and a new model for surgical training in the United States developed by Halsted at The Johns Hopkins Hospital.

The proceedings of the American Surgical Association (ASA), founded in 1880, serve as a record of the development of surgery in the United States and provide a historical perspective on the types of surgical "evidence" in use. Major advances in surgery reported from 1880 to 1930 reflect the focus of evolution of the surgical research: technologic developments such as radiation, direct examination of the urinary tract by cystoscopy, blood transfusion, and the electric cautery, and improvements in operations such as thyroidectomy, gastric resection, and craniotomy resulted in decreased mortality (1). Early research reports were descriptive and anecdotal, but reflect interest in outcomes of surgical treatment. Barnes, in a review of the ASA transactions from 1882 to 1942, examined surgical procedures that were ultimately proven to be non-beneficial and abandoned, citing the poor understanding of disease processes as enabling such procedures to endure for considerable periods before their demise. The major reasons cited for the prolonged acceptance of ineffectual operations include acceptance by surgeons, absence of ethical constraints in the development and application of new procedures, and inadequate knowledge of methods for outcome analysis and follow-up. Thus, from 1880 to 1942, new operative approaches often were developed on the basis of intuition and insight and were evaluated primarily based on trial and error.

The turning point in the evolution of evidence-based surgery can be attributed to Ernest Amory Codman who, in 1910, began efforts to reform clinical medicine and surgery. With his surgical mentor, F.B. Harrington, Codman created a case monitoring system in 1900 to record outcomes. Codman's "end-results" system proposed individual patient cards for data collection, on which a determination would be made regarding outcome and, if "perfection" had not been obtained, classification of such imperfect cases using his nosology of errors. Codman reasoned that by using his system of comparison, surgeons could specialize in operations they did best. He further proposed that each hospital would require an end-results clerk for record keeping, an efficiency committee for monitoring purposes, and publication of results in a standardized format. Codman also proposed that patients should have access to these hospital reports. Codman's approach exemplified the application of the scientific management principles of industrial efficiency techniques to the practice of medicine (2). He aggressively pursued acceptance of the end-results system but was frustrated by the difficulties encountered in gaining acceptance of this radical idea. However, Codman worked with the American College of Surgeons (ACS) and, although the ACS did not press for a quality assurance system along Codman's lines, it did push for standards for hospitals, thus bringing about hospital accreditation in the United States. The ACS also established criteria for training programs and successful examination resulting in fellowship in the ACS, thus certifying the surgeon's competence.

Since World War I, major influences on evidence-based surgery have been the public health movement and the evolution of public policy related to health care delivery, military medicine's contributions from World War II, and clinical and health services research in practice variation. The public health movement focused on social and health problems of industrialized cities and agricultural workers. The tremendous social reform after World War I raised many questions about health care delivery in the United States, especially with regard to cost, access, and quality of care. Arising from these concerns were studies of variations in health care, which, along with changes in reimbursement for health care, gave rise to contemporary health services research.

The important influence of payers on evidence-based medicine can be seen in the history of employer- and government-sponsored health care. After World War II, the government freeze on wages brought about the provision of health insurance as a form of additional compensation. By 1966, much of the non-working population was given the basic right to health benefits under the federally sponsored Medicare coverage for the elderly and the joint federal and state Medicaid program for the poor. The Medicare program brought about peer review, which gave way to performance improvement activities under the mandate of the Joint Commission on Accreditation of Health Care Organizations, further stimulating interest in outcomes research. The Medicare prospective payment system, implemented in 1983, led to the widespread use of diagnosis-related groups, creation of comprehensive claims databases now used for economic and clinical outcomes research, and the promulgation of "centers of excellence," that is, the designation of cost-effective providers based on clinical and outcomes measures for coronary artery bypass surgery and organ transplantation. In the 1980s, the Health Care Financing Administration publicly disseminated mortality data developed from Medicare claims files, a practice ultimately discontinued after debate regarding risk adjustment of data.

Study of variations in clinical practice preceded Wennberg's well known work on small area variation. In the 1920s and 1930s, tonsillectomies came under scrutiny because of the widespread use of this procedure and the anesthesia-related mortality risks. In 1973, Wennberg and Gittelsohn conducted research in surgical practice variation comparing surgical procedure rates in 13 hospital service areas in Vermont, finding that physician preferences were the greatest influence on rates of tonsillectomies, appendectomies, hysterectomies, mastectomies, hemorrhoidectomies, and surgeries for other common conditions, with considerable variation in rates of surgery across service areas (3).

Since the 1960s, increased national funding of medical research and private sector-sponsored research have supported the promulgation of clinical research. In the 1980s and 1990s, surgical outcomes research studies have focused on the efficacy and effectiveness of new surgical procedures, clinical outcomes and cost effectiveness of new versus existing procedures, surgical compared with medical treatment, the relationship between volume and outcome, and, increasingly, quality-of-life considerations. Refinements in clinical and quality-of-life outcomes measurements have contributed to these areas of study. Other burgeoning areas of research include the use and evaluation of critical pathways and practice guidelines.

The current focus on evidence-based surgery can be traced to ideals expressed and questions raised over the last century in regard to the health and welfare of the population. Public health concerns frame the resource allocation issues that comprise much of current economic debate. These concerns, along with increasingly sophisticated medical treatments and interventions, the growing availability of computer technology, the economic and political forces that brought about managed care and health care reform, and the growing interest of consumers to self-direct their personal care, give rise to current evidence-based surgery. Ultimately, evidence-based surgical research should enable stakeholders in the health care delivery process—patients, physicians, payers, and policy makers—to provide the best clinical and most cost-effective care possible.

FRAMEWORK FOR EVIDENCE-BASED SURGERY

Outcomes research focuses on measures of clinical interventions ranging from the efficacy and effectiveness of a selected treatment approach to the evaluation of systems of care delivery, with results of interest to physicians, patients, and policy makers alike. Traditional measures of the performance of health care delivery systems focus on access to care, quality, and cost. Donabedian, the foremost researcher in medical quality assessment, defined a conceptual model in which the outcomes of health care are measured by examining the structures and processes of care as well as patient factors and risks. Structural features relate to patient, provider, and payer characteristics; process of care measures describe what was done to and for the patient; and outcomes are classified as clinical and physiologic, patient-reported and economic (4).

Guice and Lipscomb (5) described the features of successful outcomes measures as follows:

- Document changes in clinical condition as a result of medical intervention.
- Collect data in a common format.
- Maintain data collected from multiple clinical sites in a single site to facilitate comparison of outcomes.
- Incorporate standardized and validated methods of accounting for a health care organization's effect on health and quality.
- Enable physicians to assess and select medical treatments on the basis of the actual results and cost of a treatment for accurate prediction of resources needed for care.
- Provide data to establish standards or guidelines for treatment, and provide patients with specific facts to help them make medical decisions, including facts concerning treatments and their cost, efficacy, and impact on quality of life.

The following sections summarize important aspects of outcomes measurement for clinical, economic, and patient-reported data.

CLINICAL OUTCOMES MEASUREMENT

Much of the evidence-based surgery literature is based on clinical and physiologic measures, which may include symptoms; anatomic descriptors and physical signs; physiologic or functional data as measured or observed by clinicians, at a specific point in time or within a specified time period; and the end results of clinical care, as measured by morbidity and mortality. Such outcome measures can be generic to a population or measured at a condition-specific level.

The most commonly used clinical measures of the consequences of surgical therapy are mortality, gains in life expectancy, relative risk and relative risk reduction, absolute risk reduction, and number needed to be treated. Mortality is the most reliably measured clinical outcome. It is most meaningfully expressed as the proportion of deaths from a particular cause over a defined time interval and most reliably measured from death certificates. *Postoperative mortality* usually refers to death within 30 days after a procedure. However, because patients today commonly have hospital stays that are far shorter than 1 month, care must be taken to differentiate between *in-hospital* versus postoperative mortality. In *mortality rates,* the denominator represents the entire population at risk of dying from the disease, that is, those with a disease or condition or at risk for the condition, including both those who have the disease and those who do not have the disease, but who are at risk for development of the disease. *Case fatality rate* includes only those with the disease in the denominator. *Gain in life expectancy* is usually discerned from life table analysis, but its interpretation can be problematic without carefully designed clinical trials. The *relative risk* is the ratio of probabilities of adverse outcomes in two treatments being compared. Alternatively, retrospective study designs commonly measure odds ratios rather than relative risk. *Relative risk reduction* is the reduction of adverse clinical outcomes due to the progres-

sion of disease, achieved by a treatment. It is expressed in the difference in event rates between the control and treatment groups, divided by the event rate in the control group. Relative risk reduction does not reflect the magnitude of the risk without therapy, and thus it overestimates or underestimates the effect of therapy when adverse events in untreated patients are very rare or very common, respectively. The *absolute risk reduction* (also known as the attributable risk reduction) is the difference in event rates between the control and treatment groups. As an expression of the consequences of giving no treatment, it provides an additional measure of clinical effect. Last, the *number needed to be treated* is the number of patients who must be treated to prevent one adverse event. The shortcomings of the foregoing measures of clinical benefit result from the properties of the measures themselves, as well as from the data used. Any measure of the benefit of treatment may vary considerably in different trials of the same or similar therapy because of different patient populations, study design, or chance; thus, the applicability of results of a study must be evaluated carefully. Because trials are of finite duration, the effects of continuing therapy beyond the period of the trial are not known. Some treatments may not be effective until long after they have been started, and there needs to be an adequate duration of follow-up (6).

Measures of Morbidity

Mortality has less meaning in the study of surgical procedures where death is an extremely rare event; therefore, it is more meaningful to report morbidity, such as complication rates. *Morbidity* measures the presence of illness and the degree of dysfunction that can be assessed as days of work missed or bed disability days. Because surgical *complications* can range in severity from simple wound infections to life-threatening conditions, they should be reported separately, considering the underlying procedure or treatment of study. Generic surgical complications (e.g., wound infection, pneumonia, urinary tract infection, and bleeding requiring blood transfusion) should be examined in addition to disease- or procedure-specific complications. Complications are coded according to the International Classification of Diseases (ICD), now in its 10th revision. Because coding categories and regulations change from one revision to another, any study of time trends in morbidity that spans more than one revision must examine the possibility that observed changes could be due entirely or in part to changes in the ICD. Changes in disease definition can also have a significant effect on the number of cases of the disease that are reported or that are reported and subsequently classified as meeting the diagnostic criteria for the disease.

Clinical signs and symptoms are important but subjective measures of morbidity. Care must be taken to standardize definitions. When reporting a test value as a clinical outcome, it is essential to define the normal range for the test because definitions might vary among laboratories or institutions. In addition, it is important clearly to define the clinical context in which the test was ordered so that interpretation of the result is appropriate. *Trends* in test results are as important as their absolute values because changes over time may represent return of disease and poor clinical outcome.

ECONOMIC OUTCOMES MEASUREMENT

As concerns about the costs of health care have risen in the 1980s and 1990s, the demand for economic outcome measures that quantify the costs or benefits of medical and surgical care has increased dramatically. In the evidence-based surgery literature, clinical measures of outcome such as mortality or treatment complications are reported much more frequently than economic measures alone or in combination with clinical measures. This may be attributed not only to the interests of investigators but to the difficulties in measuring economic outcomes.

Key parameters for economic analysis include the time period for analysis, the breadth of services provided, and the perspective from which costs are defined (i.e., the patient, the provider, or the payer). Ideally, analysis would include long-term comparisons of the cost of all services from the perspectives of all stakeholders. In practicality, the scope of analysis is much narrower; for example, an examination of the perioperative mortality for high-risk surgical procedures may limit the cost analysis to inpatient length of stay as a proxy for cost (7). Because the benefits and ultimate costs of a surgical intervention may not be realized until years later, studies of hospitalization only do not reflect all societal costs. Thus, a longer time frame of analysis is desirable, such as an episode of illness, or periods of 1 year or longer. The ideal economic measure of costs from the societal perspective is the social opportunity cost of the inputs to the health care process, that is, the highest value the inputs could earn if used for other purposes (8). Analyses that compare the utility of additional spending for health care services with the utility of other societal needs are infrequently reported. Such economic research is usually performed for purposes of making policy. An example of this is the effort of the Oregon Medicaid program in 1994 to rationalize service delivery by prioritizing all services provided to beneficiaries, based on cost and utility analysis (9).

Accounting for the costs of health care services is a complex process. Reimbursement methodologies provide incentives to classify and allocate costs differently than would be desirable for outcomes research. In addition, the data reflect what providers are paid for services rather than the true economic costs of services. Economic measures for clinical outcomes studies may be developed in several ways. Cost analysis can be completed prospectively as part of a clinical trial. Retrospective cost data can be analyzed typically based on secondary or administrative databases. In other instances, standardized or estimated costs may be applied to models of clinical outcomes. Typically reported costs include hospital and physician charges obtained from billing data. Administrative databases are also used for standard cost data from Medicare claims and cost reports.

PATIENT-REPORTED OUTCOMES MEASUREMENTS

Surgical procedures aim at improving the quality of life as well as prolonging life, and surgical studies have increasingly examined patient-reported outcome measures such as patient-reported health status or health-related quality of life, including functioning and well-being as reported by patients, and patient satisfaction with health care. These data are usually collected using standardized questionnaires or surveys. Most surgical studies conducted before the mid-1990s neglected to collect standardized data about patient-reported health status and quality of life.

Health status, functional status, quality of life, and health-related quality of life are terms used almost interchangeably to refer to the concept of patient reports of their own health. In 1948, the World Health Organization defined *health* as "a state of complete physical, mental, and social well-being, and not merely the absence of disease and infirmity" (10). This definition reflects the multidimensional nature of health, and that it has both positive and negative aspects. Bergner identified five dimensions of *health status: (a) genetic and inherited characteristics; (b) the biochemical, physiologic, and anatomic condition, including impairment of these systems, disease, signs, and symptoms; (c)* functional status, including performance of the usual activities of daily living, such as self-care, physical activities, cognition and work; (d) mental condition, which includes positive and negative emotions; and (e) health potential, including prognosis for longevity and future functioning (11).

Quality of life is a broad concept that encompasses a person's experience and assessment of aspects of life. *Health-related quality of life* encompasses several dimensions of health status that are directly experienced by the person, including physical functioning, psychological well-being, cognitive functioning, social and role functioning, and general health perceptions. The patient's symptoms are often also included under this definition.

There are two basic approaches to quality-of-life assessment: generic and disease specific (12). *Generic* instruments are designed for use across different diseases, treatments, settings, and patient groups. The major advantage is that they can be used in any population and allow comparisons of the relative impact of various health interventions. However, they may be unresponsive to changes in specific conditions and may be too general to guide clinical decision making. *Disease-specific* measures focus on dimensions of health related to a particular disease, population, symptom, or problem and may be more responsive to a change in the patient's condition than a generic instrument.

Health profiles attempt to measure multiple important dimensions of health-related quality of life. For example, the Sickness Impact Profile (13) assesses a physical dimension (including ambulation, mobility, body care, and movement), a psychosocial dimension (including social interaction, alertness behavior, communication, and emotional behavior), and domains such as eating, work, home management, sleep and rest, and recreation and pastimes. The SF-36 Health Survey (Ware, 1992) is a brief (36-item), widely used questionnaire that assesses general health perceptions, physical functioning, role limitations due to physical health, role limitations due to mental health, social functioning, pain, mental health, and energy (14). The Quality of Well-being Scale (15) is a widely used instrument that combines questions about various dimensions of functional status to generate a score.

Descriptive or *psychometric measures* are based on the patient's report or rating of his or her health state on a continuum. *Utility measures,* derived from economic and decision theory (16), refers to the value placed by the individual on a particular health state. Utility is summarized as a score ranging from 0.0, representing death, to 1.0, representing perfect health. In economic analyses, utilities are used to justify devoting resources to a treatment. Because they weight the duration of life according to its quality, they can be used to generate quality-adjusted life years. However, because they are expressed as a single score, they do not provide detail about how specific aspects of patients' lives are affected (10).

Patient satisfaction refers to patients' subjective evaluations of their health care (17). Patient ratings of care reflect what they think is important about the quality of care, including the doctor–patient relationship and their perception of the adequacy of diagnosis and therapy. They predict patients' subsequent behavior, including how well they comply with medications prescribed, whether they return or go elsewhere, and whether they recommend a physician to others (18). The Patient Satisfaction Questionnaire (PSQ) (19) and the Medical Outcomes Study 9-Item Visit Rating Form (20) are examples of instruments that assess general medical care and specific physician visits. The Consumer Assessment of Health Plans (CAHPS) surveys are intended to assess health plans and services, and help consumers to select among them (21). There are few, if any, established measures of patient satisfaction with surgical care.

Quality-of-life assessments can be relevant to surgical research and practice for defining the indication for surgery, for monitoring of the patient, and for evaluation of the impact of treatment (22). Situations in which quality-of-life assessment in surgery is important include different treatment alternatives that might have differential impacts on quality of life; when there are new interventions, scarcity of resources, or need to determine timing of an operative intervention; and when improving quality of life is the goal of intervention. In conditions for which surgery is clearly lifesaving or the only treatment alternative, quality-of-life assessment may be less important. Since early clinical trials that examined the impact of surgical treatment on quality of life, studies have helped to identify treatments that are preferable based on decreased morbidity and increased cost effectiveness. Quality-of-life assessment has evolved into a crucial component of clinical trials of new and existing treatments as well as cohort studies. Selecting an appropriate quality-of-life measure for a specific surgical problem requires a clear formulation of the question to be answered, consideration of the concepts that must be assessed, review of available instruments, review of the evidence for usefulness of instruments in a comparable population, and examination of practical considerations.

METHODOLOGIC CONSIDERATIONS

The major methodologic considerations in surgical outcomes research can be summarized as follows:

- Study design—experimental, quasiexperimental, case reports or series, metaanalysis
- Measurement—reliability and validity of measurement tool
- Sample size—sufficient to give statistical power
- Time period of study
- Original data collection versus use of available data (i.e., public databases)
- Measures of structure, process, and outcome of care
- Statistical analysis—descriptive statistics, tests of significance, trending, multivariate models, and risk adjustment

Study Design

When conducting or evaluating outcomes research, the quality of evidence and strength of the study design are critical factors. Recommended study designs for providing causal links between two variables, needed for establishing which procedures are most effective, are randomized clinical trials and matched-pair experimental studies, with blinding. The number of participants needed in a randomized, controlled trial is often greater than can be recruited at any one center. The multicenter randomized clinical trial was developed as the means to deal with such circumstances (23). In this study design, the same randomized clinical trial is conducted simultaneously at several different clinical centers. Although the clinical centers recruit the participants, collect the data, and administer the treatments, they do not conduct the randomization of assignment nor the data analysis from the trial. Those functions are performed by a coordinating center. Randomization takes place within each clinical center, and the treatments are distributed at each clinical center.

Randomized clinical trials have many strengths and weaknesses. First, randomized clinical trials are generally accepted as the definitive approach for assessing the efficacy of a new treatment. The process of randomization, when properly implemented, provides the means by which the myriad factors that may influence the results of a trial are equally distributed between the experimental treatment group and the usual care one. A second strength is the ability to provide information on the natural history of a disease during both usual care and the experimental treatment. There are also several weaknesses in the randomized clinical trial. The costs of such studies are usually considerable. It is impossible to subject all new therapies to a randomized clinical trial evaluation in part because of those costs. Such studies also require considerable time, both for recruitment and, frequently, to obtain the outcomes of interest. There are also instances in which undertaking a randomized trial is simply not ethical. For instance, it would be unethical to withhold appendectomy after a ruptured appendicitis to determine if antibiotic treatment alone (with a new wondercillin) was efficacious. Also, randomized clinical trials are not based on random samples of the population of patients. The investigators in a given trial may seek to exclude all but a very specific subset of patients with a particular disease. It is therefore often difficult for the results of a randomized clinical trial to be generalized to the population of patients with that particular disease. These weaknesses must often be carefully weighed against the considerable strengths of this type of study.

With respect to surgery, experimental studies may be impractical because the pace of the introduction of a new surgical technology or technique outstrips the ability of surgical investigators to conduct a randomized, controlled trial to evaluate its effectiveness. Other limitations of experimental study designs include the possibilities that patients recruited for a clinical study may be dissimilar to the population to which investigators wish to generalize results, and participating centers may have profound differences from nonparticipating centers (e.g., centers studying the efficacy of a new surgical procedure may have surgeons more skilled in that procedure).

When clinical trials are impractical or unavailable, quasiexperimental or observational studies can be valuable but must be interpreted with greater caution. Even if recruited randomly, patients may fail to enroll or respond because of factors that may be related to outcomes, such as the effect of illness on compliance with the study protocol.

Observational studies differ from randomized clinical trials in that exposure to the factors of interest is determined by the study subject, and the investigator merely observes the result of the exposure (i.e., the exposure is not assigned by the investigator). There are two varieties of observational studies, cohort studies and case-control studies. In cohort studies, cohorts of individuals exposed to the factor of interest and those not so exposed are recruited and followed by the investigator for the development of the outcomes of interest. In a case-control study, people with the outcomes of interest (the "cases") are recruited, as are people who do not have that outcome (the "controls"). Both groups are queried with regard to their past exposure to the factors of interest. The investigator then determines if an association exists between the exposure and subsequent outcome. Cohort studies have been part of the evaluation of surgical procedures for much of the past century.

A major component of clinical research in surgery has been the case report or the case series. In such instances, the clinician examines the response of a well characterized disease to a new treatment. The information presented in a case report or series thereby provides further data for other clinicians to consider in formulating treatment plans for their own patients. Case reports present a variety of advantages, including the speed and ease with which the data may be compiled, the facility with which most clinicians can relate to the information in a given report, and the ability of all clinicians to contribute to the corpus of medical therapeutics without intensive research training. However, there are also disadvantages to case reports, including the lack of a comparison group, the small sample size, and the lack of risk adjustment for comparisons with other studies and populations.

Regardless of the study design used, certain fundamentals apply to the analysis of data. These are best considered in the context of the new "evidence-based surgery" movement that has been described as "the conscientious, explicit, and judicious use of the current best evidence in making decisions about the care of individual patients; the integration of individual clinical expertise with the best available external clinical evidence from systemic research" (24). Such "clinical evidence" from systematic research can be of variable quality. One of the most widely used and respected classifications is that of the United States Preventive Services Task Force (25) (Table 17.1). Much of the clinical decision making performed by the average practicing surgeon falls outside the realm of evidence-based medicine. Thus, the practice of surgery represents the use of extensive clinical experience and contemporaneous research findings to determine the most appropriate treatment for an individual patient.

An excellent resource on study design and analytic considerations is the extensive series of articles published by the *Journal of the American Medical Association* to provide a primer on the critical assessment of outcomes studies (26–55). The framework for critical appraisal of the quality and applicability of a research paper to the care of an individual patient is recommended to be based on the following questions:

1. Was the assignment of patients to treatment really randomized?
2. Were all clinically relevant outcomes reported?
3. Were the study patients recognizably similar to your own?

4. Were both clinical and statistical significance considered?
5. Is this therapeutic maneuver feasible in your own practice?
6. Were all patients who entered the study accounted for at its conclusion?

Although extensive discussion of each of these questions is beyond the scope of this chapter, readers are directed to this excellent and comprehensive series of articles.

Metaanalysis

In contrast to the study designs investigators use to collect data to answer a question regarding the outcomes associated with a specific surgical procedure or a related aspect of that procedure (e.g., prophylaxis), metaanalysis assembles existing research findings to provide an aggregate view (56,57). In a metaanalysis, the investigator reviews the literature for all relevant studies regarding a given surgical procedure and a specific outcome (57). The number of subjects and the strength of the association between the procedure and the outcome are recorded for each study. Then, an aggregate strength of the association is calculated using one of the statistical techniques that have been developed for this purpose. Conceptually, the estimates are weighted by the number of subjects in each study; the larger the study, the more weight is given to that estimate in the calculation.

Metaanalysis is based on the assumptions that the quality of the individual studies is the same, that the factors examined in the studies are the same, that the data missing for any one study will not be prejudicial for the outcomes of interest, that the populations that the study subjects were drawn from are similar, and the definitions used among the studies are the same (57–59). There is also the assumption that all studies involving the factor and the outcome are known to the investigators (60). Frequently, this requirement means that the investigator must know about all studies conducted regarding a factor and an outcome (60). Because studies that do not attain statistical significance are not published as frequently as those that do reach it, some bias ("publication bias") may attend the results of the metaanalysis. Even when the investigator is aware of such studies and is able to include them in the metaanalysis, it is often difficult to be certain that all such studies have been included (61). Because all of these assumptions may not be satisfied, the degree to which they were violated must be considered when interpreting the results of any metaanalysis.

Measurement: Reliability and Validity

The quality of measurement as determined by reliability and validity is an important factor that can affect the quality of evidence. *Reliability* refers to a measure's consistency or repeatability; that is, does it give the same result repeatedly when the same thing is measured? For clinical research and quality assessment, reliability is often measured by considering the following:

Test–retest reliability: repeated use of the same measure on the same subject, yielding the same value results, when the property measured is something that should be stable over the time between the two measurements

Interrater reliability: consistent results when several observers or judges obtain the information or make judgments

Measurement bias: investigator hypotheses and beliefs, rater tendencies, recall bias, and others beyond the scope of this discussion (62)

Table 17.1. UNITED STATES PREVENTIVE SERVICES TASK FORCE CLASSIFICATION OF LEVELS OF EVIDENCE

Level	Quality of Evidence
I	Evidence obtained from at least one properly conducted randomized, controlled trial
II-1	Evidence obtained from well designed controlled trials without randomization
II-2	Evidence obtained from well designed cohort or case-control analytic studies, preferably from more than one center or research group
II-3	Evidence obtained from several time series with or without intervention, or dramatic result in uncontrolled experiments
III	Opinions of respected authorities based on clinical experiences, descriptive studies and case reports, or reports of expert committees

Random measurement error

Validity refers to whether a measure reflects what it is intended to measure (i.e., accuracy). Validity is a function of reliability; unreliable measures cannot be valid. However, reliable measures may lack validity because of built-in sources of bias. For example, a scale may reliably or repeatedly yield the same weight but be inaccurate. Tests of the validity of measures used to collect evidence about the effectiveness or quality of surgical care include:

Face validity: stakeholder perception that the measurement is likely to obtain accurate results

Content validity: whether all the important content that is part of a measure is included

Predictive validity: demonstrated to predict future events or outcomes

Criterion validity: similar to predictive validity, but relates a gold standard finding already proven or known to be related to subsequent outcomes

Convergent–discriminant validity: when there is no gold standard or future event for validation, investigators determine whether the measures agree with (or are convergent with) other similar measures and disagree with (or can be discriminated from) measures of states that theoretically should not be related to them.

To act on evidence, surgical providers should be convinced that it is valid, or accurate. Several aspects of study methods should influence whether a study is likely to be valid, including the study design, the sampling, the completeness of the conceptual model and the confounding variables that are measured and accounted for, and measurement reliability and validity. Data sources vary widely depending on the study design, ranging from original primary data collection to extraction of data from clinical databases set up to study the condition of interest or from administrative databases such as Medicare claims files. Types of data usually included for analysis range from clinical signs and symptoms, and laboratory results to measures of morbidity and mortality and economic and patient-reported measures, as previously described.

The most commonly used clinical measures—mortality, morbidity, and utilization—are frequently used because they are the most accessible from medical records, health departments, and hospital charts. Detailed clinical information can be collected unobtrusively by retrospective review of medical records. To maximize reliability, abstraction must be performed by trained reviewers with a clinical background. Patient confidentiality must be assured, and institutional review board approval must be secured before embarking on such a review.

Morbidity surveys on population samples, such as the National Health Survey and National Cancer Surveys, are helpful because they provide population-based descriptions of frequency of death and complications and can be used to monitor trends over time. Statistical power is obtained with relative ease, and data assembly and analysis is relatively inexpensive. Disease reporting—for communicable diseases and cancer registries—also is helpful for these reasons.

Claims data analysis uses data files, such as those maintained by the Medicare program or accumulated as a by-product of insurance and prepaid medical care plans, to explore patterns of clinical outcomes on a population basis. Several problems limit the value of claims data for assessing medical effectiveness or evaluating the quality of care, however. Because they are intended primarily for financial analysis, claims data may not contain enough detail about clinical features thought to affect prognosis, such as the stage of breast or colon cancer. Chart audits should be performed to confirm accuracy of coded information. The description of diagnoses and complications are often constrained by the ICD coding system, and clinical events out of hospital, in the ambulatory setting, and at free-standing surgical centers are frequently excluded from analysis (63). For confidentiality reasons, patient records often are not linked over time and across different settings. As a result, these are often cross-sectional, rather than longitudinal, analyses. Overall, it is often difficult to identify clinically relevant patient groups and to control for clinical factors likely to affect outcomes using claims data.

Statistical Analysis and Risk Adjustment

Techniques of statistical analysis are beyond the scope of this chapter. However, one important consideration to address is that of univariate versus multivariate analysis. Studies using only univariate analyses (e.g., chi-square) are limited in strength, whereas multivariate regression, key to risk adjustment, is more the gold standard. The risk adjustment process occurs as part of the main statistical analysis, usually multivariate regression analysis. In this method, multivariate regression accounts for the effects of risk variables of interest (the independent variables) on the outcome of interest (the dependent variable). There are many techniques of multivariate regression, a far superior method to another analytic approach, that of multiple chi-square or analysis of variance analyses, which are fraught with the potential to lead investigators to erroneous conclusions primarily because with these approaches, the variables are studied singularly and not simultaneously. Simultaneous adjustment of potential confounding variables is critical for "apples to apples" comparisons. Thus, risk adjustment is a critical but not the sole component in enhancing a study's validity. Other well documented study design considerations include sample size and statistical power, the distribution of data, normal or otherwise, and the effect of outliers. Adjustment for risk is essential in comparing patient outcomes because patient-specific risk factors can mask or confound the relationship between interventions or treatments and outcomes (64). It is well documented in the research literature that patient-specific characteristics and many aspects of patient health status, especially disease comorbidities (i.e., coexisting diagnoses) and severity of illness, are causally related to the outcomes of care (65–70). Therefore, risk adjustment, or, specifically, adjustment for disease comorbidity and severity of illness, is a way to remove the effects of confounding factors by accounting for pertinent patient characteristics before making inferences about the outcomes of care. These adjustments are particularly relevant to surgical studies in which the effectiveness of different procedures or approaches to care are evaluated to guide evidence-based practice.

The concept of risk defines the likelihood of a poor outcome, and the dimensions of risk are multiple. A broad set of patient risk factors can include age, sex, race, and ethnicity; clinical stability, principal diagnosis, severity of principal diagnosis, extent and severity of comorbidities, physical functional status, and psychological, cognitive, and psychosocial functioning; and cultural and socioeconomic attributes and behaviors, health status and quality of life, and patient attitudes and preferences for outcomes (70).

Comorbidities, or coexisting diagnoses, are usually coded in medical records as the secondary diagnoses, diseases unrelated in etiology to the principal diagnosis.

Often, comorbidities appear to be chronic conditions, such as diabetes mellitus, chronic obstructive pulmonary disease, or chronic ischemic heart disease. Patients with comorbidities often differ significantly from those without these conditions. Besides having a higher risk of death and complications, they are less able to tolerate treatment and slower to respond to therapy. In the case of surgery, operative risks often increase because of the presence of comorbidities (69,70).

Adjustment for severity of illness differs from that for comorbidities. The definition of severity of illness is related to disease prognosis, meaning that expectations about patients' clinical outcomes are evaluated against the extent and nature of diseases. For many diagnoses in which death is not an immediate event, defining severity involves a more subjective standard. Similarly, comparing severity among different diseases or conditions is more of a challenge. However, differentiating patients by severity levels within a single diagnostic category is important to describe the illness burden in general, and distinguishing patients by the severity of their principal diagnoses is a necessary first step. Important considerations beyond severity of the primary diagnosis are the number and severity of comorbid diagnoses, acute physiologic stability, functional status, and resource needs (68) secondary to the illness.

Relating severity and comorbidities involves translating different stages of clinical conditions into an overall risk score, which requires not only sophisticated analysis of very large databases to obtain empiric evidence, but both clinical judgment and an understanding of the limits of empiric analyses (71). To begin applying adjustments to surgical outcomes, the researcher must first determine which risk factors are important to account for in the study. These could be patient-specific characteristics such as age, sex, race, and medical conditions. In addition, risk factors relating to the patient's condition, such as comorbidities, severity, or other disease-specific conditions, or to the procedure should be adjusted for when examining the relationship between interventions and outcomes of care. These factors are usually determined by review of the literature and by data analyses examining the correlation between the outcome of interest and each risk factor.

Data Sources

There are three major sources of databases for most medical and surgical effectiveness research: administrative databases, medical records, and patient-based surveys. Administrative databases, large claims files collected for billing purposes, are very useful for outcomes studies of descriptive nature such as exploring variations in treatment patterns.

Medical records offer a rich source of information about patients and their care. In general, medical charts document patients' histories, chief complaints, presenting symptoms, physical examinations, clinical assessments and diagnoses, diagnostic laboratory results, procedures, medications, in-hospital responses to therapy, clinical courses, and discharge plans. For studies relying on medical records, investigators need to have explicit review criteria, or the study could be biased from interobserver variation and subjectivity. Risk adjustment methods that rely on clinical measures obtained from medical records such as vital signs or laboratory findings are able to measure risks not measurable using administrative data systems. However, the costs of primary data collection from medical records may be prohibitively expensive.

Patient surveys can obtain information unavailable in either the administrative files or the medical records. Survey instruments can be designed to capture subjective information such as the perception of quality, satisfaction, personal preferences, or utility. There are many survey scales available to measure health behavior and psychosocial characteristics. However, surveying patients for outcomes studies may be expensive. It requires much effort to develop an appropriate survey instrument and to validate it. The researcher needs to be aware of numerous logistical concerns about how the information is obtained from patients. Besides the cost of conducting a survey, there are potential biases relating to the process of data collection. Survey-based information should be tested for its reliability and validity.

CASE STUDY: PANCREATICODUODENECTOMY

Pancreatic cancer, the fifth leading cause of cancer death in the United States, with 28,000 new cases diagnosed each year (72), is a particularly lethal form of cancer that, once diagnosed, is often at a stage precluding any surgical treatment except palliation. Increasingly, however, potentially curative surgical treatment is performed with the radical pancreaticoduodenectomy. Generally accepted as the biggest and most complex gastrointestinal operation, this procedure is the subject of numerous research reports that have explicated the principles of patient selection, operative technique, and patient management considerations, thus enabling more patients to benefit from potentially curative surgical care.

The progression of evidence-based surgery can be seen in the study of pancreatic resection for cancer. After Halsted's case report in 1899, surgery for pancreatic resection was reported anecdotally in the literature over the next 70 years. In the 1970s, more intensive focus on periampullary tumors by a few surgeons brought about a better understanding of factors effecting mortality rates for the Whipple operation. Reports followed on improved hospital morbidity, mortality, and survival rates after the Whipple procedure, and factors influencing survival after pancreaticoduodenectomy for pancreatic cancer. During the 1960s and 1970s, most centers reported operative mortality rates for pancreaticoduodenectomy in the 20% to 40% range, with postoperative morbidity rates as high as 60%. Many physicians and some surgeons believed that pancreaticoduodenectomy should be abandoned for all periampullary carcinomas, and in particular for carcinoma of the head of the pancreas because of excessive operative mortality and few long-term survivors. In the early 1980s, a dramatic decline in operative morbidity and mortality rates was realized in a number of centers, with operative mortality rates falling to the range of 2%. In one series, 190 consecutive pancreaticoduodenectomies were performed without a death. Unless there are major contraindications to general anesthesia and surgery, the option of surgical exploration and resection should be available to all patients with periampullary cancer (73). Several factors probably account for the drop in in-hospital mortality rates: improved surgical management due to better understanding of anatomy, surgical techniques, and management principles; growth in the experience of surgeons and hospitals with this procedures; and the concomitant develop of critical pathways and specialized care teams across all disciplines to support patient care. A number of tertiary care facilities have focused on the pancreaticoduodenectomy or Whipple procedure (74), resulting in concentrated clinical experience and extensive clinical and basic science research programs at these "centers of excellence."

Despite the extensive clinical experience and encouraging results, the potential for further surgical advances came under assault when managed care dictums challenged patients' access to care at a regional center for pancreatic resection. Because of the inherent costs of teaching and research at an academic medical center, some patients were denied access to regional providers. As desperate patients sought the best place for care, they demanded payer approval of hospitals with the best outcomes, regardless of cost. This onslaught from managed care stimulated a whole new area of research into the cost-effectiveness of care. As a result of outcomes research focused on the relationship between the number of pancreaticoduodenectomy procedures performed at a hospital and in-hospital mortality and cost, research successfully demonstrated the inverse relationship between hospital volume and in-hospital mortality rates and cost for pancreaticoduodenectomy (75).

Regionalization or the aggregation of cases at the high-volume hospital with demonstrably better clinical outcomes was found to have a significant effect on reducing statewide in-hospital mortality rates, and the relationship between volume and outcome for both curative and palliative treatment of pancreatic cancer was extended beyond the concept of the original pancreaticoduodenectomy research to all surgical care for pancreatic cancer (76).

Two theories have been posited regarding the possible explanations for the volume–outcome relationship observed in the cancer studies: does "practice make perfect," or is there a selective referral process occurring that biases the results (77,78)? These questions have been addressed with careful risk adjustment techniques, as discussed in a later chapter, with results supporting the "practice makes perfect" rather than the selective referral process explanation. This finding is not unexpected, given Debakey's observation of key lessons from World War II, that concentrated experience can accelerate the determination of methods critical to enhance patient care.

Serendipitous benefits of the extensive surgical volume have been not only the considerable expertise developed in studying the pathology of pancreatic cancer, but the keen interest on the part of pathologists, oncologists, and basic scientists in the molecular events that take place in the pancreas during the development of pancreatic cancer. Molecular biologists at Johns Hopkins have written the largest body of papers to date describing the genetics of pancreatic cancer, and they are working toward a tumor marker that allows the identification of patients with adenocarcinoma of the head of the pancreas at an earlier stage (79,80). By examining the focused clinical experience and research undertaken to improve the surgical management of pancreatic cancer, provide more cost-effective care, and investigate the early molecular events in development of pancreatic cancer, this case study illustrates that evidence-based surgery can not only improve patient care but could ultimately help prevent disease. Collaborating investigators in various disciplines, through the complex interplay of their epidemiologic, clinical, and basic science research findings, have advanced the treatment of pancreatic cancer. Ultimately, evidence-based surgical research should enable stakeholders in the health care delivery process—patients, physicians, payers, and policy makers—to provide the best clinical and most cost-effective care possible.

The evidence supporting pancreatic resection for periampullary cancer has grown from case reports to extensive series of patients, from observation of the effects of treatment to sophisticated measurement of clinical outcomes, and from findings relevant to advancing the care of the single patient to improvement of the health status of the population. Most important, the extensive body of clinical experience and research has supported related basic science research leading to new information on molecular events that trigger the development of pancreatic cancer.

REFERENCES

1. Ravitch MM. *A century of surgery: the history of the American Surgical Association.* Philadelphia: JB Lippincott, 1981.
2. Reverby S. Stealing the golden eggs: Ernest Amory Codman and the science management of medicine. *Bull Hist Med* 1981;55:156–171.
3. Wennberg J, Gittelsohn A. Variations in medical care among small areas. *Sci Am* 1981;245:120–134.
4. Donabedian A. *The definition of quality and approaches to its assessment,* vol. 1. Ann Arbor, MI: Health Administration Press, 1980.
5. Guice KS, Lipscomb J. Principles of outcomes analysis. In: Stringer MD, Oldham KT, Mouriquand PDE, et al., eds. *Pediatric surgery and urology: long term outcomes.* Philadelphia: WB Saunders, 1998:23–38.
6. Lilienfeld DE. Tools and techniques: study design. In: Gordon TA, Cameron JL, eds. *Evidence-based surgery.* Toronto: BC Decker, 2000:103–116.
7. Gordon TA, Burleyson GP, Shahrokh S, et al. Cost and outcome for complex high-risk gastrointestinal surgical procedures. *Surg Forum* 1996;47:618–620.
8. Davidoff AJ, Powe NR. The role of perspective in defining economic measures for the evaluation of medical technology. *Int J Technol Assess Health Care* 1996;12(1):9–21.
9. Health Care Financing Administration. Oregon statewide health reform demonstration fact sheet [On-line]. 1999. Available at http://www.hcfa.gov/medicaid/orfact.html.
10. Wu AW. Patient-reported outcomes measures. In: Gordon TA, Cameron JL, eds. *Evidence-based surgery.* Toronto: BC Decker, 2000:221–237.
11. Bergner M. Measurement of health status. *Med Care* 1985;23: 696–704.
12. Patrick DL, Deyo RA. Generic and disease-specific measures in assessing health status and quality of life. *Med Care* 1989; 27:S217–S233.
13. Bergner M, Bobbitt RA, Carter WB, et al. The Sickness Impact Profile: development and final revision of a health status measure. *Med Care* 1981;19:787–805.
14. Ware JE, Snow KK, Kosinski M, et al. *SF-36 Health Survey: manual and interpretation guide.* Boston: The Health Institute, 1993.
15. Kaplan RM, Anderson JP. The Quality of Well-being Scale: rationale for a single quality of life index. In: Walker CS, ed. *Quality of life: assessment and application.* London: MTP Press, 1988:51–77.
16. Torrance GW, Feeny D. Utilities and quality adjusted life years. *Int J Technol Assess Health Care* 1989;5:559–575.
17. Ware JE, Snyder MK, Wright WR, et al. Defining and measuring patient satisfaction with medical care. *Eval Program Plan* 1983;6:247–263.
18. Rubin HR, Wu AW. Patient satisfaction: its importance and how to measure it. In: Gitnick G, ed. *The business of medicine: a physician's guide.* New York: Elsevier Science, 1991: 397–409.
19. Ware JE, Hays RD. Methods for measuring patient satisfaction with specific medical encounters. *Med Care* 1998;26:393.
20. Rubin HR, Gandek B, Rogers WH, et al. Patients' ratings of outpatient visits in different practice settings. *JAMA* 1993; 270:835.
21. Agency for Health Care Policy Research. Consumer Assessment of Health Plans (CAHPS) [On-line]. Available at http: //www.ahcpr.gov/qual/cahps. July 1999.
22. Neugebauer E, Troidl H, Wood-Dauphinee S, et al. Quality-of-life assessment in surgery: results the Meran Consensus Development Conference. *J Theor Surg* 1991;6:123–137.
23. Meinert CL. *Clinical trials: design, conduct and analysis.* New York: Oxford University Press, 1986.
24. Sackett DL, Rosenberg WMC, Gray JAM, et al. Evidence based medicine: what it is and what it isn't. *BMJ* 1996;312:71–72.
25. Montz FJ, Zacur HA, Fox HE, et al. Gynecologic surgery. In: Gordon TA, Cameron JL, eds. *Evidence-based surgery.* Toronto: BC Decker, 2000:549–559.
26. Oxman AD, Sackett DL, Guyatt GH. Users' guides to the med-

ical literature: I. How to get started. *JAMA* 1993;270: 2093–2095.

27. Guyatt GH, Sackett DL, Cook DJ. Users' guides to the medical literature: II. How to use an article about therapy or prevention. A. Are the results of the study valid? *JAMA* 1993;270: 2598–2601.

28. Guyatt GH, Sackett DL, Cook DJ. Users' guides to the medical literature: II. How to use an article about therapy or prevention. B. What were the results and will they help me in caring for my patients? *JAMA* 1994;271:59–63.

29. Jaeschke R, Guyatt G, Sackett DL. Users' guides to the medical literature: III. How to use an article about a diagnostic test. A. Are the results of the study valid? *JAMA* 1994;271:389–391.

30. Jaeschke R, Guyatt GH, Sackett DL. Users' guides to the medical literature: III. How to use an article about a diagnostic test. B. What are the results and will they help me in caring for my patients? *JAMA* 1994;271:703–707.

31. Levine M, Walter S, Lee H, et al. Users' guides to the medical literature: IV. How to use an article about harm. *JAMA* 1994; 271:1615–1619.

32. Laupacis A, Wells G, Richardson WS, et al. Users' guides to the medical literature: V. How to use an article about prognosis. *JAMA* 1994;272:234–237.

33. Oxman Ad, Cook DJ, Guyatt GH. Users' guides to the medical literature: VI. How to use an overview. *JAMA* 1994;272: 1367–1371.

34. Richardson WS, Detsky AS. Users' guides to the medical literature: VII. How to use a clinical decision analysis. A. Are the results of the study valid? *JAMA* 1995;273:1292–1295.

35. Richardson WS, Detsky AS. Users' guides to the medical literature: VII. How to use a clinical decision analysis. B. What are the results and will they help me in caring for my patients? *JAMA* 1995;273:1610–1613.

36. Hayward R, Wilson M, Tunis S, et al. Users' guides to the medical literature: VIII. How to use clinical practice guidelines. A. Are the recommendations valid? *JAMA* 1995;274:570–574.

37. Hayward R, Wilson M, Tunis S, et al. Users' guides to the medical literature: VIII. How to use clinical practice guidelines. B. What are the recommendations, and will they help you in caring for your patients? *JAMA* 1995;274:1630–1632.

38. Guyatt GH, Sackett DL, Sinclair JC, et al. Users' guides to the medical literature: IX. A method for grading health care recommendations. *JAMA* 1995;274:1800–1804.

39. Naylor CD, Guyatt GH, for the Evidence-Based Medicine Working Group. Users' guides to the medical literature: X. How to use an article reporting variations in the outcomes of health services. *JAMA* 1996;275:554–558.

40. Naylor CD, Guyatt GH, for the Evidence-Based Medicine Working Group. Users' guides to the medical literature: XI. How to use an article about a clinical utilization review. *JAMA* 1996;275:1435–1439.

41. Guyatt GH, Naylor CD, Juniper E, et al. Users' guides to the medical literature: XII. How to use articles about health-related quality of life. *JAMA* 1997;277:1232–1237.

42. Drummond MF, Richardson WS, O'Brien BJ, et al. Users' guides to the medical literature: XIII. How to use an article on economic analysis of clinical practice. A. Are the results of the study valid? *JAMA* 1997;277:1552–1557.

43. O'Brien BJ, Heyland D, Richardson WS, et al. Users' guides to the medical literature: XIII. How to use an article on economic analysis of clinical practice. B. What are the results and will they help me in caring for my patients? *JAMA* 1997;277:1802–1806.

44. Dans AL, Dans LF, Guyatt GH, et al. Users' guides to the medical literature: XIV. How to decide on the applicability of clinical trial results to your patients. *JAMA* 1998;279:545–549.

45. Richardson WS, Wilson MC, Guyatt GH, et al. Users' guides to the medical literature: XV. How to use an article about disease probability for differential diagnosis. *JAMA* 1999;281: 1214–1219.

46. Guyatt GH, Sinclair J, Cook DJ, et al. Users' guides to the medical literature: XVI. How to use a treatment recommendation. *JAMA* 1999;281:1836–1843.

47. Barratt A, Irwig L, Glasziou P, et al. Users' guides to the medical literature: XVII. How to use guidelines and recommendations about screening. *JAMA* 1999;281:2029–2034.

48. Randolph AG, Haynes RB, Wyatt JC, et al. Users' guides to the medical literature: XVIII. How to use an article evaluating the clinical impact of a computer-based clinical decision support system. *JAMA* 1999;282:67–74.

49. Bucher HC, Guyatt GH, Cook DJ, et al. Users' guides to the medical literature: XIX. Applying clinical trial results. A. How to use an article measuring the effect of an intervention on surrogate end points. *JAMA* 1999;282:771–778.

50. McAlister FA, Laupacis A, Wells GA, et al. Users' guides to the medical literature: XIX. Applying clinical trial results. B. Guidelines for determining whether a drug is exerting (more than) a class effect. *JAMA* 1999;282:771–777.

51. McAlister FA, Straus SE, Guyatt GH, et al. Users' guides to the medical literature: XX. Integrating research evidence with the care of the individual patient. *JAMA* 1999;283:2829–2836.

52. Hunt DL, Jaeschke R, McKibbon KA. Users' guides to the medical literature: XXI. Using electronic health information resources in evidence-based practice. *JAMA* 2000;283:1875–1879.

53. McGinn TG, Guyatt GH, Wyer PC, et al. Users' guides to the medical literature: XXII. How to use articles about clinical decision rules. *JAMA* 2000;284:79–84.

54. Giacomini MK, Cook DJ. Users' guides to the medical literature: XXIII. Qualitative research in health care. A. Are the results of the study valid? *JAMA* 2000;284:357–362.

55. Giacomini MK, Cook DJ. Users' guides to the medical literature: XXIII. Qualitative research in health care. B. What are the results and how do they help me care for my patients? *JAMA* 2000;284:478–482.

56. Lilienfeld DE, Vlahov D, Tenney JH, et al. On antibiotic prophylaxis in cardiac surgery: a risk factor for wound infection. *Ann Thorac Surg* 1986;42:670–674.

57. Sacks HS, Berrier J, Reitman D, et al. Meta-analysis of randomized controlled trials. *N Engl J Med* 1987;316:450–455.

58. Spector TD, Thompson SG. The potential and limitations of meta-analysis. *J Epidemiol Community Health* 1991;45:89–92.

59. Meinert CL. Meta-analysis: science or religion? *Control Clin Trials* 1989;10:257S–263S.

60. Dickersin K, Berlin JA. Meta-analysis: state-of-the-science. *Epidemiol Rev* 1992;14:154–176.

61. Simes RJ. Publication bias: the case for an international registry of clinical trials. *J Clin Oncol* 1986;4:1529–1541.

62. Feinstein AR. *Clinimetrics.* New Haven, CT: Yale University Press, 1987.

63. World Health Organization. *International classification of diseases—clinical modification, 9th rev.* Salt Lake City: MedIndex Publications, 1993.

64. Iezzoni LI. Risk and outcomes. In: Iezzoni LI, ed. *Risk adjustment for measuring healthcare outcomes.* Chicago: Health Administration Press, 1997:2–3;1–41.

65. Blumberg MS. Risk adjusting health care outcomes: a methodologic review. *Med Care Rev* 1986;43:351–393.

66. D'Hoore W, Sicotte C, Tilquin C. Risk adjustment in outcome assessment: the Charlson comorbidity index. *Methods Inf Med* 1993;32:382–387.

67. Charlson M. A new method of classifying prognostic comorbidity in longitudinal studies: development and validation. *J Chronic Dis* 1987;40:373–383.

68. Romano PG. Adapting a clinical comorbidity index for use with ICD-9-CM administrative databases. *J Clin Epidemiol* 1993;46(10):1075–1079.

69. Deyo R, Cherkin DC, Ciol M. Adapting a clinical comorbidity index for use with ICD-9-CM administrative databases. *J Clin Epidemiol* 1992;46:613–619.

70. Iezzoni LI. Dimension of risk. In: Iezzoni LI, ed. *Risk adjustment for measuring healthcare outcomes.* Chicago: Health Administration Press, 1997:43–167.

71. Schwartz, M, Ash A. Evaluating the performance of risk-adjustment methods: continuous outcomes. In: Iezzoni LI, ed. *Risk adjustment for measuring healthcare outcomes.* Chicago: Health Administration Press, 1997:391–426.

72. Cameron JL. Long-term survival following pancreaticoduodenectomy for adenocarcinoma of the head of the pancreas. *Surg Clin North Am* 1995;75:939–951.

73. Cameron JL, Crist DW, Sitzmann JV, et al. Factors influencing survival after pancreaticoduodenectomy for pancreatic cancer. *Am J Surg* 1991;161:120–125.

74. Crist DW, Sitzmann JV, Cameron JL. Improved hospital morbidity, mortality, and survival after the Whipple procedure. *Ann Surg* 1987;206:358–365.

75. Gordon, TA, Burleyson G, Tielsch JM, et al. The effects of re-

gionalization on cost and outcome for one high-risk general surgical procedure. *Ann Surg* 1995;221:43–49.

76. Sosa JA, Bowman HM, Gordon TA, et al. Importance of hospital volume in the overall management of pancreatic cancer. *Ann Surg* 1998;22:429–438.

77. Luft HS. The relation between surgical volume and mortality; an exploration of causal factors and alternative models. *Med Care* 1980;18:940–959.

78. Hannan EL, O'Donnell JF, Kilburn H, et al. Investigation of the relationship between volume and mortality for surgical procedures performed in New York State hospitals. *JAMA* 1989;262:503–510.

79. Allison DC, Bose KK, Hurban RH, et al. Pancreatic cancer cell DNA content correlates with long-term survival after pancreaticoduodenectomy. *Ann Surg* 1991;214:648–656.

80. Yeo CJ, Kern SH, Hruban RH, et al. New aspects of genetics and surgical management in pancreatic cancer: the Johns Hopkins experience. *Asian J Surg* 1997;20:221–228.

TWO

SURGICAL PRACTICE

SECTION A

HEAD AND NECK

SURGERY: SCIENTIFIC PRINCIPLES AND PRACTICE, Third Edition, edited by
Lazar J. Greenfield, Michael W. Mulholland, Keith T. Oldham, Gerald B. Zelenock,
and Keith D. Lillemoe. Lippincott Williams & Wilkins Publishers, Philadelphia, © 2001.

CHAPTER 18

HEAD AND NECK

THEODOROS N. TEKNOS

The head and neck is a beautifully complex region of the human body, with an equally complex range of disease processes affecting it. To cover adequately the entire subject matter in a brief chapter is impossible; therefore, highlights of the most common disease states are outlined. Specifically, discussions in this chapter center around the evaluation of patients presenting with head and neck complaints, clinically relevant head and neck anatomy, common infectious processes, benign and malignant tumors and treatment approaches.

DIAGNOSTIC EVALUATION

History

Every patient with a complaint referable to the head and neck must have a complete history and physical examination to characterize the presenting complaint and aid in making the proper diagnosis. History taking when dealing with a head and neck patient is similar to history taking when dealing with any other patient in general medicine; errors of omission account for more mistakes than errors of commission (1,2). Therefore, a thorough history with direct questioning regarding the symptoms outlined in Table 18.1 is critical. In any smoker 35 years of age or older, the presence of any signs and symptoms outlined in this table is considered indicative of head and neck cancer until proven otherwise.

After the presenting symptoms have been fully characterized, the patient must be questioned regarding potential risk factors for head and neck cancer. The best-recognized carcinogens are tobacco use and alcohol consumption.

These behaviors account for approximately 80% of all cancers in the upper aerodigestive tract, and users of these drugs have a 15-fold greater risk for development of squamous cell carcinoma than nonsmokers and nondrinkers (1,3). Aside from smoking and drinking, other, less recognized risk factors for malignancy of the head and neck do exist, and these should be included in the complete history. They include (a) ultraviolet and ionizing radiation, neoprene inorganic arsenics, burns, and riboflavin deficiencies for skin cancers; (b) wood dust, leather manufacturing, nickel refining, radium dial painting, Thorotrast and mustard gas for nose and paranasal sinus cancer; (c) nitrosamine, salted fish, Epstein-Barr virus types II and III, and vitamin deficiency for nasopharyngeal carcinoma; (d) betel nut chewing, snuff, tobacco chewing, reverse smoking, syphilis, vitamin B and riboflavin deficiencies, and chronic irritation for oral carcinoma; (e) asbestos, coke oven exposure, wood dust, and riboflavin deficiency for laryngeal and hypopharyngeal carcinoma; (f) radiation exposure, iodine deficiency, and genetic inheritance for thyroid cancer; and (g) radiation exposure and Eskimo heritage for salivary gland neoplasms (1,4). Once all the pertinent history of the present illness has been obtained, the remaining aspects of the history, as well as the review of systems, should be elicited. A host performance scale must also be assessed for each patient by inquiring about daily activities and current levels of impairment (5,6). Although time consuming to obtain, this information is critical in assessing the patient's perioperative risk status and identifying any medical illnesses that require treatment before initiating any therapeutic intervention.

Physical Examination

After completing a detailed history, the next step in appropriate management of a patient with a head and neck complaint is a complete physical examination. Adequate examination of the head and neck can often be difficult to obtain. It requires a certain amount of skill and mastery of specialized instrumentation, inasmuch as the upper aerodigestive tract is not accessible to direct visualization (1,7). An important tenet, however, is that no head and neck examination should be considered complete until all mucosal surfaces of the nasal cavity, nasopharynx, oropharynx, oral cavity, hypopharynx, and larynx have been clearly visualized. In addition to inspection of the skin and scalp, pneumatic otoscopy and a complete cranial nerve examination must clearly be documented as well. Finally, inspection, palpation, and auscultation of the neck as well as bimanual palpation of the oral cavity and oropharynx must be accomplished in each case. Performing all these steps in a routine, systematic manner provides the surgeon with the maximum amount of information and limits any errors of omission. Furthermore, a complete physical examination should be able to accomplish the following: (a) characterize the primary tumor if there is one, (b) define and characterize any neck disease, (c) rule out any synchronous tumors or other disease

Table 18.1. PROGRESSIVE SIGNS AND SYMPTOMS INDICATING HEAD AND NECK CANCER

Odynophagia	Nasal obstruction
Dysphagia	Epistaxis
Weight loss	Facial pain
Loose dentition	Cranial neuropathies
Oral fetor	Secondary infections
Trismus	Aspiration
Otalgia	Fistulization
Neck mass	Hemorrhage
Serous otitis media	Airway obstruction

Primary Site	Survival Rate (%)*			
	Stage I	Stage II	Stage III	Stage IV
ORAL CAVITY				
Tongue	70	50	40	20
Floor of mouth	70	50	25	10
Buccal mucosa	75	65	30	20
Alveolar ridge	80	65	35	15
PHARYNX				
Nasopharynx	80	60	40	20
Oropharynx	80	60	30	20
Hypopharynx	60	50	30	10
LARYNX				
Supraglottic	75	60	50	25
Glottic	95	80	50	30
Subglottic**				

* These numbers represent approximate averages; wide ranges have been reported for all sites and stages.
** Too rare for meaningful survival data.

Figure 18.1. Correlation of primary site and stage of head and neck cancer with survival rates.

processes, and (d) rule out the presence of a neoplastic process or lead the surgeon toward a diagnosis that is probably infectious in etiology. If there is a primary malignancy, it is characterized with regard to its size and extent, as manifested by bony involvement, soft-tissue extension, and cranial neuropathies. Neck disease, on the

Table 18.2. REGIONAL LYMPH NODE (N) STAGING FOR HEAD AND NECK CANCER

NX	Regional lymph nodes cannot be assessed
N0	No regional lymph node metastasis
N1	Metastasis in a single ipsilateral lymph node ≤3 cm
N2a	Metastasis in a single ipsilateral lymph node >3 cm but ≤6 cm
N2b	Metastasis in multiple ipsilateral lymph nodes, none >6 cm
N2c	Metastasis in bilateral or contralateral lymph nodes, none >6 cm
N3	Metastasis in a lymph node >6 cm

Data from American Joint Committee on Cancer. American Joint Committee on Cancer (AJCC) manual for staging of cancer, 1997.

Table 18.3. MOST COMMON PRIMARY SITES IN PATIENTS PRESENTING WITH NECK MASSES

Nodal level	Primary site
I	Oral cavity
II	Oropharynx
	Nasopharynx
	Supraglottic larynx
III	Hypopharynx
	Larynx
IV	Thyroid
	Hypopharnyx
	Larynx
	Subclavicular sites
V	Scalp
	Nasopharynx

other hand, is described by nodal size, number of nodes, level of nodes in the neck (Fig. 18.1), and fixation to skin or vascular structures (Table 18.2). The astute examiner has a thorough understanding of the anatomy of each nodal group and the patterns of spread for a particular primary site. This knowledge is critical for identifying an unknown primary tumor in a patient with known neck disease. Conversely, finding an unusual drainage pattern for a known primary tumor can alert the examiner to the presence of a second primary lesion (8,9) (Table 18.3). Clearly, a well performed and thorough examination can provide the physician with a tremendous amount of information with far-reaching therapeutic implications.

A synthesis of the information obtained from the history and physical examination then allows the head and neck surgeon, in most cases, to make the appropriate diagnosis. The most common diagnoses encountered by the surgeon in the head and neck are listed in the following sections. Infectious processes are discussed first, followed by tumors of the head and neck.

INFECTIOUS PROCESSES

Infectious processes of the head and neck are among the most common complaints seen by the medical practitioner. In most cases, the diagnosis and treatment of these conditions are fairly straightforward. However, these seemingly innocuous infections, if left undetected or untreated, can lead to profound complications, including blindness, airway obstruction, and death.

Sinusitis

Sinusitis is a common complaint that is usually self-limited, with infrequent complications. Typically, patients complain of vague discomfort in the infected cheek/upper molar region (maxillary sinusitis), forehead (frontal sinusitis), medial canthal region (ethmoid sinusitis), or retroorbital/vertex regions (sphenoid sinusitis). Often there is a purulent nasal discharge, nasal obstruction, a positional character to the discomfort, and accompanying

pus, and *Absidia* species) or *Aspergillus* species. These are fulminant, rapidly fatal diseases that must be promptly diagnosed and treated with radical surgical débridement and postoperative antifungal therapy. The classic endoscopic finding in these patients is a necrotic, blackened mucosal lining along the lateral nasal wall. The survival rate for these infections varies from 30% to 80%, with granulocytopenic patients faring worse than insulin-dependent diabetic patients.

Pharyngitis

Pharyngitis is the most common complaint a general practitioner encounters in his or her practice. It is an inflammatory disease of the mucosal and submucosal structures of the throat. Infected tissues include the tonsils, adenoids, oropharynx, and hypopharynx. Most pharyngitides are diagnosed by history and physical examination and can bc secondary to bacterial, viral, or fungal causes. Bacterial pharyngitis is typically secondary to gram-positive α- and γ-hemolytic streptococci and several anaerobic organisms. The symptoms include sore throat, fever, and odynophagia. On physical examination, there is typically intense erythema of the tonsils, with purulent exudate, symmetric tonsillar enlargement, and tender, palpable lymphadenopathy bilaterally. Effective treatment includes oral penicillin or clindamycin therapy. A dangerous and common complication of tonsillitis is the peritonsillar abscess. Specifically, a peritonsillar abscess is a collection of pus between the capsule of the tonsil and the muscle of the lateral pharyngeal wall (Fig. 18.3). Warning signs of a peritonsillar abscess include unilateral throat discomfort with severe odynophagia, hyponasal voice ("hot potato voice"), and trismus. Physical examination findings include a medialization of the affected tonsil, unilateral palatal swelling, and trismus. The diagnosis is confirmed by aspirating pus from the abscess pocket. Once the pocket has been localized, a formal incision and drainage must be performed. The mucosal surface overlying the abscess is incised with a guarded No. 11 blade, and the abscess pocket is bluntly dissected and marsupialized with a tonsil clamp. Cultures are obtained from the expressed pus, and the patient is begun on clindamycin or augmented penicillin therapy.

Another important consideration in evaluating a patient with complaints of a sore throat is not to miss an occult supraglottitis (epiglottitis being its more limited form). Adults with this condition are often misdiagnosed with pharyngitis; however, suspicion should be heightened when patients state that their sore throat is lower than usual, or when they have impressive odynophagia and hoarseness, which rarely accompany uncomplicated pharyngitis. Since the universal institution of *Haemophilus influenzae* B vaccine, the epidemiology of

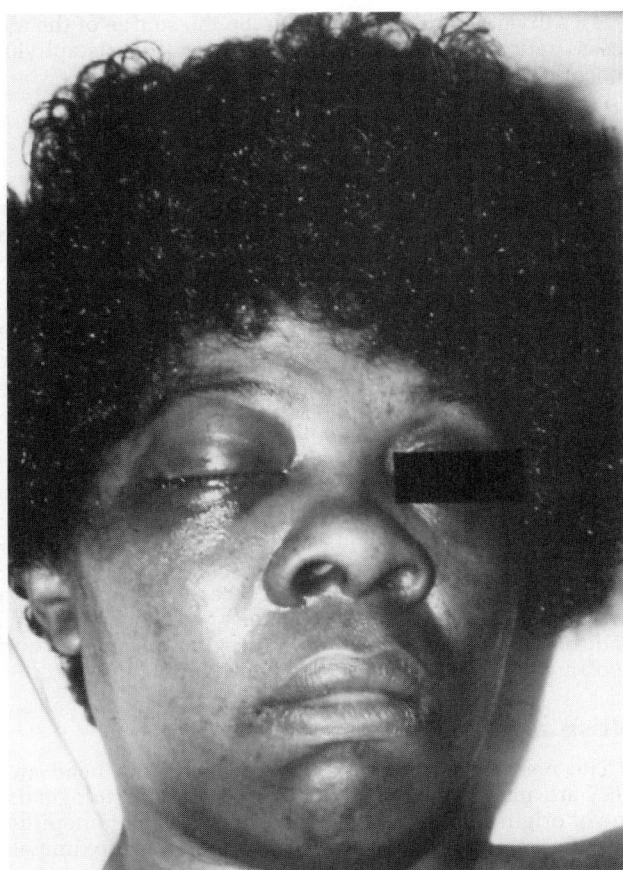

Figure 18.2. Sinusitis with extension into the orbit, causing orbital cellulitis and proptosis.

aural complaints. Diagnosis of this condition is made by history and nasal endoscopy, with visualization of purulent material at the sinus ostia. In adult patients, fever does not typically accompany sinusitis. When temperature elevation is noted, a complication of sinusitis must be suspected. Other warning signs of impending orbital and intracranial complications include severe headache, facial swelling, proptosis, or visual changes (Fig. 18.2). If any of these take place, the patient must be immediately evaluated by nasal endoscopy and high-resolution computed tomography (CT) scanning of the brain and sinuses in both the axial and coronal planes. The potential complications and emergencies related to sinusitis are listed in Table 18.4. These complications require immediate surgical intervention for abscess drainage.

A specific subgroup of patients who must always be evaluated extensively with sinusitis are those who are immunodeficient, have insulin-dependent diabetes, are transplant recipients, or are severely neutropenic patients on chemotherapy. These patients are at risk for invasive fungal sinusitis secondary to Zygomycetes (*Mucor, Rhizo-*

Table 18.4. COMPLICATIONS OF ACUTE SUPPURATIVE SINUSITIS

OPHTHALMOLOGIC	NEUROLOGIC
Orbital cellulitis	Subdural, epidural abscess
Subperiosteal abscess	Meningitis
Orbital abscess	Brain abscess
Ophthalmoplegia, blindness	Cavernous sinus thrombosis

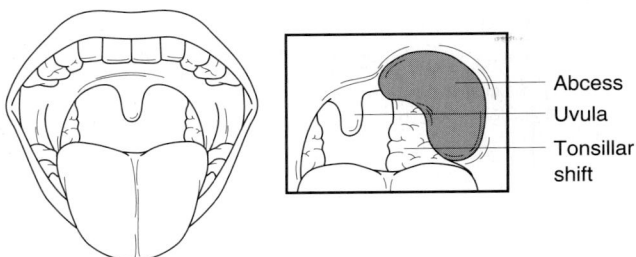

Figure 18.3. Schematic representation of peritonsillar abscess. Purulence develops between the tonsillar capsule and the superior pharyngeal constriction. As a result, the tonsil is medialized, there is a bulge in the palate, and trismus develops.

epiglottitis and supraglottitis has changed. Currently, more cases are being diagnosed in adults than in children, and the dominant organism has shifted from *H. influenzae* to *Staphylococcus aureus* and *Streptococcus pyogenes*. The disease is usually more indolent in adults. If, however, there is a rapid onset of symptoms (<4 hours) accompanied by a high fever (>102.5°F) and a white blood cell count greater than 20,000 cells/dL, these patients should have their airway secured immediately because they are most likely to experience rapid airway compromise (10). If these criteria are not met, adults can typically be treated with intravenous augmented penicillin therapy, humidification, and steroid therapy in the intensive care unit. The acute phase of inflammation responds to therapy within 48 to 72 hours.

Deep Neck Infections

The advent of antibiotics has significantly decreased the incidence and mortality rate of deep neck infections. Despite this progress, deep neck infections remain life-threatening conditions and demand prompt diagnosis and treatment. In the years before antibiotics, 70% of deep neck infections resulted from direct spread of localized abscesses from the pharyngeal–tonsillar areas. Consequently, the parapharyngeal space was the most frequently involved space in deep neck infections. An increasing percentage of currently treated infections, however, are of dental and salivary gland origin, which results in submaxillary space abscesses. The various deep neck spaces are listed in Table 18.5. Any patient with a recent history of tonsillitis, pharyngitis, an odontogenic infection, or recent dental work with onset of neck swelling and pain must be assumed to have a deep neck infection until proven otherwise. Other common findings include odynophagia, trismus, and respiratory compromise. If the diagnosis is suspected, a high-resolution CT scan must be obtained to confirm the diagnosis.

The first step in caring for these patients is securing and maintaining an adequate airway. If intubation is not possible because of airway edema or trismus, a tracheotomy under local anesthesia must be performed, remembering that the trachea may be deviated because of the inflammation (Fig. 18.4). Wide surgical drainage of the entire involved space is the required treatment for the abscess itself. After surgery, the patient is treated with intravenous ampicillin/sulbactam therapy or clindamycin with a third-generation cephalosporin.

Table 18.5. DEEP NECK SPACES

SPACES INVOLVING ENTIRE LENGTH OF NECK

Danger space (prevertebral space)
Retropharyngeal space
Visceral vascular space

SPACES LIMITED TO ABOVE THE HYOID BONE

Pharyngomaxillary space
Submandibular space
Parotid space
Masticator space
Peritonsillar space
Temporal space

SPACES BELOW HYOID BONE

Anterior visceral space

Adapted from Teknos TN, Coniglio JU, Netterville JL. Guidelines for patient management. In: Bailey BJ, ed. Head and neck surgery—otolaryngology. Philadelphia: JB Lippincott, 1993:80.

If a salivary gland is believed to be the source of the abscess, patients are treated empirically with antistaphylococcal penicillins until culture results return.

NEOPLASMS OF THE HEAD AND NECK

Despite increasing public awareness concerning the detrimental effects of tobacco and alcohol abuse, head and neck cancer remains a major contributor to the annual incidence of cancer in the United States. Each year, 78,000 people are diagnosed with a head and neck malignancy; 17,500 die of this disease (1,11). This constitutes 7% of all cancers diagnosed and 4% of all cancer deaths annually (11). Advances in tumor recognition, diagnosis, and treatment have offered hope for increased survival and functional outcomes in these patients. In truth, however, survivorship has not improved since the early 1970s, and 33% of all patients with head and neck malignancies eventually die of their disease (12). Much of this can be attributed to delays in diagnosis and inadequate initial treatment; therefore, it is imperative for the head and neck surgeon to recognize this disease process early and have a well organized plan of care. The most common neoplasms and treatment approaches for each region of the head and neck are outlined in the following sections.

Nose and Paranasal Sinuses

The neoplasms found in this region of the head and neck are among the most diverse in terms of histologic tissue of origin. They include both epithelial and nonepithelial tumors, with the former accounting for approximately 80% of all lesions. The most common symptoms associated with nasal and paranasal sinus tumors are unilateral nasal obstruction and epistaxis. The most common benign lesion is the inverting papilloma or schneiderian papilloma. These lesions arise from the lateral nasal wall and have a propensity for local recurrence. Approximately 5% to 15% of inverting papillomas contain a component of squamous cell carcinoma. For these reasons, the treatment for inverting papilloma is *en bloc* surgical resection through medial maxillectomy. More conservative resections have been attempted, but the recurrence rates have been high compared with the medial maxillectomy approach—60% versus 16%, respectively (13).

Squamous cell carcinoma is the most prevalent malignant tumor of the nose and paranasal sinuses. Approximately two thirds of these tumors arise in the maxillary sinus and one third in the ethmoid sinuses. Malignant tumors arising in the frontal or sphenoid sinuses are exceedingly rare. Cross-sectional imaging with high-resolution CT scanning or magnetic resonance imaging is mandatory for accurate staging in these lesions, as well as planning the surgical approach. Primary tumor staging in the maxillary and ethmoid sinuses is shown in Table 18.6. Curative treatment for paranasal sinus squamous cell carcinoma is primarily surgical. Maxillary sinus cancers, depending on their stage, are treated by medial maxillectomy (preserving the hard palate), subtotal maxillectomy, or total maxillectomy with or without orbital exenteration. Orbital exenteration is indicated for those tumors that invade the periorbita, orbital fat, or orbital apex. Ethmoid sinus tumors, however, often involve the anterior skull base and require (upstairs–downstairs) resection through a frontal craniotomy and lateral rhinotomy. Subcranial/midface degloving approaches can also be used effectively in such cases. The intracranial and intranasal spaces are separated by reconstructing the anterior skull base with pericranial flaps or microvascular free flaps. Postoperative ra-

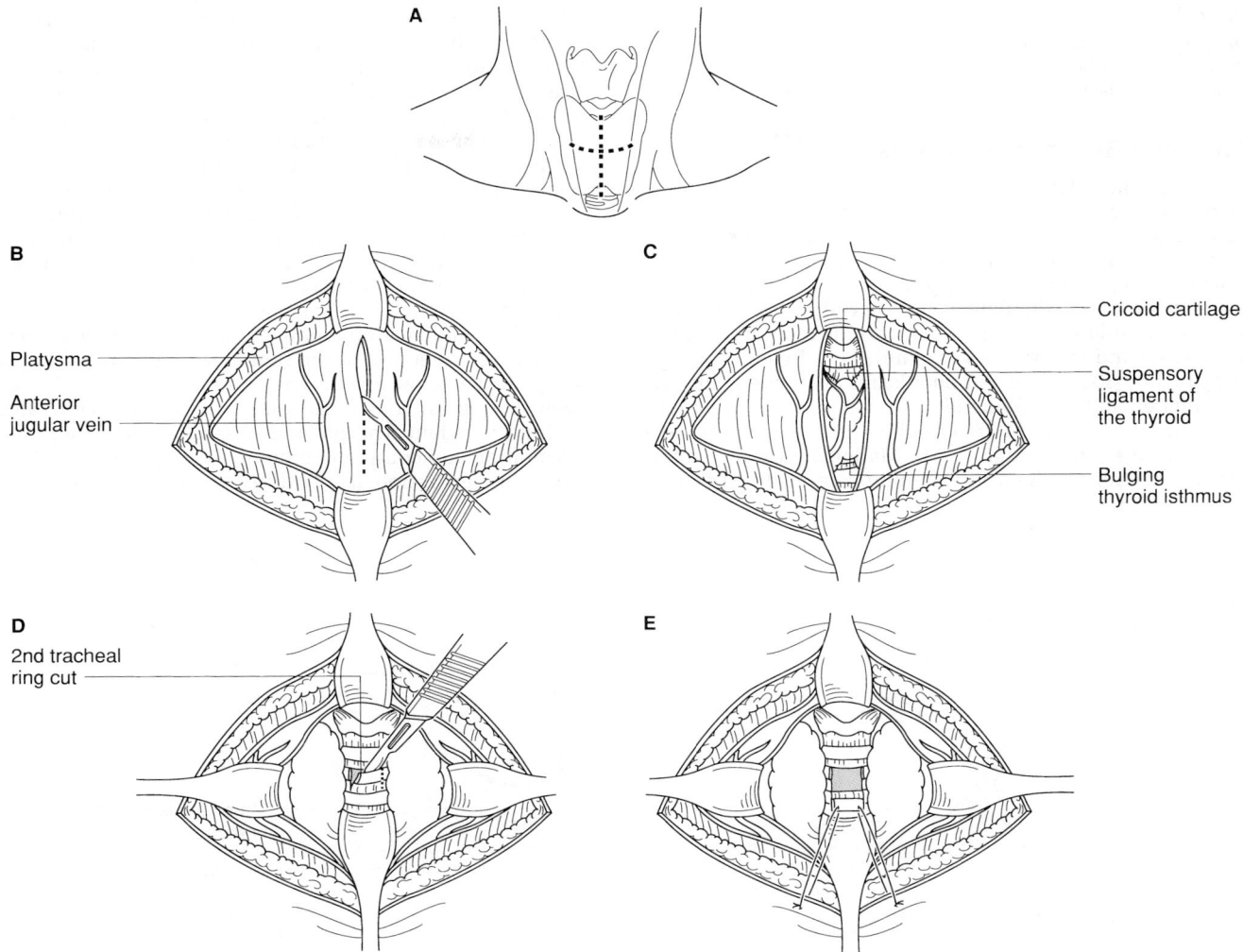

Figure 18.4. Tracheostomy. *(A)* Incision is usually made transversely for elective tracheostomy, but a vertical incision allows for less bleeding when the procedure must be performed emergently. *(B)* The strap muscles are separated in the midline. The thyroid isthmus may bulge into the wound *(C)*, necessitating inferior retraction *(D)*. *(E)* After the second tracheal ring is cleaned off, an inferiorly based flap is developed in the tracheal wall and sutured to the skin to allow easy access to the trachea while the tract is maturing.

Table 18.6. PRIMARY TUMOR STAGING OF MAXILLARY SINUS AND ETHMOID SINUS CANCERS

MAXILLARY SINUS

T1	Tumor limited to antral mucosa with no bone erosion
T2	Tumor with bone erosion, except posterior antral wall
T3	Tumor invades any of the following: bone of the posterior antral wall, subcutaneous tissues or skin of cheek, floor or medial wall of orbit, infratemporal fossa, pterygoid plates, ethmoid sinuses
T4	Tumor invades orbital contents

ETHMOID SINUS

T1	Tumor confined to ethmoid with or without bone erosion
T2	Tumor extends into the nasal cavity
T3	Tumor extends to the anterior orbit, maxillary sinus
T4	Tumor with intracranial extension, involvement of orbit, sphenoid, or frontal sinus, or skin of external nose

From American Joint Committee on Cancer. American Joint Committee on Cancer (AJCC) manual for staging of cancer, 1997.

diation therapy is given in advanced lesions, with improved long-term survival rates. The overall survival rate in paranasal sinus carcinoma is approximately 45%. A particularly poor prognostic sign is neck metastasis, which decreases the 5-year survival rate to 10% (14).

Salivary Gland Neoplasms

The salivary glands are divided into the major salivary glands (which include the parotid, submandibular, and sublingual glands), and the minor salivary glands (which include several thousand glands distributed through the upper aerodigestive tract). Approximately 80% of salivary gland neoplasms originate in the parotid gland, 10% to 15% in the submandibular gland, and the remaining in the sublingual and minor salivary glands (15). In addition, approximately 80% of parotid neoplasms are benign, and approximately 50% of submandibular neoplasms are benign. In contrast, less than 40% of sublingual and minor salivary lesions are benign (15). Malignancies are often asymptomatic, but signs and symptoms indicative of a ma-

lignancy include rapid tumor enlargement, pain, trismus, and facial or other cranial nerve paralyses. A key diagnostic test, which has 95% sensitivity in salivary gland neoplasms, is fine-needle aspiration (15,16). As a result, any patient with a mass in the salivary glands should undergo fine-needle aspiration for histologic diagnosis and surgical planning. The most common benign lesion of the major salivary glands is pleomorphic adenoma or benign mixed tumor. Grossly, these lesions appear smooth and lobular, with a well defined capsule. Histologically, however, they have epithelial and mesenchymal components, but incomplete encapsulation with pseudopod extension beyond the apparent borders of the mass. These features account for the high recurrence rate when tumors are removed by enucleation alone. Appropriate surgical therapy involves resection of the tumor with a margin of normal gland surrounding it. The intimate relationship between the parotid gland and the facial nerve necessitates facial nerve identification and dissection to ensure its preservation and complete tumor extirpation (Fig. 18.5). A second benign lesion is Warthin's tumor (papillary cys-

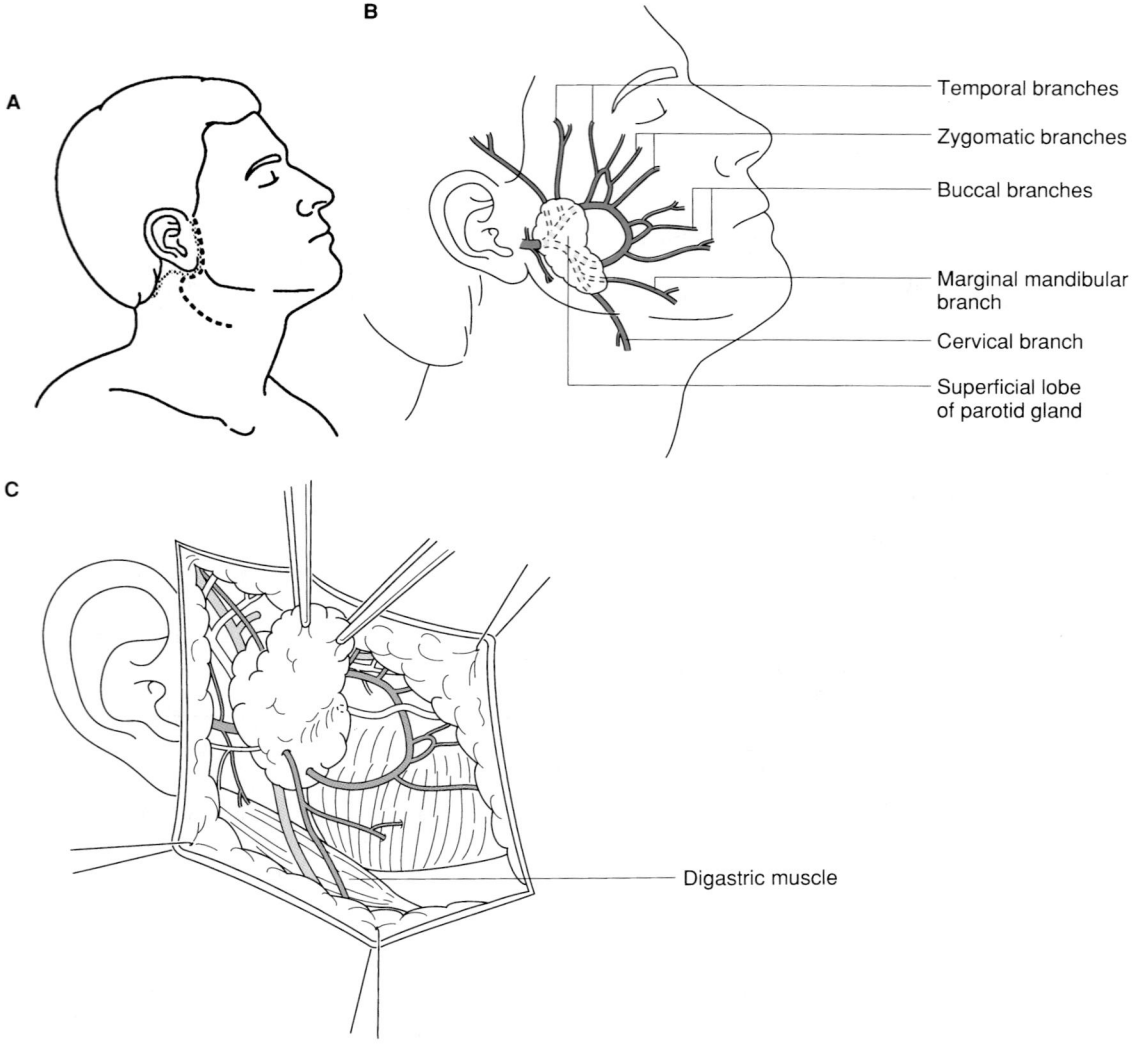

Figure 18.5. Superficial parotidectomy. *(A)* The standard Blair incision or the cosmetically superior face lift incision can be used. *(B)* Branches of the facial nerve course between the superficial and deep lobes of the parotid *(C)*. The main trunk of the facial nerve is identified 8 mm deep to the tympanomastoid suture line and at the same level as the digastric muscle. *(D)* The nerve is then dissected anteriorly, separating it from the substance of the parotid. *(E)* Schematic representation of the relationship between the parotid and surrounding structures. *(continues)*

D

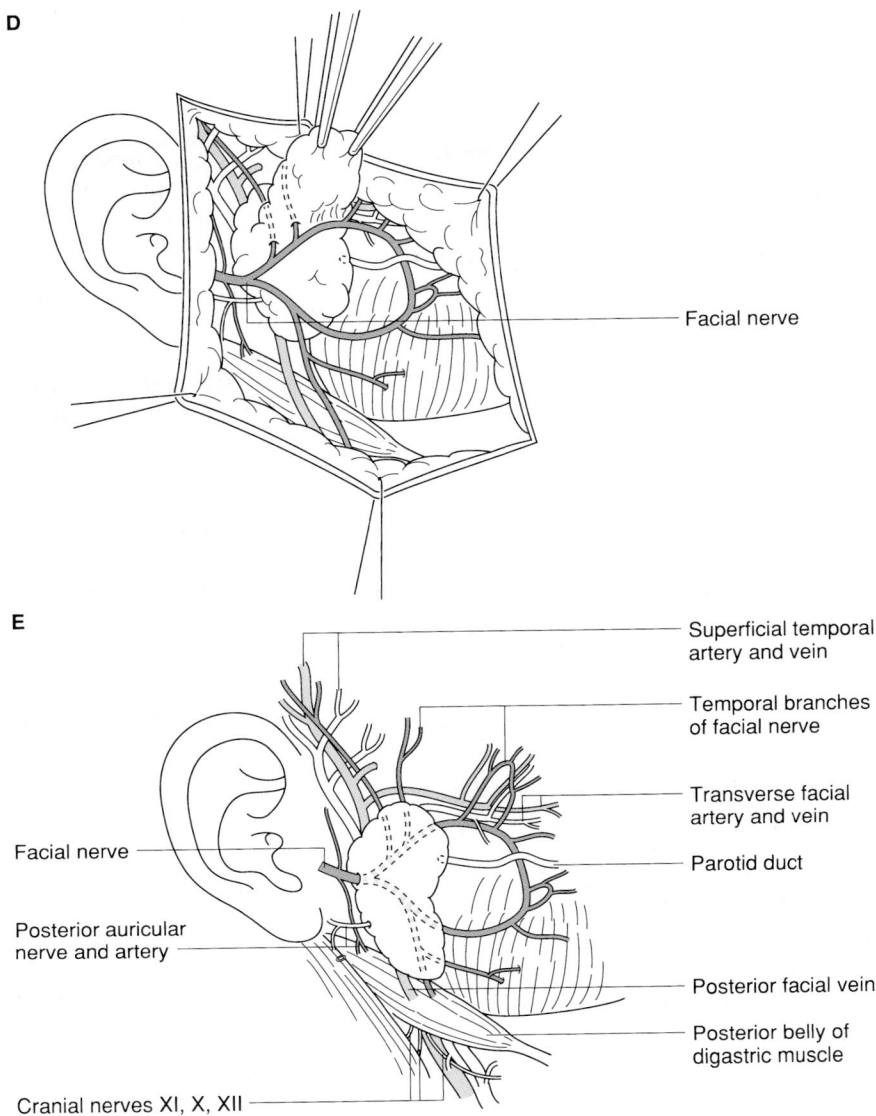

Facial nerve

E

Superficial temporal
artery and vein

Temporal branches
of facial nerve

Transverse facial
artery and vein

Parotid duct

Facial nerve

Posterior auricular
nerve and artery

Posterior facial vein

Posterior belly of
digastric muscle

Figure 18.5. *(Continued)*   Cranial nerves XI, X, XII

tadenoma lymphomatosum). These are typically cystic lesions in the tail of the parotid gland, occurring primarily in men between their fourth and seventh decades of life. They are often multicentric, and approximately 10% are bilateral. Treatment includes superficial parotidectomy, similar to pleomorphic adenoma.

Malignant lesions of the salivary glands are staged according to size and extent of local tissue invasion (Table 18.7). The most common malignant tumor is mucoepidermoid carcinoma, which histologically consists of epidermoid and mucous cells. These tumors are characterized as low, intermediate, or high grade, directly related to the proportion of epidermoid to mucoid cells found on histologic examination. High-grade mucoepidermoid carcinomas are highly aggressive, with a local recurrence rate of 60%, regional metastatic rate of 50%, and distant metastatic rate of 30%. These tumors are treated with total parotidectomy, neck dissection, and postoperative radiation therapy, with a 5-year survival rate of 50%. The most common malignancy of the submandibular gland (Fig. 18.6), and the second most common of the parotid gland is adenoid cystic carcinoma. Adenoid cystic carcinomas account for 58% of malignant submandibular and minor salivary gland tumors, and 12% of malignant

parotid tumors. This tumor has a propensity for perineural invasion and spread, as well as distant metastases. Surgical management of these tumors includes radical resection, sacrificing nerves only for direct tumor extension and postoperative radiation therapy. Despite this aggressive therapy, these tumors, which follow an indolent course, give rise to regional and distant metastases 40% of the time over a 10- to 20-year course. General

Table 18.7. PRIMARY TUMOR STAGING FOR SALIVARY GLAND CANCER

T1	Tumor ≤2 cm without extraparenchymal extension
T2	Tumor >2 cm but ≤4 cm without extraparenchymal extension
T3	Tumor with extraparenchymal extension without seventh nerve involvement and/or >4 cm but ≤6 cm
T4	Tumor invades base of skull, seventh nerve, and/or is >6 cm

Malignant tumors account for 20% of tumors arising in the parotid gland, 50% of tumors arising in the submandibular gland, and 75% of tumors arising in minor salivary glands.
From American Joint Committee on Cancer. American Joint Committee on Cancer (AJCC) manual for staging of cancer, 1997.

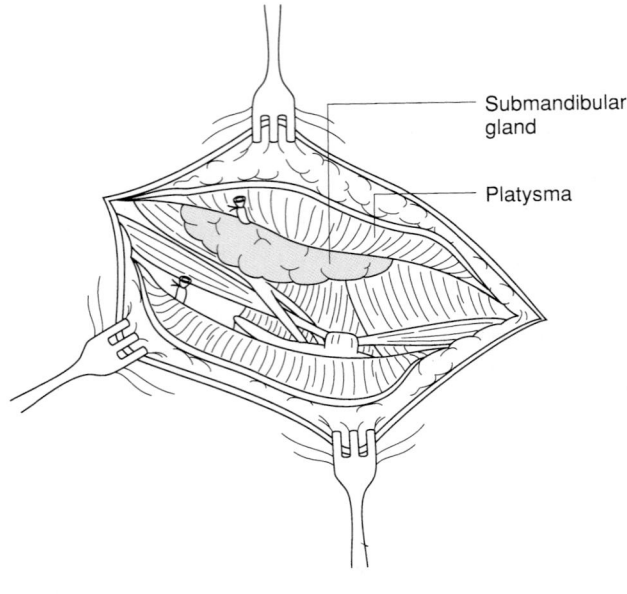

A

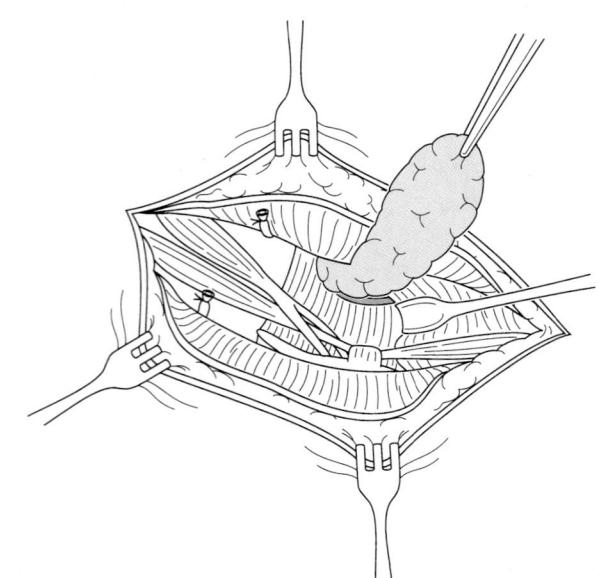

B

Figure 18.6. Resection of submandibular gland. The skin incision usually is placed in a skin crease. *(A)* After division of platysma, the ramus mandibularis is identified and retracted superiorly. *(B)* Elevation of the gland allows identification of the lingual nerve. After removal of the gland, the lingual nerve is in the base of the wound.

principles for surgical treatment of salivary gland malignancies are as follows:

1. Malignant tumors of the parotid gland warrant total parotidectomy.
2. The facial nerve should be sacrificed only for direct tumor invasion or for preexisting facial paralyses.
3. Patients with high-grade tumors should undergo elective neck dissection if there is no clinical neck disease, or a modified neck dissection for palpable adenopathy.

4. Postoperative radiation therapy is indicated for all high-grade tumors, close margins, recurrent disease, skin, bone, nerve, or extraparotid involvement, positive nodes, or unresectable disease.

Much has been written recently about fast neutron radiation beam therapy in inoperable salivary gland tumors or in adenoid cystic carcinomas of the skull base and paranasal sinuses. Early reports reveal a 100% local control rate at 2 years post-treatment but longer duration of follow-up is necessary prior to drawing definitive conclusions. There are no effective chemotherapeutic regimens for parotid neoplasms.

Squamous Cell Carcinomas of the Head and Neck

The neoplasm most commonly affecting the remaining regions of the head and neck is squamous cell carcinoma. More than 90% of head and neck cancers are of this histologic type. Early identification and treatment of squamous cell carcinoma of the upper aerodigestive tract is the most important component in reducing mortality from this devastating disease. The first step in successful treatment of these tumors is tissue confirmation of malignancy. Frequently, this can be obtained by direct biopsy of the primary lesion in the office when the tumor is in the oral cavity or oropharynx. Alternatively, fine-needle aspiration of an enlarged lymph node can also confirm squamous cell carcinoma of the head and neck if the primary is inaccessible. Once the diagnosis has been confirmed, the patient must then be adequately staged. Although the use of flexible video laryngoscopy and thorough office examination often provides an accurate staging of the tumor, there is no substitute for a thorough examination and biopsy under general anesthesia. This operative endoscopy, called *panendoscopy,* should include direct laryngoscopy (with or without microscopic assistance), esophagoscopy, and tracheobronchoscopy, and should consist of a thorough inspection of all mucous membranes of the aerodigestive tract. This is a critical part of the evaluation and is imperative because of the fairly high incidence of simultaneous primary lesions. The incidence of synchronous primary tumors varies from 2.5% to as high as 25% in the literature (17). The general consensus among otolaryngologists, however, is a synchronous tumor rate of 5% to 15%, highest in those patients with tumors of the hypopharynx (17). Panendoscopy is the only way to detect these tumors in roughly half of the cases because they are asymptomatic. Retrospective studies in the head and neck literature reveal that tumors in the digestive tract (i.e., oral cavity, oropharynx, or hypopharynx) tend to have second primary lesions in other regions of the digestive tract. Conversely, laryngeal lesions tend to have second primary tumors in other portions of the respiratory tract, predominantly the lungs and mainstem bronchi (18). Based on these data, some argue that esophagoscopy is not necessary in laryngeal carcinomas, and instead a barium swallow should be used as a screening tool, with much less morbidity and equal yield.

Regardless of the endoscopic method used, adequate biopsies of the tumor must be taken to ensure accurate histologic diagnosis. In addition, based on the panendoscopy, an accurate and detailed tumor diagram must be created and entered in the patient's permanent record. With the information gleaned from the office examination and panendoscopy, the patient's tumor is staged according to the

Table 18.8. **STAGING OF HEAD AND NECK CANCER**

Stage	Stage grouping
0	Tis, N0, M0
I	T1, N0, M0
II	T2, N0, M0
III	T3, N0, M0
	T1, N1, M0
	T2, N1, M0
	T3, N1, M0
IV	T4, N0–1, M0
	Any T, N2–3, M0
	Any T, any N, M1

TNM classification and staging system of the American Joint Committee on Cancer (19) (Table 18.8).

Treatment Guidelines

Patients with head and neck cancer present a challenge to everyone involved in their clinical care. With all the complexities of modern head and neck cancer treatment, including multiple treatment modalities, patients are best served by presenting each individual case at a multidisciplinary tumor board. After considering the tumor stage, prognostic variables, performance status of the patient, and medical and psychosocial issues, a treatment plan is formulated that is agreeable to all caregivers. The objective of any treatment is to cure the patient while maintaining optimal form and function. The specific treatments for different regions of the head and neck are discussed in the following sections, but overall treatment guidelines are essentially the same in most regions and are discussed here. The first goal of any successful treatment for head and neck cancer is to curtail alcohol and tobacco use. No therapy for the head and neck cancer can be expected to have long-term success unless this goal is accomplished. If the patient continues to abuse tobacco and alcohol, there is an approximately 40% risk of local regional recurrence, and a 10% to 40% risk for development of a second primary tumor (4). In addition, before initiating any therapy, the patient's medical, nutritional, and psychosocial status should be optimized. These steps maximize treatment benefit and limit the number of complications.

In general, stage 1 and 2 lesions can be managed equally successfully by either primary surgery or radiation therapy. For these early lesions, there is an 80% to 100% cure rate with minimal morbidity (1). The treatment modality of choice depends on tumor location and the surgeon's experience, as well as the patient's preference. The advantages of a surgical approach to stage 1 and 2 tumors include the ability fully to resect the tumor while eradicating occult or palpable nodal disease in a relatively short time. Also, successful primary surgery reserves radiation therapy for any recurrences or second primary tumors that may develop over the patient's lifetime. On the other hand, radiation therapy has the advantage of resulting in minimal functional disturbance with a comparable rate of control. For these reasons, it is ideally suited for tumors that would result in significant functional disturbance, such as those of the larynx or hypopharynx.

In contrast, stage 3 and 4 lesions typically require multimodality therapy. Initial treatment is usually surgical; however, tumors in these categories typically have more aggressive biologic behavior and can be multicentric. As a result, large areas of the upper aerodigestive tract need to be resected to clear the tumor completely. Despite the surgeon's best efforts and often massive resection, these advanced lesions tend to have close margins and frequent regional metastases with extracapsular and nodal spread. Based on these factors, postoperative radiation therapy with or without adjunctive chemotherapy has been the approach used for these high-risk patients. There are relatively few absolute contraindications to surgery for advanced lesions of the head and neck. Some of these contraindications include randomly scattered dermal metastases that cannot be completely encompassed by a full-thickness resection, solid fixation to the skull base with intracranial extension, and fixation to the cervical spine. Relative contraindications include fixation to the common or internal carotid artery, periosteal invasion of the skull base, or a clinically positive node in the root of the neck (8). Despite our best efforts to diagnose these tumors early, patients often present with or acquire distant metastases from head and neck cancer. The mainstay of therapy in these cases is palliative chemotherapy such as cisplatinum and 5-fluorouracil. A more easily tolerated regimen is of methotrexate, which can be taken with minimal side effects but equally minimal effects on tumor regression. In most cases, a low-dose, minimally toxic chemotherapeutic agent combined with analgesics is the best form of palliative care. There have been valiant attempts at surgical resection of isolated lung metastases, with essentially unchanged long-term survival (20). As a result, this is not recommended therapy unless the thoracic surgeon believes this represents a second primary rather than a true metastasis.

Treatment by Site

Oral Cavity

Malignant tumors of the oral cavity can be devastating with regard to speech and swallowing impairment after successful treatment. Principles of treatment vary according to stage. The current primary tumor staging algorithm is shown in Table 18.9.

Lip. Squamous cell carcinoma is the most common lip cancer. It arises secondary to smoking and alcohol, as well as extensive sun exposure. Approximately 90% of these lesions occur on the lower lip between the midline and lateral commissure. Stage 1 and 2 lesions of the lip can be treated with wide local excision and closure. Up to one half of the lip can be resected and closed primarily with minimal cosmetic defect. Neck dissection should be performed for known nodal disease or tumors which are stage T3 or greater. Neck metastases develop from only 10% of lip cancers, but this frequently portends a very poor prognosis. Overall, lip malignancies are among the most readily cured head and neck tumors, with a 5-year survival rate of 89% (21). This survival rate, however, drops to 25% to 50% when neck metastases are present. Aside from surgical treatment, postoperative radiation therapy should be given to patients with stage 3 and 4 disease or perineural or perivascular spread, as well as in recurrent tumors.

Tongue. Because of its rich vascularity, lesions of the oral tongue tend to grow rapidly and develop early occult nodal metastases. Approximately 30% to 40% of early T1 and T2 oral tongue lesions have occult nodal metastases at the time of presentation (22). For this reason, treatment of tongue tumors involves not only wide local excision with

Table 18.9. **PRIMARY TUMOR STAGING OF ORAL CAVITY AND OROPHARYNX CANCER**

TX	Primary tumor cannot be assessed
T0	No evidence of primary tumor
Tis	Carcinoma in situ
T1	Tumor ≤2 cm
T2	Tumor >2 cm but ≤4 cm
T3	Tumor >4 cm
T4	Tumor invades adjacent structures

From American Joint Committee on Cancer. American Joint Committee on Cancer (AJCC) manual for staging of cancer, 1997.

2-cm margins, but the appropriate neck dissection. Locally advanced oral tongue lesions may involve the mandible, and a composite resection with mandibulectomy may be required for adequate resection. In such instances, microvascular free-tissue transfer is necessary for optimal functional outcome. In general, lateral lesions of the tongue that do not involve resection of the floor of the mouth can be reconstructed with split-thickness skin grafting. If, however, the floor of the mouth, the entire hemitongue, or mandible is involved in the resection, optimal reconstruction is obtained with microvascular free-tissue transfer. The 5-year survival rate for oral tongue carcinomas is approximately 75% for stage 1 and 2 tumors, and less than 40% for stage 3 and 4 tumors (23).

Floor of the Mouth.   Surgery is the treatment of choice for patients with cancer of the floor of the mouth. Similar to tongue cancer, there is a nodal, occult metastatic rate approaching 40% in T2 tumors and 70% in T3 lesions (24). In addition, floor of mouth lesions often involve the mandible even in their early stages. Approximately 7% of T1, 55% of T2, and 63% of T3 lesions involve the mandible and require some sort of mandibulectomy (25). Based on these facts, surgery for floor of mouth carcinomas involves wide local excision, often with mandibulectomy and bilateral primary neck dissections. The reason for the bilateral neck dissections is an approximately 50% occult metastatic rate to lymph nodes in both submandibular regions. After resection of these tumors, if the floor of mouth musculature is intact and separated from the contents of the neck, the resultant defect can be reconstructed with a skin graft, with excellent functional outcome. When there are through-and-through defects of the floor of the mouth, or when mandibular defects are accompanying the floor of mouth defect, a composite microvascular flap is the most reliable and successful reconstruction in restoring form and function. Five-year survival rates for floor of mouth squamous cell carcinomas, stages 1, 2, 3, and 4, are approximately 90%, 80%, 65%, and 30%, respectively (26).

Buccal Mucosa.   Carcinomas of the buccal mucosa are uncommon and comprise only 5% of oral cavity carcinomas. The mean age for buccal carcinomas is during the seventh decade of life, and men are affected four times more frequently than women. Although buccal carcinomas are most often seen in smokers and chewers of tobacco, the use of betel nut and a history of lichen planus also predispose to this aggressive tumor. Because of the lack of symptoms in this area, patients often present late in the disease process with trismus, involvement of the bony mandible or maxilla, and neck metastases. Cervical metastases are present in approximately 50% of cases. Studies have shown that stage 1 and 2 tumors of the buccal mucosa are best treated with radiation

therapy to both the primary site and the neck. Advanced, stage 3 and 4 lesions are best treated with a combination of surgery and postoperative radiation therapy (27). Because of the thinness of the cheek, it is often necessary to perform through-and-through resections of the cheek, and these are best reconstructed with microvascular free-tissue transfer. Approximate 5-year survival rates for stages 1, 2, 3, and 4 are 75%, 65%, 30%, and 20%, respectively (28).

Oropharynx

The confines of the oropharynx extend from the soft palate to the level of the hyoid bone and include the soft palate, tonsils, lateral and posterior pharyngeal walls, and the base of the tongue. Squamous cell carcinoma of the oropharynx most commonly occurs in the fourth and fifth decades of life, with a male-to-female ratio of approximately 4:1. Traditionally, the cure rates for oropharyngeal carcinoma have been poor because most of these lesions are diagnosed at an advanced stage and they tend to metastasize early. Further clinical features of oropharyngeal carcinomas are that they spread submucosally, with early spread to the regional lymphatics. The rate of regional metastases varies from 40% for the soft palate to as high as 70% for the base of the tongue. Also, because of the rich vascularity of this region as well as the bilaterality of this vascularity, it is not unusual for patients to have bilateral cervical metastases. The tonsil and tonsillar fossa are the most common sites for primary tumors of the oropharynx. These are also the easiest tumors to diagnose because of their easy visualization. On the other hand, tongue-base tumors typically present with a neck mass, and the primary is identified on careful examination and palpation of the tongue base. Early lesions of the oropharynx (stages 1 and 2) are best treated with radiation therapy. This form of treatment results in less functional disturbance and a cure rate equivalent to that with surgery. Advanced tumors are treated with multimodality therapy, including surgery and radiation therapy or a combination of chemotherapy and radiation therapy. Survival rates for oropharyngeal tumors vary from site to site, with the best long-term prognosis seen in tonsillar cancers. The 5-year survival rate for stage 1 and 2 tonsillar carcinoma approaches 80%, but decreases to 50% in stage 3 tumors. The prognosis for tongue-base tumors is somewhat worse, with a 70% survival rate in stage 1 and 2 tumors, decreasing to approximately 40% in stage 3 and 30% in stage 4 (29).

Surgical resections of the oropharynx are the most likely of any region of the head and neck to leave the patient with impaired ability to swallow and protect the airway from secretions. Primary closure rarely can be achieved, and the use of pedicled myocutaneous flaps represents a major advance in reconstructing these defects. The pectoralis myocutaneous flap was the workhorse of head and neck reconstruction for the oropharynx in the 1970s and 1980s. However, because of pedicle retraction, unpredictability of residual bulk, and the insensate nature of these flaps, they yielded in the middle to late 1980s and early 1990s to microvascular free tissue reconstruction. Currently, microvascular free flaps, predominantly the radial forearm free flap, are used to reconstruct complex defects in the oropharynx. These flaps have the ability reliably to provide bulk, contour, and sensate capabilities to improve overall swallowing. Microvascular free flaps have resulted in approximately 80% to 90% of patients returning to a normal diet, whereas this figure is approximately 40% to 50% with myocutaneous free flaps.

Nasopharynx

The anatomic confines of the nasopharynx extend from the skull base superiorly to the level of the hard palate inferiorly. Carcinoma of the nasopharynx occurs infrequently in the United States, although it is quite common in China and Hong Kong. A number of etiologic factors have been identified in this increased incidence, and they include nitrosamines from the ingestion of salted fish, chronic sinusitis, nickel exposure, and polycyclic hydrocarbons. Furthermore, carcinoma of the nasopharynx is closely associated with Epstein-Barr virus infections. High levels of antibodies to this virus can be identified in approximately 70% of patients with this disease (30,31). The peak incidence of nasopharynx carcinoma is bimodal, either in the teenage years or between the ages of 45 and 55 years. Undifferentiated carcinomas tend to occur in a younger age group, whereas the well differentiated squamous cell carcinomas are more common in the more elderly group. The World Health Organization (WHO) has defined three histologic classes of nasopharyngeal carcinoma, denoted WHO types 1, 2, and 3. WHO type 1 tumors most closely resemble squamous cell carcinoma in the other regions of the head and neck, and they represent 25% of all nasopharyngeal carcinomas. WHO type 2 tumors are known as *transitional cell carcinomas,* and include lymphoepithelial elements as well as squamous elements. There is no keratinization in these tumors, and this allows for their identification. These tumors account for approximately 12% of all nasopharyngeal carcinomas. Finally, the most common type of nasopharyngeal carcinoma is the WHO type 3. This is also known as *undifferentiated carcinoma* or *lymphoepithelioma.* These tumors are the most radiosensitive and represent 63% of nasopharyngeal carcinomas. Because of their location, the first sign that a patient may have a nasopharyngeal carcinoma is a neck mass, and this is the presenting symptom in approximately 65% of patients (32). The next most common symptoms are ear fullness, hearing loss, and epistaxis. Furthermore, approximately one fifth of patients have bilateral neck nodes at the time of presentation, but only 3% have distant metastases (31). For all forms of nasopharyngeal carcinoma, the initial treatment is radiation therapy. These tumors are unusually radiosensitive and, even with neck metastases, the treatment should involve radiation therapy. More recently, improved long-term survival has been seen in patients receiving combined chemotherapy and radiation therapy. Five-year survival rates for patients with nasopharyngeal carcinoma are directly related to the type of nasopharyngeal carcinoma they possess. WHO type 1 tumors have an approximately 20% survival rate, whereas WHO type 3 tumors have a better prognosis, with an approximately 60% 5-year survival rate (31).

Hypopharynx

The hypopharynx is the anatomic region defined as the mucosal area lateral to the larynx inferior to the hyoid bone down to the level of the cricopharyngeus muscle. Squamous cell carcinoma of this region is an extremely aggressive disease with a poor prognosis, regardless of the therapeutic regimen instituted. Aside from smoking and drinking, etiologic factors for squamous cell carcinomas in this area include Plummer-Vinson syndrome and gastroesophageal reflux disease. This tumor most commonly occurs in men between the ages of 60 and 80 years, and the pyriform fossa is the most frequently involved site. Symptoms are not present until very late in the course of this disease, and include odynophagia, referred otalgia, dys-

Table 18.10. PRIMARY TUMOR STAGING OF HYPOPHARYNX CANCER

T1	Tumor limited to one subsite of hypopharynx and ≤2 cm
T2	Tumor involves more than one subsite of hypopharynx or adjacent site or measures >2 cm but ≤4 cm
T3	Tumor measures >4 cm or with fixation of hemilarynx
T4	Tumor invades adjacent structures

From American Joint Committee on Cancer. American Joint Committee on Cancer (AJCC) manual for staging of cancer, 1997.

phagia, and a neck mass. Occult cervical metastasis is very common, occurring in approximately 75% of these lesions at the time of presentation. Most lesions are diagnosed at stages 3 and 4 because they are often very difficult to visualize in the office. The staging of a hypopharyngeal cancer is based primarily on the subsite of the pharynx that is involved, the presence of vocal cord fixation, and the extent of lymph node metastases (Table 18.10). Surgical treatment of any hypopharyngeal lesion involves laryngectomy; therefore, early lesions, stage 1 and 2, are typically treated by primary radiation therapy. Advanced lesions are treated with surgery and postoperative radiation therapy. The surgical procedure typically involves a total laryngopharyngectomy with microvascular free tissue reconstruction of the neopharynx. Because of the morbidity of this procedure, many alternative approaches for treatment have been investigated. Lefebre and colleagues in France have published the results of a European cooperative study using induction chemotherapy followed by radiation therapy for advanced hypopharyngeal tumors. They have found comparable survival rates between the organ preservation arm and the surgery arm (33). This allows patients to preserve their larynx without a decrease in survival. Regardless of the treatment type, however, 5-year survival rates for hypopharyngeal cancer remain dismal. The overall 5-year survival rates in stages 1, 2, 3, and 4 are 50%, 40%, 25%, and 5%, respectively (34).

Larynx

The site of the head and neck that has received the greatest attention with regard to cancer therapy is the larynx. The larynx is divided into three portions, the supraglottic, glottic, and subglottic regions. The supraglottic larynx extends from the vallecula to the laryngeal ventricles. The glottis includes the true vocal cords as well as the inferior portion of the ventricles and approximately 1 cm below the true vocal cords in the superior subglottis. The subglottic larynx includes the region from 1 cm below the level of the glottis to the first tracheal ring. The hallmark symptom of laryngeal cancer is persistent hoarseness. Because of the early onset of this symptom, many laryngeal cancers are diagnosed early in their disease course, particularly at the glottic level. Other symptoms associated with laryngeal cancers include referred otalgia, dysphagia, a neck mass, weight loss, airway obstruction, hemoptysis, and odynophagia. Because of the significant role the larynx plays in speech, swallowing, and airway control, treatment decisions about cancer of the larynx involve significant quality-of-life issues. For this reason, every attempt is made to spare the patient's larynx, while providing adequate cure.

As a general rule, stage 1 and 2 disease in any region of the larynx can be managed with radiation therapy or surgery, with equal cure rates. Because of the improved functional outcome in patients after radiation therapy, this is typically the primary treatment option. Furthermore, in stage 3 and 4 disease, surgical treatment frequently requires total laryngectomy with bilateral neck dissections and postoperative radiation therapy. Because of the significant emotional and functional deficits accompanying total laryngectomy, other forms of treatment have been investigated and proven successful in stage 3 and 4 tumors.

The landmark study of advanced laryngeal cancer conducted at the Department of Veterans Affairs has changed the treatment of advanced laryngeal tumors significantly. This seminal study used induction chemotherapy (cisplatinum and 5-fluorouracil) combined with radiation therapy as an alternative to traditional laryngectomy plus radiation therapy for patients with advanced laryngeal squamous carcinoma. Analysis of the 332 patients with 60 months of median follow-up revealed that the larynx was preserved in 66% of surviving patients, without a decrease in survival rate. The estimated survival in both groups was similar at 53% and 56%, respectively (35). A 10-year follow-up study on the same study population showed no significant difference in the overall survival rate, with 30% of patients alive in the surgery arm and 25% alive in the chemotherapy arm (35). Therefore, based on this study, patients with stage 3 and 4 laryngeal cancer typically are treated with induction chemotherapy and radiation therapy in an effort to preserve their larynx. Surgery is reserved for those patients who do not respond to chemotherapy or for those with recurrence after completion of treatment.

Supraglottic Carcinoma. Primary supraglottic tumors account for 25% to 50% of all laryngeal cancers. The staging of these tumors is outlined in Table 18.11 and is based on the number of subsites involved, vocal cord fixation, and tumor invasion of laryngeal cartilage and structures outside the larynx. Not uncommonly, supraglottic tumors invade the preepiglottic space, which sits just inferior to the hyoepiglottic ligament. The rich vascularity of the supraglottis, as we have seen in other areas, predisposes this region to a high rate of occult nodal metastases. Approximately 50% to 55% of supraglottic tumors have bilateral occult nodal metastases.

Stage 1 and 2 lesions of the supraglottic larynx can be treated with primary radiation therapy, with response rates ranging from 85% to 70%, respectively. Alternatively, these early tumors may be treated with endoscopic laser resection of the supraglottic larynx as well as open supraglottic laryngectomy with neck dissections. In patients who have undergone surgical excision and have no evidence of nodal metastases, postoperative radiation therapy is not necessary, which significantly decreases patient morbidity. Stage 3 and 4 tumors may be treated with equal cure rates in one of two ways. Surgical resection requires in most instances total laryngectomy with bilateral neck dissections. The previously described Department of Veterans Affairs laryngeal cancer study protocol using induction chemotherapy with radiation therapy affords the patient an equal cure rate with a 66% chance of preserving the larynx (35). Radiation therapy alone can be used in advanced lesions; however, there is a recurrence rate of 50% to 60% with this unimodality therapy. A fourth alternative for treatment of advanced lesions is the newly described supracricoid laryngectomy for selected T1 to T3 supraglottic and transglottic cancers. These oncologically sound partial laryngeal surgeries involve removing the entire thyroid cartilage, the true vocal cords, and the entire supraglottic larynx, down to the level of the cricoid cartilage. The arytenoid cartilages and the cricoid are then suspended to the base of the tongue to allow for airway protection and phonation. Contraindications to this procedure include tumor extension inferior to the cricoid cartilage, arytenoid fixation, and extralaryngeal spread of tumor. Stage 1 and 2 supraglottic lesions are associated with excellent cure rates, approaching 75% using either surgery or radiation alone. Survival, however, decreases dramatically when lymph node metastasis is present. Stage 3 supraglottic tumors have a 5-year survival rate of approximately 60%, and stage 4 lesions decrease to 40% (36).

Glottis. Fortunately, because of the early detection afforded by persistent hoarseness, glottic tumors are frequently discovered in their early stages and have among the best cure rates of tumors of the head and neck. Early glottic cancers are amenable to treatment by radiation therapy or microsurgical resection. Vocal results tend to be slightly better with radiation therapy, although new techniques of microflap dissection of early glottic tumors may provide equal or superior results on prospective analysis. T1 and T2 glottic cancers are also amenable to more traditional open hemilaryngectomy approaches. These cause a significant disruption in normal phonation and are rarely performed for primary lesions. Contraindications to hemilaryngectomy include posterior commissure involvement, transglottic tumor spread, and cricoarytenoid joint involvement, as well as subglottic extension. Stage 1 and 2 glottic carcinomas are nearly universally treated with radiation therapy, with excellent 5-year survival data. The 5-year survival rate in stage 1 lesions is 95%, and in stage 2 lesions it is 87%. Stage 3 and 4 lesions, similar to those of the supraglottic larynx, are treated either with total laryngectomy, bilateral neck dissections, or induction chemotherapy with radiation therapy. Five-year survival rates in stages 3 and 4 are 66% and 50%, respectively (37).

Subglottis. Primary subglottic carcinomas account for less than 5% of all laryngeal cancers. Limited data do support the role of radiation therapy in stage 1 and 2 disease treatment. More advanced tumors require total laryngec-

---

Table 18.11. PRIMARY TUMOR STAGING OF LARYNX CANCER

SUPRAGLOTTIS

T1	Tumor limited to one subsite, normal vocal cord mobility
T2	Tumor involves more than one adjacent subsite or region outside the larynx, normal vocal cord mobility
T3	Tumor limited to larynx with vocal cord fixation and/or invades postcricoid or preepiglottic space
T4	Tumor invades thyroid cartilage and/or extends into soft tissues of neck, thyroid, and/or esophagus

GLOTTIS

T1	Tumor limited to the vocal cord(s) with normal mobility
T2	Tumor extends to supraglottis and/or subglottis and/or with impaired vocal cord mobility
T3	Tumor limited to the larynx with vocal cord fixation
T4	Tumor invades thyroid cartilage and/or to other tissues beyond the larynx

SUBGLOTTIS

T1	Tumor limited to subglottis
T2	Tumor extends to vocal cord(s) with normal or impaired mobility
T3	Tumor limited to larynx with vocal cord fixation
T4	Tumor invades through cricoid or thyroid cartilage and/or extends to other tissues beyond the larynx

From American Joint Committee on Cancer. American Joint Committee on Cancer (AJCC) manual for staging of cancer, 1997.

tomy, partial tracheal resection, bilateral neck dissections, paratracheal neck dissections, and superior mediastinal dissection. Subglottic tumors have occult metastases in approximately 65% of cases; therefore, the assessment of nodes is critical in appropriate treatment. The overall survival rate in stages 1 and 2 is 70%, but in more advanced tumors, survival rates are dismal (38).

Unknown Primary Tumors

Occasionally a patient presents to the surgeon with a neck mass in which a primary lesion cannot be identified. The regions most likely to present in this manner include the nasopharynx, tonsillar fossa, base of the tongue, and hypopharynx. In evaluating these patients, special attention must be paid to these areas to identify an occult primary lesion. Of the lesions that present in this manner, approximately 80% have a primary tumor identified during some point in the treatment process.

Treatment of the neck for both known and unknown primary tumors is a point of significant controversy in head and neck surgery. In a known primary with a high rate of occult metastases but no clinical evidence of metastases (N0 neck), the neck is addressed during surgical therapy by a selective neck dissection. This includes a resection of only the lymph node-bearing tissues in the regions to be staged, preserving all other structures. The types of selective neck dissection include (a) the supraomohyoid neck dissection (levels 1, 2, and 3), commonly performed for oral cavity primary tumors; (b) the anterolateral neck dissection (levels 1, 2, 3, and 4), commonly performed for oropharyngeal primary tumors; (c) the lateral neck dissection (levels 2, 3, and 4), commonly used for N0 disease of the larynx; and (d) the functional or Bocca neck dissection (levels 1 to 5), commonly used for melanoma and primary thyroid malignancies with known metastases. In the case of known nodal metastases (N-positive neck), selective neck dissections can be used as oncologic procedures if the node is small (<3 cm) and not infiltrative of any nonvital structures (sternocleidomastoid, internal jugular vein, or spinal accessory nerve). However, this is a controversial principle, and many head and neck surgeons advocate a modified radical neck dissection for anyone with known neck disease. The modified radical neck dissection is the most commonly performed procedure for known neck disease, and includes resection of the sternocleidomastoid muscle and internal jugular in addition to lymph node levels 1 to 5. The difference between a modified radical neck dissection and a radical neck dissection is that the radical neck dissection includes removal of the spinal accessory nerve, which is spared in other forms of neck dissections. Any patient with a node larger than 3 cm, multiple lymph nodes, or a node with extracapsular spread must be treated with postoperative radiation therapy. In the case of an unknown primary, the areas of greatest risk, namely, the nasopharynx, tonsillar fossa, base of tongue, and hypopharynx (Waldeyer's ring), are included in the radiation field. The overall survival rate in patients with an unknown primary is approximately 50%.

SUMMARY

As is evident from this discussion, the head and neck have a variety of disease processes affecting them, thus presenting significant diagnostic and therapeutic challenges to the practitioner. For this reason, a multidisciplinary approach to these patients provides optimal patient care. Collaboration between general surgeons, ophthalmologists, neurosurgeons, and otolaryngologists is critical in providing patients with head and neck disease not only curative treatment, but excellent functional outcome.

REFERENCES

1. Teknos TN, Coniglio JU, Netterville JL. Guidelines for patient management. In: Bailey BJ, ed. *Head and neck surgery—otolaryngology.* Philadelphia: JB Lippincott, 1993:80.
2. Gluckman JL, Waner M. Physical examination of the head and neck. In: Caparella MM, Schumrick DA, Gluckman JL, et al., eds. *Otolaryngology,* vol. 3. Philadelphia: WB Saunders, 1991:1.
3. Rice DH, Spiro RH. General management guidelines. In: *Current concepts in head and neck cancer.* New York: The American Cancer Society, 1989:1.
4. Jessie RH. General considerations. In: Suen JY, Myers EN, eds. *Cancer of the head and neck.* London: Churchill Livingston, 1981:1.
5. Goldman L, Hashimoto B, Cook EF, et al. Comparative reproducibility and validity of systems for assessing cardiovascular functional class: advantages of a new specific activity scale. *Circulation* 1981;64:1227–1234.
6. Snow GB. Evaluation and staging. In: Snow GB, Clark JR, eds. *Multimodality therapy for head and neck cancer.* New York: Thieme Medical, 1992:1.
7. McQuarry DG, Adams GL, Shons AR, et al. Objectives of care in head and neck malignancy. In: McQuarry DG, ed. *Head and neck: clinical decisions and management principles.* Chicago: Year Book Medical, 1986:1.
8. Million RR, Cassissi NJ. General principles for treatment of cancer in the head and neck. In: Million RR, Cassissi NJ, eds. *Management of head and neck cancer.* Philadelphia: JB Lippincott, 1984:64.
9. Shaw JP. Patterns of cervical lymph node metastasis from squamous carcinomas of the upper aerodigestive tract. *Am J Surg* 1990;160:405–409.
10. Senior DA, Redkowski D, McArthur D, et al. Changing patterns in pediatric supraglottitis: a multi-institutional review, 1980–1992. *Laryngoscope* 1994;104:1314–1322.
11. Goine CC, Squires TS, Tawn T. Cancer statistics, 1991. *CA Cancer J Clin* 1991;41:19.
12. McQuarry DG, Adams GL, Shons AR, et al. Objectives of care in head and neck malignancy. In: McQuarry DG, ed. *Head and neck: clinical decisions and management principles.* Chicago: Year Book Medical, 1986:1.
13. Vrabec DP. The inverted schneiderian papilloma. *Laryngoscope* 1994;104:582–605.
14. Myers EN, Fernau JL, Johnson JT, et al. Management of inverted papilloma. *Laryngoscope* 1990;100:481.
15. Eilele DW, Johns ME. Salivary gland neoplasms. In: Bailey BJ, ed. *Head and neck surgery—otolaryngology.* Philadelphia: JB Lippincott, 1993:1485.
16. Frable MAS, Frable WJ. Fine needle aspiration biopsy of salivary gland. *Laryngoscope* 1991;101:245–249.
17. Savary M, Passche R, Monner P. Endoscopic screening for multiple squamous cell carcinomas of the upper digestive and respiratory tracts. In: Wygand ME, Steiner W, Stell PM, eds. *Functional partial laryngectomy: conservation surgery for carcinoma of the larynx.* Berlin: Springer-Verlag, 1984: 51–59.
18. Sturgis EM, Miller RH. Second primary malignancies in the head and neck cancer patient. *Ann Otol Rhinol Laryngol* 1995;104:946–954.
19. American Joint Committee on Cancer. *American Joint Committee on Cancer (AJCC) manual for staging of cancer,* 4th ed. Philadelphia: Lippincott–Raven, 1997.
20. Masard G, Roeslin N, Jung GM, et al. Bronchiogenic cancer associated with head and neck tumors. *J Thorac Cardiovasc Surg* 1993;103:218–227.
21. Jesse RH. Cancer of the oral cavity: is elective neck dissection beneficial? *Am J Surg* 1970;120:505–508.
22. Spiro RH, Alfonso AE, Farr HW, et al. Cervical node metastases from epidermoid carcinoma of the oral cavity and oral pharynx: a critical assessment of current staging. *Am J Surg* 1974;128:562.
23. Faranceschi D. Improved survival in the treatment of squa-

mous cell carcinoma of the oral tongue. *Am J Surg* 1993;166: 360–365.

24. Ditroia JF. Nodal metastasis and prognosis in carcinoma of the oral cavity. *Otolaryngol Clin North Am* 1972;5:333.

25. Bradford CR, Krause CJ. Floor mouth cancer. In: Gates G, ed. *Current therapy of head and neck cancer,* 5th ed. St. Louis: Mosby, 1994:266–267.

26. Shaha AR, et al. Squamous carcinoma of the floor of the mouth. *Am J Surg* 1984;184:455–459.

27. Strome SE, Towaiyat, Strauderman M, et al. Squamous cell carcinoma of the buccal mucosa: the role of parotidectomy. *Otolaryngol Head Neck Surg* 1999;120(3):375–399.

28. Bloom ND, Spiro RH. Carcinoma of the cheek mucosa: a retrospective analysis. *Am J Surg* 1980;140:556–559.

29. Perez CA, Carmichael T, Devineni VR, et al. Carcinoma of the tonsillar fossa: a non-randomized comparison of irradiation alone or combined with surgery—long-term results. *Head Neck Surg* 1991;13:282–290.

30. Dickson RI. Nasopharyngeal carcinoma: an evaluation of 209 patients. *Laryngoscope* 1981;91:333–354.

31. Neal HB, et al. Antibodies to Epstein-Barr virus in patients with nasopharyngeal carcinoma in comparison groups. *Ann Otol Rhinol Laryngol* 1984;93:477–482.

32. Neal HB. Nasopharyngeal carcinoma: clinical presentation, diagnosis, treatment, and prognosis. *Otolaryngol Clin North Am* 1985;18:479–490.

33. Lefebre JL, Chevalier D, Luboinski B, et al. Larynx preservation in pyriform sinus cancer: preliminary results of the European Organization for Research and Treatment of Cancer Phase III Trial. *J Natl Cancer Inst* 1996;88:890–899.

34. Elbadawi SA, et al. Squamous carcinoma of the pyriform sinus. *Laryngoscope* 1982;92:357–364.

35. Wolf GT, Hawn WK, Fisher SG, et al. Induction chemotherapy plus radiation compared with surgery plus radiation in patients with advanced laryngeal cancer. *N Engl J Med* 1991; 324:1685–1690.

36. Hoekstra CJ, Lovendag PC, VanPolten WL. Squamous cell carcinoma of the supraglottic larynx without clinically detectable lymph node metastasis: problem of local relapse and influence of overall treatment time. *Int J Radiat Oncol Biol Phys* 1990;18:13.

37. Wang CC, Schulz MD, Miller D. Combined radiation therapy and surgery for carcinoma of the supraglottis and puriform sinus. *Am J Surg* 1972;124:551.

38. Ward P, Harwood A. Carcinoma of the subglottis. *Arch Otolaryngol* 1987;113:1–28.

SECTION B

ESOPHAGUS

SURGERY: SCIENTIFIC PRINCIPLES AND PRACTICE, Third Edition, edited by
Lazar J. Greenfield, Michael W. Mulholland, Keith T. Oldham, Gerald B. Zelenock,
and Keith D. Lillemoe. Lippincott Williams & Wilkins Publishers, Philadelphia, © 2001.

CHAPTER 19

ESOPHAGUS: ANATOMY, PHYSIOLOGY, AND GASTROESOPHAGEAL REFLUX DISEASE

JEFFREY H. PETERS AND TOM R. DEMEESTER

ANATOMY

A detailed knowledge of the anatomic relations of the esophagus is essential for the surgeon to be able to identify the site and significance of lesions seen by indirect studies, such as endoscopy, barium roentgenography, and computed tomography (CT), and to perform surgical procedures on the esophagus safely (1). In this section, the embryology of the esophagus is first described, then the topographic relations of the esophagus, and finally the conduct of investigations that yield anatomic information.

The *embryology* of the esophagus is important in understanding the pathogenesis of congenital malformations of the esophagus and trachea. The embryonic esophagus forms when paired longitudinal grooves appear on each side of the laryngotracheal diverticulum. These grooves subsequently grow medially and fuse to form the tracheoesophageal septum. This septum divides the foregut into the ventral laryngotracheal tube and the dorsal esophagus. Incomplete fusion of the two lateral grooves was formerly thought to be the major factor in the pathogenesis of congenital tracheoesophageal fistula, but the anomaly is now attributed to abnormal growth and differentiation of the lung buds. Initially, the esophagus is short, but elongation occurs rapidly, and the final relative length is attained by the seventh gestational week. This is followed by endodermal proliferation, which results in near obliteration of the esophageal lumen and subsequent recanalization by the development of large vacuoles that coalesce. The striated muscle of the upper esophagus is derived from the caudal branchial arches and is innervated by the vagus nerve and its recurrent laryngeal branches. The smooth muscle of the lower esophagus arises from splanchnic mesenchyme and is supplied by a visceral nerve plexus derived from neural crest cells. The adult position of the vagus nerves on the esophagus is the result of unequal growth of the greater curve of the stomach relative to the lesser curve, so that the left vagus rotates anteriorly and the right vagus posteriorly.

The *cervical esophagus* begins below the cricopharyngeus muscle, which itself is a continuation of the inferior constrictor of the pharynx. The potential space between these muscles posteriorly is the site where Zenker's diverticulum develops. The cervical esophagus is about 5 cm long. It begins at the level of C-6 and extends to the lower border of T-1, curving slightly to the left in its descent. Anteriorly, it abuts the trachea and posterior larynx and can be dissected off both organs if necessary. Posteriorly, the retroesophageal space is continuous above with the retropharyngeal space and with the superior mediastinum below. Laterally, the omohyoid muscle crosses it obliquely and is usually divided to gain access to the esophagus. The carotid sheaths lie laterally, and the lobes of the thyroid and the strap muscles anteriorly. The recurrent laryngeal nerves lie in the grooves between the esophagus and trachea. The right recurrent nerve runs a more oblique course and is more prone to anatomic variation. Consequently, although the surgical approach to this portion of the esophagus may be from either side of the neck through an incision along the anterior border of sternocleidomastoid muscle, the left side is chosen if possible.

The *thoracic esophagus* in its upper part is closely related to the posterior wall of the trachea. This close relation is responsible for the early spread of cancer of the upper esophagus into the trachea, and it limits the ability of the surgeon to perform an *en bloc* resection of such a tumor. Above the level of the tracheal bifurcation, the esophagus courses to the right of the descending aorta. It then courses to the left, passes behind the tracheal bifurcation and left main bronchus, and descends to the diaphragm. In its lower third, the esophagus courses anteriorly and to the left to pass through the diaphragmatic hiatus. The lower esophagus is covered only by flimsy mediastinal pleura on the left, and it is this portion that is most commonly the site of perforation in Boerhaave's syndrome. The azygos vein is closely related to the esophagus as it arches from its paraspinal position over the right main bronchus to enter the superior vena cava. The thoracic duct ascends behind and to the right of the distal esophagus, but at the level of T-5 it passes posterior to the aorta and ascends on the left side of the esophagus and posterior to the left subclavian artery.

Throughout its length, the attachments of the esophagus to its adjacent structures other than the posterior trachea are flimsy. This accounts for the ease with which the esophagus can be bluntly mobilized out of the mediastinum during transhiatal esophagectomy. In general, the lower esophagus is most easily approached through the left side of the chest, but access to the supraaortic esophagus is restricted. Thus, a left thoracotomy is most useful for performing Heller's myotomy, transthoracic fundoplication, or resection of an epiphrenic diverticulum. Access to the entire thoracic esophagus can be obtained only from the right side of the chest, but access to the intraabdominal organs is restricted by the liver, and

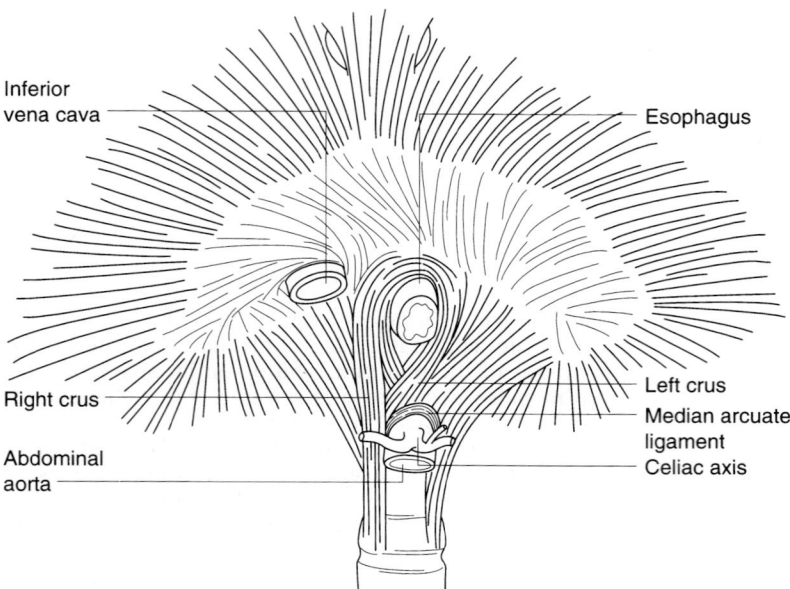

Figure 19.1. Diaphragm and esophageal hiatus viewed from below.

normally a separate upper abdominal incision is required.

The *abdominal esophagus* begins where the esophagus enters the abdomen through the diaphragmatic hiatus (Fig. 19.1). It is surrounded by a fibroelastic membrane, the phrenoesophageal ligament, which arises from the subdiaphragmatic fascia (Fig. 19.2). The lower limit of the phrenoesophageal membrane anteriorly is marked by a prominent fat pad, which corresponds to the gastroesophageal junction. The lower esophageal sphincter is a zone of high pressure 3 to 5 cm long at the lower end of the esophagus (2). It does not correspond to any macroscopic anatomic structure; rather, its function appears to be related to the microscopic architecture of the muscle fibers. The esophageal hiatus is surrounded by the right and left crura, which form a sling of muscular fibers arising by tendinous bands from the anterolateral surface of the first four lumbar vertebrae. The relative contribution of the right and left crura to the sling is variable. Surgeons name the crura from their relation to the esophagus, whereas anatomists name them from their relation to the aorta. Thus, both right and left "surgical" crura originate from the right "anatomic" crus. Caudally, the crura are united by a tendinous arch, the median arcuate ligament, just anterior to the aorta at the level of the celiac axis.

The *blood supply* and *venous drainage* are largely segmental. The inferior thyroid artery provides the main blood supply to the cervical portion of the esophagus. This becomes important in a patient with a previous thyroidectomy, although ligation is usually performed distal to the esophageal branch. The thoracic portion of the esophagus receives its blood supply from two sources. Usually, branches from two to three bronchial arteries provide the proximal arterial supply, and branches directly from the aorta supply the more distal thoracic esophagus. The upper of these aortic branches arises between the sixth and seventh thoracic vertebrae; the lower one arises between the eighth and ninth thoracic vertebrae. Intrathoracic mobilization of the esophagus during antireflux procedures often requires ligation of these branches. The abdominal esophagus receives its blood supply from branches of the left gastric artery and inferior phrenic arteries (Fig. 19.3). A particularly constant

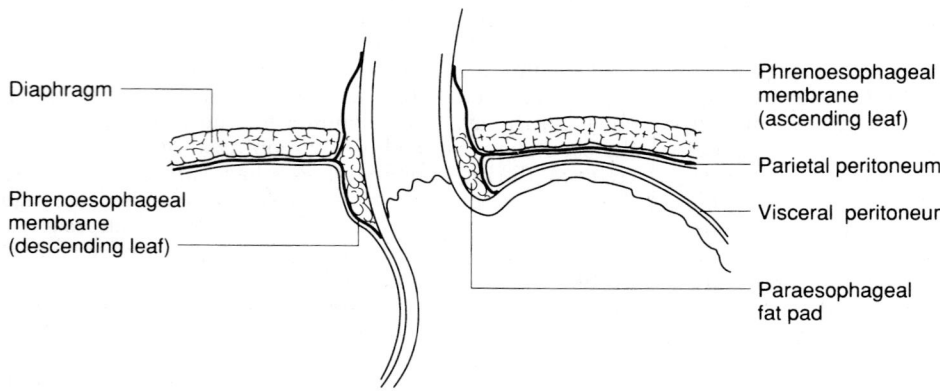

Figure 19.2. Attachments of the phrenoesophageal membrane.

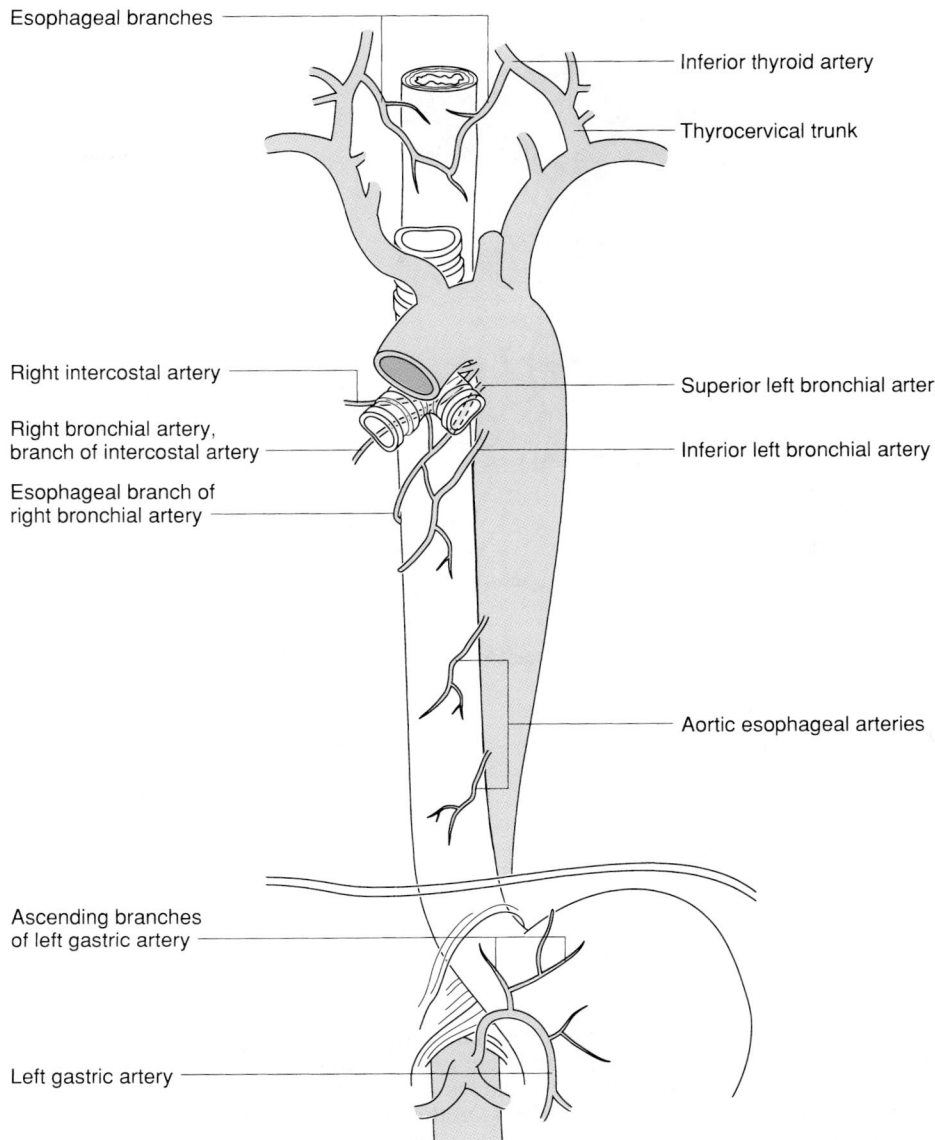

Esophageal branches

Inferior thyroid artery

Thyrocervical trunk

Right intercostal artery

Right bronchial artery,
branch of intercostal artery

Esophageal branch of
right bronchial artery

Superior left bronchial artery

Inferior left bronchial artery

Aortic esophageal arteries

Ascending branches
of left gastric artery

Left gastric artery

Figure 19.3. Arterial blood supply of the esophagus.

artery at the base of the left surgical crus connects the inferior phrenic artery to branches of the left gastric artery and is sometimes called *Belsey's artery*. It is often seen during the crural dissection performed in a laparoscopic fundoplication. Once the vessels have entered the muscular wall of the esophagus, branching occurs at right angles to provide a longitudinal vascular plexus. This anatomic arrangement allows for mobilization of the esophagus from the stomach to the aortic arch without ischemic injury.

A venous plexus in the submucosa collects capillary blood and delivers it into a periesophageal venous plexus. From this plexus, esophageal veins arise that empty into the inferior thyroid vein proximally; into the bronchial, azygos, or hemiazygos veins in the thorax; and into the left gastric vein in the abdominal region (Fig. 19.4). The left gastric vein, or coronary vein, provides the principal collateral in portal hypertension when esophageal varices develop. The submucosal veins become much more superficial in the most distal portion of esophagus, 1 to 2 cm

above the gastroesophageal junction, and are consequently the most common site of bleeding in portal hypertension. The connections between the submucosal venous networks of the esophagus and stomach provide an additional collateral pathway for portal blood to enter the superior vena cava through the azygos vein in patients with portal hypertension.

The *lymphatics* of the esophagus form a rich submucosal network draining into regional lymph nodes in the periesophageal connective tissue (Fig. 19.5). Thus, little barrier exists to the longitudinal spread of cancer in the esophagus; it is estimated that for every 1 cm of axial spread, 6 cm of longitudinal spread occurs. Lymphatic drainage from the upper two thirds of the esophagus is usually cephalad, but drainage from the lower one third is in both directions. In the cervical region, esophageal lymphatic drainage is toward the internal jugular and upper tracheal nodes. Posterior mediastinal nodes drain the thoracic portion of the esophagus dorsally. Drainage from the anterior portion of the thoracic esophagus is most often to

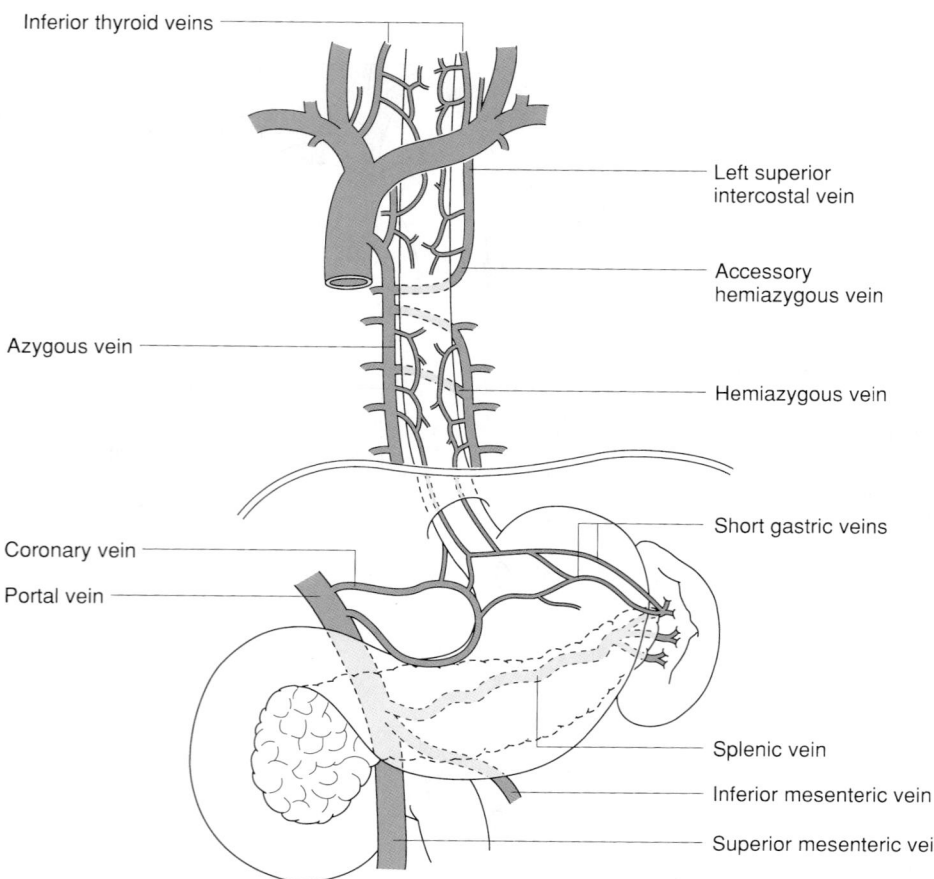

Inferior thyroid veins

Left superior intercostal vein

Accessory hemiazygous vein

Azygous vein

Hemiazygous vein

Short gastric veins

Coronary vein

Portal vein

Splenic vein

Inferior mesenteric vein

Superior mesenteric vein

Figure 19.4. Venous drainage of the esophagus.

tracheal nodes superiorly and subcarinal and paraesophageal nodes inferiorly. In the abdomen, the esophageal lymph drains to cardiac and celiac nodes, which may eventually drain into the cisterna chyli or the thoracic duct. Although lymphatic metastases in the esophagus generally involve the most proximal regional nodes, nodal involvement may develop several centimeters away from the primary lesion because of the presence of rich intramural lymphatic anastomotic channels. When a carcinoma is limited to the mucosa (above the muscularis mucosae), the incidence of lymphatic metastases is low, but once a carcinoma penetrates into the submucosa, the incidence rises to 60%. The results of three-field lymph node dissection for esophageal carcinoma have provided evidence of the widespread lymphatic connections within the esophagus.

The *innervation* of the cricopharyngeal sphincter and cervical portion of the esophagus is from both the right and left recurrent laryngeal nerves. These nerves, arising from the vagus, travel dorsally around the subclavian artery on the right and the arch of the aorta on the left. They give off branches to both the esophagus and trachea as they ascend in the tracheoesophageal groove. The nerves may be injured during dissection of the upper esophagus in the neck, or during the mediastinal dissection in transhiatal esophagectomy. Although much attention has been given to the vocal cord dysfunction that accompanies recurrent laryngeal nerve damage, it is also clear that cricopharyngeal sphincter dysfunction and

motility problems of the cervical esophagus can result from injury to these nerves. Serious episodes of aspiration following recurrent nerve injury are caused not only by cricopharyngeal dysfunction, but also by the inability to close the glottis during swallowing and loss of the protection afforded by effective coughing.

Branches from the left recurrent laryngeal nerve and from both vagus nerves innervate the upper thoracic esophagus. The esophageal plexus on the anterior and posterior walls of the esophagus innervates the lower esophagus. The esophageal plexus also receives fibers from the thoracic sympathetic chain. The single trunks located distally contain fibers from both the right and left original vagus nerves.

Efferent preganglionic sympathetic fibers supplying the esophagus arise from the fourth to sixth spinal cord segments and terminate in the cervical and thoracic sympathetic ganglia. Fibers from the superior cervical ganglion arrive at the pharyngeal plexus by way of vagal nerves. The postganglionic fibers reach the esophagus via branches from the cervical and thoracic sympathetic chain. The distal esophageal segments also receive direct sympathetic fibers from the celiac ganglion.

Afferent visceral sensory pain fibers from the esophagus terminate without synapses in the first four segments of the thoracic spinal cord, following both sympathetic and vagal pathways. Pain fibers from the heart also travel in these same pathways, which explains the similarity of symptoms in many esophageal and cardiac diseases.

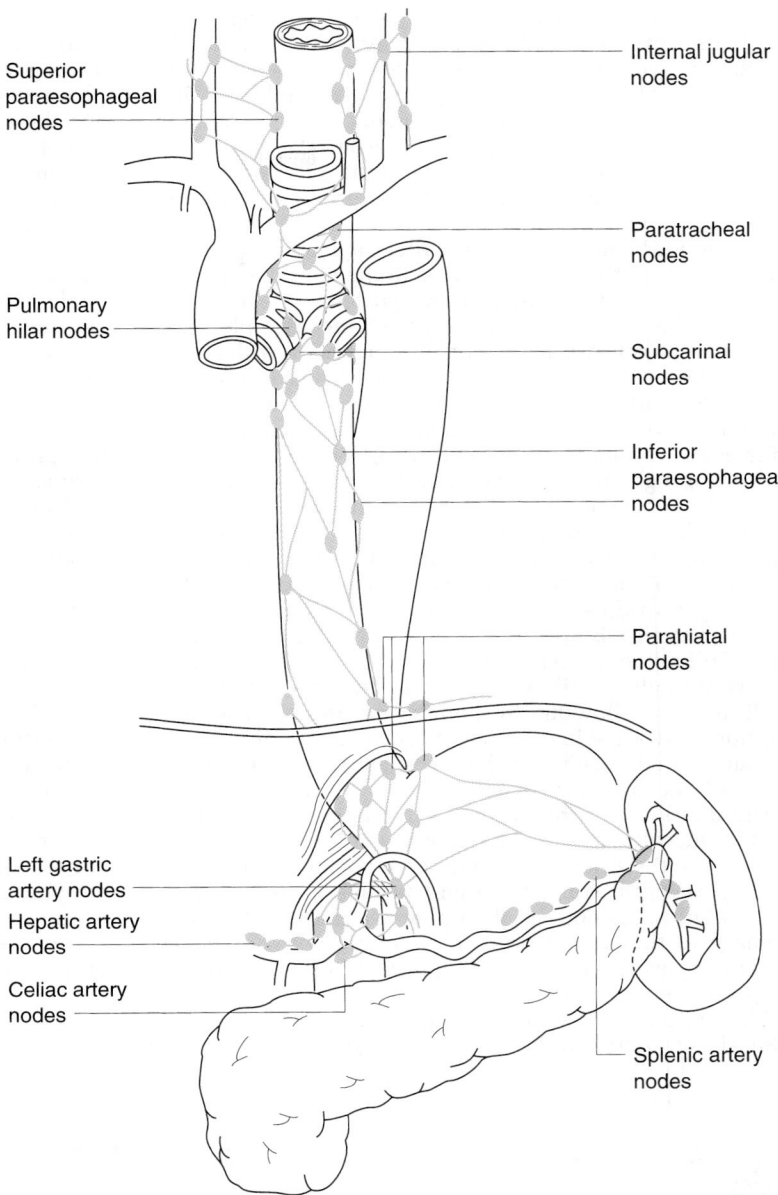

Figure 19.5. Lymphatic drainage of the esophagus.

PHYSIOLOGY

The act of alimentation requires the passage of food and drink from the mouth into the stomach. Food is taken into the mouth in a variety of bite sizes, where it is broken up, mixed with saliva, and lubricated. Swallowing, once initiated, is entirely a reflex. When food is ready for swallowing, the tongue, acting like a piston, moves the bolus into the posterior oropharynx and forces it into the hypopharynx (3). Concomitantly with the posterior movement of the tongue, elevation of the soft palate closes the passage between the oropharynx and nasopharynx. This partitioning prevents pressure generated in the oropharynx from being dissipated through the nose. When the soft palate is paralyzed, as after a cerebral vascular accident, food is commonly regurgitated into the nasopharynx. During swallowing, the hyoid bone moves upward and anteriorly, elevating the larynx, opening the retrolaryngeal space, and bringing the epiglottis under the tongue. The backward

tilted epiglottis covers the opening of the larynx to prevent aspiration. The whole pharyngeal part of swallowing occurs within 1.5 seconds.

During swallowing, the pressure in the hypopharynx rises abruptly to at least 60 mm Hg as a consequence of the backward movement of the tongue and contraction of the posterior pharyngeal constrictors. A sizable pressure difference develops between the hypopharyngeal pressure and the less-than-atmospheric midesophageal or intrathoracic pressure. This pressure gradient speeds the movement of food from the hypopharynx into the esophagus when the cricopharyngeus or upper esophageal sphincter relaxes. The bolus is both propelled by peristaltic contraction of the posterior pharyngeal constrictors and sucked into the thoracic esophagus. Critical to the bolus being received is the compliance of the cervical esophagus; when compliance is lost because of muscle disease, dysphagia can result. The upper esophageal sphincter closes within 0.5 second of the initiation of the swallow, with the immediate closing pressure reaching approximately twice the resting level of 30 mm Hg. The contraction that follows relaxation continues down the esophagus as a peristaltic wave (Fig. 19.6). The high closing pressure and initiation of the peristaltic wave prevent reflux of the bolus from the esophagus back into the pharynx. After the peristaltic wave has passed farther down the esophagus, the pressure in the upper esophageal sphincter returns to its resting level.

Swallowing can be started at will, or it can be elicited as a reflex by the stimulation of areas in the mouth and pharynx, among them the anterior and posterior tonsillar pillars and the posterior lateral walls of the hypopharynx. The afferent sensory nerves of the pharynx are the glossopharyngeal nerves and the superior laryngeal branches of the vagus nerves. Once aroused by stimuli entering via these nerves, the swallowing center in the medulla coordinates the complete act of swallowing by discharging impulses through cranial nerves V, VII, X, XI, and XII, in addition to the motor neurons of C-1 to C-3. Discharges through these nerves occur in a rather specific pattern and last for approximately 0.5 second. Little is known about the organization of the swallowing center except that it can trigger swallowing after a variety of different inputs, but the response is always a rigidly ordered pattern of outflow. Following a cerebral vascular accident, alteration of this coordinated outflow may cause mild to severe abnormalities of swallowing. In more severe injury, gross disruption of swallowing can lead to repetitive aspiration.

The striated muscles of the cricopharyngeus and upper third of the esophagus are activated by efferent motor fibers distributed through the vagus nerve and its recurrent laryngeal branches. The integrity of innervation is required for the cricopharyngeus to relax in coordination with pharyngeal contraction and resume its resting tone once a bolus has entered the upper esophagus. Operative damage to the innervation can interfere with laryngeal, cricopharyngeal, and upper esophageal function and predispose the patient to aspiration.

Pharyngeal activity in swallowing initiates the esophageal phase. Owing to the helical arrangement of its circular muscles, the body of the esophagus functions as a worm-drive propulsive pump and is responsible for transmitting a bolus of food into the stomach. The esophageal phase of swallowing represents work done by the esophagus during alimentation to move food into the stomach over a gradient of 12 mm Hg, from a negative-pressure environment (intrathoracic pressure of -6 mm Hg) to a positive-pressure environment (intraabdominal pressure of 6 mm Hg). Effective and coordinated smooth-muscle function in the lower third of the esophagus is therefore important in pumping food across this gradient.

The peristaltic wave generates an occlusive pressure varying from 30 to 120 mm Hg. The wave rises to a peak in 1 second, remains at the peak for about 0.5 second, and then subsides in about 1.5 seconds. The whole course of the rise and fall of occlusive pressure may occupy one point in the esophagus for 3 to 5 seconds (4,5). The peak of a primary peristaltic contraction initiated by a swallow (primary peristalsis) moves down the esophagus at a rate of 2 to 4 cm/s and reaches the distal esophagus about 9 seconds after swallowing starts. Consecutive swallows produce similar primary peristaltic waves, but when the act of swallowing is rapidly repeated, the esophagus remains relaxed and the peristaltic wave occurs only after the last movement of the pharynx. Progress of the wave through the esophagus is maintained by the sequential activation of esophageal muscles initiated by efferent vagal nerve fibers arising in the swallowing center.

Continuity of the esophageal muscle is not necessary for sequential activation if the nerves are intact. If the muscles, but not the nerves, are cut transversely, the pressure wave begins distally below the cut as it dies out at the proximal end above the cut. For this reason, a sleeve resection of the esophagus can be performed without destroying its normal function. Afferent impulses from receptors within the esophageal wall are not essential for progress of the coordinated wave. Afferent nerves, however, do travel to the swallowing center from the esophagus, because if the esophagus is distended at any point, a contractual wave begins with a forceful closure of the upper esophageal sphincter and sweeps down the esopha-

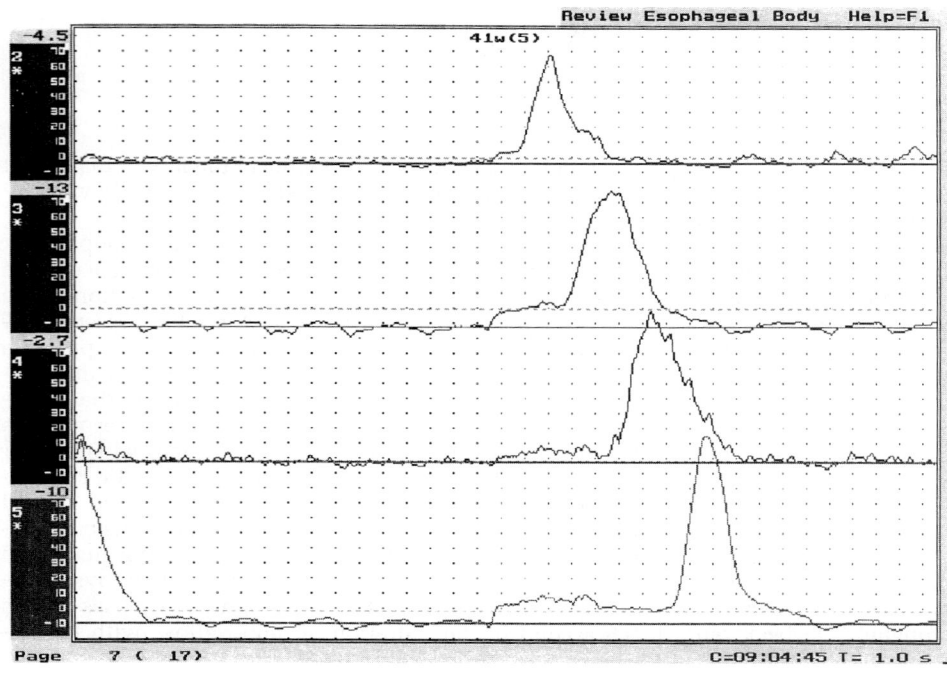

Figure 19.6. Representative example of a manometric tracing of an esophageal peristaltic wave. Channel 2 is in the proximal esophagus and channel 5 is in the distal esophagus. The channels are 5 cm apart. The wave can be seen to progress in time down the esophagus.

gus. This secondary contraction occurs without any movements of the mouth or pharynx. Secondary peristalsis can occur as an independent local reflex to clear the esophagus of ingested material left behind after the passage of the primary wave. Current studies suggest that secondary peristalsis is not as common as once thought.

Despite the rather powerful occlusive pressure, the propulsive force of the esophagus is relatively feeble. If a subject attempts to swallow a bolus attached by a string to a counterweight, the maximum weight that can be overcome is 5 to 10 g. Orderly contractions of the muscular wall and anchoring of the esophagus at its inferior end are necessary for efficient aboral propulsion to occur. Loss of the inferior anchor, as happens with a large hiatal hernia, can lead to inefficient propulsion.

The lower esophageal sphincter provides a pressure barrier between the esophagus and stomach. Although an anatomically distinct lower esophageal sphincter has been difficult to identify, microdissection studies show that in humans, the sphincter-like function is related to the architecture of the muscle fibers at the junction of the esophageal tube with the gastric pouch. The sphincter actively remains closed to prevent reflux of gastric contents into the esophagus and opens by a relaxation that coincides with a pharyngeal swallow (Fig. 19.7). The lower esophageal sphincter pressure returns to its resting level after the peristaltic wave has passed through the esophagus. Consequently, gastric juice that may flow back through the open valve during a swallow is returned to the stomach.

If the pharyngeal swallow does not initiate a peristaltic contraction, then the coincident relaxation of the lower esophageal sphincter is unguarded and reflux of gastric juice can occur. This may be an explanation for the observation of spontaneous lower esophageal relaxation, thought by some to be a causative factor in gastroesophageal reflux disease (GERD). The power of the esophageal body is insufficient to force open a valve that does not relax. In dogs, a bilateral cervical parasympathetic blockade abolishes the relaxation of the lower esophageal

sphincter that occurs with pharyngeal swallowing or distention of the esophagus. Consequently, vagal function appears to be important in coordinating the relaxation of the lower esophageal sphincter with esophageal contraction.

The lower esophageal sphincter has intrinsic myogenic tone that is modulated by neural and hormonal mechanisms (6,7). α-Adrenergic neurotransmitters or beta blockers stimulate the lower esophageal sphincter, and alpha blockers and beta stimulants decrease its pressure. It is not clear to what extent cholinergic nerve activity controls lower esophageal sphincter pressure. The vagus nerve carries both excitatory and inhibitory fibers to the esophagus and sphincter. The hormones gastrin and motilin have been shown to increase lower esophageal sphincter pressure; cholecystokinin, estrogen, glucagon, progesterone, somatostatin, and secretin decrease lower esophageal sphincter pressure. The peptides bombesin, β-enkephalin, and substance P increase lower esophageal sphincter pressure; calcitonin gene-related peptide, gastric inhibitory peptide, neuropeptide Y, and vasoactive intestinal polypeptide decrease lower esophageal sphincter pressure. Some pharmacologic agents, such as antacids, cholinergics, agonists, domperidone, metoclopramide, and prostaglandin F_2, are known to increase lower esophageal sphincter pressure; anticholinergics, barbiturates, calcium channel blockers, caffeine, diazepam, dopamine, meperidine, prostaglandins E_1 and E_2, and theophylline decrease lower esophageal sphincter pressure. Peppermint, chocolate, coffee, ethanol, and fat are all associated with decreased lower esophageal sphincter pressure and may be responsible for esophageal symptoms occurring after a sumptuous meal.

During 24-hour esophageal pH monitoring, healthy persons have occasional episodes of gastroesophageal reflux. This physiologic reflux is more common when the subject is awake and in the upright position than during sleep in the supine position. When reflux of gastric juice occurs, normal subjects rapidly clear the acid gastric juice from the esophagus regardless of their position.

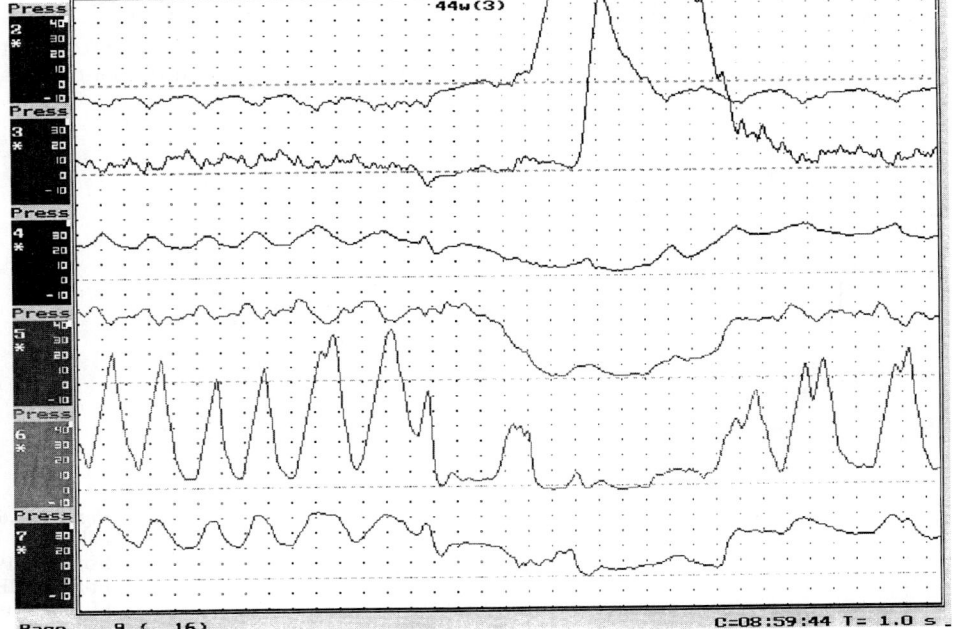

Figure 19.7. Representative example of a manometric tracing of lower esophageal sphincter relaxation. Channels 2 and 3 are in the distal esophagus and show a peristaltic wave progressing downward. The lower four channels are all at the same level within the lower esophageal sphincter and oriented radially at 12, 3, 6, and 9 o'clock. The *dotted lines* below each tracing represent gastric baseline pressures. The lower four tracings each relax to gastric baseline at the initiation of the swallow.

GASTROESOPHAGEAL REFLUX DISEASE

Epidemiology

Population-based studies have reported that one third of Western populations experience symptoms of GERD at least once a month, with 4% to 7% experiencing symptoms daily (8,9). Judging from the high prevalence of heartburn in the general population, GERD is a very common condition. Most patients with mild symptoms carry out self-medication, whereas those with more severe and persistent symptoms seek medical attention. Further, the prevalence and severity of GERD reflux are likely increasing. In contrast, the prevalence of duodenal ulcer disease has decreased markedly (10) (Fig. 19.8), possibly in part because of the effects of treatment for *Helicobacter pylori* infection (see below). The diagnosis of a columnar cell-lined esophagus is also increasing at a rapid rate, and deaths from end-stage benign esophageal disease are on an upward trend (11). These epidemiologic changes have occurred despite dramatic improvements in the efficacy of treatment options.

Studies on the natural history of GERD are rare (12,13). The few that do exist usually involve patients who were receiving some form of therapy. One of the most detailed studies of the natural history of the disease comes from Lausanne, Switzerland, where an intensive endoscopic follow-up of a defined population of 959 patients was performed during a 30-year period (12). In this study, which involved only patients who had endoscopic esophagitis and did not include those who had symptoms without mucosal injury, esophagitis developed in about 45% of patients as an isolated episode and did not return while they were taking acid suppression therapy. In the remaining patients, esophagitis intermittently recurred while they were on acid suppression therapy, and in 42% it progressed while they are on therapy to more severe mucosal injury. This latter group comprised about 23% of the initial population of patients with esophagitis. The study also showed that while they were on therapy and within as short a period as 6 weeks, a columnar cell-lined lower esophagus with intestinal metaplasia developed in 18% of the initial population.

Role of Helicobacter pylori

Recent studies suggest that *H. pylori* is not involved in the pathophysiology of GERD or the development of erosive esophagitis. Studying patients in Los Angeles, Oberg

et al. (14) found the prevalence of *H. pylori* to be similar in patients with and without erosive esophagitis. Furthermore, they found no difference in the prevalence of esophagitis in patients with acid reflux disease when they were grouped according to the presence or absence of *H. pylori* infection. Colonization with *H. pylori* may, however, have a protective effect. In the study of Labenz et al. (15), esophagitis developed significantly more frequently during the ensuing 3 years in patients with duodenal ulcer in whom *H. pylori* had been successfully eradicated than in those who remained positive for *H. pylori*. They suggested that the increased frequency of esophagitis might have resulted from increased gastric acid secretion following eradication therapy. Others have suggested, however, that gastric acid secretion may decrease following *H. pylori* eradication and have questioned the association between eradication therapy and GERD with and without erosive esophagitis.

Recent investigations have focused on the role of subpopulations of *H. pylori,* including cagA+ strains, in the development of gastroesophageal reflux and its complications. Vicari and colleagues (16) demonstrated that in patients with *H. pylori* infection, the prevalence of cagA-positive strains progressively decreases with the severity of GERD, including Barrett's esophagus and esophageal adenocarcinoma. Chow et al. (17) confirmed an inverse relationship between the presence of cagA positivity and adenocarcinoma of the esophagus and gastroesophageal junction. Both groups postulated that cagA-positive strains may provide protection from the development of adenocarcinoma by inducing more severe mucosal inflammation and atrophic gastritis and thereby decreasing acid reflux. Present data regarding gastric acid secretion are conflicting, however, and further studies are required to test if this hypothesis is true.

Clinical Presentation

The most common complaints in patients with GERD are heartburn, regurgitation, and occasionally dysphagia, or difficulty swallowing. These represent the so-called typical symptoms of GERD. Although none of these is specific to GERD, the latter is more commonly a sign of serious underlying disease, including esophageal carcinoma. Dysphagia should always be investigated promptly and thoroughly.

Heartburn is characterized as a substernal "burning" discomfort that often radiates from the epigastrium to the

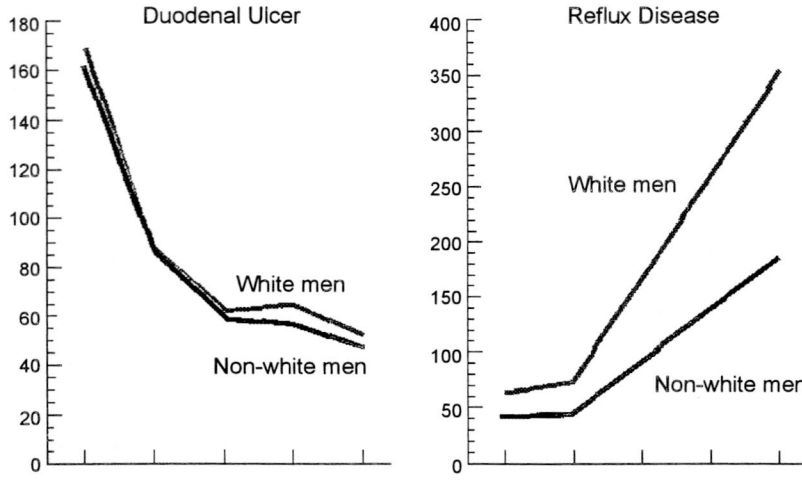

Figure 19.8. Trends in hospitalization for duodenal ulcer and gastroesophageal reflux disease from the 1970s to 1990s in U.S. veterans. (From El-Serag HB, Sonnenberg A. Opposing time trends of peptic ulcer and reflux disease. *Gut* 1998;43: 327–333, with permission.)

sternal notch. Occasionally, patients will refer to it as "chest pain" rather than as heartburn, and the two can be difficult to distinguish. Even the location can vary, with patients occasionally experiencing discomfort in the epigastrium, base of the neck, back, or other areas. Heartburn is typically made worse by "spicy" foods, such as tomato sauce, citrus juices, chocolate, coffee, and alcohol. It occurs 1 to 2 hours after eating, often at night, and is relieved by antacids and antisecretory agents, such as the over-the-counter histamine (H_2) blockers. It is well recognized that the severity of symptoms is not necessarily related to the severity of the underlying disease (Fig. 19.9).

Regurgitation is the spontaneous return of gastric contents to the area proximal to the gastroesophageal junction. Its spontaneous nature distinguishes it from vomiting. The patient often has a sensation that fluid or food is returning into the esophagus, even if it does not reach as far as the pharynx or mouth. It is typically worse when the patient lies down, at night or after a meal. Patients commonly compensate by not eating late at night and by sleeping partially upright with several pillows or in a chair. This symptom is often less effectively relieved by antacids and antisecretory agents, although it may change in character from an acid to a more "bland" nature.

Dysphagia is present in up to 40% of patients with GERD. It is generally manifested as a sensation of food hanging up in the lower esophagus (esophageal dysphagia) rather than as difficulty transferring the bolus from the mouth to the esophageal inlet (oropharyngeal dysphagia). Classically, dysphagia limited to solid food, with a normal passage of liquids, suggests the presence of a mechanical disorder, such as a large hernia, stricture, or tumor, whereas dysphagia with both solids and liquids suggests a functional or motor disorder. It often develops slowly enough that patients may adjust their eating habits and not necessarily notice it. Thus, a thorough esophageal history includes an assessment of the dietary history. Questions should be asked about the consistency of food that is typically eaten, whether liquids must be taken with the meal, and whether the patient is usually the last to finish, has interrupted a social meal, chokes or vomits while eating, or has been admitted on an emergency basis because of food impaction. These assessments, in addition to the ability to maintain nutrition, help to quantify the dysphagia and are important in determining the indications for surgical therapy.

Many patients with gastroesophageal reflux often manifest "atypical" symptoms, such as cough, asthma, hoarseness, and noncardiac chest pain. Atypical symptoms are the primary complaint in 20% to 25% of patients with GERD and are secondarily present in association with heartburn and regurgitation in many more. It is considerably more difficult to prove a cause-and-effect relationship between atypical symptoms and gastroesophageal reflux than between typical symptoms and reflux. Consequently, the results of surgical therapy have been correspondingly less satisfactory. This is not to say that patients with atypical symptoms are not good candidates for antireflux surgery, as many will benefit greatly, but that it should be applied cautiously in these patients. Often, a trial of high-dose proton pump inhibitors is helpful. Among patients with atypical symptoms, the outcome of antireflux surgery is optimal in those with a good response to medical treatment rather than in those who fail to respond.

The diagnosis of GERD based on symptoms alone is correct in only approximately two thirds of patients (18) because the symptoms are not specific for gastroesophageal reflux and can be caused by other diseases, such as achalasia, diffuse spasm, esophageal carcinoma, pyloric stenosis, cholelithiasis, gastritis, gastric or duodenal ulcer, and coronary artery disease. This fact underscores the need for objective diagnosis before surgical treatment is undertaken.

Physiology of the Antireflux Barrier

In humans, a zone of high pressure can be identified at the junction of the esophagus and stomach. This lower esophageal "sphincter" provides a barrier between the esophagus and stomach that normally prevents gastric contents from entering the esophagus. It has no anatomic landmarks, but its presence can be identified by a rise in pressure over gastric baseline pressure as a pressure transducer is pulled from the stomach into the esophagus. This high-pressure zone is normally present except in two situations: (a) after a swallow, when it momentarily relaxes to allow food to pass into the stomach, and (b) when the fundus is distended with gas, in which situation it is eliminated to allow venting of the gas (a belch). The common denominator for virtually all episodes of gastroesophageal reflux, whether physiologic or pathologic, is the loss of the normal high-pressure zone and the resistance it imposes to the flow of gastric juice from an environment of higher pressure, the stomach, to an environment of lower pressure, the esophagus. In severe disease, the high-pressure zone is usually permanently obliterated or reduced. In early disease or normal subjects, loss of the high-pressure zone is usually transient.

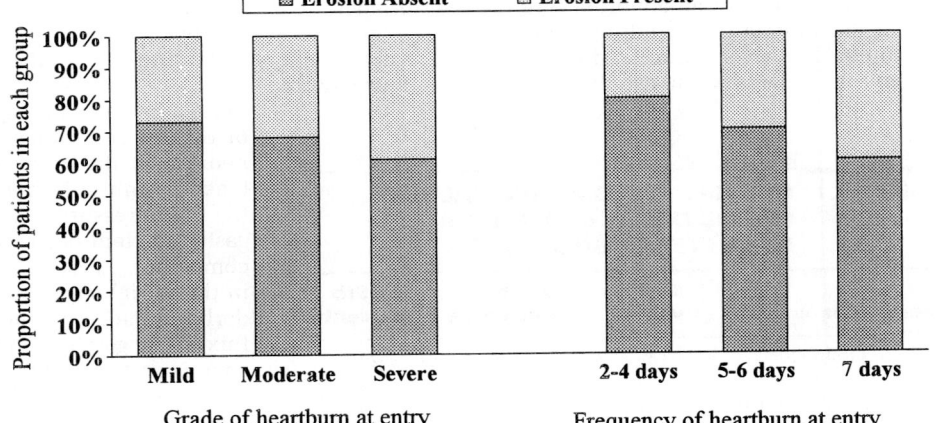

Figure 19.9. Prevalence of erosive esophagitis in 994 patients with varying severity and frequency of reflux symptoms. (From Venables TL, Newland RD, Patel AC, et al. Omeprazole 10 milligrams once daily, omeprazole 20 milligrams once daily, or ranitidine 150 milligrams twice daily, evaluated as initial therapy for the relief of symptoms of gastro-oesophageal reflux disease in general practice. *Scand J Gastroenterol* 1997;32:965–973, with permission.)

Three characteristics of the lower esophageal sphincter maintain its resistance or "barrier" function to intragastric and intraabdominal pressure challenges. These are its pressure, its overall length, and the length exposed to the positive-pressure environment of the abdomen (Table 19.1). The tonic resistance of the lower esophageal sphincter is a function of both its pressure and the length over which this pressure is exerted (19). The shorter the overall length of the high-pressure zone, the higher the pressure must be to maintain sufficient resistance for the sphincter to remain competent (Fig. 19.10). Consequently, a normal sphincter pressure can be nullified by a short overall sphincter length. Further, as the stomach fills, the length of the sphincter decreases, rather in the way the neck of a balloon shortens as the balloon is inflated. If the overall length of the sphincter is abnormally short when the stomach is empty, then with minimal gastric distention, the sphincter length will be insufficient for the existing pressure to maintain sphincter competency, and reflux will occur.

The third characteristic of the lower esophageal sphincter relates to its position, in that a portion of the overall length of the high-pressure zone should be exposed to positive intraabdominal pressure. During periods of increased intraabdominal pressure, the resistance of the lower esophageal sphincter would be overcome if the abdominal pressure were not applied equally to the high-pressure zone and stomach (20). Think of sucking on a soft soda straw immersed in a bottle of soda; the hydrostatic pressure of the fluid and the negative pressure inside the straw cause the straw to collapse instead of allowing the liquid to flow up the straw in the direction of the negative pressure. If the abdominal length is inadequate, the sphincter cannot respond to an increase in applied intraabdominal pressure by collapsing, and reflux is more liable to result.

If pressure in the high-pressure zone is abnormally low, the overall length of the zone is short, or the zone is minimally exposed to the abdominal pressure environment in the fasting state, then lower esophageal sphincter resistance is permanently lost, and the reflux of gastric contents into the esophagus is unhampered throughout the circadian cycle. A *permanently defective sphincter* is identified by the presence of one or more of the following characteristics: a high-pressure zone with an average pressure of less than 6 mm Hg, an average overall length of 2 cm or less, and an average length exposed to the positive-pressure environment of the abdomen of 1 cm or less (21). In comparison with values in normal subjects, these values are below the 2.5 percentile for each parameter. The most common cause of a permanently defective sphincter is an inadequate pressure, but the efficiency of a sphincter with a normal pressure can be nullified by an inadequate abdominal length or an abnormally short overall length.

For the clinician, the finding of a permanently defective sphincter has several implications. Foremost, it is almost always associated with esophageal mucosal injury (22)

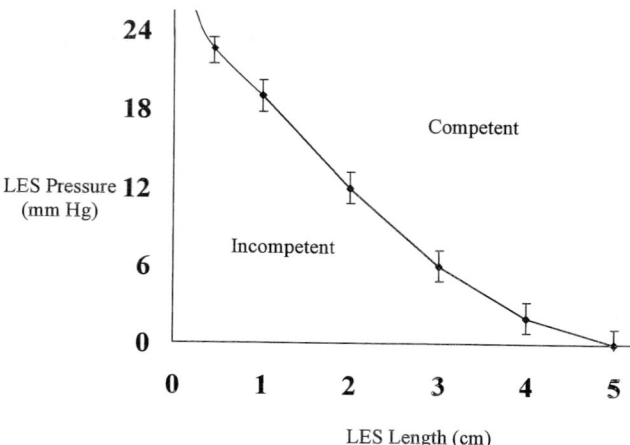

Figure 19.10. The relationship between the magnitude of pressure in the high-pressure zone measured at the respiratory inversion point and the overall length of the zone to the resistance to the flow of fluid through the zone. *Competent,* no flow. *Incompetent,* flow of varied volumes. Note that the shorter the overall length of the high-pressure zone, the higher the pressures must be to maintain sufficient resistance for competence.

and predicts that the patient's symptoms will be difficult to control with medical therapy (23). It is a signal that surgical therapy is likely to be needed for consistent and long-term control of symptoms. It is now accepted that when the sphincter is permanently defective, the condition is irreversible, even when the associated esophagitis is healed. The presence of a permanently defective sphincter is commonly associated with reduced esophageal body function, and if the disease is not brought under control, the progressive loss of effective esophageal clearance can lead to severe mucosal injury, repetitive regurgitation, aspiration, and pulmonary failure (24,25).

A transient loss of the high-pressure zone can also occur and is usually caused by a functional problem of the gastric reservoir. Excessive swallowing of air or food can result in gastric dilation and, if the active relaxation reflex has been lost, an increased intragastric pressure. When the stomach is distended, the vectors produced by gastric wall tension pull on the gastroesophageal junction with a force that varies according to the geometry of the cardia—that is, the forces are applied more directly when a hiatal hernia exists than when a proper angle of His is present. The forces pull on the terminal esophagus and cause it to be "taken up" into the stretched fundus, so that the length of the high-pressure zone, or "sphincter," is reduced. This process continues until a critical length is reached, usually about 1 to 2 cm, when the pressure drops precipitously and reflux occurs. The mechanism by which gastric distention contributes to a shortening of the high-pressure zone, so that its pressure drops and reflux occurs, provides a mechanical explanation for "transient relaxations" of the lower esophageal sphincter that occur without a neuromuscular reflex being invoked. Rather than a "spontaneous" muscular relaxation, a mechanical shortening of the high-pressure zone develops secondary to progressive gastric distention, to the point at which it becomes incompetent. These "transient sphincter" shortenings occur in the initial stages of GERD and are the mechanisms underlying the early complaint of excessive postprandial reflux. After gastric venting, the length of the high-pressure zone is restored and competence returns until distention again shortens it and encourages further venting and reflux. This sequence results in the common complaints of

---

Table 19.1. **NORMAL MANOMETRIC VALUES OF THE DISTAL ESOPHAGEAL SPHINCTER IN 50 SUBJECTS**

Parameter	Median value	2.5th percentile	97.5th percentile
Pressure (mm Hg)	13	5.8	27.7
Overall length (cm)	3.6	2.1	5.6
Abdominal length (cm)	2	0.9	4.7

repetitive belching and bloating in patients with GERD. The increased frequency of swallowing seen in patients with GERD contributes to gastric distention and is a consequence of the repetitive ingestion of saliva in an effort to neutralize the acid refluxed into the esophagus (26). Thus, GERD may begin in the stomach, secondary to gastric distention caused by overeating and the excessive ingestion of fried foods which delay gastric emptying. Both characteristics are common in Western society and may explain the high prevalence of the disease in the Western world.

If mechanical forces set in motion by gastric distention are important in pulling on the terminal esophagus and shortening the length of the high-pressure zone, or "sphincter," then the geometry of the cardia—that is, the presence of a normal acute angle of His or the abnormal dome architecture of a sliding hiatus hernia—should influence the ease with which the sphincter is pulled open. A close relationship exists between the degree of gastric distention necessary to overcome the high-pressure zone and the morphology of the cardia. A greater degree of gastric dilation, as reflected by a higher intragastric pressure, is necessary to "open" the sphincter in patients with an intact angle of His than in those with a hiatus hernia (Fig. 19.11). This is what would be expected if the high-pressure zone were shortened by mechanical forces and is the reason why a hiatal hernia is often associated with GERD.

In normal subjects, almost all episodes of reflux are precipitated by belching, which remains an important but decreasing cause of reflux as the grade of esophagitis worsens. Activities that produce a pressure gradient across the diaphragm, such as coughing, sniffing, or straining, become increasingly important in precipitating reflux as the disease, graded according to the severity of esophagitis, progresses. In patients with severe esophagitis, episodes of acid reflux occur spontaneously, which suggests that the sphincter is defective in its resting state and that the barrier is permanently lost. Episodes of reflux associated with belching are by inference caused by gastric distention and

are responsible for an increased esophageal exposure to acid in patients with early or milder mucosal disease. In this situation, the barrier is transiently lost. Mucosal damage, caused by repetitive exposure to gastric juice, results in an inflammatory injury of underlying muscle. This leads to a permanently defective high-pressure zone, or "sphincter," caused initially by the loss of abdominal length and eventually by the loss of pressure and overall length. Subsequent inflammation in the esophagus results in the loss of its clearance ability and prolonged esophageal exposure to gastric juice (27). This signals the presence of advanced disease and places the patient at risk for Barrett's metaplasia, stricture formation, and aspiration.

Integrated Hypothesis of the Pathophysiology of Gastroesophageal Reflux Disease

The data support the likelihood that GERD begins in the stomach. Fundic distention occurs because of overeating and delayed gastric emptying secondary to the high-fat Western diet. The distention causes the sphincter to be "taken up" by the expanding fundus, so that the squamous epithelium within the high-pressure zone, the distal 3 cm of the esophagus, is exposed to gastric juice. Repeated exposure causes inflammation of the squamous epithelium, the development of columnar epithelium, and carditis. This is the initial step and explains why esophagitis is mild in early disease and commonly limited to the very distal part of the esophagus. The patient compensates with an increase in swallowing, which allows saliva to bathe the injured mucosa and alleviate the discomfort induced by exposure to gastric acid. Increased swallowing results in aerophagia, bloating, and repetitive belching. The distention induced by aerophagia leads to further exposure of the terminal squamous epithelium, repetitive injury, and the development of cardiac-type mucosa. This is an inflammatory process, commonly referred to as *carditis,* and it accounts for the complaint of epigastric pain so often registered by patients with early disease. The process can lead to the development of a fibrotic mucosal ring at the squamocolumnar junction (Schatzki's ring). Extension of the inflammatory process into the muscularis propria causes a progressive loss in the length and pressure of the distal esophageal high-pressure zone; this is in turn associated with increased esophageal exposure to gastric juice and symptoms of heartburn and regurgitation. Loss of the barrier develops in a distal to proximal direction and eventually results in the permanent loss of lower esophageal sphincter resistance and the progression of disease into the esophagus, with all the clinical manifestations of severe esophagitis. This process accounts for the observation that severe esophageal mucosal injury is almost always associated with a permanently defective sphincter. At any time during the process and under specific luminal conditions or stimuli, such as exposure to a specific pH range, the development of intestinal metaplasia in the cardiac-type mucosa can set the stage for malignant degeneration.

Pathophysiology of Esophageal Mucosal Injury

The complications of gastroesophageal reflux result from the damage inflicted by gastric juice on the esophageal mucosa or respiratory epithelium. These include esophagitis, stricture, and Barrett's esophagus; in addition, repetitive aspiration causes recurrent pneumonia and progressive pulmonary fibrosis. The prevalence and severity of complications are related to the degree of loss of the gastroesophageal barrier, defects in esophageal clearance, and the content of refluxed gastric juice (22) (Fig. 19.12) The

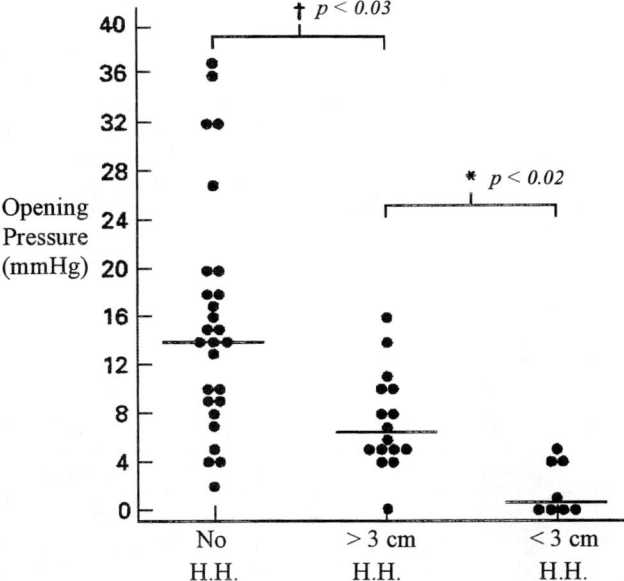

Figure 19.11. The intragastric pressure at which the lower esophagus opened in response to gastric distention by air during endoscopy. Note that the dome architecture of a hiatus hernia *(HH)* influenced how easily the sphincter could be pulled open by gastric distention. (From Ismail T, Bancewicz J, Barlow J. Yield pressure, anatomy of the cardia and gastro-oesophageal reflux. *Br J Surg* 1995;82:943–947, with permission.)

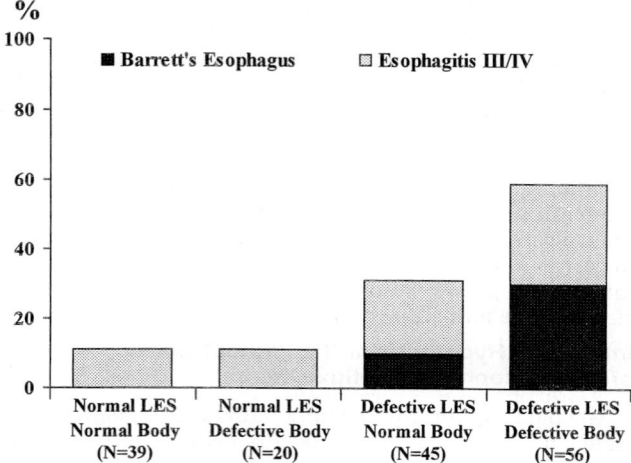

Figure 19.12. Prevalence of esophageal mucosal injury related to the presence of a defective lower esophageal sphincter, esophageal body motility, or both.

fact that nearly half of the patients without complications have a defective sphincter suggests that mucosal injury can be prevented via compensation by preserved esophageal clearance mechanisms.

The potential injurious components that flow back into the esophagus include gastric secretions, such as acid and pepsin, in addition to biliary and pancreatic secretions that return from the duodenum to the stomach. Our current understanding of the role of the various ingredients in gastric juice in the development of reflux complications is based on animal studies performed by Lillemoe and colleagues (28,29). These studies have shown that acid alone causes minimal damage to the esophageal mucosa, but the combination of acid and pepsin is highly deleterious. Hydrogen ion injury to the esophageal squamous mucosa occurs only at a pH below 2. In acidic matter that is refluxed, the enzyme pepsin appears to be the major injurious agent. Similarly, the reflux of duodenal juice alone causes little damage to the mucosa, but the combination of duodenal juice and gastric acid is particularly noxious. The reflux of bile and pancreatic enzymes into the stomach can either reduce or augment esophageal mucosal injury. For instance, the reflux of duodenal contents into the stomach may prevent the development of peptic esophagi-

tis in a patient whose gastric acid secretion maintains an acid environment because the bile salts would attenuate the injurious effect of pepsin and the acid would inactivate the trypsin. Such a patient would have bile-containing acid gastric juice that, when refluxed, would irritate the esophageal mucosa but cause a lesser degree of esophagitis than if it contained pepsin. In contrast, the reflux of duodenal contents into the stomach of a patient with limited gastric acid secretion could result in esophagitis because an alkaline intragastric environment would support optimal trypsin activity and the soluble bile salts with a high pK_a would potentiate the effect of the enzyme. Hence, duodenal–gastric reflux and the acid secretory capacity of the stomach are interrelated in that alterations in the pH and enzymatic activity of the refluxed gastric juice modulate the injurious effects of enzymes on the esophageal mucosa.

Similarly, the disparities in injury—that is, mucosal barrier abnormalities caused by acid and bile alone as opposed to gross esophagitis caused by pepsin and trypsin—provide an explanation for the poor correlation between the symptom of heartburn and the presence of endoscopic esophagitis. The reflux of acid gastric juice contaminated with duodenal contents could break the esophageal mucosal barrier, irritate nerve endings in the papillae close to the luminal surface, and cause severe heartburn. Despite the intense heartburn, the bile salts in the gastric juice would inhibit pepsin, the acidic pH would inactivate trypsin, and the patient would have little or no gross evidence of esophagitis. In contrast, the patient who refluxes alkaline gastric juice might have minimal heartburn because of the absence of hydrogen ions in the refluxed matter but would have endoscopic esophagitis because of bile salt potentiation of the effects of trypsin on the esophageal mucosa. Indeed, recent clinical studies indicate that alkaline reflux is associated with the development of mucosal injury (30).

The components of duodenal juice thought to be most damaging are the bile acids. For bile acids to injure mucosal cells, it is necessary that they be both soluble and nonionized, so that the nonionized, nonpolar form can enter mucosal cells. Before bile reaches the gastrointestinal tract, 98% of bile acids are conjugated with either taurine or glycine in a ratio of about 3:1. Conjugation increases the solubility and ionization of bile acids by lowering their pK_a. At the normal duodenal pH of approximately 7, more than 90% of bile salts are in solution and completely ionized. At pH ranges of 2 to 7, a mixture of the ionized salt and the lipophilic, nonionized acid exists (Fig. 19.13). Acidification of bile to below pH 2 results in an irreversible

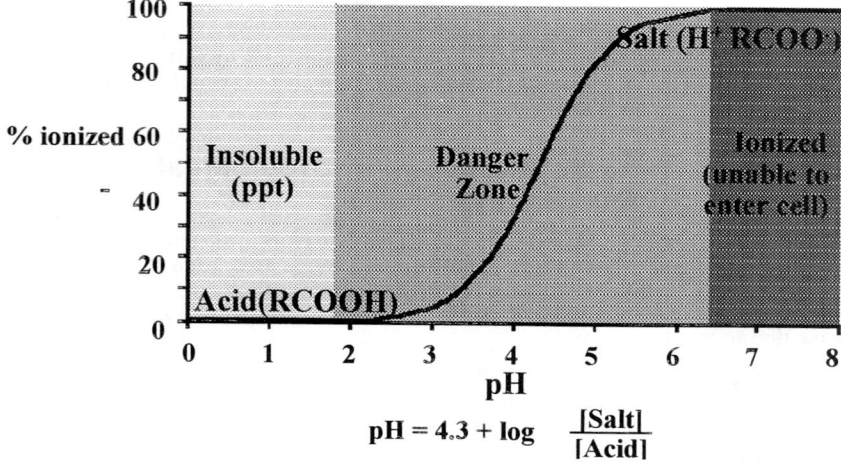

Figure 19.13. A representative ionization curve for bile acid. At a pH of 2 or less, bile acids are in their associated form (nonionized RCOOH) and insoluble, and they precipitate. Once they precipitate, they are difficult to redissolve. At a pH of 6.5 or above, bile acids are completely dissociated (ionized $H^+ + RCOO^-$), soluble, and nontoxic to the cells because their polarity prevents them from crossing the cell membrane. Between these extremes, bile acids can exist in their associated form and remain soluble. In this form, they can enter cells and cause detrimental effects. Hence, the pH range between 2 and 6.5 can be called the *danger zone*.

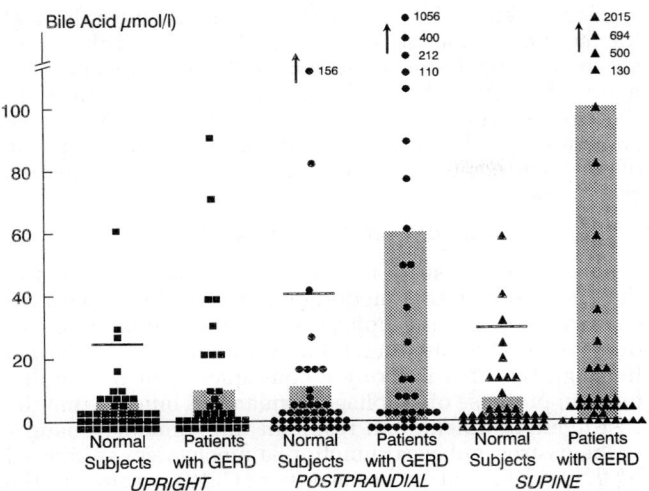

Figure 19.14. Peak bile acid concentration (μmol/L) for patients and normal subjects during upright, postprandial, and supine aspiration periods. The *shaded area* represents the mean and the *bar* the 95th percentile values.

precipitation of bile acids. Consequently, under normal physiologic conditions, bile acids precipitate and are of minimal effect in an acid gastric environment. On the other hand, in a more alkaline gastric environment, such as occurs with excessive duodenal–gastric reflux, during acid suppression therapy, or after vagotomy and partial or total gastrectomy, bile salts remain in solution and are partially dissociated, and when refluxed into the esophagus, they can cause severe mucosal injury by crossing the cell membrane and damaging the mitochondria.

Although numerous studies have suggested the reflux of duodenal contents into the esophagus in patients with GERD, few have measured this directly. Most have implied the presence of bile acids by means of pH measurements. Studies using either prolonged ambulatory aspiration techniques (Fig. 19.14) or spectrophotometric bilirubin measurement (Fig. 19.15) have shown that in patients with GERD, exposure of the esophageal mucosa to bile acid is greater than in normal subjects (31–34). This

increased exposure occurs most commonly during sleep, while the patient is supine, and after meals, while the patient is upright. Most studies have identified the glycine conjugates of cholic, deoxycholic, and chenodeoxycholic acids as the predominant bile acids aspirated from the esophagus of patients with GERD, although appreciable amounts of taurine conjugates of these bile acids are also found. Other bile salts have been identified, but in small concentrations. This is as one would expect, as glycine conjugates are three times more prevalent than taurine conjugates in normal human bile.

The fact that the combination of refluxed gastric and duodenal juice is more noxious to the esophageal mucosa than gastric juice alone may explain the consistent observation that recurrent and progressive mucosal damage develops in 25% of patients with reflux esophagitis, often despite medical therapy. A potential reason is that acid suppression therapy cannot consistently maintain the pH of refluxed gastric and duodenal juice above 6. That this is true is becoming increasingly clear. Lapses into pH ranges of 2 to 6 encourage the formation of nondissociated, nonpolarized, soluble bile acids that are capable of penetrating the cell wall and injuring mucosal cells. For bile acids to remain completely ionized in their polarized form, so that they are unable to penetrate cells, the pH of the refluxed material must be maintained above 7 for 24 hours a day, 7 days a week, for a lifetime. In practice, this is not only impractical but likely impossible unless very high doses of medications are used. The use of smaller doses allows esophageal mucosal damage to occur while the patient is relatively asymptomatic.

Barrett's Esophagus

The condition in which the tubular esophagus is lined with columnar rather than squamous epithelium was first described by Norman Barrett in 1950 (35) (Fig. 19.16). He incorrectly believed it to be congenital in origin. It is now realized that Barrett's esophagus is an acquired abnormality that occurs in 7% to 10% of patients with GERD and represents the end-stage of the natural history of this disease (36). It is also understood to be distinctly different from the congenital condition in which islands of mature gastric columnar epithelium are found in the upper half of the esophagus.

Figure 19.15. Prevalence of abnormal esophageal bilirubin exposure in healthy subjects and in patients with gastroesophageal reflux disease with varied degrees of mucosal injury. (From Kauer WKH, Peters JH, DeMeester TR, et al. Mixed reflux of gastric juice is more harmful to the esophagus than gastric juice alone: the need for surgical therapy reemphasized. *Ann Surg* 1995;222: 525–533, with permission.)

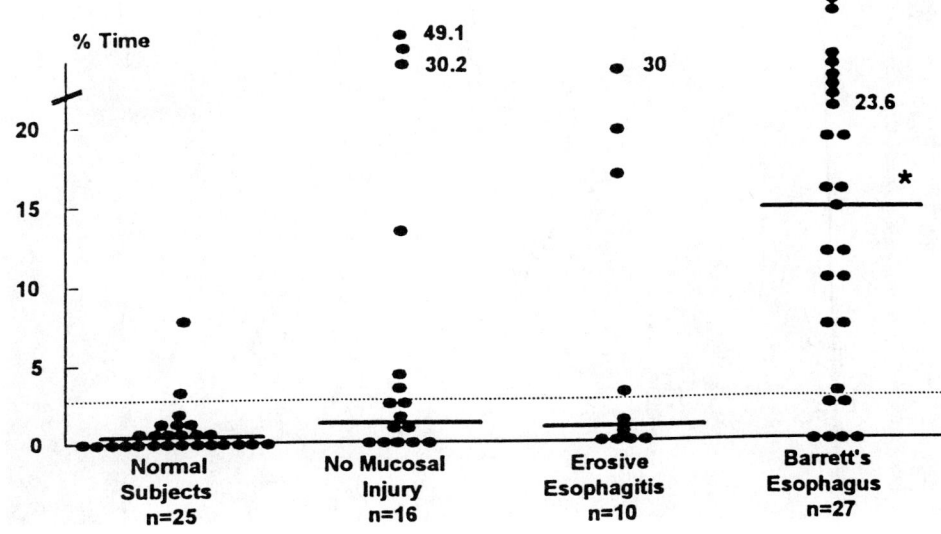

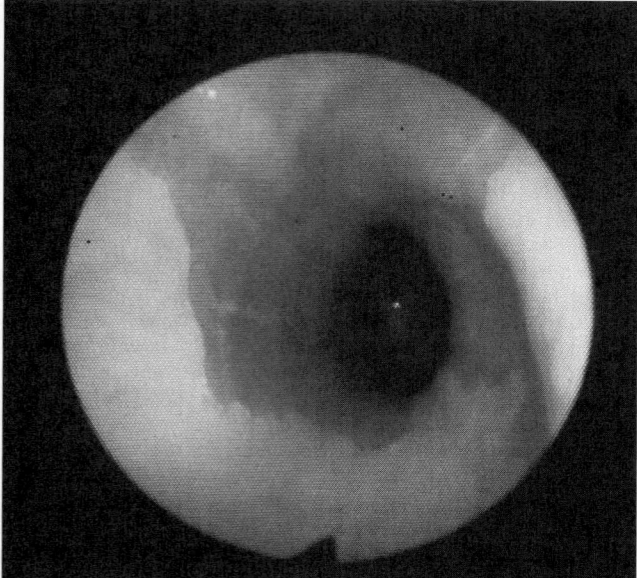

Figure 19.16. Endoscopic appearance of Barrett's esophagus. Note the pink metaplastic mucosa in contrast to the normal whitish squamous lining of the esophagus.

The definition of Barrett's esophagus has evolved considerably during the past decade (35–37). Traditionally, Barrett's esophagus was identified by the presence of any columnar mucosa extending at least 3 cm into the esophagus. Recent data indicating that specialized intestinal-type epithelium is the only tissue predisposed to malignant degeneration, coupled with the finding of a similar risk for malignancy in segments of intestinal metaplasia 3 cm long, have resulted in the diagnosis of Barrett's esophagus being given to endoscopically visible tissue of any length demonstrated to be intestinal metaplasia on histology. Whether to call long segments of columnar mucosa without intestinal metaplasia Barrett's esophagus is unclear. The hallmark of intestinal metaplasia is the presence of goblet cells (Fig. 19.17). Recent studies have identified a high prevalence of biopsy-proven intestinal metaplasia at the cardia in the absence of endoscopic evidence of columnar cells lining the esophagus. The significance and natural history of this finding remain unknown. Most authors presently use the term *Barrett's esophagus* to denote an endoscopically visible segment of intestinal metaplasia of any length, or a 3-cm or longer columnar replacement of esophageal mucosa.

Pathophysiology of Barrett's Metaplasia

Recent studies suggest that the metaplastic process at the gastroesophageal junction may actually begin with the conversion of distal esophageal squamous mucosa to cardiac-type epithelium, heretofore presumed to be a normal finding (37). This is likely a consequence of gastric distention, prolapse of esophageal squamous mucosa into the gastric environment, and resultant inflammatory changes at the gastroesophageal junction, a mechanism supported by the finding that as the severity of GERD progresses, the length of columnar lining above the anatomic gastroesophageal junction increases. This finding suggests that the presence of columnar epithelium lining the distal esophageal sphincter results from a metaplastic process associated with a loss of sphincter function and increased esophageal acid exposure. Intestinal metaplasia within the sphincter may result, as in Barrett's metaplasia of the esophageal body. This process leads to a loss of muscle function, and the sphincter becomes mechanically defective, allowing free reflux to cause progressive mucosal injury.

Factors predisposing to the development of Barrett's esophagus include early onset of GERD, abnormal lower esophageal sphincter and esophageal body physiology, and reflux of mixed gastric and duodenal contents into the esophagus (36). Direct measurement of esophageal exposure to bilirubin, as a marker for duodenal juice, has shown that esophageal exposure to duodenal juice is increased in 58% of patients with GERD, and that this exposure is most dramatically related to Barrett's esophagus.

Cellular Origin of Barrett's Epithelium

The cell of origin of Barrett's epithelium is unknown. Biochemically, Barrett's tissue resembles colonic epithelia and is characterized by the following features:

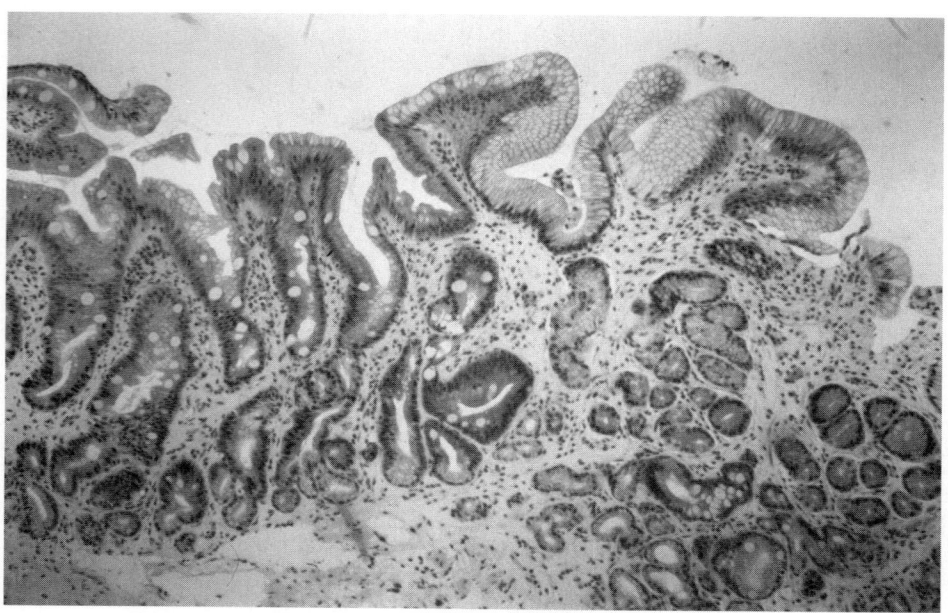

Figure 19.17. Histologic appearance of Barrett's esophagus. To the left of the photograph, columnar mucosa with abundant goblet cells is seen. This is intestinal metaplasia, which is the histologic hallmark of Barrett's esophagus. To the right of the photomicrograph, cardiac epithelium is present.

1. Lack of disaccharide activity
2. High isomaltase/sucrase activity
3. Low mucosal levels of glutathione
4. Low mucosal levels of protein synthesis
5. Abundant cytokeratin (CK-13)

Several provocative articles regarding the origin of Barrett's metaplasia have been recently published. Sawhney and colleagues (38) have described a unique surface cell at the junction of squamous and Barrett's epithelium notable for the presence of both squamous and columnar markers on its surface. In a recent study, this hybrid cell, which by electron microscopy was cuboidal with abundant microvilli and secretory vesicles, was present in 40% of patients with Barrett's esophagus (39). The authors hypothesized that this distinctive cell represents an intermediate stage in the development of Barrett's epithelium. Salo et al. (40) and Boch et al. (41) have studied the cytokeratin profile of Barrett's epithelium. Cytokeratins are a group of structural proteins present in all epithelia. Various epithelia express different cytokeratins, with the profile indicative of the differentiation pathway. Cytokeratins 4 and 13 are typical of squamous differentiation, and cytokeratins 8, 18, and 19 of glandular epithelium. Salo et al. (40) studied the cytokeratin profile in 35 patients with Barrett's esophagus and 10 normal controls. Immunohistochemistry of frozen sections showed abundant cytokeratin 13, characteristic of squamous epithelia but not found in normal gastric epithelia, in patients with Barrett's esophagus (40). Boch et al. (41) studied biopsy specimens from eight patients with Barrett's epithelium and three specimens from the gastroesophageal junction of patients without Barrett's esophagus. Staining with columnar markers was confined to either the Barrett's or the gastric epithelium, and staining with squamous markers to the adjacent squamous epithelium. In contrast, focal areas of multilayered epithelium adjacent to Barrett's epithelium stained for both types of markers, which suggests a multipotential cell as the cell of origin of Barrett's epithelium.

Evidence Supporting a Metaplasia, Dysplasia Carcinoma Sequence

Two lines of evidence support the concept of a metaplasia, dysplasia carcinoma sequence. The first is the observation that dysplasia is commonly found in areas of nondysplastic Barrett's epithelium and that high-grade dysplasia can be found adjacent to most adenocarcinomas of the esophagus. Perhaps most convincing, however, are the results of prospective studies documenting the progression from nondysplastic Barrett's epithelium to low- and high-grade dyplasia and ultimately carcinoma in individual patients. Hameeteman et al. (42) documented the progression from no or low-grade dysplasia through high-grade dysplasia to carcinoma in five patients during 1 to 10 years. In one of the few, if not only, analyses of the direct clonal relationship between metaplasia, dysplasia, and carcinoma, Zhuang et al. (43) studied *APC* gene alteration in patients with Barrett's esophagus. Twelve specimens containing areas of normal epithelium, Barrett's metaplasia, dysplasia, and invasive adenocarcinoma were selected, and deletion of the *APC* gene was identified. The *APC* locus was deleted in five patients, two of whom were women. In all five patients with a loss of heterozygosity at the *APC* gene locus, the same allele was inactivated in the invasive carcinoma and dysplasia specimens. Furthermore, loss of heterozygosity of the *APC* gene was present in Barrett's metaplasia adjacent to the dysplasia in two of the five patients.

Studies of X-chromosome inactivation and clonality analysis in these two women showed that the inactivation was from the same clone of cells in the metaplastic, dysplastic, and carcinoma sections; all contained inactivation of the same allele.

Dysplastic Barrett's Epithelium

The identification of dysplasia in Barrett's epithelium is based on the histologic examination of biopsy specimens. The cytologic and tissue architectural changes are similar to those described in ulcerative colitis. By convention, four broad categories are used:

1. No dysplasia
2. Indefinite for dysplasia
3. Low-grade dysplasia
4. High-grade dysplasia

Nondysplastic Barrett's epithelium contains cells with homogenous nuclei that lie close to the basement membrane; glandular architecture is normal. High-grade dysplasia is characterized by cells with enlarged and pleomorphic nuclei, a loss of nuclear polarity, and diminished or absent mucous production; glands are abnormally shaped (Fig. 19.18). Tissue samples in which epithelial cells similar to those of high-grade dysplasia invade beyond the basement membrane contain carcinoma.

The prevalence of dysplasia in patients presenting with Barrett's esophagus ranges from 15% to 25% if low-grade dysplasia is included and 5% to 10% if only high-grade dysplasia is considered. Few prospective studies have documented the progression of nondysplastic Barrett's epithelium to low- or high-grade dysplasia. Those available suggest that 5% to 10% of cases progress to dysplasia per year, and 1% to adenocarcinoma. Reid et al. (44) prospectively followed 62 patients with Barrett's esophagus (Table 19.2). Thirty-nine had no dysplasia on entry into the study. Low-grade dysplasia eventually developed in 10 of these patients, high-grade dysplasia in one, and invasive carcinoma in one. McCallum and colleagues (45) analyzed the longitudinal follow-up of patients with Barrett's esophagus in the registry of the American College of Gastroenterologists. All patients had nondysplastic quiescent Barrett's esophagus at initial endoscopy. One hundred nineteen patients received medical treatment, and 42 underwent antireflux surgery. Surveillance endoscopy was performed annually. Dysplasia developed in 10 patients in the medically treated group (19.7%) while they were on medical therapy, and in two following antireflux surgery (3.4%). A single adenocarcinoma was identified in a patient undergoing medical treatment. In a prospective, randomized study of Ortiz et al. (46), dysplasia developed in 6 of 27 (22%) patients while they were on medical treatment. The grade was low in five and high in one. Dysplasia developed in a single patient following antireflux surgery. Similar patterns have been documented in patients with short-segment Barrett's esophagus.

Management of Dysplastic Barrett's Esophagus

Once identified, Barrett's esophagus complicated by dysplasia should be treated aggressively (Table 19.3). Patients whose specimens are indefinite for dysplasia should be treated with an aggressive medical regimen, consisting of 60 to 80 mg of proton pump inhibitor therapy, for 3 months and then undergo a second biopsy. It is important that the esophagitis be healed with proton pump inhibitors before the presence or absence of dysplasia is determined. The presence of severe inflammation makes the microscopic interpretation of dysplasia difficult. The pur-

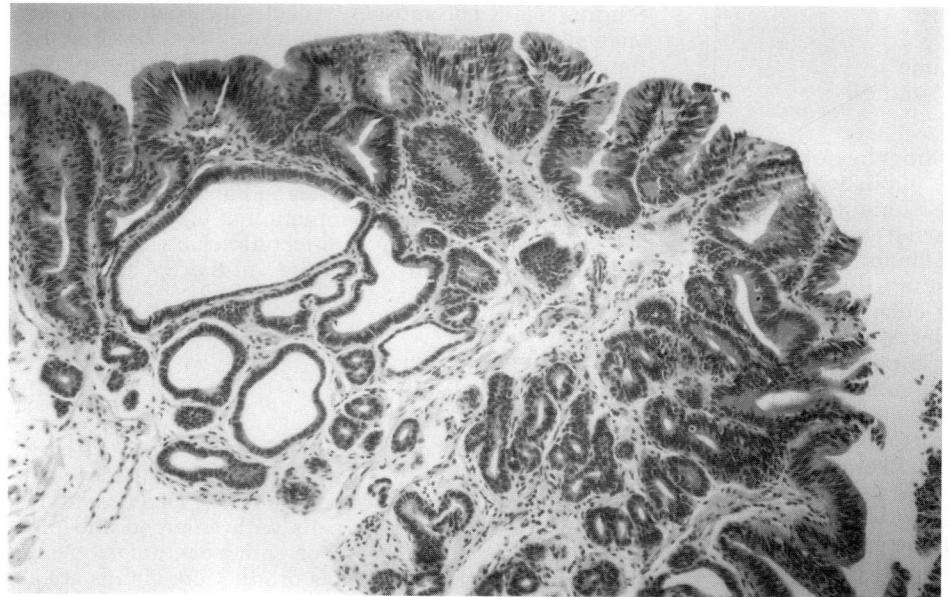

Figure 19.18. Histologic appearance of high-grade dysplasia. The cellular architecture and structure of the glands are becoming disorganized.

pose is to resolve inflammation that may complicate the interpretation of the biopsy specimen. If it remains indefinite, the patient should be treated as if low-grade dysplasia were present, with continued medical therapy or antireflux surgery and biopsy every 6 months. Patients with low-grade dysplasia are perhaps the most difficult group because of the potential difficulty in surveillance following antireflux surgery. Biopsies within the wrap may be difficult for the inexperienced to perform. Either aggressive medical treatment or antireflux surgery performed by an experienced endoscopist is appropriate.

High-grade dysplasia should be confirmed by two physicians knowledgeable in gastrointestinal pathology. Corroboration of dysplasia is important before any consideration of esophagectomy. Most would agree that it is the standard of care to proceed with esophagectomy in patients with high-grade dysplasia. On average, 45% to 50% of patients harbor invasive cancer when the specimen is removed. Thus, high-grade dysplasia is a marker for invasive carcinoma in nearly half of patients. This has been confirmed in our own studies from the University of Southern California, and also studies from the Mayo Clinic, Johns Hopkins, and many other centers around the world (47–49). This fact elevates the discussion to the

treatment of invasive adenocarcinoma, which is best carried out by esophagectomy. It is not possible with present technology, including endoscopic ultrasonography, to differentiate between patients who do and do not harbor a cancer. Furthermore, esophageal adenocarcinoma associated with high-grade dysplasia, identified with surveillance endoscopy, is highly curable (47). We and others have documented 5-year survival rates of 90% in this setting. The patient should not be denied the opportunity for cure of this highly lethal cancer. Finally, good evidence is available to suggest that high-grade dysplasia does not go away and so will almost always result in cancer given time. Although some studies suggest that low-grade dysplasia may occasionally reverse itself, the possibility of a sampling error makes this difficult to prove. As best we can tell, high-grade dysplasia, once acquired, is permanent and will almost certainly degenerate eventually into adenocarcinoma.

For these reasons, the patient is best treated by a total esophagectomy to remove all Barrett's tissue and any potential associated adenocarcinoma. Reconstruction is accomplished with either the stomach or colon; the anastomosis is located in the neck. The mortality associated with this procedure should be less than 5% and is minimal in centers experienced in esophageal surgery. Functional recovery is excellent. Nonsurgical treatments for Barrett's

Table 19.2. DEVELOPMENT OF DYSPLASIA: PROSPECTIVE EVALUATION OF 62 PATIENTS

| Initial Diagnosis | No. | Final diagnosis | | | |
		Metaplasia	Indeterminate/ LGD	HGD	CA
Metaplasia	39	27	10	1	1
I/LGD	20	4	8	3	2
HGD	3			1	2

I, indeterminate; LGD, low-grade dysplasia; HGD, high-grade dysplasia; CA, carcinoma.

From Reid BJ, Blount PL, Rubin CE, et al. Flow-cytometric and histological progression to malignancy in Barret's esophagus: prospective endoscopic surveillance of a cohort. Gastroenterology 1992;102: 1212–1219, with permission.

Table 19.3. MANAGEMENT OF BARRETT'S ESOPHAGUS WITH DYSPLASIA

INDEFINITE FOR DYSPLASIA
Aggressive antireflux therapy (60 mg PPI per day)
Repeated biopsy in 3 months

LOW-GRADE DYSPLASIA
Aggressive antireflux therapy
Medical vs. surgical treatment

HIGH-GRADE DYSPLASIA
Confirmation by two experienced pathologists
Esophagectomy (? extent)

PPI, proton pump inhibitor.

esophagus, including endoscopic ablative therapy, have been proposed. Most consider them to be investigational at the present stage of development and not standard care. Although these treatments should be investigated, few centers in the United States are capable of ablating Barrett's esophagus, the efficacy of the treatment has not been established, and clinical follow-up is not yet available to confirm efficacy. Barrett's esophagus is an increasing health concern in most Western countries. The diagnosis is usually made during the investigation of patients with symptoms of GERD. The appropriate antireflux procedure, performed in properly selected patients, will provide long-term symptomatic relief in 80% to 90% of cases. The effect of reliable and complete control of gastroesophageal reflux on the natural history of Barrett's metaplasia once it has developed, and on the prevention of Barrett's metaplasia in symptomatic patients in whom it has not yet developed, will be one of the most important areas of study during the next decade.

Gastroesophageal Reflux Disease and Respiratory Disorders

It is increasingly recognized that a significant proportion of patients with gastroesophageal reflux have associated respiratory symptoms (50). Population-based studies have reported a 10% to 15% prevalence of asthma in the community. Numerous studies have shown that up to 50% of asthmatic patients have either endoscopic evidence of esophagitis or increased esophageal acid exposure on 24-hour ambulatory pH monitoring (51). These facts suggest that the frequency of dual pathology is higher than would be expected by serendipity alone. Despite the ubiquitous nature of both diseases and the documented association between asthma and reflux disease, controversy remains regarding the ideal treatment. This reflects the relatively small number of reports, the paucity of controlled studies, and the conflicting findings of many studies.

Pathophysiology of Reflux-induced Respiratory Symptoms

Two mechanisms have been proposed in the pathogenesis of reflux-induced asthmatic symptoms. The first, the "reflux" theory, maintains that respiratory symptoms are the result of the aspiration of gastric contents. The second, or "reflex" theory, maintains that vagus-mediated bronchoconstriction follows acidification of the lower esophagus. The evidence supporting a reflux mechanism is fivefold. First, clinical studies have documented a strong correlation between idiopathic pulmonary fibrosis and hiatal hernia. Recently, complicated reflux disease was shown to be strongly associated with several pulmonary diseases, including asthma, in a recent Department of Veterans Affairs study (50). Second, pathologic acid exposure in the proximal esophagus is often identified in patients with respiratory symptoms and reflux disease. Third, scintigraphic studies have demonstrated aspiration of ingested radioactive isotope in some patients with reflux and respiratory symptoms. Fourth, simultaneous tracheal and esophageal pH monitoring in patients with reflux disease has documented tracheal acidification in concert with esophageal acidification. Finally, animal studies have shown that tracheal instillation of hydrochloric acid profoundly increases airways resistance.

A reflex mechanism is primarily supported by the fact that bronchoconstriction occurs following the infusion of acid into the lower esophagus. This can be explained by the common embryologic origin of the trachea and esophagus and their shared vagal innervation. Second, patients with respiratory symptoms and pathologic distal esopha-

geal acid exposure but normal proximal esophageal acid exposure may experience an improvement in their respiratory symptoms after antireflux therapy.

Diagnosis of Reflux-induced Respiratory Symptoms

The difficulty of this condition is establishing the diagnosis. In patients with predominantly reflux symptoms and secondary respiratory complaints, the diagnosis is straightforward. However, in a substantial number of patients with reflux-induced respiratory symptoms, the respiratory symptoms predominate in the clinical scenario. Gastroesophageal reflux in these patients is often silent and is uncovered only when an investigation is initiated. A high index of suspicion is required, notably in patients with poorly controlled asthma despite appropriate pulmonary medications. Supportive evidence for the diagnosis can be gleaned from endoscopy and stationary esophageal manometry. Endoscopy may show erosive esophagitis or Barrett's esophagus. Manometry may indicate a hypotensive lower esophageal sphincter or ineffective body motility, defined when 30% or more of contractions in the distal esophagus have an amplitude of less than 30 mm Hg.

The gold standard for the diagnosis of reflux-induced asthma is ambulatory dual-probe pH monitoring. One probe is positioned in the distal esophagus and the other at a more proximal location. Site for proximal probe placement include the trachea, pharynx, and proximal esophagus, both above and below the upper esophageal sphincter. Most would agree that the proximal esophagus is the preferred site for proximal probe location. Although ambulatory esophageal pH monitoring allows a direct correlation between esophageal acidification and respiratory symptoms, the chronologic relationship between reflux events and bronchoconstriction is complex.

Treatment of Respiratory Symptoms

Based on reported observations, relief of respiratory symptoms can be anticipated for 25% to 50% of patients with reflux-induced asthma treated with antisecretory medications (52–54). Fewer than 15%, however, can be expected to have an objective improvement in pulmonary function. The reason for this apparent paradox may be that most studies have employed relatively short courses of antisecretory therapy (< 3 months). This time period may have been sufficient for symptomatic improvement but insufficient for recovery of pulmonary function. The chances of success with medical treatment are likely directly related to the extent of reflux elimination. The conflicting findings of reports of antisecretory therapy may well be the consequence of inadequate control of gastroesophageal reflux in some studies.

The literature indicates that antireflux surgery relieves respiratory symptoms in nearly 90% of children and 70% of adults with asthma and reflux disease (55,56). Improvements in pulmonary function were demonstrated in about one third of patients. Comparisons of the results of uncontrolled studies of each form of therapy and the evidence from the two randomized, controlled trials of medical versus surgical therapy indicate that fundoplication is the most effective therapy for reflux-induced asthma (55,57). The superiority of the surgical antireflux barrier over medical therapy is probably most noticeable in a supine position, which corresponds with the period of acid breakthrough during proton pump inhibitor therapy and the time in the circadian cycle when asthma symptoms and peak expiratory flow rates are at their worst.

It is also important to realize that in an asthmatic patient with a non–reflux-induced motility abnormality of the esophageal body, an antireflux operation may result in aspiration of orally regurgitated swallowed liquid or food, which then causes respiratory symptoms and airway irritation that can elicit an asthmatic reaction. This may explain why surgical results appear to be better in children than in adults; disturbances of esophageal body motility are more common in adult patients.

Treatment of Gastroesophageal Reflux Disease

Medical Treatment

Gastroesophageal reflux disease is such a common condition that most patients with mild symptoms carry out self-medication. When first seen with symptoms of heartburn and no obvious complications, patients can reasonably be placed on 8 to 12 weeks of simple antacids before extensive investigations are carried out. In many situations, this treatment successfully aborts the attacks. Patients should be advised to elevate the head of their bed, avoid tight clothing, eat small and frequent meals, avoid eating shortly before retiring, lose weight, and avoid alcohol, coffee, chocolate, and peppermint, which may aggravate symptoms.

Alginic acid, in combination with simple antacids, may augment symptomatic relief by creating a physical barrier to reflux in addition to reducing acid. Alginic acid reacts with sodium bicarbonate in the presence of saliva to form a highly viscous solution that floats like a raft on the surface of the gastric contents. When reflux occurs, this protective layer is refluxed into the esophagus and acts as a protective barrier against the noxious gastric contents. Medications to promote gastric emptying, such as metoclopramide, domperidone, or cisapride, are beneficial in early disease but of little value in more severe disease.

The mainstay of medical therapy is acid suppression. Patients with persistent symptoms should be given hydrogen–potassium proton pump inhibitors, such as omeprazole. In daily doses as high as 40 mg, they can effect an 80% to 90% reduction in gastric acidity. This usually heals mild esophagitis, but healing may occur in only three fourths of patients with severe esophagitis. It is important to realize that in patients who reflux a combination of gastric and duodenal juice, inadequate acid suppression therapy may provide symptomatic improvement while still allowing mixed reflux to occur. This can result in an environment conducive to persistent mucosal damage in an asymptomatic patient. Unfortunately, within 6 months of discontinuation of any form of medical therapy for GERD, 80% of patients experience a recurrence of symptoms (58).

In patients with reflux disease, esophageal acid exposure is reduced by up to 80% with H_2 receptor antagonists and up to 95% with proton pump inhibitors. Despite the superiority of the latter class of drug over the former, emerging evidence suggests that periods of acid breakthrough still occur (59,60), most commonly at night, so that a split rather than a single dosing regimen is justified. Katzka et al. (59) studied 45 patients who had breakthrough reflux symptoms while taking 20 mg of omeprazole twice daily and found that 36 of them still had reflux, defined by a total distal esophageal acid exposure of more than 1.6%. Peghini et al. (60) employed intragastric pH monitoring in 28 healthy volunteers and 17 patients with reflux disease and observed nocturnal recovery of acid secretion (> 1 hour) in 75% of them. Recovery of acid secretion occurred within 12 hours of the oral evening dose of proton pump inhibitor, the median recovery time being 7.5 hours. This is particularly pertinent because it is during the night and early morning that asthma symptoms are most pronounced and that peak expiratory flow rate is lowest. In their latest study, Peghini et al. showed that 300 mg of ranitidine at bedtime is superior to 20 mg of omeprazole at bedtime in preventing acid breakthrough, and they speculate that this is because of the abolition of histamine-mediated acid secretion in the fasting state.

Patients presenting for the first time with symptoms suggestive of gastroesophageal reflux may be given initial therapy with H_2 blockers. In view of the availability of these as over-the-counter medication, many patients will have already self-medicated their symptoms. Failure of H_2 blockers to control the symptoms, or immediate return of symptoms after cessation of treatment, suggests either that the diagnosis is incorrect or that the patient has relatively severe disease. Endoscopic examination at this stage of the evaluation provides the opportunity for assessing the severity of mucosal damage and determining whether Barrett's esophagus is present. Both of these findings on initial endoscopy predict a high risk for medical failure. A measurement of the degree and pattern of esophageal exposure to gastric and duodenal juice, via 24 hour pH and bilirubin monitoring, should be obtained at this point. The status of the lower esophageal sphincter and the function of the esophageal body should also be measured. These studies identify features that predict a poor response to medical therapy, frequent relapses, and the development of complications: reflux occurring in the supine position, poor esophageal contractility, the presence of erosive esophagitis or a columnar cell-lined esophagus at initial presentation, the presence of bile in refluxed matter, and a structurally defective sphincter. Patients with these risk factors should be offered the option of surgery as a primary therapy with the expectation of long-term control of symptoms and complications.

Antireflux Surgery

Indications. Antireflux surgery is indicated for the treatment of objectively documented, relatively severe GERD. Candidates for surgery include not only patients with erosive esophagitis, stricture, and Barrett's esophagus, but also those without severe mucosal injury who are dependent on proton pump inhibitors for symptom relief. Patients with atypical or respiratory symptoms who have a good response to intensive medical treatment are also candidates. The option of antireflux surgery should be offered to all patients who have demonstrated a need for long-term medical therapy, particularly if escalating doses of proton pump inhibitors are needed to control symptoms. Antireflux surgery may be the preferred option in patients younger than 50 years of age, those who are noncompliant with their drug regimen, patients for whom medications are a financial burden, and those who favor a single intervention over long-term drug treatment (Fig. 19.19). It may be the treatment of choice for patients who are at high risk for progression despite medical therapy. Although this population is not well defined, risk factors that predict progressive disease and a poor response to medical therapy include (a) nocturnal reflux on 24-hour esophageal pH study, (b) a structurally deficient lower esophageal sphincter, (c) mixed reflux of gastric and duodenal juice, and (d) mucosal injury at presentation (61).

Preoperative Evaluation. Successful antireflux surgery is largely defined by two objectives: the achievement of long-term relief of reflux symptoms and the absence of complications or complaints after the operation. In practice, attaining these two deceptively simple goals is difficult. Both are critically dependent on establishing that the symptoms for which the operation is being undertaken are

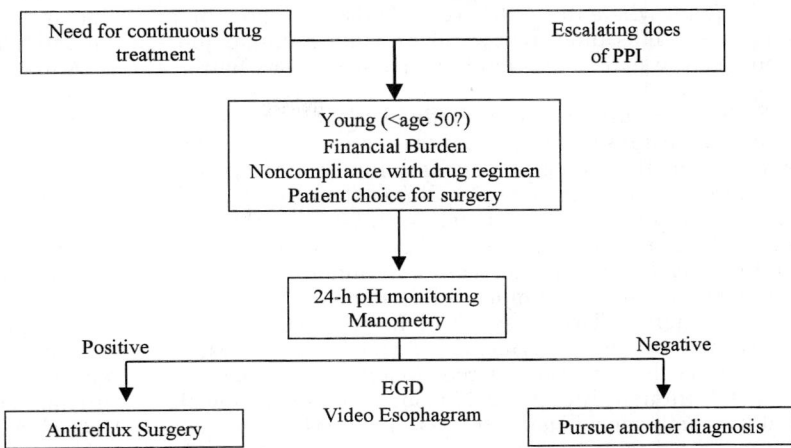

Figure 19.19. Indications for laparoscopic fundoplication.

caused by excess esophageal exposure to gastric juice and on performing the appropriate antireflux procedure correctly. Success can be expected in the vast majority of patients if these two criteria are met. The status of the lower esophageal sphincter is not as important a factor as in the days of open surgery. Patients with normal resting sphincters are often selected for antireflux surgery in the era of laparoscopic fundoplication. The outcome does not depend on sphincter function.

The important goals of the diagnostic approach to patients suspected of having GERD and being considered for antireflux surgery are fourfold:

1. Establishing that GERD is the underlying cause of the patient's symptoms
2. Estimating the risk for progressive disease
3. Determining the presence or absence of esophageal shortening
4. Evaluating esophageal body function, and occasionally gastric emptying function

Objective Documentation. The introduction of laparoscopic access, coupled with the growing recognition that surgery is a safe and durable treatment for GERD, has dramatically increased the number of patients being referred for laparoscopic fundoplication. The threshold for surgical referral is such that increasing numbers of patients without endoscopic esophagitis or other objective evidence of reflux are now considered candidates for laparoscopic antireflux surgery. These facts combine to underscore the importance of selecting patients for surgery who are likely to have a successful outcome. Although a Nissen fundoplication will reliably halt the return of gastroduodenal juice into the esophagus, little benefit is likely if the patient's symptoms are not caused by this specific pathophysiologic derangement. Thus, in large part, the anticipated success rate of laparoscopic fundoplication is directly proportional to the degree of certainty that GERD reflux is the underlying cause of the patient's complaints.

Three factors predictive of a successful outcome following antireflux surgery have emerged (62) (Table 19.4). These are (a) an abnormal score on 24-hour esophageal pH monitoring; (b) the presence of typical symptoms of GERD—namely, heartburn or regurgitation; and (c) symptomatic improvement in response to acid suppression therapy before surgery. It is immediately evident that each of these factors helps to establish that GERD is indeed the cause of the patient's symptoms and that they have little to do with the severity of disease.

ENDOSCOPIC EVALUATION. Endoscopic visualization of the esophagus corresponds to the physical examination of the foregut and is a critical part of the preoperative evaluation of patients with GERD. Its main aim is to detect complications of gastroesophageal reflux, the presence of which often influences therapeutic decisions.

In every patient, the locations of the diaphragmatic crura, gastroesophageal junction, and squamocolumnar junction are determined. These anatomic landmarks are commonly at three different sites in patients with GERD. The crura are usually evident, and their location can be

Table 19.4. PREDICTORS OF OUTCOME AFTER LAPAROSCOPIC FUNDOPLICATION: STEPWISE LOGISTIC REGRESSION RESULTS OF 199 PATIENTS

Predictor	Status	Adjusted odds ratio (95% Confidence intervals)	Wald's p value
Composite acid score	Increased	5.4 (1.9–15.3)	<.001
	Normal	—	—
Symptom	Typical	5.1 (1.9–13.7)	<.001
	Atypical	—	—
Response to medical therapy	Complete/partial	3.3 (1.3–8.7)	.02
	Minor/none	—	—

Odds ratios and corresponding p values are adjusted for age and for all other factors in the model.
From Campos GMR, Peters JH, DeMeester TR, et al. Multivariate analysis of the factors predicting outcome after laparoscopic Nissen fundoplication. J Gastrointest Surg 1999;3:292–300, with permission.

confirmed by having the patient sniff during the examination. The anatomic gastroesophageal junction is identified as the point where the gastric rugal folds meet the tubular esophagus; it is often below the squamocolumnar junction, even in patients without otherwise obvious Barrett's esophagus.

Endoscopic esophagitis is defined by the presence of mucosal erosions (Table 19.5). If these are noted, the grade and length of esophageal mucosal injury are recorded. The presence of columnar epithelium extending above the anatomic gastroesophageal junction and its length are also noted. Its presence is suspected at endoscopy if it is difficult to visualize the squamocolumnar junction at its normal location and if the mucosa has a velvety red, luxuriant appearance. The presence of Barrett's esophagus is confirmed by biopsy evidence of specialized intestinal metaplasia and is considered histologic evidence of GERD. Columnar lining that is visualized endoscopically but in which specialized intestinal metaplasia is not confirmed histologically is not considered Barrett's esophagus and likely has no premalignant potential. Multiple biopsy specimens should be taken by the endoscopist, starting distally and working cephalad, to determine the location of the junction of Barrett's epithelium and normal squamous mucosa. Barrett's esophagus is susceptible to ulceration, bleeding, stricture formation, and malignant degeneration. Dysplasia is the earliest sign of malignant change. Because dysplastic changes typically occur in a random distribution within the distal esophagus, a minimum of four biopsy specimens (one from each quadrant) should be obtained from the metaplastic epithelium at 2-cm intervals. Particular attention must be paid to the squamocolumnar junction in these patients, in whom a mass, ulcer, nodularity, or inflammatory tissue is always considered suggestive of malignancy and requires thorough investigation. The gastroesophageal junction is defined endoscopically as the place where the tubular esophagus meets the gastric rugal folds, and the squamocolumnar junction is the place where an obvious change is seen from the velvety and darker columnar epithelium to the lighter squamous epithelium.

After completion of the esophageal examination, the first and second portions of the duodenum and the stomach are systematically inspected. This is commonly done during withdrawal of the endoscope. When the antrum is visualized, the incisura angularis appears as a constant ridge on the lesser curve. Turning the lens of the scope 180 degrees allows inspection of the fundus and cardia. Attention is paid to the frenulum (angle of His) of the esophagogastric junction, and to how closely the cardia grips the scope. Hill and colleagues (63) have graded the appearance of this valve on a scale of I to IV according to the degree of unfolding or deterioration of the normal valve architecture. This grading system has been correlated with increased esophageal acid exposure, seen predominantly in patients with grade III or IV valves.

A hiatal hernia is endoscopically confirmed by finding a pouch lined with gastric rugal folds lying 2 cm or more above the margins of the diaphragmatic crura. A prominent sliding hernia is frequently associated with increased esophageal exposure to gastric juice. When a paraesophageal hernia exists, particular attention is taken to exclude a gastric ulcer or gastritis within the pouch. The intragastric retroflex or "J" maneuver is important in evaluating the full circumference of the mucosal lining of the herniated stomach. As the endoscope is removed, the esophagus is again examined and samples taken. The location of the cricopharyngeus is identified, and the larynx and vocal cords are visualized. Acid reflux may result in inflammation of the larynx. Vocal cord movement is recorded, both as a reference for subsequent surgery and an assessment of the patient's ability to protect the airway.

TWENTY-FOUR-HOUR AMBULATORY pH MONITORING. The most direct method of assessing the relationship between symptoms and GERD is to measure the esophageal exposure to gastric juice with an indwelling pH electrode. Miller (64) first reported prolonged esophageal pH monitoring in 1964, although it was not until 1973 that its clinical applicability and advantages were demonstrated by Johnson and DeMeester (65). It is considered by many to be the gold standard for the diagnosis of GERD because it has the highest sensitivity and specificity of all tests currently available. Some have suggested that 24-hour pH monitoring be used selectively, limited to patients with atypical symptoms or no endoscopic evidence of gastroesophageal reflux. Given present day referral patterns, more than half of patients referred for antireflux surgery have no endoscopic evidence of mucosal injury. For these patients, 24-hour pH monitoring provides the only objective measure of the presence of pathologic esophageal acid exposure. Although it is true that most patients with typical symptoms and erosive esophagitis will have positive results on 24-hour pH monitoring, the study provides other useful information. It quantifies the actual time that esophageal mucosa is exposed to gastric juice, measures the ability of the esophagus to clear refluxed acid, and correlates esophageal acid exposure with symptoms. It is the only way to express quantitatively the overall degree and pattern of esophageal acid exposure, which may affect the decision to perform surgery (66). Patients with nocturnal or bipositional reflux have a higher rate of complications and failure of long-term medical control (61). For these reasons, we continue to advocate the routine use of 24-hour pH monitoring in clinical practice.

The units used to express esophageal exposure to gastric juice are (a) cumulative time the esophageal pH is below a chosen threshold, expressed as a percentage of total, upright, and supine monitored time; (b) frequency of reflux episodes below a chosen threshold, expressed as number of episodes per 24 hours; and (c) duration of the episodes, expressed as the number of episodes longer than 5 minutes per 24 hours and the time in minutes of the longest episode recorded. Table 19.6 shows the normal values for these components of the 24-hour record at the whole-number pH threshold derived from 50 normal asymptomatic subjects. The upper limits of normal were established at the 95th percentile. Most centers use a pH of 4 as the threshold. To combining the six components into one expression reflecting the overall esophageal acid exposure below a pH threshold, a pH score was calculated by using the standard deviation of the mean of each of the six components measured.

Table 19.5. GRADES OF ESOPHAGITIS: "NEW" SAVARY-MILLER, 1990

Grade I	Single erosion, oval or linear
Grade II	Multiple linear erosions on more than one longitudinal fold
Grade III	Circumferential erosive lesions
Grade IV	Ulcer, stricture, or short esophagus with or without grade I–III
Grade V	Columnar cell-lined esophagus with or without I–IV

Modified from Ollyo JB, Lang F, Fontolliet Ch, et al. Savary-Miller's new endoscopic grading of reflux-oesophagitis: a simple, reproducible, logical, complete, and useful classification. Gastroenterology 1990; 89:A100, with permission.

Table 19.6. NORMAL VALUES FOR ESOPHAGEAL EXPOSURE TO PH < 4 IN 50 SUBJECTS

Component	Mean	Standard deviation	95th percentile
Total time pH < 4	1.51	1.36	4.45
Upright time pH < 4	2.34	2.34	8.42
Supine time pH < 4	0.63	1.0	3.45
No. episodes	19.00	12.76	46.9
No. > 5 min	0.84	1.18	3.45
Longest episode	6.74	7.85	19.8

From Johnson LF, DeMeester TR. Development of the 24-hour intrae-sophageal pH monitoring composite scoring system. J Clin Gastroenterol 1986;8[Suppl 1]:52-58, with permission.

Assessment of Esophageal Length. Esophageal shortening is a consequence of the scarring and fibrosis associated with repetitive esophageal injury. Anatomic shortening of the esophagus can compromise the surgeon's ability to perform an adequate, tension-free repair and may result in an increased incidence of breakdown or thoracic displacement of the repair. Esophageal length is best assessed by means of video roentgenographic contrast studies and endoscopic findings. Endoscopically, hernia size is measured as the difference between the diaphragmatic crura, identified by having the patient sniff, and the gastroesophageal junction, identified as the loss of gastric rugal folds. We consider the possibility of a short esophagus in patients with strictures or with large hiatal hernias (> 5 cm), particularly when the latter fail to reduce in the upright position on a video barium esophagram (67). These patients are best approached transthoracically and their esophageal length appraised after mobilization from the diaphragmatic hiatus up to the aortic arch. With the gastroesophageal junction marked by a suture, esophageal shortening is defined by an inability to position the repair beneath the diaphragm without tension. In this situation, a Collis gastroplasty coupled with either a partial or complete fundoplication will achieve excellent control of reflux in the majority of patients (68). In our experience, the failure to appreciate esophageal shortening is a major cause of fundoplication failure and is the explanation for the "slipped" Nissen fundoplication. In many such instances, the initial repair is incorrectly constructed around the proximal tubularized stomach rather than the terminal esophagus.

RADIOGRAPHIC EVALUATION. Radiographic assessment of the anatomy and function of the esophagus and stomach is one of the most important parts of the preoperative evaluation. Critical issues are assessed, including the presence of esophageal shortening (Fig. 19.20), the size and reducibility of a hiatal hernia, and the propulsive function of the esophagus with both liquids and solids.

The definition of radiographic gastroesophageal reflux varies depending on whether reflux is spontaneous or induced by various maneuvers. In only about 40% of patients with classic symptoms of GERD is spontaneous reflux observed by the radiologist (i.e., reflux of barium from the stomach into the esophagus with the patient in the upright position). In most patients who show spontaneous reflux on radiography, the diagnosis of increased esophageal acid exposure is confirmed by 24-hour esophageal pH monitoring. Therefore, the radiographic demonstration of spontaneous regurgitation of barium into the esophagus in the upright position is a reliable indicator that reflux is present. Failure to see this does not indicate the absence of disease.

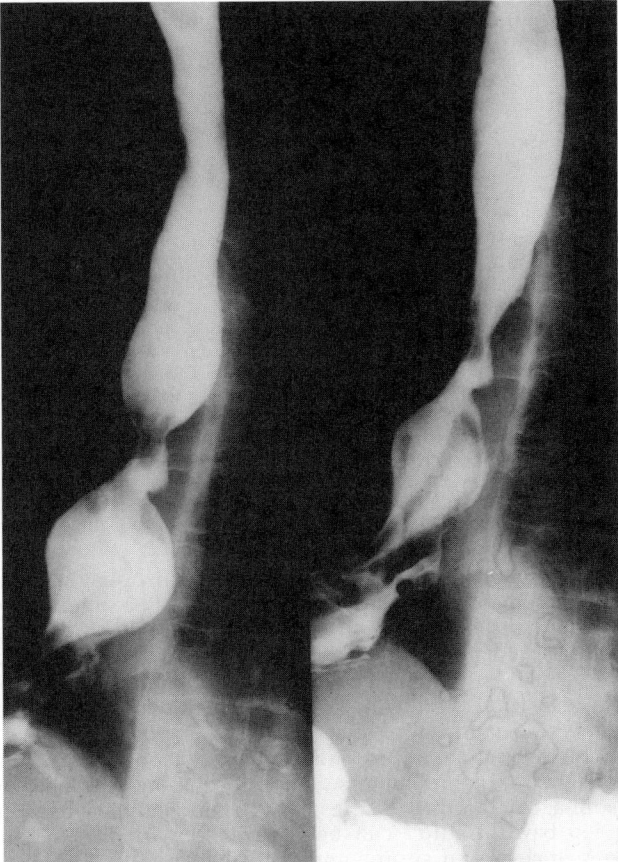

Figure 19.20. Barium-filled esophagogastric segment in a patient with a short esophagus. Note that the gastroesophageal junction is well above the hiatus.

A carefully performed video esophagram can provide an enormous amount of information about the structure and function of the esophagus and stomach. The modern barium swallow emphasizes motion recording (video), utilizes a tightly controlled examination protocol (Table 19.7), and requires an understanding of esophageal physiology.

Video taping the study greatly aids the evaluation, providing the surgeon with a real-time assessment of swallowing function, bolus transport, and the size and reducibility of hiatal hernias. Given routine review before antireflux surgery, its value becomes increasingly clear. The study provides structural information, including the presence of obstructing lesions and anatomic abnormalities of the foregut. A hiatal hernia is present in more than 80% of patients with gastroesophageal reflux. They are best demonstrated with the patient in the prone position, which causes an increase in abdominal pressure and promotes distention of the hernia above the diaphragm. The presence of a hiatal hernia is an important component of the underlying pathophysiology of gastroesophageal reflux. Other relevant findings include a large (> 5 cm) or irreducible hernia, which suggests the presence of a shortened esophagus; a tight crural "collar" inhibiting barium transit into the stomach, which suggests a possible cause of dysphagia; and a paraesophageal hernia.

Lower esophageal narrowing caused by a ring, stricture, or obstructing lesion is optimally viewed with full distention of the esophagogastric region. A full-column technique with distention of the esophageal wall can be used

Table 19.7. UNIVERSITY OF SOUTHERN CALIFORNIA PROTOCOL FOR VIDEO ESOPHAGRAM STUDIES

Patient Position	Purpose	Technique
Prone RAO	Esophageal body function	Five separate 10-mL swallows, 15 s between each, follow bolus on videotape
		Video swallow over thoracic inlet and another over distal third of esophagus without panning
	Esophageal diameter	Rapid swallow of several gulps to distend esophagus maximally
	Gastric function	Video record activity of stomach and duodenum for 30 s in prone position
Supine	Relationship of GE junction to hiatus	Two or three individual swallows focused on distal esophagus and GE junction
Erect	Cricopharyngeal function	Lateral and anteroposterior views of oropharynx and upper esophagus
	Mucosal injury	Spot of collapsed esophagus for mucosal detail
	Reducibility of hernia	Video images of one or two swallows focused on distal esophagus and GE junction
		Gas distention of distal esophagus
Erect	Solid bolus transport	Record video images of passage of two contrast-coated hamburger boluses from oropharynx to stomach

GE, gastroesophageal; RAO, right anterior oblique.

to discern extrinsic compression of the esophagus. Mucosal relief or double-contrast films should be obtained to enhance the detection of small esophageal neoplasms, mild esophagitis, and esophageal varices. The pharynx and upper esophageal sphincter are evaluated in the upright position, and an assessment of the relative timing and coordination of pharyngeal transit is possible.

The assessment of peristalsis on video esophagram often adds to, or complements, the information obtained by esophageal motility studies. This is in part because the video barium study can be performed with the patient both upright and supine and with liquid and solid bolus material, which is not true of a stationary motility examination. This is particularly valuable with subtle motility abnormalities. During normal swallowing, a stripping wave (primary peristalsis) is generated that completely clears the bolus. Residual material can stimulate a secondary peristaltic wave, but usually a second pharyngeal swallow is required. Motility disorders with disorganized or simultaneous esophageal contraction are associated with "tertiary waves" and give a segmented appearance to the barium column; this is often referred to as *beading* or *corkscrew*. In patients with dysphagia, barium-impregnated marshmallow, bread, or hamburger is a useful adjunct that can reveal a functional esophageal transport disturbance not evident on the liquid barium study. Reflux is not easily seen on video esophagram, and motility disorders that cause retrograde barium transport may be mistaken for reflux.

Assessment of the stomach and duodenum during the barium study is necessary for proper a preoperative evaluation of the patient with GERD. Evidence of gastric or duodenal ulcer, neoplasm, or poor gastroduodenal transit is obviously important in the preoperative evaluation.

Assessment of Esophageal Body and Gastric Function. The presence of poor esophageal body function, in addition to the likelihood of relieving regurgitation, dysphagia, and respiratory symptoms after surgery, may influence the decision to perform a partial rather than a complete fundoplication. When peristalsis is absent or severely disordered (> 50% simultaneous contractions), or when the amplitude of the contractions in one or more of the lower esophageal segments is below 20 mm Hg, many would opt for a partial fundoplication. The less favorable response after fundoplication of atypical than of typical reflux symptoms may be related to the persistence of poor esophageal propulsive function and the continued regurgitation of esophageal contents (69,70).

The function of the esophageal body is assessed with esophageal manometry. This is performed with five pressure transducers located in the esophagus (Fig. 19.21). To standardize the procedure, the most proximal pressure transducer is placed 1 cm below the well-defined cricopharyngeal sphincter. With this method, a pressure response along the entire esophagus can be obtained during one swallow. The study consists of recording 10 standard wet swallows with 5 mL of water. The amplitude, duration, and morphology of the contractions following each swallow are all calculated at the five discrete levels within the esophageal body (Fig. 19.22). The delay between the onset or peak of esophageal contractions at the various levels of the esophagus is used to calculate the speed of

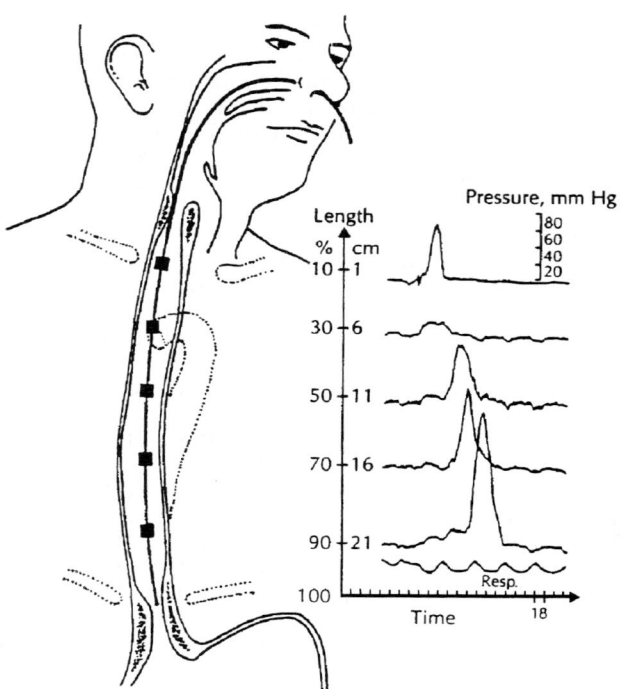

Figure 19.21. Illustration of the position of a five-channel esophageal motility catheter during the esophageal body portion of the study.

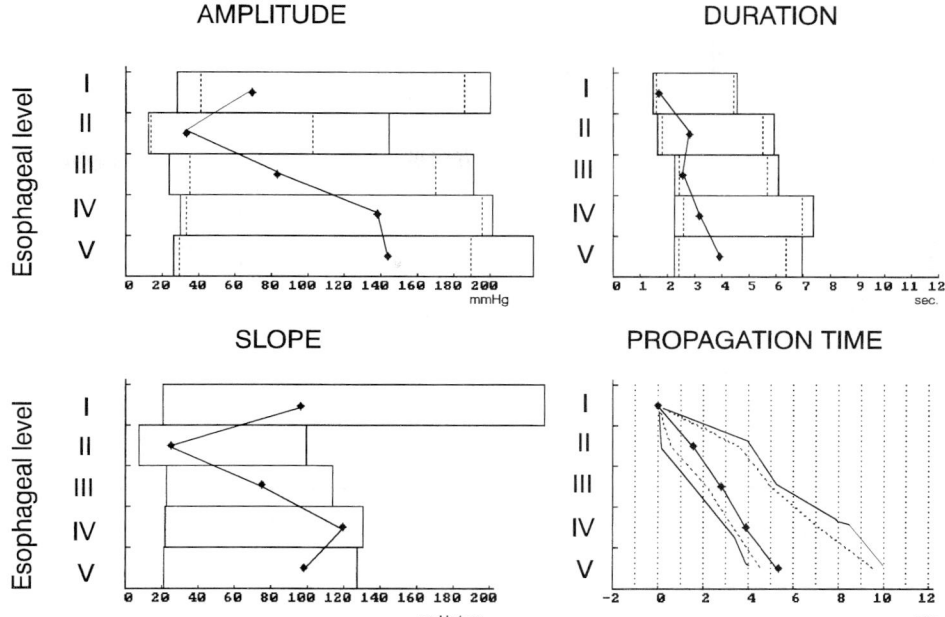

Figure 19.22. Computer-generated graphic representation of esophageal body contraction amplitudes, duration of contractions, and wave progression.

wave propagation and represents the degree of peristaltic activity.

Esophageal disorders are frequently associated with abnormalities of gastroduodenal function. Symptoms suggestive of gastroduodenal disease include nausea, epigastric pain, anorexia, and early satiety. Abnormalities of gastric motility or an increase in gastric acid secretion can be responsible for an increased esophageal exposure to gastric juice. If they are not identified before surgery, an antireflux procedure will occasionally "unmask" unrecognized gastric motility abnormalities and result in disabling postoperative symptoms (71). Considerable experience and judgment are necessary to identify the patient with occult gastroduodenal dysfunction. The surgeon should maintain a keen awareness of this possibility and investigate the stomach given any suggestion of problems. Tests of gastroduodenal function that are helpful when investigating the patient with gastroesophageal reflux include gastric emptying studies, gastric acid analysis, 24-hour gastric pH monitoring, and ambulatory bilirubin monitoring of the esophagus and stomach.

Poor gastric emptying or transit can cause reflux of gastric contents into the distal esophagus. Standard gastric emptying studies are performed with radionuclide-labeled meals. They are often poorly standardized and difficult to interpret. Emptying of solids and liquids can be assessed simultaneously when both phases are marked with different tracers. After the patient has ingested a labeled standard meal, gamma camera images of the stomach are obtained at 5- to 15-minute intervals for 1.5 to 2 hours. After correction for decay, the counts in the gastric area are plotted as a percentage of the total counts at the start of imaging. The resulting emptying curve can be compared with data obtained from normal volunteers. In general, normal subjects empty 59% of a meal within 90 minutes.

Partial versus Complete Fundoplication. The decision between partial and complete fundoplication and an open or laparoscopic approach requires considerable judgment. Two randomized studies of unselected patients undergoing laparoscopic fundoplication have shown an equivalence of complete and partial fundoplications, anterior in one study (72) and posterior in the other (73), in terms of operative time, perioperative morbidity, and hospital stay. Watson et al. (72) noted that resting and residual lower esophageal sphincter pressures were greater after complete fundoplication, and that esophageal clearance of liquid radioisotope was prolonged after complete fundoplication in comparison with partial fundoplication. Six months after operation, partial fundoplication was linked to a greater overall level of patient satisfaction, manifested by fewer episodes of dysphagia, inability to belch, and excessive flatus. Laws et al. (73) did not identify any difference in symptomatic outcome between patients treated by complete and those treated by posterior partial fundoplication at a mean follow-up time of 27 months.

These observations, however, must be weighed against recent reports questioning the durability of partial fundoplications. Jobe et al. (74) found that 51% of patients studied by 24-hour esophageal pH monitoring after Toupet fundoplication still had pathologic acid exposure. Disturbingly, only 40% of the patients with reflux were symptomatic. Two studies have identified defective lower esophageal sphincter function, an aperistaltic distal esophagus, and higher grades of esophagitis (Savary-Miller grades II through IV) as risk factors for partial fundoplication failure (75,76). Bell and Hanna (75) reported recurrent reflux in 14% of patients after Toupet fundoplication. Mild esophagitis and a normal lower esophageal sphincter were associated with a 3-year success rate of 96%, whereas complicated esophagitis and a defective lower esophageal sphincter lowered this value to 50% (Fig. 19.23).

These findings highlight an apparent paradox, in that partial fundoplication affords suboptimal reflux protection in those most at risk for the effects of unabated GERD. Moreover, current dogma holds that a partial fundoplication is the procedure of choice in patients with poor esophageal body motility. This recent evidence in addition to our own experience has led us to utilize the complete fundoplication more readily, particularly in patients with Barrett's esophagus. At the current time, partial fundoplication remains the procedure of choice for patients with named esophageal motility disorders, such as scleroderma or achalasia.

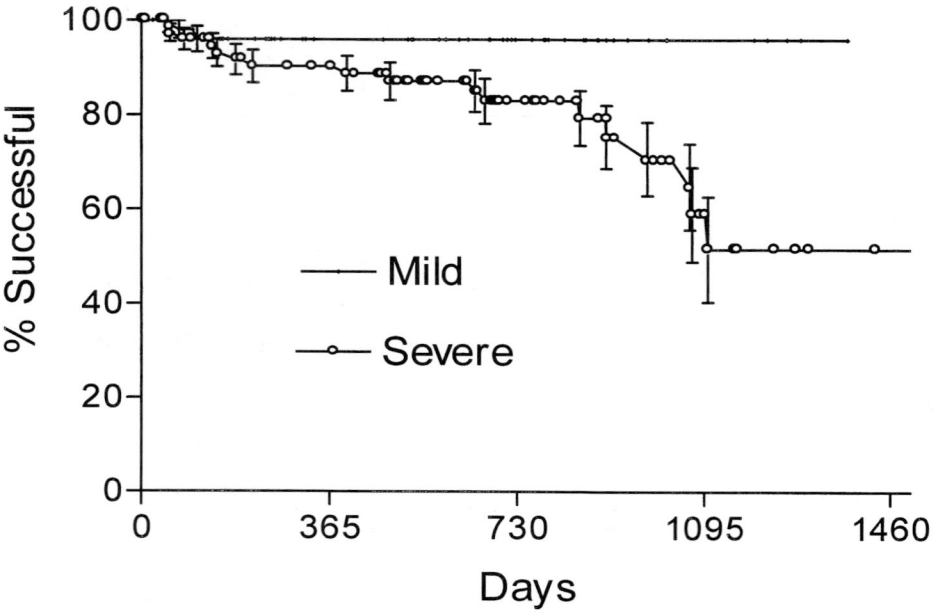

Figure 19.23. Kaplan-Meier plot indicating fundoplication success rates with time. Patients with normal lower esophageal sphincter characteristics or mild esophagitis had an actuarial success rate of 96% at 3 years, whereas those with defective lower esophageal sphincter function or complicated esophagitis had only a 50% success rate. (From Bell RC, Hanna P, Mill MR, et al. Patterns of success and failure with laparoscopic Toupet fundoplication. *Surg Endosc* 1999;13: 1189–1194, with permission.)

Laparoscopic Nissen Fundoplication. Laparoscopic fundoplication should include the following:

1. Crural dissection and identification and preservation of both vagi, including the hepatic branch of the anterior vagus
2. Circumferential dissection of the esophagus
3. Crural closure
4. Fundic mobilization by division of the short gastric vessels
5. Creation of a short, loose fundoplication by enveloping the lower esophagus with the anterior and posterior walls of the fundus

Five 10-mm ports are utilized (Fig. 19.24). The camera is placed above the umbilicus, one third of the distance to the xiphoid process. In most patients, placement of the camera in the umbilicus does not allow adequate visualization of the hiatal strictures once dissected. Two lateral retracting ports are placed in the right and left anterior axillary lines, respectively. The right-sided liver retractor is best placed in the right midabdomen (midclavicular line), at or slightly below the camera port. This creates the proper angle toward the left lateral segment of the liver, so that the instrument can be pushed toward the operating table to lift the liver. A second retraction port is placed at the level of the umbilicus, in the left anterior axillary line. The surgeon's right- and left-handed trocars are placed in the right and left midclavicular lines, 2 to 3 inches below the costal margin. When the operating trocars are placed on either side of the midline, the camera and the two instruments are arranged in a triangle, so that the difficulty associated with instruments being placed in a direct line with the camera is avoided. The falciform ligament hangs low in many patients and provides a barrier around which the left-handed instrument must be manipulated.

Initial retraction is accomplished with exposure of the esophageal hiatus. A fan retractor is placed into the right anterior axillary port and positioned to hold the left lateral segment of the liver toward the anterior abdominal wall. We prefer to utilize a table retractor to hold this instrument once it is properly positioned. Trauma to the liver should be meticulously avoided because subsequent bleeding will obscure the field. Mobilization of the left lateral segment by division of the triangular ligament is not necessary. A Babcock clamp is placed into the left anterior axillary port and the stomach retracted toward the patient's left foot. This maneuver exposes the esophageal hiatus. Commonly, a hiatal hernia will have to be reduced. An atraumatic clamp should be used, and care taken not to grasp the stomach too vigorously, as gastric perforations can occur.

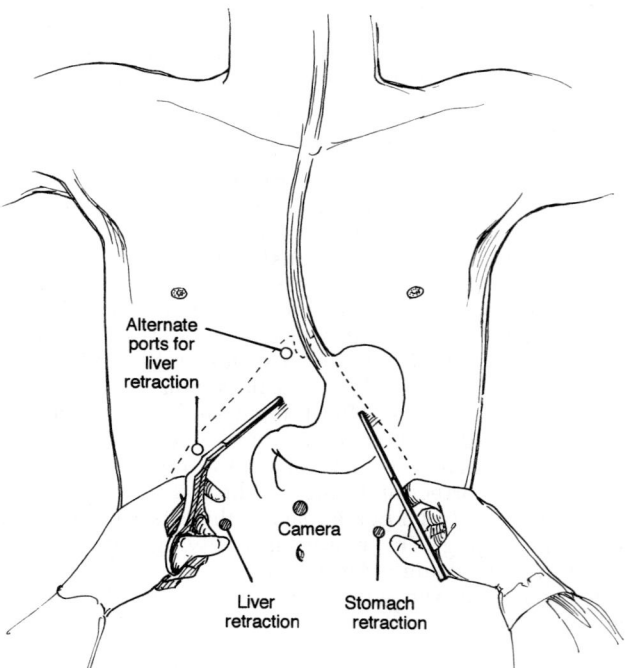

Figure 19.24. Patient positioning and trocar placement for laparoscopic antireflux surgery. The patient is placed with the head elevated 45 degrees in the modified lithotomy position. The surgeon stands between the patient's legs, and the procedure is completed via five abdominal access ports.

Hiatal Dissection. The key to the hiatal dissection is identification of the right crus. Metzenbaum-type scissors and fine grasping forceps are preferred for dissection. In all except the most obese patients, a very thin portion of the gastrohepatic omentum overlies the caudate lobe of the liver. Dissection is begun by incising the portion of the gastrohepatic omentum above and below the hepatic branch of the anterior vagus nerve, which we routinely spare. A large left hepatic artery arising from the left gastric artery is present in up to 25% of patients. It should be identified and avoided. After the gastrohepatic omentum is incised, the lateral surface of the right crus becomes evident (Fig. 19.25). The peritoneum overlying the anterior aspect of the right crus is incised with scissors and electrocautery, and the right crus is dissected as much as possible from anterior to posterior. The medial surface of the right crus leads into the mediastinum and is entered by blunt dissection with both instruments. At this juncture, the esophagus usually becomes evident. The right crus is retracted laterally, and the tissues posterior to the esophagus are dissected. No attempt is made at this point to dissect behind the gastroesophageal junction. Meticulous hemostasis is critical. Blood and fluid tend to pool in the hiatus and are difficult to remove. Irrigation should be kept to a minimum. Care must be taken not to injure the phrenic artery and vein as they course above the hiatus. A large hiatal hernia often makes this portion of the procedure easier, as it accentuates the diaphragmatic crura. On the other hand, dissection of a large mediastinal hernia sac can be difficult.

Following dissection of the right crus, attention is turned to the anterior crural confluence. The tissues anterior to the esophagus are held upward with the left-handed grasper, and the esophagus is swept downward and to the right to separate it from the left crus (Fig. 19.26). The anterior crural tissues are then divided and the left crus identified. The left crus is dissected as completely as

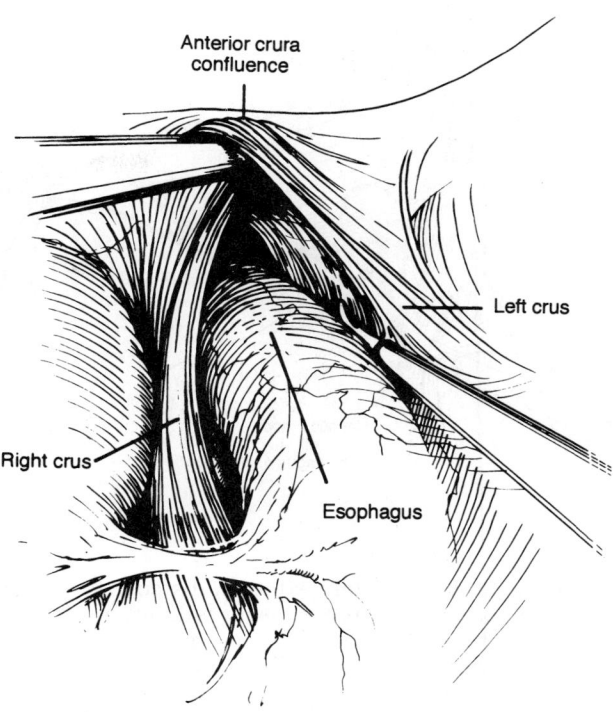

Figure 19.26. Artist's depiction of division of the anterior crural fibers and mobilization of the esophagus off the left crus.

possible; dissection includes taking down the angle of His and the attachments of the fundus to the left diaphragm. A complete dissection of the lateral and inferior aspect of the left crus and fundus of the stomach is the key maneuver allowing circumferential mobilization of the esophagus (Fig. 19.27). Failure to do so will make it difficult to encircle the esophagus, particularly if it is approached from the right. Repositioning of the Babcock retractor toward the fundic side of the stomach facilitates retraction for this portion of the procedure.

The esophagus is mobilized by careful dissection of the anterior and posterior soft tissues within the hiatus. If the

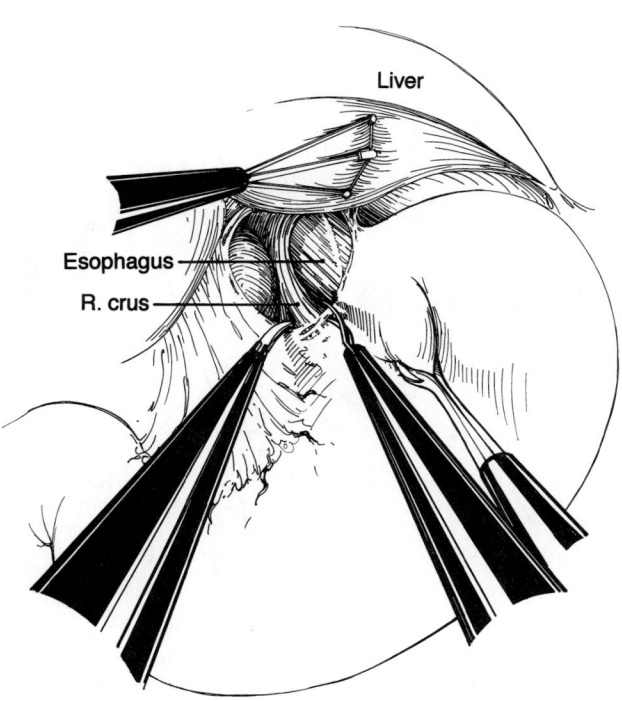

Figure 19.25. Illustration of the initial dissection of the esophageal hiatus. The right crus is identified and dissected toward its posterior confluence with the left crus.

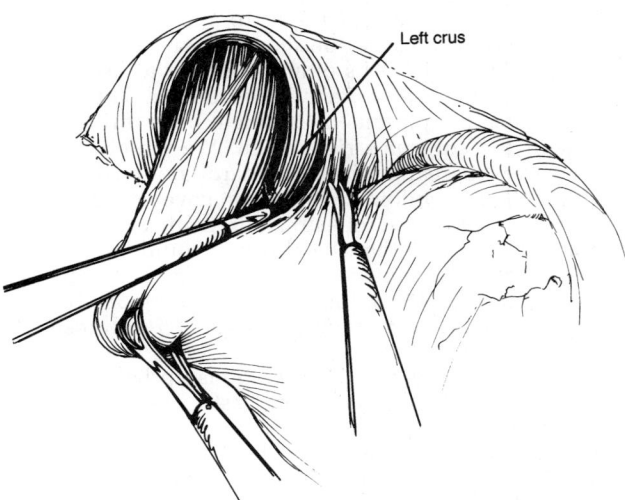

Figure 19.27. Left-sided crural dissection. The left crus is dissected as completely as possible, and the attachments of the fundus of the stomach to the diaphragm are taken down.

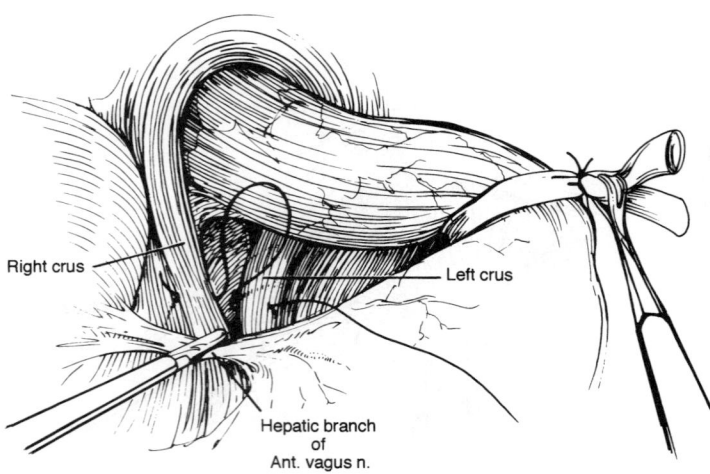

Figure 19.28. Three to six interrupted 0 silk sutures are used to close the crura. Exposure of the crura and posterior aspect of the esophagus is facilitated by traction on a Penrose drain encircling the gastroesophageal junction.

crura have been completely exposed, dissection to create a window posterior to the esophagus will not be difficult. From the patient's right side, the esophagus is retracted anteriorly, with the surgeon's left-handed instrument allowing posterior dissection with the right hand, and vice versa for the left-sided dissection. The posterior vagus nerve is left on the esophagus. The medial surface of the left crus is identified and the dissection kept caudal to it. There is a tendency to dissect into the mediastinum and left pleura. In the presence of severe esophagitis, transmural inflammation, esophageal shortening, or a large posterior fat pad, this dissection may be particularly difficult. If unduly difficult, it should be abandoned and the hiatus approached from the left side via division of the short gastric vessels. Following posterior dissection, a grasper is passed via the surgeon's left-handed port behind the esophagus and over the left crus. A Penrose drain is placed around the esophagus and used as an esophageal retractor for the remainder of the procedure.

Crural Closure.   The crura are further dissected and the space behind the gastroesophageal junction enlarged as much as possible. The esophagus is retracted anteriorly and to the left, and the crura are approximated with three to four interrupted 0 silk sutures, starting just above the aortic decussation (Fig. 19.28). We prefer a large needle (CT1) passed down the left upper 10-mm port to facilitate a durable crural closure. Because the space behind the esophagus is limited, it is often necessary to use the surgeon's left-handed instrument as a retractor. This maneuver facilitates the placement of single bites through each crus with the surgeon's right hand. We prefer tying the knots extracorporeally with a standard knot pusher.

Although no randomized studies have evaluated the role of routine crural closure, compelling evidence is available to indicate that the closure should be standard. Watson et al. (77) identified paraesophageal herniation in 17 of 253 patients (7%), the frequency being 3% in those who had undergone crural repair and 11% in those who had not.

Fundic Mobilization.   The relationship between complete fundic mobilization (short gastric vessel division) and postoperative dysphagia is a subject of debate that has continued from the open era, when fundic mobilization was linked to a lower incidence of dysphagia. Of two randomized studies comparing fundic mobilization with nonmobilization, one found no difference in outcome (78), and the other found significant reductions in the incidence of dysphagia, gas bloat, and inability to belch after

fundic mobilization (79). The beneficial effect of fundic mobilization on these parameters has also been noted by other investigators (80). Whether fundic mobilization *per se* has a direct impact on dysphagia is unclear. It may simply be that mobilization permits better visualization of the procedure and so ensures that the repair is constructed with the posterior portion of the fundus.

Replacing the liver retractor with a second Babcock forceps facilitates retraction of the gastrosplenic mesentery during division of the short gastric vessels. The gastrosplenic omentum is suspended anteroposteriorly in a clothesline fashion with both Babcock forceps, and the lesser sac is entered approximately one third the distance down the greater curvature of the stomach (Fig. 19.29). The short gastric vessels are sequentially divided with the aid of a Harmonic scalpel (Ethicon Endosurgery, Cincinnati, OH). An anterior-posterior rather than medial-to-lateral orientation of the vessels is preferred, except for those close to the spleen. The dissection includes dividing the

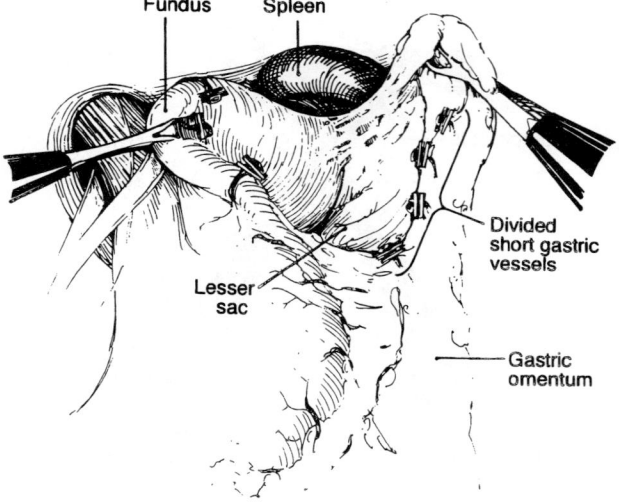

Figure 19.29. Illustration of the proper retraction of the gastrosplenic omentum to facilitate the initial steps in short gastric vessel division. Complete fundic mobilization is continued by retraction of the stomach rightward and the spleen and omentum left and downward. These maneuvers allow the lesser sac to be opened and facilitate division of the high short gastric vessels.

posterior pancreaticogastric branches that lie behind the upper portion of the stomach and continues until the right crus and caudate lobe can be seen from the left side (Fig. 19.30). With caution and meticulous dissection, the fundus can be completely mobilized in virtually all patients.

Geometry of the Fundoplication. The fundoplication is created with particular attention to the geometry of the fundus (Fig. 19.31). To ensure that the posterior fundus is used in the construction of the fundoplication, it is grasped and passed behind the esophagus from left to right rather than pulled from right to left. This is accomplished by placing a Babcock clamp through the left lower port and grasping the midportion of the posterior fundus (Fig. 19.32). The fundus is passed behind the esophagus to the right side. The Babcock clamp becomes visible on the right side with an upward and clockwise twisting motion. The anterior wall of the fundus is brought over the anterior wall of the esophagus above the supporting Penrose drain. Both the anterior and posterior fundic lips are manipulated so that the esophagus is enveloped without the fundus being twisted (Fig. 19.33). The laparoscopic visualization tends to exaggerate the size of the posterior window. Consequently, the space behind the esophagus may be smaller than it appears, so that ischemia of the fundus can result when it is passed behind the esophagus. If the posterior lip of the fundoplication has a bluish discoloration, the stomach should be returned to its original position and the posterior window enlarged. A 60F bougie is passed into the stomach, and the fundoplication is constructed around it to size its diameter properly. The anterior and posterior lips of the fundoplication are sutured together by means of a single U-stitch of 2-0 Prolene buttressed with felt pledgets. The most common error in constructing the fundoplication is to grasp the anterior

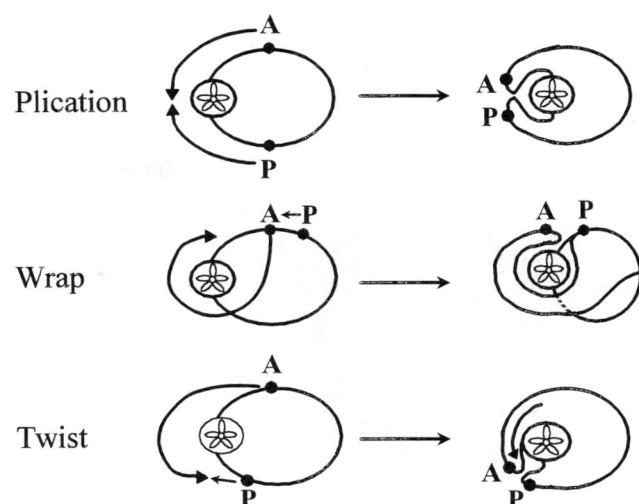

Figure 19.31. Schematic representations of the various possibilities of orientation of a Nissen fundoplication. The *top box* represents the preferred approach; in the *bottom two boxes,* twisting of the fundoplication is seen.

portion of the stomach and pull it behind the esophagus. This results in twisting of the gastric fundus around the esophagus. Rather, the esophagus should be enveloped by an untwisted fundus before suturing. Two anchoring sutures of 2-0 silk are placed above and below the U-stitch to complete the fixation of the fundoplication. When this is finished, the stomach should remain within its original plane, with the suture line of the fundoplication facing in the right anterior direction and the greater curvature in the left posterior direction. Before the ports are removed, the abdomen is irrigated, hemostasis ascertained, and the bougie removed.

Learning Curve for Laparoscopic Antireflux Surgery. In an attempt to define the learning curve for laparoscopic surgery, Watson et al. (81) evaluated their experience of 280 laparoscopic fundoplications undertaken by 11 surgeons during a 4-year period. The authors identified an institutional learning curve of 50 cases and an individual learning curve of 20 cases. Beyond these points, the rates of complications, reoperations, and conversions to an open procedure plateaued. The learning curve was particularly abrupt for the institution's first 20 cases and the individual surgeon's first five cases. Furthermore, the supervision of trainees in laparoscopic fundoplication by experienced laparoscopists resulted in fewer complications than were seen after the initial introduction of the technique. These findings have been reproduced by a number of other groups. Gotley et al. (82) noted a reduction in operative time, the rate of conversion to an open procedure, and late morbidity for their second 100 cases in comparison with their first 100.

Transthoracic Nissen Fundoplication. Performing an antireflux procedure by a transthoracic approach is appropriate in the following cases:

1. The patient has previously undergone a hiatal hernia repair. In this situation, a peripheral circumferential incision in the diaphragm is made to provide simultaneous exposure of the upper abdomen. This allows safe dissection of the previous repair from both the abdominal and thoracic sides of the diaphragm.
2. The patient requires a concomitant esophageal myotomy for achalasia or diffuse spasm.

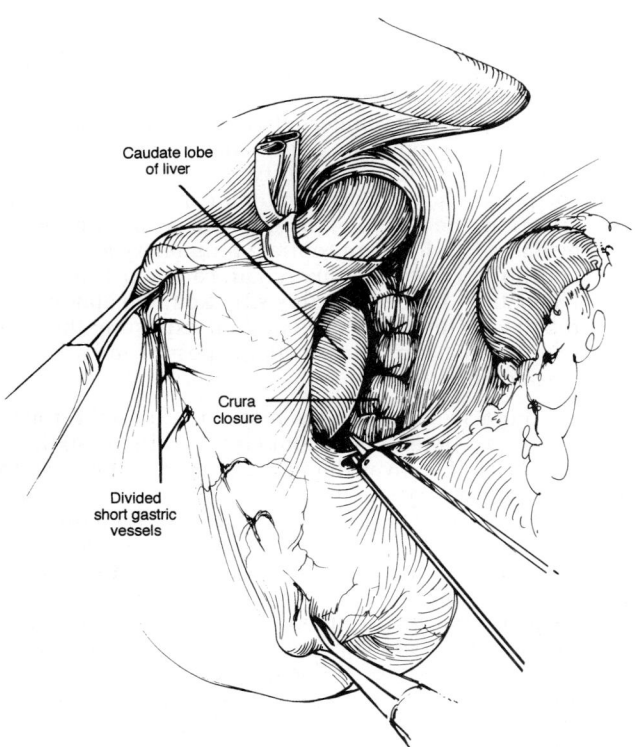

Figure 19.30. The fundic mobilization is continued to include pancreaticogastric branches and the short gastric branches. Dissection continues until the crura and the caudate lobe can be seen from the left posterior.

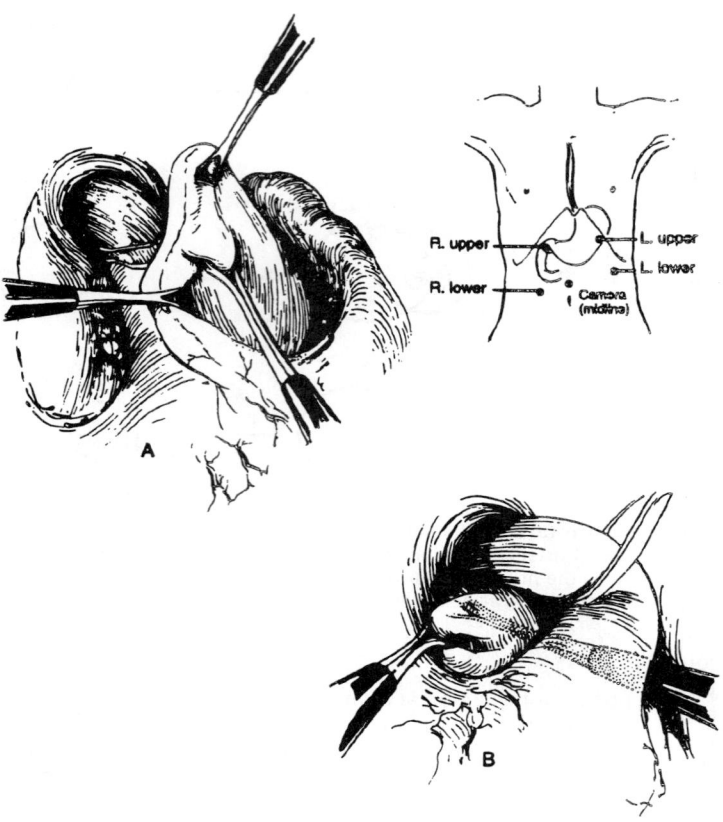

Figure 19.32. Placement of a Babcock clamp on the posterior fundus in preparation for passing it behind the esophagus to create the posterior or right lip of the fundoplication. *Inset:* To achieve the proper angle for passage, the Babcock clamp is placed through the left lower trocar. The posterior fundus is passed from left to right and grasped from the right with a Babcock clamp through the right upper trocar.

3. The patient has a short esophagus. This is usually associated with a stricture or Barrett's esophagus. In this situation, the thoracic approach is preferred to allow maximum mobilization of the esophagus, the performance of a Collis gastroplasty, or, if necessary,

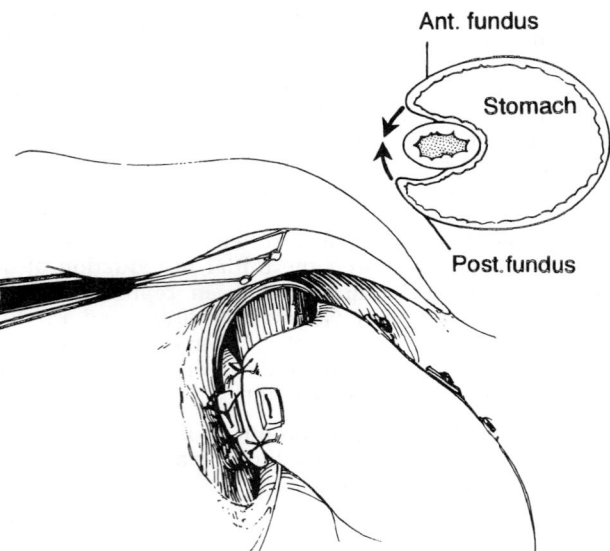

Figure 19.33. Fixation of the fundoplication. The fundoplication is sutured in place with a single U-stitch of 2-0 Prolene pledgeted on the outside. A 60F mercury-weighted bougie is passed through the gastroesophageal junction before fixation of the wrap to ensure a floppy fundoplication. *Inset* illustrates the proper orientation of the fundic wrap.

placement of the repair without tension below the diaphragm.

4. The patient has a sliding hiatal hernia that does not reduce below the diaphragm during a roentgenographic barium study in the upright position. This can indicate esophageal shortening, and again, a thoracic approach is preferred for maximum mobilization of the esophagus and, if necessary, the performance of a Collis gastroplasty.

5. The patient has associated pulmonary disease. In this situation, the nature of the pulmonary disease can be evaluated and the appropriate pulmonary surgery, in addition to the antireflux repair, can be performed.

6. The patient is obese. In this situation, the abdominal repair is difficult because of poor exposure; the thoracic approach provides better exposure and allows a more precise repair.

In the thoracic approach, the hiatus is exposed through a left posterior lateral thoracotomy incision in the sixth intercostal space (i.e., over the upper border of the seventh rib). When necessary, the diaphragm is incised circumferentially 2 to 3 cm from the lateral chest wall for a distance of approximately 10 to 15 cm. The esophagus is mobilized from the level of the diaphragm to underneath the aortic arch. Mobilization up to the aortic arch is usually necessary to place the repair in a patient with a shortened esophagus into the abdomen without undue tension. Failure to do this is one of the major causes of subsequent breakdown of a repair and a return of symptoms. The cardia is then freed from the diaphragm. When all the attachments between the cardia and diaphragmatic hiatus are divided, the fundus and part of the body of the stomach are drawn up through the hiatus into the chest. The vascular fat pad that lies at the gastroesophageal junction is excised. Crural sutures are then placed to close the hiatus,

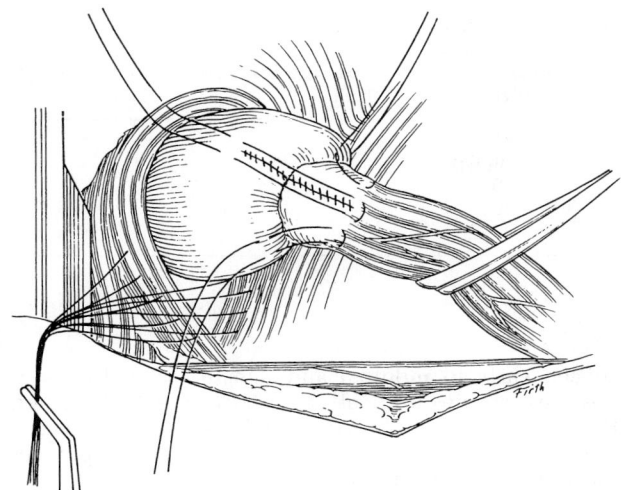

Figure 19.34. A Belsey 240-degree gastric fundic wrap. The complete repair includes posterior sutures in the crus and a first and second row of sutures to hold the partial fundoplication. Note that the second row of sutures joins the diaphragm, stomach, and esophagus. The position of the tied holding sutures is also shown.

and the fundoplication is constructed by enveloping the distal esophagus with the fundus, in a manner similar to that described for the abdominal approach. When complete, the fundoplication is placed into the abdomen by compressing the fundic ball with the hand and manually maneuvering it through the hiatus.

Belsey Mark IV Partial Fundoplication. In the presence of altered esophageal motility, when the propulsive force of the esophagus is not sufficient to overcome the outflow obstruction of a complete fundoplication, a partial fundoplication is indicated. Although a partial fundoplication may be performed laparoscopically (Toupet fundoplication), the Belsey Mark IV repair is the prototype of partial fundoplications. It consists of a 270-degree gastric fundoplication around the distal 4 cm of esophagus performed through an incision in the left side of the chest (Fig. 19.34). The dissections in the Belsey Mark IV and the transthoracic Nissen operations are the same, differing only in the technique of constructing the fundoplication.

To perform the Belsey Mark IV antireflux procedure, the esophagus is mobilized up to the aortic arch, the cardia is dissected free of the hiatus, and the fundus of the stomach is brought up through the hiatus, as described for the transthoracic Nissen procedure. The partial fundoplication is held in position by two rows of three horizontal mattress sutures placed to be equidistant between the

seromuscular layers of the stomach and the muscular layers of the esophagus. A second row of sutures is placed 1.5 to 2.0 cm above the first row, with the position of the previously placed sutures in the first row used as a guide. The diaphragmatic sutures are placed at the 4-, 8-, and 12-o'clock positions, oriented with the 6-o'clock position placed posteriorly between the right and left crura just anterior to the aorta. The reconstructed cardia is gently pushed through the hiatus and placed in the abdomen. Once in the abdomen, the cardia should remain there without exerting tension on the holding sutures.

Collis Gastroplasty. In patients with a short esophagus secondary to a stricture, Barrett's esophagus, or a large hiatal hernia, the esophagus is lengthened with a Collis gastroplasty. The esophagus is lengthened by the construction of a gastric tube along the lesser curvature. This allows the tension-free construction of a Belsey Mark IV or Nissen fundoplication around the newly formed gastric tube, with placement of the repair in the abdomen. Because a short esophagus is commonly associated with a reduction in esophageal contraction amplitude and the gastric tube is devoid of peristaltic contractions, most surgeons prefer to combine the gastroplasty procedure with a 280-degree Belsey Mark IV fundoplication rather than a 360-degree Nissen fundoplication.

Complications of Antireflux Surgery. The prevalence of complications after laparoscopic antireflux surgery are indicated in Table 19.8 (83–90). The average postoperative complication rate is 8% (range, 2% to 13%), and the rate of conversion to an open procedure is 2% (range, 1% to 10%). Mortality is uncommon. In the entire published literature, five deaths have been recorded following laparoscopic antireflux surgery.

Both pneumothorax and pneumomediastinum have been reported. The occurrence of pneumothorax is related to a breach of either pleural membrane, usually the left, during the hiatal dissection. It does not usually require insertion of a chest drain, as accumulated carbon dioxide is rapidly expelled following the release of pneumoperitoneum by a combination of positive-pressure ventilation and absorption.

As in any laparoscopic procedure, instrumental perforation of the hollow viscera is possible. Perforation tends to occur at these two sites during the course of fundoplication. Early esophageal perforation may arise during passage of the bougie, retroesophageal dissection, or suture pull-through. Late esophageal perforation is related to diathermy injury at the time of mobilization. Gastric perforation is usually related to excessive traction on the fundus for purposes of retraction. If the problem is recognized at the time of surgery, repair is required, which may be performed either laparoscopically or by an open technique.

Table 19.8. **COMPLICATIONS AND CONVERSION TO OPEN RATE AFTER LAPAROSCOPIC ANTIREFLUX SURGERY (SELECTED SERIES)**

Authors (ref.)	Year	No.	Procedure	Morbidity (%)	Conversion (%)
Cuschieri et al. (83)	1993	116	Nissen, Toupet	13	1
Hinder et al. (84)	1994	198	Nissen	12	3
Collet and Cadière (85)	1995	758	Nissen, Toupet, Angelchick	4	4
Watson et al. (86)	1995	230	Nissen	15	10
Gotley et al. (82)	1996	200	Nissen	8	5
Hunter et al. (87)	1996	300	Nissen, Toupet	12	1
Cadière et al. (88)	1997	274	Nissen	3	1
Dallemagne et al. (89)	1998	622	Nissen, Toupet	2	1
Peters et al. (90)	1998	100	Nissen	4	2

Table 19.9. RESULTS OF PRIMARY OPEN ANTIREFLUX REPAIRS: SELECTED SERIES

Authors (ref.)	Year	No. patients	Mean follow-up (y)	Good results (%)	Positive 24-h pH (%)	Dysphagia (%)
DeMeester et al. (91)	1986	100	3	91	—	3
De Haro et al. (92)	1992	51	7	90	20	
Bjerkeset et al. (93)	1992	82	6	98	2	
Loustarinen (94)	1993	109	6	70	14	
Johansson et al. (95)	1993	38	5	82	8	

One complication that appears to be more common with the laparoscopic than the open approach is herniation of the wrap through the hiatus. The explanation for this is unclear, but it may be related to the opening of tissue planes by the pneumoperitoneum; in addition, adhesions are less likely to form after laparoscopic than after open surgery. In an attempt to eliminate this complication, most surgeons routinely perform a crural repair.

Hemorrhage during the course of laparoscopic fundoplication usually arises from the short gastric vessels or spleen. Rarer causes include retractor trauma to the liver and injury to the left inferior phrenic vein, an aberrant left hepatic vein, or the inferior vena cava. Cardiac tamponade as a result of right ventricular trauma has also been reported. Major vascular injury mandates immediate conversion to an open procedure to achieve hemostasis. One complication that has been virtually eliminated since the advent of laparoscopic fundoplication is incidental splenic injury necessitating splenectomy, which occurred with a frequency of about 2% during the open era.

Outcome after Open Antireflux Surgery. Table 19.9 shows the long-term outcome of open antireflux surgery in selected series (91–96). Two studies merit specific mention. The first, by De Haro et al. (92), evaluated 51 patients with pH-proven GERD a minimum of 5 years after Nissen fundoplication. Forty-five patients (88%) reported either no or minimal reflux symptoms. Endoscopically, esophagitis remained healed in 44 patients (86%). Ten patients (20%) had positive results on 24-hour pH monitoring; only half of them were symptomatic. Johansson et al. (95) assessed 40 patients with pH-proven GERD 5 years after Nissen fundoplication. All except one patient (97%) remained free of, or had only occasional, reflux symptoms. Endoscopy revealed grade I nonerosive esophagitis in three patients. In all others, the esophagitis was healed. Three patients (8%) had positive pH scores, only one of whom was symptomatic. Importantly, no change was observed in esophageal acid exposure on 24-hour pH studies

between early (6 months) and late (5 years) follow-up. These two studies, indicating an 80% to 92% long-term, pH-proven success rate for open Nissen fundoplication, serve as the gold standard with which laparoscopic techniques should be compared.

Outcome after Laparoscopic AntiReflux Surgery

Symptomatic. Several excellent series of laparoscopic fundoplication have now been published (82–90) (Table 19.10). These reports document the ability of laparoscopic fundoplication to relieve typical reflux symptoms (heartburn, regurgitation, and dysphagia) in more than 90% of patients at a follow-up interval approaching 3 years in some studies. The results compare favorably with those of the "modern" era of open fundoplication. They also indicate the less predictable outcome of patients with atypical reflux symptoms (cough, asthma, laryngitis) after surgery, which are relieved in only two thirds of cases (97).

The goal of surgical treatment for GERD is to relieve the symptoms of reflux by reestablishing the gastroesophageal barrier. The challenge is to accomplish this without inducing dysphagia or other untoward side effects. Dysphagia that is present before surgery usually is diminished following laparoscopic fundoplication. Temporary dysphagia is common after surgery (perhaps even desirable!) and generally resolves within 3 months. Dysphagia persisting beyond 3 months has been reported in up to 10% of patients. In our experience, dysphagia (i.e., occasional difficulty in swallowing solids) was present in 7% of our patients at 3 months, 5% at 6 months, 2% at 12 months, and in a single patient at 24 months following surgery. Others have observed a similar improvement in postoperative dysphagia with time. It should be emphasized that induced dysphagia is usually mild, need not require dilation, and is temporary. It can be induced by technical misjudgments, but this explanation does not hold in all instances. When surgery is performed by experienced hands, its prevalence should be less than 3% at 1 year. Other side effects common after antireflux surgery include an inability to vomit and increased flatulence (Table 19.11). Most patients cannot vomit through an intact wrap,

Table 19.10. PHYSIOLOGIC OUTCOME AFTER LAPAROSCOPIC FUNDOPLICATION

Authors (ref.)	No. negative pH/total No. (%)	Follow-up (mo)
Cuschieri et al. (83)	88/92 (96)	3
Hinder et al. (84)	21/24 (87)	3–12
Watson et al. (86)	43/46 (93)	1.5
Gotley et al. (82)	95/96 (99)	3
Hunter et al. (87)	48/55 (87)	1.5
Hunter et al. (87)	49/54 (91)	12
Peters et al. (90)	26/28 (93)	21

Table 19.11. SIDE EFFECTS OF LAPAROSCOPIC FUNDOPLICATION

Side effect	No. patients	Percentage
Temporary swallowing	47	50
Dysphagia >3 mos	7	7
Increased flatus	45	47
Bloating	42	44
Inability to belch	19	20
Inability to vomit	24	25

Table 19.12. COMPARISON OF COSTS FOR OPEN AND LAPAROSCOPIC FUNDOPLICATION

Authors (ref.)	Access	Operative costs ($)	Hospital costs ($)	Total costs ($)[a]
Incarbone et al. (105)	Open	10,808	15,891	—
	Laparoscopic	13,871	14,651	—
Rattner et al. (106)	Open	4,060	18,394	—
	Laparoscopic	4,647	11,673	—
Blomqvist et al. (107)[b]	Open	2,100	5,900	12,400
	Laparoscopic	3,000	4,300	6,700
Heikkinen et al. (108)	Open	1,508	3,140	13,118
	Laparoscopic	2,000	2,981	7,506

[a]Includes community-related costs.
[b]Assumes the 1995 conversion rate of six Swedish crowns to one U.S. dollar.
Costs are given in U.S. dollars.

although this is rarely clinically relevant. Flatulence is a common and noticeable problem. It is likely related to increased air swallowing in most patients with reflux disease.

Physiologic. As after the open procedure, lower esophageal sphincter pressure is significantly increased after laparoscopic fundoplication. Table 19.10 indicates that at short-term follow-up, more than 90% of patients had negative pH studies. In the study with the longest follow-up, approaching 2 years, 26 of 28 patients (93%) had negative pH studies (90).

Quality of Life. Quality-of-life analysis has become an important part of surgical outcome assessment, with both generic and disease-specific questionnaires used in an attempt to quantify quality of life before and after surgical intervention. In general, these measures attempt to relate the effect of disease management to the overall well-being of the patient (98). Most studies have utilized the Short Form 36 (SF-36) instrument, as it can be rapidly administered and is well validated. This questionnaire measures 12 different health-related quality-of-life parameters encompassing mental and physical well-being. Data from Los Angeles indicated a significant improvement in scores for bodily pain and in a portion of the general health index (90). Most other measures were improved but failed to achieve statistical significance. Laycock et al. (99) have also analyzed SF-36 scores before and after laparoscopic antireflux surgery. In contrast to our data, scores in all fields were significantly better after surgery. In this study, preoperative scores were dramatically lower than those in our study. Thus, the difference is likely to be secondary to the relatively high scores of our patients before surgery (perhaps reflecting good disease control on medical therapy) and to our small sample size.

Other investigators have also reported improvement in quality of life following antireflux surgery. Glise et al. (100) utilized two standardized and validated questionnaires, the Psychological General Well-Being Index and the Gastrointestinal Symptom Rating Scale, to evaluate quality of life in a cohort of 40 patients following laparoscopic antireflux surgery. Scores with both instruments were improved following antireflux surgery and better than in untreated patients. Of particular note was that scores were as good as or better than those of patients receiving optimal medical therapy. Velonovich et al. (101), utilizing a 10-item health-related quality-of-life questionnaire specific for GERD, have also demonsrated an improvement in quality of life following antireflux surgery.

Cost Considerations. It is being increasingly recognized that antireflux treatment options should be compared prospectively in terms not only of efficacy and safety, but also of cost-effectiveness. Cost-effectiveness studies should take into account both direct costs, such as drug acquisition costs, and indirect costs, such as time lost from work. Three cost–utility analyses of long-term medical therapy versus laparoscopic fundoplication for GERD have been performed, one in the United States and two in Europe. In the United States, Heudebert et al. (102) reported that projected costs for 5 years favor medical over surgical therapy, but that after 10 years equivalence is achieved. Viljakka et al. (103), in Finland, concluded that the cost of open or laparoscopic surgery is less than that of lifelong daily therapy with proton pump inhibitors or ranitidine at a daily dose of 300 mg. Even for men ages 65 to 69 years, the cost of lifelong omeprazole at a dosage of either 20 mg or 40 mg exceeds the costs of both open and laparoscopic surgery. Van den Boom et al. (104), reporting from The Netherlands, concluded that the break-even point, when medical and surgical therapies are of similar cost, is 4 years for open surgery and 17 months for laparoscopic surgery. All three studies concluded that laparoscopic surgery is the most cost-effective form of treatment for patients likely to require lifelong therapy.

Four studies have compared the costs of open abdominal and laparoscopic fundoplication, two in the United States (105,106) and two in Europe (107,108) (Table 19.12). All concluded that laparoscopic fundoplication is associated with higher operative costs because it entails the use of more expensive instruments, but that overall the costs of laparoscopic surgery are equal to, or less than, those of open surgery. Substantial savings with minimally invasive surgery are related to a shorter hospital stay and an earlier return to work.

REFERENCES

1. Patti MG, Gantert W, Way LW. Surgery of the esophagus: anatomy and physiology. *Surg Clin North Am* 1997;77: 959–970.
2. Gray SW, Rowe JS Jr, Skandalakis JE. Surgical anatomy of the gastroesophageal junction. *Am Surg* 1979;45:575.
3. Dua KS, Ren J, Bardan E, et al. Coordination of deglutitive glottal function and pharyngeal bolus transport during normal eating. *Gastroenterology* 1997;112:73–83.
4. Pouderoux P, Shi G, Tatum RP, et al. Esophageal solid bolus transport: studies using concurrent videofluoroscopy and manometry. *Am J Gastroenterol* 1999;94:1457–1463.
5. Pouderoux P, Lin S, Kahrilis PJ. Timing, propagation, coordination, and effect of esophageal shortening during peristalsis. *Gastroenterology* 1997;112:1147–1154.
6. Mittal RK, Balaban DH. The esophagogastric junction. *N Engl J Med* 1997;336:924–932.
7. Clave P, Gonzalez A, Moreno A, et al. Endogenous cholecystokinin enhances postprandial gastroesophageal reflux in

humans through extrasphincteric receptors. *Gastroenterology* 1998;115:597–604.

8. Locke GR, Talley NJ, Fett SL, et al. Prevalence and clinical spectrum of gastroesophageal reflux: a population-based study in Olmsted County, Minnesota. *Gastroenterology* 1997;112:1448–1456.

9. Isolauri J, Laippala P. Prevalence of symptoms suggestive of gastroesophageal reflux disease in an adult population. *Ann Med* 1995;27:67–70.

10. El-Serag HB, Sonnenberg A. Opposing time trends of peptic ulcer and reflux disease. *Gut* 1998;43:327–333.

11. Panos MZ, Walt RP, Stevenson C, et al. Rising death rate from non-malignant disease of the oesophagus (NMOD) in England and Wales. *Gut* 1995;36:488–491.

12. Monnier Ph, Ollyo JB, Fontolliet C, et al. Epidemiology and natural history of reflux esophagitis. *Semin Laparosc Surg* 1995;2:2–9.

13. Spechler SJ. Epidemiology and natural history of gastro-oesophageal reflux disease. *Digestion* 1992;51:24–29.

14. Oberg S, Peters JH, DeMeester TR. *Helicobacter pylori* is not associated with the manifestations of gastroesophageal reflux disease. *Arch Surg* 1999;134:722–726.

15. Labenz J, Blum AL, Bayerdorffer E, et al. Curing *Helicobacter pylori* infection in patients with duodenal ulcer may provoke reflux esophagitis. *Gastroenterology* 1997;112:1442–1447.

16. Vicari JJ, Peek RM, Falk GW, et al. The seroprevalence of cagA-positive *Helicobacter pylori* strains in the spectrum of gastroesophageal reflux disease. *Gastroenterology* 1998;115:50–57.

17. Chow WH, Blaser MJ, Blot WJ, et al. An inverse relation between cagA+ strains of *Helicobacter pylori* infection and risk of esophageal and gastric cardia adenocarcinoma. *Cancer Res* 1998;58:588–590.

18. Costantini M, Crookes PF, Bremner RM, et al. The value of physiologic assessment of foregut symptoms in a surgical practice. *Surgery* 1993;114:780–787.

19. Bonavina L, Evander A, DeMeester TR, et al. Length of the distal esophageal sphincter and competency of the cardia. *Am J Surg* 1986;151:25–34.

20. O'Sullivan GC, DeMeester TR, Joelsson BE, et al. The interaction of the lower esophageal sphincter pressure and length of sphincter in the abdomen as determinants of gastroesophageal competence. *Am J Surg* 1982;143:40–47.

21. Zaninotto G, DeMeester TR, Schwizer W, et al. The lower esophageal sphincter in health and disease. *Am J Surg* 1988;155:104–111.

22. Stein HJ, Barlow AP, DeMeester TR, et al. Complications of gastroesophageal reflux disease: role of the lower esophageal sphincter, esophageal acid and acid/alkaline exposure, and duodenogastric reflux. *Ann Surg* 1992;216:35–43.

23. Kuster E, Ros E, Toledo-Pimentel V, et al. Predictive factors of the long-term outcome in gastro-oesophageal reflux disease: six-year follow-up of 107 patients. *Gut* 1994;35:8–14.

24. Stein HJ, Eypasch EP, DeMeester TR, et al. Circadian esophageal motor function in patients with gastroesophageal reflux disease. *Surgery* 1990;108:769–778.

25. DeMeester TR, Johnson WE. Outcome of respiratory symptoms after surgical treatment of swallowing disorders. *Semin Respir Crit Care Med* 1995;16:514–519.

26. Bremner RM, Hoeft SF, Costantini M, et al. Pharyngeal swallowing: the major factor in clearance of esophageal reflux episodes. *Ann Surg* 1993;218:364–370.

27. Rakic S, Stein HJ, DeMeester TR, et al. Role of esophageal body function in gastroesophageal reflux disease: implications for surgical management. *J Am Coll Surg* 1997;185:380–387.

28. Lillemoe KD, Johnson LF, Harmon JW. Role of the components of the gastroduodenal contents in experimental acid esophagitis. *Surgery* 1982;92:276–284.

29. Lillemoe KD, Johnson LF, Harmon JW. Alkaline esophagitis: a comparison of the ability of components of gastroduodenal contents to injure the rabbit esophagus. *Gastroenterology* 1983;85:621–628.

30. Gotley DC, Morgan AP, Cooper MJ. Bile acid concentrations in the refluxate of patients with reflux oesophagitis. *Br J Surg* 1988;75:587–590.

31. Johnnson F, Joelsson B, Floren CH. Bile salts in the esophagus of patients with esophagitis. *Scand J Gastroenterol* 1988;23:712–715.

32. Stein HJ, Feussner H, Kauer W, et al. Alkaline gastroesophageal reflux: assessment by ambulatory esophageal aspiration and pH monitoring. *Am J Surg* 1994;167:163–168.

33. Kauer WKH, Peters JH, DeMeester TR, et al. Mixed reflux of gastric juice is more harmful to the esophagus than gastric juice alone: the need for surgical therapy reemphasized. *Ann Surg* 1995;222:525–533.

34. Kauer WKH, Burdiles P, Ireland A, et al. Does duodenal juice reflux into the esophagus in patients with complicated GERD? Evaluation of a fiberoptic sensor for bilirubin. *Am J Surg* 1995;169:98.

35. Spechler SJ. The columnar lined esophagus: history, terminology, and clinical issues. *Gastroenterol Clin North Am* 1997;26:455–466.

36. Peters JH. The surgical management of Barrett's esophagus. *Gastroenterol Clin North Am* 1997;26:647–668.

37. Chandrasoma P. Norman Barrett: so close, yet 50 years away from the truth. *J Gastrointest Surg* 1999;3:7–14.

38. Sawney RA, Shields HM, Allan CH, et al. Morphological characterization of the squamocolumnar junction of the esophagus in patients with and without Barrett's epithelium. *Dig Dis Sci* 1996;41:1088–1098.

39. Shields HM, Zwas F, Antonioli DA, et al. Detection by scanning electron microscopy of a distinctive esophageal surface cell at the junction of squamous and Barrett's epithelium. *Dig Dis Sci* 1993;38:97–108.

40. Salo JA, Kivilaakso EO, Kiviluoto TA, et al. Cytokeratin profile suggests metaplastic epithelial transformation in Barrett's oesophagus. *Ann Med* 1996;28:305–309.

41. Boch JA, Shields HM, Antonioli DA, et al. Distribution of cytokeratin markers in Barrett's specialized columnar epithelium. *Gastroenterology* 1997;112:760–765.

42. Hameeteman W, Tytgat GNJ, Houthoff HJ, et al. Barrett's esophagus: development of dysplasia and adenocarcinoma. *Gastroenterology* 1989;96:1249–1256.

43. Zhuang Z, Vortmeyer AO, Mark EJ, et al. Barrett's esophagus: metaplastic cells with loss of heterozygosity at the *APC* gene locus are clonal precursors to invasive adenocarcinoma. *Cancer Res* 1996;56:1961–1964.

44. Reid BJ, Blount PL, Rubin CE, et al. Flow-cytometric and histological progression to malignancy in Barrett's esophagus: prospective endoscopic surveillance of a cohort. *Gastroenterology* 1992;102:1212–1219.

45. McCallum RW, Polepalle S, Davenport K, et al. Role of antireflux surgery against dysplasia in Barrett's esophagus. *Gastroenterology* 1991;100:A121(abst).

46. Ortiz A, Martinez de Haro LF, Parrilla P, et al. Conservative treatment versus antireflux surgery in Barrett's oesophagus: long-term results of a prospective study. *Br J Surg* 1996;83:274–278.

47. Peters JH, Clark GWB, Ireland AP, et al. Outcome of adenocarcinoma arising in Barrett's esophagus in endoscopically surveyed and non-surveyed patients. *J Thorac Cardiovasc Surg* 1994;108:813–822.

48. Pera M, Trastek VF, Carpenter HA, et al. Barrett's esophagus with high-grade dysplasia: an indication for esophagectomy. *Ann Thorac Surg* 1992;54:199–204.

49. Ferguson MK, Naunheim KS. Resection for Barrett's mucosa with high-grade dysplasia: implications for prophylactic photodynamic therapy. *J Thorac Cardiovasc Surg* 1997;114:824–829.

50. El-Serag HB, Sonnenberg A. Comorbid occurrence of laryngeal or pulmonary disease with esophagitis in United States military veterans. *Gastroenterology* 1997;113:755–760.

51. Gastal OL, Castell JA, Castell DO. Frequency and site of gastroesophageal reflux in patients with chest symptoms. *Chest* 1994;106:1793–1796.

52. Levin TR, Sperling RM, McQuaid KR. Omeprazole improves peak expiratory flow rate and quality of life in asthmatics with gastroesophageal reflux. *Am J Gastroenterol* 1998;93:1060–1063.

53. Boeree MJ, Peters FTM, Postma DS, et al. No effects of high-dose omeprazole in patients with severe airway hyperre-

sponsiveness and (a)symptomatic gastro-oesophageal reflux. *Eur Respir J* 1998;11:1070–1074.

54. Harding SM, Richter JE, Guzzo MR, et al. Asthma and gastroesophageal reflux: acid suppressive therapy improves asthma outcome. *Am J Med* 1996;100:395–405.

55. Sontag SJ, O'Connell S, Khandelwal S, et al. Antireflux surgery in asthmatics with reflux (GER) improves pulmonary symptoms and function. *Gastroenterology* 1990;98:A128(abst).

56. Perrin-Fayolle M, Gormand F, Braillon G, et al. Long-term results of surgical treatment for gastroesophageal reflux in asthmatic patients. *Chest* 1989;96:40–45.

57. Larrain A, Carrasco E, Galleguillos F, et al. Medical and surgical treatment of nonallergic asthma associated with gastroesophageal reflux. *Chest* 1991;99:1330–1335.

58. Sandmark S, Carlsson R, Fausa O, et al. Omeprozole or ranitidine in the treatment of reflux esophagitis. *Scand J Gastroenterol* 1988;23:625–632.

59. Katzka DA, Paoletti V, Leite L, et al. Prolonged ambulatory pH monitoring in patients with persistent gastroesophageal reflux disease symptoms: testing while on therapy identifies the need for more aggressive anti-reflux therapy. *Am J Gastroenterol* 1996;91:2110–2113.

60. Peghini PL, Katz PO, Bracy NA, et al. Nocturnal recovery of gastric acid secretion with twice-daily dosing of proton pump inhibitors. *Am J Gastroenterol* 1998;93:763–767.

61. Campos GM, Peters JH, DeMeester TR, et al. The pattern of esophageal acid exposure in GERD influences the severity of the disease. *Arch Surg* 1999;134:882–888.

62. Campos GMR, Peters JH, DeMeester TR, et al. Multivariate analysis of the factors predicting outcome after laparoscopic Nissen fundoplication. *J Gastrointest Surg* 1999;3:292–300.

63. Hill LD, Kozarek RA, Kraemer SJ, et al. The gastroesophageal flap valve: in vitro and in vivo observations. *Gastrointest Endosc* 1996;44:541.

64. Miller FA. Utilization of inlying pH-probe for evaluation of acid peptic diathesis. *Arch Surg* 1964;89:199–203.

65. Johnson LF, DeMeester TR. Development of the 24-hour intraesophageal pH monitoring composite scoring system. *J Clin Gastroenterol* 1986;8[Suppl 1]:52–58.

66. Jamieson JR, Stein HJ, DeMeester TR, et al. Ambulatory 24-h esophageal pH monitoring: normal values, optimal thresholds, specificity, sensitivity, and reproducibility. *Am J Gastroenterol* 1992;87:1102–1111.

67. Gastal OL, Hagen JA, Peters JH, et al. Short esophagus: analysis of predictors and clinical implications. *Arch Surg* 1999;134:633–636.

68. Ritter MP, Peters JH, DeMeester TR, et al. Treatment of advanced gastroesophageal reflux disease with Collis gastroplasty and Belsey partial fundoplication. *Arch Surg* 1998;133:523–529.

69. Stein HJ, Feussner H, Siewart JR. Failure of antireflux surgery: causes and management. *Am J Surg* 1996;171:36–40.

70. Johnson WE, Hagen JA, DeMeester TR, et al. Outcome of respiratory symptoms after antireflux surgery on patients with gastroesophageal reflux disease. *Arch Surg* 1996;131:489–492.

71. Schwizer W, Hinder RA, DeMeester TR. Does delayed gastric emptying contribute to gastroesophageal reflux disease? *Am J Surg* 1989;157:74.

72. Watson DI, Jamieson GG, Pike GK, et al. Prospective randomized double-blind trial between laparoscopic Nissen and anterior partial fundoplication. *Br J Surg* 1999;86:123–130.

73. Laws HL, Clements RH, Swillie CM. A randomized, prospective comparison of the Nissen fundoplication versus the Toupet fundoplication for gastroesophageal reflux disease. *Ann Surg* 1997;225:647–654.

74. Jobe BA, Wallace J, Hansen PD, et al. Evaluation of laparoscopic Toupet fundoplication as a primary repair for all patients with medically resistant gastroesophageal reflux. *Surg Endosc* 1997;11:1080–1083.

75. Bell RC, Hanna P. Patterns of success and failure with laparoscopic partial fundoplication. *Surg Endosc* 1998;12:S1.

76. Horvath KD, Jobe BA, Swanstrom LL. Laparoscopic Toupet is an inadequate procedure for patients with severe reflux disease. *Gastroenterology* 1998;114:A1393(abst).

77. Watson DI, Jamieson GG, Devitt PG, et al. Paraoesophageal hiatus hernia: an important complication of laparoscopic Nissen fundoplication. *Br J Surg* 1995;82:521–523.

78. Watson DI, Pike GK, Baigrie RJ, et al. Prospective double-blind randomized trial of laparoscopic Nissen fundoplication with division and without division of short gastric vessels. *Ann Surg* 1997;226:642–652.

79. Dalenbäck J, Lönroth H, Blomqvist A, et al. Improved funcional outcome after laparoscopic fundoplication by complete gastric fundus mobilization. *Gastroenterology* 1998;114:A1384(abst).

80. Hunter JG, Swanstrom L, Waring JP. Dysphagia after laparoscopic antireflux surgery: the impact of operative technique. *Ann Surg* 1996;224:51–57.

81. Watson DI, Baigrie RJ, Jamieson GG. A learning curve for laparoscopic fundoplication: definable, avoidable, or a waste of time? *Ann Surg* 1996;224:198–203.

82. Gotley DC, Smithers BM, Rhodes M, et al. Laparoscopic Nissen fundoplication—200 consecutive cases. *Gut* 1996;38:487–491.

83. Cuschieri A, Hunter J, Wolfe B, et al. Multicenter prospective evaluation of laparoscopic antireflux surgery: preliminary report. *Surg Endosc* 1993;7:505–510.

84. Hinder RA, Filipi CJ, Wetscher G, et al. Laparoscopic Nissen fundoplication is an effective treatment for gastroesophageal reflux disease. *Ann Surg* 1994;220:472–481.

85. Collet D, Cadière GB. Conversions and complications of laparoscopic treatment of gastroesophageal reflux disease. *Am J Surg* 1995;169:622–626.

86. Watson DI, Jamieson GG, Devitt PG, et al. Changing strategies in the performance of laparoscopic Nissen fundoplication as a result of experience with 230 operations. *Surg Endosc* 1995;9:961–966.

87. Hunter JG, Trus TL, Branum GD, et al. A physiologic approach to laparoscopic fundoplication for gastroesophageal reflux disease. *Ann Surg* 1996;223:673–685.

88. Cadière GB, Himpens J, Rajan A, et al. Laparoscopic Nissen fundoplication: laparoscopic dissection technique and results. *Hepatogastroenterology* 1997;44:4–10.

89. Dallemagne B, Weerts JM, Jeahes C, et al. Results of laparoscopic Nissen fundoplication. *Hepatogastroenterology* 1998;45:1338–1343.

90. Peters JH, DeMeester TR, Crookes P, et al. The treatment of gastroesophageal reflux disease with laparoscopic Nissen fundoplication: prospective evaluation of 100 patients with "typical" symptoms. *Ann Surg* 1998;228:40–50.

91. DeMeester TR, Bonavina L, Albertucci M. Nissen fundoplication for gastroesophageal reflux disease—evaluation of primary repair in 100 consecutive patients. *Ann Surg* 1986;204:9–20.

92. De Haro ML, Ortiz A, Parrilla P, et al. Long-term results of Nissen fundoplication in reflux esophagitis without strictures: clinical, endoscopic, and pH-metric evaluation. *Dig Dis Sci* 1992;37:523–527.

93. Bjerkeset T, Edna TH, Fjøsne U. Long-term results after "floppy" Nissen/Rossetti fundoplication for gastroesophageal reflux disease. *Scand J Gastroenterol* 1992;27:707–710.

94. Luostarinen M. Nissen fundoplication for reflux esophagitis: long-term clinical and endoscopic results in 109 of 127 consecutive patients. *Ann Surg* 1993;217:329–337.

95. Johansson J, Johnsson F, Joelsson B, et al. Outcome 5 years after 360° fundoplication for gastro-oesophageal reflux disease. *Br J Surg* 1993;80:46–49.

96. Orringer MB, Skinner DB, Belsey RH. Long-term results of the Mark IV operation for hiatal hernia and analyses of recurrences and their treatment. *J Thorac Cardiovasc Surg* 1972;63:25–31.

97. So JB, Zeitels SM, Rattner DW. Outcomes of atypical symptoms attributed to gastroesophageal reflux treated by laparoscopic fundoplication. *Surgery* 1998;124:28–32.

98. Testa MA, Simonson DC. Assesment of quality-of-life outcomes. *N Engl J Med* 1996;334:835–840.

99. Laycock WS, Mauren S, Waring JP, et al. Improvement in quality-of-life measures following laparoscopic antireflux surgery. *Gastroenterology* 1995;108:A1228(abst).

100. Glise H, Hallerbäck B, Johansson B. Quality-of-life assessments in evaluation of laparoscopic Rosetti fundoplication. *Surg Endosc* 1995;9:183–189.
101. Velonovich V, Vallance SR, Gusz JR, et al. Quality-of-life scale for gastroesophageal reflux disease. *J Am Coll Surg* 1996;183:217–224.
102. Heudebert GR, Marks R, Wilcox CM, et al. Choice of long-term strategy for the management of patients with severe esophagitis: a cost–utility analysis. *Gastroenterology* 1997;112:1078–1086.
103. Viljakka M, Nevalainen J, Isolauri J. Lifetime costs of surgical versus medical treatment of severe gastro-oesophageal reflux disease in Finland. *Scand J Gastroenterol* 1997;32:766–772.
104. van den Boom G, Go PM, Hameeteman W, et al. Cost effectiveness of medical versus surgical treatment in patients with severe or refractory gastroesophageal reflux disease in The Netherlands. *Scand J Gastroenterol* 1996;31:1–9.
105. Incarbone R, Peters JH, Heimbucher J, et al. A contemporaneous comparison of hospital charges for laparoscopic and open Nissen fundoplication. *Surg Endosc* 1994;9:141–145.
106. Rattner DW, Brooks DC. Patient satisfaction following laparoscopic and open antireflux surgery. *Arch Surg* 1995;130:289–294.
107. Blomqvist AM, Lönroth H, Dalenbäck J, et al. Laparoscopic or open fundoplication? A complete cost analysis. *Surg Endosc* 1998;12:1209–1212.
108. Heikkinen TJ, Haukipuro K, Koivukangas P, et al. Comparison of costs between laparoscopic and open Nissen fundoplication: a prospective randomized study with a 3-month follow-up. *J Am Coll Surg* 1999;188:368–376.

SURGERY: SCIENTIFIC PRINCIPLES AND PRACTICE, Third Edition, edited by Lazar J. Greenfield, Michael W. Mulholland, Keith T. Oldham, Gerald B. Zelenock, and Keith D. Lillemoe. Lippincott Williams & Wilkins Publishers, Philadelphia, © 2001.

CHAPTER 20

TUMORS, INJURIES, AND MISCELLANEOUS CONDITIONS OF THE ESOPHAGUS

MARK B. ORRINGER

ESOPHAGEAL TUMORS

Anatomic and Physiologic Considerations

Most esophageal tumors are malignant; fewer than 1% are benign. A knowledge of the anatomic relations between the esophagus and adjacent structures is important, both in understanding the presentation of esophageal tumors at various levels and in planning therapy. For example, tumors involving the cervicothoracic esophagus (the segment between the cricopharyngeal sphincter and the thoracic inlet at the level of the suprasternal notch) often involve the larynx, and therefore a laryngopharyngectomy may be required if resection is undertaken. This operation, combined with a pharyngeal anastomosis to reestablish alimentary continuity, is far more extensive than the usual palliative esophageal resection for carcinoma of the intrathoracic esophagus. The upper thoracic esophagus is contiguous with the posterior membranous trachea anteriorly and the aortic arch and great vessels. Thus, patients

with cancer involving the upper thoracic esophagus should routinely undergo preoperative bronchoscopy to rule out invasion of the posterior membranous trachea, which precludes resection. When an upper thoracic esophageal tumor is resected through a thoracotomy, the approach is a *right* fourth or fifth interspace incision because the aortic arch interferes with mobilization of the upper thoracic esophagus through the left side of the chest. Midthoracic esophageal tumors can involve the carina or proximal main bronchi, particularly where the esophagus passes behind the left main bronchus, a common site for the development of a malignant tracheoesophageal fistula. Once again, because of its anatomic proximity to the tracheobronchial tree, a midthoracic esophageal tumor may require a *right* thoracotomy, which provides optimal exposure to the carina and proximal bronchi. Distal esophageal tumors, if approached transthoracically, are best managed through a *left-sided* approach because the most distal portion of the esophagus and the esophagogastric junction cannot be adequately visualized through the right side of the chest.

Another important anatomic feature to be considered when an esophageal resection is performed is the unique submucosa of the esophagus, the unusual fat content of which allows a great deal of mobility of the overlying mucosa. Unless great care is taken to ensure that every anastomotic stitch transfixes the submucosa, an anastomotic leak may occur if the mucosa retracts proximally and an accurate apposition of the mucosa is not achieved (1). The esophagus is a mucosa-lined muscular tube that lacks a serosa. It is surrounded by adventitia, or mediastinal connective tissue, which is a loose fibroareolar layer. Transmural invasion by esophageal carcinoma is exceedingly common because the tumor is not limited by overlying pleura; in contrast, intestinal cancers often extend to, but not through, the adjacent peritoneum.

Although its blood supply is segmental, the esophagus is well vascularized by numerous arteries, and it has an extensive submucosal collateral circulation. The cervical esophagus receives blood from the superior and inferior thyroid arteries, both communicating through collaterals. Four to six aortic esophageal arteries supply the intrathoracic esophagus and anastomose through collaterals with the inferior thyroid, intercostal and bronchial, inferior phrenic, and left gastric arteries. Anatomic studies of the esophageal blood supply indicate that the esophageal arteries terminate in fine capillary networks before actually penetrating the esophageal muscle layer (2). In the process of transhiatal esophageal mobilization, therefore, if the dissection is kept close to the esophageal wall, the risk for serious hemorrhage from a sizable vessel is minimal.

An understanding of esophageal innervation is important in explaining the effect on swallowing of tumors and operations involving the cervicothoracic esophagus (3). The esophagus is innervated through the visceral autonomic nervous system. Efferent sympathetic innervation, which affects vasoconstriction, peristalsis, contraction of the sphincters, and muscular wall relaxation, is through the cervical and thoracic sympathetic chain. Afferent parasympathetic innervation controls increases in glandular and peristaltic activity and is through the vagus nerves, which also carry some sensory fibers. The superior laryngeal nerves arise from the vagus nerves in the neck and divide into external and internal laryngeal branches. Both the cricothyroid muscle, which is the tensor of the vocal cords, and a portion of the inferior pharyngeal constrictor are supplied by the external laryngeal nerve, whereas the internal laryngeal nerve provides sensory innervation of the larynx above the vocal cords and the base of the tongue. The parasympathetic innervation of the cervical esophagus, in addition to innervation of the upper esophageal sphincter, is through the recurrent laryngeal branches of the vagus nerves. Therefore, injury to the recurrent laryngeal nerve during construction of a cervical esophagogastric anastomosis (or any cervical or thoracic operation) may produce not only hoarseness but also upper esophageal sphincter dysfunction, which is associated with incapacitating and life-threatening aspiration during swallowing. This is a disastrous complication in a patient undergoing an operation to reestablish the ability to swallow comfortably. Similarly, delayed gastric emptying resulting from impaired motility or pylorospasm after division of the vagus nerves during an esophagectomy for cancer may result in catastrophic regurgitation and aspiration.

Finally, gastroesophageal reflux is significant not only in the development of adenocarcinoma of the lower esophagus but also in the immediate and long-term functional results of an esophagogastric anastomosis. The relation between severe gastroesophageal reflux and the development of Barrett's mucosa and subsequent adenocarcinoma has been well described. After an esophageal resection for either benign or malignant disease, gastroesophageal reflux continues to play an important role. When a low intrathoracic esophagogastric anastomosis is performed, gastroesophageal reflux is almost certain to develop because an iatrogenic hiatal hernia has been created. The higher the esophagogastric anastomosis within the thorax, the lower the incidence of subsequent gastroesophageal reflux. With a cervical esophagogastric anastomosis, after which virtually the entire stomach is within the thorax and little is below the diaphragmatic hiatus, clinically significant gastroesophageal reflux is rare. Gastroesophageal reflux is also one of the important factors responsible for the morbidity associated with an intrathoracic esophagogastric anastomotic leak. The resultant mediastinitis and empyema are a consequence not only of the extravasation of saliva and oral bacteria but also of the chemical effects of refluxed bile and gastric acid draining through the anastomosis.

Benign Esophageal Tumors and Cysts

Benign tumors of the esophagus are rare, constituting only 0.5% to 0.8% of esophageal neoplasms (4). They are classified into two major groups: epithelial (mucosal) and intramural (extramucosal) (5) (Table 20.1). Still rarer are heterotopic collections of tissue within the esophageal wall.

Leiomyomas

Leiomyomas represent the most common benign intramural esophageal tumor and characteristically occur in patients between 20 and 50 years of age. The tumors are multiple in 3% to 10% of patients, have no established predilection for either sex, and can develop at any level of the esophagus, but rarely in the cervical segment. More than 80% of esophageal leiomyomas are located in the middle and lower thirds of the esophagus. Because leiomyomas can become calcified, they must be considered in the differential diagnosis of a calcified mediastinal mass. Histologically, leiomyomas are composed of interlacing bundles of smooth-muscle cells. Tumors less than 5 cm in diameter rarely cause symptoms. When they are larger, dysphagia, retrosternal pressure, and pain are the common complaints. Most reported leiomyomas have been found incidentally at autopsy and were asymptomatic. When a leiomyoma virtually encircles the esophageal lumen, obstruction and regurgitation can occur. Bleeding is more often associated with the malignant form

TABLE 20.1. CLASSIFICATION OF BENIGN ESOPHAGEAL TUMORS

EPITHELIAL TUMORS

Papillomas
Polyps
Adenomas
Cysts

NONEPITHELIAL TUMORS

Myomas
  Leiomyomas
  Fibromyomas
  Lipomyomas
Fibromas
Vascular tumors
  Hemangiomas
  Lymphangiomas
Mesenchymal and other tumors
  Reticuloendothelial tumors
  Lipomas
  Myxofibromas
  Giant cell tumors
  Neurofibromas
  Osteochondromas

HETEROTOPIC TUMORS

Gastric mucosal tumors
Melanoblastic tumors
Sebaceous gland tumors
Granular cell myoblastomas
Pancreatic gland tumors
Thyroid nodules

From Nemir P Jr, Wallace HW, Fallahnejad M. Diagnosis and surgical management of benign disease of the esophagus. *Curr Probl Surg* 1976;13:1, with permission.

of the tumor, leiomyosarcoma. Malignant degeneration of a leiomyoma is exceedingly rare, with fewer than 10 reported cases. Occasionally, large, confluent leiomyomas involve the lower esophagus and cardia. Most leiomyomas, however, are solitary and vary from 2 to 5 cm in diameter. An interesting variation of this tumor, diffuse leiomyomatosis of the esophagus, is characterized by extensive infiltration of the entire esophagus in addition to the development of multiple leiomyomas in the stomach, uterus, major airways, and ureters. This condition has been noted in children as young as 7 years of age, tends to occur in families, and may be associated with hypertrophy of the vulva and clitoris, cataracts, and deafness.

Esophageal leiomyomas produce a characteristic smooth, concave submucosal defect with sharp borders. Abrupt sharp angles form where the tumor meets the normal esophageal wall on barium swallow examination. The tumor often appears to lie half within and half outside the esophagus (Fig. 20.1). As with every esophageal tumor, esophagoscopy is indicated to exclude the presence of carcinoma. If the radiologic impression of a leiomyoma is confirmed endoscopically, a biopsy of the mass should *not* be performed so that subsequent extramural resection will not be complicated by scarring at the biopsy site. At esophagoscopy, these tumors are characteristically mobile, have an intact overlying mucosa, and can be displaced by the advancing esophagoscope. Endoscopic ultrasonography has provided a new means for evaluating the esophageal leiomyoma, which is seen as a distinct intramural mass of characteristically low echodensity (6).

An asymptomatic leiomyoma or one discovered incidentally on a barium swallow examination can be safely observed and followed with periodic barium esopha-

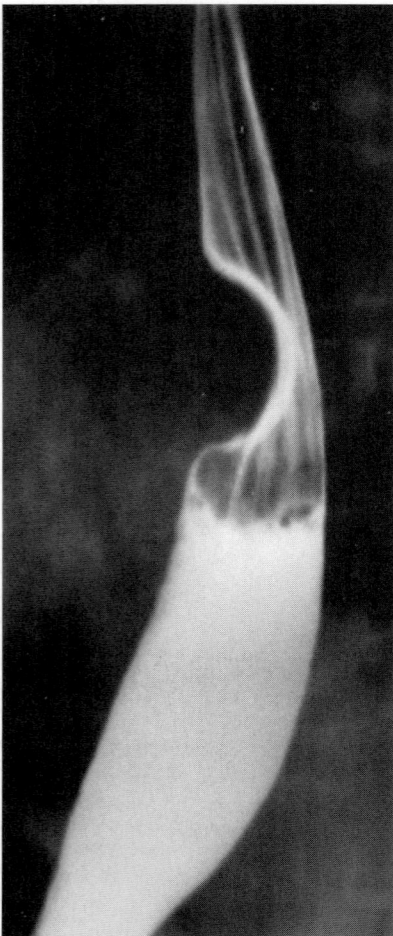

Figure 20.1. Esophagogram of a leiomyoma. The acute angle at its junction with the esophageal wall is typical. (From Orringer MB. Tumors of the esophagus. In: Sabiston DC Jr, ed. *Textbook of surgery,* 13th ed. Philadelphia: WB Saunders, 1986:736, with permission.)

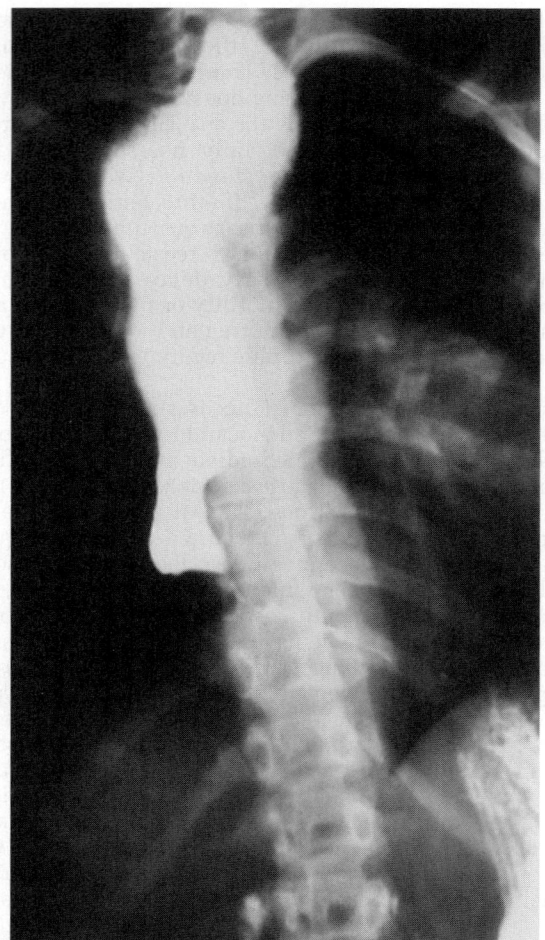

Figure 20.2. Esophagogram of a giant leiomyoma involving the distal half of the esophagus and esophagogastric junction. An esophagectomy was required to remove it. (From Orringer MB. Tumors of the esophagus. In: Sabiston DC Jr, ed. *Textbook of surgery,* 13th ed. Philadelphia: WB Saunders, 1986:737, with permission.)

gograms and endoscopic ultrasonography. Although excision of the esophageal mass provides the only definitive tissue diagnosis, the characteristic radiographic appearance, slow growth rate, and low risk for malignant degeneration, in addition to the ability to follow leiomyomas with endoscopic ultrasonography, justify conservative management. Tumors that are symptomatic or larger than 5 cm in diameter should be excised. Tumors of the middle third of the esophagus are approached through a right thoracotomy, and those in the distal third are approached through a left thoracotomy. Once the esophagus is encircled and the tumor located, the overlying longitudinal muscle is split in the direction of its fibers. The tumor is then gently dissected away from the contiguous underlying submucosa and adjacent muscle. When enucleation of the tumor is complete, the longitudinal esophageal muscle is reapproximated, although a large extramucosal defect may be left without complication. For the removal of giant leiomyomas of the cardia and adjacent stomach, esophageal resection may be required (Fig. 20.2). Alternatively, multiple enucleations may be performed. When resection is complete, leiomyomas virtually never recur.

Polyps

Benign polyps of the esophagus are rare and typically arise in the cervical portion. Traction on the polyps caused

by repeated peristaltic contractions results in progressive lengthening of their pedicles, which may be responsible for an occasionally dramatic presentation; they can intermittently extrude into and even out of the mouth or produce asphyxia as the upper airway becomes obstructed. Most benign polyps are seen in older men, frequently attached to the cricoid cartilage. The tumors typically produce dysphagia, but hematemesis or melena may occur if the overlying mucosa becomes ulcerated. The polyps tend to be solitary, with a long, cylindric configuration that can produce marked esophageal dilation. Histologically, they are composed of fibrovascular tissue with varying amounts of associated fat. Barium swallow findings may be nondiagnostic or inaccurately interpreted in these patients. The polyp may be overlooked as an air bubble or misdiagnosed as a carcinoma, or even as a foreign body or achalasia, if marked esophageal dilation is present (Fig. 20.3). Similarly, esophagoscopy may fail to define the polyp, particularly if the pedicle is not demonstrated and the mucosa overlying the polyp is normal. The endoscopist simply passes the lesion, which is soft and easily displaced with the esophagus. Although esophageal polyps have been removed endoscopically by electrocoagulation of the pedicle, the recommended approach is resection through a lateral cervical esophagotomy. The

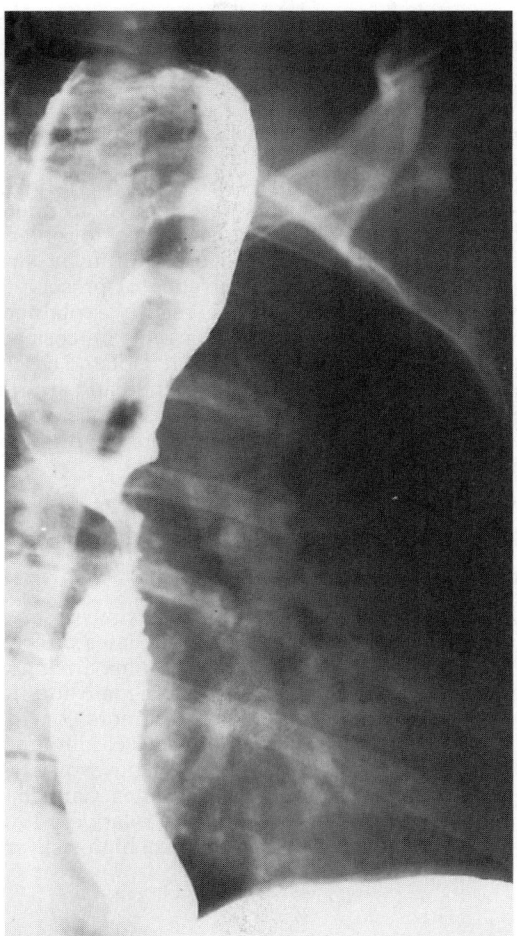

Figure 20.3. Barium esophagogram of a giant benign fibroepithelial polyp showing a large intraluminal mass distending the cervical and upper thoracic esophagus. [From Orringer MB. Miscellaneous conditions of the esophagus. In: Orringer MB, Zuidema GD, eds. *Shackelford's surgery of the alimentary tract*, vol 1 *(The esophagus)*. Philadelphia: WB Saunders, 1991:460, with permission.]

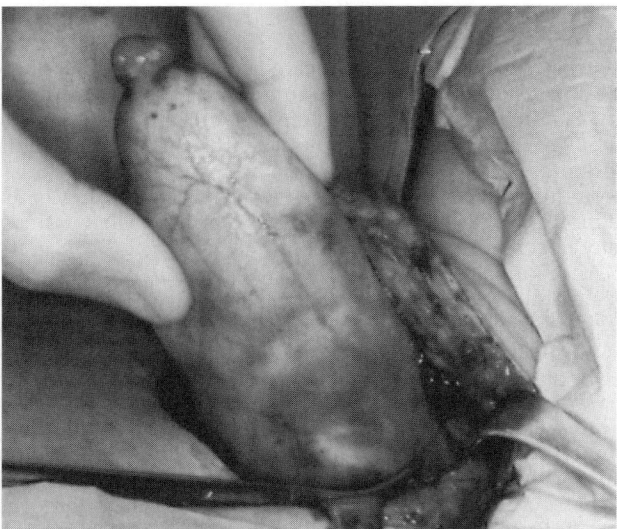

Figure 20.4. Operative photograph of the patient shown in Fig. 20.3. The giant polyp has been delivered out of the cervical esophagus through a left-sided neck incision. The patient's head is toward the right, and the retractors are against the sternocleidomastoid muscle. The hemostat indicates the base of the polyp, which was divided and oversewn without difficulty. [From Orringer MB. Miscellaneous conditions of the esophagus. In: Orringer MB, Zuidema GD, eds. *Shackelford's surgery of the alimentary tract,* vol 1 *(The esophagus)*. Philadelphia: WB Saunders, 1991:470, with permission.]

polyp is delivered from the esophagus, its mucosal base of origin is resected, and the defect is repaired under direct vision (Fig. 20.4).

Hemangiomas

Esophageal hemangiomas are rare, constituting 2% to 3% of benign tumors. Although they are generally asymptomatic, they can be responsible for periodic gastrointestinal bleeding or even massive and fatal hematemesis. Asymptomatic lesions discovered incidentally during an esophagoscopy should be followed with periodic endoscopy. Those that have bled require treatment, and although resection has been the standard approach, laser endoscopy provides an effective alternative to control small sites of bleeding visualized through the esophagoscope.

Miscellaneous Benign Tumors

Benign esophageal tumors other than leiomyomas and polyps are extremely rare. *Granular cell myoblastomas* actually arise from Schwann cells, not from muscle, as their name implies. They cause dysphagia, retrosternal pain, nausea, and vomiting. They are difficult to diagnose endoscopically because of their submucosal location and have a characteristic grayish yellow appearance. The overlying mucosa typically shows pseudoepitheliomatous hyperplasia, which may be misdiagnosed histologically as squamous cell carcinoma. Local excision is sufficient treatment for symptomatic tumors. *Papillomas,* sessile lobulated tumors that have a fibrous core and are covered by squamous mucosa, have been reported. Most occur in association with some degree of esophageal obstruction, most often in the distal portion. Papillomas have been postulated to represent localized epithelial hyperplasia or even to be premalignant lesions, but their true significance is unknown. On the basis of their size and radiographic configuration, papillomas at times warrant esophageal exploration to exclude malignancy, but a major resection should be avoided because local excision is adequate therapy. *Esophageal adenomas, carcinoid tumors,* and *inflammatory pseudotumors* also have been reported but are so rare that they are mentioned only for the sake of completeness.

Cysts

Esophageal cysts arise as outpouchings of the embryonic foregut. Embryologically, the esophagus is lined by simple columnar ciliated epithelium, which is eventually replaced by stratified squamous epithelium. Esophageal cysts can therefore contain both types of epithelium, in addition to fat and smooth muscle. The esophageal duplication cyst is a variation of the foregut cyst; it extends along the length of the thoracic esophagus and is lined by squamous epithelium. It has submucosal and muscle layers, the latter of which interdigitates with the outer, longitudinal muscle layer of the normal esophagus. Three fourths of esophageal duplication cysts present in childhood, and more than 60% are located along the right side of the esophagus. Like other foregut cysts, esophageal duplication cysts are frequently associated with vertebral anomalies (Klippel-Feil deformity or spina bifida) and spinal cord abnormalities. More than 60% of esophageal cysts cause either respiratory or esophageal symptoms in the first year of life. Those located in the upper third of the esophagus tend to present in infancy, whereas cysts in the lower third may be asymptomatic initially and present later in childhood. In adults, symptoms of dysphagia, choking, or retrosternal pain develop when a previously asymptomatic cyst enlarges as a result of bleeding or infection. The rare cyst that contains ectopic gastric mucosa may become perforated.

An esophageal cyst can usually be diagnosed on the basis of its typical radiographic appearance (Fig. 20.5). On the standard posteroanterior chest roentgenogram, the cyst may cause displacement of the trachea; on a lateral chest roentgenogram, it may appear as a retrocardiac posterior mediastinal mass. The barium esophagogram demonstrates a smooth, extramucosal esophageal mass that rarely communicates with the esophageal lumen. The cystic nature of the lesion and its relation with adjacent mediastinal structures may be delineated by computed tomography (CT), although this study is not generally necessary to make the diagnosis. When a duplication cyst is suspected, spinal radiographs should be obtained preoperatively to identify an origin of the cyst in the notochord. Because esophageal cysts tend to be associated with bleeding, ulceration, perforation, and infection, excision is generally recommended. This can generally be achieved with low morbidity by an extramucosal resection. In the rare event that the wall of the cyst cannot be separated from the common esophageal wall, it can be left behind, but the mucosa of the cyst should be stripped away to prevent recurrence. Alternative surgical treatments, such as marsupialization of the cyst, internal drainage, or cauterization of the mu-cosa, do not represent optimal management. Recurrence of the cyst after complete excision is rare.

Heterotopic Tumors

Islets of columnar mucosa may be found lining the pharynx and esophagus. These islets are much more common near the upper end than near the lower end of the esophagus. Endoscopically, they are described as an *inlet patch* of columnar mucosa. Given the embryologic replacement of the initial columnar ciliated epithelium by stratified squamous epithelium, the occurrence of preserved inlet patches of columnar epithelium is readily explained. This tissue is not to be confused with Barrett's mucosa and has little, if any, premalignant disposition. Isolated cases of sebaceous gland tumors and ectopic pancreatic and thyroid tissue within the esophagus have also been reported. These have primarily been autopsy reports with little clinical significance.

Malignant Esophageal Tumors

Squamous Cell Carcinoma

Worldwide, 95% of all esophageal cancers are squamous cell carcinomas. In the United States and Europe, however, the incidence of adenocarcinoma arising in Barrett's mucosa is increasing at an alarming rate and in many areas surpasses that of squamous cell tumors. A wide variation in the incidence of squamous cell carcinoma of the esophagus has been noted throughout the world. Among the white populations of the United States, Canada, Israel, Nigeria, and Europe, the incidence is relatively low (3 or 4/100,000 population). In contrast, in high-risk areas of

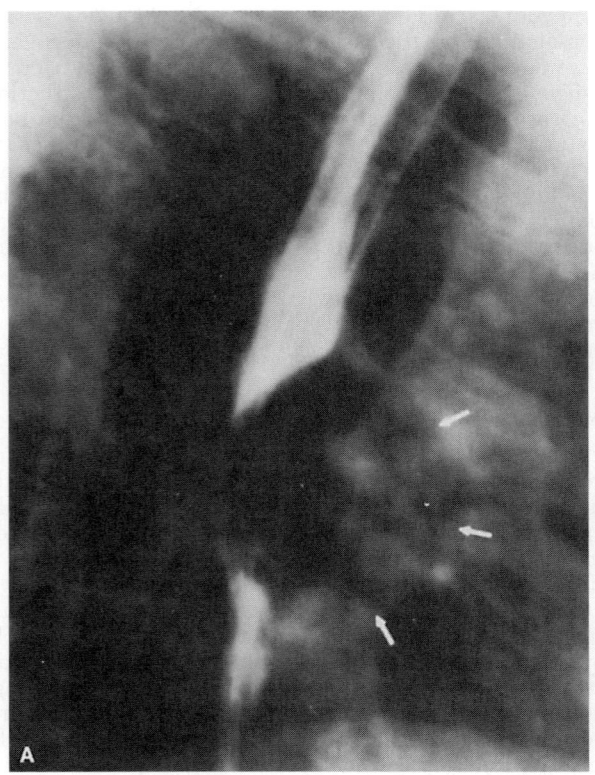
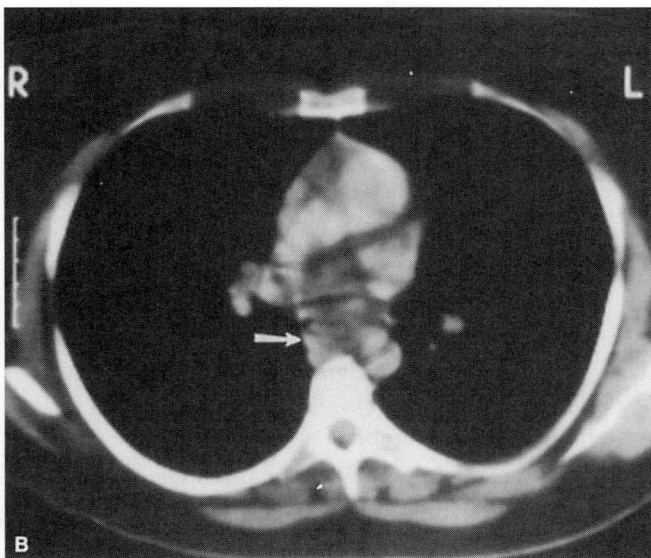

Figure 20.5. Esophageal duplication cyst presenting as a high posterior mediastinal mass. *(A)* Barium esophagogram showing the intramural, extramucosal esophageal mass. *(B)* Computed tomogram showing the cystic nature of the lesion *(arrow).*

northeastern Iran, Transkei in South Africa, Linxian County in Hunan Province in northern China, and certain areas of southern Russia that border on the Caspian Sea, the incidence is more than 35/100,000 population and is as high as 53 to 800/100,000 population in people older than 50 years of age (7,8). This disease occurs most commonly in the seventh decade of life and generally is 1.5 to 3 times more common in men than in women. The predilection for men, however, is reversed in those regions with a high incidence of Plummer-Vinson syndrome, which more commonly affects women.

The cause of esophageal carcinoma is unknown. It is thought to occur most often as a result of prolonged exposure of the esophageal mucosa to noxious stimuli in persons who have a genetic predisposition to the disease. Epidemiologic studies in endemic areas of China, for example, suggest that the presence of large amounts of carcinogenic nitrosamines in the soil and the contamination of foods by mutagenic fungi, most often *Geotrichum candidum,* and yeast are responsible for the high incidence of this tumor. In northeast Iran, esophageal carcinoma is primarily a condition of the poorest social stratum; the use of opium, which contains pyrolysates, and the ingestion of very hot tea are believed to result in repeated esophageal mucosal injury and eventual malignant degeneration. Chewing tobacco with or without betel nut, betel leaf, slaked lime, or a resin from the acacia has been linked to the development of esophageal carcinoma in India, Pakistan, and Sri Lanka. In Singapore, the ingestion of burning-hot beverages and the use of Chinese tobacco and wine are believed to be etiologic factors. The increased incidence of esophageal carcinoma among the South African Bantus and Zulus has been linked to the high nitrosamine content of the soil in that region and to the contamination of food by molds, especially the *Fusarium* species, which produces carcinogens. The most consistent risk factors among populations from Normandy, Brittany, Europe, and the United States are alcohol consumption and cigarette smoking. Carcinomas of the hypopharynx and cervical esophagus occur almost as often in women as in men, probably as the result of the higher incidence of Plummer-Vinson syndrome in women. In Sri Lanka, esophageal carcinoma is primarily a disease of women and is the most commonly encountered gastrointestinal tract malignancy. Alcohol, tobacco, zinc, nitrosamines, malnutrition, vitamin deficiencies, anemia, poor oral hygiene, dental caries, previous gastric surgery, and chronic ingestion of hot foods or beverages have all been linked to the development of esophageal cancer. In addition, certain premalignant esophageal conditions are well recognized and are discussed later.

Pathologically, esophageal carcinoma occurs over a spectrum that ranges from the early lesion, termed *early carcinoma, superficial spreading carcinoma, intramucosal carcinoma,* or *carcinoma in situ,* which is limited to the mucosa, to the more advanced form, in which the tumor penetrates the muscle layers of the esophagus or beyond. Carcinoma in situ typically is found in patients between 40 and 50 years of age and gradually progresses to invasive squamous cell carcinoma within 2 to 4 years. Microscopically, early esophageal carcinoma is defined in terms of the depth of tumor involvement: intraepithelial (carcinoma in situ), intramucosal (limited to the lamina propria), or submucosal. The histologic features of esophageal dysplasia resemble those of dysplasia in the uterine cervix, and as dysplasia becomes severe, histologic differentiation from carcinoma in situ becomes difficult. Once dysplastic cells are seen traversing the basement membrane and extending into the underlying connective tissue, the diagnosis of early invasion is made. Carcinoma in

situ of the esophagus tends to be multifocal. Early esophageal carcinoma has been well documented in China, where the high incidence of esophageal carcinoma has justified mass screening techniques, and the disease is frequently detected before it has advanced enough to cause symptoms. Thus, several macroscopic growth patterns have been defined: a coarsely granular, reddish, slightly raised, plaquelike type; an erosive type; the occult form, which is not apparent on gross inspection of the esophagus; and the papillary type, in which a slightly polypoid lesion of less than 3 cm is seen. Advanced squamous cell carcinoma of the esophagus is defined as a tumor that involves the muscle layers of the esophagus or beyond.

Adenocarcinoma

Adenocarcinomas account for 2.5% to 8% of primary esophageal cancers, but in the United States and Europe, the frequency of this tumor is increasing at a rate surpassing that of any other cancer (9–12). This increase is largely the result of the growing prevalence of adenocarcinoma arising in Barrett's mucosa. Approximately 12,300 new cases and 11,900 deaths from esophageal cancer occurred in the United States in 1998 (13). Nearly 90% of cases in the 1960s were squamous cell carcinoma, but currently, more than half of the esophageal cancers seen in this country are adenocarcinomas of the distal esophagus, gastroesophageal junction, or cardia. The annual rates of esophageal adenocarcinoma per 100,000 population increased by more than 350% between 1974 and 1994 (9). Adenocarcinomas most often involve the distal third of the esophagus, have a peak incidence in the sixth decade of life, and are three times more common in men than in woman. Risk factors include gastroesophageal reflux disease, obesity, smoking, and Barrett's metaplasia. The potential origins of esophageal adenocarcinoma are threefold: (a) metaplastic columnar epithelium (Barrett's mucosa), (b) heterotopic islands of columnar epithelium, and (c) esophageal submucosal glands. In addition, the esophagus may be involved secondarily by a gastric carcinoma growing upward.

Severe gastroesophageal reflux is a major factor in the development of a columnar epithelium-lined (Barrett's) esophagus (14). Refluxed gastric acid, proteases, and bile erode the normal squamous epithelium, and the residual pluripotent basal cells may differentiate along multiple cell lines to produce a variety of columnar epithelial cell types. Until recently, Barrett's mucosa was recognized as occurring in three characteristic histologic patterns:

1. *Gastric fundus-type epithelium,* which has a foveolar surface pattern (no villi) but contains glands with parietal cells, chief cells, and mucous cells.
2. *Junctional-type epithelium,* in which no villi are present and cardiac-type mucous glands without parietal or chief cells are seen. The mucosa has a foveolar pattern that is flat and typically is seen in normal colon and gastric cardia and in villous atrophy of the small bowel.
3. *Specialized columnar epithelium,* which is typically characterized by villiform folds lined by a single layer of glycoprotein-secreting columnar cells and mucus-secreting goblet cells. Cryptlike glands between the villi are also lined by columnar and goblet cells and contain few if any parietal or chief cells. This epithelium has also been termed *incomplete intestinal metaplasia* because only the goblet cell component of intestinal epithelium is present (Fig. 20.6).

The latter specialized or intestinal type of metaplasia has the highest association with carcinoma. It is estimated that adenocarcinoma is 40 times more likely to develop in

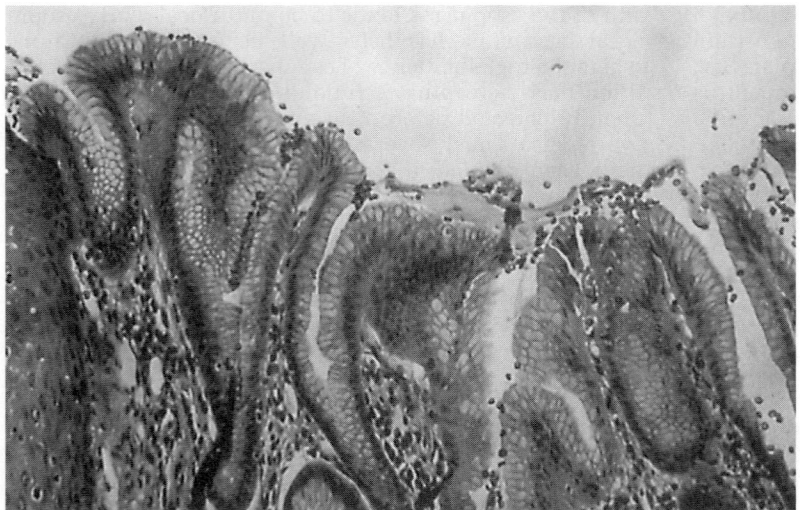

Figure 20.6. Photomicrograph of an esophageal biopsy specimen showing Barrett's mucosa with intestinal metaplasia and no dysplasia. Note the villiform folds lined by uniform goblet cells. The nuclei of all the cells are basally oriented.

patients with Barrett's esophagus than in the general population. The true incidence of Barrett's esophagus in the general population is unknown, but it is estimated that adenocarcinoma arises in up to 8% to 15% of patients with a columnar epithelium-lined esophagus. Dysplasia occurs to varying degrees in Barrett's mucosa, and dysplasia clearly is a premalignant esophageal lesion. The histologic features of dysplasia are an increased nuclear-to-cytoplasmic ratio, loss of the basilar orientation of the epithelial cells along the basement membrane, irregular chromatin clumping, hyperchromatic nuclei, and prominence of the nucleoli (Fig. 20.7). Severe dysplasia is almost always associated with carcinoma in situ and generally mandates aggressive therapy with esophagectomy.

Because gastric columnar mucosa may be found within 1 to 2 cm of the esophagogastric junction in normal anatomic variations, the traditional teaching was that the diagnosis of Barrett's mucosa is established at endoscopy by histologic documentation of columnar mucosa extending into the tubular esophagus at least 2 cm above the anatomic esophagogastric junction. New guidelines for the definition of Barrett's mucosa, however, have recently been established by the American College of Gastroenterology (15). Barrett's mucosa is now defined as changed esophageal epithelium of *any* length that (a) can be *recognized at*

endoscopy and (b) demonstrates *intestinal metaplasia* (with goblet cells) on biopsy. Although the squamocolumnar epithelial junction in Barrett's esophagus may extend to the level of the thoracic inlet, "short-segment" Barrett's mucosa within 1 to 2 cm of the esophagogastric junction has now become a well-recognized clinical entity.

Like squamous cell carcinoma, esophageal adenocarcinoma exhibits an aggressive biologic behavior that is characterized by frequent transmural invasion and lymphatic spread. Because many of these tumors arise in the lower third of the esophagus, paraesophageal, celiac axis, and splenic hilum lymph node metastases are common. The lung and liver are the viscera most frequently involved by metastases. Esophageal adenocarcinoma is associated with a 5-year survival rate of zero to 7%. Without lymph node involvement, survival of 5 years is possible; the average survival is only 9 months in patients with lymph node involvement.

Other Malignancies

Anaplastic small cell (oat cell) carcinoma arises in the esophagus from the same argyrophilic cells that give rise to this tumor in the lung. Like their pulmonary counterparts, these tumors contain neurosecretory granules on electron microscopy. They are extremely aggressive tumors, com-

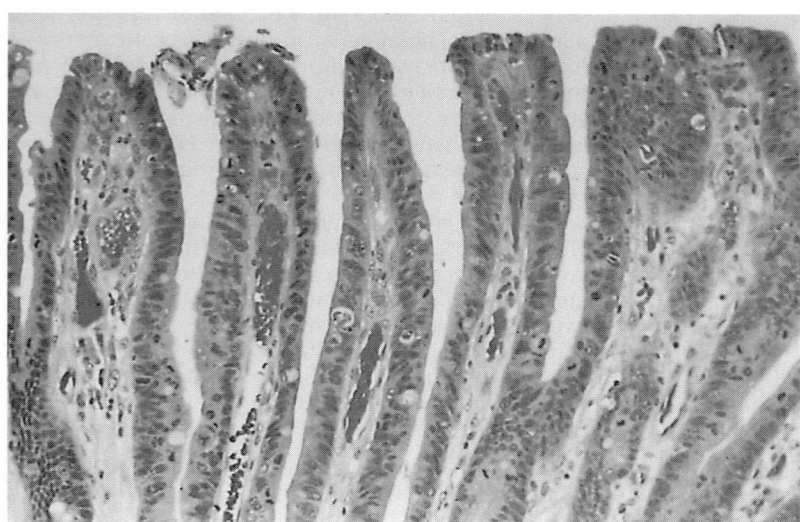

Figure 20.7. Photomicrograph of esophageal biopsy specimen showing Barrett's mucosa with intestinal metaplasia and high-grade dysplasia. In contrast to the cells in Fig. 20.6, these epithelial cells have lost their basilar orientation along the basement membrane, their nuclei are of varying sizes and hyperchromatic, and their nucleoli are prominent.

monly associated with distant spread at the time of diagnosis, and survival beyond 1 year is rare (16,17).

Adenoid cystic esophageal carcinoma is another rare lesion, and fewer than 50 cases have been reported. These tumors typically occur in the middle third of the esophagus, are discovered late in their course, metastasize widely, and are associated with a median survival of only 9 months (18).

About 100 cases of malignant melanoma of the esophagus have been reported, and these rare lesions constitute fewer than 0.1% of esophageal malignancies. Malignant melanoma may involve the esophagus either as a primary tumor or as a secondary metastasis. In the former situation, it is thought to arise from melanocytes in the esophagus. These tumors typically present as large (≥ 7 cm) polypoid masses, which may or may not be pigmented. The average survival is only 13.4 months, and fewer than 5% of patients survive 5 years. Metastasis to liver, lymph nodes, lung, and brain is common (19,20).

Carcinosarcoma is a lesion of the esophagus that has histologic features of both squamous cell carcinoma and malignant spindle cell sarcoma. These typically polypoid tumors generally occur in the distal two thirds of the esophagus, grow to large size (10 to 15 cm), and have a poor prognosis, with 2% to 6% of patients surviving 5 years (21,22).

Staging

In the tumor–node–metastasis (TNM) classification for staging esophageal cancer, the esophagus is divided into four main sections: (a) *cervical* (from the lower border of the cricoid cartilage to the thoracic inlet, or approximately 18 cm from the upper incisor teeth); (b) *upper thoracic* (from the thoracic inlet to the level of the carina at about 24 cm at endoscopy); (c) *middle third* (from the carina to half the distance to the esophagogastric junction, or about 32 cm); and (d) *lower* (to the esophagogastric junction at 40 cm) (23) (Table 20.2). When this arbitrary division of the esophagus is used, 8% of squamous cell carcinomas occur in the cervical esophagus, 55% in the upper and middle thoracic segments, and 37% in the lower thoracic segment. Microscopically, most squamous cell carcinomas of the esophagus are moderately differentiated; islands of atypical squamous cells infiltrate the underlying adjacent normal tissues, and keratin pearls and intercellular bridges are seen between the tumor cells. Macroscopically, 60% of these lesions are fungating intraluminal growths, 25% are ulcerative lesions associated with extensive infiltration of the adjacent esophageal wall, and 15% are infiltrating. Esophageal carcinoma tends to be multifocal, and a patient who survives treatment of one carcinoma has a

---

Table 20.2. TNM STAGING CLASSIFICATION FOR CANCER OF THE ESOPHAGUS

TNM DEFINITIONS

Primary tumor (T)

TX	Primary tumor cannot be assessed (cytologically positive tumor not evident endoscopically or radiographically)
T0	No evidence of primary tumor (e.g., after treatment with radiation and chemotherapy)
Tis	Carcinoma in situ
T1	Tumor invades lamina propria or submucosa, but not beyond it
T2	Tumor invades muscularis propria
T3	Tumor invades adventitia
T4	Tumor invades adjacent structures (e.g., aorta, tracheobronchial tree, vertebral bodies, pericardium)

Regional lymph node involvement (N)

NX	Regional nodes cannot be assessed
N0	No regional node metastasis
N1	Regional node metastasis

Distant metastasis (M)

MX	Presence of distant metastasis cannot be assessed
M0	No distant metastasis
M1	**Distant metastasis**

Tumors of the lower thoracic esophagus
    M1a Metastasis in celiac lymph nodes
    M1b Other distant metastasis
Tumors of the midthoracic esophagus
    M1a Not applicable
    M1b Nonregional lymph nodes and/or other distant metastasis
Tumors of the upper thoracic esophagus
    M1a Metastasis in cervical nodes
    M1b Other distant metastasis

STAGE GROUPING

Stage 0	Tis N0 M0
Stage I	T1 N0 M0
Stage IIA	T2 N0 M0
	T3 N0 M0
Stage IIB	T1 N1 M0
	T2 N1 M0
Stage III	T3 N1 M0
	T4 any N M0
Stage IV	Any T any N M1
Stage IVA	Any T any N M1a
Stage IVB	Any T any N M1b

Adapted from Fleming ID, Cooper JS, Henson DE, et al., eds. American Joint Commission on Cancer staging handbook. From the AJCC staging manual, 5th ed. Philadelphia: Lippincott–Raven, 1998:65–69.

risk for the development of a second primary esophageal neoplasm at least twice that of the normal population.

Esophageal carcinoma is notorious for its aggressive biologic behavior. It tends to infiltrate locally, involving adjacent lymph nodes and spreading along the extensive submucosal esophageal lymphatic channels. Lack of an esophageal serosa favors tumor extension into adjacent structures, such as the pericardium, aorta, tracheobronchial tree, diaphragm, stomach, and left recurrent laryngeal nerve. Mediastinal, supraclavicular, or celiac lymph node metastases are present in at least 75% of patients with esophageal cancer at the time of initial diagnosis. Cervical esophageal cancers tend to drain to the deep cervical, paraesophageal, posterior mediastinal, and tracheobronchial lymph nodes, whereas lower esophageal tumors spread to paraesophageal, celiac, and splenic hilar lymph nodes. Distant spread to the liver and lungs is seen in 90% of cases at autopsy. The overall prognosis for a patient with invasive squamous cell carcinoma is dismal; 5% to 12% of patients survive 5 years. Unfortunately, extraesophageal tumor extension is present in 70% of cases at the time of diagnosis, and when lymph node metastases are present, 5-year survival is only 3%; survival is 42% when lymph node spread is absent.

Pathophysiology of Esophageal Neoplasms

Local Effects. The symptoms of esophageal carcinoma may be insidious at onset, beginning as nonspecific retrosternal discomfort, indigestion, or transient dysphagia. Early esophageal carcinoma that is limited to the mucosa or submucosa may be completely asymptomatic or may produce localized spasm that is manifested as periodic esophageal obstruction. Because the esophagus is a distensible tube, a major portion of the circumference must be involved before obstructive symptoms develop. Many patients who sense difficulty in swallowing a bolus of meat or bread subconsciously alter their eating habits by eliminating these coarse foods, chewing their food more thoroughly, and using more liquids to wash down food. By the time of presentation to a physician with a complaint of dysphagia, symptoms have often been present for 6 to 8 months.

Dysphagia is the most common presenting symptom of esophageal carcinoma. It develops in 90% of patients and is the primary manifestation of the disease in more than 80%. Dysphagia may present in several ways. It may be a subtle retrosternal discomfort as a bolus of food is swallowed, a transient feeling of retrosternal discomfort with swallowing that may not recur for several weeks or months, painful swallowing (odynophagia), or complete esophageal obstruction. *Weight loss* is the next most common symptom and is present in about 40% of patients with esophageal carcinoma. *Pain* is the initial symptom in 10% of patients. It may be precordial, retrosternal, epigastric, or intrascapular. Transient retrosternal pain radiating to the back or neck as the solid bolus of food passes through the tumor and causes local distention or muscle contraction has a much different implication than constant, boring retrosternal or epigastric pain, which more often represents local invasion by the tumor. *Regurgitation* of undigested food that has not passed through the esophagus should not be confused with the vomiting of gastric contents. *Respiratory symptoms* may be caused by either aspiration or direct invasion of the tracheobronchial tree by the tumor. These symptoms include cough, dyspnea, pleuritic pain, and hemoptysis. *Hematemesis* is a rare, early symptom of esophageal carcinoma, but bleeding from an esophageal malignancy is seldom of sufficient quantity to cause melena. *Hoarseness* from recurrent laryngeal nerve involvement is an ominous sign of unresectability. The course of the left main bronchus

anterior to the esophagus at the level of the carina is significant in the patient with a midesophageal tumor, which may involve the common wall between the esophagus and left main bronchus and lead to the development of a malignant tracheoesophageal fistula. This is manifested clinically by paroxysmal coughing when food or liquid is swallowed.

Systemic Effects. Although the systemic effects of esophageal carcinoma are less well recognized than the local effects, they may be significant clinically. Weight loss and the negative nitrogen balance resulting from starvation are directly related to the morbidity and mortality associated with esophageal resection in these patients. Virtually every patient with advanced esophageal obstruction is dehydrated, with a depleted total body volume as a result of impaired oral intake. The patient with esophageal obstruction is prone to the development of severe hypokalemia with secondary muscle weakness. One to two liters of saliva is produced each day, and the concentration of potassium within saliva (20 mEq/mL) is higher than that in any other gastrointestinal secretions. Patients who are unable to swallow their saliva, therefore, may present with marked hypokalemia. Fever and systemic toxicity may be caused by aspiration from the obstructed esophagus.

The production of parathyroid hormone by some squamous cell esophageal carcinomas has been documented and may result in hypercalcemia, even in the absence of bone metastases. Preoperative hypercalcemia in the patient with esophageal carcinoma and no demonstrable bone metastases has been suggested to be a poor prognostic sign. The occurrence of hypertrophic osteoarthropathy in association with carcinoma of the esophagus has been reported. Dermatomyositis frequently accompanies underlying malignancy and has been seen in patients with occult esophageal carcinoma. What appears to be a vagus nerve-mediated response, "swallow syncope," has been reported in a few patients with esophageal obstruction caused by carcinoma.

Diagnostic Investigations

History and Physical Examination. Because dysphagia is the primary presenting symptom in more than 90% of patients with esophageal carcinoma (24), a complaint of dysphagia in any adult cannot be taken lightly. In most cases, particularly in patients 50 years of age or older, a complaint of dysphagia warrants *both* a barium swallow examination *and* an endoscopic evaluation to rule out the presence of carcinoma. The combination of esophageal biopsy and brushings for cytologic evaluation establishes a diagnosis of carcinoma in 95% of patients with malignant strictures. When an increase in retrosternal discomfort develops in a patient with longstanding symptoms of reflux that have previously been well controlled by medical therapy, the patient should not be presumed to have esophagitis. Rather, an appropriate radiographic and endoscopic evaluation should be performed. Aside from evidence of weight loss, most patients with esophageal carcinoma have few objective findings on physical examination to aid in the diagnosis. Nonetheless, a careful examination for cervical or supraclavicular lymph node metastases, abdominal masses, and liver nodularity is warranted. The finding of a hard supraclavicular lymph node in a patient with an intrathoracic esophageal carcinoma warrants fine-needle aspiration (FNA) biopsy. If metastatic disease is documented, the presence of a stage IV tumor has been established. Resectional therapy of the esophageal tumor in this situation is not justified because the patient's expected survival is so poor. Laboratory studies should include a complete blood cell count, measurement of blood urea nitrogen and serum creatinine levels to assess the state of hydration, and, when indicated, liver function tests, including measurement of total protein and albumin levels, to assess the nutritional status. Levels of serum electrolytes, particularly potassium and calcium, should also be determined.

In obtaining a history from the patient with dysphagia, the physician should ask the patient to localize the point at which food lodges during swallowing by placing one finger on the anterior chest or neck. The patient with a mechanical esophageal obstruction, such as a carcinoma, is able to localize the consistent point of obstruction without difficulty. In contrast, the patient with neuromotor obstruction may sense only slow esophageal emptying diffusely in the retrosternal area.

Imaging Studies. A *barium swallow examination* is the first study that should be obtained in a patient with dysphagia. Tumors of the cervical esophagus are most difficult to identify by barium swallow examination, and carcinoma of the cardia may be confused with achalasia, a benign stricture, or esophageal spasm. Nevertheless, the barium swallow examination localizes obvious esophageal disease in preparation for subsequent esophagoscopy and allows the endoscopist to predict the level at which the tumor is located and the area that requires the most careful examination. The typical esophageal carcinoma presents radiographically as an irregular, rigid narrowing of the esophageal wall (Fig. 20.8). The normal mucosal pattern is frequently destroyed. Polypoid fungating tumors present as irregular filling defects with ulcerated borders within the esophagus. An old dictum relates that an esophageal dilation proximal to a stenosis is most indicative of a benign chronic obstruction, whereas an esophageal segment proximal to a carcinoma has "not had

enough time" to dilate. This observation has proved to be incorrect on numerous occasions. Similarly, although a smooth, tapered radiographic esophageal stricture supposedly reflects benign disease, any stenosis merits esophageal biopsy and brushings for cytologic evaluation to rule out carcinoma. The barium swallow examination may also show a soft-tissue mass adjacent to the esophageal tumor, which is indicative of extraesophageal local invasion. In only half of patients with esophageal carcinoma is the appearance on the plain *chest radiograph* abnormal; the most common findings are an air–fluid level in the obstructed esophagus, a dilated esophagus, abnormal mediastinal soft tissue representing adenopathy, pleural effusions, and pulmonary metastases.

Computed tomography (CT) of the chest and upper abdomen is the standard radiographic technique for staging esophageal carcinoma. The normal esophageal wall thickness should not exceed 5 mm on CT, which is also helpful in demonstrating regional adenopathy or pulmonary, liver, adrenal, or distant nodal metastases. When distant metastases (e.g., to liver or lung) are suspected on CT, a tissue diagnosis with FNA biopsy is warranted. A positive histologic diagnosis of stage IV carcinoma translates to an average survival of only 6 to 12 months, and therefore an operation of the magnitude of esophagectomy is contraindicated. Several investigators have reported the value of CT in evaluating the resectability of esophageal carcinoma. Gastric invasion, however, is difficult to detect with CT because gastric folds usually collapse, and the coexistence of a hiatal hernia renders evaluation of both tumor length and gastric extension by CT difficult. It has also been shown that CT is not useful in assessing aortic invasion by the tumor because contiguity of the esophageal mass with the aorta does not prove invasion, and resection

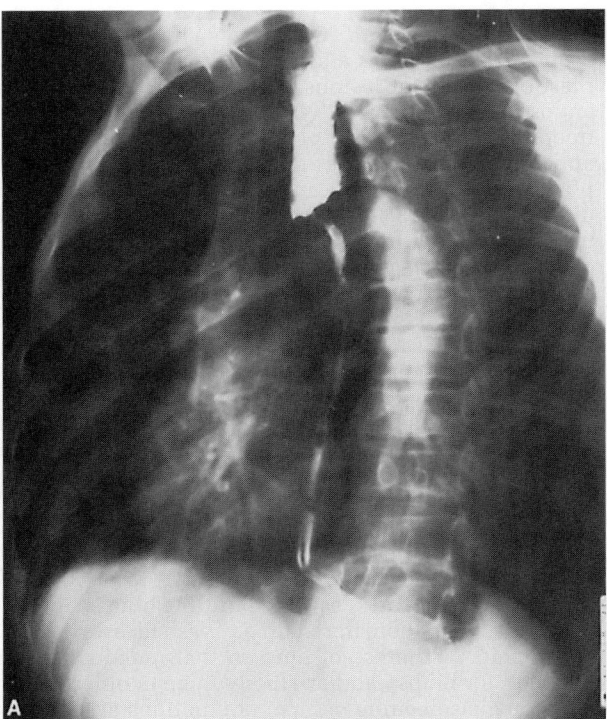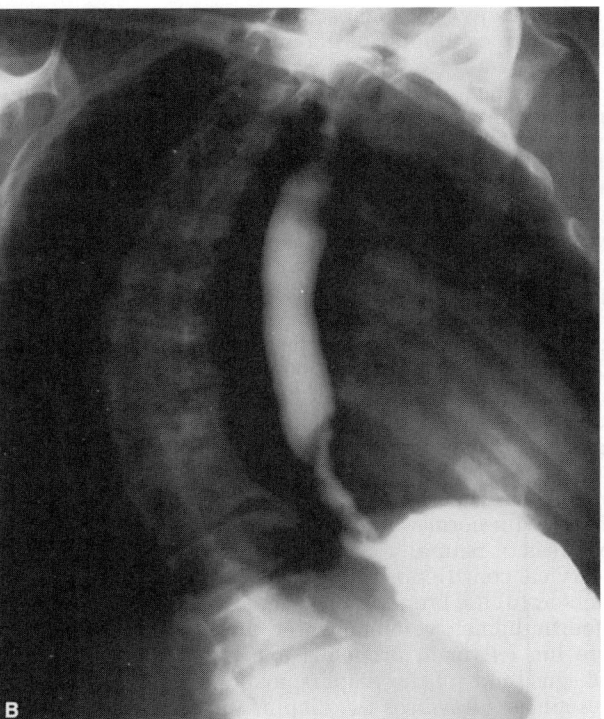

Figure 20.8. *(A)* Barium esophagogram showing an upper esophageal squamous cell carcinoma at the level of the aortic arch. Note the mucosal irregularity and shelf of tumor, which is characteristic of carcinoma. *(B)* Esophagogram showing a distal esophageal adenocarcinoma presenting as a characteristic apple core constriction above the esophagogastric junction. (From Orringer MB. Tumors of the esophagus. In: Sabiston DC Jr, ed. *Textbook of surgery,* 13th ed. Philadelphia: WB Saunders, 1986:736, with permission.)

is often possible even in patients with more than 90 degrees of contact between the esophagus and aorta (25).

Position emission tomography has recently emerged as a new modality for staging esophageal cancer and has been particularly useful in detecting distant metastases (26,27). Endoscopic ultrasonography (EUS) has become increasingly popular as a method for staging esophageal carcinoma and defining the depth of tumor invasion and involvement of mediastinal lymph nodes. The five layers of the normal esophageal wall—mucosa, lamina propria, muscularis mucosae, muscularis propria, and adventitia—are clearly identified with EUS, and tumors present as irregular, hypoechoic masses with varying depths of invasion. Mediastinal lymph nodes containing metastases are often 6 to 8 mm or larger in diameter and are more irregular and hypoechoic than normal lymph nodes. The accuracy of EUS in determining the depth of tumor invasion is approximately 85%, and its accuracy for detecting mediastinal lymph node metastases is 75% to 90% (6,28–32). Recently, EUS has been used in combination with FNA biopsy to confirm celiac lymph node metastases in patients with esophageal carcinoma (33).

Other Studies. Magnetic resonance imaging to evaluate mediastinal invasion has not gained widespread popularity. Bone scanning is not warranted unless the patient has specific complaints suggesting that bone metastases exist. Similarly, routine brain scans are not indicated because brain metastases from carcinoma of the esophagus are uncommon, seen in fewer than 4% in patients evaluated for esophagectomy (34). Minimally invasive thoracoscopic and laparoscopic staging of esophageal cancer has been advocated recently (35,36). Laparoscopic staging has been shown to be more accurate than EUS staging, and metastases that preclude resection have been detected in 10% to 20% of patients (35,37–39).

Bronchoscopy. Bronchoscopy should be performed in patients with carcinoma of the upper and middle thirds of the esophagus to exclude invasion of the posterior membranous trachea or main bronchi, which precludes a safe esophagectomy and contraindicates the operation.

Esophagoscopy. Esophagoscopy is one of the most important diagnostic tools in assessing the patient with esophageal symptoms from any cause. With the flexible fiberoptic esophagoscope, endoscopic assessment is easier than with the rigid instruments. Unfortunately, as flexible esophagoscopy has become such a commonly performed procedure, its potentially serious consequences are often forgotten. Esophagoscopy, particularly for the evaluation of an obstructing lesion, is a potentially dangerous undertaking, and a perforation in the patient with cancer is of tremendous gravity. Certain basic principles regarding esophagoscopy should always be borne in mind.

Basic Principles of Esophagoscopy and Anatomic Relations. The safe performance of esophagoscopy requires familiarity with normal esophageal anatomy, particularly the three areas of naturally occurring anatomic narrowing: (a) the cervical constriction at the level of the cricopharyngeus sphincter; (b) the bronchoaortic constriction at the level of the fourth thoracic vertebra behind the tracheal bifurcation, where the left main bronchus and aortic arch cross the esophagus; and (c) the diaphragmatic constriction, where the esophagus traverses the diaphragm. As a general rule, elective esophagoscopy should not be performed without a prior barium esophagogram displayed before the endoscopist during the procedure. Knowledge of the existing esophageal abnormality derived from the barium esophagogram assists the endoscopist in planning the procedure. It is useful to relate an esophageal abnormality on a barium

swallow examination to certain anatomic landmarks and then to extrapolate from this assessment the approximate level within the esophagus at which the abnormality should be seen. The upper esophageal sphincter is typically seen on the barium esophagogram at the level of the seventh cervical or first thoracic vertebral body, or about 15 cm from the upper incisor teeth at esophagoscopy in the adult. The sternomanubrial junction (angle of Louis) on the anterior chest wall aligns with the tracheal bifurcation, which is seen on most barium esophagograms at about the level of the fourth thoracic vertebra, corresponding to a point 25 cm from the upper incisors. The normal esophagogastric junction is typically seen endoscopically 40 cm from the upper incisors at the level of the 11th or 12th thoracic vertebra. With these landmarks in mind, a midesophageal tumor located at the level of the tracheal bifurcation on a barium esophagogram, for example, should be anticipated to be seen endoscopically at a point about 25 cm from the upper incisor teeth.

The patient suspected of having esophageal carcinoma is most often evaluated with the flexible fiberoptic esophagoscope under local anesthesia and sedation. The endoscopic assessment of an obstructing esophageal lesion may be uncomfortable for the patient, and one should not persist in attempts to obtain a biopsy specimen or dilate the stenosis in a patient who is anxious, combative, or uncooperative; at times, general anesthesia may be required. Fungating exophytic carcinomas are readily diagnosed endoscopically with biopsy specimens. Constricting esophageal tumors, however, may narrow the esophageal lumen so that only normal proximal esophageal mucosa is evident at the site of the stricture. In such cases, specimens from within the stenosis and brushings for cytologic evaluation obtained after the stricture has been gently dilated generally establish the malignant nature of the obstruction.

Vital Staining and Cytology. Vital staining of the esophageal mucosa is a useful technique in detecting dysplastic esophageal lesions that are not obvious on direct endoscopic assessment (40,41). Carcinoma in situ (intraepithelial carcinoma) or microinvasive carcinoma may appear endoscopically as flat, nondescript lesions (leukoplakia or erythroplakia) and therefore can be difficult to diagnose. Lugol (3% iodide) solution or 2% toluidine blue may be applied through the esophagoscope to the esophageal mucosa. Lugol solution stains normal glycogenic esophageal mucosa brown, whereas abnormal mucosa (early carcinoma, esophagitis, Barrett's mucosa) remains unstained. A swab of Lugol solution applied through the rigid esophagoscope stains the normal areas of esophageal mucosa and indicates the nonstaining, abnormal areas that should be sampled at biopsy. Alternatively, toluidine blue is a metachromatic stain with an affinity for cell nuclei. Therefore, tissues with a high cellular density and a high nucleus-to-cytoplasm ratio take up the stain quickly and retain it for about 1 hour. This technique is performed through the rigid esophagoscope; the esophageal mucosa is initially washed with 1% acetic acid to remove excess mucus and food particles, 1% toluidine blue is applied for 1 minute, and then the stain is washed away with 1% acetic acid. The areas of mucosa that remain stained are sampled for biopsy and are likely to be neoplastic.

Cytologic screening of large populations at high risk for the development of esophageal carcinoma is possible by means of a number of readily available outpatient techniques. In China, abrasive cytology with use of a swallowed balloon catheter (balloon cytology) has been extremely effective in screening for carcinoma. An encapsulated brush has been developed in Japan for the same purpose. The capsule, which is attached to a string, is swallowed by the patient. As the capsule dissolves, a contained polyurethane sponge ball expands, and as it is withdrawn through the esophagus, abrasive cytology can be performed. Combining abrasive cytology with vital staining of the esophageal mucosa may prove to yield the best sensitivity and specificity for screening populations.

Premalignant Esophageal Lesions

As indicated previously, chronic irritation of the esophageal mucosa by a variety of noxious stimuli (alcohol, tobacco, hot foods and liquids) eventually may lead to the development of esophageal carcinoma. A variety of esophageal lesions have a recognized premalignant nature. The risk for the development of carcinoma in a patient who survives an initial injury long enough for a *caustic esophageal stricture* to form is increased 1,000-fold in comparison with that of the normal population. This is but one reason that an esophagus that is severely strictured after caustic ingestion should be resected rather than bypassed, particularly in young patients.

The premalignant nature of *Barrett's esophagitis* was discussed earlier. When a fundoplication is performed to relieve reflux symptoms in a patient with Barrett's mucosa, the columnar epithelium within the esophagus rarely regresses. For this reason, periodic surveillance endoscopy should be performed. For the patient with Barrett's mucosa in whom dysplasia is mild or absent, endoscopy at 1- to 2-year intervals is probably adequate. For the patient with moderate dysplasia, surveillance endoscopy and biopsy at 6-month intervals is appropriate. As indicated earlier, severe dysplasia in the patient with Barrett's mucosa is virtually synonymous with carcinoma in situ and is an indication in most instances for esophageal resection.

Because *reflux esophagitis* constitutes a chronic chemical injury of the esophageal mucosa, it is regarded as a potentially premalignant abnormality of the esophagus that requires aggressive medical therapy or surgical control.

Esophageal carcinoma develops in about 10% to 12% of patients with *achalasia* of the esophagus who are observed for 15 years or longer. The cause is thought to be related to the irritating effects of the fermenting intraesophageal contents on the adjacent esophageal mucosa. These tumors are typically squamous cell carcinomas located in the middle third of the esophagus, frequently at the site of the air–fluid level seen in the obstructed organ on barium swallow examination. Carcinoma in these patients is typically diagnosed when far advanced because the patient with chronic dysphagia caused by underlying achalasia does not detect a change in swallowing as the tumor enlarges within the dilated esophagus. The prognosis for esophageal cancer in the patient with achalasia is poor. Patients who have carried a diagnosis of achalasia for 15 years or more should undergo surveillance endoscopy, perhaps with the addition of vital staining, because of their risk for the development of carcinoma.

Plummer-Vinson syndrome (Paterson-Kelly syndrome, or sideropenic dysphagia) is a premalignant esophageal condition. The term *sideropenic dysphagia* refers to the development of cervical dysphagia in patients who have iron-deficiency anemia. These patients are typically elderly women who are edentulous and have atrophic oral mucosa with glossitis and koilonychia (brittle, spoonshaped fingernails). Associated cervical esophageal webs are common (Fig. 20.9). The incidence of this syndrome is high in Scandinavia and Great Britain. Treatment consists of esophageal dilation to disrupt the web and correction of the nutritional deficiency. Squamous cell carcinoma of the hypopharynx, oral cavity, or esophagus develops in about 10% of these patients.

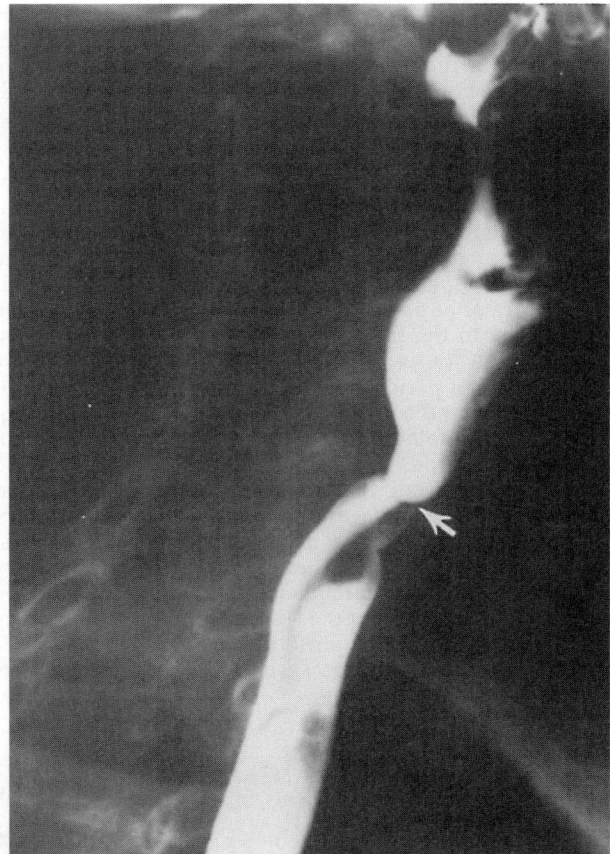

Figure 20.9. Typical cervical esophageal web *(arrow)* extending from the anterior esophageal wall. (From Orringer MB. Diverticula and miscellaneous conditions of the esophagus. In: Sabiston DC Jr, ed. *Textbook of surgery,* 13th ed. Philadelphia: WB Saunders, 1986:726, with permission.)

An increased incidence of esophageal carcinoma is found in patients who have *familial keratosis palmaris et plantaris (tylosis),* which is inherited as an autosomal dominant trait. This condition is characterized by hyperkeratosis of the interphalangeal epithelium and soles of the feet, fissures and scaling of the thickened skin of the palms and soles, and disordered sweating. Esophageal cancer occurs in these families at an earlier age than in the normal population.

Patients who have experienced *radiation esophagitis* during the course of treatment for lymphoma or lung, breast, or other mediastinal malignancies are at increased risk for the development of esophageal carcinoma years later.

Finally, several isolated cases of esophageal carcinoma found incidentally within *esophageal diverticula* have been reported; presumably carcinoma developed as a result of the irritating effects on the mucosa of stagnant, putrefying food within the pouch. Esophageal diverticula are therefore also regarded as premalignant esophageal lesions, although this occurrence is extremely rare.

Treatment of Esophageal Cancer

The therapy of esophageal carcinoma is influenced by the knowledge that in most of these patients, local tumor invasion or distant metastatic disease precludes a curative resection. Significant and consistent long-term survival has not been achieved with either chemotherapy, radiotherapy, or surgery alone in patients with esophageal carcinoma. Although certain chemotherapeutic agents, such as cisplatin, 5-fluorouracil, bleomycin, and methotrexate, either alone or in combination, have been associated with partial responses of some of these tumors, long-term remission has not been the rule (42).

Radiation.   Although squamous cell carcinoma is generally regarded as a radiosensitive and therefore potentially curable tumor, radiotherapy has not achieved cure in most of these patients (43). Radiotherapy is used in the treatment of esophageal carcinoma to provide either palliation or cure or as an adjunct to esophagectomy. Palliative radiotherapy in the range of 4,000 to 5,000 cGy administered during 3 to 4 weeks relieves dysphagia sufficiently in nearly half of patients with advanced metastatic carcinoma and severe dysphagia to allow them to swallow liquids and diet supplements. "Curative" supervoltage radiotherapy is delivered in doses of 5,000 to 7,000 cGy over 5 to 7 weeks, with rotational and oblique ports used to avoid spinal cord injury. Unfortunately, the average 5-year survival after such treatment is between 6% and 10% in most series because radiation fails to control either the primary tumor or distant metastatic disease (44,45).

Similarly, although surgical treatment most effectively relieves the esophageal obstruction, resectional therapy is local therapy, and esophageal carcinoma in most patients is unfortunately a systemic disease when it is diagnosed. Thus, reported 5-year survival rates after esophageal resection for carcinoma usually average between 10% and 15%, with more than 80% of patients dying within 1 year of diagnosis. Several Japanese reports indicate 5-year survival rates of 25% to 38% with combined preoperative radiotherapy followed by resection. Such results have not been duplicated in Western cultures, where until recently the aim of therapy has been palliation.

Intubation and Stenting.   A variety of endoesophageal tubes (Celestin, Fell, Mackler, Mousseau-Barbin, Souttar, Wilson-Cook) have been used to provide palliation for patients with esophageal carcinoma (46). Basically, these tubes are divided into two types—*pulsion* tubes, which are pushed through the tumor with the aid of an esophagoscope, and *traction* or pull-through tubes, which are pulled into place by downward traction through a gastrotomy. As is the case with many conceptually simple procedures, implementation in the clinical setting is problematic. Transoral esophageal intubation is associated with an overall mortality rate of 14% and a complication rate of at least 25%, the latter consisting of perforation of the esophagus, migration of the tubes, and obstruction of the tubes by food or tumor overgrowth. Although patients may be better able to handle their saliva after their esophageal tumors have been intubated, oral intake must be re-

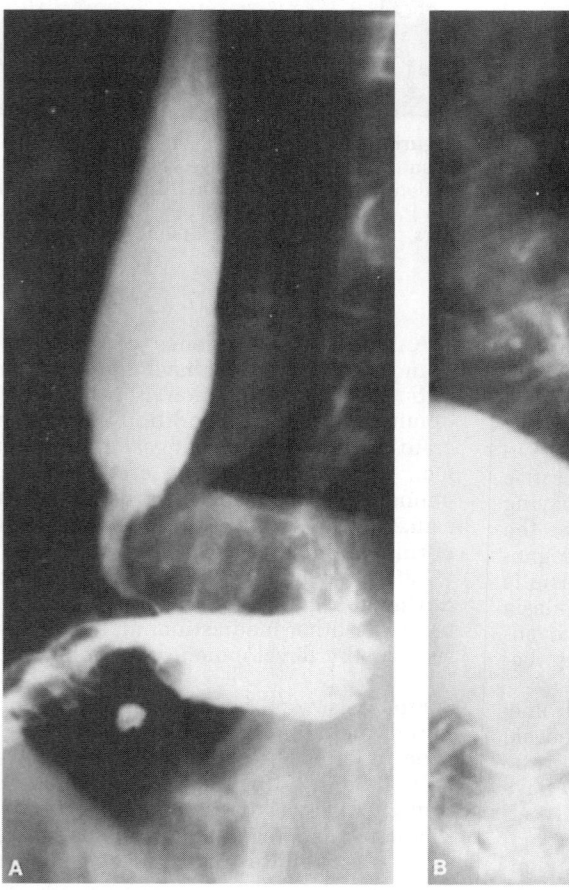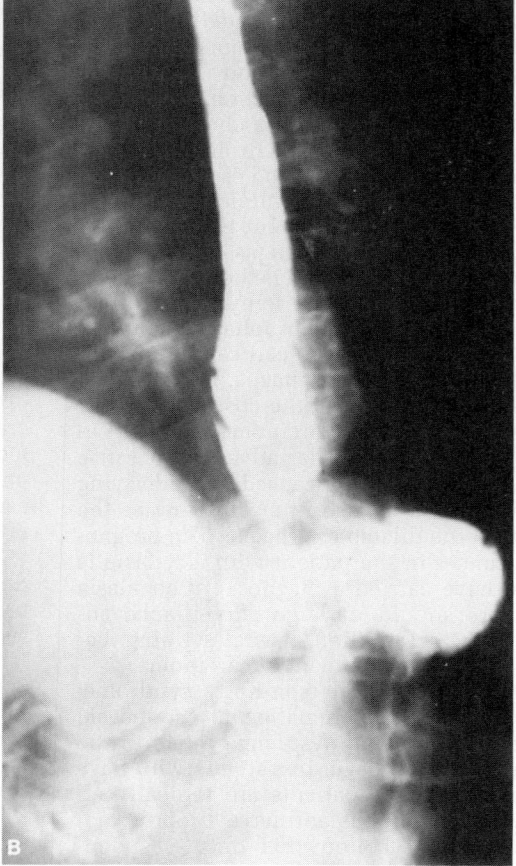

Figure 20.10. *(A)* Distal esophageal stricture that was erroneously interpreted as resulting from spasm because of its smooth, tapered contour. This proved to be an unresectable adenocarcinoma of the cardia. *(B)* Esophagogram after placement of a Celestin intraesophageal tube showing free passage of barium into the stomach. Despite relative relief of the esophageal obstruction, the patient continued to experience severe pain from esophageal spasm and local tumor invasion. Adequate palliation was not achieved. (From Orringer MB. Tumors of the esophagus. In: Sabiston DC Jr, ed. *Textbook of surgery,* 13th ed. Philadelphia: WB Saunders, 1986:736, with permission.)

stricted to a semiliquid diet, and palliation is far from optimal (Fig. 20.10). Palliative intubation for esophageal carcinoma is associated with an average survival of less than 6 months. This technique is reserved almost exclusively for patients with malignant tracheoesophageal fistulae, in whom the tube is used to occlude the esophageal side of the fistula while allowing oral alimentation.

During the past decade, a variety of expandable intraesophageal metallic stents have been used to achieve palliation in patients with unresectable esophageal carcinoma (47,48). These stents are easier to insert than the older plastic tubes, have a larger lumen, and theoretically are less likely to cause perforation. Some are coated with silicone to prevent tumor ingrowth. They are inserted under fluoroscopy by means of a flexible esophagoscope. The stents have provided good relief of esophageal obstruction, and the relief appears to last longer than that achieved with laser therapy (49,50–54).

Laser Therapy.   Endoscopic laser fulguration of esophageal carcinoma, particularly with the neodymium:yttrium-aluminum-garnet (Nd:YAG) laser, has been used to provide temporary relief of esophageal obstruction in patients with unresectable tumors. In this procedure, a flexible quartz fiber is inserted through the working channel of the esophagoscope to carry Nd:YAG laser energy at a wavelength of 1,064 nm and an energy level of up to 120 watts to vaporize the tumor. Generally, multiple sessions are required to resect sufficient tumor to achieve an adequate lumen, and functional success with restoration of comfortable swallowing and excellent palliation is achieved in 75% to 80% of properly selected patients (48,55–58). Laser fulguration may also be combined with endoluminal stenting and radiation therapy to provide palliation in these patients (49).

More recently, photodynamic therapy (PDT), an alternative form of laser therapy, has been used to restore an esophageal lumen for the palliation of inoperable carcinoma. With PDT, a hematoporphyrin is injected intravenously and is preferentially absorbed by the tumor. After 48 to 72 hours, again through quartz fibers inserted through the esophagoscope, laser energy at a wavelength of 630 nm

is delivered. This activates the hematoporphyrin, which kills the neoplastic cells by releasing singlet oxygen. Gradual sloughing of the tumor follows. Excellent palliation has been achieved with this technique (59–61).

Bypass.   A variety of surgical procedures, such as substernal gastric or colon bypass, have been developed for the palliation of unresectable esophageal carcinoma. Because the survival of patients with unresectable esophageal carcinoma averages less than 6 months, it is difficult to justify these bypass operations, which are associated with a mortality rate of between 15% and 25% (62,63). They are simply too large for patients with so advanced a malignancy. Similarly, the use of reversed gastric (Heimlich) tubes is associated with a 25% to 40% mortality rate.

Resection
Transthoracic Resection.   For the majority of patients with localized esophageal carcinoma, resection provides the most effective and reliable palliation of dysphagia. The traditional surgical approach to distal esophageal carcinoma has been a left thoracoabdominal incision (Fig. 20.11). After the distal esophagus, proximal stomach, and adjacent lymph nodes have been resected, an intrathoracic esophagogastric anastomosis is performed. Tumors involving the midportion of the esophagus are resected through either a thoracoabdominal or separate thoracic and abdominal incisions (Ivor Lewis operation), and a high intrathoracic esophagogastric anastomosis is performed (Fig. 20.12). Because a truncal vagotomy is an inevitable accompaniment of esophageal resection for carcinoma, and because gastric emptying is delayed in 15% to 30% of patients after a truncal vagotomy, a gastric drainage procedure, either a pyloromyotomy or pyloroplasty, is recommended in these cases.

Unfortunately, the standard right or left transthoracic esophagectomy and intrathoracic esophagogastric anastomosis have significant disadvantages. Weakened patients with esophageal obstruction may have difficulty tolerating combined thoracic and abdominal operations, and postoperative incisional pain and the inability to breathe deeply may lead to atelectasis and respiratory insufficiency, so

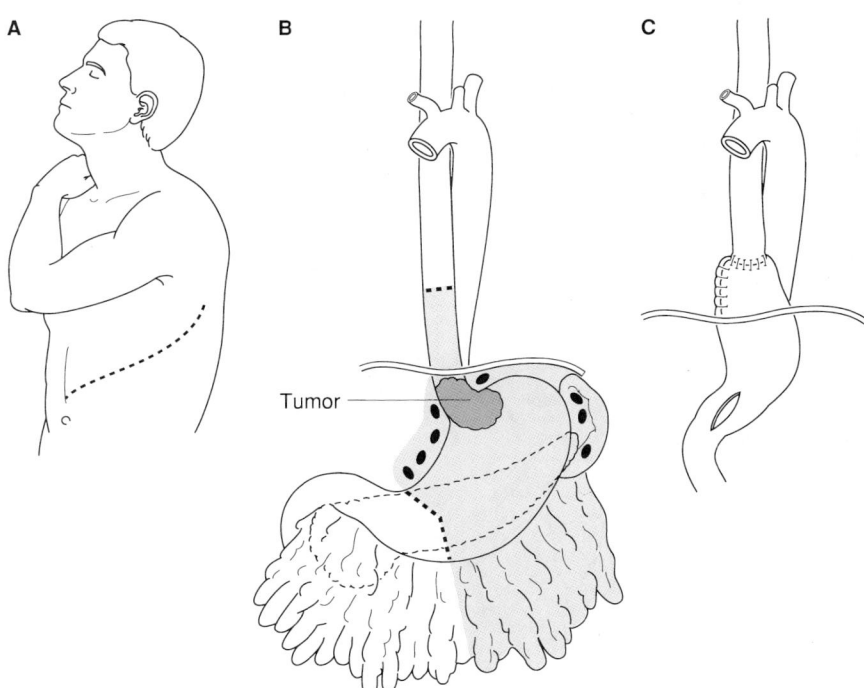

Figure 20.11. Standard thoracoabdominal esophagogastrectomy for carcinomas of the distal esophagus and cardia. *(A)* Thoracoabdominal incision. *(B)* Tissue to be resected *(colored area)*. *(C)* Completed reconstruction after intrathoracic esophagogastric anastomosis and either pyloromyotomy or pyloroplasty to prevent postvagotomy pylorospasm. (After Ellis FH Jr. Treatment of carcinoma of the esophagus and cardia. *Mayo Clin Proc* 1960;35:653, with permission.)

Tumor

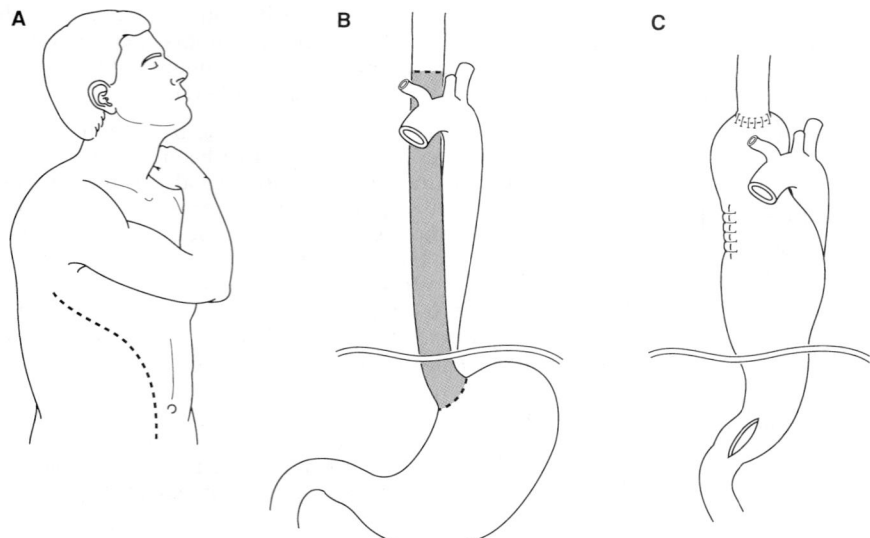

Figure 20.12. Standard thoracoabdominal esophagogastrectomy for tumors of the upper and middle thirds of the thoracic esophagus. *(A)* Either a continuous thoracoabdominal incision or separate thoracic and abdominal incisions are used. *(B)* Portion of esophagus to be resected *(colored area).* *(C)* Completed reconstruction with high intrathoracic esophagogastric anastomosis and gastric drainage procedure. (After Ellis FH Jr. Treatment of carcinoma of the esophagus and cardia. *Mayo Clin Proc* 1960;35:653, with permission.)

that mechanical ventilatory assistance is required and pneumonia often develops.

The second disadvantage of the standard operations is the potential for disruption of the intrathoracic esophageal anastomosis with resulting mediastinitis and sepsis, a fatal complication in half of patients in whom it occurs. These two factors, the physiologic impact of a combined thoracoabdominal operation and the disastrous results of an intrathoracic esophageal anastomotic disruption, are responsible for operative mortality rates for transthoracic esophagectomy and reconstruction that are occasionally

as low as zero to 3%, but generally now range from 15% to 20% (64–7,0). Further, esophageal carcinoma is often a disease of the elderly, who frequently have cardiac and renal disease, and operative mortality is higher in patients over the age of 70 years than in younger patients (68,71).

A further disadvantage of the standard intrathoracic esophagogastric anastomosis is inadequate long-term relief of dysphagia, as a result of either tumor recurrence at the anastomotic suture line or the development of reflux esophagitis above the anastomosis. Because of the notorious spread of esophageal carcinoma in submucosal lym-

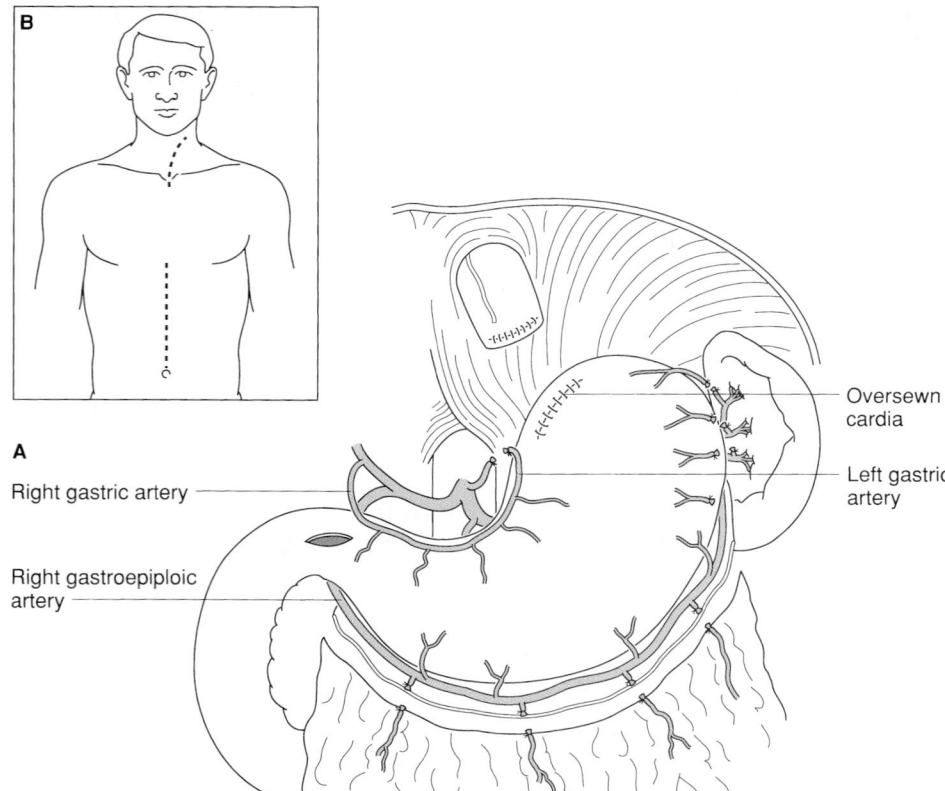

Right gastric artery

Right gastroepiploic artery

Oversewn cardia

Left gastric artery

Figure 20.13. *(A)* Standard mobilization of the stomach for esophageal replacement either in the posterior mediastinal or substernal position. The left gastric artery and left gastroepiploic vessels have been divided. The mobilized stomach is based on the remaining right gastric and right gastroepiploic arteries that are preserved. A pyloromyotomy and generous Kocher maneuver are performed. *(B)* Left cervical incision and upper midline abdominal incision used for transhiatal esophagectomy and esophageal replacement with stomach in the posterior mediastinum. (After Orringer MB, Sloan H. Substernal gastric bypass of the excluded thoracic esophagus for palliation of esophageal carcinoma. *J Thorac Cardiovasc Surg* 1975;70:836, with permission.)

phatics well beyond the gross extent of the tumor, a 10-cm proximal margin of resection is advocated whenever possible. Patients who undergo a major esophageal resection and reconstruction only to have recurrent dysphagia caused by tumor at the anastomosis several months later have received poor palliation.

Although it has long been taught that the patient with esophageal carcinoma does not live long enough for reflux esophagitis to develop after a low intrathoracic esophagogastric anastomosis has been performed, this is clearly not the case, and the development of reflux in these patients can produce not only severe pyrosis and reflux symptoms but also dysphagia from benign stenosis.

Transhiatal Resection.   During the past two decades, the technique of transhiatal esophagectomy without thoracotomy has been popularized as an operation that minimizes the factors responsible for most of the poor results of tradi-

tional transthoracic esophageal resection and reconstruction (72). In this operation, irrespective of the level of the tumor, the entire intrathoracic esophagus is resected through the diaphragmatic hiatus and a cervical incision. The mobilized stomach is repositioned in the posterior mediastinum in the original esophageal bed, and the gastric fundus is anastomosed to the cervical esophagus above the level of the clavicles. The operation is performed through an upper midline abdominal incision and a cervical incision, so that the need for a thoracotomy is eliminated. The properly mobilized stomach, based on the right gastric and right gastroepiploic vascular arcades, readily reaches above the level of the clavicles for a cervical anastomosis. A generous Kocher maneuver to mobilize the pyloroduodenal junction, pyloromyotomy, and feeding jejunostomy are performed routinely (Fig. 20.13). The thoracic esophagus is mobilized through the diaphragmatic hiatus and a neck incision (Fig. 20.14).

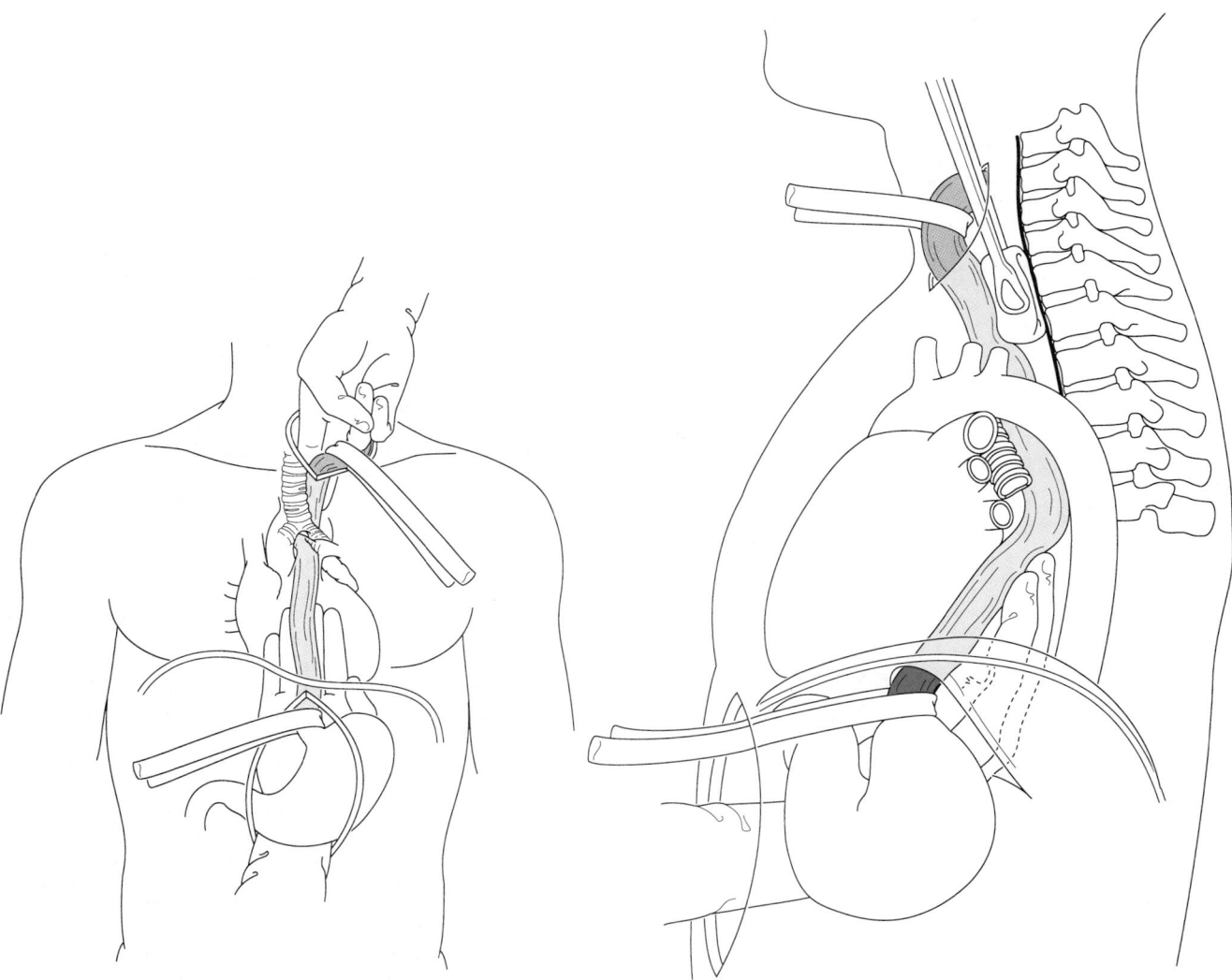

A   B

Figure 20.14. *(A)* Transhiatal mobilization of the thoracic esophagus from the posterior mediastinum with the use of blunt dissection and traction on rubber drains placed around the esophagogastric junction and cervical esophagus. The volar aspects of the fingers are kept against the esophagus to reduce the risk for injury to adjacent structures. *(B)* Lateral view showing transhiatal mobilization of the esophagus away from the prevertebral fascia. Half of a sponge on a stick is inserted through the cervical incision and advanced until it makes contact with the hand inserted from below through the diaphragmatic hiatus. Arterial pressure is monitored as the heart is displaced forward by the hand in the posterior mediastinum. (After Orringer MB. Surgical options for esophageal resection and reconstruction with stomach. In: Baue AE, Geha AS, Hammond GL, eds. *Glenn's thoracic and cardiovascular surgery,* 5th ed. Norwalk, CT: Appleton & Lange, 1991: 799–800, with permission.)

For tumors of the distal third of the esophagus that are localized to the cardia, the proximal half of the stomach is not resected; instead, the high lesser curvature of the stomach is divided 4 to 6 cm beyond the gross tumor, with preservation of the point along the high greater curvature that reaches superiorly to the neck (Figs. 20.15–20.17).

When a transhiatal esophagectomy is performed, accessible cervical, intrathoracic, and intraabdominal lymph nodes are removed for staging purposes, but no attempt is made to perform an *en bloc* resection of the esophagus and adjacent lymph node-bearing tissue. Transhiatal esophagectomy without thoracotomy and a cervical esophagogastric anastomosis have the following advantages: (a) A thoracotomy in a debilitated patient is avoided; (b) an intrathoracic esophageal anastomosis is avoided, and if a cervical anastomotic leak occurs, the resulting salivary fistula is easily managed by opening the neck wound and packing it and is not a fatal complication; (c) intraabdominal or intrathoracic gastrointestinal suture lines are avoided; and (d) subsequent clinically significant gastroe-

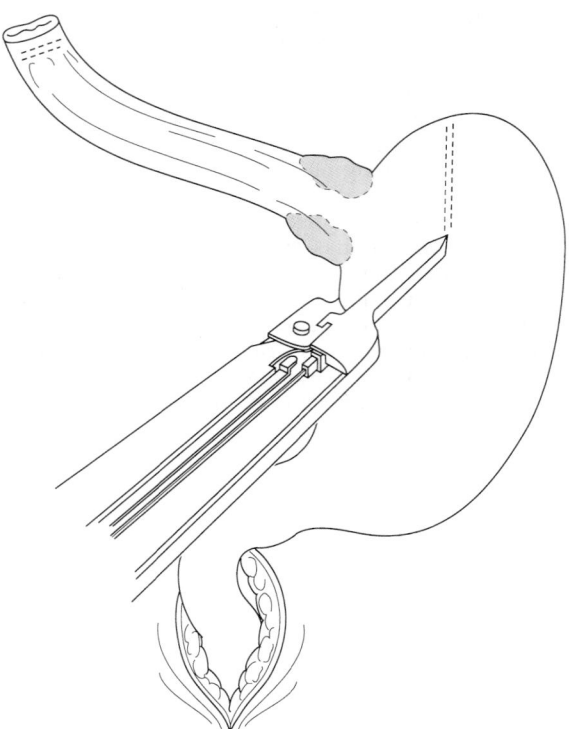

Figure 20.16. Gastric division after transhiatal mobilization of the intrathoracic esophagus for a carcinoma of the cardia. The mobilized stomach and attached distal esophagus have been delivered from the abdominal incision and are retracted superiorly as the surgical stapler is applied, beginning along the lesser curvature and proceeding toward the high greater curvature *(dashed line)*. This is the standard method used to prepare the stomach for esophageal replacement after transhiatal esophagectomy. The remaining gastric "tube" readily reaches to the neck for a cervical anastomosis. (After Orringer MB, Sloan H. Esophageal replacement after blunt esophagectomy. In: Nyhus LM, Baker RJ, eds. *Mastery of surgery.* Boston: Little, Brown, 1984:426, with permission.)

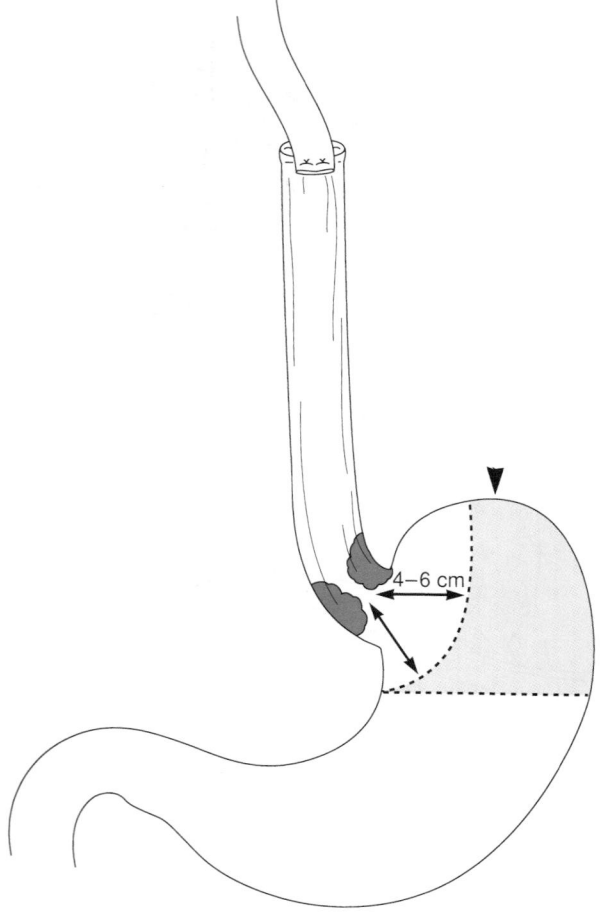

Figure 20.15. Transhiatal esophagectomy and proximal partial gastrectomy for lesions of the cardia and distal esophagus. The entire greater curvature of the stomach is preserved, including the point *(arrowhead)* that will reach farthest cephalad, to the neck. A 4- to 6-cm gastric margin is obtained while the entire greater curvature is preserved. The *colored area* indicates that portion of the stomach that is usually resected in a standard hemigastrectomy used for a distal esophageal carcinoma. Such a resection, however, eliminates the possibility of a cervical esophagogastric anastomosis. (After Orringer MB, Sloan H. Esophagectomy without thoracotomy. *J Thorac Cardiovasc Surg* 1978;76:643, with permission.)

sophageal reflux is rare. This operation has been criticized because of the limited exposure of the intrathoracic esophagus through the diaphragmatic hiatus, and therefore the risk for intraoperative bleeding from the divided aortic esophageal branches. In addition, one cannot carry out a complete mediastinal lymph node dissection through the diaphragmatic hiatus for purposes of staging or potential cure.

In the largest reported single series of transhiatal esophagectomies by the author and his associates, among 800 consecutive patients with carcinoma of the thoracic esophagus and cardia, transhiatal esophagectomy without thoracotomy was possible in 800 (98%) (72). Of the 800 resected tumors, 36 (4.5%) were located in the upper third, 177 (28%) in the middle third, and 587 (73.5%) in the lower third of the esophagus. Of the tumors, 225 (28%) were squamous cell carcinomas and 555 (69%) were adenocarcinomas. A cervical esophagogastric anastomosis was possible in 782 (98%) of these patients, a colon interposition being required in 17 patients who had undergone prior gastric resection for peptic ulcer disease. This experience clearly has demonstrated that the normal stomach, when properly mobilized, readily reaches to the neck for construction of a cervical esophagogastric anastomosis.

Of the 800 resected carcinomas, 363 (45%) were either transmurally invasive or metastatic beyond regional

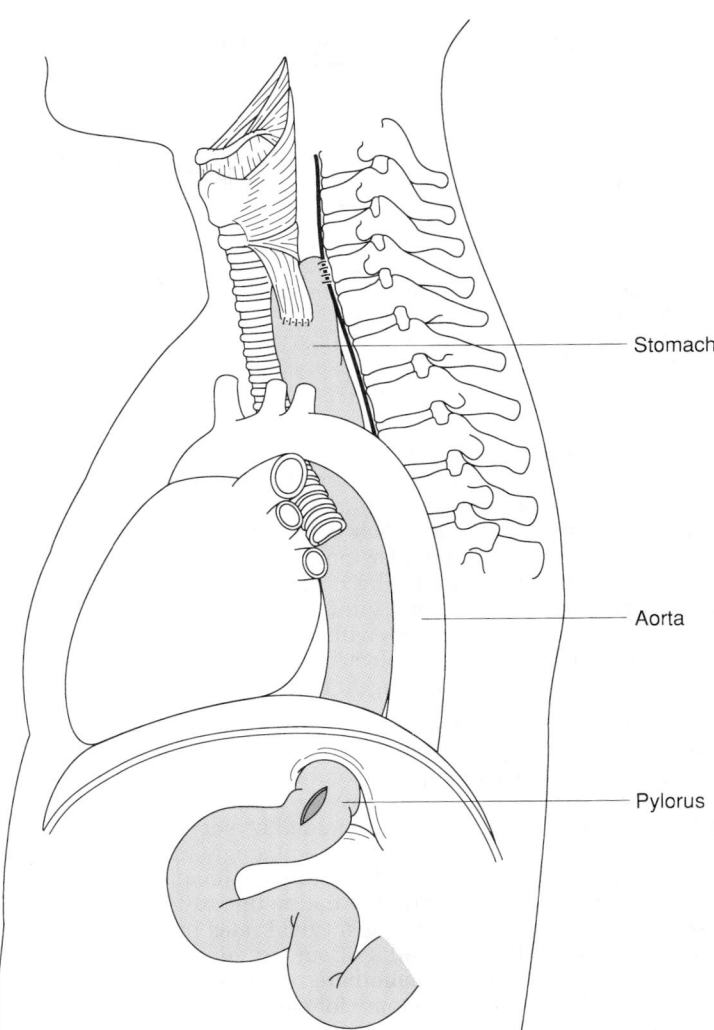

Figure 20.17. Final position of the mobilized stomach in the posterior mediastinum after transhiatal esophagectomy and cervical esophagogastric anastomosis. The gastric fundus has been suspended from the cervical prevertebral fascia, and an end-to-side cervical esophagogastrostomy has been performed. The pylorus is now located several centimeters below the level of the diaphragmatic hiatus. (After Orringer MB, Sloan H. Esophagectomy without thoracotomy. *J Thorac Cardiovasc Surg* 1978;76: 643, with permission.)

lymph nodes (stage III or IV tumors). Only 94 (11.8%) patients had tumors confined to the mucosa (stage I). Three intraoperative deaths were caused by mediastinal hemorrhage, and intraoperative blood loss averaged 794 mL. The hospital mortality rate was 2.8%. This is somewhat lower than the mortality rate of approximately 7% reported in recent collective reviews of series of transhiatal esophagectomies (73,74). The overall 2-year survival rate was 47%, and the 5-year survival rate, 23%. These survival data, although comparable with those reported in most series of transthoracic resections, were obtained with less postoperative morbidity and mortality. The introduction of a side-to-side stapled cervical esophagogastric anastomosis reduced the incidence of postoperative cervical esophagogastric anastomotic leak to below 3%, so that a safe discharge was possible 1 week after operation and the incidence of anastomotic stricture and the need for long-term dilation therapy were reduced (75). On the basis of this experience, a transhiatal esophagectomy without thoracotomy is advocated by the author whenever possible for resectable esophageal carcinomas. This approach should not be used for tumors that are judged on palpation through the diaphragmatic hiatus to have invaded the aorta or the tracheobronchial tree.

Radical Resection.   At the other end of the spectrum from transhiatal resection for esophageal carcinoma is the radical transthoracic esophagectomy with *en bloc* dissec-

tion of contiguous lymph node-bearing tissues (76–80). The goal of this procedure is complete removal of the esophagus and surrounding soft tissue and lymph nodes with a 10-cm margin on either side of the tumor. This is a much more formidable operation, the results of which, when compared with those of transhiatal esophagectomy without thoracotomy and no formal lymph node dissection, are not significantly different (Table 20.3). Comparisons such as these seem to indicate that survival after resection of esophageal carcinoma is more a function of the extent and stage of the tumor than of the size of the specimen or number of lymph nodes removed. Skinner and associates (81) subsequently reported on a group of 31 patients, half with adenocarcinoma and half with squamous cell carcinoma, undergoing radical esophagectomy under more stringent selection criteria. The overall 1- and 2-year survival rates were an encouraging 65% and 32%, respectively. Debate continues, however, over the merit of attempting to treat with a more radical resection a disease that is usually systemic. This concept has been carried even further by some surgeons with the use of a "three-field" lymph node dissection (abdominal, thoracic, and now cervical lymph nodes), particularly in Japan. Altorki and Skinner (82) recently reported the finding of occult cervical lymph node metastases in 35% of patients undergoing a three-field lymph node dissection for esophageal carcinoma that was otherwise felt to be "curable." This

Table 20.3. **EFFECT ON SURVIVAL OF EXTENT OF ESOPHAGEAL RESECTION FOR CARCINOMA**

| | 3-Year Actuarial Survival Rate (No. Patients) | |
Esophageal tumor site	Radical esophagectomy with en bloc lymph node dissection[a]	Transhiatal esophagectomy without formal lymph node dissection[b]
Middle third	14% (29)	17% (40)
Lower third	33% (37)	31% (47)

[a]From Skinner DB. En bloc resection for neoplasms of the esophagus and cardia. J Thorac Cardiovasc Surg 1983;85:59, with permission.
[b]From Orringer MB. Transhiatal esophagectomy without thoracotomy for carcinoma of the esophagus. Ann Surg 1984;200:282, with permission.

finding only reinforces the position that esophageal carcinoma is usually a systemic disease, for which systemic therapy is more appropriate than radical surgery.

As a general rule, the stomach is the preferred visceral esophageal substitute, being far more resilient than intestine and readily reaching to the neck for replacement of the entire esophagus. Colonic interposition is a major operative undertaking in patients with esophageal carcinoma and should be used only in selected cases when the stomach is not available for esophageal replacement.

Multimodality Therapy. Efforts have been made to improve survival in patients with esophageal carcinoma by using multimodality therapy in combination with surgery (24). Preoperative chemotherapy or radiation therapy alone before esophagectomy has yielded no survival benefit over surgery alone. However, several single-institution phase II trials of preoperative chemotherapy (cisplatin and 5-fluorouracil) with concurrent radiation therapy (40 to 50 Gy) have produced encouraging survival rates in comparison with the historical results of surgery alone (83–87). Combined preoperative chemotherapy and radiotherapy before transhiatal esophagectomy for carcinoma, for example, provided such encouraging survival statistics at the University of Michigan. Forty-three patients with intrathoracic esophageal carcinoma (21 with adenocarcinoma and 22 with squamous cell carcinoma) received 3 weeks of chemotherapy (cisplatin, vinblastine, and 5-fluorouracil) concurrently with 3,750 to 4,500 cGy of radiotherapy (83). After a 3-week recovery period, transhiatal esophagectomy was accomplished. Hematologic toxicity and radiation esophagitis were common. Two patients died preoperatively of sepsis resulting from bone marrow suppression, for an operability rate in this group of 95%. Two other patients were found at operation to have unresectable tumors, for an overall resectability rate of 91%. The transhiatal esophageal resection was carried out with no increased morbidity in comparison with the patients who had had no preoperative therapy. One postoperative death resulted from an unrecognized brain metastasis. Ten patients (24%) had no residual carcinoma in the resected specimen (T0 N0 status). At a mean follow-up of 36 months, the median survival time for all 43 patients was 29 months (Kaplan-Meier estimate), a clear improvement over the 12-month median survival time with transhiatal esophagectomy alone. All 10 patients with T0 N0 status (complete responders) were alive and tumor-free at a median follow-up of 36 months. At a median follow-up of 78.7 months, the 5-year survival rate of all 43 patients was 34%, and that of the complete responders, a gratifying 60%. The overall 1- and 2-year survival rates in this group of 72% and 60%, respectively, compare favorably with the figures of 65% and 32%, referred to earlier, reported by Skinner and associates (81) after radical esophagectomy.

The phase II trials cited above have produced a pathologic complete response (CR) in approximately 20% to 50% of patients and 3-year survival rates near 40%, and those who achieve a CR have a survival advantage over those who have residual tumor in the resected specimen. These preliminary results have generated hope that it may be possible to alter the natural history of esophageal carci-

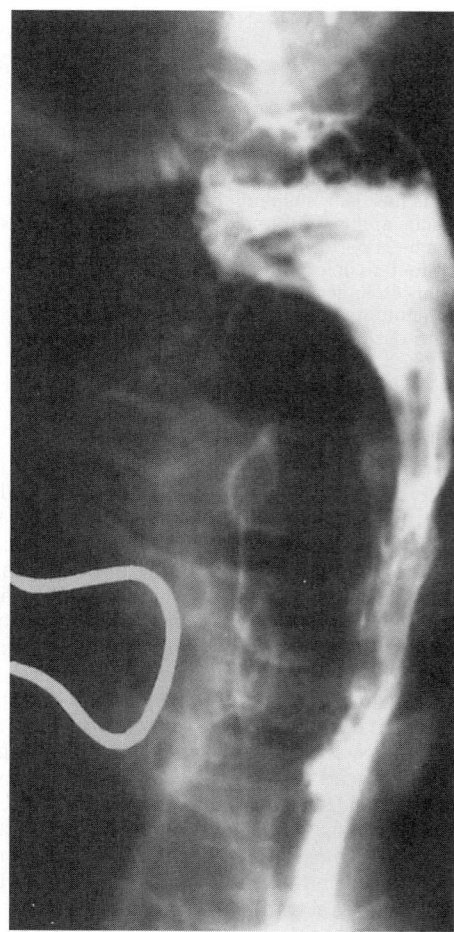

Figure 20.18. Barium esophagogram showing a large squamous cell carcinoma involving the cervicothoracic esophagus. The head of the clavicle has been highlighted to emphasize how such tumors can straddle the thoracic inlet and involve the trachea behind the sternum. [After Orringer MB. Transhiatal esophagectomy without thoracotomy. In: Orringer MB, ed. *Shackelford's surgery of the alimentary tract*, vol 1 *(The esophagus)*. Philadelphia: WB Saunders, 1991:428, with permission.]

noma and achieve long-term survival, not just palliation, in some of these patients. Three randomized, controlled trials have now been published comparing survival after chemoradiation therapy and esophagectomy with that after surgery alone (88–90). The reported CR rates after multimodality therapy were similar (approximately 25%), as were the 3-year survival rates (32% to 36%). However, only the study by Walsh et al. (90) demonstrated a statistically significant overall survival benefit for multimodality therapy. At present, although multimodality therapy seems to provide better local and regional tumor control, chemoradiation therapy before esophagectomy is associated with a superior survival benefit and should be considered investigational.

Cervicothoracic Esophageal Carcinomas. Patients with laryngotracheal, esophageal, or thyroid carcinomas that involve the cervicothoracic esophagus and adjacent larynx, either primarily or secondarily, often require esophageal reconstruction after laryngopharyngectomy (91,92). Loss of the larynx is a considerable price to pay for what is often a palliative procedure, however, and given the success of radiation and chemotherapy in the treatment of laryngeal squamous cell carcinoma, this is now the approach preferred by the author for most patients with cervicothoracic esophageal malignancies.

For those who have failed prior radiation therapy, however, a laryngopharyngectomy may be the best therapeutic option. Concomitant radical neck dissection may also be required because of regional lymph node involvement. Resection of these tumors may require division of the high retrosternal trachea, which is facilitated by removal of the anterior breast plate and construction of a mediastinal tracheostomy (Figs. 20.18–20.20). Replacement of the pharynx and cervical esophagus has been achieved with skin tubes and rotated myocutaneous flaps. These operations, however, are often multistaged, prolonged, and fraught with technical problems. Since the evolution and refinement of microvascular techniques, the isolated free jejunal transfer has become one of the most popular means of restoring alimentary continuity after the resection of proximal tumors of the hypopharynx, pharynx, and larynx above the thoracic inlet (93,94).

For tumors that involve the esophagus or trachea below the thoracic inlet, resection requires laryngopharyngoesophagectomy and mediastineal tracheostomy, as described above, and reestablishment of alimentary continuity with either a gastric (92,95) (Figs. 20.21 and 20.22) or colonic interposition. Because construction of a pharyngogastric anastomosis requires the maximal reach cephalad of the stomach that is possible, the potential for tension on the anastomosis is real and is no doubt a major contributing factor to the 30% incidence of anastomotic leak that has been reported after a pharyngogastrostomy. Another serious concern regarding the pharyngogastric anastomosis is the regurgitation of gastric contents during postural ma-

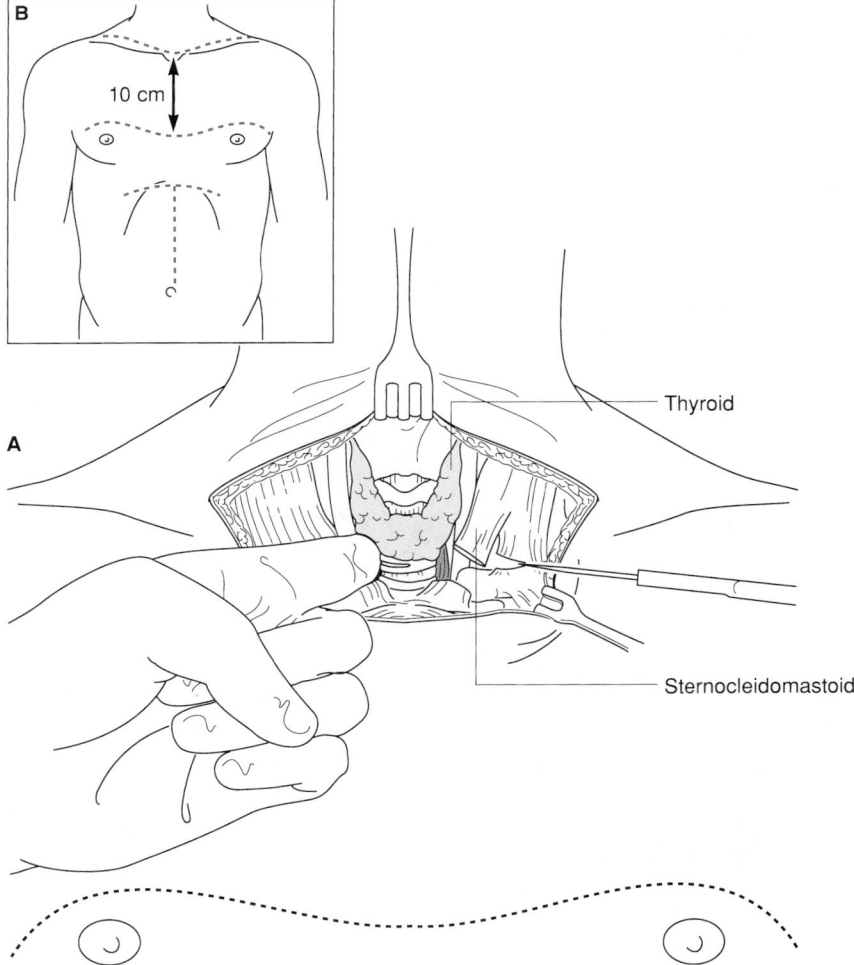

Figure 20.19. *(A)* Extended collar incision used to determine whether a cervicothoracic esophageal tumor of the type shown in Fig. 20.18 is invading the adjacent prevertebral fascia or carotid vessels. If the tumor is resectable, the anterior cervical skin and platysma flap are elevated, and the origins of the sternocleidomastoid muscles are divided from the clavicles with electrocautery. *(B)* Bipedicled upper thoracic apron flap that may be used for subsequent anterior mediastinal tracheostomy. In most cases, vigorous downward retraction of the anterior upper thoracic skin permits resection of the anterior breast plate without the need for the additional transverse incision shown. (After Orringer MB, Sloan H. Anterior mediastinal tracheostomy. *J Thorac Cardiovasc Surg* 1979;78:850, with permission.)

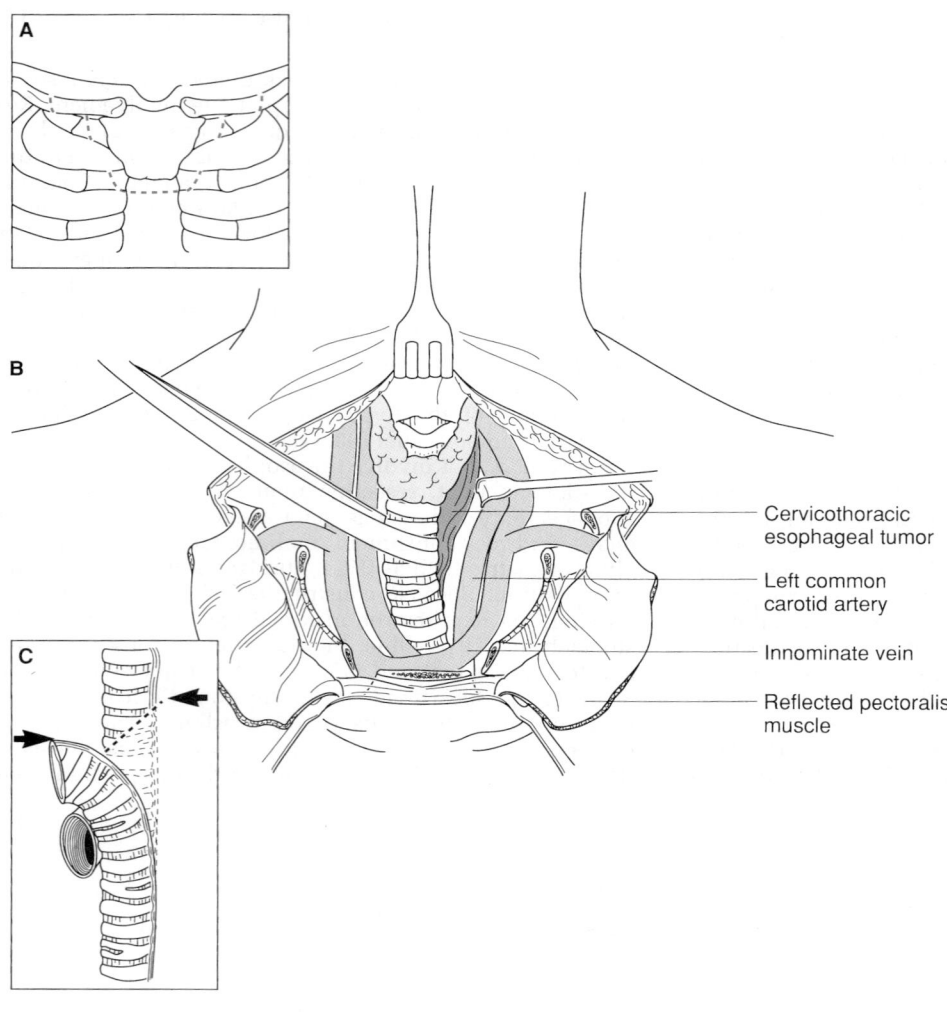

Cervicothoracic esophageal tumor

Left common carotid artery

Innominate vein

Reflected pectoralis muscle

Figure 20.20. *(A)* Removal of the anterior thoracic breast plate, including the medial clavicles and short segments of upper manubrium and adjacent first and second ribs, exposes the superior mediastinum and its contents. *(B)* The cervicothoracic esophagus with its contained tumor separated from the great vessels of the neck. *(C)* Oblique division of the trachea, with preservation of as much of the posterior membranous portion *(arrows)* as possible in preparation for construction of the anterior mediastinal tracheostomy. The trachea is brought forward over the innominate artery and sutured to the skin. (After Orringer MB, Sloan H. Anterior mediastinal tracheostomy. *J Thorac Cardiovasc Surg* 1979;78: 850, with permission.)

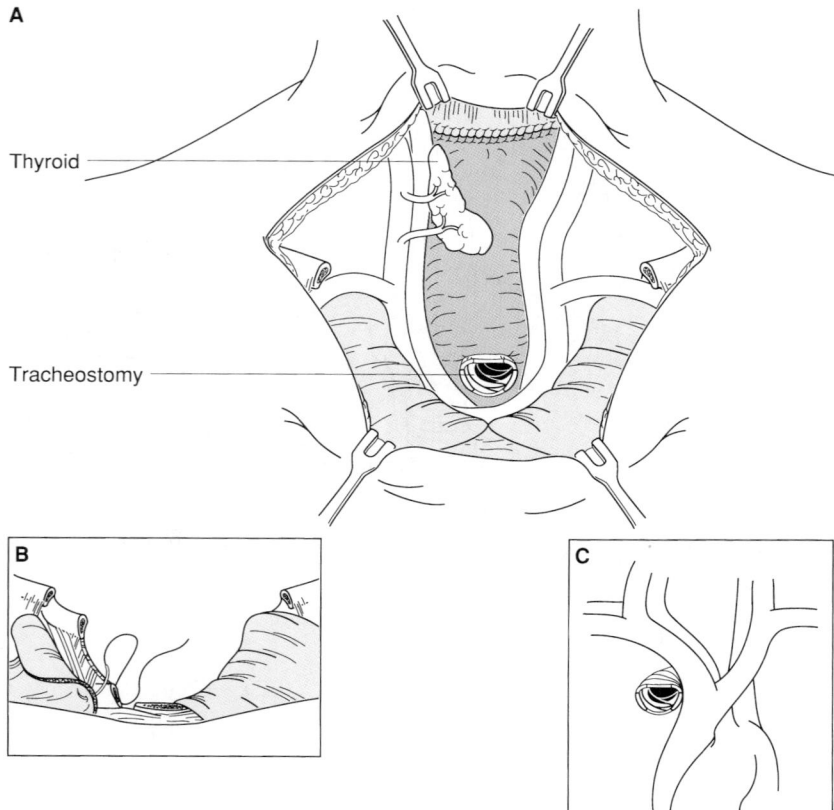

Thyroid

Tracheostomy

Figure 20.21. *(A)* After resection of the larynx, pharynx, and attached esophagus, the stomach is mobilized through the posterior mediastinum in the original esophageal bed and anastomosed to the pharynx as shown. Thyroid and parathyroid tissue are preserved whenever possible. The divided trachea is positioned over the innominate artery for construction of the mediastinal tracheostomy. *(B)* Covering the divided edge of the divided bony chest wall with remaining pectoralis muscle. *(C)* Transposition of the remaining trachea inferiorly and to the right of the innominate artery and vein to minimize tension and the risk for innominate artery erosion when the trachea is sewn to the skin. (After Orringer MB, Sloan H. Anterior mediastinal tracheostomy. *J Thorac Cardiovasc Surg* 1979;78:850, with permission.)

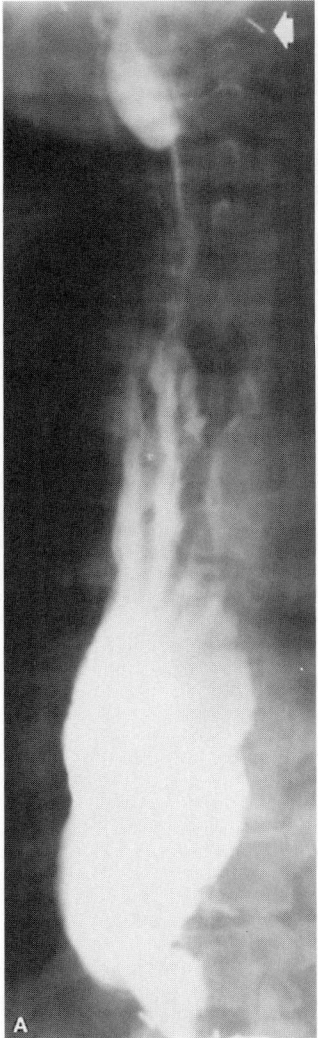

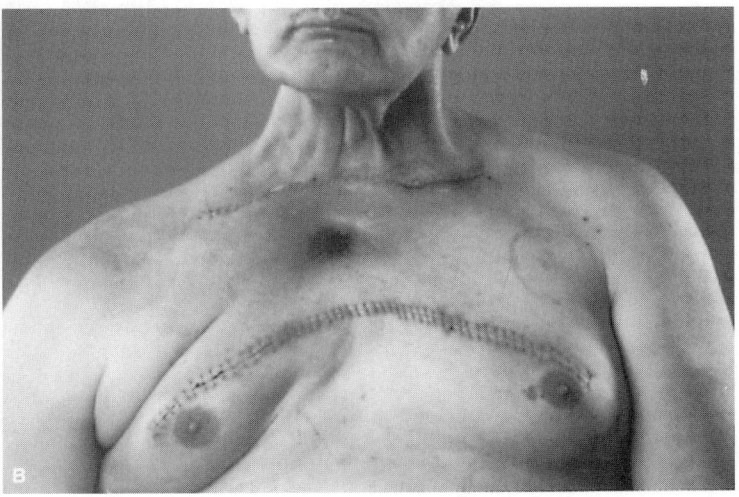

Figure 20.22. *(A)* Postoperative barium esophagogram of patient shown in Fig. 20.18 after laryngopharyngectomy, transhiatal esophagectomy, pharyngogastric anastomosis, and anterior mediastinal tracheostomy. *Large arrow* marks the pharyngogastric anastomosis. *Small arrow* is at the level of the pyloromyotomy. *(B)* Appearance of anterior mediastinal tracheostomy. This tracheostomy is several centimeters inferior to the traditional permanent cervical tracheostomy in the suprasternal notch.

neuvers that often follows and is responsible for a poor functional result in many patients. For these reasons, the author currently favors the use of a colonic interposition to reestablish alimentary continuity after a laryngopharyngoesophagectomy (96). The anastomotic leak rate is lower and the degree of postoperative regurgitation of food and bile from the colonic interposition is less than with a pharyngogastric anastomosis.

CAUSTIC INJURY

Caustic ingestion is most common in two broad categories of patients—children younger than 5 years of age who accidentally swallow these agents and adults who attempt suicide. More than 5,000 cases of caustic ingestion occur annually in the United States. The agents most frequently responsible for caustic esophageal injuries are alkalis, acids, bleach, and detergents containing sodium tripolyphosphate. Ingestion of detergents and bleach virtually always causes only mild esophageal irritation that heals without significant adverse sequelae. Acids and alkalis, on the other hand, may have devastating effects that range from acute multiple-organ necrosis and perforation to chronic esophageal and gastric strictures. Alkalis are more destructive, producing liquefaction necrosis, which almost ensures deep penetration, whereas acids usually

cause coagulation necrosis, which in part limits the depth of the injury.

In 1967, the introduction in the United States of concentrated liquid alkali preparations (e.g., Drano, Liquid Plumber) dramatically altered the nature and extent of caustic esophageal injuries. Before that time, alkali (lye) was typically available only in solid form, and lye crystals tend to adhere to the mucosa of the oropharynx and upper esophagus, producing burns in patches or linear streaks. Thus, solid alkali rarely reached the stomach in sufficient quantity to damage it. In contrast, the high viscosity of the newer liquid alkali preparations prolongs the contact between these substances and the mucous membranes and also facilitates their rapid transit into the stomach, so that severe damage to the esophagus and stomach, and also adjacent organs such as the trachea, colon, small bowel, pancreas, and aorta, is common. Ingested acids typically pass through the esophagus, quickly producing major gastric injury with relative sparing of the esophagus, although significant esophageal damage can occur.

In response to the ingestion of either acid or alkali, reflex pyloric spasm develops, with resultant pooling of these agents in the gastric antrum. Antral stenosis then produces a typical hourglass-like deformity (Fig. 20.23). Laboratory studies in a canine model have shown that cricopharyngeal and pyloric spasm occurs when concen-

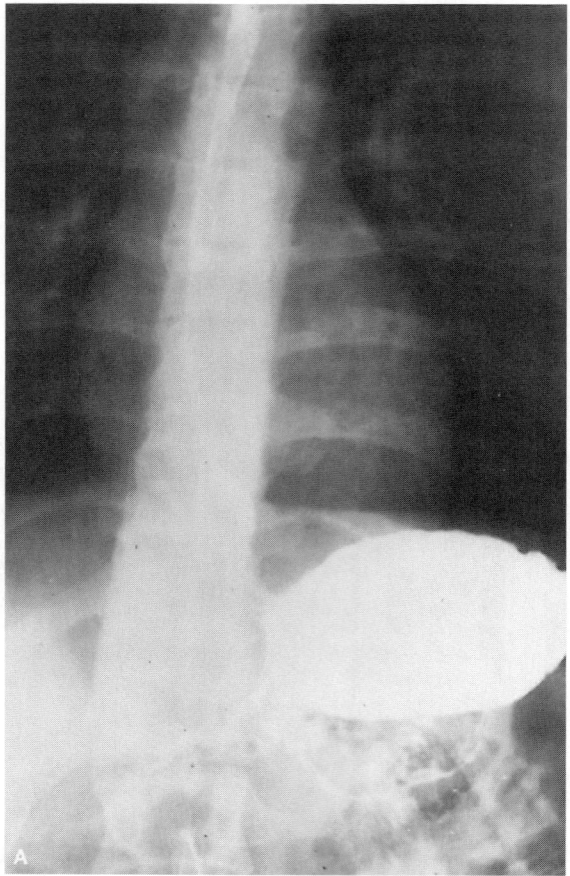

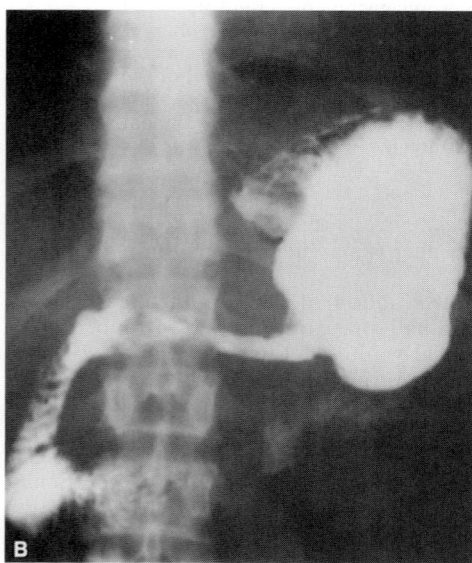

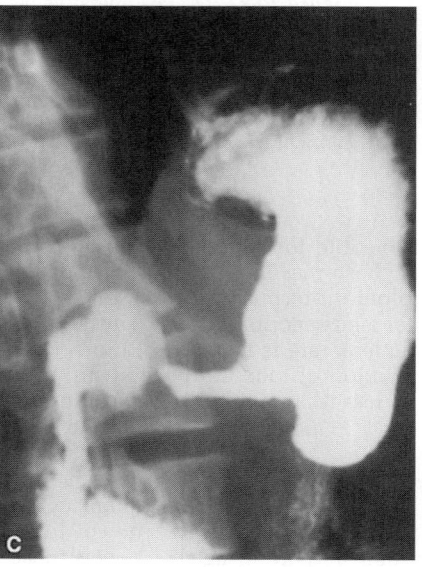

Figure 20.23. *(A)* Caustic stricture of the esophagus and stomach. *(B,C)* Detail of the stomach showing the typical hourglass deformity resulting from severe antral stenosis with sparing of the body of the stomach and duodenum.

trated lye enters the esophagus and stomach (97). The esophagus contracts vigorously, propelling the caustic agent into the stomach. Pyloric and gastric contraction follows and propels the caustic agent back up into the esophagus. This seesaw movement of the caustic agent between the esophagus and stomach continues for several minutes until gastric and esophageal atony develops as the result of extensive damage to both organs.

Clinical Features

The clinical manifestations of caustic ingestion are directly related to the amount and character of the agent ingested (98). Virtually no symptoms may be caused by mild pharyngeal, esophageal, or gastric burns (99). Solid alkali typically burns the mouth, pharynx, and upper esophagus. The resulting severe pain usually causes immediate expectoration, so that relatively little of the caustic agent is swallowed. These burns usually induce excessive salivation. On examination, the mucosa of the mouth and oropharynx shows patchy areas of white to gray–black pseudomembranes. Patients may also present with hoarseness, stridor, aphonia, and dyspnea from laryngotracheal edema or destruction. At the other end of the spectrum is liquid alkali ingestion. This form of alkali is usually swallowed quickly and produces less injury to the mouth and pharynx but more damage to the esophagus and stomach than its solid counterpart. Patients may present with dysphagia, odynophagia, and aspiration. Severe retrosternal, back, or abdominal pain and signs of peritoneal irritation suggest that mediastinitis or peritonitis resulting from esophageal or gastric perforation has developed. With acid ingestion, gastric injury is more common; therefore, signs and symptoms are frequently localized to the abdomen.

When esophageal or gastric perforation results from caustic ingestion, patients demonstrate progressively severe sepsis and hypovolemic shock until appropriate resuscitative measures are instituted. In the absence of gastric or esophageal perforation, the acute clinical manifestations typically resolve within several days, with clinical improvement lasting for several weeks. After this, symptoms of either esophageal or gastric stricture begin. Although strictures develop in only 10% to 25% of adult patients who ingest solid alkali, most patients who ingest liquid alkali sustain severe esophageal and usually gastric injury that often results in stricture formation. Children with limited exposure from accidental ingestion are less likely to have severe injuries. Acid ingestion most often results in stricture or contracture of the antrum or pylorus.

Immediate Diagnosis and Treatment

Acute caustic ingestion is an indication for hospitalization. Initial management centers on stabilizing the patient and assessing the severity of the injury. Vomiting should not be induced. Because caustic injuries produce almost instantaneous tissue damage, attempts to dilute the agent by having the patient drink water are futile. In fact, this may only aggravate the problem by causing an increase in gastric distention and vomiting. Oral intake should be withheld and hypovolemia corrected with intravenous fluids. Careful observation for evidence of airway obstruction is mandatory. Endotracheal intubation or tracheostomy may be required in cases of significant laryngeal edema or actual laryngeal destruction. Broad-spectrum antibiotics are indicated once the diagnosis of substantial esophageal injury has been established to diminish the risk for pulmonary infection resulting from aspiration and bacterial invasion through the damaged esophageal wall. Although corticosteroids have been advocated in the acute phase of caustic ingestion to minimize subsequent stricture formation, their efficacy has not been established (100,101). Because corticosteroids may mask signs of sepsis and visceral perforation and impair healing, their use in caustic esophageal injury is potentially deleterious and is therefore not recommended.

A relatively urgent contrast examination of the esophagus may provide important information in the patient with a caustic injury (102). Radiographically, acute mucosal esophageal injuries are seen as blurred, irregular margins with linear streaking of contrast in deeper ulcers. Submucosal edema may be manifested by scalloped or straightened esophagogastric junction margins. Dilation of the esophagus and stomach, gastric ulcerations, air in the gastric wall, and frank extravasation of contrast material from the esophagus or stomach are common. A contrast esophagogram is the best way to make the diagnosis of esopha-

geal perforation and should be performed if the diagnosis is suspected either at the time of admission or in subsequent follow-up. Identification of the site of perforation is vitally important in the planning of subsequent intervention. The initial esophagogram in these patients can be performed with a water-soluble agent (e.g., Gastrografin), but dilute barium provides much better mucosal detail and should be used if the diagnosis of perforation is suspected.

Management

Esophagogastroscopy should be performed soon after admission to establish whether significant esophageal injury has occurred and to permit grading of the severity of the injury (Table 20.4). Endoscopic evaluation alone, however, cannot determine with certainty the actual depth of the injury. The risk for perforation can be minimized by using a small-caliber, flexible pediatric endoscope and adequate sedation to prevent retching and movement by the patient. Although in the past it was taught that the endoscope should not be advanced beyond the first burned area, more recently, complete examination of the esophagus and stomach has been recommended, especially if severe burns are not detected proximally. This can be accomplished safely.

After the initial resuscitative and diagnostic measures have been performed, patients with caustic injuries must be observed carefully. Those with no more than first-degree burns require no other specific therapy for 24 to 48 hours. The incidence of subsequent esophageal stricture is low in patients with such injuries. Those who have second- or third-degree burns require careful and more prolonged observation for evidence of esophageal or gastric necrosis during the acute phase of the injury. Full-thickness necrosis of the esophagus, stomach, or other organs requires emergent resection. It is extremely difficult to determine on the basis of clinical, endoscopic, and radiographic information whether full-thickness necrosis has occurred. Patients with free intraperitoneal air, mediastinal air, extravasation of contrast material from the stomach or esophagus, peritonitis, or abdominal or mediastinal sepsis require immediate surgical exploration. Similarly, exploration is indicated in patients with severe persistent back or retrosternal pain, suggestive of mediastinitis, and in those with metabolic acidosis, suggestive of visceral necrosis. A gastric pH of more than 7 has been suggested as an indicator of severe gastric damage and the need for exploration. Unfortunately, this is not a reliable finding, particularly in the presence of gastric blood. Clinical evidence of peritonitis remains a much more sound indication for abdominal exploration in these patients.

Patients who have ingested caustic liquid and require operative intervention are generally best explored through the abdomen. This approach permits the assessment of injury to the intraabdominal organs and resection of areas of full-thickness gastric necrosis. Although only the lower

---

Table 20.4. **ENDOSCOPIC GRADING OF CAUSTIC ESOPHAGEAL INJURY**

Severity of injury	Endoscopic findings
First-degree	Mucosal hyperemia and edema
Second-degree	Mucosal ulceration with vesicles and exudates; pseudomembrane formation
Third-degree	Deep ulceration with charring and eschar formation; severe edema obliterating the lumen

portion of the esophagus is well visualized through the diaphragmatic hiatus, if an esophageal resection is required, transhiatal esophagectomy without thoracotomy is readily performed by the addition of a cervical incision (103,104). Before the abdominal exploration is begun, therefore, the operative field should be prepared and draped to include the area from the mandible to the pubis and anteriorly to both midaxillary lines. In patients who have sustained an acute caustic esophageal injury necessitating a resection, the surrounding periesophageal edema resulting from the caustic burn often facilitates transhiatal dissection.

When esophageal or gastric resection for acute caustic injury is required, restoration of alimentary continuity should be deferred until the patient has recovered from the acute insult and the development of chronic stricture in retained organs can be evaluated. As a rule, when the injury resulting from acid or alkali ingestion is severe enough to warrant gastric resection, esophageal resection is usually also required. Even if the esophagus has been spared, it is generally unwise simply to close off the distal esophagus and leave it as a blind pouch within the mediastinum. It is safer to perform a transhiatal dissection of the esophagus at the time of the gastrectomy. The mobilized thoracic esophagus is then delivered out of the cervical incision, and only the necrotic portion is resected, with as much potentially viable esophagus spared as possible. The remaining esophageal stump is then tunneled subcutaneously for construction of an esophagostomy on the lower neck or, preferably, on the anterior chest wall (described later).

Estrera and associates (105) have advocated a much more aggressive protocol than the approach just described, in which all patients with second- or third-degree caustic injuries identified at endoscopy undergo immediate exploratory laparotomy. Those who are found to have full-thickness injuries are treated by resection, typically esophagogastrectomy. A silicone stent is placed in those without full-thickness injuries, which is left in the esophagus for 3 weeks to prevent stricture formation. Further experience with this approach is needed before it can be advocated routinely.

Esophageal stricture formation after second- and third-degree burns is the rule, and dilation has been the traditional therapy for chronic caustic esophageal strictures. Dilation therapy should not be instituted until at least 6 to 8 weeks after the injury, when reepithelialization is complete, to minimize the risk for esophageal perforation (Fig. 20.24). If a caustic esophageal stricture is perforated during dilation, esophagectomy and visceral esophageal substitution are the best approach because repair of a perforation proximal to a stricture is rarely successful. Strictures that cannot be adequately dilated (with a 46F dilator or larger for adults) and those that remain refractory to dilation after 6 to 12 months require esophageal substitution, usually with colon. The stomach is the preferred esophageal substitute, but its use in these patients may be precluded by gastric scarring and contracture secondary to the original injury.

Severe esophageal strictures resulting from caustic ingestion were managed in the past by retrosternal colonic interposition, with the native, destroyed esophagus left in situ in the posterior mediastinum. Recent data, however, favor resection of the damaged esophagus in virtually every case, for several reasons: First, the retained obstructed esophagus can develop into a posterior mediastinal retention cyst or abscess. Second, after caustic injuries, the lower esophageal sphincter may be destroyed by fibrosis of the esophagogastric junction, and reflux esophagitis can then develop in the retained esophagus if it is still in continuity with the stomach. Finally, the risk for the de-

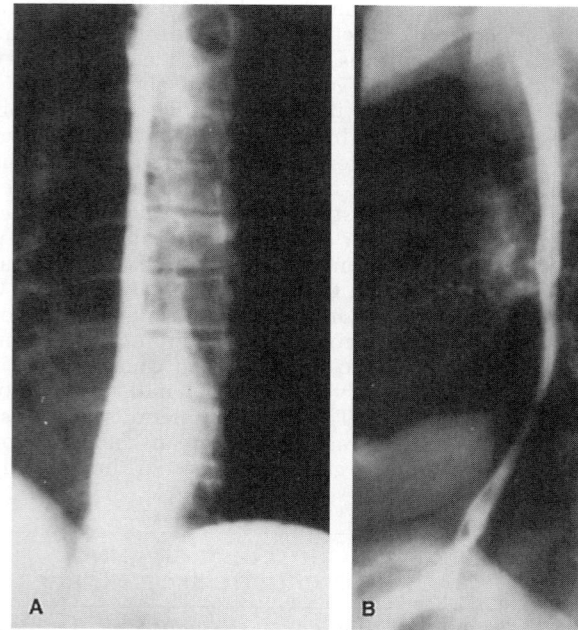
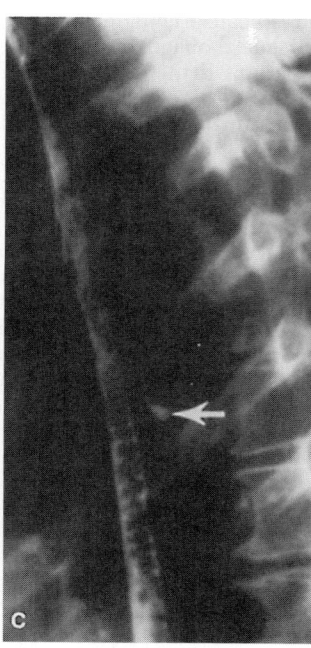

Figure 20.24. Posteroanterior *(A)* and lateral *(B)* views of a patient undergoing a Gastrografin swallow. The patient complained of chest pain after his caustic esophageal stricture was incorrectly and prematurely dilated within 10 days after his having ingested Drano, before reepithelialization of the esophagus was complete. No perforation was seen on this study. *(C)* Barium esophagogram demonstrates a perforation *(arrow)* in the middle third of the thoracic esophagus. (From Orringer MB. Complications of esophageal surgery and trauma. In: Greenfield LJ, ed. *Complications in surgery and trauma,* 2nd ed. Philadelphia: JB Lippincott, 1990:302.)

velopment of esophageal carcinoma after a caustic injury is about 1,000 times greater than the usual risk; the incidence is 0.8% to 4%, with carcinoma typically appearing after a latent period of 20 to 40 years. Therefore, a young patient whose caustic esophageal stricture is simply bypassed must be followed indefinitely for the development of carcinoma in the native esophagus, contrast studies of which are virtually impossible to obtain. Resection of the strictured esophagus also permits placement of the esophageal substitute in the posterior mediastinum in the original bed. This is the shortest and most direct route between the neck and abdominal cavity, and resection of the clavicle and adjacent sternum to enlarge the superior opening into the anterior mediastinum is not required, as it is when a retrosternal esophageal substitution is carried out.

ESOPHAGEAL PERFORATION

Esophageal perforation can be caused in various ways (106) (Table 20.5). Regardless of the specific cause, however, the pathophysiology and consequences of the resulting mediastinitis are such that prompt recognition and treatment of the esophageal disruption are required (1). Unless the perforation is contained by preexisting periesophageal fibrosis, saliva and gastric contents dissect into the fascial plains of the neck and mediastinum, and mediastinitis ensues. Except in edentulous patients, the presence of oral bacteria in these fluids initiates an infection. Esophageal and gastric contents are sucked into the mediastinum by respiratory movements and negative intrathoracic pressure. As salivary enzymes, gastric acid, bile, and food enter the mediastinum, the fulminant inflammatory response progresses. This mediastinal "burn" causes a massive accumulation of fluid that can displace the trachea, heart, or lungs. As in cases of blunt chest trauma and pulmonary contusion, the tracheobronchial tree may respond to the surrounding inflammation with a reflux bronchorrhea that results in the production of copious pulmonary secretions and noisy, wet respirations centrally, with relatively clear breath sounds peripherally. As circulating extracellular fluid volume is lost into the mediastinum, neck, or adjacent pericardial, pleural, or peritoneal spaces, hypovolemia and respiratory distress become manifest. The entire process is aggravated if preexisting esophageal disease is causing obstruction distal to the perforation.

Table 20.5. **CAUSES OF ESOPHAGEAL PERFORATION**

INSTRUMENTAL
Endoscopy
Dilation
Intubation
Sclerotherapy
Laser therapy

NONINSTRUMENTAL
Barogenic trauma
   Postemetic (Boerhaave's syndrome)
   Blunt chest or abdominal trauma
   Other (e.g., labor, convulsions, defecation)
Penetrating neck, chest, or abdominal trauma
Operative trauma
   Esophageal reconstruction (anastomotic disruption)
   Vagotomy, pulmonary resection, hiatal hernia repair, esophagomyotomy
Corrosive injuries (acid or alkali ingestion)
Erosion by adjacent infection
Swallowed foreign body

Clinical Features

Patients with esophageal perforation characteristically present with cervical or thoracic pain or difficulty swallowing, respiratory distress, and fever. Perforations of the cervical or upper thoracic esophagus generally cause cervical or high retrosternal pain, whereas those of the middle or distal esophagus produce anterior thoracic, posterior thoracic, interscapular, or epigastric pain. Upper thoracic esophageal perforations may produce signs of right pleural effusion; distal esophageal perforation is associated with left pleural effusion.

Diagnosis

Pain or fever after esophageal instrumentation or operation is indicative of an esophageal perforation until it is proven otherwise and is an indication for an immediate contrast esophagogram. Because the morbidity and mortality rates associated with esophageal perforation are directly related to the time interval between diagnosis of the injury and repair or drainage, an aggressive attitude toward diagnosing a perforation must be adopted. When the diagnosis is being considered, a water-soluble contrast agent should be administered. If the result of this study is negative, dilute barium should be administered. Barium is relatively inert, and the fear that barium will extravasate into the mediastinum through the site of injury and produce a severe reactive mediastinitis is unfounded. The risk of barium leaking into the mediastinum is far less than that of failing to recognize the perforation in a timely fashion. Also, because barium provides far better mucosal detail than water-soluble agents, only if barium has been used for the esophagogram should the result of this study to search for a perforation be considered negative (Fig. 20.24).

If the possibility of perforation after esophagoscopy is a concern, a chest roentgenogram may help to confirm the diagnosis by demonstrating air in the soft tissues of the neck or mediastinum or a hydrothorax or pneumothorax. A normal chest roentgenogram, however, does not rule out an esophageal perforation. If a perforation is suspected or considered, a contrast study of the esophagus is mandatory, both to establish the diagnosis and to demonstrate the exact site of the injury. In the exceedingly rare instance in which the esophagogram is equivocal or clinical suspicion overrides a negative study, contrast-enhanced CT may lead to the diagnosis (107).

Management

The initial treatment of an acute esophageal perforation is focused on decreasing bacterial and chemical contamination of the mediastinum and restoring intravascular volume losses. Oral intake is withheld, and the patient is instructed not to swallow saliva. A disposable oral dental suction device at the bedside is often helpful for evacuating oral secretions. Broad-spectrum intravenous antibiotics with activity against oral flora are administered: 1 g of a cephalosporin (cefazolin or cefamandole) every 4 hours and 1 to 1.5 mg of an aminoglycoside (gentamicin or tobramycin) per kilogram every 8 hours. Nasogastric tube decompression of the stomach is instituted to minimize possible gastroesophageal reflux and further soiling of the mediastinum. In the patient with a well-contained proximal perforation, however, a nasogastric tube may only interfere with the ability to breathe deeply, without providing any additional protection. The therapy of esophageal perforation is influenced by the location of the tear, its size and cause, the length of delay in diagnosis, the extent of mediastinal and pleural contamination, and the presence of intrinsic esophageal disease. Treatment must therefore be individualized.

Nonoperative Therapy

Although most esophageal perforations require operative intervention, selected patients may be managed nonoperatively with cessation of oral intake, administration of antibiotics, and intravenous hydration until the disruption heals or the small, contained cavity begins to decrease in size (108,109). Criteria for nonoperative therapy of an esophageal perforation include the following: (a) a local, contained disruption without evidence of pleural contamination (hydrothorax or pneumothorax); (b) a walled-off extravasation in which contrast material drains back into the esophagus; (c) minimal or no symptoms; and (d) minimal or no evidence of systemic infection (fever or leukocytosis). The cases that usually meet these criteria include cervical esophageal tears caused by esophagoscopy, intramural dissections that have occurred during dilation of a stricture or pneumatic dilation for achalasia, and asymptomatic esophageal anastomotic disruptions discovered on a routine postoperative contrast study. When such perforations are treated conservatively, oral hygiene should be optimized to minimize further contamination by oral bacteria by having patients brush their teeth four to six times a day. A nasogastric tube is seldom helpful. Nutrition may be maintained by a nasogastric feeding tube, gastrostomy, or jejunostomy or by intravenous hyperalimentation until oral intake can be resumed, usually 1 to 3 weeks after the injury.

When selecting patients for nonoperative therapy of an esophageal perforation, one must be certain that any cavity resulting from the tear is well contained and well drained internally into the esophagus. When a patient presents within 24 hours of an esophageal injury, it may not be possible to determine whether the leak is well contained, and a delay in surgical intervention may allow mediastinal sepsis to progress. Therefore, nonoperative therapy of an esophageal perforation is best suited for patients presenting more than 24 hours after the injury with no systemic evidence of sepsis and clearly demonstrable, contained, internally drained leaks on barium esophagogram. Infants with iatrogenic perforation can often be successfully managed without operation. Perforations complicating pneumatic dilation for achalasia occur in 4% to 6% of patients, and most are small and well managed medically with antibiotics and intravenous hyperalimentation (110–112). For the remainder of patients with a perforation, operative therapy is generally indicated.

Operative Therapy

Cervical and Upper Thoracic Esophageal Perforations. Cervical esophageal perforations lead to progressive contamination of the mediastinum as infection descends de-

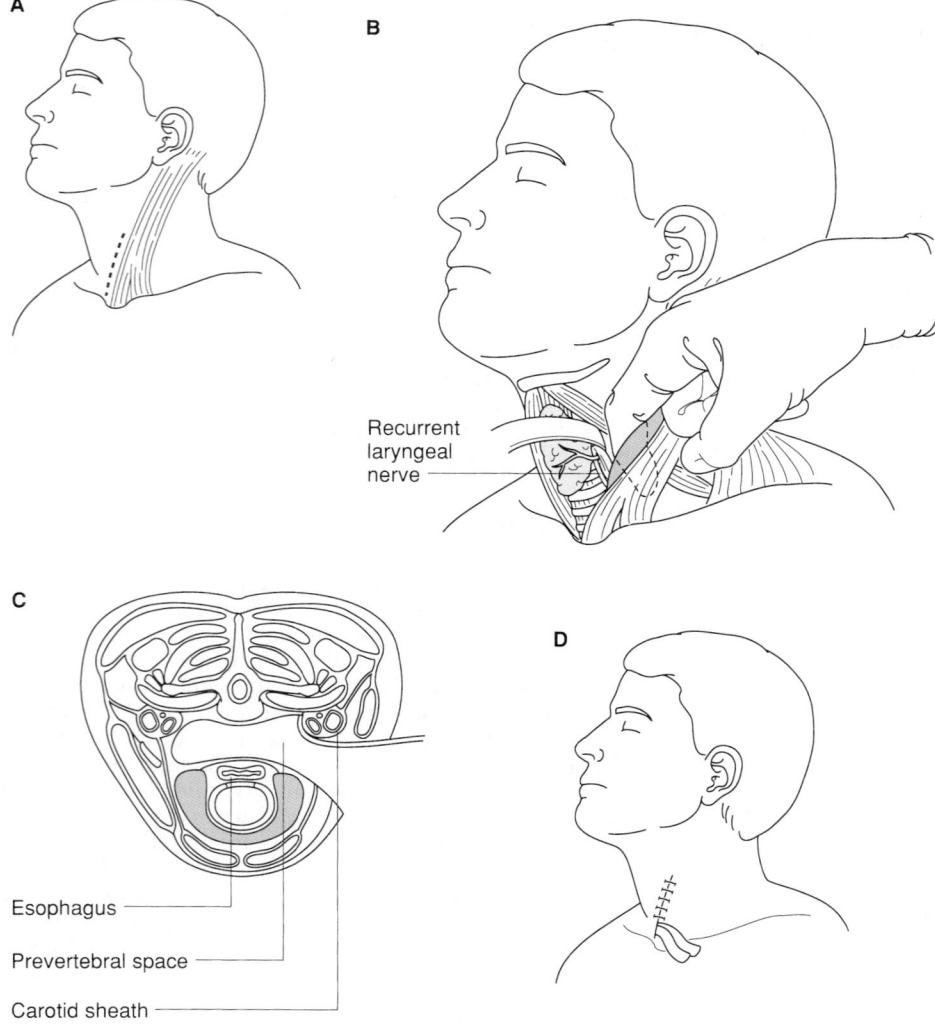

Figure 20.25. Approach for drainage of a cervical esophageal perforation. *(A)* Skin incision parallel to the anterior border of the left sternocleidomastoid muscle, extending from the level of the cricoid cartilage to the sternal notch. *(B)* With the sternocleidomastoid muscle and carotid sheath retracted laterally and the trachea and thyroid gland medially, blunt dissection along the prevertebral fascia in the superior mediastinum is carried out. Injury to the recurrent laryngeal nerve in the tracheoesophageal groove must be avoided. *(C)* Schematic drawing of the prevertebral space drained by this cervical approach. *(D)* Two 1-in rubber drains placed into the superior mediastinum are brought out through the neck wound to allow establishment of an esophagocutaneous fistula, which usually heals spontaneously. (After Orringer MB. The mediastinum. In: Nora PH, ed. *Operative surgery,* 3rd ed. Philadelphia: WB Saunders, 1990:370, with permission.)

Recurrent laryngeal nerve

Esophagus

Prevertebral space

Carotid sheath

pendently along the fascial planes from the neck. Unless adequate drainage is accomplished, death from mediastinitis follows. Most cervical and upper thoracic perforations (to the level of the carina or the fourth thoracic vertebral body) can be adequately drained through a cervical approach, with drains placed in the retroesophageal space (Fig. 20.25). An incision is made parallel to the anterior border of the sternocleidomastoid muscle, which is retracted laterally along with the carotid sheath and its contents. The trachea, thyroid gland, and strap muscles are retracted medially. It may be necessary to divide the omohyoid muscle, middle thyroid vein, and occasionally the inferior thyroid artery to reach the prevertebral fascia. Once this is identified, blunt finger dissection into the prevertebral space gives access to the abscess cavity, and appropriate drains are placed and brought out through the skin incision.

In most situations, because of the overlying trachea and larynx, it is not possible to identify the cervical esophageal tear for direct suture closure. This is seldom a problem, however, because a well-drained cervical esophageal perforation generally heals spontaneously within several days. Insufflation of air into the esophagus through a nasogastric tube or small flexible esophagoscope may be useful in identifying the tear and permitting direct closure if it is accessible. Nutrition during the first few days can be maintained with a small nasogastric feeding tube. Oral liquids can be resumed within 5 to 7 days of the injury if the fistula output is minimal. When a cervical esophageal perforation extends into either pleural cavity or the lower mediastinum, the cervical approach is inadequate, and transthoracic drainage is required.

Perforations of the Thoracic Esophagus. The earlier an esophageal perforation is recognized and treated, the better is the chance for successful primary repair. Historically, it has been taught that delay of repair beyond 6 to 8 hours after the injury is frequently associated with so much local inflammation that the torn esophageal wall is simply not amenable to suture repair. As a general rule, early esophageal perforations are those diagnosed well within 24 hours of the injury. Most agree that such perforations that are not associated with intrinsic esophageal disease are best treated with primary repair of the tear combined with wide mediastinal drainage. Mediastinal drainage is achieved by opening the mediastinal pleura from the level of the tear to the thoracic inlet superiorly and the diaphragm inferiorly, irrigating the mediastinum, and placing a large-bore chest tube that allows transpleural drainage. Perforations of the lower third of the esophagus are approached through a left thoracotomy in the sixth or seventh interspace, whereas more proximal thoracic esophageal tears are approached through a right thoracotomy. Perforations of the intraabdominal esophagus unassociated with pleural contamination are approached through the abdomen.

A change in philosophy has occurred regarding the application of primary repair to perforations in an otherwise normal esophagus *regardless of the duration of the injury.* It has now been documented that with meticulous technique, the results are good (113–115). The entire length of the mucosal injury must be exposed by extending the muscle defect 1 to 2 cm beyond the extent of the mucosal tear (Fig. 20.26). A 40F or larger dilator is placed within the esophagus to prevent undue narrowing, an endo-GIA (gastrointestinal anastomosis) stapler is applied, and the defect is closed. The staple suture line is reinforced by approximating adjacent muscle (Fig. 20.27). The perforation repair can then be reinforced with a pedicled flap of normal tissue (e.g., parietal pleura, anterior mediastinal fat, gastric fun-

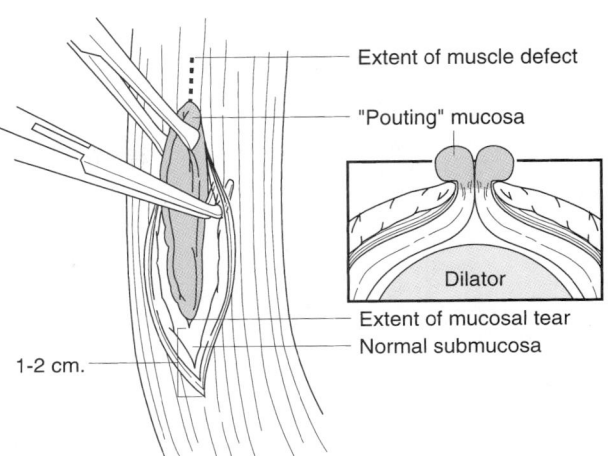

Figure 20.26. Primary repair of esophageal perforation. The edematous mucosa pouting through the muscular defect *(inset)* is grasped with Allis clamps and elevated. A 1-cm vertical esophagomyotomy is made at either end of the muscular defect to expose the entire limits of the tear. This is facilitated by using a right-angle clamp to direct muscularis away from underlying submucosa around the entire circumference of the tear. The result of this mobilization is exposure of a circumferential rim of normal submucosa that can then be closed. (After Whyte RI, Iannettoni MD, Orringer MB. Intrathoracic esophageal perforation: the merit of primary repair. *J Thorac Cardiovasc Surg* 1995;109:140, with permission.)

dus, intercostal muscle), but this is not essential if the repair has been performed well. After repair of a perforation of the lower esophagus (e.g., a postemetic rupture), a fundoplication around the repair is ideal for reinforcement of the suture line (Fig. 20.28). The fundoplication, however, should not be left in the chest to avoid subsequent compli-

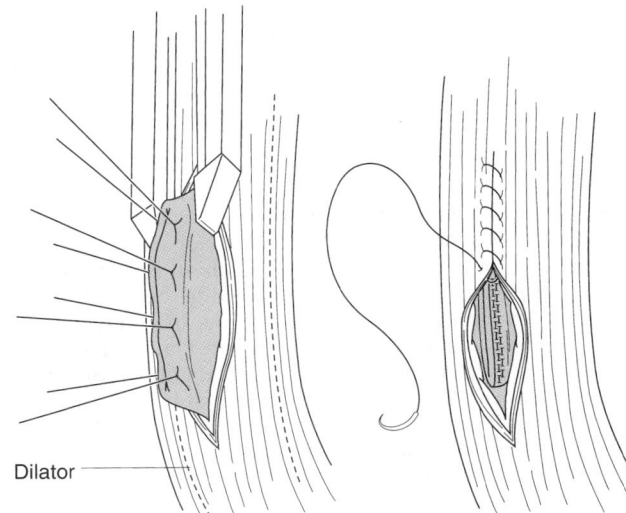

Figure 20.27. Primary repair of esophageal perforation (continued). *(Left)* Stay sutures placed into inflamed pouting mucosa elevate normal submucosa into the jaws of an endo-GIA (gastrointestinal anastomosis) stapler. The stapler is applied below inflamed edematous mucosal edges *(dashed line)*. *(Right)* After amputation of the pouting mucosal edge, the staple suture line is supported by approximating the adjacent muscle with a running suture. (After Whyte RI, Iannettoni MD, Orringer MB. Intrathoracic esophageal perforation: the merit of primary repair. *J Thorac Cardiovasc Surg* 1995;109:140, with permission.)

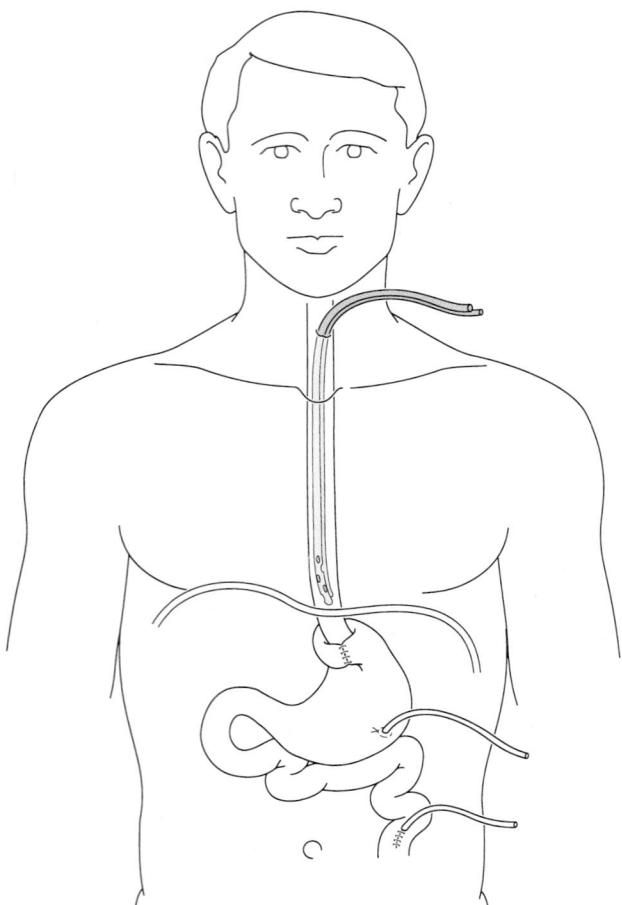

Figure 20.28. Repair of distal esophageal perforation and reinforcement with a fundoplication. To avoid potential complications of a paraesophageal hernia, the fundoplication should not be left in the chest. A decompressing gastrostomy and feeding jejunostomy, in addition to drainage of the esophagus with a nasogastric sump drain, are used. (After Orringer MB. Complications of esophageal surgery and trauma. In: Greenfield LJ, ed. *Complications in surgery and trauma,* 2nd ed. Philadelphia: JB Lippincott, 1990:302.)

cations of a paraesophageal hernia. More proximal esophageal repairs can be buttressed with intercostal muscle, parietal pleura, or a mobilized flap of anterior mediastinal fat. The intercostal muscle reinforcement should be carried out as an onlay patch rather than by encircling the esophagus to avoid subsequent esophageal obstruction that may develop as periosteum is regenerated. Omentum may be mobilized into the chest to reinforce an esophageal suture line at virtually any level. The parietal pleura must be inflamed and thickened if it is to provide adequate support of the suture line. Recently, absorbable mesh covered with fibrin glue has been used successfully to buttress a primary repair when no alternative was available (116).

After repair and drainage of the esophageal tear, a nasogastric tube is used to treat postoperative ileus, and thereafter, nasogastric tube feedings can be instituted until oral intake is resumed. It is wishful thinking to assume that the patient who is swallowing no food has a "protected" suture line, because saliva containing digestive enzymes and oral bacteria is traversing the esophagus from the moment the patient awakens from general anesthesia. Therefore, once the postoperative ileus has subsided, oral liquids may be resumed. No evidence has been found that swallowing a liquid diet results in a higher incidence of subsequent suture line disruption. A barium esophagogram is obtained 10 days after the repair to document the integrity of the esophagus, and the chest tube is not removed until after this examination. If a disruption of the esophageal repair develops, the resulting esophagopleural cutaneous fistula should heal spontaneously if external drainage through the chest tube is adequate and no associated distal esophageal obstruction is present. Such fistulae do not necessarily contraindicate oral alimentation if they are small and well drained.

Esophageal Perforation Associated with Intrinsic Disease.   Perforations associated with distal obstruction resulting from intrinsic esophageal disease constitute a much more challenging problem because breakdown of an attempted repair is common in the presence of distal obstruction. It is therefore important that the associated obstruction be relieved at the time of repair and drainage. For example, the patient with achalasia who sustains a distal perforation during balloon dilation should be treated with suture repair, esophagomyotomy to relieve the distal obstruction, and a partial fundoplication to buttress the tear if possible. A patient who sustains a small perforation during dilation of a "soft," dilatable reflux stricture may be treated successfully with repair of the tear, dilation of the stricture to relieve the obstruction, and an antireflux operation.

Patients with intrinsic esophageal disease that cannot be treated effectively by more conservative means (e.g., esophageal carcinoma; nondilatable, "hard" benign stricture; caustic injury; extensive esophageal devitalization associated with high-velocity gun shot wounds) are best treated by esophageal resection. Improvements in the techniques of esophageal replacement have resulted in a general philosophy that it is unwise to attempt to salvage a diseased esophagus simply because esophagectomy is regarded as too major an undertaking. If an esophagectomy is necessary in a patient with a perforated and diseased esophagus, a total thoracic esophagectomy, generally through a transhiatal approach, has the advantages of eliminating the source of mediastinal and pleural contamination and permitting a cervical esophageal anastomosis, which is associated with far less morbidity than an intrathoracic one (117).

If the esophageal perforation is diagnosed promptly and mediastinal contamination is not excessive, immediate restoration of alimentary continuity can be achieved at the time of transhiatal esophagectomy. This is the best approach when the stomach is healthy and available for esophageal substitution and a cervical esophagogastric anastomosis. Although immediate esophageal substitution with unprepared colon has been used successfully, it is not the preferred alternative. Patients with an esophageal perforation caused by caustic ingestion and those who are unstable or severely ill should undergo esophagectomy and cervical esophagostomy followed by later reconstruction. The preferred approach for immediate reconstruction after esophagectomy is to position the mobilized stomach in the posterior mediastinum in the native esophageal bed (Fig. 20.17). A feeding jejunostomy tube is used routinely for postoperative nutritional support until oral intake is adequate.

When a patient is so unstable that immediate esophageal reconstruction is not possible, transhiatal mobilization of the esophagus through the diaphragmatic hiatus and a cervical incision are carried out, the stomach is divided from the esophagus, and the cardia is oversewn. The mediastinum is then copiously irrigated through the cervical incision and the diaphragmatic hiatus (Fig. 20.29). The esophageal hiatus should be sutured closed to avoid herniation of abdominal viscera into the chest. The entire thoracic esoph-

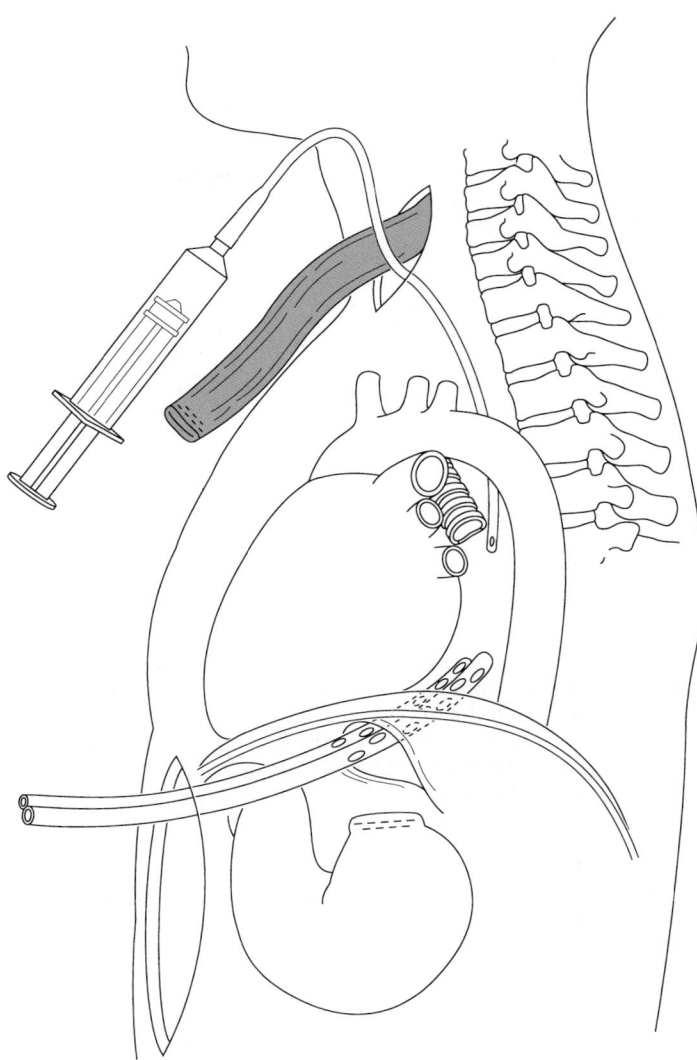

Figure 20.29. Irrigation of the posterior mediastinum after transhiatal esophagectomy for irreparable esophageal disruption. After irrigation with several liters of fluid and placement of bilateral chest tubes to drain the intentionally opened mediastinal pleura, an anterior thoracic esophagostomy (as shown in Fig. 20.30) is constructed.

agus is then delivered out of the chest through the neck wound and placed on the anterior chest wall. Only devitalized or extensively damaged esophagus should then be resected; the remaining esophageal stump is tunneled subcutaneously on the anterior chest wall, and a low cervical or high anterior thoracic esophagostomy is constructed (Fig. 20.30). An anterior thoracic esophagostomy is much easier to care for than an esophagostomy in the usual location in the supraclavicular fossa, and the extra length of remaining esophagus may facilitate later retrosternal esophageal reconstruction with stomach or colon. A feeding jejunostomy is used for enteral alimentation until reconstruction is performed several weeks later. A gastrostomy tube should also be inserted in the event that gastric atony or pylorospasm follow the vagotomy that accompanies esophagectomy. If the stomach empties well after several days, gastrostomy feedings may be used in preference to jejunostomy tube feedings, which are less amenable to bolus administration and are therefore not as convenient for the patient.

Late Esophageal Perforation. The longer the time interval between the occurrence of the perforation and operative treatment, the more inflamed are the tissues adjacent to the tear and, at least theoretically, the greater is the risk for failure of the primary suture repair. Although this may be the case, as discussed earlier, it is not the rule, and it is

well worth inspecting every esophageal tear to ascertain if primary repair might be feasible. The most difficult decision involves distinguishing between patients with a delayed esophageal perforation who are best treated with a controlled esophagopleural cutaneous fistula (or likely to be if an attempt at closure breaks down) and those who are best treated with esophageal diversion and exclusion or esophagectomy to prevent ongoing mediastinal and pleural contamination.

Patients with a late-recognized esophageal perforation have been treated in a variety of ways, including wide drainage alone, drainage and closure, drainage over a T-tube, esophageal resection, exclusion and diversion, and even nonoperative management. Clearly, this is not a uniform group of patients, and treatment must be influenced by the surgeon's experience, the condition of the patient, and the quality of the esophageal tissue at the site of the tear. Elderly patients who are edentulous often tolerate a chronic esophageal perforation because they lack substantial oral bacteria to contaminate the mediastinum and pleural cavity. Conservative management in these situations may often be successful. In most of these stable patients with a late-recognized esophageal perforation, a feeding jejunostomy and a decompressing gastrostomy to prevent gastroesophageal reflux are useful. Distal esophageal obstruction must be relieved, if necessary, by contin-

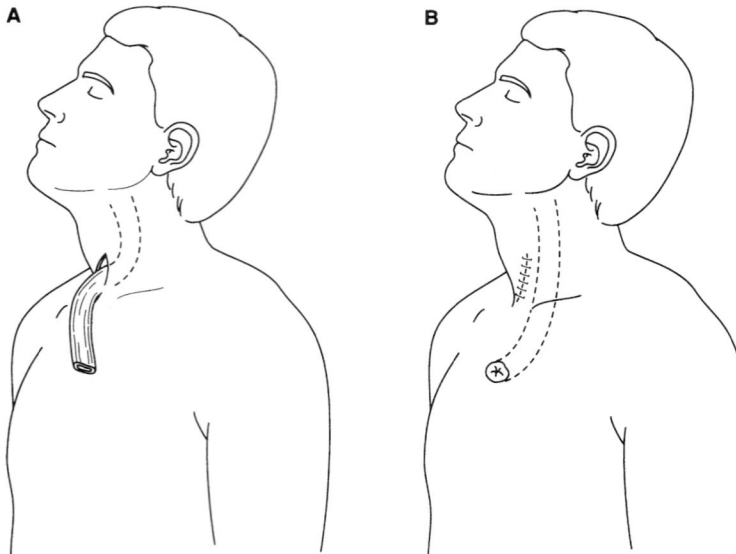

Figure 20.30. Construction of an anterior thoracic esophagostomy instead of the traditional end-cervical esophagostomy in the supraclavicular fossa. *(A)* The thoracic esophagus has been delivered out of the neck wound and placed on the anterior chest wall. Devitalized esophagus is resected, with as much remaining normal esophagus as possible left, and the distal extent is located for construction of the stoma. *(B)* The remaining esophagus has been tunneled subcutaneously and the end sutured to the skin. Stomal appliances are readily applied to the flat surface of the anterior chest, and when a colon interposition is performed at a later time, an additional 7 to 12 cm of esophageal length is available for the reconstruction. (After Orringer MB. Complications of esophageal surgery and trauma. In: Greenfield LJ, ed. *Complications in surgery and trauma,* 2nd ed. Philadelphia: JB Lippincott, 1990:302.)

uing dilations until the fistula closes. Well-drained esophagopleural cutaneous fistulae almost always heal spontaneously if no distal obstruction is present.

As discussed earlier, late-recognized esophageal perforations may be successfully closed with meticulous technique (113). For chronic esophageal defects that are too large to permit direct closure without tension, pedicled pleural flaps sutured around the edges of the defect have been used successfully to achieve closure (118). Esophageal exclusion for esophageal perforation has been used since the 1950s (119). The original technique involved division and closure of the distal thoracic esophagus through a thoracotomy or laparotomy and division of the cervical esophagus with construction of an end-cervical esophagostomy. This technique reduced mediastinal contamination and allowed the patient to recover from the septic insult. Major difficulties with subsequent esophageal reconstruction, however, are inherent in this approach. To circumvent these problems, a technique was developed for esophageal diversion and exclusion in continuity, which involved placing a removable ligature around the distal thoracic esophagus to control gastroesophageal reflux and then performing a side cervical esophagostomy to divert oropharyngeal secretions (120). Although this approach has conceptual appeal, it still entails problems with subsequent esophageal reconstruction, and control of mediastinal contamination has not been absolute. A technique has been described for stapling the esophagus above and below the perforation with absorbable staples until healing occurs and then dilating the esophagus to disrupt the staple line and restore continuity of the lumen at a later date. Further experience with this technique is needed before its efficacy can be established.

As a general rule, most patients with esophageal perforation require surgical intervention. Nonoperative therapy is contraindicated in most patients with esophageal tears, and an aggressive approach, with use of an esophagectomy if necessary, is often less radical treatment and more reliable in the long run than conservative techniques intended to preserve the esophagus.

INFECTIOUS ESOPHAGITIS

Chronic debilitation, immunosuppression, and the prolonged use of antibiotics predispose to the development of infectious esophagitis, *Candida albicans* being the most common cause. The onset of the AIDS epidemic, however, has resulted in a variety of esophageal infections caused by other fungi (*Torulopsis* and *Histoplasma* species), viruses [cytomegalovirus, herpes simplex virus (HSV), human immunodeficiency virus (HIV), Epstein-Barr virus], mycobacteria, and protozoa (*Cryptosporidium* and *Pneumocystis* species) (121).

Monilial Esophagitis

The fungus *C. albicans* is normally a commensal inhabitant of the mouth, oropharynx, and gastrointestinal tract. It may become pathogenic in patients who are severely debilitated or immunosuppressed. The use of potent broad-spectrum antibiotics, immunosuppression in organ transplant recipients, and the wide use of chemotherapeutic agents have resulted in an increased number of cases of monilial esophagitis. In its initial acute phase, monilial esophagitis with oropharyngeal involvement causes painful swallowing. As the disease progresses into the thoracic esophagus, abnormal esophageal peristalsis (decreased frequency and amplitude of primary and secondary peristaltic waves) and spasm may be seen. Radiographically, the characteristic cobblestone-like pattern of luminal nodularity is a result of inflammation and edema of the submucosa. In the advanced stages of acute monilial esophagitis, the radiographic findings on barium swallow are those of mucosal ulceration—an irregular, shaggy-appearing, narrowed esophageal lumen caused by mucosal and submucosal edema and pseudomembrane formation. The initial endoscopic findings are an erythematous, nonulcerated mucosa with an overlying whitish, cheesy exudate or pseudomembrane. The mucosa becomes granular and friable as the inflammatory reaction extends into the wall of the esophagus. Transmural invasion of the esophageal wall can be controlled with antifungal therapy if the patient survives the underlying disease, but chronic stricture formation may result after the acute esophagus heals. A characteristic radiographic pattern of intramural esophageal pseudodiverticulosis develops as the result of dilation and outpouching of the esophageal submucosal glands, which are inflamed in association with infection, stasis, or distal obstruction (Fig. 20.31). The esophageal submucosal glands are more

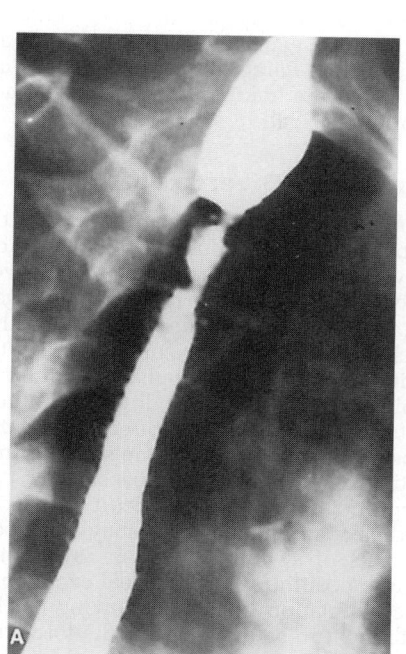
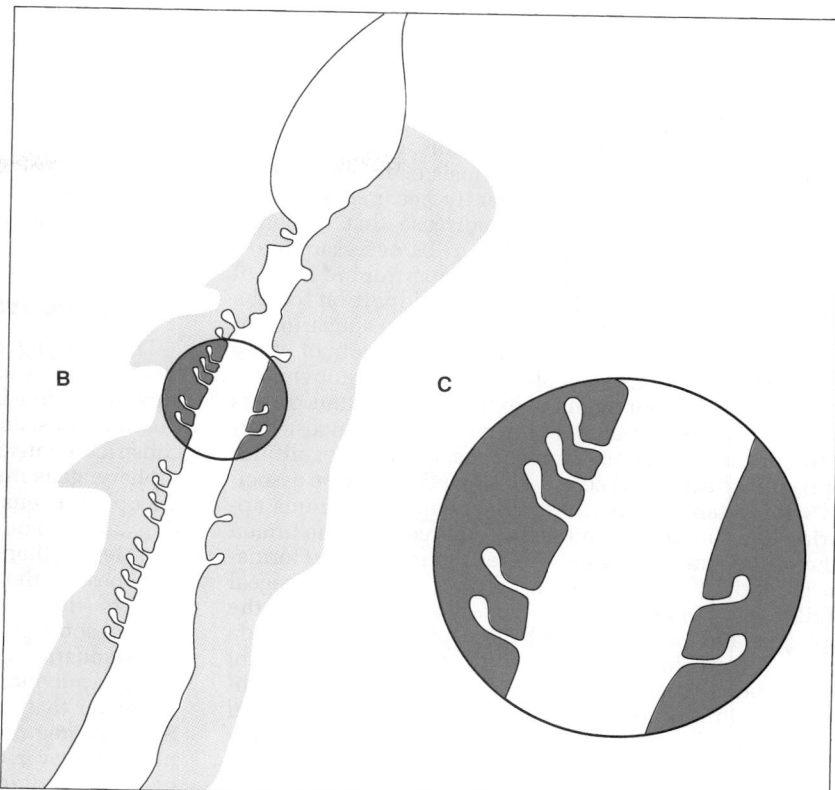

Figure 20.31. Esophagogram *(A)* and drawing *(B,C)* of an irregular upper thoracic esophageal stricture resulting from monilial esophagitis. The characteristic pattern of intramural pseudodiverticulosis is caused by dilated submucosal esophageal glands. (B and C after Orringer MB, Sloan H. Monilial esophagitis: an increasingly frequent cause of esophageal stenosis? *Ann Thorac Surg* 1978;36:364, with permission.)

numerous in the upper half of the esophagus, where monilial esophageal strictures are also encountered (122).

Minimally compromised patients with mild monilial esophagitis should receive 1 million to 3 million units of an oral nystatin suspension every 6 hours, or 100 mg of clotrimazole three to five times a day. This treatment should be continued for 1 to 3 weeks, although the infection generally subsides within 7 to 10 days. Oral amphotericin B lozenges, ketoconazole, or fluconazole may be used as an alternative. Patients with more severe immunosuppression (e.g., those with AIDS) or more severe cases warrant high-dose fluconazole (100 to 200 mg orally once a day) and ketoconazole (400 to 800 mg orally once a day). Intravenous fluconazole or amphotericin B is used for granulocytopenic patients (123). Because esophageal strictures may form after a bout of acute monilial esophagitis, patients who recover from the acute episode should be followed with periodic barium swallows during the first year to ensure the earliest possible detection of a developing stricture and prompt institution of dilation therapy if needed.

Viral Esophagitis

Viruses are the second most common cause of infectious esophagitis, HSV being the most common agent in immunosuppressed transplant recipients and cytomegalovirus in HIV-positive patients (121). Viral esophagitis causes mucosal ulceration, and patients present with dysphagia and odynophagia. The esophageal ulcers associated with viral infections appear on barium esophagogram as large lesions in cytomegalovirus disease and smaller (< 1.5 cm) ulcers in HSV infection. The diagnosis is established endoscopically by biopsy, brushings and washings for cytology, histology, and viral culture. HSV infection is diagnosed by isolation of the virus and identification in tissue culture, although the demonstration of multinucleated giant cells on Wright- or Giemsa-stained scrapings from the vesicles is presumptive evidence. The infection generally responds well to treatment with acyclovir.

Other Infections

Sporadic cases of infectious esophagitis secondary to syphilis and tuberculosis have been reported. Crohn's disease of the esophagus has also been reported as a rare cause of esophagitis. Tuberculosis of the esophagus is rare, and reported cases have invariably occurred in patients with advanced pulmonary tuberculosis who swallow copious sputum that is heavily laden with tubercle bacilli. The esophagus can become involved in several ways: implantation of swallowed bacilli, direct extension from adjacent lung or subcarinal lymph nodes, lymphatic spread from infection elsewhere, or hematogenous spread from a distant site. The midthoracic esophagus at the level of the carina is most frequently affected, probably as a result of spread from tuberculous paratracheal and subcarinal lymph nodes. Tuberculous esophagitis occurs in three forms: ulcerating, hypertrophic (stricture formation), or miliary. Esophageal symptoms may be totally absent or may range from intense pain on swallowing in the ulcerative form of the disease to dysphagia in the hypertrophic form. The barium esophagogram frequently fails to demonstrate the ulcerative or miliary forms of the disease, but the hypertrophic form appears as a midesophageal stenosis.

Fiberoptic esophagoscopy with biopsy of the stenosis establishes a diagnosis of esophageal tuberculosis by demonstrating the characteristic mucosal patterns and by retrieving specimens containing the organisms, which are identified with appropriate stains. The treatment of esophageal tuberculosis, like that of tuberculosis elsewhere in the body, is appropriate antituberculosis chemotherapy. In tuberculosis, the esophagus frequently becomes involved at an advanced stage of systemic disease that responds poorly to antituberculosis drugs. It may be necessary to dilate the esophagus in the stenosing hypertrophic form of esophageal tuberculosis. Rarely, the midportion of the esophagus is obstructed by a mass of enlarged subcarinal or paraesophageal lymph nodes, so that resection of these nodes is required to reestablish comfortable swallowing.

Syphilis of the esophagus is extremely rare and occurs in three forms: as a chancre in the esophageal mucosa during the primary stage; as an esophageal erosion or diffuse esophagitis during the secondary stage that may be associated with cutaneous manifestations; and as a gumma appearing as a submucosal mass that enlarges into the lumen of the esophagus, ulcerates, and results in stricture formation or perforation during the tertiary stage. Esophageal syphilis tends to develop in normally narrow areas of the esophagus and cause an esophagorespiratory tract fistula or an aortic erosion to form. The treatment of syphilis of the esophagus, like that of the systemic disease, is high-dose penicillin. Both the systemic disease and esophageal lesions typically respond dramatically to this treatment.

DIVERTICULA

An esophageal diverticulum is an epithelium-lined mucosal pouch that protrudes from the esophageal lumen. Most esophageal diverticula are acquired, and they occur predominantly in adults. Esophageal diverticula may be classified according to their location, the wall layers that they contain, or their presumed mechanism of formation (124). Pharyngoesophageal (Zenker's) diverticula occur at the junction of the pharynx and esophagus; parabronchial (midesophageal) diverticula develop close to the tracheal bifurcation; and epiphrenic (supradiaphragmatic) diverticula occur in the distal 10 cm of the esophagus. Diverticula containing all layers of the normal esophageal wall (mucosa, submucosa, and muscle) are termed *true diverticula,* whereas those consisting only of mucosa and submucosa are *false diverticula.* Most esophageal diverticula arise when elevated intraluminal pressure cause the mucosa and submucosa to herniate through the esophageal musculature; these are *false* diverticula. On the other hand, traction diverticula result from an external inflammatory reaction in which adjacent mediastinal lymph nodes adhere to the esophagus and then pull the wall toward them as they heal and contract; these are *true* diverticula. Pharyngoesophageal and epiphrenic diverticula are pulsion diverticula that are generally associated with abnormal esophageal motility. Parabronchial diverticula are usually but not always of the traction variety and include all layers of the esophageal wall.

Pharyngoesophageal Diverticulum

The pharyngoesophageal (Zenker's) diverticulum is the most common esophageal diverticulum and typically occurs in patients between 30 and 50 years of age. The diverticulum consistently arises within the inferior pharyngeal constrictor muscle, between the oblique fibers of the thyropharyngeus muscle and the more horizontal fibers of the cricopharyngeus muscle, the upper esophageal sphincter (Fig. 20.32). The point of transition in the direction of these muscles (Killian's triangle) represents an area of potential weakness in the posterior pharynx and is the site of formation of the diverticulum. Manometric measurement of upper esophageal sphincter function is difficult with existing standard recording equipment, which may not document rapid movements of swallowing in an asymmetric sphincter that changes position with laryngeal excursions. Some degree of incoordination in the swallowing mechanism, however, is thought to be the basis for the formation of Zenker's diverticula. Inappropriate pharyngeal contraction *after* cricopharyngeal closure has been demonstrated in these patients. Regardless of the precise motor dysfunction, a pulsion diverticulum would not occur without some cause of unusually elevated esophageal pressures. As the swallowed bolus exerts pressure within the pharynx, mucosa and submucosa herniate through the anatomically weak area above the cricopharyngeus muscle. The diverticulum may gradually enlarge with time, extending over the cricopharyngeus muscle, and dissect downward in the prevertebral space posterior to the esophagus and occasionally into the superior mediastinum.

Patients with pharyngoesophageal diverticula characteristically present with cervical dysphagia, effortless regurgitation of undigested food or pills, a gurgling sensation in the neck on swallowing, periodic choking, and aspiration (Fig. 20.33). Marked weight loss and dysphagia in an elderly patient may be misdiagnosed as an esophageal malignancy (Fig. 20.34). The diagnosis of a Zenker's divertic-

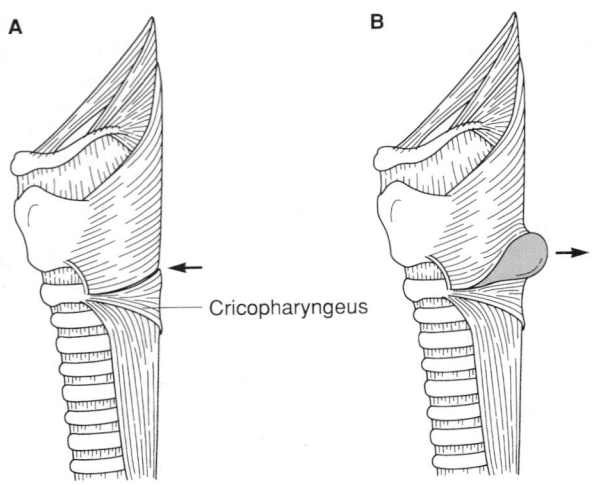

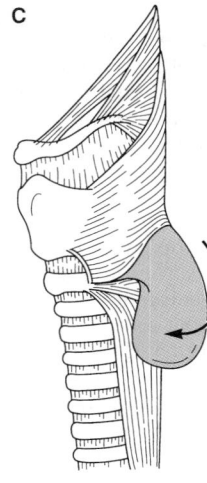

Figure 20.32. Formation of pharyngoesophageal (Zenker's) diverticulum. *(A)* Herniation of the pharyngeal mucosa and submucosa occurs at the point of potential weakness (Killian's triangle) *(arrow)* between the oblique fibers of the thyropharyngeus muscle and the more horizontal fibers of the cricopharyngeus muscle. *(B,C)* As the diverticulum enlarges, it drapes over the cricopharyngeus sphincter and descends into the superior mediastinum in the prevertebral space. (After Orringer MB. Diverticula and miscellaneous conditions of the esophagus. In: Sabiston DC Jr, ed. *Textbook of surgery,* 13th ed. Philadelphia: WB Saunders, 1986:726, with permission.)

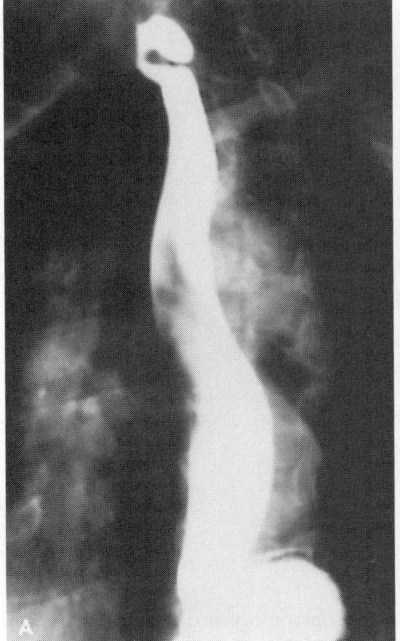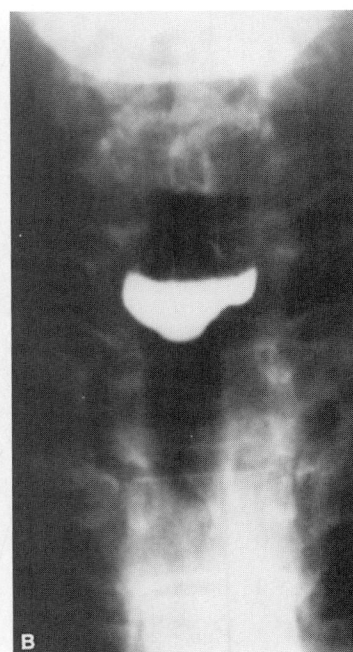

Figure 20.33. Small Zenker's diverticulum. *(A)* The 2.5-cm pouch and the esophageal narrowing distal to it representing the tight cricopharyngeus sphincter. *(B)* Detail of pouch showing retained barium. (Orringer MB. Extended cervical esophagomyotomy for cricopharyngeal dysfunction. *J Thorac Cardiovasc Surg* 1980;90:669, with permission.)

ulum is established with a barium esophagogram. In evaluating the patient with a Zenker's diverticulum, it must be realized that it is the degree of upper esophageal sphincter muscle dysfunction, not the absolute size of the pouch, that determines the severity of symptoms. In other words, a patient with a 5-mm Zenker's diverticulum may have as many or more symptoms than a patient with a 3-cm pouch. In most patients with symptoms, surgical treatment is indicated regardless of the size of the pouch to prevent additional complications (aspiration and nutritional impairment). As is the case with every pulsion diverticulum, the proper surgical treatment of a Zenker's diverticulum must be directed at relieving the underlying neuromotor functional obstruction responsible for the increased pharyngeal pressure.

The first surgical approaches to Zenker's diverticula involved simply excising the pouch and suturing the pharyngeal defect. The underlying upper esophageal sphincter dysfunction and resulting functional obstruction were not appreciated, and the incidence of suture line disruption with resulting cervical and mediastinal infection was high. Currently, a cricopharyngeal myotomy, which relieves the relative obstruction distal to the pouch, is regarded as the most important aspect of surgical treatment in these patients (Fig. 20.35). This operation is performed through a left cervical incision that parallels the anterior border of the sternocleidomastoid muscle. The sternocleidomastoid muscle and carotid sheath and its contents are retracted laterally, and the thyroid and trachea medially. The inferior thyroid artery is an important anatomic landmark in this operation. Once it is divided, the diverticulum is consistently found beneath it. The diverticulum is identified and dissected to its base, and an extramucosal esophagomyotomy is performed in either vertical direction for several centimeters from the base of the pouch to ensure that all cricopharyngeal muscle fibers are divided. Pouches of up to 2 cm in size simply are incorporated with the mucosa and submucosa, which bulge through the divided muscle at the site of the esophagomyotomy, and no resection of the pouch is needed. Larger pouches are excised with use of the surgical stapler. The results of treat-

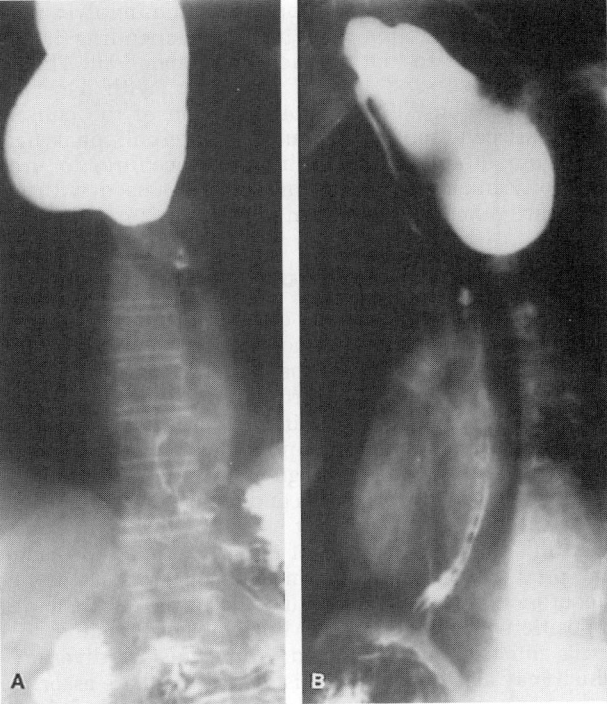

Figure 20.34. Posteroanterior *(A)* and oblique *(B)* views from barium esophagogram in an elderly woman presenting with cervical dysphagia and a 40-lb weight loss that were initially thought to be secondary to an esophageal malignancy. This 15-cm pharyngoesophageal diverticulum was treated successfully with diverticulectomy and cervical esophagomyotomy. (From Orringer MB. Diverticula and miscellaneous conditions of the esophagus. In: Sabiston DC Jr, ed. *Textbook of surgery*, 13th ed. Philadelphia: WB Saunders, 1986:726, with permission.)

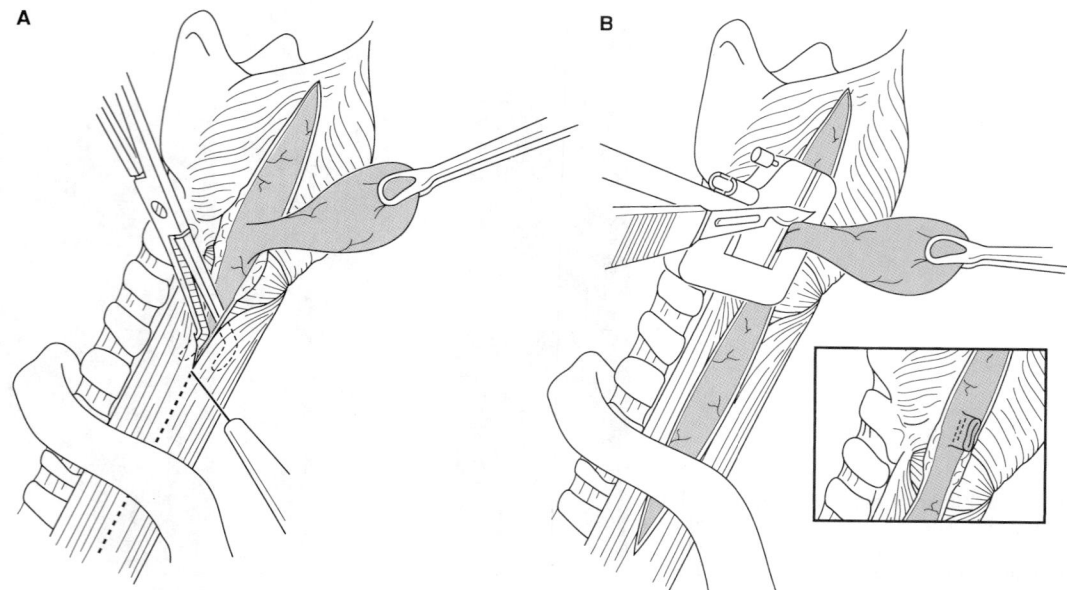

Figure 20.35. Cervical esophagomyotomy and concomitant resection of a pharyngoesophageal diverticulum. *(A)* An esophagomyotomy is performed for several centimeters in either vertical direction from the base of the mobilized diverticulum. *(B)* After completion of the esophagomyotomy, the base of the pouch is crossed with a TA-30 stapler and amputated. (After Orringer MB. Extended cervical esophagomyotomy for cricopharyngeal dysfunction. *J Thorac Cardiovasc Surg* 1980;80:669, with permission.)

ment are excellent, and recurrence is rare if the relative obstruction distal to the pouch has been relieved by complete division of the upper esophageal sphincter. An alternative approach is diverticulopexy, which involves mobilizing the pouch, inverting it, and suspending it from adjacent tissues so that the mouth is dependent. This operation is successful only if combined with a cervical esophagomyotomy. Endoscopic division of the common wall between the diverticulum (internal pharyngoesophagomyotomy, or the Dohlman procedure) for treatment of Zenker's diverticulum has been used with success, particularly by European surgeons (125,126).

Midesophageal Traction Diverticulum

Mediastinal granulomatous disease (e.g., tuberculosis or histoplasmosis) is the common cause of midesophageal traction diverticula. This type of diverticulum is much smaller than the pulsion diverticulum and has a characteristic blunt tapered tip that points toward the adjacent subcarinal and parabronchial lymph nodes to which it adheres (Fig. 20.36). It is typically diagnosed as an incidental finding on a barium esophagogram and almost always is asymptomatic. No specific treatment is indicated. At times, however, inflammatory necrosis of the granulomatous reaction may produce a fistula between the esophagus and the tracheobronchial tree requiring division of the fistula and interposition of normal tissues. Midesophageal traction diverticula must be differentiated from pulsion diverticula, which may also develop in this location and are associated with neuromotor esophageal dysfunction, as are epiphrenic diverticula.

Epiphrenic Diverticulum

An epiphrenic or supradiaphragmatic diverticulum occurs within the distal 10 cm of the thoracic esophagus. It is a pulsion diverticulum that arises because of abnormally elevated intraluminal esophageal pressure (Fig. 20.36). Al-

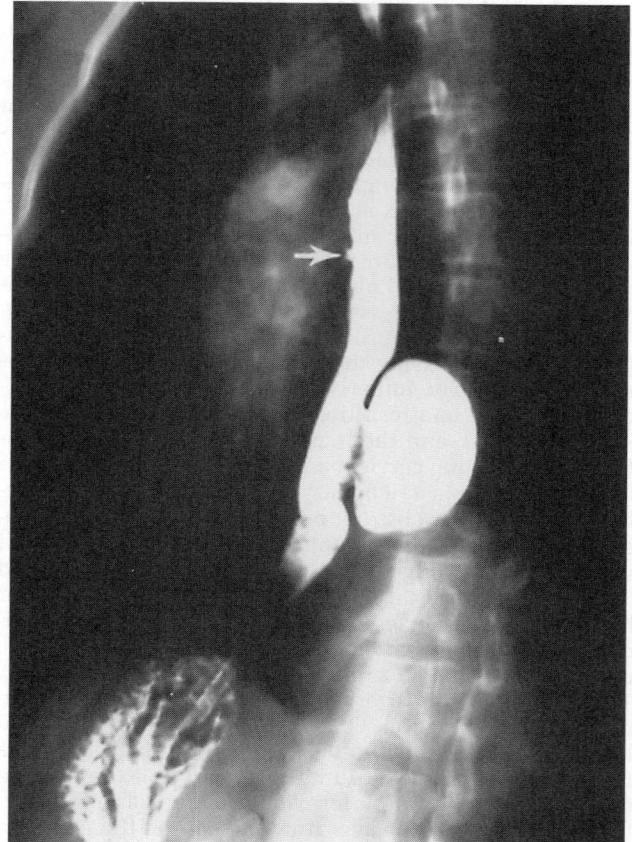

Figure 20.36. Barium esophagogram showing an epiphrenic diverticulum and a small traction diverticulum *(arrow)* of the middle esophagus. (From Orringer MB. Diverticula and miscellaneous conditions of the esophagus. In: Sabiston DC Jr, ed. *Textbook of surgery,* 13th ed. Philadelphia: WB Saunders, 1986: 726, with permission.)

though many patients have no symptoms at the time of diagnosis on barium esophagogram, others do have symptoms resulting from the frequently associated esophageal conditions: hiatal hernia, diffuse esophageal spasm, and reflux esophagitis. Dysphagia and regurgitation are the common symptoms of an epiphrenic diverticulum, and retrosternal pain may be caused by associated diffuse esophageal spasm. Esophageal manometry and acid reflux testing should be performed to define the associated motor abnormality and assess the competence of the lower esophageal sphincter mechanism (see Chapter 19). Pouches smaller than 3 cm and causing little or no symptoms require no treatment. Severe dysphagia, chest pain, or an anatomically dependent or enlarging pouch are indications for repair. Unless an associated distal esophageal stricture or tumor is present, it must be inferred that the patient with an epiphrenic diverticulum has an abnormally elevated intraesophageal pressure that has caused the pouch to form and is the result of neuromotor dysfunction. This can often, but not always, be documented manometrically.

The surgical approach to epiphrenic diverticula is through a left sixth or seventh interspace posterolateral thoracotomy. This is the case even for diverticula that present to the right of the esophagus. A long, extramucosal thoracic esophagomyotomy is performed from the level of the aortic arch to the esophagogastric junction (Fig. 20.37). If an associated hiatal hernia or incompetent lower esophageal sphincter is found, an antireflux operation should be carried out at the same operation. If an adequate esophagomyotomy is performed and the abnormally elevated intraesophageal pressure is thus relieved, suture line disruption and recurrence of the diverticulum are rare. Just as in the surgical treatment of achalasia, controversy exists regarding the distal extent of the muscle incision and the requirement for a concomitant antireflux operation. One school argues that the lower esophageal sphincter should not be disturbed if preoperative esophageal manometry and reflux testing show that it is normal. Others argue that to relieve the distal esophageal functional obstruction completely, which must be present regardless of normal manometry values, the esophagomyotomy must be carried distally through the lower esophageal sphincter and onto the stomach for 1.5 cm. The resulting incompetent lower esophageal sphincter necessitates the routine addition of an antireflux operation. Because the myotomized esophagus does not have normal propulsive force, when an antireflux procedure is added, a

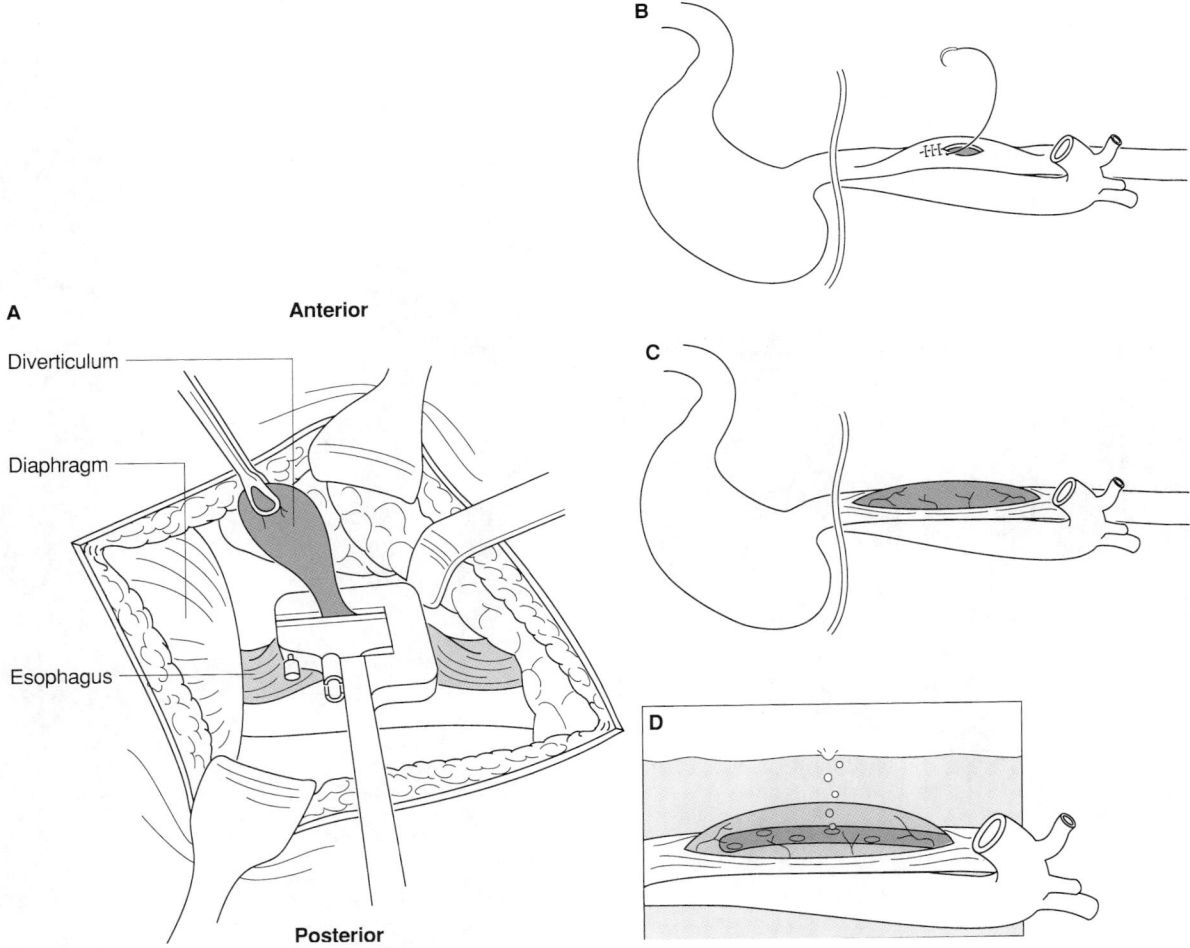

Figure 20.37. Technique of resection of epiphrenic diverticulum and concomitant esophagomyotomy. *(A)* The diverticulum is mobilized to its base and amputated with a TA-30 surgical stapler. *(B)* The staple suture line is oversewn. *(C)* A long esophagomyotomy is performed from the esophagogastric junction to the aortic arch 180 degrees on the opposite wall of the esophagus. *(D)* Air is insufflated through an intraesophageal nasogastric tube with the esophagus submerged under saline solution to be certain that the integrity of the mucosa has been maintained. (After Orringer MB. Complications of esophageal surgery and trauma. In: Greenfield LJ, ed. *Complications in surgery and trauma*, 2nd ed. Philadelphia: JB Lippincott, 1990:302.)

partial, 240-degree Belsey fundoplication, rather than a 360-degree Nissen fundoplication, is preferred so that functional obstruction is avoided. A Mayo Clinic report citing a 9% operative mortality rate associated with diverticulectomy and esophagomyotomy underscores the fact that patients with minimally symptomatic diverticula should not be subjected to surgery (127).

DISTAL ESOPHAGEAL WEB (SCHATZKI'S RING)

A Schatzki's ring is an annular constriction of the distal esophagus that forms at the esophagogastric junction in a patient with a sliding hiatal hernia. The ring characteristically projects into the lumen at a right angle to the long axis of the esophagus (Fig. 20.38). The incidence of Schatzki's ring is unknown because most patients with this abnormality do not have symptoms. Although periodic dysphagia may be experienced when the ring measures 20 mm or less on barium swallow examination, the diameter at which dysphagia almost always is experienced is 13 mm or less. The cause of a Schatzki's ring is not established. The ring occurs precisely at the squamocolumnar epithelial junction. Microscopically, it is covered by squamous epithelium over its upper surface and columnar epithelium on the gastric side. This is not a true fibrotic stricture, as usually only minimal submucosal fibrosis is present and no involvement of the esophageal muscle. Schatzki's ring can be seen only radiographically on a barium esophagogram because the squamocolumnar junction, as a consequence of the hiatal hernia, is above the diaphragm. A Schatzki's ring therefore indicates that a hiatal hernia is present, but it is *not* indicative of either associated gastroesophageal reflux or esophagitis. It may be difficult to differentiate a Schatzki's ring from a localized stricture caused by gastroesophageal reflux.

In patients with dysphagia resulting from a Schatzki's ring but no associated reflux symptoms, an excellent response often is obtained with periodic esophageal dilation. In patients who have both dysphagia and reflux symptoms, periodic dilation and an antireflux medical regimen are required. A few patients have persistent dysphagia or severe reflux symptoms despite medical therapy, and in this group, intraoperative dilation to disrupt the ring, in combination with an antireflux operation, gives good results. Resection of the distal esophageal ring alone, without repair of the associated hiatal hernia, is not adequate treatment.

RARE ESOPHAGEAL ABNORMALITIES

Esophageal Involvement in Dermatologic Disorders

A variety of dermatologic conditions involve the squamous epithelium of the esophagus (128). The development of vesicles and the subsequent formation of thin

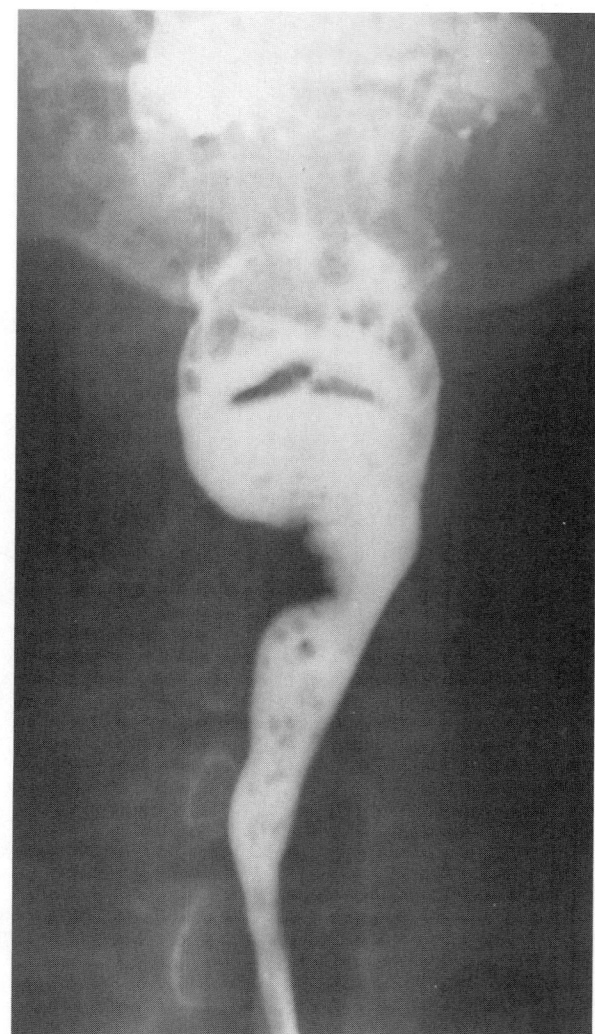

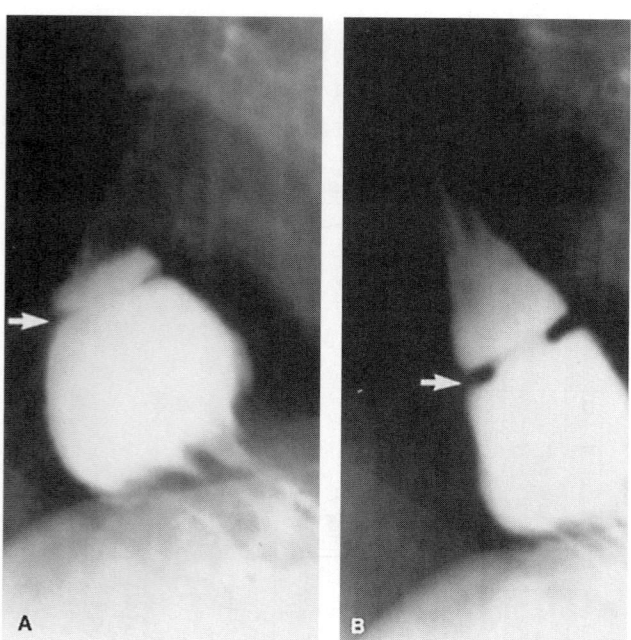

Figure 20.38. Esophagogram showing a typical distal esophageal web (Schatzki's ring) *(arrows)* projecting into the lumen at a right angle to the axis of the esophagus at the esophagogastric junction above a sliding hiatal hernia. (From Orringer MB. Diverticula and miscellaneous conditions of the esophagus. In: Sabiston DC Jr, ed. *Textbook of surgery,* 13th ed. Philadelphia: WB Saunders, 1986: 726, with permission.)

Figure 20.39. Cervical esophagogram showing an intrinsic right lateral mass that proved to be an aberrant right lobe of the thyroid gland posterolateral to the esophagus. A right thyroid lobectomy relieved the patient's dysphagia. (From Orringer MB. Diverticula and miscellaneous conditions of the esophagus. In: Sabiston DC Jr, ed. *Textbook of surgery,* 13th ed. Philadelphia: WB Saunders, 1986:726, with permission.)

esophageal webs have been reported in pemphigus vulgaris, bullous pemphigoid, and benign mucous membrane pemphigoid. These vesicles rupture, leaving denuded areas of superficial ulceration that may become secondarily infected and heal with fibrosis. In patients with pemphigus, the mucosal surfaces most commonly involved are those of the oral cavity and vagina; occasionally, the larynx, nose, and anus, and least frequently, the esophagus, are involved. The characteristic bullae on the cutaneous and mucosal surfaces are diagnostic, and the diagnosis is confirmed by examination of biopsy specimens. When these patients have dysphagia or painful swallowing, dilation therapy should be instituted early in the course of the disease to prevent the subsequent development of severe strictures. Epidermolysis bullosa dystrophica is a rare genetic skin disease that, unlike other bullous dermatoses, is inherited and generally begins early in life. The condition may be associated with severe blistering of the mucous membrane and can result in perforation or stricture formation (129). As with other dermatoses, dilation therapy is effective in maintaining comfortable swallowing in these patients.

Other Conditions

Certain rare conditions occasionally may have to be considered in the differential diagnosis of dysphagia. Marked cardiomegaly, hepatomegaly displacing the esophagus against the diaphragmatic hiatus, and tortuosity of the thoracic aorta resulting in esophageal compression all have been reported to cause dysphagia. Aberrant thyroid or parathyroid tissue may produce cervical dysphagia (Fig. 20.39). The development of cervical vertebral body osteophytic spurs, which typically involve the fifth, sixth, and seventh cervical vertebral interspaces, may displace the esophagus anteriorly and produce dysphagia (Fig. 20.40). It is important, particularly in elderly patients, to assess the cervical spine during evaluation of the esophagogram before endoscopy because the presence of exostoses makes esophagoscopy more dangerous, and the use of a pediatric flexible fiberoptic esophagoscope to exclude carcinoma is warranted in these patients with dysphagia. At times, removal of the osteophyte through an anterior cervical approach may produce excellent results.

Congenital vascular rings may compress the esophagus and produce dysphagia. The most common type of vascular ring is an aberrant right subclavian artery, which arises as the fourth branch of the aortic arch. This condition is usually asymptomatic, but it can produce esophageal obstruction in infancy or childhood or be responsible for dysphagia lusoria in adults. The classic finding on barium swallow examination is indentation of the posterior esophageal wall high in the thorax, caused by the aberrant right subclavian artery. Angiography is usually used to confirm the diagnosis. Other causes of dysphagia, especially gastroesophageal reflux with secondarily induced motor dysfunction, must be excluded. In infants, the vascular ring is approached through a left thoracotomy, and the vessel is divided and oversewn at its origin from the aortic arch. The retroesophageal portion of the vessel is oversewn and allowed to retract. In adults, this lesion has more recently been approached through a median sternotomy instead of a left thoracotomy. The origin of the aberrant right subclavian artery is identified, and the vessel is ligated and divided. The retroesophageal segment of the vessel is used for vascular reconstruction, either by creating an anastomosis to the right common carotid artery or by interposing a 10-mm vascular prosthesis between the end of the divided subclavian artery and the arch of the aorta.

The esophagus can be involved secondarily by metastases to mediastinal lymph nodes from other sites (130). Virtually any malignant tumor may metastasize to mediastinal lymph nodes, but carcinomas of the breast, lung, esophagus, and stomach predominate. Mediastinal lymphatics communicate extensively with the esophagus, and therefore any of these tumors may invade the esophageal wall from without and cause extrinsic obstruction. This is difficult to diagnose histologically with an esophageal biopsy because the tumors are submucosal. Bronchogenic carcinoma metastatic to subcarinal lymph nodes may markedly displace the esophagus and cause dysphagia (Fig. 20.41). Similarly, metastases to mediastinal lymph nodes from breast carcinoma may displace the esophagus and cause dysphagia. Therefore, any woman with a history of breast cancer, no matter how remote, who has dysphagia should be evaluated for possible mediastinal lymph node metastases.

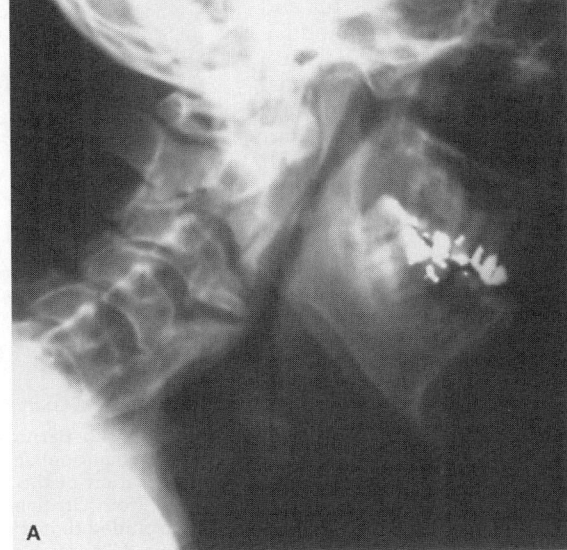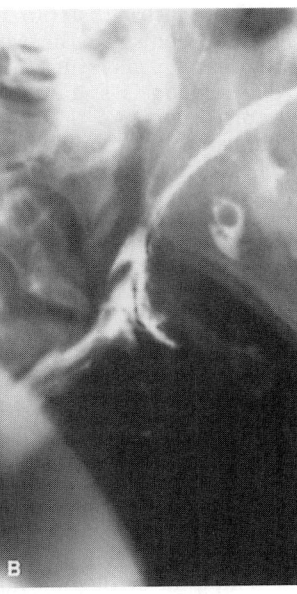

Figure 20.40. Cervical osteophytes displacing the esophagus anteriorly. *(A)* Soft-tissue radiograph of the neck. *(B)* Displacement of the barium-filled esophagus by the osteophytes. (From Orringer MB. Diverticula and miscellaneous conditions of the esophagus. In: Sabiston DC Jr, ed. *Textbook of surgery,* 13th ed. Philadelphia: WB Saunders, 1986:726, with permission.)

A   B

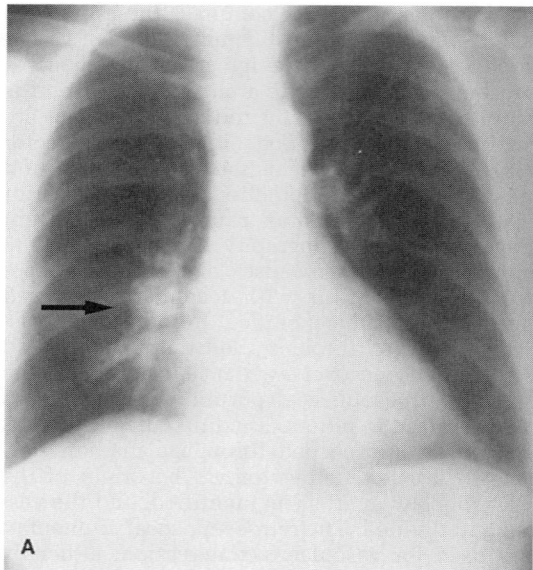
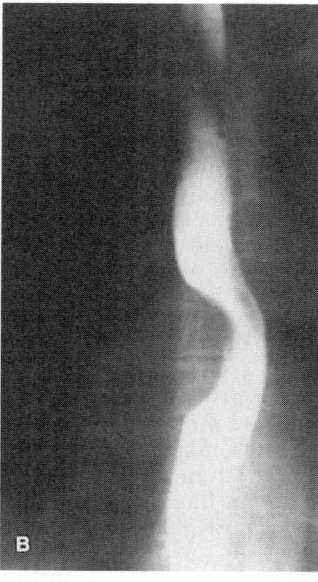

Figure 20.41. *(A)* Chest roentgenogram from a 60-year-old smoker who presented with dysphagia and a right infrahilar lung mass *(arrow)*. Bronchogenic carcinoma was diagnosed. Metastases to subcarinal lymph nodes were displacing the midportion of the esophagus, as seen on the barium esophagogram *(B)*. [From Orringer MB. Miscellaneous conditions of the esophagus. In: Orringer MB, ed. *Shackelford's surgery of the alimentary tract,* vol 1 *(The esophagus).* Philadelphia: WB Saunders, 1991:460, with permission.]

ACQUIRED TRACHEOESOPHAGEAL FISTULAE

Nonmalignant Fistulae

Only 10% of acquired fistulae between the esophagus and tracheobronchial tree are caused by benign disease (131). Nonmalignant fistulae result from erosion by contiguous infected subcarinal or mediastinal lymph nodes (e.g., tuberculosis, histoplasmosis, syphilis, actinomycosis); trauma (e.g., caustic injury, penetrating or blunt chest trauma, intubation, erosion by an aspirated foreign body, dilation of esophageal stricture); or erosion by an endotracheal or tracheostomy tube cuff in a patient requiring prolonged ventilatory support. They can also be late sequelae of a chronic midesophageal traction diverticulum. Patients present with characteristic paroxysmal coughing while eating as swallowed food or liquid enters the tracheobronchial tree. In patients who are mechanically ventilated, tracheal secretions may be reported to be excessive, ventilation may be difficult because of the loss of inspired air into the gastrointestinal tract or out of the mouth, or gastric distention may develop. Regurgitation of gastric contents into the esophagus through the fistula and into the lungs may cause fulminant aspiration pneumonia.

The diagnosis should generally be established with a contrast esophagogram. Because water-soluble contrast agents are hygroscopic and may have irritating pulmonary effects, dilute barium should be used for this study. Barium is inert and causes no harm to the lungs in small amounts. Bronchography may be useful in delineating the site of the fistula and in defining diseased pulmonary parenchyma that may need to be resected at the time of repair of the fistula. CT is used to define mediastinal adenopathy and exclude the presence of a mediastinal tumor mass. Endoscopy should be performed to exclude malignancy and assess the size and location of the fistula. Small fistulae may be difficult to localize endoscopically, and simultaneous esophagoscopy and bronchoscopy performed while air is insufflated through the flexible esophagoscope may be helpful in identifying a fistula along the posterior membranous trachea, which is inspected for bubbles of air. Biopsy specimens and brushings are taken from the tracheal and esophageal sides of the fistula for cytologic evaluation.

Benign acquired fistulae caused by mediastinal granulomatous disease are approached through a right posterolateral thoracotomy in the fourth or fifth intercostal space. The fistula is identified and divided, and the opening in the esophagus is débrided and closed. The tracheal or bronchial defect is similarly closed. Occasionally, communications with a segment of lung may necessitate a limited pulmonary resection. To prevent recurrence of the fistula, viable adjacent tissue, such as mediastinal fat, pleura, pericardium, or a rotated intercostal muscle pedicle, should be interposed between the tracheobronchial and

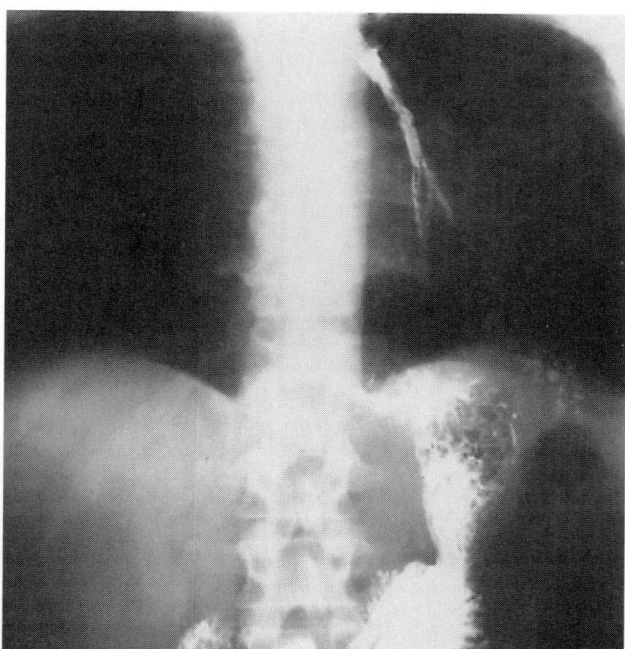

Figure 20.42. Barium esophagogram from a patient with a malignant tracheoesophageal fistula, showing the typical simultaneous opacification of the left main bronchus and the gastrointestinal tract. (From Orringer MB, Sloan H. Substernal gastric bypass of the excluded thoracic esophagus for palliation of esophageal carcinoma. *J Thorac Cardiovasc Surg* 1975;70:836, with permission.)

esophageal suture lines. Long-term results are excellent, and the recurrence of properly repaired fistulae is rare (132).

Mechanically ventilated patients in whom a tracheoesophageal fistula develops face a disastrous complication. Repair of the fistula is best deferred until the patient has been weaned from the ventilator. The fistula is managed initially by removing any nasogastric tube that is present and replacing the endotracheal or tracheostomy tube with another that has a large-volume, low-pressure cuff that is inflated below the fistula if possible. The stomach is decompressed with a gastrostomy, and a feeding jejunostomy tube is inserted for alimentation. Diversion of swallowed saliva by means of a cervical esophagostomy should be avoided if possible because this greatly complicates subsequent esophageal reconstruction.

Small fistulae, such as those resulting from an endotracheal intubation injury, are approached through a cervical collar or oblique incision anterior to the sternocleidomastoid muscle. The fistula is localized by carefully dissecting in the tracheoesophageal groove. The tracheal and esophageal openings are closed with interrupted 4-0 absorbable sutures, and the adjacent sternohyoid muscle is detached from the hyoid bone, rotated between the two suture lines, and sutured in place to prevent fistula recurrence.

Endotracheal or tracheostomy tube cuff injuries usually produce circumferential tracheal damage that necessitates a tracheal resection. This is performed through a cervical collar incision. The damaged short segment of trachea is resected, and the distal end is intubated to permit ventilation while the esophageal fistula is sutured closed and covered with mobilized cervical strap muscle. After the damaged segment of trachea has been resected, a primary tracheal anastomosis is performed. It is preferable to leave no tracheal tube in place postoperatively. The results of such repair are excellent in the patient who is no longer dependent on mechanical ventilation. Several reports have described successful endoscopic closure of tracheoesophageal fistulae, but the technique is not yet widely used (133,134).

Malignant Fistulae between the Esophagus and Airway

Ninety percent of acquired fistulae between the esophagus and tracheobronchial tree in adults are the result of malignant disease (Fig. 20.42). Tracheoesophageal fistulae complicate the course of disease in about 5% of patients with esophageal carcinoma, 0.2% of patients with lung cancer, and 15% of those with tracheal cancer. Malignant fistulae between the esophagus and respiratory tree involve the trachea in about 55% of cases, the bronchus in about 40%, and the peripheral lung

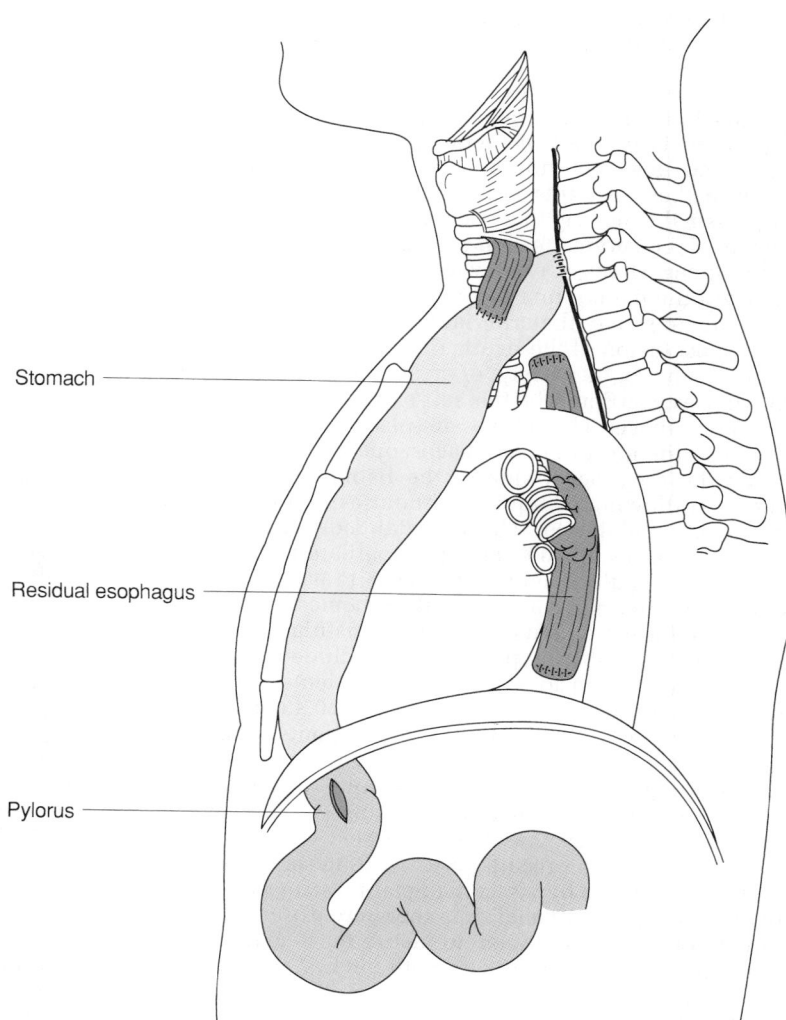

Figure 20.43. Lateral view after substernal gastric bypass of the excluded thoracic esophagus for a malignant tracheoesophageal fistula. After the cervical esophagus and esophagogastric junction have been divided and closed to exclude the diseased esophagus in the posterior mediastinum, the stomach is mobilized retrosternally in the anterior mediastinum, and an end-to-side cervical esophagogastric anastomosis is constructed. Secretions produced by the esophagus are vented into the tracheobronchial tree and periodically expectorated. (After Orringer MB, Sloan H. Substernal gastric bypass of the excluded thoracic esophagus for palliation of esophageal carcinoma. *J Thorac Cardiovasc Surg* 1975;70:836, with permission.)

Stomach

Residual esophagus

Pylorus

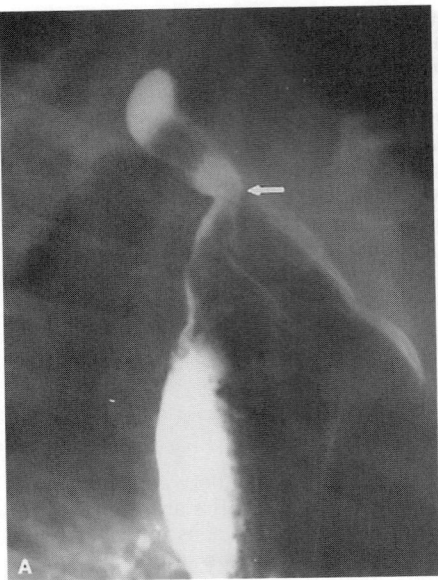
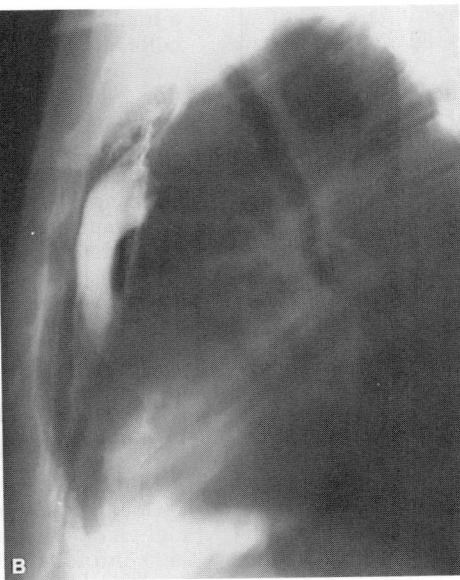

Figure 20.44. Postoperative barium esophagogram after substernal gastric bypass of the malignant tracheoesophageal fistula shown in Fig. 20.42. *(A)* The cervical esophagus angulates anteriorly at the thoracic inlet to meet the retrosternal stomach (*arrow* indicates the esophagogastric anastomosis). *(B)* Lateral view shows the retrosternal stomach in the anterior mediastinum. (From Orringer MB, Sloan H. Substernal gastric bypass of the excluded thoracic esophagus for palliation of esophageal carcinoma. *J Thorac Cardiovasc Surg* 1975;70:836, with permission.)

parenchyma in about 10%. Nearly 80% of patients with malignant tracheoesophageal fistulae die within 3 months of the onset of symptoms, and in 85% of these patients, the cause of death is aspiration pneumonia, not distant metastatic disease (135). For the most part, a malignant tracheoesophageal fistula develops in association with extensive mediastinal invasion by tumor that is incurable. Resection carries a prohibitive mortality and is seldom indicated. Because palliative relief of recurrent aspiration is the aim of therapy, insertion of a feeding tube does not constitute adequate treatment. Similarly, because these patients are unable to eat, owing to the paroxysmal coughing that occurs when they swallow, division of the cervical esophagus and creation of a cervical esophagostomy may prevent recurrent aspiration, but it leaves the patient unable to eat comfortably and therefore fails to satisfy the criteria of adequate palliation. Effective occlusion of the fistula may be achieved by insertion of one of a variety of available endoesophageal prostheses, particularly the self-expanding coated wire mesh prosthesis. These tubes are placed into the esophagus with the aid of an esophagoscope and generally occlude the esophageal side of the fistula sufficiently to allow swallowing of liquids without aspiration into the tracheobronchial tree. The hospital mortality for stent placement is 5% to 10%, and good palliation with occlusion of the fistula is achieved in 80% to 90% of patients (136–138). Stents have essentially become the treatment of choice for patients with malignant fistulae.

Substernal gastric bypass of the excluded esophagus has also been used for palliation in patients with a malignant tracheoesophageal fistula (Figs. 20.43 and 20.44). Even though excellent palliation for patients with a malignant tracheoesophageal fistula may be achieved with this technique, they usually survive only 6 months, and operative mortality rates in these patients, who have advanced malignancy, has been reported to be between 20% and 60%. The results of using long segments of jejunum or colon to bypass a malignant tracheoesophageal fistula are equally dismal. It is therefore difficult, except in extraordinary situations, to justify these major operative undertakings in patients with such a short life expectancy (60). Often, supportive care alone is the most humane treatment for them.

REFERENCES

1. Orringer MB. Complications of esophageal surgery and trauma. In: Greenfield LJ, ed. *Complications in surgery and trauma,* 2nd ed. Philadelphia: JB Lippincott, 1990:302.
2. Liebermann-Meffert DMI, Leuscher U, Neff V, et al. Esophagectomy without thoracotomy: is there a risk of intramediastinal bleeding? *Ann Surg* 1987;206:184.
3. Liebermann-Meffert D, Duranceau A. Anatomy and embryology. In: Orringer MB, Zuidema GD, eds. *Shackelford's surgery of the alimentary tract,* 4th ed, vol 1 *(The esophagus).* Philadelphia: WB Saunders, 1996:3.
4. Postlethwait RW, Lowe JE. Benign tumors and cysts of the esophagus. In: Orringer MB, Zuidema GD, eds. Shackelford's surgery of the alimentary tract, 4th ed, vol 1 *(The esophagus).* Philadelphia: WB Saunders, 1996.
5. Nemir P Jr, Wallace HW, Fallahnejad M. Diagnosis and surgical management of benign disease of the esophagus. *Curr Probl Surg* 1976;13:1.
6. Tio TL. Endoscopic ultrasonography in the evaluation of smooth muscle tumors of the upper gastrointestinal tract: a comparison with computed tomography, endoscopy, and barium meal. In: Tio TK, ed. *Endosonography in gastroenterology.* New York: Springer-Verlag, 1988:104.
7. Devitt PG, Iyer PV, Rowland R. Pathogenesis and clinical features of cancer of the esophagus. In: Jamieson GG, ed. *Surgery of the esophagus.* Edinburgh: Churchill Livingstone, 1988:551.
8. Duranceau A. Epidemiologic trends and etiologic factors of esophageal carcinoma. In: Delarue NC, Wilkins EW Jr, Wong J, eds. *International trends in general thoracic surgery,* vol 4 *(Esophageal cancer).* St. Louis: CV Mosby, 1988:3.
9. Devesa SS, Blot WJ, Fraumeni JF Jr. Changing patterns in the incidence of esophageal and gastric carcinoma in the United States. *Cancer* 1998;83:2049.
10. Hesketh PJ, Clapp RW, Doos WG, et al. The increasing frequency of adenocarcinoma of the esophagus. *Cancer* 1989; 64:526.
11. Heitmiller RF, Sharma RR. Comparison of prevalence and resection rates in patients with esophageal squamous cell carcinoma and adenocarcinoma. *J Thorac Cardiovasc Surg* 1996;112:130.
12. Cameron AJ. Epidemiology of columnar-lined esophagus and adenocarcinoma. *Gastroenterol Clin North Am* 1997;26: 487.
13. Landis SH, Murray T, Bolden S, et al. Cancer statistics, 1998. *CA Cancer J Clin* 1998;48:6.
14. Spechler SJ, Goyal RK, eds. *Barrett's esophagus: pathophysiology, diagnosis, and management.* New York: Elsevier, 1985.

15. Sampliner RE. Practice guidelines on the diagnosis, surveillance, and therapy of Barrett's esophagus. The Practice Parameters Committee of the American College of Gastroenterology. *Am J Gastroenterol* 1998;93:1028.

16. Ibrahim NBN, Briggs JC, Corbishley CM. Extrapulmonary oat cell carcinoma. *Cancer* 1984;54:1645.

17. Nicholas GL, Kelsen DP. Small cell carcinoma of the esophagus. *Cancer* 1989;64:1531.

18. Epstein JI, Sears DL, Tucker RS, et al. Carcinoma of the esophagus with adenoid cystic differentiation. *Cancer* 1984; 53:1131.

19. Chalkiadakis G, Wihlm, JM, Morand G, et al. Primary malignant melanoma of the esophagus. *Ann Thorac Surg* 1985;39: 472.

20. Sabanathan S, Eng J, Pradhan GN. Primary malignant melanoma of the esophagus. *Am J Gastroenterol* 1989;84: 1475.

21. Xu L, Sun C, Wu L, et al. Clinical and pathological characteristics of carcinoma of the esophagus: report of four cases. *Ann Thorac Surg* 1984;37:197.

22. Burt M. Unusual malignancies. In: Pearson FG, Deslauriers J, Ginsberg RJ, et al., eds. *Esophageal surgery*. New York: Churchill Livingstone, 1995:629.

23. American Joint Committee on Cancer. Esophagus. In: Fleming ID, Cooper JS, Henson DE, et al., eds. *AJCC cancer staging handbook*. From the *AJCC cancer staging manual*, 5th ed. Philadelphia: Lippincott–Raven, 1998.

24. Ferguson MK, Skinner DB. Carcinoma of the esophagus and cardia. In: Orringer MB, Zuidema GD, eds. *Shackelford's surgery of the alimentary tract*, 4th ed, vol 1 (*The esophagus*). Philadelphia: WB Saunders, 1996:305.

25. Quint LE, Glazer GM, Orringer MB, et al. Esophageal carcinoma: CT findings. *Radiology* 1985;155:171.

26. Block MI, Patterson GA, Sundaresan RS, et al. Improvement in staging of esophageal cancer with the addition of positron emission tomography. *Ann Thorac Surg* 1997;64:770.

27. Luketich JD, Schauer PR, Meltzer CC, et al. Role of position tomography in staging esophageal cancer. *Ann Thorac Surg* 1997;64:765.

28. Sugimachi K, Ohno S. Fujishima H, et al. Endoscopic ultrasonographic detection of carcinomatous invasion of lymph nodes in the thoracic esophagus. *Surgery* 1990;107:366.

29. Rosch T, Lorenz R, Zenker K, et al. Local staging and assessment of resectability in carcinoma of the esophagus, stomach, and duodenum by endoscopic ultrasonography. *Gastrointest Endosc* 1992;38:460.

30. Peters JH, Hoeft SF, Heimbucher J, et al. Selection of patients for curative or palliative resection of esophageal cancer based on preoperative endoscopic ultrasonography. *Arch Surg* 1994;129:534.

31. Fok M, Cheng SWK, Wong J. Endosonography in patient selection for surgical treatment of esophageal carcinoma. *World J Surg* 1992;16:1098.

32. Chandawarkar RY, Kakegawa T, Fujita H, et al. Endosonography for pre-operative staging of specific nodal groups associated with esophageal cancer. *World J Surg* 1996;20:700.

33. Reed CE, Mishra G, Sahai AV, et al. Esophageal cancer staging: improved accuracy by endoscopic ultrasound of celiac lymph nodes. *Ann Thorac Surg* 1999;67:319.

34. Gabrielsen TO, Eldevik OP, Orringer MB, et al. Esophageal carcinoma metastatic to the brain: clinical value and cost-effectiveness of routine enhanced CT before esophagectomy. *Am J Neuroradiol* 1995;16:1915.

35. Luketich JD, Schauer P, Landreneau R, et al. Minimally invasive surgical staging is superior to endoscopic ultrasound in detecting lymph node metastases in esophageal cancer. *J Thorac Cardiovasc Surg* 1997;114:817.

36. Krasna MJ, Flowers JL, Attar S, et al. Combined thoracoscopic/laparoscopic staging of esophageal cancer. *J Thorac Cardiovasc Surg* 1996;11:800.

37. Bemelman WA, vanDelden OM, van Lanschot JJB, et al. Laparoscopy and laparoscopic ultrasonography in staging of carcinoma of the esophagus and gastric cardia. *J Am Coll Surg* 1995;181:421.

38. O'Brien MG, Fitzgerald EF, Lee G, et al. A prospective comparison of laparoscopy and imaging in the staging of esophagogastric cancer before surgery. *Am J Gastroenterol* 1995; 90:2191.

39. Stein HJ, Kraemer SJM, Feussner H, et al. Clinical value of diagnostic laparoscopy with laparoscopic ultrasound in patients with cancer of the esophagus or cardia. *J Gastrointest Surg* 1997;1:167.

40. Endo M. Special techniques in the endoscopic diagnosis of esophageal carcinoma. In: Delarue NC, Wilkins EW Jr, Wong J, eds. *International trends in general thoracic surgery*, vol 4 (*Esophageal cancer*). St. Louis: CV Mosby, 1988:45.

41. Shiozaki H, Tahara H, Kobayashi K, et al. Endoscopic screening of early esophageal cancer with Lugol dye method in patients with head and neck cancers. *Cancer* 1990;66: 2068.

42. Roth JA, Lichter AJ, Putnam JB, et al. Cancer of the esophagus. In: Devita VT, Hehman S, Rosenberg SA, eds. *Cancer principles and practice of oncology*, ed 4.1. Philadelphia: JB Lippincott, 1993:776.

43. Turrisi AT. Esophageal cancer: the role of radiation. In: Orringer MB, Zuidema GD, eds. *Shackelford's surgery of the alimentary tract*, 4th ed, vol 1 (*The esophagus*). Philadelphia: WB Saunders, 1996:333.

44. Sykes AJ, Burt PA, Slevin NJ, et al. Radical radiotherapy for carcinoma of the oesophagus: an effective alternative to surgery. *Radiother Oncol* 1998;48:15.

45. Slabber CF, Nel JS, Schoeman L, et al. A randomized study of radiotherapy alone versus radiotherapy plus 5-fluorouracil and platinum in patients with inoperable locally advanced squamous cancer of the esophagus. *Am J Clin Oncol* 1998;21:462.

46. Game PA, Devitt PG. Intubation for carcinoma of the esophagus. In: Jamieson GG, ed. *Surgery of the esophagus*. Edinburgh: Churchill Livingstone, 1988:805.

47. Reed CE. Comparison of different treatments for unresectable esophageal cancer. *World J Surg* 1995;19:828.

48. Barnett JL. Esophageal carcinoma: palliation with intubation and laser. In: Orringer MB, Zuidema GD, eds. *Shackelford's surgery of the alimentary tract*, 4th ed, vol 1 (*The esophagus*). Philadelphia: WB Saunders, 1996:358.

49. Cottier DJ, Carter CR, Smith JS, et al. The combination of laser recanalization and endoluminal intubation in the palliation of malignant dysphagia. *J R Coll Surg Edinb* 1997;42: 19.

50. Adam A, Ellul J, Watkinson AF, et al. Palliation of inoperable esophageal carcinoma: a prospective randomized trial of laser therapy and stent placement. *Radiology* 1997;202:344.

51. Bethge N, Sommer A, Vakil N. Palliation of malignant esophageal obstruction due to intrinsic and extrinsic lesions with expandable metal stents. *Am J Gastroenterol* 1998;93:1829.

52. Raijman I, Siddique I, Ajani J, et al. Palliation of malignant dysphagia and fistulae with coated expandable metal stents: experience with 101 patients. *Gastrointest Endosc* 1998;48: 172.

53. Ramirez FC, Dennert B, Zierer ST, et al. Esophageal self-expandable metallic stents—indications, practice, techniques and complications: results of a national survey. *Gastrointest Endosc* 1997;45:360.

54. Siersema PD, Hop WCJ, Dees J, et al. Coated self-expanding metal stents versus latex prostheses for esophagogastric cancer with special reference to prior radiation and chemotherapy: a controlled, prospective study. *Gastrointest Endosc* 1998;47:113.

55. Narayan S, Sivak MV. Palliation of esophageal carcinoma: laser and photodynamic therapy. *Chest Surg Clin N Am* 1994;4:347.

56. Hurley JF, Cade RJ. Laser photocoagulation in the treatment of malignant dysphagia. *Aust N Z J Surg* 1997;67:800.

57. Reed CE, Marsh WH, Carlson LS, et al. Prospective randomized trial of palliative treatment for unresectable cancer of the esophagus. *Ann Thorac Surg* 1991;51:552.

58. Savage AP, Baigrie RJ, Cobb RA, et al. Palliation of malignant dysphagia by laser therapy. *Dis Esophagus* 1997;10:243.

59. Heier SK, Rothman KA, Heier LM, et al. Photodynamic therapy for obstructing esophageal cancer: light dosimetry and randomized comparison with Nd:YAG laser therapy. *Gastroenterology* 1995;109:63.

60. Lightdale CJ, Heier SK, Marcon NE, et al. Photodynamic therapy with porfimer sodium versus thermal ablation therapy with Nd:YAG laser for palliation of esophageal cancer: a multicenter randomized trial. *Gastrointest Endosc* 1995;42:507.

61. McCaughan JS Jr, Ellison EC, Guy JT, et al. Photodynamic therapy for esophageal malignancy: a prospective twelve-year study. *Ann Thorac Surg* 1996;62:1005.

62. Orringer MB. Substernal gastric bypass of the excluded esophagus: results of an ill-advised operation. *Surgery* 1984; 96:467.

63. Postlethwait RW. Oesophageal bypass using the colon. In: Jamieson GG, ed. *Surgery of the oesophagus.* Edinburgh: Churchill Livingstone, 1988:727.

64. Earlam R, Cunha-Melo JR. Oesophageal squamous cell carcinoma. I. An initial review of surgery. *Br J Surg* 1980;67:381.

65. King RM, Pairolero PC, Trastek VF, et al. Ivor Lewis esophagogastrectomy for carcinoma of the esophagus: early and late functional results. *Ann Thorac Surg* 1987;44:119.

66. Lazac'h P, Topart P, Etienne J, et al. Ivor Lewis operation for epidermoid carcinoma of the esophagus. *Ann Thorac Surg* 1991;52:1154.

67. Mathisen DJ, Grillo HC, Wilkins EW Jr, et al. Transthoracic esophagectomy: a safe approach to carcinoma of the esophagus. *Ann Thorac Surg* 1988;45:137.

68. Ferguson MK, Martin TR, Reeder LB, et al. Mortality after esophagectomy: risk factor analysis. *World J Surg* 1997;21: 599.

69. Law SYK, Fok M, Wong J. Risk analysis in resection of squamous cell carcinoma of the esophagus. *World J Surg* 1994;18: 339.

70. Tsutsui A, Moriguchi S, Morita M, et al. Multivariate analysis of postoperative complications after esophageal resection. *Ann Thorac Surg* 1992;53:1052.

71. Poon RTP, Law SYK, Chu KM, et al. Esophagectomy for carcinoma of the esophagus in the elderly. *Ann Surg* 1998;227: 357.

72. Orringer MB, Marshall B, Stirling MC. Transhiatal esophagectomy: clinical experience and refinements. *Ann Surg* 1999;230:392.

73. Gandhi SK, Naunheim KS. Complications of transhiatal esophagectomy. *Chest Surg Clin N Am* 1997;7:160.

74. Katariya K, Harvey JC, Pina E, et al. Complications of transhiatal esophagectomy. *J Surg Oncol* 1994;57:157.

75. Orringer MB, Marshall B, Iannettoni MD. Eliminating the cervical esophagogastric anastomotic leak with a side-to-side stapled anastomosis. *J Thorac Cardiovasc Surg* 2000;119:277.

76. Logan A. The surgical treatment of carcinoma of the esophagus and cardia. *J Thorac Cardiovasc Surg* 1963;46:150.

77. Akiyama H, Tsurumaru M, Udagawa H, et al. Radical lymph node dissection for cancer of the thoracic esophagus. *Ann Surg* 1994;220:364.

78. Altorki NK, Girardi L, Skinner DB. En bloc esophagectomy improves survival for stage III esophageal cancer. *J Thorac Cardiovasc Surg* 1997;114:948.

79. Hagan JA, Peters JH, DeMeester TR. Superiority of extended *en bloc* esophagogastrectomy for carcinoma of the lower esophagus and cardia. *J Thorac Cardiovasc Surg* 1993;106: 850.

80. Lerut T, DeLeyn P, Coosemans W, et al. Surgical strategies in esophageal carcinoma with emphasis on radical lymphadenectomy. *Ann Surg* 1992;26:583.

81. Skinner DB, Ferguson MK, Soriano A, et al. Selection of operation for esophageal cancer based on staging. *Ann Surg* 1986;204:391.

82. Altorki NK, Skinner DB. Occult cervical nodal metastasis in esophageal cancer: preliminary series of three-field lymphadenectomy. *J Thorac Cardiovasc Surg* 1997;113:540.

83. Forastiere AA, Orringer MB, Perez-Tamayo C, et al. Preoperative chemoradiation followed by transhiatal esophagectomy for carcinoma of the esophagus: final report. *J Clin Oncol* 1993;11:1118.

84. Adelstein DJ, Rice TW, Becker M, et al. Use of concurrent chemotherapy, accelerated fractionation radiation, and surgery for patients with esophageal cancer. *Cancer* 1997;80:1011.

85. Bates BA, Detterbeck FC, Bernard SA, et al. Concurrent radiation therapy and chemotherapy followed by esophagectomy for localized esophageal carcinoma. *J Clin Oncol* 1996;14:156.

86. Heath EI, Burtness BA, Heitmiller RF, et al. Phase II evaluation of preoperative chemoradiation and postoperative adjuvant chemotherapy for squamous cell and adenocarcinoma of the esophagus. *J Clin Oncol* 2000;18:868.

87. Naunheim KS, Petruska PJ, Roy TS, et al. Preoperative chemotherapy and radiotherapy for esophageal carcinoma. *J Thorac Cardiovasc Surg* 1992;5:887.

88. Bossett JF, Gignoux M, Triboulet JP, et al. Chemoradiotherapy followed by surgery compared with surgery alone in squamous cell cancer of the esophagus. *N Engl J Med* 1997; 337:161.

89. Urba S, Orringer MB, Turrisi A, et al. A randomized trial comparing surgery to preoperative concomitant chemoradiation plus surgery in patients with resectable esophageal cancer. *Proc Soc Clin Oncol* 1997;16:277.

90. Walsh TN, Noonam N, Hollywood D, et al. A comparison of multimodal therapy and surgery for esophageal adenocarcinoma. *N Engl J Med* 1996;335:462.

91. Grillo HC, Mathisen DJ. Cervical exenteration. *Ann Thorac Surg* 1990;49:401.

92. Orringer MB. Anterior mediastinal tracheostomy with and without cervical exenteration. *Ann Thorac Surg* 1992;54: 628.

93. Carlson GW, Schusteman MA, Guillamondegui OM. Total reconstruction of the hypopharynx and cervical esophagus: a 20-year experience. *Ann Plast Surg* 1992;29:408.

94. Paletta CE, Jurkiewicz MJ. Esophageal replacement: microvascular jejunal transplantation. In: Baue AE, Geha AS, Hammond GL, et al., eds. *Glenn's thoracic and cardiovascular surgery,* 6th ed. Stamford, CT: Appleton & Lang, 1996: 931.

95. Sullivan MW, Talamonti MS, Sithanandam K, et al. Results of gastric transposition for reconstruction of the pharyngoesophagus. *Surgery* 1999;126:666.

96. Orringer MB. Anterior mediastinal tracheostomy with and without cervical exenteration—updated in 1998. *Ann Thorac Surg* 1999;67:591.

97. Kirsh MM, Ritter F. Caustic ingestion and subsequent damage to the oropharyngeal and digestive passages. *Ann Thorac Surg* 1976;21:74.

98. Goldman LP, Weigert JM. Corrosive substance ingestion: a review. *Am J Gastroenterol* 1984;79:85.

99. Gorman RL, Khin-Maung-Gyi MT, Klein-Schwartz W, et al. Initial symptoms as predictors of esophageal injury in alkaline corrosive ingestions. *Am J Emerg Med* 1992;10:189.

100. Anderson KD, Rouse TM, Randolph JG. A controlled trial of corticosteroids in children with corrosive injury of the esophagus. *N Engl J Med* 1990;323:637.

101. Howell JM, Dalsey WC, Hartsell FW, et al. Steroids for the treatment of corrosive esophageal injury: a statistical analysis of past studies. *Am J Emerg Med* 1992;10:421.

102. Kuhn JR, Tunell WP. The role of initial cine-esophagography in caustic esophageal injury. *Am J Surg* 1983;146:804.

103. Gossot D, Sarfati E, Celerier M. Early blunt esophagectomy in severe caustic burns of the upper digestive tract. *J Thorac Cardiovasc Surg* 1987;84:188.

104. Orringer MB. Transhiatal esophagectomy for benign disease. *J Thorac Cardiovasc Surg* 1985;90:649.

105. Estrera A, Taylor W, Mills LJ, et al. Corrosive burns of the esophagus and stomach: a recommendation for an aggressive surgical approach. *Ann Thorac Surg* 1986;41:276.

106. Jones WG II, Ginsberg RJ. Esophageal perforation: a continuing challenge. *Ann Thorac Surg* 1992;53:534.

107. White CS, Templeton PA, Attar S. Esophageal perforation: CT findings. *AJR Am J Roentgenol* 1993;160:767.

108. Michel L, Malt RA, Grillo HC. Operative and non-operative management of esophageal perforation. *Ann Surg* 1981;194: 57.

109. Cameron JL, Kieffer RH, Hendrix TR, et al. Selective nonoperative management of contained intrathoracic esophageal disruptions. *Ann Thorac Surg* 1979;27:404.

110. Barnett JL, Eisenman R, Nostrant TT, et al. Witzel pneumatic dilation for achalasia: safety and long-term efficacy. *Gastrointest Endosc* 1990;36:482.

111. Parkman HP, Reynolds JC, Ouyang A, et al. Pneumatic dilatation or esophagomyotomy treatment for idiopathic achalasia: clinical outcomes and cost analysis. *Dig Dis Sci* 1993; 38:75.

112. Lo AY, Surick B, Ghazi A. Nonoperative management of esophageal perforation secondary to balloon dilatation. *Surg Endosc* 1993;7:529.

113. White RI, Iannettoni MD, Orringer MB. Intrathoracic esophageal perforation: the merit of primary repair. *J Thorac Cardiovasc Surg* 1995;109:140.

114. Wright CD, Mathisen DJ, Wain JC, et al. Reinforced primary repair of thoracic esophageal perforation. *Ann Thorac Surg* 1995;60:245.

115. Ohri SK, Liakakos TA, Pathi V, et al. Primary repair of iatrogenic thoracic esophageal perforation and Boerhaave's syndrome. *Ann Thorac Surg* 1993;55:603.

116. Bardaxoglou E, Manganas D, Meunier B, et al. New approach to surgical management of early esophageal thoracic perforation: primary suture repair reinforced with absorbable mesh and fibrin glue. *World J Surg* 1997;21:618.

117. Orringer MB, Stirling MB. Esophagectomy for esophageal disruption. *Ann Thorac Surg* 1990;49:35.

118. Grillo HC, Wilkins EW. Esophageal repair following late diagnosis of intrathoracic perforation. *Ann Thorac Surg* 1975;20:387.

119. Johnson J, Schwegman CW, Kirby KK. Esophageal exclusion for persistent fistula following spontaneous rupture of the esophagus. *J Thorac Surg* 1956;32:827.

120. Urschel HC, Razzuk MA, Wood RE, et al. Improved management of esophageal perforation: exclusion and diversion in continuity. *Ann Surg* 1974;179:587.

121. Wilcox MC. Esophageal disease in the acquired immunodeficiency syndrome: etiology, diagnosis, and management. *Am J Med* 1992;92:412.

122. Orringer MB, Sloan H. Monilial esophagitis: an increasingly frequent cause of esophageal stenosis? *Ann Thorac Surg* 1978;26:364.

123. McDonald GB. Esophageal disease caused by infection, systemic illness, medications, and trauma. In: Sleisenger MS, ed. *Gastrointestinal disease,* 5th ed. Philadelphia: WB Saunders, 1993:427.

124. Pairolero PC, Trastek VF. Surgical management of esophageal diverticula. In: Orringer MB, Zuidema GD, eds. *Shackelford's surgery of the alimentary tract,* 4th ed, vol 1 *(The esophagus).* Philadelphia: WB Saunders, 1996:285.

125. van Overbeck JJM, Hoeksema PE. Endoscopic treatment of the hypopharyngeal diverticulum: 211 cases. *Laryngoscope* 1982;92:88.

126. Peracchia A, Bonavina L, Narne S, et al. Minimally invasive surgery for Zenker's diverticulum. *Arch Surg* 1998;133:695.

127. Benacci JC, Deschamps G, Trastek VF, et al. Epiphrenic diverticulum: results of surgical treatment. *Ann Thorac Surg* 1993;55:1119.

128. Sherertz EF, Jorizzo JL. Cutaneous disease of the esophagus In: Castell DO, ed. *The esophagus.* Boston: Little, Brown and Company, 1992:793.

129. Horan TA, Urschel JD, MacEachern NA, et al. Esophageal perforation in recessive dystrophic epidermolysis bullosa. *Ann Thorac Surg* 1994;57:1027.

130. Herrara JL. Benign and metastatic tumors of the esophagus. *Gastroenterol Clin North Am* 1991;20:775.

131. Gudovsky LM, Koroleva NS, Biryukov YB, et al. Tracheoesophageal fistulas. *Ann Thorac Surg* 1993;55:868.

132. Mathisen DJ, Grillo HC, Wain JC, et al. Management of acquired nonmalignant tracheoesophageal fistula. *Ann Thorac Surg* 1991;52:759.

133. Antonelli M, Cicconetti F, Vivino G, et al. Closure of a tracheoesophageal fistula by bronchoscopic application of fibrin glue and decontamination of the oral cavity. *Chest* 1991;100:578.

134. Vandenplas Y, Helven R, Derop H, et al. Endoscopic obliteration of recurrent tracheoesophageal fistula. *Dig Dis Sci* 1993;38:374.

135. Burt M, Diehl W, Martini N, et al. Malignant esophagorespiratory fistula: management options and survival. *Ann Thorac Surg* 1991;52:1222.

136. Do YS, Sond HY, Lee BH, et al. Esophagorespiratory fistula associated with esophageal cancer: treatment with a Gianturco stent tube. *Radiology* 1993;187:673.

137. Dumonceau J-M, Cremer M, Lalmand B, et al. Esophageal fistula sealing: choice of stent, practical management, and cost. *Gastrointest Endosc* 1999;49:70.

138. Low DE, Kozarek RA. Comparison of conventional and wire mesh expandable prostheses and surgical bypass in patients with malignant esophagorespiratory fistulas. *Ann Thorac Surg* 1998;65:919.

STOMACH AND DUODENUM

SURGERY: SCIENTIFIC PRINCIPLES AND PRACTICE, Third Edition, edited by
Lazar J. Greenfield, Michael W. Mulholland, Keith T. Oldham, Gerald B. Zelenock,
and Keith D. Lillemoe. Lippincott Williams & Wilkins Publishers, Philadelphia, © 2001.

CHAPTER 21

GASTRIC ANATOMY AND PHYSIOLOGY

MICHAEL W. MULHOLLAND

GROSS ANATOMY

The stomach and duodenum, along with the esophagus, liver, bile ducts, and pancreas, are derived from the embryonic foregut. During the fifth week of gestation, the future stomach is marked as a dilation in the caudal portion of the foregut. Cranial to this dilation, the trachea forms as a bud from the future esophagus. At this time, the primitive stomach is invested with both ventral and dorsal mesenteries. The embryonic ventral mesentery is represented in postnatal life by the falciform ligament and by the gastrohepatic and hepatoduodenal mesenteries that form the lesser omentum. The celiac artery, the major blood supply to the foregut, passes within the dorsal mesentery. The primitive dorsal mesentery ultimately forms three structures—the gastrocolic ligament, the gastrosplenic ligament, and the gastrophrenic ligament.

During the sixth and seventh weeks of gestation, the typical morphology of the stomach is established. Accelerated growth of the left gastric wall, relative to the right, establishes the greater and lesser curvatures. This unequal growth also rotates the stomach and causes the left vagal nerve trunk to assume its anterior position, whereas the right vagal trunk is located posteriorly. The growth of structures cephalad to the stomach cause the organ to descend. During the sixth week, the primitive stomach lies between the T10 and T12 vertebral segments. By the eighth week, the stomach is located between the T11 and the L4 segments. In adult life, the stomach is most commonly located between the T10 and the L3 vertebral segments.

The stomach can be divided into anatomic regions based on external landmarks (Fig. 21.1). Although this division is commonly referred to in surgical texts and is useful in discussing gastric resective procedures, it does not necessarily reflect the secretory or motor functions of the mucosal and muscular layers of the stomach. The gastric cardia is the region of the stomach just distal to the gastroesophageal junction. The fundus is the portion of the stomach above and to the left of the gastroesophageal junction. The corpus constitutes the region between the fundus and the antrum. The margin between corpus and antrum is not distinct externally, but can be defined arbitrarily by a line from the incisura angularis on the lesser curvature to a point one fourth of the distance from the pylorus to the esophagus along the greater curvature. The gastric antrum is bounded distally by the pylorus, which can be appreciated by palpation as a thickened ring of smooth muscle.

The stomach is mobile in most people and is fixed at only two points—proximally by the gastroesophageal junction and distally by the retroperitoneal duodenum. Therefore, the position of the stomach varies and depends on the habitus of the person, the degree of gastric distention, and the position of the other abdominal organs. Anteriorly, the stomach is in contact with the left hemidiaphragm, the left lobe and the anterior segment of the right lobe of the liver, and the anterior parietal surface of the abdominal wall. The posterior surface of the stomach is related to the left diaphragm, the left kidney and left adrenal gland, the neck, tail, and body of the pancreas, the aorta and celiac trunk, and the periaortic nerve plexuses. The greater curvature of the stomach is near the transverse colon and the transverse colonic mesentery. The concavity of the spleen contacts the left lateral portion of the stomach.

The stomach is an extremely well vascularized organ, supplied by a number of major arteries and protected by a large number of extramural and intramural collaterals. Gastric viability can be preserved after ligation of all but one primary artery, an advantage that can be exploited during gastric reconstructive procedures. The rich network of anastomosing vessels also means that gastric hemorrhage cannot be controlled by the extramural ligation of gastric arteries. Most gastric blood flow is ordinarily derived from the celiac trunk (Fig. 21.2). The lesser curvature is supplied by the left gastric artery, which is the first major branch of the celiac trunk, and by the right gastric artery, which is derived from the hepatic artery. Branches of the left gastric artery also supply the lowermost portion of the esophagus. The greater curvature is supplied by the short gastric and left gastroepiploic arteries, which are branches of the splenic artery, and by the right gastroepiploic artery, a branch of the gastroduodenal artery. In instances of celiac trunk occlusion, gastric blood flow is usually maintained from the superior mesenteric artery collaterally by way of the pancreaticoduodenal arcade. In general, venous effluent from the stomach parallels the arterial supply. The venous equivalent of the left gastric artery is the coronary vein.

As a first approximation, the lymphatic drainage of the stomach parallels gastric venous return (Fig. 21.3). Lymph from the proximal portion of the stomach along the lesser curvature first drains into superior gastric lymph nodes surrounding the left gastric artery. The distal portion of the lesser curvature drains through suprapyloric nodes. The proximal portion of the greater curvature is supplied by lymphatic vessels that traverse pancreaticosplenic nodes, whereas the antral portion of the greater curvature drains into the subpyloric and omental nodal groups. Secondary

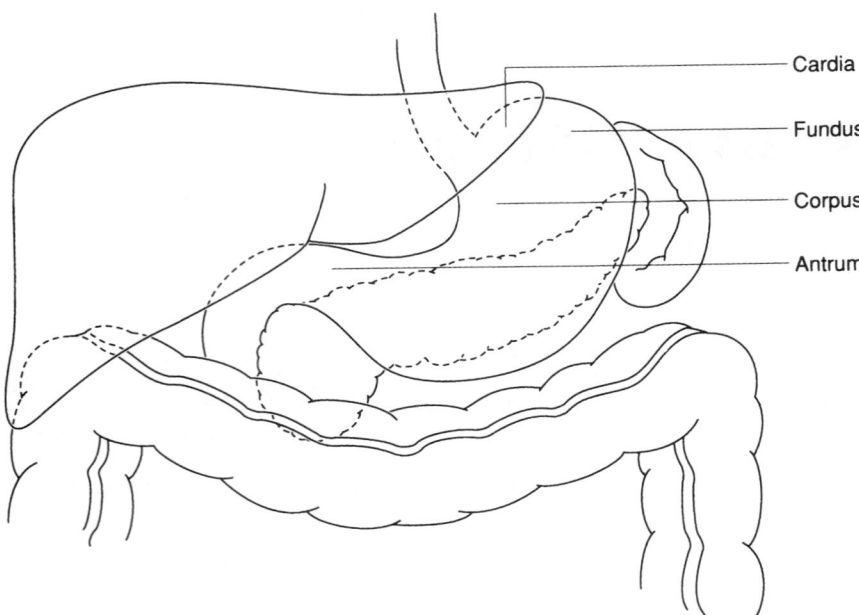

Figure 21.1. Topographic relations of the stomach.

drainage from each of these systems eventually traverses nodes at the base of the celiac axis. These discrete anatomic groupings are misleading. The lymphatic drainage of the human stomach, like its blood supply, exhibits extensive intramural ramifications and a number of extramural communications. As a consequence, disease processes that involve the gastric lymphatics often spread intramurally beyond the region of origin and to nodal groups at a distance from the primary lymphatic zone.

The left and right vagal nerves descend parallel to the esophagus within the thorax before forming a peri-esophageal plexus between the tracheal bifurcation and the diaphragm. From this plexus, two vagal trunks coa-lesce before passing through the esophageal hiatus of the diaphragm (Fig. 21.4). The left vagal trunk is usually closely applied to the anterior surface of the esophagus, whereas the posterior vagal trunk is often midway between the esophagus and the aorta. The anterior vagus supplies a hepatic division, which passes to the right in the lesser omentum before innervating the liver and biliary tract. The remainder of the anterior vagal fibers parallel the lesser curvature of the stomach, branching to the anterior gastric wall. The posterior vagus nerve branches into the celiac division, which passes to the celiac plexus, and a posterior gastric division, which innervates the posterior gastric wall.

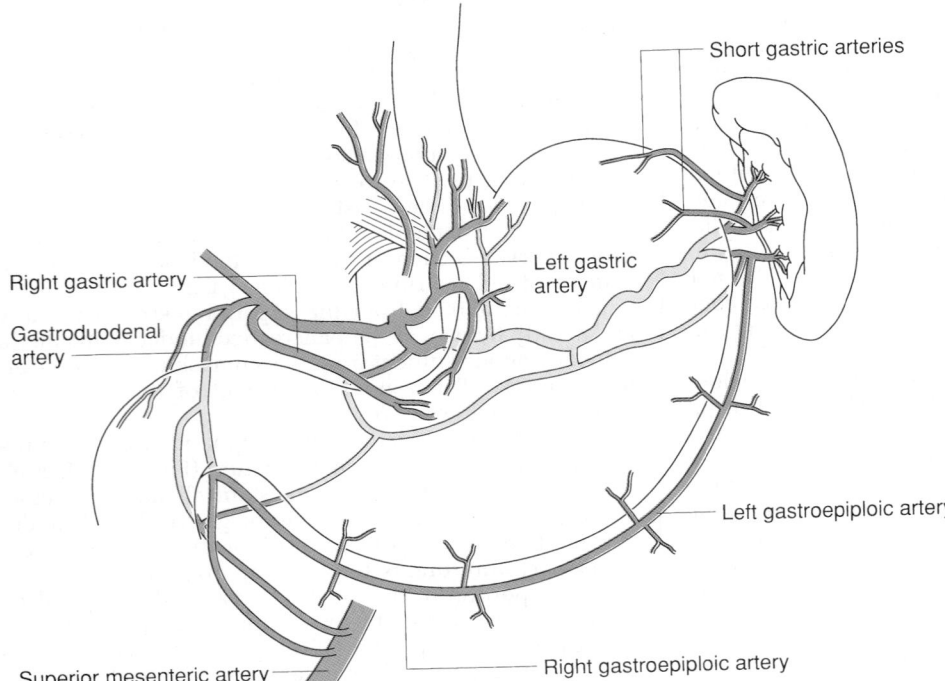

Figure 21.2. Arterial blood supply of the stomach.

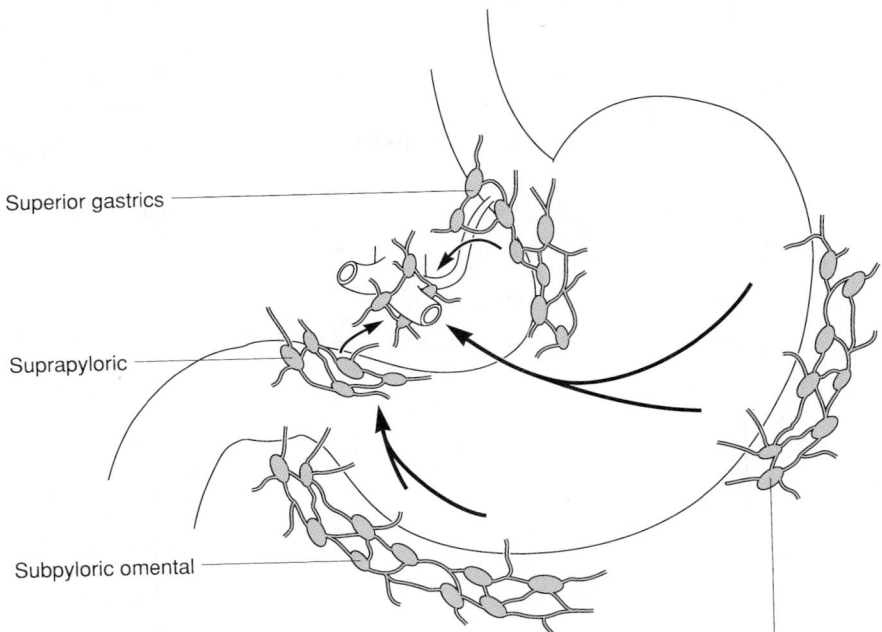

Superior gastrics

Suprapyloric

Subpyloric omental

Figure 21.3. Lymphatic drainage of the stomach.

Approximately 90% of the fibers in the vagal trunks are afferent, transmitting information from the gastrointestinal tract to the central nervous system. Parasympathetic afferent fibers are not responsible for the sensation of gastric pain. Surprisingly, only 10% of vagal nerve fibers are motor or secretory efferents. Parasympathetic efferent fibers contained in the vagus originate in the dorsal nucleus of the medulla. Vagal efferent fibers pass without synapse to contact postsynaptic neurons in the gastric wall in the myenteric and submucous plexuses. Secondary neurons directly innervate gastric smooth muscle or epithelial cells. Acetylcholine is the neurotransmitter of primary vagal efferent neurons.

The gastric sympathetic innervation is derived from spinal segments T5 through T10. Sympathetic fibers leave the corresponding spinal nerve roots by way of gray rami communicantes and enter a series of bilateral prevertebral ganglia (Fig. 21.5). From these ganglia, presynaptic fibers pass through the greater splanchnic nerves to the celiac plexus, where they synapse with secondary sympathetic neurons. Postsynaptic sympathetic nerve fibers enter the stomach in association with blood vessels. Afferent sympathetic fibers pass without synapse from the stomach to dorsal spinal roots. Pain of gastroduodenal origin is sensed through afferent fibers of sympathetic origin.

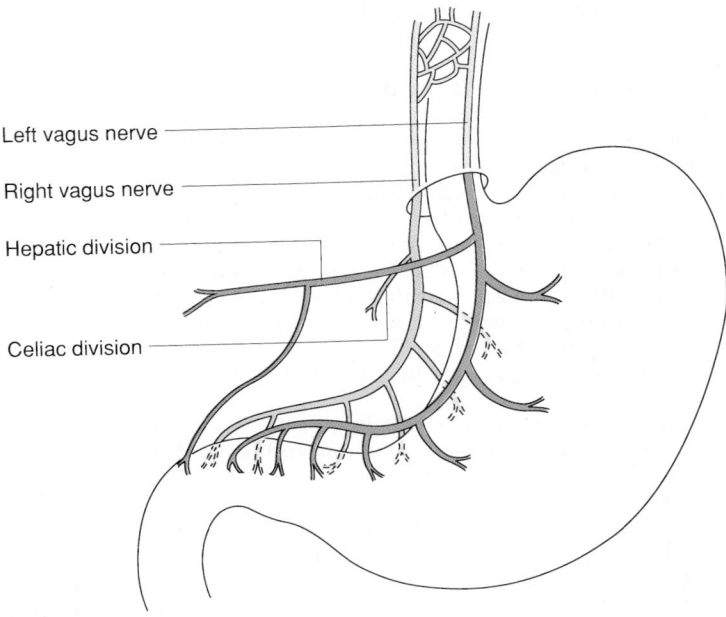

Left vagus nerve

Right vagus nerve

Hepatic division

Celiac division

Figure 21.4. Vagal innervation of the stomach.

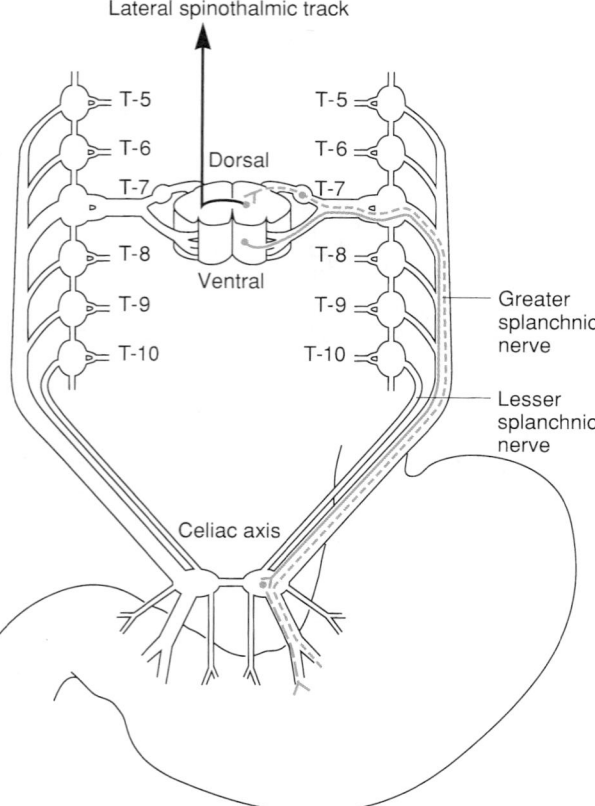

Figure 21.5. Derivation of gastric sympathetic innervation.

MICROSCOPIC ANATOMY

The glandular portions of the stomach are lined by a simple columnar epithelium composed of surface mucous cells. The luminal surface, visualized by scanning electron microscopy, appears cobblestoned, interrupted at intervals by gastric pits. Opening into the gastric pits are one or more gastric glands that impart functional significance to the gastric mucosa. The mucosa of the human stomach is composed of three distinct types of gastric glands—cardiac, oxyntic, and antral.

In humans, cardiac glands occupy a narrow zone adjacent to the esophagus and mark a transition from the stratified squamous epithelium of the esophagus to the simple columnar epithelium of the stomach. The surface and gastric pit mucous cells of the cardia are not distinguishable from those in other areas of the stomach. Cardiac glands contain mucous and undifferentiated and endocrine cells, but not the parietal or chief cells that are prominent in the adjacent oxyntic mucosa. Cardiac glands are usually branched and connect with relatively short gastric pits. The functional properties of cardiac glands are not completely understood, although the secretion of mucus is generally accepted.

Oxyntic glands are the most distinctive feature of the human stomach. They occupy the fundus and body of the stomach and contain the oxyntic or parietal cells, which are the sites of acid production. Oxyntic glands also contain chief cells, the site of gastric pepsinogen synthesis. The tubular oxyntic glands are usually relatively straight but sometimes branch; several glands may empty into a single gastric pit. The glands are divided into three regions: (a) the isthmus, containing surface mucous cells

and a few scattered parietal cells; (b) the neck, with a heavy concentration of parietal cells and a few neck mucous cells; and (c) the base of the gland, containing chief cells, undifferentiated cells, a few parietal cells, and some mucous neck cells. Endocrine cells are scattered throughout all three regions of oxyntic glands.

The most distinctive cell of the gastric mucosa is the acid-secreting parietal cell. Parietal cells have an unusual ultrastructural specialization in the form of intracellular canaliculi, a network of clefts extending to the basal cytoplasm and often encircling the nucleus, which is continuous with the gland lumen (Fig. 21.6). The surface area provided by the intracellular secretory canaliculi is large and is further magnified by microvilli lining the canaliculi. In parietal cells that are not stimulated to secrete acid, the secretory canaliculi are collapsed and inconspicuous. On stimulation, a severalfold increase in canalicular surface area occurs, the intracellular clefts become prominent, and the communication with the luminal surface is readily identified. These changes create an intracellular space in communication with the gastric lumen into which hydrogen ions are secreted at high concentration.

The cytoplasm of the parietal cell also contains an abundance of large mitochondria. Mitochondria are estimated

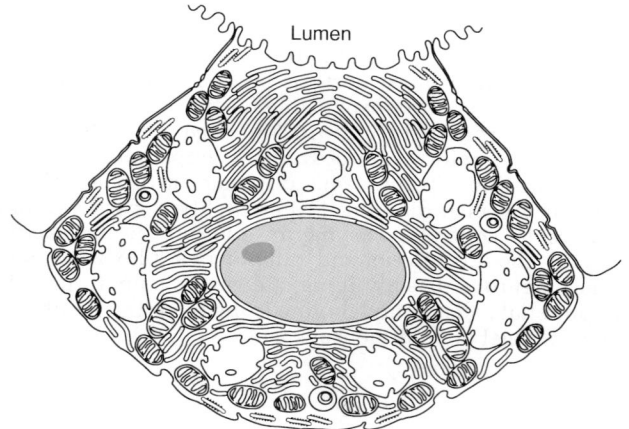

Nonsecreting parietal cell

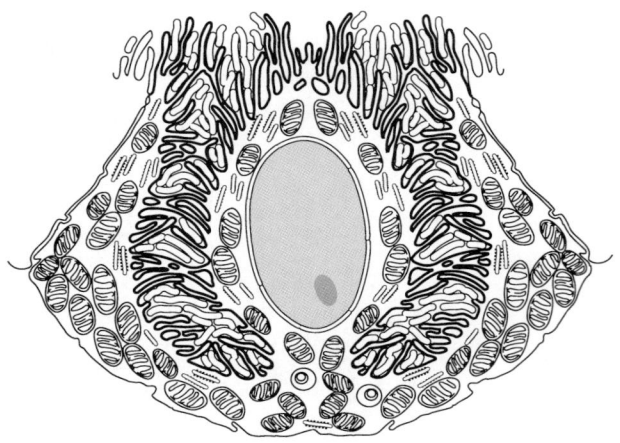

Acid-secreting parietal cell

Figure 21.6. Resting and stimulated parietal cell, emphasizing morphologic transformation with increase in secretory canalicular membrane surface area that occurs with acid secretion.

to occupy 30% to 40% of the cytoplasmic volume of unstimulated parietal cells, reflecting the extremely high oxidative activity of these cells. The oxygen consumption rate of isolated parietal cells is approximately five times higher than that of gastric mucous cells. The cytoplasm also contains a limited amount of rough endoplasmic reticulum, presumed to be the production site of intrinsic factor, which is also secreted by parietal cells.

In addition to parietal cells, the oxyntic glands contain the gastric chief cells, which synthesize and secrete pepsinogen. Chief cells are most abundant in the basal region of the oxyntic glands. The cells have a morphology typical of protein-secreting exocrine cells and are similar in ultrastructural appearance to pancreatic acinar cells. Rough endoplasmic reticulum is abundant in the cytoplasm and extends between secretory granules. Zymogen granules containing pepsinogen are most concentrated in the apical cytoplasm. Pepsinogen is released by exocytosis from secretory granules at the apical surface of chief cells.

Antral glands occupy the mucosa of the distal stomach and pyloric channel. Antral glands are relatively straight and often empty through deep gastric pits. Although most cells in the antral glands are mucus secreting, gastrin cells are the distinctive feature of this mucosa. Gastrin cells are pyramid shaped, with a narrow area of luminal contact apically and a broad surface overlying the lamina propria basally (Fig. 21.7). Gastrin cells are identified immunocytochemically by the presence of the peptide. Granules ranging from 150 to 400 nm in diameter are the sites of gastrin storage and are most numerous in the basal cytoplasm. Gastrin is released by exocytotic fusion of the secretory granule with the plasma membrane. In contrast to secretion from chief cells, emptying of gastrin-containing granules occurs at the basal membrane rather than at the apical region of the cell. Gastrin thus released diffuses to and enters submucosal capillaries in close apposition to the lamina propria.

GASTRIC PEPTIDES

The stomach contains a number of biologically active peptides in nerves and mucosal endocrine cells, including gastrin, somatostatin, gastrin-releasing peptide, vasoactive intestinal polypeptide (VIP), substance P, glucagon, and calcitonin gene-related peptide. The two peptides with the greatest importance to human disease and clinical surgery are gastrin and somatostatin.

Gastrin

The synthesis, secretion, and action of gastrin have been extensively studied, and many aspects of the biology of gastrin appear to be shared by other gastrointestinal peptide hormones (1). The gene that encodes for gastrin has been isolated using a human DNA library. The human gastrin gene contains three exons; two exons consist of coding sequences. The major active product is encoded by a single exon. In adults, the gastrin gene is expressed primarily in mucosa cells of the gastric antrum, with lower levels of expression in the duodenum, pituitary, and testis. During embryonic development, the gastrin gene is transiently active in pancreatic islets and colonic mucosa.

The human gene encompasses approximately 4,100 base pairs and directs the synthesis of a peptide of 101 amino acids (Fig. 21.8). The resulting peptide, preprogastrin, contains the sequence of gastrin within its amino acid sequence. Preprogastrin consists of a signal peptide of 21 amino acids, an intervening peptide of 37 amino acids, the 34-residue region of the gastrin molecule, and a carboxyl-terminal extension of 9 amino acids. Gastrin is derived from its preprohormone by the sequential enzymatic cleavage of the signal peptide, the intervening peptide, and the carboxyl-terminal extension.

The signal peptide region of preprogastrin consists of a series of hydrophobic amino acids that direct the nascent peptide into the endoplasmic reticulum as it is translated

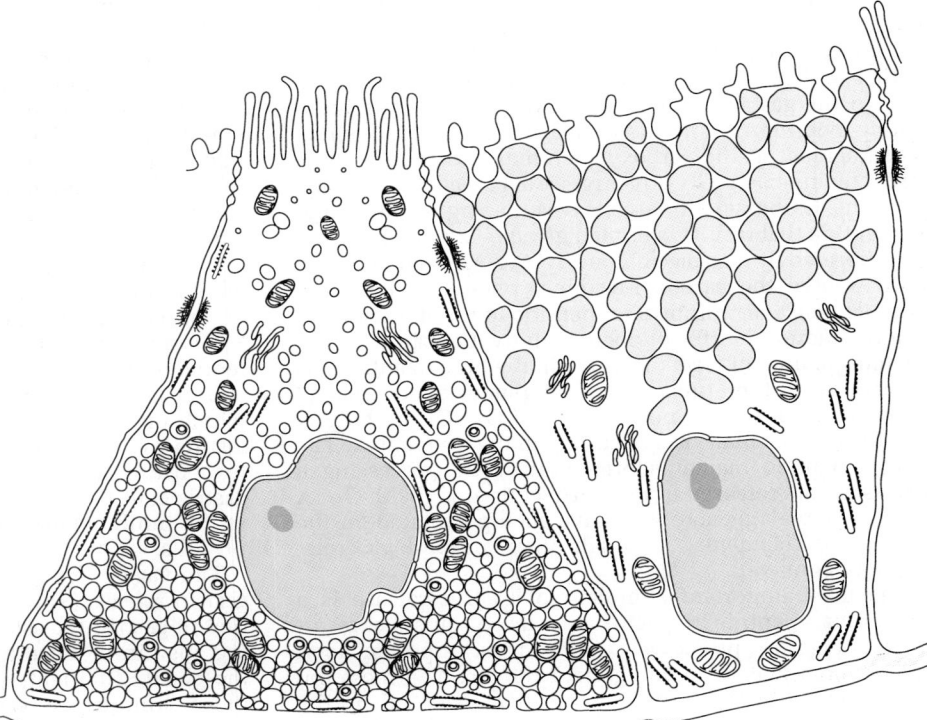

Figure 21.7. Contrasting morphology of antral gastrin cell *(left)* with basally oriented secretory granules, and gastric mucous cell *(right)* with apical mucous granules.

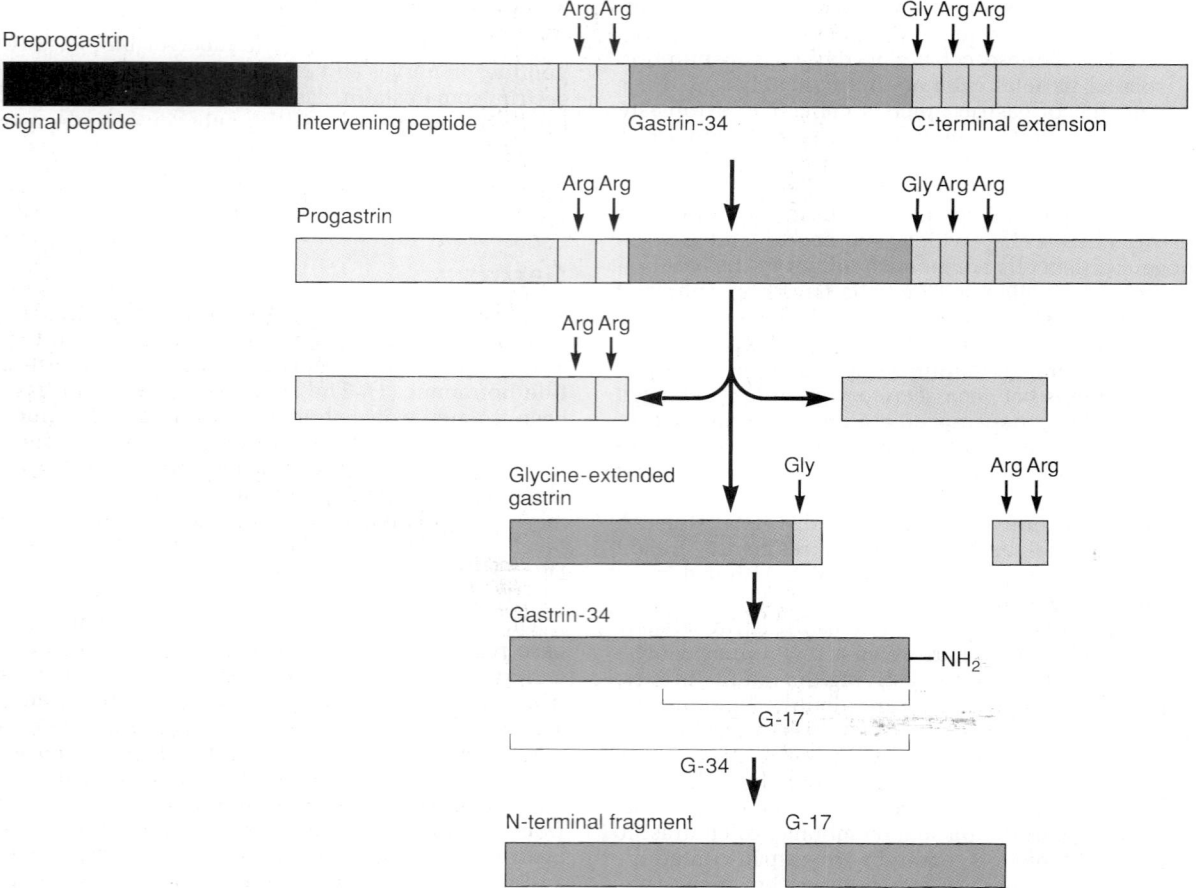

Figure 21.8. Sequential processing of preprogastrin molecule.

from messenger RNA. After directing the preprogastrin molecule into the rough endoplasmic reticulum, the signal peptide is removed. The remaining peptide is termed *progastrin*. Progastrin is further processed as it traverses the endoplasmic reticulum to mature secretory vesicles. Enzymatic cleavage at a pair of basic amino acid residues proximal to the gastrin 34 (G_{34}) sequence removes the intervening peptide. A similar cleavage removes a 6-amino acid fragment at the carboxyl-terminal end. The peptide that remains has a Gly-Arg-Arg sequence at the carboxyl terminus. Carboxypeptidase cleaves the Arg residues, and the peptide that results is termed *glycine-extended gastrin*. G_{34} is formed by cleavage of the Gly-Arg-Arg sequence and amidation of the carboxyl-terminal phenylalanine. Gastrin, like most gastrointestinal peptide hormones, requires terminal amidation for biologic activity. Gastrin 17 (G_{17}), the most abundant form of gastrin in the human antrum, is formed by further processing that removes the first 17 amino acids at the amino terminus of G_{34}. G_{34} is the predominate molecular form of gastrin in the duodenum. The various peptide fragments formed during the processing of progastrin are released from gastrin cells along with G_{17}. A number of biologic activities have been postulated for the processing fragments, although their physiologic relevance is unproved.

The most important stimulant of gastrin release is a meal. Small peptide fragments and amino acids that result from intragastric proteolysis are the most important food components that stimulate gastrin release. The most potent gastrin-releasing activities are demonstrated by the amino acids tryptophan and phenylalanine. Ingested fat

and glucose do not cause gastrin release. Dietary amino acids are transported into the gastrin cell, where decarboxylation enzymes convert them to amines. Intracellular amines promote gastrin release. Conditions that increase intracellular amine levels stimulate gastrin secretion, whereas conditions that prevent entry of amino acids into gastrin cells inhibit release of the hormone. Gastric distention by a meal activates cholinergic neurons and stimulates gastrin release. As the meal empties and distention diminishes, VIP-containing neurons are activated, which stimulate somatostatin secretion, and thus attenuate gastrin secretion.

Postprandial luminal pH also strongly affects gastrin secretion. Gastrin release is inhibited when acidification of an ingested meal causes the intraluminal pH to fall below 3.0. Conversely, maintaining intragastric pH above 3.0 potentiates gastrin secretion after ingestion of protein or amino acids (2). Pernicious anemia and atrophic gastritis, which produce chronic achlorhydria, are associated with fasting hypergastrinemia and an exaggerated gastrin meal response. Release of mucosal somatostatin occurs with gastric acidification, and this peptide has been implicated in the inhibited gastrin release that occurs when luminal pH falls.

The vagus nerve appears both to stimulate and inhibit gastrin release (3). In humans, vagally mediated stimulation of gastrin release can be demonstrated by sham feeding, insulin-induced hypoglycemia, and administration of the vagal stimulant, γ-aminobutyric acid. In contrast to these stimulatory vagal effects, hypergastrinemia, observed after vagotomy, suggests that inhibitory vagal effects on gastrin release may also exist. Cholinergic neurons stimulate gastrin secretion directly by actions on gastrin cells. By decreasing somatostatin secretion, cholinergic neurons also indirectly stimulate gastrin release. Evidence suggests that vagal stimulation of gastrin release is mediated by bombesin or its mammalian equivalent, gastrin-releasing peptide, acting as a neurotransmitter in the gastric wall. In support of this contention, vagally mediated gastrin release can be abolished by specific bombesin antisera. Adrenergic stimulation has also been noted to increase gastrin release.

Chronic gastric infection with *Helicobacter pylori* causes increased acid secretion by altering gastrin release (4,5). *H. pylori* has been observed to up-regulate proinflammatory cytokines, including interleukin (IL)-6, IL-8, and tumor necrosis factor-α (TNF-α). Several inflammatory mediators have been demonstrated to stimulate gastrin release from isolated gastrin cells. The putative gastrin secretagogues include IL-1, IL-8, TNF-α, interferon-γ, and leukotrienes C4 and D4. The same factors that affect gastrin release also influence gastrin mRNA expression. Food ingestion increases gastrin mRNA abundance, whereas fasting and somatostatin decrease gastrin mRNA production. Chronic achlorhydria, as seen in pernicious anemia, increases gastrin mRNA production.

In addition to stimulating acid secretion from gastric parietal cells (detailed later in this chapter), gastrin has important physiologic actions in the control of gastrointestinal mucosal growth. The acid-secreting oxyntic mucosa is particularly sensitive to the trophic actions of gastrin, but the mucous membranes of the duodenum, colon, and pancreatic parenchyma are also affected. In animals, removing endogenous gastrin through antrectomy results in mucosal atrophy. Mucosal hypoplasia can be prevented by administering exogenous gastrin. Responsiveness to the trophic effects of gastrin is not present at birth because of the lack of mucosal gastrin receptors. Development of mucosal receptors occurs at the time of weaning and corresponds to the development of responsiveness to the trophic effects of the hormone. Stimulation of mucosal growth by gastrin is enhanced by the presence of solid food in the diet. The 17- and 34-amino acid forms of gastrin are equipotent in stimulating mucosal growth. In humans, the relative importance of gastrin and other influences, such as the composition and form of the diet and the actions of other trophic hormones, have not been completely established. Prolonged stimulation by high levels

of gastrin, as seen in the Zollinger-Ellison syndrome, is associated with hypertrophy of the gastric mucosa. Smaller increases in circulating gastrin, such as those that follow vagotomy, do not cause mucosal hypertrophy.

Somatostatin

Somatostatin, like gastrin, is very significant in gastric physiology and has been investigated considerably. In addition, somatostatin and its biologically active analogues have important therapeutic applications in the treatment of digestive diseases and in gastrointestinal surgery. Somatostatin was first isolated from hypothalamic tissues and was named for its ability to inhibit the release of growth hormone. The peptide has subsequently been localized in neurons in central and peripheral nervous systems, and in endocrine cells in the pancreas, stomach, and intestine. The wide tissue distribution of somatostatin has suggested important regulatory functions, a concept validated by many investigations.

The human somatostatin gene is located on chromosome 3 and encodes for a precursor of 116 amino acids (Fig. 21.9). The somatostatin molecule is contained in the carboxyl-terminal sequence of this preprohormone. The first 24 amino acids of the amino terminus of preprosomatostatin constitute a signal peptide; cleavage of this signal peptide leaves prosomatostatin. Enzymatic cleavage of an additional 64-amino acid segment from prosomatostatin forms somatostatin 28. Further processing of somatostatin 28 to somatostatin 14 is tissue-specifically regulated. In the stomach, most somatostatin exists as the shorter peptide.

Gastric somatostatin release responds to luminal, hormonal, and neural signals. Luminal acidification is associated with increased somatostatin release, whereas somatostatin release decreases when luminal pH is increased. A number of peptides have been demonstrated experimentally to release somatostatin from the stomach, including gastrin, cholecystokinin, and secretin. β-Adrenergic agonists have also been shown to release somatostatin. In contrast, electrical stimulation of vagal nerves inhibits somatostatin release, as does the cholinergic agonist, methacholine.

The most important gastric function of somatostatin appears to be regulation of acid secretion and gastrin release. Circulating somatostatin appears to be important in modulating gastric acid secretion; locally released somato-

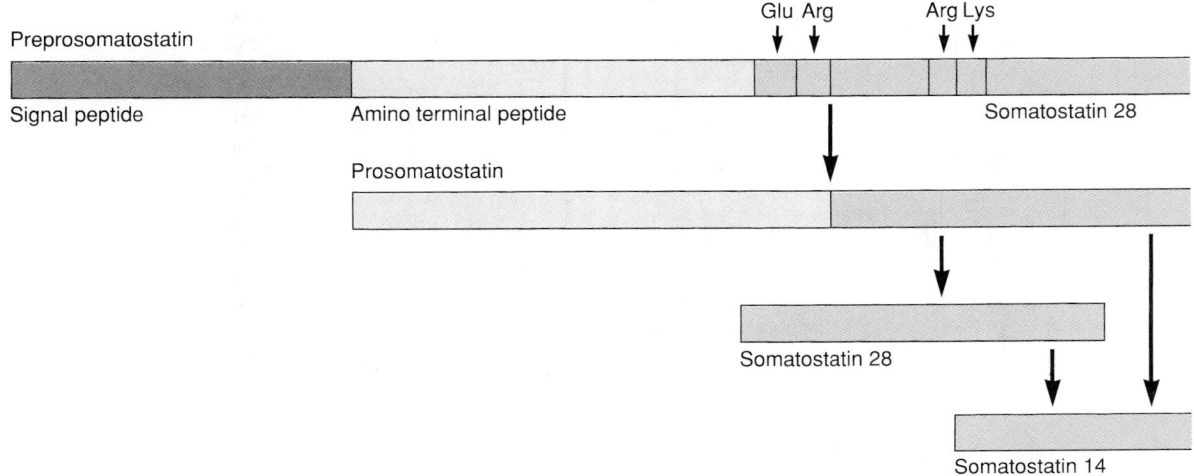

Figure 21.9. Derivation of somatostatin 14 from preprosomatostatin precursor.

statin functions to regulate gastrin release. In each instance, somatostatin serves an inhibitory function, decreasing acid secretion and diminishing the release of gastrin. In animals, antral or duodenal acidification has been associated with an increase in circulating somatostatin. Increases in circulating somatostatin are followed, in turn, by decreased gastric acid secretion. Infusion of exogenous somatostatin in doses that produce somatostatin levels similar to those observed postprandially has also been shown to inhibit acid secretion. In humans, concentrations of somatostatin capable of inhibiting acid secretion can do so without altering serum gastrin levels, indicating a direct action on the acid-secreting fundic mucosa.

Somatostatin is crucial in modulating gastrin release. Somatostatin is believed to influence gastrin secretion through a locally active intramucosal mechanism. Local actions of somatostatin are supported by ultrastructural studies of antral somatostatin cells, which demonstrate long cytoplasmic processes that make intimate cell-to-cell contact with antral gastrin cells. The presence of somatostatin at these sites of cellular contact implies that somatostatin cells influence the function of gastrin cells through local release of the peptide. Somatostatin can also reach neighboring gastrin cells through diffusion or local blood flow. A number of experiments have suggested that release of somatostatin and gastrin is functionally, although reciprocally, linked. For example, in anesthetized animals, an increase in gastric pH or ingestion of a meal is associated with increases in gastrin and decreases in somatostatin in antral venous blood. Cholinergic agents stimulate gastrin release while inhibiting somatostatin release. Prostaglandin E$_2$, in contrast, inhibits gastrin release and stimulates somatostatin secretion. These and similar observations suggest that increases in somatostatin release are often associated with decreased gastrin secretion. A family of five somatostatin receptors has been cloned. Inhibition of gastrin-stimulated gastric acid secretion is mediated by somatostatin receptor subtype 2.

GASTRIC ACID SECRETION

Cellular Events

An appreciation of the mechanisms that control the stomach's acid formation is essential to a discussion of gastric disease. An understanding of the cellular basis of acid secretion by the gastric parietal cell also provides a foundation for discussing the pharmacologic treatment of acid–peptic diseases. The basolateral membrane of the parietal cell contains specific receptors for histamine, gastrin, and acetylcholine, the three major stimulants of acid production (6). Each stimulant reaches the parietal cell by a different route. Histamine is released from mastlike cells within the lamina propria and diffuses to the mucosa; acetylcholine is released close to the parietal cells from cholinergic nerve terminals; and gastrin is delivered by the systemic circulation to the fundic mucosa from its source in the antrum and proximal duodenum (Fig. 21.10).

Histamine receptors in the gastric mucosa are classified pharmacologically as H$_2$ receptors because they may be stimulated by agonists such as 4-methylhistamine and selectively blocked by agents such as cimetidine. Occupation of the histamine receptor activates a membrane-bound enzyme called *adenylate cyclase* (Fig. 21.11). Activated adenylate cyclase catalyzes the conversion of intracellular adenosine triphosphate (ATP) to cyclic adenosine monophosphate (cAMP), and enhancement of cAMP production by histamine is closely linked to stimulation of parietal cell acid production. cAMP mediates histamine-stimulated acid production by activating protein kinase A, which in turn catalyzes protein phosphorylation. The target protein molecule for this phosphorylation and the mechanism by which this activated product stimulates acid production have yet to be defined.

Acetylcholine and related cholinergic agonists activate parietal cells after binding to muscarinic receptors. The stimulatory effects of acetylcholine and its congeners can be abolished by atropine. The action of acetylcholine are

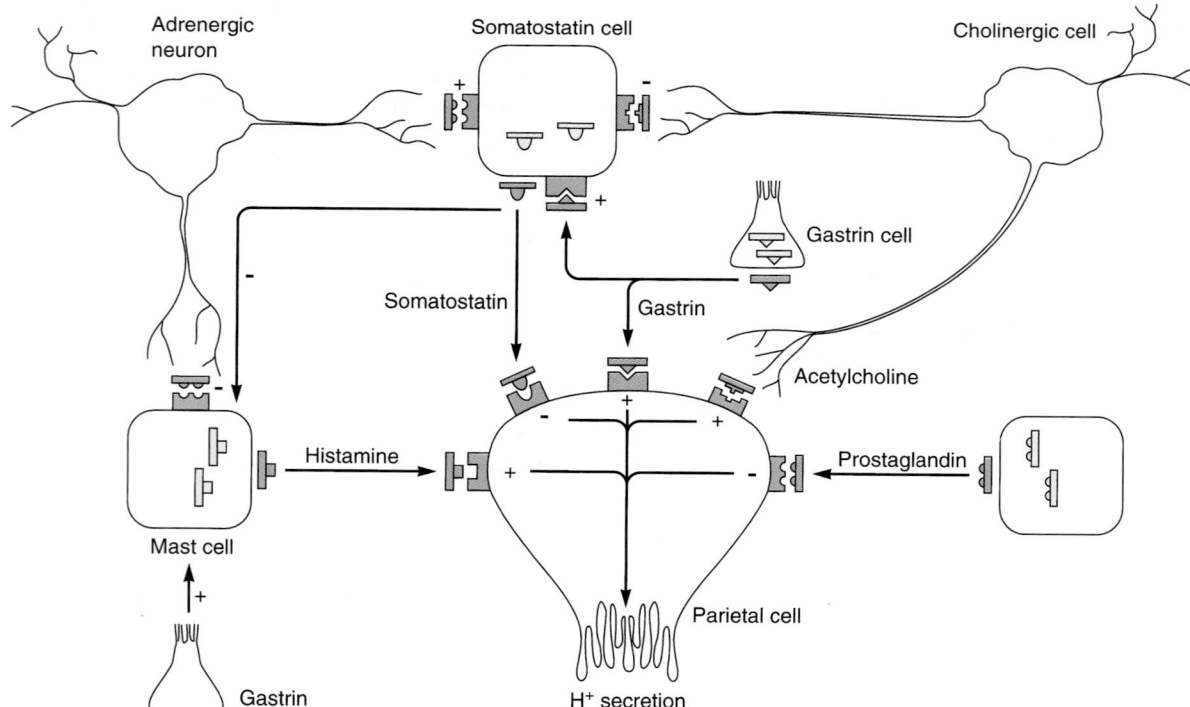

Figure 21.10. Interactions of cell types that affect parietal cell acid secretion.

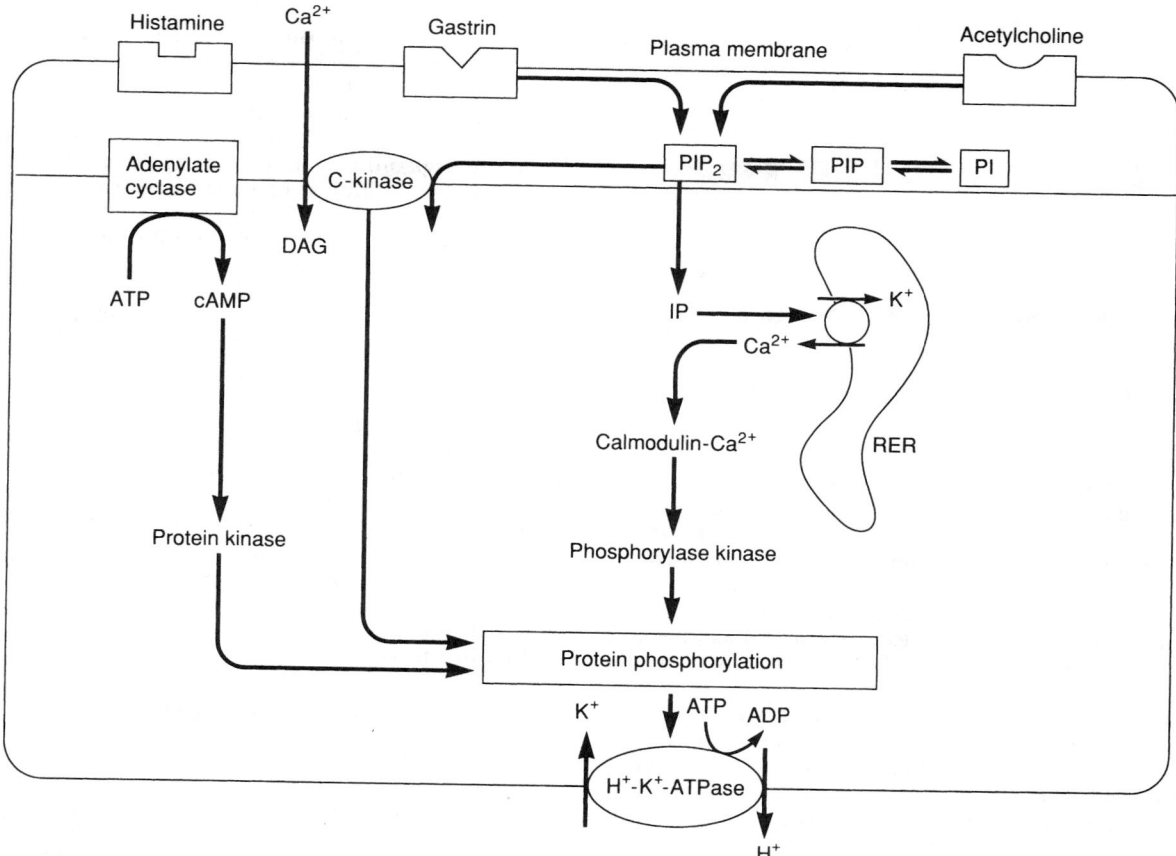

Figure 21.11. Cellular mechanisms controlling parietal cell acid secretion.

mediated by muscarinic receptor subtype 3 (M_3). Studies suggest that cholinergic stimulation of parietal cell function is coupled to enhanced mobilization of intracellular calcium. The resultant transient increases in intracellular calcium activate mechanisms that stimulate acid secretion (Fig. 21.11). Evidence also indicates that occupation of acetylcholine receptors increases turnover of specific membrane phospholipids termed *phosphatidylinositides*. Based on findings in a number of cell types, acetylcholine–receptor binding is postulated to be followed by activation of membrane-associated phospholipase C. Phospholipase C acts on phosphatidylinositol-4,5 bisphosphate (PIP_2) within the plasma membrane to liberate water-soluble inositol triphosphate (IP_3) and diacylglycerol. A major action of IP_3 is to increase intracellular calcium, mainly from intracellular stores in the endoplasmic reticulum. The resulting increased cytosolic calcium interacts with calmodulin or other calcium-binding proteins. Calmodulin kinase type II is involved in parietal cell activation by acetylcholine. Intracellular calcium in this form is postulated to modulate parietal cell function through protein phosphorylation or enzyme activation. Diacylglycerol, the second product released by hydrolysis of PIP_2, activates a class of protein kinases that are phospholipid dependent and Ca^{2+} activated, protein kinase C. Protein kinase C in turn acts to phosphorylate a set of proteins that are distinct from those affected by the calmodulin-dependent system. The ultimate result of this protein phosphorylation is parietal cell activation and hydrogen ion secretion.

Parietal cells can also be activated by occupation of specific gastrin receptors. As with cholinergic stimulation, gastrin exposure increases membrane PIP_2 turnover (Fig. 21.11). Like acetylcholine, the actions of gastrin depend highly on increases in intracellular calcium and activation of protein kinase C. The ways in which parietal cell stimulation by acetylcholine and gastrin may be similar or different remain to be completely defined.

Although histamine, acetylcholine, and gastrin occupy separate receptors on the parietal cell and activate differing second-messenger systems, each secretagogue ultimately acts by means of a specialized ion transport system called the *parietal cell proton pump*. This membrane-bound protein is located in the secretory canaliculus of the parietal cell; the peptide has not been identified in other gastric cells or in significant amounts in other organs. The proton pump is an H^+-K^+-adenosine triphosphatase (ATPase) that electroneutrally exchanges cytosolic H^+ for luminal K^+. Hydrogen ions are concentrated 2.5-million-fold within the secretory canaliculus, and the hydrolysis of ATP is the energy source for transport against the steep electrochemical gradient generated. For each H^+ ion transported to the luminal surface of the canalicular membrane, one K^+ ion is transported to the cytosolic surface (Fig. 21.12). This cotransport requires that K^+ be continuously supplied to the luminal surface of the secretory membrane. This requirement is satisfied by conductance of K^+ across the canalicular membrane from intracellular stores. Chloride ions also enter the secretory canaliculus by diffusion.

Activation of the H^+-K^+-ATPase significantly increases intracellular OH^- generation, with potential cellular toxicity. Carbonic anhydrase, which is associated with the canalicular membrane, converts OH^- to HCO_3^-. The HCO_3^-

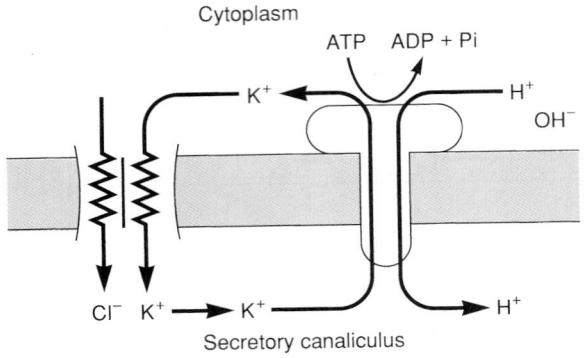

Figure 21.12. Gastric H⁺-K⁺-adenosine triphosphatase (ATPase).

produced is disposed of by exchange for Cl^- at the basolateral membrane. Intracellular Cl^- thus acquired supplies the necessary Cl^- on a one-to-one basis for each H^+ secreted. The transcellular exchange of H^+ for HCO_3^- ensures that the voluminous secretion of hydrochloride at the luminal surface of the gastric mucosa is matched by an equivalent delivery of base to submucosal capillaries. Parietal cell ionic transport pathways are shown in Fig. 21.13.

The function of the proton pump is highly regulated. In the unstimulated state, the enzyme is sequestered in cytoplasmic structures termed *tubulovesicles* that are not connected to the gastric lumen. Tubulovesicle membranes in this state have a low permeability to KCl. Stimulation of acid secretion causes tubulovesicles to fuse with apical secretory membranes and increases membrane permeability to KCl. In this way, the fusion of tubulovesicle membrane exposes the H^+-K^+ pump to the gastric lumen and simultaneously provides the K^+ substrate necessary for acid secretion.

Parietal cells also contain membrane receptors that inhibit acid secretion. Specific receptors for somatostatin have been identified using isolated gastric cells. Activation of isolated parietal cells by histamine, pentagastrin, or the cholinergic agonist carbachol can be blocked by somatostatin 28. In the case of histamine activation, the inhibitory effects appear to be mediated by the ability of so-

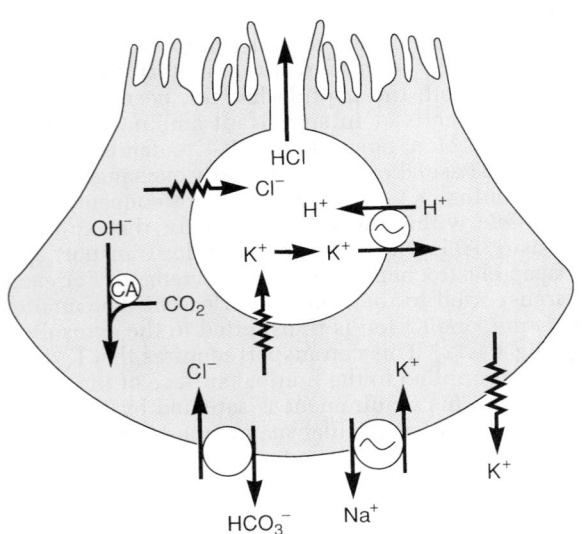

Figure 21.13. Ionic fluxes associated with acid secretion by the parietal cell.

matostatin to block the production of cAMP. The mechanisms by which somatostatin interferes with activation by pentagastrin or carbachol are not completely defined. Somatostatin appears to inhibit the actions of these agonists at a point distal to second-messenger generation. Gastric parietal cells also contain receptors for prostaglandins, notably prostaglandin E_2 and its derivatives. Prostaglandin E_2 is a potent inhibitor of histamine-stimulated parietal cell activation, probably by a mechanism that inhibits formation of cAMP. Prostaglandin inhibition is specific for histamine; the actions of gastrin or carbachol are not affected. Epidermal growth factor and transforming growth factor-a also inhibit histamine-stimulated acid secretion through effects on cAMP production.

These considerations of the cellular basis of acid production demonstrate how parietal cell function can be altered pharmacologically. Gastric acid production can be blocked by receptor antagonists for each of the three primary stimulants—gastrin, acetylcholine, and histamine. Direct inhibition of acid production can be effected by derivatives of somatostatin or prostaglandin E_2. All forms of stimulated acid production could be blocked by agents that act as inhibitors of the parietal cell proton pump. Agents that act at each of these points have been developed, and their appropriate clinical applications are discussed in subsequent chapters.

Regulation of Acid Secretion

Given the multiple receptors on parietal cells, it is not surprising that a great deal of secretagogue interdependence, both stimulatory and inhibitory, exists in humans. Parietal cell activation and the resultant acid secretion is greater in response to a combination of agonists than it is in response to the total effect of agents used singly. This increase in responsiveness is defined as *potentiation*. Potentiating interactions are most apparent when agents that act by way of different second-messenger systems are used. Thus, histamine strongly potentiates the acid-secretory response to pentagastrin or to carbachol in humans. Conversely, blockade of receptors to one stimulant also decreases responsiveness to the other agonists. For example, blocking histamine receptors with agents such as cimetidine decreases responsiveness to pentagastrin, even though gastrin receptors are not directly affected. These inhibitory interactions are exploited therapeutically in the treatment of acid–peptic diseases.

Humans normally secrete 2 to 5 mEq/h of hydrochloride in the fasting state, constituting basal acid secretion. Both vagal tone and ambient histamine secretion are presumed to be important in determining the rate of basal acid secretion. In humans, truncal vagotomy decreases basal secretion by approximately 85%. Similarly, H_2 receptor antagonists also inhibit basal acid secretion by approximately 80%. Gastrin does not have an important role in determining basal acid secretion in normal people.

Stimulated acid secretion begins with the thought, sight, or smell of food (Fig. 21.14). This cephalic phase of gastric acid secretion is mediated by the vagus nerve. Vagal discharge directs a cholinergic mechanism, and the cephalic phase of acid secretion can be inhibited by administering atropine. Vagal discharge secondary to cephalic stimulation also inhibits the release of somatostatin. Diminished secretion of somatostatin further augments stimulatory vagal effects, presumably by eliminating tonic inhibition of acid secretion exerted by somatostatin. The cephalic component of acid secretion can be measured in normal people by sham feeding and is approximately 10 mEq/h. The cephalic phase approximates 40% of the maximal acid-secretory response to gastrin infusion.

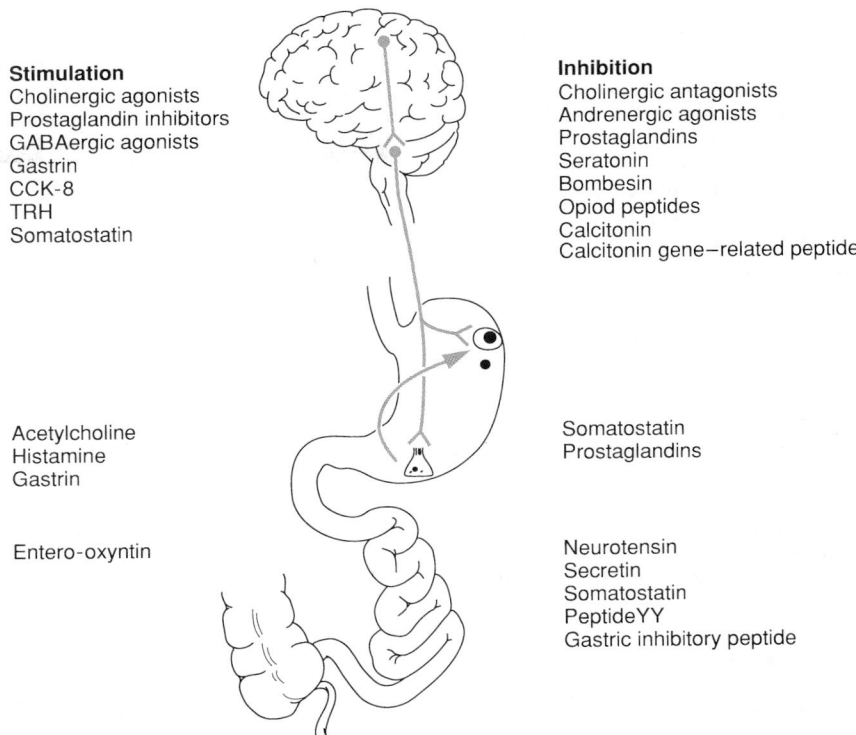

Stimulation
Cholinergic agonists
Prostaglandin inhibitors
GABAergic agonists
Gastrin
CCK-8
TRH
Somatostatin

Inhibition
Cholinergic antagonists
Andrenergic agonists
Prostaglandins
Seratonin
Bombesin
Opiod peptides
Calcitonin
Calcitonin gene—related peptide

Acetylcholine
Histamine
Gastrin

Somatostatin
Prostaglandins

Entero-oxyntin

Neurotensin
Secretin
Somatostatin
PeptideYY
Gastric inhibitory peptide

Figure 21.14. Regulation of acid secretion in vivo.

The gastric phase of acid secretion begins when food enters the stomach. The presence of partially hydrolyzed food constituents, gastric distention, and the buffering capacity of food all stimulate acid secretion. Gastrin is the most important mediator of the gastric phase of acid secretion. In normal humans, acid-secretory rates after a mixed meal average 15 to 25 mEq/h, approximately 75% of the maximal response achieved with infusion of exogenous gastrin or histamine. The meal response is less than the maximal response to exogenous stimulants because food also causes the release of somatostatin and initiates other inhibitory responses. In humans, 90% of meal-stimulated acid secretion is mediated by gastrin release (7).

The inhibitory regulation of gastric acid secretion is accomplished by central nervous system, gastric, and intestinal mechanisms. Stimulated acid secretion can be inhibited experimentally by administering various neuropeptides into the lateral cerebral ventricles, including gastrin-releasing peptide (bombesin), corticotropin-releasing factor, and calcitonin gene-related peptide. Although the relevance of these observations to human physiology remains to be determined, it is likely that central nervous system inhibition of acid secretion exists in humans. In this regard, the vagus nerve has both a stimulatory and an inhibitory role in acid secretion and gastrin release. Vagotomy causes fasting and postprandial hypergastrinemia, indicating that an inhibitory regulation of gastrin release normally exists. Hypergastrinemia is sustained long term after vagotomy by hyperplasia of antral gastrin cells. The vagal fibers to the oxyntic region of the stomach appear to mediate this inhibitory effect.

In humans, the most important and clearly established gastric inhibitory influence is the suppression of gastrin release when the antral mucosa is exposed to acid. When luminal pH falls to 2.0, gastrin release stops. Antral acidification also suppresses the gastrin response to an ingested meal. Somatostatin acting locally in the gastric mucosa as a paracrine agent may mediate this important inhibitory

response. Release of gastric somatostatin is reciprocally linked to that of gastrin; acidification of the antrum causes increases in somatostatin release and decreases in gastrin secretion. Antral distention also inhibits stimulated acid secretion.

The entry of digestive products into the intestine begins intestinal-phase inhibition of gastric acid secretion. Acidification of the duodenal bulb inhibits acid secretion, and although exogenous secretin also can inhibit acid secretion, this effect appears to be independent of the release of secretin from the duodenal mucosa. Hyperosmolar solutions and those containing fat also potently inhibit acid secretion. Several peptides, including secretin, somatostatin, peptide YY, gastric inhibitory peptide, and neurotensin, have been proposed as mediators of the intestinal phase effects. Each inhibits acid secretion experimentally. Their physiologic relevance remains to be determined.

PEPSIN

Pepsins are a heterogeneous group of proteolytic enzymes that are secreted by the gastric chief cells. Pepsin is derived under acidic conditions from pepsinogen by the autocatalytic loss of a variable amino-terminal sequence of the parent compound. This conversion occurs slowly at pH values of 5.0 to 6.0 and occurs rapidly when luminal pH approximates 2.0. Pepsin catalyzes the hydrolysis of a wide variety of peptide bonds that contain acidic residues, with a pH optimum for hydrolysis between 1.5 and 2.5. Once activated, pepsin is sensitive to ambient pH values; it is irreversibly denatured at pH 7.0 or greater.

The most important stimulus for pepsinogen secretion is cholinergic stimulation. Acetylcholine and its derivatives stimulate pepsinogen secretion by a mechanism that can be antagonized by atropine, indicating a muscarinic receptor. The receptor appears to have a high affinity for the selective muscarinic antagonist, pirenzepine, and therefore appears to be an M_1 type. Endogenous cholinergic stimulation through the vagal nerve results in the formation of a gastric secretion that is rich in pepsin. Although both exogenous histamine and gastrin can stimulate pepsin secretion, their actions appear to be indirectly due to the concomitant secretion of gastric acid rather than to direct stimulation of chief cells. Chief cells have also been shown to possess cholecystokinin receptors, and cholecystokinin-like peptides appear to have a direct stimulatory action on chief cells. The oxyntic mucosa contains somatostatin cells near chief cells. Pepsinogen secretion in response to a variety of stimuli has been demonstrated to be inhibited by somatostatin.

The major physiologic function of pepsin is to initiate protein digestion. Pepsin is highly active against collagen and may be important in the digestion of animal protein. Intragastric protein hydrolysis by pepsin is incomplete, and relatively large peptides enter the intestine, although amino acids and small peptide fragments are released. These products of partial hydrolysis are important signals for gastrin and cholecystokinin release, which in turn regulate digestive processes. In this way, pepsin also contributes to the overall coordination of the digestive process.

INTRINSIC FACTOR

The gastric mucosa is also the site of production of intrinsic factor, which is necessary for the absorption of cobalamin from the ileal mucosa. Total gastrectomy is regularly followed by cobalamin malabsorbtion, as is resection of the proximal stomach or atrophic gastritis that involves the oxyntic mucosa. Autoradiographic and immunocytochemical techniques have confirmed the parietal cell as the site of intrinsic factor synthesis and storage in humans. Intrinsic factor secretion, like acid secretion, is stimulated by histamine, acetylcholine, and gastrin. Unlike acid production, intrinsic factor secretion peaks rapidly after stimulation and then returns to baseline. The amount of intrinsic factor secreted usually greatly exceeds the amount needed to bind and absorb available dietary cobalamin.

GASTRIC BICARBONATE PRODUCTION

It is generally agreed that the gastric mucosa secretes HCO_3^- in addition to acid. The cells responsible for HCO_3^- production are presumed to be the surface mucous cells facing the gastric lumen, and HCO_3^- transport has been postulated to protect against damage from luminal acid. In theory, H^+ ions diffusing from luminal bulk fluids toward the gastric mucosa could be neutralized by secreted HCO_3^- near the surface (Fig. 21.15). In this way, nearly neutral pH can be maintained at the mucosal surface, even if the total amount of hydrochloride secreted greatly exceeded gastric HCO_3^- production. The occurrence of pH gradients at the surface of the gastric mucosa have been demonstrated in humans using microelectrodes. Drugs or chemicals that inhibit bicarbonate secretion result in acidification of the mucosal surface.

The degree of luminal acidity, reflected by pH, required to stimulate bicarbonate secretion is greater in the stomach than in the duodenum. Direct exposure of the gastric mucosa to pH levels of 2.0 or more increases bicarbonate secretion. In the duodenum, exposure of the mucosa to pH 5.0 doubles bicarbonate secretion, whereas exposure to pH 2.0 increases alkaline secretion 10-fold.

Cholinergic agonists, vagal nerve stimulation, and sham feeding have all been shown to increase gastric HCO_3^- production. The effects of cholinergic stimulation can be blocked by atropine. In the human stomach, exposure to luminal perfusates at pH 2.0 has been associated with increased release of prostaglandin E_2. Prostaglandin E_2 and its synthetic derivatives are also potent stimulants of gastric bicarbonate secretion. Because mucosal bicarbonate production can be decreased in experimental models by indomethacin, endogenous prostaglandins are thought to be important in the mucosal alkaline response.

GASTRIC BLOOD FLOW

Because the gastric mucosa is metabolically highly active, control of mucosal blood flow is of great physiologic importance. In addition, studies have implicated perfusion abnormalities in the development of mucosal lesions during periods of stress. Mucosal blood flow is regulated by neural, hormonal, and locally active influences.

Postganglionic sympathetic nerve fibers reach the stomach in association with its blood supply and richly innervate small mucosal arteries. Mucosal capillaries do not receive adrenergic innervation. Electrical stimulation of sympathetic nerves supplying the stomach is followed by decreased total gastric blood flow, decreased flow in celiac and gastroepiploic vessels, and diminished blood flow to the mucosa. With prolonged sympathetic stimulation, blood flow gradually increases to a new steady-state level. This phenomenon represents a partial escape from the

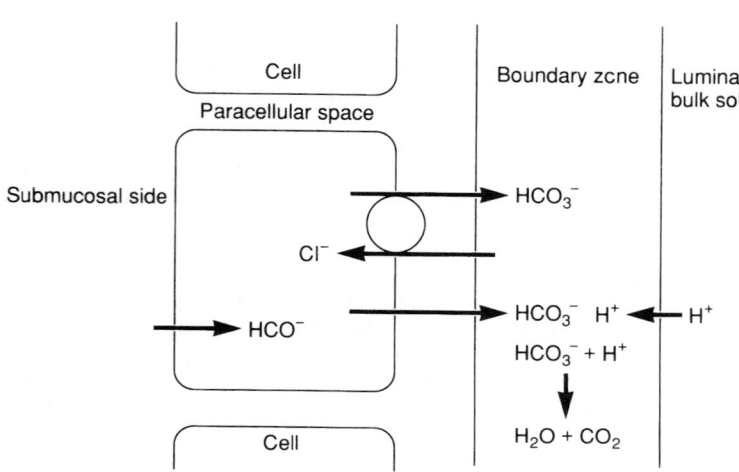

Figure 21.15. Schematic representation of mucosal bicarbonate secretion, showing neutralization of luminal hydrogen ions immediately above the mucosal surface.

vasoconstrictive adrenergic influence. Studies in animals demonstrate that vasoconstriction of the gastric vascular bed is mediated by α-adrenergic receptors, and that vasodilation, including adrenergic escape, is mediated by β-adrenergic receptors.

Stimulation of the vagus nerve is followed by a prompt increase in blood flow, suggesting a dilatory effect of parasympathetic nerves. The effects of vagal stimulation on mucosal blood flow are complicated by accompanying increases in acid secretion. Almost all stimuli that increase acid production also increase blood flow secondarily.

A number of gastrointestinal peptide hormones affect gastric blood flow, most because of their ability to increase or decrease acid secretion. Thus, gastrin, because it is a potent stimulant of acid secretion, also increases mucosal blood flow. Cholecystokinin appears to have direct vasodilatory property for gastric vasculature. Vasopressin has been well demonstrated to have direct vasoconstrictor activity. The vascular effects of other peptide hormones remain controversial.

Nitric oxide modulates basal gastric vascular tone and controls gastric vasodilation and hyperemia. Nitric oxide mediates the hyperemic response that accompanies increases in acid secretion, although the molecule has no direct stimulatory role in acid production.

Prostaglandins are important mucosally produced compounds that have clear effects on the gastric vasculature. Prostaglandins of the E class have been shown in animals and humans to increase gastric blood flow at doses that decrease acid secretion. Indomethacin, in doses sufficient to inhibit prostaglandin formation, decreases the diameter of submucosal blood vessels and reduces basal blood flow. Complete inhibition of cyclooxygenase activity causes an approximate 50% reduction in resting blood flow. These studies suggest that endogenous, locally produced prostaglandins are crucial to maintaining basal gastric blood flow in humans and probably act in concert with endogenous nitric oxide.

GASTRIC MOTILITY

Gastric Smooth Muscle

Consideration of gastric motility requires that the stomach be viewed in functional terms as two different regions—the proximal one third and the distal two thirds. These areas are distinct in terms of smooth muscle anatomy, electrical activity, and contractile function. The regions do not correspond to the traditional anatomic divisions of fundus, corpus, and antrum.

In the proximal stomach, three layers of gastric smooth muscle can be distinguished—an outer longitudinal layer, a middle circular layer, and an inner oblique layer. In the distal two thirds of the stomach, the longitudinal layer is most clearly defined and the inner oblique layer is usually not distinct. The gastric smooth muscle ends at the pylorus. A septum of connective tissue marks the change from pylorus to duodenum, separating longitudinal and circular smooth muscle bundles and providing a point of electrical and mechanical transition (Fig. 21.16).

The smooth muscle of the proximal stomach is electrically stable, whereas the smooth muscle of the distal stomach demonstrates spontaneous, repeated electrical discharges. These electrical differences can also be demonstrated using intracellular recordings from isolated gastric smooth muscle cells, indicating that gastric smooth muscle cells are somehow programmed in terms of electrical activity. Gastric smooth muscle exhibits myoelectric activity that is based on a highly regular pattern called the *slow wave* (8). In the stomach, slow waves occur with a frequency of three cycles per minute. Slow waves do not, by themselves, lead to gastric contractions, but they do set the maximum rate of contractions at three per minute. Gastric contractions occur when action potentials are phase locked with the crest of the slow wave.

Extracellular electrical recording from the serosal surface of the stomach also demonstrates the intrinsic electrical activity of the distal stomach in the form of pacesetter potentials. Pacesetter potentials reflect partial depolarization of the gastric smooth muscle cell and are recorded during relatively long periods (2 or 3 seconds). Pacesetters originate along the greater curvature at a point in the proximal third of the stomach. Pacesetter potentials, discharging at a rate of three times per minute in humans, drive cells located distally. Spread of the pacesetter potentials is faster along the greater curvature, so that a ring of electrical activity reaches the pylorus simultaneously along both curvatures. The pacesetter potentials do not result in smooth muscle contraction unless an additional depolarization is superimposed in the form of an action potential. When action potentials occur, a ring of smooth muscle contraction moves peristaltically along the distal stomach toward the pylorus.

Duodenal slow-wave frequency and maximum rate of phasic contractions is higher than observed in the stom-

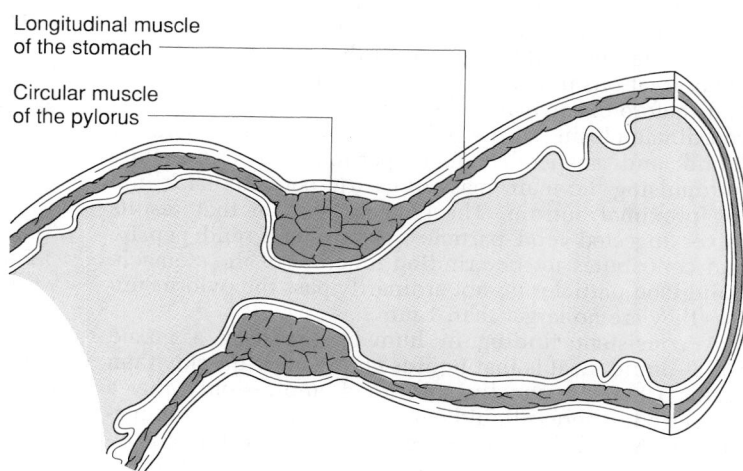

Longitudinal muscle of the stomach

Circular muscle of the pylorus

Figure 21.16. Cross-sectional anatomy of pyloric sphincter.

ach. The duodenal rate is approximately 12 cycles per minute; the contraction rate declines progressively to 9 cycles per minute in the distal ileum.

Gastric smooth muscle is affected by several neurohumoral agents that modulate contractility, both positively and negatively:

Stimulants
 Acetylcholine
 Motilin
 Macrolide antibiotics
 G_{17}
 Cholecystokinin 8
 Substance P
 Dynorphin
 Leucine enkephalin
 Methionine enkephalin
Inhibitors
 Duodenal acidification
 Ileal fat
 Rectal/colonic distention
 Pregnancy
 VIP
 Secretin
 Glucagon

The smooth muscle activity of the proximal stomach is fundamentally different from that of the distal stomach. There are no pacesetter or action potentials in the proximal stomach. As a result, peristalsis does not occur. Proximal gastric contraction is tonic and prolonged, with increases in luminal pressure often sustained for several minutes.

Coordination of Contraction

Important vagally mediated reflexes influence intragastric pressure, presumably by affecting contractile activity of smooth muscle in the proximal stomach. The most important reflex is termed *receptive relaxation* and occurs with ingestion of a meal. Increasing gastric volumes are accommodated with little increase in intragastric pressure by relaxation of the proximal stomach. This receptive relaxation allows the proximal stomach to act as a storage site for ingested food in the immediate postprandial period. Afferent impulses, presumed to originate from stretch receptors in the gastric wall, are carried along vagal fibers; efferent vagal discharges are inhibitory. Receptive gastric accommodation is lost after either truncal or proximal gastric vagotomy. After the meal has been ingested, proximal contractile activity increases; alterations in proximal gastric tone cause the compressive movement of gastric content from the fundus to the antrum.

Food that enters the antrum from the proximal stomach is propelled peristaltically toward the pylorus. A number of observations indicate that the pylorus closes 2 or 3 seconds before the arrival of the antral contraction ring. This coordinate closing of the pylorus allows a small bolus of liquid and suspended food particles to pass while retropulsing the main mass of gastric contents back into the proximal antrum. The churning action that results mixes ingested food particles, gastric acid, and pepsin, and contributes to the grinding function of the stomach. Solid food particles do not ordinarily pass the pylorus unless they are no larger than 1 mm.

A consistent finding in humans ingesting a mixed solid–liquid meal is that liquids empty more quickly than solids. Characteristically, solid food empties only after a lag period, whereas liquid emptying begins almost immediately. A traditional interpretation of these human observations has been that the proximal stomach is the dominant force in determining how quickly a liquid meal empties by the gastroduodenal pressure gradient generated by proximal gastric contractions. The actions of the proximal stomach in liquid emptying are also regulated by the sieving actions of the antropyloric segment and are modified by the nutrient composition of the ingested meal. The distal gastric segment has been postulated to control solid emptying through its grinding and peristaltic actions. This traditional concept of the two-component stomach is useful in considering observations in patients who have undergone gastric operative procedures. Patients who have undergone proximal gastric vagotomy exhibit accelerated emptying of liquids but have normal solid emptying. Because of loss of receptive relaxation, the denervation of the proximal stomach is presumed to increase intragastric pressure and accelerate liquid emptying while leaving the distal gastric segment unaffected. Conversely, vagal denervation of the antrum interrupts gastric emptying of solids to a greater degree than liquids. Although this model of gastric emptying oversimplifies the many mechanisms (gastric, pyloric, and intestinal) that work in concert to control gastric emptying, it provides a useful framework for considering the effects of gastric surgical procedures.

REFERENCES

1. Dockray GJ, Varro A, Dimaline R. Gastric endocrine cells: gene expression, processing, and targeting of active products. *Am Phys Soc* 1996;76:767–798.
2. Magee DF. Pyloric antral inhibition of gastrin release. *J Gastroenterol* 1996;31:758–763.
3. Debas HT, Carvajal SH. Vagal regulation of acid secretion and gastrin release. *Yale J Biol Med* 1994;67:145–151.
4. DeValle J. The stomach as an endocrine organ. *Digestion* 1997;58[Suppl 1]:4–7.
5. Sachs G, Meyer-Rosberg K, Scott DR, et al. Acid secretion and *Helicobacter pylori. Digestion* 1997;58[Suppl 1]:8–13.
6. Urushidani T, Forte JG. Signal transduction and activation of acid secretion in the parietal cell. *J Membr Biol* 1997;159:99–111.
7. Waldum HL, Brenna E, Kleveland PM, et al. Gastrin—physiological and pathophysiological role: clinical consequences. *Dig Dis* 1995;13:25–38.
8. Quigley EM. Gastric and small intestinal motility in health and disease. *Gastroenterol Clin North Am* 1996;25:113–145.

SURGERY: SCIENTIFIC PRINCIPLES AND PRACTICE, Third Edition, edited by Lazar J. Greenfield, Michael W. Mulholland, Keith T. Oldham, Gerald B. Zelenock, and Keith D. Lillemoe. Lippincott Williams & Wilkins Publishers, Philadelphia, © 2001.

CHAPTER 22

DUODENAL ULCER

MICHAEL W. MULHOLLAND

EPIDEMIOLOGY

Peptic ulceration remains a major public health problem worldwide (1). Some 300,000 new cases of peptic ulcer are diagnosed in the United States each year, and 4 million people receive some form of ulcer treatment. In the United States, ulcer mortality and hospitalization rates have fallen since the early 1980s, but physicians are now treating a cohort of older patients with frequent comorbidity and ulcer disease of greater chronicity. Mortality attributed to peptic ulceration remains substantial; ulcer disease is listed as a contributing cause of death in more than 10,000 cases annually.

Treatment of peptic ulcer has changed fundamentally over the 1990s. New insights into disease pathogenesis, especially the realization that gastric infection has a role in most cases of peptic ulceration, have been especially exciting. Antibiotics have become front-line antiulcer therapy. A number of powerful antisecretory drugs have been introduced into clinical practice. Medical, endoscopic, and surgical therapies are frequently integrated in the care of individual patients.

No clear racial predilection for the development of duodenal ulceration exists, but genetic factors can be important. Hyperpepsinogenemia I, with autosomal dominant inheritance, is common in duodenal ulcer, although the relation of this trait to the development of ulceration remains obscure. A number of rare familial syndromes associated with peptic ulceration have been described.

PATHOPHYSIOLOGY

The pathogenesis of peptic ulceration is complex, multifactorial, and incompletely understood. The development of peptic ulceration is often depicted as a balance between acid–peptic secretion and mucosal defense, with the equilibrium shifted toward disease. Although large increases in acid secretion alone can occasionally cause ulceration, and although acid–peptic secretion is crucial in the development of ulcers, usually a defect in mucosal defense also exists to tip the balance away from health. Mucosal infection with *Helicobacter pylori* is the factor that contributes to ulcer pathogenesis in most patients.

Helicobacter pylori

The relation between *H. pylori* infection and ulceration is inferential but overwhelmingly strong; a causal relation between *H. pylori* infection and peptic ulceration has not been tested directly (2). Because *H. pylori* infection is difficult to eradicate with certainty, and because of the potentially serious consequences of infection, the intentional exposure of humans to the organism to establish such a relation is not justified.

Many lines of circumstantial evidence establish *H. pylori* as a factor in the pathogenesis of duodenal ulceration (3–6):

1. *H. pylori* is the primary cause of chronic active gastritis, characterized by nonerosive inflammation of the gastric mucosa. Antral gastritis is nearly always present histologically in patients with duodenal ulcer, and *H. pylori* can be isolated from gastric mucosa in almost all cases.
2. Gastric metaplasia is extremely common in duodenal epithelium surrounding areas of ulceration. *H. pylori* binds only to gastric-type epithelium, regardless of location; metaplastic gastric epithelium can become colonized by *H. pylori* from gastric sources. Gastric metaplasia of the duodenal bulb is a nonspecific response to damage, and is the means by which antral gastritis with *H. pylori* is converted to active chronic duodenitis.
3. Eradication of *H. pylori* with antimicrobials that have no effect on acid secretion leads to ulcer healing rates equivalent to those seen with histamine type 2 (H_2) receptor antagonists.
4. Therapy with bismuth compounds, which eradicate *H. pylori,* is associated with reduced rates of ulcer relapse relative to conventional therapy.
5. Relapse of duodenal ulcer after antimicrobial therapy is preceded by reinfection of the gastric mucosa by *H. pylori.*

However, half of patients evaluated for dyspepsia, but without ulceration, have histologic evidence of mucosal bacterial infection. Furthermore, 20% of healthy volunteers harbor the bacteria; the incidence of bacterial carriage in the healthy, asymptomatic population increases with age. The occurrence of peptic ulcers in only a small proportion of people who carry the organism suggests that other factors must also act to induce ulceration. The ability of *H. pylori* infection to induce alterations in gastric acid secretion is a prerequisite for ulcer development in most patients.

Acid Secretory Status

The formation of duodenal ulcers depends on gastric secretion of acid and pepsin. The dictum "no acid–no ulcer" properly focuses on the importance of luminal acid in the development of the disease, although a more complete statement might be "no acid and no *H. pylori*–no ulcer." As a group, patients with duodenal ulcers have an increased capacity for gastric acid secretion relative to normal people (Table 22.1). The maximal acid output of normal men is approximately 20 mEq/h in response to intravenous histamine stimulation, whereas patients with duodenal ulcer secrete an average of approximately 40 mEq/h. Considerable overlap exists between these two groups, and the values for most people with duodenal ulcer fall within the normal range. The increase in acid secretion in some patients with duodenal ulcer has been postulated to be due to an increase in the mass of parietal cells in the acid-secreting gastric mucosa or to an increased sensitivity to circulating gastrin.

Groups of patients with duodenal ulcer demonstrate a prolonged and larger acid-secretory response to a mixed meal than do groups of normal subjects. As with histamine-stimulated acid output, overlap between patients with duodenal ulcer and normal subjects exists. Disturbances in gastric motility can exacerbate meal-stimulated acid-secretory abnormalities. Patients with duodenal ulcer have accelerated emptying of gastric contents, particularly liquids, after a meal, and duodenal acidification fails to slow emptying appropriately. In such patients, the duodenal mucosa can be exposed to low pH for prolonged periods relative to normal subjects.

Table 22.1. PATHOGENESIS OF PEPTIC ULCER

HELICOBACTER PYLORI INFECTION
Endocrine consequences
Increased basal serum gastrin
Increased gastrin response to a meal
Increased responsiveness to gastrin-releasing peptide
Production of N^a-methylhistamine
Decreased density of somatostatin cells
Decreased mucosal somatostatin content

Gastric acid secretion
Increased acid secretory capacity
Increased basal secretion
Increased pentagastrin-stimulated output
Increased meal response
Abnormal gastric emptying

Mucosal defense
Decreased duodenal bicarbonate production
Decreased gastric mucosal prostaglandin production

ENVIRONMENT
Cigarette smoking
Nonsteroidal antiinflammatory drugs

Groups of patients with duodenal ulcer also demonstrate increased basal secretion of acid. Increased basal secretion can be demonstrated by nocturnal collection of gastric secretions. Increased vagal discharge has been postulated as the responsible mechanism. In support of this contention, basal acid secretion in patients with duodenal ulcer correlates with circulating concentrations of vagally released pancreatic polypeptide. In addition, sham feeding, which is vagally mediated, does not increase acid output above basal secretion in these patients.

Studies indicate that most of these secretory abnormalities are a direct consequence of *H. pylori* infection (7). Ironically, the earliest stages of *H. pylori* infection are accompanied by a marked decrease in gastric acid secretion (8). Acute antral gastritis is followed by fundal inflammation. Fundal inflammation is associated with mucosal production of a number of cytokines, including interleukin (IL)-1β, IL-6, IL-8, and tumor necrosis factor-α (TNF-α). IL-1β is a potent inhibitor of gastric acid secretion (9). Investigators have postulated that acute reduction in gastric acid secretion facilitates further gastric colonization with *H. pylori*. Acute hypochlorhydria resolves despite persistence of *H. pylori* and is followed by a state of chronically increased acid secretion.

Basal and peak acid output are increased in patients with duodenal ulcer infected with *H. pylori* relative to uninfected healthy volunteers (10). With eradication of *H. pylori* infection, basal acid output returns to normal within 4 weeks, and peak acid output declines to the normal range by 6 months. Peak acid output reflects parietal cell mass; the slow return to normal levels suggests that *H. pylori* infection may stimulate increases in the parietal cell mass.

Abnormalities in acid secretion and parietal cell mass appear to be due to *H. pylori*-induced hypergastrinemia. *H. pylori*-infected patients have increased basal serum gastrin levels, increased gastrin responses to meal stimulation, and an augmented gastrin response to intravenous gastrin-releasing peptide. Eradication of *H. pylori* infection causes serum gastrin levels to return to baseline (11). Gastric mucosal inflammatory cells and epithelial cells are activated by *H. pylori* infection to release cytokines such as IL-8, interferon-γ, and TNF-α. These cytokines are stimulants of gastrin release from cultured canine gastrin cells.

Helicobacter pylori expresses Nα-histamine methyltransferase activity. This enzyme produces Nα-methylhistamine, an abnormal analogue of histamine that can act as a gastric acid secretory stimulant (12).

The concentration of somatostatin in the antral mucosa and the number of somatostatin-producing cells in the antrum are diminished in *H. pylori*-infected patients. Treatment of *H. pylori* infection is followed by increases in numbers of somatostatin cells and in mucosal somatostatin messenger RNA levels (13). These observations suggest that alterations in mucosal somatostatin metabolism may also contribute to the hypergastrinemia seen in *H. pylori*-infected patients by removing the inhibitory effects that somatostatin exerts on gastrin release. Somatostatin release is also suppressed by Nα-methylhistamine.

Mucosal Defense against Peptic Injury

Investigative attention has also focused on the ability of the duodenal mucosa to resist the injurious effects of luminal acid and pepsin. Because many patients with duodenal ulcer secrete normal amounts of acid and pepsin, it is attractive to postulate that abnormalities of mucosal defense might result in ulceration. In addition, several agents that are useful in the treatment of peptic ulceration are cy-

toprotective, which is defined as the ability to protect the mucosa from injury at doses lower than the threshold dose needed to inhibit acid secretion. The ability of cytoprotective agents to heal ulcers has suggested that abnormalities in mucosal defense are responsible for some instances of ulceration. Most investigative efforts have focused on the role of mucosally secreted bicarbonate and on mucosal prostaglandin production.

Gastric surface epithelial cells secrete mucus and bicarbonate, creating a pH gradient within the mucus layer that is nearly neutral at the mucous cell surface, even when the lumen is highly acidic. Failure of normal bicarbonate secretion locally would, in theory, result in exposure of surface epithelial cells to the peptic activity of gastric secretions at low pH. Patients with duodenal ulcers have been demonstrated to have significantly lower basal bicarbonate secretion in the proximal duodenum than normal subjects. In addition, in response to a physiologically relevant amount of hydrochloric acid instilled into the duodenal bulb, stimulated bicarbonate output was approximately 40% of the normal response (14). Abnormalities in duodenal bicarbonate secretion normalize after elimination of *H. pylori* in infected patients. These results suggest one mechanism by which ulceration could occur, even in patients secreting normal amounts of acid.

Diminished mucosal prostaglandin production has also been proposed to exist in subsets of patients with duodenal ulcer (15). Prostaglandins and prostaglandin analogues have been shown to exert cytoprotective effects, to accelerate healing of established duodenal ulcers, and to decrease acid secretion. In the duodenum, locally produced prostaglandins stimulate mucosal bicarbonate secretion. In patients with active duodenal ulceration, gastric mucosal production of prostaglandin E_2 and other prostanoids has been shown to be diminished. An increase in prostanoid synthesis within the gastric mucosa characterizes ulcer healing. Duodenal bicarbonate responses to prostaglandin E_2 are impaired in patients with duodenal ulcer.

Environmental Factors

Substantial evidence implicates cigarette smoking as a major risk factor in the development of duodenal ulcers. Cigarette smoking patterns parallel ulcer hospitalization and mortality rates. The sharp decline in smoking rates recorded in middle-aged American men since the early 1980s has been accompanied by a decline in ulcer incidence in this group. Unhappily, increased cigarette smoking in young and middle-aged women has been mirrored by increased peptic ulceration in the female population. Cigarette smoking impairs ulcer healing and increases the recurrence of ulcers (16). Continued smoking attenuates the effectiveness of active ulcer therapy. Cigarette smoking increases both the probability that surgery will be required and the risks of operative therapy. A variety of mechanisms have been proposed to account for the deleterious effects of smoking, including decreased prostaglandin production, increased bile reflux, stimulation of acid production, and alterations in mucosal blood flow. The actions of cigarette smoke on gastroduodenal mucosa are not yet clear and may be multifactorial. Cessation of smoking is a key element of antiulcer therapy.

The belief is widespread that diet and environmental stress are important in the development of ulcers. Systematic study of these factors has been difficult, and supportive evidence is slim. No rigorous evidence exists to suggest that alterations in diet accelerate healing of ulcers. Caffeine has not been demonstrated to be detrimental. The role of alcohol is unsettled. In experimental models, direct application of alcohol to gastroduodenal mucosa induces injury, but in humans, alcohol consumption has been variously reported to impair and to increase ulcer healing. Although cirrhosis has been associated with an increased incidence of peptic ulceration, alcohol consumption in moderation has not definitely been shown to be harmful.

Nonsteroidal antiinflammatory drugs (NSAIDs) have emerged as a significant risk factor for the development of acute ulceration. Although acute mucosal injury caused by NSAIDs is more common in the stomach than in the duodenum, NSAID-induced ulcer complications occur with equal frequency in these two sites. NSAIDs produce a variety of lesions, ranging from hemorrhage, to superficial mucosal erosions, to deeper ulcerations. In the duodenum, it appears likely that invasive, NSAID-associated ulcers result from underlying peptic ulcer diathesis compounded by the direct injurious effects of the drugs.

The ulcerogenic actions of NSAIDs have been attributed to their systemic suppression of prostaglandin production. Numerous experimental models have demonstrated the ability of NSAIDs to injure the gastroduodenal mucosa. Ulcers resembling those caused by NSAIDs can be produced experimentally by antibodies to prostaglandins. Conversely, NSAID-associated gastric ulcers can be prevented by the coadministration of prostaglandin analogues. Ulcers associated with NSAIDs usually heal rapidly when the drug is withdrawn, corresponding to the reversal of antiprostaglandin effects. All available NSAIDs appear to pose the hazard of gastroduodenal ulceration. Clinically important ulceration (of both the stomach and duodenum) is estimated by the U.S. Food and Drug Administration to occur at a rate of 2% to 4% per patient-year. The risks inherent with NSAID use appear to be increased by a history of peptic ulcer disease, by cigarette smoking, and by alcohol use. The incidence of NSAID-caused ulcer complications is highest in older patients, as is the attendant mortality rate.

DIAGNOSIS

The cardinal feature of duodenal ulceration is epigastric pain. The pain is usually confined to the upper abdomen and is described as burning, stabbing, or gnawing. Unless perforation or penetration into the head of the pancreas has occurred, referral of pain is not common. Many patients report pain on arising in the morning. Ingestion of food or antacids usually provides prompt relief. In uncomplicated cases, abnormal physical findings are minimal. The differential diagnosis is broad and includes a variety of diseases originating in the upper gastrointestinal tract. The most common disorders to be distinguished include nonulcerative dyspepsia, gastric neoplasia, cholelithiasis and related diseases of the biliary system, and both inflammatory and neoplastic disorders of the pancreas. In dyspeptic patients, the principal diagnoses that must be differentiated definitively are peptic ulceration and gastric cancer.

The evaluation of patients with suspected peptic ulceration usually involves either barium contrast examination of the stomach and duodenum or endoscopy. In most circumstances, endoscopy is the preferred method and has become the standard against which other diagnostic modalities are measured. Endoscopy is recommended because it eliminates the need for radiation, is safe, is preferred by elderly patients, and permits biopsy of the esophagus, stomach, and duodenum. In a controlled trial comparing endoscopy and barium radiography, endoscopy was both more sensitive (92% vs. 54%) and more specific (100% vs. 91%) than radiographic examination (17). Endoscopy must be recommended with discretion

because of associated morbidity (approximately 1 per 5,000 cases) and higher costs.

Duodenal ulcer is characterized by lesions that are erosive to the bowel wall. When viewed endoscopically, the ulcers have a typical appearance. The edges are usually sharply demarcated, and the underlying submucosa is exposed. The ulcer base is often clean and smooth, although acute ulcers and those with recent hemorrhage can demonstrate eschar or adherent exudate. Surrounding mucosal inflammation is common. The most frequent site for peptic ulceration is the first portion of the duodenum, with the second portion less commonly involved. Ulceration of the third or fourth portions of the duodenum is unusual, and its occurrence should arouse suspicion of an underlying gastrinoma. Ulceration in the pyloric channel or the prepyloric area is similar in endoscopic appearance to duodenal ulceration, and ulcers in these areas demonstrate other clinical features similar to duodenal ulcers. Endoscopic demonstration of a duodenal ulcer should prompt mucosal biopsy of the gastric antrum to demonstrate the presence of *H. pylori* and guide subsequent therapy.

Barium meal radiographs demonstrate retention of contrast in the ulcer. When viewed in profile, the ulcer can be seen to project beyond the level of the duodenal mucosa. Distortion of the duodenal bulb by spasm or cicatrization is a secondary sign of current or previous ulceration.

The hallmarks of the histologic appearance of duodenal ulcers are chronicity and invasiveness. Chronic injury is suggested by surrounding fibrosis; collagen is deposited in the submucosa during each round of ulcer relapse and healing. The adjacent mucosa often demonstrates evidence of chronic injury with infiltration of acute and chronic inflammatory cells. Gastric metaplasia, in which the duodenum exhibits histologic features of gastric mucosa, is common in the surrounding nonulcerated mucosa. The ulcer can extend for a variable distance through the wall of the duodenum, including the full thickness of the bowel in cases of perforation.

DRUG TREATMENT OF ULCER DISEASE

Current treatment of peptic ulceration involves a combination of an antisecretory drug, usually a proton pump inhibitor, with antibiotics. This therapy is rational for most patients who are *H. pylori* positive and results in a high rate of sustained ulcer healing.

A large number of drug regimens have been described, but the most widely used treatment protocols combine a proton pump inhibitor, usually omeprazole, with two antibiotics, usually clarithromycin and metronidazole or amoxicillin. This triple therapy is administered for 7 or 14 days. Triple drug therapy is cost effective and associated with a low rate of side effects, low rates of antibiotic resistance, and acceptable levels of patient compliance. *H. pylori* eradication rates of greater than 90% have been reported.

After elimination of *H. pylori,* ulcer recurrence rates reflect the rate of reinfection. In developed countries, reinfection rates of less than 10% at 5 years have been reported (18). Eradication of *H. pylori* improves quality of life, as measured by symptoms, drug prescriptions, physician visits, and days of missed employment.

A consideration of the cellular mechanisms regulating the production of acid by the gastric parietal cell suggests several potential sites of action for drugs that act to inhibit acid secretion (Fig. 22.1). Receptor antagonists for histamine or antagonists of the parietal cell proton pump might be expected to have therapeutic potential. In addition, agents that supplement or restore mucosal defenses might

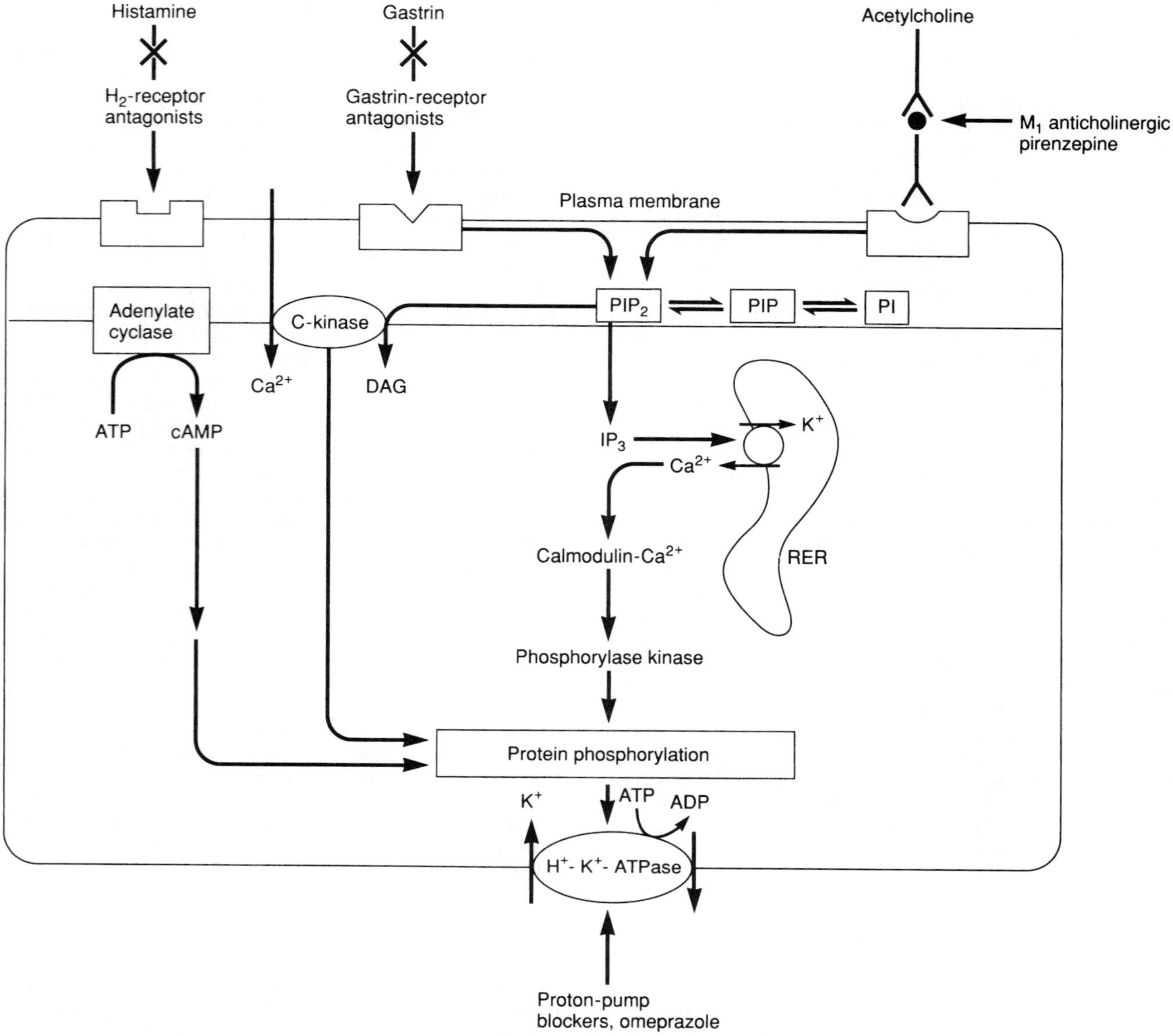

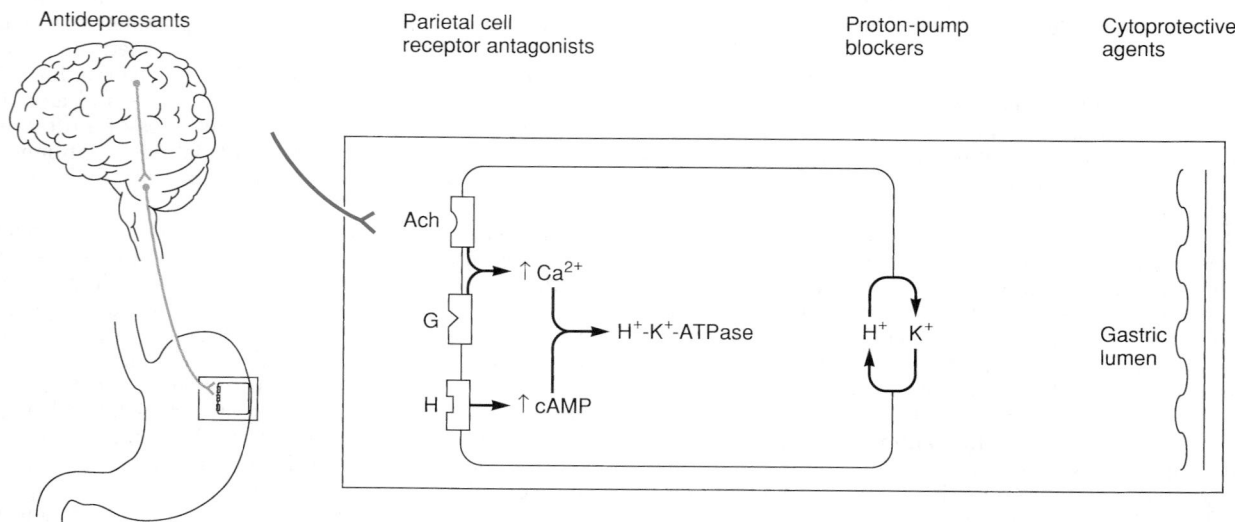

Figure 22.1. Antisecretory drugs that act on the gastric parietal cell and that are potentially useful in the treatment of duodenal ulcer. RER, rough endoplasmic reticulum; DAG, diacrylglycerol.

Figure 22.2. Overview of the sites of action of drugs with antiulcer activities.

Table 22.2. PHARMACOLOGIC PARAMETERS OF COMMONLY USED ANTIULCER DRUGS

Agent	Daily dose	Bioavailability (%)	Excretion	Side effects	Drug interactions
Cimetidine	800–1,200 mg	70	Renal	Neuropsychiatric, endocrine	Hepatically metabolized drugs
Ranitidine	300–400 mg	70	Renal	Neuropsychiatric	Warfarin
Famotidine	40 mg	70	Renal	Nonspecific	
Omeprazole	20–40 mg	40–50	Renal	Nonspecific	
Sucralfate	4 g	Unabsorbed	Unabsorbed	Constipation	

also have therapeutic importance in peptic diseases (Fig. 22.2). A number of compounds are available that have these characteristics. An appreciation of the uses and limits of drug therapy is necessary for all surgeons who treat patients with duodenal ulcer (Table 22.2).

Histamine Receptor Antagonists

Histamine, released into the interstitial fluid by cells in the fundic mucosa, diffuses to the mucosal parietal cell. Histamine stimulates acid production by occupying a membrane-bound receptor and activating parietal cell adenylate cyclase. Histamine is released in response to a number of physiologic stimuli; blockade of histamine receptors inhibits most forms of stimulated acid secretion in humans.

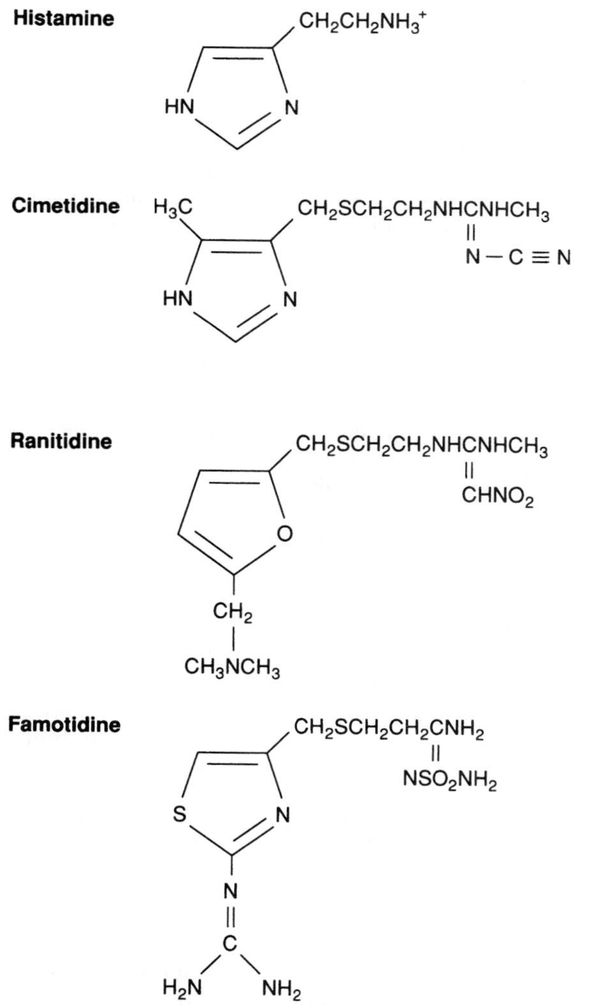

Figure 22.3. Chemical structures of selected histamine-2 (H_2) receptor antagonists and their relation to histamine.

Parietal cell histamine receptors are classified as H_2 receptors because they are activated by agonists such as 4-methylhistamine and are selectively blocked by agents such as cimetidine. Some H_2 receptor antagonists also possess nongastric actions by binding to androgen receptors, by interacting with the hepatic microsomal oxidase system, and by crossing the blood–brain barrier. All clinically useful gastric histamine receptor antagonists are of the H_2 type.

Cimetidine, ranitidine, famotidine, and newer H_2 receptor antagonists bind competitively to parietal cell H_2 receptors to produce a reversible inhibition of acid secretion. Cimetidine shares the imidazole ring of histamine; in ranitidine, the imidazole ring has been replaced with an alkyl furan ring (Fig. 22.3). In second-generation H_2 receptor antagonists, increasing structural differences compared with the parent compound have been introduced. As a result of these rearrangements, a series of compounds with increasing potency has been produced. There are two pharmacologic results: increased duration of action up to and beyond 24 hours, and improved specificity because of decreased interactions with receptors in nongastric tissues.

An enormous, worldwide experience has been accumulated with the use of H_2 receptor antagonists. The agents are effective and safe when used in the treatment of peptic ulcer. The various compounds have similar efficacy in terms of ulcer healing when used in doses that produce similar reductions in acid output. When endoscopic criteria are used to determine healing, approximately 70% of patients are ulcer free within 4 weeks of therapy. By 8 weeks, 85% to 90% of patients are pain free and without endoscopic evidence of ulceration. Most studies of maintenance therapy have used single nocturnal doses of cimetidine or ranitidine; ulcer relapse during maintenance therapy occurs in approximately 15% of patients under these circumstances. It has become increasingly clear that H_2 receptor blockers do not affect the underlying ulcer diathesis; if H_2 receptor antagonists are stopped, recurrent ulceration occurs in greater than half of patients within 1 year. The current understanding of the role of *H. pylori* in ulcer pathogenesis has changed the role of H_2 receptor antagonists from primary therapy to that of a substitute for proton pump inhibitors in conjunction with antibiotic treatment.

Proton Pump Blockers

Acid secretion by the gastric parietal cells is due to the active transport of hydrogen ions from the parietal cell cytoplasm into the secretory canaliculus in exchange for potassium. Because this so-called *proton pump* is tissue specific, being present only in gastric mucosa, its blockade would be expected to have minimal effects on nongastric functions. Omeprazole is representative of a family of compounds that selectively block the parietal cell proton pump (19).

Omeprazole is a weak base, with a pKa of approximately 4. The drug is nonionized and lipid soluble at neutral pH, but it becomes ionized and activated at a pH of less than 3. In its activated state, omeprazole binds to the membrane-bound H^+-K^+-adenosine triphosphatase (ATPase) of the parietal cell. Because the compound is a weak base, omeprazole accumulates selectively within the acidic environment of the parietal cell secretory canaliculus; 4 hours after administration, the drug is detectable in appreciable quantities only in the gastric mucosa. If enough drug is administered to occupy all parietal cell binding sites, anacidity can be produced. Omeprazole, in doses from 20 to 30 mg, causes nearly complete inhibition of stimulated gastric acid secretion within 6 hours. At 24 hours after drug administration, 60% to 70% reduction in acid secretion persists.

Omeprazole is slightly soluble in water of neutral pH but is rapidly degraded in aqueous solutions of reduced pH. As a result, various oral formulations have been developed to limit intragastric degradation and to improve systemic bioavailability. Repeated daily dosing with omeprazole results in increasing inhibitory action on gastric secretion and thus in decreased intragastric degradation of the drug. Acid suppression stabilizes after approximately 3 days. Because of tissue accumulation, the secretory actions of omeprazole do not correlate with plasma levels.

Omeprazole accelerates the healing of ulcers and provides superior symptomatic relief in patients with duodenal ulceration. Endoscopically proven ulcers demonstrate complete healing in 80% of patients after 2 weeks and in 95% of patients after 4 weeks when omeprazole is administered once daily. Several studies have demonstrated a significant inhibition of peak acid output, marked relief of epigastric pain, and decreased use of supplemental antacids during omeprazole therapy. Direct comparisons with H_2 receptor antagonists have generally favored omeprazole in terms of pain relief and rate of ulcer healing.

Toxicologic studies in animals have shown that omeprazole in high doses can produce histologic abnormalities in the gastric mucosa. Hyperplasia of enterochromaffin-like cells has been seen in chronically achlorhydric animals; the histologic changes correlate with circulating gastrin levels. Enterochromaffin-like cell hyperplasia is believed to be induced by the trophic effect of elevated gastrin. In humans, only patients with Zollinger-Ellison syndrome have received continuous high-dose omeprazole therapy, and hyperplasia of enterochromaffin-like cells has not been observed. Concerns about the development of enterochromaffin-like cell hyperplasia with long-term omeprazole use appear to have been overstated.

Sucralfate

Sucralfate is the aluminum salt of sulfated sucrose. In the acidic environment of the stomach, sucralfate polymerizes, becoming viscous and adhering to the gastroduodenal mucosa. Coating of the ulcer base by the polymer has been claimed to provide a protective barrier, binding bile salts and inhibiting the actions of pepsin. Sucralfate also stimulates the production of mucus. Sucralfate stimulates increased mucosal prostaglandin E_2 production and increases bicarbonate secretion. Sucralfate binds epidermal growth factor and may protect the mitogen from acid degradation. Sucralfate stimulates epithelial proliferation at the ulcer margin. The drug has almost no buffering capacity. Virtually no systemic absorption occurs, and because of this property, sucralfate is the recommended agent for the treatment of peptic ulcer in pregnancy.

Sucralfate is effective in promoting the healing of acute duodenal ulceration. When sucralfate is administered at a dose of 1 g four times daily, over 80% of ulcers heal by 6 weeks, a rate that is roughly equivalent to that achieved with the use of H_2 receptor antagonists (20). Pain relief with sucralfate is achieved less quickly than with antisecretory drugs. Side effects are infrequent and mild, and constipation is the most frequent complaint.

Antacids

The availability of compounds that effectively suppress acid production, combined with their greater convenience, has greatly reduced the use of antacids as the primary treatment for acute ulceration. Nonetheless, when properly used, antacids can effectively heal ulcers. Intensive treatment of acute ulcers with antacids (30 mL of liquid antacid taken seven times daily, providing approximately 1,000 mEq of buffering capacity) has been shown to heal ulcers in 78% of patients at 4 weeks (21). Although this rate compares favorably with the healing rates observed with other forms of therapy, the large and frequent dosages are unacceptable to many patients. In addition, a significant proportion of patients have diarrhea on such a regimen. Surprisingly, low-dose antacid regimens that deliver less than 200 mmol/d also promote ulcer healing. More palatable alternatives with equivalent effectiveness include low-dose antacid therapy and the use of antacids as supplements to other acid-suppressive agents.

Bismuth Compounds

Many successful antibiotic regimens are based on a bismuth compound (colloidal bismuth subsalicylate or colloidal bismuth subcitrate) plus metronidazole, alone or in combination with amoxicillin or tetracycline. An effective combination is as follows:

Bismuth subsalicylate (Pepto-Bismol; Procter & Gamble, Cincinnati, OH), two tablets with meals and at bedtime for 6 weeks
Metronidazole, 250 mg three times a day for 2 weeks
Amoxicillin, 500 mg three times a day, or tetracycline hydrochloride, 500 mg three times a day, for 2 weeks

Bismuth compounds act locally and achieve gastric concentrations above the minimum inhibitory concentration for 90% of *H. pylori* isolates.

OPERATIVE TREATMENT OF ULCER DISEASE

Surgical Goals

Operative intervention is reserved for the treatment of complicated ulcer disease. Three complications are most common and constitute the indications for peptic ulcer surgery—hemorrhage, perforation, and obstruction. The first goal in the surgical treatment of the complications of ulcer disease should be alteration of the ulcer diathesis so that ulcer healing is achieved and recurrence is minimized. The second goal is treatment of coexisting anatomic complications, such as pyloric stenosis or perforation. The third major goal should be patient safety and freedom from undesirable chronic side effects. To achieve these goals, the gastric surgeon can direct therapy through endoscopic, radiologic, or operative means, the appropriate choice depending on the clinical circumstances.

Operative Procedures

A number of operative procedures have been used to treat peptic ulcer, but three procedures—truncal vagotomy and drainage, truncal vagotomy and antrectomy, and proximal gastric vagotomy—have been most widely used. In the operative treatment of peptic ulcer disease, vagotomy has had a central role. With increasing frequency, surgical therapy of peptic ulcer is directed exclusively at correction of the immediate problem (e.g., closure of duodenal perforation) without gastric denervation. The underlying ulcer diathesis is then addressed after surgery by antibiotic therapy directed at *H. pylori*. This approach is applicable to most patients with peptic ulcer undergoing emergent operation and predicts a diminishing role for vagotomy in the future. Nonetheless, vagotomy is currently central to the surgical management of complicated ulcer disease, and an understanding of the physiologic alterations attending vagotomy is crucial to gastric surgeons.

Division of both vagal trunks at the esophageal hiatus—truncal vagotomy—denervates the acid-producing fundic mucosa as well as the remainder of the vagally supplied viscera (Fig. 22.4). Because denervation impedes normal pyloric coordination and can result in impairment of gastric emptying, truncal vagotomy must be combined with a procedure to eliminate pyloric sphincteric function. Usually, gastric drainage is ensured by performance of a pyloroplasty. Several methods of pyloroplasty have been described; often they are referred to eponymously (Fig. 22.5). The Heineke-Mikulicz pyloroplasty is performed by making a longitudinal incision of the pyloric sphincter extending into the antrum and the duodenum for approximately 2 cm on either side. The incision is closed transversely, thereby increasing the lumen of the pyloric channel. A Finney pyloroplasty is formed as a gastroduodenostomy with transection of the pyloric sphincter. The inner curve of the duodenum is approximated to the dependent aspect of the antrum and pyloric channel. A U-shaped incision is then made, crossing the pylorus. The pyloroplasty is completed by suturing the anterior duodenal wall to the antrum. For some cases in which severe pyloric scarring makes division of the pyloric channel difficult or hazardous, the Jaboulay procedure, a side-to-side gastroduodenostomy, can be used; this procedure differs from the Finney pyloroplasty only in that the incision is not completed across the pyloric sphincter.

Truncal vagotomy can also be combined with resection of the gastric antrum to effect a further reduction in acid secretion, presumably by removing antral sources of gastrin. The limits of antral resection are usually defined by external landmarks, rather than the histologic transition from fundic to antral mucosae. The stomach is divided proximally along a line from a point above the incisura angularis to a point along the greater curvature midway from the pylorus to the gastroesophageal junction. Restoration of gastrointestinal continuity by a gastroduodenostomy is termed a Billroth I reconstruction. A Billroth II procedure uses a gastrojejunostomy (Fig. 22.6).

Proximal gastric vagotomy differs from truncal vagotomy in that only the nerve fibers to the acid-secreting fundic mucosa are divided (Fig. 22.4). Vagal nerve fibers to the antrum and pylorus are left intact, and the hepatic and celiac divisions are not transected. The denervation begins approximately 5 cm from the pylorus and extends proximally along the lesser curvature. In proximal gastric vagotomy, the distal esophagus is also skeletonized for a distance of 5 to 7 cm to divide any vagal fibers traveling to the fundus intramurally within the esophagus. The operation has also been called parietal cell vagotomy to emphasize its most important functional consequence.

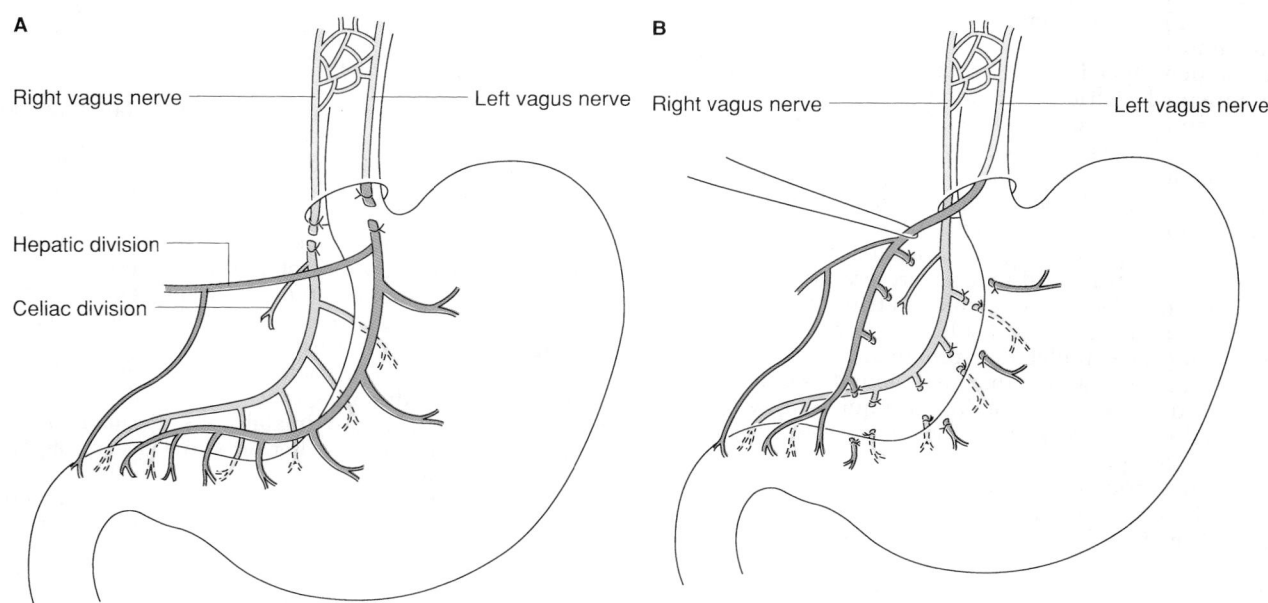

Figure 22.4. Truncal vagotomy and proximal gastric vagotomy. *(A)* With truncal vagotomy, both nerve trunks are divided at the level of the diaphragmatic hiatus. *(B)* Proximal gastric vagotomy involves division of the vagal fibers that supply the gastric fundus. Branches to the antropyloric region of the stomach are not transected, and the hepatic and celiac divisions of the vagus nerves remain intact.

Physiologic Consequences of Operation

Division of efferent vagal fibers directly affects acid secretion by reducing cholinergic stimulation of parietal cells. In addition, vagotomy also diminishes parietal cell responsiveness to gastrin and histamine. Basal acid secretion is reduced by approximately 80% in the immediate postoperative period. Basal acid secretion increases slightly within months of surgery but remains unchanged thereafter. The maximal acid output in response to exogenously administered stimulants such as pentagastrin is reduced by approximately 70% in the early period after surgery. After 1 year, pentagastrin-stimulated maximal acid output rebounds to 50% of prevagotomy values but remains at this level on subsequent testing. Acid secretion due to endogenous stimulation by a liquid meal is reduced by 60% to 70% relative to normal subjects. The acid-reducing properties of proximal gastric vagotomy and truncal vagotomy are roughly equivalent in most series (Table 22.3).

The inclusion of antrectomy with truncal vagotomy causes further reductions in acid secretion. Pentagastrin-stimulated maximal acid output is reduced by 85% relative to values recorded before surgery. Little rebound in acid secretion occurs with the passage of time.

Truncal vagotomy and proximal gastric vagotomy both cause postoperative hypergastrinemia. Fasting gastrin values are elevated to approximately twice preoperative levels, and the postprandial response is exaggerated. Immediately after vagotomy, hypergastrinemia appears to be due to decreased luminal acid, with loss of feedback inhibition of gastrin release. Loss of vagal inhibitory pathways can also be important. Chronic hypergastrinemia, sustained long term in most cases, is caused by gastrin cell hyperplasia in addition to loss of inhibitory feedback. When antrectomy is added to vagotomy, circulating gastrin levels are decreased. Basal gastrin values are reduced by approximately half and postprandial gastrin levels by two thirds. The major form of circulating hormone after antrectomy is gastrin 34, released from the duodenum.

Operations that involve vagotomy alter gastric emptying. Proximal gastric denervation abolishes vagally mediated receptive relaxation. Thus, for any given volume ingested, the intragastric pressure rise is greater and the gastroduodenal pressure gradient higher than in normal subjects. As a result, emptying of liquids, which depends critically on the gastroduodenal pressure gradient, is accelerated after proximal gastric vagotomy. Because nerve fibers to the antrum and pylorus are preserved, the function of the distal stomach to mix and triturate solid food is preserved, and emptying of solids is nearly normal in patients who have undergone proximal gastric vagotomy. Truncal vagotomy affects the motor activities of both proximal and distal stomach. Solid and liquid emptying rates are usually increased when truncal vagotomy is accompanied by pyloroplasty.

Truncal vagotomy affects a number of other gastrointestinal functions because of the removal of efferent vagal innervation. Pancreatic exocrine secretion in response to a meal is diminished, with decreased bicarbonate and enzyme outputs. Postcibal biliary secretion is decreased, and gallbladder distention is observed. Fecal fat excretion doubles after truncal vagotomy, although clinical steatorrhea is unusual. Stimulated release of a number of gastrointestinal hormones—including pancreatic polypeptide, cholecystokinin, and secretin—is decreased. In most instances, these extragastric alterations in digestive function

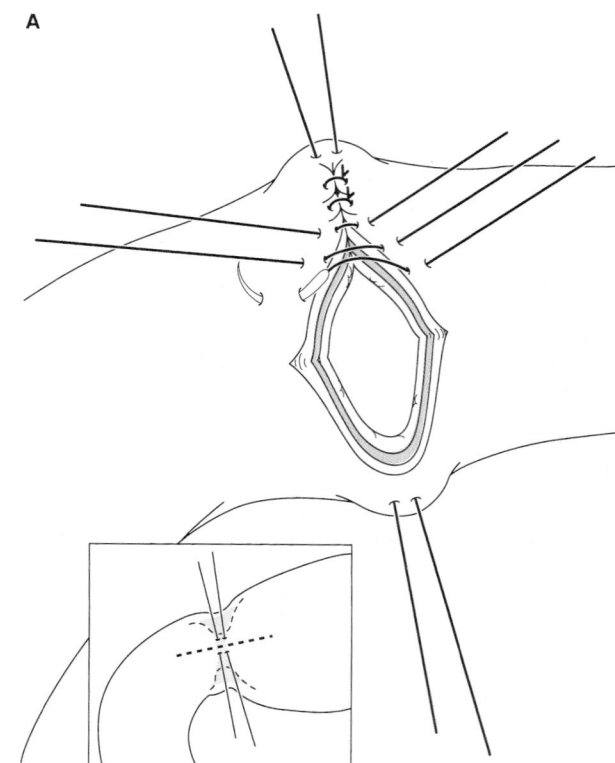

Figure 22.5. Pyloroplasty formation. A Heineke-Mikulicz pyloroplasty *(A)* involves a longitudinal incision of the pyloric sphincter followed by a transverse closure. The Finney pyloroplasty *(B)* is performed as a gastroduodenostomy with division of the pylorus. The Jaboulay pyloroplasty *(C)* differs from the Finney procedure in that the pylorus is not transected. *(continues)*

are subclinical. Proximal gastric vagotomy, in which the vagal innervation to nongastric viscera is preserved, produces fewer physiologic alterations than does truncal vagotomy.

A number of prospective, randomized trials have compared the various surgical options in terms of postoperative symptoms, including dumping, diarrhea, weight loss, and disturbance of lifestyle (Table 22.4). In most comparisons, proximal gastric vagotomy has proved superior to other operations in these measures. Dumping, a postprandial symptom complex of abdominal discomfort, weakness, and vasomotor symptoms of sweating and dizziness, occurs in 10% to 15% of patients with truncal vagotomy and antrectomy in the early postoperative period and is chronically disabling in 1% to 2%. After truncal vagotomy and pyloroplasty, dumping is present initially in 10%, and remains severe in approximately 1%. Permanent symptoms of dumping are rare after proximal gastric vagotomy. The incidence of diarrhea, which is presumably caused by denervation of the pylorus and small bowel and by elimination of pyloric function, parallels the incidence of dumping after truncal vagotomy and antrectomy or pyloroplasty. Persistent or disabling diarrhea is present in less than 1% of patients after proximal gastric vagotomy. After truncal vagotomy, weight loss averages 2 kg in the first postoperative year, whereas with proximal gastric vagotomy, a weight gain is recorded. Reoperation after proximal gastric vagotomy is rarely needed for symptoms resulting from the operation.

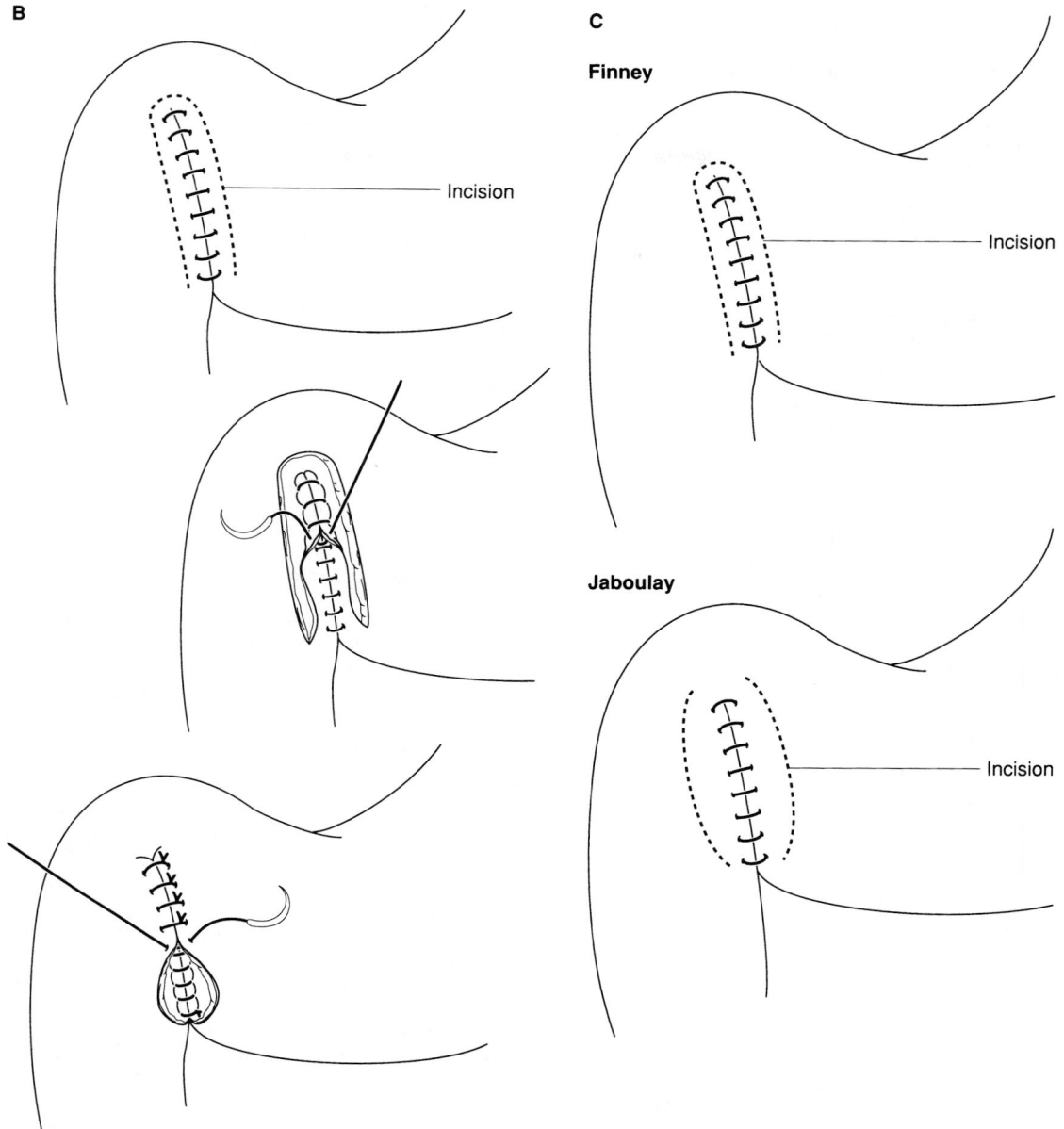

Figure 22.5. *(Continued)*

Proximal gastric vagotomy has the lowest operative mortality rate, the lowest incidence of postoperative symptoms, and an acceptable risk of recurrent ulcer. Collected series of proximal gastric vagotomies have reported an operative mortality rate of less than 0.05% (20), lower than the reported mortality rate for any other gastric procedure for peptic ulcer. Truncal vagotomy and pyloroplasty has a reported mortality rate of 0.5% to 0.8%, whereas the mortality rate after truncal vagotomy and antrectomy approximates 1.5%.

The lower incidence of postoperative symptoms is obtained at the cost of a higher postoperative ulcer recurrence rate (22). The reported recurrence rates for proximal gastric vagotomy are variable, probably reflecting differences in experience and individual surgical skill. In addition, all prospective surgical series examining ulcer recurrence rates were reported in the era before the pathogenic role of *H. pylori* was appreciated. With appropriate use of postoperative antimicrobials directed against *H. pylori,* these ulcer recurrence rates would currently be expected to be much lower. Although recurrence rates (without *H. pylori* treatment) as low as 5% have been reported, a more generally accepted figure is 10%. This rate is similar to that after truncal vagotomy and drainage (approximately 12%) but considerably greater than that reported after truncal vagotomy and antrectomy (1% to 3%). The reported ulcer recurrence rates after proximal gastric vagotomy can be adversely affected by the inclusion of prepyloric and pyloric channel ulcers. For reasons that are not clear, proximal gastric vagotomy is significantly less effective when used to treat ulcers in this position than when used for duodenal ulceration.

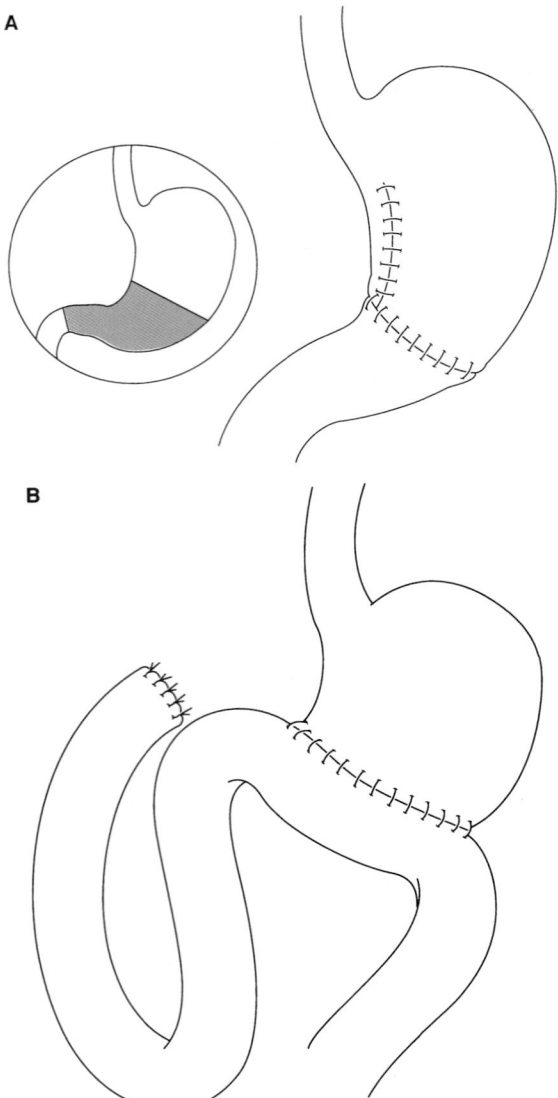

Figure 22.6. Antrectomy involves resection of the distal stomach *(blue area in inset).* Restoration of gastrointestinal continuity may be accomplished as a Billroth I gastroduodenostomy *(A)* or Billroth II gastrojejunostomy *(B)* reconstruction.

Table 22.3. PHYSIOLOGIC ALTERATIONS CAUSED BY TRUNCAL VAGOTOMY

GASTRIC EFFECTS

Decreased basal acid output
Reduced cholinergic input to parietal cells
Decreased stimulated maximal acid output
Diminished sensitivity to histamine and gastrin
Decreased meal-induced acid secretion
Increased fasting postprandial gastrin
Gastrin cell hyperplasia
Accelerated liquid emptying
Altered emptying of solids

NONGASTRIC EFFECTS

Decreased pancreatic exocrine secretion
Decreased pancreatic enzymes and bicarbonate
Decreased postprandial bile flow
Increased gallbladder volumes
Diminished release of vagally mediated peptide hormones

Table 22.4. CLINICAL RESULTS OF DUODENAL ULCER SURGERY

	PGV (%)	TV + P (%)	TV + A (%)
Mortality rate	0	0.5–1	1–2
Acid reduction			
Basal	80	70	85
Stimulated	50	50	85
Ulcer recurrence	10	12	1–2
Gastric emptying			
Liquids	Accelerated	Accelerated	Accelerated
Solids	No change	Accelerated	Slowed
Dumping			
Mild	<5	10	10–15
Disabling	0	1	1–2
Diarrhea			
Mild	<5	25	20
Disabling	0	2	1–2

PGV, proximal gastric vagotomy; TV + P, truncal vagotomy and pyloroplasty; TV + A, truncal vagotomy and antrectomy.

HEMORRHAGE

Hemorrhage is the leading cause of death associated with peptic ulcer, and the incidence of this complication has not changed since the introduction of H_2 receptor antagonists (23). The lifetime risk of hemorrhage for patients with duodenal ulcer who have not had surgery and who do not receive continuing maintenance drug therapy approximates 35%. Most hemorrhages occur during the initial episode of ulceration or during a relapse, and patients who have hemorrhaged previously have a higher risk of bleeding again. Patients with recurrent hemorrhage and elderly patients are at greatest risk of death, and these two groups should be resuscitated vigorously, investigated promptly, and treated aggressively (24,25).

Upper gastrointestinal endoscopy is the appropriate initial diagnostic test when hemorrhage from duodenal ulceration is suspected. Endoscopy can correctly determine the site and cause of bleeding in over 90% of patients. An ulcer should be accepted as the bleeding source only if it has one of the stigmata of active or recent hemorrhage. Active hemorrhage is defined by an arterial jet, active oozing, or oozing beneath an adherent clot. The signs of recent hemorrhage include an adherent clot without oozing, an adherent slough in the ulcer base, or a visible vessel in the ulcer. The ability of these endoscopic findings accurately to predict recurrent hemorrhage has been extensively validated. Approximately 30% of patients who have stigmata of recent hemorrhage experience rebleeding, and most of the patients who experience recurrent hemorrhage require emergency treatment. These stigmata are not sufficiently accurate to be used alone as indications for surgery. Rather, they serve as a warning that aggressive therapy is needed and close follow-up mandatory. The occurrence of hypovolemic shock, rebleeding during hospitalization, and a posteroinferior location of the ulcer are additional clinical features that have been associated with increased risks of recurrent bleeding. The role of gastric acidity as a cause for in-hospital rebleeding appears to be inconsequential, and reduction of acid secretion by H_2 receptor antagonists or omeprazole is not sufficient to prevent recurrent hemorrhage (26).

The ability to visualize bleeding duodenal ulcers endoscopically has led to attempts to treat hemorrhage endoscopically. There are many different methods of endoscopic therapy, but the most established consist of thermal coagulation. Thermal coagulation can be achieved by bipolar electrocoagulation or direct application of heat through a heater probe (27). Unequivocal proof of efficacy, in the form of lowered rebleeding rates and avoidance of operation, has been difficult to obtain. The analysis of reports of endoscopic treatment of hemorrhage is complicated by the 70% rate of spontaneous, although sometimes temporary, cessation of bleeding without intervention. A National Institutes of Health Consensus Development Conference has recommended endoscopic hemostatic therapy in selected patients. Hemodynamic instability, need for continuing transfusion, red stool or hematemesis, age older than 60 years, and serious medical comorbidity are clinical features that mandate endoscopic therapy. Rebleeding during hospitalization and the endoscopic findings of visible vessel, oozing, or bleeding associated with an adherent clot are other indications for endoscopic hemostasis. Ulcers with clean bases require no treatment. Failure of endoscopic hemostasis is usually due to inaccessibility because of scarring, to rapid active bleeding, or to an adherent clot. Patients treated endoscopically should be observed closely for further hemorrhage. One report indicted that patients who rebleed within 72 hours of initial endoscopic control may be successfully retreated without increasing the risk of mortality (28).

Operative intervention is appropriate for the following:

Massive hemorrhage leading to shock or cardiovascular instability
Prolonged blood loss requiring continuing transfusion
Recurrent bleeding during medical therapy or after endoscopic therapy
Recurrent hemorrhage requiring hospitalization

Operative therapy should consist of duodenotomy with direct ligation of the bleeding vessel in the ulcer base followed by a procedure to effect permanent reduction in acid production. Truncal vagotomy and pyloroplasty or truncal vagotomy and antrectomy have most commonly been used for this purpose. The need for emergency surgery significantly increases surgical risks; mortality rates are increased approximately 10-fold.

PERFORATION

The lifetime risk for perforation in patients with duodenal ulceration not receiving therapy approximates 10%. In contrast, ulcer perforation is unusual during maintenance therapy if initial ulcer healing has been achieved.

Perforation of a duodenal ulcer is usually accompanied by sudden and severe epigastric pain. The pain, caused by the spillage of highly caustic gastric secretions into the peritoneum, rapidly reaches peak intensity and remains constant. Radiation to the right scapular region is common because of right subphrenic collection of gastric contents. Occasionally, pain is sensed in the lower abdomen if gastric contents travel caudally through the paracolic gutter. Peritoneal irritation is usually intense, and most patients avoid movement to minimize discomfort.

Physical examination reveals low-grade fever, diminished bowel sounds, and rigidity of the abdominal musculature. Usually, upright abdominal radiographs reveal pneumoperitoneum, but up to 20% of perforated ulcers do not show free intraperitoneal air. Upper gastrointestinal contrast studies performed with water-soluble contrast agents can occasionally be helpful if pneumoperitoneum is not demonstrated but perforation is still suspected.

Although occasional reports have described the nonoperative treatment of this complication, perforation remains a strong indication for surgery in most circumstances. Laparotomy or laparoscopy affords the opportunity to relieve

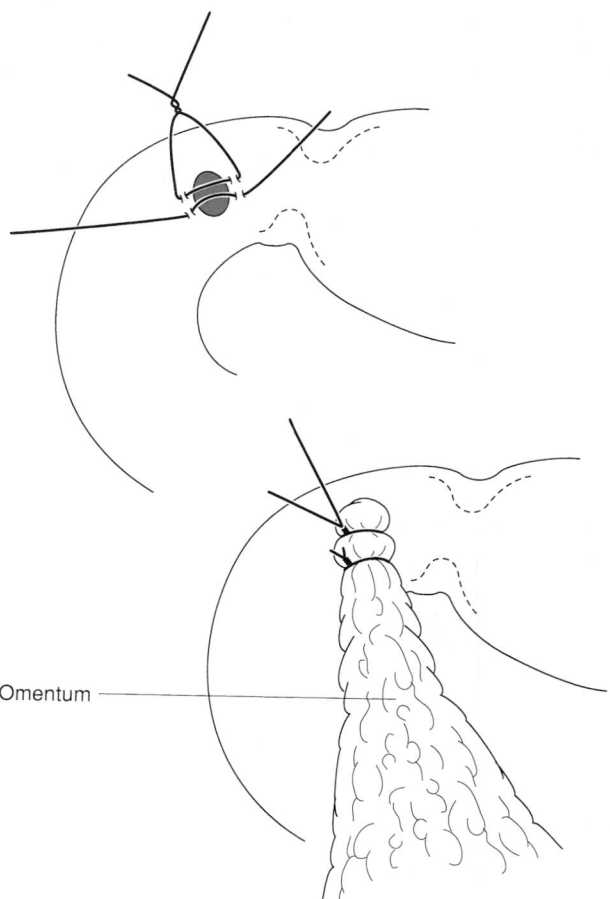

Figure 22.7. Omental patching of perforated duodenal ulcer.

intraperitoneal contamination and to close the perforation (Fig. 22.7).

Signs of antecedent duodenal ulceration, in terms of history of prior symptoms and anatomic evidence of duodenal scarring, should be sought. A lack of antecedent symptoms is not protective. Reports suggest that patients without antecedent symptoms are also at risk for recurrent ulceration. By 5 to 6 years, symptomatic ulcer recurrence in patients with acute ulcer perforation is similar to that for patients with chronic disease. Before the role of *H. pylori* was appreciated, simple omental closure of duodenal perforation resulting from chronic ulceration did not provide satisfactory long-term results; up to 80% of patients so treated had recurrent ulceration, and 10% experienced reperforation if untreated. Approximately four fifths of all patients with perforation have *H. pylori* infestation and therefore are at risk of recurrent disease.

An emergent ulcer operation may be safely performed in patients with perforation if the following circumstances apply (29,30): there has been no preoperative shock, no life-threatening medical illness coexists, and the perforation has been present for less than 48 hours. If these criteria are not met, simple omental patching of the perforation and peritoneal débridement are usually safest; definitive therapy, if necessary, can be performed at a later date, when the patient has recovered. In addition, the antiulcer operation should ideally add no additional risk of long-term sequelae and should provide excellent protection against future ulceration.

For most patients receiving prompt surgical attention, definitive antiulcer therapy can be performed with a risk equivalent to that of simple closure. The risk of recurrent ulcer and the incidence of unpleasant postoperative symptoms are similar to those seen when surgery is performed electively (31). Proximal gastric vagotomy with patch closure of the perforation is an attractive alternative in this circumstance and has been shown to be both safe and effective in preventing ulcer relapse. Incorporation of the perforation as part of a pyloroplasty or resection of the site of perforation during antrectomy can also be combined with truncal vagotomy with favorable results.

Several reports have advocated omental patch closure only, often laparoscopically, with postoperative anti-*H. pylori* therapy (32–34). This approach presumes that most duodenal ulcers are caused by *H. pylori,* that secure closure of the perforation can be obtained, and that definitive surgical therapy may await the effects of medical therapy (32). Initial reports are promising, by unconfirmed by long-term follow-up. Minimally invasive approaches are quite likely to become standard practice in the future.

OBSTRUCTION

Gastric outlet obstruction can occur acutely or chronically in patients with duodenal ulcer disease. Acute obstruction is caused by edema and inflammation associated with ulcers in the pyloric channel and the first portion of the duodenum. Pyloric obstruction is suggested by recurrent vomiting, dehydration, and hypochloremic alkalosis due to loss of gastric secretions. Acute gastric outlet obstruction is treated with nasogastric suction, rehydration, and intravenous administration of antisecretory agents. In most instances, acute obstruction resolves with such supportive measures within 72 hours.

Repeated episodes of ulceration and healing can lead to pyloric scarring and a fixed stenosis with chronic gastric outlet obstruction. In cases of untreated duodenal ulceration, the lifetime risk of chronic pyloric stenosis approximates 10%.

Upper endoscopy is indicated to confirm the nature of the obstruction and to exclude neoplasm. Endoscopic hydrostatic balloon dilatation of pyloric stenoses can also be attempted at this time (Fig. 22.8). Approximately 85% of pyloric stenoses are amenable to balloon dilatation (35). Only 40% of patients with gastric stenoses have sustained improvement by 3 months after balloon dilatation. Recurrent stenoses are presumably due to residual scarring in the pyloric channel. Thus, although pyloric dilatation is occasionally palliative, in most cases operative correction is required.

Operative management of gastric outlet obstruction should include treatment of the underlying ulcer disease and relief of the anatomic abnormality. Truncal vagotomy with antrectomy and truncal vagotomy with drainage have both been used with success in this circumstance, with ulcer recurrence rates similar to those for intractability and with satisfactory restoration of gastric emptying. There is considerable interest in the use of proximal gastric vagotomy and duodenoplasty or dilatation for the treatment of pyloric stenosis, and the experience to date must be considered promising. Ulcer recurrence rates are not reported to be increased when proximal gastric vagotomy is used in this circumstance, which is surprising in view of the higher recurrence rates associated with pyloric channel ulcers.

GASTRIC ULCER

Benign gastric ulcers are a form of peptic ulcer disease, occurring with one-third the frequency of benign duodenal ulceration. In the United States, gastric ulcer is somewhat more common in men than women and occurs in a patient cohort approximately 10 years older than for duodenal ulceration.

Endoscopic Diagnosis

Upper gastrointestinal endoscopy is the preferred method for diagnosing gastric ulceration. The ulcer base in benign disease is commonly smooth and flat and often covered by a gray, fibrous exudate. The margin is usually slightly raised, erythematous, and friable. Differentiation of benign and malignant gastric ulcers is reliably made only by histologic examination. Visual endoscopic differentiation of benign from malignant ulcers is not reliable. All gastric ulcers should have multiple biopsies taken from the perimeter of the lesion. The addition of lesional brushings to biopsy increases diagnostic accuracy to approximately 95%.

Benign gastric ulcers may occur in any location in the stomach, but approximately 60% are located along the lesser curvature proximal to the incisura angularis (Fig.

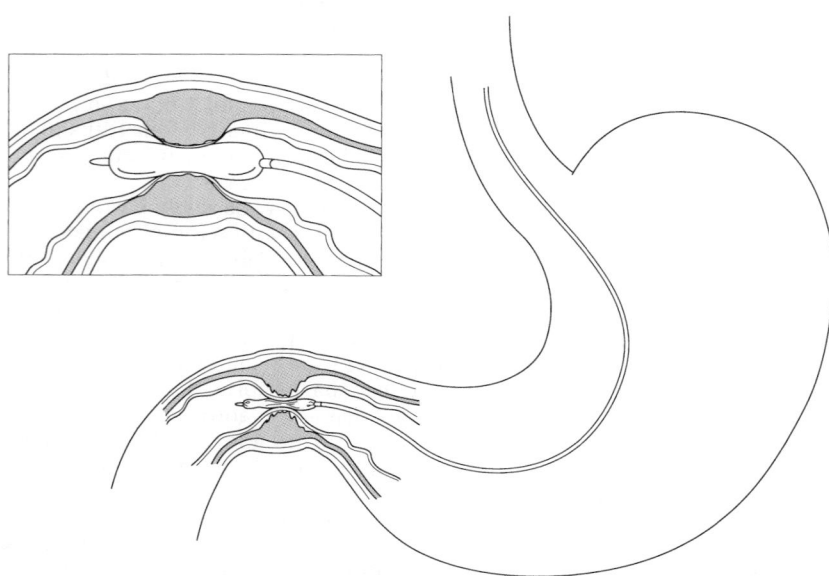

Figure 22.8. Schematic representation of balloon dilatation of pyloric stenosis.

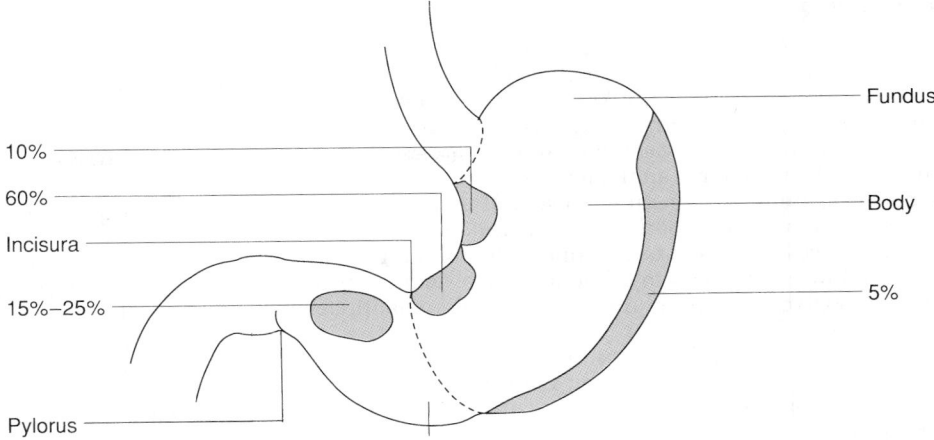

Figure 22.9. Location of gastric ulcers.

22.9). Less than 10% of benign gastric ulcers are located on the greater curvature. Virtually all gastric ulcers lay within 2 cm of the histologic transition between fundic and antral mucosa. With increasing age, this mucosal transition zone moves proximally along lesser curvature. Movement of this transition zone is reflected by the greater prevalence of proximal ulcers in elderly patients.

Ulcer location and acid-secretory status are used to classify gastric ulcers. Type I gastric ulcers are located in the body of the stomach, along the lesser curvature, and are associated with normal to low acid secretion. Type I gastric ulcers are not associated with duodenal or pyloric ulcerations. Approximately 50% of patients with gastric ulcers have type I.

Type II gastric ulcers are located in the body of the stomach, usually along the lesser curvature, but are associated with coexisting duodenal ulceration. Gastric analysis typically reveals hypersecretion of acid. Approximately one fourth of gastric ulcers are type II.

Type III gastric ulcers are prepyloric. Patients usually have gastric acid hypersecretion. Type III ulcers constitute approximately one fifth of benign gastric ulcers. Type IV gastric ulcers are located high along lesser curvature, near the gastroesophageal junction. Accounting for less than 10% of gastric ulcers, type IV ulcers are not associated with acid hypersecretion.

As with benign duodenal ulceration, *H. pylori* plays a central role in the pathogenesis of benign gastric ulcers. Benign gastric ulcers associated with *H. pylori* respond to antibiotic therapy at a rate equivalent to that of duodenal ulceration. The recurrence rate of ulcerations in these patients after *H. pylori* eradication is equal to the rate of reinfection.

In addition to *H. pylori* infection, alterations in gastric motility have been demonstrated in a small subset of patients with benign ulcers. A variety of defects have been identified, including delayed gastric emptying, incompetent pyloric sphincter function, prolonged high-amplitude gastric contractions, duodenogastric reflux, and alterations in the migrating motor complex. No defect has been demonstrated to be definitely pathogenic. A strong association of benign gastric ulceration with the use of NSAIDs has been recognized. Cigarette smoking is associated with development of gastric ulceration, and continued smoking impedes medical therapy. Gastric and duodenal ulcers have been noted in patients receiving hepatic artery chemotherapy in whom improper placement of the catheter permits perfusion of gastric and duodenal mucosae. A variety of agents, including 5-fluorouracil, cisplatin, doxorubicin, and mitomycin C, have been implicated.

Therapy

The primary therapy for benign gastric ulceration in most patients is antimicrobial treatment of *H. pylori* infection. The treatment protocols are similar to those used for benign duodenal ulceration. For many patients, cessation of NSAID therapy is also required.

Indications for surgical treatment of gastric ulcer include hemorrhage, perforation, failure of a recurrent ulcer to respond to medical therapy, and inability to exclude malignant disease.

For type I gastric ulcers, the elective operation of choice is usually a distal gastrectomy with gastroduodenal (Billroth I) anastomosis. The ulcer should be included in the gastrectomy specimen. With this approach, operative mortality rates of 2% to 3%, with ulcer recurrence rates of less than 5%, have been reported. Because type I gastric ulcers are not associated with gastric acid hypersecretion, inclusion of vagotomy does not improve recurrence rates.

In contrast, patients with type II and type III benign gastric ulcers usually demonstrate gastric hypersecretion, and vagotomy is recommended. The operation should be directed at removing the gastric mucosa at risk, encompassing the ulcer. Gastroduodenal reconstruction is preferred. If duodenal inflammation impedes healing, gastrojejunostomy is an alternative.

The occurrence of a type IV gastric ulcer, near the gastroesophageal junction, represents a difficult surgical problem. When possible, the ulcer should be excised. This usually requires a distal gastrectomy with an extension along the lesser curvature near the esophageal wall and reconstruction with gastrojejunostomy.

Emergency operations performed for hemorrhage or perforation require ulcer excision. Distal gastrectomy, performed with gastroduodenal reconstruction, is usually the procedure of choice. Operative mortality rates average 10% to 20% in the presence of hemorrhage or perforation.

POSTGASTRECTOMY SYNDROMES

A number of syndromes have been described that are associated with distressing symptoms after gastric operations performed for peptic ulcer or gastric neoplasm. The occurrence of severe postoperative symptoms is fortunately low, perhaps 1% to 3% of cases, but the disturbances can be disabling. The two most common postgastrectomy syndromes, categorized according to predominant manifestation, are dumping and alkaline reflux gastritis.

Dumping

The term *dumping* denotes a clinical syndrome with both gastrointestinal and vasomotor symptoms. The precise cause of dumping is not known but is believed to relate to the unmetered entry of ingested food into the proximal small bowel after vagotomy and either resection or division of the pyloric sphincter. Early dumping symptoms occur immediately after a meal and include nausea, epigastric discomfort, borborygmi, palpitations, and, in extreme cases, dizziness or syncope. Late dumping symptoms follow a meal by 1 to 3 hours and can include reactive hypoglycemia in addition to the aforementioned symptoms.

Although a relatively large number of patients experience mild dumping symptoms in the early postoperative period, minor dietary alterations and the passage of time bring improvement in all but approximately 1%. The somatostatin analogue octreotide has been reported to improve dumping symptoms when 50 to 100 mg is administered subcutaneously before a meal (36). The beneficial effects of somatostatin on the vasomotor symptoms of dumping are postulated to be due to pressor effects of the compound on splanchnic vessels. In addition, somatostatin analogues inhibit the release of vasoactive peptides from the gut, decrease peak plasma insulin levels, and slow intestinal transit, all effects that might be expected to ameliorate dumping symptoms. Octreotide administration before meal ingestion has been shown to prevent changes in pulse, systolic blood pressure, and packed red cell volume during early dumping and blood glucose levels during late dumping.

Alkaline Reflux Gastritis

The term *alkaline reflux gastritis* should be reserved for patients who demonstrate the clinical triad of postprandial epigastric pain often associated with nausea and vomiting, evidence of reflux of bile into the stomach, and histologic evidence of gastritis. One or more of these findings occurs transiently in 10% to 20% of patients after truncal vagotomy and drainage or resection, but they persist in only 1% to 2%.

The differential diagnosis for a patient with postoperative epigastric pain includes recurrent ulceration, biliary and pancreatic disease, afferent loop obstruction, and esophagitis in addition to alkaline reflux gastritis. Gastric acid analysis shows basal hypochlorhydria with little increase with pentagastrin stimulation. Serum gastrin measurements should be determined to exclude Zollinger-Ellison syndrome and retained gastric antrum. Endoscopic examination is essential to exclude recurrent ulcer. Endoscopy shows reflux of bile into the stomach. Quantitative assessment of enterogastric reflux can be obtained by intravenously injected radionuclides such as ^{99m}Tc Hepatic Iminodiacetic Acid (HIDA). The radionuclide is excreted in the bile, and external scintigraphy over the abdomen can be used to measure reflux of bile into the stomach.

Endoscopically, the gastric mucosa appears red, friable, and edematous. Gastric inflammation is patchy and nonulcerative. Histologic examination shows mucosal and submucosal edema and infiltration of acute and chronic inflammatory cells into the lamina propria. Glandular atrophy and intestinal metaplasia are frequent accompaniments.

No perfect solution to alkaline reflux gastritis exists. Antacids, H$_2$ receptor antagonists, bile acid chelators, and dietary manipulations have not been demonstrated definitely to be beneficial. The only proven treatment for alkaline reflux gastritis is operative diversion of intestinal contents from contact with the gastric mucosa. The most common surgical procedure used for this purpose is a Roux-en-Y gastrojejunostomy with an intestinal limb of 50 to 60 cm constructed to prevent reflux of intestinal contents (Fig. 22.10). This procedure is effective in eliminating bilious vomiting (nearly 100%), but recurrent or persistent pain is reported in up to 30% of patients, and up to 20% of patients are troubled with postoperative delayed gastric emptying.

STRESS GASTRITIS

Major trauma, accompanied by shock, sepsis, respiratory failure, hemorrhage, or multiorgan injury is often accompanied by acute stress gastritis. Acute stress gastritis is particular prevalent after thermal injury with greater than 35% total surface area burned. A similar entity is also observed as a result of central nervous system injury or intracranial hypertension. Multiple superficial ulcerations and erosions are noted in the proximal, acid-secreting portion of the stomach, with fewer lesions in the antrum, and only rare ulcerations in the duodenum.

The most sensitive diagnostic test for stress ulceration is endoscopic examination. If patients are examined within 12 hours of the onset of injury, acute mucosal ulcerations may be observed that appear as multiple, shallow areas of erythema and friability, often accompanied by focal hemorrhage. The lesions are progressive during the first 72 hours after injury. When lesions are examined histologically they are seen to consist of coagulation necrosis of the superficial endothelium with infiltration of leukocytes into the lamina propria. Chronic disease, characterized by fibrosis and scarring, is not observed. With resolution of the underlying injury or sepsis, healing is accompanying by mucosal restitution and regeneration.

Clinical observations and a large number of experimental studies suggest that mucosal ischemia is the central event underlying the development of stress gastritis. In clinical practice, most patients who contract stress gastritis do so after an episode of sepsis, hemorrhage, or cardiac dysfunction accompanied by shock. Experimental studies that cause depletion of high-energy phosphate compounds such at ATP predispose to the development of stress gastritis. Luminal gastric acid secretion, although not the sole cause of stress gastritis, appears to be a necessary concomitant. A number of experimental observations suggest that a critical concentration of luminal acid is required to initiate injury in the setting of mucosal ischemia. The fall in mucosal energy supply permits proton back-diffusion into the mucosa; the resultant decrease in mucosal pH exacerbates ischemic damage.

Clinical risk factors that predict development of stress gastritis include adult respiratory distress syndrome, multiple long bone fractures, a major burn over 35% of the body surface, transfusion requirement above 6 units, hepatic dysfunction, sepsis, hypotension, and oliguric renal failure. Scoring systems of critical illness, exemplified by the Acute Physiology and Chronic Health Evaluation (APACHE) system, accurately predict risk for acute stress gastritis.

Diagnosis

Clinical studies that use bloody nasogastric discharge as a sign of stress gastritis probably underestimate its incidence in critically ill patients. Conversely, studies based on endoscopy overestimate the incidence of clinically important stress gastritis. In one endoscopically controlled study, 100% of patients with life-threatening injuries had evidence of gastric erosions by 24 hours. Severely burned patients have endoscopic evidence of gastric erosions in greater than 90% of cases, whereas significant upper gastrointestinal hemorrhage occurs in between 25% to 50% of patients with burn wound infection.

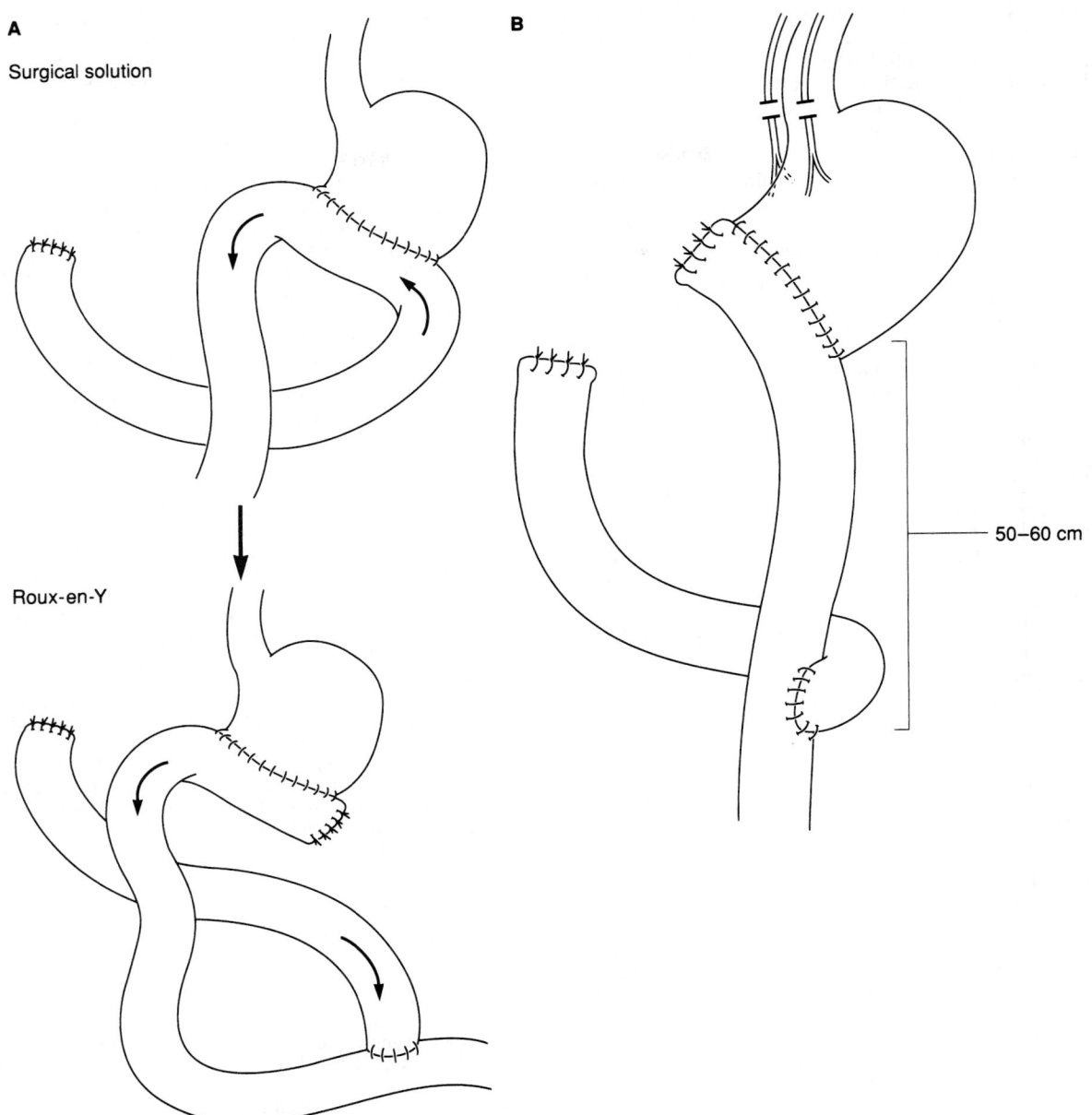

A

Surgical solution

Roux-en-Y

50–60 cm

Figure 22.10. Conversion of Billroth II gastrojejunostomy to Roux-en-Y gastrojejunostomy. The afferent limb is divided *(A)*, and intestinal continuity is reestablished by anastomosis 50 to 60 cm downstream from the original gastrojejunostomy *(B)*.

Barium contrast examinations have no role in the diagnosis of stress gastritis and interfere with subsequent endoscopic examination. Analysis of gastric contents for titration of acid production is not informative. In patients presenting with hemorrhagic stress gastritis, catheterization of the left gastric artery for selective angiography may identify the primary vessel supplying the bleeding site. This method is occasionally useful when rapid bleeding precludes safe or diagnostic endoscopic examination.

Treatment and Prophylaxis

All critically ill patients are at risk for development of acute stress gastritis. Because hemorrhage associated with stress gastritis significantly increases mortality, all such patients should be treated prophylactically.

Stress gastritis prophylaxis has focused on control of gastric luminal pH. If intragastric pH can be maintained above 3.5, effective prophylaxis can be obtained. In one study of seriously ill patients, antacid prophylaxis decreased bleeding from 25% to 4% of patients.

A number of prospective studies suggest that administration of H_2 antagonists are as effective as antacids for prophylaxis of stress gastritis. Infusion of an H_2 antagonist at a rate that maintains intraluminal gastric pH at greater than 3.5 is equally effective, relative to antacids, in terms of prevention of bleeding. Continuous-infusion H_2 receptor antagonist therapy appears to be equally effective relative to intermittent dosing with H_2 blockers or antacids.

Sucralfate as another antiulcer agent that shows efficacy as prophylactic treatment for stress gastritis. Sucralfate is not absorbed in the gastrointestinal tract and has no antisecretory activity. The agent binds to exposed collagen in areas of epithelial erosions. The mechanism of action of sucralfate is incompletely understood, but the drug prevents bacterial overgrowth by preventing intragastric pH to remain low. A lower rate of pneumonia has been observed in patients receiving sucralfate relative to prophylactic H₂ receptor antagonist therapy.

When stress gastritis causes gastrointestinal bleeding, endoscopic therapy is used as first-line treatment. Endoscopic examination is diagnostic and permits application of electrocautery or heat probe hemostasis. When severe bleeding precludes endoscopic therapy, selective angiographic catheterization of the left gastric artery for infusion of vasopressin has been used. Vasopressin is administered by continuous infusion at a rate of 0.2 to 0.4 IU/min. This methodology can be combined with selective left gastric artery embolization using metal coils, Gelfoam, or other occlusive agents.

Only a small minority of patients with acute stress gastritis and hemorrhage require operative therapy. The surgical approach should control acute bleeding, have a low risk of recurrent hemorrhage, and be associated with a low operative mortality rate. No procedure meets all of these criteria, and no large clinical experience is available to confirm the superiority of one procedure over another. Total gastrectomy is associated with the lowest risk of recurrent bleeding but has a mortality rate of approximately of 20%. Procedures such as vagotomy and pyloroplasty, vagotomy and antrectomy, and vagotomy and subtotal gastrectomy are each associated with high risks of recurrent hemorrhage.

REFERENCES

1. Logan RPH, Hirschl AM. Epidemiology of *Helicobacter pylori* infection. *Curr Opin Gastroenterol* 1996;12:1–5.
2. *Helicobacter pylori* in peptic ulcer disease. NIH Consensus Statement 1994;12:1–18.
3. Peek RM, Blaser MJ. Pathophysiology of *Helicobacter pylori*-induced gastritis and peptic ulcer disease. *Am J Med* 1997; 102;200–207.
4. Veldhuyzen van Zanten SJO, Sherman P, Hunt R. *Helicobacter pylori: new developments and treatments*. CMAJ 1997; 156:1565–1574.
5. Blaser MJ. *Helicobacter* are indigenous to the human stomach: duodenal ulceration is due to changes in gastric microecology in the modern era. *Gut* 1998;43:721–727.
6. Atherton JC. The clinical relevance of strain types of *Helicobacter pylori*. *Gut* 1997;40:701–703.
7. McGowen CC, Cover TL, Blaser MJ. *Helicobacter pylori* and gastric acid: biological and therapeutic implications. *Gastroenterology* 1996;110:926–938.
8. Morris A, Nicholson G. Ingestion of *Campylobacter pyloridis* causes gastritis and raised fasting gastric pH. *Am J Gastroenterol* 1987;82:192–199.
9. Crabtree JE, Farmery SM, Lindley IJD, et al. Cag A/cytotoxic strains of *Helicobacter pylori* and interleukin-8 in gastric epithelial cell lines. *J Clin Pathol* 1994;47:945–950.
10. Peterson WL, Barnett CC, Evans DJ, et al. Acid secretion and serum gastrin in normal subjects and patients with duodenal ulcer: the role of *Helicobacter pylori*. *Am J Gastroenterol* 1993;88:2038–2043.
11. El-Omar E, Penman I, Dorrian CA, et al. Eradication of *Helicobacter pylori* infection lowers gastrin mediated acid secretion by two thirds in patients with duodenal ulcer. *Gut* 1993;34:1060–1065.
12. Courillon-Mallet A, Launay JM, Roucayrol AM. *Helicobacter pylori* infection: pathophysiologic implication of Nα–methyl-histamine. *Gastroenterology* 1995;108:959–966.
13. Queiroz DM, Mendez EN, Rocha GA, et al. Effect of *Helicobacter pylori* eradication on antral gastrin- and somatostatin-immunoreactive cell density and gastrin and somatostatin concentrations. *Scand J Gastroenterol* 1993;28: 858–864.
14. Isenberg JI, Selling JA, Hogan DL, et al. Impaired proximal duodenal mucosal bicarbonate secretion in patients with duodenal ulcer. *N Engl J Med* 1987;316:374.
15. Bukhave K, Rask-Madsen J, Hogan DL, et al. Proximal duodenal prostaglandin E₂ release and mucosal bicarbonate secretion are altered in patients with duodenal ulcer. *Gastroenterology* 1990;99:951.
16. Sontag S, Graham DY, Belsito A, et al. Cimetidine, cigarette smoking, and recurrence of duodenal ulcer. *N Engl J Med* 1984;311:689.
17. Dooley CP, Larson AW, Stace NH, et al. Double-contrast barium meal and upper gastrointestinal endoscopy: a comparative study. *Ann Intern Med* 1994;101:538.
18. Hopkins RJ, Girardi LS, Turney EA. Relationship between *Helicobacter pylori* eradication and reduced duodenal and gastric ulcer recurrence: a review. *Gastroenterology* 1996;110: 1244–1252.
19. Massoomi F, Savage J, Destache CJ. Omeprazole: a comprehensive review. *Pharmacotherapy* 1993;13:46.
20. Lykkegaard Nielsen MC, Vagn Nielsen O, Moesgaard F. Ulcer healing after treatment with sucralfate emulsion or ranitidine: randomized controlled study in peptic ulcer disease. *J Clin Gastroenterol* 1998;10:377.
21. Berstad A, Weberg R. Antacids in the treatment of gastroduodenal ulcer. *Scand J Gastroenterol* 1986;21:385.
22. Schirmer BD. Current status of proximal gastric vagotomy. *Ann Surg* 1989;209:131.
23. Branicki FJ, Boey J, Fok PJ, et al. Bleeding duodenal ulcer: a prospective evaluation of risk factors for rebleeding and death. *Ann Surg* 1990;211:411.
24. Mueller X, Rothenbuehler J-M, Amery A, et al. Factors predisposing to further hemorrhage and mortality after peptic ulcer bleeding. *J Am Coll Surg* 1994;179:457–461.
25. Laine L, Peterson WL. Bleeding peptic ulcer. *N Engl J Med* 1994;331:717–727.
26. Peterson WL, Cook DJ. Antisecretory therapy for bleeding peptic ulcer. *JAMA* 1998;280:877–878.
27. Goh P, Tekant Y. Endoscopic hemostasis of bleeding peptic ulcers. *Dig Dis* 1993;11:216.
28. Lau FYW, Sung JJY, Lam Y-H, et al. Endoscopic retreatment compared with surgery in patients with recurrent bleeding after initial endoscopic control of bleeding ulcers. *N Engl J Med* 1999;340:751–756.
29. Boey J, Wong J, Ong GB. A prospective study of operative risk factors in perforated duodenal ulcers. *Ann Surg* 1982;195: 265.
30. Svanes C, Lie RT, Svanes K, et al. Adverse effects of delayed treatment for perforated peptic ulcer. *Ann Surg* 1994;220: 168–175.
31. Jordan PH, Thornby J. Perforated pyloroduodenal ulcers: long-term results with omental patch closure and parietal cell vagotomy. *Ann Surg* 1995;221:479–488.
32. Donovan AJ, Berne TV, Donovan JA. Perforated duodenal ulcer: an alternative therapeutic plan. *Arch Surg* 1998;133: 1166–1171.
33. Matsuda M, Nishiyama M, Hanai T, et al. Laparoscopic omental patch repair for perforated peptic ulcer. *Ann Surg* 1995; 221:236–240.
34. Lau W-Y, Leung K-L, Kwong K-H, et al. A randomized study comparing laparoscopic versus open repair of perforated peptic ulcer using suture or sutureless technique. *Ann Surg* 1996;224:131–138.
35. Hogan RB, Hamilton JK, Polter DE. Preliminary experience with hydrostatic balloon dilation of gastric outlet obstruction. *Gastrointest Endosc* 1986;32:71.
36. Lamers CBHW, Bijlstra AM, Harris AG. Octreotide, a long-acting somatostatin analog, in the management of postoperative dumping syndrome. *Dig Dis Sci* 1993;38:359.

SURGERY: SCIENTIFIC PRINCIPLES AND PRACTICE, Third Edition, edited by
Lazar J. Greenfield, Michael W. Mulholland, Keith T. Oldham, Gerald B. Zelenock,
and Keith D. Lillemoe. Lippincott Williams & Wilkins Publishers, Philadelphia, © 2001.

CHAPTER 23

MORBID OBESITY

HARVEY J. SUGERMAN

Morbid obesity has been arbitrarily defined as 100 lb above ideal body weight, as defined actuarially by the Metropolitan Life Insurance Company. Obesity may also be defined using the body mass index (BMI), which is the weight in kilograms divided by the height in meters squared; a BMI of 35 kg/m² or more is considered morbidly obese. Morbid obesity is the degree of overweight that is clearly associated with increased disability and mortality (Fig. 23.1). Severe obesity (>244 lb. for men or >225 lb. for women) has been estimated to be present in 4.9% (2.8 million) of men and 7.2% (4.5 million) of women in the United States. The causes of morbid obesity are unknown but probably include genetic factors, abnormalities of neural or humoral transmitters to the hypothalamic hunger or satiety centers, dysfunction of the hypothalamic centers themselves, and psychologically induced oral dependency drives. Morbidly obese adults have been found to have a lower basal energy expenditure (1). A genetic predisposition to obesity has been reported in several studies. In adopted children, the severity of obesity was more concordant with the natural than the adoptive parents (2). Furthermore, monozygotic twins have much more similar weights, including marked overweight, than dizygotic twins, even if they grow up in different environments (3). Other studies have shown that children born to overweight mothers have a significantly lower basal energy expenditure and more rapid weight gain than children born to normal-weight mothers (4).

Severe obesity is associated with a large number of problems that give rise to the term *morbid* obesity (Table

Table 23.1. MORBIDITY OF SEVERE OBESITY

Cardiovascular dysfunction
Hypertension
Coronary artery disease
Heart failure
Type II diabetes mellitus (adult onset or noninsulin dependent)
Nonalcoholic steatohepatitis (NASH)
Respiratory insufficiency of obesity (pickwickian syndrome)
Obesity hypoventilation syndrome
Obstructive sleep apnea syndrome
Increased intraabdominal pressure
Stress overflow urinary incontinence
   Gastroesophageal reflux
   Venous disease
   Thrombophlebitis
   Stasis ulcers
   Pulmonary embolism
   Nephrotic syndrome
   Pseudotumor cerebri
Degenerative osteoarthritis
Cholelithiasis
Infectious complications
   Difficulty recognizing peritonitis
   Necrotizing subcutaneous infections
   Wound infections or dehiscence
Sexual hormone dysfunction
   Polycystic ovary (Stein-Leventhal) syndrome
   Amenorrhea
   Infertility
   Hirsutism
   Endometrial cancer
   Breast cancer
Colon cancer
Psychosocial impairment

23.1). Several of these problems are underlying causes for the earlier mortality associated with obesity; they include coronary artery disease, hypertension, impaired cardiac ventricular function, adult-onset diabetes mellitus, obesity hypoventilation and sleep apnea syndromes, hypercoagulability leading to an increased risk of pulmonary embolism, necrotizing panniculitis, diverticulitis, and necrotizing pancreatitis. Morbidly obese patients can also die as a result of difficulties in recognizing the signs and symptoms of peritonitis. They have an increased risk for development of colon, prostate, breast, and uterine carcinoma. Premature death is much more common: there is a 12-fold excess mortality rate in morbidly obese men in the 25- to 34-year age group (5).

A number of obesity-related problems may not be associated with death but can lead to significant physical or psychological disability. These include degenerative osteoarthritis involving weight-bearing joints and the lower back, pseudotumor cerebri, cholecystitis, skin infections, chronic venous stasis ulcers, stress overflow urinary incontinence, gastroesophageal reflux, sex hormone imbalance with dysmenorrhea, hirsutism, and infertility. Many morbidly obese patients have severe psychological and social disability.

CENTRAL VERSUS PERIPHERAL OBESITY

Central obesity (android, or "apple," distribution of fat) is associated with a significantly greater morbidity than peripheral obesity (gynoid, or "pear," distribution of fat), and this increased morbidity is secondary to the increased metabolism of visceral fat. This increased visceral metabolism leads to increased blood glucose levels, hyperglycemia, increased insulin secretion, insulin-induced

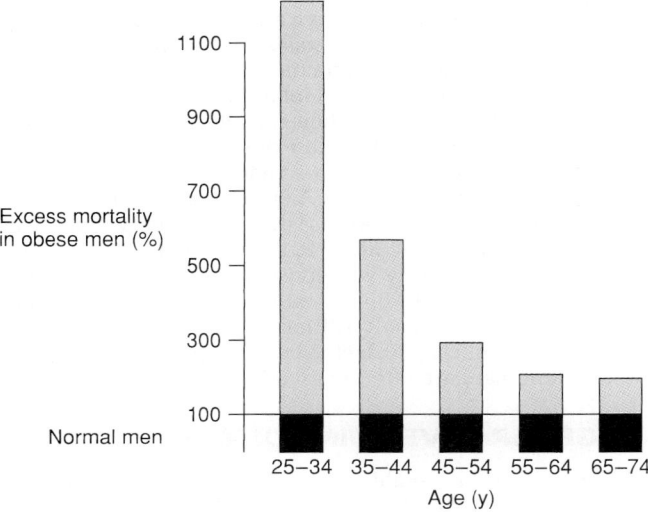

Figure 23.1. Percentage of excess probability of dying among morbidly obese men as computed for decades relative to mortality of U.S. men as a whole. (After Drenick EJ, Bale GS, Seltter F, et al. Excessive mortality and causes of death in morbidly obese men. *JAMA* 1980;243:443.)

sodium reabsorption leading to hypertension, and increased fatty acid and cholesterol turnover with an increased risk of atherosclerosis and gallstones, polycystic ovary (Stein-Leventhal) syndrome, and nonalcoholic steatohepatitis (NASH). This combination of problems is called *syndrome X* (6). Another major complication of central obesity is increased intraabdominal pressure, which can lead to venous stasis disease, gastroesophageal reflux, stress or urge urinary incontinence, obesity hypoventilation syndrome, nephrotic syndrome, incisional and inguinal hernia, and elevated pleural pressures that can markedly increase pulmonary artery and pulmonary capillary wedge pressures (7,8). The latter is probably responsible for pseudotumor cerebri seen in morbid obesity (9,10) and systemic hypertension. The increased central obesity has been assessed as an increased waist-to-hip ratio. However, severely obese patients often have both central and peripheral obesity, which cancel each other out; thus, waist-to-hip ratios can underestimate the severity of central obesity. Studies have shown that sagittal abdominal diameter is a more accurate reflection of central obesity (11).

CARDIAC DYSFUNCTION

Morbid obesity is sometimes associated with cardiomegaly and impaired left ventricular function (12). Severe obesity can be associated with a high cardiac output and a low systemic vascular resistance, leading to eccentric left ventricular hypertrophy. Obesity is also frequently associated with hypertension, which leads to concentric left ventricular hypertrophy. This combination of obesity and hypertension, with left ventricular hypertrophy, can lead to left ventricular failure. Correction of morbid obesity improves cardiac function in these patients (12). Morbid obesity is also associated with an accelerated rate of coronary atherosclerosis (13). These patients often have hypercholesterolemia and an elevated ratio of high-density lipoprotein to low-density lipoprotein. Obese women with a BMI greater than 29 have a significantly increased incidence of angina or myocardial infarction (13).

Respiratory insufficiency associated with morbid obesity can result in hypoxemic pulmonary artery vasoconstriction, which can lead to right-sided heart failure in severe cases. Correction of respiratory insufficiency after surgically induced weight loss improves the pulmonary artery hypertension within 3 months to 1 year (12). Severe obstructive sleep apnea syndrome can be associated with prolonged sinus arrest, premature ventricular contractions, and sudden death.

PULMONARY DYSFUNCTION

Respiratory insufficiency of obesity is associated with either obesity hypoventilation syndrome, obstructive sleep apnea syndrome, or a combination of the two, commonly called the *pickwickian syndrome.* The obesity hypoventilation syndrome arises from the increased weight of the chest wall and increased intraabdominal pressure leading to a high-riding diaphragm. As a result, the lungs are squeezed, producing a restrictive pulmonary defect. These patients have a markedly decreased expiratory reserve volume as well as smaller reductions in all other lung volumes. They have hypoxemia and hypercarbia while awake and a blunted ventilatory response to carbon dioxide. Chronic hypoxemia leads to pulmonary artery vasoconstriction and both right and left heart failure, as well as an increased risk of fatal arrhythmias and pulmonary embolism.

The obstructive sleep apnea syndrome is associated with severe obesity. These patients snore very loudly while asleep and have severe daytime somnolence with tendencies to fall asleep while driving or at work. The daytime somnolence is probably secondary to impaired nighttime stage III and IV and rapid-eye-movement stage sleep. The diagnosis of obstructive sleep apnea is suggested by a history of severe daytime somnolence, frequent nocturnal awakening, loud snoring, and morning headaches; it is confirmed with sleep polysomnography. This technique documents cessation of airflow during sleep associated with persistent respiratory efforts. This syndrome can be associated with sudden death and should always be considered in trauma victims who have fallen asleep while driving. Twelve percent of patients in one series who underwent gastric surgery for morbid obesity had respiratory insufficiency. Of the affected people, 25% had sleep apnea syndrome, 25% had obesity hypoventilation syndrome, and 50% had both (14). Obesity is not the only factor causing respiratory embarrassment, because many patients who underwent surgery for morbid obesity and did not have clinically significant pulmonary problems weighed more than the patients with respiratory insufficiency, although patients with this problem weighed significantly more as a group than those without it. Obstructive sleep apnea and obesity hypoventilation syndromes are associated with high mortality and serious morbidity rates; weight reduction corrects both.

DIABETES

Obesity is a frequent etiologic factor in the development of type II (adult-onset, non-insulin-dependent) diabetes mellitus. Morbidly obese patients can be resistant to insulin because of the marked down-regulation of insulin receptors. Most of these patients no longer require insulin after gastric surgery-induced weight loss (15). The tendency toward hyperglycemia manifested by obese patients is another risk factor for coronary artery disease, as well as for severe, even fatal, subcutaneous infections. Insulin resistance is also thought to be responsible for the Stein-Leventhal syndrome and NASH.

VENOUS STASIS DISEASE

Morbidly obese patients have an increased risk for deep venous thrombosis, venous stasis ulcers, and pulmonary embolism secondary to the increased intraabdominal pressure associated with central obesity. Low levels of antithrombin III can increase their risk of blood clots. The increased weight in the abdomen raises inferior vena caval pressure and the resistance to venous return, increasing the tendency for thrombosis. A similar mechanism can be responsible for the increased risk of pulmonary embolism in patients with right heart failure secondary to hypoxemic pulmonary artery vasoconstriction. Stasis ulcers are common in morbidly obese patients. These can be incapacitating and extremely difficult to treat; weight reduction can be the critical factor because pressure stockings and wound care are often ineffective.

DEGENERATIVE JOINT DISEASE

The increased weight in the morbidly obese leads to early degenerative arthritic changes of the weight-bearing joints, including the ankles, knees, hips, and spine. These patients are poor candidates for total joint replacement because of the inability of the artificial joint–bone interface to withstand the abnormal pressures. Many orthopedic surgeons refuse to insert total hip or knee prostheses in patients weighing more than 250 lb because of an unacceptable incidence of prosthetic loosening. Weight reduction after gastric surgery for obesity can permit subsequent successful joint replacement. In some instances, the decrease in pain after weight loss obviates the need for joint surgery.

OTHER OBESITY-RELATED CONDITIONS

Morbidly obese patients frequently have gastroesophageal reflux. Women often have problems with stress overflow urinary incontinence. Both of these problems are probably related to an increased intraabdominal pressure (16). Pseudotumor cerebri, also known as idiopathic intracranial hypertension, can be associated with morbid obesity. Weight loss after gastric surgery for obesity is accompanied by a significant reduction in cerebrospinal fluid pressure and the associated headaches (9). Pseudotumor has also been shown to be secondary to increased intraabdominal pressure leading to increased intrathoracic and central venous pressures (10). Women often have sexual dysfunction as a result of excessive levels of both the virilizing hormone androstenedione and the feminizing hormone estradiol. These can produce infertility, hirsutism, ovarian cysts (Stein-Leventhal syndrome), hypermenorrhea, and endometrial carcinoma. These hormonal abnormalities also resolve after weight loss.

DIETARY MANAGEMENT OF MORBID OBESITY

There are a number of dietary programs for weight reduction, including hospital-supervised programs, psychiatric behavioral modification programs, commercial organizations, commercial diets, protein-sparing fast programs, and diet pills. Unfortunately, no dietary approach has achieved uniform, long-term success for the morbidly obese. Although many people can lose weight successfully through dietary manipulation, the incidence of recidivism in the morbidly obese approaches 95% (17). A National Institutes of Health (NIH) Technology Assessment Conference in 1992 concluded that dietary management of severe obesity, with or without behavioral modification, failed to provide acceptable evidence of long-term efficacy (18). Drug therapy, using a combination of phentermine and fenfluramine, has been associated with pulmonary hypertension and cardiac valve damage (19). Newer agents include orlostat, which blocks fat absorption, and sibutramine, which works as an appetite suppressant. These agents provide only modest weight loss and are inadequate therapy for the morbidly obese patient.

SURGICAL MANAGEMENT OF MORBID OBESITY

Surgical Eligibility

According to a 1991 NIH Consensus Panel, patients are considered eligible if they have a BMI of 40 or over without comorbidity or a BMI of 35 or over with comorbidity (e.g., diabetes, respiratory insufficiency, pseudotumor cerebri).

Jejunoileal Bypass

The first popular surgical procedure for morbid obesity was the jejunoileal bypass. This operation produced an obligatory malabsorption state through bypass of a major portion of the absorptive surface of the small intestine. The

procedure connected a short length of proximal jejunum (8 to 14 inches) to the distal ileum (4 to 12 inches) as an end-to-end or end-to-side anastomosis. The end-to-end procedures, which were associated with a better weight loss, required decompression of the bypassed small intestine into the colon (Fig. 23.2). The jejunoileal bypass was associated with a number of early and late complications (20). The most serious postoperative complication was cirrhosis due to either protein–calorie malnutrition or absorption of degradation products from bacterial overgrowth in the bypassed intestine. A rheumatoid-like arthritis also occurred as a result of absorption of bacterial products from the bypassed intestine; antigen–antibody complexes to bacterial antigens can be found in the joint fluid of affected people. Rapid weight loss, as well as malabsorption of bile salts, increased the risk of cholelithiasis because of the decrease in cholesterol solubility. Hypocalcemia was frequent because of chelation of calcium with bile salts, leading to severe osteoporosis. Multiple kidney stones were seen as a result of increased oxalate absorption from the colon, where it is normally bound to calcium. Intractable, malodorous diarrhea with associated potassium and magnesium depletion, metabolic acidosis, and severe malnutrition were common, as was vitamin B_{12} deficiency. Bacterial overgrowth in the bypassed intestine also led to vitamin K deficiency, interstitial nephritis with renal failure, pneumatosis intestinalis and bypass enteritis associated with occult blood in the stools, and iron-deficiency anemia. Many of these problems, which are associated with bacterial overgrowth in the bypassed intestine, can be treated, at least temporarily, with metronidazole.

Some surgeons believe that all jejunoileal bypass procedures should be reversed because cirrhosis can develop insidiously in the absence of abnormal liver function test results. If the medical problems are severe (i.e., progressive liver or renal dysfunction), the jejunoileal bypass can be reversed. Because these patients invariably regain their lost weight, conversion to a gastric procedure for obesity

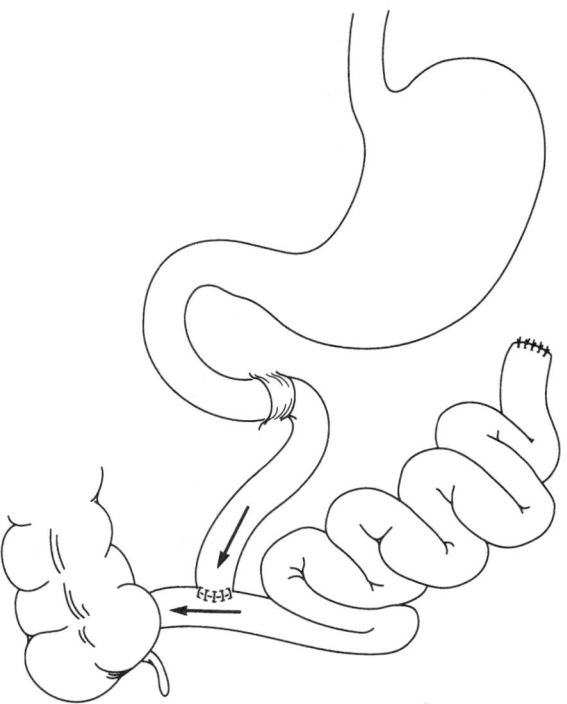

Figure 23.2. Schematic representation of jejunoileal bypass.

can be considered unless the patient is too ill (i.e., severe cirrhosis with portal hypertension). Mechanical complications of the jejunoileal bypass include small bowel obstruction and intussusception of the bypassed intestine. Randomized, prospective studies have shown that the gastric bypass operation is associated with a comparable weight loss and a significantly lower complication rate than jejunoileal bypass (21). Because of the significant complication rate, standard jejunoileal bypass should no longer be performed.

Gastric Procedures for Morbid Obesity

In 1969, investigators reported the results of weight loss after division of the stomach into a small upper pouch connected to a loop gastroenterostomy (22). The concept for this procedure was based on the observation of weight loss that sometimes followed subtotal gastrectomy for duodenal ulcer disease. There was initial concern that peptic ulcers would develop in the bypassed stomach or duodenum, and although these have occurred, the incidence is low. The technique for gastric bypass was simplified with the use of stapling instruments. The concept of gastroplasty was then proposed as a safer, easier method for restricting food intake. In gastroplasty, the stomach is only stapled and not divided, leaving a small opening to permit the normal passage of food into the distal stomach and duodenum.

Gastroplasty

Gastroplasties have been performed with either horizontal or vertical placement of the staples. Horizontal gastroplasty usually requires ligation and division of the short gastric vessels between the stomach and spleen, and it carries the risk of devascularization of the gastric pouch or splenic injury. Horizontal gastroplasties included a single application of a 90-mm stapling device without suture reinforcement of the stoma between upper and lower gastric pouches, or a double application of staples with either a central or lateral Prolene-reinforced stoma. In one study, the failure rates (loss of less than 40% excess weight) for these three horizontal gastroplasty procedures were 71%, 46%, and 42%, respectively (23). The vertical banded gastroplasty (VBGP) is a procedure in which a stapled opening is made in the stomach with the stapling device 5 cm from the cardioesophageal junction (Fig. 23.3). Two appli-

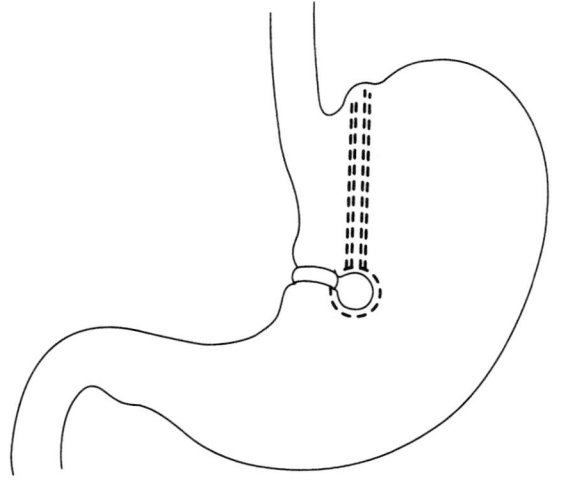

Figure 23.3. Vertical banded gastroplasty.

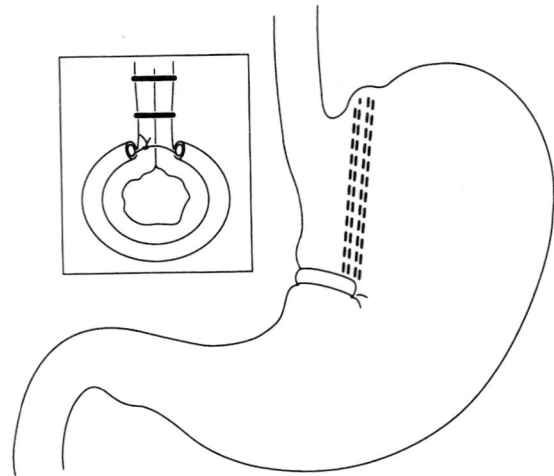

Figure 23.4. Vertical Silastic ring gastroplasty.

cations of a 90-mm stapling device are made between this opening and the angle of His, and a 1.5 × 5-cm strip of polypropylene mesh is wrapped around the stoma on the lesser curvature and sutured to itself, but not to the stomach. Erosion of the mesh into the stomach has been an unusual complication of this procedure. Pouch enlargement is much less likely to occur with a vertical staple line in the thicker, more muscular part of the stomach (as compared with the horizontal gastroplasties), and the stomal diameter is fixed with the mesh band. The Silastic ring gastroplasty is a similar procedure (Fig. 23.4) that uses a vertical staple line and a Silastic tubing-reinforced stoma. Weight loss with vertical Silastic ring gastroplasty appears to be similar to that with VBGP. Use of the four-row parallel bariatric stapler has been associated with a 35% rate of staple line disruption, leading to failure of the operative procedure. Some surgeons now recommend transecting the stomach.

Gastric Bypass

Gastric bypass can also be performed with placement of the staples in a vertical or horizontal direction; the vertical direction is preferred because there is less risk of gastric pouch devascularization or splenic injury. Because of the high incidence of staple line disruption, some surgeons also recommend transecting the stomach for gastric bypass patients. However, with three to four superimposed applications of a 90-mm stapler, the incidence of staple line disruption has been less than 2%. The gastrojejunostomy used to drain the gastric pouch can be a loop, a loop with a jejunojejunostomy constructed below the gastrojejunostomy, or a Roux-en-Y limb. The latter two techniques prevent bile reflux into the gastric pouch. The length of the Roux-en-Y jejunal limb is usually 45 cm. However, superobese patients (BMI ≥50 kg/m²) achieve a significantly better weight loss with a 150-cm Roux limb (long-limb gastric bypass) (24). The gastric pouch should be small (15 mL) and the stoma restricted to 1 cm (Fig. 23.5). The small gastric pouch has a limited volume of acid secretion and is associated with a low incidence of marginal ulcer in the absence of vagotomy.

Gastroplasty versus Gastric Bypass

In a randomized, prospective trial (Fig. 23.6), the Roux-en-Y gastric bypass resulted in a weight loss that was significantly better than that achieved with VBGP (25). VBGP can be associated with severe gastroesophageal reflux that resolves after conversion to gastric bypass. Gastric bypass

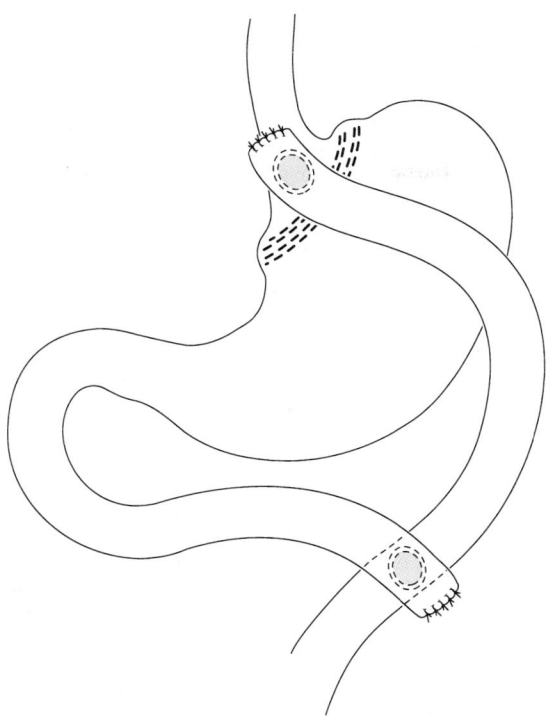

Figure 23.5. Proximal Roux-en-Y gastric bypass.

carries a higher incidence of stomal ulcer, stomal stenosis, vitamin B_{12} deficiency, and, in menstruating women, iron-deficiency anemia than does gastroplasty. Gastric bypass is, however, more effective than VBGP in correcting glucose intolerance in patients without overt type II diabetes mellitus.

Some patients can overcome the effect of a standard gastric bypass on weight loss. Although regained weight could be the result of expansion of either the stoma or pouch, this finding is not observed in most patients. Approximately 10% to 15% regain lost weight or fail to achieve an acceptable weight loss. The cause for this failure appears to be excessive, constant nibbling on foods with high caloric density. The average patient loses 66% of his or her excess weight within 2 years after gastric bypass. The percentage excess weight loss is 60% at 5 years, 50% at 10 years, and 47% at 14 years after surgery (26).

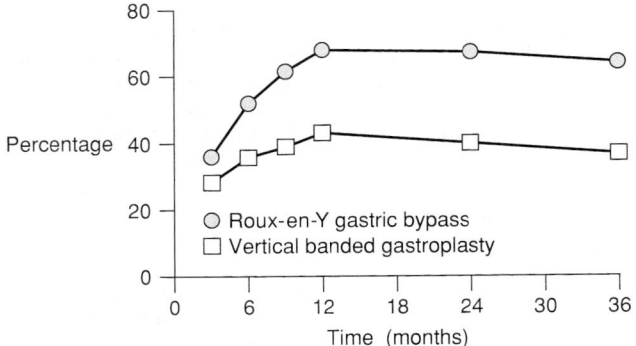

Figure 23.6. Percentage loss of excess weight over 3 years after Roux-en-Y gastric bypass compared with vertical banded gastroplasty. (After Sugerman HJ, Starkey J, Birkenhauer R. A randomized prospective trial of gastric bypass versus vertical banded gastroplasty for morbid obesity and their effects on sweets versus non-sweets eaters. *Ann Surg* 1987;205:613.)

Partial Biliopancreatic Diversion

The partial biliopancreatic diversion was developed as both a gastric restrictive procedure and a malabsorptive procedure that does not have a blind intestinal limb for bacterial overgrowth (27). In this operation, a subtotal gastrectomy is performed and the distal 2.5 m of small intestine is anastomosed with a large (2- to 3-cm) stoma to the proximal gastric remnant. The proximal, bypassed small intestine is reanastomosed to the distal ileum 0.5 m from the ileocecal valve. In this manner, the quantity of food ingested is partially restricted and then passes down the intestine mostly undigested and unabsorbed until it reaches the bile and pancreatic juices, 0.5 m from the ileocecal valve, where digestion and absorption take place. Treated patients usually pass four to six stools per day, which are foul smelling and float, reflecting malabsorption of fat. If the distal stomach is not resected, the operation is called a *distal gastric bypass.*

As with the proximal or standard gastric bypass, patients with the distal gastric bypass or partial biliopancreatic diversion are at risk for iron-deficiency anemia and vitamin B_{12} deficiency. In addition, they are also at risk for protein deficiency, osteoporosis secondary to calcium and vitamin D malabsorption, night blindness and skin eruptions secondary to vitamin A deficiency, and problems with the other fat-soluble vitamins, E and K (28). Italian patients—the operation was developed in Italy—appear to have less malabsorption and nutritional deficiencies than American patients, probably because of a much lower fat content in the Italian diet. The duodenal switch operation is a modification of the partial biliopancreatic bypass but still may be associated with malnutrition and fat-soluble vitamin and calcium deficiencies (29).

Laparoscopic Obesity Surgery

The adjustable silicone gastric band has been developed to be placed laparoscopically. The device contains a balloon that is adjusted by injecting saline into a subcutaneously implanted port. This procedure has become very popular in Europe. However, there are no long-term studies validating its safety and efficacy. A U.S. Food and Drug Administration-approved trial is in progress in the United States. There have been problems with band slippage leading to gastric obstruction and the need to revise the position of the band, band erosion into the lumen of the stomach, port infections, and inadequate weight loss.

The gastric bypass procedure is being performed laparoscopically at a number of centers, either as a totally laparoscopic procedure or as a laparoscopically assisted procedure using a device that permits insertion of the surgeon's hand for manipulation of tissues without loss of the pneumoperitoneum. This offers a marginal decrease in hospital length of stay and requires use of expensive laparoscopic devices and a longer operating time. Advantages should include a decreased frequency of incisional hernia, which currently is approximately 20% after open obesity surgery, and a decreased severity of adhesions with the potential for fewer subsequent small bowel obstructions. However, the latter may increase if the potential places for internal hernias (at the Roux anastomosis, through the mesocolon) are not closed laparoscopically.

Complications of Gastric Surgery for Morbid Obesity

The most feared complication of gastric surgery for morbid obesity is a postoperative gastric leak with the development of peritonitis. After gastroplasty, this can occur at the staple line, from the proximal gastric pouch, or from the distal stomach. Many leaks were secondary to ischemic necrosis that occurred with horizontal stapling procedures, either gastroplasty or gastric bypass, after ligation of the short gastric vessels. The distal stomach can be perforated because of marked dilatation that can occur after a gastric bypass operation as a result of afferent limb obstruction of a loop gastrojejunostomy or obstruction at the jejunojejunostomy of a Roux-en-Y procedure. This complication is usually heralded by frequent hiccups and can be diagnosed by noting a large gastric bubble on a plain abdominal roentgenogram. Impending gastric perforation requires urgent percutaneous or operative decompression. In patients converted from jejunoileal to gastric bypass or in patients with extensive adhesions from previous abdominal surgery, a gastrostomy tube should be inserted prophylactically for decompression. The gastrostomy tube also can be used for feeding until the patient's oral intake permits weight stabilization. A gastrostomy can also be used to feed patients in whom a leak develops from the proximal gastric pouch.

The most dangerous aspect of a gastric leak is the difficulty in recognizing the symptoms of peritonitis. By the third day after surgery, patients should have little pain. If patients with postoperative gastric bypass or gastroplasty experience worsening pain and complain of pain in the back or the left shoulder (consistent with inflammation of the left hemidiaphragm), urinary frequency, or rectal tenesmus (implying pelvic irritation), the clinician must suspect a leak. Tachycardia, tachypnea, fever, and leukocytosis are usually also present. A leak can often be confirmed with an emergency upper gastrointestinal roentgenographic series using water-soluble contrast. If a leak is observed, or even if the study is negative but the suspicion is high, the patient's abdomen must be urgently reexplored. An attempt to repair the leak should be made, and a large sump drain should be placed nearby because the repair frequently breaks down. This leads to a controlled fistula, which usually heals with total parenteral nutrition therapy or a distal feeding jejunostomy.

A marginal ulcer develops in approximately 10% of patients with gastric bypass. This usually responds to acid suppression therapy (histamine-2 receptor blocker or omeprazole). Stomal stenosis can develop in patients after Roux-en-Y gastric bypass or VBGP. Outpatient endoscopic balloon stomal dilatation should be attempted. This is usually successful in patients with gastric bypass but is effective in less than half of stenoses in patients who have undergone VBGP.

Rapid weight loss after either VBGP or gastric bypass is associated with a high incidence (32% to 35%) of gallstone formation, with a 10% to 20% need for subsequent cholecystectomy for acute biliary colic or cholecystitis within 3 to 5 years of obesity surgery. Some surgeons recommend routine prophylactic cholecystectomy at the time of bariatric surgery; others perform cholecystectomy only with sonographic evidence of gallstones or biliary sludge. Prophylactic ursodeoxycholic acid, 300 mg orally twice daily, has been shown to reduce the risk of gallstone formation from 32% to 2% when given for 6 months after gastric bypass surgery, and there is a very low risk of subsequent gallstone formation for the 6 months after discontinuation of the medication (30).

A rare syndrome of polyneuropathy has occurred after gastric surgery for morbid obesity. This usually occurs in association with intractable vomiting and severe protein–calorie malnutrition. Acute thiamine deficiency has been thought to be responsible for this condition. Vitamin B_{12} deficiency has been observed after gastric bypass, and this mandates long-term follow-up of these patients with annual measurement of the vitamin B_{12} level. Deficiency of this vitamin is probably due to decreased acid digestion of vitamin B_{12} from food with subsequent failure of coupling to intrinsic factor, so that these patients need to take 500 mg of oral vitamin B_{12} daily or 1 mg intramuscular vitamin B_{12} per month. Iron-deficiency anemia can occur in menstruating women after gastric bypass. This can be refractory to supplemental ferrous sulfate because iron absorption requires acid and takes place primarily in the duodenum and upper jejunum. Occasionally, iron–dextran injections may be necessary. All menstruating women should take two iron sulfate tablets (325 mg/d) after gastric bypass as long as they continue to menstruate. Magnesium deficiency may also occur and require supplementation. Patients with either a long-limb gastric or partial biliopancreatic bypass can have calcium and fat-soluble vitamin deficiencies that need to be monitored and treated.

Other complications, seen with any type of surgery in obese patients, include wound infection, wound dehiscence, incisional hernia, venous thrombosis, and pulmonary embolism. The incidence of lower leg venous thrombosis and pulmonary embolism can be significantly reduced with the use of intermittent venous compression boots. Early ambulation is also important. In addition, subcutaneous heparin should be given 30 minutes before surgery and every 8 hours after surgery until the patient is fully ambulatory. Pulmonary embolism is a not infrequent fatal complication in patients with heart failure associated with hypoxemic pulmonary hypertension and mean pulmonary artery pressure greater than 40 mm Hg. It has been recommended that a vena caval filter be placed in these patients prophylactically at the time of obesity surgery. The operative mortality rate after gastric surgery for obesity is now approximately 0.5% in most series.

Failed Gastric Surgery for Obesity

Attempts to revise a failed gastroplasty are often unsuccessful because of recurrence of stomal dilation and problems with gastric emptying. Reoperation in these patients is extremely difficult because of extensive adhesions to the liver and spleen. Results appear to be significantly better when these patients are converted to a Roux-en-Y gastric bypass. Because of the technical difficulties, these patients must understand that the risks of serious complications are far higher after a secondary than after a primary gastric bypass. It is probably inappropriate and dangerous to convert a failed gastric bypass to vertical gastroplasty. Furthermore, revision of a dilated gastrojejunal stoma has not been effective. Most patients who fail a gastric bypass do so as a consequence of excessive fat ingestion. If the patient has significant obesity comorbidity that has failed to resolve or has returned with weight regain, conversion to a malabsorptive distal gastric bypass (modified partial biliopancreatic diversion) can be performed; however, this can be associated with steatorrhea, fat-soluble vitamin deficiencies, and osteoporosis.

OVERVIEW OF GASTRIC SURGERY FOR MORBID OBESITY

Gastric procedures for morbid obesity can yield a satisfactory weight reduction, with an average loss of two thirds of excess weight within 1 to 1.5 years. Weight becomes stable at this level in most patients as the reduced caloric intake meets caloric expenditure. The patients must be followed carefully to ensure adequate protein, vitamin, and other micronutrient levels.

Weight loss completely corrects type II diabetes mellitus in almost all cases, hypertension in two thirds to three

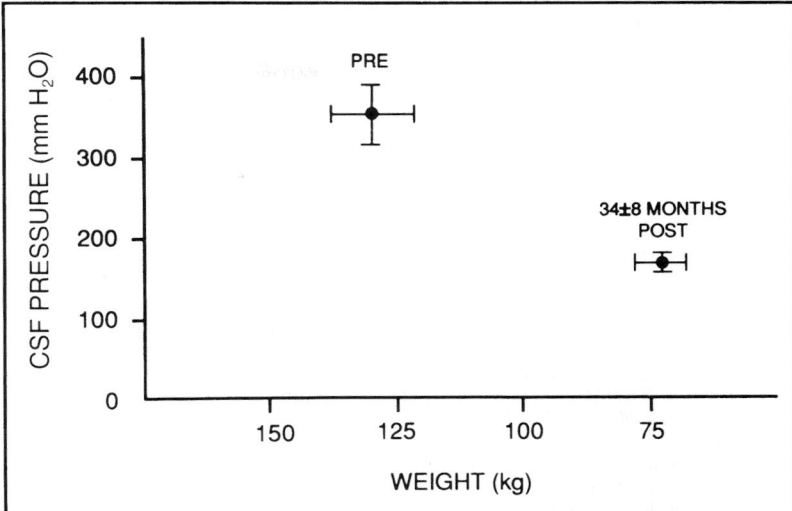

Figure 23.7. Decrease in cerebrospinal fluid (CSF) opening pressure with decreased weight when reevaluated approximately 3 years after gastric surgery-induced weight loss. (After Sugerman HJ, Felton WL, Salvant JB, et al. Effects of surgically induced weight loss on pseudotumor cerebri in morbid obesity. *Neurology* 1995;45:1655.)

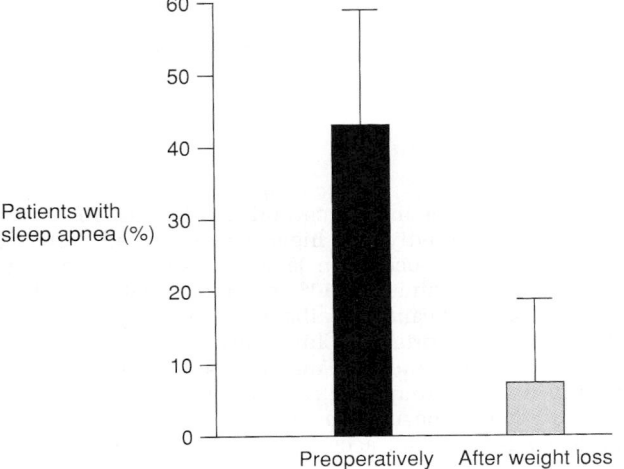

Figure 23.8. Reduction in percentage of sleep apnea (mean ± SD) in 22 patients with obstructive sleep apnea syndrome after weight loss induced by gastric surgery. (After Sugerman HJ, Fairman RP, Baron PL, et al. Gastric surgery for respiratory insufficiency of obesity. *Chest* 1986;90:82.)

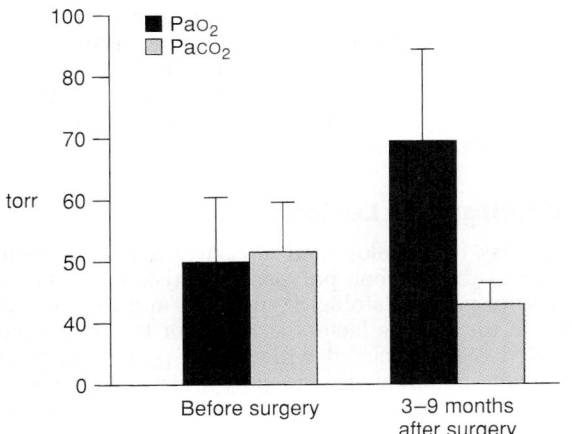

Figure 23.9. Significantly improved PaO_2 and $PaCO_2$ in 18 patients 3 to 9 months after gastric surgery-induced loss of 42% ± 19% excess weight. (After Sugerman HJ, Baron PL, Fairman RP, et al. Hemodynamic dysfunction in obesity hypoventilation syndrome and the effects of treatment with surgically induced weight loss. *Ann Surg* 1988;207:604.)

fourths of the patients, and headaches associated with cerebrospinal fluid pressure elevation in almost all patients with pseudotumor cerebri (Fig. 23.7). The obstructive sleep apnea syndrome resolves with weight loss (Fig. 23.8). Hypoxemia and hypercarbia seen in the obesity hypoventilation syndrome return toward normal with weight loss (Fig. 23.9). Elevated pulmonary artery and pulmonary capillary wedge pressures also improve significantly after weight loss with correction of abnormal arterial blood gases. The loss of weight usually corrects female sexual hormone abnormalities, permits healing of chronic venous stasis ulcers associated with venous insufficiency, prevents reflux esophagitis, relieves stress overflow urinary incontinence, and improves low back pain, as well as joint-related pain. Weight loss can permit successful total artificial joint replacement. Patient self-image is often markedly improved after gastric surgery for obesity.

REFERENCES

1. Ravussin E, Lillioja S, Knowler WC, et al. Reduced rate of energy expenditure as a risk factor for body-weight gain. *N Engl J Med* 1988;318:467.
2. Stunkard AJ, Sorensen TA, Hanis C, et al. An adoption study of human obesity. *N Engl J Med* 1986;314:193.
3. Stunkard AJ, Harris JR, Pedersen NL, et al. The body-mass index of twins who have been reared apart. *N Engl J Med* 1990;322:1483.
4. Roberts SB, Savage J, Coward WA, et al. Energy expenditure and intake in infants born to lean and overweight mothers. *N Engl J Med* 1988;318:461.
5. Drenick EJ, Bale GS, Seltter F, et al. Excessive mortality and causes of death in morbidly obese men. *JAMA* 1980;243:443.
6. Bjorntorp P. Abdominal obesity and the metabolic syndrome. *Ann Med* 1992;24:465.
7. Sugerman H, Windsor A, Bessos M, et al. Intra-abdominal pressure, sagittal abdominal diameter, and obesity co-morbidity. *J Intern Med* 1997;241:71.
8. Sugerman HJ, Kellum JM, DeMaria EJ. Effects of surgically induced weight loss on urinary bladder pressure, sagittal abdominal diameter, and obesity co-morbidity. *Int J Obes Relat Metab Disord* 1998;22:230.
9. Sugerman HJ, Felton WL, Salvant JB, et al. Effects of surgically induced weight loss on pseudotumor cerebri in morbid obesity. *Neurology* 1995;45:1655.
10. Sugerman HJ, DeMaria EJ, Felton WL III, et al. Increased intra-abdominal pressure and cardiac filling pressures in obesity associated pseudotumor cerebri. *Neurology* 1997;49:507.
11. Sjostrom L. A computer-tomography based multicompartment body composition technique and anthropometric pre-

dictions of lean body mass, total and subcutaneous adipose tissue. *Int J Obes Relat Metab Disord* 1991;15[Suppl 2]:19.

12. Sugerman HJ, Baron PL, Fairman RP, et al. Hemodynamic dysfunction in obesity hypoventilation syndrome and the effects of treatment with surgically induced weight loss. *Ann Surg* 1988;207:604.

13. Manson JE, Colditz GA, Stampfer MJ, et al. A prospective study of obesity and risk of coronary heart disease in women. *N Engl J Med* 1990; 322:882.

14. Sugerman HJ, Fairman RP, Baron PL, et al. Gastric surgery for respiratory insufficiency of obesity. *Chest* 1986;90:82.

15. Bump RC, Sugerman HJ, Fantl JA, et al. Obesity and lower urinary tract function in women: effect of surgically induced weight loss. *Am J Obstet Gynecol* 1992;167:392.

16. Pories WJ, Caro JF, Flickinger EG, et al. The control of diabetes mellitus (NIDDM) in the morbidly obese with the Greenville gastric bypass. *Ann Surg* 1987;206:316.

17. Johnson D, Drenick EJ. Therapeutic fasting in morbid obesity. *Arch Intern Med* 1977;137:1381.

18. NIH Technology Assessment Conference Panel. NIH conference: methods for voluntary weight loss and control. *Ann Intern Med* 1992;116:942.

19. Connolly HM, Crary JL, McGoon MD, et al. Valvular heart disease associated with fenfluramine-phenteramine. *N Engl J Med* 1997;337:581.

20. Hocking MP, Duerson MC, O'Leary JP, et al. Jejunoileal bypass for morbid obesity: late follow-up in 100 cases. *N Engl J Med* 1983;308:995.

21. Griffen WO, Young VL, Stevenson CC. A prospective comparison of gastric and jejunoileal bypass for morbid obesity. *Ann Surg* 1977;186:500.

22. Mason EE, Ito C. Gastric bypass. *Ann Surg* 1969;170:329.

23. Sugerman JH, Wolper JL. Failed gastroplasty for morbid obesity: revised gastroplasty versus Roux-en-Y gastric bypass. *Am J Surg* 1984;148:331.

24. Brolin RE, Kenler HA, Gorman JH, et al. Long-limb gastric bypass in the superobese: a prospective randomized study. *Ann Surg* 1992;215:387.

25. Sugerman HJ, Starkey J, Birkenhauer R. A randomized prospective trial of gastric bypass versus vertical banded gastroplasty for morbid obesity and their effects on sweets versus non-sweets eaters. *Ann Surg* 1987;205:613.

26. Yale CE. Gastric surgery for morbid obesity: complications and long-term weight control. *Arch Surg* 1989;124:941.

27. Scopinaro N, Gianetta E, Civalleri D, et al. Two years of clinical experience with bilio-pancreatic bypass for obesity. *Am J Clin Nutr* 1980;33:506.

28. Clare MW. An analysis of 37 reversals on 504 biliopancreatic surgeries over 12 years. *Obes Surg* 1993;3:169.

29. Hess DS, Hess DW. Biliopancreatic diversion with a duodenal switch. *Obes Surg* 1996;6A:122.

30. Sugerman HJ, Brewer WH, Shiffman ML, et al. A multicenter, placebo-controlled, randomized, double-blind, prospective trial of prophylactic ursodiol for the prevention of gallstone formation following gastric-bypass-induced rapid weight loss. *Am J Surg* 1995;169:91.

SURGERY: SCIENTIFIC PRINCIPLES AND PRACTICE, Third Edition, edited by Lazar J. Greenfield, Michael W. Mulholland, Keith T. Oldham, Gerald B. Zelenock, and Keith D. Lillemoe. Lippincott Williams & Wilkins Publishers, Philadelphia, © 2001.

CHAPTER 24
GASTRIC NEOPLASMS

MICHAEL W. MULHOLLAND

Gastric cancer is a relatively common, frequently lethal affliction and remains a serious and unsolved problem in general surgery. The disease often is not recognized until it is at an advanced stage. Gastric cancer usually cannot be controlled by surgery alone, and surgical cure rates have remained disappointingly low. Technical innovations and basic scientific investigations continue to be applied to this disease, however, and cautious optimism for the future is appropriate.

ADENOCARCINOMA

Epidemiology

Starting in 1930, the incidence of gastric cancer declined dramatically in the United States (Fig. 24.1). By 1980, the incidence of gastric cancer (10 cases per 100,000 population) was approximately one-fourth the incidence recorded in 1930. The incidence of the disease remained relatively constant in the decade from 1980 to 1990 (1). By 1997, reported new cases of gastric cancer had declined to 22,000, a small number relative to the 150,000 estimated deaths from cancer of the lung (2). Gastric cancer remains among the top 10 causes of cancer-related deaths for both men and women in the United States. The reasons for the early decline in the incidence of gastric cancer are unknown, but the factors contributing to its persistence are now better understood.

The worldwide incidence and death rates for gastric cancer vary markedly. The highest age-adjusted death rate for gastric cancer occurs in Japan, where the disease accounts for approximately 50% of cancer-related deaths in men and 40% of cancer deaths in women. High incidence rates are also reported in Chile, Costa Rica, Hungary, Portugal, Singapore, and Romania, a geographically and ethnically diverse group (Fig. 24.2). It has been widely assumed that exposure to environmental carcinogens, probably in the diet, accounts for the increased disease frequency observed in these populations. This supposition is supported by studies of immigrant populations. Migration from an area at high risk to one at low risk is associated with a decreased probability of development of gastric cancer. Early infection with the organism *Helicobacter pylori* now appears to predispose to subsequent development of gastric carcinoma. In animal models, ingested nitrites and metabolic derivatives such as nitrosamines can promote gastric carcinogenesis. Although nitrites in the diet have been postulated to have a role in gastric carcinogenesis in humans, specific dietary constituents that promote tumor formation in humans have not been identified.

Premalignant Lesions

The risk for development of gastric cancer is greater in stomachs that harbor polyps. This risk is related most closely to polyp histologic type, size, and number. Variations in these three factors account for the wide range in reported risk associated with gastric polyps. In terms of malignant potential, gastric polyps can be divided into two broad categories—hyperplastic polyps and adenomatous polyps.

Hyperplastic polyps are common, occurring in 0.5% to 1% of the general population and accounting for 70% to 80% of all gastric polyps. The hyperplastic polyp contains an overgrowth of histologically normal-appearing gastric epithelium. Atypia is rare. Hyperplastic gastric polyps are considered to have no neoplastic potential.

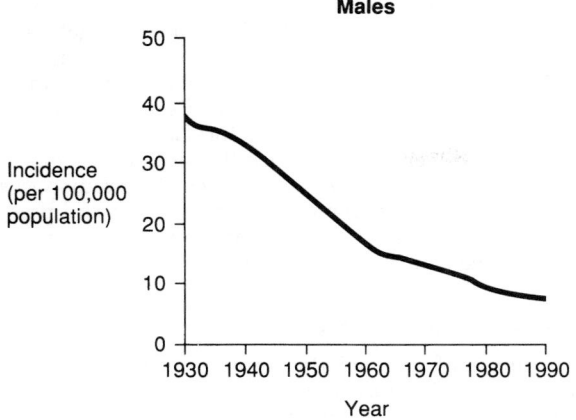

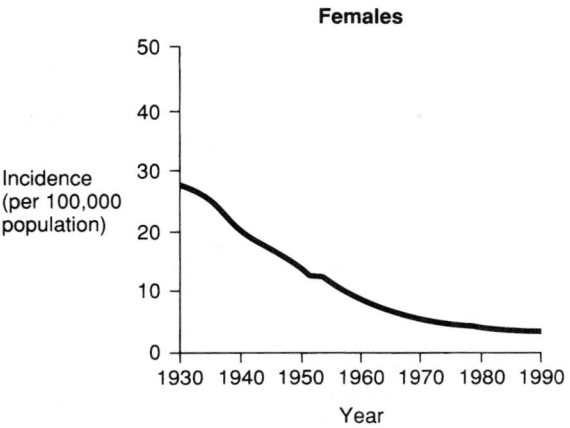

Figure 24.1. Incidence of gastric cancer deaths in the United States.

Most people with hyperplastic polyps are asymptomatic. Dyspepsia and complaints of vague epigastric discomfort are the most common complaints, although coexistent gastroduodenal disease is also frequently identified. Complications are unusual, and gastrointestinal hemorrhage occurs in less than 20%. When hyperplastic polyps are discovered, endoscopic removal for histologic examination is indicated and is sufficient treatment.

Adenomatous polyps, in contrast, have a distinct risk for the development of malignancy (3). Mucosal atypia is frequent, and mitotic figures are more common than in hyperplastic polyps. Dysplasia and carcinoma in situ have developed in adenomatous polyps observed over time. The risk for the development of carcinoma has been estimated at 10% to 20% and is greatest for polyps more than 2 cm in diameter. Multiple adenomatous polyps increase the risk of cancer. The presence of an adenomatous polyp is also a marker indicating an increased risk for the development of cancer in the remainder of the gastric mucosa.

Symptoms are similar to those for hyperplastic polyps. Endoscopic removal is indicated for pedunculated lesions and is sufficient if the polyp is completely removed and shows no evidence of invasive cancer on histologic examination. Operative excision is recommended for sessile lesions larger than 2 cm, for polyps with biopsy-proven invasive carcinoma, and for polyps complicated by pain or bleeding. After removal, endoscopic surveillance of the gastric mucosa is indicated.

Gastritis

The incidence of both gastric cancer and atrophic gastritis increases with age. Chronic gastritis is frequently associated with intestinal metaplasia and mucosal dysplasia, and these histologic features are often observed in mucosa adjacent to gastric cancer. Gastritis is frequently progressive and severe in the gastric mucosa of patients with cancer.

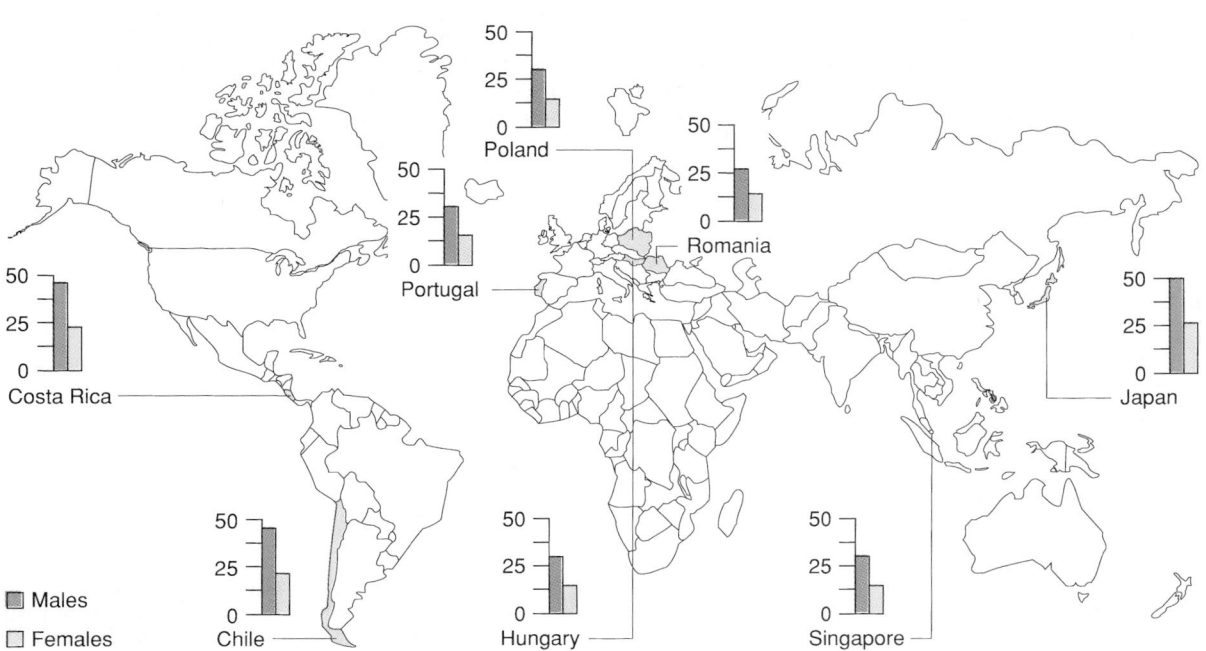

Figure 24.2. Worldwide incidence of gastric cancer.

Gastric malignancy seems to be increased in patients with chronic gastritis associated with pernicious anemia, although the risk appears to have been overstated in the past. This disease, characterized by fundic mucosal atrophy, loss of parietal and chief cells, hypochlorhydria, and hypergastrinemia, is present in 3% of people older than 60 years of age. For people in whom pernicious anemia has been active for more than 5 years, the risk of gastric cancer is twice that of age-matched control subjects. Evidence also indicates an increased risk of gastric carcinoid development in patients with pernicious anemia. This increased risk warrants aggressive investigation of new symptoms in patients with long-standing pernicious anemia, but it is not high enough to justify repeated endoscopic surveillance.

Intestinal metaplasia, the presence of intestinal glands within the gastric mucosa, is also commonly associated with both gastritis and gastric cancer. The evolution from metaplasia to dysplasia to carcinoma to invasive cancer has been demonstrated in other organs, but no direct evidence can be provided for this progression in gastric cancer.

Helicobacter pylori

Helicobacter pylori has been unequivocally associated with chronic inflammatory conditions in the stomach; this association has stimulated interest in the role of chronic infection by this organism in gastric carcinogenesis. Those areas of the world with high rates of gastric adenocarcinoma also have a high prevalence of *H. pylori* infection. Childhood acquisition of *H. pylori* infection is frequent in areas of high gastric cancer incidence, and high rates of infection have been identified in patients with premalignant lesions and invasive cancer.

In the United States, seropositivity for *H. pylori* increases the risk for cancer development approximately threefold (4). Infection with *H. pylori* is associated with an increased risk of adenocarcinoma of both major histologic types and for tumors arising in the body or antrum of the stomach. In contrast, *H. pylori* infection is not a risk factor for cancers of the gastroesophageal junction, which are frequently associated with mucosal abnormalities of Barrett's esophagus. In a separate study of Japanese-American men in Honolulu, *H. pylori*-positive subjects had an odds ratio of 6 for gastric cancer development (5).

Infection with *H. pylori* alone cannot explain the development of gastric cancer. In North America, approximately 50% of adults older than 50 years are seropositive for *H. pylori,* yet gastric cancer develops in only a small fraction. In several Asian populations, seropositivity of *H. pylori* approaches 70% to 90%. Several investigators have postulated that long-term gastric inflammation, consequent to childhood acquisition of *H. pylori,* makes the gastric mucosa more susceptible to the effects of environmental carcinogens. Dietary cofactors have been supposed to increase cancer risk, but specific carcinogens have not yet been identified. If *H. pylori* infection predisposes to gastric cancer development, then the widespread practice of treating peptic ulcer disease with antibiotics may eventually reduce cancer incidence further.

Previous Gastric Surgery

A number of uncontrolled reports have suggested that gastric cancer is more likely to develop in people who have undergone previous partial gastrectomy. The so-called *gastric remnant cancer* is a true clinical entity, although the risk for development of this gastric neoplasm appears to have been overestimated. Several large, prospective studies with long-term follow-up indicate that the relative risk is not increased for up to 15 years after gastric resection, with modest increases (three times the control value) observed only after 25 years (6–9).

Clinical Features

The symptoms produced by gastric cancer are not specific and can unfortunately closely mimic those associated with a number of nonneoplastic gastroduodenal diseases, especially benign gastric ulcer (Fig. 24.3). In early gastric cancers, epigastric pain is present in over 70% of patients (10). The pain is often constant, nonradiating, and unrelieved by food ingestion. In a surprising number of patients, pain can be relieved, at least temporarily, by antacids or gastric antisecretory drugs. Anorexia, nausea, and weight loss are present in less than 50% of patients with early gastric cancers, but become increasingly common with disease progression. Dysphagia is present in 20% of patients with proximal gastric lesions. Overt gastrointestinal hemorrhage is present in only 5%. Perforation is rare (1%).

In most patients with early gastric cancers, physical examination is negative. Stool is guaiac positive in one third. Abnormal physical findings usually reflect advanced disease (Table 24.1). Cachexia, abdominal mass, hepatomegaly, and supraclavicular adenopathy usually indicate metastasis (11). There are no simple laboratory tests specific for gastric neoplasms.

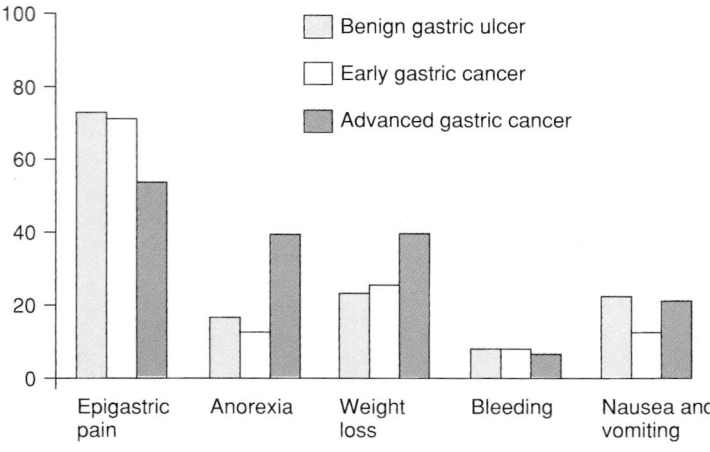

Figure 24.3. Clinical symptom frequency in benign gastric ulcer, early gastric cancer, and advanced gastric cancer. (After Meyer WC, Damiano RJ, Postlethwait RW, et al. Adenocarcinoma of the stomach: changing patterns over the past four decades. *Ann Surg* 1987;205:18.)

Table 24.1. COMMON SYMPTOMS AND PHYSICAL FINDINGS IN GASTRIC CANCER

Symptoms	Physical findings
Weight loss	Guaiac-positive stool
Pain	Cachexia
Nausea and vomiting	Abdominal mass
Anorexia	Abdominal tenderness
Dysphagia	Hepatomegaly
Melena	—

Diagnosis and Screening

Fiberoptic endoscopy is the most definitive diagnostic method when gastric neoplasm is suspected. In the initial stages, gastric cancers can appear polypoid, as flat, plaque-like lesions, or as shallow ulcers. Advanced lesions are typically ulcerated. The ulcer border can have an irregular, beaded appearance because of infiltrating cancer cells, and the base is frequently necrotic and shaggy. The ulcer can appear to arise from an underlying mass. Although each of these features suggests a malignant ulcer, differentiation of benign from malignant gastric ulcers can be made definitively only with gastric biopsy. Accuracy of diagnosis can exceed 95% if multiple biopsy specimens are obtained. False-negative results occur in approximately 10% of patients, usually as the result of sampling error; false-positive results are rare. Diagnostic accuracy can be further enhanced by the addition of direct brush cytology.

The ability to diagnose gastric adenocarcinoma endoscopically has prompted screening programs for populations at high risk. Mass screening has been performed in Japan since the 1960s with the use of fiberoptic endoscopy. The overall yield for the Japanese screening program has been 0.12% (12). The proportion of early cancers, defined as tumors whose growth is confined to the mucosa and submucosa regardless of the presence or absence of metastatic disease in the perigastric lymph nodes, steadily increased during the study period. Currently, greater than 60% of gastric malignancies detected by this program are early cancers. Early detection translates directly into improved survival (Fig. 24.4). The Japanese findings that early detection can improve survival have been confirmed by European investigations, in which patients with early gastric cancers had survival rates equivalent to those of patients with benign gastric ulcer (10) (Fig. 24.5). Mass screening for gastric adenocarcinoma has not been advocated in the United States or Canada. With incidence rates approximately one fifth of those observed in Japan, detection rates are too low to justify such a program economically.

Barium contrast radiographs have, in the past, been the standard method for diagnosing gastric neoplasm. Single-contrast examinations have a diagnostic accuracy of 80%. This diagnostic yield increases to approximately 90% when double-contrast (air and barium) techniques are used. Typical findings include ulceration, the presence of a gastric mass, loss of mucosal detail, and distortion of the gastric silhouette (Fig. 24.6). Contrast radiography has been largely supplanted by endoscopy because of the ability to obtain biopsy material by the latter technique.

Computed tomography (CT) has been used both as a primary diagnostic method and to assess extragastric spread. When performed with intraluminal contrast, CT can reliably demonstrate infiltration of the gastric wall by tumor, gastric ulceration, and hepatic metastasis (Figs. 24.7 and

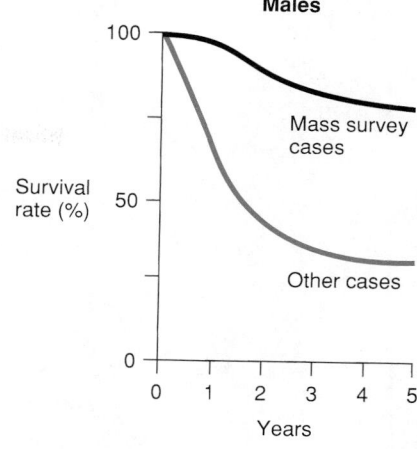

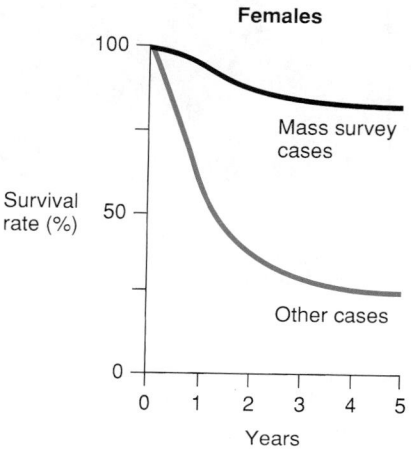

Figure 24.4. Early cancer survival rate in Japan.

24.8). The technique is less reliable with regard to invasion of adjacent organs or the presence of lymphatic metastases. In most series, involvement of adjacent organs has been overestimated by CT scanning (false-positive). Conversely, metastases to regional or distant lymph nodes have been underestimated (false-negative). One review estimated a 40% to 50% accuracy for CT scanning in preoperative local staging of gastric carcinoma (13). Because of these limitations, CT does not fulfill the requirements for

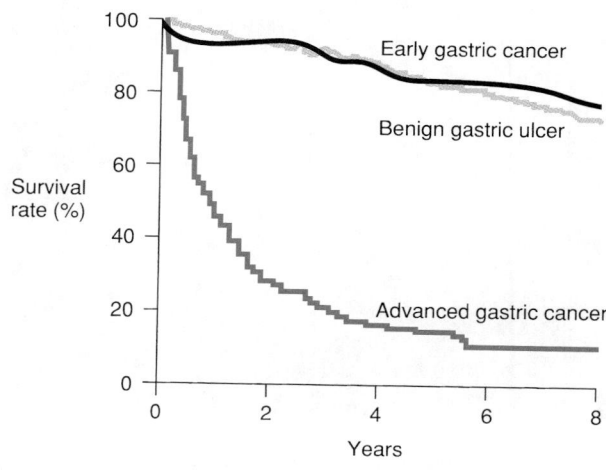

Figure 24.5. Early cancer survival rate in Europe.

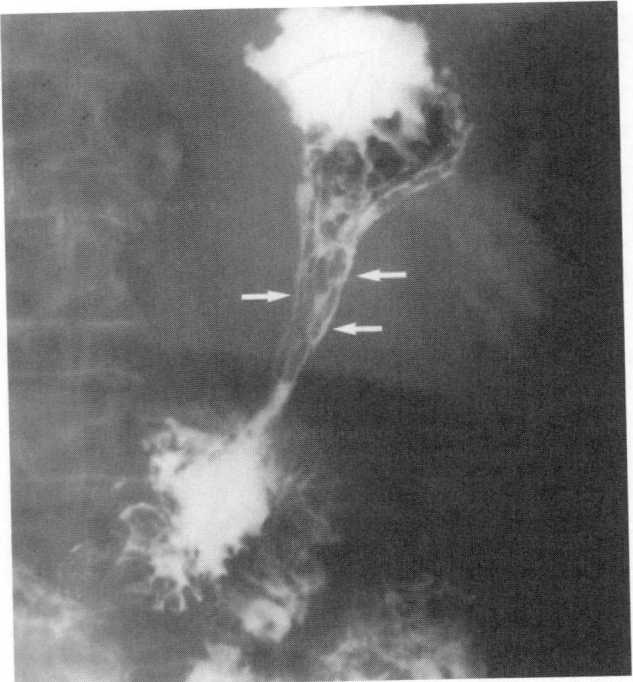

Figure 24.6. Barium contrast radiograph demonstrating extensive involvement of the gastric body by infiltrating adenocarcinoma (linitis plastica). The gastric silhouette is narrowed *(arrows)*, and the stomach is nondistensible.

a reliable staging method and usually does not eliminate the necessity for laparoscopy or laparotomy.

Endoscopically directed ultrasound is under investigation as another method of preoperative evaluation. Endoscopic ultrasound is excellent at delineating subepithelial lesions that may be confused with gastric cancer. Ultrasound-guided biopsy of subepithelial tumors is possible. Investigation of infiltrative gastric disorders, enlarged gastric epithelial folds, and differentiation of gastric lymphoma from gastric adenocarcinoma are each aided by endoscopic ultrasound. Initial reports indicate that the technique has the ability assess the depth and pattern of gastric wall penetration by gastric cancer, and has good correlation with intraoperative assessment and histologic

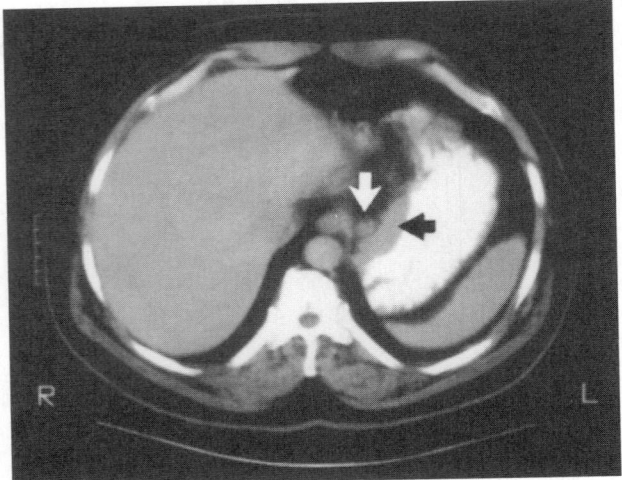

Figure 24.7. Computed tomography scan demonstrating mass along lesser curvature of the stomach *(black arrow)* and associated lymph node enlargement *(white arrow)*.

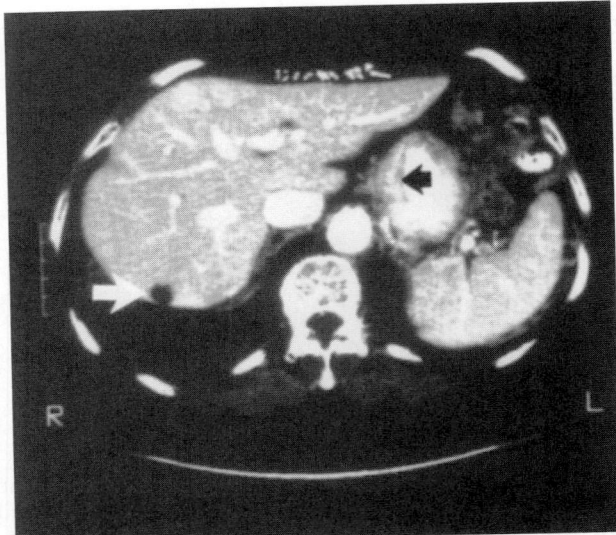

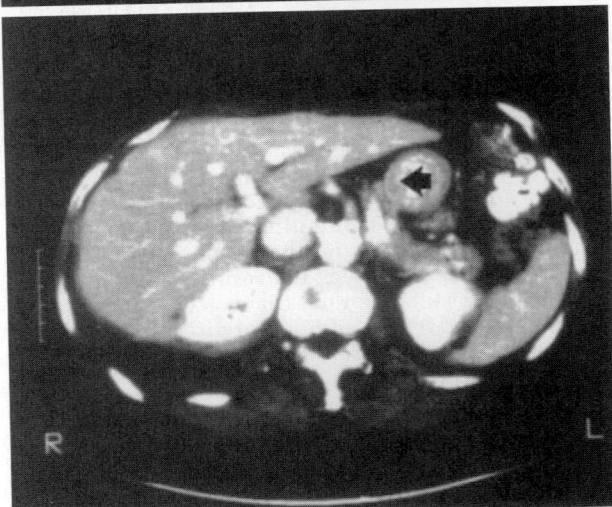

Figure 24.8. Computed tomography scans of the upper abdomen showing extensive thickening of the gastric wall *(black arrows)* caused by infiltrating adenocarcinoma and associated hepatic metastasis *(white arrow)*.

findings. Perigastric lymph nodes involved with tumor are reliably identified by endoscopic ultrasound. Because of a limited depth of tissue penetration, however, endoscopic ultrasound is unable to detect hepatic metastases; this inability is a major limitation in preoperative staging of patients with gastric cancer. Because of the inability to detect liver metastases, it seems likely that this method will continue to serve as an adjunct to standard methods of radiologic imaging.

Pathology

Gastric adenocarcinoma occurs in two distinct histologic subtypes—intestinal and diffuse. These subtypes are characterized by differing pathologic and clinical features and by differing patterns of metastatic spread.

In the intestinal form of gastric cancer, the malignant cells tend to form glands. The intestinal form of malignancy is more frequently associated with gastric mucosal atrophy, chronic gastritis, intestinal metaplasia, and dysplasia. Gastric cancer with the intestinal histologic subtype is more common in populations at high risk (e.g., Japan), and it occurs with increased frequency in men and older patients. Clinical studies suggest that this subtype more frequently demonstrates bloodborne metastases.

The diffuse form of gastric adenocarcinoma does not demonstrate gland formation and tends to infiltrate tissues as a sheet of loosely adherent cells. Lymphatic invasion is common. Intraperitoneal metastases are frequent. The diffuse form of gastric adenocarcinoma tends to occur in younger patients, in women, and in populations with a relatively low incidence of gastric cancer (e.g., the United States). The prognosis is less favorable for patients with the diffuse histologic subtype.

Efforts have been made to grade tumors on histologic criteria. Progressively anaplastic carcinomas are assigned higher grades. Not surprisingly, histologic grade correlates closely with 5-year survival; only 11% of grade IV patients survive 5 years, whereas 66% of grade I patients are alive 5 years after operation.

Gastric adenocarcinomas demonstrate a number of chromosomal and genetic abnormalities. Cytometric analysis reveals that gastric tumors with a large fraction of aneuploid cells (with a greater-than-normal amount of nuclear DNA) tend to be more highly infiltrative and have a poorer prognosis. Amplifications of both the *neu* and K-*ras* protooncogenes have been consistently detected in gastric adenocarcinomas. The mechanisms by which these genetic abnormalities contribute to gastric oncogenesis remain unclear. A number of growth factors, including epidermal growth factor, platelet-derived growth factor, and transforming growth factor-β, are overexpressed in gastric carcinoma cells (14).

In the United States, gastric adenocarcinomas occur with equal frequency in the proximal and distal regions of the stomach. In the 1990s, approximately 30% of cases have involved the proximal stomach, which is defined as the esophagogastric junction, fundus, or body, and an equal proportion have arisen in the antrum. In 10% of cases, the stomach is diffusely involved at the time of diagnosis (11). Proximal involvement is more common in elderly patients. The proportion of tumors involving the proximal stomach has dramatically increased over the

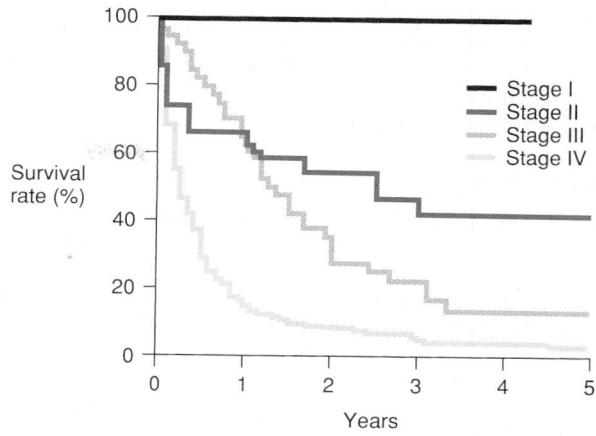

Figure 24.9. Survival rates of gastric cancer by stage.

past decades; in the 1960s, only 16% involved this region. Prognosis is distinctly less favorable for tumors arising from the proximal stomach or for those with diffuse involvement of the organ relative to antral tumors (15). The need to resect other organs in the upper abdomen, in addition to gastric resection, is also an unfavorable prognostic factor (16).

The gastric cancer staging format used by the American Joint Committee on Cancer is presented in Table 24.2. The staging system is oriented toward surgical and pathologic examinations but also accurately reflects prognosis (Fig. 24.9). A consideration of staging data illustrates the high frequency with which lymph node metastases are present at the time of diagnosis in the United States, and the severe impact lymphatic involvement has on survival. Even early gastric cancers have a 15% prevalence of nodal metastasis.

Curative Treatment

Surgical resection is the only hope for cure in gastric cancer, but an advanced stage of disease at the time of diagnosis precludes curative resection for most patients. The surgical objectives in gastric cancer must, therefore, be two: (a) to maximize chances for cure in patients with localized tumor, and (b) to provide effective and safe palliation to patients with advanced malignancy. Evolution of the surgical approach to gastric adenocarcinoma has focused on the following six issues: the ability of preoperative tests to detect metastatic disease, the extent of gastric resection needed for potentially curable lesions, the role of perigastric lymphadenectomy, the adequacy of proximal and distal resection margins, the role of splenectomy, and the implications of involvement of adjacent organs.

Laparoscopy

The ability of CT scanning to detect metastatic disease is limited, especially when tumor deposits are small. The surface of the liver, the omentum, and the peritoneal surfaces are common sites for gastric cancer metastasis that are difficult to evaluate preoperatively by CT scanning. The mean life expectancy of affected patients is 3 to 9 months, and most incurable patients can be treated with chemotherapy, radiation therapy, and nutritional support without the need for palliative surgical resection. Diagnostic laparoscopy has been used to provide accurate staging in this setting and to avoid nontherapeutic laparotomy. In approximately 25% of patients, laparoscopy detects distant disease that precludes curative resection (17,18).

Table 24.2. TNM CLASSIFICATION FOR STAGING OF GASTRIC ULCER

TNM DEFINITIONS

Primary Tumor

T1	Tumor confined to the mucosa
T2	Tumor involves the mucosa and submucosa, and extends to but does not penetrate serosa
T3	Tumor penetrates serosa with or without invasion of adjacent structures
T4	Diffuse involvement on gastric wall without obvious boundaries (linitis plastica)

Regional Lymph Node Involvement

N0	No nodal metatasis
N1	Metastasis to perigastric lymph nodes in immediate vicinity of tumor
M2	Metastasis to lymph nodes distant from primary tumor or along both curvatures of the stomach

Distant Metastasis

M0	No distant metastasis
M1	Metastasis beyond regional lymph nodes

STAGE GROUPING

Stage I	T1, N0, M0
Stage II	T2–3, N0, M0
Stage III	T1–3, N1–3, M0
Stage IV	Tumor unresectable or metastatic

The faster recovery and shorter hospitalization after laparoscopy relative to laparotomy are obvious benefits to patients with shortened life expectancy. In one study, no patients undergoing only laparoscopy required subsequent palliative surgery (19).

Laparotomy

Since the early 1980s, increasingly radical operations have been advocated for the treatment of gastric cancer, including total gastrectomy, extended subtotal gastrectomy with en bloc resection of celiac and splenic lymph nodes, splenectomy, and distal pancreatectomy. With time, it has become apparent that radical operations increase operative morbidity but do not improve survival. A prospective trial of various operations for the treatment of gastric cancer has not been performed, but reports from a number of institutions allow a consensus. For early lesions (N0–1, M0) of the antrum or middle stomach, distal subtotal gastrectomy including 80% of the stomach provides satisfactory 5-year survival rates without increasing operative morbidity. Proximal gastric lesions or larger middle stomach lesions may require total gastrectomy or esophagogastrectomy to encompass the tumor (Figs. 24.10 and 24.11). Regardless of the extent of gastric resection, patients with more advanced tumors fare poorly because of the increased likelihood of lymphatic and hematogenous spread.

The extent of gastric resection is determined, in part, by the need to obtain a resection margin free of microscopic disease. Microscopic involvement of the resection margin by tumor cells is associated with poor prognosis (11). Patients with positive surgical margins are at high risk for development of recurrent disease, and histologically positive margins are strongly correlated with the development of anastomotic recurrence. In contrast to colon cancer, gastric cancer frequently demonstrates extensive intramural spread. The propensity for intramural metastasis is related, in part, to the extensive anastomosing capillary and lymphatic network in the wall of the stomach. Retrospective studies suggest that a line of resection 6 cm from the tumor mass is necessary to ensure a low rate of anastomotic recurrence. Efforts to achieve even larger margins have not translated into improved survival.

Improvements in operative technique and in postoperative nutritional support have improved results of major gastric resection, especially total gastrectomy. Radical gastric operations can be performed with acceptable morbidity and low mortality rates in the older age groups at greatest risk for gastric cancer. Mortality rates for total gastrectomy range from 3% to 7% (20,21). Nutritional support in the immediate postoperative period is an important adjunctive measure as patients resume oral intake (22). Surgical reconstructions that interpose a small intestinal reservoir between the esophagus and the jejunum have been advocated after total gastrectomy, but provide no clear-cut nutritional benefit (23–26).

Because gastric cancer metastasizes so frequently to lymph nodes, radical extirpation of draining lymph nodes has been practiced as a therapeutic maneuver (27). The value of extended lymphadenectomy in the treatment of gastric adenocarcinoma is controversial. The first favorable experience was reported by Japanese surgeons and the Japanese Research Society for Gastric Cancer (28,29). In the original Japanese system, resections were characterized as follows:

R1—resection of stomach, omentum, and perigastric lymph nodes

R2—resection of stomach, omentum, and en bloc removal of the superior leaf of the transverse meso-

colon, the pancreatic capsule and lymph nodes along the branches of the celiac artery and in the infraduodenal and supraduodenal areas

R3—resection of the above structures plus lymph nodes along the aorta and esophagus, along with the spleen, and the tail of the pancreas, and skeletonization of vessels in the porta hepatis

Only retrospective studies of extended perigastric lymphadenectomy have been reported from Japan. Initial reports suggested an improvement of approximately 10%, stage for stage, for patients with advanced disease treated with R2 or R3 operations (28–31). The benefits of extended lymphadenectomy have not been confirmed in non-Japanese centers, and several randomized trials have failed to show a survival benefit for extended lymphadenectomy when the entire patient population was analyzed (32–36).

In addition, increasingly radical operations are accompanied by increased complication rates (37,38). One effect of extended lymphadenectomy appears to be "up-staging" of tumors; as more lymph nodes are removed, additional micrometastatic disease is discovered and patients are correctly placed in higher-stage categories with worse prognosis (39,40). Reciprocally, some patients who do not undergo extended lymphadenectomy will have undetected micrometastases and, because of progressive disease, will decrease the survivorship of the staging group to which they are assigned.

Histologically positive lymph nodes are frequently present in the splenic hilum and along the splenic artery, and routine splenectomy has been practiced in some centers. Splenectomy has not been demonstrated to improve outcome for similarly staged patients (41,42). Likewise, resection of the tail or body of the pancreas has not been demonstrated to improve survival. Resection of adjacent organs may be required for local control if direct invasion has occurred. In this circumstance, operative morbidity is increased, and the long-term survival rate is approximately 25% (43).

Palliative Treatment

When preoperative evaluation demonstrates disseminated disease, palliation of symptoms becomes a primary consideration. Palliation does not usually require surgery. Obstruction and bleeding can be managed nonoperatively by the use of endoscopic laser fulguration in selected patients. Dysphagia caused by proximal lesions and bleeding can be controlled in 80% of patients. Successful application of laser treatment requires adequate visualization, and it is hampered by circumferential tumor growth that impedes passage of the endoscope, by sharp angulation of the esophagogastric junction, and by lesions more than 6 cm long.

In the setting of metastatic gastric cancer, palliative resection does not improve survival. Nonetheless, resection appears to provide superior relief of symptoms, particularly dysphagia, compared with surgical bypass. Bypass of obstructing distal gastric cancers without resection provides relief to less than half of patients, and mean survival is less than 6 months. For proximal obstructing lesions, total gastrectomy with Roux-en-Y esophagojejunal reconstruction may be necessary. An operative mortality rate of less than 5% has been reported, and introduction of the EEA stapler has reduced the rate of anastomotic leaks to less than 5% in several series. Mean survival after palliative gastric resection approximates 9 months. For nonresectable gastric adenocarcinoma, when dysphagia is present, radiation therapy may have a significant palliative role.

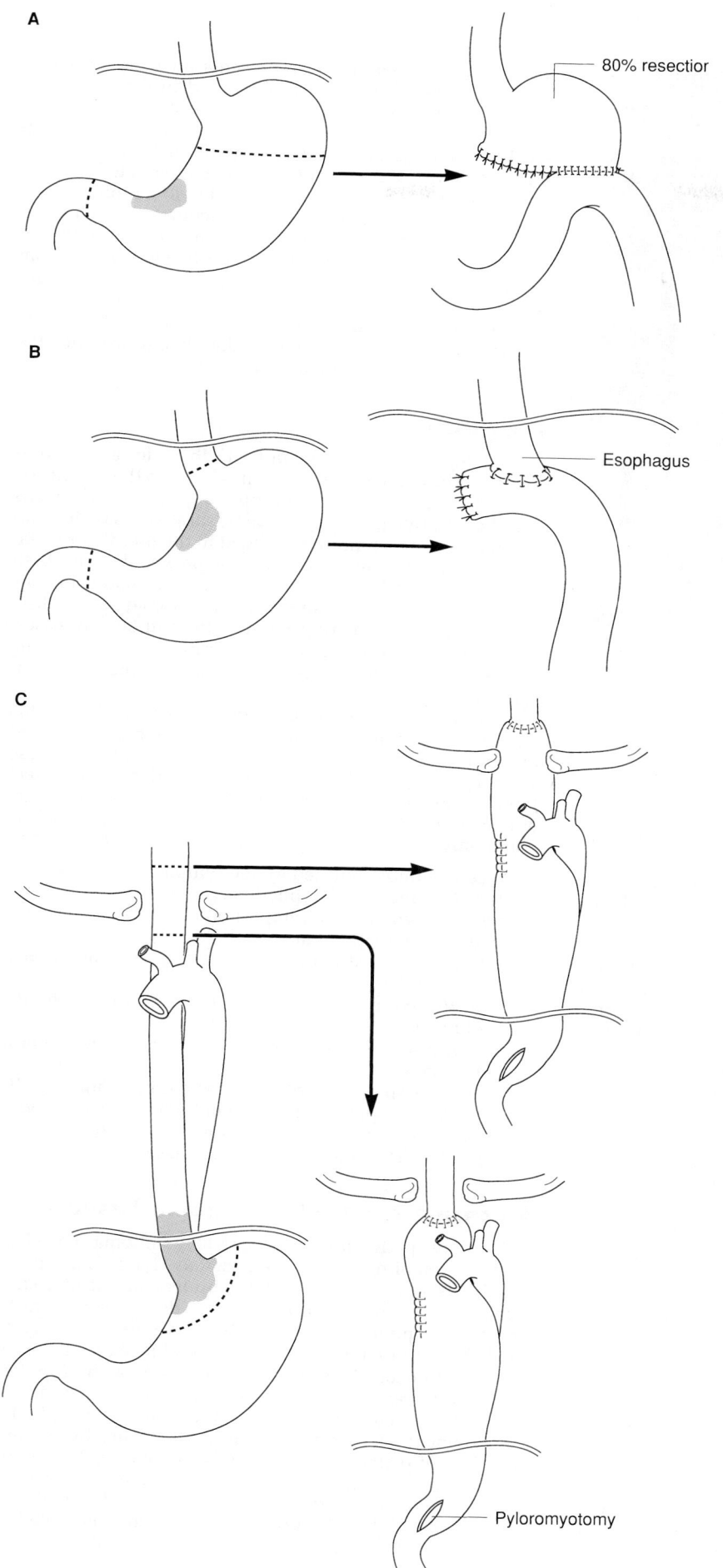

A

80% resection

B

Esophagus

C

Pyloromyotomy

Figure 24.10. Surgical options for resection of gastric neoplasms. (A) Subtotal gastrectomy with gastrojejunal reconstruction. (B) Total gastrectomy with esophagojejunostomy. (C) Esophagogastrectomy with anastomosis in cervical or thoracic position.

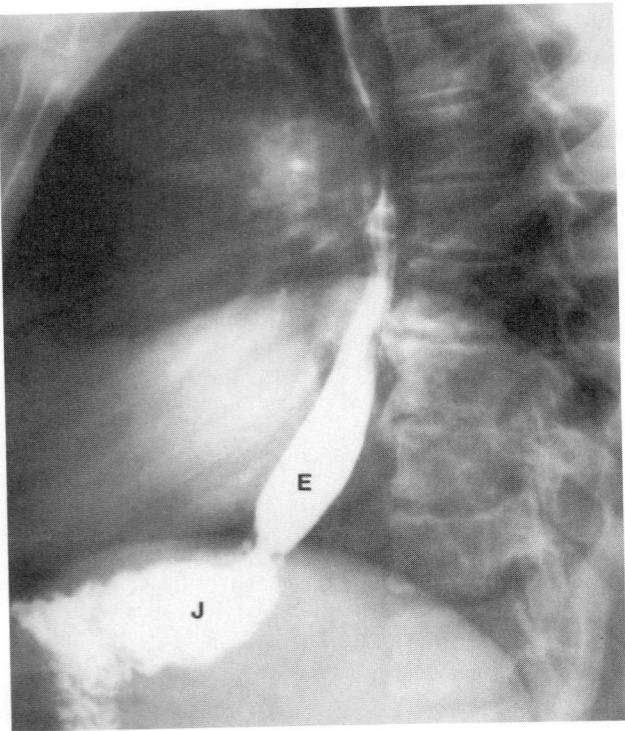

Figure 24.11. Postoperative radiograph after total gastrectomy with esophagojejunal anastomosis, showing esophagus *(E)* and jejunum *(J).*

Chemotherapy

Chemotherapy has limited efficacy in the treatment of patients with disseminated gastric adenocarcinoma. The drugs most commonly used in single-agent chemotherapy trials have been 5-fluorouracil (5-FU), mitomycin C, and doxorubicin. Few single-agent trials have partial response rates above 25% to 30%, and complete responses have not occurred (19). Because long-term survival can be expected only in patients who experience complete response, there has been no impact on patient survival from single-drug approaches. A number of trials have used FAM (the combination of 5-FU, doxorubicin, and mitomycin C) for the treatment of advanced gastric cancer, with an overall partial response rate of approximately 33%. The combination of 5-FU, doxorubicin, and cisplatin has been associated with improved response rates in some series, and complete response has been seen in 12% of treated patients. Increases in mean survival have not yet been proved with multiagent chemotherapy.

The addition of radiation therapy to chemotherapy has modest benefit. Single-agent adjuvant chemotherapy after potentially curative surgery for gastric adenocarcinoma has not proved beneficial. No definitive data are available to suggest that multiagent adjuvant combinations based on 5-FU are more effective than single agents, although several trials indicate that benefit may exist.

GASTRIC LYMPHOMA

Clinical Features

The stomach is the site of more than half of gastrointestinal lymphomas and is the most common organ involved in extranodal lymphomas. Non-Hodgkin's lymphomas account for approximately 5% of malignant gastric tumors; lymphoma represents an increasing proportion of gastric neoplasms diagnosed in the 1990s. Patients are considered to have primary gastric lymphoma if initial symptoms are gastric and the stomach is exclusively or predominantly involved with the tumor. Patients who do not fulfill these criteria are considered to have secondary gastric involvement from systemic lymphoma.

Gastric lymphoma is distinctly uncommon in children and young adults. The peak incidence is in the sixth and seventh decades. Symptoms are indistinguishable from those of gastric adenocarcinoma. Epigastric pain, weight loss, anorexia, nausea, and vomiting are common (44). Although gross bleeding is uncommon, occult hemorrhage and anemia are observed in more than half of patients. Patients rarely have spontaneous perforation.

Diagnosis

Radiologic findings are similar to those for adenocarcinoma. Endoscopic examination has become the diagnostic method of choice. The endoscopic appearance of lesions may be ulcerated, polypoid, or infiltrative. Gastric lymphoma is most commonly localized to the middle or distal stomach, and unusually involves the proximal stomach, in contrast to gastric adenocarcinoma. Endoscopic biopsy, combined with endoscopic brush cytology and ultrasonography, provides positive diagnosis in 90% of cases. Submucosal growth without ulceration of the overlying mucosa can occasionally render endoscopic biopsy nondiagnostic.

Endoscopic ultrasound-guided biopsy is useful in this circumstance. When gastric lymphoma is first diagnosed by endoscopic means, evidence of systemic disease should be sought. CT of the chest and abdomen (to detect lymphadenopathy), bone marrow biopsy, and biopsy of enlarged peripheral lymph nodes are all appropriate. The commonly used Ann Arbor staging system is as follows:

Stage I—tumor confined to one lymph node region
Stage IE—one extralymphatic organ or site
Stage II—two or more lymph node regions on the same side of the diaphragm
Stage IIE—one extralymphatic organ or site and criteria for stage II
Stage III—lymph node regions on both sides of the diaphragm
Stage IIIE—one extralymphatic organ or site and criteria for stage III
Stage IIIS—splenic involvement and criteria for stage III
Stage IIISE—splenic involvement and one extralymphatic organ or site and criteria for stage III
Stage IV—diffuse or disseminated disease

Mucosa-associated Lymphoma Tissue

The concept that low-grade gastric lymphomas have features resembling mucosa-associated lymphoid tissue (MALT) is a major advance in the understanding of gastric lymphomas. The gastric submucosa does not ordinarily contain lymphoid tissue, and the development of lymphoid tissue resembling small intestinal Peyer's patches is believed to occur in response to infection with *H. pylori* (44). A number of observations support a causal relationship between chronic *H. pylori* infection and lymphoma development. *H. pylori* is present in the stomachs of more than half of patients with gastric lymphoma (45). As with gastric adenocarcinoma, geographic regions with a high prevalence of *H. pylori* also have a high incidence of gastric lymphoma. Infection with *H. pylori* has been noted to precede development of gastric lymphoma (46).

After development of gastric lymphoid tissue, low-grade lymphoma is postulated to occur as a result of monoclonal B-cell proliferation. Initially, B-cell proliferation depends on interleukin-2 production by antigenically stimulated nonneoplastic T cells. Progressive genetic rearrangements lead to B-cell proliferation that is independent of *H. pylori*-stimulated interleukin-2. With cumulative genetic defects, low-grade MALT lymphoma progresses to high-grade MALT lymphoma.

Low-grade MALT lymphomas resemble Peyer's patches. Lymphoma cells invade between follicles and into gastric epithelium; invasion of gastric glands forms characteristic lymphoepithelial lesions. Low-grade lesions are often multifocal. Low-grade MALT lesions are less likely than high-grade tumors to invade transmurally, involve perigastric lymph nodes, or invade adjacent organs (47). High-grade MALT lymphomas cannot be distinguished histologically from non-MALT, high-grade B-cell lymphomas.

The concept that low-grade lymphoma depends on continued *H. pylori* antigenic stimulation supports eradication of *H. pylori* with antibiotics as first-line antineoplastic therapy. Complete regression of low-grade MALT lymphomas with antibiotic treatment has been reported in 70% to 100% of cases (48,49). The median time to complete response averaged 5 months (50). Most patients with partial responses were subsequently determined also to have foci of high-grade lymphoma. Radiation and chemotherapy have been proposed as salvage for antibiotic treatment failures.

Non-MALT Lymphomas

A multimodality treatment program is used in most centers for primary gastric lymphomas, with gastrectomy as the first step in the therapeutic strategy (51). This approach has evolved empirically, and prospective data to support it are lacking. Several advantages of this approach have been cited: (a) more accurate histologic evaluation is possible; (b) in cases with localized tumor, the procedure can be curative; and (c) gastrectomy eliminates the risk of life-threatening hemorrhage or perforation, which attends the treatment of tumors involving the full thickness of the gastric wall (52). The role of resection in the treatment of gastric lymphoma is controversial, and increasing numbers of patients are treated with chemoradiation therapy alone.

The risk of hemorrhage or perforation was frequently alluded to in the past as a motive for operative care, but the risk has probably been overstated. The incidence of perforation in primary gastric lymphomas that are treated with cytolytic agents in unresected patients approximates 5%. The use of endoscopic ultrasonography to detect full-thickness involvement of the gastric wall is being investigated to identify patients at risk for perforation.

If gastrectomy is performed before chemotherapy or radiation therapy, extended radical resections are not indicated. Unlike adenocarcinoma, microscopically positive resection margins do not predict local recurrence in cases of lymphoma when radiation therapy is administered after surgery. The postoperative mortality rate is under 5% and has been 0% in several recent series. In a limited number of patients with stage I disease, surgery is considered curative and no further therapy is required. Many authors have reported retrospectively that postoperative radiation to the gastrectomy bed improves local and regional control. With radiation doses ranging from 3,500 to 4,400 cGy, local recurrence was observed in less than 15% of treated patients.

In more than 30% of patients with stage II disease who undergo apparently adequate surgery and radiation therapy, the cancer recurs outside the treatment field. Patients with stage II primary gastric lymphoma should, therefore, be considered to have systemic disease and to require systemic therapy in addition to surgery or radiation therapy. The use of chemotherapy, either primarily or as postoperative adjuvant therapy, is rational and is supported by several retrospective reports. Survival for gastric lymphoma is closely linked to stage at diagnosis (Fig. 24.12).

GASTRIC CARCINOIDS

Gastric carcinoid tumors have been considered to be rare tumors, accounting for 3% to 5% of all gastrointestinal carcinoids, and only 0.3% of gastric neoplasms (53). The number of gastric carcinoids may have been underestimated in the past because of confusion with gastric carcinoma. In addition to an increased risk of adenocarcinoma, patients with pernicious anemia have an increased risk for development of gastric carcinoids. This association has suggested to several investigators that gastric carcinoids can develop as a result of chronic trophic stimulation by hypergastrinemia associated with pernicious anemia. Carcinoid tumors associated with pernicious anemia are localized to the gastric body or fundus. Histologically, the tumors appear as nests of monotonous hyperchromatic cells originating in the submucosa or in the basal area of gastric glands. Invasion, uncommon in small tumors, occurs with increasing frequency in tumors larger than 2 cm.

Most patients with small gastric carcinoids are asymptomatic. When viewed endoscopically at an early stage, carcinoids are reddish-pink to yellow submucosal nodules in the proximal stomach. Tumors are frequently multiple. Larger tumors can cause ulceration of the overlying mucosa; symptoms are similar to those of gastric ulcer or gastric adenocarcinoma. Endoscopic biopsy is usually diagnostic if deep enough to sample submucosal tumor cells.

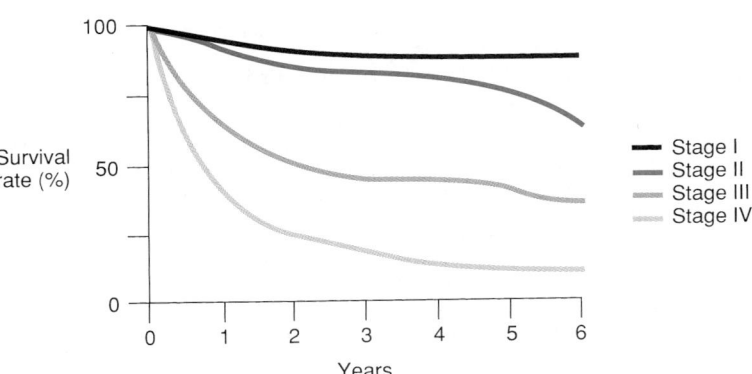

Figure 24.12. Survival rates of gastric lymphoma by stage.

Because of the potential for invasion, attempts at curative resection are indicated in almost all cases.

GASTRIC SARCOMAS

Sarcomas can arise from any of the mesenchymal components of the gastric wall, constituting approximately 3% of gastric malignancies. Leiomyosarcomas are predominant, whereas angiosarcomas and fibrosarcomas are rare. Leiomyosarcomas occur with equal frequency in both sexes in the sixth and seventh decades of life. The tumor frequently has prominent extraluminal growth and attains a large size before causing symptoms. Endoluminal growth or ulceration of the overlying mucosa due to ischemic necrosis can be associated with epigastric pain, weight loss, and gastrointestinal hemorrhage. Clinical symptoms are identical to those produced by adenocarcinoma. With large tumors, an epigastric mass can be detected by physical examination.

Leiomyosarcomas must be differentiated from their benign counterparts, leiomyomas. Benign smooth muscle tumors are often asymptomatic until they reach a large size. Symptoms related to mass effects with compression of adjacent structures are most frequent. Gastrointestinal hemorrhage can occur as a result of necrosis of overlying gastric mucosa. Endoscopic examination is usually negative if the major component of growth is extraluminal; umbilication of the mucosa can indicate an underlying mass. The presence and nature of symptoms should direct the need for surgical excision.

Grossly, the tumors are firm, gray-white masses; a pseudocapsule separating tumor from normal smooth muscle can occasionally be present. When the tumors reach a large size, central necrosis is common. Leiomyosarcomas are often graded histologically, with the frequency of mitotic figures the prime indicator of aggressive behavior. Lesions with more than 5 to 10 mitoses per 10 high-power fields demonstrate increased metastasis. With benign leiomyomas, mitoses are absent or rare.

Intraperitoneal sarcomatosis is frequent, as is local recurrence after resection. Metastasis occurs by the hematogenous route; thus, hepatic involvement is common. Lymphatic metastasis is observed in less than 10% of patients.

Leiomyosarcomas are not radiosensitive, and chemotherapy has not been shown to improve survival. Surgical resection has been the treatment of choice. *En bloc* resection of the tumor and involved structures should be attempted. Negative surgical margins must be ensured histologically, but extensive lymphadenectomy is not indicated because of the low frequency of lymphatic metastasis. The overall survival rate approximates 50%. Low-grade lesions have a significantly better prognosis (81% 5-year survival rate) than high-grade lesions (32%) (54).

REFERENCES

1. Silverberg E, Boring CC, Squires TS. Cancer statistics, 1990. *CA Cancer J Clin* 1990;40:9–26.
2. Boring CC, Squires TS, Tong T. Cancer statistics, 1993. *CA Cancer J Clin* 1993;43:19.
3. Harju E. Gastric polyposis and malignancy. *Br J Surg* 1986;73:532–533.
4. Parsonnet J, Friedman GD, Vandersteen DP, et al. *Helicobacter pylori* infection and the risk of gastric carcinoma. *N Engl J Med* 1991;325:1127–1131.
5. Nomura A, Stemmermann GN, Chyou P-H, et al. *Helicobacter pylori* infection and gastric carcinoma among Japanese Americans in Hawaii. *N Engl J Med* 1991;325:1132–1136.
6. Toftgaard C. Gastric cancer after peptic ulcer surgery: a historic prospective cohort investigation. *Ann Surg* 1989;210:159–164.
7. Lundegardh G, Adami H-O, Helmick C, et al. Stomach cancer after partial gastrectomy for benign ulcer disease. *N Engl J Med* 1988;319:195–200.
8. Greene FL. Management of gastric remnant carcinoma based on the results of a 15-year endoscopic screening program. *Ann Surg* 1996;223:701–708.
9. Newman F, Brennan MF, Hochwald SN, et al. Gastric remnant carcinoma: just another proximal gastric cancer or a unique entity? *Am J Surg* 1997;173:292–297.
10. Moreaux J, Bougaran J. Early gastric cancer: a 25-year surgical experience. *Ann Surg* 1993;217:347–355.
11. Wanebo HJ, Kennedy BJ, Chmiel J, et al. Cancer of the stomach: a patient-care study by the American College of Surgeons. *Ann Surg* 1993;218:583–592.
12. Endo M, Habu H. Clinical studies of early gastric cancer. *Hepatogastroenterology* 1990;37:408–410.
13. Rosch T, Classen M. Staging gastric cancer: the Munich experience. In: Van Dam J, Sivak MV, eds. *Gastrointestinal endosonography.* New York: WB Saunders, 1999:195–199.
14. Katano M, Nakumura M, Fujimoto K, et al. Prognostic value of platelet-derived growth factor-A (PDGF-A) in gastric carcinoma. *Ann Surg* 1998;227:365–371.
15. Harrison LE, Karpeh MS, Brennan MF. Proximal gastric cancers resected via a transabdominal-only approach. *Ann Surg* 1997;225:678–685.
16. Kodama I, Takamiya H, Mizutani K, et al. Gastrectomy with combined resection of other organs for carcinoma of the stomach with invasion to adjacent organs: clinical efficacy in a retrospective study. *J Am Coll Surg* 1997;184:16–22.
17. Lowy AM, Mansfield PF, Leach SD, et al. Laparoscopic staging for gastric cancer. *Surgery* 1996;119:611–614.
18. D'Ugo DM, Coppola R, Persiani R, et al. Immediately preoperative laparoscopic staging for gastric cancer. *Surg Endosc* 1996;10:996–999.
19. Burke EC, Karpeh MS Jr, Conlou KC. Laparoscopy in the management of gastric adenocarcinoma. *Ann Surg* 1997;225:262–267.
20. Bittner R, Butters M, Ulrich M, et al. Total gastrectomy: updated operative mortality and long-term survival with particular reference to patients older than 70 years of age. *Ann Surg* 1996;224:37–42.
21. Schwarz R, Karpeh MS, Brennan MF. Factors predicting hospitalization after operative treatment for gastric carcinoma in patients older than 70 years. *J Am Coll Surg* 1997;184:9–15.
22. Daly JM, Weintraub FN, Shou J, et al. Enteral nutrition during multimodality therapy in upper gastrointestinal cancer patients. *Ann Surg* 1995;221:327–338.
23. de Almeida ACM, dos Santos NM, Aldeia FJ. Long-term clinical and endoscopic assessment after total gastrectomy for cancer. *Surg Endosc* 1993;7:518–523.
24. Chareton B, Landen S, Manganus D, et al. Prospective randomized trial comparing Billroth I and Billroth II procedures for carcinoma of the gastric antrum. *J Am Coll Surg* 1993;183:190–194.
25. Nakane Y, Okumura S, Akehira K, et al. Jejunal pouch reconstruction after total gastrectomy for cancer: a randomized controlled trial. *Ann Surg* 1995;222:27–35.
26. Bozzetti F, Bonfanti G, Castellani R, et al. Comparing reconstruction with Roux-en-Y to a pouch following total gastrectomy. *J Am Coll Surg* 1996;183:243–248.
27. Shiu MH, Moore E, Sanders M, et al. Influence of the extent of resection on survival after curative treatment of gastric cancer: a retrospective multivariate analysis. *Arch Surg* 1987;122:1347–1351.
28. Maruyama K, Okabayashi K, Kinoshita T. Progress in gastric cancer in Japan and its limit of radicality. *World J Surg* 1987;11:418–425.
29. Noguchi Y, Imada T, Matsumoto A, et al. Radical surgery for gastric cancer: a review of the Japanese experience. *Cancer* 1989;64:2053–2062.
30. Adachi Y, Kamakura T, Mori M, et al. Role of lymph node dissection and splenectomy in node-positive gastric carcinoma. *Surgery* 1994;116:837–841.
31. Baba H, Maehara Y, Takeuchi H, et al. Effect of lymph node dissection on the prognosis in patients with node-negative early gastric cancer. *Surgery* 1994;117:165–169.
32. Maeta M, Yamashiro H, Saito S, et al. A prospective plot

study of extended (D3) and superextended para-aortic lymphadenectomy (D4) in patients with T3 or T4 gastric cancer managed by total gastrectomy. *Surgery* 1999;125:325–331.

33. Robertson CS, Chung SCS, Woods SDS, et al. A prospective randomized trial comparing R1 subtotal gastrectomy with R3 total gastrectomy for antral cancer. *Ann Surg* 1994;220; 176–182.

34. Bonekamp JJ, Hermans J, van de Velde CJH. Extended lymph-node dissection for gastric cancer. *N Engl J Med* 1999;340: 908–914.

35. Cushieri A, Fayers P, Fielding J, et al. Postoperative morbidity and mortality after D1 and D2 resections for gastric cancer. *Lancet* 1996;347:995–999.

36. Siewert JR, Bottcher K, Stein HJ, et al. Relevant prognostic factors in gastric cancer: ten-year results of the German gastric cancer study. *Ann Surg* 1998;228:449–461.

37. Adachi Y, Mimori K, Muri M, et al. Morbidity after D2 and D3 gastrectomy for node-positive gastric carcinoma. *J Am Coll Surg* 1997;184:240–244.

38. Hayer N, Ng EKW, Raimes SA, et al. Total gastrectomy with extended lymphadenectomy for "curable" stomach cancer: experience in a non-Japanese Asian center. *J Am Coll Surg* 1999;188:27–32.

39. Kodera Y, Yamamura Y, Shimizu Y, et al. The number of metastatic lymph nodes: a promising prognostic determinant for gastric carcinoma in the latest edition of the TNM classification. *J Am Coll Surg* 1998;187:579–603.

40. Clinical significance of occult micrometastasis in lymph nodes from patients with early gastric cancer who died of recurrence. *Surgery* 1996;119:397–402.

41. Stipa S, DiGiorgio A, Ferri M, et al. Results of curative gastrectomy for carcinoma. *J Am Coll Surg* 1994;179:567–572.

42. Otsuji E, Yamaguchi T, Sawai K, et al. End results of simultaneous splenectomy in patients undergoing total gastrectomy for gastric cancer. *Surgery* 1996;120:40–44.

43. Shchepotin IB, Chorny VA, Nauta RJ, et al. Extended surgical resection in T4 gastric cancer. *Am J Surg* 1998;175:123–126.

44. Isaacson PG. Gastrointestinal lymphoma. *Hum Pathol* 1994; 25:1020–1029.

45. Isaacson PG. Gastric lymphoma and *Helicobacter pylori*. *N Engl J Med* 1994;330:1310–1311.

46. Parsonnet J, Hansen S, Rodriguez L, et al. *Helicobacter pylori* infection and gastric lymphoma. *N Engl J Med* 1994;330: 1267–1271.

47. Montalban C, Castrillo JM, Abriapa V, et al. Gastric B-cell mucosa-associated lymphoid tissue (MALT): clinicopathological study and evaluation of the prognostic factors in patients. *Ann Oncol* 1995;6:798–799.

48. Bayerdorffer E, Neubauer A, Rudolph B, et al. Regression of primary gastric lymphoma of mucosa-associated lymphoid tissue type after cure of *Helicobacter pylori* infection. *Lancet* 1995;345:1591–1594.

49. Neubauer A, Thiede C, Morgner A, et al. Cure of *Helicobacter pylori* infection and duration of remission of low grade gastric mucosa associated lymphoid tissue lymphoma. *J Natl Cancer Inst* 1997;89:1350–1355.

50. Pinotti G, Zucca E, Roggero E, et al. Clinical features, treatment and outcome in a series of 93 patients with low grade gastric MALT lymphoma. *Leuk Lymphoma* 1997;26:527–537.

51. Stephens J, Smith J. Treatment of primary gastric lymphoma and gastric mucosa-associated lymphoid tissue lymphoma. *Am Coll Surg* 1998;178:312–320.

52. Bartlett DL, Karpeh MS, Filippa DA, et al. Long-term follow-up after curative surgery for early gastric lymphoma. *Ann Surg* 1996;223:53–62.

53. Creutzfeldt W. The achlorhydria–carcinoid sequence: role of gastrin. *Digestion* 1988;39:61–79.

54. Shiu M, Farr G, Papachristou D. Myosarcomas of the stomach: natural history, prognostic factors, and management. *Cancer* 1982;48:177–187.

SECTION D

SMALL INTESTINE

SURGERY: SCIENTIFIC PRINCIPLES AND PRACTICE, Third Edition, edited by
Lazar J. Greenfield, Michael W. Mulholland, Keith T. Oldham, Gerald B. Zelenock,
and Keith D. Lillemoe. Lippincott Williams & Wilkins Publishers, Philadelphia, © 2001.

CHAPTER 25

ANATOMY AND PHYSIOLOGY OF THE SMALL INTESTINE

DIANE M. SIMEONE

The small intestine is the longest organ of the gastrointestinal tract, extending from the duodenal bulb to the ileocecal valve. The functions of the small intestine are diverse. Two key functions of the small intestine are absorption of nutrients from the intestinal lumen and maintaining a balance between the absorption and secretion of water and electrolytes. By virtue of its vast surface area exposed to the outside environment, the small intestine is an important immunologic defense barrier. In addition, the small intestine serves as the largest and most complex endocrine organ in the body.

GROSS ANATOMY

Duodenum

The duodenum is the first and widest portion of the small intestine, measuring approximately 25 cm from the pylorus to the ligament of Treitz, the site where the jejunum begins. The duodenum is divided into four parts: the bulb, followed by the second (descending), third (transverse), and fourth (ascending) portions. The duodenal bulb, or cap, is invested with mesentery and slopes in a slightly cephalad direction from the pylorus. The mucosal surface of the bulb is smooth. The bulb is 5 cm long and is the site of most duodenal ulcers. Posterior to it is the head of the pancreas, portal vein, common bile duct, and the gastroduodenal artery.

The second (descending) portion of the duodenum courses posteriorly and caudally from the duodenal cap along the right side of the bodies of the L1 and L2 vertebra. The second portion of the duodenum becomes a retroperitoneal structure as it courses posteriorly. The head of the pancreas is in direct contact with the medial portion of the descending duodenum. The descending duodenum directly overlies Gerota's fascia and, more medially, the right renal vein and inferior vena cava. Incision of the peritoneum lateral to the second portion of the duodenum allows elevation of the duodenum and pancreatic head. This mobilization, referred to as the Kocher maneuver, allows palpation of the anteroposterior aspect of the head of the pancreas. The descending portion of the duodenum is approximately 10 cm long. The transition from the duodenal bulb to the descending duodenum is marked by the appearance of concentric mucosal folds known as Kerckring folds (plicae circulares), which are 1 to 3 mm high and spaced 2 to 4 mm apart with smooth mucosa intervening between the folds. The common bile duct, lying either within the substance of the pancreas or in a retropancreatic position, descends along the posteromedial surface of the duodenum; it is joined by the pancreatic duct before the two traverse the duodenal wall and open into its lumen as the major ampulla of Vater (duct of Wirsung). The ampulla of Vater is typically 7 to 10 cm from the pylorus and appears as a small, nipple-like structure marked by a longitudinal duodenal fold. The minor papilla (duct of Santorini) can be seen endoscopically in approximately half of cases, appearing as a 1- to 3-mm polypoid structure.

The third and fourth portions of the duodenum complete the duodenal sweep. The third part of the duodenum is almost completely retroperitoneal. It is intimately attached to the uncinate process of the pancreas and extends from the second part of the duodenum to the third lumbar vertebra directly over the aorta. The third portion of the duodenum is directly posterior to the hepatic flexure of the colon, and care must be taken to avoid injury to this part of the duodenum during mobilization of the hepatic flexure for colon resection. The third portion of the duodenum passes between the superior mesenteric artery anteriorly and the aorta, which lies posteriorly. This point marks the transition from the third to the fourth part of the duodenum. The fourth portion of the duodenum ascends superiorly and obliquely to the left of the aorta along the lower border of the pancreas, reaching as high as the L2 vertebra. It reaches the ligament of Treitz, which extends downward from the right crus of the diaphragm in front of the aorta and behind the pancreas to attach to the outer wall of the duodenojejunal flexure. The duodenum is separated from the jejunum by the ligament of Treitz.

Jejunum and Ileum

There is no clear anatomic boundary between the jejunum and ileum, and the proximal two fifths of the small intestine distal to the ligament of Treitz has been arbitrarily defined as *jejunum* and the distal three fifths as *ileum.* Their combined length varies from 5 to 10 m, with an average length of 7 m. Both the jejunum and ileum are invested in mesentery. The jejunum is slightly wider than the ileum and has a thicker wall because of its thick mucosal lining. The mucosa of the jejunum is characterized by prominent plicae circulares that become shorter and less frequent in the ileum. The diameter of the ileum progressively decreases as it approaches the ileocecal valve.

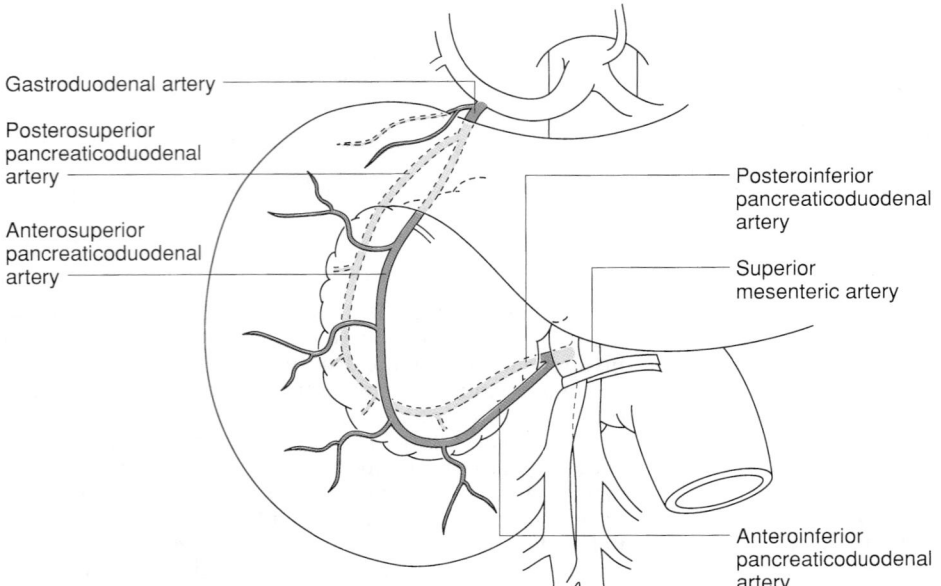

Gastroduodenal artery

Posterosuperior
pancreaticoduodenal
artery

Anterosuperior
pancreaticoduodenal
artery

Posteroinferior
pancreaticoduodenal
artery

Superior
mesenteric artery

Anteroinferior
pancreaticoduodenal
artery

Figure 25.1. Arterial supply to the duodenum.

The ileocecal valve exhibits motor characteristics separate from the terminal ileum and colon, postulated to prevent reflux of fecal material from the colon into the small intestine. The difference in bacterial flora between the terminal ileum and cecum demonstrates the ability of this region to prevent reflux. In humans, distention of the terminal ileum causes relaxation of the ileocecal valve and distention of the colon causes increased tone, suggesting that the valve may possess sphincteric function (1).

The mesentery suspends the jejunum and ileum from the posterior abdominal wall. The base, or root, of the mesentery attached to the posterior abdominal wall is approximately 15 cm long and extends from the ligament of Treitz to left of the L2 vertebra down toward the right sacroiliac joint. The broad-based mesentery tethers the small intestine, preventing kinking of its blood supply.

ARTERIAL BLOOD SUPPLY

The blood supply to the duodenal bulb comes directly from the hepatic artery as well as the gastroduodenal artery as it branches from the hepatic artery. The second and third portions of the duodenum share a common blood supply with the head of the pancreas. The anterosuperior and posterosuperior pancreaticoduodenal arteries arise from the gastroduodenal artery, and the anteroinferior and posteroinferior pancreaticoduodenal arteries branch from the superior mesenteric artery. The first jejunal branch of the superior mesenteric artery supplies the jejunum just beyond the ligament of Treitz and sends small branches back to the fourth portion of the duodenum (Fig. 25.1).

The superior mesenteric artery also supplies the jejunum and ileum through a series of branches that form arcades in the mesentery. The intestinal arteries (vasa recta) arise from the most peripheral arcades and run directly to the intestine without anastomosing. The vasa recta bifurcate as they reach the intestinal wall. The vascular pattern in the mesentery can help distinguish the jejunum from the ileum—in the jejunum, the vasa recta are straight and long, whereas in the ileum, the vasa recta are shorter with greater arborization (Fig. 25.2).

A

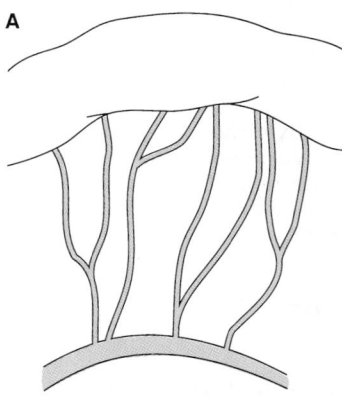

B

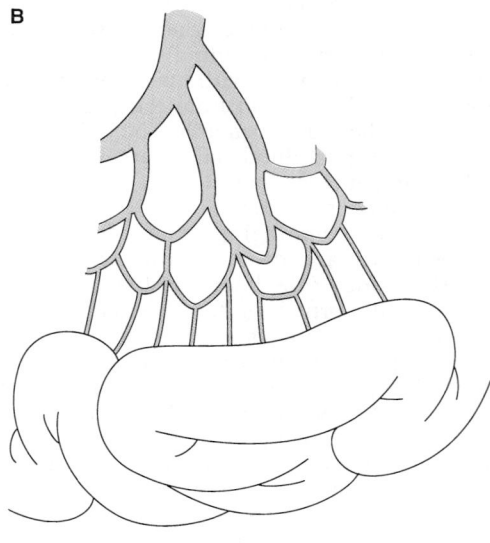

Figure 25.2. Contrasting vasa recta of jejunum *(A)* and ileum *(B)*.

VENOUS AND LYMPHATIC DRAINAGE

The venous drainage of the duodenum, in general, follows the arterial supply. There are anterior and posterior venous arcades that parallel the arterial arcades. Several small branches that drain the duodenal bulb empty into either the pancreaticoduodenal, right gastroepiploic, or portal vein. One of these venous branches, the prepyloric vein, is a landmark for the pylorus (2). The general pattern of venous drainage of the jejunum and ileum is the same as the arterial supply. The major venous drainage route is by the superior mesenteric vein, which joins the splenic vein to empty into the portal vein.

The lymphatics of the small intestine follow the blood vessels, and lymph is filtered through several levels of lymph nodes; the first set is located adjacent to the bowel wall, the second set is adjacent to the mesenteric arcades, and the third set lies along the trunk of the superior mesenteric artery. The duodenum may also drain into lymph nodes along the celiac artery. These mesenteric lymph nodes ultimately drain into the cisterna chyli and thoracic duct. Lymphatics of the small intestine are unique because they participate in absorption of fat. Lymphatics in the small intestinal mesentery may appear milky white because of the presence of emulsified fat in the lymph.

INNERVATION

The small intestine contains a complex, intrinsic nervous system referred to as the enteric nervous system (ENS). The ENS is a network of approximately 10 to 100 million neurons with cell bodies in the bowel wall, containing as many neurons as the spinal cord (3). The ENS is distinct from the autonomic nervous system, and is unique in its ability to mediate reflex activity even when isolated from the central nervous system. The ENS contains two major plexuses, the myenteric (Auerbach's) plexus, located between the longitudinal and circular muscle layers, and the submucous (Meissner's) plexus. Enteric neurons have extensive connections with each other, intestinal smooth muscle cells, epithelial cells, endocrine cells, extrinsic neurons, as well as the vasculature (Fig. 25.3). Through these connections, the ENS provides neural control of all gastrointestinal functions, including motility, blood flow, secretion, and absorption (4). The chemical mediators in the ENS were initially thought to be limited to neurotransmitters such as acetylcholine and serotonin; however, subsequent research has added purines to the list, such as adenosine triphosphate (ATP), and peptides, such as vasoactive intestinal peptide, somatostatin, and substance P. More recently, nitric oxide has also been identified as a neurotransmitter in the ENS. Over 20 candidate neurotransmitters have now been identified in enteric neurons (5).

The extrinsic autonomic innervation of the small intestine consists of components of the parasympathetic and sympathetic systems. Parasympathetic efferent fibers arise from the vagus and pass through the celiac and superior mesenteric ganglia; their postganglionic cell bodies are located in the enteric ganglia. Parasympathetic efferent fibers, in general, increase peristaltic activity and intestinal secretion. The function of the vagal afferent fibers is largely unknown, although they are believed to mediate feelings of nausea and distention and may be involved in visceral reflexes, such as the gastrocecal reflex, which activates discharge of ileal contents into the cecum when food enters the stomach (2). Sympathetic efferent fibers travel in the splanchnic nerves and synapse in the superior mesenteric ganglia. They function to inhibit motility

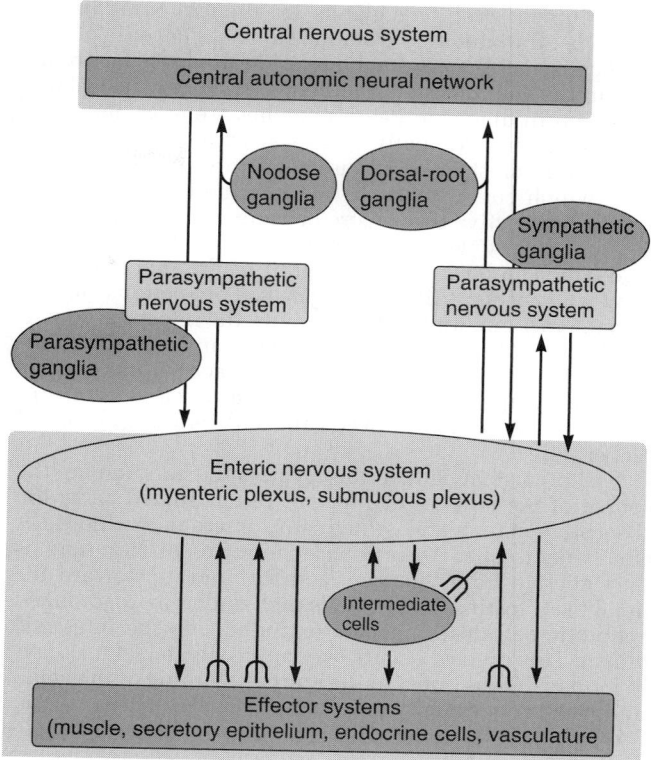

Figure 25.3. Innervation of the gastrointestinal tract. The neural plexuses in the gut represent an independently functioning network, the enteric nervous system, which is connected to the central autonomic neural network in the central nervous system by parasympathetic and sympathetic nerves. The enteric nervous system may influence the effector system in the gut directly, or indirectly through its actions on intermediate cells, which include endocrine cells and cells of the immune system. The cell bodies of the primary vagal and primary splanchnic afferent neurons are located in the nodose ganglia and dorsal root ganglia, respectively; each carries distinct information from the gut to the central nervous system. The symbol (*pitchfork*) represent afferent nerve endings, and the *arrows* show the direction of neural transmission. (From Goyal RK. Mechanisms of disease: the enteric nervous system. *N Engl J Med* 1996;334:1106.)

and secretory activity, although their most marked effect is to cause vasoconstriction. Pain from the intestine is mediated by sympathetic afferent fibers.

MICROSCOPIC ANATOMY

The wall of the small intestine is composed of four concentric layers: the serosa, muscularis, submucosa, and mucosa. The serosa, or outer coat, consists of a thin layer of mesothelial cells overlying loose connective tissue. The serosa covers only the anterior surface of the retroperitoneal segments of small bowel, but completely covers the portions of small bowel that are invested with mesentery. The muscularis consists of an inner circular and an outer longitudinal muscle layer. Between the muscle layers lies the myenteric (Auerbach's) plexus. The muscular layers are responsible for coordinating peristaltic movements.

The submucosa is a dense connective tissue layer just below the mucosa that has a rich network of blood vessels, nerves, and lymphatics. The submucosa contains Meissner's plexus. It is the strongest layer of the intestinal wall. Brunner's glands are found in the submucosa of the duodenum and secrete mucus and bicarbonate into the small bowel lumen. Brunner's glands are thought to be important in neutralizing acid from the stomach. Peyer's patches are localized collections of lymphoid follicles most prominent in the submucosa of the ileum. They may be as large as 10 mm in diameter. Peyer's patches are most abundant in early life and gradually disappear with old age.

The innermost layer of the small intestine is the mucosa, which consists of a layer of epithelial cells overlying the connective tissue core or lamina propria and resting on a narrow layer of smooth muscle, the muscularis mucosae. The basic structural unit of the mucosa is the crypt and villus. Villi are finger-like projections of mucosa 0.5 to 1 mm high extending into the intestinal lumen that have a columnar epithelial surface and a cellular connective tissue core of lamina propria. Each villus contains a central lymphatic (lacteal), a small artery and vein, and a capillary network. Between the villi are the crypts of Lieberkühn.

Anchored stem cells in the crypts of Lieberkühn are the source of the four major types of differentiated cells: the absorptive enterocyte, goblet cells, enteroendocrine cells, and Paneth cells. Absorptive enterocytes differentiate as they migrate from the crypt compartment up toward the tip of the intestinal villus. Cells then undergo programmed apoptotic cell death and are extruded into the intestinal lumen. This process occurs over approximately 4 to 5 days in humans. Thus, most of the epithelial lining of the small intestine is continually renewed at a relatively rapid rate.

Despite the rapid rate of cellular turnover, intestinal epithelial cells exhibit complex patterns of gene expression that vary according to their location on the two main spatial axes of the gut, the vertical (crypt–villus) and horizontal axis (proximal to distal). For example, cells destined to become enterocytes do not begin to express a variety of genes important in digestion and absorption until the cells have migrated out of the crypt and up the villus. In addition, many epithelial cell genes are selectively expressed in the proximal small intestine, whereas other genes are specifically expressed only in the ileum (6).

Columnar epithelial cells are responsible for absorption and secretion and constitute 90% of the cells on the villus. These cells are 22 to 26 μm high with basally located nuclei. The apices of these cells have microvilli, produced by numerous folds in the apical membrane that account for the brush border appearance. The surface of the microvilli is covered by a filamental coat called the *glycocalyx*. This coat represents external extensions of proteins and glycoproteins rooted in the cell membrane that are essential for digestion and absorption (7). The lateral membranes of neighboring enterocytes are connected by tight junctions, an apparent fusion of adjoining plasma membranes just below the level of the brush border. Movement of ions and water can occur by either a transmembrane or a paracellular route through tight junctions, which behave as selective pores.

Mucus-secreting goblet cells are present in both the crypts and villi. They are referred to as *goblet cells* because of their morphologic appearance, with a narrow base and wide apical membrane. Goblet cells have a basal nucleus and a large number of apical granules containing

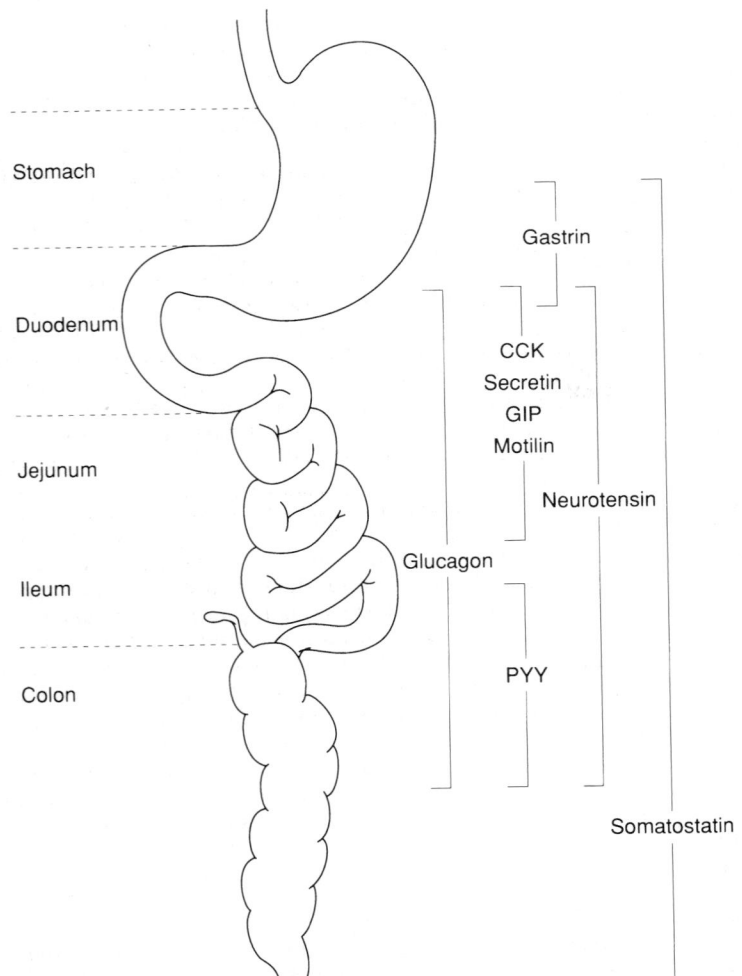

Figure 25.4. Distribution of peptide hormones in the gastrointestinal tract.

mucin. Mucin secreted by the goblet cell functions as a lubricant and has a cytoprotective function.

Paneth cells are pyramidal cells that reside in the crypt base. They contain large eosinophilic secretory granules located at their apical surface. Their life span is approximately 4 weeks, much longer than the life span of the enterocyte. It has been suggested that Paneth cells play a role in host defense based on their abundant expression of lysozyme and defensins, a family of small peptides that are found in human neutrophils. However, examination of the role of Paneth cells in the small intestine by lineage ablation in transgenic mice revealed no alteration in host defense mechanisms, and therefore the exact role of Paneth cells has yet to be determined (8).

There are multiple types of enteroendocrine cells in the mucosa that are characterized by their specific hormonal products. Enteroendocrine (also referred to as *amine precursor uptake and decarboxylation,* or *APUD*) cells may reside in the either the crypts or villi, depending on the particular neuroendocrine substance they produce. Specific areas of the small intestine have higher concentrations of specific neuroendocrine substances than other areas (Fig. 25.4). Unlike exocrine cells, which secrete apically into the lumen, endocrine cells are oriented for secretion toward the basement membrane. Their secretory granules are located below the nucleus near the basement membrane.

PHYSIOLOGY

Motility

One of the major functions of the small intestine is to process and absorb nutrients. Although neural and hormonal factors are important in modulating motility, the primary control mechanism is myogenic. The intestinal smooth muscle cell has a normal resting membrane potential of −50 to 70 mV, which is maintained by Na^+-K^+-ATPase activity (9). In humans, rhythmic fluctuations of the membrane potential of smooth muscle cells occur, resulting in slow-wave activity, also referred to as basic electrical rhythm, or pacemaker potential. The rhythmic depolarizations are thought to be generated by an oscillating electrogenic sodium pump and do not themselves cause muscle contraction. They occur 11 to 13 times per minute in the duodenum and decrease to 8 to 10 times per minute in the ileum. Specialized, low-resistance cell-to-cell connections (gap junctions or nexuses) couple electrical activity between cells, allowing the distal portion of the small intestine to be entrained by the higher frequencies of the proximal small intestine. The regional variation in velocity is advantageous for digestion. In the proximal intestine, nutrients are propelled more rapidly over a large surface area for more rapid absorption and digestion. Propulsion is slower in the ileum to permit absorption of more slowly digested substances, such as bile salts and fats. With neural or chemical stimulation, membrane depolarization exceeds a certain excitation threshold and a contraction results (Fig. 25.5). The electrical correlate of the contraction is called the *spike potential.* Spike potentials occur only during the depolarization phase of the slow-wave activity. Although both the spatial and temporal pattern of contractile activity are under myogenic control, whether a contraction occurs at all depends on local neurochemical stimulation. This allows modulation of the amplitude, duration, frequency, and distance of contractions by mechanisms outside of the gut.

After a meal, two gross patterns of small intestinal contraction result: segmentation and peristalsis. Contraction of the circular muscle divides the small intestine into seg-

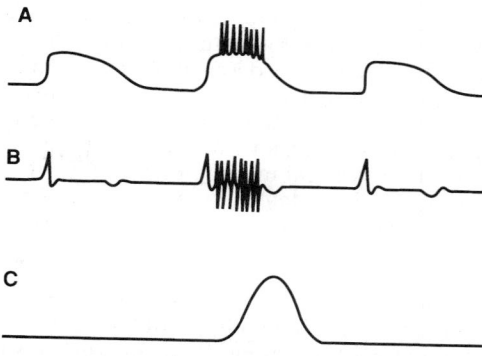

Figure 25.5. *(A)* Recording of transmembrane potential showing slow waves and superimposed spike potentials. *(B)* Extracellular recording of electrical activity represented in *(A)*. *(C)* Muscular contraction in response to electrical activity in *(A)*. (After Christianson J. The control of gastrointestinal movements: some old and new views. *N Engl J Med* 1971;285:85.)

ments, which allows local churning and circulation of chyme to promote optimal digestion and absorption. Contents of adjacent segments mix, and the process repeats itself. Peristalsis consists of a wavelike propagation of a reflex that consists of contraction proximal and relaxation distal to a bolus of food (10). Circular muscle also initiates peristalsis, with contractions propelling intestinal contents in an aboral direction. Food empties from the stomach and passes from proximal to distal small intestine.

In healthy humans, the mean transit time in the small intestine documented by scintigraphic studies is 221 ± 49 minutes, with a range of 131 to 322 minutes (11). The composition of the meal affects the rate of occurrence and propagation of contractions during the postprandial period; frequency of contraction is greatest with meals containing glucose and least after meals high in fat. Therefore, transit is regulated to optimize absorption of nutrients.

During fasting, the bowel undergoes a cyclic pattern of phasic contractions called the *migrating motor complex* (MMC). The MMC originates in either the stomach or proximal small intestine, migrates aborally along the intestine to the distal ileum, and cycles every 90 to 120 minutes. The MMC is referred to as the *intestinal housekeeper,* and the presumed role of the MMC is to propel sloughed enterocytes, undigested food particles, and mucus into the colon (12,13). The MMC is divided into four distinct phases. Phase I is an interval of contractile quiescence; phase II consists of accelerating, intermittent contractions; phase III consists of a series of high-amplitude contractions that occur at a maximum frequency for 6 to 8 minutes. Phase IV is a short transition of intermittent contractions. The overall control of the MMC seems to reside in periodic activation of the ENS. Simple transection of the small intestine disrupts the normal migration of the MMC along the length of the bowel. The central and autonomic nervous systems only modulate MMC, especially under periods of stress, because MMC cycling is not abolished with vagotomy, interruption of the splanchnic nerves, or even total extrinsic denervation (14–16).

Available evidence indicates that induction of phase III complexes results from secretion of the peptide motilin by enteroendocrine cells in the duodenum (17,18). Other peptides that have serum levels that cycle with MMC activity are somatostatin and pancreatic polypeptide; however, it is unclear whether either of these two peptides is a physiologic mediator of the cycle (19,20). Other substances that may modulate intestinal MMC activity are serotonin and opioids.

The ENS plays a vital role in the organization of contractile patterns. Most of the neurons controlling contractile activity have their cell bodies in the myenteric plexus. The submucous (Meissner's) plexus also contains ganglia, but appears to have a much smaller role in regulating motility, instead playing an important part in secretory control. Several intestinal motility disorders have been attributed to deficient or defective enteric neurons, including chronic intestinal pseudoobstruction and diabetic dysmotility.

Small intestinal motility may be modulated by gastrointestinal hormones, although their exact physiologic role is not well understood. Cholecystokinin (CCK), gastrin, and motilin stimulate intestinal motility. Gut peptides that inhibit intestinal motility include peptide YY (PYY) and enteroglucagon.

Digestion and Absorption

Absorption of Water and Electrolytes

The intestine has a remarkable ability to absorb and secrete large quantities of fluid. Absorption of water is a net result of fluxes into and out of the intestinal lumen. Approximately 8 to 10 L of fluid is presented to the small intestine each day, of which 1 to 2 L of water is oral intake, with an additional 5 to 10 L in the form of salivary (1 to 2 L), gastric (2 to 3 L), biliary (0.5 L), pancreatic (1 to 2 L), and intestinal secretions (1 L). Eighty percent of this fluid is absorbed in the small intestine, whereas the colon absorbs most of the remaining fluid, with a small amount (0.1 L) excreted in the stool. The balance between intestinal absorption and secretion of water is tightly regulated so that there is normally net absorption of fluid. Alterations in this fine balance, due to either impaired absorption or augmented secretion, can result in overall net secretion of water and diarrhea.

Water absorption is controlled indirectly through regulation of electrolyte transport. Fluid follows the direction of electrolyte movement to maintain isotonicity between the intestinal lumen and the tissue compartments. Water is absorbed passively by either a paracellular route (through tight junctions between enterocytes) or by a transcellular route. Water absorption in the proximal small intestine tends to be by paracellular transit because of higher tight junction permeability. The transcellular route is thought to be more important in the distal small bowel and colon, where tight junction permeability is decreased. Evidence suggests that an important method of transcellular water flux is through direct coupling to active transport of electrolytes and solutes (21,22).

There are three basic mechanisms of sodium absorption: (a) solute-coupled Na⁺ absorption, (b) electroneutral NaCl absorption, and (c) electrogenic Na⁺ absorption independent of other solutes or ions. Cotransport of Na⁺ with organic solutes and electroneutral NaCl absorption account for most or all of Na⁺ absorption in the small intestine. Electrogenic Na⁺ absorption through Na⁺ channels occurs primarily in the colon. In each case, Na⁺ absorbed across the apical membrane is extruded across the basolateral membrane by the Na⁺-K⁺-ATPase pump. In the presence of ATP, the Na⁺-K⁺-ATPase pump catalyzes the outward movement of three Na⁺ ions coupled with the inward movement of two K⁺ ions, maintaining a relatively low intracellular Na⁺ concentration.

The absorption of many nutrients, including glucose, amino acids, dipeptides and tripeptides, and bile acids is mediated by Na⁺ cotransporters in the small intestine (Fig. 25.6A). Luminal Na⁺ enters the cell and then exits through the basolateral Na⁺-K⁺-ATPase. The energy generated by the electrochemical gradient for Na⁺ drives intracellular accumulation of the organic solute.

Electroneutral NaCl absorption is a process that couples two neutral ion countertransport mechanisms, one that exchanges Na⁺ for H⁺ and another that exchanges Cl⁻ for HCO₃⁻ (Fig. 25.6B). This exchange results in entry of NaCl into the cell in exchange for H⁺ and HCO₃⁻ efflux. This electroneutral exchange reaction is important in intracellular pH regulation as well as Na⁺ transport. Less evidence supports direct Na⁺/Cl⁻ cotransport in mammalian small intestinal epithelial cells (23).

Chloride ion absorption occurs primarily through electroneutral Na⁺ absorption. Chloride may also be absorbed through paracellular spaces because the interstitial space is slightly electrically positive compared with the intestinal lumen. Chloride is the principal ion governing secretion. Chloride secretion occurs through apical Cl⁻ channels, and is regulated by the intracellular second messengers cyclic adenosine monophosphate and calcium. Metabolic studies reveal that approximately 85% of ingested K⁺ is absorbed in the small intestine, with passive absorption through an H⁺–K⁺ exchange pathway driven by

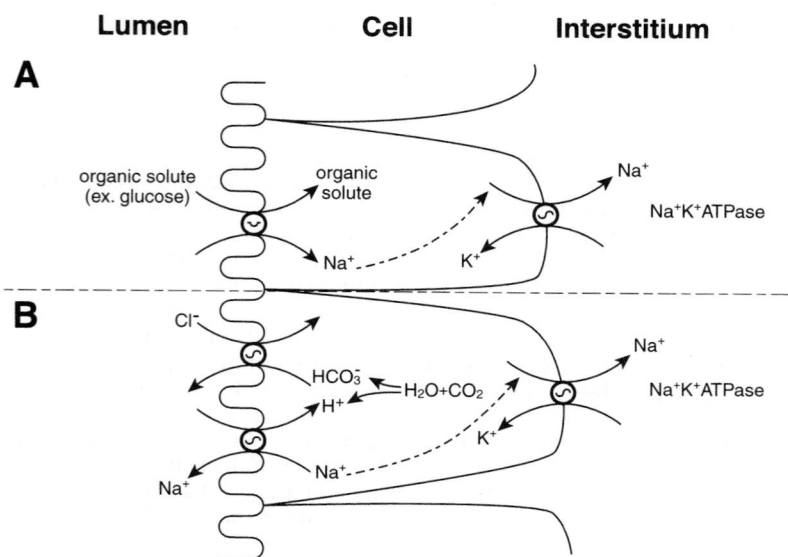

Figure 25.6. Mechanisms of sodium absorption in the small intestine: solute-coupled Na⁺ absorption (A) and electroneutral NaCl absorption (B).

preexisting electrochemical gradients (24). The accumulated K^+ may then diffuse across the basolateral membrane by a K^+ channel or K^+ carrier.

Bicarbonate absorption involves formation of carbon dioxide in the intestinal lumen from secreted hydrogen ion and bicarbonate ion. Carbon dioxide levels in the lumen exceed those in the cell, and carbon dioxide diffuses into the cell to reform hydrogen ion and bicarbonate ion through the action of carbonic anhydrase. Bicarbonate ion diffuses into the interstitium and hydrogen ion is resecreted, partly in exchange for sodium. Bicarbonate secretion occurs in the duodenum and ileum by a Cl^-–HCO_3^- exchange mechanism. Bicarbonate secretion serves to neutralize gastric acid in the duodenum. The role of HCO_3^- secretion in the distal small intestine is less clear, but it may act to conserve Cl^- at the expense of HCO_3^- secretion, thus playing a role in acid–base homeostasis.

Ion transport by the intestinal epithelium is regulated by a number of different signals, including signals supplied by hormones (both local and distant), the ENS, and the immune system. There is substantial interplay between the mediators produced by the various controlling systems. All regulatory mechanisms ultimately affect ion transport by targeting specific protein components of the transport mechanism and modifying their level of activity, abundance, or localization in the enterocyte.

Carbohydrate Digestion and Absorption

Carbohydrates constitute approximately 50% of the total daily caloric intake in humans. In Western cultures, a typical adult consumes an average of 400 g/d of carbohydrates, which yields approximately 1,600 kcal (4 kcal/g). Three major types of digestible carbohydrates are found in our diet: complex starches, the disaccharides sucrose and lactose, and simple sugars, such as glucose, galactose, and fructose. Starch accounts for most of the ingested carbohydrates (approximately 60%), and exists in two basic forms: amylopectin and amylose. Amylose is a

linear polymer of glucose joined by $\alpha(1,4)$-glycosidic bonds. Amylopectin is a branched form of amylose with $\alpha(1,6)$-glycosidic linkages at branch points, which occur every 20 to 25 molecules. Disaccharides comprise approximately one third of dietary carbohydrate. The two principal disaccharides are sucrose (glucose–fructose dimer) and lactose (glucose–galactose dimer). The remainder of dietary carbohydrate consists of undigestible fiber, such as cellulose, hemicellulose, gums, and pectin. Cellulose and hemicellulose are β-linked glucose polymers and are nondigestible because the human gastrointestinal tract does not contain digestive enzymes capable of cleaving β-glucose linkages.

Digestion of starch is initiated by salivary amylase, but this is of only minor significance because salivary amylase is rapidly inactivated in the acid environment of the stomach. Most intraluminal starch digestion is accomplished by pancreatic amylase, which has a high activity for cleavage of internal $\beta(1,4)$-glycosidic bonds. Starch digestion by amylase yields maltose (glucose dimer, 1,4 linkage), maltotriose (glucose trimer, 1,4 linkage), and α-limit dextrins, which are a series of four or more glucose molecules containing an $\alpha(1,6)$ linkage. The process of starch hydrolysis is efficient and is usually complete by the time the carbohydrate load reaches the proximal jejunum. These starch hydrolysis products, along with the ingested disaccharides sucrose and lactose, are then presented to brush border saccharidases in the jejunum for further digestion.

Brush border saccharidases are specific enzymes anchored to the apical membrane of enterocytes. They are responsible for the further breakdown of short-chain sugars into the monosaccharides glucose, galactose, and fructose. Only monosaccharides can be transported across the apical membrane of the enterocyte and absorbed into the cell (Fig. 25.7). Transport through the intestinal cell is usually the rate-limiting process for carbohydrate absorption, except for surface hydrolysis of lactose, which occurs more slowly than its transport process. Glucose and galactose

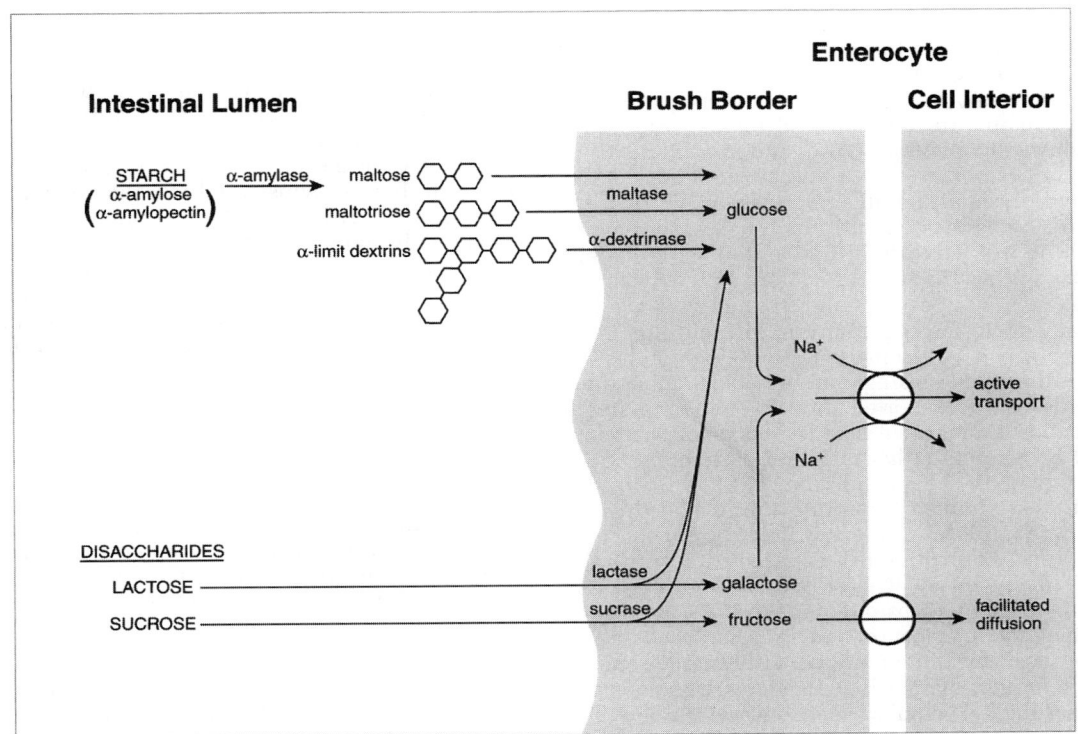

Figure 25.7. Digestion and absorption of carbohydrates.

compete for the same carrier mechanism and enter the cell by sodium-coupled active transport. Na$^+$-K$^+$-ATPase, located on the basolateral membrane, assists in the absorption of monosaccharides by maintaining a low intracellular Na$^+$ concentration, providing a large gradient for transport from the intestinal lumen into the cell. Fructose is absorbed by carrier-mediated facilitated diffusion. Although the enterocyte may use simple sugars as an energy source, most are transported across the basolateral membrane into the mesenteric venous tributaries of the portal vein.

Protein Digestion and Absorption

The recommended daily allowance for dietary proteins in adult humans is 0.75 g/kg and increases with illnesses such as sepsis, as well as in pregnancy. The average American diet consists of 70 to 100 g/d of protein. In addition, 20 to 30 g/d of endogenous protein is secreted into the intestinal lumen from gastric, biliary, pancreatic, and intestinal secretions, and an additional 30 g/d is derived from desquamated cells. These proteins are digested and assimilated in a manner similar to dietary proteins.

Protein digestion is initiated in the stomach by the action of pepsin, a protease secreted by gastric chief cells into the stomach lumen as the inactive precursor pepsinogen, which is converted to pepsin under acid conditions. Pepsin begins the process of breaking down proteins to smaller polypeptides. Most proteolysis, however, occurs in the small intestine and is mediated by pancreatic proteases. This phase begins in the duodenum, where pancreatic juice enters the small intestinal lumen. The exocrine pancreas secretes both endopeptidases (trypsin, chymotrypsin, and elastase), which are capable of cleaving internal peptide bonds, and carboxypeptidases (carboxypeptidase A and B), which hydrolyze the terminal peptide bond on the carboxyl terminus of peptides. Each of these enzymes has distinct substrate specificities. Pancreatic proteases are initially released as inactive precursors, or zymogens. Activation of the inactive zymogens is initiated in the duodenum by enterokinase, a brush border enzyme in the duodenum. Enterokinase cleaves trypsinogen to trypsin. Trypsin is then capable of cleaving additional molecules of trypsinogen as well as the other zymogens to their active forms. The action of these pancreatic enzymes on proteins in the intestinal lumen produces a mixture of short oligopeptides (70%) and free amino acids (30%).

Further hydrolysis of the oligopeptides occurs by a series of peptidases associated with the brush border membrane, resulting in a mixture of free amino acids, dipeptides, and tripeptides before absorption. Enterocytes are capable of absorbing dipeptides and tripeptides as well as free amino acids into the cell. Many amino acids are more efficiently absorbed as constituents of dipeptides or tripeptides rather than as single amino acids. Dipeptides and tripeptides are transported into the cell by a single peptide transport system that uses a transmembrane electrochemical H$^+$ gradient rather than an Na$^+$ gradient as the driving force (25,26). Once inside the cell, the dipeptides and tripeptides are broken down into amino acids by various cytosolic peptidases that are different from those in the brush border. Absorption of free amino acids into the enterocyte is mediated by at least five different transport systems with different substrate sensitivities, and is an Na$^+$-dependent active transport process. Absorbed amino acids can be used by the enterocyte either as an energy source or for protein synthesis, but most are transported across the basolateral membrane by several passive carrier-mediated amino acid transport systems into the portal circulation.

Lipid Digestion and Absorption

The average Western diet consists of 60 to 100 g/d fat, approximately 40% of the total caloric intake, and is composed primarily of triglycerides (90%), phospholipids, cholesterol, and fat-soluble vitamins. Entry of fat into the small intestine stimulates secretion of CCK from the duodenal mucosa, which is turn promotes release of lipase and its necessary cofactor colipase from the pancreas. Lipase hydrolyzes the first and third positions of triglycerides, yielding two fatty acids and β-monoglyceride (a fatty acid esterified to glycerol). Cholesterol and fat-soluble vitamins are hydrolyzed by pancreatic cholesterol esterase, and phospholipids by phospholipase A$_2$. The fat hydrolysis products are then solubilized in the aqueous contents of the intestine by aggregating with bile salts to form complexes called *micelles.* The combination of fatty acids, bile salts, and monoglycerides is referred to as *mixed micelles.* Cholesterol, phospholipids, and fat-soluble vitamins can also be be solubilized in these micelles. Bile salts possess both hydrophobic and hydrophilic regions, and when placed in an aqueous environment, orient the hydrophilic portions to face outward and the hydrophobic portions of the molecule to face inward. Free fatty acids, β-monoglyceride, as well as cholesterol, phospholipid, and fat-soluble vitamins, reside in the hydrophobic core.

Because micelles are water compatible, they can diffuse through the unstirred water layer next to the brush border membrane and empty their contents, which then traverse the plasma membrane by passive diffusion. The bile salts remain in the intestinal lumen to create new micelles. After cellular uptake, long-chain fatty acids and β-monoglyceride are transported across the cell to the smooth endoplasmic reticulum by a cytosolic carrier protein referred to as *fatty acid-binding protein.* In the endoplasmic reticulum, resynthesis of triglycerides takes place, and the triglycerides accumulate in the Golgi apparatus. Triglycerides are then packaged into structures called *chylomicrons* before exit from the cell. Chylomicrons are large particles, 80 to 600 nm in size, that contain a core of hydrophobic lipids, primarily triglycerides, but also cholesterol, phospholipid, and fat-soluble vitamins. The surface is coated with phospholipids and apoproteins, the latter of which are essential for chylomicron formation and transport. Within the Golgi, chylomicrons are packaged into secretory vesicles and exit the cell by exocytosis, where they enter the central lacteal of the villus and the intestinal lymphatic system. Smaller lipoprotein particles, called *very-low-density lipoproteins,* are also produced within enterocytes. They contain a higher cholesterol/triglyceride ratio and are the major route for entry of dietary cholesterol into the lymphatic system. Most dietary fat is absorbed in the duodenum and upper jejunum.

Short-chain fatty acids (less than eight carbon atoms) are water soluble, enter and exit the enterocyte by simple diffusion, and are taken up into the portal circulation without entering lymphatics. Medium-chain triglycerides (6 to 14 carbon atoms) are absorbed into the enterocyte by both simple diffusion and the same absorptive process used by long-chain triglycerides. These fatty acids are not reassembled into complex lipid but rather can enter the portal circulation directly as free fatty acids.

Absorption of Bile Acids

Approximately 95% of bile salts secreted into the intestine are reabsorbed and returned through the portal circulation to the liver. In the liver, bile salts are resecreted and stored in the gallbladder in preparation for release with the next meal. This cycling of bile salts is referred to as the *enterohepatic circulation.* Reabsorption of bile salts occurs by both passive and active mechanisms. A small fraction of the bile acids is absorbed passively along the entire length of the small intestine. Most of the bile salts pass to the terminal ileum, where they are absorbed by an Na^+-dependent active transport mechanism. A small amount of bile salt escapes into the colon and undergoes bacterial modification to increase solubility and promote further passive absorption. High concentrations of bile salts in the colon can promote diarrhea by inhibition of sodium and water absorption. This may occur in patients who undergo ileal resection and can be treated with the bile salt-binding resin, cholestyramine.

Vitamin Absorption

Fat-soluble vitamins (A, D, E, and K) are solubilized by bile salt micelles and are absorbed into enterocytes along with fats. Fat-soluble vitamins are packaged into chylomicrons and enter the lymph. Water-soluble vitamins are absorbed in the jejunum and ileum by a variety of mechanisms. The absorption of vitamin C (ascorbic acid), biotin, and vitamin B_2 (riboflavin) occurs by separate, Na^+-dependent brush border carriers, whereas thiamine and folate are absorbed by Na^+-independent carrier mechanisms. Niacin and vitamin B_6 (pyridoxine) are absorbed by passive diffusion.

Vitamin B_{12} (cobalamin) absorption requires intrinsic factor, a glycoprotein secreted by gastric parietal cells. In the terminal ileum, free cobalamin forms a complex with intrinsic factor and binds to a highly specific membrane receptor. Once absorbed, free cobalamin is released from the complex and exits from the cell into the portal circulation. Deficiency of cobalamin can lead to megaloblastic anemia. Factors that can inhibit absorption of cobalamin include loss of intrinsic factor, distal ileal resection or disease, and bacterial overgrowth (competition by bacteria for luminal cobalamin).

Mineral Absorption

Approximately 1 g of calcium is ingested each day, mainly in milk and dairy products. The stomach aids in calcium absorption by solubilizing nonionic calcium salts. Ionized calcium is absorbed throughout the small intestine, with greatest absorption in the ileum, followed by the jejunum and duodenum. At low concentrations, calcium absorption is an active three-step process involving transport across the apical membrane by carrier-mediated facilitated diffusion, transport across the cell by calcium-binding proteins, and extrusion of calcium into the interstitium by a Ca^{2+}-ATPase pump. This process is regulated indirectly by parathyroid hormone, which in low-calcium states promotes the conversion of vitamin D to its active form, 1,25 $(OH)_2$ vitamin D. 1,25 $(OH)_2$ Vitamin D acts directly on the intestine to increase Ca^{2+} absorption by increasing expression of both calcium-binding proteins and Ca^{2+}-ATPase (27,28). At high intraluminal calcium concentrations, the active transport process is saturated and passive Ca^{2+} absorption occurs in the distal small intestine by a paracellular route.

Most dietary iron is complexed (heme) iron that comes from ingested meat as myoglobin or hemoglobin. This form of iron is readily absorbed. Inorganic (nonheme) iron, ingested from vegetables, grains, and fruits, is preferentially absorbed in the ferrous (Fe^{2+}) form. Ascorbic acid promotes iron absorption by reducing the ferric (Fe^{3+}) ion to the more soluble ferrous ion. Absorption of iron across the apical membrane of the enterocyte involves carrier-mediated translocation. Once inside the cell, enzymes release ferrous iron from the heme moiety. Ferrous iron can

then be sequestered for intracellular storage by ferritin or transported to plasma by transferrin. Regulation is thought to occur through iron-sensing proteins called *iron-regulatory proteins* (29). Iron-regulatory peptides promote iron binding to to transferrin in low-iron states and binding to ferritin in high-iron states. Iron is absorbed in the duodenum and proximal jejunum.

IMMUNOLOGY

The small intestine represents a vast surface area that must be protected from entry of infectious and toxic materials while allowing the gut to absorb needed nutrients. The small intestine uses immunologic and nonimmunologic mechanisms to achieve this goal. The nonimmunologic defense mechanisms used by the gut to exclude, inactivate, and degrade pathologic substances include (a) gastric acid and enteric proteolytic enzymes; (b) mucin production, which coats and protects epithelial cells as well as inhibits bacterial growth; (c) secretion and peristalsis; (d) competitive inhibition between endogenous and pathologic bacteria; and (e) tight junctions between epithelial cells, which prevent penetration of bacteria.

A major component of intestinal defense against harmful substances involves immunologic mechanisms. In fact, the mucosal immune system of the gastrointestinal tract represents one of the largest immunologic compartments in the body (30). Gut-associated lymphoid tissue is a major division of the immune system and is organized into aggregated (lymphoid follicles, Peyer's patches) and nonaggregated (luminal, intraepithelial, and lamina propria) cellular components.

Nonaggregated Lymphoid Tissue

The first cells to encounter an antigenic challenge are neutrophils, lymphocytes, and macrophages located in the intestinal lumen. Increased numbers of intraluminal lymphocytes are associated with Peyer's patches during gastrointestinal infections, and there is evidence of trafficking of leukocytes through the mucosa into the lumen in inflammatory states, such as ulcerative colitis (31). Such luminal cells probably represent an effector mechanism directed toward an antigenic challenge.

The epithelium of the small intestine contains intraepithelial lymphocytes (IELs), which are found between epithelial cells along their basolateral surface. In normal health, their major biologic function is secretion of cytokines that regulate epithelial cell function and responses to luminal antigens (32). Their high level of CD8 expression suggests that they are T cells that function biologically as cytolytic effectors as a consequence of antigen recognition. In fact, their numbers can be increased dramatically in response to bacterial antigens. IELs appear to enter the epithelium from the bloodstream at the crypt, but they they do not migrate up the villus with the epithelial cells. It is presumed that they return to the circulation after exposure to luminal antigen.

The lamina propria contains a variety of nonaggregated lymphoid tissue, including B and T cells, macrophages, mast cells, and eosinophils (Fig. 25.8). B cells in the lamina propria are thought to be derived from precursors in Peyer's patches and undergo cytokine-induced differentiation in the lamina propria to become active producers of immunoglobulin A (IgA). In contrast to IELs, most T cells in the lamina propria exert a helper–inducer function for immunoglobulin production rather than a cytolytic function. Mast cells and eosinophils represent less than 1% of the cell population in the lamina propria. Mast cells and eosinophils are activated by a variety of factors, including

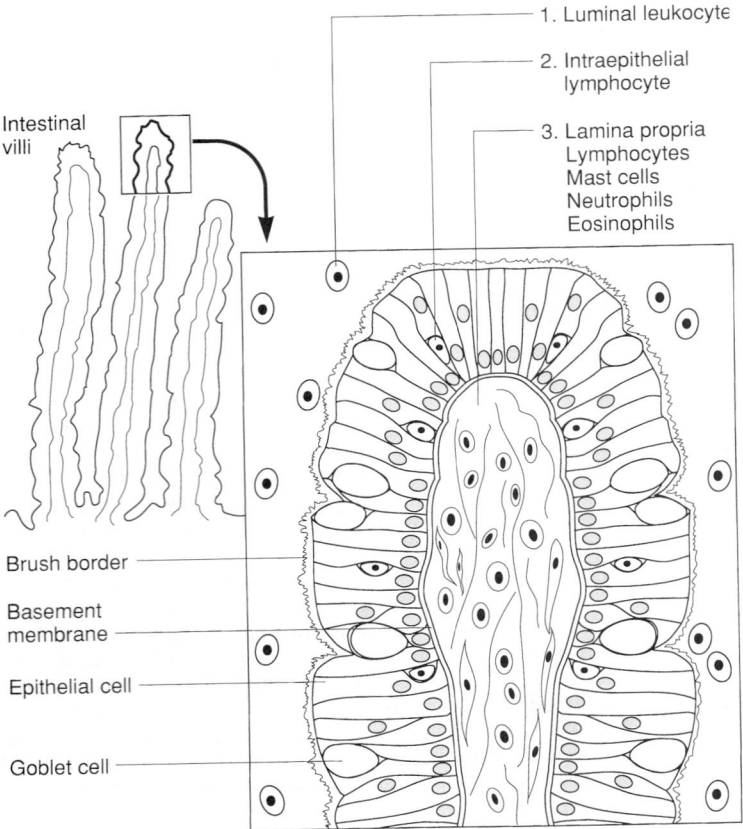

Figure 25.8. Small intestinal villus with associated immunologic cells.

IgE and IgG immune complexes, and play an important role in allergic and hypersensitivity reactions.

Aggregated Lymphoid Tissue

The aggregated lymphoid tissue in the lamina propria consists of lymphoid follicles and Peyer's patches, which represent large collections of lymphoid follicles found on the antimesenteric border of the ileum. Peyer's patches are critical structures in the recognition and processing of antigen and in the development of mucosal immunity. In Peyer's patches, there is compartmentalization of the lymphocytes with B lymphocytes in the germinal centers and T lymphocytes in the interfollicular area. Follicles have highly specialized epithelium overlying their apical dome area that contains microfold (M) cells (Fig. 25.9). M cells can be differentiated morphologically from absorptive epithelial cells by the presence of fewer, shorter, and wider microvilli. M cells cover lymphoid follicles and provide a site for selective sampling of luminal antigens (33). M cells are able to transport antigens transcellularly using a endocytotic mechanism into the underlying lymphoid tissues of Peyer's patches. M cells thus facilitate macrophage and dendritic cell processing and antigen presentation to naive lymphocytes in the lymphoid follicle.

Activated lymphocytes from intestinal lymphoid follicles migrate into afferent lymphatics, pass through mesenteric lymph nodes, and enter the circulation through the thoracic duct. During this process, the lymphocytes mature into B and T lymphoblasts with an enriched population of IgA-bearing B cells. The lymphoblasts then home in to the lamina propria of the gastrointestinal mucosa at the site of original antigenic stimulation, where B lymphoblasts mature into IgA-secreting B cells under the control of antigen-stimulated T cells that have completed the

same journey (34). These mature effector cells provide protective immunity in the lamina propria.

In addition to the gastrointestinal mucosa, activated lymphoblasts may also home to the lamina propria of other mucosa-bearing tissues, such as breast, lung, and eye, where antigen-specific antibodies are secreted (35). For example, IgA-bearing cells preferentially migrate to the mammary gland during lactation. Thus, a breast-feeding mother can passively transfer secretory IgA to her nursing infant. The secretory IgA protects the infant from bacteria and viruses in the mother's gastrointestinal tract.

The ability of activated lymphoblasts to home to specific mucosal sites is regulated by interactions with endothelial cells. Antigenic stimulation and chronic inflammation produce a rapid increase in endothelial venules. Increased expression of adhesion molecules on these endothelial cells is mediated by cytokines and stimulates an influx of antigen-specific, stimulated lymphoblasts to the effector compartment of the nonaggregated lamina propria.

Immunoglobulin Secretion

A major protective mechanism of the intestinal immune system is synthesis and secretion of IgA. Less than 5% of immunoglobulin-producing cells in the gut produce IgG. In serum, IgA exists in monomeric form. In the intestine (and other mucosal surfaces), IgA exists as a dimer that is complexed covalently with two additional molecules—the J chain, which links two IgA molecules, and polymeric immunoglobulin receptor (PIgR), which transports the IgA complex across the cell and allows release of the complex, termed *secretory component,* into the intestinal lumen (34). The J chain is a polypeptide produced in the plasma cell. PIgR, a transmembrane glycoprotein, is produced by the intestinal epithelial cell. It is thought that secretory

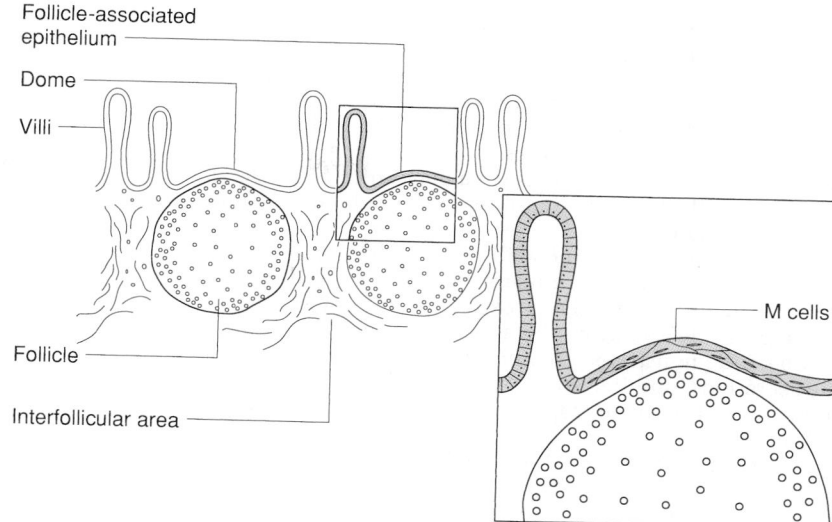

Figure 25.9. Epithelial anatomy in the area of Peyer's patches.

component may prevent proteolytic degradation of the secretory IgA molecule and may stabilize the structure of the polymeric IgA complex in an environment containing numerous proteolytic enzymes and bacteria that would otherwise rapidly degrade it (34).

Immunoglobulin A possesses functional characteristics that are distinct from other antibodies. Unlike IgG and IgM, IgA does not activate complement and does not promote cell-mediated opsonization. The major function of secretory IgA in host defense is protection against bacteria, viruses, and luminal antigens. The protective effect of secretory IgA results from its ability to effectively bind harmful substances while resisting enzymatic degradation by gut enzymes. Secretory IgA inhibits the adherence of bacteria to epithelial cells, leading to impaired colonization and proliferation. Binding of antigen to secretory IgA stimulates mucus secretion and can prevent uptake of both viruses and bacteria by entrapment in the mucus layer. Secretory IgA also binds to and blocks the absorption of antigens and toxins and may be very important in disease states where there is disruption of the mucosal barrier, such as in inflammatory bowel disease. The ability of IgA to use relatively unobtrusive mechanisms in host defense minimizes the need for an inflammatory response and thus protects the intestinal mucosa against injury.

ENDOCRINE FUNCTION

The gastrointestinal tract is the largest endocrine system in the body. Unlike other endocrine organs, which possess a solid mass of hormone-producing cells, the source of gastrointestinal hormones is scattered single cells and enteric neurons along the length of the gastrointestinal tract. These hormones play a key role in all aspects of small bowel function, including motility, secretion and absorption, blood flow, growth, and immunity.

Cholecystokinin is predominantly produced by endocrine cells in the mucosa of the proximal two thirds of the small intestine. CCK is also present in lower abundance in enteric neurons. CCK exists in multiple molecular forms (CCK-8, CCK-33, CCK-39, and CCK-58); however, no differential biologic effects among the different forms have been described. CCK is released from the small bowel mucosa in response to luminal fats and proteins. The major actions of CCK are to stimulate pancreatic acinar cell secretion of zymogens and stimulate gallbladder contractility. CCK's actions result in delivery of key digestive components into the intestinal lumen. CCK also has trophic effects on small bowel mucosa and pancreas.

Secretin is a 27-amino acid peptide synthesized in the endocrine cells (S cells) that are present in the duodenum and jejunum. The main stimulus for secretin release is acid in the duodenum, when the luminal pH decreases to 4 or lower. The major effect of secretin is secretion of bicarbonate from pancreatic and biliary ductal epithelium and Brunner's glands. The bicarbonate neutralizes luminal acid and provides a negative feedback loop for release of secretin. Secretin's ability to paradoxically induce gastrin release in patients with gastrinoma while having no effect on gastrin release in normal subjects has made the secretin stimulation test a useful tool in the diagnosis of Zollinger-Ellison syndrome. *Vasoactive intestinal peptide* is a member of the secretin family of peptides and functions exclusively as a neurotransmitter. It is a potent vasodilator and also functions to stimulate enteric smooth muscle and pancreatic exocrine and intestinal secretion, and inhibit gastric acid secretion.

Somatostatin is synthesized and secreted from both neurons and endocrine cells (D cells) found in small quantities throughout the gut mucosa. Most of the biologic effects of somatostatin are inhibitory. Somatostatin inhibits biliary, gastric, and pancreatic secretion, in addition to inhibiting release of a broad range of gastrointestinal hormones. Somatostatin also inhibits motility, presumably by inhibiting cholinergic neurons. The peptide decreases splanchnic and portal blood flow. A long-acting cyclic analogue of somatostatin, octreotide, is a very useful clinical therapeutic agent in the treatment of patients with gastrointestinal hormone-secreting tumors, carcinoid syndrome, and enterocutaneous and pancreatic fistulae.

Motilin is a 22-amino acid peptide that is produced in enteroendocrine cells in the mucosa of the upper small intestine. Motilin is released in the fasting state and is a physiologic regulator of phase III MMC activity. The initiation of motilin release is through a cholinergic-dependent pathway.

Peptide YY is a 36-amino acid peptide found predominantly in the mucosa of the terminal ileum and colon. PYY is released in response to fats in meals. The actions of PYY are largely inhibitory—PYY inhibits gastrointestinal motility and gastric and pancreatic secretion. The peptide has been given the nickname *ileal brake* because these actions promotes longer contact times when nutrients reach the distal small bowel.

Gastric inhibitory polypeptide (GIP) was originally thought to inhibit gastric acid secretion, but it has since become clear that this is not the physiologic function of this hormone. GIP is a 42-amino acid peptide that is found in highest concentration in the mucosa of the duodenum and jejunum. GIP's main physiologic function is to regulate insulin release in response to a meal (incretion effect). GIP has no effect on insulin release to parenterally administered nutrients.

Neurotensin, a 13-amino acid peptide, is produced predominantly in the ileal mucosa but is also produced in smaller quantities in the proximal small intestine and colon. It is released by a mixed meal and fats. Neurotensin has been demonstrated to stimulate pancreatic bicarbonate secretion, inhibit gastric secretion, stimulate intestinal motility, and produce trophic effects on the small intestinal mucosa.

Pancreatic glucagon and *enteroglucagon* are 29- and 37-amino acid peptides located in the pancreas and small intestine, respectively, and are the products of tissue-specific processing of the propeptide glicentin (69 amino acids). Pancreatic glucagon resides in α cells in the islet and is important in inducing glycogenolysis, lipolysis, gluconeogenesis, and ketogenesis. Enteroglucagon is produced predominantly in the distal small intestine and functions to inhibit small bowel motility.

REFERENCES

1. Cohen S, Harris LD, Levitan R. Manometric characteristics of the human ileocecal junction zone. *Gastroenterology* 1968;54:72.
2. Rosse C, Gaddum-Rosse P, eds. *Hollinshead's textbook of anatomy,* 5th ed. Philadelphia: Lippincott–Raven, 1997.
3. Furness JB, Costa M. *The enteric nervous system.* New York: Churchill Livingstone, 1987.
4. Sternini C. Functional organization of the enteric nervous system. *Regul Pept Lett* 1993;5(2):25.
5. Goyal RK, Hirano I. Mechanisms of disease: the enteric nervous system. *N Engl J Med* 1996;334:1106–1115.
6. Rubin DC. Spatial analysis of transcriptional activation in fetal rat jejunum and ileal gut epithelium. *Am J Physiol* 1992;263:G853.
7. Holmes R, Lobley RW. Intestinal brush border revisited. *Gut* 1989;30:1667.
8. Garabedian EM, Roberts LJ, Mcnevin MS, et al. Examining the role of Paneth cells in the small intestine by lineage ablation in transgenic mice. *J Biol Chem* 1997;272:23729.
9. Casteels R. Membrane potential in smooth muscle cells. In: Bulbring E, Brading AF, Jones AF, et al., eds. *Smooth muscle: an assessment of current knowledge.* Austin, TX: University of Texas Press, 1981:105.
10. Furness JB, Bornstein JC, Kunze WA, et al. The enteric nervous system and its extrinsic connections. In: Yamada T, ed. *Textbook of gastroenterology,* 3rd ed., vol 1. Philadelphia: Lippincott–Raven, 1999:11.
11. Argenyi EE, Soffer EE, Madsen MT, et al. Scintigraphic evaluation of small bowel transit in healthy subjects: inter- and intrasubject variability. *Am J Gastroenterol* 1995;90:938.
12. Carlson GM, Bedi BS, Code CF. Mechanism of propagation of intestinal interdigestive myoelectric complex. *Am J Physiol* 1972;222:1027.
13. Rees WDW, Malagelada JR, Miller LJ, et al. Human interdigestive and postprandial gastrointestinal motor and gastrointestinal hormone patterns. *Dig Dis Sci* 1982;27:321.
14. Weisbrodt NW, Copeland EM, Moore EP, et al. Effect of vagotomy on electrical activity of the small intestine of the dog. *Am J Physiol* 1975;228:650.
15. Marlett JA, Code CF. Effects of celiac and superior mesenteric ganglionectomy on interdigestive myoelectric complex in dogs. *Am J Physiol* 1979;237:E432.
16. Sarr MG, Kelly KA. Myoelectric activity of the autotransplanted canine jejunoileum. *Gastroenterology* 1981;81:303.
17. Itoh Z. Motilin and clinical application. *Peptides* 1997;18:593.
18. Tonini M. Recent advances in the pharmacology of gastrointestinal prokinetics. *Pharmacol Res* 1996;33:217.
19. Von der Ohe M, Layer P, Wollny C, et al. Somatostatin 28 and coupling of human interdigestive intestinal motility and pancreatic secretion. *Gastroenterology* 1992;103:974.
20. Malfertheiner P, Sarr MG, DiMagno EP. Role of the pancreas in the control of interdigestive gastrointestinal motility. *Gastroenterology* 1989;96:200.
21. Loo DDF, Zeuthen T, Chandy G, et al. Cotransport of water by the Na$^+$/glucose transporter. *Proc Natl Acad Sci USA* 1996;93:13367.
22. Wright EM, Loo DDF, Turk E, et al. Sodium cotransporters. *Curr Opin Cell Biol* 1996;8:468.
23. Knickerbein R, Aronson PS, Schron CM, et al. Sodium and chloride transport across the rabbit ileal brush border: II. evidence for Cl–HCO$_3$ exchange and mechanism of coupling. *Am J Physiol* 1985;249:G236.
24. Agarwal R, Afzalpurkar R, Fordtran JS. Pathophysiology of potassium absorption and secretion in the small intestine. *Gastroenterology* 1994;107:548.
25. Ganapathy V, Leibach FH. Proton-coupled solute transport in the animal cell plasma membrane. *Curr Opin Cell Biol* 1991;3:695.
26. Leibach FH, Ganapathy V. Peptide transporters in the intestine and the kidney. *Annu Rev Nutr* 1996;16:99.
27. Cai Q, Chandler JS, Wasserman RH, et al. Vitamin D and adaptation to dietary calcium and phosphate deficiencies increase intestinal plasma membrane calcium pump gene expression. *Proc Natl Acad Sci USA* 1993;90:1345.
28. Walters J. Calbindin-D$_{9k}$ stimulates the calcium pump in rat enterocyte basolateral membranes. *Am J Physiol* 1989;256:G124.
29. Ponka P, Beaumont C, Richardson DR. Function and regulation of transferrin and ferritin. *Semin Hematol* 1998;35:35.
30. Brandtzaeg P, Solli d L, Thrane P, et al. Lymphoepithelial interactions in the mucosal immune system. *Gut* 1988;29:1116.
31. Saverymuttu SH, Camilleri M, Rees H, et al. Indium 111-granulocyte scanning in the assessment of disease extent and disease activity in inflammatory bowel disease: a comparison with colonoscopy, histology, and fecal indium 111-granulocyte excretion. *Gastroenterology* 1986;90;1121.
32. Boismenu R, Harvan WL. Modulation of epithelial cell growth by intraepithelial γδ T cells. *Science* 1994;266:1253.
33. Neutra M, Frey A, Kraehenbuhl JP. Epithelial M cells: gateways for mucosal infection and immunization. *Cell* 1996;86:345.
34. Blumberg RS. The immune system. In: Yamada T, ed. *Textbook of gastroenterology,* 3rd ed., vol 1. Philadelphia: Lippincott–Raven, 1999:106.
35. McGhee JR, Mestecky J, Dertzbaugh MT, et al. The mucosal immune system: from fundamental concepts to vaccine development. *Vaccine* 1992;10:75.

SURGERY: SCIENTIFIC PRINCIPLES AND PRACTICE, Third Edition, edited by Lazar J. Greenfield, Michael W. Mulholland, Keith T. Oldham, Gerald B. Zelenock, and Keith D. Lillemoe. Lippincott Williams & Wilkins Publishers, Philadelphia, © 2001.

CHAPTER 26

ILEUS AND BOWEL OBSTRUCTION

DAVID I. SOYBEL

The modern approach to intestinal obstruction and ileus has paralleled the development of techniques for safe abdominal surgery. From 1880 to 1925, it was recognized that proximal intestinal decompression could provide relief from the symptoms of mechanical obstruction or ileus (1–3). In 1933, investigators reported the efficacy of gastrointestinal intubation in relieving symptoms of intestinal distention caused by intestinal obstruction or by the ileus that resulted from laparotomy (4,5). Subsequently, experimental evidence indicated that the source of gaseous distention in cases of obstruction or ileus was swallowed air (6). The value of intravenous fluid resuscitation in experimental models of intestinal obstruction was recognized as early as 1912 (7), and became a principle of care of patients with intestinal obstruction in the late 1920s. By 1920, plain abdominal radiographs were used in the diagnosis of intestinal obstruction (3). Thus, the principles of early diagnosis, rapid intravenous fluid resuscitation, gastrointestinal decompression, and early surgery to avoid intestinal gangrene and peritonitis were established well before the advent of antibiotic therapy, invasive hemodynamic monitoring, and parenteral nutrition (8). These early developments were most important in reducing morbidity and mortality of mechanical intestinal obstruction and ileus (9).

MECHANICAL OBSTRUCTION OF THE INTESTINE

Terminology and Classification

The term *mechanical obstruction* means that luminal contents cannot pass through the gut tube because the lumen is blocked. This contrasts with *neurogenic* or *functional* obstruction, in which luminal contents fail to pass because of disturbances in gut motility that prevent coordinated peristalsis from one region of the gut to the next. This latter form of obstruction is commonly referred to as *ileus* in the small intestine and *pseudoobstruction* in the large intestine. In *simple* obstruction, the intestinal lumen is partially or completely occluded without compromise of intestinal blood flow. Simple obstructions can be *complete*, meaning that the lumen is totally occluded (Fig. 26.1), or *incomplete*, meaning that the lumen is narrowed but permits distal passage of some fluid and air. In *stran-*

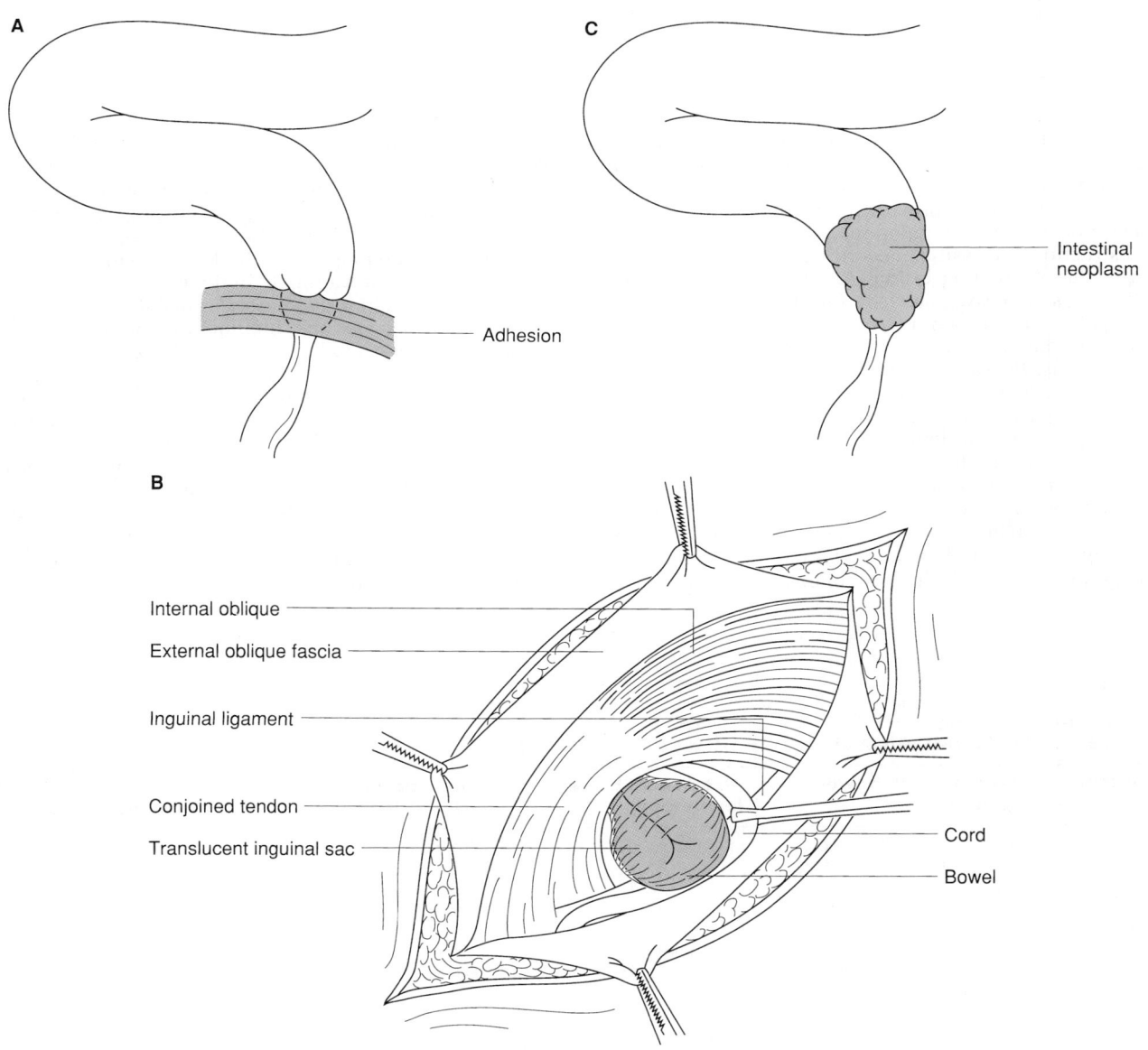

Figure 26.1. Schematic illustration of different forms of simple mechanical obstruction. Simple obstruction is most often due to adhesion *(A)*, groin hernia *(B)*, or neoplasm *(C)*. The hernia can act as a tourniquet, causing a closed-loop obstruction and strangulation.

Table 26.1. CLASSIFICATION OF ADULT MECHANICAL INTESTINAL OBSTRUCTIONS

INTRALUMINAL	INTRAMURAL	EXTRINSIC
Foreign bodies	Congenital	Adhesions
Barium inspissation (colon)	Atresia, stricture, or stenosis	Congenital
Bezoar	Web	Ladd or Meckel's bands
Inspissated feces	Intestinal duplication	Postoperative
Gallstone	Meckel's diverticulum	Postinflammatory
Meconium (cystic fibrosis)	Inflammatory process	Hernias
Parasites	Crohn disease	External
Other (e.g., swallowed objects, enteroliths)	Diverticulitis	Internal
Intussusception	Chronic intestinal ischemia or	Volvulus
Polypoid, exophytic lesions	postischemic stricture	External mass effect
	Radiation enteritis	Abscess
	Medication induced (nonsteroidal	Annular pancreas
	antiinflammatory drugs, potassium	Carcinomatosis
	chloride tablets)	Endometriosis
	Neoplasms	Pregnancy
	Primary bowel (malignant or benign)	Pancreatic pseudocyst
	Secondary (metastases, especially	
	melanoma)	
	Traumatic	
	Intramural hematoma of duodenum	

gulated obstruction, blood flow to the obstructed segment is compromised, and tissue necrosis and gangrene are imminent. Strangulation usually implies that the obstruction is complete, but some forms of partial obstruction can also be complicated by strangulation.

Obstruction is classified according to etiology and location of the obstructing lesion. As detailed in Table 26.1, distinctions are drawn between intraluminal foreign bodies or gallstones, intramural lesions such as tumors or intussusceptions, and extrinsic or extramural lesions such as adhesions. Proximal, or high, obstructions involve the pylorus, duodenum, and proximal jejunum. Intermediate levels of obstruction involve the intestine from the midjejunum to the mid-ileum. Distal levels of obstruction arise in the distal ileum, ileocecal valve, and proximal colon, whereas the most distant, or low, obstructions arise in regions beyond the transverse colon. As shown in Table 26.2, clinical symptoms and signs of obstruction (pain, vomiting, abdominal distention, gas pattern on abdominal radiographs) vary with the level of obstruction.

It is also important to distinguish *open-loop* from *closed-loop* obstructions. An open-loop obstruction occurs when intestinal flow is blocked but proximal decompression is possible through vomiting. A closed-loop obstruction occurs when inflow to the loop of bowel and outflow from the loop are both blocked. This permits gas and secretions to accumulate in the loop without a means of decompression, proximally or distally. Examples of closed-loop obstructions include torsion of a loop of small intestine around an adhesive band (Fig. 26.2), incarceration of bowel in a hernia, volvulus of the cecum or colon, and development of an obstructing carcinoma of the colon with a competent ileocecal valve. Closed-loop obstruction of the small intestine causes sudden, severe abdominal pain and vomiting, whereas obstructions of the large intestine cause pain and sudden abdominal distention. Pain often precedes associated findings of localized abdominal tenderness or involuntary guarding. When physical findings develop, viability of the bowel is often compromised.

Table 26.2. SYMPTOMS AND SIGNS OF BOWEL OBSTRUCTION

Symptom or sign	Proximal small bowel (open loop)	Distal small bowel (open loop)	Small bowel (closed loop)	Colon and rectum
Pain	Intermittent, intense, colicky; often relieved by vomiting	Intermittent to constant	Progressive, intermittent to constant; rapidly worsens	Continuous
Vomiting	Large volumes, bilious and frequent	Low volume and frequency; progressively feculent with time	May be prominent (reflex)	Intermittent, not prominent; feculent when present
Tenderness	Epigastric or periumbilical; quite mild unless strangulation is present	Diffuse and progressive	Diffuse, progressive	Diffuse
Distention	Absent	Moderate to marked	Often absent	Marked
Obstipation	May not be present	Present	May not be present	Present

Adapted from Schuffler MD, Sinanan MN. Intestinal obstruction and pseudo-obstruction. In: Sleisenger MH, Fordtran JS, eds. Gastrointestinal disease, 5th ed. Philadelphia: WB Saunders, 1993:898.

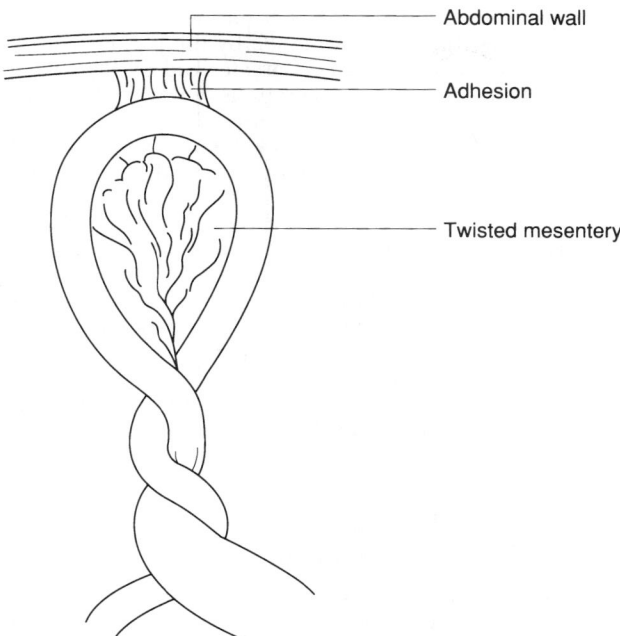

Abdominal wall

Adhesion

Twisted mesentery

Figure 26.2. Schematic illustration of a closed-loop obstruction. The small intestine twists around its mesentery, compromising inflow and outflow of luminal contents from the loop. Also, the vascular supply to the loop may be compromised because of the twisting of the mesentery. The risk of strangulation is high.

Pathophysiology of Intestinal Obstruction

Local Effects of Bowel Obstruction

When a loop of bowel becomes obstructed, intestinal gas and fluid accumulate. The rate at which symptoms and complications develop depends on luminal volume, bacterial proliferation, and alterations in motility and perfusion.

Intestinal Gas

Approximately 80% of the gas seen on plain abdominal radiographs is attributable to swallowed air (6). Approximately 70% of the gas in the obstructed gut is inert nitrogen (10). Oxygen accounts for 10% to 12%, carbon dioxide 6% to 9%, hydrogen 1%, methane 1%, and hydrogen disulfide 1% to 10%. In the setting of acute pain and anxiety, patients with intestinal obstruction may swallow excessive amounts of air. Passage of such swallowed air distally is prevented by nasogastric suction.

Intestinal Flora

An important contribution to normal digestive function comes from the resident bacterial population. In patients with normal gastric acid secretion, the chyme entering the duodenum is nearly sterile. The small numbers of bacteria that are found in stomach and proximal intestine are aerobic, gram-positive species similar to those found in the oropharynx. Distally, in the ileum and colon, gram-negative aerobes are present, and anaerobic organisms predominate. Total bacterial counts in normal feces reach 10^{11} organisms per gram of fecal matter. Control of the bacterial populations depends on intact motor activity of the intestines and the interactions of all species present. This ecology can be disturbed by antibiotic therapy or by surgical reconstructions that result in stasis in intestinal segments. Intestinal bacteria serve several functions, including the following:

1. Metabolism of fecal sterols, releasing the short-chain fatty acids that are an important food source for colonocytes
2. Metabolism of fecal bile acids, fat-soluble vitamins, and vitamin B_{12}
3. Breakdown of complex carbohydrates and organic matter, leading to the formation of carbon dioxide, hydrogen, and methane gases (8)

Evidence suggests that the normal flora contributes to baseline levels of intestinal secretion and normal intestinal motility. The small intestines in germ-free animals are frequently dilated, fluid filled, and without peristalsis (11,12).

The role of bacterial toxins in mediating the mucosal response to obstruction has received increasing attention. In germ-free dogs, luminal accumulation of fluid is not observed, and absorption continues (11). In addition, it is well recognized that bacterial endotoxins can stimulate secretion, possibly causing release or potentiation of neuroendocrine substances and prostaglandins (12). Because a substantial number of systemic microvascular and hemodynamic responses to endotoxemia appear to be attributable to heightened synthesis of nitric oxide (13,14), it seems likely that mucosal responses to local inflammation and endotoxin release also are altered by conditions modifying the synthesis or activity of nitric oxide. The role of nitric oxide in mucosal fluid and electrolyte movements is under active investigation (15,16).

Intestinal Fluid

Fluid accumulates intraluminally with open- or closed-loop small intestinal obstruction because of the following:

1. Intraluminal distention and pressure
2. Release of prosecretory and antiabsorptive hormones and paracrine substances
3. Changes in mesenteric circulation
4. Elaboration and luminal release of bacterial toxins (8,17)

Experimental studies and clinical investigation (18,19) have demonstrated that elevation of luminal pressures above 20 cm H_2O inhibits absorption and stimulates secretion of salt and water into the lumen proximal to an obstruction. In closed-loop obstruction, luminal pressures can exceed 50 cm H_2O and may account for a substantial proportion of luminal fluid accumulation (20). In simple open-loop obstruction, distention of the lumen by gas rarely leads to luminal pressures higher than 8 to 12 cm H_2O (21). Thus, in open-loop obstruction, the contributions of high luminal pressures to hypersecretion may not be important.

The release of endocrine and paracrine substances is suggested to occur in mechanical bowel obstruction (22,23). Vasoactive intestinal polypeptide may be released from the submucosal and myenteric plexuses in the gut wall, promoting epithelial secretion and inhibiting absorption (22). Excess release of prostaglandins can also occur (23).

Intestinal Blood Flow

Microvascular responses to intestinal obstruction also can play an important role in determining hydrostatic gradients for fluid transfer across the mucosa into the lumen. In response to heightened luminal pressure, total blood flow to the bowel wall may initially increase (24). Enzymatic breakdown of stagnant intestinal contents leads to increased osmolality of luminal contents. Along with secretory stimulation and absorptive inhibition of the mucosa, the simultaneous changes in hydrostatic and osmotic pressures on the blood and lumen sides of the mucosa favor flow of extracellular fluid into the lumen. Subsequently, blood flow is compromised as luminal pressures increase, bacteria invade, and inflammation leads to edema within the bowel wall.

Intestinal Motility

Obstruction of the intestinal lumen does not simply block distal passage of luminal contents. The accumulation of fluid and gas in the obstructed lumen also elicits changes in the myoelectrical function of the gut, proximal and distal to the obstructed segment. In response to this distention, the obstructed segment itself may dilate, a process known as *receptive relaxation* (25). Such changes ensure that, despite accumulation of air and fluid, intraluminal pressures do not rise easily to the point of compromising blood flow to the intestinal mucosa. At sites proximal and distal to the obstruction, changes in myoelectrical activity are time dependent. Initially, there may be intense periods of activity and peristalsis. Subsequently, myoelectrical activity is diminished, and the interdigestive migrating myoelectrical complex pattern is replaced by ineffectual and seemingly disorganized clusters of contractions (26–28). Similar alterations have been observed in experimental models of large bowel obstruction (29,30). Subsequent patterns of myoelectrical quiescence may correspond to an increasing accumulation of fluid and air proximally and act to prevent luminal pressures from rising.

Complications of Bowel Obstruction

Closed-loop Obstruction

The complications of closed-loop obstructions evolve rapidly. The reasons for this rapid evolution are best understood by considering the simplest and most common form of closed-loop obstruction, appendicitis. When a fecalith or hypertrophied lymph nodule obstructs the mouth of the blind-ended appendix, secretion of mucus and enhanced peristalsis represent the initial attempt to clear the blockage. Intense, crampy abdominal pain focused at the umbilicus results. Nausea and vomiting are not uncommon as a reflexive response to hyperperistalsis and stretching of the mesentery. During the next 8 to 18 hours, continued secretion of mucus leads to high intraluminal pressures, stasis, bacterial overgrowth, and mucosal disruption. When luminal pressure exceeds mural venous pressure and then capillary perfusion pressures, inflammatory cells are recruited from surrounding peritoneal structures. This sequence of events leads to intense inflammation, release of exudate in the area of the appendix, and the first localization of pain from the umbilicus to the area of peritoneum lying nearest the inflamed appendix. Peritoneal findings (localized tenderness, involuntary guarding, rebound or referred tenderness) and fever appear. Subsequently, 20 to 24 hours into the illness, the blood supply of the appendix is compromised. Gangrene and perforation follow, and, if not contained by surrounding structures, free perforation leads to peritonitis. Toxins from necrotic tissue and bacterial overgrowth are released into the systemic circulation, and shock ensues. Torsion of a loop of small intestine around an adhesive band or inside a hernia leads to a similar sequence of events. Torsion of the large bowel is usually accompanied by massive distention of the loop by air and feces.

Open-loop Obstruction

Complications of open-loop obstruction do not evolve as rapidly as those in closed-loop obstruction. Not un-commonly, an open-loop obstruction located in the proximal jejunum can be decompressed by the patient's ability to vomit. The obstruction is characterized by loss of gastric, pancreatic, and biliary secretions, with resulting electrolyte disturbances, including dehydration, metabolic alkalosis, hypochloremia, hypokalemia, and usually hyponatremia. In contrast, obstruction of the distal ileum may lead only to a slowly progressive distention of the small intestine, with accommodation by intestinal myoelectrical function and minor alterations in fluid and electrolyte balances. Open-loop obstruction located in the midgut is often characterized by events similar to those seen in closed-loop obstruction or combinations of events seen in high and low obstruction (Table 26.2). Thus, patients with distal jejunal obstruction may present with a combination of complications resulting from loss of intestinal contents from vomiting, as well as distention and compromise of intestinal wall perfusion.

Clinical Presentation and Differential Diagnosis

The four key symptoms that are associated with acute mechanical bowel obstruction include abdominal pain, vomiting, distention, and obstipation. Colon obstruction is usually accompanied by varying levels of pain, with massive abdominal distention, and obstipation. Other abdominal conditions, such as appendicitis, diverticulitis, perforated peptic ulcer, cholecystitis, or choledocholithiasis, can usually be distinguished from small bowel obstruction by clinical examination and basic laboratory data. Bowel obstruction can complicate *any* of these abdominal conditions. Thus, the presence of another abdominal process does not exclude the complication of small bowel obstruction, and the symptoms of bowel obstruction do not exclude other conditions.

Numerous attempts have been made to use groupings of clinical criteria to establish the diagnosis of complete and irreversible intestinal obstruction, and to distinguish complete obstruction from partial intestinal obstruction. In more recent studies, computer-assisted analysis has been used to identify such criteria (31). Key factors in the history and clinical examination include the following:

1. Previous abdominal surgery
2. Quality of pain (colicky and intermittent vs. steady)
3. Abdominal distention
4. Hyperactivity of bowel sounds

Not surprisingly, the use of such computer-assisted algorithms confirms that the most important clues to the diagnosis of simple obstruction of the small intestine result from a complete and careful history and physical examination. The role of plain abdominal radiographs and other imaging studies is to confirm the clinical diagnosis of simple obstruction. In simple obstruction, laboratory studies do not play a direct role in diagnosis, but are helpful in evaluating complications such as dehydration, strangulation, and sepsis.

Strangulation obstruction of the small or large intestine is accompanied by symptoms and signs that suggest peritonitis. Large fluid shifts and systemic toxicity are imminent or have already occurred. These signs include abdominal tenderness or involuntary guarding localized to the area of the strangulated loop of bowel, decreased urine output, fever, and tachycardia. There have been attempts to use common clinical and laboratory test criteria to identify the likelihood that the obstruction is associated with strangulation. Clinical intuition suggests that the risk of strangulation is low in patients with incomplete or complete small bowel obstruction as long as fever, tachycardia, localized abdominal tenderness, and leukocytosis are not present (32). However, these clinical features, considered individually or in combination, are not specific in distinguishing simple from strangulated obstruction. When complete obstruction is present, no satisfactory criteria are available reliably to exclude the possibility of strangulation (32–34). Metabolic acidosis and increases in serum amylase, inorganic phosphate, hexosaminidase, intestinal fatty acid-binding protein, and serum d-lactate levels have all been associated with intestinal ischemia, and it has been hoped the such laboratory abnormalities would be helpful in diagnosing strangulation when the symptoms and signs are not obvious (35,36). Unfortunately, a noninvasive and rapid test that can provide information to suggest that tissue necrosis is not yet available (37).

Radiographs and Imaging

Plain Films

The role of plain abdominal radiographs and imaging studies is to confirm the diagnosis of bowel obstruction, locate the site of obstruction, and provide insight into the lesion responsible for the obstruction. On plain radiographs of the abdomen, the findings that suggest the diagnosis of small bowel obstruction reflect the accumulation of air and fluid proximal to, and clearance of fluid and air distal to, the point of obstruction. Such findings include dilated loops of small bowel on the flat plate and multiple air–fluid levels located at different areas on the upright film or lateral decubitus film (Fig. 26.3). Dilated loops of small intestine are defined as those larger than 3 cm in diameter. Free air represents perforation of a viscus and mandates immediate operation. In the presence of complete small bowel obstruction, colon loops do not con-

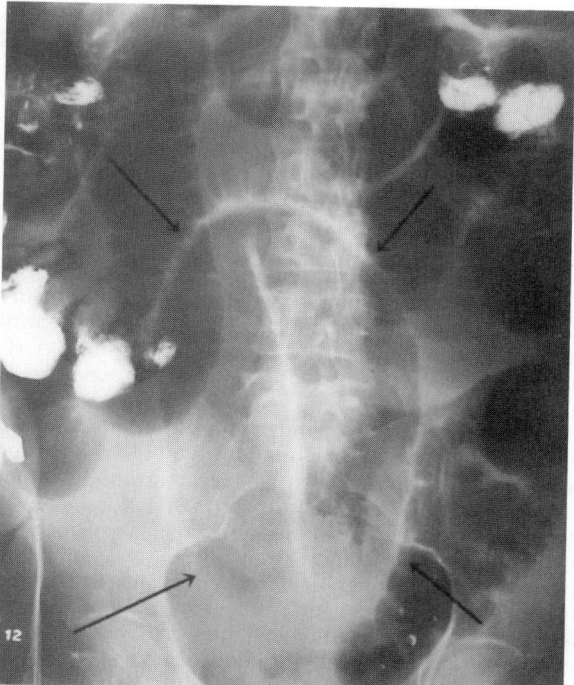

Figure 26.4. Plain supine abdominal film of a patient with sigmoid volvulus. The centrally located sigmoid loop is outlined by trapped air. The proximal small intestine is dilated as well, suggesting that the volvulus has been present for sufficient time to cause accumulation of air and fluid proximally. (Courtesy of John Braver, M.D., Department of Radiology, Brigham and Women's Hospital, Harvard Medical School, Boston, MA.)

tain air. If there is air in the colon, the small bowel obstruction may be complete but early, or it may be incomplete.

In the colon, tightly closed loop obstructions, such as volvulus of the cecum, transverse colon, and sigmoid colon, are accompanied by distention of the obstructed segment (Fig. 26.4). The proximal colon is considered dilated when it reaches 8 to 10 cm, and the sigmoid colon is dilated at 4 to 5 cm. In contrast, obstruction by carcinoma or diverticulitis presents with massive distention of the entire colon from the point of obstruction to the ileocecal valve. From this standpoint, any large bowel obstruction represents a closed loop as long as the ileocecal valve is competent. Although it is usually possible to differentiate obstruction of the small bowel from that of the large bowel, it is not usually possible to localize the region of obstruction within these organs.

Two points should be stressed about the appearance of plain films in patients with a closed-loop obstruction: first, a closed loop may contain mostly fluid and very little gas, and may be barely visible as a minimally dilated "sentinel loop" that remains unchanged over time. Second, because such patients usually present early after the onset of symptoms, the upstream regions of small intestine may not have had time to fill with air and the remainder of the abdomen may appear gasless. Thus, in contrast to patients presenting with open-loop obstructions, the plain films may be characterized by less air than normal.

Contrast Studies

Contrast studies (small bowel follow-through, enteroclysis, contrast enema) can provide specific localization of the point of obstruction and may identify the nature of

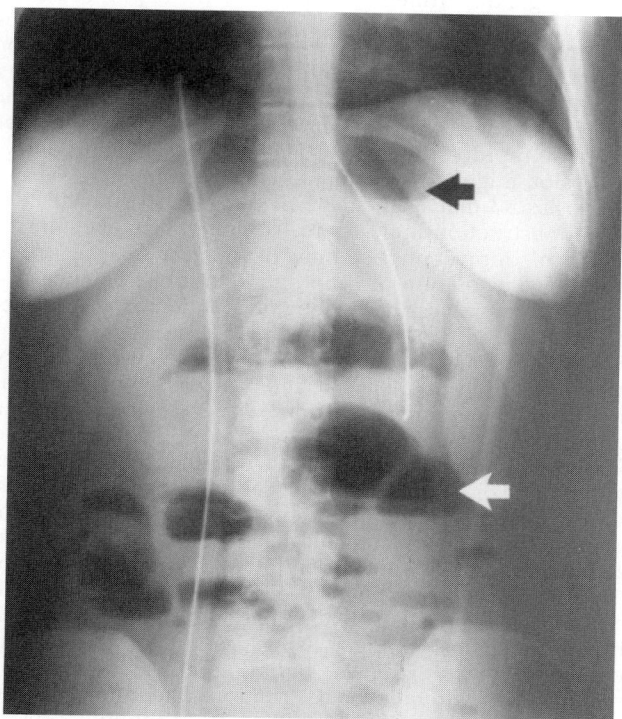

Figure 26.3. Plain upright abdominal film of a patient with small intestinal obstruction. Note the air–fluid levels in the stomach *(black arrow)*, multiple dilated loops of small intestine *(white arrow)*, and absence of air in the colon or rectum.

the underlying lesion. When obstruction of the small intestine is not progressing or resolving, a small bowel follow-through is indicated to confirm the presence and location of the obstruction. Also, even under acute circumstances, diagnosis and management of colonic obstruction are usually enhanced by the use of a contrast enema. Under some circumstances, contrast studies are unnecessary and may be contraindicated. For example, in the classic setting of abdominal pain, nausea, vomiting, and a plain film indicating multiple air–fluid levels in the small intestine and colonic collapse, the diagnosis of acute obstruction can be made clinically. Failure to improve in a short time mandates surgery, and contrast studies are unnecessary. When strangulation or perforation is strongly suspected, contrast studies are contraindicated.

The choice of contrast materials includes water-insoluble suspensions of barium and water-soluble agents such as Gastrografin (Bristol-Myers Squibb, Princeton, NJ) or Hypaque (Sanofi Winthrop, New York, NY). Barium studies provide the clearest images in both small bowel studies, in which the contrast is given from above, and colorectal studies, in which the contrast is given by enema. If barium leaks into the peritoneum, it elicits intense peritonitis. If there is any possibility of bowel perforation or gangrene, barium should not be used. Water-soluble agents are hyperosmotic and can elicit fluid translocation into the gut. When the obstruction of the small intestine is incomplete, these agents can facilitate resolution (38).

Computed Tomography and Other Imaging Modalities

The potential benefits of computed tomographic (CT) scanning in the diagnosis of bowel obstruction include the following:

1. With dilute barium used for luminal contrast, the obstructing segment can be localized and characterized as complete or incomplete (39,40).
2. The nature of the obstructing lesion, especially if it is malignant, can be established.
3. Additional abdominal disease (e.g., metastases, ascites, parenchymal liver abnormalities) can be identified.

Evidence also suggests that CT can improve preoperative detection of strangulation in certain circumstances (41, 42). Findings at the site of obstruction include beaklike narrowing, mesenteric edema or engorged veins, moderate to severe wall thickening, and intramural air (pneumatosis). Studies also have suggested that real-time abdominal sonography can aid in the diagnosis of strangulation obstruction. The presence of significant amounts of peritoneal fluid and of an akinetic and dilated loop of bowel is strongly associated with strangulation. In patients who had strangulation but who were thought to have simple obstruction only, these findings helped to make the preoperative diagnosis of infarction (43). Thus, when the clinical picture is not clear, CT and real-time ultrasound may each have a role in the early detection of strangulation. When the clinical picture clearly points to strangulation, imaging studies should not delay resuscitation or expeditious transfer to the operating room. Such studies are not necessarily helpful when clinical criteria and basic abdominal radiographs indicate the presence of a simple and complete obstruction. By itself, this diagnosis mandates urgent exploration, and the information sought should be weighed against the risk of delaying surgery.

General Considerations in Management of the Patient with Bowel Obstruction

The presentation of small bowel obstruction depends on the level of obstruction, the open- or closed-loop nature, and the interval since the onset of symptoms. Pain, vomiting, obstipation, and distention are present in variable degrees. Patients with obstruction of the large bowel present with abdominal pain, distention, and obstipation. Vomiting and acute fluid and electrolyte imbalances are sometimes prominent. Elderly patients are prone to dehydration. The overall picture, however, is usually one of a patient with abdominal symptoms that are evolving and getting worse. In the settings described here, the following questions must be addressed as expeditiously as possible:

1. Is the pain out of proportion to the physical findings?
2. How rapidly are the symptoms and signs evolving (minutes, hours, or more slowly)?
3. Does the patient have dehydration and serum electrolyte and pH imbalances?
4. Is the obstruction complete or incomplete?
5. Is there a possibility of strangulation?

Clinical data and basic laboratory studies provide reliable information to answer the first three questions. Answering questions 4 and 5 often depends on close clinical observation and reexamination in the first hours or days after presentation. Abdominal radiographs and imaging studies are frequently used to provide additional information to help answer the last questions; they also provide information to identify the obstructing lesion.

The principles of diagnosis and management of bowel obstruction begin with clinical information. Laboratory studies and plain abdominal films are used to confirm the diagnosis of obstruction and to determine the extent of physiologic impairment. The patient's history and clinical course in the first few hours of observation are used to determine the likelihood of strangulation. Indications for surgery include rapid evolution of symptoms and signs and diagnosis that the obstruction is complete. Contrast or imaging studies are used only when symptoms are not evolving rapidly and when identification of the underlying lesion might alter the operative strategy.

The initial management of all patients with suspected bowel obstruction includes restricting oral intake and infusion of intravenous isotonic Ringer's or normal saline solution. Restoration of fluid and electrolyte balance is a priority, often requiring frequent evaluation of serum electrolytes and pH. In rapidly evolving cases or in patients with significant dehydration, an indwelling urinary catheter should be placed to monitor urine output. Invasive hemodynamic monitoring (e.g., with a Swan-Ganz catheter) may be necessary to monitor the response to fluid resuscitation in patients with underlying cardiac, pulmonary, or renal insufficiency. Nasogastric decompression is indicated in all but the most mild cases. The nasogastric tube serves to prevent distal passage of swallowed air and minimizes the discomfort of refluxing intestinal content. The use of longer tubes has been advocated in certain settings, especially for patients with chronic but intermittent obstruction arising from Crohn's disease, peritoneal carcinomatosis, radiation enteritis, or many previous laparotomies for obstruction. The underlying rationale is that advancement of the tip of the long tube to the obstructed loop permits more effective decompression, perhaps resulting in relaxation of the loop and relief of the obstruction. Although this concept is appealing, no well designed trials have been performed to support the use of the long tube in such settings (44).

Studies in humans have demonstrated that, even in simple obstruction, bacteria can translocate across the intestinal mucosa, passing into lymph channels (45). Furthermore, experimental studies have demonstrated that germ-free animals can survive strangulation obstruction longer than normal animals and that luminal fluid taken from obstructed segments in germ-free animals is much less toxic than fluid taken from normal animals (46,47). It is well established that perioperatively administered antibiotics reduce wound infection and abdominal sepsis rates in patients undergoing surgery to relieve intestinal obstruction, simple or strangulated. Once the decision has been made to proceed with surgery, broad-spectrum antibiotics covering gram-negative aerobes and anaerobes should be administered. The use of antibiotics in patients who have not yet been committed to surgery has not been evaluated systematically.

The decision to perform abdominal exploration to relieve intestinal obstruction should be made expeditiously, but not in the absence of critical information or before adequate resuscitation. When the diagnosis of bowel obstruction is likely or certain, indications for surgery include the following:

1. Rapidly progressing abdominal pain or distention, with or without peritoneal findings
2. Development of peritoneal findings, fever, diminished urine output, leukocytosis, hyperamylasemia, metabolic acidosis
3. Failure of the obstructive picture to resolve in 24 to 48 hours, even in the absence of evolving symptoms or peritoneal findings

Once a diagnosis of complete obstruction is made, whether simple or strangulated, surgery should proceed without undue delay. It is reasonable to commit the patient to a period of observation if the diagnosis is uncertain, if there is a possibility of a nonsurgical diagnosis, or if the obstruction is not complete. A practical point is that obstruction occurring in a patient without a previous history of laparotomy is not likely to be caused by peritoneal adhesions. This is known as *de novo obstruction* and, whatever the underlying cause, usually does not resolve without surgery.

Specific Types of Bowel Obstruction

Adhesions

Peritoneal adhesions account for more than half of small bowel obstruction cases. Lower abdominal procedures such as appendectomy, hysterectomy, and abdominoperineal resection are common precursor operations to adhesive obstruction. Adhesions form after any abdominal procedure, including cholecystectomy, gastrectomy, and abdominal vascular procedures. In long-term follow-up, approximately 5% of patients undergoing laparotomy acquire adhesive obstruction; of these, 10% to 30% experience additional episodes (48). Simple adhesive obstruction is distinguished from most other forms of obstruction by its capacity to resolve without surgical intervention. According to recent surveys, up to 80% of episodes of small bowel obstruction caused by adhesions resolve without surgery (32,33,38,42,44,49). This observation makes it difficult to distinguish a complete mechanical obstruction that resolves without surgery from a partial obstruction that never was complete. From a practical standpoint, the distinction does not matter. A history of a

laparotomy simply provides a reasonable basis for expectant management of patients in whom it is not yet possible to diagnose a complete obstruction. Ultimately, patients who present with signs and symptoms of bowel obstruction are treated according to the clinical course.

The pathobiology of adhesion formation has been the subject of considerable investigation. Histologic examination of chronic adhesions reveals foreign body reaction, usually to talc, starch, lint, intestinal content, or suture. Talc and starch are found less often than previously because of improvements in the techniques of surgical glove manufacture and sterilization. Mesothelial cells are the presumed origin of tissue plasminogen activator (tPA). tPA binds fibrin and plasminogen, thereby preventing adhesion formation. Inflammatory cells, including mast cells, appear to be significant in the process that produces adhesions, possibly through production of modulators of fibrinolysis and growth factors such as transforming growth factor-β. However, the cell biology of these pathways is not fully defined (50). A number of experimental approaches have been tried to reduce adhesion formation, including peritoneal exposure to tPA, phosphatidylcholine, vitamin E, polyethylene glycol, high-molecular-weight dextrans, and polypentapeptide of elastin (50). The benefit of such strategies in reducing the incidence of small bowel obstruction has not been proved. The most reasonable approach to reducing adhesion formation includes meticulous attention to hemostasis, gentle surgical technique, and removal of foreign material from the peritoneal cavity. It is also possible that the use of monofilament sutures for fascial closure and avoidance of closure of the peritoneum as a separate layer lower the formation of adhesions between viscera and the abdominal wall (51).

Early Postoperative Adhesions

Obstruction immediately after abdominal surgery is uncommon but occurs in up to 1% of patients during the 4 weeks after laparotomy. Adhesions are responsible for approximately 90% of such cases and hernias for approximately 7%. Intussusception, abscess, and technical errors are responsible for the remainder of cases (52,53). Most cases occur after surgery of the colon, especially abdominoperineal resections or operations in the lower abdomen. It is rare for upper abdominal surgery to cause such obstructions. Patients with acutely evolving symptoms and signs represent cases of complete obstruction and should be treated as such. In this setting, the mortality rate may be as high as 15% because of delays in recognition and operative intervention. The loss of bowel sounds after a short period of normal or hyperactive activity is worrisome for ischemia of the obstructed segment. Most cases can be treated as partial intestinal obstruction; with use of nasogastric suction and intravenous fluids, symptoms usually resolve within a few days (Fig. 26.5). When the clinical course does not demand earlier intervention, a nonoperative approach can be tried for 10 to 14 days; this corrects the obstruction in over 75% of cases (54,55).

Hernia

Hernias of all types are second only to adhesions as the most frequent causes of obstruction. External hernias, such as inguinal or femoral hernias, may present with the symptoms of obstruction. Femoral hernias are particularly prone to incarceration and bowel necrosis because of the small size of the hernia inlet (56). Internal hernias, including obturator hernias, paraduodenal hernias, and hernias through the foramen of Winslow or mesenteries, are usually diagnosed at laparotomy for obstruction.

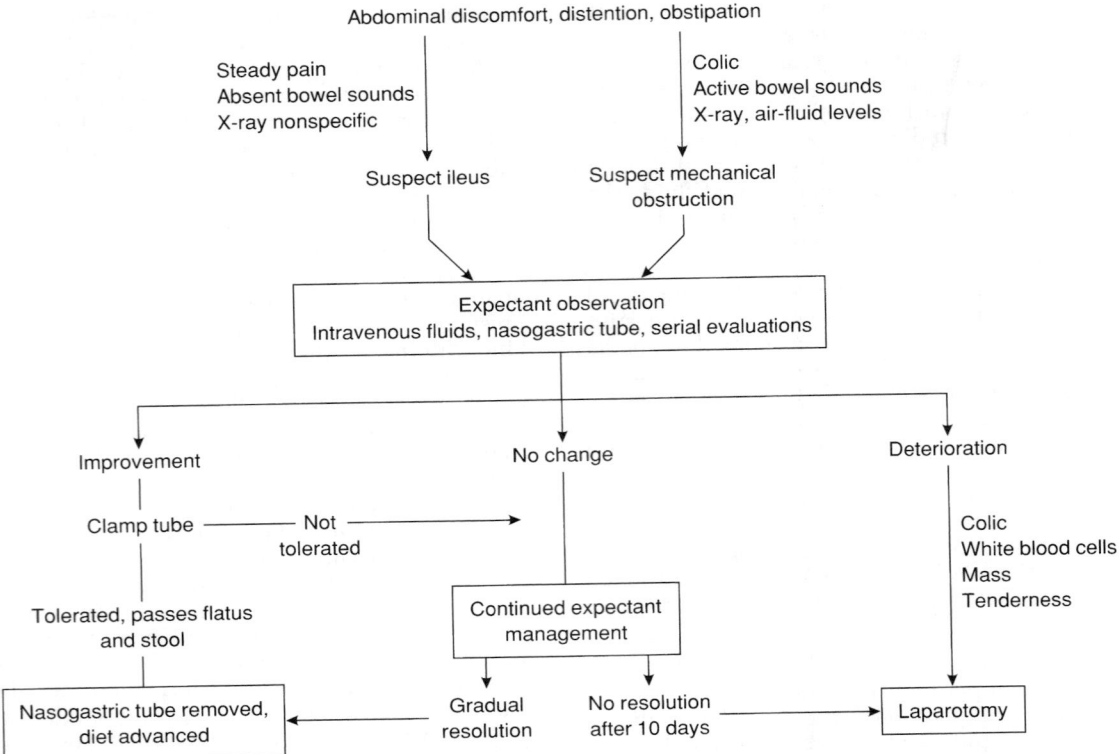

Figure 26.5. An approach to postoperative intestinal obstruction. (Adapted from Welch JP. *Bowel obstruction: differential diagnosis and clinical management.* Philadelphia: WB Saunders, 1989.)

When herniation is the cause of the obstruction, the patient is quickly resuscitated and taken to the operating room. The hernia is reduced and the viability of the bowel assessed. If viable, the bowel is left alone; if not, it is resected. The hernial defect is then repaired. One important consideration is Richter's hernia. In this variant, only a portion of the wall of the bowel is incarcerated. These hernias occur most frequently in association with femoral or inguinal hernias. Complete obstruction can occur if more than half to two thirds of the bowel circumference is incarcerated.

Gallstone Ileus

As a result of intense inflammation surrounding a gallstone, a fistula may develop between the biliary tree and the small or large intestine. Most fistulae develop between the gallbladder fundus and duodenum. If the stone is more than 2.5 cm in diameter, it can lodge in the narrowest portion of the terminal ileum, which is just proximal to the ileocecal valve. This complication is rare, accounting for fewer than 6 in 1,000 cases of cholelithiasis and no more than 3% of cases of intestinal obstruction. Typically, the patient is elderly and presents with intermittent symptoms over several days, as the stone tumbles distally toward the ileum. The classic findings on plain radiographs include intestinal obstruction, a stone lying outside the right upper quadrant, and air in the biliary tree (Fig. 26.6).

Treatment includes removal of the stone and resection of the obstructed bowel segment if there is evidence of tissue necrosis. The difficult decisions in management relate to the biliary tract. Arguments in favor of resecting the biliary fistula and removing the gallbladder include the possibility of recurrence of gallstone ileus and the risk of cholangitis because of reflux of intestinal content

into the biliary tree. When surgery on the biliary fistula is performed, the mortality rate doubles relative to that of simple removal of the gallstone. The long-term incidence of biliary tract infections has not been high enough to warrant an aggressive approach at the initial operation. Some clinicians have advocated cholecystectomy at a second operation, especially if the patient is young and fit. Except in highly selected patients, cholecystectomy should not be performed at the initial operation for gallstone ileus. The entire intestine should be carefully searched to exclude the possibility of additional large stones. The risk of a recurrent gallstone ileus is approximately 5% to 10% (57). Recurrences typically occur within 30 days of the initial episode and are usually caused by stones in the small intestine that were missed at the original operation.

Intussusception

Approximately 5% of intussusception cases occur in adults. An intussusception occurs when one segment of bowel telescopes into an adjacent segment, resulting in obstruction and ischemic injury to the intussuscepting segment (Fig. 26.7). The obstruction may become complete, particularly if tissue inflammation and necrosis occur. Ninety percent of adult cases are associated with pathologic processes. Tumors, benign or malignant, act as the lead point of intussusception in over 65% of adult cases. A significant proportion of cases have been reported to occur after abdominal surgery for other lesions. In the postoperative period, 20% relate to the suture line, 30% to adhesions, and 50% to intestinal tubes (58). Intussusception related to long tubes can occur when the tube is withdrawn, but most frequently occurs with the tube in place. Perioperative intussusception frequently subsides without intervention (58).

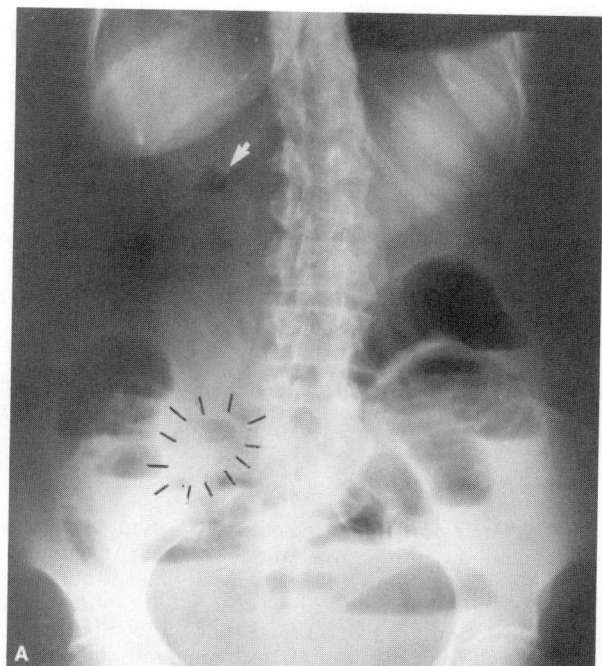

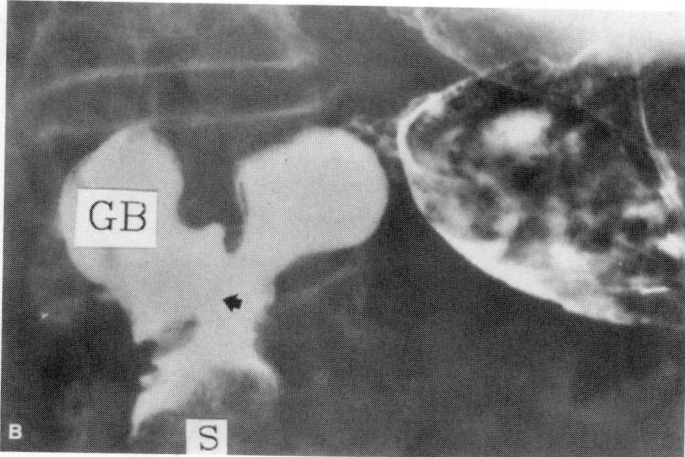

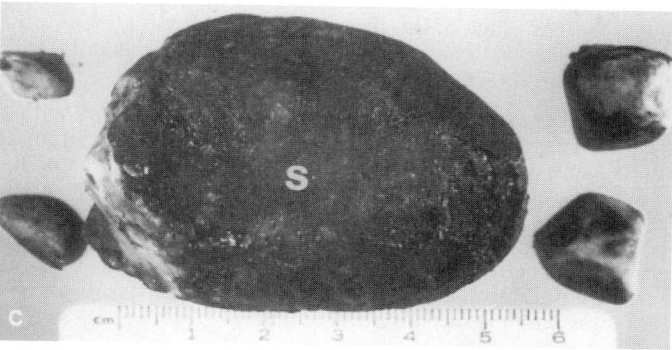

Figure 26.6. *(A)* Plain radiograph of a patient with gallstone ileus, showing air in the biliary tree and a gallstone *(highlights)* outside the right upper quadrant. *(B)* Upper gastrointestinal radiograph showing a cholecystoduodenal fistula *(arrow)* with a large stone (S) obstructing the duodenum. *(C)* Stones recovered from the duodenum and small stones found distally in the small intestine.

Four types of intussusception are recognized: enteric, ileocolic, ileocecal, and colonic. In the ileocolic form, the ileum telescopes into the colon past a fixed ileocecal valve. In the ileocecal form, the valve itself is the lead point of the intussusception.

Radiographic features of intussusception are not specific. Plain films reveal evidence of partial or complete obstruction. Occasionally, a sausage-shaped soft-tissue density, outlined by two strips of air, is seen. It has been suggested that sonography may be useful in diagnosis in both pediatric and adult cases. The mainstays of diagnosis are contrast studies (Fig. 26.8). Because of the high incidence of tumors, surgery is recommended. Reduction by hydrostatic pressure, which is the standard of care in pediatric cases, should not be attempted.

Crohn's Disease

Intestinal obstruction is the most frequent indication for surgery in patients with Crohn's disease (59,60). In this disease, obstruction occurs under two different sets of circumstances. When the disease flares acutely, the lumen may be narrowed by a reversible inflammatory process. The result is an open-loop obstruction that may respond to intravenous hydration and nasogastric decompression and to therapy with corticosteroids. Alternatively, obstruction can occur in the setting of a chronic stricture. Chronic strictures do not respond to conservative measures; when they are diagnosed, operative therapy should not be delayed. Affected bowel may not dilate proximal to the obstruction but can develop a small perforation. Such a microperforation may not be large enough to be associated with free air on plain films. The patient may present with significant abdominal pain and tenderness. A CT scan is sensitive in differentiating conditions that require immediate surgery (closed-loop obstruction, microperforation) from simple obstruction that would otherwise be managed without surgery. In the absence of clinical progression of symptoms and signs, extended conservative management is warranted before the patient is committed to surgery.

Malignant Obstruction

Obstruction can complicate malignancies of the small and large bowel in a number of settings. Most commonly, a primary lesion such as an adenocarcinoma or a lymphoma enlarges until the lumen of the intestine is

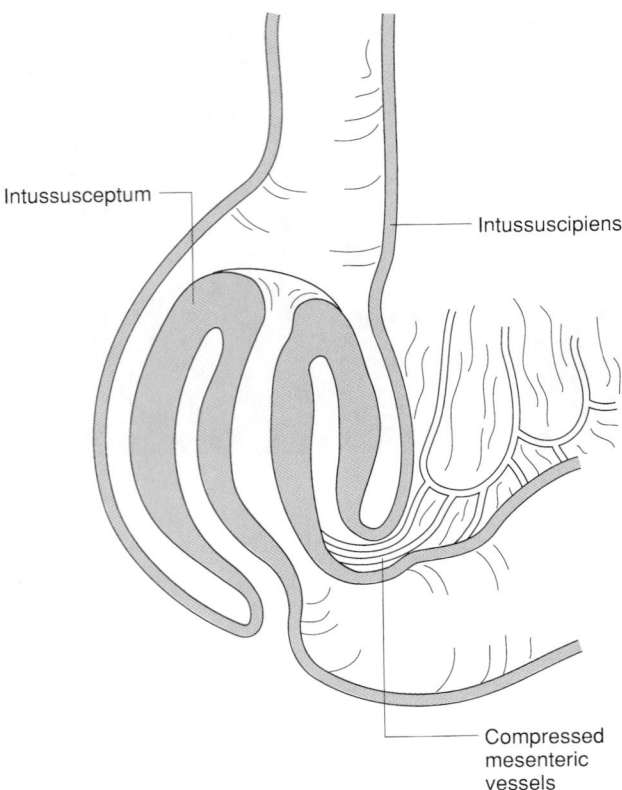

Figure 26.7. Anatomy of intussusception. The intussusceptum is the segment of bowel that invaginates into the intussuscipiens.

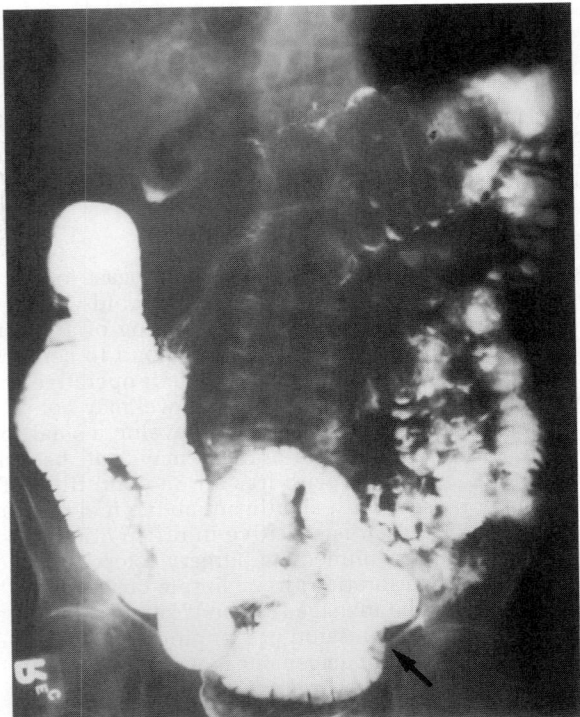

Figure 26.8. Barium enema, showing intussusception of ileum *(arrow)* into ascending colon, shortly after a cecectomy for tumor with ileal to ascending colon anastomosis. (Courtesy of John Braver, M.D., Department of Radiology, Brigham and Women's Hospital, Harvard Medical School, Boston, MA.)

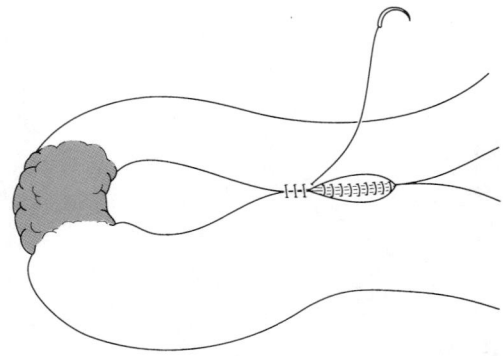

Figure 26.9. Significant palliation can be achieved in a patient with obstructing but unresectable malignancy. Enteroenterostomy is performed to bypass the obstructing segment.

blocked. The lesion then presents with symptoms and signs associated with the level of obstruction. Another setting involves a patient who previously has undergone surgery for malignancy and now returns with evidence of bowel obstruction. The likelihood that the obstruction is caused by recurrent disease relates to several factors:

1. The origin of the primary malignancy
2. The stage of the primary malignancy
3. The designation of the original surgery as curative or palliative

Gastric and pancreatic carcinomas often present with or are subsequently complicated by peritoneal carcinomatosis and ensuing obstruction. With respect to colon and rectal carcinomas, as many as half of cases of obstruction after resection of the primary tumor are caused by adhesions and not recurrent malignancy (61). In addition, even if obstruction is caused by unresectable disease, significant palliation can be obtained through bypass or enterostomy in 75% of patients (Fig. 26.9).

Volvulus

The term *volvulus* indicates that a loop of bowel is twisted more than 180 degrees about the axis of its mesentery. Volvulus has been reported for the cecum, transverse colon, splenic flexure, and sigmoid colon. A special variant of volvulus, complicating a condition known as *Chilaiditi's syndrome,* can occur when redundant loops of the transverse colon slip between the liver and diaphragm and then become twisted (62). The most common site for volvulus is the sigmoid colon, accounting for 65% of cases (63). By definition, a volvulus is a form of closed-loop obstruction of the colon. Volvulus of any segment of the colon is associated with abdominal distention and, usually, severe abdominal pain. As shown in Fig. 26.4, the most common radiographic features include the "bent innertube" appearance of the sigmoid. The preferred method of management involves endoscopic decompression. A flexible sigmoidoscope is advanced gently into the rectum until a rush of air and feces indicates that the loop has been detorsed. A rectal tube is then advanced into the loop as a stent to prevent twisting again. Gangrene of the colon does not usually develop if the patient is treated promptly. This conservative approach resolves the volvulus in 85% to 90% of cases, and elective resection of the redundant segment can then be planned. After endoscopic decompression, the recurrence rate of the volvulus is higher than 60% if sigmoid resection is not performed (64). Semielective operation to remove the sigmoid should be performed if the patient is fit for surgery (64,65). Most of these patients are elderly and infirm, and 15% of all patients with sigmoid volvulus have histories of psychiatric disorder. If the patient presents with peritoneal findings, sepsis, and shock, rapid resuscitation followed by urgent resection and colostomy is warranted. Other forms of volvulus usually cannot be detorsed without surgery. Fixation of the twisted segment is in general a less satisfactory solution than resection of the involved segment.

Radiation Enteritis

Radiation injury elicits an underlying vasculitis and fibrosis that lead to chronic, recurring, low-grade partial obstruction of the small intestine, or cicatrization and bleeding in the colon and rectum. Surgery is indicated for incapacitating symptoms but is associated with increased risk. Attempts to suture scarred loops can result in chronic inflammation and the formation of interloop abscesses and fistulas. The incidence of suture line leak is high.

Role of Laparoscopy in the Management of Mechanical Small Bowel Obstruction

Since the advent of laparoscopically assisted techniques for general abdominal surgery, a number of investigators have reported the feasibility of laparoscopic approaches to obstruction of the small or large bowel. Laparoscopy has been used for lysis of adhesions, enterolithotomy for gallstone ileus, and fixation of volvulus segments. Laparoscopic approaches to all forms of abdominal surgery have been advocated as a way of reducing the formation of adhesions and thus reducing the long-term risk for adhesive small bowel obstruction. This benefit has not yet been documented. In a number of anecdotal case reports, bowel obstruction has been observed as a complication of laparoscopic procedures. Specific lesions causing obstruction include Richter's hernias resulting from entrapment of bowel in trocar entry sites or unrecognized internal or abdominal wall hernias. Conversion to open laparotomy is required right away in approximately 40% of patients and, of those in whom laparoscopic treatment is started, only approximately 50% may actually be treated without subsequent conversion to an open procedure. Bowel injuries occur in as many as 5% of patients in whom placement of ports is attempted (66,67). These outcomes should improve as experience increases.

ILEUS AND PSEUDOOBSTRUCTION

Ileus

Etiologic Factors

Ileus reflects underlying alterations in motility of the gastrointestinal tract, leading to functional obstruction. From a practical standpoint, ileus represents the interval between abdominal exploration and the reappearance of flatus and bowel movements. Our understanding of the physiology of ileus has been hindered by the insensitivity of techniques for studying gastrointestinal motility. Clinically, bowel sounds and passage of flatus have been used to follow postoperative progress. Electromyographic or intraluminal pressure recordings have proved to be reproducible and more objective but have not necessarily correlated with the ability of the different segments of the bowel to coordinate propulsion of gas and liquid from the stomach to the rectum. More recently, the distribution of radiolabeled $^{51}CrO_4$, as it is propelled aborally, has been used as a marker of intestinal transit. When radioactive markers are given orally after laparotomy, they remain in

Table 26.3. POTENTIAL CONTRIBUTIONS TO PROLONGED ILEUS

NEUROGENIC
Spinal cord lesions or injury
Retroperitoneal process, hematoma, tumor
Ureteral colic

METABOLIC
Hypokalemia
Uremia
Ca^{2+}, Mg^{2+} imbalance
Hypothyroidism
Diabetic coma or ketoacidosis

PHARMACOLOGIC
Anticholinergics
Opiates
Autonomic blockers
Calcium channel blockers
Antihistamines
Psychotropics
Phenothiazines
Haloperidol
Tricyclic antidepressants
Clonidine
Vincristine

INFECTIOUS
Systemic sepsis
Pneumonia
Peritonitis
Herpes zoster
Tetanus
Bacterial overgrowth of bowel

the stomach for 12 to 24 hours. Although such markers move into the small intestine rapidly, and electromyographic activity seems normal by 4 to 6 hours after laparotomy, the markers can remain in the small intestine for 3 to 5 days before moving to the transverse colon and beyond for defecation (68). Peritonitis or spillage of noxious material (acid, bile, stool) leads to increases in delay of marker passage.

A number of factors have been implicated in the development and persistence of ileus (Table 26.3). These include sympathetic neuronal hyperactivity and increases in the release of endogenous opioid and other peptides, such as calcitonin gene-related peptide or motilin (68–71). Use of calcium channel blockers and, most important, anticholinergic medications or narcotics can delay recovery from ileus (72,73). In clinical studies, the use of patient-controlled analgesia delivered intravenously delays recovery from ileus compared with the intramuscular route (73). Also implicated are solute and electrolyte disturbances such as hypokalemia and hypercalcemia or hypocalcemia and hypomagnesemia, uremia, diabetic ketoacidosis, and metabolic conditions such as hypothyroidism. In the current era of laparoscopically assisted general abdominal surgery, it appears that less invasive access and manipulation of the bowel may decrease the interval between operation and the passage of flatus and stool (74). There is also evidence that the interval to toleration of oral diets is shorter than previously thought for patients undergoing laparotomy or laparoscopy (75).

Diagnosis

Because ileus is a predictable consequence of laparotomy, it is important to distinguish normal *postoperative* ileus from what some authors have termed *paralytic* ileus. The distinction is based on time since operation and clin-

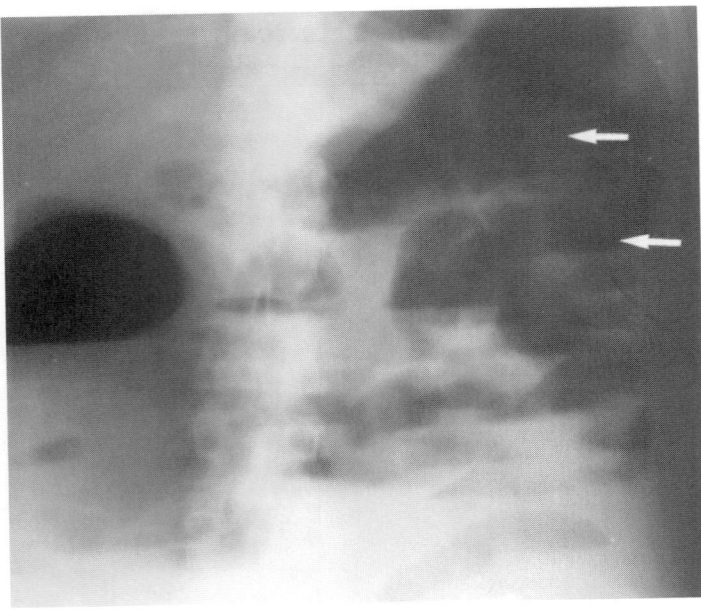

Figure 26.10. Plain upright abdominal radiograph of a patient with ileus. Air–fluid levels are present in the stomach and small intestine *(arrows)*. Gas is seen in the colon. These findings are characteristic of, but not specific for, ileus.

ical circumstances. For example, for a patient who has undergone elective open cholecystectomy, the normal period for the ileus should not be more than 48 hours. For the patient who has undergone a low anterior resection of the colon, 3 to 5 days before passage of flatus would not be unexpected. Thus, the absence of bowel sounds, flatus, or bowel movements beyond the expected period indicates delayed resolution.

When the patient's postoperative ileus has extended beyond the expected period, plain films of the abdomen reveal gas in segments of both the small and large bowel (Fig. 26.10). The patient may experience discomfort and distention as swallowed air fills loops that do not have effective peristalsis. The differential diagnosis includes mechanical obstruction from early postoperative adhesions (see earlier). To differentiate early postoperative obstruction from ileus, contrast studies or CT scan may be helpful (76). The latter may be useful if other abdominal disease, such as an abscess, could be contributing to the clinical picture. The flow of contrast to the large bowel excludes the diagnosis of complete small bowel obstruction but does not necessarily exclude a partial obstruction.

Management

A number of interventions have been advocated for reducing the period of ileus. Prokinetic agents such as metoclopramide, cisapride, and erythromycin have been evaluated in this clinical setting. For certain forms of upper gastrointestinal ileus (e.g., after a Whipple procedure), such medications may be effective in promoting gastric emptying (77). There has been little success in using these agents to shorten recovery times after lower abdominal procedures (78,79). Experimental studies have used pharmacologic interventions specifically directed at abnormal release of neurotransmitters or hormones that might prolong ileus. Agents as diverse as opioid antagonists, a somatostatin analogue, sympatholytic agents, local anesthetics, and nonsteroidal antiinflammatory drugs such as ketorolac are said to promote faster recovery to normal myoelectric activity and shorten intestinal transit times (69–71,74,80,81). Few of these interventions have been evaluated systematically in the clinical setting. Measures to prevent prolongation of ileus include meticulous technique in the operating room, minimal use of narcotics for

analgesia, correction of electrolyte or metabolic imbalances, and early recognition of septic complications that may contribute to prolongation beyond the expected period for ileus.

Colonic Pseudoobstruction

Etiologic Factors

Acute pseudoobstruction of the colon, also known as Ogilvie's syndrome, is an often painless paralytic ileus of the large bowel characterized by rapidly progressive abdominal distention. Plain radiographs of the abdomen may reveal air in the small bowel and distention of discrete segments of the colon (cecum or transverse colon) or of the entire abdominal colon. Although the distention of the colon is not caused by mechanical obstruction, the wall of the bowel, particularly that of the cecum, can become sufficiently distended so that its blood supply is compromised. Gangrene, perforation, peritonitis, and shock can follow. Major risk factors for the development of Ogilvie's syndrome include severe blunt trauma, orthopedic trauma or procedures, acute cardiac events or coronary bypass surgery, acute neurologic events or neurosurgical procedures, and acute metabolic derangements (82). Only 5% of cases occur in the absence of other conditions. Several lines of evidence suggest that Ogilvie's syndrome is related, at least partly, to sympathetic nervous overactivity or interference with sacral parasympathetic efferents.

Diagnosis

The diagnosis is usually apparent from plain films. In doubtful cases, and when bowel necrosis is not a significant worry, a gentle Hypaque contrast enema can establish the nonmechanical nature of the dilatation. Colonoscopy can be both therapeutic and diagnostic. Features suggesting the complication of bowel ischemia include localized tenderness, leukocytosis, metabolic acidosis, evidence of sepsis, and a rapidly deteriorating clinical course.

Management

Initial management includes resuscitation and correction of underlying metabolic or electrolyte imbalances. A nasogastric tube is helpful if the patient is vomiting and can prevent swallowed air from passing distally. When bowel ischemia is suspected, surgery is indicated. If bowel necrosis is found, the affected segment is resected and an ileostomy or colostomy established. If the bowel is viable, a cecostomy is placed to vent the colon and prevent distention.

If distention is painless and the patient shows no signs of toxicity or bowel ischemia, expectant management is successful in approximately 50% of cases (83,84). If the distention worsens so that the cecal diameter increases beyond 10 to 12 cm, or if it persists for more than 48 hours, colonoscopy is recommended. Endoscopic decompression is successful in 60% to 90% of cases (83,84) but colonic distention can recur in up to 40%. Rectal tubes are ineffective in managing distention of the proximal colon. Such tubes can be useful in promoting passage of air and feces after colonoscopy, but should not be used as temporizing measures to avoid colonoscopic decompression. In anecdotal reports, prokinetic agents such as cisapride and erythromycin have been used to treat Ogilvie's syndrome with success. Successful resolution of pseudoobstruction has been reported with sympatholytic agents or spinal sympathetic block. The efficacies of these modalities have not been systematically evaluated.

In the most recent studies, the sympatholytic agent, neostigmine, has been advocated if a 24-hour interval of conservative measures (nasogastric suction, intravenous fluids, nothing by mouth) has failed to improve symptoms (85,86). Serious cardiovascular complications can occur and patients require telemetry. In addition, underlying factors (sepsis, electrolyte abnormalities, ileus-promoting medications) should be addressed to obtain the earliest and maximum benefit.

REFERENCES

1. Treves F. *Intestinal obstruction: its varieties, with their pathology, diagnosis, and treatment.* Philadelphia: HC Lea's Son, 1884.
2. Ballantyne GH. The meaning of ileus: its changing definition over three millennia. *Am J Surg* 1984;148:252.
3. Welch JP. History. *Bowel obstruction: differential diagnosis and clinical management.* Philadelphia: WB Saunders, 1990: 3.
4. Wangensteen OH, Paine JR. Treatment of acute intestinal obstruction by suction with a duodenal tube. *JAMA* 1933;101: 1532.
5. Paine JR, Carlson HA, Wangensteen OH. Postoperative control of distension, nausea, and vomiting: clinical study with reference to employment of narcotics, cathartics, and nasal catheter suction-siphonage. *JAMA* 1933;100:1910.
6. Wangensteen OH, Rea CE. The distension factor in simple intestinal obstruction: an experimental study with exclusion of swallowed air by cervical esophagostomy. *Surgery* 1939;5: 327.
7. Hartwell HJ, Hoguet JP. Experimental intestinal obstruction in dogs with special reference to the cause of death and the treatment by large amounts of normal saline solution. *JAMA* 1912;59:82.
8. Milamed DR, Hedley-White J. Contributions of the surgical sciences to a reduction of the mortality rate in the United States for the period 1968–1988. *Ann Surg* 1994;219:94.
9. Wangensteen OH. *Intestinal obstructions,* 3rd ed. Springfield, IL: Charles C Thomas, 1955.
10. Ellis H. Pathology. In: *Intestinal obstruction.* New York: Appleton-Century-Crofts, 1982:11.
11. Heneghan J, Robinson J, Menge H, et al. Intestinal obstruction in germ-free dogs. *Eur J Clin Invest* 1981;11:285.
12. Roscher R, Oettinger W, Berger HG, et al. Bacterial microflora, endogenous endotoxin, and prostaglandins in small bowel obstruction. *Am J Surg* 1988;155:348.
13. Stark ME, Szurszewski JH. Role of nitric oxide in gastrointestinal and hepatic function and disease. *Gastroenterology* 1992;103:1928.
14. Caplan MS, Hedlund E, Hill N, et al. The role of endogenous nitric oxide and platelet-activating factor in hypoxia-induced intestinal injury in rats. *Gastroenterology* 1994;106:346.
15. Kubes P. Nitric oxide modulates epithelial permeability in the feline small intestine. *Am J Physiol* 1992;262:G1138.
16. Barry MK, Aloisi JD, Pickering SP, et al. Nitric oxide modulates water and electrolyte transport in the ileum. *Ann Surg* 1994;219:382.
17. Shields R. The absorption and secretion of fluid and electrolytes by obstructed bowel. *Br J Surg* 1965;52:774.
18. Sung DT, Williams LF. Intestinal secretion after intravenous fluid infusion and small bowel obstruction. *Am J Surg* 1971; 121:91.
19. Wright HK, O'Brien JJ, Tilson MD. Water absorption in experimental closed segment obstruction of the ileum in man. *Am J Surg* 1971;121:96.
20. Ruf W, Suehiro G, Suehiro A, et al. Intestinal blood flow at various intraluminal pressures in the piglet with closed abdomen. *Ann Surg* 1980;191:157.
21. Ohman U. Studies on small intestinal obstruction. I. Intraluminal pressure in experimental low obstruction in the cat. *Acta Chir Scand* 1975;141:413.
22. Basson M, Fielding LP, Bilchik A, et al. Does vasoactive intestinal polypeptide mediate the pathophysiology of bowel obstruction? *Am J Surg* 1989;157:109.
23. Ohman U. The effects of luminal distension and obstruction on the intestinal circulation. In: Shepherd AP, Granger DN, eds. *Physiology of the intestinal circulation.* New York: Raven Press, 1984:321.
24. Enochsson L, Nylander G, Ohman U. Effects of intraluminal pressure on regional blood flow in obstructed and unobstructed small intestines in the rat. *Am J Surg* 1982;144:558.
25. Fondacaro JD. Intestinal blood flow and motility. In: Shepherd AP, Granger DN, eds. *Physiology of the intestinal circulation.* New York: Raven Press, 1984:107.
26. Camilleri M. Jejunal manometry in distal subacute mechanical obstruction: significance of prolonged simultaneous contractions. *Gut* 1989;30:468.
27. Frank JW, Sarr MG, Camilleri M. Use of gastroduodenal motility to differentiate mechanical and functional intestinal obstruction: an analysis of clinical outcome. *Am J Gastroenterol* 1994;89:339.
28. Summers RW, Yanda R, Prihoda M, et al. Acute intestinal obstruction: an electromyographic study in dogs. *Gastroenterology* 1983;85:1301.
29. Fraser I. Motility changes associated with large bowel obstruction and its surgical relief. *Ann R Coll Surg Engl* 1984; 66:321.
30. Coxon JE, Dickson C, Taylor I. Changes in colonic motility during the development of large bowel obstruction. *Br J Surg* 1985;72:690.
31. Eskelinen M, Ikonen J, Liponen P. Contributions of history-taking, physical examination, and computer assistance to diagnose small bowel obstruction: a prospective study of 1,333 patients with acute abdominal pain. *Scand J Gastroenterol* 1994;29:715.
32. Stewardson RH, Bombeck CT, Nyhus LM. Critical operative management of small bowel obstruction. *Ann Surg* 1978;187: 189.
33. Sarr MG, Bulkley GB, Zuidema GD. Preoperative recognition of intestinal strangulation obstruction: prospective evaluation of diagnostic capability. *Am J Surg* 1983;145:176.
34. Pain JA, Collier DS, Hanka R. Small bowel obstruction: computer-assisted prediction of strangulation at presentation. *Br J Surg* 1987;74:981.
35. Murray MJ, Barbose JJ, Cobb CJ. Serum D-lactate levels as a predictor of acute intestinal ischemia in a rat model. *J Surg Res* 1993;54:507.
36. Gollin G, Marks WH. Early detection of small intestinal ischemia by elevated circulating intestinal fatty acid binding protein (I-FABP). *Surg Forum* 1991;42:118.
37. Kazmierczak SC, Lott JA, Caldwell JH. Acute intestinal infarction or obstruction: search for better laboratory tests in an animal model. *Clin Chem* 1988;34:281.
38. Assalia A, Schein M, Kopelman D, et al. Therapeutic effect of oral Gastrografin in adhesive, partial small bowel obstruction: a prospective randomized trial. *Surgery* 1994;115:433.

39. Frager D, Medwid SW, Baer JW, et al. CT of small bowel obstruction: value in establishing the diagnosis and determining the degree and cause. *Am J Roentgenol* 1994;162:37.

40. Balthazar EJ. George W. Holmes lecture: CT of small bowel obstruction. *AJR Am J Roentgenol* 1994;162:255.

41. Donckier V, Closset J, Van Gansbecke D, et al. Contribution of computed tomography to decision making in the management of adhesive small bowel obstruction. *Br J Surg* 1998;85: 1071–1074.

42. Ha HK, Park CH, Kim SK, et al. CT analysis of intestinal obstruction due to adhesions: early detection of strangulation. *J Comput Assist Tomogr* 1993;17:386.

43. Ogata M, Mateer JR, Condon RE. Prospective evaluation of abdominal sonography for the diagnosis of bowel obstruction. *Ann Surg* 1996;223:237–241.

44. Brolin RE, Krasna MJ, Mast BA. Use of tubes and radiographs in the management of small bowel obstruction. *Ann Surg* 1987;206:126.

45. Deitch EA. Simple intestinal obstruction causes bacterial translocation in man. *Arch Surg* 1989;124:699.

46. Cohn I Jr, Floyd CE, Dresden CF, et al. Strangulation obstruction in germ-free animals. *Ann Surg* 1962;156:692.

47. Amundsen E, Gustafsson BE. Results of experimental intestinal strangulation obstruction in germfree rats. *J Exp Med* 1963;117:823.

48. Ellis H, Moran BJ, Thompson JN, et al. Adhesion-related hospital readmissions after abdominal and pelvic surgery: a retrospective cohort study. *Lancet* 1999;353:1476–1480.

49. Krebs HB, Goplerud DR. Mechanical intestinal obstruction in patients with gynecological disease. *Am J Obstet Gynecol* 1987;157:577.

50. Holmdahl L, Risberg B. Adhesion prevention and complications in general surgery. *Eur J Surg* 1997;163:169–174.

51. O'Leary DP, Coakley JB. The influence of suturing and sepsis on the development of post-operative peritoneal adhesions. *Ann R Coll Surg Engl* 1992;74:134.

52. Coletti L, Bossart PA. Intestinal obstruction in the early post-operative period. *Arch Surg* 1989;55:385.

53. Stewart RM, Page CP, Brender J, et al. The incidence and risk of early post-operative small bowel obstruction: a cohort study. *Am J Surg* 1987;154:643.

54. Pickleman J, Lee RM. The management of patients with suspected early post-operative small bowel obstruction. *Ann Surg* 1989;210:216.

55. Serror D, Feigin E, Szold A, et al. How conservatively can post-operative small bowel obstruction be treated? *Am J Surg* 1993;165:121.

56. Chamary VL. Femoral hernia: intestinal obstruction is an unrecognized source of morbidity and mortality. *Br J Surg* 1993;80:230.

57. Reisner RM, Cohen JR. Gallstone ileus: a review of 1,001 reported cases. *Am Surg* 1994;60:441.

58. Sarr MG, Nagorney DM, McIlrath DC. Post-operative intussusception in the adult. *Arch Surg* 1981;116:144.

59. Mekhijan HS, Switz DM, Watts HD, et al. National Cooperative Crohn's Disease Study: factors determining recurrence of Crohn's disease after surgery. *Gastroenterology* 1979;77: 907.

60. Farmer RG, Whelan G, Fazio VW. Long-term follow-up of patients with Crohn's disease. *Gastroenterology* 1985;88:1818.

61. Soybel D, Bliss D, Wells S. Colorectal carcinoma. *Curr Probl Cancer* 1987;11:259.

62. Orangio GR, Fazio VW, Winkelman E, et al. The Chilaiditi syndrome and associated volvulus of the transverse colon: an indication for surgical therapy. *Dis Colon Rectum* 1986;29: 653.

63. Gibney EJ. Volvulus of the sigmoid colon. *Surg Gynecol Obstet* 1991;173:243.

64. Wertkin MG, Aufses AH. Management of volvulus of the colon. *Dis Colon Rectum* 1978;21:40.

65. Peoples JB, McCafferty JC, Scher KS. Operative therapy for sigmoid volvulus: identification of risk factors affecting outcome. *Dis Colon Rectum* 1990;33:643.

66. Navez B, Arimont JM, Guiot P. Laparoscopic approach in acute bowel obstruction: a review of 68 patients. *Hepatogastroenterology* 1998;45:2146–2150.

67. Strickland P, Lourie DJ, Suddleson EA, et al. Is laparoscopy safe and effective for treatment of acute small bowel obstruction. *Surg Endosc* 1999;13:695–698.

68. Nadrowski L. Paralytic ileus: recent advances in pathophysiology and management. *Curr Surg* 1983;40:260.

69. Zittel TT, Reddy SN, Plourde V, et al. Role of spinal afferents and CGRP in the postoperative gastric ileus in anesthetized rats. *Ann Surg* 1994;219:79.

70. Cullen JJ, Eagon JC, Kelly KA. Gastrointestinal peptide hormones during postoperative ileus. *Dig Dis Sci* 1994;39:1179.

71. Riviere PJ, Pascaud X, Chevalier E, et al. Fedotozine reverses ileus induced by surgery or peritonitis: action at peripheral kappa opioid receptors. *Gastroenterology* 1993;104:724.

72. Frantzides CT, Cowles V, Salaymeh B. Morphine effects on human colonic myoelectric activity in the post-operative period. *Am J Surg* 1992;163:144.

73. Stamley BK, Noble MJ, Gilliland C, et al. Comparison of patient controlled analgesia vs. intramuscular narcotics in resolution of postoperative ileus after retropubic prostatectomy. *J Urol* 1993;150:1434.

74. Garcia-Caballero M, Vara-Thorbeck C. The evolution of post-operative ileus after laparoscopic cholecystectomy: a comparative study with conventional cholecystectomy. *Surg Endosc* 1993;7:416.

75. Binderow SR, Cohen SM, Wexner SD, et al. Must early post-operative intake be limited to laparoscopy? *Dis Colon Rectum* 1994;37:584.

76. Peck JJ, Milleson T, Phelan J. The role of computed tomography with contrast and small bowel follow-through in management of small bowel obstruction. *Am J Surg* 1999;1777: 375–378.

77. Yeo CJ, Barry MK, Sauter PK, et al. Erythromycin accelerates gastric emptying after pancreaticoduodenectomy: a prospective, randomized, placebo-controlled trial. *Ann Surg* 1993; 218:229.

78. Bonacini M, Quiason S, Reynolds M, et al. Effect of intravenous erythromycin on postoperative ileus. *Am J Gastroenterol* 1993;88:208.

79. Cheape JD, Wexner SD, James K, et al. Does metoclopramide reduce the length of ileus after colorectal surgery? *Dis Colon Rectum* 1991;34:437.

80. Cullen JJ, Eagon JC, Dozois EJ, et al. Treatment of acute post-operative ileus with octreotide. *Am J Surg* 1993;165:113.

81. Kelley MC, Hocking MP, Marchand SD, et al. Ketorolac prevents postoperative small intestinal ileus in rats. *Am J Surg* 1993;165:107.

82. Vanek VW, Al-Salti M. Acute pseudoobstruction of the colon (Ogilvie's syndrome): an analysis of 400 cases. *Dis Colon Rectum* 1986;29:203.

83. Love R, Starling JR, Sollinger HW, et al. Colonoscopic decompression of acute colonic pseudo-obstruction (Ogilvie's syndrome). *Gastrointest Endosc* 1988;34:426.

84. Strodel WE, Nostrant TT, Eckhauser FE, et al. Therapeutic and diagnostic colonoscopy in nonobstructive colonic dilatation. *Ann Surg* 1983;197:416.

85. Ponec RJ, Saunders MD, Kimmey MB. Neostigmine for the treatment of acute colonic pseudo-obstruction. *N Engl J Med* 1999;341:137–141.

86. Laine L. Management of acute colonic pseudo-obstruction [Editorial]. *N Engl J Med* 1999;341:192–193.

SURGERY: SCIENTIFIC PRINCIPLES AND PRACTICE, Third Edition, edited by
Lazar J. Greenfield, Michael W. Mulholland, Keith T. Oldham, Gerald B. Zelenock,
and Keith D. Lillemoe. Lippincott Williams & Wilkins Publishers, Philadelphia, © 2001.

CHAPTER 27

CROHN'S DISEASE

FABRIZIO MICHELASSI AND ROGER D. HURST

Crohn's disease is of unknown etiology. It occurs in persons of both sexes at any age, with a peak in the third decade. Although Crohn's disease was originally described as a chronic granulomatous inflammatory condition of the terminal ileum, it has become clear that it can involve any part of the gastrointestinal tract and cause varying symptoms and complications. Medical treatment is administered with the intent of alleviating symptoms and improving the patient's quality of life. Surgical treatment becomes necessary when medical treatment fails or when complications of the underlying disease develop. The surgical options vary according to the location and extent of the disease and the nature of the complications. The optimal management of Crohn's disease requires an understanding of the pathologic characteristics of this entity in addition to the indications for medical and surgical treatment.

EPIDEMIOLOGY

Crohn's disease was first identified as a unique clinical entity in 1932 (1). Since the original description, the number of reported cases has increased greatly, and Crohn's disease is no longer seen as a rare disorder, although it remains relatively uncommon (2). Precise trends in incidence have been difficult to determine because early epidemiologic data were limited to hospital admissions. The first population-based studies were not undertaken until the 1960s. The available data indicate that within the Western world, the incidence of Crohn's disease increased rapidly at least through the 1980s. More recently, the incidence of Crohn's disease appears to have stabilized, with no increase noted during the past decade. In the United States, the incidence of Crohn's disease currently approximates four new cases per 100,000 population per year. The prevalence of Crohn's disease is between 80 and 120 cases per 100,000 population.

Crohn's disease is most common in North America and Europe. It is seldom seen in Asia, South America, or Japan. Few data are available regarding the incidence of Crohn's disease in Africa, but it is thought to be rare in this part of the world. When immigrants from areas with a low incidence of Crohn's disease move to countries where the incidence is higher, their risk for Crohn's disease increases to the level of the native population in the new residence, which suggests that environmental factors influence the incidence. Crohn's disease appears to be slightly more common in women than in men. The onset occurs most commonly between the ages of 15 and 25, with a second, much smaller peak between 55 and 65 years of age. Crohn's disease is very uncommon in children under the age of 6 years.

The incidence of Crohn's disease is highest among whites, lower among blacks, and lowest among Asians. The disease is three to four times more common among ethnic Jews than in non-Jewish whites. This increased risk is greater for Ashkenazi Jews of European descent than for Sephardic Jews of North African or Asian origin. It has been reported that Crohn's disease is more common among persons of higher socioeconomic status, although several epidemiologic studies indicate no predilection of Crohn's disease for the affluent or well educated (2).

Familial clusters of disease have been observed, with a sixfold to 10-fold increase in the risk for Crohn's disease in first-order relatives of patients affected by the disorder. Although familial aggregations are common, distributions within families do not indicate a pattern of mendelian inheritance.

ETIOLOGY AND PATHOGENESIS

The etiology of Crohn's disease is unknown, and possible causes have been the subject of many theories and much speculation (3). In the last decade, basic scientific research has contributed to an understanding of the pathophysiology of Crohn's disease (4).

An altered immune response contributes to the pathogenesis of Crohn's disease. Although no specific primary defect in the systemic or mucosal immune systems has been identified, various immunologic alterations have been described. Lymphocytes within the lamina are substantially increased in Crohn's disease. This increase in submucosal and mucosal lymphocytes is most pronounced among mast cells producing immunoglobulin G. Proinflammatory cytokines such as interleukin-1 and interleukin-6 are also elevated in Crohn's disease. The genesis of the immunologic alterations seen in Crohn's disease is not known. Specifically, it is unclear whether Crohn's disease is a true autoimmune response driven by host antigens or an exaggerated inflammatory response to exogenous antigens or infection.

As suggested by the observed familial aggregations and the variability of risk among differing ethnic and racial groups, a genetic predisposition is likely to play at least a part in the etiology of Crohn's disease. The distribution of Crohn's disease within families is complex and defies a simple mendelian transmission of disease, but recent laboratory studies have suggested a linkage of susceptibility to Crohn's disease to chromosomes 3, 7, 12, and 16 (5).

Numerous infectious agents have been investigated as potential causes of Crohn's disease, with mycobacteria receiving the most attention. Since the original description of Crohn's disease, an association with mycobacteria has been postulated. *Mycobacterium paratuberculosis* has been isolated from the resected specimens of some patients with Crohn's disease. This association has not been a consistent finding, and even sensitive polymerase chain reaction studies have failed to provide definitive evidence of the presence of *M. paratuberculosis*-specific DNA in bowel affected by Crohn's disease. Other specific agents that have been extensively studied include measles virus and *Helicobacter pylori*. To date, no single infectious agent has been identified as a cause of Crohn's disease (6).

Environmental factors, including diet and smoking, have also been investigated as potential causes of Crohn's disease. Although dietary modification can affect the severity of the symptoms of Crohn's disease, no dietary factor has been identified as a cause of the disease. Smokers are at a higher risk for contracting Crohn's disease than nonsmokers are (7). Additionally, smoking is known to exacerbate existing disease. The component of cigarette smoke that is responsible for the deleterious affect on the clinical course of Crohn's disease is not known, but it seems likely that chemical components of cigarette smoke represent an aggravating factor rather than a causative agent for Crohn's disease.

Studies of intestinal transport have demonstrated an increased intestinal permeability in both patients with Crohn's disease and their symptom-free first-degree relatives (8). This has led some investigators to speculate that Crohn's disease is the result of an altered mucosal barrier function that allows abnormal interactions to take place between the multitude of antigenic substrates normally found in the gut lumen and the immunocompetent tissue of the submucosa.

Epidemiologic data, along with clinical observations and the results of basic scientific investigation, suggest that the pathogenesis of Crohn's disease is complex and that no one single genetic abnormality or environmental factor is responsible. Instead, Crohn's disease is more likely the result of a combination of multiple predisposing factors and environmental or infectious triggers that set an immunologic derangement into motion (3).

PATHOLOGY

The gross and microscopic features of Crohn's disease can occur in any segment of the gastrointestinal tract. The disease tends to be discontinuous and segmental, affecting isolated segments of the gastrointestinal tract. Disease of the terminal ileum with or without some involvement of the cecum is the most common pattern, representing approximately 60% of cases (9). Crohn's disease is limited to the colon in 15% to 20% of cases. In 10% of cases, the proximal small bowel is involved, and in approximately 15% of patients, a pattern of multiple sites of disease is found. Perianal manifestations of Crohn's disease, including perianal fistulae, abscesses, and stenoses, occur in about one third of patients with Crohn's disease. In half of these cases, perianal disease occurs simultaneously with active disease elsewhere in the gastrointestinal tract.

Gross Pathology

The earliest gross manifestation of Crohn's disease is the development of small aphthous ulcers (10). Aphthous ulcers are small areas of mucosal ulceration that generally develop over microscopic lymphoid aggregates. Aphthous ulcers appear as red spots or focal mucosal depressions in

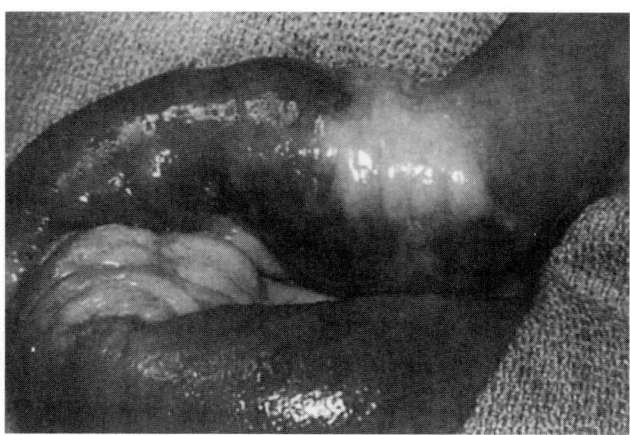

Figure 27.1. Fat wrapping or "creeping fat" of the terminal ileum. (From Scott S, Fazio VW. The surgical management of Crohn's disease. In: Kirsner JB, ed. *Inflammatory bowel disease,* 5th ed. Philadelphia: WB Saunders, 2000:658–709, with permission.)

the fresh specimen. As the disease progresses, the aphthous ulcers enlarge and become stellate. The ulcerations coalesce to form longitudinal mucosal ulcerations. In Crohn's disease of the small bowel, these linear ulcerations always occur along the mesenteric aspect of the bowel wall. Further development of disease leads to a serpiginous network of thin, linear ulcerations that surround islands of edematous mucosa; these produce the classic "cobblestone" appearance. Mucosal ulcerations may penetrate through the submucosa and coalesce to form intramural channels that can bore through the bowel wall and produce abscesses, fistulae, or sinuses (11).

The inflammation of Crohn's disease extends through all layers of the bowel wall. The inflammation also involves the mesentery and regional lymph nodes, so that the mesentery can become massively thickened. During early or acute intestinal inflammation, the bowel wall is hyperemic and boggy. As the inflammation becomes chronic, fibrotic scarring develops, and the bowel becomes thickened and leathery (Fig. 27.1).

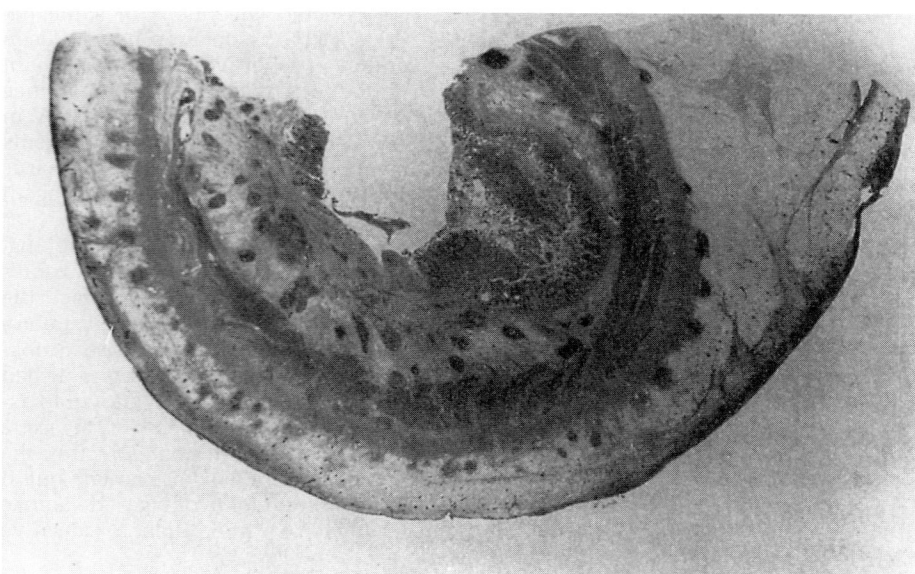

Figure 27.2. Classic distribution of lymphoid aggregates in Crohn's disease, which are scattered across all layers of the bowel wall but are visible primarily as "rosary beads" in the submucosa and subserosa. (From Block GE, Michelassi FM, Tanaka M, et al. Crohn's disease. *Curr Probl Surg* 1993; 30:173–272, with permission.)

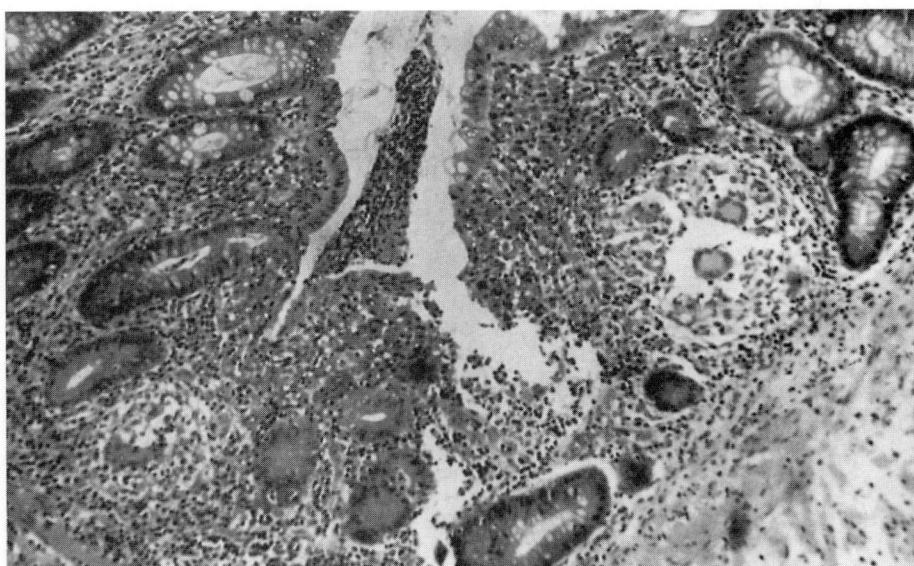

Figure 27.3. Aphthoid ulcer with two adjacent noncaseating granulomas containing giant cells. (From Block GE, Michelassi FM, Tanaka M, et al. Crohn's disease. *Curr Probl Surg* 1993;30:173–272, with permission.)

Microscopic Pathology

Crohn's disease results in a transmural inflammation characterized by multiple lymphoid aggregates that thicken and expand the submucosa. In some cases, the lymphoid aggregates are not limited to the submucosa but extend through the muscularis propria. The presence of well-developed lymphoid aggregates in an edematous or fibrotic submucosa or subserosa is virtually diagnostic of Crohn's disease (Fig. 27.2). A sentinel microscopic feature of Crohn's disease is the presence of noncaseating granulomas (Fig. 27.3). They are found in up to 50% of surgically resected specimens but are only rarely seen in specimens obtained endoscopically. Although granulomas are a valuable diagnostic feature of Crohn's disease, their presence is not pathognomonic, and they do not imply activity (10).

CLINICAL FEATURES

The clinical features of Crohn's disease vary according to the location of the involved intestinal segments and the development of related complications, which include intestinal obstruction, inflammatory mass, fistula, abscess, free perforation, hemorrhage, and cancer.

Patterns of Disease

Crohn's disease can be loosely categorized based on the gross pattern of disease that gives rise to the clinical manifestations and associated complications. The three categories of Crohn's disease are *stricturing, perforating,* and *inflammatory.* These three categories do not represent distinct forms of disease; rather, they provide a means to describe and categorize the predominant gross manifestation of disease (12). Although features of more than one pattern often occur in the same patient or even in the same segment of intestine, one pattern tends to predominate in most cases. The predominant pattern of disease often determines the clinical presentation and affects management and treatment options.

Inflammatory Pattern

Uncomplicated inflammation is manifested by mucosal ulceration and thickening of the bowel wall caused by inflammatory infiltration and edema. This process can result in narrowing of the intestinal lumen and even partial intestinal obstruction. Intestinal luminal narrowing resulting from inflammation and edema can often be relieved with medical treatment.

Stricturing Pattern

In the stricturing pattern of disease, the intestinal lumen is narrowed by fibrotic scar tissue. These cicatricial strictures are referred to as *"fibrostenotic" lesions.* Patients with a predominantly stricturing pattern of Crohn's disease have primarily obstructive symptoms. Fibrotic strictures are not reversible with medical treatment, so that symptomatic stricturing disease often requires surgical management.

Perforating Pattern

The perforating pattern of disease is characterized by the development of fistulae and abscesses. Small sinus tracts, which typically originate from the mesenteric portion of the intestinal lumen, bore through the bowel wall. They may simply penetrate for a short distance, in which case they are seen as blind tracts on small bowel radiographs, or they may give rise to abscesses or fistulae (Fig. 27.4). As perforating disease develops, the inflammatory response about the boring sinus typically results in the formation of adhesions, most often to an adjoining segment of intestine, the urinary bladder, or the abdominal wall. The boring sinus then advances through the adhesion and into the adjacent structure, so that a fistula forms. Only rarely does this process result in free perforation with spillage of intestinal contents into the abdominal cavity. Frequently, perforating disease is accompanied by some degree of stricture formation, but the pattern of fistulae and abscesses generally dictates the surgical strategy.

Crohn's Disease of the Small Bowel

The symptoms of small bowel Crohn's disease include chronic abdominal pain, weight loss, fever, and anorexia (13). The predominant symptom is pain, which occurs in up to 90% of cases. Abdominal pain related to partial intestinal obstruction is intermittent and cramping and is often brought on by meals. More persistent pain can be the result of acute exacerbations of inflammation or the development of septic complications, such as abscesses. Patients with perforating small bowel disease may have

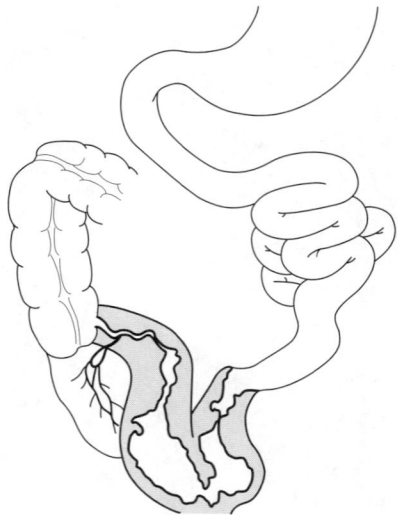
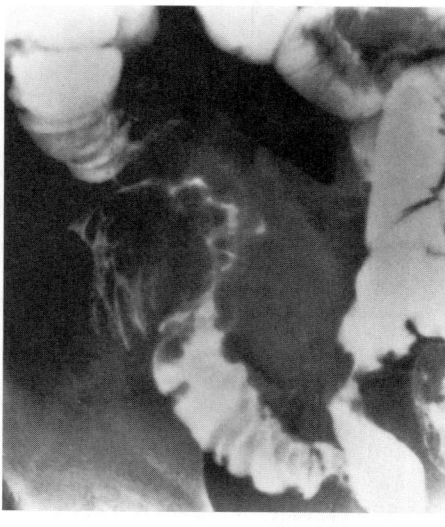

Figure 27.4. Small bowel follow-through study showing a right psoas abscess originating from a walled-off perforation of the terminal ileum. (From Michelassi F. Crohn's disease. In: Bell RH, Rikkers LF, Mulholland MW, eds. *Digestive tract surgery.* Philadelphia: Lippincott–Raven, 1996:1201–1227.)

fever or a tender palpable mass associated with an abscess or phlegmon. Fistulization to the skin, urinary bladder, or vagina may also occur. An enlarged inflammatory mass that adheres to the retroperitoneum can compress the right ureter and cause symptomatic ureteral obstruction and hydronephrosis. Diarrhea, a hallmark of Crohn's colitis, is not often a predominant symptom in Crohn's disease limited to the small bowel. However, many patients with small bowel Crohn's disease report an increased frequency of bowel movements. Many patients with small bowel disease lose weight because of anorexia or avoidance of food for fear of initiating abdominal pain. Malnutrition and weight loss may also result from malabsorption and protein loss in cases of extensive Crohn's disease affecting a long segment of small bowel.

Crohn's Colitis

Patients with Crohn's disease of the colon typically have diarrhea along with abdominal pain and hematochezia. Crohn's colitis can give rise to manifestations of perforating disease, with the formation of abscesses and intestinal fistulae. Stricture can also occur in chronic Crohn's colitis and give rise to symptoms of colonic obstruction, including abdominal pain and distention. Toxic megacolon can develop in Crohn's colitis, but this potentially life-threatening complication is much less frequent in Crohn's colitis than in ulcerative colitis.

Perianal Crohn's Disease

Perianal Crohn's disease results in the formation of perianal fistulae, abscesses, and strictures that are often associated with hypertrophic perianal skin tags, fissures, and perineal scarring. Perianal manifestations of Crohn's disease include acute pain (abscess), purulent drainage and chronic discomfort (fistula), and laborious defecation (anal stenosis).

It is important to distinguish perianal from rectal Crohn's disease. In rectal Crohn's disease, the rectal mucosa is inflamed and ulcerated, whereas in perianal Crohn's disease, inflammation and fistulization develop in the anal crypt glands. This distinction is key in planning therapy for patients with perianal Crohn's disease.

Extraintestinal Disease

Crohn's disease is associated with a variety of extraintestinal manifestations. They include dermatologic, ocular, hepatobiliary, and joint disorders. Dermatologic disorders in Crohn's disease include erythema nodosum and pyoderma gangrenosum. Ocular manifestations include uveitis and episcleritis. Ankylosing spondylitis, sacral ileitis, and a seronegative peripheral polyarthropathy are associated with Crohn's disease. Patients with Crohn's disease are also at risk for the development of primary sclerosing cholangitis, but this very serious complication is less common in Crohn's disease than in ulcerative colitis. The manifestations of peripheral arthritis, uveitis, episcleritis, erythema nodosum, and possibly pyoderma gangrenosum associated with Crohn's disease generally parallel the activity of the intestinal disease, and symptoms typically regress with successful medical management or complete surgical resection of the affected segments of bowel. Ankylosing spondylitis and primary sclerosing cholangitis do not correlate with bowel disease activity, and so their clinical course is not attenuated by surgical resection of intestinal Crohn's disease.

DIAGNOSIS

Many patients go for months or years after the onset of symptoms before the diagnosis of Crohn's disease is made. No specific laboratory test allows the diagnosis of Crohn's disease to be made; rather, the diagnosis is most often based on the results of a thorough clinical history, complete physical examination, and small bowel radiography and colonoscopy. Occasionally, tissue obtained during endoscopic biopsy can be diagnostic. Other studies, such as computed tomography (CT), can assist in the detection and diagnosis of the intraabdominal septic complications of Crohn's disease.

Radiography of the Small Bowel

Evaluation of the small bowel is best undertaken with contrast radiography, either small bowel follow-through or enteroclysis. The radiographic abnormalities of small bowel Crohn's disease are often distinctive (14). In early disease, mucosal granularity with ulceration and nodularity are typically apparent. Both the mucosal folds and the

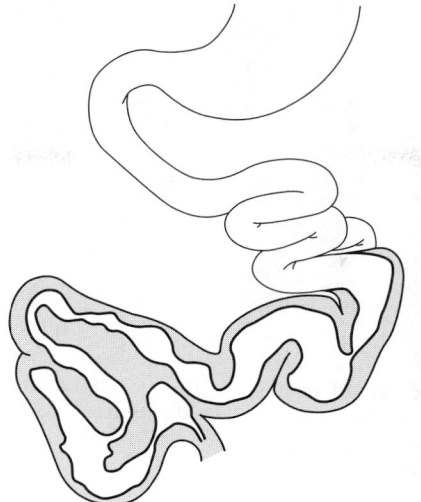
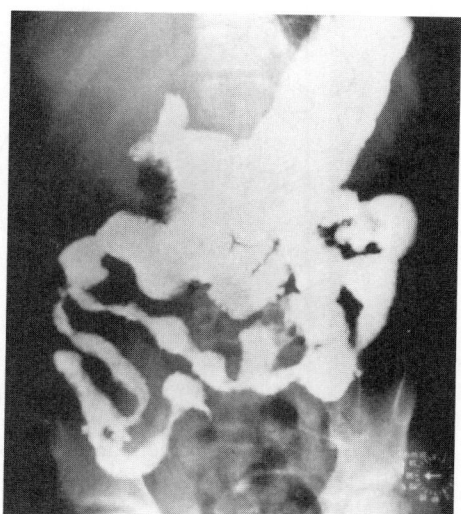

Figure 27.5. Typical radiographic appearance of extensive jejunoileal Crohn's disease. (From Block GE, Michelassi F, Tanaka M, et al. Crohn's disease. *Curr Probl Surg* 1993;30:173–272, with permission.)

bowel wall are often thickened. Luminal narrowing, fissures, and "cobblestoning" are radiographically apparent with more severe disease (Fig. 27.5).

Small bowel studies can in many cases demonstrate the complications of Crohn's disease, including high-grade strictures and fistulae. It is important to note that many enteric fistulae are not apparent by radiographic contrast studies, and the absence of radiographic evidence of fistulization does not exclude this possibility. Small bowel contrast studies also provide information regarding enlargement of the mesentery by phlegmon and the formation of inflammatory masses or abscesses, demonstrated as a mass effect separating or displacing contrast-filled loops of bowel (Fig. 27.6).

Small bowel radiographs should be studied to determine the location of disease and to estimate both the length of small intestine affected by the disease process and the length of uninvolved bowel. It is also important to note the pattern of small bowel involvement; small bowel disease may be continuous, or it may display a discontinuous pattern in which skip lesions are separated by areas of normal intestine.

Colonoscopy

The colon and rectum are best evaluated with colonoscopy. Colonoscopy allows mucosal disease to be visualized and also provides the opportunity for mucosal biopsy and histologic evaluation. In many cases, the terminal ileum can be entered and evaluated. Characteristic features of Crohn's disease seen on colonoscopy include aphthoid ulcers, discrete serpiginous ulcerations that usually track along the long axis of the bowel, diseased mucosa separated by areas of normal mucosa, rectal sparing, and strictures (15).

Computed Tomography

The most typical CT finding of uncomplicated Crohn's disease is thickening of the bowel wall. Bowel wall thickening correlates with disease activity and tends to dissipate with successful medical management (16). The CT findings of uncomplicated Crohn's disease are nonspecific, and routine abdominal CT does not assist in confirming the diagnosis of Crohn's disease. CT can be useful

Figure 27.6. Crohn's disease of the terminal ileum. Resultant mass effect has displaced several loops of small bowel from the right lower quadrant. (From Michelassi F, Balestracci T, Chappell R, et al. Primary and recurrent Crohn's disease: experience with 1,379 patients. *Ann Surg* 1991;214:230–238.)

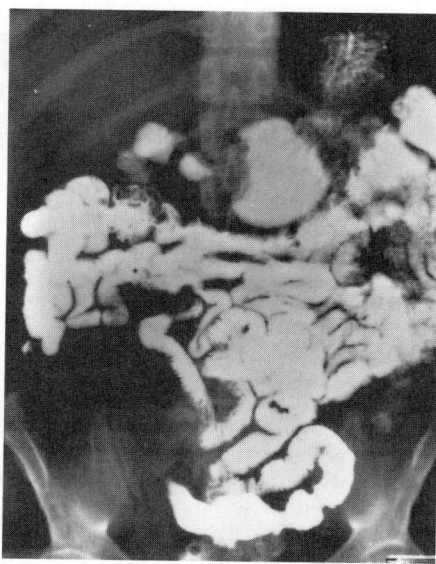

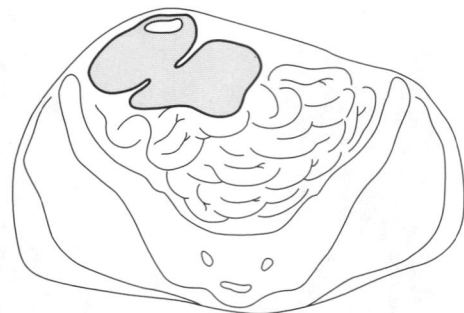
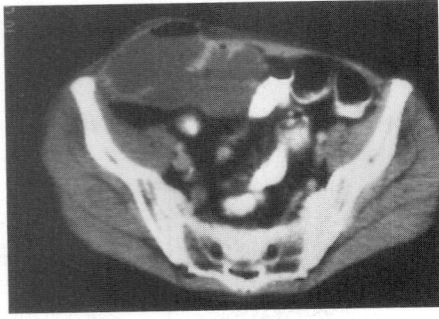

Figure 27.7. Computed tomogram showing an abscess of the right lower quadrant resulting from Crohn's disease of the terminal ileum. (From Michelassi F, Balestracci T, Chappell R, et al. Primary and recurrent Crohn's disease: experience with 1,379 patients. *Ann Surg* 1991;214: 239.)

in identifying the complications associated with Crohn's disease, and when an abscess or inflammatory mass is suspected, CT of the abdomen and pelvis should be performed (17). Most abscesses related to Crohn's disease are readily detectable with CT (Fig. 27.7). Additionally, CT allows for the assessment of possible ureteral obstruction resulting from compression by a retroperitoneal inflammatory mass. Enterovesical fistulae can be detected on CT by the presence of air within the urinary bladder.

DIFFERENTIAL DIAGNOSIS

The differential diagnosis for Crohn's disease of the small bowel includes irritable bowel syndrome, acute appendicitis, intestinal ischemia, and gynecologic disorders, such as pelvic inflammatory disease, endometriosis, and even gynecologic malignancies. Other entities within the differential diagnosis include radiation enteritis, *Yersinia* infections, intestinal tuberculosis, and small bowel tumors. Occasionally, the distinction between Crohn's disease and small bowel malignancies may be difficult to make by small bowel roentgenography. When the diagnosis of Crohn's disease versus tumors is uncertain, the question should be resolved with surgical resection. Nonsteroidal antiinflammatory drugs (NSAIDs) can cause a focal enteritis with ulceration and stricture formation that can be very difficult to distinguish from Crohn's disease.

For Crohn's disease limited to the colon, the differential diagnosis includes infectious colitis, microscopic or collagenous colitis, ischemic colitis, diverticular disease, Behçet's disease, colonic neoplasms, solitary rectal ulcer syndrome, and NSAID colopathy. The condition that can be most difficult to distinguish from Crohn's colitis is idiopathic ulcerative colitis. In the vast majority of cases of Crohn's disease, the unique manifestations of Crohn's disease are readily apparent, and the distinction from ulcerative colitis is not difficult. In only a small percentage of patients does Crohn's disease present in such a manner that it cannot be distinguished from ulcerative colitis. Evidence to support the diagnosis of Crohn's colitis over ulcerative colitis includes small bowel involvement, sparing of the rectal mucosa, cobblestoning of the colonic mucosa, and the presence of skip lesions, perianal abscesses, fistulae or fissures, transmural inflammation, and noncaseating granulomas.

MEDICAL MANAGEMENT

The medical treatment of Crohn's disease is often a challenging endeavor. Because the etiology of Crohn's disease is unknown, no therapy directed against the primary cause of Crohn's disease is available; rather, medical treatment consists of supportive symptomatic care along with a variety of antiinflammatory drugs. Because of the variable course of disease and the differing clinical presentations

and associated complications, medical therapy must be individualized to each clinical situation.

To assess the relative response to therapy, various systems of scoring clinical disease activity have been utilized to allow some degree of objective assessment of overall disease activity. The most commonly used is the Crohn's Disease Activity Index (CDAI) (18,19). Assigned values for the CDAI parameters are weighted by derived regression coefficients (Table 27.1). A CDAI below 150 is indicative of quiescent disease, and a CDAI above 450 signifies severe disease.

Supportive Care

Supportive care includes antidiarrheals, antispasmodics, and nutritional support. Antidiarrheals such as diphenoxylate and loperamide are commonly used. These agents are often effective in relieving diarrhea when the patient has chronic subacute disease or when the diarrhea is related to previous intestinal resection. In the face of a severe acute flare of disease, antidiarrheals should be used with caution because they may precipitate intestinal obstruction or even toxic megacolon. Antispasmodics lessen cramping abdominal pain by decreasing intestinal hypermotility. In the presence of severe acute colitis, antispasmodics should also be avoided because they may precipitate toxic megacolon.

Although no correlation between dietary agents and disease activity has been identified, dietary modification can

Table 27.1. CROHN'S DISEASE ACTIVITY INDEX

Variable	Multiplication factor
No. of liquid or soft stools (each day for 7 days)	2
Sum of 7 daily abdominal pain scores (0, none; 1 or 2, intermediate; 3, severe)	6
Sum of 7 daily general well-being scores (0, good; 1, 2, or 3, intermediate; 4, poor)	6
No. of complications:	30
Arthralgia or arthritis	
Iritis or uveitis	
Erythema nodosum, pyoderma gangrenosum, or aphthous stomatitis	
Anal fissure, fistula, or abscess	
Other fistula	
Fever (>37.8°C) during previous week	
Use of opiates for diarrhea (0, no; 1, yes)	4
Abdominal mass (0, none: 2, questionable; 5, definite)	10
47 minus hematocrit (men), 42 minus hematocrit (women)	6
Percentage deviation from standard weight	1
Crohn's disease activity index (CDAI)	SUM

lessen the severity of symptoms in some cases. For instance, patients with obstructive symptoms often benefit from a low- or minimal-residue diet as a short-term means of relief. Many patients report fewer symptoms with an exclusionary diet based on personal experience with food.

Nutritional support in the form of total parenteral nutrition can (TPN) be of value in malnourished patients with Crohn's disease. TPN has been shown to increase body weight and improve nitrogen balance in patients with severe disease. Prolonged bowel rest combined with TPN can result in a significant reduction in disease activity, and in rare instances, "resting" the gastrointestinal tract with TPN nutritional support is indicated as a means of preparing a malnourished patient for surgery. Although bowel rest may relieve symptomatic Crohn's disease, the disease activity frequently recurs when oral intake is resumed.

Corticosteroids

Systemic corticosteroids are the mainstay of treatment in acute exacerbations of Crohn's disease. In up to 60% of patients with acutely active small bowel disease, clinical remission can be achieved with a short course of oral prednisone in a dosage of 0.25 to 0.75 mg/kg per day (20). For adult patients unable to take oral medication, 40 to 60 mg of methylprednisolone can be given as a continuous daily infusion. More than 75% of patients respond within a week to intravenous methylprednisolone (21).

Long-term systemic corticosteroid therapy is associated with substantial side effects, including osteonecrosis, osteoporosis, cataracts, diabetes, myopathy, systemic infection, and adrenal suppression. Because of the high risk for these serious side effects, systemic steroids should not be given on a long-term basis to treat Crohn's disease. Systemic steroids should be utilized to treat acute exacerbations of Crohn's disease and then tapered and discontinued within a matter of weeks. If symptoms do not adequately respond to a short course of systemic steroids or if the patient cannot be successfully weaned from steroid therapy during a 3- to 6-month period, then alternative treatments or surgery is indicated.

Budesonide, a synthetic glucocorticoid with reduced systemic absorption, has been shown to be effective in moderately acute exacerbations of Crohn's disease (22). Because of its reduced bioavailability, budesonide is less likely to cause the severe side effects observed with systemic corticosteroids. Budesonide can be administered in an oral controlled-release preparation for direct topical application to the ileum and proximal colon. Although the absorption of budesonide is minimal, some systemic absorption through inflamed mucosa does occur, and hypothalamic–pituitary–adrenal suppression may develop. Budesonide is an effective treatment for active disease but has not been shown to have any benefit as a maintenance treatment to prevent recurrent disease.

Aminosalicylates

Aminosalicylates include sulfasalazine and 5-aminosalicylic acid (5-ASA) derivatives (mesalamine). These compounds are commonly used to treat patients with moderately active Crohn's disease or quiescent disease. The antiinflammatory mechanisms of the aminosalicylates are not fully understood, but they likely inhibit the cyclooxygenase and lipoxygenase pathways, along with thromboxane synthetase and platelet-activating factor synthase. Sulfasalazine at a dosage of 3 to 5 g/d has been shown to be beneficial for mild to moderate ileocolitis or colitis. Sulfasalazine, however, has no beneficial effect when disease is limited to the small bowel.

Pentasa capsules (mesalamine encapsulated in ethylcellulose microspheres) provide a continuous release of mesalamine to the small and large intestine and are effective against mild to moderate disease. Continuous-release mesalamine is also effective as maintenance therapy to prevent relapse after medically induced remission or surgical resection (23).

The 5-ASA derivatives should not be confused with acetylsalicylic acid (aspirin) or other NSAIDs. Classic NSAIDs can exacerbate Crohn's disease activity and should not be prescribed for these patients.

Immunomodulators (Azathioprine and 6-Mercaptopurine)

Azathioprine and 6-mercaptopurine (6-MP) are immunosuppressive agents that act by inhibiting DNA synthesis. The result is suppression of cytotoxic T-cell and natural killer cell function. Azathioprine and 6-MP are effective in treating active and quiescent Crohn's disease (24). A 50% to 60% response rate is seen in patients with active Crohn's disease when they are given 1.0 to 1.5 mg of 6-MP per kilogram daily or 2 to 2.5 mg of azathioprine per kilogram daily (21). Both 6-MP and azathioprine are also effective in maintaining remission and suppressing recurrent disease.

As experience with these agents has increased, concerns over possible long-term side effects have lessened somewhat, and their use is appropriate in selected patients. Nevertheless, many potential and serious side effects can occur, and these agents should be used with caution. Close observation is required. Serious potential side effects include bone marrow suppression, hepatotoxicity, and pancreatitis. Bone marrow suppression with 6-MP and azathioprine is dose-related, so that weekly monitoring of blood counts is necessary during initial treatment, and continued monitoring is required every 2 to 3 months during therapy for chronic stable disease. The most concerning toxicity is the potential for iatrogenically induced lymphoma. Accumulating data suggest, however, that the risk for lymphoma in patients with Crohn's disease who are taking 6-MP or azathioprine is low.

In addition to the many potential side effects of 6-MP and azathioprine, which limit their use, these agents have a greatly delayed onset of action. Typically, 3 to 6 months of therapy is required before a clinical response occurs, so they they are not appropriate to treat acute flares of disease. However, 6-MP and azathioprine are often useful for their steroid-sparing effect, and they can be used to maintain remission as systemic steroid therapy is withdrawn.

Metronidazole

Although no infectious agent has been identified as a cause of Crohn's disease, the antibiotic metronidazole is somewhat effective in the treatment of mild to moderately active Crohn's disease. The mechanism of action of metronidazole in active Crohn's disease is not known. The effects are often marginal, and rarely can active disease be managed with metronidazole alone. The long-term use of metronidazole is associated with many side effects, including peripheral neuropathy, which occurs in up to 50% of patients. In some cases, peripheral neuropathy associated with the long-term use of metronidazole is irreversible.

Tumor Necrosis Factor Antibody

Infliximab (Remicade), a monoclonal chimeric anti-tumor necrosis factor antibody, represents a novel approach to the management of Crohn's disease. This agent actively blocks tumor necrosis factor (TNF), a proinflammatory cytokine thought to be important in the pathogenesis of Crohn's disease. Trials have shown clinical response rates of up to 80% within 1 week of a single infusion of infliximab (25,26). Infliximab is indicated for moderately active Crohn's disease that has not adequately responded to more conventional treatment. Infliximab is also effective against persistent perianal fistulae associated with Crohn's disease (27). Initial infusions are typically well tolerated, but a serum sickness-like syndrome has occurred in some patients after repeated infusions. Additionally, it is thought that infusions of anti-TNF antibody may expose the patient to an increased risk for the development of lymphoma.

Other Medical Therapy

Other medical therapies that have been applied in the treatment of Crohn's disease include methotrexate, cyclosporine, ciprofloxacin, omega-3 fatty acids, and thalidomide (21).

Selecting the optimal medical regimen for each patient requires experience and special expertise. Although most patients respond to initial measures of medical management, ultimately three fourths of patients with Crohn's disease require surgery. It is important to emphasize that the goal of medical treatment of Crohn's disease is to alleviate symptoms and improve the quality of life and overall health of the patient. This can often be a difficult balance to attain, given the many potential side effects observed with the most commonly utilized therapies. The patient, the gastroenterologist, and the surgeon should not mistakenly assume that avoidance of surgery is a primary goal of medical treatment. Otherwise, the patient may unduly suffer from inadequately controlled Crohn's disease, be at risk for side effects and complications related to ineffective medical treatment, and be denied the significant and typically long-term benefits seen in the vast majority of patients who undergo surgical treatment for Crohn's disease.

SURGICAL TREATMENT

Crohn's disease is a recurring disorder that cannot be cured with surgical resection. As such, surgery is intended to provide palliation. The surgeon must strive to alleviate symptoms as effectively as possible without exposing the patient to excessive morbidity. Nonresectional techniques, such as strictureplasty, may be required to avoid excessive loss of intestine, or it may be necessary to remove only portions of the gastrointestinal tract affected by severe disease while leaving segments with mild, asymptomatic disease intact. To manage Crohn's disease optimally, the surgeon must always keep in mind the natural history of the disease, with its high risk for recurrence and the need for repeated surgery.

Indications for Operation

Failure of Medical Management

Failure of medical management to control symptoms and disease activity adequately is the most common indication for surgery (28). Medical treatment fails when symptoms of an acute flare do not improve or new complications of Crohn's disease develop during optimal treatment. Some patients fail medical therapy because significant side effects develop that are related to the medical therapy; in other cases, symptoms may resolve during sys-

temic steroid therapy only to recur with each attempt to withdraw the steroids. Because severe complications are inevitable with prolonged steroid use, surgery is indicated if the patient cannot be weaned from corticosteroids within 3 to 6 months.

Intestinal Obstruction

Partial or complete intestinal obstruction is a common indication for surgery in Crohn's disease (9). Chronic partial obstruction of the small bowel is much more common than acute complete obstruction. Luminal narrowing and partial small bowel obstruction in Crohn's disease is the result of acute inflammation and bowel wall thickening or chronic scarring with fixed stricture formation. Partial small bowel obstruction related to acute inflammation and bowel wall edema can often be managed with medical therapy. Failure of medical treatment to relieve obstructive symptoms in these patients obviously indicates a need for surgery. Patients with obstructive symptoms that result from fibrotic, fixed strictures do not benefit from medical therapy and are best treated with surgery.

Enteric Fistulae

Asymptomatic enteroenteric fistulae do not require surgical treatment. However, the presence of asymptomatic fistulae may indicate the presence of severe, complicated disease associated with other indications for surgical treatment. A fistula by itself is usually an indication for surgery if it causes discomfort or embarrasses the patient (e.g., enterocutaneous or enterovaginal fistula) or has the potential to induce significant complications (e.g., enterovesical fistula causing repeated urinary tract infections and deteriorating renal function) (29).

Abscess and Inflammatory Mass

Intraabdominal abscesses and inflammatory masses occur less frequently than fistulae but are more often an indication for surgical therapy. Abscesses do not respond to medical treatment and require drainage. An abscess from Crohn's disease that has been drained percutaneously is very likely to recur or result in an enterocutaneous fistula, so that surgical resection is warranted even after successful drainage. Inflammatory masses indicate severe disease and often harbor an unrecognized abscess (30). Thus, inflammatory masses are considered an indication for surgical treatment.

Hemorrhage

Hemorrhage is an uncommon complication of Crohn's disease. Massive gastrointestinal hemorrhage occurs more frequently in Crohn's colitis than in small bowel Crohn's disease. Hemorrhage in small bowel Crohn's disease tends to be more indolent, with episodes of chronic bleeding that require intermittent transfusion (31).

Perforation

Free perforation with peritonitis is a rare complication of Crohn's disease, occurring in approximately 1% of patients. Free perforation is a clear indication for urgent operation (32).

Cancer and Suspected Cancer

Patients with Crohn's disease are at increased risk for the development of adenocarcinoma of the colon and small intestine. Current estimates indicate an observed prevalence of 0.3% for small bowel adenocarcinoma and 1.8% for large-intestinal adenocarcinoma (33,34). The preoperative diagnosis of carcinoma of the small bowel is difficult because the symptoms, physical signs, and radiologic findings of small bowel cancer are similar to those of the underlying Crohn's disease. Adenocarcinomas complicating Crohn's disease tend to be multifocal (10%) and poorly differentiated. Nonfunctional bowel seems to be at particular risk for malignancy. Therefore, bypass surgery should not be performed for Crohn's disease of the small bowel, and rectal stumps should either be restored to their function or excised.

Small intestinal carcinoma should be suspected in patients with long-standing disease whose symptoms change suddenly, especially after a lengthy quiescent period. Small bowel cancer should also be considered when high-grade obstruction fails to resolve with conservative treatment.

Although surveillance of the large bowel is feasible, it is difficult to distinguish neoplastic from inflammatory stricture and is thus difficult to make an early diagnosis of adenocarcinoma. When adenocarcinoma is suspected or histologically proven, surgical treatment is indicated.

Growth Retardation

Growth is retarded in up to 25% of children affected by Crohn's disease (35). If growth retardation persists despite adequate medical and nutritional therapy, prompt surgical treatment should be carried out before puberty; meaningful growth will not occur after epiphyseal closure.

Preoperative Evaluation and Preparation

A complete preoperative assessment of the gastrointestinal tract should be undertaken before elective surgery for abdominal Crohn's disease. The small bowel should be studied with contrast radiography. The colon and rectum are best evaluated with colonoscopy. Patients with suspected abscesses or inflammatory masses should undergo preoperative CT of the abdomen and pelvis to determine the extent of the septic complication, the feasibility of percutaneous drainage, and the relationship of the septic process to retroperitoneal structures. Occasionally, contrast injected into the cutaneous opening of an enterocutaneous fistula can help in determining the extent of disease, the presence of complicating abscess, and the anatomy of diseased segments.

Meticulous mechanical preparation of the colon should be undertaken in all patients before abdominal surgery for Crohn's disease. Even in cases thought to be limited to the small bowel, the surgeon must always be prepared to perform surgery on the colon because secondary involvement of the colon by fistulae or an adherent inflammatory mass cannot always be excluded by preoperative studies.

Abdominal Exploration

At initial laparotomy, the contents of the abdomen should be thoroughly examined and the location and extent of disease identified. When exploring the abdomen, the surgeon should closely examine the entire small bowel from the ligament of Treitz to the ileocecal valve, taking note of the precise locations of disease. This often requires division of areas of adhesion. The surgeon should make note of areas of possible fistulization. Any inflammatory adhesions should be suspected of harboring a fistulous tract. Although separation of inflammatory adhesions is appropriate, adhesions that may be a result of cancer should be left intact and the affected area resected *en bloc*.

In most cases, the areas affected by Crohn's disease are readily apparent, with the bowel wall thickened and indurated. Serosal hyperemia with a "corkscrew" appearance of the serosal vessels is typical. Also seen in areas of disease is encroachment of the mesentery fat along the serosal surface of the bowel, often referred to as "fat wrapping" or "creeping fat" (Fig. 27.1). The mesentery of grossly diseased bowel is often massively thickened and stiff. Serosal manifestations of less severe disease are more subtle and can be more difficult to identify. In mild Crohn's disease, some degree of induration of the mesenteric bowel wall is typically present that can be detected with palpation.

Resection

Small bowel resection is the most common surgical procedure utilized to treat small bowel Crohn's disease. For many years, the optimal extent of resection necessary to provide the lowest risk for recurrence has been a subject of controversy. It was once thought that wide resection with generous margins of normal bowel combined with radical mesenteric excision would result in lower recurrence rates. The accumulated clinical data, however, do not support the need for wide or radical resection for Crohn's disease. Resection should be wide enough to encompass the limits of gross disease; wider resections offer no benefit in terms of lessening the risk for recurrence, even when the mucosal margins of the resected portion are positive for microscopic features of Crohn's disease (36). The extent of mesenteric resection does not affect the rate of disease recurrence. It is now generally accepted that resection to grossly normal intestinal margins is sufficient and that frozen section to exclude microscopic disease at the resection margins is not warranted because microscopically positive margins do not adversely affect long-term results.

Division of the small bowel mesentery that has been affected by Crohn's disease is often challenging. The mesentery in Crohn's disease is typically massively thickened, with indurated fat, hypertrophied lymphatics, and engorged blood vessels. Standard techniques of simple clamping of mesenteric vessels and ligation are inadequate to handle the thickened mesentery because it is often impossible to fashion vascular pedicles for simple ligation. Inadequate control of mesenteric vessels may result in the development of large mesenteric hematomas, which further complicate the ability to gain vascular control and may even result in a compromise of mesenteric perfusion and resultant bowel ischemia. The preferred technique for dividing the thickened mesentery without losing vascular control is to apply overlapping clamps on either side of the intended line of transection. The mesentery is incised and the tissue within the clamps is suture-ligated (Fig. 27.8). To increase the efficacy and safety of mesenteric control in the case of an extremely thickened mesentery, mattress sutures can be applied through the mesentery on the patient's side of the proposed transection line before hemostatic clamps are applied.

Once the resection is complete, the proximal and distal margins of the resected specimen should be examined to ensure that they are free of gross disease. The entire specimen is closely examined for areas that may be suspected of harboring an occult cancer. Should any areas of the specimen be suspected of harboring an adenocarcinoma, a frozen section should be obtained. If the specimen is found to contain an area of adenocarcinoma, further mesenteric resection may be necessary.

A wide variety of techniques for performing intestinal anastomoses have been applied in the treatment of Crohn's disease. These include end-to-end, side-to-end, end-to-side, and side-to-side anastomoses. Standard staple techniques can be utilized on healthy, pliable bowel. Hand-sewn techniques provide more versatility for edematous or hypertrophied small intestine. Regardless of the techniques employed, it is important to follow the basic re-

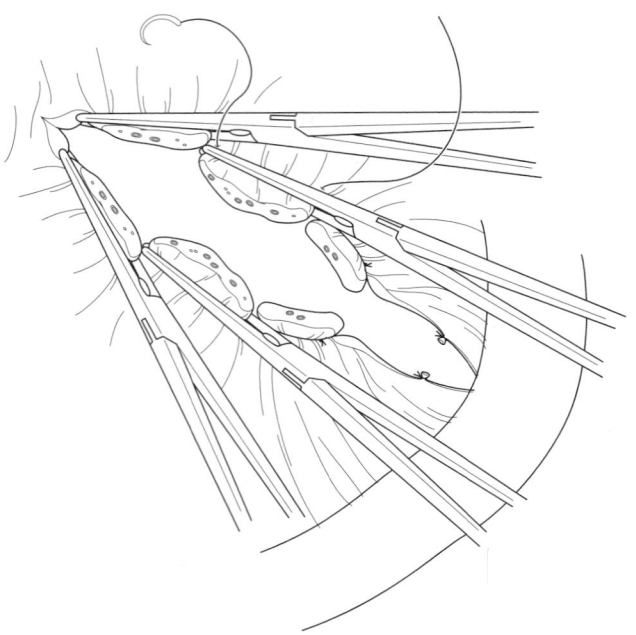

Figure 27.8. Technique for suture ligation and division of a thickened and friable mesentery in a patient with Crohn's disease. (From Walsh CJ, Lavery IC. Ileocecectomy. In: Michelassi F, Milsom JW, eds. *Operative strategies in inflammatory bowel disease.* New York: Springer-Verlag, 1999:294–302, with permission.)

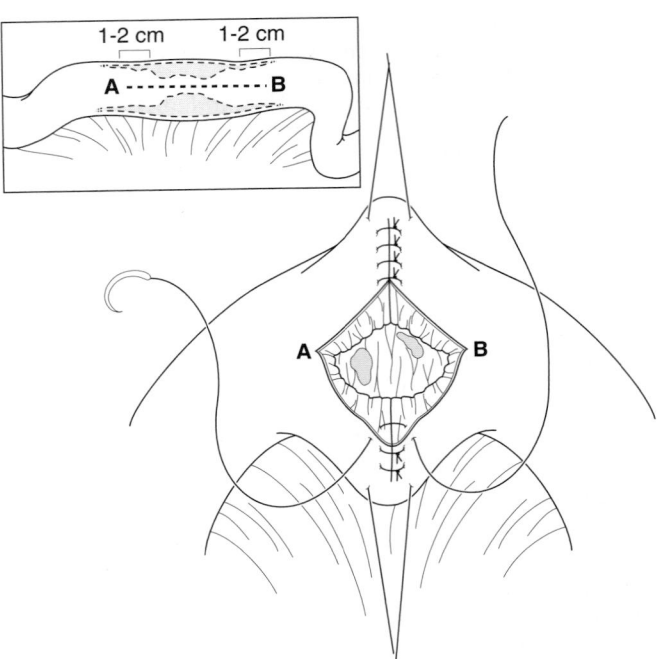

Figure 27.9. Heineke-Mikulicz strictureplasty. (From Milsom JW. Strictureplasty and mechanical dilation in strictured Crohn's disease. In: Michelassi F, Milsom JW, eds. *Operative strategies in inflammatory bowel disease.* New York: Springer-Verlag, 1999: 259–267, with permission.)

quirements for performing a safe intestinal anastomosis (adequate blood supply, no gross contamination or sepsis, no tension on the anastomosis, no distal obstruction, and adequate bowel cleansing). So long as these basic requirements are met and the patient does not have profound malnutrition, resection and primary anastomosis can be performed in Crohn's disease with a high degree of safety (28).

Strictureplasty

Intestinal strictureplasty is a surgical technique that relieves intestinal obstruction while preserving the length of the small bowel. Although strictureplasty is not appropriate for all surgical cases of Crohn's disease, strictureplasty techniques are being utilized with increasing frequency. Strictureplasty is indicated for jejunoileitis with single or multiple fibrotic strictures. Strictureplasty should be considered if the patient has a history of multiple prior resections or rapidly recurring disease. Strictureplasty has also been applied to isolated strictures of the duodenum.

Although strictureplasty is an excellent option in selected cases of small bowel Crohn's disease, intestinal resection is required in most cases. Strictureplasty is contraindicated for segments with acute inflammation and phlegmon. It is also contraindicated in patients with generalized peritonitis or profound malnutrition. Additionally, long, high-grade strictures resulting from extremely thickened and rigid intestinal wall are often not amenable to strictureplasty and therefore require resection.

The two most common strictureplasty methods, the Heineke-Mikulicz and the Finney, are named after the pyloroplasty methods from which they are derived. The Heineke-Mikulicz strictureplasty technique is appropriate for strictures less than 7 cm long (37). With this technique, a longitudinal incision is made along the antimesenteric border of the stricture. The longitudinal enterotomy is then closed in a transverse fashion to increase the width of the bowel at the point of the stricture (Fig. 27.9). Once the

enterotomy is made, the mucosal surface of the stricture is closely examined, and specimens are taken from areas of the stricture where adenocarcinoma is suspected to rule out the possibility of an occult cancer.

The Finney strictureplasty can be utilized for longer strictures, up to 15 cm in length (38). With this technique, the affected bowel is folded onto itself in a U shape and the two limbs are sutured together (Fig. 27.10). A longitudinal enterotomy is then made halfway between the mesenteric and antimesenteric borders, following the course of the U. Again, the mucosal surface is examined and samples are taken as necessary. Sutures are then placed on the posterior wall of the enteroenterostomy, beginning at the apex of the strictureplasty. This suture line is continued anteriorly and is reinforced with an outer layer of interrupted nonabsorbable sutures. For long strictures, the Finney strictureplasty may result in a functional intestinal bypass, with a sizable lateral diverticulum at risk for bacterial overgrowth. For this reason, Finney strictureplasties are utilized far less frequently than Heineke-Mikulicz strictureplasties.

Patients with multiple strictures in close proximity to one another are better treated with a "side-to-side isoperistaltic strictureplasty" (39). With this technique, the loop of diseased bowel is divided at its midpoint between bowel clamps, and the mesentery is incised (Fig. 27.11). The proximal intestinal loop is moved over the distal loop in a side-to-side fashion. With the stenotic areas of one loop placed adjacent to dilated areas of the other loop, the two limbs are approximated by a layer of seromuscular interrupted, nonabsorbable sutures. A longitudinal enterostomy is performed on both loops, and the intestinal ends are tapered to avoid blind stumps. Suspected areas of disease are sampled for frozen section to exclude the presence of occult malignancy. The outer suture line is reinforced with an internal row of running, full-thickness absorbable sutures, continued anteriorly. This layer is reinforced by an outer layer of seromuscular interrupted,

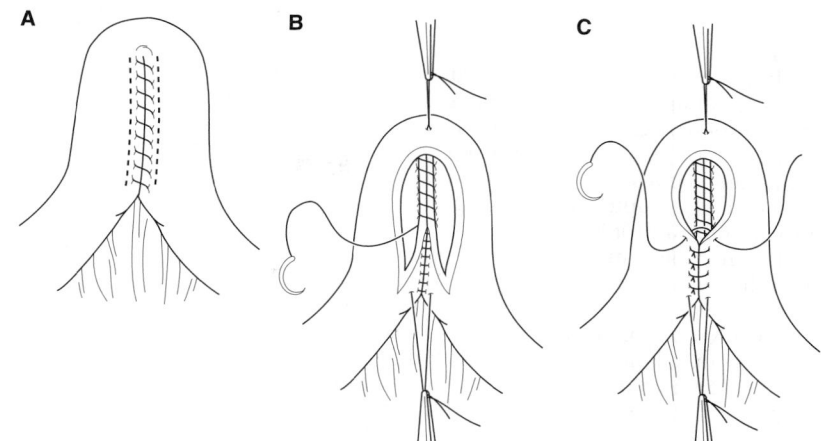

Figure 27.10. Finney strictureplasty. (From Hurst RD, Michelassi F. Management of small bowel Crohn's disease. *World J Surg* 1998;22:359–363, with permission.)

nonabsorbable sutures. The side-to-side isoperistaltic strictureplasty is a very recent advance in the surgical management of difficult cases of extensive Crohn's disease, and initial experience with the technique indicates that it is a safe and effective procedure in appropriately selected patients (40).

In resections, diseased tissue is removed and anastomotic sutures are placed in healthy intestine, whereas in strictureplasties, diseased segments are retained and suture lines are placed in diseased tissue. This has raised concerns regarding the risk for early postoperative morbidity and recurrent symptomatic disease. The available data indicate that in appropriately selected patients, pe-

rioperative morbidity after strictureplasty is similar to that after resection (37,41,42). The most common postoperative complication directly related to strictureplasty is hemorrhage from the suture line. Hemorrhage occurs in up to 9% of the cases. Fortunately, gastrointestinal hemorrhage following strictureplasty is typically minor and can usually be managed conservatively with blood transfusions alone. Occasionally, arteriography with selected infusion of vasopressin into the branches of the superior mesenteric artery is required to control bleeding. Only in rare instances is reoperation required to control hemorrhage following strictureplasty. Septic complications such as dehiscence, intraabdominal abscess, and fistula

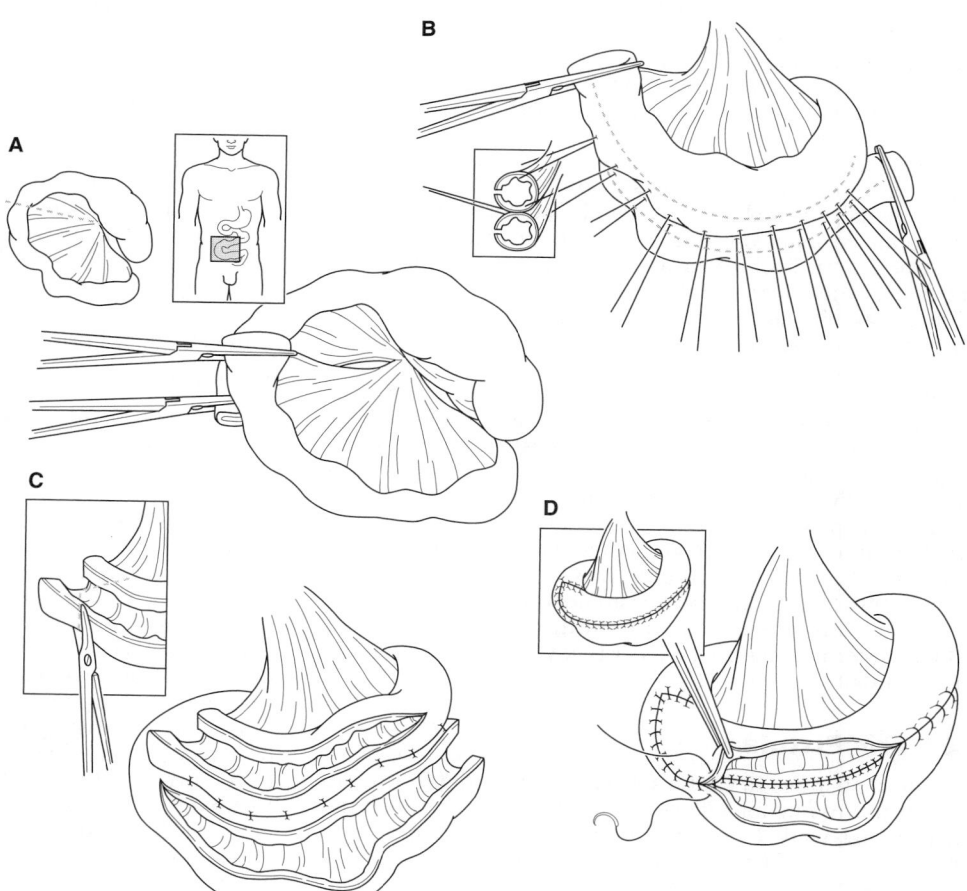

Figure 27.11. Side-to-side isoperistaltic strictureplasty. (From Michelassi F. Side-to-side isoperistaltic strictureplasty for multiple Crohn's strictures. In: *Diseases of the colon and rectum.* Baltimore: Williams & Wilkins, 1996;39:345–349.)

formation occur in only 2% to 3% of strictureplasty cases (37,43).

Although no randomized, controlled studies have directly compared recurrence rates after resection versus those after strictureplasty, the observed recurrence rates after strictureplasty in several reports compare well with published recurrence rates after resection, and rapid recurrence of symptoms following strictureplasty has not proved to be a problem (43–45).

Epidemiologic studies have shown an increased risk for small bowel adenocarcinoma in patients with Crohn's disease. Persistently diseased intestine and continued long-term inflammation at the strictureplasty site may increase the risk for adenocarcinoma. Although isolated cases of adenocarcinoma developing close to or at the site of strictureplasty have been reported, the precise risk for neoplastic degeneration is not currently known.

MANAGEMENT OF COMPLICATED CROHN'S DISEASE

Intestinal Obstruction

Small bowel stricturing disease can range from chronic low-grade obstruction, with symptoms of cramping abdominal pain, bloating, avoidance of food, and weight loss, to high-grade partial or even complete small bowel obstruction.

Intestinal obstruction resulting from Crohn's disease does not pose the same degree of surgical urgency as small bowel obstruction caused by adhesions or herniation. Most patients who have high-grade partial or complete small-bowel obstruction associated with Crohn's disease can be treated initially with nasogastric decompression, intravenous hydration, and steroid therapy. This regimen, in which acutely distended and edematous bowel is decompressed, in most cases results in resolution of the obstruction, so that appropriate bowel preparation and safer conditions for surgery are possible. When there is concern that the obstruction may not be related to Crohn's disease but rather to adhesions or herniation, or if intestinal ischemia or injury is a possibility, then conservative management should be abandoned and the abdomen explored. In addition, if a high-grade or complete bowel obstruction in Crohn's disease fails to resolve, one must consider a neoplastic cause.

Patients with complete obstruction who respond well to initial therapy with nasogastric decompression and intravenous steroids remain at high risk for persistent or recurrent symptoms of obstruction and are best managed with surgery once adequate decompression has been achieved.

Stricturing disease of the small intestine can be managed with either resection, strictureplasty, or a combination of both techniques (46). Patients with short-segment stricturing disease are best managed with simple resection and anastomosis because a relatively short resection does not place the patient at risk for the sequelae of short-bowel syndrome. Resection with anastomosis obviates the short-term concern of hemorrhage from the strictureplasty and the long-term concern of cancer risk when diseased tissue is left in situ.

Enteric Fistulae

Enteric fistulae in Crohn's disease result from full-thickness rupture into an adjacent hollow viscus or through the abdominal wall. Fistulae are present in more than one third of cases of Crohn's disease, but only rarely do they represent the primary indication for operative intervention. Most patients with fistulous disease come to surgery with coexisting stricture or abscess. Although fistulae are not often the primary reason for recommending surgery, when they develop in combination with other complications of Crohn's disease, they generally pose challenging problems to the surgeon (47).

Enteroenteric Fistulae

Enteroenteric fistulae are a common manifestation of Crohn's disease. They are typically asymptomatic and are often not identified by small bowel radiography. Hence, many are not appreciated before operation and are discovered at the time of abdominal exploration or during inspection of the resected specimen (48). Many enteroenteric fistulae, especially ileoileal or ileocecal fistulae, are completely contained within the diseased segments of the intestine and can thus be managed by simple *en bloc* resection. In cases involving distant fistulization, when *en bloc* resection would required extensive sacrifice of uninvolved intestine, the surgeon should attempt to separate normal loops adherent to the diseased segment.

Ileosigmoid Fistulae

Because of the proximity of the terminal ileum to the sigmoid colon, ileosigmoid fistulae often develop in perforating Crohn's disease of the terminal ileum. Typically, active Crohn's disease is limited to the terminal ileum, and the sigmoid colon is only secondarily involved by the ileal inflammatory adhesion and fistulization. Most ileosigmoid fistulae are asymptomatic. However, large-diameter fistulae, particularly those originating proximal to a high-grade stricture, can result in a functional bypass of the colon and cause significant diarrhea.

Two thirds of ileosigmoid fistulae are not recognized before operation (49). For this reason, the surgeon must always be prepared for the possibility of encountering an ileosigmoid fistula in all cases of small bowel Crohn's disease. Most ileosigmoid fistulae can be managed by dividing the fistulous adhesion, resecting the diseased small bowel, and then performing a simple closure of the colonic defect after appropriate débridement of the edges of the colonic fistula opening (49,50). Sigmoid resection is necessary in the following circumstances: (a) The sigmoid is primarily involved with active Crohn's disease, (b) the sigmoid is extensively involved in an inflammatory ileal adhesion and is thus thickened and rigid, (c) débridement of the edges of the fistula results in a large sigmoid defect, and (d) the fistulous opening involves the mesenteric side of the colon and primary closure is difficult.

Ileovesical Fistulae

Ileovesical fistulae are encountered in approximately 5% of patients with Crohn's disease (28). Two thirds of patients with ileovesical fistulae will have a history of pneumaturia, fecaluria, or both. Small bowel radiographs and cystograms often do not demonstrate the fistula between the small bowel and the bladder. CT of the pelvis can provide indirect evidence for an enterovesical fistula when air is present within the bladder. Ileosigmoid and ileovesical fistulae often occur together. Up to 60% of patients with an ileovesical fistula also have an ileosigmoid fistula (50). Thus, the presence of an ileovesical fistula is often an indicator of complex fistulous disease (Fig. 27.12).

The timing of surgery for enterovesical fistulae is controversial. Some physicians consider enteric fistulization to the urinary tract as an absolute indication for surgical treatment, whereas others have argued that patients with enterovesical fistulae can be managed safely with conservative management for extended periods of time (48). Most surgeons and gastroenterologists agree that the effects of chronic urinary tract infection on renal function,

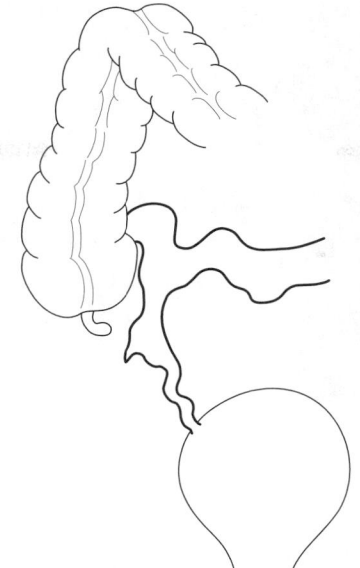

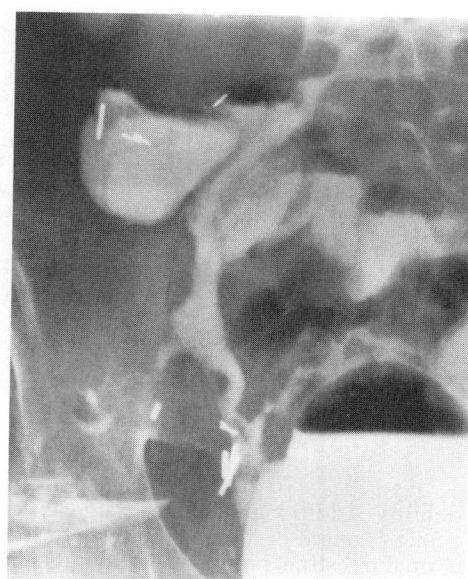

Figure 27.12. Cystogram demonstrating an ileovesical fistula resulting from Crohn's disease of the terminal ileum. (From Michelassi F, Balestracci T, Chappell R, et al. Primary and recurrent Crohn's disease: experience with 1,379 patients. *Ann Surg* 1991;214: 230–238.)

in addition to symptoms of the primary ileal Crohn's disease, indicate operation. As with other Crohn's fistulae, the surgical treatment is based on resection of the diseased segment of intestine and extirpation of the fistulous tract. With ileovesical fistulae, the connection to the bladder is most commonly located at the dome, and débridement and primary closure can be effected without endangering the trigone.

Enterocutaneous Fistulae

Enterocutaneous fistulae occur in approximately 4% of patients with Crohn's disease (29). Enterocutaneous fistulae result from either direct penetration of a sinus through the abdominal wall or external drainage of an abscess that communicates with the diseased intestinal tract. The most common site of spontaneous drainage of an enterocutaneous fistula in Crohn's disease is through a previous abdominal scar or the umbilicus.

The presence of an enterocutaneous fistula does not necessarily dictate the need for surgical intervention. If the patient's underlying disease is under satisfactory control and the output of the enterocutaneous fistula is minimal, then a period of conservative management may be appropriate. The nonoperative management of fistulae related to Crohn's disease includes clearance of sepsis, aggressive nutritional support, and appropriate medical therapy. Anti-TNF chimeric monoclonal antibody (infliximab) may be of particular value in this situation (25,27). Even with aggressive nonoperative management, enterocutaneous fistulae related to Crohn's disease are slow to heal, and surgery is often ultimately required. Surgical therapy is based on resection of the diseased intestinal segment, extirpation of the fistula, and débridement of the entire fistulous tract through the abdominal wall.

Enterogenital Fistulae

Enterogenital fistulae, including enterovaginal, enterosalpingeal, and enterouterine fistulae, are very rare complications of Crohn's disease. Enterovaginal fistulae most commonly occur in patients who have undergone a previous hysterectomy (51). Symptoms include a malodorous discharge and the passage of air through the vagina. Surgical treatment involves resection of the diseased intestine and extirpation of the fistulous tract along with drainage of any intervening abscess.

Enterosalpingeal and enterouterine fistulae are extremely rare. They are difficult to identify preoperatively and are most often recognized only at the time of surgical exploration. Enterosalpingeal fistulae should be managed by removal of the affected tube. If the fistula gives rise to a tuboovarian abscess, then resection of both the ovary and the tube is necessary. With enterouterine fistulae, attempts to salvage the uterus may be undertaken should the patient wish to preserve fertility; otherwise, hysterectomy with resection of the affected small bowel is the best surgical option.

Abscesses

Intraabdominal abscesses that form in Crohn's disease tend to be chronic, with an indolent clinical course of modest fever, abdominal pain, and leukocytosis. Abscesses related to Crohn's disease only rarely present with overwhelming systemic sepsis. A tender palpable abdominal mass is very likely to be an intraabdominal abscess, as more than 50% of inflammatory masses harbor an abscess collection. In up to one third of abscesses related to Crohn's disease, no preoperative clinical signs of localized infection are present, and the abscesses are discovered only by intraoperative exploration. When an abscess is suspected or a mass palpated, preoperative CT should be performed (Fig. 27.7). CT provides information regarding the size and location of the abscess, the feasibility of percutaneous drainage, and the relationship of the septic process to retroperitoneal structures, such as the ureters, duodenum, and inferior vena cava.

Many abscesses in Crohn's disease are small collections that are nearly completely contained within the area of diseased intestine. This is particularly true for intramesenteric and intraloop abscesses (Fig. 27.13). In these cases, resection of the affected segment of intestine extirpates the abscess cavity, so that the placement of drains is not necessary and primary anastomosis can be performed without risk.

Small abscesses can be readily managed at the time of surgical exploration, but larger abscesses are best managed with preoperative CT-guided percutaneous drainage (52). The preoperative drainage of larger abscesses facilitates subsequent surgical intervention by controlling sepsis that might otherwise result in perioperative hemodynamic in-

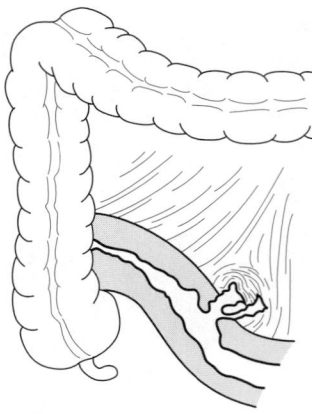

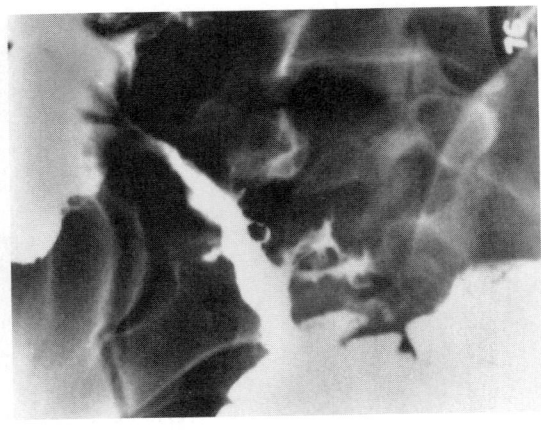

Figure 27.13. Small bowel follow-through study demonstrating an intramesenteric abscess originating from a perforation of the terminal ileum into the mesentery. (From Michelassi F. Crohn's disease. In: Bell RH, Rikkers LF, Mulholland MW, eds. *Digestive tract surgery.* Philadelphia: Lippincott–Raven, 1996: 1201–1227.)

stability. Additionally, when a large abscess is adherent to a long segment of normal intestine or to the mesentery of normal intestine, preoperative percutaneous drainage may allow for sufficient healing that sacrifice of normal intestine can be avoided and a more limited resection accomplished. Percutaneous drainage may also allow for resection and primary anastomosis when the degree of sepsis and inflammation would otherwise dictate the need for a temporary ileostomy (53).

CROHN'S DISEASE OF THE DUODENUM

Symptomatic Crohn's disease of the duodenum is a rare entity, and the need for surgical intervention is uncommon (54). When the duodenum is involved with Crohn's disease, special surgical strategies must be employed. Unlike jejunal or ileal resections, resection of the duodenum is an extreme undertaking. Fortunately, because of the peculiar manifestations of duodenal Crohn's disease, resection of the duodenum is almost never necessary.

The duodenum can be involved either primarily with Crohn's disease or secondarily by inflammatory adhesions or fistulae originating from disease elsewhere in the gastrointestinal tract. Primary Crohn's disease of the duodenum typically manifests with an inflammatory pattern that results in ulceration and edema. The inflammation may cause strictures to form, but fistulae, sinuses, abscesses, and free perforation almost never develop (Fig. 27.14). Crohn's fistulae involving the duodenum are almost always the result of perforating disease originating elsewhere, in the small bowel or colon (55).

Primary Disease of the Duodenum

Because the predominant complication of duodenal Crohn's disease is the formation of strictures rather than fistulae, nonresectional techniques such as strictureplasty and bypass procedures are applicable in most cases. The optimal surgical strategies for managing duodenal strictures in Crohn's disease depend on the pattern of disease. Most of these strictures are focal and can be managed with a Heineke-Mikulicz strictureplasty (56).

If the duodenal stricture is lengthy or the tissues are too rigid and unyielding, then strictureplasty is not suitable, and an intestinal bypass procedure should be performed. A simple side-to-side retrocolic gastrojejunostomy can be performed for obstructing disease of the duodenum. This procedure effectively relieves the symptoms of duodenal obstruction but has the drawback of being inherently ulcerogenic. To lessen the likelihood that stomal ulcerations will develop, vagotomy is performed along with the gastrojejunostomy. After truncal vagotomy, the frequency of soft stools is often increased, and in some cases frank diarrhea develops. This possible side effect is particularly concerning in patients with Crohn's disease, who often have an altered baseline bowel function. For this reason, highly selective vagotomy, which is much less likely to cause diarrhea, is preferred over truncal vagotomy.

If the first and second portions of the duodenum are spared from Crohn's disease, a Roux-en-Y duodenojejunostomy can be performed to bypass obstructing disease of the more distal duodenum (57). This procedure allows the strictured duodenum to be bypassed and obviates concerns about acid-induced marginal ulceration and the need for vagotomy.

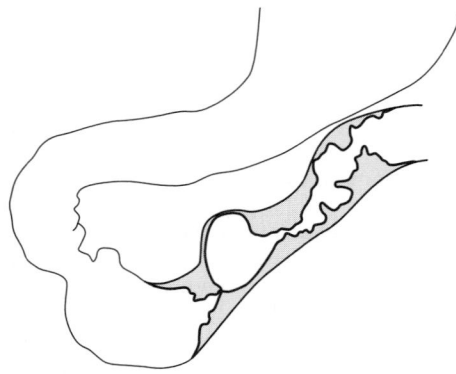

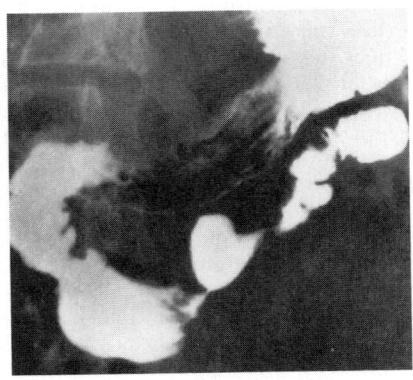

Figure 27.14. Crohn's disease affecting the third and fourth portions of the duodenum. (From Block GE, Michelassi F, Tanaka M, et al. Crohn's disease. *Curr Probl Surg* 1993;30:173–272, with permission.)

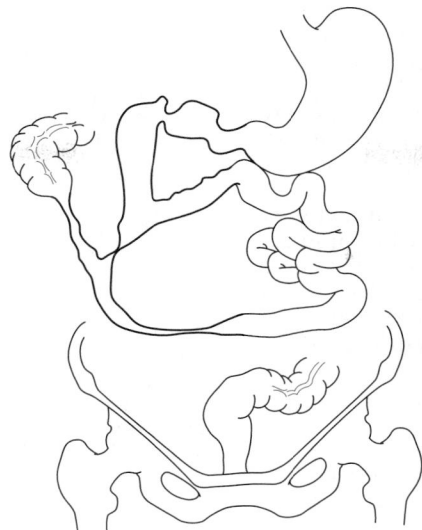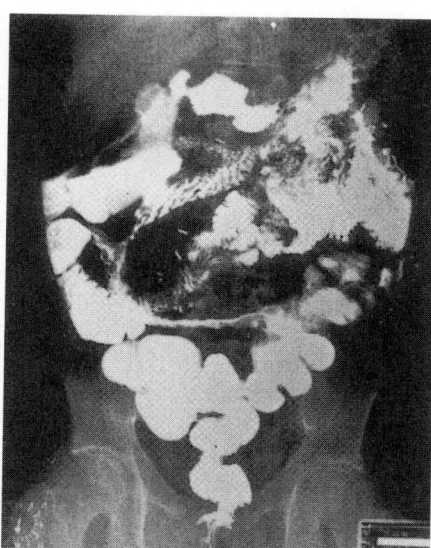

Figure 27.15. Upper gastrointestinal series showing an ileoduodenal fistula in patient with recurrent Crohn's disease proximal to an ileocolonic anastomosis. (From Michelassi F, Balestracci T, Chappell R, et al. Primary and recurrent Crohn's disease: experience with 1,379 patients. *Ann Surg* 1991;214:230–238.)

Secondary Involvement of the Duodenum

Fistulous Crohn's disease of the jejunum, ileum, or colon may secondarily involve the duodenum. This is most commonly seen in recurrent Crohn's disease at the site of a previous ileocolonic anastomosis that has become adherent to the duodenum (Fig. 27.15). Most duodenal fistulae are asymptomatic; others may shunt duodenal content to the distal small bowel or colon, so that malabsorption and diarrhea result. In a majority of cases, duodenoenteric fistulae are identified with preoperative small bowel radiography, yet many are discovered only at the time of surgery.

The surgical management of duodenal-enteric fistulae entails resection of the primary disease with repair of the duodenal defect. Most duodenal fistulae are located away from the juncture of the duodenal wall with the head of the pancreas, and thus they can be managed by simple débridement and primary closure without difficulty. Larger fistulae or fistulae associated with more significant inflammatory adhesion may require more extensive débridement; the resulting sizable duodenal defects require closure with a Roux-en-Y duodenojejunostomy or with a jejunal serosal patch (58). Duodenal resections are almost never necessary and should be considered the surgical option of last resort.

CROHN'S DISEASE OF THE COLON

The surgical management of Crohn's disease of the large intestine depends on a variety of factors, including the distribution and pattern of disease, the extent of rectal involvement, and the adequacy of fecal continence. The surgical procedures commonly required include segmental colectomy or ileocolectomy with primary anastomosis, total abdominal colectomy with ileoproctostomy, and total proctocolectomy with permanent end-ileostomy. Because of the recurrent nature of Crohn's disease, a restorative procedure such as ileal pouch–anal anastomosis or continent ileostomy is not appropriate for patients with an established diagnosis of Crohn's disease.

Ileocolitis

The management of ileocecal or ileocolonic disease is similar to the management of disease limited to the terminal ileum. Resection to grossly normal margins with primary anastomosis is often the best surgical option. The long-term clinical course of terminal ileal disease with limited involvement of the proximal colon resembles the clinical course of Crohn's disease involving only terminal ileum. Disease tends to recur at the anastomosis and preanastomotic ileum. The risk for recurrent disease in the distal colon or rectum is low, so the long-term chance that a permanent stoma will be required is low.

Extensive Crohn's Colitis with Rectal Sparing

Crohn's disease that predominates in the colon often involves long segments of the colon. Extensive Crohn's colitis that does not respond to medical treatment requires total colectomy. Commonly, the rectum is spared, and an ileorectal anastomosis can be performed and a permanent stoma avoided or at least delayed. Unfortunately, recurrence after total abdominal colectomy with ileorectal anastomosis is common, and many of these patients ultimately require proctectomy with permanent ileostomy (59). Even with a high risk for recurrence, a permanent stoma can be avoided for several years in most patients whose rectum is not affected by disease (60). For patients with Crohn's colitis who also have anal incontinence, removal of the colon and rectum with permanent ileostomy is required, even though the rectum itself may be free of disease.

Segmental Crohn's Colitis

In segmental Crohn's colitis, a short length of diseased colon is surrounded by normal colon both proximally and distally. This is a relatively uncommon pattern. Segmental resection of the diseased portion of the colon with colocolonic anastomosis has been advocated, and several reports have demonstrated good long-term results (61,62). However, segmental colectomy is controversial because of the high risk for recurrence, which at times develops rapidly in the preanastomotic colon. Many believe that the rate of recurrence can be lowered by resecting the entire proximal colon, with subsequent anastomosis of the terminal ileum to the normal colon distal to the area of disease. This approach results in an extensive loss of normal colonic mucosa when disease is limited to the distal left colon or sigmoid, which may result in frequent watery stools or even incontinence. A reasonable approach for the surgical management of segmental Crohn's disease of the colon is to perform a segmental resection with colocolonic anastomosis for disease isolated to the distal descending or sigmoid colon and resection to normal ileum with ileocolonic anastomosis for segmental colitis of the more proximal colon. With this approach, the significant absorptive capacity of the proximal colon is not sacrificed in patients with limited left-sided disease, and the risk for rapid recurrence in the proximal colon is avoided in patients with more extensive proximal disease. Regardless of the extent of resection, patients with focal Crohn's colitis are at high risk for long-term recurrent Crohn's disease of the colon and rectum.

Rectal Crohn's Disease

The surgical treatment of Crohn's disease of the rectum requires proctectomy with a permanent stoma. Commonly, Crohn's proctitis occurs with extensive Crohn's colitis, and so a total proctocolectomy is performed. When disease is isolated to the rectum, an abdominoperineal resection with end-colostomy will suffice. Unlike removal of the rectum for malignant disease, proctectomy for Crohn's disease does not require and should not involve a wide excision of perirectal tissue. To avoid injury to pelvic sympathetic and parasympathetic nerves, the dissection should be undertaken close to the rectal wall (63). In the absence of significant perianal disease, the perineal dissection is carried out with an intersphincteric dissection between the internal and external anal sphincter muscles. The intersphincteric dissection results in a smaller wound, and healing is faster than after the wide perineal excision required for malignant disease. If significant perianal disease with abscesses, complex fistulae, and dense scarring is present, then a wide perineal excision is required. In more severe cases, the perineal wound may require closure with tissue transfer grafts.

PERIANAL CROHN'S DISEASE

Perianal manifestations are found in approximately one third of patients with Crohn's disease. These include abscesses, fistulae, fissures, anal stenosis, and hypertrophic skin tags (64). Except in very rare cases, perianal Crohn's disease does not occur in isolation; most patients have some evidence of active or quiescent disease elsewhere in the gastrointestinal tract. Unlike isolated idiopathic perianal abscess or fistula-in-ano, which can occur in patients without Crohn's disease, perianal disease Crohn's disease tends to be recurrent, complex, and occasionally progressive. As a general rule, the treatment of perianal Crohn's disease should be conservative. Repeated operations with recurring disease can lead to significant injury to the anal sphincters, with a risk for incontinence.

Medical therapies that have been shown to be effective in the management of perianal Crohn's disease include antibiotics, particularly metronidazole and ciprofloxacin; antimetabolites, such as 6-MP and azathioprine; and cyclosporine. More recently, anti-TNF antibody (infliximab) has been shown to be effective in promoting the healing of complex Crohn's perianal fistulae, with apparently few side effects (27). The surgical procedures commonly employed include incision and drainage of abscesses, simple fistulotomy, incision and opening of fistulous tracts, application of "draining" setons or mushroom catheters, and the creation of rectal mucosal advancement flaps.

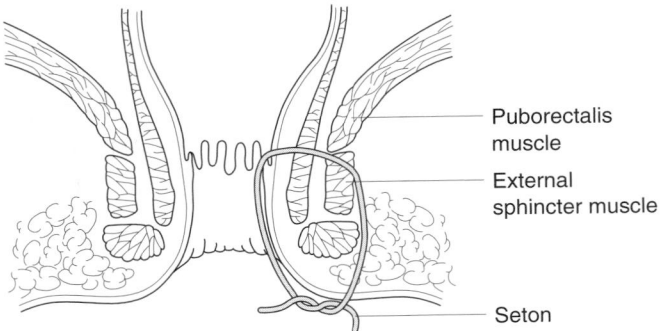

Figure 27.16. Placement of a seton suture through a transsphincteric fistula-in-ano. (From Gordon PH. Anorectal abscesses and fistula-in-ano. In: Gordon PH, Nivatvongs S, eds. *Principles and practice of surgery for the colon, rectum, and anus.* St. Louis: Quality Medical, 1992:221–265, with permission.)

Surgical incision and drainage are mandated for perianal abscesses. Perianal sepsis requires surgical drainage; attempts at treating purulent collections with medical therapy are invariably unsuccessful. Uncomplicated low-lying fistulae are best treated initially with metronidazole or ciprofloxacin (65,66). These agents are moderately effective in promoting the healing of fistulae related to Crohn's disease and are associated with a very low risk for complications. If the response to antibiotic therapy is inadequate, then simple fistulotomy should be performed for uncomplicated low-lying fistulae. Low-lying Crohn's fistulae typically heal well after fistulotomy, and the risk for incontinence is low. More complex perianal fistulae carry a higher risk for postsurgical complications, and so attempts at more aggressive medical treatment with anti-TNF antibody or 6-MP are warranted before surgery is recommended.

Surgical options in the treatment of complex perianal fistulae include the extensive opening of complex fistulous tracts with setons (Fig. 27.16). In the management of these difficult cases, careful judgment is required, as surgical fistulotomy or the application of cutting setons can result in incontinence with high-lying Crohn's fistulae. To prevent incontinence in these patients, a rectal mucosal advancement flap procedure is often the best option for high-lying, suprasphincteric, complex fistulae (67) (Fig. 27.17). Rectal advancement flaps are not appropriate when the rectal mucosa itself is affected by active Crohn's disease.

A temporary stoma to divert the fecal stream is created only in selected cases of complicated perianal disease. Fecal diversion is occasionally appropriate to help in the healing of rectovaginal fistulae. Temporary fecal diversion is sometimes employed in conjunction with rectal advancement flaps to assist in the healing of particularly difficult cases. In severe cases of perianal disease that do not respond to aggressive medical and surgical treatment, fecal diversion typically results in significant relief of local sepsis and inflammation. Unfortunately, disease activity typically recurs rapidly in these cases after reestablishment of the fecal stream.

LONG-TERM MORBIDITY AND RECURRENCE OF DISEASE

Because of the recurrent nature of Crohn's disease, repeated operations are often required. Serial, massive, or injudicious resections of the small bowel in patients with

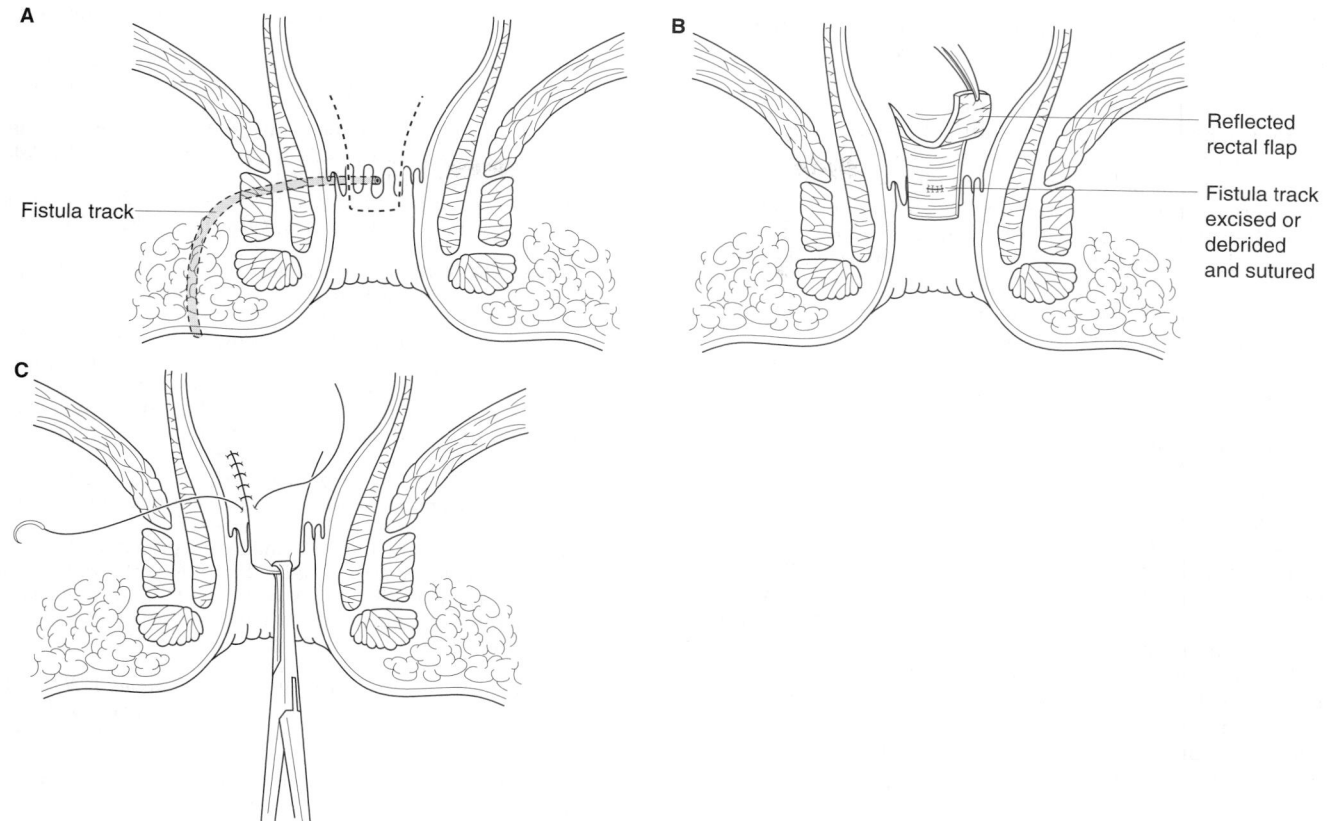

Figure 27.17. Rectal advancement flap procedure can be performed to treat fistula-in-ano and rectovaginal fistula. (From Strong S, Fazio VW. The surgical management of Crohn's disease. In: Kirsner JB, ed. *Inflammatory bowel disease,* 5th ed. Philadelphia: WB Saunders, 2000:658–709, with permission.)

Crohn's disease can result in permanent impairment of intestinal absorption. Important factors influencing the absorptive capacity of the bowel include the following:

Anatomic site of resection
Length of resection
Presence of the ileocecal valve
Condition of the remaining bowel and related digestive organs
Adaptation of the remaining bowel after resection

Resection of one half to two thirds of the small bowel represents the upper limit of safety. When resections exceed this limit, particularly in the absence of the colon, absorption is markedly altered and poses significant management problems. In addition, loss of the specialized function of the ileum can lead to vexing diarrhea and nutrient-specific malabsorption, even after seemingly "conservative" resections. Fortunately, only in rare instances does a true short-gut syndrome occur. In many such cases, the short-gut syndrome can be managed with dietary manipulations, and fewer than 1% of patients with Crohn's disease become dependent on long-term hyperalimentation.

The loss of ileal function leads directly to malabsorption of bile salts and vitamin B_{12}. After resection of the terminal ileum, particularly if the ileocecal valve is lost, bile salts normally absorbed by the terminal ileum are delivered to the colon. Bile salts interfere with the colonic absorption of fluid and electrolytes. In many patients, this results in an increased frequency of stools, which tend to be soft or pasty. Some patients have frank diarrhea. This so-called bile salt diarrhea may be treated with oral cholestyramine,

which binds unabsorbed bile acids so that they do not affect the colon. Significant malabsorption of vitamin B_{12} does not develop in most patients who undergo resection of the terminal ileum, but patients who have undergone lengthy or repeated resections of the terminal ileum should be monitored for possible B_{12} deficiency.

The most common long-term complication following surgery for Crohn's disease is recurrent disease. Reported crude and cumulative recurrence rates vary greatly. Endoscopic evidence of recurrence has been reported to vary from 28% to 73% at 1 year and from 77% to 85% at 3 years after ileal resection (68). In most instances, endoscopically detected recurrence is minor and asymptomatic and therefore not of great clinical significance. The recurrence rate of symptomatic Crohn's disease is approximately 60% at 5 years, and the recurrence rate increases with time, so that symptomatic recurrence is noted after 20 years in 75% to 95% of cases (69). Hence, the long-term risk for recurrence of the symptoms of Crohn's disease is very high. Reports vary, but the rate of reoperation to treat recurrent disease is about 20% at 5 years, 33% at 10 years, and 50% at 20 years (9,70,71).

Crohn's disease is most likely to recur close to the previously resected intestinal segment, typically at the anastomosis and in the preanastomotic bowel. This is particularly true for terminal ileal disease. Additionally, the length of small bowel involved with recurrent disease corresponds to the length of bowel originally resected (72). Short-segment disease tends to recur within a short segment of the preanastomotic bowel, and lengthy segments of disease typically recur in lengthy segments. Also, with a lesser degree of concordance, stenotic disease tends to recur as stenotic disease and perforating disease tends to recur as perforating disease.

Many putative risk factors for recurrence have been studied. The cumulative literature has validated few of them as true risk factors for postsurgical recurrence of disease. A growing body of evidence indicates that smoking can increase the risk for recurrence. Some evidence indicates that the use of NSAIDs may also promote recurrence of disease. All patients with Crohn's disease should be strongly advised to refrain from smoking cigarettes or taking NSAIDs. It does not appear that diet has any influence on the likelihood of recurrence.

The results of recent trials indicate that recurrent disease can be diminished with postoperative maintenance therapy. The most common maintenance therapies recommended are controlled-release 5-ASA (Pentasa) and 6-MP (23,73,74). Maintenance with 5-ASA is associated with few side effects, but up to 12 pills per day are required, and the drug is expensive. 6-Mercaptopurine is less expensive and is taken on a once-a-day basis, but it is associated with potential bone marrow suppression, so that patients on 6-MP maintenance must be followed with periodic blood cell counts. The degree to which postsurgical maintenance therapy lessens the risk for recurrent disease is in some cases only marginal. The effects on long-term quality of life and the cost-effectiveness of postoperative maintenance therapy have not been fully determined. Thus, the decision to recommend maintenance therapy must be individualized for each patient.

REFERENCES

1. Crohn BB, Ginzburg L, Oppenheimer GD. Regional ileitis: a pathological and clinical entity. *JAMA* 1932;99:1323–1329.
2. Sandler RS, Glenn ME. Epidemiology of inflammatory bowel disease. In: Kirsner JB, ed. *Inflammatory bowel disease.* Philadelphia: WB Saunders, 2000:89–112.
3. Kirsner JB. Etiologic concepts of inflammatory bowel disease; past, present, and future. In: Michelassi F, Milsom JW, eds. *Operative strategies in inflammatory bowel disease.* New York: Springer-Verlag, 1999:3–20.
4. Fiocchi C. Inflammatory bowel disease: etiology and pathogenesis. *Gastroenterology* 1998;115:182–205.
5. Schreiber S, Hampe J. Genetics and inflammatory bowel disease. *Curr Opin Gastroenterol* 1999;15:315–321.
6. Mayer L. Current concepts of inflammatory bowel disease etiology and pathogenesis. In: Kirsner JB, ed. *Inflammatory bowel disease.* Philadelphia: WB Saunders, 2000:280–296.
7. Thomas GAO, Rhodes J, Green JT. Inflammatory bowel disease and smoking—a review. *Am J Gastroenterol* 1998;93:144–149.
8. May GR, Sutherland LR, Meddings JB. Is small intestinal permeability really increased in relatives of patients with Crohn's disease? *Gastroenterology* 1993;104:1627–1632.
9. Michelassi F, Balestracci T, Chappell R, et al. Primary and recurrent Crohn's disease: experience with 1,379 patients. *Ann Surg* 1991;214:230–236.
10. Block GE, Michelassi F, Tanaka M, et al. Crohn's disease. *Curr Probl Surg* 1993;2:173–272.
11. Riddell RH. Pathology of idiopathic inflammatory bowel disease. In: Kirsner JB, ed. *Inflammatory bowel disease.* Philadelphia: WB Saunders, 2000:427–450.
12. Steinhart AH, Girrah N, McLeod RS. Reliability of a Crohn's disease clinical classification scheme based on disease behavior. *Inflamm Bowel Dis* 1998;4:228–234.
13. Mekhjian HS, Switz DM, Melnyk CS, et al. Clinical features and natural history of Crohn's disease. *Gastroenterology* 1979;77:898–906.
14. Carlson HC. The small bowel examination in the diagnosis of Crohn's disease. *AJR Am J Roentgenol* 1986;147:63–65.
15. Rutgeerts D, Vantrappen G, Geboes K. Endoscopy in inflammatory bowel disease. *Scand J Gastroenterol* 1989;170:12–19.
16. Gossios KJ, Tsianos EV. Crohn disease: CT findings after treatment. *Abdom Imaging* 1997;22:160–163.
17. Wheller JG, Slack NF, Duncan A, et al. The diagnosis of intraabdominal abscesses in patients with severe Crohn's disease. *Q J Med* 1992;82:159–167.
18. Best WR, Becktel JM, Singleton JW. Rederived values of the eight coefficients of the Crohn's disease activity index (CDAI). *Gastroenterology* 1979;77:843–846.
19. Best WR, Becktel JM, Singleton JW, et al. Development of a Crohn's disease activity index. *Gastroenterology* 1976;70:439–444.
20. Summers RW, Switz DM, Sessions JTJ, et al. National Cooperative Crohn's Disease Study: results of drug treatment. *Gastroenterology* 1979;77:847–869.
21. Hanauer SB, Stein RB. Medical therapy. In: Michelassi F, Milsom JW, eds. *Operative strategies in inflammatory bowel disease.* New York: Springer-Verlag, 1999:138–149.
22. Campieri M, Ferguson A, Doe W, et al. Oral budesonide is as effective as oral prednisolone in active Crohn's disease. *Gut* 1997;41:209–214.
23. McLeod RS, Wolf BG, Steinhart AH, et al. Prophylactic mesalamine decreases postoperative recurrence of Crohn's disease. *Gastroenterology* 1995;109:404–413.
24. Choi PM, Targan SR. Immunomodualatory treatment in inflammatory bowel disease. *Dig Dis Sci* 1994;39:1885–1892.
25. Targan SR, Hanauer SB, van Deventer SJ, et al. A short-term study of chimeric monoclonal antibody cA₂ to tumor necrosis factor alpha for Crohn's disease. *N Engl J Med* 1997;337:1029–1035.
26. Van Dulleman HM, Van Deventer SJH, Hommes DW, et al. Treatment of Crohn's disease with anti-tumor necrosis factor chimeric monoclonal antibody (cA₂). *Gastroenterology* 1995;109:129–135.
27. Present DH, Rutgeerts P, Targan S, et al. Infliximab for the treatment of fistulas in patients with Crohn's disease. *N Engl J Med* 1999;340:1398–1405.
28. Hurst RD, Molinari M, Chung TP, et al. Prospective study of the features, indications, and surgical treatment in 513 consecutive patients affected by Crohn's disease. *Surgery* 1997;122:661–668.
29. Michelassi F, Stella M, Balestracci T, et al. Incidence, diagnosis, and treatment of enteric and colorectal fistulas in patients with Crohn's disease. *Ann Surg* 1993;218:660–666.
30. Michelassi F. Incidence, diagnosis, and treatment of abdominal abscesses in Crohn's disease. *Res Surg* 1996;8:35–39.
31. Sparberg M, Kirsner JB. Recurrent hemorrhage in regional enteritis: report of 3 cases. *Am J Dig Dis* 1966;2:652–657.
32. Greenstein J, Mann D, Heimann T, et al. Spontaneous free perforation and perforated abscess in 30 patients with Crohn's disease. *Ann Surg* 1987;205:72–75.
33. Ribeiro MB, Greenstein AJ, Sachar DB, et al. Colorectal adenocarcinoma in Crohn's disease. *Ann Surg* 1996;223:186–193.
34. Darke SG, Parks AG, Grogono JL, et al. Adenocarcinoma and Crohn's disease: a report of 2 cases and analysis of the literature. *Br J Surg* 1973;60:169–175.
35. Telander RL, Schmeling DJ. Current surgical management of Crohn's disease in childhood. *Semin Pediatr Surg* 1994;3:19–24.
36. Fazio VW, Marchetti F, Church J, et al. Effect of resection margins on the recurrence of Crohn's disease in the small bowel: a randomized controlled trial. *Ann Surg* 1996;224:563–573.
37. Fazio VW, Galandiuk S, Jagelman DG, et al. Strictureplasty in Crohn's disease. *Ann Surg* 1989;210:621–625.
38. Sharif H, Alexander-Williams J. The role of strictureplasty in Crohn's disease. *Int Surg* 1992;77:15–18.
39. Michelassi F. Side-to-side isoperistaltic strictureplasty for multiple Crohn's strictures. *Dis Colon Rectum* 1996;39:345–349.
40. Michelassi F, Hurst RD, Melis M, et al. Side-to-side isoperistaltic strictureplasty in extensive Crohn's disease: a prospective longitudinal study. *Ann Surg* 2000;232:401–408.
41. Nivatvongs S. Strictureplasty for Crohn's disease of small intestine. Present status in Western countries. *J Gastroenterol* 1995;30:139–142.
42. Alexander-Williams J, Haynes IG. Conservative operations for Crohn's disease of the small bowel. *World J Surg* 1985;9:945–951.
43. Hurst RD, Michelassi F. Strictureplasty for Crohn's disease:

techniques and long-term results. *World J Surg* 1998;22: 359–363.

44. Fazio VW, Tjandra JJ, Lavery IC, et al. Long-term follow-up of strictureplasty in Crohn's disease. *Dis Colon Rectum* 1993;36: 355–361.

45. Spencer MP, Nelson H, Wolff BG, et al. Strictureplasty for obstructive Crohn's disease: the Mayo experience. *Mayo Clin Proc* 1994;69:33–36.

46. Milsom JW. Strictureplasty and mechanical dilation in strictured Crohn's disease. In: Michelassi F, Milsom JW, eds. *Operative strategies in inflammatory bowel disease.* New York: Springer-Verlag, 1999:259–267.

47. Broe PJ, Bayless TM, Cameron JL. Crohn's disease: are enteroenteral fistulas an indication for surgery? *Surgery* 1982; 91:249–253.

48. Glass RE, Ritchie JK, Lennard-Jones JE, et al. Internal fistulas in Crohn's disease. *Dis Colon Rectum* 1985;28:557–561.

49. Block GE, Schraut WH. The operative treatment of Crohn's enteritis complicated by ileosigmoid fistula. *Ann Surg* 1982; 196:356–360.

50. Schraut WH, Chapman C, Abraham VS. Operative treatment of Crohn's ileocolitis complicated by ileosigmoid and ileovesical fistulae. *Ann Surg* 1988;207:48–51.

51. Heyen F, Winslet MC, Andrews J, et al. Vaginal fistulas in Crohn's disease. *Dis Colon Rectum* 1989;32:379.

52. Doemeny JM, Burke DR, Meranze SG. Percutaneous drainage of abscesses in patients with Crohn's disease. *Gastrointest Radiol* 1988;13:237–241.

53. Bernini A, Spencer MP, Wong WD, et al. Computed tomography-guided percutaneous abscess drainage in intestinal disease. *Dis Colon Rectum* 1997;40:1009–1013.

54. Schoetz DJ. Gastroduodenal Crohn's disease. In: Michelassi F, Milsom JW, eds. *Operative strategies in inflammatory bowel disease.* New York: Springer-Verlag, 1999:389–393.

55. Harold KL, Kelly KA. Duodenal Crohn disease. *Probl Gen Surg* 1999;16:50–57.

56. Poggioli G, Stocchi L, Laureti S, et al. Duodenal involvement of Crohn's disease. *Dis Colon Rectum* 1997;40:179–183.

57. Alexander-Williams J, Haynes IG. Up-to-date management of small bowel Crohn's disease. *Adv Surg* 1987;20:245–246.

58. Pichney L, Fantry G, Graham S. Gastrocolic and duodenocolic fistulas in Crohn's disease. *J Clin Gastroenterol* 1992;15: 205–211.

59. Lefton HB, Farmer RG, Fazio V. Ileorectal anastomosis for Crohn's disease of the colon. *Gastroenterology* 1975;69: 612–617.

60. Longo WE, Oakley JR, Lavery IC, et al. Outcome of ileorectal anastomosis for Crohn's colitis. *Dis Colon Rectum* 1992;35: 1066–1071.

61. Sanfey H, Bayless TM, Cameron JL. Crohn's disease of the colon: is there a role for limited resection? *Am J Surg* 1984; 147:38–42.

62. Allan A, Andrews MB, Hilton CJ, et al. Segmental colonic resection is an appropriate operation for short skip lesions due to Crohn's disease of the colon. *World J Surg* 1989;13:611–616.

63. Berry AR, Campos RDE, Lee ECG. Perineal and pelvic morbidity following perimuscular excision of the rectum for inflammatory bowel disease. *Br J Surg* 1986;73:675–677.

64. Homan WP, Tang CK, Thorbjarnarson B. Anal lesions complicating Crohn's disease. *Arch Surg* 1976;111:1333–1336.

65. Turunen U, Farkkila M, Seppala K. Long-term treatment of perianal or fistulous Crohn's disease with ciprofloxacin. *Scand J Gastroenterol* 1989;24[Suppl]:144(abst).

66. Bernstein LH, Frank MS, Brandt LJ, et al. Healing of perineal Crohn's disease with metronidazole. *Gastroenterology* 1980; 79:357–365.

67. Kodner IJ, Mazor A, Shemesh EI, et al. Endorectal advancement flap repair of rectovaginal and other complicated anorectal fistulas. *Surgery* 1993;114:682–690.

68. Rutgeerts P, Geboes K, Vantrappen G, et al. Predictability of the postoperative course of Crohn's disease. *Gastroenterology* 1990;99:956–963.

69. Mekhjian HS, Switz DM, Watts HD, et al. National Cooperative Crohn's Disease Study: factors determining recurrence of Crohn's disease after surgery. *Gastroenterology* 1979;77: 907–913.

70. Post S, Herfath C, Bohm E, et al. The impact of disease pattern, surgical management, and individual surgeons on the risk for relaparotomy for recurrent Crohn's disease. *Ann Surg* 1996;223:253–260.

71. Greenstein AJ, Sachar DB, Pasternack BS, et al. Reoperation and recurrence in Crohn's colitis and ileocolitis: crude and cumulative rates. *N Engl J Med* 1975;392:685–690.

72. D'Haens G, Baert F, Gasparaitis A, et al. Length and type of recurrent ileitis after ileal resection correlate with presurgical features in Crohn's disease. *Inflamm Bowel Dis* 1997;3: 249–253.

73. Lochs H, Mayer M, Fleig WE, et al. Prophylaxis of postoperative relapse in Crohn's disease with mesalamine (Pentasa) in comparison to placebo. *Gastroenterology* 1997;112:A1027(abst).

74. Korelitz B, Hanauer S, Rutgeerts P, et al. Post-operative prophylaxis with 6-MP, 5-ASS, or placebo in Crohn's disease: a 2-year multicenter trial. *Gastroenterology* 1998;114:A1011(abst).

SURGERY: SCIENTIFIC PRINCIPLES AND PRACTICE, Third Edition, edited by Lazar J. Greenfield, Michael W. Mulholland, Keith T. Oldham, Gerald B. Zelenock, and Keith D. Lillemoe. Lippincott Williams & Wilkins Publishers, Philadelphia, © 2001.

CHAPTER 28

SMALL INTESTINAL NEOPLASMS

MARGARET L. SCHRIEBER AND BARBARA LEE BASS

Small bowel tumors, both benign and malignant, are uncommon. Although the small bowel accounts for 75% of the length and 90% of the mucosal surface of the gastrointestinal tract, it is the site of only 1% to 3% of gastrointestinal malignancies. In the year 2000, it is estimated that 4,700 new cases of small bowel malignancy will be diagnosed; two-and-a-half–fold more esophageal malignancies and twenty-eight–fold more colorectal cancers will be diagnosed in 2000. Although benign lesions are unusual, autopsy series have demonstrated them in 0.2% to 0.3% of hospital deaths, a rate 15 times the operative incidence, which attests to the frequently asymptomatic nature of these neoplasms (1). Table 28.1 lists the wide variety of

Table 28.1. PRIMARY SMALL BOWEL TUMORS AND REPORTED FREQUENCY RATES

	Frequency (%)
BENIGN NEOPLASMS	
GIST/leiomyoma	40–50
Lipoma	13–24
Adenoma	11–18
Lymphangioma	0–12
Fibroma	0–6
Hamartoma	0–6
Hemangioma	0–6
Aberrant pancreas, dermoid cyst, eosinophilic granuloma, angiodysplasia, hyperplastic polyp	Rare
MALIGNANT NEOPLASMS	
Adenocarcinoma	29–50
Carcinoid	10–49
Non-Hodgkin's lymphoma	13–42
GISS/leiomyosarcoma	8–27
Liposarcoma, myxoliposarcoma, lymphangiosarcoma	Rare

GIST, gastrointestinal stromal tumor; GISS, gastrointestinal stromal sarcoma.

primary tumors in the small bowel. Small intestinal tumors may originate in cells of the epithelium—adenomas, adenocarcinomas, or carcinoid; the lymphatic tissues—lymphomas; or mesenchymal and neural elements—the gastrointestinal stromal tumors, including leiomyomas, lipomas, hemangiomas, neuromas, and a wide variety of sarcomas. The small intestine is also a rare site for metastasis from other primary tumors.

EPIDEMIOLOGY

Little consensus has been reached regarding the relative incidence rates of small bowel tumors in the United States or worldwide. Clearly, geographic variations are found around the world. For example, carcinoid tumor is rare to nonexistent in Asian reviews, yet represents 15% to 35% of malignant neoplasms in Western series (2,3). The percentage of small bowel tumors that are benign varies from 14% to 52%, a disparity perhaps explained by failure to detect typically asymptomatic benign lesions. Among malignant tumors, reported rates of non-Hodgkin's lymphoma (NHL) vary from 27% to 72% in different series, a discrepancy that is partly a consequence of the inconsistent categorization of lymphomas as primary or metastatic tumors, but also of true geographic variation. Given the rarity of small bowel tumors and the wide variety of histologic types, the actual reported numbers for given histologic types are small even in the largest series, so that reliable comparisons are difficult and definitive incidence rates impossible to confirm (4).

Although generalizations regarding these rare tumors can be difficult to formulate, certain patterns can be discerned. Small bowel neoplasms are less common in women than in men. A male preponderance (ratio of 3:2) is reported for both benign and malignant neoplasms. Most patients with small bowel neoplasms present in their sixth to seventh decade of life. Except for adenocarcinoma, which has a predilection for the duodenum, malignant small bowel tumors become progressively more common toward the distal portions of the small bowel. Approximately 20% of tumors arise in the duodenum, 30% in the jejunum, and 50% in the ileum (5).

PATHOGENESIS

Several hypotheses have been proposed to explain the low incidence of small bowel tumors, particularly those derived from cells of the intestinal epithelium. Although none of these hypotheses has been proved, they provide a plausible explanation relative to our understanding of the pathogenesis of other gastrointestinal tumors.

The dilute, alkaline liquid contents of the small bowel are potentially less capable of causing direct mechanical mucosal injury and disruption than the more solid contents of the colon. Bacterial counts in the luminal contents of the healthy small bowel are lower than in the colon; bacteria and their potentially toxic metabolites are less likely to induce the genetic alterations implicated in colon carcinogenesis. Rapid transit time through the small bowel lumen, normally 30 minutes to 2 hours, may limit mucosal exposure to potential carcinogens, and the presence of the enzyme benzopyrene hydroxylase in the brush border of the small intestine may provide protection against mucosal damage by detoxifying the carcinogen benzopyrene. The greater concentration and distribution of lymphoid tissue in the intestinal epithelium and submucosa and high levels of luminal immunoglobulin A may provide an immunologic protective mechanism. Some investigators suggest that the high rate of metachronous primary malignancies, observed in up to 20% of patients, and the frequency of multicentric small bowel malignancies support an alteration in host defenses or a breakdown in this immunologic protective mechanism as an important etiologic factor. Unlike the well-defined adenoma–carcinoma genetic sequence described for colorectal malignancies, a consistent pattern of gene mutations or deletions has not been identified for small bowel carcinomas.

CONDITIONS ASSOCIATED WITH INCREASED RISK FOR SMALL BOWEL TUMORS

Although few tumors develop in the small bowel, risk factors for the development of malignant lesions have been identified. As shown in Table 28.2, several conditions carry an increased risk of neoplasia.

Crohn's Disease

Crohn's disease is associated with up to a 100-fold increase in the risk for adenocarcinoma; carcinoma develops in diseased segments of the bowel with preexisting dysplasia (6). Three fourths of these cancers arise in the ileum, the segment of small bowel most commonly involved with Crohn's disease but least commonly affected by adenocarcinoma. The remaining tumors are found in the duodenum and jejunum, following the usual distribution of sporadic carcinoma, which tends to develop in the duodenum. Carcinomas associated with Crohn's disease carry a particularly poor prognosis because the tumors are frequently diagnosed at an advanced stage, likely because the abdominal symptoms of the tumor are attributed to the underlying inflammatory bowel disease.

Familial Adenomatous Polyposis

Also at risk for the development of adenocarcinoma, primarily of the duodenum, are patients with familial adenomatous polyposis (7). Between 27% to 92% of these patients have duodenal adenomas that can undergo malignant transformation. Duodenal and periampullary adenocarcinomas are the leading cause of cancer deaths in patients with familial adenomatous polyposis previously treated by colectomy. Careful screening with periodic esophagogastroduodenoscopy and prompt local resection of adenomas are of paramount importance in this patient population. Endoscopic polypectomy is appropriate for small or pedunculated lesions, whereas pancreaticoduo-

Table 28.2. CONDITIONS ASSOCIATED WITH AN INCREASED RISK FOR NEOPLASIA

Preexisting condition	Potential malignancy
Adenomatous polyps	Adenocarcinoma
Familial adenomatous polyposis	Adenocarcinoma
Peutz-Jeghers syndrome/ hamartomatous polyps	Adenocarcinoma
Leiomyomas	Possible leiomyosarcoma
Neurofibromatosis	Leiomyosarcoma, carcinoid, adenocarcinoma
Crohn's disease	Adenocarcinoma
Celiac sprue	Lymphoma, adenocarcinoma
Immunosuppression	Lymphoma
HIV infection	Lymphoma, Kaposi's sarcoma
Helicobacter pylori infection	Low-grade lymphoma (MALToma)
EBV infection	Lymphoma

EBV, Epstein-Barr virus; MALT, mucosa-associated lymphoid tissue.

denectomy may be required for adequate treatment of larger villous tumors, particularly in the periampullary region.

Other Conditions with Increased Risk for Malignancy of the Small Bowel

Celiac sprue is associated with lymphoma, and to a lesser degree adenocarcinoma; malignancy occurs in up to 14% of patients (8). It remains unclear whether a gluten-free diet decreases this risk. The neurofibromas of von Recklinghausen's disease may undergo malignant transformation, as may leiomyomas of the small bowel. In Peutz-Jeghers syndrome, hamartomas develop throughout the gastrointestinal tract and may undergo malignant transformation to adenocarcinoma. Whether these malignancies, especially in the duodenum, actually arise from preexisting hamartomas has been poorly documented. Benign adenomatous polyps can undergo malignant transformation and should be resected when identified.

Bile acids and their metabolites may have a role in the pathogenesis of small bowel adenocarcinoma. In one study of patients with small intestinal malignancy, 12% had a history of cholecystectomy, and of those with duodenal adenocarcinoma, 25% had had a prior cholecystectomy. A causative relationship between cholecystectomy and small intestinal adenocarcinoma remains unproven, however. Within the duodenum, the periampullary region is the most frequent site of primary carcinoma, although a link between this finding and pancreaticobiliary secretions is unexplored.

Immunosuppression, either iatrogenic following organ transplantation or secondary to disease, places a patient at increased risk for small bowel malignancy, primarily lymphoma and sarcoma. Patients maintained on immunosuppressive regimens after transplantation of a solid organ have an incidence rate of non-Hodgkin's lymphoma (NHL) 45 to 100 times higher than that of persons who have not undergone transplantation; this condition is termed *posttransplant lymphoproliferative disorder* (9). Posttransplant lymphoproliferative disorder accounts for 30% of all malignancies in patients treated with cyclosporine, but for only 12% when cyclosporine is not a component of the regimen. Posttransplant lymphoproliferative disorder tends to develop rapidly, often within 12 months of transplantation, in patients treated with cyclosporine, and the level of immunosuppression appears to be related to the development of lymphoma. In patients who require a high degree of suppression to sustain a graft, as in small bowel, heart, liver, or lung transplantation, the incidence of lymphoma rises as high as 30%. In contrast, lymphoproliferative tumors develop in only 5% of kidney transplant recipients, who generally require less immunosuppression.

Another form of immunosuppression, HIV infection, is also associated with lymphoma. Lymphoma is the second most common malignancy, after Kaposi's sarcoma, in these patients. As life expectancy for patients with HIV infection has lengthened with improved antiviral medications, the rates of lymphoma have increased, so that the risk at 3 years now approaches 30%. Two thirds of these lymphomas are extranodal, and the gastrointestinal tract is involved in 10% to 25% of cases. More than 90% of patients present with stage IV disease, and the median survival is only 6 months.

CLINICAL PRESENTATION

No signs or symptoms are pathognomonic for small bowel tumors. Complaints, if reported at all by the patient, are nonspecific. As shown in Table 28.3, the most com-

Table 28.3. CLINICAL PRESENTATION OF PRIMARY SMALL BOWEL TUMORS

	Percentage
BENIGN NEOPLASMS	
Asymptomatic	47–60
Abdominal pain	24–50
Acute GI hemorrhage	29–44
Anemia	28–58
Intermittent obstruction	12–28
MALIGNANT NEOPLASMS	
Asymptomatic	6–12
Abdominal pain	62–83
Weight loss	38–55
Nausea/vomiting	23–64
Acute GI hemorrhage	6–31
Anemia	12–38
Abdominal mass	5–32

GI, gastrointestinal.

mon symptoms—abdominal pain, weight loss, anemia, nausea, and vomiting—do not suggest specific localization and are present in only 40% to 80% of patients (10,11). The vague complaints can lead to erroneous diagnoses, such as irritable bowel syndrome and even neurosis, before the correct diagnosis of small bowel neoplasm is established. As tumors grow, symptoms are more likely to develop. Seventy-five percent of all lesions measuring at least 4 cm cause symptoms, whereas 92% of malignant lesions of that size are symptomatic. Smaller lesions may be associated with symptoms in the ileum, where the lumen is narrower and obstruction more likely to develop. Overall, malignant lesions tend to be more symptomatic than benign lesions, particularly causing abdominal pain and weight loss. In contrast, benign tumors more often present with acute hemorrhage as the primary symptom, or they are identified as an incidental finding on a radiologic examination or at laparotomy.

Because of their ill-defined symptoms, both benign and malignant small bowel tumors frequently present late in their course. Tumors are often diagnosed at the time of emergency surgical exploration for intestinal obstruction, perforation, or massive gastrointestinal hemorrhage. Only in hindsight may a history of abdominal complaints be elicited.

DIAGNOSIS

Many factors contribute to the well-recognized difficulty of diagnosing a small bowel tumor. In most series, the average duration of symptoms before diagnosis ranges from weeks to many months. Diagnosis is hindered by the infrequency of these tumors and omission of the diagnosis from the differential diagnosis in patients with nonspecific abdominal complaints. More importantly, the diagnosis is delayed because the imaging modalities available to study the small bowel are limited. An accurate preoperative diagnosis is established in only 19% to 53% of cases (12,13).

Plain abdominal radiography is rarely helpful unless the patient presents with obstructive symptoms. For patients being evaluated for gastrointestinal bleeding or other symptoms, the diagnosis of small bowel tumor is usually considered after evaluation of the stomach and colon has demonstrated no pathology to explain the symptoms. Following negative findings on esophagogastroduodenoscopy and colonoscopy, the diagnostic work-up should begin with computed tomography (CT) of the abdomen. In addition to readily identifying bulky mass lesions, CT imaging allows subtle findings to be detected that are highly suggestive of small bowel tumors. Neoplastic disease must be strongly suspected if the scan shows the small bowel wall to be thicker than 1.5 cm, or if discrete mesenteric masses larger than 1.5 cm in diameter are present. CT may reveal a transition zone demarcating dilated proximal bowel from decompressed distal bowel. If associated with bowel-wall thickening, a tumor is likely except in patients with clinical presentations more typical of Crohn's disease.

Tumors of the distal small bowel may be associated with the finding of ileocolic or jejunoileal intussusception on CT. This characteristic finding is sufficient to proceed with surgical exploration in adult patients. During intussusception, the small bowel tumor serves as the lead point to pull a portion of the small bowel into the distal small bowel or colonic lumen; the mass lesion precludes spontaneous reduction. In adults, reduction of an intussusception should not be attempted radiographically. Rather, prompt surgical exploration and resection of the nonreduced intussuscepted bowel segment should be completed.

If abdominal CT fails to reveal evidence of a small bowel tumor, the next diagnostic study should be an upper gastrointestinal contrast series with small bowel follow-through (SBFT). Barium meals demonstrate a duodenal lesion in 70% to 80% of cases, and when an air double-contrast technique is used, the diagnostic rate rises to 85% to 90%, although esophagogastroduodenoscopy has essentially replaced this study for duodenal evaluation. The sensitivity of barium studies declines significantly in the mesenteric small bowel. The SBFT study reveals an abnormality in 53% to 83% of cases, although direct evidence of a tumor is detected in only 30% to 44% of cases. Given these poor detection rates, some radiologists support enteroclysis as the primary study of choice for imaging the small bowel distal to the ligament of Treitz. Enteroclysis is a dynamic contrast technique in which a combination of barium and methylcellulose is infused into the small bowel via a nasoduodenal tube to distend the small bowel uniformly without abolishing peristalsis. Expertise in this procedure is important for success, and enteroclysis may not be available in all radiology departments. Enteroclysis is clearly a superior modality for identifying small luminal tumors. In one series, enteroclysis identified 90% of cases, whereas SBFT identified 33% in the same cohort of patients.

Other lesions may mimic small bowel tumors on these imaging studies. An inflammatory reaction secondary to a sealed perforation will thicken the bowel wall and may appear neoplastic. An annular pancreas may appear on an upper gastrointestinal contrast series as an "apple core" lesion in the duodenum and be mistaken for a malignancy. Thickening of the bowel wall is common in Crohn's disease. The clinical presentation may clarify the diagnosis, although the diagnosis may not be confirmed until surgical exploration.

Enteroscopy

Endoscopic modalities are helpful where the expertise is available. In push enteroscopy, a pediatric colonoscope is passed orally into the proximal small bowel for direct examination of the mucosa. Identified lesions can be sampled with this instrument, although the examination is limited as only the proximal 2 to 3 feet of small bowel can be visualized. Push enteroscopy is performed in the endoscopy suite with the patient under intravenous sedation; the procedure is not well tolerated by all patients. In contrast, Sonde small bowel enteroscopy relies on peristalsis for the passive transport of an enteroscope with a wide-angled lens into the distal ileum or colon. Passage requires up to 8 hours, after which the enteroscope is slowly withdrawn for visual examination of the tumor. The small diameter of the device precludes a biopsy port for tissue sampling. The procedure can be poorly tolerated, and only 50% to 70% of the intestinal mucosa is fully examined because fine control of the scope tip is difficult during withdrawal and the deflection capacity of the enteroscope is minimal. In one study of 258 patients with obscure gastrointestinal bleeding that could not be diagnosed by standard modalities, a combination of push and Sonde enteroscopy ultimately achieved a diagnosis in 50% of patients and demonstrated a small bowel neoplasm in 5% of them (14). These findings were subsequently confirmed at laparotomy.

Intraoperative enteroscopy allows full visualization of the small bowel mucosal surface and the opportunity to treat identified lesions surgically. Rarely, however, is it necessary to resort to this procedure to identify a tumor. Except in very obese patients, once surgical exploration is initiated, small bowel tumors can usually be identified readily by careful palpation of the bowel.

In addition to these techniques, which attempt to visualize intraluminal pathology, other modalities are useful in specific situations. Selective visceral angiography may be helpful in the diagnosis of acute or chronic gastrointestinal hemorrhage. Massive hemorrhage is most common with benign smooth-muscle tumors, and arteriography may provide both diagnostic and temporizing therapeutic advantages if selective embolization of a bleeding vessel can be achieved. Benign vascular lesions, including hemangiomas, are more likely to present with occult gastrointestinal blood loss. For patients who present with jaundice or upper gastrointestinal hemorrhage and in whom a duodenal tumor is suspected, endoscopic ultrasonography or magnetic resonance cholangiopancreatography (MRCP) may be helpful to delineate the pathology if gastroduodenoscopy is not revealing.

Despite the availability of multiple diagnostic modalities, more than half of patients with small bowel neoplasms present with a surgical emergency, and metastasis has developed in more than half of patients with malignant disease at the time of operation.

BENIGN TUMORS OF THE SMALL INTESTINE

Accounting for 30% to 50% of primary neoplasms of the small bowel, benign tumors are poorly characterized. Half of patients with benign tumors are symptom-free, even in retrospect, until the need for emergency surgery arises. Up to 60% of benign small bowel tumors are diagnosed at the time of presentation with a surgical emergency, such as obstruction, massive gastrointestinal hemorrhage, or perforation. For those patients who do present with symptoms that require evaluation, vague abdominal pain and recurrent gastrointestinal bleeding are the most common. Acute hemorrhage was the presentation of 29% of benign lesions in one series (1) and of 40% in another (5). This presentation may help differentiate benign from malignant lesions; malignant tumors bleed less often. Many benign tumors are never identified because they cause no symptoms.

As noted above, the diagnostic work-up is challenging. In patients with symptoms, the investigation should proceed as outlined above. The secondary effects of the neoplasms—obstruction, hemorrhage, perforation—dictate the pathway of evaluation.

Regardless of their location, the treatment of benign small bowel tumors is local excision or limited resection. Endoscopic resection, submucosal excision via operative enterotomy, or segmental limited resection may be appropriate, depending on the size and location of the lesion. Intraoperative examination of the small bowel with careful palpation, including the possible use of intraoperative enteroscopy to evaluate suspected abnormalities, is essential to rule out synchronous lesions.

Adenomas

Brunner's gland adenomas are rare tumors of the proximal duodenum (15,16). Brunner's glands, normally found in the duodenal submucosa, secrete an alkaline, bicarbonate-rich fluid and mucus that aids in the neutralization of gastric acid. The pathogenesis of the glandular hyperplasia that is linked to adenoma formation remains unknown. Brunner's gland adenomas appear to have minimal if any malignant potential. Once identified, local resection via endoscopic means or duodenotomy with submucosal excision should be performed to prevent intussusception or biliary obstruction as the adenoma grows.

Like adenomas in the colon, small bowel adenomas may be histologically classified as tubular, tubulovillous, or villous. Adenomas occur predominantly in the duodenum, with the majority found in the periampullary region, but they may also be found in the proximal jejunum. Because roughly 25% of these villous and tubulovillous adenomas harbor malignancy, it is important to identify and resect them when they are identified (17). All are associated with a potential for malignant transformation, a risk that increases with size, although the relative risks of various-sized adenomas to undergo such transformation are difficult to determine given the low total number of cases. Adenomas larger than 2 cm should be considered worrisome for malignancy.

Approximately one third of adenomas in the duodenum present with obstructive jaundice or small bowel obstruction, in which case ultrasonography and abdominal radiography are the initial diagnostic studies. Without these physical signs to direct the work-up, an appropriate initial diagnostic study of the duodenum is a double-contrast upper gastrointestinal series or esophagogastroduodenoscopy; both of these are equally sensitive in most series. Adenomas appear usually as small intraluminal filling defects and are frequently pedunculated on a stalk (Fig. 28.1). For those few patients who undergo a contrast series before esophagogastroduodenoscopy, the pathognomonic finding for villous adenoma is a "soap bubble" or "paint brush" sign, in which one sees rounded radiolucent areas intermixed with a meshwork of radiopaque material. Esophagogastroduodenoscopy with biopsy is appropriate following a positive result on an upper gastrointestinal contrast series. CT may be helpful to differentiate an adenoma from a carcinoma because an adenoma is not associated with thickening of the bowel wall. Similarly, endoscopic ultrasonography may detect invasive disease or lymphadenopathy. Treatment requires either endoscopic excision or surgical resection. The surgical choices include transduodenal local excision for small lesions, pancreas-sparing duodenectomy, or pylorus-preserving pancreaticoduodenectomy for larger lesions or periampullary tumors. A recent review of locally resected duodenal villous tumors demonstrated local recurrence rates of 40% at 10 years; 25% of the recurrences were malignant. Based on these retrospective data, pancreaticoduodenectomy is recommended as an appropriate surgical option for benign lesions in selected patients. Because of this high risk for local recurrence, those patients who undergo

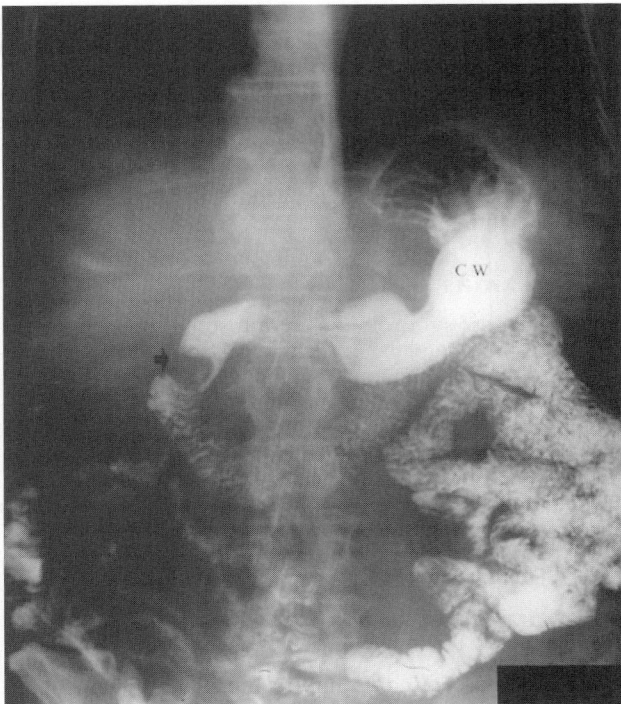

Figure 28.1. Polypoid lesion of the second portion of the duodenum *(arrow)*, representing a benign adenoma in a 64-year-old woman.

local excision require annual surveillance with endoscopy (18).

Gastrointestinal Stromal Tumors

Gastrointestinal stromal tumors are the most common nonepithelial cell tumor of the small bowel. Gastrointestinal stromal tumors may arise from pluripotential mesenchymal cells within the muscular wall of the gastrointestinal tract, most commonly those destined to be smooth-muscle or neural cells. Well-differentiated gastrointestinal stromal tumors include leiomyomas and schwannomas.

In many series, leiomyoma is the most common benign small bowel tumor. Leiomyoma is also the benign lesion most likely to bleed. Located primarily in the jejunum or ileum, leiomyomas can be submucosal, subserosal, or rarely intraluminal, each with characteristic findings on small bowel contrast imaging studies. Submucosal lesions appear as a smooth filling defect, whereas the subserosal lesions typically displace adjacent loops of bowel. Large tumors are readily detected on abdominal CT. Intraluminal leiomyomas are often hypervascular, and ulceration and bleeding may be initial presenting signs. All should be treated with segmental small bowel resection because they are often difficult to differentiate from low-grade sarcomas, even on final pathologic examination.

Lipomas

Lipomas are fatty tumors that may be found throughout the small bowel. They are typically asymptomatic. Because they are polypoid, compressible, intraluminal lesions, lipomas are likely to cause intussusception. They are most often found incidentally on abdominal CT completed to evaluate a different clinical condition. Lipomas are identified as well-circumscribed lesions of fat density on CT. On barium contrast study, they appear radiolucent. Unless associated with bleeding or obstruction, small tumors under 2 cm can be safely observed; larger or growing lesions should be resected to rule out malignant liposarcoma. If surgery is performed either for a complication of the lipoma or for an unrelated condition, local excision is adequate treatment.

Hamartomas

Peutz-Jeghers syndrome is an autosomal dominant condition characterized by multiple gastrointestinal hamartomas and mucocutaneous pigmentation. The polyps arise predominantly in the jejunum and ileum and often present as an intussusception. Although hamartomas rarely if ever undergo malignant transformation, they have been associated with the synchronous development of adenocarcinoma. Local resection is indicated for intussusception or bleeding, although the widespread nature of the hamartomas precludes complete extirpation.

Hemangiomas

Hemangiomas are rare congenital lesions of the small bowel that affect predominantly the jejunum and ileum. They grow slowly, typically coming to medical attention in the third decade of life because of acute or chronic blood loss. Arising from the submucosal vascular plexuses, hemangiomas are classified as capillary, cavernous, or mixed, depending on the size of the vessels primarily affected. Hemangiomas are usually solitary, and malignant degeneration is exceedingly rare. Depending on their size, hemangiomas may be locally excised or resected with a limited small bowel resection. Efforts to manage hemangiomas with endoscopic or operative sclerotherapy or coagulation and operative or angiographic interruption of arterial supply have been minimally successful.

MALIGNANT NEOPLASMS

Malignant neoplasms in the small bowel can be either primary or metastatic. Primary malignancies include adenocarcinoma, leiomyosarcoma, NHL, and carcinoid. Rarely reported other lesions include liposarcoma, myxoliposarcoma, and lymphangiosarcoma. Metastatic tumors of the small bowel have been reported from many primary solid tumors, but melanoma and lymphoma are the most common. Patients with malignant lesions are more likely to present with pain, weight loss, and anorexia than are patients with benign tumors. Although nonspecific, these findings are more ominous than the symptoms shared with benign tumors, such as nausea and vomiting and acute or chronic blood loss. As a group, patients with malignant small bowel tumors present at advanced stages and have a poor prognosis. High rates of metastatic spread are noted at initial surgical operation.

The diagnosis of small bowel malignancy should prompt a thorough diagnostic evaluation. Second primary malignancies are found in 20% to 30% of patients. This is especially true for patients with carcinoid tumors, in whom the incidence rate of second primaries is as high as 30% to 50%, but also applies to patients with adenocarcinomas and leiomyosarcomas. The second primary cancer may arise in any organ, but the most frequent second primary sites are the colorectum and breast (19,20).

Adenocarcinoma

Epidemiology

Adenocarcinoma accounts for 30% to 50% of small bowel tumors, so that it is the most common primary malignancy. Regional prevalence rates correlate with prevalence rates for colon cancer rather than for gastric cancer, a finding that also holds true internationally. Like adenomas, sporadic adenocarcinomas have a predilection for the duodenum; a marked decrease in frequency is noted toward the more distal portions of the small bowel. Approximately 80% of tumors are located in the duodenum or proximal jejunum. Most studies demonstrate a slight male predominance.

Several factors increase a person's risk for the development of adenocarcinoma. Malignant transformation of villous and tubulovillous adenomas is likely the most important and occurs predominantly in the periampullary region of the duodenum. Crohn's disease increases the risk up to 100-fold and predisposes to cancer in the more distal portions of the small bowel in regions of dysplasia.

Clinical Presentation

The presenting symptoms of small bowel adenocarcinoma depend on the location and size of the tumor. Because tumors tend to arise in the proximal small bowel and to encompass the bowel wall, adenocarcinomas cause obstruction, with associated anorexia. Most of the tumors cause cramping abdominal pain. Periampullary duodenal adenocarcinomas may cause obstructive jaundice or pancreatitis as they grow. In this case, the physical complaints and findings help guide the diagnostic evaluation. Often, the only complaint is vague, persistent abdominal pain.

Diagnosis

If obstruction is present, plain abdominal films may reveal gastric distention or nearly complete obstruction of the proximal small bowel. More commonly, these films are unrevealing. In a jaundiced patient, ultrasonography, abdominal CT, or MRCP may demonstrate the duodenal mass and site of biliary obstruction. Upper gastrointestinal contrast studies or esophagogastroduodenoscopy demonstrate duodenal adenocarcinomas equally well, with diagnostic rates of 85% to 90%. Endoscopy offers the advantage of tissue biopsy. For duodenal lesions, these rates compare favorably with those of CT, which can establish the diagnosis in roughly 50% of cancers.

Seventy percent of small bowel adenocarcinomas are polypoid, 20% ulcerated, and 10% infiltrative. Like those in other segments of the gastrointestinal tract, adenocarcinomas of the jejunum and ileum are usually annular, constricting tumors, seen as apple core lesions on luminal contrast studies (Fig. 28.2). Their appearance may be indistinguishable from that of metastatic lesions. Compression during fluoroscopic examination shows these tumors to be rigid and non-deformable. Long lesions, especially when ulcerated, may be mistaken for lymphomas. On CT, adenocarcinomas may exhibit heterogeneous attenuation and moderate contrast enhancement. Again, usually only a short segment of small bowel is involved, occasionally in association with an ulcer. Despite the array of diagnostic modalities, preoperative diagnosis remains infrequent, achieved in only 20% to 50% of cancers.

Management

The only potential cure for adenocarcinoma is complete surgical resection. At operation, the resectability rate for cure lies between 50% and 65%. For lesions in the proxi-

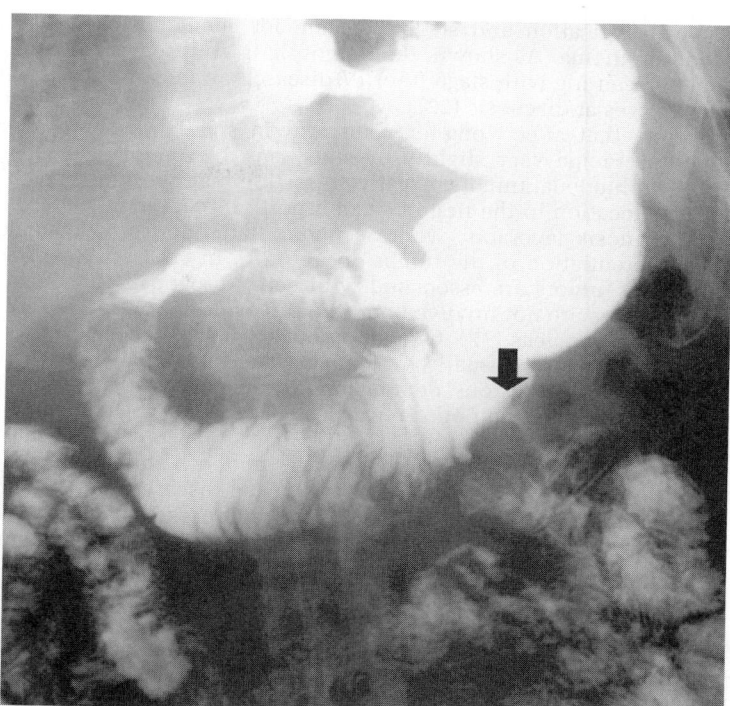

Figure 28.2. Results of upper gastrointestinal endoscopy were negative in a 73-year-old woman with early satiety and bilious vomiting. This upper gastrointestinal barium contrast study shows an "apple core" lesion *(arrow)* in the proximal jejunum, characteristic of adenocarcinoma.

mal and middle portions of the duodenum, pancreatico-duodenectomy is necessary to resect the tumor and lymphatic basin completely. In the third and fourth portions of the duodenum and in the mesenteric small bowel, a segmental resection with lymphadenectomy should be performed to attempt surgical cure. In patients with metastatic or unresectable disease, palliative procedures to relieve obstruction or control hemorrhage should be considered. Segmental resection or intestinal bypass is appropriate pending operative findings. Duodenal obstruction may be palliated with endoscopic placement of expandable stents, although recurrent obstruction and hemorrhage may complicate this procedure. The placement of a gastrojejunal or gastrostomy tube should be considered in patients with carcinomatosis or unresectable disease for long-term decompression or nutritional support.

Staging and Prognosis

The American Joint Committee on Cancer (AJCC) staging system for small bowel adenocarcinoma is similar to the systems used for gastric and colon carcinoma (21). The staging system applies only to adenocarcinomas of the small bowel, not to other malignant neoplasms of the small intestine. Carcinoma of the ampulla of Vater is also staged separately. As in other gastrointestinal malignancies, the tumor (T) classification describes the depth of invasion; T1 and T2 are both contained within the bowel wall, whereas T3 and T4 describe gradations of penetration through the wall. The node (N) classification in small bowel carcinoma depends only on the presence or absence of lymph node metastases, not on the numbers of positive nodes. Distant metastases are classified under M. Table 28.4 illustrates the

Table 28.4. TNM CLASSIFICATION AND STAGING OF SMALL BOWEL ADENOCARCINOMA

TNM	Carcinoma penetration	Stage	Five-year survival
TX	Unknown primary		
T0	No evidence of primary		
Tis	Carcinoma in situ	Stage 0	
T1	Tumor invades lamina propria or submucosa	Stage I	70%
T2	Tumor invades muscularis propria		
T3	Tumor extends <2 cm into subserosa or into nonperitonealized perimuscular tissue (mesentery in jejunum or ileum, retroperitoneum in duodenum)	Stage II	50%
T4	Tumor penetrates visceral peritoneum or directly invades >2 cm into adjacent structures		
NX	Regional lymph nodes not assessed		
N0	No regional lymph node involvement		
N1	Regional lymph nodes involved	Stage III	20%
MX	Distant metastases not assessed		
M0	No distant metastases		
M1	Distant metastases present	Stage IV	10%

TNM, tumor–node–metastasis.

TNM classification and staging system for small bowel adenocarcinoma. As shown, the prognosis is grim for patients presenting with stage III or IV disease, the most frequent stages at diagnosis (22).

Factors that affect long-term survival in small bowel adenocarcinoma vary slightly by study and tumor location. For duodenal tumors, negative resection margins and a tumor location in the first or second portion seem to affect prognosis favorably, whereas nodal status and size and differentiation of the tumor do not (23). In contrast, ampullary tumors are associated with better prognosis if lymph nodes are not involved and the tumor does not infiltrate the pancreas (17). One study evaluating the prognostic factors for all small bowel malignancies exclusive of periampullary lesions demonstrated poor survival in patients with positive nodes regardless of curative resection.

Chemotherapy or radiation therapy has not been shown to confer a survival advantage or a prolonged disease-free interval. At this time, the role of adjuvant therapies is within clinical trials. Wide surgical resection remains the mainstay of therapy.

Non-Hodgkin's Lymphoma

Non-Hodgkin's lymphoma of the gastrointestinal tract represents 4% to 20% of all cases of NHL, with the gastrointestinal tract the most common extranodal site. The stomach harbors the largest number of lymphomas, followed by the small bowel and then the colon. Twenty-five to thirty-five percent of gastrointestinal non-Hodgkin's lymphomas occur within the small bowel. The distribution pattern is marked by relative sparing of the duodenum and an equal frequency in the jejunum and ileum.

Many retrospective reviews of small bowel malignancy exclude primary NHL from analysis because of the difficulties in differentiating primary from secondary lymphomas in chart review data. Specific criteria must be met to establish the diagnosis of primary gastrointestinal NHL. No superficial adenopathy must be detected on physical examination, and no mediastinal adenopathy on chest radiography. Peripheral blood cell counts must be normal, and no evidence of splenic or hepatic involvement must be present. Finally, at laparotomy, disease must be restricted to the primary tumor with mesenteric lymph node involvement (24).

Multiple histologic variations of lymphoma exist and show significant geographic variability. Most primary intestinal NHLs are of the B-cell type, with T-cell lymphomas comprising only 10% to 25%. Further classifications of B- and T-cell tumors have been proposed, but none has been uniformly adopted. A significant number of gastrointestinal lymphomas appear to be low-grade lymphomas derived from mucosa-associated lymphoid tissue (MALT). These arise predominantly in the stomach but also occur in the small bowel. In the stomach, they are associated with *Helicobacter pylori* infection and may regress when this infection is treated (25). In the small bowel, they should be resected. The most common high-grade B-cell histologic type is diffuse large cell lymphoma. Less common and more lethal subtypes of B-cell lymphoma include immunoproliferative small intestinal disease (IPSID), alpha heavy-chain disease, and Mediterranean lymphoma. Patients with these conditions often present with severe malabsorption and have a poor prognosis. Regression of duodenal IPSID has been reported after treatment for *H. pylori* infection and suggests an infectious etiology, as in MALT lymphoma (26).

Patients with T-cell lymphomas tend to have a worse prognosis than those with B-cell tumors. Enteropathy-associated T-cell lymphoma is most commonly associated with celiac sprue and may result from a disordered response to gluten in the initial reactive T-cell population. Epstein-Barr virus has also been implicated in enteropathy-associated T-cell lymphoma.

Clinical Presentation

Like patients with other small bowel malignancies, the majority of patients present with abdominal pain that is nonspecific and unlocalized. Malabsorption, obstruction, and evidence of a palpable mass may be present. Although rare, perforation is a more common presentation in gastrointestinal NHL than in adenocarcinoma and is possibly related to the lack of a vigorous desmoplastic response in lymphoma. Signs that are common in nodal lymphoma, such as adenopathy and splenomegaly, are unusual in primary gastrointestinal NHL.

Diagnosis

Most small bowel lymphomas are demonstrable on CT. Lymphomas may grow to be quite large. CT demonstrates the mass and also marked luminal dilatation, thickening of the bowel wall, and displacement of neighboring loops (Fig. 28.3). Short strictures are more suggestive of adenocarcinoma but may be seen in lymphoma at times. SBFT reveals multifocal lesions in 10% to 25% of patients. For a tissue diagnosis to be made, biopsy specimens must be obtained from the submucosa, as the overlying mucosa often demonstrates no tumor infiltration. CT-guided biopsy may be diagnostic, although proximal lesions are best diagnosed with endoscopic submucosal biopsy. Additional tests to stage gastrointestinal NHL include a complete blood cell count with manual differential, serum liver chemistries, chest radiography to rule out mediastinal adenopathy, and a bone marrow biopsy.

Staging and Prognosis

The TNM system does not apply in the staging of gastrointestinal NHLs. Rather, staging is based on site involvement (Table 28.5). In stage I disease, only a single site is involved. Stage II confines disease to below the diaphragm but allows extension beyond the primary gastrointestinal site. The stage is subdivided into II_1 and II_2 to differentiate between involvement of regional and distant nodes, respectively. Stage IIE is a further subdivision of stage II that represents penetration of the serosa and involvement of adjacent organs. Disease on both sides of the diaphragm is stage III, and wide dissemination involving the liver and spleen is stage IV (27). The distinction between stages III and IV may be irrelevant clinically, as they both describe advanced disease and carry a dismal prognosis.

Treatment

With no randomized series and small numbers of cases at single institutions, the optimal treatment of gastrointestinal NHL remains controversial. Most agree that surgical resection of isolated small bowel lymphoma is the cornerstone of treatment. Resection is important for local control and prevents perforation and bleeding. A segmental small bowel resection with lymphadenectomy should be performed to attempt cure. Surgery rarely eradicates disease, but the prognosis after complete resection appears to be better than that following incomplete resection.

Small bowel lymphoma is the only small intestinal malignancy that responds to currently available adjuvant therapy (28). Again because of the small numbers, the ideal postoperative regimen has not been standardized. Debate continues over whether adjuvant therapy is necessary after curative resection for stage I disease, but most investigators advocate adjuvant chemotherapy to control

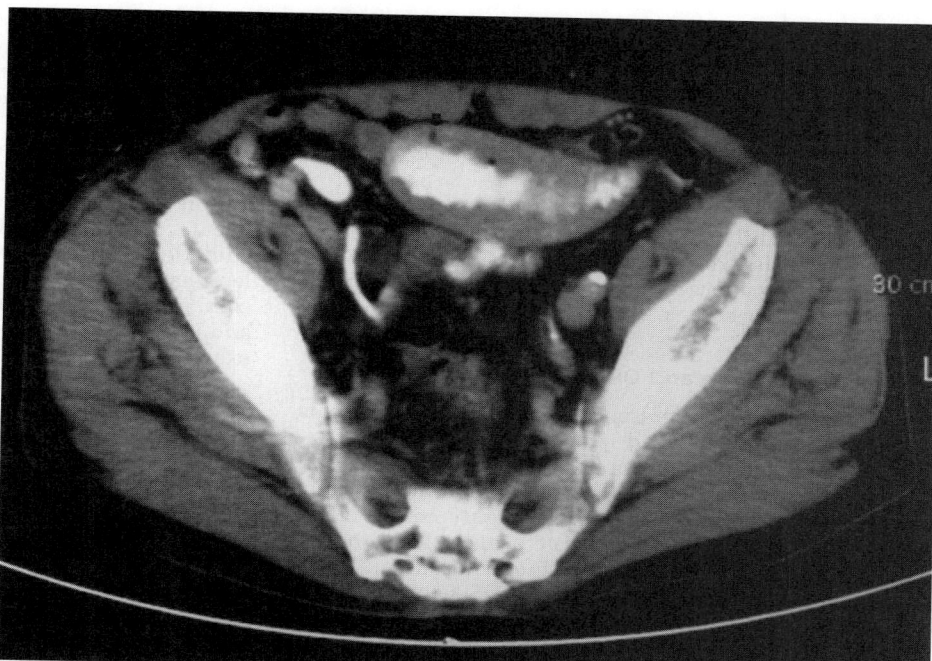

Figure 28.3. In a 71-year-old man with weight loss, episodic vomiting, and cramping abdominal pain, computed tomography of the abdomen reveals a dilated loop of distal ileum with thickened bowel wall *(arrow),* determined to be a primary small-bowel lymphoma.

presumed systemic disease. For more extensive gastrointestinal lymphoma, no evidence-based consensus on optimal management is available. Treatment options based on existing clinical trial data include limited resection of symptomatic lesions followed by adjuvant chemotherapy and radiation, or extensive surgical debulking to improve local control and reduce the potential local complications associated with adjuvant therapy. Reported rates of perforation following chemotherapy are as high as 5% to 15% when chemotherapy is administered after incomplete resection or in the neoadjuvant setting. Presumably, perforation is a consequence of chemotherapy-induced tumor necrosis.

The most important factor in the prognosis of small bowel NHL is the stage at diagnosis. Like tumors elsewhere in the gastrointestinal tract, lymphomas are typically diagnosed late, almost half of patients presenting with stage III or IV disease. Fewer than 30% of patients have surgically resectable tumors. Patients with stage I tumors have a 5-year survival of 40% to 60%, and those with stage II disease have a 5-year survival of 20%. The long-term survival for patients with stages III and IV remains

negligible despite the aggressive use of chemotherapy and radiation therapy.

In children, NHL, typically the Burkitt type of small B-cell lymphoma, is the most common tumor of the small bowel. More than 50% of tumors in children are diagnosed at emergency surgery for intussusception or presumed appendicitis. Because dissemination occurs early in children, especially to the central nervous system, it is important to include CT of the head, lumbar puncture, and bone marrow biopsy in the staging work-up. Pediatric intestinal lymphomas are more sensitive to chemotherapy than the lymphomas of adults, so that limited resection is appropriate, followed by adjuvant chemotherapy.

Carcinoids

Carcinoids are indolent malignant neuroendocrine tumors that arise from the enterochromaffin cells at the base of the crypts of Lieberkühn. These cells are part of the amine precursor uptake and decarboxylation (APUD) system and can secrete peptides responsible for the carcinoid syndrome. Although 80% of carcinoids arise in the gastrointestinal tract, 10% of primary carcinoids occur in the bronchus or lung. Other sites, such as the ovaries, testicles, pancreas, and kidney, are far less common. Within the gastrointestinal tract, carcinoids are most often identified in the appendix, followed by the small bowel, which harbors approximately 30% of all gastrointestinal carcinoids. Almost half of these arise in the distal 2 feet of ileum.

Accounting for 5% to 35% of small bowel neoplasms, carcinoids are found slightly more often in men than in women. The mean age at presentation is 60 years. The tumors are frequently asymptomatic; the autopsy rate in one study was more than 2,000 times the annual incidence rate, which indicates the potential for long-term slow growth. When symptomatic, carcinoids typically present with pain or obstructive symptoms. Because these tumors are typically slow-growing, symptoms may be present for 2 to 20 years before diagnosis. Ulceration is rare in carcinoids, so gastrointestinal bleeding is uncommon. Patients present with carcinoid syndrome in up to 40% of cases,

Table 28.5.	STAGING OF NON-HODGKIN'S LYMPHOMA OF THE GASTROINTESTINAL TRACT

Stage	Extent of lymphomatous disease
I	Tumor confined to the GI tract, either at single primary site or as multiple noncontiguous lesions.
II	Tumor extends from primary GI site, either to lymph nodes or as direct invasion. Confined to below the diaphragm.
*IIE	*Tumor penetrates serosa to involve adjacent structures.
*II₁	*Local nodal involvement.
*II₂	*Distant nodal involvement.
III	Evidence of supradiaphragmatic disease.
IV	Disseminated disease above and below the diaphragm.

GI, gastrointestinal.

and only when the symptoms of carcinoid syndrome are present is the diagnosis consistently made preoperatively.

Five histologic patterns correlate embryologically with the location of the tumor (29). Foregut, or duodenal, lesions usually demonstrate a trabecular or ribbon pattern. An insular pattern predominates in the midgut, or small bowel, and a mixed pattern is typical of the hindgut, or colorectum. The least common patterns are glandular or tubular and undifferentiated, both of which carry a much poorer prognosis than the three more common variations. The histologic pattern does not affect treatment but, together with other factors, appears to determine long-term survival.

Clinical Presentation and Diagnosis

The most common presenting symptom for patients with small bowel carcinoid is abdominal pain. As carcinoids grow, the polypoid lesions may serve as a lead point for intussusception (Fig. 28.4). Intussusception is characterized by intermittent symptoms and signs of obstruction. Abdominal films often demonstrate a distal small bowel obstruction. On CT, the appearance of intussusception is distinctive—a multilayered ring in the ileocolic region (Fig. 28.5). If the patient does not have a complete small bowel obstruction, a contrast study may be helpful, but it yields a diagnosis in only 20% to 50%.

In the appendix, multicentricity is rare, but carcinoids of the small bowel are multiple 30% to 40% of the time. In addition, 30% to 50% of small bowel carcinoids are associated with second primary malignancies, most frequently of the breast or colon. Gastrointestinal carcinoids have the capacity to elicit a marked desmoplastic reaction. Fibrosis and foreshortening of the mesentery of the small bowel lead to kinking of the bowel or even intestinal ischemia, as a result of sclerosis of the mesenteric blood vessels. This finding is readily identified on CT and is sometimes associated with calcifications. The small bowel appears fixed and angulated.

Staging and Prognosis

The risk for metastatic spread increases with tumor size at initial diagnosis and must be considered when surgical strategies are being planned. Unlike appendiceal carcinoids, which may cause appendicitis while they are small

and before lymph node metastasis develops, small bowel lesions often remain asymptomatic long enough for lymph node and also hepatic metastases to develop. With lesions smaller than 1 cm, the incidence of nodal and hepatic spread is 20% to 30%. Tumors 1 to 2 cm in size are associated with nodal spread in 60% to 80% of cases and with hepatic disease in 20%. The rate of nodal metastases for tumors larger than 2 cm is more than 80%, and the rate of hepatic metastases is 40% to 50% (30). These figures must guide the choice of operation. Whereas a small lesion of less than 1 cm may be adequately treated with local excision, anything larger must be presumed to be metastatic, and a wide resection with lymphadenectomy and careful examination of the liver is necessary.

Carcinoid Syndrome

The term *carcinoid syndrome* refers to the vasomotor, gastrointestinal, and cardiac manifestations induced by the systemic circulation of a variety of peptide and non-peptide molecules elaborated by carcinoid tumors. The APUD cells of carcinoid tumors can produce vasoactive products, including serotonin, histamine, kallikrein, bradykinin, and prostaglandins, although the specific mediator or mediators of the syndrome remain unknown. Carcinoid syndrome is most reliably confirmed by the finding of an elevated 24-hour urinary excretion of 5-hydroxyindoleacetic acid (5-HIAA), the primary stable metabolite of serotonin.

Attacks are initiated by stimuli such as stress, alcohol, a large meal, or sexual intercourse. Flushing is the most common finding and affects approximately 80% of patients with carcinoid syndrome. The flush varies slightly according to the location of the tumor, but with midgut carcinoids, the flush is usually short-lived, lasting 5 to 10 minutes. Classically, the erythematous flush begins on the face and spreads to the trunk and limbs. Diarrhea, which occurs in 75% of patients, seems to be caused by the release of serotonin. The diarrhea is intermittent, watery, and at times explosive. It may be associated with abdominal cramps, and malabsorption may be present to some degree. Although the diarrhea can be the most bothersome symptom to a patient, the cardiac manifestations present in 60% to 70% of cases are the most serious. Endocardial fibrosis develops in the tricuspid and pulmonary valves,

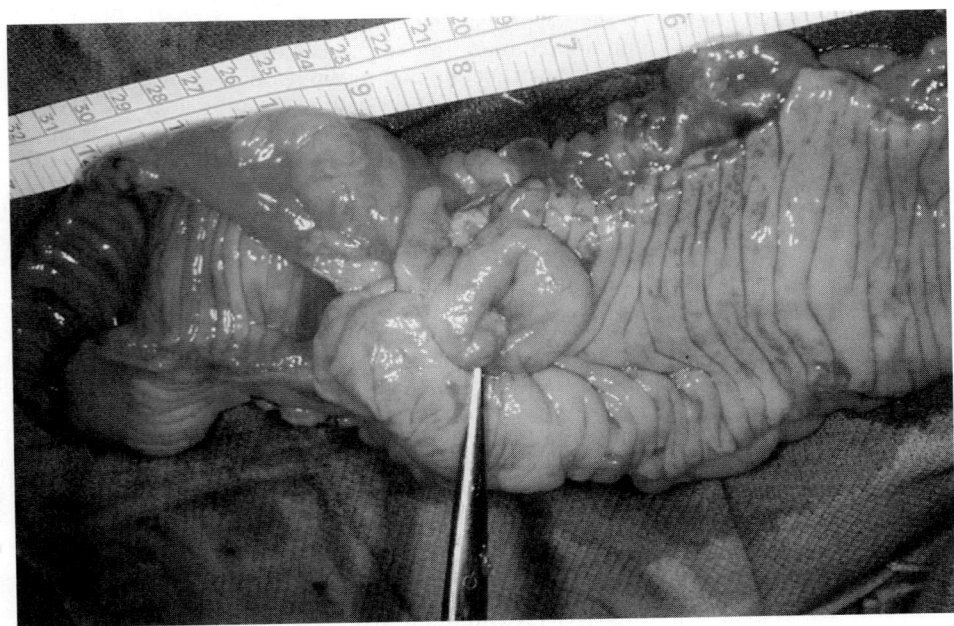

Figure 28.4. Resected ileocolonic specimen from the patient in Fig. 28.5. The clamp identifies the tip of a carcinoid tumor that has served as the lead point of an intussusception though the ileocecal valve.

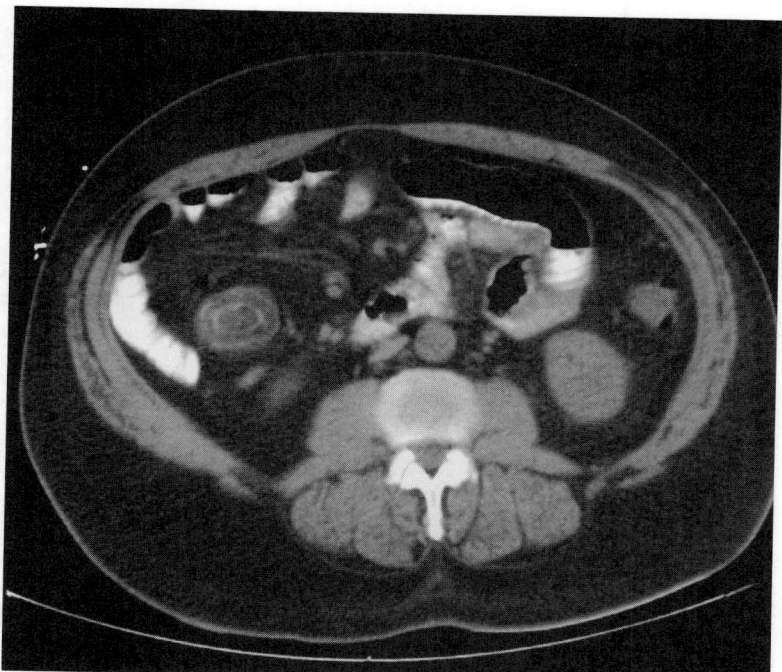

Figure 28.5. Abdominal computed tomogram from a 63-year-old man presenting with a 3-week history of intermittent cramping abdominal pain. No abdominal masses or tenderness was detected on physical examination. Result of Hemoccult test was positive. The scan demonstrates a mass of the right lower quadrant with the distinct appearance of a multilayered ring, characteristic of small-bowel intussusception *(black arrow)*. At surgical exploration, the patient was found to have an ileocolic intussusception with an ileal carcinoid tumor serving as the lead point (Fig. 28.4).

possibly secondary to high levels of 5-HIAA. As the disease progresses, stiffening of the fibrotic plaque leads eventually to right-sided heart failure.

Patients with gastrointestinal carcinoid tumors who present with carcinoid syndrome have metastatic disease. The liver contains large amounts of monoamine oxidase, which deactivates serotonin, one of the major effector hormones. Hence, for the carcinoid syndrome to develop, a patient must have either a tumor in a location that does not primarily drain into the portal circulation, such as a bronchial carcinoid, or hepatic metastases that overwhelm the capacity of the hepatic monoamine oxidase. The bioactive products from a small volume of hepatic metastases may be cleared by the hepatocytes, but with a larger tumor burden, products are released into the hepatic veins and systemic circulation. It follows that patients with bronchial and ovarian carcinoids, which drain directly into the systemic circulation, can manifest carcinoid syndrome with primary disease. Patients with gastrointestinal carcinoids, which drain into the portal circulation, must have metastatic disease before the syndrome develops.

Patients with carcinoid syndrome may be managed surgically, radiologically, or medically, and often a combination of all three modalities is required. Surgical debulking of extensive hepatic disease may relieve symptoms and prolong life. Hepatic artery embolization or radiofrequency ablation may be more appropriate for patients with widespread hepatic metastases, and in small series, these methods have been shown to provide marked symptomatic relief and durable tumor control. Medical therapy relies primarily on the use of the inhibitory peptide octreotide, a long-acting somatostatin analogue. Octreotide inhibits the release of peptides from carcinoid tumors, and 5-HIAA levels are markedly reduced. Symptoms are effectively palliated in 90% of patients treated with octreotide, and some studies have even demonstrated tumor inhibition and shrinkage after the administration of somatostatin, although these findings have not been consistently reproduced.

Potential chemotherapeutic agents for the treatment of metastatic carcinoid tumor have been used singly and in combination in an effort to halt progression of disease. Common single agents include Adriamycin, 5-fluorouracil, dacarbazine, and interferon alfa, with response rates of approximately 20%. Interferon alfa has been shown to relieve the symptoms of carcinoid syndrome and possibly prolong life. Combination protocols most often utilize streptozotocin and 5-fluorouracil.

Gastrointestinal Stromal Sarcomas

Gastrointestinal stromal tumors comprise a poorly defined continuum of benign to malignant neoplasms. The well-differentiated gastrointestinal stomal tumors, leiomyomas, have been discussed previously. Poorly differentiated malignant tumors, formerly called *leiomyosarcomas,* are now referred to as *gastrointestinal stromal sarcomas.* The distinction is often not clear, and tumors with the cellular features of sarcomas (poorly differentiated cells with a high mitotic index rate) have been described that fail to manifest an aggressive metastatic phenotype (31).

In most series, gastrointestinal stromal sarcomas are the least common primary small bowel malignancy. They tend to develop in the fifth and sixth decades of life and arise slightly more often in men than in women. Unusual in the duodenum, gastrointestinal stromal sarcomas develop predominantly in the distal small bowel. Like other small bowel tumors, stromal tumors may present with abdominal pain and obstructive symptoms, but acute hemorrhage may be the herald sign more often than in other primary malignancies. Like their benign counterparts, gastrointestinal stromal sarcomas may be submucosal, subserosal, or rarely intraluminal, and therefore they may grow to a large size before presenting as an abdominal mass.

Diagnosis

Vague abdominal complaints or the presence of a mass leads to diagnostic evaluation. On CT, a well-defined mass may be appreciated that is homogenous or shows evidence

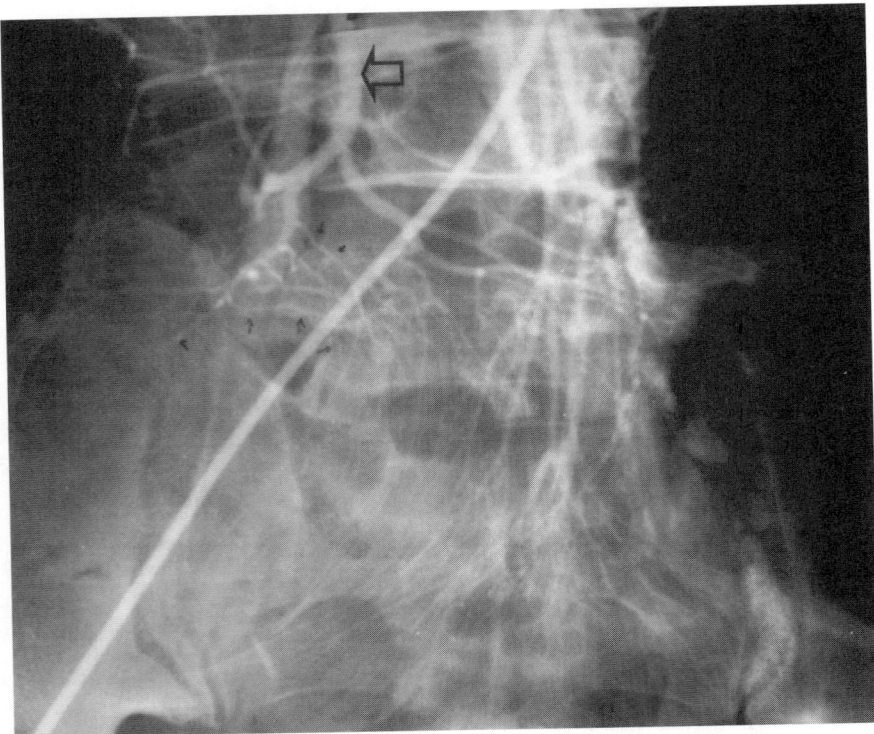

Figure 28.6. Selective visceral angiography in a patient with an 8-cm leiomyosarcoma of the distal small bowel. The ileocolic artery *(open arrow)* gives rise to a large ileal feeding vessel. Multiple small branches lead to the tumor *(small arrows).*

of central necrosis, occasionally with calcifications. Evidence of direct extension into adjacent structures and vascular encasement suggest a malignant neoplasm. Because these are often hypervascular tumors, angiography may reveal neovascularization of the tumor with feeding vessels (Fig. 28.6), although this finding does not aid in differentiating benign from malignant smooth-muscle tumors, both of which are prone to hemorrhage. Magnetic resonance imaging outlines tumor relationships to adjacent organs but is less able than CT to characterize the primary tumor. Because of the usual submucosal site, endoscopic biopsy usually yields normal mucosa.

Treatment

At operation, wide local excision of the primary tumor is the primary goal. In-continuity resection of adherent organs is appropriate to attain curative resection. Lymph node metastasis is rare, so that wide mesenteric resection is not required. A benign leiomyoma can be difficult to differentiate from a leiomyosarcoma at operation, and late

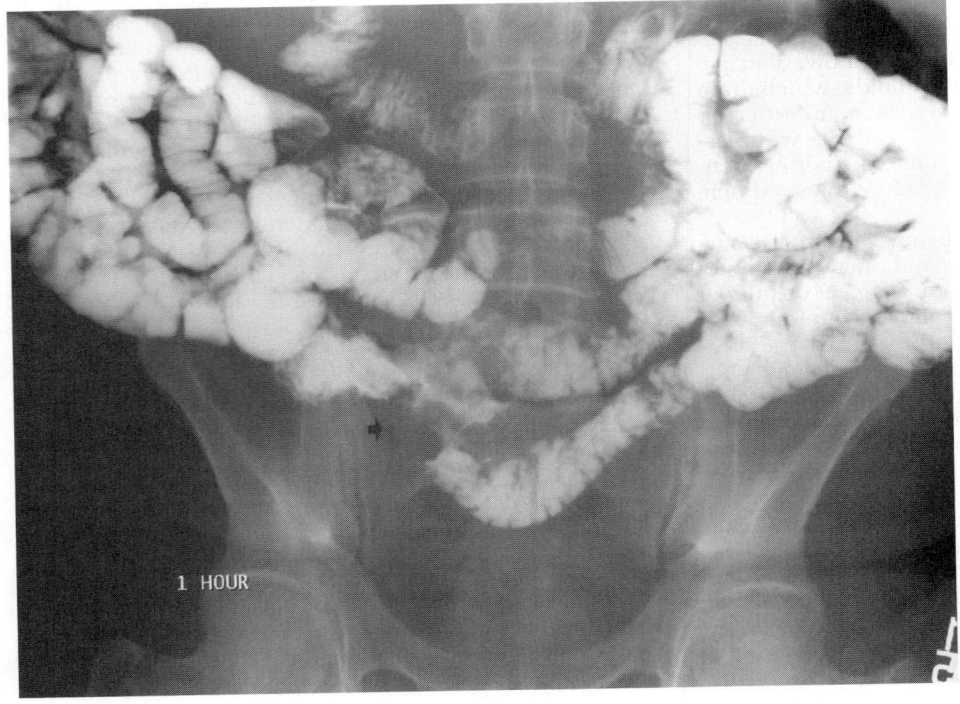

Figure 28.7. Small bowel follow-through study from a 75-year-old man with weight loss and iron deficiency. He had a remote history of stage I melanoma of the back. At exploration, the lesion *(arrow)* was determined to be a metastatic melanoma.

liver metastases from presumed benign leiomyomas have been reported (32). Therefore, excisions should be wide, even if the lesion appears benign.

Histologic differentiation between benign and malignant stromal tumors remains difficult, and no method has proved to distinguish between the two reliably. At this time, the strongest predictors of malignant behavior remain size larger than 5 cm and mitotic count above five per high-power field, although the relevance of these parameters as independent predictors has been questioned (33,34). Until better molecular biologic markers become available, tumor size and mitotic count together provide the best guidelines for follow-up after resection. Although adjuvant therapy has been reported in the literature, no consistent benefit has been demonstrated, and surgical resection has provided the only long-term cures.

Metastatic Lesions to the Small Bowel

The majority of malignant small bowel tumors are metastatic lesions from other primary sites rather than primary small bowel neoplasms. Metastatic spread can occur by direct invasion, hematogenous spread, or intraperitoneal seeding. Direct invasion by a colon or pancreatic cancer represents the most common mode of involvement. Hematogenous spread arises most frequently from bronchogenic or breast carcinoma or malignant melanoma. Peritoneal seeding has been documented from primary tumors of the stomach, liver, ovary, appendix, and colon.

Computed tomography often demonstrates not only the degree of involvement of the small bowel, but also the primary tumor. In metastatic small bowel tumors, one may see thickening of the bowel wall in addition to lesions in the mesentery or retroperitoneal fat. For small lesions, CT findings may be negative, whereas an SBFT study may reveal an irregular luminal filling defect (Fig. 28.7). Carcinomatosis is frequently not specifically identifiable on imaging studies.

Optimal management is based on clinical criteria. Palliative intestinal resection or bypass to relieve hemorrhage, obstruction, or pain is indicated except for patients in the most terminal stages of disease. Case reports of prolonged survival after intestinal resection of solitary metastases have been reported, although progression of metastatic disease is more common.

The management of patients with carcinomatosis remains difficult. Palliative measures to maintain intestinal continuity and the liberal use of decompressive gastrostomy tubes are indicated.

REFERENCES

1. Ciresi DL, Scholten DJ. The continuing clinical dilemma of primary tumors of the small intestine. *Am Surg* 1995;61: 698–703.
2. Matsuo S, Eto T, Tsunoda T, et al. Small bowel tumors: an analysis of tumor-like lesions, benign and malignant neoplasms. *Eur J Surg Oncol* 1994;20:47–51.
3. Minardi AJ Jr, Zibari GB, Aultman DF, et al. Small bowel tumors. *J Am Coll Surg* 1998;186:664–668.
4. Johnson AM, Harman PK, Hanks JB. Primary small bowel malignancies. *Am Surg* 1985;51:31–36.
5. Serour F, Dona G, Birkenfeld S, et al. Primary neoplasms of the small bowel. *J Surg Oncol* 1992;49:29–34.
6. Sigel JE, Petras RE, Lashner BA, et al. Intestinal adenocarcinoma in Crohn's disease: a report of 30 cases with a focus on coexisting dysplasia. *Am J Surg Pathol* 1999;23:651–655.
7. Alarcon FJ, Burke CA, Church JM, et al. Familial adenomatous polyposis: efficacy of endoscopic and surgical treatment for advanced duodenal adenomas. *Dis Colon Rectum* 1999;42: 1533–1536.
8. O'Boyle CJ, Kerin MJ, Feeley K, et al. Primary small intestinal tumours: increased incidence of lymphoma and improved survival. *Ann R Coll Surg Engl* 1998;80:332–334.
9. Crump M, Gospodarowicz M, Shepherd FA. Lymphoma of the gastrointestinal tract. *Semin Oncol* 1999;26:324–337.
10. Baillie CT, Williams A. Small bowel tumors: a diagnostic challenge. *J R Coll Surg Edinb* 1994;39:8–12.
11. Naef M, Buhlmann M, Baer HU. Small bowel tumors: diagnosis, therapy, and prognostic factors. *Langenbecks Arch Chir* 1999;384:176–180.
12. Maglinte DDT, Reyes BL. Small bowel cancer: radiologic diagnosis. *Radiol Clin North Am* 1997;35:361–380.
13. Buckley JA, Jones B, Fishman EK. Small bowel cancer: imaging features and staging. *Radiol Clin North Am* 1997;35: 381–402.
14. Lewis BS, Kornbluth A, Waye JD. Small bowel tumours: yield of enteroscopy. *Gut* 1991;32:763–765.
15. Adeonigbagbe O, Lee C, Karowe M, et al. A Brunner's gland adenoma as a cause of anemia. *J Clin Gastroenterol* 1999;29: 193–196.
16. Zangara J, Kushner H, Drachenberg C, et al. Iron deficiency anemia due to a Brunner's gland hamartoma. *J Clin Gastroenterol* 1998;27:353–356.
17. Beger HG, Treitschke F, Gansange F, et al. Tumor of the ampulla of Vater. *Arch Surg* 1999;134:526–532.
18. Farnell MB, Sakorafas GH, Sarr MG, et al. Villous tumors of the duodenum: reappraisal of local vs. extended resection. *J Gastrointest Surg* 2000;4:13–21.
19. Cunningham JD, Aleali R, Aleali M, et al. Malignant small bowel neoplasms: histopathologic determinants of recurrence and survival. *Ann Surg* 1997;225:300–306.
20. Marcilla JAG, Bueno FS, Aquilar J, et al. Primary small bowel malignant tumors. *Eur J Surg Oncol* 1994;20:630–634.
21. American Joint Committee on Cancer and TNM Committee of the International Union Against Cancer. Small intestine. In: Beakers OH, Henson DE, Hutter RVP, et al., eds. *Handbook for the staging of cancer.* Philadelphia: JB Lippincott, 1993: 89–93.
22. Contant CME, Dambuis RAM, van Geel AN, et al. Prognostic value of the TNM-classification for small bowel cancer. *Hepatogastroenterology* 1997;44:430–434.
23. Sohn TA, Lillemoe KD, Cameron JL, et al. Adenocarcinoma of the duodenum: factors influencing long-term survival. *J Gastrointest Surg* 1998;2:79–87.
24. Case Records of the Massachusetts General Hospital. Case 30-1999. *N Engl J Med* 1999;341:1063–1071.
25. Cooper DL, Daria R, Salloum E. Primary gastrointestinal lymphomas. *Gastroenterologist* 1996;4:54–64.
26. Fischbach W, Jacke W, Greber A, et al. Regression of immunoproliferative small intestinal disease after eradication of *Helicobacter pylori. Lancet* 1997;349:31–32.
27. Turowski GA, Basson MD. Primary malignant lymphoma of the intestine. *Am J Surg* 1995;169:433–441.
28. Pandey M, Wadhwa MK, Patel HP, et al. Malignant lymphoma of the gastrointestinal tract. *Eur J Surg Oncol* 1999;25:164–167.
29. Memon MA, Nelson H. Gastrointestinal carcinoid tumors: current management strategies. *Dis Colon Rectum* 1997;40: 1101–1118.
30. Rothmund M, Kisker O. Surgical treatment of carcinoid tumors of the small bowel, appendix, colon, and rectum. *Digestion* 1994;55:86–91.
31. Lev R, Karir Y, Issakov J, et al. Gastrointestinal stromal sarcomas. *Br J Surg* 1999;86:545–549.
32. Salari GR, Peny MO, van de Stadt J, et al. Late liver metastases of small bowel leiomyoma: the difficulty in assessing malignancy in gastro-intestinal smooth muscle tumors and their clinical behavior. *Am J Surg* 1997;173:390–394.
33. Ludwig DJ, Traverso LW. Gut stromal tumors and their clinical behavior. *Am J Surg* 1997;173:390–394.
34. Emory TS, Sobin LH, Lukes L, et al. Prognosis of gastrointestinal smooth-muscle (stromal) tumors: dependence on anatomic site. *Am J Surg Pathol* 199;23:82–87.

SECTION E

PANCREAS

SURGERY: SCIENTIFIC PRINCIPLES AND PRACTICE, Third Edition, edited by
Lazar J. Greenfield, Michael W. Mulholland, Keith T. Oldham, Gerald B. Zelenock,
and Keith D. Lillemoe. Lippincott Williams & Wilkins Publishers, Philadelphia, © 2001.

CHAPTER 29

PANCREATIC ANATOMY AND PHYSIOLOGY

F. CHARLES BRUNICARDI AND WILLIAM E. FISHER

ANATOMY

Precise knowledge of pancreatic anatomy and physiology is critical for pancreatic surgeons. Pancreatic anatomy explains the unique presentation of patients with pancreatic disease. The pancreas is situated deep within the abdomen in the retroperitoneum at the level of the second lumbar vertebra. It extends in an oblique, transverse position from the duodenal C loop to the hilum of the spleen (Fig. 29.1). The pancreas is a relatively small organ, weighing only 75 to 100 g, and is 15 to 20 cm long. These factors account for the silent clinical course and late clinical manifestation and diagnosis of many pancreatic diseases. The pancreas is divided into three portions: (a) the head, which fits snugly into the duodenal C loop; (b) the neck, which lies over the superior mesenteric vessels; and (c) the body and tail, which are closely adherent to the posterior wall of the stomach and spleen. Resection of the pancreas at the level of the neck results in a 50% reduction in pancreatic mass.

Embryology

The pancreas is of endodermal origin and develops from ventral and dorsal pancreatic buds. The ventral bud arises from the hepatic diverticulum, and the dorsal bud arises from the developing duodenum. During the fifth week of life, the dorsal bud appears first and grows rapidly. The ventral bud rotates clockwise behind the duodenum and fuses with the dorsal bud (Fig. 29.2). The ventral bud becomes the uncinate process and inferior head of the pancreas; the dorsal bud becomes the neck, body and tail, and superior head of the pancreas. The ventral bud duct fuses with the dorsal bud to become the *main pancreatic duct,* or duct of Wirsung, which drains most of the pancreas. The proximal duct of the dorsal bud, known as the *lesser pancreatic duct,* or duct of Santorini, usually persists and drains into the duodenum through the lesser papilla (Fig. 29.3). Abnormalities in the rotation or fusion of the developing pancreas can result in specific congenital disorders.

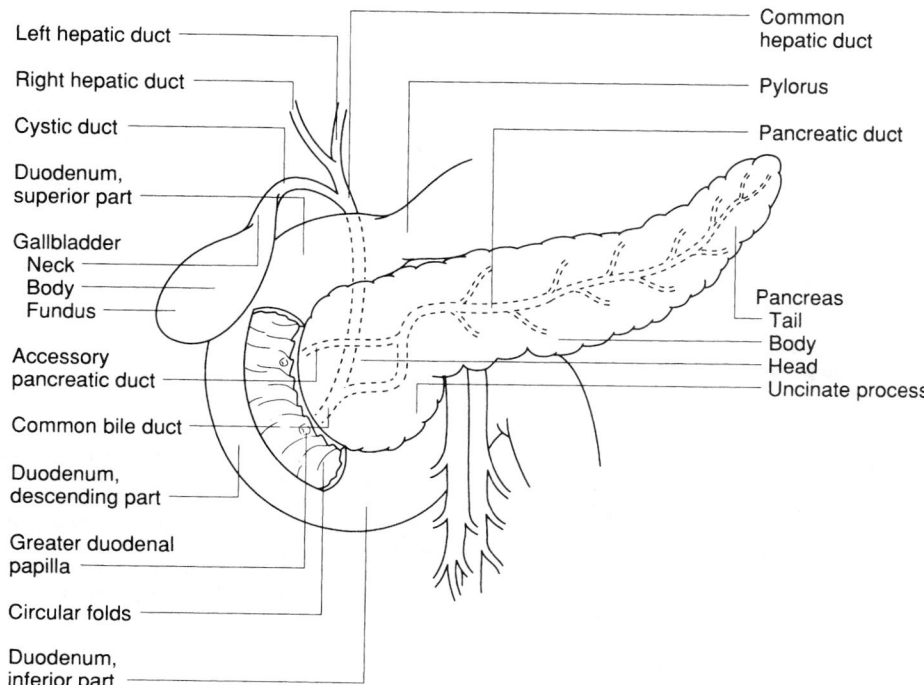

Figure 29.1. Relation of the pancreas to the duodenum and extrahepatic biliary system. (After Woodburne RT. *Essentials of human anatomy.* New York: Oxford University Press, 1973, with permission.)

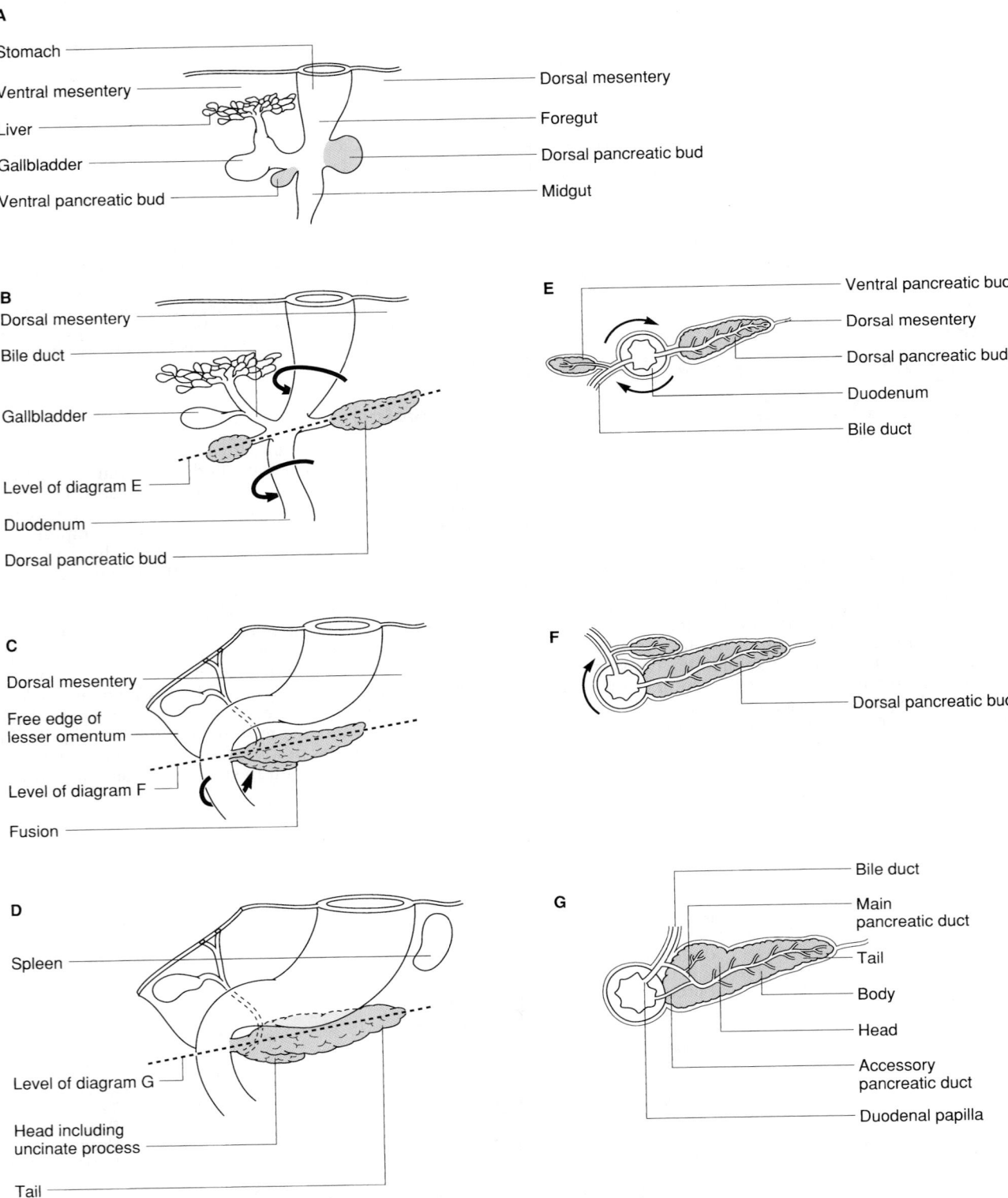

Figure 29.2. *(A–D)* Schematic drawings of the successive stages in the development of the pancreas from the fifth through the eighth weeks. *(E–G)* Diagrammatic transverse sections through the duodenum and the developing pancreas. Growth and rotation *(arrows)* of the duodenum bring the ventral pancreatic bud toward the dorsal bud, and they subsequently fuse. The bile duct initially attaches to the ventral aspect of the duodenum and is carried around to the dorsal aspect as the duodenum rotates. The main pancreatic duct is formed by the union of the distal part of the dorsal pancreatic duct and the entire ventral pancreatic duct. (From Moore KL. *The developing human*, 3rd ed. Philadelphia: WB Saunders, 1982, with permission.)

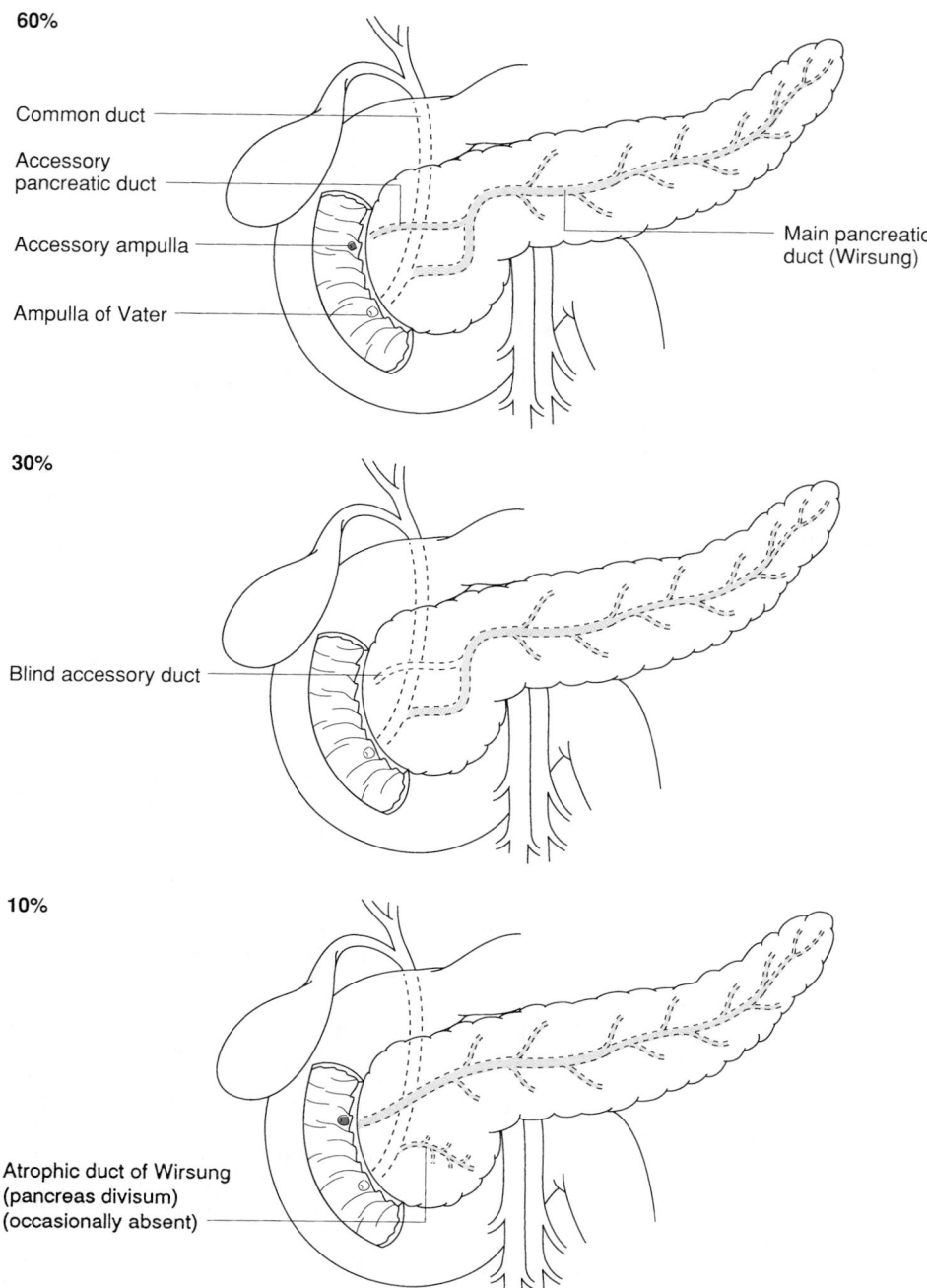

60%

Common duct

Accessory
pancreatic duct

Accessory ampulla

Ampulla of Vater

Main pancreatic
duct (Wirsung)

30%

Blind accessory duct

10%

Atrophic duct of Wirsung
(pancreas divisum)
(occasionally absent)

Figure 29.3. Anatomic configuration of the intrapancreatic ductal system. A lack of communication between the two ducts, which occurs in 10% of cases, is referred to as *pancreas divisum*. (After Silen W. Surgical anatomy of the pancreas. *Surg Clin North Am* 1964;44:1253, with permission.)

Surgical Anatomy

Relations to Other Structures

The pancreas is almost entirely retroperitoneal and lies close to a number of organs (Fig. 29.4). The head of the pancreas fits closely into the curve of the duodenum and lies to the right of the superior mesenteric vessels. The head is crossed anteriorly by the root of the transverse mesocolon and lies anterior and adjacent to the vena cava, renal veins, and right renal artery. The uncinate process, which is part of the head, wraps around and extends posteriorly to the superior mesenteric vessels. The intrapan-

creatic portion of the common bile duct descends in the posterior surface of the pancreatic head to join the main pancreatic duct at the ampulla of Vater.

The neck is defined as that portion of the pancreas overlying the superior mesenteric vessels and is identifiable from the head of the pancreas by a notch that contains the superior mesenteric vessels. This part of the pancreas is sometimes referred to as the *incisura pancreatis*. Usually, no anterior venous tributaries of the superior mesenteric or portal vein extend from the pancreatic neck. A plane can be developed between these vessels and the pancreas during pancreatic resection.

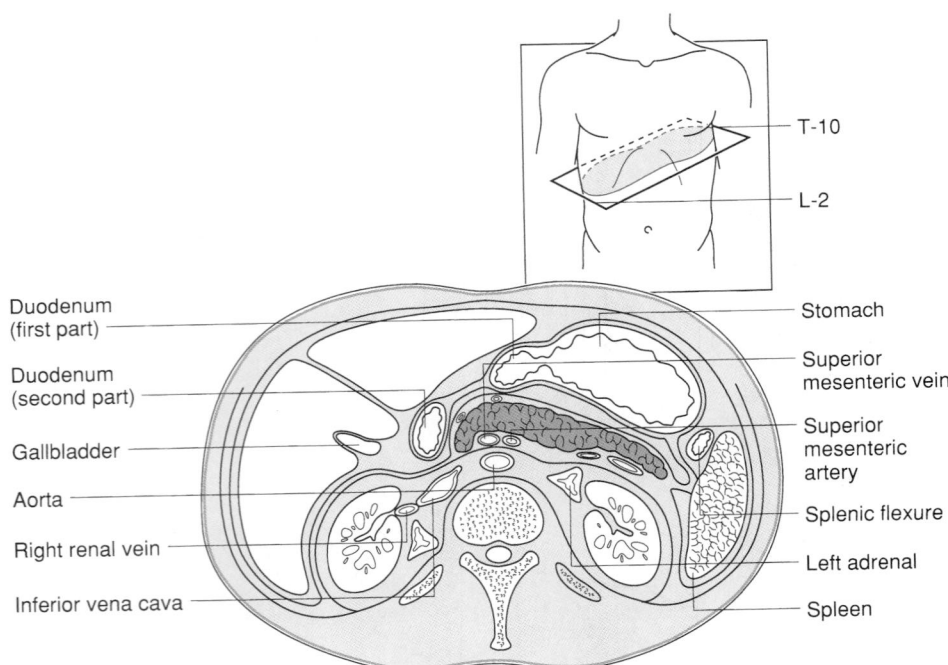

Figure 29.4. Cross-sectional relation of the pancreas to other abdominal structures in an oblique plane through the long axis of the pancreas extending from the level of L-2 on the right to T-10 on the left. (After Mackie CR, Moossa AR. Surgical anatomy of the pancreas. In: Moossa AR, ed. *Tumors of the pancreas.* Baltimore: Williams & Wilkins, 1980.)

The body begins to the left of the neck. Its anterior surface is covered with peritoneum that forms the posterior floor of the lesser sac. The transverse mesocolon attaches to its inferior margin. The body lies behind the posterior wall of the stomach and overlies the aorta at the origin of the superior mesenteric artery. These anatomic relationships explain why an inflammatory processes like pancreatitis is sometimes contained within the lesser sac.

The small portion of the pancreas anterior to the left kidney is referred to as the *tail.* The tail of the pancreas lies close to the spleen, left colic flexure, and lienorenal ligament, so that it is susceptible to injury during splenectomy. An understanding of these complex relations can help avoid injury during surgery performed on the pancreas or any of its adjacent organs and structures.

Pancreatic Ducts

The main pancreatic duct, or duct of Wirsung, runs the entire length of the pancreas and joins the common bile duct to empty into the duodenum at the ampulla of Vater. The duct usually runs midway between the superior and inferior borders and is usually closer to the posterior than to the anterior surface. The pancreatic duct is only 2 to 3.5 mm in diameter and contains 20 secondary branches, which drain the tail, body, and uncinate process. Pancreatic ductal pressure is 15 to 30 mm Hg, whereas that in the common bile duct is only 7 to 17 mm Hg. This normal pressure differential is thought to prevent damage to the pancreatic duct by reflux of bile. The drainage of the lesser duct, or duct of Santorini, is variable. The lesser duct commonly drains the superior portion of the head of the pancreas. It empties separately into the second portion of the duodenum through the lesser papilla, which is 2 cm proximal to the ampulla of Vater. Usually, the lesser duct patently communicates with the main duct. When the ducts do not communicate, a nonpatent connection is frequently present; less frequently, the lesser duct does not communicate at all with the major duct. Another variation

is a lesser duct that empties into the main duct and does not communicate with the duodenum. All the variations in the ductal system are secondary to differences in embryologic development and can be of clinical significance. Pancreas divisum results from an incomplete fusion of the ventral pancreatic duct with the dorsal duct during fetal development and is present in 5% of patients. In this anomaly, the lesser duct drains the entire pancreas; inadequacy of this pattern of drainage can result in chronic pain.

The main pancreatic duct joins with the common bile duct and empties at the ampulla of Vater. The surrounding sphincter of Oddi controls pancreatic and biliary secretions into the duodenal lumen. This sphincter, which is a complex set of muscular fibers surrounding the common bile duct and pancreatic duct, is regulated by neural and hormonal factors. The sphincter prevents reflux of duodenal contents into the ducts and can prevent reflux of bile into the pancreatic duct because of the differential in pancreatic and biliary ductular pressures. A short *common channel,* containing flow from both secretory systems, is seen in a significant number of patients (Fig. 29.5).

Arterial Supply

The unique arterial supply to the pancreas must be considered during pancreatic resection. The pancreas receives its blood supply from a variety of major arterial sources. The celiac and superior mesenteric arteries supply blood to the pancreas through their major branches (Fig. 29.6). Collateral vessels generally form between arcades in the anterior and posterior surfaces of the head of the pancreas. These arcades arise from branches of the gastroduodenal and superior mesenteric arteries. The gastroduodenal artery is a branch of the common hepatic artery and is divided when a pancreaticoduodenectomy is performed. Just distal to the first portion of the duodenum, the gastroduodenal artery becomes the superior pancreaticoduodenal artery, which divides into anterior and posterior

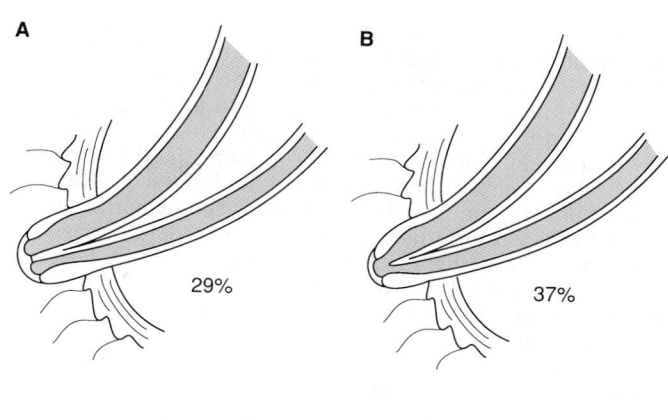

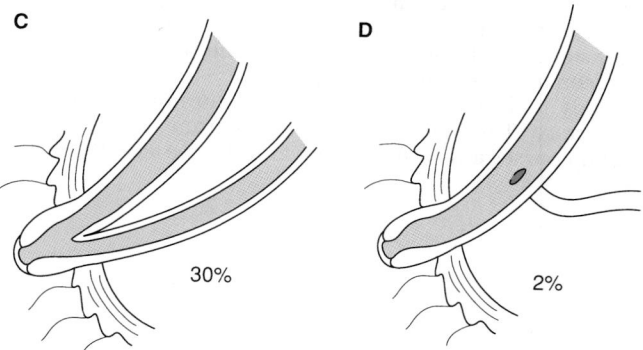

Figure 29.5. Variations in the relation between the intrapancreatic portion of the common bile duct and the main pancreatic duct at the ampulla of Vater. A common channel *(C)* is found in almost one third of subjects. (After Rienhoff WF Jr, Pickrell KL. Pancreatitis: anatomic study of pancreatic and extrahepatic biliary systems. *Arch Surg* 1945;51: 205, with permission.)

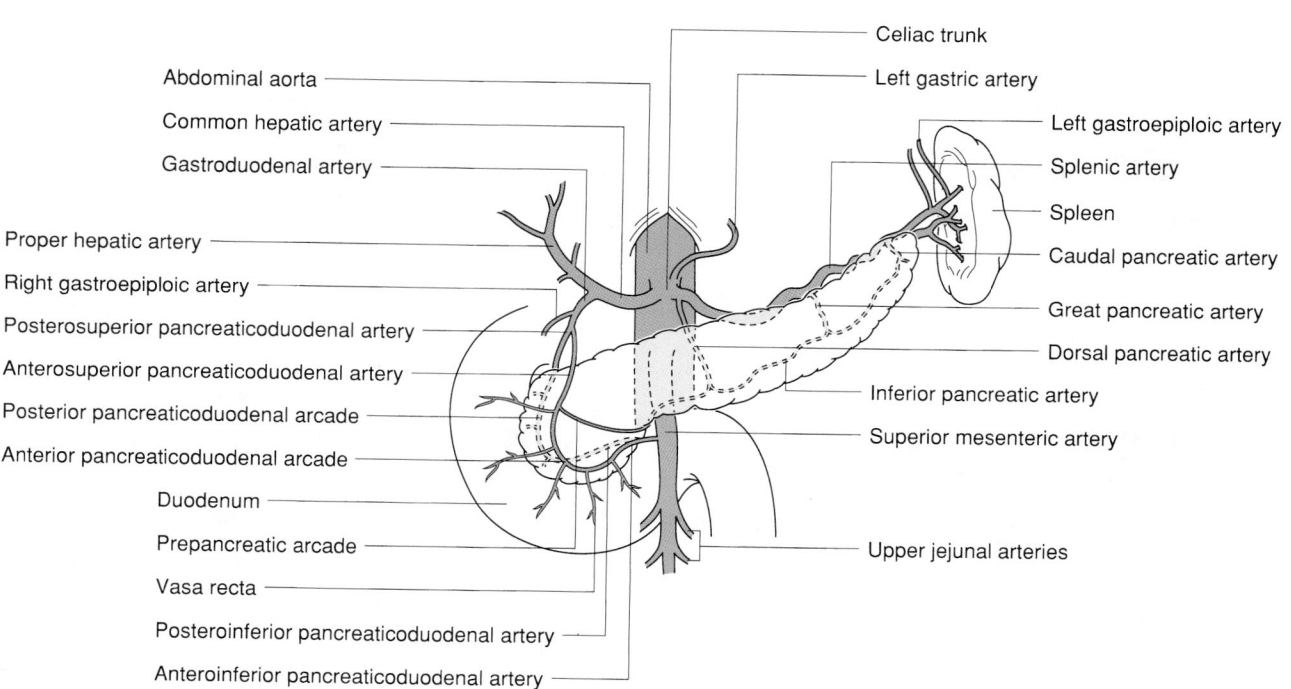

Figure 29.6. Arterial supply to the pancreas. (After Woodburne RT. *Essentials of human anatomy.* New York: Oxford University Press, 1973, with permission.)

branches. The inferior pancreaticoduodenal artery is the first branch of the superior mesenteric artery and divides into anterior and posterior branches. The anterosuperior pancreaticoduodenal artery lies in the anterior head of the pancreas, and collateral vessels usually extend between this artery and the anteroinferior pancreaticoduodenal artery. The posterosuperior pancreaticoduodenal artery crosses the common bile duct and forms the posterior arcade with the posteroinferior pancreaticoduodenal artery. These arcades provide a rich vascular supply to the head and second and third portions of the duodenum. The duodenum and head of the pancreas share a vascular supply; the two structures must be resected together. Anomalies in the vascular supply to the head of the pancreas are found in 20% of patients; the common hepatic, right hepatic, or gastroduodenal artery can arise from the superior mesenteric artery. When the right hepatic artery arises from the superior mesenteric, it usually runs along the portal vein posterior to the neck of the pancreas. Knowledge of these variations and careful attention to detail help the pancreatic surgeon avoid serious mistakes.

The body and tail of the pancreas are supplied by the splenic artery. The splenic artery arises from the celiac trunk and courses along the posterosuperior surface of the pancreas to the spleen. About 10 branches of the splenic artery supply the body and tail of the pancreas. Three of the larger branches are (a) the dorsal pancreatic artery, which lies close to the celiac trunk; (b) the great pancreatic artery, or pancreatica magna, which supplies the midportion of the body; and (c) the caudal pancreatic artery, which supplies the tail. These three arteries course through the length of the pancreas and form collateral vessels with the inferior pancreaticoduodenal artery, which arises from the superior mesenteric artery.

Venous Drainage

The venous drainage of the pancreas and duodenum follows the arterial supply (Fig. 29.7). The veins are usually superficial to the arteries, and the frequency of anomalies is similar. The anterior and posterior venous arcades drain the head, and the body and tail drain into the splenic vein. All venous effluent from the pancreas ultimately drains into the portal vein. The major venous drainage areas are the suprapancreatic portal vein, retropancreatic portal vein, splenic veins, and infrapancreatic superior mesenteric vein. The anterior and posterior venous arcades in the head of the pancreas drain directly into the suprapan-

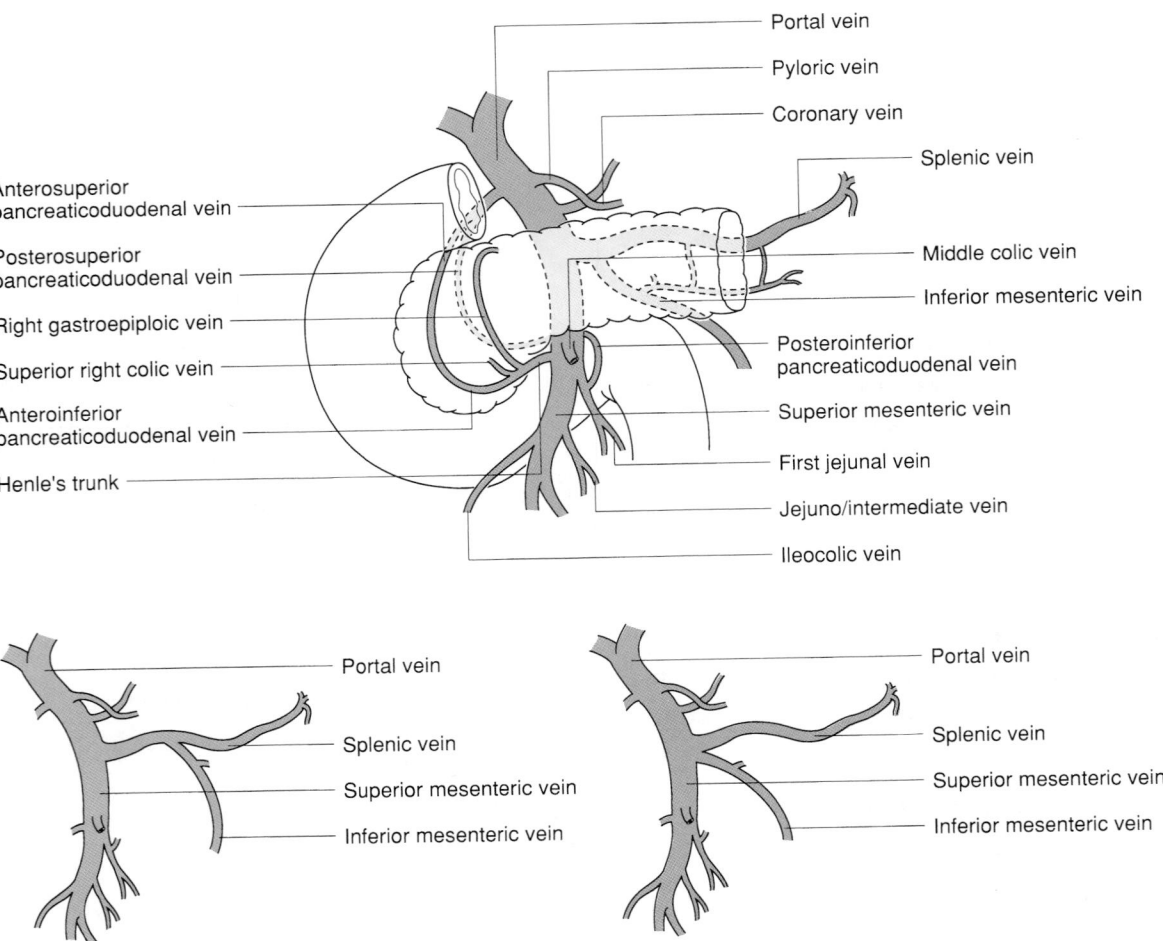

Figure 29.7. Venous drainage of pancreas. Variations in the relation of the portal, splenic, superior mesenteric, and inferior mesenteric veins are shown at the bottom. (After Mackie CR, Moossa AR. Surgical anatomy of the pancreas. In: Moossa AR, ed. *Tumors of the pancreas.* Baltimore: Williams & Wilkins, 1980.)

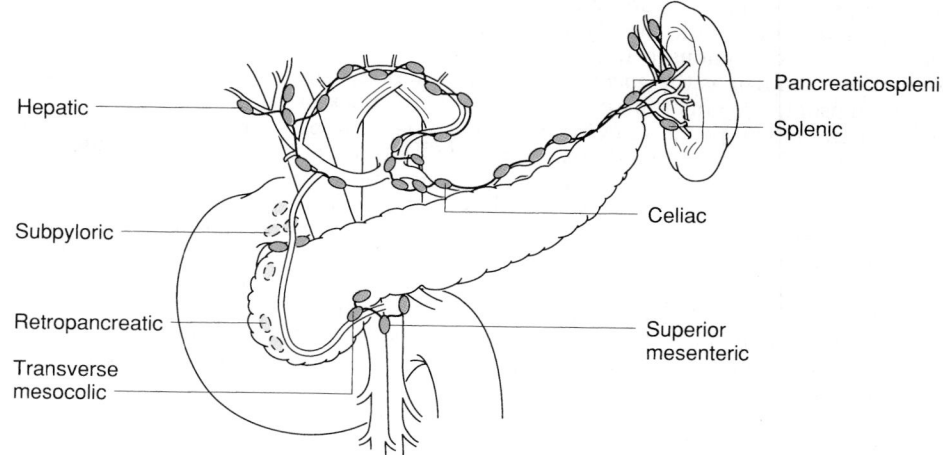

Figure 29.8. Lymph node groups receiving drainage from the pancreas. (After Mackie CR, Moossa AR. Surgical anatomy of the pancreas. In: Moossa AR, ed. *Tumors of the pancreas.* Baltimore: Williams & Wilkins, 1980.)

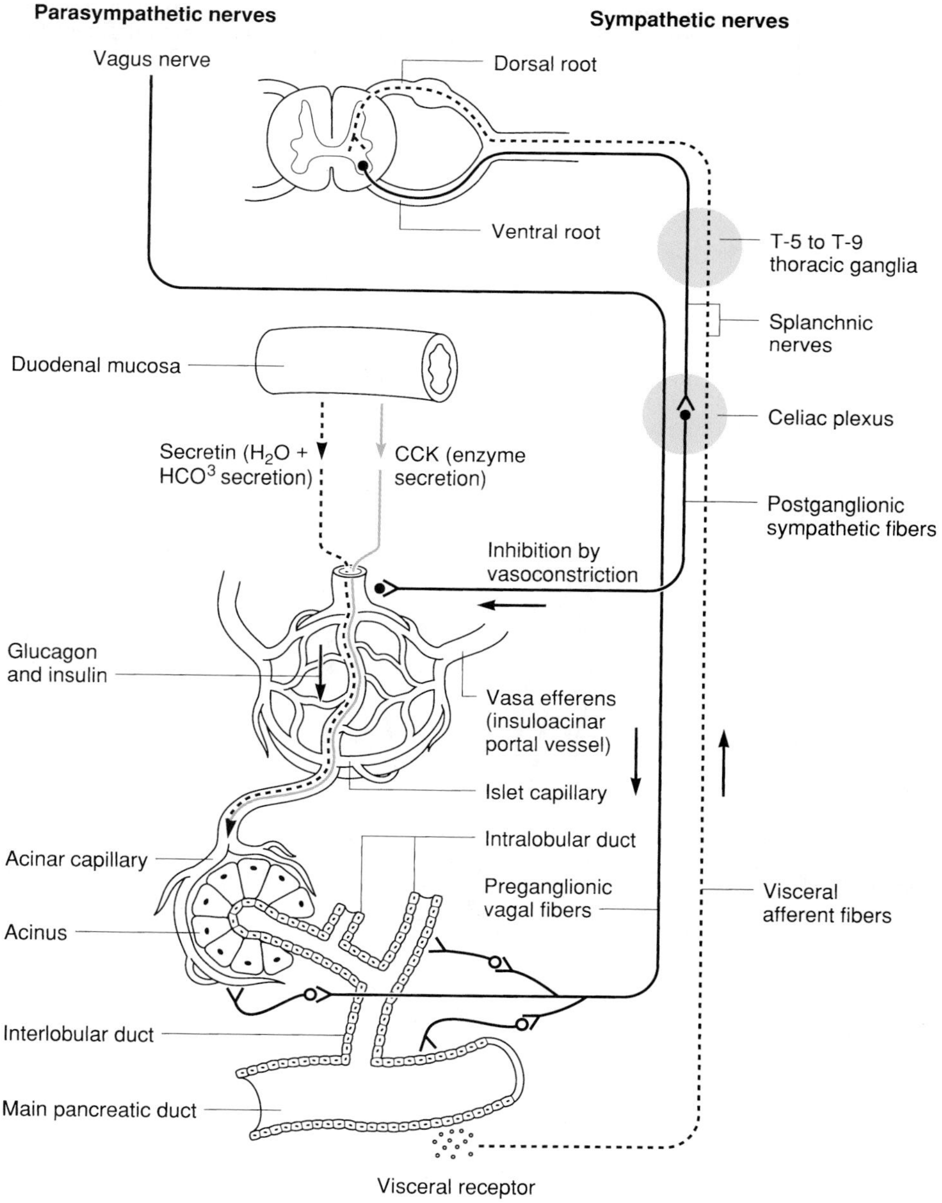

Figure 29.9. Schematic diagram of the neurohormonal control of the exocrine cells. Visceral receptors line the ductule system and carry the sensation of pain to the spinal cord. Sympathetic fibers first synapse in the celiac plexus after traveling through the thoracic ganglia and splanchnic nerves. Postganglionic fibers then synapse on intrapancreatic arterioles. Parasympathetic preganglionic fibers travel through the celiac plexus after leaving the vagus nerves and course with vessels and ducts to synapse on postganglionic fibers near acinar cells, islet cells, and the smooth muscle of major ducts. Stimulation of these parasympathetic fibers results in an immediate release of pancreatic enzymes. Secretin and cholecystokinin *(CCK)* first enter the pancreas through the capillary network of the islet cells, then enter the separate capillary network of the acinar tissue through the insuloacinar portal vessels. Glucagon, somatostatin, pancreatic polypeptide, and insulin from the islet cells reach the acinar tissue immediately after release. In this way, the islet cells can influence the acinar tissue responses to CCK and secretin. (After Tompkins RK, Traverso LW. The exocrine cells. In: Keynes WM, Keith RG, eds. *The pancreas.* New York: Appleton-Century-Crofts, 1981, with permission.)

creatic portal vein. The anteroinferior pancreaticoduodenal arcades drain with the right gastroepiploic vein to form a common venous trunk with the right colic vein. This trunk, known as the *gastrocolic trunk,* enters the superior mesenteric vein at the inferior border of the neck of the pancreas. The posteroinferior venous arcade empties directly into the superior mesenteric vein. The veins of the head drain laterally into the superior mesenteric and portal veins. For this reason, it is safe to dissect the neck of the pancreas directly anterior to the portal vein during a pancreaticoduodenectomy.

Three major venous branches drain the body and tail of the pancreas. These are (a) the inferior pancreatic vein, (b) the caudal pancreatic vein, and (c) the great pancreatic vein. All these branches drain into the splenic vein. The inferior mesenteric vein courses behind the pancreas and joins either with the splenic vein or directly with the superior mesenteric vein.

Lymphatic Drainage

The abundant and diffuse lymphatic drainage of the pancreas is most likely is responsible for the high incidence of metastases associated with pancreatic cancer (Fig. 29.8). The pancreatic head and duodenum drain into the celiac and superior mesenteric lymph nodes, which constitute the predominant drainage. The anterior lymphatics drain to the peripyloric nodes, and the tail and body drain into the pancreaticolienal nodes along the splenic vessels. The other regional lymphatic groups include the splenic, transverse mesocolic, subpyloric, hepatic, lesser gastric omental, jejunal, and colonic mesenteric nodes. When the entire pancreas is resected, usually 70 nodes can be found with the pancreatic specimen. For a Whipple procedure, 35 nodes are usually recovered (1). The absence of a peritoneal barrier on the posterior surface of the pancreas results in a direct communication of the intrapancreatic lymphatics with the retroperitoneal tissues, and this probably contributes to the high incidence of recurrence after presumably curative resections of pancreatic cancer.

Innervation

The exocrine and endocrine secretion of the pancreas is regulated by a rich neural supply that includes sympathetic fibers from the splanchnic nerves, parasympathetic fibers from the vagus, and peptidergic neurons that secrete amines and peptides (2). The sympathetic and parasympathetic fibers give rise to intrapancreatic periacinar plexuses, which send neural fibers to the bases of acinar cell groups (Fig. 29.9). The pancreatic islets are innervated by similar

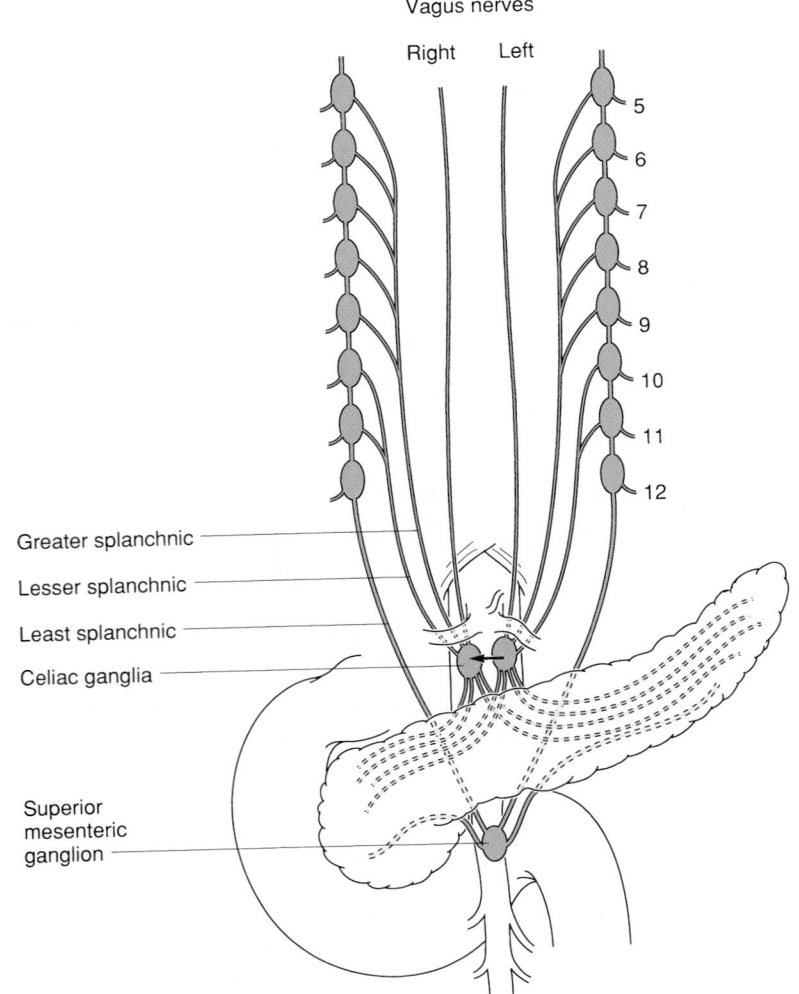

Vagus nerves

Right   Left

Greater splanchnic
Lesser splanchnic
Least splanchnic
Celiac ganglia
Superior
mesenteric
ganglion

Figure 29.10. Diagram of the automomic nerve supply to the pancreas. (After Skandalakis JE, Gray SW, Rowe JS Jr, et al. Anatomical complications of pancreatic surgery. *Contemp Surg* 1979;15:17, with permission.)

plexuses that communicate with both the islet vasculature and the islet cells. In general, parasympathetic fibers stimulate both exocrine and endocrine secretion, whereas sympathetic fibers have a predominantly inhibitory effect (3). The peptidergic neurons that innervate the pancreas secrete hormones such as somatostatin, vasoactive intestinal peptide (VIP), calcitonin gene-related peptide (CGRP), and galanin. Although the peptidergic neurons influence exocrine and endocrine function, their precise physiologic role is unknown. The pancreas also has a rich afferent sensory fiber network, which probably contributes to the intrinsic pancreatic pain associated with pancreatic cancer and chronic pancreatitis (Fig. 29.10). Although results have been equivocal, ganglionectomy or celiac ganglion blockade can be performed in an effort to interrupt these somatic fibers. The best results have been reported after combined bilateral thoracic sympathectomy and celiac ganglionectomy (4).

STRUCTURE AND HISTOLOGY

Exocrine Structure

The two major components of the exocrine pancreas are the acinar cells and the ductular network. Together, they constitute 80% to 90% of the pancreatic mass. The acinar cells secrete the enzymes responsible for digestion. The cells are pyramidal and have an apex that faces the lumen of the duct. Within the apex of the cell are numerous zymogen granules, which contain the digestive enzymes. Twenty to 40 acinar cells coalesce into a unit called the acinus (Fig. 29.11). A second cell type in the acinus is the centroacinar cell, which is responsible for fluid and electrolyte secretion by the pancreas. These cells contain carbonic anhydrase and other enzymes necessary for bicarbonate and electrolyte transport (5).

The ductular system is composed of a network of conduits that carry the exocrine secretions into the duodenum. The acinus drains into small, intercollated ducts. Several small, intercollated ducts join to form an interlobular duct. The interlobular ducts contribute to fluid and electrolyte secretion along with the centroacinar cells. The interlobular ducts form secondary ducts that empty into the main duct. Progressive destruction of the ductular network during recurrent episodes of pancreatitis contributes in part to exocrine insufficiency and pain. Research is under way to identify the precursor cell that gives rise to pancreatic ductal adenocarcinoma. Many assume that this cancer arises from ductal cells simply be-

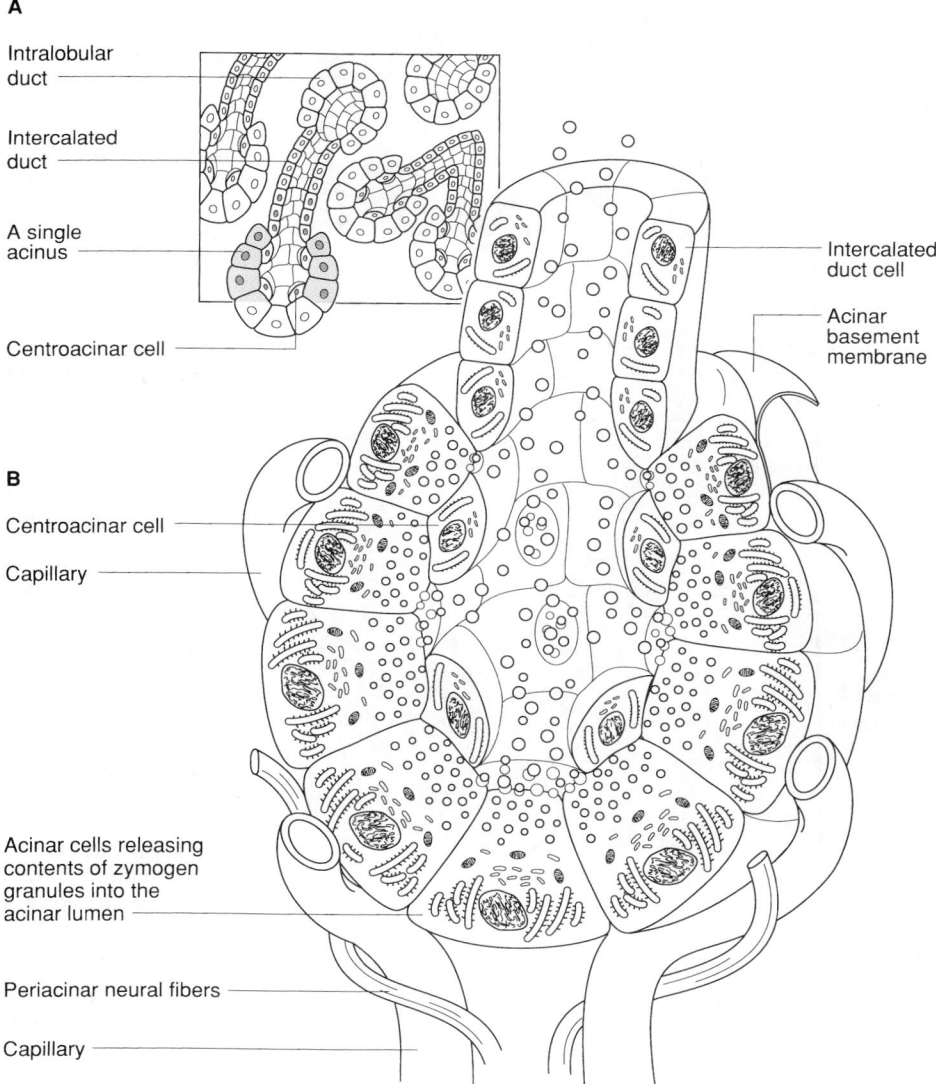

Figure 29.11. Histologic anatomy of the acinus. *(A)* Low-magnification view of a portion of the pancreas. *(B)* High-magnification view of a single acinus. (After Krstic RV. *Die Gewebes des Menschen und der Saugetiere.* Berlin: Springer-Verlag, 1978, with permission.)

Intralobular duct
Intercalated duct
A single acinus
Centroacinar cell
Intercalated duct cell
Acinar basement membrane
Centroacinar cell
Capillary
Acinar cells releasing contents of zymogen granules into the acinar lumen
Periacinar neural fibers
Capillary

cause the tumors exhibit a ductal structure. Some investigators believe pancreatic cancer arises from transdifferentiated acinar cells (6). Others are convinced that pancreatic cancer arises more frequently from islets, most probably from reserve stem cells (7). These cells are thought to be progenitor cells that can differentiate into endocrine or exocrine cells. The genetic mechanisms involved in this normal differentiation process and abnormal transformation into pancreatic cancer cells is under investigation.

Endocrine Structure

Within the pancreas are small nests of cells responsible for the secretion of hormones that control glucose homeostasis. These nests are called islets of Langerhans. In contrast to the exocrine cells, the endocrine pancreas ac-

counts for only 2% of the pancreatic mass; the remaining portion of the gland consists of extracellular matrix, blood vessels, and major ducts. The islets contain an average of 3,000 cells and range in diameter from 40 to 900 μm. The islets are composed of four major cell types—alpha (A), beta (B), delta (D), and pancreatic polypeptide (PP) or F cells, which secrete glucagon, insulin, somatostatin, and PP, respectively. The B cells are centrally located within the islet and constitute 70% of the islet mass, whereas the PP, A, and D cells are located at the periphery of the islet (Fig. 29.12). D cells have also been shown to be located within the core of human islets (8). The PP, A, and D cells constitute roughly 15%, 10%, and 5% of the islet cell mass, respectively. Islet cells can secrete more than one hormone. For example, in addition to insulin, the B cells secrete amylin, which can also regulate glucose metabolism (9). The cellular composition of the islets varies throughout the pancreas. Islets in the uncinate process are rich in PP cells and poor in A cells, whereas the islets in the body and tail are rich in A cells and poor in PP cells (Fig. 29.12). The B cells and D cells are evenly distributed throughout the pancreas (10). The physiologic significance of this distribution remains largely unknown. As a consequence, certain operations can remove a specific islet population. For example, removal of 95% of the functioning PP cell mass during pancreaticoduodenectomy can contribute to subsequent glucose intolerance (11).

Islets contain small numbers of additional cells that secrete hormones such as VIP, serotonin, and pancreastatin. The islets also secrete numerous neuropeptides, such as CGRP, neuropeptide Y, gastrin-releasing peptide, and somatostatin, which probably exert local regulatory effects on endocrine and exocrine secretion. Islet cells are physiologically and chemically distinct and are related to other neuroendocrine cells derived from the neural crest of the embryo. These groups of cells share the capacity of amine precursor uptake and decarboxylation and can give rise to tumors called APUDomas.

Intravascular Pattern

The blood flow to the pancreas has a distinctive pattern. The islets represent 2% of the pancreatic tissue but receive 20% to 30% of the pancreatic arteriolar flow. The distribution of blood flow can change after a meal, when blood flow to different parts of the pancreas is redirected (12).

Research is under way to determine the possible existence of different microvascular patterns within the islets depending on location (periductular or intralobular). In one pattern, the arteriole of the islet penetrates the islet and first perfuses the center, where the B cells are located (13). The blood then flows toward the periphery, or mantle, of the islet, where the non-B cells are located, so that high concentrations of insulin modulate secretion of the non-B cells through a paracrine action (Fig. 29.13). In another pattern, the arteriole perfuses the mantle, then the core (14,15). The collecting vessels drain the islets and then perfuse the acinar tissue. Perfusion of the acinar tissue with venous blood from the islet, known as the *insuloacinar portal system*, permits endocrine regulation of the exocrine pancreas. This regulation is principally effected by insulin, but the other islet hormones, such as PP and somatostatin, are also known to influence exocrine secretion (16). Much of the acinar tissue is perfused directly by pancreatic arterial blood that bypasses the endocrine tissue.

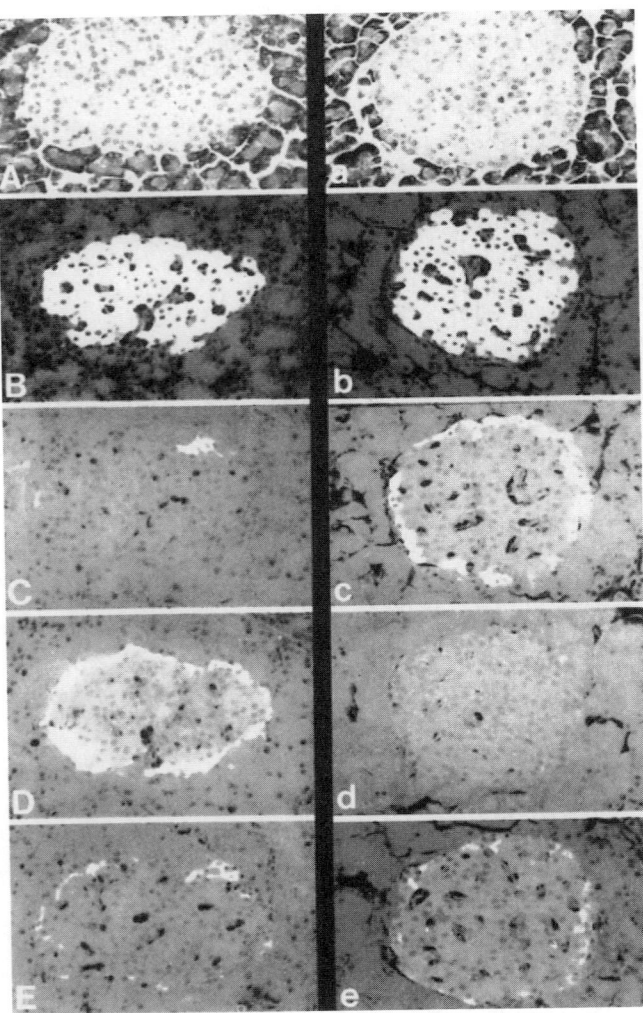

Figure 29.12. Histologic anatomy of the islet. Serial sections of a representative islet found in the ventral *(A–E)* and dorsal *(A–E)* portions of the pancreas. *(A,a)* Cells stained with hematoxylin and eosin. *(B,b)* B cells immunohistochemically stained with antiinsulin antisera. *(C,c)* A cells stained with antiglucagon antisera. *(D,d)* Pancreatic polypeptide cells stained with antipancreatic polypeptide antisera. *(E,e)* D cells stained with antisomatostatin antisera. (From Orci L. Macro- and micro-domains in the endocrine pancreas. *Diabetes* 1982;31:538, with permission.)

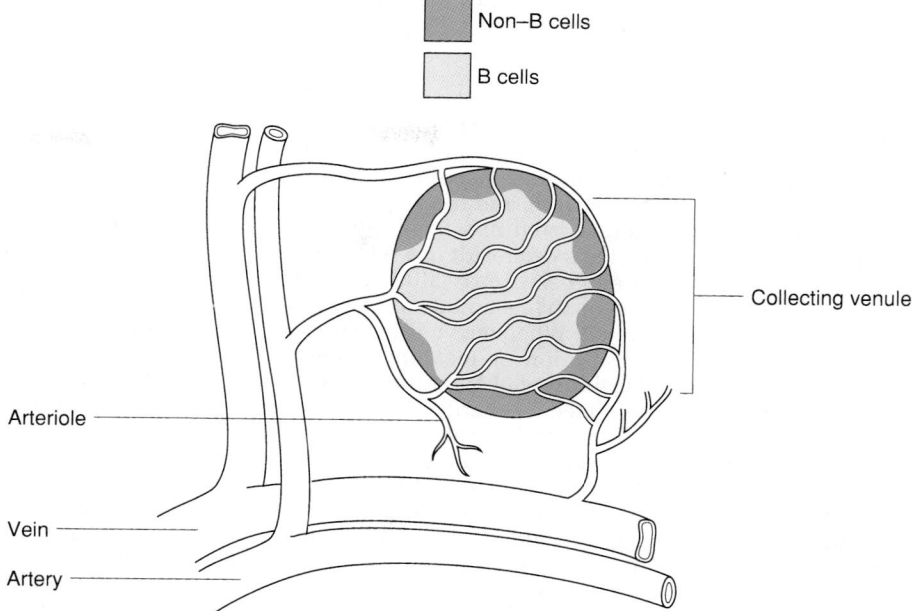

Figure 29.13. Diagram of a typical islet. Afferent arterioles enter the islet through discontinuities of the mantle of non-B cells and break into capillaries, most of which traverse the B-cell mass and pass through the mantle as efferent vessels. Occasionally, a capillary passes at the interface of the B cells and non-B cells and never enters the B-cell core. In the larger islets, the efferent capillaries coalesce at the edge of the islet and pass along the mantle as collecting venules before draining into a vein. (After Bonner-Weir S, Orci L. New perspectives on the microvasculature of the islets of Langerhans in the rat. *Diabetes* 1982;31:883, with permission.)

PHYSIOLOGY

Exocrine Function

Early discoveries related to the exocrine pancreas were entirely separate from those involving the endocrine pancreas, as if the exocrine and endocrine pancreas were two separate organs (17). Only recently has the intimate relation between exocrine and endocrine function been recognized. Islet peptide products are now known to influence the function of the exocrine pancreas. The final secretory product of the exocrine pancreas derives from the combination of ductal and acinar cell functions. The secretion of water and electrolytes originates in the centroacinar and intercalated duct cells. Pancreatic enzymes originate in the acinar cells. The final product is an alkaline fluid (or juice) that contains digestive enzymes; 500 to 800 mL of the fluid is secreted daily. The alkaline pH results from secreted bicarbonate, which serves to neutralize gastric acid and regulate the pH of the intestine, where the enzymes digest carbohydrates, proteins, and fats. Pancreatic fluid is colorless, odorless, and isosmotic. It contains 0.2% protein, mostly enzymes such as amylase, lipase, and trypsinogen.

Bicarbonate Secretion

The centroacinar cells and ductular epithelium secrete fluid containing 20 mmol of bicarbonate per liter in the basal state and up to 150 mmol of bicarbonate per liter under maximal stimulation. The fluid, with a pH that varies from 7.6 to 9.0, acts as a vehicle to carry inactive proteolytic enzymes to the duodenal lumen. Sodium and potassium concentrations are constant and equal those of plasma. Chloride secretion varies inversely with bicarbonate secretion, and the sum of these two cations remains constant and equal to that of plasma (18) (Fig. 29.14).

Bicarbonate is formed from carbonic acid by the enzyme carbonic anhydrase. Secretin, the major stimulant for bicarbonate secretion, is released from the duodenal mucosa in response to a duodenal luminal pH of less than 3.0. Cholecystokinin (CCK) only weakly stimulates bicarbonate secretion but potentiates secretin-stimulated bicarbonate secretion. Gastrin and acetylcholine are also weak stimulants of bicarbonate secretion (19). Although cholinergic innervation appears to play a permissive role, bicarbonate secretion is inhibited by atropine and can be reduced 50% by a truncal vagotomy (20). Islet peptide

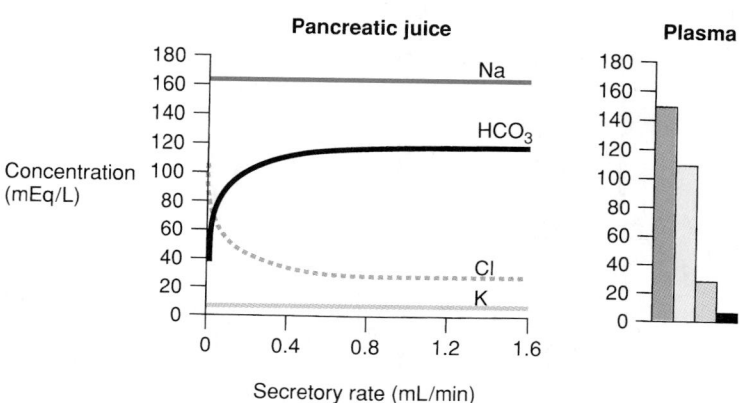

Figure 29.14. Relation of pancreatic secretion and concentration of electrolytes. (From Bro-Rasmussen F, Kilman SA, Thaysen JH. The composition of pancreatic juice as compared to sweat, parotid saliva, and tears. *Acta Physiol Scand* 1956;37:97, with permission.)

products such as somatostatin, PP, and glucagon are all thought to inhibit exocrine secretion.

Enzyme Secretion

The acinar cells secrete isozymes that fall into three major enzyme groups—amylases, lipases, and proteases. These enzymes include amylase, lipase, trypsinogen, chymotrypsinogen, procarboxypeptidases A and B, ribonuclease, deoxyribonuclease, proelastase, and trypsin inhibitor. The enzyme groups are not secreted in a fixed ratio, and stimulation by specific nutrients can result in a relative increase of one enzyme over another. Dietary alterations can also result in changes in the relative amounts of amylases, lipases, and proteases secreted. When enzyme secretion is absent or impaired, malabsorption or incomplete digestion occurs, resulting in fecal losses of fat and protein.

Enzyme secretion is regulated primarily through hormonal and neural factors. The enteric hormone CCK is the predominant regulator and stimulates acinar cells through specific membrane-bound receptors. The intracellular effectors or second messengers are calcium and diacylglycerol. Acetylcholine strongly stimulates acinar cells when released from postganglionic fibers of the pancreatic plexus and acts in synergy with CCK to potentiate enzyme secretion (Fig. 29.15). Secretin and VIP weakly stimulate acinar cell secretion, but they potentiate the effect of CCK on the acinar cells. Acinar cell secretion also is influenced by islet hormones in the insuloacinar portal system. The enzymes are synthesized in the endoplasmic reticulum of the acinar cells and are packaged in the zymogen granules. These are released from the apical portion of the acinar cells into the lumen of the acinus and are then transported into the duodenal lumen, where the enzymes are activated.

Enzyme Groups

Amylase is secreted within the human body from both pancreatic and salivary tissue. Pancreatic amylase represents isoamylase type P. A pancreatic source of excess levels of amylase, as in pancreatitis, can be determined by the results of isoamylase studies. Amylase hydrolyzes starch and glycogen to glucose, maltose, maltotriose, and dextrins. Amylase is the only digestive enzyme secreted by the pancreas in an active form, although it functions optimally at a pH of 7.0.

Lipases emulsify and hydrolyze fat in the presence of bile salts. They hydrolyze insoluble esters of glycerol, alcohol esters, and water-soluble esters. Lipases function optimally at a pH of 7.0 to 9.0, and steatorrhea can result from excessive acidification of the duodenum and jejunum, as in gastric hypersecretory states. There are two phospholipases, A and B. Phospholipase A cleaves the fatty acid off lecithin or cephalin to form lysolecithin or lysocephalin. Phospholipase B cleaves the fatty acid off lysolecithin to form glycerol phosphatidylcholine.

The proteolytic enzymes are essential for protein digestion. These enzymes are secreted as proenzymes and require activation for proteolytic activity. The proenzymes

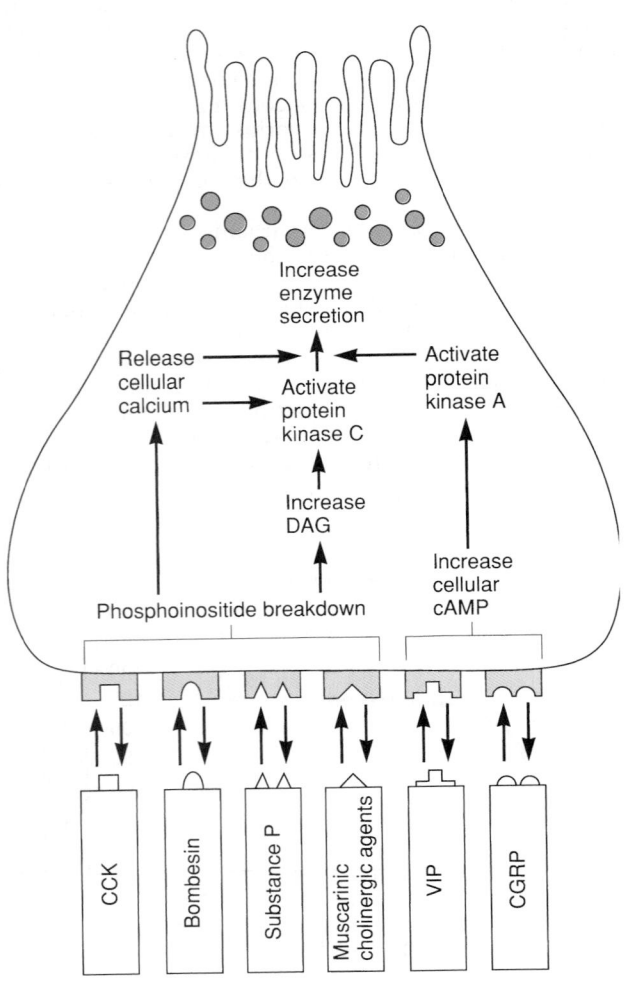

Figure 29.15. Schematic diagram of an acinar cell, demonstrating receptors for exocrine secretagogues and their intracellular bases of action. Six distinct classes of receptors are known, with principal ligands shown. *CCK*, cholecystokinin; *VIP*, vasoactive intestinal polypeptide; *CRGP*, calcitonin gene-related peptide; *DAG*, diacylglycerol.

of trypsin and chymotrypsin are trypsinogen and chymotrypsinogen. They are activated primarily by a duodenal enzyme, enterokinase, which converts trypsinogen to trypsin. Trypsin, in turn, activates chymotrypsin, elastase, carboxypeptidase, and phospholipase. Trypsinogen can also be activated by a fall in pH below 7.0. Within the pancreas, enzyme activation is prevented by an antiproteolytic enzyme secreted by the acinar cells. This enzyme inactivates trypsin by direct binding and thereby protects the pancreatic tissue from autodigestion.

Trypsinogen is a 229-amino acid polypeptide that hydrolyzes proteins and also acts as a thrombokinase, accelerating coagulation of the blood. Trypsinogen can convert spontaneously to trypsin, but the change is accelerated by enterokinase, by acid, or by active trypsin itself. Chymotrypsinogen is a 246-amino acid polypeptide. Chymotrypsinogen is converted to the active form, chymotrypsin, by trypsin or, indirectly, by enterokinase. The enzyme hydrolyzes proteins by a mechanism similar to that of trypsin but cleaves the proteins at a different site. The optimal activity of chymotrypsin and trypsin occurs at a pH of 8.0 to 9.0. Other proteolytic enzymes, such as carboxypeptidases A and B, further digest proteins that have been digested by trypsin and chymotrypsin. The nucleolytic enzymes, ribonuclease and deoxyribonuclease, hydrolyze nucleic acids into mononucleotides. Thus, through the secretion of the three classes of enzymes, the pancreas regulates the complete digestion of fats, carbohydrates, and proteins.

Endocrine Function

Insulin Synthesis, Secretion, and Action

Insulin is a 56-amino acid polypeptide with a molecular weight of 6 kd. It consists of two polypeptide chains, an A and a B chain, joined by two disulfide bridges. Although species variation occurs in the amino acid sequence, the positions of the disulfide bridges are constant and important for biologic activity. Insulin is synthesized in the B cells of the islets of Langerhans. Destruction of the B cells in type I, or insulin-dependent, diabetes results in an absolute insulin deficiency. A considerable capacity exists for secretory reserves of insulin; 80% of the islet cell mass must be surgically removed before diabetes becomes clinically apparent (21).

When the B cell is stimulated, a newly synthesized single-chain peptide, proinsulin, is transported from the endoplasmic reticulum to the Golgi complex. At this site, proinsulin is packaged into granules and cleaved into insulin and a residual connecting peptide, or C peptide (Fig.

29.16). The granules then move toward the outer membrane by way of microtubules and are released into the intervascular space through emiocytosis. Defects in the synthesis and cleavage of insulin can lead to rare forms of diabetes mellitus, such as Wakayama syndrome and the proinsulin syndromes (22).

Insulin is secreted in two phases. The first phase consists of a burst of stored insulin that lasts 4 to 6 minutes. This is followed by a second phase of sustained secretion, attributed to an ongoing synthesis of insulin. The secretion of insulin is regulated by nutrient, neural, and hormonal factors. Glucose is the predominant nutrient regulator. The B cell is exquisitely sensitive to small changes in glucose concentration, with the maximal stimulation of insulin secretion occurring at a glucose concentration of 400 to 500 mg/dL.

Glucose is transported actively across cell membranes throughout the body by 55-kd membrane-bound facilitator peptides called *glucose transporters* (Fig. 29.17). Several classes of glucose transporters have been identified. The type of glucose transporter located on the B cell (GLUT-2) has a low affinity (or high K_m) for glucose, which results in a modest rate of glucose transport at lower physiologic concentrations but an increased rate of transport and therefore an increase in subsequent insulin secretion at higher concentrations of glucose (23). Studies suggest that a loss of B-cell GLUT-2 glucose transporters can precede, and therefore contribute to, the development of diabetes (24).

Orally administered glucose stimulates a greater insulin response than an equivalent amount of glucose administered intravenously because of the release of enteric hormones that potentiate insulin secretion. This effect is known as the *enteroinsular axis*. Gastric inhibitory polypeptide (GIP) appears to be an important regulator of this incretion effect (25), although other gut peptides, such as glucagon-like peptide-1, also contribute. Additional nutrients that regulate insulin secretion are amino acids, such as arginine, lysine, and leucine, and free fatty acids. Hormones that stimulate insulin secretion include glucagon, GIP, and CCK, whereas somatostatin, amylin, and pancreastatin are inhibitory. Insulin secretion is also stimulated by sulfonylurea compounds, which act independently of the glucose concentration and form the basis of treatment of type II, or non–insulin-dependent, diabetes.

The B cell is neurally regulated by cholinergic fibers that stimulate insulin secretion. β-Sympathetic fibers are also stimulatory, whereas α-sympathetic fibers strongly inhibit insulin secretion. A loss of pancreatic innervation, as after pancreatic transplantation, results in changes in the

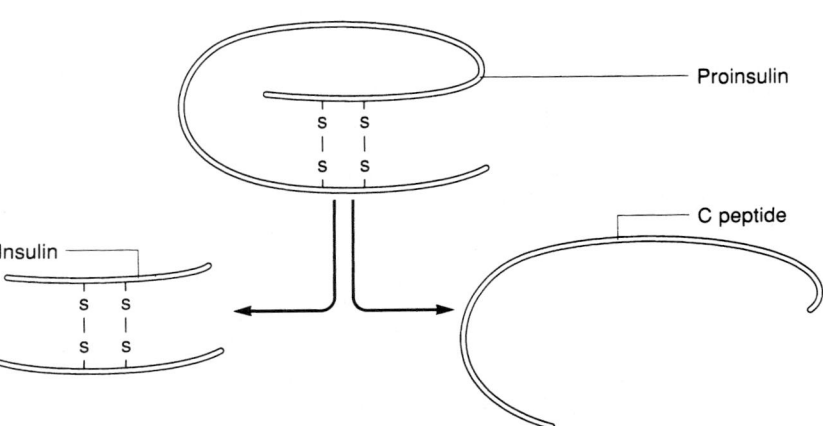

Figure 29.16. Synthesis of insulin. Proinsulin is synthesized by the endoplasmic reticulum and packaged within secretory granules of the B cell, where it is cleaved into insulin and C peptide. Equimolar amounts of insulin and C peptide are secreted into the bloodstream.

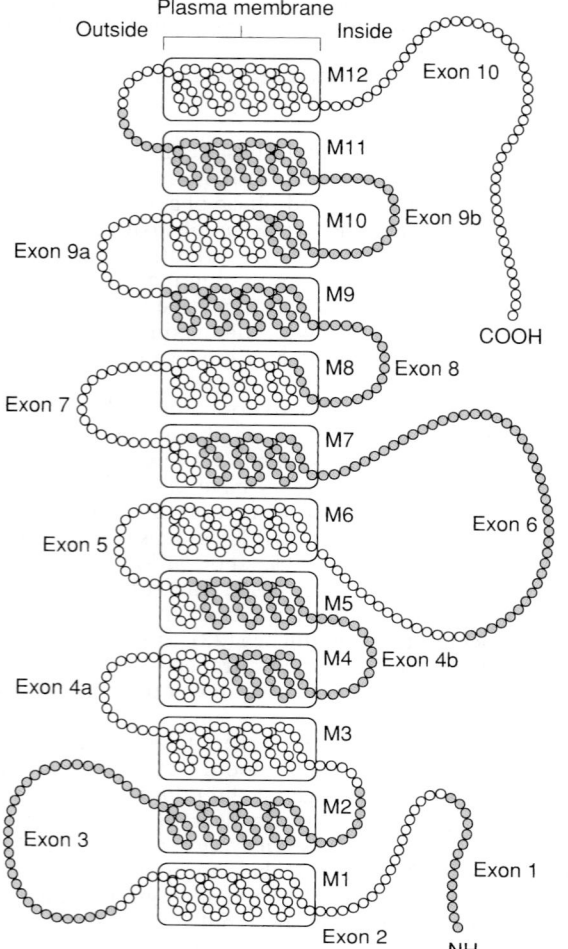

Figure 29.17. Model of the basic structure of a membrane-bound glucose transporter peptide, encoded by a gene divided into 10 exon regions. Membrane-spanning β-helical peptide chains are numbered M1 through M12. Mutations of the promoter region of the gene or the synthesis of an abnormal form of the protein could result in altered transport of glucose. For the B-cell GLUT-2 transporter, this could cause reduced sensitivity to glucose. For the muscle and fat cell GLUT-4 transporter, this could result in decreased peripheral uptake of glucose. (After Bell GI, Kayano T, Buse JB, et al. Molecular biology of mammalian glucose transporters. *Diabetes Care* 1990;86:1615, with permission.)

pattern or quantity of insulin secretion. Research is under way to define the role of neuropeptides such as CGRP and galanin in the regulation of insulin secretion.

Insulin is released in an oscillatory or pulsatile pattern, and release is controlled by an internal pacemaker, present even in isolated islets (26). Once secreted, insulin has a half-life of 7 to 10 minutes and is metabolized primarily by the liver. Of the insulin secreted into the portal vein, 40% to 70% is cleared by the hepatocytes during the first pass. The brain and red blood cells take up no insulin. The liver, kidneys, and skeletal muscles slowly metabolize insulin and remove it from the circulation. Little insulin is excreted in the urine.

Insulin promotes glucose transport in all cells, except B cells, hepatocytes, and cells of the central nervous system. Insulin-stimulated glucose transport in muscle and adipose tissue can also result from insulin regulation of membrane-bound glucose transporters. Insulin inhibits glycogenolysis but stimulates protein synthesis. Insulin also inhibits fatty acid breakdown and therefore inhibits ketone formation.

Like all endocrine hormones, insulin binds to specific receptors. These receptors have been isolated and characterized. The insulin receptor is a glycoprotein with a molecular weight of 300 kd. Stimulation of the receptor depends on the insulin concentration. Insulin resistance can be the result of either a decreased number of receptors or a decreased affinity for insulin, whereas excessive receptors can result in hypoglycemia. Defects in insulin receptors can lead to the insulin resistance seen in type II diabetes mellitus and in rare forms of diabetes, such as the type A syndrome, leprechaunism, and lipotrophic diabetes (27).

Glucagon Synthesis, Secretion, and Action

Glucagon is a single-chain, 29-amino acid polypeptide with a molecular weight of 3.5 kd. Glucagon is secreted by the A cells of the islet and promotes hepatic glycogenolysis. Other forms of glucagon are released from the gut, including gastric glucagon, enteroglucagon, and glucagon-like peptides. Their physiologic role remains unclear.

Pancreatic glucagon secretion is controlled by neural, hormonal, and nutrient factors. Glucose is the primary regulator and has a potent suppressive effect on glucagon secretion. Glucagon and insulin respond in reciprocal fashion to changes in glucose concentrations; therefore, glucagon is considered a counterregulatory hormone to insulin. In a balance of actions, the two hormones work together to maintain basal glucose levels. Exaggerated or excess glucagon secretion can contribute to hyperglycemia, whereas a failure of glucagon secretion or an absence of glucagon-rich portions of the pancreas can contribute to profound hypoglycemia. Glucagon is stimulated by the amino acids arginine and alanine. Hormones such as GIP have been shown to have a stimulatory effect on glucagon secretion in vitro but not in vivo. Insulin and somatostatin have a potent suppressive effect on glucagon secretion and can regulate glucagon secretion through paracrine effects within the islet.

The neural regulation of glucagon is similar to that of insulin (28). Cholinergic fibers have a strong stimulatory effect. α-Sympathetic fibers inhibit glucagon secretion, and β-sympathetic fibers are weakly stimulatory. The role of neuropeptides in glucagon secretion is unknown. Glucagon elevates blood glucose levels through the stimulation of glycogenolysis and gluconeogenesis. Along with epinephrine, cortisol, and growth hormone, glucagon is considered a stress hormone because it provides metabolic fuel during stress. The peptide is metabolized by the kidney and, to a lesser extent, by the liver.

Some authors consider dysfunctional A-cell secretion to play a major role in the elevation of blood sugar in diabetes. In the bidysfunctional theory of diabetes, absent or impaired insulin secretion and deranged glucagon secretion result in hyperglycemia, ketoacidosis, and accelerated lipolysis (29). Suppression of glucagon secretion with somatostatin has resulted in improved glucose homeostasis in insulin-dependent, type I diabetes (30).

Somatostatin Synthesis, Secretion, and Action

In 1973, Brazeau et al. (31) reported the isolation of a hypothalamic peptide that inhibits the release of growth hormone (somatotropin) and named it *somatostatin*. Somatostatin is a 14-amino acid polypeptide that inhibits the release of almost all peptide hormones; it also inhibits gastric, pancreatic, and biliary secretion. Found in the D cell of the islet, the role of the hormone within the pancreas remains unclear. Although exogenous infusion of somatostatin has been shown to inhibit the release of insulin, glucagon, and PP, endogenous somatostatin has not been proved to influence the secretion of the adjacent islet cells directly. Therefore, the D cell is probably responsible for the paracrine regulation of islet cell hormone secretion (32). Some researchers have suggested that the D cells regulate exocrine secretion as part of the insuloacinar portal system. Somatostatin has also been found in the neurons of the islet and can act as an inhibitory neuropeptide. The potent inhibitory effect of the peptide has been used to treat both endocrine and exocrine disorders (33).

Pancreatic Polypeptide Synthesis, Secretion, and Action

Pancreatic polypeptide is a 36-amino acid peptide that is secreted by the F cells of the islet. The F cells are located predominantly in the uncinate process of the pancreas and represent 5% to 15% of the islet cell mass. The physiologic role of PP remains unclear. The peptide has been shown to inhibit exocrine secretion in addition to choleresis and gallbladder emptying. The release of PP is regulated predominantly by cholinergic innervation. The rise in PP levels after a meal is ablated by vagotomy, and the ablation of this rise can be used as a marker of completion of vagotomy. Circulating PP levels are increased in diabetes and in normal aging because of increased secretion. Other studies suggest that PP is involved in glucose homeostasis and that a deficiency of PP in chronic pancreatitis or after pancreaticoduodenectomy contributes to glucose intolerance, so that PP deficiency has been linked to pancreatogenic diabetes (34).

Many of the pathophysiologic responses observed in chronic pancreatitis are thought to be partly a consequence of either a disruption of the insuloacinar axis, destruction of islet cell mass, or both. Each of the four types of hormone-secreting islet cells is affected by the destructive process of chronic pancreatitis. The insulin-secreting B cells appear to be affected both qualitatively and quantitatively. Directly related to the changes in the B cells are the physiologic responses of the glucagon-secreting A cells. Their physiologic response in chronic pancreatitis appears to be related to the residual B-cell function. Recently, PP has been implicated as a contributor to abnormal glucose metabolism in pancreatogenic diabetes. The deficiency of this peptide appears to influence the expression of hepatocyte insulin receptors in chronic pancreatitis. Also, PP deficiency and pancreatic exocrine insufficiency appear to be closely correlated. Although somatostatin appears to have a significant role within the insuloacinar axis, the effects of chronic pancreatitis on the role of somatostatin in the insuloacinar axis are still poorly understood. Further exploration of the relationship between the endocrine and exocrine pancreas is needed so that better methods can be developed to manage the alterations in glucose metabolism related to chronic pancreatitis (35).

Other Peptide Products

Other peptides have been found to be secreted within the islet. These include neuropeptides, such as VIP, galanin, and serotonin, which are believed to play a role in the regulation of islet cell secretion. Amylin is a 36-amino acid polypeptide that was discovered in 1988. It is secreted by the B cell, but not in equimolar amounts to C peptide and insulin. Amylin inhibits insulin secretion and insulin uptake peripherally. It has been found in amyloid deposits within the pancreas of patients with type II diabetes and has been implicated in the development of type II diabetes mellitus. Furthermore, the peptide is absent in type I diabetes mellitus because the B cells are ablated in this disease. The significance of amylin deficiency is unknown.

Pancreastatin is another peptide found in large amounts in the pancreas. It is a derivative of a larger, ubiquitous endocrine tissue-related peptide, chromogranin A, and has been shown to inhibit insulin secretion. Its physiologic role is unknown.

Regulation of Hormone Secretion within the Islet

Because exogenous infusions of insulin, glucagon, and somatostatin have profound effects on islet hormone secretion, the paracrine regulation of islet hormone secretion has been an area of intense investigation. In 1982, it was demonstrated that the blood flow of the islet is centripetal—that is, a central artery penetrates into the islet and perfuses the centrally located B-cell mass first. The blood then flows outward toward the peripherally located A, D, and F cells, allowing a paracrine cascade. By using antibodies specific for each hormone, it has been possible to demonstrate that insulin secretion within the islet regulates the secretion of glucagon and somatostatin. This observation suggests that the suppression of glucagon during hyperglycemia is not regulated by glucose, but rather by an increase in insulin secretion (Fig. 29.18). Intra-islet somatostatin is known to regulate insulin secretion (32). The overall physiologic significance of the paracrine cascade is unknown, but it can result in the hyperglucagonemia and hypersomatostatinemia seen in insulin-dependent, type I diabetes.

Recent observations made during in vivo microscopic studies of the isolated perfused human pancreas have contributed to our understanding of the physiology of the endocrine pancreas (36). The human endocrine pancreas is composed of approximately 1 million islets that act as end-neurons of the central nervous system to secrete the appropriate hormonal milieu for glucose homeokinesis. To accomplish this, the endocrine pancreas secretes a hormonal milieu regulated by the microcirculation, nitric oxide, and neural and hormonal mechanisms. Changes in the arterial concentrations of nutrients and hormones are recognized simultaneously by all islets of the endocrine pancreas and by the central nervous system. Responses occur at two levels. At one level, the central nervous system sends neural signals to the endocrine pancreas to alter the microcirculation, which is regulated by internal and external gates. One of the final regulators of the gates is nitric oxide. Blood flow to the endocrine pancreas and within the islets is optimized to expose the appropriate cell type required to respond to the changes in the arterial milieu. The other level of response is within the islet. The islet cells respond directly to changes in the arterial concentrations of nutrients and hormones. Considerable communication between the cells within the islet is regulated by hormonal feedback loops and nitric oxide. These two levels of response result in secretion of the hormonal milieu necessary for glucose homeokinesis into the portal vein.

For example, when an increase in arterial glucose is sensed by the endocrine pancreas and the brain, a two-tiered response occurs. The central nervous system sends a cholinergic signal to the endocrine pancreas that is mediated by nitric oxide. Both external gates, which shunt blood flow to the entire endocrine pancreas, and internal gates, which shunt flow to B cells in the core of the islet and away from A cells in the mantle, are opened. In addition, B cells and A cells respond directly to the increase in capillary glucose, and these responses are locally modified by hormonal feedback loops and nitric oxide. The two-tiered response results in two-phase insulin secretion and a decrease in glucagon secretion. Alterations in the hormonal milieu secreted from the endocrine pancreas into the portal circulation ultimately result in glucose

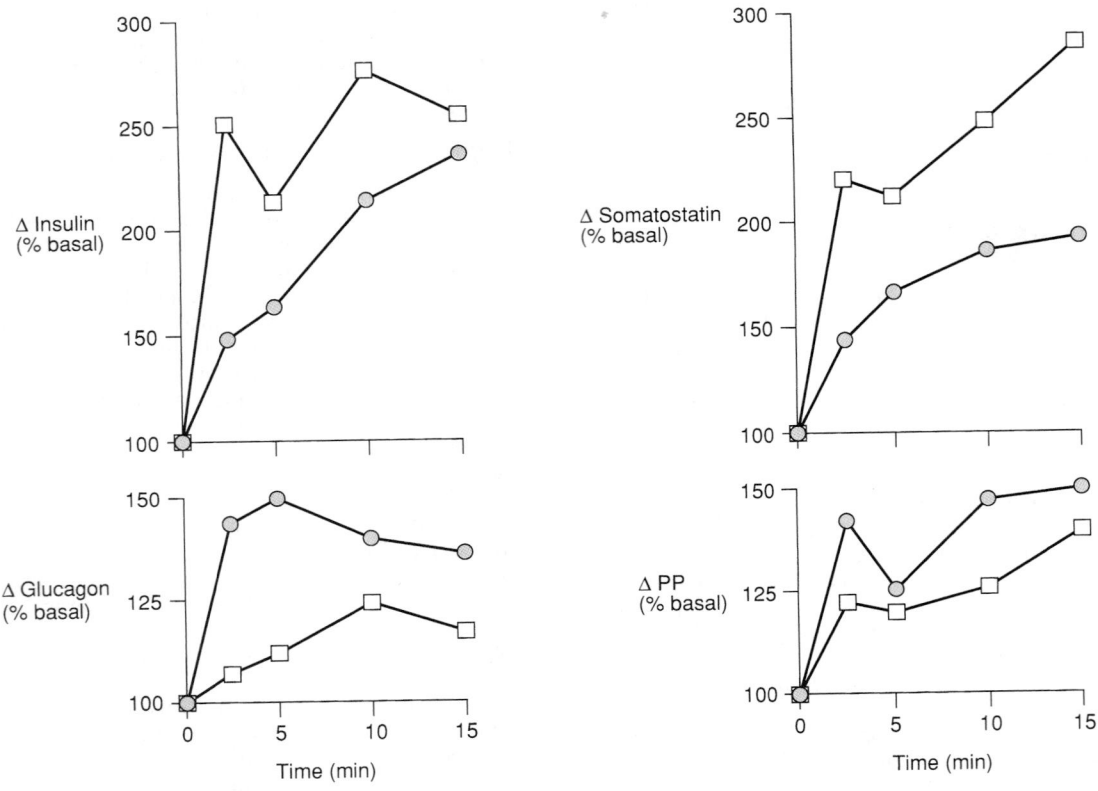

Figure 29.18. Paracrine modulation of islet secretion by insulin. The islet cell response to combined glucose (16 mmol) and gastric inhibitory polypeptide (1 nmol) perfusion in the isolated human pancreas is shown with *(circles)* and without *(squares)* the addition of 20 μU of insulin per milliliter to the arterial circuit. Venous insulin concentrations ranged from 1,500 to 3,000 μU/mL. Insulin and somatostatin secretion are inhibited, whereas glucagon and pancreatic polypeptide secretion are enhanced. These data suggest that insulin exerts negative feedback on insulin secretion from the islet, and that insulin released from the B-cell core of the islet enhances somatostatin release from the D cells in the perimeter of the islet. (After Brunicardi FC, Druck P, Sun YS, et al. Regulation of pancreatic polypeptide secretion in the isolated perfused human pancreas. *Am J Surg* 1988;155:63, with permission.)

homeokinesis. In this theoretical model of the endocrine pancreas, an effective physiologic response is possible to a wide variety of changes in the arterial milieu, and the appropriate portal venous hormonal milieu required for glucose homeokinesis is maintained.

Tests of Pancreatic Function

Exocrine Function

The secretin test is the classic test for pancreatic exocrine function (37). After the patient has fasted overnight, a double-lumen tube is placed in the duodenum. After 20-minute basal collections have been obtained, an intravenous bolus of 2 U of highly purified secretin per kilogram is administered, and four 20-minute collections of duodenal fluid are aspirated and analyzed for total volume, bicarbonate output, and enzyme secretion. The lower limits of normal for this study are 1.8 mL of pancreatic fluid per kilogram per hour, 6.2 mEq of bicarbonate output per hour, and 82 mEq of maximal bicarbonate content per hour. Amylase secretion normally ranges from 6 to 18 IU/kg. The test result is considered positive when abnormal values indicate pancreatic exocrine insufficiency (Table 29.1). In chronic pancreatitis, bicarbonate secretion is decreased because of stasis in the ducts. In pancreatic malignancy, volume is decreased because of replacement of normal pancreatic tissue with cancerous tissue. After cholecystectomy, the pancreatic juice can be diluted by bile, and results must be cautiously interpreted.

The fecal fat test is used to distinguish between pancreatic dysfunction and malabsorption secondary to enteric disease. Steatorrhea secondary to pancreatic disease is the result of lipase deficiency and is usually not present until lipase secretion is reduced by 90%. With a marked reduction of lipase secretion, the 24-hour fecal fat content is elevated to more than 20 g. Conversely, steatorrhea in the presence of low levels of fecal fat indicates intestinal dysfunction. A reduction in fecal fat indicates efficacy of pancreatic enzyme replacement in patients with exocrine insufficiency.

The dimethadione (DMO) test is based on the observation that the pancreas degrades trimethadione (Tridione), an anticonvulsant drug, and secretes its metabolite, DMO. The measurement of secreted DMO can be used as an assessment of exocrine function. Trimethadione is given to the patient orally; the dosage is 0.45 g three times a day for 3 days. A double-lumen tube is placed in the duodenum, and the secretin test is performed. The duodenal output of DMO correlates well with exocrine function and is impaired in patients with exocrine insufficiency (38).

The Lundh test measures pancreatic enzyme secretion in response to a meal of carbohydrate, fat, and protein. The test relies on endogenous secretion of secretin and CCK in addition to pancreatic secretion; therefore, the test

Table 29.1. CHARACTERISTIC RESULTS OF SECRETIN TESTING: FLOW, BICARBONATE, AND ENZYME CHANGES OBSERVED IN PATIENTS WITH VARIOUS PANCREATIC AND OTHER DISORDERS

Disorder	Pattern	Flow rate	Maximum bicarbonate concentration	Enzyme secretion
End-stage pancreatitis, advanced pancreatic cancer	Total insufficiency	Decreased	Decreased	Decreased
Chronic pancreatitis	Qualitative insufficiency	Normal	Decreased	Normal
Pancreatic cancer	Quantitative insufficiency	Decreased	Normal	Normal
Malnutrition*	Isolated enzyme deficiency	Normal	Normal	Decreased
Hemochromatosis, Zollinger-Ellison syndrome, various cirrhoses	Hypersecretion	Increased	Normal	Normal

*Sprue, ulcerative colitis, and regional enteritis.
From Dreiling DA, Wolfson P. New insights into pancreatic disease revealed by the secretin test. In: Berk JE, ed. Developments in digestive diseases, vol 2. Philadelphia: Lea & Febiger, 1979:155, with permission.

result can be abnormal in diseases involving the gastrointestinal mucosa. After an overnight fast, a double-lumen tube is placed in the duodenum and a basal collection of duodenal fluid is taken. The patient is given a mixed meal of 18 g of corn oil, 15 g of casein, and 40 g of glucose in 300 mL of water. Thirty-minute collections of the duodenal fluid are taken for 2 hours and are analyzed for trypsin, amylase, and lipase. The result of this test is abnormal in patients with chronic pancreatitis and diminished pancreatic reserve. Like the secretin and DMO tests, the Lundh test is limited by the need for duodenal intubation.

The triolein breath test is a noninvasive test of exocrine insufficiency (39). Radiolabeled triglycerides are given orally, and the metabolite, 14C-carbon dioxide, can be measured in the breath. Twenty-five grams of corn oil containing 5 µCi of [14C]triolein is given orally, and breath samples are obtained 4 hours later. The radioactivity of the breath samples is then measured. Patients with disorders of fat digestion or absorption exhale less than 3% of the [14C]triolein dose per hour. The test is repeated after oral pancreatic enzyme replacement. Patients with exocrine insufficiency achieve a normal rate of excretion of 14C-carbon dioxide, whereas patients with enteric disorders show no improvement.

The paraaminobenzoic acid test is another noninvasive test of pancreatic insufficiency (40). N-benzoyl-l-tyrosyl-paraaminobenzoic acid (BT-PABA) is cleaved by chymotrypsin to form PABA. PABA is excreted in the urine after being absorbed from the small intestine. One gram of BT-PABA in 300 mL of water is given orally, and urine collections are obtained for 6 hours. Patients with chronic pancreatitis excrete less than 60% of the ingested dose of BT-PABA. This test is useful in cases of moderate or severe pancreatic insufficiency.

The PP response to a test meal allows suspected pancreatic disease to be confirmed based on plasma levels of the islet hormone PP. Although no circulating peptide or compound changes specifically with pancreatic exocrine insufficiency, basal and meal-stimulated levels of plasma PP are reduced in severe chronic pancreatitis or after extensive pancreatic resection. After an overnight fast, a test meal consisting of 20% protein, 40% fat, and 40% carbohydrate is ingested. Basal levels of immunoreactive PP (normal, 100 to 250 pg/mL) are frequently less than 50 pg/mL in severe chronic pancreatitis (41). PP levels normally rise to 700 to 1,000 pg/mL for 2 to 3 hours after the meal, but they are reduced to 250 pg/mL or less in severe disease. Because PP release depends on intact pancreatic innervation, the PP response can be depressed in cases of diabetic autonomic neuropathy or after truncal vagotomy or antrectomy (Table 29.2).

Endocrine Function

The oral glucose tolerance test, which is the most widely used test of pancreatic endocrine function, is an indirect assessment of the insulin response to an oral glucose load. After the patient has fasted overnight, two basal blood samples are drawn for glucose determination. An oral glucose load of 40 g/m^2 is given over 10 minutes. Blood samples are drawn every 30 minutes for 2 hours (Table 29.3). This test is used to help confirm the diagnosis of diabetes (42). Caution must be used in interpreting

Table 29.2. DIFFERENTIAL DIAGNOSIS OF INTESTINAL AND PANCREATIC STEATORRHEA

Parameter	Intestinal steatorrhea	Pancreatitis
Fecal fat	<20 g monoglycerides and diglycerides; soapy consistency	>20 g triglycerides; oily seepage
D-Xylose	Low	Normal
Secretin test	Normal	Abnormal
Small-bowel series	Abnormal	Normal
Small-bowel biopsy	Abnormal	Normal
Lunch meal	Normal	Abnormal
PABA test	Normal	Abnormal
PP response to test meal	Normal	Low
Vitamin B$_{12}$ and folate	Low	Normal
Treatment with pancreatic enzymes	No change	Improvement

PABA, paraaminobenzoic acid; PP, pancreatic polypeptide.
Modified from Brandt LJ. Gastrointestinal disorders of the elderly. New York: Raven Press, 1984:470.

Table 29.3. INTERPRETATION OF ORAL GLUCOSE TOLERANCE TEST RESULTS

Interpretation	Fasting glucose value (mg/dL)		Intermediate glucose value (mg/dL)		2-Hour glucose value (mg/dL)
Normal	<115	and	All values <200	and	<140
Impaired glucose tolerance	<140	and	Any value ≥200	and	140–199
Diabetic	≥140 or		(Glucose tolerance test not necessary)		
	<140	and	Any value ≥200	and	≥200
Nondiagnostic	Any combination of glucose values that does not fit into another category				

Modified from National Diabetes Data Group. Classification and diagnosis of diabetes mellitus and other categories of glucose intolerance. Diabetes 1979;28:1039, with permission.

the results because the oral glucose tolerance test measures the glucose profile and not the actual insulin response. The insulin response to oral glucose is affected by enteric factors, especially those hormones involved in the enteroinsular axis (e.g., GIP, glucagon-like peptide-1, CCK). The test result can also be affected by antecedent diet, drug use, exercise, and the age of the patient. Although a diagnosis of diabetes can be based on the result of the oral glucose tolerance test, insulin secretion *per se* is but one factor that affects the test result.

The intravenous glucose tolerance test reflects the pancreatic endocrine response to a bolus of intravenous glucose (43). The test measures the disappearance of plasma glucose after administration of the glucose bolus, which indirectly reflects both the secretion and action of insulin. With this test, the gastrointestinal influences on glucose metabolism that affect the oral glucose tolerance test result are eliminated. After an overnight fast, two basal samples of blood are drawn. The patient is then given an intravenous bolus of 0.5 g of glucose per kilogram over 2 to 5 minutes. Blood samples are drawn every 10 minutes for 1 hour. The decline in glucose concentration (percentage of disappearance per minute) is called the *K value*. A K value of 1.5 or higher is normal. The intravenous glucose tolerance test response decreases with age, and results should be evaluated with age-adjusted criteria.

The intravenous arginine test is useful for the diagnosis of hormone-secreting tumors. The amino acid arginine stimulates the secretion of islet hormones. After an overnight fast, the patient is given a 30-minute infusion of 0.5 g of arginine per kilogram. Blood samples are taken every 10 minutes, and radioimmunoassays are performed for the specific hormones in question. This test is particularly useful for the diagnosis of glucagon-secreting tumors; elevations of plasma glucagon to above 400 pg/mL usually indicate a glucagonoma.

The tolbutamide response test is also useful in detecting hormone-secreting tumors. Tolbutamide is a sulfonylurea that stimulates insulin secretion. After the patient has fasted overnight, basal blood samples are drawn. One gram of sodium tolbutamide is given intravenously, and the blood glucose level is monitored for 1 hour. Blood samples are also drawn for radioimmunoassay of insulin or other suspected hormones, such as somatostatin. In normal patients, the blood glucose level falls to 50% of basal values after 30 minutes. Sustained hypoglycemia with hypersecretion of insulin is consistent with an insulinoma. In the case of a somatostatinoma, somatostatin levels are more than twice as high as the prevailing normal values for the particular somatostatin radioimmunoassay used.

REFERENCES

1. Cubilla AC, Fortner JC, Fitzgerald PJ. Lymph node involvement in carcinoma of the head of the pancreas area. *Cancer* 1978;41:880.
2. Ahren B, Taborsky GJ Jr, Porte D Jr. Neuropeptidergic versus cholinergic and adrenergic regulation of islet hormone secretion. *Diabetologia* 1986;29:827.
3. Havel PJ, Taborsky GJ Jr. The contribution of the autonomic nervous system to changes in glucagon and insulin secretion during hypoglycemic stress. *Endocr Rev* 1989;10:332.
4. Sadar ES, Cooperman AM. Bilateral thoracic sympathectomy-splanchnicectomy in the treatment of intractable pain due to pancreatic carcinoma. *Cleve Clin Q* 1974;41:185.
5. Gorelick FS, Jamieson JD. Structure–function relationship of the pancreas. In: Johnson LR, ed. *Physiology of the gastrointestinal tract.* New York: Raven Press, 1981:773.
6. Longnecker DS, Shinozuka H, Dekker A. Focal acinar cell dysplasia in human pancreas. *Cancer* 1980;45:534–540.
7. Pour PM, Schmied B. The link between exocrine pancreatic cancer and the endocrine pancreas. *Int J Pancreatol* 1999;25:77–87.
8. Kleinman R, Gingerich R, Wong H, et al. The use of the Fab fragment for immunoneutralization of somatostatin in the isolated perfused pancreas. *Am J Surg* 1994;167:114.
9. Cooper GJ, Day AJ, Willis AC, et al. Amylin and the amylin gene: structure, function, and relationship to islet amyloid and to diabetes mellitus. *Biochem Biophys Acta* 1989;1014:247.
10. Stefan Y, Orci L, Malaisse-Legae F, et al. Quantitation of endocrine cell content in the pancreas of non-diabetic and diabetic humans. *Diabetes* 1982;31:694.
11. Seymour NE, Brunicardi FC, Chaiken RL, et al. Reversal of abnormal glucose production after pancreatic resection by pancreatic polypeptide administration in man. *Surgery* 1988;104:119.
12. Jansson L, Hellerstrom C. Glucose-induced changes in pancreatic islet blood flow mediated by central nervous system. *Am J Physiol* 1986;25:E644.
13. Bonner-Weir S, Orci L. New perspectives on the microvasculature of the islets of Langerhans in the rat. *Diabetes* 1982;31:883.
14. Murakami T, Fujita T, Ohtsuka A, et al. The insulino-acinar portal and insulino-venous drainage systems in the pancreas of the mouse, dog, monkey, and certain other animals: a scanning electron microscopic study of corrosion casts. *Arch Histol Cytol* 1993;56:127.
15. Liu Y, Guth PH, Kaneko K, et al. Dynamic in vivo observation of rat islet microcirculation. *Pancreas* 1993;8:15.
16. Lee W, Kazunori M, Funakoshi A. Effects of somatostatin and pancreatic polypeptide on exocrine and endocrine pancreas in the rats. *Gastroenterol Jpn* 1988;23:49.
17. Busnardo AC, Didio L, Tidrick R, et al. History of the pancreas. *Am J Surg* 1983;146:539.
18. Davenport HW. Pancreatic secretion. In: Davenport HN, ed. *Physiology of the digestive tract,* 5th ed. Chicago: Year Book Medical Publishers, 1982:143.
19. Valenzuela JE, Weiner K, Saad C. Cholinergic stimulation of human pancreatic secretion. *Dig Dis Sci* 1986;31:615.
20. Konturek SJ, Becker HD, Thompson JC. Effect of vagotomy on hormones stimulating pancreatic secretion. *Arch Surg* 1974;108:704.
21. Leahy JL, Bonner-Weir S, Weir GC. Abnormal glucose regulation of insulin secretion in models of reduced B-cell mass. *Diabetes* 1984;33:667.
22. Nanjo K, Sanke T, Mujano M, et al. Diabetes due to secretion of a structurally abnormal insulin (insulin Wakayama): clinical and functional characteristics of Leu-A3 insulin. *J Clin Invest* 1986;77:514.
23. Bell GI, Kayano T, Buse JB, et al. Molecular biology of mammalian glucose transporters. *Diabetes Care* 1990;13:198.

24. Orci L, Unger RH, Ravazzola M, et al. Reduced beta-cell glucose transporter in new onset diabetic BB rats. *J Clin Invest* 1990;86:1615.
25. Ebert R, Creutzfeldt W. Gastrointestinal peptides and insulin secretion. *Diabetes Metab Rev* 1987;3:1.
26. Opara EC, Atwater I, Go VLM. Characterization and control of pulsatile secretion of insulin and glucagon. *Pancreas* 1988;3:484.
27. Eisenbarth GS. Type I diabetes mellitus: a chronic autoimmune disease. *N Engl J Med* 1986;314:1360.
28. Brunicardi FC, Sun YS, Druck P, et al. Splanchnic neural regulation of insulin and glucagon secretion in the isolated perfused human pancreas. *Am J Surg* 1987;153:34.
29. Unger RH, Dobbs RE. Insulin, glucagon, and somatostatin in the regulation of metabolism. *Ann Rev Physiol* 1978;40:307.
30. Gerich JE. Somatostatin and diabetes. *Am J Med* 1981;70:619.
31. Brazeau P, Vale N, Burgus R, et al. Hypothalamic polypeptide that inhibits the secretion of immunoreactive pituitary growth hormone. *Science* 1973;179:77.
32. Kleinman R, Watt P, Ohning G, et al. The regulatory role of intraislet somatostatin on insulin secretion in the isolated perfused human pancreas. *Pancreas* 1993;9:172.
33. Mulvihill SJ, Pappas TN, Passaro E, et al. The use of somatostatin and its analogs in the treatment of surgical disorders. *Surgery* 1986;100:467.
34. Kennedy FP. Pathophysiology of pancreatic polypeptide secretion in human diabetes mellitus. *Diabetes Nutr Metab* 1990;2:155.
35. Fagan SP, Anderson DK, Brunicardi FC. Islet cell hormones and chronic pancreatitis. *Probl Gen Surg* 1998;15:7–16.
36. Moldovan S, Brunicardi FC. The endocrine pancreas: a summary of observations generated by surgical fellows. *World J Surg* 2000 (in press).
37. Dreiling DA, Wolfson P. New insights into pancreatic disease revealed by the secretin test. In: Berk JE, ed. *Developments in digestive diseases,* vol 2. Philadelphia: Lea & Febiger, 1979;155.
38. Noda A, Hayakowa T, Kondo T, et al. Clinical evaluation of pancreatic excretion test with dimethadione and oral BT-PABA test in chronic pancreatitis. *Dig Dis Sci* 1983;30:230.
39. Goff JS. Two-stage triolein breath test differentiates pancreatic insufficiency from other causes of malabsorption. *Gastroenterology* 1982;83:44.
40. Arvanitakis C, Greenberger NJ. Diagnosis of pancreatic disease by a synthetic peptide: a new test of exocrine pancreatic function. *Lancet* 1976;1:663.
41. Nealon WH, Beauchamp RD, Townsend CM, et al. Diagnostic role of gastrointestinal hormones in patients with chronic pancreatitis. *Ann Surg* 1986;204:430.
42. National Diabetes Data Group. Classification and diagnosis of diabetes mellitus and other categories of glucose intolerance. *Diabetes* 1979;30:1039.
43. Andres R, Tobin JD. Endocrine systems. In: Finch CE, Hayflick L, eds. *Handbook of the biology of aging.* New York: Van Nostrand Reinhold, 1977:357.

SURGERY: SCIENTIFIC PRINCIPLES AND PRACTICE, Third Edition, edited by Lazar J. Greenfield, Michael W. Mulholland, Keith T. Oldham, Gerald B. Zelenock, and Keith D. Lillemoe. Lippincott Williams & Wilkins Publishers, Philadelphia, © 2001.

CHAPTER 30

ACUTE PANCREATITIS

MICHEL M. MURR AND JAMES NORMAN

Acute pancreatitis is a potentially reversible, acute inflammatory condition of the pancreas. The clinical manifestations of acute pancreatitis range from mild and isolated local inflammation of the pancreas to a dramatic systemic inflammatory response associated with end-organ damage. This chapter, a comprehensive review of acute pancreatitis, provides the reader with treatment algorithms based on our current understanding of the pathophysiology of acute pancreatitis. This understanding has evolved during the last decade as molecular biology techniques have been applied to elucidate the complex and occasionally unpredictable events of pancreatitis. Because many of the exact pathogenic mechanisms are still unclear, specific and directed treatment is not available, and empiric support remains the mainstay of therapy.

INCIDENCE

The incidence of acute pancreatitis appears to have increased recently for reasons that are as yet unclear. It is estimated that acute pancreatitis develops in approximately 250,000 people in the United States each year. Although the overall mortality of acute pancreatitis approaches 5%, more than 50% of the deaths are in patients with severe acute pancreatitis.

CLASSIFICATION OF PANCREATITIS

For many years, physicians have had difficulties describing and classifying pancreatic disease in a reasonably understandable and predictable manner. In response to this confusion, a number of expert pancreatologists reached a consensus regarding the classification and nomenclature of acute pancreatitis in 1993 (1). This clinically based system, which has since become known as the *Atlanta classification,* has been adopted by pancreas experts worldwide and is used throughout this text.

Mild acute pancreatitis is an acute inflammation of the pancreas with minimal distant organ dysfunction and an uneventful recovery.

Severe acute pancreatitis is an acute inflammation of the pancreas associated with organ failure and local complications, such as necrosis, abscess, and pseudocyst.

Acute fluid collections occur early in the course of acute pancreatitis, are located in or near the pancreas, and always lack a wall of granulation or fibrous tissue. This is the most misunderstood term and is commonly confused with a pseudocyst. Fluid collections may regress spontaneously or persist to form pseudocysts.

Pancreatic necrosis denotes diffuse or focal areas of nonviable pancreatic parenchyma, typically associated with peripancreatic fat necrosis.

Pseudocyst is a collection of pancreatic juice enclosed by a wall of fibrous or granulation tissue arising as a consequence of acute pancreatitis, chronic pancreatitis, or trauma to the pancreas.

Pancreatic abscess is a collection of pus, usually in proximity to the pancreas, containing little or no pancreatic necrosis. It arises as a consequence of acute pancreatitis or trauma to the pancreas.

Participants in the Atlanta symposium recommended discarding such terms as *phlegmon, infected pseudocyst, hemorrhagic pancreatitis,* and *persistent acute pancreatitis* because of their ambiguity and lack of specificity.

PATHOPHYSIOLOGY OF LOCAL INJURY

Normal pancreatic anatomy and physiology are presented in detail in Chapter 29. Relevant to this discussion are the features of acinar cell morphology and normal function; these are represented schematically in Fig. 30.1, which illustrates the important ultrastructural features and the normal cytosolic processing of digestive proenzymes. The process culminates in the orderly apical dis-

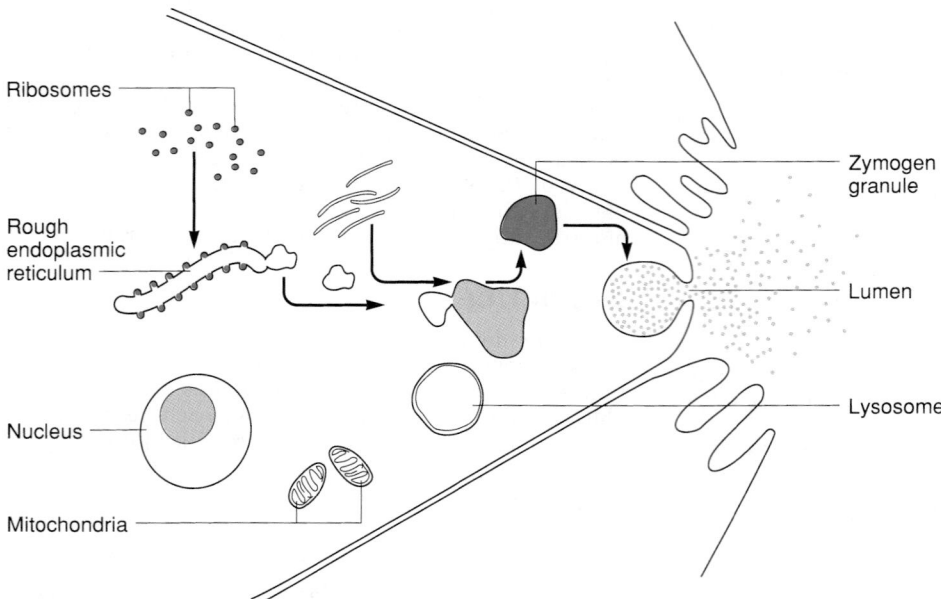

Figure 30.1. Normal acinar cell ultrastructure. Cytoplasmic processing of the proenzymes is depicted, with apical discharge into the acinar ductule by means of zymogen granule exocytosis.

charge of zymogen granules into the duct lumen. Acute pancreatitis is characterized by alterations in acinar cell structure and function and by the development of acute regional and systemic inflammatory responses. The fundamental pathologic event is injury to the acinar cell.

It is generally believed that the cellular event that leads to acute pancreatitis is colocalization of the digestive enzymes and lysozymes in the cytoplasm of acinar cells (Fig. 30.2). Normally, digestive enzymes and proteases are packaged into zymogen granules, which are exported to the ductal lumen by exocytosis at the apical membrane of the acinar cells (Fig. 30.1). The mechanisms by which lysosomes (containing lysozymes) fuse with zymogen granules and migrate to the basolateral membrane of the acinar cell in acute pancreatitis are still elusive. Cathepsin B, which is abundant in lysosomes, is presumed to activate trypsinogen to form trypsin, which in turn activates the rest of the proteases in zymogen granules. Most probably, colocalization occurs under normal conditions to a very limited degree and is thus unnoticed because en-

dogenous antiproteases protect the pancreatic parenchyma from autodigestion. These protective mechanisms are overwhelmed in acute pancreatitis, and the pancreatic enzymes are activated.

The events of intracellular activation of proteases result in acinar cell injury that perpetuates itself by inducing neighboring acinar cell injury. This leads to a local inflammatory reaction characterized by the rapid formation of interstitial edema and inflammatory cell infiltration. Grossly, the gland becomes enlarged and edematous, with small areas of focal necrosis involving either pancreatic tissue or adjacent areas of retroperitoneal fat. Acute inflammation develops rapidly, even within minutes in experimental animal models. This initial inflammatory response involves the influx of polymorphonuclear leukocytes into the perivascular regions of the pancreas. Within hours, mononuclear cells, including macrophages and lymphocytes, accumulate. A significant amount of experimental evidence has been accumulated recently showing that these invading inflammatory cells are hyperacti-

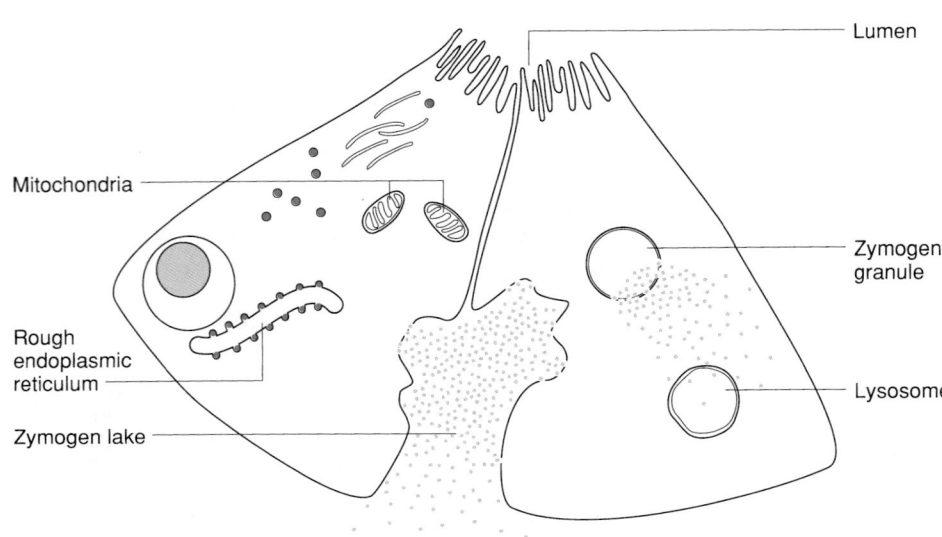

Figure 30.2. Schematic diagram illustrating the loss of acinar cell polarity and the process of cytoplasmic fusion of lysosomes and zymogen granules. Disordered basolateral discharge of activated proteases from the acinar cell follows.

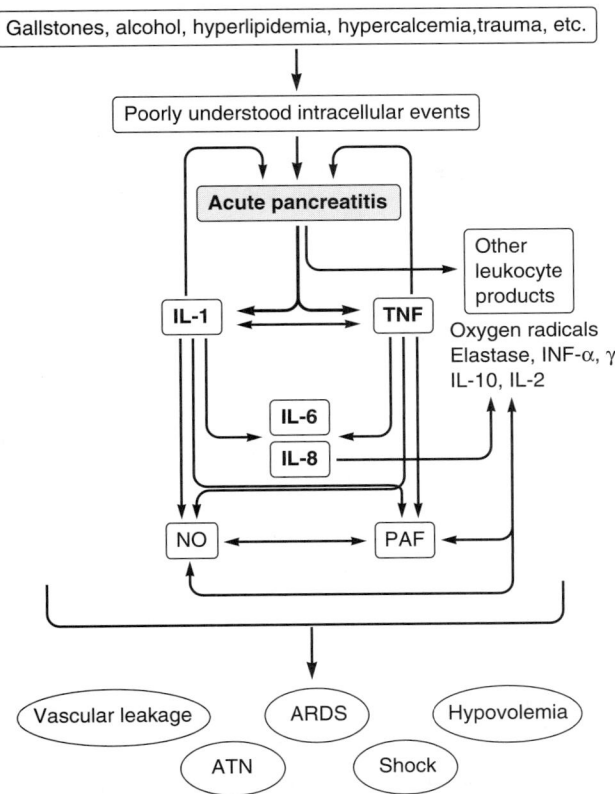

that exert their effects through specific cell receptors, and they possess the ability to amplify their own closely regulated production. The inflammatory cytokines interleukin-1 (IL-1), IL-6, IL-8, and tumor necrosis factor (TNF) are produced locally and systemically during acute pancreatitis. IL-1 and TNF are proximal inflammatory mediators that can induce nearly all the manifestations of a sepsis syndrome, including shock and end-organ damage. Circulating monocytes, lymphocytes, and neutrophils from patients with severe pancreatitis become hyperstimulated and are capable of secreting large amounts of cytokines (4,5). It has been demonstrated that neither IL-1 nor TNF can induce the acinar cell derangements associated with acute pancreatitis, but there seems to be little doubt that inflammatory cytokines play a central role in the progression of pancreatitis and the development of its systemic manifestations (6) (Fig. 30.3).

A tremendous amount of experimental evidence has accumulated during the past 15 years to suggest that macrophage- and neutrophil-derived mediators are responsible for the progression of acute pancreatitis from a localized inflammation of the retroperitoneum to a systemic illness. We now know that IL-1, TNF, PAF, nitric oxide, and other mediators are initially produced in the pancreatic parenchyma within 30 minutes after the initiation of pancreatitis in different animal models (2,6). The major source of these inflammatory substances is the leukocytes that invade the pancreatic parenchyma early in acute pancreatitis. After a latent period, cytokines and other mediators are then produced to a larger extent in specific distant organs, such as the lungs, liver, and spleen. In addition to initiation of the production of systemic cytokines, cytokine receptors are upregulated in various target tissues, so that their deleterious systemic effects are amplified.

The signal(s) that cause the systemic and intraparenchymal activation of inflammatory cells and the production of cytokines in severe pancreatitis are still unknown. For years, it was thought that the noxious effects of pancreatic enzymes on tissues resulted in the systemic manifestations of pancreatitis. However, recent evidence now suggests that macrophages and neutrophils throughout the body are activated in response to certain circulating pancreatic enzymes through specific cell surface receptors. Activated pancreatic enzymes may in fact play the dominant role in this process, but there seems little doubt that the actual systemic illness that is the hallmark of acute pancreatitis is the result of an overzealous production of cytokines and other inflammatory molecules throughout the body. The therapeutic implications of these findings are extremely important and are discussed in the section on management.

Figure 30.3. Inflammatory mediators of acute pancreatitis. Regardless of the inciting event, a number of inflammatory mediators are produced locally and systematically during acute pancreatitis. Cascades develop quickly, and the process is rapidly amplified to involve mediators of various classes. Interleukin-1 beta (IL-1) and tumor necrosis factor-alpha (TNF) have the ability to induce nearly all of the other mediators while feeding back to produce a direct noxious effect within the pancreas itself. Although some are likely to play a much more significant role, each of these mediators plays a part in the development of the systemic manifestations of pancreatitis. Importantly, notice the lack of activated enzymes, bacteria, and endotoxin in this scheme. ARDS = adult respiratory distress syndrome; NO = nitric oxide; NF = interferon; PAF = platelet activating factor. (From Norman J. Role of cytokines in the pathogenesis of acute pancreatitis. *Am J Surg* 1998;175:76, with permission.)

vated and produce a large number of inflammatory mediators, which propagate the damage taking place within the pancreatic parenchyma. The inflammatory reaction is amplified by ongoing acinar cell damage that leads to hyperinflammation, with local and systemic overproduction of kinins, complement, nitric oxide, oxygen-derived free radicals, cytokines, and platelet-activating factor (PAF). The eventual presence of these inflammatory mediators within distant tissues of the body is primarily responsible for the systemic effects and manifestations of acute pancreatitis such as ARDS, hypovolemia and shock, acute tubular necrosis and multi-system organ failure (2,3) (Fig. 30.3).

PATHOPHYSIOLOGY OF SYSTEMIC DISEASE

The role of cytokines and other inflammatory mediators during bouts of severe acute pancreatitis has become apparent during the past decade. Cytokines are regulatory proteins produced by numerous cell types as a means of cellular communication. They are very potent compounds

ETIOLOGY

A number of conditions associated with the development of acute pancreatitis share the feature of obstruction of the main pancreatic duct. However, acute pancreatitis develops in the absence of ductal obstruction or any other identifiable cause in 10% to 15% of patients. More than 80% patients with acute pancreatitis have either choledocholithiasis (stones in the common bile duct) or a history of alcohol use. Other conditions associated with acute pancreatitis are listed in Table 30.1. Previous reports have suggested the etiology of acute pancreatitis differs significantly between the United States and Great Britain. A recently completed multicenter trial that enrolled more than 700 patients from each country, however, shows that this may not be so. It is likely that the greater use of invasive monitoring and testing in the United States provides a better assessment of the etiology, especially in that an etiology is not assigned to as many as a third of British patients.

Table 30.1. CLINICAL ASSOCIATIONS WITH ACUTE PANCREATITIS

Biliary tract stone disease
Ethanol
Other
Trauma
   Postprocedural
      Postoperative
      Post-ERCP
   Direct
Mechanical (nongallstone) obstruction
   Tumors of the pancreas, duodenum, or bile duct
   Duodenal obstruction
   Pancreas divisum
Infection
Hyperlipidemia
Hyperparathyroidism
Drugs
   Steroids
      Estrogen
      Glucocorticoids
   Diuretics
      Furosemide
      Thiazides
      Ethacrynic acid
      Diazoxide
   Calcium
   Warfarin
   Cimetidine
   Quinidine
   Phenformin
   Azathioprine
   Mercuric chloride
   Paracetamol
   Sulfonamides
   Tetracyclines
   L-Asparaginase
   Methyldopa
   Clonidine
Pregnancy
Idiopathic

ERCP, endoscopic retrograde cholangiopancreatography.

Biliary Tract Stones

The particular anatomy of the pancreatic and biliary ductal systems has been subjected to many interpretations because of the existence of a common channel in the intrapancreatic portion of these ducts (Fig. 30.4). It has long been held that this common channel allows a reflux of bile or duodenal contents into the pancreatic duct. Many studies have not been able to resolve the question of whether an impacted stone in the ampulla results in pancreatitis by inducing a reflux of bile into the pancreatic duct or by causing pancreatic ductal hypertension. Central to this controversy is the fact that choledocholithiasis can be demonstrated in only 20% of patients with pancreatitis, and an impacted stone in the ampulla can be found in only 2% of patients. Nevertheless, gallstones can be found in the stools of 90% of patients with acute gallstone pancreatitis. It appears that by the time patients seek medical attention, the offending gallstones have already passed into the gastrointestinal tract. These are important considerations because therapeutic interventions such as endoscopic retrograde cholangiopancreatography (ERCP) may be necessary to extract an impacted stone in only a minority of patients.

Alcohol

Alcohol consumption is a common cause of acute pancreatitis worldwide, although it may be more common in

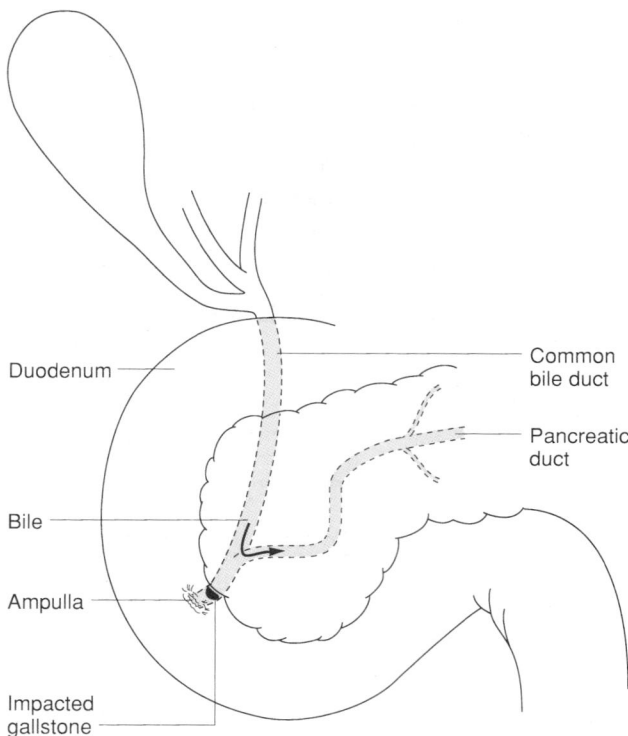

Figure 30.4. Illustration of the common channel concept. A gallstone at the ampulla of Vater causes reflux of bile into the pancreatic duct.

the United States. The reasons for this variation are unclear, but it may have to do with certain societal differences in the perception of alcoholism. The mechanisms by which alcohol induces pancreatitis in humans are not fully elucidated. However, several mechanisms based on experimental observations are plausible. Ethanol increases the secretion of pancreatic fluid and protein and increases the resistance of the ampulla (Fig. 30.5). This results in the formation of proteinaceous precipitates and plugs, which lead to pancreatic ductal hypertension and pancreatitis.

Postprocedural Pancreatitis

Many surgical procedures in the upper abdomen can be associated with postoperative pancreatitis. The incidence of acute pancreatitis after gastric resection is between 0.6% and 1.3%. After biliary tract surgery, particularly after common bile duct exploration, acute pancreatitis occurs with an incidence of 0.5% to 3%. Direct manipulation or retraction of the pancreas or pancreatic duct appears to be the most common cause. Acute pancreatitis develops in about 3% to 4% of patients after ERCP. This is a predictable event, and the risk can be minimized, although not eliminated, by limiting the pressure used for contrast injection of the pancreatic duct. Acute pancreatitis also occurs in patients after coronary artery bypass surgery and a variety of other procedures performed in regions remote from the pancreas. Although pancreatitis in this circumstance is thought to result from ischemia, hypotension is not always noted. It has been suggested that the systemic consequences of activation of the inflammatory system may contribute to changes in the microvascular blood flow in these cases.

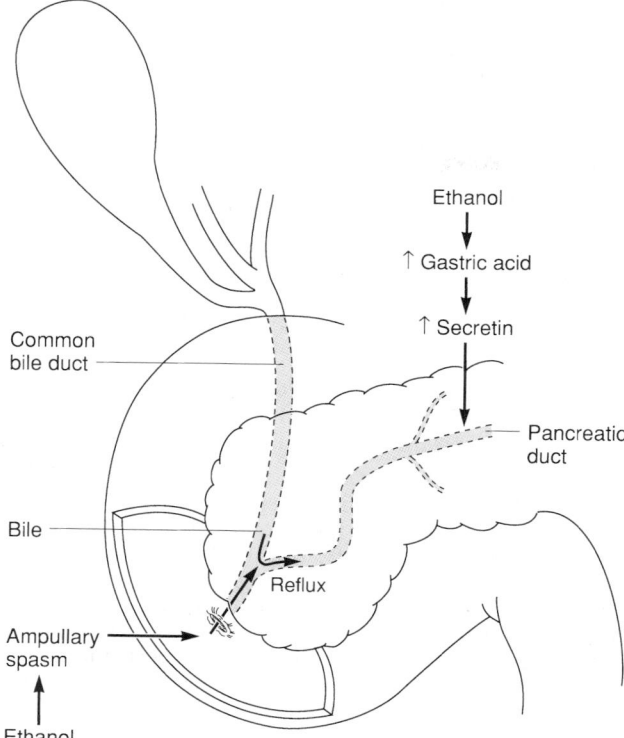

Figure 30.5. Ethanol-induced increases in ampullary resistance may exacerbate the reflux of bile into the pancreatic duct. Coupled with acid-stimulated, secretin-mediated increases in pancreatic secretion, such reflux may contribute to pancreatic duct hypertension and the development of acute pancreatitis.

Trauma

Hyperamylasemia is common after major abdominal trauma; however, the full clinical picture of pancreatitis is much less common and occurs in fewer than 5% of patients who sustain major blunt trauma (7). Trauma to the pancreas is covered in Chapter 11.

Hyperlipidemia

Rare causes of acute pancreatitis are the hyperlipoproteinemias, types I and V. The initial acinar cell injury is thought to result from the liberation of free fatty acids from circulating triglycerides by the local action of lipases within the pancreatic microcirculation. The microvascular endothelium may also be physically disrupted by cholesterol crystals.

Hyperparathyroidism and Hypercalcemia

These are very uncommon but well documented causes of pancreatitis. Calcium is a secretagogue and may cause pancreatitis when it precipitates in the pancreatic duct. Pancreatitis may develop in patients with hyperparathyroidism because of associated hypercalcemia or increased serum levels of parathyroid hormone.

Drugs

A multitude of drugs are suspected of causing acute pancreatitis, but a clear and defined association has been found with very few (Table 30.1). The mechanisms of drug-induced pancreatitis are largely elusive and most probably involve different pathways.

Infection

The recent epidemic of AIDS has uncovered many cases of pancreatitis, most commonly caused by cytomegalovirus infection. In addition, certain medications used to treat AIDS, such as pentamidine, may also result in pancreatitis. Pancreatitis has been described after infection with many bacterial, fungal, and viral agents.

Tumors

Tumors of the head of the pancreas and the periampullary region can present as acute pancreatitis as a result of obstruction of the pancreatic duct in 1% to 3% of patients. A high index of suspicion should be maintained, especially when elderly patients are treated for pancreatitis.

Pancreas Divisum

This is a normal variant in 5% to 7% of people, in which the ducts of the ventral and dorsal pancreas fail to fuse during embryonic life. The association with acute pancreatitis is not absolute because pancreatitis never develops in the majority of persons with pancreas divisum. However, in those patients with no other identifiable causes of pancreatitis, an association with this ductal anomaly is likely, and they may obtain relief from recurrent attacks after dorsal duct sphincterotomy.

Idiopathic Pancreatitis

In some series, the incidence of idiopathic pancreatitis is as high as 20%. However, alterations in the composition of bile resulting in microlithiasis and "sludge" formation were noted in about two thirds of these patients. Recent large clinical trials have shown that a cause can be identified in the majority of cases of "idiopathic pancreatitis" if appropriate diagnostic testing is performed.

Pregnancy

Acute pancreatitis has been linked to pregnancy with an incidence of 0.01% to 0.1%. Because most reports include patients with gallstones, ethanol use, or other risk factors, it is unclear whether pregnancy is an independent risk factor.

CLINICAL PRESENTATION

The cardinal clinical symptom of acute pancreatitis is epigastric pain of a visceral nature that radiates to the back. The pain can have an insidious onset, but often patients can tell exactly when the pain started. The pain is constant and at times can be poorly localized. Other clinical findings include fever, nausea, vomiting, ileus, and abdominal distention (Table 30.2) The clinical presenta-

Table 30.2. COMMON SIGNS AND SYMPTOMS OF UNCOMPLICATED ACUTE EDEMATOUS PANCREATITIS

Sign or symptom	Frequency (%)
Abdominal pain	85–100
Nausea and vomiting	54–92
Anorexia	83
Fever	12–80
Abdominal mass	6–20
Ileus	50–80

tion can be quite variable and primarily depends on the severity of the disease process.

Clinical signs of *severe* necrotizing pancreatitis include jaundice and hypotension. In addition, retroperitoneal hemorrhage may become apparent as blood dissects into the subcutaneous tissues, producing blue discoloration of the flanks (Grey Turner's sign), umbilicus (Cullen's sign), or inguinal ligament (Fox's sign).

DIAGNOSIS

The diagnosis of acute pancreatitis ultimately depends on clinical judgment and is generally based on the finding of epigastric abdominal pain and hyperamylasemia. No single laboratory or physical finding is pathognomonic. Most experts agree that computed tomography (CT) is the most specific test for acute pancreatitis, but, as is discussed below, the timing of the scan is a critical factor in determining its accuracy.

Laboratory Tests

Amylase

Amylase is released from the acinar cells into the pancreatic microcirculation in conjunction with the pathophysiologic events described earlier. The laboratory finding of hyperamylasemia in a patient with clinical signs and symptoms of acute pancreatitis is the usual means of confirming the diagnosis. Efforts to correlate the degree of hyperamylasemia with disease severity or prognosis have been consistently unsuccessful, and common prognostic criteria, such as Ranson's signs, are notable for the absence of serum amylase levels. An important reason for this relates to the relatively rapid clearance of amylase from plasma, the half-life being about 130 minutes. Pancreatitis resulting from a discrete event, such as transient obstruction of the pancreatic duct with gallstone passage, is characterized by a single serum amylase peak with a rapid rise and prompt clearance, both measured in terms of hours. Given the inherent delays in seeking clinical care and obtaining diagnostic studies, this peak may have passed and the serum amylase may be relatively normal within 24 hours of the event. A minimally or modestly elevated serum amylase level may also be found in a patient with necrotizing pancreatitis or chronic pancreatitis; in these instances, complete or nearly complete destruction of the acinar cell population may have occurred, reducing the plasma amylase level. Additionally, a number of nonpancreatic sources of amylase exist, so that hyperamylasemia may result from other pathology. Salivary glands, fallopian tubes, and the small bowel are important alternative sources of amylase. Clinical conditions associated with hyperamylasemia including the following:

- Salivary gland injury
- Burns
- Cerebral trauma
- Multiple trauma
- Diabetic ketoacidosis
- Macroamylasemia
- Renal transplantation
- Renal dysfunction
- Pneumonia
- Pregnancy
- Fallopian tube disease
- Drugs
- Afferent loop syndrome
- Acute appendicitis
- Dissecting aortic aneurysm

- Small-bowel injury
- Perforated ulcer
- Small-bowel obstruction
- Mesenteric infarction

In the case of salivary gland disease, plasma amylase isoenzyme determinations may differentiate the source, but clinical findings or abdominal CT findings make these unnecessary in most instances.

Because plasma amylase levels reflect renal clearance, renal dysfunction may also contribute to hyperamylasemia. Indeed, determination of the ratio of amylase (A) clearance to creatinine (Cr) clearance is a potentially useful diagnostic test for acute pancreatitis. This fractional excretion (Fe) is calculated as follows:

$$Fe_A = \frac{U_A \times S_{Cr}}{U_{Cr} \times SA} \times 10$$

The normal fractional urinary excretion of amylase is between 1% and 4%. Clearance in excess of 4% to 4.5% is considered abnormal but is not specific for acute pancreatitis. Renal dysfunction (particularly if associated with impaired tubular reabsorption), diabetic ketoacidosis, the formation of amylase macroconjugates, and thermal injuries are clinical conditions that limit the specificity of this test. In the correct clinical setting, the determination of an increased amylase clearance may be a method of confirming hyperamylasemia that is useful after initial plasma elevations have cleared.

Lipase

Serum lipase is also increased in acute pancreatitis and is cleared at a slower rate by the kidneys. Serum lipase determinations have not been found to be more useful clinically than serum amylase measurements; however, the sensitivity and specificity of a concomitant increase in serum amylase and lipase are 90% to 95% in detecting acute pancreatitis in patients with abdominal pain (8). The measurement of other enzymes or products of acinar cell injury, such as trypsin, chymotrypsin, elastase, phospholipase, and methalbumin, has not been shown to provide any useful information beyond that obtained by the simple determination of serum amylase. Other biochemical features of acute pancreatitis are listed in Table 30.3.

Table 30.3. BIOCHEMICAL FEATURES OF ACUTE PANCREATITIS

Increased
Hematocrit, hemoglobin (hemoconcentration)
White blood cell count
Blood urea nitrogen
Creatinine
Bilirubin
Lipids, triglycerides
Glucose
Alkaline phosphatase
SGOT, SGPT
Decreased
Hematocrit, hemoglobin (hemorrhage)
Calcium
Magnesium
Pao$_2$
Other
Respiratory alkalosis (early)
Metabolic alkalosis (early)
Consumptive coagulopathy
Metabolic acidosis (late)
Respiratory acidosis (late)

SGOT, serum glutamic–oxaloacetic transaminase; SGPT, serum glutamic–pyruvic transaminase; Pao$_2$, arterial oxygen pressure.

Radiologic Tests

Although a diffuse ileus and a solitary left upper abdominal sentinel loop are classic and often seen on abdominal roentgenograms, neither is specific for acute pancreatitis. The psoas muscle margins may be obscured by retroperitoneal edema, pancreatic ascites may be apparent, and pancreatic calcifications imply preexisting chronic disease. About one third of patients with acute pancreatitis have abnormal findings on chest radiographs at the time of diagnosis. An upright chest radiograph may demonstrate segmental atelectasis, an elevated hemidiaphragm, pleural effusions, or the presence of early pulmonary parenchyma infiltrates. Barium studies of the gastrointestinal tract often demonstrate narrowing or spasm of the duodenum, with widening of the C loop secondary to pancreatic inflammation and edema.

Ultrasonography is a rapid, inexpensive, and noninvasive tool for evaluating patients with presumed pancreatitis. It can demonstrate edema of the pancreas and furnish information on the status of the gallbladder (cholecystitis, cholelithiasis) and biliary ductal system (dilatation, choledocholithiasis). The examination is limited by the presence of dilated bowel loops overlying the area of the pancreas. In recently completed trials, ultrasonography often yielded an inadequate examination in comparison with concurrently performed CT, and often no assessment of the pancreas could be made. Furthermore, ultrasonography often underestimates the amount of parenchymal damage and cannot detect parenchymal necrosis in patients with severe pancreatitis. The most common use for ultrasonography in the clinical setting of pancreatitis is not evaluation of the pancreas *per se*, but rather examination of the biliary system for the presence of dilated ducts and gallstones.

Contrast-enhanced dynamic CT has become the most widely used test to evaluate patients with acute pancreatitis and is now the standard with which all other investigative measures are compared. It is more sensitive than ultrasonography for detecting parenchymal changes in the pancreas and peripancreatic tissues, but less sensitive for detecting cholelithiasis and choledocholithiasis. Findings on CT include edema of the pancreas, peripancreatic fluid collections, and edema of the surrounding viscera and mesentery. Absence of enhancement of the pancreatic parenchyma by intravenous contrast denotes pancreatic necrosis. Extravisceral gas is pathognomonic of infection but is a rare finding.

Endoscopic retrograde cholangiopancreatography is of little use, if any, as a diagnostic modality in acute uncomplicated pancreatitis. In fact, most gastroenterologists feel that ERCP is contraindicated if no clinical or radiologic evidence of ongoing ductal obstruction is found. ERCP may provide useful anatomic information in patients with recurrent "idiopathic" or complicated pancreatitis and so is indicated in such patients once the acute phase of the disease has resolved. The therapeutic role of ERCP is discussed in the section on management.

The experience with magnetic resonance imaging (MRI) and cholangiopancreatography (MRCP) in the diagnostic workup of acute pancreatitis is limited, and therefore the use of these techniques has not become routine. In centers where they are being used regularly, preliminary results appear promising in the noninvasive assessment of biliary and pancreatic duct pathology.

PROGNOSTIC CRITERIA AND DETERMINATION OF SEVERITY

Because of the wide spectrum of presentations of acute pancreatitis and its propensity to progress into multisystem organ failure, a mechanism of predicting the severity and outcome of pancreatitis is essential. The most commonly known and used system is that of Ranson, which takes into consideration 11 clinical findings measured during a 48-hour period (Table 30.4). The total score based on these criteria accurately predicts mortality; patients with only one or two criteria have a predicted mortality of 1%, which increases to 10% when three criteria are present. Predicted mortality is almost 50% for patients with seven or more criteria. The major limitations of Ranson's criteria are that complete assessment requires data that are not available until 48 hours after admission, and that they cannot be calculated serially at later times during hospitalization.

The APACHE II (acute physiology score and chronic health evaluation) scoring system overcomes the limitations of Ranson's criteria but is cumbersome to calculate. It utilizes 12 physiologic and laboratory parameters available at admission, age, and preexisting comorbid conditions (Table 30.5). The APACHE II score can be calculated on a daily basis, so that it provides a mechanism to evaluate the disease process sequentially. An APACHE II score above 9 denotes severe acute pancreatitis. Recent clinical trials used the APACHE II scoring system as an eligibility criterion, assuming a higher incidence of organ system failure with higher scores. Although this was unquestionably true, several flaws in this scoring system became apparent in the setting of acute pancreatitis. The APACHE II score tends to overestimate the effect of age, and therefore mildly ill patients can be labeled as severely ill simply as a function of advanced age. In addition, this scoring system tends to overemphasize some "low normal" values, such as a low heart rate and serum creatinine level.

With the possible exception of IL-6 and IL-8, many biochemical markers of acute pancreatitis and inflammation have not proved superior to the clinical scoring systems in predicting the severity of pancreatitis at the time of presentation (9,10). Despite their predictive value, the clinical use of IL-6 and IL-8 levels has been hampered by the unavailability of a rapid assay. A rapid assay for trypsinogen activation peptide is currently being evaluated in European studies as a predictor of severity in acute pancreatitis. It is likely that one of these assays will find its way to the patient's bedside in the next decade.

Table 30.4. RANSON'S CRITERIA

	Nonbiliary pancreatitis	Biliary pancreatitis
Admission		
Age (y)	>55	>70
WBC count (per mm³)	>16,000	>18,000
Glucose (mg/dL)	>200	>220
LDH (IU/L)	>350	>400
AST (IU/L)	>250	>250
Within 48 hours		
Hematocrit decrease (points)	>10	>10
BUN increase (mg/dL)	>5	>2
Calcium (mg/dL)	<8	<8
Pao₂ (mm Hg)	<60	<60
Base deficit (mEq/L)	>4	>5
Fluid requirement (L)	>6	>4

WBC, white blood cell; LDH, lactate dehydrogenase; AST, aspartate aminotransferase; BUN, blood urea nitrogen; Pao₂, arterial oxygen pressure.

Table 30.5. APACHE II CLASSIFICATION OF SEVERITY OF DISEASE

A. Physiologic variable
Temperature (°C)
MAP (mm Hg)
Pulse
Respirations
PaO_2
Arterial pH
Serum Na^+
Serum K^+
Serum creatinine (mg/dL)
Hematocrit (%)
WBC count
Glasgow Coma Score
Serum HCO_3^- (mmol/L)
B.   Age points
C.   Chronic health points
APACHE II score is equal to A + B + C.

APACHE, acute physiology score and chronic health evaluation; MAP, mean arterial pressure; PaO_2, arterial oxygen pressure.

MANAGEMENT

Specific therapeutics to treat acute pancreatitis are not yet available. Based on newly acquired information about the role of cytokines and other inflammatory mediators during acute pancreatitis, mediator antagonism seems to be the next frontier to explore in the treatment of pancreatitis. The concept of inflammatory mediator blockade capitalizes on the therapeutic window that occurs between the onset of symptoms (prompting hospitalization) and the systemic production of mediators and the resultant dysfunction of distant organs (Fig. 30.6). The beneficial results of using a PAF antagonist (Lexipafant) that were demonstrated in two clinical trials in Europe were not confirmed by a larger multiinstitutional, multinational study that was recently con-

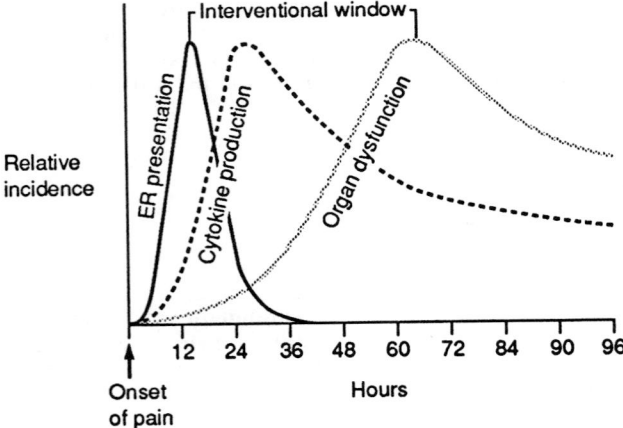

Figure 30.6. Time course of pancreatitis progression demonstrating a therapeutic window for inflammatory mediator antagonism. The majority of patients with acute pancreatitis will present within 18 hours after the onset of pain. This is followed closely by inflammatory cytokine production typically lasting several days. Although distant organ dysfunction is occasionally manifest at the time of presentation, the vast majority of patients develop severe systemic manifestations of pancreatitis 2 to 4 days later. This type of presentation allows for an interventional window during which time specific inflammatory mediator antagonists could be administered to attenuate or block the development of distant organ dysfunction/failure. (From Norman J. Role of cytokines in the pathogenesis of acute pancreatitis. *Am J Surg* 1998:175:76, with permission.)

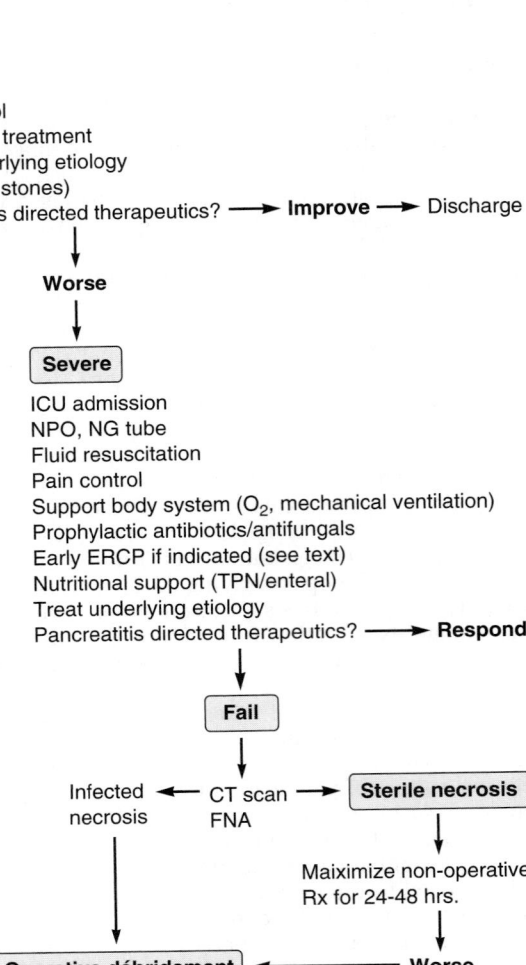

Figure 30.7. Algorithm for the treatment of acute pancreatitis.

cluded. The failure of this particular trial has demonstrated how difficult it is to enroll a large, homogeneous group of patients in a well-controlled study of pancreatitis. Further studies that are planned to address the role of other mediators must take into consideration the valuable lessons learned in these large anti-PAF trials, in which more than 2,000 patients were enrolled.

Currently, treatment in acute pancreatitis is mainly supportive (Fig. 30.7). The term *bowel rest* is misleading and is not based on a current understanding of pancreatitis. The pancreas is in a state of hyperinflammation and autodigestion, and further stimulation by food may be clinically insignificant. In this regard, the treatment of acute pancreatitis has changed during the past decade, with most experts advocating resumption of oral intake as soon as patients can tolerate it. However, patients should be given nothing by mouth until any associated ileus resolves, and in some patients, oral intake may be delayed by persistent or recurrent pain. Routine nasogastric tube decompression should be reserved for patients with severe pancreatitis or those demonstrating signs of gastric outlet obstruction. Aggressive fluid and electrolyte resuscitation should be undertaken to prevent hypovolemia and prerenal azotemia, which is associated with a poor outcome. Serial monitoring of electrolytes and serum glucose is necessary to direct fluid resuscitation. Supplemental oxygen should be administered and mechanical ventilation instituted in the event of respiratory insufficiency. Invasive monitoring should be undertaken as clinical circumstances dictate.

Pain control is an important aspect of management and should be carried out diligently. Narcotics are usually needed, and the theoretical disadvantage of morphine-induced spasm of the sphincter of Oddi has not been shown to be of any clinical significance.

Prophylactic antibiotics are believed to reduce the morbidity and mortality of acute severe pancreatitis and are used by many experts for these severely ill patients (11). Their benefit in acute mild pancreatitis, however, is not well established. Nevertheless, most experts believe that antibiotics should not be given routinely to all patients, but rather on a selective case-by-case basis depending on the severity of the pancreatitis and the presence of necrosis on CT. Imipenem is the antibiotic of choice because of its superior concentration in the pancreatic parenchyma and its ability to cover multiple pathogens. Newer-generation antibiotics with similar penetration in the pancreas have not been evaluated clinically, but they are likely to find a role. Prophylaxis for deep venous thrombosis and stress ulceration is also required.

Nutritional support should be instituted promptly after hemodynamic stability has been established. Because of many considerations, including ileus and fluid and electrolyte shifts, the parenteral route is the most practical one initially. However, enteral feeding should be started as soon as it can be tolerated. The normal increase in pancreatic secretions in response to intravenous lipid infusions has not been shown to worsen the disease process. Once ileus has resolved, the patient can be fed orally or through a jejunal feeding tube. Recent studies have demonstrated that enteral feeding is an important component in maintaining the integrity of the gastrointestinal tract, and patients fed enterally are less susceptible to bacterial translocation and subsequent infection.

Considerable debate surrounds the issue of whether biliary obstruction resulting from choledocholithiasis should be decompressed and whether removal of impacted stones reduces the severity of pancreatitis. This question has been addressed by two prospective, randomized clinical studies, which have demonstrated that endoscopic sphincterotomy can effectively relieve biliary obstruction and reduce the morbidity of biliary sepsis, although its effects on overall mortality from pancreatitis are not as clear. To achieve these outcomes, ERCP should be carried out in the first 24 hours after the onset of severe pancreatitis in an appropriate clinical setting that suggests biliary obstruction. The risk of routine early ERCP outweighs its benefit in most patients with acute biliary pancreatitis.

The concept of reducing pancreatic secretions and inhibiting pancreatic enzymes has been the subject of many trials that failed to demonstrate any clinical benefit from using anticholinergic agents, calcitonin, glucagon, or a somatostatin analogue. With our evolving understanding of the role of inflammatory mediators in propagating the systemic manifestations of acute pancreatitis, it is becoming clear why interventions aimed at reducing pancreatic secretions, rather than the hyperinflammatory response, have failed to improve the outcome of pancreatitis.

Factors precipitating acute pancreatitis should be eliminated regardless of the etiology. Treatment of hyperlipidemia in affected persons should prevent recurrences in most cases. Cholecystectomy for cholelithiasis should be performed in all patients with gallstone pancreatitis. Most surgeons recommend laparoscopic cholecystectomy during the same hospitalization as soon as the pancreatitis has resolved and the patient is nearing discharge. Abstinence from alcohol should reduce the recurrences of alcoholic pancreatitis; however, it is not known why some patients never have another bout while others have recurrent attacks.

Most episodes of acute pancreatitis are mild and resolve with minimal specific interventions; thus, the role of surgery in these patients is limited to correcting any underlying associated biliary tract disease. However, in approximately 2% to 5% of patients, severe pancreatic necrosis develops that may require operative intervention. As with mild forms of pancreatitis, treatment in severe pancreatitis is mainly supportive, as outlined in the algorithm. Because of advances in intensive care, larger numbers of patients survive the initial hemodynamic instability of severe pancreatitis only to suffer the late infectious and systemic complications of the disease. The role of operative treatment in this subset of patients continues to evolve; however, it is generally agreed that operative treatment is indicated for patients in whom infected necrotizing pancreatitis develops or who continue to deteriorate despite maximal nonoperative treatment, whether or not they have infected necrosis. When the development of infected necrosis is suspected, sampling the necrotic areas in the lesser sac via CT-directed fine-needle aspiratation can secure the diagnosis. Other CT findings, such as the presence of extravisceral air, would indicate the need for surgical débridement in the appropriate clinical setting.

The rationale for the operative treatment of necrotizing pancreatitis is the removal of necrotic peripancreatic and pancreatic tissue, which acts as a reservoir for infection and sepsis. This can be accomplished by a necrosectomy, which is the common feature of the various operative approaches. After the initial necrosectomy, surgeons have drained the lesser sac with multiple drains (closed drainage), or lavaged the lesser sac with a large volume of dialysate (closed lavage), or packed the lesser sac through an open abdomen (open packing) (12). Others have adopted a more aggressive approach of repeated planned necrosectomy every 48 hours and closure of the abdominal wall with a zipper, which resulted in a low rate of recurrent abdominal abscesses and incisional hernias (13). The mortality of operative treatment of necrotizing pancreatitis ranges from 7% (closed packing) to 22% (planned necrosectomy); although significant, this mortality rate is still more favorable than the uniformly fatal outcome of untreated infected pancreatic necrosis. It has become clear that in the appropriate clinical setting, postponement of necrosectomy may be associated with a more favorable outcome. Waiting more than 28 days, however, seems to be of no further benefit (14).

Simple percutaneous catheter aspiration or drainage achieves little in the evacuation of thick necrotic material and augments the risk for infection and thus is not recommended. Pancreatic resection and peritonenal lavage have no role in the treatment of necrotizing pancreatitis. The long-term outcome after necrosectomy is characterized by pancreatic insufficiency (endocrine, exocrine, or both) in half of the patients (15).

PANCREATIC PSEUDOCYSTS

Perhaps the most commonly misunderstood term in the study of the pancreas is *pseudocyst*. Pseudocysts of the pancreas most often occur as a result of pancreatitis and disruption of the pancreatic duct. The extravasated pancreatic fluid is walled off by a dense inflammatory reaction in the lesser sac. Thus, the lining of a pseudocyst, which takes weeks to form, consists of nonepithelial granulation tissue and is formed from the surrounding viscera. Pseudocyst fluid invariably contains pancreatic enzymes in high concentrations. Acute collections of peripancreatic fluid that are found within 4 weeks after the onset of

Table 30.6. RESULTS OF PSEUDOCYST DRAINAGE PROCEDURES

Type	Complication rate (%)	Recurrence rate (%)	Mortality rate (%)
Percutaneous aspiration	0	63	0
Percutaneous catheter	16	8	3
Surgical external drainage	35	20–25	7–27
Surgical internal drainage	23–35	5–9	3–9

pancreatitis should not be mistaken for pseudocysts and should not be treated as such.

Pseudocysts occur in fewer than 10% of all patients with acute pancreatitis and are more often associated with alcoholic than with biliary pancreatitis. Multiple pseudocysts are uncommon but can appear as such on CT because they may assume odd shapes.

The natural history of pseudocysts has not been completely elucidated, but it has recently become apparent that not all pseudocysts require operative treatment. Pseudocysts often persist because of continued pancreatitis and more importantly because of a continued disruption of the pancreatic duct. One might assume that once the ductal disruption heals and seals, the fluid in the pseudocyst would be cleared by the body. However, what happens clinically is much more complex and at times not as clear. Symptoms of abdominal pain, nausea, vomiting, or jaundice are caused by compression of adjacent organs.

The treatment of pseudocysts has evolved over the years; at one time, operative drainage was recommended for all pseudocysts larger than 6 cm, but the approach is now more selective. With the widespread use of CT, it became apparent that many acute peripancreatic fluid collections and pseudocysts resolve spontaneously. In two reports of the selective management of pseudocysts, from Johns Hopkins and the Mayo Clinic, nonoperative management was successful in 50% to 60% of asymptomatic patients irrespective of pseudocyst size (16,17). Complications of expectant management occurred in only 9% of patients in one series. These data contrast sharply with the prevailing dictum and support the selective and nonoperative management of patients with asymptomatic pseudocysts. Patients who are treated in this manner should be monitored closely for the development of complications and changes in the character or size of their pseudocysts. It follows that the management of pseudocysts after acute pancreatitis takes into consideration the clinical presentation (symptomatic vs. asymptomatic, presence of complications, resolution of pancreatitis) and the age of the pseudocyst. Because it is impossible to determine the age of a pseudocyst with certainty, 6 weeks is generally allowed between the onset of pancreatitis and elective operative drainage. In that period of time, the pseudocyst wall "matures," meaning that a capsule of granulation tissue develops that allows internal drainage.

Generally, infected pseudocysts are drained externally. Percutaneous drainage is inadequate because the contents are typically too viscous to be drained effectively. Enteric internal drainage of sterile pseudocysts can be achieved by anastomosing the pseudocyst wall to the stomach, jejunum, or duodenum. New endoscopic approaches to drain appropriately located pseudocysts have yielded encouraging results, but the long-term outcome is not known (Table 30.6).

Neoplastic cystic lesions can be mistaken for simple pseudocysts; therefore, a biopsy of the pseudocyst wall should be performed if a clear history of recent pancreatitis cannot be established.

The role of ERCP in the management of pseudocysts after an attack of acute pancreatitis is less clear than its role in chronic pancreatitis. Ductal abnormalities that may change the treatment plan or drainage route can be demonstrated by pancreatography; however, MRCP is quickly evolving as an effective means to address these issues. The role of somatostatin analogue in the management of pancreatic fistulae and pseudocysts is highly controversial and requires further evaluation.

Complications of pseudocysts require prompt treatment. Rupture of a pseudocyst can result in an acute abdomen and may be accompanied by intraabdominal hemorrhage and sepsis. Bleeding into a pseudocyst can result in severe abdominal pain and shock, and emergency angiographic control of the bleeding vessel has become widely accepted. Pancreatic ascites and pleural effusion are more common in chronic pancreatitis and result from a pancreatic ductal disruption that communicates with the abdominal or pleural cavity. Treatment is mainly nonoperative and includes hyperalimentation and aspiration of the accumulated ascitic fluid or effusion. Stenting the pancreatic ductal disruption has improved the outcome of nonoperative treatment.

REFERENCES

1. Bradley EL. A clinically based classification system for acute pancreatitis. *Arch Surgery* 1993;128:586.
2. Norman J. The role of cytokines in the pathogenesis of acute pancreatitis. *Am J Surg* 1998;175:76.
3. Norman J, Fink G, Denham W, et al. Tissue-specific cytokine production during experimental acute pancreatitis: a probable mechanism for distant organ dysfunction. *Dig Dis Sci* 1997;42:1783.
4. de Beaux AC, Ross JA, Maingay JP, et al. Pro-inflammatory cytokine release by peripheral blood mononuclear cells from patients with acute pancreatitis. *Br J Surg* 1996;83:1071.
5. McKay CJ, Gallagher G, Brooks B, et al. Increased monocyte cytokine production in association with systemic complications in acute pancreatitis. *Br J Surg* 1996;83:919.
6. Denham W, Yang J, Norman J, et al. TNF but not IL-1 decreases pancreatic acinar cell survival without affecting exocrine function: a study in the perfused human pancreas. *J Surg Res* 1998;74:3.
7. Ryan S, Sandler A, Trenhaile S, et al. Pancreatic enzyme elevations after blunt trauma. *Surgery* 1994;116:622.
8. Calvien PA, Burgan S, Moosa AR. Serum amylase and other laboratory tests in acute pancreatitis. *Br J Surg* 1989;76:1234.
9. Golloway SW, Kingsnorth AN. Reduction in circulating levels of CD4-positive lymphocytes in acute pancreatitis: relationship to endotoxin, interleukin-6, and disease severity. *Br J Surg* 1994;81:312.
10. Pezilli R, Billi P, Miniero R, et al. Serum interleukin-6, interleukin-8, and beta 2-microglobulin in early assessment of severity of acute pancreatitis: comparison with C-reactive protein. *Dig Dis Sci* 1995;40:2341.
11. Golub R, Siddiqi F, Pohl D. Role of antibiotics in acute pancreatitis: a meta-analysis. *J Gastrointest Surg* 1998;2:496.
12. Uhl W, Büchler MW. Approach to management of necrotizing pancreatitis. *Probl Gen Surg* 1997;13:67.
13. Murr MM, Tsiotos GG, Sarr GM. Operative management of necrotizing pancreatitis by repeated planned necrosectomy and delayed primary closure of the abdominal wall. *Probl Gen Surg* 1997;13:131.
14. Fernandez del-Castillo C, Rattner DW, Makary MA, et al. Débridement and closed packing for the treatment of necrotizing pancreatitis. *Ann Surg* 1998;228:676.
15. Tsiotos GG, Luque-de-leon E, Sarr MG. Long-term outcome of necrotizing pancreatitis treated by necrosectomy. *Br J Surg* 1998;85:1650.

16. Yeo CJ, Bastidas JA, Lynch-Nyham A, et al. The natural history of pancreatic pseudocysts documented by computed tomography. *Surg Gynecol Obstet* 1990;170:411.

17. Vitas GJ, Sarr MG. Selected management of pancreatic pseudocysts: operative versus expectant management. *Surgery* 1992;111:123.

SURGERY: SCIENTIFIC PRINCIPLES AND PRACTICE, Third Edition, edited by Lazar J. Greenfield, Michael W. Mulholland, Keith T. Oldham, Gerald B. Zelenock, and Keith D. Lillemoe. Lippincott Williams & Wilkins Publishers, Philadelphia, © 2001.

CHAPTER 31

CHRONIC PANCREATITIS

KENRIC M. MURAYAMA AND RAYMOND J. JOEHL

Pancreatitis is an inflammatory disorder that encompasses a spectrum of pancreatic derangement. Although numerous attempts have been made to classify and subdivide the types of pancreatitis, at present the disease should be categorized simply as acute or chronic, with each type being subject to acute exacerbations. Acute pancreatitis is characterized by clinical and histologic improvement after the underlying cause has been treated or removed; conversely, the changes of chronic pancreatitis are persistent and progressive. Chronic pancreatitis is characterized by pancreatic exocrine and endocrine insufficiency and suggests irreversible and chronic damage; however, subclinical parenchymal changes are likely to be present long before this occurs. Destruction of the pancreatic parenchyma and fibrosis of the gland are characteristic, and these lead to strictures of the pancreatic duct, dilations, and calcifications. Although numerous attempts to classify chronic pancreatitis have been made, the wide range of presentations has made classification difficult.

Most epidemiologic information about chronic pancreatitis has been obtained from retrospective data, and therefore the exact incidence and prevalence are unknown. However, autopsy data suggest that prevalence ranges from 0.04% (1) to 5% (2). The only prospective evaluation of chronic pancreatitis, performed in Denmark, demonstrated an incidence of 8.2 cases per 100,000 and a prevalence of 26.4 cases per 100,000 (3). Alcohol consumption is the most important predisposing factor for chronic pancreatitis, and therefore the incidence and prevalence of the disease are partly related to the rate of alcohol intake in a population. Interestingly, although alcohol consumption contributes to the disease, it is but one of many associated factors. As an example, alcohol consumption is higher in Sweden than in Denmark, but the incidence of chronic pancreatitis is higher in Denmark, which suggests that environmental and hereditary factors are also important.

ETIOLOGY

The causes of chronic pancreatitis are numerous. Alcohol abuse is responsible for 70% to 80% of cases in developed countries. Interestingly, although the pathologic lesions (loss of acinar cell mass, parenchymal fibrosis, inflammatory cell infiltration, and intraductal lithiasis) are remarkably similar regardless of the cause, the relationship between these lesions and the pathophysiology of the disease is uncertain.

Alcoholic Pancreatitis

Although alcohol is the major cause of chronic pancreatitis, the mechanism of injury is not known. The type of alcohol and the manner of consumption do not seem to correlate with disease severity, but the severity of chronic pancreatitis does appear to increase with the amount and duration of alcohol consumption (4). Additionally, susceptibility and disease severity appear to vary significantly between individual people, and chronic pancreatitis can progress even after the cessation of alcohol consumption. Chronic pancreatitis develops in only 10% of alcoholics, but autopsy series reveal an incidence of chronic pancreatitis that is 50 times greater in alcoholics than in nondrinking controls.

The mechanisms of alcohol-induced cellular injury are unknown, but inferences can be drawn by examining the effects of alcohol on pancreatic secretion. It appears that long-term alcohol intake causes changes in the composition of pancreatic juice, including increased protein concentration, decreased flow, and decreased bicarbonate concentration (5). These changes produce a juice with increased viscosity that is prone to forming stones and protein plugs. Ductal obstruction produces progressive injury and destruction of parenchyma, with a deterioration of both exocrine and endocrine function.

Hereditary Pancreatitis

Hereditary pancreatitis is one of the most fascinating forms of chronic pancreatitis. A point mutation of the cationic trypsinogen gene on chromosome 7 has been identified as the cause (6). The genetic defect is inherited as an autosomal dominant disorder with a penetrance of 80% (7). The mutation interferes with one of the regulatory mechanisms of trypsin deactivation, so that "longer-acting" trypsin is able to autodigest the pancreas. Approximately 80% of persons with the mutation exhibit the phenotype and become symptomatic at an average age of 10 to 12 years. Although the effects of identifying a genetic cause for one type of chronic pancreatitis have yet to be fully realized, the prospect for future gene therapy is real.

Nutritional Pancreatitis

The pathophysiology of nutritional pancreatitis, otherwise known as *tropical pancreatitis,* is poorly understood, except that it is probably related to chronic malnutrition. In tropical Africa and much of Asia, this is the most common form of chronic pancreatitis, which typically affects children (8). Endocrine and exocrine insufficiency is generally present by adolescence, and death frequently ensues by early adulthood. The exact cause is unknown, but protein-calorie malnutrition and deficiencies in zinc, copper, and selenium may contribute. Recently, the cassava fruit, which is common in the diet of many tropical cultures, has been implicated because it contains toxic glycosides that are converted to cyanogens when exposed to hydrochloric acid. Cyanogens can subsequently inhibit a variety of antioxidant enzymes, and it is therefore postulated that ingestion of cassava leads to injury of the pancreas by unopposed free radicals (9).

Obstruction-induced Pancreatitis

Obstruction of the main pancreatic duct by strictures, scars, tumors, or pseudocysts leads to a distinct form of chronic pancreatitis characterized by acinar atrophy and fibrosis. In contrast to alcohol-induced chronic pancreatitis, obstruction-induced pancreatitis is rarely associated with the formation of intraductal stones, and parenchymal changes may regress with relief of the obstruction. Additionally, the pancreatic duct proximal to the obstruction is diffusely dilated; in contrast, segmental ductal stricture and dilation are characteristic of the other forms of chronic pancreatitis.

Hyperparathyroidism

Pancreatitis develops in approximately 10% to 15% of patients with hyperparathyroidism, and if inadequately treated, it becomes chronic, presumably as a result of the effects of persistent hypercalcemia (10). Calcium is a potent stimulator of pancreatic exocrine secretion. An increase in the concentration of calcium in pancreatic juice leads to intraductal precipitation (11).

Pancreas Divisum

Pancreas divisum, the most common congenital abnormality of the pancreas (4% to 11% of the population), results from incomplete or absent fusion of the ducts of the ventral and dorsal pancreas in embryologic development. It is postulated that the minor papilla is inadequate to handle all the exocrine secretion from the main body of the gland, so that the main duct becomes relatively obstructed. Whether or not pancreas divisum can cause chronic pancreatitis remains controversial. In an early report by Cotton (12), the incidence of pancreas divisum on endoscopic retrograde cholangiopancreatography (ERCP) was 25.6% in patients with idiopathic pancreatitis and only 3.6% in patients undergoing ERCP for biliary tract disease. More recently, however, several studies have found the incidence of pancreas divisum to be similar in patients with and without pancreatitis (13).

Traumatic Pancreatitis

Blunt and penetrating trauma to the pancreas can lead to pancreatic injury. Parenchymal injury with duct disruption can lead to the formation of pseudocysts, pancreatic ascites, and pancreatic fistulae. Additionally, injury to the blood supply of the pancreas may result in ischemia and stricture of the pancreatic duct. Inadequate or delayed treatment can lead to persistent injury and ultimately chronic pancreatitis.

Idiopathic Pancreatitis

The majority of cases of nonalcoholic chronic pancreatitis in North America and Europe is idiopathic (10% to 40% of cases), and these can be divided into two broad groups with a bimodal age distribution. The juvenile type generally begins in the teenage years, and the predominant presenting symptom is pain. In the senile type of idiopathic pancreatitis, the age of onset is most commonly between 50 and 60 years, and the disease is often painless, presenting only after the changes of exocrine insufficiency and calcification appear (14). This group of patients with chronic pancreatitis underscores our lack of understanding regarding the pathophysiology of the disease.

CLINICAL PRESENTATION

Pain

Patients with chronic pancreatitis most commonly present with constant pain that is usually epigastric and dull and radiates to the back (Fig. 31.1). Frequently, sitting upright and tilting the torso forward or lying prone alleviates the discomfort, whereas the supine position tends to ag-

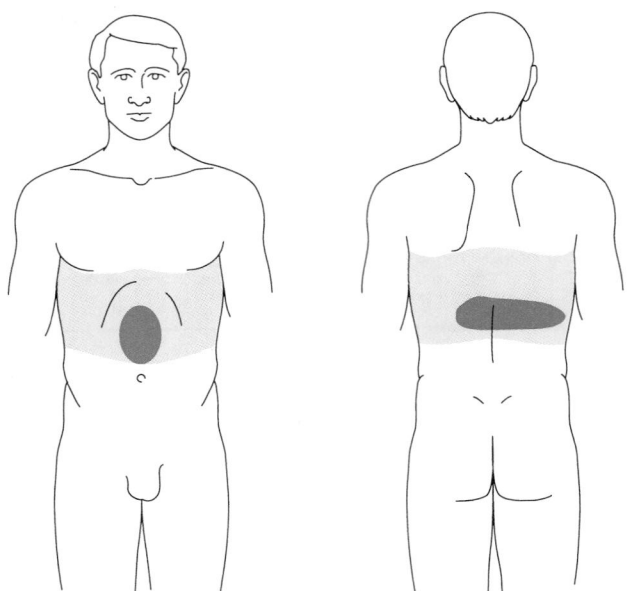

Figure 31.1. Topographic locations of pancreatic pain.

gravate the discomfort. The pain may continue, decrease, or disappear completely, and it has been reported that the pain actually diminishes as the disease worsens as a consequence of mechanisms that remain unclear (15,16). Pain is most often the complaint that brings a patient with chronic pancreatitis to a physician, and it often leads to absence from work, frequent hospitalization, and narcotic addiction.

The pathophysiology of the pain associated with chronic pancreatitis is poorly understood, but several explanations have been proposed, including increased intrapancreatic and intraductal pressures, neural inflammation, and associated conditions such as pseudocysts, bile duct strictures, and duodenal obstruction. The pain of chronic pancreatitis may be related to the increase in intraductal and parenchymal pressures resulting from continued exocrine secretion with persistent duct obstruction. As a corollary, a decrease in pain is usually experienced with the onset of pancreatic insufficiency in patients with chronic alcoholic pancreatitis. Bradley (17) demonstrated that in 19 patients with pain and elevated intraductal pancreatic pressures, the pain was relieved after a duct decompression procedure. In addition, patients with pain and dilated pancreatic ducts or pseudocysts have higher interstitial pancreatic pressures; these are decreased after duct decompression or cyst drainage, with a resulting decrease in pain (18).

Parenchymal pancreatic nerves appear to be larger and more numerous in patients with chronic pancreatitis. The intracellular organelles of these neurons appear abnormal, and damage to the perineural protective sheath is apparent (19). Theoretically, this breach in the perineurium permits noxious stimuli to reach the neurons and cause pain. Additionally, pain may result from the degranulation of perineural inflammatory cells (e.g., eosinophils) (20).

Inflammation of surrounding tissues and organs, such as the retroperitoneum and duodenum, may contribute to the pain of chronic pancreatitis. Continued or recurrent inflammation of the head of the pancreas may result in duodenal narrowing and, more commonly, stenosis and obstruction of the distal common bile duct, both of which can be associated with abdominal pain.

Malabsorption

With sufficient loss of functional exocrine pancreas, diarrhea, steatorrhea, and azotorrhea can develop. Because of the 10-fold reserve of exocrine pancreatic enzymes, malabsorption occurs only after more than 90% of the functioning exocrine cell mass is lost (21). Pancreatic insufficiency resulting from alcohol-induced chronic pancreatitis usually takes 10 to 20 years to develop. The secretion of lipase is usually diminished earlier than the secretion of the proteolytic enzymes, and as a result, steatorrhea generally precedes proteinaceous diarrhea. Patients with fat malabsorption report loose, greasy, and foul-smelling stools associated with cramping abdominal pain and excessive flatus. Weight loss almost always occurs with malabsorption, and occasionally significant deficiencies of the fat-soluble vitamins develop. In general, however, clinically important vitamin deficiencies are relatively uncommon, although body stores of the fat-soluble vitamins may be diminished. Postprandial pancreatic bicarbonate secretion is similarly diminished in long-standing, severe chronic pancreatitis. The duodenal pH may decrease (pH < 4) within 90 minutes after ingestion of a meal, and when the bicarbonate concentration is inadequate, an acidic milieu with precipitation of bile salts and inactivation of pancreatic enzymes results in a further decrease in lipid and protein digestion.

Although persistent malabsorption inevitably results in weight loss, many patients with chronic pancreatitis experience significant weight loss before the onset of malabsorption. Patients with chronic pancreatitis usually decrease their caloric intake significantly to avoid exacerbating abdominal pain. Because weight loss is fairly unusual in most other painful abdominal conditions, the combination of chronic upper abdominal pain and significant weight loss should suggest a pancreatic process, such as chronic pancreatitis.

Endocrine Insufficiency

Although the derangement of pancreatic exocrine function is the most common clinical concern in chronic pancreatitis, glucose intolerance frequently develops early in the course of chronic pancreatitis, and clinically evident diabetes occurs later (Table 31.1). Altered insulin secretion is observed in these patients, as is a blunted insulin and C-peptide response to oral or intravenous glucose. Endocrine insufficiency develops in up to 60% of patients, but in general not until after the diagnosis of chronic pancreatitis has been made. Diabetic ketoacidosis and nephropathy are rare, but diabetic neuropathy and

retinopathy can occur in chronic pancreatitis-associated diabetes if the patient lives long enough.

DIAGNOSIS

The clinical history suggests the diagnosis of chronic pancreatitis. Numerous tests have been described to aid in making the diagnosis, but most are of limited clinical value. An important caveat is that most of the standard modalities used to make the diagnosis are effective, with good sensitivity and specificity if moderate to severe disease is present. However, the ideal test would permit chronic pancreatitis to be diagnosed at an earlier stage and would be effective in differentiating between the changes of chronic pancreatitis and those of pancreatic adenocarcinoma. Tests of blood or serum are usually of little help, and frequently the diagnosis can be made on the basis of the history and simple radiographs.

Routine Laboratory Findings

Although anemia secondary to malnutrition can occur in chronic pancreatitis, it is much less common than in other malabsorptive disorders, such as celiac disease. Deficiencies of the fat-soluble vitamins secondary to the steatorrhea of chronic pancreatitis are also uncommon. Leukocytosis can occur during acute exacerbations of chronic pancreatitis, but if it develops without such an exacerbation, investigation for another source should be initiated.

Serum amylase and lipase concentrations may be elevated in chronic pancreatitis, but they are generally normal or low except in the presence of an acute exacerbation. Even during an acute attack with seemingly significant abdominal pain, the amylase and lipase levels may be only slightly elevated because of depletion of the exocrine pancreatic parenchyma. In contrast, acute pancreatitis in patients without chronic pancreatitis is often associated with significantly elevated amylase and lipase levels.

Abnormalities of liver function, manifested by elevations in the liver enzymes, may be a result of either coexistent liver disease or obstruction of the common bile duct. Obstruction of the common bile duct in chronic pancreatitis may be secondary to the fibrotic process or may result from extrinsic compression by a pseudocyst or mass in the head of the pancreas. Although liver disease is frequently associated with alcoholism, the pattern of liver enzyme elevations is usually different from that seen with obstruction of the common duct. The presence of an obstructive pattern of the liver enzyme abnormalities warrants further investigation to identify the cause, primarily to exclude a concomitant pancreatic malignancy and determine the best method for bile duct decompression.

Tests of Pancreatic Exocrine Function

Tests of pancreatic exocrine function fall into two categories. The first group directly measures exocrine function, and the second group evaluates the secondary effects of impaired enzyme secretion.

Direct measurements of pancreatic exocrine function require the collection and assay of one or more components of pancreatic juice. Earlier attempts at this required collection of enteric contents in the duodenum or proximal jejunum; however, results were inaccurate because of the difficulties involved in collecting a consistent percentage of the luminal contents. More recently, direct endoscopic cannulation of the pancreatic duct has made the collection of pure pancreatic juice more feasible, although this pro-

---

Table 31.1. **HORMONAL AND METABOLIC ASPECTS OF PANCREATIC DIABETES, IDDM, AND NIDDM**

	Pancreatic diabetes	IDDM	NIDDM
Insulin secretion	↓↓	↓↓↓	↓
Insulin sensitivity	N	↓	↓↓
Glucagon secretion	↓↓	↑/↓	↑/↓
Plasma amino acids	↑↑	↑ or N	↑ or N
Ketosis-prone	↑↑	↑↑↑	↑
Glucose counterregulation	↓	N or ↓	N or ↓
Lipids	N	↑	↑↑

↑, increased; ↓, decreased; N, normal; IDDM, insulin-dependent diabetes mellitus; NIDDM, non–insulin-dependent diabetes mellitus. Adapted from Sjoberg RJ, Kidd GS. Pancreatic diabetes mellitus. Diabetes Care 1989;12:715, with permission.

cedure is invasive and uncomfortable. A number of pancreatic juice components have been evaluated, and studies suggest that all the components are equally depressed in chronic pancreatitis, and that no advantage is derived by assaying any one particular component. Moreover, none of the components differentiates chronic pancreatitis from pancreatic cancer.

In humans, the basal secretory rate of the pancreas is extremely variable, and meaningful measurement of exocrine function requires some form of pancreatic stimulation. The most common methods to stimulate the pancreas directly include the administration of secretin, cholecystokinin (CCK), or bombesin, none of which seems to be superior to the others. Indirect stimulation can be achieved by feeding a standard meal (Lundh test), although this method is thought to be inferior to direct stimulation.

Decreased levels of pancreatic enzymes and bicarbonate in pancreatic juice are considered to be the most sensitive indicators of chronic pancreatitis, provided pancreatic carcinoma can be excluded. Unfortunately, pancreatic tissue is rarely obtained to verify the diagnosis and determine severity, so these measurements of pancreatic juice are most accurate in the presence of severe disease. Additionally, the direct measurement of pancreatic exocrine function is unreliable in patients with concomitant diabetes mellitus or cirrhosis. Because of patient discomfort and the inability to diagnose early disease consistently, and because relatively few centers perform the necessary studies, direct measurements of exocrine function are not commonly performed.

Most of the indirect tests of pancreatic exocrine function measure the absorption of a compound that first must be digested by pancreatic enzymes. Unfortunately, malabsorption does not become detectable until pancreatic secretion has diminished to less than 10% of normal, and therefore the indirect tests of pancreatic exocrine function cannot detect early chronic pancreatitis. Interestingly, most of the indirect tests were first evaluated in patients with severe chronic pancreatitis and normal controls. The tests appeared promising until they were performed in patients with less severe disease, in whom the results were found to be much less sensitive and specific than originally thought.

In the bentiromide test, the patient ingests N-benzoyl-L-tyrosyl-p-aminobenzoic acid (NBT-PABA), which is digested by chymotrypsin to release PABA. Free PABA is absorbed in the small intestine and is excreted by the kidney. The quantity of excreted PABA is a measure of pancreatic exocrine function. The sensitivity of the bentiromide test is directly related to disease severity; in patients with end-stage chronic pancreatitis, the test can be almost 100% sensitive, but in patients with mild disease, the test may only be 40% to 50% sensitive. In addition, the test can be inaccurate in the presence of coexistent diabetes mellitus, renal insufficiency, liver disease, or malabsorption states. The bentiromide test may be most useful in determining the severity of the chronic pancreatitis, not in making the diagnosis.

Malabsorption of fat occurs in patients with significant chronic pancreatitis, and several tests have been directed at detecting this defect. Most of them involve ingestion of the triglyceride [^{14}C]olein. Subsequently, the [^{14}C]olein is hydrolyzed, and the breakdown product, [^{14}C]oleate, is absorbed, with resultant production and pulmonary excretion of carbon dioxide C 14. The level of carbon dioxide C 14 in the exhaled gas is a simple measure of triglyceride digestion.

Imaging Studies

Imaging studies have essentially replaced both direct and indirect tests of pancreatic function in making the diagnosis of chronic pancreatitis. These can be divided into non-invasive and invasive studies. Noninvasive studies include plain abdominal roentgenography, transabdominal ultrasonography, computed tomography (CT), and, more recently, magnetic resonance imaging (MRI). Invasive studies that have been used to aid in making the diagnosis of chronic pancreatitis include endoscopic retrograde pancreatography (ERP) and endoscopic ultrasonography (EUS).

The presence of diffuse, speckled pancreatic calcifications is diagnostic of chronic pancreatitis; however, calcification is not a predictor of functional reserve. Although the sensitivity of this finding is only 30% to 40% in chronic pancreatitis, plain abdominal roentgenography should be the first diagnostic test performed because it obviates the need for other tests.

Transabdominal ultrasonography is the simplest and least invasive of the remaining noninvasive tests. Additionally, ultrasonography has a sensitivity of 60% to 70% and a specificity of 80% to 90%. Ultrasonographic findings of a dilated main pancreatic duct (> 4 mm), large cavitary dilations (> 1 cm), and calcifications correlate well with changes seen on ERCP and confirm the diagnosis of chronic pancreatitis (22).

Computed tomography is up to 20% more sensitive than ultrasonography for making the diagnosis of chronic pancreatitis; however, the specificity of the studies is roughly equal. The most common findings include duct dilation (Fig. 31.2), calcifications, and cystic lesions (Fig. 31.3). CT frequently detects pancreatic calcifications missed by other imaging modalities, and recent technologic advances have increased the accuracy of CT in making the diagnosis of chronic pancreatitis.

Magnetic resonance imaging can produce detailed images of the pancreas without ionizing radiation, and recent improvements in image acquisition times have decreased the motion artifacts that previously limited the value of MRI of the pancreas. The image of the pancreatic duct system can be reconstructed by using a heavily T$_2$-weighted scan. Magnetic resonance cholangiopancreatography is proving to be useful as an alternative to ERCP (23), especially in patients with a disrupted main pancreatic duct, contrast allergy, or an inaccessible pancreatic papilla.

Invasive imaging is performed as an adjunct to upper gastrointestinal endoscopy. ERP has become the "gold standard" for making the diagnosis of chronic pancreatitis (Fig. 31.4) It is widely recognized as the most sensitive (90%) diagnostic test, with an equally good specificity (90%). In moderate to severe chronic pancreatitis, the de-

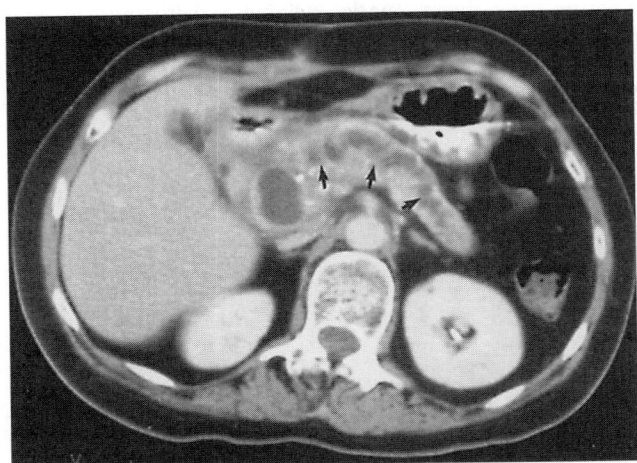

Figure 31.2. Abdominal computed tomography in a patient with chronic pancreatitis shows dilatation of the main pancreatic duct *(arrows)*.

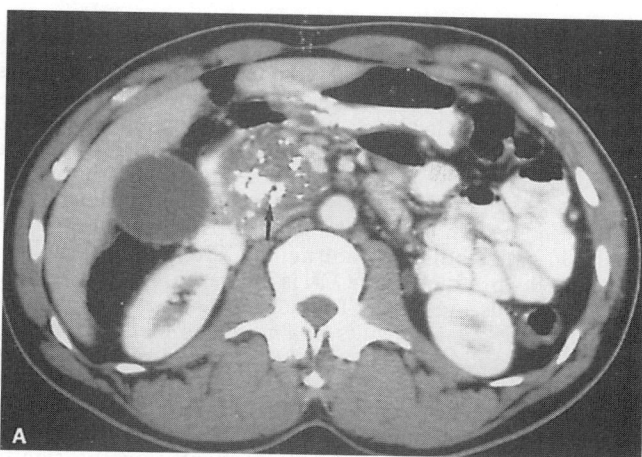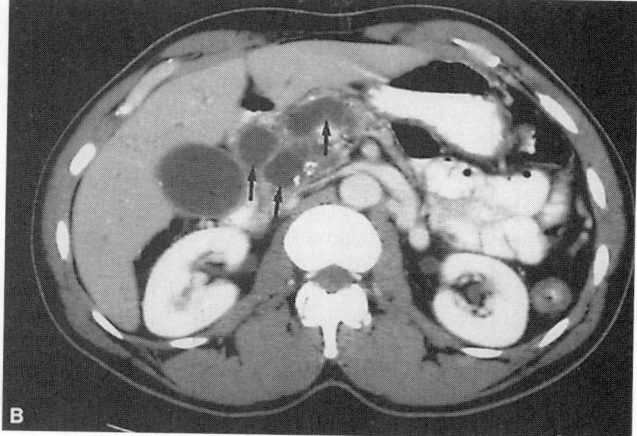

Figure 31.3. Abdominal computed tomography demonstrates pancreatic calcifications *(arrow, A)* and associated cystic lesions *(arrows, B).*

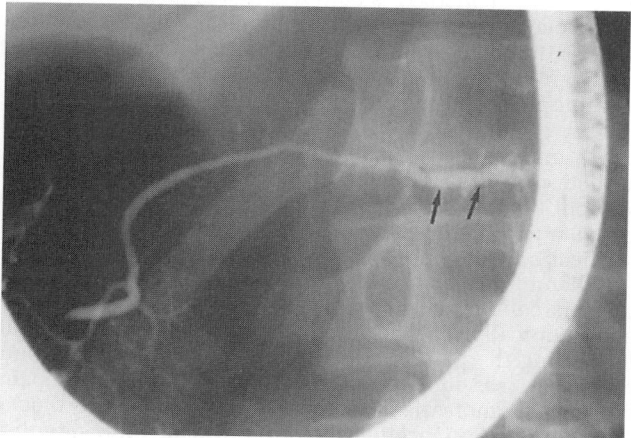

Figure 31.4. Endoscopic retrograde cholangiopancreatography illustrates early changes of chronic pancreatitis, with ductal ectasia confined to the pancreatic tail *(arrows).*

gree of ductal distortion (Figs. 31.5 and 31.6) correlates strongly with functional pancreatic reserve and histologic grade (24). Unfortunately, the correlation is poor with milder ERP grades of chronic pancreatitis (24). The specificity of ERP is extremely high in advanced chronic pancreatitis, but with less severe disease, the peripheral duct abnormalities (stricture, ectasia, and dilation) associated with chronic pancreatitis are relatively nonspecific. Although ERP provides valuable information, particularly in patients for whom surgical treatment of chronic pancreatitis is being considered, it is costly and requires technical expertise. In addition, ERP is associated with an overall risk for induction of acute pancreatitis of up to 4% and should be used only if the results will conceivably alter the treatment plan or help identify a complication.

Endoscopic ultrasonography is a relatively new technology that is being used to aid in making the diagnosis of chronic pancreatitis with increasing frequency. The diagnostic criteria with EUS include a hyperechogenic parenchymal focus, hyperechogenic stranding, glandular lobularity, pancreatic cysts, ductal dilation, and pancreatic stones. The use of endoscopic high-frequency ultrasonographic probes permits imaging of the pancreas

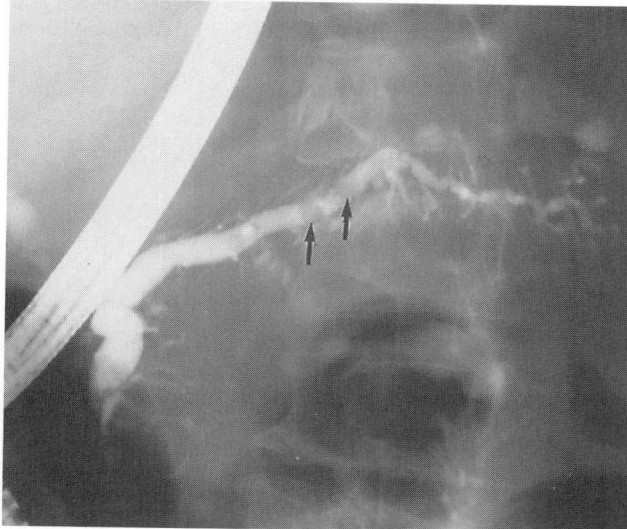

Figure 31.5. Endoscopic retrograde cholangiopancreatography illustrates moderate dilation of the main pancreatic duct and ectasia of the secondary ducts associated with moderately advanced chronic pancreatitis. *Arrows* indicate intraductal pancreatic stones.

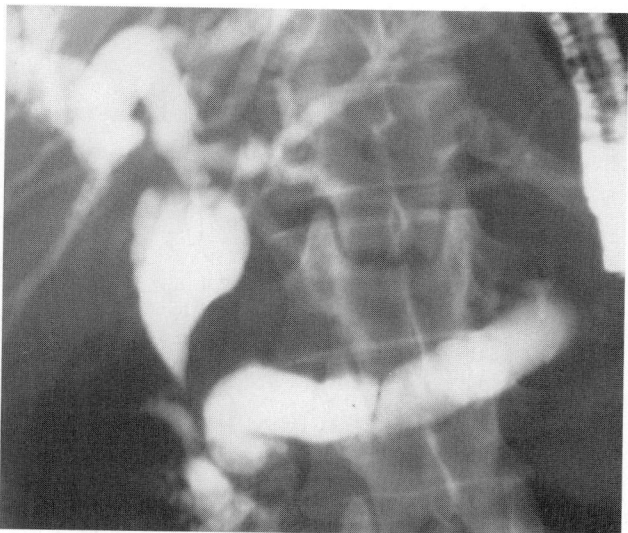

Figure 31.6. Endoscopic retrograde cholangiopancreatography demonstrates florid pancreatic ductal dilatation associated with end-stage chronic pancreatitis.

through the walls of the duodenum and stomach without interference from intestinal gas. Although EUS appears to be as effective as other imaging modalities in making the diagnosis of moderate to severe chronic pancreatitis, its utility in identifying mild pancreatic changes has yet to be determined.

TREATMENT

Unfortunately, the management of patients with chronic pancreatitis is aimed at the treatment of complications rather than the prevention of disease progression. The two most frequent sequelae requiring treatment are chronic pain and malabsorption, but pseudocysts, pancreatic ascites and fistulae, biliary tract complications, and vascular complications can occur and often require intervention.

Pain

The most frequent complication of chronic pancreatitis for which patients seek medical care is intractable pain. Our understanding of the mechanism for this pain is incomplete, but it is likely multifactorial. The commonly hypothesized mechanisms, one or all of which may be involved, include inflammation, duct obstruction, encasement of parenchymal pancreatic sensory nerves, inflammatory injury to neural sheaths, and elevated intraductal pressures. It is generally believed that pain subsides as organ "burnout" occurs, but the amount of time necessary for this to happen is extremely variable, and some believe that spontaneous pain relief is unlikely (25). In fact, in a study by Lankisch et al. (26), even with exocrine insufficiency requiring enzyme replacement, 54% of alcoholics and 73% of nonalcoholics still experienced significant pain.

If alcohol abuse is the cause of chronic pancreatitis, the treatment of pain should begin with abstinence. Alcohol acts as a pancreatic secretagogue, and if patients have significant residual exocrine function, pain may be provoked or exacerbated by alcohol intake. Conversely, in patients with little remaining exocrine function, levels of secretion and pain do not vary with alcohol intake. Although some report up that up to 75% of alcoholic patients with chronic pancreatitis experience at least partial relief with abstinence (27), others report no greater likelihood of pain relief (28). Warshaw et al. (25) concluded that spontaneous pain relief is unreliable and that telling patients with

chronic pancreatitis and severe pain to wait for this to happen may be unreasonable advice.

The administration of oral pancreatic pancreatic enzymes is thought to relieve pain by inhibiting the pancreas through negative feedback (Fig. 31.7). Normally, pancreatic trypsin denatures a CCK-releasing factor (CCK-RF) in the duodenum and prevents continued hormonal stimulation of the exocrine pancreas. It is theorized that because of the decreased secretion of pancreatic trypsin in patients with chronic pancreatitis, denaturing of CCK-RF is insufficient. In turn, the production of CCK is increased, and so exocrine stimulation is increased. The administration of exogenous pancreatic enzymes results in a more complete breakdown of CCK-RF and diminishes the subsequent release of CCK (29). Six prospective, randomized trials have been published in which the benefit of exogenous oral enzyme replacement was examined (25). Unfortunately, because of the heterogeneous population of patients and the significant placebo effect in the studies, it is difficult to draw conclusions about the benefits of this form of therapy. In summary, the role of pancreatic enzyme replacement therapy to treat chronic pancreatitis pain remains unclear.

The mainstay of medical therapy for the pain of chronic pancreatitis is the administration of analgesics. Generally, treatment begins with non-narcotic analgesics, such as acetaminophen and nonsteroidal agents; the doses and frequency of administration should be increased before narcotics are prescribed. Once narcotics become necessary, addiction is almost inevitable, and the evaluation of subsequent treatment is extremely difficult. It is common for patients with chronic pancreatitis to request narcotic pain medication from multiple physicians.

Celiac plexus blockade can be performed surgically, either via celiotomy or laparoscopy under CT guidance, or endoscopically. This form of therapy has been beneficial in treating the pain resulting from pancreatic cancer, but results are less consistent when it is used to treat the pain of chronic pancreatitis. The benefit of celiac plexus blockade in this group rarely lasts for more than a few months, and repeated treatments are not as effective (30).

Endoscopic therapy has been used to treat the pain of chronic pancreatitis when it is related to pancreatic duct narrowing or blockage resulting from pancreatic duct stones, strictures, or papillary stenosis. If a stricture is present, endoscopic dilation and stent placement can be successfully performed in more than 80% of patients, with re-

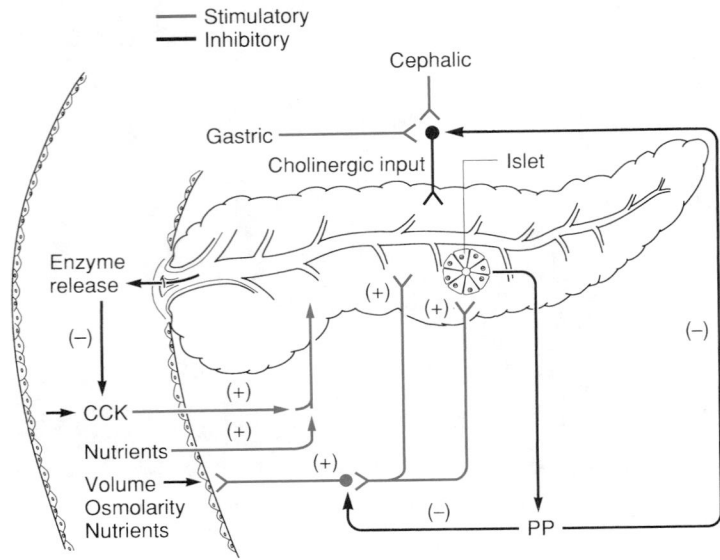

Figure 31.7. Schematic diagram of stimulatory and inhibitory influences on pancreatic exocrine secretion. CCK, cholecystokinin; PP, pancreatic polypeptide.

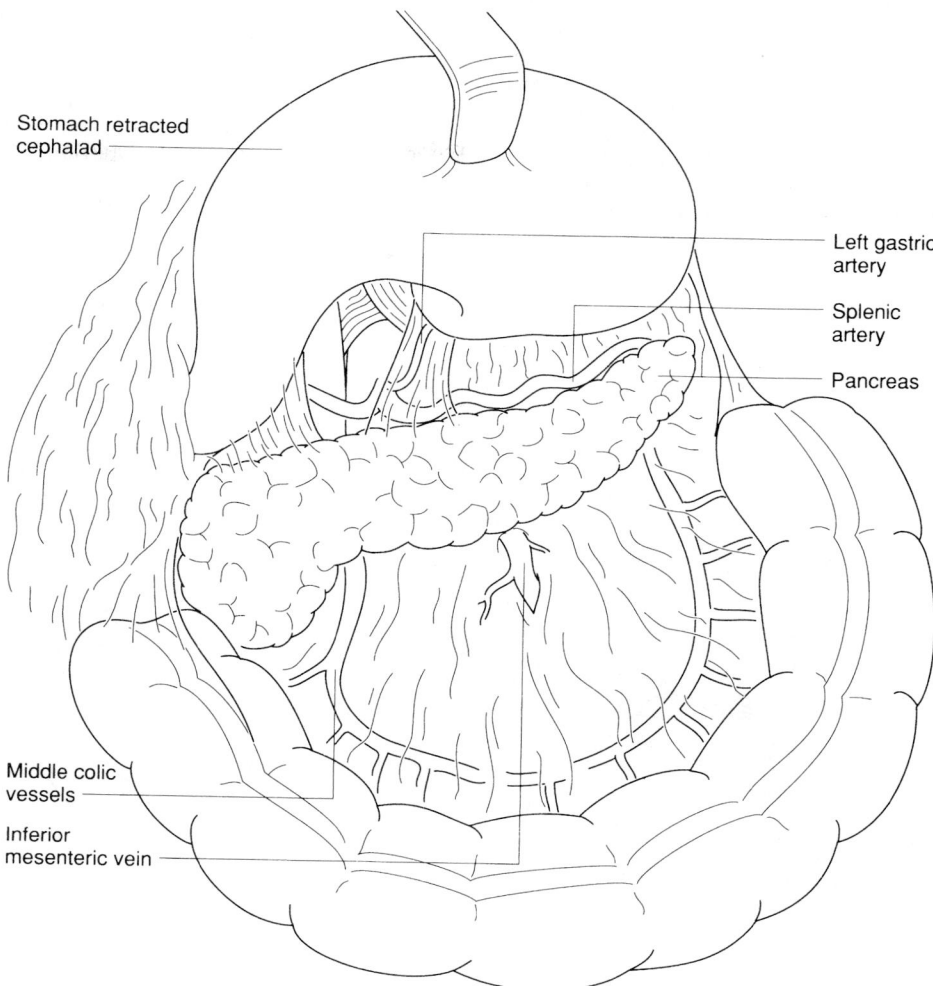

Figure 31.8. Exposure of the anterior surface of the pancreas through the lesser sac.

lief of pain in 55% to 100% during 8 to 39 years of follow-up (31). Unfortunately, significant ductal or parenchymal injury occurs in 50% to 80% of patients when polyethylene stents are placed endoscopically in the pancreatic duct (25), and the injury resolves in only two thirds of these patients after stent removal (32). Occasionally, relief of pain after short-term stent drainage is used to identify patients who will benefit from surgical drainage of the pancreatic duct.

Surgery is indicated for several reasons in patients with chronic pancreatitis, but pain is the most common. Patients being considered for surgery must have failed medical management of their pain, and their pancreatic anatomy must be completely delineated. Operations to relieve the pain of chronic pancreatitis can be divided into two categories: drainage procedures for patients with ductal dilation and obstruction, and resective procedures for patients with a diseased pancreas but normal ductal size. The long-term postoperative relief of pain is the standard by which all operations for chronic pancreatitis are measured.

Drainage Procedures

Longitudinal Pancreaticojejunostomy (Puestow Procedure). In the presence of a dilated main pancreatic duct (> 7 mm), longitudinal pancreaticojejunostomy is the most commonly performed operation. The gastrocolic ligament is divided to access the lesser sac, and the entire anterior surface of the pancreas is exposed (Fig. 31.8). The main pancreatic duct is identified by palpation of a soft central area in the body of the gland representing the duct or by in-

traoperative ultrasonography. A 25-gauge needle can be placed into the duct and pancreatic fluid can be aspirated to confirm the duct location. Duct size is important because pain will be relieved in 65% to 80% of patients after longitudinal pancreaticojejunostomy if the duct is wider than 7

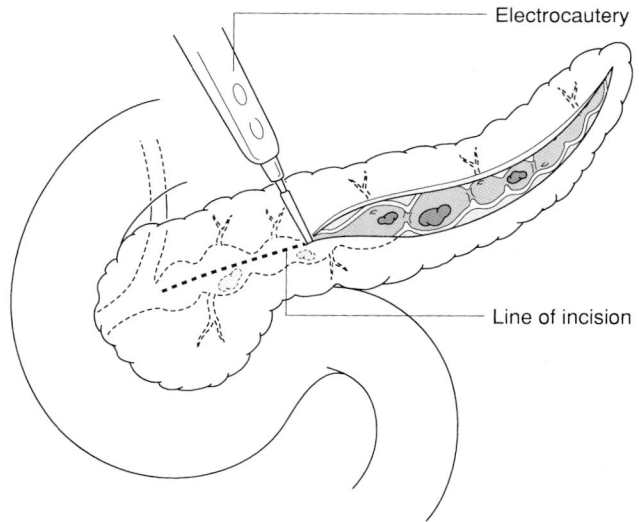

Figure 31.9. Longitudinal incision of the main pancreatic duct in preparation for lateral pancreaticojejunostomy.

mm. If the operation is performed with a smaller duct, the long-term patency rate of the anastomosis is decreased. The pancreas is opened longitudinally, and pancreatic duct stones are removed. The main pancreatic duct is opened (Fig. 31.9) as far into the head as possible (preferably to within 1 cm of the duodenum) to ensure that segments of the duct do not remain undrained. A standard Roux-en-Y loop of jejunum is created, and an anastomosis is made between the Roux limb and the length of the opened pancre-

atic duct (Fig. 31.10). The anastomosis can be made with either a single- or double-layer interrupted technique according to the surgeon's preference. Immediate pain relief with the longitudinal pancreaticojejunostomy can be expected in more than 80% of patients. Operative mortality is less than 5%. Unfortunately, pain recurs in 25% to 50% of patients within 5 years (Fig. 31.11). The remaining pancreatic exocrine and endocrine function can be preserved because no pancreatic tissue is resected.

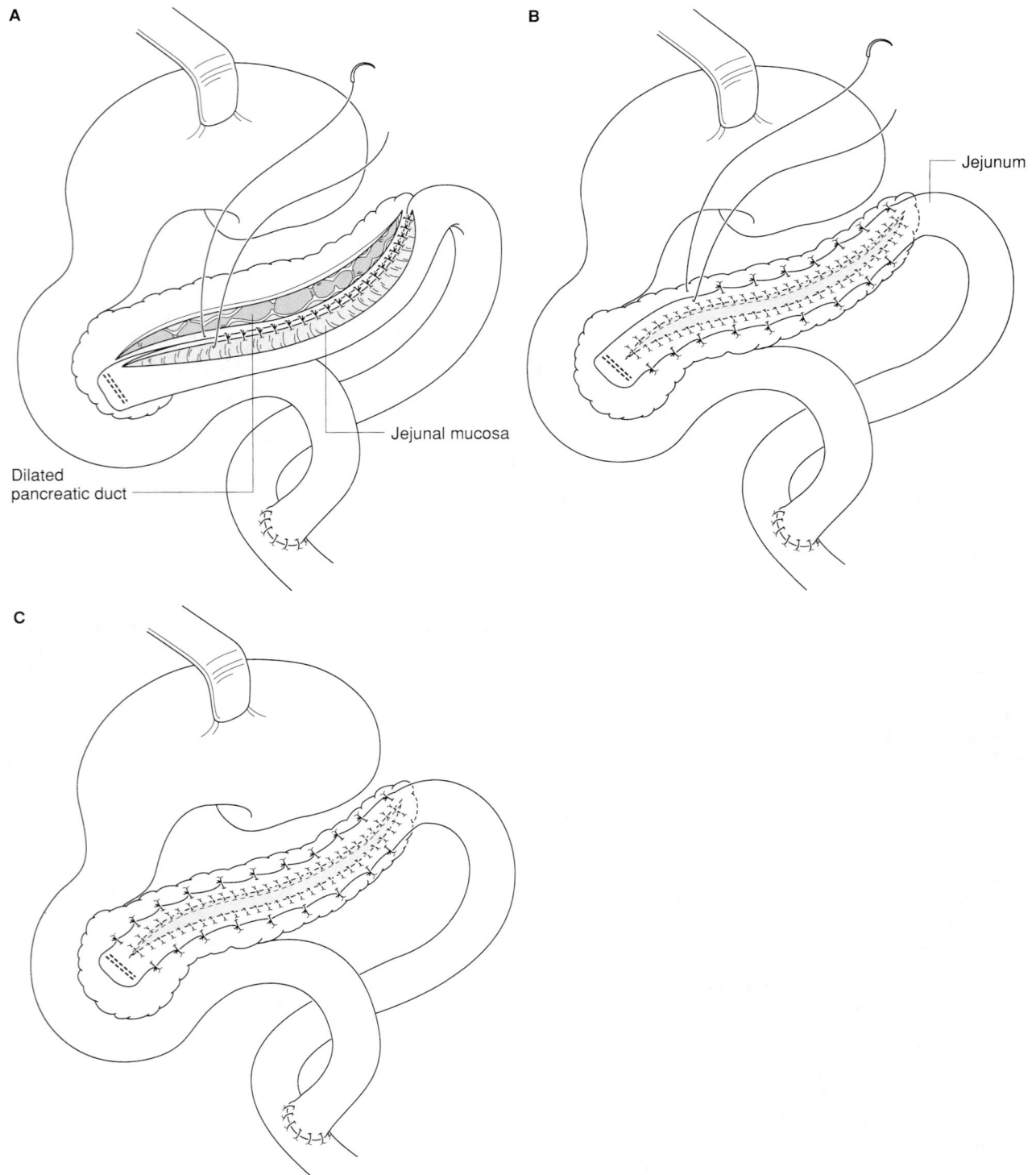

Figure 31.10. Lateral pancreaticojejunostomy.

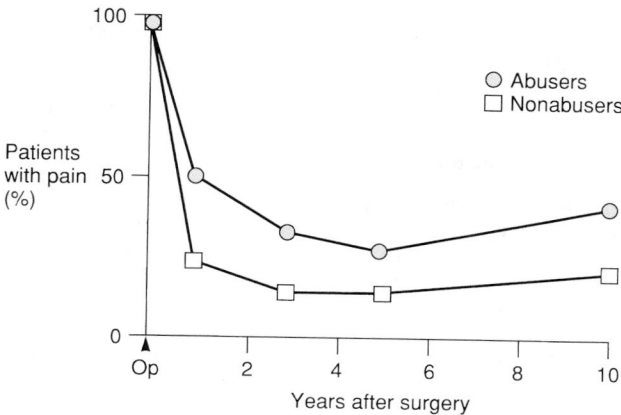

Figure 31.11. Long-term pain relief after pancreaticojejunostomy. (From Ihse I, Borch K, Larsson J. Chronic pancreatitis: results of operations for relief of pain. *World J Surg* 1990;14:53, with permission.)

Local Resection of the Pancreatic Head with Longitudinal Pancreaticojejunostomy (Frey Procedure).

This procedure was developed to facilitate drainage of the three main ducts in the head and uncinate process of the pancreas (33). A standard longitudinal pancreaticojejunostomy may provide inadequate drainage of the pancreatic head and uncinate process, where the ducts of Wirsung and Santorini join the duct from the uncinate process. In the Frey procedure, the head and uncinate process of the pancreas are "shelled out," and the resultant cavity is connected to the main pancreatic duct. As in the standard longitudinal pancreaticojejunostomy, the Roux limb of the jejunum is sutured to the opened pancreatic duct in the pancreatic body and tail for drainage. Because Frey reported excellent pain relief in 75% of patients after 3 years, this modification may replace the standard Puestow-type lateral pancreaticojejunostomy in selected patients, although more experience with this new operation is needed.

Resection Procedures

Patients with chronic pancreatitis whose duct size is less than 4.5 to 5 mm are uniformly considered poor candidates for drainage procedures, and pancreatic resection should be considered in some circumstances. Pancreatic resection is most beneficial if the disease is confined to one portion of the gland. Removing the diseased portion of the gland theoretically reduces chronic pain and the risk for complications.

Distal Pancreatectomy.   If changes of chronic pancreatitis are confined to the tail and body of the pancreas, a distal pancreatectomy may provide relief. If resection occurs at the level of the superior mesenteric vessels, approximately 50% of the gland is removed (Fig. 31.12). Because of recurrent inflammation and scarring, it is common for splenectomy to be performed because splenic vein tributaries from the posterior aspect of the pancreas are difficult to dissect. Thus, the preoperative administration of vaccines is indicated to prevent overwhelming postsplenectomy infections caused by encapsulated organisms (pneumococci, *Haemophilus influenzae*, meningococci).

Pancreaticoduodenectomy (Whipple Procedure).   Resection of the pancreatic head may be indicated when the disease is confined predominantly to this region. Appropriate indications include the following: (a) a chronic in-

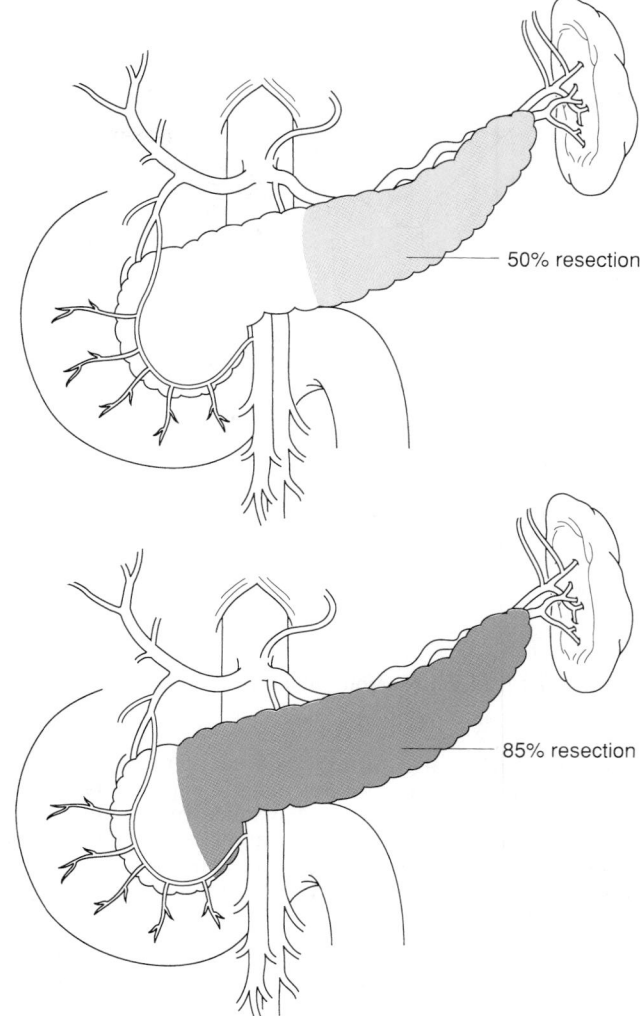

Figure 31.12. Points of parenchymal transection for 50% and 85% distal pancreatectomies.

flammatory mass that cannot be differentiated from a malignancy, (b) chronic inflammation associated with duodenal narrowing, (c) multiple pseudocysts confined to the head of the gland, and (d) failure of a pancreaticojejunostomy to drain the head and uncinate process adequately. Standard pancreaticoduodenectomy involves resection of the pancreatic head, duodenum, gallbladder, distal common duct, and antrum (Fig. 31.13). In the pylorus-preserving modification of the procedure, the antrum and proximal 1 to 2 cm of duodenum are preserved (Fig. 31.14). Regardless of the type of pancreaticoduodenectomy, the reported success rate for pain relief is between 60% and 80% after 5 years. If a mass in the head of the pancreas is identified and malignancy cannot be excluded, pancreaticoduodenectomy is indicated, and frequently an occult malignancy is identified on histologic examination (34).

Ninety-five Percent Distal Pancreatectomy.   The 95% distal pancreatectomy involves removal of the entire pancreas except for a small rim of gland adjacent to the duodenum. As previously mentioned for distal pancreatectomy, attempts at splenic preservation are often futile because the splenic vessels are difficult to dissect from the chronically inflamed and scarred pancreas. Although pain relief can be achieved in up to 80% of patients undergoing

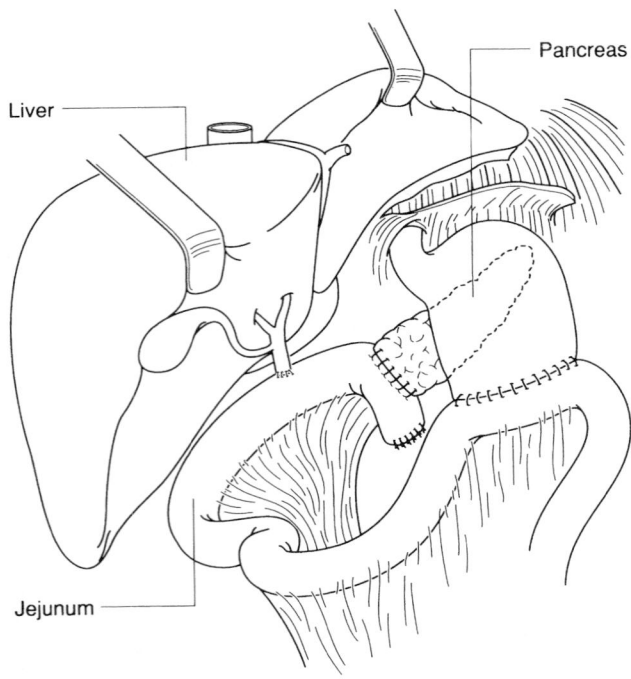

Figure 31.13. Reconstruction after standard pancreaticoduodenectomy.

this procedure, the resulting high incidence of insulin-dependent diabetes and its complications prevents it from being performed frequently. Advances in techniques to isolate and transplant human pancreatic islet cells offer the potential for simultaneous islet cell autotransplantation during pancreatic resective procedures in selected patients.

Total Pancreatectomy. Because of the morbid sequelae, total pancreatectomy is rarely performed for chronic

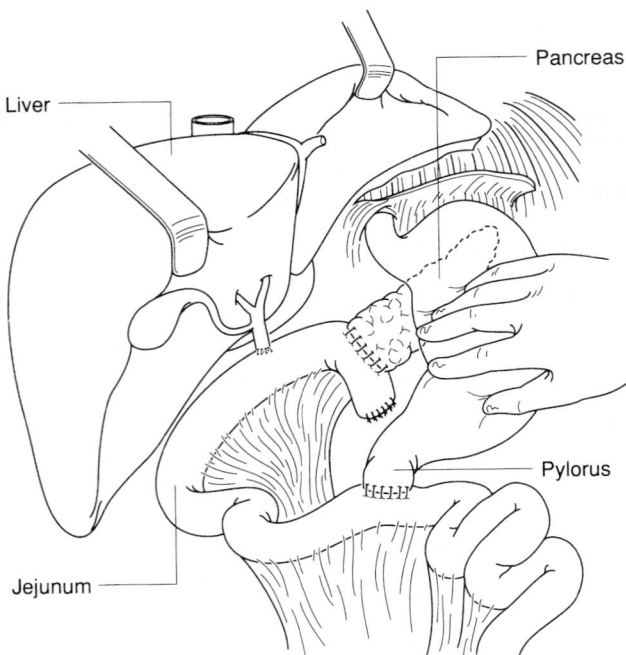

Figure 31.14. Reconstruction after pylorus-preserving pancreaticoduodenectomy.

pancreatitis. In general, the procedure is reserved for patients who have undergone one resective procedure and have either persistent symptoms or a complication requiring further resection. All patients are insulin-dependent diabetics and require enzyme replacement postoperatively. Even with all the pancreatic tissue removed, pain relief is not uniform.

Duodenum-preserving Resection of Pancreatic Head (Beger Procedure). Candidates for this procedure are the same as those who are candidates for a standard pancreaticoduodenectomy except when duodenal stenosis is present. The operation requires transection of the pancreas at its neck and removal of the head and uncinate process except for a rim of parenchyma between the common bile duct and the duodenum. A Roux-en-Y limb is created and sewn to the open end of the body of the pancreas and the portion of pancreas adjacent to the duodenum. Although Beger reports pain relief in approximately 80% of patients, the operation is technically challenging and may offer little advantage in comparison with standard pancreaticoduodenectomy (35).

Malabsorption

Two major consequences of pancreatic insufficiency include steatorrhea and azotorrhea, and on initial consideration, both would seem easy to prevent with the administration of commercially available oral pancreatic enzyme supplements. Unfortunately, for a variety of reasons, complete correction of steatorrhea is infrequently achieved. Oral enzyme supplements (Table 31.2) must contain adequate amounts of lipase, and delivery must be such that sufficient amounts reach the proximal small intestine. Fat absorption is adequate if 25,000 IU of lipase activity can be provided during the 4-hour postprandial period. Acid pepsin inactivates pancreatic enzymes, and gastric acidity is a major impediment to the delivery of active enzymes to the duodenum. Duodenal samples demonstrate recovery of less than 8% of ingested lipase and less than 22% of ingested trypsin. Pancreatic lipase is irreversibly denatured at a pH of less than 4, and attempts to circumvent this problem have included the administration of large amounts of enzyme with meals and the inhibition of acid secretion with histamine (H_2) receptor antagonists. Enteric coating of pancreatic enzyme supplements is effective if the supplements are delivered to the duodenum with food and if sufficient intraduodenal dissolution occurs.

In general, the administration of adequate numbers of enzyme tablets to eliminate azotorrhea and decrease steatorrhea is ideal. This requires that multiple tablets be taken with meals and snacks; if symptoms persist, the number of tablets should be increased or the fat content of meals decreased. With this regimen, most patients can achieve ad-

Table 31.2. COMMERCIALLY AVAILABLE PANCREATIC ENZYME PREPARATIONS

Preparation[a]	Lipase content (IU per pill)
Donnazyme	8,000
Ilozyme	3,600
Ku-Zyme HP	2,300
Cotazym-S	2,000
Pancrease	4,500
Viokase	3,800

[a]Each in capsule formulation.
Adapted from Owyang C, Levitt M. Chronic pancreatitis. In: Yamada T, Alpers DH, Powell DW, et al., eds. Textbook of gastroenterology. Philadelphia: JB Lippincott, 1991:1888.

equate nutritional status and maintain their weight. The addition of histamine (H₂) receptor antagonists or proton pump inhibitors should be reserved for patients who are relatively resistant to this regimen or who have documented acidic duodenal contents.

Pseudocysts

The most common complication of chronic pancreatitis is the formation of pseudocysts. Unfortunately, pseudocysts in patients with chronic pancreatitis are less likely to resolve spontaneously because of underlying ductal abnormalities. Percutaneous drainage can be used to decompress symptomatic pseudocysts rapidly, but recurrence rates are as high as 25% once the drain is removed. In particular, if the pseudocyst remains in communication with the pancreatic ductal system, the removal of a percutaneous drain may result in re-formation of the pseudocyst, even if it has been completely decompressed. In all likelihood, this occurs when resistance to the normal flow of pancreatic juice flow resulting from partial or complete obstruction in the pancreatic ducts causes the cyst cavity to refill, and a patent fistulous communication with the pseudocyst is maintained.

If pseudocysts recur after removal of a percutaneous drain in a patient with chronic pancreatitis, the treatment should be internal surgical drainage. Pseudocyst drainage rarely results in alleviation of the pain of chronic pancreatitis. If the pseudocysts are large enough to cause gastrointestinal symptoms or become infected, then percutaneous or external surgical drainage is indicated. Asymptomatic cysts less than 5 cm in size do not necessarily require therapy in patients with chronic pancreatitis.

Biliary Tract Complications

The distal common bile duct is intimately associated with the head of the pancreas in up to 90% of the population. In two thirds of people, the common bile duct actually runs through the posterior portion of the pancreatic head, and in approximately 25%, the duct runs in a posterior groove in the parenchyma. Significant fibrosis of the pancreatic head can lead to stenosis of the retropancreatic or intrapancreatic portion of the common bile duct. As in most forms of bile duct obstruction, elevation of serum alkaline phosphatase is the most sensitive marker, and the level is usually increased before the appearance of jaundice. Although ultrasonography, CT, and percutaneous transhepatic cholangiography can all provide valuable information, ERCP is commonly used to define the anatomy of the common duct (Fig. 31.15) and frequently can provide a tissue diagnosis. Bile duct stenosis associated with pancreatic head fibrosis is often characterized by a long segment of narrowing, whereas malignant stenosis or stricture is generally characterized by abrupt termination of the bile duct lumen.

Treatment options for bile duct stenosis caused by chronic pancreatitis include endoscopic stent placement and surgical drainage of the bile duct. Although the long-term use of stents to alleviate common duct obstruction has been reported, emphasis must be placed on ensuring that no malignancy is present. With the associated risk for malignancy, stent placement should be reserved for those patients who have cholangitis requiring immediate duct drainage or who are poor risks for surgical drainage.

Either choledochoduodenostomy or choledochojejunostomy (Fig. 31.16) is an excellent choice for long-term surgical drainage of the biliary tract in patients with strictures of the common duct. At the time of surgery, if malignancy has not been sufficiently excluded, the pancreatic head should be explored and samples should be taken to be certain that an undiagnosed malignancy is not present. If malignancy is suspected because of a mass and biopsy specimens are not diagnostic, pancreaticoduodenectomy should be contemplated because pancreatic cancer is reported to occur in 4% of patients with chronic pancreatitis observed for 20 years.

Management of Other Complications

Several other complications can arise, such as splenic vein thrombosis, pancreatic ascites, and pancreatic fistula. These are covered in detail in other chapters.

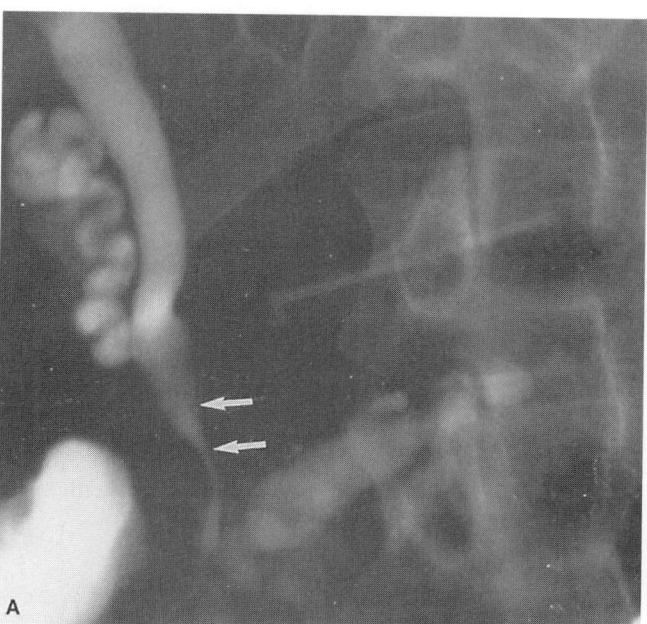
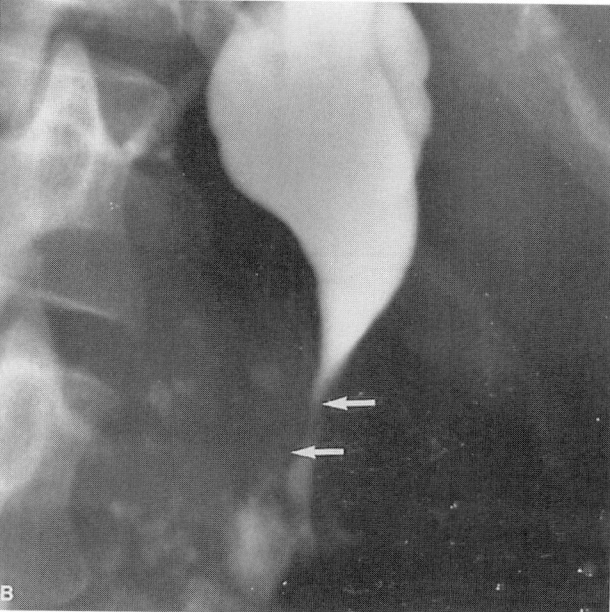

Figure 31.15. Endoscopic cholangiograms of early *(A)* and advanced *(B)* biliary stricture accompanying chronic pancreatitis. Smooth, tapering strictures *(arrows)* can be seen confined to the intrapancreatic portion of the bile duct.

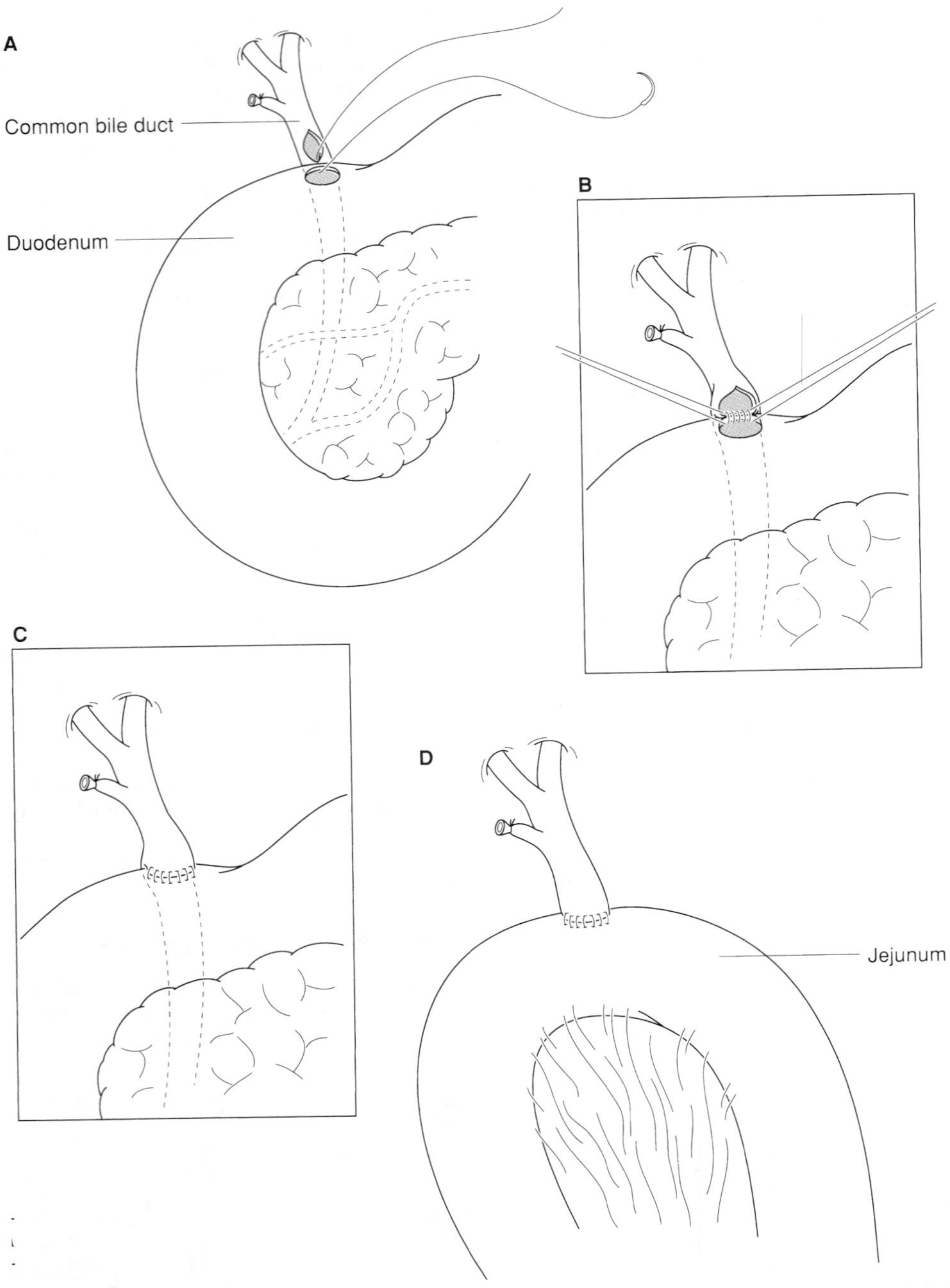

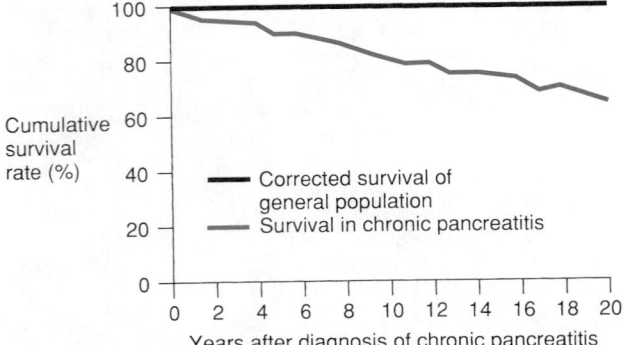

A

Common bile duct

Duodenum

B

C

D

Jejunum

Figure 31.16. Operative construction of choledochoduodenostomy *(A–C)* and choledochojejunostomy *(D)*.

Figure 31.17. Long-term survival in patients with chronic pancreatitis. (From Petrozza JA, Sudhir KD, Latham PS, et al. Prevalence and natural history of distal common bile duct stenosis in alcoholic pancreatitis. *Dig Dis Sci* 1984;29:890, with permission.)

Cumulative survival rate (%)

Corrected survival of general population
Survival in chronic pancreatitis

Years after diagnosis of chronic pancreatitis

PROGNOSIS

Patients with chronic pancreatitis have an excess mortality of 36% during 20 years (Fig. 31.17) and a decreased life expectancy in comparison with the general population. Fewer than 20% of patients with chronic pancreatitis die of direct complications of their disease. The majority of patients die of complications of tobacco or alcohol overuse. Also, aerodigestive cancers, diabetic complications, and cirrhosis are frequent causes of death in patients with chronic pancreatitis.

REFERENCES

1. Sarles H. An international survey on nutrition and pancreatitis. *Digestion* 1972;9:389.
2. Skyhoj Olsen T. The incidence and clinical relevance of chronic inflammation in the pancreas in autopsy material. *Acta Pathol Microbiol Scand* 1978;86:361.

3. Copenhagen Pancreatic Study. An interim report from a prospective epidemiological multicenter study. *Scand J Gastroenterol* 1981;16:305.

4. Gastard J, Jobaud F, Farbos T, et al. Etiology and course of primary chronic pancreatitis in western France. *Digestion* 1973; 9:416.

5. Sahel J, Sarles H. Modifications of pure human pancreatic juice induced by chronic alcohol consumption. *Dig Dis Sci* 1979;24:897.

6. Whitcomb DC, Gorry MC, Preston RA, et al. Hereditary pancreatitis is caused by a mutation in the cationic trypsinogen gene. *Nat Genet* 1996;14:141.

7. Sossenheimer MJ, Aston CE, Preston RA, et al. Clinical characteristics of hereditary pancreatitis in a large family based on high-risk haplotype. *Am J Gastroenterol* 1997;92:1113.

8. Pitchumoni CS. Special problems of tropical pancreatitis. *Clin Gastroenterol* 1984;13:541.

9. Pitchumoni CS, Jain NK, Lowenfels AF, et al. Chronic cyanide poisoning: unifying concept for alcoholic and tropical pancreatitis. *Pancreas* 1988;3:220.

10. Bess MA, Edis AJ, van Heerden JA. Hyperparathyroidism and pancreatitis. *JAMA* 1980;243:246.

11. Layer P, Hotz J, Eysselein VE, et al. The effects of acute hypercalcemia on exocrine pancreatic secretion in the cat. *Gastroenterology* 1985;88:1168.

12. Cotton PB. Congenital anomaly of pancreas divisum as cause of obstructive pain and pancreatitis. *Gut* 1980;21:105.

13. Burtin P, Person B, Charneau J, et al. Pancreas divisum and pancreatitis: a coincidental association. *Endoscopy* 1991;23: 55.

14. Layer P, Kalthoff L, Clain JE, et al. Nonalcoholic chronic pancreatitis: two diseases? *Dig Dis Sci* 1985;30:980.

15. Amman RW, Akovbiantz A, Largiader F, et al. Course and outcome of chronic pancreatitis: longitudinal study of a mixed medical–surgical series of 245 patients. *Gastroenterology* 1984;86:820.

16. Gridwood AH. Does progressive pancreatic insufficiency limit pain in calcific pancreatitis with duct stricture or continued alcohol insult? *J Clin Gastroenterol* 1981;3:241.

17. Bradley EL III. Pancreatic duct pressure in chronic pancreatitis. *Am J Surg* 1982;144:313.

18. Ebbehoj N, Borly L, Madsen P, et al. Pancreatic tissue pressure and pain in chronic pancreatitis. *Pancreas* 1986;1:556.

19. Bockman DE, Buchler M, Malfertheiner P, et al. Analysis of nerves in chronic pancreatitis. *Gastroenterology* 1988;94;1459.

20. Keith RG, Keshavjee SH, Kereni NR. Neuropathology of chronic pancreatitis in humans. *Can J Surg* 1985;28:207.

21. DiMagno EP, Go VLW, Summerskill WHJ. Relations between pancreatic enzyme outputs and malabsorption in severe pancreatic insufficiency. *N Engl J Med* 1973;288:813.

22. Jones SN, Lees WR, Frost RA. Diagnosis and grading of chronic pancreatitis by morphological criteria derived by ultrasound and pancreatography. *Clin Radiol* 1988;39:43.

23. Ueno E, Takada Y, Yoshida I, et al. Pancreatic diseases: evaluation with MR cholangiopancreatography. *Pancreas* 1998; 16:418.

24. Braganza JM, Hunt LP, Warwick R. Relationship between exocrine function and ductal morphology in chronic pancreatitis. *Gastroenterology* 1982;82:1341.

25. Warshaw AL, Banks PA, Fernandez-Del Castillo C. AGA technical review: treatment of pain in chronic pancreatitis. *Gastroenterology* 1998;115:765.

26. Lankisch PG, Seidensticker F, Lohr-Happe A, et al. The course of pain is the same in alcohol- and non–alcohol-induced chronic pancreatitis. *Pancreas* 1995;10:338.

27. Trapnell JE. Chronic relapsing pancreatitis: a review of 64 cases. *Br J Surg* 1979;66:471.

28. Lankisch PG, Lohr-happe A, Otto J, et al. Natural course in chronic pancreatitis: pain, exocrine and endocrine pancreatic insufficiency, and prognosis of the disease. *Digestion* 1993; 54:148.

29. Layer P, Janson JBMJ, Cherian L, et al. Feedback relation of human pancreatic secretion: effective protease inhibition of duodenal, liver, and small intestinal transit of pancreatic enzymes. *Gastroenterology* 1990;98:1311.

30. Leung JWC, Bowen-Wright M, Aveling W, et al. Celiac plexus block for pain control in pancreatic cancer and chronic pancreatitis. *Br J Surg* 1983;70:730.

31. Geenen JE, Rolny P. Endoscopic therapy of acute and chronic pancreatitis. *Gastrointest Endosc* 1991;37:377.

32. Smith MT, Sherman S, Ikenberry SO, et al. Alterations in pancreatic ductal morphology following polyethylene pancreatic stent therapy. *Gastrointest Endosc* 1996;44:268.

33. Frey CF, Amikura K. Local resection of the head of the pancreas combined with longitudinal pancreaticojejunostomy in the management of patients with chronic pancreatitis. *Ann Surg* 1994;220:492.

34. Thompson JS, Murayama KM, Edney JA, et al. Pancreaticoduodenectomy for suspected but unproven malignancy. *Am J Surg* 1994;169:571.

35. Beger HG, Buchler M. Duodenum-preserving resection of the head of the pancreas in chronic pancreatitis with inflammatory mass in the head. *World J Surg* 1990;14:83.

SURGERY: SCIENTIFIC PRINCIPLES AND PRACTICE, Third Edition, edited by Lazar J. Greenfield, Michael W. Mulholland, Keith T. Oldham, Gerald B. Zelenock, and Keith D. Lillemoe. Lippincott Williams & Wilkins Publishers, Philadelphia, © 2001.

CHAPTER 32

NEOPLASMS OF THE EXOCRINE PANCREAS

ATTILA NAKEEB, KEITH D. LILLEMOE, CHARLES J. YEO, AND JOHN L. CAMERON

In the United States, more than 28,000 people die each year of pancreatic cancer; it is the fifth leading cause of cancer death in this country. The nonspecific symptoms associated with early pancreatic cancer, the inaccessibility of the pancreas to examination, the aggressiveness of the tumors, and the technical difficulties associated with pancreatic surgery make pancreatic cancer one of the most challenging diseases treated by general surgeons. In recent years, significant advances have been made in our understanding of the pathogenesis and clinical management of pancreatic cancer. This chapter reviews the epidemiology and risk factors associated with pancreatic cancer, discusses recent developments in the field of molecular genetics, and provides an update on the current management of pancreatic cancer.

EPIDEMIOLOGY AND RISK FACTORS

In the United States, approximately nine new cases of pancreatic cancer are diagnosed per 100,000 population annually (1). Although the incidence rate of pancreatic cancer has been relatively stable during the last two decades, it has increased nearly threefold since the beginning of the last century (Fig. 32.1). It has been argued that the apparent increase in the incidence of pancreatic cancer may represent a misclassification of pancreatic cancer as other types of upper gastrointestinal cancer, particularly gastric cancer, in the past. However, several analyses indicate that a portion of the threefold increase in the incidence of pancreatic cancer has been real.

The risk for the development of pancreatic cancer is related to age, race, sex, tobacco use, diet, and specific genetic syndromes (Table 32.1). The incidence increases with advancing age. More than 80% of cases occur in persons between the ages of 60 and 80 years, and pancreatic cancer is rare in people less than 40 years of age. The incidence and mortality rates for pancreatic cancer in African-Americans of both sexes are higher than those in whites. The gender differences in pancreatic cancer have been equalizing during recent years. Pancreatic cancer is

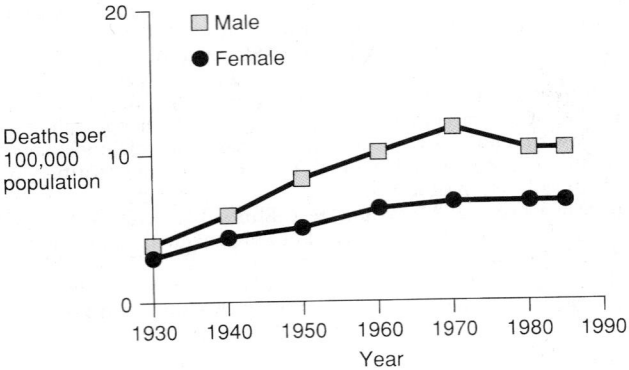

Figure 32.1. Age-adjusted death rates for pancreatic carcinoma.

still more common in men than in women, but the incidence and mortality rates have increased in women while they have stabilized or slightly decreased for men.

Environmental and dietary factors have also been implicated as risk factors for the development of pancreatic cancer. The most consistently observed environmental risk for the development of pancreatic cancer is cigarette smoking. It has been estimated that cigarette smoking can increase the risk for pancreatic cancer between one and a half and five times. The mechanism is unknown, but carcinogens in cigarette smoke have been shown to produce pancreatic cancers in laboratory animals. In addition, autopsy studies have documented hyperplastic changes in pancreatic ductal cells with atypical nuclear patterns in smokers. Alcohol consumption does not seem to be a risk factor for pancreatic cancer despite conflicting past reports. Recent studies suggest that past studies linking pancreatic cancer to alcohol use may have been confounded by tobacco use. Similarly, coffee consumption and exposure to ionizing radiation have been shown not to be associated with an increased pancreatic cancer risk.

Several epidemiologic investigations have suggested that diet may play an important role in the development of pancreatic cancer. An apparent association has been noted between pancreatic cancer and an increased consumption of total calories, carbohydrate, cholesterol, meat, salt, dehydrated food, fried food, refined sugar, soy beans, and nitrosamines. The risks are unproven for the ingestion of fat, beta carotene, and coffee. A protective effect has been reported for dietary fiber, vitamin C, fruits, and vegetables (2).

In addition to well-defined genetic syndromes, a number of common conditions have been thought to be etiologic factors in the development of pancreatic cancer. An apparent association between diabetes and pancreatic cancer has been suggested. Although the data are somewhat inconsistent, mostly they suggest that long-standing diabetes is not a risk factor for pancreatic cancer. Diabetes may actually be an early symptom of pancreatic cancer and not a causative factor. Chronic pancreatitis of any cause has been associated with a 25-year cumulative risk for the development of pancreatic cancer of approximately 4%. Other conditions for which a possible association with pancreatic cancer has been demonstrated include thyroid and other benign endocrine tumors, cystic fibrosis, and pernicious anemia.

Most cases of pancreatic cancer have no obvious predisposing factors. However, six genetic syndromes have been associated with an increased risk for the development of pancreatic cancer (3). These include (a) hereditary nonpolyposis colon cancer, (b) familial breast cancer associated with the *BRCA2* mutation, (c) Peutz-Jeghers syndrome, (d) ataxia–telangiectasia syndrome, (e) familial atypical multiple mole–melanoma syndrome, and (f) hereditary pancreatitis.

MOLECULAR GENETICS

Tremendous advances have been made in understanding the molecular genetics of pancreatic cancer in recent years. In general, the genes involved in the pathogenesis of pancreatic cancer can be divided into three categories: (a) tumor-suppressor genes, (b) oncogenes, and (c) DNA mismatch-repair genes.

Tumor-suppressor genes normally function to control cellular proliferation. When these genes are inactivated by genetic events such as mutation, deletion, chromosome rearrangements, or mitotic recombination, their function as growth suppressors can be lost, and abnormal growth regulation is the result. The tumor-suppressor genes *p53, p16,* and *DPC4* are frequently inactivated in sporadic adenocarcinoma of the pancreas (Table 32.2). The function of *p53* appears to be inactivated in up to 75% of all pancreatic cancers. The *p53* gene product is a DNA-binding protein that acts as both a cell cycle checkpoint and an inducer of apoptosis. Inactivation of the *p53* gene in pancreatic cancer leads to the loss of two important controls of cell growth: regulation of cellular proliferation and induction of cell death. The *p16* gene encodes a protein that binds cyclin to cyclin D–Cdk4 complexes. When the *p16* gene product binds these complexes, it inhibits the phosphorylation of a number of growth and regulatory proteins. Inactivation of *p16* leads to the loss of an important cell cycle checkpoint and therefore relatively unchecked proliferation. *DPC4* is a tumor-suppressor gene that has been identified on chromosome 18q. This chromosome has been shown to be missing

Table 32.1. RISK FACTORS FOR PANCREATIC CANCER

	Increased risk	Possible risk	Unproven risk
Demographic factors	Advancing age Male sex Black race	Geography	Socioeconomic status Migrant status
Host factors	Hereditary nonpolyposis colorectal cancer Familial breast cancer Peutz-Jeghers syndrome Ataxia–telangectasia Familial atypical multiple-mole melanoma Hereditary pancreatitis		Peptic ulcer surgery Cholecystectomy
Environmental factors	Tobacco	Diet Occupation	Alcohol Coffee Radiation

Modified from Gold EB, Goldin SB. Epidemiology of and risk factors for pancreatic cancer. Surg Oncol Clin N Am 1998;7:67–91, with permission.

Table 32.2. TUMOR-SUPPRESSOR GENES IN PANCREATIC CANCER

Gene	Chromosome location	Frequency (%)
p53	17p	75
p16	9p	95
DPC4	18q	50
BRCA2	13q	4–7

Modified from Hruban RH, Petersen GM, Ha PK, et al. Genetics of pancreatic cancer: from genes to families. Surg Oncol Clin N Am 1998;7:1–23, with permission.

Table 32.3. HISTOLOGIC CLASSIFICATION OF 645 CASES OF PRIMARY NONENDOCRINE CANCER OF THE PANCREAS

Classification	Number
Duct cell origin	572 (89%)
Duct cell adenocarcinoma	494
Giant cell carcinoma	28
Adenosquamous carcinoma	20
Microadenocarcinoma	16
Mucinous carcinoma	9
Mucinous cystadenocarcinoma	5
Acinar cell origin	8 (1%)
Acinar cell carcinoma	7
Cystadenoma	1
Uncertain histogenesis	61 (9%)
Pancreaticoblastoma	1
Papillary and cystic neoplasm	1
Mixed type—duct and islet cells	1
Unclassified	58
Connective tissue origin	4 (1%)

From Bell RH. Neoplasms of the exocrine pancreas. In: Greenfield LJ, Mulholland MW, Oldham KT, eds. Surgery: scientific principles and practice, 2nd ed. Philadelphia: Lippincott–Raven, 1997:901–918.

in nearly 90% of pancreatic cancers. The *DPC4* gene is inactive in almost 50% of pancreatic carcinomas. The mutation appears to be a homozygous deletion in 30% of pancreatic cancers, and a point mutation in another 20% of tumors. *DPC4* mutations are more specific than *p53* or *p16* mutations for pancreatic cancer.

Oncogenes are derived from normal cellular genes called *protooncogenes*. When overexpressed or activated by mutation, oncogenes encode proteins with transforming properties. Activating point mutations in the K-*ras* oncogene is the most common genetic alteration in pancreatic cancer. Point mutations in codons 12, 13, or 61 of the K-*ras* oncogene impair the intrinsic guanosine triphosphatase activity of its gene product; the result is a protein that is constitutively active in signal transduction. Mutations of K-*ras* have been found in 80% to 100% of pancreatic cancers and therefore may prove useful in the development of a molecular screening test for pancreatic cancer.

Mismatch-repair genes function to ensure the accuracy of DNA replication, and when these genes are mutated, errors in DNA replication are not repaired. The human mismatch-repair genes are *hMSH2*, *hMLH1*, *hPMS1*, *hPMS2*, *hMSH6/GTBP*, and *hMSH3*. The enzymes encoded by these genes repair single base pair changes and small insertions and deletions that occur during DNA replication. Approximately 4% of pancreatic cancers can be characterized by disorders of DNA mismatch-repair genes (4).

PATHOLOGY

Tumors of the exocrine pancreas can be classified based on their cell of origin (Table 32.3). The most common neoplasms of the exocrine pancreas are ductal adenocarcinomas. Approximately 65% of pancreatic ductal cancers arise in the head, neck, or uncinate process of the pancreas; 15% originate in the body or the tail of the gland, and 20% diffusely involve the whole gland.

Solid Epithelial Tumors

Ductal Adenocarcinomas

Ductal adenocarcinomas account for 75% of all nonendocrine pancreatic cancers. Grossly, they are white–yellow, poorly defined, hard masses that often obstruct the distal common bile duct or main pancreatic duct. They are often associated with a desmoplastic reaction that causes fibrosis and chronic pancreatitis. Microscopically, they contain infiltrating glands of varying size and shape surrounded by dense, reactive fibrous tissue (Fig. 32.2). The epithelial cells sometimes form papillae and cribriform structures, and they frequently contain mucin. The nuclei of the cells can show marked pleomorphism, hyperchromasia, loss of polarity, and prominent nucleoli.

Ductal adenocarcinomas tend to infiltrate into vascular, lymphatic, and perineural spaces. At the time of resection, most ductal carcinomas have already metastasized to regional lymph nodes. In addition to the lymph nodes, pancreatic ductal adenocarcinoma frequently metastasize to the liver (80%), peritoneum (60%), lungs and pleurae (50% to 70%), and adrenal glands (25%). They also can directly invade the duodenum, stomach, transverse mesocolon, colon, spleen, and adrenal glands.

The histologic examination of a pancreas resected for cancer frequently reveals the presence of lesions in the pancreatic ducts and ductules adjacent to the cancers (5). This suggests that much like colon cancer, which arises from benign adenomas, pancreatic cancer may also arise from precursor lesions. Flat ductal lesions may progress to papillary ductal lesions without atypia, then to papillary ductal lesions with atypia, and finally to invasive adenocarcinoma. In these abnormal ducts, the normal cuboidal cells are replaced by a mucin-producing proliferative epithelium with varying degrees of atypia. Several lines of evidence suggest that the ductal lesions are precursors of infiltrating pancreatic cancer, including their association with cancer. In addition, three-dimensional mapping techniques have demonstrated a stepwise transformation from mild dysplasia to severe dysplasia in pancreatic duct lesions. Finally, ductal lesions display some of the same genetic changes seen in infiltrating adenocarcinomas, most notably activating point mutations in codon 12 of K-*ras* and mutations in the *p16* and *p53* tumor-suppressor genes.

Adenoaquamous Carcinomas

Adenosquamous carcinoma is a rare variant of ductal adenocarcinoma that shows both glandular and squamous differentiation. This variant appears to be more common in patients who have undergone previous chemoradiation therapy. The biologic behavior of adenosquamous carcinoma appears to be similar to that of ductal adenocarcinoma, with similar rates of perineural invasion, lymph node metastases, and dissemination.

Acinar Cell Carcinomas

Acinar cell carcinomas account for only 1% of pancreatic exocrine tumors. Acinar tumors are typically smooth, fleshy, lobulated, hemorrhagic, or necrotic. Histologically, they form acini, and the cells display an eosinophilic, granular cytoplasm. Immunohistochemical staining demonstrates ex-

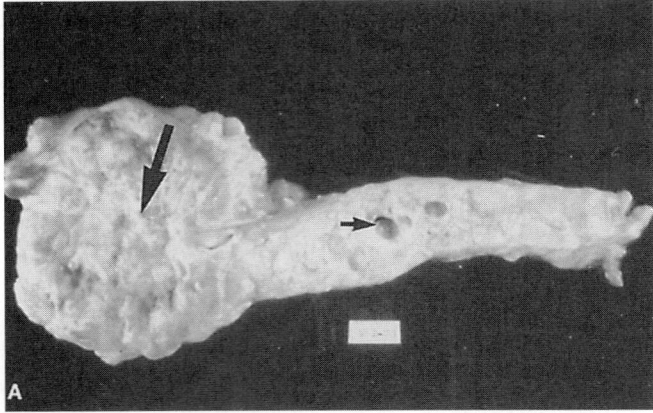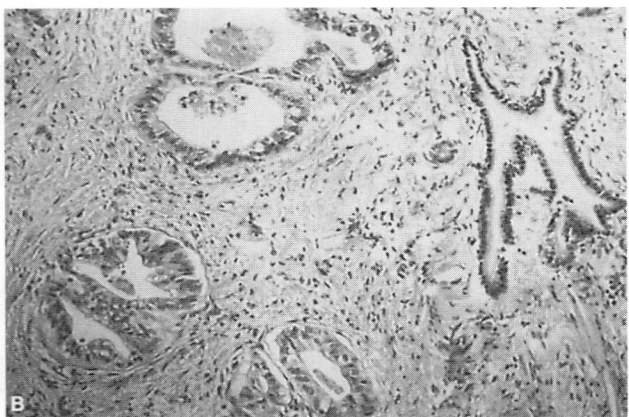

Figure 32.2. Gross and microscopic appearance of ductal adenocarcinoma of the head of the pancreas. In the gross specimen *(A)*, the scirrhous reaction in the head of the pancreas *(arrow)* and the dilation of the pancreatic duct in the body of the gland *(small arrow)* are notable. Microscopic section *(B)* demonstrates glands from a well-differentiated adenocarcinoma *(lower left)* embedded in a fibrous matrix. Some residual normal residual ductal structures remain *(right)*.

pression of trypsin, lipase, chymotrypsin, or amylase. These tumors tend to be larger than ductal adenocarcinomas, often being larger than 10 cm. Although data are limited, it appears that patients with acinar cell carcinoma have a slightly better prognosis than patients with ductal carcinoma.

Giant Cell Carcinomas

Giant cell carcinomas account for fewer than 5% of nonendocrine pancreatic cancers. They tend to be large, with average diameters greater than 10 cm. Microscopically, they contain large, uninucleated or multinucleated tumor cells, many of which are pleomorphic. The nuclei contain prominent nucleoli and numerous mitotic figures. Giant cell carcinomas are associated with a poorer prognosis than ductal adenocarcinomas.

Pancreatoblastoma

Pancreatoblastomas occur primarily in children ages 1 to 15 years. Pancreatoblastomas contain both epithelial and mesenchymal elements. The epithelial component appears to arise from acinar cells. The tumors are typically larger than 10 cm and often contain areas of degeneration and hemorrhage. The prognosis appears to be more favorable than that for typical ductal adenocarcinoma if the tumor can be resected.

Cystic Epithelial Tumors

Cystic neoplasms also arise from the exocrine pancreas. Cystic neoplasms are much less common than ductal adenocarcinomas, tend to occur in women, and are evenly distributed throughout the gland. The vast majority of pancreatic and peripancreatic cysts are benign pseudocysts. However, it is important to recognize cystic neoplasms because their management is very different from that for non-neoplastic cysts.

Serous Cystic Neoplasms

Serous cystadenomas or microcystic adenomas are more common in women than in men. These tumors can vary from a few centimeters to more than 10 cm in size. Grossly, they appear as spongy, well-circumscribed, multiloculated cysts. Microscopically, they consist of a layer of simple cuboidal cells separated by dense fibrous bands. Most serous cystic neoplasms are benign, although malignant behavior has been reported rarely (i.e., metastases to the liver or peripancreatic lymph nodes).

Mucinous Cystic Neoplasms

These neoplasms range from benign tumors with small cysts to larger tumors associated with an infiltrating carcinoma. Mucinous cystic neoplasms are also more common in women than in men. They can be divided into three types: (a) mucinous cystadenoma, (b) the intermediate or borderline tumor, and (c) mucinous cystadenocarcinoma. Mucinous cystadenomas contain a single layer of columnar epithelium without atypia. In borderline tumors, the epithelium may form papillae and a more complex architecture, and the cells show atypia. Mucinous cystadenocarcinomas demonstrate invasion of the neoplastic epithelium into the surrounding stroma. Otherwise benign-appearing mucinous cystic neoplasms may contain small foci of carcinoma. Therefore, it appears that all mucinous cystic neoplasms should be completely resected. The prognosis for patients with resected benign or borderline tumors is excellent. Patients with mucinous cystadenocarcinoma tend to do better than patients with ductal adenocarcinoma, with a 5-year survival of approximately 50%.

Intraductal Papillary–Mucinous Neoplasms

Intraductal papillary–mucinous neoplasms are soft villous tumors that are often found within mucus-filled, dilated pancreatic ducts. Microscopically, they consist of papillary projections lined by columnar mucin-secreting cells. They show varying degrees of cellular atypia. Intraductal papillary–mucinous neoplasms appear to be more common in the head, neck, and uncinate process of the pancreas but can be found diffusely throughout the whole gland. They are often diagnosed when mucin is seen oozing from the ampulla of Vater during endoscopic retrograde cholangiopancreatography (ERCP). They may contain areas of invasive carcinoma and therefore should be resected if possible.

Solid and Cystic Papillary Neoplasms

Solid and cystic papillary neoplasms, also termed *Hamoudi tumors*, occur primarily in women in their third to fourth decade of life. Grossly, the masses range from 5 to 15 cm in diameter. The tumors show solid, cystic, and papillary components. Although most patients are cured after resection, metastases have been reported.

CLINICOPATHOLOGIC STAGING

Accurate pathologic staging of pancreatic cancer is important for providing prognostic information to patients

Table 32.4. AMERICAN JOINT COMMITTEE ON CANCER STAGING OF PANCREATIC CANCER

Stage Grouping	T	N	M	5-Year survival (%)
Stage I	T1 or T2	N0	M0	20–40
Stage II	T3	N0	M0	10–25
Stage III	Any T	N1	M0	10–15
Stage IVA	T4	Any N	M0	0–5
Stage IVB	Any T	Any N	M1	—

Tumor (T)
  TX: primary tumor cannot be assessed
  T0: no evidence of primary tumor
  Tis: in situ carcinoma
  T1: tumor limited to the pancreas; 2 cm or less in greatest dimension
  T2: tumor limited to the pancreas; more than 2 cm in greatest dimension
  T3: tumor extends directly into any of the following: duodenum, bile duct, or peripancreatic tissues
  T4: tumor extends directly into any of the following: stomach, spleen, colon, or adjacent large vessels
Regional lymph nodes (N)
  NX: regional lymph nodes cannot be assessed
  N0: no regional lymph node metastasis
  N1: regional lymph node metastasis
Distant metastasis (M)
  MX: distant metastasis cannot be assessed
  M0: no distant metastasis
  M1: distant metastasis

Adapted from the American Joint Committee on Cancer staging manual, 5th ed. Philadelphia: Lippincott–Raven, 1997: 121–126.

and for comparing the results of various therapeutic trials. The American Joint Committee on Cancer (AJCC) staging for pancreatic cancer is shown in Table 32.4. This system, based on the TNM classification, takes into account the extent of the primary tumor (T), the presence of absence of regional lymph node involvement (N), and the presence or absence of distant metastatic disease (M).

DIAGNOSIS

Clinical Presentation

Many of the difficulties associated with the management of pancreatic cancer result from our inability to make the diagnosis at an early stage. The early symptoms of pancreatic cancer include anorexia, weight loss, abdominal discomfort, and nausea. Unfortunately, the nonspecific nature of these symptoms often leads to a delay in the diagnosis. Specific symptoms usually develop only after invasion or obstruction of nearby structures has occurred. Most pancreatic cancers arise in the head of the pancreas, and obstruction of the intrapancreatic portion of the common bile duct leads to progressive jaundice, acholic stools, darkening of the urine, and pruritus. Pain is a common symptom of pancreatic cancer. The pain usually starts as vague upper abdominal or back pain that is often ignored by the patient or attributed to some other cause. It is usually worse in the supine position and is often relieved by leaning forward. Pain may be caused by invasion of the tumor into the splanchnic plexus and retroperitoneum, and by obstruction of the pancreatic duct. Other digestive symptoms are also common in pancreatic cancer (Table 32.5).

Occasionally, pancreatic cancer may be discovered in an unusual manner. The onset of diabetes may be the first clinical feature in 10% to 15% of patients. An episode of acute pancreatitis may also be the initial presentation of pancreatic cancer if the tumor partially obstructs the pancreatic duct. It is important to consider a pancreatic cancer in patients presenting with acute pancreatitis, especially those without an obvious cause for their pancreatitis (alcohol or gallstones).

The most common physical finding at the initial presentation is jaundice (Table 32.6). Hepatomegaly and a palpable gallbladder may be present in some patients. In cases of advanced disease, cachexia, muscle wasting, or a nodular liver, consistent with metastatic disease, may be evident. Other physical findings in patients with disseminated cancer include left supraclavicular adenopathy (Virchow's node), periumbilical adenopathy (Sister Mary

Table 32.5. SYMPTOMS OF PANCREATIC CANCER

Symptom	Patients (%)
Head	
Weight loss	92
Jaundice	82
Pain	72
Anorexia	64
Dark urine	63
Light stools	62
Nausea	45
Vomiting	37
Weakness	35
Pruritus	24
Diarrhea	18
Melena	12
Constipation	11
Fever	11
Hematemesis	8
Body and tail	
Weight loss	100
Pain	87
Weakness	43
Nausea	43
Vomiting	37
Anorexia	33
Constipation	27
Hematemesis	17
Melena	17
Jaundice	7
Fever	7
Diarrhea	3

From Bell RH. Neoplasms of the exocrine pancreas. In: Greenfield LJ, Mulholland MW, Oldham KT, et al., eds. Surgery: scientific principles and practice, 2nd ed. Philadelphia: Lippincott–Raven, 1997: 901–918.

Table 32.6. **SIGNS OF PANCREATIC CANCER**

Sign	Patients (%)
Head	
Jaundice	87
Palpable liver	83
Palpable gallbladder	29
Tenderness	26
Ascites	14
Abdominal mass	13
Body and tail	
Palpable liver	33
Tenderness	27
Abdominal mass	23
Ascites	20
Jaundice	13

From Bell RH. Neoplasms of the exocrine pancreas. In: Greenfield LJ, Mulholland MW, Oldham KT, et al., eds. Surgery: scientific principles and practice, 2nd ed. Philadelphia: Lippincott–Raven, 1997: 901–918.

Joseph's node), and pelvic drop metastases (Blumer's shelf). Ascites can be present in 15% of patients.

Laboratory Studies

In patients with cancer of the head of the pancreas, laboratory studies usually reveal a significant increase in serum total bilirubin, alkaline phosphatase, and γ-glutamyl transferase. The transaminases can also be elevated, but usually not to the same extent as the alkaline phosphatase. In patients with localized cancer of the body and tail of the pancreas, laboratory values are frequently normal early in the course. Patients with pancreatic cancer may also demonstrate a normochromic anemia and hypoalbuminemia secondary to the nutritional consequences of the disease. In patients with jaundice, the prothrombin time can be abnormally prolonged. This usually is an indication of biliary obstruction, which prevents bile from entering the gastrointestinal tract and leads to malabsorption of fat-soluble vitamins and decreased hepatic production of vitamin K-dependent clotting factors. The prothrombin time can usually be normalized by the ad-

ministration of parenteral vitamin K. Serum amylase and lipase levels are usually normal in patients with pancreatic cancer.

A wide variety of serum tumor markers have been proposed for use in the diagnosis and follow-up of patients with pancreatic cancer. The most extensively studied of these is CA 19-9, a Lewis blood group-related mucin glycoprotein. Approximately 5% of the population lacks the Lewis gene and therefore cannot produce CA 19-9. When a normal upper limit of 37 U/mL is used, the accuracy of the CA 19-9 level in identifying patients with pancreatic adenocarcinoma is only about 80%. When a higher cutoff value of more than 90 U/mL is used, the accuracy improves to 85%, and increasing the cutoff value to 200 U/mL increases the accuracy to 95% (6). The combined use of CA 19-9 and either ultrasonography, computed tomography (CT), or ERCP can improve the accuracy of the individual tests, so that the combined accuracy approaches 100% for the diagnosis of pancreatic cancer. Levels of CA 19-9 have also been correlated with prognosis and tumor recurrence. In general, higher CA 19-9 values before surgery indicate an increased size of the primary tumor and increased rate of unresectability. In addition, the CA 19-9 level has been used to monitor the results of neoadjuvant and adjuvant chemoradiation therapy in patients. Increasing CA 19-9 levels usually indicate recurrence or progression of disease, whereas stable or declining levels indicate a stable tumor burden, absence of recurrence on imaging studies, and an improved prognosis.

Radiologic Investigations

The early diagnosis of pancreatic cancer requires a low index of suspicion and appropriate aggressiveness in pursuing the diagnosis. Ultrasonography, CT, and magnetic resonance imaging (MRI) are all useful noninvasive tests in the patient suspected of having a pancreatic cancer.

Transabdominal ultrasonography is the most sensitive test for detecting gallstones, an ever-present issue in the elderly patient who is jaundiced. Ultrasonography is operator-dependent but can demonstrate dilated intrahepatic and extrahepatic bile ducts, liver metastases, pancreatic

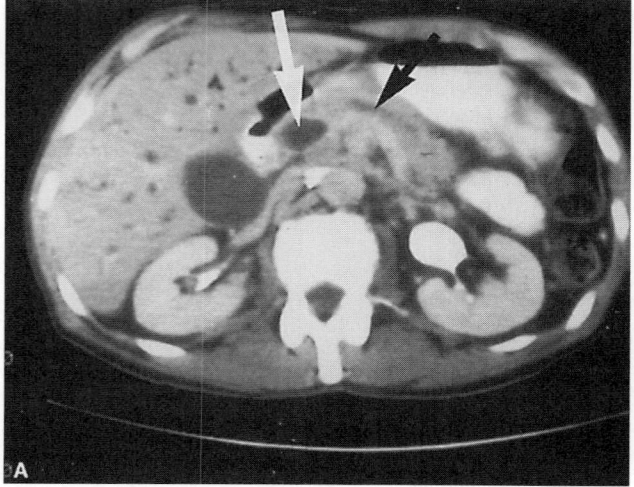
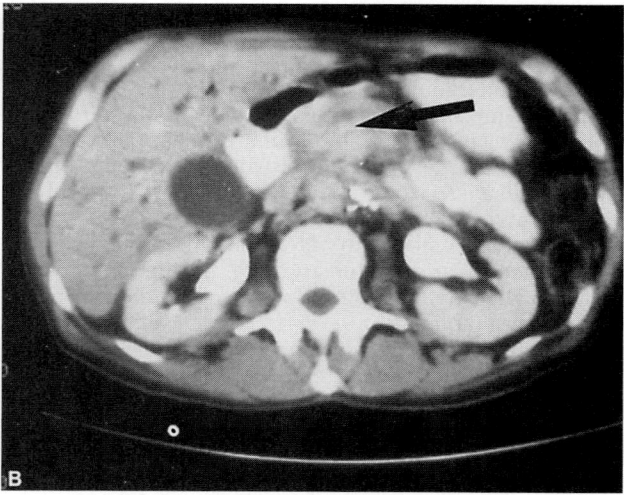

Figure 32.3. Computed tomogram of the abdomen of a patient with adenocarcinoma of the pancreas. *(A)* The obstructed and dilated common bile duct *(light arrow)* and pancreatic duct *(dark arrow)* can be seen. In the adjacent cross section *(B)*, a large mass is present in the head of the pancreas *(arrow)*.

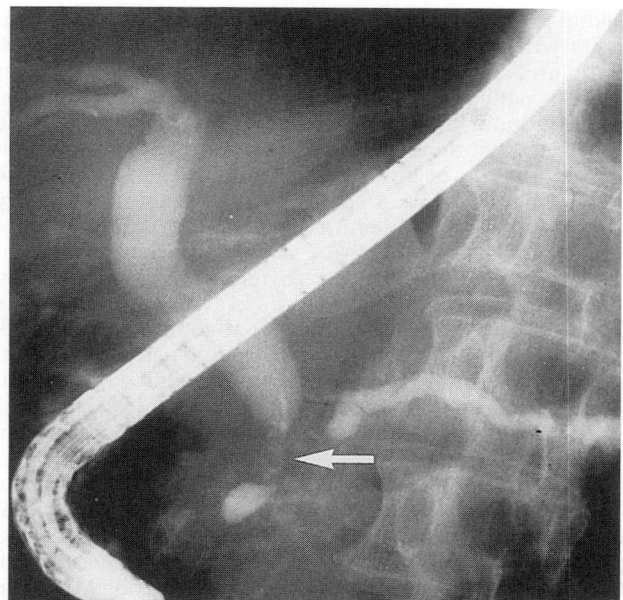

Figure 32.4. Endoscopic retrograde cholangiopancreatography in a patient with adenocarcinoma of the pancreas demonstrates a stricture of both the distal common bile duct and the pancreatic duct *(arrow)*.

masses, ascites, and enlarged peripancreatic lymph nodes. Pancreatic cancer typically appears as a hypoechoic mass on ultrasonography. Ultrasonography will reveal a pancreatic mass in 60% to 70% of patients with cancer. Because helical CT is just as sensitive as ultrasonography and provides more complete information about surrounding structures and the local and distant extent of the disease, ultrasnography has been largely replaced by CT.

Helical or spiral CT is currently the preferred noninvasive imaging test for the diagnosis of pancreatic cancer. Pancreatic cancer usually appears as an area of pancreatic enlargement with a localized hypodense lesion (Fig. 32.3). For pancreatic lesions, a dual-phase intravenous contrast study is ideal. Thin cuts are obtained through the pancreas and liver during both an arterial phase and portal venous phase after the administration of intravenous contrast. In addition to determining the primary tumor size, CT is used to evaluate invasion into local structures or metastatic disease.

In general, MRI offers no significant advantages over CT because of a low signal-to-noise ratio, motion artifacts, lack of bowel opacification, and low spatial resolution. More recently, however, the introduction of magnetic resonance cholangiopancreatography (MRCP) has offered a promising noninvasive technique that can visualize both the bile duct and the pancreatic duct; images are similar to those obtained with ERCP.

Traditionally, the next step in the evaluation of the jaundiced patient has been cholangiography, either by the endoscopic or percutaneous route. If the endoscopic approach is used, the duodenum and ampulla can be visualized and and biopsy specimens obtained if necessary. In addition, ERCP allows for direct imaging of the pancreatic duct. The sensitivity of ERCP for the diagnosis of pancreatic cancer approaches 90%. The finding of a long, irregular stricture in an otherwise normal pancreatic duct is highly suggestive of a pancreatic cancer (Fig. 32.4). Often, the pancreatic duct will be obstructed with no dis-

tal filling. Although ERCP is reliable in confirming the presence of a clinically suspected pancreatic cancer, it should not be used routinely. Diagnostic ERCP should be reserved for patients with presumed pancreatic cancer and obstructive jaundice in whom no mass is demonstrated on CT, symptomatic but nonjaundiced patients without an obvious pancreatic mass, and patients with chronic pancreatitis in whom the development of a pancreatic mass is suspected based on clinical evidence or the development of jaundice.

PREOPERATIVE STAGING

The goal of preoperative staging of pancreatic cancer is to determine the feasibility of surgery and the optimal treatment for each individual patient. In many cases, dynamic CT with oral and intravenous contrast may provide all the information necessary by demonstrating liver metastasis or major vascular invasion. The use of dual-phase CT with both arterial and venous timed injection is currently the best noninvasive technique available for determining the proximity of the primary neoplasm to major peripancreatic vascular structures, such as the celiac axis, superior mesenteric artery, and the superior mesenteric, splenic, and portal veins. Preservation of the fat planes around each of these vessels suggests a lack of direct invasion by the tumor and is consistent with resectability. For tumors of the head, neck, or uncinate process of the pancreas, occlusion of the superior mesenteric vein or portal vein along with the presence of periportal collateral vessels is a sign of unresectability and typically precludes resection for cure. In contrast, for tumors of the body and tail of the pancreas, occlusion of the splenic vein with perigastric collaterals does not always preclude resection and should not be considered a sign of unresectability.

The extent of further staging to be performed depends on the individual patient and the surgeon's preference. If the surgeon's philosophy is to pursue a surgical treatment for all patients, either to attempt resection or provide palliation, then further staging is not necessary. However, if the findings of staging could preclude an operation and lead to nonoperative palliation, then these efforts are worthwhile.

Endoscopic ultrasonography (EUS) is a minimally invasive technique in which a high-frequency ultrasonographic probe is placed into the stomach and duodenum endoscopically and the pancreas is imaged. Tumors appear as hypoechoic areas in the pancreatic substance (Fig. 32.5). The main uses for EUS are to detect small pancreatic lesions (< 2 cm) and lymph node and vascular involvement. EUS is not effective in assessing metastatic disease to the liver. In patients for whom a tissue diagnosis is required (poor operative candidates or undergoing neoadjuvant therapy), EUS-guided fine-needle aspiration (FNA) has been used to acquire tissue samples for cytologic analysis. This approach may avoid the risks of tumor seeding. In a large international multicenter experience comprising a total of 124 patients, EUS-guided FNA had a sensitivity of 86%, a specificity of 94%, a positive predictive value of 100%, a negative predictive value of 86%, and an accuracy of 88% (7).

The technique of staging laparoscopy has been advocated by some surgeons for patients with potentially resectable pancreatic cancers (8). The liver and peritoneum are the most common sites of distant spread of pancreatic carcinoma. Once distant metastases have developed, survival is so limited that a conservative approach is usually indicated. Liver metastases larger than 2 cm in diameter can usually be detected by CT, but approximately 30% of

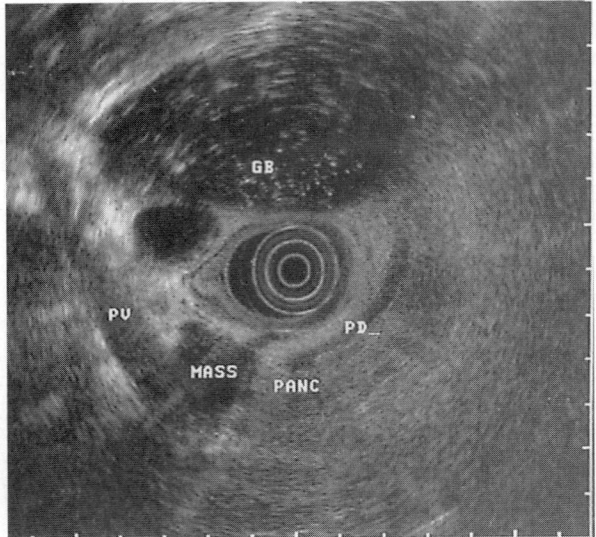

Figure 32.5. Endoscopic ultrasonogram of a 2.2-cm mass in the head of the pancreas. The transducer tip is located in the duodenum. The dilated common bile duct and gallbladder *(GB)* can be seen at the top of the image. The pancreatic duct *(PD)* is also dilated. The mass involves the portal vein *(PV)*.

these metastases are smaller and therefore may not be routinely detected. Moreover, peritoneal and omental metastases are usually only 1 to 2 mm in size and frequently can be detected only by direct visualization. With the recent improvements in CT imaging, the rate of positive peritoneal findings approaches 20% to 25% for all patients with pancreatic cancer and is significantly higher for patients with cancers of the body and tail. For example, patients presenting with obstructive jaundice secondary to tumors in the head of the pancreas typically have only a 15% to 20% incidence of unexpected intraperitoneal metastasis after routine staging studies. In contrast, unex-

pected peritoneal metastasis is found in up to 50% of patients with cancer of the body and tail of the pancreas. Therefore, staging laparoscopy appears to be justified for patients with cancers of the body and tail, in whom the primary tumor does not typically cause biliary or gastric outlet obstruction and who therefore do not routinely require palliation of biliary or gastric obstruction. In these cases, laparoscopy can spare the patient an unnecessary laparotomy because operative palliation is seldom appropriate. However, the role of preoperative staging is not clear in patients with localized tumor on spiral CT who present with obstructive jaundice, symptoms of gastric outlet obstruction, and tumor-related abdominal and back pain. Many surgeons believe that such patients are best managed via surgical palliation that includes biliary–enteric bypass, gastrojejunostomy, and alcohol celiac nerve block. Preoperative staging laparoscopy would serve no purpose in such a setting.

Percutaneous FNA of pancreatic masses is helpful in selected patients. The technique is safe and generally reliable but is of limited use in patients in whom surgical exploration for attempted resection or palliation is planned. The reasons for not using FNA or percutaneous biopsy in potentially resectable lesions are twofold. First, even after repeated sampling, a negative result does not exclude malignancy; in fact, it is the smaller and likely more curable tumors that are likely to be missed by the needle. The second concern is seeding of the tumor, either along the needle tract or with intraperitoneal spread. Percutaneous biopsy is primarily indicated in patients with unresectable cancers according to preoperative staging. The results can be used to direct palliative chemoradiation therapy. The technique is also useful in patients with cancer in the head of the pancreas for whom neoadjuvant protocols are being considered.

The information gained from preoperative staging provides the basis for planning therapy for each individual patient. If the results of preoperative staging with CT, angiography, and laparoscopy show localized disease, resectability rates may approach 80% for tumors in the head of the pancreas. An algorithm for the clinical staging of suspected pancreatic cancer is shown in Fig. 32.6.

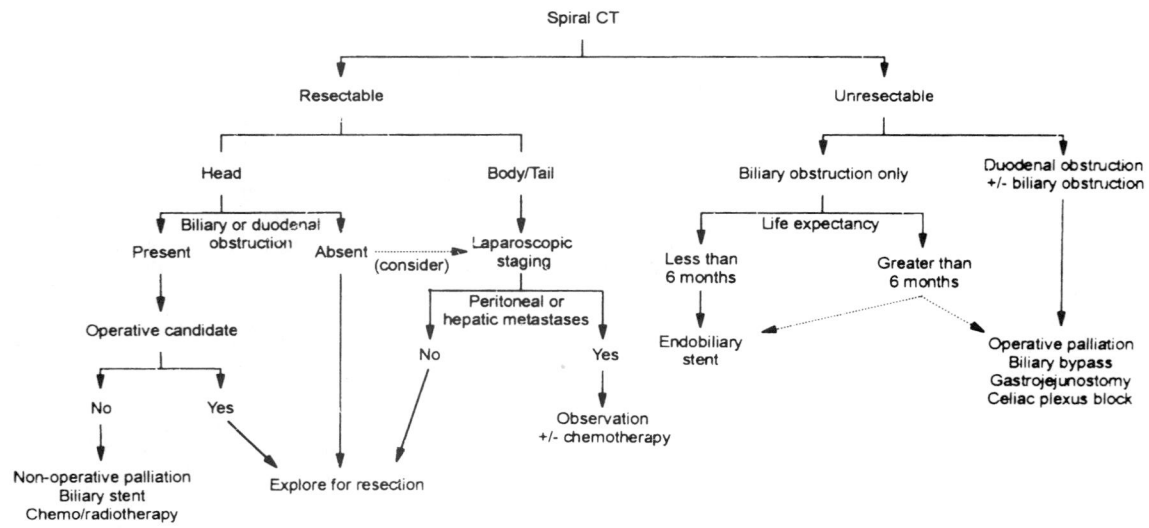

Figure 32.6. Algorithm for use in the clinical setting of presumptive pancreatic cancer. (From Tsiotis GG, Sarr MG. Diagnosis and clinical staging of pancreatic cancer. In: Howard JM, Idezuki Y, Ihse I, et al., eds. *Surgical disease of the pancreas,* 3rd ed. Baltimore: Williams & Wilkins, 1998: 510.)

RESECTION OF PANCREATIC CARCINOMA

Carcinoma of the Head, Neck, or Uncinate Process

In 1912, Kaush (9) reported the first successful resection of the duodenum and a portion of the pancreas for an ampullary cancer. In 1935, Whipple and associates (10) described a technique for radical excision of a periampullary carcinoma. The operation was originally performed in two stages. A cholecystogastrostomy to decompress the obstructed biliary tree and a gastrojejunostomy to relieve gastric outlet obstruction comprised the first stage. The second stage was performed several weeks later when the jaundice had resolved and the nutritional status had improved. During the second stage, an *en bloc* resection of the second portion of the duodenum and head of the pancreas was performed without reestablishing pancreatic–enteric continuity. Although earlier contributions had been made, the report by Whipple and colleagues began the modern-day approach to the treatment of pancreatic carcinoma.

Since Whipple's original description, pancreaticoduodenal resection has undergone numerous modifications and technical refinements. Unfortunately, during most of the first 50 years when the procedure was performed, the reported morbidity and mortality rates were unacceptably high, and long-term survival rates were disappointing. During the late 1960s and 1970s, the high operative morbidity and mortality and poor long-term survival rates led some surgeons to suggest that the Whipple procedure be abandoned. However, during the last decade, a number of reports have documented improved operative results and long-term survival rates for patients with periampullary tumors following the Whipple procedure, so that a resurgence in its popularity has occurred.

The operative management of pancreatic cancer consists of two phases: first, assessing tumor resectability and then, if the tumor is resectable, completing a pancreaticoduodenectomy and restoring gastrointestinal continuity. After the abdomen has been opened through an upper midline or bilateral subcostal incision, a careful search for tumor outside the limits of a pancreaticoduodenal resection should be carried out. The liver, omentum, and peritoneal surfaces are inspected and palpated, and suspect lesions are sampled and specimens submitted for frozen section analysis. Next, regional lymph nodes are evaluated for tumor involvement. The presence of tumor in the periaortic lymph nodes of the celiac axis indicates that the tumor is beyond the limits of normal resection. However, the presence of tumor-bearing lymph nodes that normally would be incorporated within the resection specimen do not constitute a contraindication to resection.

Once distant metastases have been excluded, the primary tumor is assessed in regard to resectability. Local factors that preclude pancreaticoduodenal resection include retroperitoneal extension of the tumor to involve the inferior vena cava or aorta, or direct involvement or encasement of the superior mesenteric artery, superior mesenteric vein, or portal vein. The technical aspects of determining local resectability begin with a Kocher maneuver and mobilization of the duodenum and head of the pancreas from the underlying inferior vena cava and aorta. Once the duodenum and head of the pancreas are mobilized sufficiently, the surgeon's hand can be placed under the duodenum and head of the pancreas to palpate the relationship of the tumor mass to the superior mesenteric artery. Inability of the surgeon to identify a plane of normal tissue between the mass and the arterial pulsation indicates direct tumor in-

volvement of the superior mesenteric artery, and the possibility of complete tumor resection is eliminated.

The final step to determine resectability involves dissection of the superior mesenteric and portal veins to rule out tumor invasion. Identification of the portal vein can be simplified greatly if the common hepatic duct is divided and reflected early in the dissection. Once the hepatic duct has been divided, the posteriorly located portal vein can be identified easily. After the anterior surface of the portal vein is dissected posterior to the neck of the pancreas, the next step is to identify the superior mesenteric vein and dissect its anterior surface. This is done most easily by extending the Kocher maneuver past the second portion of the duodenum to include the third and fourth portions of the duodenum. During this extensive kocherization, the first structure that one encounters anterior to the third portion of the duodenum is the superior mesenteric vein. The anterior surface of the vein then can be cleaned rapidly and dissected under direct vision by retracting the neck of the pancreas anteriorly. The dissection is continued until it connects to the portal vein dissection from above.

Most experienced pancreatic surgeons, at this point, proceed with a pancreaticoduodenectomy without obtaining a tissue diagnosis. The clinical presentation, results of preoperative CT and cholangiography, and operative findings of a palpable mass in the head of the pancreas surpass the ability of an intraoperative biopsy to define the diagnosis of malignancy.

Having excluded regional and distant metastases and demonstrated no tumor involvement in major vascular structures, the surgeon can proceed with pancreaticoduodenectomy with a high degree of certainty that the tumor is resectable. In the pylorus-preserving modification of pancreaticoduodenectomy, the duodenum is first mobilized and divided approximately 2 cm distal to the pylorus. If a classic Whipple procedure is to be performed, the stomach is divided to include approximately 40% to 50% of the stomach with the resected specimen. The gastroduodenal artery is exposed, ligated, and divided near its origin at the common hepatic artery. It is always important to confirm, before ligation, that the structure to be ligated is indeed the gastroduodenal artery and not a replaced right hepatic artery. Next, the neck of the pancreas is divided, with care taken to avoid injury to the underlying superior mesenteric and portal veins. The portal and superior mesenteric veins are then dissected from the uncinate process and head of the pancreas. At this point, the fourth portion of the duodenum and the proximal jejunum are mobilized, with the proximal jejunum divided approximately 10 cm distal to the ligament of Treitz. The proximal jejunum and fourth portion of the duodenum are passed under the superior mesenteric vessels to the right, and the uncinate process is dissected from the superior mesenteric artery. The course of the superior mesenteric artery should be identified clearly to avoid injury to this structure. At this point, the specimen—consisting of the gallbladder and common bile duct, the head, neck, and uncinate process of the pancreas, the entire duodenum, and the proximal jejunum (and the distal stomach for a traditional Whipple procedure)—is freed completely and removed from the operative field (Fig. 32.7).

A number of techniques are used to restore gastrointestinal continuity after a pancreaticoduodenal resection. In the most common technique, the end of the divided jejunum is placed in a retrocolic position, with creation of a pancreaticojejunostomy, followed by a hepaticojejunostomy and a duodenojejunostomy or gastrojejunostomy. The pancreaticojejunostomy is the most problematic anastomosis in the reconstruction. Traditionally, much of the morbidity and mortality associated with this operation are

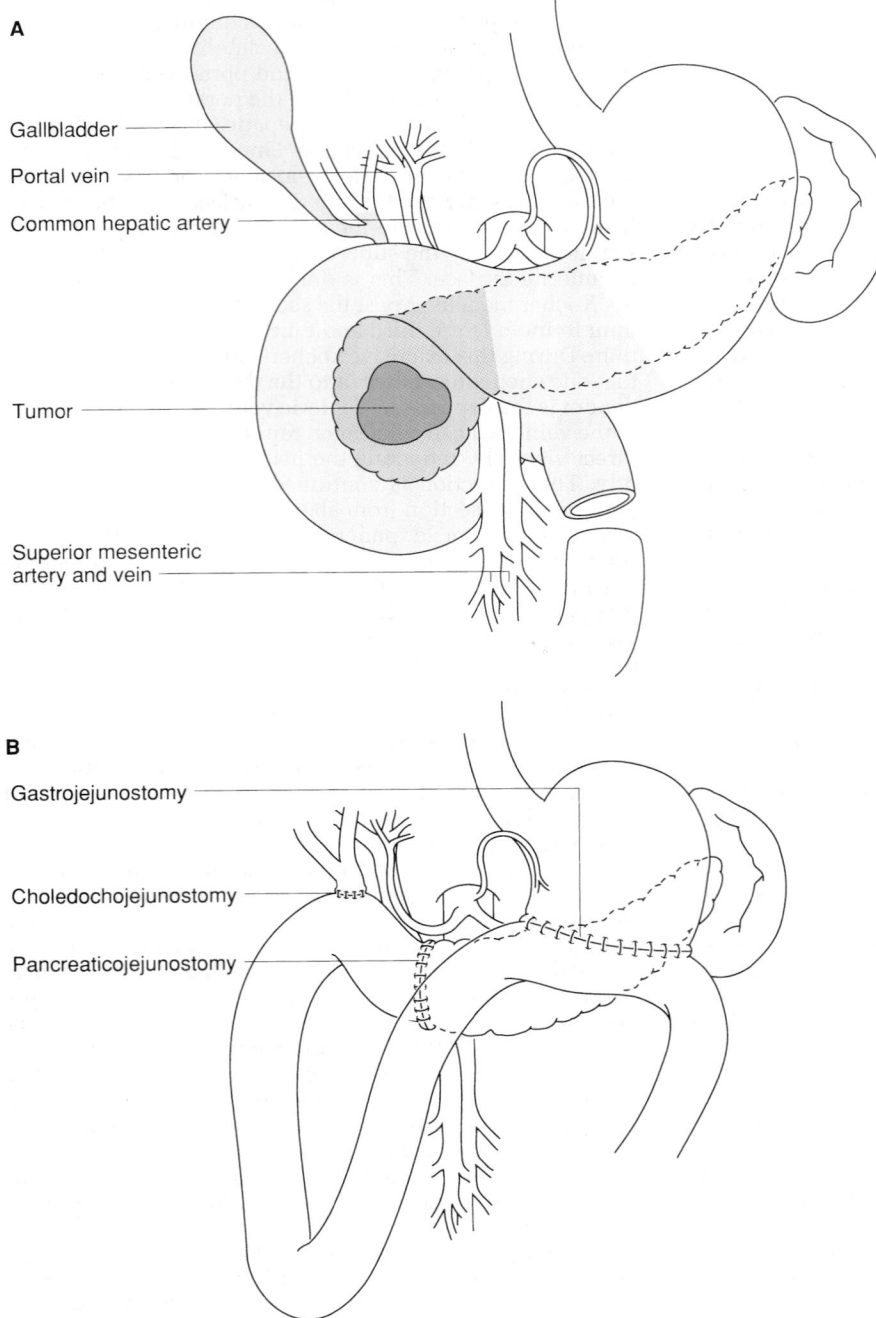

A

Gallbladder

Portal vein

Common hepatic artery

Tumor

Superior mesenteric
artery and vein

B

Gastrojejunostomy

Choledochojejunostomy

Pancreaticojejunostomy

Figure 32.7. Pancreaticoduodenectomy.
(A) The tissue to be resected in a standard
pancreaticoduodenectomy. *(B)* Reconstruction after a standard pancreaticoduodenectomy. *(continues)*

related to problems associated with this anastomosis. Several techniques to manage the pancreatic remnant can be
used, including end-to-end and end-to-side pancreaticojejunostomy, or pancreaticogastrostomy. The biliary–enteric
anastomosis is performed approximately 10 cm distal to
the pancreaticojejunostomy. Approximately 15 cm distal
to the biliary–enteric anastomosis, an end-to-side duodenojejunostomy or gastrojejunostomy is performed.

Extent of Resection

The classic pancreaticoduodenectomy performed for
decades included a distal gastrectomy. In 1978, Traverso
and Longmire (11) described the pylorus-preserving modification of the Whipple procedure. By preserving the
antrum and pylorus, the pylorus-preserving Whipple procedure may reduce the incidence of troublesome postgas-

trectomy problems, including marginal ulceration. However, a concern regarding the use of the pylorus-preserving
Whipple procedure for the management of periampullary
tumors is the possibility of compromising the already
small surgical margins of resection. Nonetheless, in a comparison of patients treated with the pylorus-sparing Whipple procedure and those managed by the traditional Whipple resection for pancreatic cancer, no difference in
survival has been noted (12).

An extension of the Whipple procedure to include a total
pancreatectomy with removal of the spleen and more extensive regional lymph nodes has been advocated by some
surgeons. The overall poor long-term survival following
the standard Whipple operation was the impetus for the
concept of extending resection to a total pancreatectomy.
Advocates also cite the advantages of eliminating multicentric disease and preventing the spread of disease to the

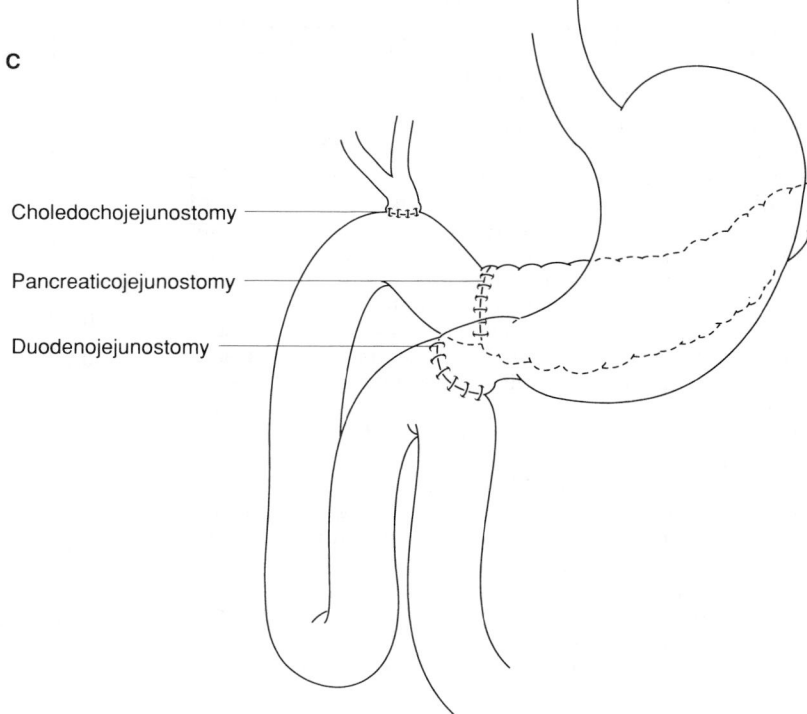

C

Choledochojejunostomy

Pancreaticojejunostomy

Duodenojejunostomy

Figure 32.7. *(Continued) (C)* Reconstruction after the pylorus-sparing variation.

distal pancreas by direct extension, intraductal seeding, or lymphatic spread. In addition, it is felt that this is a better cancer operation, including a wider *en bloc* resection of the pancreas in addition to regional lymph nodes. Another advantage is elimination of the pancreaticojejunal anastomosis, which is a major cause of morbidity and mortality following the Whipple operation. Despite these rational arguments, no evidence has accumulated that a total pancreatectomy offers any survival advantage for patients with carcinoma of the head of the pancreas who are undergoing the procedure. Furthermore, no reduction in morbidity and mortality has been noted for those patients managed by a total pancreatectomy. The major disadvantage of the total pancreatectomy is the inevitable complete loss of pancreatic endocrine function, resulting in the development of diabetes that can be difficult to control. Total pancreatectomy should be reserved for those patients with histologic evidence of tumor at the margin of resection or those with gross multicentric disease.

The concept of an even wider resection, or radical pancreatectomy, has also been suggested. These procedures include resection of the portal vein with reconstruction and an extensive regional lymph node dissection. Reports from Japanese centers have suggested a potential improvement in long-term survival with extended lymphadenectomy. However, these results have been uncontrolled and do not appear significantly better than those in recent Western reports (13). Furthermore, two recent multicenter prospective, randomized trials have not shown a significant survival advantage for the wider resection (14,15). Finally, although major vascular resection in experienced hands is not associated with increased perioperative morbidity and mortality (16), the procedure does increase operative time, blood loss, and, in most series, length of hospital stay.

Carcinoma of the Body and Tail

The surgical management of adenocarcinoma of the body and tail of the pancreas is much more limited than that of the head of the pancreas because of the extent of the disease usually present at the time of symptomatic presentation.

Most patients are unable to undergo resection, based on findings of major vascular involvement on CT or peritoneal or liver metastases on laparoscopy. If an attempt at open exploration for possible cure is undertaken, the exploration should be started with a search for evidence of either metastatic disease to the liver or peritoneal implants. If this is not the case, the lesser sac is opened, and the superior mesenteric vein is identified as it passes under the neck of the pancreas. If this vessel is normal, and if the splenic vein does not appear to be obstructed preoperatively, a distal pancreatectomy with splenectomy is performed. The spleen is mobilized, as is the distal pancreas, and an *en bloc* resection of the structure, including the mass, is obtained. The resection should be extended as proximally as possible, with the transected pancreas simply oversewn. The tumor bed should be marked with the placement of clips for postoperative radiation therapy. If, as in most cases, the tumor cannot be resected, a tissue biopsy should be performed, in addition to a chemical splanchnicectomy with alcohol for pain management. In some cases, a prophylactic gastrojejunostomy may be indicated because of the potential for obstruction by tumor at the ligament of Treitz.

Postoperative Results

During the 1960s and 1970s, many centers reported operative mortality following pancreaticoduodenectomy in the range of 20% to 40%, with postoperative morbidity rates as high as 40% to 60%. During the last decade, a dramatic decline in operative morbidity and mortality following pancreaticoduodenectomy has been reported at a number of centers, with operative mortality rates in the range of 2% to 3% (17–19). The reasons behind this decline appear to be the following: (a) Fewer, more experienced surgeons are performing the operation on a more frequent basis; (b) preoperative and postoperative care has improved; (c) anesthetic management has improved; and (d) large numbers of patients are being treated at high-volume centers (20).

Although the operative mortality rates for pancreatic cancer have been reduced significantly, the complication rates remain high (approximately 40%) (Table 32.7). Pancreatic fistula remains the most frequent serious complication following pancreaticoduodenectomy, with an incidence ranging from 5% to 20%. In the past, the development of pancreatic fistula after pancreaticoduodenectomy was associated with mortality rates of 10% to 40%. Although the incidence of pancreatic fistula following pancreaticoduodenectomy remains stable, the overall associated mortality rate has diminished owing to improved management. Control of the anastomotic leak with careful placement of drains in the area of the pancreatic anastomosis is a major step in minimizing the morbidity of a pancreatic leak. Important supportive measures include careful maintenance of fluid and electrolyte balance, parenteral nutrition, and meticulous care of the drainage site to avoid skin excoriation and autodigestion by activated pancreatic enzymes.

The most frequent complication following pylorus-preserving pancreatic resection is delayed gastric emptying, with an incidence in the range of 20% to 40%. The cause of this complication is unknown, and in most patients mechanical obstruction should be ruled out by either contrast studies or endoscopic evaluation. The management of delayed gastric emptying includes gastric decompression and maintenance of parenteral or enteral nutrition. In most cases, delayed gastric emptying is temporary and resolves spontaneously. The use of prokinetic agents such as metoclopramide or erythromycin, a motilin agonist, may be useful in the treatment of postoperative delayed gastric emptying.

Long-term Survival

Historically, 5-year survival rates for patients undergoing resection for adenocarcinoma of the head of the pancreas were reported to be in the range of 5%. However, a number of recent studies have suggested an improved survival for patients following pancreaticoduodenectomy (17–19). In 1995, Yeo and associates (13) reported on 201 patients with adenocarcinoma of the head of the pancreas managed by pancreaticoduodenectomy. The actuarial 5-year survival for these patients was 21%, with a median survival of 15.5 months (Fig. 32.8). In this study, factors found to be important predictors of survival included tumor diameter (< 3 cm), lymph node status, and resection margin status. Patients who underwent resection with negative margins had a median survival of 18 months and a 5-year survival of 26%, whereas those with positive margins fared significantly worse, with a median survival of 10 months and a 5-year survival of 8%. The outcome was particularly favorable in the subgroup of patients who underwent pancreaticoduodenectomy with both negative lymph nodes and negative resection margins; the median survival was 32 months and the 5-year survival was 40%.

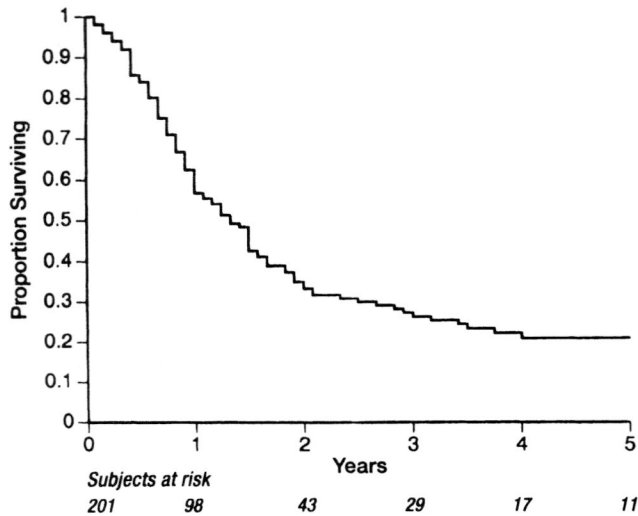

Figure 32.8. The actuarial survival curve for 201 patients who underwent pancreaticoduodenectomy for pancreatic adenocarcinoma. (From Yeo CJ, Cameron JL, Lillemoe KD, et al. Pancreaticoduodenectomy for cancer of the head of the pancreas: 201 patients. *Ann Surg* 1995;221:721–733, with permission.)

NEOADJUVANT AND ADJUVANT THERAPY

At present, the general consensus of most surgeons treating patients with pancreatic carcinoma is that any future improvement in the management of this disease will involve improvements in adjuvant therapy. The role of adjuvant radiation therapy is emphasized by the pattern of relapse after surgical resection, as more than half of the patients undergoing resection experience local regional recurrence without evidence of distant metastases (21).

In 1985, the Gastrointestinal Tumor Study Group reported encouraging results from a prospective, randomized trial to evaluate the efficacy of adjuvant radiation and chemotherapy following curative resection for adenocarcinoma of the head of the pancreas (22). Forty-three patients were randomized to either adjuvant therapy with radiation and 5-fluorouracil (5-FU) or no adjuvant therapy. The median survival for the 21 patients who received adjuvant therapy was 20 months, and three (14%) survived 5 years or longer. For the 22 patients who received no adjuvant therapy, the median survival was 11 months, and only one patient (4.5%) survived 5 years. These results have been subsequently confirmed and provide strong support for the concept of postoperative combined adjuvant therapy (23).

In a recent study from Johns Hopkins (24), 174 patients with resected, pathologically confirmed adenocarcinoma of the head, neck, or uncinate process of the pancreas who had undergone resection were prospectively evaluated. In this group, all resections were standard pancreaticoduodenectomies without extended retroperitoneal lymph node dissection. Postoperatively, the patients were evaluated by a multidisciplinary group that included surgeons, radiation oncologists, medical oncologists, and pathologists, and they were offered three options for postoperative treatment after pancreaticoduodenectomy: (a) standard therapy that consisted of external beam radiation to the pancreatic bed (4,000 to 4,500 cGy) given with two 3-day courses of 5-FU followed weekly by a bolus of 5-FU for an additional 4 months; (b) intensive therapy that consisted of external beam radiation to the pancreatic bed (5,040 to 5,760 cGy) with prophylactic hepatic irradiation (2,340 to

Table 32.7. **COMPLICATIONS AFTER PANCREATICODUODENECTOMY**

Common	Uncommon
Delayed gastric emptying	Fistula
Pancreatic fistula	Biliary
Intraabdominal abscess	Duodenal
Hemorrhage	Gastric
Wound infection	Organ failure
Metabolic	Cardiac
Diabetes	Hepatic
Pancreatic exocrine insufficiency	Pulmonary
	Renal
	Pancreatitis
	Marginal ulceration

From Yeo CJ, Cameron JL. Pancreatic cancer. Curr Probl Surg 1999;36:61–152, with permission.

2,700 cGy) followed by infusional 5-FU plus leucovorin for 5 of 7 d/wk for 4 months; (c) no therapy. All patients who had a satisfactory recovery from pancreaticoduodenectomy by postoperative day 60 were encouraged to accept either standard therapy or the more intensive regimen. In the 4-year period of this study, 174 patients underwent pancreaticoduodenectomy for pancreatic carcinoma. The median survival for the entire cohort of 174 patients was 19 months, with actuarial 1-, 2-, and 3-year survivals of 68%, 36%, and 29%, respectively. No difference in survival was observed based on age, sex, or race. Patients who received either type of adjuvant therapy had a median survival of 19.5 months and a 2-year survival of 39%, significantly better than the survival rate of the patients who received no therapy (13.5 months and 30%) (Fig. 32.9). Based on these data and the earlier results from the Gastrointestinal Tumor Study Group, standard chemotherapy based on 5-FU with external beam radiation appears to be indicated after pancreaticoduodenectomy for adenocarcinoma of the pancreas.

At present, a number of clinical trials are under way that are utilizing preoperative chemoradiation protocols for the treatment of pancreatic cancer. Preliminary results suggest that neoadjuvant therapy can be completed without increasing the subsequent morbidity and mortality of surgical resection. The group from the M.D. Anderson Cancer Center has recently reported on the multimodality treatment of 142 consecutive patients with localized adenocarcinoma of the pancreatic head (25). A subset of 41 patients treated by preoperative chemoradiation and pancreaticoduodenectomy were compared with 19 patients receiving pancreaticoduodenectomy and postoperative adjuvant chemoradiation. Surgery did not have to be delayed for any patient who received preoperative chemoradiation because of chemoradiation toxicity, but 24% of the eligible patients did not receive their intended postoperative chemoradiation because of delayed recovery following pancreaticoduodenectomy. The patients treated with rapid fractionation were reported to have a significantly shorter duration of treatment (median, 62.5 days) than patients who received postoperative chemoradiation (median, 98.5 days). In early follow-up, no patient who received preoperative chemoradiation experienced a local recurrence, and peritoneal recurrence developed in only 10% of these patients. Local or regional recurrence developed in 21% of patients who received postoperative chemoradiation. The overall survival curves were similar for both cohorts. The use of neoadjuvant therapy remains controversial, with some groups reserving neoadjuvant therapy for patients with evidence of locally unresectable tumors (as defined by imaging studies or laparotomy).

PALLIATION

Unfortunately, it has been the experience nationwide that only a minority of patients with carcinoma of the pancreas can undergo resection for possible cure at the time diagnosis is made. Thus, the optimal palliation of symptoms to maximize quality of life is of primary importance in most patients with pancreatic cancer. Both operative and nonoperative options are available for the palliation of pancreatic cancer.

Jaundice

Obstructive jaundice is present in most patients who have pancreatic cancer. If left untreated, it can result in progressive liver dysfunction, hepatic failure, and early death. In addition, the pruritus associated with obstructive jaundice can be debilitating and usually does not respond to medication. When patients undergo exploration for possible cure and are found to have unresectable disease, a biliary bypass should be performed.

Traditionally, surgeons have performed either choledochojejunostomy or cholecystojejunostomy for the relief of malignant biliary obstruction. Both procedures are effective in relieving jaundice, but it appears that the rate of recurrent jaundice after cholecystojejunostomy is approximately 10%. Therefore, our preference for the palliation of obstructive jaundice is a hepaticojejunostomy or choledochojejunostomy reconstructed with a Roux-en-Y limb of jejunum. The surgical palliation of jaundice can be accomplished safely, with a mortality rate of less than 3% and an overall morbidity rate of 30% to 40% (26). The gallbladder is usually removed at the time of choledochojejunostomy to prevent the development of late cholecystitis if the cystic duct becomes obstructed by tumor. In certain circumstances, however, it may be appropriate to use the gallbladder. These include the presence of large bulky tumors that have invaded the porta hepatis or of large periductal varices that have developed as a result of portal vein thrombosis. If the gallbladder is to be used, the patency of the cystic duct should be confirmed, and the cystic duct should enter the common bile duct at least 2 cm away from any tumor.

In recent years, nonoperative palliation has become available as an option for managing these patients. Plastic or metal stents can be placed across the biliary obstruction by either an endoscopic or a percutaneous technique. For pancreatic cancer, the endoscopic approach is usually preferred. The overall morbidity rate for endoscopic stenting ranges up to 35%, but the rate of major procedure-related morbidity is less than 10%. Early complications include cholangitis, pancreatitis, and bile duct or duodenal perforation. The major late complications of stent placement are cholecystitis, duodenal perforation, and stent migra-

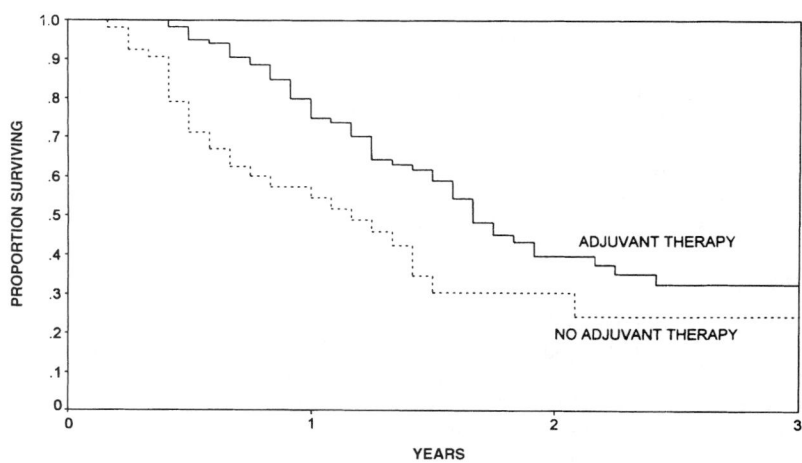

Figure 32.9. Actuarial survival curves for 173 patients who underwent pancreaticoduodenectomy. Patients who received adjuvant therapy (*n* = 120) are compared with those who declined adjuvant therapy (*n* = 53). (From Yeo CJ, Abrams RA, Grochow LB, et al. Pancreaticoduodenectomy for pancreatic adenocarcinoma: postoperative adjuvant chemoradiation improves survival: a prospective, single-institution experience. *Ann Surg* 1997;225:621–636, with permission.)

Table 32.8. **PROSPECTIVE RANDOMIZED TRIAL OF PROPHYLACTIC GASTROJEJUNOSTOMY IN PATIENTS WITH UNRESECTABLE PERIAMPULLARY CANCER**

	Patients (No.)	Morbidity (%)	Mortality (%)	Postoperative length of stay (d)	Late gastric outlet obstruction (%)
Gastrojejunostomy	44	32	0	8.5	0
No gastrojejunostomy	43	33	0	8.0	19

Adapted from Lillemoe KD, Cameron JL, Hardacre JM, et al. Is prophylactic gastrojejunostomy indicated for unresectable periampullary cancer? Ann Surg 1999;230:322–330, with permission.

tion. Stent occlusion can result in episodes of cholangitis and recurrent jaundice. For most patients, an exchange of stents is required every 3 to 6 months. The newer metal stents appear to remain patent for longer periods of time.

Nonoperative palliation appears to be associated with lower complication rates, lower procedure-related mortality rates, and shorter initial periods of hospitalization in comparison with surgical palliation. However, the rate of recurrent jaundice is higher. No advantage with respect to long-term survival has been noted for either approach. Therefore, nonoperative palliation should be offered to patients with advanced disease or poor performance status. Surgical palliation should be considered for patients with an anticipated life expectancy of at least 3 months.

Duodenal Obstruction

At the time that pancreatic cancer is diagnosed, approximately one third of patients have symptoms of nausea or vomiting. Although true mechanical obstruction of the duodenum seen by radiologic or endoscopic examination is much less frequent, duodenal obstruction develops in almost 20% of patients before they die as the disease progresses (27). Duodenal obstruction can be caused in the C-loop by cancers of the head or at the ligament of Trietz by cancers of the body and tail. In patients with evidence of duodenal obstruction or impending obstruction, a gastrojejunostomy is indicated for palliation. This is typically performed as a retrocolic, isoperistaltic loop gastrojejunostomy with a loop of jejunum 20 to 30 cm distal to the ligament of Trietz.

In patients with unresectable pancreatic cancer who do not have symptoms of gastric outlet obstruction, whether or not to perform a prophylactic gastric bypass at the time of biliary bypass is a matter of debate. Surgeons who do not perform a prophylactic bypass feel that it needlessly increases the postoperative length of stay and can be associated with delayed gastric emptying and increased morbidity and mortality. However, data from a recent prospective, randomized trial of prophylactic gastrojejunostomy in patients with unresectable cancer do not support this view (28). In this study, 44 patients were randomized to a gastrojejunostomy, and 43 did not undergo gastric bypass. No mortality occurred in either group. No difference was observed in either the complication rate or the postoperative length of stay (Table 32.8). However, late duodenal obstruction developed in 19% of the patients who did not undergo bypass. Therefore, we believe that a prophylactic gastrojejunostomy should be performed in patients undergoing surgical palliation for unresectable pancreatic carcinoma.

Pain

Tumor-associated pain can be incapacitating in patients with unresectable pancreatic cancer. The postulated causes of tumor-associated pain are many and include tumor infiltration into the celiac plexus, increased parenchymal pressure caused by pancreatic duct obstruction, pancreatic inflammation, gallbladder distention resulting

from biliary obstruction, and gastroduodenal obstruction. The management of pain in patients dying of carcinoma of the pancreas is one of the most important aspects of their care. The appropriate use of oral agents can be successful in most patients. Patients with significant pain should receive their medication on a regular schedule and not an "as-needed" basis. The use of long-acting morphine derivative compounds appears to be best suited for such treatment. Percutaneous neurolytic block of the celiac axis, performed under either fluoroscopic or CT guidance, is also successful in the majority of patients at eliminating pain. Patients with unresectable cancer at the time of surgical exploration should receive a chemical splanchnicectomy, with 20 mL of 50% alcohol injected on either side of the aorta at the level of the celiac axis (29).

SUMMARY

The decision to perform nonoperative versus surgical palliation for pancreatic cancer is influenced by a number of factors, including the patient's symptoms, overall health status, predicted procedure-related morbidity and mortality, and projected survival. Surgical palliation can be completed with acceptable perioperative morbidity and mortality and postoperative length of stay. The avoidance of late complications of recurrent jaundice, duodenal obstruction, and disabling pain would strengthen the argument in favor of surgical palliation in those patients expected to survive 6 months or more. Nonoperative methods of palliation should be considered for patients in whom preoperative staging suggests distant metastatic disease or a locally unresectable tumor, patients who are not candidates for operative intervention, and those not expected to survive more than 3 months.

Radiation and Chemotherapy for Unresectable Pancreatic Carcinoma

Specific antitumor therapies in patients with advanced pancreatic carcinoma have been studied for years, with limited success. Trials evaluating the use of chemotherapy and radiation therapy both alone and in combination have shown a marginal improvement in survival, often with relatively high toxicity rates and some negative impact on quality of life. Recently, a novel chemotherapeutic agent, gemcitabine, a deoxycytidine analogue capable of inhibiting DNA replication and repair, has been released by the Food and Drug Administration for patients with advanced pancreatic carcinoma. Following a phase I study, gemcitabine was evaluated in a multicenter trial of 34 patients with advanced pancreatic cancer, with the finding of frequent subjective symptomatic benefit, often in the absence of an objective tumor response (30). The currently available data suggest that chemotherapy with gemcitabine appears to be more effective than chemotherapy with 5-FU in patients with advanced pancreatic cancer; improvements in median survival (generally a few weeks to a month or two), pain control, performance status, and weight gain have been observed with gemcitabine in comparison with 5-FU. Additionally, preliminary data have demonstrated that gemcitabine is a potent radiation sensitizer of human pancreatic cancer cells in vitro (31). This effect is being evaluated in various trials of gemcitabine plus radiation therapy worldwide.

In addition to gemcitabine, other agents are currently being studied for a role in the palliation of patients with pancreatic adenocarcinoma. Examples of such agents are paclitaxel (Taxol), matrix metalloproteinase inhibitors (e.g., marimastat, perillyl alcohol), and inhibitors of angiogenesis, such as TNP-470. The results of such studies are eagerly awaited.

CONCLUSION

Carcinoma of the pancreas remains a disease with a generally dismal prognosis. Potentially curable lesions are typically confined to the head of the pancreas and present early with obstructive jaundice. Aggressive evaluation with appropriate staging should be performed. Either resection for cure by a pancreaticoduodenectomy or operative palliation should be performed by surgeons experienced in the management of this disease to minimize morbidity and mortality. Following resection, adjuvant radiation and chemotherapy should be offered to most patients for improved long-term survival.

REFERENCES

1. Greenlee RT, Murray T, Bolden S, et al. Cancer statistics, 2000. *CA Cancer J Clin* 2000;50:7–33.
2. Yeo CJ, Cameron JL. Pancreatic cancer. *Curr Probl Surg* 1999;36:61–152.
3. Hruban RH, Petersen GM, Ha PK, et al. Genetics of pancreatic cancer: from genes to families. *Surg Oncol Clin N Am* 1998;7:1–23.
4. Goggins M, Oferhaus GJA, Hilgers W, et al. Adenocarcinoma of the pancreas with DNA replication errors (RER+) are associated with a characteristic histopathology: poor differentiation, a syncytial growth pattern, and pushing borders suggest RER+. *Am J Pathol* 1998;152:1501–1507.
5. Wilentz RE, Hruban RH. Pathology of cancer of the pancreas. *Surg Oncol Clin N Am* 1998;7:43–65.
6. Ritts RE, Pitt HA. CA 19-9 in pancreatic cancer. *Surg Oncol Clin N Am* 1998;7:93–101
7. Wiersema MJ, Vilman P, Giovannini M, et al. Endosonography-guided fine-needle aspiration biopsy: diagnostic accuracy and complication assessment. *Gastroenterology* 1997;112:1087–1089.
8. Fernandez-del Castillo C, Rattner DW, Warshaw AL. Further experience with laparoscopy and peritoneal cytology in staging for pancreatic cancer. *Br J Surg* 1995;82:1127–1129.
9. Kausch W. Das Carcinom der Papilla Duodeni und seine radikale Entfeinung. *Beitrage zur Klinische Chirurgie* 1912;78:439–486.
10. Whipple AO, Parsons WB, Mullins CR. Treatment of carcinoma of the ampulla of Vater. *Ann Surg* 1935;102:763–779.
11. Traverso LW, Longmire WP Jr. Preservation of the pylorus in pancreaticoduodenectomy. *Surg Gynecol Obstet* 1978;146:959–962.
12. Tsao JI, Rossi RL, Lowell JA. Pylorus-preserving pancreatoduodenectomy: is it an adequate cancer operation? *Arch Surg* 1994;129:405–412.
13. Yeo CJ, Cameron JL, Lillemoe KD, et al. Pancreaticoduodenectomy for cancer of the head of the pancreas: 201 patients. *Ann Surg* 1995;221:721–733.
14. Pedrazzoli S, DiCarlo V, Dionigi R, et al. Standard versus extended lymphadenectomy associated with pancreaticoduodenectomy in the surgical treatment of adenocarcinoma of the head of the pancreas: a multicenter, prospective, randomized study group. Lymphadenectomy Study Group. *Ann Surg* 1998;222:508–517.
15. Yeo CJ, Cameron JL, Sohn TA, et al. Pancreaticoduodenectomy with or without extended retroperitoneal lymphadenectomy for periampullary adenocarcinoma: comparison of morbidity, mortality, and short-term outcome. *Ann Surg* 1999;229:613–614.
16. Fuhrman GM, Leach SD, Staley CA, et al. Rationale for *en bloc* vein resection in the treatment of pancreatic adenocarcinoma adherent to the superior mesenteric–portal vein confluence. *Ann Surg* 1996;223:154–162.
17. Trede M, Schwall G, Saeger H. Survival after pancreaticoduodenectomy: 118 consecutive resections without an operative mortality. *Ann Surg* 1990;211:447–458.
18. Fernandez-del Castillo, Rattner DW, Warshaw AL. Standards for pancreatic resection in the 1990s. *Arch Surg* 1995;130:295–300.
19. Yeo CJ, Cameron JL, Sohn TA, et al. Six hundred fifty consecutive pancreaticoduodenectomies in the 1990s: pathology, complications, outcomes. *Ann Surg* 1997;226:248–260.
20. Sosa JA, Bowman HM, Gordon TA, et al. Importance of hospital volume in the overall management of pancreatic cancer. *Ann Surg* 1998;228:320–370.
21. Tepper J, Nardi G, Suit H. Carcinoma of the pancreas: review of MGH experience from 1963–1973: analysis of surgical failure and implications for radiation therapy. *Cancer* 1977;37:1519–1524.
22. Kaiser MH, Ellenberg SS. Pancreatic cancer: adjuvant combined radiation and chemotherapy following curative resection. *Arch Surg* 1985;97:28–35.
23. Gastrointestinal Tumor Study Group. Further evidence for effective adjuvant combined radiation and chemotherapy following curative resection of pancreatic cancer. *Cancer* 1987;59:2006–2010.
24. Yeo CJ, Abrams RA, Grochow LB, et al. Pancreaticoduodenectomy for pancreatic adenocarcinoma: postoperative adjuvant chemoradiation improves survival: a prospective, single-institution experience. *Ann Surg* 1997;225:621–636.
25. Spitz FR, Abbruzzese JL, Lee JE, et al. Preoperative and postoperative chemoradiation strategies in patients treated with pancreaticoduodenectomy for adenocarcinoma of the pancreas. *J Clin Oncol* 1997;15:928–937.
26. Sohn TA, Lillemoe KD, Cameron JL, et al. Surgical palliation of unresectable periampullary carcinoma in the 1990s. *J Am Coll Surg* 1999;188:658–669.
27. Sarr MG, Cameron JL. Surgical management of unresectable carcinoma of the pancreas. *Surgery* 1982;91:123–133.
28. Lillemoe KD, Cameron JL, Hardacre JM, et al. Is prophylactic gastrojejunostomy indicated for unresectable periampullary cancer? *Ann Surg* 1999;230:322–330.
29. Lillemoe KD, Cameron JL, Kaufman HS, et al. Chemical splanchnicectomy in patients with unresectable pancreatic cancer: a prospective randomized trial. *Ann Surg* 1993;217:447–457.
30. Casper ES, Green MR, Kelsen DP, et al. Phase II trial of gemcitabine (2′,2′-difluorodeoxycytidine) in patients with adenocarcinoma of the pancreas. *Invest New Drugs* 1994;12:29–34.
31. Lawrence TS, Chang EY, Hahn TM, et al. Radiosensitization of pancreatic cancer cells by 2′,2′-difluoro-2′-deoxycytidine. *Int J Radiat Oncol Biol Phys* 1996;34:867–872.

SURGERY: SCIENTIFIC PRINCIPLES AND PRACTICE, Third Edition, edited by Lazar J. Greenfield, Michael W. Mulholland, Keith T. Oldham, Gerald B. Zelenock, and Keith D. Lillemoe. Lippincott Williams & Wilkins Publishers, Philadelphia, © 2001.

CHAPTER 33

NEOPLASMS OF THE ENDOCRINE PANCREAS

CHARLES J. YEO

Neoplasms of the endocrine pancreas are rare, with an annual clinically recognized incidence in the United States of about five cases per million persons and per year. In unselected autopsy material, however, the prevalence of these tumors approximates 1/100 person-years, and they are typically noted as incidental findings. Cells of the pancreatic islets are presumed to originate from neural crest cells. Cells of this origin are called *amine precursor uptake and decarboxylation (APUD) cells* because they have a high content of amine, are capable of amine precursor uptake, and contain an amino acid decarboxylase. A generalized derangement of the APUD system can cause abnormalities of multiple endocrine cells, as is observed in the multiple endocrine neoplasia (MEN) syndromes. Evidence suggests that some APUD cells may not originate from neural crest cells but rather have an endodermal origin (1).

Neoplasms of the endocrine pancreas can be divided into functional and nonfunctional varieties. Most pancreatic endocrine neoplasms discovered clinically are functional; they elaborate one or more hormonal products into the blood, which lead to a recognizable clinical syndrome. Functional tumors are named according to their predominant clinical syndrome and hormonal product (Table 33.1). Patients with endocrine tumors of the pancreas but no recognizable clinical syndrome and normal serum hormone levels (excluding pancreatic polypeptide) are considered to have nonfunctional pancreatic endocrine tumors.

All neoplasms of the endocrine pancreas have a similar appearance under the light microscope. Routine histologic examination does not predict the biologic behavior or the endocrine manifestations of these neoplasms. Immunofluorescence techniques and the peroxidase–antiperoxidase procedure allow the demonstration of specific hormones within neoplastic cells. Malignancy is typically determined by the presence of local invasion that has spread to regional lymph nodes or by the existence of hepatic or distant metastases.

Recent observations in the fields of classic and molecular genetics have added to our knowledge of pancreatic endocrine neoplasms. For example, up to half of malignant pancreatic endocrine tumors have been found to have clonal chromosomal abnormalities (2), whereas *ras* oncogene mutations are absent in most of these tumors (3). Gastrinoma has been shown to be associated with amplification of the *HER-2/neu* protooncogene (4), and a high level of expression of mRNA for the alpha subunit of G_s protein has been demonstrated in insulinoma (5). Furthermore, sporadic pancreatic endocrine tumors and tumors arising as a manifestation of MEN-I have both been shown to have mutations leading to genetic loss on chromosome 11 that inactivates a putative tumor-suppressor gene on that chromosome (6).

Much progress has been made in the genetic understanding of MEN-I (7). Chromosomal linkage studies have localized the genetic defect to the 11q13 locus, and studies of DNA markers have localized the MEN-I gene between PYGM and D11S97. The gene contains 10 exons that code for a 610-amino acid protein called *menin,* whose function is unknown. Recent studies in patients with MEN-I have shown allelic deletions at chromosome 11q13 in nearly 100% of parathyroid tumors, 85% of non-

gastrinoma islet cell tumors, and up to 40% of gastrinomas. In patients with sporadic tumors (without MEN-I), the 11q13 deletions are seen in about 25%, 20%, and almost 50% of parathyroid, nongastrinoma islet cell tumors, and gastrinomas, respectively.

Three general principles apply to the treatment of patients with suspected functional neoplasms of the endocrine pancreas. First is the recognition of the abnormal physiology or characteristic syndrome. Characteristic clinical syndromes are well described for insulinoma, gastrinoma, VIPoma, and glucagonoma. The somatostatinoma syndrome is nonspecific, much more difficult to recognize, and exceedingly rare. Second is the detection of hormone elevations in serum by radioimmunoassay. Radioimmunoassays are widely available for measuring insulin, gastrin, vasoactive intestinal peptide (VIP), and glucagon. Assays for somatostatin, pancreatic polypeptide (PP), prostaglandins, and other hormonal markers are not widely available but can be obtained from certain laboratories and investigators. The third step in patient evaluation involves localizing and staging the tumor in preparation for possible operative intervention.

LOCALIZATION AND STAGING

The initial imaging technique used to localize a pancreatic neoplasm and stage the disease is high-quality spiral (helical) computed tomography (CT) (8–11). The accuracy of CT in detecting the primary islet cell tumor varies considerably, from about 35% to 85%, and depends largely on the scanning technique and the size and location of the primary tumor (Fig. 33.1). The accuracy of CT and tumor localization has been improved by modern, highly sophisticated techniques, with the use of focused scanning through the pancreas at 3- to 5-mm intervals. CT is also used to assess for peripancreatic lymph node enlargement and the presence or absence of hepatic metastases.

Recent data suggest that somatostatin receptor scintigraphy (SRS) should play an increasingly important role as an early imaging modality for patients with various pancreatic endocrine tumors (12–18). In this novel technique, octreotide labeled with indium 111 is administered via intravenous injection to patients in whom a pancreatic endocrine tumor is suspected. The tracer preferentially identifies such tumors because they express large numbers of somatostatin receptors on their cell surfaces (Fig. 33.2). Numerous studies have evaluated SRS in the evaluation of pancreatic endocrine disease. For example, Termanini et al. (12) prospectively studied 122 consecutive patients with gastrinoma by means of various conventional imaging studies. They found SRS to be superior to any single imaging study; it led to an alteration in management in 47% of patients overall. Another report, by Meko et al.

Table 33.1. CLASSIFICATION OF FUNCTIONAL PANCREATIC ENDOCRINE TUMORS

Tumor (syndrome)	Clinical features	Extrapancreatic location	Malignancy rate
Insulinoma	Hypoglycemia	Rare	10%
Gastrinoma (Zollinger-Ellison)	Peptic ulcer Diarrhea	Frequent	50%
VIPoma (Verner-Morrison; WDHA; pancreatic cholera)	Watery diarrhea Hypokalemia Achlorhydria/Acidosis	10%	Most
Glucagonoma	Hyperglycemia Dermatitis	Rare	Most
Somatostatinoma	Hyperglycemia Steatorrhea Gallstones	Rare	Most

WDHA: watery diarrhea, hypokalemia, achlorhydria or acidosis.

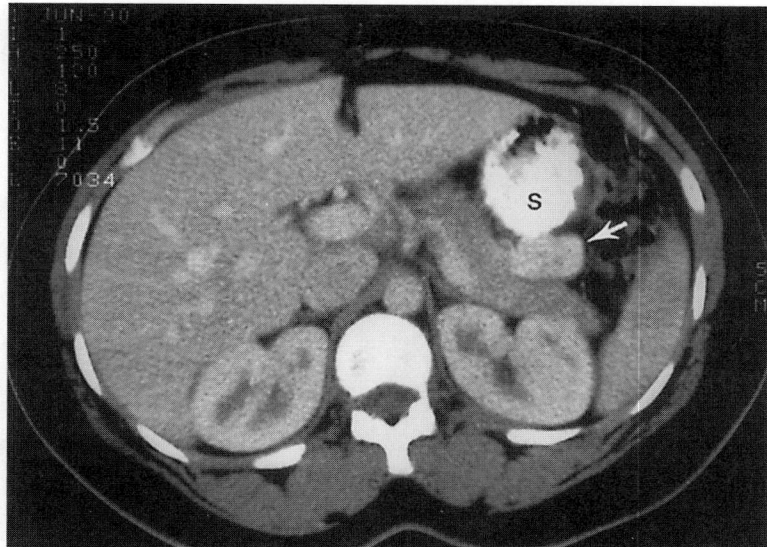

Figure 33.1. Computed tomography with oral and intravenous contrast in a patient with biochemical evidence of insulinoma. The neoplasm *(arrow)* is seen as a contrast-enhancing structure, 3 cm in diameter, in the tail of the pancreas posterior to the stomach *(S)*. (From Yeo CJ. Islet cell tumors of the pancreas. In: Niederhuber JE, ed. *Current therapy in oncology.* St. Louis: Mosby, 1993:272, with permission.)

(13), evaluated the results of SRS in 35 patients and found the overall sensitivity of SRS to be 74% for detecting local disease and 67% for detecting distant disease. Importantly, the negative predictive value ranged from 33% to 100%, which indicates that negative SRS findings in patients with pancreatic endocrine tumors must be viewed cautiously because the false-negative rate is somewhat high. Kisker et al. (14), in a prospective study of 55 patients, compared SRS with CT and abdominal ultrasonography. None of the insulinomas were localized by SRS, and nonfunctional tumors were localized less frequently by SRS than by CT or ultrasonography. In the group of patients with gastrinoma, SRS was superior to CT and ultrasonography for determining the extent of disease. In all, the accumulated evidence suggests that SRS should play an important role in the preoperative localization and staging of gastrinoma (12,16–18), but that the role of SRS in other pancreatic endocrine tumors is not as clear.

A particularly important role for SRS appears to be in the evaluation of patients with liver metastases from pancreatic endocrine tumors, especially in identifying extrahepatic tumor spread. In a 5-year study by Frilling et al. (18) of 35 patients with liver metastases, 54% of patients had extrahepatic tumors detected by SRS that were not detected by other imaging techniques. Of these patients, most had extensive abdominal or thoracic lymph node metastases, and three had bony metastases. Patients with extrahepatic disease were excluded from hepatic surgery or evaluation for hepatic transplantation.

A further technique that has shown clear promise for improving the preoperative localization of pancreatic endocrine neoplasms is endoscopic ultrasonography (EUS) (19–21). Rosch and colleagues (20) were able to localize 32 of 39 tumors (82%) correctly with EUS after CT had failed to locate the tumor (Fig. 33.3). In their experience, EUS

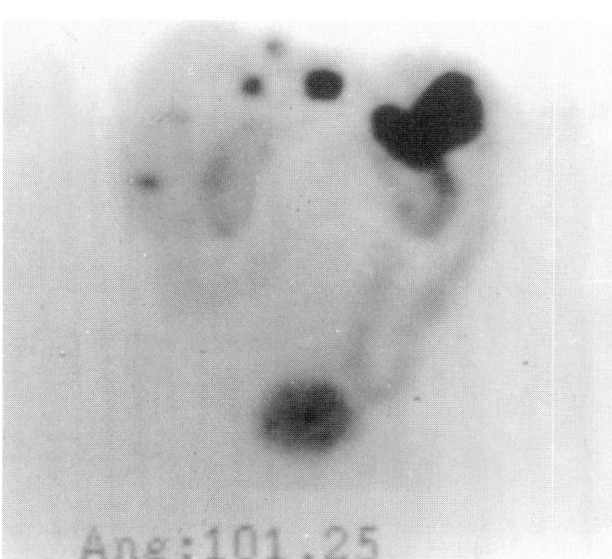

Figure 33.2. Octreotide scan (anterior view) in a patient with a large endocrine tumor in the tail of the pancreas *(large dark mass, upper right)* and several hepatic metastases. A small amount of the tracer is seen in the bladder *(lower midline)*.

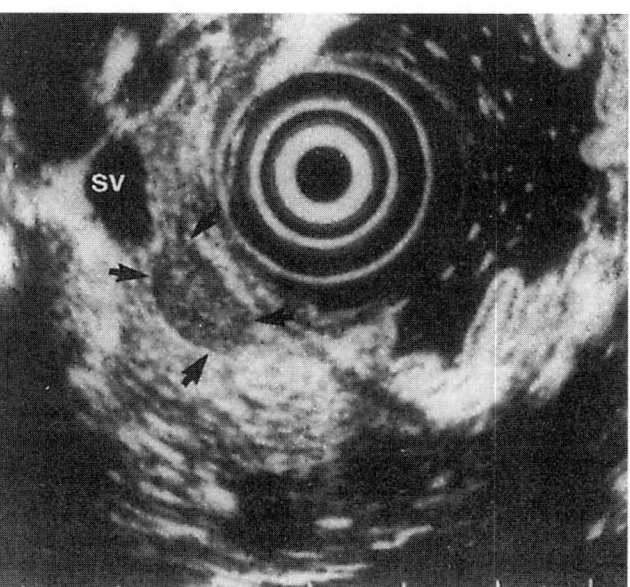

Figure 33.3. Endoscopic ultrasonographic image from a patient with an insulinoma *(arrows)* in the body of the pancreas. *SV,* splenic vein. (From Rosch T, Lightdale CJ, Botet JF, et al. Localization of pancreatic endocrine tumors by endoscopic ultrasonography. *N Engl J Med* 1992;326:1721, with permission.)

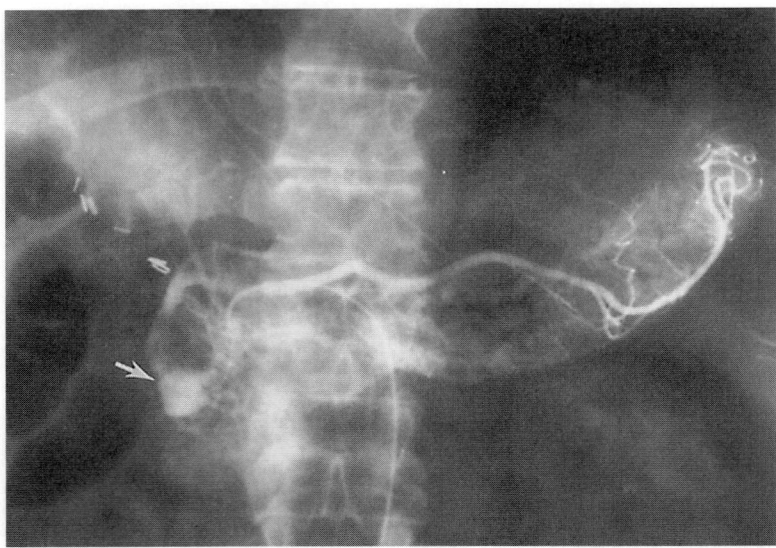

Figure 33.4. Selective celiac angiogram in a patient with gastrinoma. During the late phase of the angiogram, a 2-cm neoplasm is demonstrated as a vascular blush *(arrow)*. (From Yeo CJ. Islet cell tumors of the pancreas. In: Niederhuber JE, ed. *Current therapy in oncology*. St. Louis: Mosby, 1993:272, with permission.)

was more sensitive than the combination of CT and visceral angiography. A more recent study, by Proye et al. (22), evaluated preoperative EUS and SRS in 41 patients with insulinoma and gastrinoma. The sensitivity and positive predictive value of EUS were 77% and 94%, respectively, for pancreatic tumors, 40% and 100% for duodenal gastrinomas, and 58% and 78% for metastatic lymph nodes. These results have been duplicated by others and have led some to suggest that EUS should serve as the initial localization procedure in patients with insulinoma and gastrinoma. Of note, the drawback to EUS is that it does not evaluate for hepatic metastatic disease; rather, it is most sensitive for imaging the duodenal wall, pancreatic parenchyma, and peripancreatic lymph nodes.

One imaging test that is less useful now, with the advent of SRS and EUS, is visceral angiography. Such imaging was used in the past for selective visualization of the arterial supply to the pancreas and peripancreatic regions (23). The accuracy of angiography in detecting the primary islet cell tumor reportedly varied from 45% to 85%, depending on radiographic technique and expertise (Fig. 33.4).

In a minority of patients with pancreatic endocrine neoplasms, the primary tumor may not be localized with initial imaging studies such as CT, SRS, or EUS. This happens most often in patients with insulinoma or gastrinoma. In these cases, selective transhepatic portal venous hormone sampling may help to assist in localizing the occult neoplasm (24–28). This invasive technique is designed to demonstrate an increase in hormone concentration at the site where the tumor drains its hormonal product into the portal venous system (Fig. 33.5). The results of portal venous hormone sampling are used to define the region of the pancreas (or duodenum in the case of a gastrinoma) that harbors the occult tumor. The overall accuracy of this test ranges from 70% to more than 95%, depending on factors such as the number of portal venous samples obtained, the persistence of autonomous production of the hormone by the tumor, and the careful handling and assaying of all specimens.

In addition to selective transhepatic portal venous hormone sampling, a newer technique has been described for localizing occult gastrinomas and insulinomas. This is the *selective arterial secretin stimulation* or *calcium stimulation* test; it is also referred to as *provocative angiography*. The technique involves the selective visceral arterial injection of secretin or calcium and concurrent hepatic venous sampling for either gastrin or insulin (29,30). The

procedure takes advantage of the unique biology of both gastrinomas and insulinomas; gastrinoma cells are known to respond both in vitro and in vivo to secretin by releasing gastrin (31,32), and insulinoma cells respond to calcium by releasing insulin. The provocative secretogogue is serially injected through an arterial catheter into at least three sites—the splenic, gastroduodenal, and inferior pancreaticoduodenal arteries—and samples are drawn from a hepatic vein catheter before and immediately after the three or more arterial injections of secretogogue. The arterial supply to the occult tumor can then be determined based on which selective secretogogue injection is followed by a large increment in hepatic vein hormone concentration. An example of a secretin stimulation test is shown in Fig. 33.6. Several recent studies have evaluated provocative angiography in patients with gastrinoma or insulinoma (33–37). Overall, arterial stimulation with hepatic venous sampling is simpler than selective transhepatic portal venous sampling, and it appears to be effective in localizing pancreatic endocrine tumors that cannot be localized with other preoperative imaging tests.

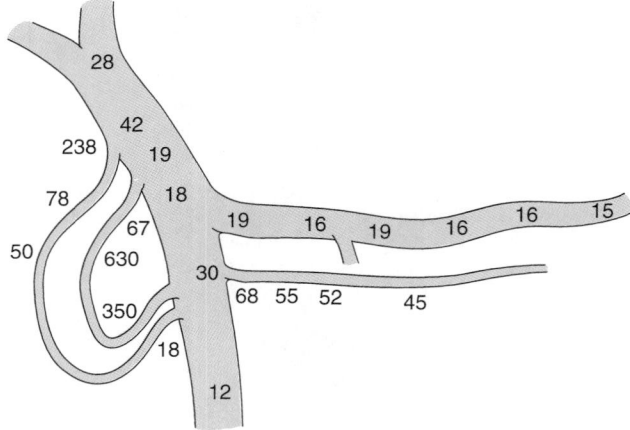

Figure 33.5. Schematic depiction of data from transhepatic portal venous insulin sampling in a patient with an insulinoma. Insulin levels are given in microunits per milliliter. These data localize the neoplasm to the head of the pancreas. (From Norton JA, Sigel B, Baker AR, et al. Localization of an occult insulinoma by intraoperative ultrasonography. *Surgery* 1985;97:381, with permission.)

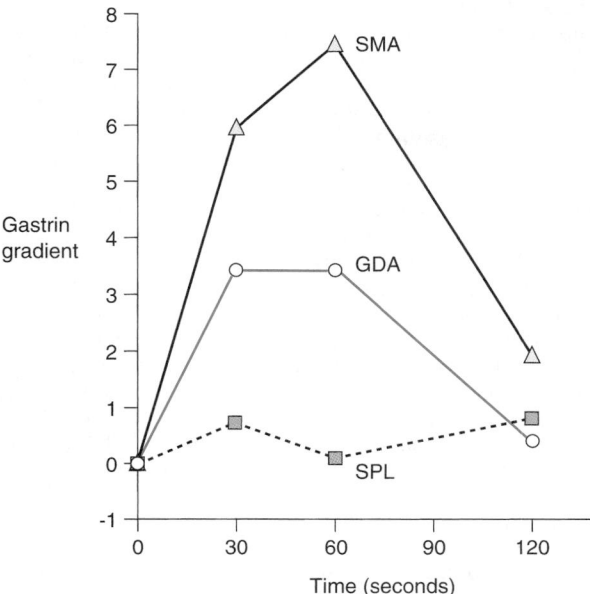

Figure 33.6. Graphic depiction of the results of a selective arterial secretin stimulation test in a patient with gastrinoma. The rise in hepatic vein gastrin concentration (gastrin gradient) is plotted on the y-axis, and basal values are plotted on the x-axis: *1,* 100% rise; *2,* 200% rise; and so forth. A rise in the hepatic vein gastrin concentration observed after the injection of secretin into the superior mesenteric artery *(SMA)* and gastroduodenal artery *(GDA)* localizes the neoplasm to the head of the pancreas or duodenum. *SPL,* splenic artery. (From Thom AK, Norton JA, Doppman JL, et al. Prospective study of the use of intraarterial secretin injection and portal venous sampling to localize duodenal gastrinomas. *Surgery* 1992;112:1002, with permission.)

SURGICAL EXPLORATION

At the time of surgical exploration for pancreatic endocrine neoplasm, a complete evaluation of the pancreas and peripancreatic regions is performed. The body and tail of the pancreas are exposed by dividing the gastrocolic ligament. This portion of the pancreas can be partially elevated out of the retroperitoneum by dividing the inferior retroperitoneal attachments to the gland. After the second portion of the duodenum has been elevated out of the retroperitoneum by means of the Kocher maneuver, the pancreatic head and uncinate process are palpated bimanually. The liver is carefully assessed for evidence of metastatic disease. Potential extrapancreatic sites of tumor are evaluated in all cases, with particular attention paid to the duodenum, splenic hilum, small intestine and its mesentery, peripancreatic lymph nodes, and the reproductive tract in women. One technique that provides additional information in the operating room is intraoperative real-time ultrasonography, which can assist in tumor identification (38,39). The goals of surgical therapy for pancreatic endocrine neoplasms include controlling the symptoms of hormone excess, safely resecting maximal tumor mass, and preserving maximal pancreatic parenchyma. Management strategies, including preoperative, intraoperative, and postoperative considerations, vary for the different types of endocrine neoplasms of the pancreas. There have been scattered reports of laparoscopic resection of pancreatic endocrine tumors.

INSULINOMA

Insulinoma is the most common neoplasm of the endocrine pancreas. The insulinoma syndrome is associated

Table 33.2. INSULINOMA

Parameter	Description
Symptoms	Neuroglycopenia causes confusion, personality change, coma. Catecholamine surge causes trembling, diaphoresis, tachycardia.
Diagnostic tests	Monitored fast Insulin-to-glucose ratio C-peptide and proinsulin blood levels
Anatomic localization	Evenly distributed throughout pancreas

with the following features, known as the *Whipple triad:* (a) symptoms of hypoglycemia during fasting; (b) documentation of hypoglycemia, with a serum glucose level below 50 mg/dL; and (c) relief of hypoglycemic symptoms following administration of exogenous glucose (40). Autonomous insulin secretion in insulinomas leads to spontaneous hypoglycemia, with symptoms that can be classified into two groups (Table 33.2). Neuroglycopenic symptoms include confusion, seizure, obtundation, personality change, and coma. Hypoglycemia-induced symptoms, related to a surge in catecholamine levels, include palpitations, trembling, diaphoresis, and tachycardia. In most cases, patients consume carbohydrate-rich meals and snacks to relieve or prevent these symptoms.

The Whipple triad is not specific for insulinoma. The differential diagnosis of adult hypoglycemia is extensive and includes the following:

Reactive hypoglycemia
Functional hypoglycemia associated with gastrectomy or gastroenterostomy
Nonpancreatic tumors
Pleural mesothelioma
Sarcoma
Adrenal carcinoma
Hepatocellular carcinoma
Carcinoid
Hypopituitarism
Chronic adrenal insufficiency
Extensive hepatic insufficiency
Surreptitious self-administration of insulin or ingestion of oral hypoglycemic agents

A comprehensive review of hypoglycemic disorders has been presented by Service (41). Reactive hypoglycemia is the most common form, in which symptoms of hypoglycemia develop 3 to 5 hours after meals, not typically after long periods of fasting. In some cases, nonendocrine tumors cause hypoglycemia (42), with recent evidence implicating insulin-like growth factor II as one humoral causative factor (43). A recent report by Seckl et al. (44) documents a case of hypoglycemia caused by an insulin-secreting small cell carcinoma of the cervix, further underscoring the fact that not all insulin-secreting tumors localize to the pancreas.

A common error made in evaluating a patient with suspected insulinoma is to begin with an oral glucose tolerance test. Instead, insulinoma is most reliably diagnosed by means of a monitored fast. During a monitored fast, blood is sampled for glucose and insulin determinations every 4 to 6 hours and when symptoms appear. Hypoglycemic symptoms typically occur when glucose levels are below 50 mg/dL, with concurrent serum insulin levels often exceeding 25 μU/mL. Additional support for the diagnosis of insulinoma comes from the calculation of the insulin-to-glucose ratio at different times during the monitored fast. Normal persons have insulin-to-glucose ratios below 0.3, whereas patients with insulinoma typically demonstrate insulin-to-glucose ratios above 0.4 after a prolonged fast. Other measurable beta-cell products synthesized in excess in patients with insulinoma include C peptide and proinsulin. Elevated levels of both are typically found in the peripheral blood of patients with insulinoma.

The possibility of the surreptitious administration of insulin or oral hypoglycemic agents should be considered in all patients with suspected insulinoma. Levels of C peptide and proinsulin are not elevated in patients who self-administer insulin. Additionally, patients self-administering either bovine or porcine insulin may demonstrate antiinsulin antibodies in circulating blood. The ingestion of oral hypoglycemic agents, such as sulfonylureas, can be assessed by means of standard toxicologic screening.

After the diagnosis of insulinoma has been confirmed by biochemical analysis, the appropriate localization and staging studies described earlier are performed. For insulinoma, the standard imaging studies include abdominal CT, EUS, and provocative angiography. The treatment of insulinoma is surgical in nearly all cases. Insulinomas are evenly distributed in the pancreas, with one third found in the head and uncinate process, one third in the body, and one third in the tail of the gland (45). Of patients diagnosed with insulinoma, 90% are found to have benign solitary adenomas amenable to surgical cure. Fewer than 10% of patients with insulinoma have some form of the MEN-I syndrome. In patients with MEN-I, the possibility of multiple insulinomas must be suspected, and the recurrence rate is higher than in sporadic cases (46). In about 10% of all cases, insulinoma is metastatic to peripancreatic lymph nodes or the liver, in which case a diagnosis of malignant insulinoma is justified.

During surgical exploration, the pancreas is assessed not only by operative palpation but also by intraoperative real-time ultrasonography. This makes it possible to evaluate the entire pancreas more thoroughly and search for the site of the primary tumor (38,39). Small, benign insulinomas that are not close to the main pancreatic duct can be removed by enucleation (47), regardless of their location in the gland (Fig. 33.7). In the body and tail of the pancreas, insulinomas more than 2 cm in diameter and those close to the pancreatic duct are most commonly excised by distal pancreatectomy. Large insulinomas deep in the head or uncinate process of the pancreas may not be amenable to local excision, and pancreaticoduodenectomy may be required (48,49).

In rare instances, patients undergo exploration for insulinoma without definite preoperative tumor localization. At surgery, no tumor may be identified intraoperatively by visualization, palpation, and real-time ultrasonography. In these circumstances, a management dilemma exists. Some authors have recommended a "blind" distal (left-sided) pancreatic resection to the level of the superior mesenteric vein (60% to 70% pancreatectomy), in the hope of excising a previously unidentified insulinoma residing in the body or tail of the pancreas. Others have suggested that a blind pancreaticoduodenectomy would be more appropriate because the thickness of the head and uncinate process render this region of the pancreas most likely to harbor an unidentifiable insulinoma. The favored option in this situation of an occult insulinoma is to defer any type of blind resection and to perform postoperative selective arterial calcium stimulation with hepatic venous insulin sampling to allow for specific tumor localization and directed surgical excision at a second operation (50).

About 10% of insulinomas are malignant, typically with evidence of lymph node or hepatic metastases. Under these circumstances, cautious and safe resection of the primary tumor and accessible metastases should be considered

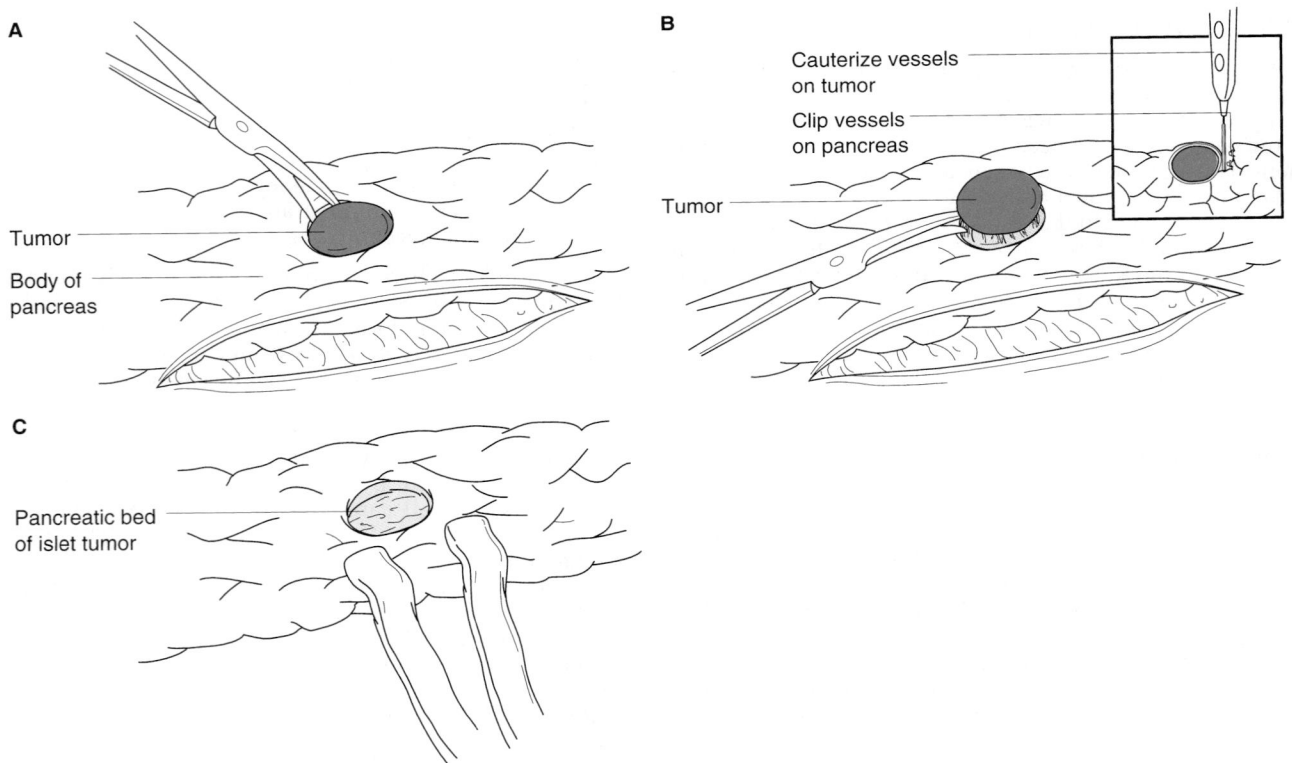

Figure 33.7. The technique for enucleating a benign pancreatic endocrine neoplasm with scissors *(A)* or electrocautery *(B). (C)* After enucleation, the site of excision is drained. (From Cameron JL. *Atlas of surgery,* vol 1. Philadelphia: BC Decker/Mosby, 1990:441, with permission.)

(51–53). Such tumor debulking can be helpful in reducing hypoglycemic symptoms, which can threaten long-term survival. The average patient survives several years after the diagnosis and treatment of malignant islet cell tumors, which indicates that the natural history of these malignant tumors typically follows an indolent course (11,54). In patients with unresectable insulinoma, dietary manipulations, such as the judicious spacing of carbohydrate-rich meals and the consumption of night-time snacks, can be helpful to minimize dangerous hypoglycemic episodes. Medications such as diazoxide and octreotide can be used to inhibit insulin release, raise serum glucose levels, and further minimize hypoglycemia. Chemotherapeutic agents with some efficacy against malignant insulinoma include streptozotocin, dacarbazine, doxorubicin, and 5-fluorouracil (55–57). The highest response rates to chemotherapy have been observed with the use of combination therapy.

GASTRINOMA (ZOLLINGER-ELLISON SYNDROME)

In 1955, Zollinger and Ellison described two patients with severe peptic ulcer disease and pancreatic endocrine tumors and postulated that an ulcerogenic agent originated from the pancreatic tumor (58,59). It is currently estimated that 1 in 1,000 patients with primary duodenal ulcer disease and 2 in 100 patients with recurrent ulcer after ulcer surgery harbor gastrinomas (60). Seventy-five percent of gastrinomas occur sporadically, and 25% are associated with the MEN-I syndrome. In the past, most gastrinomas were found to be malignant, based on the findings of metastatic disease at the time of work-up or exploration. More recently, with increased awareness and earlier screening for hypergastrinemia, the diagnosis of gastrinoma is made earlier, so that a higher percentage of the neoplasms discovered are benign and curable (61,62). The clinical symptoms of patients with gastrinoma are a direct result of excessive levels of circulating gastrin (Table 33.3). Abdominal pain and peptic ulceration of the upper gastrointestinal tract are seen in up to 90% of patients. Fifty percent of patients have some degree of diarrhea, and about 10% have diarrhea as the only symptom. Esophageal symptoms or endoscopic abnormalities resulting from gastroesophageal reflux are seen in more than 50% of patients; esophagitis typically occurs in association with peptic ulcer disease or diarrhea (63).

The diagnosis of gastrinoma should be suspected in several clinical settings, and the liberal use of serum gastrin measurement for screening is encouraged. The indications for measuring gastrin include the following:

Initial diagnosis of peptic ulcer disease
Recurrent ulcer
Failure of medical therapy
Postoperative ulcer
Postbulbar ulcer
Family history of ulcer disease
Ulcer with diarrhea
Prolonged undiagnosed diarrhea
MEN-I kindred
Nongastrinoma pancreatic endocrine tumor (because of the high association of secondary hormone elevations) (64,65)
Prominent gastric rugal folds on upper gastrointestinal series (reflecting the trophic effect of gastrin on the gastric fundus)

In most patients with gastrinomas, the fasting serum gastrin level is elevated to at least 200 pg/mL. Gastrin values above 1,000 pg/mL are virtually diagnostic of gastrinoma, particularly when they are accompanied by hyperchlorhy-

Table 33.3. GASTRINOMA

Parameter	Description
Symptoms	Peptic ulcer disease
	Diarrhea
	Esophagitis
Diagnostic tests	Serum gastrin measurement
	Gastric acid analysis
	Secretin stimulation test
Anatomic localization	Duodenum and head of pancreas (gastrinoma triangle)

dria or well-established ulcer disease. Fasting hypergastrinemia alone, however, is not sufficient for the diagnosis of gastrinoma; hypergastrinemia can exist in other pathophysiologic states because gastrin is the normal secretory product of antral G cells (Table 33.4). Gastric acid analysis is important in evaluating patients with suspected gastrinoma; it can differentiate between ulcerogenic (high levels of gastric acid) causes of hypergastrinemia and nonulcerogenic (low levels of gastric acid) causes of hypergastrinemia. To obtain an accurate gastric acid analysis, patients must abstain from antisecretory medications, such as histamine (H_2) receptor antagonists or proton pump inhibitors (omeprazole, lansoprazole). The diagnosis of gastrinoma is supported by a basal acid output above 15 mEq/h in nonoperated patients, a basal acid output exceeding 5 mEq/h in patients with previous vagotomy or ulcer operations, or a ratio of basal to maximal acid output that exceeds 0.6.

Once it has been documented that hypergastrinemia is associated with excessive acid secretion, provocative testing with secretin should be performed to differentiate between gastrinoma, antral G-cell hyperplasia or hyperfunction, and the other causes of ulcerogenic hypergastrinemia. The secretin stimulation test is performed in the fasting state by obtaining peripheral serum samples for gastrin measurement in the basal period, administering 2 U of secretin per kilogram as an intravenous bolus, and obtaining serum samples for gastrin measurement at 5-minute intervals for 30 minutes. An increase in the gastrin level of more than 200 pg/mL above the basal level supports the diagnosis of gastrinoma (Fig. 33.8). This conventional secretin stimulation test performed on peripheral blood differs markedly from the doubly invasive selective arterial secretin stimulation test, which is designed to localize the site of a primary tumor in patients with gastrinomas that have already been documented by biochemical testing.

After the biochemical confirmation of the diagnosis of gastrinoma, two steps are important in patient treatment. First, gastric acid hypersecretion is pharmacologically controlled. The proton pump inhibitors are now considered the drugs of choice for antisecretory therapy in patients with

Table 33.4. DISEASE STATES ASSOCIATED WITH HYPERGASTRINEMIA

Nonulcerogenic causes (normal to low acid secretion)
Atrophic gastritis
Pernicious anemia
Previous vagotomy
Renal failure
Short-gut syndrome
Ulcerogenic causes (excess acid secretion)
Antral G-cell hyperplasia or hyperfunction
Gastric outlet obstruction
Retained excluded antrum
Zollinger-Ellison syndrome

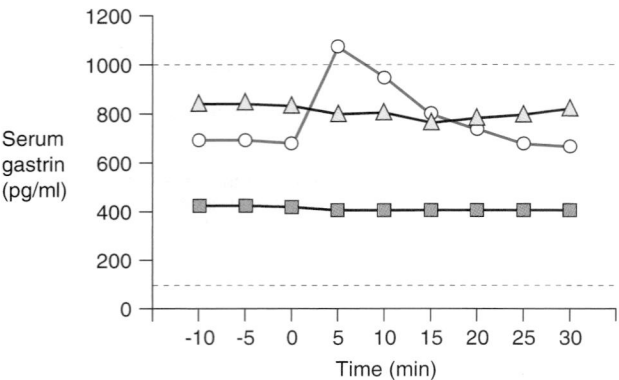

Figure 33.8. Results of intravenous secretin stimulation tests in patients with atrophic gastritis *(triangles),* gastric outlet obstruction *(squares),* and gastrinoma *(circles).* A positive test result, consistent with the presence of gastrinoma, is indicated by an increase over basal serum gastrin levels of at least 200 pg/mL. (From Wolfe MM, Jensen RT. Zollinger-Ellison syndrome: current concepts in diagnosis and management. *N Engl J Med* 1987;317:1200, with permission.)

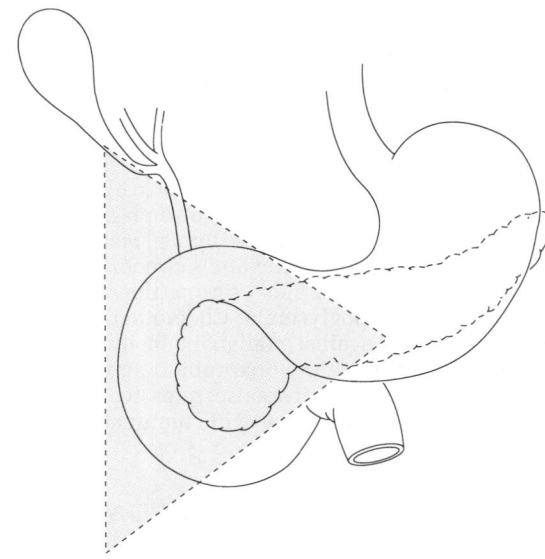

Figure 33.9. Most gastrinomas are found within the gastrinoma triangle. (From Stabile BE, Morrow DJ, Passaro E. The gastrinoma triangle: operative implications. *Am J Surg* 1984;147:26, with permission.)

gastrinoma (66,67). The dose is adjusted to achieve a nonacidic gastric pH during the hour immediately before the next dose of the drug. Second, after the initiation of therapy, all patients with gastrinomas should undergo imaging studies to localize the primary tumor and assess for metastatic disease. The modalities appropriate for the localization and staging of gastrinoma have already been discussed: spiral abdominal CT, EUS, SRS, percutaneous transhepatic portal venous sampling for gastrin, and the selective arterial secretin stimulation test. A recent study by Alexander and colleagues (68) prospectively evaluated 35 consecutive patients with gastrinoma and compared the ability of various localization modalities to locate the tumor in each patient. SRS was able to identify the tumor correctly in 78% of the patients, MRI and conventional angiography in 57%, and CT in 51%. Overall, SRS detected 30% of gastrinomas 1.1 cm or smaller in size, 64% of those between 1.1 and 2 cm, and 96% of those larger than 2 cm; it missed mainly small duodenal tumors. The authors concluded that SRS is the most sensitive preoperative imaging study for extrahepatic gastrinomas, although the use of SRS before surgery did not increase the disease-free rate after exploration.

Patients whose localization and staging studies indicate unresectable hepatic metastases should undergo percutaneous or laparoscopically directed liver biopsy for absolute histologic verification. If unresectable gastrinoma is confirmed, open surgical exploration is not performed, and the patient is maintained on long-term proton pump inhibitor therapy. Virtually all patients can be rendered achlorhydric with an appropriate dose of omeprazole or lansoprazole. Noncompliant patients who refuse to take appropriate doses of acid secretory inhibitors and who experience complications related to their ulcer diathesis may require total gastrectomy. Total gastrectomy removes the end-organ (parietal cell mass) and was once the procedure of choice for gastrinoma. Today, its use in patients with gastrinomas has markedly declined.

In most patients, unresectable disease is not identified by staging studies, and patients should be offered surgical exploration with a curative intent. At the time of exploration, the entire abdomen is carefully assessed for areas of extrapancreatic and extraduodenal gastrinoma (69). Most gastrinomas are found to the right of the superior mesenteric vessels, in the head of the pancreas or the duodenum. This area is called the *gastrinoma triangle* (45,70)

(Fig. 33.9). Intraoperative ultrasonography should be available to assist in tumor localization. In addition, intraoperative upper gastrointestinal endoscopy may be helpful by allowing transillumination of the duodenal wall and identification of small duodenal gastrinomas (71,72). At exploration, any suspect peripancreatic lymph nodes are excised and submitted for frozen section. Primary tumors located in the substance of the pancreas that are small (< 2 cm) and well encapsulated can be carefully enucleated. Pancreatic tumors without defined capsules or that are situated deep in the pancreatic parenchyma may require partial pancreatic resection by either distal pancreatectomy or pancreaticoduodenectomy (48,73). In the absence of an identifiable pancreatic or duodenal tumor, a longitudinal duodenotomy can be performed at the level of the second portion of the duodenum to allow for eversion of the duodenum in a search for duodenal microgastrinomas (71,74). Primary gastrinomas identified in the duodenal wall are resected locally with primary closure of the duodenal defect (75,76). In a small percentage of patients, gastrinoma is found only in peripancreatic lymph nodes, with these lymph nodes harboring the primary tumor. Resection of these apparent lymph node primary gastrinomas has been associated with long-term eugastrinemia and biochemical cure in up to half of cases (77).

An important recent article by Norton and coworkers (78) provides excellent support for the role of surgery in patients with sporadic gastrinoma. Because the gastric hypersecretion can now be controlled in virtually every patient with appropriate medications, the natural history of the tumor is now the major determinant of survival. In this series of 151 patients followed at the National Institutes of Health, 123 had sporadic gastrinoma and 28 had tumors associated with MEN-I. Gastrinomas were found in 140 of the patients (93%): 49% in the duodenum, 24% in the pancreas, 11% as primary tumors in lymph nodes, and 9% in other locations. Of the patients with sporadic gastrinoma, 34% were free of disease at 10 years. None of the MEN-I patients were free of disease at follow-up. These data, summarized by Wells (79), provide compelling evidence that patients with localized sporadic gastrinoma benefit from expert surgical exploration and tumor resection. The management of gastrinoma associated with MEN-I is not as clear. The surgical treatment of hypercalcemia caused by parathyroid hyperplasia should precede any surgery for hypergastrinemia in patients with MEN-I. In these patients, pancreatic tumors are routinely multicentric, duodenal tumors may be multiple and are often associated with regional lymph node metastases, and hepatic metastases appear to be somewhat related to primary tumor size in most studies (78,80), but not all (81). Although some groups have favored exploration only when MEN-I gastrinoma tumors exceed 3 cm (78), it seems that earlier intervention may be warranted (81,82). Unfortunately, more data from an appropriate clinical trial are needed to define better the timing of surgery for MEN-I gastrinoma.

Occasionally, preoperative localization studies, such as portal venous gastrin sampling or the selective arterial secretin stimulation test, localize the tumor in the gastrinoma triangle; however, no tumor may be demonstrable at laparotomy. In the face of such a negative exploration, several surgical options are available. First, parietal cell vagotomy has been proposed as a way to reduce antisecretory drug dose requirements in patients on high-dose antisecretory drug therapy but without prior life-threatening complications (83). The usefulness of parietal cell vagotomy in decreasing dose requirements has not been well established in patients treated with proton pump inhibitors, however, and such an operative procedure leaves behind potentially resectable gastrinoma. For these reasons, parietal cell vagotomy has lost favor as an option. The second surgical option for patients with negative results on exploration is total gastrectomy. Although total gastrectomy was the most reliable way to control the ulcer diathesis in the past (84), the introduction and availability of proton pump inhibitors has drastically reduced the need for total gastrectomy. Total gastrectomy may still have a limited role in patients whose tumors cannot be localized, if they cannot or will not take adequate doses of proton pump inhibitors. Unfortunately, like parietal cell vagotomy, total gastrectomy leaves the primary tumor behind, with the potential for subsequent growth, metastasis, and causing patient death from tumor burden. A third, albeit controversial, surgical option in patients with a clear biochemical documentation of hypergastrinemia and hyperchlorhydria and tumor localization in the gastrinoma triangle involves blind pancreaticoduodenectomy. In a small number of patients, these blind resections have yielded pathologically verified primary gastrinomas in the duodenal wall or head of the pancreas that were not apparent at laparotomy. Blind resections should be performed as classic pancreaticoduodenectomies, including a distal gastric resection, because duodenal gastrinomas may arise close to the pylorus and be inadvertently left behind with a pylorus-sparing pancreaticoduodenectomy. In a limited number of cases reported, patients have been rendered eugastrinemic by blind resection, and most continue to be eugastrinemic at postoperative follow-up (49).

The overall results in patients with gastrinoma have improved markedly since the initial description of the syndrome. In the 1950s and 1960s, most gastrinomas were diagnosed late in the course of the disease, when the tumor burden was already significant. At that time, effective medical therapy for hyperchlorhydria was not available, and sophisticated radiographic localization and staging techniques did not exist. Patients often suffered multiple ulcer complications, required total gastrectomy to control the ulcer diathesis, and typically succumbed to continued tumor growth following total gastrectomy. Reviews of patients with gastrinoma treated surgically provide room for optimism (85–87). Up to 35% of patients who undergo exploration for gastrinoma with curative intent have been rendered eugastrinemic at follow-up. When only those patients who underwent exploration and whose resections were thought to be successful are considered, the cure rates approach 60% to 70%. These recent results represent a major improvement in the treatment of gastrinoma during the past few decades and support the practice of initial pharmacologic control of gastric hypersecretion with proton pump inhibitors, followed by tumor localization and staging, in the hope of achieving a curative resection.

Most patients with incurable metastatic gastrinoma succumb eventually to tumor growth and dissemination. Multiple modalities have been used to treat patients with such metastatic gastrinoma. The overall objective response rate to chemotherapy appears to be less than 50%. A prospective study of monthly cycles of streptozotocin, 5-fluorouracil, and doxorubicin in 10 patients with metastatic gastrinoma showed a partial response rate of 40%; 60% had no response (88). Chemotherapy did not improve the length of survival. Hormonal therapy with octreotide has been reported to relieve symptoms, reduce hypergastrinemia, and diminish hyperchlorhydria in patients with metastatic gastrinoma (89,90). Anecdotal reports suggest that octreotide may occasionally reduce tumor volume, although this response is clearly uncommon. The role of octreotide remains somewhat limited, however, because the drug must be administered parenterally and because omeprazole can control hyperchlorhydria and peptic symptoms in nearly all patients. Aggressive resection and palliative debulking of metastatic gastrinoma have been performed in a small number of patients, with apparent improvement in the clinical course (51–53). Hepatic transplantation, hepatic artery embolization, and interferon therapy have all been used in a small number of patients with gastrinoma metastatic to the liver (91–96). None of these therapies appears to be associated with reproducible improvements in survival.

VIPOMA (VERNER-MORRISON SYNDROME)

Since their report of two cases in 1958, Verner and Morrison (97) have been credited with defining this secretory type of diarrhea syndrome. Synonyms include *WDHA syndrome* (watery diarrhea, hypokalemia, and either achlorhydria or acidosis) and *pancreatic cholera syndrome*. Patients characteristically present with intermittent severe diarrhea, typically of a watery nature and averaging 5 L/d (Table 33.5). Malabsorption and steatorrhea are not common. Hypokalemia results from the fecal loss of large amounts of potassium (up to 400 mEq/d), and low serum potassium levels are associated with muscular weakness, lethargy, and nausea. A metabolic acidosis may be present, with a low serum bicarbonate level. Half of the patients have some degree of hyperglycemia and hypercalcemia, and cutaneous flushing can be observed in a minority. The diagnosis of VIPoma is typically made after other, more common causes

Table 33.5. VIPOMA

Parameter	Description
Symptoms	Watery diarrhea
	Weakness
	Lethargy
	Nausea
Diagnostic tests	Hypokalemia
	Achlorhydria
	Metabolic acidosis
	Serum VIP levels
Anatomic localization	Most in body or tail of pancreas

VIP, vasoactive intestinal peptide.

Table 33.6. DIFFERENTIAL DIAGNOSIS OF VERNER-MORRISON SYNDROME

Entity	Workup
Villous adenoma	Lower GI endoscopy
Laxative abuse	Stool examination for phenolphthalein
Celiac disease	Fecal fat measurement
	D-Xylose tolerance test
	Small-bowel biopsy
Parasitic and infectious diseases	Stool culture
	Ovum and parasite analysis
	Clostridium difficile toxin assay
Inflammatory bowel disease	Lower GI endoscopy
	Upper GI and small-bowel series
Carcinoid syndrome	Urinary 5'-HIAA
	Upper GI and small-bowel series
	Abdominal CT
	Serum serotonin measurement
Gastrinoma	Serum gastrin measurement
	Gastric acid analysis
	Secretin stimulation test

CT, computed tomography; GI, gastrointestinal; 5'-HIAA, 5'-hydroxy-indoleacetic acid.

of diarrhea have been excluded (Table 33.6). The active agent in VIPoma syndrome is usually VIP (98); in a minority of patients, other candidate mediators, such as peptide histidine–isoleucine or prostaglandins, are elevated (99). Because VIP secretion can be episodic in patients with VIPomas, several fasting VIP levels should be measured because a single low level of VIP does not rule out the syndrome.

After biochemical documentation of elevated VIP levels, tumor localization and staging begin with spiral abdominal CT (Fig. 33.10). In addition, because 10% of patients with VIPomas may have extrapancreatic tumors located in the retroperitoneum or thorax, thoracic CT is indicated if the abdominal scan fails to identify a tumor. In most reported cases, abdominal CT identified the tumor, and further imaging studies, such as visceral angiography or portal venous hormone sampling, were unnecessary. SRS may demonstrate the primary tumor in addition to metastatic lesions.

When patients with VIPomas are prepared for surgical exploration, fluid and electrolyte balances must be corrected by vigorous intravenous fluid administration and appropriate electrolyte replacement. Therapy with parenterally administered octreotide can be an important adjunct in the preoperative setting because octreotide effects a reduction in circulating VIP levels, with a resultant decrease in the volume of diarrhea.

A recent report from the Mayo Clinic reviewed 18 patients with VIPoma seen during a 15-year period (100). Nine men and nine women were included whose mean age was 51 years. Nine tumors were in the tail of the pancreas, four in the body, and two in the head; three were not localized. Liver metastases were identified in 14 of the 18 patients. Eight patients underwent either curative or palliative resection. The mean survival for the group was 3.6 years.

Surgical excision of the VIPoma is appropriate in nearly all patients with the Verner-Morrison syndrome. Most VIPomas have been located in the distal pancreas, where they are amenable to resection by distal pancreatectomy. If no tumor is found in the pancreas, a careful exploration of the retroperitoneum, including both adrenal glands, should be performed. Metastatic disease to the lymph nodes and liver have been reported in the majority of cases. In the presence of metastatic disease, safe palliative debulking of the metastatic tumor is indicated (101).

In patients with recurrent or unresectable VIPoma, octreotide therapy is used to reduce circulating VIP levels and control diarrhea. Chemotherapy specific for VIPoma has not been well studied, although small numbers of patients have appeared to respond partially to streptozotocin, combination chemotherapy, or interferon.

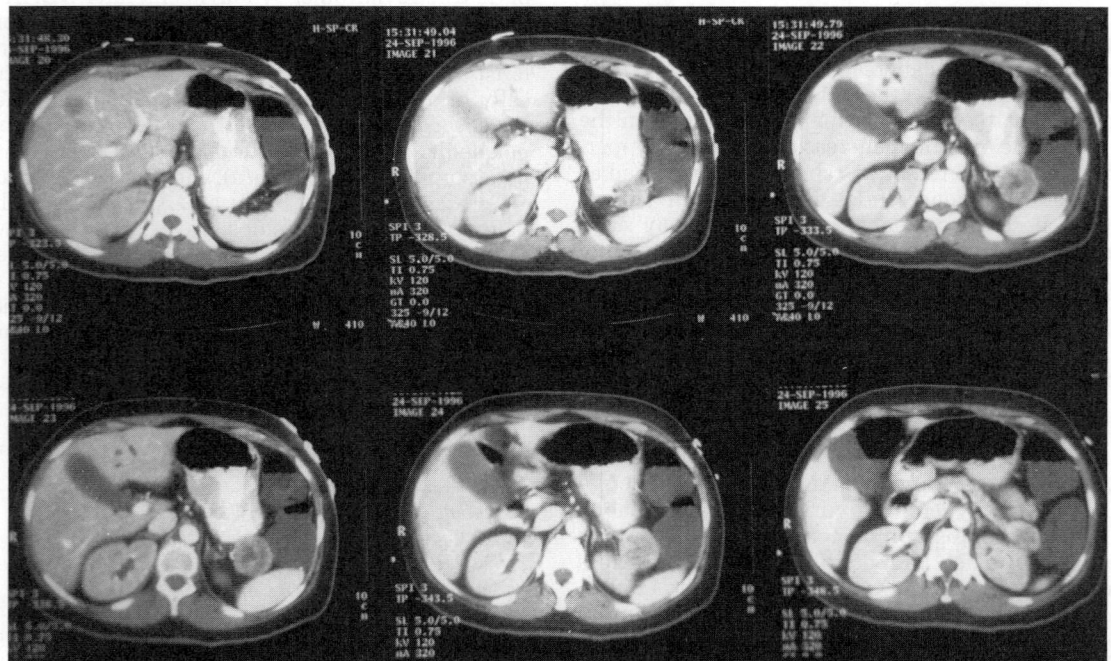

Figure 33.10. Several computed tomographic images from a patient with a primary VIPoma in the tail of the pancreas. The tumor is nearly spherical. Its location is posterior to the stomach and adjacent to the spleen.

Table 33.7. GLUCAGONOMA

Parameter	Description
Symptoms	Dermatitis manifested as necrolytic migratory erythema
	Stomatitis
	Weight loss
Diagnostic tests	Hyperglycemia
	Hypoproteinemia
	Serum glucagon measurement
	Serum amino acid profile
Anatomic localization	Most in body or tail of pancreas

GLUCAGONOMA

The most common findings in the glucagonoma syndrome are severe dermatitis, mild diabetes, stomatitis, anemia, and weight loss (102) (Table 33.7). The dermatitis manifests as a characteristic skin rash termed *necrolytic migratory erythema*. This rash exhibits cyclic migrations, with erythematous patches that spread serpiginously and central healing points of resolution. It has been theorized that the hypoaminoacidemia seen in patients with glucagonoma is responsible for the dermatitis. Because glucagon is a catabolic hormone, patients with glucagonoma typically demonstrate malnutrition and hypoproteinemia.

The diagnosis of glucagonoma may be suggested by the clinical presentation and biopsy of the skin lesions but is secured by the documentation of elevated levels of fasting serum glucagon. Normal fasting levels of glucagon peak at 150 pg/mL. The diagnosis of glucagonoma can be confirmed by the demonstration of hypoaminoacidemia; however, such testing is expensive and is not necessary in most cases.

Patients with biochemical documentation of hyperglucagonemia in the appropriate clinical setting should undergo radiographic localization and staging with spiral abdominal CT. Because these tumors are usually large and solitary, CT localizes the tumor in most cases (Fig. 33.11). Before exploration, attention should be directed to managing the malnutrition. Total parenteral nutrition has been used to reverse the catabolic state resulting from hyper-glucagonemia, reverse the malnutrition, and relieve the dermatitis. Octreotide has been used to reduce the circulating glucagon levels and improve the response to total parenteral nutrition.

Most glucagonomas have been located in the body and tail of the pancreas. These tumors are typically large and bulky, and surgical resection requires distal pancreatectomy. Metastases have been found in most patients, and safe debulking of these metastatic lesions should be considered.

In patients with incurable or recurrent glucagonoma, the response rates to standard chemotherapeutic agents, such as streptozotocin and dacarbazine, appear to be low (103). Octreotide can be successful in reducing elevated glucagon levels and controlling the hyperglycemia and dermatitis associated with incurable glucagonoma (104,105).

SOMATOSTATINOMA

The somatostatinoma syndrome is the least common of the five generally accepted functional pancreatic endocrine neoplasia syndromes, with an estimated annual incidence of less than 1 in 40 million people. The clinical features of the somatostatinoma syndrome, which are nonspecific, include steatorrhea, diabetes, hypochlorhydria, and cholelithiasis (Table 33.8). A fasting plasma somatostatin level can be used to confirm the diagnosis of a somatostatinoma. The normal plasma level of somatostatin is below 100 pg/mL, and patients with somatostatinoma have been found to have high levels of circulating somatostatin, often measurable in nanograms per milliliter (106,107). Most somatostatinomas have been located in the head of the pancreas and the periampullary region. The most useful test for localization and staging is abdominal CT, which has been used to identify and stage these typically large tumors. The preoperative management of patients with somatostatinoma involves treatment of hyperglycemia and malnutrition. Surgical resection for cure has been uncommon because metastatic disease is present in most cases. Safe resection of the primary tumor and careful debulking of hepatic metastases appear to be indicated. At the time of exploration, cholecystectomy is indicated, even in the absence of documented gallstones, because of the concern about the development of cholelithiasis with persistently elevated somatostatin levels.

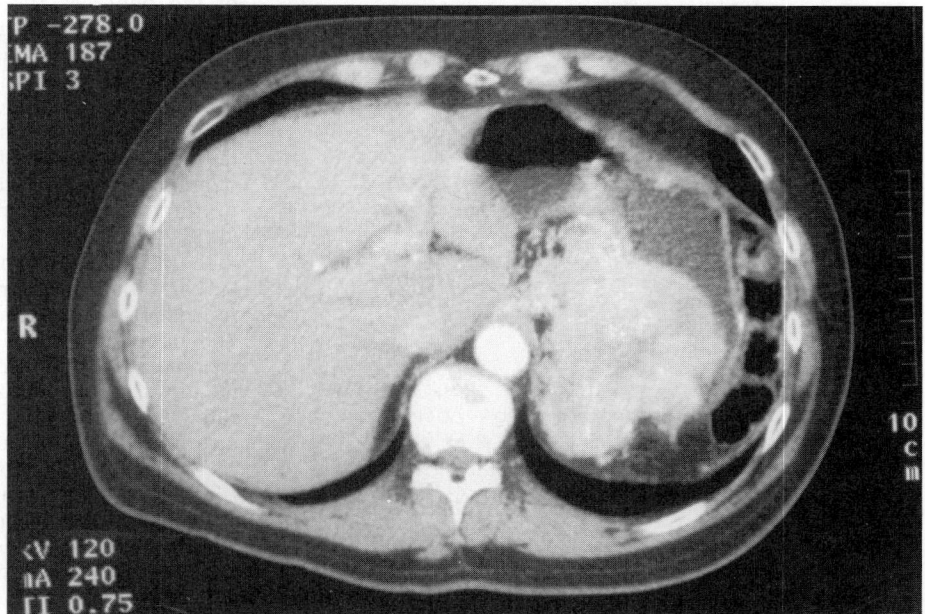

Figure 33.11. Computed tomography with oral and intravenous contrast in a patient with a glucagonoma. The large tumor appears to be posterior to the stomach and to the right of the aorta from the viewer's perspective.

RARE CANDIDATE FUNCTIONAL PANCREATIC ENDOCRINE NEOPLASMS

Several rare clinical syndromes have been proposed as candidate functional endocrine syndromes associated with pancreatic neoplasms (Table 33.9). These include calcitoninoma (108,109), parathyrinoma (110), GRFoma, ACTHoma, and neurotensinoma (111). Calcitonin-secreting pancreatic endocrine neoplasms are associated with watery diarrhea. Parathyrinomas are accompanied by elevations in parathyroid hormone-related protein (PTH-rp) and clinical features of hypercalcemia. PTH-rp activates the PTH receptor and causes hypercalcemia by increasing bone resorption and renal tubular resorption of calcium (112). PTH-rp is the predominant cause of hypercalcemia in cancer patients, and this protein is found in many tissues, including epithelia, mesenchymal tissues, endocrine glands, and the central nervous system. The identification of elevated PTH-rp levels appears to be increasing in certain patients with pancreatic endocrine tumors.

GRFoma is marked by elevations of serum growth hormone-releasing factor (GRF) and clinical features of acromegaly. ACTHoma is associated with features of Cushing's syndrome and elevated serum levels of adrenocorticotropic hormone (ACTH). Neurotensinoma appears to be characterized by tachycardia, hypotension, and malabsorption, and serum levels of neurotensin are elevated. As further cases are reported and clinical experience broadens, these rare and unusual functional pancreatic exocrine neoplasms and others may someday be recognized along with the classic five syndromes of insulinoma, gastrinoma, VIPoma, glucagonoma, and somatostatinoma.

NONFUNCTIONAL ISLET CELL TUMORS

About a third of patients with neoplasms of the endocrine pancreas have no defined clinical syndrome and no evidence of elevated serum insulin, gastrin, VIP, glucagon, or somatostatin levels. These patients are considered to have nonfunctional endocrine neoplasms. The one hormone that may be elevated in the serum of patients with nonfunctional tumors is PP. It appears to be a marker for some pancreatic endocrine tumors without being the mediator of any specific PP-related clinical syndrome (113). A recent study by Mutch et al. (114) determined a relationship between fasting plasma PP levels in patients with MEN-I and the presence of a radiographically detectable pancreatic endocrine tumor. According to their results, a PP level that is more than three times the normal age-specific value is 95% sensitive and 88% specific for an islet cell tumor that can be imaged. Patients with nonfunctional endocrine neoplasms present with clinical manifestations such as abdominal pain, weight loss, and jaundice, which are caused by space-occupying lesions in the pancreas (115,116). These clinical manifestations are similar to those in patients with ductal adenocarcinoma of the pancreas. Nonfunctional tumors are most commonly located in the head, neck, or uncinate process of the pancreas (117). The malignancy rate for these tumors ranges from 50% to 90%. However, in contrast to ductal adenocarcinoma of the pancreas, which carries a poor prognosis, these nonfunctional tumors tend to grow in a more indolent fashion and are associated with a longer survival.

Localization and staging studies are similar to those performed in patients with the more common diagnosis of ductal adenocarcinoma of the exocrine pancreas. Abdominal CT is used to evaluate the primary tumor and assess for hepatic metastases. Preoperative cholangiography may be indicated in the setting of jaundice, with the potential for imaging by endoscopic or percutaneous transhepatic routes. At surgery, most of these nonfunctional neoplasms are larger than 2 cm and are not safely excised by local techniques. Tumors in the head, neck, or uncinate process of the pancreas typically require pancreaticoduodenectomy for safe resection, whereas tumors arising in the body or tail of the pancreas are treated by distal pancreatectomy. Patients with unresectable tumors in the head of the pancreas are candidates for surgical palliation of obstructive jaundice and gastric outlet obstruction by biliary–enteric and gastroenteric bypass, respectively. The overall 5-year survival rate in all patients with resected nonfunctional pancreatic neoplasms approaches 50% (118).

In patients with unresectable disease, partial responses to combination chemotherapy have been reported. In a multicenter trial reported by Moertel and associates (55), 105 patients with advanced islet cell carcinoma, half of whom had nonfunctional tumors, were randomly assigned to one of three treatment regimens. The lowest response rate (30%) was in the group receiving chlorozotocin alone; an intermediate response rate (45%) was seen in patients receiving the combination of streptozotocin plus 5-fluorouracil, and the highest response rate (69%) was noted in patients receiving streptozotocin plus doxorubicin. The streptozotocin-plus-doxorubicin therapy was associated with a significant survival advantage in comparison with the other two treatments. The most common toxic reactions to the chemotherapy were nausea and vomiting, leukopenia, and mild renal insufficiency.

REFERENCES

1. Andrew A. Further evidence that enterochromaffin cells are not derived from the neural crest. *J Embryol Exp Morphol* 1974;31:589.
2. Long PP, Hruban RH, Lo R, et al. Chromosome analysis of nine endocrine neoplasms of the pancreas. *Cancer Genet Cytogenet* 1994;77:55.
3. Yashiro T, Fulton N, Hara H, et al. Comparisons of mutations of *ras* oncogene in human pancreatic exocrine and endocrine tumors. *Surgery* 1993;114:758.
4. Evers BM, Rady PL, Sandoval K, et al. Gastrinomas demonstrate amplification of the *HER-2/neu* protooncogene. *Ann Surg* 1994;219:596.
5. Zeiger MA, Norton JA. Gs alpha: identification of a gene highly expressed by insulinoma and other endocrine tumors. *Surgery* 1993;114:458.
6. Eubanks PJ, Sawicki MP, Samara GJ, et al. Putative tumor-suppressor gene on chromosome 11 is important in sporadic endocrine tumor formation. *Am J Surg* 1994;167:180.
7. Marx S, Spiegel AM, Skarulis MC, et al. Multiple endocrine neoplasia type 1: clinical and genetic topics. *Ann Intern Med* 1998;129:484–494.
8. Fedorak IJ, Ko TC, Gordon D, et al. Localization of islet cell tumors of the pancreas: a review of current techniques. *Surgery* 1993;113:242.
9. Frucht H, Doppman JL, Norton JA, et al. Gastrinomas: comparison of MR imaging with CT, angiography, and US. *Radiology* 1989;171:713.
10. Wank SA, Doppman JL, Miller DL, et al. Prospective study of the ability of computed axial tomography to localize gastrinomas in patients with Zollinger-Ellison syndrome. *Gastroenterology* 1987;92:905.
11. Yeo CJ, Wang BH, Anthone GJ, et al. Surgical experience with pancreatic islet-cell tumors. *Arch Surg* 1993; 128:1143.
12. Termanini B, Gibril F, Reynolds JC, et al. Value of somatostatin receptor scintigraphy: a prospective study in gastrinoma of its effect on clinical management. *Gastroenterology* 1997;112:335–347.
13. Meko JB, Doherty GM, Siegel BA, et al. Evaluation of somatostatin-receptor scintigraphy for detecting neuroendocrine tumors. *Surgery* 1996;120:975–984.
14. Kisker O, Bartsch D, Weinel RJ, et al. The value of somatostatin-receptor scintigraphy in newly diagnosed endocrine gastroenteropancreatic tumors. *J Am Coll Surg* 1997;184: 487–492.
15. Schirmer WJ, O'Dorisio TM, Schirmer TP, et al. Intraoperative localization of neuroendocrine tumors with ^{125}I-tyr^3-octreotide and a hand-held gamma-detecting probe. *Surgery* 1993;114:745.
16. Modlin IM, Tang LH. Approaches to the diagnosis of gut neuroendocrine tumors: the last word (today). *Gastroenterology* 1997;112:583–590.
17. Krausz Y, Bar-Ziv J, deJong RBJ, et al. Somatostatin-receptor scintigraphy in the management of gastroenteropancreatic tumors. *Am J Gastroenterol* 1998;93:66–70.
18. Frilling A, Malago M, Martin H, et al. Use of somatostatin receptor scintigraphy to image extrahepatic metastases of neuroendocrine tumors. *Surgery* 1998;124:1000–1004.
19. Glover JR, Shorvon PJ, Lees WR. Endoscopic ultrasound for localisation of islet cell tumours. *Gut* 1992;33:108.
20. Rosch T, Lightdale CJ, Botet JF, et al. Localization of pancreatic endocrine tumors by endoscopic ultrasonography. *N Engl J Med* 1992;326:1721.
21. Thompson NW, Czako PF, Fritts LL, et al. Role of endoscopic ultrasonography in the localization of insulinomas and gastrinomas. *Surgery* 1994;116:1131.
22. Proye C, Malvaux P, Patton F, et al. Noninvasive imaging of insulinomas and gastrinomas with endoscopic ultrasonography and somatostatin receptor scintigraphy. *Surgery* 1998; 124:1134–1144.
23. Maton PN, Miller DL, Doppman JL, et al. Role of selective angiography in the management of patients with Zollinger-Ellison syndrome. *Gastroenterology* 1987;92:913.
24. Norton JA, Shawker TH, Doppman JL, et al. Localization and surgical treatment of occult insulinomas. *Ann Surg* 1990; 212:615.
25. Vinik AI, Moattari AR, Cho K, et al. Transhepatic portal vein catheterization for localization of sporadic and MEN gastrinomas: a ten-year experience. *Surgery* 1990;107:246.
26. Pedrazzoli S, Pasquale C, Miotto D, et al. Transhepatic portal sampling for preoperative localization of insulinomas. *Surg Gynecol Obstet* 1987;165:101.
27. Vinik AI, Delbridge L, Moattari R, et al. Transhepatic portal vein catheterization for localization of insulinomas: a ten-year experience. *Surgery* 1991;109:1.
28. Fraker DL, Norton JA. Localization and resection of insulinomas and gastrinomas. *JAMA* 1988;259:3601.
29. Imamura M, Minematsu S, Suzuki T, et al. Usefulness of selective arterial secretin injection test for localization of gastrinoma in the Zollinger-Ellison syndrome. *Ann Surg* 1987; 205:230.
30. Rosato FE, Bonn J, Shapiro M, et al. Selective arterial stimulation of secretin in localization of gastrinomas. *Surg Gynecol Obstet* 1990:171:196.
31. Gower WR Jr, Buzogany JA, Ellison EC, et al. Control of gastrin release in cultured gastrinoma-derived G cells. *Surgery* 1988;104:424.
32. Chiba T, Yamatani T, Yamaguchi A, et al. Mechanism for increase of gastrin release by secretin in Zollinger-Ellison syndrome. *Gastroenterology* 1989;96:1439.
33. Thom AK, Norton JA, Doppman JL, et al. Prospective study of the use of intraarterial secretin injection and portal venous sampling to localize duodenal gastrinomas. *Surgery* 1992;112:1002.
34. Pereira PL, Roche AJ, Maier GW, et al. Insulinoma and islet cell hyperplasia: value of the calcium intraarterial stimulation tests when findings of other preoperative studies are negative. *Radiology* 1998;206:703–709.
35. Cohen MS, Picus D, Lairmore TC, et al. Prospective study of provocative angiograms to localize functional islet cell tumors of the pancreas. *Surgery* 1997;122:1091–1100.
36. Brown CK, Bartlett DL, Doppman JL, et al. Intraarterial calcium stimulation and intraoperative ultrasonography in the localization and resection of insulinomas. *Surgery* 1997;122: 1189–1194.
37. Aoki T, Sakon M, Ohzato H, et al. Evaluation of preoperative and intraoperative arterial stimulation and venous sampling for diagnosis and surgical resection of insulinoma. *Surgery* 1999;126:968–973.
38. Grant CS, van Heerden J, Charboneau JW, et al. Insulinoma: the value of intraoperative ultrasonography. *Arch Surg* 1988; 123:843.
39. Norton JA, Sigel B, Baker AR, et al. Localization of an occult insulinoma by intraoperative ultrasonography. *Surgery* 1985;97:381.
40. Whipple AO, Frantz VK. Adenoma of islet cells with hyperinsulinism: a review. *Ann Surg* 1935;101:1299.
41. Service FJ. Hypoglycemic disorders. *N Engl J Med* 1995;332: 1144–1152.
42. Kahn CR. The riddle of tumour hypoglycemia revisited. *J Clin Endocrinol Metab* 1980;9:335.
43. Daughaday WH, Emanuele MA, Brooks MH, et al. Synthesis and secretion of insulin-like growth factor II by a leiomyosarcoma with associated hypoglycemia. *N Engl J Med* 1988; 319:1434.
44. Seckl MJ, Mulholland PJ, Bishop AE, et al. Hypoglycemia due to an insulin-secreting small-cell carcinoma of the cervix. *N Engl J Med* 1999;341:733–736.
45. Howard TJ, Stabile BE, Zinner MJ, et al. Anatomic distribution of pancreatic endocrine tumors. *Am J Surg* 1990;159:258.
46. Service FJ, McMahon MM, O'Brien PC, et al. Functioning insulinoma: incidence, recurrence, and long-term survival of patients—a 60-year study. *Mayo Clin Proc* 1991;66:711.
47. Menegaux F, Schmitt G, Mercadier M, et al. Pancreatic insulinomas. *Am J Surg* 1993;165:243.
48. Udelsman R, Yeo CJ, Hruban RH, et al. Pancreaticoduodenectomy for selected pancreatic endocrine tumors. *Surg Gynecol Obstet* 1993;177:269.

49. Phan GQ, Yeo CJ, Cameron JL, et al. Pancreaticoduodenectomy for selected periampullary neuroendocrine tumors: fifty patients. *Surgery* 1997;122:989–997.

50. Thompson GB, Service FJ, van Heerden JA, et al. Reoperative insulinomas, 1927 to 1992: an institutional experience. *Surgery* 1993;114:1196.

51. Carty SE, Jensen RT, Norton JA. Prospective study of aggressive resection of metastatic pancreatic endocrine tumors. *Surgery* 1992;112:1024.

52. Modlin IM, Lewis JJ, Ahlman H, et al. Management of unresectable malignant endocrine tumors of the pancreas. *Surg Gynecol Obstet* 1993;176:507.

53. McEntee GP, Nagorney DM, Kvols LK, et al. Cytoreductive hepatic surgery for neuroendocrine tumors. *Surgery* 1990; 108:1091.

54. Thompson GB, van Heerden JA, Grant CS, et al. Islet cell carcinomas of the pancreas: a twenty-year experience. *Surgery* 1988;104:1011.

55. Moertel CG, Lefkopoulo M, Lipsitz S, et al. Streptozocin-doxorubicin, streptozocin-fluorouracil, or chlorozotocin in the treatment of advanced islet-cell carcinoma. *N Engl J Med* 1992;326:519.

56. Moertel CG, Hanley JA, Johnson LA. Streptozocin alone compared with streptozocin plus fluorouracil in the treatment of advanced islet-cell carcinoma. *N Engl J Med* 1980;303:1189.

57. Altimari AF, Badrinath K, Reisel HJ, et al. DTIC therapy in patients with malignant intra-abdominal neuroendocrine tumors. *Surgery* 1987;102:1009.

58. Zollinger RM, Ellison EH. Primary peptic ulcerations of the jejunum associated with islet cell tumors of the pancreas. *Ann Surg* 1955;142:709.

59. Zollinger RM, Ellison EC, Fabri PJ, et al. Primary peptic ulcerations of the jejunum associated with islet cell tumors: twenty-five-year appraisal. *Ann Surg* 1980;192:422.

60. Wolfe MM, Jensen RT. Zollinger-Ellison syndrome: current concepts in diagnosis and management. *N Engl J Med* 1987; 317:1200.

61. Yeo CJ. ZES: current approaches. *Contemp Gastroenterol* 1990;:17.

62. Andersen DK. Current diagnosis and management of Zollinger-Ellison syndrome. *Ann Surg* 1989;210:685.

63. Miller LS, Vinayek R, Frucht H, et al. Reflux esophagitis in patients with Zollinger-Ellison syndrome. *Gastroenterology* 1990;98:341.

64. Chiang HCV, O'Dorisio TM, Huang SC, et al. Multiple hormone elevations in Zollinger-Ellison syndrome. *Gastroenterology* 1990;99:1565.

65. Wynick D, Williams SJ, Bloom SR. Symptomatic secondary hormone syndromes in patients with established malignant pancreatic endocrine tumors. *N Engl J Med* 1988;319:605.

66. Maton PN, Vinayek R, Frucht H, et al. Long-term efficacy and safety of omeprazole in patients with Zollinger-Ellison syndrome: a prospective study. *Gastroenterology* 1989;97:827.

67. Metz DC, Pisegna JR, Fishbeyn VA, et al. Currently used doses of omeprazole in Zollinger-Ellison syndrome are too high. *Gastroenterology* 1992;103:1498.

68. Alexander HR, Fraker DL, Norton JA, et al. Prospective study of somatostatin receptor scintigraphy and its effect on operative outcome in patients with Zollinger-Ellison syndrome. *Ann Surg* 1998;228:228–238.

69. Sawicki MP, Howard TJ, Dalton M, et al. The dichotomous distribution of gastrinomas. *Arch Surg* 1990;125:1584.

70. Stabile BE, Morrow DJ, Passaro E Jr. The gastrinoma triangle: operative implications. *Am J Surg* 1984;147:25.

71. Sugg SL, Norton JA, Fraker DL, et al. A prospective study of intraoperative methods to diagnose and resect duodenal gastrinomas. *Ann Surg* 1993;218:138.

72. Frucht H, Norton JA, London JF, et al. Detection of duodenal gastrinomas by operative endoscopic transillumination: a prospective study. *Gastroenterology* 1990;99:1622.

73. Delcore R, Friesen SR. Role of pancreatoduodenectomy in the management of primary duodenal wall gastrinomas in patients with Zollinger-Ellison syndrome. *Surgery* 1992;112:1016.

74. Thompson NW, Vinik AI, Eckhauser FE. Microgastrinomas of the duodenum: a cause of failed operations for the Zollinger-Ellison syndrome. *Ann Surg* 1989;209:396.

75. Farley DR, van Heerden JA, Grant CS, et al. Extrapancreatic gastrinomas: surgical experience. *Arch Surg* 1994;129:506.

76. Chiarugi M, Pucciarelli M, Goletti O, et al. Outcome of surgical treatment for extrapancreatic gastrinomas. *Surg Gynecol Obstet* 1993;177:153.

77. Arnold WS, Fraker DL, Alexander HR, et al. Apparent lymph node primary gastrinoma. *Surgery* 1994;116:1123.

78. Norton JA, Fraker DL, Alexander HR, et al. Surgery to cure the Zollinger-Ellison syndrome. *N Engl J Med* 1999;341: 635–644.

79. Wells SA Jr. Surgery for the Zollinger-Ellison syndrome. *N Engl J Med* 1999;341:689–690.

80. Cadiot G, Vuagnat A, Doukhan I, et al. Prognostic factors in patients with Zollinger-Ellison syndrome and multiple endocrine neoplasia type 1. *Gastroenterology* 1999;116: 286–293.

81. Lowney JK, Frisella MM, Lairmore TC, et al. Pancreatic islet cell tumor metastasis in multiple endocrine neoplasia type 1: correlation with primary tumor size. *Surgery* 1999;125: 1043–1049.

82. Lairmore TC, Chen VY, DeBenedetti MK, et al. Duodenopancreatic resections in patients with multiple endocrine neoplasia type 1 (MEN 1). *Ann Surg* 2000;231:909–918.

83. Richardson CT, Peters MN, Feldman M, et al. Treatment of Zollinger-Ellison syndrome with exploratory laparotomy, proximal gastric vagotomy, and H_2-receptor antagonists: a prospective study. *Gastroenterology* 1985;89:357.

84. Thompson JC, Lewis BG, Weiner I, et al. The role of surgery in the Zollinger-Ellison syndrome. *Ann Surg* 1983;197:594.

85. Norton JA, Doppman JL, Jensen RT. Curative resection in Zollinger-Ellison syndrome: results of a 10-year prospective study. *Ann Surg* 1992;215:8.

86. Fraker DL, Norton JA, Alexander HR, et al. Surgery in Zollinger-Ellison syndrome alters the natural history of gastrinoma. *Ann Surg* 1994;220:320.

87. Delcore R, Friesen SR. The place for curative surgical procedures in the treatment of sporadic and familial Zollinger-Ellison syndrome. *Curr Opin Gen Surg* 1994;2:69.

88. von Schrenck T, Howard JM, Doppman JL, et al. Prospective study of chemotherapy in patients with metastatic gastrinoma. *Gastroenterology* 1988;94:1326.

89. Mozell E, Woltering EA, O'Dorisio TM, et al. Effect of somatostatin analog on peptide release and tumor growth in the Zollinger-Ellison syndrome. *Surg Gynecol Obstet* 1990; 170:476.

90. Mozell E, Cramer AJ, O'Dorisio TM, et al. Long-term efficacy of octreotide in the treatment of Zollinger-Ellison syndrome. *Arch Surg* 1992;127:1019.

91. Makowka L, Tzakis AG, Mazzaferro V, et al. Transplantation of the liver for metastatic endocrine tumors of the intestine and pancreas. *Surg Gynecol Obstet* 1989;168:107.

92. Ajani JA, Carrasco CH, Charnsangavej C, et al. Islet cell tumors metastatic to the liver: effective palliation by sequential hepatic artery embolization. *Ann Intern Med* 1988;108:340.

93. Pisegna JR, Slimak GG, Doppman JL, et al. An evaluation of human recombinant α-interferon in patients with metastatic gastrinoma. *Gastroenterology* 1993;105:1179.

94. Knechtle SJ, Kalayoglu M, D'Alessandro AM, et al. Proceed with caution: liver transplantation for metastatic neuroendocrine tumors. *Ann Surg* 1997;225:345–346.

95. Lang H, Oldhafer KJ, Weimann A, et al. Liver transplantation for metastatic neuroendocrine tumors. *Ann Surg* 1997;225: 347–354.

96. LeTreut YP, Delpero JR, Dousset B, et al. Results of liver transplantation in the treatment of metastatic neuroendocrine tumors: a 31-case French multicentric report. *Ann Surg* 1997;225:355–364.

97. Verner JV, Morrison AB. Islet cell tumor and a syndrome of refractory watery diarrhea and hypokalemia. *Am J Med* 1958;25:374–380.

98. Rood RP, DeLellis RA, Dayal Y, et al. Pancreatic cholera syndrome due to a vasoactive intestinal polypeptide-producing tumor: further insights into the pathophysiology. *Gastroenterology* 1988;94:813.

99. Jaffe BM, Kopern DF, DeSchryver-Kecskemeti K, et al. Indomethacin-responsive pancreatic cholera. *N Engl J Med* 1977;297:817.

100. Smith SL, Branton SA, Avino AJ, et al. Vasoactive intestinal polypeptide-secreting islet cell tumors: a 15-year experience and review of the literature. *Surgery* 1998;124:1050–1055.

101. Nagorney DM, Bloom SR, Polak JM, et al. Resolution of recurrent Verner-Morrison syndrome by resection of metastatic VIPoma. *Surgery* 1983;93:348.

102. Higgins GA, Recant L, Fischman AB. The glucagonoma syndrome: surgically curable diabetes. *Am J Surg* 1979;137:142.

103. Prinz RA, Badrinath K, Banerji M, et al. Operative and chemotherapeutic management of malignant glucagon-producing tumors. *Surgery* 1981;90:713.

104. Boden G, Ryan IG, Eisenschmid BL, et al. Treatment of inoperable glucagonoma with the long-acting somatostatin analogue SMS 201-955. *N Engl J Med* 1986;314:1686.

105. Altimari AF, Bhoopalam N, O'Dorisio T, et al. Use of a somatostatin analog (SMS 201-955) in the glucagonoma syndrome. *Surgery* 1986;100:989.

106. Ganda OP, Weir GC, Soeldner JS, et al. Somatostatinoma: a somatostatin-containing tumor of the endocrine pancreas. *N Engl J Med* 1977;296:963.

107. Kregs GJ, Orci L, Conlon JM, et al. Somatostatinoma syndrome: biochemical, morphologic, and clinical features. *N Engl J Med* 1979;301:285.

108. McLeod MK, Vinik AI. Calcitonin immunoreactivity and hypercalcitoninemia in two patients with sporadic, nonfamilial, gastroenteropancreatic neuroendocrine tumors. *Surgery* 1992;111:484.

109. Howard JM, Gohara AF, Cardwell RJ. Malignant islet cell tumor of the pancreas associated with high plasma calcitonin and somatostatin levels. *Surgery* 1989;105:227.

110. Mao C, Carter P, Schaefer P, et al. Malignant islet cell tumor associated with hypercalcemia. *Surgery* 1995;117:37.

111. Meko JB, Norton JA. Endocrine tumors of the pancreas. *Curr Opin Gen Surg* 1994;2:186.

112. Strewler GJ. The physiology of parathyroid hormone-related peptide. *N Engl J Med* 2000;342:177–185.

113. Langstein HN, Norton JA, Chiang HCV, et al. The utility of circulating levels of human pancreatic polypeptide as a marker for islet cell tumors. *Surgery* 1990;108:1109.

114. Mutch MG, Frisella MM, DeBenedetti MK, et al. Pancreatic polypeptide is a useful plasma marker for radiographically evident pancreatic islet cell tumors in patients with multiple endocrine neoplasia type 1. *Surgery* 1997;122:1012–1020.

115. Kent RB III, van Heerden JA, Weiland LH. Nonfunctioning islet cell tumors. *Ann Surg* 1981;193:185.

116. Eckhauser FE, Cheung PS, Vinik AI, et al. Nonfunctioning malignant neuroendocrine tumors of the pancreas. *Surgery* 1986;100:978.

117. White TJ, Edney JA, Thompson JS, et al. Is there a prognostic difference between functional and nonfunctional islet cell tumors? *Am J Surg* 1994;168:627.

118. Evans DB, Skibber JM, Lee JE, et al. Nonfunctioning islet cell carcinoma of the pancreas. *Surgery* 1993;114:1175.

SECTION F

LIVER AND PORTAL VENOUS SYSTEM

SURGERY: SCIENTIFIC PRINCIPLES AND PRACTICE, Third Edition, edited by Lazar J. Greenfield, Michael W. Mulholland, Keith T. Oldham, Gerald B. Zelenock, and Keith D. Lillemoe. Lippincott Williams & Wilkins Publishers, Philadelphia, © 2001.

CHAPTER 34

HEPATOBILIARY ANATOMY

DAVID R. BYRD

The general and hepatobiliary surgeon confronts the challenges of hepatic anatomy in any of the following four situations: (a) elective partial hepatic resection to remove a primary or secondary neoplasm, (b) elective or emergent decompression for portal venous hypertension or management of a hepatic arterial aneurysm; (c) whole- and split-liver surgical transplantation in donors and recipients, and (d) emergent control of hemorrhage with or without liver resection in cases of hepatic trauma.

Several unique anatomic features of the liver pose formidable obstacles to safe and successful surgery. The liver is a large, transversely oriented, fragile organ that is prone to fracture and bleeding on manipulation. A dual afferent blood supply is intertwined with delicate afferent biliary ducts in a crowded hepatic hilum. The three large hepatic veins that drain the liver empty directly into the inferior vena cava (IVC) posterior to the liver and are completely obscured from view without extensive retrohepatic dissection.

Every surgeon contemplating an operation that exposes or resects all or part of the liver should have a thorough understanding of the general hepatic anatomy and an absolute understanding of each individual patient's hepatic anatomy. A knowledge of segmental hepatic anatomy and the relations of structures within the liver parenchyma is required, in addition to the correlation of preoperative imaging studies with an operative plan for each patient.

TOPOGRAPHIC ANATOMY AND RELATIONS TO PERIHEPATIC STRUCTURES

The normal adult liver is a large, wedge-shaped organ occupying the right upper quadrant of the abdomen, extending vertically on the right side from the undersurface of the right hemidiaphragm to the anterior costal margin and horizontally to the left midclavicular line at the superior pole of the spleen. The anterior surface of the liver is invested by visceral peritoneum that extends to the anterior abdominal wall in the midline from the ligamentum teres, or round ligament (the obliterated umbilical vessels), and by an obliquely oriented fusion of peritoneum known as the *falciform ligament*. Posteriorly, the investing peritoneum becomes contiguous with the peritoneum of the diaphragm at the coronary and triangular attachments, so that a rhomboidal retroperitoneal "bare area" is not covered by peritoneum (Fig. 34.1). Glisson's capsule is a thin, fibrous covering that closely envelops the entire liver deep to the peritoneum and sends thin fibrous septa into the hepatic parenchyma.

Ordinarily, the liver can be surgically separated from adjacent organs and structures by dividing areolar tissue planes (Fig. 34.2). Neoplasms or inflammatory conditions in the liver or surrounding structures may obliterate these tissue planes and may be difficult to appreciate on preoperative imaging studies. Superiorly and anteriorly, the diaphragm or abdominal wall may be invaded by cancer or

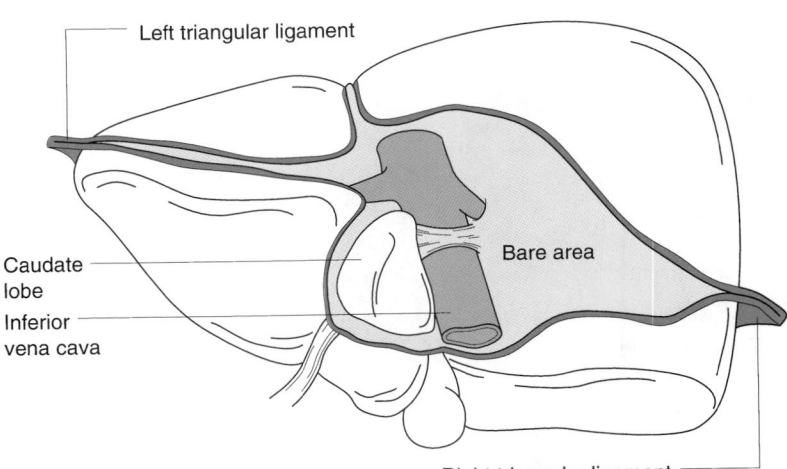

Figure 34.1. Posterior view of liver, showing the level of peritoneal reflections.

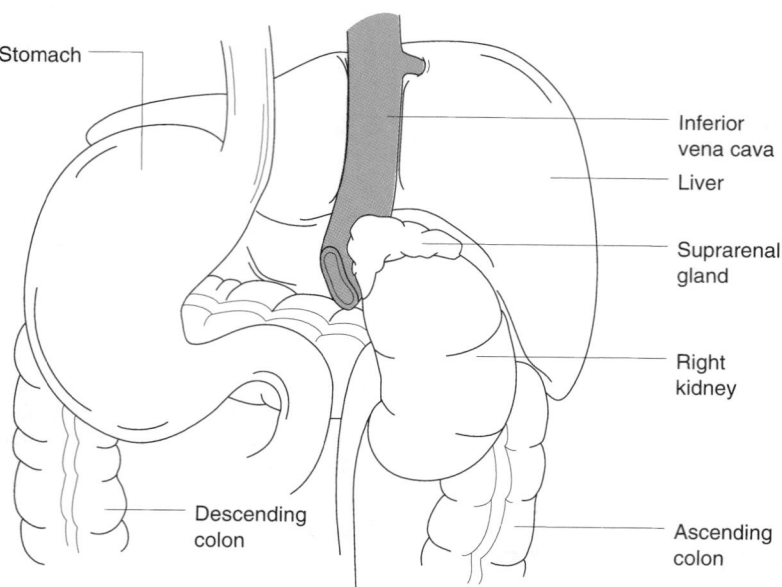

Figure 34.2. Posterior view of the liver, showing organs that produce impressions on its inferior surface.

abscess. Posteriorly, neoplasms of the right adrenal gland or superior pole of the right kidney may densely adhere to the right hepatic lobe. Inferiorly, the gallbladder, hepatic flexure of the colon, duodenum, or periportal lymph nodes may be inseparable from the liver edge. On the left side, cancers of the stomach or gastroesophageal junction may invade the left hepatic lobe. Preoperative recognition of potential adjacent involvement is essential to help guide the choice of incision, determine the preoperative function of both kidneys should nephrectomy become necessary, and initiate a mechanical bowel preparation to allow a safe colon or gastric resection if required.

MORPHOLOGIC AND FUNCTIONAL ANATOMY

The description and definition of the anatomic divisions of the liver have been revised numerous times in the past 40 years. The revisions have been based on detailed autopsy studies and more recently on correlation with hepatic imaging by computed tomography (CT) and ultrasonography. The original morphologic division of the liver into right and left lobes separated by the falciform ligament has now been replaced by detailed descriptions of functional divisions based on hepatic venous drainage and portal pedicles (branches of the hepatic artery, portal vein, and bile duct) to individual segments. Extensively detailed descriptions and diagrams of hepatic anatomy form the modern understanding of the functional anatomy of the liver and should be carefully reviewed by all hepatic surgeons (1–8).

Differences in the hepatic anatomic nomenclature in the English and French literature are confusing. Until recently, anatomic descriptions in the English literature began with a major division of the liver into right and left hepatic lobes, separated by a vertical line drawn from the gallbladder fossa to the IVC (Fig. 34.3). The middle hepatic vein can be found within the hepatic parenchyma along this line, and there is little portal pedicle crossover

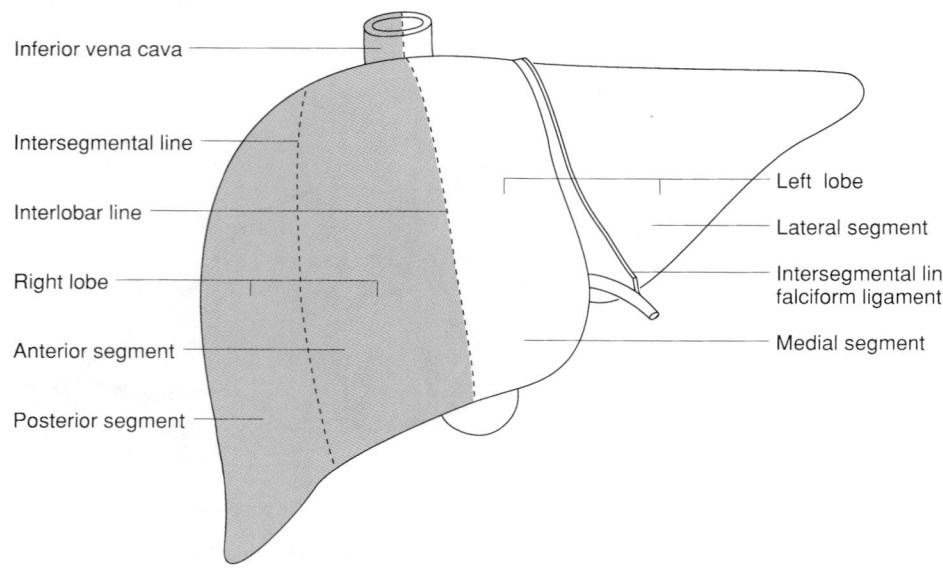

Figure 34.3. Anatomic division of the liver into right and left lobes by a line extending from the gallbladder fossa posteriorly to the inferior vena cava.

when this division is used. The left lobe is further divided by the falciform ligament (continuous with the umbilical fissure) into a medial segment (quadrate lobe) and a lateral segment. The main left hepatic vein courses to the left of the umbilical fissure. The right lobe is further divided into anterior and posterior segments by an intersegmental line without any reliable topographic landmarks or intraparenchymal septa to allow easy identification. The caudate lobe is generally considered separately because it usually receives portal pedicle branches from both the right and left sides and has an isolated hepatic venous drainage through multiple short veins that enter directly into the IVC.

In the now widely accepted French nomenclature, the liver can be divided into eight discrete segments based on portal pedicle branches and hepatic venous drainage. The most surgically relevant rendition of Couinaud's "blowout" segmental diagram is shown in Fig. 34.4. It demonstrates that segments VI and VII most accurately reside posteriorly in vivo but are often drawn to appear lateral in Couinaud's ex vivo description. In these descriptions, the left, middle, and right hepatic veins course in three vertical connective planes called *scissurae*, which divide the liver into four sectors, each receiving a major portal pedicle. Each of the four sectors can be further subdivided into two segments, based on a transverse line drawn through the main right and left portal veins within these sectors, known as the *transverse scissura.*

Enumeration of the segments begins left to right, beginning with segment I, the caudate lobe. The left lateral sector (lobe) consists of a superior segment II and an inferior segment III and is synonymous with the left lateral segment in the older terminology. The left vertical scissura separates the left lateral sector from segment IV, which may be subdivided into a superior segment IVa and an inferior segment IVb and is synonymous with the quadrate lobe or medial segment of the left lobe. The main scissura separates the right and left hepatic lobes. The right vertical scissura divides the right lobe into an anteromedial sector and a posterolateral sector. The anteromedial sector is further subdivided into an inferior segment V and a superior segment VIII. The posterolateral sector is further subdivided into an inferior segment VI and a superior segment VII.

The major advantages of using this detailed segmental anatomy based on discrete portal pedicle branches are to locate individual lesions in the hepatic substance accurately by preoperative imaging and intraoperative ultrasonography and to allow the possibility of less-than-lobar, segmental anatomic resections that minimize blood loss and functional loss of hepatic reserve.

Hepatic Veins

Three major hepatic veins carry blood from the central veins of the hepatic substance to the IVC. Branches of these veins generally drain obliquely from inferior to superior and posterior regions within the hepatic parenchyma. Two thirds of patients have a single, large right hepatic vein that joins the right anterior wall of the IVC and a middle and a left hepatic vein that converge 1 to 2 cm from the IVC and enter the left anterior wall of the IVC as a single vessel, adjacent to the confluence of the right hepatic vein and IVC (Fig. 34.5). In one third of patients, each major hepatic vein joins the IVC at the same horizontal level as a separate trunk. In some patients, a short but definable extraparenchymal segment of one or more of the hepatic veins is found at the confluence with the IVC. More frequently, the entire length of the hepatic veins is within the parenchyma, which may preclude early, safe hepatic venous isolation during hepatic resection. These veins have fragile, thin walls, and inadvertent injury may result in rapid hemorrhage that is difficult to isolate and control.

The venous drainage of the liver begins in the central vein of the hepatic lobule. The left hepatic vein drains segments II, III, and IV. The middle hepatic vein drains a portion of segment IV and anterior segments V and VIII. The right vein drains the posterior segments VI and VII and a portion of the anterior segments.

Venous drainage of the caudate lobe is through multiple short posterior veins that empty directly into the IVC. In addition, several posterior accessory veins (up to 10) drain the medial aspect of the right lobe and empty directly into the right anterior surface of the IVC (Fig. 34.6). It is essential that the surgeon know and identify these accessory veins during right hepatic lobectomy, caudate lobe resection, and right adrenalectomy.

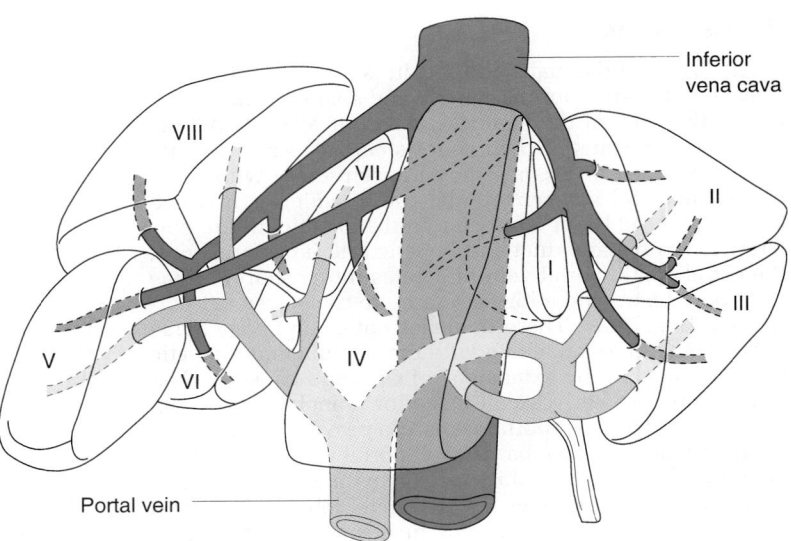

Inferior vena cava

Portal vein

Figure 34.4. Functional division of the liver and liver segments according to Couinaud's nomenclature.

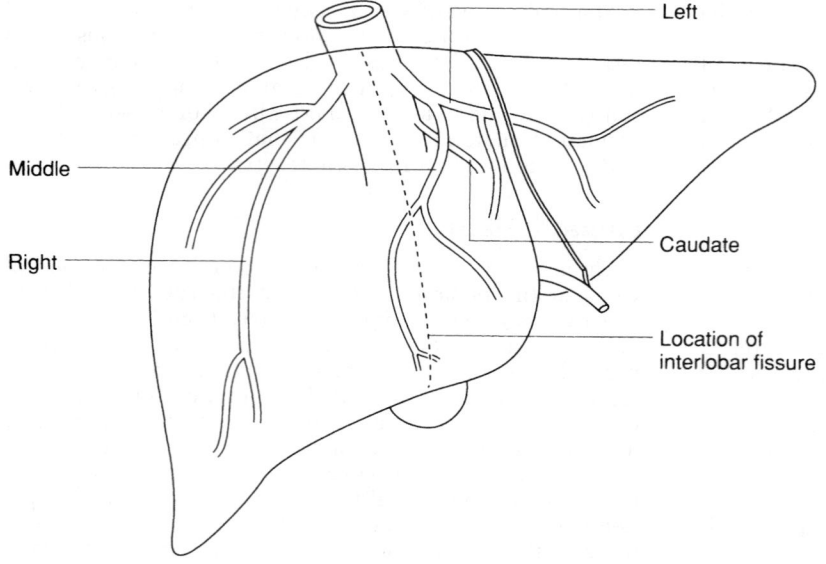

Figure 34.5. Three major hepatic veins drain the liver. The caudate segment of the liver usually drains directly into the inferior vena cava.

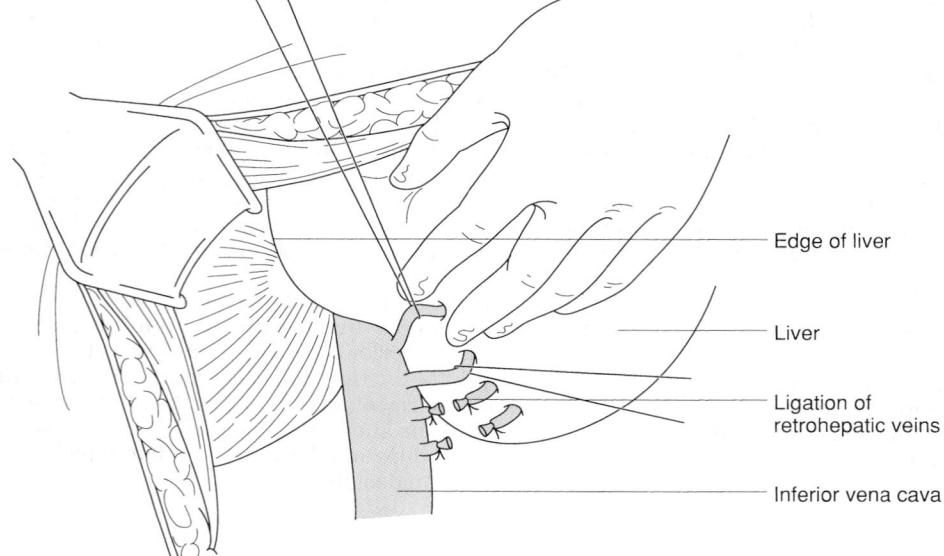

Figure 34.6. Retraction of right hepatic lobe medially exposes small venous tributaries that drain the right lobe directly into the retrohepatic vena cava. Several branches are ligated.

Portal Veins

The origin of the main portal vein is formed by the confluence of the superior mesenteric and splenic veins posterior to the neck of the pancreas, where it receives pyloric and coronary veins. It then courses cephalad and slightly obliquely to form the most posterior structure within the hepatoduodenal ligament (portal triad), which is invested by leaves of the lesser omentum. In the hepatic hilum, posterior to the hepatic duct and hepatic arterial bifurcations, the extrahepatic portal vein bifurcates into a short oblique right portal vein and a longer and more transverse left portal vein (Fig. 34.7). These branches enter the parenchyma and become invested, along with the bile duct and hepatic arterial branches, by extensions of Glisson's capsule. Usually, one or two early, small posterior branches arise from both the right and left portal veins and provide a dual blood supply to the caudate lobe. The left portal vein then courses anteriorly in the pars umbilicus to give off a medial branch or branches to segment IV (quadrate lobe) and lateral branches to the left lateral sector, further subdividing into a

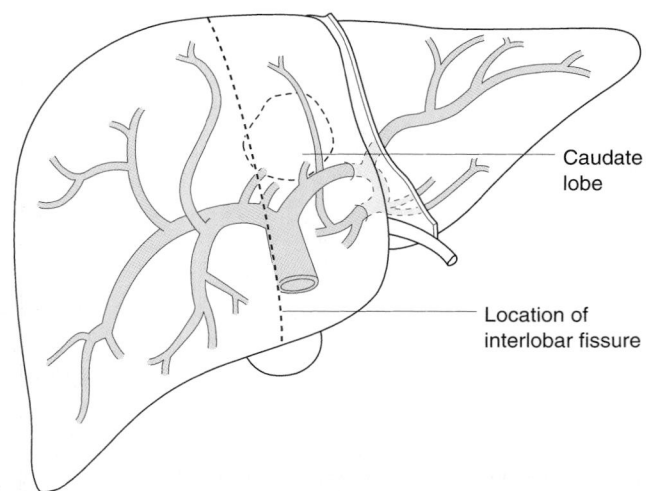

Figure 34.7. Intrahepatic divisions of the portal vein.

Table 34.1. DESCRIPTION AND FREQUENCY OF HEPATIC ARTERIAL VARIATIONS

Description	Occurrence (%)
Right, left, middle	55
Right, middle, replaced left (off left gastric)	10
Left, middle, replaced right (off superior mesenteric)	11
Middle, replaced right and left	1
Right, left, middle, accessory left	8
Right, left, middle, accessory right	7
Right, left, middle, accessory right and left	1
Combined replaced right, accessory left or replaced left, accessory right	2
No celiac trunk, common hepatic origin off superior mesenteric	2
No celiac trunk, common hepatic origin off left gastric	0.5

From Michels NA. Newer anatomy of the liver and its variant blood supply and collateral circulation. Am J Surg 1966;112:337, with permission.

superior branch to segment II and an inferior branch to segment III. The right portal vein further branches within 1 to 2 cm of the main portal bifurcation into an anterior division, which gives off an inferior branch to segment V and a superior branch to segment VIII, and a posterior division, which gives off an inferior branch to segment VI and a superior branch to segment VII.

Hepatic Arteries

The origin and course of the right and left hepatic arteries vary considerably. The most common finding is a transverse common hepatic artery from the celiac trunk that gives off the gastroduodenal, right gastric, and supraduodenal arteries and then courses obliquely in the left anterior aspect of the hepatoduodenal ligament as the proper hepatic artery. After the cystic artery to the gallbladder is given off, a fairly low trifurcation of the proper hepatic artery gives rise to single right, middle, and left hepatic arteries. The middle hepatic artery may arise from either the right or left hepatic arteries after bifurcation of the proper hepatic artery. This arterial pattern is found only 55% of the time. The descriptions and frequency of hepatic arterial variants have been well characterized by Michels (5) (Table 34.1). Knowledge of the most common variations is extremely important because vessels can be divided inadvertently during gastric, pancreatic, and hepatobiliary procedures. A replaced or accessory left hepatic artery may arise from the left gastric artery and course transversely in the lesser omentum (Fig. 34.8). Nearly as often, a replaced or accessory right hepatic artery may also arise from the superior mesenteric artery near its origin and course posteriorly or through the head of the pancreas and obliquely along the right posterior border of the hepatoduodenal ligament. Within the hepatic parenchyma, the hepatic arterial branches course closely with bile duct branches and fairly closely with portal venous branches, in-

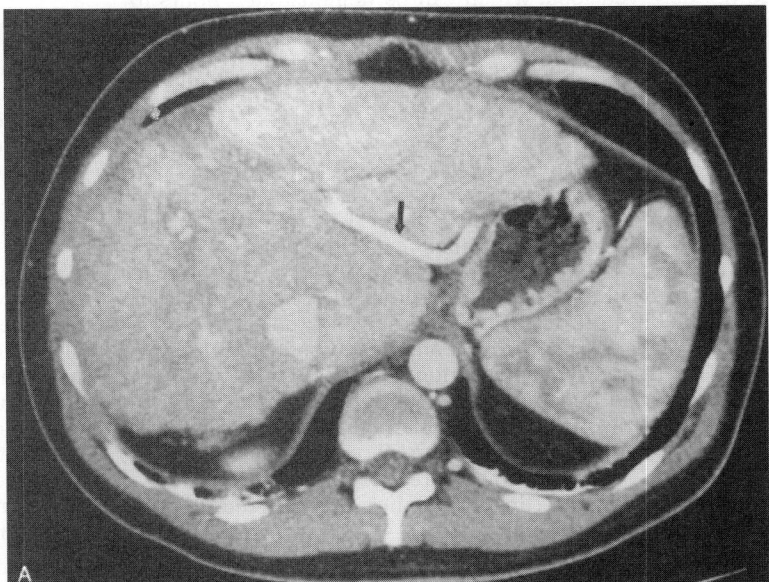

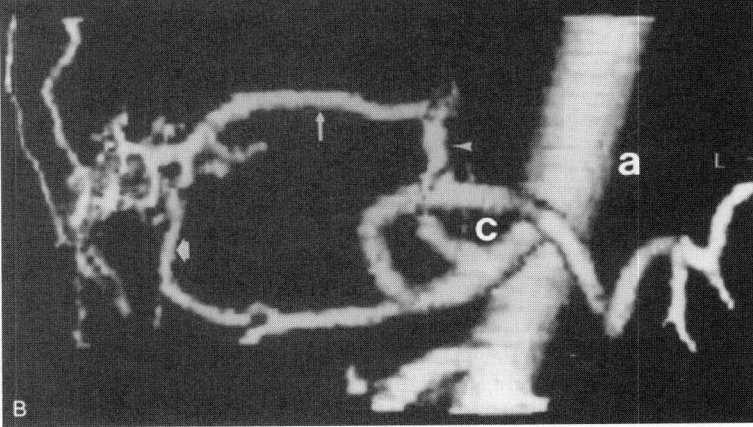

Figure 34.8. Replaced left hepatic artery arising from the left gastric artery. *(A)* Conventional transaxial images from spiral helical computed tomography *(CT)* during the arterial contrast phase show the replaced left hepatic artery *(dark arrow)* coursing in the lesser omentum. *(B)* Spiral helical CT allows detailed visceral arterial reconstruction, as in this oblique projection of the aorta *(a)* and celiac axis *(c)*, which shows the replaced left hepatic artery *(thin arrow)* arising from the left gastric artery *(arrowhead)* and the right hepatic artery coursing in the portal triad *(thick arrow)*. (Courtesy of T. Winter, M.D., Department of Radiology, University of Washington, Seattle, WA.)

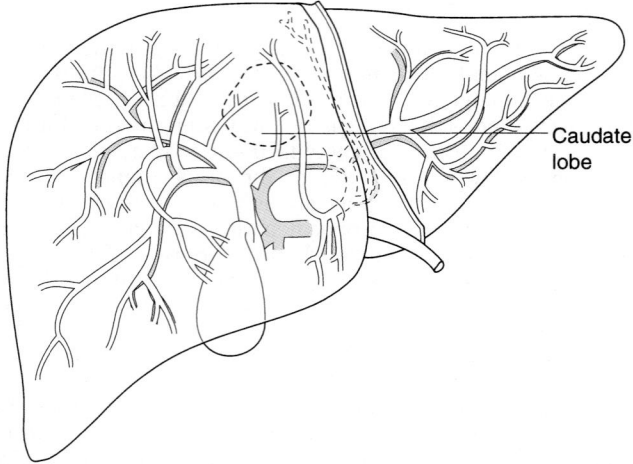

Caudate lobe

Figure 34.9. Intrahepatic divisions of bile ducts and hepatic arteries. Arteries and ducts in the liver parenchyma run in parallel.

vested by Glisson's capsule, to supply portal pedicle branches to each hepatic segment (Fig. 34.9). Although the original anatomic descriptions denied the existence of collateral vessels to the opposite hepatic lobe, imaged perfusion studies after ligation of main or replaced hepatic arteries have clearly demonstrated the presence of collateral flow to the deprived lobe, which can be demonstrated hours to days after ligation.

IMAGING THE LIVER

Ultrasonography

Hepatic ultrasonography has been used for the past 20 years to identify lesions in the parenchyma, describe the consistency and homogeneity of the liver (the fatty or cirrhotic liver), and identify dilatation of the biliary tree and any abnormalities or stones in the gallbladder. In the past 10 years, it has become possible to acquire detailed anatomic descriptions of the hepatic veins, portal pedicles, and IVC by means of intraoperative ultrasonography and probes with improved resolution. Cooperation between the radiologist and hepatic surgeon in the application of intraoperative ultrasonography has made it possible to identify lesions during surgery that were formerly not visible by conventional transcorporeal ultrasonography or CT. Probes with horizontal or vertical orientation and different depths of resolution can be placed directly on the surface of the liver to allow a complete definition of the hepatic anatomy. Laparoscopic ultrasonographic probes are now available that can be used to direct ablational therapies of hepatic tumors with minimally invasive techniques. In addition, a number of ultrasonographic contrast agents are being developed that may improve the utility of hepatic ultrasonography. Beginning superiorly at the IVC, the confluence and course of each of the hepatic veins can be easily determined (Fig. 34.10). More inferiorly, the main right and left portal pedicles can be seen coursing in the transverse scissura. The left portal pedicle can be seen to course anteriorly as the pars umbilicus in the ligamentum teres. Portal structures are easily differentiated from hepatic veins by the hyperechoic extensions of Glisson's capsule that surround these structures. If a circular structure is encountered and a mass or metastasis is suspected, scanning away from the mass may reveal a tubular vascular shape that was imaged in cross section. Flattening a circular mass by external compression with the ultrasonographic probe differentiates a vascular structure from a solid mass.

Computed Tomography

The entire abdomen and pelvis cannot be imaged with ultrasonography because some intraabdominal regions are distorted by gastric, small-bowel, and colonic air. Thus, CT has been increasingly used to screen for hepatic and other intraabdominal or retroperitoneal lesions. Conventional CT includes 0.5- to 1-cm transectional images of the liver acquired after oral administration of barium and bolus injection of intravenous contrast. Although resolution has improved, hepatic lesions smaller than 1 cm or lesions that are of the same density as the hepatic parenchyma may be missed.

Until recently, the resolution of hepatic lesions was greatly enhanced by a combination of visceral angiography and CT, known as *CT arterioportography*. Most primary or secondary hepatic lesions are supplied mainly by branches of the hepatic artery. CT performed immediately after the injection of contrast directly into the common hepatic artery (CT arteriography) may identify small hepatic lesions, which usually appear more dense than the surrounding hepatic parenchyma. CT portography includes the injection of contrast directly into the splenic or superior mesenteric arteries, with CT imaging performed during the portal venous phase of this injection. Hepatic lesions supplied by the hepatic artery appear as discrete hypodense lesions surrounded by normal hepatic parenchyma enhanced by portal venous contrast. Determination of the anatomic relations between hepatic lesions and portal structures also becomes possible and is useful to aid in preoperative planning and assess the feasibility of surgical resection. In many centers, CT portographic imaging of the liver is a standard procedure before resection of hepatomas or colorectal metastases to the liver is attempted. In other centers, conventional CT followed by intraoperative ultrasonography during exploration is preferred.

Single- or multiple-phase double-helical (spiral) CT is becoming more widely available and shows considerable promise to complement or replace CT arterioportography in preoperative imaging. This scanning technique allows total hepatic imaging in both the arterial and arteriovenous phases after a single rapid low- or high-dose bolus injection of intravenous contrast has been administered during a single breath-hold by the patient (Fig. 34.11). This technique also allows visualization of the portal structures and hepatic veins on a single scan and provides high resolution for small hepatic lesions. In addition, three-dimensional reconstructions in different planes can be created to further delineate the hepatic parenchyma and demonstrate a CT-constructed hepatic arteriogram (Fig. 34.8). This technique may completely replace invasive angiography in fully characterizing the blood supply to the liver before hepatic resection or after hepatic transplantation.

Magnetic Resonance Imaging

Magnetic resonance imaging (MRI) of the liver after enhancement with iron oxide or gadolinium has yielded results similar to those of helical CT. However, it has not demonstrated sufficient superiority to justify its higher cost, although its role in hepatic imaging is becoming more prominent. It does not provide optimal images of the intestine and retroperitoneum. Refinements in MRI technique to improve resolution or decrease cost may increase its utility in the future. Magnetic resonance cholangiopancreatography (MRCP) is rapidly evolving as a new, noninvasive imaging test to evaluate pancreatobiliary abnormalities, including stones, strictures, and neoplasms (Fig. 34.12). Heavily T_2-weighted scans that maximize the signal from the ducts are acquired while patients hold their breath. No injections of contrast agents are needed. With three-dimensional reconstructions, ducts can be viewed from different angles.

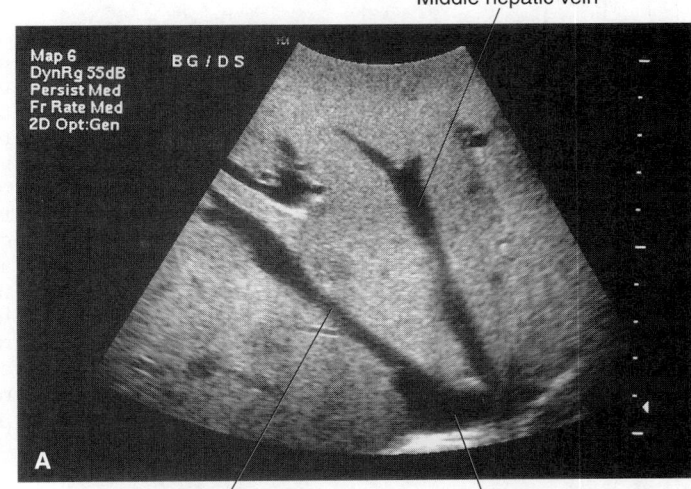

Middle hepatic vein

Right hepatic vein   Inferior vena cava (IVC)

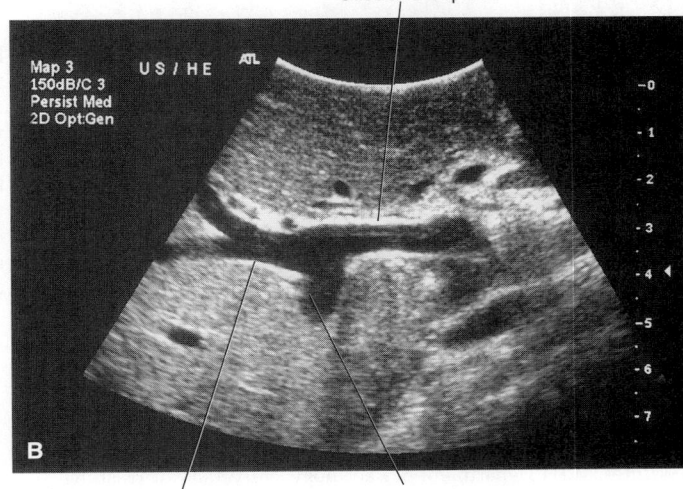

Glisson's capsule

Anterior division   Posterior division

Pars umbilicus

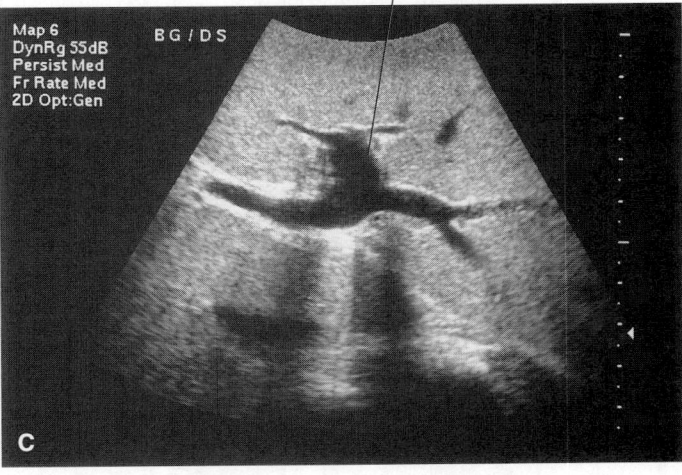

Figure 34.10. Intraoperative ultrasonography of the liver. *(A)* Confluence of the middle and right hepatic veins and entry into the inferior vena cava. *(B)* Right portal structures invested by hyperechoic Glisson's capsule. *(C)* Left portal structures showing the anterior direction of the pars umbilicus. Hyperechoic parenchymal lesion can be seen straddling segments VII and VIII. (Courtesy of T. Winter, M.D., and U. Schmiedl, M.D., Department of Radiology, University of Washington, Seattle, WA.)

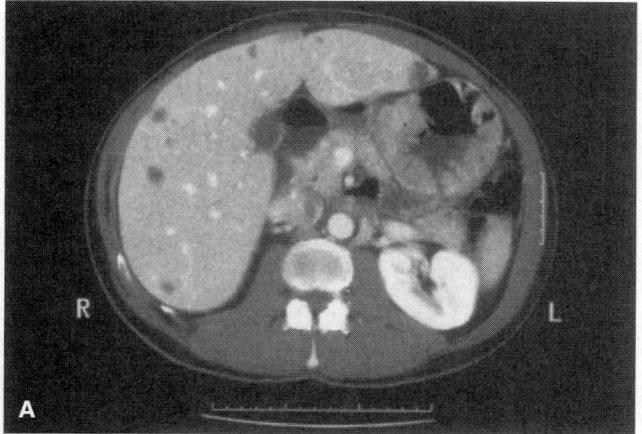

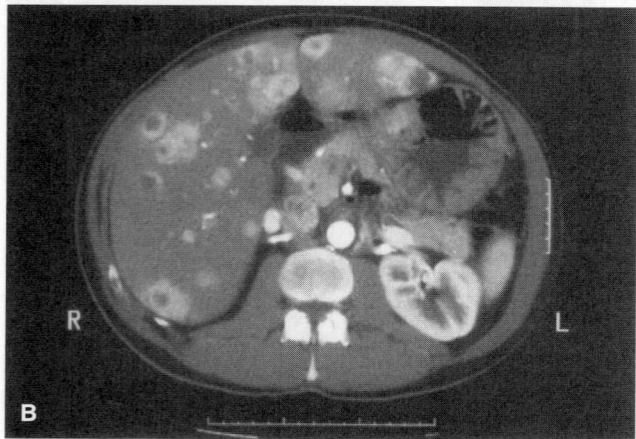

Figure 34.11. Double helical (spiral) computed tomography in a 50-year-old man with hypervascular lesions from metastatic gastrinoma. *(A)* Conventional venous contrast phase demonstrates a few poorly defined parenchymal lesions. *(B)* Hepatic arterial phase more clearly demarcates lesions from surrounding normal parenchyma and reveals several additional lesions. (Courtesy of T. Winter, M.D., Department of Radiology, University of Washington, Seattle, WA.)

Positron Emission Tomography

Recent advances in total-body imaging with positron emission tomography (PET) have made it possible to obtain images of hepatic primary and secondary tumors with better resolution. This technique is based on the increased metabolism of compounds such as glucose in tumors. A glucose analogue that is retained longer in tumor cells than glucose, fluorodeoxyglucose tagged with fluorine 18, is injected intravenously before scanning. Areas of increased uptake may be imaged not only in the liver but also, equally important, in other areas, such as the primary tumor basin, regional nodes, and distant sites like the lung. Preoperative PET is playing an increasing important role in the staging of patients presumed to have disease confined to the liver before surgery. The current and future roles of this technique in the surgical management of hepatomas and metastatic lesions to the liver are under active investigation.

PREOPERATIVE EVALUATION OF HEPATIC RESERVE

Although the preoperative assessment and prediction of hepatic reserve after resection are critical in determining the safety of a procedure, only modest progress has been made in obtaining these measurements during the past 20 years. Tests of liver function that measure synthetic ability (albumin and prothrombin time) and bile excretory function (total bilirubin and alkaline phosphatase) and prognostic scores such as the Child-Pugh score have been helpful only to evaluate hepatic dysfunction before any intervention. More sophisticated dynamic tests include the following:

1. Measurement of hepatic perfusion based on the clearance of galactose or organic anionic dyes, such as indocyanin green and sulfobromophthalein
2. Tests of microsomal function, such as the aminopyrine breath test, caffeine clearance, or lidocaine clearance
3. Specific measurements of mitochondrial oxidative metabolism of the liver based on ketone body ratio or redox tolerance index

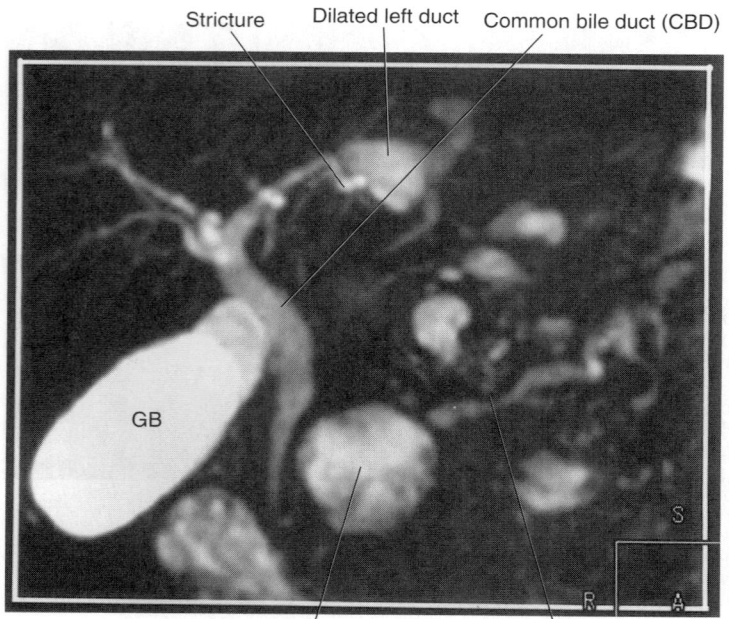

Stricture   Dilated left duct   Common bile duct (CBD)

GB

Pseudocyst   Pancreatic duct (PD)

Figure 34.12. Magnetic resonance cholangiopancreatography of the entire pancreatobiliary tree demonstrates a pseudocyst of the pancreatic head *(arrow)* and a dilated left hepatic duct behind a stricture *(arrow). PD,* pancreatic duct; *GB,* gallbladder. (Courtesy of U. Schmiedl, M.D., Department of Radiology, University of Washington, Seattle, WA.)

None of these techniques has thus far proved reliable or been universally accepted. The previous surgical dicta regarding the safety of resection are still reasonably accurate. In other words, up to 75% to 80% of the hepatic volume may be safely resected if no evidence of hepatitis or cirrhosis is found. For a cirrhotic liver, wedge resections or segmental resections may be considered in some circumstances. Full lobar resection of a cirrhotic liver should be discouraged except in special circumstances and must be performed by experienced hepatic surgeons.

Correlation of Computed Tomographic Images with Segmental Anatomy

Preoperative CT remains the primary imaging technique to determine the location of hepatic lesions and estimate the extent of resection required to remove all disease. Very few descriptive reports are available that correlate the location of a hepatic lesion with CT images. Figure 34.13 is provided to help guide the hepatic surgeon to the ex-

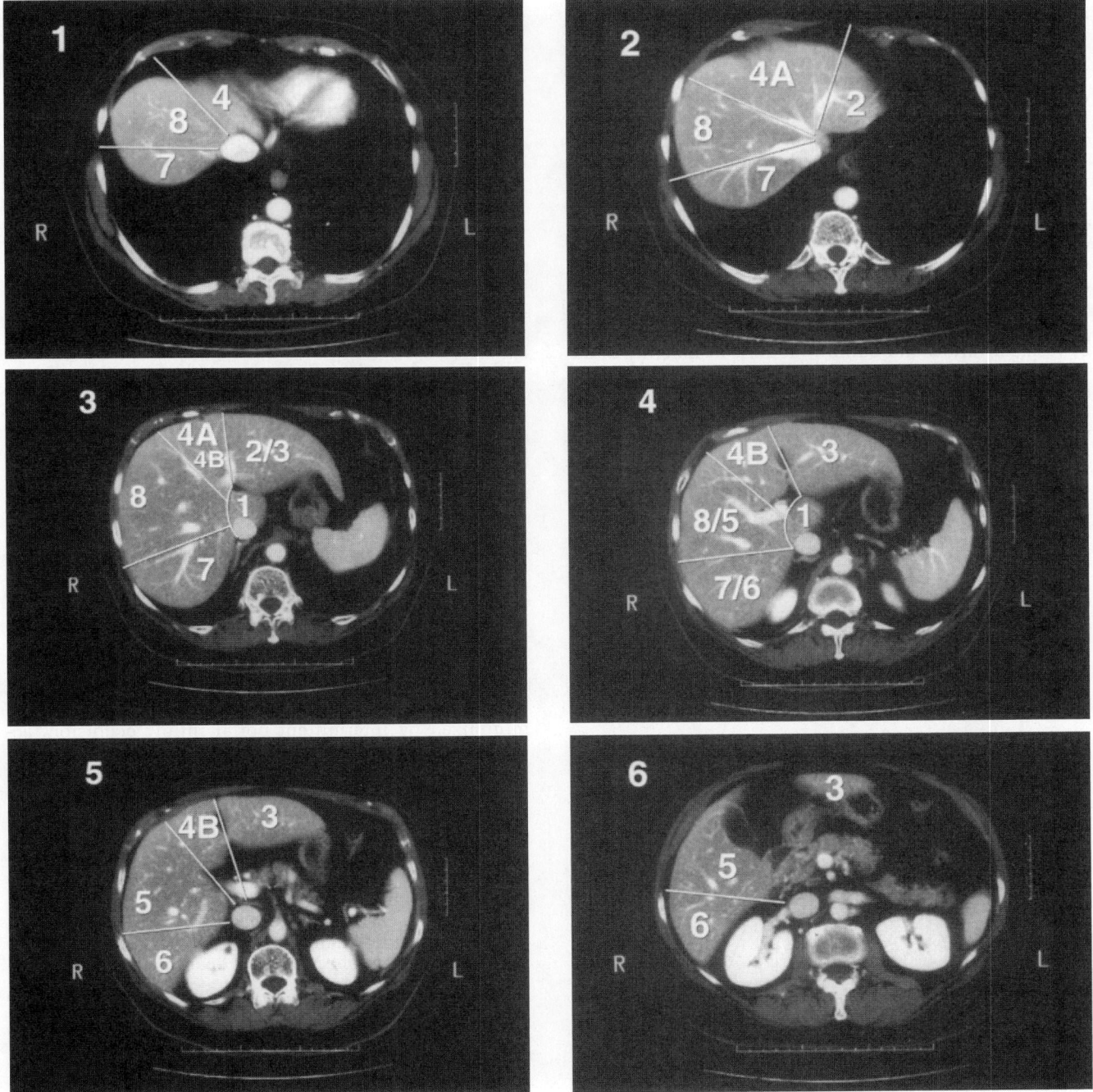

Figure 34.13. Correlation of transaxial computed tomography images with hepatic segmental anatomy by Couinaud's nomenclature. Note the posterior location of segments VI and VII, and compare with Fig. 34.4.

pected segment or segments of liver affected by a lesion and to provide an imaging technique that complements intraoperative ultrasonography in defining hepatic anatomy. The sectors of the liver can be easily defined by noting the location and course of the major hepatic veins that separate them. Individual segments within each sector may be identified by a superior or inferior location relative to the main portal structures within the transverse scissura. When a lesion straddles two or more segments, a bisegmentectomy may be feasible.

Oncologic Considerations in Hepatic Resection

The goals in the operative management of primary or secondary neoplasms of the liver should be clearly delineated before any attempt at resection is made. Several questions should be answered: What is the diagnosis? What is the biology of the tumor in this patient? Is the goal of resection curative or palliative? Has other distant disease been excluded with a reasonable number of preoperative tests? What is the comorbid status of the patient? What other treatments are effective, and what is the optimal sequence of these treatments?

INTRAOPERATIVE ASSESSMENT

The principles of safe hepatic resection are simple: wide operative exposure with a generous incision and the use of self-retaining retractors; a clear operative plan with capable surgical and anesthesia assistants; potential rapid control of vascular inflow and outflow; and the availability of autologous and banked blood products if necessary. The incisions most commonly used for major hepatic resections include an extended right subcostal incision with potential vertical or intercostal extensions if necessary (Fig. 34.14). A

generous vertical incision is occasionally used for left-sided resections, and a right thoracoabdominal incision may be used for right-sided resections. Several versions of self-retaining costal margin retractors are currently available that provide wide access to the entire subdiaphragmatic surface, and these may be combined with other self-retaining ringed retractors to keep the stomach, colon, and small bowel away from the operative field.

For major resections or for complete intraoperative ultrasonography, complete mobilization of the liver may be required. After the hepatic flexure of the colon is detached and the falciform ligament ligated and divided, both the left and right triangular ligaments may be sharply taken down to mobilize the liver fully. During division of the left triangular ligament, care must be taken to avoid injury to the spleen, left phrenic vein, left hepatic vein, and IVC. During division of the right triangular ligament, care must be taken to avoid injury to the right hemidiaphragm, right adrenal gland and adrenal vein, right phrenic vein, several moderate-sized accessory right hepatic veins draining into the right lateral wall of the vena cava, main right hepatic vein, and IVC. After mobilization, digital and bimanual palpation is performed and intraoperative ultrasonography may also be performed.

Recognition of two of the three vertical scissurae is fairly reliable. The left lateral scissura courses just to the left of the umbilical fissure, and the main scissura courses along a line drawn from the gallbladder fossa anteriorly to the IVC posteriorly. The right vertical scissura is not reliably identified by external landmarks but has been described as a vertical line running parallel to the right side of the liver about three fingers' breadths from it, on a plane inclined from 40–45 degrees from the horizontal plane. The posterior limit of the scissura is the right side of the vena cava.

The porta hepatis is dissected by many hepatic surgeons to identify the main bifurcations of the hepatic artery, bile duct, and portal vein. This allows individual ligation of unilateral branches of each of these structures during hepatic lobectomy but before parenchymal dissection. Ligation delineates the surface line of devascularization and eliminates the portal contribution of blood loss during parenchymal dissection. This technique requires tedious dissection and may take a considerable amount of time. An alternative approach has been recently described in which the main portal structures are left undisturbed and branches to a given lobe are ligated during parenchymal transection. Hemorrhage can be minimized by intermittent portal inflow occlusion, accomplished by clamping or compressing the portal triad (Pringle maneuver). Greater exposure of the superior aspect of the hepatic hilum and exposure of a high or intraparenchymal bifurcation of a portal structure may be aided by careful exposure of the hilar plate (Fig. 34.15) and division of Glisson's capsule transversely at the most inferior border of segment IV (the quadrate lobe). Details of this technique have been described elsewhere in the literature (9).

Early versus late isolation and ligation of a given hepatic vein during lobectomy has been the subject of considerable debate because the extraparenchymal component of a hepatic vein may be quite short or absent. Because hemorrhage in this location may be difficult to expose and control, a safe strategy is always to avoid early isolation of a given hepatic vein or to attempt isolation only if a considerable length of vein is found on mobilization of the respective triangular ligament (Fig. 34.16).

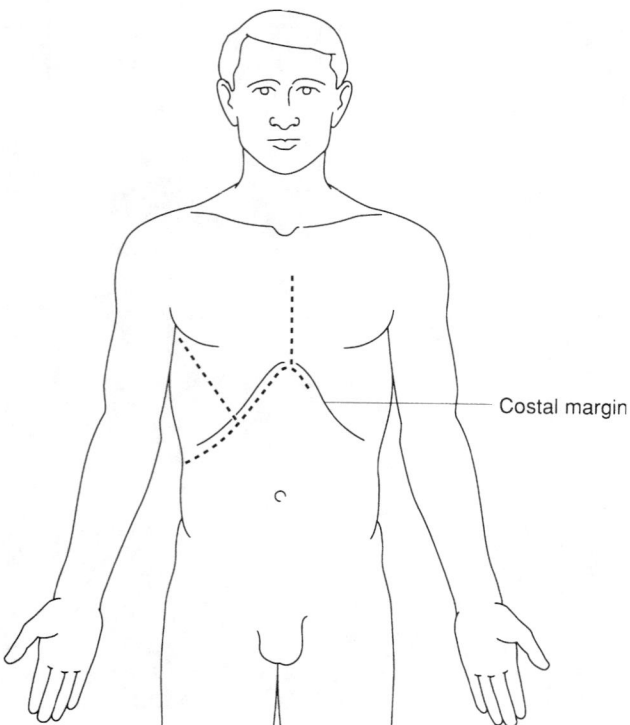

Costal margin

Figure 34.14. Incisions commonly used for hepatic resection.

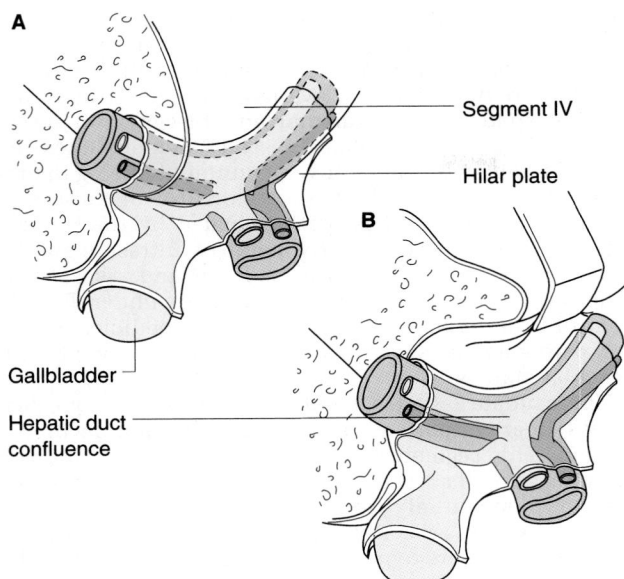

Figure 34.15. Lowering the hilar plate. *(A)* The inferior border of segment IV (quadrate lobe) overlies the hepatic duct confluence. *(B)* Division of the connective issue investment allows elevation of segment IV, which results in a "lower" hilar plate and surgical exposure to the hepatic duct confluence. (After Blumgart LH, ed. *Surgery of the liver and biliary tract.* New York: Churchill Livingstone, 1994, with permission.)

MAJOR LOBECTOMY

Major lobectomy or hemihepatectomy includes segments V, VI, VII, and VIII (right hepatic lobectomy) or resection of segments II, III, and IV (left hepatic lobectomy). Extended resections of each major lobe have been described that include segments V, VI, VII, VIII, and IV (right trisegmentectomy in older nomenclature) or segments II, III, IV, and anterior segments V and VIII (left trisegmentectomy). The caudate lobe may or may not be included in the major resections, but care must be taken to preserve portal pedicle branches to this lobe if it is to be saved. A cholecystectomy is included in all these hepatic resections.

The steps involved in each of these major resections are similar and adhere to the tenets of optimal operative exposure and control of vascular inflow and outflow. In select circumstances, control of the vena cava may be desired. The infrahepatic vena cava may be safely encircled superior to the junction of the renal veins. The suprahepatic vena cava may be encircled with caution just inferior to the diaphragm or within the pericardium. Preparation for the Pringle maneuver is accomplished by encircling the main portal vein and proper hepatic artery with individual umbilical tape tourniquets or a noncrushing vascular clamp. Division of the hepatic parenchyma is begun by scoring Glisson's capsule with cautery or knife; the hepatic substance is then divided with the use of blunt dissection by finger fracture, the blunt end of an instrument or suction tip, or an ultrasonic dessicator–dissector. Individual vessels and bile ducts are cauterized, sutured, or clipped in rapid succession from anterior to posterior. Constant reevaluation of the direction of transection prevents inadvertent division of vital vascular structures in adjacent segments. If temporary portal inflow occlusion is used, intermittent 10- to 20-minute intervals of clamping with 3 to 5 minutes to reestablish blood flow is recommended. The hepatic

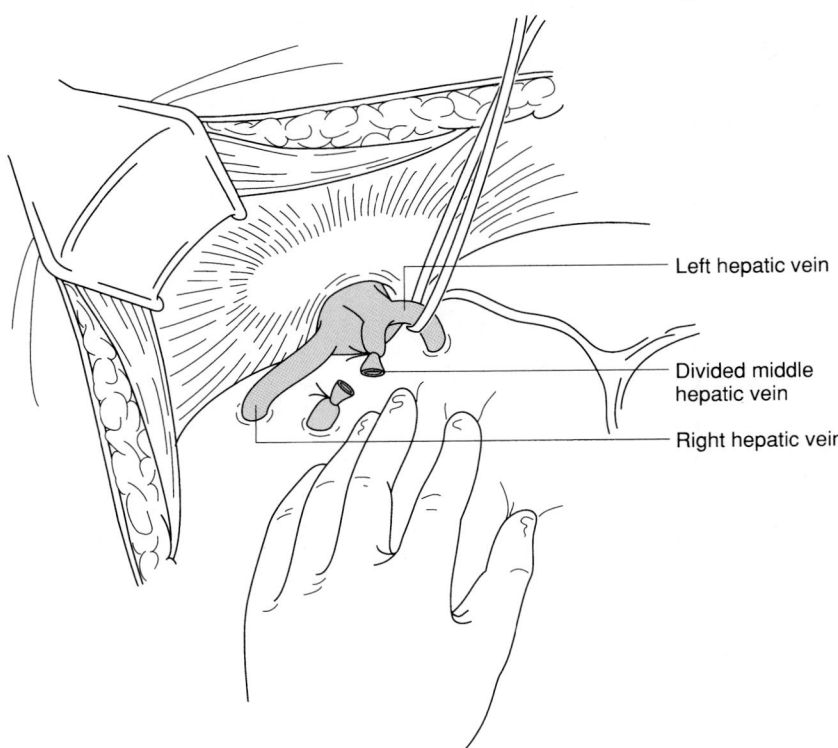

Figure 34.16. Caudal retraction of the left hepatic lobe with division of middle and left hepatic veins during left hepatic lobectomy.

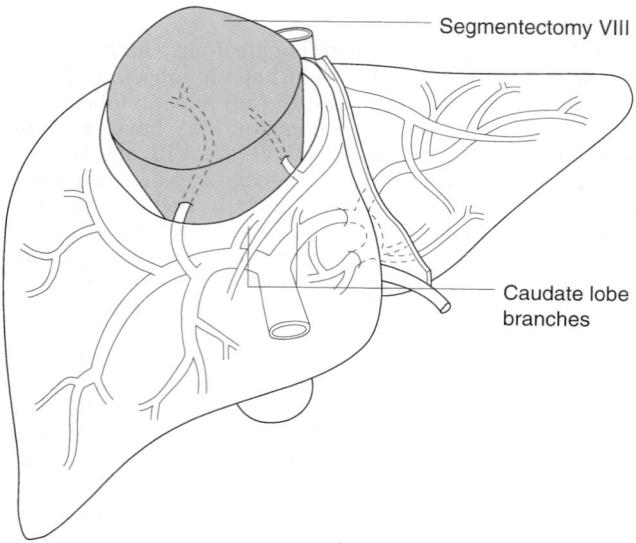

Segmentectomy VIII

Caudate lobe branches

Figure 34.17. Isolated resection of segment VIII. The lack of dependable anterior topographic landmarks and the complex posterior relationships to the portal pedicles of segment I (caudate process and caudate lobe) make isolated resection of this segment extremely difficult. (From Bismuth H, Houssin D, Castaing D. Major and minor segmentectomies "réglées" in liver surgery. *World J Surg* 1982;6:10–24, with permission.)

veins are encountered in the hepatic substance near the vena cava and are carefully clamped and ligated with sutures to complete the resection. The raw hepatic surface is carefully inspected for bleeding and bile leaks; these can be controlled by individual suture ligation, argon beam coagulator, or fibrin glue. The greater omentum can be used to buttress the transected liver edge. Perihepatic closed suction drains are often placed to monitor for unrecognized postoperative bile leaks (10).

SEGMENTAL RESECTIONS

Recent hepatic resection stagies have focused on maximizing functional reserve without compromising

safety. Segmental, bisegmental, and subsegmental or nonanatomic partial resections have been performed with increasing frequency and are now well described. Excellent reviews are now available that describe in detail the anatomy of segmental and bisegmental resections (8,11). For example, Fig. 34.17 demonstrates the vascular and biliary anatomy encountered during the resection of segment VIII. Vascular control of these segmental resections is best accomplished by the pedicle ligation technique (12). Intraoperative ultrasonography is critical to locate the portal pedicles and assess their relationship to the lesion. Hepatotomy under Pringle control is necessary to gain access to the pedicles within the parenchyma. Mass ligation is best performed with vascular staples.

The caudate lobe (segment I) has several unique features that are important to consider before and during resection. This segment can essentially be thought of as a separate, smaller liver. Although segment I receives its afferent blood supply from both the right and left portal pedicles, which arise early after the main portal bifurcation, the only parenchymal attachment to the rest of the liver is via the thin caudate process, which extends from the posterior aspect of the right lobe (Fig. 34.18). The anterior surface of segment I is completely separated from the left lobe by the extension of the lesser omentum known as the *ligamentum venosum* (Fig. 34.19). The route of hepatic venous drainage is completely different, through multiple short veins that pass directly posteriorly into the left and anterior surfaces of the vena cava. It is often unnecessary to remove this segment during hemihepatectomy unless its blood supply is compromised or it is involved by malignancy. Recently, isolated resection of segment I has been described for solitary lesions in this segment (13,14).

Complete familiarity with the anatomic features of the liver is essential for safe hepatic resection. Current standards for major hepatic resections should include a perioperative mortality rate of 5% or less, an infrequent need for blood transfusions during or after straightforward hemihepatectomy, and the use of autologous blood replacement when needed and when prior donation is feasible. An interdisciplinary strategy is essential to define the goals of resection, the minimal volume of liver to be removed to accomplish those goals, and the most cost-

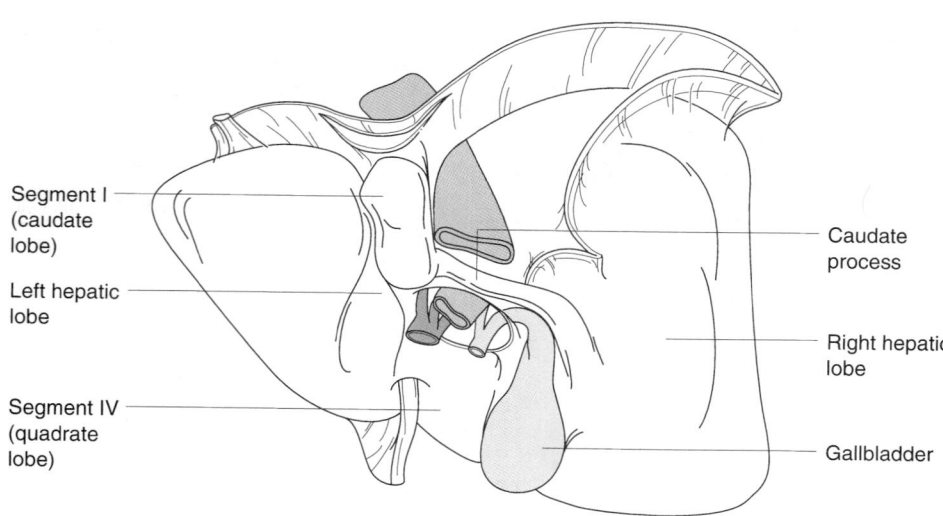

Segment I (caudate lobe)

Left hepatic lobe

Segment IV (quadrate lobe)

Caudate process

Right hepatic lobe

Gallbladder

Figure 34.18. Inferior aspect of the liver, demonstrating relation of the caudate lobe to other hepatic structures.

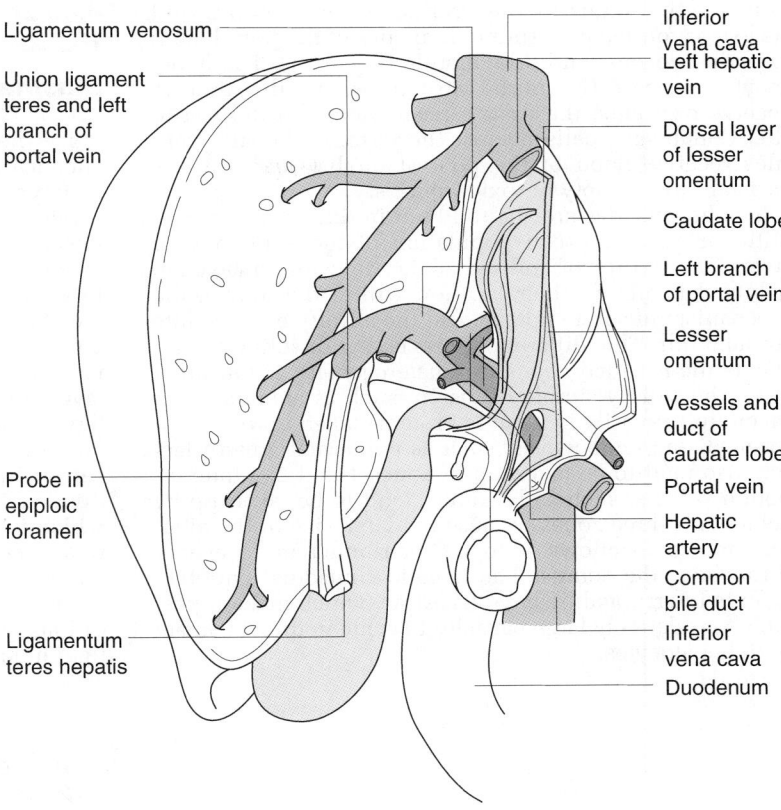

Figure 34.19. Relation of the caudate lobe to the right and left hepatic lobes and structures in the hepatic hilum.

effective use of preoperative and intraoperative imaging studies.

REFERENCES

1. Cantlie J. On a new arrangement of the right and left lobes of the liver. *J Anat* 1897;32:4.
2. McIndoe AH, Counseller VS. The bilaterality of the liver. *Arch Surg* 1927;15:589.
3. Goldsmith NA, Woodburne RT. The surgical anatomy pertaining to liver resections. *Surg Gynecol Obstet* 1975;105:310.
4. Healey JE Jr. Clinical anatomic aspects of radical hepatic surgery. *J Int Coll Surg* 1954;22:542.
5. Michels NA. Newer anatomy of the liver and its variant blood supply and collateral circulation. *Am J Surg* 1966;112:337.
6. Tung TT. *Les résections majeures et mineures du foie.* Paris: Masson, 1979.
7. Couinaud C. *Le foie. Études anatomiques et chirurgicales.* Paris: Masson, 1957.
8. Bismuth H, Houssin D, Castaing D. Major and minor segmentectomies "réglées" in liver surgery. *World J Surg* 1982; 6:10.
9. Hepp J, Couinaud C. L'abord et l'utilisation du canal hépatique gauche dans les réparations de la voie biliaire principale. *Presse Med* 1956;64:947.
10. Adson MA, Beart RW. Elective hepatic resections. *Surg Clin North Am* 1977;57:339.
11. Billingsley KG, Jarnagin WR, Fong Y, et al. Segment-oriented hepatic resection in the management of malignant neoplasms of the liver. *J Am Coll Surg* 1998;187:471.
12. Launois B, Jamieson GG. The posterior intrahepatic approach for hepatectomy or removal of segments of the liver. *Surg Gynecol Obstet* 1992;174:155.
13. Launois B, Jamieson GG. The posterior intrahepatic approach for hepatectomy or removal of segments of the liver. *Surg Gynecol Obstet* 1992;174:155.
14. Yanaga K, Matsumata T, Hayashi H, et al. Isolated hepatic caudate lobectomy. *Surgery* 1994;115:757.

SURGERY: SCIENTIFIC PRINCIPLES AND PRACTICE, Third Edition, edited by Lazar J. Greenfield, Michael W. Mulholland, Keith T. Oldham, Gerald B. Zelenock, and Keith D. Lillemoe. Lippincott Williams & Wilkins Publishers, Philadelphia, © 2001.

CHAPTER 35

HEPATIC PHYSIOLOGY

STEVEN E. RAPER

HISTOLOGIC ORGANIZATION OF THE LIVER

The free surface of the liver is invested by a single layer of mesothelial cells. Beneath this cell layer is Glisson's capsule, which is composed of collagen bundles, fibroblasts, and small blood vessels. At the hepatic hilus, Glisson's capsule joins with dense connective tissue inside the liver. Intrahepatic connective tissue provides support for the hepatic parenchyma; surrounds vessels, bile ducts, and nerves; and subdivides the parenchyma into its characteristic lobular structure. The dense connective tissue disappears within the lobules and is replaced by a more loosely organized reticular network, which provides a framework for orderly regeneration after hepatic injury.

The lobular structure of the mammalian liver has been recognized since the 17th century. In humans, the classic lobule, a polygonal or hexagonal arrangement of the sinusoids and their associated cell plates, is poorly defined. The smallest functional unit of the liver is the acinus (1), which is defined as a small oval or diamond-shaped mass of hepatic parenchyma. The apices of the acinus are the terminal hepatic venules, and its axis is formed by terminal branches of the portal vein, hepatic arteriole, and bile ductule (Fig. 35.1). The hepatocytes nearest the portal structures are the first to receive nutrients, the first to regenerate, and the last to die. Conversely, cells nearest the terminal hepatic venules receive blood of the poorest quality and are less resistant to a variety of toxic injuries.

The hepatocytes are about 30 μm in diameter and constitute 80% of the cell population of the adult human liver. The ability of individual hepatocytes to take up solute depends on their location within the lobule, the mechanism of solute uptake, and the affinity of the solute for albumin. This differential processing of solute within the lobule is called *hepatocyte heterogeneity.* Solutes that enter the cell by simple diffusion, such as ammonia, are taken up primarily in zone 1. Proteins taken up by receptor-mediated endocytosis, such as epidermal growth factor, also tend to be taken up in zones 1 and 2. Albumin-bound solutes, such as bilirubin, tend to be taken up by cells of all three zones because the large size of the albumin molecule allows it to be distributed more evenly throughout the acinus. The hepatic sinusoidal endothelium is interrupted by large fenestrae, which make it possible for relatively large particles to come in direct contact with hepatocytes.

PARENCHYMAL CELL ULTRASTRUCTURE

Plasma Membrane

The hepatocyte is capable of carrying out 2,000 biochemical reactions simultaneously, and function is intimately related to structure. An understanding of the hepatocyte organelles that allow the liver to perform its many metabolic functions is important (Fig. 35.2). The hepatocyte plasma membrane consists of a phospholipid bilayer in which hydrophobic fatty acid tails are oriented to the membrane interior and hydrophilic phospholipid head groups are oriented to the exterior (sinusoidal or cytoplasmic) membrane (Fig. 35.3). Within this phospholipid bilayer are proteins, often complexed with sugar molecules (glycoproteins), which perform either structural functions (e.g., tight junctions) or metabolic functions (e.g., receptor, carrier, or enzyme). The hepatocyte plasma membrane is divided into three domains: (a) the sinusoidal domain, which is studded with microvilli to increase the absorptive area in contact with sinusoidal blood; (b) the basolateral domain, which is in contact with other liver cells; and (c) the bile canalicular domain, which under normal conditions is completely separated from the bloodstream by tight junctional complexes (2).

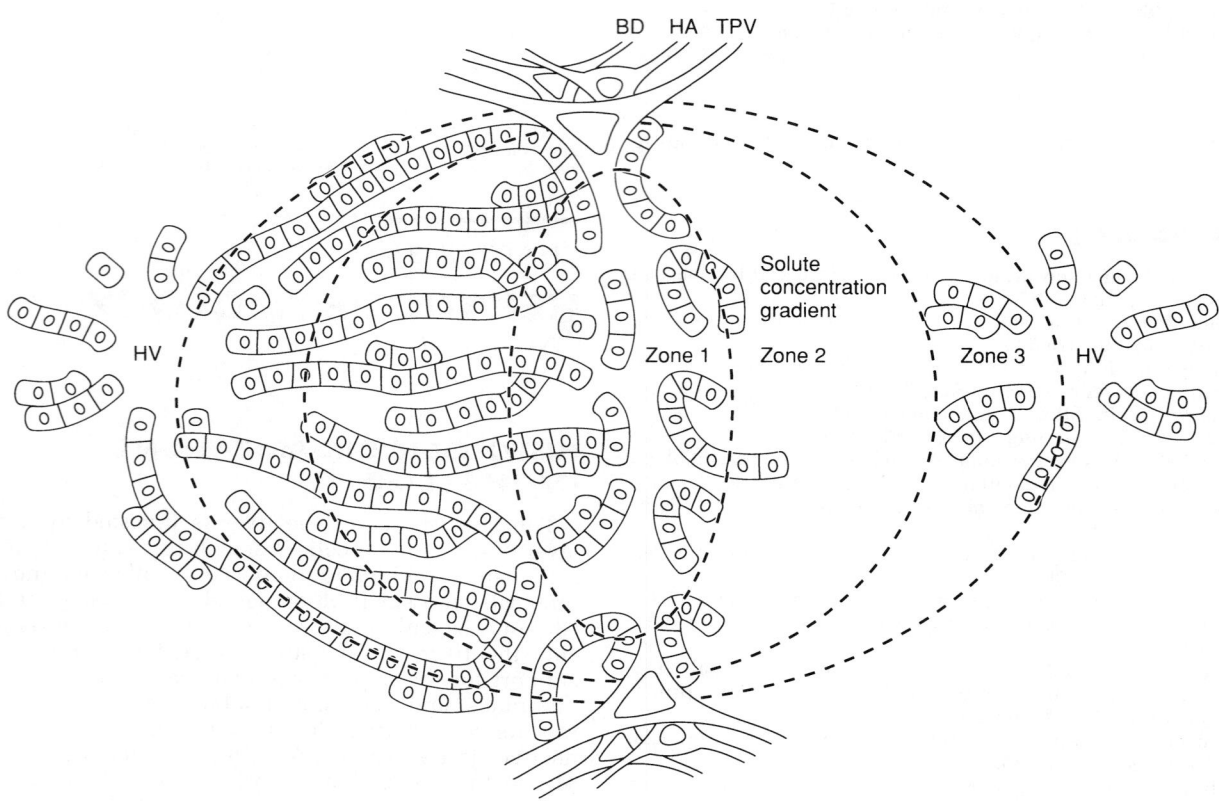

Figure 35.1. The hepatic acinus. Unidirectional perfusion of the hepatocytes within the acinus causes a gradient of solute concentration as blood moves from the terminal portal venule *(TPV)* to the hepatic venule *(HV)*. Hepatocytes nearest the portal tract are in zone 1, midacinar cells are in zone 2, and centrilobular cells are in zone 3. The TPV-to-HV oxygen gradient is 50 μmol/L. This implies that zone 1 cells have a higher oxygen tension than zone 3 cells. The concept of acinar zones fits well, therefore, with observations of histologic injury for a variety of toxins. *BD,* bile ductule; *HA,* hepatic arteriole. (After Rappaport AM. The acinus: microvascular unit of the liver. In: Lautt WW, ed. *Hepatic circulation in health and disease.* New York: Raven Press, 1981:175.)

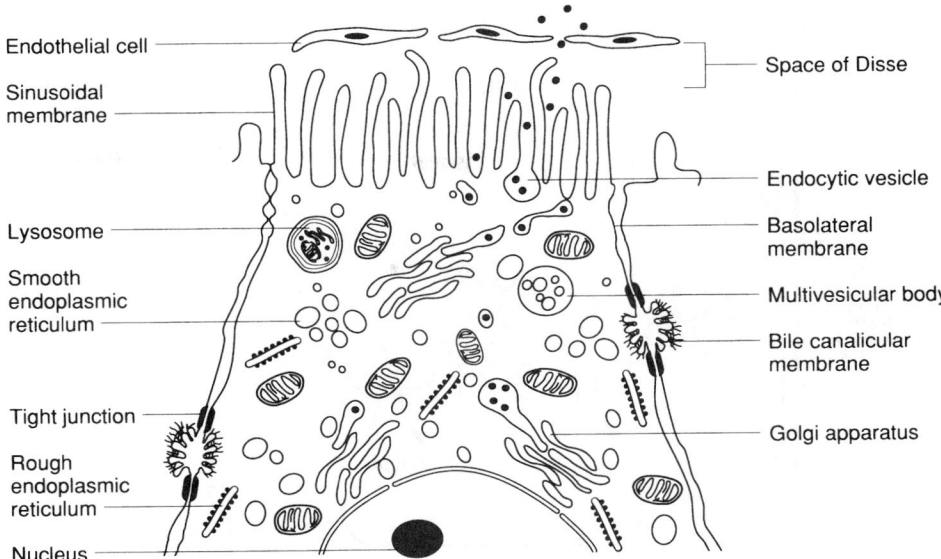

Endothelial cell

Sinusoidal membrane

Lysosome

Smooth endoplasmic reticulum

Tight junction

Rough endoplasmic reticulum

Nucleus

Space of Disse

Endocytic vesicle

Basolateral membrane

Multivesicular body

Bile canalicular membrane

Golgi apparatus

Figure 35.2. Major ultrastructural features of the hepatocyte.

Cell membranes, by virtue of their high lipid content, allow lipid-soluble molecules to enter the cell by simple diffusion. Polar molecules are brought into the cells by membrane transport proteins (Fig. 35.4). Some transport proteins carry solute in a single direction and are called *uniports*. Cotransport carriers involve the transfer of a second solute. Two molecules transported in the same direction use a symport, whereas two molecules transported in opposite directions use an antiport. Passive transport can occur by simple or facilitated diffusion. Channel proteins allow molecules to diffuse simply into cells without binding, whereas carrier proteins first bind the solute and, by conformational change, allow it to be transported into the cell. The glucose carrier in hepatocytes is an example of carrier-facilitated diffusion. Active transport requires an energy source, usually adenosine triphosphate (ATP), to transport molecules against a thermodynamically unfavorable electrochemical or concentration gradient.

The various membrane regions perform specific functions. The sinusoidal membrane is the site of active bidirectional transport of proteins, water, and organic and in-

organic solutes. Transport of large protein-bound substances into liver cells is facilitated by fenestrations of about 1,000 nm in the endothelial cell membrane. The basolateral membrane extends from the sinusoid to the edge of the bile canaliculus. This portion of the membrane is almost flat and contains structural proteins that allow attachment and communication between cells. Tight junctional complexes separate the basolateral surface from the canalicular surface. The bile canalicular membrane surface area is also increased by the presence of microvilli. In humans, the total canalicular surface area can reach 10 m². The bile canalicular membrane is intimately associated with microfilaments, which appear to be responsible for the canalicular shape and bile formation. Each plasma membrane domain contains characteristic membrane proteins. Alkaline phosphatase and 5'-nucleotidase are found predominantly in the canalicular membrane, whereas membrane receptors for various proteins are localized to the sinusoidal membrane.

The plasma membrane is also directly responsible for endocytosis, the process by which hepatocytes take up extracellular fluids and macromolecules. The three types of endocytosis are pinocytosis, phagocytosis, and receptor-mediated endocytosis. Pinocytosis is a process by which water and solute are nonspecifically taken up into vesicles of 0.1 to 0.2 μm. Phagocytosis involves the uptake of large particles, such as malaria sporozoites. Receptor-mediated endocytosis is a special form of pinocytosis and occurs when extracellular macromolecules bind to specific cell surface receptors before internalization.

Cell Surface Receptors

The sinusoidal membrane is studded with receptors, which are large glycoprotein molecules that span the plasma membrane lipid bilayer. Regions of the receptor molecule project into the space of Disse. When such regions bind a specific molecule, or ligand (peptide hormone, steroid, or other regulatory molecule), the entire ligand can be internalized for intracellular degradation or biliary transport. The ligand can transmit a signal to the interior of the hepatocyte by a number of intracellular sec-

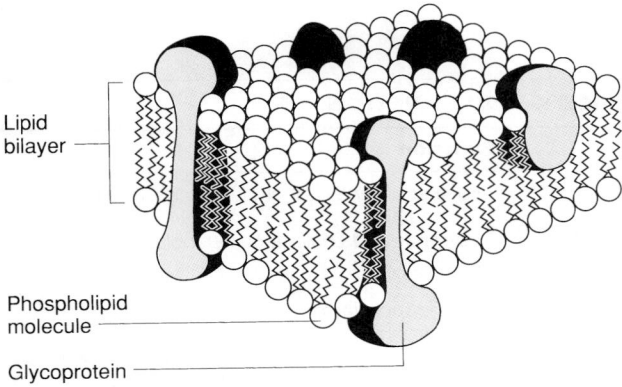

Lipid bilayer

Phospholipid molecule

Glycoprotein

Figure 35.3. Schematic three-dimensional view of a small section of a hepatocyte membrane, illustrating the lipid bilayer and integral glycoproteins.

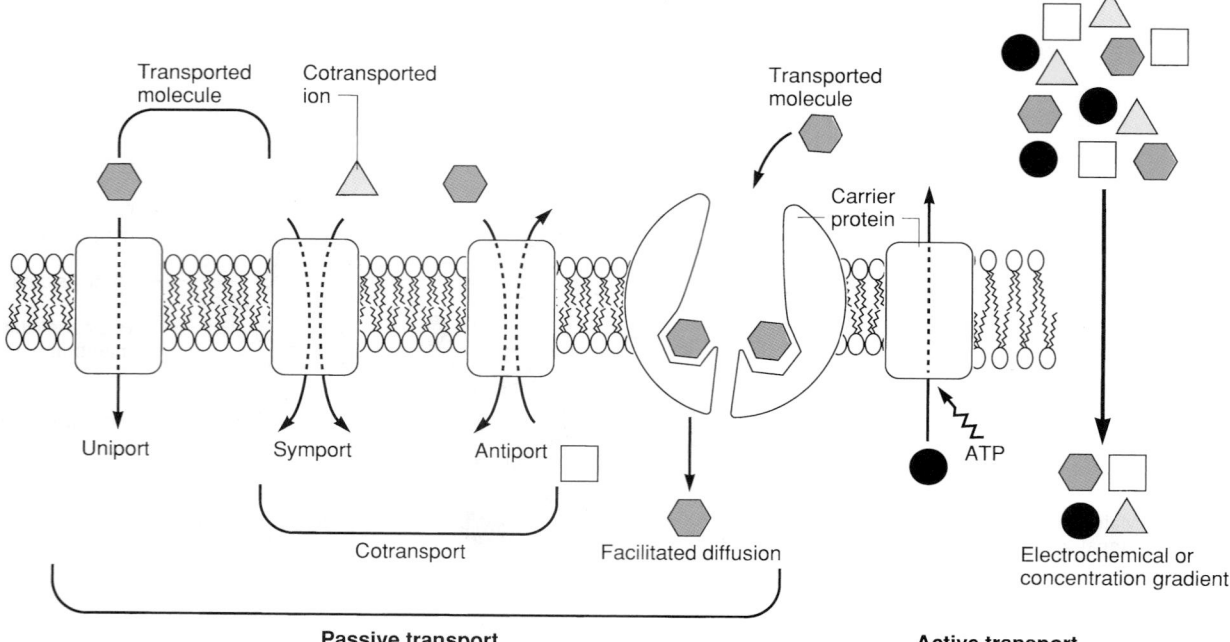

Figure 35.4. Schematic representation of the major types of membrane transport proteins, which are crucial for the transport of polar solutes. Passive transport involves the passage of molecules in the direction of a concentration gradient. Uniports, symports, and antiports are examples of channel proteins, which allow molecules to pass by simple diffusion. Some carrier proteins facilitate diffusion by specifically binding to individual molecules. Other carrier proteins actively transport molecules against a concentration or electrochemical gradient, a thermodynamically unfavorable event that requires adenosine triphosphate or some other form of exogenous energy.

ond-messenger systems (3). Table 35.1 lists many important hepatocyte receptors with their ligands and functions. Novel methods of delivering genes to hepatocytes are based on the use of receptor-mediated endocytosis. For example, by chemically coupling a biochemical antagonist to normally internalized proteins, normal liver cells can be protected from the toxic effect of a chemotherapeutic agent while the malignant cells are killed (4). Similarly, a DNA carrier system has been devised that can target selected DNA fragments to hepatocytes by way of the membrane asialoglycoprotein (ASGP) receptor.

Although ligands undergo receptor binding and internalization at the plasma membrane, they can follow a number of different intracellular pathways (Fig. 35.5). In the intracellular compartments responsible for the processing of receptor-bound proteins, molecular sorting takes place, which in effect targets proteins to various intracellular destinations. Some of the ligand–receptor vesicles are coated with clathrin, a small protein that can encode sorting information (5). Receptor phosphorylation may be another mechanism by which the liver can sort receptors to their final destinations (6).

Some cell surface receptors initiate a cascade of intracellular events by acting to generate intracellular second messengers, a process known as *signal transduction.* Such second messengers include cyclic adenosine monophosphate, inositol triphosphate, and diacylglycerol (7). Each of these structurally simple chemicals can

Table 35.1. **KNOWN HEPATIC RECEPTORS, LIGAND SPECIFICITY, AND FUNCTION**

Receptor	Ligand	Function
Asialoglycoprotein	Desialylated proteins with exposed terminal galactose residues	Targeting of senescent proteins to lysomes for degradation
Chylomicron remnant	Lipoproteins containing apolipoprotein B-48	Triglyceride and cholesterol metabolism
Epidermal growth factor	Epidermal growth factor; transforming growth factor-α	Hepatic growth
c-kit	Hepatocyte growth factor	Hepatotrophic factor
Growth hormone	Growth hormone	Hepatotrophic factor
Immunoglobulin A	Polymeric immunoglobulin A	Secretory component formation; intestinal immunity
Insulin	Insulin	Hepatotrophic factor; glycogenesis
Insulin-like growth factor-1	Insulin-like growth factor-1	Hepatotrophic factor; lysosomal enzyme processing
Low-density lipoprotein	Lipoproteins containing apolipoprotein B-100 or E	Triglyceride and cholesterol metabolism
Transferrin	Transferrin-iron complexes	Iron uptake and storage

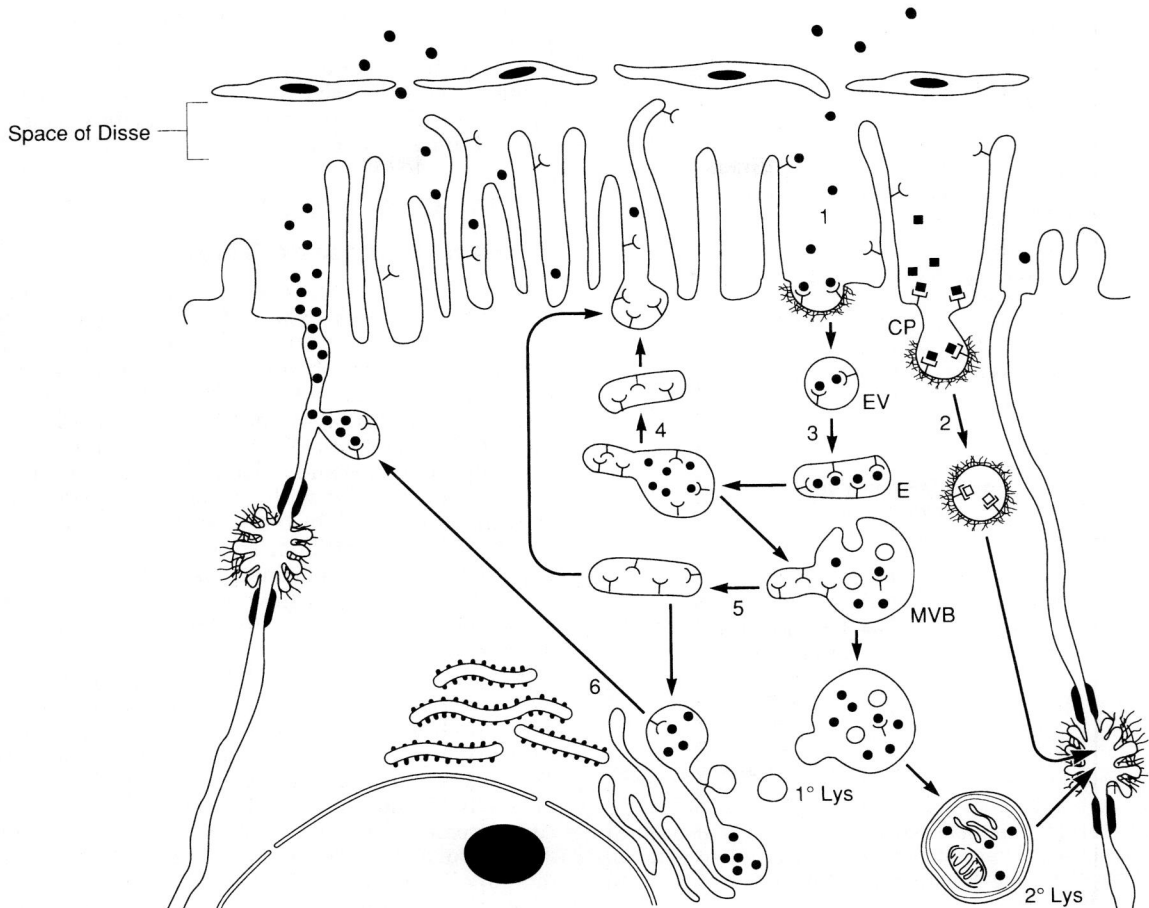

Figure 35.5. Possible routes for the intracellular processing of proteins by receptor-mediated endocytosis. *(1)* Ligands in the space of Disse bind specific receptors. *(2)* Ligand–receptor complexes are internalized in coated pits *(CPs)* to become endocytic vesicles *(EVs)*. Some endocytic vesicles are transported directly to the bile canaliculus to secrete intact protein (i.e., polymeric immunoglobulin A). *(3)* Other coated vesicles lose their clathrin coat and fuse to become endosomes *(Es)*. *(4)* Acidified endosomes become the compartment of uncoupling of receptor and ligand. Receptors are recycled to the plasma membrane, while the ligands remain in multivesicular bodies *(MVBs)*. *(5)* Multivesicular bodies fuse with primary lysosomes *(1° Lys)* to become secondary lysosomes *(2° Lys)*, in which ligands are degraded and excreted into bile (i.e., the asialoglycoproteins). *(6)* New receptors are synthesized in the rough endoplasmic reticulum and processed through the Golgi complex before insertion into the plasma membrane.

amplify cell membrane events and bring about major changes in cellular physiology (Fig. 35.6).

Mitochondria

Liver mitochondria are self-replicating organelles that contain an independent complement of DNA. The outer membrane is freely permeable to all molecules of 10 kd. The inner membrane contains the enzymes of the electron transport chain and ATP synthetase. The mitochondrial matrix contains hundreds of enzymes responsible for the interconversion of a wide variety of small molecules. Mitochondria are more numerous in the zone 1 cells, where oxygen tension is higher. The primary role of mitochondria is to generate large amounts of ATP through the citric acid cycle and oxidative phosphorylation. Electron transport enzymes of the inner membrane create a large electrochemical gradient, which drives ATP synthase to form new ATP.

Endosomes, Multivesicular Bodies, and Lysosomes

After the clathrin coat falls away from endocytosed vesicles, the vesicles coalesce to form endosomes (5). The endosomal membrane contains an ATP-driven hydrogen ion pump that acidifies the endosome and thereby causes the ligand and receptor to dissociate. Endosomal components may return to the cell surface, the receptors in effect being recycled, or may enter multivesicular bodies, which are aggregates of endosomal remnants. Primary lysosomes are vesicles full of newly synthesized degradative enzymes that are capable of fusing with multivesicular bodies. Under acidic conditions, the lysosomal enzymes are activated and secondary lysosomes form that are full of degraded intracellular components. Lysosomes are numerous in the liver and are found in the cytoplasm adjacent to the bile canaliculus and Golgi complex. Secondary lyso-

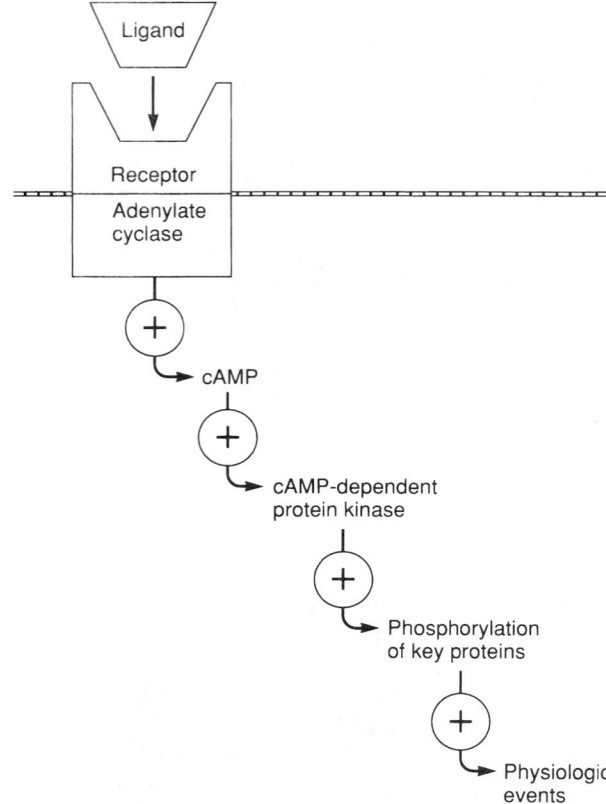

Figure 35.6. Role of cyclic adenosine monophosphate-dependent protein kinase in signal transduction. A single ligand–receptor interaction at the membrane is amplified many times by the stimulation of adenyl cyclase.

somes fuse with the bile canalicular membrane and discharge their contents into the bile (Fig. 35.5).

Endoplasmic Reticulum and Golgi Complex

The liver is unique in that both smooth- and rough-surfaced endoplasmic reticula are well developed. The smooth endoplasmic reticulum (ER) is composed of a complex meshwork of branching tubules that communicate with the rough ER and the Golgi complex. Rough ER usually forms aggregates of parallel, flattened cisternae scattered throughout the cytoplasm. The granules that give the rough appearance to rough ER are ribosomes. The Golgi complex consists of three to five closely packed, parallel, smooth cisternae associated with some vesicular structures. The smooth ER, rough ER, and Golgi complex are collectively referred to as the *liver microsomal fraction.*

The liver microsomes are known to participate in the following mechanisms: (a) synthesis of albumin, fibrinogen, and other proteins destined for export to the plasma; (b) synthesis of cholesterol and bile salts; (c) glucuronidation of bilirubin, drugs, and steroids; (d) esterification of free fatty acids to triglycerides; and (e) glycogenolysis.

The Nucleus

The nucleus is the largest of the cellular organelles and is separated from the cytoplasm by a nuclear envelope consisting of an inner and outer membrane. All the chromosomal DNA is packaged into chromatin fibers in association with DNA-binding proteins called *histones.* Ribosomes are synthesized in the nucleolus to aid in protein synthesis. The cytoplasm and nucleus communicate through nuclear pores.

HEPATIC BLOOD FLOW

Control of Hepatic Blood Flow

The liver constitutes about 2.5% of the total body weight but receives 25% of the cardiac output. Total hepatic blood flow is 100 to 130 mL/min per kilogram. About two thirds of the total hepatic flow is derived from the portal vein and one third from the hepatic artery. To a large extent, portal venous flow into the liver is regulated by extrahepatic factors, such as the rate of flow from the intestines and spleen. Thus, hepatic flow might be expected to vary with the metabolic state of the organism. Blood flow in the liver, however, is remarkably unaffected by nutritional status. The constancy of total hepatic blood flow is primarily a consequence of changes in the hepatic arterial flow. Both intrinsic and extrinsic mechanisms of flow regulation are operative in the hepatic artery (8).

Flow is regulated intrinsically through arterial autoregulation, which is based on the local concentration of adenosine surrounding the hepatic arteriole and portal venule. Adenosine is a potent vasodilator of the hepatic arteriole. The vessels are surrounded by a limiting plate and a microenvironment called the *space of Mall* (Fig. 35.7). An increase in portal venous flow causes an increased washout of adenosine and hepatic arteriolar constriction. If the portal venous flow is reduced, local concentrations of adenosine increase and cause the hepatic arteriole to dilate; a compensatory increase in hepatic arterial flow thereby maintains a constant level of total hepatic blood flow (9).

Less is known about extrinsic flow regulation. Both humoral and neural mechanisms have been demonstrated. Although the hepatic artery can dilate in response to pharmacologic doses of many vasoactive compounds, the physiologic relevance of this observation is unknown. The hepatic artery does not constrict in the postprandial state despite marked increases in portal flow; some agents apparently can overcome the intrinsic regulatory control exerted by the adenosine washout response. Possible humoral mediators of extrinsic regulation include gastrin, glucagon, secretin, and bile salts. The hepatic artery is also densely innervated by sympathetic nerves, which are known to cause vasoconstriction mediated by α-adrenergic receptors.

Resistance to portal blood flow is thought to occur primarily across a distinct hepatic venous sphincter-like zone. Several investigators have documented histologically the presence of such sphincters in humans. This anatomic evidence is supported by detailed physiologic studies in several animal species. In normal liver, no resistance is attributable to either the portal venule or the sinusoid. The hepatic venous sphincters constrict in response to histamine, norepinephrine, angiotensin, and nerve stimulation (in cats and dogs).

The liver serves as a physiologic blood reservoir. Blood accounts for about 25% to 30% of the liver volume, and in cases of acute blood loss, up to 30% (as much as 300 mL) of the hepatic blood volume can be released into the systemic circulation without adverse effects on liver function. Conversely, in cases of right-sided heart failure or other causes of systemic volume overload, as much as 1 L of extra blood can be stored in the liver before passive congestion and injury occur.

A

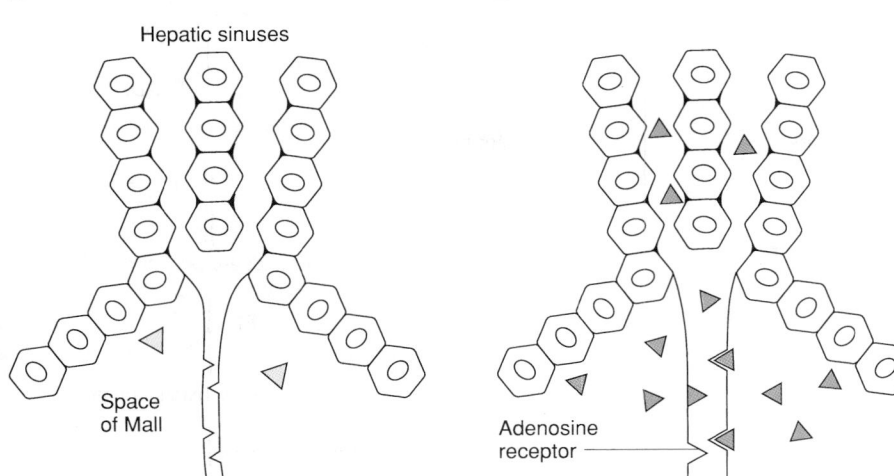

B

Figure 35.7. Adenosine washout hypothesis. Terminal branches of the portal vein, hepatic artery, and bile duct lie within the space of Mall, delimited by a plate of hepatocytes. Adenosine is continuously secreted into the space of Mall and determines the hepatic arteriolar tone. A decrease in portal vein flow causes an increase in levels of adenosine and hepatic arteriolar dilation. An increase in flow causes a decrease in adenosine and vasoconstriction, the so-called hepatic arterial buffer response.

Blood Cleansing

Hepatic sinusoids are lined by an endothelium punctuated with pores that allow proteins as large as albumin to diffuse out of the vascular tree and into proximity with hepatocytes. Sinusoidal pressure is only 6 to 8 mm Hg, so that proteins can also diffuse back into the vasculature. Much of the extravasated protein enters the lymphatics, and hepatic lymph contains as much protein as plasma. This extreme permeability of the liver allows of a diverse number of nutrients, hormones, and environmental agents to be exchanged between the blood and the hepatocyte. The liver also acts as a filter for particulate debris, which enters the portal circulation through intestinal capillaries. Particles such as bacteria are ingested by Kupffer's cells through the process of phagocytosis. Kupffer's cells line the hepatic sinusoidal endothelium, where formed blood elements and particulate matter may come in direct contact with these phagocytic cells. Once particulate matter is internalized, the Kupffer's cells contain a wide variety of degradative enzymes to neutralize any threat to the host.

CARBOHYDRATE METABOLISM

The products of intestinal carbohydrate digestion are glucose (80%) and fructose and galactose (20%). Fructose and galactose are rapidly converted to glucose, and the body uses glucose for transport and for uptake of carbohydrates by cells throughout the body. The blood glucose level is tightly regulated by the liver despite wide fluctuations in dietary ingestion. The liver can take up as much as 100 g of glucose per day and convert it into glycogen by the process of glycogenesis. The liver can also release glucose into the blood by glycogenolysis, which is the breakdown of glycogen, or by gluconeogenesis, which is the formation of new glucose from substrates such as alanine, lactate, glycerol, or certain dietary amino acids. Hormones play a key role in the hepatic regulation of glucose metabolism. Insulin, for example, stimulates glycogenesis, and glucagon stimulates glycogenolysis and gluconeogenesis. The liver metabolizes glucose primarily to provide substrates for biosynthetic reactions. Most other tissues use glucose to generate ATP for energy (10).

Glycogen Storage and Metabolism

Glycogen is a complex polymer of glucose with an average molecular weight of 5 million. Liver cells can store up to 8% of their weight as glycogen. The first step in glycogen storage is the transport of glucose through the hepatocyte plasma membrane. About 90% of portal venous glucose is removed from the blood by liver cells through carrier-facilitated diffusion. Large numbers of carrier molecules on the sinusoidal domain of the hepatocyte are capable of binding glucose and transferring it to the cytoplasm. The rate of glucose transport is enhanced (up to 10-fold) by insulin.

Glycogenesis and Glycogenolysis

Once in the hepatocyte, glucose and ATP are converted by the enzyme glucokinase to glucose-6-phosphate (G6P), the first intermediate in the synthesis of glycogen (Fig. 35.8). Because complete oxidation of one molecule of G6P generates 37 molecules of ATP, and storage uses only one molecule of ATP, the overall efficiency of glucose storage in glycogen is a remarkable 97%.

Glycogenolysis does not occur by simple reversal of glycogenesis. Each succeeding glucose on a glycogen chain is released by glycogen phosphorylase (Fig. 35.9).

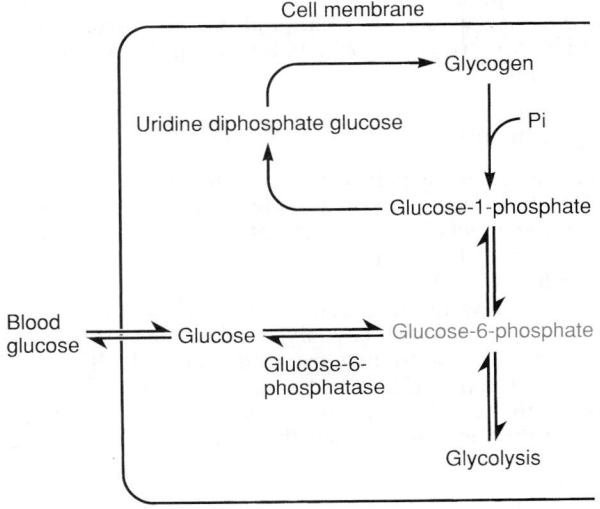

Figure 35.8. The chemical reactions of glycogenesis and glycolysis. Glucose-6-phosphatase allows hepatic glucose to be transported out of the hepatocyte for use in other tissues. Glucose-6-phosphate plays a central role in carbohydrate metabolism.

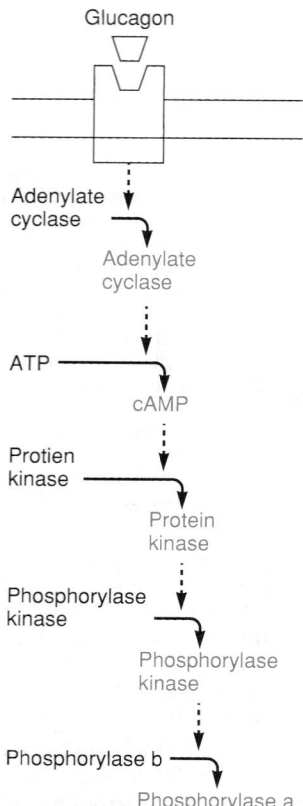

Figure 35.9. Glucagon-stimulated enzyme cascade, responsible for the control of glycogen metabolism. Inactive forms are shown in black, active forms in blue.

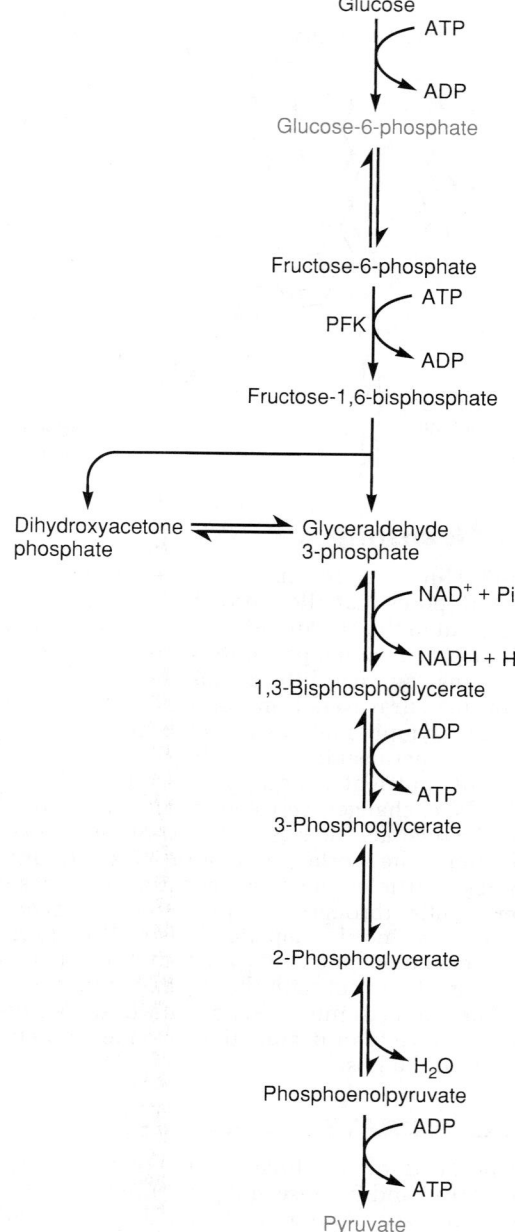

Figure 35.10. The glycolytic pathway. There is a net gain of two adenosine triphosphate molecules per glucose molecule. Phosphofructokinase is the key regulatory enzyme in this pathway.

Eventually, G6P is re-formed. G6P cannot exit from cells and must first be converted back to glucose. This reaction is catalyzed by glucose-6-phosphatase, found only in hepatocytes, kidney, and intestinal epithelial cells. Neither brain nor muscle cells, which use glucose as a primary fuel source, contain the phosphatase enzyme. This lack of glucose-6-phosphatase ensures a ready supply of glucose for the energy needs of brain and muscle. Liver does not use glucose primarily for fuel, but as a precursor for other molecules.

Glycolysis

Glycolysis is the pathway by which glucose is converted to two molecules of pyruvate (Fig. 35.10). This conversion has three effects: (a) a net gain of two ATP molecules, (b) generation of two molecules of nicotinamide adenine nucleotide, and (c) conversion of pyruvate to acetyl coenzyme A (CoA) and degradation of acetyl CoA in the citric acid cycle (see later). Glycolysis takes place in the cytoplasm, in contrast to the citric acid cycle, which occurs in the mitochondria (Fig. 35.11). During times of glucose excess, as in the fed state, hepatic glycolysis can generate energy in the form of ATP, but the oxidation of ketoacids is preferred.

Phosphogluconate Pathway

When glucose enters the liver, glycogen is formed until the hepatic glycogen capacity is reached (about 100 g). If excess glucose is still available, the liver converts it to fat

by the phosphogluconate pathway (Fig. 35.12). Up to 30% of hepatic glucose metabolism occurs by this pathway. Hydrogen atoms released in the phosphogluconate pathway combine with NADP+ (oxidized nicotinamide adenine dinucleotide phosphate) to form NADPH (reduced nicotinamide adenine dinucleotide phosphate) (11).

Gluconeogenesis

When glucose becomes scarce, as in the fasting state, glycogenolysis occurs. Once glycogen stores have been depleted, the liver is capable of synthesizing new glucose by the process of gluconeogenesis. About 60% of the naturally occurring amino acids, glycerol, or lactate can be

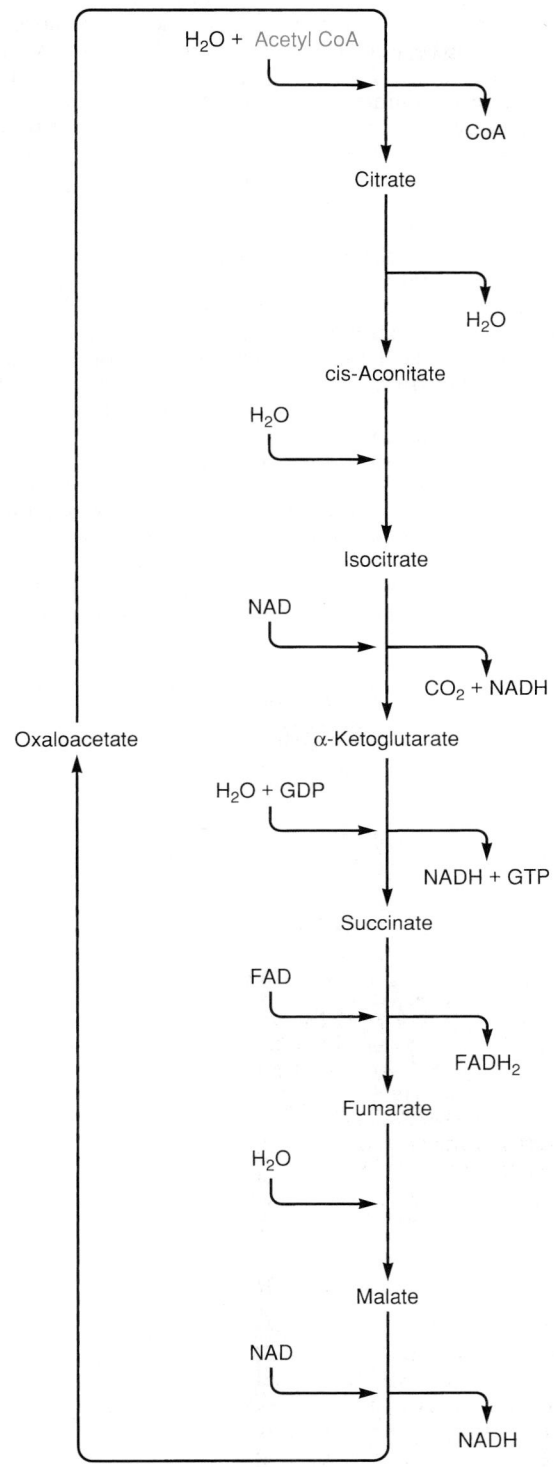

Figure 35.11. The citric acid cycle. Reduced nicotinamide adenine dinucleotide and reduced flavin adenine dinucleotide, formed in the citric acid cycle, are subsequently oxidized in mitochondria by means of the electron transport chain to generate adenosine triphosphate. Acetyl coenzyme A plays a key role.

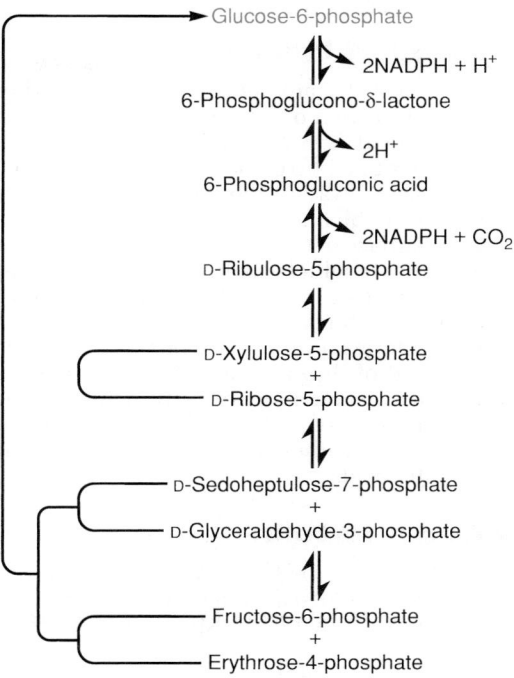

Figure 35.12. The phosphogluconate pathway. One of the major purposes of this pathway is to generate reduced nicotinamide adenine dinucleotide, which can serve as an electron donor and allow the liver to perform reductive biosynthesis.

used as substrates for glucose production. Alanine is the amino acid most easily converted into glucose. Simple deamination allows conversion to pyruvic acid, which is subsequently converted to glucose. Other amino acids can be converted into three-, four-, or five-carbon sugars and then enter the phosphogluconate pathway.

Gluconeogenesis is enhanced by fasting, critical illness, and periods of anaerobic metabolism. Active skeletal muscle and erythrocytes form large quantities of lactate. In patients with large wounds, lactate also accumulates. The liver can convert lactate to glucose (Fig. 35.13).

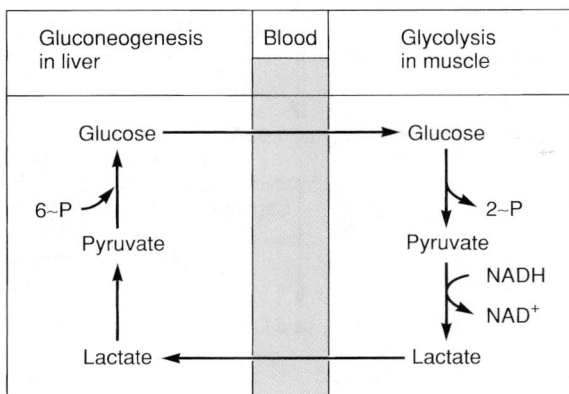

Figure 35.13. The Cori cycle, an elegant mechanism for the hepatic conversion of muscle lactate into new glucose. Pyruvate plays a key role in this process.

LIPID METABOLISM

Lipid Transport into Liver

Dietary triglycerides are split into monoglycerides and fatty acids by the action of intestinal lipases. After absorption into the small intestinal cells, triglycerides are reformed and aggregate into chylomicrons, which then enter the bloodstream by way of the lymph. Chylomicrons are removed from the blood by the liver and adipose tissue. The capillary surface of the liver contains large amounts of lipoprotein lipase, which hydrolyzes triglycerides into fatty acids and glycerol. The fatty acids freely diffuse into the hepatocytes for further metabolism.

The liver performs a number of important functions in the metabolism of lipids, including the synthesis of apolipoproteins, degradation of fatty acids into energy substrates, synthesis of triglycerides from carbohydrates and proteins, and synthesis of cholesterol and phospholipids from fatty acids.

Fatty Acid Metabolism

Most human fatty acids found in plasma are long-chain acids (C-16 to C-20). Because long-chain fatty acids are not readily absorbed by the intestinal mucosa, they must first be incorporated into chylomicrons. In contrast, short-chain and medium-chain fatty acids are absorbed directly into the portal circulation and are avidly taken up by hepatocytes. Free fatty acids in the circulation are noncovalently bound to albumin and are transferred to the hepatocyte cytosol by way of fatty acid-binding proteins. Under basal conditions, most free fatty acids are catabolized for energy by cardiac and skeletal muscle. Under conditions of adipocyte lipolysis, the liver can take up and metabolize fatty acids. The liver is unique in that it contains dehydrogenases that can unsaturate essential dietary fatty acids. Structural elements of all tissues contain significant amounts of unsaturated fats, and the liver is responsible for the production of these unsaturated fatty acids. The best example is the production of the prostaglandin precursor, arachidonic acid. Dietary linoleic acid is elongated and dehydrogenated to arachidonic acid by the liver.

Fatty acid CoA esters are also synthesized in the cytosol after hepatic uptake. These fatty acid CoA esters can be converted into triglyceride, transported into mitochondria for the production of acetyl CoA and ATP, or stored in the liver as triglycerides. Figure 35.14 illustrates the essential pathways of hepatic lipid metabolism. The rate-limiting step in the synthesis of triglyceride is the conversion of

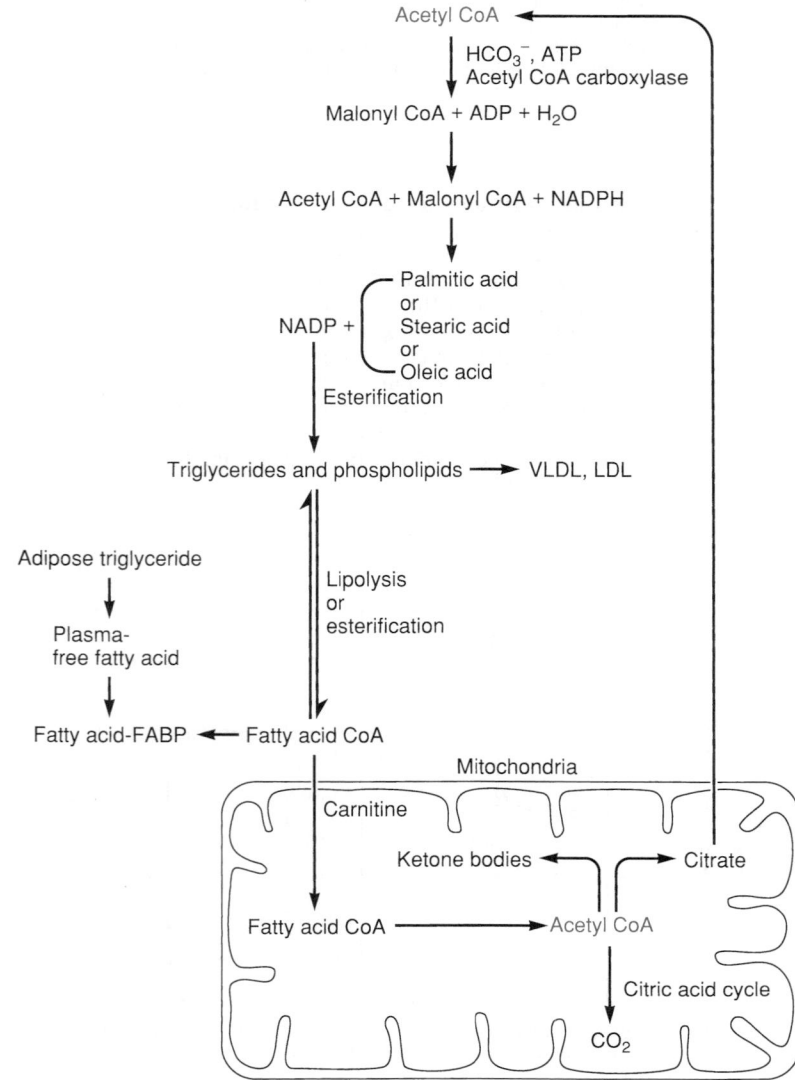

Figure 35.14. Diagram of hepatic fatty acid metabolism. Both dietary and newly synthesized fatty acids are esterified and subsequently degraded in the mitochondria for energy.

acetyl CoA to malonyl CoA. Malonyl CoA in turn inhibits the mitochondrial uptake of fatty acid CoA ester.

Fatty acid CoA esters bind carnitine, a carrier molecule, and in the absence of cytosolic malonyl CoA, they enter the hepatic mitochondria, where they undergo β-oxidation to acetyl CoA and ATP (Fig. 36.14). Acetyl CoA can then take one of the following routes: (a) enter the tricarboxylic acid cycle and be degraded to carbon dioxide; (b) be converted to citrate for fatty acid synthesis; or (c) be converted into 3-hydroxy-3-methylglutaryl CoA (HMG-CoA), a precursor of cholesterol and ketone bodies. The mitochondrial hydrolysis of fatty acids is a source of large quantities of ATP. The conversion of stearic acid to carbon dioxide and water, for instance, generates 136 molecules of ATP and demonstrates the highly efficient storage of energy in fat.

In times of unrestrained lipolysis, such as starvation, uncontrolled diabetes, or other conditions of triglyceride mobilization from adipocyte stores, the ability of liver to perform β-oxidation may be inadequate. Under such circumstances, hepatic storage of triglyceride or fatty infiltration of the liver can be significant. Triglyceride storage by itself does not appear to be a cause of hepatic fibrosis or necrosis, but fatty infiltration may be a marker for the derangement of normal processes by alcohol or drug toxicity, diabetes, long-term total parenteral nutrition, or morbid obesity. A specific type of microvesicular fatty accumulation is seen in a variety of diseases, such as Reye's syndrome and acute fatty liver of pregnancy.

Cholesterol Metabolism

Cholesterol is an important regulator of membrane fluidity and is a substrate for bile acid and steroid hormone synthesis. Cholesterol may be available by dietary intake or by de novo synthesis. In mammals, about 90% of new cholesterol is synthesized in the liver from its precursor, acetyl CoA. Dietary cholesterol intake can suppress endogenous synthesis by inhibiting the rate-limiting enzyme in the cholesterol biosynthetic pathway, HMG-CoA reductase (12). A competitive antagonist, lovastatin, can also block HMG-CoA reductase and effectively lower plasma cholesterol by blocking cholesterol synthesis, stimulating low-density lipoprotein (LDL) receptor synthesis, and allowing an increased hepatic uptake and metabolism of cholesterol-rich LDL lipoproteins. The structure of the LDL receptor is known and serves as a model for other cell membrane receptors (Fig. 35.15).

Cholesterol is lipophilic and hydrophobic, and most plasma cholesterol is found in lipoproteins esterified with oleic or palmitic acid. The liver can process cholesterol esters from all classes of lipoproteins. Hepatocytes can also take up chylomicron remnants containing dietary cholesterol esters. Newly synthesized hepatic cholesterol is used primarily to synthesize bile acids for further intestinal absorption of dietary fats.

Phospholipids

The three major classes of phospholipid synthesized by the liver are lecithins, cephalins, and sphingomyelins. Although most cells in the body are capable of some phospholipid synthesis, the liver produces 90%. Phospholipid formation is controlled by the overall rate of fat metabolism and also by the availability of choline and inositol. The main role of phospholipids of all types is to form plasma and organelle membranes. The amphiphilic nature of phospholipids makes them essential for reducing surface tension between membranes and surrounding fluids. Phosphatidylcholine, one of the lecithins, is the major bil-

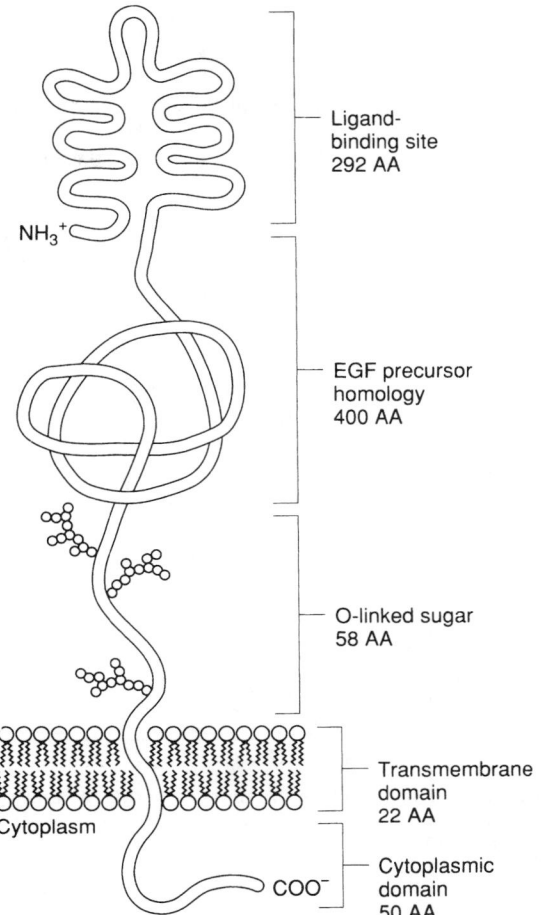

Figure 35.15. The low-density lipoprotein *(LDL)* receptor, an example of a transmembrane receptor that participates in receptor-mediated endocytosis. The LDL receptor specifically binds lipoproteins that contain apolipoprotein B-100 or E. Once internalized, the lipoproteins are degraded. Some receptors, such as the insulin receptor, have a larger cytoplasmic domain that is catalytically active. On binding insulin, the receptor is able to phosphorylate itself and other as yet unidentified proteins; as a result, biologic activity is altered. *AA,* amino acids.

iary phospholipid and is important in promoting the secretion of free cholesterol into bile. Thromboplastin, one of the cephalins, is needed to initiate the clotting cascade. The sphingomyelins are necessary for the formation of the myelin nerve sheath.

PROTEIN METABOLISM

Amino Acid Transport and Storage

Essentially all the end products of dietary protein digestion are amino acids, which are absorbed by the enterocytes into the portal circulation in ionized states. Amino acids are taken up by hepatocytes by one of several active transport mechanisms (Fig. 35.4). Amino acids are not stored in the liver but are rapidly used in the production of plasma proteins, purines, heme proteins, and hormones. Under certain conditions, the amine group is removed from amino acids, and the carbon chain is used for carbohydrate, lipid, or nonessential amino acid synthesis.

The ammonia formed as a result of the deamination of amino acids is detoxified by one of two routes (13). The

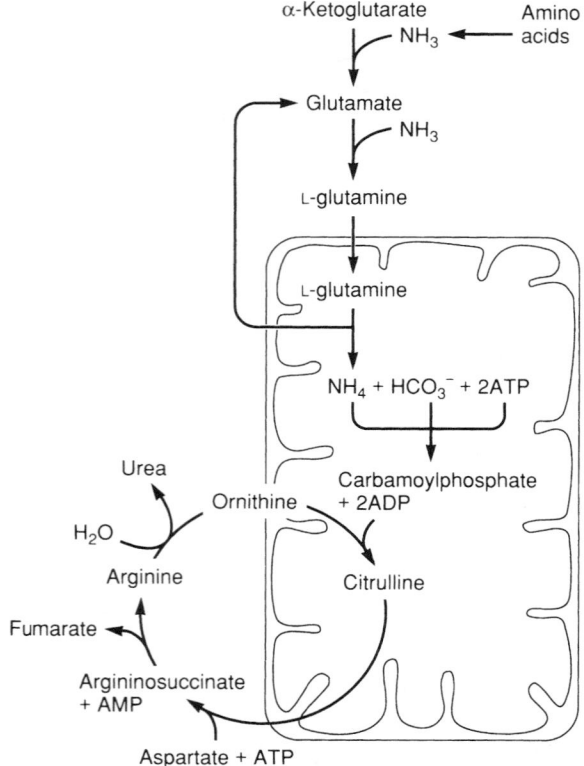

Figure 35.16. The urea cycle. Ammonia entering the urea cycle is derived from protein and amino acid degradation in tissues (endogenous) and the colonic lumen (exogenous).

most important pathway involves the conversion of ammonia to urea by enzymes of the Krebs-Henseleit cycle, found only in the liver (Fig. 35.16). A second route of ammonia metabolism involves deamination of L-glutamine by the kidney, with excretion of ammonia into the urine, important for urinary acidification.

Formation of Plasma Proteins

Essentially all albumin, fibrinogen, and apolipoproteins are derived from the liver, which can add up to 50 g of protein to the plasma a day. Of the total hepatic protein synthesized, 75% is destined for export in plasma. Most newly synthesized proteins are not stored in the liver, and the rate of protein synthesis is primarily determined by the intracellular levels of amino acids. A partial list of major plasma proteins synthesized by the liver is found in Table 35.2.

The synthesis and export of albumin has been intensively studied. Human albumin is a single-chain polypeptide consisting of 584 amino acids. The 17 disulfide bridges give albumin its tertiary structure and expose both electrostatic and hydrophobic binding sites, allowing albumin to bind with a variety of smaller molecules. Albumin does not contain terminal galactose residues and therefore is not rapidly cleared by ASGP receptors. As a result, the half-life of albumin in plasma is 19 days (14). Decreased hepatic protein synthesis is only partially responsible for the low plasma levels of albumin seen in cirrhosis or malnutrition. The long half-life of albumin makes it an insensitive indicator of hepatic synthetic function.

The tertiary structure of many proteins undergoes post-translational modification after they have been synthesized in the liver rough ER. Glycosylation, or the addition of carbohydrate moieties, occurs in the smooth ER. Sialation, or the addition of sialic acid, occurs in the

Table 35.2. MAJOR PROTEINS SYNTHESIZED BY THE LIVER

Broad category	Protein	Molecular weight	Function
Transport proteins	Albumin	66,000	Multiple
	Transferrin	57,000	Transport iron
	Hemopexin	80,000	Transport heme to liver
	Ceruloplasmin	132,000	Transport copper
	Haptoglobin	90,000	Transport free hemoglobin
	Thyroxine-binding globulin	55,000	Transport thyroid hormone
	Thyroxine-binding prealbumin	50,000	Transport thyroid hormone
	Testosterone-estradiol-binding globulin	90,000	Facilitate testosterone action
	Retinol-binding protein	21,000	Transport vitamin A
	Vitamin D-binding protein	52,000	Transport vitamin D
Coagulation proteins	Fibrinogen (factor I)	340,000	Form fibrin
	Prothrombin (factor II)	73,000	Convert fibrinogen to fibrin
	Factors V, VII, IX, X, XI, XII	50,000–75,000	Extrinsic and intrinsic pathways
	Plasminogen	90,000	Form plasmin
	α_2-Antiplasmin	70,000	Inhibit plasmin
	Antithrombin III	60,000	Protease inhibitor
	Protein S	50,000	Protein C cofactor
	Protein C	55,000	Anticoagulant
Acute-phase reactants	α_2-Macroglobulin	720,000	Bind endopeptidases
	α_1-Antitrypsin	54,000	Inhibit serine proteases
	C-reactive protein	105,000	Modify inflammation
	Orosomucoid	40,000	Unknown
Lipoprotein metabolism	Apolipoprotein A-I, A-II	17,000–30,000	LCAT cofactors
	Apolipoprotein C-I, C-II, C-III	6,000–10,000	Inhibit binding to liver
	Apolipoprotein E	34,000	Receptor recognition
	Apolipoprotein B-100	510,000	VLDL synthesis and secretion
	LCAT	—	Cholesterol synthesis in blood

LCAT, lecithin-cholesterol acetyl transferase; VLDL, very low-density lipoprotein.

Golgi. Glycosylation is important in allowing some proteins to bind with specific receptors for subsequent hepatic uptake and processing. Removal of sialic acid residues, or desialation, from the terminal galactose molecules of glycoproteins allows them to bind the ASGP receptor in the liver and undergo degradation. Desialation, therefore, is important in the clearance of senescent proteins from the plasma.

Protein Uptake and Degradation

Proteins such as ASGP are generally taken up by receptor-mediated processes. ASGPs are proteins from which sialic acid residues have been removed by tissue neuraminidases. Terminal galactose residues are exposed and recognized by the ASGP receptor, so that hepatic receptor-mediated endocytosis can take place (Fig. 35.5). Protein degradation occurs primarily in lysosomes. The lysosomal enzymes are nonselective in their activities; more than 20 known hydrolytic enzymes are present in lysosomes.

HEPATIC METABOLISM

Metabolic processes in the liver are essential for the production of fuel substrates for other organs. The liver, by virtue of its terminal position in the portal system, is the organ that must regulate intestinally absorbed nutrients for tissue consumption or storage. The liver accomplishes its task by synthesizing three key metabolites—G6P, pyruvate, and acetyl CoA (Fig. 35.17). Each of these three simple chemical molecules can be extensively modified by the liver to allow an almost limitless number of metabolic fates.

Glucose-6-phosphate can be stored as glycogen or converted into glucose, pyruvate, or ribose-5-phosphate (a nucleotide precursor). Pyruvate can be converted into lactate, alanine (and other amino acids), and acetyl CoA, or it can enter the tricarboxylic acid cycle. Acetyl CoA is converted to HMG-CoA (a cholesterol and ketone body precursor) or citrate (for fatty acid and triglyceride synthesis), or it is degraded to carbon dioxide and water for energy. In mammals, acetyl CoA cannot be converted into pyruvate. Thus, lipids cannot be converted into carbohydrates.

The preferred energy substrates for liver are ketoacids derived from amino acid degradation. Glucose produced by the dephosphorylation of G6P rapidly diffuses out of the cell and is taken up by the brain, muscles, and other organs. Hepatic glycolysis is used primarily for the production of intermediates of metabolism, not for energy. Hepatic fatty acid degradation for energy is also inhibited under most circumstances and is seen only during adipocyte lipolysis.

BILE FORMATION

Composition and Secretion

The adult human liver secretes about 1.5 L of bile daily. Eighty percent of this volume is secreted by the hepatocytes (canalicular bile), and 20% is secreted by the bile duct epithelial cells (ductular bile). Solutes constitute about 3% of bile. The major solutes are conjugated bile acids, phosphatidylcholine, cholesterol, protein, and bilirubin. The organic solutes have transport systems, and the most important solutes are the bile acids. Bile acids are the main determinant of bile production, and canalicular bile flow is traditionally divided into bile acid-dependent and bile acid-independent components.

Bile acid-dependent flow is that portion of bile flow resulting from the active secretion of bile acids. The bile acid concentration in hepatic bile is usually between 1 and 5 mmol. The concentration in plasma is 1 to 5 µmol, a 1,000-fold difference. Bile flow is linearly related to bile acid output; hence, bile acids are one of the most important determinants of hepatic bile flow and account for about half of canalicular bile production (15).

Conjugated bile acids enter the hepatocyte at the sinusoidal surface via a saturable membrane transport protein (Fig. 35.4). The driving force for bile acid uptake is the electrochemical sodium gradient between sinusoidal blood and the cytoplasm. As sodium enters, conjugated bile acids passively move along with the sodium. Intracellular transport is less well understood than the uptake of bile acids.

The ability of bile acids to stimulate bile acid-dependent flow depends on bile acid structure. Most bile acids form micelles when present in solution above a critical micellar concentration. When micelles form, the concentration of free, osmotically active bile acids decreases. Bile acids, such as dehydrocholate, that do not form micelles stimulate more bile flow than micelle-forming bile acids, such as taurocholate. Because bile formation is an active secretory process, bile secretory pressure can be higher than hepatic perfusion pressure. Bile, therefore, is fundamentally different from glomerular urine, which is essentially a pressure-driven ultrafiltrate of plasma.

The hepatic uptake of conjugated and unconjugated bilirubin, sulfobromophthalein, indocyanin green, and certain radiologic contrast media also appears to be carrier-mediated. The process is saturable but does not appear to be sodium-dependent, and these organic ions can compete with each other but not with bile acids for uptake. Unconjugated bilirubin is bound in plasma to albumin. Bilirubin is then released from albumin and subsequently internalized. After internalization, bilirubin binds to intracellular carrier proteins. Once in the hepatocyte, bilirubin is conjugated with glucuronic acid to bilirubin diglucuronide before biliary secretion. Less than 1% of biliary bilirubin is secreted in the unconjugated form.

Figure 35.17. A summation of the key regulatory molecules used by the liver during diverse metabolic functions. Essentially, any compound found in the body can be synthesized in the liver from glucose-6-phosphate, acetyl coenzyme A, or pyruvate. As a consequence of the inability of mammalian liver to convert acetyl coenzyme A to pyruvate, fats cannot be converted to carbohydrates.

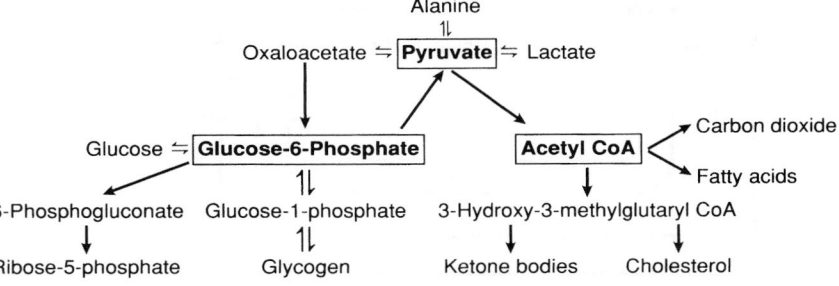

Bile Acid Metabolism

In discussing bile acid metabolism, it is useful to distinguish primary from secondary bile acids. Primary bile acids are synthesized from cholesterol in the liver; in humans, these consist of cholic acid and chenodeoxycholic acid. Secondary bile acids, formed in the intestinal lumen by bacterial dehydroxylation, consist of deoxycholic acid and lithocholic acid, derived from cholic acid and chenodeoxycholic acid, respectively. Essentially all the primary and secondary bile acids are conjugated with the amino acids glycine or taurine. Amino acid conjugation lowers the pKa of bile acids so that they remain ionized in the intestinal lumen and are not passively reabsorbed through nonionic diffusion. Conjugated bile acids also form micelles, which more effectively facilitate lipid digestion and absorption from the small intestine (16).

The human liver synthesizes 300 to 400 mg of bile acids per day from cholesterol, or about 10% of the total bile salt pool. The rate of bile acid synthesis is tightly linked to bile acid loss through the colon. Bile acid synthesis is the major mechanism for cholesterol degradation in the body, and the rate-limiting enzymatic step is catalyzed by cholesterol 7-α-hydroxylase. By the dietary ingestion of resins that bind bile acids, such as cholestyramine, it is possible to increase the fecal excretion of bile acids and thus the degradation of cholesterol. Intestinal bile acids are efficiently (about 95%) taken up by the enterohepatic circulation (Fig. 35.18). Luminal bile acids are transported by carrier proteins in the distal ileum and appear in the portal venous effluent. The hepatocyte extracts more than 95% of portal venous bile acids for re-secretion into the bile.

Biliary Lecithin and Cholesterol Secretion

The main biliary phospholipid is lecithin, or phosphatidylcholine. Lecithin is amphipathic, which means it contains both hydrophilic and hydrophobic domains. Lecithin serves two main purposes in bile—to solubilize free biliary cholesterol and emulsify dietary fats in the intestines. Free cholesterol is not soluble in water or simple micelles of bile acids but is readily solubilized in mixed micelles of both bile acids and lecithin. Although most biliary cholesterol appears to be derived from plasma lipoproteins, biliary lecithin is predominantly synthesized in the liver. Biliary secretion of both lecithin and cholesterol is tightly linked to the rate of bile acid secretion, so that as bile acid output increases, so does biliary lipid secretion. Lecithin is also found in chylomicrons and other lipoproteins responsible for the intravascular transport of dietary lipids.

Biliary Proteins

Proteins constitute about 5% of the total biliary solute. Immunoglobulin A is an example of a protein that is secreted into bile intact. After binding to plasma membrane receptors, undegraded proteins are transported through the hepatocyte in endocytic vesicles. The functions of intact proteins in bile can be related to intestinal immunity, as in secretory immunoglobulin A, or to the prevention of gallstone nucleation, as in apolipoproteins. A variety of proteins are also degraded in lysosomes before biliary excretion. This mechanism serves as a means of eliminating senescent plasma proteins, as in haptoglobin. Some regulatory peptides can use both pathways (e.g., insulin and epidermal growth factor) (17).

HEPATIC BIOTRANSFORMATION

Biotransformation is defined as the intracellular metabolism of endogenous organic compounds (e.g., heme proteins and steroid hormones) and exogenous compounds (e.g., drugs and environmental compounds). The liver contains enzyme systems that can expose functional groups, such as hydroxyl ions (phase I reactions), or alter the size and solubility of a wide variety of organic and inorganic compounds by conjugation with small polar molecules (phase II reactions). The general strategy of the liver is to convert hydrophobic, potentially toxic compounds into hydrophilic conjugates that can then be excreted into bile or urine.

The four general enzyme families responsible for hepatic biotransformation are the cytochromes P-450, the uridine diphosphate-glucuronyl (UDP-glucuronyl) transferases, the glutathione (GSH) S-transferases, and the sulfotransferases. Biotransforming enzymes are not distributed uniformly within the cells of the hepatic lobule. This heterogeneity may account for the ability of some drugs to cause damage preferentially in zone 3 hepatocytes (Fig. 35.1).

Cytochromes P-450

The cytochromes P-450 are named for their ability to absorb light maximally at 450 nm in the presence of carbon monoxide. These enzymes are bound to the ER and collectively catalyze reactions by using NADPH and oxygen. The P-450 isozymes present in mammalian liver catalyze reactions such as oxidation, hydroxylation, sulfoxide formation, oxidative deamination, dealkylation, and dehalogenation. Such reactions allow further phase II conjugation with polar groups such as glucuronate, GSH, and sulfate.

The cytochromes P-450 can also create potentially toxic metabolites. Drugs such as acetaminophen, isoniazid,

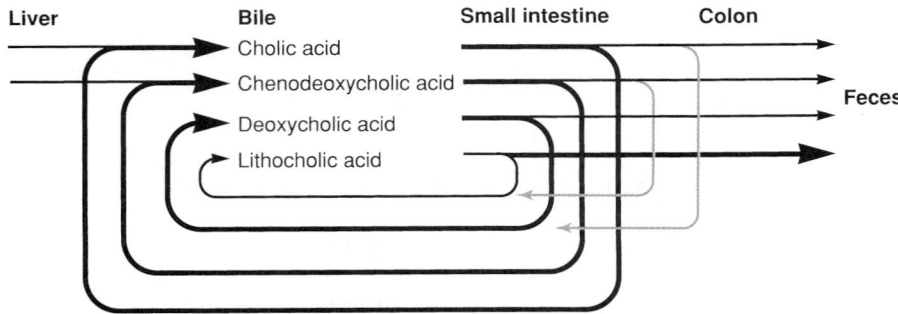

Figure 35.18. The enterohepatic circulation of bile acids. The primary bile acids, cholic acid and chenodeoxycholic acid, are synthesized in the liver from cholesterol. Deoxycholic acid and lithocholic acid are formed in the colon (*blue lines*) during bacterial degradation of the primary bile acids. All four bile acids are conjugated with glycine or taurine in the liver. Most of the lithocholic acid is also sulfated, which decreases reabsorption and increases fecal excretion. Bile acids are absorbed passively in the epithelium of the small and large intestine and actively in the distal ileum.

halothane, and the phenothiazines can be converted into reactive forms that cause cellular injury and death. The cytochromes also are responsible for the formation of organic free radicals, reactive metabolites that can directly attack and injure cellular components or act as a hapten in the generation of an autoimmune response. Several of the most potent known carcinogens are aromatic hydrocarbons, which are modified by cytochrome P-450.

Uridine Diphosphate-Glucuronyl Transferases

Glucuronidation is the conjugation of UDP-glucuronic acid to a wide variety of xenobiotics by either ester (acyl) or ether linkages. The transferases catalyzing these reactions reside in the ER. Many common compounds are metabolized in this way, including bilirubin, testosterone, aspirin, indomethacin, acetaminophen, chloramphenicol, and oxazepam. Clinically significant loss of activity can occur with acute ethanol exposure or acetaminophen overdose, when formation of UDP-glucuronic acid from UDP-glucose is outstripped by use. Some acyl linkages lead to the generation of electrophilic centers that can react with other proteins. The covalent linkage of conjugated bilirubin to albumin is believed to occur by this mechanism.

Glutathione S-Transferases

The GSH transferases are more selective in the biotransformations they perform. GSH conjugation occurs only with compounds that have electrophilic and potentially reactive centers. The role of GSH conjugation catalyzed by the GSH S-transferases is best seen with acetaminophen. In this drug, cytochrome P-450 creates an electrophilic center that reacts with protein thiol groups or GSH (18). The presence of GSH S-transferase allows the preferential detoxification of acetaminophen rather than the potentially injurious binding to thiol groups. A class of GSH S-transferases, known as *ligandins,* appears to facilitate the uptake and intracellular transport of bilirubin, heme, and bile acids from plasma to liver. In addition to the detoxification of potential toxins, GSH is a substrate for GSH peroxidase, an enzyme important in the metabolism of hydrogen peroxide.

Sulfotransferases

The sulfotransferases catalyze the transfer of sulfate groups from 3'-phosphoadenosine-5'-phosphosulfate (PAPS) to compounds such as thyroxine, bile acids, isoproterenol, α-methyldopa, and acetaminophen. They are located primarily in the cytosol. Although many P-450 derivatives can be further conjugated by either the sulfotransferases or the glucuronyl transferases, a limited ability of the liver to synthesize PAPS makes glucuronidation the predominant mechanism.

HEME AND PORPHYRIN METABOLISM

Heme is formed from glycine and succinate and is the functional iron-containing center of hemoglobin, myoglobin, cytochromes, catalases, and peroxidases. From glycine and succinate precursors, δ-aminolevulinic acid (δ-ALA) is synthesized by the rate-limiting enzyme ALA synthase. The porphyrinogens are intermediates in the pathway from δ-ALA to heme, and porphyrins are oxidized forms of porphyrinogen (Fig. 35.19). Inherited enzyme defects in the heme synthetic pathway cause the overproduction of various porphyrinogens, which can in turn cause clinical manifestations known as the *porphyrias* (19). Acquired porphyria can be caused by heavy metal intoxication, estrogens, alcohol, or environmental exposure to chlorinated hydrocarbons.

Bilirubin IXα is the predominant heme degradation product in humans and is derived mostly from hemoglobin. The enzyme heme oxygenase, found in cells of the reticuloendothelial system, is primarily responsible for this conversion. Heme oxygenase is located in the ER and requires NADPH as a cofactor. Hepatic processing of bilirubin is further detailed in the section on bile formation.

METAL METABOLISM

Iron uptake in liver cells appears to occur by two distinct processes: (a) receptor-mediated endocytosis of iron–transferrin complexes and (b) facilitated diffusion across the plasma membrane. More iron is taken up and stored by the liver than by any other organ, with the exception of the bone marrow. Transferrin is synthesized in the liver and has

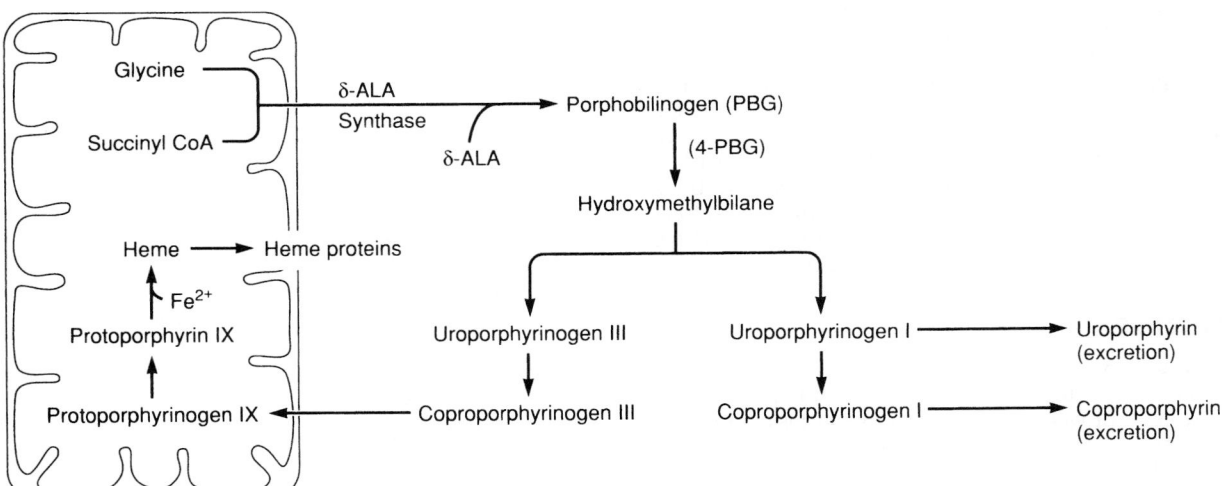

Figure 35.19. The heme biosynthetic pathway. Inherited defects of each of the heme biosynthetic enzymes except δ-aminolevulinic acid synthase have been described and lead to the clinical disorders known as the *porphyrias.*

specific plasma membrane receptors on a number of different tissues. After endocytosis, the transferrin and iron dissociate and the transferrin and transferrin receptor return to the cell surface for recycling. A pathway appears to involve the dissociation of iron and transferrin at the plasma membrane and subsequent internalization by carrier-mediated diffusion. Once internalized, iron is stored and complexed to apoferritin. Each apoferritin molecule is capable of storing several thousand iron molecules. The iron–apoferritin complex, called *ferritin,* is responsible for iron storage under physiologic conditions. Iron storage in a protein-bound form is essential because free iron can catalyze free radical formation, leading to cell injury (20).

Copper is transported to the liver bound to albumin or histidine and enters the hepatocytes by a process of facilitated diffusion. Once inside the cell, copper can bind to several intracellular proteins for storage or as a necessary enzyme cofactor. Copper-binding proteins include metallothionein, monoamine oxidase, cytochrome *c* oxidase, and superoxide dismutase. *Ceruloplasmin* is a liver-derived protein that binds hepatic copper for transport to other tissues. The low levels of ceruloplasmin seen in patients with Wilson's disease suggest a pathogenetic defect.

Zinc is taken up by and competes for the same binding sites as copper. In hepatocytes, zinc binds predominantly to metallothionein and is excreted into bile, in which it enters the enterohepatic circulation. Other metals, usually found in trace amounts, are lead, cadmium, selenium, mercury, and nickel. These metals are usually bound to metallothionein or GSH, and intoxication is associated with free radical formation and liver injury.

VITAMIN METABOLISM

The liver plays an important role in the metabolism of the fat-soluble vitamins A, D, and K. Hepatic bile salt secretion is necessary for the solubilization and absorption of dietary fat-soluble vitamins from the intestine. The liver also stores significant amounts of the fat-soluble vitamins and synthesizes transport proteins for the various vitamins. Vitamin A is exclusively stored in the liver, and excessive ingestion of vitamin A can be associated with significant liver injury. Retinol-binding protein, synthesized by the liver, is responsible for the plasma transport of vitamin A.

Vitamin D must be metabolized in the liver to 25-hydroxyvitamin D, a necessary step in the conversion from dietary to biologically active vitamin D. Vitamin D undergoes biliary secretion, intestinal absorption, and hepatic uptake or enterohepatic circulation in a sequence similar to that of bile acid metabolism. Vitamin D-binding globulin is synthesized in the liver and is responsible for the transport of all forms of vitamin D. Vitamin K_1 is ingested with food, and vitamin K_2 is formed as a product of bacterial action in the gut lumen. Vitamin K is required for the the γ-carboxylation of glutamic acid residues, a necessary step in the hepatic synthesis of biologically active coagulation factors II, VII, XI, and X. Of the water-soluble vitamins, only vitamin B_{12} is stored to any appreciable extent in the liver.

CYTOKINES

Cytokines, long the exclusive domain of the immune response, are now known to be important in hepatic physiology and pathophysiology. Now that cytokines are known to be important, many direct effects on the liver cell will be discovered. Several important observations have already been made. Interleukin-6 (IL-6) is known to be essential in the liver-mediated acute-phase response to trauma or inflammation. The acute-phase response is associated with rapid increases in haptoglobin, α_1-acid glycoprotein, and serum amyloid A (21). IL-6 also activates the transcription factor STAT-3, which is important in the regenerative process (22). The antiinflammatory cytokine IL-10 is produced in response to hepatic ischemia reperfusion. Tumor necrosis factor-α (TNF-α) has been shown to be important in liver regeneration. Elimination of transforming growth factor-α (TGF-α) before hepatectomy blocks the increase of a variety of nuclear transcription factors, including *jun* kinase, c-*jun,* and AP-1 (23). Lastly, inducible nitric oxide synthase (iNOS) is expressed by hepatocytes in response to a number of stimuli and is important in a number of physiologic conditions, especially cytoprotection (24).

LIVER REGENERATION

The rapid, controlled proliferation of liver cells after surgical resection or toxic injury of the liver is a fundamental response almost unique among solid organs (23). The regenerative response is proportional to the amount of liver resected. All cells of the liver participate, including mature hepatocytes, biliary epithelial cells, endothelial cells, Kupffer's cells, and Ito or stellate cells. An additional remarkable feature of the hepatocyte is its ability to proliferate rapidly while continuing to perform all the duties required of a differentiated cell, including secretion of proteins (albumin, clotting factors), glucose homeostasis, and biotransformation. Within 30 minutes, several new genes are turned on, including those noted in Table 35.3, and others not yet identified (25). Many growth factors and cytokines are important in the stimulus to liver regeneration. Solid experimental evidence suggests that hepatocyte growth factor, epidermal growth factor, TGF-α, IL-6, TNF-α, insulin, and epinephrine are all necessary for a full proliferative response and intact signaling pathways. Additional factors are probably also necessary, as shown by experiments involving parabiotic rats. If hepatectomy is performed in one of a pair, the liver in the unresected mate also grows, demonstrating the presence of a circulating mitogenic signal that has not yet been completely characterized. Stop signals to end the regenerative process are also required for orderly regeneration; the best characterized is TGF-β.

Table 35.3. MAJOR GENES INDUCED DURING LIVER REGENERATION*

GROWTH-REGULATED

β-Actin
Fibronectin
junB
c-jun
c-myc
c-ets
Albumin
CCAAT/enhancer-binding protein-α (C/EBPα)
Phosphoenolpyruvate carboxykinase (PEPCK)
Thrombospondin-1

CELL CYCLE-REGULATED

Insulin-like growth factor-binding protein-1 (IGFBP1)
c-fos
LRF1
Epidermal growth factor
Glucose-6-phosphatase
α-Fetoprotein (AFP)
Thymidine kinase (TK)
Cyclin D1
Cyclin-dependent kinase (CDK)

---

*For a total of more than 70, further detail is available in Taub R. Transcriptional control of liver regeneration. FASEB J 1996;10:413.

In normal circumstances, mature hepatocytes are capable of the rapid proliferative response necessary for growth or repair. The fumarylacetoacetate hydrolase (FAH) knockout mouse has been used to study the ability of hepatocytes to proliferate. In humans, FAH deficiency leads to hereditary tyrosinemia. In this disorder, succinylacetone causes hepatocyte death in FAH-deficient cells, whereas cells that contain FAH survive. Transplanting as few as 1,000 normal congenic hepatocytes into the FAH knockout mouse led to repopulation of the liver with normal FAH activity (26). To underscore further the remarkable regenerative capacity of these mature hepatocytes, cells from the repopulated livers were serially transplanted up to six times, which corresponded to about 70 cell doublings or 10^{21} cells (27). Despite the fact that mature hepatocytes are capable of almost unlimited proliferation, a hepatic stem cell compartment is probably also involved. These stem, or oval, cells have been studied extensively in rats and are characterized by the expression of the stem cell factor receptor c-*kit* (28). Recently, cells positive for c-*kit* have been seen in recipient hepatectomy specimens in pediatric patients with fulminant hepatic failure. The significance of two such different mechanisms is not yet completely understood but is presumably of fundamental importance.

ACKNOWLEDGMENTS

I acknowledge grant NIH DK 47811 for partial support.

REFERENCES

1. Rappaport AM. The acinus: microvascular unit of the liver. In: Lautt WW, ed. *Hepatic circulation in health and disease.* New York: Raven Press, 1981:175.
2. Jones AL, Spring-Mills E. The liver and gallbladder. In: Weiss L, ed. *Histology: cell and tissue biology.* New York: Elsevier Science, 1983:707.
3. Burwen SJ, Jones AL. Hepatocellular processing of endocytosed proteins. *J Electron Microsc Tech* 1990;14:140.
4. Wu GY, Wu CH, Stockert RJ. A model for the specific rescue of normal hepatocytes during methotrexate treatment of hepatic malignancy. *Proc Natl Acad Sci USA* 1983;80:3078.
5. Geuze HJ, Van der Donk HA, Simmons CF, et al. Receptor mediated endocytosis in liver parenchymal cells. *Int Rev Exp Pathol* 1986;29:113.
6. Casanova JE, Breitfeld PP, Ross SA, et al. Phosphorylation of the polymeric immunoglobulin receptor required for its efficient transcytosis. *Science* 1990;248:742.
7. Bourne HR. Summary: signals past, present, and future. In: *Cold Spring Harbor symposia on quantitative biology. LIII. Molecular biology of signal transduction.* Cold Spring Harbor, NY: Cold Spring Harbor Laboratory, 1988:1019.
8. Lautt WW, Greenway CV. Conceptual review of the hepatic vascular bed. *Hepatology* 1987;7:952.
9. Lautt WW, Legare DJ, Ezzat WR. Quantitation of the hepatic arterial buffer response to graded changes in portal blood flow. *Gastroenterology* 1990;98:1024.
10. Hetenyi G, Perez G, Vranic M. Turnover and precursor–product relationships of non-lipid metabolites. *Physiol Rev* 1983; 63:606.
11. Styrer L. Pentose phosphate pathway and gluconeogenesis. In: Styrer L, ed. *Biochemistry,* 3rd ed. New York: WH Freeman, 1988:427.
12. Havel RJ, Hamilton RL. Hepatocytic lipoprotein receptors and intracellular lipoprotein catabolism. *Hepatology* 1988;8:1869.
13. Meijer AJ, Lamers WH, Chamuleau RAFM. Nitrogen metabolism and ornithine cycle function. *Physiol Rev* 1990;70:701.
14. Margarson M, Soni N. Serum albumin: touchstone or totem? *Anaesthesia* 1998;53:789–803.
15. Boyer J. Isolated hepatocyte couplets and bile duct units: novel preparations for the in vitro study of bile secretory function. *Cell Biol Toxicol* 1997;13:289–300.
16. Lowe M, Dawson S. New insights into bile acid transport. *Curr Opin Lipidol* 1998;9:225–229.
17. LaRusso NF. Proteins in bile: how they get there and what they do. *Am J Physiol* 1984;247:G199.
18. Lee T, Li L, Ballatori N. Hepatic glutathione and glutathione S-conjugate transport mechanisms. *Yale J Biol Med* 1997;70: 287–300.
19. Bissell DM, Schmid R. The hepatic porphyrias. In: Schiff L, Schiff ER, eds. *Diseases of the liver,* 7th ed. Philadelphia: JB Lippincott, 1993:1061.
20. Morley CGD, Bezkorovainy A. Cellular iron uptake from transferrin: is endocytosis the only mechanism? *Int J Biochem* 1985;17:553.
21. Kopf M, Baunann H, Freer G, et al. Impaired immune and acute-phase responses in interleukin-6–deficient mice. *Nature* 1994;368:339.
22. Bradham C, Plumpe J, Manns MP, et al. Mechanisms of hepatic toxicity I: TNF-induced injury. *Am J Physiol* 1998; 275[Gastrointest Liver Physiol 38]:G387–G392.
23. Michalopoulos G, DeFrances M. Liver regeneration. *Science* 1997;276:60.
24. Taylor B, Alarcon L, Billiar T. Inducible nitric oxide synthase in the liver: regulation and function. *Biochemistry (Moscow)* 1998;63:766.
25. Taub R. Transcriptional control of liver regeneration. *FASEB J* 1996;10:413.
26. Overturf K, alDhalimy M, Tanguay R, et al. Hepatocytes corrected by gene therapy are selected in vivo in a murine model of hereditary tyrosinemia type I. *Nat Genet* 1996;12: 266.
27. Overturf K, alDhalimy M, Ou CN, et al. Serial transplantation reveals the stem-cell like potential of adult mouse hepatocytes. *Am J Pathol* 1997;151:1273.
28. Fujio K, Evarts RP, Hu Z, et al. Expression of stem cell factor and its receptor, c-kit, during liver regeneration from putative stem cells in adult rats. *Lab Invest* 1994;70:511.

SURGERY: SCIENTIFIC PRINCIPLES AND PRACTICE, Third Edition, edited by Lazar J. Greenfield, Michael W. Mulholland, Keith T. Oldham, Gerald B. Zelenock, and Keith D. Lillemoe. Lippincott Williams & Wilkins Publishers, Philadelphia, © 2001.

CHAPTER 36

HEPATIC INFECTION AND ACUTE HEPATIC FAILURE

MICHAEL R. LUCEY

PYOGENIC HEPATIC ABSCESS

Pyogenic hepatic abscesses are rare and account for fewer than 0.2% of adult admissions to hospitals in the United States, where most of these abscesses occur secondary to other infections. Underlying causes of pyogenic hepatic abscess include benign or malignant biliary obstruction accompanied by cholangitis, extrahepatic abdominal sepsis, and trauma or surgery to the right upper quadrant. In special circumstances, pyogenic hepatic abscess is associated with hepatic arterial occlusion in liver transplant recipients (Fig. 36.1) or with the treatment of hepatoma by intraarterial chemotherapy or direct injection of ethanol. The method by which bacteria reach the hepatic parenchyma reflects these underlying causes. For example, in pyogenic hepatic abscess complicating biliary obstruction and cholangitis, bacteria spread directly through the biliary radicles to the hepatic parenchyma. Pyogenic hepatic abscess after intraabdominal sepsis (e.g., diverticulitis) is most likely to be caused by a hematogenous spread through the portal bloodstream. Similarly, hematogenous spread by hepatic arterial inflow may occur

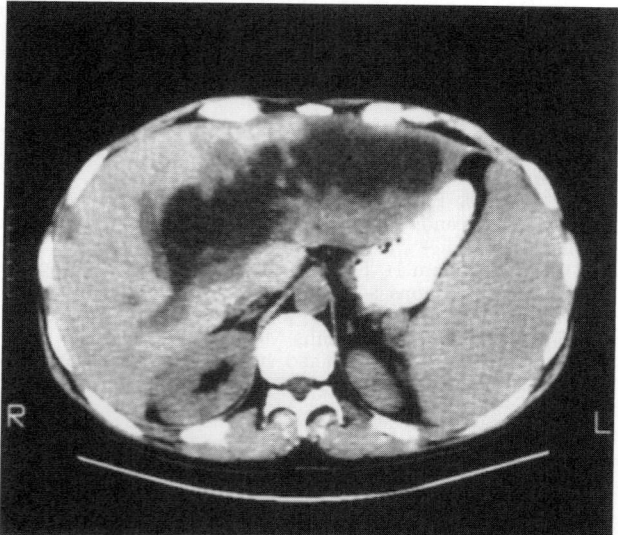

Figure 36.1. Computed tomogram of a pyogenic hepatic abscess in a liver transplant recipient with occlusion of the hepatic artery.

in infectious endocarditis. Abscesses arising from hematogenous transmission are usually unifocal, whereas those resulting from biliary obstruction are more often multifocal. Metastatic cancer in the liver, diabetes mellitus, and alcoholism predispose patients to the development of pyogenic hepatic abscess.

The organisms that predominate in pyogenic hepatic abscesses are gram-negative aerobic rods, streptococci, and anaerobes, including *Bacillus fragilis*. When careful anaerobic cultures are performed, anaerobes or microaerophilic organisms are present in half of all pyogenic hepatic abscesses.

Pyogenic hepatic abscesses occur with equal frequency in men and women, and the median age at presentation is in the fifth decade. Pyogenic hepatic abscesses lead to death in about 15% of affected patients, usually as a result of uncontrolled sepsis. A typical presentation consists of fevers, chills, abdominal pain, and weight loss. Although 60% of patients have symptoms of 2 weeks' duration or less at diagnosis, delayed recognition is common because of the nonspecific symptoms. Some 40% of patients have abdominal tenderness. Overt jaundice is present in 20% of all cases. Almost all patients have a polymorphonuclear leukocytosis and nonspecific abnormal results of biochemistry tests, including elevated alkaline phosphatase, elevated transaminases, and hypoalbuminemia.

The differential diagnosis is broad and includes ascending cholangitis, amebic hepatic abscess, and sepsis elsewhere in the body associated with hepatic dysfunction. It can sometimes be difficult to distinguish between pneumonia with accompanying abnormal liver chemistries and hepatic abscess with accompanying pulmonary changes. About 40% of patients with pyogenic hepatic abscess have right lower lobe abnormalities on chest radiographs, including atelectasis, pulmonary infiltrate, or elevated right hemidiaphragm [1].

The key to a correct diagnosis in suspected pyogenic hepatic abscess is the early use of appropriate hepatobiliary imaging tests. These tests include real-time ultrasonography, computed tomography (CT), radioisotope scans, and contrast-enhanced magnetic resonance imaging (MRI). Although a radioisotope scan is an accurate method of outlining abscesses larger than 2 cm in diameter, it is no longer the preferred test. Both ultrasonography and CT

more accurately define intrahepatic lesions, permit an assessment of accompanying intraabdominal pathology, and allow needle aspiration of the abscess when appropriate. Because biliary obstruction and cholangitis are often part of the differential diagnosis, the hepatic parenchyma, biliary tree, and gallbladder should be inspected. Occasionally, the sonographic appearance of a pyogenic abscess is poorly defined early in the patient's clinical course, and a second sonogram taken a few days later shows more characteristic features of a hepatic abscess. Sonography does not distinguish pyogenic from amebic abscess. CT, especially with intravenous contrast, is as sensitive a diagnostic method as sonography and may be better in identifying an abscess in the area of the hepatic dome. Both real-time ultrasonography and contrast-aided CT may fail to distinguish multiple microabscesses from diffuse fatty infiltration of the hepatic parenchyma or from hepatic metastases. Contrast-aided MRI is an accurate method for recognizing hepatic abscesses.

Once a unifocal or multifocal hepatic abscess has been demonstrated on sonography or CT, diagnostic percutaneous aspiration is advisable unless clear indications are present that the abscess may be amebic [1,2]. Diagnostic aspiration allows the causative organism to be identified, even after antibiotics have been started. The antibiotic regimen can be modified based on subsequent culture results.

Although antibiotic therapy alone may be advisable for some patients in whom attempted drainage is judged to be excessively hazardous or in whom multiple abscesses appear small, the administration of antibiotics along with drainage is the preferred treatment for most pyogenic hepatic abscesses [2]. In many cases, percutaneous drainage under ultrasonographic or CT guidance is sufficient to evacuate pus. Surgical exploration is advised for unstable patients exhibiting signs of continued sepsis despite attempted nonsurgical treatment, and for stable patients who have fevers that persist for longer than 2 weeks after percutaneous catheter drainage and the institution of appropriate antibiotics. Occasionally, surgical drainage is required if viscous pus cannot be aspirated percutaneously, if pus coexists with solid debris, or if the abscess is multilocular.

Before formal identification of the causative organism, antibiotic coverage should be started to treat aerobic gram-negative bacilli, microaerophilic streptococci, and anaerobic bacilli, including *Bacteroides* species. A commonly used combination is ampicillin, an aminoglycoside, with either metronidazole or clindamycin. Third-generation cephalosporins (e.g., ceftriaxone) can be substituted for the aminoglycoside in patients at risk for renal toxicity. Once the causative organisms are identified, the antibiotic regimen should be modified to match sensitivities. Intravenous antibiotics should be administered for 14 days and then replaced with oral preparations to complete a 6-week course. Defervescence occurs within the first week of intravenous antibiotics in most patients with pyogenic hepatic abscesses, although up to 20% of cases are febrile into the second week of therapy. When possible, therapy directed at correcting the underlying pathology (e.g., cholelithiasis and biliary ductal obstruction) should be implemented simultaneously with antibiotics and drainage.

AMEBIC HEPATIC ABSCESS

Entamoeba histolytica is the only ameba that invades human tissue. The parasite is endemic throughout the world and is particularly troublesome in societies with poor sanitation. *E. histolytica* exists in two forms—a cyst, which is the infective form, and a trophozoite. The infection is spread by the fecal–oral route. *E. histolytica* causes two distinct clinical syndromes, amebic colitis and amebic hepatic abscess. About 10% of adults in the United States are entamebic carriers who shed cysts in their feces without evidence of either colitis or abscess formation. This discussion is limited to amebic hepatic abscess.

Amebic hepatic abscess remains a diagnostic challenge. Effective therapy is available, and recovery is expected if therapy is started promptly. The presentation of amebic hepatic abscess can be indistinguishable from that of pyogenic abscess, with acute onset of fever, abdominal pain (often in the right upper quadrant), and disturbed liver chemistries (1). In cases with this presentation, a liver sonogram and serologic tests for amebic infection can be used to make the diagnosis. Features that should prompt consideration of amebic hepatic abscess are a history of travel to or origin from a high-risk area or a history of alcoholism. Homosexual men are particularly at risk because they have a high frequency of bowel carriage of *E. histolytica* and because they are at a higher-than-average risk for AIDS. About half of all patients presenting with amebic abscesses have abnormalities in the right lower lung field (e.g., atelectasis, infiltrate, effusion, or elevated hemidiaphragm). The duration of illness at presentation of amebic hepatic abscess varies, and an acute form with symptoms that last for less than 2 weeks can be distinguished from a chronic form. Nonetheless, some patients with the chronic form have an acute decompensation that is then indistinguishable from a typical acute case. Although up to one third of patients with amebic hepatic abscess describe diarrhea, amebic colitis is rare.

Clinical examination does not separate amebic from pyogenic abscess (1). Although subtle differences between the patterns of hematologic and serum liver values in pyogenic and amebic abscess have been described, these are of little discriminatory value. Moderate elevations in the levels of serum aminotransferases and alkaline phosphatase are common in both conditions. Significant increases in levels of serum bilirubin are uncommon in amebic hepatic abscess. A significant reduction in serum albumin levels (<3 g/dL) is rare in amebic hepatic abscess but is observed in half of patients with pyogenic hepatic abscess.

No specific features on imaging reliably distinguish amebic abscess from pyogenic abscess. Liver ultrasonography and CT are accurate methods to detect amebic hepatic abscess (Fig. 36.2). Serologic tests for the presence of antibody to *E. histolytica* [e.g., indirect hemagglutination, enzyme-linked immunosorbent assay (ELISA), counterim-

mune immunofluorescence, and indirect immunofluorescence] are specific and sensitive in amebic hepatic abscess and yield positive results in 95% of cases. Antibody titers in invasive bowel disease without hepatic involvement can vary. A negative serologic test result encountered in circumstances that are strongly suggestive of an amebic hepatic abscess may be caused by the lack of a particular reactive epitope, and the diagnosis can then be made by using an alternative serologic test. The combination of an appropriate clinical setting, the sonographic appearance of a hepatic abscess, and a positive result on *E. histolytica* serology confirms the diagnosis of amebic hepatic abscess and is sufficient to warrant proceeding immediately to medical therapy.

The drug of choice for amebic hepatic abscesses is metronidazole in a dosage of 750 mg three times daily. Chloroquine phosphate can be added to metronidazole for acutely ill patients. Glucose-6-phosphate dehydrogenase activity should be checked before chloroquine therapy is initiated. Alternative therapeutic regimens include dehydroemetine, iodoquinol, and emetine. Most uncomplicated amebic hepatic abscesses do not require aspiration. Superinfection of an amebic abscess rarely occurs with this protocol and is usually a complication of invasive aspiration procedures or abscess rupture. Therapeutic aspiration should be performed in the occasional patient who is unresponsive to both metronidazole and chloroquine to exclude pyogenic abscess, and in patients with large amebic abscesses of the left lobe, which can rupture into the pericardium, a complication that is frequently fatal.

HYDATID DISEASE OF THE LIVER

Echinococcosis in humans is caused by infection with the tapeworms *Echinococcus granulosis* and *Echinococcus multilocularis.* The more common pathogen in humans is *E. granulosis.* Echinococcosis is a rare infection in North America. The dog is the definitive host, although the disease is endemic in sheep- and cattle-farming regions. Humans are intermediate hosts and acquire echinococcal eggs by ingesting contaminated food. The egg is digested in the duodenum and yields an embryo, which travels through the portal bloodstream and lodges in the liver. Less commonly, the echinococcal embryo may lodge in the lungs, and rarely it comes to rest in the spleen, central nervous system, or bone. An echinococcal embryo that has survived host defenses and is lodged in a capillary develops into a hydatid cyst. This slow-growing structure, which comprises the *Echinococcus* organism and

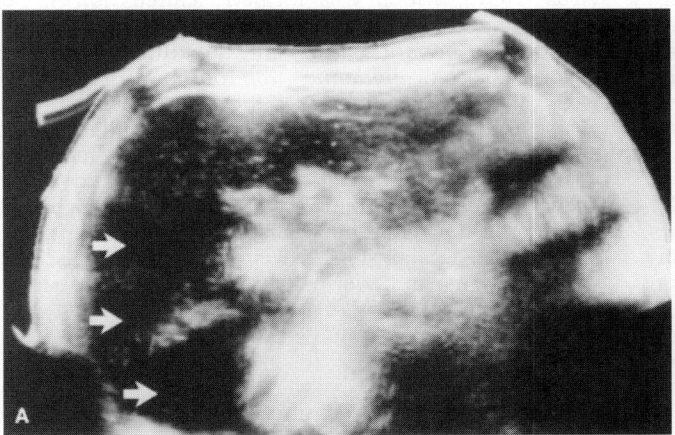
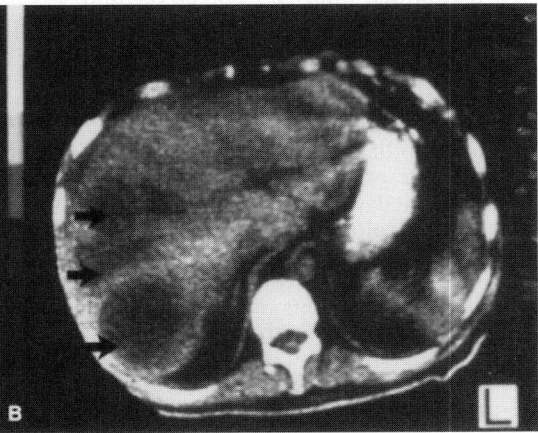

Figure 36.2. Sonogram *(A)* and computed tomogram *(B)* in a patient with multiple amebic abscesses *(arrows).*

host tissue, has three layers: (a) an outer pericyst, which is 2 to 4 mm thick and composed of fibroblasts that produce a capsule of fibrous and connective tissue; (b) a middle hyaline layer up to 2 mm thick and devoid of nuclei; and (c) an inner germinal layer from which the echinococcal scoleces develop. The life cycle of the organism is complete when the definitive host ingests infected viscera; the scoleces are released in its intestine, where they develop into adult worms.

The most frequent site of hydatid cysts is the liver (50% to 70% of cases), followed by the lungs (20% to 30% of cases). Because hydatid cysts grow slowly, a protracted asymptomatic stage is typical. Indeed, in endemic areas, many cases are discovered in persons without earlier symptoms. When they develop, symptoms are caused by enlarging cysts that lead to abdominal pain (the most common presenting symptom), biliary obstruction and jaundice, and, rarely, portal hypertension. Hydatid cysts may be associated with biliary tract pathology, either as a result of communication between the pericyst and biliary ducts or because of rupture of the cyst into the biliary tract. Communication with the biliary tract may lead to secondary bacterial infection of the cyst, cholangitis, or biliary obstruction. Occasionally, cysts spontaneously rupture into the peritoneal cavity and cause abdominal pain and anaphylaxis. Multiple intraabdominal cysts occasionally develop, presumably as the result of a previous unrecognized intraperitoneal leakage. Hepatic hydatid cysts may perforate the diaphragm and cause empyema, pulmonary cysts, biliary–bronchial fistulae, or pericardial collection. Alternatively, pulmonary hydatid cysts can develop when the embryo migrates to the lung. The only typical clinical finding of hepatic hydatid cyst is a palpable hepatic mass.

The results of routine laboratory tests in patients with hydatid cysts may be normal or nonspecifically abnormal (e.g., showing features of obstructive jaundice). Eosinophilia may be absent. Serologic tests (e.g., indirect hemagglutination, complement fixation, dot immunobinding, and ELISA) are specific and sensitive, yielding positive results in 80% or more of cases of hepatic hydatid cyst. Although routine chest or abdominal radiographs can show a mass, sometimes with a calcific rim, sonography and CT are favored for imaging hydatid cysts. The presence of calcification and daughter cysts within the parent cyst suggests echinococcosis. In endemic areas, serologic testing should precede needling of any likely hydatid cyst.

The classic treatment of hydatid cysts is operative. The surgical aim is to remove any cysts without disseminating the organism. At operation, the cyst is drained of fluid through a cannula, after the operative field is carefully protected from fluid leakage. If the aspirate is clear, a parasiticidal fluid (e.g., ethyl alcohol or 20% sterile saline solution) is injected into the cyst to kill any adherent scoleces. If the cyst fluid is bilious, ethyl alcohol or hypertonic saline solution is not injected to avoid infusing irritant solution into the biliary tree. The cyst contents and pericystic wall are then removed with careful dissection. Surgery is often combined with administration of the scolecidal agent benzimidazole albendazole. Recently, investigators reported a randomized controlled trial in which the combination of albendazole (10 mg/kg per day for 8 weeks) plus careful percutaneous drainage under sonographic guidance was compared with surgical cystectomy plus albendazole (3). They found albendazole plus sonographic drainage to be just as effective as albendazole and surgical cystectomy in reducing cyst size, causing cysts to disappear, and reducing echinococcal antibody titers during a mean follow-up period of 17 months (3). Furthermore, the less invasive course was associated with fewer side effects and shorter hospital stays. It appears that percutaneous drainage and albendazole should now be considered the treatment of first choice for hydatid cysts.

SCHISTOSOMAL HEPATIC DISEASE

Schistosomiasis resulting from invasion by *Schistosoma mansoni* and *Schistosoma japonicum* is an important cause of portal hypertension worldwide. Two distinct syndromes can be recognized. Acute schistosomiasis occurs soon after cercariae enter the human host by penetrating the skin. Early manifestations include an irritating maculopapular rash that lasts for several days. After an incubation period of 1 to 2 months, a systemic syndrome of lassitude, anorexia, and gastrointestinal upset with intermittent fevers, chills, sweating, headache, diarrhea, muscle aches, and bronchospasm develops. In rare cases, an acute abdomen and jaundice may develop. On clinical examination, hepatomegaly, moderate splenomegaly, and generalized lymphadenopathy are recognized. Sigmoidoscopy shows a red edematous mucosa with fine granulation, petechiae, and ulcers. Diagnosis is established by revealing ova in the stool or ova trapped within the submucosa of the rectum. Acute syndromes are seen most frequently in nonimmune visitors to endemic areas. Occasionally, acute infection can produce widespread granulomatous necrosis and even death.

In contrast, chronic schistosomiasis is usually asymptomatic until variceal hemorrhage occurs. Ascites is less common. Hepatosplenomegaly is progressive, and the spleen can become large, with resultant hypersplenism. The typical manifestations of chronic liver insufficiency (e.g., jaundice, spider angiomas, palmar erythema, gynecomastia) are unusual in chronic schistosomiasis unless an additional cause of parenchymal liver disease is present, such as chronic hepatitis C infection. Laboratory features include eosinophilia, hypoalbuminemia, hypergammaglobulinemia, and elevated serum alkaline phosphatase. Serum transaminase levels are usually normal. Inspecting the feces for ova is the diagnostic test of choice.

Praziquantel is the preferred agent for treating schistosomiasis in adults and children. Bleeding esophageal varices associated with schistosomiasis should be treated with the same variety of therapies used to manage variceal hemorrhage of other causes.

VIRAL HEPATITIS

The five viruses that cause acute viral hepatitis are hepatitis A virus (HAV); hepatitis B virus (HBV); hepatitis C virus (HCV), which was formerly called *non-A, non-B (NANB) hepatitis virus;* hepatitis D virus (HDV), formerly called *delta hepatitis virus;* and hepatitis E virus (HEV), formerly called *epidemic waterborne NANB hepatitis virus.* Table 36.1 summarizes the characteristics of these viruses, their modes of transmission, and the consequences of infection. Two other candidate hepatotropic viruses, designated *hepatitis G virus (HGV)* and *TT virus,* do not appear to be injurious to the liver and will not be considered further. Other viruses that can cause acute hepatitis (e.g., Epstein-Barr virus, cytomegalovirus, herpes simplex virus, and varicella virus) are described elsewhere in the text.

Hepatitis A Virus

Although epidemic community-acquired jaundice was recognized centuries ago, HAV was not identified until 1973. Since then, HAV has been propagated in cell culture, and the complete genome has been cloned (4). HAV

Table 36.1. **CHARACTERISTICS OF VIRUSES**

Virus	Genus	Genome	Genome length (kb)	Mode of transmission	Incubation* (d) Mean	Incubation* (d) Range	Consequences of Infection Acute hepatitis	Consequences of Infection Fulminant hepatic failure	Consequences of Infection Chronic hepatitis	Consequences of Infection Hepatoma	Post-transplantation Infection Recipient to allograft	Post-transplantation Infection New acquisition
Hepatitis A	Picornavirus	RNA	7.5	Fecal–oral Parenteral	28	15–50	Yes	Yes	No	No	No	No
Hepatitis B	Hepadnavirus	DNA	3.2	Parenteral Venereal ? Fecal–oral	84	28–160	Yes	Yes	Yes	Yes	Yes	Yes
Hepatitis C	Flavivirus	RNA	10.2	Parenteral ? Venereal ? Fecal–oral	56	14–160	Yes	Probable	Yes	Yes	Yes	Yes
Hepatitis D	Viroid	RNA	1.67	Parenteral	—	—	Yes	Yes	Yes	No	Yes	Uncertain
Hepatitis E	Probably calicivirus	RNA	7.6	Fecal–oral	40	22–60	Yes	Yes†	No	No	Uncertain	No

*Time from exposure to clinical hepatitis.
†Especially in pregnant women in third trimester.

is a member of the picornavirus family, which also includes poliovirus, coxsackievirus, echovirus, and rhinovirus. HAV is a nonenveloped particle about 27 nm in diameter. It contains a single-stranded RNA genome, 7.5 kb (kilobases) in size, that encodes a number of proteins. It is a robust virus and is stable at 60°C for 1 hour. Only one serotype is known for HAV.

Humans appear to be the only host for HAV infection, although other primates have been infected experimentally. The principal mode of transmission of HAV infection is fecal–oral, although parenteral transmission is also possible. Occasional outbreaks in the developed world have been attributed to contaminated foodstuffs and shellfish. The liver is the only organ of injury for HAV, and HAV genomic replication occurs exclusively in the cytoplasm of the infected hepatocyte. HAV is shed from the hepatocyte into the bile canaliculi, with passage of free virus into the feces. The mechanisms whereby HAV causes liver injury are incompletely understood. An initial phase of viral replication, in which the virus is not cytopathic, may be followed by a phase of immune-mediated liver injury associated with the emergence of anti-HAV immunoglobulin M (IgM) and a decline in HAV production.

Hepatitis A viral infections can produce either anicteric or icteric clinical syndromes (Fig. 36.3). In general, the frequency of anicteric infection is greater in children than in

adults. Similarly, when the icteric form of HAV infection develops in children, the illness is often milder than in adults. The incubation period is usually about 28 days. The initial prodrome consists of malaise, arthralgia, myalgia, anorexia, and loss of taste for food. In HAV infection, the prodrome may also include coryza, headache, photophobia, fever, and pharyngitis. Before the onset of jaundice, the patient may notice dark urine and pale stools. In many patients, epigastric or right upper quadrant pain develops that is accompanied by diarrhea. This anicteric prodrome may persist from 2 days to 3 weeks. When it subsides without progression to overt jaundice, as it may in young patients, the illness is often attributed to influenza. With the onset of jaundice, the described constitutional features subside. On examination, the liver may be enlarged and slightly tender. Spider angiomas may develop acutely but disappear with the resolution of the hepatitis. Clinical jaundice persists for 1 to 6 weeks. Lassitude is commonly described in adults after hepatitis A and may last for months.

Fecal shedding of HAV usually occurs for about 7 to 10 days before and after the onset of jaundice (Fig. 36.3). Measurement of serum transaminases usually reveals levels above 1,000 IU/mL. The differential diagnosis includes any acute viral hepatitis and the many forms of acute toxic, autoimmune, or ischemic hepatic injury. Serum anti-HAV IgM is usually detectable when jaundice appears and strongly indicates the diagnosis. Elevated titers of anti-HAV IgM may persist for months. The IgG fraction of anti-HAV rises as jaundice subsides, and this elevation persists for years. Liver biopsy is rarely required to make the diagnosis, but if performed, it demonstrates periportal and lobular infiltration by lymphocytes and macrophages associated with parenchymal injury. Hepatocellular injury is characterized by balloon degeneration of hepatocytes, acidophil bodies (apoptotic hepatocytes), and hepatocyte dropout. These changes lead to a loss of the normal hepatic lobular architecture.

Serious consequences of HAV infections are uncommon. Fulminant hepatic failure can develop rarely in patients with HAV infection (see later discussion). Although occasional patients who have recovered from a typical HAV infection relapse 7 to 10 weeks after the initial rapid recovery, no chronic carrier state of HAV infection has been identified, and HAV does not cause chronic active hepatitis or cirrhosis. HAV infection is not associated with the development of hepatoma. Recently, acute HAV infection has been implicated in the development of liver failure in

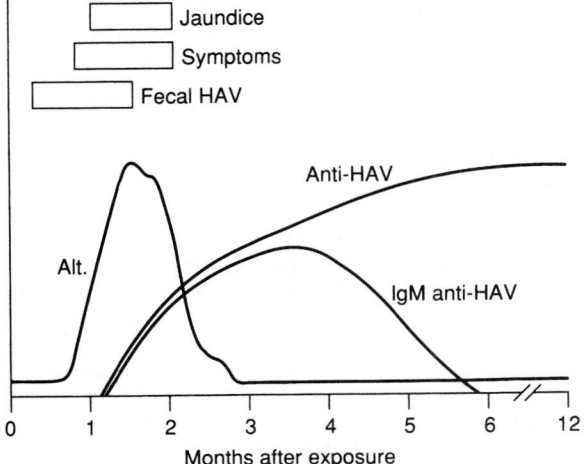

Figure 36.3. Clinical course of hepatitis A infection.

patients with chronic HCV infection. All that is required for treating most patients with HAV infection is simple nursing care, adequate nutrition, and attention to hygiene after defecation.

A formalin-inactivated HAV vaccine, in which immunogenicity has been enhanced by conjugation with alum, has been licensed in many countries. Studies of this and another similar vaccine have shown that it is highly immunogenic, inducing an immune response in 95.7% and 99.8% of persons after one and two doses, respectively (5). The recommended dosage protocol is for two doses to be given 2 to 4 weeks apart. A booster injection given 6 to 12 months later provides longer protection, perhaps for many years. Field trials among at-risk children have shown that the vaccine is highly effective in preventing clinical HAV infection. The vaccine is safe, and only minor side effects have been reported. The availability of HAV vaccination makes redundant previous advice about HAV prophylaxis with immunoglobulin. Vaccination should be recommended for travelers to endemic areas and for persons, such as sewage workers, whose occupation places them at high risk for exposure to HAV. Investigators have advocated routine vaccination of all children above the age of 2 years (4).

Passive prophylaxis with intramuscular injection of immune globulin is recommended for susceptible (negative for anti-HAV IgG and anti-HAV IgM) persons, such as employees of day care centers and custodial homes where acute HAV infection has been diagnosed in the people with whom they have contact. The Centers for Disease Control does not recommend administering immune globulin to susceptible persons more than 2 weeks after exposure.

Hepatitis B Virus

Hepatitis B virus is a member of the hepadnavirus family, which includes the closely related woodchuck hepatitis virus, ground squirrel hepatitis virus, and duck hepatitis virus (6). All hepadnaviruses contain a partially double-stranded DNA genome of 3,200 base pairs and are packaged in a virion that contains an outer surface coat and an inner core nucleocapsid. HBV is similar to retroviruses in that viral replication is accomplished by a process in which viral DNA polymerase acts as a reverse transcriptase. As a result of overlapping reading frames, the genome encodes multiple proteins, including the core protein called *hepatitis B core antigen (HBcAg),* a second protein product of the reading frame encoding the core protein called *hepatitis B early antigen (HBeAg),* a surface coat protein called *hepatitis B surface antigen (HBsAg),* DNA polymerase, and a transactivating protein called *protein X* (Fig. 36.4). The initiation of transcription at one of two upstream initiation sites can generate longer forms of HBsAg: pre-S2, which has an extra 88-amino acid segment, and pre-S1, which has an extra 128-amino acid segment. Both HBcAg and HBeAg are encoded by a common gene having two initiation codons for protein synthesis. The product of protein synthesis initiated at the first (pre-C) codon is HBeAg, which undergoes posttranslational processing in the endoplasmic reticulum and is then actively secreted out of the hepatocyte. HBeAg is useful clinically as a serum marker of viral replication. In contrast, protein synthesis initiated at the second start (C) codon yields HBcAg, which accumulates in the cytoplasm of the infected hepatocyte and is utilized for incorporation in complete virions.

Mutant forms of HBV arise from spontaneous alterations in the genome (7). In perhaps the most frequent type, sometimes called the *precore mutant virus,* the mutation affects the precore region of the genome. In patients in-

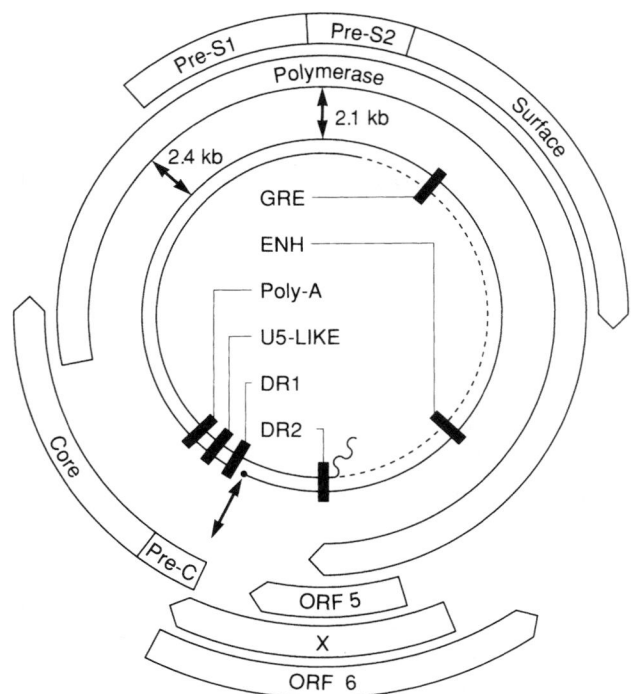

Figure 36.4. Hepatitis B viral genome.

fected with precore mutant viruses, transcription of the precore region is prevented as the result of a base pair alteration in that region of the genome, and consequently, elaboration of HBeAg does not occur. Instead, anti-HBe antibody is usually present. Nonetheless, despite the precore mutation, as a result of the initiation of transcription at the C start codon, active viral replication occurs without the formation of HBeAg. In these circumstances, active viral replication is recognizable, despite the absence of HBeAg, by the recognition of serum HBV DNA by standard hybridization methods. When precore (or HBeAg-nonsecreting) viral mutants were first identified, they were thought to be associated with aggressive hepatitis and fulminant hepatic failure. More recently, it has become clear that precore mutants are more widespread and frequently coexist with wild-type HBV forms, particularly during seroconversion from HBeAg-positive to anti-HBe–positive status.

A mutation in the tyrosine methionine aspartate aspartate (YMDD) locus of the RNA-dependent DNA polymerase gene has been recognized in patients receiving the antiviral agent lamivudine (8). This mutation has also been observed HIV-infected patients treated with lamivudine. Other mutant forms of HBV that involve amino acid substitution in the *a* determinant of HBsAg have been described as occurring during "immune pressure" from passive or active immunization.

Hepatitis B virus is spread by parenteral routes and by intimate personal contact. Vertical transmission from mother to infant is an important problem in the developing world. HBV is hepatotropic, and the hepatocyte is the principal site of viral replication. The mechanism whereby HBV enters the hepatocyte is unknown. Extrahepatic cellular infection can occur and may account for persistence of infection in some circumstances, such as after hepatic transplantation. In general, HBV does not appear to be cytopathic to the hepatocyte. Rather, HBV hepatitis begins as an antigen-specific antiviral cellular immune response that initiates a sequence of nonspecific cellular and molecular immune effector mechanisms that combine to cause liver damage. Current research is focused on the nature of the immune mechanisms that dictate the course of acute infection, the factors that influence the development of viral clearance or persistence, the progression to either benign chronic carriage of the virus or progressive injury, including cirrhosis and hepatoma, and finally the genesis of escape mutants. In some circumstances, such as hepatitis B in liver allografts, the virus appears to have a direct cytopathic effect.

The onset of acute hepatitis B is often insidious (Fig. 36.5). Many cases are asymptomatic and are recognized by serologic survey of asymptomatic persons during an outbreak. Commonly, a diagnosis of previous acute HBV infection is made in a patient with newly diagnosed chronic hepatitis B. The incubation of HBV is about 8 weeks. The first serum indicator of infection by HBV is serum HBsAg, which may precede the onset of jaundice. When anicteric hepatitis develops, it is indistinguishable from acute HAV infection, described previously. Acute HBV infection is accompanied by the certain serum and liver markers of viral replication: serum HBV DNA, serum HBV DNA polymerase, serum HBeAg, liver HBV DNA, and liver HBcAg. With the onset of clinical hepatitis, serum anti-HBc IgM becomes detectable. In most persons, when HBV infection is self-limited and does not progress to chronic hepatitis, anti-HBc IgM does not persist for more then 6 months after HBV is acquired. Thus, serum anti-HBc IgM is used to distinguish acute from chronic hepatitis B. Unfortunately, anti-HBc IgM occasionally persists for years after acute infection or may recur as an amnestic phenomenon in reactivating chronic active hepatitis B. It is therefore an imperfect marker for acute infection.

The outcome of acute HBV infection of adults in the Western world (low carrier rate) is shown in Fig. 36.6. Most patients have subclinical infections with complete recovery. About 25% experience clinical jaundice that resolves without development of the carrier state. After recovery, patients retain antibodies to one or more hepatitis B epitopes; anti-HBc and anti-HBs are the most common. These patients are negative for HbsAg and HBV DNA on standard assays. Patients with acute HBV infection rarely proceed to fulminant hepatic failure. In some 10% of patients with acute HBV infection, whether subclinical or clinical, a chronic carrier state develops. The carrier state

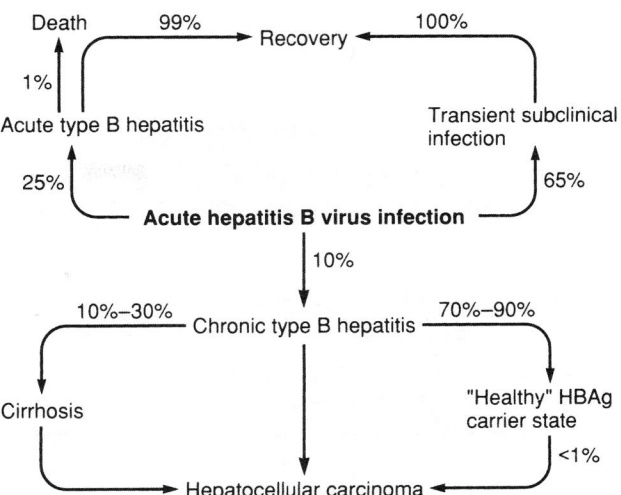

Figure 36.6. Common outcomes of acute hepatitis B.

is defined by the presence of HBsAg in serum for longer than 6 months.

A characteristic of hepadnaviruses is the ability to cause chronic infections in which viral particles persist in the liver. Chronic HBV infection exists in two interrelated forms. Most patients have a benign carrier state, in which an excess of HBsAg is produced in the liver but no evidence of ongoing liver injury or active viral replication is found on standard testing. A smaller proportion of HBV carriers has evidence of ongoing active viral replication and clinical features of chronic active hepatitis (Fig. 36.7).

Hepatic histology in benign chronic HBV carriers with chronic hepatitis shows hepatocytes with a ground-glass appearance as a result of excess cytoplasmic HBsAg proteins (Fig. 36.8). Inflammation may not be present, or it may be confined to the portal triad without evidence of liver injury. In contrast, chronic HBV carriers with progressive liver injury (previously called *chronic active hepatitis*) usually have serum markers of active viral replication (e.g., HBeAg or HBV DNA) and ongoing liver injury (e.g., elevation of serum transaminase levels), and a histologic pattern of active inflammation. Molecular hybridization studies of liver tissue demonstrate HBV DNA sequences integrated into the native genome in benign chronic carriers. In contrast, patients with chronic HBV infection associated with active replication and ongoing hepatitis have HBV sequences existing as free episomal HBV DNA in addition to genomic integration.

Chronic replicative hepatitis B can progress to cirrhosis. Patients with chronic hepatitis B can sometimes spontaneously become benign chronic carriers. This seroconversion is often accompanied by an acute exacerbation of hepatitis, with a typical viral syndrome and elevated levels of transaminases. A similar phenomenon is observed when seroconversion is induced by interferon therapy. Spontaneous reactivation of chronic HBV infection resulting in seroconversion from the benign chronic carrier state to chronic liver injury with serum markers of active viral replication also occurs. This may be accompanied by elevated transaminases and progressive liver damage. Consequently, acute hepatitis might develop in a patient with HBV infection for several reasons. These include acute onset of HBV infection, acute exacerbation of chronic hepatitis B, seroconversion of chronic hepatitis B with acute replication to the benign chronic HBV carrier state, reactivation of chronic benign HBV carriage, and acquisition of other infections (e.g., HAV, HCV, CMV). One example of

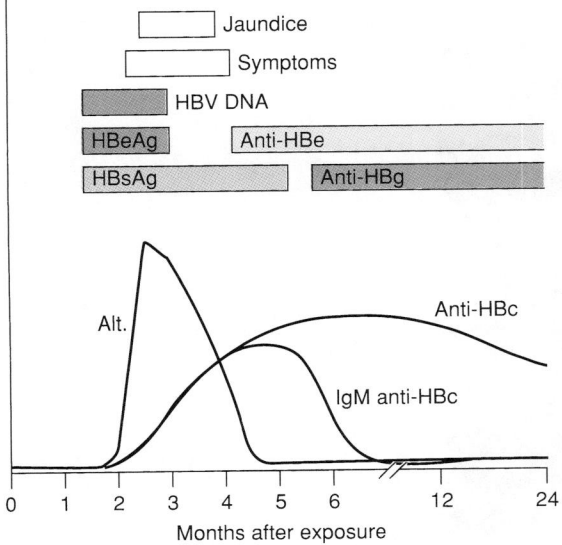

Figure 36.5. Clinical course of acute hepatitis B infection.

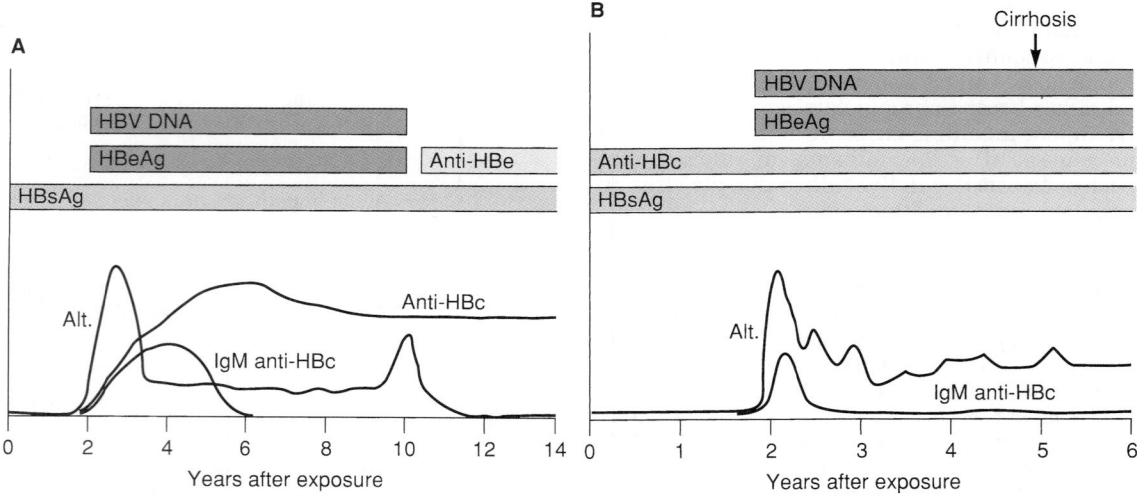

Figure 36.7. Clinical course of chronic hepatitis B. *(A)* A benign chronic carrier has continued production of hepatitis B surface antigen but an absence of serum markers of viral replication. *(B)* A pattern of continuing liver injury and serum markers of active viral replication.

the latter phenomenon is superinfection by HDV in chronic HBV carriers (see later discussion).

Hepatoma is an important consequence of chronic HBV infection, usually after a lead time of 10 to 20 years. It appears to result from concordance of the following factors:

Male sex
Cirrhosis
Infection with HBV or HCV
Inherited disorders, such as hemochromatosis or tyrosinemia
Environmental exposure to the procarcinogen aflatoxin

Hepatoma also complicates chronic HCV infection, and HCV may contribute to hepatoma development in areas where HBV is endemic.

The best treatment for HBV infection is primary prevention by vaccination. High-risk persons include all health care workers, those who have had sexual contacts with an acutely infected person or chronic carrier, those who share a household with persons at risk for parenteral exposure to HBV (e.g., patients with thalassemia, hemophiliacs, intra-

venous drug abusers), and visitors to areas where the disease is highly endemic. All people who have had susceptible household or sexual contact with a person having a positive serum test result for HBsAg should be unequivocally advised to receive a full course of HBV vaccine, whether or not the index case expresses serum markers of viral replication. Sexual contacts of an index case should also receive passive prophylaxis with hepatitis B immunoglobulin (HBIG) and should use condoms during sexual intercourse until the contact has demonstrated an adequate immune response to HBV vaccination. Similarly, susceptible contacts who have had a recent potential parenteral exposure (e.g., accidental needle stick, shared needles) should receive HBIG. The risk for transmission of HBV to intimate contacts from persons with serologic evidence of previous HBV infection but no markers of chronic carriage (i.e., anti-HBs–positive, anti-HBc–positive, or HBsAg-negative status) is low except in special circumstances, such as immunosuppression for solid organ transplantation.

Hepatitis B vaccines are so safe and efficacious that universal HBV vaccination in North America is appropriate.

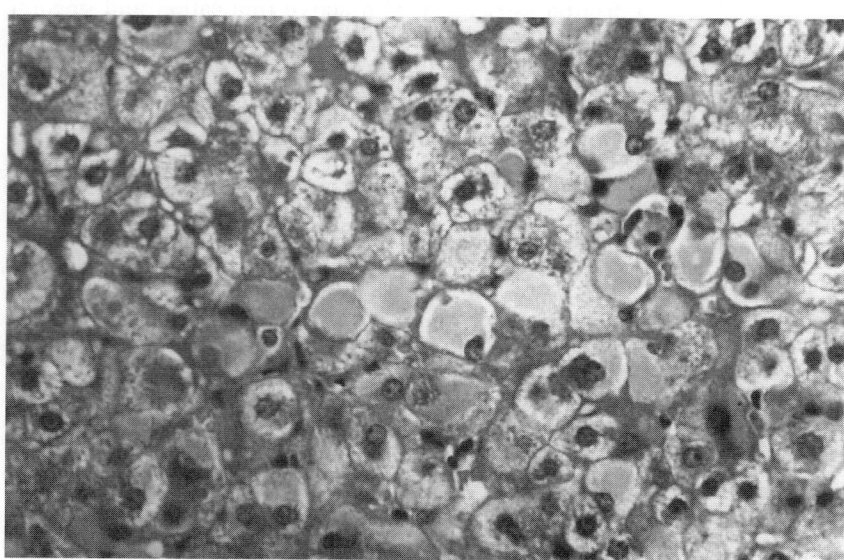

Figure 36.8. Photomicrograph of ground-glass hepatocytes. H&E stain.

Vertical transmission from a chronically infected mother during parturition can almost always be prevented by early recognition of the mother's carrier status and administration of HBIG and vaccine to the newborn infant.

No established treatment strategies ameliorate acute HBV infection or prevent its progression to chronic infection. Patients with HBV-induced fulminant hepatic failure may require liver transplantation. The utitity of lamivudine and similar antiviral agents (famciclovir, adefovir) in patients with acute hepatitis B is uncertain. Because most patients clear the virus without specific therapy and become immune to further infection, antivirals are not usually necessary. Chronic HBV carriers with no markers of active viral replication should not receive interferon therapy. Clinical trials have demonstrated that 500 million IU of interferon alfa per day given subcutaneously for 3 to 4 months induces seroconversion from HBeAg and HBV DNA positivity to anti-HBe positivity and HBV DNA negativity in about one third of stable patients with chronic active hepatitis B. In 10% of these patients, HBsAg is cleared from the serum. An initial response is more common in patients with a moderate viral load, an active inflammatory response [i.e., alanine aminotransferase (ALT) level >200 IU/L], and an absence of HIV. Asian patients with chronic HBV infection are infrequent responders to interferon alfa. The role of antiviral agents in managing replicative chronic hepatitis B infection remains in doubt. However, the chances that lamivudine will induce a complete seroconversion from HBV DNA and HBeAg positivity to HBV DNA negativity and anti-HBe positivity are greatest in patients with high serum levels of ALT, indicative of an ongoing T lymphocyte-mediated immune response to the infected hepatocytes (9). The optimal duration of lamivudine therapy, the utility of combining lamivudine with interferon or other antiviral agents, and the clinical significance of the YMDD mutants that arise during long-term lamivudine administration to immunocompetent patients with chronic HBV infection have yet to be clarified.

Liver transplantation is the treatment of choice for patients with chronic HBV infection that has led to liver failure. Recurrence of HBV infection is effectively controlled by the serial administration of hyperimmune gamma globulin (HBIG) for life (10). Most programs add lamivudine to the protocol, although the data to support its use in this setting are largely anecdotal. Many transplant programs use livers from HBsAg-negative, anti-HBc–positive donors for transplantation into HBV-naïve recipients. If prophylaxis with HBIg and lamivudine is not given, the chance for active HBV replication being stimulated in these livers under the influence of immunosuppression is 50%.

Hepatitis C

Infection with HCV is responsible for more than 90% of cases of posttransfusion NANB hepatitis and for most sporadic cases of NANB hepatitis throughout the world. It presents a public health catastrophe of enormous proportions. Recent estimates suggest that 1.8% of the U.S. population, accounting for 3.9 million persons, is currently or has been chronically infected with HCV and that 2.7 million persons are viremic (11).

Hepatitis C virus is a lipid-enveloped, single-stranded positive-sense RNA virus with a genome of 9.4 kb. It is a member of the flavivirus family. A single, large, open reading frame encodes a large viral precursor polyprotein from which individual viral proteins are cleaved. These proteins are both structural and nonstructural. The structural proteins include a nucleocapsid core protein and two envelope proteins, termed *E1* and *E2*, which coat the

virus. The nonstructural proteins are essential to viral replication and include a viral protease, helicase, and an RNA-dependent RNA polymerase. Based on nucleic acid sequencing, six major genotypes have been identified, with further subdivision into at least 15 subtypes. Patients are infected by one genotypic form of the virus only. Worldwide geographic variation has been noted with regard to the predominant genotypic forms of HCV in different areas. More than 70% of patients in the United States are infected with genotype 1 virus. The most important clinical impact of genotype status appears to be that it influences responsiveness to interferon alfa therapy.

The most common identifiable sources of HCV acquisition in the United States are a prior transfusion of blood or blood-derived products and a history of illicit intravenous drug use (12). Sexual transmission of HCV is less commonly observed than of HBV, although a history of multiple sexual partners is associated with chronic HCV infection. The Centers for Disease Control do not advise monogamous couples to modify their sexual practices when one partner is infected with HCV. Rare anecdotal cases of transmission of HCV have been reported in renal dialysis units, by contaminated endoscopic instruments, or by an HCV-infected surgeon. No source can be identified in as many as 40% of chronically infected persons (13,14).

The usual incubation period of posttransfusion HCV infection is from 5 to 10 weeks (14). The initial elevated ALT level ranges from 500 to 1,000 IU/L and may be associated with little or no clinical disturbance. Viral replication coincides with this initial episode of hepatitis, often with very high viral RNA titers (Fig. 36.9). Commonly, anti-HCV antibody does not appear until 18 weeks after the initial posttransfusion hepatic illness. In some persons, acute HCV infection does not progress to chronic infection, and anti-HCV antibody may or may not appear in the serum. Chronic infection develops in between 55% and 70% of persons who contract HCV infection from blood products (and probably in sporadic cases also) (15). Chronic HCV infection is usually characterized by an indolent clinical syndrome in which the transaminase levels fluctuate from normal to 200 to 400 IU/L (Fig. 36.10), and at this time, viral replication is usually detectable by polymerase chain reaction amplification of HCV in serum. The quantitative levels of HCV RNA vary, however, and even qualitative HCV RNA can become undetectable for periods, only to reappear later. Patients can harbor HCV for many years

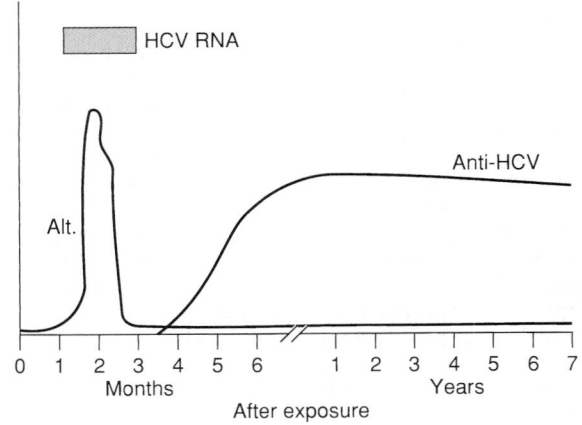

Figure 36.9. Clinical course in acute posttransfusion non-A, non-B hepatitis (hepatitis C).

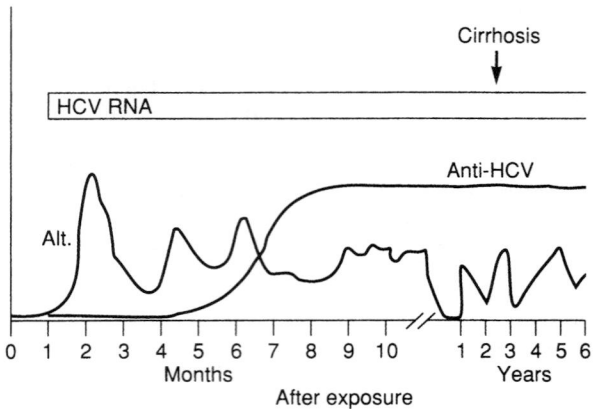

Figure 36.10. Clinical course in chronic posttransfusion non-A, non-B hepatitis (hepatitis C).

without apparent clinical ill effects, even in the absence of fluctuating mild elevations of liver enzymes. Almost invariably, a liver biopsy shows some degree of chronic hepatitis. Typical histologic features of chronic HCV infection include a lymphocytic infiltrate in the portal triads, bile duct injury, acidophil bodies, and macrovesicular fat deposition.

Although it is traditional to think of chronic HCV infection as a *chronic hepatitis,* chronic HCV infection is more appropriately considered a disease of *progressive fibrosis* (13,16). The main harmful effects on the liver of chronic HCV infection are caused by fibrosis progressing to cirrhosis and liver failure. The development of hepatocellular carcinoma is also a consequence of fibrosis/cirrhosis. Many factors can predispose a patient to the development of fibrosis. Poynard et al. (16) used a cross-sectional study technique to identify three independent factors associated with an increased rate of progression of fibrosis: age at acquisition of HCV infection exceeding 40 years, daily alcohol intake exceeding 50 g, and male sex. HCV genotype did not correlate with degree or rate of fibrosis. On average, the interval from acquisition to recognition of cirrhosis is on the order of 20 to 30 years. However, in the data of Poynard et al., the interval to the development of cirrhosis declines to 13 years in men infected after age 40 and extends to 42 years in women, abstinent from alcohol, infected before age 40.

Mortality in chronic HCV infection is influenced by many of the same factors associated with development of fibrosis. In a prospective study of 838 persons positive for both anti-HCV antibodies and HCV RNA who were followed for an average of 4 years, mortality was increased by cirrhosis, long duration of infection, a history of intravenous drug abuse, or excessive alcohol consumption (13). Survival was increased by treatment with interferon alfa. In that cohort study, serum levels of ALT and bilirubin, patient sex, and viral genotype had no effect on survival. Understanding the factors that promote fibrogenesis helps explain the conflicting data regarding whether HCV infection alters life expectancy. For example, the Irish cohort of women infected by contaminated gamma globulin have many favorable factors for a slow rate of progression to fibrosis (female sex, exposure at a young age, lack of exposure to alcohol, absence of intravenous drug abuse), so it is not surprising that they have yet to manifest significant mortality despite nearly 20 years of follow-up (15,16).

Infection with HCV has been associated with many extrahepatic clinical phenomena, including the following:

Leukocytoclastic vasculitis
Membranoproliferative glomerulonephritis
Mixed cryoglobulinemia
Thyroiditis
Sjögren's syndrome
Porphyria cutanea tarda
Mooren's ulcer
Lichen planus

Some of these phenomena occur in combination, such as mixed cryoglobulinemia, leukocytoclastic vasculitis, and glomerulonephritis. In addition, B-cell lymphomas have been reported in patients with cryoglobulinemia associated with chronic HCV infection. Recent studies have noted an unexpected prevalence of insulin-dependent diabetes among patients with HCV infection.

The most concerning complications of chronic HCV infection are advancing liver failure and primary hepatocellular carcinoma (13,17). Cirrhosis must be present for either to occur. Cirrhosis is the most important factor in determining reduced survival in chronic HCV infection. Hepatic decompensation, as indicated by the onset of ascites, jaundice, variceal hemorrhage, or hepatic encephalopathy, occurs in approximately 20% of compensated cirrhotic patients within 5 years (13). Cirrhosis is the key element in the progression of HCV infection to hepatocellular carcinoma (13). The duration of infection before the development of hepatocellular carcinoma depends on the rate of progression of fibrosis. The accrual rate is 7% at 5 years among patients with chronic HCV infection and established cirrhosis (17).

All HCV-infected persons should be advised to abstain from alcohol. Interferon alfa, in the standard dosage schedule of 3 million IU given three times per week, was the first therapy for chronic hepatitis C to be approved by the Food and Drug Administration. At first, interferon alfa was associated with a restoration of liver enzymes to the normal range, loss of detectable HCV RNA in serum, and clinical improvement in extrahepatic manifestations, such as cryoglobulinemia or membranoproliferative glomerulonephritis. Unfortunately, the biochemical and virologic response to interferon alone was usually transient, and the liver enzyme and serum HCV RNA levels usually relapsed either during therapy or after interferon had been stopped. This was particularly true of patients infected by genotype 1 virus. Consequently, in more recent studies, response to therapy has been defined more stringently as end-treatment response and sustained response. End-treatment response indicates that no viral RNA can be measured in serum and that liver enzymes are in the normal range when the treatment period is complete. Sustained response indicates the same features 6 months after treatment is finished. It appears that most patients with a true sustained response have eradicated the virus.

Ribavirin is an oral antiviral agent that has no measurable antiviral effect when used as a single agent in infected persons. However, many studies have indicated that a combination of interferon alfa and ribavirin has increased efficacy against chronic hepatitis C (18,19). The genotype of the virus predicts the likelihood of a sustained response to combination therapy. Approximately 30% of interferon-naïve patients infected with genotype 1 virus demonstrate a sustained response after 48 weeks of therapy. A sustained response rate of nearly 70% is achieved in interferon-naïve patients infected with genotype 2 or 3 who are treated with combination therapy for 24 weeks. Interferon alfa plus ribavirin has achieved a sustained clearance of virus in patients who previously relapsed on interferon alone, the best results once again being observed with genotype 2 or 3 (20). Interferon and ribavirin are associated with many unwanted effects, including hemolysis, flulike symptoms, malaise, irritability, and autoimmune thyroiditis. No consensus exists on how best to proceed once an HCV-infected patient has relapsed or failed to respond to interferon plus ribavirin, or who is unable to tolerate the side effects. Options include consensus interferon, experimental agents including depot interferon linked to polyethylene glycol, and doing nothing while waiting for better agents.

The previous discussion has been limited to eradication of the virus as the sole goal of therapy. However, suggestive data indicate that interferon alfa may arrest or reverse fibrosis, even when the virus is not eradicated. Finally, emerging data suggest that interferon alfa reduces the rate of development of hepatocellular carcinoma (21).

Liver transplantation is the treatment of choice for patients with incapacitating liver failure caused by chronic HCV infection, or with localized but unresectable hepatocellular carcinoma. HCV always infects the allograft. Survival in the first 5 years is unchanged in comparison with the survival of other transplant recipients (22). The rate of fibrosis in liver transplant recipients infected with hepatitis C is increased at 5 years, and it is likely that this will affect long-term survival. In occasional patients, a progressive hepatitis with cholestasis and fibrosis develops that is usually fatal unless re-transplantation is performed. The outcome of re-transplantion for HCV infection is mixed, and sometimes the subsequent graft is rapidly lost.

Hepatitis D

Hepatitis D (or delta hepatitis) is caused by an incomplete viruslike particle similar to viroids and related satellite RNAs of plants. Like viroids, the genome of HDV is a covalently closed RNA circle consisting of 1.67 kb. This is smaller than the genome of any conventional virus. HDV is found worldwide, and humans appear to be the only natural host.

Because of an association with HBV infection, HDV affects the same populations at risk for HBV infection. HDV requires simultaneous infection with HBV to complete its life cycle. HD antigen (HDAg) has been recovered from liver tissue infected by both viruses. Unlike HBV, however, HDV infects only the hepatocyte, and no other sites of replication have been identified. When detectable in serum, HDAg exists within HBsAg particles. The mechanism by which HDV gains access to HBV-infected hepatocytes is unknown. Similarly, the mechanisms of HDV-induced liver injury are unknown. Curiously, HDV appears to suppress HBV replication.

Hepatitis D viral infection acquired simultaneously with HBV infection is termed *coinfection* (Fig. 36.11). HDV may also infect a host in whom HBV infection already exists. This is called *superinfection* (Fig. 36.12). In general, coinfection is a mild, transient clinical phenomenon, sometimes recognizable only by later detection of anti-HBc IgM and anti-HDV IgM. A biphasic pattern of elevated transaminases may be noted, the first peak corresponding to acute HBV replication and the second peak corresponding to acute HDV replication. One circumstance in which the host receives a large inoculum of HBV and HDV is acute coinfection in an intravenous drug addict. In two community-based studies of acute coinfection associated with intravenous drug use, clinical hepatitis was common, and fulminant hepatic failure developed in some patients. Most patients with acute coinfection of HBV and HDV do not progress to chronic carriage of HDV, and some lose carriage of HBsAg also. Similarly, reinfection does not often develop after liver transplantation for

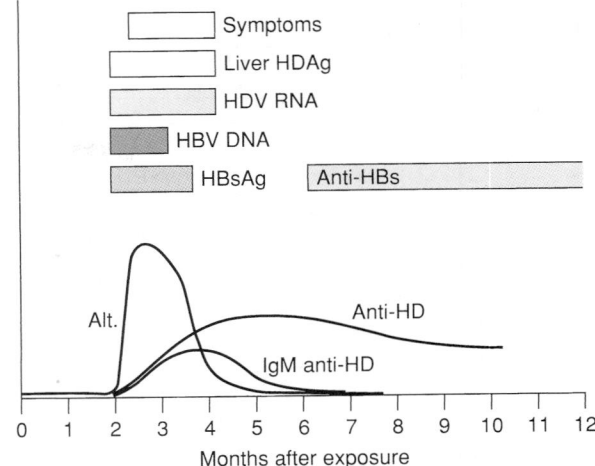

Figure 36.11. Synchronous infection with hepatitis B virus and hepatitis D virus.

fulminant hepatic failure caused by HBV and HDV, probably because of the suppressant effect of HDV on HBV.

Superinfection by HDV is an important cause of acute hepatitis in persons who already have chronic HBV infection. Superinfection may result from exposure to a small inoculum of HDV. Acquisition of acute HDV infection may result in seroconversion of HBsAg to anti-HBs and consequently loss of HDV infection also. Alternatively, chronic HDV and HBV infection may coexist (Fig. 36.13). Chronic hepatitis with progression to cirrhosis is one of the consequences of chronic HDV infection. Chronic hepatitis caused by HDV is associated with persistent HDV replication, which may be accompanied by HDV-induced suppression of HBV replication. An association of HDV with primary hepatocellular carcinoma has not been found.

Tests for HDV infection are limited in most centers to measurement of anti-HD IgM and IgG. In research settings, HDAg and HDV RNA can be measured in the serum and liver. In typical cases, after an incubation period of 4 to 20 weeks, a short period of viral replication and shedding of HDAg into serum occurs. Measurements of anti-HD IgM

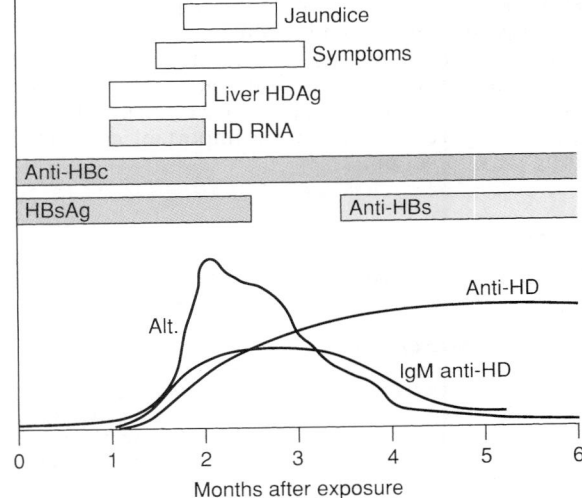

Figure 36.12. Superinfection of chronic hepatitis B carrier with hepatitis D.

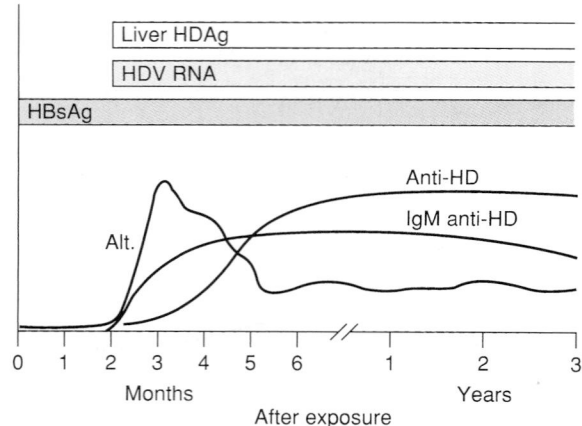

Figure 36.13. Clinical course of chronic hepatitis D infection.

has been reported to be variable in acute infection. Anti-HD IgG appears late in acute infection.

Interferon alfa has been used to treat chronic HDV infection (23). It appears that eradication of HBV and HDV is rare, even with high-dose therapy. A recrudescence of both viruses after interferon has been stopped is common, except in the rare instances in which HBsAg is cleared during or soon after therapy. HDV and HBV coinfection can recur after liver transplantation, although less often than HBV infection alone after transplantation.

Hepatitis E

Hepatitis E is a form of epidemic viral hepatitis previously called *waterborne NANB hepatitis* (24). It is an ecologically determined disease associated with fecal contamination of drinking water. Large epidemics have been reported in the Indian subcontinent, Africa, and Central America. Studies suggest that hepatitis E is caused by a unique virus with a single-stranded RNA genome of 7.6 kb that should probably be classified with the caliciviruses. It does not appear to be related to HAV or other picornaviruses.

The usual incubation period is 40 days. Transient cholestatic jaundice develops, followed by a complete recovery without chronic sequelae. An important exception is HEV infection during pregnancy. HEV has a predilection for pregnant women, in whom both the frequency and severity of infection are increased. Fulminant hepatic failure from to HEV infection is common in pregnant women during the third trimester. A clean water supply and the hygienic disposal of excreta are important goals in controlling HEV infection.

ACUTE HEPATIC FAILURE

Definitions

Acute hepatic injury refers to a sudden loss of hepatocyte mass, most usually caused by a toxin, ischemia, or an inflammatory reaction in the liver (25). Acute hepatic failure is manifested by a sudden increase in previously normal levels of liver transaminases. Typically, the serum level of ALT is more than 10 to 25 times the upper limits of the normal range. *Fulminant hepatic failure,* seen in a specific subgroup of patients with severe acute hepatic injury, is defined as the development of acute hepatic encephalopathy within 8 weeks after the onset of symptomatic hepatocellular disease in a previously healthy person. Submassive hepatic necrosis is similar to fulminant hepatic failure except that it is slower in onset. *Submassive hepatic necrosis* (synonyms: subfulminant hepatic failure, subacute hepatic failure) is defined as the development of acute hepatic encephalopathy within 9 to 24 weeks after the onset of symptomatic hepatocellular disease in a previously healthy person.

Clinical Features

Acute hepatic injury in the absence of hepatic encephalopathy always resolves, except when it is caused by other ongoing systemic disease or when the elevated transaminase levels represent the first manifestation of previously covert chronic liver disease. The incidence of acute hepatic injury is unknown. It is estimated that 2,000 cases of fulminant hepatic failure and submassive hepatic necrosis occur in the United States annually and that 80% of these patients die. Outcome is determined by the course of encephalopathy, which is classified according to four grades (Table 36.2). Cerebral edema, leading to increased intracranial pressure, is a common feature of severe fulminant hepatic failure and may cause permanent cerebral injury and death. Fulminant hepatic failure and submassive hepatic necrosis are always accompanied by severe coagulopathy.

The causes of fulminant hepatic failure are listed in Table 36.3. Wilson's disease is usually included among the causes of fulminant hepatic failure despite the fact that it is a covert chronic disorder. A history of heavy alcohol use also suggests chronic injury, even though alcoholics are at particular risk for acetaminophen-induced hepatic failure. A characteristic clinical scenario is the development of hepatic failure when an alcohol abuser stops drinking and 24 to 48 hours later has abdominal pain from gastritis or pancreatitis or headache from a hangover. This person then takes a standard dose of acetaminophen to soothe the symptoms and unwittingly produces acute hepatic injury. When presented with an apparent case of acute hepatic injury, the physician must always answer two questions: Is

Table 36.2. CLINICAL GRADES OF ACUTE HEPATIC ENCEPHALOPATHY

Grade	Mental state	Asterixus	Electroencephalogram result
I	Altered affect, subtle loss of mental acuity, slurred speech	Slight or none	Normal
II	Accentuation of stage I, confusion, drowsiness, inappropriate behavior, loss of sphincter control	Easily elicited	Abnormal, generalized slowing
III	Sleepy but rousable, marked confusion, can answer simple questions only	Present when patient can cooperate	Always abnormal
IV	Coma	Cannot cooperate	Always abnormal
	IVa—responds to pain		
	IVb—no response to pain		

Table 36.3. CAUSES OF FULMINANT HEPATIC FAILURE

VIRAL INFECTION

Hepatitis A
Hepatitis B
Hepatitis D
Other viruses (less common)
    Cytomegalovirus
    Epstein-Barr virus
    Varicella virus
    Herpesvirus

POISONS, CHEMICALS, AND DRUGS

Amanita phalloides
Acetaminophen
Tetracycline
Phosphorus
Halogenated volatile anesthetics (especially halothane)
Isoniazid
Methyldopa
Valproate
Monoamine oxidase inhibitors

ISCHEMIA AND HYPOXIA

Hepatic vascular occlusion
Acute circulatory stroke
Heat stroke
Gram-negative sepsis

MISCELLANEOUS

Acute fatty liver of pregnancy
Reye's syndrome
Wilson's disease
Hodgkin's disease and other lymphomas
Hereditary fructose intolerance
Galactosemia, tyrosinemia
Idiopathic (also called non-A non-B)

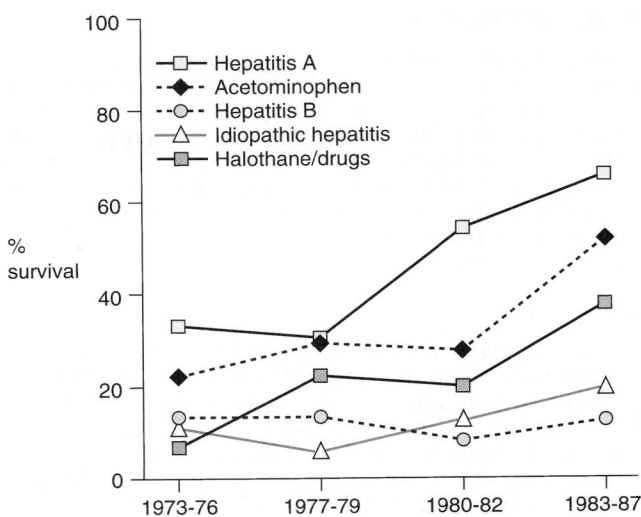

Figure 36.14. Survival of patients with fulminant hepatic failure leading to grade III or IV encephalopathy. The survival of patients with hepatitis A or B and acetaminophen-induced failure has improved with time, but not that of patients with halothane-induced failure or idiopathic hepatitis. (After O'Grady JG, Gimson AES, O'Brien CJ, et al. Controlled trials of charcoal hemoperfusion and prognostic factors in fulminant hepatic failure. *Gastroenterology* 1989;97:439, with permission.)

this really an acute illness or rather the first presentation of a previously unrecognized chronic disorder? Are single or multiple factors contributing to the acute hepatic injury?

Predicting Outcome in Fulminant Hepatic Failure and Subacute Hepatic Necrosis

In general, the deeper the coma, the worse the outcome. For example, patients in whom a grade III or IV coma develops have a higher mortality rate than patients with hepatic failure in whom encephalopathy never progresses beyond grade II. Paradoxically, the rapid onset of encephalopathy is a favorable prognostic sign (Fig. 36.14). Consequently, most patients with acetaminophen-induced fulminant hepatic failure who experience grade III coma recover spontaneously. Delay in the onset of encephalopathy after the onset of jaundice indicates a lack of spontaneous recovery and is an unfavorable prognostic factor. For this reason, submassive hepatic necrosis has a particularly poor outcome.

The criteria for determining the prognosis of fulminant hepatic failure are shown in Table 36.4 (26). This classification distinguishes between acetaminophen-induced fulminant hepatic failure and that from all other causes. Drug-induced hepatic failure, other than that caused by acetaminophen, has a poor prognosis. Examples include hepatic failure caused by phenytoin or halothane. HBV- and HAV-induced hepatic failure has a better outcome than idiopathic (presumed viral) fulminant hepatic fail-

ure. It is unclear whether HCV causes hepatic failure. Patients younger than 2 years or older than 40 years have a poor prognosis. Renal failure is also a poor prognostic factor. As mentioned, coagulopathy is always present. Some have recommended serum factor V levels as an indicator of when to proceed to transplant. A factor V level of less than 20% is a poor prognostic indicator (25). Acidosis is a poor prognostic factor, particularly in acetaminophen-induced fulminant hepatic failure.

Table 36.4. PROGNOSTIC CRITERIA FOR PREDICTING REQUIRED LIVER TRANSPLANTATION IN PATIENTS WITH FULMINANT HEPATIC FAILURE

Cause of liver failure	Criteria
Acetaminophen toxicity	pH <7.3 (irrespective of grade of encephalopathy) or Prothrombin time >50 s and serum creatinine >3.4 mg/dL (300 μmol/L) in patients with grade III or IV encephalopathy
All other causes	Prothrombin time >50 s (irrespective of grade of encephalopathy) or Any three of the following variables (irrespective of grade of encephalopathy): Age <10 y or >40 y Liver failure from halothane or other drug idiosyncrasy or idiopathic hepatitis Duration of jaundice before encephalopathy >7 d Prothrombin time >25 s Serum bilirubin >17.5 mg/dL (300 μmol/L)

Adapted from O'Grady JG, Alexander GJM, Hayllar KM, et al. Early indicators of prognosis in fulminant hepatic failure. Gastroenterology 1989;97:439, with permission.

Management

Patients with uncomplicated acute hepatic injury can be treated in their local hospitals, but their physicians may alert a transplant center so that expeditious transfer can be arranged should encephalopathy develop. All patients with fulminant hepatic failure should be transferred to an intensive care unit at a liver transplant center. Management of acute hepatic injury, including fulminant hepatic failure and submassive hepatic necrosis, should be directed as follows:

Diagnosis

Anti-HBc IgM, HBsAg, and anti-HAV IgM should be checked to identify patients with acute HBV and HAV infection. Antibodies to cytomegalovirus, Epstein-Barr virus, herpes simplex virus, and varicella virus should also be checked. Serum ceruloplasmin levels should be determined, and the eyes should be examined by slit lamp for corneal rings. A family history of early onset of liver or neurologic failure or a history of gradual intellectual deterioration may be a clue to Wilson's disease. An unusually low serum alkaline phosphatase level (<80 IU) may also indicate underlying Wilson's disease. The physician should look for toxic insults (e.g., *Amanita,* drugs) and consider the acute onset of chronic disease.

Specific Therapy

Patients with hepatic failure who have ingested acetaminophen should receive a full course of *N*-acetylcysteine (27,28). Unconfirmed evidence suggests that *N*-acetylcysteine may be beneficial even in hepatic failure that is unrelated to acetaminophen. Although considerable data are available to support a role for circulating benzodiazepines in the development of acute (and chronic) hepatic encephalopathy, flumazenil has no place in the treatment of fulminant hepatic failure except within a defined research protocol.

Avoidance of Renal Failure

Aminoglycosides, radiographic dye, and other potentially nephrotoxic agents should be used cautiously. Some practitioners advocate early introduction of dialysis for better management of fluid balance.

Metabolic Fluxes

Hepatic failure may be complicated by hypoglycemia and coma, which can be misinterpreted as cerebral edema. Correcting hypoglycemia in hepatic failure may require large amounts of dextrose. Hypokalemia and acidosis may also complicate hepatic failure.

Hematologic Stability

Coagulopathy should be corrected by the administration of fresh frozen plasma before invasive procedures are performed (placement of central lines, placement of intracranial pressure monitor) or whenever evidence of hemorrhage is present (intracranial hemorrhage, gastrointestinal bleeding). In most circumstances, it is not necessary to give fresh frozen plasma simply to correct a prolonged prothrombin time of up to 30 seconds.

Cardiorespiratory Status

Hypotension is common in fulminant hepatic failure despite a high cardiac output because of associated low systemic vascular resistance. Hypotension may exacerbate low cerebral perfusion pressure consequent to raised intracranial pressure. Assisted ventilation should be undertaken in patients with grade IV coma or with any evidence of hypoxia or respiratory distress because pulmonary edema and adult respiratory distress syndrome are features of deteriorating hepatic failure. Ventilation also maintains hypocapnea as an adjunct to controlling elevated intracranial pressure.

Infection

Patients with fulminant hepatic failure or subacute hepatic necrosis are at high risk for sepsis. Daily cultures of blood, urine, and other body fluids are advisable. This is particularly important because sepsis may prevent liver transplantation. The syndrome of high-output hypotension mimics septicemia. Unexplained fever despite broad-spectrum antibiotic coverage warrants consideration of an antifungal prophylaxis.

Cerebral Edema

Cerebral edema is the single most dangerous complication of fulminant hepatic failure. In such patients, positional changes and movement may precipitate rapid and extreme changes in cerebral perfusion pressure. An acute elevation in intracranial pressure may present as seizures, changes in pupillary responses, and cerebral posturing. The immediate response to clinical signs of increased intracranial pressure should exclude hypoglycemia, as it may mimic acute changes in mental status. Hypoglycemia is a particular risk for patients with acetaminophen-related fulminant hepatic failure or with disorders of microvesicular fat deposition (e.g., Reye's syndrome, acute fatty liver of pregnancy, valproate poisoning). Only mannitol has been shown to offer a therapeutic benefit in the hepatic failure syndrome of elevated intracranial pressure and reduced cerebral perfusion pressure. Dexamethasone is of no value. The ability of barbiturate coma and ventilator-driven hypocapnea to reverse elevations of intracranial pressure associated with hepatic failure is unknown, but these are often tried on an empiric basis. Because the intracranial pressure is subject to rapid changes, the use of intracranial pressure monitoring in the treatment of severely ill patients with fulminant hepatic failure has received much attention. However, it is associated with side effects and is of uncertain clinical utility (29,30).

Liver Transplantation

Liver transplantation is a life-saving procedure for patients with hepatic failure or submassive hepatic necrosis that does not respond to medical management (31). Notwithstanding the aforementioned prognostic factors, the most important indicators that liver transplantation is required are the level of encephalopathy and the trend of change in encephalopathy. Unfortunately, because acute hepatic encephalopathy can vary between grades II and III in a matter of minutes, making a decision based on these factors remains difficult. Even when a patient is given highest-emergency status, it is not unusual in North America to wait 72 hours or longer for a suitable donor. During this time, further deterioration, especially worsening cerebral edema, may make transplantation impossible. For this reason, human heterotopic auxiliary transplants, live donor segmental liver transplantation, extracorporeal perfusion through human or pig livers or artificial hepatocyte perfusion devices, and xenografts have been attempted to sustain the patient until spontaneous recovery occurs or a suitable organ is found.

The outcome of liver transplantation in patients with fulminant hepatic failure is somewhat worse than the outcome of transplantation performed for other causes. One-year survival rates of 50% to 60% are common.

REFERENCES

1. Barnes PF, DeCock KM, Reynolds TN, et al. A comparison of amebic and pyogenic abscess of the liver. *Medicine* 1987;66:472.
2. Bertel CK, van Heerden JA, Sheedy PF. Treatment of pyogenic hepatic abscesses. *Arch Surg* 1986;121:554.
3. Khuroo MS, Nazir WA, Gul J, et al. Percutaneous drainage compared with surgery for hepatic hydatid cysts. *N Engl J Med* 1997;337:881.
4. Koff RS. Hepatitis A. *Lancet* 1998;351:1643.
5. Innes BL, Snitbhan R, Kunasol P, et al. Protection against hepatitis A by an inactivated vaccine. *JAMA* 1994;271:1328.
6. Lau JYN, Wright TL. Molecular virology and pathogenesis of hepatitis B. *Lancet* 1993;342:1335.
7. Carman W, Thomas H, Domingo E. Viral genetic variation: hepatitis B virus as a clinical example. *Lancet* 1993;34:349.
8. Lai CL, Chien RN, Leung NWY, et al. A one-year trial of lamivudine for chronic hepatitis B. *N Engl J Med* 1998;339;61.
9. Chien R-N, Liaw Y-F, Atkins M. Pretherapy alanine transaminase level as a determinant for hepatitis B e antigen seroconversion during lamivudine therapy in chronic hepatitis B infection. *Hepatology* 1999;30:770.
10. Samuel D, Muller R, Alexander G, et al. Liver transplantation in European patients with the hepatitis B surface antigen. *N Engl J Med* 1993;329:1842.
11. Alter MJ, Kruszon-Moran D, Nainan OV, et al. The prevalence of hepatitis C virus infection in the United States, 1988 through 1994. *N Engl J Med* 1999;341:556.
12. Conry-Cantilena C, VanRaden M, Gibble J, et al. Routes of infection, viremia, and liver disease in blood donors found to have hepatitis C virus infection. *N Engl J Med* 1996;334:1691.
13. Niederau C, Lange S, Heintges T, et al. Prognosis of chronic hepatitis C: results of a large prospective cohort study. *Hepatology* 1998;28:1687.
14. Farci P, Alter HF, Wong D, et al. A long-term study of hepatitis C virus replication in non-A, non-B hepatitis. *N Engl J Med* 1991;325:98.
15. Kenny-Walsh E, and the Irish Hepatology Research Group. Clinical outcomes after hepatitis C infection from contaminated anti-D immune globulin. *N Engl J Med* 1999;340:1228.
16. Poynard T, Bedossa P, Opolon P. Natural history of liver fibrosis progression in patients with chronic hepatitis C. *Lancet* 1997;349:825.
17. Fattovich G, Giustina G, Degos F, et al. Morbidity and mortality in compensated cirrhosis type C: a retrospective follow-up study of 384 patients. *Gastroenterology* 1997;112:463.
18. Poynard T, Marcellin P, Lee SS, et al. Randomised trial of interferon alpha-2b plus ribavirin for 48 weeks or for 24 weeks versus interferon alpha-2b plus placebo for 48 weeks for treatment of chronic infection with hepatitis C. *Lancet* 1998;352:1426.
19. McHutchison JG, Gordon SC, Schiff ER, et al. Interferon alfa-2b alone or in combination with ribavirin as initial treatment for chronic hepatitis C. *N Engl J Med* 1998;339:1485.
20. Davis GL, Esteban-Mur R, Rustgi V, et al. Interferon alfa-2b alone or in combination with ribavirin for the treatment of relapse of chronic hepatitis C. *N Engl J Med* 1998;339:1493.
21. International Interferon Alpha Hepatocellular Carcinoma Study Group. Effect of interferon alpha on progression of cirrhosis to hepatocellular carcinoma: a retrospective cohort study. *Lancet* 1998;351:1535.
22. Feray C, Caccamo L, Alexander GJM, et al. European collaborative study on factors influencing outcome after liver transplantation for hepatitis C. *Gastroenterology* 1999;117:619.
23. Farci P, Mandas A, Coiana A, et al. Treatment of chronic hepatitis D with interferon alfa-2a. *N Engl J Med* 1994;330:88.
24. Krawczynski K. Hepatitis E. *Hepatology* 1993;17:932.
25. Lee WM. Acute liver failure. *N Engl J Med* 1993;329:1862.
26. O'Grady JG, Alexander GJM, Hayllar KM, et al. Early indicators of prognosis in fulminant hepatic failure. *Gastroenterology* 1989;97:439.
27. Smilkstein MJ, Knapp GL, Kulig KW, et al. Efficacy of oral *N*-acetylcysteine in the treatment of acetaminophen overdose. *N Engl J Med* 1988;319:1557
28. Harrison PM, Keays R, Bray GP, et al. Improved outcome of paracetamol-induced fulminant hepatic failure by late administration of acetylcysteine. *Lancet* 1990;335:157.
29. Lidofsky SD, Bass NM, Prager MC, et al. Intracranial pressure monitoring and liver transplantation for fulminant hepatic failure. *Hepatology* 1992;16:1.
30. Blei AT, Olafsson S, Webster S, et al. Complications of intracranial pressure monitoring in fulminant hepatic failure. *Lancet* 1993;341:157.
31. Bismuth H, Samuel D, Gugenheim J, et al. Emergency liver transplantation for fulminant hepatitis. *Ann Intern Med* 1987;107:337.

SURGERY: SCIENTIFIC PRINCIPLES AND PRACTICE, Third Edition, edited by Lazar J. Greenfield, Michael W. Mulholland, Keith T. Oldham, Gerald B. Zelenock, and Keith D. Lillemoe. Lippincott Williams & Wilkins Publishers, Philadelphia, © 2001.

CHAPTER 37

CIRRHOSIS AND PORTAL HYPERTENSION

MICHAEL R. MARVIN AND JEAN C. EMOND

CIRRHOSIS

Background and Definition

The term *cirrhosis*, derived from the Greek word *kirrhos* ("orange-yellow"), was first coined by Laennec in 1826. In 1911, Mallory described the disease as a "progressive, destructive lesion with reparative activity and contraction of the connective tissue, resulting in obstruction of the bile ducts and interference of portal blood flow" (1). Multiple definitions of cirrhosis can be found in the literature, but all reflect the underlying pathology of injury, repair, regeneration, and fibrosis. Cirrhosis is not a localized process but one that, by definition, involves the entire liver. One may define cirrhosis as the end result of multiple, varied, repeated/chronic pathologic insults to the liver with subsequent repair that cause an irreversible derangement in the hepatic architecture; the primary histologic features are marked fibrosis, destruction of vascular and biliary elements, regeneration, and nodule formation.

Pathophysiology

Cirrhosis can be caused by a wide range of pathologic entities, including the viral hepatitides, alcohol, metabolic disorders, drug toxicity, and biliary obstruction, among others (Table 37.1). Regardless of the cause, the primary event that leads to cirrhosis is injury to hepatocellular elements. Injury initiates an inflammatory response with associated cytokine release; elaboration of toxic substances; destruction of hepatocytes, bile duct cells, and vascular endothelial cells; repair through cellular proliferation and regeneration; and formation of fibrous scar (Fig. 37.1).

The primary cell implicated in the formation of this fibrous scar is the stellate cell (Ito cell, lipocyte, perisinusoidal cell), located in the perisinusoidal space of Disse (2) (Fig. 37.2). In the normal liver, these cells are primarily responsible for the storage of vitamin A (3). In response to various stimuli, they become activated, as evidenced by cellular enlargement and proliferation, an increase in rough endoplasmic reticulum, loss of vitamin A droplets, expression of actin filaments, and increased expression of

Table 37.1. CLASSIFICATION OF CIRRHOSIS

Alcohol
Viral hepatitis
Biliary obstruction
   Primary
   Secondary
Venoocclusive disease
Hemochromatosis
Wilson's disease
Autoimmune
Syphilis
Drugs and toxins
α_1 = Antitrypsin deficiency
Cystic fibrosis
Glycogen storage disease
Other metabolic diseases
Sarcoidosis
Copper
Small-bowel bypass
Idiopathic

"fibril-forming" collagen types I, III, and V (4,5). They also express components of the extracellular matrix, including heparan sulfate, dermatan, chondroitin sulfate (6), laminin (7), and fibronectin (8).

The activation process may be influenced by Kupffer cells within the liver, which have been shown to enhance the activation of stellate cells in vitro (9), perhaps by eliciting the production of cytokines such as transforming growth factor-β (TGF-β), platelet-derived growth factor (PDGF), tumor necrosis factor-α (TNF-α), interleukin-1 (IL-1), interleukin-6 (IL-6), and epidermal growth factor, in addition to their cellular receptors (9–12). Both TGF-β and PDGF have been shown to enhance proliferation and fibrogenesis in animal models (9,10), with TGF-β being the primary stimulator of collagen synthesis and fibrosis. Further evidence implicating TGF-β in the production of hepatic fibrosis is the observation that levels of TGF-β are reduced after patients who are positive for hepatitis C virus are treated with interferon alfa. This reduction has been correlated with a regression of hepatic fibrosis (13). As a result of the activation of stellate cells and a subsequent enhancement in collagen and extracellular matrix synthesis, the space of Disse becomes thickened, so that "capillarization" develops and the normal fenestrated architecture of the sinusoidal endothelium is lost (14). Obliteration of sinusoidal fenestrations may be the essential component of fibrosis-induced hepatocellular dysfunction in cirrhosis, preventing the normal flow of nutrients to hepatocytes and increasing vascular resistance (15). In addition, stellate cell production of endothelin-1, a potent vasoconstrictor, can cause contraction of the myofilaments within the stellate cell, influencing blood flow to injured areas and contributing to portal hypertension. Initially, fibrosis may be reversible if the inciting agents are removed. With sustained injury, the process of fibrosis becomes irreversible and leads to cirrhosis.

Classification Systems

Morphology

In 1977, the World Health Organization divided cirrhosis into three categories based on the morphologic characteristics of hepatic nodules (16) (Fig. 37.3).

Micronodular Pattern. Nodules are almost always less than 3 mm in diameter, are relatively uniform in size and regularly distributed throughout the liver, and rarely contain portal tracts or efferent veins. Micronodular livers are usually of normal size or are mildly enlarged, and the fibrous septa vary in thickness. These changes reflect relatively early disease and are characteristic of a wide range of disease processes, including alcoholism, biliary obstruction, venous outflow obstruction, hemochromatosis, and Indian childhood cirrhosis.

Macronodular Pattern. In this category, nodules vary considerably in size and are larger than 3 mm in diameter, with some nodules measuring several centimeters. Portal structures and efferent veins are present but display architectural distortion. These livers are usually coarsely scarred with variably thick and thin septa and may be either normal or reduced in size. Two separate subcategories are recognized based on the nature of the fibrous septa. In the first one, characteristic of "posthepatitis" pathology and found in Wilson's disease, fine, sometimes incomplete septa link portal tracts; these are difficult to see on gross inspection of the liver. The second is characteristic of "postnecrotic" disease, is commonly found in patients with viral hepatitis, and is characterized by coarse, thick septa that are readily apparent on gross examination. Because of the relatively large size of the nodules relative to the size of biopsy specimens, diagnosis by biopsy may be difficult in macrodnodular cirrhosis.

Mixed Pattern. This description is applied to livers in which both micronodules and macronodules are present in approximately equal proportions.

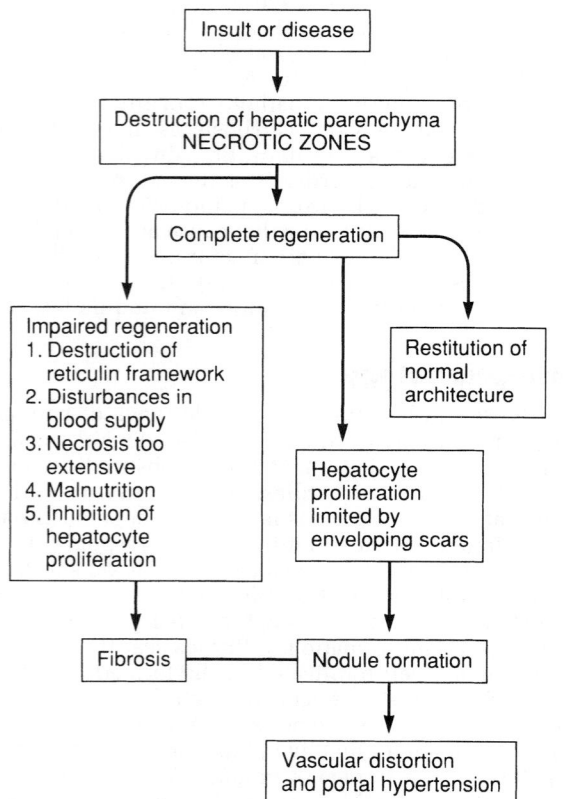

Figure 37.1. Evolution of cirrhosis. Fibrosis develops in nonregenerative necrotic areas, producing scars. The pattern of nodularity and scars reflects the type of response to injury (e.g., uniform vs. nonuniform necrosis) and the extent of injury.

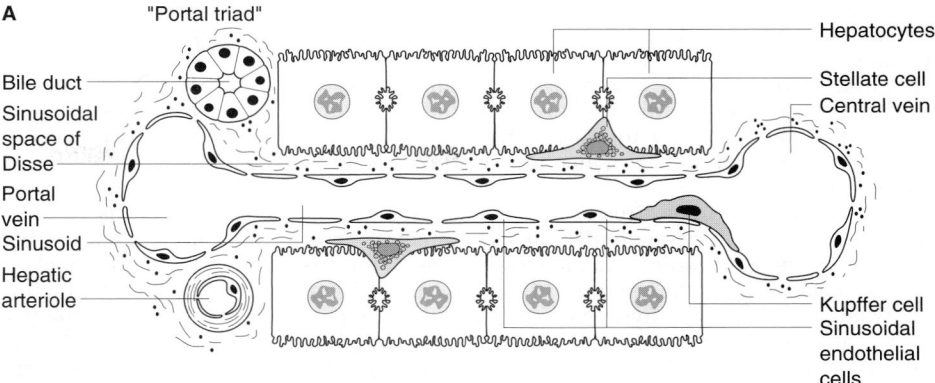

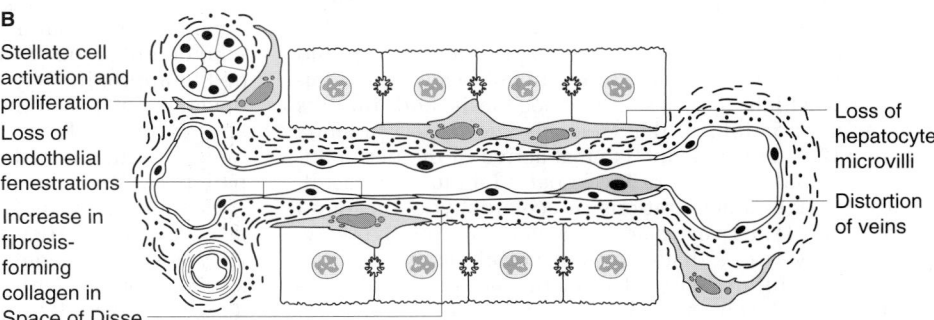

Figure 37.2. Matrix and cellular alterations in hepatic fibrosis. *(A)* In normal liver, a modest amount of low-density matrix is present in the subendothelial space of Disse. *(B)* In the fibrotic liver, the accumulation of fibril-forming matrix in this region leads to "capillarization" of the sinusoid and functional changes in all neighboring cell types. (Redrawn from Friedman SL, Arthur MJP, Millward-Sadler. Cirrhosis and hepatic fibrosis. In: Wright R, et al., eds. *Liver and biliary disease,* 3rd ed. London: Bailliere Tindall, 1992: 822–881, with permission.)

Etiology

Another commonly used method for classifying cirrhosis is by etiology. Unfortunately, the causes of cirrhosis and the morphologic and histologic characteristics of the liver overlap significantly.

Alcohol. The relationship between alcohol and liver disease has been well established. In 1849, Rokitansky, referring to the association of alcohol intake and liver disease, coined the term *Laennec's cirrhosis* (17). More than 50% of alcoholics with cirrhosis and two thirds of patients with alcoholic hepatitis and cirrhosis die within 4 years of diagnosis (18). However, cirrhosis develops in only 10% to 30% of heavy drinkers (19). The reasons why cirrhosis develops in some alcoholics but not in others are not clear and may depend on a variety of factors, such as genetic predisposition, nutritional effects, concomitant drug use, and viral infection.

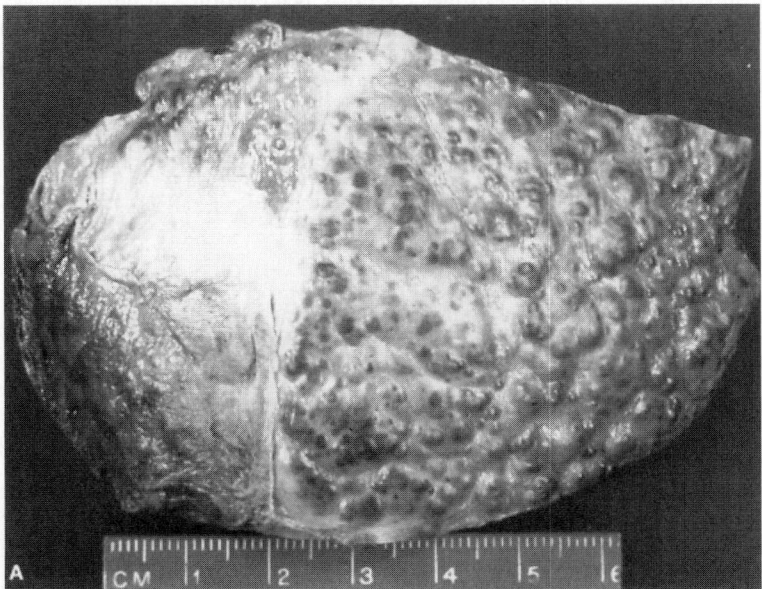

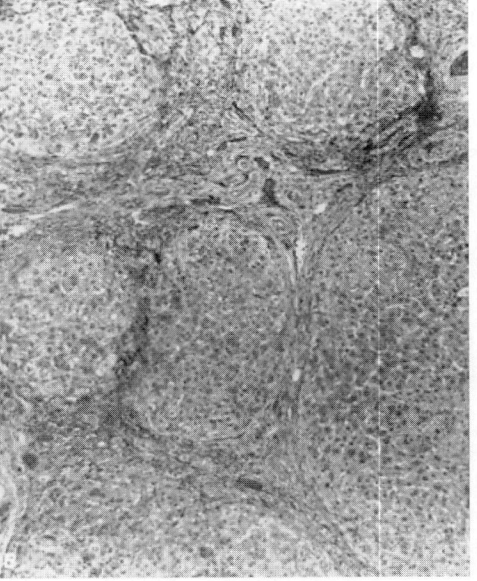

Figure 37.3. *(A)* Small, shrunken liver and a fairly regular pattern of nodularity. This appearance is rather typical of end-stage cirrhosis, regardless of the cause. *(B)* Photomicrograph of cirrhotic liver tissue, showing irregular nodules of regenerating hepatocytes surrounded by scar. Trichrome stain, ×60.

Alcoholic liver disease usually begins with a transition of normal architecture to fatty liver and alcoholic hepatitis, indicated histologically by the presence of megamitochondria, Mallory bodies (eosinophilic accumulations of intermediate filaments with cytokeratin proteins), inflammation and necrosis, and ultimately fibrosis (Fig. 37.4). Classically, the morphology of alcoholic cirrhosis is a micronodular pattern.

Although alcohol may directly activate stellate cells to produce collagen independently of inflammation and necrosis (5), the key mediator in alcohol-induced liver disease is acetaldehyde, the product of alcohol metabolism by the enzyme alcohol dehydrogenase. Acetaldehyde produces numerous deleterious effects on the liver, including the following: direct activation of stellate cells (20); inhibition of DNA repair (21); depletion of glutathione, which impairs mitochondrial function and the ability to handle free radical production (19); damage to microtubles, which causes protein and water sequestration (22); and formation of NADH (reduced nicotinamide adenine dinucleotide), which opposes gluconeogenesis and inhibits fatty acid oxidation, so that steatosis and hyperlipidemia develop (23). This enzyme is most active in the perivenular/centrilobular zone 3 of the hepatic lobule; as a result, relatively high concentrations of acetaldehyde are found in this area of the liver. In addition, zone 3 is relatively hypoxic relative to its distance from portal venous and hepatic arterial inflow. These two factors are presumably responsible for the characteristic initial perivenular location of alcohol-induced liver disease.

Other effects of acetaldehyde include induction of lipid peroxidation with subsequent loss of integrity of cell membranes, which causes the characteristic "ballooning degeneration" of alcohol-induced liver disease (24). Necrosis and inflammation in the perivenular region activate the stellate cells in the space of Disse, so that fibrosis develops. With continued ingestion of alcohol and hepatic injury, expansion of the areas of fibrosis expand toward the periportal regions leads to bridging fibrosis and ultimately cirrhosis.

Hepatitis. Viral hepatitis is the most common cause of cirrhosis worldwide, accounting for at least 50% of cases. Hepatitis A, B, C, D, and E have all been proven to cause acute hepatitis, characterized histologically by lymphocytic parenchymal and portal inflammation, focal necrosis, ballooning degeneration, cholestasis, Kupffer cell and macrophage hypertrophy and hyperplasia, and lobular dis-

array (25). Only hepatitis B, C, and D have been shown to progress to chronic hepatitis, defined by persistent liver cell necrosis and inflammation lasting longer than 6 months.

Chronic infection with hepatitis B virus (HBV) develops in fewer than 5% of patients who experience acute HBV infection. The development of cirrhosis in approximately 10% to 20% of chronically infected persons produces an overall rate of cirrhosis of approximately 1%. Of patients with hepatitis C, 90% become chronically infected, and chronic hepatitis develops in 60% of these. Thirty percent of patients with chronic hepatitis progress to cirrhosis (17), so that the incidence of cirrhosis in patients initially infected with hepatitis C is approximately 10%.

Treatment of HCV hepatitis with interferon-α can completely eradicate infection in a small portion of patients (15% to 30%) (25,26). In patients who respond to interferon therapy, progression to cirrhosis is eliminated, and hepatocellular carcinoma does not develop. In patients who do not respond to interferon therapy, cirrhosis develops in approximately 40%, and hepatocellular carcinoma develops in 16% of these (27). Recently, combination therapy with interferon and ribavirin has improved these rates, producing sustained remissions in 30% to 40% of patients (28).

Hepatitis D virus (HDV) is an RNA virus that requires the presence of HBV to be pathogenic. Superinfection of HBV-positive patients with HDV leads to a more rapid clinical course, with progression to cirrhosis in 70% to 80% of patients (29).

Among patients with compensated cirrhosis of viral origin, hepatocellular carcinoma developed in approximately 20% with HCV, 9% with HBV, and 41% with both HBV and HCV (17).

Cholestasis. Cholestasis, defined as a decrease or absence of bile flow into the duodenum, may be caused by intrahepatic or extrahepatic biliary obstruction or defects in the ability of hepatocytes to excrete bile. Causes of cholestasis are presented in Table 37.2. Prolonged biliary obstruction leads to proliferation of bile ducts, formation of bile lakes caused by disruption of bile ducts, fibrosis, and ultimately secondary biliary cirrhosis as a result of the direct toxic effects of bile salts on hepatobiliary elements.

Primary biliary cirrhosis is a chronic, slowly progressive disease that most commonly affects middle-aged women; it is characterized by portal inflammation, destruction of intrahepatic bile ducts, and progression to cirrhosis (30). Ap-

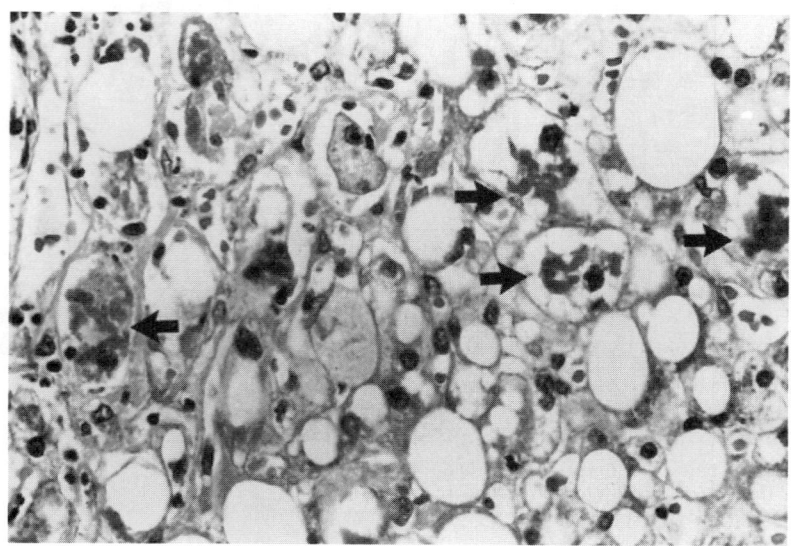

Figure 37.4. Alcoholic hepatitis. Mallory bodies *(arrows)* are evident within the swollen, clear cytoplasm of several hepatocytes. This hyaline material is chemotactic for leukocytes, many of which are seen within the field. H&E, ×470.

Table 37.2. CAUSES OF CHOLESTASIS

Extrahepatic	Intrahepatic	Hepatocellular cholestasis
Common bile duct stones	Primary biliary cirrhosis	Genetic
Cancers	Space-occupying lesions	α-Antitrypsin deficiency
Pancreas	Primary or metastatic hepatic tumors	Benign recurrent intrahepatic cholestasis
Ampulla of Vater	Lymphoma	Blyer's syndrome
Bile duct	Amyloidosis	Cholestasis of pregnancy
Cysts	Vanishing bile duct syndrome	Abnormal bile acid synthesis
Pancreatic	Allograft rejection	Porphyrias
Choledochal	Graft-vs.-host disease	Acquired
Infections	Alagille's syndrome	Viral hepatitis
Parasites	Idiopathic adult ductopenia	Drugs
AIDS	Primary sclerosing cholangitis	Alcoholic hepatitis
Chronic pancreatitis	Hodgkin's disease	Bacterial infections
Bile duct strictures	Cystic fibrosis	Total parenteral nutrition
Benign		Renal carcinoma
Ischemic		Hodgkin's disease
Hodgkin's disease		Postoperative cholestasis
Biliary atresia		

proximately 95% of patients are women, and 95% of these women express antimitochondrial antibodies in serum (31). The autoimmune inflammatory process damages not only the bile ducts but eventually the hepatocytes as a result of leakage of bile acids into surrounding parenchyma (32). Patients present with fatigue, jaundice, and pruritus, but as many as 50% to 60% of patients may be asymptomatic (33). Primary biliary cirrhosis progresses in the majority of patients; median survival times are approximately 10 to 15 years in asymptomatic and 7 years in symptomatic patients (34,35). Poor prognostic factors include hyperbilirubinemia, advanced age, hepatosplenomegaly, and symptomatic disease. Treatment options include cholestyramine, colchicine and methotrexate for pruritus and fatigue, and ursodiol for slowing progression of the disease and delaying the need for transplant (35,36). Orthotopic liver transplantation is the only known curative treatment (37).

Primary sclerosing cholangitis (PSC) is a chronic, progressive cholestatic liver disease of unknown cause characterized by diffuse segmental intrahepatic or extrahepatic biliary ductular strictures with associated fibrosis and inflammation. The disease has no cure and often leads to secondary biliary cirrhosis, portal hypertension, hepatic failure, and cholangiocarcinoma if hepatic transplantation is not performed. PSC is strongly associated with inflammatory bowel diseases, most commonly ulcerative colitis. Approximately 70% of patients with PSC also have ulcerative colitis (38). Conversely, approximately 5% of patients with ulcerative colitis have PSC. The cause of PSC is thought to be autoimmune in nature; elevated levels of autoantibodies and an increased expression of HLA class II molecules on biliary epithelial cells have been observed (39,40). Approximately two thirds of patients are male and less than 45 years of age at the time of diagnosis (41,42). Patients with PSC may be completely asymptomatic (up to 50%) or have signs of advanced disease at the time of diagnosis (43). Commonly, the diagnosis is made in symptomatic patients after endoscopic retrograde cholangiopancreatography has been performed to evaluate elevated liver enzymes, including alkaline phosphatase and γ-glutamyltransferase. Symptomatic patients have a waxing and waning course and may present with complaints of fatigue (75%), pruritus (25% to 70%), jaundice (30% to 69%), abdominal pain (16% to 37%), and weight loss (10% to 34%) (38,44). Complications secondary to pro-

gression to cirrhosis are less common and include ascites, variceal bleeding, and acute cholangitis.

The diagnosis is suggested by a history of inflammatory bowel disease in the setting of elevated liver enzymes and established by cholangiography, which reveals diffuse multifocal sclerosis of the intrahepatic and extrahepatic bile ducts in the absence of other etiologic factors (choledocholithiasis, congenital liver disease, trauma/ischemia, cholangiocarcinoma). Pathologically, bile ductular proliferation, periductal fibrosis and inflammation, ductopenia, and less commonly obliterative fibrous cholangitis may be present. PSC may be considered a premalignant condition. One of the most deadly complications of PSC, cholangiocarcinoma, occurs in up to one third of patients (45,46). Although the only effective treatment for PSC is hepatic transplantation, the presence of cholangiocarcinoma is a contraindication to transplantation.

Metabolic/Genetic Disorders. Some of these diseases are listed in Table 37.1. A description of all the metabolic disorders causing liver disease is beyond the scope of this chapter.

In hemochromatosis of the liver, an inborn error of metabolism causes an increased absorption of iron from the gastrointestinal tract. The pathophysiology of iron-induced hepatotoxicity is related to lipid peroxidation induced by iron in periportal regions of the liver. Activation of stellate cells by cytokines released from Kupffer cells that have phagocytosed necrotic hepatocytes injured by iron toxicity is also contributory (47). Over time, the reaction progresses to bridging fibrosis and eventually to a mixed micronodular–macronodular cirrhosis. Treatment includes reduction of iron intake, repeated phlebotomy, and orthotopic liver transplantation.

Wilson's disease is an autosomal, recessively inherited disease caused by a deficiency in hepatocyte transport of copper into the bile. The disease is characterized biochemically by low serum ceruloplasmin levels, and clinically by corneal pigmentation (Kayser-Fleischer rings), neuropsychiatric disease, and hepatic cirrhosis (48). As copper accumulates in the liver, periportal inflammation develops that leads to piecemeal and lobular necrosis, bridging fibrosis, and a mixed micronodular–macronodular cirrhosis (49). Treatment options include chelating penicillamine, trientine, zinc salts, and orthotopic liver transplantation.

Venous Outflow Obstruction. Cirrhosis may also result from obstruction of the hepatic veins. Causes include chronic right-sided heart failure as a result of severe tricuspid regurgitation, constrictive pericarditis, and the Budd-Chiari syndrome.

Hepatic dysfunction secondary to passive vascular congestion in the setting of right-sided heart failure and increased right-sided heart pressures is caused by the transmission of increased pressure to the hepatic venous system. This increased pressure leads to sinusoidal congestion, perivenular atrophy, hemorrhagic necrosis, and distortion and enlargement of sinusoidal fenestrations (50). Increased pressure also causes perisinusoidal edema that eventually exceeds the clearance capabilities of hepatic lymphatics, so that ascites develops (51). Grossly, the liver is described as having a "nutmeg" appearance in which areas of hemorrhage are interspersed with relatively normal yellowish parenchyma (51). Histologically, perivenular fibrosis progresses to bridging fibrosis that spares the portal regions. Portal sparing is characteristic of "cardiac cirrhosis." In addition to causing ascites, chronic vascular congestion can lead to fibrosis in the space of Disse, which compromises nutrient delivery and contributes to portal hypertension and zone 3 hepatocellular injury (52).

Budd-Chiari syndrome is a rare disease caused by mechanical obstruction of the hepatic veins (Table 37.3). Obstruction may occur at the level of the terminal hepatic veins, the major hepatic veins, or the vena cava and may be caused by obstructing webs or membranes (most commonly in Africa and Asia) or thrombosis secondary to hypercoagulable states and neoplasms (most commonly in the West).

The range of presentations is wide; some patients are completely asymptomatic, where as acute hepatic failure or cirrhosis develops in others (53). These variations in symptoms are related to the degree and rate of progression of hepatic outflow obstruction. Patients classically present with abdominal pain, hepatomegaly, and ascites. The diagnosis can be made by duplex Doppler ultrasonography, which has a sensitivity of 85% to 95% (54). Computed tomography (CT) is another diagnostic option.

Table 37.3. ETIOLOGIC FACTORS IN BUDD-CHIARI SYNDROME

Idiopathic
Hematologic disorders
  Polycythemia vera
  Paroxysmal nocturnal hemoglobinuria
  Myeloproliferative disorders
  Antithrombin III deficiency
  Circulating lupus anticoagulants
Oral contraceptives
Pregnancy and postpartum
Tumors
  Hepatocellular carcinoma
  Renal cell carcinoma
  Adrenal carcinoma
  Leiomyosarcoma of the inferior vena cava
Vena caval webs
Infections
  Amebic abscess
  Aspergillosis
  Hydatid cyst
Phlebitis
Trauma
Venoocclusive disease

Table 37.4. PHYSICAL FINDINGS IN CIRRHOSIS

Physical findings	Cases (%)
Palpable liver	96
Jaundice	68
Ascites	66
Spider angiomas	49
Dilated abdominal wall veins	47
Palpable spleen	46
Testicular atrophy	45
Palmar erythema	24
Noninfectious fever	22
Hepatic coma	18
Gynecomastia	15
Dupuytren's contractures	5

Diagnosis of Cirrhosis

Significant information can be obtained by performing a thorough history and physical examination. A history of alcohol abuse, hepatitis, toxin or drug exposure, upper gastrointestinal bleeding, enlarging hemorrhoids, infections, and alteration in mental status suggest the possibility of liver disease. Physical findings associated with cirrhosis are listed in Table 37.4. In addition to these findings, fetor hepaticus, purpura and bruising, decreased body hair, and white nails are common.

Laboratory tests of liver function are indicated if liver disease is suggested by the history and physical examination. Although levels of bilirubin, aspartate aminotransferase, alanine aminotransferase, and alkaline phosphatase are elevated in hepatic disease, the increases are not specific for liver pathology, and levels may be normal even in the setting of significant disease. A very common finding in patients with cirrhosis is thrombocytopenia, caused by hypersplenism and portal hypertension. The platelet growth factor thrombopoietin, which is produced by the liver, has been shown to be decreased in patients with cirrhosis, and this deficit may contribute to the thrombocytopenia associated with hepatic disease (55).

The definitive diagnosis of cirrhosis usually requires biopsy, either percutaneous or operative, or gross inspection during laparoscopy or laparotomy. Noninvasive methods to diagnose cirrhosis include ultrasonography, CT, and magnetic resonance imaging (MRI). Ultrasonographic criteria for cirrhosis include the demonstration of multiple nodular irregularities on the ventral liver surface that are clearly separate from the anterior abdominal wall. When these criteria are used, ultrasonography has been shown to have a sensitivity, specificity, and accuracy of approximately 90% in the diagnosis of cirrhosis (56). Indirect evidence of cirrhosis includes endoscopically discovered variceal disease, and the presence of splenomegaly detected by CT or MRI.

Manifestations of Cirrhosis

Renal

Renal insufficiency may develop in a patient with cirrhosis as a direct consequence of the underlying condition (i.e., primary biliary cirrhosis, amyloidosis), as a consequence of excessive diuretic use in the treatment of ascites and fluid overload, or as a secondary reaction to the release of cytokines or hormones by the liver that alter renal function. Renal dysfunction is characterized by avid sodium retention despite normovolemia or hypervolemia, dilutional hyponatremia secondary to free water overload, ascites, and ultimately renal failure and the hepatorenal syndrome. An unresolved question is which of the above problems is a primary pathologic entity and which are the secondary consequences of circulatory dysfunction.

Observations that support a secondary effect theory include the lack of anatomic abnormalities in patients with cirrhosis-related renal dysfunction, the normal function of previously dysfunctional kidneys transplanted into otherwise healthy recipients, and resolution of renal abnormalities after successful hepatic transplantation. The exact pathophysiology behind this process remains to be defined.

Sodium Retention. Patients with cirrhosis who do not have ascites have relatively normal sodium handling capabilities. Patients in whom ascites develops have a marked inability to excrete sodium. Because of this deficit, sodium intake in excess of renal excretion contributes to fluid overload. Three theories attempt to explain the cause of sodium retention and development of ascites in cirrhotic patients. The first is the "underfill" theory, whereby portal hypertension causes an increase in pressure in the splanchnic circulation. Ascites occurs when hepatic lymph production exceeds lymphatic return, with subsequent contraction of the blood volume and renal sodium retention. The second is the "overflow" theory, which suggests that the primary defect is inherent to the kidney. Abnormal renal retention of sodium leads to concomitant water retention, expansion of plasma volume, and subsequently edema and ascites (57). The third explanation is the "arterial vasodilation hypothesis," which suggests that the responsible defect lies within the vascular system, with arterial hypotension as the primary event (58). Arterial vasodilation in the splanchnic circulation leads to relative peripheral hypovolemia and activation of the renin–angiotensin–aldosterone and sympathetic nervous systems. The effects, in turn, are a release of antidiuretic hormone (arginine vasopressin), enhancement of sodium and water conservation, an increase in effective circulating volume, and edema and ascites (59). Most evidence supports the latter hypothesis.

The cause of the splanchnic vasodilation is unclear. Some evidence suggests that nitric oxide may be the key mediator. Elevations in portal venous nitric oxide have been reported in both animal and human studies (60,61), and inhibitors of nitric oxide production have been shown to reduce the activity of vasoconstrictor systems and enhance renal hemodynamics (60). The exact role of nitric oxide activity in the pathophysiology of renal disease in cirrhosis remains to be determined.

Water Retention. Patients with cirrhosis and ascites may have a marked inability to handle free water. An increased production of antidiuretic hormone, decreased delivery of fluid to the diluting segments of the nephron, and reduced renal production of prostaglandins all may contribute (38). Retention of water leads to dilutional hyponatremia (serum sodium < 130 mEq/L), which can cause nausea, vomiting, lethargy, and seizures.

Hepatorenal Syndrome. Hepatorenal syndrome is a complication of cirrhosis, most often with ascites, characterized by progressive renal failure in the absence of intrinsic renal disease. This syndrome occurs in 10% of hospitalized patients with cirrhosis and ascites (62). Manifestations of the disease include progressive oliguria, with urine outputs of 400 to 800 mL/d, a rising serum creatinine level, increased cardiac output, and decreased arterial pressure. The disease process is highly variable and is associated with marked renal cortical vasoconstriction induced by activity of the renin–angiotensin–aldosterone and sympathetic nervous systems. In addition, the powerful endothelium-derived vasoconstrictor endothelin-1, in addition to decreased renal production of vasodilator prostaglandins, may play a role. Endothelin-1 has been shown to be elevated in patients with cirrhosis (63,64).

Hepatorenal syndrome may develop in patients who were previously well compensated as a result of infection, use of nonsteroidal antiinflammatory drugs, variceal hemorrhage, or excessive diuretic use. The differentiation of hepatorenal syndrome from acute renal failure is possible by the laboratory evaluation of urine and serum samples. However, hepatorenal syndrome is virtually indistinguishable by laboratory testing from prerenal azotemia. Both prerenal azotemia and hepatorenal syndrome are characterized by extremely low sodium concentrations in the urine, high urine osmolality, high urine-to-plasma ratios of creatinine, and normal urinary sediment (Table 37.5). Criteria for the diagnosis of hepatorenal syndrome are listed in Table 37.6.

The treatment of ascites in patients with cirrhosis requires sodium and water restriction in addition to the use of diuretics. Excessive use of these treatment modalities may lead to increases in serum creatinine that can be difficult to distinguish from those of hepatorenal syndrome. A failure to respond to cessation of diuretics and fluid challenge suggests hepatorenal syndrome. Patients with hepatorenal syndrome usually die within months of the development of severe disease, defined as a serum creatinine level above 2 mg/dL (65). The only effective treatment for hepatorenal syndrome is orthotopic liver transplantation, after which the kidneys usually revert to normal function.

Pulmonary

Many pathologic processes in patients with cirrhosis affect pulmonary function. Some reflect an underlying condition that causes both hepatic and pulmonary disease (i.e., cystic fibrosis, α_1-antitrypsin deficiency); others are primary pulmonary processes, such as interstitial lung disease, primary pulmonary hypertension, and obstructive airway disease. Of the two main pulmonary manifestations of cirrhosis that are discussed here, one is related to increased intraabdominal pressure secondary to ascites, and the other, caused by intrapulmonary shunting, is known as the *hepatopulmonary syndrome*.

The presence of copious ascitic fluid can lead to pulmonary dysfunction by compromising diaphragmatic excursion secondary to increases in intraabdominal and intrapleural pressures. Ascites may also induce large pleural effusions because of the presence of lymphatic transdi-

Table 37.5. DIFFERENTIAL DIAGNOSIS OF ACUTE AZOTEMIA IN PATIENTS WITH LIVER DISEASE

	Prerenal azotemia	Hepatorenal syndrome	Acute renal failure
Urinary sodium	< 10 mEq/L	< 10 mEq/L	> 30 mEq/L
Urine/plasma creatinine ratio	> 30:1	> 30:1	< 20:1
Urine osmolality	100 mOsm, or more than plasma osmolality	100 mOsm, or more than plasma osmolality	Equal to plasma osmolality
Urine sediment	Normal	Normal	Casts: cellular debris

Table 37.6. DIAGNOSTIC CRITERIA FOR HEPATORENAL SYNDROME[a]

MAJOR CRITERIA

1. Low glomerular filtration rate, as indicated by serum creatinine >1.5 mg/dL or 24-hour creatinine clearance <40 mL/min.
2. Absence of shock, ongoing bacterial infection, fluid losses, and current treatment with nephrotoxic drugs.
3. No sustained improvement in renal function (decrease in serum creatinine to ≤1.5 mg/dL or increase in creatinine clearance to 340 mL/min) following diuretic withdrawal and expansion of plasma volume with 1.5 L of a plasma expander.
4. Proteinuria <500 mg/d and no ultrasonographic evidence of obstructive uropathy or parenchymal renal disease.

ADDITIONAL CRITERIA

1. Urine volume <500 mL/d.
2. Urine sodium <10 mEq/L.
3. Urine osmolality greater than plasma osmolality.
4. Urine red blood cells <50 per high-power field.
5. Serum sodium concentration <130 mEq/L.

[a]All major criteria must be present for the diagnosis of hepatorenal syndrome. Additional criteria are not necessary for the diagnosis but provide supportive evidence.
From Arroyo V, Gines Ginés P, Gerbes A, et al. Definition and diagnostic criteria of refractory ascites and hepatorenal syndrome in cirrhosis. Hepatology 1996;23:164, with permission.

aphragmatic communications between the abdomen and thorax (66). Effusions can compress the pulmonary parenchyma and impair gas exchange, so that ventilation–perfusion mismatch and hypoxemia develop. Patients present with worsening pulmonary symptoms in the setting of increasing abdominal girth. Pulmonary function testing reveals decreases in functional residual capacity and total lung capacity (67). Marked improvement in pulmonary function results from large-volume paracentesis (68). This intervention decreases the work of breathing and relieves symptoms. With control of ascites, even in the presence of pleural effusions, no other interventions may be necessary.

Hepatopulmonary syndrome occurs in patients with mild to severe hepatic disease and in approximately 10% to 50% of patients with hepatic dysfunction (69,70). The criteria for diagnosis include hepatic dysfunction, an oxygen tension below 70 mm Hg and/or a diffusion gradient above 20 mm Hg, and the presence of pulmonary vascular dilation (71). Other manifestations include platypnea (increased shortness of breath with movement from a supine to an erect position) and othodeoxia (decreased oxygen tension on moving from a supine to an erect position). These two positional deficits in pulmonary function are related to the increased number of dilated capillaries in the basal areas of the lung; flow is increased in these vessels while the subject is standing, so that shunting is increased. Physical findings include clubbing and cyanosis of the nail beds and spider nevi.

While the underlying cause of hypoxemia in these patients is right-to-left intrapulmonary shunting, ventilation–perfusion mismatch and impaired hypoxic vasoconstriction also play a role. Patients usually present with dyspnea and worsening hypoxemia without evidence of a primary pulmonary process. Initial diagnostic tools include pulse oximetry and arterial blood gas analysis. When significant hypoxemia is found, pulmonary function testing is useful to rule out obstructive or restrictive airway disease (72). A definitive diagnosis can be obtained by the use of contrast-enhanced echocardiography (bubble study), spiral CT, or angiography, which will confirm the presence of a shunt. The only effective therapy for this disease is orthotopic liver transplantation.

Hepatic Encephalopathy

Etiology. Hepatic encephalopathy is a neuropsychiatric syndrome that occurs in the setting of hepatic disease. It is characterized by variable alterations in mental status ranging from deficits detectable only by detailed psychometric tests to confusion, lethargy, and ultimately frank coma. The disease may present in association with acute hepatic failure, as a consequence of progression of chronic liver disease, or after the creation of a surgical portosystemic shunt. Usually, a precipitating cause, such as an acute variceal hemorrhage or infection, can be found.

The causative agent in hepatic encephalopathy has been the subject of much debate. Most evidence implicates ammonia in the development of this condition (73). Ammonia is produced during the bacterial digestion of proteins in the gut, is absorbed into the portal circulation, and usually undergoes extensive degradation in the liver (74). Most researchers believe that encephalopathy is caused by products, such as ammonia, derived from the gastrointestinal tract that are usually metabolized by the liver. These agents reach the peripheral circulation as a result of poor hepatic metabolism or through portosystemic shunts that may be physiologic or the result of surgical procedures. In patients with cirrhosis, in addition to the accumulation of ammonia in the blood, the permeability of the brain to ammonia appears to be increased (75). Other suggested etiologic agents for hepatic encephalopathy include γ-aminobutyric acid (76), endogenous benzodiazepines (77), branched-chain amino acids such as tryptophan (78), neurotoxic short-chain fatty acids, mercaptans, phenols (79), and endogenous opiates (80).

The following observations suggest that ammonia is the key mediator in hepatic encephalopathy: (a) Ammonia levels are increased in 80% to 90% of patients with the condition (81); (b) factors that precipitate hepatic encephalopathy cause increases in ammonia levels; and (c) treatments that relieve hepatic encephalopathy lower ammonia levels (82). Arguments against this hypothesis include the following: (a) Levels of ammonia correlate poorly with the severity of hepatic encephalopathy; (b) high ammonia levels alone do not cause encephalopathy (83); (c) administration of ammonia to patients with cirrhosis but not hepatic encephalopathy does not cause encephalopathy (84); and (d) treatments that reduce ammonia levels also reduce the levels of other putative toxins (85).

Clinical Features. A wide range of neurologic symptoms may occur in patients with hepatic dysfunction. Subtle deficits may include changes in personality, memory loss, alterations in sleep patterns, and minor decreases in intellectual function. Defects may be detectable only by detailed psychometric testing. If no known underlying liver disease is suspected, establishing the cause of an alteration in mental status may be difficult.

With progression of disease, asterixis, a rapid repetitive flexion/extension of the wrist that occurs in response to sustained extension of the forearm and fingers, may occur. In addition, stigmata of liver disease are usually evident, including fetor hepaticus and spider angiomas. The combination of asterixis, elevated ammonia levels, and altered mental status in a patient with known liver disease strongly suggests the diagnosis. Electroencephalographic changes are nonspecific and may occur in patients with a variety of other conditions.

Factors that commonly precipitate hepatic encephalopathy include impaired renal function, variceal hemorrhage, constipation, infection, excessive dietary protein, and drugs, especially benzodiazepines and barbiturates.

Treatment. Treatment options for hepatic encephalopathy include correction of the precipitating factors, alterations in diet, bowel cleansing, medications that reduce ammonia production and neutralize its effects, and medications to treat possible neurotransmitter and nutrient deficiencies.

A search for precipitating factors is imperative and includes cultures of urine, sputum, and ascitic fluid; determination of electrolyte abnormalities; screening for viral infection; assessment of overall volume status; drug history; and endoscopy (Table 37.7).

Therapy begins with a trial of volume expansion via intravenous hydration to relieve azotemia and reduce concentrations of toxic substances by dilution. The mainstays of treatment are directed at the removal of nitrogenous compounds from the gut. Most ammonia is produced within the small and large bowel by bacterial metabolism of dietary and endogenous protein (86). Orally administered cathartics and enemas are the best methods to achieve bowel cleansing (87), and these are combined with marked dietary restriction of protein.

The cathartic of choice is lactulose, a nonabsorbable disaccharide that reaches the distal ileum and colon essentially unmetabolized. Many theories regarding the mechanism of action of lactulose have been proposed. Initially, the presumed mechanism of action was that on reaching the colon, lactulose is metabolized by colonic bacteria to acidic products that lower the pH of the colon. Lowering the pH inhibits the growth of ammonia- and urea-producing bacteria and promotes the growth of *Lactobacillus,* a bacterium with little proteolytic activity (88). The validity of this theory has been questioned (89). It appears now that lactulose alters the metabolism of intestinal bacteria by providing carbohydrate, which enhances the bacterial uptake of ammonia. Combined with the osmotic diarrhea caused by the cathartic activities of lactulose, this effect leads to an increased excretion of ammonia (82,90–92).

The dosage of lactulose, 45 to 90 g/d, is administered orally divided into three or four doses. The dosage can be adjusted to produce two or three soft stools daily. Hourly doses of 30 to 45 mL can be used to induce more rapid improvement during the initial phase of therapy. Symptoms usually abate within 24 hours, but more than 48 hours may be required. Doses can be adjusted if side effects such as flatulence, diarrhea, and electrolyte abnormalities occur.

Nonabsorbable antibiotics have also been used to decrease the number and concentration of ammonia-forming bacteria in the gut. Most experience has accrued for neomycin and metronidazole. These antibiotics are active against gram-negative anaerobes such as *Bacteroides,* which are considered to be a major source of ammonia production (93). The dosage of neomycin, 2 to 8 g/d, is divided into four doses and is continued for 4 to 10 days. Multiple double-blinded, randomized trials have determined the efficacy of antibiotics alone or in combination with lactulose. (For a complete review, see reference 82.) For acute hepatic encephalopathy, studies have shown that neomycin for 4 days is equally as effective as lactulose (94), and metronidazole for 7 days is as effective as neomycin (95). In addition, for chronic hepatic encephalopathy, neomycin for 10 days was equal to lactulose (96). Although only small amounts (1% to 3%) of neomycin are absorbed, a risk for nephrotoxicity and ototoxicity still exists (97,98). Rifamixin, a macrolide antibiotic not approved for use in the United States, has similar efficacy when compared with lactulose and neomycin (99–101).

PORTAL HYPERTENSION

Portal hypertension is defined as a portal vein pressure above the normal range of 5 to 8 mm Hg (102). Portal hypertension may also be defined by the hepatic vein–portal vein pressure gradient, which is greater than 5 mm Hg in portal hypertensive states. Pressures in the portal venous system are usually measured indirectly via the wedged hepatic venous pressure. The technique is similar to that used to determine pulmonary capillary wedge pressure by pulmonary arterial (Swan-Ganz) catheterization.

Anatomy

The venous anatomy of the portal system is relatively constant, with the "usual" anatomy present in 98% of the population (Fig. 37.5). The portal vein is formed by the confluence of the superior mesenteric and splenic veins behind the neck of the pancreas. The inferior mesenteric vein most often joins the splenic vein before the portal vein is formed, but approximately one third of the time the inferior mesenteric vein joins the superior mesenteric vein. The superior mesenteric vein may not be present, and the

---

Table 37.7. TREATMENT OF HEPATIC ENCEPHALOPATHY

Identify precipitating factors
  Disordered carbohydrate metabolism
  Narcotics
  Infection
  Hypotension
  Hypoxia
  Excess exogenous protein
  Gastrointestinal bleeding
  Electrolyte abnormalities
  Alkalosis
Supportive therapy
  Eliminate dietary nitrogen
  Purge gastrointestinal tract to removal blood and other
    nitrogenous compounds
  Nonabsorbable antibiotics (neomycin or metronidazole)
  Lactulose or lactitol
Dopamine receptor agonists
  L-Dopa and bromocriptine[a]
Branched-chain amino acids[b]
Temporary liver support
Orthotopic liver transplantation

[a]Arousal effect in selected patients may be secondary to enhanced renal function.
[b]High cost and equivocal benefits of intravenous amino acid mixtures make it difficult to justify routine use.

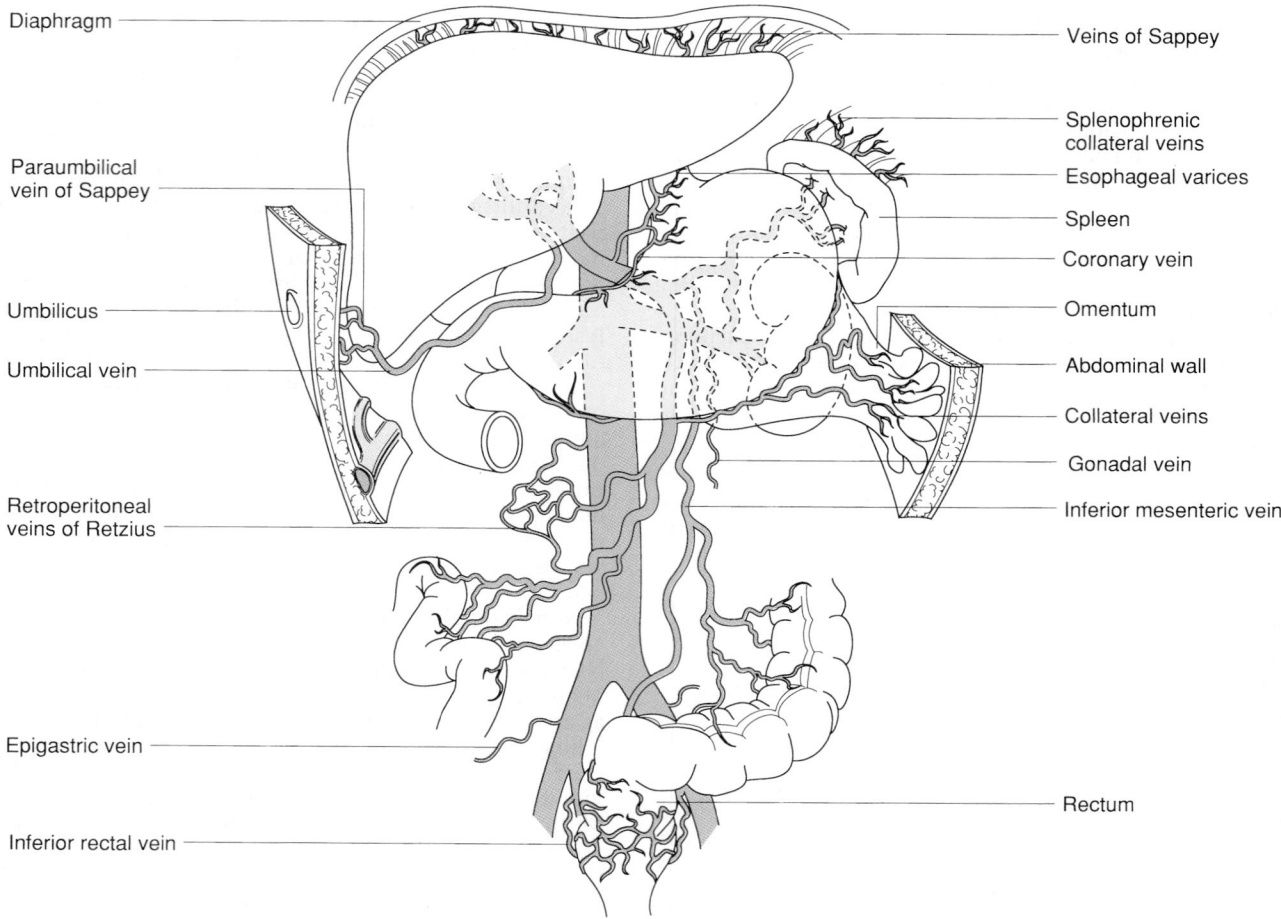

Figure 37.5. Potential venous collaterals that develop with portal hypertension. The veins of Sappey drain portal blood through the bare areas of the diaphragm and through paraumbilical vein collaterals to the umbilicus. The veins of Retzius form in the retroperitoneum and shunt portal blood from the bowel and other organs to the vena cava.

portal vein may be formed by multiple small branches from the mesenteric system that join the splenic vein.

Many branches of the portal venous system are affected when portal pressure rises. As pressure increases, blood flow decreases and the pressure in the portal system is transmitted to its branches. This transmission of pressure through branches of the portal system is beneficial in that it decreases overall portal pressure, but it also is responsible for many of the complications of portal hypertension in that it distends venous tributaries.

Significant branches of the portal system include the coronary or left gastric vein, which communicates with esophageal veins and is the main vessel responsible for the formation of esophageal varices. The inferior mesenteric vein connects with its rectal branches, which when distended form hemorrhoids. The umbilical vein in the ligamentum teres of the falciform ligament joins the left portal vein, and an increase in portal pressure causes abdominal wall veins around the paraumbilical plexus to dilate (caput medusae). The short gastric veins, branches of the splenic vein, communicate with gastric veins and contribute to gastric varices. The retroperitoneal veins of Retzius communicate with the gastrointestinal veins through the bare areas of the liver where no peritoneal layer separates the abdominal viscera from the retroperitoneum.

Physiology

Portal hypertension is caused by increased resistance to portal blood flow secondary to cirrhosis, portal vein thrombosis, or hepatic venous obstruction. Normally, the liver offers little resistance to portal flow because of the porous nature of the hepatic sinusoids. Moreover, the liver has no intrinsic control over portal blood flow; it is a merely a passive recipient of splanchnic flow, the primary regulation of which occurs at the level of the splanchnic arterioles (103). As discussed earlier, the deposition of collagen in the space of Disse (capillarization), in addition to the contractile properties of stellate cells, causes an increased resistance to portal blood flow in cirrhosis. In addition, various cytokines and hormones contribute to elevated portal pressures by inducing splanchnic vasodilation and an increase in splanchnic flow.

The increased blood flow through collateral vessels and subsequently increased venous return cause the characteristic hemodynamic features of portal hypertension, which include an increase in cardiac output and total blood volume (104) and a decrease in systemic vascular resistance. Arteriovenous shunts within the liver, stomach, and small intestine contribute to the augmented venous return and decreased peripheral vascular resistance. Early in the course of portal hypertension, blood pressure may be normal, but with progression of disease, blood pressure usually falls (105).

The portal venous concentration of nitric oxide, a potent vasodilator, has been shown to be elevated in patients with cirrhosis and portal hypertension (106). In addition to nitric oxide, many other vasodilators are elevated in portal hypertension, including prostacyclins, endotoxins, and glucagon (107).

Etiology

Many pathologic processes can cause portal hypertension (Table 37.8). These are usually classified as prehepatic, hepatic, or posthepatic (presinusoidal, sinusoidal, or postsinusoidal) conditions. In prehepatic and posthepatic conditions, portal hypertension is the result of mechanical venous obstruction at the level of the portal or hepatic veins, respectively, whereas cirrhosis is the main cause of hepatic portal hypertension (108).

Budd-Chiari Syndrome and Venoocclusive Disease

The Budd-Chiari syndrome is caused by hepatic venous obstruction. The name of the syndrome is derived from two investigators, the first of whom (Budd) (109) described the classic presentation of abdominal pain, ascites,

---

Table 37.8. COMMON CAUSES OF PORTAL HYPERTENSION

DISORDERS THAT PRIMARILY INCREASE RESISTANCE TO FLOW:

Prehepatic
Congenital atresia
Extrinsic compression
Portal, superior mesenteric, or splenic vein thrombosis

Hepatic

CIRRHOSIS
α_1-Antitrypsin deficiency
Cryptogenic cirrhosis
Cystic fibrosis
Hemochromatosis
Nutritional (alcoholic)
Wilson's disease

CONGENITAL HEPATIC FIBROSIS
Focal regenerative hyperplasia
Hepatic venoocclusive disease
Idiopathic
Metastatic carcinoma
Sarcoidosis
Schistosomiasis
Toxin and drug injuries

ACUTE DISEASE
Acute fatty liver
Alcoholic hepatitis
Fulminant hepatic failure

Posthepatic
Budd-Chiari syndrome
Chronic heart failure
Constrictive pericarditis
Vena cava webs

DISORDERS THAT PRIMARILY INCREASE FLOW:

Hepatocellular carcinoma
Mesenteric arteriosclerotic or aneurysmal vascular disease
Osler-Weber-Rendu syndrome

Splenomegaly

---

and hepatomegaly, and the second of whom (Chiari) (110) described the pathologic characteristics of the liver. The obstruction may occur at the level of the inferior vena cava, the hepatic veins, or the central veins within the liver itself and may be the result of congenital webs (most common in Africa and Asia), acute/chronic thrombosis (most common in the West), and malignancy. With occlusion of the hepatic veins, pressure increases in the central veins. As a result, centrilobular congestion, necrosis, and, with chronic disease, fibrosis and cirrhosis with portal hypertension develop.

In the West, the most common causes of this syndrome are hypercoagulable states associated with polycythemia vera, myeloproliferative disorders, paroxysmal nocturnal hemoglobinuria, and defects in the coagulation cascade, as in conditions associated with high estrogen levels (e.g., pregnancy and administration of birth control pills) (111–114). Neoplasms may cause hepatic venous obstruction by direct invasion and occlusion of the vessels; or by establishment of a prothrombotic milieu secondary to the malignancy itself. In the East, the major causes of obstruction of the vena cava and hepatic veins are membranous webs that directly occlude the vessels. The etiology of vena cava webs is unknown.

Venoocclusive disease is characterized by obliterative endophlebitis of the intrahepatic veins (Table 37.3). Causes of venoocclusive disease include medications, toxins, and pyrrolizidine alkaloids.

Budd-Chiari syndrome may present with either acute, subacute, or chronic symptoms. More than 50% of patients have had symptoms for less than 3 months (115). Acute symptoms include hepatomegaly, right upper quadrant abdominal pain, nausea, vomiting, and ascites. In the chronic form of the disease, patients may present with the sequelae of cirrhosis and portal hypertension, including variceal bleeding, ascites, spontaneous bacterial peritonitis, fatigue, and encephalopathy. In the chronic form, the entire liver atrophies except for the caudate lobe. The caudate lobe may be enlarged because its hepatic vein enters the vena cava separately, so that venous outflow is not impeded (116).

The diagnosis is most often made by ultrasonographic evaluation of the liver and its vasculature, which has a sensitivity of 85% to 95% (117). Duplex scanning may reveal the location of the obstruction and characterize the flow within the vena cava and hepatic, portal, mesenteric, and splenic veins. CT is also useful in evaluating the patency of portal vessels and assessing the status of the liver and its individual lobes; it can also assess the spleen and the amount of ascitic fluid. The "gold standard" for the diagnosis is angiography, which provides detailed information on the location and degree of obstruction.

The management of patients with this syndrome usually requires surgical intervention. Liver biopsies are usually performed preoperatively. The response rates to medical therapy, which does not relieve the obstruction to portal outflow, are poor (118,119), and survival rates without surgical intervention are approximately 10%. Antithrombotic agents may be used in the rare patient who presents early with acute venous occlusion. The mainstay of therapy is surgical decompression with a portosystemic shunt, which may not be an option if the vena cava is completely occluded. This circumstance requires anastomosis of the shunt to the right atrium via a mesoatrial shunt. The rates of postprocedural encephalopathy are usually not increased in patients with Budd-Chiari syndrome, as they are in patients who undergo portosystemic shunting for esophageal bleeding. In patients with end-stage liver disease, liver transplantation may be performed (120). The 5-year survival rate for patients with good hepatic function before the shunt procedure is approximately 60%, with a 34% to 88% survival for patients after liver transplantation (115,121–123). Postoperatively, patients are treated with long-term anticoagulation to prevent recurrent thrombosis (121).

A new potential treatment for this syndrome is the transjugular intrahepatic portosystemic shunt (TIPS). Case reports and small series have suggested efficacy for this technique (124,125), but follow-up has been too short to recommend this method as a routine form of treatment. In addition, in most patients, shunts become occluded, and further angiographic manipulation is required to maintain patency. The most useful role for TIPS in the treatment of Budd-Chiari syndrome is as a temporizing measure in anticipation of a liver transplant.

Portal Vein Thrombosis

Portal vein thrombosis is the cause of portal hypertension in fewer than 10% of adult patients but is the most common cause in children (126). In contrast to patients with cirrhosis-induced portal hypertension, these patients have normal liver function and are not as susceptible to the development of complications, such as encephalopathy. Causes of portal vein thrombosis include umbilical vein infection (the most common cause in children), coagulopathies (protein C and antithrombin III deficiency), hepatic malignancy, myeloproliferative disorders, inflammatory bowel disease, pancreatitis, trauma, and previous splenorenal shunt (127,128). Most cases in adults are idiopathic.

The diagnosis can be made by sonography, which reveals an echogenic lesion in the lumen of the portal vein and an absence of portal venous flow on duplex examination (129). With time, cavernous transformation of the portal vein may occur, in which channels develop within the clotted portal vein (130). CT and MRI are also useful in establishing the diagnosis. Often, the initial manifestation of portal vein thrombosis is variceal bleeding in a noncirrhotic patient with normal liver function. Splenomegaly is another common finding.

Therapeutic options for the control of hemorrhage caused by portal vein thrombosis are esophageal variceal ligation and sclerotherapy. If unsuccessful, the distal splenorenal shunt is the preferred surgical treatment for patients with isolated portal vein thrombosis. However, in patients whose left portal vein is patent (most commonly children), a shunt created by placing an internal jugular vein graft between the superior mesenteric vein and the patent left portal vein within the parenchyma of the liver (Rex shunt) may be the optimal therapeutic procedure for reestablishing physiologic portal flow (130).

Splenic Vein Thrombosis

Splenic vein thrombosis is most often caused by disorders of the pancreas, including acute and chronic pancreatitis, trauma, pancreatic malignancy, and pseudocysts. This association is related to the location of the splenic vein behind and close to the pancreas. Other causes include retroperitoneal masses, abscesses, and inflammatory bowel disease; the remaining cases are idiopathic. Gastric varices are present in approximately 80% of patients, and esophageal varices in 30% to 40% (131). Isolated "sinistral" or left-sided portal hypertension occurs in the setting of normal liver function, and patients are readily cured with splenectomy, although observation for asymptomatic patients is acceptable (131). The main indication for splenectomy is variceal hemorrhage.

Complications of Portal Hypertension

The most important complications of portal hypertension are gastrointestinal bleeding secondary to esophageal and gastric varices, ascites, and hepatic encephalopathy. The severity of portal hypertension and its complications and how amenable these conditions are to treatment with surgical intervention have been graded by a scoring scale initially called the *Child-Turcotte score* and subsequently modified to the *Child-Turcotte-Pugh score* (Table 37.9). These indices incorporate clinical and laboratory data as a means to assess the functional status of the liver, estimate hepatic reserve, and predict morbidity and mortality (132). They have been adopted by the United Network for Organ Sharing (UNOS) as a tool for determining the need for liver transplantation. Child A patients have adequate hepatic reserve and survival rates similar to those of noncirrhotic patients, whereas Child C patients have mortality rates in excess of 50% and may not tolerate any intervention short of hepatic transplantation. Although initially utilized to determine the potential success of surgical interventions, these scores are now used globally to assess the prognosis for all patients with hepatic dysfunction.

Table 37.9. CHILD-TURCOTTE CRITERIA FOR HEPATIC FUNCTIONAL RESERVE

Criterion	Class A	Class B	Class C
Encephalopathy	None	Minimal	Advanced
Ascites	None	Easily controlled	Poorly controlled
Bilirubin (mg/dL)	<2	2–3	>3
Albumin (g/dL)	>3.5	3–3.5	<3
Nutrition	Excellent	Good	Poor, "wasting"

CHILD-TURCOTTE-PUGH GRADING OF SEVERITY OF LIVER DISEASE

Score	1	2	3
Encephalopathy	None	1 or 2	3 or 4
Ascites	None	Mild	Moderate
Bilirubin (mg/dL)	1–2	2.1–3	≥3.1
Albumin (g/dL)	≥3.5	2.8–3.5	≤2.7
Protime (s)	1–4	4.1–6	≥6.1
or INR	<1.7	1.7–2.3	>2.3
Grade A, 5–6; grade B, 7–9; grade C, 10–15.			

INR, international normalized ratio.
From Wantz GE, Payne MA. Experience with portacaval shunt for portal hypertension. N Engl J Med 1961;265:721, with permission.

Varices

One of the most life-threatening complications of portal hypertension is bleeding from esophageal varices. Esophageal varices are dilated veins found most commonly in the distal 5 cm of the esophagus. In the normal esophagus, a venous plexus is located in the submucosa; it becomes more superficially located to the lamina propria in the distal esophagus (133,134). This more superficial location in the distal esophagus is consistent with the known increased occurrence of bleeding varices in that location. In addition, 10% to 15% of patients with esophageal varices have gastric varices.

The pressure in the portal system is an important determinant of the likelihood for varices to develop. Varices do not develop in persons with hepatic vein–portal vein gradients below 12 mm Hg. Pressure gradients above 12 mm Hg are invariably present in patients with varices, but this pressure does not necessarily produce varices in all patients. Other, undetermined factors must play a role. The prevalence of varices in patients with cirrhosis varies from 25% to 70%, depending on the severity of their liver disease (135).

In approximately 10% of all patients presenting with acute upper gastrointestinal bleeding, esophageal varices are the cause of bleeding. Rates of bleeding from varices vary among studies. In a study of the natural history of varices in which patients were prospectively followed for 6 years, esophageal varices developed in approximately 8% of patients with cirrhosis each year during the first 2 years of observation; the percentage increased to 30% by 6 years. Of the patients who had small varices detected at initial endoscopy, large varices developed in 25% (136). Other studies show an incidence of varices of up to 90% for patients with cirrhosis (137,138). Once varices are present, bleeding occurs in 25% to 35% of cases, with the highest risk occurring within the first year after diagnosis (139). Of patients who survive an episode of bleeding, 30% experience rebleeding within 6 weeks, and 70% at 1 year (140,141). Mortality rates from bleeding varices range from 5% to 50%, with rates of 5%, less than 25%, and more than 50% for Child A, B, and C patients, respectively (135,140).

The following equation (a modification of Laplace's law) has been used to study the pressure–flow–resistance relationship in blood vessels:

$$T = \frac{P \times R}{W}$$

where T = tension, P = pressure, R = radius, and W = wall thickness (142). As portal pressure increases, dilation and thinning of venous collaterals leads to increased vascular tension and a predisposition to bleeding.

The propensity for varices to bleed has been extensively studied. When combined with clinical data, certain endoscopic characteristics of varices have been correlated with initial episodes of bleeding (Table 37.10) These factors include variceal size, Child-Pugh class, and the presence of red wale markings (longitudinal dilated venules that resemble whip marks) (139), in addition to active alcohol consumption. Direct and indirect measurements of portal pressure have been used to predict the likelihood of bleeding, with hemorrhage occurring only in patients with portal–hepatic venous gradients above 12 mm Hg (143). These predictors have been prospectively validated by numerous studies, but the patients with the highest risk for bleeding comprised only 40% of the total group of patients who bled; low-risk patients constituted 25% of those with bleeding.

Bleeding esophageal varices have an associated mortality rate of up to 50% after the first episode, and the tendency for further bleeding within the first year is 60% or greater (144). Mortality is related to the severity of liver disease, with Child C patients having a 1-year survival rate of 10%; in contrast, Child A patients have a 5-year survival of 50% (145).

Prevention of Initial Variceal Bleeding. Because of the severe consequences of variceal bleeding, methods to prevent first (primary prophylaxis) and recurrent (secondary prophylaxis) episodes of bleeding have been developed. These include control of the underlying cause of cirrhosis (i.e., alcohol consumption) and pharmacologic and surgical interventions to lower portal pressure. The next section discusses methods of primary prophylaxis for the prevention of initial episodes of bleeding (Table 37.11).

Beta Blockade. The use of nonspecific β-adrenergic blockade has been studied extensively in randomized, controlled trials of the primary prophylaxis of variceal bleeding. The mechanism of action of these drugs (propranolol, nadolol) involves effects of both β_1-adrenergic and β_2-adrenergic blockade, including decreased cardiac output and increased splanchnic arteriolar vasoconstriction as a result of the loss of opposing β_2-adrenergic dilation (145,146). The combined effects decrease portal blood flow and subsequently portal pressure.

These drugs are effective in portal hypertension associated with prehepatic, intrahepatic, and posthepatic conditions (147,148), regardless of whether ascites is present (149). However, not all patients respond to therapy. Two

---

Table 37.10. ENDOSCOPIC SIGNS THAT CORRELATE WITH RISK FOR VARICEAL RUPTURE

Category	Subcategory
Basic color	White varices
	Blue varices
Signs	Red color sign
	Red wale marking
	Cherry red spot
	Hematocystic spot
	Diffuse redness
Form	Linear
	Tortuous
	Large

From Japanese Research Society for Portal Hypertension.

Table 37.11. PREVENTION/TREATMENT OPTIONS FOR VARICEAL BLEEDING

Propranolol
    10–20 mg bid titrated weekly
    maximum of 160 mg bid
Nadolol
    20 mg orally qd
    titrate to: reduction of HR by 20%–25%
        absolute HR of 55–60
        symptoms
Isosorbide-5-mononitrate
    20 mg orally tid
Vasopressin with nitroglycerin
    0.4 U/min to maximum of 1.0 U/min
    titrated to maintain SBP at approximately 100 mm Hg
Octreotide
    50 µg bolus, followed by 50 mg/h for 5 days or until definitive
        treatment

HR, heart rate; SBP, systolic blood pressure.
Adapted from Rikkers LF. Variceal hemorrhage: surgical therapy. Gastroenterol Clin North Am 1993;22(4):821–842, with permission.

metaanalyses have evaluated seven randomized, controlled trials comparing propranolol or nadolol with placebo in the prevention of initial variceal bleeding. Both analyses concluded that beta blockade is significantly correlated with a reduced incidence of bleeding. A reduction of 40% was noted overall after all trial results were combined, with bleeding developing in approximately 16% of treated and 27% of untreated patients. The goal of therapy is to reduce the hepatic vein–portal vein gradient to below 12 mm Hg or to more than 20% below baseline (150).

In addition to reducing the number of first episodes of bleeding, beta blockade therapy has been shown to reduce mortality in most clinical trials (151–155). However, the differences were significant in only one study (154). A metaanalysis of these studies concluded that mortality from bleeding is reduced in patients with large varices (156).

Nitrates. Organic nitrates such as isosorbide-5-mononitrate, a vasodilator, have been used to reduce portal pressures. The possible mechanisms of action may include the following: (a) reflex splanchnic vasoconstriction secondary to peripheral venodilation and venous pooling; (b) decreased collateral resistance by arterial vasodilation; and (c) decreased intrahepatic resistance, possibly as a result of inhibition of stellate cell contractility (157). These agents may be used alone in patients with contraindications to beta blocker therapy, such as chronic obstructive pulmonary disease and congestive heart failure, or in combination with beta blockade in patients who do not have contraindications but respond inadequately to beta blocker therapy alone. Studies have indicated an enhanced reduction of portal pressure and a decreased incidence of bleeding in patients who receive combination therapy (158,159). In the only study that compared combination therapy with beta blocker therapy alone, approximately 8% of patients treated with the combined regimen experienced bleeding, compared with 18% of patients treated with beta blocker therapy alone (160). Thus, combination therapy may become the mainstay for prevention of bleeding in cirrhotic patients with varices.

Surgical Intervention. In the 1950s and 1960s, surgeons created prophylactic portosystemic shunts in an attempt to prevent variceal bleeding. These procedures were studied in a randomized, controlled fashion, and although effective in preventing variceal bleeding, they caused an increased incidence of hepatic failure and encephalopathy and had no effect on overall survival (161,162). Therefore, they are no longer performed for this indication.

Endoscopic Sclerotherapy and Variceal Ligation. In the past, prophylactic sclerotherapy to prevent variceal bleeding was an accepted practice. A recent study demonstrated an increased mortality in alcoholic patients treated with sclerotherapy (163). This therapeutic option is no longer used for the primary prevention of variceal bleeding. Investigations of the effectiveness of variceal ligation as a method of primary prophylaxis to prevent initial bleeding in high-risk patients with esophageal varices have reported mixed results (164,165). In one study, no statistically significant differences in the incidence of initial bleeding and mortality were found in a comparison of patients after variceal ligation with controls (164). A subgroup analysis revealed a significant decrease in the incidence of initial bleeding for Child-Pugh class B patients. In another report, a comparison of patients undergoing sclerotherapy or ligation with controls demonstrated a significant difference between both the sclerotherapy group and the ligation group versus the controls. Further research is needed before this therapeutic intervention can be endorsed.

Treatment of Esophageal Variceal Bleeding

Initial Management. Initial management of the patient with acute variceal includes the following: (a) establishment and maintenance of an airway; (b) hemodynamic monitoring; (c) placement of large-bore intravenous lines; (d) full laboratory investigation, including measurement of hemoglobin and hematocrit, coagulation profile, liver function tests, measurement of electrolytes, and assessment of renal function; (e) administration of blood products as needed, including packed red cells, platelets, and fresh frozen plasma; and (f) intensive care unit monitoring.

Pharmacologic Therapy. Administration of vasoactive medications may be commenced almost immediately after patient presentation if the history and physical findings suggest variceal bleeding. This practice decreases the rate of bleeding and enhances the endoscopic ability to visualize the site(s) of bleeding.

Vasopressin (antidiuretic hormone) has potent splanchnic vasoconstrictive properties that decrease portal venous and collateral flow and reduce portal pressure. In randomized, prospective trials, as well as in a metaanalysis, continuous intravenous administration of vasopressin has proved to reduce variceal bleeding. When vasopressin was compared with placebo, bleeding stopped in an average of 52% of patients who received vasopressin and 18% of patients who received placebo (166–168). However, rates of rebleeding as high as 45% were noted. Because of coronary vasoconstrictive effects, vasopressin must be used in combination with a vasodilator, such as nitroglycerin (169). The combination provides protection from adverse cardiac events and increases the effectiveness of vasopressin by decreasing intrahepatic and collateral resistance (170,171). A metaanalysis of three randomized, controlled trials (172–174) confirmed the increased effectiveness of vasopressin/nitroglycerin in comparison with vasopressin alone. A derivative of vasopressin, terlipressin, has similar efficacy with fewer side effects (172), but this drug is not available in the United States.

Somatostatin and octreotide, its longer acting eight-amino acid derivative, have been used extensively for the treatment of variceal bleeding. These agents decrease splanchnic blood flow indirectly by reducing the levels of other factors, such as glucagon, vasoactive intestinal peptide, and substance P, rather than by direct vasoconstriction (175,176). The effects of somatostatin are limited to the splanchnic circulation, so that side effects are minimized (177). Somatostatin/octreotide has proved to be as effective as vasopressin, sclerotherapy, and balloon tamponade in multiple studies (178–184). Because of the lack of complications related to somatostatin therapy, octreotide is the initial drug of choice for the treatment of acute variceal hemorrhage.

Endoscopic Interventions. The two main nonpharmacologic interventions for the treatment of variceal bleeding are endoscopic sclerotherapy and endoscopic variceal ligation. Both can be performed at the bedside. The technique of sclerotherapy (Fig. 37.6) entails performing upper gastrointestinal endoscopy with a flexible endoscope, visualizing the varices, and injecting 1 to 5 mL of sclerosing agent into or in close proximity to each varix. Sclerosing agents include sodium morrhuate, ethanolamine, polidocanol, and sodium tetradecyl sulfate. Total injection volume is 20 to 30 mL. The injections are begun at the distal esophagus and are continued circumferentially and proximally until all clinically relevant varices have been injected. Complications of sclerotherapy occur in 10% to 30% of patients and include fever, retrosternal chest pain (most common), dysphagia, and, more significantly, perforation with mediastinitis, bleeding from sclerosant-induced ulcers, esophageal stenosis, and sepsis. Overall, the

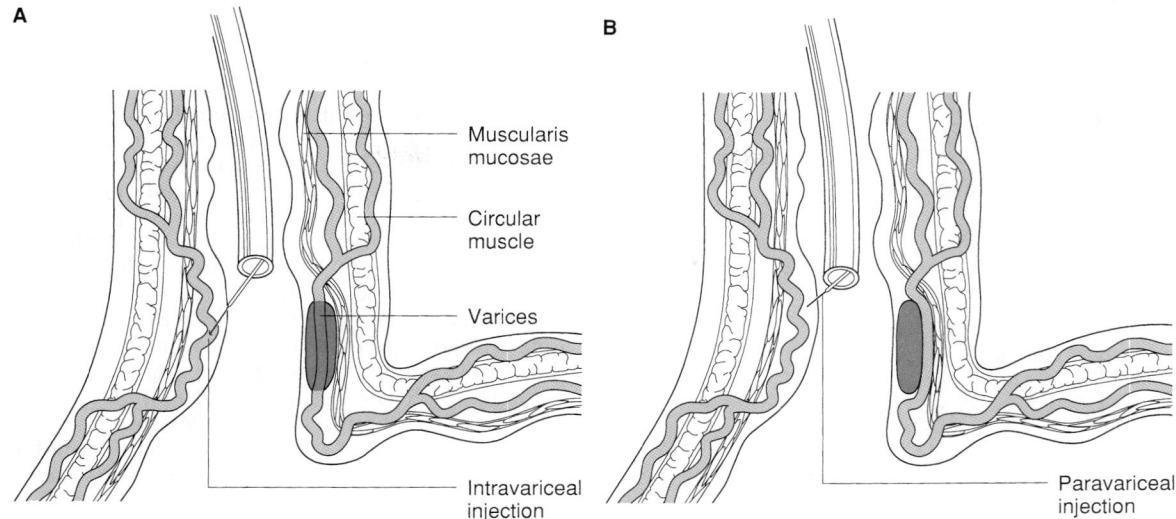

Figure 37.6. Techniques of intravariceal *(A)* and paravariceal *(B)* injection of esophageal varices.

treatment-related mortality rate is less than 2%. In the approximately 1% of patients in whom perforation occurs, the mortality rate may be as high as 50%. Success rates for initial control of variceal bleeding by sclerotherapy range from 60% to 90% (185), but more than one session is required to stop bleeding completely in up to 95% of cases.

In the past, sclerotherapy was considered the initial intervention of choice. Currently, the initial therapy of choice is endoscopic variceal ligation. The technique of ligation (Fig. 37.7) includes placement of an endoscope over a sheath (which allows multiple insertions and removal of the endoscope), suctioning of a varix into the lumen of a plastic channel, and then placement of a rubber band around the tissue. The procedure is similar to the ligation of hemorrhoids. The tissue then sloughs in 1 to 3 days, leaving a shallow ulcer. Up to six bands can be placed at each session. Newer endoscopes allow for the placement of multiple bands without removal of the endoscope. The placement of bands follows the same pattern as in sclerotherapy.

Success rates for variceal ligation range from 80% to 100%, in comparison with 77% to 94% for sclerotherapy, in controlled trials (186–190). A metaanalysis (191) that examined these data and compared the results of seven randomized, controlled trials (186–190,192,193) indicated an equal or better success rate for variceal ligation than for sclerotherapy in eliminating esophageal variceal bleeding, with fewer complications. When patients who underwent ligation therapy were compared with patients who underwent sclerotherapy, a reduction of approximately 50% in the incidence of rebleeding (50% vs. 25%) and death from bleeding (17% vs. 10%) and a reduction of 30% in overall mortality (32% vs. 24%) were noted in the ligation group. In addition, the incidence of esophageal stricture, bleeding from treatment-related ulceration, and the number of treatment sessions were decreased with ligation. In patients with profuse bleeding, the type of endoscope used for variceal ligation may make visualization of the bleeding varices difficult. Some investigators choose to perform sclerotherapy in these patients and utilize variceal ligation once bleeding is somewhat controlled.

Balloon Tamponade. The vast majority of patients (75% to 90%) with bleeding esophageal varices respond to endoscopic or pharmacologic therapy. For patients who fail these interventions, balloon tamponade (Fig. 37.8) is

an alternative therapy with a high success rate in controlling bleeding. It entails the placement of a specialized nasogastric tube with two balloons that can be inflated separately and to different pressures. The most commonly used tubes are the Sengstaken-Blakemore tube and the Minnesota tube. The former consists of a gastric balloon and an esophageal balloon with a sump port for gastric suctioning. The latter tube has an additional port above the esophageal balloon for the aspiration of saliva and other material from the esophagus and pharynx.

Placement of these tubes begins with the establishment of a safe airway by endotracheal intubation. The tube is then passed through the nose and into the stomach. Radiographic confirmation that the tip of the tube is in the stomach is required before balloon inflation to prevent inadvertent intraesophageal inflation of the gastric balloon and resultant perforation. The gastric balloon is inflated

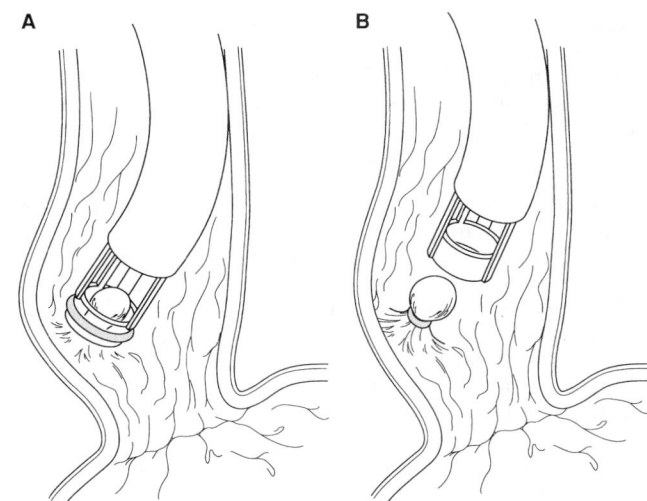

Figure 37.7. Endoscopic ligation of esophageal varices. The device used for ligation is based on the standard Barron-type ligator for the treatment of anal hemorrhoids. The esophageal varix is drawn up into the ligating device with suction *(A)*, and the base of the varix is ligated with an O-ring *(B)*. Up to six varices can be treated at a single session.

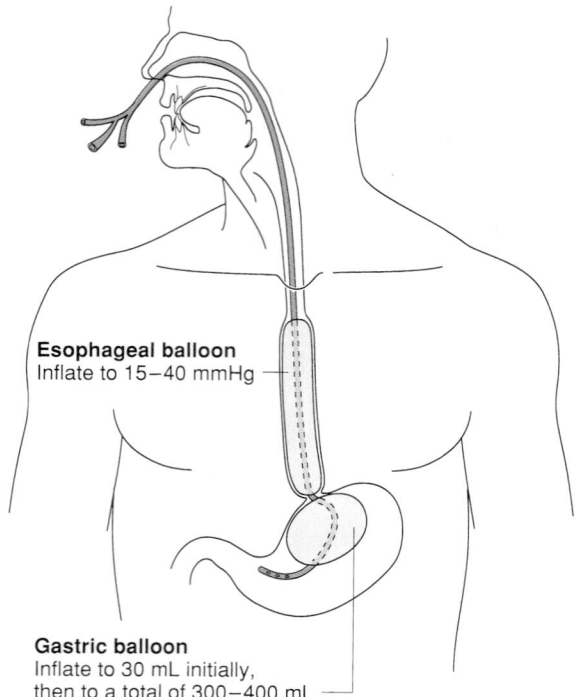

Esophageal balloon
Inflate to 15–40 mmHg

Gastric balloon
Inflate to 30 mL initially,
then to a total of 300–400 mL

Figure 37.8. The Sengstaken-Blakemore tube is used to tamponade acutely bleeding gastroesophageal varices. The tube has three lumina—one to aspirate the stomach, another to inflate the gastric balloon, and a third to inflate the esophageal balloon. Patients treated with balloon tamponade should be in an intensive care unit, and endotracheal tubes should be placed in almost all to prevent aspiration.

with 200 mL of air and firmly pulled backward against the gastroesophageal junction to tamponade any proximal gastric bleeding. The esophageal balloon is then inflated to a pressure of 30 to 40 mm Hg, and the tube is secured to the patient by means of a catcher's mask or football helmet to ensure adequate stability of the tube and prevent inadvertent removal.

Because of the possible complications of balloon tamponade (e.g., aspiration, esophageal and gastric perforation and necrosis), which occur in 10% to 20% of patients, its use is restricted to approximately 24 hours. Success rates for cessation of bleeding are 70% to 80%, but more than half of all patients rebleed when the balloons are deflated. Although this method is highly effective in the initial control of bleeding, with an efficacy similar to that of pharmacologic agents, because of its transient effects it can be used only as a temporizing measure in anticipation of a more definitive procedure, such as TIPS, placement of a surgical shunt, or transplantation and is used only after endoscopic and pharmacologic therapies have failed.

Transjugular Intrahepatic Portasystemic Shunt. In the 10% to 20% of patients who continue to bleed or who have early rebleeding, a shunt procedure (to bypass the high-pressure hepatic vascular bed) may be indicated. The mortality rate associated with failure to control bleeding can be as high as 90% (194), and surgically created shunts in this setting are associated with a high morbidity and mortality rate.

The transjugular intrahepatic portosystemic shunt (Fig. 37.9) is a recent addition to the nonoperative armamentarium of treatments for bleeding esophageal varices. After

ultrasonographic confirmation of patency of the portal vein, the procedure is performed in the interventional radiology suite, where a wire-guided stent (8 to 12 mm in diameter) is placed percutaneously into the jugular vein. The wire is then guided through the superior vena cava, right atrium, and inferior vena cava into a hepatic vein, after which the catheter traverses the hepatic parenchyma and joins the hepatic vein to a portal vein. This connection effectively creates a side-to-side portacaval shunt. Success rates in the cessation of variceal bleeding are as high as 90% to 100%, with an incidence of recurrent bleeding of approximately 10% (195,196).

The therapeutic goal is to reduce the hepatic–portal venous pressure gradient to below 12 mm Hg. TIPS reduces the portosystemic pressure gradient to a mean of approximately 9 to 15 mm Hg (average, 10 mm Hg), or to 40% to 62% below baseline (197,198). Mortality rates are high (40% to 60% at 6 to 7 weeks) despite the relative noninvasiveness of the procedure and reflect the gravity of the clinical condition of most patients requiring this intervention (195,196). One potential cause of the high mortality is a delay in instituting the TIPS until multiple unsuccessful attempts at sclerotherapy or banding have been made. This delay allows the patient's hepatic function and overall stability to deteriorate.

As with all portosystemic shunts, a significant complication of TIPS is the development of hepatic encephalopathy. After placement of a TIPS, the incidence of hepatic encephalopathy rises from 10% before treatment to 25% (199), and the incidence of progression to accelerated liver failure is approximately 3% to 5% (194).

In addition, stenoses or occlusion of the stent develops in up to 50% to 60% of patients. Shunt stenosis can be managed angiographically with thrombolytic therapy, dilation, or replacement of the stent. Patients are usually followed at 3-month intervals by ultrasonography to assess the patency of the shunt. At 6 months of follow-up, 92% of patients had had no episodes of rebleeding, and 82% are free of hemorrhage at 1 year (124).

Two clear indications for TIPS are emerging from clinical trials. In Child C patients with cirrhosis, in whom placement of a surgical shunt is considered too risky, TIPS is clearly indicated. In addition, in relatively low-risk patients who are likely to receive a liver transplant as definitive therapy, TIPS is helpful in decompressing the portal system and halting bleeding while leaving the external hepatobiliary anatomy undisturbed and free of postoperative adhesions.

Surgical Decompression

BACKGROUND. Surgeons have been performing shunt procedures since the 1800s. The first was an end-to-side portacaval shunt with ligation of the distal portal vein, performed by Nicolai Eck (Eck fistula) in dogs. In 1945, Whipple and Blakemore at the Columbia-Presbyterian Medical Center in New York performed this shunt for the first time for the indication of variceal bleeding (200). This group was also responsible for the development of the tube for the tamponade of bleeding esophageal varices, which adopted the name of Blakemore, as discussed above.

Surgical interventions for the treatment of bleeding varices are divided into three main types: (a) liver transplantation, (b) shunt procedures, and (c) devascularization procedures. The only definitive procedure for the treatment of portal hypertension caused by cirrhosis is orthotopic liver transplantation, and the success of this option during the past two decades has revolutionized the treatment of portal hypertension and its complications in patients with end-stage liver disease. However, for the treatment of portal hypertension in patients without cirrhosis, or in those whose liver function does not warrant

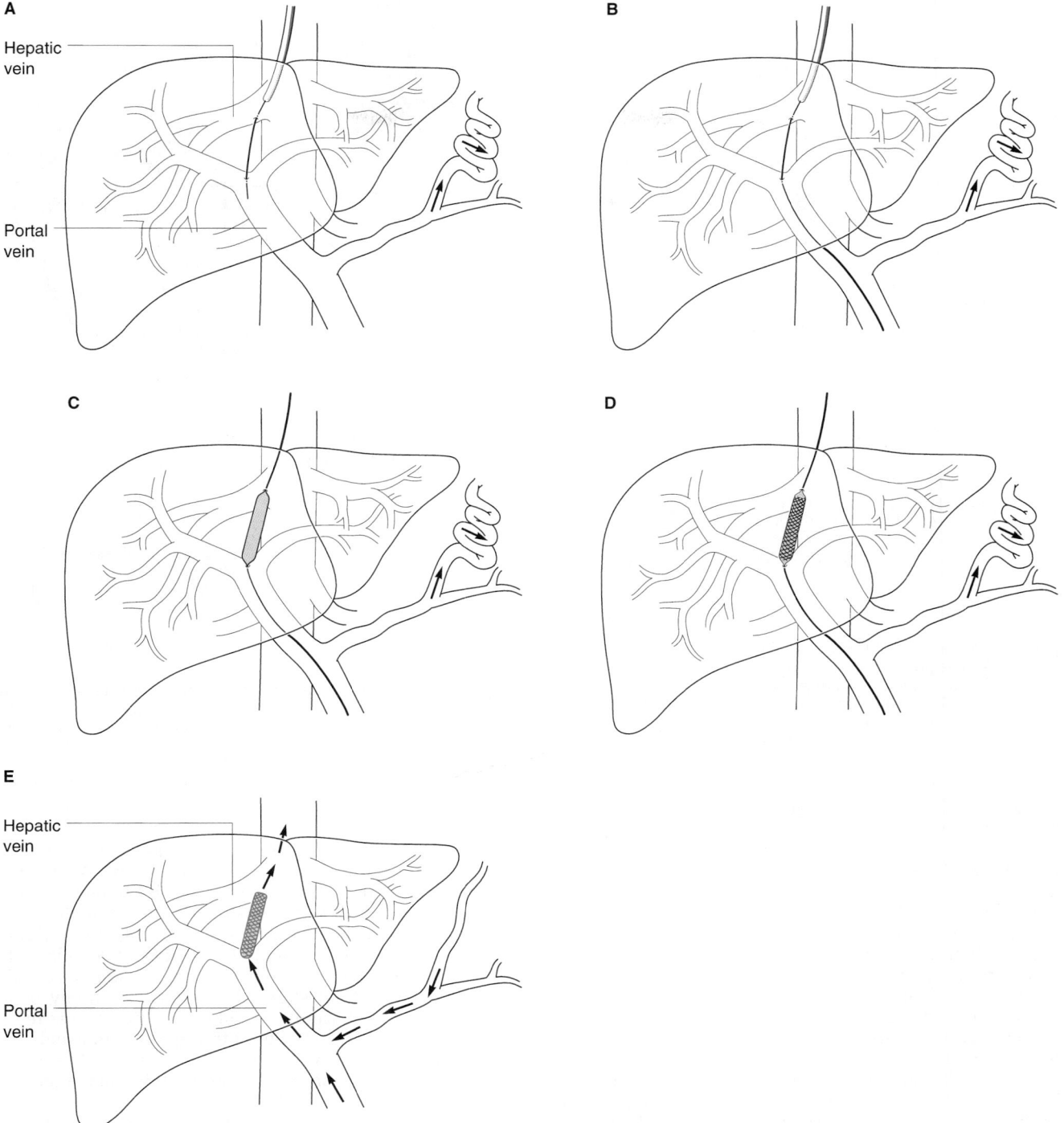

A

Hepatic vein

Portal vein

B

C

D

E

Hepatic vein

Portal vein

Figure 37.9. Schematic representation of the steps used to create a transjugular intrahepatic portosystemic shunt. (After Zemel G, Katzen BT, Becker GJ, et al. Percutaneous transjugular portosystemic shunt. *JAMA* 1991;266:390, with permission.)

a transplant (e.g., patients with portal vein thrombosis), decompressive surgically created shunts or devascularization procedures may be performed.

SHUNTS. Surgical shunts can be divided into three categories: (a) totally diverting shunts, (b) partially diverting shunts, and (c) selective shunts. Total shunts are created by completely bypassing the flow of blood away from the liver. Examples include the end-to-side portacaval shunt (Eck fistula) (Fig. 37.10) and the large-diameter (> 10 mm)

side-to-side portacaval (Fig 37.11), mesocaval, and central splenorenal shunts. These large side-to-side shunts divert all blood flow through the path of least resistance, so that flow in the portal vein, which becomes the outflow tract for portal blood flow, is reversed. One of the causes of ascites in patients with portal hypertension is high pressure at the level of the hepatic sinusoids. The main difference between end-to-side and side-to-side shunts is that maintenance of high pressure with end-to-side shunts may

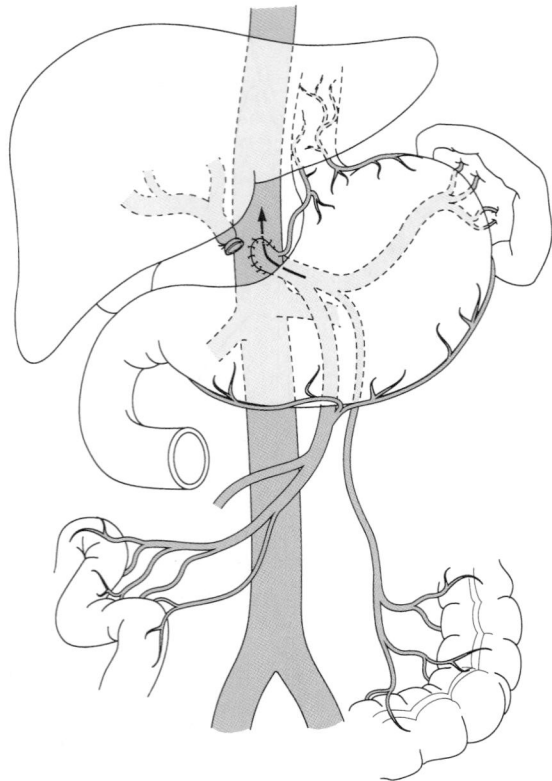

Figure 37.10. End-to-side portacaval shunt, also referred to as an *Eck fistula*. The portal vein is divided, the hepatic limb of the portal vein is ligated, and the splanchnic end of the portal vein is anastomosed end-to-side to the vena cava. All portal blood is necessarily diverted into the vena cava, and the hepatic limb of the portal vein cannot serve as an outflow tract.

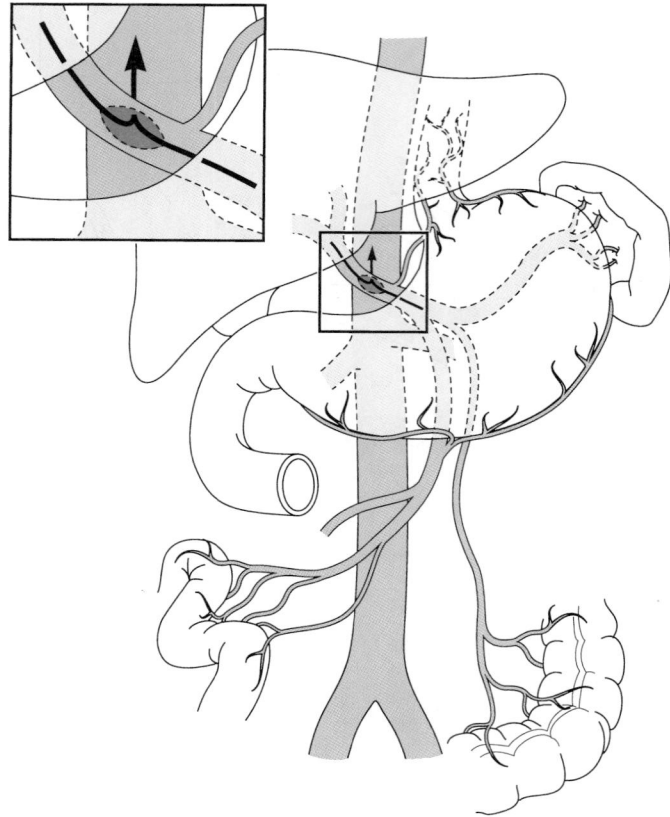

Figure 37.11. Side-to-side portacaval shunt. An anastomosis is made between the side of the portal vein and the side of the inferior vena cava. With a shunt of standard diameter, almost all splanchnic blood is diverted around the liver into the low-pressure vena cava. The hepatic limb of the portal vein serves as an outflow tract from the liver toward the low-pressure vena cava.

worsen ascites, whereas side-to-side procedures effectively relieve this problem by reducing sinusoidal pressure. Complete portal blood flow diversion lowers portal pressure and is highly effective in the treatment of bleeding esophageal varices.

The main complications of totally diverting shunts are a worsening of liver function and hepatic encephalopathy as a result of decreased flow through the liver and loss of hepatotrophic factors from the mesenteric venous system. Another disadvantage of portacaval shunts is that the porta hepatis must be dissected, so that future surgical procedures in the area, such as liver transplantation, are more difficult.

Partially diverting shunts allow for the maintenance of hepatopetal flow while decompressing the high pressures in the portal system. The original shunts were larger than 10 mm in diameter and were able to create a gradient between the portal vein and vena cava that maintained some prograde hepatic flow. However, all these shunts dilated over time and became complete shunts in that the portal vein-to-inferior vena cava pressure gradient disappeared. The small-diameter (8 mm) side-to-side mesocaval (Fig. 37.12) and portacaval (Sarfeh) (Fig. 37.13) shunts are performed with an interposition graft made of either expanded polytetrafluoroethylene (ePTFE) or Dacron. A significant component of the Sarfeh procedure is ligation of the coronary (left gastric), gastroepiploic, and other collateral veins. Bleeding from varices resolves in more than 90% of patients (201,202). This smaller-diameter shunt has a higher resistance than the larger shunt, is synthetic and therefore does not dilate, can

maintain hepatic perfusion, and is associated with a lower incidence of hepatic encephalopathy. With these shunts, portal pressure gradients can be reduced to the critical 12 mm Hg while hepatopetal flow is maintained in up to 80% to 90% of patients (203,204). In addition, the maintenance of mesenteric pressure at or relatively close to normal levels may prevent the hyperammonemia associated with total shunts (205). One relatively common complication is graft thrombosis, which occurs in up to 16% of patients (202). Shunt thrombosis can usually be treated angiographically. Dissection at the porta hepatis leads to the formation of adhesions, which may compromise later liver transplantation.

Selective shunts are designed to create two separate drainage systems within the portal venous network. A high pressure is maintained within the mesenteric system, and a low pressure is created in the esophagogastric system by shunting blood from the latter into the systemic circulation without decompressing the mesenteric network. The most frequently used selective shunt is the distal splenorenal shunt (206) (Fig. 37.14). Another rarely used selective shunt is the coronary–caval shunt (203). The distal splenorenal shunt selectively decompresses the gastroesophageal venous system through an anastomosis between the distal end of the splenic vein and the side of the renal vein. Decompression occurs through the short gastric veins, which are in continuity with the splenic vein. In addition, as in the small side-to-side shunts described above, collateral veins must be ligated.

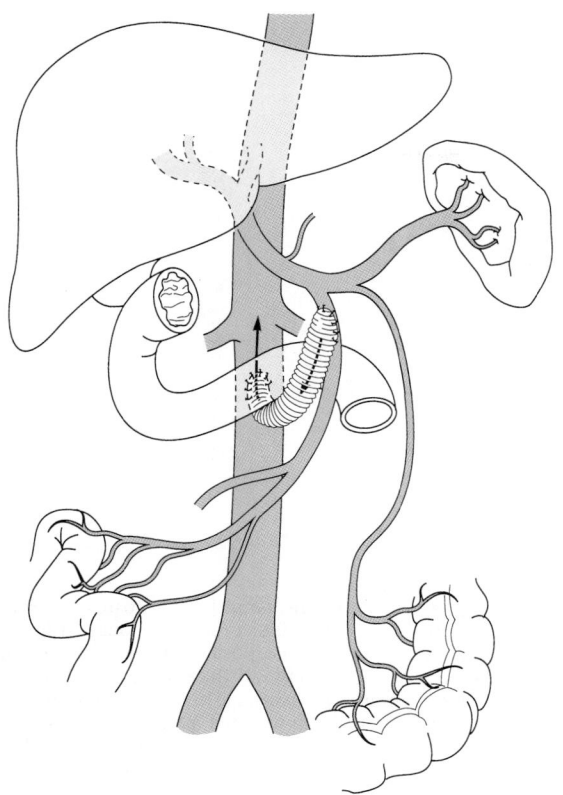

Figure 37.12. Interposition mesocaval shunt. A plastic prosthesis or an autogenous internal jugular vein is used for the shunt. One end is anastomosed to the inferior vena cava, and the other end is anastomosed to the trunk of the superior mesenteric vein. The shunt curves around the lower edge of the third portion of the duodenum and is sometimes called a *C-shunt*.

Advantages to this procedure are the following: (a) Control of bleeding is excellent in more than 90% of patients; (b) no dissection of the porta hepatis is required; (c) hepatopetal flow is maintained; and (d) the incidence of encephalopathy (5% to 24%) and progressive liver failure is lower (207–210). Experience with this shunt has revealed that most patients have hepatopetal flow, with 84% of alcoholic and 90% of nonalcoholic patients having prograde flow at 4 years after surgery (211,212). Some loss of prograde portal flow does occur as a result of either portal vein thrombosis (approximately 10% of patients) or increased flow through collaterals located along the pancreas. This latter mechanism can be prevented by complete dissection of the splenic vein from the posterior aspect of the pancreas (splenopancreatic disconnection) (212), but this additional technique adds to the complexity of the operative procedure and to the incidence of complications.

The distal splenorenal shunt is relatively contraindicated in patients with significant ascites. Because no portal venous decompression occurs, ascites may increase after a distal splenorenal shunt is created. In addition, ligation of collateral vessels and lymphatics during the procedure contributes to increased portal pressures and subsequent increase in ascites. Patients with small splenic veins (< 8 mm) have a relatively high incidence of shunt thrombosis (213).

Several trials comparing side-to-side total shunts with the distal splenorenal shunt found that they are equally effective (> 90%) in stopping variceal hemorrhage (214).

The incidence of hepatic encephalopathy is lower after the distal splenorenal shunt, with rates of 36% and 15% for the total and selective shunts, respectively. Rates of rebleeding were similar and ranged from zero to 30%, with no survival advantage for either procedure.

Investigators have also utilized the side-to-side nonselective total shunt for the emergency treatment of bleeding varices (215). Bleeding stopped in more than 90% of patients with medical therapy alone, although bleeding often restarted shortly thereafter. Bleeding stopped in all patients after surgery, and 99% of patients were completely free of episodes of rebleeding. The 5-year survival was approximately 80%, with the majority of deaths occurring during the first year after surgery as a result of progressive hepatic failure. Hepatic encephalopathy requiring recurrent intervention, including dietary restriction and lactulose/neomycin therapy, occurred in 8% of patients. These data support an aggressive, systematic approach to caring for these patients before, during, and after surgery.

DEVASCULARIZATION PROCEDURES. Devascularization procedures are nonshunting techniques in which the venous drainage of the stomach and esophagus is disconnected from the liver and intestinal vessels. These procedures are relatively less technically demanding than shunting procedures and can be performed in patients with extensive portal thromboses that preclude other options. They do not interfere with hepatopetal blood flow and therefore do not increase the incidence of hepatic encephalopathy.

The procedures range in complexity from simple esophageal transection and reanastomosis with an end-to-end anastomosis (EEA) stapler combined with ligation of the coronary vein (Fig. 37.15) to the Sugiura procedure (Fig. 37.16). The Sugiura procedure requires both abdominal and thoracic incisions, through which a splenectomy, devascularization of the proximal stomach and esophagus, transection of the esophagus with reanastomosis, and ligation of all gastroesophageal collaterals is performed (216). The latter procedure can also be performed via a single abdominal incision (217). Bleeding recurs in fewer than 5% of patients in Japan, but rates of rebleeding range from 10% to 54% in other countries (216,218). Operative mortality rates range from 10% to 35% (218).

Four controlled trials have compared devascularization procedures with sclerotherapy (214,219–221). Although esophageal transection appeared to be associated with a lower incidence of rebleeding, the mortality rates were higher.

HEPATIC TRANSPLANTATION. Liver transplantation is the definitive therapy for portal hypertension and cirrhosis and the complications thereof. The limited number of organs and the potential complications of this procedure make it one of last resort. Only patients with end-stage liver disease (Child C patients with cirrhotis) are candidates for transplantation. When successful, transplantation treats both the underlying disease and any acute complication.

Algorhythm for the Treatment of Variceal Bleeding. The following recommendations assume the following: (a) adequate expertise in all aspects of caring for cirrhotic patients, including endoscopy and interventional radiology; (b) the availability of trained surgeons capable of performing the indicated surgical procedures; (c) the availability of hepatic transplantation or transfer to a center where it is available (Fig. 37.17).

RESUSCITATION AND PRIMARY CONTROL. At presentation, patients should immediately undergo resuscitation and hemodynamic monitoring, followed by establishment of the diagnosis of variceal bleeding. A pharmacologic agent should be commenced immediately in the emergency department, consisting of octreotide and/or beta blockade.

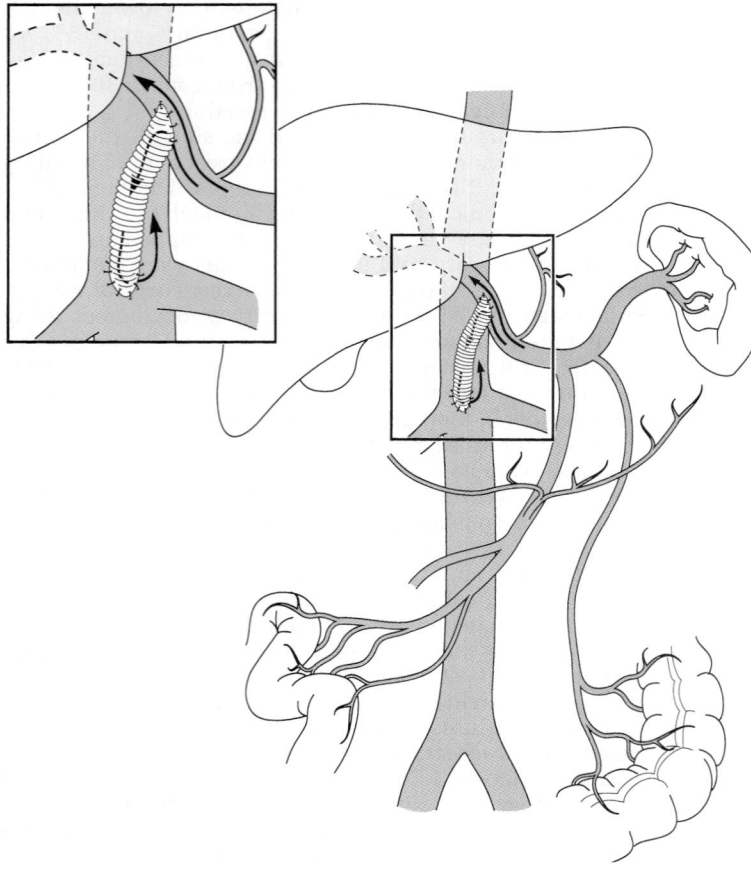

Figure 37.13. Small-diameter interposition portacaval Sarfeh shunt. A vascular prosthesis measuring 8 to 10 mm in diameter is interposed between the side of the vena cava and the side of the portal vein. The goal is to reduce portal pressure partially and thereby prevent variceal hemorrhage but still maintain sufficient pressure to permit the prograde flow of portal blood to the liver. This procedure is simpler to perform than that for the Warren shunt and theoretically avoids the problem of diversion of an increasing proportion of portal blood away from the liver over time, as occurs with the Warren shunt.

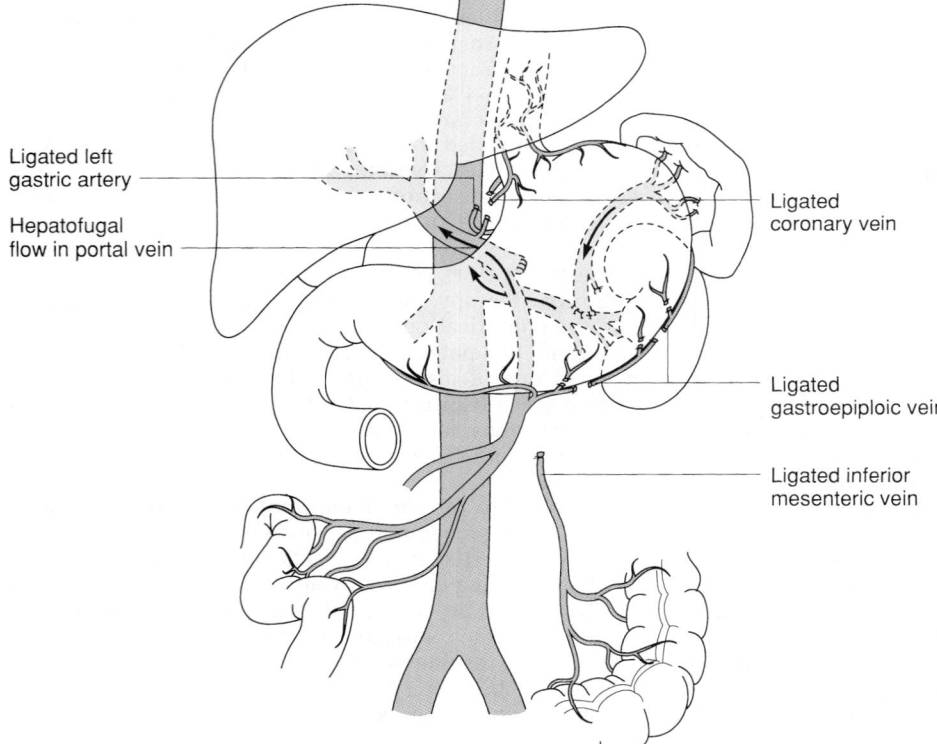

Ligated left gastric artery

Hepatofugal flow in portal vein

Ligated coronary vein

Ligated gastroepiploic vein

Ligated inferior mesenteric vein

Figure 37.14. Distal splenorenal Warren shunt. The splenic vein is divided near its junction with the superior mesenteric vein. The distal end of the splenic vein is anastomosed to the renal vein. Varices are selectively decompressed through the stomach and short gastric veins into the splenic vein and then into the vena cava through the renal vein. Portal hypertension is maintained in the portal and superior mesenteric veins to provide enough pressure to drive portal blood through the diseased liver.

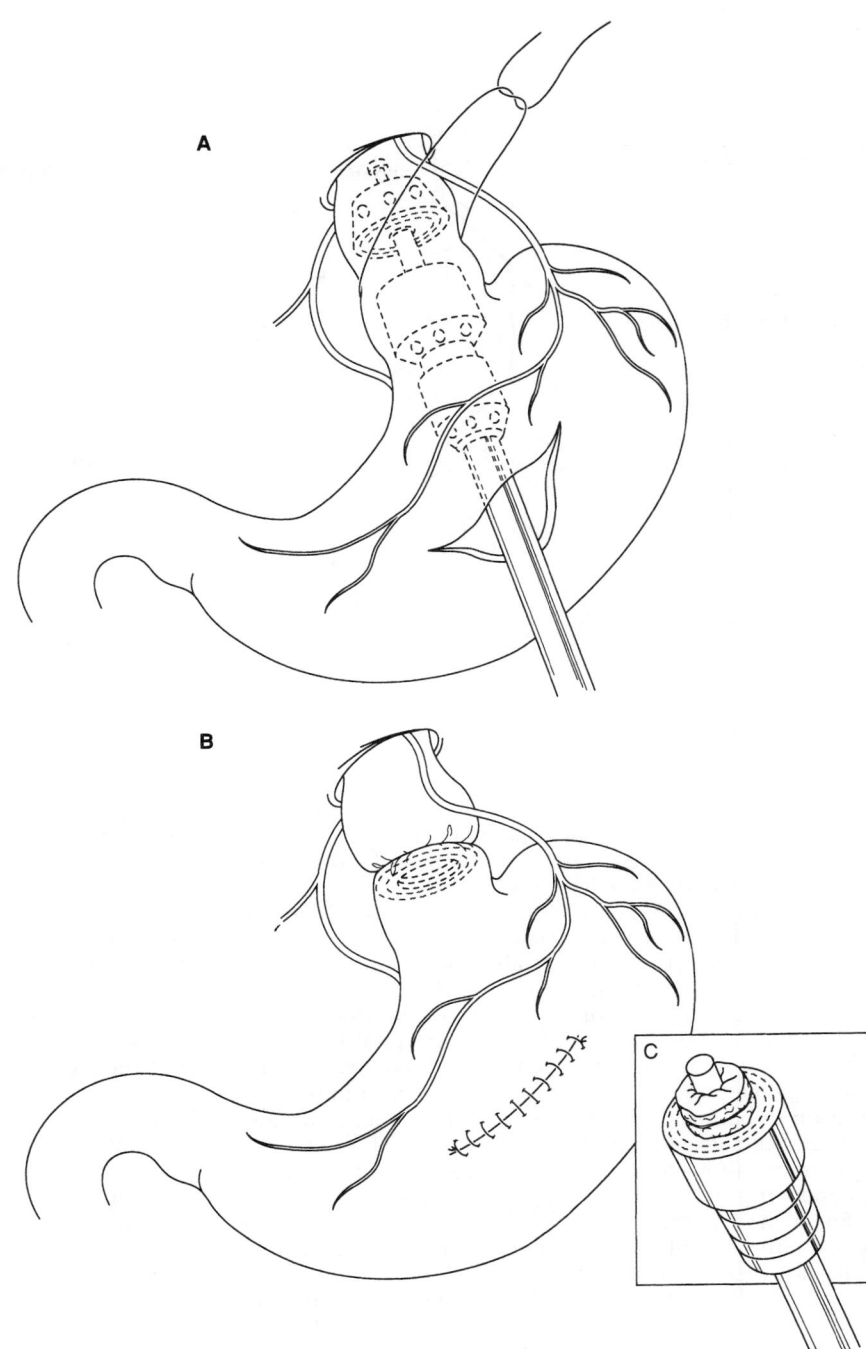

Figure 37.15. Transection and reanastomosis of the distal esophagus with the stapling device to control variceal hemorrhage. *(A)* A stapling device is inserted through a small gastrotomy incision. *(B)* When the device is fired, the esophagus is simultaneously transected and reanastomosed with staples. *(C)* If the device fires correctly, a complete ring of esophageal tissue is excised.

Second-tier agents include vasopressin/nitroglycerin. Upper gastrointestinal endoscopy should be performed expeditiously in the appropriate setting for attempts at variceal ligation. Sclerotherapy is a second choice. Rapid triage is imperative, and repeated attempts at endoscopic therapy in the setting of continued bleeding may lead to worsening of the patient's overall status and increased morbidity and mortality. For the majority of patients (75% to 90%), these interventions will be effective in controlling the hemorrhage. If rebleeding occurs, another attempt at endoscopic therapy is warranted while preparations are made for one of the alternative therapies in the event of treatment failure. In the relatively small number of patients in whom primary control is not achieved, balloon tamponade is usually the next immediate procedure of choice to stop the hemorrhage, albeit temporarily.

DEFINITIVE CONTROL. The failure of primary measures mandates definitive interventions, which include TIPS, surgical shunts, devascularization procedures, and emergent liver transplantation. These methods introduce permanent mechanical alterations that may adversely affect liver function and are of varying practical utility in the emergency setting. Proper decision making requires primary stratification based on hepatic function and secondary stratification according to treatment setting (emergent vs. elective). It is critical that the issue of eligibility for hepatic transplantation be addressed before these interventions are undertaken because portal decompression

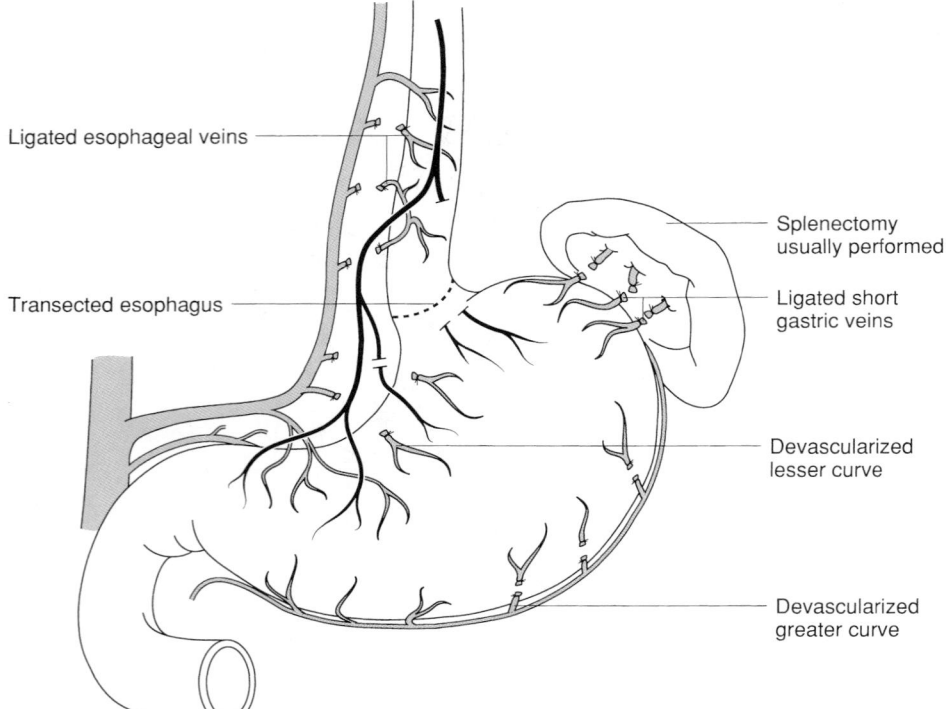

Ligated esophageal veins

Transected esophagus

Splenectomy
usually performed

Ligated short
gastric veins

Devascularized
lesser curve

Devascularized
greater curve

Figure 37.16. Sugiura esophageal transection and devascularization operation.

can provoke hepatic failure. In patients who are not transplant candidates, the development of postoperative hepatic failure is a lethal event, and this must be discussed in detail with patients before intervention.

The question of which of the various types of surgical procedures should be used for emergency variceal bleeding has been studied in multiple trials. The number of publications on a given topic is not necessarily correlated with the general applicability of a specific surgical intervention and may reflect the referral pattern or hospital system in which the studies were performed. As in all complex operative procedures, the technical ability of each individual surgeon to perform a given procedure is crucial to its success and is correlated with complications. The following recommendations are based on the assumption that well-trained surgeons are performing these procedures.

For hemodynamically stable Child A cirrhotic patients who continue to bleed and are potential transplant candidates, are bleeding from gastric varices, or have portal gastropathy, a distal splenorenal shunt is the procedure most commonly performed worldwide. Excellent results have also been reported in this setting with small-diameter por-

tacaval H-graft shunts. The arguments for the H-graft are that it is technically easier to perform and provides excellent control of bleeding. In addition, it is associated with high rates of long-term maintenance of prograde portal flow and patency and low rates of hepatic encephalopathy and mortality. Similar arguments can be made for the small-diameter mesocaval H-graft shunts. Mesocaval shunts have the added advantage of eliminating the need for portal dissection with the subsequent formation of adhesions, which can significantly prolong operative time and increase blood loss during liver transplantation performed later. In addition, some hepatic transplantation protocols utilize femoral–axillary venovenous bypass to prevent significant elevations in portal and vena caval pressures during venous clamping; mesocaval shunts effectively serve that purpose and can easily be ligated at the termination of the transplant procedure. The role of TIPS in this setting is yet to be determined.

In the hemodynamically unstable Child A cirrhotic patient, a nonselective side-to-side portacaval or mesocaval shunt is the procedure of choice for immediate control of bleeding. TIPS is another option. For patients who are

Variceal Bleeding with Endoscopic/Pharmacologic Failure

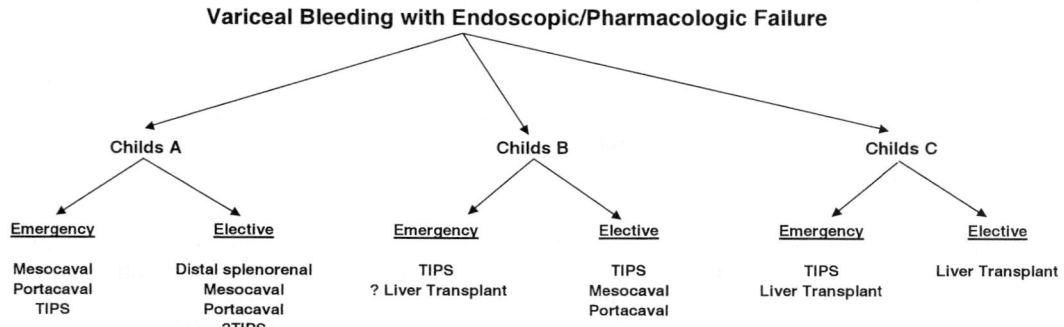

Childs A		Childs B		Childs C	
Emergency	Elective	Emergency	Elective	Emergency	Elective
Mesocaval	Distal splenorenal	TIPS	TIPS	TIPS	Liver Transplant
Portacaval	Mesocaval	? Liver Transplant	Mesocaval	Liver Transplant	
TIPS	Portacaval		Portacaval		
	?TIPS				

Figure 37.17. This algorithm represents the suggested treatment options, in order of preference, for patients who fail medical management for variceal bleeding.

noncompliant or live far from tertiary care medical centers capable of performing and maintaining the TIPS, a single operation such as the side-to-side shunt, which requires comparatively little follow-up, may be more appropriate.

Hemodynamically stable Child B cirrhotic patients without medically untreatable ascites who are transplant candidates can be treated with a TIPS or with a distal splenorenal or mesocaval shunt to avoid dissection in the porta hepatis. Unstable patients may undergo the same procedures, with the caveat that the distal splenorenal shunt should be avoided. If the patient has medically uncontrollable ascites, a TIPS is the procedure of choice. Small-diameter shunts are less effective for patients with ascites.

For Child C cirrhotic patients, the options are much more limited. All patients should undergo TIPS with the expectation that liver function will deteriorate and hepatic encephalopathy may worsen unless urgent transplant can be performed. In nontransplant candidates who fail nonoperative therapy and continue to bleed, TIPS may be lifesaving in the short term, but many patients will die of progressive liver failure.

An interesting consideration is the use of TIPS in patients with alcoholic cirrhosis. With abstinence, liver function may improve sufficiently that the shunt will no be longer needed. The approximately 50% occlusion rate requiring angiographic intervention to maintain patency may be of benefit in this patient population. Patients can undergo maintenance procedures for their TIPS until such time that their liver function improves to the degree that the shunt is not needed. After that time, no further intervention would take place and thrombosis would develop in the shunt. Thus, temporary self-limited support would be provided until liver function improved.

Currently, the only indication for devascularization procedures is the presence of extensive thrombosis in the portal vessels, which precludes the use of a shunt.

In conclusion, surgical intervention for patients with portal hypertension is becoming a rarity except in those with end-stage liver disease, in whom hepatic transplantation is indicated. With the advent of TIPS, the indications for surgically created shunts are dwindling. Child A cirrhotic patients may become the only true candidates for surgically created shunts in the setting of esophageal variceal bleeding, with most Child B patients undergoing the TIPS procedure. A randomized, prospective, multicenter trial of TIPS and partial and selective shunts would be the only method to determine the relative effectiveness of these therapies. The choice of a surgical procedure, if any, to treat bleeding varices depends most importantly on the expertise of the surgeon performing the procedure.

Prevention of Recurrent Variceal Bleeding. The risk for rebleeding in untreated patients with a history of prior variceal bleeding ranges from 47% to 70%, with an associated mortality rate of 20% to 70% (163). The risk factors for subsequent bleeding from esophageal varices are the same as those for initial bleeding and include continued alcohol abuse, size of varices, Child class, and the presence of red markings on endoscopic evaluation.

Multiple randomized trials (222–232), including a meta-analysis (163), have shown a reduction in rebleeding rates with the use of beta blocker therapy in comparison with placebo. Mortality rates were reduced in most of those trials. All patients without a contraindication to beta blocker therapy should be treated with one of these agents. In addition, combination therapy with beta blockade and nitrates reduces rates of rebleeding in comparison with either agent alone (233).

As indicated in the section on treatment of bleeding varices, endoscopic variceal ligation has surpassed sclerotherapy in effecting a cessation of bleeding. Moreover, in preventing rebleeding, variceal ligation has proved to be at least as effective as sclerotherapy, with fewer complications, and has become the endoscopic intervention of choice (234).

Almost 10 randomized trials have been performed to compare endoscopic intervention with TIPS (235–243). The vast majority of data support the use of TIPS, which is associated with significantly decreased rates of rebleeding (approximately 25% less) and no increase in mortality. However, because the incidence of significant encephalopathy is doubled, TIPS should be reserved for patients who fail other means of therapy.

Many randomized trials have compared endoscopic sclerotherapy with elective shunt surgery to prevent recurrent bleeding from esophageal varices (244–248). The majority utilized the distal splenorenal shunt. Rates of rebleeding varied from 3% to 17% for shunts and from 35% to 60% for sclerotherapy, with no difference in overall survival. For good-risk patients without medically intractable ascites, the distal splenorenal shunt appears to be a better option to prevent recurrent variceal bleeding than repetitive sclerotherapy.

Gastropathy and Gastric Varices. Approximately 10% of patients with esophageal varices also have gastric varices. Conversely, about 90% of patients with gastric varices have esophageal varices (249–252). Bleeding from gastric varices occurs in approximately 25% of affected patients, is usually more severe than bleeding from esophageal varices, and is poorly controlled by sclerotherapy. Rebleeding occurs in up to 30% of patients after an initial bleed (252). The same pharmacologic interventions utilized for esophageal varices are used for the treatment of gastric varices. Balloon tamponade may also be used. The surgical procedure of choice for bleeding gastric varices is the distal splenorenal shunt.

Portal hypertensive gastropathy is a condition characterized by dilation of the venules and capillaries of the gastric mucosa without associated inflammation (253,254). The major complication of gastropathy is bleeding; gastropathy accounts for 4% to 38% of all episodes of acute bleeding in patients with cirrhosis (255,256).

Ascites

One of the most important consequences of hepatic dysfunction in cirrhosis and portal hypertension is ascites. This development portends a significant worsening of the patient's condition, with markedly decreased survival rates. Ascites is defined as the accumulation of free fluid within the abdominal cavity (normally < 150 mL). Causes of ascites are listed in Table 37.12. In cirrhosis, the fluid is derived from a combination of hepatic (high in protein) and splanchnic (low in protein) lymph that cannot be absorbed as a result of the increased hydrostatic pressures within the liver and splanchnic systems secondary to cirrhosis and capillarization of the space of Disse. Because of the loss of sinusoidal fenestrations and a subsequent decrease in their permeability, splanchnic lymph is more abundant than hepatic lymph in cirrhotic patients with advancing disease, so that the protein content of ascitic fluid is relatively low (257). The main underlying pathophysiology in the development of ascites is renal sodium retention and associated water retention, which lead to fluid overload. Peripheral vasodilation and lower pressures are thought to be secondary to the dilator effects of nitric oxide, glucagon, and prostaglandins (136) on nascent arteriovenous shunts present throughout the splanchnic

Table 37.12. DIFFERENTIAL DIAGNOSIS OF ASCITES

PORTAL HYPERTENSION
Cirrhosis and other intrahepatic diseases
Hepatic congestion
   Congestive heart failure
   Constrictive pericarditis
   Inferior vena cava obstruction
   Budd-Chiari syndrome
Portal vein occlusion

HYPOALBUMINEMIA
Nephrotic syndrome
Protein-losing enteropathy
Malnutrition

MISCELLANEOUS DISORDERS
Myxedema
Ovarian disease (Meigs' syndrome, struma ovarii)
Peritoneal carcinomatosis
End-stage renal disease
Chylous ascites
Bile ascites
Urine ascites

From Sleisenger MH, Fordran JS. *Gastrointestinal disease: pathophysiology, diagnosis and management,* 4th ed. Philadelphia: WB Saunders, 1989:433, with permission.

vascular system, as well as in muscle, skin, and brain (258). The severity of liver disease is not uniformly correlated with the presence or absence of ascites.

Clinical and Laboratory Features. Ascites may be present in patients with cirrhosis who have no other overt signs or symptoms. Patients may present with subtle signs of weight gain and an inability to fit into clothes. Physical examination reveals shifting dullness to percussion (1.5 L of ascitic fluid), fluid waves (10 L), and bulging flanks (258). With progression of disease and massive ascites, respiratory status may be compromised secondary to increased intraabdominal pressure and pleural effusions, which are often present and usually located on the right side. The progression may be slow or more rapid after an inciting event such as a variceal bleed or infection.

Stigmata of poor liver function include peripheral muscle wasting, palmar erythema, spider angiomas, peripheral edema, a palpable liver, and caput medusae (dilated periumbilical veins). With progressive ascites and increased abdominal pressure, umbilical and inguinal hernias often develop and may be difficult to manage. Abdominal distention may be caused by gastrointestinal gas rather than ascites. Gas may be differentiated from fluid by eliciting hyperresonance to percussion, secondary to gas, as opposed to dullness with fluid. The most widely used test for the diagnosis of ascites is ultrasonography, which can also be helpful in determining the best location for therapeutic and diagnostic paracentesis.

Diagnostic Paracentesis. The differential diagnosis of ascites is presented in Table 37.12. Determination of the character of the ascitic fluid is helpful in establishing the diagnosis. Paracentesis may be performed in the midline, midway between the umbilicus and the pubic symphysis. The fluid from patients with cirrhosis is usually straw-colored and clear; measurements of protein (usually < 2 g/dL), quantitative cell counts, microbiologic culture, and determination of pH and amylase, glucose and albumin levels should be obtained. The serum-to-ascitic fluid albumin gradient is calculated. This gradient is helpful in de-

termining the cause of ascites; high values (> 1.1 g/dL) are generally associated with portal hypertension.

Treatment. Initial therapy is usually directed at control of renal sodium and water retention, with bed rest and dietary manipulation. The upright position exacerbates sodium retention as a result of venous pooling and relative hypovolemia. Up to 15% of patients respond to this therapy alone with a natriuresis. A low-sodium diet is a critical part of the management of patients with cirrhosis (1 to 2 g of sodium per day or 45 to 90 mEq/d). A major problem with a strict low-sodium diet is lack of palatability and poor compliance. Fluid restriction is also an essential component of therapy in patients in whom hyponatremia develops (sodium concentration < 125 mEq/L), with only 1,000 to 1,500 mL of fluid allowed each day.

For the 85% to 95% of patients who do not respond to bed rest and fluid and salt restriction, the mainstay of treatment is diuresis (Table 37.13). The loop diuretic furosemide and the potassium-sparing diuretic spironolactone are the two most widely utilized agents, and they may be combined to minimize side effects and maximize effectiveness. Spironolactone is a relatively weak natriuretic agent whose mechanism of action is competitive inhibition of aldosterone at the receptor level. It prevents the sodium retention and potassium loss that occur in the setting of high aldosterone levels. Spironolactone is the initial diuretic of choice for patients with mild ascites. Because of the long half-life of the drug, effects may take days to become evident. Furosemide is a faster-acting loop diuretic that inhibits sodium and chloride reabsorption from the thin ascending limb of the loop of Henle. A diuresis of approximately 500 mL/d is the goal for patients with mild ascites, and of up to 1 to 2 L/d for patients with both ascites and peripheral edema. More than 90% of patients respond to the combination of dietary manipulation and diuretics (259).

Complications of the use of spironolactone include hyperkalemia, gynecomastia, and metabolic acidosis. Complications of the more potent furosemide include prerenal azotemia, which occurs in approximately 20% of patients as a result of excessive diuresis and hypovolemia (258). Additional complications include hyponatremia and encephalopathy.

Table 37.13. TREATMENT OF ASCITES

Bed rest
Sodium restriction
   1–2 g/d (45–90 mEq/d)
Fluid restriction
   1–1.5 L/d
Diuretics
   Spironolactone
      50 mg po q8h
         maximum of 100 mg q6h
   Furosemide
      40–370 mg/d
Antibiotics
   Cefotaxime
      2 q IV q12h
   Ofloxacin
      400 mg po q12h
   Prophylaxis
   Norfloxacin
      400 mg/d while hospitalized
   Ciprofloxacin
      750 mg po weekly
   Norfloxacin
      400 mg/d for 6 mo
   Trimethoprim/sulfamethoxazole
      One double-strength table 5 times a week

Large-volume paracentesis (removal of 4 to 6 L of ascitic fluid per day) and total paracentesis are techniques that may be utilized for patients with large amounts of fluid who are experiencing symptoms and are not responding to the above-mentioned therapeutic endeavors. Patients requiring paracentesis usually have severe underlying liver disease and a 1-year survival rate of 25% (260). The technique of paracentesis involves placing a catheter into the abdominal cavity, either in the lower midline or in one of the lower quadrants. Care is taken to enter lateral to the rectus muscle and avoid the inferior epigastric artery. More than 30 L of fluid can be removed by means of total paracentesis, with 6 to 10 g of albumin infused for each liter of ascitic fluid removed (258). The albumin commonly is administered in the form of 25% albumin (12.5 g/50 mL). Other possible replacement solutions include normal saline solution, low-molecular-weight dextran 70, and 5% synthetic polymerized gelatin. Controversy exists regarding the need for albumin replacement therapy in patients undergoing total paracentesis and repetitive large-volume paracentesis. Patients who have less than 5 L of ascitic fluid removed do not require albumin replacement (261).

The efficacy of paracentesis in the treatment of tense ascites has been studied extensively. Repetitive large-volume paracentesis has been shown to be as effective as diuretics in the treatment of moderate to severe ascites, with fewer systemic complications. A decreased length of hospital stay with no increase in the incidence of spontaneous bacterial peritonitis has been noted (262–264). Paracentesis has become the therapy of choice for severe ascites.

Peritoneovenous shunts are surgically placed tubes that connect the peritoneal cavity with the superior vena cava via the internal jugular vein (Fig. 37.18). The two main types are the LeVeen shunt and the Denver shunt, both of which have a one-way valve that allows unidirectional movement of ascitic fluid from the peritoneal cavity into the systemic circulation. Although these shunts are effective in decreasing the volume of ascitic fluid, a significant number of major complications have been noted, including disseminated intravascular coagulation, heart failure, and sepsis (260,265), and associated mortality rates are high (approximately 20%) (266). The shunt is occluded in approximately 50% of patients at 1 year, and no improvement in survival is noted (260). The use of these shunts has drastically decreased with the development of the TIPS procedure.

Surgically created portosystemic shunts have been used in the past for the treatment of ascites. Because of high morbidity and mortality rates, an increase in encephalopathy and progression to liver failure, and the recent addition of the TIPS procedure to treatment options, surgically created shunts are now used infrequently for this indication alone. As discussed earlier, the TIPS is a total nonselective shunt that completely decompresses the portal system and reduces pressure at the hepatic sinusoids, thereby eliminating the drive for the production of ascitic fluid. In a study evaluating the use of TIPS for the treatment of medically refractory ascites, the ascites resolved completely in almost 75% of patients, and a partial response was noted in an additional 20% (267). In addition, renal function improved during the 6 months of follow-up. TIPS in this group of patients was associated with an increase in the number of cases of encephalopathy. Survival was related to the effectiveness of TIPS in treating ascites. Patients who experienced a complete resolution of ascites had a median survival of 558 days; those with a partial response survived for a median of 382 days, and those with no response for a median of 75 days.

Spontaneous bacterial peritonitis is a potentially lethal complication of portal hypertension with ascites that oc-

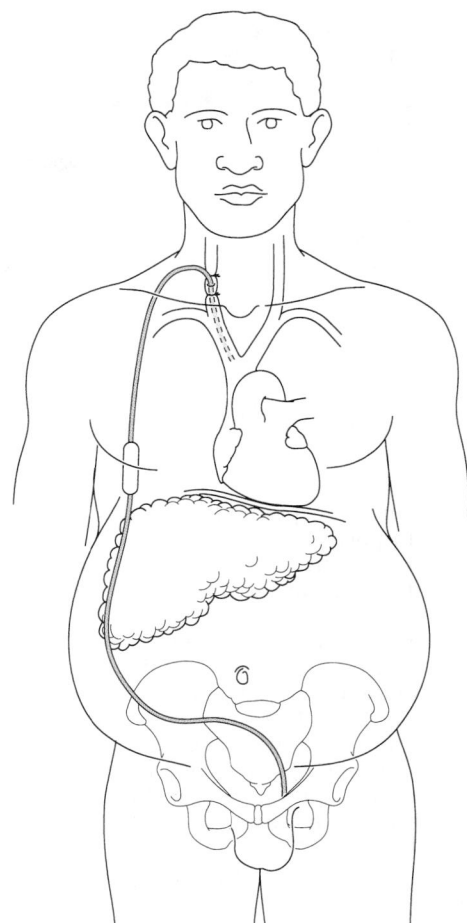

Figure 37.18. LeVeen peritoneovenous shunt used for routing ascitic fluid into the systemic circulation. The shunt consists of fenestrated tubing for insertion into the peritoneal cavity, a one-way valve, and a length of venous tubing for insertion into the superior vena cava.

curs in up to 10% of patients. The etiology of spontaneous bacterial peritonitis is unknown. Antecedent gastrointestinal hemorrhage is common, and spontaneous bacterial peritonitis in this setting may be related to bacterial translocation from the gut. Deficits in immune function, both systemically and within the abdomen, including depressed reticuloendothelial function (268), low ascitic protein concentration (269), and deficient ascitic opsonic activity (270), may play a role. Patients often present with abdominal pain and fever, but 10% to 20% of cases are discovered on routine paracentesis (265,271). In addition, patients may present with other signs not clearly related to spontaneous bacterial peritonitis, including worsening encephalopathy and deteriorating renal function. The diagnosis is easily made by examination of the ascitic fluid obtained by paracentesis. An elevated number of white blood cells (> 250/mm^3) is diagnostic. The vast majority of cases of spontaneous bacterial peritonitis are caused by a single organism, most commonly gram-negative enteric bacteria. Hematogenous spread may lead to infection with *Streptococcus pneumoniae* (265) (Table 37.14). If more than one organism is present, the diagnosis of spontaneous bacterial peritonitis must be questioned, and a search for intraabdominal disease (secondary peritonitis), such as a perforated viscus or diverticulitis, should be performed.

Table 37.14. **BACTERIOLOGY OF SPONTANEOUS BACTERIAL PERITONITIS**

Organisms	Percentage of total
Escherichia coli	40
Pneumococci	15
Streptococci	14
Klebsiella	7
Pseudomonas	3
Proteus	3
Staphylococci	3
Anaerobes	5
Other	20
Multiple isolates	10

Adapted from Targan S, Chow A, Gluze L. Role of anaerobic bacteria in spontaneous peritonitis of cirrhosis. Am J Med 1977;62:397, with permission.

The treatment of spontaneous bacterial peritonitis consists of supportive care and broad-spectrum antibiotics, most commonly cefotaxime, a third-generation cephalosporin. Other antibiotics with proven efficacy include ofloxacin, a quinolone. This antibiotic has potent activity against gram-negative organisms and reaches high levels in ascitic fluid. For patients who are clinically stable and able to take oral medications, this is the drug of choice (272). Cure can be achieved in 75% to 90% of cases, but mortality rates are high, ranging from 20% to 40% (272–276). The poor prognosis associated with spontaneous bacterial peritonitis warrants consideration of liver transplantation.

Prophylactic oral or intravenous antibiotics are indicated for two distinct groups of cirrhotic patients with ascites: (a) those with gastrointestinal hemorrhage, and (b) those with low protein counts in the ascitic fluid (< 10 to 15 g/L) (273). The antibiotics used in patients with hemorrhage are neomycin, colistin, and nystatin in combination, and ofloxacin alone (277,278). These antibiotics reduce the incidence of spontaneous bacterial peritonitis from approximately 15% to 20% to 3% to 9% and cause few side effects. A recent metaanalysis evaluating the use of prophylactic antibiotics in patients with gastrointestinal hemorrhage confirmed the utility of prophylaxis, with approximately a 30% decrease in the incidence of infection, a 20% decrease in the incidence of spontaneous bacterial peritonitis and bacteremia, and a 10% improvement in overall survival (279). In patients with low protein levels in the ascitic fluid, multiple regimens have proved effective in reducing the incidence of spontaneous bacterial peritonitis, from approximately 20% to less than 5% (280–283).

Hernias and Ascites. Hernias of the anterior abdominal wall occur in up to 20% of patients with cirrhosis. The causes include increased intraabdominal pressure and nutritional deficits with muscular wasting and thinning of the fascia. If the hernias are left untreated, complications include incarceration, rupture, strangulation, and leakage. Hernias should be treated electively, with preoperative paracentesis to decrease intraabdominal pressure. No increase in complication rates was noted in a study comparing the outcome of umbilical hernia repair in patients with and without ascites. However, a longer hospital stay and a significantly higher recurrence rate (73% vs. 14%) was noted in the group of patients with ascites (284).

REFERENCES

1. Mallory FB. Cirrhosis of the liver: five different types of lesions from which it may arise. *Bull Johns Hopkins Hosp* 1911;22:69–75.
2. Friedman SL, Roll FJ, Boyles J, et al. Hepatic lipocytes: the principle collagen-producing cells of normal rat liver. *Proc Natl Acad Sci USA* 1985;82:8681–8685.
3. Wake K. "Sternzellen" in the liver: perisinusoidal cells with special reference to storage of vitamin A. *Am J Anat* 1971;132:429–462.
4. Takahara T, Kojima T, Miyabayashi C. Collagen production in fat-storing cells after carbon tetrachloride intoxication in the rat: immunoelectron microscopic observation of type I, type III collagens, and prolyl hydroxylase. *Lab Invest* 1988;59:509–521.
5. Friedman SL. The cellular basis of hepatic fibrosis. *N Engl J Med* 1993;328:1828–1835.
6. Gressner AM, Bachem MG. Cellular sources of noncollagenous matrix proteins: role of fat-storing cells in fibrogenesis. *Semin Liver Dis* 1990;10:30–46.
7. Loreal O, Levasseur F, Rescan PY, et al. Differential expression of laminin chains in hepatic lipocytes. *FEBS Lett* 1991;290:9–12.
8. Ramadori G, Knittel T, Odenthal M, et al. Synthesis of cellular fibronectin by rat liver fat-storing (Ito) cells: regulation by cytokines. *Gastroenterology* 1992;103:1313–1321.
9. Friedman SL, Arthur MJP. Activation of cultured rat hepatic lipocytes by Kupffer cell conditioned medium: direct enhancement of matrix synthesis and stimulation of cell proliferation via induction of platelet-derived growth factor receptors. *J Clin Invest* 1989;84:1780–1785.
10. Pinzani M, Gesualdo L, Sabbah GM, et al. Effects of platelet-derived growth factor and other polypeptide mitogens on DNA synthesis and growth of cultured rat liver fat-storing cells. *J Clin Invest* 1989;84:1786–1793.
11. Matsuoka M, Pham N-T, Tsukamoto H. Differential effects of interleukin-1 alpha, tumor necrosis factor alpha, and transforming growth factor beta-1 on cell proliferation and collagen formation by cultured fat-storing cells. *Liver* 1989;9:71–78.
12. Gressner AM. Cytokines and cellular crosstalk involved in the activation of fat-storing cells. *J Hepatol* 1995;22:28–36.
13. Tsushima H, Kawata S, Tamura S. Reduced plasma transforming growth factor-β_1 levels in patients with chronic hepatitis C after interferon-α therapy: association with regression of hepatic fibrosis. *J Hepatol* 1999;30:1–7.
14. Schaffner F, Popper H. Capillarization of hepatic sinusoids in man. *Gastroenterology* 1963;44:239–242.
15. Friedman SL. Hepatic fibrosis. In: Schiff ER, Sorrell MF, Maddrey WC, eds. *Diseases of the liver*, 8th ed. Philadelphia: JB Lippincott, 1999:371–386.
16. Anthony PP, Ishak KG, Nayak NC, et al. The morphology of cirrhosis: definition, nomenclature, and classification. *Bull World Health Organ* 1977;55:521–540.
17. Chiaramonte M, Stroffolini T, Vian A, et al. Rate of incidence of hepatocellular carcinoma in patients with compensated viral cirrhosis. *Cancer* 1999;85:2132–2137.
18. Chedid A, Mendenhall CL, Garside P, et al. Prognostic factors in alcoholic liver disese. *Am J Gastroenterol* 1991;86:210–216.
19. Lieber CS. Medical disorsders of alcoholism. *N Engl J Med* 1995;333:1058–1065.
20. Moshage H, Casini A, Lieber CS. Acetaldehyde selectively stimulates collagen production in cultured rat liver fat-storing cells but not in hepatocytes. *Hepatology* 1990;12:511–518.
21. Espina N, Lima V, Lieber CS, et al. In vitro and in vivo inhibitory effect of ethanol and acetaldehyde on O-6-methylguanine transferase. *Carcinogenesis* 1988;9:761–766.
22. Wondergem R, Davis J. Ethanol increases hepatocyte water volume. *Alcohol Clin Exp Res* 1994;18:1230–1236.
23. Lieber CS, ed. *Medical and nutritional complications of alcoholism: mechanisms and management*. New York: Plenum, 1992.
24. Flier JS, Underhill LH. Medical disorders of alcoholism. *N Engl J Med* 1995;333:1058–1065.
25. Davis GL, Balart LA, Schiff ER, et al. Treatment of chronic hepatitis C with recombinant interferon alpha: a multicenter randomized, controlled trial. *N Engl J Med* 1989;321:1501–1506.
26. Di Bisceglie AM, Martin P, Kassianides C, et al. Recombinant interferon alpha therapy for chronic hepatitis C: a random-

ized, double-blind, placebo-controlled trial. *N Engl J Med* 1989;321:1506–1510.

27. Shindo M, Ken A, Okuno T. Varying incidence of cirrhosis and hepatocellular carcinoma in patients with chronic hepatitis C responding differently to interferon therapy. *Cancer* 1999;85:1943–1950.

28. Davis GL. Treatment of chronic hepatitis C: combination treatment with interferon and ribavirin for chronic hepatitis C. *Clin Liver Dis* 1999;3:811–826.

29. Szakacs JG, Szakacs JE. Progress in diagnosis of hepatitis and the cirrhotic liver. *Ann Clin Lab Sci* 1999;29:87–103.

30. Kaplan MM. Primary biliary cirrhosis. *N Engl J Med* 1996; 335:1570–1580.

31. Van De Water J, Cooper A, Surh CD, et al. Detection of autoantibodies to recombinant mitochondrial proteins in patients with primary biliary cirrhosis. *N Engl J Med* 1989;320: 462–466.

32. Portmann B, Popper H, Neuberger J, et al. Sequential and diagnostic features in primary biliary cirrhosis based on serial histologic study in 209 patients. *Gastroenterology* 1985;88: 1777–1790.

33. Tornay AS Jr. Primary biliary cirrhosis: natural history. *Am J Gastroenterol* 1980;73:223–226.

34. Balasubramaniam K, Grambasch PM, Wiesner RH, et al. Diminished survival in asymptomatic primary biliary cirrhosis: a prospective study. *Gastroenterology* 1990;98:1567–1571.

35. Mahl TC, Shockcor W, Boyer JL. Primary biliary cirrhosis: survival of a large cohort of symptomatic and asymptomatic patients followed for 24 years. *J Hepatol* 1994;20:707–713.

36. Heathcote EJ, Lindor KD, Poupon R, et al. Combined analysis of French, American, and Canadian randomized controlled trials of ursodeoxycholic acid therapy in primary biliary cirrhosis. *Gastroenterology* 1995;108[Suppl]:A1082 (abst).

37. Markus BH, Dickson ER, Grambsch PM, et al. Efficacy of liver transplantation in patinets with primary biliary cirrhosis. *N Engl J Med* 1989;320:1709–1713.

38. Angulo P, Lindor KD. Primary biliary cirrhosis and primary sclerosing cholangitis. *Clin Liver Dis* 1999;3:529–570.

39. Broome U, Glaumann H, Hultcrantz R, et al. Distribution of HLA-DR, HLA-DP, HLA-DQ antigens in liver tissue from patients with primary sclerosing cholangitis. *Scand J Gastroenterol* 1990;25:54.

40. Zauli D, Schrumpf E, Crespi C, et al. An autoantibody profile in primary sclerosing cholangitis. *J Hepatol* 1987;5:14.

41. Wiesner RH. Current concepts in primary sclerosing cholangitis. *Mayo Clin Proc* 1994;69:969.

42. Martin FM, Braasch JW. Primary sclerosing cholangitis. *Curr Probl Surg* 1992;29:133.

43. Okolicsanyi L, Fabris L, Viaggi S, et al. Primary sclerosing cholangitis: clinical presentation, natural history, and prognostic variables—an Italian multicenter study. *Eur J Gastroenterol Hepatol* 1996;8:685.

44. Bergquist A, Broome U. Primary biliary cirrhosis, primary sclerosing cholangitis, and adult cholangiopathies. *Clin Liver Dis* 1998;2:283–301.

45. Broome U, Lofberg R, Veress R, et al. Primary sclerosing cholangitis and ulcerative colitis: indicator of increased neoplastic potential. *Hepatology* 1995;22:1404.

46. Pasha TM, Petz J, Ludwig J, et al. Incidence of cholangiocarcinoma in patients with primary sclerosing cholangitis. *Hepatology* 1997;26:170A(abst).

47. Stal P, Broome U, Scheynius A. Kuppfer cell iron overload induced intercellular adhesion molecule-1 expression on hepatocytes in genetic hemochromatosis. *Hepatology* 1995; 21:1301–1316.

48. Schilsky ML, Tavill AS. Wilson's disease. In: Schiff ER, Sorrell MF, Maddrey WC, eds. *Diseases of the liver*, 8th ed. Philadelphia: JB Lippincott, 1999:1091.

49. Leggett BA, Halliday JW, Brown NN, et al. Prevalence of haemochromatosis amongst asymptomatic Australians. *Br J Haematol* 1990;74:525–530.

50. Safran AP, Schaffner F. Chronic passive congestion of the liver in man: electron microscopic study of cell atrophy and intralobular fibrosis. *Am J Pathol* 1967;50:447–463.

51. Dunn GD, Hayes P, Breen KJ, et al. The liver in congestive heart failure: a review. *Am J Med Sci* 1973;265:174–189.

52. Rosenberg PM, Friedman LS. The liver in circulatory failure.

In: Schiff ER, Sorrell MF, Maddrey WC, eds. *Diseases of the liver*, 8th ed. Philadelphia: JB Lippincott, 1999:1217.

53. Tilanus HW. Budd-Chiari syndrome. *Br J Surg* 1995;82: 1023–1030.

54. Gupta S, Barter S, Pillips GW, et al. Comparison of ultrasonography, computed tomography, and ^{99m}Tc liver scan in diagnosis of Budd-Chiari syndrome. *Gut* 1987;28:242–247.

55. Ishikawa T, Ichida T, Matsuda Y, et al. Reduced expression of thrombopoietin is involved in thrombocytopenia in human and rat liver cirrhosis. *J Gastroenterol Hepatol* 1998; 13:907–913.

56. Simonovsky V. The diagnosis of cirrhosis by high resolution ultrasound of the liver surface. *Br J Radiol* 1999;72:29–34.

57. Lieberman FL, Denison EK, Reynolds TB. The relationship of plasma volume, portal hypertension, ascites, and renal sodium retention in cirrhosis: the overflow theory of ascites formation. *Ann N Y Acad Sci* 1970;170:202.

58. Schrier RW, Arroyo V, Bernardi M, et al. Peripheral arterial vasodilation hypothesis: a proposal for the initiation of renal sodium and water retention in cirrhosis. *Hepatology* 1988;8: 1151.

59. Ginès P, Arroyo V, Rodes J. Renal complications. In: Schiff ER, Sorrell MF, Maddrey WC, eds. *Diseases of the liver*, 8th ed. Philadelphia: JB Lippincott, 1999:453.

60. Martin PY, Ginès P, Schrier RW. Nitric oxide as a mediator of hemodynamic abnormalities and sodium and water retention in cirrhosis. *N Engl J Med* 1998;339:533–541.

61. Sarela AI, Mihaimeed FMA, Batten JJ, et al. Hepatic and splanchnic nitric oxide activity in patients with cirrhosis. *Gut* 1999;44:749–753.

62. Rodes J, Bosch J, Arroyo V. Clinical types and drug therapy of renal impairment in cirrhosis. *Postgrad Med J* 1975;55: 492.

63. Asbert M, Ginès A, Ginès P, et al. Circulating levels of endothelin in cirrhosis. *Gastroenterology* 1993;104:1485.

64. Moore K, Wendon J, Frazer M, et al. Plasma endothelin immunoreactivity in liver disease and the hepatorenal syndrome. *N Engl J Med* 1992;327:1774.

65. Gines A, Escorsell A, Ginès P, et al. Incidence, predictive factors, and prognosis of the hepatorenal syndrome in cirrhosis with ascites. *Gastroenterology* 1993;105:229.

66. Singer JA, Kaplan MM, Katz RL. Cirrhotic pleural effusion in the absence of ascites. *Gastroenterology* 1977;73:575.

67. Fitz G. Systemic complications of liver disease. In: Feldman M, ed. *Sleisenger and Fordtran's gastrointestinal and liver disease*, 6th ed. Philadelphia: WB Saunders, 1998:1340–1342.

68. Berkowitz KA, Butensky MS, Smith RL. Pulmonary function changes after large volume paracentesis. *Am J Gastroenterol* 1993;88:905.

69. Hopkins WE, Waggoner AD, Brazilai B. Frequency and significance of intrapulmonary right-to-left shunting in endstage hepatic disease. *Am J Cardiol* 1992;70:516–519.

70. Hourani JM, Bellamy PE, Tashkin DP, et al. Pulmonary dysfunction in advanced liver disease: frequent occurrence of an abnormal diffusing capacity. *Am J Med* 1991;90:693–700.

71. Scott VL, Dodson SF, Kang Y. The hepatopulmonary syndrome. *Surg Clin North Am* 1999;79:23–41.

72. Fitz G. Systemic complications of liver disease. In: Feldman M, ed. *Sleisenger and Fordtran's gastrointestinal and liver disease*, 6th ed. Philadelphia: WB Saunders, 1998:1340–1342.

73. Mousseau DD, Butterworth RF. Current theories on the pathogenesis of hepatic encephalopathy. *Proc Soc Exp Biol Med* 1994;206:329–344.

74. Nomura F, Ohnishi K, Terabayashi J, et al. Effect of intrahepatic portal–systemic shunting on hepatic ammonia extraction in patients with cirrhosis. *Hepatology* 1994;20: 1478–1481.

75. Lockwood AH, Yap EW, Wong WH. Cerebral ammonia metabolism in patients with severe liver disease and minimal hepatic encephalopathy. *J Cereb Blood Flow Metab* 1991;11: 337–341.

76. Schafer DF, Jones EA. Hepatic encephalopathy and the γ-aminobutyric acid neurotransmitter system. *Lancet* 1982;1: 18–19.

77. Mullen KD, Martin JV, Mendelson WB, et al. Could an endogenous benzodiazepine ligand contribute to hepatic encephalopathy? *Lancet* 1988;1:457–459.

78. Bengtsson F, Gage FH, Jeppson B, et al. Brain monoamine

metabolism and behavior in portacaval shunted rats. *Exp Neurol* 1985;70:21–35.

79. Zieve L, Doizaki WM, Zieve J. Synergism between mercaptans and ammonia or fatty acids in the production of coma: a possible role for mercaptans in the pathogenesis of hepatic coma. *J Lab Clin Med* 1974;83:16–28.

80. Yurdaydin C, Li Y, Ha JH, et al. Brain and plasma levels of opioid peptides are altered in rats with thioacetamide-induced fulminant hepatic failure: implications for the treatment of hepatic encephalopathy with opioid antagonists. *J Pharmacol Exp Ther* 1995;273:185–192.

81. Schenker S, Bay MK. Portal systemic encephalopathy. *Clin Liver Dis* 1997;1:157–184.

82. Mullen KD, Dasarathy S. Hepatic encephalopathy. In: Schiff ER, Sorrell MF, Maddrey WC, eds. *Diseases of the liver,* 8th ed. Philadelphia: JB Lippincott, 1999:545.

83. Flannery DB, Hsia YE, Wolf B. Current status of hyperammonemia syndrome. *Hepatology* 1982;2:495–506.

84. Eichler M, Bessman SP. A double-blind study of the effects of ammonium infusion on psychological functioning in cirrhotic patients. *J Nerv Ment Dis* 1962;134:539–542.

85. Zeneroli ML, Venturini I, Stefanilli S, et al. Antibacterial activity of rifaximin reduces the levels of benzodiazepine-like compounds in patients with liver cirrhosis. *Pharmacol Res* 1997;35:537–560.

86. Lockwood AH. Ammonia. In: Lockwood AH, ed. *Hepatic encephalopathy.* Boston: Butterworth-Heineman, 1992:65–72.

87. Conn HO, Lieberthal MM. Management of acute portal systemic encephalopathy. In: Conn HO, Lieberthal MM, eds. *The hepatic coma syndrome and lactulose.* Baltimore: Williams & Wilkins, 1978:189–219.

88. Conn HO, Floch MH. Effects of lactulose and *Lactobacillus acidophilus* on the fecal flora. *Am J Clin Nutr* 1970;23:1588–1594.

89. Price JB, Sawoda M, Voorhees AB. Clinical significance of intraluminal pH in intestinal ammonia transport. *Am J Surg* 1970;119:595–598.

90. Fessel JM, Conn HO. Lactulose in the treatment of acute hepatic encephalopathy. *Am J Med Sci* 1973;266:103–110.

91. Mortensen PB. The effect of orally administered lactulose on colonic nitrogen metabolism and excretion. *Hepatology* 1992;16:1350–1356.

92. Weber FL Jr, Banwell JG, Fresard KM, et al. Nitrogen in fecal bacteria, fiber, and soluble fractions of cirrhotic patients: effects of lactulose and lactulose plus neomycin. *J Lab Clin Med* 1987;110:259–263.

93. Vince AJ, Burridge SM. Ammonia production by intestinal bacteria: effects of lactose, lactulose, and glucose. *J Med Microbiol* 1980;13:177–191.

94. Atterbury CE, Maddrey WC, Conn HO. Neomycin, sorbitol, and lactulose in the treatment of acute portal systemic encephalopathy: a controlled double-blind clinical trial. *Am J Dig Dis* 1978;23:398–406.

95. Morgan M, Read AE, Speller PCE. Treatment of hepatic encephalopathy with metronidazole. *Gut* 1982;23:1–7.

96. Conn HO, Leevy CM, Vlahcevic ZR, et al. Comparison of lactulose and neomycin in the treatment of chronic portal systemic encephalopathy. *Gastroenterology* 1977;72:573–583.

97. Kunin CM, Chalmers TC, Leevy CM, et al. Absorption of orally administered neomycin and kanamycin with special reference to patients with severe hepatic and renal disease. *N Engl J Med* 1960;262:380–385.

98. Berk DP, Chalmers T. Deafness complicating antibiotic therapy of hepatic encephalopathy. *Ann Intern Med* 1970;73:393–396.

99. DiPiazza S, Filippazzp MC, Valenza LM, et al. Rifaximin vs. neomycin in the treatment of portosystemic encephalopathy. *Ital J Gastroenterol* 1991;23:403–407.

100. Pedretti G, Calzetti C, Missale C, et al. Rifaximin versus neomycin on hyperammonemia in chronic portal systemic encephalopathy of cirrhosis: a double-blind randomized trial. *Ital J Gastroenterol* 1991;23:175–178.

101. Fera G, Agostinacchio F, Nigro M, et al. Rifaximin in the treatment of hepatic encephalopathy. *Eur J Clin Res* 1992;4:57–66.

102. Reynolds TB, Redecker AG, Geller HM. Wedged hepatic vein pressure. *Am J Med* 1957;22:341.

103. Greenway C, Stark R. Hepatic vascular bed. *Physiol Rev* 1971;51:23.

104. Vorobioff J, Bredfeldt JE, Groszmann RJ. Increased blood flow through the portal system in cirrhotic rats. *Gastroenterology* 1984;87:1120–1126.

105. Moller S, Christensen E, Henriksen JH. Continuous blood pressure monitoring in cirrhosis: relations to splanchnic and systemic haemodynamics. *J Hepatol* 1997;27:284–294.

106. Battista S, Bar F, Mengozzi G, et al. Hyperdynamic circulation in patients with cirrhosis: direct measurement of nitric oxide levels in hepatic and portal veins. *J Hepatol* 1997;26:75–80.

107. Jaffe DL, Chung RT, Friedman LS. Management of portal hypertension and its complications. *Med Clin North Am* 1996;80:1021–1034.

108. Gupta TK, Chen L, Groszmann RJ. Pathophysiology of portal hypertension. *Clin Liver Dis* 1997;1:1–12.

109. Budd G. *On diseases of the liver.* London: John Churchill, 1845:146.

110. Chiari H. Über die selbstandige phlebitis obliterans der hauptstamme der venae hepaticae als todesursache. *Beitr Z Pathol Anat* 1899;26:1–18.

111. Tilanus HW. Budd-Chiari syndrome. *Br J Surg* 1995;82:1023–1030.

112. Gordon SC, Polson DJ, Shirkoda A. Budd-Chiari syndrome complicating preeclampsia: diagnosis by magnetic resonance imaging. *J Clin Gastroenterol* 1991;13:460–462.

113. Ilan Y, Oren R, Shouval D. Postpartum Budd-Chiari syndrome with prolonged hypercoagulability state. *Am J Obstet Gynecol* 1990;162:1164–1165.

114. Valla D, Le MG, Poynard T, et al. Risk of hepatic vein thrombosis in relation to recent use of oral contraceptives: a case-control study. *Gastroenterology* 1986;90:807–811.

115. Mitchell MC, Boitnott JK, Kaufman S, et al. Budd-Chiari syndrome: etiology, diagnosis, and management. *Medicine* 1982;61:199–218.

116. Faust TW, Sorrell MF. Budd-Chiari syndrome. In: Schiff ER, Sorrell MF, Maddrey WC, eds. *Diseases of the liver,* 8th ed. Philadelphia: JB Lippincott, 1999:1207–1214.

117. Gupta S, Barter S, Phillips GW, et al. Comparison of ultrasonography, computed tomography, and ^{99m}Tc liver scan in diagnosis of Budd-Chiari syndrome. *Gut* 1987;28:242–247.

118. Langer B, Stone RM, Colapinto RF, et al. Clinical spectrum of the Budd-Chiari syndrome and its surgical management. *Am J Surg* 1975;129:137–145.

119. McCarthy PM, vanHeerden JA, Adson MA, et al. The Budd-Chiari syndrome: medical and surgical management of 30 patients. *Arch Surg* 1985;120:657–662.

120. Halff G, Todo S, Tzakis AG, et al. Liver transplantation for the Budd-Chiari syndrome. *Ann Surg* 1990;211:43–49.

121. Hemming AW, Langer B, Greig P, et al. Treatment of Budd-Chiari syndrome with portosystemic shunt or liver transplantation. *Am J Surg* 1996;171:176–181.

122. Campbell DA, Rolles K, Jamieson N, et al. Hepatic transplantation with perioperative and long-term anticoagulation as treatment for Budd-Chiari syndrome. *Surg Gynecol Obstet* 1988;166:511–518.

123. Shaked A, Goldstein RM, Klintmalm GB, et al. Portosystemic shunt versus orthotopic liver transplantation for the Budd-Chiari syndrome. *Surg Gynecol Obstet* 1992;174:453.

124. Uhl MD, Roth DB, Reily CA. Transjugular intrahepatic portosystemic shunt (TIPS) for Budd-Chiari syndrome. *Dig Dis Sci* 1996;41:1494–1499.

125. Ryu RK, Durham JD, Drysl J, et al. Role of TIPS as a bridge to hepatic transplantation in Budd-Chiari syndrome. *J Vasc Interv Radiol* 1999;10:799–805.

126. Belli L, Romani F, Riolo F, et al. Thrombosis of portal vein in absence of hepatic disease. *Surg Gynecol Obstet* 1989;169:46.

127. Orozco H, Takahashi T, Mercado MA, et al. Surgical management of extrahepatic portal hypertension and variceal bleeding. *World J Surg* 1994;18:246–250.

128. Choen J, Edelman RR, Chopra S. Portal vein thrombosis: a review. *Am J Med* 1992;92:173–182.

129. Parvey HR, Raval B, Sandler CM. Portal vein thrombosis: imaging findings. *AJR Am J Roentgenol* 1994;152:77–81.

130. de Ville de Goyet J, Alberti D, Clapuyt P, et al. Direct by-

passing of extrahepatic portal venous obstruction in children: a new technique for combined hepatic portal revascularization and treatment of extrahepatic portal hypertension. *J Pediatr Surg* 1998;33:597–601.

131. Loftus FP, Nagorney DM, Ilstrup D, et al. Sinistral portal hypertension: splenectomy or expectant management. *Ann Surg* 1993;217:35–40.

132. Child CG, Turcotte JG. Surgery and portal hypertension. In: Child CG II, ed. *Major problems in clinical surgery: the liver and portal hypertension,* vol 1. Philadelphia: WB Saunders, 1964:1.

133. Spence R. The venous anatomy of the lower esophagus in normal subjects and patients with varices: an image analysis study. *Br J Surg* 1984;71:739.

134. Noda T. Angioarchitectural study of esophageal varices with special reference to variceal rupture. *Virchows Arch [A]* 1984;404:381.

135. Roberts LR, Kamath PS. Pathophysiology and treatment of variceal hemorrhage. *Mayo Clin Proc* 1996;71:973–983.

136. Pagliaro L, D'Amico G, Pasta L, et al. Portal hypertension in cirrhosis: natural history. In: Bosch J, Groszmann R, eds. *Portal hypertension: pathophysiology and treatment.* Oxford: Blackwell Science, 1994:72–92.

137. Cales P, Desmorat H, Vinel J, et al. Incidence of large esophageal varices in patients with cirrhosis: application to prophylaxis of first bleeding. *Gut* 1990;31:1298–1302.

138. Christensen E, Fauerholdt L, Schlichting P, et al. Aspects of the natural history of gastrointestinal bleeding in cirrhosis and the effects of prednisone. *Gastroenterology* 1981;81:944–952.

139. North Italian Endoscopic Club. Prediction of the first variceal hemorrhage in patients with cirrhosis of the liver and esophageal varices. *N Engl J Med* 1988;319:983.

140. Graham D, Smith J. The course of patients after variceal hemorrhage. *Gastroenterology* 1981;80:800–809.

141. Grace ND, Bhattacharya K. Pharmacologic therapy of portal hypertension and variceal hemorrhage. *Clin Liver Dis* 1997;1:59–75.

142. Polio J, Groszmann RJ. Hemodynamic factor in the development and rupture of esophageal varices: a pathophysiologic approach to treatment. *Semin Liver Dis* 1986;6:318.

143. Garcia-Tsao G, Groszmann RJ, Fisher RL, et al. Portal pressure, presence of gastroesophageal varices, and variceal bleeding. *Hepatology* 1985;5:419.

144. Boyer TD. The natural history of portal hypertension. *Clin Liver Dis* 1997;1:31.

145. Kroeger R, Groszmann R. The effect of selective blockade of β_2-adrenergic receptors on portal and systemic hemodynamics in a portal hypertensive model. *Gastroenterology* 1985;88:896.

146. Price H, Cooperman L, Warden J. Control of the splanchnic circulation in man: role of beta-adrenergic receptors. *Circ Res* 1967;1(21):333.

147. Braillon A, Moreau R, Hadengue A, et al. Hyperkinetic circulatory syndrome in patients with presinusoidal portal hypertension: effect of propranolol. *J Hepatol* 1989;9:312.

148. Kiire C. Controlled trial of propranolol to prevent recurrent variceal bleeding in patients with non-cirrhotic portal fibrosis. *BMJ* 1989;298:1363.

149. Poynard T, Cales P, Pasta L, et al. Beta-adrenergic-antagonist drugs in the prevention of gastrointestinal bleeding in patients with cirrhosis and esophageal varices: an analysis of data and prognostic factors in 589 patients from four randomized clinical trials. *N Engl J Med* 1991;324:1532–1538.

150. Feu F, Garcia-Pagan J, Bosch J, et al. Relation between portal pressure response to pharmacotherapy and risk of recurrent variceal haemorrhage in patients with cirrhosis. *Lancet* 1995;346:1056–1059.

151. Conn H, Grace N, Bosch J, et al. Propranolol in the prevention of the first hemorrhage from esophagogastric varices: a multicenter, randomized clinical trial. *Hepatology* 1991;13:902.

152. Andreani T, Poupon R, Balkau B, et al. Preventive therapy of first gastrointestinal bleeding in patients with cirrhosis: results of a controlled trial comparing propranolol, endoscopic sclerotherapy, and placebo. *Hepatology* 1990;12:1413.

153. Ideo G, Bellati G, Fesce E, et al. Nadolol can prevent the first gastrointestinal bleeding in cirrhotics: a prospective, randomized study. *Hepatology* 1988;8:6.

154. Pascal J, Cales P, Multicenter Study Group. Propranolol in the prevention of first upper gastrointestinal tract hemorrhage in patients with cirrhosis of the liver and esophageal varices. *N Engl J Med* 1987;317:856.

155. PROVA. Prophylaxis of first hemorrhage from esophageal varices by sclerotherapy, propranolol or both in cirrhotic patients: a randomized multicenter trial. *Hepatology* 1991;14:1016–1024.

156. Poynard T, Cales P, Pasta L, et al. β-Adrenergic antagonists in the prevention of first gastrointestinal bleeding in patients with cirrhosis and esophageal varices: an analysis of data and prognostic factors in 589 patients from four randomized clinical trials. *N Engl J Med* 1991;324:1532–1538.

157. Groszmann RJ, de Franchis R. Portal hypertension. In: Schiff ER, Sorrell MF, Maddrey WC, eds. *Diseases of the liver,* 8th ed. Philadelphia: JB Lippincott, 1999:387–442.

158. Angelica M, Carli R, Piat C, et al. Isosorbide-5-mononitrate versus propranolol in the prevention of first bleeding in cirrhosis. *Gastroenterology* 1993;104:1460–1465.

159. Vorobioff J, Picabea E, Gamen M. Propranolol compared with propranolol plus isosorbide dinitrate in portal-hypertensive patients: long-term hemodynamics and renal effects. *Hepatology* 1993;18:477–484.

160. Merkel C, Marin R, Enzo E, et al. Randomized trial of nadolol alone or with isosorbide mononitrate for primary prophylaxis of variceal bleeding in cirrhosis. *Lancet* 1996;348:1677–1681.

161. Conn HO. The rational evaluation and management of portal hypertension. In Schaffner F, Sherlock S, Leevey CM, eds. *The liver and its diseases.* New York: Intercontinental, 1974:289–306.

162. Grace ND, Muench H, Chalmers TC. The present status of shunts for portal hypertension in cirrhosis. *Gastroenterology* 1966;50:684–691.

163. D'Amico G, Pagliaro L, Bosch J. The treatment of portal hypertension: a meta-analytic review. *Hepatology* 1995;22:332.

164. Lo GH, Lai KH, Cheng JS, et al. Prophylactic banding ligation of high-risk esophageal varices in patients with cirrhosis: a prospective, randomized trial. *J Hepatol* 1999;31:451–456.

165. Svoboda P, Kantorova I, Ochmann J, et al. A prospective randomized controlled trial of sclerotherapy vs. ligation in the prophylactic treatment of high-risk esophageal varices. *Surg Endosc* 1999;13:580–584.

166. Fogel M, Knauer C, Andres L, et al. Continuous intravenous vasopressin in active upper gastrointestinal bleeding. *Ann Intern Med* 1982;96:565.

167. Chojkier M, Groszmann R, Atterbury C, et al. A controlled comparison of continuous intra-arterial and intravenous infusions of vasopressin in hemorrhage from esophageal varices. *Gastroenterology* 1979;77:540.

168. Merigan TP, Plotkin GR, Davidson CS. Effect of intravenously administered posterior pituitary extract on hemorrhage from bleeding esophageal varices. *N Engl J Med* 1962;266:134.

169. Zito RA, Diez AR, Groszmann RJ. Comparative effects of nitroglycerin and nitroprusside on vasopressin-induced cardiac dysfunction in the dog. *J Cardiovasc Pharmacol* 1983;5:586.

170. Groszmann R, Kravetz D, Bosch J, et al. Nitroglycerin improves the hemodynamic response to vasopressin in portal hypertension. *Hepatology* 1982;2:757.

171. Iwao T, Toyonaga A, Ikegami M, et al. Portohepatic pressures, hepatic function, and blood gases in the combination of nitroglycerin and vasopressin: search for additive effects in cirrhotic portal hypertension. *Am J Gastroenterol* 1992;87:719–724.

172. Gimson A, Westaby D, Hegarty J, et al. A randomized trial of vasopressin and vasopressin plus nitroglycerin in the control of acute variceal hemorrhage. *Hepatology* 1986;6:410.

173. Bosch J, Groszmann R, Garcia-Pagan J, et al. Association of transdermal nitroglycerin to vasopressin infusion in the treatment of variceal hemorrhage: a placebo-controlled clinical trial. *Hepatology* 1989;10:962.

174. Tsai Y, Lay C, Lai K, et al. Controlled trial of vasopressin

plus nitroglycerin vs. vasopressin alone in the treatment of bleeding esophageal varices. *Hepatology* 1986;6:406–409.

175. Sonneburg G, Keller U, Perruchoud A, et al. Effect of somatostatin on splanchnic hemodynamics in patients with cirrhosis of the liver and in normal subjects. *Gastroenterology* 1981;80:526–532.

176. Sieber C, Mosca P, Groszmann R. Effect of somatostatin on mesenteric vascular resistance in normal and portal hypertensive rats. *Am J Physiol* 1992;262:274–277.

177. Bosch J, Kravetz D, Rodes J. Effects of somatostatin on hepatic and systemic hemodynamics in patients with cirrhosis of the liver: comparison with vasopressin. *Gastroenterology* 1981;80:518–525.

178. Jenkins S, Baxter J, Corbett W, et al. A prospective randomized controlled clinical trial comparing somatostatin and vasopressin in controlling acute variceal hemorrhage. *BMJ* 1985;290:275.

179. Burroughs A, McCormick P, Hughes M, et al. Randomized, double-blind, placebo-controlled trial of somatostatin for variceal bleeding: emergency control and prevention of early variceal rebleeding. *Gastroenterology* 1990;99:1388.

180. Kravetz D, Bosch J, Teres J, et al. Comparisons of intravenous somatostatin and vasopressin infusions in the treatment of acute variceal hemorrhage. *Hepatology* 1984;4:442.

181. Saari A, Klvilaakso E, Inberg M, et al. Comparison of somatostatin and vasopressin in bleeding esophageal varices. *Am J Gastroenterol* 1990;85:804.

182. Hsia H, Lee F, Tsai Y, et al. Comparison of somatostatin and vasopressin in the control of acute esophageal variceal hemorrhage: a randomized, controlled study. *Chin J Gastroenterol* 1990;7:71–78.

183. Jaramillo J, de la Mata M, Mino G, et al. Somatostatin versus Sengstaken balloon tamponade for primary haemostasis of bleeding esophageal varices. *J Hepatol* 1991;12:100–105.

184. Avgerinos A, Klonis C, Rekoumis G, et al. Controlled trial of somatostatin and balloon tamponade in bleeding esophageal varices. *J Hepatol* 1991;13:78–83.

185. Burroughs AK, Hamilton G, Phillips A, et al. A comparison of sclerotherapy with staple transection of the esophagus for the emergency control of bleeding from esophageal varices. *N Engl J Med* 1989;321:857–862.

186. Stiegmann G, Goff J, Michaletz-Onody P, et al. Endoscopic sclerotherapy as compared with endoscopic ligation for bleeding oesophageal varices. *N Engl J Med* 1992;326:1527–1532.

187. Young M, Sanowski R, Rasche R. Comparison and characterization of ulcerations induced by endoscopic ligation of esophageal varices versus endoscopic sclerotherapy. *Gastrointest Endosc* 1993;39:119–122.

188. Mundo F, Mitrani C, Rodriquez G, et al. Endoscopic variceal treatment: is band ligation taking over sclerotherapy? *Am J Gastroenterol* 1993;88:1493(abst).

189. Laine L, El-Newihi H, Migikowsky B, et al. Endoscopic ligation compared with sclerotherapy for the treatment of bleeding oesophageal varices. *Ann Intern Med* 1993;119:1–7.

190. Gimson A, Ramage J, Panos M, et al. Randomized trial of variceal banding ligation versus injection sclerotherapy for bleeding oesophageal varices. *Lancet* 1993;342:391–394.

191. Laine L, Cook D. Endoscopic ligation compared with sclerotherapy for treatment of esophageal variceal bleeding: a meta-analysis. *Ann Intern Med* 1995;123:280–287.

192. Jensen D, Kovacs T, Randall G, et al. Initial results of a randomized prospective study of emergency banding vs. sclerotherapy for bleeding gastric or oesophageal varices. *Gastrointest Endosc* 1993;39:279(abst).

193. Lo G, Lai K, Cheng J, et al. A prospective, randomised trial of injection sclerotherapy versus banding ligation in the management of bleeding oesophageal varices. *Hepatology* 1995;22:466–471.

194. McCormick PA, Dick R, Panagou EB, et al. Emergency transjugular intrahepatic portasystemic stent shunting as salvage treatment for uncontrolled variceal bleeding. *Br J Surg* 1994;81:1324–1327.

195. LaGerge JM, Ring EJ, Gordon RL, et al. Creation of transjugular intrahepatic portosystemic shunts with the Wallstent endoprosthesis: results in 100 patients. *Radiology* 1993;187:413–420.

196. Sanyal A, Freedman A, Luketic V, et al. Transjugular intrahepatic portosystemic shunts for patients with active variceal hemorrhage unresponsive to sclerotherapy. *Gastroenterology* 1996;111:138–146.

197. Miller-Catchpole R. Transjugular intrahepatic portosystemic shunt (TIPS): diagnostic and therapeutic technology assessment (DATTA). *JAMA* 1995;21:1824–1830.

198. Kerlan RK Jr, LaBerge JM, Gordon RL, et al. Transjugular intrahepatic portosystemic shunts: current status. *AJR Am J Roentgenol* 1995;164:1059–1066.

199. Rossle M, Haag K, Ochs A, et al. The transjugular intrahepatic portosystemic stent–shunt procedure for variceal bleeding. *N Engl J Med* 1994;330:165–171.

200. Whipple AO. The problem of portal hypertension in relation to the hepatosplenopathies. *Ann Surg* 1945;122:449–475.

201. Sarfeh IJ, Rypins EB. Partial versus total portacaval shunt in alcoholic cirrhosis: results of a prospective, randomized clinical trial. *Ann Surg* 1994;219:353–361.

202. Rosemurgy AS, Goode SE, Zwiebel BR, et al. A prospective trial of transjugular intrahepatic portasystemic stent shunts versus small-diameter prosthetic H-graft portacaval shunts in the treatment of bleeding varices. *Ann Surg* 1996;224:378–384.

203. Sarfeh IJ, Rypins EB, Mason GR. A systemic appraisal of portocaval H-graft diameters: clinical and hemodynamic perspectives. *Am Surg* 1986;204:356–363.

204. Sarfeh IJ, Rypins EB. Partial versus total portacaval shunt in alcoholic cirrhosis: results of a prospective, randomized, clinical trial. *Ann Surg* 1994;219:353–361.

205. Johansen KH, Girod C, Lee SS, et al. Mesenteric venous stenosis reduces hyperammonemia in the portacaval-shunted rat. *Eur Surg Res* 1990;22:170–174.

206. Inokuchi K. A selective portacaval shunt. *Lancet* 1968;2:51–52.

207. Hermann RE, Henderson JM, Vogt DP, et al. Fifty years of surgery for portal hypertension at the Cleveland Clinic Foundation: lessons and prospects. *Ann Surg* 1995;221:459–466.

208. Henderson JM, Gilmore GT, Hooks MA, et al. Selective shunt in the management of variceal bleeding in the era of liver transplantation. *Ann Surg* 1992;216:248–254.

209. Rikkers LF. Is the distal splenorenal shunt better? *Hepatology* 1988;8:1705–1707.

210. Orozco H, Mercado MA, Garcia JG, et al. Selective shunts for portal hypertension: current role of a 21-year experience. *Liver Transpl Surg* 1997;3:475–480.

211. Warren WD, Millikan WJ Jr, Henderson JM, et al. Ten years' portal hypertensive surgery at Emory. *Ann Surg* 1982;195:530.

212. Henderson JM, Warren WD, Millikan WJ, et al. Distal splenorenal shunt with splenopancreatic disconnection: a 4-year assessment. *Ann Surg* 1989;210:332–339.

213. Jin G, Rikkers LF. Etiology and management of upper gastrointestinal bleeding after distal splenorenal shunt. *Surgery* 1990;112:719.

214. Henderson JM. Variceal bleeding: which shunt? *Gastroenterology* 1986;91:1021–1023.

215. Orloff MJ, Orloff MS, Orloff SL, et al. Three decades of experience with emergency portacaval shunt for acutely bleeding esophageal varices in 400 unselected patients with cirrhosis of the liver. *J Am Coll Surg* 1995;180:257–272.

216. Sugiura M, Futagawa S. Esophageal transection with paraesophagogastric devascularizations (the Sugiura procedure) in the treatment of esophageal varices. *World J Surg* 1984;8:673–679.

217. Yamamoto S, Hidemura R, Sanada M, et al. The late results of terminal esophago-proximal gastrectomy (TEPG) with extensive devascularization and splenectomy for bleeding esophageal varices in cirrhosis. *Surgery* 1976;80:106.

218. Wexler MJ, Stein BL. Nonshunting operations for variceal hemorrhage. *Surg Clin North Am* 1990;70:425.

219. Cello JP, Crass R, Trunkey DD. Endoscopic sclerotherapy versus esophageal transection in Child's class C patients with variceal hemorrhage: comparison with results of portacaval shunt—preliminary report. *Surgery* 1982;91:333.

220. Hamilton G, Burroughs AK, McIntyre N, et al. The final report on prospective randomized trial of endoscopic scle-

rotherapy versus esophageal stapled transection in uncontrolled variceal bleeding. Presented at the Second World Congress on Hepato-pancreato-biliary Surgery, Amsterdam, May 29–April 3, 1988.

221. Huizinga WKJ, Angorn IB, Baker LW. Esophageal transection versus injection sclerotherapy in the management of bleeding esophageal varices in patients of high risk. *Surg Gynecol Obstet* 1985;160:539.

222. Colombo M, de Franchis F, Tommasini M, et al. Beta-blockade prevents recurrent gastrointestinal bleeding in well-compensated patients with alcoholic cirrhosis: a multicenter randomized controlled trial. *Hepatology* 1989;9:433–438.

223. Villeneuve J, Pomier-Layrargues G, Infante-Rivard C, et al. Propranolol for the prevention of recurrent variceal hemorrhage: a controlled trial. *Hepatology* 1986;6:1239.

224. Lebrec D, Poynard T, Berneau J, et al. A randomized controlled study of propranolol for prevention of recurrent gastrointestinal bleeding in patients with cirrhosis: a final report. *Hepatology* 1984;4:355.

225. Burroughs A, Jenkins W, Sherlock S, et al. Controlled trial of propranolol for the prevention of recurrent variceal hemorrhage: a controlled trial. *N Engl J Med* 1983;309:1539.

226. Queuniet A, Czernichow P, Lerebours E, et al. Étude controlée du propranolol dans la prévention des récidives hémorragiques chez les patients cirrhotiques. *Gastroenterol Clin Biol* 1987;11:41.

227. Gatta A, Merkel C, Sacerdoti D, et al. Nadolol for prevention of variceal rebleeding in cirrhosis: a controlled clinical trial. *Digestion* 1987;37:22.

228. Ink O, Servent L, Attali P, et al. Propranolol prevention of hemorrhagic recurrence caused by rupture of esophageal varices: worsened prognosis in ascites and jaundice. *Gastroenterologie Clinique et Biologique* 1985;9:819–823.

229. Garden O, Mills P, Birnie G, et al. Propranolol in the prevention of recurrent variceal hemorrhage in cirrhotic patients. *Gastroenterology* 1990;98:185.

230. Sheen I, Chen T, Liaw Y. Randomized controlled study of propranolol for prevention of recurrent esophageal bleeding in patients with cirrhosis. *Liver* 1989;9:1.

231. Rossi V, Cales P, Pascal B, et al. Prevention of recurrent variceal bleeding in alcoholic cirrhotic patients: prospective controlled trial of propranolol and sclerotherapy. *J Hepatol* 1991;12:283–289.

232. Colman J, Jones P, Finch C, et al. Propranolol in the prevention of variceal hemorrhage in alcoholic cirrhotic patients. *Hepatology* 1990;12:851(abst).

233. Villanueva C, Balanzo J, Novella M, et al. Nadolol plus isosorbide mononitrate compared with sclerotherapy for the prevention of variceal rebleeding. *N Engl J Med* 1996;334:1624–1629.

234. Westaby D, Binmoller K, de Franchis R, et al. Baveno II consensus statements: the endoscopic management of variceal bleeding. In: de Franchis R, ed. *Portal hypertension II. Proceedings of the Second International Consensus Workshop on definitions, methodology, and therapeutic strategies.* Oxford: Blackwell Science, 1996:126.

235. Sauer P, Theilmann L, Benz T, et al. Transjugular intrahepatic portosystemic stent shunt (TIPS) vs. sclerotherapy in the prevention of variceal rebleeding: a randomized study. *Gastroenterology* 1996;110:A1313(abst).

236. Sanyal A, Freedman A, Luketic V, et al. Transjugular intrahepatic portosystemic shunts compared with endoscopic sclerotherapy for the prevention of recurrent variceal hemorrhage: a randomized controlled trial. *Ann Intern Med* 1997;126:849–857.

237. Cabera J, Maynar M, Granados R, et al. Transjugular intrahepatic portosystemic shunt (TIPS) vs. sclerotherapy in the elective treatment of variceal bleeding. *Gastroenterology* 1996;110:832–839.

238. Cello J, Ring E, Elcott E, et al. Transjugular intrahepatic portosystemic shunt vs. sclerotherapy for variceal hemorrhage. *Gastroenterology* 1995;108:A1045(abst).

239. Jalan R, Forrest E, Stanley A, et al. TIPS vs. variceal band ligation for the prevention of variceal rebleeding in cirrhosis: a randomized controlled study. *Hepatology* 1996;24:247A(abst).

240. Rossle M, Deibert P, Haag K, et al. TIPS versus sclerotherapy and β-blockage: preliminary results of a randomized study

in patients with recurrent variceal hemorrhage. *Hepatology* 1994;20:107A(abst).

241. Garcia-Villarreal L, Martinez-Lagares F, Sierra A, et al. TIPS vs. sclerotherapy for the prevention of variceal rebleeding: preliminary results of a randomized study. *Hepatology* 1996;24:208A(abst).

242. Groupe d'Étude des Anastomoses Intra-Hepatiques. TIPS vs. sclerotherapy + propranolol in the prevention of variceal rebleeding: preliminary results of a multicenter randomized trial. *Hepatology* 1995;22:297A(abst).

243. Merli M, Riggio O, Capocaccia L, et al. Transjugular intrahepatic portosystemic shunt (TIPS) vs. endoscopic sclerotherapy (ES) in preventing variceal rebleeding: preliminary results of a randomized controlled trial. *Hepatology* 1994;20:107A(abst).

244. Henderson J, Kutner M, Millikan WJ, et al. Endoscopic variceal sclerosis compared with distal splenorenal shunt to prevent recurrent variceal bleeding in cirrhosis: a prospective, randomized trial. *Ann Intern Med* 1990;112:262.

245. Planas R, Boix J, Broggi M, et al. Portacaval shunt versus endoscopic sclerotherapy in the elective treatment of variceal hemorrhage. *Gastroenterology* 1991;100:1078–1086.

246. Rikkers L, Burnett D, Valentine G, et al. Shunt surgery versus endoscopic sclerotherapy for long-term treatment of variceal bleeding: early results of a randomized trial. *Ann Surg* 1987;206:261.

247. Spina G, Santambrogio R, Opocher E, et al. Distal splenorenal shunt vs. endoscopic sclerotherapy in the prevention of variceal rebleeding: first stage of a randomized controlled trial. *Ann Surg* 1990;211:178.

248. Teres J, Bordax J, Rodes J. Sclerotherapy versus distal splenorenal shunt in the elective treatment of variceal hemorrhage: a randomized controlled trial. *Hepatology* 1987;7:430.

249. Watanabe K, Kimura K, Matsutani S, et al. Portal hemodynamics in patients with gastric varices: a study in 230 patients with oesophageal or gastric varices using portal vein catheterization. *Gastroenterology* 1988;95:434–440.

250. Sarin S, Lahoti D, Saxena S, et al. Prevalence, classification, and natural history of gastric varices: long-term follow-up study in 568 patients with portal hypertension. *Hepatology* 1992;16:1343–1349.

251. Sarin S, Kumar A. Gastric varices: profile, classification, and management. *Am J Gastroenterol* 1989;84:1244.

252. Kim T, Shijo H, Kokawa H, et al. Risk factors for hemorrhage from gastric fundal varices. *Hepatology* 1997;25:307–312.

253. Quintero F, Pique J, Bombi J, et al. Gastric mucosal vascular ectasias causing bleeding in cirrhosis. *Gastroenterology* 1987;93:1054–1061.

254. Sarfeh I, Tarnawsky A. Gastric muscosal vasculopathy in portal hypertension. *Gastroenterology* 1987;93:1129–1131.

255. D'Amico G, Montalbano L, Pagliaro L, et al. Natural history of congestive gastropathy in cirrhosis. *Gastroenterology* 1990;99:1558.

256. McCormack T, Sims J, Eyre-Brook I, et al. Gastric lesions in portal hypertension: inflammatory gastritis or congestive gastropathy? *Gut* 1985;26:1226.

257. Huet P-M, Goresky CA, Villeneuve J-P, et al. Assessment of liver microcirculation in human cirrhosis. *J Clin Invest* 1982;70:1234–1244.

258. Roberts LR, Kamath PS. Ascites and hepatorenal syndrome: pathophysiology and management. *Mayo Clin Proc* 1996;73:874–881.

259. Stanley MM, Ochi S, Lee KK, et al. Peritoneovenous shunting as compared with medical treatment in patients with alcoholic cirrhosis and massive ascites. *N Engl J Med* 1989;321:1632–1638.

260. Bories P, Compean DG, Michel H, et al. The treatment of refractory ascites by the LeVeen shunt: a multi-centre controlled trial (57 patients). *J Hepatol* 1986;2:212–218.

261. Aiza I, Perez GO, Schiff ER. Management of ascites in patients with chronic liver disease. *Am J Gastroenterol* 1994;89:1949–1956.

262. Ginès P, Arroyo V, Quintero E, et al. Comparison of paracentesis and diuretics in the treatment of cirrhotics with tense ascites. *Gastroenterology* 1987;93:234–241.

263. Salerno F, Badalamenti S, Incerti P, et al. Repeated paracen-

tesis and i.v. albumin infusion to treat "tense" ascites in cirrhotic patients: a safe alternative therapy. *J Hepatol* 1987;5: 102–108.

264. Sola R, Andreu M, Coll S, et al. Spontaneous bacterial peritonitis in cirrhotic patients treated using paracentesis or diuretics: results of a randomized study. *Hepatology* 1995;21:340.

265. Olafsson S, Blei AT. Diagnosis and management of ascites in the age of TIPS. *AJR Am J Roentgenol* 1995;165:9–15.

266. Greig PD, Langer B, Blendis LM, et al. Complications after peritoneovenous shunting for ascites. *Am J Surg* 1980;139: 125–131.

267. Ochs A, Rossle M, Haag K, et al. The transjugular intrahepatic portasystemic stent–shunt procedure for refractory ascites. *N Engl J Med* 1995;332:1192–1197.

268. Rimola A, Soto R, Bory F, et al. Reticuloendothelial system phagocytic activity in cirrhosis and its relation to bacterial infections and prognosis. *Hepatology* 1984;4:53–58.

269. Runyon BA. Low-protein-concentration ascitic fluid is predisposed to spontaneous bacterial peritonitis. *Gastroenterology* 1986;91:1343–1346.

270. Almdal TP, Skinhoj RG, Craxi A, et al. Spontaneous bacterial peritonitis in cirrhosis: incidence, diagnosis, and prognosis. *Scand J Gastroenterol* 1987;22:295–300.

271. Ginès P, Arroyo V, Rodes J. Portal hypertension, pathophysiology, complications, and treatment of ascites. *Clin Liver Dis* 1997;1:129–155.

272. Rimola A, Salmeron JM, Clemente G, et al. Two different dosages of cefotaxime in the treatment of spontaneous bacterial peritonitis in cirrhosis: results of a prospective, randomized, multicenter study. *Hepatology* 1995;21:674–679.

273. Felisart J, Rimola A, Arroyo V, et al. Cefotaxime is more effective than is ampicillin-tobramycin in cirrhotics with severe infections. *Hepatology* 1985;5:457–462.

274. Runyon BA, McHutchison JG, Antillon MR, et al. Short-course versus long-course antibiotic treatment of spontaneous bacterial peritonitis. *Gastroenterology* 1991;100:1737–1742.

275. Runyon BA. Patients with deficient ascitic fluid opsonic activity are predisposed to spontaneous bacterial peritonitis. *Hepatology* 1988;8:632–635.

276. Toledo C, Salmeron JM, Rimola A, et al. Spontaneous bacterial peritonitis in cirrhosis: predictive factors of infection resolution and survival in patients treated with cefotaxime. *Hepatology* 1993;17:251–257.

277. Rimola A, Bory F, Teres J, et al. Oral, nonabsorbable antibiotics prevent infection in cirrhotics with gastrointestinal hemorrhage. *Hepatology* 1985;5:463–467.

278. Soriano G, Guarner C, Tomas A, et al. Norfloxacin prevents bacterial infection in cirrhotics with gastrointestinal hemorrhage. *Gastroenterology* 1992;103:1267–1272.

279. Bernard B, Grange JD, Khac EN, et al. Antibiotic prophylaxis for the prevention of bacterial infections in cirrhotic patients with gastrointestinal bleeding: a meta-analysis. *Hepatology* 1999;29:1655–1661.

280. Grange JD, Roulot D, Pelletier G. Primary prophylaxis of bacterial infections with norfloxacin in cirrhotic patients with ascites: results of a double-blind, placebo-controlled trial. *Gastroenterology* 1994;106:901A(abst).

281. Rolachon A, Cordier L, Bacq Y, et al. Ciprofloxacin and long-term prevention of spontaneous bacterial peritonitis: results of a prospective controlled trial. *Hepatology* 1995;22:1171–1174.

282. Singh N, Gayowski T, Yu VL, et al. Trimethoprim-sulfamethoxazole for the prevention of spontaneous bacterial peritonitis in cirrhosis: a randomized trial. *Ann Intern Med* 1995;122:595–598.

283. Soriano G, Guarner C, Teixido M, et al. Selective intestinal decontamination prevents spontaneous bacterial peritonitis. *Gastroenterology* 1991;100:477–481.

284. Runyon BA, Juler GL. *Am J Gastroenterology* 1985;80:38–39.

SURGERY: SCIENTIFIC PRINCIPLES AND PRACTICE, Third Edition, edited by Lazar J. Greenfield, Michael W. Mulholland, Keith T. Oldham, Gerald B. Zelenock, and Keith D. Lillemoe. Lippincott Williams & Wilkins Publishers, Philadelphia, © 2001.

CHAPTER 38

HEPATIC NEOPLASMS

JAMES V. SITZMANN AND LUKE O. SCHOENIGER

HISTORY AND PHYSICAL EXAMINATION

Most patients who present with hepatic masses are asymptomatic, and the mass is found on imaging performed to evaluate other abdominal problems or as the result of abnormal liver function tests. When they are symptomatic, patients usually present with vague right upper quadrant pain. Those with left-sided hepatic lesions may experience epigastric pain or early satiety. The history may include fever associated with malaise and weight loss. Patients often present with palpable masses, and laboratory investigation reveals elevated levels of serum enzymes (alkaline phosphatase, transaminases) and tumor markers. The examiner should question the patient about prior travel experience, high-risk behavior for hepatitis exposure (intravenous drug abuse, skin tattoo), residence in areas endemic for hepatitis (Africa and Asia), alcohol use, exposure to environmental toxins associated with liver tumors (carbon tetrachloride, aromatic solvents), or possible exposure to hepatotoxins (Thorotrast, arsenic, aflatoxin, vinyl chloride). A history of the use of oral contraceptives, hormone replacement therapy, or steroid supplements is an important factor for patients suspected of having hepatocellular carcinoma (HCC) or hepatic adenoma. Familial diseases, such as hereditary polycystic disease, neurofibromatosis, glycogen storage disease, Wilson's disease, and iron storage disease, are associated with an increased risk for primary hepatocellular lesions. A history of HIV infection or long-term immunosuppression is also associated with an increased incidence of infectious mass or primary hepatic lymphoma.

The physical examination should include a careful search for characteristic skin lesions associated with cirrhosis and portal hypertension, such as spider angioma or caput medusae. Evidence of ascites and leg swelling can indicate fluid overload resulting from portal hypertension. An elevated right hemidiaphragm or a palpable abdominal mass on physical examination is consistent with a lesion of the right lobe. Examination of the head and neck should include a careful search for icterus or cervical adenopathy, particularly left supraclavicular adenopathy. A survey of the skin may reveal petechiae or other signs of thrombocytopenia, easy bruising, or ecchymoses, which are indicators of coagulation abnormalities. Evidence of superficial thrombophlebitis can be indicative of perineoplastic syndrome, which is commonly associated with HCC and metastatic tumors.

DIAGNOSIS

The diagnostic modalities available for imaging the liver include computed tomography (CT), magnetic resonance imaging (MRI), sonography, radionuclide scanning, angiography, and cholangiography. CT, MRI, sonography, and radionuclide scanning represent three-dimensional imaging studies (Table 38.1). These tests are used principally to (a) characterize and anatomically locate the lesion; (b) deter-

Table 38.1. EVALUATION OF THE PATIENT WITH A HEPATIC TUMOR

BASIC COMPONENTS

History, physical examination
CBC count—hemoglobin, hematocrit, white blood cell count
Coagulation profile—PT, PTT, platelet count
AST—aspartate aminotransferase
ALT—alanine aminotransferase
Albumin
Bilirubin
Alkaline phosphatase
GGT—γ glutamyl transferase
Hepatitis serologies
Tumor markers CEA, CA 19-9, α-fetoprotein (AFP)
CT with IV contrast

ADDITIONAL TESTING

Ultrasound—cystic vs. solid; most tumors are hyperechoic
MR—vascular anatomy
Technetium-labeled RBC scan—prove hemangioma
Technetium sulfur colloid scan—support diagnosis of focal nodular hyperplasia
ERCP or PTC to define biliary involvement of cholangiocarcinoma if suspected

BIOPSY

Use if safe and result would change therapy

CBC, complete blood cell; CEA, carcinoembryonic antigen; CT, computed tomography; ERCP, endoscopic retrograde cholangiopancreatography; IV, intravenous; MRI, magnetic resonance imaging; PTC, percutaneous transhepatic cholangiography; RBC, red blood cell.

mine the number of lesions; (c) define the relationship of the lesion to the biliary tree, portal venous anatomy, and hepatic venous anatomy; and (d) screen for extrahepatic disease. Ultrasonography of the liver is the least costly imaging study and is the most frequently used test for three-dimensional imaging of the liver. Transabdominal ultrasonography has a low sensitivity but a high specificity for liver lesions and can accurately determine the anatomy of the extrahepatic bile ducts and gallbladder. Intraoperative ultrasonography is the most sensitive and specific indicator of hepatic mass lesions and their position relative to the intrahepatic venous and biliary anatomy. Intraoperative ultrasonography in many centers is considered a routine element in the evaluation of the liver before resection or biopsy of suspected hepatic lesions (Fig. 38.1).

Computed tomography can be useful in the assessment of hepatic lesions if intravenous contrast is used. Failure to use intravenous contrast results in scans of low sensitivity that fail to aid in the evaluation of hepatic lesions. The addition of intravenous contrast significantly improves the sensitivity and specificity of CT. Although the bolus administration of intravenous contrast improves CT imaging, multiphase contrast-enhanced spiral CT is the most sensitive method for lesion detection.

Hepatic MRI is considered to be the most accurate method of assessing hepatic mass lesions and is useful in establishing the relationship to vascular structures. T_1- and T_2-weighted images with contrast enhancement (gadolinium or superparamagnetic iron oxide) must be included if MRI is to achieve maximum sensitivity and specificity. The use of superparamagnetic iron oxide decreases the liver signal intensity significantly and consequently increases the number of detected lesions. Gadolinium enhancement improves the detection of many metastatic lesions, and it is especially valuable differentiating hemangiomas or highly vascular lesions from other mass lesions (Fig. 38.2).

Radionuclide imaging is the least sensitive and least specific of three-dimensional imaging modalities of the liver (Fig. 38.3). Radionuclide imaging serves as an adjunct to spiral CT or MRI in the evaluation of liver lesions but fails to identify lesions that are 2 cm or less in size, and it lacks sensitivity. Radionuclide imaging is most helpful when used to differentiate various types of masses. Three frequently used radionuclides are technetium 99m, technetium pertechnetate Tc 99m, and gallium 67. Sulfur colloid labeled with technetium 99m, the agent used most often, is taken up by the reticuloendothelial cells of the spleen and liver (Fig. 38.4). Radionuclide imaging allows for a gross assessment of the liver parenchyma. Scanning with technetium pertechnetate Tc 99m-labeled red blood cell helps to determine the vascularity of a lesion and is used to confirm that a lesion is a hemangioma. Gallium 67 concentrates in malignant and inflammatory cells; this radiopharmaceutical is useful in detecting focal nodular hyperplasia (FNH), evidenced by uptake in Kupffer cells. The

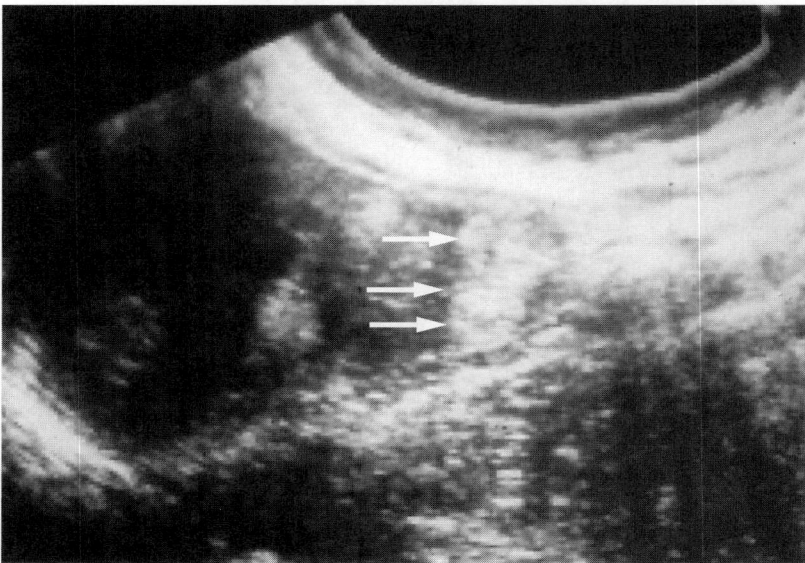

Figure 38.1. An ultrasonographic image displaying the hyperechoic nature of hemangioma.

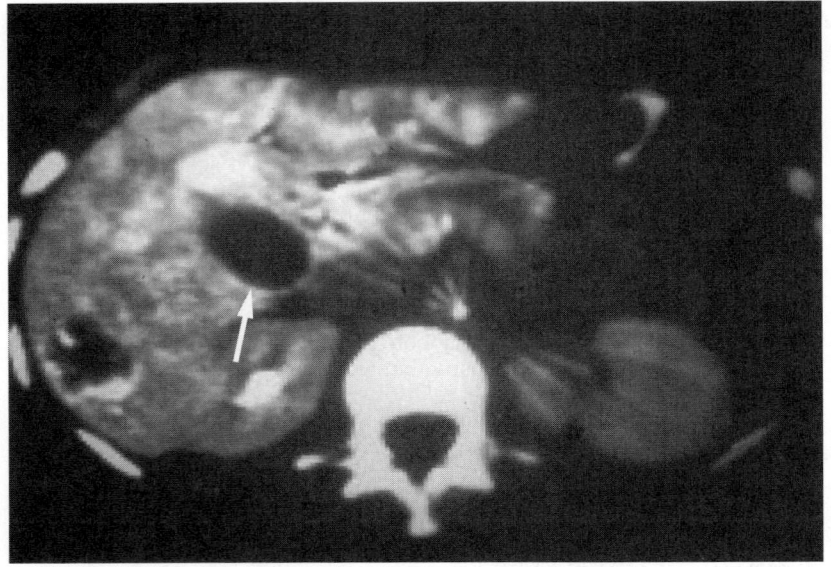

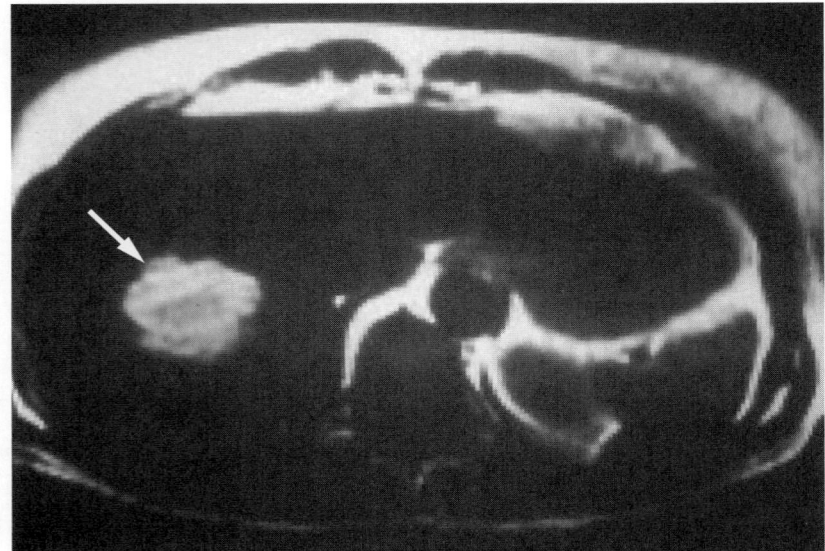

Figure 38.2. *(A)* Computed tomographic image of a hepatic hemangioma demonstrating peripheral enhancement. *(B)* Magnetic resonance image of a hemangioma of the right lobe.

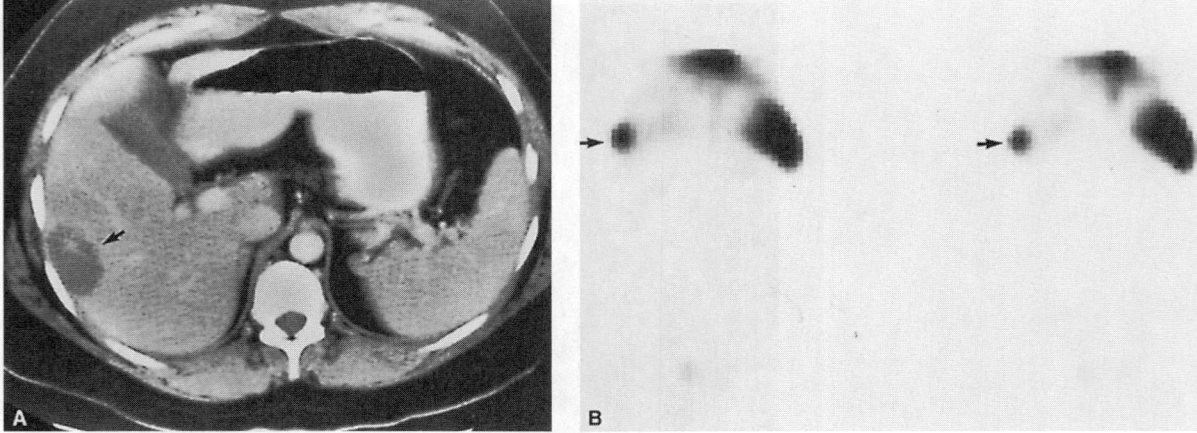

Figure 38.3. *(A)* Computed tomography of the liver demonstrates a 3- to 3.5-cm mass in the lateral aspect of the right lobe *(arrow)* with the characteristics of a hemangioma (peripheral enhancement with centripetal filling). *(B)* A tagged red blood cell scan *(arrow)* confirms the diagnosis. The two confirmatory tests obviate the need for arteriographic evaluation of these lesions.

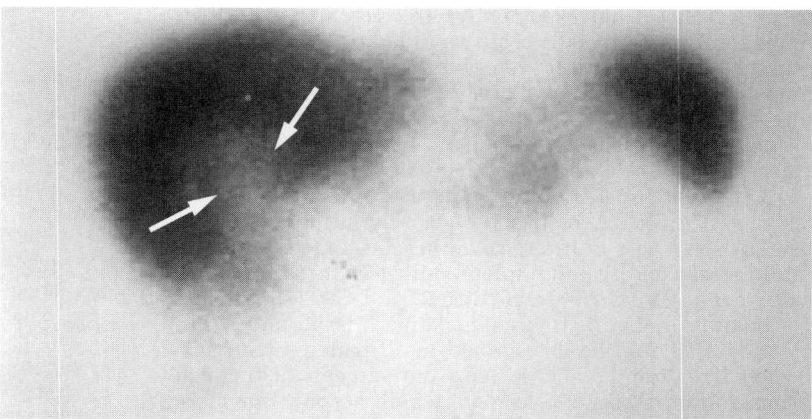

Figure 38.4. Technetium sulfur colloid scan demonstrating a lesion devoid of reticular endothelial cells—in this case, a hemangioma.

use of radionuclide scanning has decreased since advances in MRI have made it possible to determine the histology of many hepatic lesions with a high degree of accuracy.

Ancillary tests in the evaluation of liver lesions include angiography, cholangiography, and biopsy. The role of angiography is of historical interest only for the diagnosis of hepatic neoplasms. Before the advent of dynamic contrast enhancement or spiral CT and contrast-enhanced MRI, angiography was the only means available to assess lesion vascularity (Fig. 38.5). Angiography does not have the specificity or sensitivity of MRI or CT; its primary use, with regard to hepatic neoplasms, is to delineate extrahepatic vascular anatomy more accurately when the surgeon places hepatic arterial infusion devices. Cholangiography can be used to demarcate the relationship of hepatic masses to the biliary tree and the degree of biliary tree involvement. The

cholangiographic technique used most often is endoscopic retrograde cholangiopancreatography (ERCP), which clearly depicts the hepatic biliary tree. Percutaneous transhepatic cholangiography (PTC) may be indicated in patients with tumors that are known to involve the biliary tree and in whom a biliary stent will be placed to aid the surgeon in the dissection and reconstruction. PTC is not indicated for the routine determination of hepatic anatomy in patients with liver tumors because of the risks associated with needle puncture to the tumor. The risks of failure to identify bile ducts in patients with an abnormal biliary anatomy and of hepatic injury when the biliary anatomy is displaced by tumor are significant.

The role of biopsy is an issue of debate among hepatic surgeons. Three types of biopsy are (a) measurement of serum markers, which serve as a "biopsy" of the lesion be-

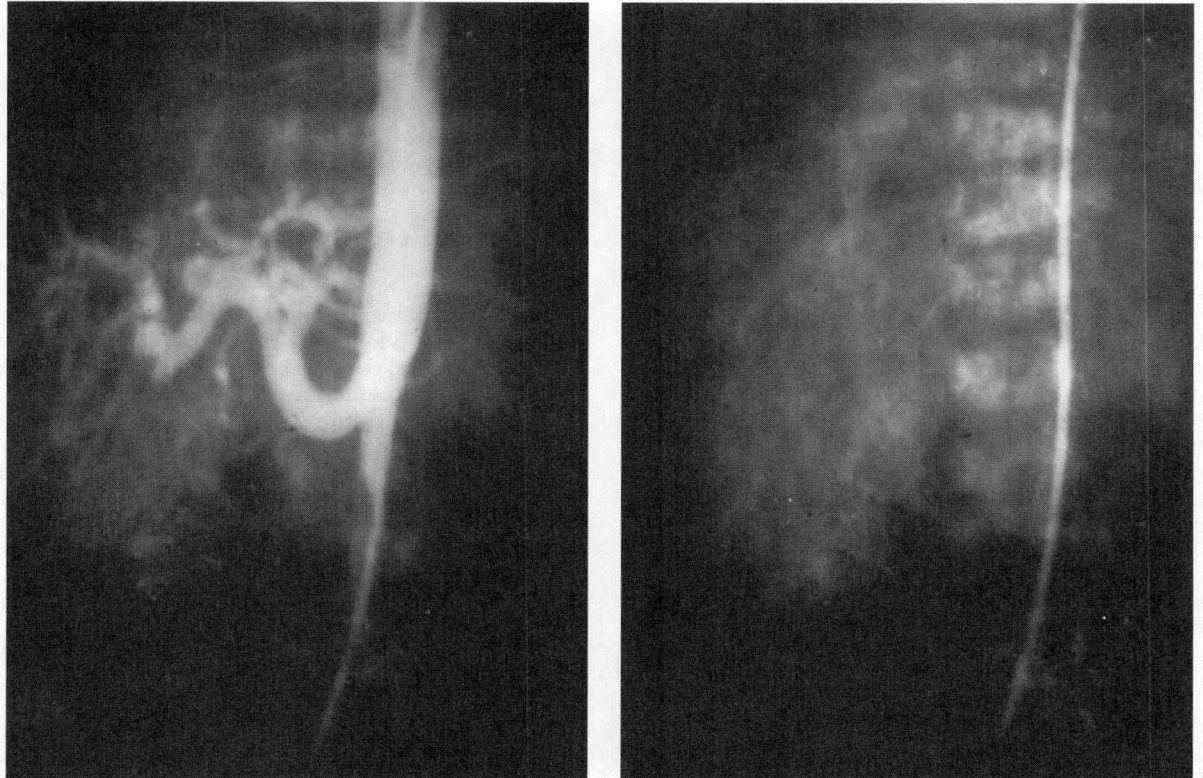

A   B

Figure 38.5. Appearance of hemangioma at arteriography. *(A)* Early injection and *(B)* persistence of "cotton wool" after injection.

cause of their high specificity; (b) percutaneous liver biopsy, either core needle biopsy (guided by CT or sonography) or fine-needle aspiration biopsy; and (c) open hepatic biopsy, either at the time of laparoscopy or during open exploration. Tumor markers should be measured routinely in all patients with suspected hepatic lesions. Markedly elevated levels of α-fetoprotein (> 500 mg/mL) are diagnostic of HCC; these patients do not require additional diagnostic tests to characterize the tissue type. Any further investigation is useful only in regard to aiding the surgeon in determining resectability and implementing treatment. Levels of carcinoembryonic antigen, CA 19-9, and CA 125 and hepatitis titers (hepatitis B virus, hepatitis C virus, and 5'-nucleotidase) should be determined in all patients with suspected liver tumors. These help the surgeon distinguish primary from metastatic lesions, which account for more than 80% of liver tumors. Knowledge of prior extrahepatic malignancy can diminish the need for tissue biopsy. Tumor markers should also be measured before percutaneous biopsy is considered. Percutaneous biopsy is performed when surgical options have been eliminated or when knowledge of the tissue type would alter therapy. Biopsy can establish the histologic type and allow for appropriate nonsurgical therapy in the patient with multiple liver lesions. The risks of biopsy include mortality, tumor seeding of the needle track, intraperitoneal spread of tumor, and bleeding. Exploration rather than biopsy should be used in patients with isolated resectable lesions.

Other infrequently used imaging tests include positron emission tomography (PET) and single-photon emission computed tomography (SPECT), in which tracers that are selectively metabolized by malignant cells are used to distinguish metastatic lesions from primary hepatic lesions or other benign hepatitic masses. These tests are included as part of the diagnostic program for patients who have elevated tumor markers or are at high risk for recurrence. Screening programs for liver tumors in asymptomatic persons are controversial, and they have been used extensively only to screen high-risk populations for HCC.

Surveillance

The advantage of surveillance in the treatment of HCC is that it provides the opportunity to detect lesions early in the course of this rapid disease. If lesions are discovered when they are less than 5 cm in diameter, the chances of survival are improved. Surveillance can be cost-effective when applied to populations of cirrhotic patients who are at high risk for the development of HCC. Surveillance procedures, performed every 6 months, include ultrasonography and measurement of α-fetoprotein levels. The disadvantages of screening programs are that only 50% of patients with HCC test positive for α-fetoprotein, and fewer than 20% of cases of HCC are amenable to curative resection. Initial screening of high-risk populations who test positive for hepatitis B virus or hepatitis C virus and who have established cirrhosis has demonstrated that HCC develops in approximately 8.6% of them annually. The predicted survival benefit is more than 5 years when screening is applied to populations at high risk. The survival benefit is less than 3 to 12 months when screening is applied to populations at low risk (no evidence of cirrhosis) or to patients with end-stage liver disease (severe cirrhosis).

BENIGN HEPATIC LESIONS

Masses in the liver are most frequently benign hepatic lesions (Table 38.2). Generally, benign processes can be accurately diagnosed by a combination of spiral CT and contrast-enhanced MRI with or without radionuclide imaging

---

Table 38.2. HISTOPATHOLOGY OF HEPATIC NEOPLASMS

BENIGN

Hepatic adenoma
Hepatic hemangioma
Focal nodular hyperplasia
Simple cysts
Angiomyolipoma
Regenerative nodule

MALIGNANT

Hepatic cyst adenoma (papillary, cystic)
Hepatic cystic adenocarcinoma
Hepatic angiosarcoma
    Epithelial hemangioendothelioma
Leiomyosarcoma
Hepatocellular carcinoma
Cholangiocarcinoma
Hepatoblastoma
Metastatic hepatic tumors

---

studies. Most benign lesions can be classified as being derived from one of the three major cell types of the liver: hepatocyte or parenchymal lesions; vascular lesions, derived from the blood vessels of the liver; and biliary lesions, associated with the bile ducts. Hepatic parenchymal lesions display various regenerative phenomena that present as mass lesions on scans; these include regenerative nodules and fatty infiltration.

Normal hepatocytes respond to a number of different stimuli with proliferative responses. Hepatocyte injury may be a result of extraneous toxins (aromatic solvents and alcohol) or environmental stimuli (high-fat diets, diabetes, total parenteral nutrition, starvation). The earliest response of the liver is fatty infiltration, which is a reversible process that occurs in a number of disease states. Fat alters the observed pattern of blood supply within the liver, especially if the fatty deposits are variable. Fatty infiltration can appear as a loss of homogeneity on contrast-enhanced CT with various areas of echogenic texture. It is rare for the radiologist to misconstrue anatomic variations, such as persistent fetal lobulation, Riedel's lobe, or caudate lobe hypertrophy, as a neoplastic process, but it is not uncommon for a fatty liver or liver regeneration to be interpreted as a mass lesion.

The liver response to injury after hepatocellular death is regrowth of hepatocytes. Fibrosis develops if regrowth is associated with bridging necrosis, in which case a more exuberant and localized hepatocellular proliferative response results in nodule formation. The liver is relatively small and shrunken if the cirrhosis is micronodular. On radiographic examination, the appearance of the liver mimics that of a neoplastic mass if the cirrhosis is macronodular. These "regenerative" nodules can be confused with a moderately vascularized mass on routine contrast-enhanced CT or sonography. MRI usually distinguishes regenerative nodules from neoplastic masses. Significant portal hypertension associated with extensive cirrhosis can occur and is evidenced by a reduction in total liver blood flow and the appearance of gastric varices, splenomegaly, and retroperitoneal varices.

Hepatic Adenoma

Hepatic adenoma is a benign proliferative lesion that arises from the hepatocyte. Hepatic adenomas occur primarily in women between 20 to 40 years of age but may occur in men and children. The tumor is associated with exogenous estrogen or progesterone use and typically develops in women after 30 years of age. In men, hepatic adenomas are usually associated with anabolic steroid use. The incidence of hepatic adenoma is increased in patients with glycogen storage disease, especially type 1A. Despite an etiologic association with estrogen use, hepatic adenomas often do not express estrogen or progesterone receptors.

Adenomas can produce symptoms of acute abdominal pain as a result of rapid growth or bleeding within the tumor, which can be followed by rupture with hemoperitoneum. The risk for rupture is associated with a rapid increase in the size of the tumor. Rupture can occur in patients using estrogen or during pregnancy.

The tumor presents as a single mass or as multiple lesions on pathologic examination. On gross examination, an adenoma is smooth and soft, with an orange or yellow color, and is most often circumscribed by a capsule. The adenoma is comprised of hepatocytes with a specific absence of bile ducts. The tumor can be misconstrued for primary HCC because it may contain mitotic figures. The radiographic appearance is variable. A hyperintense lesion may appear on the T_1-weighted image, and most lesions are hyperintense on the T_2-weighted image. Approximately 10% to 20% of the lesions are hemorrhagic. On PET, an adenoma may show evidence of decreased uptake in comparison with metastatic disease or HCC, and PET can be a valuable tool in differentiating adenomas from malignant lesions. On CT, an adenoma can demonstrate an early intense enhancement, but because of bleeding within the tumor, enhancement is often heterogenous. In the absence of this occurrence, early enhancement can be confused with FNH or HCC.

Liver adenomatosis, the presence of multiple adenomas of varying sizes throughout the liver, is rare. Extramedullary hematopoiesis or intrahepatic splenosis rarely mimics a hepatic adenoma. Adenomas associated with familial adenomatous polyposis have been reported in infants and children.

The management of hepatic adenomas is controversial in patients whose tumors are smaller than 4 cm. The most common option is to stop all oral contraceptives or androgenic steroids and observe the patient, especially as the risk for bleeding is small. For patients with lesions larger than 5 cm, most centers recommend resection if the lesions are causing symptoms. Lesions should be resected, regardless of size, if the α-fetoprotein level is increased. Liver transplantation for hepatic adenomatosis has been reported, but this approach is controversial.

Hepatic Hemangioma

Hepatic hemangioma is the most common benign tumor of the liver, affecting 7% of the population. Hemangioma occurs most frequently in the third and fourth decades of life and affects women more often than men. Hemangioma is associated with estrogen use in women and can grow rapidly during pregnancy. Several variations of this tumor exist. Cavernous hemangioma is the most common type and appears as a single mass or multiple large, vascular tumors (Fig. 38.6). Hemangiomatosis can occur in adults or children, in whom it is known as *infantile hemangiomatosis*. Infantile hemangiomatosis can result in Kasabach-Merritt syndrome or neonatal hemangiomatosis, which is a coagulopathy syndrome of high-output cardiac failure resulting from massive arteriovenous shunting within the hemangioma. On pathologic examination, the tumor is a soft, compressible lesion that is dark blue to red in color with a thin and somewhat friable texture. A clear plane between the lesion and the normal liver parenchyma allows for dissection (Fig. 38.7). Microscopically, the lesion consists of cystic dilated vas-

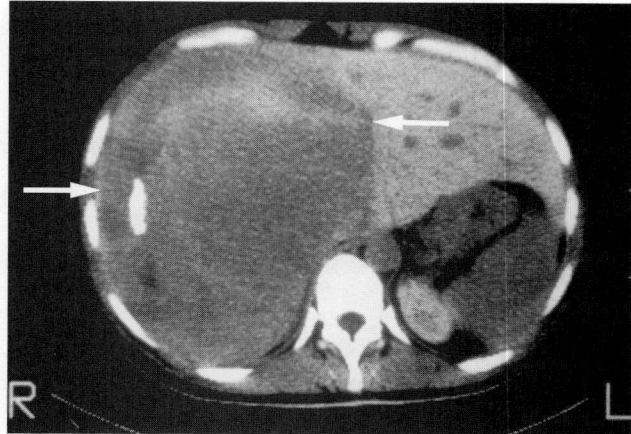

Figure 38.6. Computed tomographic view of a "giant hemangioma."

cular spaces that are lined with endothelial cells. Multiple septa of fibrous tissue are seen, and a greater amount of fibrous tissue can give rise to a harder mass that appears less vascular. In the hyalinized variant of hemangioma, vascular spaces are filled with hyaline material and an abundance of fibrous stroma. Needle biopsy tends to cause hemorrhage, and hemangioma can be confused with sarcoma or other neoplasms (Fig. 38.8).

Most hemangiomas present as an asymptomatic mass found incidentally during routine CT, MRI, or sonography. When symptoms develop, the lesion generally is large. Lesions of the left lobe can cause early satiety; lesions of the right lobe can present with right upper quadrant pain. Bleeding within the tumors is rare, and they usually do not enlarge to the point at which significant arteriovenous shunting occurs.

Laboratory testing may show evidence of thrombocytopenia or hyperfibrinogenemia. Biliary pigment crystal formation may be seen with large tumors or multiple lesions because of hemolysis resulting from trapping of red blood cells within the tumor vascular bed.

Imaging modalities used to diagnosis hemangiomas include Doppler ultrasonography, CT, MRI, scanning with tagged red blood cells, and angiography. Ultrasonography may reveal a hyperechoic mass that is sharply demarcated from the surrounding parenchyma. Blood flow can be identified on ultrasonographic examination in large lesions. However, the sensitivity of ultrasonography is poor (approximately 60%), and hemangiomas can frequently be confused with other hypoechoic lesions, such adenoma, FNH, HCC, or solitary metastases. For this reason, ultrasonography is rarely used as a definitive test for identifying hemangioma.

Computed tomography is useful if intravenous contrast is administered. On CT without contrast, a hypodense, well-demarcated lesion is seen most often. After the administration of contrast, a peripheral zone of enhancement with a corrugated inner margin appears; the center of the lesion is hypodense, and the size remains constant throughout the study. These are classic findings for hemangioma on CT. However, hemangioma is consistently misinterpreted as a lesion with another histology on CT if the lesion fills in during the contrast phase and the peripheral enhancement is missed. The hemangioma can also be misinterpreted if inadequate precontrast and postcontrast views are obtained. After the administration of contrast, the characteristic vascular pattern often is obscured if the lesion is small (< 2 cm). If the lesion is

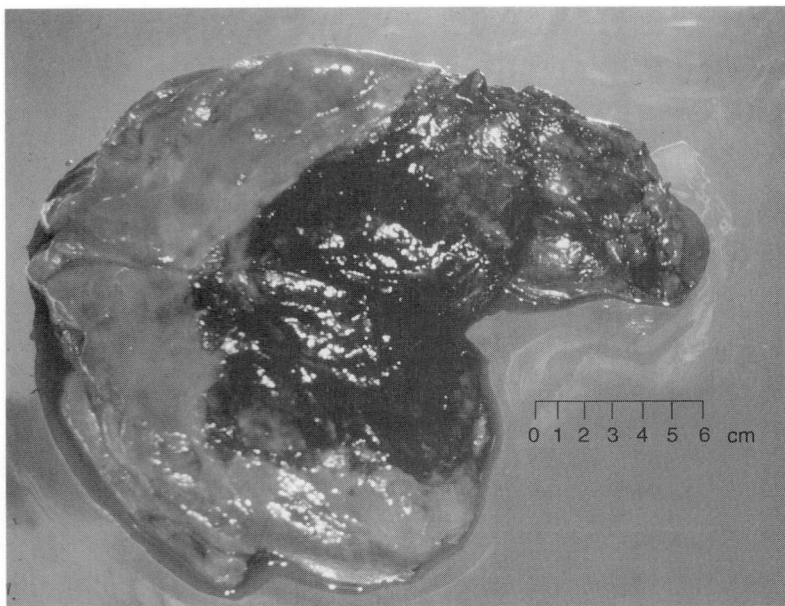

Figure 38.7. Gross view of a resected hemangioma. The blood-filled nature of the tumor is apparent. Many hemangiomas can be enucleated.

hyalinized, it does not enhance and will subsequently be misinterpreted on CT. Hemangiomas also may be confused with other lesions, such as hypervascular metastases or even focal fatty infiltration. Dynamic or spiral CT is the preferred examination because it is the most accurate screening test available, with a sensitivity between 75% and 80% and a specificity between 80% and 88%. MRI can also be used to diagnose hemangiomas on T_1-weighted images; typically, a clearly defined mass is shown. On T_2-weighted images that are isodense to hyperintense, the use of gadolinium (flash sequence) improves lesion detection. Peripheral rim enhancement with or without lesion enhancement is the usual finding. The accuracy of MRI (approximately 90%) is equal to or better than that of CT, but MRI is more expensive. The overall sensitivity of MRI is 80%, and its specificity is 99%.

In the past, when a lesion could not be identified as a hemangioma on CT or ultrasonography, hepatic scintigraphy was the study of choice. Scintigraphy with technetium 99m-labeled sulfur colloid is considered to have the greatest sensitivity (86%) in comparison with ultrasonography but is reported to have a low specificity (approximately 79%). A false-negative result can be obtained on scintigraphy when the lesion is smaller than 2 cm or located deeply in the hepatic parenchyma. Hepatic scintigraphy does not adequately delineate the mass if the lesion is thrombosed or hyalinized. Angiography is of historical interest and is rarely used in the diagnosis of hemangiomas. Typical angiographic findings include normal hepatic arterial vessels with central contrast pooling and an intense vascular blush. The vascular blush gives rise to the so-called cotton wool appearance. Angiography is not as accurate as CT or MRI, is costly to perform, and is not used for staging or planning. Most surgeons use multiple modalities to evaluate hemangiomas, including ultrasonography, CT, and scanning with tagged red blood cells. This combination can increase the sensitivity to 85%, with a specificity of 100% and an overall diagnostic accuracy of 91%. Biopsy should not be per-

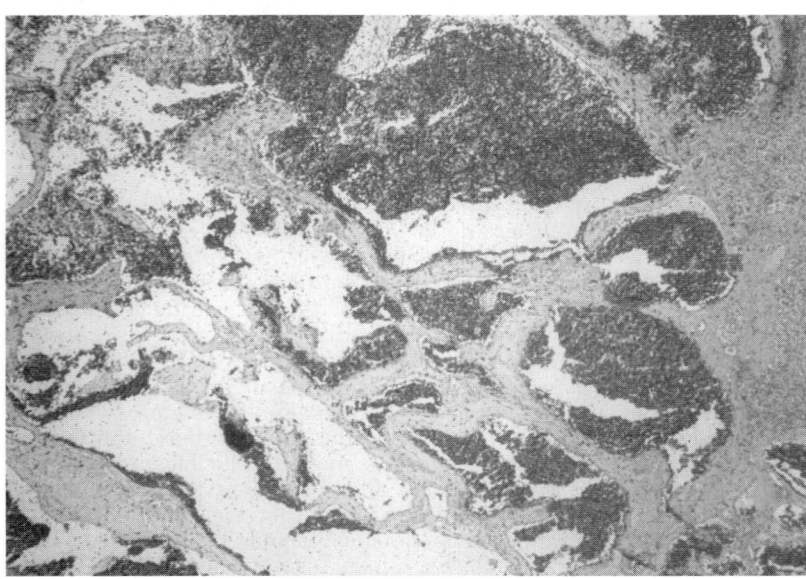

Figure 38.8. Photomicrograph demonstrating the histology of hemangioma. Red blood cells are trapped within enlarged irregular endothelial-lined vascular spaces.

formed in the management of hepatic hemangiomas because it carries a significant risk for hemorrhage.

The clinical course of hemangiomas is benign. Several larger studies have demonstrated no change in the size of lesions during a 5- to 10-year period in most patients. In one study, approximately 10% of lesions followed for 3 years enlarged, and new lesions developed in 12% of patients. Most surgeons agree that asymptomatic patients with fewer than three lesions smaller than 4 cm should be discharged from follow-up. Asymptomatic patients with lesions 4 to 7 cm in size or with more than three lesions should undergo imaging studies periodically. Resection is indicated only for those patients who are symptomatic, as in cases of intratumoral bleeding, or whose diagnosis is uncertain. Few surgeons would recommend resection based solely on the size of the lesion(s).

The surgical treatment of hemangiomas is accomplished with enucleation. This method avoids lobar and segmental resection and the subsequent loss of normal parenchyma. Enucleation has proved to incur less blood loss, require less operative time, shorten length of stay, and result in fewer complications. Hepatic transplantation has also been reported in patients with hemangiomatosis, giant hemangioma, or hemangiomas associated with adenomas. However, liver transplantation is not advocated for patients with benign lesions because of a shortage of donor organs. Some surgeons have advocated intraarterial therapy for patients with hepatic hemangiomas if they are bleeding or, in the case of infants, with hemangiomatosis and Kasabach-Merritt syndrome. This procedure, which consists of hepatic ligation or embolization, has not been shown to decrease the size of hemangiomas; the confirmed reports of resolution of symptoms of hypofibrinogenemia and congestive heart failure are few in number.

Medical therapy of hemangiomatosis is of little benefit. Steroids have been described as a treatment of infantile hemangiomatosis, but no reduction in lesion size or symptoms has been documented. A benefit is possible for patients with hemangioma-associated coagulopathy. The use of cryotherapy or thermal ablation to treat hemangiomas has been reported anecdotally. In theory, the increased blood flow within a hemangioma counteracts the therapeutic effect of thermal intervention.

In summary, hemangioma is a benign neoplasm. Usually, no surgical intervention is required for asymptomatic lesions smaller than 4 cm in size and fewer than three in number. Careful follow-up is recommended for patients who have asymptomatic lesions larger than 4 cm or who present with more than three or four lesions. Symptomatic lesions should be resected by enucleation if possible.

Focal Nodular Hyperplasia

Focal nodular hyperplasia is a common benign tumor of the liver. An etiologic relationship with oral contraceptive use is suggested by a marked female predominance. FNH generally is discovered during three-dimensional imaging studies performed for other reasons. It differs from hepatic adenomas, which tend to present as symptomatic lesions.

Focal nodular hyperplasia may represent a hepatic parenchymal hyperplastic response to an initial vascular malformation. Demonstration of the presence of an X chromosome in most cases of FNH indicates a clonal etiology. Other researchers believe that FNH is polyclonal, which would suggest that it is a reactive process rather than a process of cellular tumoral proliferation. The natural history of FNH is widely regarded to be benign. Only scattered cases of bleeding from FNH tumors have been reported. On pathologic analysis, FNH usually displays a central stellate scar surrounded by highly fibrous tissue. The lesion rarely hemorrhages. Gross histologic examination reveals a firm, fibrous nodular lesion that is subcapsular (Fig. 38.9).

The differential diagnosis of these lesions based on imaging studies can be difficult, and it is not uncommon for them to be confused with adenoma or other mass lesions. Because of the Kupffer cell activity of FNH, scanning with technectium 99m-labeled sulfur colloid or MRI with superparamagnetic iron oxide is useful in the diagnosis. Ultrasonography usually shows a hyperechoic lesion with a sharply defined margin between the mass and hepatic parenchyma. MRI with superparamagnetic iron oxide shows uptake of iron oxide particles. CT of FNH demonstrates marked enhancement with washout on delayed images. The lesion can be confused with hepatic adenoma, but hepatic adenoma is more homogenous. FNH appears het-

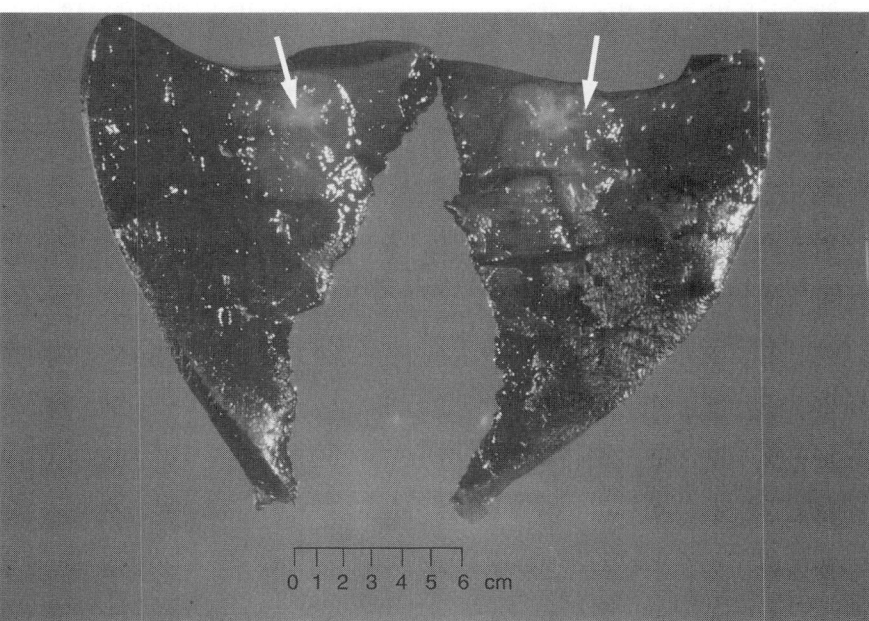

Figure 38.9. Resected liver specimen opened to show the characteristic central scarring of focal nodular hyperplasia.

erogenous when gadolinium-enhanced MRI is used. Most lesions are hyperintense, but they may be homogenous and isointense. The appearance of a central scar on CT or MRI increases specificity.

If FNH is clearly diagnosed on CT in an asymptomatic patient, the patient should not undergo a resection but should halt external estrogen or steroid use and remain under observation. If the lesion is symptomatic or shows signs of having bled, it should be resected. FNH is resected when a diagnosis is in question and the lesion is difficult to distinguish from hepatic adenoma or other neoplasms. Some physicians have suggested needle biopsy to aid in the diagnosis of FNH, but this should be undertaken with caution because of the risk for bleeding from an adenoma or other vascular lesion.

Simple Cysts

Cysts of the liver are common and generally benign. They present as asymptomatic masses or as symptomatic space-occupying lesions if they grow to a large size. Hepatic cysts are believed to be congenital, but they can enlarge and compress liver substance or cause biliary obstruction. If the patient has multiple cysts, they can increase in size and cause hepatic failure, as in polycystic kidney disease. Most cysts are pathologically simple, unilocular structures that are covered with a secretory epithelium. The cysts may communicate with the biliary tract.

Cysts are the easiest of all hepatic mass lesions to diagnose on radiographic examination because of a characteristic water intensity signal from the lesions. Infectious cysts of the liver, especially hydatid, amebic, or chronic abscesses, are distinguished from simple cysts by the presence of septa or calcification, or the finding of "hydatid sand" on CT or MRI. Simple cysts can be diagnosed with ultrasonography, CT, or MRI; no additional radiographic examinations are needed.

The treatment of hepatic cysts is straightforward. Cysts should be followed without intervention if they are asymptomatic. If hepatic cysts are symptomatic as a result of mass effects, they should be operatively marsupialized or resected by open or laparoscopic techniques. Needle aspiration of hepatic cysts should not be performed because the cyst will inevitably recur. Needle aspiration is associated with significant complications, including infection of the cyst or perforation of a small vessel or bile duct, which causes hemorrhage or conversion of the cyst to a biloma.

MALIGNANT LESIONS OF THE LIVER

Primary Hepatic Malignant Lesions

Primary lesions occur in about 10,000 to 12,000 patients per year in the United States. This group includes malignancies of the liver, biliary tree, and gallbladder. Despite a relatively low incidence in the United States, HCC represents the most common malignancy worldwide because of an extraordinarily high incidence in Africa, Asia, and India.

The four predominant histologic types of primary hepatic cancer include HCC, a tumor derived from the hepatocyte; cholangiocarcinoma, a tumor derived from the bile duct epithelium; hepatoblastoma, which occurs mainly in children; and angiosarcoma. Less common histologic types include fibrosarcoma, rhabdosarcoma, leiomyosarcoma, teratoma, hepatic neurofibromatosis, Kaposi's sarcoma, and primary hepatic lymphoma. All these latter tumor types are very rare.

Hepatic Cyst Adenoma and Adenocarcinoma

Hepatic cyst adenoma is a rare and relatively low-grade neoplasm of the liver. Hepatic cyst adenocarcinoma and hepatic mucinous cyst adenoma can mimic simple hepatic cysts. These lesions present incidentally or as mildly symptomatic right upper quadrant masses. Occasionally, they may present with jaundice because of direct involvement or compression of the biliary tract. Papillary cyst adenoma and mucinous cyst adenoma are believed to arise from the bile duct epithelium. Septa are present in the lesions or lobulated cystic mass. The ultrasonographic appearance is that of a hypoechoic, central mass with or without septa and a thicker than normal wall. CT and MRI show a thickened wall and an associated adjacent mass. ERCP can show a biliary communication or direct compression or involvement of a deep bile duct by the tumor. The treatment should always be resection, not enucleation, and marsupialization should be avoided because it will cause neoplastic cyst contents to spill into the abdominal cavity and increase the risk for recurrence.

Angiosarcoma

Angiosarcoma is a rare, malignant tumor of the liver. Angiosarcoma has been described in adults but is more common in children. Etiologic factors include exposure to toxins, including vinyl fluoride monomer, arsenic, and androgenic steroids such as methyltestosterone. The latency period between exposure to the carcinogen and the development of cancer can be as long as 30 years. These tumors are highly malignant and very aggressive. They present as a large, unilobar hepatic mass and tend to metastasize via the bloodstream.

A variant of angiosarcoma is the epithelial hemangioendothelioma. When this tumor occurs in children, it is called *pediatric hemangioendothelioma* and is somewhat less aggressive than adult hepatic angiosarcoma. Radiographically, angiosarcoma presents as a solid tumor with an intense vascular blush; central necrosis may be develop because of rapid growth. If necrosis develops in a significant proportion of the tumor and liquefies, the mass can be confused with a hepatic abscess, especially if "tumor fever" is present. The suggested treatment of these lesions is resection. Some authors have suggested doxorubicin as a postoperative adjuvant therapy because of the high likelihood of recurrence.

Leiomyosarcoma and Angiomyolipoma

Primary leiomyosarcoma and angiomyolipoma have been known to occur in the liver. Angiomyolipomas do not have metastatic potential but are difficult to distinguish from a malignant lesion on CT. The tumor is often defined as a well-demarcated homogeneous mass on ultrasonography, CT, or MRI, but it appears hypervascular after contrast administration or on arteriography. Angiomyolipoma of the kidney can safely be observed. Most authors suggest resection because of the difficulty of obtaining a definitive diagnosis.

Hepatocellular Carcinoma

Hepatocellular cancer typically arises in a liver that has been subjected to chronic stimulation, usually by environmental or biologic toxins that result in hepatocellular death, chronic regeneration, and cirrhosis. The most common causes are hepatitis B, hepatitis C, and exposure to hepatotoxins, notably aflatoxin B_1 (the mycotoxin of the fungus *Aspergillus flavus*) and ethanol. HCC worldwide disproportionately affects Asians and Africans because of the high prevalence of hepatitis B and hepatitis C in these populations. Other diseases and conditions that cause cir-

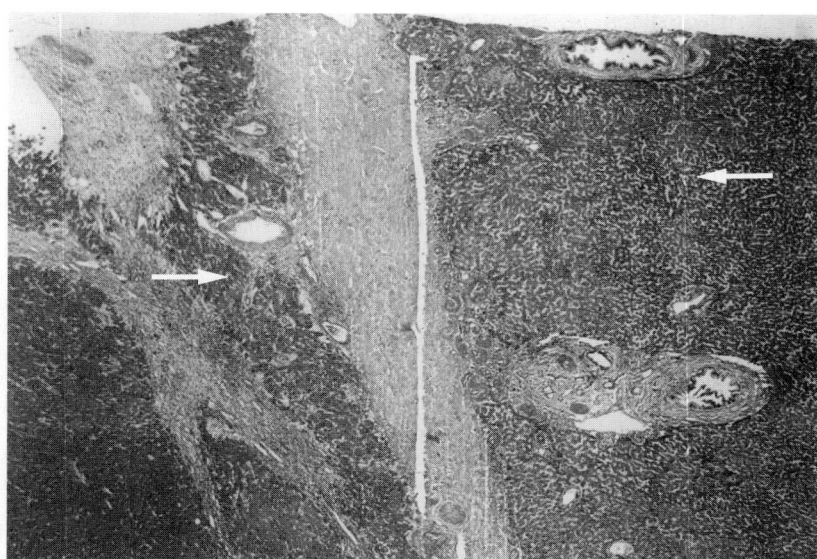

Figure 38.10. Photomicrograph demonstrating a well-differentiated hepatocellular carcinoma *(left upper corner)* and normal hepatic parenchyma *(right half of image)*. These can be impossible to distinguish on small biopsy samples.

rhosis also predispose to the development of HCC. These include hemochromatosis, type 1 glycogen storage disease, α_1-antitrypsins deficiency, tyrosinemia, androgenic steroid use, and primary biliary cirrhosis. Dietary carcinogens include cycasin from the cycad nut.

From 60% to 80% of HCCs arise in livers with preexisting cirrhosis. Although investigators have attempted to document the integration of hepatitis B viral DNA into the host genome, a direct relationship has not been conclusively proved.

Hepatocellular carcinoma occurs in three distinct histologic types (Figs. 38.10 and 38.11). The fibrolamellar type presents as a single large lesion in the liver. The nodular type presents with multiple, bilobar, scattered nodules of tumor. The diffuse type is associated with an infiltrative pattern that is dispersed throughout the liver with no single developed foci. On pathologic examination, these tumors contain cells that resemble hepatocytes. If the tumor is well differentiated, the cells form cords and may be separated by fibrous septa, and the tumors can even elaborate

bile. As the cells become less differentiated, they contain more cytoplasm and multiple nuclei.

Patients with HCC usually are asymptomatic, or HCC is found as a mass on a scan performed to evaluate vague abdominal complaints. Another clinical presentation is sudden deterioration in an otherwise stable cirrhotic patient. Such deterioration can manifest as the onset of gastrointestinal bleeding with rapidly increasing portal hypertension, Budd-Chiari syndrome resulting from hepatic venous obstruction by rapidly growing tumor, or tumor thrombosis in the hepatic veins. Patients also can present with acute hepatic failure and encephalopathy as a result of the loss of parenchymal cell volume caused by tumor growth, or with new-onset ascites as a result of portal vein thrombosis caused by tumor involvement or tumor thrombus. All these acute clinical scenarios indicate advanced end-stage hepatic dysfunction and render surgical intervention difficult or unwise. Other presentations include early satiety and epigastric masses with lesions of the left lobe, pleuritic or diaphragmatic pain, or right upper quad-

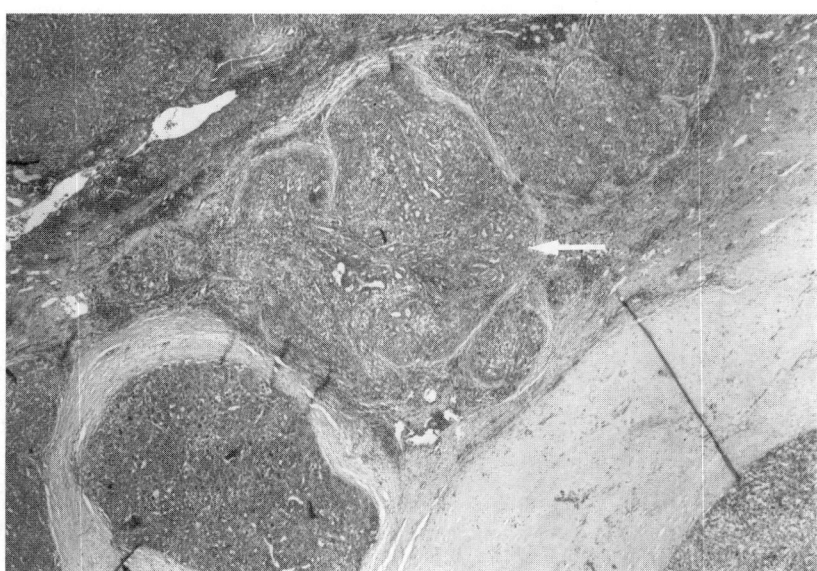

Figure 38.11. Photomicrograph of poorly differentiated hepatocellular carcinoma. Contrast with specimen in Fig. 38.12.

rant pain with large lesions of the right lobe. HCC is frequently associated with weight loss, and hypoproteinemia and hypoalbuminemia are common on laboratory studies. An associated thrombocytopenia is frequently present, a consequence of hypersplenism secondary to portal hypertension. A perineoplastic syndrome may also be associated with HCC, characterized by polycythemia, dysfibrinogenemia, hypoglycemia, and possible autonomic up-regulation, including hypertension, diarrhea, and palpations secondary to ectopic hormone production.

Diagnostic tests include spiral CT and MRI (Fig. 38.12). It is difficult with either of these modalities to differentiate HCC completely from adenomas and other malignant tumors of the liver. Lesions on contrast CT appear as hypointense, isointense, or mildly intense. Some calcification may be present, with thrombus in the portal or hepatic veins. After the administration of gadolinium contrast, the lesions also appear as hypointense, isointense, or hyperintense. Elevation of the tumor marker α-fetoprotein is highly specific and occurs in approximately 50% of patients. Biopsy can yield a diagnosis in many cases, but it is important to use core needle aspiration to obtain an adequate sample size so that hepatic architecture can be determined. Adenomas and poorly differentiated HCC can frequently be confused with clear cell carcinomas or cholangiocarcinomas. Percutaneous biopsy carries a significant risk in this patient population because of associated portal hypertension and hematologic abnormalities, thrombocytopenia, and hypofibrinogenemia. Similarly, the presence of portal hypertension and associated hematologic abnormalities complicates the use of laparoscopic biopsy in the evaluation of these tumors. Nonetheless, this modality is popular, especially when used in conjunction with laparoscopic intraoperative sonography. Percutaneous biopsy may also cause needle track seeding, which increases the risk for local recurrence.

Patients with HCC are one identifiable high-risk group that can benefit from screening programs because of the close association of HCC with hepatitis B and cirrhosis. Typical screening programs enroll patients who have a significant history of chronic, active hepatitis B and commence with serial α-fetoprotein measurements and sonographic evaluation of the liver. These programs have assisted in the early detection and treatment of lesions, especially in patients with a significant hepatocellular reserve and thus a longer life expectancy.

The treatment of HCC depends on the degree of liver dysfunction, the anatomic location and size and number

of tumors, and any associated medical illnesses. Regardless of the modality used, better results are obtained in patients with intact hepatocellular function than in those with poor hepatic function. Thus, Child group A patients have the best outcomes for any given stage of tumor. Patients in Child group C rarely benefit from any therapeutic modality short of transplantation. The modalities available include surgical excision, hepatic transplantation, operative cryotherapy, and radiofrequency ablation. Nonoperative modalities include percutaneous ethanol injection, percutaneous radiofrequency ablation, chemoembolization, and intraarterial chemotherapy. Some interest is still shown in radiotherapy with implanted isotopes (brachytherapy) or external beam radiation. External beam radiotherapy must be skillfully planned to reduce the risk for radiation-induced hepatitis or biliary injury. Chemoembolization involves the use of a chemotherapeutic agent, usually 5-fluorouracil, mitomycin, Adriamycin, or cisplatin, administered with an embolic agent such Gelfoam or Lipiodol. Lipiodol is the preferred agent because it embolizes small vessels and allows for repeated treatments during many months. Gelfoam tends to occlude larger vessels and does not permit sequential therapeutic sessions. In general, response rates are upward of 50% for intraarterial chemoembolic therapy, but no cures have been reported with this therapy.

Percutaneous ethanol injection has received increasing attention, especially for patients with small HCCs and poor liver function. Survival rates at 1 year of 80% have been achieved by treating lesions up to 2 cm with repeated injections of ethanol. The therapy is not useful with multinodular disease (at least five nodules) or for large fibrolamellar lesions.

Hepatic transplantation is used rarely for HCC in North America. It is appealing because in addition to the hepatic tumor, it treats the underlying hepatic disease that, in most cases, contributes to the development of HCC. Tumor growth is rapid, and the average wait for donor organs in the United States exceeds 3 to 6 months. Consequently, the disease progresses significantly while the patient awaits transplantation. Furthermore, immunosuppression after transplantation significantly increases the rate of HCC growth, so that any residual disease recurs early and rapidly. Nonetheless, for a patient with severe liver dysfunction and early HCC (< 2 cm in diameter and fewer than three nodules), hepatic transplantation is an important treatment that significantly increases long-term survival.

Surgical extirpation is the mainstay of therapy and, besides transplantation, the only definitive therapy. A 5-year disease-free survival of approximately 50% can be expected for patients whose tumors are completely excised. Numerous studies have shown that lobar, segmental, and nonanatomic parenchyma-sparing resections yield equal survival rates. Mortality rates for the operative procedure are between 2% and 5%; a major cause of mortality is liver failure resulting from inadequate underlying hepatic reserve. Hepatic resection is the single best therapy for patients with reasonable hepatic function and fibrolamellar tumors.

Cholangiocarcinoma

Cholangiocarcinoma, the second most common primary malignancy of the liver, arises from the biliary epithelium and presents histologically as an adenocarcinoma. Cholangiocarcinoma is classified based on location and may be intrahepatic, perihilar, or distal (common bile duct). Approximately 10% to 25% of cholangiocarcinomas present as intrahepatic lesions. Intrahepatic cholangiocarcinomas are associated with several disease states,

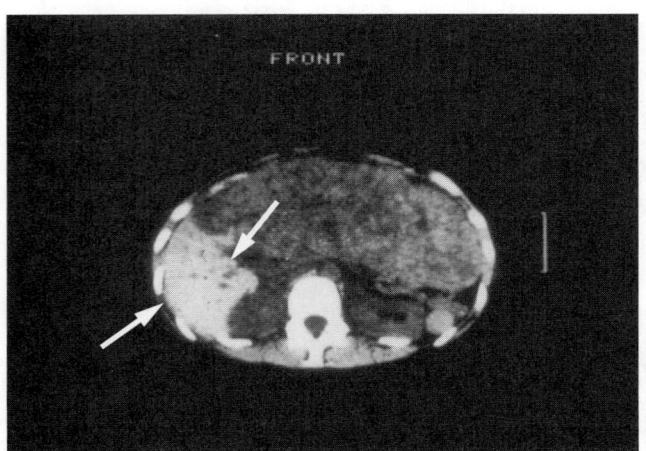

Figure 38.12. Computed tomographic images of a large hepatoma that was rendered resectable by neoadjuvant treatment.

especially ulcerative colitis, sclerosing cholangitis, hemochromatosis, and cystic biliary tract disease, including *Clonorchis sinensis* infection, oriental cholangiohepatitis, choledochal cysts, and chronic biliary obstruction. Confusing pathologic nomenclature includes cholangiohepatocellular cancer, a pathologic entity with features that closely resemble those of HCC and cholangiocarcinoma.

Patients with intrahepatic cholangiocarcinoma typically present with asymptomatic hepatic masses or with vague symptoms of weight loss, early satiety, and anorexia. Occasionally, they present with signs and symptoms of cholangitis, which include fever and upper abdominal pain without jaundice. Jaundice may be absent if the tumor is associated with a segmental bile duct obstruction and only partial biliary stasis. Perihilar tumors arise in the extrahepatic biliary tree at the hepatic ductal bifurcation (Klatskin tumor), and painless jaundice is the presenting sign. The diagnosis of intrahepatic cholangiocarcinoma is difficult because tumors can present as a single, peripheral hepatic mass. Percutaneous biopsy will document an adenocarcinoma. In these cases, the tumor most frequently suspected is a metastatic adenocarcinoma, and an extensive work-up is needed to rule out an extrahepatic source of tumor. Cholangiography usually demonstrates an obstructed or involved bile duct, which confirms a cholangiocarcinoma. Typically, metastatic tumors do not cause biliary obstruction but rather distend or deform the bile duct. Cholangiocarcinomas usually result in biliary obstruction earlier than metastatic lesions do.

The preferred treatment of cholangiocarcinomas is excision. Chemoembolization has not proved to be of benefit in this patient population. Conformal external beam radiotherapy may be palliative.

Primary Hepatic Sarcomas

Primary hepatic sarcomas and angiomyolipomas are vascular tumors of the liver that behave differently. Angiomyolipomas are mostly benign. They have a high fat content and are easily distinguished on CT or MRI from sarcomas and other primary liver tumors. Hepatic sarcoma is a rare tumor that is highly lethal and grows rapidly. It is frequently associated with exposure to carcinogens, including vinyl chloride, Thorotrast, arsenic, and methyltestosterone. The latency period between toxin exposure and tumor development is prolonged (10 to 20 years). Presenting signs are similar to those observed in HCC and cholangiocarcinoma—an asymptomatic abdominal mass associated with vague right upper quadrant pain, weight loss, and anorexia.

Angiohemangioendothelioma is an intermediate-grade tumor that is similar to an angiosarcoma but has less malignant potential. Angiosarcoma and angiohemangioendothelioma can be metastatic from other sites or may arise as a primary hepatic tumor. An extensive search for other tumor sites, including the abdomen and extremities, should be made before resectional surgery is undertaken. A chest CT is recommended to eliminate pulmonary involvement because of the high risk for metastatic disease.

Metastatic Disease

The liver is a common site for metastatic cancer, particularly gastrointestinal malignancies, because of its function as a portal venous "sieve" for all alimentary organs. The liver tumor can represent an isolated, indirect "downstream" metastasis from gastrointestinal organs or can be one of many metastatic sites. Isolated hepatic metastases from favorable biologic tumors have the most promising prognosis and represent potentially curable metastatic disease. The liver is also a site for "systemic metastases"; in this case, tumor cells reach the liver through the arterial circulation, rather than the closed portal circulation, and presumably become established because of a favorable hepatic microenvironment. Tumors that metastasize to the liver via the systemic circulation include melanomas, sarcomas, and breast, lung, prostate, kidney, and endocrine tumors.

Hepatic resection has been used to treat both local, regional, portal metastatic disease and systemic metastatic disease. The benefit derived from surgical resection of metastatic disease depends on (a) the primary tumor biology, with more rapidly dividing, aggressive tumors having a less favorable prognosis than well-differentiated, more slowly growing tumors; (b) the site of metastases, with portal metastatic spread having a better prognosis than systemic metastatic spread; and (c) chronicity, with single tumors that appear metachronously having a better prognosis than multiple lesions that are discovered at the same time as the primary tumor.

The most widely accepted use of hepatic metastasectomy is in patients with colorectal cancer. In one of the largest early series of hepatic resection for metastatic cancer, investigators demonstrated the close relationship between number of lesions and timing of the diagnosis of metastatic disease to treatment of the primary tumor and prognosis. Patients with synchronous lesions did less well than patients with metachronous lesions. Patients with multiple tumors had poorer survival rates than those with single lesions. This work indicated the need for a 1-cm margin around the tumor to achieve 20% to 30% long-term, disease-free survival. The results of the study, confirmed by many other investigators, also indicated that approximately 20% of patients have only hepatic disease and no remaining systemic disease; hepatic resection in these patients can be curative. Approximately 150,000 cases of colon cancer occur each year in the United States; hepatic metastases develop in 60,000 patients, who represent the potential group to be evaluated for resectional therapy. Other sites of tumor metastasis must be excluded when a patient is evaluated for hepatic metastasectomy. The evaluation should include chest roentgenography, chest CT, colonoscopy to exclude another primary lesion or local recurrence, and full abdominal and pelvic CT to eliminate any other extrahepatic disease. Alkaline phosphatase levels should be determined, and if elevated, a bone scan should be considered. A careful neurologic history should be obtained, and any new neurologic symptom, such as headache, disorientation, or dizziness, should prompt further evaluation with MRI.

Resection should be considered if it is determined that disease is confined to the liver and the patient has four or fewer lesions. The patient should be considered to be at high risk for other regional recurrence or systemic recurrence if more than four lesions are present. Surgeons should be more reluctant to offer metastasectomy to these patients.

The role of palliative cytoreductive therapy in hepatic metastatic disease is controversial (Fig. 38.13). The theory behind this form of treatment is that reduction of the total tumor mass significantly prolongs life in patients with slowly growing tumors. Modalities available include cryoablation, radiofrequency thermal ablation, and interstitial radiation. None of these therapies is known to provide the same local–regional control or long-term cure rates as resection. In general, palliative cytoreductive therapies are used for tumors that are nonresectable by conventional techniques because of proximity to major vessels or bile ducts. These modalities, like resection, are limited by the size of the lesion. Thermal ablation cannot be applied to lesions larger than 5 cm, and cryoablation is rarely effective in lesions larger than 7 to 8 cm.

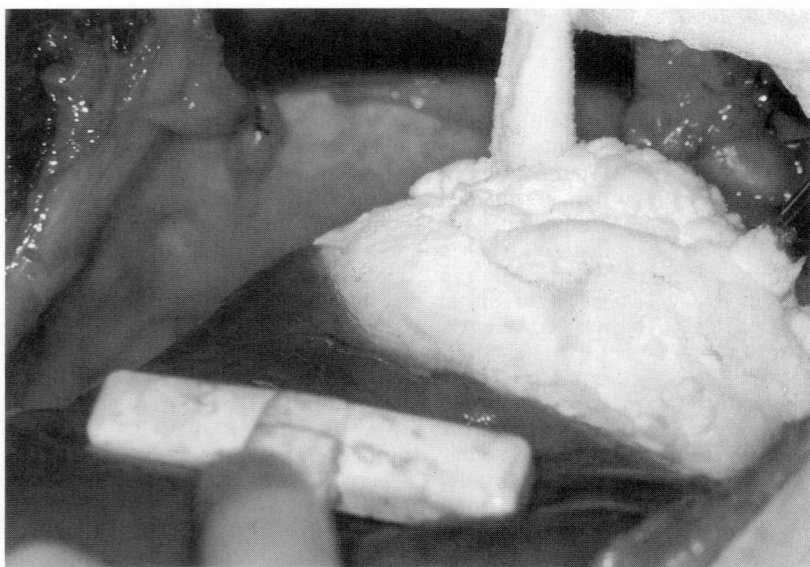

Figure 38.13. Intraoperative view of cryoablation of a hepatic tumor. The cryoprobe is inserted into the liver and with a superficial lesion is covered with ice crystals. Progress is continuously monitored with an ultrasonic probe placed on the surface of the liver.

Other treatments available for patients with hepatic metastases include systemic chemotherapy and intraarterial chemotherapy. Intraarterial chemotherapy usually includes the surgical implantation of an infusion pump with a catheter that leads to the hepatic artery. The most commonly used agent is fluorodeoxyuridine, a prodrug for 5-fluorouracil that is 90% extracted by the liver. Regional chemotherapy has been shown to improve the response rates of hepatic metastases to chemotherapy but does not improve survival.

Other portally derived metastatic tumors for which hepatic resection has been used on rare occasions include gastric cancer, small-intestinal neoplasms, and pancreatic cancer. The use of hepatic resection for metastatic gastric cancer has been described only for patients with fewer than four metachronous lesions. It appears that the life of several patients has been prolonged significantly, but no randomized, controlled trials have compared hepatic resection with chemotherapy. The use of hepatic resection for metastatic pancreatic cancer or cancer of the small intestine has been anecdotally reported, but it is not believed to be successful because of the rapid growth rates of pancreatic and small-intestinal cancers; in these cases, most hepatic disease is inoperable because of the synchronous presence of systemic or extrahepatic disease.

Tumors that seed the liver by systemic spread and that are amenable to surgical resection include sarcomas and neuroendocrine tumors. Hepatic resection has also been described for metastatic breast cancer, melanoma, renal cell cancer, and endocrine tumors. In general, resection is indicated for patients with large, symptomatic, and isolated tumors who have had a long, disease-free interval between diagnosis of the primary tumor and appearance of the metastasis. In this circumstance, disease-free intervals in excess of 2 years or, in many cases, of 5 years indicate suitable tumor biology for resection. Most centers have not been able to report a significant prolongation of life despite the use of these criteria but do report survivals of up to 2 to 3 years.

The use of resectional therapies such as a palliative cytoreduction is controversial. In these situations, the surgeon is asked to remove the bulk of tumor even though the risk for recurrence or residual extrahepatic disease may be overwhelming. This strategy is used only to treat extraordinarily slow-growing tumors that are highly symptomatic—most commonly, neuroendocrine tumors. Tissue types include carcinoid, islet cell, metastatic medullary thyroid, and other neuroendocrine tumors. These tumors can become symptomatic when they produce hormones, and resection of the tumor bulk results in significant control of tumor-related paraneoplastic symptoms.

The technical aspects of hepatic resection have been described in many reports. In many large centers, the mortality associated with these procedures is less than 2%, with a morbidity of 20% to 30%. Risk factors include the need for hepatic lobar or segmental resection, which may carry a higher risk than nonanatomic resection. A relatively large hepatocellular mass and elevated bilirubin levels increase the risk for complications. Age or associated medical conditions are not known to be risk factors. The complexity of the resection and amount of blood loss have been shown to be associated with complications, and many authors have focused on technical methods to control intraoperative hemorrhage. Several investigations have studied whether the liver should be vascularly excluded before resection, and none has shown a benefit for this particular technique. Technical measures that can decrease blood loss include lowering the portal venous pressure, either with vasoactive agents or portal blood flow occlusion (Pringle maneuver). Isovolemic hemodilution or autologous transfusion has been recommended to control blood loss and reduce the total number of units transfused.

Many centers report a relatively high risk for morbidity, above 20%. Predominant complications include pulmonary atelectasis and pneumonia, perihepatic sepsis (including biloma, subhepatic abscess, or subphrenic abscess), uncontrolled hemorrhage, and primary liver failure as a result of failure of liver regeneration. Infection is the most common cause of morbidity and death after hepatic resection. The maximum limit of hepatic resection is believed to be 60% of the functional hepatic mass. Many surgeons use the terminology of Couinaud to describe tumor location and resection size. Trisegmentectomy includes the anatomic anterior and posterior segments of the right lobe and the medial segment of the left lobe, which leaves the left lateral segment and caudate lobe. Some surgeons have reported removal of the entire liver with the exception of the left lateral segment, and the patients have survived. Patients who have undergone larger resections are at risk for hypoglycemia resulting from the loss of hepatic gluconeogenesis. These patients must be maintained on glucose infusions perioperatively. The remnant liver is dependent on hepatic arterial and remnant portal flow. Vasoactive agents or hypotension should be avoided because of the severe impact on arterialized flow to the remaining liver. Hypovolemia or arterial vasospasm leads to significant impairment of the regenerative response of the liver. Other agents that typically limit liver regeneration include the nonsteroidal antiinflammatory drugs.

REFERENCES

Akaki S, Mitsumori A, Kanazawa S, et al. Lobar decrease in ^{99m}Tc-GSA accumulation in hilar cholangiocarcinoma. *J Nucl Med* 1999;40:394–398.

Arsenault TM, Johnson CD, Gorman B, et al. Hepatic adenomatosis. *Mayo Clin Proc* 1996;71:478–480.

Ault GT, Wren SM, Ralls PW, et al. Selective management of hepatic adenomas. *Am Surg* 1996;62:825–829.

Awan S, Davenport M, Portmann B, et al. Angiosarcoma of the liver in children. *J Pediatr Surg* 1996;31:1729–1732.

Bala S, Wunsch PH, Ballhausen WG. Childhood hepatocellular adenoma in familial adenomatous polyposis: mutations in adenomatous polyposis coli gene and *p53*. *Gastroenterology* 1997;112:919–922.

Becker YT, Raiford DS, Webb L, et al. Rupture and hemorrhage of hepatic focal nodular hyperplasia. *Am Surg* 1995;61:210–214.

Bismuth H, Nakache R, Diamond T. Management strategies in resection for hilar cholangiocarcinoma. *Ann Surg* 1992;215:31–38.

Cohen C. Lawson D, DeRose PB. Sex and androgenic steroid receptor expression in hepatic adenomas. *Hum Pathol* 1998;29:1428–1432.

Cristaldi M, Rovati M, Conte D, et al. Primary liver adenomatosis. Report of two cases and literature review. *Dig Surg* 1998;15:75–78.

Daller JA, Dueno J, Gutierrez J, et al. Hepatic hemangioendothelioma: clinical experience and management strategy. *J Pediatr Surg* 1999;34:98–105.

DeCarlis L, Pirotta V. Rondinara GF, et al. Hepatic adenoma and focal nodular hyperplasia: diagnosis and criteria for treatment. *Liver Transpl Surg* 1997;3:160–165.

Ferrucci JT. Liver tumor imaging. Current concepts. *Radiol Clin North Am* 1994;32:39–54.

Gaffey MJ, Iezzoni JC, Weiss LM. Clonal analysis of focal nodular hyperplasia of the liver. *Am J Pathol* 1996;148:1089–1096.

Gates LK Jr, Cameron AJ, Nagorney DM, et al. Primary leiomyosarcoma of the liver mimicking liver abscess. *Am J Gastroenterol* 1995;90:649–652.

Gedaly R, Pomposelli JJ, Pomfret EA, et al. Cavernous hemangioma of the liver: anatomic resection vs. enucleation. *Arch Surg* 1999;134:407–411.

Gruen DR, Gollub MJ. Intrahepatic splenosis mimicking hepatic adenoma. *AJR Am J Roentgenol* 1997;168:725–726.

Hayasaka K, Tanaka Y, Satoh T, et al. Hepatic hemangioblastoma: an unusual presentation of von Hippel-Lindau disease. *J Comput Assist Tomogr* 1999;23:565–566.

Horton KM, Bluemke DA, Hruban RH, et al. CT and MR imaging of benign hepatic and biliary tumors. *Radiographics* 1999;19:431–451.

Hultcrantz R, Olsson R, Danielsson A, et al. A 3-year prospective study on serum tumor markers used for detecting cholangiocarcinoma in patients with primary sclerosing cholangitis. *J Hepatol* 1999;30:669–673.

Hytiroglou P, Thiese ND. Differential diagnosis of hepatocellular nodular lesions. *Semin Diagn Pathol* 1998;15:285–299.

Idilman R, Domkmeci A, Beyler AR, et al. Successful medical treatment of an epithelioid hemangioendothelioma of the liver. *Oncology* 1997;54:171–175.

Karak PK, Karak AK, Singh SP, et al. Biliary cystadenoma mistaken as hydatid cysts. *Trop Gastroenterol* 1993;14:109–113.

Kim KH, Kim CD, Lee HS, et al. Biliary papillary hyperplasia with clonorchiasis resembling cholangiocarcinoma. *Am J Gastroenterol* 1999;94:514–417.

Kim YB, Suh JS, Park TR, et al. A case of huge solitary angiomyolipoma of the liver. *Korean J Intern Med* 1995;10:73–77.

Lauffer JM, Zimmermann A, Krahenbuhl L, et al. Epithelioid hemangioendothelioma of the liver. A rare hepatic tumor. *Cancer* 1996;78:2318–2327.

Loh A, Kamar S, Dickson GH. Solitary benign papilloma (papillary adenoma) of the cystic duct: a rare cause of biliary colic. *Br J Clin Pract* 1994;48:167–168.

Longeville JH, de la Hall P, Dolan P, et al. Treatment of a giant hemangioma of the liver with Kasabach-Merritt syndrome by orthotopic liver transplant: a case report. *HPB Surg* 1997;10:159–162.

Looser C, Stain SC, Baer HU, et al. Staging of hilar cholangiocarcinoma by ultrasound and duplex sonography: a comparison with angiography and operative findings. *Br J Radiol* 1992;65:871–877.

Makhlouf HR, Ishak KG, Goodman ZD. Epithelioid hemangioendothelioma of the liver: a clinicopathologic study of 137 cases. *Cancer* 1999;85:562–582.

Nadig DE, Wade TP, Fairchild RB, et al. Major hepatic resection. Indications and results in a national hospital system from 1988 to 1992. *Arch Surg* 1997;132:115–119.

Nagorney DM. Benign hepatic tumors: focal nodular hyperplasia and hepatocellular adenoma. *World J Surg* 1995;19:13–18.

Nakajima T, Sugano I, Matsuzaki O, et al. Biliary cystadenocarcinoma of the liver. A clinicopathologic and histochemical evaluation of nine cases. *Cancer* 1992;69:2426–2432.

Ojanguren I, Ariza A, Casterlla EM, et al. P53 immunoreactivity in hepatocellular adenoma, focal nodular hyperplasia, cirrhosis and hepatocellular carcinoma. *Histopathology* 1995;26:63–68.

Ona FV, Dtytoc JN. *Clonorchis*-associated cholangiocarcinoma: a report of two cases with unusual manifestations. *Gastroenterology* 1991;101:831–839.

Paradis V, Laurent A, Flejou JF, et al. Evidence for the polyclonal nature of focal nodular hyperplasia of the liver by the study of X-chromosome inactivation. *Hepatology* 1997;26:891–895.

Paulson EK, McClellan JS, Washington K, et al. Hepatic adenoma: MR characteristics and correlation with pathologic findings. *AJR Am J Roentgenol* 1994;163:113–116.

Pazdur R, Royce ME, Rodriguez GI, et al. Phase II trial of docetaxel for cholangiocarcinoma. *Am J Clin Oncol* 1999;22:78–81.

Peterson MS, Murakami T, Baron RL. MR imaging patterns of gadolinium retention within liver neoplasms. *Abdom Imaging* 19988;23:592–599.

Ribeiro A, Burgart LJ, Nagorney DM, et al. Management of liver adenomatosis: results with a conservative surgical approach. *Liver Transpl Surg* 1998;4:388–398.

Rosh JR, Collins J, Groisman GM, et al. Management of hepatic adenoma in glycogen storage disease Ia. *J Pediatr Gastroenterol Nutr* 1995;20:225–228.

Ruszniewski P, Rougier P, Roche A, et al. Hepatic arterial chemoembolization in patients with liver metastases of endocrine tumors. A prospective phase II study in 24 patients. *Cancer* 1993;71:2624–2630.

Sakamoto M, Hirohashi S. Natural history and prognosis of adenomatous hyperplasia and early hepatocellular carcinoma: multi-institutional analysis of 53 nodules followed up for more than 6 months and 141 patients with single early hepatocellular carcinoma treated by surgical resection or percutaneous ethanol injection. *Jpn J Clin Oncol* 1998;28:604–608.

Samuel M, Spitz L. Infantile hepatic hemangioendothelioma: the role of surgery. *J Pediatr Surg* 1995;30:1425–1429.

Shirkhoda A, Farah MC, Bernacki E, et al. Hepatic focal nodular hyperplasia: CT and sonographic spectrum. *Abdom Imaging* 1994;19:34–38.

Shortell CK, Schwartz SI. Hepatic adenoma and focal nodular hyperplasia. *Surg Gynecol Obstet* 1991;173:426–431.

Thomas JA, Scriven MW, Puntis MC, et al. Elevated serum CA 19-9 levels in hepatobiliary cystadenoma with mesenchymal stroma. Two case reports with immunohistochemical confirmation. *Cancer* 1992;70:1841–1846.

Urego M, Flickinger JC, Carr BI. Radiotherapy and multimodality management of cholangiocarcinoma. *Int J Radiat Oncol Biol Phys* 1999;44:121–126.

Van Thiel DH, Carr B, Iwatsuki S, et al. The 11-year Pittsburgh experience with liver transplantation for hepatocellular carcinoma. *J Surg Oncol Suppl* 1993;3:78–82.

Yun EJ, Choi BI, Han JK, et al. Hepatic hemangioma: contrast-enhancement pattern during the arterial and portal venous phases of spiral CT. *Abdom Imaging* 1999;24:262–266.

SURGERY: SCIENTIFIC PRINCIPLES AND PRACTICE, Third Edition, edited by
Lazar J. Greenfield, Michael W. Mulholland, Keith T. Oldham, Gerald B. Zelenock,
and Keith D. Lillemoe. Lippincott Williams & Wilkins Publishers, Philadelphia, © 2001.

CHAPTER 39

BILIARY ANATOMY AND PHYSIOLOGY

MARY T. HAWN

EMBRYOLOGY

The biliary system begins to develop during the fifth gestational week as a ventral diverticulum of the primitive gastrointestinal tract (1). This ventral bud divides into a cranial portion, which gives rise to the liver and intrahepatic ducts, and a caudal portion, which develops into the gallbladder and cystic duct (Fig. 39.1). A third, more caudal bud develops into the ventral pancreas. The common bile duct is formed from the base of the diverticulum. The ventral pancreas rotates 180 degrees to form the uncinate process and posterior aspect of the pancreatic head. In this process, the distal common bile duct is brought to a position posterior to the duodenum and transverses the pancreas before opening into the medial wall of the duodenum.

ANATOMY

Gallbladder

The gallbladder resides on the inferior surface of the liver between the right and left lobes (2). It is attached to the liver bed by loose connective tissue containing lymphatics, veins, and occasionally small accessory bile ducts, the so-called ducts of Luschka. The free surface of the gallbladder is covered by peritoneum. The gallbladder wall is composed of four layers: mucosa, muscularis, perimuscular subserosal connective tissue, and serosa. The gallbladder is anatomically divided into four parts: fundus, body, infundibulum, and neck (Fig. 39.2).

The fundus is the rounded blind end of the gallbladder and extends beyond the liver bed. The fundus can often be palpated when the gallbladder becomes dilated during a pathologic process, such as acute cholecystitis or malignant obstruction of the bile duct. The body is the largest part of the gallbladder. Where the body tapers to form the neck, an outpouching is often found on the inferior and lateral aspect of the gallbladder, referred to as the infundibulum or Hartmann's pouch. The neck of the gallbladder has an S-shaped course and terminates in the cystic duct. The infundibulum and neck are covered by a peritoneal reflection from the free edge of the hepatoduodenal ligament (3).

The cystic duct, which is 1 to 4 mm in diameter and 0.5 to 4.0 cm in length, joins the common hepatic duct to form the common bile duct. The cystic duct usually joins the common hepatic duct at an acute angle 2 to 4 cm distal to the confluence of the right and left hepatic ducts, but it may run parallel to the common hepatic duct and enter it anywhere along its course to the duodenum. Rarely, it enters directly into the right hepatic duct (4) (Fig. 39.3). The cystic duct contains the valves of Heister, which are folds of mucosa that project into its lumen and occasionally make it difficult to insert a catheter during cholangiography.

Arterial blood reaches the gallbladder via the cystic artery, which originates from the right hepatic artery. The course of the cystic artery is normally posterior to the common hepatic duct, superior to the cystic duct and enters the hepatocystic triangle created by the cystic duct, common hepatic duct, and inferior edge of the right lobe of the liver (5). Other important structures that sometimes pass through this area are a replaced right hepatic artery and accessory bile ducts, so that it is essential to define structures clearly before ligating them. Several known variations in the origin and course of the cystic artery are illustrated in Fig. 39.4. The venous drainage of the gallbladder is via multiple small channels that drain either directly into the liver bed or the common bile duct plexus. The lymphatic drainage parallels the venous drainage. The gallbladder receives both sympathetic and parasympathetic innervation. The sympathetic innervation is from the celiac plexus, and afferent fibers mediate visceral pain signals. The parasympathetic fibers originate from the anterior and posterior branches of the vagus nerve and may play a minor role in gallbladder contractility.

Common Bile Duct

The cystic and common hepatic ducts join to form the common bile duct. The common bile duct is approximately 8 to 10 cm in length and 0.4 to 0.8 cm in diameter, and it can be divided into three anatomic segments: supraduodenal, retroduodenal, and intrapancreatic (Fig. 39.5). The supraduodenal segment resides in the hepatoduodenal ligament lateral to the hepatic artery and anterior to the portal vein (Fig. 39.6). The highly variable anatomy of the hepatic artery leads to many common variations in the relationship of these two structures and should be familiar to all surgeons operating in this area (Fig. 39.7). Only 55% of people have the standard anatomy (4). The course of the retroduodenal segment is posterior to the first portion of the duodenum, anterior to

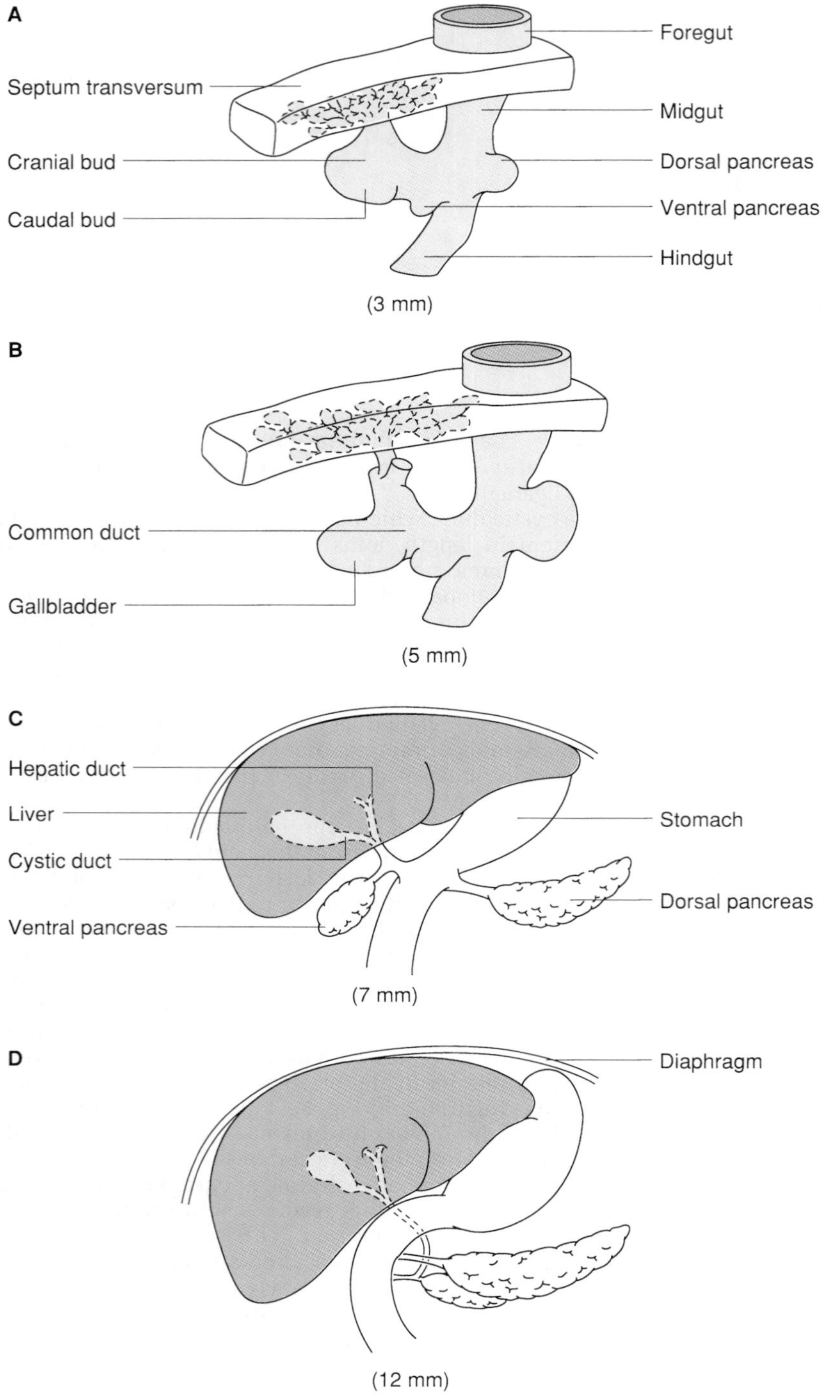

A

Septum transversum

Cranial bud

Caudal bud

Foregut

Midgut

Dorsal pancreas

Ventral pancreas

Hindgut

(3 mm)

B

Common duct

Gallbladder

(5 mm)

C

Hepatic duct

Liver

Cystic duct

Ventral pancreas

Stomach

Dorsal pancreas

(7 mm)

D

Diaphragm

(12 mm)

Figure 39.1. Sequence of steps in the embryonic development of the biliary tract.

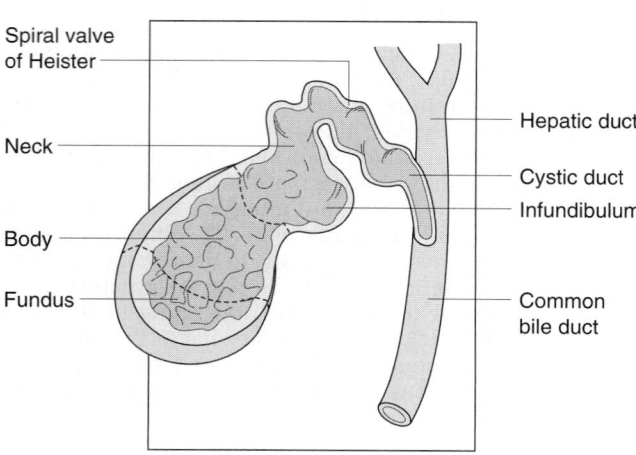

Spiral valve
of Heister

Neck

Body

Fundus

Hepatic duct

Cystic duct

Infundibulum

Common
bile duct

Figure 39.2. Cross section of the gallbladder and cystic duct.

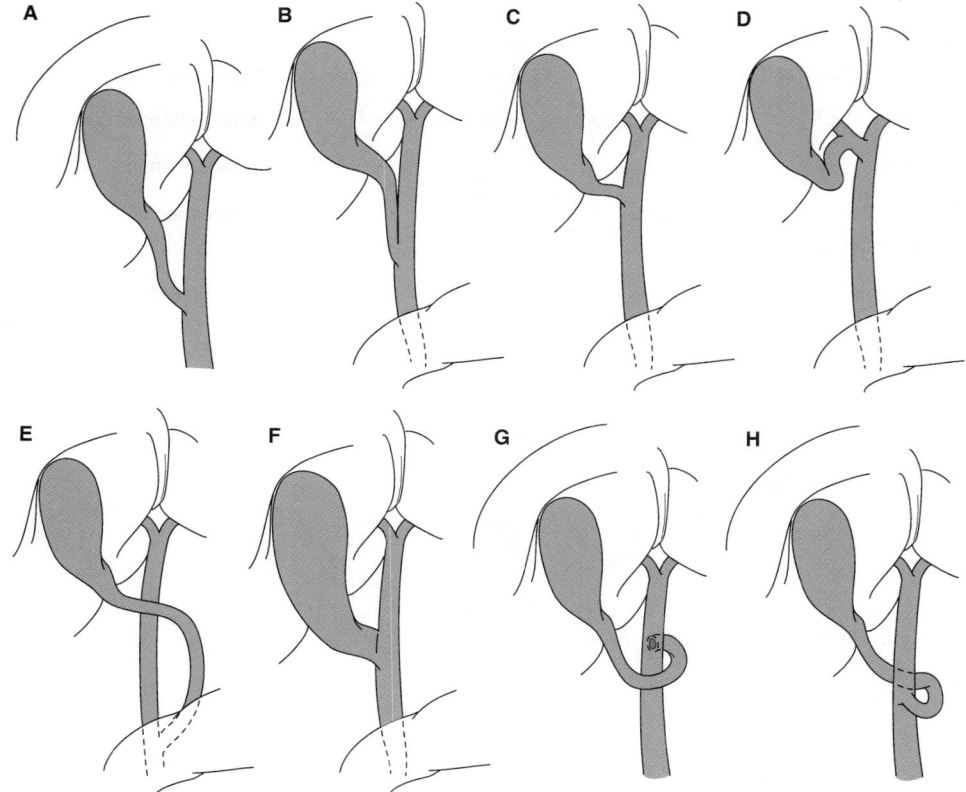

Figure 39.3. Variations in the junction of the cystic duct and common hepatic duct.

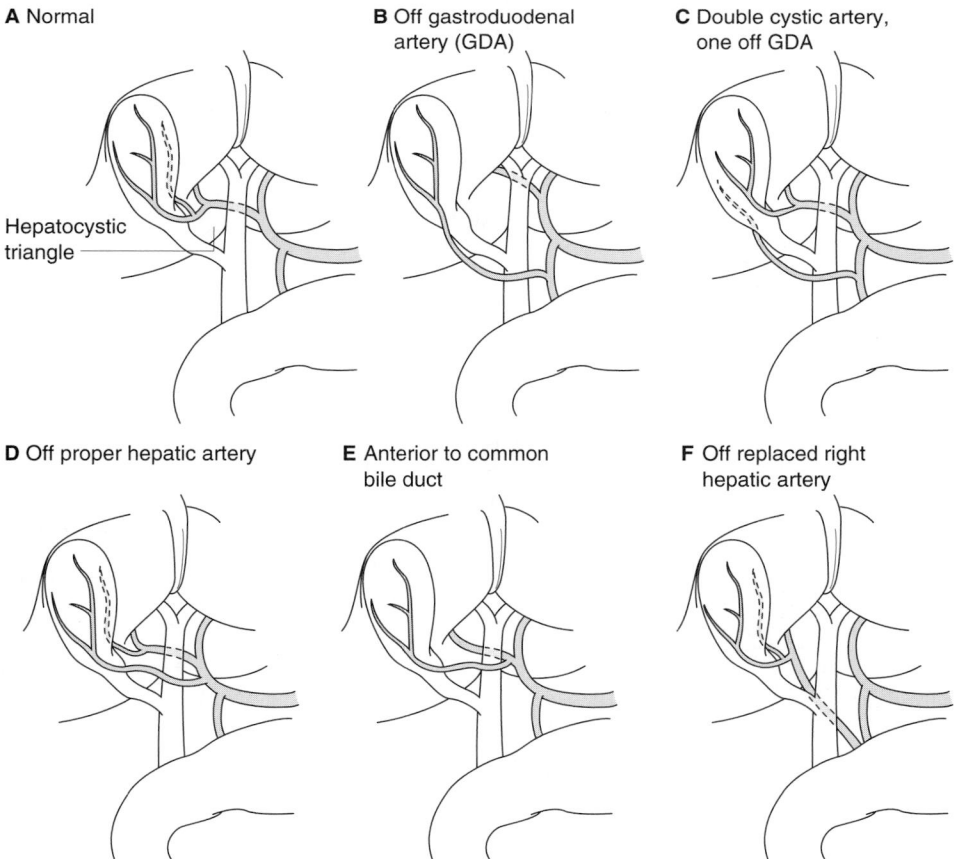

Figure 39.4. Variations in the origin and course of the cystic artery.

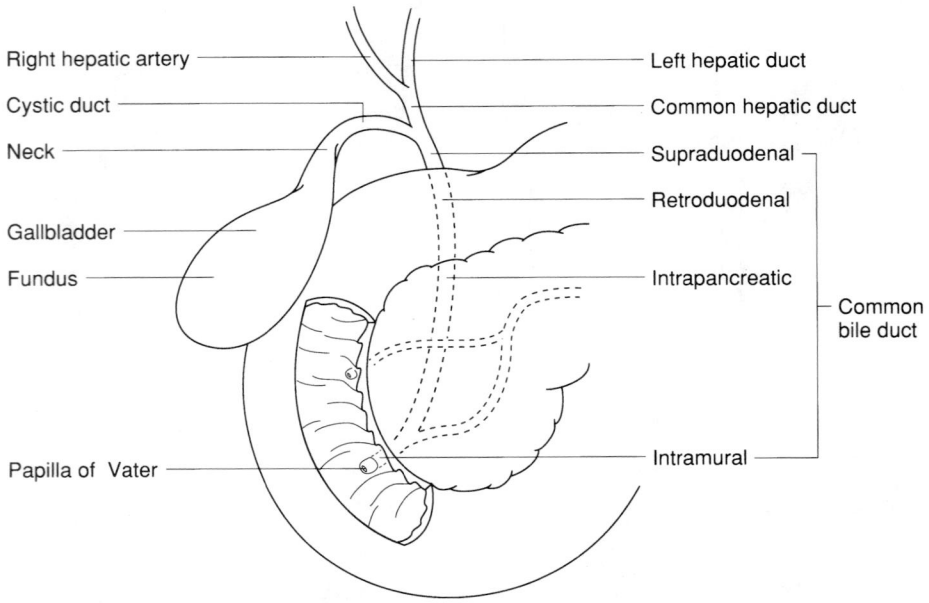

Figure 39.5. Anatomic divisions of the common bile duct.

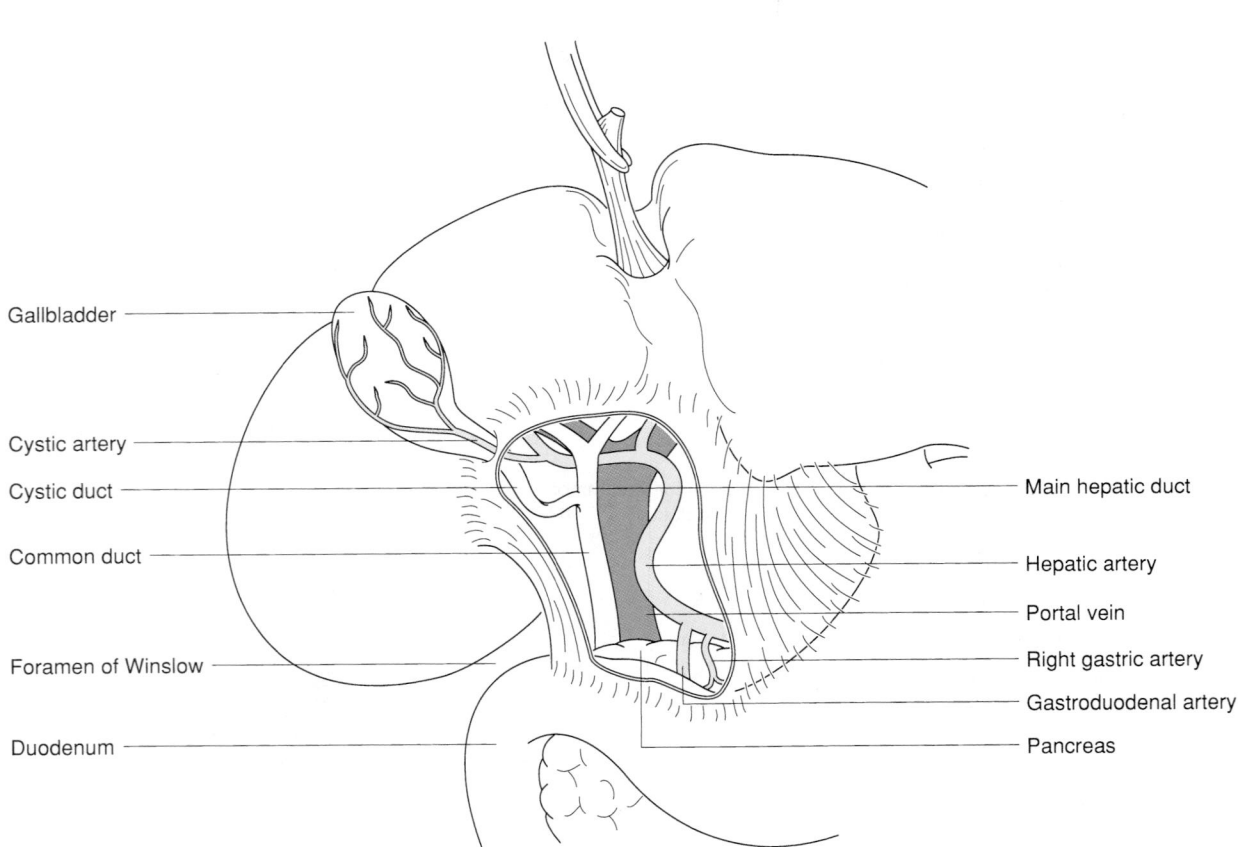

Figure 39.6. Relationship of structures within the hepatoduodenal ligament.

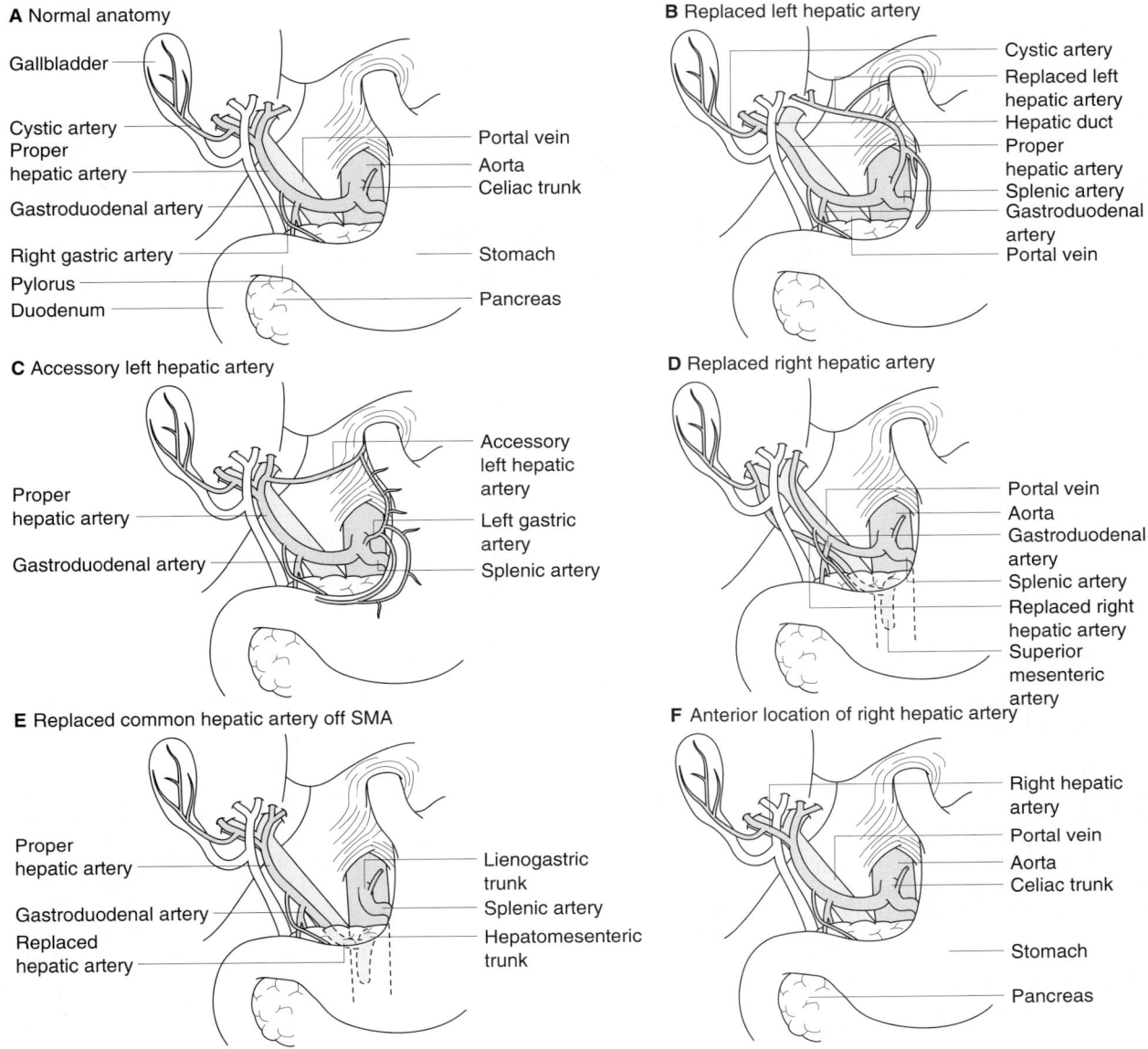

Figure 39.7. Variations in the origin and course of the hepatic artery and its relationship to the bile ducts.

the inferior vena cava, and lateral to the portal vein. The pancreatic portion of the duct lies within a tunnel or groove on the posterior aspect of the pancreas; it then enters the medial wall of the duodenum, courses tangentially through the submucosal layer for 1 to 2 cm, and terminates in the major papilla in the second portion of the duodenum (Fig. 39.8). The distal portion of the duct is encircled by smooth muscle that forms the sphincter of Oddi. The common bile duct may enter the duodenum directly (25%) or join the pancreatic duct (75%) to form a common channel, termed the ampulla of Vater.

The blood supply of the common bile duct is segmental in nature and consists of branches from the cystic artery, hepatic artery, and gastroduodenal arteries. These meet to form collateral vessels that run in the 3- and 9-o'clock positions relative to the common bile duct. The venous and lymphatic drainage forms a plexus on the anterior surface of the common bile duct. The venous drainage enters the portal system, and the lymphatic drainage follows the course of the hepatic artery to the celiac nodes.

PHYSIOLOGY

Bile Composition

Bile is composed of an isoosmotic solution of water, inorganic electrolytes, and organic solutes (Table 39.1). The principal organic components are bile acids. Bile is formed at the canalicular membrane of the hepatocyte and the bile ducts. Three fourths of bile is secreted at the canalicular membrane and is divided equally into bile acid-dependent and bile acid-independent components. Cholic acid and chenodeoxycholic acid are synthesized from cholesterol in the liver. Deoxycholic, lithocholic, and ursodeoxycholic

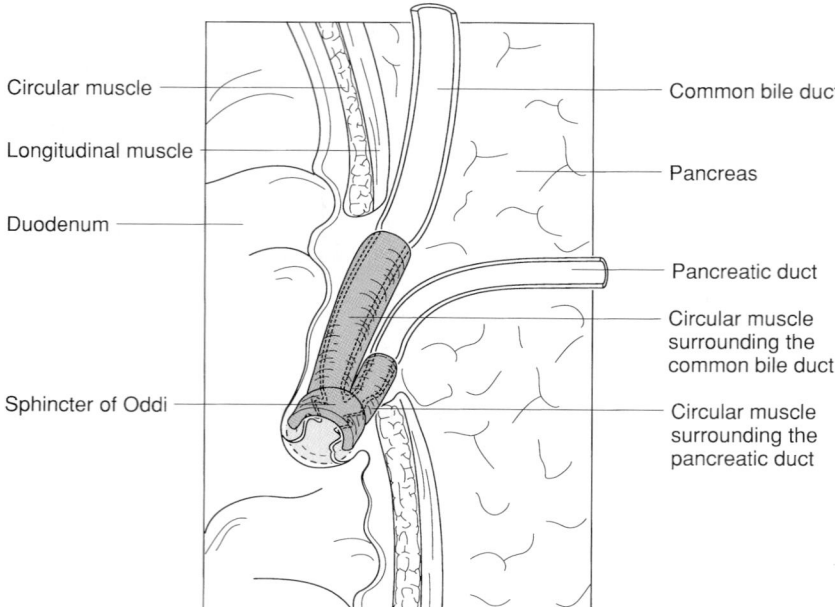

Figure 39.8. Terminal course of the common bile duct and sphincter of Oddi.

acids are produced during enzymatic modification of the bile acids by intestinal bacteria and returned to the liver by the portal vein. Bile acids are transported into the hepatocyte at the sinusoidal surface by Na^+-coupled and Na^+-independent carrier mediated mechanisms (6). Primary and secondary bile acids undergo conjugation with glycine and taurine in the liver, which renders them more efficient in facilitating fat digestion and absorption. Bile acids are then actively transported into bile at the canalicular membrane of the hepatocyte. Cholesterol and lecithin are secreted into bile at a rate proportional to bile acid secretion. Protein accounts for a small percentage of the organic solutes and is secreted in a bile acid-independent fashion. The hepatocyte also contributes electrolytes and water to the composition of bile. Bile duct secretion of electrolytes and water accounts for the remaining 25% of bile produced in the fasting state (6). The choleretic response to secretin and vasoactive intestinal peptide occurs at the level of bile duct epithelium (7–9). Secretin stimulation results in opening of the chloride channel and activation of the Cl^-/HCO_3^- exchanger.

Table 39.1. COMPOSITION OF HEPATIC BILE

Component	Concentration
Inorganic electrolytes	
Na^+	140–165 mEq/L
K^+	3.8–5.8 mEq/L
Cl^-	93–123 mEq/L
HCO_3^-	15–55 mEq/L
Ca^{2+}	1.4–5.0 mEq/L
Mg^{2+}	1.5–3.0 mEq/L
Organic solutes	
Bile acids	5–50 mmol/L
Bilirubin	50–170 mg/dL
Cholesterol	100–340 mg/dL
Lecithin	150–800 mg/dL
Proteins	25–500 mg/dL

Regulation of Bile Flow

The gallbladder performs the following functions: storage and concentration of bile in the interdigestive state, expulsion of bile in response to cholecystokinin (CCK), and moderation of hydrostatic pressure within the biliary system. The normal adult secretes 250 to 1,000 mL of bile per day. Bile is secreted continuously and is diverted into the gallbladder, depending on resistance in the bile duct secondary to sphincter of Oddi (SO) function. Normal pressure in the common bile duct is approximately 12 mm Hg, and the average in the SO is 12 to 15 mm Hg. SO activity correlates with duodenal activity during the interdigestive period but is independent of duodenal smooth-muscle contraction (10). In phase 1 and early phase 2 of the migrating motility complex, tonic contraction of the SO results in a mean pressure gradient between the duodenal lumen and SO of 10 mm Hg (11). This resistance to flow combined with active relaxation of the gallbladder leads to accumulation of bile within the gallbladder. During late phase 2 and phase 3, active contractions of the SO take place, with amplitudes measuring 100 to 120 mm Hg (12). The gallbladder reaches its maximal intraluminal pressure of 16 mm Hg at the end of phase 2 and also exhibits contractile activity during phases 2 and 3 (13). Bile is intermittently released into the duodenum during this phase. Gallbladder filling is not completely dependent on SO function, as demonstrated by the observation that gallbladder filling still occurs in patients who have undergone sphincterotomy, most likely secondary to resistance to bile flow as a result of duodenal contractions (13).

Gallbladder and SO motility are under hormonal and neural control. CCK is a peptide hormone released from I cells of the small intestine in response to intraluminal acid, fat, and amino acids. Several isoforms of the peptide (CCK-8, CCK-33, CCK-39, CCK-58) exist (14). The eight amino acids at the C-terminus are necessary and sufficient for its CCK-like activity. Pancreatic hormones, primarily trypsin, and the presence of bile in the duodenum inhibit the release of CCK. CCK mediates gallbladder contraction in a dose-dependent fashion via direct interaction with re-

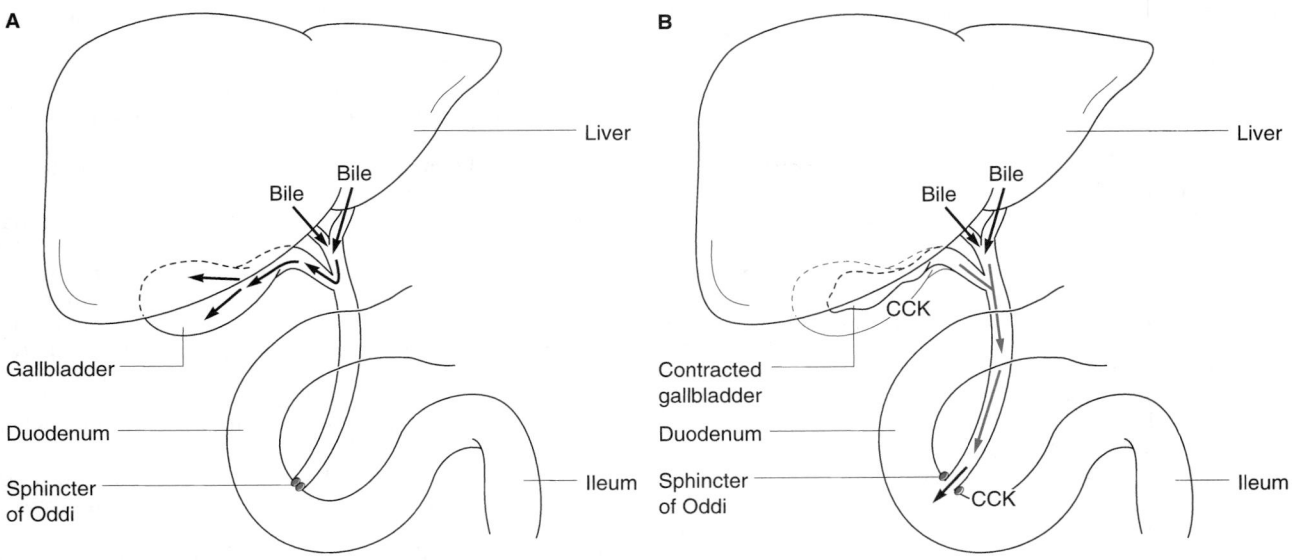

Figure 39.9. Effect of cholecystokinin on the gallbladder, sphincter of Oddi, and bile flow.

ceptors in gallbladder smooth muscle (15). Approximately 50% to 70% of bile is ejected from the gallbladder in response to CCK. CCK also causes a simultaneous decrease in the basal pressure and phasic activity of SO (16) (Fig. 39.9).

Vagal stimulation does not mediate gallbladder motility, but it does lower the threshold for CCK activity. Secretin is also released in response to a meal and potentiates the effect of CCK, although it has no intrinsic effect on gallbladder motility (17). Pancreatic polypeptide (PP) is released following a meal or CCK infusion and remains mea-surable in the serum for 6 hours. PP causes gallbladder relaxation and may facilitate gallbladder filling during the interdigestive phase (18). Similarly, peptide YY is released from the distal small intestine and colon and also causes gallbladder relaxation. Vasoactive intestinal polypeptide (VIP) and somatostatin inhibit CCK-mediated gallbladder contraction (19). Morphine is a potent stimulator of SO activity and can completely block bile flow into the duodenum (20). Gallbladder distention independent of common bile duct hypertension mediates SO inhibition by an undefined mechanism (21).

Motilin, a gastrointestinal polypeptide, has also been shown to mediate gallbladder contraction and may regulate activity during the interdigestive state. Gallbladder contractions that occur spontaneously during phase 3 of the migrating motility complex are associated with peaks in endogenous motilin levels. Erythromycin, a motilin agonist, produces gallbladder contraction independently of CCK. Blocking the CCK receptor with the specific antagonist loxiglumide has no effect on erythromycin-induced contractions, whereas atropine can abrogate the effect (22). Therefore, the effects of motilin appear to be mediated via cholinergic mechanisms.

The gallbladder capacity is 35 to 50 mL. Bile is rapidly concentrated by the gallbladder via Na^+ coupled Cl^- transport and the passive diffusion of water (23). Approximately 90% of water is absorbed by the gallbladder mucosa within four hours. The relative concentration of bile components during storage in the gallbladder is shown in Fig. 39.10. The regulation of absorption is under neurohormonal control. VIP released from adrenergic neurons inhibits net fluid absorption and leads to bile duct secretion (24). This process can be blocked by inhibiting α-adrenergic ganglionic release of VIP or by infusing somatostatin (25,26). Alterations in gallbladder absorption and motility have been implicated in stone formation.

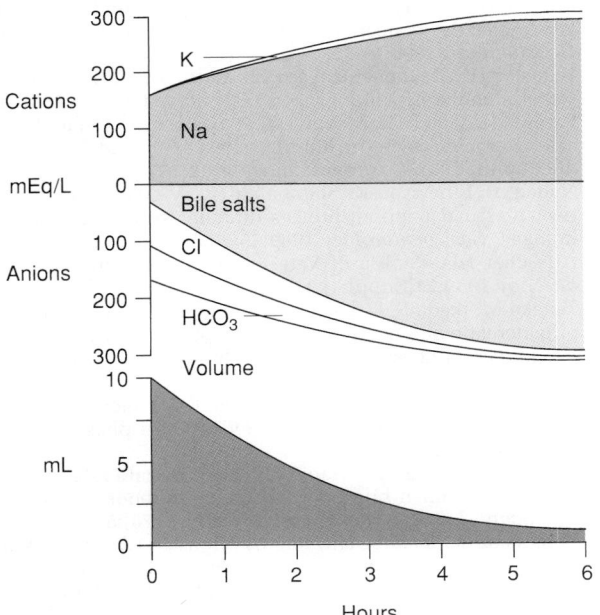

Figure 39.10. Relative changes in gallbladder bile composition (top) and volume (bottom) during the fasting state.

DYSMOTILITY SYNDROMES

Defining the mechanisms that regulate gallbladder and SO motility has led to an investigation of these patterns as the cause of disease processes. Patients who have biliary pain in the absence of gallstones or after cholecystectomy often undergo a myriad of diagnostic tests, most of which yield inconclusive results and leave patients frustrated.

Gallbladder Dyskinesia

Approximately 5% of patients who present with classic biliary colic do not have gallstones on imaging studies. Diagnostic evaluation of these patients has led to an identifiable subset with chronic acalculous cholecystitis who may benefit from cholecystectomy. Provocative CCK infusion may reproduce symptoms, and cholecystectomy in these patients results in long-term pain relief (27). CCK-hepatobiliary iminodiacetic acid (HIDA) is a quantitative test that evaluates the gallbladder ejection fraction in response to CCK infusion. The normal ejection fraction in response to CCK is 75%. In one series, patients with biliary symptoms in the absence of gallstones and an ejection fraction of less than 40% (3 standard deviations below the mean) achieved excellent relief of symptoms following cholecystectomy (28).

Sphincter of Oddi Dysfunction

Dysfunction of the SO is thought to be responsible for 1% to 10% of biliary symptoms that persist after cholecystectomy. Two distinct clinical entities exist: papillary stenosis and SO dyskinesia. Both disorders have a vague presentation and are often diagnoses of exclusion. They primarily affect middle-aged women and typically present with abdominal pain. The pain is usually postprandial, sharp, and located in the epigastrium or right upper quadrant. The pain may radiate to the shoulder or back and be associated with nausea or vomiting, but rarely with fever or jaundice. Laboratory analysis may show transient elevations of serum liver enzymes, especially in association with symptoms. Amylase and lipase may also be transiently elevated.

No classic radiographic findings are associated with SO dysfunction. The most useful diagnostic tool is endoscopic retrograde cholangiopancreatography (ERCP) with biliary manometry. ERCP may show a dilated common bile duct or delayed emptying of contrast from the common bile duct to the duodenum (>45 minutes). These findings are more likely to be associated with papillary stenosis. A triple-lumen catheter with recording channels 2 mm apart and the most distal orifice 5 mm from the catheter tip is used to perform biliary manometry. Duodenal pressures are measured and then the catheter is inserted into the distal common bile duct. Pull-back pressures are measured every 2 mm for the common bile duct and the SO. The mean basal pressure is calculated from an average of the maximal basal pressures recorded from all three catheter channels. A mean basal pressure that is 40 mm Hg above intraduodenal pressure is considered abnormal (29). Elevation in basal SO pressure has been observed in some patients with SO dysfunction. CCK or glucagon may decrease SO pressure, and a lack of response to these agents is more indicative of papillary stenosis.

Several noninvasive tests for SO dysfunction are available and may help delineate patients with SO dysfunction. Secretin ultrasonography measures a change in the caliber of the pancreatic duct in response to intravenous secretin. An increase in diameter of 1 to 2 mm is suggestive of SO dysfunction (30). Similarly, fatty meal ultrasonography measures changes in the caliber of the common bile duct in response to the administration of Lipomul. An increase of 2 mm or more is indicative of SO dysfunction but can also occur with partial bile duct obstruction (31). Quantitative hepatobiliary scintigraphy measures isotope distrib-

ution in the liver, bile duct, and intestine. A delay in isotope clearance is consistent with SO dysfunction or partial bile duct obstruction. Further modifications of this study with the use of morphine sulfate or CCK to provoke sphincter spasm or enhance relaxation have been reported to increase its diagnostic efficacy.

Spasmolytic therapy is the first line of treatment for suspected SO dysfunction. Sublingual nitroglycerin and nifedipine have both been reported to relieve biliary symptoms after cholecystectomy. Bile acid substitutes and pancreatic enzyme replacement therapy, when administered continuously, have also been reported to relieve symptoms (32). However, no long-term series have documented the effects of medical therapy for SO dysfunction.

Endoscopic sphincterotomy and surgical transduodenal sphincteroplasty and septectomy have been reported to relieve symptoms in 50% to 80% of carefully selected patients with pain after cholecystectomy. When performed in patients with elevated basal SO pressures, endoscopic sphincterotomy has been shown to relieve symptoms in 50% to 75% of patients during long-term follow-up (33). Transduodenal sphincteroplasty with transampullary septectomy has yielded similar encouraging results in patients with persistent biliary pain after cholecystectomy (34). This procedure underscores the importance of pancreatic ductal hypertension as a contributor to the symptom complex in such patients.

REFERENCES

1. Moore KL, Persaud TVN. *The developing human: clinically oriented embryology*, 6th ed. Philadelphia: WB Saunders, 1998:218.
2. Clemente CD. *Gray's anatomy*, 13th ed. Philadelphia: Lea & Febinger, 1985:132.
3. Crist DW, Gadacz TR. Laparoscopic anatomy of the biliary tree. *Surg Clin North Am* 1993;73:785.
4. Benson EA, Page RE. A practical reappraisal of the anatomy of the extrahepatic bile ducts and arteries. *NBr J Surg* 1976;63:854.
5. Rocko JM, Swan KG, DiGioia JM. Calot's triangle revisited. *Surg Gynecol Obstet* 1981;153:410.
6. Boyer JL. Bile secretion—models, mechanism, and malfunctions: a perspective on the development of modern cellular and molecular concepts of bile secretion and cholestasis. *J Gastroenterol* 1996;1:475.
7. Wheeler HO, Mancusi-Ungaro PL. Role of bile ducts during secretin choleresis in dogs. *Am J Physiol* 1966;210:1153.
8. Farouk M, Vigna SR, McVey DC, et al. Localization and characterization of secretin binding sites expressed by rat bile duct epithelium. *Gastroenterology* 1992;102:963.
9. Nyberg B, Einarsson K, Sonnenfeld T. Evidence that vasoactive intestinal peptide induces ductular secretion of bile in humans. *Gastroenterology* 1989;96:920.
10. Allescher HD. Papilla of Vater: structure and function. *Endoscopy* 1989;21[Suppl 1]:324.
11. Tanaka M, Ikeda S, Nakayama F. Nonoperative measurement of pancreatic and common bile duct pressures with a microtransducer catheter and effects of duodenoscopic sphincterotomy. *Dig Dis Sci* 1981;26:545.
12. Torsoli A, Corazziari E, Habib FI, et al. Frequencies and cyclical pattern of the human sphincter of Oddi phasic activity. *Gut* 1986;27:363.
13. Torsoli A, Corazziari E, Habib FI, et al. Pressure relationships within the human bile tract: normal and abnormal physiology. *Scand J Gastroenterol* 1990;25[Suppl 175]:52.
14. Thompson JC, Fender HR, Ramus NI, et al. Cholecystokinin metabolism in man and dogs. *Ann Surg* 1975;182:496.
15. Steigerwalt RW, Goldfine JD, Williams JA. Characterization of cholecystokinin receptors on bovine gallbladder membranes. *Am J Physiol* 1984;247:709.
16. Toouli J, Hogan WJ, Geenen JE, et al. Action of cholecystokinin octapeptide on sphincter of Oddi basal pressure and phasic activity in humans. *Surgery* 1982;92:497.

17. Ryan J, Cohen S. Interaction of gastrin I, secretin, cholecystokinin on gallbladder smooth muscle in vitro. *Am J Physiol* 1976;230:533.

18. Conter R, Roslyn JJ, Muller El, et al. Effect of pancreatic polypeptide on gallbladder filling. *J Surg Res* 1985;38:461.

19. Strah KM, Melendez RL, Pappas TN, et al. Interactions of vasoactive intestinal polypeptide and cholecystokinin octapeptide on the control of gallbladder contraction. *Surgery* 1986; 99:469.

20. Pedersen SA, Oster-Jorgensen E, Kraglund K. The effects of morphine on biliary dynamics: a scintigraphic study with (99m)Tc-HIDA. *Scand J Gastroenterol* 1987;22:982.

21. Thune A, Saccone GTP, Scicchitano JP, et al. Distention of the gallbladder inhibits sphincter of Oddi motility in man. *Gut* 1991;32:690.

22. Jebbink MC, Masclee AA, van der Kleij GC, et al. Effect of loxiglumide and atropine on erythromycin-induced reduction in gallbladder volume in human subjects. *Hepatology* 1992;16: 937.

23. Rose RC. Absorptive functions of the gallbladder. In: Johnson LR, ed. *Physiology of the gastrointestinal tract*, 2nd ed. New York: Raven Press, 1987.

24. Sundler F, Alumets J, Hakanson R, et al. VIP innervation of the gallbladder. *Gastroenterology* 1977;72:1375.

25. O'Grady SM, Wolters PJ, Hildebrand K, et al. Regulation of ion transport in porcine gallbladder: effects of VIP and norepinephrine. *Am J Physiol* 1989;257:52.

26. Bjork S, Svanvik J. The influence of somatostatin on gallbladder response to intraduodenal acid and autonomic nerve stimulation in the cat. *Scand J Gastroenterol* 1984;19:173.

27. Rhoades M, Lennard TWJ, Farndon JR, et al. Cholecystokinin provocation test: long-term follow-up after cholecystectomy. *Br J Surg* 1988;75:951.

28. Yap L, Wycherley AG, Morphett AD, et al. Acalculous biliary pain: cholecystectomy alleviates symptoms in patients with abnormal cholescintigraphy. *Gastroenterology* 1991;101:786.

29. Greenen JE, Hogan WJ, Toouli J, et al. A prospective randomized study of the efficacy of endoscopic sphincterotomy for patients with presumptive sphincter of Oddi dysfunction. *Gastroenterology* 1984;86:1086.

30. Warshaw AL, Simeone J, Schapiro RH, et al. Objective evaluation of ampullary stenosis with ultrasonography and pancreatic stimulation. *Am J Surg* 1985;149:65.

31. Darweesh R, Dodds WJ, Hogan WJ, et al. Efficacy of quantitative hepatobiliary scintigraphy and fatty-meal sonography for detecting partial common bile duct obstruction. *Gastroenterology* 1987;92:1363.

32. Lasson A. The postcholecystectomy syndrome: diagnostic and therapeutic strategy. *Scand J Gastroenterol* 1987;22: 897.

33. Greenen JE, Hogan WJ, Dodds WJ, et al. The efficacy of endoscopic sphincterotomy after cholecystectomy in patients with sphincter of Oddi dysfunction. *N Engl J Med* 1989;320:82.

34. Moody FG, Becker JM, Potts JR. Transduodenal sphincteroplasty and transampullary septectomy for postcholecystectomy pain. *Ann Surg* 1983;197:627.

SURGERY: SCIENTIFIC PRINCIPLES AND PRACTICE, Third Edition, edited by Lazar J. Greenfield, Michael W. Mulholland, Keith T. Oldham, Gerald B. Zelenock, and Keith D. Lillemoe. Lippincott Williams & Wilkins Publishers, Philadelphia, © 2001.

CHAPTER 40

CALCULOUS BILIARY DISEASE

STEVEN STRASBERG AND JEFFREY DREBIN

DEDICATION

This chapter is dedicated to Joel Rosslyn, who was the author of the chapter in the previous edition of *Surgery: Scientific Principles and Practice*. Dr. Rosslyn was an outstanding surgeon and scientist, and a colleague and friend to many working in the field of gallstone disease. Readers will recognize his imprint in the current chapter.

Gallstone disease is one of the most common digestive health problems. It may develop in the gallbladder, where it is called *cholelithiasis* or *cholecystolithiasis,* or in the bile ducts, where it is called *choledocholithiasis.* Stones may exist in both sites simultaneously. *Gallstones* are solid concretions varying in size from tiny, sandlike particles to large stones several centimeters in diameter. Gallstones of different chemical compositions are formed as a result of several distinct pathologic processes. The type of gallstone may be related to some clinical factors, such as age at the onset of symptoms and site of the stone in the biliary tree, although frequently different types of stones give rise to similar symptoms. Consequently, it is useful to consider the major stone types as different diseases with clinical similarities.

The last hundred years or so have seen the introduction and advancement of rational treatments for gallstone disease. Major diagnostic, technical, and scientific advances have been made. Before the late 19th century, no reliable method of diagnosing cholelithiasis was available. Crystal analysis by percutaneous biliary drainage was the first diagnostic method and was the initial guide for patient selection. Oral cholecystography, introduced by surgical scientists Graham and Cole in 1930, greatly facilitated the ease and reliability of diagnosis, with a sensitivity of about 95%. Ultrasonography replaced oral cholecystography in the 1970s; it is even more sensitive than oral cholecystography and is well tolerated by patients. A technique for surgical removal of the gallbladder, *cholecystectomy,* was introduced by Langenbuch in 1882 on the heels of advances in general anesthesia and asepsis. Over 100 years, it evolved from a dangerous procedure with a mortality rate of 10% to an extremely safe procedure with a mortality rate of 0.1%. In 1990, it was supplanted by laparoscopic cholecystectomy, a technique that has made it possible to treat cholelithiasis on an outpatient basis. The other great technical advance was the endoscopic treatment of choledocholithiasis, which revolutionized the treatment of *cholangitis,* a severe bacterial inflammation of the biliary tract often associated with choledocholithiasis; it also eliminated the need in some cases for open surgery to treat choledocholithiasis. Finally, experimental studies in the last 30 years have led to a greatly improved, although still incomplete, understanding of the metabolic basis for stone formation. However, so much has been learned recently that scientific inquiry will in all likelihood solve the problem of stone formation in the future.

GALLSTONES AND GALLSTONE DISEASES

Types of Gallstones

Gallstones may be grouped into cholesterol and pigment (bilirubin) types, although stones are rarely composed of just one of these elements.

Cholesterol Gallstones

Cholesterol gallstones are 70% cholesterol or more. The two types of cholesterol stones are the pure cholesterol stone and the mixed cholesterol stone.

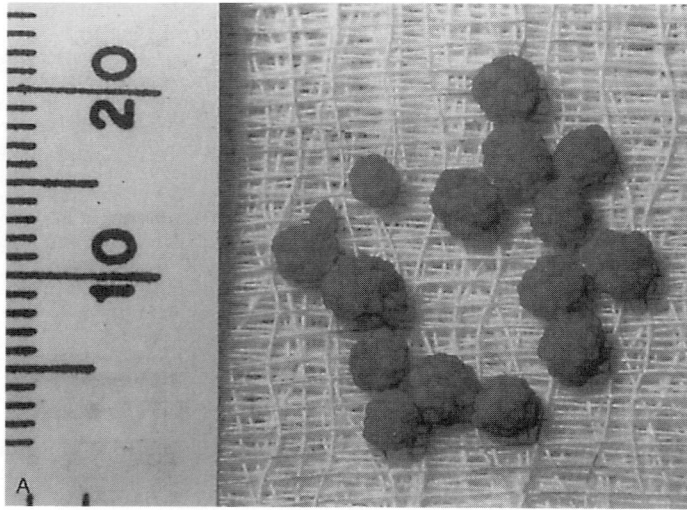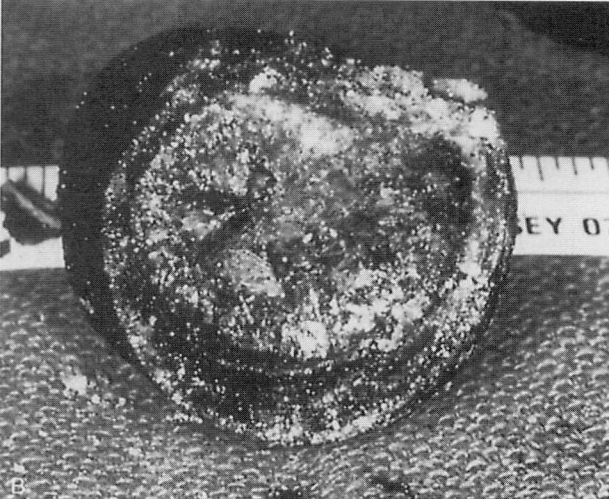

Figure 40.1. Gallstones from patients include multiple small cholesterol calculi *(A)* and a single large mixed stone *(B)*.

The pure stone is almost 100% cholesterol. It is characteristically single, ovoid or spherical in shape, and 0.5 to 4 cm in diameter (Fig. 40.1). On cut section, it has a white to slightly yellow color, with a more pigmented center, and a radiating crystalline pattern. This type of stone is often called a *cholesterol solitaire.*

The mixed cholesterol stone, usually 0.1 to 2 cm in diameter, contains variable amounts of pigment but is always more than 70% cholesterol by weight. These stones are usually multiple and may have a mulberry (bumpy spheroid) (Fig. 40.1) or faceted shape. Dark brown pigment is often found in the center of such stones and in ringlike zones, the other parts of the stones being various shades of yellow. Gallstones are porous structures, and it appears that bilirubin can precipitate inside them as a secondary event over years (1).

The primary common event in the formation of both types of cholesterol gallstone is supersaturation of bile with cholesterol. Both types of stones almost always form in the gallbladder and give rise to similar clinical problems, with some variations. Therefore, cholesterol gallstones may be considered as one disease.

Pigment Stones

Pigment stones may be black or brown. Except that both types of stones are dark, because of the presence of calcium bilirubinate, they have little in common and should be considered as two separate diseases. Both types of pigment stones contain less than 20% cholesterol. Stones containing between 20% to 70% cholesterol are rare (i.e., stones are either cholesterol or pigment types on this basis).

Black Stones. These are usually less than 1 cm in diameter, jet black, brittle, and often spiculated. They are formed by the supersaturation of calcium salts of bilirubin, carbonate, and phosphate, most often secondary to hemolysis. They almost always form in the gallbladder.

Brown Stones. These are usually small stones, less than 1 cm in diameter. They are brown or brownish yellow and are soft and often deformable or mushy. They develop secondary to bacterial contamination of the biliary tract, caused by bile stasis, and as such may form either in the bile ducts or gallbladder. They are largely composed of bacterial cell bodies and precipitated calcium bilirubinate.

Brown stones contain calcium palmitate derived from the bacterial cell wall.

Types of Gallstone Disease

In summary, the three types of gallstone disease are the following: cholesterol gallstone disease, caused by the pathologic supersaturation of bile with cholesterol, which leads to cholecystolithiasis; black stone disease, caused by pathologic supersaturation with calcium salts, especially calcium bilirubinate, which also results in the formation of stones in the gallbladder; and lastly brown stone disease, caused by stasis-induced bacterial contamination of bile, in which stones form in both the gallbladder and bile duct. Cholesterol and black stones may move from the gallbladder to the bile ducts and cause biliary stasis, so that such stones are sometimes the proximate cause of brown stones.

INCIDENCE AND RISK FACTORS

Cholesterol Gallstones

Cholesterol gallstones account for 85% of all stones in Western industrialized countries. Their prevalence increases with age. Stones are uncommon below age 25, but a sharp increase is noted with each decade to about age 70. The disease is epidemic, with about 20% of women and 10% of men having stones by age 60. Recent studies have shown that about 14 million American women and 6 million American men harbor stones (2). In certain populations, such as American Indians, the incidence is extremely high, especially in women. In Chileans and Bolivians of Indian ancestry, the incidence of gallstones is also very high and is associated with a high incidence of gallbladder cancer. In fact, gallbladder cancer is the most common gastrointestinal cancer in these countries. The prevalence of stones is higher in Mexican American women (26%) than in American white women (17%), in whom the prevalence is higher than in American black women (14%) (2). Gallstones are more common in women, especially those who have had multiple pregnancies, in persons taking birth control pills, in the obese, in persons undergoing rapid weight loss, and in some persons with hyperlipidemia. Diet plays an important role in cholesterol supersaturation. Cholesterol gallstones do not form in vegetarians. Cholesterol gallstones are common in populations consuming a Western diet, which is relatively high in animal fat. The incidence of cholesterol gallstones rises in a population as it shifts to a higher consumption of dietary fat.

Black Stones

Black stones account for 10% to 15% of stones in Western industrialized countries but for a much higher percentage of stones in Asian countries, such as Japan. Black stones are common in hemolytic disorders, such as hereditary spherocytosis and sickle cell anemia, but these disorders cause only a small percentage of black stones, the remainder being the consequence of an unknown metabolic defect. Black stones are also more common in persons with cirrhosis, those who have undergone ileal resection, or people on long-term hyperalimentation.

Brown Stones

Brown stones are uncommon in Western industrialized countries and account only for a small percentage of stones. In these countries, the bile stasis that causes brown stones to form is usually secondary to biliary strictures or to the passage of cholesterol or black stones into the bile ducts. Brown stones are more common in geographic regions, such as southeast Asia, where biliary parasites, including *Clonorchis sinensis, Opisthorchis viverrini,* and *Ascaris lumbricoides,* are endemic. In these locations, the biliary stasis induced by the worms leads to stone formation and then sometimes to repeated bouts of cholangitis—a disease called *oriental cholangiohepatitis.*

PATHOGENESIS

Bile is a complex aqueous solution produced by hepatocytes that undergoes modification as it passes through the bile ducts and while it resides in the gallbladder. The liver is capable of excreting or secreting highly insoluble lipids from the body through the bile. It does so by associating these lipids with water-soluble components that make their transport in bile possible. In the case of bilirubin, this is accomplished by conjugation with glucuronide molecules. Cholesterol is solubilized by multimolecular associations with bile salts and lecithin. Cholesterol and bilirubin are the least water-soluble common components of bile. It is not surprising, therefore, that failure of the solubilizing systems of these constituents leads to the formation of cholesterol and pigment stones.

Pathogenesis of Cholesterol Gallstones

Structure and Behavior of Biliary Lipids in Aqueous Solutions

The main biliary lipids are cholesterol, phospholipids, and bile salts. All are amphipaths—that is, they have hydrophobic (nonpolar) and hydrophilic (polar) components. They differ mainly in the strength of their polar components.

Cholesterol is a sterol obtained in the diet or synthesized, mainly in the liver. Structurally, it consists of a large sterol nucleus and a side chain, both of which are hydrophobic, and a hydrophilic hydroxyl group (Fig. 40.2). Rather than projecting from the molecule, the hydroxyl group is internalized, which reduces any beneficial effect on aqueous solubility. Thus, cholesterol is very sparingly soluble in water; its aqueous solubility is 10^{-8} M (3), and at any concentration above this very low level of aqueous solubility, cholesterol self-associates into solid cholesterol monohydrate crystals—the stuff of cholesterol gallstones.

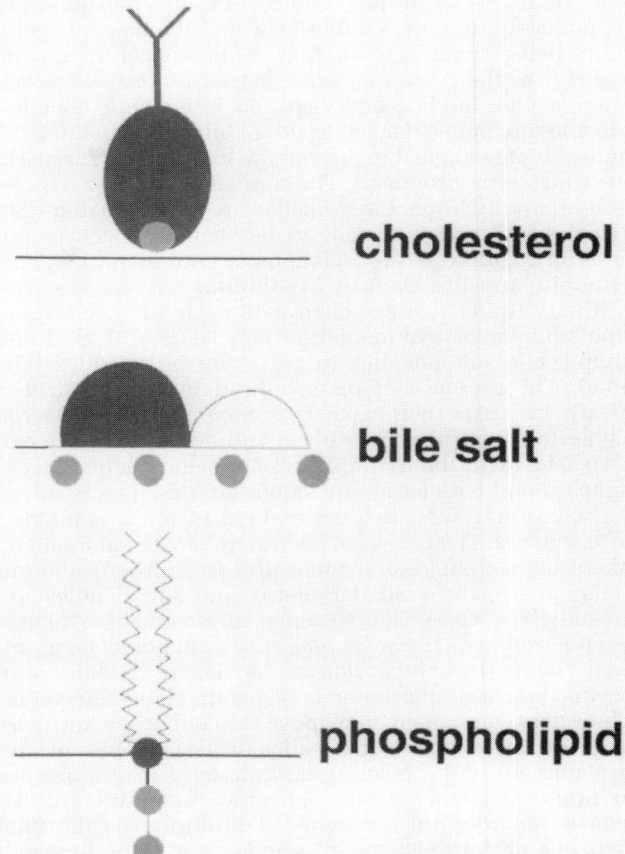

Figure 40.2. Structural representation of the major biliary lipids. Polar portions of the molecules are shown in *light shading.* Nonpolar portions are shown in *darker shading.*

Therefore, cholesterol carriers are required for cholesterol to be transported in bile at its usual concentration.

Phosphatidyl choline (lecithin) is the major phospholipid of bile. Structurally, it has glycerol backbone, to which two fatty acid chains and a choline group are linked (Fig. 40.2). The two fatty acid chains are hydrophobic, but the choline group is strongly polar. Spatially, lecithin is a linear amphipathic molecule, with a hydrophilic head and a hydrophobic body and tail (Fig. 40.2). Phospholipids predictably have a somewhat higher aqueous solubility than cholesterol. However, at relatively low concentrations, phospholipids also come out of solution in self-association. They form a molecular *bilayer* in which the hydrophobic ends of the molecules are turned in, away from the aqueous environment, and the hydrophilic ends are turned out, toward the aqueous environment. This familiar structure is the basis of cell membranes. These sheets of molecular bilayers close naturally to form hollow spheres called *vesicles.* Vesicles are visible with specialized light microscopy, such as phase-contrast microscopy, and are very easily seen by electron microscopy. Vesicles are not in solution but are a solid phase. They are highly deformable and therefore are often called *liquid crystals.*

Bile salts are synthesized from cholesterol in the liver. In the course of synthesis, hydroxyl groups are added to the sterol ring of the cholesterol molecule, and a carboxyl group to the side chain (Fig. 40.2). The spatial orientation of these polar groups, in most physiologic bile salts, is along one side of the molecule (Fig. 40.2). The bile salt molecule may therefore be thought of as a plate, one side of which is hydrophilic and the other hydrophobic. Bile salt monomers, unlike cholesterol or phospholipid monomers, are quite soluble in water, the aqueous solubility being about 10^{-3} M. Above this concentration, referred to as the *critical micellar concentration,* self-association begins, and bile salts aggregate into *simple* micelles. Micelles are molecular aggregates of bile salts in which the molecules are aligned to present the hydrophilic surface to the aqueous environment. The core of the micelle is therefore highly hydrophobic. Micelles are much smaller than vesicles and are too small to be seen by electron microscopy. Unlike self-associations of cholesterol or phospholipid, micelles are fully in solution.

Biliary lipids also associate with each other. Phospholipid and cholesterol monomers may be incorporated into simple bile salt micelles to create *mixed* micelles (Fig. 40.3). The presence of phospholipid in mixed micelles greatly increases their capacity to incorporate cholesterol. Cholesterol may also enter phospholipid vesicles, where it associates with the hydrophobic fatty acid chains. Mixed micelles and vesicles are the cholesterol carriers in bile.

Each form in which cholesterol exists in bile is referred to as a *phase.* The phases of cholesterol are the monomeric phase (single cholesterol molecules in solution), the micellar phase, the vesicular phase, and solid cholesterol crystals (Fig. 40.4). The vesicular and crystalline phases are referred to as the *solid phases,* the monomers and micelles being the *soluble phases.* Movement of cholesterol occurs between phases and is governed by energetics. Cholesterol monomers may move into either the vesicular or the micellar phase. If micelles or vesicles become supersaturated with cholesterol, cholesterol may move out to form cholesterol crystals. This process continues until a *state of equilibrium* is reached. Equilibrium is the final state of a physical–chemical system, a condition in which all acting influences are canceled by others, so that a stable, unchanging system results. The phases present at equilibrium are predicted by the *equilibrium phase diagram* (Fig. 40.5). The monomeric phase is not depicted in this diagram. By definition, a solution is *supersaturated* with respect to cholesterol when a solid phase is present at equilibrium—either vesicles, solid cholesterol monohydrate crystals, or both. Unsaturated solutions contain only monomers and micelles. The range of bile composition in humans is such that bile is either unsaturated or supersaturated, and if supersaturated, cholesterol crystals are present with or without vesicles (i.e., human bile is never supersaturated at equilibrium as a result of the presence of vesicles without cholesterol crystals).

Whether bile is supersaturated with cholesterol can be determined by measuring the concentration of the lipids in bile and plotting its *relative composition* on the phase diagram. As this is cumbersome, the information on the phase diagram has been mathematically converted to a *cholesterol saturation index* (4). If bile has a cholesterol saturation index above 1.0, it is supersaturated with cholesterol and will contain cholesterol crystals *when it reaches equilibrium.*

Bile is not in a state of equilibrium when it is secreted into the canaliculus. Therefore, such bile may be supersaturated with cholesterol yet not contain cholesterol crystals. Crystals will appear only if the bile progresses to equilibrium. Some supersaturated bile reaches equilibrium while still in the biliary tree, but in other cases, it does not. Whether cholesterol crystals form in supersaturated bile while it is still in the biliary tree depends on certain kinetic factors, to be discussed later.

Biliary Secretion and Transport of Cholesterol

Hepatic cholesterol is derived either from preformed cholesterol taken up from the serum by hepatocytes or is

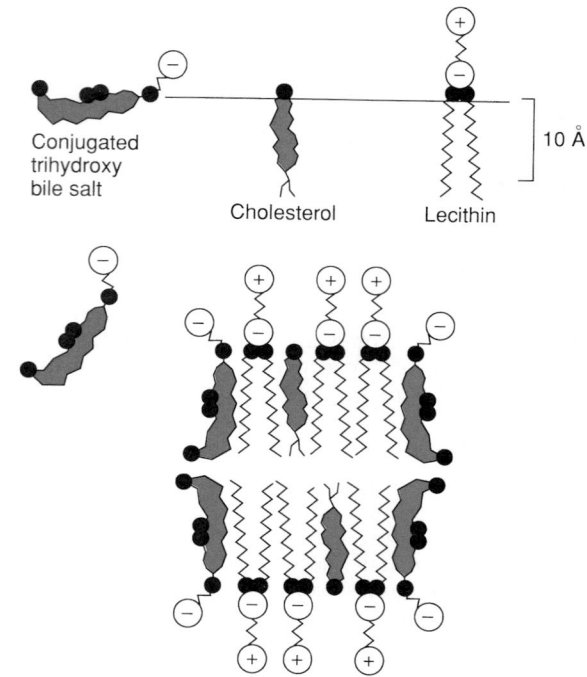

Figure 40.3. Bile acid–lecithin–cholesterol mixed micelle. The polar ends of bile acids and lecithin are oriented outward, and hydrophobic, nonpolar portions make up the interior. Cholesterol is solubilized within the hydrophobic, nonpolar center.

PHASES OF CHOLESTEROL IN BILE

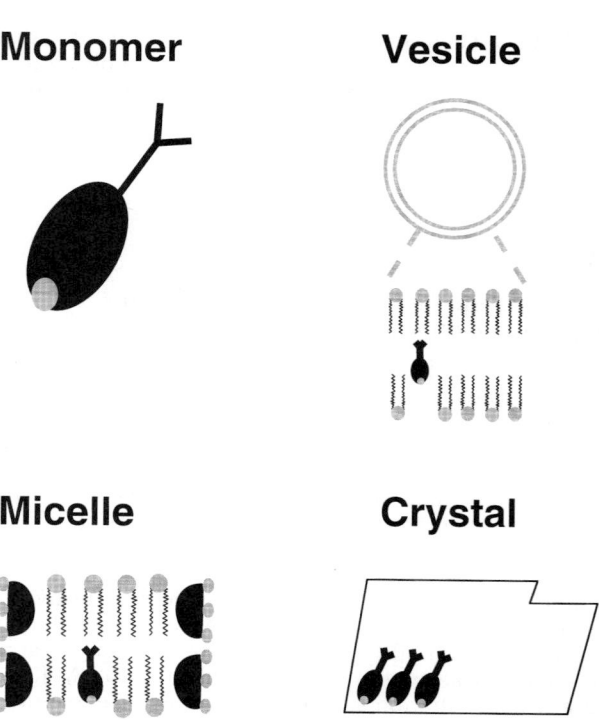

Figure 40.4. Phases of cholesterol in bile.

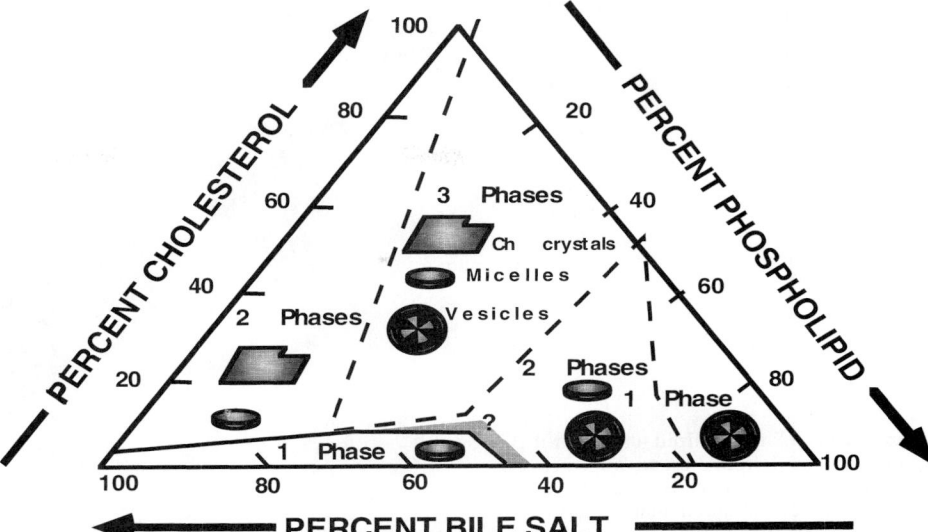

Figure 40.5. Equilibrium phase diagram for bile salt–lecithin–cholesterol–water at a concentration of 10% solids, 90% water. The monomeric phase is not depicted as a phase because it exists at the same concentration throughout. The one-phase zone contains only micelles. Several other zones exist, but only the two on the left above the one-phase zone apply to human gallbladder bile, and both contain cholesterol monohydrate crystals at equilibrium.

synthesized by hepatocytes (Fig. 40.6). Hepatic cholesterol may be exported into bile, synthesized into bile salts, or converted into cholesterol esters. Bile salts are secreted into bile, and cholesterol esters are either exported from the liver into serum or stored in the liver. Many of the enzymes and receptors involved in these steps are known. Certain of the risk factors associated with gallstone formation affect the activity of these enzymes or the expression of receptors governing these steps (Fig. 40.6).

Cholesterol is secreted into bile as cholesterol–phospholipid vesicles (5) (Fig. 40.7). Bile salts are probably needed for vesicles to bud off from the canalicular membrane. Bile salts are secreted into the canaliculus in monomeric form and associate to form simple micelles. Supersaturation of bile is determined largely at the moment of secretion and depends on the amount of cholesterol packaged in vesicles relative to the amount of phospholipid. Some modification may occur as a result of lipid absorption in the gallbladder, but this appears to be a minor influence on the state of saturation.

The presence of vesicles and micelles in the same aqueous compartment provides an opportunity for the movement of lipid between carriers. The process by which vesicles are changed in the presence of micelles after secretion into bile is *vesicular maturation* (Figs. 40.8 and 40.9). The net effect is the incorporation of vesicular lipid into simple micelles to form mixed micelles. Unsaturated bile is characterized by micellar excess, and eventually all vesicular lipid enters micelles (Fig. 40.8). Vesicular phospholipid is incorporated into micelles more readily than vesicular cholesterol. As a result, during maturation, vesicles become enriched in cholesterol. When the cholesterol-to-phospholipid ratio in the vesicles exceeds 1.0, the vesicles tend to become

Figure 40.6. Intermediary metabolism of hepatic cholesterol. A central cholesterol pool is shown. Cholesterol enters the pool after synthesis or receptor-mediated uptake from the serum. It leaves the pool to be exported directly into bile, used for bile salt synthesis, or converted into cholesterol esters that are stored in the liver or exported. Some of the enzymes and receptors involved in these steps are shown. Bile salts stimulate cholesterol and phospholipid secretion. Cholesterol to be excreted into bile is first packaged into phospholipid vesicles.

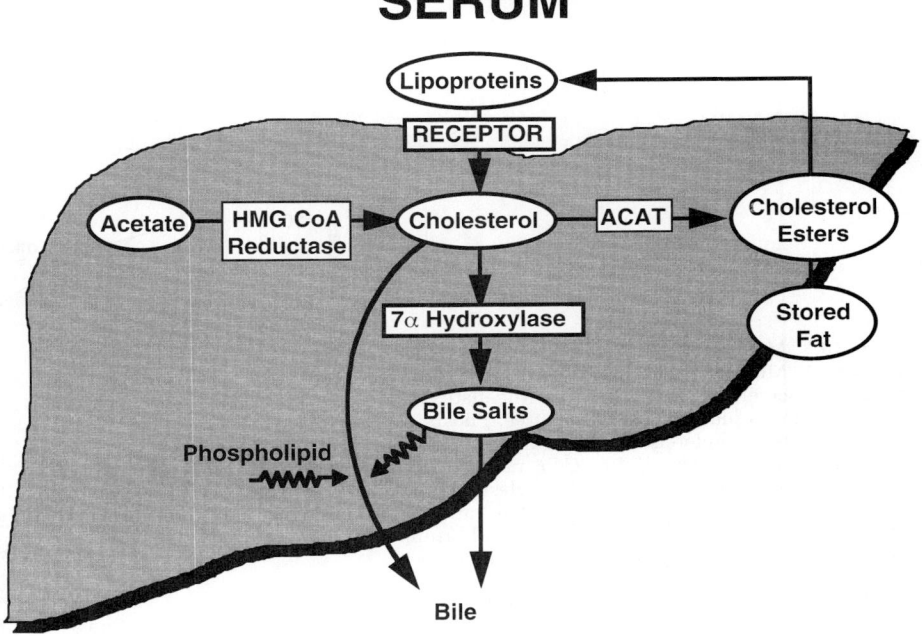

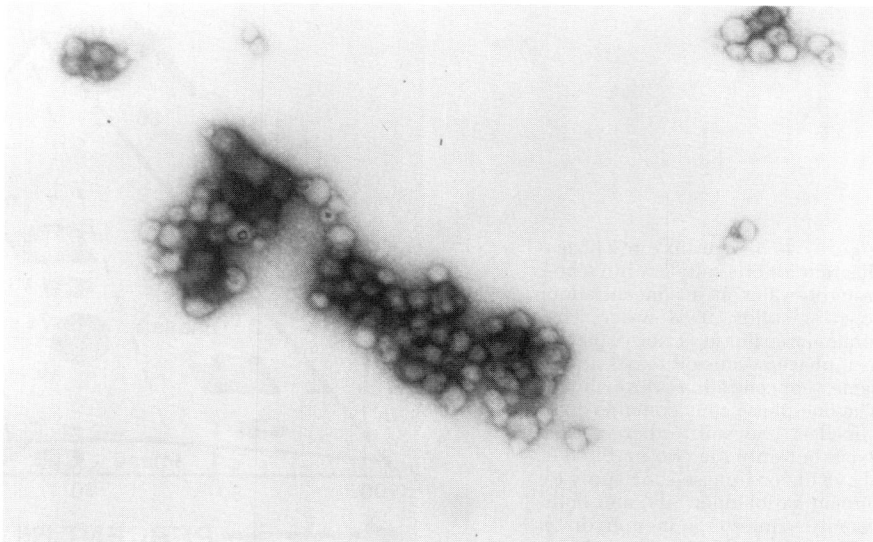

Figure 40.7. Phospholipid–cholesterol vesicles obtained from human bile. The diameter of these vesicles is about 1 μm. Note aggregation. Original magnification × 1,000.

unstable and nucleate cholesterol crystals. In unsaturated bile, cholesterol enrichment of vesicles is inconsequential because eventually all vesicular lipid is incorporated into micelles, but in supersaturated bile not all vesicles are micellized (Fig. 40.9). In the remaining cholesterol-enriched vesicles, cholesterol-dense zones develop on the surface. The subsequent steps leading to the appearance of cholesterol monohydrate crystals consist of vesicular *aggregation, fusion, nucleation,* and *crystal growth.* Aggregation and fusion bring cholesterol-rich zones on the vesicles into apposition, so that the nucleation of cholesterol monohydrate crystals is facilitated (Fig. 40.10). Initially, crystals are small and unstable, but with growth, they attain a stable size. Sometimes, the initial crystal is a classic cholesterol monohydrate crystal, but at other times, the initial crystals are filaments, coils, or tubes that subsequently are transformed into classic cholesterol monohydrate crystals (6).

The Three Stages of Cholesterol Gallstone Formation: Supersaturation, Accelerated Crystallization, and Stone Formation from Crystals

Supersaturation and Its Relation to Known Risk Factors for Gallstone Formation. Supersaturation is almost always caused by cholesterol hypersecretion rather than by a reduced secretion of phospholipid or bile salts. Multiple mechanisms produce cholesterol hypersecretion, and many of these are related to known risk factors for cholesterol stone formation.

Age. Supersaturation of bile increases with age because cholesterol secretion increases (7). Cholesterol 7-α-hydroxylation, the rate-limiting step in the synthesis of bile salts from cholesterol, is significantly decreased in older persons in comparison with middle-aged subjects. This suggests that increased cholesterol secretion in older

Figure 40.8. Maturation of vesicles in unsaturated bile—case 1. Micellar excess. Cholesterol and phospholipid are secreted in vesicular form. Micellation of these lipids takes place in the biliary tree. Phospholipid is micellated preferentially, with the result that the cholesterol-to-phospholipid *(C:P)* ratio of the residual vesicles rises. However, all cholesterol and phospholipid are eventually incorporated into micelles, and only this phase exists at equilibrium. (From Strasberg SM, Harvey PR. Biliary cholesterol transport and precipitation: introduction and overview of conference. *Hepatology* 1990;12:1S–5S, with permission.)

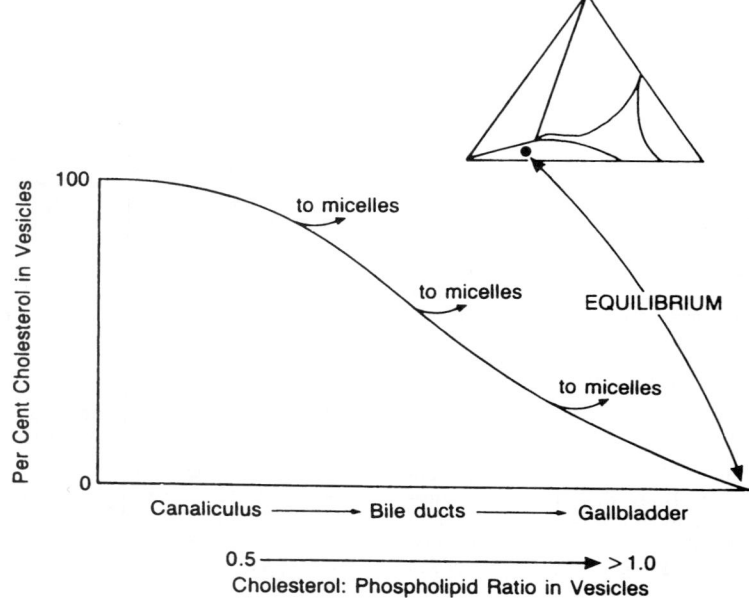

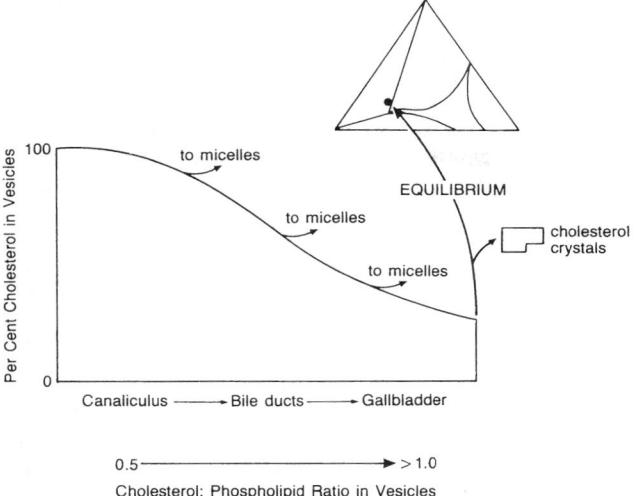

Figure 40.9. Maturation of vesicles in saturated bile—case 2. Micellar insufficiency. The same process of micellation takes place, including the preferential micellation of phospholipid. The residual "mature" vesicles are rich in cholesterol relative to phospholipid (high C:P ratio). These vesicles persist after all micelles are saturated with cholesterol. Processes of vesicle aggregation and fusion promote the formation of cholesterol microcrystals. At equilibrium, cholesterol monohydrate crystals are present. (From Strasberg SM, Harvey PR. Biliary cholesterol transport and precipitation: introduction and overview of conference. *Hepatology* 1990;12:1S–5S, with permission.)

subjects is linked to a decreased utilization of hepatic cholesterol for bile salt synthesis (8).

Obesity. Cholesterol synthesis increases with increasing weight. The correlation between body weight and cholesterol secretion into bile is linear (9). Neither reduced bile salt synthesis nor reduced esterification of cholesterol contributes to the excessive cholesterol secretion in obesity (10). The hepatocytes of patients with gallstones contain an intracellular vesicular fraction rich in lecithin. The cholesterol-to-phospholipid ratio in this vesicular fraction and the cholesterol-to-phospholipid ratio in bile canalicular membranes and in bile are correlated. In the obese, the transport of this fraction into bile is more rapid (11). Rapid weight loss in the obese patient also contributes to gallstone formation because during rapid weight loss, the se-

cretion of cholesterol into bile is sharply increased (9). Altered gallbladder motility and accelerated crystallization rates may also contribute to gallstone formation during rapid weight loss.

Female Sex, Pregnancy, and Exogenous Hormones. Estrogen promotes the secretion of cholesterol into bile. Premarin causes this effect by enhancing hepatic lipoprotein uptake and by inhibiting bile salt synthesis (12). During the last two trimesters of pregnancy, cholesterol secretion into bile increases relative to bile salt and phospholipid secretion, with the result that the cholesterol saturation index rises (13). Animal studies suggest that this is a consequence of increasing rates of cholesterol synthesis late in pregnancy. Also, the percentage of chenodeoxycholic acid in the bile salt pool decreases progressively during pregnancy as the rate of chenodeoxycholic acid synthesis decreases; chenodeoxycholic acid is an inhibitor of cholesterol synthesis. In pregnant women and those taking contraceptive steroids, the rate of gallbladder emptying is reduced and the gastrointestinal transit time is prolonged (14). As is discussed later, slower gallbladder emptying is a critical kinetic factor in gallstone formation.

Diet. The relationship between diet and gallstones is complex. Cholesterol gallstones do not form in vegetarians. Cholesterol gallstones are common in populations that consume a Western diet, which is relatively high in animal fat. Stone formers and control patients handle cholesterol feeding very differently (13). During cholesterol feeding, absorption decreases in both controls and patients with stones. Cholesterol synthesis decreases in both groups, as would be expected because of negative feedback inhibition. Bile salt synthesis and pool size tend to increase in the controls; however, in gallstone subjects, bile salt synthesis and pool size actually decrease. Biliary cholesterol secretion increases only in the gallstone group. This set of findings strongly suggests a genetic mechanism at work.

Genetic Mechanisms. A large interstrain variability in gallstone formation has been observed in cholesterol-fed mice (15). During genetic analysis, susceptibility to gallstone formation was found to be a dominant trait, determined by at least two genes. Susceptible strains fail to down-regulate cholesterol synthesis during cholesterol feeding.

Deoxycholate Enrichment of Bile Salt Pool. Persons with stones often have higher deoxycholate levels in bile. The rates of cholesterol and deoxycholate secretion into

Figure 40.10. Schematic depicting how aggregation and fusion provide ideal conditions for contact between cholesterol-rich zones on unilamellar or multilamellar vesicles. (From Strasberg SM, Harvey PR. Biliary cholesterol transport and precipitation: introduction and overview of conference. *Hepatology* 1990;12:1S–5S, with permission.)

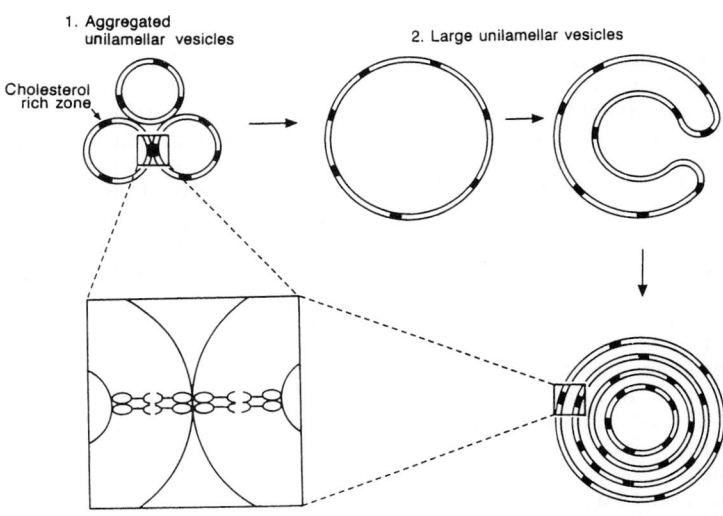

bile appear to be correlated. Presumably, deoxycholate is more efficient in stimulating cholesterol secretion by the liver than other bile salts. Deoxycholate enrichment may be a consequence of slower intestinal transit, which allows more time for the conversion of cholate to deoxycholate in the bowel or of increased cholic acid 7-α-dehydroxylation activity of the intestinal microflora, which has the same effect (16).

Accelerated Crystallization. The second stage of stone formation is crystallization from supersaturated bile. Virtually all patients with cholesterol gallstones have supersaturated bile, but many normal persons also have supersaturated bile (17). In other words, supersaturation is required for stone formation but does not guarantee stone formation. The difference between persons with supersaturated bile who form stones and those who do not is that bile from patients with stones reaches equilibrium while in the biliary tree, whereas bile from supersaturated controls does not. In other words, bile from patients with gallstones crystallizes more rapidly (18). Two mechanisms permit bile to reach equilibrium within a pathophysiologically relevant time frame. The first is a defect in gallbladder motility that results in prolonged retention of bile in the gallbladder. This provides time for maturation, aggregation, fusion, nucleation, and crystal growth to occur. The second is a defect in kinetics that results in acceleration of the steps in the crystallization pathway. As a result maturation, aggregation, and the other steps occur more rapidly.

Cholesterol Crystallization and the Gallbladder Motility Defect. Some patients with cholesterol stones have a motility defect in which gallbladder emptying is slow and incomplete (19). Also, gallbladder emptying is reduced during pregnancy, and residual volumes are increased. Likewise, obesity impairs gallbladder motility. The motility defect precedes crystal formation in animal models (20). Human gallbladder muscle from patients with crystals but no stones demonstrates impaired contractility (i.e., the motility defect is not secondary to stone-induced inflammation of the gallbladder wall) (21). In animal models, cholesterol feeding results in an increase in the cholesterol content and cholesterol-to-phospholipid molar ratio in gallbladder muscle plasma membranes, and a reduction in muscle cell contraction in response to cholecystokinin octapeptide (22). Incubation of normal gallbladder muscle cells with cholesterol-rich liposomes produces similar effects (22). Therefore, supersaturation of bile with cholesterol appears to expose gallbladder myocytes to higher cholesterol levels. Presumably, this occurs through absorption of cholesterol by the gallbladder and results in impaired motility. Why these events selectively affect only some persons with supersaturated bile is uncertain.

Cholesterol Crystallization and the Kinetic or "Nucleation" Defect. Gallbladder bile from patients with cholesterol stones produces crystals much more rapidly than equally supersaturated bile from control patients (18). Such a kinetic defect capable of accelerating crystallization must act by influencing one of the elements in the crystallization pathway leading to equilibrium—vesicle maturation, aggregation, fusion, nucleation, and crystal growth. Substances that potentially influence these mechanisms have been referred to as procrystallizing (23) and anticrystallizing factors (antinucleating and pronucleating factors). Several procrystallizing substances have been identified, including mucous glycoproteins (24), immunoglobulins (25), aminopeptidase N (26), phospholipase C (27), alpha acid glycoprotein (28), haptoglobin (29), and an 84-kd glycoprotein (30). Of these, immunoglobulin G and alpha acid glycoprotein have been shown to be more abundant in bile from patients with cholesterol gallstones. In an attempt to determine the relative importance of the different proteins, comparative studies were performed, but these often yielded differing results regarding the potency of these compounds because of different experimental methods. Procrystallizing proteins might act at any point on the crystallization pathway. Afdahl et al. (31) showed that mucin greatly accelerates vesicle fusion. Yamashita et al. (32) have demonstrated that haptoglobin exerts its procrystallizing effect by increasing the cholesterol content of vesicles. More studies of this type are required to refine further our understanding of proteins and crystallization.

In patients with cholesterol gallstones, the total protein concentration in gallbladder bile also appears to be increased (33). Total biliary protein increases in animal models before stone formation (34). Multiple gallbladder stones seem to be associated with a shorter nucleation time and higher biliary concentrations of total protein and glycoprotein than solitary stones (35). Furthermore, the total protein concentration is higher in gallbladder bile from patients with crystals but no stones and higher in patients with gallstones who have crystals in their bile at the time of cholecystectomy; both these observations indicate that the high protein concentration in humans is not secondary to stone formation. The high protein concentration might simply be secondary to a general increase in the concentration of bile, which by increasing the chance for contact between cholesterol carriers would accelerate vesicle maturation and aggregation and perhaps other steps in the crystallization pathway. Indeed, an early increase in bile concentration in animal models of gallstones is caused by enhanced absorption of water and electrolytes (36).

The common feature of many of the procrystallizing proteins, such as immunoglobulins and mucous glycoprotein, is that they are secreted as a result of inflammation. Cholesterol supersaturation appears to be the insult capable of initiating inflammation (37). Cholesterol supersaturation, especially when coupled with deoxycholate excess (38), may lead to gallbladder inflammation (39) and the secretion of procrystallizing proteins (38), which in turn lead to crystal formation in the gallbladder. The associated dysmotility extends the time in which crystallization can occur.

Other agents in bile, including apolipoprotein A, a 120-kd glycoprotein, and a 15-kd protein, have anticrystallizing effects (40). Several anticrystallizing proteins appear to bind to cholesterol crystals, which suggests that they inhibit crystal growth. Stimulation of the production of anticrystallizing agents (e.g., by dietary modification or additives) is potentially a means of preventing gallstones.

It is not surprising that gallstones form in the gallbladder because many of the factors required for stone formation, such as increases in the retention time of bile in the bilary tree, the concentration of bile, and the secretion of procrystallizing factors, are based on gallbladder activity or abnormalities of gallbladder function.

Formation of Stones from Crystals

The third and final stage of cholesterol stone formation occurs when cholesterol crystals form into stones. A schema for the growth of cholesterol stones has been described by Wolpers and Hofmann (41). Solitary gallstones form from free-floating crystal laminae of cholesterol. These laminae aggregate loosely and undergo external compaction and internal remodeling by movement of cholesterol molecules to form compact spheroids. Multiple gallstones form as a result of the abrupt aggregation of innumerable, very thin cholesterol crystals into spheres up to 1 mm in diameter. A second aggregation takes place within 3 months, in which these spheres coalesce to form mulberry stones. Mulberry stones are transformed into either faceted stones or barrel stones.

Sludge, Sediment, and Stone Formation. The term *sludge* has been used to describe various entities: necrotic collagen that obstructs bile ducts after liver transplantation, material that precipitates in bile ducts in association with cholangiohepatitis or stents, and echogenic material that layers out in the gallbladder, especially in some fasting patients. The latter is now the usual meaning of the term. The term *sludge* used in this way denotes *echogenic gallbladder sludge* (i.e., material detectable in the gallbladder on ultrasonography). *Sludge* must be distinguished from *sediment,* which is solid material detectable in the bile by microscopy. Bile normally has sediment, but it is sparse, consisting mainly of dead cells. Pathologic sediment contains microcrystals of cholesterol, calcium bilirubinate, or both. Pathologic sediment is usually not detectable by ultrasonography, but if sludge is detected, then pathologic sediment will always be present.

Sludge is usually composed of bilirubinate microcrystals (42) and mucus; however, cholesterol crystals are also sometimes present. Sludge is a precursor of bilirubinate stones (43) and has been proposed as a precursor of cholesterol stones. This is an attractive hypothesis, but little direct evidence is available to show that it applies to most instances of cholesterol stone formation.

Pathogenesis of Pigment Gallstones

Black Pigment Stones

Black pigment stones contain three calcium salts—calcium bilirubinate as a polymer, calcium carbonate, and calcium phosphate. The factors governing the solubility of calcium salts in bile are complex. In simple aqueous solutions, calcium solubility may be predicted by whether the ion product in the solution $[Ca^{2+}] \bullet [anion]$ exceeds the "solubility product." The solubility product is the highest value of the ion product at which the calcium salt will be in solution at equilibrium and is determined experimentally. Bile is a complex solution in which calcium is bound to bile salt monomers and micelles in addition to proteins. These "buffers" increase the capacity for transport of calcium salts. Acidification of bile, a normal function of the gallbladder, has the same effect, and defective acidification may contribute to the formation of black stones. Adding to the complexity is the fact that unconjugated bilirubin is much less soluble than conjugated bilirubin. Deconjugation normally occurs in bile at a very slow rate via alkaline hydrolysis or by the action of human β-glucuronidase. Congenital or acquired hemolytic states result in excessive levels of conjugated bilirubin in bile, which increase the rate of production of unconjugated bilirubin. Certain intestinal conditions that are associated with bile salt malabsorption, such as Crohn's disease and ileal resection, apparently result in the cycling of bilirubin and increased secretion into bile, much as in hemolytic states. Cirrhosis may cause the direct secretion of unconjugated bilirubin into bile.

Stasis of bile within the gallbladder has also been implicated as an important etiologic factor in the pathogenesis of black pigment gallstones. This is underscored by the finding that calcium bilirubinate stones tend to form in patients on total parenteral nutrition, a clinical setting characterized by gallbladder stasis.

Brown Pigment Stones

When a foreign body such as a parasite or stone lodges in the bile duct, bile stasis and bacterial contamination follow. The same happens in the presence of a biliary stricture. The precise mechanisms of these events are unclear. Bile normally is sterile, and it is maintained in this state by the mechanical action of bile flow in addition to some of the constituents of bile, such as immunoglobulin A and perhaps bile salts. Presumably, these and other bacterial defense mechanisms are impaired in partial biliary obstruction. Once bacterial contamination occurs, organisms such as *Escherichia coli* secrete a β-glucuronidase that enzymatically cleaves bilirubin glucuronide, to produce insoluble unconjugated bilirubin. This substance precipitates and, along with dead bacterial cell bodies, produces a thick sludge that forms soft brown stones throughout the biliary tree and gallbladder. A vicious cycle ensues, with further stasis and contamination. Eventually, frank infection in the form of cholangitis develops.

NATURAL HISTORY OF GALLSTONES

Understanding the natural history of cholelithiasis is central to the rational management of patients with gallstones. Gallstone disease may be divided into three clinical stages: asymptomatic gallstones, symptomatic gallstones, and complicated gallstone disease. When stones first form, they are asymptomatic, and most patients remain in this clinical stage throughout life. The stones do not obstruct the opening into the cystic duct, and the gallbladder is able to fill and empty; if the gallbladder does become obstructed, this may not cause pain. For unknown reasons, some cases of asymptomatic disease progress to the symptomatic stage, in which pain, *biliary colic,* develops. Pain is caused when the gallbladder contracts against an obstructing gallstone lodged at its outlet, at or in the cystic duct. Disease in the symptomatic stage may then progress to the complicated stage of *cholelithiasis,* in which complications develop in the gallbladder or bile ducts. The main complication in the gallbladder is *acute cholecystitis,* an inflammation of the gallbladder wall. Acute cholecystitis if untreated may resolve or result in gallbladder perforation, with resultant abscess, fistula, or generalized peritonitis. If a fistula forms, stones may enter the gastrointestinal tract. When the stones are large and enter the small intestine via a *cholecystoduodenal fistula,* they may lodge in the ileum and produce small-bowel obstruction, a condition called *gallstone ileus.* The presence of gallstones in the bile ducts is termed *choledocholithiasis.* The stones usually originate in the gallbladder. They may pass asymptomatically from the bile duct into the duodenum, especially if they are less than 3 mm in diameter. They may obstruct the biliary tree and cause biliary colic or jaundice, usually intermittent or incomplete jaundice. Choledocholithiasis may also lead to *acute cholangitis,* also called *acute suppurative cholangitis,* a severe and life-threatening bacterial inflammation that affects the whole biliary system. Repeated bouts of cholangitis may lead to *bile duct strictures,* abscesses, and eventually destruction of the liver, a condition called *secondary biliary cirrhosis. Acute gallstone pancreatitis* is another severe complication of choledocholithiasis. It develops when stones obstruct the free flow of pancreatic juice; usually, they obstruct the *common channel* formed by the union of the bile and pancreatic ducts close to their entry into the duodenum.

The pool of asymptomatic patients is huge, about 20 million in the United States, because the disease is so common. Annually, about 3% of asymptomatic persons, or about 600,000 people, become symptomatic (i.e., biliary colic develops). Symptomatic patients tend to have recurring bouts of biliary colic. Complicated gallstone disease develops in 3% to 5% of symptomatic patients per year. It is unusual (< 0.5% annually) for complicated gallstone disease to develop in an asymptomatic person who has not previously had an interval of symptomatic disease without complications.

ASYMPTOMATIC GALLSTONES

The diagnosis of asymptomatic stones is incidental, as screening is not performed or indicated for this disease. Fifteen percent of stones are radioopaque and may be seen on abdominal radiographs or even chest radiographs obtained to evaluate nonbiliary symptoms. Stones may also be detected by computed tomography (CT), although this is not a sensitive technique, or when ultrasonography of the upper abdomen is performed for nonbiliary symptoms. Asymptomatic gallstones are found occasionally during "pelvic" ultrasonography in women. Gallstones may also be discovered in asymptomatic patients during abdominal surgery for unrelated conditions. Patients with abdominal symptoms may still have asymptomatic gallstones. Classic studies have demonstrated that dyspeptic symptoms, such as nausea, bloating, eructation, and flatulence, are equally common in all persons of the same age, whether or not gallstones are present. Nor can symptoms in the lower bowel in the absence of pain be attributed to gallstones.

Several studies have followed asymptomatic patients for many years (44,45). Between 20% and 30% of patients become symptomatic within 20 years. In very few patients do complications develop before a period without symptoms, so prophylactic cholecystectomy is not indicated to prevent sudden, unexpected complications in persons with asymptomatic stones. Death resulting from a complication arising in a previously asymptomatic patient is extremely rare. Gallbladder cancer occurs only in association with gallstones, but it is so uncommon in the United States that screening programs and prophylactic cholecystectomy are not indicated. Diabetic patients with asymptomatic gallstones have the same natural history as other persons in that symptoms appear, presenting a window of opportunity for treatment, before complications develop.

Cholecystectomy during the asymptomatic stage is indicated in a few uncommon situations. *Porcelain gallbladder,* a rare, premalignant condition in which the wall of the gallbladder becomes calcified, is an *absolute* indication for cholecystectomy. Malignant transformation occurs in about 25% of untreated patients (46). The calcification of gallstones is not associated with a cancer risk. There are also a few *relative* indications for prophylactic cholecystectomy. North and South American Indian and European–American Indian admixed populations have an increased risk for gallstones and gallbladder cancer. In this population, cancer may develop in 3% to 5% of patients with asymptomatic gallstones, and prophylactic cholecystectomy may be advisable. Patients with gallstones larger than 3 cm may also be at increased risk for cancer. Patients who have a family history of gallbladder cancer sometimes request ultrasonographic examinations, and when stones are found, cholecystectomy is a reasonable choice, often partly for psychological reasons. To date, no screening program is available for those who may be at higher risk for genetic reasons. Gallstone disease in children is a relative indication for cholecystectomy. The management of gallstones discovered at laparotomy is controversial. Conflicting reports have been published regarding the inci-

dence of biliary symptoms after surgery in patients whose gallbladder is not removed, and the incidence of longer recovery times and perioperative complications in patients who do undergo *incidental cholecystectomy,* also called *cholecystectomy en passant.* Incidental cholecystectomy should be avoided when vascular grafts are to be placed in the abdomen during the same surgery, when the procedure is likely to be hazardous, or when incisions must be greatly extended to expose the gallbladder.

SYMPTOMATIC GALLSTONES

The diagnosis of symptomatic gallstones depends on the presence of characteristic symptoms and the demonstration of stones on diagnostic imaging. The chief symptom is biliary colic, which develops when pressure in the gallbladder is increased by contraction of the gallbladder against an obstructing stone. The pain, which is transmitted along visceral nerves and is not associated with peritoneal signs, has typical features, but in many patients, biliary colic has atypical features (47). Four traits are characteristic of typical biliary colic. It is episodic; patients suffer discrete attacks of pain, between which they feel well. It is severe, bringing the patients to care quickly; the pain is often so severe that patients cry or compare the pain to labor. It is located in the epigastrium or right upper quadrant, and it comes on in the middle of the night or after a meal, often a fatty or heavy meal. Patients whose *attacks of pain* have the characteristic *location, severity,* and *timing* and who have gallstones demonstrated on ultrasonography may be confidently advised that they have symptomatic cholelithiasis. Other common features of the pain are that it is steady, increases in severity during 30 minutes and lasts 2 to 4 hours, often radiates to the back, is associated with nausea and vomiting, and may be followed by an episode of diarrhea. Patients usually walk or roll around in an attempt to relieve the pain.

Atypical pain is common. Sometimes the pain is continuous rather than episodic, lasting days or more. This may happen when a stone is impacted in the cystic duct. The pain may be located predominantly in the back or the left upper or right lower quadrant. Not all attacks are necessarily severe, and some patients do not relate their pain to meals or time of day. There is no formula to determine when pain is arising from stones. The less typical the pain, the more carefully the clinician should search for another cause, even in the presence of stones—causes such as renal colic, peptic ulcer disease, hiatal hernia, esophageal spasm, abdominal tumor, abdominal wall hernia, liver disease, and disease of the small and large intestine, including irritable bowel disease. Diaphragmatic problems and extraabdominal diagnoses, such as pleuritic and myocardial pain, must also be considered. Treatment of atypical biliary colic is appropriate when other causes of pain have been eliminated.

Because biliary colic is a mechanically induced pain transmitted along visceral nerves, an attack produces few abdominal findings. Mild right upper quadrant tenderness may be present.

Diagnostic imaging is used to confirm the presence of gallstones. *Abdominal ultrasonography* is the standard diagnostic test. Stones are acoustically dense and return strong echoes to an ultrasonic transducer. They also prevent the passage of sound into the region of view behind the stone, thereby producing an *acoustic shadow.* Echoes without shadows may be caused by gallbladder polyps. A definitive sonographic diagnosis requires both echogenic structures and posterior acoustic shadows (Fig. 40.11). The patient should be fasting for several hours so that gallbladder filling is maximal; a full gallbladder greatly fa-

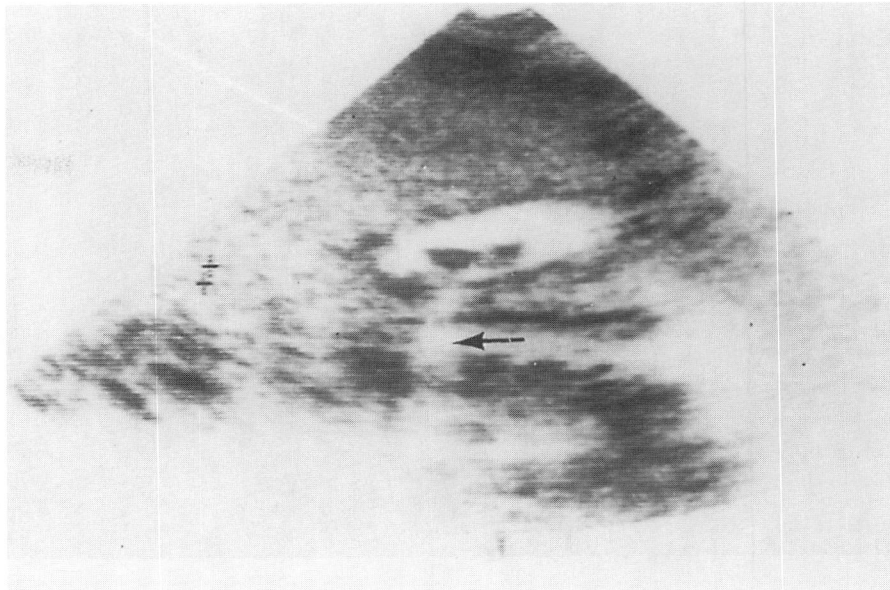

Figure 40.11. On abdominal ultrasonogram, echogenic foci within the gallbladder cause acoustic shadowing *(arrow),* typical of cholelithiasis.

cilitates the demonstration of these features. Sometimes, the stones are so dense that all sound is reflected from the tops of the stones, and they appear as inverted Us rather than round objects. Usually, little or no associated gallbladder wall thickening is seen. The biliary ducts are assessed for evidence of dilatation or choledocholithiasis. *Oral cholecystography* is an older test. A radioopaque dye, administered orally, is absorbed by the intestine, secreted by the liver, and concentrated by the gallbladder. When the gallbladder is imaged 12 hours later, the stones appear as filling defects (Fig. 40.12). Another sign indicative of stones is nonvisualization of the gallbladder, provided the pills were taken and intestinal and hepatic function is normal. This indicates that the cystic duct is obstructed or that gallbladder wall inflammation has progressed to a point at which the gallbladder cannot concentrate the dye. Cholecystography is slightly less sensitive than ultrasonography (95% vs. 98%). Other disadvantages are that it entails radiation exposure and requires patient compliance. Also, digestive, hepatic, and gallbladder function must be intact.

Occasionally, patients may have typical attacks of biliary pain but no evidence of stones on ultrasonography. This pain may be caused by sludge, or very small stones not detectable by ultrasonography. It is reasonable to treat patients who have sludge and who also have recurrent disabling and typical pain. It is the authors' practice to require the demonstration of sludge on two occasions several weeks apart at times when the patient is on a normal diet. It should be remembered that sludge may appear if a patient stops eating because of pain of any cause. Small stones and other biliary disease may be detected by *biliary drainage.* Gallbladder bile is aspirated after a tube or endoscope is placed in the duodenum and cholecystokinin octapeptide is slowly injected intravenously in the recommended dose. The gallbladder bile, or "b" bile, which is characteristically very dark, is centrifuged and the sediment examined microscopically. The presence of cholesterol crystals (Fig. 40.13) or calcium bilirubinate crystals indicates the presence of small stones or other biliary disease (48).

Sludge and gallstones are not the only conditions capable of inducing biliary colic. Cholesterolosis is a condition in which cholesterol accumulates within macrophages in the gallbladder mucosa, either diffusely or locally as

polyps. It may sometimes cause biliary colic. The polypoid form is often detected by ultrasonography. Adenomyomatosis is a non-neoplastic condition characterized by the ingrowth of gallbladder mucosal glands into the muscle layer, either diffusely or focally in the fundus (fundal adenomyoma). It may also cause biliary colic. Functional abnormalities of gallbladder contraction may lead to pain. Hypomotility is detectable by measuring the gallbladder ejection fraction with the cholecystokinin/biliary scintigraphy test. The authors consider the result of this

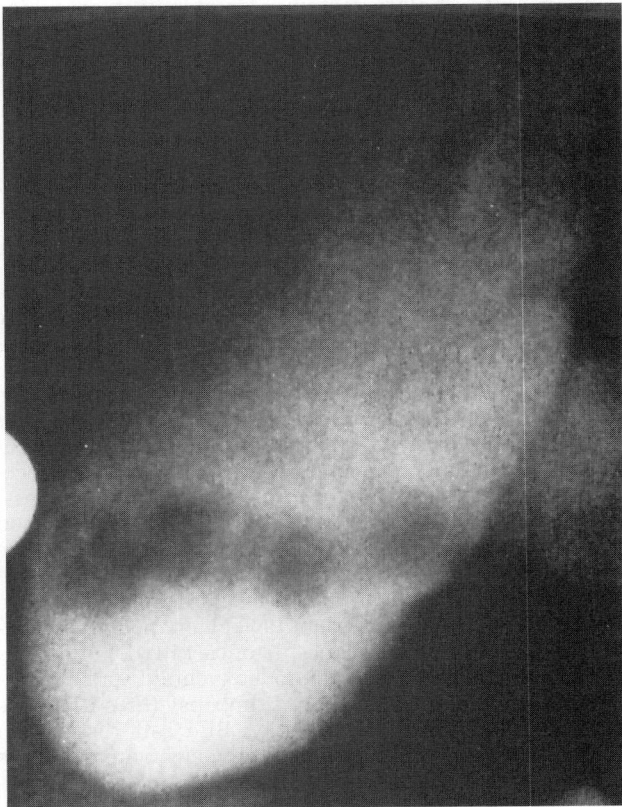

Figure 40.12. Oral cholecystogram demonstrating multiple radiolucent, free-floating stones in the gallbladder.

Figure 40.13. Cholesterol crystals as they appear in gallbladder bile sediment under polarized light. Original magnification × 100.

test to be positive only when it has been repeated after an interval and the ejection fraction is reduced (40%) on both tests. Patients with sludge, crystals, cholesterolosis, adenomyomatosis, or a reduced ejection fraction and pain that is *recurrent, typical,* and *disabling* may be treated by the same approaches as a patient with symptomatic gallstones, and good results can be expected. On the other hand, if the pain is atypical, other sources of pain should be sought because cholecystectomy is much less likely to alleviate the symptoms.

Symptomatic cholelithiasis is an indication for treatment, usually *cholecystectomy,* an operation in which the gallbladder and the contained gallstones are removed. Before 1990, the operation was performed through an abdominal incision—*open cholecystectomy.* Today, the operation is almost always performed laparoscopically—*laparoscopic cholecystectomy.* In a third technique, *minicholecystectomy,* the gallbladder is removed through a very small abdominal incision (5 to 7 cm). Minicholecystectomy is performed in a few centers. Laparoscopic cholecystectomy is discussed separately in the next section.

In *cholecystostomy,* the gallbladder is opened, the stones are removed, and the gallbladder is drained; the drain is later removed. It is now never used to treat symptomatic stones because the rate of stone recurrence is high.

Variants of cholecystostomy include *contact dissolution* of stones with methyl tert butyl ether and *percutaneous cholecystolithotripsy* with extraction. Both require percutaneous intubation of the gallbladder. In the former procedure, stones are bathed in a cholesterol solvent for several hours until they dissolve; the technique is not widely used today. In the latter technique, the tract is enlarged and the stones are destroyed by direct lithotripsy and mechanically extracted. This technique is available in centers with advanced interventional radiology. Nonoperative treatments include dissolution of gallstones with the bile acids ursodeoxycholic acid and chenodeoxycholic acid and extracorporeal shock wave biliary lithotripsy (ESWL). These treatments are rarely used today. Bile salt dissolution works consistently well only in patients who are not obese and who have small cholesterol gallstones (5% to 10% patients presenting with stones), and the stones eventually re-form in more than 50% of these patients. ESWL is a reasonable therapy for patients with single stones 0.5 to 2 cm

in diameter; single stones have a lower recurrence rate, of about 20%. Again, only a small percentage of patients with stones fit these criteria. The method has never been approved by the Food and Drug Administration in the United States.

Patients who become symptomatic should undergo elective laparoscopic cholecystectomy without long delay to avoid the onset of complications—days to a few weeks is an appropriate time span. During that time, dietary fats and large meals should be avoided to reduce the chance of another attack. Diabetic patients are a special case (47). They are no more prone to become symptomatic; however, once biliary colic begins, acute cholecystitis is more likely to develop, the cholecystitis is often severe, and they are less well able to tolerate the insult. Therefore, once these patients become symptomatic, treatment should be prompt. Patients who have biliary colic should undergo treatment before becoming pregnant. The treatment of biliary colic arising during pregnancy depends on the trimester. Laparoscopic cholecystectomy is undesirable in the first trimester because of the chance of inducing abortion; also, it is inadvisable to expose the embryo to drugs or anesthetic agents at this early stage of development. In the third trimester, the concern is early onset of labor. The second trimester is a window of opportunity in which laparoscopic cholecystectomy is relatively safe. When biliary colic arises during pregnancy, it should be managed expectantly with diet. If the colic is recurrent or if the patient is unable to maintain nutrition because of fear of pain or actual pain, then laparoscopic cholecystectomy should be performed in the second trimester. Patients in the first trimester should be carried into the second trimester whenever possible and those in the third trimester brought to delivery before surgery. Rarely, laparoscopic cholecystectomy must be performed in the first trimester and open cholecystectomy in the third trimester. Laparoscopic cholecystectomy is safe and effective in children who require it, as attested by a number of case series. Laparoscopic cholecystectomy is also safe in the elderly and in persons with intercurrent disease provided their cardiopulmonary status permits administration of a general anesthetic. When cardiac and pulmonary status is so poor that a general anesthetic is contraindicated, percutaneous cholecystolithotripsy with extraction is a useful technique.

LAPAROSCOPIC CHOLECYSTECTOMY AND OPEN CHOLECYSTECTOMY

Laparoscopic cholecystectomy revolutionized the treatment of gallstones. It rapidly displaced open cholecystectomy, and also ESWL and bile salt therapy. The remarkable demand for this procedure can be attributed to its ability to cure cholelithiasis with a minimum of inconvenience, pain, and loss of activity.

Symptomatic cholelithiasis is the main indication for laparoscopic cholecystectomy, which is the accepted first-line therapy for this disease. Contraindications are uncommon and may be divided into patient-based and surgeon-based categories. Patient-based contraindications include the inability to withstand a general anesthetic, intractable bleeding disorder, and end-stage liver disease. Few patients have such severe cardiac or pulmonary disease (e.g., cardiac ejection fraction < 20%) that the procedure cannot be performed. The presence of a ventriculoperitoneal shunt is not a contraindication. Surgeon-based contraindications relate to the anticipated difficulty of a procedure, as determined by the presence of certain preoperative factors. Previous and current attacks of cholecystitis are a risk factor for difficult cholecystectomy. Male sex, advanced age, and multiple previous attacks of pain are additive risk factors for difficult cholecystectomy (49). The probability of complications rises with inexperience and difficulty of the procedure. If the operator is inexperienced, these factors are relative contraindications to the procedure. Cholecystoenteric fistula is a relative contraindication, even if the laparoscopist is highly experienced. Laparoscopic cholecystectomy should not be attempted in a patient with acute cholecystitis if the inflammation has been present for longer than 72 hours because vascularity and tissue edema will be increased. Conversion rates of 10% or less are possible with proper patient selection.

Technique of Laparoscopic Cholecystectomy

The goal of dissection in laparoscopic cholecystectomy is the conclusive identification of the cystic artery and duct, as these are the structures to be divided. During the dissection leading up to the conclusive identification, normal structures must not be injured. These surgical principles govern the conduct of this operation (50).

A pneumoperitoneum is created by entering the abdomen via a small incision at the umbilicus and inserting a Hasson trocar. This open method is safer than the blind Veress needle technique. Three other trocars are inserted under direct vision. Mechanical devices that lift the abdominal wall ("laparolift") have been used to create room for laparoscopic cholecystectomy, with very good results. When the patient has previously undergone surgery, great care must be taken in entering the peritoneal cavity. The gallbladder is grasped with instruments placed through ports on the right side of the abdomen. Traction on the fundus should be upward and to the right, and traction on the pouch of Hartmann laterally to the right. This combination "disaligns" the common duct and cystic duct, so that they appear as distinct structures. Incorrect traction aligns the ducts so that they appear as a continuous structure, and as a consequence the chance of biliary injury is increased (Fig. 40.14). During dissection, portions of the gallbladder without peritoneum may appear; these should not be grasped by instruments because they tear easily when this is done, with consequent rupture of the gallbladder.

The goal of conclusive identification of the cystic structures can be achieved in several ways. In the critical view technique (50), the triangle of Calot is dissected free of fatty, fibrous, and areolar tissue and the lower one fourth to one third of the gallbladder is dissected off the liver bed (Fig. 40.15). The latter is an essential step to exclude the possibility that one is dissecting around the common bile duct (see below). It also precludes injury to an aberrant duct. At the completed dissection, only two structures should be seen entering the gallbladder, and the lower part of the liver bed should be visible (Fig. 40.15). It is not necessary to see the common duct. At this point, the surgeon has achieved the "critical view of safety," and the cystic structures may be occluded, as they have been conclusively identified. These principles are similar in rationale to those enunciated for years by expert biliary surgeons for open cholecystectomy, the difference being that it was recommended to free the entire gallbladder from the liver bed from above *after identifying, but before dividing* the cystic structures. It is sometimes difficult to do this during laparoscopic cholecystectomy, and the same goal can be achieved by freeing the base of the gallbladder off the liver bed, which is actually much easier to do laparoscopically than during open surgery. The cystic artery rather than the cystic duct may appear in the free edge of the peritoneal fold running between the gallbladder and the hepatoduodenal ligament. This does not alter the procedure. Not infrequently, no distinct cystic artery is seen because with a dissection plane right on the gallbladder, only small arterial branches are divided, much as in adrenalectomy. In that case, only one structure is seen to enter the gallbladder at the completion of dissection. Rarely, a short cystic artery tethers the gallbladder and prevents dissection of the hepatocystic triangle. In these cases, the artery is cleared of surrounding tissues, and if it can be demonstrated both to enter the gallbladder and be pulsatile, it is divided before the complete clearance of the hepatocystic triangle.

Another technique is to rely on displaying the junction of the cystic duct with the infundibulum of the gallbladder. The cystic duct is circumferentially cleared where it joins the gallbladder, with the surgeon working on both sides of the hepatocystic triangle to identify the point where the cystic duct widens to form the infundibulum. The characteristic shape of the widening infundibulum is used as the key to identifying the cystic duct. Based on the authors' experience with biliary injuries, this approach is highly questionable. Especially in the presence of inflammation and a short cystic duct, the exact point where the

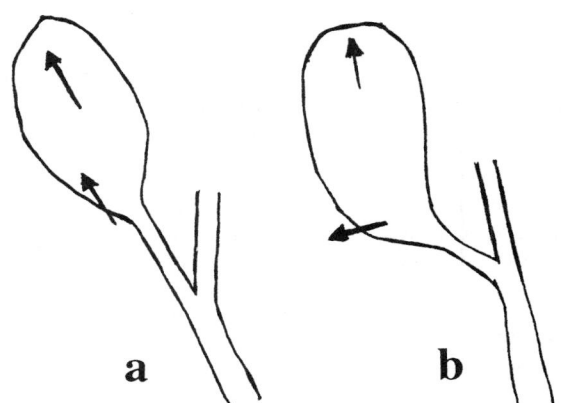

Figure 40.14. (a) Incorrect method of retracting the gallbladder brings the cystic and common ducts into alignment and makes them appear as one. (b) Correct method of retraction.

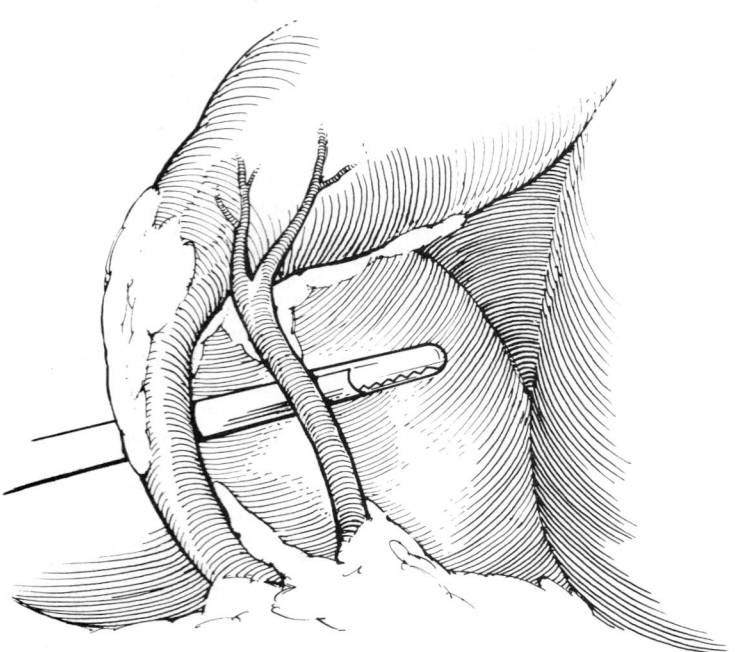

Figure 40.15. The "critical view of safety." The triangle of Calot is dissected free of all tissue except for the cystic duct and artery, and the base of the liver bed is exposed. When this view is achieved, the two structures entering the gallbladder can only be the cystic duct and artery. It is not necessary to see the common bile duct. (From Strasberg SM, Hertl M, Soper NJ. An analysis of the problem of biliary injury during laparoscopic cholecystectomy. *J Am Coll Surg* 1995;180:101–125, with permission.)

gallbladder becomes the cystic duct is difficult to discern at the beginning of a dissection. The common bile duct may be mistaken for the cystic duct, and it can be cleared circumferentially up to the point where it appears to widen as it divides into the cystic duct and the common hepatic duct. This widening apparently has fooled surgeons into thinking that they have reached the infundibulum. It is possible to clear around both sides of the common bile duct, much as one clears both sides of the hepatocystic triangle, and gain the impression that the infundibular technique is being properly applied. Having reached the false infundibulum, the surgeon believes that the cystic duct has been conclusively identified and then proceeds to divide the common bile duct. This technique also seems sometimes to fail to identify aberrant right ducts that are closely applied to the underside of the gallbladder. These appear to be more readily identified if the transection of cystic structures is delayed until the hepatocystic triangle is cleared, as described above. This method also lacks the definitive end point of the critical view technique. It has the further disadvantage that the cystic duct is divided before the artery. In the authors' opinion that the infundibular technique should be abandoned in favor of the critical view technique, which in fact is a laparoscopic adaptation of the classic way of performing a cholecystectomy safely.

Once the cystic structures have been identified, they may be clipped and divided. It is at this time, just before the cystic duct is divided, that a selective or routine operative cholangiogram may be performed. When the cystic duct is divided, care must be taken not to tent up and occlude the common bile duct ("tenting injury"). Thick ducts are occluded with preformed catgut loops rather than clipped because clips are insecure under these circumstances. After the ducts are divided, the gallbladder is dissected off the liver bed and then extracted.

Routine operative cholangiography has been advocated to avoid ductal injury. Opinion on the subject is sharply divided. Biliary injuries appear to be less frequent in the hands of surgeons who perform operative cholangiography routinely. In about 50% of ductal injuries, a cholangiogram fails to prevent the injury although abnormal anatomy is present (i.e., cholangiograms are often incor-

rectly interpreted). The indications for intraoperative cholangiography, when it is performed selectively, are known choledocholithiasis, a history of jaundice, a history of pancreatitis, a large cystic duct and small gallstones, any abnormality in preoperative liver function tests, and dilated biliary ducts on preoperative sonography. Provided these indications are carefully followed, selective cholangiography is as effective in detecting clinically relevant stones as routine cholangiography. Laparoscopic sonography is as accurate as intraoperative cholangiography in the detection of common bile duct stones (51).

The superiority of laparoscopic cholecystectomy over open cholecystectomy has been demonstrated in randomized controlled trials comparing laparoscopic cholecystectomy with minicholecystectomy (52,53). In the two studies, the hospital stay was shorter in the laparoscopic group, as was the duration of convalescence and the time before a normal diet could be resumed. Patients who underwent laparoscopic cholecystectomy had lower pain scores, returned to work earlier, and were more satisfied with the cosmetic results of the procedure. The benefits of laparoscopic cholecystectomy also seem to extend to direct costs and cost-effectiveness, although this depends on the incidence of biliary injury. Patient satisfaction with the procedure is extremely high because of the combination of convenience, lack of pain, minimal scarring, and permanent resolution of cholelithiasis. The point has been made that patient satisfaction is so much greater with the laparoscopic technique that patients would choose it even if it were less cost-effective.

The most common complication of laparoscopic cholecystectomy is a wound infection, which occurs in 1% to 2% of patients; this is a minor problem compared with infection of a laparotomy incision. Hernias at the umbilical trocar site have been reported; these can be avoided by suturing this incision when the trocar is removed.

Serious complications of laparoscopic cholecystectomy are rare, the mortality rate being less than 0.1%. However, as cholecystectomy rates have risen (54), the total number of deaths has not decreased. Similarly, cardiopulmonary complication rates have fallen, but not the total number of these complications (54). The single greatest problem in laparoscopic cholecystectomy is biliary injury. The most reliable data available place the rate of major bile duct injury between 0.3% and 0.6%, but if all biliary injuries are considered, the injury rate in these reports ranges from 0.6% to 1.5%, which is three to four times the injury rate at open surgery (50). Laparoscopic biliary injuries are somewhat different from those that were sustained in the era of open surgery, and for this reason a new classification has been introduced (50) (Fig. 40.16). Major vascular injuries to the hepatic arteries, especially the right hepatic artery, may occur in association with biliary injuries and sometimes lead to intraoperative blood loss. Hepatic infarction has not been a major problem, presumably because of the dual blood supply of the liver. Isolated vascular injuries to hepatic vessels are rare. Avoidance of injuries with use of the techniques described above is of paramount importance. Although the increase in cholecystectomy rates means that the total number of deaths from cholecystectomy has not decreased, an individual patient's risk for death is smaller.

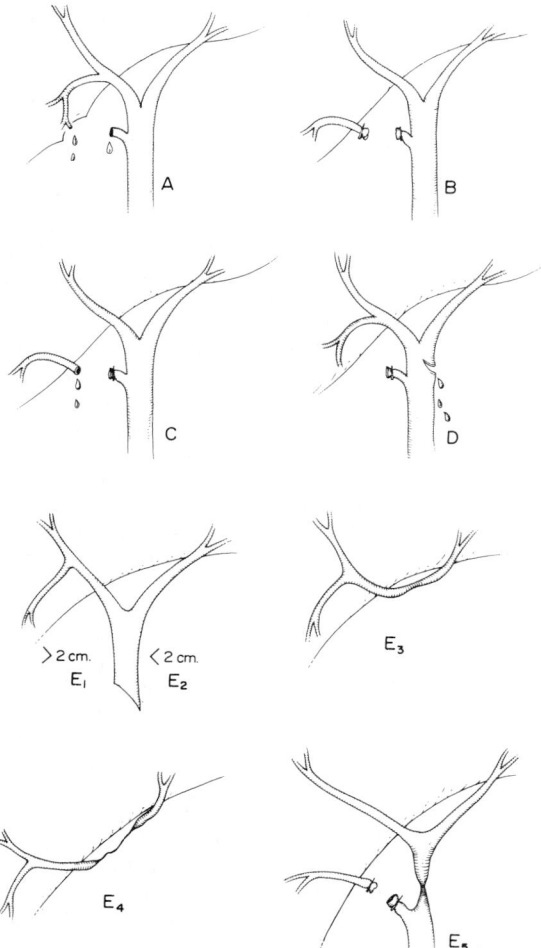

Figure 40.16. Classification of laparoscopic injuries to the biliary tract. Types A through E injuries are illustrated. Type E injuries are subdivided according to the Bismuth classification. Type A injuries occur when there is insecure closure of the cystic duct or when small bile ducts are entered in the liver bed. Types B and C injuries almost always involve aberrant right hepatic ducts. Types A, C, D, and some E injuries may cause bilomas or fistulae. Type B and other type E injuries occlude the biliary tree and bilomas do not occur. (From Strasberg SM, Hertl M, Soper NJ. An analysis of the problem of biliary injury during laparoscopic cholecystectomy. *J Am Coll Surg* 1995;180:101–125, with permission.)

Spillage of stones into the peritoneal cavity during laparoscopic cholecystectomy occurs in 10% or more of cases. Leaving stones in the peritoneal cavity may not be innocuous (55). Intraabdominal abscess, subcutaneous abscess, and later discharge of stones through the abdominal wall or through the lung and trachea have all been described. Every attempt should be made to remove spilled stones by picking and irrigating them out. Clearance is usually quite successful with the use of retractors to lift the liver and the 30-degree laparoscope, which allows the depths of the recess between liver and kidney to be visualized. Laparoscopic ultrasonography may be useful to detect stones. Large stones or massive spills should be cleaned up by laparotomy if necessary. If there is any chance that stones have been left behind, the patient should be informed.

As in open cholecystectomy, a gallbladder containing an unsuspected cancer is excised one to three times per 1,000 laparoscopic cholecystectomies. It is good practice to open the gallbladder and inspect it and obtain frozen sections in suspect circumstances. If cancer is suspected, the gallbladder should be extracted in an impermeable bag. If a cancer is discovered, it should be treated at that time. The tissue surrounding the umbilical trocar port is excised as part of the treatment because seeding at that site may have occurred. When the tumor is discovered on later pathologic examination, early reoperation is the approach of choice. Gallbladder carcinomas that have clear resection margins probably require no further surgical treatment other than excision of the umbilical port site. Those that have penetrated more deeply or that have positive resection margins require further surgery.

Open Cholecystectomy

Open cholecystectomy is performed in the minority of patients for whom laparoscopic cholecystectomy is contraindicated, who require conversion intraoperatively, or who require laparotomy for another operation. The gallbladder is dissected free of the hepatic bed from the "top down" after identification but before division of the cystic structures. This allows definitive demonstration of the cystic duct and cystic artery and prevents damage to the remaining biliary tree or hepatic arterial circulation. Drains are no longer used routinely after this procedure.

COMPLICATED GALLSTONE DISEASE

Acute Calculous Cholecystitis

Acute calculous cholecystitis is an inflammatory complication of cholelithiasis. It is usually a sterile chemical inflammation, but secondary bacterial inflammation may occur. The two conditions that seem to be necessary for inflammation to develop are an obstructed cystic duct and altered bile chemistry—particularly the supersaturation of bile with cholesterol. Both these conditions are potentially associated with cholesterol cholelithiasis. Why inflammation develops only occasionally when biliary colic is present is uncertain; it is perhaps related to the duration of obstruction of the gallbladder by a stone. The mediators of the inflammation are not known. Lysolecithin, a highly detergent product of lecithin, appears to be important and may damage and increase the permeability of mucosal cell membranes. Other potential mediators of importance are bile salts and platelet-activating factor. With obstruction, the gallbladder becomes a secretory rather than an absorptive organ, and it becomes full and tense. Hyperemia and edema of the gallbladder wall cause it to thicken and take on a reddish external aspect; pericholecystic fluid is often present. Gangrene may supervene when secondary contamination with putrefactive organisms occurs. Perforation is more common under these circumstances. Emphysematous cholecystitis is another severe variant in which gas produced by gas-forming organisms accumulates in the wall and lumen of the gallbladder. The gas is detected on images and at surgery.

An attack of acute cholecystitis begins as an attack of biliary colic—a mechanical problem that evolves into an inflammatory problem. As in biliary colic, the initial event in acute cholecystitis is obstruction of the cystic duct by an impacted gallstone. Although the resulting pain is similar in onset and character to the pain associated with biliary colic, it is unremitting and may persist for several days. In a limited number of cases, the cystic duct remains obstructed, and one of the complications of acute cholecystitis may develop. These include empyema, gangrene, and contained or free perforation of the gallbladder with abscess formation.

The diagnosis of cholecystitis depends on the constellation of symptoms, signs, and characteristic findings on diagnostic imaging modalities. The pain of acute cholecystitis is similar to, but more severe than, the pain of biliary colic. The pain is typically in the right upper quadrant or epigastrium and is unremitting in comparison with the time-limited pain of biliary colic. The inflammatory process progresses to affect the parietal peritoneum, and patients become reluctant to move. In most patients, systemic complaints, such as anorexia, nausea, vomiting, and chills, are also present. The signs of acute cholecystitis include the systemic manifestations of inflammation, such as fever and tachycardia; rigors are uncommon. Local inflammatory signs, including tenderness and guarding, and peritoneal signs are usually present in the right upper quadrant or more diffusely. A mass, the inflamed gallbladder, is occasionally palpable, but guarding often prevents the appreciation of mass formation. Murphy's sign—inspiratory arrest during deep palpation of the right upper quadrant—is characteristic of acute cholecystitis. This is most informative when the acute inflammation has subsided and direct tenderness is absent. Severe jaundice is rare, but mild jaundice may be present—up to 6 mg/dL. Severe jaundice suggests the presence of common bile duct stones, cholangitis, or obstruction of the common hepatic duct by severe pericholecystic inflammation resulting from impaction of a large stone in Hartmann's pouch, which mechanically obstructs the bile duct (Mirizzi's syndrome). Some patients, especially the elderly, may have acute cholecystitis with minimal signs and symptoms, such as anorexia without spoken complaints of pain. Many patients do not have fever. It is not uncommon for acute cholecystitis to coexist with choledocholithiasis or it complications (acute cholangitis and acute pancreatitis). The coexistence of two of these conditions often explains an unusual or atypical clinical presentation.

Laboratory abnormalities may include leukocytosis (typically a white blood cell count of 12,000 to 15,000/mm^3). However, many patients have a normal white blood cell count. A white cell count above 20,000 should suggest further complication of cholecystitis, such as gangrene, perforation, or cholangitis. Serum liver chemistries, including bilirubin (usually < 3 mg/dL), alkaline phosphatase, and amylase, also may be abnormal.

Diagnostic imaging confirms the clinical impression of acute calculous cholecystitis. Ultrasonography is the most sensitive and specific test for diagnosing acute cholecystitis. Ultrasonographic findings include stones, thickening of the gallbladder wall (≥ 4 mm), and pericholecystic fluid. A sonographic Murphy's sign has also been described

(which in this case means direct tenderness over the gallbladder when it is compressed by the ultrasonic probe).

Radionuclide cholescintigraphy occasionally is needed to provide additional information in cases that are not well defined by ultrasonography. Scintigraphic scanning is performed with derivatives of aminodiacetic acid [hepatic 2,6-dimethyliminodiacetic acid (HIDA), paraisopropyliminodiacetic acid (PIPIDA), diisopropyliminodiacetic acid (DISIDA)]. Concentration of the radionuclide in the bile by the liver allows the demonstration of bile flow from the liver into the common hepatic duct, filling or nonfilling of the gallbladder, and emptying of the gallbladder and biliary tree into the duodenum. Because they depend on hepatic excretion of bile, these tests are not useful when the serum bilirubin exceeds 3 mg/dL. However, newer agents such as 99mTc-mebrofenin may image the biliary tract when the serum bilirubin level is above 20 mg/dL. Nonfilling of the gallbladder after 4 hours of observation in the appropriate clinical setting is good evidence of acute cholecystitis. A completely normal test result is filling within 30 minutes. The sensitivity and specificity of the test may be increased by administering morphine to put the sphincter of Oddi into spasm and thereby encourage gallbladder filling.

Computed tomography occasionally is performed in evaluating the patient with abdominal pain and acute illness. CT may demonstrate evidence of acute cholecystitis, including gallbladder wall thickening, pericholecystic fluid and edema, gallstones, and air in the gallbladder or gallbladder wall (emphysematous cholecystitis), although it is less sensitive for these conditions than ultrasonography.

The initial management for patients with acute cholecystitis includes hospitalization, intravenous fluid resuscitation, and systemic antibiotics. The antibiotic regimen should be appropriate for typical bowel flora (gram-negative rods and anaerobes). Typical regimens are (a) a third-generation cephalosporin with good anaerobic coverage, (b) a second-generation cephalosporin combined with metronidazole, and (c) an aminoglycoside with metronidazole. Although enterococci are frequently cultured from the gallbladder in acute cholecystitis, it is not necessary to cover these organisms separately because they are rarely a solitary pathogen. In many cases, the inflammation is sterile; however, antibiotics have become standard because it is difficult to determine who has become secondarily infected. In some countries, antibiotics are withheld unless systemic signs of sepsis are present or the patient is elderly or immunosuppressed (e.g., diabetics).

The definitive treatment of acute cholecystitis is cholecystectomy, but the timing of the procedure is controversial. Early cholecystectomy is performed soon after the patient is admitted with the diagnosis of acute cholecystitis, usually the same day or the next day. Interval or delayed cholecystectomy is performed 2 to 3 months after nonoperative treatment of the acute attack. The interval is intended to allow the acute inflammation to settle. The results of randomized controlled trials performed in the era of open cholecystectomy attested to the benefits of early versus interval cholecystectomy for acute cholecystitis (56,57). Two trials performed in the laparoscopic era support this position, citing a prolonged hospital stay (58,59) and recuperation period (59) in the delayed group. However, these studies were performed in cohorts of about 100 patients and cannot determine whether the number of bile duct injuries is increased when the procedure is performed acutely. Laparoscopic cholecystectomy in acute cholecystitis was found to be associated with a higher rate of biliary injury in a statewide experience involving more than 30,000 cholecystectomies (60). Furthermore, percutaneous cholecystostomy was either not used or used infrequently in these trials, so that it was necessary to perform urgent surgery in an unusually large number of patients in the delayed group as a result of failed conservative management that might not have failed had percutaneous cholecystostomy been used.

Early cholecystectomy has the advantage of resolving the illness in a shorter time frame. However, the laparoscopic approach must be used early in the course of the disease, while inflammation around the gallbladder is still minimal. This operation is best performed within 48 hours after the onset of symptoms and in the same fashion as for symptomatic gallstones. Overall conversion rates are higher because of inflammation but are not significantly lowered by delayed cholecystectomy. Conversion rates are higher in patients with a longer duration of symptoms, higher white blood cell counts, higher levels of alkaline phosphatase, and higher APACHE II scores (acute physiology and chronic health evaluation) (61). Approximately 80% of attempts at laparoscopic cholecystectomy during acute cholecystitis can be completed successfully. Patients enjoy the same postoperative benefits as after elective laparoscopic cholecystectomy, and generally laparoscopic cholecystectomy can be performed safely during the phase of acute inflammation. Open cholecystectomy is also an option in acute cholecystitis and can probably be performed safely somewhat later (up to 72 hours) after the onset of the illness. Perioperative antibiotics are universally recommended.

When interval cholecystectomy is selected, the acute attack is managed with intravenous fluids and antibiotics. The response to treatment must be assessed frequently, and assessment should include physical examination and monitoring of the patient's fever curve and laboratory values. If the patient's condition does not improve, then the treatment must be altered—to a different antibiotic regimen, percutaneous cholecystostomy, or operative cholecystectomy, or cholecystostomy, usually percutaneous cholecystostomy (Fig. 40.17). In most patients, acute cholecystitis resolves with nonoperative treatment, and delayed cholecystectomy can be performed after 2 to 3 months, usually laparoscopically. This regimen is occasionally the only option for patients who present after 3 to 4 days of continuous symptoms of acute cholecystitis.

Cholecystostomy can be performed in patients with acute cholecystitis who are failing systemic therapy but are not candidates for cholecystectomy because of locally severe illness or concomitant medical problems. Cholecystostomy can be performed either operatively or percutaneously. The latter is less invasive and allows the gallbladder to be drained, which almost uniformly resolves the episode of acute cholecystitis. However, the patient must be observed closely, and if improvement does not occur within 24 hours, laparotomy is indicated. Failure to improve after percutaneous cholecystostomy is usually caused by gangrene of the gallbladder or perforation. After the acute episode resolves, the patient can undergo either cholecystectomy or percutaneous stone extraction and removal of the cholecystostomy tube. The latter is an option in elderly or debilitated patients for whom a general anesthetic is contraindicated.

Gallstone Ileus

Gallstone ileus is a rare complication of acute cholecystitis in which the lower small bowel is obstructed by a large gallstone. The gallstone generally has eroded from the gallbladder into the duodenum and passed through the small bowel until it reaches the narrower ileum, where it can no longer pass. The patient presents with small-bowel obstruction and air in the biliary tree from the passage of bowel gas through the cholecystoduodenal fistula. At

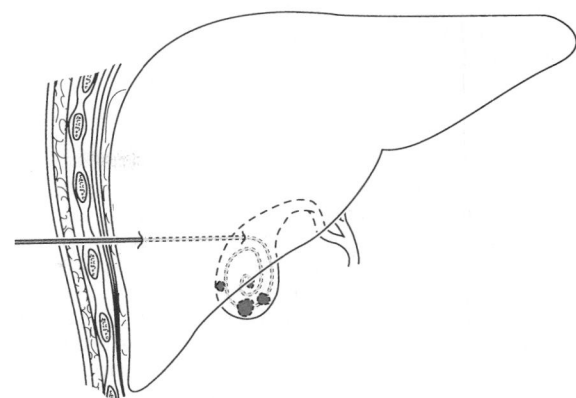

Figure 40.17. Schematic demonstration of the technique of percutaneous placement of a pigtail catheter into the gallbladder.

operation, the stone(s) is milked back into an area of normal bowel and removed by enterotomy. Rarely, segmental small-bowel resection is required. The bowel should be searched for other stones.

The management of cholecystoduodenal fistula is controversial. Because these patients are usually elderly, with a single large stone that has passed and with marked scarring around the gallbladder from chronic biliary tract disease, some surgeons recommend not addressing the biliary enteric fistula at all. Others recommend dividing the fistula, removing the gallbladder, and appropriately closing the duodenum after débridement; this is most appropriate when large stones remain in the gallbladder. Management should be individualized, based on the patient's clinical status at the time of surgery and the presence or absence of residual stones in the gallbladder.

Choledocholithiasis and Its Complications

Choledocholithiasis is generally caused by gallstones that have passed from the gallbladder through the cystic duct into the common duct. There, they can become lodged and obstruct the biliary tree, causing symptoms. In Western countries, stones rarely form primarily in the hepatic or common ducts. Patients with choledocholithiasis are on average about 10 years older than patients with uncomplicated gallbladder disease, presumably because it takes some time for stones to pass into the bile duct.

Patients with choledocholithiasis may be asymptomatic, or they may present with jaundice (bilirubin typically < 10 mg/dL), pain, or both. The first manifestation of disease may also be cholangitis or gallstone pancreatitis. The pain caused by a stone in the bile duct is virtually identical to the biliary colic caused by impaction of a stone in the gallbladder. Nausea and vomiting are common; pruritus is uncommon, probably because the obstruction is usually incomplete and of short duration. Physical signs commonly are limited to icterus. Ultrasonography is a useful test, although it directly demonstrates the stone(s) in only 20% to 30% of cases. Frequently, gallstones in the lower common bile duct cannot be demonstrated by ultrasonography because of overlying bowel gas. However, indirect ultrasonographic signs are usually present, consisting of bile duct dilatation and gallbladder stones in a patient with jaundice and perhaps pain. The alkaline phosphatase level is often highly elevated. Acute impaction of a gallstone in the bile duct may cause a sharp rise in serum transaminases that lasts 24 to 48 hours. Because obstruction by gallstones is usually incomplete and often intermittent, urine urobilin is usually elevated, as is urine bilirubin; in complete obstruction, urobilin is absent from the urine. Generally, the diagnosis depends on the demonstration of enlarged common bile and intrahepatic ducts in association with abnormal serum liver chemistries. The diagnosis often is confirmed by endoscopic retrograde cholangiopancreatography (ERCP) or sometimes by percutaneous transhepatic cholangiography (PTC), both of which opacify the biliary tree and demonstrate the intraductal stones.

It is routine to search for asymptomatic choledocholithiasis in a patient who is about to undergo a cholecystectomy. A dilated bile duct (> 6 mm) on ultrasonography or abnormal serum liver chemistries (alkaline phosphatase, transaminase, or bilirubin) suggest the presence of bile duct stones, as do previous attacks of jaundice or pancreatitis. Management of suspected or actual choledocholithiasis in a patient who also has gallbladder stones and requires a cholecystectomy depends on the available expertise. Unless they are elderly or have prohibitive concomitant medical problems, all patients should undergo cholecystectomy. Jaundiced patients should undergo preoperative ERCP to rule out malignancy. Cholelithiasis is a common condition and may coexist with periampullary cancers; one should be particularly suspicious of cancer when the jaundice is not associated with pain and is complete, and the patient is more than 60 years of age. Patients known to have many, large, or intrahepatic stones should undergo endoscopic extraction preoperatively because such stones are difficult to extract laparoscopically. With other types of stones, or when stones are suspected, at centers with experienced laparoscopic biliary surgeons, a laparoscopic cholecystectomy is performed, and operative cholangiography or intraoperative laparoscopic ultrasonography (Fig. 40.18) is performed to determine the site and number of stones actually present at the time of surgery. If stones are present, laparoscopic bile duct exploration follows, by means of fluoroscopic cholangiography, biliary balloon catheters, stone baskets, or direct laparoscopic common bile duct exploration. All this re-

quires an institutional commitment to equipment and expertise that is not available at every site.

If the patient's common bile duct cannot be cleared of stones at the laparoscopic operation, ERCP with sphincterotomy and clearance of the common bile duct is performed postoperatively. It is possible that the bile duct cannot be cleared by either laparoscopic exploration or ERCP, and a subsequent open reoperation may be required to effect this, but this situation is very rare in experienced hands. Small stones less than 3 mm in diameter often pass spontaneously. Larger stones do not and may cause serious complications; if a patient has had gallstone pancreatitis, even a very small stone should be considered dangerous. Stones larger than 5 mm and a stone of any size in a patient who has had gallstone pancreatitis should be removed soon after surgery, usually the day after. There is a small chance that pancreatitis will develop in the interval between failed extraction and ERCP. An alternative but overall more morbid approach is to perform an open bile duct exploration. It is good practice to explain these alternatives to the patient. It should be noted that a randomized controlled trial has not compared the treatment of stones diagnosed during operative cholangiography by laparoscopic exploration of the bile duct versus postoperative ERCP.

An alternative strategy in centers where this expertise is not available is preoperative ERCP with sphincterotomy in all patients who are at high risk for common bile duct stones or in whom common bile duct stones have been demonstrated. ERCP with sphincterotomy carries a 1% risk of mortality and 10% risk of morbidity. When ERCP is based simply on ultrasonographic and laboratory risk factors, the negative rate exceeds 50%. For this reason, preoperative ERCP based on risk factors for stones has fallen out of favor and has been replaced with a regimen of operative cholangiography to diagnose stones followed by postoperative ERCP in centers where laparoscopic bile duct exploration is not performed. In such centers, when preoperative ERCP is unsuccessful at clearing the common bile duct of stones, the patient may require open cholecystectomy and common bile duct exploration because one cannot rely on postoperative extraction. With widen-

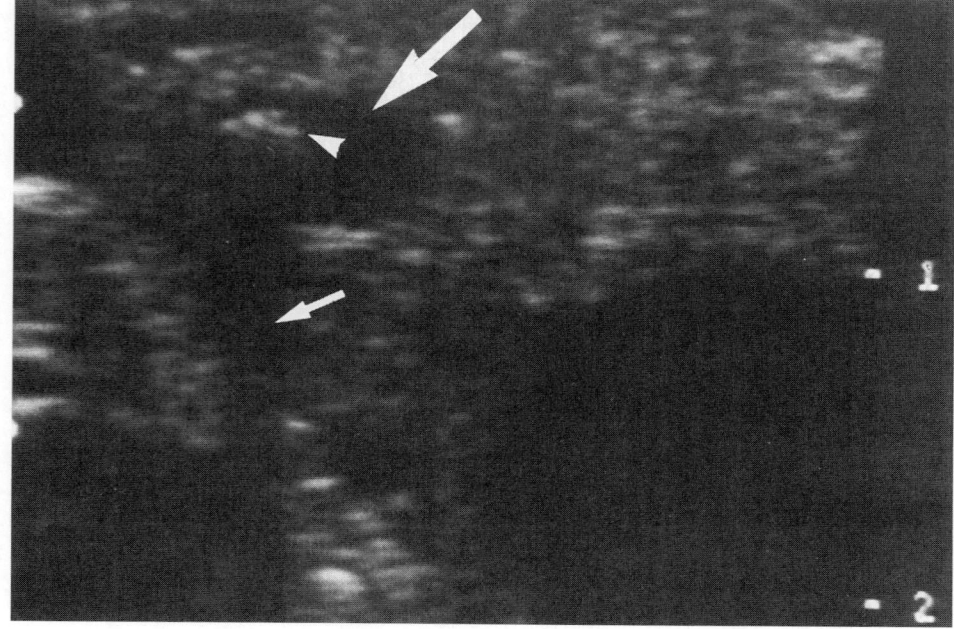

Figure 40.18. Laparoscopic sonography of bile duct *(large arrow)* showing calculus *(arrowhead)* and acoustic shadow *(small arrow)*.

ing expertise in laparoscopic exploration and ERCP, these considerations are becoming less important.

Patients over the age of 70 presenting only with symptoms of choledocholithiasis or cholangitis need not undergo cholecystectomy after the stones are cleared from the bile duct by ERCP. Symptoms attributable to residual cholecystolithiasis develop later in only about 15% of these elderly patients, and they can be treated as the need arises by cholecystectomy or percutaneous methods.

In some cases, choledocholithiasis is diagnosed days to years after a cholecystectomy, and these stones are removed whenever possible by nonoperative techniques, usually endoscopic sphincterotomy and extraction. Occasionally, percutaneous transhepatic methods or ESWL is needed for large or impacted stones in this postcholecys-

tectomy group. Stones can also be treated through a T-tube tract if one has been placed at surgery (Fig. 40.19).

Cholangitis

Cholangitis is one of the two main complications of choledocholithiasis, the other being acute gallstone pancreatitis. Gallstones are the most common cause of cholangitis, but cholangitis can be caused by parasites, instrumentation or indwelling stents, benign and malignant strictures, and partially obstructed biliary–enteric anastomoses. Unlike acute cholecystitis, acute cholangitis is nearly always a bacterial infection. In acute cholangitis, infection develops behind a partially obstructing stone. It

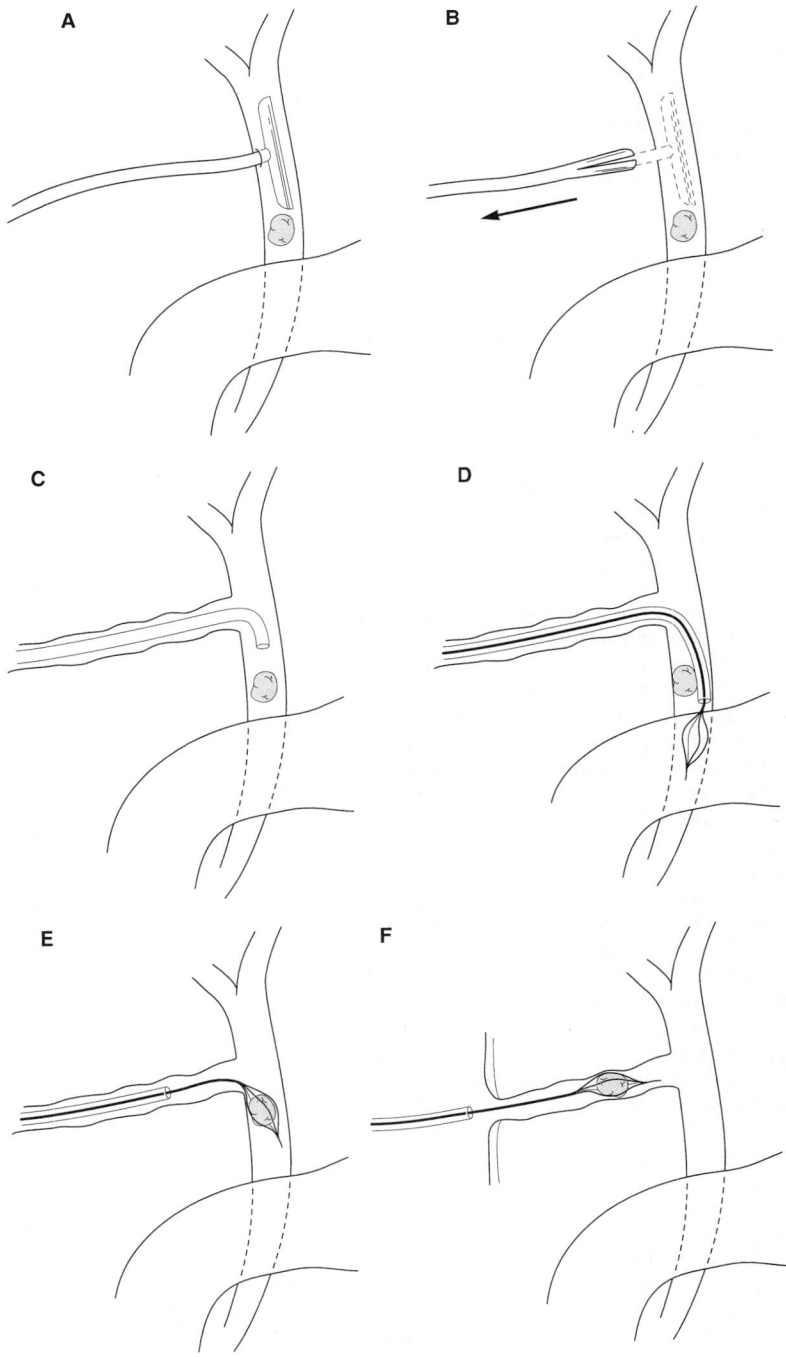

A **B** **C** **D** **E** **F**

Figure 40.19. Illustration of Burhenne technique, with placement of basket down matured tract and stone extraction.

is likely that bacteria intermittently enter the biliary tree through the ampulla, bloodstream, or lymphatics. Bacteria are cleared mechanically by bile flow and by the presence of antibacterial substances in bile, such as immunoglobulin A; hepatic bile is normally sterile. In the presence of a stone, mechanical clearance is interrupted, bile formation is inhibited, and contamination may become infection. The infection spreads rapidly throughout the biliary tree, a huge surface area, and bacteria readily enter the systemic circulation to cause septicemia. These factors explain why acute cholangitis is usually a much more serious inflammation than acute cholecystitis. Acute cholangitis should always be considered to be potentially life-threatening, although cholangitis encompasses a spectrum of diseases ranging from subclinical illness to acute toxic cholangitis.

Patients presenting with gallstone-induced cholangitis are often older and female. They often present with a combination of systemic and local symptoms. Commonly, the illness commences with a sudden shaking chill (rigor), followed by the high fever of septicemia. The patient may become disoriented secondary to septic shock. Jaundice and right upper quadrant pain are frequent symptoms. These symptoms have been categorized in two well-known eponymous groups. Charcot's triad is the combination of fever, jaundice, and right upper quadrant pain, present in 50% to 70% of patients. Reynolds' pentad is Charcot's triad plus hemodynamic instability and mental status changes. Local signs are indistinguishable from those of acute cholecystitis.

Ultrasonography is a useful investigation in the patient who is not known to have gallstone disease because it usually establishes the presence of cholecystolithiasis and dilated bile ducts, but the definitive diagnostic measure is ERCP. If ERCP is not available or fails, PTC is indicated. These studies demonstrate the level of obstruction and allow culture of bile, removal of stones, and placement of drainage catheters if necessary. Blood should be drawn for culture from all patients.

The initial management of cholangitis includes intravenous antibiotics appropriate for the coverage of the most commonly cultured organisms: *Escherichia coli, Klebsiella pneumoniae, Streptococcus faecalis,* and less commonly *Bacteroides fragilis.* For patients with acute toxic cholangitis or who fail to respond to antibiotic therapy, emergency decompression of the biliary tree is required. This is typically accomplished by endoscopic sphincterotomy and nasobiliary drainage or temporary stenting. Percutaneous transhepatic drainage is used when ERCP fails or is unavailable. If decompression by these less invasive means is not available or possible, then operative intervention to decompress the biliary tree is indicated. In such an unstable patient, operative intervention should be restricted to insertion of a T tube in the common bile duct. Stone extraction should be limited to those stones that can be extracted easily within a short period of time. In cases of cholangitis with a cause other than stones, a similar policy should be followed. Definitive operative therapy for benign or malignant biliary tract stricture should be deferred until a later date. Indwelling tubes or stents in patients who have cholangitis generally require repeated imaging and exchange over guide wire. Internal stents, whether placed percutaneously or endoscopically, may require a revision of the previous procedure or a new approach to biliary drainage to achieve decompression.

Oriental cholangiohepatitis, also known as *recurrent pyogenic cholangitis,* is a special form of cholangitis. It is endemic to the Orient and is caused by biliary parasites such as *Clonorchis sinensis, Opisthorchis viverrini,* and *Ascaris lumbricoides.* These parasites are associated with bacterial contamination of the biliary tree. As outlined in the section on brown stones, bacterial contamination results in the deconjugation of bilirubin, which precipitates in the bile as sludge. The sludge and dead bacterial cell bodies form brown stones. Unlike the stones in Western disease, these stones form throughout the biliary tree, including the intrahepatic biliary tree, and cause a partial obstruction, which in turn leads to repeated bouts of cholangitis. The consequences of cholangitis are biliary strictures (which themselves promote stone formation and infection), hepatic abscesses, and eventually complete destruction of the liver (secondary biliary cirrhosis). Strictures may be found anywhere in the biliary tree but are common in the main hepatic ducts. The left duct is more frequently and severely affected than the right. Symptoms and signs are those of recurrent cholangitis. The patients are typically young and thin and present with right upper quadrant pain, fever, and jaundice. The episodes vary in severity from chronic subclinical illness, leading gradually to generalized symptoms of hepatic insufficiency and malnutrition, to severe acute suppurative cholangitis with hypotension, mental status changes, acidosis, and death in the absence of acute intervention.

Diagnostic imaging demonstrates the typical diffuse biliary findings and multiple stones. Ultrasonography can reveal biliary obstruction, stones in the biliary tree, pneumobilia from infection with gas-forming organisms, liver abscesses, or occasionally strictures. Intrahepatic stones are very well demonstrated by their characteristic posterior acoustic shadowing. In contrast, ultrasonography is not the best means for demonstrating strictures, although some may be evident with this modality.

Computed tomography can demonstrate similar findings and can also provide detailed information about the hepatic anatomy and amount of hepatic parenchyma remaining in more advanced disease. In addition, it can help guide liver resection. ERCP and PTC are the mainstays of biliary imaging for oriental cholangiohepatitis. As in more conventional forms of cholangitis, these studies can detect biliary obstruction, define the level of biliary strictures and stones, and allow acute decompression of the biliary tree.

The management of oriental cholangiohepatitis consists of treatment of biliary strictures and extraction of stones or resection of the involved area when the disease is localized to one part of the liver. During acute episodes of cholangitis, temporary percutaneous or endoscopic drainage must be achieved to alleviate sepsis. In occasional patients known to have oriental cholangiohepatitis and stricture of the lower duct, acute surgical intervention with drainage of the common bile duct by T-tube placement is appropriate. Typically, management of the acute episode involves biliary drainage and systemic supportive care, including intravenous antibiotics and hydration. On a long-term basis, the multiple biliary strictures and stones must be treated; generally, multiple percutaneous or endoscopic approaches to the biliary tree with dilatation are required. In specialized centers, percutaneous access to the biliary tree can be established through a large tract. Through this tract, strictures can be dilated and stones extracted by applying a combination of radiologic and percutaneous endoscopic techniques during multiple sessions.

Another approach is to perform surgery in which the gallbladder is removed and a wide hepaticojejunostomy with a Roux limb is created. Stone extraction and stricture dilation are performed at the time of surgery, but only rarely can all stones be removed or strictures dilated at this time. Intrahepatic stones may also pass postoperatively through the large anastomosis, but this also usually is not sufficient. Therefore, the blind end of the Roux limb is brought into a subcutaneous position in the right flank and marked with a radiopaque ring. Postoperatively, multiple interventional procedures, in which strictures are dilated and stones removed, can be performed through this limb. The limb should not be brought to the surface anteriorly because this puts the radiologist's hands directly under the roentgen rays. In cases in which the disease is very extensive, it is simpler to establish a jejunostomy at this point and close it after treatment, usually 1 to 2 years later. Not infrequently, the damaged area is completely or mainly confined to one portion of the liver, usually the left half or left lateral section, and in these cases, liver resection is appropriate and highly effective.

Biliary Pancreatitis

Biliary pancreatitis is caused by obstruction of the pancreatic duct by a common duct stone, although the mechanism by which temporary obstruction of the pancreatic duct leads to pancreatitis is still not completely clear (see Chapter 30). The management of biliary tract disease in this entity includes ERCP with sphincterotomy if the patient has severe acute pancreatitis, which may be caused by an impacted stone at the ampulla. Otherwise, ERCP in the acute setting probably is not indicated. Once the episode of acute pancreatitis has resolved, the gallbladder should be removed while the patient is still hospitalized to prevent recurrent acute biliary pancreatitis. Exceptionally, the pancreatitis is so severe that several weeks must elapse before cholecystectomy is performed. Preoperative ERCP is unnecessary because most of the time the causative stone has passed, but an operative cholangiogram should always be obtained to prove that this is so. If a patient with gallstone pancreatitis requires surgical exploration (e.g., in the case of infected necrosis), cholecystostomy with stone extraction is recommended. Cholecystectomy is often difficult in these circumstances and should not be attempted unless it is obviously straightforward

Acalculous Cholecystitis

Acalculous cholecystitis typically occurs in a patient with other acute systemic illness (e.g., after major burns, major trauma, or significant abdominal or thoracic operation; during or after prolonged parenteral nutrition; in association with an episode of systemic sepsis; or during multiple organ system failure).

Symptoms and signs depend largely on the patient's concurrent medical conditions. Alert patients often complain of right upper quadrant or diffuse upper abdominal pain and tenderness. Laboratory evaluation may demonstrate an elevated white blood cell count and bilirubin and alkaline phosphatase levels may also be increased. The patient may also have less specific findings of transaminase elevations. In patients with more severe systemic illness, the symptoms and signs may not be evident because of sedation or alteration of consciousness because of the illness. In such patients, elevated alkaline phosphatase or bilirubin levels are indications for further investigation.

Diagnostic imaging is the key to establishing the diagnosis of acalculous cholecystitis. Ultrasonography is inexpensive and can be performed at the bedside of a critically ill patient. It can demonstrate the typical findings of acalculous or calculous cholecystitis, including gallbladder wall thickening, pericholecystic fluid, and abscess formation in the right upper quadrant. The study can be limited, however, by overlying bowel gas or concomitant abdominal wounds or dressings, and it does suffer from some false-negative outcomes. Abdominal CT is as sensitive as ultrasonography for this condition and allows imaging of the remainder of the abdominal cavity from

the lung bases to the pelvis. This modality can investigate other intraabdominal problems that may be a part of the differential diagnosis, particularly in postoperative patients. CT generally is not impaired by overlying dressings, wounds, or bowel gas. The disadvantage of CT is that the patient must be moved to the radiology department, which adds risk for a critically ill person. If the diagnosis is in doubt, percutaneous cholecystostomy is both diagnostic and therapeutic.

The management of acalculous cholecystitis must be tailored to the individual patient. Definitive management includes urgent cholecystectomy. However, most affected patients are not fit to tolerate a major abdominal operation. In these cases, percutaneous cholecystostomy is the procedure of choice; it resolves the cholecystitis in more than 90% of patients and generally is well tolerated. Concomitant management must include systemic antibiotics, maintenance of NPO (nothing by mouth) status, and treatment of the concomitant illnesses that have placed the patient at risk for this disease. The response to treatment must be monitored, and if improvement is not apparent within 24 hours, then other steps must be taken. Failure is usually caused by gangrene with perforation or a mistaken diagnosis. Cholecystectomy is performed after the patient has recovered from concomitant illnesses, if needed.

REFERENCES

1. Sanabria JR, Upadhya GA, Harvey RP, et al. Diffusion of substances into human cholesterol gallstones. *Gastroenterology* 1994;106:749–754.
2. Everhart JE, Khare M, Hill M, et al. Prevalence and ethnic differences in gallbladder disease in the United States. *Gastroenterology* 1999;117:632–639.
3. Chijiiwa K, Kiyosawa R, Nakayama F. Cholesterol monomer activity correlates with nucleation time in model bile. *Clin Chim Acta* 1988;178:181–191.
4. Carey MC, Small DM. The physical chemistry of cholesterol solubility in bile: relationship to gallstone formation and dissolution in man. *J Clin Invest* 1978;61:998–1026.
5. Ulloa N, Garrido J, Nervi F. Ultracentrifugal isolation of vesicular carriers of biliary cholesterol in native human and rat bile. *Hepatology* 1987;7:235–244.
6. Konikoff FM, Chung DS, Donovan JM, et al. Filamentous, helical, and tubular microstructures during cholesterol crystallization from bile: evidence that cholesterol does not nucleate classic monohydrate plates. *J Clin Invest* 1992;90:1155–1160.
7. Einarsson K, Nilsell K, Leijd B, et al. Influence of age on secretion of cholesterol and synthesis of bile acids by the liver. *N Engl J Med* 1985;313:277–282.
8. Bertolotti M, Abate N, Bertolotti S, et al. Effect of aging on cholesterol 7-alpha-hydroxylation in humans. *J Lipid Res* 1993;34:1001–1007.
9. Bennion LJ, Grundy SM. Effects of obesity and caloric intake on biliary lipid metabolism in man. *J Clin Invest* 1975;56: 996–1011.
10. Stahlberg D, Rudling M, Angelin B, et al. Hepatic cholesterol metabolism in human obesity. *Hepatology* 1997;25:1447–1450.
11. Ahmed HA, Jazrawi RP, Goggin PM, et al. Intrahepatic biliary cholesterol and phospholipid transport in humans: effect of obesity and cholesterol cholelithiasis. *J Lipid Res* 1995;36: 2562–2573.
12. Everson GT, McKinley C, Kern F Jr. Mechanisms of gallstone formation in women: effects of exogenous estrogen (Premarin) and dietary cholesterol on hepatic lipid metabolism. *J Clin Invest* 1991;87:237–246.
13. Kern F Jr. Effects of dietary cholesterol on cholesterol and bile acid homeostasis in patients with cholesterol gallstones. *J Clin Invest* 1994;93:1186–1194.
14. Everson GT, McKinley C, Lawson M, et al. Gallbladder function in the human female: effect of the ovulatory cycle, pregnancy, and contraceptive steroids. *Gastroenterology* 1982;82: 711–719.
15. Khanuja B, Cheah YC, Hunt M, et al. Lith1, a major gene af-

fecting cholesterol gallstone formation among inbred strains of mice. *Proc Natl Acad Sci USA* 1995;92:7729–7733.

16. Berr F, Kullak-Ublick GA, Paumgartner G, et al. 7-Alpha-dehydroxylating bacteria enhance deoxycholic acid input and cholesterol saturation of bile in patients with gallstones. *Gastroenterology* 1996;111:1611–1620.

17. Holzbach RT, Marsh M, Olszewski M, et al. Cholesterol solubility in bile: evidence that supersaturated bile is frequent in healthy man. *J Clin Invest* 1973;52:1467–1479.

18. Holan KR, Holzbach RT, Hermann RE, et al. Nucleation time: a key factor in the pathogenesis of cholesterol gallstone disease. *Gastroenterology* 1979;77:611–617.

19. Pomeranz IS, Shaffer EA. Abnormal gallbladder emptying in a subgroup of patients with gallstones. *Gastroenterology* 1985;88:787–791.

20. Fridhandler TM, Davison JS, Shaffer EA. Defective gallbladder contractility in the ground squirrel and prairie dog during the early stages of cholesterol gallstone formation. *Gastroenterology* 1983;85:830–836.

21. Behar J, Lee KY, Thompson WR, et al. Gallbladder contraction in patients with pigment and cholesterol stones. *Gastroenterology* 1989;97:1479–1484.

22. Yu P, Chen Q, Biancani P, et al. Membrane cholesterol alters gallbladder muscle contractility in prairie dogs. *Am J Physiol* 1996;271:G56–G61.

23. Burnstein MJ, Ilson RG, Petrunka CN, et al. Evidence for a potent nucleating factor in the gallbladder bile of patients with cholesterol gallstones. *Gastroenterology* 1983;85:801–807.

24. Lee SP, LaMont JT, Carey MC. Role of gallbladder mucus hypersecretion in the evolution of cholesterol gallstones. *J Clin Invest* 1981;67:1712–1723.

25. Harvey PR, Upadhya GA, Strasberg SM. Immunoglobulins as nucleating proteins in the gallbladder bile of patients with cholesterol gallstones. *J Biol Chem* 1991;266:13996–14003.

26. Offner GD, Gong D, Afdhal NH. Identification of a 130-kilodalton human biliary concanavalin A-binding protein as aminopeptidase N. *Gastroenterology* 1994;106:755–762.

27. Pattinson NR, Willis KE. Effect of phospholipase C on cholesterol solubilization in model bile: a concanavalin A-binding nucleation-promoting factor from human gallbladder bile. *Gastroenterology* 1991;101:1339–1344.

28. Abei M, Kawczak P, Nuutinen H, et al. Isolation and characterization of a cholesterol crystallization promoter from human bile. *Gastroenterology* 1993;104:539–548.

29. Yamashita G, Secknus R, Chernosky A, et al. Comparison of haptoglobin and apolipoprotein A-I on biliary lipid particles involved in cholesterol crystallization. *J Gastroenterol Hepatol* 1996;11:738–745.

30. Lipsett PA, Fox-Talbot MK, Falconer SD, et al. Biliary nonmucin glycoproteins in patients with and without gallstones. *J Surg Res* 1995;58:386–390.

31. Afdhal NH, Niu N, Nunes DP, et al. Mucin–vesicle interactions in model bile: evidence for vesicle aggregation and fusion before cholesterol crystal formation. *Hepatology* 1995;22:856–865.

32. Yamashita G, Corradini SG, Secknus R, et al. Biliary haptoglobin, a potent promoter of cholesterol crystallization at physiological concentrations. *J Lipid Res* 1995;36:1325–1333.

33. Gallinger S, Harvey PR, Petrunka CN, et al. Biliary proteins and the nucleation defect in cholesterol cholelithiasis. *Gastroenterology* 1987;92:867–875.

34. Moser AJ, Abedin MZ, Roslyn JJ. Increased biliary protein precedes gallstone formation. *Dig Dis Sci* 1994;39:1313–1320.

35. Tudyka J, Kratzer W, Kuhn K, et al. Solitary versus multiple gallstones: the importance of total biliary protein concentration and other factors. *Hepatogastroenterology* 1995;42:638–644.

36. Roslyn JJ, Conter RL, DenBesten L. Altered gallbladder concentration of biliary lipids during early cholesterol gallstone formation. *Dig Dis Sci* 1987;32:609–614.

37. Haley-Russell D, Husband KJ, Moody FG. Morphology of the prairie dog gallbladder: normal characteristics and changes during early lithogenesis. *Am J Anat* 1989;186:133–143.

38. Sanabria JR, Upadhya A, Mullen B, et al. Effect of deoxy-

cholate on immunoglobulin G concentration in bile: studies in humans and pigs. *Hepatology* 1995;21:215–222.

39. Rege RV, Prystowsky JB. Inflammation and a thickened mucus layer in mice with cholesterol gallstones. *J Surg Res* 1998;74:81–85.

40. Kibe A, Holzbach RT, LaRusso NF, et al. Inhibition of cholesterol crystal formation by apolipoproteins in supersaturated model bile. *Science* 1984;225:514–516.

41. Wolpers C, Hofmann AF. Solitary versus multiple cholesterol gallbladder stones: mechanisms of formation and growth. *Clin Invest* 1993;71:423–434.

42. Allen B, Bernhoft R, Blanckaert N, et al. Sludge is calcium bilirubinate associated with bile stasis. *Am J Surg* 1981;141:51–56.

43. Conter RL, Roslyn JJ, Pitt HA, et al. Carbohydrate diet-induced calcium bilirubinate sludge and pigment gallstones in the prairie dog. *J Surg Res* 1986;40:580–587.

44. Friedman GD, Raviola CA, Fireman B. Prognosis of gallstones with mild or no symptoms: 25 years of follow-up in a health maintenance organization. *J Clin Epidemiol* 1989;42:127–136.

45. Ransohoff DF, Gracie WA, Wolfenson LB, et al. Prophylactic cholecystectomy or expectant management for silent gallstones: a decision analysis to assess survival. *Ann Intern Med* 1983;99:199–204.

46. Berk RN, Armbuster TG, Saltzstein SL. Carcinoma in the porcelain gallbladder. *Radiology* 1973;106:29–31.

47. Strasberg SM, Clavien PA. Cholecystolithiasis: lithotherapy for the 1990s. *Hepatology* 1992;16:820–839.

48. Burnstein MJ, Vassal KP, Strasberg SM. Results of combined biliary drainage and cholecystokinin cholecystography in 81 patients with normal oral cholecystograms. *Ann Surg* 1982;196:627–632.

49. Sanabria JR, Gallinger S, Croxford R, et al. Risk factors in elective laparoscopic cholecystectomy for conversion to open cholecystectomy. *J Am Coll Surg* 1994;179:696–704.

50. Strasberg SM, Hertl M, Soper NJ. An analysis of the problem of biliary injury during laparoscopic cholecystectomy. *J Am Coll Surg* 1995;180:101–125.

51. Teefey SA, Soper NJ, Middleton WD, et al. Imaging of the common bile duct during laparoscopic cholecystectomy: sonography versus videofluoroscopic cholangiography. *AJR Am J Roentgenol* 1995;165:847–851.

52. McMahon AJ, Russell IT, Baxter JN, et al. Laparoscopic versus minilaparotomy cholecystectomy: a randomised trial. *Lancet* 1994;343:135–138.

53. Barkun JS, Barkun AN, Sampalis JS, et al. Randomised controlled trial of laparoscopic versus minicholecystectomy: the McGill Gallstone Treatment Group. *Lancet* 1992;340:1116–1119.

54. Steiner CA, Bass EB, Talamini MA, et al. Surgical rates and operative mortality for open and laparoscopic cholecystectomy in Maryland. *N Engl J Med* 1994;330:403–408.

55. Leslie KA, Rankin RN, Duff JH. Lost gallstones during laparoscopic cholecystectomy: are they really benign? *Can J Surg* 1994;37:240–242.

56. Jarvinen HJ, Hastbacka J. Early cholecystectomy for acute cholecystitis: a prospective randomized study. *Ann Surg* 1980;191:501–505.

57. Lahtinen J, Alhava EM, Aukee S. Acute cholecystitis treated by early and delayed surgery: a controlled clinical trial. *Scand J Gastroenterol* 1978;13:673–678.

58. Lai P, Kwong K, Leung K, et al. Randomized trial of early versus delayed laparoscopic cholecystectomy for acute cholecystitis. *Br J Surg* 1998;85:764–767.

59. Lo CM, Liu CL, Fan ST, et al. Prospective randomized study of early versus delayed laparoscopic cholecystectomy for acute cholecystitis. *Ann Surg* 1998;227:461–467.

60. Russell JC, Walsh SJ, Mattie AS, et al. Bile duct injuries, 1989–1993: a statewide experience. Connecticut Laparoscopic Cholecystectomy Registry. *Arch Surg* 1996;131:382–388.

61. Rattner DW, Ferguson C, Warshaw AL. Factors associated with successful laparoscopic cholecystectomy for acute cholecystitis. *Ann Surg* 1993;217:233–236.

SURGERY: SCIENTIFIC PRINCIPLES AND PRACTICE, Third Edition, edited by
Lazar J. Greenfield, Michael W. Mulholland, Keith T. Oldham, Gerald B. Zelenock,
and Keith D. Lillemoe. Lippincott Williams & Wilkins Publishers, Philadelphia, © 2001.

CHAPTER 41

BILIARY NEOPLASMS

SHARON WEBER AND YUMAN FONG

Tumors arising in the gallbladder and biliary tree are often asymptomatic until late in the course of the disease. Consequently, these tumors commonly present in an advanced, often unresectable, stage. Surgery remains the only curative option for biliary malignancies. Resection of biliary neoplasms, however, often requires radical resections and complex biliary reconstructions that have only recently become safe in routine practice. Surgery also offers effective palliation for these cancers, including biliary bypasses for jaundiced patients with unresectable tumors. Both the late diagnosis and the complex operative techniques required for potentially curative resection contribute to the challenge of these cases. In addition, there are no proven effective options for adjuvant treatment. This chapter reviews the incidence, diagnosis, and therapy of these malignancies as well as the outcome of treatment.

GALLBLADDER CARCINOMA

Gallbladder cancer is a rare malignancy with a dismal outlook because of its insidious onset, propensity for local invasion, and rapid disease progression. Overall, most series report a 5-year survival rate of less than 5%. The extent of surgical resection remains ill defined because of the rarity of this lesion and its poor prognosis.

Incidence

Only 6,000 to 7,000 new cases of gallbladder cancer are diagnosed nationally each year (1). Attesting to the rarity of this lesion, after routine screening abdominal ultrasonography (US) in asymptomatic patients in Japan, only 19 of 194,767 people screened (0.01%) were found to have gallbladder cancer (2). This tumor occurs more frequently in women (female-to-male ratio = 3 : 1) and the peak incidence is in the seventh decade (1). There is an increased risk of gallbladder cancer in Native American populations of the United States and Mexico. The increased risk of gallbladder cancer with cholelithiasis is well established; 70% to 90% of all patients with carcinoma also have gallstones. However, less than 0.5% of patients with gallstones are found to have gallbladder cancer. After elective cholecystectomy for gallstones, gallbladder cancer is found incidentally in 1% of patients. The association of gallstones with carcinoma is probably related to chronic inflammation. Larger stones (>3 cm) are associated with a 10-fold increased risk of cancer.

This association of gallbladder cancer with gallstone disease has prompted the question of whether all patients with gallstones should undergo cholecystectomy. The use of cholecystectomy for symptomatic patients only, thus leaving the gallbladder in place in patients with asymptomatic gallstones, has not led to an increase in the prevalence of gallbladder cancer. Also, epidemiologic studies have found the 20-year risk for development of cancer in patients with gallstones is less than 0.5% for the overall population and 1.5% for high-risk groups. Therefore, rou-

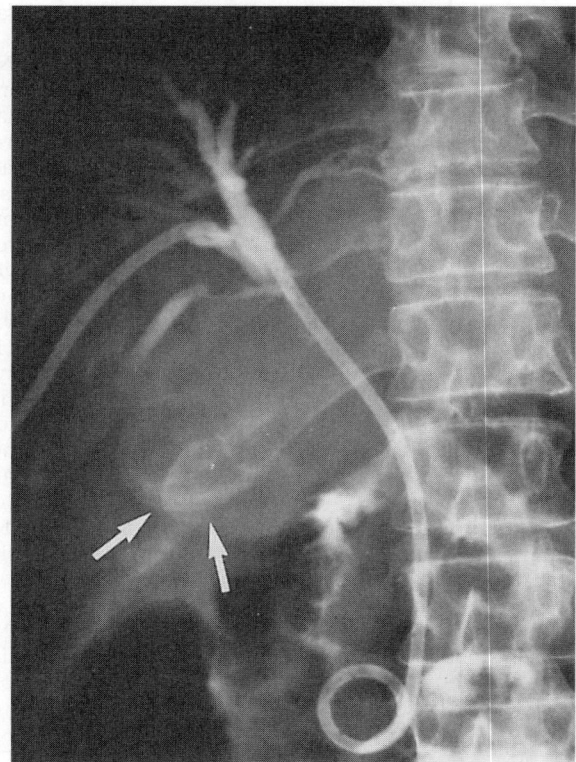

Figure 41.1. Unresectable gallbladder cancer demonstrating palliative transhepatic percutaneous stent placed to relieve jaundice. Porcelain gallbladder is present *(arrows)*.

tine cholecystectomy for asymptomatic gallstones because of concern about gallbladder cancer does not appear to be warranted. However, because of the 25% to 60% incidence of cancer in those with "porcelain gallbladder," or calcification of the gallbladder wall, all patients with this finding should undergo cholecystectomy, even if asymptomatic (Fig. 41.1). Patients with choledochal cysts have an increased risk of carcinoma developing anywhere in the biliary tree, but the incidence is highest in the gallbladder. This risk increases with age. Therefore, complete surgical resection is recommended for all patients with choledochal cysts at the time of diagnosis.

Pathology and Staging

More than 80% of gallbladder cancers are adenocarcinomas; there are several histologic subtypes, including papillary, nodular, and tubular. Prognostically, grade is important because patients with well differentiated tumors have an improved prognosis (3). Less than 5% of cases are squamous cell carcinomas, and the remaining 10% are anaplastic lesions.

Gallbladder cancer spreads through the lymphatic and venous drainage. Because the cholecystic veins drain directly into the adjacent liver, these tumors often involve hepatic parenchyma, most often portions of segments IV and V. Lymphatic spread first involves the cystic duct (Calot's) node, then the pericholedochal and hilar nodes, and finally the peripancreatic, duodenal, periportal, celiac, and superior mesenteric artery nodes. Nodal disease in the porta often causes common bile duct (CBD) obstruction and resultant jaundice, which is the first clinical symptom in 30% of patients. Jaundice may also be caused by tumors arising in the infundibulum, which may spread directly to the cystic duct and common hepatic duct. Although peritoneal metastases are frequent, distant extraperitoneal metastases are not.

The American Joint Committee on Cancer's (AJCC) TNM staging system (Table 41.1) reflects prognostic characteristics of tumor depth, regional nodal disease, or distant spread. The gallbladder differs histologically from the rest of the gastrointestinal tract in that it lacks a muscularis mucosa and submucosa. The gallbladder wall is composed of (a) a single layer of columnar cells, the mucosa, and lamina propria; (b) a fibromuscular layer; (c) a perimuscular, subserosal layer containing lymphatics and neurovascular structures; and (d) a serosal surface, except where the gallbladder is embedded in the liver. Because lymphatics are present in the subserosal layer only, tumors invading less than the full thickness of the muscular layer have minimal risk of nodal spread. Thus, disease invading into but not through the muscular layer of the gallbladder is stage I disease. Stage II disease has invaded the perimuscular, subserosal layer without spread to the liver and without nodal disease. Nodal disease or infiltration less than 2 cm into the liver without nodal involvement is stage III, with stage IV disease including liver invasion greater than 2 cm or distant metastases.

The most useful alternative staging system is the modified Nevine classification (4). One problem with the TNM staging system is that it includes tumors with invasion into the liver but without positive nodes as stage III. How-

Table 41.1. AJCC STAGING SYSTEM FOR GALLBLADDER CARCINOMA

Stage	Tumor	Nodes	Metastasis
0	Tis	N0	M0
I	T1	N0	M0
II	T2	N0	M0
III	T1	N1	M0
	T2	N1	M0
	T3	N0	M0
	T3	N1	M0
IVA	T4	N0	M0
	T4	N1	M0
IVB	Any T	N2	M0
	Any T	Any N	M1

Definition of TNM
Primary Tumor (T)
TX   Primary tumor cannot be assessed
T0   No evidence of primary tumor
Tis   Carcinoma in situ
T1   Tumor invades the lamina propria or muscle layer
  T1a   Tumor invades the lamina propria
  T1b   Tumor invades the muscle layer
T2   Tumor invades the perimuscular connective tissue; no extension beyond the serosa or into the liver
T3   Tumor perforates the serosa or directly invades one adjacent organ (extends <2 cm into the liver)
T4   Tumor extends more than 2 cm into the liver, or into two or more adjacent organs (stomach, duodenum, colon, pancreas, omentum, extrahepatic bile ducts, any involvement of liver)
Regional lymph nodes (N)
NX   Regional lymph nodes cannot be assessed
N0   No regional lymph node metastasis
N1   Metastasis in the cystic duct, pericholedochal, or hilar lymph nodes (i.e., in the hepatoduodenal ligament)
N2   Metastasis in the peripancreatic (head only), periduodenal, periportal, celiac, superior mesenteric, or superior mesenteric lymph nodes
Distant metastasis (M)
MX   Presence of distant metastasis cannot be assessed
M0   No distant metastasis
M1   Distant metastasis

Table 41.2. MODIFIED NEVINE CLASSIFICATION FOR GALLBLADDER CANCER

Stage	Extent of tumor
I	Mucosa only
II	Mucosa and muscular invasion
III	Transmural direct liver invasion
IV	Regional lymph node involvement
V	Distant spread

ever, because patients with liver invasion alone have better outcomes than those with involved nodes, staging systems have been advocated that correlate more closely with prognostic factors such as lymph node metastases (Table 41.2). This will likely result in a change in the TNM classification system in the future.

Clinical Findings and Diagnosis

In patients with symptoms, abdominal pain consistent with biliary colic or acute cholecystitis is most common. Most patients are found to have gallbladder cancer during work-up or treatment of cholelithiasis or choledocholithiasis. Patients also present with jaundice, weight loss, anorexia, or an increase in abdominal girth secondary to ascites. Physical findings include right upper quadrant tenderness or a palpable mass, hepatomegaly, and ascites. Laboratory investigation results, if abnormal, are most often consistent with biliary obstruction. Because of its nonspecific presentation and the lack of reliable screening tests, gallbladder cancer is not diagnosed before surgery in over half the cases.

Imaging evaluation often reveals a thickened gallbladder wall or a mass within or replacing the gallbladder on US examination. Because polyps and carcinoma can have an echogenicity similar to that of the gallbladder wall, these lesions are often difficult to distinguish. This distinction is even more difficult when inflammation is present from gallstones. At times, US can visualize invasion of the liver, adjacent adenopathy, and a dilated biliary tree. The ability of US to differentiate benign from neoplastic disease is enhanced with the use of endoscopic US, which may be more specific than computed tomography (CT) or magnetic resonance imaging (MRI) (5).

CT scan may identify a gallbladder mass or invasion into the liver parenchyma or adjacent organs. The sensitivity and specificity of contrast-enhanced CT in diagnosing neoplastic lesions is close to 90% (6). However, staging of gallbladder carcinoma using CT is limited by poor sensitivity in identifying nodal spread (7). Angiography may be necessary to assess the extent of vascular involvement. Also, in patients who are jaundiced, direct cholangiography may be useful to delineate the extent of biliary involvement. A mid-bile duct obstruction not due to gallstones is suspect for gallbladder cancer (Fig. 41.2). More recently, with the improvements in MRI technology, magnetic resonance cholangiopancreatography has evolved into a single noninvasive imaging modality that allows complete assessment of biliary, vascular, hepatic parenchymal, and nodal involvement, as well as involvement of adjacent organs (7–9) (Fig. 41.3).

Surgery

Cholecystectomy with or without Partial Hepatectomy

Gallbladder cancer, if not completely surgically removed, results in rapid local progression and death. In a

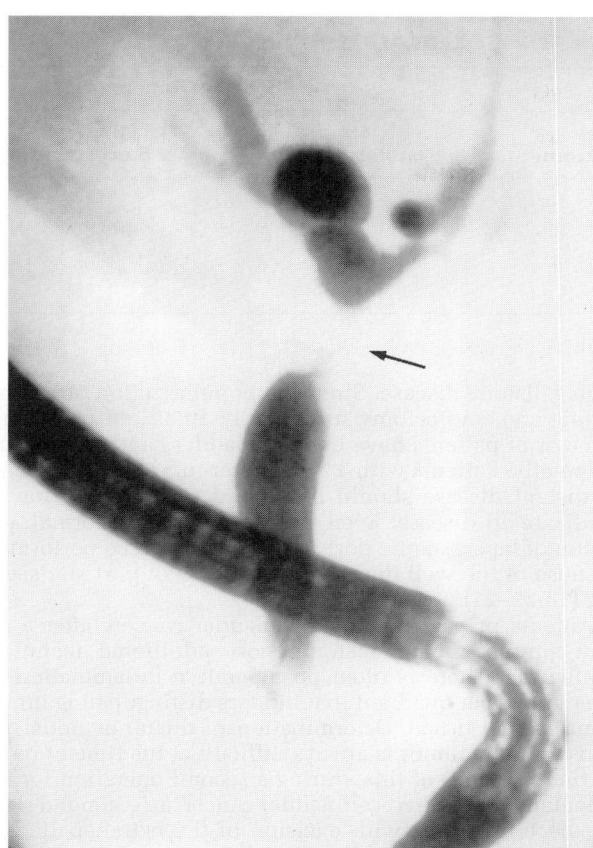

Figure 41.2. Endoscopic retrograde cholangiopancreatogram obtained from a patient with gallbladder cancer. Mid-bile duct obstruction *(arrow)* is due to direct extension of tumor to the cystic and common hepatic duct.

collected review of 5,836 patients with gallbladder cancer, the overall mean survival time was between 2 and 5 months, whereas the 5-year survival rate was 4% (10). The 5-year survival rate of patients undergoing resection with curative intent was 17%. Of the 2,115 unresectable patients, there was only one 5-year survivor. Although surgi-

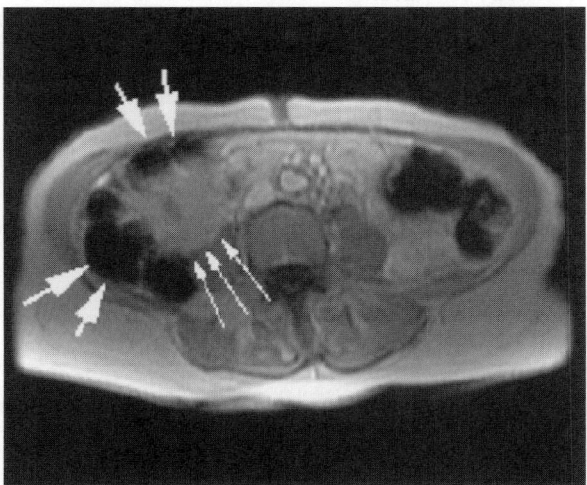

Figure 41.3. T$_1$-weighted magnetic resonance imaging scan of a patient with gallbladder cancer *(small arrows)* with extension into the duodenum and the hepatic flexure of the colon *(large arrows)*.

cal resection represents the treatment of choice and the only potentially curative therapy available, resection is possible in only 25% of patients at presentation because of the advanced stage of the disease (10).

There is little doubt that the results of treatment, as well as the scope of operation, are related to depth of penetration of the tumor (Table 41.3). For tumors limited to the muscular layer of the gallbladder (T1), there is near-universal agreement that simple cholecystectomy is adequate (11–14). T1 tumors have not yet invaded the subserosal layer, which contains lymphatics, and therefore lymphadenectomy is not required. Attesting to the fact that early gallbladder carcinoma is completely curable, simple cholecystectomy has resulted in near 100% survival rates when early cancer is an incidental finding after elective cholecystectomy (14,15).

The extent of surgical resection for T2 or greater tumors is controversial, with recommendations ranging from simple cholecystectomy to radical excision including hepatectomy. For advanced local disease, some groups have advocated radical resections including hepatectomy and pancreatectomy. Although it is clear that major hepatic resection can be performed safely with a mortality rate of less than 5% (12–17) (Table 41.4), it has not been universally accepted that more aggressive resections improve survival. To understand the rationale for extensive resections, it is necessary to understand the pattern of spread of gallbladder cancer. Direct extension to the adjacent liver parenchyma often occurs first, followed by adjacent organ involvement, including duodenum, colon, and stomach (Fig. 41.3). Lymphatic spread of gallbladder cancer is routine, often involving nodes in the porta hepatis, peripancreatic region, celiac axis, and the aortocaval nodal basins.

For tumors with full-thickness invasion of the muscular layer into the perimuscular connective tissue, but not to the serosa (T2), radical cholecystectomy, with resection of segments 4b and 5 of the liver parenchyma, is required. Because the gallbladder is not surrounded by serosa where it is attached to the liver, even T2 tumors may invade into the plane of dissection on the hepatic side of the gallbladder for a simple cholecystectomy. Therefore, T2 tumors cannot be completely removed with cholecystectomy alone. Complete excision of tumor is more likely with a procedure involving resection of segments 4B and 5, the segments immediately surrounding the gallbladder bed, where direct tumor extension into the liver occurs. Regional lymphadenectomy is an important part of this procedure. Half the patients with T2 tumors are found to have nodal spread after resection (16). Dissection of lymph nodes should include all tissue from the bifurcation of the hepatic ducts to the distal CBD and include nodes along the hepatic artery to the celiac axis. Proponents of this approach advocate liver resection on the basis that it is the only way to obtain an adequate margin on the hepatic side of the gallbladder, and resection of the regional nodes allows the best chance for tumor clearance. For all of these reasons, simple cholecystectomy is inadequate.

When segments 4b and 5 have been resected in patients with T2 tumors, it has increased the 5-year survival rate from 25%–40% after simple cholecystectomy to 70%–100% after radical resection (11,12,14,16,18,19). For T3 and T4 lesions, there is a high likelihood of intraperitoneal and hematogenous spread and significant morbidity from the radical procedures that are often necessary for excision of local disease. Recent series, however, support an aggressive approach to resection of these large tumors, particularly if no indication of nodal involvement is found (Table 41.4). Local recurrence after resection of gallbladder cancer usually occurs in segments 4, 5, and 8 because of the venous drainage of the gallbladder into intrahepatic

Table 41.3. **FIVE-YEAR SURVIVAL RATES AFTER RESECTION FOR GALLBLADDER CANCER**

Institution	T1 or T2 Tumors		T3 or T4 Tumors	
	Simple cholecystectomy	Radical cholecystectomy	Simple cholecystectomy	Radical cholecystectomy
University of Virginia 1982[18]	33%	—	3%	13%
Tohoku University 1987[11]	57%	100%	0%	23%
Hamamatsu University 1989[17]	—	100%	—	15%
Mayo Clinic 1990[12]	—	—	0%	29%
Nigata University 1992[13]	—	72%	—	37%

right portal branches (66% of patients), left portal branches (6%), or both right and left (28%) (20). Therefore, some have advocated hepatectomy of segments 4, 5, and 8. Most often, however, a right extended hepatectomy (trisegmentectomy, segments 4, 5, 6, 7, and 8) is necessary for complete excision of tumor. With aggressive resection, long-term survival can be achieved for patients with stage III or IV disease (12–14,16,17,21).

Surgical exploration should be performed for all patients with no medical contraindications. If a T1 tumor is suspected, a cholecystectomy and biopsy of regional nodes should be performed after thorough examination of the abdominal cavity for any signs of tumor dissemination. The pathologic type and depth of penetration should be confirmed by frozen section, and the procedure terminated if a T1 tumor with negative margins is confirmed. For T2 lesions, a resection of segments 4b and 5 with lymphadenectomy should be performed (16). For T3 and T4 lesions, a more radical excision of the liver, such as extended right hepatectomy, usually must be performed for adequate tumor clearance.

Location of the tumor may be important in determining the extent of resection. If the tumor arises in the gallbladder infundibulum, the CBD is often involved with tumor, either by direct extension or external invasion of the hepatoduodenal ligament. In this case, an extended liver resection and removal of a portion of the CBD should be performed. Reconstruction is then performed by Roux-en-Y hepaticojejunostomy. Tumor arising in the fundus of the gallbladder can be treated with limited hepatic resection without excision of the CBD. Complete lymphadenectomy should include posterior superior pancreatic nodes and nodes in the hepatoduodenal ligament. To clear the porta hepatis nodes, the CBD, hepatic artery, and portal vein should be fully exposed. Skeletonizing the CBD, hepatic artery, and portal vein is absolutely essential to perform an adequate lymphadenectomy. Often, excision of the CBD is necessary to facilitate nodal clearance.

Incidentally or Laparoscopically Discovered Gallbladder Cancer

Gallbladder cancer is often discovered during pathologic examination after cholecystectomy for presumed be-

nign gallstone disease. Since the popularization of laparoscopic cholecystectomy in the early 1990s, an increasing number of patients have had gallbladder cancer found incidentally. Patients with T2 or greater tumors and no signs of distant disease should be offered radical resection to eradicate all disease. Even if they are grossly normal, excision of laparoscopic port sites should also be performed because of the well documented history of port site seeding (18,22–24).

Patients presenting with gallbladder cancers after a recent simple cholecystectomy pose additional technical challenges. There is often postoperative inflammation in the right upper quadrant that hinders distinguishing tumor from normal tissue. Determination of ductal or nodal involvement by tumor is always difficult at the time of reoperation. Because of this, during a second operation for incidentally discovered gallbladder cancer, an extended right hepatectomy along with excision of the extrahepatic biliary tree and periductal lymphatic tissues is almost always necessary. This resection allows adequate excision of the lymphatic tissues at the confluence of the bile ducts, provides greater confidence of a negative margin on the bile duct, and permits biliary reconstruction to only one side of the liver. The disadvantage is that a large portion of normal liver parenchyma is sacrificed and, consequently, transient postoperative liver dysfunction is common.

When a patient presents with T1 gallbladder cancer discovered after simple cholecystectomy, histopathologic study should determine if the entire gallbladder has been removed and if the cystic duct margin is clear of tumor. If the cystic duct margin is positive, the patient requires local bile duct excision. If all margins are negative, no further therapy is warranted. If the tumor is proven to be T2 or greater, the patient should undergo a radical excision if the extent of disease evaluation is negative. Patients with a known or suspected early gallbladder carcinoma should not undergo laparoscopic cholecystectomy. Rather, open exploration and cholecystectomy should be performed.

Adjuvant Therapy

No study has shown efficacy of radiation or chemotherapy in the treatment of gallbladder cancer. Response to

Table 41.4. **RESULTS AFTER RADICAL RESECTION FOR GALLBLADDER CANCER**

Institution	Operative mortality	No. resected	Stage III–IV	5-Year survival rate
Hamamatsu University 1989[17]	0	15	87%	25%
Mayo Clinic 1990[12]	2	42	40%	33%
Japan Multicenter 1991[13]	5	1,686	50%	51%
Nigata University 1992[14]	0	40	53%	65%
Kyushu University 1994[21]	0	32	75%	53%
Memorial Sloan-Kettering Cancer Center 1996[16]	0	23	78%	58%

chemotherapy has consistently been less than 10%. Radiation therapy has been attempted, but results are unclear because of the limited sample sizes of the published series.

Prognosis

The 5-year survival rate of all patients with gallbladder cancer is less than 5% in most series, with a median survival of 6 months. This is primarily because most patients present with unresectable disease. Of those patients undergoing resection, survival depends on depth of penetration and nodal status. Near 100% survival rates are reported after simple cholecystectomy for T1 disease, whereas T2 and T3 tumors without nodal disease have a 5-year survival rate greater than 50% (14–20). Node positivity is an ominous finding, with few series reporting 5-year survivors.

Follow-up after Resection for Gallbladder Cancer

The most common site of recurrence after resection of gallbladder cancer is intraabdominal, specifically in the liver or the celiac or retropancreatic nodal basins. Jaundice is a common sign, but recurrence may also present with carcinomatosis. If recurrent disease is found after resection, prognosis is exceedingly poor. Death occurs secondary to biliary sepsis or liver failure.

Because gallbladder cancer is usually treated by a radical surgical resection and complex reconstruction, diagnosis of locally recurrent disease is difficult and excision of a recurrence even more so. The only exception is in patients with T1 gallbladder cancer previously treated with a simple cholecystectomy. A local recurrence in these patients may be treatable with a more radical resection. For most tumors, however, local recurrence is found synchronously with diffuse intraabdominal spread. Therefore, treatment of recurrence has little potential for cure. No study has proven the efficacy of chemotherapy or radiation therapy in the treatment of recurrent disease. Consideration of chemotherapy or radiation in patients with recurrent disease must take into account their limited life span.

The main goal of follow-up after resection of gallbladder cancer is to provide palliation of symptomatic recurrences. The main symptoms associated with recurrence requiring palliation are pruritus or cholangitis associated with jaundice, and bowel obstruction associated with carcinomatosis. The other goals of follow-up are to detect benign complications of surgical treatment (e.g., biliary stricture, peptic ulcer disease) and to provide patient reassurance. When jaundice or cholangitis is found, a nonsurgical palliative approach using percutaneous transhepatic cholangiography (PTC) and stenting is usually favored unless a benign postsurgical stricture is suspected. Because of the rapid growth of tumor and impending demise of the patient, the hospitalization and recovery time from a surgical bypass is usually not justified for recurrences resulting in biliary obstruction.

Therefore, the routine follow-up of a patient after resection of gallbladder cancer includes office visits every 3 months with physical examination and measurement of liver function tests. Although carcinoembryonic antigen (CEA) is often produced by gallbladder cancer and serum CEA levels have been advocated as a tool in the diagnosis of this malignancy, use of this tumor marker in follow-up is not recommended. We also do not favor using complex imaging studies to assess for recurrence. Because it is unlikely that an asymptomatic recurrence will be treated, the financial cost of measuring tumor markers or conducting imaging studies is not justified. When patients become symptomatic with jaundice, an abdominal sonogram should be obtained. This allows for assessment of intrahepatic ductal dilatation as well as portal vein patency. Need for further imaging with CT or direct cholangiography is usually dictated by the sonographic findings.

BILE DUCT CARCINOMA

Incidence

Cholangiocarcinoma is a rare cancer that arises from the biliary epithelium and occurs in less than 4,500 patients in the United States each year. Cholangiocarcinoma has a relatively even distribution between men and women with a male : female ratio of 1.3 : 1. The average age of patients presenting with bile duct cancer is between 50 and 70 years. Risk factors for this disease include primary sclerosing cholangitis, ulcerative colitis, choledochal cysts, and biliary tract infection, either with *Clonorchis* or in chronic typhoid carriers. Surgical resection is the most effective treatment option and the only curative option.

Pathology and Staging

Similar to gallbladder cancer, bile duct tumors tend to invade locally. Over 95% of these tumors are adenocarcinomas. They are morphologically described as nodular, which is the most common, scirrhous, diffusely infiltrating, or papillary. Histologic subtypes include acinar, ductular, trabecular, alveolar, and papillary. Much less common types of bile duct tumors include cystadenocarcinomas, hemangioendotheliomas, and mucoepidermoid carcinomas.

Historically, cholangiocarcinomas have been classified according to their location in the upper (60%), middle (15% to 20%), or lower third (15% to 20%) of the bile duct. Middle-third lesions arise between the cystic duct and the superior border of the duodenum. Lower-third lesions are found below the superior border of the duodenum but above the ampulla. The problem with this classification is that the anatomic landmarks are somewhat arbitrary and not clinically useful. Most mid-bile duct malignant obstructions are due to gallbladder cancers. Even when the tumor is truly a mid-bile duct cholangiocarcinoma, very few of these tumors are amenable to treatment by local excision of the bile duct. A more useful classification is to divide these lesions into upper-half or lower-half tumors (based on the location of the cystic duct as it enters the common duct). This allows the surgeon to delineate whether a hepatic or pancreatic resection, respectively, is required for clearance of tumor. The AJCC TNM staging system for bile duct cancers is described in Table 41.5.

Cholangiocarcinoma occurring at the hepatic hilus is commonly referred to as *hilar cholangiocarcinoma* or *Klatskin's tumors*. These tumors have been further classified into four types, based on the modified Bismuth-Corlette classification (25) (Fig. 41.4). Other staging systems have been created that attempt to incorporate clinically important indicators of resectability, such as hepatic lobe atrophy or portal vein involvement (26). Most important, with the increasing acceptance of major hepatic resection for these tumors, these systems attempt to define whether there is ipsilateral involvement alone, because tumors with bilateral extension past the primary biliary radicles are not resectable.

Clinical Findings and Diagnosis

Most patients with cholangiocarcinoma present with painless jaundice, although mild right upper quadrant

Table 41.5. AJCC STAGING SYSTEM FOR BILE DUCT CARCINOMA

Stage	Tumor	Nodes	Metastasis
0	Tis	N0	M0
I	T1	N0	M0
II	T2	N0	M0
III	T1	N1	M0
	T1	N2	M0
	T2	N1	M0
	T2	N2	M0
IVA	T3	Any N	M0
IVB	Any T	Any N	M1

Definitions of TNM

Primary tumor (T)
- TX Primary tumor cannot be assessed
- T0 No evidence of primary tumor
- Tis Carcinoma in situ
- T1 Tumor invades subepithelial connective tissue or fibromuscular layer
  - T1a Tumor invades subepithelial connective tissue
  - T1b Tumor invades fibromuscular layer
- T2 Tumor invades perifibromuscular connective tissue (invades tissue beyond the confines of the bile duct)
- T3 Tumor invades adjacent structures: liver, pancreas, duodenum, gallbladder, colon, stomach

Regional lymph nodes (N)
- NX Regional lymph nodes cannot be assessed
- N0 No regional lymph node metastasis
- N1 Metastasis in cystic duct, pericholedochal, or hilar lymph nodes (i.e., in the hepatoduodenal ligament)
- N2 Metastasis in peripancreatic (head only), periduodenal, periportal, celiac, superior mesenteric, or posterior pancreaticoduodenal lymph nodes

Distant metastasis (M)
- MX Presence of distant metastasis cannot be assessed
- M0 No distant metastasis
- M1 Distant metastasis

pain, pruritus, anorexia, malaise, and weight loss may also be reported. Cholangitis is the presenting symptom in 10% to 30% of patients. Some patients have cancer discovered on evaluation for otherwise asymptomatic elevations of alkaline phosphatase and γ-glutamyltransferase.

Abdominal US is noninvasive, easily available, and inexpensive, and thus is commonly used as a first-line imaging modality. It can establish the level of biliary obstruction while ruling out cholelithiasis or choledocholithiasis as the etiology. CT scans frequently reveal dilated intrahepatic biliary ducts with a normal, collapsed gallbladder and, depending on the level of the tumor, a nondilated or partially dilated extrahepatic biliary tree (Fig. 41.5). Portal vein patency can be determined with US or helical CT. In addition, signs of hepatic lobar atrophy should be sought because this is associated with a high incidence of ipsilateral portal vein involvement by tumor.

In most centers, selective celiac angiography and percutaneous cholangiography are used to evaluate the extent of vascular and biliary involvement. Endoscopic retrograde cholangiopancreatography (ERCP) plays a little role in high biliary obstruction because opacification of the proximal biliary tree is difficult. ERCP is used to image more distal lesions. During cholangiography, some authors advocate the routine preoperative placement of biliary drainage catheters for palliation and to aid in intraoperative identification of the bile ducts (27). Others have found a higher incidence of infectious complications (28) and mortality (29), and a longer hospital stay (30) after preoperative placement of biliary drainage catheters.

Magnetic resonance cholangiopancreatography offers the potential of evaluating parenchymal, vascular, biliary, and nodal involvement with a single, noninvasive examination (7–9). Frequently, it is possible to visualize the tumor itself with MRI (Figs. 41.6 and 41.7). In many cases, it is difficult to obtain pathologic confirmation of cholangiocarcinoma except in very advanced cases. For most cases, patients are offered surgical therapy based on clinical suspicion and radiographic appearance.

Surgery

Proximal Cholangiocarcinomas

Untreated, most patients with bile duct cancers die within a year of diagnosis. Surgical excision is the treatment of choice, with no other potentially curative therapy. The immediate causes of death are most commonly hepatic failure or cholangitis related to tumor growth and inadequate drainage of the biliary tree. Therefore, the objectives of management for patients with cholangiocarcinoma include both complete removal of tumor and adequate biliary drainage. It has become clear over the experience since the early 1970s that curative treatment of tumors involving the upper half of the bile duct depends on aggressive excision that often requires a major liver resection. Until as recently as the early 1990s, treatment of hilar cholangiocarcinomas was associated with mortality rate as high as 30% (31–33, 35,36). More recently, major improvements in the safety of these operations have been demonstrated, and resection of hilar tumors now results in a mortality rate of less than 10%, even when liver resections are required (31–35).

Assessment of Resectability and Surgical Procedure. Surgical exploration is often the only means of assessing resectability. Tumors are considered unresectable because of both local factors and metastatic spread. Local invasion of the main portal vein or both the right and left portal vein or hepatic arteries is considered unresectable disease, as is a tumor in the second-order biliary radicals of both right and left hepatic lobes. By contrast, tumors extending into second- or third-order biliary radicals on one side (with or without vascular involvement) can be resected with curative outcome. Peritoneal implants are often the

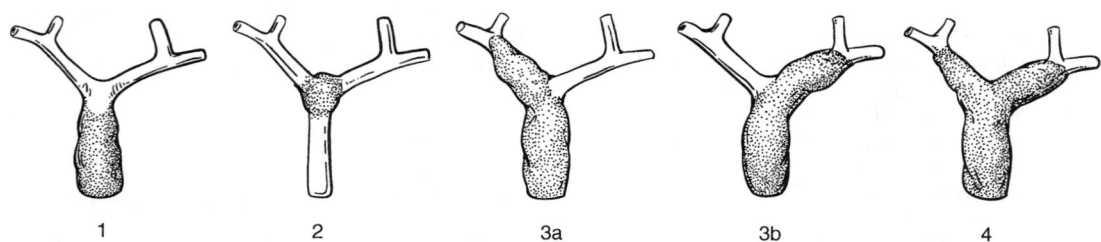

Figure 41.4. Modified Bismuth-Corlette classification for hilar cholangiocarcinomas.

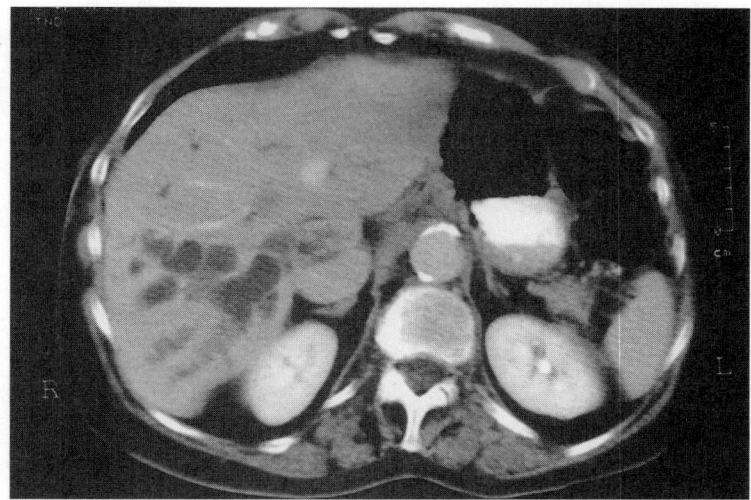

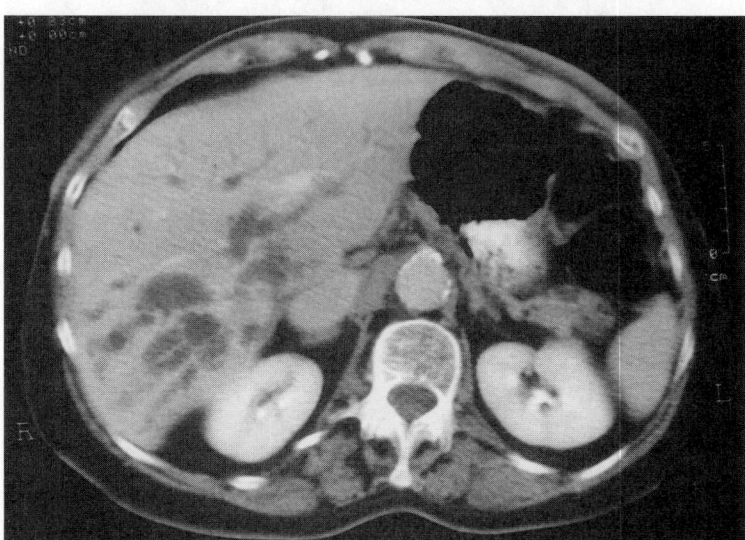

Figure 41.5. Computed tomography scan in a patient with hilar cholangiocarcinoma, demonstrating dilated intrahepatic ducts in the right lobe but inability to visualize tumor directly.

only evidence of metastatic disease, thereby suggesting a role for staging laparoscopy. Imaging studies such as angiography, cholangiography, and CT scan may suggest unresectable disease, but exploration should be offered to all patients with potentially resectable tumors. Most patients are unresectable at presentation, which is reflected in the poor overall survival rate.

The goals of surgical management for cholangiocarcinomas are eradication of tumor and establishment of adequate biliary drainage. Complete surgical excision accomplishes both these goals and is the treatment of choice for cholangiocarcinoma. Tumors of the biliary confluence are particularly difficult to treat because symptoms often appear late in the course of disease when the lesion has already involved adjacent structures, including the portal vein or adjacent hepatic parenchyma. Complete resection, therefore, requires biliary and hepatic resection and often major vascular reconstruction. Therefore, it is not surprising that, until recently, the surgical therapy for proximal biliary malignancies consisted mainly of biliary-enteric bypass as palliation for jaundice and cholangitis. The therapeutic approach to cholangiocarcinomas was largely nihilistic because of lack of familiarity with the disease, difficulty in delineating the extent of disease, and the technical challenge of resecting such lesions.

In the 1990s, surgical approaches became more aggressive, as demonstrated by the increasing number of hepatic resections that have been performed for bile duct cancers (31–33,35,36). Improvements in US, CT, MRI, and angiography have greatly facilitated preoperative diagnosis and staging of cholangiocarcinoma, allowing improved patient selection and surgical planning. The location and local extension of tumors dictate the extent of resection, with most lesions requiring an extended right or left hepatectomy for complete excision. Caudate resection is often required because of direct extension into caudate biliary radicals or parenchyma (31,35,36). CBD excision and portal lymphadenectomy are also essential for tumor clearance.

Prognosis after Resection. Results of major studies on resection of hilar cholangiocarcinoma are summarized in Table 41.6. Five-year survival rates for this group range from 10% to 30% (27,31,32,36–39). Surgical resection provides not only improved survival but improved quality of life (40). The greatest risk factors for recurrence include the presence of positive margins (40) and node-positive tumors (34).

In patients with distal cholangiocarcinomas, resection with primary reanastomosis is rarely possible, even for

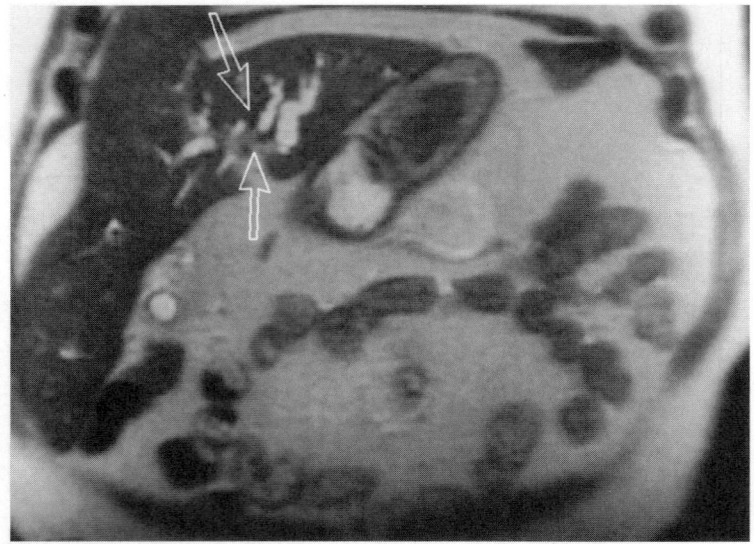

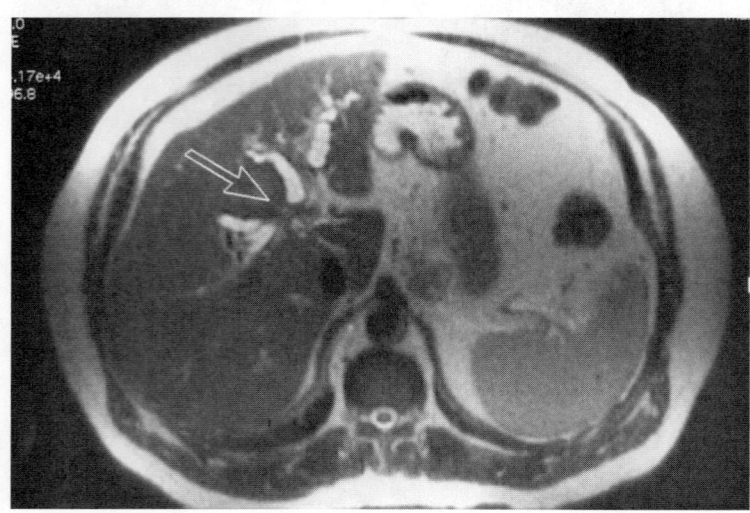

Figure 41.6. Coronal *(A)* and axial *(B)* magnetic resonance imaging scans in patient with hilar cholangiocarcinoma. Dilated intrahepatic ducts are present with a soft-tissue density consistent with tumor *(arrows).*

small lesions. For most of the lesions arising below the cystic duct, pancreaticoduodenectomy (Whipple procedure) is required to obtain adequate clearance of tumor because of the intrapancreatic location of the distal CBD. Patients with cholangiocarcinomas arising in the distal bile duct have both an increased resectability rate and an improved prognosis over those with hilar cholangiocarcinomas (42). Patients with resectable distal bile duct cancer have a 5-year survival rate of 30% to 50% (43,44), with decreased survival if nodes are involved with tumor.

Surgical Treatment of Unresectable Cholangiocarcinoma

For patients with unresectable hilar cholangiocarcinomas, significant improvement in quality of life can occur with surgical bypass. Palliative bypass can be performed in several ways. A partial excision of the left lateral segment and biliary-enteric anastomosis to the left hepatic duct (Longmire procedure) was used commonly in the past, but more recent surgical techniques have become available that are less complicated and do not require hepatic parenchymal transection. One technique involves biliary decompression through the left duct, approached through the round ligament, which is a segment III bypass

(Fig. 41.8). Opening the bridge of tissue just beneath the ligamentum teres allows access to the duct. In this position, a long anastomosis can be performed from the segment III duct to a jejunal limb because of the horizontal course of the duct in this location. Although less commonly used, the right hepatic duct can be approached at the base of the gallbladder fossa. This is technically more difficult and results in a higher rate of late bypass failure (45).

Nonoperative palliative biliary decompression can be accomplished with percutaneous or endoscopic stenting, depending on the level of obstruction. Proximal lesions are usually approached percutaneously with placement of expandable stents or drainage catheters (Fig. 41.9). Internal stents result in fewer electrolyte abnormalities and improvement in patient comfort, although morbidity and mortality occur in up to 30% of patients and stent occlusion is common (46–48). There is a significant risk of cholangitis with external and internal drainage, occurring in 11 of 12 patients with metallic expandable internal stents in one series (47). Bleeding and bile leaks are also frequent complications.

Patients who are clearly unresectable on preoperative imaging should undergo percutaneous internal or external drainage. In patients who are explored and found to be un-

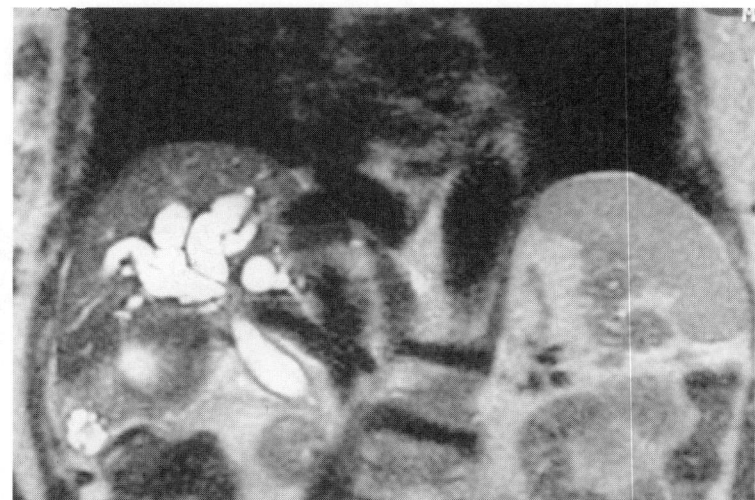

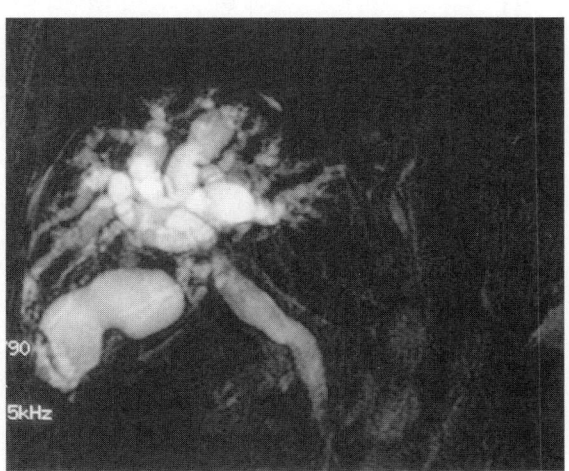

Figure 41.7. Coronal magnetic resonance image *(A)* and magnetic resonance cholangiopancreatogram *(B)* in a patient with hilar cholangiocarcinoma, demonstrating dilated intrahepatic ducts narrowing off at the area of obstruction.

resectable, surgical bypass offers fewer episodes of cholangitis, with an improved quality of life. In some series, surgical bypass for unresectable patients is the only biliary drainage procedure ever required by the patient.

In patients with unresectable distal cholangiocarcinomas, palliation can be achieved with surgical bypass, percutaneous biliary drains, or ERCP-placed stents. The most simple and effective way to relieve jaundice is usually with an ERCP-placed stent. Although surgical bypass offers improved patency and fewer episodes of cholangitis,

the morbidity of the procedure is not warranted in patients with metastatic disease.

Adjuvant Therapy

To date, no chemotherapeutic regimen has consistently shown activity against cholangiocarcinoma. Although 5-fluorouracil (5 -FU)-based chemotherapy is often offered to patients with unresectable disease, the likelihood of response is less than 10%. The use of mitomycin C and dox-

Table 41.6. RESULTS AFTER RESECTION FOR HILAR CHOLANGIOCARCINOMA

Author	N	Percent resected	Postoperative mortality rate	5-Year survival rate	Survival (mo) Mean	Median
Iwasaki et al., 1986[37]	46	22%	0	20%	—	25
Iida et al., 1987[38]	41	56%	4%	30%	—	8
Cameron et al., 1990[27]	96	55%	2%	8%	—	18
Hadjis et al., 1990[36]	131	21%	7%	12%	25	—
Altaee et al., 1991[31]	70	21%	—	19%	—	12
Baer et al., 1993[32]	48	44%	4%	23%	34	—
Nagorney et al., 1993[42]	79	15%	5%	16%	—	13
McMasters et al., 1997[39]	91	44%	0	26%	—	22
Burke et al., 1998[26]	69	43%	7%	45%	40	

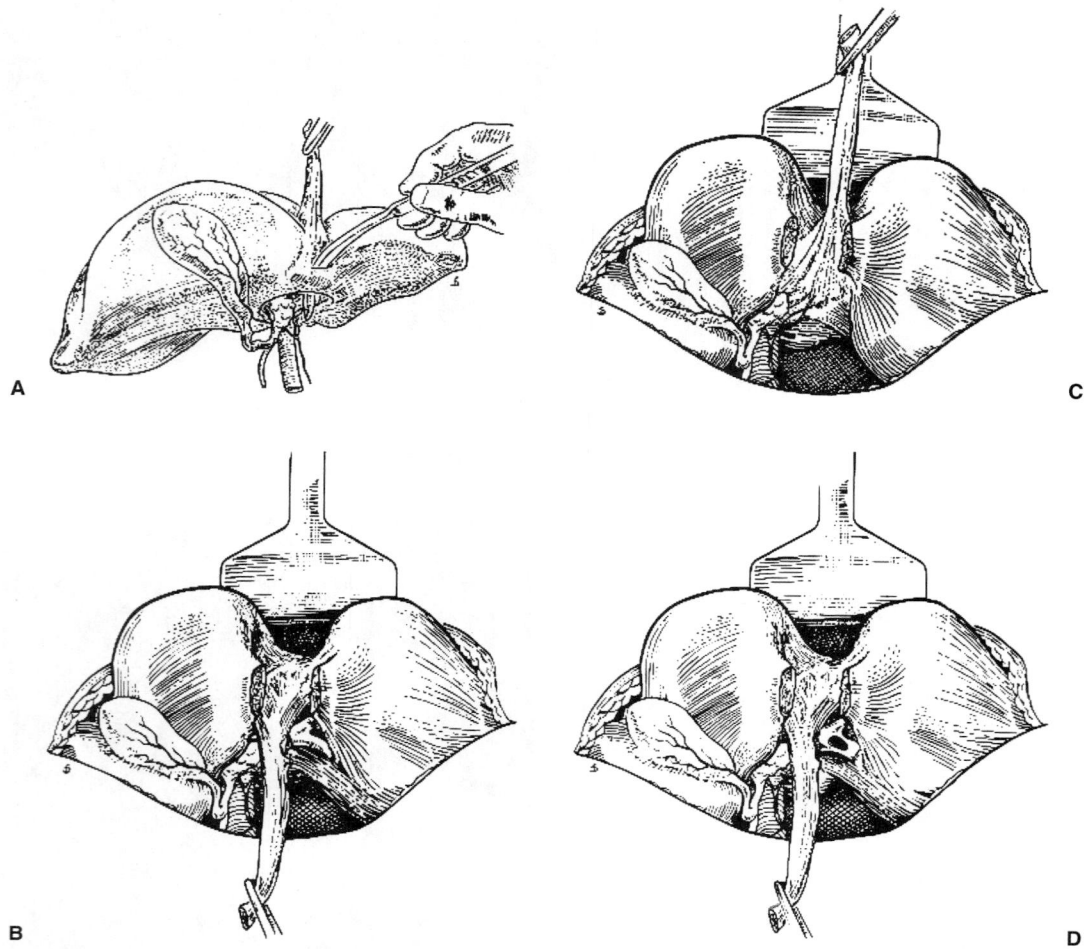

Figure 41.8. Surgical approach to segment III duct. *(A)* The bridge of tissue present at the base of the liver is divided. *(B)* The ligamentum teres is held superiorly to expose the tissue overlying the segment III duct. *(C)* The segment III duct is exposed. *(D)* The duct is opened in preparation for anastomosis with a Roux-en-Y jejunal limb. (Courtesy of Dr. L. H. Blumgart, M.D.)

orubicin, in combination with 5-FU, has resulted in combined response rates of less than 30%, with higher toxicity than 5-FU alone (49). There is no proven role for adjuvant chemotherapy in the treatment of cholangiocarcinoma.

In cases of unresectable cholangiocarcinoma, the use of external beam radiation therapy has been explored (50–52). To date, no study has clearly demonstrated efficacy for this modality. Anecdotal reports of long-term survivors after external beam radiation therapy show that some patients may benefit from such treatment, but this must be weighed against the potential complications such as duodenal or bile duct stenosis, and duodenitis. The most encouraging results involve use of intraoperative or interstitial radiation. Our current practice is to use combined interstitial radiation and external beam radiation in unresectable cases after palliative bypass. In patients who are resected, adjuvant radiation therapy has not been shown to increase quality of life or survival (53).

Follow-up after Resection of Cholangiocarcinoma

The most likely site of recurrence after resection of a hilar cholangiocarcinoma is locally in the bile duct, regional lymph nodes, or liver. Therapy for recurrence is palliative. Surgical reexcision is usually impossible because

of the challenging anatomic location and the radical procedures that are required for resection of the primary tumor. Therefore, the goal of follow-up is diagnosis of symptomatic recurrences to direct palliative therapy and diagnosis of benign complications of surgical treatment such as biliary strictures. The main symptoms of recurrence that demand palliation are pruritus or cholangitis associated with jaundice. For biliary drainage to relieve jaundice or cholangitis, either surgical drainage (47) or drainage by PTC can be effective (54). Endoscopic drainage has little role in the relief of jaundice in patients who have had Roux-en-Y biliary reconstruction. For limited recurrences, intraluminal brachytherapy or external beam radiation therapy may improve palliation and, potentially, survival.

Routine follow-up consists of office visits every 3 months with physical examination and measurement of liver function tests. Although a rising alkaline phosphatase is a good indicator of evolving biliary obstruction, patients recovering from liver resection and biliary obstruction may have persistent elevations of alkaline phosphatase. However, a benign anastomotic stricture may develop in up to 10% of patients with biliary surgical reconstruction. Most patients with recurrence or a benign stricture present with jaundice or cholangitis. Because there is a low likelihood of effective therapy for recurrences, the routine use of tumor markers is not recommended, although a fair per-

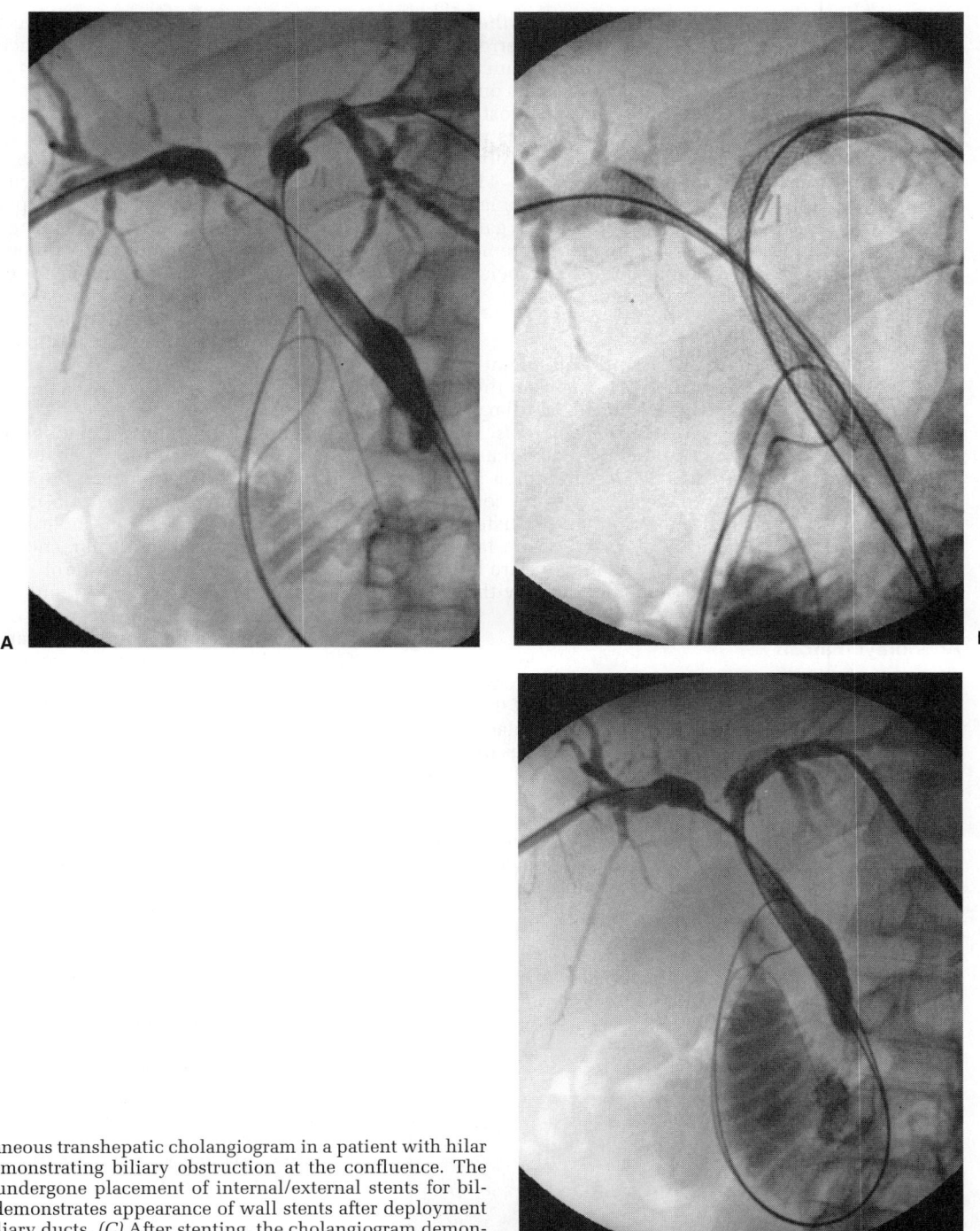

Figure 41.9. *(A)* Percutaneous transhepatic cholangiogram in a patient with hilar cholangiocarcinoma, demonstrating biliary obstruction at the confluence. The patient has previously undergone placement of internal/external stents for biliary drainage. *(B)* Film demonstrates appearance of wall stents after deployment into the left and right biliary ducts. *(C)* After stenting, the cholangiogram demonstrates adequate biliary drainage, with contrast filling the duodenum.

centage of biliary malignancies express CEA or CA 19-9. The routine use of imaging studies to follow patients with cholangiocarcinoma after resection should be limited for the same reasons. When patients become symptomatic with jaundice, an abdominal US should be obtained. Other imaging is usually dictated by the sonographic findings.

BENIGN GALLBLADDER NEOPLASMS

Incidence

Benign tumors of the biliary tract are rare, but have been reported more frequently as imaging modalities such as US and CT scan have come into widespread and frequent use. In patients undergoing cholecystectomy, the reported incidence of benign gallbladder tumors is 0.5% to 3.0% (55).

Pathology

Polyps and Pseudotumors

Benign gallbladder tumors are most frequently polyps or polypoid lesions. The incidence of polyps in asymptomatic patients is approximately 5% (2). Cholesterol polyps (cholesterolosis), accounting for half of all gallbladder polypoid lesions (56), result from epithelium-covered, cholesterol-laden macrophages in the lamina propria. These lesions are likely a result of an error in cholesterol metabolism. They extend from the mucosa on a narrow stalk, grossly appearing as yellow spots on the mucosal surface. Nearly all are multiple and most are less than 10 mm in size (6,56,57). When a polyp is pedunculated, it is benign in most cases; alternatively, sessile "polyps" are most often malignant (57) (Fig. 41.10). Inflammatory polyps result from chronic inflammation and extend by a narrow vascularized stalk into the gallbladder lumen. None of these lesions is considered premalignant, although isolated cases of cholesterolosis associated with in situ carcinoma have been reported.

Adenomas

Gallbladder adenomas are found infrequently. They may be tubular or papillary, both arising from the epithelial layer of the gallbladder. Multiple papillary adenomas, or papillomas, are called *papillomatosis*. A direct association between benign adenoma, adenoma containing carcinoma in situ, and invasive carcinoma has been demonstrated, and therefore these lesions are considered premalignant (58). However, malignant transformation has been reported only rarely, primarily from large adenomas. In one series, all benign adenomas were less than 12 mm in diameter, whereas the adenomas with cancerous foci were greater than 12 mm (59).

Adenomyomatosis

Adenomyomatosis of the gallbladder is characterized by localized or diffuse hyperplastic extensions of the mucosa into, and often beyond, a hypertrophied gallbladder muscular layer. Hyperplasia occurs at outpouchings of the mucosa of the gallbladder through the wall (Rokitansky-Aschoff sinuses) and through the crypts of Luschka. This can result in focal thickening of the gallbladder wall, resembling gallbladder adenocarcinoma. The etiology is unknown. This lesion may be premalignant because cases of adenocarcinoma arising in or near adenomyomatosis have been reported (59,60).

Other Benign Gallbladder Tumors

Other benign lesions include tumors arising from the tissue of the gallbladder wall, such as leiomyomas, lipo-

mas, hemangiomas, and granular cell tumors, and heterotopic tissue, including gastric, pancreatic, or intestinal epithelium.

Clinical Findings

Patients with benign gallbladder tumors typically present with symptoms consistent with choledocholithiasis, including right upper quadrant pain, fatty food intolerance, and nausea. Many benign gallbladder lesions are also discovered incidentally after elective cholecystectomy, and therefore symptoms due to benign lesions are difficult to separate from those due to gallstones. Most lesions, are, however, asymptomatic and are discovered incidentally during imaging for other abdominal conditions.

Diagnosis

Diagnosis of benign gallbladder polyps is usually made when US is obtained to evaluate a patient for symptoms consistent with gallstones. On US, a filling defect that does not change with position is likely a polyp or carcinoma and not a gallstone. Cholesterol polyps are typically small, submucosal, multiple, and hyperechoic on US because of their high cholesterol content. Other than this typical appearance, it is difficult to differentiate benign from malignant polyps.

Both intravenous contrast-enhanced and unenhanced CT may be important in distinguishing benign from malignant polyps. In one series examining 31 polypoid lesions of the gallbladder, contrast-enhanced CT detected all of the lesions. Benign polyps were not visualized with unenhanced CT, unlike neoplastic tumors, thus improving the ability to distinguish these lesions when both enhanced and unenhanced CT scans are obtained (6). Endoscopic US has also been used to image these lesions, and may be more accurate than transabdominal US in differentiating benign from malignant tumors (5).

Treatment

Large polyps, greater than 10 mm, have the greatest malignant potential (6,56,57). However, without evidence of invasion or metastatic disease, no radiologic test can reliably differentiate benign from malignant lesions. Therefore, if large (>1 cm) polyps are present, even in asymptomatic patients without stones, cholecystectomy is warranted (61). Smaller pedunculated lesions with the gross characteristics of a benign cholesterol polyp may be observed and resected only if symptomatic. These lesions should be carefully followed with US every 3 to 6 months. Cholecystectomy is required if there is any increase in size.

BENIGN BILE DUCT NEOPLASMS

Incidence

Benign bile duct tumors, at times clinically resembling hilar cholangiocarcinoma, are less common, occurring in less than 1% of patients (1).

Pathology

Attesting to the rarity of these lesions, of 4,200 biliary tract operations in one institution, only 2 were for benign extrahepatic bile duct disease (62). The most common benign tumors of the extrahepatic biliary tree arise from the glandular epithelium lining the ducts; approximately two thirds of benign tumors are polyps, adenomatous papillomas, or bile duct adenomas (63). Most are found in the pe-

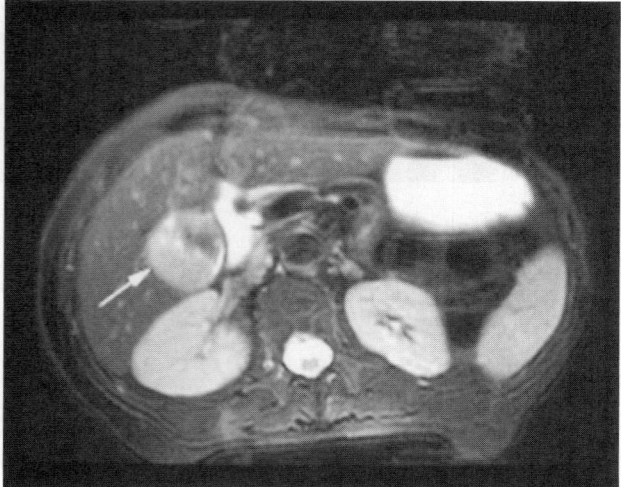

Figure 41.10. T$_2$-weighted magnetic resonance imaging scan showing a sessile polyp in the gallbladder *(arrow)* that proved malignant on histologic examination.

riampullary region, but they can be distributed throughout the entire biliary tree (Fig. 41.11). Multiple papillomas also have been reported throughout the intrahepatic and extrahepatic biliary tree, termed *multiple biliary papillomatosis.* Although local recurrence and progression to death from obstructive jaundice and cholangitis occur frequently in these rare cases, these tumors have little, if any, malignant potential. Other benign tumors such as cystadenoma, granular cell myoblastoma, leiomyoma, and heterotopic tissue have also been reported.

One condition that deserves consideration is the case of "malignant masquerade," a fibrotic lesion clinically resembling hilar cholangiocarcinoma but pathologically consisting only of extensive fibrosis without evidence of dysplasia or preneoplastic change (64). In patients being considered for palliative treatment alone with presumed hilar cholangiocarcinoma, it is essential to obtain a tissue diagnosis. It is inappropriate to treat benign lesions by percutaneous stenting because of the excellent outcome after resection of these lesions.

Clinical Findings

Biliary obstruction, with resultant jaundice or cholangitis, is frequently the presenting symptom in patients with benign bile duct tumors. Symptoms may also include epigastric pain or nausea. Because these tumors are indolent, symptoms may be intermittent or gradually progressive.

Diagnosis

Because of the presence of jaundice, benign bile duct tumors are usually initially evaluated with US. Many patients then undergo ERCP or PTC and CT scan. A diagnosis of malignant masquerade should be suspected in patients with mass lesions that resemble hilar cholangiocarcinomas, but without lobar atrophy or portal vein involvement.

Treatment

Resection and reconstruction are performed to relieve jaundice and cholangitis. Primary reanastomosis can usu-

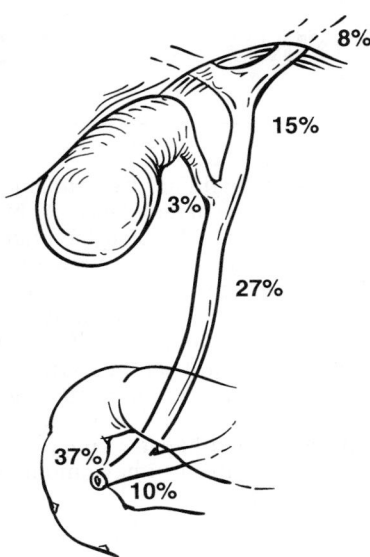

Figure 41.11. Distribution of papillomas and adenomas of the biliary tree. The ampulla and common bile duct are the most frequent sites.

ally be performed without tension if less than 2 cm of the duct is sacrificed. If longer segments of the duct are removed, reconstruction with a choledochoduodenostomy, or, more commonly, a Roux-en-Y choledochojejunostomy, is performed.

REFERENCES

1. Diehl AK. Epidemiology of gallbladder cancer: a synthesis of recent data. *J Natl Cancer Inst* 1980;65:1209–1213.
2. Okamoto M, Okamoto H, Kitahara F, et al. Ultrasonographic evidence of association of polyps and stones with gallbladder cancer. *Am J Gastroenterol* 1999;94:446–450.
3. Yamamoto M, Nakajo S, Tahara E. Carcinoma of the gallbladder: the correlation between histogenesis and prognosis. *Arch Pathol Anat* 1989;414:83–90.
4. Nevine JE, Moran TJ, Day S, et al. Carcinoma of the gallbladder: staging, treatment, and prognosis. *Cancer* 1976;37:141–148.
5. Sugiyama M, Xie XY, Atomi Y, et al. Differential diagnosis of small polypoid lesions of the gallbladder: the value of endoscopic ultrasonography. *Ann Surg* 1999;229:498–504.
6. Shinkai H, Kimura W, Muto T. Surgical indications for small polypoid lesions of the gallbladder. *Am J Surg* 1998:175;114–117.
7. Soto JA, Barish MA, Yucel EK, et al. Magnetic resonance cholangiography: comparison with endoscopic retrograde cholangiopancreatography. *Gastroenterology* 1996;110:589–597.
8. Demachi H, Matsui O, Hoshiba K, et al. Dynamic MRI using a surface coil in chronic cholecystitis and gallbladder carcinoma: radiologic and histopathologic correlation. *J Comput Assist Tomogr* 1997;21:643–651.
9. Schwartz LH, Coakley FV, Sun Y, et al. Neoplastic pancreaticobiliary duct obstruction: evaluation with breath-hold MR cholangiopancreatography. *AJR Am J Roentgenol* 1998;170:1491–1495.
10. Piehler JM, Crichlow RW. Primary carcinoma of the gallbladder. *Surg Gynecol Obstet* 1978;147:929–942.
11. Ouchi K, Owada Y, Matsuno S, et al. Prognostic factors in the surgical treatment of gallbladder carcinoma. *Surgery* 1987;101:731–737.
12. Donohue JH, Nagorney DM, Grant CS, et al. Carcinoma of the gallbladder: does radical resection improve outcome? *Arch Surg* 1990;125:237–241.
13. Ogura Y, Mizumoto R, Isaji S, et al. Radical operations for carcinoma of the gallbladder: present status in Japan. *World J Surg* 1991;15:337–343.
14. Shirai Y, Yoshida K, Tsukada K, et al. Radical surgery for gallbladder carcinoma. *Ann Surg* 1992;216:565–568.
15. Yamaguchi K, Tsuneyoshi M. Subclinical gallbladder carcinoma. *Am J Surg* 1993;25:86.
16. Bartlett DL, Fong Y, Fortner JG, et al. Long-term results after resection for gallbladder cancer. *Ann Surg* 1996;224:639–646.
17. Nakamura S, Sakaguchi S, Suzuki S, et al. Aggressive surgery for carcinoma of the gallbladder. *Surgery* 1989;106:467–453.
18. Shirai Y, Yoshida K, Tsukada K, et al. Inapparent carcinoma of the gallbladder: an appraisal of a radical second operation after simple cholecystectomy. *Ann Surg* 1992;:215:326–331.
19. Wanebo HJ, Castle WN, Fechner RE. Is carcinoma of the gallbladder a curable lesion? *Ann Surg* 1982;196:624–631.
20. Wanebo HJ, Vezeridis MP. Carcinoma of the gallbladder. *J Surg Oncol* 1993;[Suppl 3]:134.
21. Chijiiwa K, Tanaka M. Carcinoma of the gallbladder: an appraisal of surgical resection. *Surgery* 1994;115:751–756.
22. Fong Y, Brennan MF, Turnbull A, et al. Gallbladder cancer discovered during laparoscopic surgery: potential for iatrogenic tumor dissemination. *Arch Surg* 1993;128:1054–1056.
23. Drouard F, Delamarre J, Capron JP. Cutaneous seeding of gallbladder cancer after laparoscopic cholecystectomy. *N Engl J Med* 1991;325:1316.
24. Pezet D, Fondrinier E, Rotman N, et al. Parietal seeding of carcinoma of the gallbladder after laparoscopic cholecystectomy. *Br J Surg* 1992;79:230.
25. Bismuth H, Nakache R, Diamond T. Management strategies in resection for hilar cholangiocarcinomas. *Ann Surg* 1992;21 5:31.

26. Burke EC, Jarnagin WR, Hochwald SN, et al. Hilar cholangiocarcinoma: patterns of spread, and the importance of hepatic resection for curative operation, and a presurgical clinical staging system. *Ann Surg* 1998;228:385–394.

27. Cameron JL, Pitt HA, Zinner MJ, et al. Management of proximal cholangiocarcinomas by surgical resection and radiotherapy. *Am J Surg* 1990;159:91–97.

28. Hochwald SN, Burke EC, Jarnagin WR, et al. Association of preoperative biliary stenting with increased postoperative infectious complications in proximal cholangiocarcinoma. *Arch Surg* 1999;134:261–266.

29. McPherson GA, Benjamin IS, Hodgson HJ, et al. Pre-operative percutaneous transhepatic biliary drainage: the results of a controlled trial. *Br J Surg* 1982;69:261.

30. Pitt HA, Gomes AS, Lois JF, et al. Does preoperative percutaneous biliary drainage reduce operative risk or increase hospital cost? *Ann Surg* 1985;201:545.

31. Altaee MY, Johnson PJ, Farrant JM, et al. Etiologic and clinical characteristics of peripheral and hilar cholangiocarcinoma. *Cancer* 1991;68:2051–2055.

32. Baer HU, Stain SC, Dennison AR, et al. Improvements in survival by aggressive resections of hilar cholangiocarcinoma. *Ann Surg* 1993;217:20–27.

33. Bengmark S, Ekberg H, Evander A, et al. Major liver resection for hilar cholangiocarcinoma. *Ann Surg* 1988;207:120–125.

34. Reding R, Buard JL, Lebeau G, et al. Surgical management of 552 carcinomas of the extrahepatic bile ducts (gallbladder and periampullary tumors excluded): results of the French Surgical Association Survey. *Ann Surg* 1991;213:236–241.

35. Bismuth H, Nakache R, Diamond T. Management strategies in resection for hilar cholangiocarcinoma. *Ann Surg* 1992;215:31–38.

36. Hadjis NS, Blenkharn JI, Alexander N, et al. Outcome of radical surgery in hilar cholangiocarcinoma. *Surgery* 1990;107:597–604.

37. Iwasaki Y, Okamura T, Ozaki A, et al. Surgical treatment for carcinoma at the confluence of the major hepatic ducts. *Surg Gynecol Obstet* 1986;162:457–463.

38. Iida S, Tsuzuki T, Ogata Y, et al. The long-term survival of patients with carcinoma of the main hepatic duct junction. *Cancer* 1987;60:1612–1619.

39. McMasters KM, Tuttle TM, Leach SD, et al. Neoadjuvant chemoradiation for extrahepatic cholangiocarcinoma. *Am J Surg* 1997;174:605–608.

40. Blumgart LH, Hadjis NS, Benjamin IS, et al. Surgical approaches to cholangiocarcinoma at confluence of hepatic ducts. *Lancet* 1984;1:66–69.

41. Yeo CJ, Pitt HA, Cameron JL. Cholangiocarcinoma. *Surg Clin North Am* 1990;70:1429–1447.

42. Nagorney DM, Donohue JH, Farnell MB, et al. Outcomes after curative resections of cholangiocarcinoma. *Arch Surg* 1993;128:871–877.

43. Nakeeb A, Pitt HA, Sohn TA, et al. Cholangiocarcinoma: a spectrum of intrahepatic, perihilar, and distal tumors. *Ann Surg* 1996;224:463–473.

44. Fong Y, Blumgart LH, Lin E, et al. Outcome of treatment for distal bile duct cancer. *Br J Surg* 1996;83:1712–1715.

45. Jarnagin WR, Burke E, Powers C, et al. Intrahepatic biliary enteric bypass provides effective palliation in selected patients with malignant obstruction at the hepatic duct confluence. *Am J Surg* 1998;175:453–460.

46. Glattli A, Stain SC, Baer HU, et al. Unresectable malignant biliary obstruction: treatment by self-expandable biliary endoprostheses. *Hepatobil Surg* 1993;6:175–184.

47. Kuvshinoff BW, Armstrong JG, Fong Y, et al. Palliation of irresectable hilar cholangiocarcinoma with biliary drainage and radiotherapy. *Br J Surg* 1995;82:1522–1525.

48. Lee BH, Choe DH, Lee JH, et al. Metallic stents in malignant biliary obstruction: prospective long-term clinical results. *AJR Am J Roentgenol* 1997;168:741–745.

49. Oberfield RS, Rossi RL. The role of chemotherapy in the treatment of bile duct cancer. *World J Surg* 1988;12:105.

50. Cameron JL, Broe P, Zuidema GD. Proximal bile duct tumors. Surgical management with silastic transhepatic biliary stents. *Ann Surg* 1982;196:412–419.

51. Fletcher MS, Brinkley D, Dawson JL, et al. Treatment of high bile duct carcinoma by internal radiotherapy with iridium-192 wire. *Lancet* 1981;2:172–174.

52. Kopelson G, Gunderson LL. Primary and adjuvant radiation therapy in gallbladder and extrahepatic biliary tract carcinoma. *J Clin Gastroenterol* 1983;5:43–50.

53. Pitt HA, Nakeeb A, Abrams RA, et al. Perihilar cholangiocarcinoma: postoperative radiotherapy does not improve survival. *Ann Surg* 1995;221:788–797.

54. Polydorou AA, Cairns SR, Dowsett JF, et al. Palliation of proximal malignant biliary obstruction by endoscopic endoprosthesis insertion. *Gut* 1991;32:685–689.

55. Nahrwold DL. Benign tumors and pseudotumors of the biliary tract. In: Way LW, Pellegrini CA, eds. *Surgery of the gallbladder and bile ducts.* Philadelphia: WB Saunders, 1987:459.

56. Koga A, Watanabe K, Fukuyama T, et al. Diagnosis and operative indications for polypoid lesion of the gallbladder. *Arch Surg* 1988;123:26.

57. Furukawa H, Kosuge T, Shimada K, et al. Small polypoid lesions of the gallbladder: differential diagnosis and surgical indications by helical computed tomography. *Arch Surg* 1998;133:735–739.

58. Kozuka S, Tsubone M, Yasui A, et al. Relation of adenoma to carcinoma in the gallbladder. *Cancer* 1982;50:2226.

59. Aldridge MC, Gruffaz R, Castaing D, et al. Adenomyomatosis of the gallbladder: a premalignant lesion? *Surgery* 1991;109:107–110.

60. Kurihara K, Mizuseki K, Ninomiya T, et al. Carcinoma of the gallbladder arising in adenomyomatosis. *Acta Pathol Jpn* 1993;43:82–85.

61. Aldridge MC, Bismuth H. Gallbladder cancer: the polyp cancer sequence. *Br J Surg* 1990;77:363–364.

62. Farris KB, Faust BF. Granular cell tumors of the biliary ducts. *Arch Pathol Lab Med* 1979;103:510–512.

63. Beazley RM, Blumgart LH. Benign tumours and pseudotumours of the biliary tract. In: Blumgart LH, ed. *Surgery of the liver and biliary tract.* Edinburgh: Churchill Livingstone, 1994:941.

64. Hadjis NS, Collier NA, Blumgart LH. Malignant masquerade at the hilum of the liver. *Br J Surg* 1985;71:72–74.

SURGERY: SCIENTIFIC PRINCIPLES AND PRACTICE, Third Edition, edited by Lazar J. Greenfield, Michael W. Mulholland, Keith T. Oldham, Gerald B. Zelenock, and Keith D. Lillemoe. Lippincott Williams & Wilkins Publishers, Philadelphia, © 2001.

CHAPTER 42

BILIARY STRICTURES AND SCLEROSING CHOLANGITIS

KEITH D. LILLEMOE

Benign strictures of the biliary tree are among the most difficult challenges that a surgeon faces. Although numerous technologic developments have facilitated diagnosis and management, bile duct strictures remain a significant clinical problem. If they go unrecognized or are managed improperly, life-threatening complications, such as biliary cirrhosis, portal hypertension, and cholangitis, can develop. To avoid these complications, virtually every patient with a bile duct stricture should undergo evaluation and treatment with the goal of relieving the obstruction to bile flow and its associated hepatic injury.

Benign bile duct strictures can have numerous causes:

Postoperative Strictures

Injury at primary biliary operations
    Laparoscopic cholecystectomy
    Open cholecystectomy
    Common bile duct exploration
Injury at other operative procedures

Gastrectomy
Hepatic resection
Portacaval shunt
Stricture of a biliary-enteric anastomosis
Blunt or penetrating trauma

Strictures Due to Inflammatory Conditions

Chronic pancreatitis
Cholelithiasis and choledocholithiasis
Primary sclerosing cholangitis
Stenosis of the sphincter of Oddi
Duodenal ulcer
Crohn's disease
Viral infections
Toxic drugs

Most biliary strictures occur after primary operations on the gallbladder or biliary tree. With the introduction of laparoscopic cholecystectomy, bile duct injuries and associated strictures have been seen with increased frequency. Operative injury to the bile ducts can also occur during nonbiliary operations on the gallbladder or biliary tree or as a result of external penetrating or blunt abdominal trauma. Inflammatory conditions and fibrosis due to chronic pancreatitis, gallstones in the gallbladder or the bile duct, stenosis of the sphincter of Oddi, or biliary tract infections can also cause benign bile duct strictures. Finally, primary sclerosing cholangitis, a rare disease of unknown cause, can result in multiple strictures of the intrahepatic and extrahepatic bile ducts. This chapter focuses primarily on postoperative bile duct strictures and primary sclerosing cholangitis.

POSTOPERATIVE BILE DUCT STRICTURES

Pathogenesis

Most benign bile duct strictures result from operations in or near the right upper quadrant. Over 80% of strictures occur after injury to the bile ducts during cholecystectomy. The exact incidence of bile duct injury is unknown because many cases may go unreported in the literature. Data suggest that the incidence of bile duct injury during open cholecystectomy is 1 in 500 to 1,000 cases. The incidence of bile duct injury during laparoscopic cholecystectomy is clearly higher. Although a wide range in the incidence of injury can be found in reported series, the most accurate data most likely come from surveys encompassing thousands of patients. These reports reflect the results from a large number of surgeons in both community and teaching hospitals. The results of such series suggest an incidence of bile duct injury during laparoscopic cholecystectomy ranging from 0.3% to 0.6%.

A number of factors are associated with bile duct injury during either open or laparoscopic cholecystectomy, including acute or chronic inflammation, inadequate exposure, patient obesity, and failure to identify structures before clamping, ligating, or dividing them. More specific causes of bile duct injury also exist. Bleeding from the cystic or hepatic arteries can lead to bile duct injury during attempts to gain hemostasis. The generous application of Liga clips at either open or laparoscopic cholecystectomy to hilar areas not well visualized can result in placing a clip on or across a bile duct, with resultant injury (Fig. 42.1). Failure to recognize congenital anatomic anomalies of the bile ducts, such as insertion of the right hepatic duct into the cystic duct or a long common wall between the cystic duct and the common bile duct, can also lead to injury (Fig. 42.2). A number of technical factors are associated with laparoscopic cholecystectomy that can also in-

crease the risk of bile duct injury compared with the open procedure. These include the use of an end-viewing laparoscope, which alters the surgeon's perspective of the operative field. Excessive cephalad retraction of the gallbladder fundus can cause the cystic duct and common bile duct to become aligned in the same plane. This distortion often results in the classic laparoscopic injury, in which the common bile duct is mistaken for the cystic duct and clipped and divided (1) (Fig. 42.3). The role of intraoperative cholangiography in preventing bile duct injury during laparoscopic cholecystectomy is controversial. Based on a number of published series advocating either routine or selective cholangiography, it appears that cholangiography does not prevent bile duct injury. The procedure, however, can minimize the extent of injury. Finally, ample evidence exists to support the conclusion that the experience of the surgeon in performing laparoscopic cholecystectomy can be correlated with the risk of bile duct injury.

The importance of ischemia of the bile duct in the formation of postoperative strictures has been emphasized. Unnecessary dissection around the bile duct during cholecystectomy or bile duct anastomosis can divide or injure the major arteries of the bile duct that run in the 3- and 9-o'clock positions (Fig. 42.4). Another important factor contributing to the formation of biliary strictures is the intense connective tissue response with fibrosis and scarring that can occur after bile duct injury. Experimental studies of bile duct ligation in a canine model have demonstrated immediate and sustained elevation of bile duct pressure

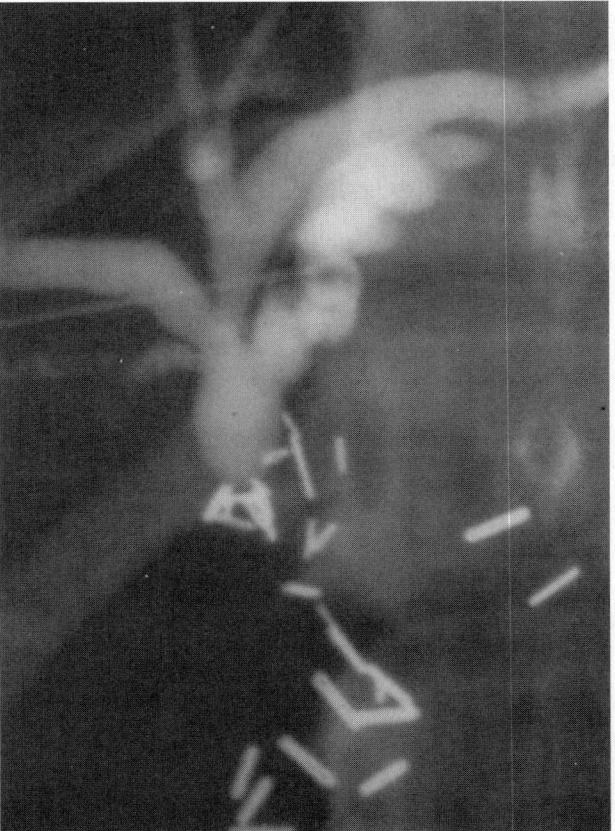

Figure 42.1. Percutaneous transhepatic cholangiogram in a patient with a bile duct stricture secondary to iatrogenic injury during cholecystectomy. Numerous surgical clips can be seen in the area of the stricture. (From Lillemoe KD, Pitt HA, Cameron JL. Postoperative bile duct strictures. *Surg Clin North Am* 1990;70: 1356, with permission.)

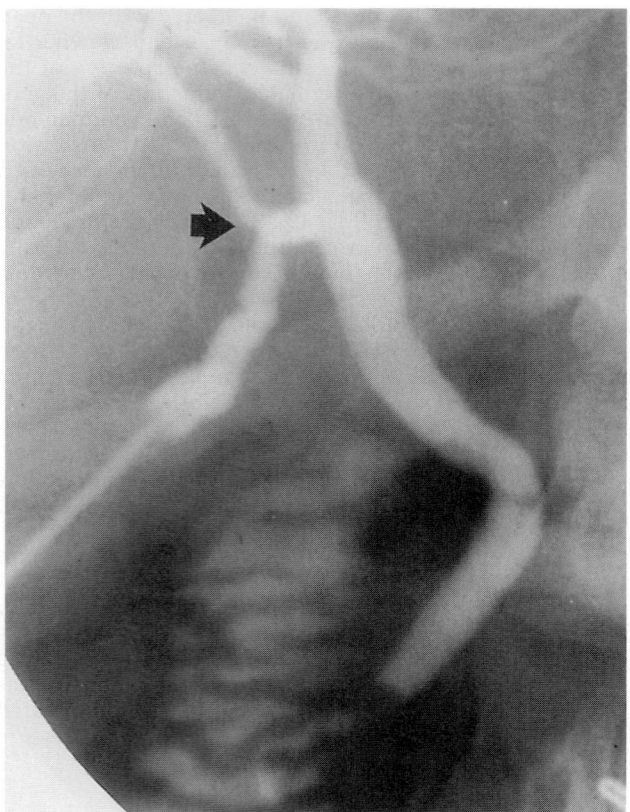

Figure 42.2. Operative cholangiogram demonstrating a right lobe segmental bile duct entering the cystic duct *(arrow)*. Division of the cystic duct proximal to this insertion can result in a bile leak or obstruction of bile flow from a significant segment of the liver.

and progressive increase in bile duct diameter. Histologic changes at 1 month after ligation have shown that the bile duct wall is thickened, with a reduction of mucosal folds and loss of surface microvilli, associated with a well defined epithelial degeneration. Biochemical analysis of

connective tissue response to ligation showed that collagen synthesis and prolene hydroxylase activity is increased within 2 weeks in the obstructed bile duct and is sustained throughout the period of observation. Finally, a marked local inflammatory response can develop in the adjacent tissue in association with bile leakage, which occurs with many bile duct injuries. This inflammation can be further intensified in the face of infection. This inflammation results in fibrosis and scarring in the periductal tissue, further contributing to stricture formation. These factors can be of major importance in bile duct injuries during laparoscopic cholecystectomy, which are frequently associated with bile leaks.

After cholecystectomy and common bile duct exploration, the two most common operations associated with bile duct injury are gastrectomy and hepatic resection. The most common situation resulting in bile duct injury during gastrectomy involves dissection of the pyloric region and the first portion of the duodenum in the face of inflammation from peptic ulcer disease. The injury occurs during mobilization of the duodenum either for creation of a Billroth I gastroduodenostomy or for closure of the duodenal stump. Biliary injury during liver resection is most likely to occur during dissection of the hepatic hilum.

In addition to iatrogenic bile duct injury occurring during cholecystectomy or other operations, bile duct strictures can also occur at biliary anastomoses. Such strictures can occur at a biliary-enteric anastomosis performed for reconstruction after resection for benign or malignant disease of the pancreaticobiliary system, or after end-to-end

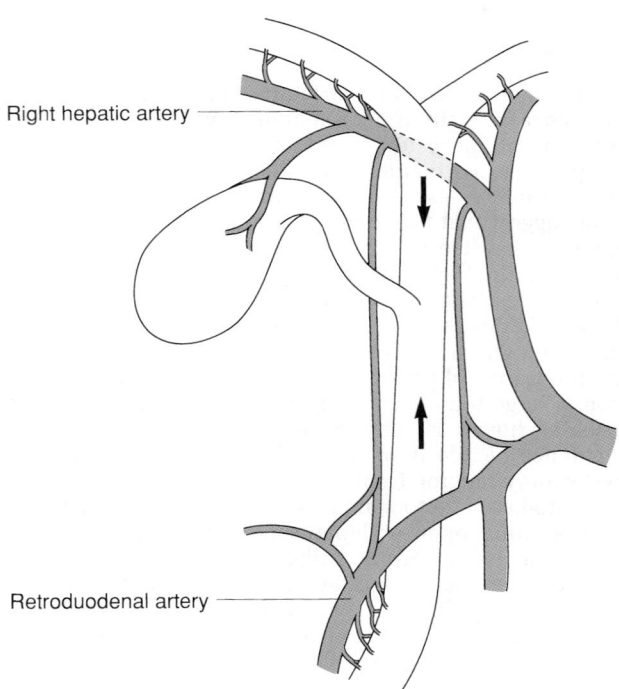

Figure 42.4. Diagrammatic view of the blood supply of the human bile duct. The blood supply to the bile ducts in the hilum of the liver *(above)* and to the intrapancreatic bile duct *(below)* from adjacent arteries is profuse. The supraduodenal bile duct blood supply is axial and tenuous, with 60% from below and 38% from above. The small main axial vessels (3- and 9-o'clock arteries) are vulnerable and easily damaged. (After Terblanche J, Allison HF, Northover JMA. An ischemic basis for biliary strictures. *Surgery* 1983;94:52, with permission.)

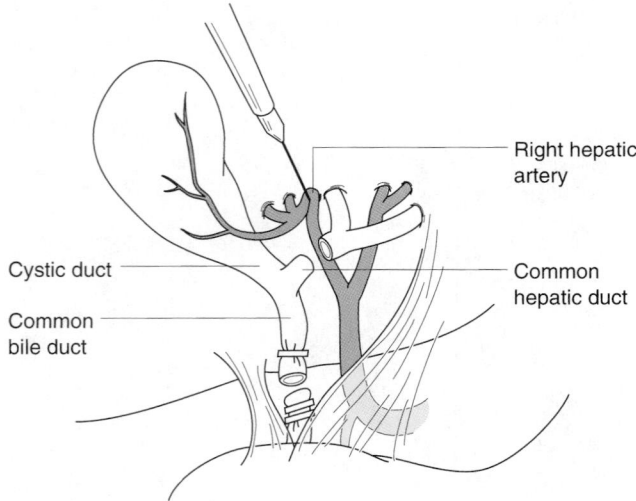

Figure 42.3. Classic laparoscopic bile duct injury. The common bile duct is mistaken for the cystic duct and transected. A variable extent of the extrahepatic biliary tree is resected with the gallbladder. The right hepatic artery, in background, is also often injured. (After Branum G, Schmidt C, Baile J, et al. Management of major biliary complications after laparoscopic cholecystectomy. *Ann Surg* 1993;217:532, with permission.)

bile duct anastomosis performed for hepatic transplantation or for repair of traumatic injury. Ischemia of the anastomosis due to excessive skeletonization of the duct in preparation for the anastomosis is an important factor in many such strictures.

Unfortunately, the recurrence of bile duct strictures after an initial attempt at repair is not uncommon and can also account for a number of anastomotic strictures (2,3). A number of other factors have been evaluated in patients who have a recurrent bile duct stricture, including the location of the stricture, the length of follow-up, the influence of previous operations, the type of operation performed, the type of sutures used, and the use and duration of postoperative stenting (2). Previous attempts at repair and performance of a procedure other than choledochojejunostomy or hepaticojejunostomy and stricture location higher in the biliary tree appear to be associated with a higher incidence of recurrent stricture. The type of suture material used for repair does not influence the outcome. When postoperative biliary stents are used, a longer period of stenting appears to be favorable. Finally, long-term follow-up of a bile duct anastomosis is important because strictures can develop years after the original anastomosis.

Clinical Presentation

Most patients with benign postoperative bile duct strictures present early after their initial operation (Fig. 42.5). After open cholecystectomy, only approximately 10% of postoperative strictures are actually suspected within the first week, but nearly 70% are diagnosed within the first 6 months, and over 80% are diagnosed within 1 year of surgery (2). In series reporting bile duct injuries during laparoscopic cholecystectomy, the injury is usually recognized either during the procedure or, more commonly, in the early postoperative period.

Patients suspected of having a postoperative bile duct stricture within days to weeks of initial operation usually present in one of two ways. One presentation is the progressive elevation of liver function test results, particularly total bilirubin and alkaline phosphatase levels. These changes can often be seen as early as the second or third postoperative day. The second mode of early presentation is with leakage of bile from the injured bile duct. This presentation appears to occur most often in patients presenting with bile duct injuries after laparoscopic cholecystectomy. Bilious drainage from operatively placed drains or through the wound after cholecystectomy is abnormal and represents some form of biliary injury. In patients without drains (including patients in whom the drains have been removed), the bile can leak freely into the peritoneal cavity, or it can loculate as a collection. Free accumulation of bile into the peritoneal cavity results in either biliary as-

cites or bile peritonitis. Similarly, a loculated bile collection can result in sterile biloma (Fig. 42.6) or in an infected subhepatic or subdiaphragmatic abscess.

Patients with postoperative bile duct strictures who present months to years after the initial operation frequently have evidence of cholangitis. The episodes of cholangitis are often mild and respond to antibiotic therapy. Repetitive episodes usually occur before the definitive diagnosis. Less commonly, patients may present with painless jaundice and no evidence of sepsis. Finally, patients with markedly delayed diagnoses may present with advanced biliary cirrhosis and its complications.

Laboratory Investigations

Liver function tests usually show evidence of cholestasis. The serum bilirubin can fluctuate; occasionally, it is normal. In patients with bile leakage, the bilirubin can be normal or minimally elevated owing to absorption from the peritoneal cavity. When elevated, serum bilirubin usually ranges from 2 to 6 mg/dL unless secondary biliary cirrhosis has developed. Serum alkaline phosphatase is usually elevated. Serum aminotransferase levels can be normal or minimally elevated except during episodes of cholangitis. If advanced liver disease exists, hepatic synthetic function can be impaired, with lowered serum albumin and a prolongation of prothrombin time. Serum electrolytes and complete blood count are typically normal unless there is associated biliary sepsis.

Radiologic Examinations

The imaging techniques of abdominal ultrasound and computed tomography (CT) play an important initial role in the evaluation of patients with benign postoperative biliary strictures. In patients who present in the early postoperative period with evidence of a bile leak or biliary sepsis, these studies are useful to rule out the presence of intraabdominal collections that might require drainage (Fig. 42.6). CT and ultrasound are also important in the initial evaluation of the patient presenting with a bile duct stricture months to years after initial operation. Both studies can confirm biliary obstruction by demonstrating a dilated biliary tree. CT is especially useful in identifying the level of obstruction of the extrahepatic bile duct.

In patients suspected of having early postoperative bile duct injury, a radionucleotide biliary scan can confirm bile leakage. In patients with postoperative external bile fistula, injection of water-soluble contrast media through the drainage tract (sinography) can often define the site of leakage and the anatomy of the biliary tree. Sinography can also identify intraabdominal collections and facilitate nonoperative drainage.

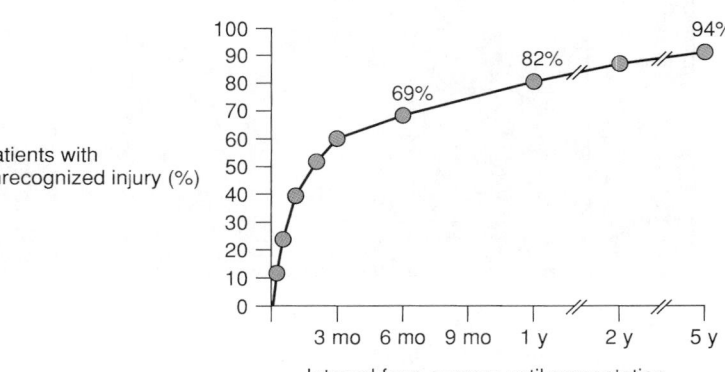

Figure 42.5. The cumulative percentage of patients in whom symptoms develop is shown with respect to the time from the procedure during which the injury occurred until the presentation of the symptoms. (After Pitt HA, Miyamoto T, Parapatis SK, et al. Factors influencing outcome in patients with postoperative biliary strictures. *Am J Surg* 1982;144:14, with permission.)

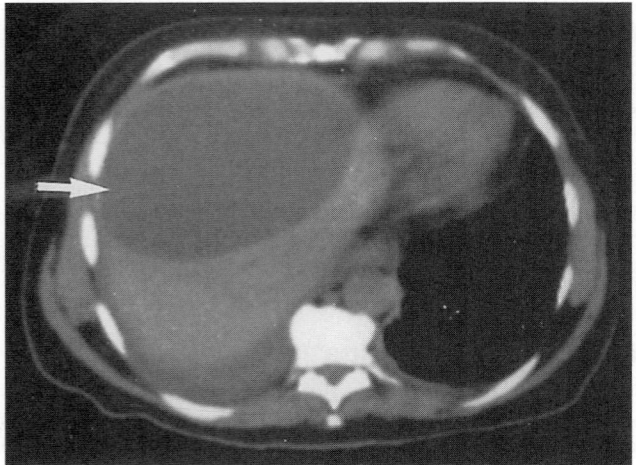

Figure 42.6. Large bile duct collection (biloma; *arrow*) occurring after bile duct injury. (From Lillemoe KD, Pitt HA, Cameron JL. Post-operative bile duct strictures. *Surg Clin North Am* 1990;70: 1362, with permission.)

The gold standard for evaluation of patients with bile duct strictures is cholangiography. Percutaneous transhepatic cholangiography (PTC) is usually more valuable than endoscopic retrograde cholangiography (ERC). PTC is more useful in that it defines the anatomy of the proximal biliary tree that is to be used in the surgical reconstruction (Fig. 42.7). Furthermore, PTC can be followed by placement of percutaneous transhepatic catheters, which can be useful in decompressing the biliary system either to treat or prevent cholangitis. These catheters can also be of assistance in surgical reconstruction and provide access to the biliary tree for nonoperative dilation. ERC is often less useful than PTC because the discontinuity of the extrahepatic bile duct usually prevents adequate filling of the proximal biliary tree (Fig. 42.8). Often, ERC can demonstrate a normal-sized distal bile duct up to the site of the stricture without visualization of the proximal biliary system (Fig. 42.9). This is frequently the case in patients with injury during laparoscopic cholecystectomy, when the distal bile duct is often clipped and divided. The development of magnetic resonance cholangiopancreatography has provided a noninvasive technique that provides excellent delineation of the biliary anatomy. The quality of these images has led some surgeons to advocate this technique as the initial step in the evaluation of patients with suspected bile duct injuries and may eliminate the need for a diagnostic ERC in many patients.

Preoperative Management

The preoperative management of a patient with a postoperative bile duct stricture depends primarily on the timing of the presentation. Patients presenting in the early postoperative period can be septic with either cholangitis or intraabdominal bile collections. Sepsis must be controlled first with broad-spectrum parenteral antibiotics, percutaneous biliary drainage, and percutaneous or operative drainage of biliary leaks. Once sepsis is controlled, there is no hurry in proceeding with surgical reconstruction of the bile duct stricture. The combination of proxi-

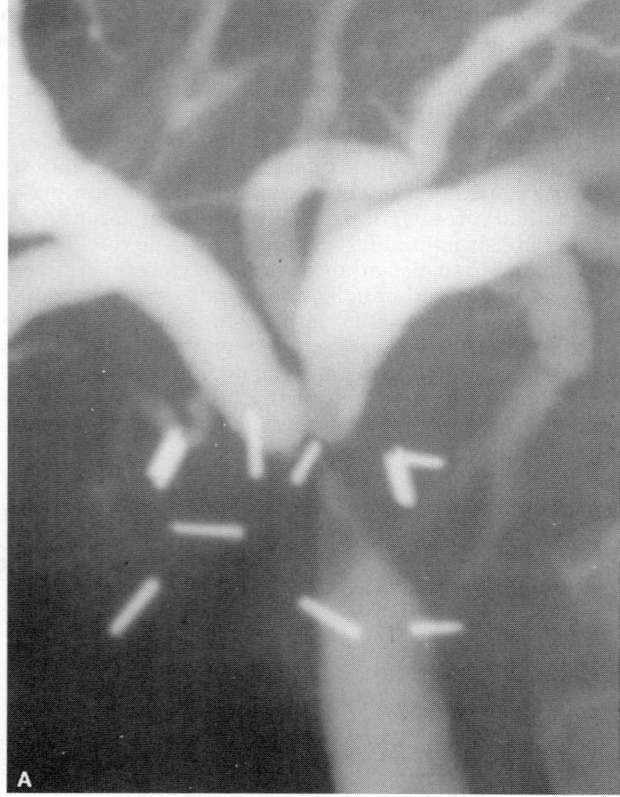

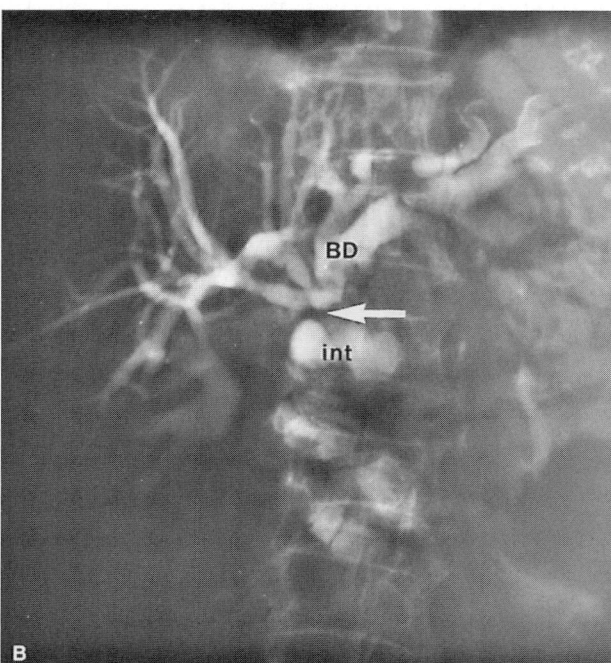

Figure 42.7. *(A)* Percutaneous transhepatic cholangiogram demonstrating bile duct stricture *(arrow)* at hepatic duct bifurcation with proximal duct dilatation. *(B)* Percutaneous transhepatic cholangiogram demonstrating stricture at a hepaticojejunostomy anastomosis. BD, bile duct; int, intestine.

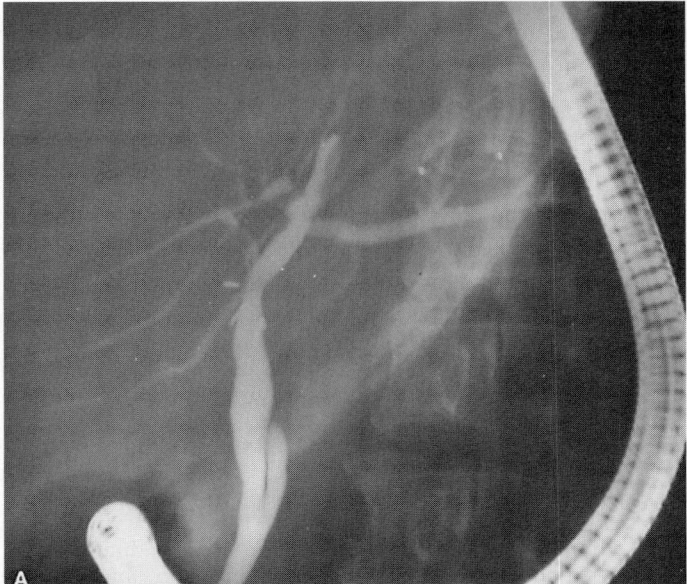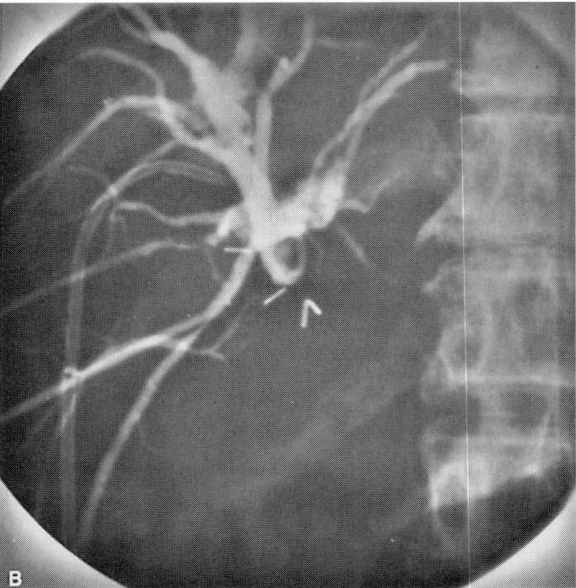

Figure 42.8. *(A)* Endoscopic retrograde cholangiogram showing a relatively normal biliary tree in a patient with a postoperative bile collection (see Fig. 42.6). *(B)* Percutaneous transhepatic cholangiogram of same patient, showing entire right hepatic posterior lobe segment obstructed as the result of ligation of the segmental duct. The patient had an unrecognized anatomic variant similar to that shown in Fig. 42.2.

mal biliary decompression and external drainage allows most biliary fistulae to be controlled or even to close. The patient can then be discharged home to allow several weeks to elapse for resolution of the inflammation in the periportal region and recovery of overall health.

The management of a suspected bile duct injury after laparoscopic cholecystectomy presenting with a bile leak

deserves special mention. Often, when bile leakage is suspected, the surgeon believes that urgent surgical exploration is necessary. Unfortunately, at laparotomy, the marked inflammation associated with bile spillage and the small decompressed biliary tree that appears retracted high into porta hepatis make recognition of the injury and repair virtually impossible. In such cases, every attempt should be made to define the biliary anatomy by preoperative cholangiography and to control the bile leak with either percutaneous or endoscopic stents. In many cases, early operative intervention is not required because the bile either can be drained percutaneously or simply is absorbed from the peritoneal cavity. Delayed reconstruction, aided by percutaneous biliary catheters, then allows optimal surgical results.

In patients who present with a biliary stricture remote from the initial operation, symptoms of cholangitis can necessitate urgent cholangiography and biliary decompression. Biliary drainage is best accomplished by the transhepatic method, although successful endoscopic stent placement can also be accomplished. Parenteral antibiotics and biliary drainage should be continued until sepsis is controlled. In patients who present with jaundice but without cholangitis, cholangiography should be performed to define the anatomy. Preoperative biliary decompression in patients without cholangitis has not been demonstrated to improve outcome.

Surgical Management

The goal of operative management of bile duct stricture is the establishment of bile flow into the proximal gastrointestinal tract in a manner that prevents cholangitis, sludge or stone formation, restricture, and biliary cirrhosis. This goal is best accomplished with a tension-free anastomosis between healthy tissues. A number of surgical alternatives exist for primary repair of bile duct strictures, including end-to-end repair, Roux-en-Y hepaticojejunostomy or choledochojejunostomy, choledochoduodenostomy, and

Figure 42.9. Endoscopic retrograde pancreaticocholangiogram showing filling of a normal pancreatic duct (PD). The common bile duct (CBD), however, does not fill beyond the large clip that appears to be placed across the duct. (From Lillemoe KD, Pitt HA, Cameron JL. Postoperative bile duct strictures. *Surg Clin North Am* 1990;70:1363, with permission.)

mucosal grafting. The choice of repair depends on a number of factors, including the extent and location of the strictures, the experience of the surgeon, and the timing of the repair.

Immediate Repair of Intraoperative Bile Duct Injury

In many cases, initial proper management of bile duct injury recognized at the time of cholecystectomy can avoid the development of a bile duct stricture. Unfortunately, recognition of a bile duct injury is uncommon during either open or laparoscopic cholecystectomy. If bile leakage is observed or atypical anatomy is encountered during laparoscopic cholecystectomy, early conversion to an open technique and prompt cholangiography are imperative. If a segmental or accessory duct less than 3 mm has been injured and cholangiography demonstrates segmental or subsegmental drainage of the injured ductal system, simple ligation of the injured duct is adequate. If the injured duct is 4 mm or larger, however, it is likely to drain multiple hepatic segments or the entire right or left lobe and thus requires operative repair.

If the injury involves the common hepatic duct or the common bile duct, repair should also be carried out at the time of injury. The aims of any repair should be to maintain ductal length and not to sacrifice tissue as well as to effect a repair that will not result in postoperative bile leakage. To accomplish these goals, all repairs at the time of initial operation should involve some sort of external drainage. If the injured segment of the bile duct is short (<1 cm), and the two ends can be opposed without tension, an end-to-end anastomosis can be performed with placement of a T-tube through a separate choledochotomy either above or below the anastomosis. Generous mobilization of the duodenum out of the retroperitoneum (Kocher maneuver) can be useful to help approximate the injured ends of the bile duct. An end-to-end repair, however, should be avoided if the ductal injury is near the hepatic duct bifurcation.

For proximal injuries or if the injured segment of bile duct is greater than 1 cm in length, an end-to-end bile duct anastomosis should be avoided because of the excessive tension that usually exists in these situations. In these circumstances, the distal bile duct should be oversewn, and the proximal bile duct should be débrided of injured tissue and anastomosed in an end-to-side fashion to a Roux-en-Y jejunal limb. The use of a Roux-en-Y jejunal limb is preferable to anastomosis to the duodenum because, in the latter case, an anastomotic leak results in a duodenal fistula.

The long-term results of immediate repair of common bile duct injuries is uncertain. Most injuries occur away from major centers, and therefore even the successes are unlikely to be reported in the literature. In a Swedish report, early primary repair with end-to-end anastomosis resulted in good results in only 22% of patients. Anastomotic leak requiring reoperation occurred in 32% of patients, and late stricture occurred in another 37% of patients. In patients undergoing immediate repair with a biliary-enteric anastomosis, good results were seen in 54% of patients, with strictures occurring in only 12% of patients. Similar poor late results were observed in another series in which 29 of 36 patients with primary end-to-end repair had postoperative strictures within 4 years.

Elective Repair of Established Strictures

Several principles are associated with successful repair of a biliary stricture: exposure of healthy proximal bile ducts that provide drainage of the entire liver; preparation of a suitable segment of intestine that can be brought to the area of the stricture without tension, most frequently a Roux-en-Y jejunal limb; and creation of a direct biliary-enteric mucosal-to-mucosal anastomosis. A number of alternatives for elective repair of bile duct strictures exist. The choice of procedure is dictated by the location of the stricture, the history of previous unsuccessful attempts at repair, and the surgeon's personal preference. Simple excision of a bile duct stricture and end-to-end bile duct anastomosis or repair of the damaged duct can rarely be accomplished because of the invariable loss of duct length as a result of fibrosis associated with the injury. Similarly, anastomosis of the proximal bile duct to the duodenum as a choledochoduodenostomy is not suitable for most postcholecystectomy strictures because an adequate length of bile duct for creating a tension-free anastomosis to the duodenum usually cannot be obtained. Thus, in almost all cases, hepaticojejunostomy constructed to a Roux-en-Y limb of jejunum is the preferred procedure.

Many surgeons believe that a transanastomotic stent is helpful in almost all cases. In the early postoperative period, a stent is used to decompress the biliary tree and provide access for cholangiography. If the injury involves the common bile duct or the common hepatic duct at least 2 cm distal to the hepatic duct bifurcation, and adequate proximal bile duct mucosa can be defined, the use of long-term biliary stents is not necessary. In these situations, the preoperatively placed percutaneous transhepatic catheter or operatively placed T-tube is used to decompress the biliary-enteric anastomosis for 4 to 6 weeks after surgery. When adequate proximal bile duct is not available for a good mucosa-to-mucosa anastomosis, long-term stenting of the biliary-enteric anastomosis with a Silastic transhepatic stent is recommended. For strictures involving the hepatic duct bifurcation, both the right and left main hepatic ducts should be individually stented.

An operative technique for biliary reconstruction with transhepatic stents uses the preoperatively placed percutaneous transhepatic catheters (4,5). The porta hepatis is dissected, which usually involves separating adhesions of the duodenum and hepatic flexure of the colon to Glisson's capsule and the gallbladder fossa. Identification of the proximal biliary segment can be difficult and can be aided by the presence of the transhepatic biliary catheter. The bile duct is then divided at the lowest extent of the stricture and dissected proximally. A segment of the strictured duct should be resected and submitted for pathologic examination. The distal duct is then oversewn, and the bile duct proximal to the stricture is carefully dissected circumferentially in a cephalad direction for a distance not to exceed 5 mm. Excessive dissection should be avoided to prevent vascular compromise of this segment of duct, which will be used for the anastomosis. After mobilization and division of the bile duct, the biliary catheters protrude through the proximal end (Fig. 42.10A). A radiologic guide wire is then placed through these catheters. A series of progressively larger coudé catheters are then passed over the guide wire, dilating the system to allow the placement of a Silastic stent. The Silastic stents are 70 cm long and come in 12F to 22F sizes. Multiple side holes are present along 40% of the length of the stent. These side holes are left to reside within the intrahepatic biliary tree and the portion of the Roux-en-Y jejunal limb used for the biliary anastomosis. The end of the stent without the side holes exits through the hepatic parenchyma and is brought out through a stab wound in the upper anterior abdomen. After stent placement, a Roux-en-Y jejunal limb is prepared, and the anastomosis is then performed as an end-to-side hepaticojejunostomy (Fig. 42.10B).

An alternative technique has been described for management of bile duct strictures involving the bifurcation

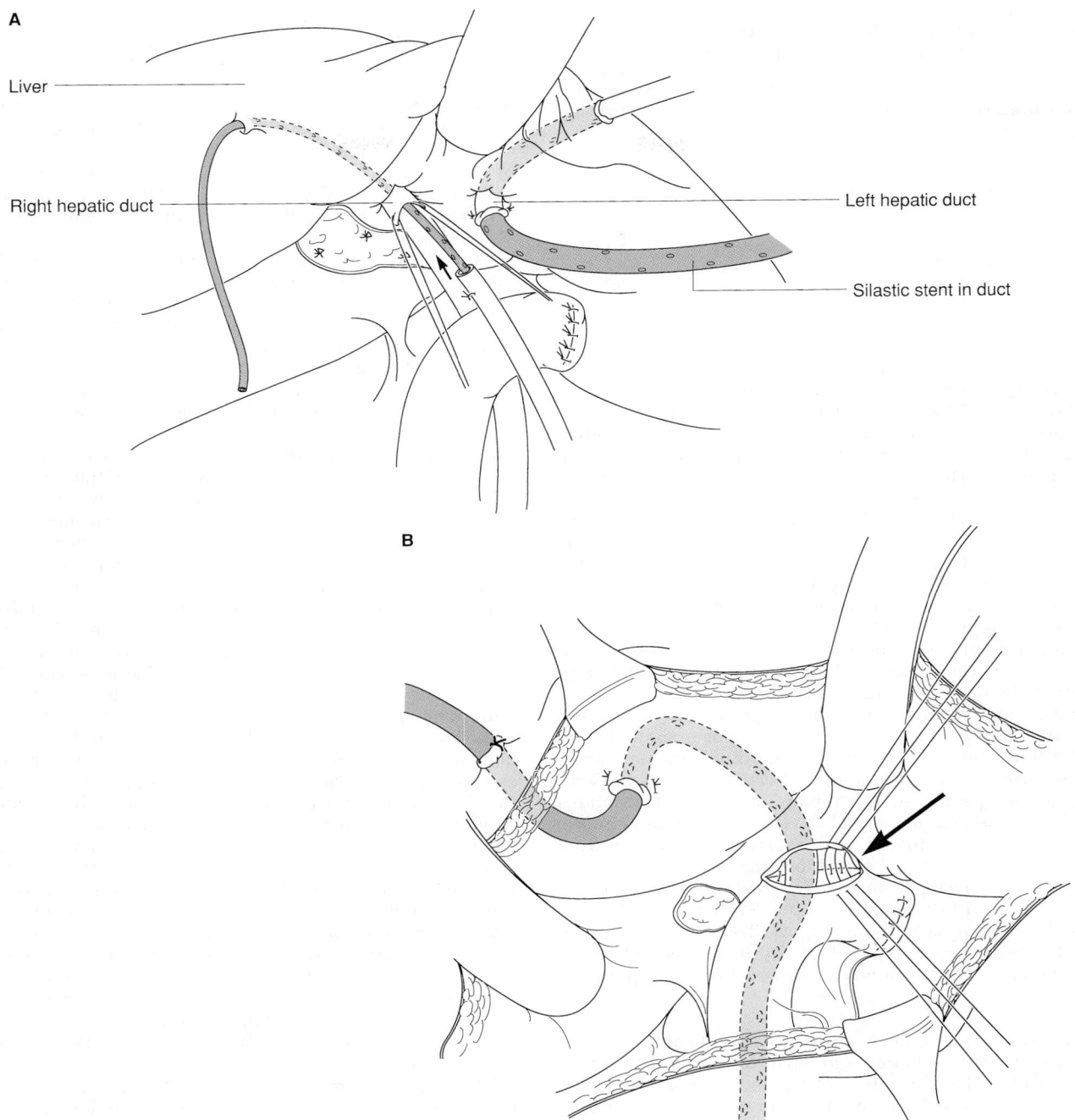

Figure 42.10. *(A)* A coudé catheter is sutured to the preoperatively placed transhepatic catheter, which protrudes through the transected hepatic duct. The coudé catheter and subsequently the Silastic stent can then be pulled through the catheter tract in the hepatic parenchyma. *(B)* A Roux-en-Y jejunal loop is then anastomosed to the hepatic duct at the egress site of the Silastic stent in the hilum of the liver. The portion of the stent that passes through the liver and into the jejunum contains multiple side holes. (After Cameron JL, Gayler BW, Zuidema GD. The use of Silastic transhepatic stents in benign and malignant strictures. *Ann Surg* 1978;188:552, with permission.)

and one or both of the hepatic ducts in which a side-to-side anastomosis of the left hepatic duct to the Roux-en-Y limb is constructed. A long opening along the anterior surface of the left hepatic duct is anastomosed to the side of the Roux-en-Y limb. Because it is possible to dissect the anterior surface of the left hepatic duct high up into the hepatic parenchyma, this procedure permits anastomosis to normal mucosa, even though there can be fibrosis and stricture at the bifurcation of the ducts and in the distal

portion of the hepatic duct. This technique can avoid the need for postoperative stenting.

Results

Morbidity and Mortality

Repairs of bile duct strictures are performed primarily in major medical centers by experienced surgeons, yet

Table 42.1. **RESULTS OF SURGICAL MANAGEMENT OF BILE DUCT STRICTURES**

Investigators	Patients	Success (%)	Follow-up (mo)
Pitt et al., 1982[2]	66	86	60
Pelligrini et al., 1984[3]	60	78	102
Genest, 1986	105	82	60
Innes, 1988	22	95	72
Pain, 1988	163	72	133
Pitt et al., 1989[5]	25	88	57
David et al., 1993[12]	35	83	50
Lillemoe et al., 2000[8]	142	91	58

these operations are still associated with significant morbidity and mortality. In 1982, a review of 38 series published since 1900, containing over 7,643 procedures performed on 5,586 patients, reported an overall operative mortality rate of 8.3% (6). In the 1990s, however, most series have reported mortality rates of less than 5%. Factors frequently associated with operative mortality include advanced age, coexistent disease, and a history of major biliary tract infection. The state of underlying liver disease, however, is the most important determinant of operative morbidity and mortality. In patients with advanced biliary cirrhosis and portal hypertension, operative mortality rates can approach 30%, with most deaths due to liver failure. Bile duct strictures located proximally are also associated with increased technical difficulty and thus also contribute to slightly increased risk.

Postoperative morbidity rates approach 20% to 30%. Complications may include the usual postoperative complications, such as hemorrhage, cardiopulmonary problems, urinary tract infection, and wound infection. Complications specific to the repair of bile duct strictures include anastomotic leaks at the site of the biliary-enteric anastomosis, cholangitis, and hepatic insufficiency from preexisting biliary cirrhosis. Most anastomotic leaks documented by postoperative cholangiography or by bilious drainage from intraoperatively placed drains can be successfully managed without surgery. Transhepatic stenting diverts biliary secretions externally in the face of a leak and is one of the major advantages of this technique.

Long-term Results

Excellent long-term results can be achieved in 70% to 90% of patients who undergo repair of bile duct strictures (Table 42.1). The definition of satisfactory results in most series requires that patients have no symptoms, jaundice, or cholangitis. Length of follow-up is important in analyzing final results because recurrent strictures can occur up to 20 years after the initial procedure (2,3) (Fig. 42.11). Approximately two thirds of restrictures are evident within 2 years, and 90% are seen within 7 years. The percentage of patients with good results is inversely related to the number of previous repairs. Other factors that favor a good outcome include young age at the time of stricture repair, use of a Roux-en-Y biliary-enteric anastomosis, absence of infection and hepatic fibrosis, and use of transhepatic stents.

It had been well established in the era before laparoscopic cholecystectomy that excellent long-term results were obtainable in tertiary care centers, specializing in the management of these problems. Questions had arisen as to whether the excellent results of bile duct strictures after open cholecystectomy could be directly transferred to patients sustaining laparoscopic bile duct injuries. Some had suggested that the mechanism of bile duct injury during laparoscopic cholecystectomy, the complex nature of many of these injuries, and the frequent association of significant inflammation and fibrosis secondary to sustained, unrecognized bile leakage might result in poor long-term results. Furthermore, the high percentage of these patients who have undergone unsuccessful operations, often performed by the primary laparoscopic surgeon, might also lead to a poor long-term outcome. Evidence for the latter hypothesis was provided by a recent report (7). In this report, the records of 85 patients who underwent a total of 112 biliary repairs were analyzed. Four factors determined the success or failure of treatment in this series. These factors included performance of preoperative cholangiography, the choice of surgical repair, details of the operative repair, and experience of the surgeon performing the repair. The importance of preoperative delineation of anatomy was clear, in that 96% of procedures in which cholangiograms were not obtained before surgery were unsuccessful, and 69% of repairs were not successful when the cholangiographic data were incomplete. When cholangiographic data were complete, the initial repair was successful in 84% of patients. The type of repair was also of significance in influencing outcome. A primary end-to-end ductal repair over a T-tube was unsuccessful in all patients in whom a complete transection of the bile duct had taken place, whereas 63% of Roux-en-Y hepaticojejunostomies were successful. Attempts at repair by the primary surgeon were successful only in 17% of cases, and in no case was a secondary repair by the primary surgeon successful. In those cases in which the first repair was performed by a tertiary care biliary surgeon, a 94% success rate was obtained.

The outcome of management of 142 patients with major bile duct injuries treated during the 1990s has been reported (8). Laparoscopic cholecystectomy was the initial

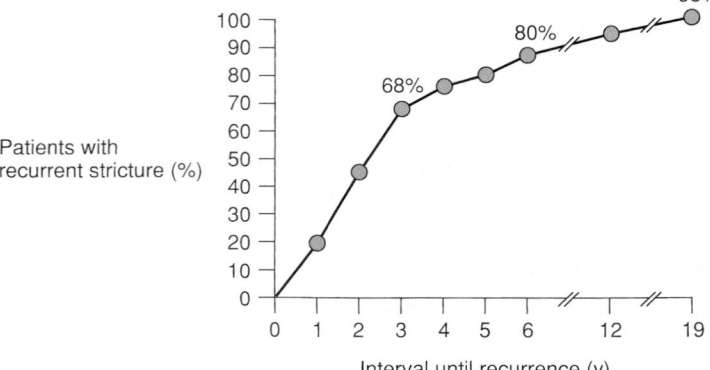

Figure 42.11. The cumulative percentage of recurrent strictures with respect to the time from the initial repair until the next repair. (After Pitt HA, Miyamoto T, Parapatis SK, et al. Factors influencing outcome in patients with postoperative biliary strictures. *Am J Surg* 1982; 144:14, with permission.)

operation in 75% of these patients, and 41% had undergone a previous attempt or attempts at surgical repair before referral. In this series with a median follow-up of 58 months (range, 11 to 119 months), a successful outcome was obtained in 91% of patients. These results suggest that surgical reconstruction of major bile duct injuries after laparoscopic cholecystectomy can still result in excellent long-term results.

Nonoperative Management

Operative management of bile duct strictures is technically difficult and continues to be associated with significant postoperative morbidity and mortality. Moreover, in all series, recurrent strictures develop in a proportion of patients. These factors, in addition to technical advances in the fields of therapeutic radiology and endoscopy, have led to the development of nonoperative techniques for management of bile duct strictures.

Percutaneous Balloon Dilation

The largest nonoperative experience in the management of benign bile duct strictures is using the percutaneous transhepatic route. The procedure in many cases can be performed with a combination of local anesthesia and intravenous sedation. In this technique, access to the proximal biliary tree is gained and the stricture is traversed with a guide wire under fluoroscopic guidance. At this point, the stricture is dilated using angioplasty-type balloon catheters, chosen on the basis of the location of the stricture and the diameter of the normal duct (Fig. 42.12). After the procedure, a transhepatic stent is left in place across the stricture to allow access to the biliary tree for follow-up cholangiography, repeat dilation, and maintenance of a lumen during the healing process. In most series, numerous dilations are required.

The early results in a number of series have been encouraging (Table 42.2). In a multicenter review, 3-year follow-up showed a 67% patency rate for anastomotic and a 76% patency rate for iatrogenic primary bile duct strictures, yielding an overall 70% success rate (9). Others have achieved successful dilatation in 87.5% of patients with primary ductal strictures and in 72.5% of patients with biliary-enteric anastomotic strictures, with an overall success rate of 78% (10). A report of 25 patients with bile duct strictures after laparoscopic cholecystectomy managed with percutaneous dilation showed a success rate of 64% with a mean follow-up of 28 months (11).

Complications of balloon dilation are frequent. Cholangitis, hemobilia, and bile leaks can occur in up to 20% of patients. Bleeding, usually from the hepatic parenchyma, has been reported, with transfusions often necessary. Sepsis due to cholangitis can occur despite antibiotic prophylaxis. Sepsis and significant bleeding seldom occur in patients dilated by a T-tube tract, suggesting that much of the morbidity is the result of traversing the hepatic parenchyma by the large percutaneously placed catheters.

Endoscopic Balloon Dilation

The experience with endoscopic balloon dilation is more limited. This technique is technically possible only in patients with primary bile duct strictures or with strictures at a choledochoduodenal anastomosis. This technique begins with ERC and endoscopic sphincterotomy. The stricture is traversed retrograde with an atraumatic guide wire, and sequential balloon dilation is used. Reevaluation with cholangiography is performed every 3 to 6 months. Redilation is performed as necessary. In most cases, an endoprosthesis is left in place after dilation for at least 6 months.

The reported experience with endoscopic dilation of benign bile duct strictures is shown in Table 42.3. The largest experience comes from the group in The Netherlands and is discussed in the following section (Comparative Data) (12). A similar experience was reported in the United States (13). In this series, 18 of 25 strictures were postoperative. Strictures were located at the cystic duct junction in 17 patients and in the distal bile duct in the remaining 8 patients. Twenty-two of 25 patients (88%) had significant clinical benefit from the therapy. Only two complications occurred in this series—one case each of pancreatitis and cholangitis.

Comparative Data

Comparison of results of nonoperative dilation with those of surgery have been difficult. Few centers have a significant experience with both operative and nonoperative management. Furthermore, the definition of a successful procedure, the reporting of complications, and the length of follow-up have not been consistent in the literature. There are no prospective, randomized studies to compare these techniques. However, two retrospective comparative studies exist. In the first study, a retrospective review of the results at the Johns Hopkins Hospital between 1979 and 1987 compared percutaneous balloon dilation and surgery in 43 patients with benign postoperative bile duct strictures (5). Twenty-five patients underwent surgical repair with Roux-en-Y choledochojejunostomy or hepaticojejunostomy with postoperative transhepatic stenting for a mean of 13 ± 1.3 months. Twenty patients had percutaneous balloon dilation, a mean of 3.9 times, and were stented transhepatically for a mean of 13.3 ± 2 months. Three patients were managed with both surgery and balloon dilation. The two groups were similar with respect to multiple parameters that might have influenced outcome, including age, sex, associated medical problems, and presentation with either obstructive jaundice or biliary fistulas.

No patients died after any of the procedures. Procedure-related morbidity occurred in 20% of surgical patients and in 35% of the patients undergoing balloon dilation. For both groups, a successful outcome was defined as no evidence of cholangitis or jaundice requiring another procedure more than 12 months from the onset of treatment. A failed treatment was defined as the need for crossover to the other treatment modality, either operation or dilation, or late death from liver failure, biliary sepsis, or portal hypertension. A successful repair was achieved in 89% of the surgical patients and in only 52% of the balloon dilation patients (Fig. 42.13). The overall late mortality rate in this series was 10%. One late death occurred in the surgical group, whereas three late deaths followed balloon dilation (4% vs. 15%, respectively). No deaths, however, were attributed to liver failure, biliary sepsis, or portal hypertension associated with the bile duct stricture.

To define further the relative benefits of the two procedures, total hospital stay and total procedural costs were determined. As expected, initial hospitalization was longer for surgery than for balloon dilation. When rehospitalization for further dilation, complications, or recurrences were considered, total hospital stay did not differ significantly between the two groups. Cost data paralleled hospitalization data and did not differ significantly between the groups. Thus, the authors concluded that until properly designed, randomized, prospective, controlled trials can be performed, surgical repair for benign postoperative strictures appears to be associated with fewer problems and a greater success rate.

In the second comparative study, the group from The Netherlands compared endoscopic versus surgical treat-

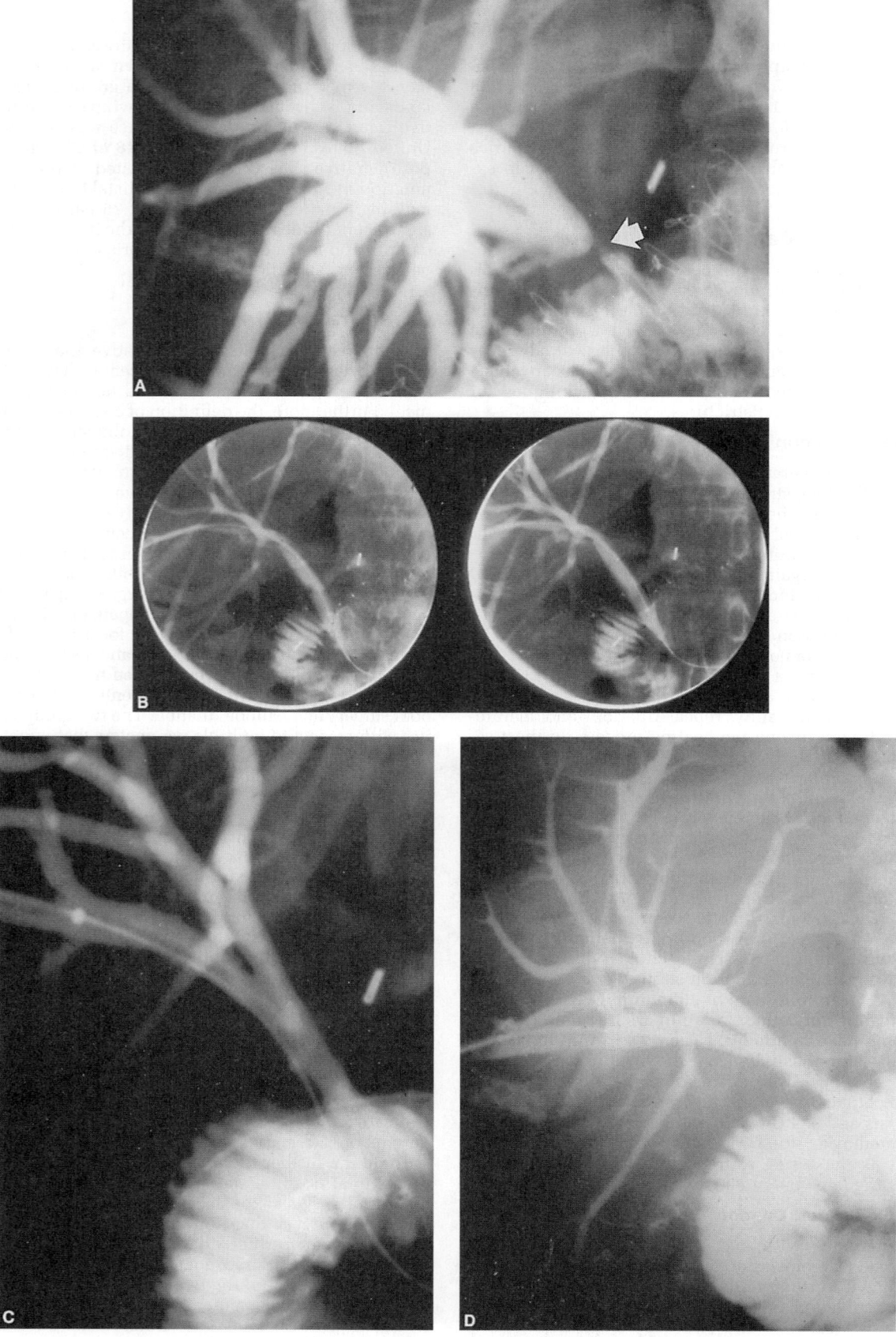

Figure 42.12. *(A)* Transhepatic cholangiogram demonstrating stricture *(arrow)* at a previous chole-dochojejunostomy. *(B)* Progressive dilation of the strictured anastomosis with an angioplasty bal-loon catheter. *(C)* Postdilation stenting of the anastomotic stricture for prolonged periods. *(D)* Sub-sequent cholangiogram demonstrating resolution of the anastomotic stricture. (From Pitt HA, Kaufman SL, Coleman J, et al. Benign postoperative biliary strictures: operate or dilate? *Ann Surg* 1989;210:417, with permission.)

Table 42.2. RESULTS OF TRANSHEPATIC BALLOON DILATION OF BILE DUCT STRICTURES

Investigators	Patients	Success (%)	Follow-up (mo)
Mueller et al., 1986[9]	61	70	36
Williams, 1987	64	78	28
Moore, 1987	18	83	33
Pitt et al., 1989[5]	20	55	59
Citron et al., 1991	28	93	38
Lillemoe et al., 1997[11]	25	64	28

Table 42.3. RESULTS OF ENDOSCOPIC BALLOON DILATATION OF BILE DUCT STRICTURES

Investigators	Patients	Success (%)	Follow-up (mo)
Foutsch, 1985	9	55	6
Geenen et al., 1989[13]	25	88	48
David et al., 1993[12]	46	83	48

ment of benign bile duct strictures (12). Thirty-five patients were treated surgically, and 66 were treated by endoscopic stenting. Patient characteristics, initial injury, previous repairs, and the level of obstruction were comparable in both groups. Surgical therapy consisted of Roux-en-Y hepaticojejunostomy, and endoscopic therapy consisted of placement of an endoprosthesis with trimonthly elective exchange for 1 year. Successful stent placement was accomplished in 94% of patients managed endoscopically. Six of the 66 endoscopic patients, however, underwent surgical reconstruction either for failed stent placement or for other reasons. Early complications occurred more frequently in the surgically treated group (26% vs. 8%; $p < .03$). However, the only procedure-related death occurred in a patient in whom severe pancreatitis developed after endoscopic stent placement. Late complications, which included primarily episodes of cholangitis, occurred only in the endoscopic group (27%). The overall complication rates, therefore, were similar at 26% for surgical patients and 35% for endoscopic patients. The mean follow-up and definition of success were similar to those in the aforementioned study. After surgery, excellent results were observed in 83% of patients, with a recurrent

stricture developing in 6 patients at a mean of 40 months after the initial operation. After endoscopic stenting, excellent results were observed in 72% of patients, with restricture developing in 18% of patients at a mean of 3 months after stent removal. The investigators concluded that endoscopic stenting should be considered for the initial attempt at definitive management in suitable patients in the hope of avoiding reoperation.

PRIMARY SCLEROSING CHOLANGITIS

Primary sclerosing cholangitis is an idiopathic disease characterized by intrahepatic and extrahepatic inflammatory strictures of the bile ducts that cannot be attributed to other specific causes. The cause of primary sclerosing cholangitis is unknown. Many experts consider primary sclerosing cholangitis to be an autoimmune reaction because it is associated with other autoimmune diseases, such as ulcerative colitis, retroperitoneal fibrosis, and Riedel's thyroiditis (Table 42.4). It is likely that a number of causes, including viral or bacterial infections, toxic drug reactions, and congenital anomalies, can all result in the same end-stage injury that is recognized as primary sclerosing cholangitis.

The usual clinical presentation of patients with primary sclerosing cholangitis involves intermittent jaundice, which begins insidiously in the fourth or fifth decade of life. Right upper quadrant pain, pruritus, fever, weight loss, and fatigue can also occur. The disease is characterized by cyclic remissions and exacerbations. Despite the nomenclature, acute cholangitis is uncommon without previous biliary manipulation or surgery. The diagnosis is suggested by clinical presentation associated with cholestatic liver function test abnormalities. The levels of bilirubin often fluctuate with respect to the remissions and exacerbations of the disease and the extent of hepatic injury. Alkaline phosphatase is usually elevated out of proportion to the serum bilirubin, and is a more persistent finding. The diagnosis, however, usually is confirmed by cholangiography, which reveals multiple dilatations and strictures (beading) of the intrahepatic and extrahepatic bile ducts (Fig. 42.14). ERC is the preferred procedure because of difficulties in cannulation of the intrahepatic ducts by the percutaneous transhepatic route, because the ducts are usually nondilated and fibrotic. The disease should be followed closely by cholangiography and liver biopsy to provide appropriate management before the development of biliary cirrhosis.

No known specific medical therapy is effective for primary sclerosing cholangitis. The most encouraging results,

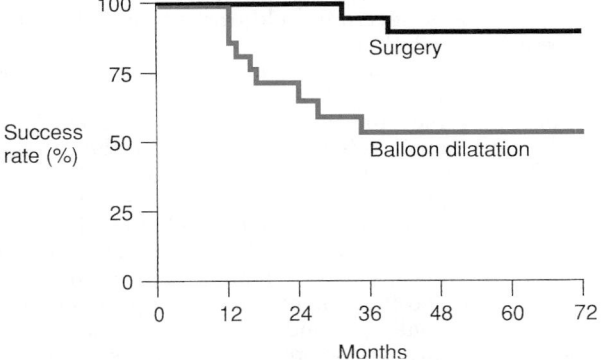

Figure 42.13. Actuarial success rates over 72 months for surgery (89%) and balloon dilation (52%). The difference is statistically significant ($p < .01$). (After Pitt HA, Kaufman SL, Coleman J, et al. Benign postoperative biliary strictures: operate or dilate? *Ann Surg* 1989;210:417, with permission.)

Table 42.4. DISEASES ASSOCIATED WITH PRIMARY SCLEROSING CHOLANGITIS

Disease	Frequency (%)
Ulcerative colitis	40–60
Pancreatitis	12–25
Diabetes mellitus	5–10
Retroperitoneal fibrosis	Rare
Riedel's thyroiditis	Rare
Crohn's disease	Rare
Histiocytosis X	Rare
Sicca complex	Rare
Rheumatoid arthritis	Rare
Hypertrophic osteoarthropathy	Rare
Sarcoidosis	Rare
Angioimmunoblastic lymphadenopathy	Rare
Acquired immunodeficiency syndrome	Rare

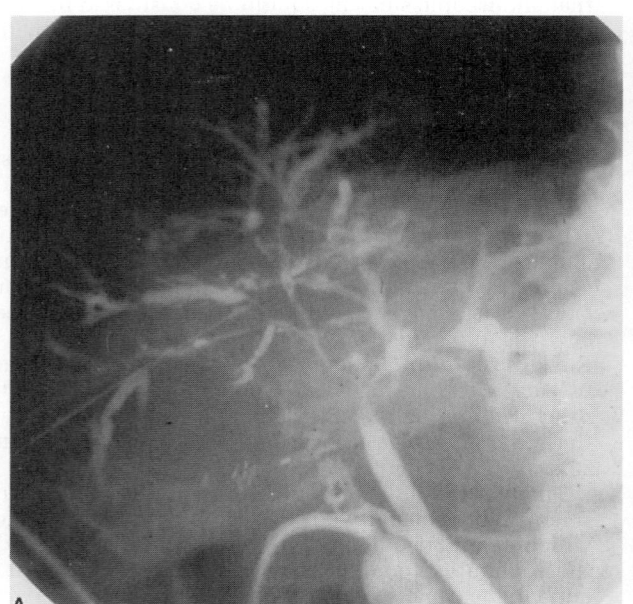
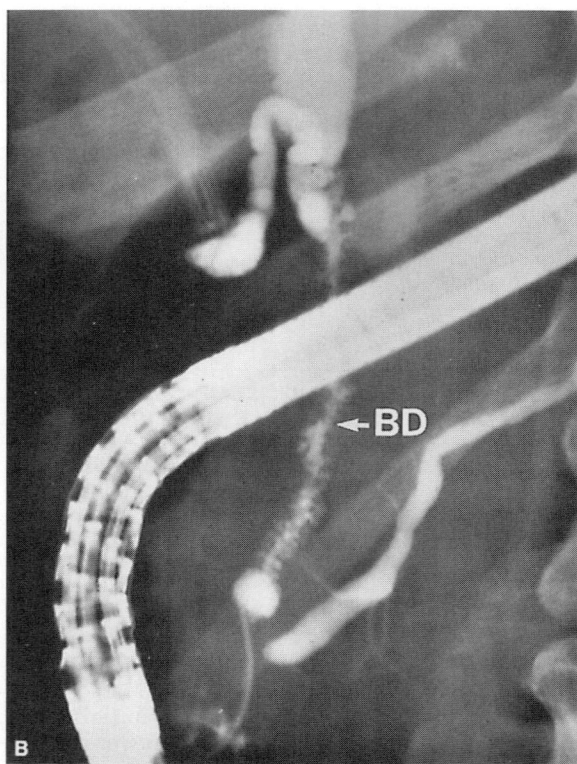

Figure 42.14. *(A)* Cholangiogram of a patient with primary sclerosing cholangitis. Multiple irregular strictures and dilatation (beading) of intrahepatic bile ducts can be seen. *(B)* Endoscopic retrograde cholangiogram showing extensive involvement of extrahepatic bile duct (BD) with primary sclerosing cholangitis. *(B* from Lillemoe KD, Pitt HA, Cameron JL. Primary sclerosing cholangitis. *Surg Clin North Am* 1990;70:1390, with permission.)

from a prospective, randomized, placebo-controlled trial, suggest that ursodeoxycholic acid significantly improves serum liver function tests and liver histologic appearance. Unfortunately, there were no significant differences in clinical outcome between the two groups at up to 6 years of follow-up (14). Nonoperative dilation therapy (discussed earlier), by either the transhepatic or endoscopic route, has been used for dominant strictures. In a multicenter review of percutaneous balloon dilation, only 43% of patients with primary sclerosing cholangitis had successful long-term results (9). The results of endoscopic dilation and stenting may be more favorable.

Because of the lack of effective medical therapy, an aggressive surgical approach is advocated for most symptomatic patients with primary sclerosing cholangitis. One surgical approach, in patients with a dominant stricture at the hepatic duct bifurcation, uses resection of the bifurcation and long-term transhepatic stenting with Silastic stents. This mode of therapy was reported in 31 patients (15). Indications for operation included persistent jaundice in 29 patients and recurrent cholangitis in 2 patients. Five of the 31 patients had secondary biliary cirrhosis before surgery, with the remaining 26 having varying degrees of fibrosis without cirrhosis. The 1- and 5-year actuarial survival rates for patients with fibrosis were 92% and 71%, respectively, whereas the actuarial survival rate at 1 and 5 years was 20% in patients with established biliary cirrhosis (Fig. 42.15). Four patients have undergone hepatic transplantation for progressive disease. A more recent report of this form of surgical therapy has demonstrated a greater and longer biochemical improvement, improved survival until death or liver transplantation, and

a lower incidence of cholangiocarcinoma than was observed in patients treated medically or with endoscopic or percutaneous dilation (16).

The role of biliary surgery in primary sclerosing cholangitis, however, has decreased considerably with the growing success of liver transplantation. Primary sclerosing cholangitis has become one of the most common indications for liver transplantation in the United States, with a cumulative 1-year survival rate after transplantation of greater than 85%, with many programs achieving 90% to 97% 1-year survival rates, and better than an 85% 5-year survival rate (17). Liver transplantation should be considered before the disease is too advanced. The development of a poor quality of life as a result of disabling fatigue, intractable pruritus, severe muscle wasting, and chronic or recurrent bacterial cholangitis or persistent elevations in serum bilirubin are primary indications for referral for liver transplantation.

Preoperative recognition of cholangiocarcinoma is extremely important in this population in that the development of this complication significantly worsens the result after liver transplantation. The presence of known malignancy results in patients being refused transplantation. The microscopic identification of intrahepatic cholangiocarcinoma in the absence of lymph node involvement often demonstrated in the explanted liver specimen, however, does not usually portend a poor prognosis.

Patients with primary sclerosing cholangitis have a significantly higher rate of development of nonanastomotic biliary strictures after liver transplantation, with histologic features on posttransplantation biopsy consistent with recurrence of the disease. Other causes of stricture, such as

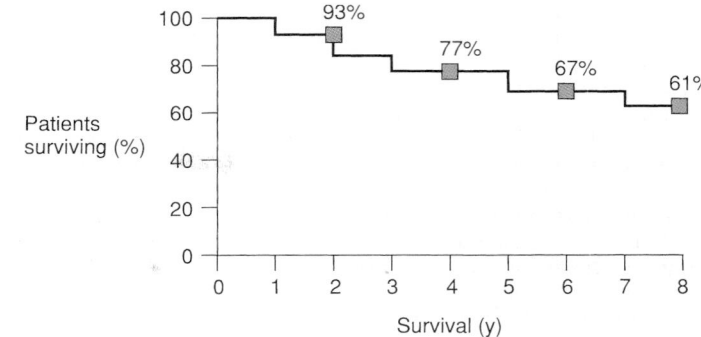

Figure 42.15. Actuarial survival rates among 31 noncirrhotic patients with primary sclerosing cholangitis who underwent resection of the hepatic bifurcation and long-term transhepatic stenting. (From Lillemoe KD, Pitt HA, Cameron JL. Primary sclerosing cholangitis. *Surg Clin North Am* 1990;70: 1397, with permission.)

hepatic artery thrombosis, preservation-related ischemia, cytomegalovirus infection, and chronic ductopenic rejection, can cause similar lesions. Recurrent primary sclerosing cholangitis usually does not have an aggressive course.

Resection of the hepatic duct bifurcation and long-term transanastomotic stenting in selected patients can preclude or delay the need for hepatic transplantation. Moreover, this operation does not eliminate or influence the results of hepatic transplantation. Resection of the hepatic bifurcation and long-term transhepatic stenting can be recommended for selected patients with primary sclerosing cholangitis with severe strictures at or distal to the hepatic duct bifurcation but without established biliary cirrhosis. In patients with biliary cirrhosis, hepatic transplantation is recommended.

BILE DUCT STRICTURES SECONDARY TO CHRONIC PANCREATITIS

Chronic pancreatitis is an uncommon cause of benign bile duct strictures, resulting in less than 10% of such cases. Transient partial obstruction of the distal common bile duct due to inflammation and edema frequently occurs in patients with acute pancreatitis. With chronic pancreatitis, however, the clinical problem is distal bile duct obstruction due to inflammation and parenchymal fibrosis of the gland. These strictures classically involve the entire intrapancreatic segment of the common bile duct and are associated with dilatation of the entire proximal biliary tree (Fig. 42.16). In most cases, the cause of the chronic pancreatitis is alcoholism. Often, advanced disease is present in that the incidence of pancreatic calcification, diabetes, and malabsorption is increased at the time of presentation with jaundice compared with patients with chronic pancreatitis without jaundice. Common bile duct strictures have been reported to occur in 3% to 29% of patients with chronic alcoholic pancreatitis. In a review of a number of clinical series, the overall incidence of common bile duct strictures in patients with chronic pancreatitis was 5.7% (18). The exact incidence of common bile duct strictures is not known, however, because cholangiography is not routinely performed in patients with chronic pancreatitis.

The clinical presentation of patients with common bile duct strictures secondary to chronic pancreatitis is variable. Some patients have no symptoms, with the diagnosis of bile duct strictures suggested only by abnormal liver function test results. The serum alkaline phosphatase appears to be the most sensitive laboratory finding and is elevated in over 80% of patients. Abdominal pain with or without jaundice is another common presentation. In some cases, the abdominal pain can be difficult to distinguish from the pain associated with chronic pancreatitis. Failure to recognize and address a bile duct stricture, how-

ever, can lead to ultimate failure of operative procedures performed for chronic pain in patients with chronic pancreatitis. Finally, the development of jaundice in patients with chronic pancreatitis must be differentiated from underlying periampullary malignancy.

The definitive evaluation of patients with a bile duct stricture due to chronic pancreatitis is cholangiography. Either endoscopic retrograde cholangiopancreatography (ERCP) or PTC can be useful. ERCP offers the advantage of demonstrating pancreatic ductal anatomy and possible abnormality, which is essential in optimal surgical management of chronic pancreatitis. Both techniques allow decompression of the obstructed biliary tree if necessary for cholangitis or severe jaundice. A long (usually 2 to 4 cm),

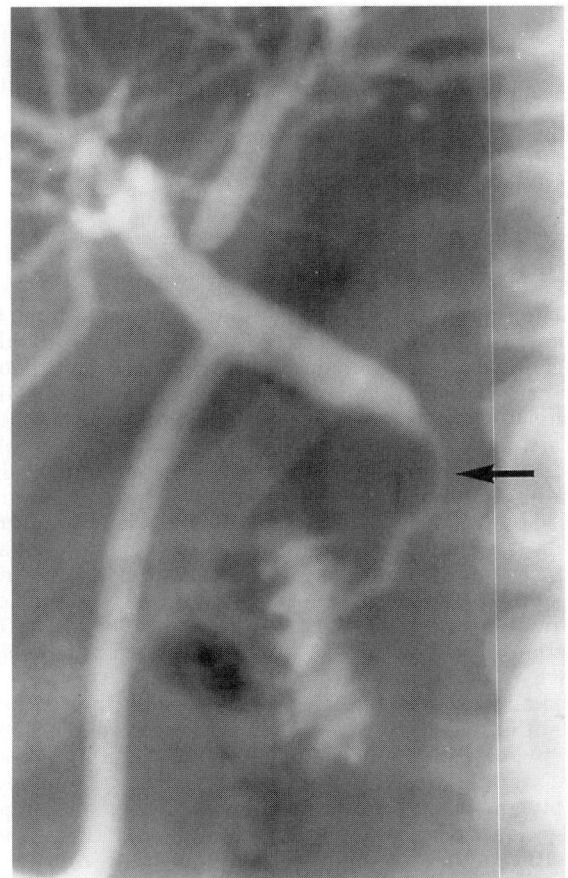

Figure 42.16. Cholangiogram of a patient with a long distal common bile duct stricture *(arrow)* due to chronic pancreatitis.

smooth, gradual tapering of the common bile duct is most compatible with a benign stricture due to chronic pancreatitis (Fig. 42.16).

The indications for surgical management of common bile duct strictures due to chronic pancreatitis are clear in patients with significant pain, jaundice, or cholangitis. Controversy exists, however, concerning the necessity of biliary decompression in patients with an asymptomatic elevation of serum alkaline phosphatase. In general, biliary bypass is indicated because changes from obstructive biliary cirrhosis have been observed in liver biopsy specimens obtained from patients with long-standing, functionally significant biliary obstruction due to chronic pancreatitis (19,20).

Choledochoduodenostomy and Roux-en-Y choledochojejunostomy are acceptable methods of biliary bypass in patients with bile duct strictures due to chronic pancreatitis. Choledochoduodenostomy is preferred by many surgeons because it does not divert bile from the duodenum, is technically easier to perform, and leaves the jejunum intact for any associated procedures required for decompression of an obstructed gastrointestinal tract or pancreatic duct. Finally, in patients in whom periampullary malignancy cannot be completely ruled out by the clinical course or imaging studies, or in patients with significant chronic pain thought secondary to proximal pancreatic duct disease, pancreaticoduodenectomy offers an excellent treatment option. The results of surgical management of distal bile duct structures due to chronic pancreatitis are usually excellent, with a low rate of perioperative complications and excellent long-term results.

Transduodenal sphincteroplasty is not recommended for the management of common bile duct strictures due to chronic pancreatitis because the stricture is too long to be managed adequately by this technique. Similarly, endoscopic sphincterotomy has no role in the management of biliary obstruction due to chronic pancreatitis. Limited experience has been reported with balloon dilation of distal bile duct strictures secondary to pancreatitis, with little long-term follow-up.

MISCELLANEOUS CAUSES OF BILE DUCT STRICTURES

Benign strictures of the bile duct can result from the chronic inflammation associated with gallstones in either the gallbladder or common bile duct. This is an uncommon cause of bile duct strictures and a rare complication of gallstone disease. Bile duct strictures due to cholelithiasis are usually associated with a narrowing at the level of the common hepatic duct caused by a stone impacted in the infundibulum of the gallbladder. The narrowing can be caused by two means. First, simple compression can occur from a large stone lying adjacent to the common hepatic duct. Second, chronic or acute inflammation arising from the gallbladder or cystic duct can extend to the contiguous bile duct, resulting in stricture formation. The biliary obstruction associated with either of these conditions is known as *Mirizzi's syndrome*.

The clinical presentation of a bile duct stricture due to cholelithiasis is often associated with acute cholecystitis and hyperbilirubinemia. In some long-standing cases, these findings exist in the face of chronic gallbladder symptoms. If hyperbilirubinemia is present and urgent cholecystectomy is not indicated, ERCP or PTC can help to delineate the preoperative biliary anatomy. Most cases that are associated with acute cholecystitis, however, are recognized at the time of cholecystectomy and operative cholangiography. When the duct compression is associated with acute inflammation, the common hepatic duct almost always returns to normal after the offending stone has been removed by cholecystectomy and the inflammatory process has resolved. Care must be taken during the dissection to avoid creation of a defect in the common hepatic duct. Rarely, after the acute episode has resolved, a well established stricture presents months to years after the acute episode. In such cases, management by Roux-en-Y hepaticojejunostomy is appropriate.

Strictures due to choledocholithiasis are also rare. The presumed mechanism is erosion of the epithelium of the distal duct, creating inflammation with subsequent fibrosis and stricture. Because of the anatomic tapering of the common bile duct, nearly all stones are entrapped in the intrapancreatic portion of the duct and are often difficult to remove by the supraduodenal route.

Excessive intraoperative manipulation at the time of bile duct exploration with forceps, scoops, and catheters can often create additional trauma to an already friable distal duct. After the stone has been removed, the distal bile duct should be gently sized with a soft rubber catheter to be sure that no stricture exists. If a stricture persists after stone removal, it may not be recognized until the time of postoperative T-tube cholangiography. If recognized in the postoperative period, time should be allowed for resolution of inflammation before considering stricture repair. If a distal bile duct stricture does persist, a biliary-enteric anastomosis with either Roux-en-Y choledochojejunostomy or a choledochoduodenostomy is indicated. If the proximal duct is adequately dilated (>2 cm in diameter) to allow a large choledochoduodenal anastomosis, this procedure is usually preferable because of its technical ease and excellent results.

Stenosis of the sphincter of Oddi, or papillitis, is a benign intrinsic obstruction of the outlet of the common bile duct, usually associated with inflammation, fibrosis, or muscular hypertrophy. Sphincter stenosis can result in any of three clinical conditions: (a) common bile duct obstruction due to fibrotic stenosis of the papilla, (b) recurrent pancreatitis, or (c) recurrent right upper quadrant pain without jaundice or pancreatitis. The pathogenesis of the inflammation of sphincter stenosis is unclear. In many cases, it is thought to be due to the trauma of the passage of multiple small stones from the common duct through the ampulla. This trauma results in inflammation, scarring, and stricture formation. Many patients with papillary stenosis have no gallstones. Other potential mechanisms include primary sphincter motility disorders and congenital anomalies. The clinical presentation is usually either jaundice or cholangitis. In some cases, an impacted common bile duct stone may be present. The diagnosis can be supported with either PTC or ERC. This condition can be managed by sphincterotomy performed either endoscopically or operatively. If a cholecystectomy was performed previously, endoscopic papillotomy is the initial procedure of choice.

Cholangiohepatitis is an unusual infection of the biliary tree frequently associated with *Clonorchis sinensis* and other parasites. These infections are most commonly seen in natives of Asia. Most patients present with recurrent episodes of cholangitis. Cholangiography can demonstrate multiple strictures of both the intrahepatic and extrahepatic biliary tree, with the bile ducts filled with sludge and stones (Fig. 42.17). Surgical management consists of cholecystectomy and improved biliary drainage with either Roux-en-Y choledochojejunostomy or choledochoduodenostomy. Access to the biliary tree for postoperative management of intrahepatic stones or sludge should be maintained with either transhepatic biliary stents or a choledochojejunocutaneous or subcutaneous fistula. No specific medical management is available for this condition.

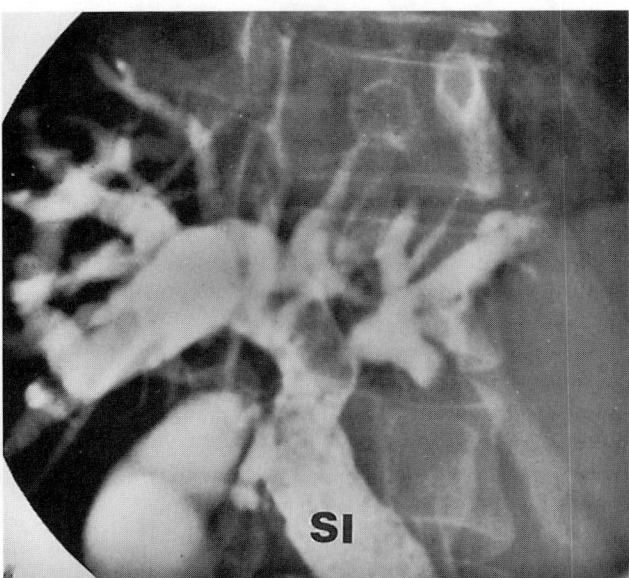

Figure 42.17. Cholangiogram of a patient with cholangiohepatitis with diffuse bile duct dilatation. The biliary tree is filled with sludge (Sl) and stones.

Finally, rare causes of benign intrahepatic and extrahepatic bile duct strictures have been reported secondary to intrahepatic arterial infusion of 5-fluorouracil used in the treatment of hepatic metastases of colorectal carcinoma. The clinical picture closely resembles primary sclerosing cholangitis but usually can be managed by simple discontinuation of infusion and, in some cases, percutaneous transhepatic drainage. Surgery should be reserved for patients with persistent evidence of biliary obstruction. A similar cholangiographic appearance has been reported in patients with acquired immunodeficiency syndrome. The pathogenesis of this injury is believed to be viral and related to cytomegalovirus infection. No experience in the surgical management of this condition has been reported.

REFERENCES

1. Branum G, Schmitt C, Baille J, et al. Management of major biliary complications after laparoscopic cholecystectomy. *Ann Surg* 1993;17:53.

2. Pitt HA, Miyamoto T, Parapatis SK, et al. Factors influencing outcome in patients with postoperative biliary strictures. *Am J Surg* 1982;144:14.

3. Pelligrini CA, Thomas MJ, Way LW. Recurrent biliary stricture: patterns of recurrent and outcome of surgical therapy. *Am J Surg* 1984;147:175.

4. Cameron JL, Gayler BW, Zuidema GD. The use of Silastic transhepatic stents in benign and malignant biliary strictures. *Ann Surg* 1978;188:552.

5. Pitt HA, Kaufman SL, Coleman J, et al. Benign postoperative biliary strictures: operate or dilate? *Ann Surg* 1989;210:417.

6. Warren KW, Christophi C, Armendari ZR. The evolution and current perspectives of the treatment of benign bile duct strictures: a review. *Surg Gastroenterol* 1982;1:141

7. Stewart L, Way LW. Bile duct injuries during laparoscopic cholecystectomy. *Arch Surg* 1995;130:1123.

8. Lillemoe KD, Melton GB, Cameron JL, et al. Postoperative bile duct strictures: management and outcome in the 1990s. *Ann Surg* 2000;232:430–441.

9. Mueller PR, van Sonnenberg E, Ferrucci Jr T, et al. Biliary stricture dilatation: multicenter review of clinical management in 73 patients. *Radiology* 1986;160:17.

10. Williams HF, Bender CE, May GR. Benign postoperative biliary strictures: dilatation with fluoroscopic guidance. *Radiology* 1987;163:629.

11. Lillemoe KD, Martin SA, Cameron JL, et al. Major bile duct injuries during laparoscopic cholecystectomy: follow-up after combined surgical and radiologic management. *Ann Surg* 1997;225:459.

12. David PHP, Tanka AKF, Rauws EAJ, et al. Benign biliary strictures: surgery or endoscopy? *Ann Surg* 1993;217:237.

13. Geenen DJ, Geenen JE, Hogan WJ, et al. Endoscopic therapy for benign bile duct strictures. *Gastrointest Endosc* 1989;35:367.

14. Lindor KD. Ursodiol for primary sclerosing cholangitis. *N Engl J Med* 1997;336:691.

15. Lillemoe KD, Pitt HA, Cameron JL. Primary sclerosing cholangitis. *Surg Clin North Am* 1990;70:1381.

16. Ahrendt SA, Pitt HA, Kalloo AN, et al. Primary sclerosing cholangitis: resect, dilate, or transplant. *Ann Surg* 1998;227:412.

17. Gross JA, Shackelton CR, Farmer DG, et al. Orthotopic liver transplantation for primary sclerosing cholangitis: a 12-year single center experience. *Ann Surg* 1997;225:472.

18. Stahl TJ, O'Connor A, Ansel M, et al. Partial biliary obstruction caused by chronic pancreatitis: an appraisal of indications for surgical biliary drainage. *Ann Surg* 1988;207:26.

19. Warshaw AL, Schapiro RH, Ferrucci JT Jr, et al. Persistent obstructive jaundice, cholangitis, and biliary cirrhosis due to common bile duct stenosis in chronic pancreatitis. *Gastroenterology* 1976;70:562.

20. Afroudakis A, Kaplowitz N. Liver histopathology in chronic bile duct stenosis due to chronic alcoholic pancreatitis. *Hepatology* 1981;1:65.

SECTION H

COLON, RECTUM, AND ANUS

SURGERY: SCIENTIFIC PRINCIPLES AND PRACTICE, Third Edition, edited by
Lazar J. Greenfield, Michael W. Mulholland, Keith T. Oldham, Gerald B. Zelenock,
and Keith D. Lillemoe. Lippincott Williams & Wilkins Publishers, Philadelphia, © 2001.

CHAPTER 43

COLONIC ANATOMY AND PHYSIOLOGY

JOHN F. SWEENEY

EMBRYOLOGY

The primitive gut begins to form during the fourth week of gestation. For descriptive purposes, it is divided into the foregut, midgut, and hindgut. In this chapter, the discussion will focus only on the midgut and hindgut.

Midgut derivatives include the entire small intestine distal to the ampulla of Vater, the cecum and appendix, the ascending colon, and the right half to two thirds of the transverse colon. These structures receive their blood supply from branches of the superior mesenteric artery. At the beginning of the sixth week of gestation, the midgut loop undergoes a physiologic umbilical herniation and migrates into the extraembryonic coelom. During the next 4 weeks the midgut loop elongates considerably and also undergoes a series of counterclockwise rotations around the axis of the superior mesenteric artery. During the 10th week of gestation, the midgut structures return into the abdomen, having undergone a total counterclockwise rotation of 270 degrees. At this point, the cecum and appendix lie in a subhepatic position. During the final months of gestation, the cecum grows down into the right iliac fossa.

The hindgut structures include the left one third to one half of the transverse colon, the descending colon, the sigmoid colon, the rectum, and the superior portion of the anal canal. Branches of the inferior mesenteric artery supply all these hindgut structures.

ANATOMY OF THE COLON

General Considerations

The large intestine, or colon, begins in the right lower quadrant of the abdomen where the distal ileum empties into posteromedial aspect of the cecum at the ileocecal valve (Fig. 43.1). The colon extends from the ileocecal valve to the anal canal and can range between 3 to 6 feet in total length. The approximately 7.5- to 8.5-cm diameter of the cecum makes it the widest portion of the colon. The appendix projects from the lowest portion of the cecum. From the cecum, the colon ascends along the right side of the abdomen for a distance of approximately 20 to 30 cm to a level overlying the inferior pole of the right kidney. At this point, the colon forms a medial, anterior, and downward angulation, the right colic or hepatic flexure, which is the portion of the ascending colon that joins the transverse colon. During mobilization of the hepatic flexure in a right hemicolectomy, it is important to stay in the plane close to the colon to avoid mobilization and injury of the right kidney and duodenum.

The transverse colon extends from the hepatic flexure to the splenic flexure and is the longest segment of colon, ranging between 30 and 60 cm in length. The transverse colon is suspended by the transverse mesocolon and is considered to be completely intraperitoneal. It is the most mobile portion of the colon and can be located anywhere from the upper abdomen down to the pelvis. The greater omentum descends from the greater curve of the stomach in front of the transverse colon and then ascends to attach to the transverse colon on its anterosuperior edge. The left colic or splenic flexure is the angle between the distal transverse colon and the descending colon. The splenic flexure is situated high in the left upper quadrant, more cephalad than the hepatic flexure. The flexure lies anterior to the midportion of the left kidney and also closely abuts the lower pole of the spleen. The attachments to the diaphragm and spleen (phrenocolic and splenocolic ligaments) should be carefully identified and divided during mobilization of the splenic flexure to avoid unnecessary injury to the spleen.

The descending colon is approximately 20 to 30 cm in length and courses from the splenic flexure to its junction with the sigmoid colon at the pelvic brim. The anterior, lateral, and medial portions of the descending colon are covered by peritoneum, but the posterior surface is adherent to the posterior abdominal wall and frequently lies in close contact with the left ureter. The sigmoid colon extends from the pelvic brim to the sacral promontory, where it continues as the rectum. The sigmoid colon can vary from 15 to 50 cm in length. The sigmoid colon is extremely mobile and has a generous mesentery that extends along the pelvic brim from the iliac fossa across the sacroiliac joint to the second or third sacral segment. When the sigmoid colon is mobilized, care should be taken to identify the left ureter as it runs in the intersigmoid fossa and crosses the point where the common iliac artery bifurcates into the internal and external iliac arteries.

Anatomists have classically described the beginning of the rectum at the level of the third sacral vertebra. Surgeons often consider the rectum to begin at the level of the sacral promontory. From here, the rectum proceeds posteriorly and downward along the curvature of the sacrum and coccyx and ends by passing through the levator ani muscles, at which point it turns abruptly downward and backward to become the anal canal. As the rectum proceeds distally, the lumen enlarges; the most distal segment is called the *rectal ampulla*.

The four layers of the colonic wall include the mucosa, submucosa, circular muscle layer, and longitudinal muscle layer (Fig. 43.2). The mucosal surface of the colon consists of columnar epithelium made up of regularly

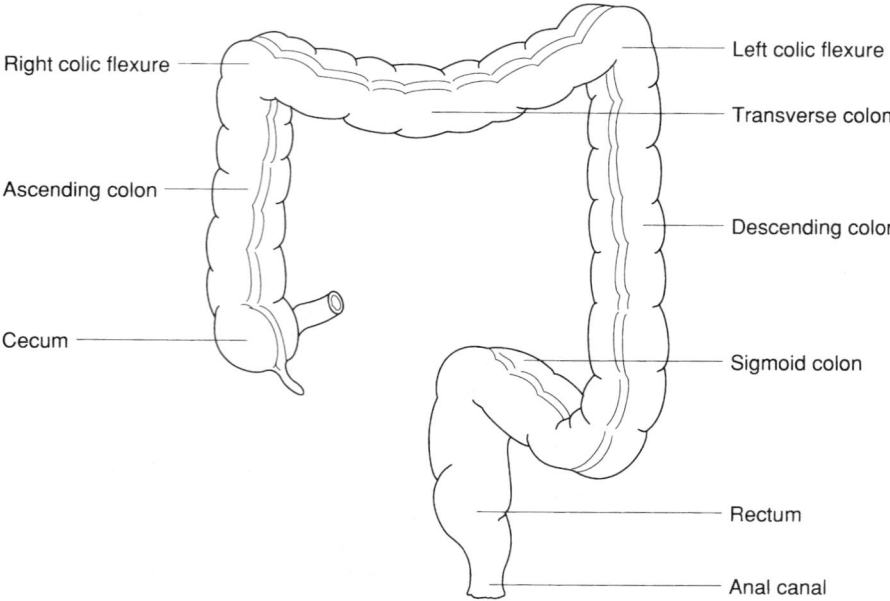

Figure 43.1. General anatomic components of the colon.

arranged crypts and numerous goblet cells. Unlike that of the small intestine, the columnar epithelium of the colon does not possess villi. The muscularis propria of the colon consists of an inner circular layer and an outer longitudinal layer. The thick circular muscle forms a continuous layer around the entire circumference of the colon. In contrast, the outer longitudinal muscle layer is grouped into three bands known as *taeniae*. These bands are positioned approximately 120 degrees apart about the circumference of the colon, with one taenia along the mesenteric border and the other two found on the antimesenteric border of the colon. Although some longitudinal muscle is located between the taeniae, the bulk of the muscle is found within the taeniae. The taeniae begin proximally at the appendix and disappear as distinct bands at the level of the upper rectum. At this point, the longitudinal muscle

layer coalesces to form a continuous layer around the circumference of the rectum. The sacculations seen between the taeniae are called the *haustra coli*.

Arterial Blood Supply

The superior mesenteric artery arises from the aorta, runs posterior to the pancreas, and passes anterior to the third portion of the duodenum (Fig. 43.3).The superior mesenteric artery gives rise to the ileocolic and middle colic branches that supply the cecum, ascending colon, and proximal transverse colon. The right colic artery, which also supplies the ascending colon, can originate as a branch of the ileocolic artery or may arise directly from the superior mesenteric artery. The inferior mesenteric artery arises from the infrarenal aorta and supplies the distal transverse colon, descending colon, sigmoid colon, and upper rectum via its left colic, sigmoid, and superior hemorrhoidal branches. The middle and inferior hemorrhoidal arteries arise from the hypogastric arteries and supply the distal two thirds of the rectum. A series of arterial arcades along the mesenteric border of the entire colon, known as the marginal *artery of Drummond,* connect the superior mesenteric and inferior mesenteric arterial systems. This important collateral circulation allows the left colon to remain viable while the inferior mesenteric artery is ligated during an extended sigmoid resection.

Venous Drainage

The veins that drain the large intestine bear the same terminology and follow a course similar to that of their corresponding arteries (Fig. 43.4). The veins from the right colon and transverse colon, along with the veins draining the small intestine, drain into the superior mesenteric vein. The superior mesenteric vein runs slightly anterior to and to the right of the superior mesenteric artery. The superior mesenteric vein courses beneath the neck of the pancreas, where it joins with the splenic vein to form the portal vein. The inferior mesenteric vein drains blood from the left colon, sigmoid colon, rectum, and superior anal canal. The inferior mesenteric vein ascends over the psoas muscle in a retroperitoneal plane. The vein courses under the body of the pancreas to drain into the splenic

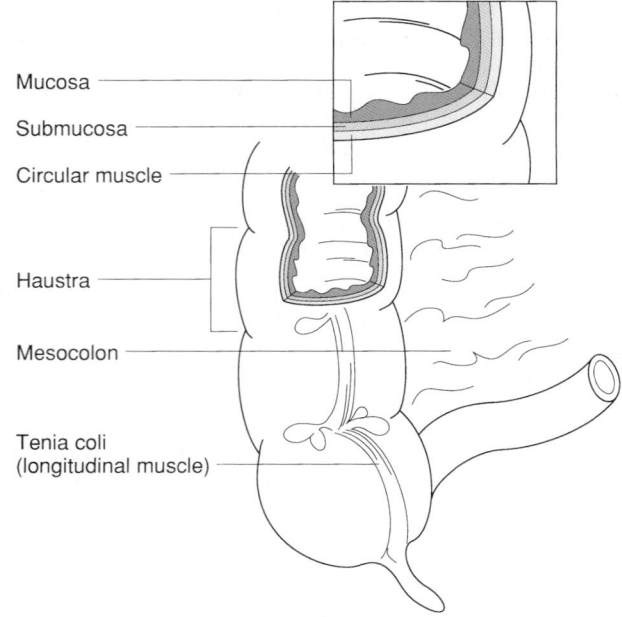

Figure 43.2. Layers of the colonic wall.

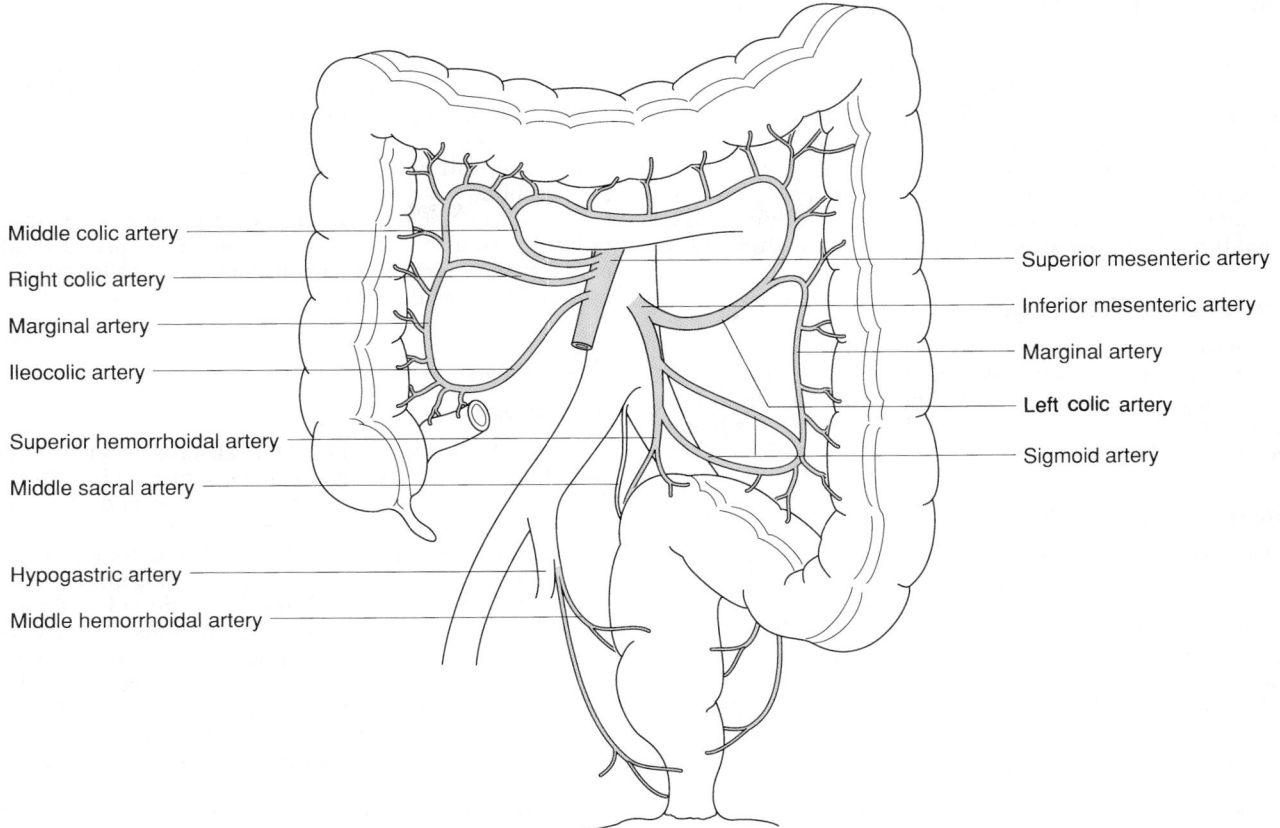

Figure 43.3. Arterial blood supply of the colon.

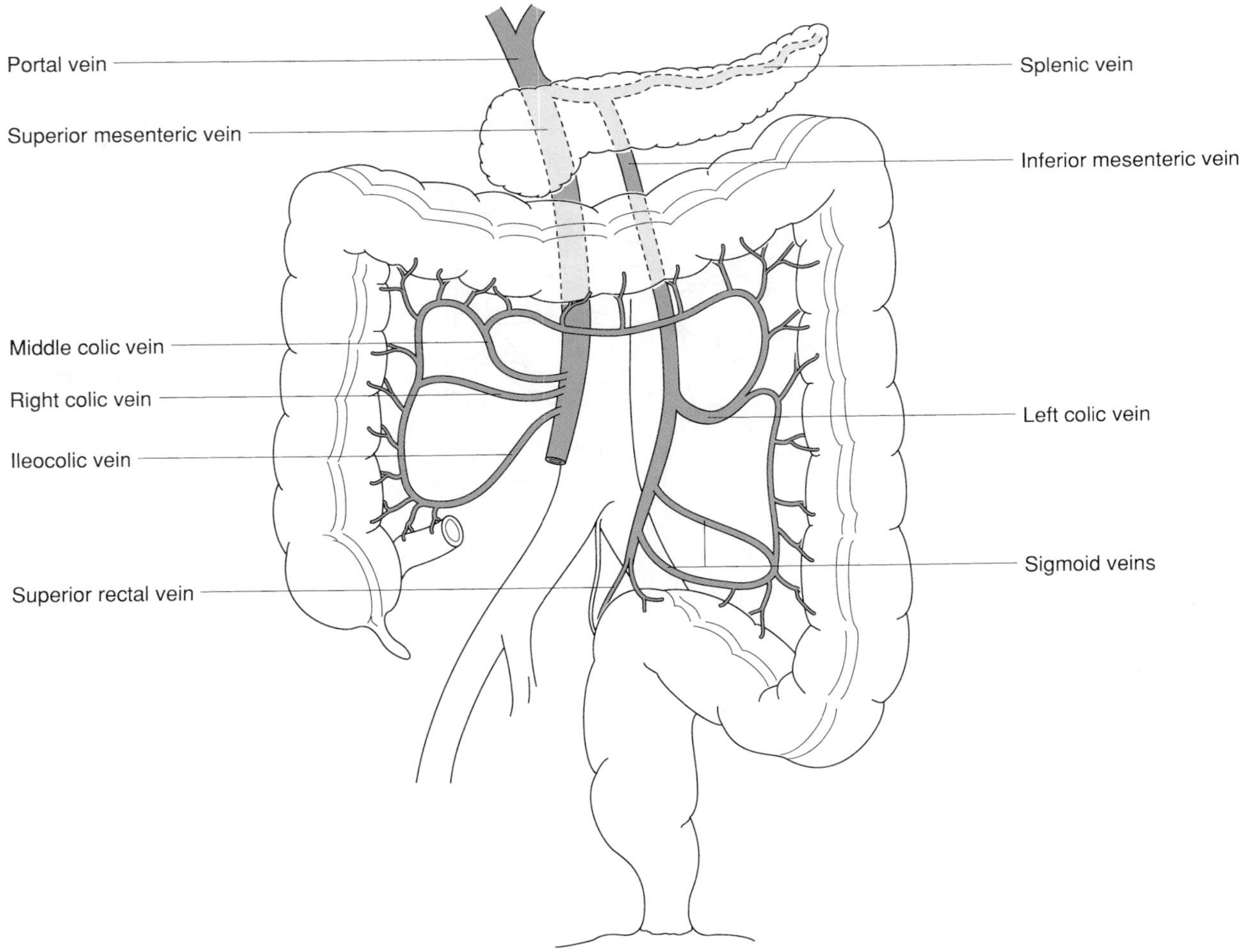

Middle colic artery

Right colic artery

Marginal artery

Ileocolic artery

Superior hemorrhoidal artery

Middle sacral artery

Hypogastric artery

Middle hemorrhoidal artery

Superior mesenteric artery

Inferior mesenteric artery

Marginal artery

Left colic artery

Sigmoid artery

Portal vein

Superior mesenteric vein

Middle colic vein

Right colic vein

Ileocolic vein

Superior rectal vein

Splenic vein

Inferior mesenteric vein

Left colic vein

Sigmoid veins

Figure 43.4. Venous drainage of the colon by the portal vein.

vein. The superior hemorrhoidal veins drain blood from the rectum into the portal system via the inferior mesenteric vein. The middle and inferior hemorrhoidal veins drain blood from the lower rectum and anal canal into the systemic venous circulation via the internal iliac veins. In the setting of portal hypertension, the superior, middle, and inferior hemorrhoidal veins interact to shunt venous blood from the portal system into the systemic circulation.

Lymphatic Drainage

Lymphatic drainage generally follows the arterial blood supply of the colon and rectum (Fig. 43.5). In the anal canal, lesions above the dentate line ultimately drain into inferior mesenteric lymph nodes. However, lesions below the dentate line drain into the internal iliac nodes.

Neural Components

The colon possesses extrinsic and intrinsic (enteric) neuronal systems. The extrinsic system consists of sympathetic and parasympathetic nerves that generally inhibit or stimulate colonic peristalsis, respectively. The sympathetic nerves to the right side of the colon originate from the lower thoracic segments of the spinal cord and travel in the thoracic splanchnic nerves to the celiac and superior mesenteric plexuses. Postganglionic fibers emerge from here and course along the superior mesenteric artery and its branches to the right side of the colon. The parasympathetic innervation originates from the right vagus nerve and travels along with the sympathetic nerves to the right side of the colon. The left side of the colon and the rectum receive sympathetic fibers that arise from L-1

through L-3. The parasympathetic supply to the left side of the colon and the rectum arises from S-2 through S-4.

The intrinsic, or enteric, nervous system consists of two groups of plexuses that are identified by their location within the wall of the colon. Meissner's plexus is located in the submucosa between the muscularis mucosae and the circular muscle of the muscularis propria. The myenteric plexus, also known as *Auerbach's plexus*, is located between the inner circular muscle and outer longitudinal muscle layers of the colon.

PHYSIOLOGY

Absorption

In healthy persons, the colon absorbs water, sodium, and chloride while it secretes potassium and bicarbonate. The physiologic control of colonic water and electrolyte transport requires careful integration of neural, endocrine, and paracrine components. Although the colonic epithelium does not actively absorb glucose or amino acids, as the small-intestinal epithelium does, the colon does absorb short-chain fatty acids and vitamins that are produced by the bacterial breakdown of nonabsorbed sugars and amino acids. These short-chain fatty acids, which include acetate, butyrate, and propionate, are absorbed in a concentration-dependent fashion. They are a major energy substrate for the colonic epithelial cells and are the major fecal anions (1,2).

Approximately 1,500 mL of ileal effluent reaches the cecum during a 24-hour period, of which 90% is water. Of this amount, only 100 to 150 mL of water appears in the stool. The colon has a tremendous reserve capacity that al-

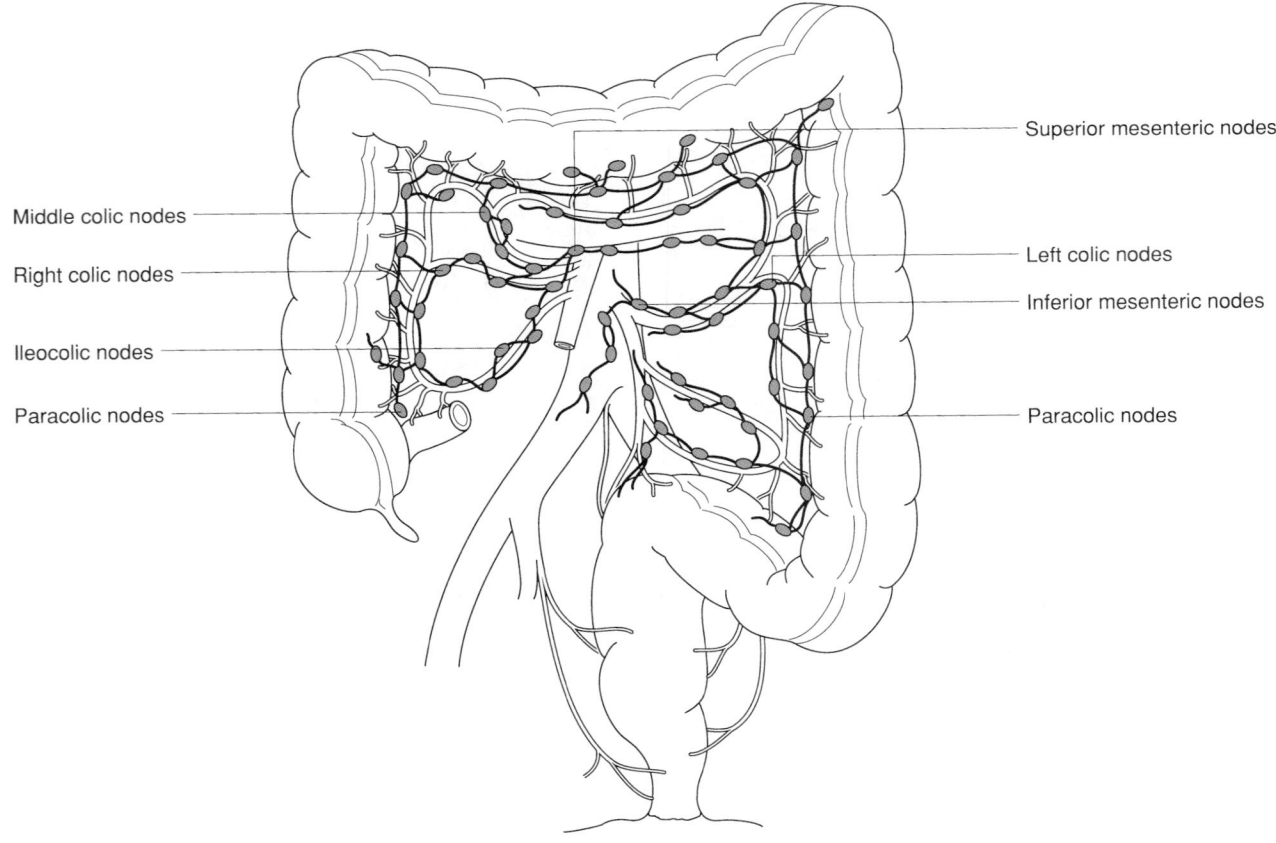

Figure 43.5. Lymphatic drainage of the colon.

Superior mesenteric nodes

Middle colic nodes

Right colic nodes

Ileocolic nodes

Paracolic nodes

Left colic nodes

Inferior mesenteric nodes

Paracolic nodes

lows it to absorb as much as 5 to 6 L of water within a 24-hour period (3). Normally formed feces consist of 70% water and 30% solid material. Almost half of the solid material is made up of bacteria, with the other half composed of undigested food material and desquamated epithelium. Water absorption in the colon is a passive process that depends primarily on the osmotic gradient established by the active transport of sodium across the colonic epithelium. The composition of ileal effluent and luminal flow rates also play an important role in water absorption. Upsetting the balance of these three factors results in diarrhea. The absorptive capacity is not the same throughout each segment of the colon. Salt and water absorption is greater in the right side of the colon than in the left side and the sigmoid colon. Patients undergoing a right hemicolectomy should therefore be counseled preoperatively that they may experience loose bowel movements or frank diarrhea in the early postoperative period. Patients should also be reassured that this will resolve with time as the remaining colon adapts.

Sodium absorption by the colonic epithelium is an active cellular transport process that is very similar in nature to that seen in small-intestinal and kidney epithelial cells (4). Initially, sodium absorption involves the passive movement of sodium across the apical membrane into the mucosal cell down an electrochemical gradient. To maintain an adequate electrochemical gradient, intracellular sodium is then removed from the cell into the interstitial space in exchange for potassium. This is an energy-dependent process that is controlled by Na^+-K^+-ATPase at the basolateral membrane of the colonic epithelium. Mineralocorticoids (aldosterone) and glucocorticoids accelerate sodium absorption and potassium excretion in the colon by increasing Na^+-K^+-ATPase activity (5). Potassium movement into the colonic lumen is primarily a passive process that depends on the electrochemical gradient generated by the active transport of sodium across colonic epithelial cells. Chloride absorption in the colon is generally thought to be an energy-independent process that is associated with reciprocal exchange for bicarbonate at the luminal border of the mucosal cell (6).

Colonic Flora

The bacterial flora of the colon is established soon after birth and depends in large part on dietary and environmental factors. Approximately 400 different species of bacteria have been identified in the human colon. Bacteria constitute between 40% to 55% of fecal solids in a person who consumes a normal Western diet. The vast majority of the normal colonic flora consists of anaerobic bacteria, with *Bacteroides* species, especially *B. fragilis*, the most prevalent (7). Other anaerobic bacteria include *Lactobacillus bifidus*, *Clostridium* species, and *Eubacterium* species (7). Aerobic colonic bacteria are mainly coliforms and enterococci. *Escherichia coli* is the predominant coliform (7). Other aerobic coliforms include *Klebsiella*, *Proteus*, and *Enterobacter*. The principal enterococcus is *Streptococcus faecalis* (7).

The fecal flora plays an important role in many physiologic processes. The host absorbs vitamin K, which is produced by many colonic microorganisms. The degradation of bile pigments by colonic bacteria gives stool its characteristic brown color. The enterohepatic circulation of bilirubin and bile acids depends greatly on bacterial enzymes produced by fecal flora. Colonic bacteria also influence colonic motility and absorption, generate intestinal gases, and play an important role in the prevention of infection by keeping the growth of pathogenic bacteria like *Clostridium difficile* in check.

Colonic Motility

The motor activity of one segment of the colon varies markedly in comparison with another. Three patterns of colonic smooth-muscle contraction are known to exist: retrograde movement, segmental contractions, and mass movements. *Retrograde movements* are a unique pattern of antiperistaltic contractions that originate in the distal right side of the colon and travel toward the cecum, slowing the movement of the luminal contents (8,9). These contractions facilitate a thorough mixing of the ileal effluent and prolong exposure of the luminal contents to the mucosa of the right side of the colon, thereby promoting microbial metabolism and water and electrolyte absorption (10). *Segmental contractions* are intermittent contractions of the longitudinal and circular muscles that result in the segmented appearance of the colon (11). Segmental contractions are most commonly seen in the transverse and descending colon. These contractions propel luminal contents in a back-and-forth pattern over short distances to cause further mixing of fecal matter. The final type of colonic activity is termed *mass movement*, consisting of strong, propulsive contractions of the smooth muscle that involve a long segment of colon (12). The contractions move the luminal contents forward at a rate of 0.5 to 1.0 cm/s and typically last for 20 to 30 seconds (13). Mass movement contractions occur three to four times per day, primarily after awakening and after meals.

The orderly progression of colonic luminal contents from cecum to anus requires the coordination of smooth-muscle contractions. The cyclic depolarization and repolarization of the colonic smooth-muscle cell membrane generates a basic electrical pattern of slow-wave activity that allows each smooth-muscle cell to control its own contraction and to couple with adjacent smooth-muscle cells (14). The mechanism for this spontaneous depolarization of the colonic smooth-muscle cell membrane is calcium-dependent. The extrinsic and intrinsic (enteric) neuronal systems also interact to influence colonic motility. The extrinsic system consists of preganglionic parasympathetic neurons and postganglionic sympathetic neurons.

Defecation

As the fecal mass enters the rectum, the internal anal sphincter relaxes while the external anal sphincter contracts to maintain anal continence. Distention of the rectum in this setting is the primary stimulus for the initiation of defecation. At this point, the urge to defecate may be suppressed by further conscious contraction of the external anal sphincter. Receptive relaxation of the rectal ampulla accommodates the fecal mass and the urge to defecate passes unless the volume of feces is extremely large or the sphincter mechanism is impaired. If the subject voluntarily accedes to the urge to defecate, a squatting position is assumed, which straightens the anorectal angle. A Valsalva's maneuver is then performed, which increases the intraabdominal and intrathoracic pressure and overcomes the resistance of the external anal sphincter. Relaxation of the pelvic muscles causes the pelvic floor to descend and the anorectal angle to straighten further. Conscious inhibition of the external anal sphincter then allows passage of the fecal bolus. On completion, the pelvic floor returns to its resting position and the anal sphincter muscles return to their resting activity, closing the anal canal. Under normal circumstances, this process occurs once every 24 hours; however, the interval between bowel movements may vary between 8 and 12 hours and 2 to 3 days in normal subjects. The frequency of defecation is influenced by multiple environmental and dietary factors.

DISORDERS OF COLONIC MOTILITY

Constipation

To the lay person, constipation means infrequent stools or difficulty in passing stools. However, the Rome definition requires two or more of the following criteria to be present before a diagnosis of constipation can be assigned: (a) straining on more than 25% of bowel movements; (b) incomplete evacuation of the rectum after more than 25% of bowel movements; (c) hard stool consistency on more than 25% of bowel movements; (d) infrequent defecation, with three or fewer bowel movements reported weekly (15). The causes of constipation are numerous and include faulty dietary and life-style habits; structural/functional, neurologic, and endocrine/metabolic disorders; and iatrogenic causes/medication (Table 43.1). The recent onset of constipation in an otherwise healthy adult is a warning sign and should prompt a search to exclude an obstructing anatomic lesion.

The standard initial treatment for patients with constipation involves dietary manipulation with bulk-forming agents to increase dietary fiber. Patients should also be encouraged to increase their fluid intake. Patients who fail an initial trial of bulk-forming agents may respond to stool softeners such as docusate (Colace). These increase the

Table 43.1. CAUSES OF CONSTIPATION

FAULTY DIETARY AND LIFESTYLE HABITS

Inadequate dietary fiber
Inadequate fluids
Lack of exercise
Environmental changes (e.g., travel, hospitalization)

STRUCTURAL/FUNCTIONAL

Slow transit
Pelvic floor dysfunction (e.g., rectocele, procidentia)
Immobilization
Depression
Irritable bowel syndrome
Diverticulosis
Colonic obstruction (e.g., neoplasm, volvulus, inflammation)
Scleroderma
Amyloidosis

NEUROLOGIC DISORDERS

Central nervous system (e.g., stoke, Parkinson's disease, Alzheimer's disease)
Spinal cord (e.g., multiple sclerosis, tumor, herniated disk, trauma)
Nervi erigentes damage
Aganglionosis (Hirschsprung's disease, Chagas' disease)

IATROGENIC/MEDICATION

Narcotics
Anticholinergics
Antacids
Antihypertensives
Antidepressants
Iron
Barium

ENDOCRINE/METABOLIC

Hypothyroidism
Hypercalcemia
Pheochromocytoma
Diabetes
Pregnancy
Uremia
Dehydration

stool water content by inhibiting the normal water-absorptive capacity of the colon. Although they soften the stool, they do not promote defecation. If bulk-forming agents and stool softeners do not successfully treat the constipation, the next preferred therapy involves osmotic laxatives. These agents (which include magnesium citrate, sodium sulfate, phosphate, and potassium tartrate) are poorly absorbed chemicals that increase the stool water content through an osmotic effect. Caution should be exercised in prescribing them for patients with significant underlying cardiac, renal, or hepatic disease. Polysaccharides such as lactulose or sorbitol are also poorly absorbed substances that have an osmotic effect and increase stool water. They can cause excess cramping, bloating, flatulence, and fluid loss. Stimulant laxatives act on the mucosa to reduce water and electrolyte secretion; they also increase colonic motility. Examples include diphenylmethane derivatives (e.g., bisacodyl) and anthraquinone cathartics (senna, cascara sagrada).

Treatment of constipation should result in a normal frequency and consistency of stools and freedom from associated discomfort. This goal is achieved in most patients simply by increasing dietary fiber and water intake. Additional agents should be added in a graded fashion at the lowest effective dose. Long-term laxative abuse should be avoided. Surgical treatment should be reserved for patients with the new onset of constipation with an underlying anatomic cause (e.g., diverticular stricture or obstructing colon carcinoma). The surgical treatment of chronic constipation is poorly defined and should not be considered until a complete workup has been completed.

Postoperative Ileus

Postoperative ileus is most commonly seen in patients who have undergone intraabdominal operative procedures, but it can also occur after major extraabdominal (e.g., cardiothoracic or orthopedic) surgical procedures. The colon appears to be most profoundly affected by the postoperative ileus, with the stomach and small intestine recovering function earlier. The causes of this phenomenon are not clear and are likely to be multifactorial. Bowel manipulation is one factor that has often been cited (16). The observation that postoperative ileus is less severe after minimally invasive surgical approaches to intraabdominal diseases adds credence to this theory (17). Anesthetic agents utilized intraoperatively and postoperative analgesia can also influence the duration of postoperative ileus (18). Electrolyte abnormalities, including deficits in potassium, magnesium, and calcium, are also known to alter intestinal motility following surgery.

Irritable Bowel Syndrome

Irritable bowel syndrome is defined as abdominal pain that is not associated with an anatomic abnormality and may or may not be associated with alterations in bowel habits. The causes of this disorder are uncertain. Emotional stress and psychiatric illness have been implicated in the pathogenesis and may exacerbate symptoms (19). Physiologic abnormalities have also been demonstrated in patients with irritable bowel syndrome (20,21). Abnormal colonic motility in response to an ingested meal has been demonstrated in some patients with irritable bowel syndrome. Other studies have cited altered myoelectric activity and abnormal gut hormone secretion as causes.

Because no one clear cause of irritable bowel syndrome has been demonstrated, no specific treatment regimen has been defined for this disorder. Most patients have asymptomatic periods interrupted by intervals of symptoms. The approach to treatment begins with an evaluation of the factors associated with irritable bowel syndrome. Diagnosis and treatment of an underlying psychiatric problem may resolve the patient's symptoms. A careful dietary history should also be taken, and factors that contribute to constipation or diarrhea should be adjusted appropriately. If these management strategies are not successful, a gradual introduction of anticholinergic medications may be helpful. Anticholinergic agents can reduce the rate of myoelectric activity and decrease tonic contractions in the colon, thereby relieving the cramping and bloating that many patients experience. Low doses of tricyclic antidepressants, including imipramine, amitriptyline, and nortriptyline, often decrease or eliminate abdominal symptoms. Constipation is known to be one major side effect of these agents, which may be helpful in patients with irritable bowel syndrome and underlying diarrhea but a problem in patients with preexisting constipation. The myriad of treatment options described for irritable bowel syndrome reinforces the poor understanding of the etiology of this clinical entity.

Colonic Pseudoobstruction

Colonic pseudoobstruction is a clinical entity in which signs and symptoms of bowel obstruction are present without an actual mechanical obstruction. Pseudoobstruction is usually observed in patients with serious underlying medical conditions who have undergone a major (usually extraabdominal) surgical procedure. The most frequent presenting symptoms include abdominal pain and distention. Constipation/obstipation or diarrhea may be present. Nausea and vomiting may also be seen. Physical examination usually demonstrates tympany to percussion and mild tenderness on palpation. Abdominal radiographic findings are significant for marked colonic distention that is typically localized to the right side of the

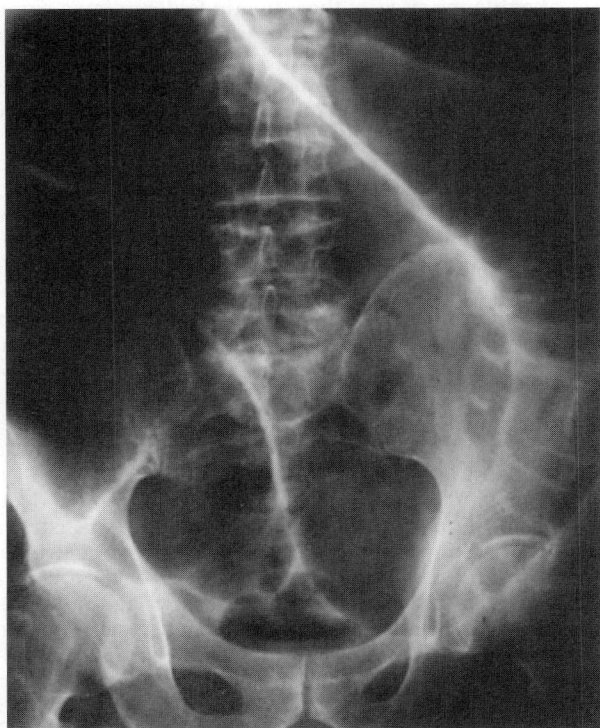

Figure 43.6. Pseudoobstruction of the colon (Ogilvie's syndrome).

colon (Fig. 43.6). The management of colonic pseudoobstruction is nonoperative initially and consists of nasogastric decompression, correction of fluid and electrolyte imbalances, gentle enemas, rectal tube placement, and avoidance of narcotics and anticholinergics. With these conservative measures, colonic pseudoobstruction usually resolves in more than 75% of cases (22). In cases in which conservative measures fail or the luminal diameter of the cecum reaches 10 to 12 cm, a more aggressive approach is warranted because of the risk for cecal perforation. Decompressive colonoscopy has historically been the method of choice in this setting (23). More recently, the intravenous administration of 2.5 mg of neostigmine during 2 to 3 minutes has been found to decompress the colon promptly in nearly all patients (24). Surgery is reserved for patients with obvious peritoneal signs or who fail all forms of nonoperative therapy. In the latter setting, when the possibility of cecal perforation is high, a cecostomy is warranted.

REFERENCES

1. Cummings JH, Macfarlane GT. The control and consequences of bacterial fermentation in the colon. *J Appl Bacteriol* 1991;70:443–459.
2. Latella G, Caprilli R. Metabolism of the large bowel mucosa in health and disease. *Int J Colorectal Dis* 1991;6:127–132.
3. Pemberton JH, Phillips SF. Colonic absorption. *Perspect Colon Rectal Surg* 1988;1:89–103.
4. Grady GF, Duhamel RC, Moore EW. Active transport of sodium by human colon in vitro. *Gastroenterology* 1970;59:583–588.
5. Giller J, Phillips SF. Electrolyte absorption and secretion in the human colon. *Am J Dig Dis* 1972;17:1003–1011.
6. Powell DW. Transport in the large intestine. In: Giebisch G, Tosteson DC, Ussing HH, eds. *Membrane transport in biology*. New York: Springer-Verlag, 1978:318–327.
7. Dunn DL. Autochthonous microflora of the gastrointestinal tract. *Perspect Colon Rectal Surg* 1989;2:105–119.
8. Cannon WB. The movements of the intestine studied by means of roentgen rays. *Am J Physiol* 1902;6:251–277.
9. Elliott TR, Barclay-Smith E. Antiperistalsis and other muscular activities of the colon. *J Physiol* 1904;31:272–304.
10. Cohen S, Snape WJ. Movement of the small and large intestine. In: Fordtran J, Sleisinger M, eds. *Gastrointestinal disease,* 3rd ed. New York: McGraw-Hill, 1983:56–71.
11. Ritchie JA. Movements of segmental constrictions in the human colon. *Gut* 1971;6:251–277.
12. Herz AF. The passage of food along the human alimentary canal. *Guy's Hosp Rep* 1907;61:389–427.
13. Ritchie JA. Mass peristalsis in the human colon after contact with oxyphenisatin. *Gut* 1972;13:211–219.
14. Daniel EE. Electrophysiology of the colon. *Gut* 1975;16:298–329.
15. Drossman DA, Thompson WG, Talley NJ, et al. Identification of sub-groups of functional gastrointestinal disorders. *Gastroenterol Int* 1990;3:159–172.
16. Benson MJ, Roberts JP, Wingate DL, et al. Small bowel motility following major intra-abdominal surgery: the effects of opiates and rectal cisapride. *Gastroenterology* 1994;106:924–936.
17. Bohm B, Milsom JW, Fazio VW. Postoperative intestinal motility following conventional and laparoscopic intestinal surgery. *Arch Surg* 1995;130:415–419.
18. Olgilvy AJ, Smith G. The gastrointestinal tract after anaesthesia. *Eur J Anaesthesiol* 1995;12[Suppl 10]:35–42.
19. Walker EA, Byrnne PP, Katon WJ. Irritable bowel syndrome and psychiatric illness. *Am J Psychiatry* 1990;147:565–572.
20. Munakata J, Naliboff B, Harraf F, et al. Repetitive sigmoid stimulation induces rectal hyperalgesia in patients with irritable bowel syndrome. *Gastroenterology* 1997;112:55–63.
21. Snape WJ Jr, Carlson GM, Cohen S. Colonic myoelectric activity in the irritable bowel syndrome. *Gastroenterology* 1976;70:326–330.
22. Sloyer A, Panella V, Demas B. Ogilvie's syndrome: successful

management with colonoscopy. *Dig Dis Sci* 1988;33: 1391–1396.

23. Nakhgevany KB. Colonoscopic decompression of the colon in patients with Olgivie's syndrome. *Am J Surg* 1984;148: 317–320.

24. Hutchinson R, Griffiths C. Acute colonic pseudo-obstruction: a pharmacological approach. *Ann R Coll Surg Engl* 1992;74: 364–367.

SURGERY: SCIENTIFIC PRINCIPLES AND PRACTICE, Third Edition, edited by Lazar J. Greenfield, Michael W. Mulholland, Keith T. Oldham, Gerald B. Zelenock, and Keith D. Lillemoe. Lippincott Williams & Wilkins Publishers, Philadelphia, © 2001.

CHAPTER 44

ULCERATIVE COLITIS

JAMES M. BECKER AND ARTHUR F. STUCCHI

Ulcerative colitis is a chronic, diffuse inflammatory disease of unknown cause that affects the mucosa of the rectum and colon. Periods of remission alternate with exacerbations characterized by rectal bleeding and diarrhea. No etiology has been clearly identified, nor is any specific medical therapy available for ulcerative colitis, which typically affects patients during youth or early middle age. The disease has serious local and systemic long-term effects. Although medical therapy can ameliorate the inflammatory process and control most symptomatic flares, it provides no definitive treatment for the disease. Total removal of the colon and rectum provides complete cure. Newer surgical alternatives have eliminated the need for a permanent ileostomy after definitive resection of the involved colon and rectum.

Diarrheal illnesses have been described since the early writings of Hippocrates; however, it was not until 1875 that ulcerative colitis was more specifically characterized and distinguished by clinical and pathologic criteria from common infectious enteritis. With the description of regional enteritis in the 1930s by Crohn, the separation of ulcerative colitis from Crohn's disease of the intestine seemed relatively straightforward. The two diseases appeared initially to have distinct pathologic features, and each affected a different organ system. During the past several decades, a marked overlap between the two conditions has become appreciated, not only in pathologic features but also in anatomic distribution. The fact that a clear diagnosis cannot be made in more than 10% of patients can be extremely important because the surgical approaches to ulcerative colitis and Crohn's colitis are quite different.

Sigmoid colostomy was the first well-documented surgical procedure for inflammatory bowel disease. Not until 1940 did it become clear that definitive treatment of chronic ulcerative colitis required either total proctocolectomy or at least subtotal abdominal colectomy with ileostomy. The ostomy was associated with a high complication rate until Brooke and others proposed immediate maturation of the stoma in the 1950s. Proctocolectomy with the Brooke ileostomy emerged as the procedure of choice for ulcerative colitis. Since these early attempts, numerous techniques have been proposed for the restoration of continence after colectomy. The continent ileostomy, or Kock pouch, was used in the 1970s with moderate success. This has been challenged in the past two decades with the development of anal sphincter-sparing operations.

EPIDEMIOLOGY

The incidence of ulcerative colitis varies greatly within particular geographic regions and within distinct populations. These differences within and between populations have provided valuable insights into the etiology and pathogenesis of ulcerative colitis. Recent studies have suggested that the annual incidence is about 6 to 12/100,000 in northern countries, such as the United Kingdom, Norway, Sweden, and the United States, and about 2 to 8/100,000 in southern regions, such as Australia, South Africa, and the countries of southern Europe. The incidence in Asia and South America is considerably lower (1). These trends suggest that the incidence of ulcerative colitis is highest in developed or urban regions of the world and lowest in developing regions, although there are signs that the incidence rates of inflammatory bowel disease may be leveling off in the developed countries and starting to increase in the developing nations (2). Although still quite low, cases of ulcerative colitis are being reported with increasing frequency in Japan, India, Thailand, and other countries in Asia. Epidemiologic studies have also supported the earlier impression of a higher incidence of ulcerative colitis among Jews (two to four times the incidence versus non-Jews) and in whites (four times the incidence in nonwhites). The patients are more commonly Western than Asian; in the Western population, they are much more often northern European, Anglo Saxon, or from the northern portion of eastern Europe. An increasing incidence has also been observed in non-Jewish, black, and Hispanic populations (3).

Although the onset of ulcerative colitis typically occurs between the ages of 15 and 40 years, the age range can extend from infancy to old age. In fact, 3% to 5% of new cases occur after age 60. Throughout the age range, male and female subjects are affected about equally. Several lines of evidence suggest that genetic factors play a significant role in the pathogenesis of ulcerative colitis. Of patients with ulcerative colitis, 10% to 25% have first-degree relatives with the disease. A number of families have been reported with up to eight members affected over several generations. Both Crohn's disease and ulcerative colitis can occur within the same family, but concordance for the same disease category within the family appears to be 80% to 90% (4). The concordance for inflammatory bowel disease is higher in monozygous than in dizygous twins. In addition, the HLA phenotypes AW24 and BW35 are associated with ulcerative colitis, particularly in Israeli Jews of European origin. The frequency of the AW24 phenotype is increased in patients with an early onset of chronic ulcerative colitis and moderate to severe disease. Both geographic and racial differences can influence the occurrence of the disease, and no conclusive evidence has been found regarding the genetic versus the environmental determination of familial patterns.

A recent study analyzing age- and sex-specific death rates in addition to total mortality data from Australia, Canada, England and Wales, The Netherlands, Sweden, and the United States showed that mortality from ulcerative colitis has decreased continuously during the past 40 years. In contrast, mortality from Crohn's disease has increased between 1950 and the mid-1970s until reaching a level similar to that for ulcerative colitis. Since then, the death rates of both diseases have followed a parallel time course. A similar trend was found when male and female data were analyzed separately, again showing that the incidence of ulcerative colitis is similar for both sexes (5).

ETIOLOGY

The etiology of ulcerative colitis remains unknown despite intensive investigations. Considerable scientific attention has been devoted to infectious and immunologic hypotheses, and other avenues of investigation have included dietary, environmental, vascular, neuromotor, allergic, and psychogenic causes. A number of recent treatises explore these topics extensively (6–8).

The investigation of bacterial and viral agents continues to be an area of active research, although the fundamental role that infectious agents play in the pathogenesis of ulcerative colitis is far from certain. Whether the infectious agents are more likely to trigger or perpetuate the disease is a topic of great controversy. To act as a trigger, an infectious agent would have to initiate or reactivate the disease. Agents could initiate an autoimmune response by altering antigens, affecting molecular immunity, or increasing immune responsiveness. The microbial agent might also trigger the pathologic response by increasing mucosal permeability or stimulating epithelial injury or localized ischemia. The microbial agent could reactivate the inflammatory process directly, by secondary infection, or by the release of endotoxins. Although it has been recently postulated that ulcerative colitis is caused by one as yet unknown microbial pathogen (9), much of the evidence implicating microbial agents as triggers in inflammatory bowel disease is only indirect. No consistent evidence has been found that ulcerative colitis in humans is caused by any known microbial pathogen, although resident luminal bacterial components could initiate a chronic intestinal inflammation in a susceptible host following a breach in the mucosal barrier function or an environmental trigger (10). Dysentery has also been associated with flares of ulcerative colitis. In countries with high rates of dysentery, the incidence of ulcerative colitis appears to be increased. Upper respiratory infections have been associated with apparent reactivation or flares of ulcerative colitis. The seasonal pattern observed in many patients with ulcerative colitis suggests a pattern of initiation and reactivation.

Even though the microbial initiation of inflammation is the subject of much speculation, other investigators have suggested that infectious agents act primarily to perpetuate the disease. The full clinical expression of ulcerative colitis requires an intact mucosal immune system and also depends on normal intestinal flora and their products. Thus, alterations in the disease may result from subtle changes in intestinal flora. In addition, treatment interventions may affect disease activity by altering the flora and therefore the energetic or immunologic environment. As discussed later in this chapter, short-chain fatty acids are effective in treating diversion colitis and are natural products of the intestinal flora. Metronidazole may have a therapeutic effect in ulcerative colitis by altering the flora. Finally, remissions of inflammatory bowel disease have been observed anecdotally in patients with AIDS.

Studies suggesting that particular pathogens, including *Chlamydia* species, cytomegalovirus, and *Yersinia* species, are primary agents in the pathogenesis of ulcerative colitis have not been substantiated by further work. *Clostridium difficile* toxin activity has been associated with relapses of ulcerative colitis but appears to be correlated more with prior antibiotic administration than with disease activity. Specific strains of *Escherichia coli* have been identified in patients with ulcerative colitis. A viral cause also appears unlikely because the disease cannot be transmitted, and viral particles have not been identified; however, the limited presence of cells infected with Epstein-Barr virus in the affected areas of colonic specimens with inflammatory bowel disease indicates that Epstein-Barr viral infection may be related to such disease (11).

Speculation that chronic ulcerative colitis is an autoimmune disease has been considerable. A number of immunologic studies have supported this concept, and the role of cytokines and immunoregulatory molecules in the control of the immune response in patients with inflammatory bowel disease is a matter of great interest (12). For example, many patients with ulcerative colitis have circulating antibodies to normal colonic epithelium that cross-react with specific enterobacterial lipopolysaccharide antigens. Although autoantibodies to intestinal constituents have been reported, the evidence to support an autoimmune defect in the pathogenesis of ulcerative colitis is not compelling. However, it was demonstrated that more than 95% of patients with ulcerative colitis tested positive for a 40-kd antibody reactive to tropomyosin, an actin-binding protein localized in colonic epithelial cells (13). This epithelial autoantigen purportedly plays a role in complement activation mediated by immunoglobulin (Ig) G1 and may be a pathogenic mechanism for epithelial damage and persistent inflammation. More recently, patients with ulcerative colitis, but not Crohn's disease, were found to have high titers of mucosal autoantibodies to certain tropomyosin isoforms (14). In addition, antibodies against polymorphonuclear neutrophils or antineutrophil cytoplasmic antibodies (pANCAs) were identified in the serum of up to 86% of patients with ulcerative colitis, and distinct subsets may have important differential diagnostic, pathophysiologic, and treatment implications (15). Although the role of pANCAs and other autoantigens in the pathogenesis of inflammatory bowel diseases is unclear, their presence emphasizes the immunopathologic differences between ulcerative colitis and Crohn's disease and suggests that both disorders are heterogeneous inflammatory disease processes. Whether pANCAs have any value in the diagnosis of ulcerative colitis remains unclear (16).

Lymphocytes may be rendered cytotoxic to colonic epithelium by incubation with serum from patients with ulcerative colitis. Affected patients have also been found to have alterations of T- and B-lymphocyte activation and homing properties. Although total lymphocyte and T-lymphocyte counts are generally normal in patients with ulcerative colitis, the thymosine-dependent T-lymphocyte response may be abnormal, suggesting an immune-deficient state.

A number of investigators have argued that the immunologic events that have been observed in patients with ulcerative colitis are nonspecific epiphenomena and are not clinically useful disease markers. Little correlation exists between systemic immunity and the clinical status of the patient. The changes are nonspecific, particularly those in regard to heat shock proteins and lymphocyte function. The changes in the systemic immune system may simply reflect inflammation, rather than being specific for the disease. In contrast, many investigators believe that mucosal immunity plays a key role in mucosal defense and repair (17), and support is growing for the importance of altered mucosal immunity in the pathogenesis of inflammatory bowel diseases (18). Although a fully functional mucosal immune system appears vital to host defense, it is argued that the intestinal epithelial cell, equipped with a host of constitutive and inducible defense mechanisms, is the key element in host defense (19). More than likely, epithelial and mucosal immune cells function synergistically to sustain barrier function and mucosal integrity.

Thus, the intestinal immune system appears to play a pivotal role in the pathophysiology of mucosal inflammation. Normal gastrointestinal immune function appears to be regulated, in part, by cytokines, bioactive proteins secreted by activated immunocytes, in addition to other inflammatory cells, that influence the activity, differentiation, or rate of proliferation of other cells. Because cytokines are thought to modulate the gastrointestinal immune response, it appears that the balance between proinflammatory and antiinflammatory cytokines may be dysregulated in inflammatory bowel disease. In Crohn's disease, it appears that an excessive Th-1 T-cell response to an antigenic stimulus leads to increased levels of proinflammatory cytokines, such as interferon-γ (IFN-γ), interleukin (IL)-12, IL-1, IL-6, and tumor necrosis factor-α (TNF-α). In contrast, in ulcerative colitis, a Th-2 T-cell response appears to be the pathologic process responsible for inflammatory disease (20). Cytokines exert their biologic activities by autocrine, paracrine, and endocrine effects. They have both inflammatory and immunoregulatory activities and may amplify the immune response by activating the proliferation or chemotactic activity of effector cells or by stimulating mesenchymal cells to proliferate and increase production of eicosanoids, cytokines, and growth factors.

Specific activities of interleukins that are potentially relevant to ulcerative colitis have been identified recently (21). The most important of these may be IL-1, which activates T and B lymphocytes in addition to macrophages and neutrophils. IL-1 stimulates the production of eicosanoids, cytokines, growth factors, and destructive enzymes; increases adhesion of neutrophils and monocytes to endothelial cells; induces the acute-phase response in addition to fever, anorexia, and sleep; and stimulates collagen production and thus fibrosis. IL-1 has been shown to be elevated in ulcerative colitis and in experimental models of colitis. Increased IL-1 levels appear to correlate with severity of disease, which suggests that *IL1B* gene polymorphisms may participate in determining the course and severity of ulcerative colitis (22). In addition, alterations in IL-2, IL-4, IL-6, IL-8, IFN-γ, and the cytokines associated with the Th-2 T-cell response have been identified in tissues from patients with ulcerative colitis (20). The production of IFN during inflammation could play a significant role in the differentiation of mature memory and effector cells within the intestine. TNF may also be particularly important in the activation of mesenchymal cells but has not been fully evaluated in ulcerative colitis. Recent findings also suggest that IL-4, in combination with other Th-2–like cytokines, may play a pivotal role in active ulcerative colitis (23). Thus, it appears that cytokines are integrally involved in the pathogenesis of inflammatory bowel disease, having both immunoregulatory and proinflammatory properties. A better understanding of the pathogenic role of certain cytokines in intestinal inflammation can lead to potential new therapies such as infliximab, a monoclonal antibody directed against the proinflammatory cytokine TNF-α that shows promise in the treatment of Crohn's disease (24).

It has been proposed that ulcerative colitis represents an energy-deficient state of the colonic epithelium, in which levels of free coenzyme A are decreased and the rate of oxidation of butyrate to carbon dioxide is lower in colonic mucosal cells (25). Based on this theory, it has been suggested that short-chain fatty acids might be therapeutically beneficial. In patients with diversion colitis (occurring after the creation of a bypassed rectal segment), levels of short-chain fatty acid were found to be reduced within the bypassed segments. Treatment with intraluminal instillation of an isotonic short-chain fatty acid solution resulted in complete endoscopic healing in all patients. Recurrence resulted when saline solution was substituted for the short-chain fatty acid solution (26). Luminal short-chain fatty acids have also been shown to accelerate the healing of surgical anastomoses and increase regional blood flow and oxygen uptake. Impaired short-chain fatty acid metabolism by the colonocyte has been suggested as a pathogenic factor in ulcerative colitis; however, recent studies have demonstrated that although colonic butyrate oxidation is decreased in patients with active ulcerative colitis, the fact that remission was associated with normal oxidation suggests that the mucosa is not intrinsically altered in butyrate oxidation, which makes this unlikely to be a primary defect in ulcerative colitis (27). Although short-chain fatty acids may play a role in the pathogenesis and treatment of ulcerative colitis, this issue requires further study in the clinical setting.

Despite imperfections and differences, the accumulated evidence (especially the presence of chronic ulcerative colitis in three or more members of a family spanning several generations, the increased frequency among first-degree relatives, and the increased concordance rates of inflammatory bowel disease in monozygous twins) strongly suggests a genetic influence (4). The genetic mechanisms involved are poorly understood, although multiple gene alterations are likely. Genetic possibilities in ulcerative colitis include a polygenetic mode of inheritance, a specific form of somatic gene mutation in mesenchymal stem cells, the growth of a forbidden clone of cells producing mutant humoral factors that attack the colonic mucosa, and a rare additive major gene (28). The identification of specific biologic markers of chronic ulcerative colitis would greatly facilitate genetic epidemiologic studies and further clarify the nature of the disorder. The study of genetically modified (transgenic) rodent models and genetic deletion ("knockout") animal models may provide important clues to the genetic nature of ulcerative colitis.

Further experimental and clinical work is necessary to evaluate the etiologic possibilities in ulcerative colitis. During the past decade, animal models of intestinal inflammation have substantially augmented our understanding of the pathogenesis of ulcerative colitis, particularly in the areas of inflammatory mediators and cytokine regulation, genetic susceptibility, and the influence of ubiquitous luminal bacterial constituents (29–31). Inducible models utilizing the administration of acetic acid, trinitrobenzenesulfonic acid, and indomethacin to rats and the feeding of dextran sodium sulfate to mice are inexpensive, easily accomplished, and reproducible, so that these models are the preferred routes for testing novel pharmaceutical agents (29). Submucosal injection of the bacterial cell wall with polymer peptidoglycan polysaccharide (32) and intravenous administration of preformed immune complexes after rectal instillation of formalin (33) elicit more immunologically and environmentally relevant inflammatory responses than the toxin-induced models and permit more in-depth dissection of immunoregulatory mechanisms of acute and chronic intestinal inflammation. The cotton-top tamarin is unique in that it exhibits spontaneous colitis with associated adenocarcinoma of the colon, which allows this association to be studied in humans (34). Interestingly, in vitro models of inflammatory bowel disease are also being utilized to study the interactions of various cells and suspected inflammatory agents with intestinal epithelia (35) and colonic microvascular endothelium (36).

Unprecedented advances in molecular biology have provided techniques to overexpress or delete selected genes associated with spontaneous intestinal inflammation in rodents. The creation of in vivo models of overexpression (transgenic modification) or deletion (knockout) of genes encoding targeted cytokines, T-cell receptors, HLA molecules, and intracellular messengers by basic scientists working outside the field of inflammatory bowel disease has unexpectedly provided us with a whole new class of animal models of inflammatory bowel disease. Spontaneous intestinal inflammation in these genetically engineered rodents, in addition to the colitis that follows a spontaneous genetic mutation in C3H/HeJ mice and restoration of T-lymphocyte subsets in immunocompromised hosts, now permit the development of exciting new approaches to the exploration of mechanisms of chronic, spontaneous gastrointestinal inflammation.

PATHOLOGY

Ulcerative colitis, for the most part, is a disease confined to the mucosal and submucosal layers of the colonic wall. Ulcerative colitis is a continuous disease, with the rectum essentially always involved and the remainder of the colon diseased to a greater or lesser extent. Occasionally, with severe pancolitis, the terminal ileum shows secondary mild inflammation and dilation, a process that has been called *backwash ileitis*. On gross inspection, healed granular superficial ulcers are superimposed on a friable and thickened colonic mucosa with increased vascularity. Superficial fissures and small and regular pseudopolyps may also be noted (37). This appearance is in contradistinction to the transmural inflammatory changes found in Crohn's disease of the colon, in which all layers of the colonic wall may be involved in a granulomatous inflammatory process (Table 44.1). In their earlier stages, typical lesions consist of an infiltration of round cells and polymorphonuclear leukocytes into the crypts of Lieberkühn at the base of the mucosa to form crypt abscesses. Light microscopy reveals poor staining and vacuolization of overlying epithelial cells. Swelling of mitochondria, widening of intercellular spaces, and broadening of the endoplasmic reticulum are observed by transmission electron microscopy. As the lesions progress, coalescence of the crypt abscesses and desquamation of overlying cells result in the formation of an ulcer. This cryptitis is associated with the undermining of adjacent, relatively normal mucosa, which becomes edematous and assumes a polypoid configuration as it becomes isolated between adjacent ulcers (38). Collagen and a luxurious growth of granulation tissue occupy the areas of ulceration, which extend down to, but rarely through, the muscularis. Although ulcerative colitis is generally confined to the mucosa and submucosa, in the most severe forms of the disease, especially in toxic megacolon, the disease process may extend to the deeper muscular layers of the colon and even to the serosa. Rarely, crypt abscesses penetrate the muscularis propria, often extending along a blood vessel. In this situation, the colon may perforate, with resultant confusion about the diagnosis.

Table 44.1. PATHOLOGIC FEATURES OF CROHN'S DISEASE AND ULCERATIVE COLITIS

	Crohn's disease	Ulcerative colitis
Transmural inflammation	Yes	Uncommon
Granulomas	50%–75%	No
Fissures	Common	Rare
Submucosal thickening, fibrosis	Common	No
Submucosal inflammation	Common	Uncommon

CLINICAL FEATURES

Ulcerative colitis usually presents with bloody diarrhea, abdominal pain, and fever. Sixty percent of patients present with a relatively mild attack that occurs as a segmental colitis involving the distal colon (80%) or as a pancolitis (20%). In 5% to 15% of patients with disease limited to the rectosigmoid area, the disease eventually progresses to involve most, if not all, of the length of the colon. Twenty-five percent of all patients present with a moderate attack in which bloody diarrhea is the major symptom. In a small number of patients (15%), ulcerative colitis has an acute and catastrophic fulminating course. These patients have a relatively sudden onset of frequent bloody bowel movements, high fever, weight loss, and diffuse abdominal tenderness (39).

Physical findings are directly related to the duration and presentation of the disease. Weight loss and pallor are usually present, with a detectable alteration in numerous metabolic functions (40). In the active phase, the abdomen in the region of the colon is tender to palpation. During acute attacks or in the fulminating form of the disease, signs of an acute surgical abdomen may be accompanied by fever and decreased bowel sounds. In patients with toxic megacolon, abdominal distention may be identified. Examination of the integument, tongue, joints, and eyes is important because the presence of disease in these areas may suggest inflammatory bowel disease as a likely cause of the diarrheal illness.

Extraintestinal manifestations of ulcerative colitis are observed in a number of organ systems (41). The extracolonic manifestations of ulcerative colitis can be categorized as the *colitic group*, the *pathophysiologic group*, and the *miscellaneous group* of disorders. The activity of the colitic group of extracolonic manifestations parallels the activity of the underlying bowel disease, being present and most active when the colitis is active and subsiding when the colitis goes into remission. Included in this group are ocular lesions, including iritis or uveitis (seen in 0.5% to 3% of patients), conjunctivitis, episcleritis, keratitis, retinitis, and retrobulbar neuritis. With the exception of ulcerative panophthalmitis, ocular symptoms are closely related to disease activity and respond to therapy with steroids or other immunosuppressive agents.

Articular disorders, including peripheral joint disease, arthralgias, swelling, pain, and redness with migratory involvement, usually parallel the intensity of the colitis and respond to medical or surgical treatment. The joints of the lower extremities are most frequently involved. Overall, 15% to 20% of patients manifest endopathologic peripheral arthritis. Ankylosing spondylitis is seen in 1% to 6% of patients, and sacroiliitis is observed in 4% to 18% of patients. Both these conditions can result in permanent fixation of the spine and should be treated aggressively. Bone involvement specific to the axial skeleton is less closely related to the inflammatory state of the colon and may precede clinical evidence of ulcerative colitis.

Lesions of the skin and oral cavity are frequently observed in patients with ulcerative colitis. Aphthous stomatitis and gingivitis and erythema nodosum are observed less frequently in ulcerative colitis than in Crohn's disease. In contrast, pyoderma gangrenosum is more frequently observed in ulcerative colitis (0.6%) than in Crohn's disease.

Liver and biliary tract disorders occur commonly in patients with chronic ulcerative colitis (42). Up to 80% of patients demonstrate histologic evidence of pericholangitis on liver biopsy, with hepatic involvement more common in patients with pancolitis. Between 50% and 90% of patients with ulcerative colitis have fatty infiltration of the liver.

Chronic active hepatitis affects 1% to 10% of patients, and biliary cirrhosis develops in about 1%. One of the most difficult complications, sclerosing cholangitis, is observed in 1% to 4% of patients with ulcerative colitis. Affected patients present with pruritus, alkaline phosphatase elevation, right upper quadrant pain and tenderness, and jaundice. The diagnosis is confirmed by endoscopic retrograde cholangiopancreatography or transhepatic cholangiography. Controversy surrounds the treatment of this disorder (43). Although some patients respond to colectomy, hepatic disease progresses in most even after colon resection. Surgical drainage, internal stent placement, and antibiotics have all been reported to be of value in the treatment of symptomatic sclerosing cholangitis. Patients with progressive liver failure ultimately require orthotopic liver transplantation. Affected patients are also at greater risk for the development of carcinoma of the bile duct, although this may also develop de novo in patients with ulcerative colitis.

Patients with ulcerative colitis are at slightly greater risk for the development of thromboembolic disease and vasculitis. Rarely, renal disease, clubbing, bronchial and pulmonary abnormalities, and amyloidosis develop in association with inflammatory bowel disease.

DIAGNOSIS

The diagnosis of acute ulcerative colitis is one of exclusion. No laboratory, radiographic, or histologic features are pathognomonic. In all patients presenting with diarrhea or bloody diarrhea, an infectious cause must be excluded. Stool samples and biopsy specimens should be evaluated for *Campylobacter* species, *Salmonella* species, pathogenic *E. coli, Aeromonas* species, *Plesiomonas* species, amebae, and *C. difficile.* Particularly important and difficult to exclude are pseudomembranous colitis, the proctocolitis seen increasingly in homosexual men, and traveler's diarrhea. It has become increasingly important to distinguish ulcerative colitis from granulomatous colitis. Major distinguishing clinical characteristics of Crohn's colitis and ulcerative colitis are shown in Table 44.2.

Flexible sigmoidoscopy is the first step in diagnosis because ulcerative colitis involves the distal colon and rectum in 90% to 95% of cases (37). Mild cases may show only a loss of the normal vascular pattern, a granular texture, and microhemorrhages when the friable mucosa is touched or wiped (Fig. 44.1) (see color insert following page 1190). In more advanced cases, when the disease is moderately active, the mucosa becomes more grossly pitted and spontaneous bleeding is seen (Fig. 44.2) (see color insert following page 1190). In severe cases, macro-ulcera-

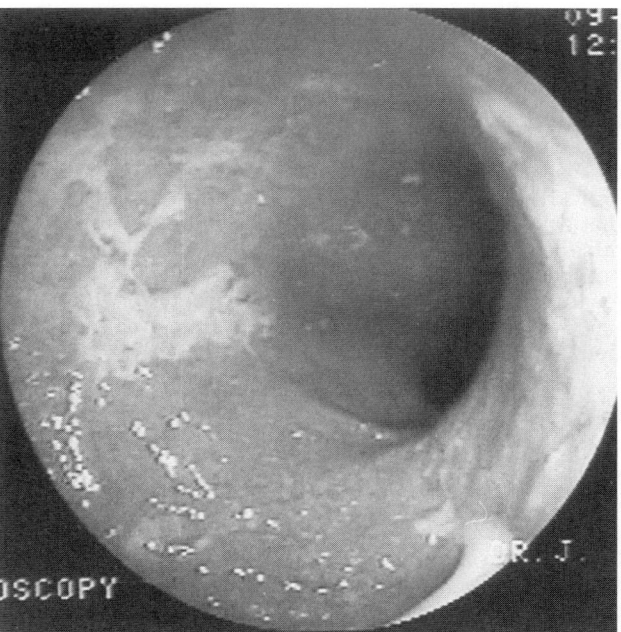

Figure 44.1. Endoscopic appearance of the rectum in a patient with mild ulcerative colitis, with mucosal granularity and loss of the normal vascular pattern.

tions with profuse bleeding and a purulent exudate is seen (Fig. 44.3) (see color insert following page 1190). In advanced disease, areas of ulceration may surround areas of heaped-up granulation tissue and edematous mucosa, so-called pseudopolyps. The use of flexible sigmoidoscopy and other imaging modalities has greatly improved diagnostic accuracy and patient acceptability (44). Colonoscopy may be useful in determining the extent and activity of disease, particularly in patients in whom the diagnosis

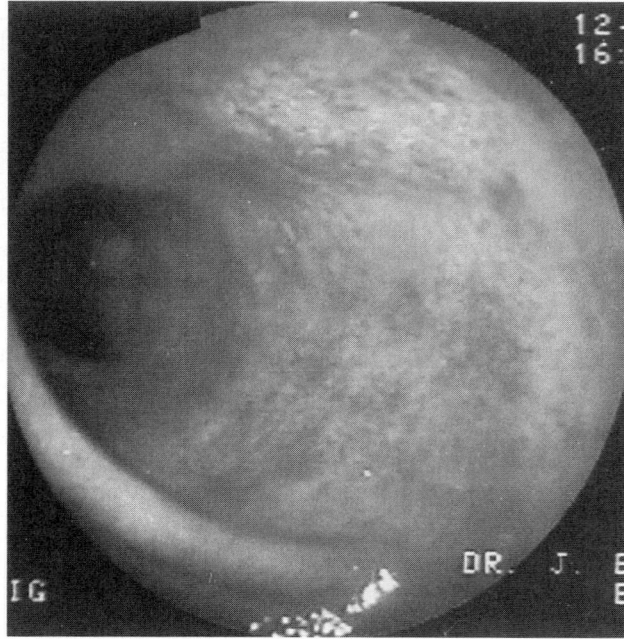

Figure 44.2. Endoscopic appearance of the rectum in a patient with moderate ulcerative colitis, with pitted mucosa and spontaneous hemorrhage.

Table 44.2. **DISTINGUISHING CHARACTERISTICS OF CROHN'S DISEASE AND ULCERATIVE COLITIS**

Characteristics	Crohn's disease	Ulcerative colitis
Location	Small-bowel involvement	Colon only (rare backwash ileitis)
Anatomic distribution	Asymmetric distribution (skip lesions)	Contiguous involvement beginning distally
Rectal involvement	Rectal sparing common	Involved in 90%
Gross bleeding	Absent in 25%–30%	Universal
Perianal disease	≤75%	Rare, may be severe
Fistulization	Yes	No
Granulomas	50%–75%	No

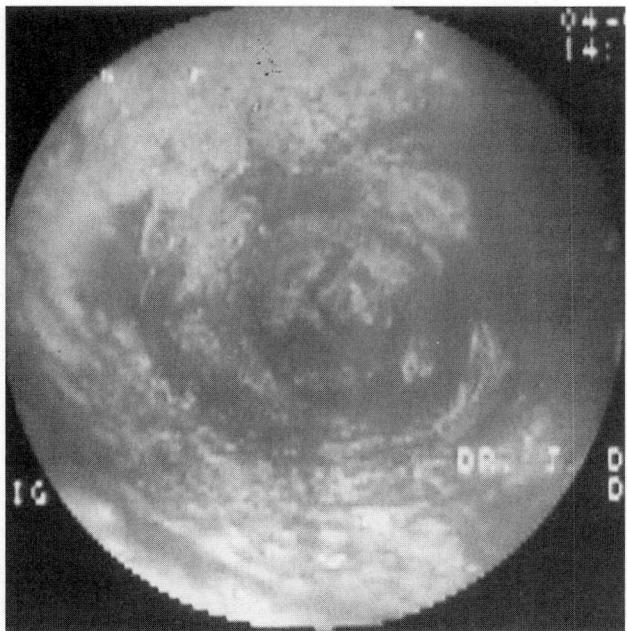

Figure 44.3. Endoscopic appearance of the rectum in a patient with severe ulcerative colitis, with frank ulceration, bleeding, and a purulent exudate.

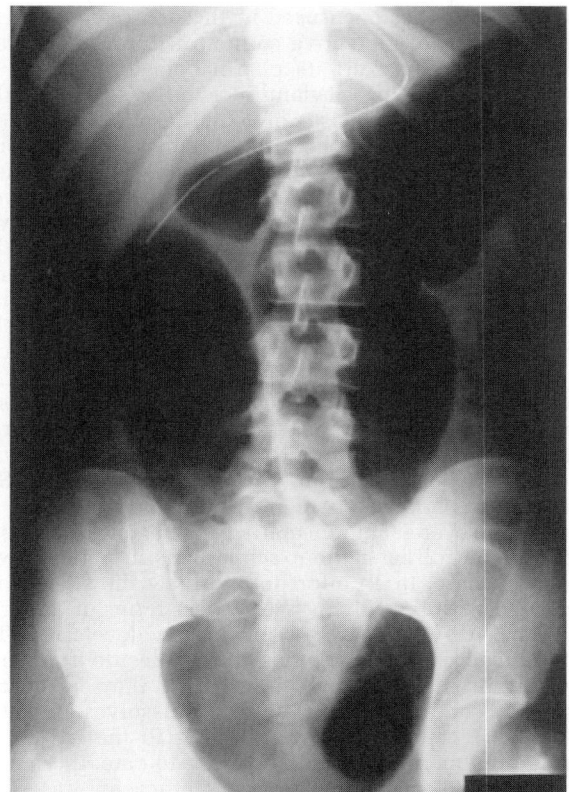

Figure 44.4. Colonic dilation, particularly of the transverse colon, in a patient with toxic megacolon.

is unclear or cancer is suspected. Endoscopy can be useful in distinguishing between ulcerative colitis and Crohn's colitis (Table 44.3).

Barium enema examination of the colon is useful in most patients, although potentially dangerous in those with toxic megacolon. When ulcerative colitis develops, mucosal granularity and microhemorrhages produce a diffusely reticulated pattern, on which are superimposed countless punctate collections of contrast material lodged in micro-ulcerations. A mild case of acute ulcerative colitis may be manifested by a diffusely granular appearance, which is best seen on air-contrast barium enema. In more advanced cases, irregular margins develop in the colon with spiculated and undermining "collar button" ulcers that can be well demonstrated on full-column barium enema. End-stage, or burned-out, ulcerative colitis is characterized by shortening of the colon, loss of normal redundancy in the sigmoid region and at the splenic and hepatic flexures, disappearance of the haustral pattern, a featureless mucosa, absence of discrete ulceration, and narrowed caliber of the bowel. Chronic inflammation may lead to diffuse mucosal atrophy, leaving behind hyper-

trophic islands of inflamed mucosa and granulation tissue, which assume a polypoid shape and are called *pseudopolyps.* These pseudopolyps may carpet the colon, simulating the polyposis syndrome, or they may be discrete, as in the case of filiform pseudopolyposis.

A plain abdominal radiograph may also be useful in patients with severe ulcerative colitis. An abdominal film may demonstrate colonic dilation, which has been called *toxic megacolon,* in 3% to 5% of patients (Fig. 44.4). Most frequently, dilation is observed in the transverse colon. Free air may be seen within the peritoneal cavity as a result of perforation of the diseased colon.

MEDICAL MANAGEMENT

The principal categories of drug treatment for ulcerative colitis include symptomatic antidiarrheal and antispasmodic agents, sulfasalazine and its analogues, corticosteroids and adrenocorticotropic hormone (ACTH), immunosuppressive antimetabolites, and certain antibiotics (45,46). Future treatments may also include such novel therapies as antigen-directed and immune mediator blockade, antiinflammatory cytokines, neuroimmune modulators such as substance P antagonists, nitric oxide synthase inhibitors, oxygen radical scavengers, antisense blockade of gene expression, and probiotic manipulation of luminal bacteria (47). Although many of these therapies are in experimental and developmental stages, their effectiveness may provide valuable insight into the pathogenesis of ulcerative colitis. Once the diagnosis of ulcerative colitis has been clearly established, the decision regarding treatment depends on the severity of symptoms and on the severity and extent of disease as indicated by radiographic and endoscopic studies.

Table 44.3. ENDOSCOPIC FEATURES OF CROHN'S DISEASE AND ULCERATIVE COLITIS

Endoscopic features	Crohn's disease	Ulcerative colitis
Mucosal involvement	Discontinuous	Contiguous
Discrete ulcers (aphthous ulcers)	Common	Rare
Surrounding mucosa	Relatively normal	Abnormal
Longitudinal ulcer	Common	Rare
Cobblestoning	In severe cases	No
Rectal involvement	Sparing common	Involved in 90%
Mucosal friability	Uncommon	Common
Vascular pattern	Normal	Distorted

Sulfasalazine has been used in the management of the chronic phases of ulcerative colitis for the past 50 years. Sulfasalazine may exert its pharmacologic effect by inhibiting mucosal prostaglandin synthesis. The sulfasalazine molecule consists of 5-aminosalicylic acid (5-ASA), linked by an azo bond to sulfapyridine. Evidence suggests that 5-ASA is the therapeutically active moiety, with the sulfapyridine acting as a vehicle for drug delivery to the lower gastrointestinal tract. Most of the toxicity of the drug is attributable to the sulfapyridine. Reversible hypospermia and infertility are observed in male patients. About 25% to 30% of patients experience headaches, nausea, anorexia, and dyspepsia, and fever and rash develop in patients allergic to sulfa drugs. Less common side effects include hemolysis and neutropenia, which are related to serum sulfapyridine levels. In some patients, sulfasalazine may actually exacerbate the disease. Overall, sulfasalazine has been found to be effective in treating mild to moderate disease in 75% to 80% of patients. Sulfasalazine has not been of significant value in treating patients with severe acute ulcerative colitis, but it may play a role in controlling acute exacerbations in patients with chronic disease. In an effort to eliminate the side effects associated with the sulfa carrier, newer forms of the drug, such as 5-ASA and 4-ASA, have been developed. The basic concept is to prevent the active molecule from being absorbed in the proximal bowel. This may be accomplished by coating the tablet so that it dissolves only at an alkaline pH of 6 or 7, corresponding to the pH in the terminal ileum or colon. In all studies to date, these compounds have been shown to be as efficacious as sulfasalazine in treating acute ulcerative colitis and in preventing relapse.

The other common therapeutic modality for the treatment of mild distal ulcerative colitis is topical steroids. Steroid enemas are effective for patients with proctitis and proctosigmoiditis but are of little value for patients with more extensive left-sided disease or pancolitis. In an attempt to avoid systemic effects of steroid enemas, tixocortol pivalate was synthesized by adding a thiol ester group at position 21 on the hydrocortisone molecule. In trials, this agent has been useful for treating patients with left-sided colitis and has resulted in a reduction in systemic steroid side effects.

Patients with moderate ulcerative colitis, whether left-sided or universal, require some form of systemic therapy. These patients initially can be managed with topical steroid therapy and oral sulfasalazine. If they do not respond to this regimen, oral corticosteroids are introduced. Corticosteroids remain the mainstay of therapy during acute attacks. Between 40 and 60 mg of prednisone in a single daily dose is effective in most cases in terms of inducing remission. If the patient's clinical symptoms and sigmoidoscopic findings improve, the steroid dose can be tapered after several weeks. Although maintenance steroids may be useful in controlling symptoms in patients with continuing activity, maintenance therapy with low-dose corticosteroids for patients with inactive disease has not been demonstrated to prevent relapse. Patients must be monitored carefully for the long-term adverse sequelae of corticosteroid use, including hypertension, hyperglycemia, cataracts, osteoporosis, and osteomalacia.

Some 10% to 20% of patients with ulcerative colitis have a more severe clinical course and require hospitalization. These patients must have nutritional support, generally with intravenous hyperalimentation or total parenteral nutrition (48), and their anemia must be corrected. Patients with more active disease or toxicity require parenteral steroids in the form of hydrocortisone. Whether intravenous ACTH plays any role in the treatment of severe ulcerative colitis has been a matter of controversy. In general, the response rate for ACTH appears to be similar to that for hydrocortisone, although ACTH may be more effective in patients not previously treated with corticosteroids. The usual doses recommended are in the range of 300 mg of hydrocortisone per day or 40 IU of ACTH per day. Total parenteral nutrition plays no primary role in ameliorating the inflammatory response in ulcerative colitis but allows nutritional maintenance and repletion during the treatment phase (49). During an acute episode of severe colitis, narcotic pain medications and antidiarrheal agents should be avoided to prevent provocation of toxic megacolon. Once the patient has responded clinically, oral foods can be started, and the patient can begin receiving oral steroids as parenteral steroids are tapered.

A number of immunosuppressive agents have been used for the management of ulcerative colitis, including azathioprine (50) and its metabolite, 6-mercaptopurine (51). Because these drugs do not produce a clinical response for several months, they have no role in the treatment of acute flares of ulcerative colitis. Cyclosporine, which has a more rapid onset of action, has been advocated for the treatment of severe, refractory acute ulcerative colitis. The results of both uncontrolled trials and one controlled study suggest that high-dose cyclosporine is efficacious for severe ulcerative colitis. However, the theoretic risk for irreversible cyclosporine-associated nephropathy after treatment of ulcerative colitis with high-dose cyclosporine is significant. Severe infectious complications may also occur (52).

Although widely prescribed for both ulcerative colitis and Crohn's disease, metronidazole and other antibiotics are of no proven value in the treatment of inflammatory bowel disease. In addition, the drugs have associated side effects. The major problem with metronidazole is patient intolerance secondary to side effects, such as a metallic taste and paresthesias.

SURGICAL CONSIDERATIONS

Nearly half of patients with chronic ulcerative colitis undergo surgery within the first 10 years of their illness, mainly because of the chronic nature of the disease and the tendency for relapse. In addition, occasional fulminant complications occur in ulcerative colitis, and the risk for malignant degeneration is significant. The indications for surgery vary widely, and these differing indications have different implications for the timing of surgery and the choice of operative procedure. Indications for surgical intervention include the following: (a) massive unrelenting hemorrhage, (b) toxic megacolon with impending or frank perforation, (c) fulminating acute ulcerative colitis that is unresponsive to steroid therapy, (d) obstruction resulting from stricture, (e) suspicion or demonstration of colonic cancer, (f) systemic complications, and (g) intractability (53). An additional indication for surgery in children is failure to mature at an acceptable rate. For most patients with ulcerative colitis, a colectomy is performed when the disease enters an intractable, chronic phase and becomes a physical and social burden. With sphincter-sparing operations available for patients with ulcerative colitis, it has become critically important to avoid standard proctectomy whenever possible and make a diagnostic distinction between patients with ulcerative colitis and those with Crohn's disease.

Indications for Surgery

Intractable Disease

A failure of medical management, reflected by chronic physical disability and physiologic dysfunction, is by far the most common indication for surgery in chronic ulcerative colitis (54). This indication is also the hardest to define. Intractability can best be characterized as the severe and persistent impairment of quality of life, created by the underlying disease or by the treatment required for that disease. Elective operations for medically intractable ulcerative colitis include total proctocolectomy with Brooke ileostomy or continent ileostomy (Kock pouch), subtotal colectomy with ileostomy or ileorectal anastomosis, and colectomy with mucosal proctectomy and ileoanal anastomosis (55). In the past, when total proctocolectomy combined with ileostomy was the only definitive alternative, patients frequently delayed surgery for as long as possible, often to the point at which their life-style and health were remarkably restricted. With the availability of newer surgical alternatives, patients and their physicians are electing surgery much earlier in the course of the disease. Criteria regarding the timing of operation and indications for surgery are therefore undergoing considerable revision.

Extracolonic Disease

The relation between systemic extracolonic manifestations of ulcerative colitis and colectomy is not entirely clear. Except for extreme retardation of growth and development, the extracolonic complications of ulcerative colitis rarely provide an independent indication for operation. Although the arthritis and skin lesions associated with chronic ulcerative colitis do respond to colectomy, ankylosing spondylitis and liver dysfunction or failure may remain unresponsive. Studies suggest that progression of sclerosing cholangitis bears no relation to the presence or absence of the colon or to the degree of the inflammatory process within the diseased mucosa. A colitis-related extraintestinal manifestation that occasionally emerges as a potential surgical indication is a progressively destructive pyoderma gangrenosum. In approximately 50% of the patients with active colitis, colectomy is followed by resolution of the skin lesions. A rare but urgent extracolonic indication for colectomy is massive hemolytic anemia, usually Coombs' test-positive, that is unresponsive to steroid and immunosuppressive therapy. In this case, colectomy is generally accompanied by splenectomy. The most common extraintestinal indication for surgery in ulcerative colitis is the retardation of growth and development in children and adolescents. Colectomy can be of dramatic benefit in children with ulcerative colitis.

Cancer Prophylaxis

Most authors agree that significant dysplasia or suspected cancer is a clear indication for colectomy. Ulcerative colitis is clearly associated with an increased risk for colorectal cancer (56–58). Although the risk may be as low as 2% to 3% for the first 10 years after the onset of ulcerative colitis, the risk can increase at a rate of 1% to 2% per year (59). Thus, by the time the patient has had the disease for 20 years, the risk for colon cancer may be as high as 20%, climbing to as high as 30% in patients who have had ulcerative colitis for longer than 35 years (60,61). Many epidemiologists believe that earlier studies overestimated the risk for malignancy because of referral and ascertainment biases inherent in retrospective surveys from tertiary referral hospital centers.

The question of timing of surgery for cancer prophylaxis remains controversial. In fact, this is the sole indication for operation in few patients. The role of rectal or colonic biopsy in directing the timing of colectomy also remains controversial. Several studies have demonstrated that more than 20% of patients have a more proximally located colonic malignancy at the time that a random rectal biopsy shows severe dysplasia. In a patient with long-standing colitis, an unequivocal high-grade dysplasia or a dysplasia-associated lesion or mass is certainly an indication for colectomy. Some newer evidence suggests that even low-grade dysplasia, if it is unequivocal and not associated with inflammation, should prompt colectomy.

The presence of carcinoma is not a contraindication to mucosal proctectomy with ileoanal anastomosis unless the tumor is found to be of an advanced stage or is located within the rectum. If the stage of the tumor at the time of the initial operation is uncertain, subtotal colectomy with ileostomy and Hartmann closure of the rectum can be performed. This operation allows a subsequent conversion to ileoanal anastomosis if the patient remains disease-free.

Surgical Emergencies

Only 15% of patients with ulcerative colitis present initially with catastrophic illness. Several well-identified complications require urgent operation if a patient with ulcerative colitis is to survive. These include (a) massive, unrelenting hemorrhage; (b) toxic megacolon with impending or frank perforation; (c) fulminating acute ulcerative colitis that is unresponsive to steroid therapy; (d) acute colonic obstruction resulting from stricture; and (e) suspicion or demonstration of colon cancer.

Acute perforation occurs infrequently, with the incidence directly related to both the severity of the initial attack and the extent of disease in the bowel. Although the overall incidence of perforation during a first attack is less than 4%, if the attack is severe, the incidence rises to about 10%. If the patient has pancolitis, the perforation rate is 15%; if the pancolitis is associated with a clinically severe attack, the perforation rate rises to nearly 20%. Perforation is the most lethal complication of acute colitis, with an associated mortality rate of 40% to 50%. Although free colon perforation occurs much more frequently when toxic megacolon is present than when it is not, it is important to remember that toxic megacolon is not a prerequisite for the development of perforation. In the presence of colonic perforation, the operation should be definitive without being overly aggressive. Abdominal colectomy with ileostomy and Hartmann closure of the rectum is the procedure of choice.

Obstructions caused by benign stricture formation develop in 11% of patients, with 34% of the strictures occurring in the rectum. Strictures are usually the result of submucosal fibrosis and occasionally mucosal hyperplasia. Although these lesions do not usually cause acute obstruction, they must be differentiated from carcinoma by biopsy or excision, and particular attention should be given to ruling out Crohn's disease. Strictures caused by carcinoma are less common than those caused by benign disease and are more prone to perforate.

Massive hemorrhage secondary to ulcerative colitis is rare, occurring in fewer than 1% of patients and accounting for about 10% of urgent colectomies performed for ulcerative colitis. Prompt surgical intervention is indicated after hemodynamic stabilization. Uncontrollable hemorrhage from the entire colorectal mucosa may be the one clear indication for emergency proctocolectomy. If possible, the rectum should be spared for later mucosal proctectomy with ileoanal anastomosis, with the realization that about 12% of patients will have continued hemorrhage from the retained rectal segment.

Anorectal complications of ulcerative colitis are more common than generally appreciated, occasionally confusing the differential diagnosis between Crohn's colitis and ulcerative colitis. Most rectal symptoms occur within the first year after the onset of symptoms and, in part, correlate with the severity of the disease. Overall, perirectal or ischiorectal abscesses and associated anal fistulae develop in up to 18% of patients with ulcerative colitis.

Acute toxic megacolon occurs in 6% to 13% of patients with ulcerative colitis. The initial treatment for toxic megacolon includes intravenous fluid and electrolyte resuscitation, nasogastric suction, broad-spectrum antibiotics to include anaerobic and aerobic gram-negative coverage, and total parenteral nutrition to improve nutritional status. Although the therapeutic role of steroids in toxic megacolon is controversial, most patients presenting with a severe attack of ulcerative colitis are already on steroid therapy and thus need stress doses of corticosteroids to prevent adrenal crisis. When toxic megacolon is promptly treated, subsequent surgery is not inevitable. Even among patients in whom prompt resolution has occurred, about half require surgery within a year, and most eventually require colectomy.

In the presence of acute toxic megacolon caused by ulcerative colitis, surgery can be associated with a high operative morbidity and mortality rate. Postoperative complications, including sepsis, wound infection, abscess, fistula, or delayed wound healing, have been reported in up to half of patients (62). Postoperative mortality rates range between 11% and 16% and, for the subset of patients with perforation, between 27% and 44%. The overall mortality rate after emergency surgery is 9%; the mortality rate is 6% for total abdominal colectomy and 15% for proctocolectomy. These numbers suggest that more conservative surgery is appropriate in the acute setting. With the popularity of anal sphincter-sparing procedures, the surgeon should always weigh the possibility of the need for later surgery to restore continence. Specifically, leaving the rectum intact allows it to be used for subsequent mucosal proctectomy and ileoanal anastomosis.

Surgical Approaches

Because chronic ulcerative colitis is cured once the colon and rectum are removed, single-stage total proctocolectomy with permanent ileostomy has historically been the procedure of choice for elective surgical treatment. Despite the fact that this operation eliminates all diseased tissue and the risk for malignant transformation, it has remained controversial and is poorly accepted by patients and their physicians, primarily because a permanent abdominal ileostomy is required after standard proctocolectomy. Although immediate maturation of the stoma (Fig. 44.5) eliminates many of the mechanical problems associated with ileostomy, patients receiving even the most carefully constructed ileostomies are incontinent of gas and stool and must wear an external collecting bag day and night. Several studies have demonstrated that although 90% of patients with a Brooke ileostomy are able to adjust

to the stoma, between 25% and 50% of patients with ileostomies complain of appliance-related problems (63). These include skin irritation or excoriation, discomfort, leakage and odor, the financial burden of caring for an ileostomy with modern disposable stomal devices, and the time and effort that are required. Perhaps more important than these problems are the significant psychological and psychosocial implications of a permanent ileostomy, particularly for young and physically active patients. It is for this reason that surgeons have long sought other alternatives to total proctocolectomy and ileostomy.

Proctocolectomy and Ileostomy

Until about 20 years ago, single-stage total proctocolectomy with ileostomy was the operation of choice when complications of ulcerative colitis were treated electively (64). Currently, proctocolectomy is the procedure of choice in relatively few patients with ulcerative colitis. Advantages of the operation are that it is curative, there is no anastomosis to heal, and no further surgery is required. The patient is provided with a predictable functional result, and the fear of anal incontinence is eliminated.

The disadvantage of total proctocolectomy is that it results in permanent fecal incontinence. Patients require an external ileostomy device, which may need emptying four to eight times per day. Also, significant complications are associated with the operation. A 20% overall morbidity rate is reported for elective, 30% for urgent, and 40% for emergency proctocolectomy. The risks are primarily hemorrhage, contamination, sepsis, and neural injury. Revision of the stoma is required in 10% to 25% of patients. Perineal wound problems develop after a standard abdominal perineal proctectomy in 10% to 20%, and bowel obstruction occurs at some point in the postoperative period in 15% to 20%. Of major concern is bladder and sexual dysfunction associated with parasympathetic nerve injury. Impotence is reported to develop in to up to 5% of male patients after proctectomy for benign disease.

Subtotal Colectomy

Subtotal colectomy, Brooke ileostomy, and Hartmann closure of the rectum, or ileorectal anastomosis (Fig. 44.6), have been employed in the surgical treatment of ulcerative colitis for decades. The operation eliminates an abdominal stoma if ileorectal anastomosis is performed, and because the pelvic autonomic nerves are not disturbed, impotence and bladder dysfunction are not a risk. As described earlier, subtotal colectomy with ileostomy is the procedure of choice in the emergency setting or if the diagnosis of ulcerative colitis, as opposed to Crohn's disease, cannot be clearly established. Although abdominal colectomy with ileorectal anastomosis is a less extensive procedure that usually leaves the patient with full continence, it has not

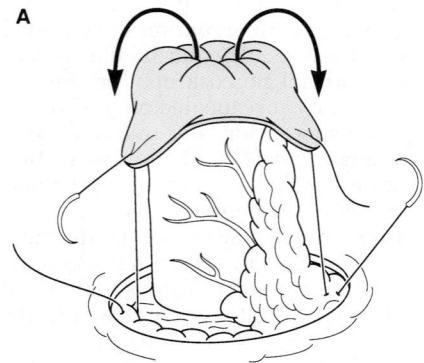

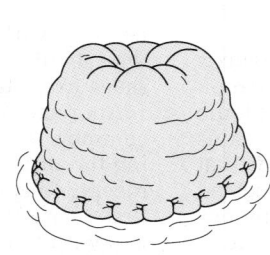

Figure 44.5. Construction of an end-ileostomy. The terminal ileum is brought 5 cm through an abdominal wall defect *(A)*, everted, and sutured *(B)* to the more proximal ileal seromuscularis and then dermis to mature the ileostomy.

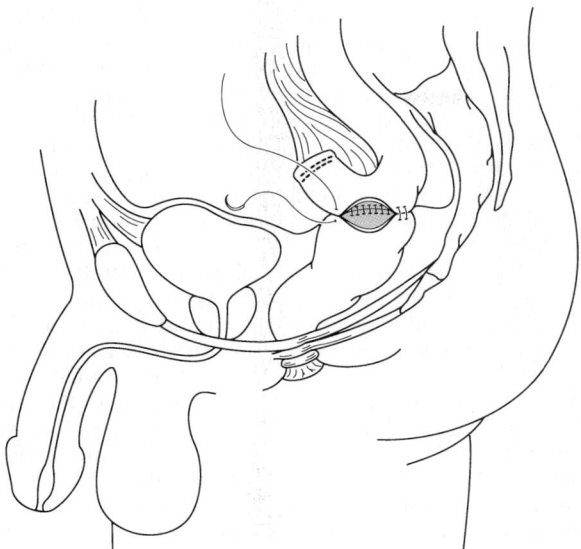

Figure 44.6. Ileorectal anastomosis after abdominal colectomy. This represents a nondefinitive operation for selected patients with chronic ulcerative colitis.

gained wide popularity because it is not a curative operation. The inflammatory process persists in the retained rectum in essentially all patients, and the ongoing risk for malignancy may be as high as 17% after 20 years (65). At least 10% of patients require subsequent proctectomy for uncontrollable proctitis, and another 10% require proctectomy because of a poor functional result. Even in patients who do well, the stool frequency is high in the early postoperative period, eventually averaging four or five stools per 24 hours. The operation is also associated with a number of operative complications, including small-bowel obstruction, which has been reported in 10% to 20% of patients. In addition, leakage of the anastomosis between the ileum and the disease-bearing rectum is a possibility. The operation is clearly contraindicated in patients with anal sphincter dysfunction, severe rectal disease, rectal dysplasia, or frank cancer. Subtotal colectomy with ileorectal anastomosis is clearly a compromise operation (66). With the availability and success of the definitive mucosal proc-

tectomy and ileoanal anastomosis, ileorectal anastomosis is applicable in few patients.

Continent Ileostomy

Kock (67) first described the continent ileostomy, constructed entirely from terminal ileum and consisting of an intestinal pouch that serves as a reservoir for stool, with an ileal conduit connecting the pouch to a cutaneous stoma (Fig. 44.7). The operation was modified several years later to include an intestinal nipple valve between the pouch and the stoma. For construction of the pouch and the valve, 45 to 50 cm of terminal ileum is used. The proximal 30 to 35 cm is formed into a pouch, and a nipple valve is constructed by intussuscepting the outflow tract from the pouch and then securing it with sutures or staples. The reservoir is sutured to the peritoneum and fascia, and the efferent limb is brought out through the abdominal wall as a flush stoma. Patients empty the pouch by passing a soft plastic tube through the valve by way of the stoma. The advantage of this operation is that it is curative because a total proctocolectomy is performed. The technique offers the patient a potentially new life-style because the ileostomy is continent, so that the need for an external appliance is avoided (68).

The continent ileostomy has been associated with a high complication rate (69). Most of the complications are related to displacement of the nipple valve, which produces fecal incontinence, and difficulty in intubating and emptying the pouch. Valve failure has been reported to occur in between 4% and 40% of patients. Bowel obstruction develops in 10% to 20% of patients. The operation carries the same risk for bladder dysfunction, impotence, and perineal wound problems as standard proctocolectomy and ileostomy. Several syndromes of ileostomy dysfunction related to the Kock pouch have also been reported. These are variably described as stagnant loop syndrome, enteritis, nonspecific ileitis, and pouchitis. Clinical features include diarrhea, malabsorption of fat and vitamin B_{12}, proliferation of anaerobic bacteria, inflammation of the pouch, and incontinence. In addition, fistulae may develop between the pouch and the skin or other enteric organs. Crohn's disease is a clear contraindication to this operation. Despite these complications, patient satisfaction with the continent ileostomy is high.

Although the Kock ileostomy has advantages over the Brooke ileostomy, its high rate of mechanical, functional,

A

B

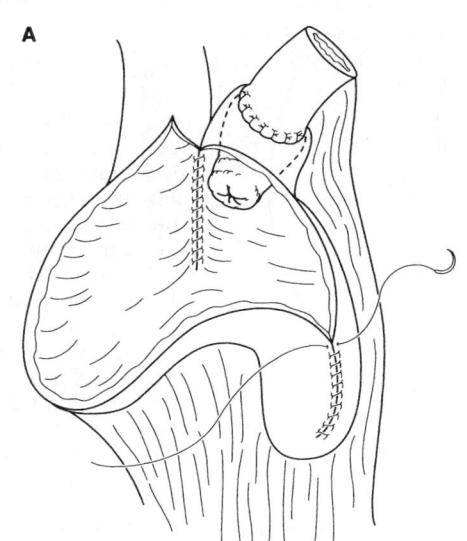
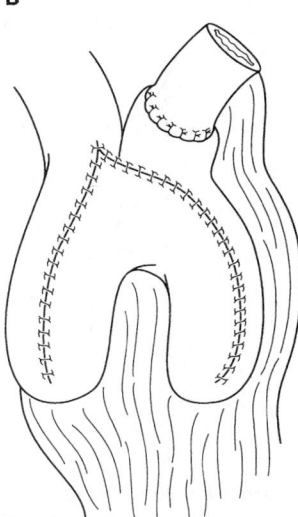

Figure 44.7. The continent ileostomy (Kock pouch) consists of an ileal reservoir and nipple valve constructed by (A) intussuscepting the efferent limb and fixing it in place with sutures or staples. (B) The pouch itself is then closed with sutures. This provides a continent internal intestinal reservoir that the patient can drain by intubating the pouch through the flush cutaneous stoma several times throughout the day.

and metabolic complications has limited its clinical usefulness. In centers that offer all surgical alternatives to patients with ulcerative colitis requiring colectomy, few Kock pouches are being constructed. The continent ileostomy may be useful in patients who have already undergone total proctocolectomy and ileostomy and, after careful counseling, are extremely desirous of an attempt at a continence-restoring procedure.

Ileoanal Anastomosis

To avoid ablating the entire rectum, anus, and anal sphincter, it is possible to take advantage of the fact that ulcerative colitis is a mucosal disease. The rectal mucosa can be selectively dissected out and removed down to the dentate line of the anus (70,71). This preserves an intact rectal muscular cuff and anal sphincter apparatus. Continuity of the intestinal tract can be reestablished by extending the ileum into the pelvis endorectally, and circumferentially suturing it to the anus in an end-to-end fashion (Fig. 44.8). The potential advantages of this approach are that it eliminates all diseased tissue and is as definitive an operation as total proctocolectomy. Because the pelvic dissection is confined to the endorectal plane, it preserves parasympathetic innervation to the bladder and genitalia and eliminates the problem of urinary dysfunction or impotence. Because the abdominal perineal proctectomy is eliminated, a long-term draining perineal wound is avoided. A permanent abdominal stoma is unnecessary because of the ileoanal anastomosis. Finally, if performed carefully, it preserves the anorectal sphincter and maintains continence.

During the past 20 years, clinical application of the ileal pouch–anal anastomosis procedure has increased (53). This interest developed in part because other alternatives, such as the Kock pouch, were not as successful as originally had been hoped. In addition, important technical advances had been made. By the mid-1980s, larger reports from various centers suggested that acceptable morbidity could be achieved (72). Although the functional result was encouraging, it was still variable and unpredictable. Attempts were made to identify factors associated with improved outcome and parameters that could be used in selecting patients for the pull-through procedure. It was found that patients had to have adequate anal sphincter

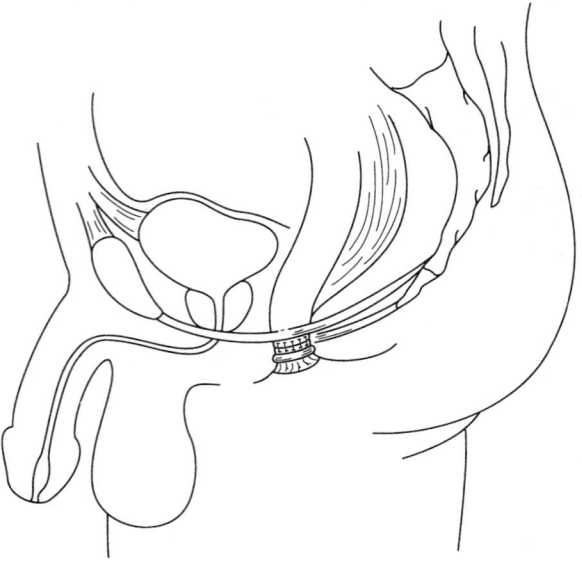

Figure 44.8. End-to-end ileoanal anastomosis after colectomy, mucosal proctectomy, and endorectal ileoanal pull-through.

function preoperatively to have acceptable continence postoperatively. Manometric techniques were developed to quantify anal sphincter function. In addition, an inverse correlation was found between ileal compliance and capacity and stool frequencies in patients after the end-to-end ileoanal anastomosis (73). This process of ileal adaptation and dilation could be hastened by the surgical construction of an ileal pouch or reservoir proximal to the ileoanal anastomosis. Several types of ileal reservoirs were proposed, including the J-pouch (74), S-pouch (75), W-pouch (76), and lateral side-to-side isoperistaltic pouch (77) (Fig. 44.9). Several studies comparing functional results after ileoanal anastomosis with and without an ileal reservoir demonstrated a reduction in stool frequency in adult patients in whom an ileal pouch was constructed, particularly in the early postoperative period (78). Another important technical addition to the operation was the temporary diverting loop ileostomy. This allows fecal diversion during the early weeks of ileal pouch and ileoanal anastomotic healing, thereby reducing the incidence of pelvic sepsis and ileal pouch and ileoanal anastomotic dehiscence. Some surgeons have eliminated the loop ileostomy in "good-risk" patients.

Although it was thought initially that only patients who were young and had relatively quiescent disease were candidates for ileoanal anastomosis, the indications have been considerably liberalized during the past 10 to 15 years. Patients are not candidates if other medical problems or the severity of the colitis precludes a 4- to 6-hour operation. Although some series reported better results in younger than in older patients, others have not found this to be the case. Many surgeons are comfortable in offering ileoanal anastomosis to patients in their sixth decade if they are in relatively good health and have adequate anal sphincter function. Obesity significantly increases the technical difficulty of ileoanal anastomosis but is only a relative contraindication to the operation. Severity of disease severity has not been found to correlate with operative morbidity or with subsequent functional results. Although Crohn's disease would appear to be an absolute contraindication to the operation, the procedure has been proposed for selected patients with no history of anal manifestations and no evidence of small-bowel involvement for whom rectal resection is mandatory, as an alternative to coloproctectomy with definitive end-ileostomy (79,80). The most important criterion for electing ileoanal anastomosis is that the patient fully understand the physiology and technique of the operation and have realistic expectations about the outcome. If possible, all potential candidates for ileoanal anastomosis should be seen several weeks before the proposed surgery. Flexible sigmoidoscopic examination is performed to confirm the diagnosis and assess the status of the inflammatory process in the rectal mucosa. Anorectal manometry is performed with either a pneumohydraulic perfused catheter system or solid-state transducers (81,82). In patients with active disease of the rectum, steroid or salicylate treatment is accelerated in the immediate preoperative period.

For most patients, the operation is performed in two stages. The first stage consists of abdominal colectomy, mucosal proctectomy, endorectal ileal pouch–anal anastomosis, and diverting loop ileostomy. During the second stage, performed at least 8 weeks after the initial operation, the loop ileostomy is closed. For patients who require an emergency colectomy, the operation is staged. The first stage consists of abdominal colectomy, ileostomy, and Hartmann closure of the rectum. During the second stage, the rectal mucosa is dissected free, and the ileal pouch–anal anastomosis is performed with loop ileostomy. Finally, the loop ileostomy is closed. A group of pa-

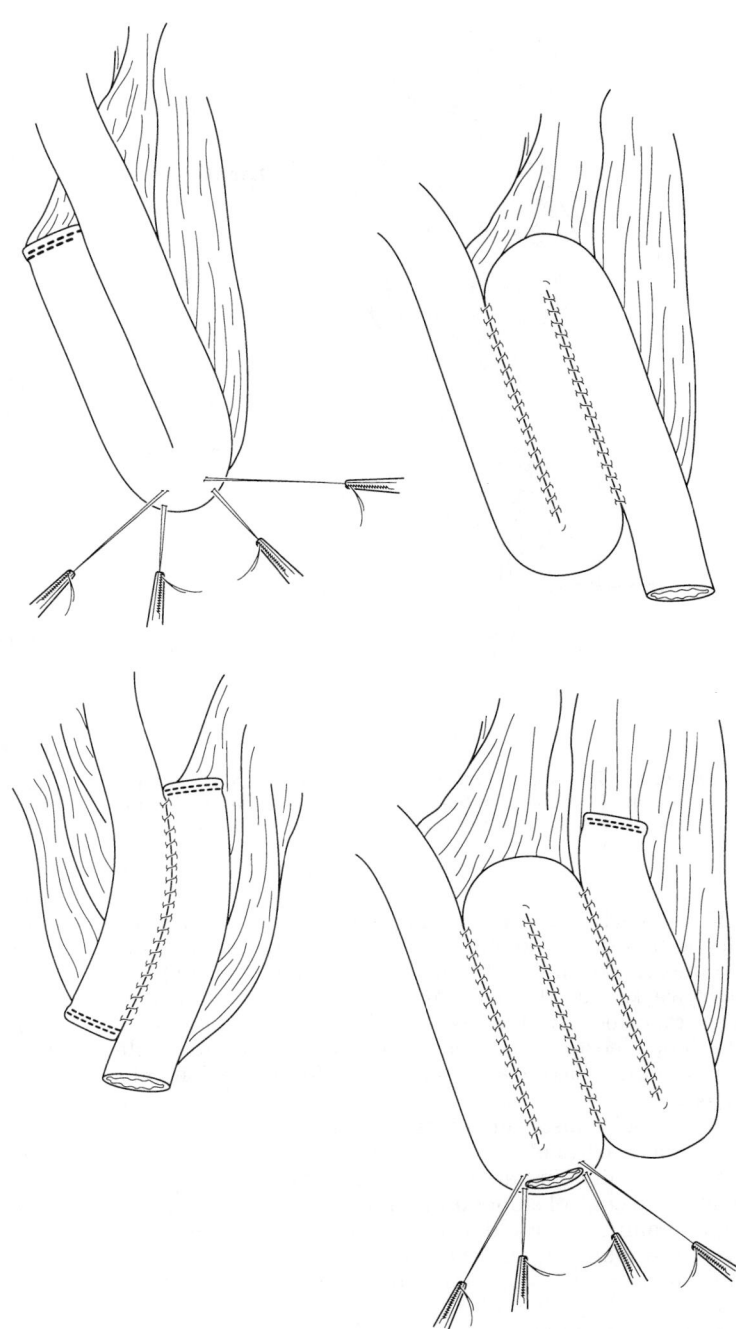

Figure 44.9. Ileal pouch configurations in patients undergoing ileal pouch–anal anastomosis.

tients who required prior abdominal colectomy followed by a staged mucosal proctectomy with ileal pouch–anal anastomosis were compared with matched patients who had undergone colectomy with ileoanal anastomosis at a single operative setting (83,84). Previous abdominal colectomy was associated with a higher cumulative operative morbidity rate, a prolonged hospital stay, increased costs, and a less optimal functional result. Aggressive and extended medical therapy, including cyclosporine, has been associated with an increased number of patients requiring staged subtotal colectomy with delayed ileoanal anastomosis. Therefore, patients with ulcerative colitis who have relative indications for urgent colectomy (bleeding, intractability, or toxic megacolon) should be given a full medical trial in an attempt to perform partially elective surgery in a single stage.

Colectomy with mucosal proctectomy and ileoanal anastomosis is performed with the patient in a modified lithotomy position (85,86). An abdominal colectomy is performed in a standard fashion through a midline incision. The entire rectal mucosal dissection is performed transanally. A circumferential incision is made at the dentate line, and the rectal mucosa is carefully dissected away from the anal sphincter and then the rectal muscularis (Fig. 44.10).

With the mucosal dissection completed, the ileal pouch is constructed with suturing techniques or mechanical staplers (Fig. 44.11). The ileal pouch is extended into the pelvis endorectally, and its apex is opened and sutured circumferentially to the dentate line (Fig. 44.12). A loop ileostomy is then constructed 40 cm proximal to the pouch (Fig. 44.13).

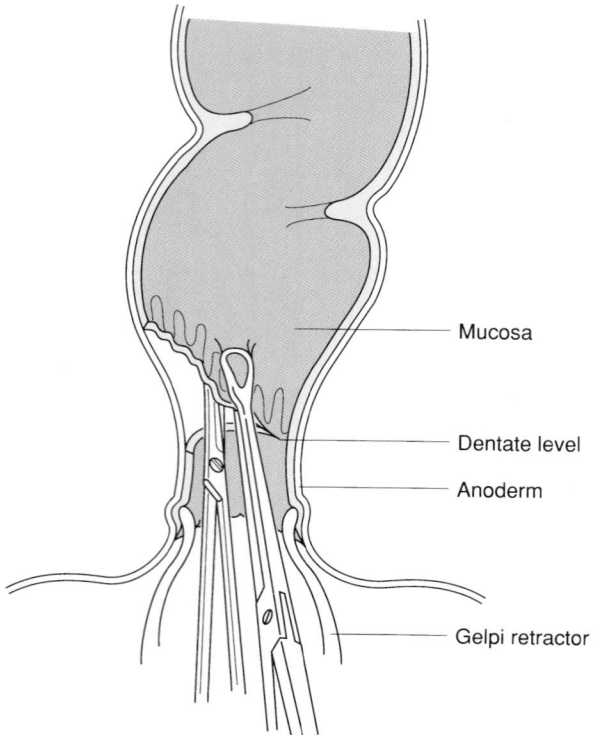

Mucosa

Dentate level

Anoderm

Gelpi retractor

Figure 44.10. Transanal mucosal proctectomy. A circumferential incision is made at the dentate line, and the rectal mucosa is carefully dissected away from the anal sphincter and the rectal muscularis.

Four weeks after the initial operation, standardized radiographic studies are performed to assess continence and the integrity of the ileal pouch and ileoanal anastomosis. Eight weeks after the ileoanal anastomosis, anal manometry is repeated, and the ileal pouch capacity is measured. The loop ileostomy is then closed with a stapling technique, which has greatly simplified this operation (Fig. 44.14).

Poor stool consistency, increased stool frequency, and nocturnal leakage of stool are the most common postoperative complaints in patients after ileoanal anastomosis. In an effort to control stool output, patients have been placed on loperamide hydrochloride, a synthetic opioid antidiarrheal agent, and supplementary fiber in the form of psyllium hydrophilic mucilloid. In addition, patients are placed on a high-fiber diet.

The postoperative morbidity and functional results in most large series after ileal pouch–anal anastomosis have been encouraging (72). In the author's experience with nearly 600 patients (J.M.B.), 86% of the patients underwent surgery for ulcerative colitis and 14% for familial polyposis coli. The mean age was 36 years, with a range of 11 to 76 years. Fifty-five percent of the patients were male. Experience with ileal pouch–anal anastomosis supports that this operation can be associated with a low rate of morbidity and no mortality provided that it is performed frequently, carefully, and with a standard operative technique. No operative deaths occurred in the series, and the overall operative morbidity after the ileal pouch–anal anastomosis portion of the operation was about 10%. The major operative morbidity was bowel obstruction, both after the initial operation and after loop ileostomy closure. The bowel obstruction rate requiring reoperation compares favorably with the 7% to 13% incidence of reoperation reported after proctocolectomy and ileostomy. An ob-

struction rate of 10% to 25% is reported in most series of patients undergoing ileal pouch–anal anastomosis (Fig. 44.15). Recent evidence suggests that the high incidence of postoperative adhesions associated with ileal pouch–anal anastomosis can be markedly reduced by the use of a sodium hyaluronate-based bioresorbable membrane (87). Pelvic and wound infections have been reported to occur in 10% to 20% of patients undergoing ileoanal anastomosis, although the overall infection rate was reduced to about 5% in several more recent large series. A 1% to 5% failure rate necessitating conversion to permanent ileostomy has been reported in several series. Similar satisfactory results have been reported in several large clinical series that showed a significant improvement in bowel function and quality of life following restorative proctocolectomy in patients with disabling chronic symptoms of distal ulcerative colitis (88). Other series stress that increased experience decreases the risk for postoperative and pouch-related complications and improves long-term outcome (64).

Although results with mucosal proctectomy and ileal pouch–anal anastomosis have been excellent, divergent points of view have arisen regarding the operative technique and its effect on anal physiology and functional result (89,90). A number of surgeons have advocated an alternative approach to conventional endoanal rectal mucosal resection that eliminates distal mucosal proctectomy (91–93). Instead, the distal rectum is divided near the pelvic floor, with the anal canal left largely intact. The ileal pouch is then stapled to the top of the anal canal. The rationale for this approach is that by preserving the mucosa of the anal transition zone, the anatomic integrity of the anal canal is preserved and the rate of fecal incontinence decreased. Although several studies have suggested that sensation and functional results are better when the anal transition zone is preserved, this has not been documented by prospective study. Several prospective, randomized clinical trials have compared ileal pouch–anal anastomosis with or without mucosectomy (94) and have demonstrated no functional or technical advantage of the stapled low rectal anastomosis over standard rectal mucosectomy with ileal anastomosis (95,96). The obvious concern is that when disease-bearing mucosa is left in the anal canal, the patient is exposed to a lifelong risk for persistent or recurrent inflammatory disease and the potential for malignant transformation.

Among 50 patients treated with proctocolectomy for ulcerative colitis at the Mayo Clinic, 90% had disease in the mucosa within 1 cm of the dentate line when the specimens were carefully examined histologically (97). This inflamed mucosa is left behind by ileal pouch–distal rectal anastomosis. In addition, dysplasia and adenocarcinoma have been described in the mucosa of the anal canal in patients with ulcerative colitis. Although these studies indicate that rectal mucosal resection is beneficial in patients undergoing colectomy with ileal pouch–anal anastomosis, care must be taken regarding the extent of anorectal smooth muscle resected at the time of mucosal proctectomy to preserve postoperative bowel and anal sphincter function. A recent series demonstrated that a loss of resting pressure of the internal anal sphincter could be correlated with the extent of smooth muscle resected during rectal mucosectomy, and that these factors in turn correlated with an increased stool frequency and a greater likelihood of nocturnal stool leakage. Consequently, an optimal functional result requires care in identifying and preserving as much anorectal smooth muscle as possible during mucosectomy (98). Until this technique is further evaluated, patients who have anorectal mucosa left behind will require careful lifetime surveillance. Mucosectomy

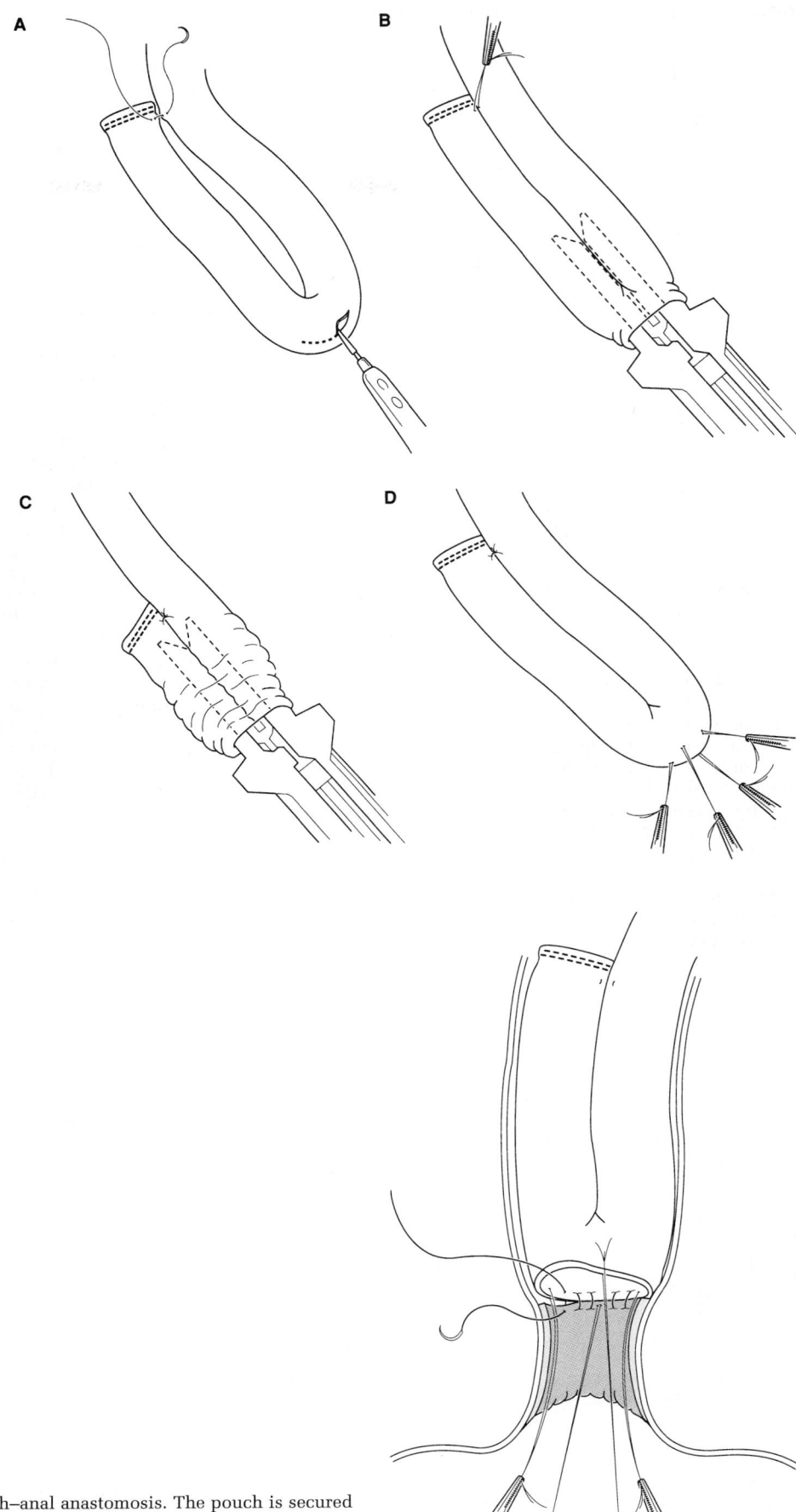

Figure 44.11. Ileal J-pouch construction. *(A)* An electrocautery is used to create an enterotomy at the apex of the 15-cm loop of terminal ileum. *(B)* The forks of an intestinal anastomosing stapler are pressed into the intestinal limbs, and the instrument is fired. *(C)* This is repeated once or twice while the limbs are telescoped onto the stapler, until a 15-cm side-to-side anastomosis is completed. *(D)* The apical enterotomy is closed with a simple purse string stitch.

Figure 44.12. Creating the ileal pouch–anal anastomosis. The pouch is secured to the sphincter in each quadrant with a suture. The purse string stitch closing the enterotomy is cut to allow the apex of the pouch to open. An anastomosis is then created between the apex of the pouch and the anoderm with interrupted absorbable sutures.

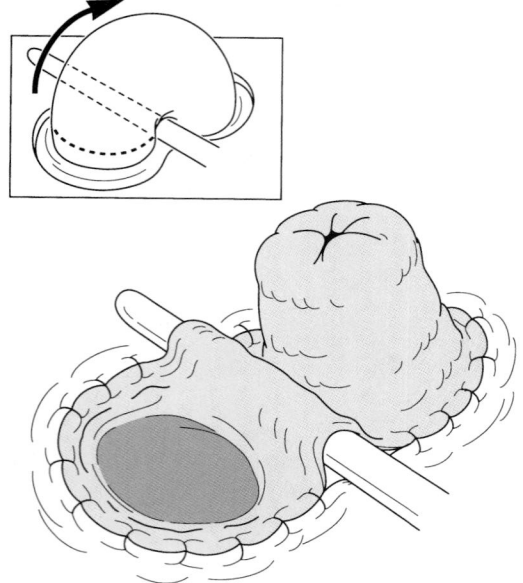

Figure 44.13. A loop ileostomy is constructed 40 cm proximal to the ileal pouch and matured over a rod.

must be recommended for patients with rectal dysplasia, proximal rectal cancer, diffuse colonic dysplasia, and familial polyposis (92).

Several reports have questioned the need for a diverting ileostomy at the time of ileal pouch–anal anastomosis for ulcerative colitis (74). The avoidance of a diverting loop ileostomy has several theoretic advantages: it eliminates the additional surgery needed to close the ileostomy, it eliminates the complications of ileostomy and ileostomy closure, and it may reduce diversion enteritis. A diverting ileostomy, however, reduces the risk for leakage from the ileal pouch or ileoanal anastomosis, a serious complication associated with significant morbidity and the poten-

tial for total loss of the ileal pouch. Only prospective, randomized, controlled trials will answer this question.

The pelvic pouch procedure remains an excellent option for most patients requiring surgery for ulcerative colitis (99), especially as larger series have shown that the overall morbidity and mortality rates are low (64,88,100). Despite significant surgical advances, nonspecific, idiopathic inflammation of the ileal pouch or pouchitis has become the most common late postoperative complication following restorative proctocolectomy for ulcerative colitis (101). A recent review of 23 clinical studies between 1984 and 1996 reported the incidence of acute and chronic pouchitis in patients following restorative proctocolectomy to be between 10% and 50% (102). Although pouchitis can occur at any time following ileal pouch construction, most patients experience the initial episode within the first 2 years. Pouchitis has been reported to occur primarily in patients undergoing the procedure for ulcerative colitis and rarely develops in patients undergoing the procedure for familial polyposis (103). Pouchitis can present with any number of symptoms, including increased stool frequency, watery diarrhea, fecal urgency, incontinence, rectal bleeding, abdominal cramping, fever, and malaise. The syndrome is similar to that found in patients with Kock continent ileostomy pouches. In some patients, pouchitis can be accompanied by extraintestinal manifestations, such as primary sclerosing cholangitis (104), arthritis, skin lesions, and eye problems (102). Patients with preoperative extraintestinal manifestations are likely to experience a higher incidence of pouchitis (105). The cause of this condition is unknown, but suggestions include early undetected Crohn's disease, bacterial overgrowth or bacterial dysbiosis, primary or secondary malabsorption, stasis, ischemia, and nutritional or immune deficiencies (106,107). Investigators have described axonal necrosis of enteric autonomic nerves in continent ileal pouches (108). Axonal necrosis, an ultrastructural diagnosis, was previously demonstrated in samples of small intestine obtained from patients with Crohn's disease. These same findings were demonstrated in patients with pouchitis associated with mucosally invasive bacteria,

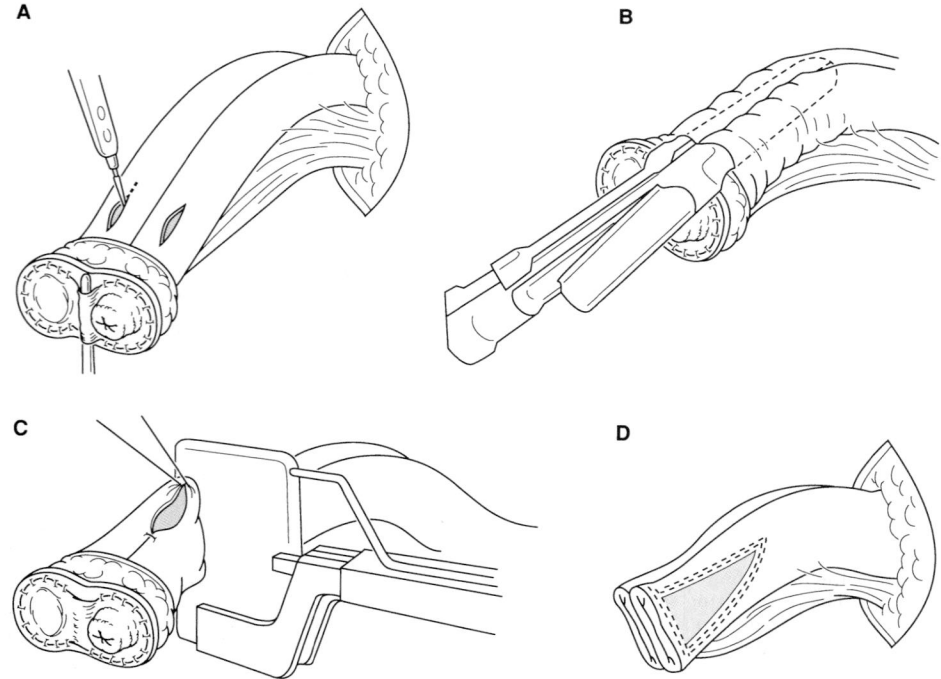

Figure 44.14. Closure of loop ileostomy. *(A)* A transverse elliptic incision is made around the stoma, and the limbs are dissected free. *(B)* The antimesenteric surfaces of the limb are tacked together, and the jaws of an anastomosing stapler are passed through enterotomies and down into the lumen of each of the intestinal limbs. The stapler is then fired to create a side-to-side anastomosis between the afferent and efferent ileal limbs. *(C)* A linear stapler is placed and fired below the former stoma and below the edges of the enterotomy. The stoma and distal limbs are amputated, and the stapler is released. *(D)* The anastomosis is dropped back into the peritoneal cavity, and the peritoneum, fascia, and skin are closed.

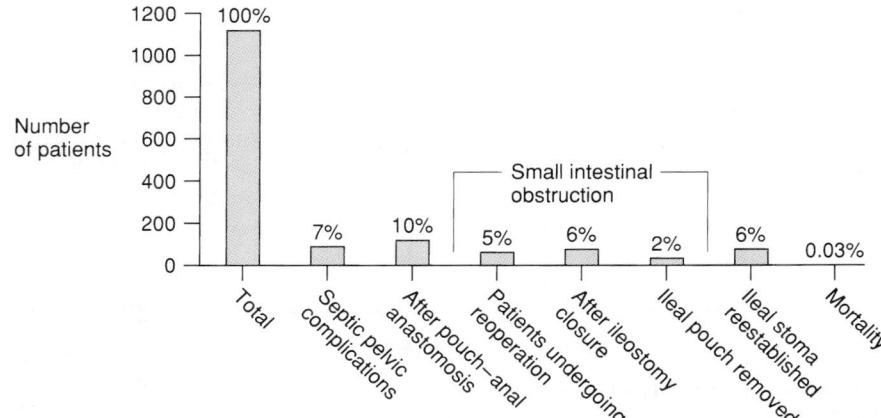

Figure 44.15. Operative morbidity after colectomy and ileoanal anastomosis in 12 clinical series.

which suggests mechanistic similarities for the pathogenesis of Crohn's disease and pouchitis.

The role of stasis in pouchitis is confused by the fact that it occurs to some degree in nearly all ileal pouches, and most authors fail to differentiate pouchitis from pouch dysfunction. Most available evidence suggests that stasis is not directly responsible for pouchitis; however, patients with poor pouch function must be identified accurately, and this can be accomplished with scintigraphic emptying studies (109). Perturbation of the bacterial flora, or bacterial dysbiosis, may be responsible for pouchitis, but no link has been found between a specific microbial pattern and pouchitis. Although a cause-and-effect relation is purely speculative, short-chain fatty acid concentrations are decreased in patients with pouchitis (110,111), and low concentrations of butyric acid correlate with severe villous atrophy. Another possible cause of pouchitis is a relative deficit of glutamine (112). Based on these preliminary observations, nutritional repletion with either butyrate or glutamine may be an option for the prevention or management of pouchitis. Ischemia may likewise cause pouchitis (113). Under conditions of hypoperfusion, xanthine oxidase activity may act as a potent source of oxygen free radicals that can damage tissue. The fact that oxidative stress has been demonstrated in human ileal pouch mucosal biopsy specimens suggests that oxygen free radicals may play a role in the pathogenesis of pouchitis (114).

As mentioned earlier, an important clinical clue to the etiology of pouchitis may be the observation that the incidence of pouchitis is significantly higher in patients with extraintestinal manifestations of inflammatory bowel disease before colectomy (105). In a recent series, the cumulative risk for pouchitis in 1,097 patients who had ulcerative colitis without preoperative primary sclerosing cholangitis after restorative proctocolectomy at the Mayo Clinic at 1, 2, 5, and 10 years postoperatively was 16%, 23%, 36%, and 45%, respectively. However, in patients with preoperative primary sclerosing cholangitis, the risk for pouchitis rose to 22%, 43%, 61%, and 79% at 1, 2, 5, and 10 years, respectively. More than 60% of the patients with primary sclerosing cholangitis experienced repeated episodes of pouchitis, in comparison with only 15% of the patients without associated primary sclerosing cholangitis (115). This leads to the speculation that pouchitis may be a further manifestation of inflammatory bowel disease. A striking clinical observation has been the difference in frequency of pouchitis between patients operated on for ulcerative colitis and those operated on for familial polyposis coli. In one series of more than 400 patients evaluated for a period of 10 years, no cases of pouchitis were ob-

served in those with familial polyposis, whereas a rate of 19% was noted in patients with chronic ulcerative colitis.

Pouchitis remains a clinically defined syndrome. Much of the controversy surrounding pouchitis revolves around the fact that no clear diagnostic criteria have been established. Clinical, endoscopic, and histologic criteria have all been applied without clear controls or norms; a pouchitis disease activity index encompassing these diagnostic parameters and providing a simple, objective, and quantitative criterion for pouch inflammation has been proposed recently (116). Endoscopically, inflamed ileal pouches appear edematous, hyperemic, and granular. The mucosa is typically friable and may exhibit contact bleeding, submucosal hemorrhage, and superficial ulceration (117). Even mild pouchitis can be characterized by swelling, friability, and erythema of the mucosa. Superficial ulcers occur in moderate pouchitis, whereas severe pouchitis is characterized by diffuse erythema, copious exudate, extensive superficial ulceration, and even necrosis. Endoscopic findings do not always correlate well with clinical symptoms; patients have been observed with inflammation who lacked clinical symptoms (118). Thus, the relationships among endoscopic appearances, clinical symptoms, and histologic changes are unclear. Although investigators have shown a significant relation between the endoscopic and histologic features of acute inflammation, specimens from 24 of 46 patients with endoscopic abnormalities appeared normal microscopically (119). Similarly, others have been unable to define morphologic abnormalities that distinguish patients with pouchitis from those without (85).

Histologic assessment alone is not adequate to diagnose pouchitis because even in the absence of pouchitis, villous atrophy, crypt and goblet cell hyperplasia, and chronic inflammatory cell infiltration may be present and represent nonspecific, metaplastic changes that commonly occur in the mature pouch (120). These chronic inflammatory changes observed in essentially all ileal pouches may be an unavoidable response to fecal stasis and are unrelated to clinical results in terms of stool frequency and incontinence. Moreover, some degree of acute inflammation is present in up to two thirds of pouches, although more severe and extensive infiltrates with acute inflammatory cells are seen in association with symptomatic pouchitis. Investigators have attempted to quantify inflammatory infiltrates in patients with pouchitis by means of a white cell-scanning technique (121). These studies confirmed that the inflammatory infiltrate in pouchitis, whether acute or chronic, is characterized by neutrophil accumulation and is usually localized to the pouch mucosa. When

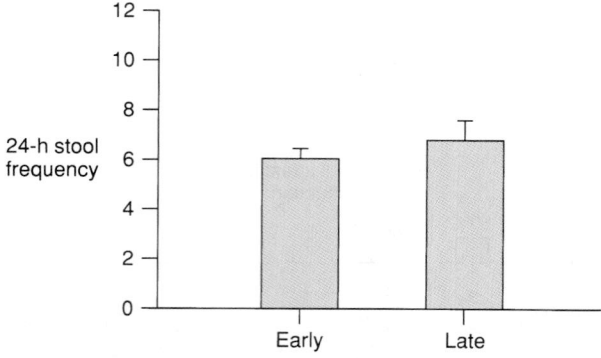

Figure 44.16. Early and late postoperative daily stool frequency in patients after colectomy and ileal pouch–anal anastomosis as reported in 12 clinical series.

a positive indium granulocyte scan result and an increased 4-day fecal indium granulocyte excretion rate were combined, all patients with severe pouchitis were identified and treated. A number of false-positive scans were observed. The role of such scanning techniques is unclear, although they may help distinguish nonspecific postoperative pouch dysfunction from acute mucosal inflammation and help quantify the response to therapy.

Fortunately, a short course of ciprofloxacin and metronidazole is successful in treating about two thirds of patients with pouchitis. The remaining patients have recurrent pouchitis, which responds to repeated therapy with ciprofloxacin and metronidazole, or a chronic, unresponsive form (122). It has been argued that with the high incidence of pouchitis observed in some patients after ileoanal anastomosis, one disease (ulcerative colitis) is simply being replaced by another (pouchitis). Pouch failure and excision for unremitting pouchitis are rare, and of those pouches that fail for any reason, up to 60% can be successfully salvaged, so that permanent ileostomy is avoided. These results suggest that a continued effort to salvage failed pouches, including the use of total reconstruction, is a viable alternative to permanent ileostomy (123).

The functional result after ileoanal anastomosis has been consistent in the larger series with adequate late follow-up data. These studies have demonstrated the number of bowel movements to be in the range of four to nine daily, with an average of six per day (Fig. 44.16). Nocturnal bowel movements occurred one to two times nightly, with a mean of slightly more than one. Nocturnal seepage of stool or staining was observed in 20% of patients in the early postoperative period, but was infrequently observed by 1 year. Overall, mean 24-hour and nocturnal stool fre-

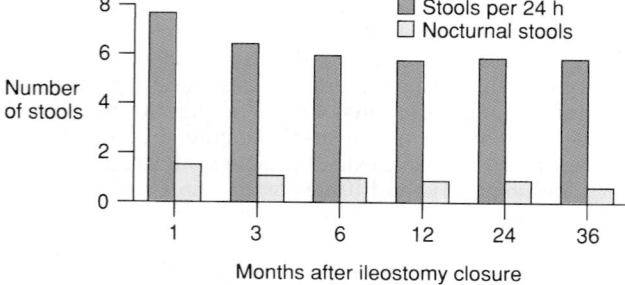

Figure 44.17. Twenty-four-hour and nocturnal stool frequencies after colectomy and ileoanal anastomosis in the author's (J.M.B.) series of patients.

quencies averaged five or six bowel movements per 24 hours and 0.5 bowel movements at night in the late follow-up period (Fig. 44.17). The most important determinants of outcome appear to be the diagnosis of ulcerative colitis rather than familial polyposis, the preoperative stool frequency and pattern of stools, and the capacity of the ileal pouch 1 year after surgery. Several studies have demonstrated that patients' level of satisfaction and performance after ileoanal anastomosis is extremely high, particularly when they are compared with those who have undergone conventional Brooke ileostomy.

CONCLUSION

Ulcerative colitis is a chronic inflammatory disease of the mucosa of the colon and rectum of uncertain etiology. It can be effectively controlled with diet, salicylates, and steroids. In the near future, more selective pharmacologic manipulation of the immune system can be anticipated. Eventually, a significant proportion of patients require operation, with the realization that colectomy does not reflect a therapeutic failure but rather a permanent cure. Colectomy with mucosal proctectomy and endorectal ileal pouch–anal anastomosis is the operation of choice for young patients and for most adults requiring elective proctocolectomy for chronic ulcerative colitis. Total proctocolectomy with Brooke ileostomy should be reserved for patients who are not candidates for ileoanal anastomosis or who, after careful counseling about all the surgical alternatives, elect that alternative. Subtotal colectomy with ileostomy and Hartmann closure of the rectum should be performed when emergency colectomy is indicated or if the diagnosis of ulcerative colitis, as opposed to Crohn's colitis, is uncertain. Because of the added morbidity associated with this staged approach and the possibility of a less-than-optimal functional result, attempts should be made to prepare the patient for a single-stage colectomy, mucosal proctectomy, and ileal pouch–anal anastomosis. The continent ileostomy should be considered in patients desirous of an attempt to restore continence who are not candidates for ileal pouch–anal anastomosis or in whom total proctocolectomy with ileostomy has already been performed.

REFERENCES

1. Andres PG, Friedman LS. Epidemiology and the natural course of inflammatory bowel disease. *Gastroenterol Clin North Am* 1999;28:225–281.
2. Langman MJS. Epidemiological overview of inflammatory bowel diseases. In: Allan RN, Rhodes JM, Hanauer SB, et al., eds. *Inflammatory bowel diseases*, 3rd ed. New York: Churchill Livingstone, 1997:35–39.
3. Hugot JP, Zouali H, Lesage S, et al. Etiology of the inflammatory bowel diseases. *Int J Colorectal Dis* 1999;14:2–9.
4. Binder V. Genetic epidemiology in inflammatory bowel disease. Dig Dis 1998;16:351–355.
5. Delco F, Sonnenberg A. Commonalities in the time trends of Crohn's disease and ulcerative colitis. *Am J Gastroenterol* 1999;94:2171–2176.
6. Papadakis KA, Targan SR. Current theories on the causes of inflammatory bowel disease. *Gastroenterol Clin North Am* 1999;28:283–296.
7. Stucchi AF, Becker JM. Pathogenesis of inflammatory bowel disease. In: Becker JM, ed. *Problems in general surgery*. Philadelphia: Lippincott Williams & Wilkins, 1999:1–11.
8. Fiocchi C. Inflammatory bowel disease: etiology and pathogenesis. *Gastroenterology* 1998;115:182–205.
9. Blaser MJ. Microbial causation of the chronic idiopathic inflammatory bowel diseases. *Inflamm Bowel Dis* 1997;3: 225–229.
10. Sartor RB. Enteric microflora in IBD: pathogens or commensals? *Inflamm Bowel Dis* 1997;3:230–235.

11. Yanai H, Shimizu N, Nagasaki S, et al. Epstein-Barr virus infection of the colon with inflammatory bowel disease. *Am J Gastroenterol* 1999;94:1582–1586.

12. Amati L, Caradonna L, Jirillo E, et al. Immunological disorders in inflammatory bowel disease and immunotherapeutic implications. *Ital J Gastroenterol Hepatol* 1999;31: 313–325.

13. Das KM, Dasgupta A, Mandal A, et al. Autoimmunity to cytoskeletal protein tropomyosin: a clue to the pathogenetic mechanism for ulcerative colitis. *J Immunol* 1993;150: 2487–2493.

14. Geng X, Biancone L, Dai HH, et al. Tropomyosin isoforms in intestinal mucosa: production of autoantibodies to tropomyosin isoforms in ulcerative colitis. *Gastroenterology* 1998;114:912–922.

15. Sandborn WJ, Landers CJ, Tremaine WJ, et al. Association of antineutrophil cytoplasmic antibodies with resistance to treatment of left-sided ulcerative colitis: results of a pilot study. *Mayo Clin Proc* 1996;7:431–436.

16. Targan SR. The utility of ANCA and ASCA in inflammatory bowel disease. *Inflamm Bowel Dis* 1999;5:61–63.

17. Podolsky DK. Innate mechanisms of mucosal defense and repair: the best offense is a good defense. *Am J Physiol* 1999; 277:G495–G499.

18. De Winter H, Cheroutre H, Kronenberg M. Mucosal immunity and inflammation. II. The yin and yang of T cells in intestinal inflammation: pathogenic and protective roles in a mouse colitis model. *Am J Physiol* 1999;276:G1317–G1321.

19. Hecht G. Innate mechanisms of epithelial host defense: spotlight on intestine. *Am J Physiol* 1999;277:C351–C358.

20. McClane SJ, Rombeau JL. Cytokines and inflammatory bowel disease: a review. *J Parenter Enter Nutr* 1999;23: S20–S24.

21. Rogler G, Andus T. Cytokines in inflammatory bowel disease. *World J Surg* 1998;22:382–389.

22. Nemetz A, Nosti-Escanilla MP, Molnar T, et al. IL1B gene polymorphisms influence the course and severity of inflammatory bowel disease. *Immunogenetics* 1999;49:527–531.

23. Inoue S, Matsumoto T, Iida M, et al. Characterization of cytokine expression in the rectal mucosa of ulcerative colitis: correlation with disease activity. *Am J Gastroenterol* 1999; 94:2441–2446.

24. Hanauer SB, Cohen RD, Becker RV, et al. Advances in the management of Crohn's disease: economic and clinical potential of infliximab. *Clin Ther* 1998;20:1009–1028.

25. Roediger WEW. The starved colon: diminished mucosal nutrition, diminished absorption, and colitis. *Dis Colon Rectum* 1990;33:858–862.

26. Harig JM, Soergel HH, Koworowski RA, et al. Treatment of diversion colitis with short chain fatty acid irrigation. *N Engl J Med* 1989;230:23–28.

27. DenHond E, Hiele M, Evenepoel P, et al. In vivo butyrate metabolism and colonic permeability in extensive ulcerative colitis. *Gastroenterology* 1998;115:584–590.

28. Kirsner JB. The historical basis of the idiopathic inflammatory bowel diseases. *Inflamm Bowel Dis* 1995;1:2–26.

29. Elson CO, Sartor RB, Tennyson GS, et al. Experimental models of inflammatory bowel disease. *Gastroenterology* 1995; 109:1344–1367.

30. Sartor RB. Review article: How relevant to human inflammatory bowel disease are current animal models of intestinal inflammation? *Aliment Pharmacol Ther* 1997;11:89–96.

31. Dieleman LA, Pena AS, Meuwissen SG, et al. Role of animal models for the pathogenesis and treatment of inflammatory bowel disease. *Scand J Gastroenterol Suppl* 1997;223: 99–104.

32. McCall RD, Haskill S, Zimmermann EM, et al. Tissue interleukin-1 and interleukin-1 receptor antagonist expression in enterocolitis in resistant and susceptible rats. *Gastroenterology* 1994;106:960–972.

33. Cominelli F, Nast CC, Clark BD, et al. Interleukin-1 (IL-1) gene expression, synthesis, and effect on specific IL-1 receptor blockade in rabbit immune complex colitis. *J Clin Invest* 1990;86:972–980.

34. Bertone ER, Giovannucci EL, King NWJ, et al. Family history as a risk factor for ulcerative colitis-associated colon cancer in cotton-top tamarin. *Gastroenterology* 1998;114:669–674.

35. Madara JL. Review article: Pathobiology of neutrophil interactions with intestinal epithelia. *Aliment Pharmacol Ther* 1997;11:57–62.

36. Welton ML. Human colonic microvascular endothelial cells is a model of inflammatory bowel disease. *Am J Surg* 1997; 174:247–250.

37. Irvine EJ, Hunt RH. Endoscopy—lower intestinal tract. In: Allan RN, Rhodes JM, Hanauer SB, et al., eds. *Inflammatory bowel diseases*, 3rd ed. New York: Churchill Livingstone, 1997:273–284.

38. Riddell RH. Histopathology of ulcerative colitis. In: Allan RN, Rhodes JM, Hanauer SB, et al., eds. *Inflammatory bowel diseases*, 3rd ed. New York: Churchill Livingstone, 1997: 291–309.

39. Spence DT, Mayberry JF. Clinical indices in inflammatory bowel disease. In: Allan RN, Rhodes JM, Hanauer SB, et al., eds. *Inflammatory bowel diseases*, 3rd ed. New York: Churchill Livingstone, 1997:335–341.

40. Capristo E, De Gaetano A, Mingrone G, et al. Multivariate identification of metabolic features in inflammatory bowel disease. *Metabolism* 1999;48:952–956.

41. Lichtenstein DR, Park PD, Lichtenstein GR. Extraintestinal manifestations of inflammatory bowel disease. In: Becker JM, ed. *Problems in general surgery*. Philadelphia: Lippincott Williams & Wilkins, 1999:23–39.

42. Raj V, Lichtenstein DR. Hepatobiliary manifestations of inflammatory bowel disease. *Gastroenterol Clin North Am* 1999;28:491–513.

43. van den Berg A, Jansen PL. Pathogenesis and medical therapy of primary sclerosing cholangitis: any news? *Eur J Gastroenterol Hepatol* 1999;11:121–124.

44. Scotiniotis I, Rubesin SE, Ginsberg GG. Imaging modalities in inflammatory bowel disease. *Gastroenterol Clin North Am* 1999;28:391–421.

45. Stein RB, Hanauer SB. Medical therapy for inflammatory bowel disease. *Gastroenterol Clin North Am* 1999;28: 297–321.

46. Lichtiger S. New trends in medical therapy for inflammatory bowel disease. In: Becker JM, ed. *Problems in general surgery*. Philadelphia: Lippincott Williams & Wilkins, 1999:12–22.

47. Sands BE. Novel therapies for inflammatory bowel disease. *Gastroenterol Clin North Am* 1999;28:323–351.

48. Han PD, Burke A, Baldassano RN, et al. Nutrition and inflammatory bowel disease. *Gastroenterol Clin North Am* 1999;28:423–443.

49. Seo M, Okada M, Yao T, et al. The role of total parenteral nutrition in the management of patients with acute attacks of inflammatory bowel disease. *J Clin Gastroenterol* 1999; 29:270–275.

50. Sandborn WJ. Azathioprine: state-of-the-art in inflammatory bowel disease. *Scand J Gastroenterol Suppl* 1998;225:92–99.

51. Lamers CB, Griffioen G, van Hogezand RA, et al. Azathioprine: an update on clinical efficacy and safety in inflammatory bowel disease. *Scand J Gastroenterol Suppl* 1999; 230:111–115.

52. Sandborn WJ. A critical review of cyclosporine therapy in inflammatory bowel disease. *Inflamm Bowel Dis* 1995;1: 48–63.

53. Becker JM. Surgical therapy for ulcerative colitis and Crohn's disease. *Gastroenterol Clin North Am* 1999;28: 371–390.

54. Sacher DB. Colectomy in ulcerative colitis: indications. In: Bayless TM, ed. *Current management of inflammatory bowel disease*. Philadelphia: BC Decker, 1989:100–103.

55. Sitzmann JV. Surgical alternatives for ulcerative colitis. In: Becker JM, ed. *Problems in general surgery*. Philadelphia: Lippincott Williams & Wilkins, 1999:115–123.

56. Bernstein CN. Ulcerative colitis and colon cancer: epidemiology, surveillance, diagnosis, and treatment. In: Becker JM, ed. *Problems in general surgery*. Philadelphia: Lippincott Williams & Wilkins, 1999:107–114.

57. Lewis JD, Deren JJ, Lichtenstein GR. Cancer risk in patients with inflammatory bowel disease. *Gastroenterol Clin North Am* 1999;28:459–477.

58. Becker JM. Consensus statement. Ulcerative colitis and colon carcinoma: epidemiology, surveillance, diagnosis, and treatment. The Society for Surgery of the Alimentary Tract,

American Gastroenterological Association, American Society for Liver Diseases, American Society for Gastrointestinal Endoscopy, American Hepato-Pancreato-Biliary Association. *J Gastrointest Surg* 1998;2:305–306.

59. Collins RH, Feldman M, Fordtran JS. Colon cancer, dysplasia, and surveillance in patients with ulcerative colitis: a critical review. *N Engl J Med* 1987;316:1654–1658.

60. Ekbom A, Helmick C, Zack M, et al. Ulcerative colitis and colorectal cancer: a population-based study. *N Engl J Med* 1990;323:1228–1233.

61. Ekbom A. Risk of cancer in ulcerative colitis. *J Gastrointest Surg* 1998;2:312–313.

62. Block GE, Moossa AR, Simonowitz D, et al. Emergency colectomy for inflammatory bowel disease. *Surgery* 1977;82:531–536.

63. Roy PH, Sauer WG, Beahrs OH, et al. Experience with ileostomies: evaluation of long-term rehabilitation in 497 patients. *Am J Surg* 1970;119:77–86.

64. Meagher AP, Farouk R, Dozois RR, et al. J ileal pouch–anal anastomosis for chronic ulcerative colitis: complications and long-term outcome in 1,310 patients. *Br J Surg* 1998;85:800–803.

65. Baker WN, Glass RE, Ritchie JK, et al. Cancer of the rectum following colectomy and ileorectal anastomosis for ulcerative colitis. *Br J Surg* 1978;65:862–868.

66. Hawley PR. Surgical treatment of ulcerative colitis—subtotal colectomy and ileorectal anastomosis. In: Allan RN, Rhodes JM, Hanauer SB, et al., eds. *Inflammatory bowel diseases,* 3rd ed. New York: Churchill Livingstone, 1997:741–745.

67. Kock NG. Continent ileostomy. *Prog Surg* 1973;12:180–201.

68. Peiser JG, Cohen Z, McLeod RS. Surgical treatment of ulcerative colitis—continent ileostomy. In: Allan RN, Rhodes JM, Hanauer SB, et al., eds. *Inflammatory bowel diseases*, 3rd ed. New York: Churchill Livingstone, 1997:753–760.

69. Dozois RR, Kelly KA, Beart RW, et al. Improved results with continent ileostomy. *Ann Surg* 1980;192:319–324.

70. Ravitch MM, Sabiston DLJ. Anal ileostomy with preservation of the sphincter: a proposed operation in patients requiring total colectomy for benign lesions. *Surg Gynecol Obstet* 1947;84:1095–1099.

71. Dean PA, Dozois RR. Surgical options—ileoanal pouch. In: Allan RN, Rhodes JM, Hanauer SB, et al., eds. *Inflammatory bowel diseases*, 3rd ed. New York: Churchill Livingstone, 1997:761–772.

72. Becker JM, Raymond JL. Ileal pouch–anal anastomosis: a single surgeon's experience with 100 consecutive cases. *Ann Surg* 1986;204:375–383.

73. Heppell J, Kelly KA, Phillips SF, et al. Physiologic aspects of continence after colectomy, mucosal proctectomy, and endorectal ileo-anal anastomosis. *Ann Surg* 1982;195:435–443.

74. Utsunomiya J, Iwama T, Imajo M, et al. Total colectomy, mucosal proctectomy, and ileoanal pull-through. *Dis Colon Rectum* 1980;23:459–466.

75. Parks AG, Nicholls RJ, Belliveau P. Proctocolectomy with ileal reservoir and anal anastomosis. *Br J Surg* 1980;67:533–538.

76. Nicholls RJ, Pezim ME. Restorative proctocolectomy with ileal reservoir for ulcerative colitis and familial adenomatous polyposis: a comparison of three reservoir designs. *Br J Surg* 1985;72:470–474.

77. Fonkalsrud EW. Endorectal ileoanal anastomosis with isoperistaltic ileal reservoir after colectomy and mucosal proctectomy. *Ann Surg* 1984;199:151–157.

78. Taylor BM, Beart RWJ, Dozois RR, et al. Straight ileoanal anastomosis vs. ileal pouch–anal anastomosis after colectomy and mucosal proctectomy. *Arch Surg* 1983;118:696–701.

79. Phillips RKS. Ileal pouch–anal anastomosis for Crohn's disease. *Gut* 1998;43:303–304.

80. Panis Y. Is there a place for ileal pouch–anal anastomosis in patients with Crohn's colitis? *Neth J Med* 1998;53:S47–S51.

81. Becker JM. Anal sphincter function after colectomy, mucosal proctectomy, and endorectal ileoanal pull-through. *Arch Surg* 1984;119:526–531.

82. Becker JM, Hillard AE, Mann FA, et al. Functional assessment after colectomy, mucosal proctectomy, and endorectal ileoanal pull-through. *World J Surg* 1985;9:589–605.

83. Zenilman ME, Soper NJ, Dunnegan D, et al. Previous abdominal colectomy affects functional results after ileal pouch–anal anastomosis. *World J Surg* 1990;14:594–599.

84. Ferzoco SJ, Becker JM. Does aggressive medical therapy for acute ulcerative colitis result in a higher incidence of staged colectomy? *Arch Surg* 1994;129:420–423.

85. Becker JM, Parodi JE. Total colectomy with preservation of the anal sphincter. *Surg Annu* 1989;21:263–302.

86. Becker JM, Soper NJ. Colectomy, mucosal proctectomy, endorectal ileal pouch–anal anastomosis. *Perspect Gen Surg* 1990;1:107–132.

87. Becker JM, Dayton MT, Fazio VW, et al. Prevention of postoperative abdominal adhesions by a sodium hyaluronate-based bioresorbable membrane: a prospective, randomized, double-blind multicenter study. *J Am Coll Surg* 1996;183:297–306.

88. Brunel M, Penna C, Tiret E, et al. Restorative proctocolectomy for distal ulcerative colitis. *Gut* 1999;45:542–545.

89. Becker JM. What is the better surgical technique in ileal pouch–anal anastomosis? Mucosectomy. *Inflamm Bowel Dis* 1996;2:151–154.

90. Fazio VW. What is the better surgical technique in ileal pouch–anal anastomosis? Stapled anastomosis. *Inflamm Bowel Dis* 1996;2:148–150.

91. Tuckson W, Tavery I, Fazio V, et al. Manometric and functional comparison of ileal pouch–anastomosis with and without anal manipulation. *Am J Surg* 1991;161:90–95.

92. Pemberton JH, Kelly KA, Beart RWJ, et al. Ileal pouch–anal anastomosis for chronic ulcerative colitis. *Ann Surg* 1987;206:504–513.

93. Sugerman HJ, Newsome HH, DeCosta G, et al. Stapled ileoanal anastomosis for ulcerative colitis and familial polyposis without a temporary diverting ileostomy. *Ann Surg* 1991;213:606–617.

94. Choen S, Tsunoda A, Nicholls RJ. Prospective randomized trial comparing anal function after hand-sewn ileoanal anastomosis with mucosectomy versus stapled ileoanal anastomosis without mucosectomy in restorative proctocolectomy. *Br J Surg* 1991;78:430–434.

95. Luukkonen P, Jarvinen H. Stapled vs. hand-sutured ileoanal anastomosis in restorative proctocolectomy. *Arch Surg* 1993;128:437–440.

96. Reilly WT, Pemberton JH, Wolff BG, et al. Randomized prospective trial comparing ileal pouch–anal anastomosis performed by excising the anal mucosa to ileal pouch–anal anastomosis performed by preserving the anal mucosa. *Ann Surg* 1997;225:666–676.

97. Ambroze WL, Pemberton JH, Dozois R, et al. The histological pattern and pathological involvement of the anal transition zone in patients with ulcerative colitis. *Gastroenterology* 1993;104:514–518.

98. Becker JM, LaMorte W, St Marie G, et al. Extent of smooth muscle resection during mucosectomy and ileal pouch–anal anastomosis affects anorectal physiology and functional outcome. *Dis Colon Rectum* 1997;40:653–660.

99. McLeod RS. The pelvic pouch procedure remains an excellent option for most patients with ulcerative colitis requiring surgery. *Inflamm Bowel Dis* 1997;3:236–238.

100. DeSilva HJ, Millard PR, Kettlewell M, et al. Mucosal characteristics of pelvic ileal pouches. *Gut* 1991;32:61–65.

101. Heppell J, Kelly K. Pouchitis. *Curr Opin Gastroenterol* 1998;14:322–326.

102. Schouten WR. Pouchitis. *Mediators Inflamm* 1998;7:175–181.

103. Madden MV, Farthing MJ, Nicholls RJ. Inflammation in ileal reservoirs: pouchitis. *Gut* 1990;31:247–249.

104. Aitola P, Matikainen M, Mattila J, et al. Chronic inflammatory changes in the pouch are associated with cholangitis found on peroperative liver biopsy specimens at restorative proctocolectomy for ulcerative colitis. *Scand J Gastroenterol* 1998;33:289–293.

105. Lohmuller JL, Pemberton JH, Dozois RR, et al. Pouchitis and extraintestinal manifestations of inflammatory bowel disease after ileal pouch–anal anastomosis. *Ann Surg* 1990;211:622–627.

106. Pemberton JH. The problem with pouchitis. *Gastroenterology* 1993;104:1209–1211.

107. Stucchi AF, Becker JM. Pathogenesis of pouchitis. In: Becker JM, ed. *Problems in general surgery*. Philadelphia: Lippincott Williams & Wilkins, 1999:139–150.
108. Dvorak AM, Onderdonk AB, McLeod RS, et al. Axonal necrosis of enteric autonomic nerves in continent ileal pouches. *Ann Surg* 1993;217:260–271.
109. O'Connell PR, Rankin DR, Weiland LH, et al. Enteric bacteriology, absorption, morphology, and emptying after ileal pouch–anal anastomosis. *Br J Surg* 1986;73:909–914.
110. Clausen MR, Tvede M, Mortensen PB. Short-chain fatty acids in pouch contents from patients with and without pouchitis after ileal pouch–anal anastomosis. *Gastroenterology* 1992;103:1144–1153.
111. Sagar PM, Taylor BA, Godwin P, et al. Acute pouchitis and deficiencies of fuel. *Dis Colon Rectum* 1995;38:488–493.
112. Wischmeyer P, Pemberton JH, Phillips SF. Chronic pouchitis after ileal pouch–anal anastomosis: responses to butyrate and glutamine suppositories in a pilot study. *Mayo Clin Proc* 1993;68:978–981.
113. Levin KE, Pemberton JH, Phillips SF, et al. Role of oxygen free radicals in the etiology of pouchitis. *Dis Colon Rectum* 1992;35:452–456.
114. Stucchi AF, Materne O, Beer E, et al. Evidence for oxidative stress in the etiology of pouchitis. *Gastroenterology* 1999;116:A1359(abst).
115. Penna C, Dozois R, Tremaine W, et al. Pouchitis after ileal pouch–anal anastomosis for ulcerative colitis occurs with increased frequency in patients with associated primary sclerosing cholangitis. *Gut* 1996;38:234–239.
116. Sandborn WJ, Tremaine WJ, Batts KP, et al. Pouchitis after ileal pouch–anal anastomosis: a pouchitis disease activity index. *Mayo Clin Proc* 1994;69:409–415.
117. DiFebo G, Miglioli M, Lauri A, et al. Endoscopic assessment of acute inflammation of the ileal reservoir after restorative ileo-anal anastomosis. *Gastrointest Endosc* 1990;36:6–9.
118. Rubenstein MC, Fisher RL. Pouchitis: pathogenesis, diagnosis, and management. *Gastroenterologist* 1996;4:129–133.
119. Moskowitz RL, Shepherd NA, Nicholls RJ. An assessment of inflammation in the reservoir after restorative proctocolectomy with ileoanal ileal reservoir. *Int J Colorectal Dis* 1986;1:167–174.
120. Garcia-Armengol J, Hinojosa J, Lledo S, et al. Prospective study of morphologic and functional changes with time in the mucosa of the ileoanal pouch: functional appraisal using transmucosal potential differences. *Dis Colon Rectum* 1998;41:846–853.
121. Kmiot WA, Hesslewood SR, Smith N, et al. Evaluation of the inflammatory infiltrate in pouchitis with ^{111}In-labeled granulocytes. *Gastroenterology* 1993;104:981–988.
122. Becker JM, Stucchi AF, Bryant DE. How do you treat refractory pouchitis and when do you decide to remove the pouch? *Inflamm Bowel Dis* 1998;4:167–169.
123. Saltzberg SS, DiEdwardo C, Scott TE, et al. Ileal pouch salvage following failed ileal pouch–anal anastomosis. *J Gastrointest Surg* 1999;3:633–641.

SURGERY: SCIENTIFIC PRINCIPLES AND PRACTICE, Third Edition, edited by Lazar J. Greenfield, Michael W. Mulholland, Keith T. Oldham, Gerald B. Zelenock, and Keith D. Lillemoe. Lippincott Williams & Wilkins Publishers, Philadelphia, © 2001.

CHAPTER 45

COLONIC POLYPS AND POLYPOSIS SYNDROMES

ROBERT S. BRESALIER AND C. RICHARD BOLAND

The gastrointestinal tract accounts for more neoplastic disease than any other organ system in the body. In North America, carcinomas of the colon and rectum have attracted the greatest interest because of their relatively high incidence and because appropriate intervention can dramatically modify the morbidity and mortality associated with them. The adenoma is the usual precursor of colorectal cancer, and early removal of adenomatous polyps can interrupt the natural history of the disease and prevent death. A variety of pathologic lesions can present as polyps within the colon, but the adenoma is the only lesion that is truly neoplastic and carries a risk for the development of cancer. During the past decade, understanding of the genetic events that lead to the development of colorectal polyps has advanced greatly, and progress in the clinical management of these lesions has been equally brisk. It is imperative that the biology, natural history, and clinical behavior of premalignant lesions in the colon, in addition to the genetic basis of the polyposis syndromes, be well understood because these have important impact on patient treatment.

CLASSIFICATION OF COLORECTAL POLYPS

The term *polyp* (from the Greek *polypous*, "morbid excrescence") refers to a macroscopic protrusion of the colonic mucosa into the bowel lumen. This can result from abnormal growth of the mucosa or from a submucosal process that causes the mucosa to protrude into the lumen. Mucosal polyps can be *sessile*, protruding directly from the colonic wall, or *pedunculated*, extending from the mucosa through a fibrovascular stalk.

Mucosal polyps in the colon can be categorized as *neoplastic*, with malignant potential, and *non-neoplastic*, with no malignant potential (Table 45.1). Neoplastic polyps include benign adenomatous polyps that may evolve to carcinoma, adenomatous polyps that contain foci of intramucosal carcinoma (carcinoma in situ), and adenomatous polyps in which carcinoma has penetrated the muscularis mucosae (invasive carcinoma). Sometimes a polyp is found in which carcinoma has completely obliterated the adenomatous tissue from which it arose (polypoid carcinoma). Non-neoplastic mucosal polyps include hyperplastic polyps, juvenile polyps, Peutz-Jeghers hamartomas, and a variety of inflammatory polyps, including those associated with idiopathic inflammatory bowel disease. Any submucosal lesion can expand to push the mucosa into the bowel lumen and thus appear as a polypoid lesion. Examples include lipomas, colitis cystica profunda, pneumatosis cystoides intestinalis, lymphoid aggregates, primary or secondary lymphomas, carcinoid tumors, and other metastatic neoplasms.

NEOPLASTIC MUCOSAL POLYPS

Most colorectal cancers arise in preexisting adenomatous polyps. These are macroscopic neoplastic lesions consisting of dysplastic epithelium that has the potential

Table 45.1. **CLASSIFICATION OF COLORECTAL POLYPS**

MUCOSAL POLYPS

Neoplastic

BENIGN

Adenomatous polyps (dysplastic mucosa)
Tubular
Tubulovillous
Villous

MALIGNANT

Carcinoma in situ
Invasive carcinoma
Polypoid carcinoma

Non-neoplastic

Hyperplastic polyps
Juvenile polyps
Peutz-Jeghers polyps
Inflammatory polyps
Normal epithelium

SUBMUCOSAL POLYPS

Lipomas
Leiomyomas
Colitis cystica profunda
Pneumatosis cystoides intestinalis
Lymphoid aggregates
Lymphoma (primary or secondary)
Carcinoids
Metastatic neoplasms

to evolve to malignancy. Carcinomas of the colon and rectum do not arise de novo. The mucosal epithelium progresses through a series of molecular and cellular events that lead to altered proliferation, cellular accumulation, and glandular disarray, processes that become macroscopically evident in the form of the adenomatous polyp. Further genetic alterations result in the evolution to higher degrees of cellular atypia and glandular disorganization (dysplasia), which may evolve to carcinoma. This is known as the *adenoma-to-carcinoma sequence*.

Several pieces of evidence support the assumption that colorectal adenocarcinomas arise from adenomatous polyps. The descriptive epidemiology of colonic adenomas parallels that of carcinomas. Adenomas are rare in geographic regions with a low prevalence of colon cancer, and the distribution of adenomas in the colon parallels that of carcinomas. Adenomas often occur in anatomic proximity to colon cancers, and cancer risk is proportional to the number of adenomas present synchronously or metachronously in a patient. Cancer is often present in polyps removed endoscopically or surgically, and the risk for cancer is proportional to the degree of dysplasia or atypia in the polyp. Conversely, histologically evident residual adenomatous tissue may be found within carcinomas. Most important, results from several studies indicate that removal of adenomatous polyps during surveillance proctosigmoidoscopy decreases the risk for subsequent death from colorectal cancer.

Pathogenesis

Molecular Biology

Genetic changes that lead to the development of adenomas (and carcinomas) can be loosely organized into three major classes: alterations in protooncogenes, loss of tumor-suppressor gene activity, and abnormalities of genes involved in DNA repair (Fig. 45.1). Much of what is known about the molecular genetic events that occur

during the adenoma-to-carcinoma sequence has come from the study of familial colon cancer syndromes. It is now clear, however, that the development of adenoma and carcinoma is always associated with the accumulation of genetic changes (1). In familial adenomatous polyposis (FAP), hereditary nonpolyposis colorectal cancer (HNPCC), and other familial syndromes, genetic alterations are inherited in the germline. Environmental factors may lead to additional genetic mutations that lead to malignant transformation. "Sporadic" polyps and cancers are associated with multiple somatic mutations caused by environmental insults. Adenomas and cancers that develop in both cases arise in the context of genomic instability, whereby epithelial cells acquire the number of mutations needed to attain a neoplastic state (2). Destabilization of the genome is a prerequisite to carcinogenesis. This may involve (most commonly) chromosomal instability with subsequent allelic losses, chromosomal amplifications and translocations, or increased rates of intragenic mutation in tandemly repeated DNA sequences known as *microsatellites* (microsatellite instability; see below) (3).

Cellular protooncogenes are a group of evolutionarily conserved genes that play a role in signal transduction and normal regulation of cell growth. Inappropriate activation of these genes leads to abnormal transmission of growth regulatory messages from the cell surface to the nucleus, resulting in altered cellular proliferation. Mutations of the K-*ras* oncogene, for example, can be found in about 65% of sporadic colorectal neoplasms and appear to play a role in the transition from the early adenoma to more advanced stages of adenomatous change. Only 9% of small adenomas have *ras* gene mutations, whereas 58% of adenomas larger than 1 cm have altered K-*ras* genes. Although activation of *ras* alone is not sufficient for progression to carcinoma, understanding its role in stimulating proliferation may lead to the development of antitumor therapies aimed at interrupting signals that induce tumor cell growth.

Allelic losses of chromosome 5q occur early during carcinogenesis in the colon. Originally described in association with familial adenomatous polyposis coli (APC), mutations of the *APC* gene on chromosome 5 are found in more than 60% of sporadic adenomas (4). *APC* acts as the "gatekeeper" of colonic epithelial proliferation, and inactivation of this gene is required for net cellular proliferation and initiation of neoplasia in the colon. *APC* functions to modulate extracellular signals that are transmitted to the nucleus through the cytoskeletal protein β-catenin. One such pathway, the Wnt-1 signaling pathway, activates a protein (Tcf-4) in the nucleus, which in turn activates various target genes (5). *APC* is a tumor-suppressor gene that binds to β-catenin and causes its degradation. Loss of *APC* function therefore leads to unopposed stimulation through the Wnt/Tcf signaling pathway. Abnormalities in *APC* may also lead to disruption of normal cell–cell adhesion through interactions with the cellular adhesion molecule E-cadherin.

Other genetic changes occur later in the adenoma-to-carcinoma sequence. Stepwise tumor progression is associated in more than 75% of cases with loss of the tumor-suppressor gene activity located on chromosome 18q. Several candidate genes are present on this chromosome, and loss of chromosome 18 is associated with a poor prognosis (6). One gene, designated *DCC* (deleted in colorectal cancer), was originally thought to be important because its loss from a stage II (Dukes B) cancer is associated in some studies with a significantly worse prognosis. Recent studies, however, have questioned its role as an important tumor-suppressor gene. Deletions of chromosome 17p involve the *p53* tumor-suppressor gene, whose product normally

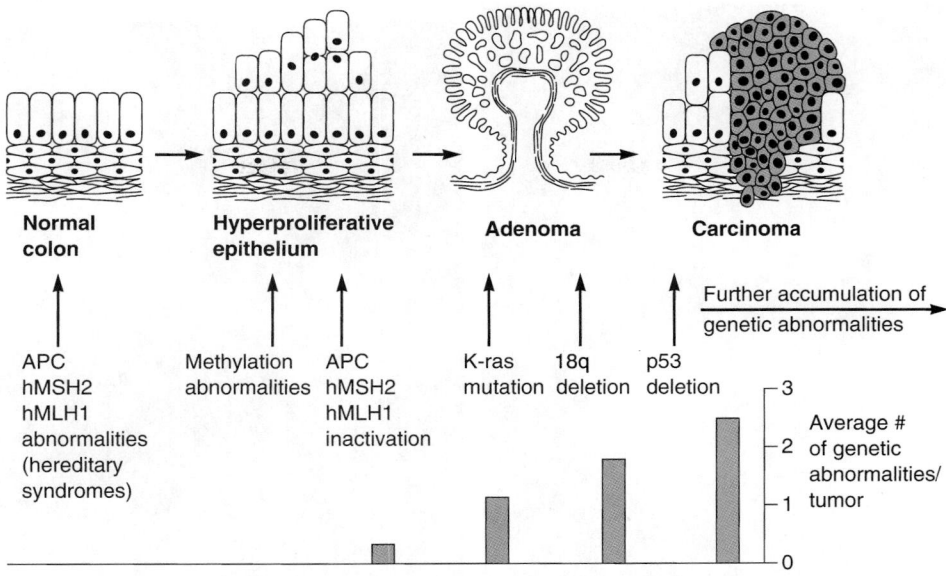

Figure 45.1. Molecular genetic events during the adenoma-to-carcinoma sequence. The progression to adenoma and carcinoma is associated with an accumulation of alterations in oncogenes (K-*ras*), tumor-suppressor genes *(APC,* genes on chromosome 18q, *p53),* and genes involved in maintaining the fidelity of DNA synthesis (DNA repair genes *hMSH2, hMLH1*). Alterations in *APC,* K-*ras,* and the DNA repair genes occur as early events in the development of adenomas, whereas deletions of genes on 18q and *p53* occur during the evolution from adenoma to carcinoma. The exact sequence of events is approximate. (Modified from Bresalier RS, Toribara NW. Familial colon cancer. In: Eastwood GL, ed. *Premalignant conditions of the gastrointestinal tract.* New York: Elsevier Science, 1991:227–244, with permission.)

prevents cells with damaged DNA from progressing from the G_1 to the S phase in the cell cycle. Loss of *p53* may also be associated with abnormal apoptosis (programmed cell death) of damaged cells. Inactivation of the *p53* gene mediates the conversion from adenoma to carcinoma.

Alterations in genes that help maintain DNA fidelity during replication are characteristic of patients with HNPCC (7). Alterations in mismatch repair genes designated *hMLH1, hPMS1* and *hPMS2,* and *hMSH2, hMSH3,* and *hMSH6* may lead to the inability to repair base pair mismatches and result in DNA replication errors or microsatellite instability. Microsatellite instability involves mutations or instability in short tandemly repeated DNA sequences such as $(A)^n$, $(CA)^n$, and $(GATA)^n$. Such DNA sequences are found in several key genes that are important for maintaining normal cellular function. The receptor for transforming growth factor-β (TGF-βRII), for example, is often mutated as the result of microsatellite instability. Multiple lines of evidence suggest that the TGF-β pathway is an important tumor-suppressing pathway in the colon, and that alterations in this pathway lead to tumor development (8). Although this high frequency of microsatellite instability (instability at 40% or more of microsatellite loci) is characteristic of HNPCC, similar alterations can be found in about 15% of sporadic colorectal cancers and also in premalignant lesions. Patients whose tumors demonstrate microsatellite instability may have a better prognosis than those whose tumors are characterized by chromosomal instability.

Abnormal Proliferation

The development of adenomatous polyps is associated with abnormal cellular proliferation, a hallmark of neoplasia. In the normal colon, DNA synthesis and cellular proliferation occur only in the lower and middle regions of the crypt. Cells that have migrated to the upper crypt become terminally differentiated and can no longer divide. Disordered proliferation and aberrant crypt development are characteristic of adenomas. Abnormal proliferation can be detected throughout the crypt even in the grossly normal-appearing mucosa of some patients at especially high risk for adenoma development, such as those with FAP or HNPCC. This increased proliferative rate may be associated with alterations in biochemical markers of cellular proliferation, such as ornithine decarboxylase and protein kinase C. The initiating event in the development of an adenoma, however, is thought to be inactivation of the *APC* tumor-suppressor gene, which has led to its designation as the "gatekeeper" for colorectal neoplasia.

Histopathology and Malignant Potential

Adenomatous polyps are characterized according to their physical features, size, glandular structure, and degree of dysplasia, which all have important implications for clinical management. Polyps may be sessile, with a broad-based attachment to the colonic wall, or pedunculated, attached to the colonic wall by way of a fibrovascular stalk (Fig. 45.2). Whether a polyp is sessile or pedunculated typically determines whether the endoscopist can remove the polyp completely by snare polypectomy. Diminutive polyps that measure 5 mm or less in diameter are not likely to contain high-grade dysplasia or invasive carcinoma. Malignant potential increases with polyp size in all histologic groups of adenoma.

Adenomas are classified histologically according to their glandular structure. Aberrant (dysplastic) crypts and microadenomas may be the earliest lesions detected in the

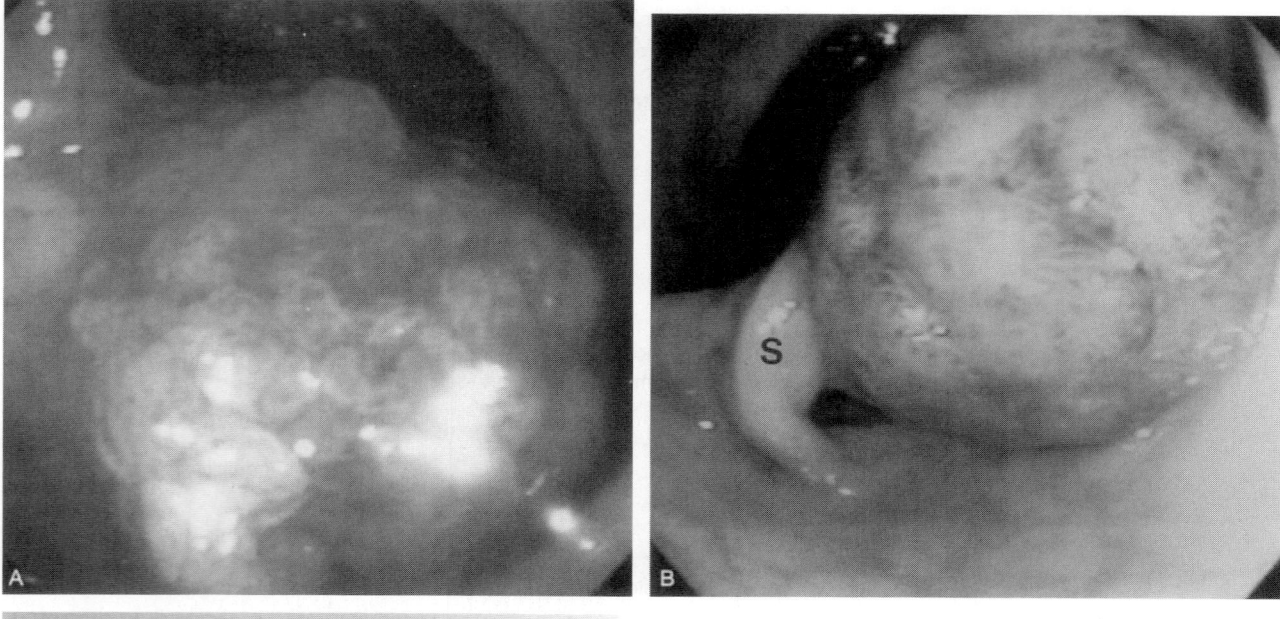

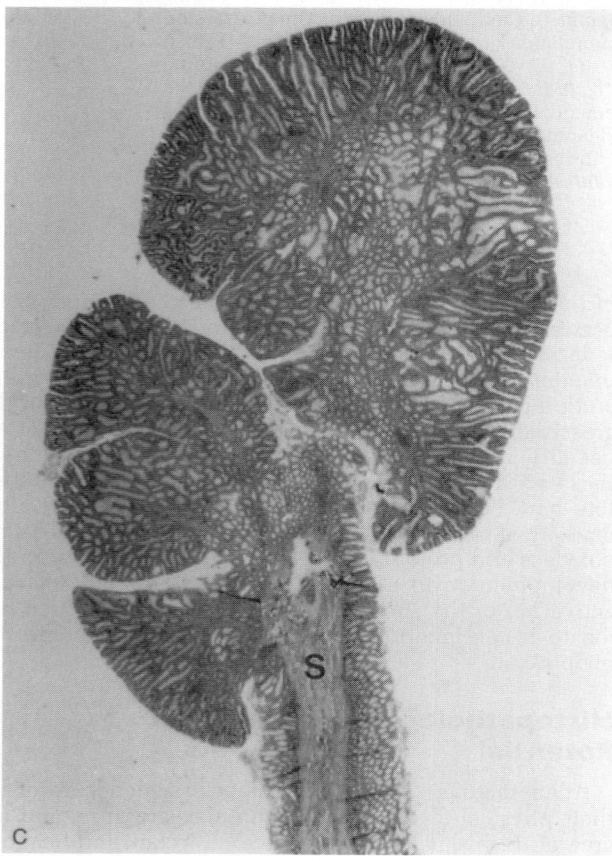

Figure 45.2. Mucosal polyps of the colon may be sessile, protruding directly from the colonic wall, or pedunculated, extending from the mucosa through a fibrovascular stalk. *(A)* Large sessile polyp seen at colonoscopy. The polyp has a broad-based attachment to the mucosa. *(B)* Large pedunculated polyp seen at colonoscopy. The polyp is attached to the mucosa through a distinct stalk *(S)*. *(C)* Low-power photomicrograph of a pedunculated polyp (a tubular adenoma) cut in cross section to demonstrate its fibrovascular stalk *(S)*.

flat mucosa of patients at risk. These enlarge and progress to macroscopic adenomatous polyps. Tubular adenomas are characterized by a complex network of branching adenomatous glands, whereas villous adenomas contain glands that extend straight down from the surface to the base of the polyp (Fig. 45.3). Often, both histologic types coexist in a mixed tubulovillous adenoma. The malignant potential of an adenomatous polyp correlates with its degree of villous architecture.

All adenomas by definition consist of dysplastic mucosa. The term *dysplasia* refers to abnormalities in crypt architecture (such as irregular branching or crowded "back-to-back" glands) and cytologic detail (enlarged pleomorphic and hyperchromatic nuclei with multiple mitoses and pseudostratification; Fig. 45.4). Dysplasia may be mild, moderate, or severe, depending on the degree to which these characteristics are present. Severe, or high-grade, dysplasia represents carcinoma in situ when the basement membrane is intact. Extension into the lamina propria denotes intramucosal carcinoma. Invasion into the muscularis mucosae defines invasive carcinoma and the malignant polyp. The degree of dysplasia often

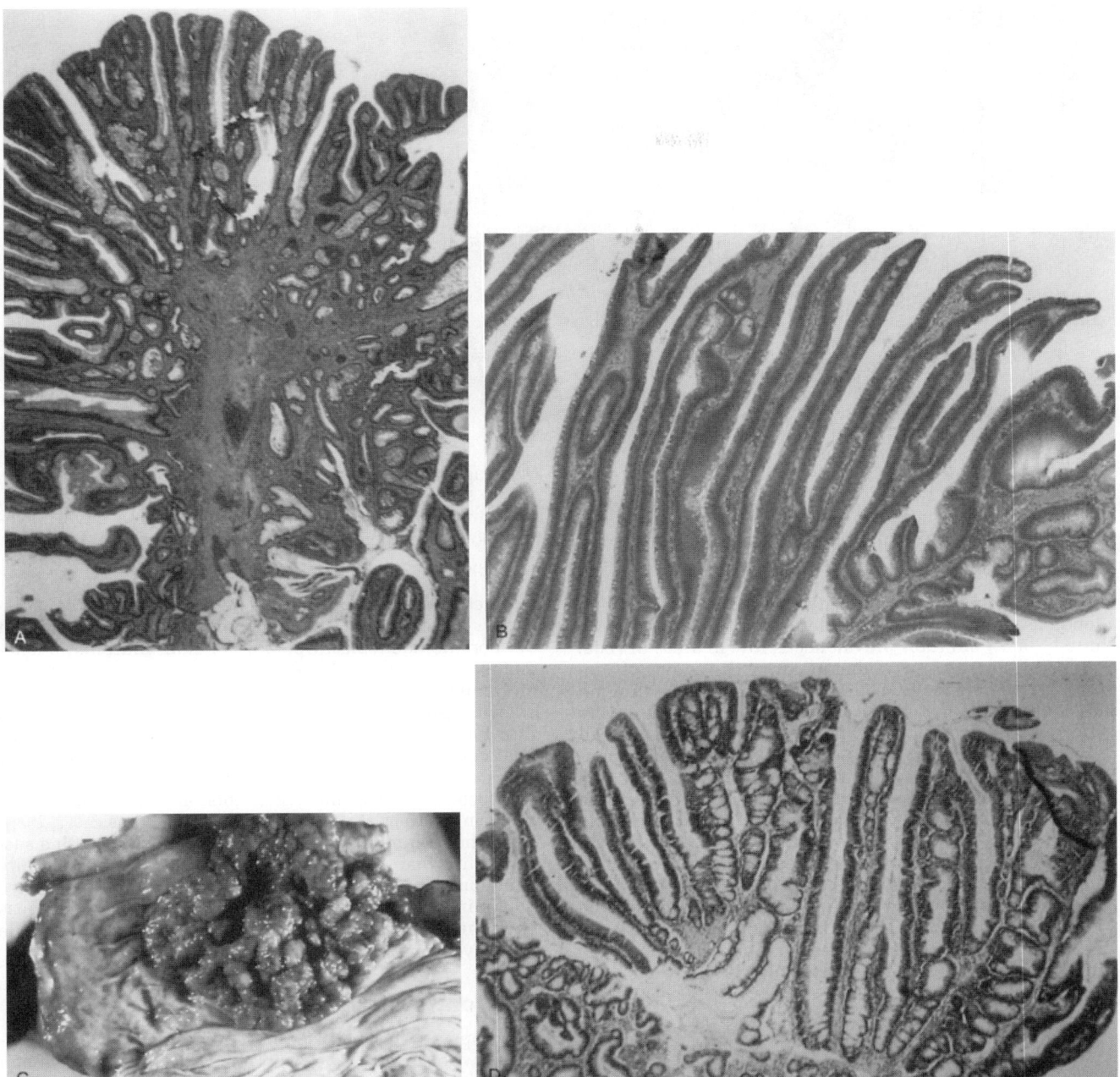

Figure 45.3. Histology of adenomatous polyps. *(A)* Tubular adenomas are characterized by a complex network of branching adenomatous glands *(see also D).* (B) Villous adenomas consist of glands that extend straight down from the surface to the base as fingerlike projections; this pattern may be suggested by the gross appearance of these polyps. *(C)* Surgical specimen demonstrating a large sessile polyp with fingerlike fronds, typical of a villous adenoma. *(D)* Tubulovillous adenoma. Many polyps contain both tubular and villous components on histologic examination.

correlates with polyp size and extent of villous architecture.

Even though all adenocarcinomas of the colon and rectum arise in adenomatous polyps, not all polyps evolve into carcinoma. The malignant potential of adenomatous polyps is related to polyp size and histologic characteristics (9). Large polyps and those with predominantly villous architecture are more likely to contain coincident carcinoma (Fig. 45.5). These features are interdependent, however, because large polyps are more likely

to be villous and dysplastic. Adenomas that measure 0.5 cm or less are most often tubular adenomas and rarely contain severe dysplasia or carcinoma (<0.5% in autopsy series). Likewise, only 1% to 2% of adenomatous polyps smaller than 1 cm contain carcinoma, but autopsy studies suggest that 40% of adenomas larger than 2 cm contain cancer. Data derived from the examination of colonoscopic polypectomy specimens indicate similar trends but suggest a lower incidence of cancer-containing polyps.

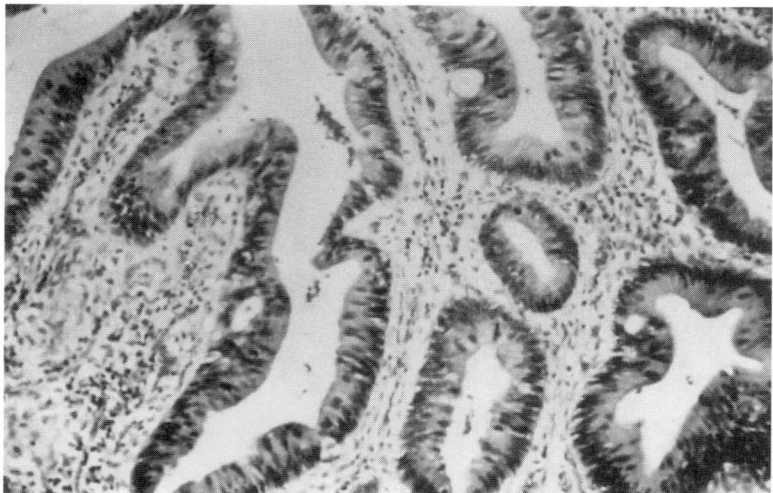

Figure 45.4. Moderate dysplasia. Dysplastic mucosa is characterized by crowded, irregular glands and cells with enlarged, hyperchromatic nuclei of varied size and shape that do not line up uniformly on the basement membrane (pseudopalisading). Adenomas are composed of dysplastic mucosa in which the degree of atypia may vary. These changes precede the development of invasive carcinoma.

Epidemiology

Prevalence

The descriptive epidemiology of adenomatous polyps of the colon and rectum parallels that of colorectal carcinoma with relation to geographic distribution, age prevalence, and genetic susceptibility. Like colorectal cancer, adenomas are common in Western countries such as the United States, but their prevalence is low in areas of Asia, South America, and sub-Saharan Africa. Estimates of adenoma prevalence in the United States vary depending on the mode of data collection. Data from older studies were collected from autopsies and sometimes grouped all polyps together, whereas more recent studies have examined adenoma prevalence in the context of endoscopic screening. Studies using colonoscopy suggest an adenoma prevalence in patients without symptoms who are older than 50 years that ranges between 20% and 40%. Prevalence rates from autopsy studies are 50% higher. Based on autopsy studies, one half to two thirds of people older than 65 years may have colonic adenomas. Adenoma prevalence increases with age in all populations. Age-associated prevalence rates suggest that adenomas precede carcinomas in a given population by 5 to 10 years. Ad-

vancing age also correlates with multiplicity of polyps, polyp size, and higher degrees of dysplasia. In addition, 30% to 50% of patients with one adenoma have a synchronous adenoma elsewhere in the colon (10).

Heredity

Heredity plays a role not only in the gastrointestinal polyposis syndromes and HNPCC but also in the development of sporadic adenomas. Sporadic or nonsyndromic adenomatous polyps and colon cancers represent more than 90% of colorectal neoplasms. Clinical studies, including case-control and prospective analyses, indicate a twofold to threefold increased risk for colon cancer among first-degree relatives of patients with a history of colonic adenoma or carcinoma (11). The relative risk increases with the number of affected relatives and when adenomas and carcinomas occur in relatives at a younger age (12). In some cases, it appears that common adenomas may be inherited with a susceptibility that is autosomal dominant but only partially penetrant. Therefore, it has been suggested that inheritance determines individual susceptibility to neoplasia, whereas environmental factors determine which susceptible people will have adenomas and carcinomas of the colon.

Anatomic Distribution

Autopsy series and colonoscopic examination of patients who do not have symptoms suggest that although adenomas are uniformly distributed throughout the colon, the distribution of clinically important larger adenomas is more similar to that of carcinomas, with a left-sided predominance.

Natural History

Although adenomas are common in people older than 50 years, and although most carcinomas arise in adenomatous polyps, relatively few adenomas progress to carcinoma. Few precise data are available on what percentage of adenomas evolve to carcinomas. In Norway, an example of a high-risk Western population, it has been estimated that colorectal adenomas are present in 29% of the population older than 35 years. The annual conversion rate from adenoma to carcinoma in this group (based on cancer incidence from multiple tumor registries) has been calculated to be 0.25%. In other words, the risk that a colorectal cancer will develop in a polyp-bearing person within 10 years is 2.5%. The annual conversion rates to invasive cancer for people with adenomas larger than 1 cm, villous compo-

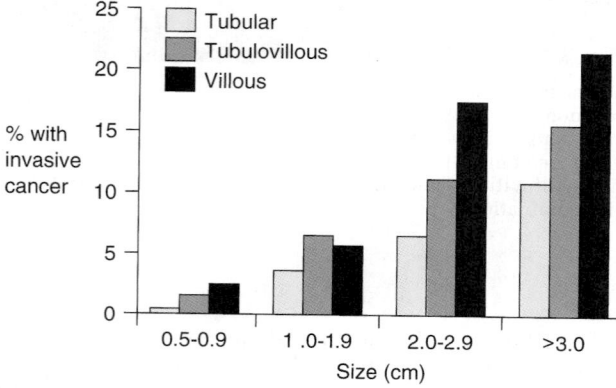

Figure 45.5. The relation of adenoma size and histology to malignant potential based on an analysis of 7,000 endoscopically removed polyps. The incidence of polyp-associated carcinoma determined from examination of polypectomy specimens is lower than that derived from early autopsy studies. (Data derived from Shinya H, Wolff WI. Morphology, anatomic distribution, and cancer potential of colonic polyps. *Ann Surg* 1979;1990:675, with permission.)

nents, and severe dysplasia have been estimated to be 3%, 17%, and 37%, respectively, based on these inferences.

Both longitudinal follow-up of a small number of people with unresected adenomas and studies of age distribution provide indirect evidence that the evolution from adenoma to carcinoma takes at least 5 to 10 years. Age prevalence data from the National Polyp Study, for example, suggest that it may take as long as 5 to 10 years for normal-appearing mucosa to develop into a macroscopically visible adenomatous polyp, and an additional 3 to 5 years for invasive carcinoma to develop. Case-control studies also support that the development of adenomas in the colon and the evolution to carcinoma occur slowly. Several studies have estimated that the protective effect of screening sigmoidoscopy may last at least 10 years.

Associated Disease States

A number of clinical situations have been associated with a greater than average risk for adenoma development, but the evidence in most cases is tenuous. Although adenomas and carcinomas develop frequently in patients who have undergone urinary diversion by way of ureterosigmoidoscopy, this is largely of historical interest. Nonetheless, patients who have undergone this procedure require periodic colonoscopic surveillance for adenoma and carcinoma development. An increased prevalence of colonic adenomas and carcinomas has been reported in patients with acromegaly, and patients with elevated gastrin levels have been reported to be at risk for neoplasia. Alleged associations between colorectal adenomas and a history of prior cholecystectomy, atherosclerosis, acrochordons (skin tags), and hyperplastic polyps remain unproven.

Clinical Features

Adenomatous polyps of the colon and rectum are highly prevalent in Western societies, but most patients with colonic adenomas do not have symptoms directly referable to these lesions. Overt bleeding manifesting as hematochezia may occur with larger polyps, which may be evident when the polyps are located distally in the rectum. More commonly, blood loss from adenomas is minimal and clinically occult. Although colorectal polyps are the most common lesions detected in patients without symptoms undergoing colonoscopy because of the presence of fecal occult blood, it is unclear whether the presence of occult blood results from polyp bleeding or is coincidental because of the high prevalence of polyps in the population at large. Blood loss from adenomas and a positive fecal occult blood test result are related to polyp size. Very large colonic polyps may be associated with obstructive symptoms, such as lower abdominal cramping or alterations in bowel habits, but this is unusual. Secretory diarrhea with accompanying hypokalemia and hypochlorhydria has been associated with very large villous adenomas of the distal colon and rectum. This is a rare syndrome, and the search for secretagogues such as vasoactive intestinal polypeptide or prostaglandins in patients with polyps and diarrhea is infrequently productive.

Adenomas Associated with Hereditary Nonpolyposis Colorectal Cancer and Its Variants

Hereditary nonpolyposis colorectal cancer (Lynch's syndrome) is a disease of autosomal dominant inheritance in which cancers arise in discrete adenomas but polyposis (i.e., hundreds of polyps) does not occur. This entity is most narrowly defined by the Amsterdam criteria: Families must have at least three relatives with colorectal cancer, one of whom is a first-degree relative of the other two. Colorectal cancer must involve at least two generations, and at least one cancer case must occur before 50 years of age. Broader definitions of HNPCC take into account the occurrence of extracolonic tumors and smaller kindreds (13). Adenomas and carcinomas in HNPCC arise at an early age (adenomas may occur in patients in their 20s and 30s, with a mean age for carcinoma development of 40 to 45 years) and are often proximal in location and multiple. Some families with HNPCC (Lynch's syndrome II, cancer family syndrome) are prone to cancers of the female genital tract (endometrium and ovary) and other sites in addition to colorectal neoplasms.

The frequency of HNPCC in the general population is yet to be determined, but HNPCC may account for as many as 4% to 6% of colorectal cancer cases. Germline mutations in genes that play a role in DNA mismatch repair occur in patients with HNPCC and lead to microsatellite instability in a variety of genes important in maintaining normal cell function (14) (see above).

Turcot's syndrome is characterized clinically by the concurrence of primary brain tumors and multiple colorectal adenomas. Evidence suggests that this can result from two distinct types of germline defects: mutation of the *APC* gene (i.e., a variant of FAP) or mutation of a mismatch repair gene (i.e., a variant of HNPCC).

Diagnosis

Most colorectal adenomas are asymptomatic and are often detected in the setting of an evaluation for unrelated colonic symptoms or occult blood in the stool. Similarly, adenomatous polyps are frequently detected when patients without symptoms are screened for colorectal neoplasia. Nevertheless, data strongly suggest that the detection and removal of adenomatous polyps are important in reducing colorectal cancer-related mortality.

Fecal Occult Blood Tests

Screening studies from both Europe and the United States indicate that a polyp is detected in about 30% of patients without symptoms who are 50 years of age or older and who undergo colonoscopy for follow-up of a positive fecal occult blood test result. Blood loss from polyps and positive fecal occult blood test results are related to polyp size. In one study in which rehydrated Hemoccult slides were used (rehydration results in greater sensitivity but also increases the number of false-positive findings), only 15% of polyps smaller than 1 cm were associated with a positive Hemoccult test result, whereas 80% of polyps larger than 2 cm were associated with a positive result. In another study, standard testing with Hemoccult cards detected 17% of adenomas smaller than 1 cm and 42% of adenomas larger than 1 cm. An immunochemical fecal occult blood test is promising, but not yet widely tested. This test detected 36% of adenomas smaller than 1 cm and 76% of adenomas larger than 1 cm in a small group of patients. A prospective, randomized study of fecal occult blood tests in which rehydrated Hemoccult cards were used suggested that annual tests reduce colorectal cancer-related deaths by 33% through 18 years of follow-up (15). This study in addition to two European trials have also demonstrated a 15% to 21% reduction in colon cancer-related death from biennial fecal occult blood testing (16). How much of this impact resulted from detection and removal of adenomas *per se* (as opposed to detection of early cancers) is unclear. Results from the National Polyp Study, however, strongly indicate that the removal of index polyps detected by fecal occult blood testing and other methods, together with subsequent colonoscopic surveillance, results in a lower than expected incidence of colon cancer in comparison with historical reference groups (17).

Sigmoidoscopy

The National Cancer Institute, the American Cancer Society, the American College of Physicians, the American Gastroenterological Association, and the World Health Organization Collaborating Center for Prevention of Colorectal Cancer all advocate screening sigmoidoscopy every 5 years in conjunction with yearly fecal occult blood tests beginning at 50 years of age (18,19). The benefit of sigmoidoscopy in interrupting the adenoma-to-carcinoma sequence is suggested by a number of studies. Investigators compared the use of rigid sigmoidoscopy in 261 members of the Kaiser Permanente Medical Care Program who died of cancer of the rectum or distal colon versus that in 868 matched controls (20). Only 8.8% of those with cancer had undergone screening sigmoidoscopy, compared with 24.2% of controls. The impact of sigmoidoscopy was limited to the development of fatal colon cancer within reach of the sigmoidoscope and was long-standing (at least 10 years). Other investigators determined the long-term risk of colorectal cancer development after rigid sigmoidoscopy and polypectomy in 1,618 patients with rectosigmoid adenomas. The overall risk for subsequent rectal cancer in these patients was similar to that in the general population, but subject analysis revealed that risk depended on histologic type, size, and number of adenomas removed (19,21,22). Based on existing data, the Health Care Financing Administration decided to provide coverage for colon cancer screening procedures to Medicare beneficiaries beginning January 1, 1998. This includes yearly fecal occult blood testing and flexible sigmoidoscopy every 4 years in persons at average risk.

The 60-cm flexible sigmoidoscope has supplanted the rigid scope because it causes less discomfort to the patient, visualizes 2.5 times more surface area, and detects two to three times more adenomas. Flexible sigmoidoscopy can be learned by paramedical personnel and has been successfully used in screening programs by nurse-practitioners (23).

Other Screening Modalities

Given the high cost of repeated screening of average-risk, asymptomatic patients for adenomas and carcinomas and the long natural history of the adenoma-to-carcinoma sequence, some have advocated a single air-contrast barium enema or colonoscopy at 50 years of age, with no further screening in patients without symptoms who have negative examination results. The appropriateness of this alternative to yearly fecal occult blood tests plus periodic sigmoidoscopy is unclear, and it has not gained wide acceptance. However, the American Cancer Society and other groups do consider colonoscopy every 10 years or barium enema every 5 to 10 years beginning at age 50 as a screening option in average-risk individuals (18).

Hydrocolonic sonography (instillation of water in the colon followed by extracorporeal ultrasonographic examination) has been suggested as a means of detecting large adenomas in the colon, but this test is insensitive and not an accepted screening tool. In "virtual colonoscopy," thin-section helical computed tomography of an air-distended, clean colon is used to generate high-resolution images (24). Computer-generated three-dimensional images are then constructed off-line. The overall sensitivity of this modality as a screening test for polyps is low (70% in one study), but evolving technology may make this a more effective option. Detection of adenoma-associated antigens or mutated protooncogenes such as K-*ras* in stool is possible, but the effectiveness of such methods as a screening measure is doubtful.

Management of Adenomas

Index Polypectomy

Once detected, adenomas should be completely removed, preferably by endoscopic snare polypectomy (Fig. 45.6). Polypectomy is relatively safe and easily performed when adenomas are small or pedunculated but is more difficult when polyps are large or sessile. Potential complications include bleeding and perforation of the polypectomy site. Large sessile villous adenomas (>2 cm) have a great potential for malignant degeneration. If such lesions cannot be completely removed by snare polypectomy, segmental surgical resection may be necessary. Diminutive polyps, on the

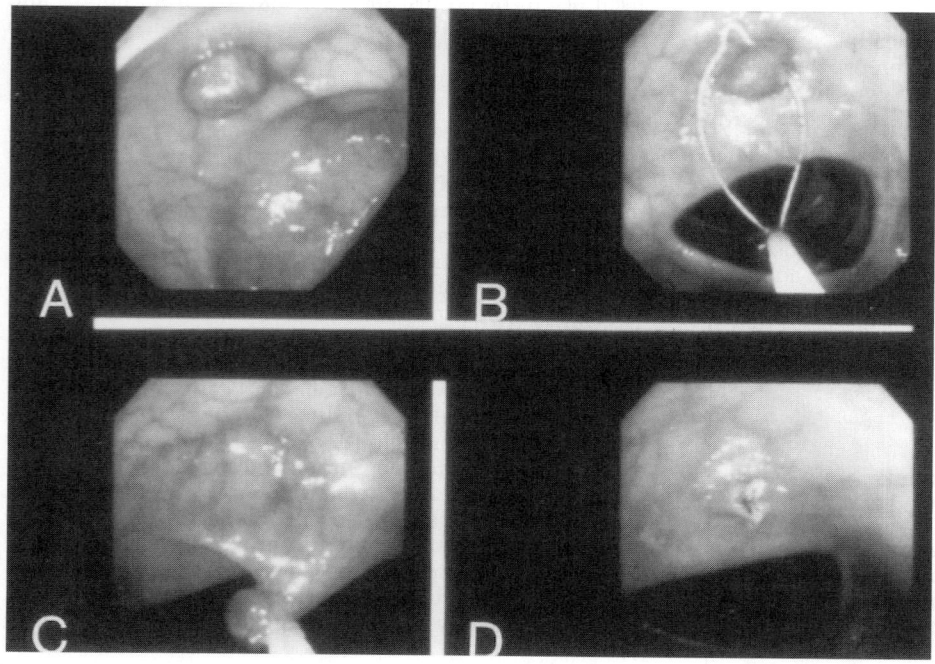

Figure 45.6. Endoscopic snare polypectomy. *(A)* A small colonic polyp. *(B)* The polypectomy snare is placed around the polyp. *(C)* The snare is closed around the base of the polyp, and the head of the polyp is gently pulled away from the wall and into the lumen. Current is applied to cut the stalk and cauterize the site. *(D)* The postpolypectomy site.

other hand, carry little malignant potential. If they are too small for snare polypectomy, ablation with a hot biopsy forceps is a reasonable approach. Because 30% to 50% of patients with one adenoma have a synchronous adenoma elsewhere in the colon, the entire colon should be "cleared" by colonoscopy in polyp-bearing patients.

Follow-up

Additional metachronous adenomas are likely to develop in patients who have had adenomas removed. Colonoscopic surveillance studies have provided estimates of the frequency and time course of recurrence in these patients. Data from the National Polyp Study suggested a recurrence rate of 32% to 42% by 3 years after index polypectomy. A prospective colonoscopic analysis also demonstrated a cumulative recurrence rate at 3 years of 42%. Most adenomas detected at this 3-year interval were small tubular adenomas. Age above 60 years, multiple adenomas at index polypectomy, and large size of the index adenoma predicted polyp recurrence in the National Polyp Study, but only multiplicity predicted recurrence of polyps with advanced pathologic features (larger than 1 cm, high-grade dysplasia or invasive cancer) at follow-up. The 3-year recurrence rate in patients with a known history of adenoma (42%) was higher than the incidence rate of adenoma appearance de novo during this period in patients who had no adenomas detected on index colonoscopy (16%) (25).

The high recurrence rate of adenomas after index polypectomy supports the use of postpolypectomy surveillance in patients with known histories of adenoma. Colonoscopy is the preferred means of follow-up in these patients. Air-contrast barium enemas may detect most large polyps in the colon but may miss smaller lesions. The published sensitivity of air-contrast barium studies for detecting colorectal polyps is 85% to 95%, but data from the National Polyp Study suggest a substantially lower sensitivity, probably because of failure to detect small polyps. Colonoscopy is the most accurate means of evaluating the colonic mucosa and allows biopsy and removal of suspect lesions.

The National Polyp Study was organized in 1978 by the American Gastroenterological Association, the American Society of Gastrointestinal Endoscopy, and the American College of Gastroenterology as a long-term randomized, prospective multicenter study to assess postpolypectomy surveillance. Data from the National Polyp Study indicate that colonoscopy need not be repeated at intervals shorter than 3 years in patients whose index polyp demonstrates no evidence of high-grade dysplasia or carcinoma. Although patients undergoing postpolypectomy surveillance at both 1 and 3 years after index polypectomy had a greater number of polyps detected in this study than did those undergoing colonoscopy at 3 years only, the percentage of patients whose adenomas had advanced pathologic features was similarly low in both groups (3.3%). Subsequent studies have confirmed the low incidence of recurrent advanced adenomas 3 to 5 years after polypectomy. Recent recommendations suggest an initial follow-up interval of 3 years after polypectomy. If the result of this colonoscopy is negative, the interval can be extended to every 5 years.

The National Polyp Study has demonstrated that colonoscopic polypectomy and surveillance result in a 76% to 90% reduction in colorectal cancer in comparison with historical reference groups. This and other studies have demonstrated, however, that in patients with no family history of colorectal cancer, most adenomas detected at interval follow-up are small tubular adenomas. In addition, when the index polyp is a small tubular adenoma, the risk for the subsequent development of a histologically important lesion is low. This is especially true of the diminutive polyp (<6 mm in diameter). Given the high cost of repeated colonoscopy procedures, clearly it will be necessary to establish better who may benefit most from colonoscopic surveillance and who may require less rigorous follow-up.

Management of Malignant Polyps

Endoscopic polypectomy is adequate treatment for an adenomatous polyp containing cancer if it can be demonstrated that the cancer is confined to the head of the polyp (i.e., carcinoma in situ or intramucosal carcinoma; Fig. 45.7). The adequacy of simple polypectomy has been controversial in cases in which malignant cells have invaded the polyp stalk (Fig. 45.8), but most studies now indicate that polypectomy is adequate treatment provided that a margin of more than 2 mm is present, the cancer is not poorly differentiated, and no vascular or lymphatic inva-

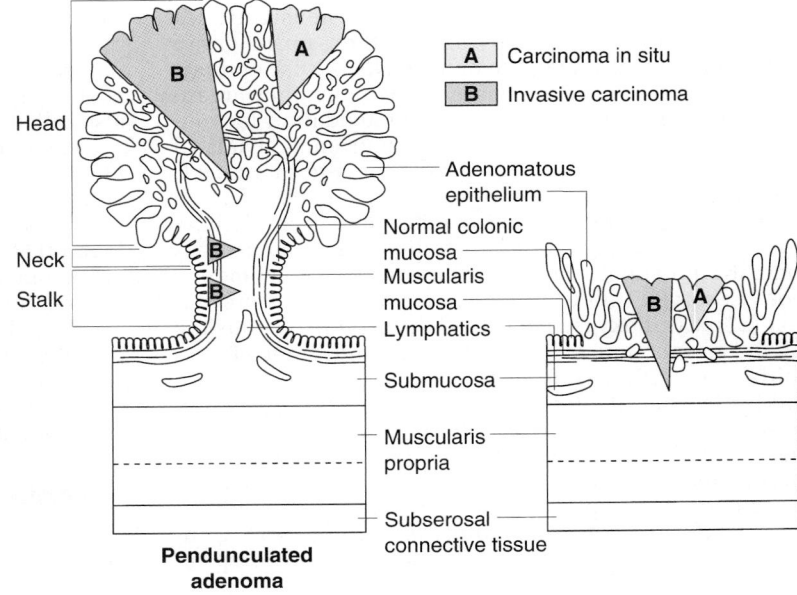

Figure 45.7. Diagrammatic representation of cancer-containing polyps. Pedunculated adenoma is described on the left and a sessile adenoma on the right. In carcinoma in situ, malignant cells are confined to the mucosa. These lesions are adequately treated by endoscopic polypectomy. Polypectomy is adequate treatment for invasive carcinoma only if the margin is sufficient (perhaps 2 mm), the carcinoma is not poorly differentiated, and no evidence of venous or lymphatic invasion is found. (After Haggitt RC, Glotzbach RE, Soffen EE, et al. Prognostic factors in colorectal carcinomas arising in adenomas: implications for lesions removed by endoscopic polypectomy. *Gastroenterology* 1985;89:328, with permission.)

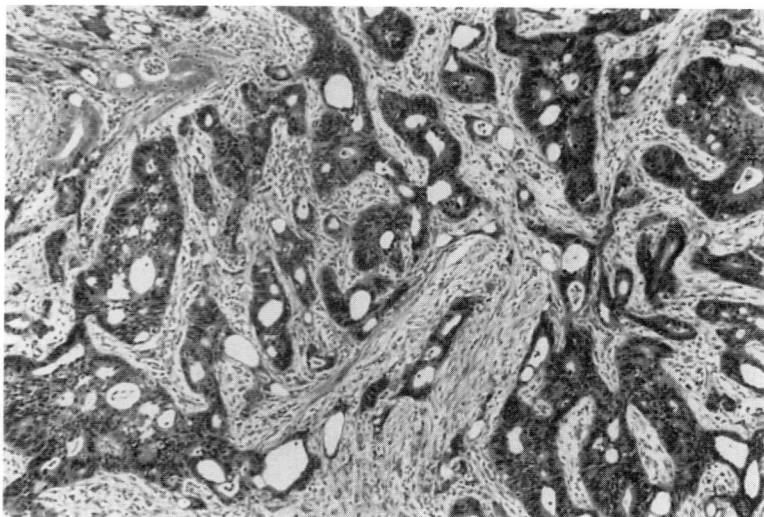

Figure 45.8. Invasive carcinoma in the stalk of an adenomatous polyp.

sion is noted. The presence of cancer at or near the margin is significantly associated with adverse outcome, even in the absence of other unfavorable parameters. On the other hand, in the absence of unfavorable histology and with a negative margin, the incidence of residual cancer is low (<1%). These criteria are more difficult to assess in sessile polyps. If an adequate margin cannot be demonstrated or negative histologic parameters are present, surgery is recommended to treat the possibility of regional lymph node metastases.

Primary Prevention of Adenoma Recurrence

Primary prevention relates to the ability to identify genetic, environmental, and biologic factors that cause cancer and to alter their effects. Laboratory, clinical, and epidemiologic evidence suggests that the regular use of nonsteroidal antiinflammatory drugs (NSAIDs), including aspirin, is associated with a decreased risk for the development of colorectal cancer. The number of colorectal adenomas discovered among regular NSAID users is lower than that in nonusers in most observational studies. The only published randomized trial to assess the effect of NSAIDs on colorectal cancer development in an average-risk population (the Physicians Health Study) demonstrated a small but nonsignificant decrease in incident polyps among the aspirin group (26). Therefore, although the data on NSAID use and primary prevention of adenomas are promising, they are insufficient to support a clinical recommendation for routine NSAID use to prevent polyp recurrence. Trials of antioxidant vitamins such as β-carotene and vitamins C and E have not convincingly demonstrated any effect on adenoma recurrence. Experimental data from animal studies and limited data from studies of human cancers suggest a potential role for inhibitors of the enzyme cyclooxygenase-2 (COX-2) in adenoma and cancer prevention (27). Cyclooxygenase is the key enzyme responsible for the production of prostaglandins and other eicosanoids. The COX-2 isoform is induced by inflammation and is elevated in adenomas and colorectal cancers. Experimental trials are under way to evaluate the use of COX-2 inhibitors in preventing adenoma recurrence. Supplemental calcium reduces proliferative activity in the mucosa of experimental animals and patients at high-risk for the development of colorectal cancer. Clinical evidence suggests a modest reduction in polyp recurrence in patients taking supplemental daily calcium (28).

NON-NEOPLASTIC MUCOSAL POLYPS

Hyperplastic Polyps

Hyperplastic polyps are small, usually sessile lesions most frequently encountered in the distal colon and rectum (Fig. 45.9A). Although grossly indistinguishable from small adenomas, they carry no potential for malignant degeneration. Microscopically, hyperplastic polyps are characterized by a serrated epithelial pattern representing micropapillary luminal in-foldings of columnar absorptive cells and mature, frequently hyperdistended goblet cells (Fig. 45.9B). Elongation and subsequent in-folding of the epithelium may be caused by an expanded, but otherwise normally located, replication zone in the crypt. The cytologic atypia found in adenomatous polyps is not seen in these lesions. Hyperplastic and adenomatous glands occasionally coexist in a polyp and in some cases even share the same basement membrane. This is not strong evidence that adenomas derive from hyperplastic polyps. Abundant evidence documents the divergent growth and differentiation patterns of hyperplastic polyps and adenomas. Another entity, the so-called mixed hyperplastic adenomatous polyp, exhibits the architectural, but not the cytologic, features of hyperplastic polyps. These lesions demonstrate the cytologic features of adenomas and are considered adenoma variants; they are also called *serrated adenomas.*

Hyperplastic polyps are common age-related lesions found in about one third of the population older than 50 years. Although they often coexist with adenomas in polyp-bearing patients, no convincing evidence has been found that hyperplastic polyps are harbingers of adenoma development. They are most common in the distal colon and rectum and are usually diminutive. Because hyperplastic polyps are asymptomatic and carry no malignant potential, no specific treatment is required for these lesions. If a hyperplastic polyp is the only lesion detected on index flexible sigmoidoscopy or colonoscopy, no further evaluation is indicated.

Juvenile Polyps

Juvenile polyps, also known as *retention polyps,* can occur sporadically or as part of a familial polyposis syn-

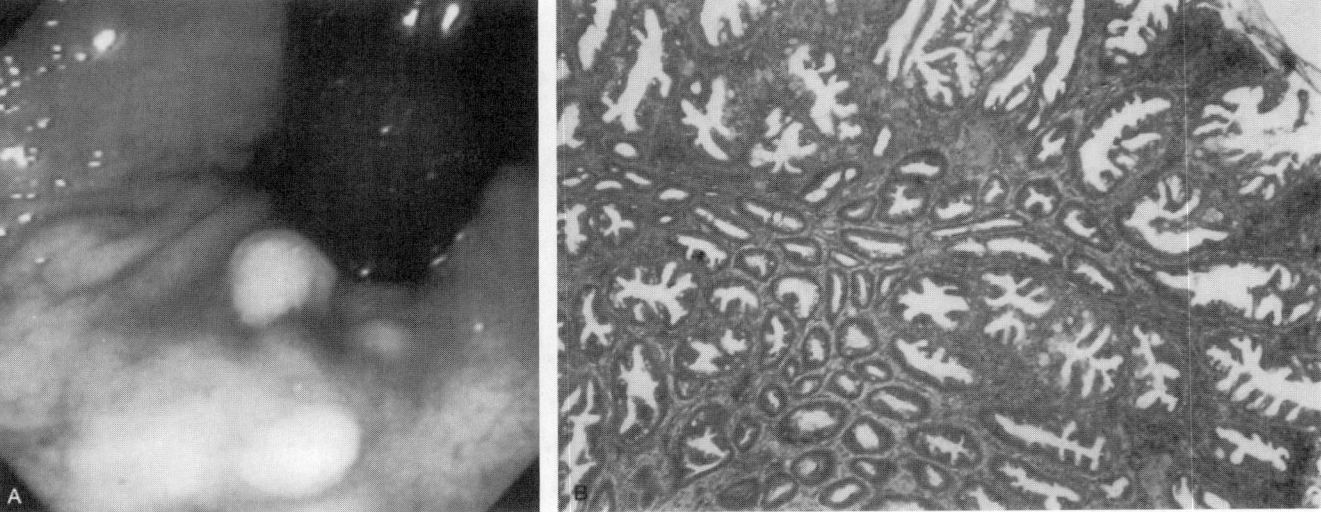

Figure 45.9. Hyperplastic polyps. *(A)* Several diminutive hyperplastic polyps seen in the rectum during flexible sigmoidoscopy. *(B)* Photomicrograph of a hyperplastic polyp, characterized by elongated glands with papillary in-foldings that have a typical serrated epithelial pattern.

drome. These mucosal polyps consist of dilated cystic mucus-filled glands, abundant lamina propria, and inflammatory infiltrates. Seventy-five percent occur in children younger than 10 years of age, often appearing as single pedunculated cherry-red polyps with a smooth surface and contour. The exact prevalence of such lesions has not been determined, but they appear to be acquired lesions detected in about 2% of children who do not have symptoms. Juvenile polyps often present in the form of hematochezia because they are highly vascularized lesions. Rectal prolapse and autoamputation may occur with distal lesions, whereas intussusception may be precipitated by proximal juvenile polyps found in the context of familial syndromes. Individually, these polyps have no malignant potential, but symptomatic polyps should be removed to prevent further complications. Juvenile polyposis, on the other hand, is associ-ated with an increased risk for the early development of cancer.

Inflammatory Polyps

Inflammatory mucosal polyps are common in the setting of idiopathic inflammatory bowel disease. Marked inflammation and ulceration coexist with granulation tissue in a distorted mucosal architecture that appears polypoid (Fig. 45.10A). Subsequent healing leads to residual islands of mucosa interspersed with denuded epithelium (so-called pseudopolyps; Fig. 45.10B). Severe chronic inflammation of any kind, including a variety of infectious diseases (tuberculosis, amebiasis, schistosomiasis, amebic colitis), may result in inflammatory polyps that resemble those found in the active stages of idiopathic inflammatory bowel disease.

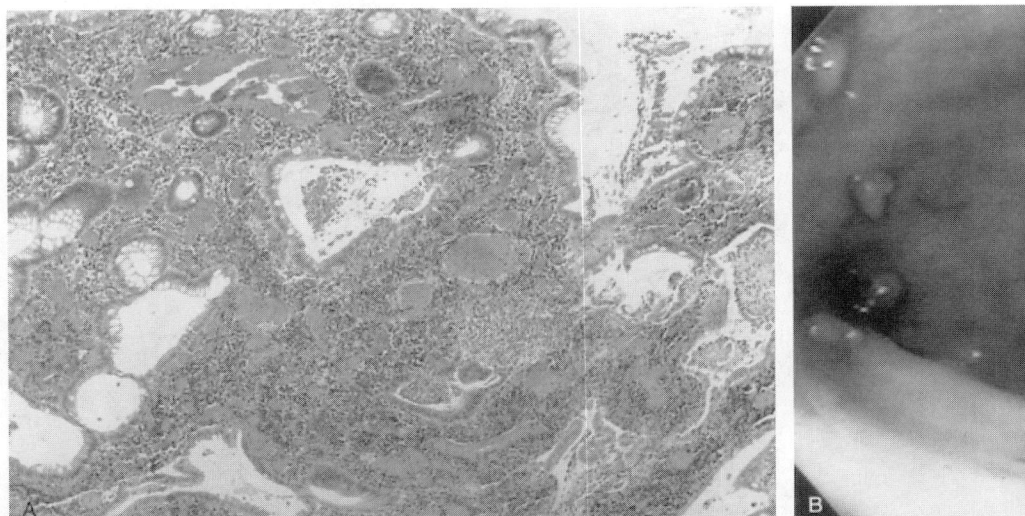
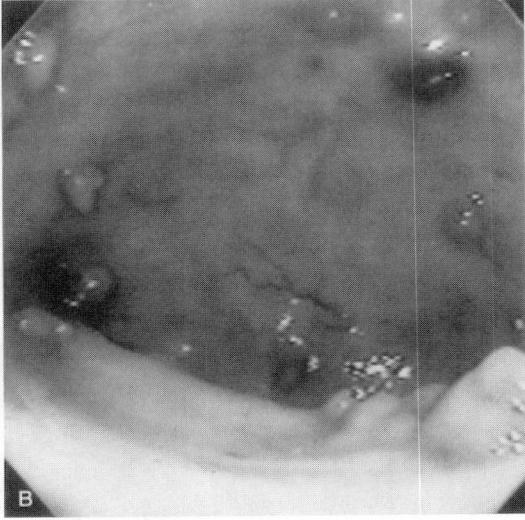

Figure 45.10. Inflammatory polyps. *(A)* Severe mucosal inflammation with infiltrates and granulation tissue shown here microscopically can appear clinically with a polypoid configuration. *(B)* Resolution of inflammation can leave islands of intact mucosa among large areas of denuded epithelium, resulting in pseudopolyps.

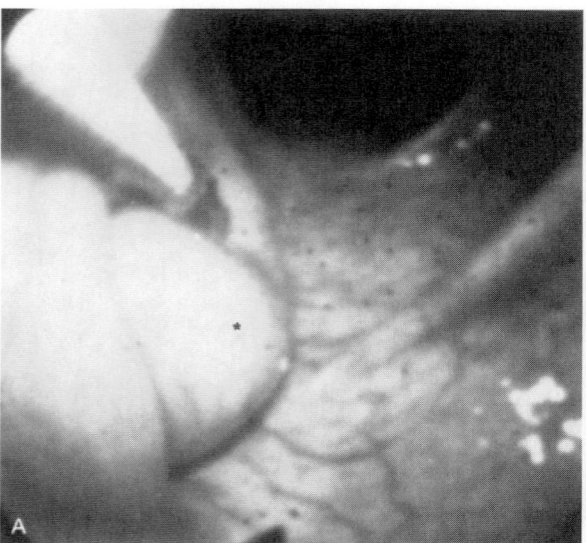
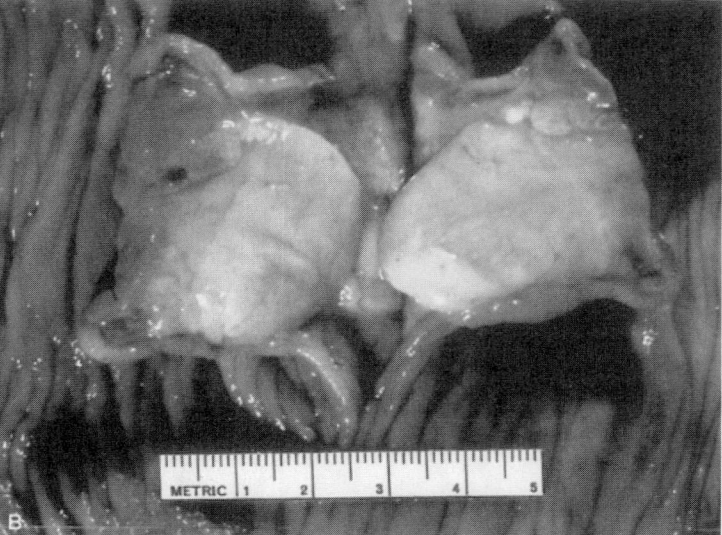

Figure 45.11. Submucosal lipoma. *(A)* Cecal lipoma seen at colonoscopy *(asterisk).* Submucosal fatty tissue causes the mucosa to protrude into the lumen; such protrusion appears as a polyp. *(B)* Colectomy specimen demonstrating a large submucosal lipoma cut in cross section.

SUBMUCOSAL POLYPS

Submucosal masses can expand to push the colonic mucosa into the bowel lumen and thus appear as polypoid lesions. Many submucosal lesions (e.g., lipomas, leiomyomas) are clinically asymptomatic and must be differentiated from neoplastic lesions. Others are malignant lesions that require early detection, such as lymphomas and metastatic tumors. Many submucosal lesions are not detected on endoscopic mucosal biopsy because standard biopsy forceps do not reach beyond the mucosa. If a submucosal lesion is suspected, multiple biopsy specimens of the same site sometimes provides tissue for diagnosis.

Lipomas are benign fatty tumors that occur throughout the gastrointestinal tract but are most commonly found in the cecum near the ileocecal valve (Fig. 45.11). They appear endoscopically as soft, smooth polyps that are pliable

and deformable. The overlying mucosa is intact but may be light yellow in appearance. These are benign lesions that have little clinical significance.

Isolated lymphoid nodules consisting of benign lymphoid tissue may appear as sessile smooth polyps of various sizes, with a predilection for the distal colon and rectum. These are usually asymptomatic. Diffuse nodular lymphoid hyperplasia also occurs in children as an incidental finding. The nodules must be distinguished from primary or secondary lymphoma of the large intestine, which may present as mucosal nodularity resembling the pseudopolyposis of inflammatory bowel disease or even polyposis (Fig. 45.12).

Pneumatosis cystoides intestinalis has the appearance of multiple air-filled cysts within the submucosa. This may be an incidental finding in patients with chronic obstructive pulmonary disease, scleroderma, or asympto-

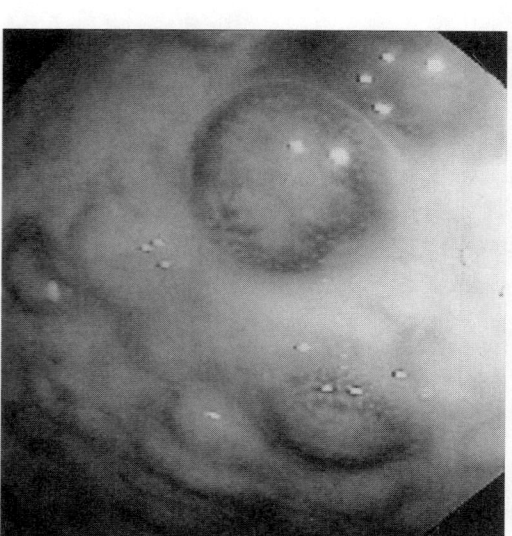
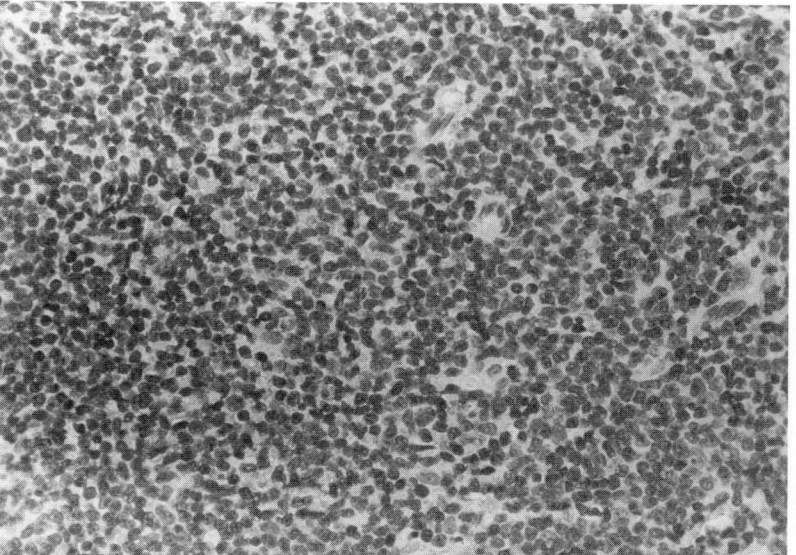

Figure 45.12. Lymphomatous polyposis of the colon. *(A)* Colonoscopic view of B-cell lymphoma presenting as multiple colonic polyps. *(B)* Histology of lymphoma in one of the polyps.

matic pneumoperitoneum secondary to recent surgery or instrumentation, in which air or colonic gas diffuses into the cysts. These sometimes resolve with administration of oxygen. A far more virulent form of pneumatosis is associated with fulminant mucosal inflammation, ischemia, or necrotizing enterocolitis in children. These cysts are thought to result from mucosal invasion by gas-producing bacteria.

Colitis cystica profunda is a rare condition in which the intestinal wall is thickened by submucosal mucus-filled cysts of various sizes and an accumulation of fibroblasts in the lamina propria. It can present as an ulcerating or mass lesion in the rectosigmoid in association with the solitary rectal ulcer syndrome. Although the pathogenesis of this condition is unknown, it may result from the downward displacement of colonic glands during chronic inflammation and healing. The appearance of aberrant submucosal glandular epithelium and acellular mucous lakes should not be mistaken for colloid carcinoma because this lesion has no malignant potential.

Carcinoid tumors of the rectum appear as isolated, small, yellow-gray submucosal nodules. These are often incidental findings during sigmoidoscopy. Most are smaller than 1 cm and have little malignant potential. These are amenable to local excision. Lesions larger than 2 cm are more commonly malignant but seldom give rise to metastases. They should, however, be treated aggressively with complete excision. Rectal carcinoid tumors are usually asymptomatic but may present with hematochezia. They are not associated with the carcinoid syndrome. Carcinoid tumors in the proximal colon may be locally invasive or metastasize to the liver, liberating vasoactive peptides into the systemic circulation and producing the carcinoid syndrome.

Other lesions that can present as submucosal polyps include metastatic tumors, such as malignant melanoma, and benign lesions, such as leiomyomas, fibromas, lymphangiomas, hemangiomas, and endometriosis.

GASTROINTESTINAL POLYPOSIS SYNDROMES

Gastrointestinal polyposis indicates the presence of a systemic process that promotes the development of multiple polyps throughout the gastrointestinal tract. In some instances, the polyps are located predominantly in the colon; however, in many syndromes, polyps may be found in the stomach, small intestine, colon, and rectum. The classification of the polyposis syndromes has traditionally been based on the histologic characteristics of the polyps, but gradually an awareness of the genetic basis for the most important of these syndromes has permitted more precise diagnosis and individualized approaches to treatment.

Familial Adenomatous Polyposis

Familial adenomatous polyposis is an inherited disease characterized by the development of multiple adenomatous polyps throughout the colon and rectum (Fig. 45.13). The polyps first appear in adolescence, with the median age of onset being about 16 years. The number of polyps in each patient is variable, and they increase in number and size with advancing age. The genetic basis for this disease is a germline mutation in the APC gene located on chromosome 5q. In part, the age of onset, number of polyps, and age at which cancer develops are determined by the location of the mutation in the APC gene. More than 5,000 polyps eventually develop in patients with the most severe types of mutation, and cancer develops in these patients at a mean age of 35 years. Additional factors not related to the mutation on the APC gene, some genetic and some environmental, also modify the clinical characteristics of the disease (29,30).

Gastrointestinal Features

Polyps in the stomach and small intestine develop in about 90% of patients with FAP. The gastric polyps primarily consist of fundic gland hyperplasia, which is not a premalignant lesion. Occasionally, gastric adenomas are found, but stomach cancer is only rarely reported as a complication of FAP in North America, where the incidence of gastric cancer is low.

Small-intestinal neoplasia is not rare in FAP and principally occurs in the periampullary region of the duodenum. Duodenal adenomatous polyps, which typically appear later than the colonic lesions, may be multiple but tend not to carpet the proximal small intestine. The ampulla of Vater is a particular target for neoplastic development. With time, carcinoma develops in up to 5% of these patients, so that surveillance is required in this area. Adenomas and carcinomas occur in the jejunum and ileum, but these are rare. Polyps in the terminal ileum are more likely to represent lymphoid aggregates than adenomas and should be sampled for diagnostic purposes.

Classically, it has been stated that the natural history of FAP is for cancer to develop at a median age of 40 to 45 years. In fact, the development of cancer is variable and again is based in part on the location of the germline mutation in the APC gene. Colon cancer is rare before 30 years of age, and cancer may not develop in patients with the attenuated form of FAP until they are in their 50s or 60s. Thus, the treatment of these patients relies increasingly on a genetic characterization of the disease.

Extraintestinal Features

Traditionally, patients with manifestations of FAP together with extraintestinal manifestations were considered to have Gardner's syndrome. It is now appreciated that families with FAP all have extraintestinal manifestations and that no distinction can be made between families with Gardner's syndrome and other families with FAP. FAP is characterized by osteomas of the mandible, skull, and long bones and a variety of other benign soft-tissue tumors, such as fibromas and lipomas (Fig. 45.14). Osteomas are commonly found in the skull and may be multiple. Some of these lesions have been reported to regress and later reappear. Osteomas may also be found in the mandible, and radiographs of the mouth may reveal impacted or supernumerary teeth. Congenital hypertrophy of the retinal pigmented epithelium (CHRPE) is present in some families with FAP, depending on the location of the mutation in the APC gene. CHRPE lesions may be seen in the general population but are small and usually single. Multiple, bilateral, and large CHRPE lesions are essentially diagnostic of FAP.

Malignant tumors in the colon are considered to be nearly inevitable, and they may occur occasionally in the duodenum or (less commonly) elsewhere in the gastrointestinal tract. Patients with FAP are also at increased risk for brain tumors (particularly medulloblastomas), thyroid tumors, adrenal tumors, and benign and malignant tumors of the hepatobiliary tree. The occurrence of a malignant brain tumor in conjunction with intestinal polyposis was traditionally referred to as *Turcot's syndrome*. Medulloblastomas are a rare complication of FAP, but the risk for this tumor is increased 99-fold in FAP families. Interestingly, one of the index families initially reported by Turcot

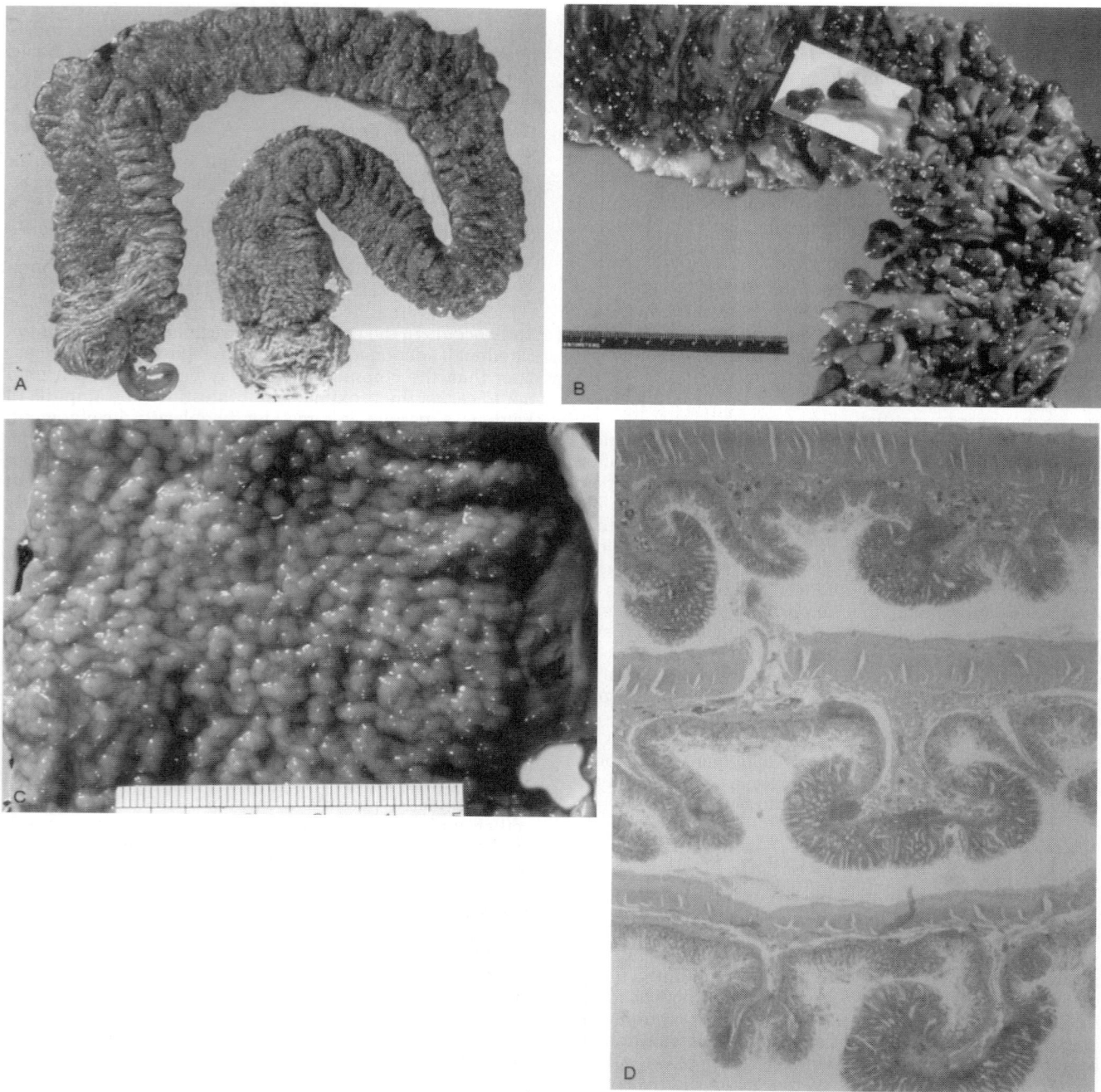

Figure 45.13. Familial adenomatous polyposis *(FAP)*. *(A)* Gross specimen of a resected colon from a patient with FAP. *(B)* Sessile and pedunculated adenomatous polyps in the colon of a patient with FAP. *(C)* Close-up view of a profuse type of FAP, in which the mucosa is carpeted with innumerable polyps. *(D)* Photomicrograph demonstrating profuse FAP with both sessile and pedunculated adenomatous polyps.

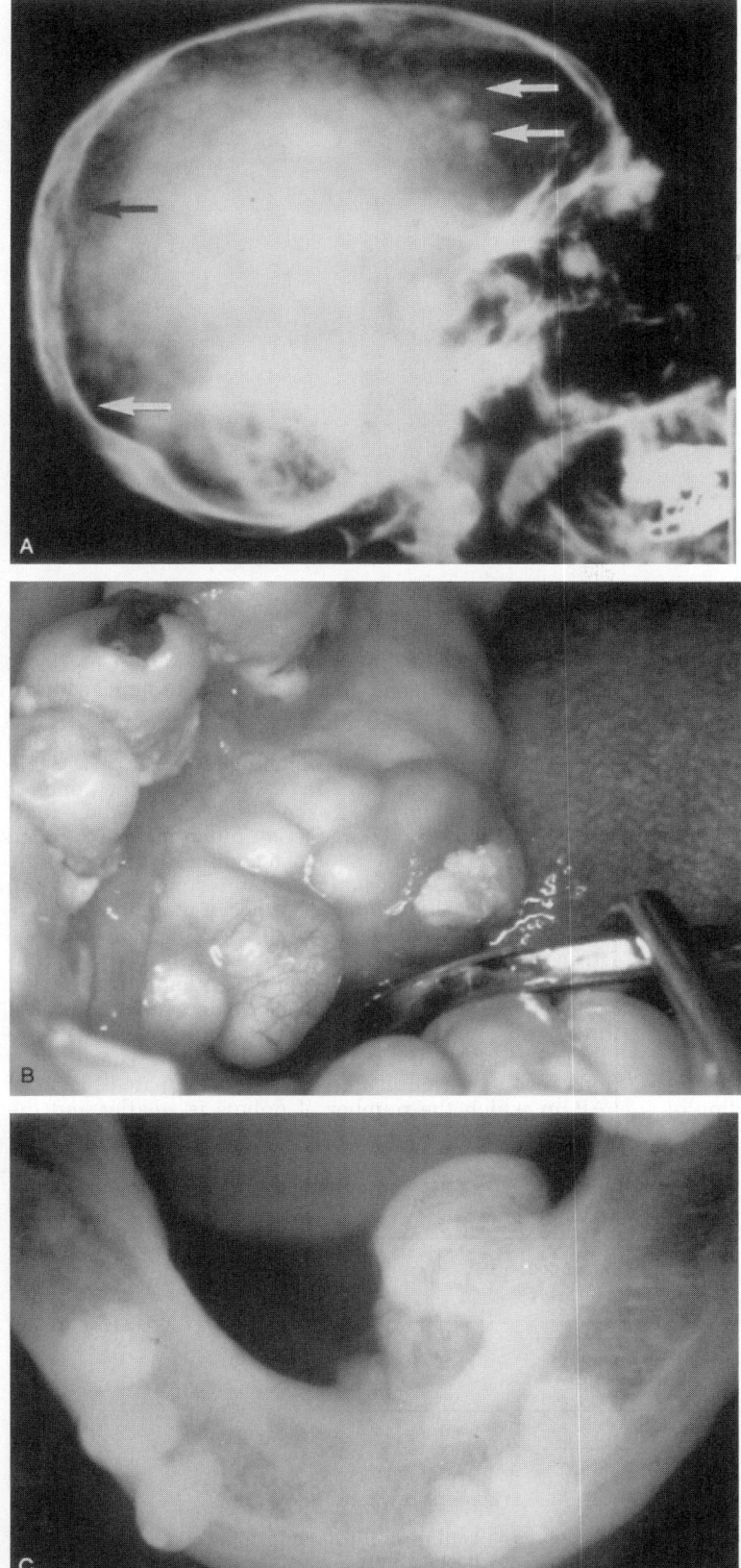

Figure 45.14. Extraintestinal manifestations of familial adenomatous polyposis *(FAP)*. *(A)* Skull film demonstrating osteomas of the calvarium *(arrows)*. *(B)* Photograph of the mandible demonstrating protuberant mandibular osteomas. *(C)* Mandibular radiograph demonstrating a large osteoma of the mandible. *(D)* Chest radiograph demonstrating multiple fibromas *(arrows)* in a patient with FAP. *(continues)*

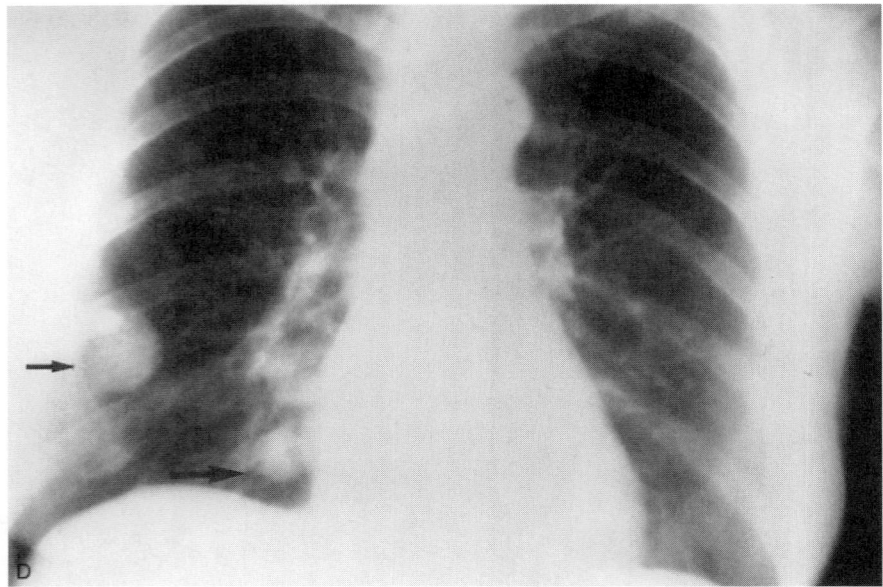

Figure 45.14. *(Continued)*

in 1959 did not have FAP but rather HNPCC characterized by an excess of astrocytomas, such as glioblastoma multiforme.

Desmoid Tumors

When FAP is recognized, a colectomy should be performed long before cancer develops, and strategies are available to reduce the likelihood of the development of cancer in the upper gastrointestinal tract. Desmoid tumors, however, develop later in 10% to 15% of patients with FAP, often as a complication of laparotomy but sometimes spontaneously. These are benign but aggressive tumors of mesenteric fibroblasts that can envelop and obstruct the gastrointestinal tract, arteries, veins, or ureters. In some instances, desmoid tumors virtually fill the abdominal cavity with tissue, so that additional abdominal exploration is impossible. Desmoid tumors can be lethal.

Genetic Basis

Familial adenomatous polyposis occurs when a germline mutation in the *APC* gene inactivates the function of

the *APC* gene product (29). In most instances, the genetic lesion creates a premature stop codon in the *APC* gene, which in turn leads to the translation of a truncated APC protein. The *APC* gene encodes a large protein (311 kd) that binds to other intracellular proteins—namely the catenins and E-cadherin. Depending on the location of the premature stop codon, the mutant protein is of variable length. The *APC* gene encodes 2,844 codons (i.e., one for each amino acid) and is broken into 15 translated exons. The structure of the *APC* gene is unique in that the 15th exon makes up about 75% of the coding sequences of the gene. Because it is unusually large, this long, open reading frame is a natural target for the types of mutations that result in premature stop codons (30).

The location of the germline mutation is of some clinical significance (Fig. 45.15). For example, mutations that occur at the 5' end of the gene, particularly in the first three exons, encode products that are intrinsically unstable and typically not detectable in tissues. These mutations result in a clinically mild or "attenuated" form of FAP, in which the number of polyps is smaller and the

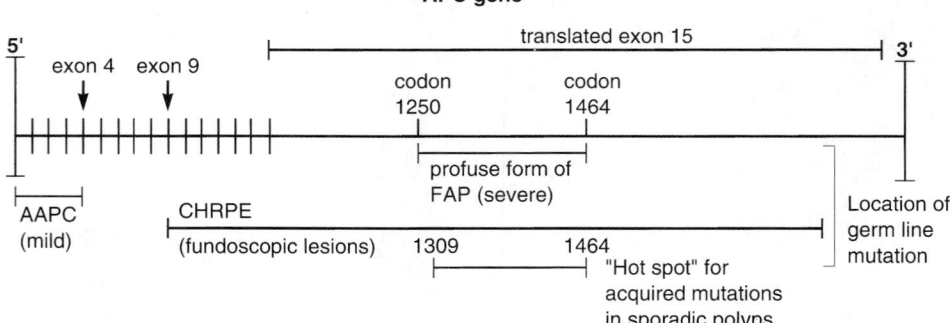

Figure 45.15. This scheme of the *APC* (adenomatous polyposis coli) gene illustrates the genotype–phenotype correlations. Most mutations of *APC* result in premature stop codons; therefore, the site of the mutation usually indicates the relative length of the mutant protein product. Mutations at the 5' end of the gene produce "attenuated" adenomatous polyposis coli, a milder form of the disease. The retinal lesions (congenital hypertrophy of retinal pigmented epithelium) occur when the mutations are between exons 9 and 15. The portion of the *APC* gene that binds to other cytoskeletal elements in the cell (β-catenins) is represented in the 15th exon. Mutations in a hot spot immediately downstream from the β-catenin–binding site result in a more virulent, profuse form of familial adenomatous polyposis. This site is also the location of most of the acquired mutations in sporadic colorectal neoplasms.

onset of disease later, with cancer developing in the sixth or seventh decade. To complicate matters, however, family members with the same mutation may have variable manifestations of the disease. Indeed, some members who inherit this mutation have few polyps yet can pass on an increased risk for cancer to their progeny. In contrast, mutations that occur at the 58 end of the 15th exon, particularly in a segment between codons 1,250 and 1,464, are associated with a particularly virulent form of the disease, in which the number of polyps is larger and the risk for the development of colorectal cancer at an early age is increased (median age, 34 years). A large proportion of acquired mutations that occur in sporadic cancers are also located in this "hot spot," typically between codons 1,309 and 1,464. It appears that these mutations occur downstream (i.e., toward the carboxyl terminus) in a portion of the APC protein that associates with other cytoskeletal proteins. Thus, mutations in this region result in abnormal proteins that interfere with the wild-type protein and prevent the APC protein from regulating β-catenin normally. Mutant proteins that are truncated before this region are less capable of this function, and proteins that are truncated but nearly complete in length may be less deleterious to cellular behavior.

In families who have FAP with CHRPE lesions, the mutations are usually in exons 9 to 15, and this manifestation rarely occurs in families with mutations in any of the first eight exons. Thus, detailed knowledge of the location of the germline mutation can be used to predict the clinical manifestations and guide therapy.

Diagnosis

The clinical diagnosis of FAP is usually not difficult. When FAP is known in a family, the relatives at risk should undergo surveillance sigmoidoscopy on an annual basis beginning in their middle teens. The entire colon is at risk for the development of neoplasia, so sigmoidoscopy is sufficient to detect carriers of the abnormal gene. If a single adenoma appears in a teenager at risk, the disease is strongly suspected; however, because of its typically slow progression, patients can be observed until multiple adenomas appear. After the first adenoma is noted, diffuse adenoma typically develops during the next few years. The lesions must be sampled to confirm that they are adenomas. No other disease produces multiple adenomatous polyps in young patients.

The diagnosis of FAP is often made in adults in whom it has not previously been suspected. In some instances, the disease is present in relatives, but the proper diagnosis has not been appreciated. About 25% of patients, however, have a germline lesion in the *APC* gene that is not present in either parent. These new mutations are more frequent in FAP than in some other diseases because the large size of the 15th exon of the *APC* gene makes it a likely target for nucleotide insertions or deletions. These create frame shifts and subsequent downstream premature stop codons. In ambiguous cases, which often include patients who have attenuated adenomatous polyposis coli (with fewer polyps and a later onset), it may be useful to confirm a suspected diagnosis with an in vitro truncated protein test. This test is about 60% to 80% sensitive in patients who have FAP, depending on the laboratory. Although its lack of sensitivity is a problem, the test is highly specific and reproducible. Therefore, once a positive test result has been obtained, the mutant *APC* gene can be sought in other relatives. Unrelated FAP families all have mutations in the *APC* gene, but most families have unique mutations. Although many families have CHRPE lesions, osteomas, or other extraintestinal manifestations of the disease, the appearance of these is sufficiently variable that they are an inadequate substitute for endoscopic examination or direct genetic testing. Genetic testing must be accompanied by proper counseling of patients and their families, so that they understand the implications of the findings (31).

In a family with FAP, each first-degree relative of an affected patient has a 50% likelihood of inheriting the mutated gene. By age 16, about half of affected patients have polyps. With each passing year, a negative sigmoidoscopic examination result reduces further the likelihood that a patient carries the gene. Carriage of the gene can be ruled out with greater certainty if the family's germline lesion can be identified and excluded in an at-risk family member.

Management

Surgery is the only reasonable management option in FAP, and the clinical decision involves the selection and timing of the operation. The diagnosis of FAP is often made in adolescence, but a delay of 20 years or more is typical from the appearance of the first adenomas until the development of cancer. Thus, it is usually prudent to wait until the patient has reached full physical maturity before surgery is planned.

The safest surgical approach is a total proctocolectomy with an ileoanal anastomosis. Any residual rectal mucosa that is left behind is at risk for the development of neoplasia. Even with careful endoscopic surveillance of the rectal segment, invasive carcinomas may develop.

The fact that small adenomatous polyps of the rectum can spontaneously regress after a subtotal colectomy and ileorectal anastomosis underscores the reversible nature of the benign adenoma. Additionally, it has been found that adenomas can regress in FAP in response to treatment with sulindac (Clinoril). Several reports have confirmed that even large numbers of polyps regress in patients on 150 to 200 mg of sulindac twice per day (32). Similar results have recently been obtained with COX-2 inhibitors. Unfortunately, the polyps reappear when the drug is stopped, and development of cancer despite treatment with sulindac has been reported. Medical treatment is therefore not a safe first-line treatment for FAP, but it may be of some benefit in patients who refuse operative intervention. Although no data are available to support this approach, sulindac may be a useful adjunct in patients with milder forms of FAP (i.e., smaller numbers of polyps with relative rectal sparing) and in circumstances in which residual rectal tissue must be left behind. Sulindac is not effective in the management of upper gastrointestinal tract neoplasia. Furthermore, no role has been found for sulindac in the management of sporadic adenomatous polyps or advanced colorectal neoplasia in any setting.

Management of Extracolonic Disease

In addition to the risks for colorectal neoplasia, patients with FAP are at risk for the development of osteomas, lipomas, fibromas, and a variety of other lesions. Although the osteomas, fibromas, and lipomas can degenerate into sarcomas, this is a sufficiently rare event that prophylactic surveillance and surgery are not indicated. Likewise, the CHRPE lesions do not require therapy. Gastric carcinoma is distinctly uncommon in North American populations, and it is not necessary to provide endoscopic surveillance of the stomach.

The two major management issues after removal of the colon and rectum are periampullary neoplasia and desmoid tumors. One or more adenomas are found in the duodenum in 90% of patients with FAP, usually close to the ampulla of Vater. These lesions should be excised for biopsy and destroyed by electrocautery, laser, or other ablative approaches. Although no data are available to indicate the optimal intervals for safe surveillance, it seems prudent to examine the duodenum about every 2 years. Complex neoplasms, including adenomas with varying degrees of dysplasia, may require individualized management, including the use of biliary stents while extensive ablative therapy of the periampullary region is performed. Surgical approaches may be required for advanced neoplasms (i.e., carcinoma in situ or frank carcinoma), but therapeutic endoscopy remains the first option. Duodenotomy with local surgical excision is an option for these lesions.

Desmoid tumors are aggressive benign tumors of fibroblasts that can cause multiple clinical complications; they are a significant cause of morbidity and mortality in FAP. They typically grow slowly and can surround or compress vascular structures, nerves, or the abdominal viscera. Surgical management is generally avoided unless simple local excision of an abdominal wall lesion is possible, and postoperative recurrences are common. Radiotherapy has been used to control the growth of some of these, but it is not always successful. No medical approach to this disease has been uniformly successful. A combination of sulindac plus tamoxifen may be tried for intraabdominal tumors and has been successful in some patients. Cytotoxic chemotherapy with doxorubicin was successful in a patient whose tumor was refractory to other treatment.

Variants

A number of names, especially *Gardner's syndrome*, have been attached to variations of FAP to emphasize the presence of particular extracolonic findings. Actually, Gardner's syndrome is the same entity as FAP; all families with Gardner's syndrome have mutations in the *APC* gene, and virtually all families with FAP have the stigmata previously attributed to Gardner's syndrome. A few families with prominent sebaceous cysts were formerly said to have Oldfield's syndrome, and families with brain tumors were said to have Turcot's syndrome. All these syndromes represent the variable expression of germline mutations in the *APC* gene and are largely of historical interest. The current mode of classifying FAP families is based on the *APC* gene mutation.

Peutz-Jeghers Syndrome

Peutz-Jeghers syndrome is an autosomal dominant familial syndrome associated with multiple gastrointestinal polyps and characteristic skin pigmentation. The gene responsible for this disease has been mapped to chromosome 19p13.3 and encodes a serine/threonine kinase (Table 45.2); carriers of the gene are predisposed to a number of early-onset cancers.

Gastrointestinal Features

The gastrointestinal polyps in Peutz-Jeghers syndrome are non-neoplastic hamartomas consisting of a supportive framework of smooth muscle tissue covered by somewhat hyperplastic epithelium (Fig. 45.16). These are histologically distinct from juvenile polyps and show no inflammatory cell infiltrate. Polyps may be found in the stomach, small intestine, or colon, and in each instance they have a distinctive appearance. Peutz-Jeghers polyps can usually be identified as such by the pathologist, and the characteristic cutaneous pigmentation makes this syndrome easily detected.

Skin Lesions

The cutaneous manifestations of Peutz-Jeghers syndrome may be found early in life and consist of dark, macular lesions on the mouth (both on the skin and in the buc-

Table 45.2. GENETIC ALTERATIONS IN COLONIC POLYPOSIS SYNDROMES

Polyposis syndrome	Chromosome	Gene
Familial adenomatous polyposis	5q21	APC
Gardner's	5q21	APC
Turcot	5q21, 7p22, 3p21.3–23	APC, hPMS2, hMLH1
Peutz-Jeghers	19p13.3	LKB1/STK1
Hereditary mixed polyposis	6q	Unknown
Juvenile polyposis coli	10q22.3–24.1, 18q21.1	PTEN plus SMAD4
Bannayan-Riley-Ruvalcaba	10q23	PTEN; possibly others
Cowden's disease	10q22–23	PTEN

cal mucosa), nose, lips, hands, feet, genitalia, and anus. These lesions tend to become less obvious by the time of puberty. Unlike ordinary freckles, the cutaneous lesions of Peutz-Jeghers syndrome are present from birth. Moreover, ordinary freckles typically do not extend beyond the vermilion border of the lips, nor is the buccal mucosa involved, as it is in Peutz-Jeghers syndrome.

Clinical Complications

The principal complication of Peutz-Jeghers syndrome is intestinal obstruction, which may develop in infancy or childhood. This complication is most prominent in the small intestine because of its narrower diameter. Gastrointestinal bleeding may also be seen in this disease.

Cancer in the small intestine or colon can occur in Peutz-Jeghers syndrome; however, this is an uncommon complication (33). It is thought that neoplasia may arise from foci of adenomatous epithelium found in some Peutz-Jeghers polyps. The risk for cancer is such that prophylactic surgery is not recommended.

Patients with Peutz-Jeghers syndrome are also at increased risk for cancers outside the gastrointestinal tract. Cancer developed in about half of the patients in one large study at a median age of about 50 years. At risk are the gastrointestinal tract, gonads, breasts, pancreas, and biliary tree. Ovarian cysts and sex cord tumors are seen in 5% to 12% of female patients, and boys are at risk for endocrinologically active Sertoli's cell testicular tumors that may produce feminizing features before puberty. No internal organ is at sufficiently high risk for cancer that a specific screening regimen or prophylactic surgery is indicated. The clinician should be aware of these risks, however, and should be particularly alert to gonadal tumors (which are otherwise rare) and breast cancer (for which screening should start at an early age, and bilateral disease should be suspected).

Management

The management of Peutz-Jeghers syndrome is limited to the removal of polyps; endoscopic techniques should be used when possible. Surgery may be required for intussusception caused by small-intestinal polyps. The risk for neoplastic development should be kept in mind, but these patients are not candidates for prophylactic removal of any section of the gastrointestinal tract. As mentioned earlier, gonadal neoplasms and breast cancer are potential complications that may require surgery.

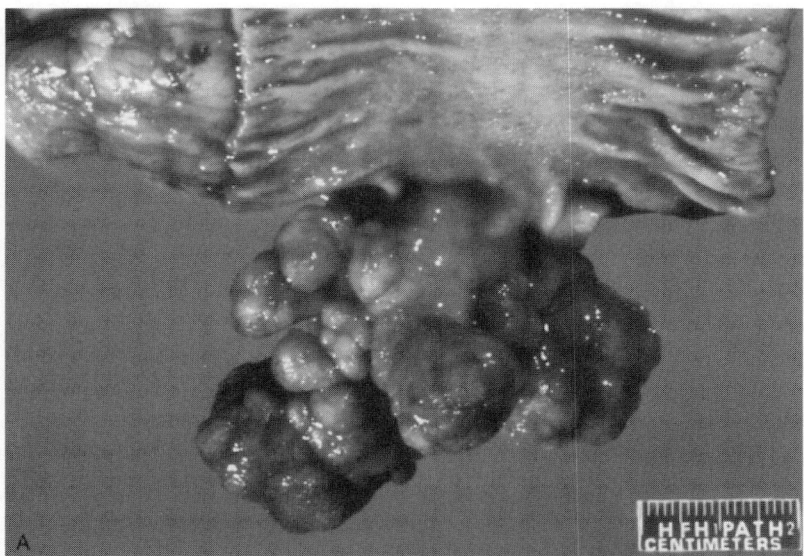

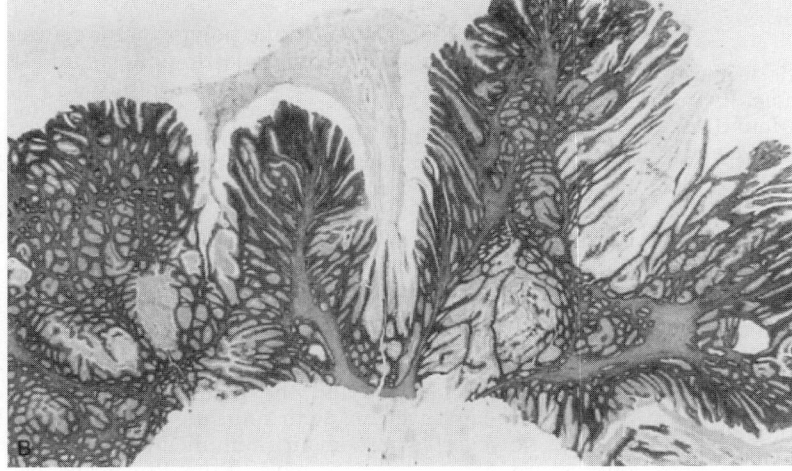

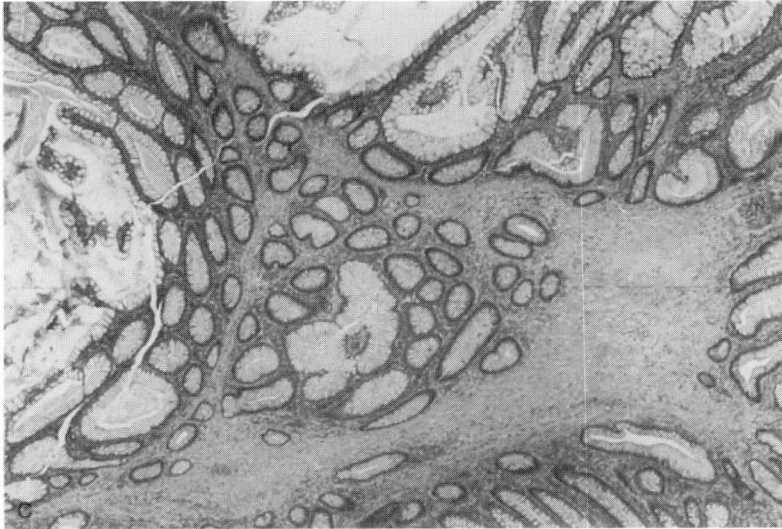

Figure 45.16. Peutz-Jeghers syndrome. *(A)* Gross specimen of a Peutz-Jeghers polyp illustrating a large, multilobular lesion. *(B)* Low-power photomicrograph of a Peutz-Jeghers polyp of the colon revealing smooth-muscle stroma covered by non-neoplastic colonic epithelium. *(C)* Photomicrograph of the Peutz-Jeghers polyp at higher power indicates that the stroma contains arborizing bands of smooth muscle.

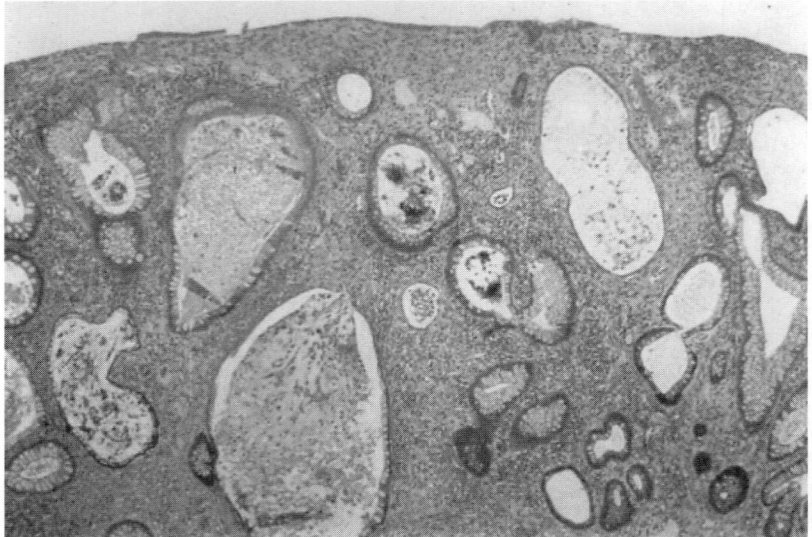

Figure 45.17. Photomicrograph of a juvenile polyp reveals an attenuated surface epithelium overlying an edematous lamina propria with fluid- and mucus-filled cystic structures.

Juvenile Polyposis

Juvenile polyps are pathologically characteristic lesions that can be solitary or part of a polyposis syndrome. Juvenile polyps are most commonly solitary lesions found in the rectum during childhood. The lesions may be large and are made up of an edematous, mildly inflamed lamina propria covered by normal colonic epithelium (Fig. 45.17). If multiple polyps are found, a familial juvenile polyposis syndrome should be suspected. Three different syndromic presentations have been reported; it is not known, however, whether these are truly distinctive syndromes. They may consist of familial juvenile polyposis limited to the colon, familial juvenile polyposis throughout the gastrointestinal tract, and familial juvenile polyposis limited to the stomach. The genetic basis of this syndrome is not understood, but germline mutations in a gene *(SMAD4)* located on chromosome 18q21.1 that encodes an intracellular mediator in the TGF-β signaling pathway has been identified in some affected patients (Table 45.2). The *PTEN* gene located on chromosome 10 has also been linked to some cases.

The manifestations of juvenile polyposis can vary but are largely limited to bleeding, intussusception, obstruction, and the passage of autoamputated lesions. In some children, a life-threatening protein-losing enteropathy may develop that requires surgical resection of the affected segment of intestine. Patients with familial juvenile polyposis are at some increased risk for the development of colorectal cancer. It has been suggested that the presence of mixed juvenile and adenomatous polyps indicates which lesions are premalignant. It is important that the pathologist examine lesions carefully for the presence of adenomatous tissue in such polyps. When mixed lesions are found, patients in these families should be subjected to colonoscopic surveillance, perhaps as often as every 2 years.

Other Familial Polyposis Syndromes

A variety of other rare syndromes may give rise to multiple gastrointestinal polyps (34). Cowden's syndrome consists of multiple gastrointestinal hamartomas and may be complicated by multiple lesions of the face that arise from follicular epithelium and are pathologically trichilemmomas. The diagnosis of Cowden's syndrome should be considered for patients with multiple trichilemmomas. Gastrointestinal polyps, which are usually asymptomatic, may develop in these patients. The polyps include a variety of hamartomas, such as hyperplastic polyps and ganglioneuromas of the colon. Glycogenic acanthosis of the esophagus may also occur and usually is found incidentally as multiple, diminutive, flat polyps of the esophagus. These patients are at increased risk for the development of breast cancer and a variety of benign and malignant complications of the thyroid gland. No specific therapy need be directed toward the gastrointestinal tract. It is of interest that a germline mutation of the *PTEN* gene on chromosome 10q has been identified in most families with Cowden's syndrome; this is the same locus affecting some families with juvenile polyposis.

Other diseases, such as neurofibromatosis (von Recklinghausen's syndrome) and the basal cell nevus syndrome, may be associated with multiple gastrointestinal polyps; however, symptomatic complications of these polyps are uncommon. Bannayan-Riley-Ruvalcaba syndrome is a generalized hamartoma syndrome inherited in an autosomal dominant manner that is characterized by ileal and colonic polyps and lingual lesions. Other characteristics include ocular abnormalities, delayed motor development, lipid storage myopathy, and Hashimoto's disease. This disease is also linked to germline mutations in the *PTEN* gene and appears to be a variant of familial juvenile polyposis.

Nonfamilial Gastrointestinal Polyposis Syndromes

Multiple gastrointestinal polyps are occasionally seen in nonfamilial syndromes. The Cronkhite-Canada syndrome is an acquired, nonfamilial syndrome characterized by cutaneous lesions (Fig. 45.18), chronic diarrhea, protein-losing enteropathy, and gastrointestinal polyps. The enteropathy may produce progressive inanition that can result in death. The diarrhea is attributable to diffuse mucosal injury of the small intestine but may be complicated by bacterial overgrowth. Gastrointestinal polyps are present in most patients and occur in the stomach, small intestine, colon, and rectum. These polyps are pathologically similar to juvenile retention-type polyps. The lamina propria is edematous and contains an inflammatory infiltrate. As has been reported in juvenile polyps, the lesions in this syndrome may contain adenomatous epithelium, and occasionally carcinomas have

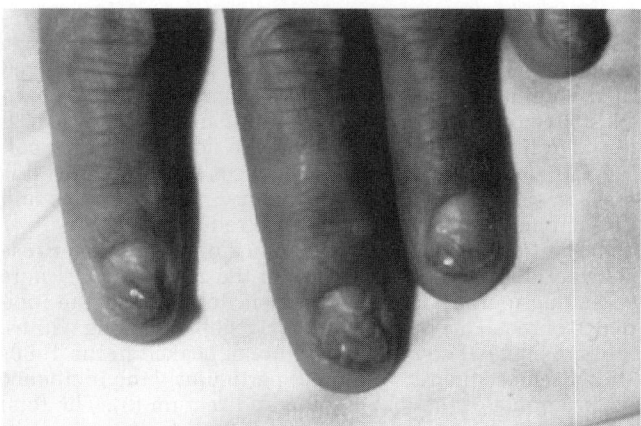

Figure 45.18. Cronkhite-Canada syndrome. Onycholysis and hyperpigmentation are characteristic cutaneous manifestations of Cronkhite-Canada syndrome, a nonfamilial, poorly understood, acquired condition in which multiple juvenile, inflammatory-type gastrointestinal polyps and characteristic cutaneous features are found.

complicated this disease. A variety of medical and surgical measures have been used as treatment, and primary attention should be drawn to the treatment of the diarrhea and maintenance of the nutritional status. The cutaneous lesions consist of onycholysis, alopecia, and hyperpigmentation. In a number of cases, treatment of the bacterial overgrowth with antibiotics and maintenance of the nutritional status have resulted in complete resolution of the cutaneous features. Curiously, the cutaneous features may resolve despite persistence of the gastrointestinal polyps.

Other acquired lesions that may present with multiple gastrointestinal polyps include inflammatory pseudo-polyps in the setting of inflammatory bowel disease, lymphoma, pneumatosis cystoides intestinalis, and multiple lipomas or hyperplastic polyps. None of these syndromes requires specific surgical treatment.

REFERENCES

1. Kinzler KW, Vogelstein B. Lessons from hereditary colon cancer. *Cell* 1996;87:159.
2. Grady WM, Markowitz S. Genomic instability and colorectal cancer. *Curr Opin Gastroenterol* 2000;16:62–67.
3. Gryfe R, Hyejc K, Hsieh ETK, et al. Tumor microsatellite instability and clinical outcome in young patients with colorectal cancer. *N Engl J Med* 2000;342:69.
4. Spirio L, Olschwang S, Groden J, et al. Alleles of the APC gene: an attenuated form of familial polyposis. *Cell* 1993;755:951.
5. Morin P, Sparks AB, Korinek V, et al. Activation of β-catenin-Tcf signaling in colon cancer by mutations in β-catenin or APC. *Science* 1997;275:1787.
6. Martinez-Lopez E, Abad A, Fort A, et al. Allelic loss on chromosome 18q as a prognostic marker in stage II colorectal cancer. *Gastroenterology* 1998;114:1180.
7. Boland CR. Hereditary non-polyposis colorectal cancer. In: Vogelstein B, Kinzler K, eds. *The genetic basis of human cancer.* New York: McGraw-Hill, 1998:333–346.
8. Grady W, Myerhoff LL, Swinler SE, et al. Mutational inactivation of transforming growth factor-b receptor type II in microsatellite stable cancers. *Cancer Res* 1999;59:320.
9. Shinya H, Wolff WI. Morphology, anatomic distribution, and cancer potential of colonic polyps. *Ann Surg* 1979;1990:675.
10. Neugat AO, Jacobson JS, Ahsan H, et al. Incidence and recurrence rates of colorectal adenomas: a prospective study. *Gastroenterology* 1995;108:402.
11. Fuchs CS, Giovanni EC, Colditz GA, et al. A prospective study of family history and the risk of colorectal cancer. *N Engl J Med* 1994;331:1669.
12. Winawer SJ, Zauber AG, Gerdas H, et al. Risk of colorectal cancer in families of patients with adenomatous polyps. *N Engl J Med* 1996;334:82.
13. Syngal S, Fox EA, Li C, et al. Interpretation of genetic test results for hereditary nonpolyposis colorectal cancer. *JAMA* 1999;282:247.
14. Boland CR, Thibodeau SN, Hamilton SR, et al. A National Cancer Institute Workshop on microsatellite instability for cancer detection and familial predisposition: development of international criteria for the determination of microsatellite instability in colorectal cancer. *Cancer Res* 1998;58:5248.
15. Mandel JS, Bond JH, Church TR, et al. Reducing mortality from colorectal cancer by screening for fecal occult blood. *N Engl J Med* 1993;328:1365.
16. Mandel J, Church TR, Ederer F, et al. Colorectal cancer mortality: effectiveness of biennial screening for fecal occult blood. *J Natl Cancer Inst* 1999;91:434.
17. Winawer SJ, Zauber AG, Ho MN, et al. Prevention of colorectal cancer by colonoscopic polypectomy. *N Engl J Med* 1993;329:1977.
18. Byers T, Levin B, Rothenberger D, et al. American Cancer Society guidelines for screening and surveillance for early detection of colorectal polyps and cancer: update 1997. *CA Cancer J Clin* 1997;47:154.
19. Winawer SJ, Fletcher RH, Miller L, et al. Colorectal cancer screening guidelines and rationale. *Gastroenterology* 1997;112:594.
20. Selby JV, Friedman GD, Quesenberry C, et al. A case-control study of screening sigmoidoscopy and mortality for colorectal cancer. *N Engl J Med* 1992;326:653.
21. Cooper HS, Deppisch LM, Gourley WK, et al. Endoscopically removed malignant polyps: clinicopathologic correlations. *Gastroenterology* 1995;108:1657.
22. Atkin WS, Morson BC, Cuzick J. Long-term risk of colorectal cancer after excision of rectosigmoid adenomas. *N Engl J Med* 1992;326:658.
23. Schoenfeld PS, Ash B, Kita J, et al. Effectiveness and patient satisfaction with screening flexible sigmoidoscopy by registered nurses. *Gastrointest Endosc* 1999;341:158.
24. Fenlon HM, Nunes DP, Schroy PC, et al. A comparison of virtual and conventional colonoscopy for detection of colorectal polyps. *N Engl J Med* 1999;341:1996.
25. Winawer SJ, Zauber AG, O'Brien MJ, et al. Randomized comparison of surveillance intervals after colonoscopic removal of newly diagnosed adenomatous polyps. *N Engl J Med* 1993;328:901.
26. Giavannucci E, Rimm EB, Stampfer MJ, et al. Aspirin use and the risk for colorectal cancer and adenoma in male health professionals. *Ann Intern Med* 1994;121:241.
27. Oshima M, Dinchuk JE, Oshima H, et al. Suppression of intestinal polyposis in Apc^{D716} knockout mice by inhibition of cyclooxygenase-2 (COX-2). *Cell* 1996;87:803.
28. Baron J, Beach M, Mandel JS, et al. Calcium supplements for prevention of colorectal adenomas. *N Engl J Med* 1999;340:101.
29. Nagase H, Miyoshi Y, Horii A, et al. Correlation between the location of germ-line mutations in the APC gene and the number of colorectal polyps in familial adenomatous polyposis patients. *Cancer Res* 1992;52:4055.
30. Powell SM, Petersen GM, Krush AJ, et al. Molecular diagnosis of familial adenomatous polyposis. *N Engl J Med* 1993;329:1982.
31. Giardello FM, Brensinger JD, Petersen GM, et al. The use and interpretation of commercial APC gene testing for familial adenomatous polyposis. *N Engl J Med* 1997;336:823.
32. Giardiello FM, Hamilton SR, Krush AJ, et al. Treatment of colonic and rectal adenomas with sulindac in familial adenomatous polyposis. *N Engl J Med* 1993;328:1313.
33. Giardiello FM, Welsh SB, Hamilton SR, et al. Increased risk of cancer in the Peutz-Jeghers syndrome. *N Engl J Med* 1987;316:1511.
34. Marra G, Armelao F, Vecchio FM, et al. Cowden's disease with extensive gastrointestinal polyposis. *J Clin Gastroenterol* 1994;18:42.

SURGERY: SCIENTIFIC PRINCIPLES AND PRACTICE, Third Edition, edited by
Lazar J. Greenfield, Michael W. Mulholland, Keith T. Oldham, Gerald B. Zelenock,
and Keith D. Lillemoe. Lippincott Williams & Wilkins Publishers, Philadelphia, © 2001.

CHAPTER 46

COLORECTAL CANCER

ALAN M. YAHANDA AND ALFRED E. CHANG

Adenocarcinoma of the large intestine is the fourth most common malignancy in the United States, with approximately 130,000 new cases diagnosed annually (1). Malignancies more prevalent than colorectal cancer are those of the prostate, breast, and lung, in decreasing order. Nevertheless, colorectal carcinoma is the second leading cause of all cancer-related deaths after lung cancer. Approximately 57,000 persons die each year in the United States of colorectal cancer. If diagnosed in its early stages, however, this malignancy is curable by surgical treatment with minimal morbidity and mortality.

Because of the potential for cure of early-stage disease, the definition of populations at risk and screening of asymptomatic patients are important considerations. Controlled clinical trials have demonstrated that the multidisciplinary approach to the treatment of localized colorectal cancer has decreased the morbidity and mortality associated with this disease. For recurrent disease, various therapeutic approaches are reviewed. Other colorectal tumors, such as lymphomas, sarcomas, and carcinoid tumors, are distinct from adenocarcinoma and are discussed separately at the end of the chapter.

EPIDEMIOLOGY

Worldwide, colorectal cancer ties with breast cancer as the third most frequent cancer, after gastric and lung cancers (2). An important feature of colorectal cancer is the wide variation in incidence (as much as 30-fold) noted between population groups according to geographic region (Fig. 46.1). These differences do not appear to be solely the result of genetic factors because populations migrating from low- to high-incidence regions experience an increase in the rate of colorectal cancer. Such data provide indirect evidence that environmental factors are involved in the pathogenesis of this disease. Industrialized countries have the highest incidence rates, and numerous studies have linked dietary factors to the development of colorectal cancer (see later). Evidence suggests that this disease may be responsive to dietary manipulations and that its incidence may therefore be reducible.

In the United States, the incidence of colon cancer rose substantially in the second half of the 20th century, more so among men than among women. In contrast, the incidence of rectal carcinoma was fairly stable. Among whites, the incidence of colorectal carcinoma peaked in the 1980s and has subsequently declined, particularly the incidence of carcinoma of the distal colon and rectum (3). The total rates for colorectal carcinoma shifted from an excess among whites to an excess among blacks by the late 1980s. Blacks have not experienced the recent decline in incidence observed in whites. Within a study period of 1975 to 1994, the rates of carcinoma of the proximal colon were higher than those of the distal colon or rectum (3). Furthermore, the rates of carcinoma of the proximal colon in black Americans were considerably higher than those in whites and continue to increase, whereas the rates in whites showed signs of declining during the period of 1975 to 1994. The decline in incidence rates among whites has been attributed to widespread screening for colorectal carcinoma. The explanation for the increased incidence of proximal cancers in blacks is unknown at this time.

In North America, the pattern of geographic regions with a substantially increased risk does not suggest the presence of an important carcinogenic agent, although the incidence of colorectal cancers tends to be greater in urban populations and people of higher socioeconomic status. In addition, no high-risk occupations have been found consistently, and smoking does not play an etiologic role.

ETIOLOGY

Dietary Factors

Evidence from epidemiologic studies suggests that dietary factors play important causative and protective roles in the development of large-bowel cancers. Fat intake has

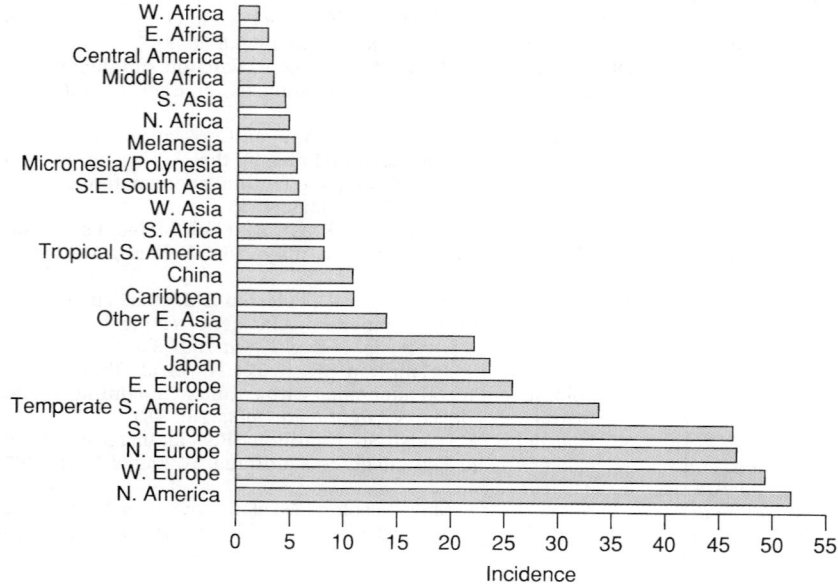

Figure 46.1. Incidence of colorectal cancer per 100,000 persons in 23 geographic regions during 1980. (After Parkin DM, Laara E, Muir CS. Estimates of the worldwide frequency of sixteen major cancers in 1980. *Int J Cancer* 1988;41:184, with permission.)

been the most consistently positive association and fiber intake the most consistently inverse association noted in the incidence of colorectal cancer.

In comparisons between countries, the rates of colon cancer are strongly associated with the intake of animal fat and meat (4) (Fig. 46.2). The associations between per capita consumption of total fat, saturated fat, and cholesterol and the national incidence rates of colon cancer are strongly positive (5). The proposed mechanism by which dietary fat increases the risk for colonic cancer is its interaction with bile acids, discussed in more detail later.

The relation between fiber intake and colon cancer was initially noted by Burkitt (6), who reported low rates of colon cancer in areas of Africa where fiber consumption and stool bulk are high. In general, epidemiologic studies have demonstrated that fiber intake is higher in nonindustrialized countries with lower incidence rates of colon cancer. However, in countries where fiber intake is high, the intake of fat and frequently the life expectancy also tend to be lower, so that confounding variables are introduced. The role of fiber was originally seen simply as the provision of bulk to dilute potential carcinogens and speed their transit through the colon. Data now suggest that this is an oversimplification and that the relation between fiber intake and colon cancer is more complex. Certain fibers can bind mutagens, reducing their contact with colonic epithelium; others can favorably change the fecal pH or participate in other complex interactions.

The difficulty in sorting out the association of fiber intake with risk for colon cancer reflects the heterogeneous nature of fiber, the nondigestible component of carbohydrates. Fiber is derived from cereal products, vegetables, and fruit. Dietary fiber comprises a diverse collection of carbohydrates that are unlikely to have identical physiologic effects. Although the role of fiber in protecting against colorectal cancer is strong, the specific foods related to this effect are poorly defined.

Mutagenesis

Carcinogenesis in the colon and rectum has been described in terms of an initiation–promotion model based on experimental observations in laboratory animals. According to this model, the first step involves initiating factors that directly interact with cellular DNA to induce mutations in the genome. Afterward, the process is driven by promotional factors, which are not mutagenic by themselves but enhance cellular proliferation of previously mutated cells. Although this concept represents an oversim-

plification of a complex, multiple-step process, it serves as a useful framework to understand data generated from animal models examining the pathogenesis of large-bowel cancer. One can enhance or reduce tumorigenesis in experimental animals both by maneuvers that modify the generation of a mutagen (or carcinogen) and by those that alter promotional factors long after the administration of an initiating agent.

The human diet contains a myriad of naturally occurring mutagens or substances that can be metabolized into mutagens. A wide range of such substances are generated from interactions between the diet, microbial flora, and colonic mucosal enzymes. In addition, protective mechanisms are present throughout the mucosa to detoxify these compounds. The action of carcinogens on DNA appears not to be an entirely random process. Mutagens typically alkylate DNA at specific carbon residues and cause nucleotide misreading during the next cycle of DNA replication. A mutation commonly seen early in colonic carcinogenesis results in activation of the *ras* protooncogene, one of several genetic events presumed to occur during malignant transformation (7). The activation of *ras* may be involved in the initiation or promotion of carcinogenesis. Because of the ubiquitous presence of mutagens in the gut, many strategies that aim to reduce colon cancer attempt to interfere with the interaction between mutagens and the target colonic cells.

In animal studies, the role of fat in the pathogenesis of colon cancer appears to be that of a promotional factor. With increasing fat intake, total fecal bile acid increases significantly. Available data suggest that bile acids stimulate the generation of reactive oxygen metabolites that enhance the conversion of unsaturated fatty acids to compounds that promote cellular proliferation. Theoretically, this would facilitate the emergence of a mutated clone of neoplastic cells. Enhanced proliferation of these transformed cells can either compress the time required for carcinogenesis or, perhaps, make the process more efficient. An extension of this concept is the observation that increased dietary calcium has been associated with a decreased risk for colorectal cancer. Experimental data demonstrate that an increase in dietary calcium tends to inhibit colonic proliferative indices.

Molecular Genetics

The molecular genetic events that lead to colorectal cancer have served as a paradigm for the multiple-step process of tumorigenesis. This concept arose from frequently clinical and pathologic observations of an orderly

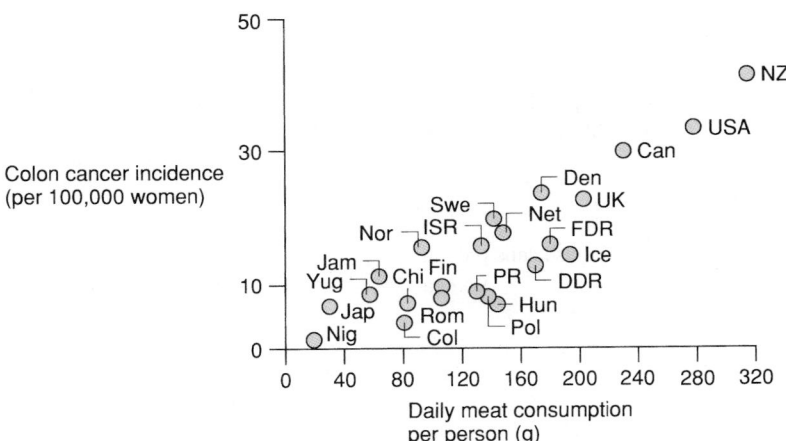

Figure 46.2. Correlation between meat intake and the incidence of colon cancer among women in 23 countries. (After Willett W. The search for the causes of breast and colon cancer. *Nature* 1989;338: 389, with permission.)

progression of cellular transformation from normal colonic or rectal epithelium to small adenoma, then to large adenoma, and finally to carcinoma. These rather distinct stages have allowed scientists to elucidate the genetic alterations that may be responsible for the progression of the neoplastic process. Coincident with this line of investigation was the discovery of the genetic basis of several familial cancer syndromes in which colorectal cancer is a prominent feature of the phenotype. When taken together, the evidence suggests that colorectal cancers result from a series of genetic alterations leading to progressive disordering of the normal mechanisms that control cellular growth and differentiation (Fig. 46.3). It should be recognized that not every colorectal tumor will acquire each of the mutations described. Furthermore, other genetic events are likely to be necessary for cancer formation, and each tumor may have a unique genetic profile. Such a model of multiple-step tumorigenesis, however, helps us to understand better the complex molecular genetics of cancer. Within this paradigm, mutations in three distinct types of genes are known to contribute to colorectal cancer formation: oncogenes, tumor-suppressor genes, and DNA mismatch repair genes.

In colon cancer, an important genetic alteration that has been demonstrated is a mutation of the K-*ras* protooncogene. The *ras* protooncogenes are a family of normal genes (N-*ras*, H-*ras*, and K-*ras*) that are highly conserved in nature and encode the production of guanosine triphosphate-binding proteins (G proteins), which are important for signal transduction. G proteins are involved in the transduction of proliferative signals induced by growth factors or factors involved in cell differentiation. The product of a mutated *ras* gene is an abnormal G protein that becomes constitutively activated and continuously stimulates autonomous cell growth. Experimentally, transfection of normal fibroblasts by mutated *ras* genes confers neoplastic properties to those cells.

About half of colorectal carcinomas and a similar percentage of adenomas larger than 1 cm in diameter have been found to have the *ras* gene mutation (7,8). By contrast, fewer than 10% of adenomas smaller than 1 cm have this mutation. The *ras* gene mutation may be the initiating event in some colorectal carcinomas or, alternatively, may promote the clonal expansion of a mutated cell population. It appears that the *ras* gene mutation alone is not responsible for tumorigenesis. Other molecular events are required in addition to *ras* gene mutations.

The concept of tumor-suppressor genes arose from several observations. Cytogenetic studies demonstrated that tumor cells often have losses of specific chromosomal regions and suggested that loss of a particular gene or genes could contribute to tumor formation and progression. Conversely, experimental evidence documented that replacement of specific chromosomes or portions of chromosomes in tumor cells could result in inhibition of growth. It was thus deduced that genes exist that function to keep cellular growth and proliferation in check, and that their loss results in unregulated growth and neoplastic transformation. One such tumor-suppressor gene associated with colon cancer is the *APC* (adenomatous polyposis coli) gene, mutations in which result in the familial cancer syndrome, familial adenomatous polyposis (FAP). In persons affected with FAP, hundreds to thousands of colorectal adenomatous polyps develop, all of which have the potential to progress to a cancer. The lifetime risk for the development of colon cancer is virtually 100% (9). When linkage analysis was performed in families with FAP, the *APC* gene was mapped to chromosome 5q21 and was subsequently cloned by several groups (10,11). The *APC* gene encodes a large protein of 2,843 amino acids that contains a number of functional domains. A key function of the protein is to bind and thereby decrease intracellular levels of β-catenin. Mutations of the *APC* gene that result in loss of this binding function lead to an increase in free β-catenin, which then activates the expression of other genes involved in cellular growth (12,13).

Mutations of the *APC* gene are also commonly found in sporadic cases of colorectal cancer. Approximately 70% of all sporadic cases of colorectal cancer have such mutations. Among those cancers in which *APC* is not mutated, a number have mutations in β-catenin that disrupt its ability to bind to the APC protein, and as such, they are phenotypically similar to those in which *APC* is mutated (13,14). Mutations in the *APC* gene appear to be an early or initiating event in sporadic colorectal cancer, as mutations in the gene have been identified in aberrant crypt foci, one of the earliest events in the neoplastic proliferation of colonic mucosa (15).

Mutation or loss of the *p53* tumor-suppressor gene, located on chromosome 17p, is another common genetic event in colorectal cancer. Although *p53* mutations have been found in 75% of sporadic colorectal cancers, they are seen infrequently in earlier lesions, which suggests that inactivation of *p53* is an important event in the transition

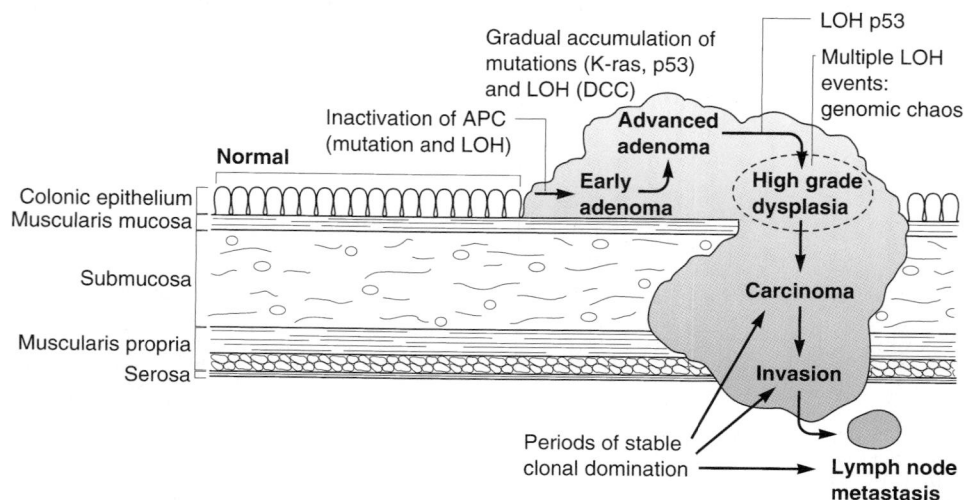

Figure 46.3. Model of genetic events mediating neoplastic progression in the colon. *LOH,* loss of heterozygosity. (After C. R. Boland, University of Michigan, Ann Arbor, MI, with permission.)

from adenoma to carcinoma. The *p53* gene codes for a 393-amino acid phosphoprotein that has the ability to bind to DNA in a sequence-specific manner. When bound to DNA, the p53 protein can activate the expression of certain genes that are presumed to participate in growth inhibition. Mutations that disrupt this ability to bind DNA result in a decrease in the expression of growth-inhibitory genes and an increase in cellular proliferation (16). Germline mutations in *p53* are responsible for the Li-Fraumeni syndrome. Interestingly, colorectal cancer is not a prominent feature of the phenotype.

Chromosome 18q21 appears to have an important role in the development of colorectal cancer, as allelic loss of this region is observed in many cases. The clinical importance of such a loss is controversial; one report has identified 18q21 allelic loss as an independent negative prognostic factor in patients with stage II tumors, whereas others have failed to identify such an association (17,18). Several candidate tumor-suppressor genes have been identified on chromosome 18q21, including deleted in colon cancer *(DCC),* deleted in pancreatic cancer locus 4 *(DPC4)* and mad-related *(smad2)* genes. The role of these genes and others in the 18q21 region in colorectal tumorigenesis is not well defined. Investigation has been hampered by the inability to identify a significant number of mutations in any of these genes in sporadic colon cancers and by the lack of any familial syndromes in which germline mutations can be identified.

A third mechanism that has been implicated in colorectal tumorigenesis involves disruption of the normal surveillance for and repair of DNA damage. Maintaining the fidelity of the genome during DNA replication and cell division is of paramount importance for the normal growth and development of an organism. Ordinarily, cells have numerous mechanisms that constantly survey DNA for damage or replication errors and, if present, repair them. In this manner, the integrity of the genome is ensured, and the accumulation and propagation of mutations is minimized. If these survey and repair mechanisms are defective, genetic instability and accelerated rates of mutation follow. If such mutations result in the activation of oncogenes or the inactivation of tumor-suppressor genes, affected cells gain a growth advantage.

In the early 1990s, several investigators observed that a subset of colorectal tumors have widespread instability in microsatellite repeats in tumor DNA, and that such instability is present in the tumors of many patients affected by familial nonpolyposis colorectal cancer (HNPCC) (19–21). Simultaneously, bacterial and yeast geneticists described a set of DNA repair enzymes, termed *DNA mismatch repair enzymes,* that function to excise and repair nucleotide base mismatches that occur during DNA replication. The connection between DNA mismatch repair enzymes and HNPCC was solidified when it was found that tumor cells from patients with HNPCC lack DNA mismatch repair activity in vitro (22). Subsequently, the first human mismatch repair homologue, *hMSH2,* was cloned and was found to be mutated in many patients with HNPCC (23,24). Soon thereafter, a second human homologue of a mismatch repair enzyme, *hMLH1,* was cloned and demonstrated to be altered in a subset of patients with HNPCC who had normal *hMSH2* (25,26).

It is now thought that DNA mismatch repair in the eukaryotic cell requires the participation of at least four other enzymes in addition to *hMSH2* and *hMLH1.* These additional enzymes include *hPMS1, hPMS2, hMSH6* (formerly called *GTBP*), and *hMSH3* (27). Together, these enzymes form a complex that performs the many aspects of the DNA mismatch repair process. The strongest mutator phenotypes, as measured by microsatellite instability, are observed with mutations in either *hMSH2* or *hMLH1,*

which suggests that the other enzymes play a less significant role in the process or that some redundancy in their function may exist. This, in fact, is the case with *hMSH3* and *hMSH6;* functional overlap between the two may attenuate the mutator phenotype resulting from a mutation in one or the other (28,29). Also consistent with this concept is the observation that more than 60% of the mutations found in HNPCC kindreds are in either *hMSH2* or *hMLH1.*

Delineation of the molecular genetic alterations responsible for colorectal tumor development has defined much of our current understanding of the multiple-step process of tumorigenesis. Yet despite these discoveries, an even greater number of questions remain to be answered. For example, among individuals who carry mutations in the APC gene, there is a wide variability in the phenotype; those affected with mutations that preserve the β-catenin binding domain may manifest a much more attenuated, or even absent, polyposis phenotype. What accounts for such variability, and how will this impact on clinical management? Clearly, there are a myriad of interacting and modifying factors that contribute to the ultimate phenotype, with each being expressed to varying degrees in affected individuals. It is the elucidation of these interacting pathways that will be paramount to our understanding of colorectal cancer and to the design of more specific treatment or prevention strategies.

CLINICAL RISK FACTORS

Familial Cancer Syndromes

The vast majority of colorectal cancer cases have no apparent familial association and, as such, are considered truly sporadic. Epidemiologic studies have suggested that at least 15% of all colorectal cancers occur in a dominantly inherited pattern, and that an inherited susceptibility to polyps and cancer could account for up to 90% of the total number of colorectal cancers in the population (30,31). The two best-described familial colorectal cancer syndromes are FAP and HNPCC. Currently, it is estimated that 3% to 5% of all colorectal cancers occur in persons affected with one of these two syndromes (Table 46.1).

Table 46.1. CLINICAL RISK FACTORS FOR COLORECTAL CANCER

GENETIC

Polyposis syndromes

Familial polyposis coli
Gardner's syndrome
Turcot syndrome (CNS tumors)
Oldfield's syndrome (sebaceous cysts)
Peutz-Jeghers syndrome (hamartomas)

Nonpolyposis syndromes

Lynch syndrome I
Lynch syndrome II (associated extracolonic cancers)

Preexisting disease

Ulcerative colitis
Crohn's disease
Prior colorectal cancer
Neoplastic polyps
Pelvic irradiation
Breast or genital tract cancer

GENERAL

Age >40 y
Family history of colorectal cancer

CNS, central nervous system.

Familial adenomatous polyposis is an autosomal, dominantly inherited disease caused by mutations in the *APC* gene. In affected subjects, hundreds to thousands of adenomatous polyps typically develop throughout the colon and rectum, each of which has the potential to progress to an invasive cancer. The average age for the diagnosis of colorectal cancer is 42 years, markedly earlier than the average age of 63 years in sporadic cases. Cancer develops in virtually all affected persons by age 55. Polyps are also found in other regions of the gastrointestinal tract in patients with FAP, the most common locations being the duodenum and stomach. Polyps of the stomach have little propensity to progress to cancer. The duodenal and periampullary polyps, however, are associated with an increased risk for the development of cancer (32,33). Additionally, a number of extraintestinal manifestations of FAP have been described, including congenital hypertrophy of the retinal pigment epithelium (CHRPE), osteomas, and desmoid tumors. This and other polyposis syndromes are discussed in more detail in the preceding chapter.

The first description of HNPCC kindreds was made by Aldred Warthin, a pathologist at the University of Michigan, in 1913. One of these kindreds, referred to as *family G*, has been followed extensively through the years and represents a classic example of the HNPCC syndrome (34,35). A more systematic collection of families and analysis of their pedigrees was performed by Henry Lynch and coworkers at Creighton University. It was recognized that although colorectal cancer is the most predominant cancer in the syndrome, an associated polyposis phenotype is not seen, as it is in patients with FAP. For this reason, the syndrome was given the "nonpolyposis" designation. Two phenotypic variants of HNPCC have been described: Lynch syndromes I and II. Lynch syndrome I families manifest only colon cancer. Lynch syndrome II families manifest colon cancer in addition to a number of others, including endometrial, gastric, small-bowel, breast, liver and biliary tract, upper urologic tract, and central nervous system cancers. The median age for the development of either colorectal or endometrial cancer in HNPCC patients is 46 years (36). The penetrance of HNPCC is not accurately known, although with respect to colorectal cancer, it is certainly less than that of FAP. An unusual clinical variant of HNPCC is the Muir-Torre syndrome, in which affected members have sebaceous tumors (both benign and malignant) and keratoacanthomas in addition to the spectrum of tumors found in Lynch syndrome II.

The clinical criteria necessary for identifying a family as an HNPCC kindred were established by an international collaborative group meeting in Amsterdam in 1990. These criteria, termed the *Amsterdam criteria,* include the following: at least three relatives with histologically verified colorectal cancer, with at least one being a first-degree relative of the other two; exclusion of FAP; at least two successive generations affected; and diagnosis of colorectal cancer in one of the relatives before the age of 50 years (37). These criteria have been criticized for their failure to recognize the extracolonic cancers that may be found in HNPCC kindreds and, as such, are felt to be too narrow. This is supported by the finding that not all genetically proven HNPCC families satisfy the Amsterdam criteria.

What patients, then, should one suspect to be part of an HNPCC kindred? Certainly, the likelihood of having a mutation in a mismatch repair gene is high if all Amsterdam criteria are strictly met. Conversely, the frequency of mutations is low in families in which the criteria are not fully met (38). Other clinical factors not included in the Amsterdam criteria that are associated with an increased likelihood of mismatch repair gene mutations include the following: diagnosis of colorectal cancer at an early age, occurrence of endometrial or small-bowel cancer in the kindred, occurrence of colorectal cancer or endometrial cancer in multiple members, and the presence of multiple colorectal cancers or both colorectal cancer and endometrial cancer in the same family member (39). The tumors of patients in families that do not strictly meet the Amsterdam criteria, yet have any of these other risk factors, should be tested for microsatellite instability, and if the result is positive, should be subjected to further genetic analysis (40).

Recently, a novel type of mutation was described that by itself does not result in a tumor phenotype but indirectly confers a predisposition for the development of colorectal cancer. A single base pair alteration was identified in the *APC* gene that results in the substitution of a lysine for an isoleucine at codon 1,307. This mutation does not alter the function of the encoded protein but does produce an extended mononucleotide tract that becomes a hypermutable region of the gene. It was hypothesized that this unstable region of the gene leads to a higher rate of detrimental somatic mutations and cancer. The 1,307 mutation has been found in 6% of Ashkenazi Jews and in 28% of Ashkenazim with a family history of colorectal cancer (41).

In the future, more and more patients with cancer will be determined to have a responsible hereditary defect in either a specific tumor gene or in a modifying gene that imparts a predisposition to cancer. Obtaining a thorough family history is now a necessity in the workup of any patient with cancer, especially one with onset at a young age or with multiple tumors. The easy availability of genetic testing by many commercial laboratories has been problematic, as most physicians are not prepared to interpret the results or to counsel patients regarding their cancer risk and treatment. In a study of patients undergoing genetic testing for familial polyposis by a commercial company, it was found that only 19% of patients received genetic counseling before the test, and in 32% of cases, the physician ordering the test misinterpreted the results (42). Although most problems with misinterpretation are encountered with negative results, the interpretation of a positive result also can be difficult. It must be emphasized that a negative result can provide reassurance only if the predisposing mutation in the family is already known. Otherwise, a negative result may mean that the mutation was missed, that it occurred in a promoter or intronic sequence not evaluated, or that a cancer predisposition still exists because of a mutation in another known or unknown disease gene (43). In the case of a positive result, one must be sure that the mutation does in fact confer a cancer risk and that it is not merely a benign polymorphism. Therefore, when identified, patients suspected of having an inherited cancer syndrome should be offered counseling by a cancer geneticist or experienced genetic counselor, both before the test is ordered and after the results are known.

Inflammatory Bowel Disease

A strong association exists between inflammatory bowel disease and bowel cancer. For patients with ulcerative colitis, the incidence of malignancy is proportional to the extent of colonic involvement, age at onset, and severity and duration of disease. The duration of inflammatory bowel disease is a critical factor in predicting the likelihood of adenocarcinoma. Cancer develops in about 3% of patients during the first 10 years after the onset of colitis, and in an additional 20% during each of the next two decades. The cure rate in patients with ulcerative colitis who are treated for cancer is similar to that in noncolitic patients treated for cancer (44).

Patients with Crohn's disease are also at increased risk for colon cancer in addition to small-bowel cancer. The risk for malignancy is lower than that reported for ulcerative colitis. Like the cancers associated with ulcerative colitis, the cancers associated with Crohn's disease tend to occur at an earlier age than those in patients without inflammatory bowel disease.

Polyps

Colorectal polyps can be divided into two broad categories: neoplastic and non-neoplastic. Non-neoplastic polyps include hyperplastic, inflammatory, juvenile, and hamartomatous polyps, none of which are precursors to colorectal cancer. Neoplastic polyps are adenomas and have the potential to develop into malignant cancers. The incidence of colorectal malignancy is two to five times higher in patients with adenomatous polyps than in those without them. Carcinoma is twice as likely to develop in patients with multiple polyps as in patients with a single polyp. Evidence suggests the existence of a common inherited susceptibility toward both sporadic colonic adenomatous polyps and colorectal cancer (30).

Adenomas can be classified as tubular (75% to 100% tubular components), tubulovillous (25% to 75% villous components), or villous (75% to 100% villous components). Tubular adenomas, or adenomatous polyps, are the most common type and constitute about 75% of neoplastic polyps (45) (Table 46.2). Tubulovillous adenomas account for 15% and purely villous adenomas for 10% of neoplastic polyps. All adenomas contain some degree of dysplasia or cellular atypia, which can be graded from mild to severe. Carcinoma in situ and severe dysplasia have been grouped together under the classification of high-grade dysplasia. In contrast to invasive carcinoma, carcinoma in situ has not invaded the muscularis mucosae (Fig. 46.4). The incidence of invasive malignancy differs markedly for the three types of adenomas and increases with the size of the adenoma. In general, malignancies are seen in 5% of adenomatous polyps, in 22% of tubulovillous adenomas, and in 40% of villous lesions. Although villous lesions are much less common, they are more likely to harbor a malignancy.

Other Risk Factors

People older than 40 years of age have an increased risk for colorectal cancer, and this risk increases proportionally to the eighth decade. Patients who have received irradiation for gynecologic cancer have a twofold to threefold increased risk for the development of colorectal cancer. Patients with previously resected colorectal cancer have a threefold increased risk for the development of a second

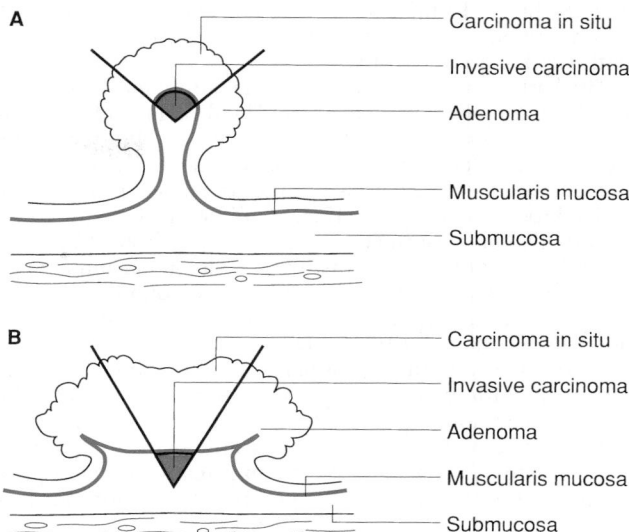

Figure 46.4. Anatomic distinction between carcinoma in situ and invasive malignancy in a pedunculated *(A)* and a sessile *(B)* adenomatous polyp. Carcinoma in situ is characterized by the absence of invasion into the muscularis mucosae.

primary large-bowel cancer. Women with breast or genital tract cancer also are at increased risk for large-bowel cancer.

DIAGNOSIS

Symptoms

The diagnosis of colorectal cancer can be based on the evaluation of a symptomatic patient or on the results of screening programs. The symptoms of colorectal cancer can be nonspecific, such as intermittent pain, bleeding, nausea, and vomiting. Bleeding may present as melena, which is more commonly associated with right-sided colon cancers, or as gross red blood, associated with left-sided colon and rectal cancers. Lesser amounts of bleeding may be detected on a fecal occult blood test. Iron-deficiency anemia associated with fatigue may develop in Patients with chronic blood loss.

Malignant obstruction can result in abdominal pain with nausea and vomiting. In the presence of obstruction, a perforation may develop either at the site of the tumor or through the proximal uninvolved intestine. With rectal tumors, compromise of the rectal reservoir can cause a change in bowel habits, such as constipation or a decreased stool caliber. With locally advanced rectal cancers, symptoms of tenesmus, urgency, and perineal pain can occur.

Diagnostic Tests

A broad range of diagnostic studies can be employed in the evaluation of a suspected large-bowel cancer. The least expensive and potentially most informative study for rectal tumors is the digital examination. This permits the localization of distal rectal and anal neoplasms. In addition, stool can be obtained for the evaluation of bleeding.

Rigid sigmoidoscopy with a 25-cm instrument is comparatively inexpensive but is limited by the length of intestine that can be examined and by patient compliance. Flexible fiberoptic sigmoidoscopy has gained more acceptance. Instruments measuring 35 and 65 cm are available, and an examination of the sigmoid colon and rectum can

---

Table 46.2. **NEOPLASTIC COLORECTAL POLYPS**

Type	Histologic features	Incidence (%)	Invasive malignancy (%)
Adenomatous (tubular adenoma)	Branching tubules embedded in lamina propria	75	5
Villous (villous adenoma)	Finger-like projections of epithelium over lamina propria	10	40
Intermediate (tubulovillous adenoma	Mixture of adenomatous and villous patterns	15	22

usually be performed after cleansing enemas have been administered. Patient acceptance is much higher than with rigid sigmoidoscopy.

The barium enema is the traditional study for the diagnosis of colonic polyps and cancers. The double-contrast technique in which air insufflation is used is superior to the standard single-contrast barium enema to detect early polyps or cancers. The classic apple core defect has been described for colonic cancers (Fig. 46.5). Proctosigmoidoscopy should also be performed to exclude rectal lesions because visualization of the rectum is inadequate on barium enema. One advantage of barium enema over colonoscopy is the routine visualization of the right side of the colon, which is not possible in 5% to 10% of colonoscopic examinations.

Colonoscopy with the 180-cm fiberoptic instrument is the most widely used diagnostic study to evaluate the colon. A valuable aspect of this procedure is the ability to obtain mucosal biopsy specimens and perform polypectomies. The incidence of severe complications that require surgical intervention (e.g., hemorrhage, perforation) is 0.1% to 0.3%.

Increasingly, the diagnosis of colorectal cancer is based on the evaluation of a positive fecal occult blood test result. The most commonly employed test to detect occult blood uses guaiac-impregnated paper slides that change color in the presence of peroxidase activity from hemoglobin. Several factors affect the utility of this test. First, not all colonic cancers or polyps are associated with bleeding, and even in those that are, bleeding is often intermittent in nature. Second, patients must be instructed to remain on diets low in peroxidase (no rare beef) before testing to avoid false-positive results. Third, certain medications, such as iron, cimetidine, antacids, and ascorbic acid, may interfere with the peroxidase reaction and lead to a false-negative result. The experience with unhydrated fecal occult blood testing in asymptomatic populations has shown that about 2.5% of tested patients have positive results. Among these, only 10% to 15% have colorectal cancer (46).

Screening

For screening purposes, asymptomatic patients can considered to be at high risk or classified with the general population. People in the high-risk group have been described previously. First-degree relatives of patients with known hereditary colon cancer syndromes should undergo colonoscopy by age 20 and regularly thereafter. Patients who have had adenomatous polyps removed should undergo colonoscopy yearly until no further polyps are seen and then every 3 to 5 years thereafter. Patients with ulcerative colitis should have surveillance colonoscopy after 8 to 10 years of disease activity. Based on the findings, a subsequent surveillance program can be formulated.

In the asymptomatic general population, several prospective, randomized, controlled trials have evaluated the efficacy of fecal occult blood testing (FOBT) in reducing mortality from colorectal cancer. The results of four separate trials comprising more than 400,000 persons are summarized in Table 46.3 (47–51). Follow-up was substantial, ranging from 8 to 18 years. With unhydrated FOBT, performed in two trials, the rate of positive test results was approximately 2%. With rehydrated FOBT, the rate of positive test results was 5% to 10%. All these studies reported a higher percentage of earlier-stage (i.e., Dukes A) cancers detected in the screened group than in the control group. These studies demonstrated a 15% to 21% decrease in mortality from colorectal cancer with biennial FOBT. Annual FOBT was associated with a 33% decrease in colorectal cancer mortality. Because not all patients were compliant with FOBT, the reductions in mortality from colorectal cancer are thought to be an underestimate. If one were to exclude the noncompliant patients from the Minnesota study, it is estimated that a 50% reduction in colorectal cancer mortality would be observed. Interestingly, even though colorectal cancer mortality is decreased with screening, the overall mortality of the screened populations has been no different from that of

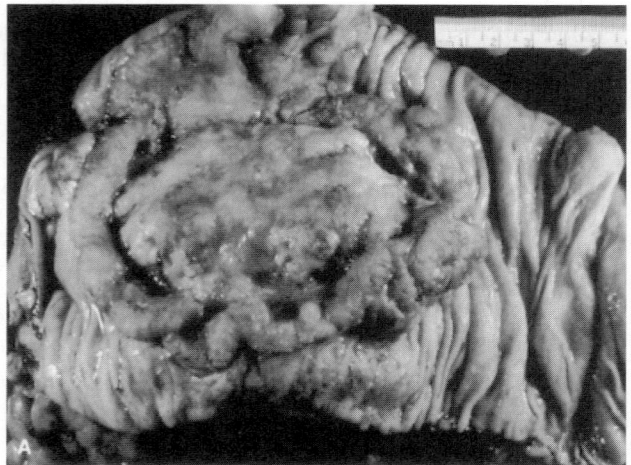
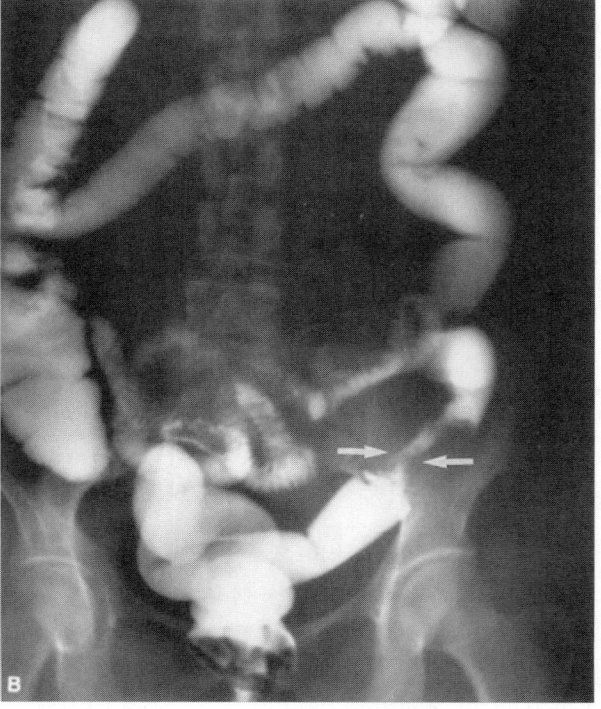

Figure 46.5. Surgical specimen with correlating barium enema examination of an invasive sigmoid carcinoma. *(A)* The tumor is a circumferential lesion. *(B)* The barium enema study demonstrates features of the apple core defect *(arrows)*.

Table 46.3. **SUMMARY OF PROSPECTIVE RANDOMIZED TRIALS OF FECAL OCCULT BLOOD TESTING**

Study	No. of patients	Randomized groups	Type of FOBT	Cancers follow-up period (y)	Detected by FOBT (%)	RR of CRC Dukes A cancers (%)	Death with screening (95% CI)
Mandel et al. (47,48) Minnesota, U.S.	46,551	Annual Biennial Control	Rehydrated	18	Annual 50 Biennial 39	Annual 33 Biennial 29 Control 25	Annual 0.67 (0.51–0.89) Biennial 0.79 (0.62–0.97)
Hardcastle et al. (49) Nottingham, U.K.	152,850	Biennial Control	Unhydrated	7.5 (median)	27	Screen 21 Control 12	0.85 (0.74–0.98)
Kronburg et al. (50) Funen, Denmark	140,000	Biennial Control	Unhydrated	10	25	Screen 23 Control 12	0.82 (0.68–0.99)
Kewenter et al. (51) Gothenburg, Sweden	63,308	Two screens, 16–22 mo. apart Control	Rehydrated	8.2 (median)	28	Screen 26 Control 9	0.88 (0.69–1.12)

FOBT, fecal occult blood testing; CRC, colorectal cancer; CI, confidence interval; RR, relative risk.

the control groups. It appears that mortality is shifted to other causes (i.e., cardiovascular deaths) in the screened population. Cost-effective analyses performed by the Congressional Office of Technology Assessment and the National Cancer Institute indicate that FOBT screening would cost about $15,000 to $20,000 per year of life saved, which is substantially less than the cost for currently recommended preventive measures (i.e., mammography).

No randomized, controlled trials have evaluated endoscopic procedures as a modality of screening the asymptomatic population. However, in a cohort and case-control study, screening sigmoidoscopy reduced the mortality from distal colorectal cancers between 60% to 80% (52). Approximately 70% of all large-bowel polyps and cancers should be within reach of a flexible sigmoidoscope. Data for colonoscopy suggest that this procedure can be an effective screening tool. In the National Polyp Study, patients who underwent colonoscopy and subsequent removal of benign polyps were followed with periodic colonoscopy for an average period of 6 years (53). A 90% decrease in colorectal cancer in patients participating in the National Polyp Study was noted in comparison with a general population registry. These data indicate that colonoscopy can be a very effective tool in reducing the inci-

dence of colorectal cancer. However, the potential complications, limited patient acceptance, and high cost make this test more difficult to institute on a large scale.

Current guidelines for the screening of asymptomatic men and women beginning at the age of 50 years have been endorsed by the American Cancer Society and five professional societies (54). These guidelines are listed in Table 46.4.

STAGING

Pathology

Of all large-bowel cancers, 90% to 95% are adenocarcinomas, with the remaining histologic types being squamous cell carcinomas, adenosquamous carcinomas, lymphomas, sarcomas, and carcinoid tumors. Most colonic adenocarcinomas are moderately differentiated or well-differentiated tumors. About 20% of adenocarcinomas are poorly differentiated or undifferentiated, and these are associated with a poorer prognosis. Another commonly described characteristic of adenocarcinomas is the relative amount of mucin that is produced. Ten percent to 20% of tumors are described as mucinous or colloid carcinomas based on the abundant production of mucin. These tumors are associated with a poorer 5-year survival rate in comparison with nonmucinous tumors. Other histologic features associated with a poorer prognosis include blood vessel invasion, lymphatic vessel invasion, and the absence of a lymphocytic response to the tumor.

Dukes Classification

The most important prognostic factor in colorectal cancer is the depth of invasion of the primary tumor. The first practical staging system to incorporate this observation was described by Dukes, who classified the depth of invasion of rectal tumors in stages from A to C. In his original classification, stage A indicated penetration through the muscularis propria but not through the intestinal wall (Fig. 46.6). Stage B represented penetration through the muscularis propria into the perirectal fat. Stage C represented metastasis to lymph nodes regardless of the extent of intestinal wall penetration. This application of this classification was strictly confined to rectal tumors lying be-

Table 46.4. **GUIDELINES FOR COLORECTAL CANCER SCREENING***

Asymptomatic men or women beginning at age 50 years should undergo screening with one or more of the following:
- Annual fecal occult blood test,
- Flexible sigmoidoscopy every 5 years, or
- Double-contrast barium enema every 5 to 10 years, or
- Colonoscopy every 10 years

Diagnostic evaluation with colonoscopy or double-contrast barium enema (preferably accompanied by flexible sigmoidoscopy) should be performed in any patients with either positive findings on screening with fecal occult blood testing or symptoms suggestive of colorectal cancer or polyps.

*Endorsed by the American Cancer Society, American College of Gastroenterology, American Society of Colon and Rectal Surgeons, American Society for Gastrointestinal Endoscopy, Oncology Nursing Society, and Society of American Gastrointestinal Endoscopic Surgeons.

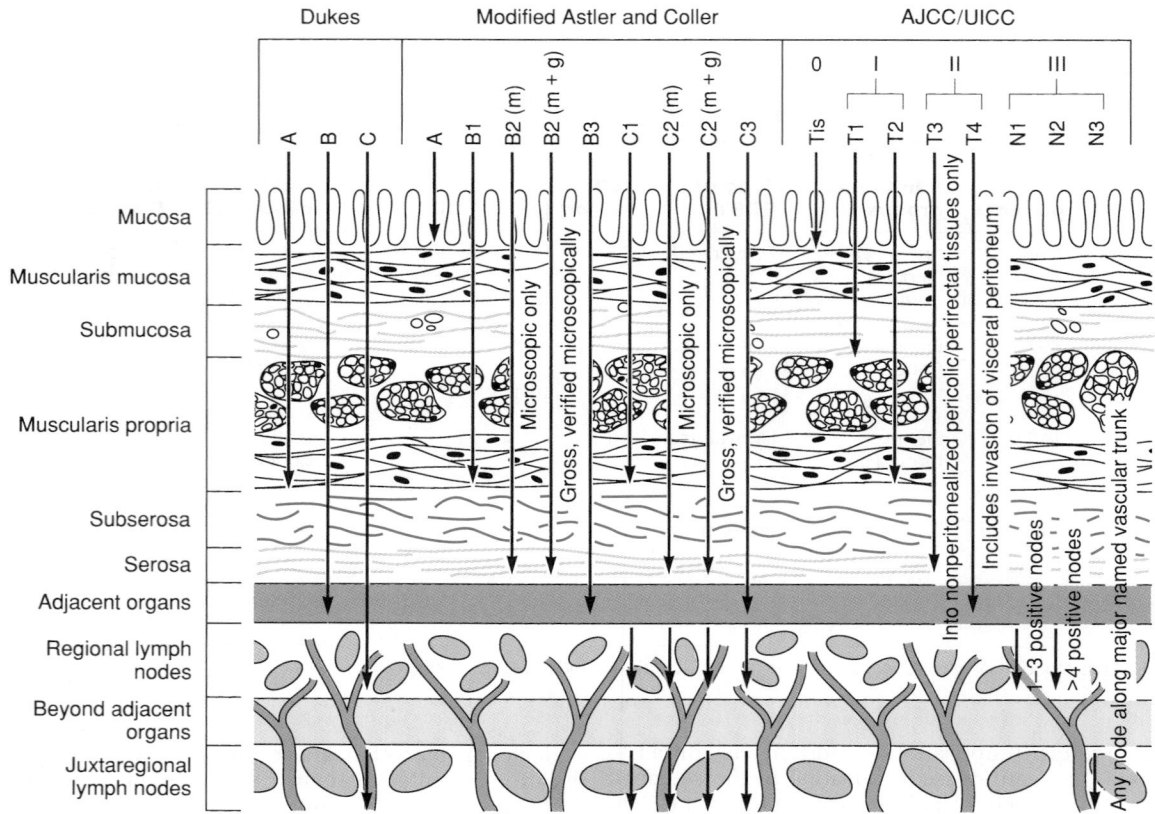

Figure 46.6. Schematic description of the staging systems with respect to depth of invasion.

Table 46.5. **FIVE-YEAR SURVIVAL RATES OF PATIENTS WITH OPERABLE COLORECTAL CANCER**

Investigators (ref.)	No. Patients	5-Year Actuarial Survival Rate by Stage (%)								
		A	**B**	**B1**	**B2**	**B3**	**C**	**C1**	**C2**	**C3**
Corman et al., 1973 (79)	244	98	79	—	—	—	42	—	—	—
Eisenberg et al., 1982 (80)	1,704	82	73	—	—	—	40	—	—	—
Pihl et al., 1980 (81)*	615	88	78	—	—	—	60	—	—	—
Willett et al., 1984 (82)*	533	90	—	75	70	64	—	63	45	38
Minsky et al., 1988 (83)*	294	92	—	93	90	66	—	78	56	33
	Total 3,390	Mean 90	77				47			

*Restricted to colon cancers.

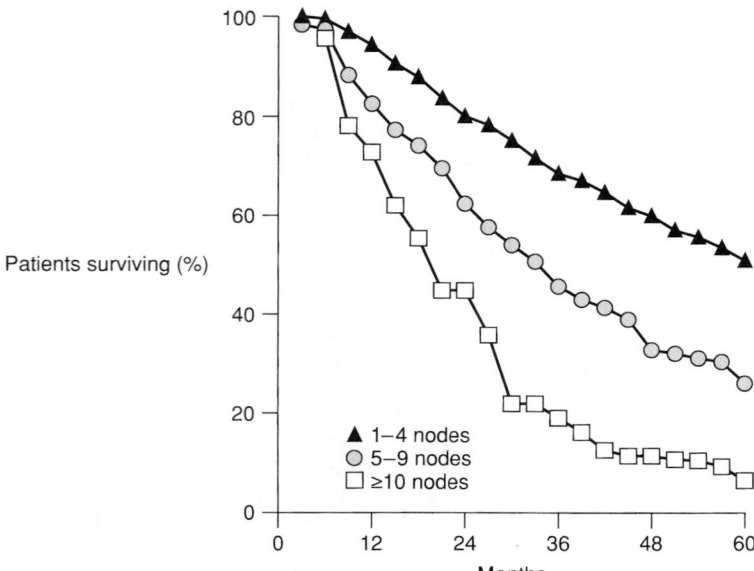

Figure 46.7. Survival of Dukes stage C patients according to the number of positive nodes.

neath the peritoneal reflection, and therefore the concept of serosal involvement was not relevant.

Since Dukes' original description, various modifications of this system have been described to stage tumors in the rectum and throughout the colon. Because of these variations, the specific classification system used in a particular instance must be identified.

Modified Astler-Coller Staging System

One of the more commonly used staging systems is the modified Astler-Coller system (Fig. 46.6). According to this system, stage A represents tumors that invade into the mucosa only. Stage B1 tumors invade into but not through the muscularis propria. Stage B2 lesions invade through the intestinal wall without involving adjacent organs, whereas stage B3 tumors involve adjacent organs. Stage C tumors involve regional lymph nodes and are subgrouped into stages C1, C2, and C3 according to the depth of intestinal wall penetration. Stage D represents evidence of distant organ involvement. In general, the 5-year survival rate for patients with stage D disease is less than 10%. Survival rates after curative resection for the other stages of colorectal cancer are summarized in Table 46.5. Overall, the 5-year survival rates for stages A, B, and C are 90%, 77%, and 47%, respectively. Additional studies have revealed that among Dukes stage C patients, the number of involved lymph nodes is a significant predictor of survival and should be incorporated into the staging of colorectal tumors (55) (Fig. 46.7).

Tumor–Node–Metastasis Classification

The American Joint Committee on Cancer and the International Union Against Cancer (AJCC/UICC) have proposed an alternative staging system based on the extent of the primary tumor (T), regional node involvement (N), and metastasis (M). In contrast to the modified Astler-Coller system, the TNM system includes carcinoma in situ (Tis) and stratifies according to number of positive nodes (Fig. 46.6). Stage 0 represents Tis tumors that do not metastasize, stage I includes T1 and T2 tumors, stage II includes T3 and T4 tumors, and stage III includes any tumors with nodal involvement (N1 to N3). Stage IV includes any cancer with distant metastases. The TNM system is correlated with equivalent Dukes and modified Astler-Coller stages in Table 46.6. The TNM method has been generally adopted in the field of oncology as the universal colorectal cancer staging system.

PROGNOSTIC FACTORS

Although the pathologic stage is the major determinant of prognosis, many clinical and pathologic features have been described to correlate with survival. Many of these factors are interrelated and may reflect the same characteristics. Table 46.7 summarizes some of the reported factors and how they are associated with survival.

More recently, genetic markers have been identified that relate to prognosis. Tumor DNA content has been shown to be a significant prognostic factor. With the use of flow cytometry, tumors can be categorized as aneuploid (abnormal DNA content) or diploid (normal DNA content). Patients with aneuploid tumors have been reported to have higher recurrence rates and decreased survival rates than patients with diploid tumors (56). By amplification of microsatellite markers, the allelic loss of chromosome 18q has been found to have a significant prognostic effect in patients with node-negative colorectal cancer (i.e., stage II tumors) (17). The *DCC* gene located on chromosome 18q is hypothesized to be a tumor-suppressor gene in colorectal tumor formation (see section on molecular genetics). In a

Table 46.6. **STAGING CLASSIFICATION OF COLORECTAL CANCER***

Stage	Description
TUMOR–NODE–METASTASIS (TNM) SYSTEM	
Primary Tumor	
TX	Primary tumor cannot be assessed
T0	No evidence of tumor in resected specimen (prior polypectomy or fulguration)
Tis	Carcinoma in situ
T1	Invades into submucosa
T2	Invades into muscularis propria
T3/T4	Depends on whether serosa is present
SEROSA PRESENT	
T3	Invades through muscularis propria into subserosa Invades serosa (but not through) Invades pericolic fat within the leaves of the mesentery
T4	Invades through serosa into free peritoneal cavity or through serosa into a continuous organ
NP SEROSA (distal two thirds of rectum, posterior left or right colon)	
T3	Invades through muscularis propria
T4	Invades other organs (vagina, prostate, ureter, kidney)
Regional Lymph Node Involvement	
NX	Nodes cannot be assessed (e.g., local excision only)
N0	No regional node metastases
N1	1–3 positive nodes
N2	4 or more positive nodes
N3	Central nodes positive
Distant Metastasis	
MX	Presence of distant metastases cannot be assessed
M0	No distant metastases
M1	Distant metastases present
DUKES STAGING SYSTEM CORRELATED WITH TNM SYSTEM	
Dukes A	T1, N0, M0 (stage I) T2, N0, M0 (stage I)
Dukes B	T3, N0, M0 (stage II) T4, N0, M0 (stage II)
Dukes C	T (any), N1, M0; T (any), N2, M0 (stage III)
Dukes D	T (any), N (any), M1 (stage IV)
MODIFIED ASTLER-COLLER (MAC) SYSTEM CORRELATED WITH TNM SYSTEM	
MAC A	T1, N0, M0 (stage I)
MAC B1	T2, N0, M0 (stage I)
MAC B2	T3, N0, M0 (stage II)
MAC B3	T4, N0, M0 (stage II)
MAC C1	T2, N1, M0; T2, N2, M0 (stage III)
MAC C2	T3, N1, M0; T3, N2, M0 (stage III) T4, N1, M0; T4, N2, M0 (stage III)
MAC C3	T4, N1, M0; T4, N2, M0 (stage III)

*In all pathologic staging systems, particularly those applied to rectal cancer, the abbreviations m and g may be used; m denotes microscopic transmural penetration; g or m + g denotes transmural penetration visible on gross inspection and confirmed microscopically.

retrospective analysis, the 5-year survival rate among patients with stage II disease and no evidence of allelic loss of 18q was 93%. By contrast, stage II patients with allelic loss of 18q had a 5-year survival rate of 54%, which was similar to that of node-positive patients (i.e., stage III). In the same study, the survival rate of stage III patients was not affected by the status of chromosome 18q. However, these findings were not confirmed in a separate study (18). Recently, 8p allelic imbalance in stages B2 and C colorectal cancers was found to be an independent prognostic factor predicting poor outcome (57). Genetic markers have an increasingly important role in the evaluation of patients with cancer.

Table 46.7. PROGNOSTIC FACTORS FOR PRIMARY COLORECTAL CANCER

Factor	Association
Age	Patients <40 y old often present with more advanced stage of disease.
Symptoms	Symptomatic patients tend to have more advanced stage of disease.
Obstruction and perforation	Poorer prognosis when present.
Location of primary	Rectosigmoid and rectal cancers have lower cure rates compared with cancers elsewhere in the colon.
Tumor configuration	Exophytic tumors are associated with less advanced stage of cancer compared with ulcerative tumors.
Blood vessel invasion	Poorer prognosis when present.
Lymphatic vessel invasion	Poorer prognosis when present.
Perineural invasion	Poorer prognosis when present.
Lymphocytic infiltration	Improved prognosis when present.
Carcinoembryonic antigen study	Poorer prognosis when elevated before primary tumor resection.
Aneuploidy	Poorer prognosis when present.

NATURAL HISTORY

The natural progression of colorectal cancer comprises three processes: local invasion, lymphatic spread, and hematogenous spread. Studies described by Dukes in the 1930s led to the theory of an orderly progression from local tumor invasion to subsequent lymphatic and hematogenous spread after the tumor had penetrated the intestinal wall. Today, we know that these observations are not entirely correct because in some subsets of patients with tumors that do not invade through the intestinal wall, lymphatic metastases or distant disease develops nonetheless. In this regard, even patients who undergo curative resection of apparently localized colorectal cancers should be viewed as harboring blood-borne metastases. The risk for the development of disseminated disease can be predicted by the depth of tumor invasion into the intestinal wall and the involvement of draining lymph nodes. Therapies designed to reduce the development of recurrent disease after surgical resection are discussed in later sections of this chapter.

Local growth of an adenocarcinoma is initially characterized by intramural expansion of the tumor into the bowel lumen. Subsequent lateral invasion into the intestinal wall usually progresses in a transverse direction rather than longitudinally and thereby leads to circumferential involvement of the intestine. The incidence of lymphatic metastasis increases with extent of local invasion through the intestinal wall; however, 10% to 20% of patients with cancer limited to the intestinal wall are found to have positive lymph nodes.

The liver is the most common site of hematogenous spread of colorectal cancer; liver metastasis occurs in about half of all cases (58). The liver is the first capillary network exposed to tumor emboli traveling through the portal system and represents the major site of venous drainage of the colon and upper rectum. The liver can be the sole site of tumor metastasis, as evidenced by the successful resection of liver metastases for cure in selected patients. By contrast, the lower rectum has a dual drainage system, draining into the portal system and the vena cava by way of the middle and inferior hemorrhoidal veins, respectively. Some think that isolated lung metastases can develop from lower rectal tumors when tumor emboli travel through the systemic venous drainage system. The lung is the second most common site of metastasis from colorectal tumors. Tumor involvement of other sites in the absence of liver and lung metastases is unusual. In certain circumstances, isolated bone metastases to the sacrum or vertebral bodies can arise when tumor emboli travel through portal–vertebral venous communications known as *Batson's plexus*.

Another potential mode of spread is by intraluminal or extraluminal exfoliation of tumor cells with subsequent implantation. Tumor implantation may occur during surgical resection; spillage of tumor cells can cause recurrences in bowel anastomoses, abdominal incisions, or other intraabdominal sites. When tumors penetrate the intestinal wall, shed tumor cells can be implanted intraperitoneally and cause peritoneal carcinomatosis.

A summary of the natural history of patients who present with colorectal cancer is depicted in Fig. 46.8 (58).

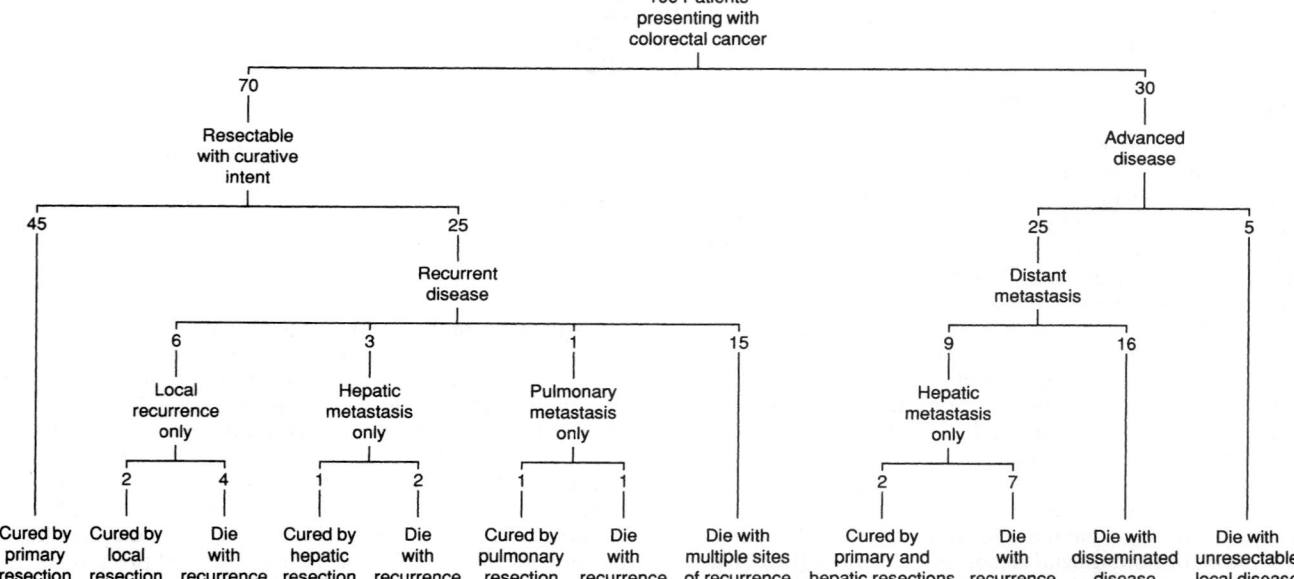

Figure 46.8. Algorithm depicting the natural history of colorectal cancer.

For every 100 patients initially evaluated, 30 have clinically evident distant spread, and the remaining 70 undergo resection for localized disease. Among these 70 patients, 45 are cured and disease recurs in the remainder. Extrapolation of these figures to the approximately 130,000 patients in whom colorectal cancer is diagnosed each year in the United States implies that 58,500 patients can be cured with surgical resection alone; disease recurs in the remaining 71,500 patients after resection, or they have disseminated tumor at the time of diagnosis.

TREATMENT OF PRIMARY COLORECTAL TUMORS

Neoplastic Polyps

With the availability of colonoscopy, endoscopic polypectomy has become the standard approach for the treatment of neoplastic polyps unless it is medically contraindicated. The risk of this procedure is extremely low, with a complication rate of less than 1%. Almost all pedunculated polyps can be removed endoscopically with a snare. Sessile lesions can frequently be removed piecemeal, but several sessions may be required. A dilemma in treating colonic polyps occurs if a resected lesion contains a malignant focus. A decision must then be made about the need for a colectomy. If the lesion does not penetrate the muscularis mucosae, it should be considered a malignancy in situ that does not have the propensity to metastasize and therefore does not require further surgery. If the lesion penetrates the muscularis mucosae, it is an invasive cancer and may require surgery (Fig. 46.2). In general, if evidence of invasion is found, colectomy with resection of paracolonic lymph nodes is indicated. In selected cases of pedunculated polyps, conservative management without colectomy may be undertaken if the lesion does not contain poorly differentiated tumor cells or show evidence of vascular invasion and if a negative resection margin has been obtained at the level of the stalk. Lesions that are poorly differentiated or have evidence of vascular invasion, regardless of a negative surgical margin, should be treated by colectomy.

Large villous tumors of the rectum can pose a challenge. Total excision is required to assess the presence of invasive cancer accurately. Transanal excision with sphincteric muscle and mucosal approximation is preferred; however, other approaches, such as low anterior resection, coloanal procedures, or abdominoperineal resection, may have to be employed to excise extensive benign rectal lesions totally.

Invasive Colorectal Cancers

Surgery

The surgical options for colorectal cancer depend on the location of the primary tumor. These surgical procedures are summarized as follows:

Intraperitoneal colon and upper third of the rectum
  Resection and anastomosis
Middle third of the rectum
  Abdominoperineal resection
  Low anterior resection
  Abdominosacral resection
  Coloanal resection
  Local excision or fulguration
  Primary radiation therapy
Lower third of the rectum
  Abdominoperineal resection
  Local excision or fulguration
  Primary radiation therapy

Before surgical resection, evaluation for sites of metastatic disease is important. A careful physical examination determines the presence of hepatomegaly, ascites, or adenopathy. For rectal tumors, the distance of the tumor from the anal verge and its mobility are important in assessing resectability and the type of operation required. Rectal ultrasonography can be helpful in assessing the extent of local invasion and the presence of enlarged lymph nodes within the mesorectum. Laboratory studies should include a complete blood cell count, determination of serum liver enzymes, and a carcinoembryonic antigen (CEA) assay. Determination of a baseline CEA level can be useful in subsequent follow-up of the patient (see below). Abnormal results of liver function studies may indicate the need to perform abdominal computed tomography (CT) to assess the presence of liver metastases. It is not unreasonable to perform preoperative abdominal CT in all patients with colorectal cancer. The presence of metastatic disease may alter the planned surgical procedure—that is, a low rectal cancer with evidence of hepatic metastases may be better palliated with fulguration than with abdominoperineal resection. A full colonoscopy or air-contrast barium enema should be performed to rule out the presence of other primary colorectal polyps or cancers.

The surgical goals in the resection of a primary colorectal cancer are to achieve an *en bloc* resection that encompasses an adequate amount of normal colon proximal and distal to the tumor, to obtain adequate lateral margins if the tumor is adherent to contiguous structures, and to remove regional lymph nodes. Accomplishment of these goals optimizes the chance of preventing locoregional recurrence of the disease. The extent of bowel resection has been the subject of numerous debates. In pathologic studies, tumor rarely extends intramurally more than 2 cm beyond the area of gross involvement. Traditionally, 5 cm of normal large intestine proximal and distal to the tumor has been advocated as a margin that is adequate to encompass intramural spread completely. The actual margin of intestine removed is often determined by the extent of the lymphadenectomy. The paracolic and intermediate draining lymph nodes should be removed as part of a curative resection (Fig. 46.9). Extensive resections of bowel along with more central or retroperitoneal lymph nodes are not indicated because they add minimal oncologic benefit and substantially increase operative complications. At the time of surgical resection, the abdominal viscera, particularly the liver and peritoneal surfaces, should be thoroughly investigated. If evidence of disseminated disease is apparent, a less extensive resection of the primary lesion for palliation to avoid complications of obstruction or bleeding may be indicated.

Intraperitoneal Colon and Upper Third of the Rectum. The surgical resection of cancers in different sites in the colorectum requires attention to specific anatomic details. Resection plus primary anastomosis is the surgical procedure of choice for cancers of the colon and upper third of the rectum. Whenever possible, a mechanical bowel preparation, along with oral antibiotics, should be instituted preoperatively to reduce infectious complications. The choice of anastomotic technique (i.e., stapling vs. hand sewing) depends on the surgeon's preference.

Tumors of the cecum and ascending colon should be resected by a right hemicolectomy. Ligation of the ileocolic, right colic, and right branches from the middle colic artery is required (Fig. 46.9). For tumors in the hepatic flexure, an extension of a right hemicolectomy is performed with ligation of the middle colic artery near its origin. Care must be taken during the mobilization of the ascending colon and hepatic flexure because the right ureter and tes-

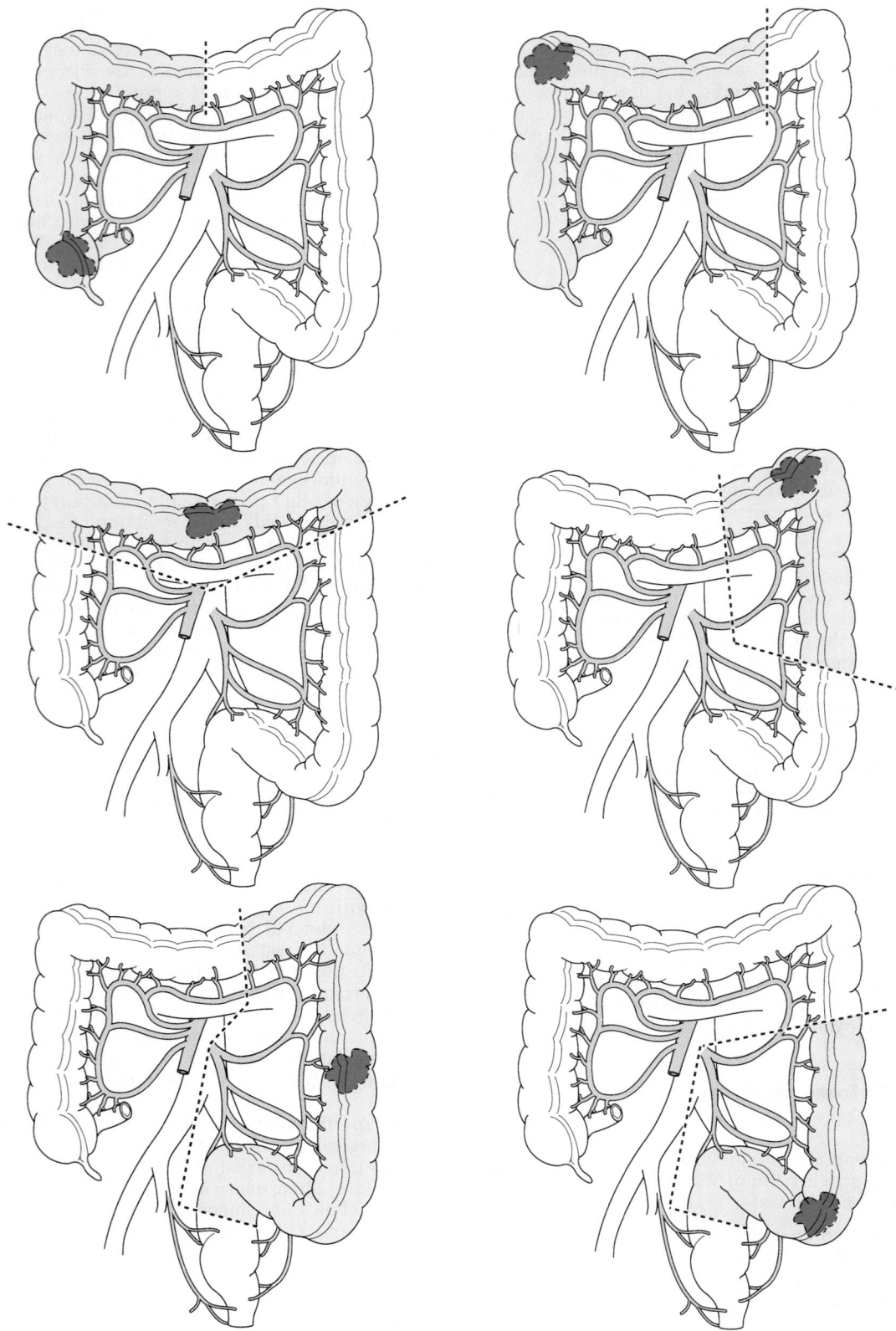

Figure 46.9. Segmental resections for cancers of the colon and upper third of the rectum.

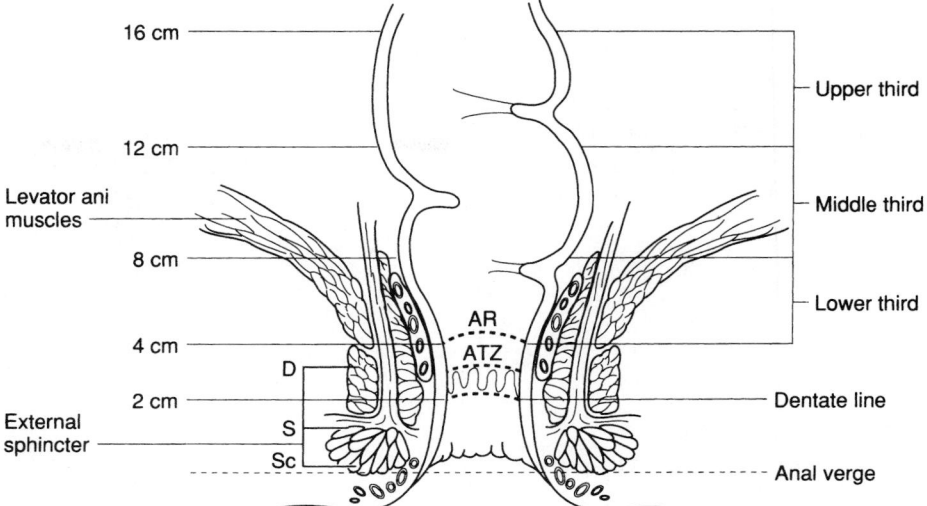

Figure 46.10. Anorectal anatomy with important landmarks. Approximate measurements are relative to the anal verge. *D,* deep; *S,* superficial; *Sc,* subcutaneous; *AR,* anorectal ring; *ATZ,* anal transition zone.

ticular or ovarian vessels, inferior vena cava, superior mesenteric vein, and duodenum are all close together.

For lesions of the transverse colon, a transverse colectomy is accomplished by proximal ligation of the middle colic artery (Fig. 46.9). Cancer of the splenic flexure can be treated with a segmental resection in which the middle transverse colon is anastomosed to the middle descending colon. For this procedure, the left colic artery is divided and the middle colic artery is preserved. Mobilization of the splenic flexure requires care to avoid injury to the spleen.

A left hemicolectomy with removal of intestine from the middle transverse to the distal sigmoid colon can be used for tumors of the descending colon (Fig. 46.9). High ligation of the inferior mesenteric artery is necessary in this operation. For cancers of the sigmoid colon, a segmental resection can be performed with ligation of the sigmoid artery near its origin. Rectosigmoid cancers and tumors confined to the upper third of the rectum are removed by an anterior resection. The upper third of the rectum is about 12 to 16 cm from the anal verge and is located above the peritoneal reflection (Fig. 46.10). The pelvic peritoneum is incised circumferentially around the rectum, and the intestine is mobilized from the presacral fascia. Laterally, the middle hemorrhoidal vessels are ligated, and anteriorly, the rectum is mobilized from the seminal vesicles and prostate or the vagina. The mesenteric vessels are divided at the origin of the sigmoid artery or higher, at the origin of the inferior mesenteric artery, if further mobilization of the splenic flexure is required to obtain a tension-free anastomosis.

Middle and Lower Third of the Rectum. Cancers located in the lower third of the rectum, between the anorectal ring and 7 to 8 cm from the anal verge, are reliably treated by abdominoperineal resection (Fig. 46.10). The procedure involves wide excision of the rectum to include the lateral attachments and pelvic mesocolon and establishment of a colostomy. The extent of surgery for an abdominoperineal resection is illustrated in Fig. 46.11. With the patient in a modified lithotomy position, the abdominal and perineal procedures can be performed simultaneously by two teams or sequentially by one team. Alternatively, the abdominal procedure can be completed with the patient in the supine position, and the perineal portion completed afterward, with the patient turned in the lateral position. On opening of the abdomen, evidence of

intraabdominal spread is ascertained. The discovery of extensive disseminated disease may eliminate the need for an abdominoperineal resection because a local excision or fulguration to preserve anal function may be more appropriate for palliation. If an abdominoperineal resection is performed, ligation of the superior hemorrhoidal vessels at their origin from the left colic artery is required. Occasionally, if extensive nodal disease is present, higher arterial ligation may be necessary. The rectum is mobilized in a fashion similar to that described for an anterior resec-

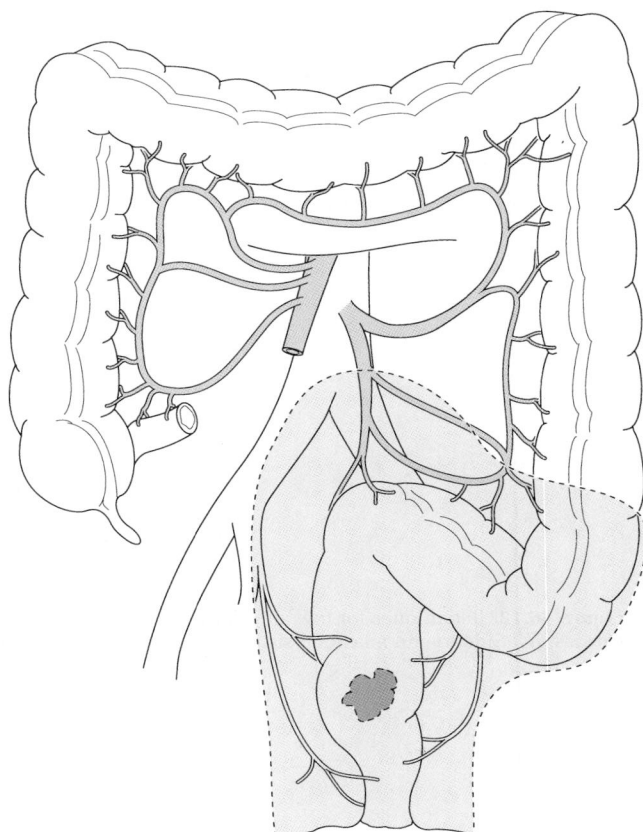

Figure 46.11. Extent of surgery in abdominoperineal resection.

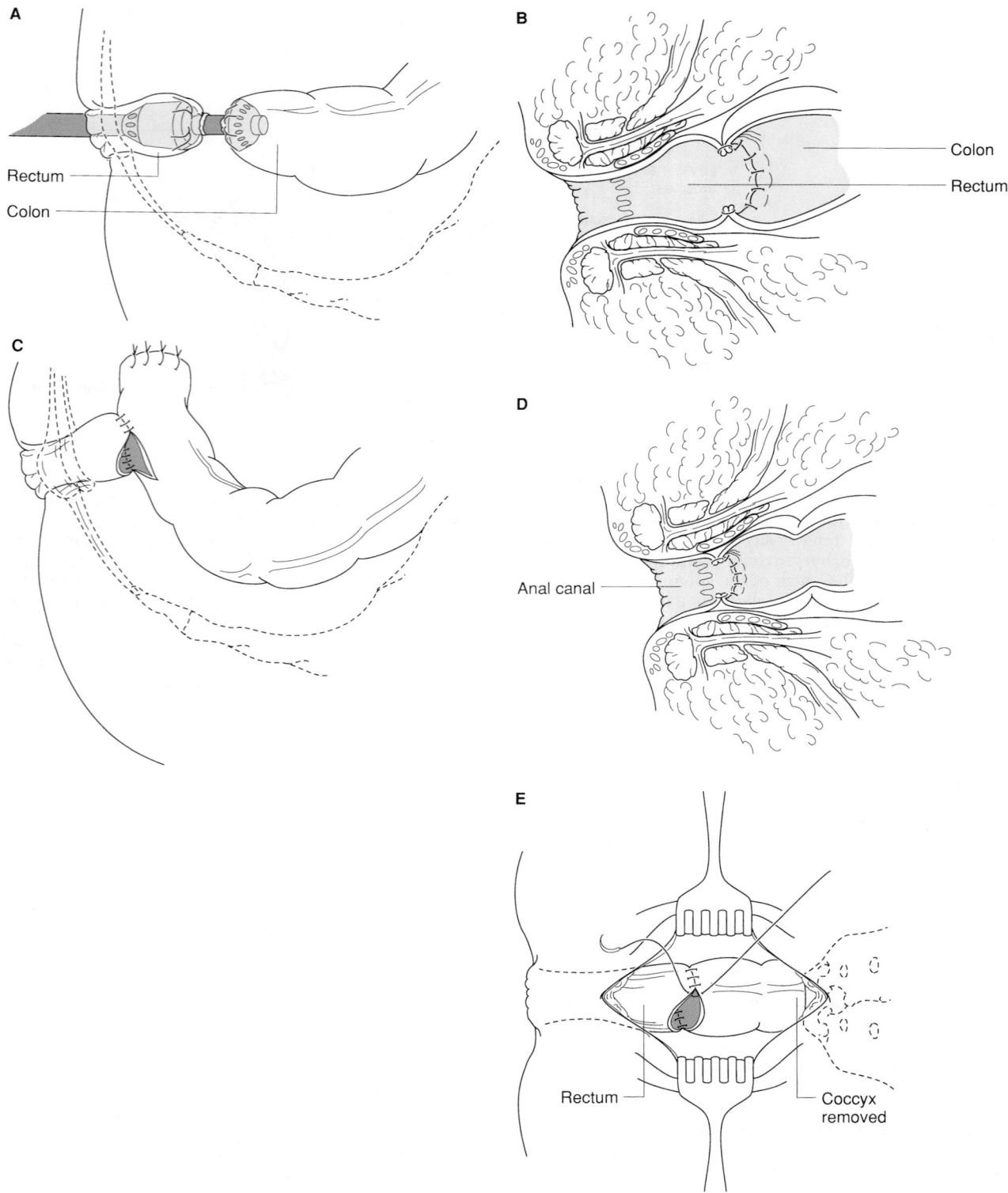

Figure 46.12. Techniques for low anterior resections. *(A)* End-to-end stapler. *(B)* Single layer with sutures. *(C)* Side-to-end anastomosis. *(D)* Pull-through. *(E)* Transsacral resection.

tion, but the dissection is carried down to the pelvic floor muscles, which are excised *en bloc* with the anus. An end-sigmoid colostomy is brought out through the rectus sheath. Efforts to exclude small intestine from a future radiation field by use of the uterus, omentum, peritoneum, or absorbable mesh should be considered. Primary closure of the perineal wound over drains can usually be accomplished without complications.

Cancer of the middle third of the rectum, between 8 and 12 cm from the anal verge (Fig. 46.10), can be managed by a variety of techniques. For these tumors, abdominoperineal resection does not yield results superior to those of other procedures that spare the anal sphincter. Therefore, an effort should be made to maintain intestinal continuity. Low anterior resection is a commonly used technique that involves resection of the middle rectum with primary anastomosis. The introduction of the end-to-end anastomosis stapler has increased the use of this sphincter-saving procedure (Fig. 46.12A). If a transanal reconstruction with a stapler is contemplated, the patient should be placed in the lithotomy position. The initial stages of the operation, with complete mobilization of the rectum to the level of the pelvic floor, are identical to those for an abdominoperineal resection. After removal of the tumor, the anastomosis, which can be end-to-end or end-to-side, is joined with sutures or staples (Fig. 46.12B,C). A temporary transverse colostomy should be employed if the integrity of the anastomosis is a concern.

Other sphincter-saving approaches have been described for middle rectal cancers (59). Coloanal anastomosis involves restoring bowel continuity by bringing the colon to the level of the anus and dentate line (Fig. 46.12D). Abdominosacral resections were described in the 1940s and allowed surgeons more direct visualization of low, hand-sewn anastomoses. The rectum is mobilized through an abdominal approach, and a second incision is made above the anus, with resection of the coccyx for visualization into the pelvis. A hand-sewn anastomosis is completed through the transsacral incision (Fig. 46.12E). This procedure has largely been supplanted by the use of stapling devices.

One of the controversies concerning sphincter-saving procedures for rectal tumors concerns the length of an adequate distal mucosal margin. The traditional dictum of 5 cm for a margin is not substantiated by any studies. Only 2.5% of patients have intramural spread beyond 2 cm from the palpable tumor, and these patients usually have dissemination of tumor despite aggressive local therapy. No correlation has been found between local recurrence and extent of the distal margin when it is greater than 2 cm. Ideally, a surgical margin of 3 cm, measured on the fresh specimen, should be achieved. If the end-to-end anastomosis stapler is used, then a margin of 2 cm plus the additional "doughnut" specimen obtained by the stapler should be adequate. If, in the surgeon's judgment, this length of margin cannot be obtained, then abdominoperineal resection should be performed. The segment of rectum located between the tumor and the pelvic floor, determined preoperatively, can be lengthened as much as 4 cm after the rectum is mobilized from its pelvic attachments (Fig. 46.13).

As with many oncologic surgical procedures, increased interest has been shown in less radical types of surgery to manage cancers of the middle and lower third of the rectum in an effort to preserve the anal sphincters and avoid an abdominoperineal resection. Initially, these local procedures, such as excision, ablation, and irradiation, were reserved for patients with advanced disease or with med-

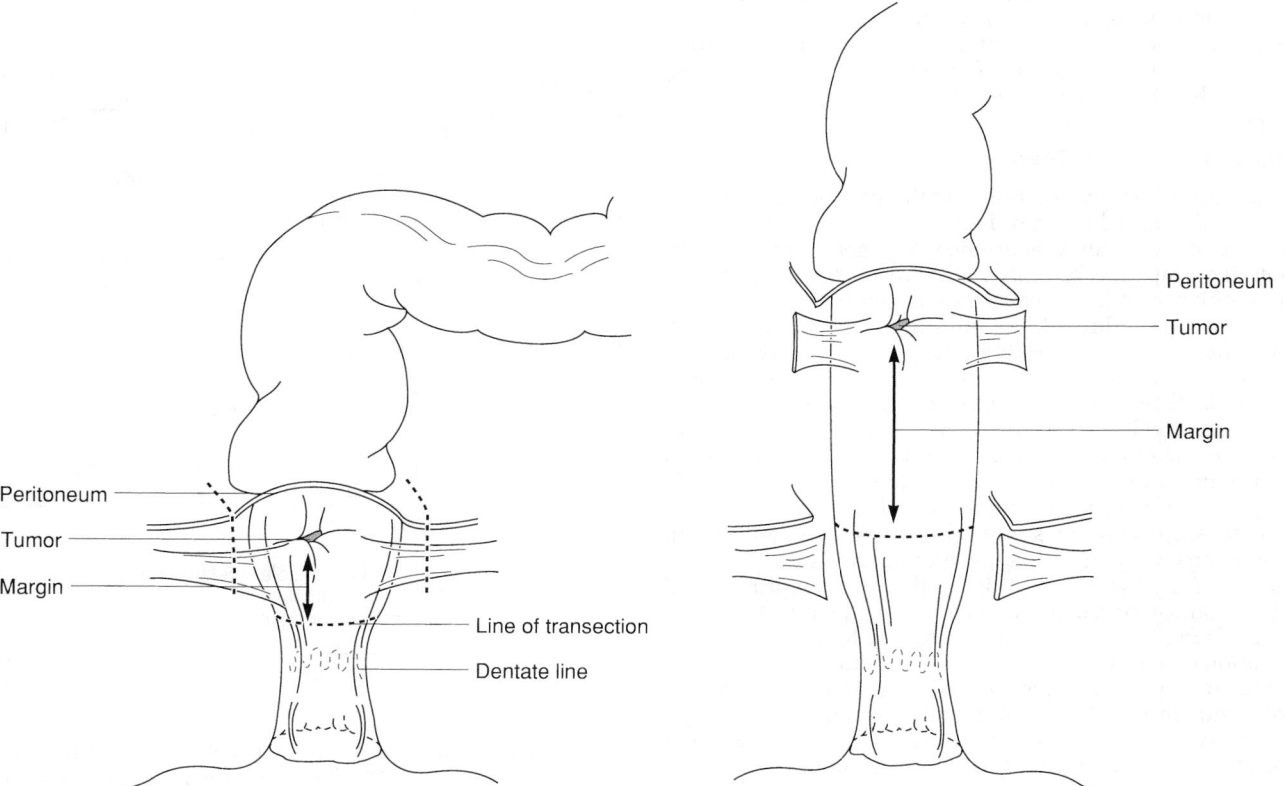

Figure 46.13. Dissection of the rectum from pelvic attachments lengthens distal tumor-free margins and may permit a sphincter-saving procedure.

ical contraindications to radical surgery. Evidence is increasing, however, that for selected patients with low rectal cancers local excision is an acceptable treatment option that is associated with rates of local recurrence and survival similar to those seen after radical surgery. A multicenter, prospective study addressing this question was recently published (60). To be eligible, patients had to have an adenocarcinoma of the rectum that was 10 cm or less from the dentate line and 4 cm or less in diameter, and that involved 40% or less of the rectal lumen. All patients registered underwent local excision of their tumor. Those determined to have T1 tumors with negative surgical margins received no further treatment, and those with T2 tumors underwent postoperative radiation and chemotherapy. The 6-year disease-free survival rates were 83% and 87%, respectively, and the overall survival rates were 71% and 85%, respectively, for T1 and T2 tumors. Of those patients who had a local recurrence, 78% were salvaged by an abdominoperineal resection. It was unclear from this study whether salvage abdominoperineal resection performed for local recurrences provides the same chance for survival as abdominoperineal resection performed at the time of primary cancer treatment (60). The data are supported by several retrospective studies confirming that local excision alone for well-differentiated T1 tumors, and local excision with postoperative radiation with or without chemotherapy for T2 tumors, are appropriate treatments for selected patients with rectal cancer (61–63).

Other forms of local treatment for low rectal cancers should still be reserved for patients who are not candidates for abdominoperineal resection or local excision. Ablation by transanal electric fulguration of the tumor in multiple stages has been reported to be an acceptable treatment in patients who are poor surgical candidates; however, this procedure cannot be used for circumferential tumors (64). Endocavitary irradiation as a primary curative therapy for early cancers has been reported with some success. The neodymium:yttrium-aluminum garnet laser has been found to be effective in palliating obstructive or bleeding lesions of locally advanced colorectal tumors.

Adjuvant Radiation Therapy

Radiation therapy combined with surgical resection for colorectal cancer has been demonstrated to reduce the incidence of local tumor recurrence. In general, the use of radiation therapy has been limited to rectal tumors in which the incidence of local recurrence is significant, including those extending through the intestinal wall or with lymph node involvement. Overall, for stage II (Dukes B2 and B3) rectal tumors, the incidence of local recurrence is about 30% to 35% but can be reduced to 5% with adjuvant radiation therapy. For stage III (Dukes C2 and C3) rectal cancers, the use of adjuvant radiation therapy decreases local recurrences from the range of 45% to 65% down to 10%. Despite improved local tumor control, distant metastases still develop, and no studies have documented an improved survival rate with adjuvant radiation therapy alone. Nevertheless, the use of this modality to improve local tumor control for rectal tumors invading the intestinal wall or involving lymph nodes is warranted to avoid the complications associated with tumor recurrence in the pelvis.

The technical aspects of radiation therapy relate to dose and timing. The effectiveness of radiation therapy is directly proportional to the total dose. It appears that the most effective dose of radiation to eradicate microscopic disease is at least 5,000 cGy. Adjuvant radiation therapy can be delivered preoperatively, postoperatively, or in a combined "sandwich" approach, in which small doses of preoperative treatment are followed by postoperative treatment to a high total cumulative dose. No studies clearly indicate that one approach is superior.

Less experience has been reported for adjuvant radiation therapy of resected colon cancer. Adjuvant radiation therapy for colon cancer is associated with special problems of toxicity because of the large amount of small intestine that may lie within the treatment field. Nevertheless, several reports indicate that in high-risk cases, such as tumors involving adjacent viscera or perforated lesions, adjuvant radiation therapy can decrease local and regional recurrences.

Adjuvant Chemotherapy

Even if local tumor control is adequate, patients with colorectal cancer die of disseminated disease. In about 25% of patients with stage II tumors, and 50% of those with stage III tumors, the growth of micrometastatic disease present at the time of primary tumor resection eventually causes death. Several randomized, prospective studies have demonstrated that postoperative adjuvant systemic chemotherapy benefits certain subgroups of patients.

A national cooperative intergroup study reported results in 1,296 patients with stage II or III colon cancer who were randomly assigned to receive either no chemotherapy, levamisole alone, or 5-fluorouracil (5-FU) plus levamisole therapy after resection (65). This study did not include patients with rectal cancer. Patients with stage III disease had improved disease-free and overall survival rates if treated with the combination of 5-FU and levamisole (Fig. 46.14). The survival curve of patients treated with levamisole

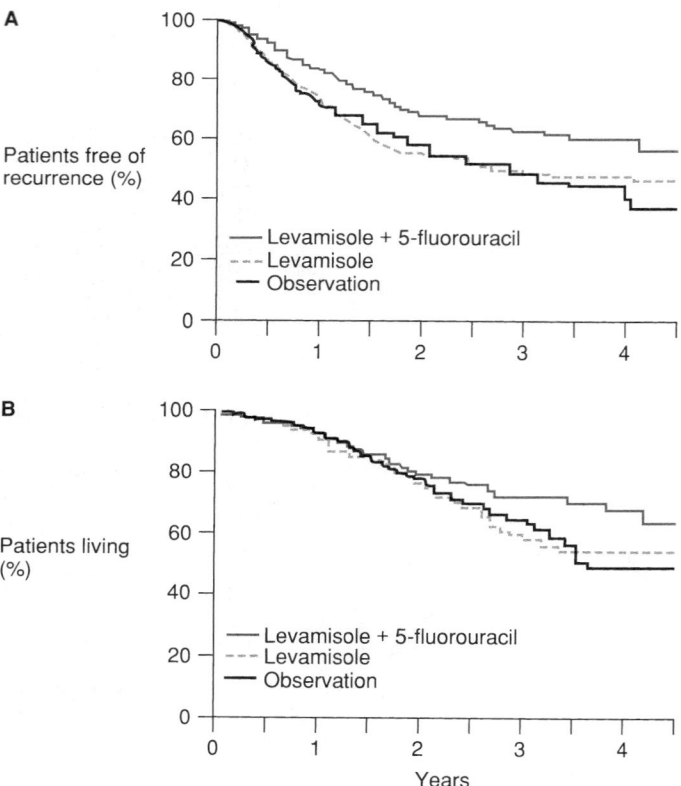

Figure 46.14. Improved disease-free and overall survival in patients with colon cancer who received adjuvant chemotherapy. (After Moertel CG, Fleming TR, MacDonald JS, et al. Levamisole and fluorouracil for adjuvant therapy of resected colon carcinoma. *N Engl J Med* 1990;322:352, with permission.)

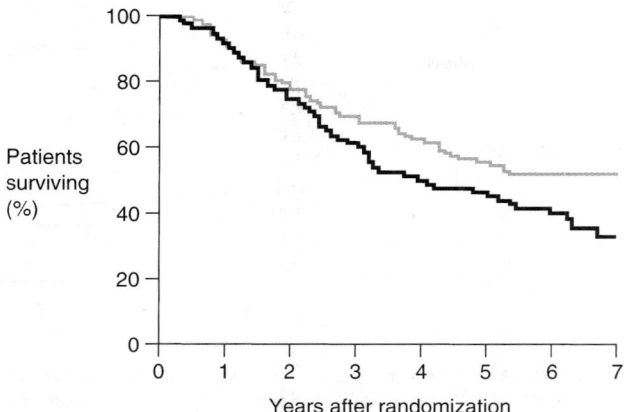

Figure 46.15. Improved overall survival in patients with stage II or III rectal cancer who received adjuvant chemotherapy plus radiation *(blue line)* or radiation alone *(black line)* postoperatively (*p* = .025). (After Krook J, Moertel C, Gunderson L, et al. Effective surgical adjuvant therapy for high-risk rectal carcinoma. *N Engl J Med* 1991;324:709, with permission.)

alone was similar to that of the control population. The results in patients with stage II tumors were equivocal and too preliminary to allow definitive conclusions.

In another study, comprising 1,166 patients with stage II or III colon cancers, the National Surgical Adjuvant Breast and Bowel Project (NSABP) reported a better survival rate in patients randomly assigned to receive adjuvant chemotherapy (5-FU, semustine, and vincristine) than in those who received no further treatment after resection (66). In a follow-up study, the NSABP evaluated the efficacy of therapy with 5-FU, semustine, and vincristine versus 5-FU plus leucovorin in patients with stage II or III colon cancer (67). Treatment with 5-FU plus leucovorin resulted in significantly improved survival rates, and they appeared to be the better combination of drugs. Semustine, which has been reported to have a leukemogenic effect, is no longer administered in this setting. Based on an evaluation of prospective, randomized studies, the National Institutes of Health recommended that patients with stage III colon cancer be offered adjuvant chemotherapy as standard treatment to improve the survival rate (68).

In colon cancer, local recurrence is infrequent; in rectal cancer, the use of adjuvant chemotherapy combined with radiation has proved effective in improving local control and increasing the survival rate. In rectal cancer, it is almost as important to prevent local failure and ensuing symptoms as it is to prevent death from distant metastasis. As noted in the previous section, radiation therapy is routinely recommended for patients with stage II or III rectal cancers. In a randomized, prospective study, 204 patients with stage II or III rectal cancer were randomly assigned to receive either postoperative radiation alone or radiation plus chemotherapy with 5-FU and semustine (69). The group that received chemotherapy had better local tumor control and an increased overall survival rate (Fig 46.15). In another prospective study, semustine was found not to be an essential component for effective adjuvant therapy (70). Based on these and other clinical studies, the National Institutes of Health has recommended that patients with stage II or III rectal cancer should receive postoperative chemotherapy and radiation as standard care (68).

Other Adjuvant Therapies

Adjuvant Portal Vein Chemotherapy. The liver is the most common site of metastatic disease in colorectal can-

cer. Metastasis is established by tumor cells embolized into the portal vein. From anatomic studies, it is known that micrometastases to the liver are initially fed by portal blood flow. These observations form the rationale for the administration of adjuvant chemotherapy with intraportal 5-FU in an attempt to decrease the incidence of liver metastasis. In an initial study, 244 patients who had undergone resection of Dukes A, B, or C colorectal tumors were randomly assigned to receive or not receive continuous intraportal 5-FU with heparin immediately after surgery (71). In patients with Dukes B and C tumors, the survival rate appeared to improve with intraportal 5-FU and the incidence of liver metastases to decrease. To confirm these results, the NSABP conducted a prospective, randomized study in which 1,158 patients with Dukes A, B, or C colon carcinoma (rectal cancers were excluded) were randomly assigned to either observation or treatment with intraportal 5-FU in the postoperative period (72). The study demonstrated an increased survival advantage in the group receiving intraportal 5-FU compared with the control group; however, the incidence of hepatic metastasis did not differ between the two groups. These results suggest that the intraportal 5-FU confers a systemic rather than a regional effect in reducing the incidence of metastatic disease; because the incidence of hepatic metastasis was not decreased by intraportal 5-FU, the application of regional therapy in this setting does not appear to be justified.

Adjuvant Immunotherapy. An increasing interest in immunotherapy for cancer is based on animal studies indicating that tumor regression can be mediated by modulation of the host immune system. One approach has been to use bacillus Calmette-Guérin (BCG) as a nonspecific immunostimulatory agent, but randomized studies have demonstrated that adjuvant BCG therapy does not improve the survival rate of patients with resected colorectal cancer. Another approach has been active specific immunization with the use of autologous irradiated tumor cells admixed with BCG (73). This treatment was promising in a small, single-institution clinical trial. A prospective, randomized trial of 254 patients with either stage II or III colon cancer was recently reported (74). Patients were randomly assigned to vaccination with autologous tumor cells plus BCG or no adjuvant treatment. After a median of 5 years, a survival benefit was noted for vaccine therapy in patients with stage II but not stage III disease. Until confirmatory trials are performed, this therapy should still be considered investigational.

Another form of immunotherapy that has been reported in colorectal cancer is the administration of monoclonal antibody. For example, 17-1A is murine monoclonal antibody that recognizes a 34-kd glycoprotein of the cell membrane on epithelial cells. A randomized trial involving 189 patients with Dukes C colorectal cancer has been reported (75). At 7 years of follow-up, 17-1A monoclonal antibody therapy was associated with improved survival in comparison with observation after surgical resection. Confirmatory trials need to be performed before this therapy can be considered as standard.

TREATMENT OF RECURRENT COLORECTAL CANCER

A subset of patients with recurrent colorectal cancer can be cured, so that a comprehensive follow-up program in patients who have undergone resection of their primary tumor is appropriate. Fifty percent of cancers that recur do so within 18 months after surgery, and 90% of recurrences are evident by 3 years. Therefore, careful follow-up is important during the 3-year period after primary tumor resection. Be-

Table 46.8. GUIDELINES FOR SURVEILLANCE STUDIES AFTER RESECTION OF STAGE II OR III COLORECTAL CANCER*

Test	Recommendations
CEA	If patient is medically fit to undergo liver resection for liver metastases, the CEA should be evaluated every 2 to 3 months for 2 years or more. An elevated CEA warrants further evaluation for metastatic disease but does not justify systemic therapy for presumed disease.
History and physical examination	Every 3 to 6 months for first 3 years, and yearly thereafter.
Colonoscopy	Every 3 to 5 years to detect new cancers and polyps.
Computed tomography	Not indicated.
Chest roentgenography	Not indicated.
Complete blood cell count	Not indicated.
Liver chemistries	Not indicated.
Fecal occult blood	Not indicated.

*Endorsed by the American Society of Clinical Oncology.
CEA, carcinoembryonic antigen.

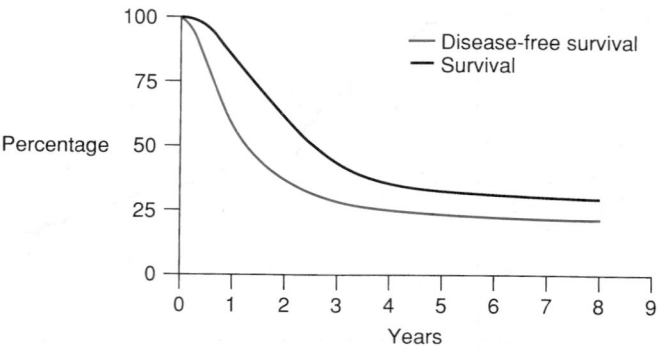

Figure 46.16. Disease-free and overall survival in patients who underwent hepatic resection for colorectal carcinoma metastases to the liver. (After Hughes KS, Simon R, Songhorabodi S, et al. Registry of hepatic metastases: resection of the liver for colorectal carcinoma metastases—a multiinstitutional study of indications for resection. *Surgery* 1988;103:278, with permission.)

sides identifying recurrences, a careful follow-up program also identifies the 5% of patients in whom a metachronous primary tumor of the large intestine develops.

The CEA assay is a sensitive serologic test in the diagnosis of recurrent colorectal cancer. CEA is a glycoprotein that was originally described as a tumor-specific antigen derived from neoplasms of the gastrointestinal tract. It is now known that CEA is not tumor-specific because its concentration can be elevated in a variety of malignancies from different sites and in some benign conditions. CEA is an oncofetal antigen that is also expressed by early embryonic or fetal cells. CEA is not useful as a screening or diagnostic test but is useful as a tumor marker. The CEA concentration is elevated in more than 90% of patients with disseminated colorectal cancer and in about 20% of patients with localized disease. Serum levels usually are elevated in proportion to the mass of the tumor present and often correlate with response to therapy. CEA measurement provides useful information when elevated levels fall to normal after curative resection. In about two thirds of patients with recurrent disease, an increased CEA level is the first indicator of tumor recurrence; therefore, serial CEA testing, combined with regular physical examinations, is one of the most useful means for detecting recurrent colorectal cancer. In fact, the CEA determination, along with the history and physical examination, is the only surveillance test recommended for patients during the first 3 years after curative resection of stage II or III disease. An expert panel organized by the American Society of Clinical Oncology reviewed the published data on surveillance studies and established guidelines; these are summarized in Table 46.8 (76). The only other surveillance study recommended is colonoscopy every 3 to 5 years.

Hepatic Metastases

The liver is the most frequent site of blood-borne metastases from primary colorectal cancers. In a subgroup of patients, the liver is the only site of recurrent disease, and surgical excision of the metastases is the only curative option for these patients. Overall, surgical resection is asso-

ciated with a 5-year survival rate of 25% to 30% (77) (Fig. 46.16). Patients eligible for hepatic resection of metastatic disease are those who have no evidence of extrahepatic tumor, no medical contraindications to surgery, and fewer than four lesions that are amenable to resection with negative surgical margins.

Patients who have unresectable hepatic metastases that appear to be confined to that organ have been treated with regional chemotherapy through the hepatic artery (e.g., 5-FU, 5-FU-deoxyribonucleoside). Several studies have demonstrated significantly higher tumor response rates with regional chemotherapy than with systemic chemotherapy, but an improved survival rate with this therapy has not been demonstrated clearly in randomized trials.

Pulmonary Metastases

Pulmonary metastases develop in about 10% of all patients with colorectal cancer, usually in association with widespread metastatic disease. Because the colon is drained solely by the portal system, one would not expect metastases to the lung without evidence of tumor in the liver. In contrast, rectal cancers may spread through the portal or systemic venous systems and can theoretically give rise to isolated pulmonary metastases. In selected patients, particularly those with rectal cancers, resection of pulmonary recurrences can result in a 5-year survival rate of 20% (78).

Local Recurrence

Colon cancer recurs locally in about 20% of cases, and the local lesion is the only site of recurrence in about one third of these cases. If the recurrent tumor is isolated to the suture line, resection of such recurrence can be curative. Locoregional failure occurs in 30% to 65% of patients with transmural or node-positive rectal cancers. Often, pelvic recurrences of rectal cancer after a low anterior or abdominoperineal resection are diffuse and associated with disseminated disease. If pelvic recurrences are localized, they should be resected if negative surgical margins can be achieved. Surgical procedures necessary to accomplish this include *en bloc* partial sacrectomy or total pelvic exenteration.

Disseminated Disease

Recurrent colorectal cancer is not usually localized to one site that is amenable to surgical resection. More commonly, colorectal cancer recurs in multiple sites. In these cases, systemic therapy may be considered. No studies have clearly documented that systemic therapies for disseminated colorectal cancer improve the survival rate; however, systemic treatment is commonly used for palliation.

The most commonly employed agent is 5-FU, a fluoropyrimidine. As a single agent, 5-FU produces an objective response rate of 10% to 20%. Studies have shown that the antitumor activity of 5-FU can be enhanced by folinic acid (leucovorin). Tumor response rates to this combination of drugs have been in the range of 30% to 40%. The combination of 5-FU and leucovorin is the first-line regimen for the treatment of disseminated colorectal cancer. A second-line chemotherapeutic regimen for patients who have failed 5-FU regimens is irinotecan (CPT-11, Camptosar). As a second-line therapy, it is associated with 15% response rate.

OTHER COLORECTAL TUMORS

Carcinoid Tumors

Carcinoid tumors are neoplasms derived from cells that are capable of synthesizing a wide variety of hormones. Most gastrointestinal tract carcinoids occur in the ileum and the appendix. The rectum is the next most common site, and occasionally carcinoid tumors occur in the colon. Tumor size is an extremely important prognostic factor. About 60% of rectal carcinoids present as asymptomatic submucosal nodules measuring less than 2 cm in diameter. Transanal local excision suffices for definitive therapy because small tumors rarely metastasize. Malignant potential is seen almost exclusively in tumors larger than 2 cm. More radical excisions of larger rectal lesions may be required for local control; however, the results of radical excisions for large rectal carcinoids are poor because these tumors are prone to metastasize.

Lymphomas

Colorectal lymphomas are rare and account for fewer than 0.5% of all colorectal malignancies. The documentation of widespread dissemination of lymphoma in most cases underscores the concept that lymphoma of the gastrointestinal tract is a systemic disease in which tumor cells are present in other organ sites. Because this disease is highly responsive to chemotherapy and radiation, surgery is not the primary mode of therapy. If the clinical workup reveals a focal site of disease in the large intestine, surgical resection may be considered. Usually, for localized, low-grade colorectal lymphomas, radiation therapy is considered first-line therapy. For intermediate- and high-grade lymphomas, chemotherapy combined with radiation therapy should be the primary treatment modality. Surgery for colorectal lymphomas has been primarily for diagnostic and staging purposes and for the management of treatment-related complications (i.e., perforation or bleeding).

Sarcomas

Colorectal sarcomas are extremely rare and account for fewer than 0.1% of all large-bowel malignancies. The most common histologic sarcoma subtype is leiomyosarcoma. With these tumors, the most significant prognostic indicator is the tumor grade. Patients with high-grade tumors do poorly. These tumors usually metastasize to the liver and peritoneal surfaces. If the tumors are clinically localized at initial presentation, a radical *en bloc* excision should be performed to obtain a margin of uninvolved normal tissue.

Because of the rarity of this tumor, no studies have addressed whether adjuvant radiation therapy or chemotherapy is beneficial.

REFERENCES

1. Landis SH, Taylor M, Bolden S, et al. Cancer statistics 1990. *CA Cancer J Clin* 1999;49:8.
2. Parkin DM, Laara E, Muir CS. Estimates of the worldwide frequency of sixteen major cancers in 1980. *Int J Cancer* 1988;41:184.
3. Troisi RJ, Freedman AN, Devesa SS. Incidence in colorectal carcinoma in the U.S.: an update of trends by gender, race, age, subsite, and stage, 1975–1994. *Cancer* 1999;85:1670.
4. Willett WC. The search for the causes of breast and colon cancer. *Nature* 1989;338:389.
5. Willett WC, MacMahon B. Diet and cancer: an overview. *N Engl J Med* 1984;310:697.
6. Burkitt DP. Epidemiology of cancer of the colon and rectum. *Cancer* 1971;28:3.
7. Bos JL, Fearon ER, Hamilton SR, et al. Prevalence of *ras* gene mutations in human colorectal cancers. *Nature* 1987;327:293.
8. Fearon ER, Vogelstein B. A genetic model for colorectal tumorigenesis. *Cell* 1990;61:759.
9. Arvanitis ML, Jagelman DG, Fazio VW, et al. Mortality in patients with familial adenomatous polyposis. *Dis Colon Rectum* 1990;33:639–642.
10. Kinzler KW, Nilbert MC, Su L-K, et al. Identification of FAP locus genes from cromosome 5q21. *Science* 1991;253:661–665.
11. Groden J, Thliveris A, Samowitz W, et al. Identification and characterization of the familial adenomatous polyposis coli gene. *Cell* 1991;66:589–600.
12. Gorinek V, Barker N, Morin P, et al. Constitutive transcriptional activation by a β-catenin-Tcf complex in APC$^{-/-}$ colon carcinoma. *Science* 1997;275:1784–1787.
13. Morin PJ, Sparks AB, Korinek V, et al. Activation of β-catenin-Tcf signaling in colon cancer by mutations in β-catenin or APC. *Science* 1997;275:1787–1790.
14. Powell SM, Zilz N, Beazer-Barclay Y, et al. APC mutations occur early during colorectal tumorigenesis. *Nature* 1992;359:235–237.
15. Smith A, Stern H, Penner M, et al. Somatic APC and K-*ras* codon 12 mutations in aberrant crypt foci from human colons. *Cancer Res* 1994;54:5527–5530.
16. Vogelstein B, Kinzler KW. *p53* function and dysfunction. *Cell* 1992;70:523–526.
17. Jen J, Kim H, Piantadosi S, et al. Allelic loss of chromosome 18q and prognosis in colorectal cancer. *N Engl J Med* 1994;331:213–221.
18. Carethers JM, Hawn MT, Greenson JK, et al. Prognostic significance of allelic loss of chromosome 18q21 for stage II colorectal cancer. *Gastroenterology* 1998;114:1–8.
19. Thibodeau SN, Bren G, Schaid D. Microsatellite instability in cancer of the proximal colon. *Science* 1993;260:816–819.
20. Ionov Y, Peinado MA, Makhosyan S, et al. Ubiquitous somatic mutations in simple repeated sequences reveal a new mechanism for colonic carcinogenesis. *Nature* 1993;363:558–561.
21. Aaltonen LA, Peltomaki P, Leach FS, et al. Clues to the pathogenesis of familial colorectal cancer. *Science* 1993;260:812–816.
22. Parsons R, Li GM, Longley MJ, et al. Hypermutability and mismatch repair deficiency in RER+ tumor cells. *Cell* 1993;75:1227–1236.
23. Leach FS, Nicolaides NC, Papadopoulos N, et al. Mutations of a *mutS* homolog in hereditary nonpolyposis colorectal cancer. *Cell* 1993;75:1215–1225.
24. Fishel R, Lescoe MK, Rao MRS, et al. The human mutator gene homolog *MSH2* and its association with hereditary nonpolyposis colon cancer. *Cell* 1993;75:1027–1038.
25. Papadopoulos N, Nicolaides NC, Wei Y-F, et al. Mutation of a *mutL* homolog in hereditary colon cancer. *Science* 1994;263:1625–1629.
26. Bronner CE, Baker SM, Morrison PT, et al. Mutation in the DNA mismatch repair gene homologue *hMLH1* is associated

with hereditary non-polyposis colon cancer. *Nature* 1994; 368:258–261.

27. Kolodner R. Biochemistry and genetics of eukaryotic mismatch repair. *Genes Dev* 1996;10:1433–1442.

28. Marsischky GT, Filosi N, Kane MF, et al. Redundancy of *Saccharomyces cerevisiae* MSH3 and MSH6 in MSH2-dependent mismatch repair. *Genes Dev* 1996;10:407–420.

29. Umar A, Risinger JI, Glaab We, et al. Functional overlap in mismatch repair by human MSH3 and MSH6. *Genetics* 1998;148:1637–1646.

30. Cannon-Albright L, Skolnick M, Bishop D, et al. Common inheritance of susceptibility to colonic adenomatous polyps and associated colorectal cancers. *N Engl J Med* 1988;319: 533–537.

31. Houlston R, Collins A, Slack J, et al. Dominant genes for colorectal cancer are not rare. *Ann Hum Genet* 1992;56:99–103.

32. Offerhaus GJA, Giardiello FM, Krush AJ, et al. The risk of upper gastrointestinal cancer in familial adenomatous polyposis. *Gastroenterology* 1992;102:1980–1982.

33. Tonelli F, Nardi F, Bechi P, et al. Extracolonic polyps in familial polyposis and Gardner's syndrome. *Dis Colon Rectum* 1985;28:664–668.

34. Warthin AS. Heredity with reference to carcinoma. *Arch Intern Med* 1913;12:546–555.

35. Lynch HT, Krush AJ. Cancer family G revisited: 1895–1970. *Cancer* 1971;27:1505–1511.

36. Watson P, Lynch HT. Extracolonic cancer in hereditary non-polyposis colorectal cancer. *Cancer* 1993;71:677–685.

37. Vasen HFA, Mecklin J-P, Khan PM, et al. The International Collaborative Group on Hereditary Non-Polyposis Colorectal Cancer. *Dis Colon Rectum* 1991;34:424–425.

38. Wijnen J, Khan PM, Vasen H, et al. Hereditary nonpolyposis colorectal cancer families not complying with the Amsterdam criteria show extremely low frequency of mismatch-repair gene mutations. *Am J Hum Genet* 1997;61:329–335.

39. Wijnen JT, Vasen HFA, Khan PM, et al. Clinical findings with implications for genetic testing in families with clustering of colorectal cancer. *N Engl J Med* 1998;339:511–518.

40. Aaltonen LA, Salovaara R, Kristo P, et al. Incidence of hereditary nonpolyposis colorectal cancer and the feasibility of molecular screening for the disease. *N Engl J Med* 1998;338: 1481–1487.

41. Laken SJ, Petersen GM, Gruber SB, et al. Familial colorectal cancer in Ashenazim due to a hypermutable tract in APC. *Nat Genet* 1997;17:79–83.

42. Giardiello FM, Brensinger JD, Petersen GM, et al. The use and interpretation of commercial APC gene testing for familial adenomatous polyposis. *N Engl J Med* 1997;336:823–827.

43. Ponder B. Genetic testing for cancer risk. *Science* 1997;278: 1050–1054.

44. Gyde SN, Prior P, Thompson H, et al. Survival of patients with colorectal cancer complicating ulcerative colitis. *Gut* 1984;25:228.

45. Muto T, Bussey HJR, Morson BC. The evolution of cancer of the colon and rectum. *Cancer* 1975;36:2251.

46. Hardcastle JD, Armitage NC, Chamberlin J, et al. Fecal occult blood screening for colorectal cancer in the general population. *Cancer* 1986;58:397.

47. Mandel JS, Bond JH, Church TR, et al. Reducing mortality from colorectal cancer by screening for fecal occult blood. *N Engl J Med* 1993;328:1365.

48. Mandel JS, Church TR, Ederer F, et al. Colorectal cancer mortality: effectiveness of biennial screening for fecal occult blood. *J Natl Cancer Inst* 1999;91:434.

49. Hardcastle JD, Chamberlain JO, Robinson MH, et al. Randomized controlled trial of faecal-occult-blood screening for colorectal cancer. *Lancet* 1996;348:1472.

50. Kronberg O, Fenger C, Olsen J, et al. Randomized study of screening for colorectal cancer with faecal-occult-blood test. *Lancet* 1996;1467.

51. Kewenter J, Brevinge H, Engaras B, et al. Results of screening, rescreening, and follow-up in a prospective randomized study for detection of colorectal cancer by fecal occult blood testing: results for 68,308 subjects. *Scand J Gastroenterol* 1994;29:468.

52. Selby JV, Friedman GD, Quesenberry CP Jr, et al. A case-control study of screening sigmoidoscoy and mortality from colorectal cancer. *N Engl J Med* 1992;326:653.

53. Winawer SJ, Zauber AG, Ho MN, et al. Prevention of colorectal cancer by colonoscopic polypectomy. *N Engl J Med* 1993; 329:1977.

54. Winawer SJ, Fletcher RH, Miller L, et al. Colorectal cancer screening: clinical guidelines and rationale. *Gastroenterology* 1997;112:594.

55. Wolmark N, Fisher B, Wieand HS. The prognostic value of the modifications of the Dukes' C class of colorectal cancer. *Ann Surg* 1986;203:115.

56. Kokal WA, Gardine RL, Sheibani K, et al. Tumor DNA content in resectable, primary colorectal carcinoma. *Ann Surg* 1989; 209:188.

57. Halling KC, French AJ, McDonnell SK, et al. Microsatellite instability and 8p allelic imbalance in stage B2 and C colorectal cancers. *J Natl Cancer Inst* 1999;91:1295.

58. August DA, Ottow RT, Sugarbaker PH. Clinical perspective of human colorectal cancer metastasis. *Cancer Metastasis Rev* 1984;3:303.

59. Yeatman TJ, Bland KI. Sphincter-saving procedures for distal carcinoma of the rectum. *Ann Surg* 1989;209:1.

60. Steele GD, Hendon JE, Bleday R, et al. Sphincter-sparing treatment for distal rectal adenocarcinoma. *Ann Surg Oncol* 1999;5:433–441.

61. Wagman R, Minsky BD, Cohen AM, et al. Sphincter preservation in rectal cancer with preoperative radiation therapy and coloanal anastomosis: long-term follow-up. *Int J Radiat Oncol Biol Phys* 1998;42:51–57.

62. Chakravarit A, Compton CC, Shellito PC, et al. Long-term follow-up of patients with rectal cancer managed by local excision with and without adjuvant irradiation. *Ann Surg* 1999; 230:49–54.

63. Temple LKC, Maimark D, McLeod RS. Decision analysis as an aid to determining the management of early low rectal cancer for the individual patient. *Clin Oncol* 1999;17:312–318.

64. Madden JL, Kandalft SI. Electrocoagulation as a primary curative method in the treatment of carcinoma of the rectum. *Surg Gynecol Obstet* 1983;157:164.

65. Moertel CG, Fleming TR, MacDonald JS, et al. Levamisole and fluorouracil for adjuvant therapy of resected colon carcinoma. *N Engl J Med* 1990;322:352.

66. Wolmark N, Fisher B, Rockette H, et al. Postoperative adjuvant chemotherapy or BCG for colon cancer: results from NSABP protocol C-01. *J Natl Cancer Inst* 1988;80:30.

67. Wolmark N, Rockette H, Fisher B, et al. The benefit of leucovorin-modulated fluorouracil as postoperative adjuvant therapy for primary colon cancer: results from National Surgical Adjuvant Breast and Bowel Project protocol C-03. *J Clin Oncol* 1993;11:1879.

68. Steele GD Jr, Augenlicht LH, Begg CB, et al. National Institutes of Health Consensus Development Conference statement: adjuvant therapy for patients with colon and rectal cancer. *JAMA* 1990;264:1444.

69. Krook JE, Moertel CG, Gunderson LL, et al. Effective surgical adjuvant therapy for high-risk rectal carcinoma. *N Engl J Med* 1991;324:709.

70. Gastrointestinal Tumor Study Group. Radiation therapy and fluorouracil with or without semustine for the treatment of patients with surgical adjuvant adenocarcinoma of the rectum. *J Clin Oncol* 1992;10:549.

71. Taylor I, Machin D, Mullee M, et al. A randomized controlled trial of adjuvant portal vein cytotoxic perfusion in colorectal cancer. *Br J Surg* 1985;72:359.

72. Wolmark N, Rockette H, Wickerham DL, et al. Adjuvant therapy of Dukes' A, B, and C adenocarcinoma of the colon with portal-vein fluorouracil hepatic infusion: preliminary results of National Surgical Adjuvant Breast and Bowel Project protocol C-02. *J Clin Oncol* 1990;8:1466.

73. Hoover HC, Brandhorst JS, Peters LC, et al. Adjuvant active specific immunotherapy for human colorectal cancer: 6.5-year median follow-up of a phase III prospectively randomized trial. *J Clin Oncol* 1993;11:390.

74. Vermorken JB, Claessen AM, van Tinteren H, et al. Active specific immunotherapy for stage II and stage III human colon cancer: a randomized trial. *Lancet* 1999;353:345.

75. Riethmuller G, Holz E, Schlimok G, et al. Monoclonal antibody therapy for resected Dukes' C colorectal cancer: seven-year outcome of a multicenter randomzied trial. *J Clin Oncol* 1998;16:1788.

76. Desch CE, Benson AB, Smith TJ, et al. Recommended colorectal cancer surveillance guidelines by the American Society of Clinical Oncology. *J Clin Oncol* 1999;17:1312.

77. Hughes KK, Simon R, Songhorabodi S, et al. Registry of hepatic metastases. Resection of the liver for colorectal carcinoma metastases: a multi-institutional study of indications for resection. *Surgery* 1988;103:278.

78. Kern KA, Pass HI, Roth JA. Surgical treatment of pulmonary metastases. In: Rosenberg SA, ed. *Surgical treatment of metastatic cancer.* Philadelphia: JB Lippincott, 1987:69.

79. Corman ML, Swinton NW, O'Keefe DD, et al. Colorectal carcinoma at the Lahey Clinic, 1962–1966. *Am J Surg* 1973;125:424.

80. Eisenberg B, Decosse JJ, Harford F, et al. Carcinoma of the colon and rectum: the natural history reviewed in 1,704 patients. *Cancer* 1982;49:1131.

81. Pihl E, Hughes ESR, McDermott FT, et al. Carcinoma of the colon: cancer-specific long-term survival—a series of 615 patients treated by one surgeon. *Ann Surg* 1980;192:114.

82. Willett CG, Tepper JE, Cohen AM, et al. Failure patterns following curative resection of colonic carcinoma. *Ann Surg* 1984;200:685.

83. Minsky BD, Mies C, Rich TA, et al. Potentially curative surgery of colon cancer: patterns of failure and survival. *J Clin Oncol* 1988;6:106.

SURGERY: SCIENTIFIC PRINCIPLES AND PRACTICE, Third Edition, edited by Lazar J. Greenfield, Michael W. Mulholland, Keith T. Oldham, Gerald B. Zelenock, and Keith D. Lillemoe. Lippincott Williams & Wilkins Publishers, Philadelphia, © 2001.

CHAPTER 47

ANAL CANCER

SANTHAT NIVATVONGS

Anal cancers, which are uncommon, comprise cancers of the perianal skin and the anal canal. Although the literature is replete with reports on this subject, the use of terminology and classification has not been uniform; consequently, interpreting the results of treatment is difficult because malignant neoplasms at different locations with different behaviors were formerly grouped together. To overcome this confusion, the World Health Organization and the American Joint Committee on Cancer have developed a universally accepted description terminology for the histologic typing and staging of intestinal neoplasms of the anal region (1,2).

ANATOMIC LANDMARKS

The anal canal from the anorectal ring to the anal verge comprises the "surgical" anal canal. The mucosal lining is divided into three zones: upper or rectal, middle or transitional, and lower or squamous. The transitional zone extends proximally from the dentate line for a distance of approximately 1 cm (1,2). This definition contrasts with the one found in many series in the literature, which use the dentate line as the dividing point and describe the anal canal as the area above the dentate line and the anal margin as the area below the dentate line (3–6). The perianal skin starts at the lateral border of the anal verge (7,8). The lateral or distal extent of the perianal skin is reasonably defined as being 5 to 6 cm from the anal verge (8,9).

The lymphatic drainage of the area above the dentate line up to the anorectal ring (the first 6 to 10 mm referred to as the *transitional zone*) is primarily cephalad via the superior rectal lymphatics to the inferior mesenteric nodes. This area also drains laterally along both the middle rectal vessels and inferior rectal vessels through the ischioanal fossa to the internal iliac nodes. Lymphatic drainage from the anal canal below the dentate line is directed to the inguinal nodes. Secondary drainage may follow the inferior rectal lymphatics to the ischioanal nodes and internal iliac nodes, and along the superior rectal nodes. Lymphatic drainage of the perianal skin is entirely to the inguinal nodes.

INCIDENCE

Anal carcinoma represents 1% to 6% of all carcinomas of the anus and rectum. Eighty-five percent of anal carcinomas arise in the anal canal. The mean age of patients at presentation averages from 58 to 67 years. Carcinomas of the anal canal show a marked female predominance, with a female-to-male ratio of approximately 5:1. In areas with a large proportion of male patients at high risk (e.g., homosexuals), the female-to-male ratio approaches 1:1 (10).

ETIOLOGY AND PATHOGENESIS

Infection with human papillomavirus (HPV) increases the risk for anal carcinoma in a manner that closely parallels the role of HPV infection in the genesis of cervical carcinoma.

Human papillomavirus types 6 and 11 are associated with benign lesions such as warts and with low-grade anal intraepithelial neoplasia, a dysplastic lesion that rarely progresses to invasive carcinoma. In contrast, HPV types 16, 18, 31, 33, 34, and 35 are most commonly associated with high-grade anal intraepithelial neoplasia and carcinomas of the anus and cervix. HPV types 6 and 11 are maintained as extrachromosomal episomes, whereas HPV types 16 and 18 are integrated into host DNA, which explains the different propensity for the development of carcinoma (11). HPV types 16 and 18 also have a predilection for the less stable epithelium of the upper anal canal (transitional zone) rather than for the modified skin of the lower anal canal (anoderm) (10). The risk for anal carcinoma is increased in immunosuppressed patients, such as renal transplant and cardiac allograft recipients, and in patients who have undergone chemotherapy. Approximately 50% of patients positive for HIV have detectable HPV DNA (10).

To manage patients with anal carcinomas properly, it is essential for clinicians to know and understand the staging system. The prognosis and approaches to management of these patients differ according to the stage of the disease. Unlike carcinomas of the colon and rectum, anal carcinomas cannot be classified according to the Dukes staging system because part of the lymphatic drainage is to the inguinal region and outside the extent of the resection. The TNM (tumor–node–metastasis) system has now become the standard classification. The World Health Organization in its most recent edition of standards and the unified American Joint Committee on Cancer have introduced major changes in the staging of the primary carcinoma (1,2). The *T* category is now determined by the largest diameter of the primary carcinoma measured in centimeters. Formerly, it was necessary to estimate clinically the circumferential extent of the anal carcinoma and whether the external sphincter was invaded (Table 47.1).

The best means of staging anal carcinoma remains a careful examination, under general anesthesia if necessary, supplemented by endorectal ultrasonography, computed tomography (CT), or magnetic resonance imaging (MRI). These procedures make it possible to perform biopsies and decide on the best mode of treatment. If the patient receives

Table 47.1. TUMOR–NODE–METASTASIS (TNM) CANCER STAGING SYSTEM

Anal canal		Perianal skin	
T1	= 2 cm	T1	= 2 cm
T2	>2 to 5 cm	T2	>2 to 5 cm
T3	>5 cm	T3	>5 cm
T4	Adjacent organ(s)	T4	Deep extradermal structures
N1	Perirectal		(e.g., cartilage, skeletal muscle,
N2	Unilateral internal		bone)
	iliac/inguinal	N1	Regional
N3	Perirectal and inguinal,		
	bilateral internal		
	iliac/inguinal		

From Fleming ID, Cooper JS, Henson DE, et al. American Joint Committee on Cancer. Cancer Staging Manual, 5th ed. Philadelphia: Lippincott–Raven, 1997:91–95, 157–161.

radiotherapy or chemotherapy, further staging should be carried out 8 weeks later to assess the results of treatment.

PERIANAL NEOPLASMS

Squamous Cell Carcinoma

Squamous cell carcinomas of the perianal area resemble those occurring in skin elsewhere. They grow slowly and typically have rolled, everted edges with central ulceration. Any chronic unhealed or indurated ulceration in the perianal area should be considered squamous cell carcinoma until biopsy proves otherwise. Squamous cell carcinomas are usually well differentiated histologically, with well-developed patterns of keratinization (Fig. 47.1). Lymphatic spread from squamous carcinomas of the perianal area is mainly to inguinal lymph nodes. Despite their superficial location, most lesions are diagnosed late, with half of cases detected more than 22 months after the onset of symptoms. The tumor is often discovered at a late stage, when it is 5 cm or larger in diameter (12).

Wide local excision is the cornerstone of treatment of perianal squamous cell carcinoma in properly selected cases. For in situ or microinvasive carcinoma, the cure rate with local excision is 100% (7,13). For other, less favorable

lesions, chemoradiation should be used (8). Abdominoperineal resection is reserved for patients who cannot tolerate chemoradiation and those with anal incontinence. The size of the carcinoma determines the survival rate. The 5- and 10-year survival rates for T1 lesions are both 100%, and for T2 lesions they are 60% and 40%, respectively (9).

Basal Cell Carcinoma

Basal cell carcinoma of the perianal area is rare and occurs more frequently in men than in women, usually during the sixth decade. The lesions are characterized by central ulceration and irregular, raised edges. Basal cell carcinomas are usually superficial and not fixed to deeper structures, and they rarely metastasize. Inguinal lymphadenopathy develops frequently from reactive inflammation. The patient most frequently presents with complaints of mild discomfort, itching, or bleeding.

A wide local excision is the treatment of choice. Local recurrence after excision is common, however, and occurs in almost one third of patients. Repeated excision is indicated. Abdominoperineal resection is reserved for patients with large lesions and uncontrollable local recurrence and those with anal incontinence. The 5-year survival is around 70% (14).

Bowen's Disease

Bowen's disease of the perianal skin is a rare, slow-growing intraepidermal squamous cell carcinoma (carcinoma in situ) (Fig. 47.2). Bowen's disease occurs in relatively young people with an average age of 46 to 50 years (15,16). The lesions appear as a discrete scaly or crusted plaque that sometimes exhibits a moist surface. The patient may report itching, burning, or spotty bleeding. Although symptoms and gross appearance are suggestive, only a biopsy can confirm the diagnosis. Untreated, the disease eventually progresses to invasive squamous cell carcinoma (15). Wide local excision is the treatment of choice (15,16). The extent of involvement should be mapped by obtaining multiple biopsy specimens 1 cm from the lesion all around the perianal area, including the dentate line, anal verge, and perineum. Bowen's disease can be extensive, involving the entire perianal skin and

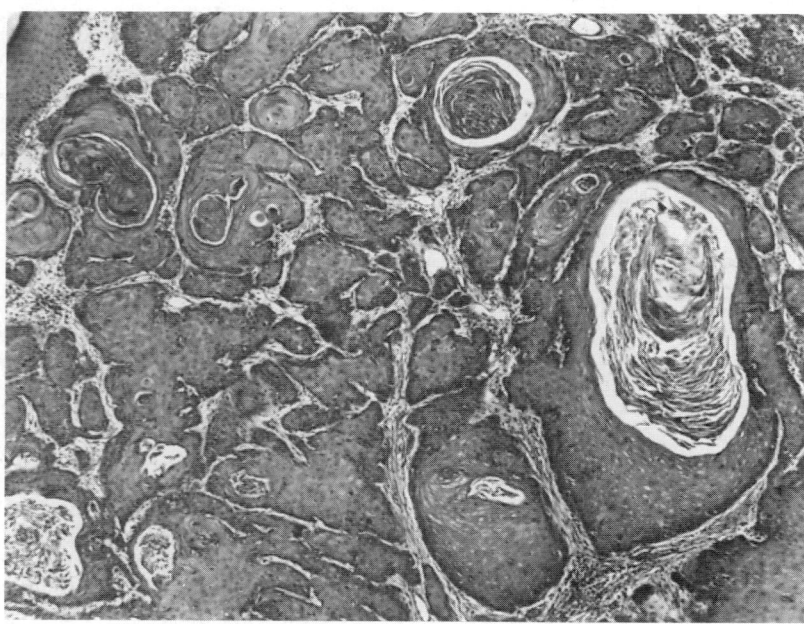

Figure 47.1. Photomicrograph of squamous cell carcinoma of the perianal skin. Note the presence of keratin.

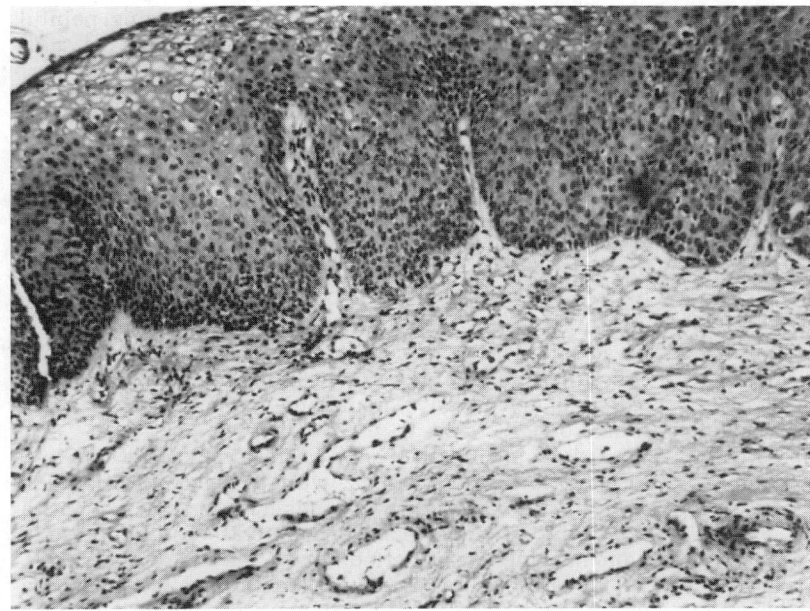

Figure 47.2. Bowen's disease. Atypical epithelial cells involve the full thickness of the epidermis (carcinoma in situ).

anoderm. In this circumstance, sliding V-Y flaps are required to cover the wound.

Perianal Paget's Disease

In 1874, Sir James Paget first described this disease in relationship to the nipple of the breast in female patients. Extramammary Paget's disease can be found in the axilla and the anogenital region (labia majora, penis, scrotum, groin, pubic area, perineum, perianal region, thigh, and buttock). The histogenesis of perianal Paget's disease is not fully understood, but ultrastructural and immunohistochemical studies have helped to clarify the debate. Most authors agree with the concept that Paget's cells are of glandular, probably apocrine, origin (17,18). An alternative hypothesis implicating pluripotential intraepidermal cells cannot be excluded, but evidence for such a histogenesis is lacking (17). In contrast to Paget's disease of the nipple, which is invariably associated with an underlying invasive or in

situ ductal adenocarcinoma, perianal Paget's disease starts as a benign neoplasm. It may eventually become invasive and give rise to an adenocarcinoma.

Perianal Paget's disease occurs mostly in elderly people with an average age of 68 years (19). The lesions appear as a slowly enlarging erythematous, eczematous, and often sharply demarcated anal skin rash that may ooze or scale and is usually accompanied by pruritus. Because of the similarity of perianal Paget's disease to other perianal conditions, such as idiopathic pruritus ani, hidradenitis suppurativa, condyloma acuminatum, Crohn's disease, Bowen's disease, and squamous cell carcinoma, the diagnosis is often delayed because of clinical diagnostic error. In almost one third of cases, the lesion involves the entire circumference of the perianal skin and anus (20).

The diagnosis must be confirmed by biopsy and by identification of the characteristic Paget's cells—large, pale, vacuolated cells with hyperchromatic, eccentric nuclei (Fig. 47.3). The cells invariably contain acid muco-

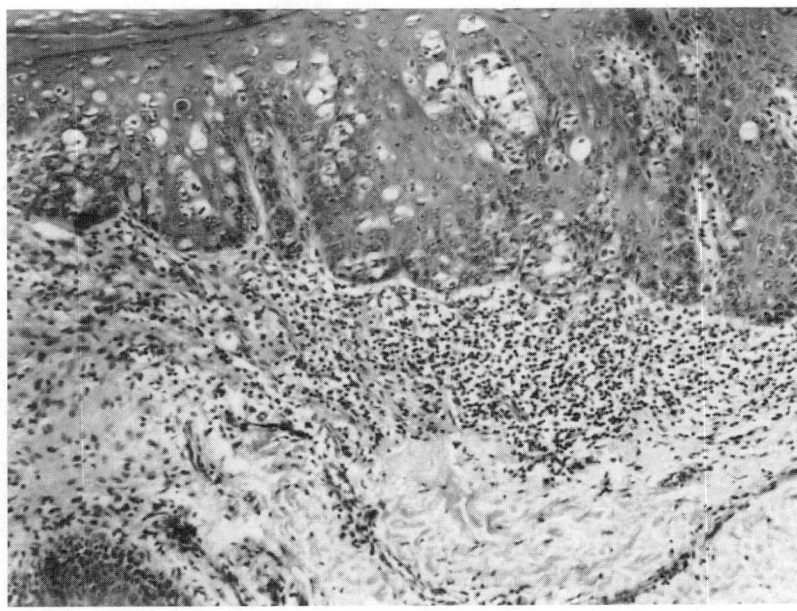

Figure 47.3. Perianal Paget's disease. Paget's cells are above the basal layer.

protein, an important feature in distinguishing this lesion from Bowen's disease and melanoma. True Paget's disease of the perianal skin must not be confused with the downward intraepidermal spread of a signet ring-cell carcinoma of the rectum or with Bowen's disease of the perianal skin. A complete large-bowel investigation with emphasis on thorough examination of the rectum and anal canal should be performed. The coexistence of visceral carcinomas is well-known, with an incidence as high as 50% (19,21).

In the absence of invasive carcinoma, wide excision is the treatment of choice. Obtaining an adequate microscopically clear margin is important. Because perianal Paget's disease may extend beyond the gross margin of the lesion, the extent of involvement is mapped by obtaining multiple biopsy specimens 1 cm from the edge of the lesion all around the perianal area, including the dentate line, anal verge, and perineum. The large wound defect of the perianal area and anal canal can be reconstructed with sliding V-Y subcutaneous skin flaps. Successful radiation therapy has also been reported for perianal Paget's disease (20,22).

For more advanced lesions with an underlying invasive carcinoma, an abdominoperineal resection along with inguinal lymph node dissection is necessary. Whether preoperative chemoradiation is helpful remains unproven. Because of the commonly delayed diagnosis (average of 4 years), metastasis has already occurred in approximately 25% of patients with invasive adenocarcinoma in Paget's disease (23,24). The sites of metastasis in order of frequency are the inguinal and pelvic lymph nodes, liver, bone, lung, brain, bladder, prostate, and adrenal gland (24).

Long-term follow-up is essential to detect local recurrence and development of invasive Paget's disease or intercurrent invasive carcinoma of the rectum and anal canal (20,25,26). A patient with invasive perianal Paget's disease has a poor prognosis despite abdominoperineal resection because in most cases distant metastasis has already occurred at the time of diagnosis (24).

Verrucous Carcinoma

It is now generally felt that the entity previously termed *giant condyloma acuminatum* or *Buschke-Löwenstein tumor* represents verrucous carcinoma. These lesions typ-ically present as large (8 × 8 cm), slowly enlarging, painful, wartlike growths that are relatively soft and have a cauliflower-like appearance. The lesions may arise in the perianal skin, anal canal, or distal rectum and are frequently indistinguishable from condylomata acuminata. Although they are histologically benign, their clinical behavior is malignant.

The clinical course is one of relentless progression and expansion of the neoplasm by extensive erosion and pressure necrosis of surrounding tissues; invasion of the ischioanal fossa, perirectal tissues, and even the pelvic cavity is seen. The invasive nature of these lesions can cause multiple sinuses and fistulous tracts to form, which may invade the fascia, muscle, rectum, and uterus and cause subsequent inflammation, infection, and hemorrhage. The extent of local and regional involvement can be determined by CT.

Microscopically, the lesion bears a marked resemblance to condylomata acuminata, with papillary proliferation, keratinization, acanthosis, parakeratosis, and vacuolization of superficial layers. Distant metastasis from these tumors has not been reported.

The basic treatment is wide local excision. If the carcinoma involves the anal sphincters, an abdominoperineal resection should be performed. The use of multimodality therapy in the treatment of verrucous carcinoma has not been reported. Squamous cell carcinoma associated with condyloma acuminatum has been treated effectively with chemoradiation. The difference in the two entities may be simply one of nomenclature (27,28).

NEOPLASMS OF THE ANAL CANAL

Squamous Cell Carcinoma

This general category encompasses a number of different microscopic appearances, including large cell keratinizing, large cell nonkeratinizing (transitional), and basaloid. The term *cloacogenic carcinoma* has been used for the basaloid and large cell nonkeratinizing (transitional) forms of squamous carcinoma. Most squamous cell carcinomas of the anal canal above the dentate line are nonkeratinizing (Fig. 47.4). Mucoepidermoid carcinoma is extremely rare.

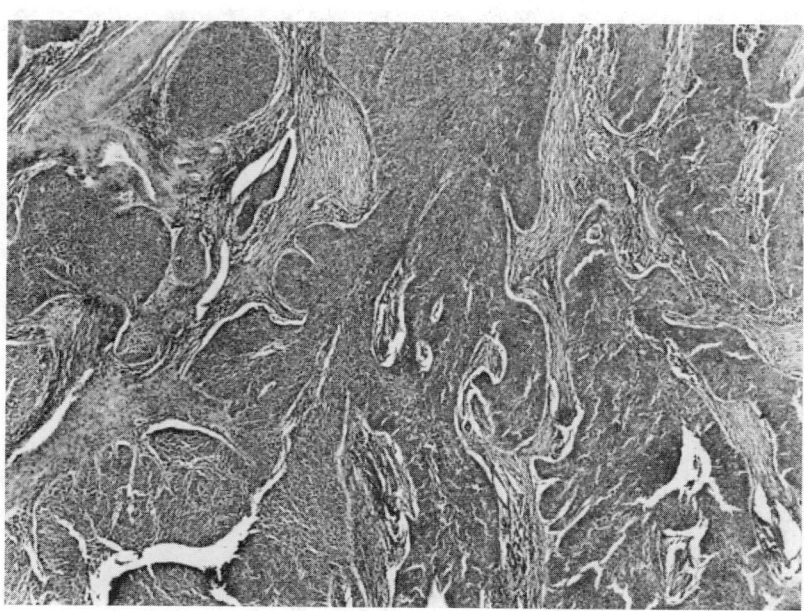

Figure 47.4. Squamous cell carcinoma of the anal canal. Note the absence of keratin.

The presentation of squamous cell carcinomas generally follows a long history of minor perianal problems, such as bleeding. Other signs and symptoms include pruritus, discharge, pain, and an indurated anal mass. In almost one third of patients with anal canal squamous cell carcinoma, benign or inflammatory disease is initially incorrectly diagnosed.

The most important part of the diagnosis is a digital examination of the anal canal. The size, consistency, and fixation of the primary lesion and the presence or absence of pararectal lymph nodes can be determined. Proctoscopy should be performed to confirm the digital findings and determine the exact location of the neoplasm in the anal canal. A biopsy must be performed to determine the histologic type. A colonoscopic examination is indicated to rule out more proximal associated lesions. Endorectal ultrasonography is useful in evaluating the depth of invasion and detecting lymph node metastasis. Both groins must be examined carefully to identify any enlargement of lymph nodes. Enlarged or suspect lymph nodes in the groin area should be assessed by excision or biopsy because reactive lymphadenopathy is common.

The anal canal has extensive lymphatic pathways. If the carcinoma is situated above the dentate line, metastases are found along the superior rectal vessels; if the carcinoma is at the dentate line, the lymphatic drainage is toward the internal pudendal, hypogastric, and obturator nodes; if the carcinoma is below the dentate line, the lymphatic drainage is via the inguinal nodes. About 40% of lymph node metastases are in lymph nodes less than 5 mm in diameter (29). Most lymph nodes in the anal region drain above the peritoneal reflection. Lymph nodes are scant in the perianal zones.

Inguinal metastasis is found in 15% to 20% of patients at the time of diagnosis and becomes apparent later in an additional 10% to 25% (30). The risk for lymphatic metastasis is correlated with the depth of invasion, size, and histologic grade. Nodal metastasis is present in 30% of patients when the smooth muscle is infiltrated and in 58% when infiltration is beyond the external sphincter. Lymph node metastasis in found in only 3% of patients with a carcinoma less than 2 cm in diameter (31). Although distant metastasis is uncommon at presentation, subsequent metastasis is common: 40% of carcinoma-related deaths are caused by disease identified outside the pelvis.

Local excision is the treatment of choice for carcinoma in situ or microscopic invasive carcinoma in the anal canal. Unfortunately, only small numbers of the lesions are suitable for this option; most are too large or too advanced at the time of diagnosis. Abdominoperineal resection is no longer the primary treatment for invasive squamous cell carcinoma of the anal canal and most perianal carcinomas. The recurrence rate is high after this treatment, and local recurrence after abdominoperineal resection has a less favorable prognosis. At the present time, abdominoperineal resection is reserved for patients with local treatment failure after chemoradiation or anorectal complications of treatment, especially fecal incontinence, and for those who cannot tolerate chemoradiation.

The combination of 5-fluorouracil, mitomycin C, and pelvic radiation therapy was pioneered by Nigro (32) and has now become the standard treatment for squamous cell carcinoma of the anus. The regimen is as follows:

External radiation—30 Gy to the primary carcinoma and pelvic inguinal nodes; start—day 1 (2 Gy/d, 5 d/wk).

Systemic chemotherapy with 5-fluorouracil—1,000 mg/m^2 per 24 hours as a continuous infusion for 4 days; start—day 1; repeat 4-day infusion starting day 28.

Mitomycin C—15 mg/m^2 as an intravenous bolus; start—day 1 only.

Protocols vary among institutions, particularly the dose of radiation. In most, a dose of 40 to 50 Gy has been used. Complete regression with treatment has been in the neighborhood of 90%. The 5-year survival ranges from 76% to 90% (5,33–35).

The simultaneous appearance of inguinal metastasis is an ominous sign. Because of its associated high morbidity and low success rate in preventing the dissemination of carcinoma, prophylactic groin dissection is no longer recommended. The treatment of inguinal node metastasis is chemoradiation to the inguinal area (34,36). Whether prophylactic groin radiation should be performed is controversial, but it has been recommended by many authorities. Elective radiation to clinically normal inguinal nodes reduces the risk for lymph node failure and carries little morbidity. In one series, only 1 of 38 patients had late recurrence in the inguinal area after undergoing combination chemotherapy and radiotherapy (37). In series in which inguinal nodes were not treated electively, the late nodal recurrence rate was 15% to 25% (31,38, 39).

Adenocarcinoma

Adenocarcinomas of the anus are rare, constituting 3% to 9% of all anal carcinomas (40,41). The World Health Organization classifies these malignancies into rectal type, anal glands, and those within an anorectal fistula (1).

Rectal type: The tumor arises within the upper zone lined by colorectal-type mucosa. The histology is similar to that of an adenocarcinoma of the large intestine. It is generally difficult to separate adenocarcinoma of the anal canal from adenocarcinoma of the lower rectum.

Anal glands: The ducts of the anal glands are lined by stratified columnar epithelium with mucin-secreting or goblet cells. The histologic picture of these lesions, therefore, may be one of adenocarcinoma or mucoepidermoid carcinoma. The most characteristic feature of anal duct carcinoma is extramucosal adenocarcinoma without involvement of the surface epithelium, except when the lesion has become advanced.

Anorectal fistula: Well-differentiated mucinous adenocarcinomas occasionally develop within an anorectal fistula that may be developmental or acquired (1). Most often, these carcinomas arise in patients with long-standing perianal disease (42). Some authors believe that the tumors originate in the anal glands and ducts (43,44).

To treat small and well-differentiated rectal-type adenocarcinomas that have not invaded the muscular layer of the anorectum, a wide local excision can be performed; otherwise, an abdominoperineal resection is indicated. An abdominoperineal resection is indicated for adenocarcinomas of the anal gland or an anal fistula. The role of adjuvant therapy is not yet defined because of the uncommon nature of the disease. The Nigro chemoradiation regime has been used successfully; of nine patients who were treated with this protocol, six patients were free of disease at follow-up of 2 to 4 years (45).

Small Cell Carcinoma

This very rare carcinoma may arise in the anorectal region. Small cell carcinoma is similar in histology, behavior, and histochemistry to small cell (oat cell) carcinoma of the lung. The tumor is often widely disseminated at the time of discovery. The term *neuroendocrine* has been applied to this carcinoma, but this implies an embryologic derivation that is unproven (1). The treatment of these carcinomas is the same as for adenocarcinomas. The prognosis can be expected to be poor.

Undifferentiated Carcinoma

Also very rare, this type of malignant lesion has no glandular structure or other features to indicate definite differentiation. The treatment is the same as for adenocarcinomas. The prognosis is poor.

MELANOMA

Anal melanoma, a rare malignant tumor of the anal canal, accounts for 1% to 3% of all melanomas. Nevertheless, the anal canal is the third most common site for melanomas, exceeded only by the skin and eyes. Almost all anal melanomas arise from the epidermoid lining of the anal canal. Most melanomas occur adjacent to the dentate line, although a few tumors arising in the rectum have been reported. The female-to-male ratio is approximately 2:1, and the average age at presentation is approximately 63 years (46).

Rectal bleeding is the most common symptom. Melanoma is suspected when a deeply pigmented lesion is seen, but most tumors are lightly pigmented or not pigmented and are often mistakenly diagnosed as polyps or squamous cell carcinomas. In amelanotic melanomas, a tissue biopsy result can be misinterpreted as poorly differentiated or undifferentiated squamous cell carcinoma.

Anal canal melanomas have a marked tendency to spread submucosally into the rectum, but they rarely invade adjacent organs, probably because most patients die before this occurs. Lymphatic spread to the mesenteric nodes is seen in about one third of patients at the time of diagnosis; spread to the inguinal nodes is less common. Hematogenous spread to the liver and lung is early and rapid, accounting for most of the deaths (47).

Melanomas of the anal canal are radioresistant and do not respond to chemotherapy or immunotherapy. The surgical approach to this malignant neoplasm is controversial. No statistical difference in survival has been found when patients treated by abdominoperineal resection are compared with those treated by wide local excision. Both 5-year survival rates are about 15% to 17% (46,48). Local control of the disease after operation is not as much a problem as distant metastasis, which remains the major cause of death. A reasonable approach is to perform local excision if this can be accomplished with wide margins and full thickness without causing fecal incontinence. Otherwise, an abdominoperineal resection should be performed.

REFERENCES

1. Jass JR, Sobin LH. *Histologic typing of intestinal tumors,* 2nd ed. World Health Organization. New York: Springer-Verlag, 1989:32–33, 41–46.
2. Fleming ID, Cooper JS, Henson DE, et al. American Joint Committee on Cancer. *Cancer Staging Manual,* 5th ed. Philadelphia: Lippincott–Raven, 1997:91–95, 157–161.
3. Brown DK, Ogelsby AB, Scott DH, et al. Squamous cell carcinoma of the anus: a twenty-five year retrospective. *Am Surg* 1988;54:337–342.
4. Greenall MJ, Quan SHQ, Urmacher C, et al. Treatment of epidermoid carcinoma of the anal canal. *Surg Gynecol Obstet* 1985;161:509–517.
5. Pintor MP, Northover JMA, Nicholls RJ. Squamous cell carcinoma of the anus at one hospital from 1948 to 1984. *Br J Surg* 1989;76:806–810.
6. Nigro ND. Multidisciplinary management of cancer of the anus. *World J Surg* 1987;11:446–451.
7. Beahrs OH, Wilson SM. Carcinoma of the anus. *Ann Surg* 1976;184:422–428.
8. Cummings BJ. Editorial. *Oncology* 1996;10:1853–1854.
9. Jensen SL, Hagen K, Shokouh-Amiri MH, et al. Does an erroneous diagnosis of squamous-cell carcinoma of the anal canal and anal margin at first physician visit influence prognosis? *Dis Colon Rectum* 1987;30:345–351.
10. Deans GT, McAlee JJA, Spence RAJ. Malignant anal tumors. *Br J Surg* 1994;81:501–508.
11. Saclarides TJ, Klem D. Genetic alterations and virology of anal cancer. *Semin Colon Rectal Surg* 1995;6:131–134.
12. Papillon J, Chassard JL. Respective roles of radiotherapy and surgery in the management of epidermoid carcinoma of the anal margin. *Dis Colon Rectum* 1992;35:422–429.
13. Schrout WH, Wang C, Dawson PJ, et al. Depth of invasion, location, and size of cancer of the anus dictate operative treatment. *Cancer* 1983;51:1291–1296.
14. Nielsen OV, Jensen SL. Basal cell carcinoma of the anus—a clinical study of 34 cases. *Br J Surg* 1981;68:856–857.
15. Sarmiento JM, Wolff BG, Burgart LJ, et al. Perianal Bowen's disease: associated tumors, human papilloma virus, surgery, and other controversies. *Dis Colon Rectum* 1997;40:912–918.
16. Marchesa P, Fazio VW, Oliart S, et al. Perianal Bowen's disease: a clinicopathologic study of 47 patients. *Dis Colon Rectum* 1997;40:1286–1293.
17. Morson BC, Dawson IMP, Day DW, et al. *Morson and Dawson's gastrointestinal pathology.* London: Blackwell Science, 1990:673–675.
18. Rosai J. *Ackerman's surgical pathology,* 8th ed. St. Louis: Mosby, 1996:808–809.
19. Sarmiento JM, Wolff BG, Burgart LJ, et al. Paget's disease of the perianal region—an aggressive disease? *Dis Colon Rectum* 1997;40:1187–1194.
20. Jensen SL, Sjolin KE, Shokouh-Amiri MH, et al. Paget's disease of the anal margin. *Br J Surg* 1988;75:1089–1092.
21. Beck DE. Paget's disease and Bowen's disease of the anus. *Semin Colon Rectal Surg* 1995;6:143–149.
22. Brown SD, Spittle MF. Radiotherapy for perianal Paget's disease [Letter to the Editor]. *J R Soc Med* 1998;91:114–115.
23. Grodsky L. Uncommon nonkeratinizing cancers of the anal canal and perianal region. *N Y State J Med* 1965;65:894–901.
24. Helwig EG, Graham JH. Anogenital (extramammary) Paget's disease: a clinicopathological study. *Cancer* 1963;16:387–403.
25. Tjandra J. Perianal Paget's disease: report of three cases. *Dis Colon Rectum* 1988;31:462–466.
26. Armitage NC, Jass JR, Richman PI, et al. Paget's disease of the anus: a clinicopathological study. *Br J Surg* 1989;76:60–63.
27. Cintron J. Buschke-Löwenstein tumor of the perianal and anorectal region. *Semin Colon Rectal Surg* 1995;6:135–139.
28. Gordon PH. Current status—perianal and anal canal neoplasms. *Dis Colon Rectum* 1990;33:799–808.
29. Wade DS, Herrera L, Castillo NB, et al. Metastases to the lymph nodes in epidermoid carcinoma of the anal canal studied by a clearing technique. *Surg Gynecol Obstet* 1989;169:238–242.
30. Cummings BJ. Treatment of primary epidermoid carcinoma of the anal canal. *Int J Colorectal Dis* 1987;2:107–112.
31. Boman BM, Moertel CG, O'Connell MJ, et al. Carcinoma of the anal canal: a clinical and pathologic study of 188 cases. *Cancer* 1984;54:114–125.
32. Nigro ND. An evaluation of combined therapy for squamous cell cancer of the anal canal. *Dis Colon Rectum* 1984;27:763–766.
33. Cummings BJ, Keane TJ, O'Sullivan B, et al. Epidermoid anal cancer: treatment by radiation alone or by radiation and 5-fluorouracil with and without mitomycin C. *Int J Radiat Oncol Biol Phys* 1991;21:1115–1125.
34. Flam MS, John MJ, Mowry PA. Definitive combined modality therapy of carcinoma of the anus: a report of 30 cases including results of salvage therapy in patients with residual disease. *Dis Colon Rectum* 1987;30:495–502.
35. Beck DE, Karulf RE. Combination therapy for epidermoid carcinoma of the anal canal. *Dis Colon Rectum* 1994;37:1118–1125.
36. Doci R, Zucali R, Bombelli L, et al. Combined chemoradiation therapy for anal cancer. *Ann Surg* 1992;215:150–156.
37. Cummings BJ, Thomas GM, Keane TJ. Primary radiation therapy in the treatment of anal canal carcinoma. *Dis Colon Rectum* 1982;25:778–782.
38. Papillon J, Montbarbon JF. Epidermoid carcinoma of the anal

canal: a series of 276 cases. *Dis Colon Rectum* 1987;30: 324–333.

39. Stearns MW, Urmacher C, Sternborg SE, et al. Cancer of the anal canal. *Curr Probl Cancer* 1980;4:1–44.

40. Basik M, Rodriguez-Bigas MA, Penetrante R, et al. Prognosis and recurrence patterns of anal adenocarcinoma. *Am J Surg* 1995;169:233–237.

41. Tarazi R, Nelson R. Adenocarcinoma of the anus. *Semin Colon Rectal Surg* 1995;6:169–173.

42. Jensen SL, Shokouh-Amiri MH, Hagen K, et al. Adenocarcinoma of the anal ducts: a series of 21 cases. *Dis Colon Rectum* 1988;31:268–272.

43. Jensen SL, Nielsen OV. Anal duct carcinoma [Editorial]. *Dis Colon Rectum* 1989;32:355–357.

44. Getz SB Jr, Ough YD, Patterson RB, et al. Mucinous adenocarcinoma developing in chronic anal fistula: report of two cases and review of the literature. *Dis Colon Rectum* 1981;24: 562–566.

45. Tarazi R, Nelson RL. Anal adenocarcinoma: a comprehensive review. *Semin Colon Rectal Surg* 1994;10:235–240.

46. Thibault C, Sagar P, Nivatvongs S, et al. Anorectal melanoma: an incurable disease? *Dis Colon Rectum* 1997;40:661–668.

47. Cooper PH, Mills SE, Allen MS Jr. Malignant melanoma of the anus: report of 12 patients and analysis of 255 additional cases. *Dis Colon Rectum* 1982;25:693–703.

48. Brady MS, Kavolius JP, Quan SHQ. Anorectal melanoma: a 64-year experience at Memorial Sloan-Kettering Cancer Center. *Dis Colon Rectum* 1995;38:146–151.

SURGERY: SCIENTIFIC PRINCIPLES AND PRACTICE, Third Edition, edited by Lazar J. Greenfield, Michael W. Mulholland, Keith T. Oldham, Gerald B. Zelenock, and Keith D. Lillemoe. Lippincott Williams & Wilkins Publishers, Philadelphia, © 2001.

CHAPTER 48

DIVERTICULAR DISEASE

MARY F. OTTERSON AND GORDON L. TELFORD

Diverticular disease of the colon includes both diverticulosis and diverticulitis. *Diverticulosis* is an abnormal state in which noninflamed diverticula are present with or without symptoms. *Diverticulitis* occurs when one or more diverticula become inflamed. Inflammation can lead to perforation of the diverticulum with pericolic infection *(peridiverticulitis)* or abscess formation, free perforation with peritonitis, fistula formation, or obstruction. Hinchey et al. (1) devised a classification system for the inflammatory conditions encountered under the term *diverticulitis.*

Stage I is a small, confined pericolonic abscess; stage II indicates a larger collection; stage III is suppurative peritonitis, and stage IV denotes fecal peritonitis.

Before 1940, diverticulosis of the colon was infrequently recognized. Retrospective reviews of colon radiographs and examinations of pathologic specimens from this period recorded an incidence of diverticulosis of 5% to 10% (2). Diverticulosis is now more commonly identified in Western countries. The incidence depends on the age of the population studied, varying from less than 2% in patients younger than 30 years to 30% to 50% in patients older than 50 years (3). Although most patients with diverticulosis of the colon have no or only mild symptoms, complications of hemorrhage or infection occur in 15% to 30% of affected patients, and about 30% of these patients require operative treatment. Thus, colonic diverticular disease remains a major public health problem in the United States and a continuing challenge for general surgeons.

PATHOLOGIC ANATOMY

True diverticula involve all layers of the bowel wall: mucosa, submucosa, and muscularis externa. False diverticula involve only mucosa and submucosa that herniate through the muscularis externa. Most diverticula of the colon are false diverticula. True diverticula are rare. Most false diverticula emanate from weak points in the colonic wall where mesenteric blood vessels penetrate the circular muscle layer (Fig. 48.1). Diverticula also can develop along the antimesenteric border in the area between the taeniae (4).

Most colonic diverticula are found in the sigmoid colon, although they can be scattered throughout the intraabdominal colon (2–4). In up to 65% of patients, diverticulosis is limited to the sigmoid colon. In about 35% of patients, at least one other area of the colon is involved. Only 1% to 4% of patients have no involvement of the sigmoid colon.

PATHOPHYSIOLOGY

Diverticulosis has been described as a disease of Western industrialized civilization, although it may better be described as a disease of affluence and refined food products. As the people of Western nations have decreased their intake of dietary fiber, the incidence of diverticulosis has increased. A decrease in fiber is the most consistent factor associated with the high incidence of diverticulosis in Western populations (5). In contrast, diverticulosis is rare in less affluent, nonindustrialized countries. Diverticulosis is also unusual in Japan, however, where the population continues to consume a diet high in fiber.

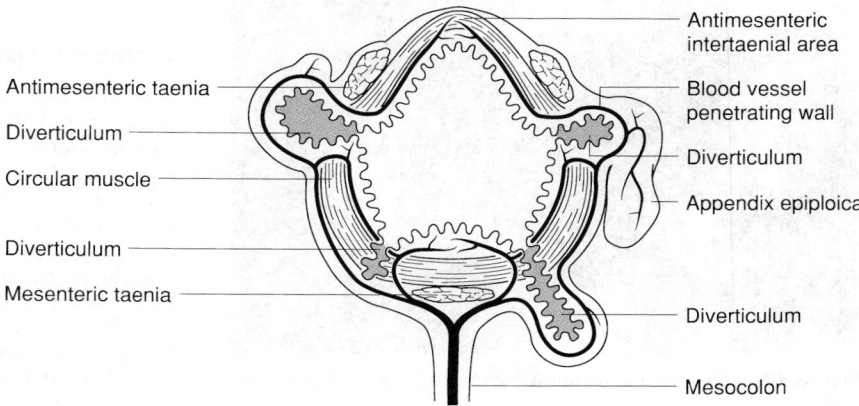

Figure 48.1. Cross section of the colon showing the relation of diverticula to the blood vessels penetrating the circular muscle layer, the taeniae, and the appendices epiploicae.

It is unclear how a low-fiber diet results in the formation of diverticula. One hypothesis states that during circular muscular contractions in patients with small amounts of stool in the colon, as in patients on low-fiber diets, the colonic lumen can be totally occluded. When two such contractions occur close together, the lumen of the intervening segment of colon is isolated from the remainder of the colon, and high pressure is generated in that segment. Theoretically, increased pressure results in the formation of diverticula because tension on the colonic wall is increased. In some people, the tensile strength of the colonic wall also appears to be decreased. Pressure–volume curves in patients with diverticulosis indicate a decrease in colonic wall tension in comparison with controls. The combination of colonic segmentation and decreased wall tension may be more important than either factor in isolation.

CLINICAL PRESENTATION AND DIFFERENTIAL DIAGNOSES

Diverticulosis

Most patients with evidence of colonic diverticula on barium enema have mild or no symptoms. In patients with abdominal pain and evidence of noninflamed diverticula on barium enema, the diverticula are not usually the cause of symptoms (Fig. 48.2). Noninflamed colonic diverticula are not a noted cause of pain or discomfort. A more plausible explanation for pain in patients with diverticula is the excessive pressure generated by segmentation of the colon. Although diverticulosis should be considered in the differential diagnosis of a patient with intermittent, mild to moderate pain of the lower abdomen, it is imperative that other causes of the pain be considered. Other diagnoses that should be eliminated include chronic constipation, diverticulitis, irritable bowel syndrome, and adenocarcinoma of

the colon. If pain is severe and constant, a diagnosis of diverticulitis should be considered. Irritable bowel syndrome is thought by some to be a condition that precedes the development of diverticula and a diagnosis made by exclusion. In patients in whom barium enema does not demonstrate diverticula, irritable bowel or chronic constipation should not be diagnosed until colonoscopy has definitively ruled out carcinoma.

Diverticulitis

The usual symptoms of diverticulitis include fever, lower abdominal pain, and lower abdominal tenderness. A lower abdominal mass, tachycardia, and an elevated white blood cell count with a left shift are frequently noted. Abdominal pain and tenderness can vary markedly, depending on the precise location of the inflammation and whether free perforation into the abdominal cavity is present. When free perforation and generalized peritonitis are present, it is often difficult to differentiate diverticulitis from other causes of perforated viscus. Suspicion of diverticular complications is heightened when the process is localized to the left lower quadrant and a palpable, tender mass is noted. The differential diagnosis for diverticulitis without free perforation includes perforated colon cancer, acute appendicitis, perforated peptic ulcer, acute-onset ulcerative colitis, acute-onset Crohn's colitis, and ischemic colitis.

Perforated colon cancer is difficult to differentiate from diverticulitis. Both diseases frequently involve the sigmoid colon, and both can produce a tender mass in the left lower quadrant. Patient histories are frequently similar because both diseases can cause vague, poorly defined lower abdominal pain. Although helpful, colonoscopy is not always diagnostic. The inflammation that results from the perforation can make colonoscopy difficult, and it may be impossible to see the involved area. Therefore, if carcinoma cannot be eliminated preoperatively, a thorough examination must be performed intraoperatively. Evidence of pericolic lymph nodes on computed tomography (CT) is seen more frequently in patients with colonic cancer than in patients with diverticulitis. Detection of pericolic lymph nodes in patients suspected of having diverticulitis should raise the suspicion of underlying colonic cancer (6). The patient's history is usually helpful in differentiating appendicitis from diverticulitis unless the diverticula are right-sided in origin. Inflammatory bowel disease and ischemic colitis can be diagnosed by colonoscopy or flexible sigmoidoscopy. With ulcerative colitis or Crohn's disease, the patient's history usually includes a diagnosis of inflammatory bowel disease, but when the onset is acute, diverticulitis may be difficult to distinguish. The inflammatory changes that occur with diverticulosis may mimic inflammatory bowel disease. Caution should be exercised in diagnosing Crohn's disease in the presence of diverticular disease (7).

Hemorrhage

Hemorrhage can occur as a result of either diverticulosis or diverticulitis, although massive bleeding is more typically associated with diverticulosis (Fig. 48.3). It is important to distinguish hemorrhage as a complication of diverticulosis from colonic angiodysplasia (8). Like patients with bleeding caused by diverticulosis, patients with bleeding resulting from angiodysplasia are usually asymptomatic before hemorrhage, and the blood loss can be massive. Carcinoma of the colon is seldom a cause of acute massive bleeding. Patients in whom massive bleeding develops secondary to inflammatory bowel disease usually have a history of colitis. Occasionally, a patient with colitis presents with a fulminant course and no history of the

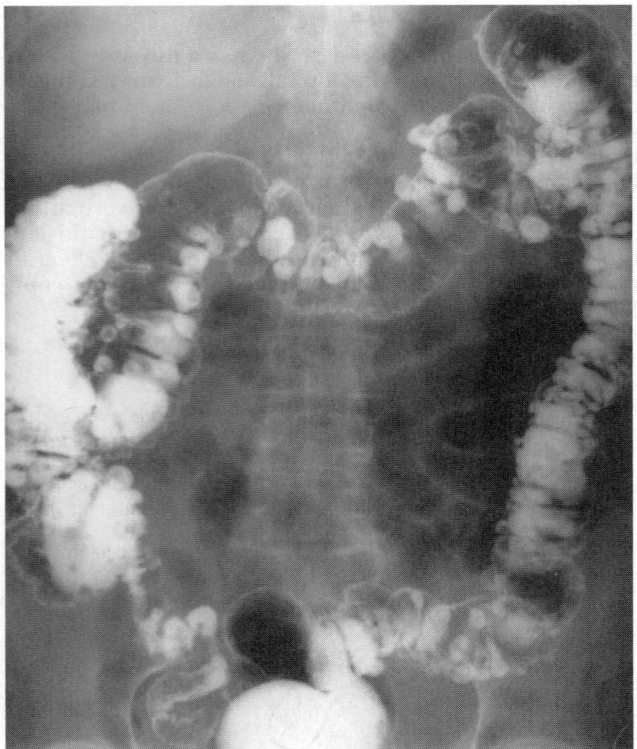

Figure 48.2. Barium enema showing multiple diverticula of the colon.

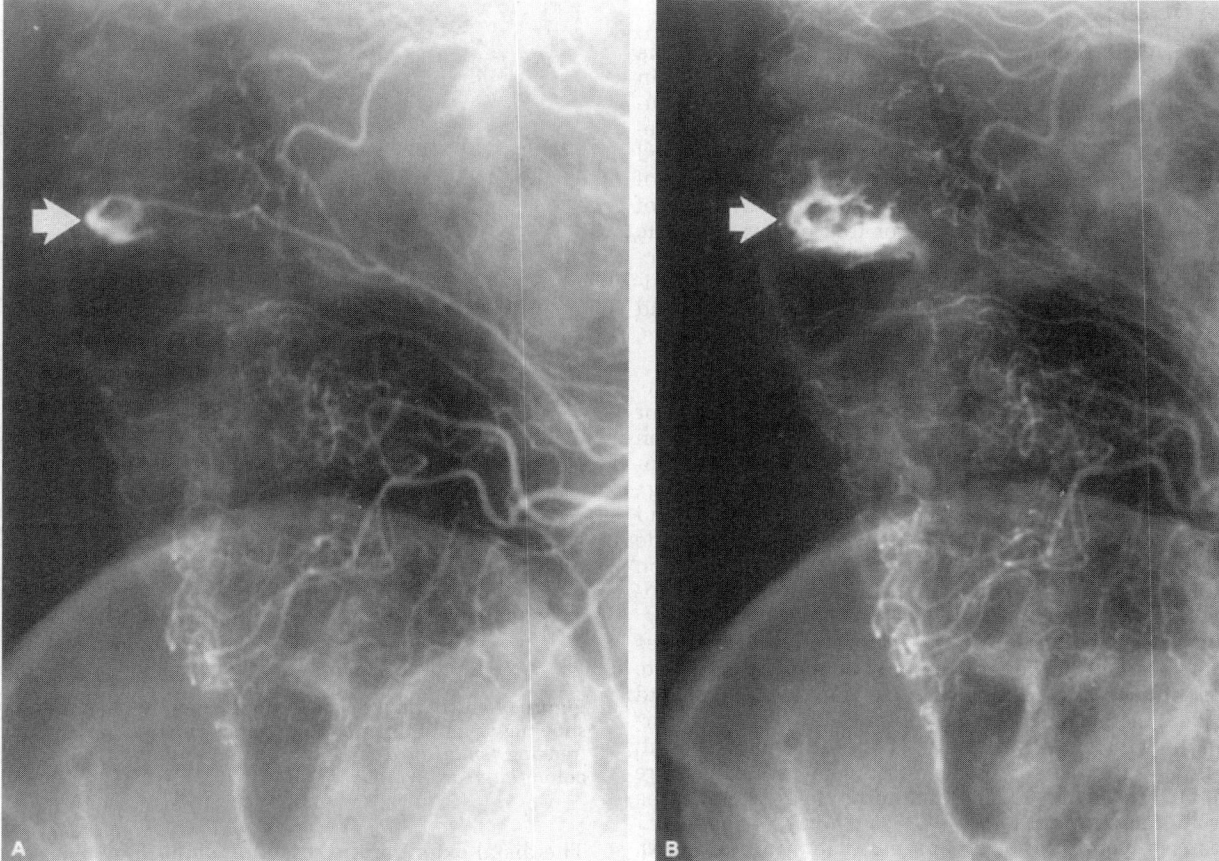

Figure 48.3. Superior mesenteric arteriogram from a patient with bleeding from a right-sided colonic diverticulum. *(A)* Early roentgenogram with contrast material outlines the diverticulum *(arrow).* (B) Late roentgenogram demonstrates overflow of contrast material into the colonic lumen.

disease. Ischemic colitis is usually accompanied by a history of abdominal pain, diarrhea, and vascular occlusive disease. The differential diagnosis of lower gastrointestinal bleeding must always include the various causes of massive upper gastrointestinal bleeding.

Obstruction

Diverticulitis and its complications account for about 13% of cases of large-bowel obstruction. Significant problems in evaluating patients with obstruction of the sigmoid colon are the relatively high incidence (7%) of carcinoma in patients with symptomatic sigmoid diverticular disease and the relative difficulty of making the diagnosis of carcinoma of the colon when a large phlegmonous mass is present (6). Colonoscopy is helpful only when the endoscope can pass the area of obstruction and biopsy specimens can be obtained. Negative findings on distal colonoscopy in a patient with obstruction, inflammation, and edema do not eliminate carcinoma.

DIAGNOSIS AND THERAPY

Diverticulosis

Patients with a combination of chronic, intermittent pain in the lower abdomen and diverticula on barium enema should be treated symptomatically. The diverticula are not considered to be the cause of the pain, and surgical therapy is not indicated. Colectomy should be reserved for the treatment of complications of diverticular disease.

Population studies have demonstrated that diverticula can be prevented by consuming a diet high in fiber, and such a diet has been widely prescribed for the treatment of symptomatic diverticulosis. No study, however, has shown that a diet high in fiber prevents the complications of diverticulosis. Likewise, the efficacy of fiber supplements or bulk laxatives to treat the pain associated with diverticula is controversial. Studies have demonstrated that an increase in dietary fiber can relieve symptoms related to constipation. Vegetarians have a lower incidence of diverticulosis than nonvegetarians do. Recommendations for increasing dietary fiber are probably worthwhile.

In more than 70% of patients with diverticular hemorrhage, bleeding stops spontaneously, and 75% of these patients do not have recurrent bleeding. In the 25% of patients whose bleeding recurs, even if the bleeding is managed successfully by nonoperative means, segmental colectomy should be performed because most of these patients have subsequent hemorrhage. The management of diverticular hemorrhage is discussed in more detail in Chapter 49.

Reports suggest that angiodysplasia of the right side of the colon is a more common cause of massive lower gastrointestinal bleeding than previously appreciated (8). In one series, half the patients with angiodysplasia had diverticula, which is not surprising because both diseases occur predominantly in the elderly. All the bleeding angiodysplastic lesions were in the right side of the colon, which explains why massive colonic hemorrhage tends to be right-sided in origin.

Diverticulitis

Diverticulitis is a complication of diverticulosis. One theory is that diverticulitis occurs when impacted feces in a single diverticulum obstructs the neck of the diverticulum or abrades its thin walls, so that invasive infection results. Another theory states that microperforation caused by increased intraluminal pressure leads to spillage of colonic contents. Either event could result in infection of the surrounding pericolic tissues or free perforation. The process, once initiated, could cause a self-limiting infection without clinical symptoms or could progress to clinically significant infection requiring hospitalization and surgical intervention. When the infection is progressive, other complications can develop.

If a clinical diagnosis of mild diverticulitis is made, therapy should be initiated immediately. Treatment for mild distress in a patient who can tolerate oral hydration should include 7 to 10 days of oral broad-spectrum antimicrobial therapy, including anaerobic coverage (e.g., trimetholoprim/sulfamethoxazole or ciprofloxacin and metronidazole) (9,10). Most patients with an acute episode of diverticulitis severe enough to require hospitalization can be treated with intravenous fluids, bowel rest, broad-spectrum antibiotics, and analgesics. Older studies suggest that morphine sulfate should be avoided as it causes colonic spasm (11). Meperidine may be more appropriate because it decreases intracolonic pressure (12). Signs and symptoms of severe diverticulitis include fever, tachycardia, leukocytosis with left shift of the differential count, abdominal pain (usually in the left lower quadrant) severe enough to require analgesics, abdominal tenderness, and a lower abdominal mass.

If nausea, vomiting, or abdominal distention develops, nasogastric suction should be instituted. The patient should be reexamined frequently for progression of disease. If, despite maximal therapy, the patient does not improve within 48 hours, complications of diverticulitis probably exist, and further therapy is necessary. Complications develop in only about 20% of patients having a first episode of diverticulitis; this incidence rises to 60% with recurrent episodes. Although a water-soluble contrast enema radiograph frequently provides the diagnosis of diverticulitis (Fig. 48.4), CT has become the preferred diagnostic test for those patients whose condition does not improve within 48 hours, who are assumed to have a complication of diverticulitis (Fig. 48.5). Some controversy surrounds the management of patients under the age of 35 years with diverticulitis. Certain authors have suggested that these patients should undergo elective surgical resection because of the recurrent nature and frequency of serious complications. Others think that the increased frequency of complications requiring surgery is secondary to a delayed or inaccurate diagnosis (9,13).

In patients with presumed diverticulitis, CT and ultrasonography have replaced the use of contrast studies. CT is the safest and most cost-effective method and has the additional potential benefit of allowing percutaneous drainage to treat abscess (9). Radiologically guided percutaneous drainage has been recommended as the initial therapeutic maneuver in patients with diverticular abscesses larger than 5 cm in diameter. Most smaller abscess regress with antibiotics and do not require radiologic drainage. After CT drainage of an abscess, 50% to 90% of patients undergo a successful one-stage procedure of segmented colectomy and primary anastomosis (14). If percutaneous drainage is not feasible or an abscess is not identified, surgical intervention is recommended.

At the time of exploratory laparotomy, if the disease is localized, a segmental colectomy should be performed.

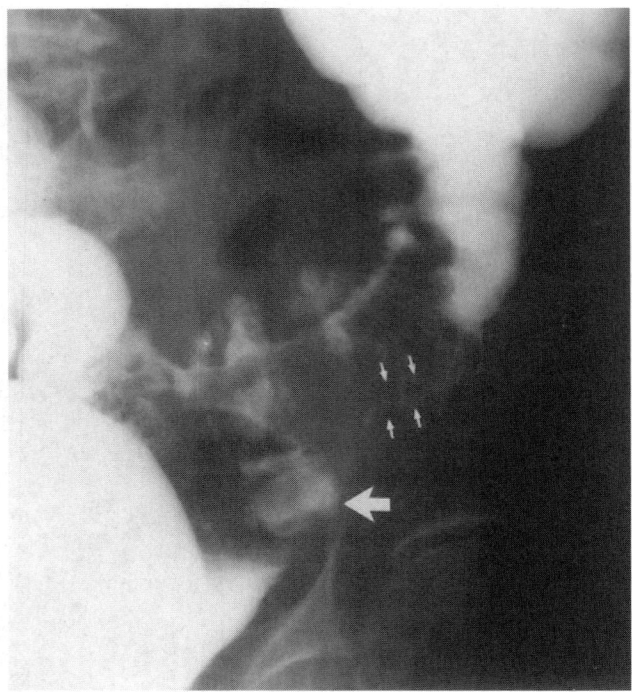

Figure 48.4. Barium enema examination of a sigmoid colon showing signs of diverticulitis: persistent narrowing, intramural tracking *(small arrows),* and an abscess inferior to the sigmoid colon *(large arrow).*

The distal extent of the resection should always extend to the proximal rectum to decrease the chance of recurrence. The proximal extent of resection should include the segment involved with the acute disease plus any additional portion of colon with signs of chronic disease or many diverticula. When this approach is used, the recurrence rate after surgical resection is less than 10%. The only absolute contraindications to primary anastomosis are free perforation with generalized peritonitis, obstruction with an unprepared bowel, and intraoperative conditions that preclude primary anastomosis, such as septic shock, ureteral injury, and other medical conditions that make a prolonged operation inadvisable. If resection is thought to be unsafe in the presence of a massive phlegmon, or if the patient is too unstable to undergo a resection, a diverting end-colostomy with mucous fistula and drainage may be appropriate, with colonic resection planned at a later date, after inflammation subsides. This approach is seldom necessary, however, and most patients can undergo resection of the diseased segment of bowel at the initial operation. Current trends suggest that laparoscopic resection of the diseased sigmoid colon may be possible (15–18). The laparoscopic approach has primarily been utilized for elective operations, and the conversion rate to an open procedure is higher in emergent or urgent cases (ranging from 10% to 53%).

Most patients improve on a regimen of intravenous fluids, bowel rest, and broad-spectrum antibiotics, and emergency surgery is not necessary. Intravenous antibiotics should be continued for 7 to 10 days, and intravenous fluids and bowel rest should be continued until colonic function has normalized. A contrast enema should be performed subsequently to confirm the presumed diagnosis and evaluate the extent of disease. If disease is minimal and no sign of obstruction, fistula formation, or abscess is present, the patient can be discharged and followed as an outpatient. If any of these

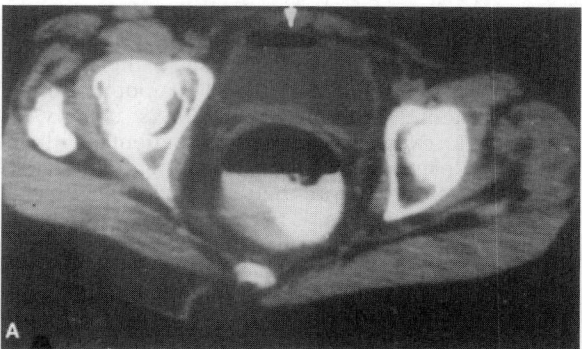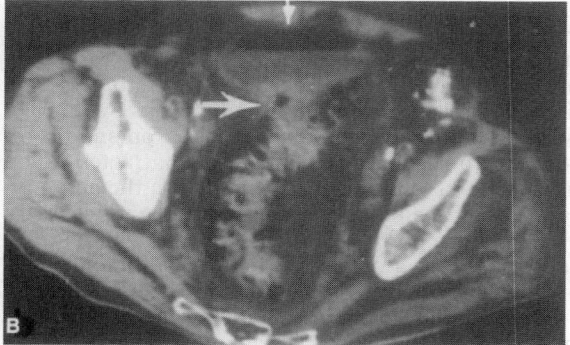

Figure 48.5. *(A)* Computed tomography demonstrates air in the urinary bladder *(arrow)* in the presence of a colovesical fistula secondary to diverticulitis. *(B)* Air in the urinary bladder *(small arrow)* is associated with a paravesical inflammatory mass *(large arrow).* (From Sarr MG, Fishman EK, Goldman SM. Enterovesical fistula. *Surg Gynecol Obstet* 1987;164:2, with permission.)

complications are present, a segmental resection should be performed before the patient is discharged. After a second episode of diverticulitis, a resection should be performed because the risk for further episodes of diverticulitis increases with each episode.

Obstruction

A fibrotic colonic stricture and large-bowel obstruction can develop in patients who have experienced one or more episodes of diverticulitis. When obstruction is diagnosed, it is important to differentiate between diverticulitis, colon carcinoma, and colonic volvulus. All patients should undergo sigmoidoscopy or colonoscopy to allow biopsy of any masses. Water-soluble contrast radiographs of the colon should be obtained to define the degree of obstruction. The extent of the workup depends on the condition of the patient and the degree of obstruction. Patients with an incomplete obstruction should be given a thorough but rapid preoperative evaluation in an attempt to secure an exact diagnosis. Because patients with a complete obstruction require urgent operation, it is not always feasible to finish all tests before surgery.

If the obstruction is partial, a complete preoperative bowel preparation should be carried out, including the administration of oral antibiotics. Patients with a high-grade colonic obstruction cannot tolerate a rapid bowel preparation with laxatives or polyethylene glycol. Such patients should be prepared slowly, with extra time allowed for the completion of bowel cleansing. Once the bowel has been prepared, the patient with incomplete obstruction can undergo one-stage resection and primary anastomosis. Some authors have suggested that intraoperative colonic lavage may be a safe method for accomplishing a single-stage resection of the colon in selected patients with diverticulitis who require an urgent operation (19). This technique involves occlusion of the bowel lumen proximal to the pathologic process. Sterile corrugated plastic tubing is inserted through a colotomy proximal to the occlusion and secured. The distal end of the tubing is passed off the field. The cecum is cannulated through the stump of the appendix and colonic lavage with warm saline solution is continued until the effluent is clear. The rectum is irrigated through a proctoscope to clear the remaining fecal material. Following resection of the pathologic process, a primary anastomosis is performed (20,21). This technique is most safely utilized in patients with bleeding and obstruction rather than infectious complications of diverticulitis. Only 35% to 75% of patients who undergo colostomy for diverticular disease go on to colostomy closure,

probably because of the debilitated condition of many of these patients (9). Nevertheless, a staged procedure is virtually mandated in the presence of generalized peritonitis. Unless colon carcinoma has been eliminated as a possible diagnosis, a cancer operation should be performed for this circumstance.

Patients with complete obstruction who cannot undergo bowel preparation, and in whom a one-stage operation is not feasible, should undergo an urgent diverting colostomy to relieve the obstruction. Resection of the diseased, obstructed segment of bowel can be performed during this operation or can be delayed until additional workup has been completed. The workup to differentiate between carcinoma and diverticulitis should be completed after the patient has recovered from the initial surgery.

When the patient has recovered from the first operation, which usually takes at least 1 month, the next procedure can be performed. Depending on placement of the colostomy, the second operation can be a resection of the colostomy and diseased segment of colon and reestablishment of bowel continuity by colocolostomy. When the diseased segment of bowel has been removed during the first operation, the secondary procedure can include colostomy closure.

Fistulae

Diverticular disease can also be complicated by the development of fistulae from the diseased colon to other viscera or to skin. Colovesical fistulae account for about half of fistulae associated with diverticulitis. Most patients with colovesical fistulae present with urinary tract symptoms, including urgency, dysuria, pneumaturia, and fecaluria. Despite what in retrospect often appear to be obvious symptoms, the diagnosis of a colovesical fistula can be difficult to establish conclusively. Recurrent urinary tract infections in an elderly man should arouse suspicion. Barium enema usually demonstrates diverticula and occasionally shows sigmoid narrowing. Only rarely is the fistulous tract actually filled. Cystoscopy demonstrates hyperemia and inflammation consistent with chronic cystitis. Although these findings can be localized to some extent to suggest the diagnosis, the fistulous opening is seldom seen. CT with intraluminal contrast material has emerged as the most sensitive test to detect the presence of a colovesical fistula. In addition, after the rectal administration of barium, the patient's urine sediment should be checked for barium by radiograph of a spun urine sample. The presence of barium in the urine is diagnostic of a colovesical fistula. In more than 90% of patients, air is present in the urinary bladder, and an indurated segment of sigmoid colon is observed adjacent to a locally thickened bladder wall (22).

Most patients with colovesical fistulae are treated effectively with a one-stage procedure consisting of segmental colectomy and closure of the fistulous opening in the bladder. The proximal margin of resection should include the entire segment of thickened, contracted colon and any additional colon that is involved in the acute inflammation. As stated earlier, although it is not necessary to resect the entire portion of the colon involved with diverticulosis, the resection should include sufficient colon to allow the anastomosis to be performed in an area of colon relatively free of diverticula. The distal resection margin should be the proximal rectum. If the fistulous opening cannot be identified because it is small in diameter, nothing needs to be done to identify the bladder fistula. Urinary catheter drainage for 7 to 10 days, followed by cystographic verification of closure of the fistula, is sufficient therapy. Depending on the severity of the related complications of diverticulitis (obstruction, inflammation, abscess, sepsis, other fistulae), it may occasionally be necessary to perform a two-stage procedure, the first stage being segmental colectomy and colostomy formation and the second stage consisting of closure of the colostomy. Either the one- or two-stage procedure can be carried out with low rates of morbidity and mortality and with less than a 5% recurrence rate. The three-stage approach of creation of a diverting colostomy, then resection, and finally colostomy closure is not recommended because the inflammatory process and the fistula are not removed at the first operation, so that potential sources of sepsis are left.

Although they were rare in the past, recent reports indicate an increase in the occurrence of colovaginal fistulae. Almost all patients with colovaginal fistulae have had a hysterectomy. The only consistent symptom is feculent vaginal discharge. About 40% of patients have intermittent abdominal pain and distention. A mass may be felt on pelvic examination; on examination of the vagina with a speculum, the fistula opening is visible in 85% of cases. The diagnosis is confirmed in 50% of cases by barium enema. Vaginal contrast studies may also be helpful.

Unless other complications of diverticulitis are present, a one-stage procedure is appropriate. The involved colon is resected and a primary anastomosis is formed. The vaginal defect is closed if this can be easily accomplished, but such a defect usually closes spontaneously if left open.

Diarrhea, abdominal pain, and constitutional symptoms are frequently observed in patients with diverticular coloenteric fistulae. The usual signs of coloenteric fistula are abdominal tenderness, abdominal distention, and pelvic mass. Barium enema is diagnostic in 40% to 100% of patients. The preferred operative management of an uncomplicated coloenteric fistula is *en bloc* resection of the involved segment of small intestine, the fistula, and the diseased segment of colon. Primary anastomoses of both the small intestine and colon are then performed. If complicating factors are present, such as other fistulae, intraabdominal abscess, or inadequate bowel preparation secondary to obstruction, primary anastomosis of the small intestine, combined with colostomy formation, is performed as the first stage of a two-stage procedure.

DIVERTICULITIS OF THE CECUM AND ASCENDING COLON

The actual incidence of right-sided diverticula is not known; estimates based on barium enema examinations are between 5% and 10% (3). The incidence of true diverticula is higher in the cecum and ascending colon than in the remainder of the colon, but false diverticula still predominate. True diverticula tend to be solitary and originate in the anterior cecum close to the ileocecal valve. They occur in only 1% to 2% of the population. Most are asymptomatic, and the diagnosis is usually made by pathologic examination. Among patients with left-sided diverticulosis, 7% to 30% have right-sided diverticula (23). In a study of more than 250 patients with right-sided colonic diverticulitis, 81% had a solitary diverticulum and 19% had multiple diverticula (24). The incidence of right-sided colonic diverticula and diverticulitis is increased and the incidence of left-sided diverticulitis is lower than expected in Asian patients (25).

When diverticulitis develops in patients with right-sided diverticula, the symptom complex is similar to that in acute appendicitis, and misdiagnosis is frequent (24,26). Patients with right-sided diverticulitis are generally younger than patients with left-sided disease and are older than most patients with appendicitis (26). Patients with right-sided diverticulitis are usually in their late 30s or 40s; patients with left-sided diverticulitis are usually more than 50 years of age (26). Patients with right-sided diverticulitis have a longer duration of illness than patients with appendicitis, infrequently vomit, and feel pain initially in the right lower quadrant rather than the mid-abdomen. Despite these dissimilarities, acute appendicitis is incorrectly diagnosed in more than 60% of patients who are later found to have right-sided diverticulitis (24,26). In only 20% of cases is the correct diagnosis made preoperatively. CT can be helpful in the diagnosis of right-sided diverticulitis. CT findings include thickening of the colonic wall, the presence of an extraluminal mass involving the cecum or ascending colon, and signs of pericolic inflammation. CT is recommended in patients with atypical appendicitis who are elderly and in whom right-sided diverticulitis is being considered as a diagnosis. Barium enema examination is seldom helpful because many patients have a single diverticulum that is not visible on barium studies. Associated findings, such as compression of the colon, are nonspecific and usually nondiagnostic.

At the time of operation, it may be difficult to establish a diagnosis of diverticulitis of the cecum or ascending colon. Most series report a correct intraoperative diagnosis in fewer than 60% of cases (26). The presence of an intact, normal appendix eliminates appendicitis as the diagnosis in almost all circumstances. Usually, a large inflammatory mass involves the cecum and ascending colon. In many cases, however, it is difficult to distinguish the mass from a perforated carcinoma, and a right hemicolectomy should be performed. If the resection can be accomplished without contaminating the peritoneal cavity and a mechanical bowel preparation has been accomplished preoperatively, a primary anastomosis is acceptable. If spillage of abscess contents occurs or bowel preparation has not been feasible, an end-ileostomy and mucous fistula can be performed. When the only abnormality noted at laparotomy is an inflamed diverticulum, a few authors propose leaving the diverticulum in situ and treating the patient with broad-spectrum antibiotics. If this therapy is undertaken, an appendectomy should be performed to avoid confusion if right lower quadrant symptoms recur. Diverticulitis does not recur in most patients treated in this manner.

If right-sided diverticulitis is diagnosed before operation, the patient should be given the same treatment as for sigmoid diverticulitis. If improvement is noted with intravenous fluids, broad-spectrum antibiotics, bowel rest, and analgesics, therapy should be continued and further testing performed when the patient recovers. If the patient's condition does not improve or deteriorates, laparotomy is recommended.

GIANT COLONIC DIVERTICULUM

Although uncommon, giant colonic diverticulum is a well-described clinical entity. Giant diverticula usually occur in the sigmoid colon, although they have been described in other areas of the left side of the colon. Giant diverticula almost always arise from the antimesenteric border of the colon, unlike most left-sided diverticula, which develop where the vascular supply passes through the muscularis externa. Most are filled with gas and therefore visible on plain abdominal radiographs. They range in size from 3 to 35 cm, with an average size of 13.5 cm.

The pathogenesis of giant diverticula is not understood; they are assumed to be a complication of diverticulosis and not a separate entity. The most widely accepted explanation is that inflammation of a diverticulum causes its neck to narrow; as a result, a ball-valve mechanism develops that entraps gases that pass into the diverticulum from the colon.

The predominant symptoms are abdominal pain, bloating, nausea, vomiting, and diarrhea. Physical findings include abdominal tenderness and a movable mass in the lower abdomen. Perforation causes abdominal pain, leukocytosis, fever, and signs of localized or generalized peritonitis. Although the diagnosis can be suspected based on plain radiographs of the abdomen, barium enema and CT confirm the diagnosis. On barium enema, the diverticula fills with barium in 50% to 70% of cases, and other diverticula are frequently demonstrated (Fig. 48.6). CT of giant diverticula performed with intraluminal contrast usually demonstrates apposition of the colon and giant diverticulum in addition to the presence of barium in the diverticulum. On CT, wall thickness is variable and has not proved to be diagnostic.

Giant colonic diverticula are managed surgically. The patient should undergo standard mechanical bowel preparation, including oral antibiotics. The diverticulum, along with the adjacent colon, should be resected in continuity. Bowel continuity can usually be restored with an end-to-end primary anastomosis.

REFERENCES

1. Hinchey EJ, Schaal PGH, Richards GK. Treatment of perforated diverticular disease of the colon. *Adv Surg* 1978;12:85.
2. Spriggs EI, Marxer OA. Intestinal diverticula. *Q J Med* 1925; 19:1.
3. Hughes LE. Postmortem survey of diverticular disease of the colon. *Gut* 1969;10:336.
4. Slack WW. The anatomy, pathology, and some clinical features of diverticulitis of the colon. *Br J Surg* 1962;50:185.
5. Mendeloff AI. Thoughts on the epidemiology of diverticular disease. *Clin Gastroenterol* 1986;15:855.
6. Chintapalli KN, Esola Cc, Chopra S, et al. Pericolic mesenteric lymph nodes: an aid in distinguishing diverticulitis from cancer of the colon. *AJR Am J Roentgenol* 1997;169: 1253.
7. Geldhill A, Dixon MF. Crohn's-like reaction in diverticular disease. *Gut* 1998;42:392.
8. Welch CE, Athanasoulis CA, Galdabini JJ. Hemorrhage from the large bowel with special reference to angiodysplasia and diverticular disease. *World J Surg* 1978;2:73.
9. Ferzoco LB, Raptopoulos V, Silen W. Acute diverticulitis. *N Engl J Med* 1998;338:1521.
10. Freeman SR, McNally PR. Diverticulitis. *Med Clin North Am* 1993;77:1149.
11. Painter NS, Truloce SC. The intraluminal pressure patterns in diverticulosis of the colon. *Gut* 1964;5:201.
12. Arfwidsson S. Pathogenesis of multiple diverticula of the sigmoid colon in diverticular disease. *Acta Chir Scand* 1964; 342[Suppl]:1.
13. Spivak H, Weinrauch S, Harvey JC, et al. Acute colonic diverticulitis in the young. *Dis Colon Rectum* 1997;49:570.
14. Stabile BE, Puccio E, Van Sonnenberg E, et al. Preoperative percutaneous drainage of diverticular abscesses. *Am J Surg* 1990;159:99.
15. Memon MA, Fitzgibbons RJ. The role of minimal access surgery in the acute abdomen. *Surg Clin North Am* 1997;77: 1333.
16. Bruce CJ, Coller JA, Murray JJ, et al. Laparoscopic resection for diverticular disease. *Dis Colon Rectum* 1996;39[Suppl]:S1.
17. Eijsbouts QA, Cuesta MA, deBrauw LM, et al. Elective laparoscopic-assisted sigmoid resection for diverticular disease. *Surg Endosc* 1997;11:750.
18. Sher ME, Agachan F, Bortul M, et al. Laparoscopic surgery for diverticulitis. *Surg Endosc* 1997;11:264.
19. Lee EC, Murray JJ, Coller JA, et al. Intraoperative colonic lavage in nonelective surgery for diverticular disease. *Dis Colon Rectum* 1997;40:669.
20. Murray JJ, Schoetz DJ, Coller JA, et al. Intraoperative colonic lavage and primary anastomosis in nonelective colon resection. *Dis Colon Rectum* 1991;34:527.
21. Scott HJ, Lane IF, Glynn MJ. Colonic hemorrhage: a technique for rapid intraoperative bowel preparation and colonoscopy. *Br J Surg* 1986;73:390.
22. Woods RJ, Lavery IC, Fazio VW, et al. Internal fistulas in diverticular disease. *Dis Colon Rectum* 1988;31:591.
23. Beranbaum SL, Zausner J, Lane B. Diverticular disease of the right colon. *Radiology* 1972;115:334.
24. Graham SM, Ballantyne GH. Cecal diverticulitis: a review of the American experience. *Dis Colon Rectum* 1987;30:821.
25. Katz DS, Lane MJ, Ross BA, et al. Diverticulitis of the right colon revisited. *AJR Am J Roentgenol* 1998;171:151.
26. Gouge TH, Coppa GF, Eng K, et al. Management of diverticulitis of the ascending colon: 10 years' experience. *Am J Surg* 1983;145:387.

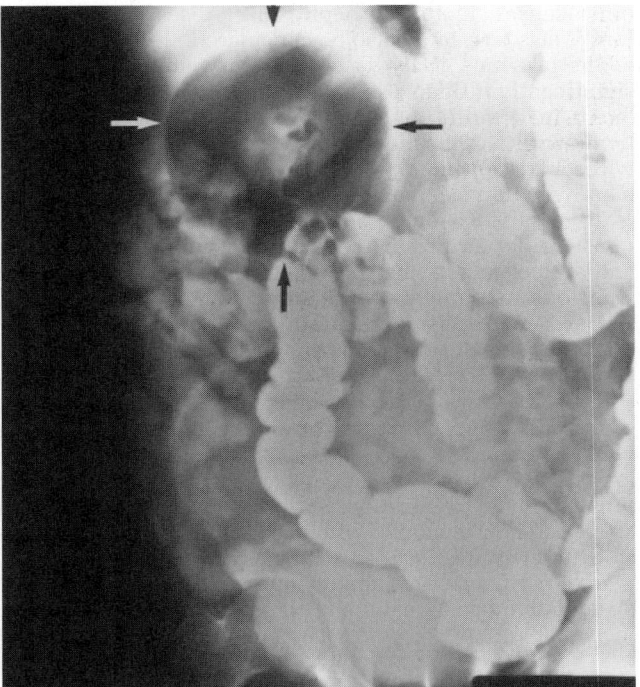

Figure 48.6. Barium enema examination following evacuation demonstrates a giant colonic diverticulum *(arrows)* partially filled with barium. (From McNutt R, Schmitt D, Schulte W. Giant colonic diverticula. *Dis Colon Rectum* 1988;31:624, with permission.)

SURGERY: SCIENTIFIC PRINCIPLES AND PRACTICE, Third Edition, edited by
Lazar J. Greenfield, Michael W. Mulholland, Keith T. Oldham, Gerald B. Zelenock,
and Keith D. Lillemoe. Lippincott Williams & Wilkins Publishers, Philadelphia, © 2001.

CHAPTER 49

ACUTE GASTROINTESTINAL HEMORRHAGE

LAWRENCE T. KIM AND RICHARD H. TURNAGE

Acute hemorrhage from the gastrointestinal (GI) tract is a common clinical problem encountered in a variety of medical and surgical disciplines. The morbidity and potential mortality risk associated with this condition necessitate that all physicians who care for these patients have a working knowledge of the principles of volume replacement, diagnostic evaluation, and therapeutic options. Although a complete differential diagnosis of GI hemorrhage is expansive, relatively few conditions comprise the most common causes. Localizing the site of hemorrhage relative to the ligament of Treitz directs the evaluation and ultimately therapy. Hemorrhage from the esophagus, stomach, and duodenum accounts for about 80% of cases of GI hemorrhage, with nearly all of the remainder coming from the colon. The small intestine is the site of hemorrhage in about 1% of cases. Causes of overt upper and lower GI hemorrhage are listed in Tables 49.1 and 49.2, respectively.

CLINICAL PRESENTATION

Patients with GI hemorrhage generally present with one of two clinical complaints. The first is the observed passage of blood, either by vomiting or per rectum. The second type of complaint reflects the manifestations of acute intravascular volume depletion (i.e., light-headedness, dizziness, orthostatic syncope or near-syncope, or palpitations from tachycardia). An upper GI source of hemorrhage is generally suggested by hematemesis (the vomiting of blood), melena, or the presence of a material resembling "coffee grounds" within the nasogastric aspirate. Melena is the passage per rectum of blood that has been converted by enteric bacteria to form a black, sticky, tarry stool. Melena may be seen after hemorrhage of 50 to 200 cc of blood (1,2). Although melena is generally indicative of an upper GI source of hemorrhage, bleeding from the small intestine or right

Table 49.1. DIFFERENTIAL DIAGNOSIS OF ACUTE UPPER GASTROINTESTINAL HEMORRHAGE

Peptic ulcer disease
  Duodenal ulcer
  Gastric ulcer
Gastroesophageal varices
Mallory-Weiss tear
Stress gastritis
Dieulafoy's disease
Esophageal, gastric, or duodenal tumors
Aortoduodenal fistula
Esophagitis
Angiodysplasia
Hemobilia
Pancreatitis-induced pseudoaneurysm

Table 49.2. DIFFERENTIAL DIAGNOSIS OF ACUTE LOWER GASTROINTESTINAL HEMORRHAGE

Colonic diverticular disease
Colonic vascular ectasia
Small-intestinal diverticular disease
  Meckel's diverticulum
  Pseudodiverticula
Inflammatory bowel disease
  Chronic ulcerative colitis
  Crohn's disease
Neoplasms
  Colonic neoplasms
  Small-intestinal neoplasms
Aortoenteric fistula
Colitis
  Infectious
  Ischemic
  Radiation-induced
Hemorrhoids

side of the colon may also appear black if it has remained in the GI tract for a period of time, usually longer than about 14 hours (3). Hematochezia is the passage of bright red blood per rectum. Although hematochezia is generally indicative of a colonic or perianal source, massive upper GI bleeding may also be associated with the passage of bright red blood or maroon-colored stools per rectum.

The medical history and physical examination may provide important clues to the cause of hemorrhage and the potential risk to the patient's life. The onset of hemorrhage following several days of worsening epigastric or upper abdominal pain suggests peptic ulcer disease, whereas, hematemesis or melena following vomiting or retching strongly suggests a Mallory-Weiss tear. Massive, painless upper GI hemorrhage in a patient with cirrhosis should suggest the diagnosis of variceal hemorrhage, although other causes, including peptic ulcer disease and a Mallory-Weiss tear, must also be considered.

The presence of cardiac, pulmonary, and renal disease significantly influences outcome and may be an important factor in determining therapy. For example, elderly patients with significant chronic illnesses will be unable to withstand continued blood loss as well as a younger healthy patient, so that earlier definitive operative therapy is necessary. Commonly utilized medications, such as nonsteroidal antiinflammatory agents (NSAIDs), aspirin, and anticoagulants, have all been shown to be important contributors to the development of GI hemorrhage.

A systematic physical examination should document the magnitude of the hemorrhage and the patient's ability to compensate. Massive hemorrhage is associated with signs and symptoms of hypovolemic shock, including cool, clammy, mottled skin, tachycardia, tachypnea, flat jugular veins, oliguria, and perhaps hypotension. These responses may be altered by the patient's age, concomitant medical problems, and medications. Physical examination should also document evidence of cirrhosis and portal hypertension (e.g., ascites, spider angiomas, hepatosplenomegaly, palmar erythema, and large hemorrhoidal veins). A rectal examination can reveal the presence of bright red blood or melena.

INITIAL EVALUATION AND VOLUME REPLACEMENT

At presentation, two large-bore intravenous lines should be placed in peripheral veins and intravascular volume restored begun with an isotonic saline solution. Lactated Ringer's solution is often preferred to 0.9% normal saline solution because the amount of sodium and chloride administered in the former more closely approximates the electrolyte composition of whole blood. In most patients, bleeding stops spontaneously, and crystalloid volume replacement is all that is required. The patient with massive bleeding should receive packed red blood cells to restore the intravascular volume and oxygen-carrying capacity. The decision to transfuse blood or blood products depends on the individual needs of the patient and the disease process encountered. The risks of the blood product (i.e., infection and allergic reactions) must be carefully weighed against the risks of withholding transfusion (i.e., anemia, decreased oxygen-carrying capacity, coagulopathy).

The propensity of the lesion to rebleed or to continue bleeding is an important factor in the decision to transfuse blood. Esophageal varices are associated with a significant risk for recurrent or continued hemorrhage, and blood should be transfused earlier in the treatment of patients with bleeding from this source. Although most gastric and duodenal ulcers cease bleeding spontaneously, endoscopic findings of active hemorrhage or a visible vessel identify a lesion in which rebleeding or continued bleeding is likely. In contrast, if a condition in which continued hemorrhage or rebleeding is unlikely has been identified (e.g., Mallory-Weiss tear), one should hesitate to give blood to a stable patient whose bleeding appears to have stopped. The hemodynamic reserve of a patient should also be carefully considered in the decision to use blood products. Compromised cardiac reserve, pulmonary disease, and vascular disease necessitate optimizing oxygen delivery, often with the use of blood products. In such patients, the risk for myocardial ischemia and infarction may be greater than the infectious risk from the transfusion of blood products.

On presentation, blood is drawn for type and cross-match, complete blood cell count with platelet count, electrolyte determination, liver function tests, and coagulation profiles. It is important to emphasize that on presentation, the hematocrit or hemoglobin level does not accurately reflect the magnitude of acute blood loss. Estimates of the severity of hemorrhage must be based on clinical parameters.

A nasogastric tube should be placed shortly after presentation and the presence of gastric blood determined. The absence of blood in bilious gastric fluid suggests a lower intestinal source. However, caution in interpreting the appearance of the nasogastric aspirate is warranted. In one study, only 6 of 10 yellow-green nasogastric aspirates actually tested positive for bile, whereas 5 of 8 clear aspirates tested positive for bile (4). If no bilious fluid is obtained, esophagogastroduodenoscopy (EGD) is necessary to exclude a duodenal source of hemorrhage because nearly 20% of patients with a clear nasogastric aspirate are bleeding from an upper GI source (5). If upper GI hemorrhage has been significant, orogastric lavage through a large-bore tube is used to clear the stomach of clot to facilitate endoscopy. Nasogastric tubes are not sufficiently large to permit the evacuation of large clots and particulate gastric contents. In many cases, bleeding stops before or during volume replacement and cleansing of retained blood from the stomach. Lavage of the stomach with iced solutions plays no role in the management of upper GI hemorrhage because of the potential for systemic hypothermia with attendant adverse effects on coagulation, oxygen delivery, and hemodynamic stability.

Careful hemodynamic monitoring of these potentially critically ill patients is vital to successful management. Patients who are actively bleeding and those who have re-

cently sustained significant hemorrhage should be admitted to an intensive care unit for close monitoring of hemodynamic parameters and for signs of continued or recurring hemorrhage. The presence of significant underlying illnesses, such as cardiac, renal, hepatic, or pulmonary insufficiency, may necessitate invasive cardiac monitoring with central cardiac and arterial catheters. The information gained from these devices allows cardiac performance to be optimized during intravascular volume replacement. Of note, central venous catheterization should be performed only after initial volume restoration through peripheral sites. The placement of a urinary catheter and frequent monitoring of heart rate, blood pressure, gastric aspirate, and mentation are the minimum steps necessary for patients who have had a GI hemorrhage. The importance of prompt, adequate volume restoration and diligent observation cannot be overemphasized as cornerstones in the management of these potentially mortally ill patients.

DIAGNOSTIC APPROACH

Following restoration of the circulating blood volume, the next step is to identify the source of hemorrhage so that definitive therapy may be instituted. If the patient presents with hematemesis, localization of the bleeding to the upper GI tract is straightforward. A more difficult problem occurs when patients present with lower GI hemorrhage. The first step in determining the cause of bleeding is to place a nasogastric tube and examine the gastric aspirate. If blood is found in the stomach, an immediate EGD will often define the site of hemorrhage. In those instances in which EGD is unsuccessful, and for those patients with a lower GI hemorrhage, other diagnostic techniques are required to define the site and cause of the hemorrhage and plan appropriate, definitive therapy. A general algorithm for evaluating acute upper and lower GI hemorrhage is presented in Figs. 49.1 and 49.2, respectively.

Esophagogastroduodenoscopy

The initial diagnostic (and often therapeutic) modality for patients sustaining upper GI hemorrhage (or in whom an upper GI source cannot be excluded) is EGD. Numerous studies have documented the unequivocal diagnostic superiority of endoscopy over contrast radiography in demonstrating sites of upper GI hemorrhage, so that barium studies do not have a role today in the evaluation of acute GI hemorrhage (6). The benefits of EGD in patients sustaining an upper GI hemorrhage include the following: (a) It plays an important therapeutic role, with improved outcome noted in patients with variceal bleeding or hemorrhage from peptic ulcers (7,8); (b) endoscopic identification of the source of bleeding facilitates operative intervention (e.g., the operative management of a bleeding duodenal ulcer is substantially different from that of gastroesophageal varices or a Mallory-Weiss tear); and (c) the endoscopic findings may allow an estimate of the risk of subsequent rebleeding or continued hemorrhage and thereby facilitate the appropriate timing of definitive operative management (e.g., the likelihood of continued bleeding is greatest for gastroesophageal varices, intermittent for duodenal ulcerations, and least for a Mallory-Weiss tear).

Endoscopy is highly sensitive in demonstrating the site of hemorrhage. This may be particularly important for patients with more than one disease process identified at endoscopy. Factors that limit the diagnostic efficacy of endoscopy in actively bleeding patients are primarily related to impaired visibility, abnormal anatomy, and processes

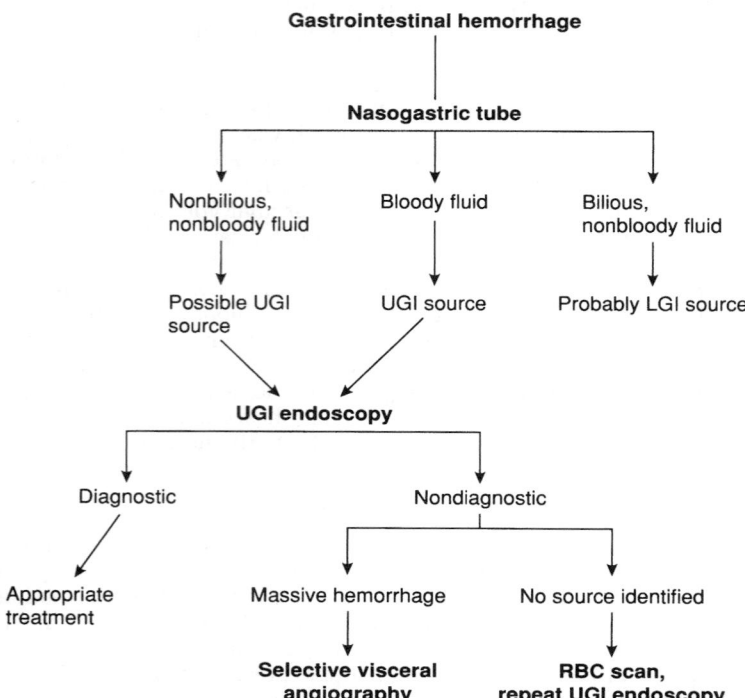

Figure 49.1. Diagnostic steps in the evaluation of acute gastrointestinal hemorrhage.

that simulate ulcers. The most common cause of diagnostic failure is retention of blood in the stomach and duodenum, which prevents adequate inspection of the mucosal surfaces. Pathologic changes, such as scarring of the duodenal bulb from chronic peptic ulcer disease, may also prevent adequate inspection and lead to diagnostic failure. In addition, the endoscopist may be misled by a number of factors that can simulate an ulcer or occur concomitantly with the lesion responsible for the hemorrhage (e.g., antacid suspensions adherent to normal mucosa, nasogastric tube suction artifacts, and endoscopic trauma).

When an emergent or urgent esophagogastroscopy is performed in a patient with active or recent bleeding, the incidence of complications associated with the procedure is increased. In one survey, the complication rate was 0.9%, about eight times higher than the 0.13% complication rate found in a survey of elective procedures (5,9). Potential complications include aspiration, recurrent or increased hemorrhage, respiratory depression from sedatives, and perforation of the esophagus, stomach, or duodenum. The risks of endoscopy can be minimized by performing the procedure in the intensive care unit with adequate monitoring of the patient's respiratory and hemodynamic parameters. Endoscopy should be performed in a hemodynamically stable patient after volume replacement.

Colonoscopy

The three commonly utilized diagnostic modalities for lower GI hemorrhage (colonoscopy, scintigraphy with red blood cells tagged with radioactive isotopes, and selective visceral arteriography) are complementary in that each is best suited to a particular group of patients. Colonoscopy is most appropriate for patients with minimal to moderate bleeding at the time of the study. In general, colonic lavage with a polyethylene glycol solution clears the lumen of clot and stool to provide adequate visualization of the mucosa. Patients who are massively bleeding or hemodynamically unstable present a situation in which the diagnostic yield is minimal and the potential for complications is significant.

The use of colonoscopy in the evaluation of patients with lower GI hemorrhage has some important limitations. Although this technique can be invaluable in detecting unusual causes of acute colonic hemorrhage (e.g., colitis, polyps, and cancer), its ability to determine the site of hemorrhage in patients bleeding from the most common lower GI sources is much more limited. Given the high frequency of diverticulosis in the general population, the visualization of a diverticulum at the time of colonoscopy does not establish it as the site of hemorrhage unless bleeding at that site is evident (e.g., active bleeding or adherent clot). Fur-

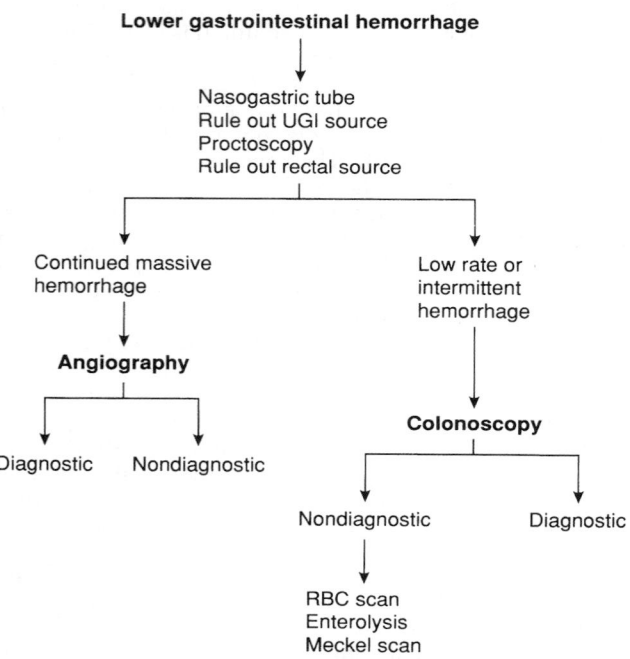

Figure 49.2. Diagnostic steps in the evaluation of acute lower gastrointestinal hemorrhage.

thermore, the massive nature of diverticular hemorrhage and the intermittent nature of bleeding in vascular ectasia further complicate the utility of this procedure. The shunting of blood flow away from the colonic mucosa that accompanies hemodynamically significant hemorrhage and hypovolemic shock further limits the diagnostic capacity of this procedure, particularly in patients with vascular ectasia. Lastly, it should be realized that the presence of blood throughout the colon does not prove the presence of a right-sided lesion because the reflux of blood from the left side of the colon to the right is not unusual.

Radionuclide Scanning

Abdominal scintigraphy with red blood cells labeled with technetium 99m is the most sensitive but least precise method for localizing bleeding. Although lacking the spatial resolution and diagnostic precision of angiography and endoscopy, this test can be extremely valuable in localizing intermittently bleeding lesions or those with very low rates of hemorrhage, as in vascular ectasia. Abdominal scintigraphy with labeled erythrocytes has been shown to detect bleeding at rates as low as 0.04 to 0.1 mL/min (10,11). The precise localization of the site of hemorrhage may be complicated by the rapid distribution of isotope throughout the intestine by peristalsis or by accumulation in the right side of the colon. The accuracy of scanning with tagged red blood cells localizing lower GI bleeding remains controversial; some groups have concluded that scintigraphy is of no use in evaluating colonic bleeding (12–14), whereas others have found it quite helpful (15). More recent techniques of cine-scintigraphy may improve diagnostic accuracy (16) (Fig. 49.3).

One area in which radionuclide scanning has a clear role is in the diagnosis of Meckel's diverticulum. Pertechnetate Tc 99m is secreted by ectopic gastric mucosa in Meckel's diverticula (17). This study should be considered early in the evaluation of young patients with lower GI bleeding.

Selective Visceral Angiography

Selective visceral arteriography is primarily useful in those patients in whom endoscopy cannot be performed or in whom endoscopy has been unsuccessful in determining the site of ongoing, rapid hemorrhage. Successful angiographic identification of the source of bleeding depends primarily on the presence of active arterial bleeding at the time of the study. The extravasation of contrast may be detected if the patient is bleeding at a rate above 0.5 to 1 mL/min (18); this rate correlates clinically with the requirement for continuous volume infusion to maintain hemodynamic stability. Selective visceral angiography and endoscopy can be complementary in evaluating an actively bleeding patient. For example, when bleeding is massive, endoscopic visualization is often severely limited, whereas selective mesenteric arteriography is most effective in cases of rapid extravasation of blood (Fig. 49.4). Selective visceral angiography may be particularly valuable in elucidating the cause of lower GI hemorrhage. Angiography may detect vascular patterns diagnostic of vascular ectasia (described later), or it may demonstrate extravasation of contrast into the lumen of the bowel, as in hemorrhage from diverticula. The risks of angiography are primarily related to technical complications of the procedure (e.g., arterial thrombosis and embolism) and to acute renal insufficiency resulting from intravascular administration of the contrast agent.

Intraoperative Enteroscopy

Intraoperative endoscopy has been shown to be valuable in the rare patient in whom the site of bleeding cannot be clearly defined before laparotomy. The procedure can be performed without undue difficulty and may allow localization of the site of hemorrhage, thus limiting the extent of resection. Localization of Dieulafoy's lesions and angiodysplastic lesions in the stomach may allow precise

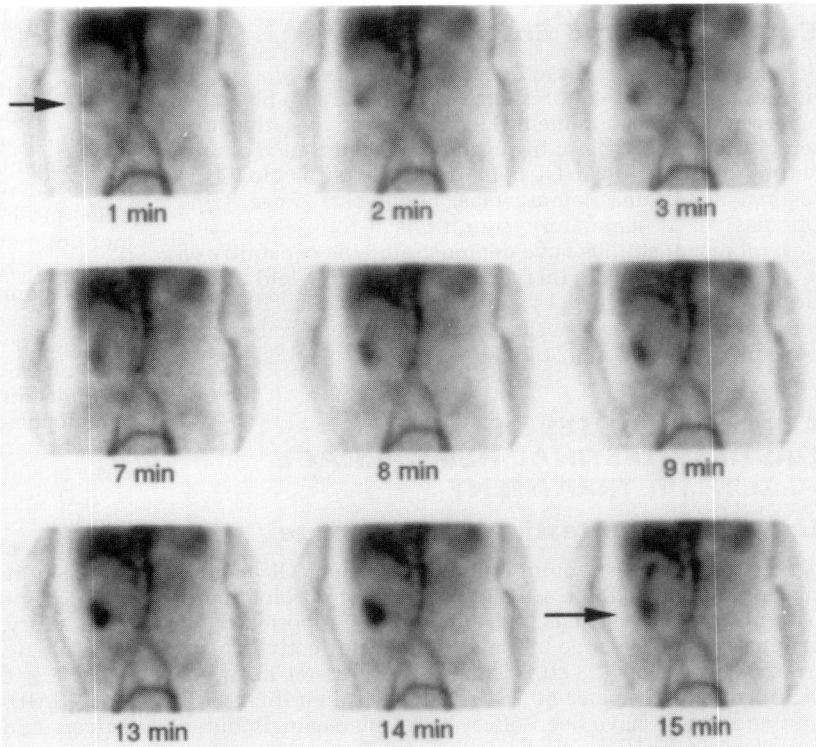

Figure 49.3. Cine-scintigraphy with erythrocytes labeled with technetium 99m shows extravasation of isotope in the right side of the colon. Only a small portion of the image set is shown. *Arrows* point to accumulation of isotope in the right side of the colon. The bleeding was a delayed hemorrhage following endoscopic polypectomy.

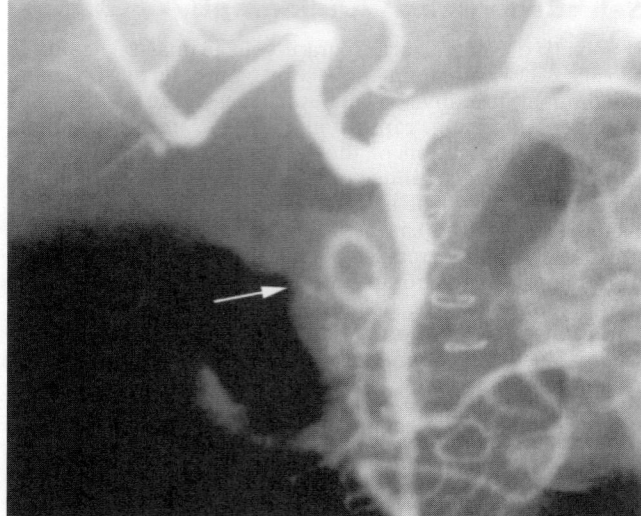

Figure 49.4. Selective celiac arteriography with injection into the common hepatic artery in a patient with a bleeding duodenal diverticulum. Extravasation of contrast from a branch of the gastroduodenal artery can be seen *(arrow)*.

resection or ligation. Transillumination of the intestine during intraoperative enteroscopy may demonstrate angiodysplastic lesions, and insufflation of the intestine may aid in the demonstration of small-bowel diverticula. In cases in which diagnostic tests failed to find a source of bleeding, diagnostic laparotomy with intraoperative enteroscopy successfully identified lesions in 83% of patients. It is disappointing to note, however, that rebleeding was common, particularly in the case of small-intestinal vascular anomalies (19). This procedure should be performed before patients are committed to subtotal colectomy without a clear documentation of the source of lower GI hemorrhage.

Enteroscopy and Enteroclysis

Enteroscopy and enteroclysis may occasionally be needed when a patient presents with intermittent bleeding and results of the aforementioned studies are negative. Enteroclysis may be useful in suggesting the presence of rare causes of overt lower GI hemorrhage, such as small-intestinal neoplasms (leiomyomas, leiomyosarcomas, lymphomas) or inflammatory conditions (Crohn's disease). Several recent studies have demonstrated the capability of a video-enteroscope to increase the diagnostic yield by approximately one third in small-bowel lesions (20). Enteroscopy may also be used as treatment for focal small-bowel angiodysplasia (21,22).

COMMON CAUSES OF GASTROINTESTINAL HEMORRHAGE AND THEIR TREATMENT

Upper Gastrointestinal Hemorrhage

A list of the most common causes of upper GI hemorrhage is found in Table 49.1. The mortality rate for acute upper GI hemorrhage has traditionally been reported to be about 10%, with a large number of deaths directly related to exsanguination (23–26). This figure has not changed significantly in the past 40 years. Advances in critical care and endoscopy have been offset by an increasingly older and chronically ill population.

Age is a significant prognostic factor that influences outcome in nearly every report. In a national survey of patients bleeding from a variety of upper GI sources, the mortality rate was 8.7% for patients younger than 60 years and 13.4% for those over 60 (5). Concurrent chronic illness also markedly affects morbidity and mortality; the death rates of patients bleeding from upper GI sources who have a history of congestive heart failure, cardiac arrhythmias, central nervous system diseases, cirrhosis, cancer, pneumonia, chronic obstructive pulmonary disease, and renal disease are significantly increased. The risk for death was found to be particularly high in patients who were bleeding during admission to the hospital for other medical conditions. In one survey, the mortality rate for patients who bled while hospitalized for other conditions was 33%, whereas those presenting to the hospital with hemorrhage had a 7.1% mortality rate (5). Patients sustaining hemorrhagic shock are also at high risk for death. Hypotension and transfusion requirement of more than 5 units have both been identified as independent predictors of mortality (5,25). In addition, bleeding from esophageal varices usually portends a worse prognosis than nonvariceal upper GI bleeding (25,26).

Peptic Ulcer Disease

Peptic ulcer disease is the most common cause of acute upper GI hemorrhage, accounting for nearly 40% of cases in most series. About 15% to 20% of patients with peptic ulcer disease experience bleeding during the course of their disease, and in as many as 20% of these patients, bleeding is the initial manifestation. Hemorrhage is the principal cause of death from peptic ulcer disease and has replaced intractable pain as the most frequent indication for surgery. Complications of peptic ulcer disease occur more commonly in older patients, who often have medical problems that profoundly influence their risk for morbidity and mortality.

Duodenal ulcers occur slightly more frequently than gastric ulcers. Penetration of the ulcer through the posterior wall of the duodenal bulb is associated with erosion into the gastroduodenal artery or one of its branches, resulting in brisk hemorrhage. Patients may present with hematemesis of bright red blood and clots or with melena alone. Bleeding stops spontaneously in 80% to 90% of patients during the initial stages of therapy with volume replacement and gastric lavage.

In general, when compared with patients who have duodenal ulcers, patients who have gastric ulcers tend to be older and have coexisting medical problems that increase morbidity and mortality. Bleeding may be from any site in the stomach, although bleeding from ulcers at the incisura is most common. At this site, involvement of the branches of the left gastric artery may result in brisk, if not torrential, hemorrhage. The clinical presentation of patients with bleeding gastric ulcers is similar to that of patients with bleeding duodenal ulcers: hematemesis, melena, and hematochezia.

An important risk factor for the development of GI hemorrhage and gastroduodenal ulcers is the use of NSAIDs. NSAID use has been associated with a range of mucosal injuries comprising small, acute mucosal hemorrhages and large, chronic ulcers. It has been estimated that 10% to 15% of regular NSAID users have chronic gastric ulcers (27). Symptoms correlate poorly with the degree of mucosal injury, evidenced by the observation that as many as 20% of ulcers penetrating the muscularis are asymptomatic (28). Case-control and cohort studies have suggested that NSAIDs are associated with a relative risk for GI hemorrhage and ulceration ranging from about 2 to 9.1 (29). Ketorolac, in particular, has been associated with a high risk for GI bleeding (relative risk approaching 25) (30). The risk for NSAID-associated complications is highest in patients with a history of upper GI bleeding, the elderly, and patients taking oral anticoagulants (31) or corticosteroids. Patients with a prior history of peptic ulcer disease also appear to be at increased risk for NSAID-associated GI hemorrhage. A number of studies have documented a significantly worse outcome among users of NSAIDs than among nonusers (32,33).

The tremendous frequency with which NSAIDs are used by the elderly underscores the magnitude of this problem. Those patients at increased risk for NSAID-induced hemorrhage should probably receive the prostaglandin E1 analogue misoprostol, which has been shown to prevent NSAID-induced gastric erosions and ulcers (34). Histamine (H_2) receptor blockers (ranitidine and cimetidine) are effective in preventing NSAID-induced duodenal ulcers but appear to have little effect in preventing gastric lesions (28,35,36). Omeprazole has recently been shown to be protective in patients on NSAIDs, with greater efficacy than the H_2 blockers (37). NSAIDs are also associated with lower GI bleeding, including bleeding from lesions not generally considered related to NSAID-induced ulcers, such as diverticula (38–40).

Medical Treatment.   Once bleeding has stopped, either spontaneously or through intervention, treatment should be instituted with a proton pump inhibitor. Omeprazole has been shown to reduce the risk for rebleeding significantly in patients with nonbleeding, visible vessels or adherent clots, but not in those with arterial spurting or oozing (41). Omeprazole was shown to be more effective than cimetidine in the prevention of rebleeding after endoscopic treatment of peptic ulcers (42). *Helicobacter pylori* infection may be less common in patients with bleeding ulcers than in those with nonbleeding ulcers. In one study, the risk for bleeding in ulcer patients with *H. pylori* infection was lower than the risk in those without *H. pylori* infection (43). If *H. pylori* infection is found, however, treatment of the infection significantly reduces the recurrence of hemorrhage in comparison with no treatment or with long-term antisecretory treatment alone (44).

Endoscopic Treatment.   During the initial endoscopic evaluation of a bleeding ulcer, the lesion may be categorized to facilitate treatment decisions and communication among physicians. A commonly used scheme is a modification of that described by Forrest (45) (Table 49.3), in which category I findings are those of active bleeding and type II findings are stigmata of recent bleeding. In general, only actively bleeding ulcers are treated endoscopically (Forrest category I). A variety of endoscopic techniques are available to arrest hemorrhage from bleeding ulcers. All stop hemorrhage by inducing coagulation necrosis of the bleeding vessel and surrounding tissue with thermal or laser energy or by inducing thrombosis or sclerosis of the bleeding vessels. The precise method of treatment is less important than the correct selection of patients and experience of the endoscopist.

Table 49.3. FORREST CLASSIFICATION OF ENDOSCOPIC APPEARANCE OF BLEEDING ULCERS

Ia	Spurting bleeding
Ib	Nonspurting, active bleeding
IIa	Visible vessel
IIb	Nonbleeding ulcer with overlying clot
IIc	Ulcer with hematin-covered (black) base
III	Clean ulcer base

Heater probes and monopolar and bipolar electrocoagulation probes can effectively control upper GI hemorrhage. Monopolar probes apply high-frequency electric current to the tissue, which results in localized heating to 100°C and sealing of the bleeding vessel by coagulation necrosis of the surrounding tissue and vessel wall. To control bleeding, gentle pressure is applied to compress the vessel wall and occlude the lumen during coagulation. In uncontrolled trials, monopolar electrocoagulation probes have been shown to arrest nonvariceal hemorrhage effectively in 80% to 95% of patients, with about 12% rebleeding and ultimately requiring operative treatment (46). The depth of thermal injury is unpredictable with dry electrodes and varies with the amount of contact pressure and tissue adherence. Irrigating the tip of the electrode with water limits the area and depth of coagulation, prevents tissue adherence, and limits the risk for clot dislodgement. The risk for perforation is about 2%.

Multipolar electrocoagulation (bicap) probes consist of three equally spaced pairs of bipolar microelectrodes. This orientation of electrodes allows the use of tangential approaches and eliminates some of the disadvantages of the monopolar probe, such as the unpredictable depth of thermal injury, adherence of tissue, and clot dislodgement. Electrocoagulation is carried out circumferentially around a vessel, with a depth of tissue coagulation between 1 and 5 mm, depending on the power used and the pressure applied to the probe. This method of electrocoagulation appears promising; randomized studies of patients with active bleeding have demonstrated significant reductions in emergency operations, transfusion requirements, duration of hospital stay, and overall treatment cost (47).

Direct thermal coagulation of a source of bleeding can be applied with a heater probe consisting of an aluminum tip coated with Teflon. The tip is rapidly heated to 250°C by an inner coil. The tip can be irrigated with a water jet to prevent the accumulation of debris and clot. Heat conducted from the probe produces tissue coagulation to a depth of 1 to 5 mm. *En face* and tangential applications are effective in achieving hemostasis as long as the bleeding vessel is precisely identified. Clinical use of this technique has yielded excellent results, with an initial hemostatic efficacy that exceeds 90% and a reduction in the rate of rebleeding.

Injection of epinephrine to induce vasoconstriction has been used successfully, particularly as an adjunct measure with some form of cautery. In one study, epinephrine injection alone, bipolar coagulation, and injection plus coagulation were compared. Epinephrine injection alone was as effective as the other treatments in initial control of bleeding. However, epinephrine injection plus bipolar coagulation resulted in fewer episodes of rebleeding and a smaller transfusion requirement than either treatment alone (48). Another report found no difference between epinephrine injection and epinephrine plus heater probe except in a subgroup of patients with spurting hemorrhage (49).

The injection of sclerosants has been well described as a method of treating esophageal varices and has recently been popular for controlling nonvariceal sites of bleeding. Sodium morrhuate and ethanolamine oleate are most commonly used to treat esophageal varices, whereas ethanol and polidocanol are most commonly used for nonvariceal sites. These agents act by inducing thrombosis in bleeding vessels and necrosis and subsequent fibrosis of surrounding tissue. The clinical results with sclerosants have been similar to those obtained with electrocoagulation. In one large multicenter study of 332 patients with active bleeding or with stigmata of recent hemorrhage, after 98% alcohol was injected around the lesions, only two patients continued to bleed, 20 rebled, and 10 required emergency operative intervention (50). Similar success has been achieved with polidocanol, either alone or with epinephrine. Fibrin glue (51) or thrombin (52) may also be useful in the treatment of bleeding peptic ulcers.

A 1989 National Institutes of Health consensus statement concluded that the two most promising forms of endoscopic hemostatic therapy for bleeding gastroduodenal ulcers are the heater probe and multipolar electrocautery (53). A metaanalysis of 25 randomized trials of endoscopic therapy for bleeding ulcers concluded that endoscopic treatment methods have a beneficial effect on survival by reducing the rate of recurrent hemorrhage. This analysis suggested that endoscopic therapy results in a relative reduction of 69% in recurrent bleeding, 62% in emergent surgery, and 30% in mortality rate, with the greatest benefit seen in patients with actively bleeding ulcers and ulcers with nonbleeding visible vessels (8). The effectiveness of early aggressive endoscopic diagnosis and treatment is further supported by a report of 562 patients with various causes of bleeding; only 2.5% required emergency operations to control hemorrhage (25).

Surgical Treatment. The successful use of endoscopic therapies has relegated operative procedures to a rescue role for those cases in which endoscopy is unsuccessful in arresting hemorrhage. If endoscopic treatment cannot arrest hemorrhage, operative intervention is mandated. However, endoscopic therapy appears to be successful in many cases until rebleeding develops. Most episodes of rebleeding occur within 96 hours (54,55).

During the past two decades, numerous studies have attempted to identify those patients at greatest risk for continued or recurrent bleeding. Of the many factors examined, those associated with the highest risk for rebleeding included hypovolemic shock during initial endoscopy, ulcers greater than 2 cm in diameter, and endoscopic stigmata of recent or ongoing hemorrhage (Forrest types I and II lesions) (56). Many studies have demonstrated the ability of endoscopy to identify those patients at greatest risk for rebleeding. In one review, the presence of active bleeding was associated with a 90% to 100% chance of continued or recurrent hemorrhage. A nonbleeding visible vessel was associated with a 40% to 50% chance, adherent clot with 20% to 30%, oozing without visible vessel 10%, flat spot 5% to 10%, and clean-based ulcer 1% to 2% (57). Even among patients who rebleed following initial endoscopic therapy, two thirds may be successfully re-treated endoscopically so that operative intervention can be avoided (27). Despite these data, factors that must be considered in the decision regarding the timing of operative intervention should include the magnitude of the initial (or recurrent) hemorrhage, the physiologic ability of the patient to withstand continued or recurrent hemorrhage, and the likelihood of recurrent or continued hemorrhage. Lastly, it is generally accepted that elderly patients and those with significant concurrent medical problems should undergo operative intervention earlier during the course of the hemorrhage because they can poorly tolerate continued hemorrhage, recurrent hypotension, and repeated transfusions.

The type of operation depends on the pathology encountered. For bleeding gastric ulcers, the operation of choice depends on the patient's condition and location of the ulcer. For favorably located ulcers in stable patients, the preferred procedure is gastric resection (to include the ulcer in the resected specimen) with or without vagotomy, depending on the ulcer type (see Chapter 22). In patients who are hemodynamically unstable, excision of the ulcer with closure of the gastrotomy provides hemostasis, and tissue can be obtained for histologic evaluation without the need for a more formal gastric resection in these criti-

cally ill patients. If the ulcer is unfavorably located (e.g., near the gastroesophageal junction), simple undersewing of the bleeding ulcer may adequately control bleeding (58). Subsequent endoscopic biopsy may allow a neoplastic cause to be excluded. Extensive gastric resections, such as subtotal or total gastrectomies, are generally unwise in these unstable patients. For patients with bleeding from duodenal ulcers, the most widely used operation comprises truncal vagotomy, pyloroplasty, and oversewing of the bleeding vessel. Highly selective vagotomy with duodenotomy and oversewing of the bleeding vessel has also been recommended. Direct ligation of the bleeding vessel through the duodenotomy should incorporate the pancreaticoduodenal artery proximal and distal to the ulcer and also the transverse pancreatic artery.

Stress Gastritis

Although studies in the 1960s and 1970s demonstrated acute erosions of the gastric mucosa in as many as 60% to 100% of critically ill patients, the incidence has markedly decreased during the past two decades. Factors postulated to have been important in this phenomenon include the following: (a) widespread use of prophylactic gastric alkalinization; (b) improvements in the ability to detect and treat sepsis; (c) improvements in the ability to monitor and correct hemodynamic instability; and (d) the ability to provide adequate nutritional support to critically ill patients.

In general, stress gastritis is characterized by the appearance of multiple superficial gastric ulcerations within 12 to 14 hours of an acute injury. These lesions, initially localized to the fundus and body of the stomach, later involve the entire gastric surface. Patients at greatest risk include those with sepsis, major burns, or severe trauma. Critically ill patients with a coagulopathy and respiratory insufficiency appear to be at highest risk for the development of stress gastritis (59,60). In this setting, the disease appears to represent the gastric component of the multiple organ failure syndrome.

The primary defect is in the protective processes that maintain the integrity of the gastric mucosal barrier. Although some gastric acid secretion is required for the development of stress gastritis, it is clear that the hypersecretion of acid is not the cause of mucosal injury. Altered gastric mucosal blood flow and impaired clearance of hydrogen ions from the mucosa appear to be of particular importance. Stress gastritis should be differentiated from the deep, often solitary ulcerations occurring in patients with severe central nervous system lesions (Cushing's ulcers).

Generally, hemorrhage is the only symptom that patients with stress gastritis experience. Overt bleeding is often heralded by the appearance of flecks of blood in the gastric aspirate. The superficial nature of the lesions makes perforation unlikely.

Prophylactic therapy is directed toward preventing hemorrhage, primarily by neutralizing gastric acid, augmenting mucosal defenses, and removing or preventing physiologic stress. Antacids, H_2-receptor antagonists, and sucralfate have all been used successfully to prevent stress gastritis. Alkalinization of the gastric contents is associated with colonization of the stomach with oral and fecal flora and has raised concerns about an increased risk for nosocomial pneumonia. This concern has prompted the use of sucralfate as a preferred prophylactic agent instead of antacids or cimetidine (61). However, in one recent large, blinded study, 1,200 patients were randomized to receive either ranitidine or sucralfate for stress ulcer prophylaxis. The group receiving ranitidine had a lower rate of bleeding (1.7%) than the sucralfate group (3.8%). No difference was noted in mortality or incidence of ventilator-assisted pneumonia (62).

The success of these prophylactic measures has led to a dearth of recent experience in managing patients with bleeding resulting from stress gastritis. Based on early reports, attention to blood replacement, intravascular volume restoration, and correction of coagulation defects are associated with the cessation of hemorrhage in nearly 80% of cases and so are the principal means of initial treatment. A variety of nonoperative techniques have been employed with variable success in arresting hemorrhage caused by stress gastritis, including endoscopic and embolization techniques and the selective catheterization of the left gastric artery with continuous infusion of vasopressin (63).

Based on these same early experiences, very few patients with bleeding from erosive gastritis require operative intervention to arrest hemorrhage. A variety of surgical treatment options had been reported, including vagotomy and pyloroplasty with oversewing of sites of bleeding, vagotomy and hemigastrectomy, total gastrectomy, and gastric devascularization. The dilemma facing the surgeon is that these critically ill patients poorly tolerate extensive procedures, yet lesser operations often fail to control hemorrhage. Regardless of the operation performed, mortality risk depends on the underlying illness, particularly in the presence of multiple organ failure. Mortality rates between 30% and 60% are commonly quoted, with as many as one fourth of the deaths resulting from continued hemorrhage. Rates of rebleeding ranging from 25% to 61% have been reported (64). The combination of vagotomy, hemigastrectomy, and oversewing of points of bleeding has been touted as more successful in these patients; however, rates of rebleeding of 11% to 44% and operative mortality rates ranging from 33% to 63% have been associated with this procedure (64). More extensive operations, such as near-total gastrectomy or total gastrectomy, are associated with significant mortality, although they successfully stop hemorrhage.

Gastroesophageal Varices

Cirrhosis is a leading cause of death in the United States, and variceal hemorrhage is a common cause of death in these patients. Gastroesophageal varices develop in about 30% of people with cirrhosis, and of these patients, about 30% bleed as a result, usually within 1 to 2 years of diagnosis. Gastroesophageal varices are a significant cause of upper GI hemorrhage, accounting for about 20% of such cases. In patients with bleeding gastroesophageal varices, rates of rebleeding, transfusion requirements, length of hospitalization, and risk for death tend to be much higher than in patients with nonvariceal causes of bleeding (25,26,65).

Although the basic tenets of restoration of volume in patients with massive variceal hemorrhage are similar to those for patients with massive hemorrhage from any other source, intravenous volume replacement should be particularly judicious. The hyperaldosteronism associated with cirrhosis promotes sodium and water retention, with aggravation of ascites and peripheral edema. Accurate blood replacement is imperative because excessive transfusion increases the central venous pressure, worsens portal hypertension, and so exacerbates hemorrhage. Invasive cardiac monitoring with Swan-Ganz catheterization may be particularly useful for guiding volume replacement. Coagulation deficits should be aggressively corrected by administering fresh frozen plasma. Thrombocytopenia, secondary to hypersplenism or dilution, should be treated promptly with pooled platelet transfusions. Sedatives are best avoided or used sparingly because cirrhosis impairs the ability of the liver to metabolize many of these drugs. Adequate prophylaxis for delirium tremens should be administered to alcoholics.

As with other sources of upper GI hemorrhage, early endoscopy is imperative for successful diagnosis and therapy (Fig. 49.5). The identification of varices alone is not ade-

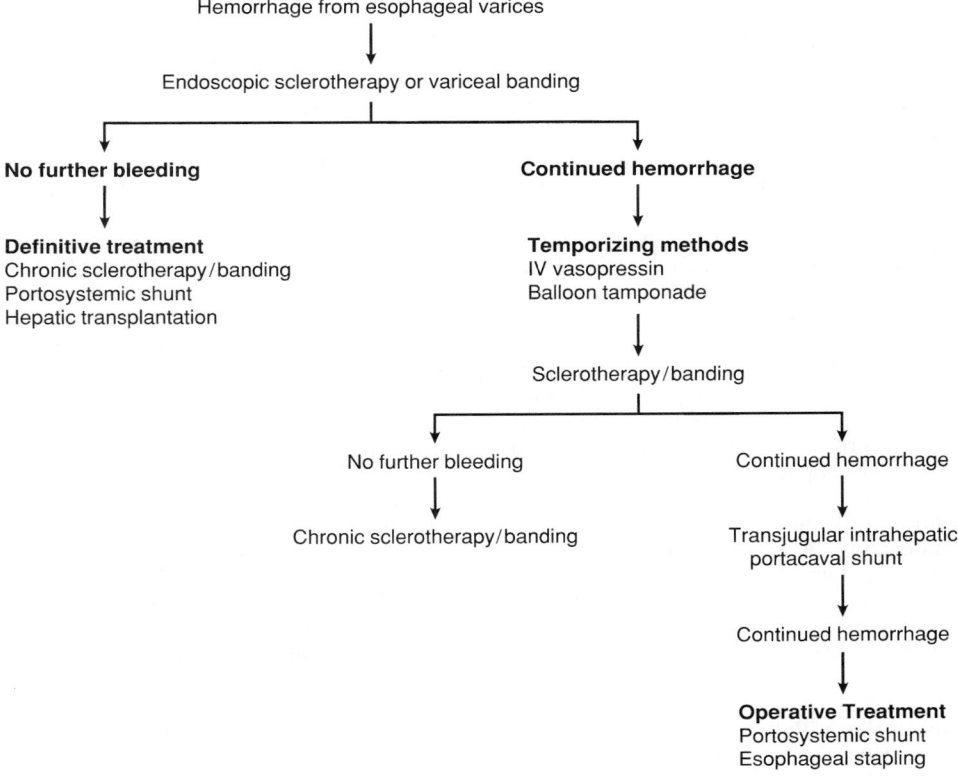

Figure 49.5. Diagnostic and therapeutic algorithm for the management of esophageal varices.

quate to explain the hemorrhage because up to half of patients with cirrhosis bleed from a source other than varices. Furthermore, endoscopy may identify factors associated with a heightened risk for variceal hemorrhage, such as an increased size and number of varices and the presence of red, blue, or other colored spots on the varix. The presence of gastric and duodenal varices and portal hypertensive changes in the gastric mucosa (portal gastropathy) will influence therapeutic decisions and prognosis.

Although vasopressin has commonly been used in the management of variceal hemorrhage, recent reports suggest the superiority of somatostatin or its synthetic analogue, octreotide. Metaanalyses have shown that somatostatin infusion is more effective and safer than vasopressin infusion in the pharmacologic control of variceal hemorrhage (66,67). Other studies have shown that somatostatin or octreotide can improve the results of sclerotherapy or endoscopic variceal ligation (68–70). In addition to enhancing the control of hemorrhage, the use of octreotide eliminates the cardiac risks of vasopressin infusion (i.e., coronary artery vasoconstriction, myocardial ischemia, and infarction). Although neither somatostatin nor vasopressin plus nitroglycerin is efficacious in definitively treating bleeding esophageal varices, these modalities may initially control hemorrhage and so reduce transfusion requirements and provide time for adequate volume replacement before definitive treatment.

Another temporizing method used for patients with massive bleeding is balloon tamponade with a Sengstaken-Blakemore tube or a Minnesota tube. These devices consist of a gastric tube with esophageal and gastric balloons. With the Minnesota tube, a proximal esophageal lumen is available for aspirating swallowed secretions. The inflated gastric and esophageal balloons compress the bleeding varices and control hemorrhage in more than 80% of cases. Hemorrhage recurs in 25% to 50% of patients on deflation of the balloons, so that this technique is limited to a temporizing role (71). The greatest value of these tubes is for arresting massive hemorrhage that has been unresponsive to other measures, so that time is gained for volume replacement and angiographic definition of the portal system before definitive treatment is instituted.

When used inappropriately, these tubes can be associated with significant morbidity and mortality. Complications occur in 4% to 9% of patients, most frequently aspiration pneumonitis. Measures to prevent pulmonary complications include endotracheal intubation before tube insertion and the placement of an esophageal tube to remove swallowed salivary secretions. Other significant complications include esophageal rupture or necrosis and airway occlusion during the attempted removal of an incompletely deflated gastric balloon.

Endoscopic sclerotherapy or banding has become the most widely used modality for the initial definitive control of bleeding esophageal varices. Several controlled trials have confirmed that sclerotherapy arrests acute variceal hemorrhage in the majority of patients. In general, a patient bleeding from esophageal varices should undergo urgent sclerotherapy or banding of the varices at the time of the first emergency endoscopy. A single treatment controls variceal bleeding in more than 70% of patients, and a second treatment increases the rate of control to between 90% and 95%. Continued or recurrent hemorrhage after sclerotherapy requires temporary control with balloon tamponade and somatostatin, usually followed by urgent operative intervention.

Following control of the initial hemorrhage, sclerotherapy is repeated in 5 to 10 days and then at 1- to 3-week intervals until the varices have been obliterated. In general, from three to five sessions are required. During this period, the risk for recurrent bleeding is at its highest. Overall, long-term sclerotherapy appears to be at least as effective as portacaval or selective splenorenal shunt surgery in terms of preventing hemorrhage, preserving hepatic function, and preventing death from variceal hemorrhage. A metaanalysis of seven trials suggests that overall survival for patients with variceal bleeding is improved by treatment with sclerotherapy (72). Complications following sclerotherapy occur in 10% to 20% of patients and include local manifestations, such as perforation, stricture formation, and ulceration. Systemic complications, including fever and sepsis, have also been reported.

A more recent method of endoscopic control of variceal hemorrhage involves the mechanical ligation of variceal channels by applying small, elastic O-rings similar to those used for banding internal hemorrhoidal veins. A recent analysis of available studies comparing endoscopic variceal ligation and sclerotherapy for variceal bleeding found that endoscopic variceal ligation was associated with a lower incidence of rebleeding, lower mortality, lower mortality from bleeding, and lower incidence of esophageal stricture (73).

Recently, a large experience with nonoperative decompression of the portal venous system by means of a percutaneously created channel between a hepatic vein and the portal vein was reported. In this procedure, termed *transjugular intrahepatic portosystemic shunting* (TIPS), expandable 8- to 10-mm metallic stents are used to maintain shunt patency. By supporting the shunt wall, the metallic stent prevents elastic recoil of the hepatic parenchyma from occluding the shunt lumen. A number of studies have documented the short-term effectiveness of this procedure in controlling hemorrhage, although the long-term durability is poor, with a stenosis or occlusion rate of almost 50% at 2 years (74). Many of these shunts, however, can be salvaged by careful surveillance and repeated percutaneous techniques. As with other nonselective shunts, the risk for hepatic encephalopathy is substantial, which has limited enthusiasm for this therapy in patients with good hepatic reserve. Transjugular intrahepatic portosystemic shunting may be particularly useful in the management of continued or recurrent variceal bleeding in poor-risk patients, such as those with Child class C cirrhosis. In addition to the lesser physiologic insult, TIPS avoids the upper abdominal dissection associated with operative shunts in patients who will ultimately require hepatic transplantation. The mean operative blood loss, length of surgery, and intensive care unit and hospital stays for patients undergoing hepatic transplantation after portacaval shunting have been reported to be significantly greater than those of patients undergoing transplantation after TIPS (75).

Mallory-Weiss Tears

In the Mallory-Weiss syndrome, acute upper GI hemorrhage occurs after retching or vomiting. The stereotypic patient is an alcoholic who begins to retch and vomit after a binge. Recently, this syndrome has been noted in a significant number of nonalcoholics with bouts of emesis. Initially, the vomitus consists of gastric contents without blood; subsequently, hematemesis and melena develop. Overall, these lesions account for about 5% to 10% of patients with upper GI bleeding (25,26,65).

Mallory and Weiss (76) described a laceration of the gastric cardia and postulated the mechanism of injury to be violent emesis against an unrelaxed cardia. Similar mucosal tears were produced in cadavers by forcing gastric contents against an occluded gastroesophageal junction. Other studies have demonstrated that vomiting raises intragastric pressure to levels capable of causing mucosal laceration.

The initial management of these patients is similar to that of patients with other sources of upper GI hemorrhage and includes volume replacement, gastric lavage, and de-

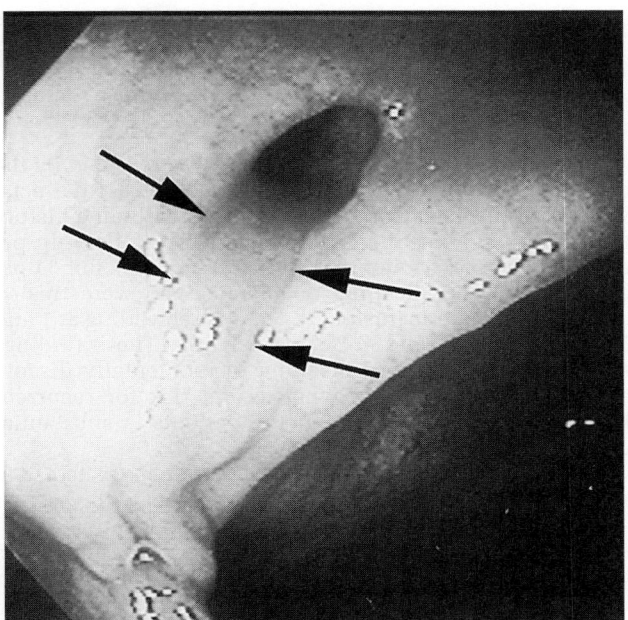

Figure 49.6. Colonoscopic view of a colonic diverticulum. A vas rectum is seen entering the diverticulum and forming one of the walls.

compression. In most patients with Mallory-Weiss tears, bleeding stops spontaneously, either before treatment or after these early measures. Once bleeding has stopped, rebleeding is rare.

In patients who continue to bleed despite these maneuvers, nonoperative and operative therapeutic options are available. Nonoperative management, consisting of endoscopic electrocoagulation or injection therapy, has been successfully applied to these lesions. In cases not amenable to endoscopic therapy, operative management consists of oversewing the laceration through an anterior longitudinal gastrotomy in the middle third of the stomach.

Lower Gastrointestinal Hemorrhage

Although the passage of maroon or bright red blood per rectum may occur in the presence of a massive upper GI hemorrhage, this finding suggests a source distal to the ligament of Treitz. The absence of blood in bilious nasogastric aspirate further supports a distal location of hemorrhage. Although the potential causes of lower GI hemorrhage are numerous (Table 49.2), colonic diverticulosis and vascular ectasia of the colon are by far the most common. The relative frequency with which these two conditions lead to lower GI hemorrhage is difficult to ascertain because both are common in the general population and are typically asymptomatic. Small-bowel sources and other colonic lesions, such as colon cancer, are relatively unusual causes of acute GI hemorrhage.

Colonic Diverticulosis. In Western society, the prevalence of colonic diverticula increases with age such that about 60% of people in their seventh decade of life are affected. The incidence increases roughly 1% annually. Only about 20% of patients with diverticulosis have symptoms attributable to this condition, and fewer than 5% experience hemorrhage (77). Hemorrhage from diverticular disease is most often massive, associated with hematochezia and varying degrees of hemorrhagic shock. Classically, patients present with a sudden onset of mild lower abdominal discomfort, rectal urgency, and the subsequent passage of a large maroon or melenic stool. Because the colon can con-

tain large volumes of blood, neither the volume nor the frequency of bloody stools is a reliable guide to the rate of hemorrhage. Despite the massive nature of the hemorrhage, in most cases of diverticular disease bleeding stops spontaneously. In a recent series, bleeding stopped spontaneously in 76% of patients initially, although rebleeding developed in 38% of them. Of the 28 patients with rebleeding, only six required surgery (78).

Bleeding associated with diverticular disease comes from a perforated vas rectum located at the neck or apex of a diverticulum. The vas rectum penetrates the colonic wall from the serosa to the submucosa through obliquely oriented connective tissue septa. Protrusion of colonic mucosa through this connective tissue plane results in apposition of the diverticulum and the vas rectum (Fig. 49.6) (see color insert following page 1190). Ulceration of the mucosa within the neck of the diverticulum and disruption of the arterial wall produces hemorrhage into the lumen of the bowel. Although diverticular disease is more prevalent in the left side of the colon, right-sided lesions account for half or more episodes of bleeding (78,79).

The massive nature of the hemorrhage associated with colonic diverticula limits the diagnostic usefulness of colonoscopy. Rarely is a bleeding vessel seen within a diverticulum, and the presence of blood or clot within diverticula is of no diagnostic benefit. Selective mesenteric arteriography may demonstrate the luminal extravasation of contrast; however, in one study of patients with bleeding from diverticulosis, angiographic localization was effective in fewer than 20% of them (80). Failure to visualize a point of bleeding is usually the consequence of cessation of active bleeding at the time of angiography.

Given the relatively low risk for recurrent hemorrhage, patients in whom bleeding stops should be treated expectantly. In about 10% of patients with bleeding from colonic diverticula, the bleeding continues, and ultimately operative intervention is required. Nonoperative methods of arresting GI hemorrhage, such as angiographic embolization and endoscopic electrocoagulation, have been reported to be successful, although experience with either of these modalities is very limited. Embolization of bleeding vessels in the colon has been reported to be safe and effective in the majority of patients; however, the substantial risk for ischemic complications limits the enthusiasm of most surgeons for this procedure (81,82). The rapid nature of the hemorrhage and the difficulty in defining the site of hemorrhage through the endoscope have prevented endoscopic treatments from being beneficial for bleeding diverticula.

Patients with continued bleeding from diverticular disease should undergo resection of the colon segment that contains the site of hemorrhage. Even after successful localization of a source of bleeding, the least drastic operation that can usually be contemplated is a hemicolectomy or wide segmental colectomy. Scanning with tagged red blood cells, although sensitive, cannot pinpoint a site of bleeding with great accuracy. Although angiography usually provides a more precise localization, correlation between the vascular pattern and the anatomic location is sufficiently imprecise that at least a segmental resection is warranted.

Although a subtotal colectomy for *nonlocalized, ongoing* colonic hemorrhage may occasionally be necessary, it should be performed only after exhaustive attempts have been made to localize the site of hemorrhage. Subtotal colectomy is associated with higher rates of perioperative morbidity than segmental resection is, and postoperative diarrhea may present a significant problem in elderly patients. However, if massive bleeding from the colon continues and all attempts at preoperative and intraoperative localization are unsuccessful, subtotal colectomy with ileoproctostomy may be required.

Colonic Angiodysplasia

Sometimes called *vascular ectasia* or *arteriovenous malformations,* these lesions are believed to arise from the age-related degeneration of previously normal intestinal submucosal veins and overlying mucosal capillaries. Angiodysplasia is located most frequently in the cecum and ascending colon, although it may be found more distally in 20% to 30% of cases. Multiple lesions are present in 40% to 75% of cases (83). Endoscopically, they appear as flat or slightly raised red lesions that are 2 to 10 mm wide. They may be round or stellate, or they may have sharply circumscribed, fernlike margins. A prominent feeding vessel may be evident in addition to a surrounding halo.

Microscopically, angiodysplasia consists of dilated, thin-walled vessels that appear to be ectatic veins and venules localized within the submucosa. A dilated submucosal vein is often found, and occasionally an enlarged artery. Smooth muscle is usually absent. It is believed that this variability of histologic patterns represents different stages in the development of this disease, with early changes being ectatic capillaries and venules and later lesions composed of arteriovenous communications. Angiodysplasia in the colon is generally thought to be an acquired lesion associated with aging, but the exact cause is unknown.

The prevalence of colonic angiodysplasia in the general population is difficult to determine because most patients who undergo evaluation are experiencing symptoms. Investigators have found colonic vascular ectasia in 2% to 6% of patients undergoing colonoscopy, depending on the indication for endoscopy (83). In one study of asymptomatic patients undergoing colonoscopic screening for neoplasms, the incidence of vascular ectasia was 0.83% (83,84). These lesions may present with hematochezia, melena, occult blood loss, or iron-deficiency anemia. Bleeding lesions are almost always found in the right side of the colon. In comparison with diverticular bleeding, episodes of hemorrhage in vascular ectasia are usually less severe and are somewhat more likely to recur. After the initial episode of hemorrhage, bleeding stops spontaneously in the majority of patients (85).

Vascular ectasia may be diagnosed by either colonoscopy or selective mesenteric angiography. Colonoscopy has been reported to have a sensitivity of 80% (86). Colonoscopic diagnosis of these lesions patients with active bleeding may be confounded by the presence of other, incidental lesions, including traumatic and suction artifacts produced during the examination. In addition, in patients with significant bleeding and hypovolemia, the shunting of blood flow away from the intestinal mucosa may obscure lesions when volume replacement is inadequate. Colonoscopy can be used effectively to treat vascular ectasia, either with coagulation or with injection of sclerosants (87,88).

Selective mesenteric angiography may complement colonoscopy, particularly in patients with massive bleeding or in whom colonoscopy is unrevealing or incomplete. Characteristic angiographic findings include the following:

1. A densely opacified and slowly emptying, dilated, tortuous vein. This is seen in 90% of patients and is best observed during the late venous phase of the angiogram.
2. A vascular tuft. This cluster of vessels, which empties slowly with opacification persisting into the venous phase, is seen in 66% to 75% of patients.
3. An early-filling vein. This is usually a segmental vein in the cecum or right side of the colon, although at

times, it may be the ileocolic vein. Early-filling veins can characteristically be visualized within 5 seconds after injection of contrast. Extravasation of contrast material into the lumen of the bowel during angiography is seen in a minority of cases.

The natural history of these lesions was revealed by the clinical course of 101 patients with colonic vascular ectasia (86). In the 15 asymptomatic patients without a history of bleeding, no bleeding occurred during a follow-up period lasting up to 68 months (mean, 23 months). For 31 patients with overt bleeding or anemia who were treated only with blood transfusion, the rate of rebleeding at 1 and 3 years was 26% and 46%, respectively. These findings suggest that the risk for bleeding in incidentally discovered lesions is minimal, whereas the risk for recurrent hemorrhage in most symptomatic patients is substantial and may increase with time.

Bleeding in colonic vascular ectasia can be treated with endoscopy. Nonrandomized trials of patients with vascular ectasia managed with monopolar electrocoagulation, endoscopic injection sclerotherapy, contact probes, and lasers have reported good results. All methods appear to be effective for treating bleeding in vascular ectasia, and all are associated with procedure-related morbidity rates of 2% to 10%. Perforation rates of 2% to 3% have been reported.

Patients with bleeding from vascular ectasia in whom endoscopic hemostatic methods are unsuccessful or unavailable can be treated with resection of the colon following preoperative localization of the site of bleeding. For the usual patient with bleeding from vascular ectasia in the cecum or ascending colon, a right colectomy with ileotransverse colostomy is the treatment of choice. The value of preoperative localization of the site of bleeding cannot be overstated, and every effort should be made to determine the site of hemorrhage before laparotomy is undertaken.

UNUSUAL CAUSES OF ACUTE GASTROINTESTINAL HEMORRHAGE

As outlined in Tables 49.1 and 49.2, a wide variety of pathologic processes may present with acute GI hemorrhage. Although these lesions generally account for a relatively small percentage of the total number of cases of overt GI hemorrhage, they can present vexing problems to the clinician faced with a patient with bleeding in whom the usual causes have been excluded. The following lesions occur commonly enough that an individual clinician is likely to encounter them.

Dieulafoy's Vascular Malformation

In Dieulafoy's vascular malformation, an unusual cause of recurrent hematemesis, bleeding originates from an unusually large (1- to 3-mm diameter) artery running through the gastric submucosa for a variable distance. Erosion of the gastric mucosa overlying the vessel results in necrosis of the arterial wall and brisk hemorrhage. The mucosal defect is usually small (2 to 5 mm) and without evidence of chronic inflammation.

Painless hematemesis and melena are typical. Recurrent bleeding with spontaneous cessation is also common. In a collective review of 101 cases, the mean age of the patients was 52 years, and the lesion occurred twice as frequently in men as in women. No significant association was found with alcohol abuse or antecedent symptoms (89).

The diagnosis is most frequently made endoscopically by demonstrating arterial bleeding from a pinpoint mucosal defect. Occasionally, a small arterial vessel may be seen protruding from the gastric mucosa. Characteristically, the lesions are located within 6 cm of the esophagogastric junction along the lesser curvature, although they may also occur at other sites.

Most patients can be managed with endoscopic electrocoagulation of the bleeding vessel (90). If operative excision is required, a combined endoscopic and surgical approach may be useful (91).

Angiodysplasia of the Stomach and Small Intestine

Angiodysplastic lesions may occur throughout the GI tract. Like colonic lesions, they appear as minute, flat or slightly raised red lesions with round or stellate shapes. The margins are characteristically sharp, with a pale mucosal halo surrounding the lesion. The lesions are frequently multiple and are found most commonly in the stomach and duodenum, although esophageal and small-intestinal involvement has also been described.

These lesions may be diagnosed by endoscopy, although their minute size and sessile nature complicate detection. The lesions may be mistaken for submucosal hemorrhage associated with acute gastritis or trauma artifact from a nasogastric tube or endoscope. The lesions may also be demonstrated arteriographically, as they have many of the features described for colonic vascular ectasia.

Endoscopic injection of sclerosants, electrocoagulation, and laser photocoagulation have all been used to treat gastroduodenal angiodysplasia, with good results. The multiplicity of lesions often necessitates several courses of therapy to eliminate recurring hemorrhage. Surgical resection of the gastric or intestinal wall containing the lesion and also oversewing of the bleeding lesion have been reported to control hemorrhage successfully.

Aortoenteric Fistula

Although communication between the aorta and the intestine may occur as a result of aneurysmal disease or infectious aortitis *(primary aortoenteric fistula),* most aortoenteric fistulae are caused by erosion of an aortic vascular prosthesis through the wall of the distal duodenum *(secondary aortoenteric fistula).* The incidence of aortoenteric fistula following aortic reconstructive surgery is about 1%, with most of these fistulae arising from the proximal graft anastomosis. Secondary aortoenteric fistulae are believed to develop after prolonged contact of a prosthetic graft with a fixed segment of intestine. Ultimately, erosion of the graft through the bowel wall results in the development of a low-grade infection around the graft; involvement of the suture line leads to dehiscence of the anastomosis and massive hemorrhage.

The interval between aortic reconstructive surgery and the onset of GI hemorrhage may range from a few days to many years; the median interval is about 3 years (92). Most patients have an initial episode of GI bleeding, called a *herald bleed,* that is followed in hours, days, or weeks by catastrophic hemorrhage. Patients may also complain of back or abdominal pain and less commonly have fever or signs of sepsis from infection of the graft.

The diagnosis of an aortoenteric fistula must be considered in any patient with an aortic prosthesis or an abdominal aortic aneurysm who presents with GI hemorrhage. Endoscopy should be performed urgently following volume restoration to eliminate another cause of bleeding (e.g., peptic ulcer disease). If endoscopy fails to demonstrate an aortoenteric fistula or another convincing source

of blood loss and the bleeding is not massive, computed tomography may be helpful in detecting infection involving the graft or other evidence of an aortoenteric fistula. In patients with actively bleeding, exploratory laparotomy with exposure of the proximal graft should be undertaken. If an aortoenteric fistula or erosion is identified, resection of the graft with extraanatomic bypass and repair of the duodenal wall is required.

Meckel's Diverticulum

Meckel's diverticulum is an unusual cause of acute GI hemorrhage, particularly in adults. About 25% of patients with symptomatic Meckel's diverticula present with hemorrhage (93). In a series of 17 patients with bleeding from Meckel's diverticula, 11 experienced frank hemorrhage and six had chronic occult blood loss. The incidence of GI hemorrhage is greatest in the first decade of life and steadily decreases thereafter. In one series, no patient older than 40 years of age, and only one patient older than 31 years, had bleeding from a Meckel's diverticulum (93). The pathogenesis of bleeding involves the presence of ectopic gastric mucosa and peptic ulceration of adjacent bowel wall. Although these lesions may be demonstrated by enteroclysis, abdominal scintigraphy following the intravenous injection of radioactive technetium demonstrates the ectopic gastric mucosa within the diverticulum and suggests the correct diagnosis. Treatment consists of resecting the diverticulum along with a cuff of adjacent bowel.

Diverticulum of the Small Intestine

Diverticular disease of the small intestine is another uncommon cause of either upper GI (duodenal diverticula) or lower GI (jejunoileal diverticula) hemorrhage. The pathogenesis is similar to that of colonic diverticula, with erosion of a vas rectum through the diverticular wall and the acute onset of massive hemorrhage. Depending on the location of the diverticulum, patients may present with either hematemesis, melena, or hematochezia. Hemorrhage from this source can be a vexing diagnostic problem because jejunoileal lesions are beyond the reach of the gastroscope and bleeding from duodenal diverticula may be difficult to discern. Mesenteric angiography or intraoperative enteroscopy may localize the site of hemorrhage in patients with active bleeding. Segmental resection of the involved intestine is the treatment of choice.

Hemorrhage after Endoscopic Procedures

Significant hemorrhage can occur following endoscopic biopsy, sphincterotomy, and other traumatic procedures. Hemorrhage following endoscopic biliary sphincterotomy occurs in approximately 2% of patients (94–96). Mild immediate bleeding is common and is usually self-limited. Late hemorrhage usually develops within 48 hours of the procedure but can occur many days after sphincterotomy (97). More severe hemorrhage can be controlled by epinephrine injection (97,98), so that a need for operative treatment is uncommon.

Biopsy of lesions in the GI tract may also cause bleeding, which is usually minor and self-limited. Clinically significant hemorrhage after colonic polypectomy is seen in approximately 0.2% of biopsies and may occur up to 12 days after the procedure (99). The site of bleeding can be confirmed by scanning with tagged red cells, arteriography, or colonoscopy. Arteriography and colonoscopy can be used therapeutically, as described previously. The endoscopic placement of bands, such as those used for esophageal varices, has also been reported to be successful in arresting hemorrhage (37). Surgical treatment is rarely required.

REFERENCES

1. Daniel WA Jr, Egan S. The quantity of blood required to produce a tarry stool. *JAMA* 1939;113:2232.
2. Schiff L, Stevens RJ, Shapiro N, et al. Observations on the oral administration of citrated blood in man. II. The effect on the stools. *Am J Med Sci* 1942;203:409–412.
3. Hilsman JH. The color of blood-containing feces following the instillation of citrated blood at various levels of the small intestine. *Gastroenterology* 1999;15:131–134.
4. Cuellar RE, Gavaler JS, Alexander JA, et al. Gastrointestinal tract hemorrhage: the value of a nasogastric aspirate [see comments]. *Arch Intern Med* 1990;150:1381–1384.
5. Gilbert DA, Silverstein FE, Tedesco FJ, et al. The national ASGE survey on upper gastrointestinal bleeding. III. Endoscopy in upper gastrointestinal bleeding. *Gastrointest Endosc* 1981;27:94–102.
6. Morris DW, Levine GM, Soloway RD, et al. Prospective, randomized study of diagnosis and outcome in acute upper-gastrointestinal bleeding: endoscopy versus conventional radiography. *Am J Dig Dis* 1975;20:1103–1109.
7. Cook DJ, Guyatt GH, Salena BJ, et al. Endoscopic therapy for acute nonvariceal upper gastrointestinal hemorrhage: a meta-analysis. *Gastroenterology* 1992;102:139–148.
8. Sacks HS, Chalmers TC, Blum AL, et al. Endoscopic hemostasis: an effective therapy for bleeding peptic ulcers. *JAMA* 1990;264:494–499.
9. Silvis SE, Nebel O, Rogers G, et al. Endoscopic complications: results of the 1974 American Society for Gastrointestinal Endoscopy Survey. *JAMA* 1976;235:928–930.
10. Smith R, Copely DJ, Bolen FH. ^{99m}Tc RBC scintigraphy: correlation of gastrointestinal bleeding rates with scintigraphic findings. *Am J Roentgenol* 1987;148:869–874.
11. Thorne DA, Datz FL, Remley K, et al. Bleeding rates necessary for detecting acute gastrointestinal bleeding with technetium-99m-labeled red blood cells in an experimental model. *J Nucl Med* 1987;28:514–520.
12. Garofalo TE, Abdu RA. Accuracy and efficacy of nuclear scintigraphy for the detection of gastrointestinal bleeding [see comments]. *Arch Surg* 1997;132:196–199.
13. Hunter JM, Pezim ME. Limited value of technetium 99m-labeled red cell scintigraphy in localization of lower gastrointestinal bleeding. *Am J Surg* 1990;159:504–506.
14. Voeller GR, Bunch G, Britt LG. Use of technetium-labeled red blood cell scintigraphy in the detection and management of gastrointestinal hemorrhage. *Surgery* 1991;110:799–804.
15. Suzman MS, Talmor M, Jennis R, et al. Accurate localization and surgical management of active lower gastrointestinal hemorrhage with technetium-labeled erythrocyte scintigraphy [see comments]. *Ann Surg* 1996;224:29–36.
16. Maurer AH, Rodman MS, Vitti RA, et al. Gastrointestinal bleeding: improved localization with cine scintigraphy [see comments]. *Radiology* 1992;185:187–192.
17. Singh PR, Russell CD, Dubovsky EV, et al. Technique of scanning for Meckel's diverticulum. *Clin Nucl Med* 1978;3:188–192.
18. Nusbaum M, Baum S. Radiographic demonstration of unknown sites of GI bleeding. *Surg Forum* 1963;14:374–375.
19. Lewis MP, Khoo DE, Spencer J. Value of laparotomy in the diagnosis of obscure gastrointestinal haemorrhage. *Gut* 1995;37:187–190.
20. Bouhnik Y, Bitoun A, Coffin B, et al. Two-way push videoenteroscopy in investigation of small-bowel disease. *Gut* 1998;43:280–284.
21. Schmit A, Gay F, Adler M, et al. Diagnostic efficacy of push-enteroscopy and long-term follow-up of patients with small-bowel angiodysplasias. *Dig Dis Sci* 1996;41:2348–2352.
22. Davies GR, Benson MJ, Gertner DJ, et al. Diagnostic and therapeutic push-type enteroscopy in clinical use. *Gut* 1995;37:346–352.
23. Blatchford O, Davidson LA, Murray WR, et al. Acute upper gastrointestinal haemorrhage in west of Scotland: case ascertainment study. *BMJ* 1997;315:510–514.
24. Rockall TA, Logan RF, Devlin HB, et al. Incidence of and mortality from acute upper gastrointestinal haemorrhage in the United Kingdom: Steering Committee and members of the National Audit of Acute Upper Gastrointestinal Haemorrhage [see comments]. *BMJ* 1995;311:222–226.
25. Sugawa C, Steffes CP, Nakamura R, et al. Upper GI bleeding in an urban hospital: etiology, recurrence, and prognosis. *Ann Surg* 1990;212:521–526.
26. Wilcox CM, Clark WS. Causes and outcome of upper and lower gastrointestinal bleeding: the Grady Hospital experience. *South Med J* 1999;92:44–50.
27. Hirschowitz BI, Lanas A. NSAID association with gastrointestinal bleeding and peptic ulcer [Review] [33 refs]. *Agents Actions Suppl* 1991;35:93–101.
28. Ehsanullah RS, Page MC, Tildesley G, et al. Prevention of gastroduodenal damage induced by non-steroidal anti-inflammatory drugs: controlled trial of ranitidine. *BMJ* 1988;297:1017–1021.
29. Strom BL, Taragin MI, Carson JL. Gastrointestinal bleeding from the nonsteroidal anti-inflammatory drugs [Review] [21 refs]. *Agents Actions Suppl* 1990;29:27–38.
30. Garcia RL, Cattaruzzi C, Troncon MG, et al. Risk of hospitalization for upper gastrointestinal tract bleeding associated with ketorolac, other nonsteroidal anti-inflammatory drugs, calcium antagonists, and other antihypertensive drugs. *Arch Intern Med* 1998;158:33–39.
31. Shorr RI, Ray WA, Daugherty JR, et al. Concurrent use of nonsteroidal anti-inflammatory drugs and oral anticoagulants places elderly persons at high risk for hemorrhagic peptic ulcer disease. *Arch Intern Med* 1993;153:1665–1670.
32. Armstrong CP, Blower AL. Non-steroidal anti-inflammatory drugs and life-threatening complications of peptic ulceration. *Gut* 1987;28:527–532.
33. Klein WA, Krevsky B, Klepper L, et al. Nonsteroidal antiinflammatory drugs and upper gastrointestinal hemorrhage in an urban hospital. *Dig Dis Sci* 1993;38:2049–2055.
34. Lanza FL, Fakouhi D, Rubin A, et al. A double-blind placebo-controlled comparison of the efficacy and safety of 50, 100, and 200 micrograms of misoprostol QID in the prevention of ibuprofen-induced gastric and duodenal mucosal lesions and symptoms. *Am J Gastroenterol* 1989;84:633–636.
35. Robinson MG, Griffin JWJ, Bowers J, et al. Effect of ranitidine on gastroduodenal mucosal damage induced by nonsteroidal antiinflammatory drugs. *Dig Dis Sci* 1989;34:424–428.
36. Roth SH, Bennett RE, Mitchell CS, et al. Cimetidine therapy in nonsteroidal anti-inflammatory drug gastropathy: double-blind long-term evaluation. *Arch Intern Med* 1987;147:1798–1801.
37. Pfaffenbach B, Adamek RJ, Wegener M. Endoscopic band ligation for treatment of post-polypectomy bleeding. *Z Gastroenterol* 1996;34:241–242.
38. Wilcox CM, Alexander LN, Cotsonis GA, et al. Nonsteroidal antiinflammatory drugs are associated with both upper and lower gastrointestinal bleeding. *Dig Dis Sci* 1997;42:990–997.
39. Lanas A, Sekar MC, Hirschowitz BI. Objective evidence of aspirin use in both ulcer and nonulcer upper and lower gastrointestinal bleeding. *Gastroenterology* 1992;103:862–869.
40. Holt S, Rigoglioso V, Sidhu M, et al. Nonsteroidal antiinflammatory drugs and lower gastrointestinal bleeding. *Dig Dis Sci* 1993;38:1619–1623.
41. Khuroo MS, Yattoo GN, Javid G, et al. A comparison of omeprazole and placebo for bleeding peptic ulcer [see comments]. *N Engl J Med* 1997;336:1054–1058.
42. Lin HJ, Lo WC, Lee FY, et al. A prospective randomized comparative trial showing that omeprazole prevents rebleeding in patients with bleeding peptic ulcer after successful endoscopic therapy. *Arch Intern Med* 1998;158:54–58.
43. Pilotto A, Leandro G, Di Mario F, et al. Role of *Helicobacter pylori* infection on upper gastrointestinal bleeding in the elderly: a case-control study. *Dig Dis Sci* 1997;42:586–591.
44. Laine LA. *Helicobacter pylori* and complicated ulcer disease [Review] [47 refs]. *Am J Med* 1996;100:52S–57S.
45. Schiano TD, Adrain AL, Vega KJ, et al. High-resolution endoluminal sonography assessment of the hematocystic spots of esophageal varices. *Gastrointest Endosc* 1999;49:424–427.
46. Moreto M, Zaballa M, Ibanez S, et al. Efficacy of monopolar electrocoagulation in the treatment of bleeding gastric ulcer: a controlled trial. *Endoscopy* 1987;19:54–56.

47. Jessen K, Gilbert GA, Tytgat GN, et al. [Bipolar electrocoagulation in active upper gastrointestinal hemorrhage: results of a prospective, non-controlled, multicenter study] (in German). *Z Gastroenterol* 1983;21:268–272.

48. Lin HJ, Tseng GY, Perng CL, et al. Comparison of adrenaline injection and bipolar electrocoagulation for the arrest of peptic ulcer bleeding. *Gut* 1999;44:715–719.

49. Chung SS, Lau JY, Sung JJ, et al. Randomised comparison between adrenaline injection alone and adrenaline injection plus heat probe treatment for actively bleeding ulcers [see comments]. *BMJ* 1997;314:1307–1311.

50. Asaki S. Endoscopic haemostasis by local absolute alcohol injection for UGI tract bleeding: a multicentre study. In: Okabe H, Honda T, Ohshiba S, eds. *Endoscopic surgery*. New York: Elsevier Science, 1984:105–116.

51. Rutgeerts P, Rauws E, Wara P, et al. Randomised trial of single and repeated fibrin glue compared with injection of polidocanol in treatment of bleeding peptic ulcer [see comments]. *Lancet* 1997;350:692–696.

52. Kubba AK, Murphy W, Palmer KR. Endoscopic injection for bleeding peptic ulcer: a comparison of adrenaline alone with adrenaline plus human thrombin. *Gastroenterology* 1996;111: 623–628.

53. Anonymous. Consensus conference: therapeutic endoscopy and bleeding ulcers [Review] [0 refs]. *JAMA* 1989;262:1369–1372.

54. Hsu PI, Lin XZ, Chan SH, et al. Bleeding peptic ulcer—risk factors for rebleeding and sequential changes in endoscopic findings. *Gut* 1994;35:746–749.

55. Mueller X, Rothenbuehler JM, Amery A, et al. Factors predisposing to further hemorrhage and mortality after peptic ulcer bleeding. *J Am Coll Surg* 1994;179:457–461.

56. Lau JY, Sung JJ, Lam YH, et al. Endoscopic retreatment compared with surgery in patients with recurrent bleeding after initial endoscopic control of bleeding ulcers [see comments]. *N Engl J Med* 1999;340:751–756.

57. Gupta PK, Fleischer DE. Nonvariceal upper gastrointestinal bleeding [Review] [117 refs]. *Med Clin North Am* 1993;77: 973–992.

58. Teenan RP, Murray WR. Late outcome of undersewing alone for gastric ulcer haemorrhage. *Br J Surg* 1990;77:811–812.

59. Schuster DP, Rowley H, Feinstein S, et al. Prospective evaluation of the risk of upper gastrointestinal bleeding after admission to a medical intensive care unit. *Am J Med* 1984;76: 623–630.

60. Cook DJ, Fuller HD, Guyatt GH, et al. Risk factors for gastrointestinal bleeding in critically ill patients: Canadian Critical Care Trials Group [see comments]. *N Engl J Med* 1994; 330:377–381.

61. Driks MR, Craven DE, Celli BR, et al. Nosocomial pneumonia in intubated patients given sucralfate as compared with antacids or histamine type 2 blockers: the role of gastric colonization. *N Engl J Med* 1987;317:1376–1382.

62. Cook D, Guyatt G, Marshall J, et al. A comparison of sucralfate and ranitidine for the prevention of upper gastrointestinal bleeding in patients requiring mechanical ventilation: Canadian Critical Care Trials Group [see comments]. *N Engl J Med* 1998;338:791–797.

63. Athanasoulis CA. Therapeutic applications of angiography (first of two parts) [Review] [103 refs]. *N Engl J Med* 1980;302: 1117–1125.

64. Robert A, Kauffman GL Jr. Stress ulcers, erosions, and gastric mucosal injury. In: Sleisenger MH, Fordtran JS, eds. *Gastrointestinal disease: pathophysiology, diagnosis, management*. Philadelphia: WB Saunders, 1989:772–792.

65. Silverstein FE, Gilbert DA, Tedesco FJ, et al. The national ASGE survey on upper gastrointestinal bleeding. II. Clinical prognostic factors. *Gastrointest Endosc* 1981;27:80–93.

66. Imperiale TF, Teran JC, McCullough AJ. A meta-analysis of somatostatin versus vasopressin in the management of acute esophageal variceal hemorrhage. *Gastroenterology* 1995;109: 1289–1294.

67. Burroughs AK. Octreotide in variceal bleeding. *Gut* 1994;35: S23–S27.

68. Avgerinos A, Nevens F, Raptis S, et al. Early administration of somatostatin and efficacy of sclerotherapy in acute oesophageal variceal bleeds: the European Acute Bleeding Oesophageal Variceal Episodes (ABOVE) randomised trial [see comments]. *Lancet* 1997;350:1495–1499.

69. Besson I, Ingrand P, Person B, et al. Sclerotherapy with or without octreotide for acute variceal bleeding. *N Engl J Med* 1995;333:555–560.

70. Sung JJ, Chung SC, Yung MY, et al. Prospective randomised study of effect of octreotide on rebleeding from oesophageal varices after endoscopic ligation [see comments]. *Lancet* 1995;346:1666–1669.

71. Hermann RE, Traul D. Experience with the Sengstaken-Blakemore tube for bleeding esophageal varices. *Surg Gynecol Obstet* 1970;130:879–885.

72. Terblanche J, Krige JE, Bornman PC. The treatment of esophageal varices [Review] [47 refs]. *Annu Rev Med* 1992;43: 69–82.

73. Laine L, Cook D. Endoscopic ligation compared with sclerotherapy for treatment of esophageal variceal bleeding: a meta-analysis [see comments]. *Ann Intern Med* 1995;123: 280–287.

74. LaBerge JM, Somberg KA, Lake JR, et al. Two-year outcome following transjugular intrahepatic portosystemic shunt for variceal bleeding: results in 90 patients. *Gastroenterology* 1995;108:1143–1151.

75. Menegaux F, Keeffe EB, Baker E, et al. Comparison of transjugular and surgical portosystemic shunts on the outcome of liver transplantation. *Arch Surg* 1994;129:1018–1023.

76. Mallory GK, Weiss S. Hemorrhages from lacerations of the cardiac orifice of the stomach due to vomiting. *Am J Med Sci* 1929;178:506–515.

77. McGuire HHJ, Haynes BW Jr. Massive hemorrhage for diverticulosis of the colon: guidelines for therapy based on bleeding patterns observed in fifty cases. *Ann Surg* 1972;175:847–855.

78. McGuire HH Jr. Bleeding colonic diverticula: a reappraisal of natural history and management. *Ann Surg* 1994;220:653–656.

79. Casarella WJ, Kanter IE, Seaman WB. Right-sided colonic diverticula as a cause of acute rectal hemorrhage. *N Engl J Med* 1972;286:450–453.

80. Boley SJ, DiBiase A, Brandt LJ, et al. Lower intestinal bleeding in the elderly. *Am J Surg* 1979;137:57–64.

81. Nicholson AA, Ettles DF, Hartley JE, et al. Transcatheter coil embolotherapy: a safe and effective option for major colonic haemorrhage [see comments]. *Gut* 1998;43:79–84.

82. Gordon RL, Ahl KL, Kerlan RK, et al. Selective arterial embolization for the control of lower gastrointestinal bleeding. *Am J Surg* 1997;174:24–28.

83. Foutch PG. Angiodysplasia of the gastrointestinal tract [see comments] [Review] [110 refs]. *Am J Gastroenterol* 1993;88: 807–818.

84. Foutch PG, Rex DK, Lieberman DA. Prevalence and natural history of colonic angiodysplasia among healthy asymptomatic people. *Am J Gastroenterol* 1995;90:564–567.

85. Sharma R, Gorbien MJ. Angiodysplasia and lower gastrointestinal tract bleeding in elderly patients [Review] [75 refs]. *Arch Intern Med* 1995;155:807–812.

86. Richter JM, Hedberg SE, Athanasoulis CA, et al. Angiodysplasia: clinical presentation and colonoscopic diagnosis. *Dig Dis Sci* 1984;29:481–485.

87. Gupta N, Longo WE, Vernava AM. Angiodysplasia of the lower gastrointestinal tract: an entity readily diagnosed by colonoscopy and primarily managed nonoperatively. *Dis Colon Rectum* 1995;38:979–982.

88. Benvenuti GA, Julich MM. Ethanolamine injection for sclerotherapy of angiodysplasia of the colon. *Endoscopy* 1998;30: 564–569.

89. Veldhuyzen VZS, Bartelsman JF, Schipper ME, et al. Recurrent massive haematemesis from Dieulafoy vascular malformations—a review of 101 cases. *Gut* 1986;27:213–222.

90. Baettig B, Haecki W, Lammer F, et al. Dieulafoy's disease: endoscopic treatment and follow-up. *Gut* 1993;34:1418–1421.

91. Grisendi A, Lonardo A, Della CG, et al. Combined endoscopic and surgical management of Dieulafoy vascular malformation. *J Am Coll Surg* 1994;179:182–186.

92. Nagy SW, Marshall JB. Aortoenteric fistulas: recognizing a potentially catastrophic cause of gastrointestinal bleeding [Review] [32 refs]. *Postgrad Med* 1921;93:211–212.

93. Mackey WC, Dineen P. A fifty-year experience with Meckel's diverticulum. *Surg Gynecol Obstet* 1983;156:56–64.

94. Halme L, Doepel M, von Numers H, et al. Complications of diagnostic and therapeutic ERCP. *Ann Chir Gynaecol* 1999;88: 127–131.

95. Freeman ML, Nelson DB, Sherman S, et al. Complications of endoscopic biliary sphincterotomy [see comments]. *N Engl J Med* 1996;335:909–918.

96. Gholson CF, Favrot D, Vickers B, et al. Delayed hemorrhage following endoscopic retrograde sphincterotomy for choledocho-cholithiasis. *Dig Dis Sci* 1996;41:831–834.

97. Vasconez C, Llach J, Bordas JM, et al. Injection treatment of hemorrhage induced by endoscopic sphincterotomy [see comments]. *Endoscopy* 1998;30:37–39.

98. Leung JW, Chan FK, Sung JJ, et al. Endoscopic sphincterotomy-induced hemorrhage: a study of risk factors and the role of epinephrine injection. *Gastrointest Endosc* 1995;42:550–554.

99. Gibbs DH, Opelka FG, Beck DE, et al. Postpolypectomy colonic hemorrhage. *Dis Colon Rectum* 1996;39:806–810.

SURGERY: SCIENTIFIC PRINCIPLES AND PRACTICE, Third Edition, edited by Lazar J. Greenfield, Michael W. Mulholland, Keith T. Oldham, Gerald B. Zelenock, and Keith D. Lillemoe. Lippincott Williams & Wilkins Publishers, Philadelphia, © 2001.

CHAPTER 50

ANORECTAL DISORDERS

SANTHAT NIVATVONGS

ANATOMY OF THE RECTUM AND ANAL CANAL

Rectum

The rectum extends from the level of the promontory of the sacrum to the level of the levator ani muscle and varies in length from 12 to 15 cm. The rectum differs from the colon in that the outer layer is covered circumferentially by longitudinal muscle rather than the three taeniae bands. The rectum has two or three lateral curves that form submucosal folds in the lumen, known as the *valves of Houston*. The posterior part of the rectum is devoid of peritoneum and is covered with the endopelvic fascia. The presacral fascia is a strong, endopelvic fascia that covers the entire anterior surface of the sacrum and also the underlying vessels and nerves. At about the level of S-4, the presacral fascia runs forward and downward and attaches to the rectum (1). This portion is referred to as the *rectosacral fascia* (Fig. 50.1). It is necessary to cut this fascia for full mobilization of the rectum, as in abdominoperineal resection or low anterior resection. Peritoneum covers the upper two thirds of the rectum anteriorly, and the upper one third of the rectum is covered by peritoneum laterally. The lower third of the rectum is entirely devoid of peritoneum. In general, the anterior peritoneal reflection is about 6 to 8 cm from the anal verge. The extraperitoneal portion of the rectum is covered by the endopelvic fascia, which, on the anterior surface, is called *Denonvilliers' fascia*. The lateral endopelvic fascia, which is thicker, is referred to as the *lateral rectal stalks*, which must also be divided for full mobilization of the rectum.

Anal Canal

The anal canal, about 4 cm in length, is the terminal portion of the large bowel that passes through the levator ani muscle and opens to the anal verge. The muscular wall of the anal canal, as a continuation of the circular muscular layer of the rectum, is thickened and forms the internal sphincter. The anal canal is wrapped by the external sphincter muscle and the puborectal muscle, which are arranged in three U-shaped loops (2). The top loop is formed by the puborectal muscle, which originates from the pubis. The intermediate loop is the superficial external sphincter muscle; the origin of this loop, at the tip of the coccyx, is known as the *anococcygeal ligament*. The basal loop is composed of the subcutaneous portion of the external sphincter muscle (Fig. 50.2).

The upper portion of the anal canal, where the internal sphincter muscle becomes thickened and the puborectal muscle wraps around (felt on digital examination of the lateral and posterior quadrants), is called the *anorectal ring*. From the level of the anorectal ring distally and between the internal and external sphincter muscles, the longitudinal muscle coat of the rectum is joined by fibers of the levator ani and puborectal muscles to form the conjoined longitudinal muscle (Fig. 50.3). These muscle

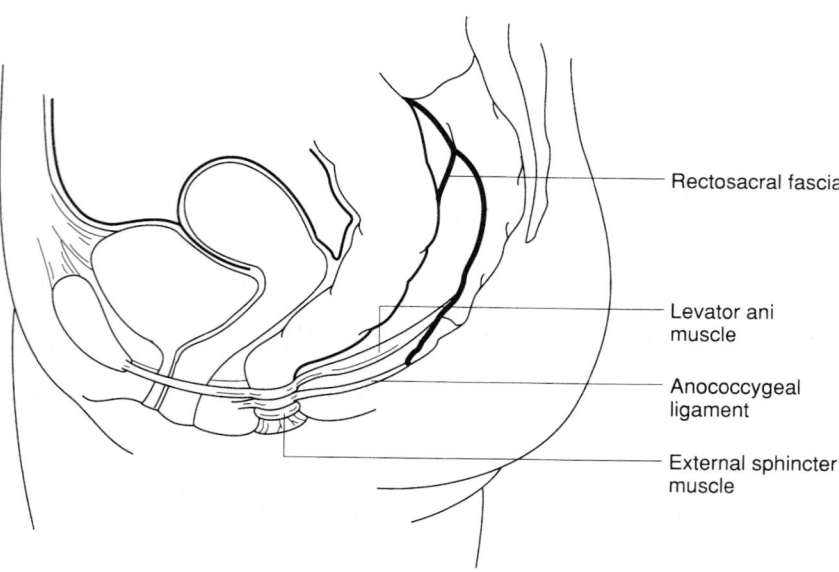

Rectosacral fascia

Levator ani muscle

Anococcygeal ligament

External sphincter muscle

Figure 50.1. Fascial attachments of the rectum.

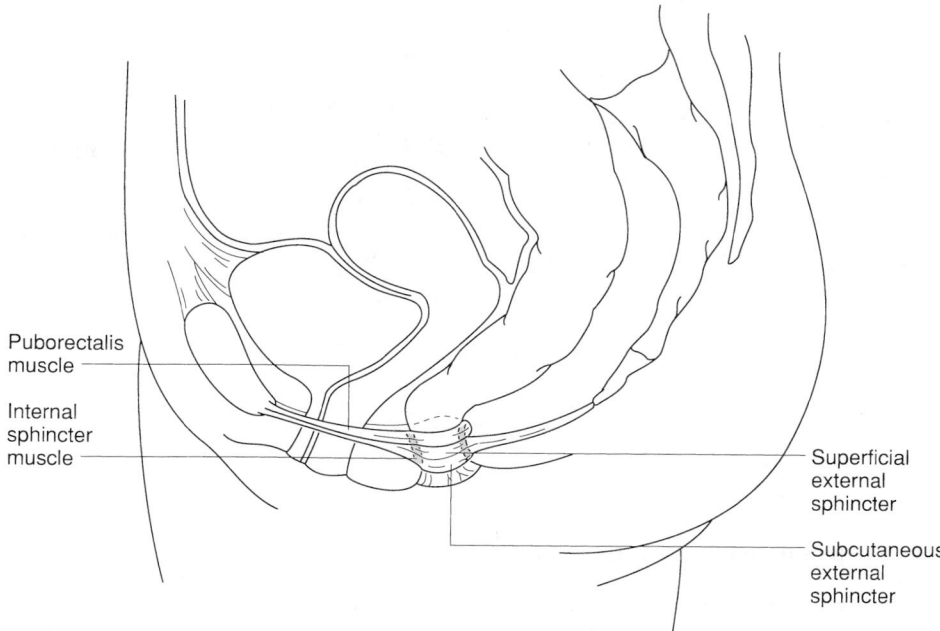

Figure 50.2. Arrangement of the external sphincter muscles.

fibers, which may traverse the lower portion of the distal external sphincter to insert in the perianal skin and cause wrinkling of the anal verge, are referred to as the *corrugator cutis ani*.

At about the midpoint of the anal canal, 2 cm from the anal verge, is an undulating demarcation called the *dentate* or *pectinate line*. Longitudinal folds of the mucosa above the dentate line are known as the *columns of Morgagni*. For a distance of about 1 cm above the dentate line, the epithelial lining may be columnar, transitional, or stratified squamous epithelium; this area is referred to as the *transitional* or *cloacogenic zone*. The area above the transitional zone is lined by columnar epithelium, and the area below the dentate line is lined by squamous epithe-

lium (Fig. 50.3). This is also the area where the internal hemorrhoidal plexus lies.

Pelvic Floor Muscles

The pelvic floor muscles consist of the levator ani and the iliococcygeal muscle. The levator ani is a broad, thin muscle that forms the floor of the pelvic cavity and is innervated by the fourth sacral nerve. This muscle has traditionally been considered to consist of three muscles—iliococcygeal, pubococcygeal, and puborectal. Studies suggest that it consists only of the iliococcygeal and pubococcygeal muscles, and that the puborectal muscle is ac-

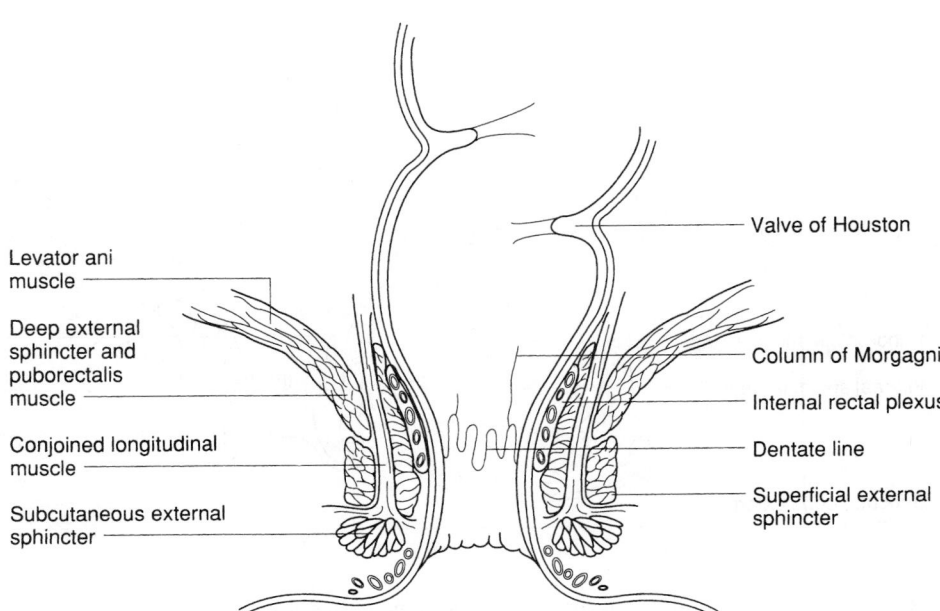

Figure 50.3. Anatomy of the anal canal.

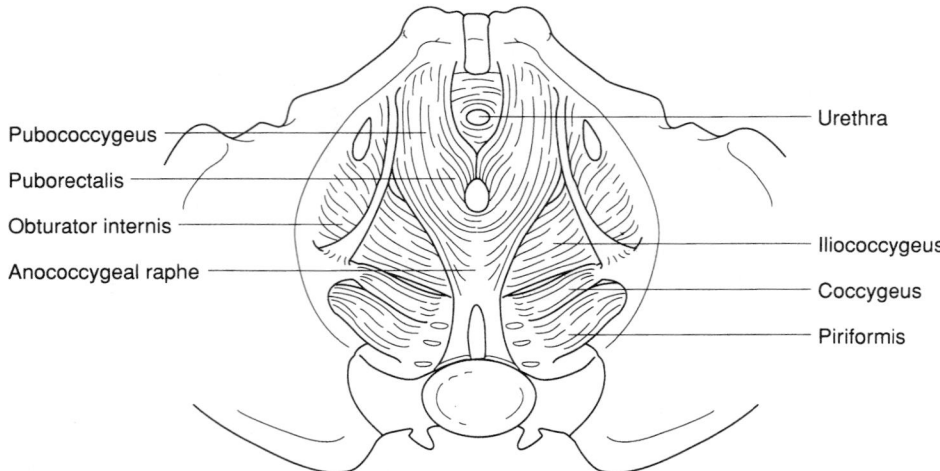

Figure 50.4. Muscles of the pelvic floor.

tually a part of the deep portion of the external sphincter (3,4).

The iliococcygeal muscle arises from the ischial spine and posterior part of the obturator fascia; it passes downward, backward, and medially and inserts on the last two segments of the sacrum and the anococcygeal raphe (Fig. 50.4). The pubococcygeal muscle arises from the anterior half of the obturator fascia and the back of the pubis. The fibers of the pubococcygeal muscle are directed backward, downward, and medially, where they decussate with fibers of the opposite side. The line of decussation is called the *anococcygeal raphe* (Fig. 50.4). Some fibers that lie more posteriorly are attached directly to the tip of the coccyx and the last segment of the sacrum. This muscle also contributes fibers to the conjoined longitudinal muscle. The puborectal and levator ani muscles have reciprocal actions;

as one contracts, the other relaxes. During defecation, puborectal relaxation is accompanied by levator ani contraction, which widens the hiatus and elevates the lower rectum and anal canal. When a person is in an upright position, the levator ani muscle supports the viscera.

Perianal and Perirectal Spaces

Surrounding the anorectum are several potential spaces that are normally filled with areolar tissues or fat. These spaces are clinically important because they are sites where abscesses can form. The perianal space immediately surrounds the anus. Laterally, the perianal space is contiguous with the subcutaneous fat of the buttocks. Medially, it is bound by the anoderm to the level of the dentate line. The ischioanal space is a triangular region below the

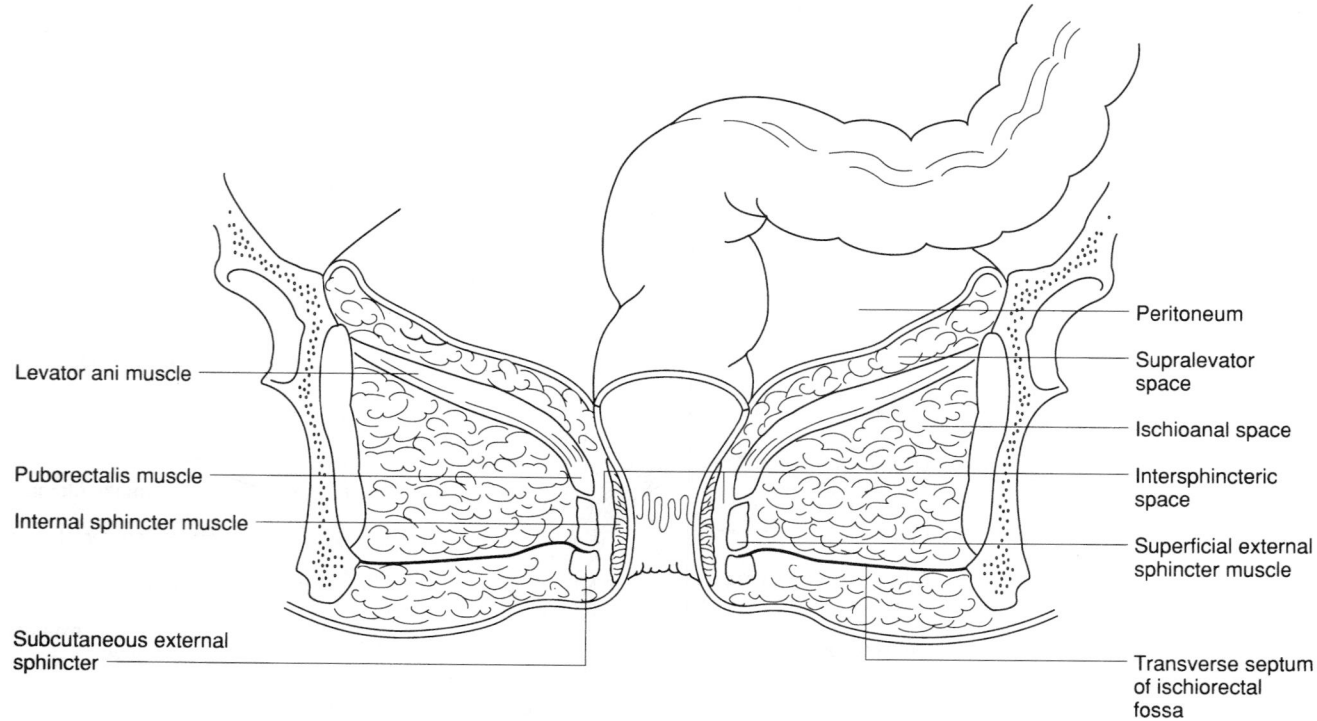

Figure 50.5. Anatomy of the perianorectal spaces (anteroposterior view).

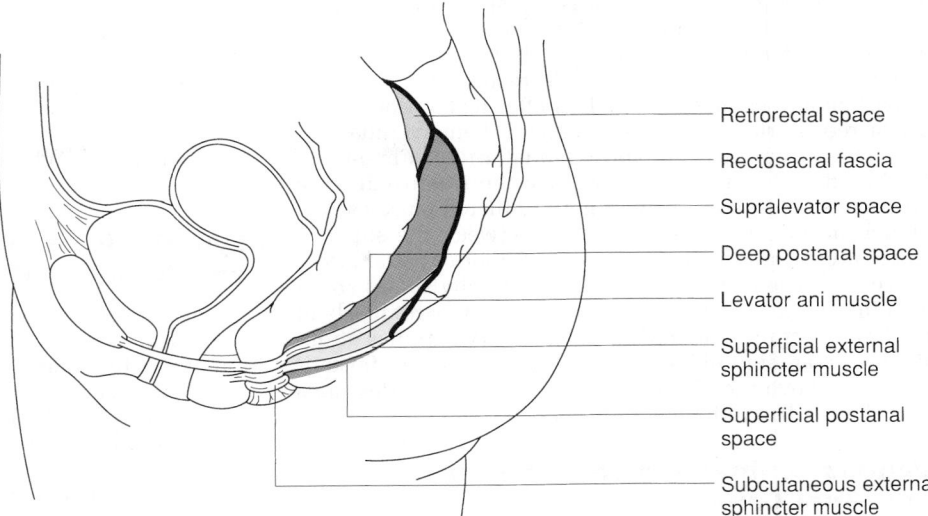

Figure 50.6. Anatomy of the peri-anorectal spaces (lateral view).

Retrorectal space

Rectosacral fascia

Supralevator space

Deep postanal space

Levator ani muscle

Superficial external sphincter muscle

Superficial postanal space

Subcutaneous external sphincter muscle

levator ani muscle, bound medially by the external sphincter muscle, laterally by the ischium, and inferiorly by the transverse septum of the ischiorectal fossa (Fig. 50.5). The ischioanal space on each side is filled with fat and contains the inferior rectal vessels and lymphatics. The deep postanal space connects the ischioanal space on each side posteriorly and lies between the levator ani muscle above and the anococcygeal ligament below (Fig. 50.6). The deep postanal space is an important pathway in the formation of abscess; spread from one ischiorectal fossa to the other may result in a so-called horseshoe abscess. The intersphincteric space lies between the internal and external sphincter muscles. It is continuous with the perianal space below

and extends above into the wall of the rectum. The supralevator spaces are situated on each side of the rectum above the levator ani (Fig. 50.5). The supralevator spaces communicate posteriorly and may allow spread of infection cephalad into the retroperitoneum (Fig. 50.6).

Arterial Supply of the Rectum and Anal Canal

The superior rectal (hemorrhoidal) artery is a continuation of the inferior mesenteric artery; it descends posteriorly to the rectum, where it bifurcates to supply the rectum and upper portion of the anal canal (Fig. 50.7). The middle

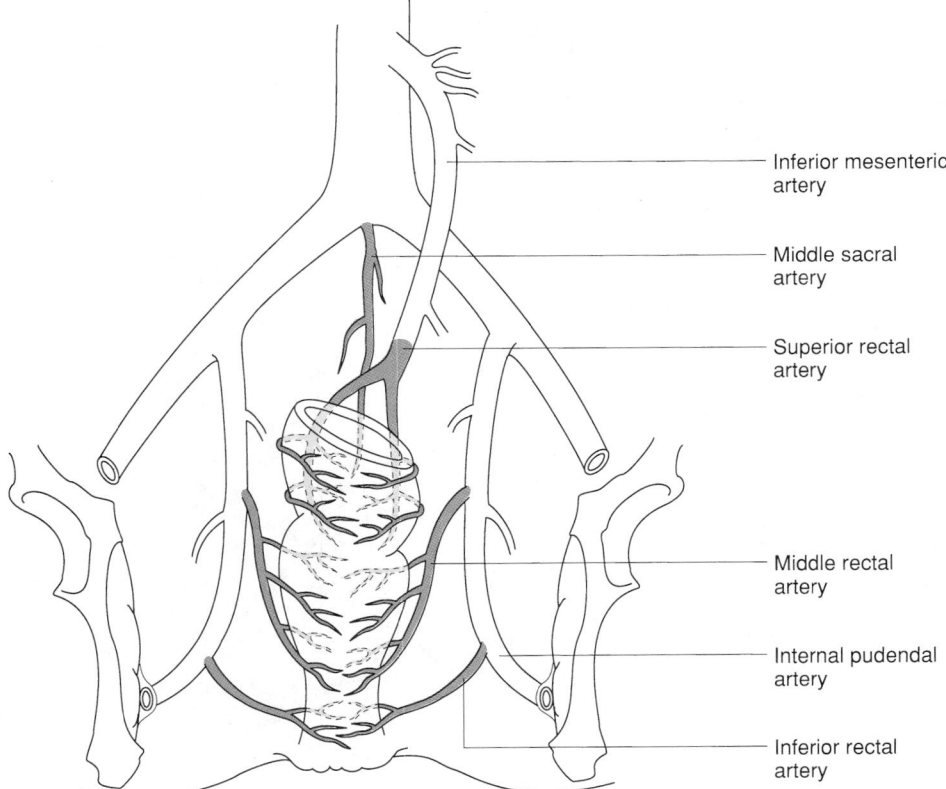

Inferior mesenteric artery

Middle sacral artery

Superior rectal artery

Middle rectal artery

Internal pudendal artery

Inferior rectal artery

Figure 50.7. Arterial supply of the rectum and anal canal.

rectal (hemorrhoidal) arteries arise from the internal iliac artery on each side and enter the lower portion of the rectum anterolaterally at variable points but usually in the lower third of rectum. The middle rectal arteries are inconsistent and cannot be relied on after ligation of the superior rectal artery. The inferior rectal (hemorrhoidal) arteries arise from the internal pudendal artery, a branch of the internal iliac artery, and traverse the ischioanal fossa on each side to supply the anal sphincter muscles. Although no extramural anastomoses between the superior rectal artery, middle rectal artery, and inferior rectal artery are seen on cadaver dissection, arteriography shows abundant intramural anastomoses between them, particularly in the lower rectum. The middle sacral artery supplies an insignificant amount of blood to the rectum. It arises posteriorly, just above the bifurcation of the aorta, and descends over the lumbar vertebrae, sacrum, and coccyx.

Venous Drainage of the Rectum and Anal Canal

Blood returns from the rectum and anal canal through two systems—portal and systemic (Fig. 50.8). The superior rectal (hemorrhoidal) vein drains the rectum and upper part of the anal canal into the portal system through the inferior mesenteric vein. The middle rectal veins drain the lower part of the rectum and upper part of the anal canal; they accompany the middle rectal arteries and terminate in the internal iliac veins. The inferior rectal veins, following the corresponding arteries, drain the lower part of the anal canal by way of the internal pudendal veins, which empty into the internal iliac veins.

Lymphatic Drainage of the Rectum and Anal Canal

Lymph from the upper and middle portions of the rectum ascends along the superior rectal artery and subsequently to the inferior mesenteric lymph nodes. The lower part of the rectum drains cephalad by way of the superior rectal lymphatics to the inferior mesenteric nodes, and laterally by way of the middle rectal lymphatics to the internal iliac nodes (Fig. 50.9). Lymphatics from the anal canal above the dentate line drain cephalad through the superior rectal lymphatics to the inferior mesenteric nodes, and laterally along both middle rectal vessels and inferior rectal vessels through the ischioanal fossa to the internal iliac nodes. Lymph from the anal canal below the dentate line

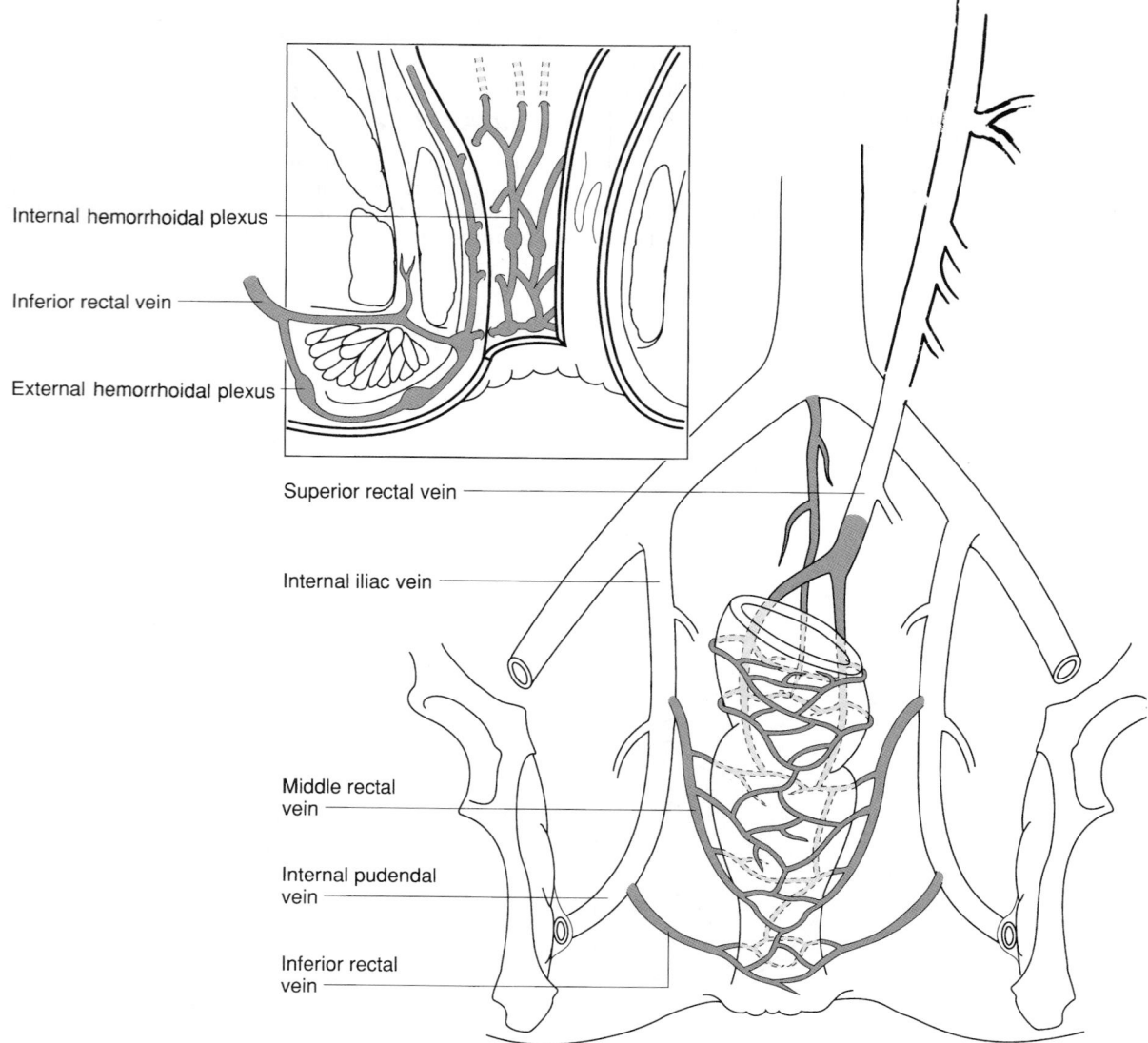

Internal hemorrhoidal plexus

Inferior rectal vein

External hemorrhoidal plexus

Superior rectal vein

Internal iliac vein

Middle rectal vein

Internal pudendal vein

Inferior rectal vein

Figure 50.8. Venous drainage of the rectum and anal canal.

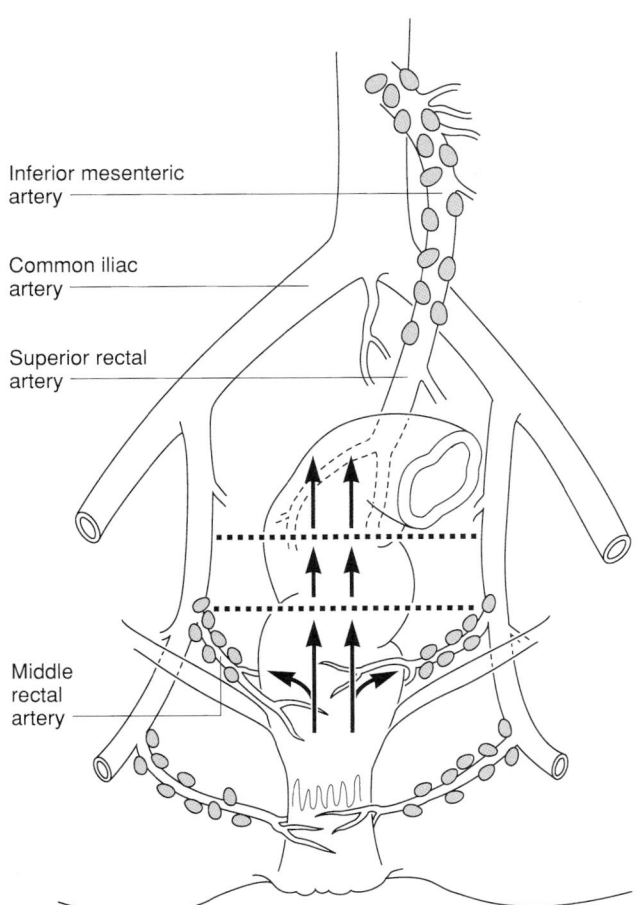

Figure 50.9. Lymphatic drainage of the rectum.

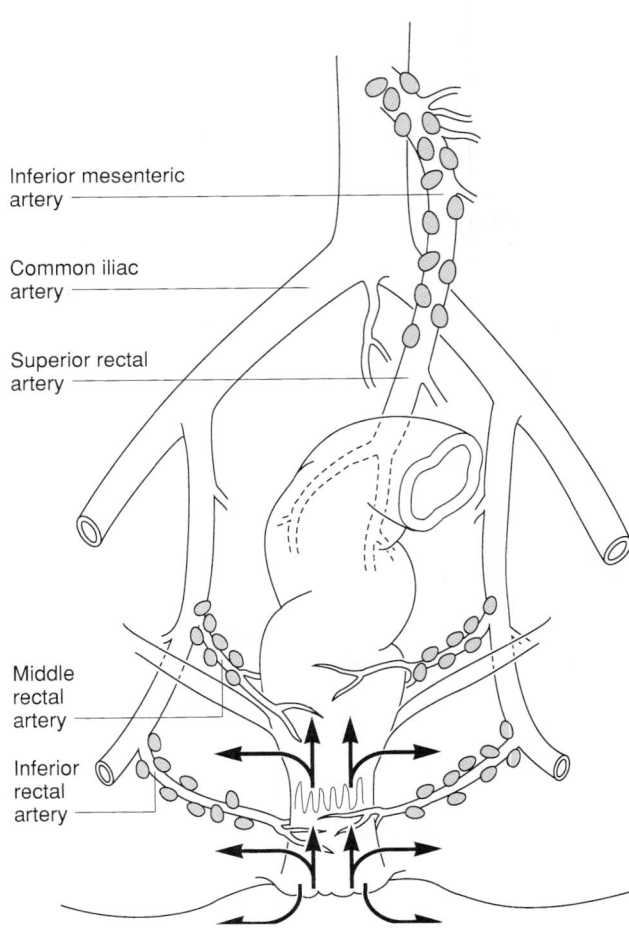

Figure 50.10. Lymphatic drainage of the anal canal.

usually drains to the inguinal nodes, although it can also drain to the superior rectal lymph nodes or along the inferior rectal lymphatics to the ischioanal fossa if the primary drainage is obstructed (Fig. 50.10). Retrograde lymphatic spread of carcinoma of the rectum and anal canal occurs only in cases of extensive involvement of the perirectal structures, serosal surfaces, veins, and perineural lymphatic and proximal lymphatic channels (5).

Nerve Supply of the Rectum and Urogenital Organs

Sympathetic and parasympathetic nerves of the autonomic nervous system supply the anorectum and also send branches to the adjacent urogenital organs. Nerve trunks are close to the rectum and are prone to injury during mobilization of the rectum unless specific precautions are taken.

Sympathetic nerve fibers to the rectum are derived from the first three lumbar segments of the spinal cord. Sympathetic fibers pass through ganglionated sympathetic chains before forming the preaortic plexus. Preaortic fibers extend below the bifurcation of the aorta to form the hypogastric plexus or the presacral nerve (Fig. 50.11). The plexus thus formed divides into left and right branches on each side of the pelvis, where they are joined by the parasympathetic nerves.

The pelvic parasympathetic nerve supply is from the nervi erigentes, which originate from the second, third, and fourth sacral nerve roots. The fibers pass inward and

forward to join the sympathetic nerve fibers and form the pelvic plexus. The pelvic plexus on each side is encased in the midportion of the lateral stalk, which is located just above the levator ani muscle (Fig. 50.11). From each pelvic, both types of nerve fibers are distributed to urinary and genital organs.

In women, the sympathetic nerve fibers from the hypogastric plexus are directed toward the uterosacral ligament close to the rectum. In men, the nerve fibers from the hypogastric plexus pass immediately adjacent to the anterolateral wall of the rectum in the retroperitoneal tissue.

The pelvic plexus gives rise to the periprostatic plexus, an important subdivision that is essential to sexual function in men. The periprostatic plexus distributes fibers to the prostate, seminal vesicles, corpora cavernosa, terminal part of the vas deferens, prostatic and membranous urethra, ejaculatory ducts, and bulbourethral glands. Both parasympathetic and sympathetic nervous systems are involved in erection. Nerve impulses from the parasympathetic nerves, which lead to erection, produce vasodilation and increase blood flow in the cavernous spaces of the penis. Activity of the sympathetic system adds to vascular engorgement and sustained erection. Moreover, sympathetic activity causes contraction of the ejaculatory ducts, seminal vesicles, and prostate, with subsequent expulsion of semen into the posterior urethra. Depending on which nerves have been damaged, deficiencies may include incomplete erection, lack of ejaculation, retrograde ejaculation, or total impotence (6).

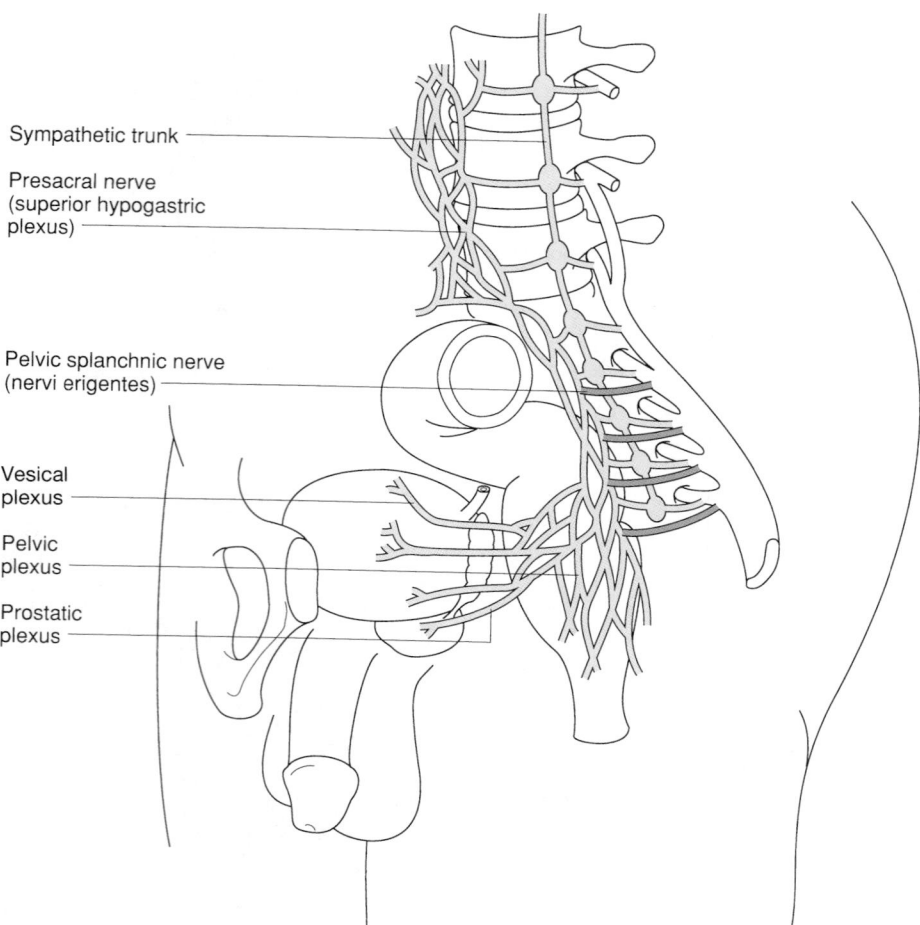

Sympathetic trunk

Presacral nerve
(superior hypogastric
plexus)

Pelvic splanchnic nerve
(nervi erigentes)

Vesical
plexus

Pelvic
plexus

Prostatic
plexus

Figure 50.11. Sympathetic and parasympathetic nerve supply of the rectum.

The following precautions can be exercised during operations on the pelvic colon to avoid nerve injuries:

1. When mobilizing the rectosigmoid colon and upper rectum for nonmalignant disease, dissect close to the bowel wall posteriorly and do not disturb the retroperitoneal tissue, to avoid injury to the hypogastric plexus.
2. Cut the peritoneum on each side close to the rectum and brush off the retroperitoneal tissue laterally to avoid injury to the left and right branches of the hypogastric plexus.
3. Divide the lateral stalks close to the rectum to avoid injury to the nervi erigentes and the pelvic plexus.
4. Note that the bulk of the pelvic plexus is lateral and posterior to the seminal vesicles (7). Separation of the rectum from the seminal vesicle should start at the midline. This is carried laterally to the edge of the seminal vesicle, then curves inferiorly to avoid injury to the neurovascular bundle.

The pudendal nerve arises from the sacral plexus (S-2 to S-4). It leaves the pelvis through the greater sciatic foramen, crosses the ischial spine, and then continues in the pudendal canal toward the ischial tuberosity in the lateral wall of the ischioanal fossa on each side. Three of its important branches are the inferior rectal, perineal, and dorsal nerves of the penis or clitoris. The pudendal nerve is anatomically protected from injury during mobilization of the rectum. Sensory stimuli from the penis and clitoris are mediated by a branch of the pudendal nerve and thus are preserved after proctectomy.

Nerve Supply of the Anal Canal

Motor Innervation

The internal sphincter is supplied by both sympathetic and parasympathetic nerves. The sympathetic and parasympathetic nerves inhibit the internal anal sphincter. The external sphincter is supplied by the inferior rectal branch of the internal pudendal nerve and the perineal branch of the fourth sacral nerve. The levator ani is supplied not only by the pudendal nerve but also by direct branches of the third, fourth, and often the fifth sacral nerves, the fifth lying above the pelvic floor.

Sensory Innervation

The sensory nerve supply of the anal canal comes from the inferior rectal nerve, a branch of the pudendal nerve. The epithelium of the anal canal is profusely innervated with sensory nerve endings, especially in the vicinity of the dentate line. Painful sensations in the anal canal can be felt at sites up to 1.5 cm proximal to the dentate line.

PHYSIOLOGY OF THE ANORECTUM

Sensation of the Anorectum

Complete anal continence cannot be achieved unless the subject can sense the presence of material in the rectum and can discriminate the quality of the substances (feces or gas). The receptors responsible for the appreciation of rectal fullness and impending evacuation lie outside the anorectal wall, probably within the levator ani. The epithelium of the anal canal is rich with sensory nerve endings, and although this sensitive area plays an important role in discriminating between flatus and feces, it is not a critical factor in preserving anal continence. When the anoderm is anesthetized with a topical anesthetic, the ability to differentiate between air and water is impaired, but the continence of rectally infused saline solution is maintained (8).

Mechanism of Anal Continence

Stool can accumulate in the rectum for a variable period of time before the urge to retain defecate is experienced. The ability of the rectum to retain stool is known as *reservoir continence*. Continence is favored by the influence of pelvic muscles on rectal shape. The anal canal is pulled forward by the puborectal muscle, a U-shaped sling, at an angle of 80 to 90 degrees to the rectum. This anorectal angle, maintained by the continuous tonic activity of the puborectal muscle, effectively prevents stool in the rectum from entering the anal canal. Although it has been postulated that the mucosa of the anterior wall of the lower rectum is pressed firmly into the anal canal to create a flap valve effect, recent studies have suggested that continence is maintained by sphincteric action rather than such a valvular mechanism. In the upper part of the anal canal, three submucosal anal cushions are usually present, which may contribute to the mechanism of anal closure and create high pressure in the anal canal.

The internal sphincter, because it is innervated by the autonomic nervous system, is not subject to voluntary control. This powerful muscle exists in a continuously tonic state and is responsible for maintaining closure of the resting anal canal. The high-pressure zone of the anal canal at rest is maintained by the actions of the internal sphincter. The external sphincter contributes to anal pressure only when a bolus of stool is present within the anal canal. The increase in pressure during voluntary contraction (squeeze pressure) is caused exclusively by the activity of the external sphincter. The high resting pressure in the anal canal acts as a barrier to prevent leakage of mucus and gas.

When the rectum is distended, the internal sphincter relaxes (rectoanal reflex). This relaxation allows the rectal contents to move down to the anal canal. In contrast, the external sphincter contracts when the rectum is distended. Reflex contraction of the external sphincter prevents rectal contents from leaking through the anus. A marked distention of the rectum, however, inhibits external sphincter contraction, and the voluntary act of straining also inhibits the external sphincter and pelvic floor muscles. Although volitional contraction of the external sphincter can be sustained only for short periods, it is the most important mechanism of voluntary continence.

Defecation

Defecation, the act of evacuating fecal material from the rectum, is a complex process that involves both a reflex response and voluntary performance. When a fecal bolus enters the rectum, the stretch receptors, believed to reside within the muscles of the pelvic floor, register a sensation and an urge to defecate. Distention of the rectum causes a reflex relaxation of the internal sphincter and contraction of the external sphincter and puborectal muscle, which allow the rectal contents to make contact with the anal canal. This contact allows the sensory epithelium of the anal canal to sense and discriminate the nature of the material. If rectal distention is maintained, the rectal muscu-

lature adapts to decrease the rectal pressure, the accommodation response. The act of defecation proceeds with the subject assuming a squatting or sitting position to straighten out the angle between the rectum and anal canal. Expulsion of feces is accomplished by contraction of the rectum and by the Valsalva maneuver, which increases intraabdominal pressure. After defecation is completed, voluntary sphincters contract actively and the normal postural tone is restored.

HEMORRHOIDS

In the upper anal canal are cushions of submucosal tissue that consist of connective tissue containing venules and smooth-muscle fibers. Usually, three cushions—left lateral, right anterior, and right posterior—are found. This anatomic arrangement is remarkably constant and bears no relation, as previously thought, to the terminal branches of the superior rectal vein. The function of these cushions is to aid in anal continence. During the act of defecation, when they become engorged with blood, they cushion the anal canal and support the anal canal lining. The anal cushions are supported by muscles that arise partly from the internal sphincter and partly from the conjoined longitudinal muscles. *Hemorrhoid* is the pathologic term used to describe the downward displacement of the anal cushion, which causes the contained venules to dilate (9,10). Hence, hemorrhoids develop when the supporting tissues of the anal cushion deteriorate (11).

Classification

External hemorrhoids are dilated venules of the inferior hemorrhoidal plexus located below the dentate line. Thrombosed external hemorrhoids are intravascular clots in the venules of the external hemorrhoids. Internal hemorrhoids are anal cushions located above the dentate line that have become prolapsed. The appearance and symptoms of internal hemorrhoids depend on their severity. For practical purposes, internal hemorrhoids are graded according to the degree of prolapse.

First degree: The anal cushions slide down beyond the dentate line on straining.

Second degree: The anal cushions prolapse through the anus on straining but reduce spontaneously.

Third degree: The anal cushions prolapse through the anus on straining or exertion and require manual replacement into the anal canal.

Fourth degree: The prolapse is not manually reducible.

Clinical Manifestations

The most common complaints of burning, itching, swelling, and pain usually are not caused by hemorrhoids but by pruritus ani, anal abrasion, anal fissure, thrombosed external hemorrhoids, or a prolapsed anal papilla. The most common manifestation of hemorrhoids is painless rectal bleeding of bright red blood that is associated with a bowel movement. A patient with severe hemorrhoids commonly describes the episode of bleeding as blood dripping into the toilet bowl. A feeling of incomplete evacuation is also common. In chronic prolapse, exposed rectal mucosa often causes perianal irritation and mucous staining on the underwear. Congestion of external hemorrhoids or skin tags can cause discomfort or pain. Symptoms are aggravated by constipation and diarrhea.

Examination

The definitive diagnosis of hemorrhoids is made by examination. An enema administered shortly before examination will make a complete inspection easier and more thorough. The examination can be performed in the left lateral or prone jackknife position. Anal skin tags, an external fistula opening, perianal excoriation from anal discharge, and anal fissure can be easily detected. The best and most accurate method of diagnosis of hemorrhoids is to ask the patient to sit and strain on the toilet and watch for the prolapse.

Internal hemorrhoids cannot be palpated. Digital examination may detect anal stenosis or an anal scar. The anal sphincter tone and sphincter squeeze can be subjectively evaluated. A mass in the anal canal can be detected, and prostatic hypertrophy can be diagnosed in male patients.

Anoscopy is the ideal method to examine the anal canal. For patients in the prone jackknife position, the table should not be tilted during the examination. The patient is asked to strain to estimate the degree of prolapse of the hemorrhoids. During anoscopy, one must exclude a coexisting anal fissure or fistula. Proctoscopy or flexible sigmoidoscopy should be performed in all cases to rule out coexisting rectal abnormalities, particularly carcinoma and inflammatory bowel disease, both of which can cause symptoms similar to those of hemorrhoidal complaints. In young patients, if the rectal bleeding is obviously from the hemorrhoids, a complete colonic examination is not indicated. In patients older than 50 years, particularly those with a family history of cancer, a complete colonoscopy or barium enema should be performed.

Treatment

According to modern concepts, the prolapse of anal cushions is initiated by the shearing effect of the passage of a large, hard stool or by the precipitous act of defecation, as in urgent diarrhea. If prolapse of the vascular cushions can be prevented or if the congestive effect of a tight anal canal can be abolished, the anal cushions return to their normal state and symptoms are relieved without removal of the cushions themselves. Therefore, the rationale of adding bulk to the diet is to eliminate straining at defecation. A high-fiber diet usually reduces symptoms of

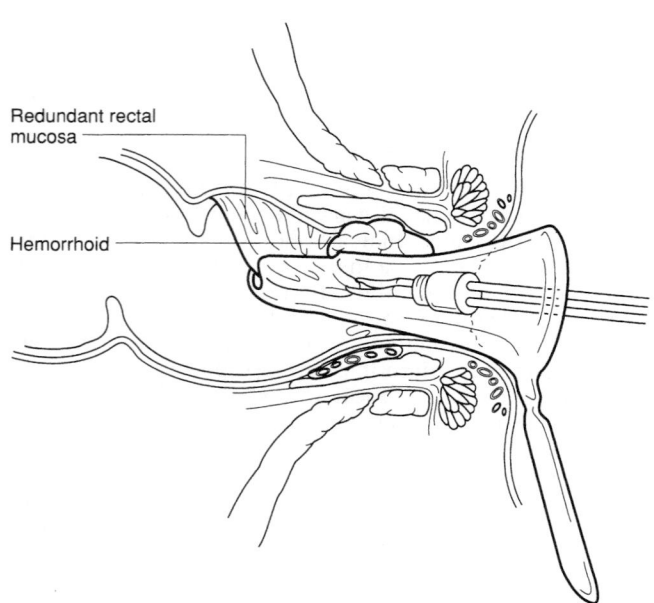

Figure 50.12. Rubber band ligation of an internal hemorrhoid.

hemorrhoids and is ideal for patients with first- and second-degree hemorrhoids.

Rubber Band Ligation

Rubber band ligation is suitable for patients with second-degree and first-degree hemorrhoids whose condition does not respond to bulk-forming agents, and it is suitable for patients with third-degree hemorrhoids in some cases. The procedure may be performed in the office after the patient has been prepared with an enema. Aspirin, nonsteroidal antiinflammatory drugs, and anticoagulants should be discontinued at least 1 week before and for 2 weeks after the procedure, which is performed through an anoscope. The band should be placed on the rectal mucosa just above the internal hemorrhoid (Fig. 50.12). Usually, one hemorrhoid is ligated per session, with additional ligation performed 4 to 6 weeks later; however, ligation of two or three hemorrhoids at one session has been practiced with good results.

Rubber band ligation is not painless. The patient should be warned of anal discomfort or even pain, usually from anal sphincter spasm. Warm sitz baths reduce the pain, and an appropriate analgesic should be prescribed. Patients should increase the amount of fruits and vegetables in their diet or take a bulk-forming agent with plenty of water for at least 6 to 8 weeks. Immediate severe or progressive pain is an indication of misplaced rubber band ligation, too close to the dentate line, and requires immediate removal of the rubber band. The safety of rubber band ligation has been a matter of concern because deaths from acute perianal sepsis have been reported. Symptoms of delayed anal pain, urinary retention, and fever are clues to the development of perianal infection. Prompt and aggressive treatment should include antibiotics, drainage of abscesses, and excision of necrotic tissues. Severe infection after rubber band ligation is rare. Because of these potentially severe complications, rubber band ligation should not be performed in patients with immune deficiencies.

Infrared Photocoagulation

Infrared photocoagulation coagulates tissue protein or evaporates water in the cells, depending on the intensity and duration of the application. An infrared probe is applied just proximal to the internal hemorrhoids through an anoscope. The results of infrared photocoagulation in first- and second-degree hemorrhoids are comparable with those of rubber band ligation. Pain and complications occur infrequently. A regular electrocautery unit with a flat or ball tip works as well or even better. For the treatment to be effective, it is essential to coagulate the submucosa at the top of the internal hemorrhoids.

Hemorrhoidectomy

Hemorrhoidectomy should be considered when hemorrhoids are severely prolapsed through the anus, requiring manual replacement, or when they are complicated by associated pathology, such as ulceration, fissures, fistulae, hypertrophic anal papilla, or extensive skin tags. In most cases, hemorrhoidectomy can be performed under local anesthesia with mild sedation. For muscular or obese patients, general or regional block anesthesia may be preferable. The procedure is performed with the patient in the prone jackknife position. The cheeks of the buttocks are taped apart. An elliptic excision starts at the perianal skin, includes external and internal hemorrhoids, and ends at the anorectal ring. The mucosa and submucosa are dissected off the underlying internal

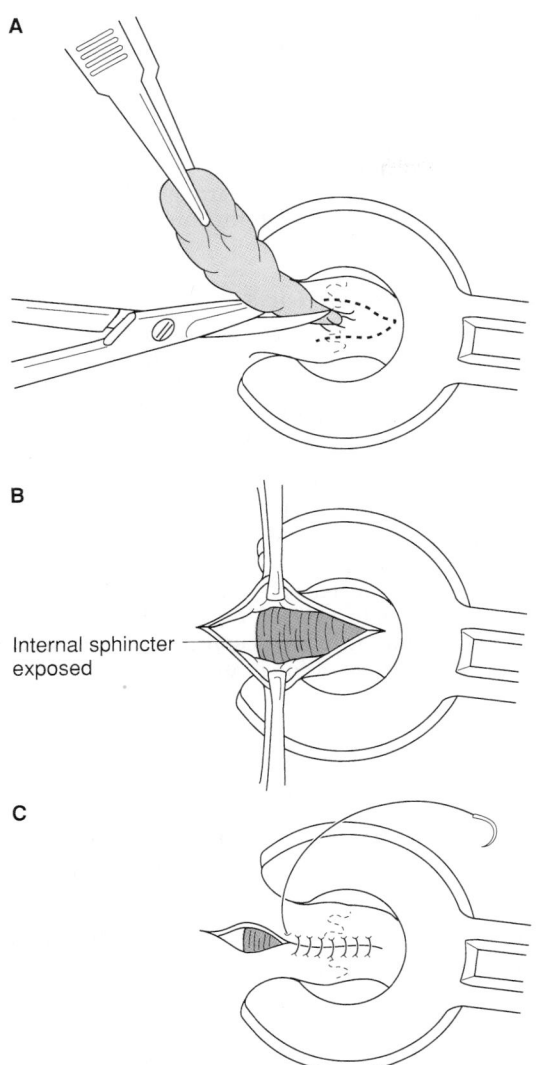

Figure 50.13. Technique of intraanal closed hemorrhoidectomy. *(A)* Exposure of hemorrhoid with elliptic excision started at the perianal skin and extended to the anorectal ring. *(B)* Submucosal hemorrhoidal plexus dissected from the internal sphincter, anoderm, and mucosa. *(C)* Wound closed with a running suture.

sphincter muscle (Fig. 50.13). Unless an associated anal stenosis or chronic anal fissure is present, internal sphincterotomy is not performed. The entire wound is closed with running absorbable sutures, preferably with 3-0 chromic catgut. The largest and most redundant hemorrhoid should be excised first. No packing is placed in the anal canal.

Urinary retention is a common complication of hemorrhoidectomy unless intravenous fluids are restricted during the procedure and minimized for the next 6 to 8 hours (12). Warm sitz baths are started the next morning, as is bran or psyllium seed. A mild laxative is given the following night. Laser hemorrhoidectomy not only adds to the cost but also provides no advantage over conventional hemorrhoidectomy (13).

Management of Special Situations

Thrombosed External Hemorrhoids. Thrombosis is a fairly common complication of hemorrhoidal disease. Most patients give no history of straining or physical ex-

ertion and do not have a history of hemorrhoidal disease. The complication develops as an abrupt onset of anal mass and pain that peaks within 48 hours. Usually, the pain becomes minimal after the fourth day. Occasionally, the skin overlying the hematoma becomes necrotic and causes bleeding and discharge or infection, which in turn causes further necrosis and more pain. Treatment should be aimed at relief of severe pain, prevention of recurrent clot, and prevention of residual skin tags. If the patient is examined during an episode of severe pain, the clot should be excised. Conversely, if the pain is already subsiding and the clot is starting to shrink, thrombosis may be managed conservatively with warm sitz baths for comfort, proper anal hygiene, and bulk-producing agents such as bran or psyllium seed. The entire clot must be removed if operation is chosen. The procedure can often be performed with local anesthesia, and the wound can be left open without packing. Relief of pain is usually immediate. Postoperative care is simple and is aimed at keeping the wound clean with warm sitz baths and washing. An analgesic drug may be required during the first 24 hours.

Strangulated Hemorrhoids. Strangulation results from prolapsed third- or fourth-degree hemorrhoids that have become irreducible. History reveals a long-standing hemorrhoidal prolapse on straining. On examination, one may observe marked edema of both external and internal hemorrhoids everting through the anus. Untreated, strangulation may progress to ulceration and necrosis. Pain is usually severe and urinary retention is common. Proper treatment requires an urgent or emergent hemorrhoidectomy. The operation should be performed in the operating room or ambulatory surgical center and can usually be carried out under local anesthesia. Antibiotics are not indicated. The wound can be closed as in other hemorrhoidectomy procedures.

Postpartum Hemorrhoids. This condition can occur as the result of prolonged labor. The patient may or may not have had previous problems with hemorrhoids. The problem may manifest as thrombosed external and internal hemorrhoids or strangulated hemorrhoids. The treatment should be directed accordingly. If an excision or a hemorrhoidectomy is indicated, one should not hesitate to operate because complications and healing are the same as in other patients.

Acute Hemorrhoidal Bleeding Resulting from Portal Hypertension. Despite the communication between the systemic and portal systems in the anal canal, the incidence of hemorrhoidal disease in patients with portal hypertension is no greater than that in the normal population. Although uncommon, massive bleeding from hemorrhoids in patients with portal hypertension can be life-threatening. Anoscopic examination is essential to identify the site of bleeding; proctoscopy or flexible sigmoidoscopy may miss the point of bleeding entirely.

Suture of the site of bleeding must incorporate the mucosa, submucosa, and internal sphincter. It is essential to correct any coexisting coagulopathy. Hemorrhoidectomy should be reserved for the rare situation in which the stick-tie method fails to control the bleeding.

Hemorrhoids in Inflammatory Bowel Disease. Hemorrhoidal problems in inflammatory bowel disease are uncommon. Most anal problems are the result of diarrhea, which causes perianal irritation and swelling, rather than of hemorrhoids themselves. The treatment is anal hygiene and symptomatic relief of pain. Hemorrhoidectomy can be safely performed in patients with ulcerative colitis. However, in patients with Crohn's disease, it should be avoided because problems with unhealed wounds are frequent.

RECTAL PROLAPSE

Prolapse of the rectum (procidentia) is an uncommon condition in which the full thickness of the rectal wall turns inside out, into or through the anal canal. Typically, the extruded rectum is seen as concentric rings of mucosa.

Pathophysiology

Although the cause of rectal prolapse is poorly understood, the disorder is best considered a form of intussusception. The intussusception usually starts in the lower rectum anteriorly, at a level about 8 cm from the anal verge, although the starting point may be at the rectosigmoid junction. Although childbearing has been proposed to cause prolapse, about half of patients with prolapse are men or nulliparous women. Many patients with rectal prolapse have a clear history of straining associated with intractable constipation, and some have had chronic diarrhea. A high incidence of rectal prolapse has been noted in patients affected by mental retardation.

Studies of anorectal function and defecation dynamics in patients with rectal prolapse have revealed impaired resting and voluntary sphincter activity, decreased functional rectal capacity, and impaired continence. A failure of normal relaxation of the external sphincter and pelvic floor musculature during defecation attempts is also characteristic.

Anatomic Abnormalities

Prolapse of the rectum predominates in female patients, with a female-to-male ratio of 5:1 or 6:1. Several anatomic defects or abnormalities are consistently demonstrated in patients with chronic rectal prolapse:

Abnormally deep rectovaginal or rectovesical pouch
Lax and atonic musculature of the pelvic floor
Lack of normal fixation of the rectum and an elongated mesorectum
Redundant sigmoid colon
Lax and atonic anal sphincter

These defects are most likely the consequence of long-standing prolapse rather than the cause.

Classification

Rectal prolapse is classified in the following manner (14):

Incomplete (partial): prolapse of the rectal mucosa only
Complete: prolapse involving all layers
Grade 1: occult prolapse
Grade 2: prolapse to, but not through, the anus
Grade 3: protrusion through the anus for a variable distance

Clinical Manifestations

One of the early symptoms of rectal prolapse is anorectal discomfort during defecation. Difficulty in initiating bowel movements and the feeling of incomplete evacuation are common. Some patients require digital evacuation of the stool in the rectum. In many patients, the prolapse causes obstruction that leads to chronic constipation. In an overt prolapse, initially the protrusion occurs only during or after defecation. As the problem becomes more pronounced, the protrusion may be precipitated by coughing, exertion, or walking. In patients with grade 1 (occult) and grade 2 prolapse, perineal pressure, difficult with defecation, and incomplete evacuation may be the only complaints. Fecal and urinary incontinence are associated symptoms in prolapse of long duration.

Diagnosis

Rectal prolapse is easy to diagnose if the prolapse has protruded through the anus. Typically, the protrusion has circumferential mucosal folds. When the prolapse remains in the rectum or anal canal (occult prolapse), the diagnosis is difficult. Redness of the rectal mucosa, especially anteriorly at 7 to 10 cm from the anal verge, provides a clue. In grade 2 prolapse, in which the protrusion extends to but not through the anus, the rectal prolapse is often confused with prolapsed hemorrhoids.

Evaluation

Although not useful for the diagnosis of rectal prolapse, colonoscopy is indicated in certain patients to rule

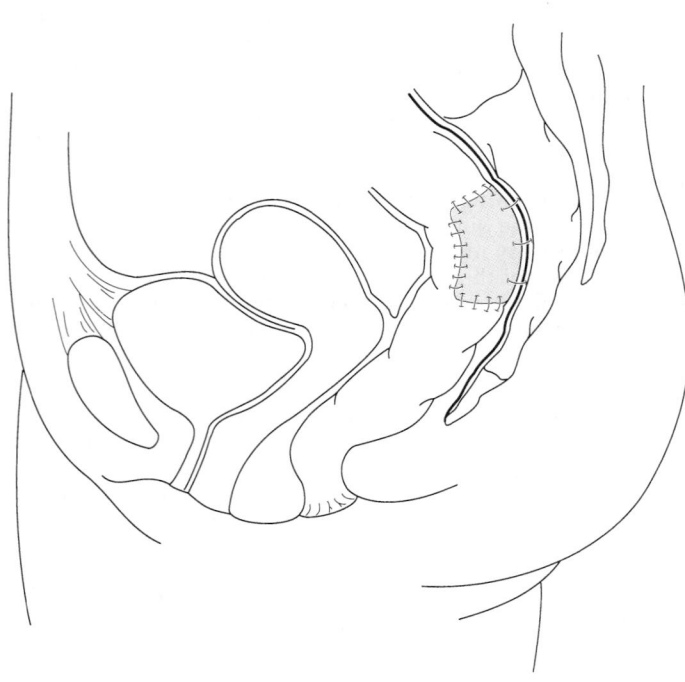

Figure 50.14. Marlex or Teflon mesh is sutured to the presacral fascia, then wrapped around the rectum posteriorly to three fourths of the circumference.

out an associated lesion, particularly in patients who have family history of colorectal cancer. Barium enema should be avoided because it may cause straining and strangulation. Anal manometry is helpful for the evaluation of patients with incontinence and for follow-up of anal sphincteric function after the repair. Manometry does not help to predict the outcome of surgery and therefore is not an essential part of the work-up. A defecating proctogram is useful to confirm the diagnosis of grade 1 and grade 2 rectal prolapse if an intussusception can be demonstrated.

Complications

Complications of rectal prolapse are rare. Ulceration from chronic trauma to the prolapsed rectum is frequent but rarely severe. Strangulation is uncommon. Spontaneous rupture of the prolapsed rectum with evisceration of small bowel through the anus is even more rare.

Treatment

The modern concept of repair of rectal prolapse involves removal of the intussusception and the application of measures to prevent intussusception from recurring. Most methods of repair are carried out by the transabdominal approach, although in most elderly or unfit patients a transperineal approach is more appropriate.

The rectal sling operation, a method introduced by Ripstein, is the technique used most often for rectal prolapse in the United States. The operation consists of the construction of a sling of Teflon or Marlex that wraps the fully mobilized rectum anteriorly and attaches to the presacral fascia.

The anterior rectal wrap was plagued with problems of defecation and obstruction. Ripstein later abandoned this technique and changed to posterior wrap (15), the technique described by Wells in 1959 (15a) (Fig. 50.14). Although mechanical rectal obstruction has been elimi-

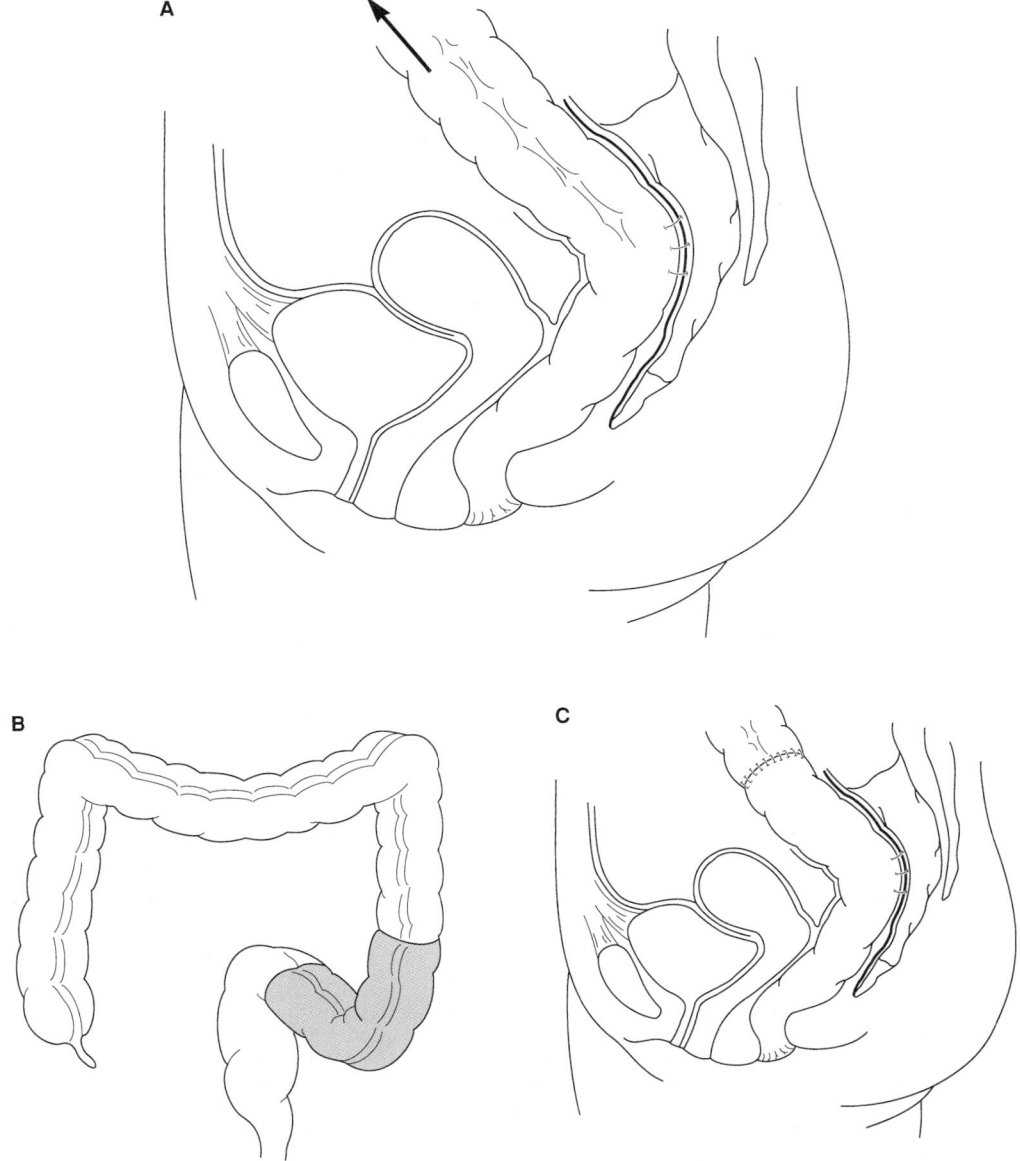

Figure 50.15. Transabdominal proctopexy. *(A)* After full mobilization of the rectum, the endorectal fascia and peritoneum on each side are sutured to the presacral fascia below the promontory of the sacrum. *(B)* Resection of redundant rectosigmoid colon. *(C)* Completed colonic anastomosis.

nated, the problems with defecation and constipation continue (16).

Transabdominal rectosigmoid resection with suture rectopexy is a composite surgical procedure in which the rectum is fully mobilized to the level of the pelvic floor musculature. The redundant sigmoid and the rectum are resected with primary anastomosis. The endorectal tissue and peritoneum on each side of the midrectum are then sutured to the presacral fascia (Fig. 50.15). The recurrence rate has been reported to be 6% to 9% with up to 10 years of follow-up (17,18). Transabdominal rectosigmoid resection with suture rectopexy has become the preferred choice among the abdominal approaches. Like mesh wrap, suture rectopexy is associated with significant problems of defecation and constipation, which occur in about 50% of cases (18,19).

Perineal rectosigmoidectomy is a transperineal approach in which the prolapsed rectum and redundant sig-moid colon are excised endorectally. The prolapse must protrude at least 3 cm through the anus. The operation is performed with the patient in the lithotomy (Fig. 50.16) or prone jackknife position. The operation is well tolerated, and postoperative pain is minimal. Several recent series report a recurrence rate of about 10% with a relatively short-term follow-up (18,20,21). Perineal rectosigmoidectomy is an excellent choice for patients with a prolapse extruded at least 3 cm, particularly elderly patients. In patients with severe fecal incontinence, an anal sphincteroplasty and levatoroplasty can be performed simultaneously without an additional incision (21).

The modified Delorme procedure is another transperineal approach. This technique is used for rectal prolapse that comes down to but not through the anus, or for overt prolapse that protrudes less than 3 cm through the anus. The procedure is conducted with the patient in the prone jackknife position. The submucosa from the dentate line is

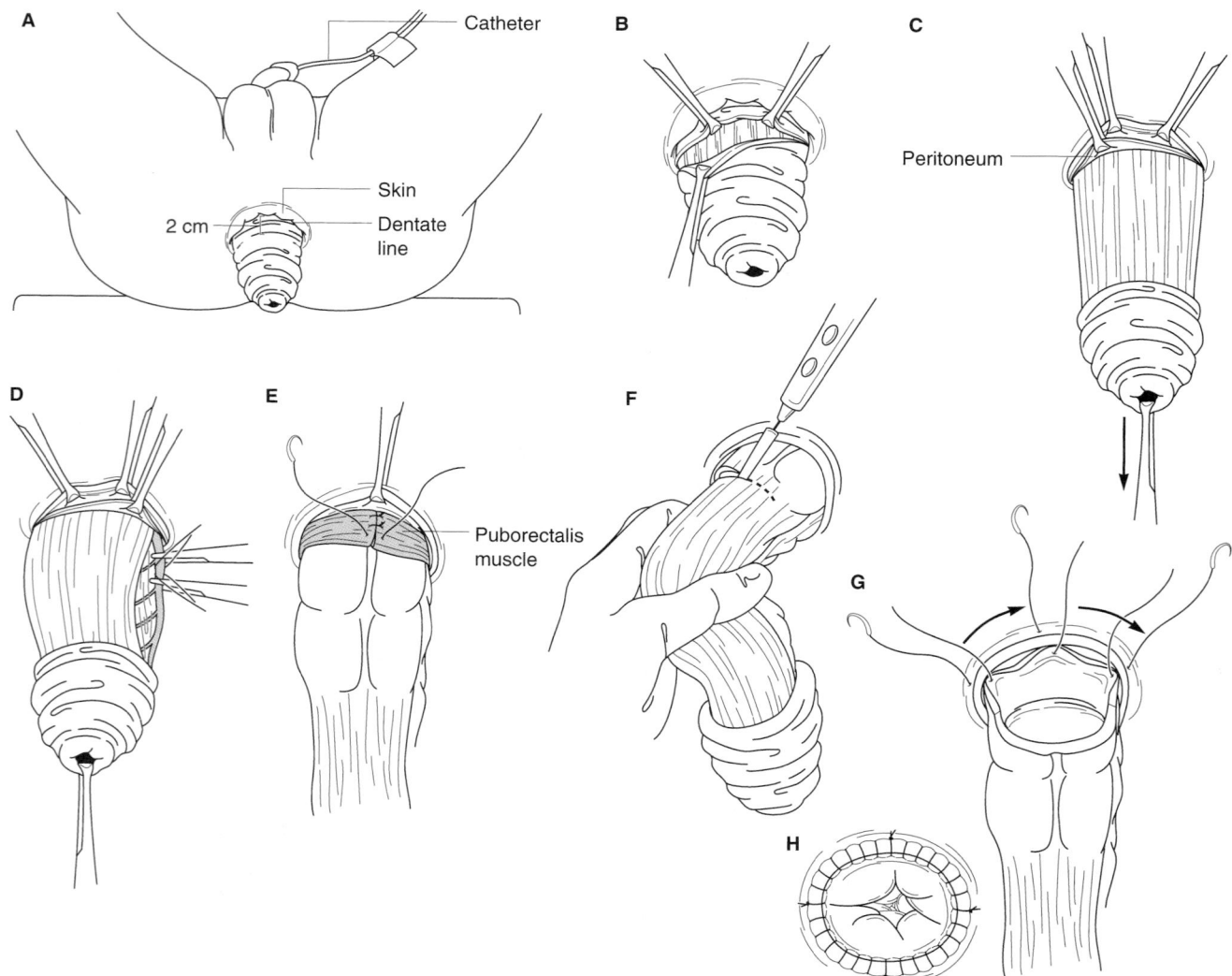

Figure 50.16. Perineal rectosigmoidectomy. The patient is placed in the lithotomy position with both legs in gynecologic stirrups. *(A,B)* A circular incision is made on the prolapsed rectum 2 cm proximal to the dentate line. *(C)* Dissection of the peritoneal attachment from the anterior rectal wall creates an opening into the peritoneal cavity. *(D)* The mesorectum or mesosigmoid is clamped and divided laterally and posteriorly. *(E)* The previously opened peritoneum is sutured to the anterior wall of the rectum or sigmoid colon as high as possible. This is followed by approximation of the puborectalis (optional). *(F)* The anterior wall of the protruding rectum is cut 1 cm distal to the anal verge. *(G)* Stay sutures of 3-0 synthetic absorbable material are placed in four quadrants. *(H)* Anastomosis with running stitches.

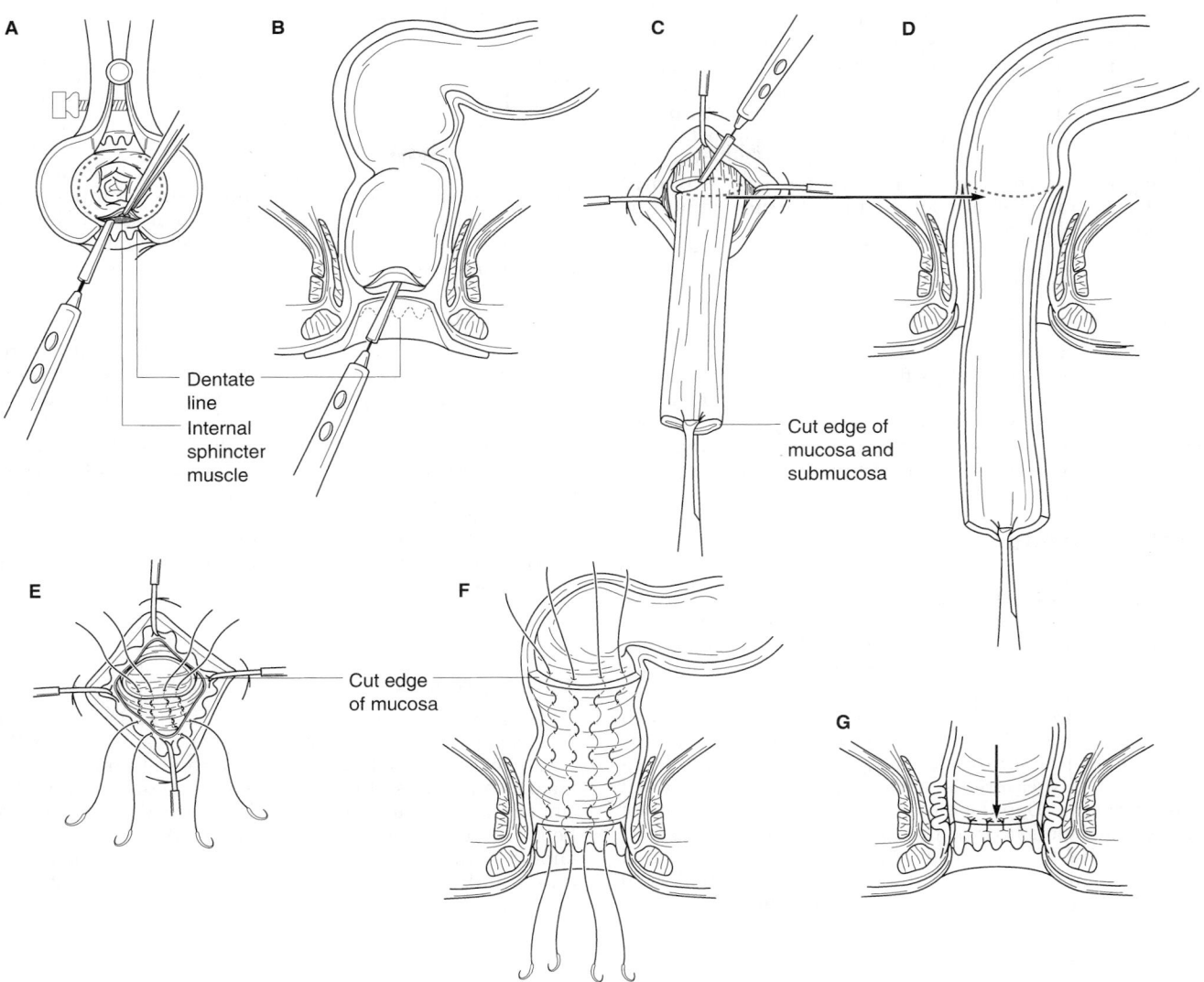

Figure 50.17. Modified Delorme procedure. The patient is placed in the prone position. *(A,B)* With a Pratt speculum used for exposure, a circumferential incision is made 1 cm proximal to the dentate line. The submucosa is dissected from the underlying internal sphincter. At the level of the anorectal ring, the Pratt speculum is replaced by Gelpi retractors placed at a right angle to the dentate line. *(C,D)* Proximal to the anorectal ring, the dissection continues in the submucosal plane until it resists being pulled down. The submucosal tube is then cut. *(E,F)* With 3-0 synthetic absorbable sutures, the mucosa–submucosa at the upper cut end is brought down to the mucosa–submucosa at the lower cut end; the denuded anorectal wall is taken along. Eight such sutures are placed all around. *(G)* At completion of the anastomosis, the anorectum is plicated.

stripped circumferentially with the use of electrocautery. This is continued proximally until it is taut. At this point, the submucosal tube is transected. The proximal cut end is then brought down and anastomosed to the dentate line. The denuded rectal wall is incorporated into the stitches to eliminate the dead space (Fig. 50.17). Like perineal rectosigmoidectomy, it is well tolerated by patients and causes little postoperative pain. The recurrence rate is about 10% at 3 years of follow-up (22,23).

The surgeon must tailor the operation to fit the patient. Abdominal rectopexy with or without resection is a major operation associated with potentially higher morbidity and mortality, but the recurrence rate is low. Perineal approaches (perineal rectosigmoidectomy and Delorme procedure) provide the benefits of less morbidity, less pain, and a shorter hospital stay, but recurrence rates are ultimately much higher. The perineal approach has appeal as

a lesser procedure for elderly patients or patients who are high surgical risks. For younger patients, the benefits of the perineal approach, as a lesser procedure, must be weighed against the disadvantage of a higher recurrence rate (18).

Laparoscopically assisted resection rectopexy has been shown to be feasible and safe, with acceptable short-term recurrence rates and functional results. Intestinal function returns rapidly, so that an early discharge from the hospital is possible (24). This approach should be limited to a small group of surgeons who are properly trained. The long-term results are not yet available.

Incontinence in Rectal Prolapse

By the time rectal prolapse is diagnosed, half of the patients already are anally incontinent. Loss of continence is not caused solely by prolonged protrusion and mechanical stretching of the sphincter. Incontinence in rectal prolapse is also caused by damage to the pudendal nerve that supplies the sphincter muscles, probably as a result of prolonged stretching (25). In about 50% of patients with fecal incontinence resulting from rectal prolapse, the condition improves after repair of the prolapse. Because the return of continence takes as long as 6 to 12 months, operative treatment for incontinence should be postponed for a year.

ANAL FISSURE

Definition

Anal fissure is an ulcer in the lower portion of the anal canal. Fissures can be classified as acute or chronic and further subdivided as primary or secondary. A primary fissure is not associated with other local or systemic disease. Secondary fissure develops in association with other systemic diseases, such as Crohn's disease, leukemia, aplastic anemia, or agranulocytosis.

Pathophysiology

Most tears of the anal canal can be traced to the passage of a large, hard stool or explosive diarrhea, trauma to the anus, or tearing during vaginal delivery. In men, almost all fissures are located in the posterior midline, whereas 10% of fissures in women are in the anterior midline. Numerous studies on anal sphincteric function reveal that the resting anal pressure (internal sphincter) in patients with anal fissure is significantly higher than normal, whereas the squeeze pressure (external sphincter) is normal. Increased anal pressure is caused by increased internal sphincter tone. Doppler flowmetry shows a lower rate of anodermal blood flow at the fissure site, which suggests that unhealed fissure is caused by ischemia. Reduction of anal pressure by sphincterotomy improves anodermal blood flow and results in fissure healing (26).

Clinical Manifestations

Anal pain, particularly during and after bowel movement, is the most prominent symptom. The pain is described as burning, throbbing, or dull aching. In acute anal fissure, the pain can be severe and incapacitating and may last for many hours. If fever is present, fissure may mimic an anorectal abscess, especially intersphincteric abscess. Bleeding is common and, as a rule, stains the toilet paper during wiping. Constipation is a common association because the pain may make patients reluctant to have a bowel movement.

Diagnosis

Although pain and bleeding are typical of anal fissure, the diagnosis is confirmed by examination. Inspection of the anus by gently spreading the buttocks reveals the fissure in most cases. On digital examination, the fissure can be appreciated as a small fibrotic defect. Digital examination can also detect tightness of the anal canal, another clue indicating an anal fissure. A small anoscope is useful to visualize the fissure. Proctoscopy or flexible sigmoidoscopy should be performed to exclude any associated abnormalities of the anal canal and rectum, especially inflammatory bowel disease. Occasionally, the examination must be performed under general anesthesia because of severe pain.

Management

The initial treatment of acute anal fissure is pain relief, with proper anal hygiene and warm sitz baths to relax the anal canal. Of equal importance are bulk-forming agents, such as bran or psyllium seed, to relieve constipation. Application of a topical anesthetic jelly directly to the fissure before a bowel movement is helpful. Acute anal fissure should heal within 6 weeks. Surgery is not usually required unless the fissure is an exacerbation of a chronic anal fissure.

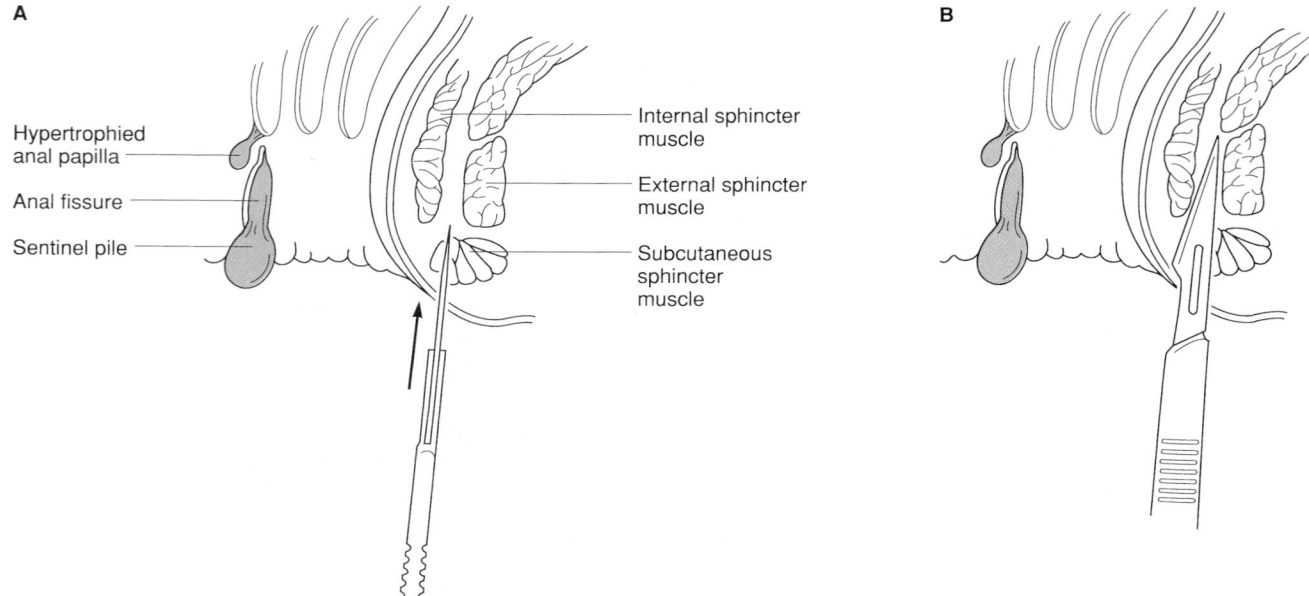

Figure 50.18. Lateral internal sphincterotomy (closed technique). *(A)* Triad of fissure, sentinel pile, and hypertrophic anal papilla. With an anal speculum used for exposure of the lateral quadrant, a No. 11 scalpel blade stabs into the subcutaneous tissue from the anal verge to the dentate line, with the knife in the horizontal position. *(B)* The knife is turned 90 degrees and the internal sphincter muscle is cut while the anal canal is stretched open.

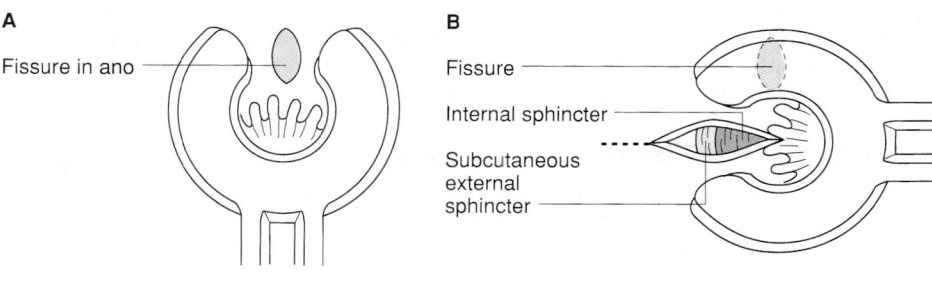

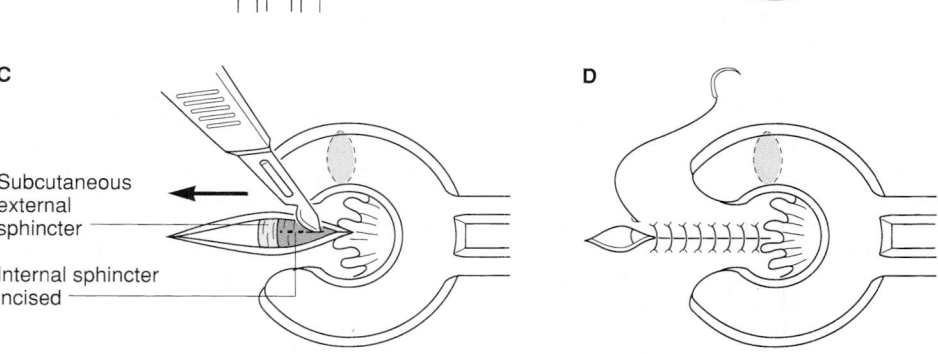

Figure 50.19. Lateral internal sphincterotomy (open method). *(A)* The fissure in the midline is left alone. *(B)* With a speculum used to expose the left lateral quadrant, an incision is made through the subcutaneous tissue to expose both the subcutaneous external sphincter and the internal sphincter. *(C)* The internal sphincter is incised to its full thickness; care is taken not to cut the external sphincter. *(D)* The wound is closed.

Chronic anal fissure is usually deep, exposing the internal anal sphincter. Occasionally, chronic anal fissure consists of a triad of fissure, sentinel skin tag, and hypertrophic anal papilla. The sentinel tag is the fibrotic or edematous skin adjacent to the fissure. A relatively new conservative treatment for chronic anal fissure is the application of 0.2% to 0.3% nitroglycerin paste directly to the anal fissure twice a day. Nitroglycerin reduces the anal resting pressure and increases the anodermal blood flow. Patients should be warned about headache. In about 50% of patients, the fissure is healed at 6 weeks (27). Long-term results with this medication are not available.

Lateral internal sphincterotomy has become the treatment of choice for the unhealed chronic anal fissure (28). The procedure can be performed under local, regional, or general anesthesia. Most patients can return home on the day of surgery.

In the closed method, the left or right lateral quadrant of the anal canal is exposed with an anal speculum. The speculum is gently and gradually opened maximally. The stretched internal sphincter can be easily felt, like a bow string. A knife blade is passed through the skin at the lateral border of the internal sphincter muscle, in the subcutaneous plane, with the blade in the horizontal position. The knife blade is then advanced to the level of the dentate line. At this point, the blade is turned 90 degrees, with the cutting edge on the muscle. The internal sphincter muscle is then cut to its full thickness by gentle pressure on the blade while it is withdrawn. The stab wound is left open (Fig. 50.18). The fissure in the posterior or anterior midline is left undisturbed, but the redundant skin or the hypertrophic anal papilla can be excised as appropriate.

With the open technique, the skin and subcutaneous tissue from the dentate line to the anal verge are incised; an anal speculum is used to expose the left or right lateral quadrant. The internal sphincter muscle is identified and incised to its full thickness. The wound is closed with running sutures (Fig. 50.19).

Fissurectomy with anoplasty, with use of a skin flap to cover the wound, is suitable for cases in which markedly redundant skin tags are present around the fissure. A triangular skin flap with the apex at the fissure and the wide base at the perianal skin is created. Internal sphincterot-

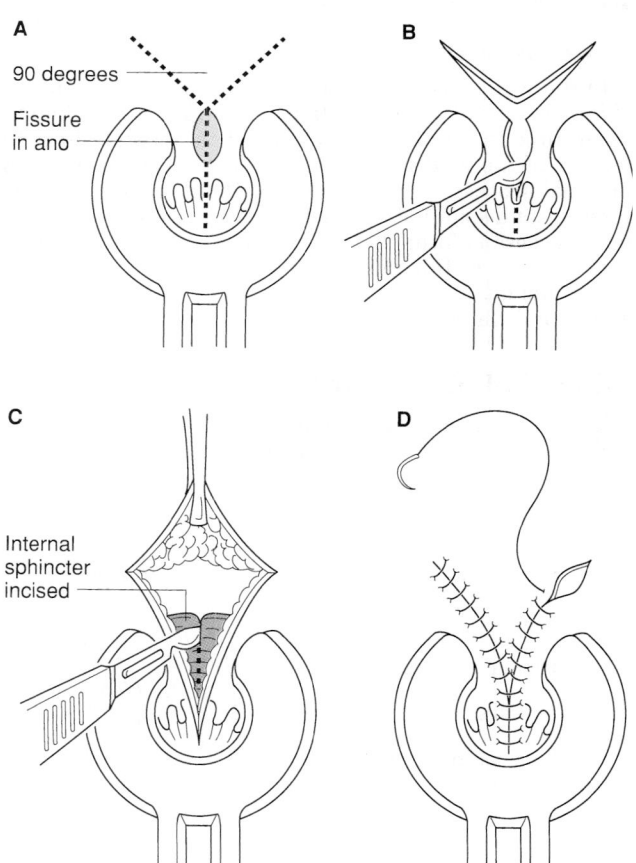

Figure 50.20. Internal sphincterotomy with V-Y anoplasty. *(A)* The skin flap is outlined, with the apex at the fissure, at a right angle. *(B)* A full-thickness skin flap is created. *(C)* An internal sphincterotomy is made through the fissure in its full thickness to the dentate line. *(D)* The skin flap is advanced to cover the wound and is sutured.

omy is performed in the bed of the fissure from the dentate line to its lateral border. If preferred, the fissure can be excised. The full-thickness flap is then slid to cover the wound and is closed with running sutures (Fig. 50.20).

Secondary Anal Fissure

Fissures or ulcers in Crohn's disease are larger and deeper than primary anal fissures. The skin around the ulcer is edematous, macerated, and erythematous. As a rule, pain is not as severe as that associated with idiopathic primary fissure; severe pain from a fissure in Crohn's disease may be a sign of abscess formation. The treatment of fissure associated with Crohn's disease is proper anal hygiene, local care of the lesion, and control of constipation or diarrhea. Surgery should be avoided and is contraindicated in the presence of active Crohn's disease.

Anal fissure or ulcer often occurs in patients with leukemia, aplastic anemia, or agranulocytosis. The fissure usually follows a bout of diarrhea or constipation at a time when the patient is neutropenic. The ulcer is extremely painful and often necrotic at its base. Fever or septicemia is common; if present, broad-spectrum antibiotics should be given. Treatment is directed at perineal hygiene and relief of pain with a nonconstipating analgesic drug. The ulcer usually heals when the white blood cell count rises above 1,000/mL. Surgery should be avoided.

ANORECTAL ABSCESS

Pathogenesis

In the wall of the anal canal, a variable number of anal glands (4 to 10) lined by stratified columnar epithelium open directly into the anal crypts at the dentate line. Infection of the anal glands is the most common origin of perianal abscess. Because the anal glands lie between the internal and external sphincter muscles, an intersphincteric abscess is formed. The infection may then spread to different spaces (Fig. 50.21). The sites of abscess, in order of frequency, are perianal, ischioanal, intersphincteric, and supralevator.

Clinical Manifestations

The initial symptom of most anorectal abscesses is severe pain in the anal region. The pain is throbbing or dully aching in character and is aggravated by walking, straining, coughing, and sneezing. Depending on the location of the abscess, a swollen mass may be felt. Fever or even septicemia may be present. In some patients, urinary retention develops.

Management

Like an abscess in any other part of the body, an anorectal abscess must be drained as soon as possible. In general, antibiotics are not necessary after the abscess is adequately drained, but appropriate antibiotics should be considered for immunodeficient patients and those with prostheses or cardiac valvular abnormalities.

Perianal abscesses are the most superficial and the easiest to treat. The abscess is usually small and can be drained under local anesthesia. A cruciate incision is made on the most prominent part of the skin and subcutaneous tissue overlying the abscess cavity. Redundant skin edges are excised to prevent premature closure of the abscess. It is important that the incision be deep to the base of the abscess cavity. The cavity is thoroughly curetted and irrigated. No packing is necessary.

An ischioanal abscess causes a diffuse swelling of the ischioanal fossa. The drainage is the same as in perianal abscess. Bilateral ischioanal or horseshoe abscess originates in the deep postanal space and spreads to both sides of the ischioanal space. A horseshoe abscess should be drained through the deep postanal space. A longitudinal incision is made in the skin between the tip of the coccyx and the anus to expose the anococcygeal ligament. The anococcygeal ligament is incised along its fibers, and the deep postanal space is entered. After the abscess cavity is drained, curetted, and irrigated, a counterdrainage incision is made on one or both limbs of the ischioanal space. No packing is needed.

With intersphincteric abscesses, signs of swelling or induration are not apparent in the perianal area, as they are with perianal and ischioanal abscesses. The diagnosis is suspected when anorectal pain is so severe that rectal examination is impossible. A deep-seated tenderness is present when pressure is applied around the anus. Most intersphincteric abscesses are located in the posterior quadrant. An indurated or bulging mass can be felt in the anal wall above the dentate line and can extend into the rectum for a variable distance. Intersphincteric abscesses are drained by incising the anal canal lining and incising through the internal sphincter muscle. The abscess cavity

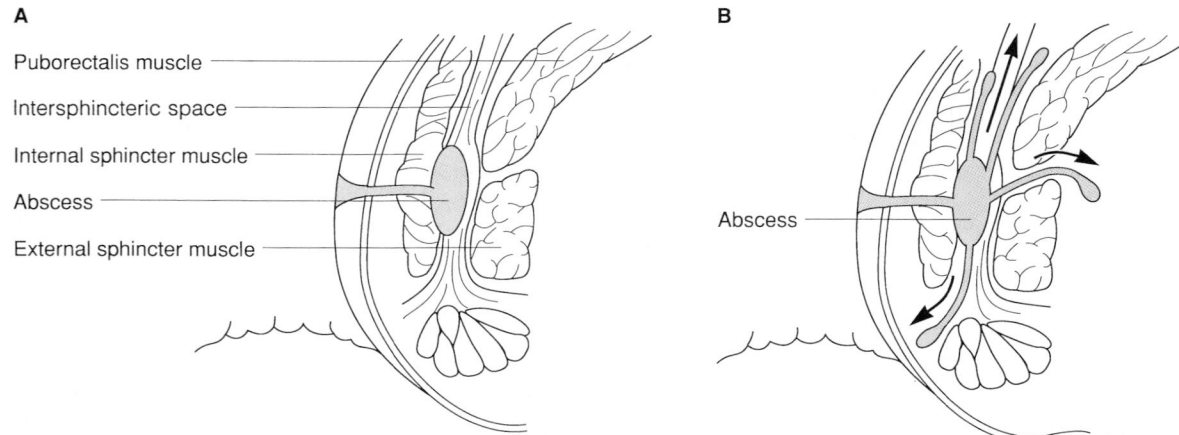

A

Puborectalis muscle
Intersphincteric space
Internal sphincter muscle
Abscess
External sphincter muscle

B

Abscess

Figure 50.21. Pathways of infection start in the intersphincteric space *(A)* and then spread to the perianal spaces, causing perianal abscesses to form *(B)*.

is curetted and irrigated with saline solution until clean. No packing is placed. Postoperative care consists of warm sitz baths for comfort. A bulk-producing agent is started the next day.

Supralevator abscess is uncommon and can be difficult to diagnose. Because of its proximity to the abdominal cavity, a supralevator abscess can mimic acute intraabdominal conditions. Digital examination reveals an indurated or bulging tender mass on either side of the lower rectum or posteriorly above the level of the anorectal ring. A supralevator abscess may arise in one of three ways: through upward extension of an intersphincteric abscess, by upward extension of an ischioanal abscess, or by extension from an intraabdominal process, such as diverticular abscess, appendiceal abscess, or abscess associated with Crohn's disease. It is essential to determine the origin of the abscess before treatment. If the abscess is secondary to upward extension of an intersphincteric abscess, it should be drained into the rectum. If such an abscess is drained through the ischioanal fossa, a complicated suprasphincteric fistula can form. If a supralevator abscess arises from the upward extension of an ischiorectal abscess, it should be drained through the ischioanal fossa. Attempts at draining this kind of abscess into the rectum may result in an extrasphincteric fistula. If the abscess is secondary to an intraabdominal disease, the primary disease is treated and the supralevator abscess is drained into the rectum, through the ischioanal fossa, or through the abdominal wall.

FISTULA-IN-ANO

Fistula-in-ano is a chronic form of perianal abscess in which the abscess cavity does not heal completely after spontaneous or surgical drainage. Instead, an inflammatory track forms, with a primary (internal) opening in the anal crypt at the dentate line and a secondary (external) opening in the perianal skin.

Classification

Four main forms of fistula-in-ano have been described, based on the relation of the fistula to the sphincter muscles (29) (Fig. 50.22).

Intersphincteric fistula: The fistulous track is in the intersphincteric plane. The external opening is usually in the perianal skin close to the anal verge.

Transsphincteric fistula: The fistula starts in the intersphincteric plane or in the deep postanal space. The fistulous track traverses the external sphincter, with the external opening at the ischioanal fossa. Horseshoe fistulae are also in this category.

Suprasphincteric fistula: The fistula starts in the intersphincteric plane in the midanal canal and then passes upward to a point above the puborectal muscle. The fistula passes laterally over this muscle and downward between the puborectal muscle and the levator ani into the ischioanal fossa.

Extrasphincteric fistula: The fistula passes from the perineal skin through the ischioanal fossa and the levator ani and finally penetrates the rectal wall. Extrasphincteric fistulae may have a cryptoglandular origin, or they may be caused by trauma, a foreign body, or a pelvic abscess, such as a diverticular or appendiceal abscess.

Clinical Manifestations

Most patients have a previous history of anorectal abscess subsequently associated with intermittent drainage. Recurrence of a perianal abscess suggests the presence of a fistula-in-ano. The external opening is usually visible as a red elevation of granulation tissue with purulent or serosanguineous drainage on compression. In the simple or superficial fistula, the track can be palpated as an indurated cord. Deeper fistulae usually are not palpable.

Anoscopy should be performed to identify the internal opening. Proctoscopy or flexible sigmoidoscopy is performed to rule out other lesions and inflammatory bowel disease. A fistula probe can be introduced into the fistulous track to determine its direction, although it is not always possible to pass the probe through the internal opening.

Several disorders must be considered in the differential diagnosis of fistula-in-ano. Hidradenitis suppurativa is differentiated by the presence of multiple perianal skin openings and surrounding leather-like skin. A pilonidal sinus with perianal extension and infected perianal sebaceous cysts must be considered. It is important to exclude fistulae associated with ulcerative colitis and Crohn's dis-

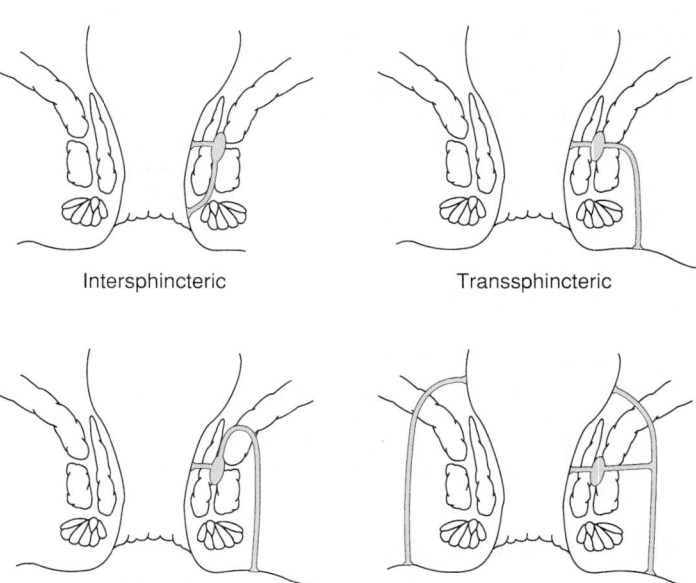

Intersphincteric   Transsphincteric

Suprasphincteric   Extrasphincteric

Figure 50.22. The four main anatomic types of fistula.

ease. Diverticulitis of the sigmoid colon, with perforation and fistulization to the perineum, rarely occurs. Low rectal and anal canal carcinomas may present as a fistula in the perineum.

Management

The principles of fistula surgery include unroofing the fistula, eliminating the primary opening (infective source), and establishing adequate drainage. Failure to open the entire track may lead to recurrence. With most fistulae, the treatment of choice involves opening the entire fistulous track, with a fistulous probe in place. Granulation tissues are curetted and the edges of the wound marsupialized. Fistulectomy, the excision of the fistulous track, has no advantages over fistulotomy, which is a laying open of the track. Horseshoe fistula, an uncommon form of fistula-in-ano, is a direct extension of an intersphincteric abscess and usually starts in the deep postanal space. Radical unroofing results in a large wound and is not necessary. Incision of the deep postanal space combined with excision or curettage of the lateral tracks is the procedure of choice.

In young patients, transection of the internal and external sphincter muscle in the posterior half, when performed in the course of a fistulotomy, does not always jeopardize anal continence. In older patients and in women, however, transection of the external sphincter muscle, particularly in the anterior half, risks incontinence. When sphincter transection appears likely, some authors recommend the use of a seton. A seton is a suture, usually silk, a rubber band, or a strip of Penrose drain, that is drawn through a fistula. Setons are tied around the muscles covering the fistula to create fibrosis, or to cut the muscles. The seton is threaded through the fistulous track and tied over the muscles. In the second stage (average interval, 6 to 8 weeks), fistulotomy is performed. Incontinence after the proper use of a seton is uncommon, even when the fistula is deep.

Anal Fistula Associated with Crohn's Disease

Fistulae associated with Crohn's disease are often asymptomatic. They resemble the ordinary fistulae seen in patients without Crohn's disease in that an indurated opening in the skin exudes pus and a palpable track passes toward the anal canal. The fistulae can be simple and superficial, or complex, with multiple tracks, or deep, with an origin in the upper anal canal or lower rectum.

The most important part of treatment is adequate and aggressive medical therapy, including medications for active Crohn's disease. Metronidazole has been found to be useful in some patients. The basic principle of surgery is to curette the granulation tissue locally in the fistulous tracks, lay open the superficial tracks, and open and clean the abscess cavity.

PILONIDAL SINUS

Most authors now accept the fact that pilonidal sinuses start with infection of the hair follicle in the sacrococcygeal area. Reports of pilonidal sinus in unusual positions, such as the umbilicus, healed amputation stumps, and interdigital clefts, all support the acquired etiology of this disease. Pilonidal sinuses are more likely to occur in the hirsute patient.

Clinical Manifestations

The average patient with pilonidal disease is a hirsute, moderately obese man in his second or third decade. Pi-

lonidal disease is rare in people under age 15; the incidence rises sharply to peak between 16 and 20 years and remains high until age 25, when it declines quickly. Pilonidal disease occurs less frequently in women, almost always in teenagers or young adults. Pilonidal disease may present as an acute abscess at the sacrococcygeal area that ruptures spontaneously, leaving unhealed sinuses with chronic drainage. When sinuses develop, pain is usually minimal.

Diagnosis

A painful and fluctuant mass is the most common presentation of the acute process. In the earliest stage, only cellulitis may be present, whereas in the chronic state, the diagnosis is confirmed by identifying the sinus opening in the intergluteal fold, about 5 cm above the anus. Most sinus tracks run cephalad (93%); the rest run caudad (7%) and may be confused with fistula-in-ano or suppurative hidradenitis. On careful examination, one can always find a pit or pits in the midline, which represent infected hair follicles. The differential diagnoses include furuncles of the skin, anal fistula, syphilitic or tuberculous granulomas, and osteomyelitis with multiple draining sinuses in the skin. Actinomycosis in the sacral region has been described as virtually indistinguishable from pilonidal disease.

Treatment

A pilonidal abscess can almost always be drained under local anesthesia. A longitudinal incision is made lateral to the midline in the coccygeal area. The incision is deepened into the subcutaneous tissue, and the abscess cavity is entered. All the hairs in the abscess cavity, if present, must be removed, and the wound is lightly packed with fine gauze. The patient is instructed to clean the wound at least once a day and to apply light packing. An antibiotic is not usually indicated.

For chronic pilonidal sinuses, the chronically infected cavity is opened lateral to the midline. The sinus tracks to the midline pits are probed and laid open. The granulation tissue in the cavity is curetted and the wound packed. Healing is rapid, and usually the wound is completely closed within 4 weeks (30). This is the technique of choice for most primary pilonidal sinuses with or without abscess.

Excision of pilonidal sinuses in the midline with marsupialization, primary closure, or Z-plasty is unnecessary and is plagued by delayed healing, unhealing, or recurrence.

Postoperative Care

The postoperative care is as important as the operation. The wound should be washed in the bathtub or shower at least once a day. If the cavity is large, it should be packed with fine gauze. If it is small, it should be swabbed to remove any foreign body, especially hair, at least once a day. The patient should return for follow-up at 1- to 2-week intervals until the wound is completely healed.

Pilonidal Sinus Complicated by Carcinoma

Carcinoma arising from chronic pilonidal sinus is rare; 44 cases had been reported in the world literature up to 1994 (31). Almost all are well-differentiated squamous cell carcinomas. The average duration of pilonidal disease in these patients was 23 years. The appearance of the wound should alert one to suspect carcinoma. Usually, an ulcer with a friable, bleeding, and fungating margin is seen. Wide excision is the treatment of choice. When inguinal node metastasis is present, the prognosis is poor.

RECTOVAGINAL FISTULA

A rectovaginal fistula is a communication between the anterior wall of the anal canal or rectum and the posterior wall of the vagina. Causes of rectovaginal fistula include the following:

Congenital maldevelopment
Trauma
Obstetric injury
Operative injury
Blunt or penetrating injury
Foreign body
Infection of anal canal or vaginal septum
Pelvic irradiation
Neoplasm

Obstetric injury accounts for the majority of rectovaginal fistulae. Rectovaginal fistulae are considered low if they can be repaired from a perineal approach and high if they must be repaired transabdominally (Fig. 50.23).

Rectovaginal fistulae can be classified as simple or complex, based on location, size, and cause:

Simple
    Low vaginal or midvaginal septum
    Diameter of 2.5 cm or less
    Traumatic or infectious cause
Complex
    High vaginal septum
    Diameter of 2.5 cm or more
Caused by inflammatory bowel disease, irradiation, or
    neoplasm

The symptoms of rectovaginal fistulae depend on location, size, and cause. With low or small fistulae, the most common complaint is passage of gas per vagina. With large fistulae, symptoms include vaginal discharge with a fecal odor, passage of flatus and stool through the vagina, and vaginitis. Some patients also have fecal incontinence.

The definitive diagnosis is made by examination. With a low fistula, digital examination of the anal canal reveals scar and a defect in the anterior wall. Bimanual examination with one finger in the rectum and a finger of the other hand in the vagina is helpful. Anoscopy can also detect the opening in the anal canal. Middle and high fistulae require proctoscopy. If the fistula cannot be seen, a tampon is placed in the vaginal canal and 100 mL of diluted methylene blue is instilled into the anorectum. After a time, the tampon is removed and checked for evidence of blue staining. Barium enema is usually not helpful but may be indicated in certain patients with inflammatory bowel disease or previous irradiation.

Spontaneous or nonoperative healing of a rectovaginal fistula depends primarily on its cause and, to a lesser extent, its size. About half of small rectovaginal fistulae secondary to obstetric trauma heal spontaneously.

Removal of a foreign body is often followed by healing. Similarly, proper treatment of an infectious process may allow the fistula to heal. Fistulae caused by Crohn's disease or irradiation rarely heal spontaneously. For a low, simple fistula and some mid-rectovaginal fistulae, endorectal advancement of an anorectal flap gives the best results. The rectal flap, which consists of mucosa, submucosa, internal sphincter, and the circular muscle of the lower rectum, is outlined lateral and distal to the fistula. It is important to base the flap at least 4 cm cephalad to the fistula, and the base should be about twice the length of the flap to ensure adequate blood supply. After the flap is raised from the apex to the base, the underlying fistula and the excess flap are excised. The cut edges of the internal sphincter and the circular muscle of the lower rectum are approximated to obliterate the opening of the fistula in the anal canal. The opening in the vagina is left open for drainage. The anorectal flap is then advanced over the repaired area and sutured (Fig. 50.24). If the rectovaginal fistula is associated with incontinence resulting from injury to the external sphincter, a sphincteroplasty is also performed. In this technique, the ends of the transected muscle are identified and mobilized. The fistula is excised, and the muscle ends are then overlapped and sutured. The results of endorectal flap advancement to treat simple rectovaginal fistula are good,

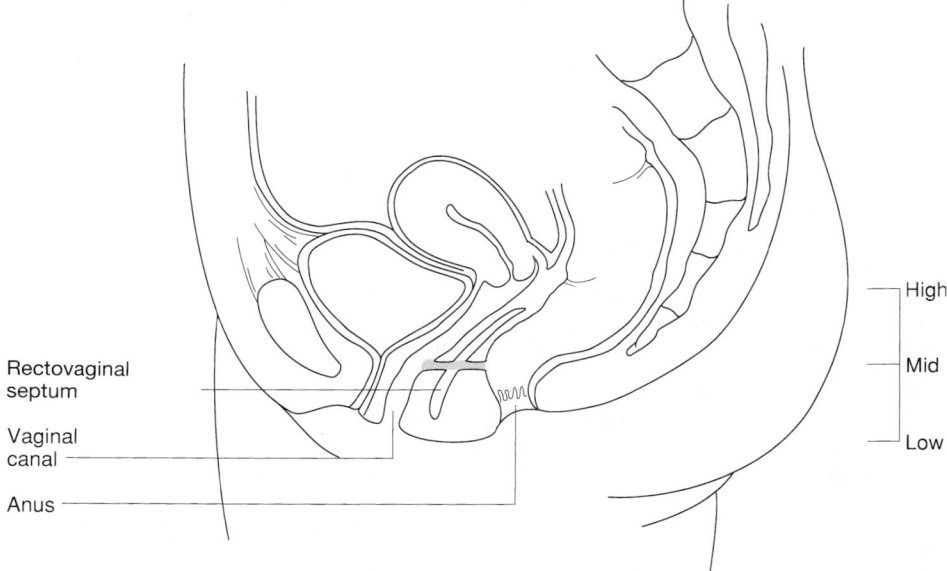

Figure 50.23. Rectovaginal fistula classified by location. Fistulae are low when situated at or just cephalad to the dentate line, high when located near the cervix, and middle when located in between.

Rectovaginal
septum

Vaginal
canal

Anus

High

Mid

Low

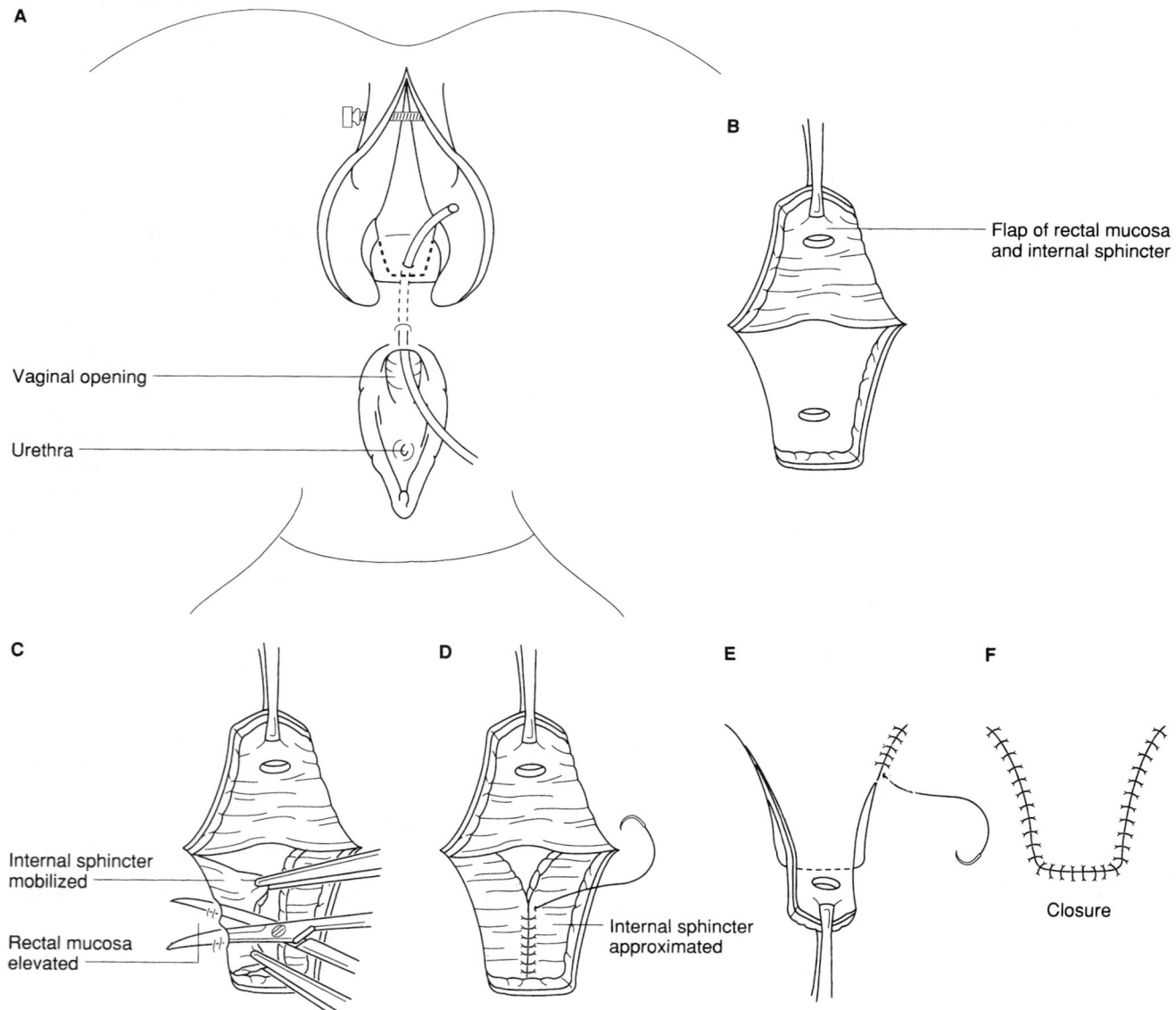

Figure 50.24. Endorectal advancement of anorectal flap. *(A)* Exposure is gained with an anal speculum and the fistula is identified. Outline of endorectal flap, extending proximally to 7 cm from the anal verge. *(B)* The full-thickness flap is created to include the internal sphincter muscle. *(C)* Lateral mobilization is performed on each side in the submucosal plane. *(D)* Anorectal wall on each side is approximated. *(E,F)* The endorectal flap is pulled down to cover the wound and sutured. The fistula is excised. The aperture in the vagina is not sutured but is left open for drainage.

with primary healing of the fistula achieved in 83% of treated patients (32). It is important to wait, usually 3 to 6 months, until the inflammation has subsided before a surgical repair is considered. An alternative repair is to lay open the rectovaginal fistula and convert it to a fourth-degree perineal tear. A layer closure of the anal and vaginal defect is performed with synthetic absorbable sutures.

High fistulae and some mid-rectovaginal fistulae require a transabdominal approach. Simple fistulae with healthy surrounding tissues can be repaired by mobilization of the rectovaginal septum, division of the fistula, and layer closure of the rectal defect without bowel resection. If the local tissues are damaged by irradiation, infection, or inflammatory disease, an extended low anterior resection with coloanal anastomosis should be performed.

Although most simple rectovaginal fistulae do not require a diverting colostomy, complex rectovaginal fistulae are best managed by a preliminary colostomy. For elderly or unfit patients, most patients with radiation-induced fistulae, and patients with rectovaginal fistulae associated with Crohn's disease, a permanent colostomy may be the procedure of choice.

ANAL INCONTINENCE

The term *anal incontinence* covers many forms of anorectal functional impairment, ranging from simple involuntary passage of flatus to complete loss of sphincteric tone and involuntary passage of formed stool.

Anal incontinence results when the normal anorectal anatomy or physiology is lost or disturbed. A contracted rectum, poor rectal compliance, or a resection of the rectum with loss of normal rectal reservoir function may result in incontinence. A neurologic problem may disturb anorectal sensation, which provides awareness of the presence of stool in the anorectum. About half of patients with long-standing rectal prolapse have anal incontinence, presumably resulting from stretching of the pudendal nerve, which causes the sphincter muscles to dysfunction. A large volume of diarrheal stool emptying rapidly into the anorectum may overcome the continence mechanism, even in healthy persons. Direct mechanical injuries to the sphincter muscles include obstetric tear, fistulotomy, hemorrhoidectomy, internal sphincterotomy, anal stretching, and perianal trauma.

Examination of the patient starts with observation of any fecal materials in the undergarments and the degree of perianal skin excoriation. Obvious gaping or laxity of the anus indicates neurogenic dysfunction of the sphincteric muscles. Abnormal perineal descent, in which the downward movement of the anus on straining extends more than 2 cm below the plane of the ischial tuberosities, may indicate damage to the levator ani muscle. A scar or defect in the anal region may indicate surgical injuries to the sphincter muscle. Digital examination can accurately sense the tone of the internal sphincter muscle, and voluntary squeezing of the anal canal can allow one to estimate the function of the external sphincter muscle, especially the puborectal muscle. Flexible sigmoidoscopy should always be performed. A total colonoscopy or barium enema is usually indicated. Anal manometry is useful to evaluate the status of the internal and external sphincteric muscles and may also be helpful in evaluating the results of operation. Anal endosonography has added a new dimension to the investigation of the anal sphincter. The sonographic probe or endoscope provides a clear image of the internal and external sphincters all around. Ultrasonography has lessened the need for other investigations, such as electromyography, because the ultrasonographic image can accurately localize defects and asymmetry. It provides an equally reliable method for mapping external sphincter defects and is more comfortable for the patient than electromyographic mapping (33).

Regulation of bowel habit, particularly decreasing the number of bowel movements to once a day or once every other day, usually relieves the condition. Adherence to a high-fiber diet results in a formed and bulky stool, so that it is easier for patients to evacuate and empty the rectum. Antidiarrheal drugs may be prescribed judiciously.

Biofeedback is used in the treatment of anal incontinence, to retrain the anorectum to sense rectal fullness and to retrain the sphincteric muscles to contract. Biofeedback training helps 85% of patients with various causes of anal incontinence (34). In the most commonly used system, a triple-balloon catheter is attached to a pressure transducer. While the patient watches the rectal manometer tracings, the balloon is inflated, and the patient is coached to contract the sphincter muscle to elevate the sphincter tracing. Several sessions may be required before the patient is aware of the sensation in the rectum and can specifically contract the anal sphincter. Eventually, the patient can learn to contract the sphincter muscle without the instrument. A small, portable anorectal biofeedback system can be used for practice at home.

Operative treatment is reserved for patients resistant to conservative management. Sphincteroplasty is most suitable for incontinence secondary to obstetric injury or injury sustained during anorectal surgery. The procedure involves a curved incision in the perianal skin where the sphincter muscle has been transected. The sphincter mus-

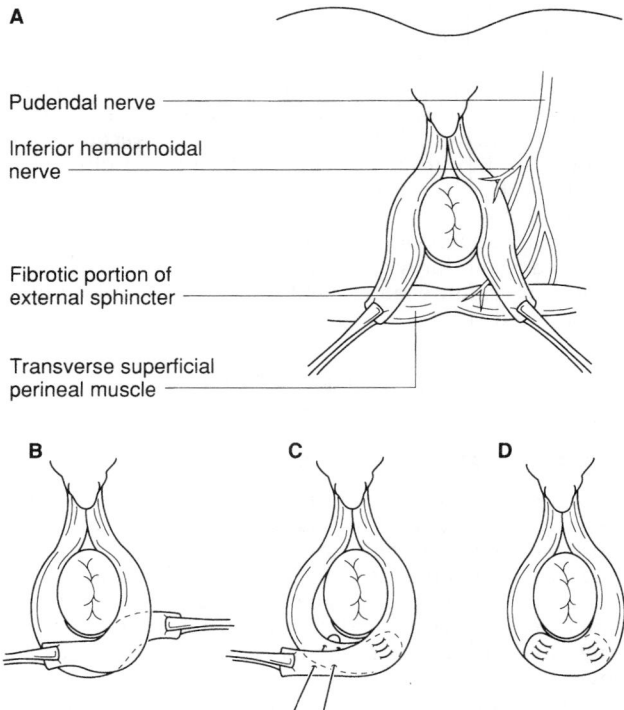

Figure 50.25. Overlap anal sphincteroplasty.

cle, including the puborectal muscle, is mobilized enough so that it can be wrapped over itself with modest tension (Fig. 50.25). This operation is successful on a short-term basis in about 85% of patients (35).

Postanal intersphincteric sphincteroplasty was designed for incontinence caused by prolapse of the rectum and for certain cases of idiopathic incontinence. The approach is through the intersphincteric plane posteriorly. The levator ani muscle is approximated to restore the anorectal angle to normal. The puborectal muscle and the external sphincter muscles are also tightened with sutures. The procedure also lengthens the anal canal to a significant degree. Although 80% of patients experience short-term improvement, long-term improvement after the repair has been noted in only 25% (36,37).

Gracilis muscle transposition can be used when significant loss of the anal sphincter muscle mass has occurred or when other techniques have failed. These striated muscles are capable of producing a voluntary contraction to occlude the anal canal. However, the gracilis muscles are unable to maintain a closed lumen at all times because of the lack of an inherent tone within the muscles; in contrast, the internal sphincter muscle generates a resting anal tone. This operation has fallen out of favor because of unsatisfactory short-term success rates of about 50% (38,39). Gluteal muscle transposition has yielded similar results (40). The electrically stimulated graciloplasty, in which the gracilis muscle is stimulated by an implanted electric stimulating device, provides short-term positive results in 75% of cases (41). The constant low-frequency electric stimulation of skeletal muscle converts a fast-twitch muscle into a slow-twitch muscle capable of sustained activity. This operation is expensive and is still experimental.

More recently, an artificial anal sphincter has generated enthusiasm. The sphincter consists of an inflatable cuff of silicone rubber that is placed around the upper anal canal via two small perianal incisions. The pressure-regulating balloon is placed extraperitoneally to the left or right of the bladder, and the pump by which the patient can inflate and deflate the cuff is placed in the labia majora or the scrotum (42). In a series of 17 patients with a follow-up of 5 to 10 years, Christiansen et al. (42) reported good functioning results of 50% despite neurogenic incontinence in 10 of 17 patients. This operation has been received with enthusiasm in Europe but is not approved for clinical applications by the Food and Drug Administration in the United States.

For patients who are incapacitated by complete fecal incontinence and for whom anal sphincter repair is unlikely to be successful, a permanent end-sigmoid colostomy is the best choice.

SEXUALLY TRANSMITTED DISEASES OF THE ANORECTUM

Anal Condylomata Acuminata

Anal condylomata acuminata are caused by the human papillomavirus (HPV), primarily HPV-6 and HPV-11. In most patients, the warts involve the perianal skin, anal verge, and anoderm. Occasionally, the lesions also involve the mucosa of the upper anal canal and lower rectum. The extent of the disease varies from a few small warts to a large mass occluding the anus. The diagnosis is usually obvious by the characteristic papillary appearance. Anoscopic examination is essential to detect intraanal involvement. Because most cases are transmitted by sexual contact, other venereal diseases, especially gonorrhea and syphilis, should be excluded.

Small perianal warts can be destroyed by applying podophyllin solution or bichloracetic acid. Both podophyllin and bichloracetic acid are caustic; therefore, the uninvolved skin should be protected with petroleum jelly before these agents are applied so that caustic injury can be prevented. Extensive warts in the perianal area or in the anal canal are best treated by excision with a small iris scissors, followed by electrocoagulation of the bases.

Frequent postoperative follow-up is necessary because the recurrence rate is as high as 65%. The patient should be seen every 2 to 4 weeks until at least 3 months have passed without disease recurrence. Immunotherapy (with the use of autogenous wart tissue vaccine) in conjunction with excision of the lesions has been found effective, but the role of immune mechanisms in the recurrence of warts has yet to be determined.

Malignant transformation of condylomata acuminata is rare and is usually associated with long-standing disease. The microscopic picture includes squamous dysplasia with proliferation and disorganization of epidermal cells, keratinization of individual cells, keratin pearl formation, an increased number of normal and abnormal mitoses, and, most important, invasion into the underlying tissue. Anal condylomata acuminata with invasive carcinoma should be treated in the same manner as squamous cell carcinoma of the anus (see Chapter 47).

Gonococcal Proctitis and Syphilis

Patients with gonococcal proctitis are generally asymptomatic but may have mild anal burning, pain, discharge, or bleeding in the acute phase. Proctoscopic examination reveals hyperemic and edematous anorectal mucosa with purulent discharge in the anal crypts at the dentate line. In the chronic phase, the anorectum may appear normal. Diagnosis is confirmed by observing *Neisseria gonorrhoeae* on stained smears of the discharge and by plating the exudate immediately onto Thayer-Martin culture medium. In the United States, antimicrobial resistance of the gonococcus continues to evolve, and coinfection with *Chlamydia trachomatis* is a serious problem. Chlamydial infection may be documented in up to 45% of gonorrhea cases when adequate chlamydial cultures are performed.

The recommended treatment is 250 mg of ceftriaxone administered once intramuscularly plus 100 mg of doxycycline given orally twice a day for 7 days (43). For those patients who cannot take ceftriaxone, 500 mg of ciprofloxacin administered orally once plus 100 mg of doxycycline given orally twice a day for 7 days is a good alternative (44). Doxycycline or tetracycline alone is not adequate, but these drugs can be added to counter possible coexisting chlamydial infection.

All patients treated for gonorrhea should have a serologic test for syphilis. *Treponema pallidum* is still sensitive to penicillin. The intramuscular administration of 2.4 million units of benzathine penicillin G will maintain treponemicidal levels for 2 weeks. For latent syphilis, 2.4 million units is given weekly for 3 weeks. Patients who are allergic to penicillin may be treated with 500 mg of tetracycline or erythromycin four times a day for 30 days (43).

Follow-up cultures should be obtained from the anorectum 3 to 7 days after completion of treatment. Recurrent gonococcal infections after treatment with recommended schedules commonly represent reinfection rather than treatment failure and indicate a need for improved tracing of sex partners and patient education. Because antimicrobial resistance is a cause of treatment failure, all posttreatment isolates should be tested for antimicrobial susceptibility.

Chlamydial Proctitis

Chlamydia trachomatis is the most common cause of sexually transmitted disease in the United States, affecting 4 million Americans each year. Although most chlamydial infections affect the urethra, anorectal involvement among male homosexuals is common. Proctoscopy reveals nonspecific proctitis with friable, granular, and edematous mucosa. Immunofluorescent microscopy provides an accurate and rapid diagnosis. The specimen should be collected by swabbing the anorectal mucosa.

Treatment includes 500 mg of tetracycline hydrochloride by mouth four times daily for 7 days or 100 mg of doxycycline by mouth twice daily for 7 days. For patients in whom tetracyclines are contraindicated, 500 mg of erythromycin base or stearate by mouth four times daily for 7 days or 800 mg of erythromycin ethylsuccinate by mouth four times daily for 7 days may be used. When taken as directed, the tetracycline and erythromycin regimens listed above are highly effective (>95% cure rate). Therefore, posttreatment *C. trachomatis* test-of-cure cultures may be omitted if laboratory resources are limited. Although cultures may not become positive until 3 to 6 weeks after treatment, when they are positive, patients should be re-treated with one of the above regimens, and any interim sex partners should also be contacted.

Two new drugs have been approved by the Food and Drug Administration for the treatment of *Chlamydia* infection: 1 g of oral azithromycin in a single dose and 300 mg of oral ofloxacin two times a day for 7 days. A substantial advantage of azithromycin, in comparison with all other therapies, is that a single dose is effective; this antimicrobial may prove most useful for situations in which compliance with a 7-day regimen of another antimicrobial cannot be ensured. In view of the high efficacy of tetracycline and doxycycline, cost should also be considered when a treatment regimen is selected (45).

Herpes Simplex Viral Proctitis

Anorectal herpes is caused by herpesvirus hominis type 2, the same organism implicated in genital herpes. The usually severe anorectal pain is associated with fever, inguinal adenopathy, tenesmus, constipation, anorectal discharge, and bleeding. Neurologic symptoms in the distribution of the sacral roots are noted in some patients. These may include urinary retention, dyspareunia, and impotence. Examination reveals erythematous areas with small groups of vesicles that rupture and become ulcerated. Proctoscopic examination may reveal a nonspecific proctitis (46,47).

The diagnosis can be made by staining the exudate with the Papanicolaou or Giemsa method. A finding of multinucleated giant cells is diagnostic. One may also use immunofluorescence or immunoperoxidase staining of lesion scrapings to detect the herpes simplex virus antigens. Both techniques are rapid and useful when results are positive but are less sensitive than viral isolation in tissue culture from the vesicles or ulcers.

For the first episode, 200 mg of acyclovir by mouth five times daily for 7 to 10 days is effective if initiated within 6 days of the onset of lesions. This treatment shortens the median duration of first-episode eruptions by 3 to 5 days and may reduce systemic symptoms in primary episodes. For patients with severe symptoms or complications that necessitate hospitalization, 5 mg of acyclovir per kilogram given intravenously every 8 hours for 5 to 7 days is recommended. This treatment shortens the median course of first episodes by about 7 days. Topical acyclovir ointment is of marginal benefit in decreasing virus shedding but has no significant effect on symptoms or healing time.

For recurrent anorectal herpes, because the benefit may be minimal, treatment should be limited to those patients who typically have severe symptoms and who are able to begin therapy at the beginning of the prodrome or within 2 days of the onset of lesions. Oral acyclovir in a dosage of 200 mg five times a day for 5 days is used. It shortens the mean clinical course by about 1 day. Intravenous or topical acyclovir is not indicated for recurrences.

ANORECTAL DISEASES IN PATIENTS WITH AIDS AND HIV POSITIVITY

Kaposi's Sarcoma

Kaposi's sarcoma, normally a rare tumor of the skin, is one of the most common malignant tumors in AIDS patients. In most cases, Kaposi's sarcoma of the colon and rectum is asymptomatic, but bleeding, diarrhea, and obstruction may occur. The characteristic lesion is a red, round, submucosal nodule with central umbilication. A deep biopsy is required to yield an accurate result. The diagnosis is useful as a prognostication because no effective medical treatment is available. Surgery is indicated only to control massive bleeding, perforation, or obstruction.

Cytomegalovirus Infection

Although cytomegalovirus (CMV) has been found in virtually every human organ system, its presence is not uniformly associated with pathologic changes. Symptomatic CMV proctocolitis occurs in at least 10% of AIDS patients. CMV infection in immunocompromised patients, however, leads to serious complications. In about 50% of the AIDS patients who harbor the virus, the infection is serious. Disseminated CMV has been identified at postmortem examination in 90% of patients with AIDS, with 30% having CMV in the gastrointestinal tract. CMV enteroproctocolitis occurs in 5% to 10% of AIDS patients but is re-

sponsible for 70% of all deaths in AIDS patients who undergo major abdominal surgery on an emergency basis (48,49). Symptoms of CMV enterocolitis are diarrhea, fever, right lower quadrant abdominal pain, and weight loss. Not uncommon is coinfection with one or more opportunistic agents, such as *Salmonella, Shigella, Campylobacter, Clostridium difficile, Cryptosporidium, Microsporida, Entamoeba,* and *Giardia.*

The morphologic hallmarks of CMV enteroproctocolitis are sharply demarcated areas of shallow ulcers, frequently covered with fibrin. Biopsy gives an accurate diagnosis. The pathognomonic histopathologic features include large basophilic intranuclear CMV inclusions. The problems that most commonly necessitate emergent or urgent surgical intervention are bleeding and perforation of the CMV ulcers. These complications occur in 60% to 100% of emergency exploratory celiotomies performed in AIDS patients. Medical treatment consists of ganciclovir (49).

Lymphoma

The incidence of non-Hodgkin's lymphoma is increased in patients with HIV positivity and AIDS. In the United States, about 3% of AIDS cases present with lymphoma. When the gastrointestinal tract is the primary site, the stomach is affected more than the colon. The identification of anorectal lymphoma is difficult because the disease is extraluminal in most cases. Most patients are brought to the operating room with perianal abscesses as a preoperative diagnosis (49). The diagnosis relies on the microscopic identification of the B-cell immunoblastic configuration of extranodular lymphoma. A consideration in the treatment of AIDS-related lymphoma is that radiation and chemotherapy may actually accelerate the demise of the patient through further immunosuppression. It is worthwhile, in patients with resectable tumors, to excise the lesion (50).

Anal Carcinoma

Although anal carcinoma is uncommon in general population, anal carcinoma and its precursor lesion, anal intraepithelial neoplasia, are increased in homosexual men. The association of these lesions with HPV is clear. A good deal of evidence is available to suggest that the incidence of invasive anal carcinoma has risen since the onset of the HIV epidemic. Few data have been published on the morbidity and mortality associated with anal carcinoma among HIV-infected men. It is likely that if the life span of HIV-infected persons is prolonged by even a few years, anal carcinoma will become a frequent complication of HIV infection, with considerable morbidity and mortality (50).

Relatively little is known about the prevalence of anal intraepithelial neoplasia, primarily because until recently screening has never been performed for what are generally subclinical, asymptomatic lesions. Anal intraepithelial neoplasia can be detected by means of cytologic smears (Papanicolaou staining). With the use of this approach, it has become apparent that such pathology is exceedingly common. Low-grade anal intraepithelial neoplasia regresses and can simply be followed. High-grade anal intraepithelial neoplasia is the counterpart of carcinoma in situ; ablation of visible lesions is recommended (50).

Anorectal Ulcers

The anal-receptive male homosexual is at increased risk for various viral, bacterial, and parasitic diseases of the anorectum. Anal ulcers are common among HIV-positive patients. About half of the anal ulcers are idiopathic. Most ulcers are located in the posterior midline of the anus, somewhat closer to the dentate line than the ordinary anal fissure. Idiopathic ulcers in HIV-positive patients are extremely erosive, dissecting along the submucosal and intersphincteric planes and many times skeletonizing the internal sphincter muscle. These erosions create pockets in which stool and pus collect; severe pain results, especially during defecation (51).

Examination of the anorectum under general anesthesia is usually necessary. Biopsy specimens should be taken and sent for viral culture and dark-field examination if indicated. If lymphoma is suspected, the tissue should be sent for typing. Pocketing of the ulcers should be corrected by division of a portion of the internal sphincter muscle along with débridement. In patients with intolerable pain from anal ulcers, a sigmoid colostomy gives symptomatic relief. Specific ulcers in HIV-positive patients are usually caused by syphilis, tuberculosis, herpes simplex, cytomegalovirus infection, or bacterial pathogens.

REFERENCES

1. Crapp AR, Cuthbertson AM. William Waldeyer and the rectosacral fascia. *Surg Gynecol Obstet* 1974;138:252–256.
2. Shafik A. A new concept of the anatomy of the anal sphincter mechanism and the physiology of defecation: the external anal sphincter—a triple-loop system. *Invest Urol* 1975; 12:412–419.
3. Oh C, Kark AE. Anatomy of the external sphincter. *Br J Surg* 1972;59:717–723.
4. Shafik A. A new concept of the anatomy of the anal sphincter mechanism and the physiology of defecation. II. Anatomy of the levator ani muscle with special reference to puborectalis. *Invest Urol* 1975;13:175–182.
5. Miscusi G, Masoni L, Dell'Anna A, et al. Normal lymphatic drainage of the rectum and the anal canal revealed by lymphoscintigraphy. *Coloproctology* 1987;9:171–174.
6. Bauer JJ, Gelernt IM, Salky B, et al. Sexual dysfunction following proctectomy for benign diseases of the colon and rectum. *Ann Surg* 1983;197:363–367.
7. Lepor H, Gregerman M, Crosby R, et al. Precise localization of the autonomic nerves from the pelvic plexus to the corpora cavernosa: a detailed anatomical study of the adult male pelvis. *J Urol* 1985;133:207–212.
8. Cherry DA, Rothenberger DA. Pelvic floor physiology. *Surg Clin North Am* 1988;68:1217–1230.
9. Thomson WHF. The nature of hemorrhoids. *Br J Surg* 1975; 62:542–552.
10. Loder PB, Kamm MA, Nicholls RJ, et al. Hemorrhoids: pathology, pathophysiology, and etiology. *Br J Surg* 1994;81: 946–954.
11. Bernstein WC. What are hemorrhoids and what is their relationship to the portal venous system? *Dis Colon Rectum* 1983;26:829–834.
12. Buls JG, Goldberg SM. Modern management of hemorrhoids. *Surg Clin North Am* 1978;58:469–478.
13. Senagore A, Mazier WP, Luchtefeld MA, et al. Treatment of advanced hemorrhoidal disease: a prospective, randomized comparison of cold scalpel vs. contact Nd:YAG laser. *Dis Colon Rectum* 1993;36:1042–1049.
14. Beahrs OH, Theuerkauf FJ Jr, Hill JR. Procidentia: surgical treatment. *Dis Colon Rectum* 1972;15:337–346.
15. McMahan JD, Ripstein CB. Rectal prolapse: an update on rectal sling procedure. *Am Surg* 1987;53:37–40.
15a. Wells C. New operation for rectal prolapse. *Proc R Soc Med* 1959;52:602–604.
16. Aitola P, Hiltunen KM, Matikainen MJ. Functional results of operative treatment of rectal prolapse over an 11-year period. *Dis Colon Rectum* 1999;42:655–660.
17. Wolff BG, Dietzen C. Abdominal resectional procedures for rectal prolapse. *Semin Colon Rectal Surg* 1991;2:184–186.
18. Kim DS, Tsang CBS, Wong WD, et al. Complete rectal prolapse: evolution of management and results. *Dis Colon Rectum* 1999;42:460–469.
19. Huber FT, Stein H, Siewert JR. Functional results after treatment of rectal prolapse with rectopexy and sigmoid resection. *World J Surg* 1995;19:138–143.
20. Finlay IG, Aitchison M. Perineal excision of the rectum for prolapse in the elderly. *Br J Surg* 1991;78:687–689.
21. Agachan F, Reissman P, Pfeifer J, et al. Comparison of three perineal procedures for the treatment of rectal prolapse. *South Med J* 1997;90:925–932.
22. Uhlig BE, Sullivan ES. The modified Delorme operation: its place in surgical treatment of massive rectal prolapse. *Dis Colon Rectum* 1979;22:513–521.
23. Nivatvongs S. Rectal prolapse: techniques of transperineal repair. *Perspect Colon Rectal Surg* 1991;4:101–109.
24. Andrew RL, Stevenson RL, Stitz RW, et al. Laparoscopic-assisted resection rectopexy for rectal prolapse: early and medium follow-up. *Dis Colon Rectum* 1998;41:46–54.
25. Parks AG, Swash M, Urich H. Sphincter denervation in anorectal incontinence and rectal prolapse. *Gut* 1977;18: 656–665.
26. Schouten WR, Briel JW, Auwerda JJA, et al. Ischemic nature of anal fissure. *Br J Surg* 1996;83:63–65.
27. Watson SJ, Kamm MA, Nicholls RJ, et al. Topical glyceryl trinitrate in the treatment of chronic anal fissure. *Br J Surg* 1996;83:771–775.
28. Gordon PH, Vasilevsky CA. Lateral internal sphincterotomy: rationale, technique, and anesthesia. *Can J Surg* 1985;28: 28–30.
29. Parks AG, Gordon PH, Hardcastle JE. A classification of fistula-in-ano. *Br J Surg* 1976;63:1–12.
30. Bascom J. Pilonidal disease: long-term results of follicle removal. *Dis Colon Rectum* 1983;26:800–807.
31. Davis KA, Mock CN, Versaci A, et al. Malignant degeneration of pilonidal cyst. *Am Surg* 1994;60:200–204.
32. Lowry AC, Thorson AG, Rothenberger DA, et al. Repair of simple rectovaginal fistula: influence of previous repairs. *Dis Colon Rectum* 1988;31:676–678.
33. Sentovich S, Wong WD, Blatchford G, et al. Accuracy and reliability of transanal ultrasound for anterior anal sphincter injury. *Dis Colon Rectum* 1998;41:1000–1004.
34. Patankar S, Ferrara A, Levy JR, et al. Biofeedback in colorectal practice: a multicenter, statewide, three-year experience. *Dis Colon Rectum* 1997;40:827–831.
35. Young CJ, Mathur MN, Egers AA, et al. Successful overlapping anal sphincter repair: relationship to patient age, neuropathy, and colostomy formation. *Dis Colon Rectum* 1998; 41:344–349.
36. Parks AG. Anorectal incontinence. *Proc R Soc Med* 1975;68: 681–690.
37. Jameson JS, Speakman CT, Darze A, et al. Audit of postanal repair in the treatment of fecal incontinence. *Dis Colon Rectum* 1994;37:369–372.
38. Christiansen J, Sevensen M, Rasmussen OO. Gracilis muscle transposition for fecal incontinence. *Br J Surg* 1990;77: 1039–1040.
39. Foucheron JL, Hannoun L, Thome C, et al. Is fecal continence improved by nonstimulated gracilis muscle transposition? *Dis Colon Rectum* 1994;37:979–983.
40. Devesa JM, Fernandez JM. Bilateral gluteoplasty for anal incontinence. *Semin Colon Rectal Surg* 1997;8:103–109.
41. Baeten CGMI, Geerdes BP, Adang EMM, et al. Anal dynamic graciloplasty in the treatment of intractable fecal incontinence. *N Engl J Med* 1995;32:1600–1605.
42. Christiansen J, Rasmussen OO, Lindorff-Larsen K. Long-term results of artificial anal sphincter implantation for severe anal incontinence. *Ann Surg* 1999;230:45–48.
43. U.S. Department of Health and Human Services. Sexually transmitted disease treatment guidelines. *MMWR Morb Mortal Wkly Rep* 1993;42(RR14):1–102.
44. Echols RM, Heyd A, O'Keefe BJ, et al. Single-dose ciprofloxacin for the treatment of uncomplicated gonorrhea: a worldwide summary. *Sex Transm Dis* 1994;24:345–352.
45. Minnesota Department of Health. Disease control newsletter 1994;22:1–8.
46. Jacobs E. Sexually transmitted diseases of the anorectum and intestine. *Perspect Colon Rectal Surg* 1989;2:27–43.
47. Milsom JW. Herpes simplex infections of the anorectum. *Semin Colon Rectal Surg* 1992;3:222–226.

48. Soderlund C, Brett GA, Engstrom L, et al. Surgical treatment of cytomegalovirus enterocolitis in severe human immunodeficiency virus infection: report of eight cases. *Dis Colon Rectum* 1994;37:63–72.

49. Wexner SD. AIDS: what the colorectal surgeon needs to know. *Perspect Colon Rectal Surg* 1989;2:19–54.

50. Surawicz CM, Kiviat NB. A rational approach to anal intraepithelial neoplasia. *Semin Colon Rectal Surg* 1998;9:99–106.

51. Bernstein M. Benign human immunodeficiency virus/acquired immune deficiency syndrome—specific anorectal conditions. *Semin Colon Rectal Surg* 1998;9:94–98.

SECTION I

HERNIA, ACUTE ABDOMEN, AND SPLEEN

SURGERY: SCIENTIFIC PRINCIPLES AND PRACTICE, Third Edition, edited by
Lazar J. Greenfield, Michael W. Mulholland, Keith T. Oldham, Gerald B. Zelenock,
and Keith D. Lillemoe. Lippincott Williams & Wilkins Publishers, Philadelphia, © 2001.

CHAPTER 51

ABDOMINAL WALL HERNIAS

ALAN T. RICHARDS, THOMAS H. QUINN,
AND ROBERT J. FITZGIBBONS, JR.

One of the most frequently performed operations by general surgeons worldwide is the repair of an abdominal wall hernia. In the United States, approximately 1 million hernia operations are performed each year (1). Because hernias are far less age-dependent than other conditions, a large proportion of the patients undergoing hernia repair are relatively young.

ANATOMY OF THE ABDOMINAL WALL AND GROIN

The abdominal muscles, their aponeuroses, and the associated peritoneal and fascia layers admirably function in most circumstances to prevent eventration from the abdominal or pelvic cavity. Although this extensive muscular and aponeurotic system may withstand great pressures from within the abdominal cavity, it is subject to predictable failure at a number of sites in both sexes. The failure or weakness of any component of the abdominal wall or inguinal region often causes neighboring structures to be weakened also, so that hernias of varying degrees of complexity result. A positive outcome for a herniorrhaphy, whether by conventional or laparoscopic technique, depends on a detailed knowledge of the anatomy to be encountered.

This chapter describes the surgical anatomy of the abdominal wall and the inguinal region, first from the viewpoint of the surgeon using open techniques and subsequently from the perspective of the surgeon utilizing the laparoscope. The abdominal wall is discussed in its entirety, rather than with a limited focus on inguinal anatomy. Anatomic terms for which synonyms and eponyms are commonly used are listed in Table 51.1. Specific anatomic nomenclature can now be found in *Terminologia Anatomica*, the successor to *Nomina Anatomica*.

The abdominal wall spans the prodigious gap between the lower ribs and the pelvis; the lowest ribs, pelvic brim, and lumbar spine comprise its only skeletal support. The muscular and aponeurotic structures that provide much of the integrity of the wall must not only compress and con-

Table 51.1. ANATOMIC TERMS WITH COMMON SYNONYMS AND EPONYMS

FASCIAL STRUCTURES/SPACES
Fatty layer of superficial fascia; panniculus adiposus; Camper's fascia
Investing fascia of external abdominal oblique; fascia innominata
Membranous layer of superficial fascia; Scarpa's fascia
Retroinguinal space; space of Bogros
Retropubic space; space of Retzius

LIGAMENTOUS STRUCTURES
Iliopectineal ligament; iliopectineal arch
Iliopubic tract; Thompson's ligament (band)
Inguinal ligament; Poupart's ligament
Lacunar ligament; Gimbernat's ligament
Pectineal ligament; Cooper's ligament

APONEUROSIS-DERIVED STRUCTURES
Arcuate line; semicircular line; linea semicirculars; line of Douglas
Falx inguinalis (often incorrectly referred to as conjoined tendon)
Reflected inguinal ligament; reflex ligament; Colles' ligament
Semilunar line; linea semilunaris; Spigelius' line

tain abdominal viscera, but also contribute to the support and movement of the spine and pelvis.

The sheets of relatively thin muscles and aponeuroses that make up the abdominal wall would, individually, seem to predispose to visceral eventration. The lamination of most of the wall precludes this in most cases. The most common sites of hernia formation are found between laminations, where only peritoneum and fascia are found between the viscera and skin. These weak areas are most important to the hernia surgeon and will be described in detail in the subsequent sections dealing with the anterior and posterolateral abdominal wall and the inguinal region.

Anterior Abdominal Wall

Superficial Fascia, Vessels, and Nerves

The anterior abdominal wall does not consist solely of muscle and aponeurosis; it can also be the repository for copious amounts of adipose tissue (panniculus adiposus) in its superficial fascial layer, often called *Camper's fascia*. This layer, which is continuous inferiorly with the outer layer of fascia covering the perineum and genitalia, also contains the dartos muscle fibers of the scrotum. The major blood vessels of the superficial fatty layer are the superficial epigastric vessels and superficial circumflex iliac vessels, which are tributaries of the femoral vessels. The superficial fascia is also replete with lymphatic vessels that drain into the inguinal lymph nodes inferior to the umbilicus. The lymphatic structures cross the inguinal ligament,

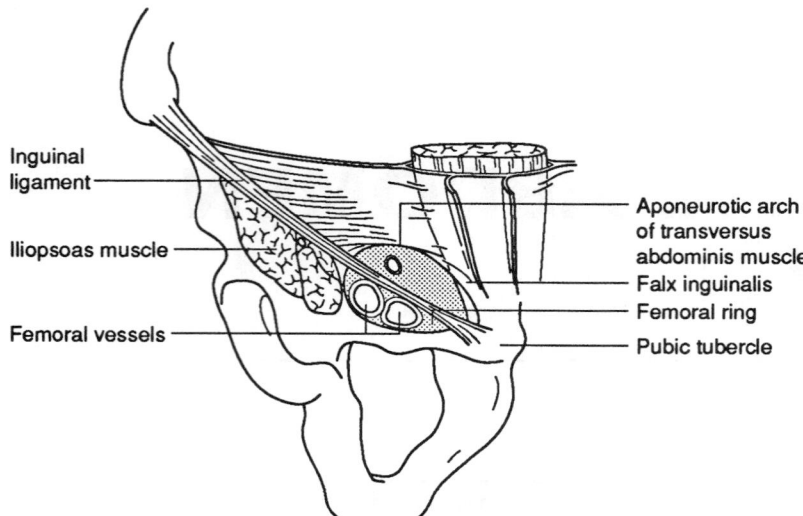

Inguinal ligament

Iliopsoas muscle

Femoral vessels

Aponeurotic arch of transversus abdominis muscle

Falx inguinalis

Femoral ring

Pubic tubercle

Figure 51.1. The myopectineal orifice. Superior to the inguinal ligament, this area includes the inguinal (Hesselbach's) triangle. Inferior to the ligament, the orifice transmits the iliopsoas muscle, the femoral nerve and vessels, and the femoral canal and sheath. (From Wantz GE. *Atlas of hernia surgery.* New York: Raven Press, 1991: 4–5, with permission.)

so that they are potentially placed in the surgical field during open herniorrhaphy (2–6).

A second fascial layer in the superficial abdominal wall is the deep fascia of Scarpa. Although most commonly considered a distinct anatomic layer, Scarpa's fascia actually consists of compressed fibrous components of the superficial fascia (7). The deeper fibrous tissue of the superficial fascia forms the fundiform ligament of the penis (suspensory ligament of the female clitoris), continues onto the penis and scrotum, and ultimately fuses with the superficial fascia of the perineum.

The superficial fascia also fuses with the layer of fascia (fascia innominata) investing the external abdominal oblique muscle. This fascia is bound inferiorly to the inguinal ligament and pubis before continuing onto the thigh, where it blends with the fascia lata to seal the space beneath and inferior to the inguinal ligament, which is the inferior portion of the myopectineal orifice (Fig. 51.1). This portion of the inguinal region includes Hesselbach's (inguinal) triangle superiorly and therefore constitutes the weakest aspect of the groin.

The skin of the anterior abdominal wall is segmentally innervated in the familiar dermatome pattern. The nerve branches to this area are derived from the anterior and lateral cutaneous branches of the ventral rami of the seventh to 12th intercostal nerves, and from the ventral rami of the first and second lumbar nerves. Disruption of one of these nerves is rarely noted by the postoperative patient because the dermatome fields overlap significantly. The anterior and lateral cutaneous branches reach the subcutaneous layer by coursing between the flat lateral muscles and by piercing the sheath of the rectus abdominis.

Anterior Musculature and Ligaments

The division of the wall into anterior and posterior segments is somewhat artificial because the anterior muscles, with the exception of the rectus abdominis, arise posteriorly and also form part of the posterior wall.

The three muscles of the lateral aspect of the anterior abdominal wall (Fig. 51.2) are composed of a variable amount of muscle with a large aponeurosis. The aponeurosis is the tendon of insertion for the lateral muscles, and it also

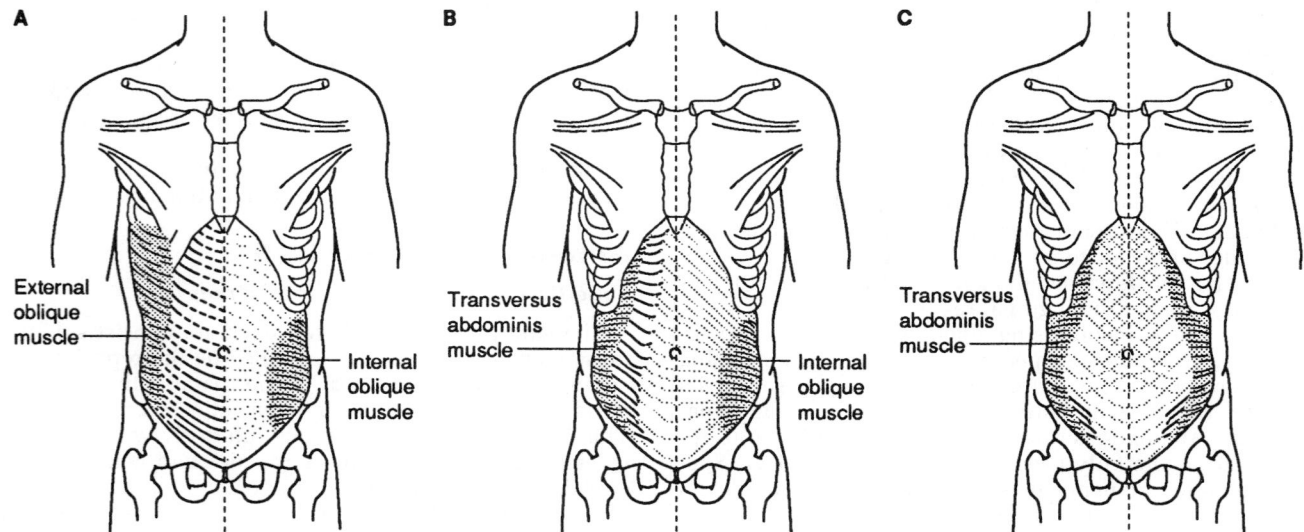

A

External oblique muscle

Internal oblique muscle

B

Transversus abdominis muscle

Internal oblique muscle

C

Transversus abdominis muscle

Figure 51.2. Pattern of crossing of the aponeurotic fascicles of the abdominal wall musculature. *(A)* Fascicles from the right external oblique and anterior lamina of the left internal oblique. *(B)* Fascicles from the right transversus abdominis and posterior lamina of the left internal oblique. *(C)* Fascicles between the right and left transversus abdominis muscles.

forms the sheath of the rectus abdominis. The midline decussation of the three aponeuroses forms the linea alba.

External Abdominal Oblique Muscle and Associated Ligaments

The external abdominal oblique muscle (Figs. 51.2, 51.3A,B) is the most superficial of the three lateral abdominal muscles. The external abdominal oblique arises from the posterior aspects of the lower eight ribs and interdigitates with both the serratus anterior and the latissimus dorsi at its origin. The direction of the muscle fibers varies from nearly horizontal in its upper portion to oblique in the middle and lower portions. The mostly horizontal fibers, which originate posteriorly, insert onto

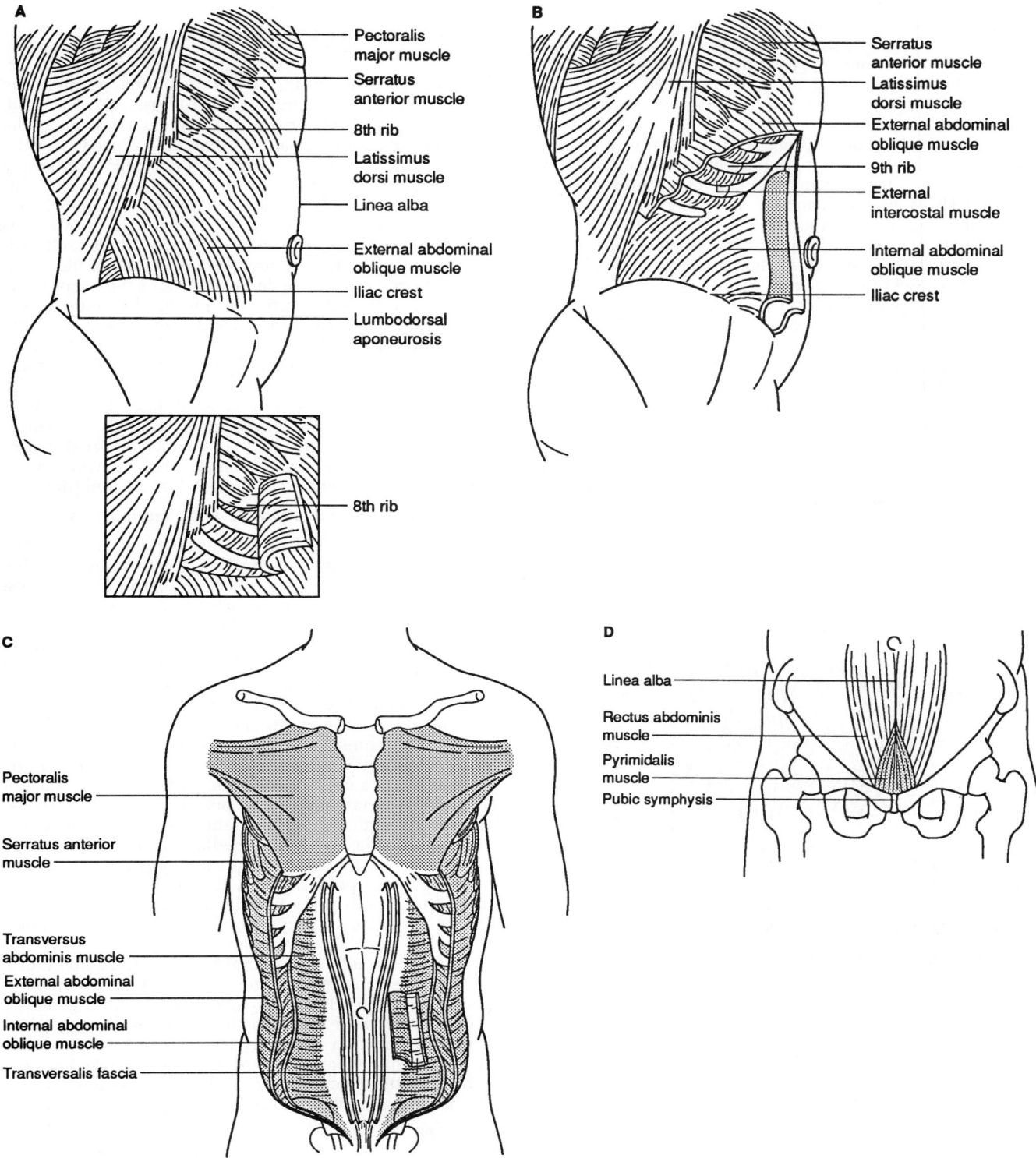

Figure 51.3. *(A)* External oblique muscle and aponeurosis. *(B)* Internal oblique muscle and aponeurosis. *(C)* Transversus abdominis muscle and aponeurosis. *(D)* Lower rectus abdominis and pyramidalis muscle. The linea alba is formed by the intermeshed fibers of the aponeuroses of the lateral muscle layers; it is tensed by the pyramidalis, which inserts into it.

the anterior portion of the iliac crest. The obliquely arranged anteroinferior fibers of insertion fold upon themselves to form the inguinal ligament. The remaining portion of the aponeurosis inserts into the linea alba after contributing to the anterior portion of the rectus abdominis sheath. Some fibers cross the linea alba to reinforce further the anterior rectus sheath of the opposite side.

The more medial fibers of the aponeurosis of the external oblique divide into a medial and a lateral crus to form the external or superficial inguinal ring. The spermatic cord (or round ligament) and branches of the ilioinguinal and genitofemoral nerves pass through this opening. The superolateral portion of the ring is reinforced by horizontal intercrural fibers, which presumably prevent spreading of the crural fibers.

The *inguinal ligament* (Fig. 51.4) is worthy of special consideration because of its important role as both a landmark and an integral component of many groin hernia repairs. The inguinal ligament is formed by obliquely oriented anteroinferior aponeurotic fibers of the external abdominal oblique. The ligament is formed when the aponeurosis folds beneath itself. Its lateral attachment is to the anterior superior iliac crest; its medial insertion is primarily on the pubic tubercle. The ligament is better described as an inferiorly directed arc rather than as a taut cord. This is in part a consequence of the connection of the ligament to the overlying investing fascia of the external abdominal oblique and the subsequent attachment of this tissue to the fascia lata of the thigh. The inguinal ligament bridges the muscular and vascular structures to leave the pelvis inferiorly (with the exception of those components contained in the spermatic cord). The area deep to the inguinal ligament and just above the inguinal ligament, including the inguinal (Hesselbach's) triangle, is often called the *myopectineal orifice* (Fig. 51.1).

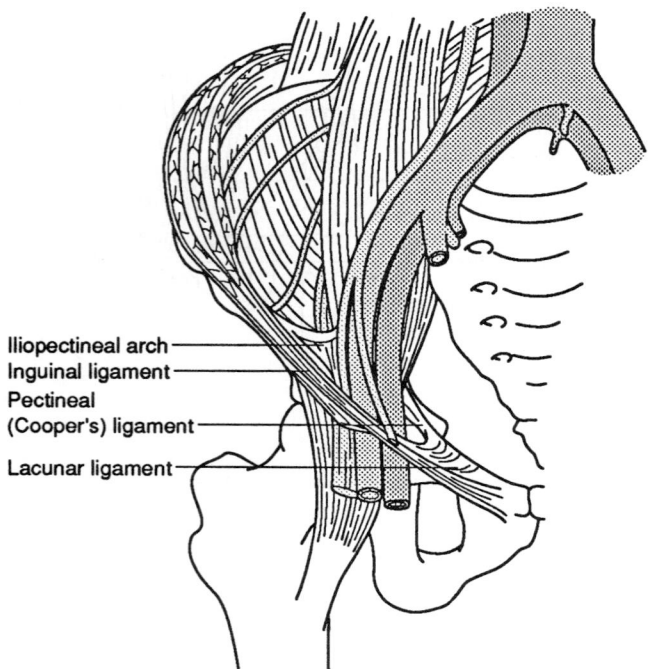

Iliopectineal arch
Inguinal ligament
Pectineal
(Cooper's) ligament
Lacunar ligament

Figure 51.4. Ligamentous structures of the inguinal region. The iliopubic tract is not seen in this view because it is obscured by the inguinal ligament. The lacunar ligament is the expanded medial end of the inguinal ligament; on the pecten pubis, it blends with the inguinal (Cooper's) ligament.

The medial insertion of the inguinal ligament in most persons is dual. One portion runs along the superior surface of the pubic tubercle and symphysis to form (or at least reinforce) the superior pubic ligament. The other portion is fan-shaped and spans the distance between the inguinal ligament proper and the pectineal line of the pubis. This fan-shaped portion of the ligament is called the *lacunar ligament* (Fig. 51.4). It blends laterally with the pectineal (Cooper's) ligament.

Internal Abdominal Oblique Muscle and Aponeurosis

The middle layer of the lateral abdominal group is the internal abdominal oblique muscle (Figs. 51.2, 51.3B,C). This muscle primarily arises from the iliac fascia along the iliac crest and forms a band of iliac fascia fused with the inguinal ligament. The uppermost fibers course obliquely toward the distal ends of the lower three or four ("floating") ribs. The muscle fibers of the internal oblique fan out following the shape of the iliac crest, so that the lowermost fibers are directed inferiorly. These fibers arch over the round ligament, or spermatic cord. Some of the lower muscle bundles in the male join fibers of the transversus abdominis to form the cremaster muscle. The aponeurosis of the internal oblique (Fig. 51.5A) above the level of the umbilicus splits to envelop the rectus abdominis, re-forming in the midline to join and interweave with the fibers of the linea alba. Below the level of the umbilicus (Fig. 51.5B), the aponeurosis does not split, but rather runs anterior to the rectus muscle, continues medially as a single sheet, joins the anterior rectus sheath, and finally contributes to the linea alba. The aponeurotic portion of the internal oblique is widest at the level of the umbilicus.

Transversus Abdominis Muscle and Aponeurosis

The transversus abdominis muscle (Figs. 51.2, 51.3C) arises from the fascia along the iliac crest and inguinal ligament and from the lower six costal cartilages and ribs, where it interdigitates with the lateral diaphragmatic fibers. The muscle bundles of the transversus abdominis for the most part run horizontally. The lower medial fibers, however, may continue in a more inferomedial course toward the site of insertion on the crest and pecten of the pubis.

The aponeurosis of the transversus abdominis joins the posterior lamina of the internal abdominal oblique, forming above the umbilicus a portion of the posterior rectus sheath. Below the umbilicus, the transversus abdominis aponeurosis is a component of the anterior rectus sheath. The gradual termination of aponeurotic tissue on the posterior aspect of the rectus abdominis forms the arcuate line (of Douglas) (Fig. 51.6). The medial aponeurotic fibers of the transversus abdominis insert on the pecten pubis and the crest of the pubis to form the falx inguinalis. These fibers infrequently are joined by a portion of the internal oblique aponeurosis; only then is a true conjoined tendon formed (8).

The arch formed by the termination of the aponeurotic fibers of the transversus abdominis is called the *aponeurotic arch* (Fig. 51.6). The area beneath the arch varies. A high arch may be a predisposing factor in direct inguinal hernia. Contraction of the transversus abdominis causes the arch to move down toward the inguinal ligament in a kind of shutter mechanism, which reinforces the weakest area of the groin when intraabdominal pressure is raised.

Rectus Abdominis

The rectus abdominis (Figs. 51.3D, 51.5) forms the central and anchoring muscle mass of the anterior abdomen. The rectus muscle arises from the fifth to the seventh costal cartilages and inserts on the pubic symphysis and

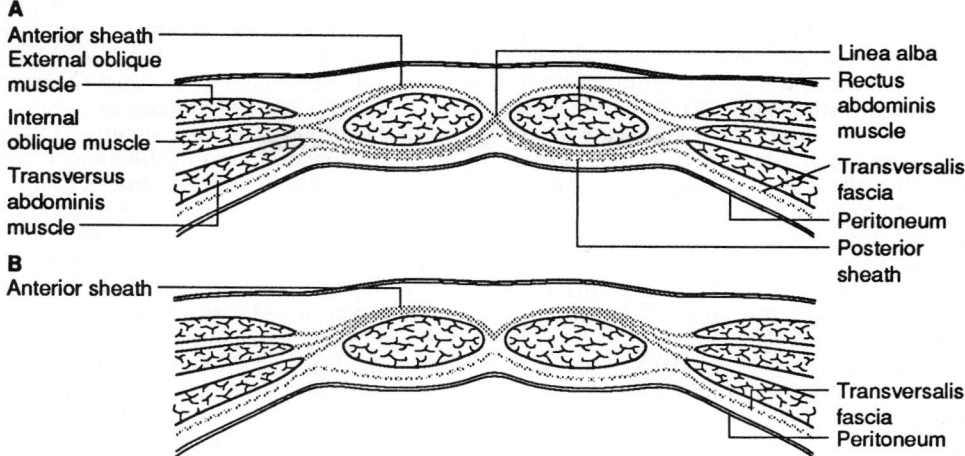

A

Anterior sheath
External oblique muscle
Internal oblique muscle
Transversus abdominis muscle

Linea alba
Rectus abdominis muscle
Transversalis fascia
Peritoneum
Posterior sheath

B

Anterior sheath

Transversalis fascia
Peritoneum

Figure 51.5. *(A)* Immediately superior to the umbilicus, the rectus sheath consists of anterior and posterior components. The anterior sheath is composed of the aponeuroses of the external and internal abdominal oblique muscles, and the posterior sheath consists of the posterior aponeurotic lamina of the internal oblique and the aponeurosis of the transversus abdominis muscle. *(B)* The rectus sheath inferior to the arcuate line (of Douglas) consists of an anterior portion made up of fibers from all aponeurotic layers; the posterior portion at this point comprises only transversalis fascia covered internally by peritoneum.

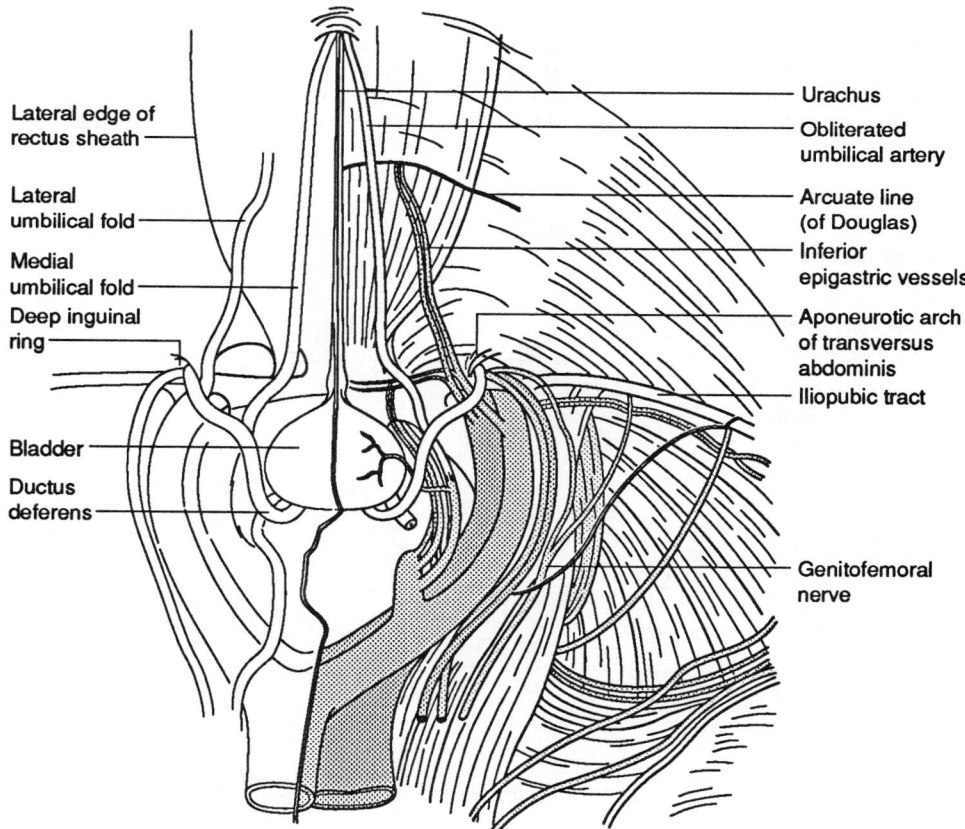

Lateral edge of rectus sheath
Lateral umbilical fold
Medial umbilical fold
Deep inguinal ring
Bladder
Ductus deferens

Urachus
Obliterated umbilical artery
Arcuate line (of Douglas)
Inferior epigastric vessels
Aponeurotic arch of transversus abdominis
Iliopubic tract

Genitofemoral nerve

Figure 51.6. The deep inguinal region, pelvis, and anterior abdominal wall from the viewpoint of a surgeon using a laparoscopic technique. The anterior wall folds upward approximately at the iliopubic tract in this illustration.

pubic crest. Each rectus muscle is segmented by tendinous intersections at the levels of the xiphoid process and the umbilicus, and at a point midway between these two. The principal blood supply reaches the muscle from the superior and inferior epigastric arteries (Fig. 51.5), which anastomose just superior to the umbilicus. Other vessels are anterior branches of the intercostal arteries; these reach the muscle by entering the lateral aspect of the rectus sheath. The innervation of the muscle is from the seventh to the 12th intercostal nerves, which laterally pierce the aponeurotic sheath of the muscle. The lateral edge of the muscle is demarcated by a slight depression in the aponeurotic fibers coursing toward the muscle; this depression is the *semilunar line*.

The small pyramidalis muscle (Fig. 51.3D) accompanies the rectus abdominis at its origin in a minority of people. The pyramidalis arises from the pubic symphysis. It lies within the rectus sheath and tapers to attach to the linea alba, the conjunction of the two rectus sheaths and the major site of insertion of three aponeuroses from all three lateral muscle layers.

Rectus Sheath

Although the components of the rectus sheath individually have been discussed in relation to the three lateral abdominal muscles, it should also be considered as a distinct entity. Three features of the rectus muscle and its sheath can be observed even topographically in well-muscled or very thin subjects: (a) The semilunar line is a slight depression in the aponeurotic fibers corresponding to the lateral edge of the rectus muscle. It marks the site of initial lateral insertion of the aponeurotic tendons of the lateral abdominal muscles. (b) The tendinous inscriptions divide each muscle into three parts (9). These are the basis of the expression "six pack," popularized by bodybuilders. (c) The linea alba is the midline confluence of the aponeuroses of the rectus muscles and also the internal and external oblique muscles.

The composition of the rectus sheath varies depending on the level sampled. The anterior sheath superior to the umbilicus is composed of the aponeurosis of the external abdominal oblique and the anterior lamina of the internal abdominal oblique. The transversalis aponeurosis does not participate in the formation of the anterior sheath at this level. At a variable level inferior to the umbilicus, the anterior sheath is a composite of all the aponeurotic layers.

The posterior sheath of the rectus muscle superior to the umbilicus is a lamination of the posterior lamina of the aponeurosis of the internal abdominal oblique and the transversus abdominis aponeurosis. The external abdominal oblique does not participate in the formation of the posterior portion of the rectus sheath. At a highly variable site inferior to the umbilicus, all the aponeurotic tendons pass anteriorly to form the anterior rectus sheath. The fibers of the posterior sheath are seen to attenuate gradually. The aponeurotic fibers do not end abruptly at the arcuate line. This transfer of connective tissue away from the posterior rectus sheath causes the arcuate line (of Douglas) to form on the posterior surface of the muscle (Fig. 51.6). The tissue covering the deep surface of the rectus muscle inferior to the arcuate line is primarily the transversalis fascia.

Some have questioned this traditional scheme of rectus sheath composition, contending that each of the aponeurotic layers superior to the umbilicus is actually bifid, with both contributing to the anterior and posterior sheaths (10). The fibers of the posterior sheath are seen to attenuate

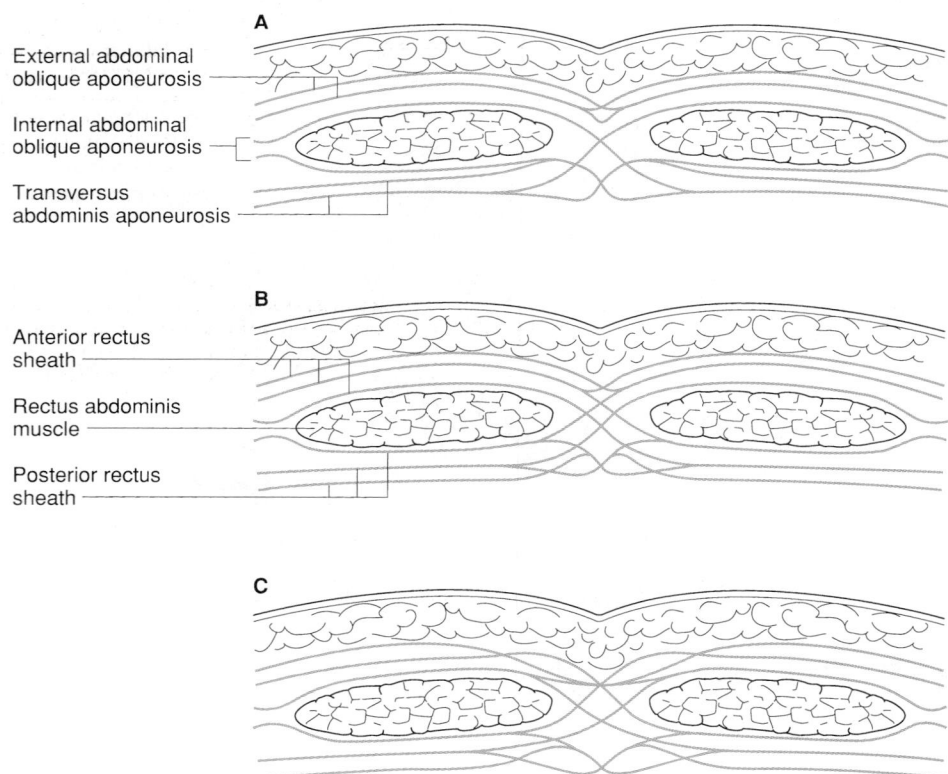

Figure 51.7. Patterns of midline decussation of the aponeuroses. *(A)* Single anterior and posterior lines of decussation. *(B)* Single anterior and triple posterior lines of decussation. *(C)* Triple anterior and posterior lines of decussation. (After Askar O. Surgical anatomy of the aponeurotic expansions of the anterior abdominal wall. *Ann R Coll Surg Engl* 1977;59:313, with permission.)

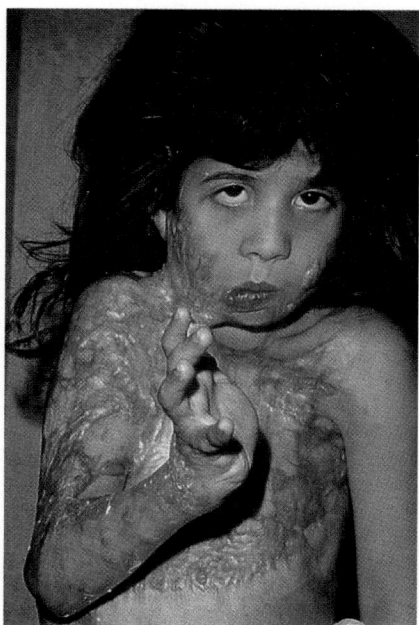

Color Figure 12.1. Suboptimal management of small burns can have major adverse functional and cosmetic implications.

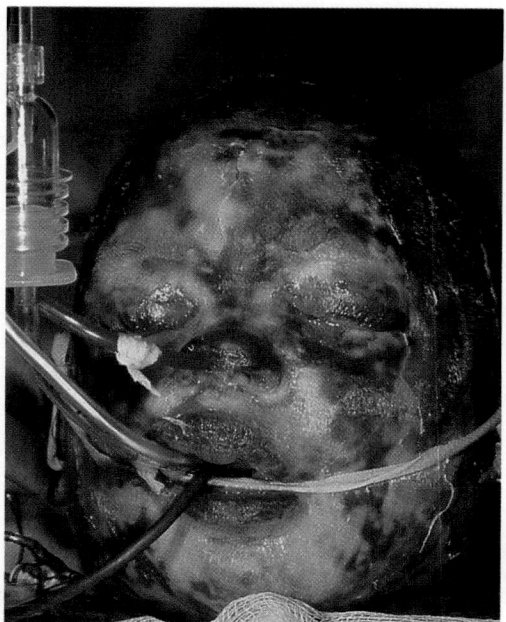

Color Figure 12.2. Endotracheal tube security is of the utmost importance during the first few postburn days, because airway edema can result in significant difficulty when one is attempting to reinsert displaced endotracheal tubes. Secure airway control is facilitated by the use of umbilical ties, rather than adhesive tape, to anchor endotracheal tubes.

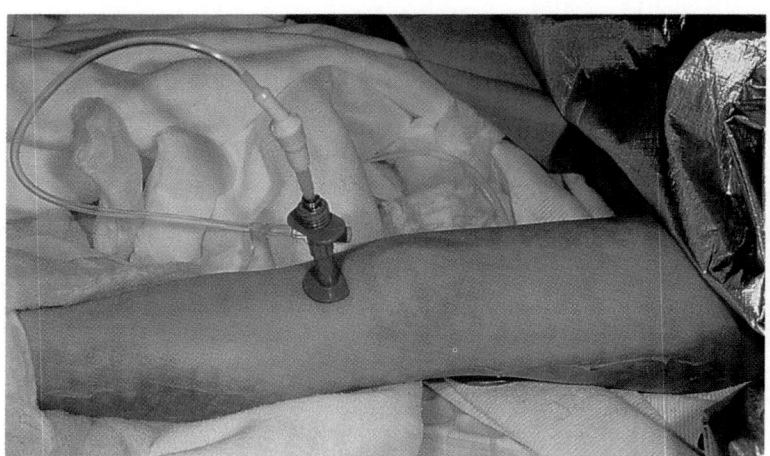

Color Figure 12.3. Intraosseous infusion can be life-saving in children in whom vascular access cannot be promptly achieved.

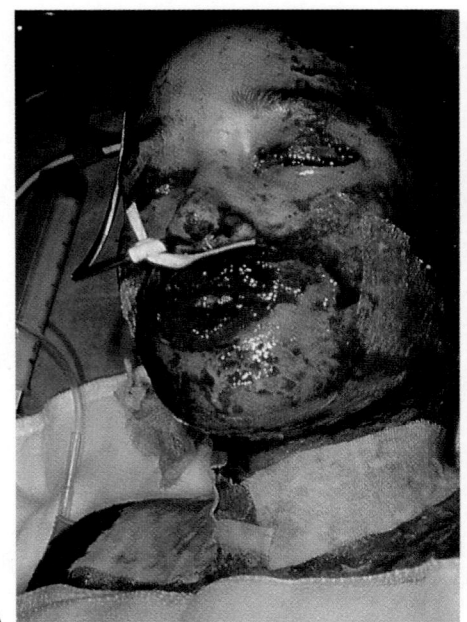
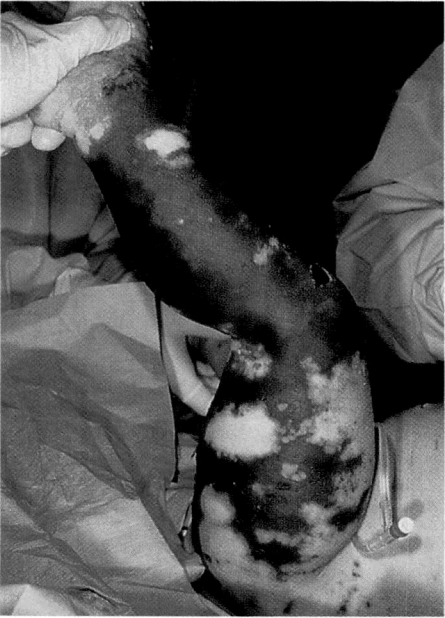

Color Figure 12.4. *(A)* Toxic epidermal necrolysis is a severe variant of erythema multiform. When there is major mucous membrane involvement, as in this patient, it is described as Stevens-Johnson syndrome. *(B)* Purpura fulminans describes a syndrome in which extensive soft tissue necrosis results from transient protein C or protein S deficiency complicating meningococcal sepsis.

A
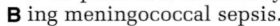B

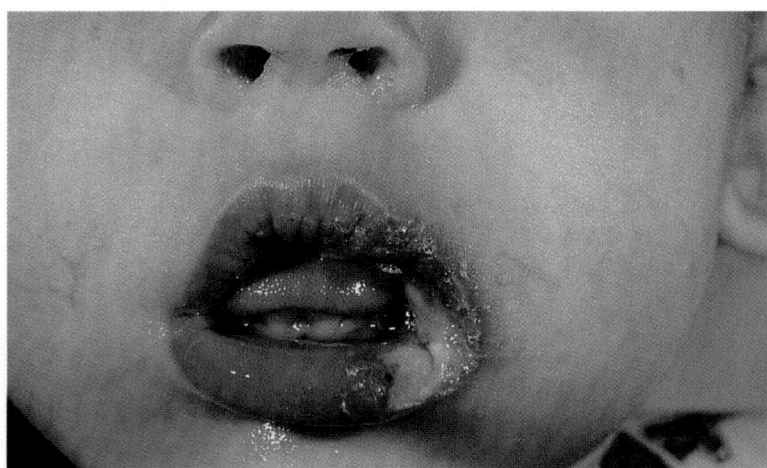

Color Figure 12.5. Low- and intermediate-voltage injuries can be locally destructive, as in this child who suffered a 110-volt commissure burn to the mouth by biting the cord of an electrical appliance. These injuries are rarely associated with serious systemic sequelae.

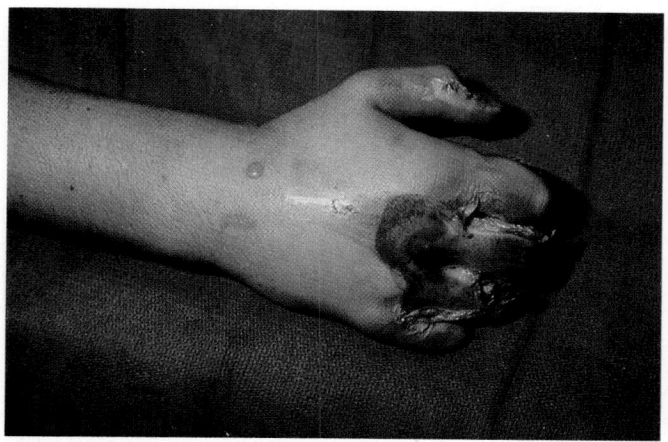
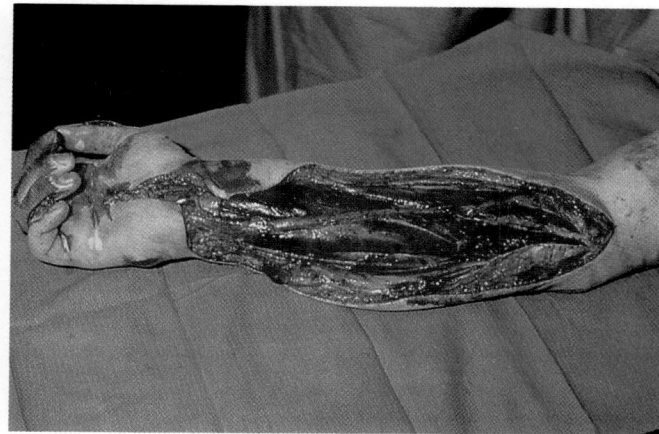

A

B

Color Figure 12.6 *(A)* This patient made contact with a 20,000-volt power line, resulting in a locally destructive entrance wound and occult muscle injury in the proximal extremity, leading to a compartment syndrome. *(B)* Prompt fasciotomy of the forearm and hand prevented the development of an additional ischemic injury secondary to high intracompartmental pressures.

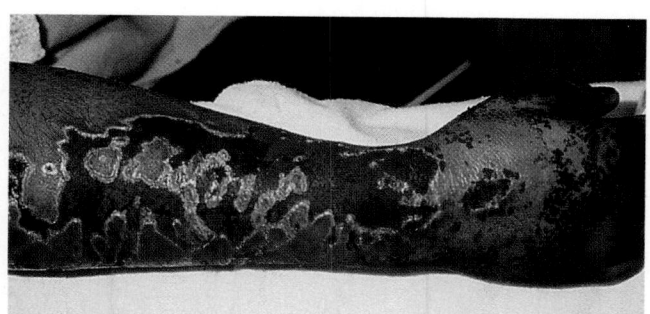

Color Figure 12.7. Chemical burns are often deeper than they appear on initial examination, as in this patient who suffered a sulfuric acid splash injury. Copious irrigation remains the mainstay of initial therapy.

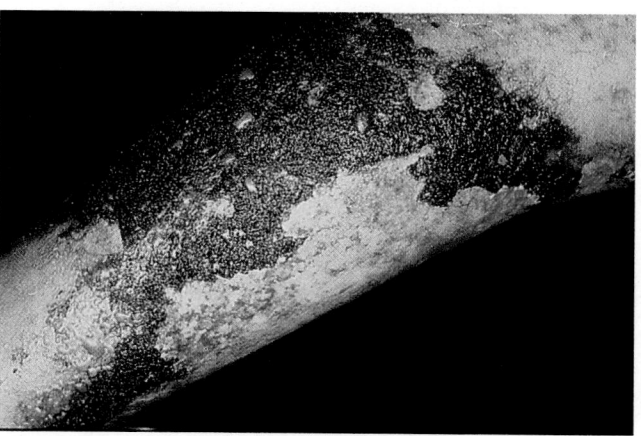

Color Figure 12.8. Tar burns are managed with initial cooling irrigation followed by later tar removal. In this patient, residual tar is being removed after softening in a lipophyllic solvent. Such burns are usually deep and generally require resurfacing.

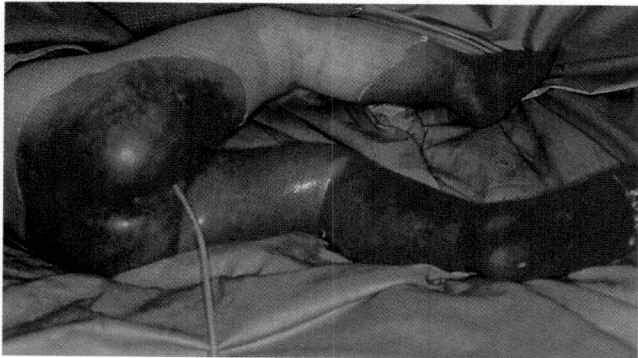

Color Figure 12.9. This child's wound is consistent with an intentional immersion in scalding water, demonstrating both flexor sparing and sharply defined margins around a deep burn of uniform depth.

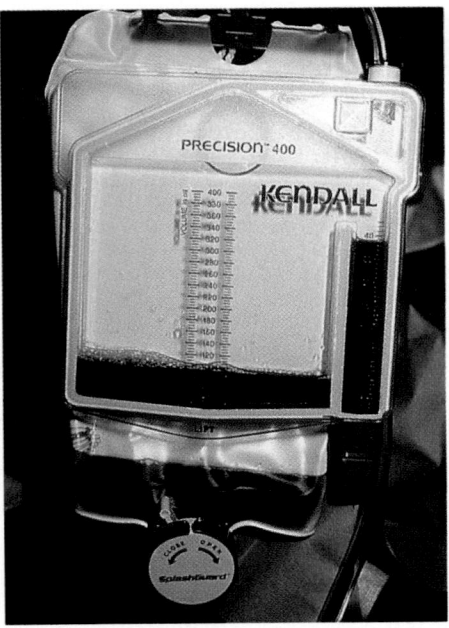

Color Figure 12.10. Heavily pigmented urine must be cleared of hemochromogens to avoid acute tubular necrosis.

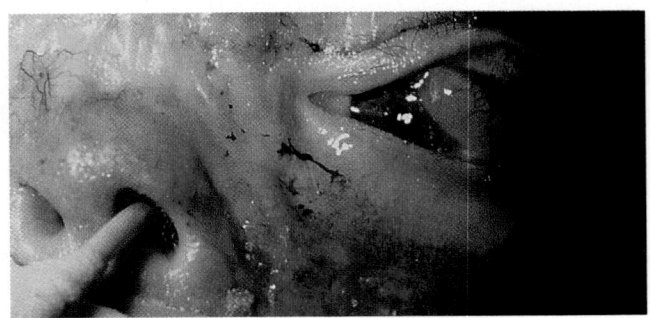

Color Figure 12.11. Contracture of burned ocular adnexae results in exposure and desiccation of the globe. When ocular lubrication is inadequate, lid release is mandatory.

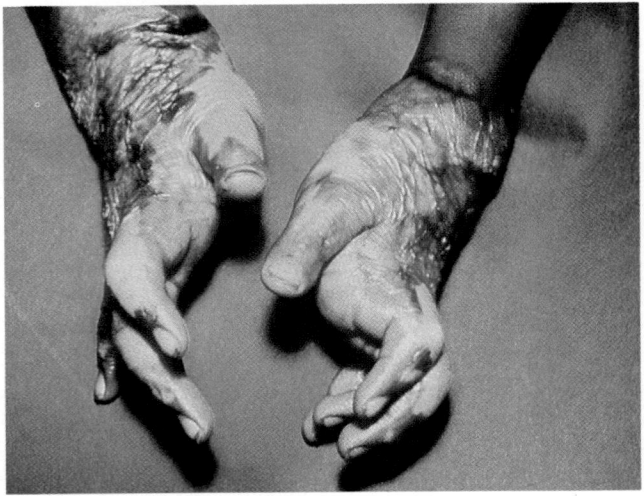

Color Figure 12.12. Spontaneous healing of deep dermal hand burns can result in a poor functional result.

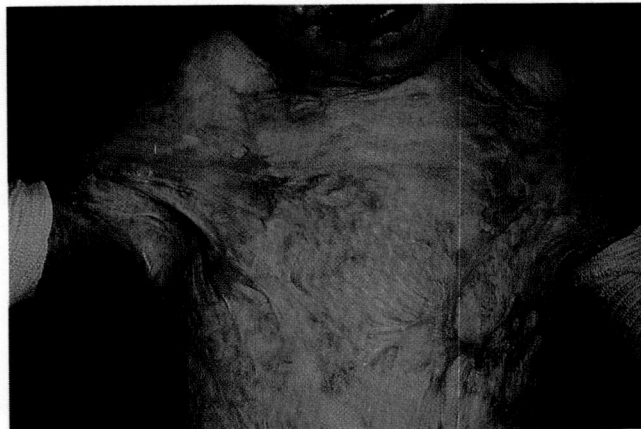

Color Figure 12.13. Hypertrophic scar formation has major adverse functional and cosmetic implications.

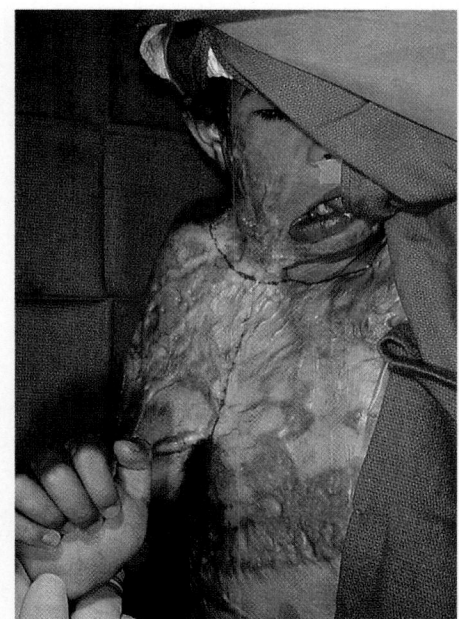

A

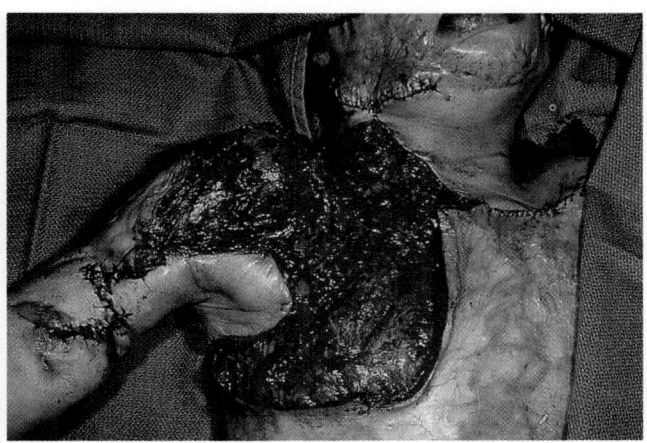

B

Color Figure 12.14. Prompt release and autografting is indicated when hypertrophic scar formation threatens to limit function.

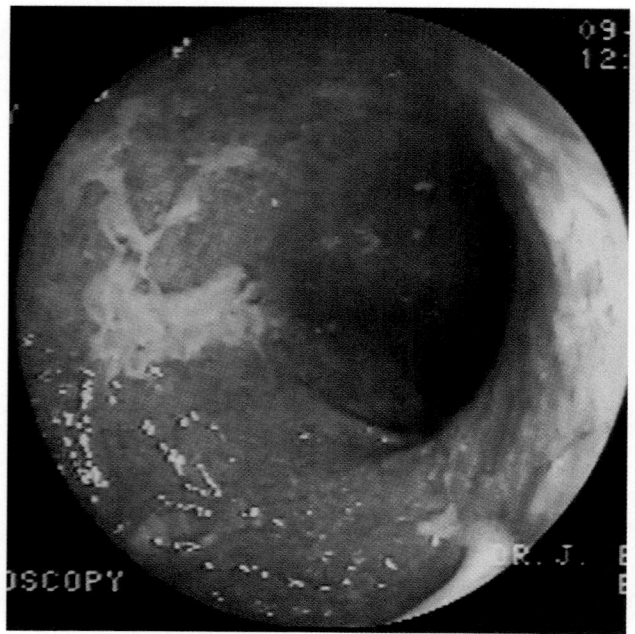

Color Figure 44.1. Endoscopic appearance of the rectum in a patient with mild ulcerative colitis, with mucosal granularity and loss of the normal vascular pattern.

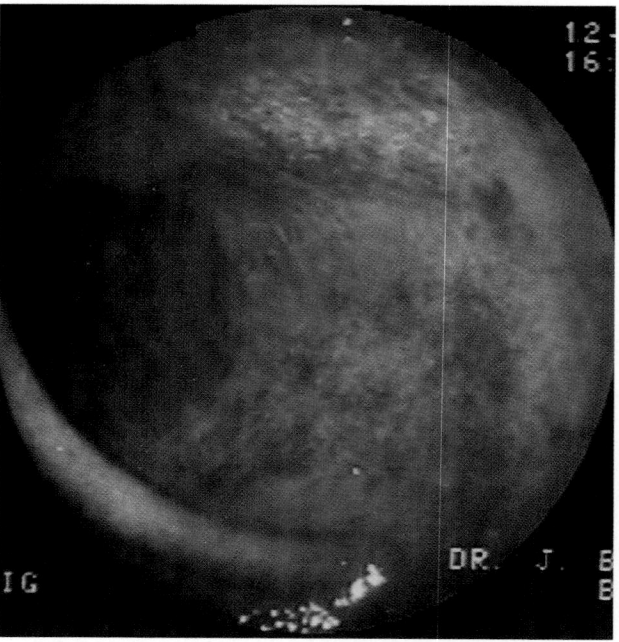

Color Figure 44.2. Endoscopic appearance of the rectum in a patient with moderate ulcerative colitis, with pitted mucosa and spontaneous hemorrhage.

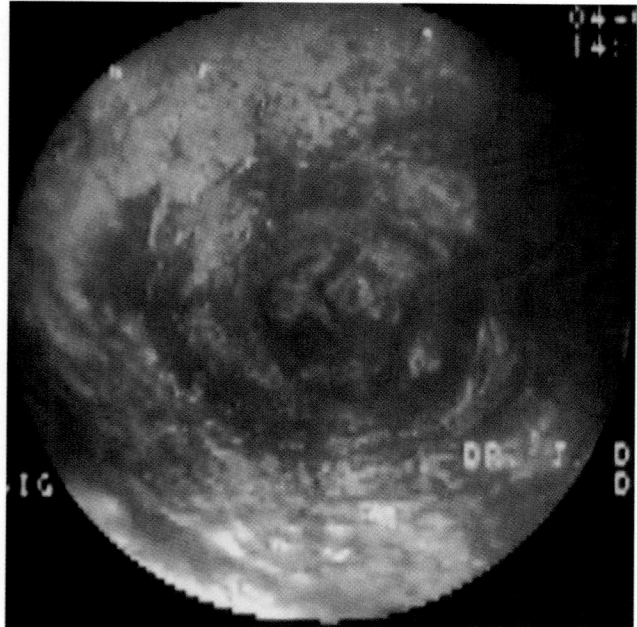

Color Figure 44.3. Endoscopic appearance of the rectum in a patient with severe ulcerative colitis, with frank ulceration, bleeding, and a purulent exudate.

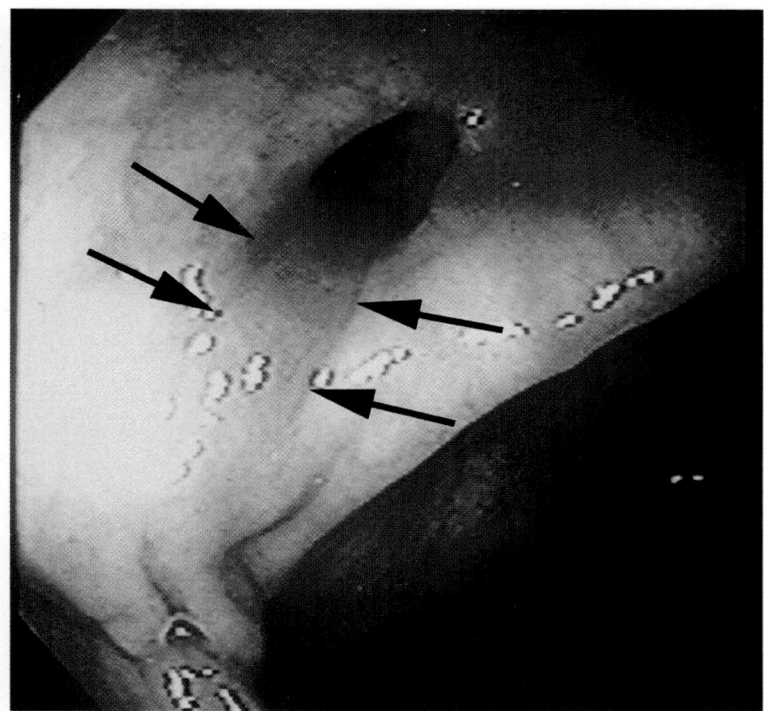

Color Figure 49.1. Colonoscopic view of a colonic diverticulum. A vas rectum is seen entering the diverticulum and forming one of the walls.

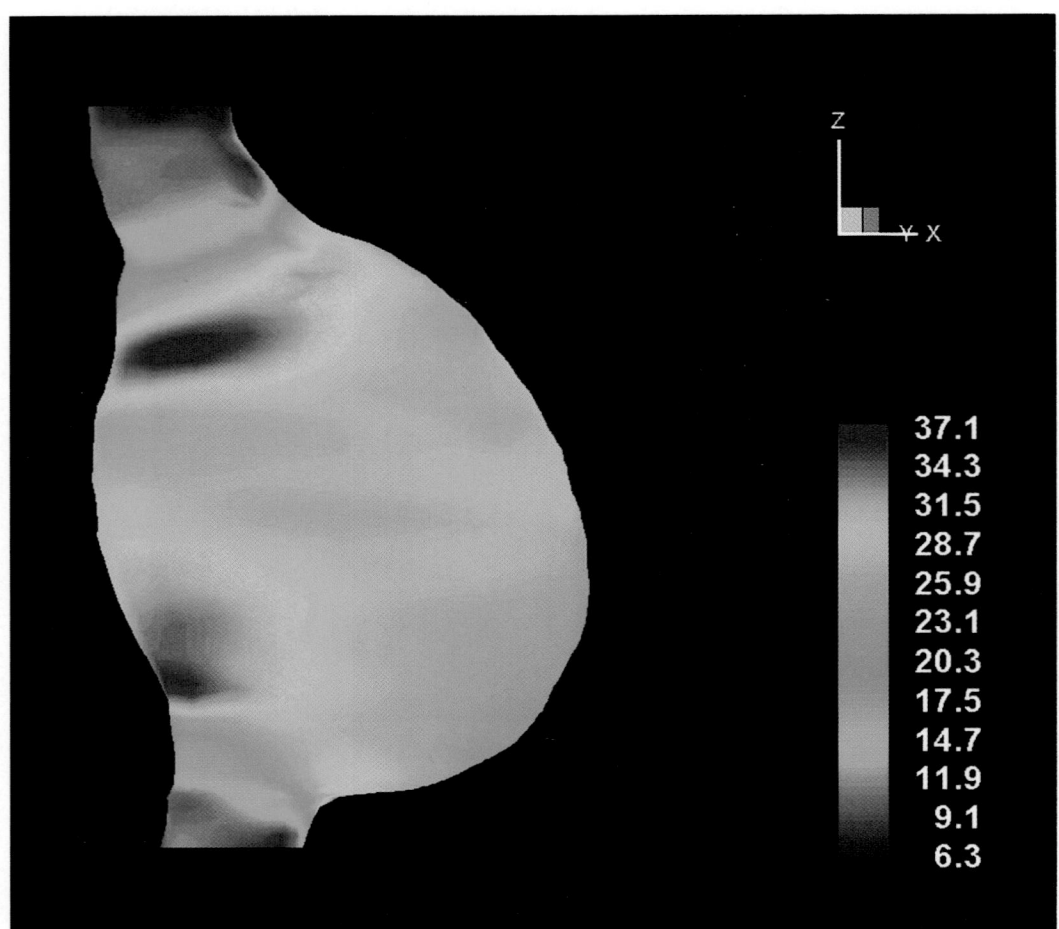

Color Figure 70.1. Wall stress distribution in an actual abdominal aortic aneurysm. *Colors* represent levels of tensile stress within the aortic wall at that location (correlation of color and stress level is displayed in the *bar* on the right). A three-dimensional reconstruction of the aneurysm was generated from computed tomographic data and transformed into the wall stress distribution by means of finite element analysis and the patient's blood pressure values (see text). This is a lateral view (see three-dimensional framework, upper right). Note that the highest levels of stress are not at the maximal diameter but along the posterolateral wall, where ruptures most commonly occur in clinical experience and autopsy series. Thus, stresses induced by the shape of the abdominal aortic aneurysm appear to be at least as important as the stresses induced by diameter alone.

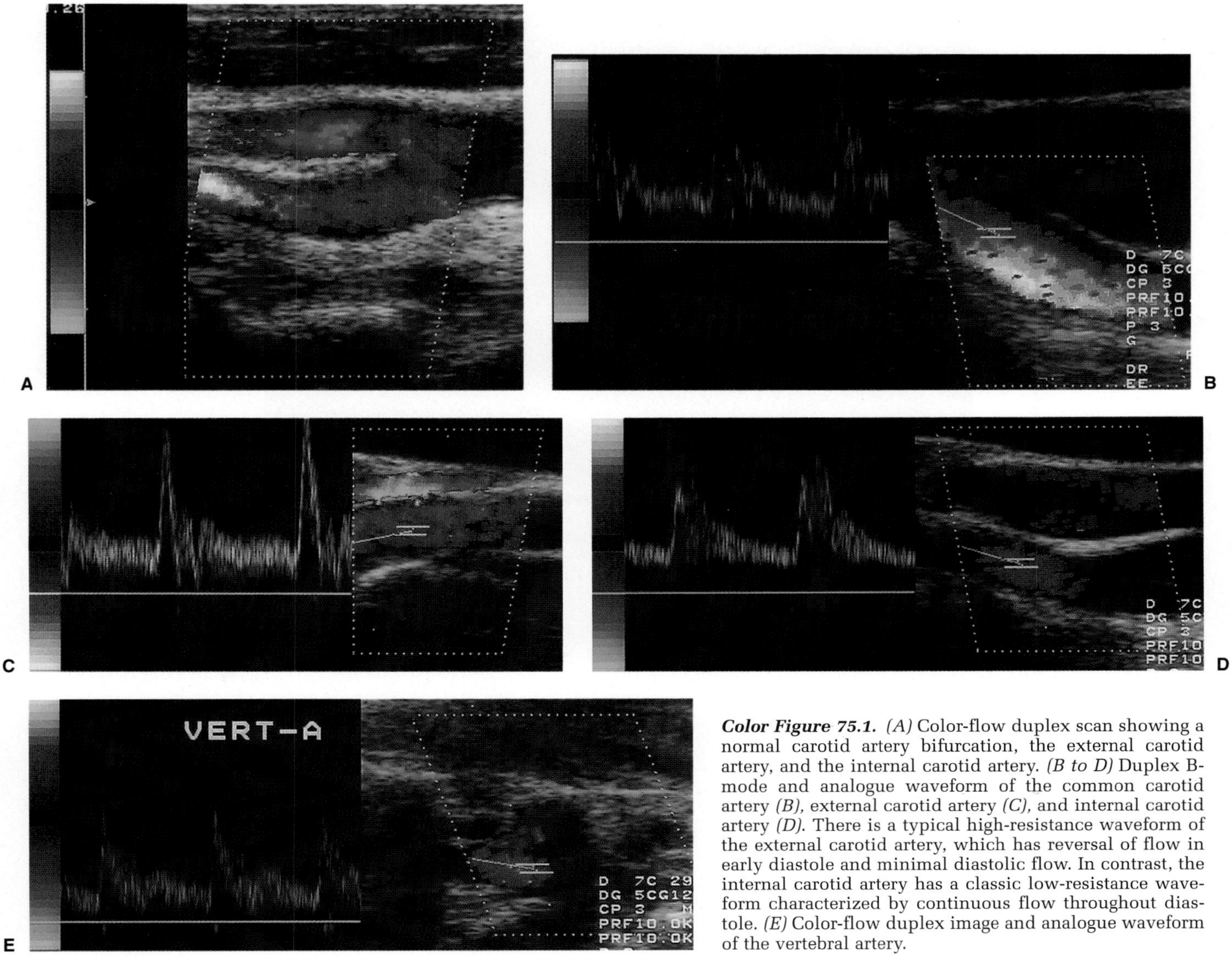

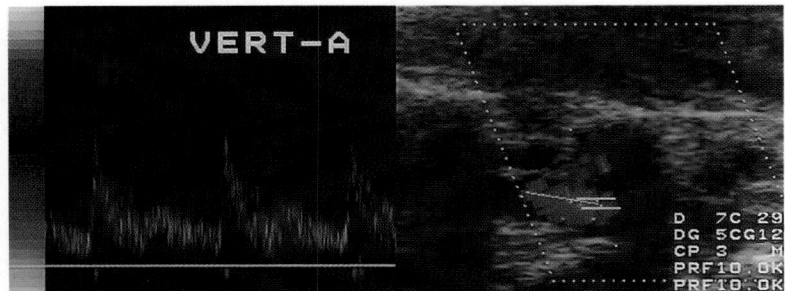

Color Figure 75.1. *(A)* Color-flow duplex scan showing a normal carotid artery bifurcation, the external carotid artery, and the internal carotid artery. *(B to D)* Duplex B-mode and analogue waveform of the common carotid artery *(B)*, external carotid artery *(C)*, and internal carotid artery *(D)*. There is a typical high-resistance waveform of the external carotid artery, which has reversal of flow in early diastole and minimal diastolic flow. In contrast, the internal carotid artery has a classic low-resistance waveform characterized by continuous flow throughout diastole. *(E)* Color-flow duplex image and analogue waveform of the vertebral artery.

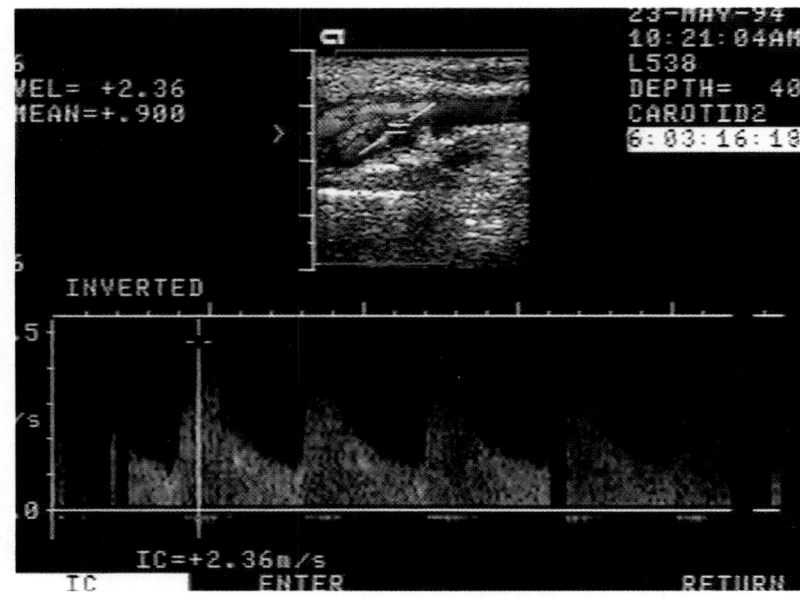

Color Figure 75.2. Color-flow duplex scan and analogue waveform of a high-grade internal carotid artery stenosis. Note acoustic shadowing in the region of the stenosis caused by calcification of the artery wall. Doppler taken at midstream of the jet of flow through the stenosis shows marked elevation of the peak systolic velocity (236 cm/s).

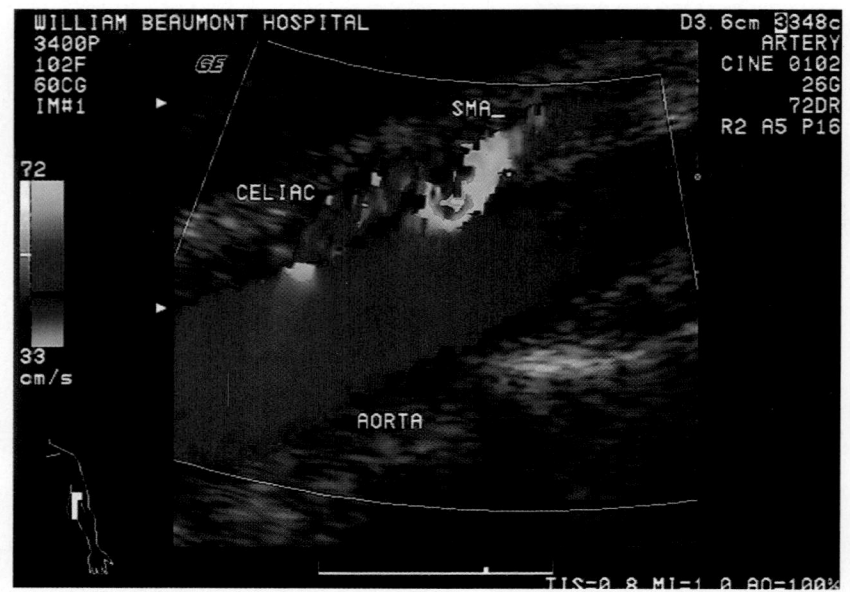

Color Figure 77.1. Color-flow Doppler scanning allows rapid identification of flow disturbances. (Courtesy of Dr. Phillip Bendick, William Beaumont Hospital, Royal Oak, MI.)

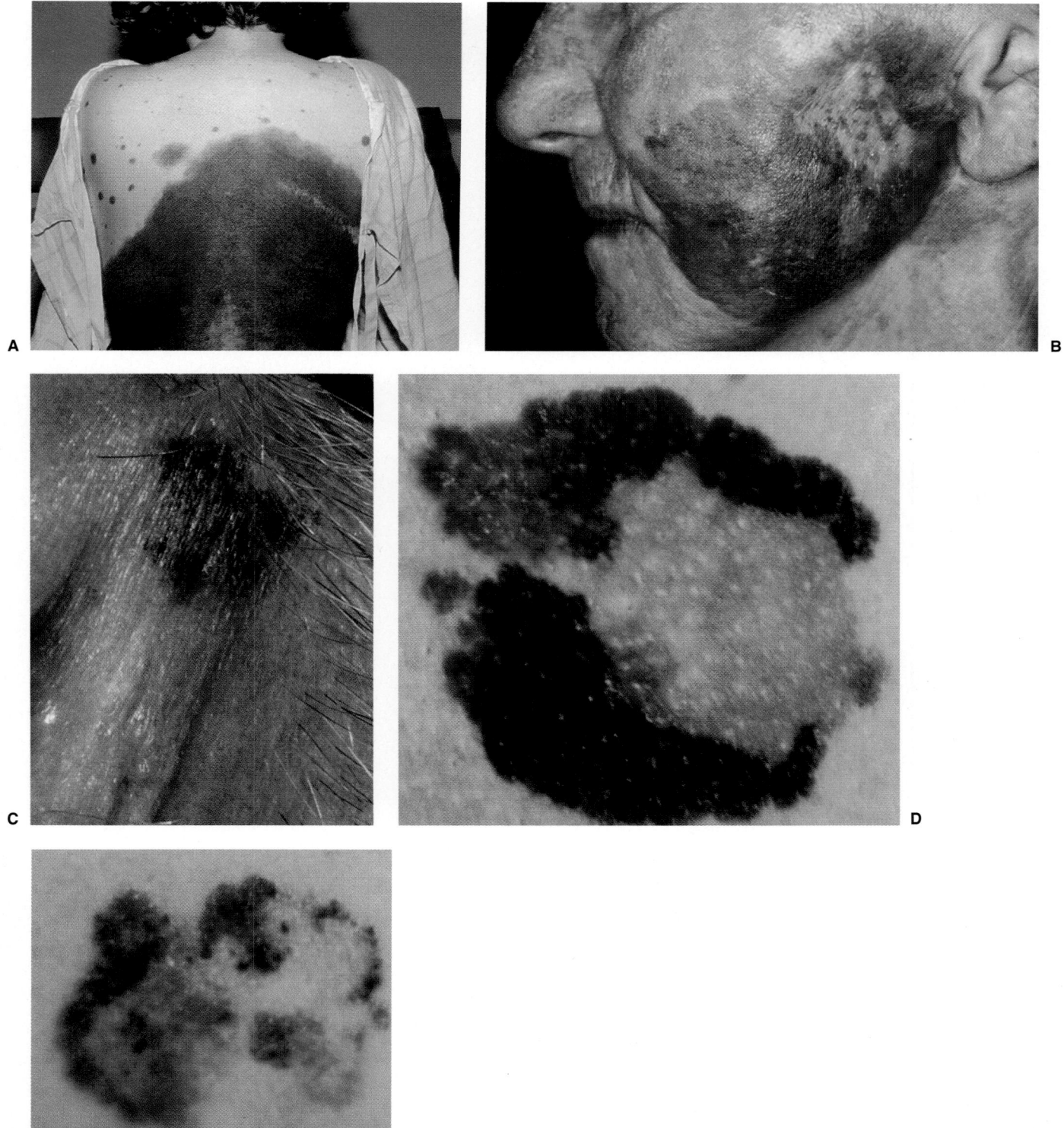

Color Figure 105.1. Examples of skin lesions. *(A)* Giant congenital nevus. *(B)* Lentigo maligna (Hutchinson freckle). *(C)* Melanoma arising in a lentigo maligna (lentigo maligna melanoma). *(D and E)* Superficial spreading melanoma. *(continues)*

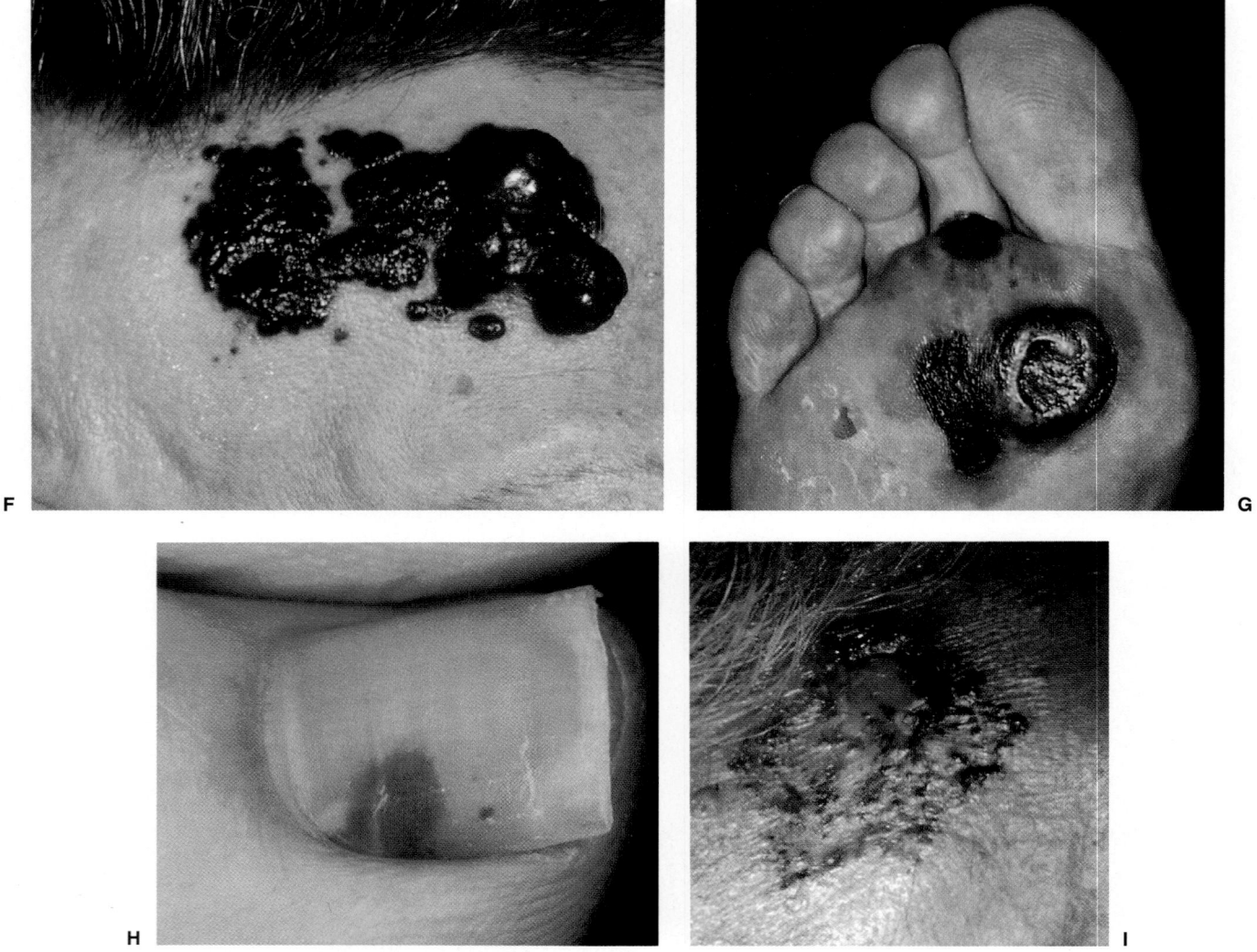

Color Figure 105.1. *(Continued)* *(F)* Nodular melanoma. *(G)* Acral lentiginous melanoma (ulcerated nodular plantar melanoma with satellite lesions). *(H)* Subungual melanoma. *(I)* Pigmented basal cell carcinoma.

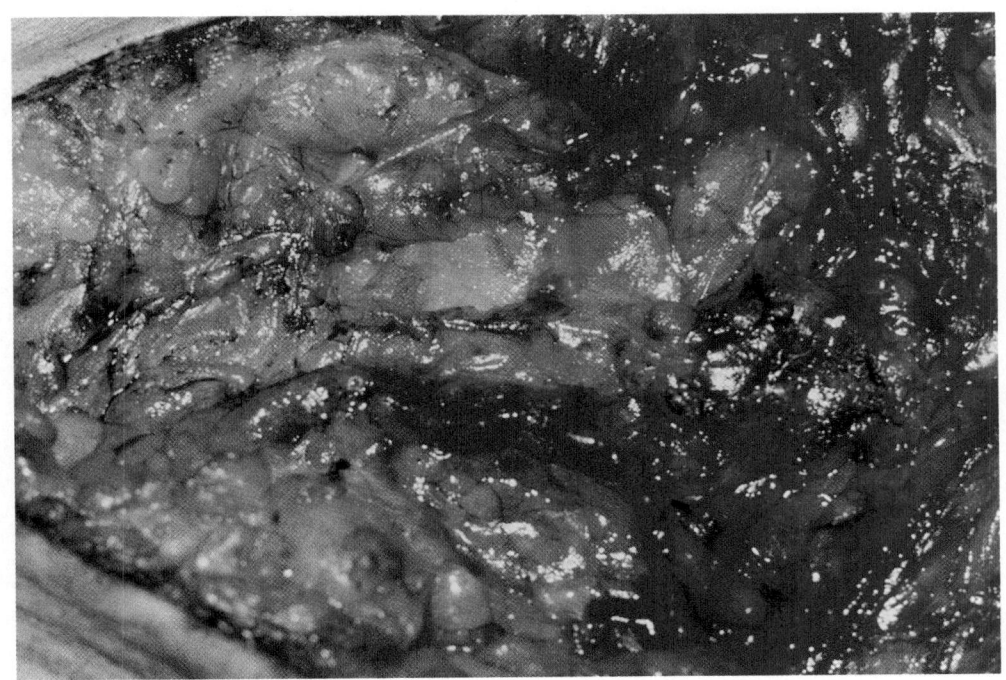

Color Figure 105.2. Blue dye tracking up a lymphatic vessel to a blue-stained lymph node.

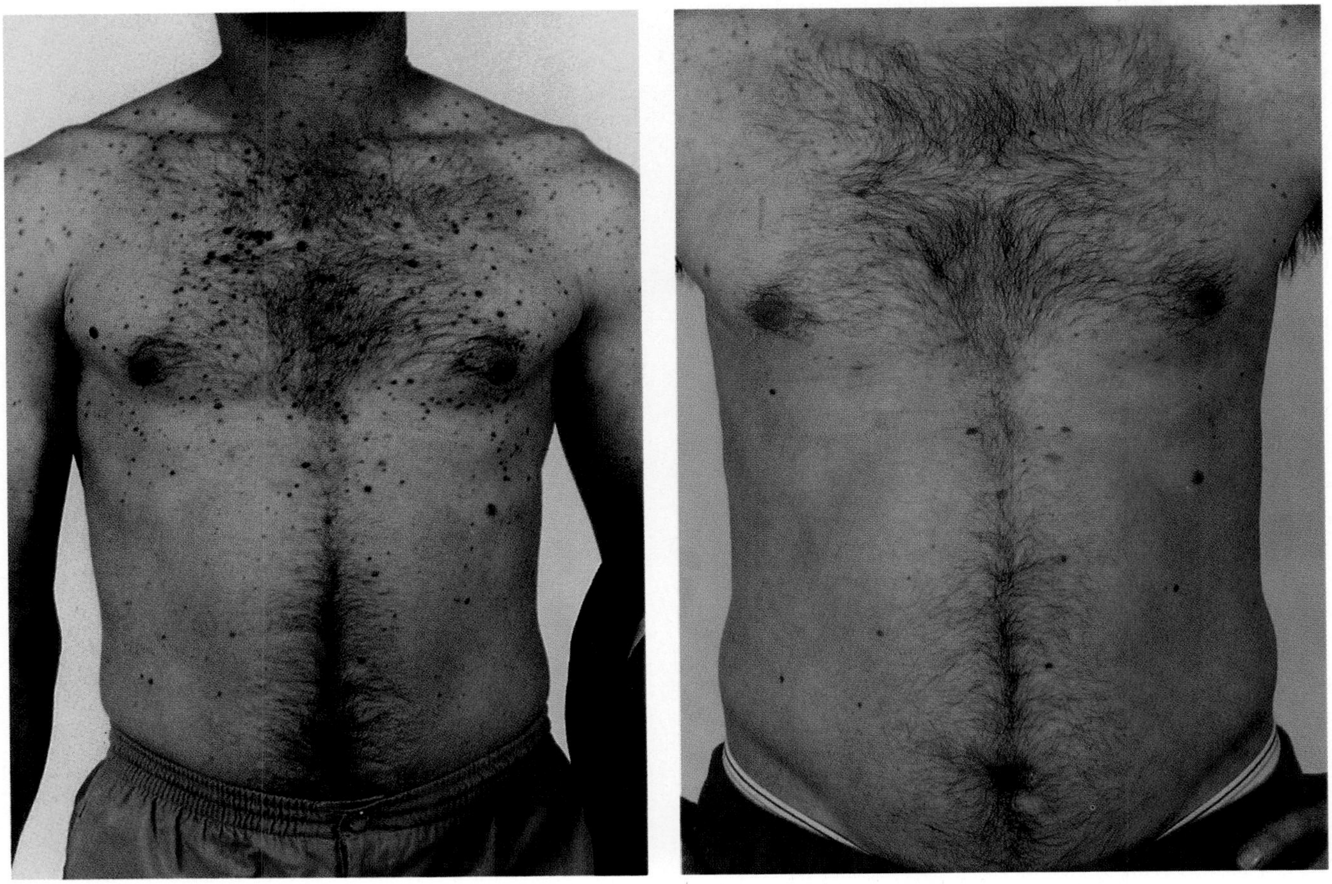

A

B

Color Figure 105.3. *(A)* Patient with disseminated melanoma metastatic to multiple cutaneous sites. *(B)* After several courses of therapy with lymphokine-activated killer cells and interleukin-2, the patient had a complete response. (Courtesy of Steven A. Rosenberg, M.D., Surgery Branch, National Cancer Institute, Bethesda, MD.)

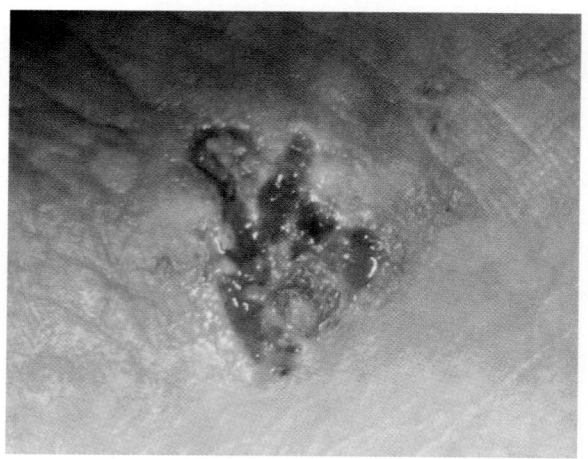

Color Figure 105.4. Squamous cell carcinoma of the hand secondary to exposure to arsenic in welding flux.

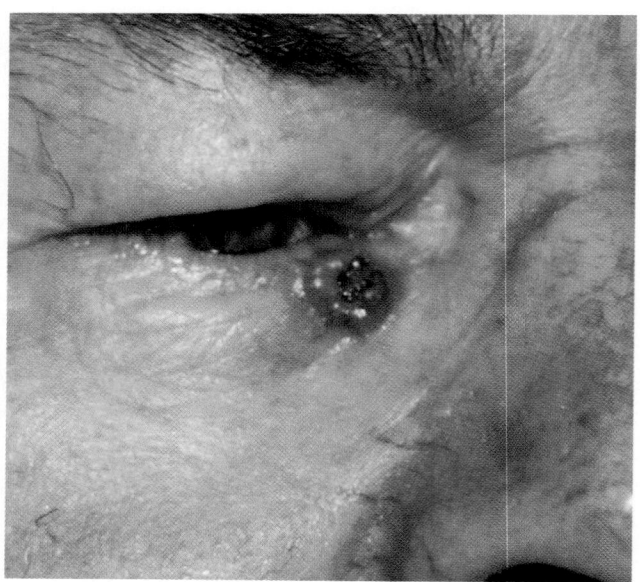

Color Figure 105.5. Basal cell carcinoma near the eye.

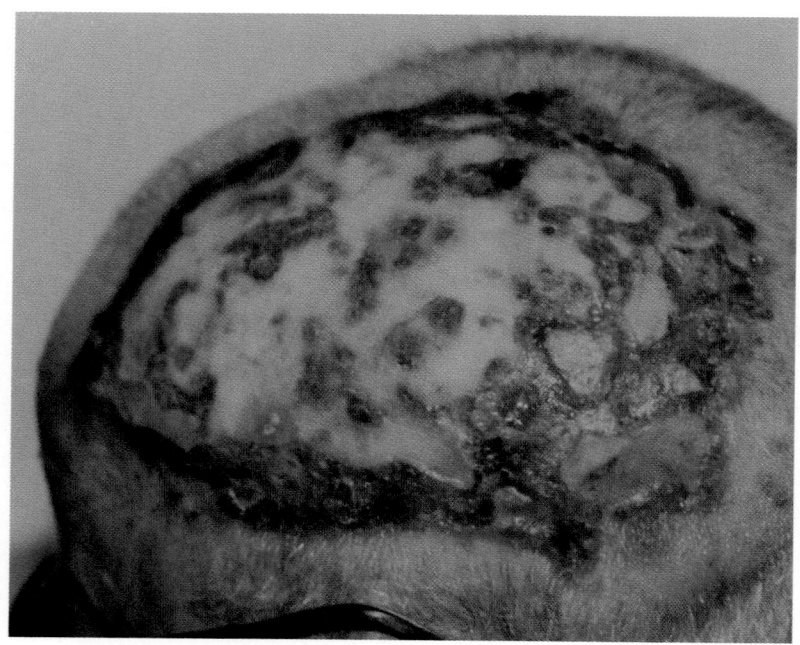

Color Figure 105.6. Morpheaform basal cell carcinoma of the scalp.

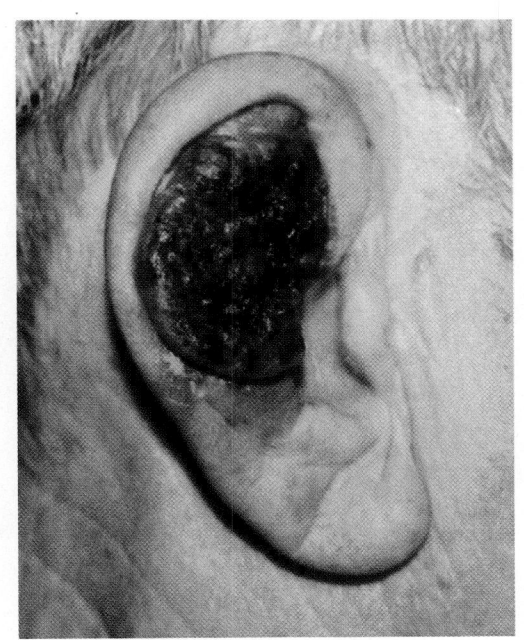

Color Figure 105.7. Ulcerative squamous cell carcinoma.

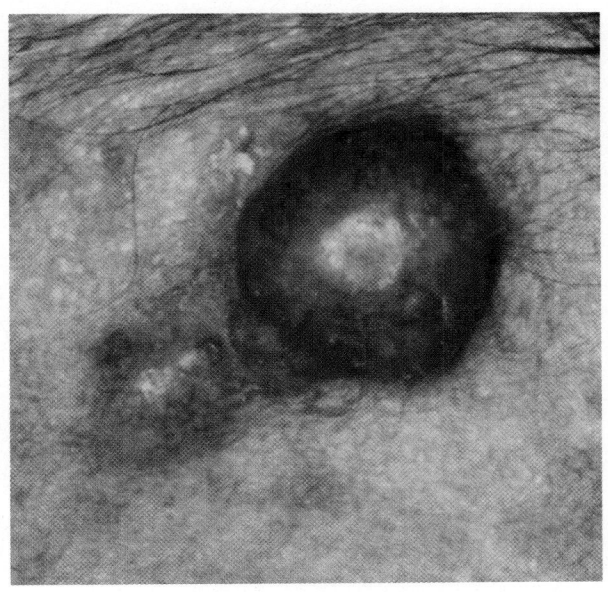

Color Figure 105.8. Merkel cell carcinoma.

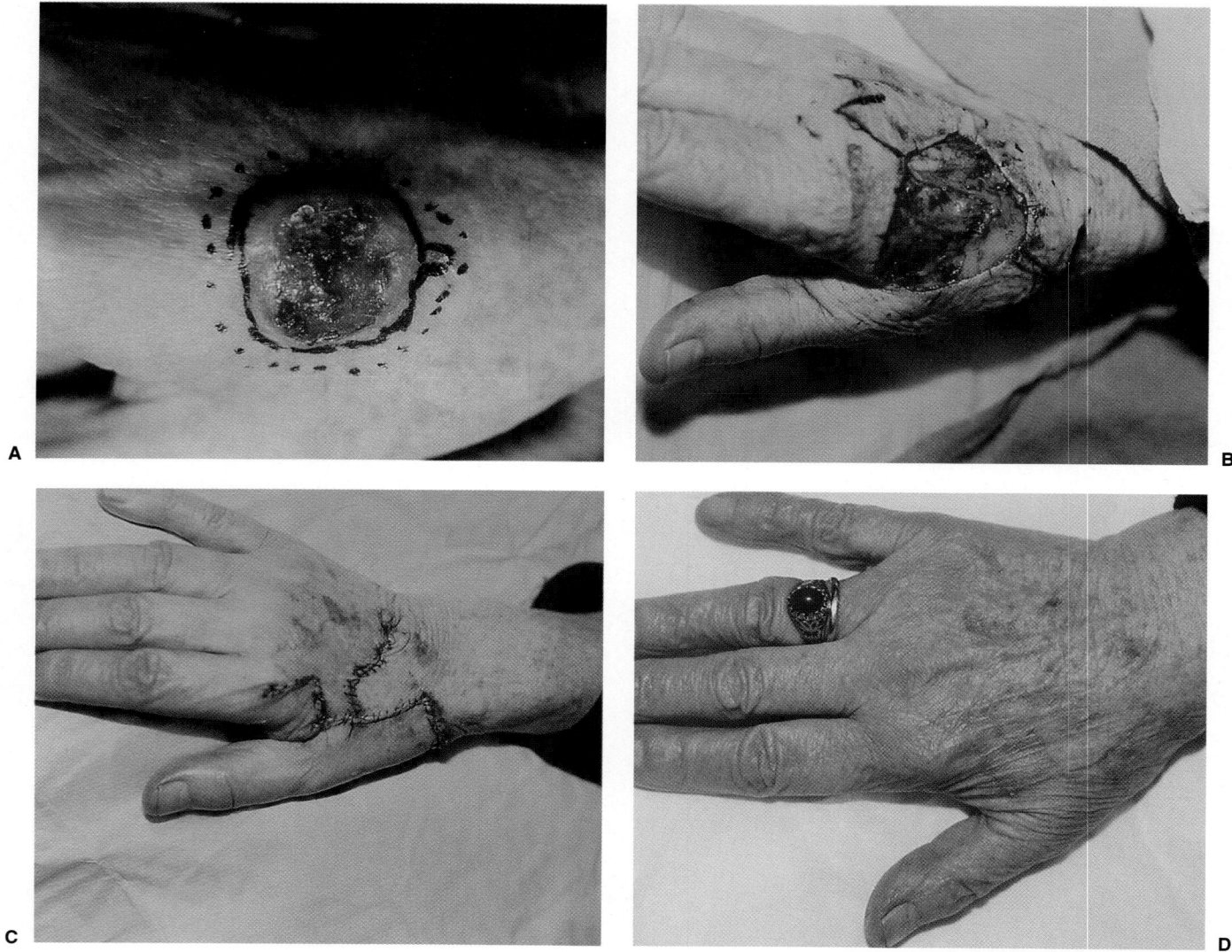

Color Figure 105.9. *(A)* Patient with a 3 × 3-cm basal cell carcinoma on the right dorsal hand with mixed nodular and aggressive growth histologic pattern. *(B)* Final Mohs surgery defect measuring 4 × 4.8 cm to the underlying tendon with preservation of tendon and nerve structures. Complete excision of the tumor required two Mohs stages (10 frozen sections). *(C)* The defect was reconstructed immediately after achievement of clear margins under local anesthesia in the Mohs Surgery Unit using birhombic flap soft tissue reconstruction. *(D)* Result 3 months after surgery.

gradually. The concept of rectus sheath composition favored by most is shown in Fig. 51.7 (11).

Innervation and Blood Supply of the Anterior Abdominal Wall

The innervation of the anterior wall muscles is multiple. The lower intercostal and upper lumbar nerves (T-7 to T-12, L-1, L-2) contribute most of the innervation to the lateral muscles and to the rectus abdominis and overlying skin. The nerves pass anteriorly in a plane between the internal abdominal oblique and the transversus abdominis, eventually piercing the lateral aspect of the rectus sheath to innervate the muscle therein. The external oblique muscle receives branches of the intercostal nerves, which penetrate the internal oblique. The anterior ends of the nerves form part of the cutaneous innervation of the abdominal wall. The first lumbar nerve divides into the ilioinguinal and iliohypogastric nerves. These may divide within the psoas major muscle or between the internal oblique and transversus abdominis muscles. The ilioinguinal nerve may communicate with the iliohypogastric nerve before innervating the internal oblique. The ilioinguinal nerve then passes through the external inguinal ring to run with the spermatic cord, whereas the iliohypogastric nerve pierces the external oblique to innervate the skin above the pubis. The cremaster muscle fibers, which are derived from the internal oblique muscle, are innervated by the genitofemoral nerve (L-1, L-2).

The blood supply of the lateral muscles of the anterior wall is primarily from the lower three or four intercostal arteries, the deep circumflex iliac artery, and the lumbar arteries. The rectus abdominis has a complicated blood supply derived from the superior epigastric artery (a terminal branch of the internal thoracic, or internal mammary, artery), the inferior epigastric artery (a branch of the external iliac artery), and the lower intercostal arteries. The latter arteries enter the sides of the muscle after traveling between the oblique muscles. The superior and inferior epigastric arteries enter the rectus sheath and anastomose near the umbilicus.

Posterolateral (Lumbar) Abdominal Wall

The posterolateral or lumbar portion of the abdominal wall (Fig. 51.8) often is overlooked in discussions of abdominal hernia, perhaps because of the much more common occurrence of groin and femoral hernias. The configuration of the muscle layers in the lumbar area also predisposes to hernia formation. For the purposes of this discussion, the lumbar portion of the abdominal wall is defined as the area bounded superiorly by the 12th rib, inferiorly by the iliac crest, and medially by the erector spinae group. Eight muscles arrayed in three layers constitute the posterolateral or lumbar portion of the abdominal wall.

The most superficial layer is composed of the external abdominal oblique muscle, which arises from the posteroinferior portion of the lower ribs and inserts in part along the posterior iliac crest. Closely associated with the external oblique in this area is the latissimus dorsi, which arises from the posterior iliac crest, the spinous processes of the sacrum and lumbar vertebrae, and the lumbodorsal fascia. The muscle courses obliquely toward its insertion on the medial aspect of the intertubercular groove of the humerus. The triangular space formed by the two muscles just described and the iliac crest is called the *inferior lumbar (Petit's) triangle* (Fig. 51.8A).

The middle layer of lumbar abdominal muscles consists of the erector spinae, the internal abdominal oblique, and the extremely thin insignificant serratus posterior inferior. The erector spinae forms a significant portion of the abdominal wall in the lumbar region, with fibers extending nearly the length of the spinal column. The internal abdominal oblique muscle forms the remainder of the layer. The serratus posterior inferior arises from the lumbodorsal fascia and inserts on the lower four ribs. The middle layer of lumbar muscle is associated with the superior lumbar triangle, a more common site of hernia than the inferior lumbar triangle described above. The superior triangle (Fig. 51.8B) is formed superiorly by the 12th rib, the serratus posterior inferior, and the superior lumbocostal liga-

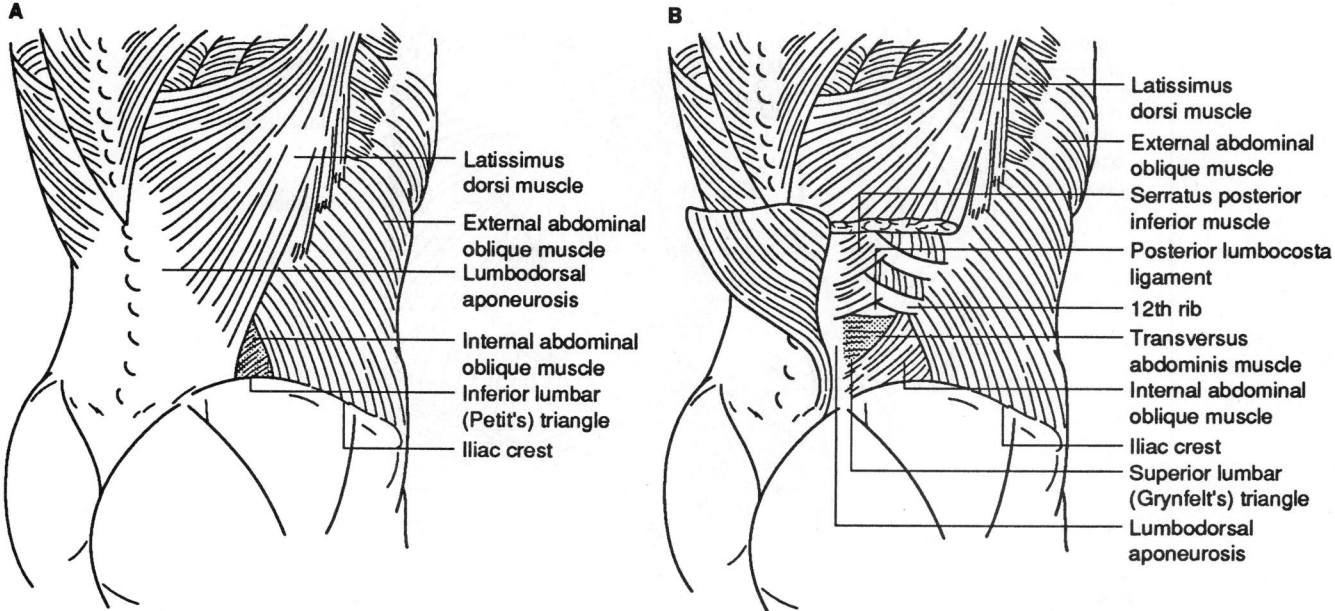

A
— Latissimus dorsi muscle
— External abdominal oblique muscle
— Lumbodorsal aponeurosis
— Internal abdominal oblique muscle
— Inferior lumbar (Petit's) triangle
— Iliac crest

B
— Latissimus dorsi muscle
— External abdominal oblique muscle
— Serratus posterior inferior muscle
— Posterior lumbocosta ligament
— 12th rib
— Transversus abdominis muscle
— Internal abdominal oblique muscle
— Iliac crest
— Superior lumbar (Grynfelt's) triangle
— Lumbodorsal aponeurosis

Figure 51.8. The lumbar abdominal wall with the inferior lumbar triangle *(A)* and the superior lumbar triangle *(B)*.

ment; inferiorly by the upper border of the internal abdominal oblique; and medially by the erector spinae.

The deep layer of the lumbar abdominal wall includes three muscles: the quadratus lumborum, the psoas major, and the transversus abdominis. The quadratus lumborum primarily arises from the posterior iliac crest and inserts on the 12th rib. The psoas major arises from vertebrae T-12 through L-5 and passes beneath the inguinal ligament to insert on the lesser trochanter of the femur.

Deep Inguinal Region

Laparoscopic View

A thorough knowledge of the deep inguinal region and the posterior aspect of the anterior abdominal wall has assumed great importance to a growing number of laparoscopic surgeons who, without the ability to palpate directly, must orient their instruments with only the aid of a two-dimensional image on a monitor. Many who are not accustomed to the unique viewpoint encountered during laparoscopic procedures find the images to be quite disorienting. The area in which anterior wall and groin hernias occur can be easily mastered if several relatively consistent landmarks are noted.

Deep Aspect of the Anterior Abdominal Wall, Peritoneal Folds, and Associated Structures

If one creates a space in the abdominal cavity by distending it with gas, an excellent view of the anterior wall can be obtained. The umbilical peritoneal folds (Fig. 51.9)

in most subjects are very prominent and provide easily identified landmarks. The folds (ligaments) primarily exist because the peritoneum covers underlying structures.

The single median umbilical fold extends from the umbilicus to the urinary bladder and covers the urachus, the fibrous remnant of the fetal allantois. The urachus may be patent for a short distance in adults or may open into the umbilical scar in newborns. The medial umbilical fold is formed by the underlying obliterated portion of the fetal umbilical artery. This normally cordlike structure, like the urachus, may be patent for a portion of its length. Indeed, the proximal, patent portion of the artery normally supplies the superior vesicular arteries to the bladder. The lateral fold covers the inferior epigastric arteries as they course toward the posterior rectus sheath, which they enter approximately at the level of the arcuate line.

Between the median and the medial ligaments, a depression is usually found that is called the *supravesical fossa*. This is the site of hernias of the same name. The fossa formed between the medial and lateral ligaments is the medial fossa; this is the site of direct inguinal hernias. The lateral fossa is less well delineated than the others. The medial border of the fossa is formed by the lateral umbilical ligament and the rectus abdominis. This fossa does not have a lateral border; rather the concavity slowly attenuates. The deep inguinal ring is located in the lateral fossa and therefore is the site of the congenital or indirect inguinal hernia.

Transversalis Fascia

The transversalis fascia (endoabdominal fascia) is perhaps the most commonly misunderstood structure in the

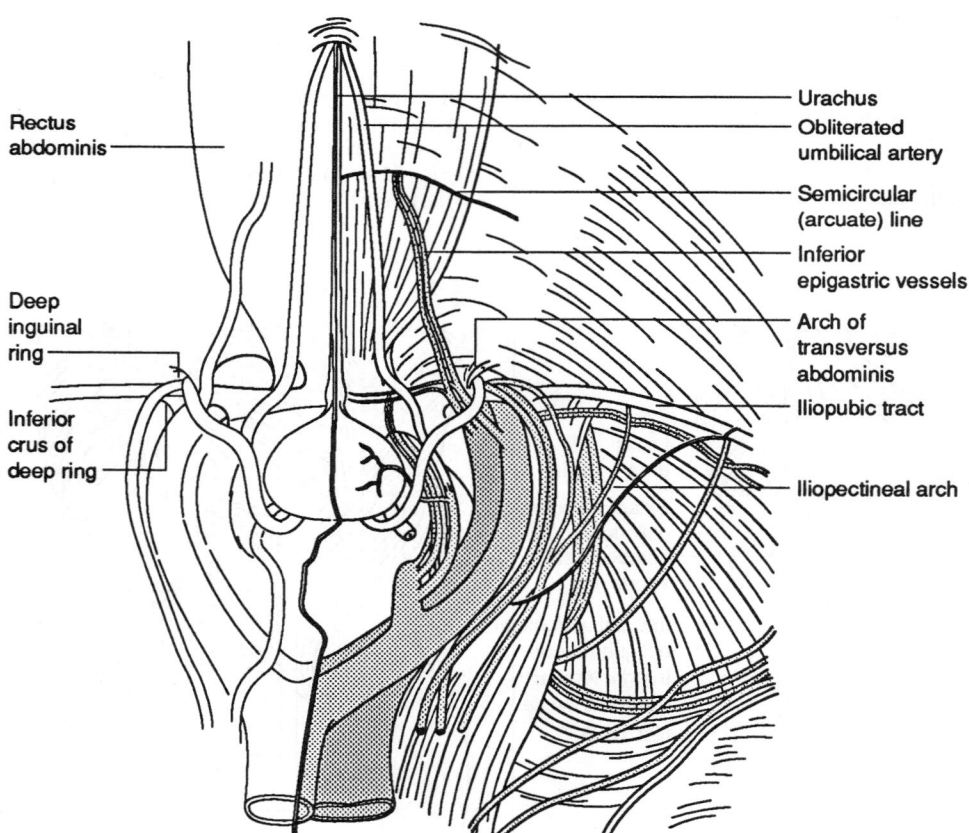

Figure 51.9. The deep inguinal region and the anterior abdominal wall seen from within the abdomen. The urachus, the obliterated portion of the umbilical artery, and the inferior epigastric vessels are covered by peritoneal folds, respectively called the *median, medial,* and *lateral umbilical folds.*

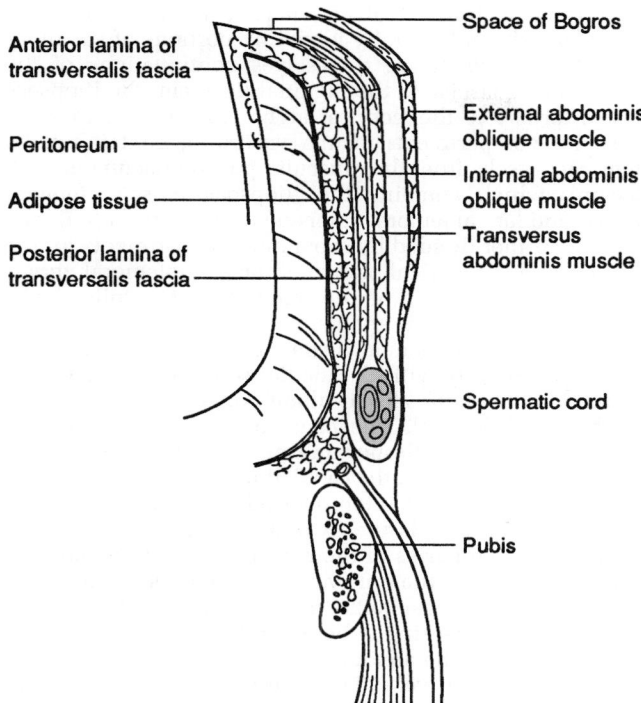

Figure 51.10. A parasagittal section through the layers of the anterior abdominal wall and groin. Observe that the transversalis fascia is depicted as a bilaminar structure.

literature devoted to groin hernia. Confusion results because surgeons may actually be referring to very different anatomic structures when discussing various hernia repairs, yet each may use the same anatomic term or eponym. Indeed, perhaps the biggest reservation among surgeons intent on performing a Shouldice repair is a precise definition of what is being sewn to what.

The transversalis fascia proper is a continuous sheet that extends throughout the extraperitoneal space. The term *transversalis fascia* generally is defined as the deep or endoabdominal fascia covering the internal surface of the transversus abdominis, the iliacus, the psoas muscles, and the obturator internus and portions of the periosteum. One variant of this convention is the use of terms specific to the muscle covered by the fascia (e.g., iliac fascia).

Most authors feel that only one layer of transversalis fascia exists, whereas others maintain that the transversalis fascia comprises two layers, or laminae (12–16). The posterior lamina is a layer of fibrous connective tissue that widely varies in density and continuity and is interspersed with adipose tissue, as seen in Fig. 51.10. This layer is often referred to simply as the *preperitoneal fascia.* The anterior lamina is more uniform and is adherent to the deep surface of the transversus abdominis and the rectus abdominis. The posterior lamina is contained within the preperitoneal space, which is defined as the space between the peritoneum and the anterior lamina of the transversalis fascia. The inferior epigastric vessels are enclosed by, or interspersed with, the adipose tissue and the fibrous tissue of the posterior lamina of the transversalis fascia. The vessels are in contact anteriorly with the anterior lamina of the transversalis fascia as they course upward to enter the rectus abdominis sheath.

Transversalis Fascia Derivatives

The transversalis fascia analogues or derivatives are the iliopectineal arch, iliopubic tract, and crura of the deep inguinal ring. The superior and inferior crura form a transversalis fascia sling, a structure shaped like a "monk's hood," around the deep inguinal ring (Fig. 51.9). The transversalis fascia also contributes the internal spermatic fascia to the spermatic cord at this point. This "sling" has functional significance; when the transversus abdominis contracts, the crura of the ring are pulled upward and laterally, which results in a valvular action that helps to prevent the indirect formation of a hernia.

The iliopubic tract (Figs. 51.9, 51.11) has become an increasingly important landmark for surgeons as the use of laparoscopic technology has increased (17,18). The iliopubic tract is the thickened band of transversalis fascia formed at the zone of transition between the deep surfaces

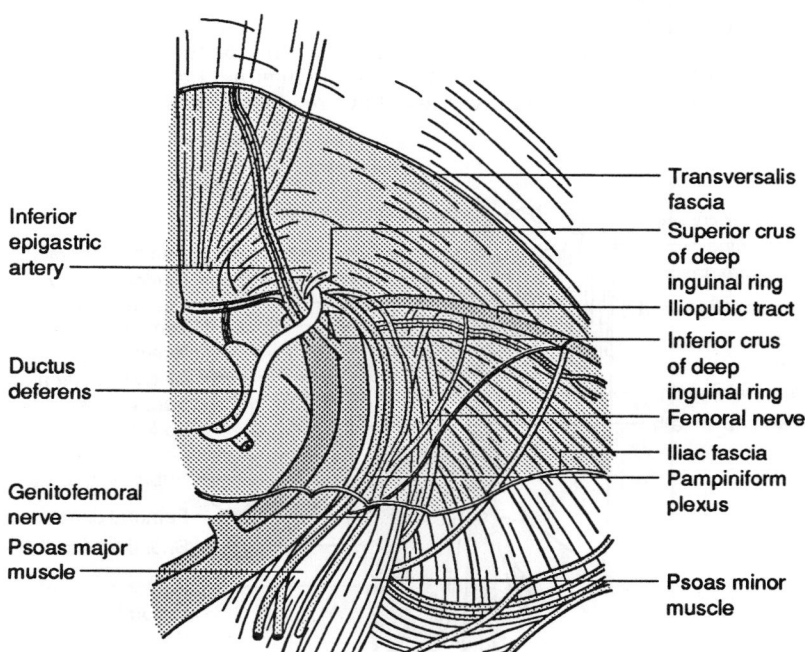

Figure 51.11. A schematic representation of the deep inguinal region. The iliopubic tract is shown as a thickening of the transversalis fascia, inferior to which many of the branches of the lumbar plexus exit the pelvis.

of the iliac and transversus abdominis muscles. The structure courses parallel to the more superficially located inguinal ligament, is attached to the iliac crest laterally, and inserts on the pubic tubercle medially. The tract forms along its course a portion of the inferior crus of the deep inguinal ring and then contributes to the anterior and medial walls of the femoral sheath. The tract fuses with the inguinal ligament to form a component of the inferior wall of the inguinal canal. At its insertion on the pubic tubercle, it curves backward slightly to blend with Cooper's pectineal ligament. The pectineal ligament actually is a condensation of periosteum and is not a true analogue of the transversalis fascia, but it is reinforced by fibers from the iliopubic tract and inguinal ligament.

The iliopubic tract contains not only fibrous connective tissue but also some elastic fibers (19). In one series, the iliopubic tract was a substantial structure, suitable for use in hernia repairs, in 42% of the specimens examined. The tract, whether substantial or not, can be used as a readily identified landmark.

The iliopubic tract has particular significance because of its importance as a landmark to the laparoscopic surgeon. Many of the branches of the lumbar plexus run inferior to the tract, and damage to these nerves may be the result of aggressive dissection or the placement of tacks or staples to affix a prosthesis below this structure. The tract is not obviously visible in every patient from a laparoscopic view, but its location should always be immediately known to the surgeon because of its constant relationship to the other landmarks in this area.

The iliopectineal arch (Fig. 51.9) is also a condensation of the transversalis fascia. The iliopectineal arch commences at the medial border of the iliacus muscle, where it is continuous with the iliac fascia, itself a portion of the transversalis (endoabdominal) fascia. The arch separates the vascular compartment containing the femoral vessels from the neuromuscular compartment containing the iliopsoas muscle, femoral nerve, and lateral femoral cutaneous nerve. The iliopectineal arch also contributes to the proximal portion of the femoral sheath, thereby joining the iliopubic tract in the formation of the femoral sheath.

Femoral Sheath, Canal, and Ring

The femoral sheath (Fig. 51.12) is composed primarily of extensions of the transversalis fascia. The sheath is best understood in terms of the structures contained within. As the external iliac artery and vein pass beneath the inguinal ligament to become the femoral vessels, they are covered an-teriorly by the transversalis fascia proper. This fascial layer is posteriorly and laterally joined by portions of the iliopsoas fascia, which are themselves continuations of the transversalis fascia. At the inguinal ligament, the iliopsoas fascia forms the iliopectineal arch. This arch divides the vascular compartment (lacuna vasorum), containing the femoral vessels, from the muscular portion (lacuna musculorum), which contains the iliopsoas muscle, femoral nerve, and lateral femoral cutaneous nerve. The vascular lacuna is further divided by septa into compartments for the vessels and the femoral branch of the genitofemoral nerve.

The medial border of the femoral sheath follows the transversus abdominis aponeurosis to its insertion just lateral to that of the lacunar ligament and extends inferiorly to fuse eventually with the medial septum and adventitia of the femoral vein. The resultant cone-shaped cul-de-sac is the femoral canal. The canal normally contains only wisps of connective tissue and small lymphatic nodes. The wider proximal part of the canal, the femoral ring, contains a large node, which is often referred to as *Cloquet's node*.

The femoral ring is the extraperitoneal opening of the canal. The boundaries of the ring are formed medially by the curved edge of the transversus abdominis aponeurosis, not the lacunar ligament, which inserts more medially (20). Laterally, the ring is bounded by the connective tissue septum and the adventitia that is interposed between it and the femoral vein. The anterior boundary is the inguinal ligament; posteriorly, the ring is reinforced by the iliopubic tract and iliopectineal ligament. The canal is not in direct communication with the pelvic cavity. The transversalis fascia is not a component of the roof of the canal because it is diverted at this point to form the femoral sheath. This weakened area is therefore quite prone to hernia formation, especially in female subjects.

Inguinal (Hesselbach's) Triangle

The inguinal triangle is the site of direct inguinal hernias. This triangle is most often described from the anterior aspect (Fig. 51.13), in which case the inguinal ligament forms the base of the triangle, the rectus abdominis the medial border, and the inferior epigastric vessels the superolateral border. The triangle as originally described by Hesselbach had the pectineal ligament as its base. The latter description is quite useful to the surgeon viewing the abdomen from within because the inguinal ligament cannot be seen from this viewpoint. When the inguinal triangle is transilluminated, the thinness and translucency of the area of abdominal wall within the triangle underscores

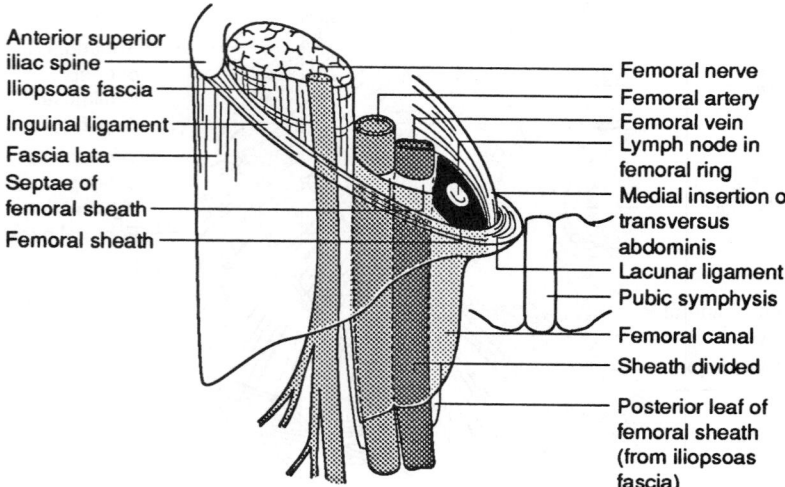

Anterior superior iliac spine
Iliopsoas fascia
Inguinal ligament
Fascia lata
Septae of femoral sheath
Femoral sheath

Femoral nerve
Femoral artery
Femoral vein
Lymph node in femoral ring
Medial insertion of transversus abdominis
Lacunar ligament
Pubic symphysis
Femoral canal
Sheath divided
Posterior leaf of femoral sheath (from iliopsoas fascia)

Figure 51.12. Schematic view of the femoral sheath, ring, and canal. The transversalis fascia forms the anterior portion of the sheath, and the iliopsoas fascia forms the posterior portion. Septa separate the vessels from each other and the vein from the femoral canal. The femoral ring contains a lymph node. The ring is formed medially by the aponeurosis of the transversus abdominis aponeurosis, anteriorly by the inguinal ligament, posteriorly by the pubic bone, and laterally by the femoral sheath.

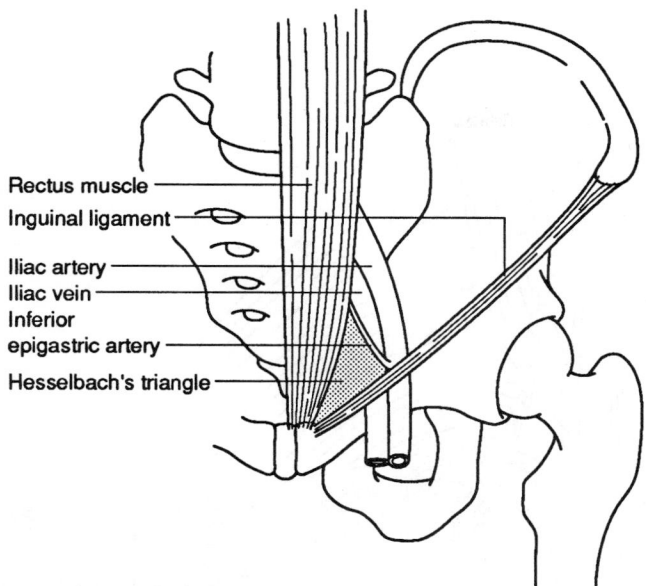

Figure 51.13. The inguinal (Hesselbach's) triangle.

its importance in hernia development and repair. In the most translucent area, little or no muscle is present. Only the peritoneum and the transversalis fascia cover the triangle here. The aponeurotic arch of the transversus abdominis crosses the triangle just below the apex in most people. A high aponeurotic arch affords less reinforcement to the triangle and may therefore predispose a person to the formation of a direct inguinal hernia.

Components of the Spermatic Cord

The spermatic cord (Figs. 51.11, 51.14) is closely associated with the deep inguinal ring. The spermatic cord is most appropriately described at this point because the deep ring itself is formed by derivatives of transversalis fascia, as is the innermost covering layer of the spermatic cord, the internal spermatic fascia. The middle covering layer is called the *cremasteric fascia* and contains the cremasteric muscle bundles; both are derived from the internal abdominal oblique muscle and fascia. The outermost covering of the spermatic cord is the external spermatic fascia, which is continuous with the investing fascia of the external abdominal oblique muscle.

The tunica vaginalis is initially a component of the cord, but normally it atrophies and closes early in neonatal life. This structure is an evagination of peritoneum. The testicle descends retroperitoneally in fetal life and is merely in contact with the posterior aspect of the tunica. An indirect congenital hernia enters the patent tunica vaginalis.

The cord structures enclosed by the coverings described above are the ductus (vas) deferens, the pampiniform venous plexus, the testicular artery, and the genital branch of the genitofemoral nerve, a branch of the lumbar plexus (Figs. 51.9, 51.11, 51.15).

Branches of the Lumbar Plexus

The nerves crossing the iliac fossa are some of the most variable in the body. This variability may be the cause of frequent intraoperative injury to the fragile nerves. The lumbar plexus is formed by roots from the 12th thoracic nerve and the first through fourth lumbar nerves. Cutaneous territories innervated by branches of the lumbar plexus are seen in Fig. 51.15A. The five terminal branches commonly encountered in laparoscopic herniorrhaphy can be discerned in many people as they course across the iliacus muscle covered by peritoneum and the iliac fascia (a portion of the transversalis–endopelvic fascia). The nerves form within or deep to the psoas major muscle (Fig. 51.15B), often ramifying with other nerves within or close to the muscle. The nerve branches initially lie within the so-called triangle of pain (21), bordered medially by the psoas muscle, anteriorly and inferiorly by the iliopubic tract, and laterally by the iliac crest. With the exception of the genital branch of the genitofemoral nerve, the branches of the lumbar plexus destined for the thigh run beneath the iliopubic tract.

The most anterior of the nerves encountered, the genitofemoral nerve, is also the most variable (22). This nerve may occur as a single trunk lying deep to the peritoneum and fascia on the anterior surface of the psoas muscle. The nerve may also divide into its component genital and femoral branches within the muscle. The genital branch travels with the spermatic cord, entering at the deep inguinal ring; it ultimately innervates the cremaster muscle and the lateral scrotum. The femoral branch of the nerve innervates the skin of the proximal midthigh.

The lumbar plexus branch encountered immediately deep to the lateral aspect of the psoas muscle is the large femoral nerve. Although not routinely encountered during laparoscopy, the femoral nerve has been injured in some cases (23). The lateral femoral cutaneous nerve crosses the iliac fossa under the iliac fascia to run deep

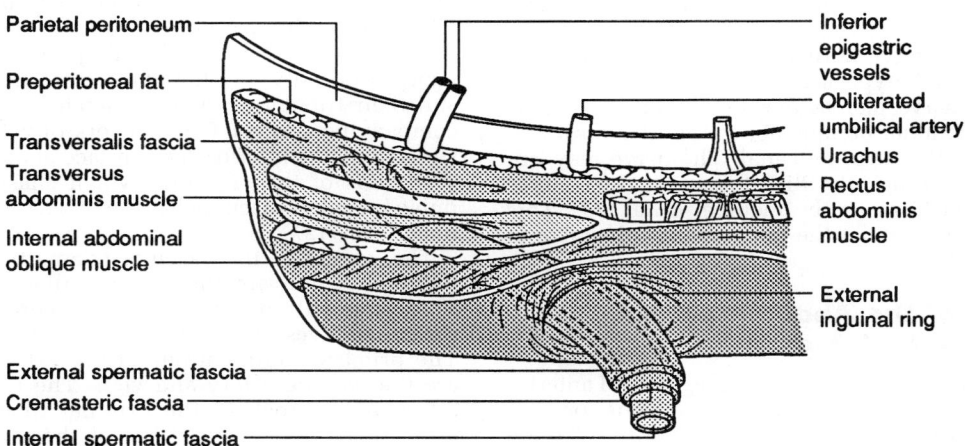

Figure 51.14. The component layers covering the contents of the spermatic cord.

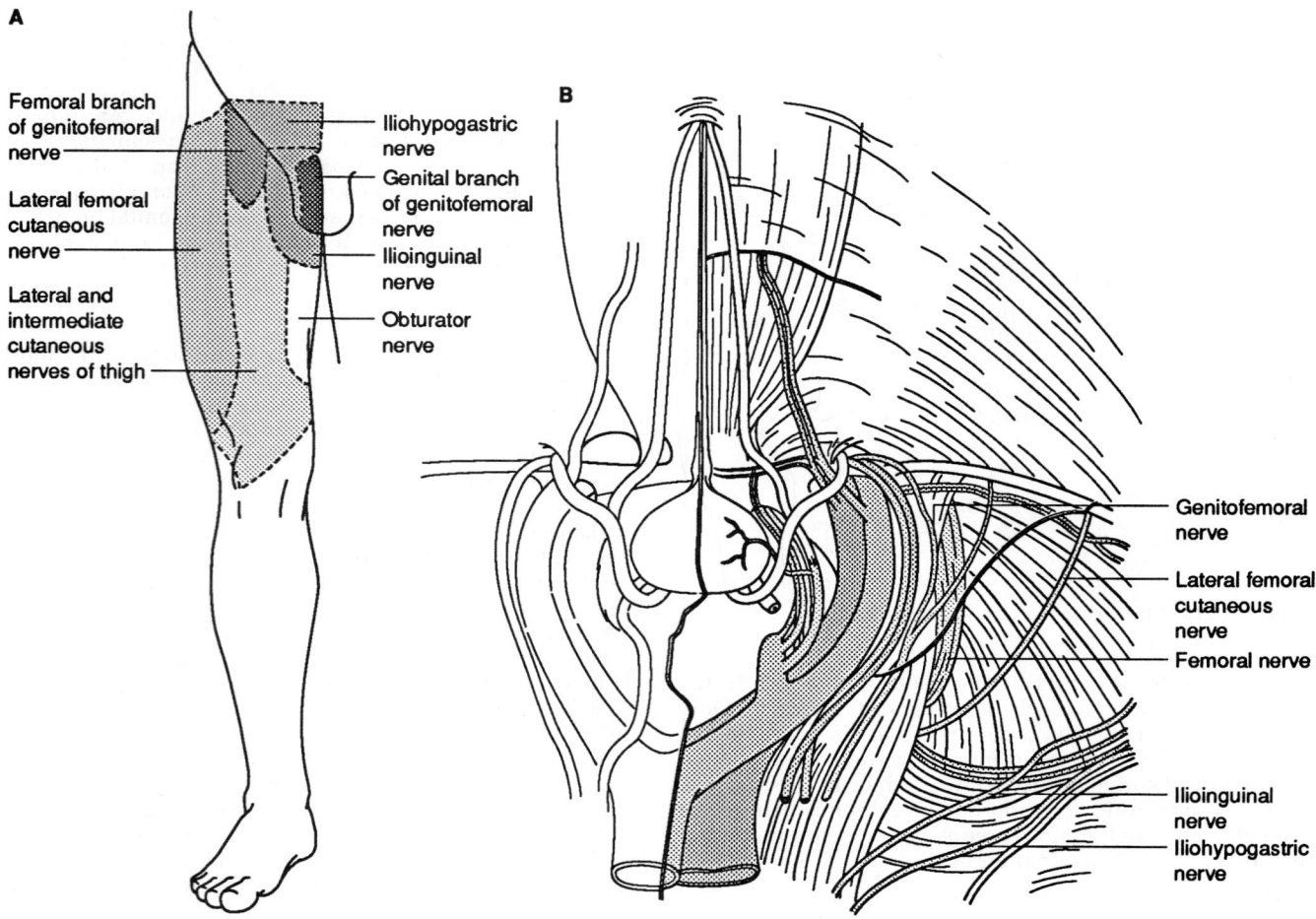

Figure 51.15. *(A)* The cutaneous territories innervated by several branches of the lumbar plexus. *(B)* Some of the branches of the lumbar plexus seen from within the abdomen.

to the iliopubic tract and the inguinal ligament, which it pierces to enter the thigh.

The iliohypogastric nerve typically arises with the ilioinguinal by a common trunk from the first lumbar nerve. They may exchange fibers within the muscle, but they usually diverge immediately to form individual nerves. The iliohypogastric nerve crosses the iliac fossa just inferior to the kidney and pierces the transversus abdominis. The subsequent course of the nerve carries it between the transversus and the internal abdominal oblique until it pierces the aponeuroses of both obliques just above the external inguinal ring.

The ilioinguinal nerve normally crosses the iliac fossa just inferior to the iliohypogastric nerve. In its typical further course, the nerve pierces the transversus abdominis and internal abdominal oblique above the iliac crest and eventually enters the inguinal canal. The nerve may run more diagonally through the iliac fossa and then pierce the iliopubic tract to reach the inguinal canal (24). This path "can obviously render the nerve more vulnerable to iatrogenic injury" (24).

Vasculature of the Abdominal Wall and Deep Inguinal Region

The vasculature of the deep inguinal region and anterior abdominal wall has been analyzed by surgeons for well over 100 years. The importance and variability of these vessels has been underscored by the ominous mnemonics used to refer to them—"crown of death" (*corona mortis*)

and "triangle of doom." The primary blood supply to the deep anterior wall is from the inferior epigastric artery. This artery is a branch of the external iliac artery. In many cases, an artery called the "aberrant" obturator artery arises from the inferior epigastric, which joins the "normal" obturator artery and thereby forms a circle—the corona mortis—before entering the obturator foramen. Injury to the circle, usually sustained while the surgeon is working in the area of Cooper's ligament, causes copious bleeding. Recent studies have indicated that aberrant obturator vessels are present in between 60% and 90% of whole pelves studied (25,26).

The veins in this area also are prone to injury because many, especially the iliopubic veins and obturator veins and their tributaries, may be much larger than their accompanying arteries. One network of veins in the area is situated on the inferior deep surface of the rectus muscles. The veins of this network, which anastomose with the pubic branches discussed above, have been called the *rectusial veins* (27).

The vessels in the vascular compartment of the deep inguinal region are the external iliac artery and vein. They arise within a triangular area bordered laterally by the gonadal vessels and medially by the ductus deferens. The primary continuations of the external iliac vessels are the femoral artery and vein. The inferior epigastric artery is a branch of the external iliac. The obturator artery may arise from either of these arteries as a replacement or accessory to the obturator branch of the internal iliac artery.

A final vessel to consider in this review is the deep circumflex iliac artery (Fig. 51.10). The origin of this artery is an extremely variable, but its course is predictable along the iliopubic tract. It pierces the transversalis fascia and runs along the iliac fossa to anastomose eventually with a deep lumbar artery. Because the deep circumflex artery runs along the iliopubic tract, it can inadvertently be stapled or otherwise injured during laparoscopic herniorrhaphy.

Pelvic Floor and Obturator Muscles

The pelvic musculature normally affords remarkable support to the structures within the true pelvis. Although a myoaponeurotic hammock-like sheet forms the pelvic diaphragm, obturator muscles and membrane, and urogenital diaphragm, herniation of fat or viscera through or around any of these layers occurs. The potential for hernia formation is increased because of the openings through which many structures exit or enter the pelvis.

The Latin term *obturator* is translated as "stopper for a bottle." The aptly named obturator internus, along with its membrane and the obturator externus, closes off nearly all the large obturator foramen. The small superolateral aperture through which the obturator vessels and nerve pass is the site where obturator hernias form. The obturator internus arises from the deep surface of parts of all three pelvic bones. The muscle fibers converge on a tendon, which leaves the pelvis through the lesser sciatic foramen to insert on the greater trochanter. The dense internal obturator fascia covers the muscle and is thickened to form the arcuate ligament, from which the levator ani muscles (the pelvic diaphragm) are in part suspended. The obturator internus fascia splits to enclose the pudendal vessels in the pudendal canal. The external obturator muscle arises from the pelvic bones surrounding the obturator foramen and from the anterior portion of the obturator membrane. The external obturator muscle is supplied by the obturator nerve and vessels.

The component muscles of the bowl-shaped pelvic diaphragm, the pubococcygeus, iliococcygeus, and puborectalis, along with the coccygeus form the floor of the pelvis. The pubococcygeus arises from the posterior aspect of the pubis and the thickened portion of the internal obturator fascia, called the *tendinous arch* (Fig. 51.16), that spans the distance between the pubis and ischial spine. The puborectalis, the midportion of the diaphragm, arises from

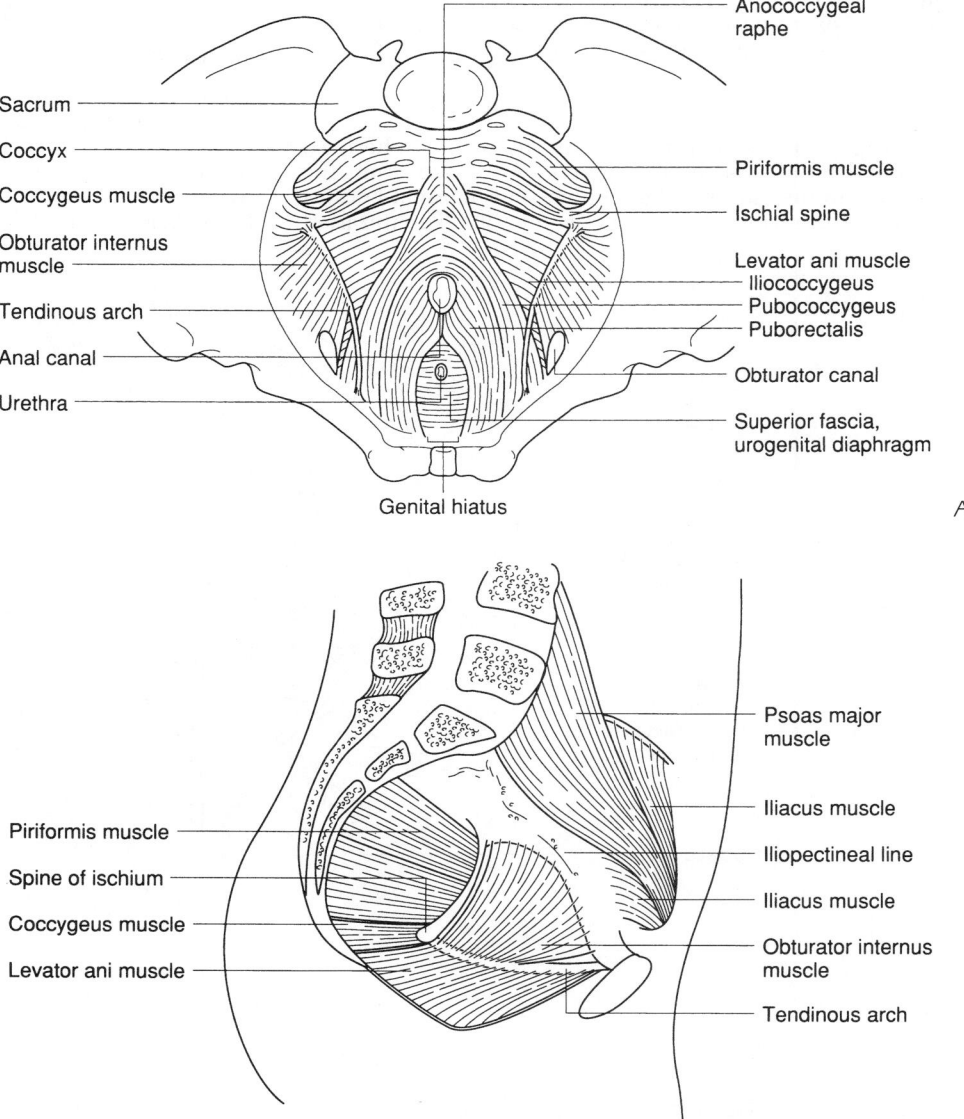

Figure 51.16. *(A)* The pelvic diaphragm (levator ani and the piriformis) and the urogenital diaphragm viewed from within the pelvis. *(B)* Hemisection of the pelvis revealing the levator ani, piriformis, obturator internus, and psoas muscles.

the pubis and loops around the rectum as the puborectal sling. The iliococcygeus is suspended at its origin from the tendinous arch and inserts on the coccyx. The coccygeus muscle completes the diaphragm posteriorly, arising from the ischial spine and inserting on the sides of the coccyx.

The area remaining between the sacrum and the greater sciatic foramen is filled for the most part by the piriformis muscle. The piriformis arises from the anterior surface of the second through fourth sacral vertebrae and the sacrotuberous ligament. This muscle exits the pelvis through the greater sciatic foramen, which is thereby divided into suprapiriform and infrapiriform portions (Figs. 51.16, 51.17). The superior gluteal nerves and vessels pass through the suprapiriform foramen, whereas the inferior gluteal nerves and vessels in company with the sciatic nerve pass through the infrapiriform foramen.

The most pronounced deficit in the pelvic diaphragm is situated anteriorly, where an aperture must allow the urogenital structures to pass out of the pelvis. This area is reinforced by the urogenital diaphragm, a structure primarily consisting of the superficial and deep transverse perineal muscles. The deep transverse perineal muscle is enclosed by a weak superior fascia and a sturdier inferior perineal fascia. The urogenital diaphragm recently has been shown to be more funnel-shaped than sandwich-like, as previously depicted in many atlases (28). The urogenital diaphragm exists only in humans because the human pelvic outlet faces inferiorly, unlike that of quadrupeds (29).

CLINICAL FEATURES OF HERNIAS

No age group is immune to the development of hernias. Inguinal hernias occur in persons of all ages, from the neonate to the elderly. The incidence of inguinal hernias in premature babies is approximately 10%. The duration of symptoms varies from individual to individual; some patients have had a hernia for many years at the time of presentation, whereas in others the development of a strangulated hernia is the initial presentation. The patient will give a history of a lump or swelling that develops on straining. This may be painful if it occurs suddenly after straining, with stretching of a preexisting processus vaginalis.

On clinical examination, a swelling is noted that has a cough impulse. An uncomplicated hernia reduces spontaneously when the patient relaxes or lies down. When the upright position is assumed, the hernia becomes more prominent because the abdominal viscera fall forward. With hernias about the umbilicus or incisional hernias, the edges of the defect in the abdominal wall can be palpated easily, and the size of the neck of the hernia can be assessed accurately. When the hernia is reduced, a gurgle of the intestinal contents in the abdomen can be heard and felt by the examiner. Auscultation of the hernia elicits bowel sounds. A hernia does not transmit light, as opposed to a hydrocele, which usually transilluminates brilliantly. After the hernia is reduced, if the hand is placed over the defect and the patient strains or coughs, the hernia does not protrude.

COMPLICATIONS OF HERNIAS

Incarceration

Incarcerated means "trapped" or "imprisoned." Clinically, an incarcerated hernia is an irreducible hernia. Incarceration does not denote obstruction. The contents of the hernia may be omentum, nonobstructed bowel, or ovary, and its irreducibility is associated with adhesions to the hernial sac.

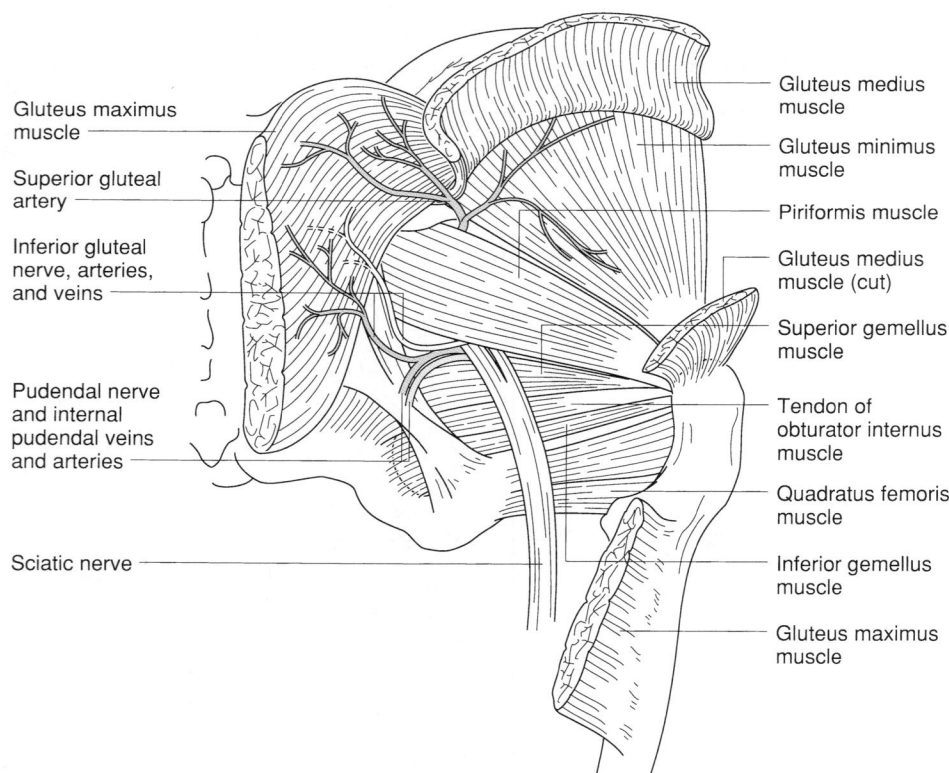

Figure 51.17. The gluteal muscles and lateral rotators of the hip. External relations of the sciatic foramen are also evident.

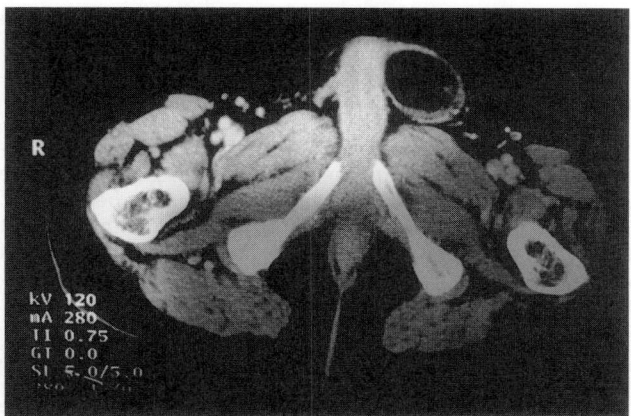

Figure 51.18. Computed tomogram showing a left-sided inguinal hernia.

The hernia itself is not necessarily tense to palpation, and the overlying skin appears normal. Normal bowel sounds may be heard within the hernia. It is important to differentiate an incarcerated hernia from a hydrocele of the cord. One can get above the hydrocele with the examining fingers. One cannot get above a hernia, however, as it communicates with the abdominal cavity. A hydrocele will transilluminate clearly, but a hernia will not.

The recommended treatment of an incarcerated hernia is surgical, but the need for treatment is not urgent because no life-threatening complications are present. This routine recommendation is currently being tested in a multicenter, randomized trial of watchful waiting versus operation that is being sponsored by the National Institutes of Health.

Intestinal Obstruction

One hundred years ago, the most common cause of intestinal obstruction was a hernia. At the present time, hernia is third, after adhesive obstructions and cancer. Hernia is an important cause of obstruction that is not infrequently missed on clinical examination. When a patient with an intestinal obstruction is examined, great emphasis should be placed on adequate exposure of the entire abdominal wall and groin area (from nipples to knees). Proper lighting is essential because previous scars can fade with time and become barely perceptible. The patient with intestinal obstruction as a result of a hernia will have a tense hernia that is irreducible. The abdomen itself will be distended, and high-pitched bowel sounds with frequent rushes will be heard. If the process continues to the

complication of strangulation, these signs will disappear. Unlike adhesive small-bowel obstructions, partial small-bowel obstructions secondary to hernia are rare. Most patients will have had vomiting and obstipation.

A plain roentgenogram of the abdomen will reveal the signs of an intestinal obstruction—dilated loops of bowel with air–fluid levels and no bowel gas distal to the obstruction. Frequently on a plain roentgenogram, one can see bowel shadows in the region of the hernia. A lateral view is often useful to demonstrate this feature more clearly. Contrast studies are not usually necessary in this instance. Computed tomography reliably demonstrates the hernia with characteristic features of obstruction and should be considered if the clinical diagnosis is not certain (Fig. 51.18) because a distal intestinal obstruction secondary to another cause (e.g., adhesions) may result in significant distention of a coincidental nonobstructing hernia of the abdominal wall. Should the examiner focus attention exclusively on the hernia, the real cause of the obstruction may be missed when the hernia is repaired.

The patient is sedated and placed in bed. The Trendelenburg position should facilitate reduction of a groin hernia. An attempt should be made at the initial examination to reduce the hernia. The maneuver of taxis entails grasping the neck of the hernia with the fingers of one hand and then applying intermittent pressure on the most distal part of the hernia with the other hand. Taxis has the effect of elongating the neck of the hernia so that the contents of the hernia may be guided through this area back into the abdominal cavity with a rocking movement. Mere pressure on the most distal part of the hernia causes bulging of the hernial sac around the neck, which can occlude the neck and prevent it from being reduced (Fig. 51.19). The maneuver of taxis should not be performed with excessive pressure or too vigorously. If the hernia is strangulated, gangrenous bowel might be reduced into the abdomen or perforated in the process. One or two gentle attempts should be made at taxis. If they are unsuccessful, this procedure should be abandoned. Rarely, the hernia together with its peritoneal sac and constricting neck may be reduced into the abdomen (reduction *en masse*). The patient would then have persistent obstruction after reduction of the hernia.

The next steps in management include resuscitation followed by urgent surgery. At surgery, an approach directly over the hernia is used. In all patients, the entire gastrointestinal tract must be assessed to eliminate causes of obstruction other than the hernia itself. This is done before the hernia is repaired. The bowel, if viable, is reduced into the abdomen. If difficulty is encountered in reducing the hernia, the neck of the hernia can be widened. In the case of an inguinal hernia, division of the neck with or without ligation and division of the inferior epigastric vessels, is

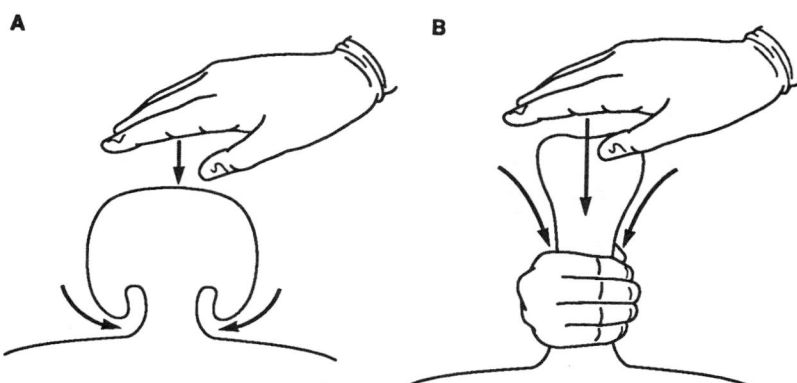

Figure 51.19. Reduction of a hernia by taxis. *(A)* Applying pressure on the hernia directly occludes the neck. *(B)* Elongating the neck of the hernia while applying pressure allows reduction.

safe, and the hernia contents can be reduced into the abdomen. In the case of a femoral hernia, the inguinal ligament can be split anteriorly and the hernia contents reduced into the abdomen. If the bowel is nonviable, then a bowel resection can be performed with anastomosis. The hernia is then repaired.

Strangulation

Strangulation of a hernia is a serious and life-threatening condition in which the hernial contents become ischemic and nonviable. The pathogenesis of this condition involves bowel within the hernia sac. Straining may push more bowel into the sac, and the tense sac then causes pressure at the neck. This pressure initially produces venous congestion, as a result of which the bowel becomes edematous. Eventually, the pressure is so great that the arterial supply is obstructed and the bowel becomes gangrenous.

In addition to having an irreducible hernia and intestinal obstruction, the patient is toxic, dehydrated, and febrile. Examination of the abdomen reveals the signs of an intestinal obstruction, with distention and increased bowel sounds. Absolute constipation and vomiting are other manifestations. The hernia itself is tense, irreducible, and very tender, and the overlying skin may be discolored with a reddish or bluish tinge. No bowel sounds are heard within the hernia itself. The patient commonly manifests a leukocytosis with a predominance of polymorphonuclear leukocytes. Blood gases may reveal metabolic acidosis.

Management of these patients requires urgent attention to detail. No attempt should be made to reduce the hernia. Rapid resuscitation should commence immediately, with nasogastric suction and replacement of fluids and electrolytes. The patient should be given antibiotics. Once the patient is resuscitated, urgent surgery commences to expose the hernia, open the sac, and assess the viability of the bowel. More bowel can be pulled into the hernia so that viable bowel can be transected and the gangrenous portion removed. An end-to-end anastomosis should be performed and the bowel then reduced into the abdominal cavity. The hernia is then repaired.

Richter's Hernia

In this interesting complication, part of the bowel wall herniates through the defect and may become ischemic and gangrenous. However, intestinal obstruction does not occur (Fig. 51.20). The overlying skin may be discolored.

The herniated bowel wall is exposed by opening the sac. The neck of the sac is enlarged to allow delivery of the bowel into the wound. The gangrenous patch is excised and the bowel wall reconstituted. The hernia is then repaired.

Massive Hernia

In these defects, a large portion of the abdominal contents is situated within the hernia. These hernias have usually been present for many years, and because of chronicity, the contents of the hernia have lost their "right of domicile" within the abdomen. Reduction of the hernia with replacement of contents into the abdominal cavity and repair of the hernia can increase the intraabdominal tension tremendously, with the effect of pushing up the diaphragm and impairing respiratory function. In addition, compression of the inferior vena cava may decrease venous return and cause renal insufficiency, and the hernia repair itself is subject to a high degree of tension. Problems often affect the skin overlying a massive hernia. The skin can become edematous and cellulitis can develop (28). It is imperative that the skin over the hernia be in healthy condition before the hernia is repaired.

Some authors recommend the use of pneumoperitoneum when returning contents to the abdominal cavity is likely to be difficult (29). The maneuver involves injecting 500 to 1,500 cc of air every 1 to 3 days for about 3 weeks before the repair. This technique is designed to stretch the abdominal wall so that it can accommodate the bowel that has lost its right of domicile. However, the injected gas can enter the hernial sac, distending the sac and stretching the abdominal cavity but little.

The repair of these hernias requires opening the sac and reducing the contents into the abdomen. Because the defect is usually large, a prosthetic repair is most appropriate.

GROIN HERNIAS

Edoardo Bassini described the principle of reinforcement of the posterior wall of the inguinal canal in 1887 (30). It is generally agreed that Bassini ushered in the modern era of inguinal hernia repair. His scientific approach to the problem led to the development of several distinct steps essential for the procedure. These include the following:

1. Complete division of the external oblique aponeurosis and the transversalis fascia
2. Differentiation between indirect and direct defects
3. Isolation of the spermatic cord
4. Ligation and removal of the sac at the deep inguinal ring flush with the peritoneum
5. Oblique reconstruction of the inguinal canal with an anterior and posterior wall and an internal and external ring

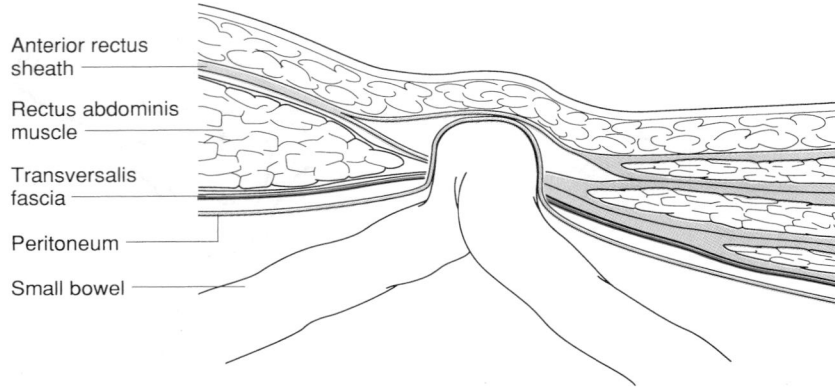

Anterior rectus sheath

Rectus abdominis muscle

Transversalis fascia

Peritoneum

Small bowel

Figure 51.20. Richter's hernia. Part of the bowel wall herniates through the defect in the abdominal wall.

The desire to reduce recurrence rates led to the development of numerous variations of Bassini's operation that have undergone phases of popularity. The fact that so many types of repair have been described attests to the frequency of the major complication of the surgical procedure, recurrence of the hernia. In the mid-20th century, a variety of repairs were developed; strengthening of the endoabdominal fascia was claimed to be an integral component of all of them. As noted in the section on anatomy, a consistent definition of the endoabdominal fascia was then and is now still lacking. Nevertheless, McVay (Cooper's ligament) and Shouldice repairs became especially popular and were until recently the most commonly used and most successful (lowest rate of recurrence) techniques. Although it is true that the Bassini repair and its modifications were associated with a much lower incidence of recurrence than historical controls, surgeons realized that the results were far from perfect, particularly when performed outside specialty centers. Indeed, population-based studies, such as those conducted by the Rand Corporation, confirmed recurrence rates to be in the 10% to 30% range, with the lesser figure applying to the repair of simple, small hernias and the higher rate to the repair of recurrent hernias (31).

The excessive recurrence rate is not surprising because the Bassini repair and its modifications all create tension at the suture line when muscle and fascia are sutured to close the defect. Purely sutured repairs inevitably result in distortion of the anatomy and tissue approximation under tension. The tension thus created has been considered the root cause of late failure (recurrence). Many surgeons feel that tension causes the pain and disability that commonly occur in the postoperative period.

Four developments in the latter half of the 20th century significantly decreased morbidity and favorably influenced the recurrence rate to the currently accepted level of less than 5%:

1. Routine use of prosthetic materials
2. Widespread acceptance of the "tension-free" concept
3. Realization that the preperitoneal space can be used for hernia repair
4. Therapeutic laparoscopy

Prosthetic materials: The use of plastic prostheses for many medical applications increased during the 20th century. The term *plastic* refers to a family of materials, synthesized by polymerizing carbon rings, that can be fashioned to replace many natural substances, such as wood or metal.

Several materials have emerged as suitable for routine use in hernia surgery, as they fulfill the characteristics of an ideal prosthesis:

1. Not modified physically by tissue fluid
2. Chemically inert
3. Does not cause an inflammatory or foreign body reaction
4. Does not cause carcinogenesis
5. Does not cause allergic or hypersensitivity responses
6. Resistant to mechanical strain
7. Conformable
8. Sterilizable

These materials included polypropylene, either monofilament (Marlex, Prolene) or polyfilament (Surgipro); Dacron (Mersilene); and expanded polytetrafluoroethylene, or e-PTFE (Gore-Tex).

Widespread acceptance of the "tension-free" concept: For a consistently successful inguinal hernia repair to be achieved, the reconstruction of the posterior wall of the inguinal canal is necessary in addition to closure of the defect through which the hernia protrudes. Techniques, both conventional and laparoscopic, have been developed that avoid the creation of tension by using a nonabsorbable prosthesis to reconstruct the inguinal floor, with or without closure of the defect itself. In the technique described by Lichtenstein, the prosthesis is inserted in a traditional open surgical procedure that can be performed under local anesthesia. Most patients leave the hospital or outpatient surgical center on the day of the operation. Proponents of this procedure claim that patients have little pain and disability in the postoperative period because the procedure is "tension-free." Reported rates of recurrence are lower than those with previous techniques that include tension at muscle and fascia suture lines. In their series of 4,000 patients, Lichtenstein and colleagues (32,33) recorded a recurrence rate of 0.1%, including procedures for recurrent hernias; other complications occurred only rarely. Studies in which this technique was used by surgeons outside Lichtenstein's clinic have confirmed a low recurrence rate, which indicates that the good results were not necessarily related to the fact that the operation was performed by an enthusiastic proponent in a highly specialized hernia unit (34–36).

Use of the preperitoneal space: The key to the preperitoneal hernia repair is the placement of a large prosthesis in the preperitoneal space on the abdominal side of the defect in the transversalis fascia rather than on the external oblique aponeurosis. The preperitoneal space can be entered through a variety of conventional incisions (i.e., lower midline, paramedian, or Pfannenstiel). The hernia defect itself may or may not be closed, depending on the preference of the surgeon. Unlike the extraperitoneal repair, in which abdominal pressure is a major contributing factor in recurrence, the preperitoneal repair makes use of the abdominal pressure to help fix the mesh material against the abdominal wall, which adds strength to the repair (37,38). A variety of sutured and nonsutured repairs have been introduced that are based on the theory that "... by covering the hernia defect and adjacent areas far beyond the limits of the defect with the mesh, the intraabdominal pressure becomes an efficient means of fixation of the mesh over the site of the hernia rather than a factor in recurrence" (39).

Laparoscopic techniques: At about the same time that surgeons were beginning to accept the routine use of a prosthetic mesh for repair of an inguinal hernia, laparoscopic cholecystectomy was introduced. With laparoscopy, the intraabdominal space can be accessed with minimal perioperative discomfort—hence the interest in intraabdominal herniorrhaphy under laparoscopic guidance. The advantage of laparoscopic herniorrhaphy over a conventional, open procedure is a matter of intense study at the present time.

Etiology, Epidemiology, and Natural History

Spontaneous abdominal hernias occur in about 5% of the world population over a lifetime. The prevalence may be as high as 10% (31). Inguinal hernias are the most common of all the abdominal wall hernias and constitute about 80% of cases. Femoral hernias occur in about 5% of instances. Incisional, umbilical, epigastric, and a host of miscellaneous hernia types make up the other 15%. The majority of inguinal hernias occur in male subjects, with a male-to-female ratio of 7:1. With femoral hernias, a female predominance of about 1.8:1 is seen.

The prime cause of an indirect inguinal hernia is a patent processus vaginalis. The processus vaginalis is the direct result of the migration of the testis from its abdominal location to the scrotum, which is completed by about 28 weeks of gestation. Normally, the processus becomes obliterated in the first few months of life. If all or part of the processus remains patent, the defect can give rise to an indirect inguinal hernia, a scrotal hydrocele, or an encysted hydrocele of the cord or hydrocele of the canal of Nuck in a female patient. The congenital etiology of indirect inguinal hernias has resulted in controversy over the incidence of bilaterality of groin hernias. In a 38-year follow-up of 1,944 patients, investigators found a contralateral lesion in 15.8% (40). In a large series of patients with hernias occurring in childhood, others reported that the patent processus vaginalis closed over a period of time in most cases (41). In premature babies, both sides were patent. In the neonatal period, the contralateral side was patent in 60% of cases, but by the age of 2 years, only 40% of the children had a patent processus vaginalis. This 40% rate persists into adult life, but in only 20% of these cases does symptomatic hernia develop; the other 20% have a lifelong patent processus that does not produce any symptoms (40,41).

The myopectineal orifice of Fruchaud (Fig. 51.1) is an area of transversalis fascia that is not protected by the posterior rectus sheath or by muscle. This is an area of potential weakness through which all groin hernias emerge. Some degree of protection is afforded by the shutter mechanism, whereby with increased intraabdominal pressure the curved fibers of the internal oblique and the falx inguinalis flatten and move toward the inguinal ligament. Contraction of the transversus abdominis muscle also pulls up and tenses the crura of the internal ring.

Hernias are also caused by a mechanical disparity between visceral pressure and resistance of the abdominal musculature. Causes of increased abdominal pressure include coughing, constipation, prostatism, pregnancy, and unusual exertion (especially lifting heavy weights). Under these circumstances, when a patent processus vaginalis is present or the endoabdominal fascia is attenuated, hernia results. The sudden onset of a painful hernia in a young person after lifting a heavy weight is usually associated with a patent processus vaginalis. This potential space expands suddenly like a collapsed balloon, giving rise to the notion the patient "ruptured" himself. In older persons, the abdominal muscles and fascia weaken with the aging process, so even moderate effort may be sufficient to produce a hernia. Although obesity has traditionally been regarded as a causative factor, this is probably not as true for inguinal hernias as it is for other abdominal hernias.

The fascia transversalis, like other fascial tissue, derives its strength from collagen fibers that are continually being produced and reabsorbed. A disturbance of this balance results in attenuation of the fascia. Congenital defects, such as occur in Marfan, Ehlers-Danlos, and Hunter-Hurler syndromes, can predispose to hernia formation. It appears that certain life-styles can lead to defective collagen production, including the now rare condition of lathyrism, in which a patient ingests large quantities of foods, particularly peas, that contain ε_1–aminopropionitrile (42). This substance prevents covalent cross-linking between and within forming collagen molecules, so that collagen is produced that is reduced in tensile strength. An association between cigarette smoking and groin hernias has also been demonstrated (43). Levels of circulating serum elastolytic activity have been shown to be significantly greater in patients who smoke.

The natural history of an untreated inguinal hernia is poorly understood, with almost no modern data available. This lack of information is a consequence of the commonly held opinion that all inguinal hernias should be repaired when diagnosed to prevent complications. In fact, the risk of a major complication, such as incarceration, obstruction, or strangulation, is very low. It has been estimated that an 18-year-old man has a 0.272 lifetime risk of strangulation, and that the risk for a 75-year-old is 0.034 (44). This extremely low incidence of major complications may offset the ninefold to 10-fold increase in mortality in patients presenting with intestinal obstruction in comparison with nonobstructed patients. Other investigators have reported the annual risk of a major complication to be 0.002 to 0.0037 (45). Based on this incidence, coupled with the life expectancy in 1971 and the operative mortality rates for uncomplicated and complicated hernia repair in the Medicare population in 1971, elective operation was associated with a greater loss of life than no operation was. A randomized, prospective trial is currently accruing patients to compare operative management versus careful observation for minimally symptomatic patients with inguinal hernias. This study will provide the data needed to understand the natural history of an inguinal hernia, so that the indications for elective repair can be better defined.

Classification

Groin hernias may be primary or recurrent. Hernias are classified as inguinal and femoral, the inguinal hernias being further subdivided into direct and indirect hernias (Fig. 51.21) (Table 51.2). An indirect hernia occurs as a protrusion of abdominal contents through the internal ring, lateral to the inferior epigastric vessels, into the inguinal canal. Indirect inguinal hernias are situated within the spermatic cord and therefore may extend into the scrotum. In female patients, the hernia follows the round ligament and may present as a swelling in the labium. A direct hernia is a protrusion through the triangle of Hesselbach medial to the inferior epigastric vessels. These hernias develop through an area where the endoabdominal fascia is not protected by overlying muscle. Direct hernias do not usually involve the cord, as they tend to protrude forward. However, they occasionally track alongside the cord down the entire length of the inguinal canal and even enter the scrotum. For this reason, the only absolute distinction between a direct and an indirect hernia is the relationship to the inferior epigastric vessels. A femoral hernia protrudes through the femoral canal, which is bordered by the inguinal ligament superiorly, the pubic ramus medially and inferiorly, and the femoral vein laterally. This hernia presents below the inguinal ligament. In a sliding hernia, part of the sac is formed by the viscera, on the left side the sigmoid colon or bladder and on the right side the cecum or bladder (46) (Fig. 51.22).

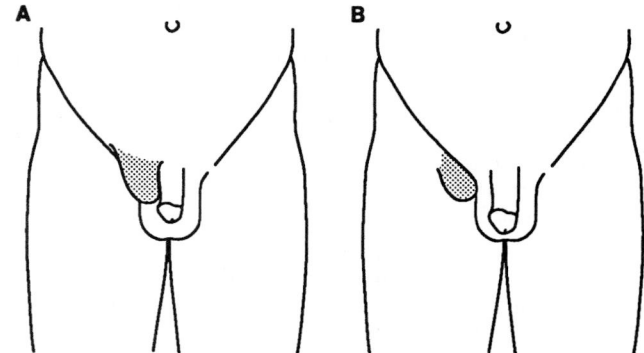

Figure 51.21. (A) Inguinal hernia. This presents above the inguinal ligament and extends below it. (B) Femoral hernia. This presents below the inguinal ligament.

Table 51.2. NYHUS CLASSIFICATION OF GROIN HERNIAS

Type I	Indirect hernia
	Normal-size internal ring
	Typically in infants, children, small adults
Type II	Indirect hernia
	Dilated internal ring
	Posterior wall intact
	Inferior epigastric vessels not displaced
	Does not extend to the scrotum
Type III	Posterior wall defect
	A. Direct hernia
	Size not taken into account
	B. Indirect hernia
	Dilated internal ring encroaching on Hesselbach's triangle (Massive scrotal, sliding or pantaloon type)
	C. Femoral hernia
Type IV	Recurrent hernia
	A. Direct
	B. Indirect
	C. Femoral
	D. Combined

Clinical Diagnosis

Groin hernias present with a swelling that has a cough impulse. With indirect hernias, the swelling may extend down into the scrotum. The swelling reduces when the patient lies down. Sometimes, the hernia does not reduce easily and the patient has to reduce it manually. Applying pressure over the mid-inguinal point (midway between the anterior superior iliac spine and the pubic tubercle and just above the inguinal ligament) with the fingertip will control an indirect hernia and prevent it from protruding when the patient strains. A direct hernia will not be controlled with this maneuver. Similarly, if the scrotum is invaginated with the index finger and the tip of the finger is placed through the external inguinal ring into the canal, and the patient is then asked to strain, an indirect hernia will push against the fingertip, whereas a direct hernia will push against the pulp of the finger. It should be

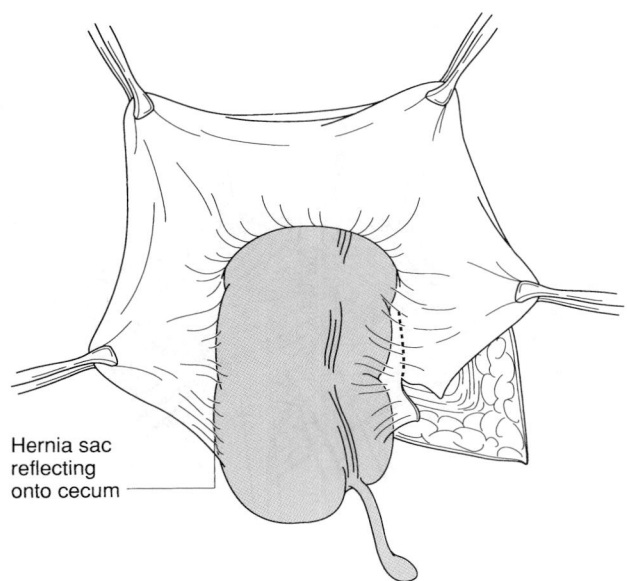

Hernia sac reflecting onto cecum

Figure 51.22. Sliding hernia (right indirect inguinal).

noted that the accuracy of this clinical assessment is questioned by many authorities. A femoral hernia presents as a swelling below the inguinal ligament and just lateral to the pubic tubercle (Fig. 51.21).

Differential Diagnosis

The clinical presentation of a groin hernia, especially when large, is frequently obvious to the examiner. Smaller hernias and recurrent hernias can be confused with a number of different conditions that can be mistaken for a hernia (Table 51.3).

A hydrocele extending into the scrotum or an encysted hydrocele of the cord can involve the groin area. The distinguishing features are that the examining hand can get above a hydrocele but not above a hernia, and that a hydrocele transilluminates very clearly. A varicocele does not transilluminate, has the characteristic feel of a "bag of worms," and is more tubelike in conformation. Lesions of the testicle may sometimes mimic a hernia, particularly in inflammatory conditions, such as epididymoorchitis. The distinguishing features are intense pain extending down into the scrotum. The testicle itself is enlarged and tender, as is the epididymis. On rectal examination, the seminal vesicles are tender. This condition may be bilateral. Torsion of the testicle is distinguished by the fact that the testicle is absent from the scrotum and the swelling in the groin feels firm. A sonogram reveals a solid mass in the testicle, which has been pulled up because of the torsion. Testicular tumors, if large enough, may extend up to the groin area, but they have a solid feel and sonography can distinguish them.

Pseudohernia is a condition that occurs in patients with denervation of the abdominal wall musculature—for example, after polio. The abdominal wall muscles bulge forward on straining and have the appearance of a hernia. An aneurysm of the femoral artery may present as a groin swelling, but with an expansile impulse and sometimes a bruit. If thrombosis develops in the aneurysm, pulsation may be lost. In this instance, the aneurysm becomes tender. Femoral aneurysms move from side to side but not up and down. A saphena varix usually presents below the inguinal ligament and represents a varicosity of one of the branches of the long saphenous vein as it emerges from the hiatus. Like a hernia, the varix has a cough impulse and becomes more prominent when the patient is standing. Compression over the femoral hiatus obliterates this lesion. The varix is sometimes associated with varicose veins farther down the lower limb. The overlying skin has an associated bluish discoloration.

Table 51.3. DIFFERENTIAL DIAGNOSIS OF A GROIN HERNIA

Hydrocele
Encysted hydrocele of the cord
Varicocele
Epididymoorchitis
Torsion of the testis
Undescended testis
Ectopic testis
Testicular tumor
Pseudohernia
Femoral artery aneurysm
Saphena varix
Lipoma of spermatic cord
Inguinal lymphadenopathy
Psoas abscess
Cutaneous lesions (e.g., sebaceous cyst, skin tumor)

A lipoma within the spermatic cord is a very common condition that may masquerade as a hernia and be misdiagnosed as such or may be found incidentally during repair of a hernia. If found at surgery, the lipoma is removed to avoid a persistent bulge in the inguinal region despite a successful hernia repair.

Enlargement of inguinal lymph nodes may also be mistaken for herniation. Inflammatory nodes are usually tender; metastatic lymphadenopathy is usually not tender. If inguinal lymph nodes are replaced by metastasis, a primary lesion can arise in the skin in any part of the lower limb. A primary source should be looked for very carefully, particularly between the toes and on the undersurface of the foot. The perineum and anal canal should also be examined. Lymphadenopathy can also be caused by lymphoma, and groin nodes may be the only site. Lymphadenopathy characteristically appears as a well-circumscribed mass below the inguinal ligament that one can get above with the examining hand. Lymph nodes are solid on ultrasonography, and for this reason, it may be difficult to differentiate nodes from a femoral hernia containing omentum.

Treatment

The current surgical literature suggests that all inguinal hernias should be repaired unless specific contraindications are present. This recommendation is based on the presumption that complications of incarceration, obstruction, and strangulation are greater threats than are the risks of operation. The operative mortality, especially in the elderly, is increased at least ninefold to 10-fold when obstruction occurs (47–53). However, because of the low incidence of life-threatening complications of groin hernias and the possibility of the development of chronic groin pain in 10% to 12% of patients after herniorrhaphy, the notion that the presence of an inguinal hernia is an indication for repair has come under scrutiny. Until more data are available, the treatment of a groin hernia is surgical unless a serious medical condition precludes repair. Because of the ease with which groin hernias can be repaired under local anesthesia, very few conditions preclude surgery. If it is impossible for the patient to undergo surgery, a truss can be worn. This is a type of belt with an appliance that compresses the area through which the hernia protrudes. Trusses are successful in controlling symptoms in a certain percentage of patients, but complications can develop despite their use.

Open Approach

In the first of the three basic types of hernia repair, the *herniotomy,* the patent processus vaginalis is ligated at its origin at the internal ring and divided, so-called high ligation of the sac. This procedure is used for Nyhus type I hernias, such as those that occur in children. The skin incision starts at the pubic tubercle and is extended laterally. The external oblique aponeurosis is opened in the line of its fibers through the external ring and the lower leaf is freed from the spermatic cord. The spermatic cord is freed from the floor of the inguinal canal and the pubic bone. The genital branch of the genitofemoral nerve and the spermatic vessels are included with the cord. The ilioinguinal and iliohypogastric nerves are usually preserved. The cremasteric fibers are separated, and the hernia sac is dissected from the cord structures to a point proximal to the internal ring. Ligation can be performed at this point (high ligation), followed by division of the neck of the sac. The sac can be opened to allow a digital examination of the abdominal cavity and femoral ring. No form of repair is necessary, and an excellent result can be expected.

The second type of hernia operation is the *herniorrhaphy,* which is used to repair Nyhus type II or III hernias. The sac is ligated at its origin. Large scrotal hernias are transected at the midpoint of the canal, and the distal sac is left in situ. The area of weakness in the posterior wall is then reinforced with the patient's own tissues. The Bassini, Shouldice, and McVay repairs are good examples of this type of operation.

In the Bassini repair, the transversus abdominis aponeurosis together with the transversalis fascia is sutured to the shelving edge of the inguinal ligament with nonabsorbable interrupted sutures (Fig. 51.23). In the Shouldice repair, the transversalis fascia is divided from the internal ring to the pubic tubercle and lifted from the peritoneum. The fascia is then overlapped with two rows of running sutures (Fig. 51.24). Two further rows of sutures are applied to bring the transversus abdominis muscle to the shelving edge of the inguinal ligament. Although the suture material originally used for this repair was stainless steel wire, other nonabsorbable materials, such as Prolene, are now

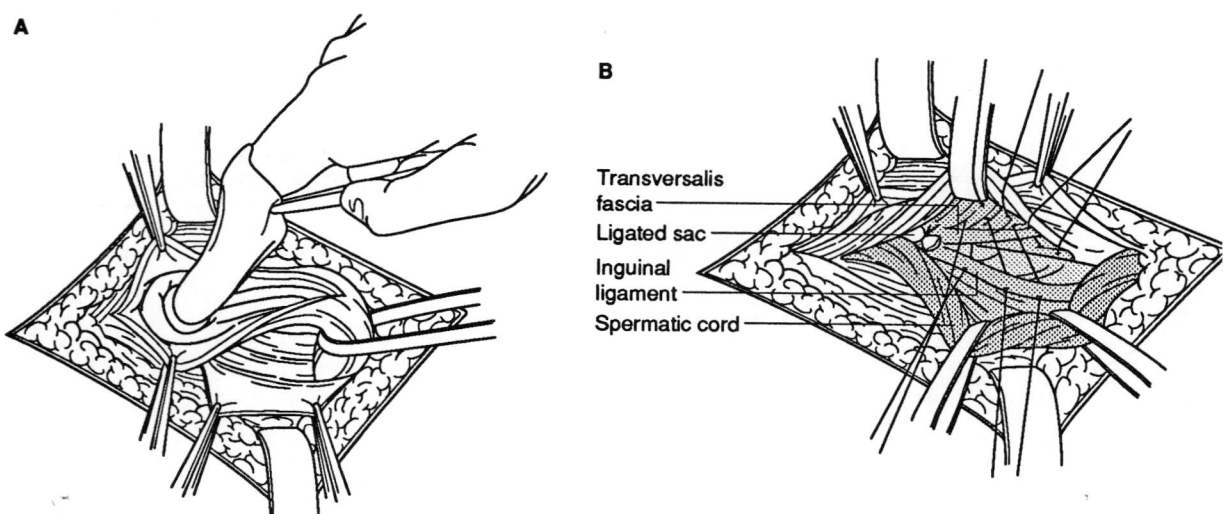

A

B

Transversalis fascia
Ligated sac
Inguinal ligament
Spermatic cord

Figure 51.23. Bassini repair.

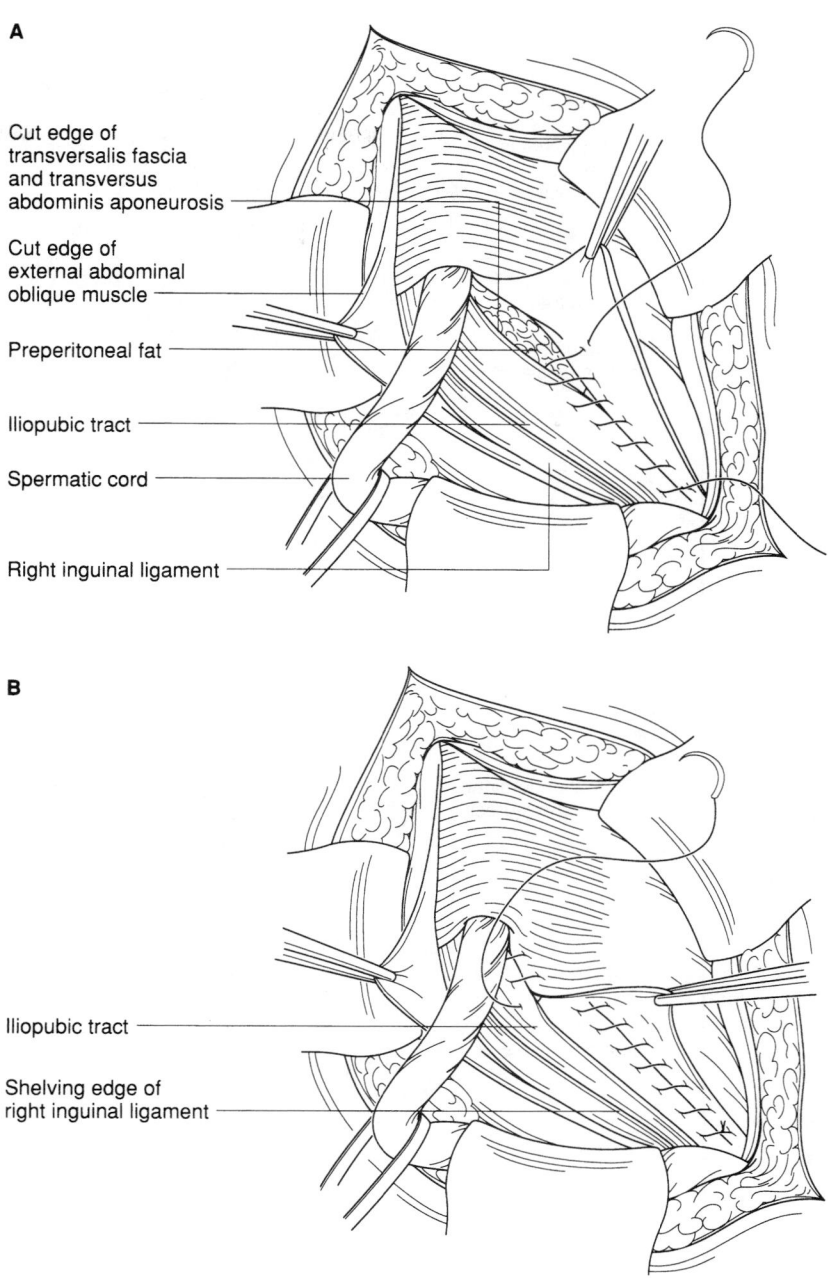

A

Cut edge of
transversalis fascia
and transversus
abdominis aponeurosis

Cut edge of
external abdominal
oblique muscle

Preperitoneal fat

Iliopubic tract

Spermatic cord

Right inguinal ligament

B

Iliopubic tract

Shelving edge of
right inguinal ligament

Figure 51.24. Shouldice repair.

used. The McVay repair (Fig. 51.25) addresses both inguinal and femoral hernias. The central attenuated portion of the inguinal floor is excised. Cooper's ligament must be clearly identified. The inguinal floor is then repaired by approximating the transversus abdominis aponeurosis and transversalis fascia to Cooper's ligament between the pubic tubercle and the femoral vein. More laterally, the transversus abdominis muscle and transversalis fascia are approximated to the iliopubic tract and femoral sheath up to the internal ring.

A relaxing incision is necessary for repairs of large indirect hernias and whenever the McVay repair is used. Failure to make a relaxing incision has been implicated in a greater incidence of recurrence. The relaxing incision is made in the internal lamina of the anterior rectus sheath in a vertical direction and is extended 1 to 2 cm above the pubis to a level opposite the internal ring (Fig. 51.25). The

resulting defect in the sheath is protected posteriorly by the body of the rectus muscle, which prevents herniation at that site.

In the third type of repair, *hernioplasty,* the hernial sac is ligated at the neck, as described above. Alternatively, the sac may be simply inverted. The proponents of not opening the sac feel that with this method the patient experiences less pain because the highly innervated peritoneum has not been violated (54). The repair then consists of reinforcement of the posterior abdominal wall defect with synthetic material. The prosthesis can be placed either as a plug to invert the hernial sac or as a patch, which may be an underlay, overlay, or a combined type (Fig. 51.26). The overlay patch technique is currently the most popular (32,35,54–56).

In the Lichtenstein operation (32) (Fig. 51.27), the incision starts at the pubic tubercle and is extended laterally

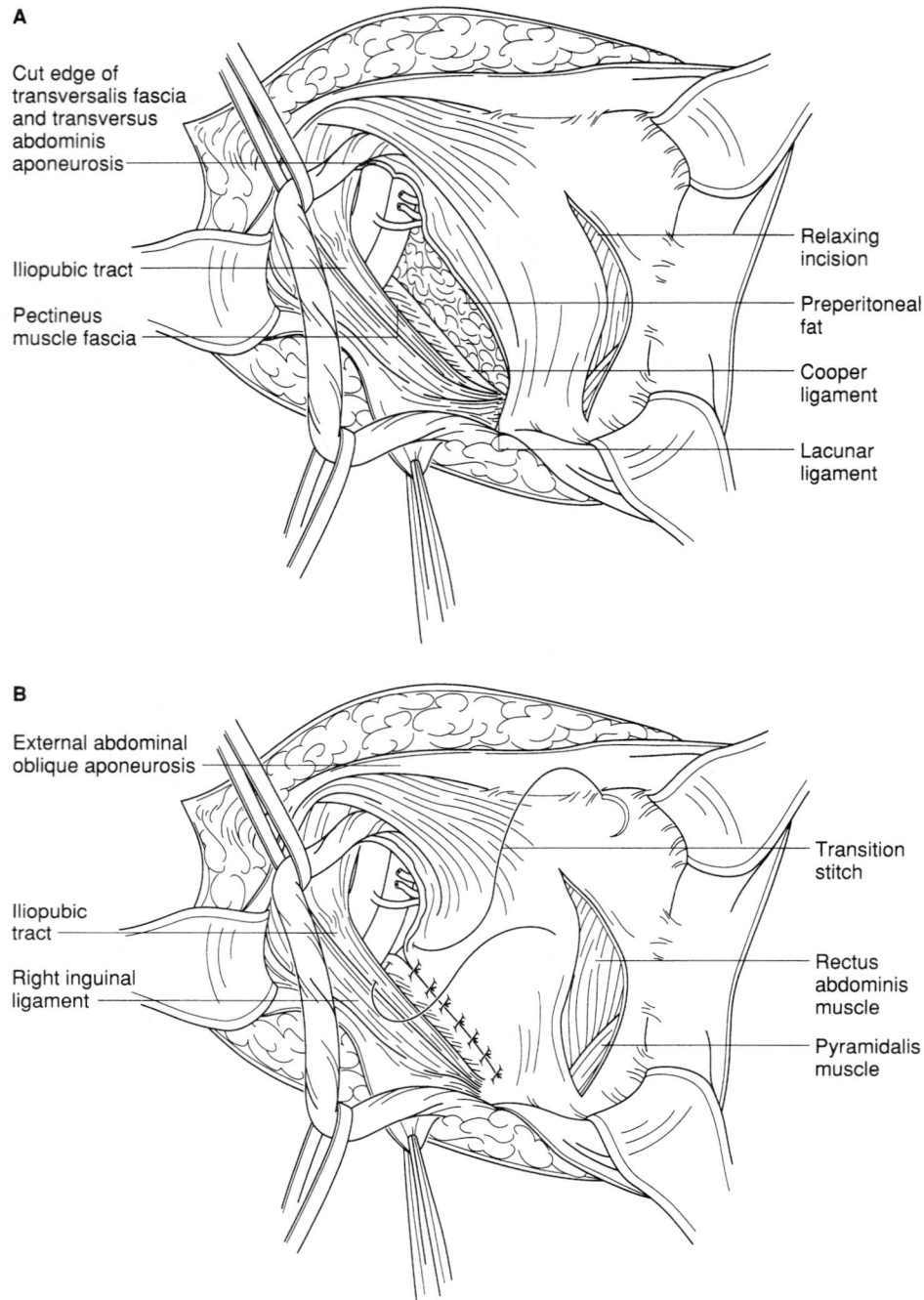

A

Cut edge of
transversalis fascia
and transversus
abdominis
aponeurosis

Iliopubic tract

Pectineus
muscle fascia

Relaxing
incision

Preperitoneal
fat

Cooper
ligament

Lacunar
ligament

B

External abdominal
oblique aponeurosis

Iliopubic
tract

Right inguinal
ligament

Transition
stitch

Rectus
abdominis
muscle

Pyramidalis
muscle

Figure 51.25. McVay (Cooper's ligament) repair.

for about 10 cm. The exposure of the cord is as described above. The hernial sac is dealt with and then the defect is repaired with synthetic mesh. The upper leaf of the external oblique aponeurosis is separated from the underlying internal oblique muscle and anterior rectus sheath so that the mesh will be able to overlap 2 to 3 cm above the upper border of Hesselbach's triangle. A 6 × 8–cm sheet of polypropylene mesh is used, the medial end of which is rounded to the shape of the medial corner of the inguinal canal. This medial end is sutured to the aponeurotic tissue over the pubic bone with a 2-0 polypropylene suture so that it overlaps the pubic bone by 2 cm. The periosteum of

the bone is avoided. The suture is continued to attach the lower edge of the prosthesis to the shelving edge of the inguinal ligament up to a point just lateral to the internal ring. If a femoral hernia is present, the posterior surface of the mesh is sutured to Cooper's ligament after the inferior edge has been attached to the inguinal ligament. This closes the femoral canal. The repair is then continued by securing the superior border of the mesh to the internal oblique aponeurosis and the anterior rectus sheath. A slit is cut in the lateral end of the mesh to produce a narrow (1/3-width) tail below and a wider (2/3-width) tail above. The spermatic cord is positioned between the two tails.

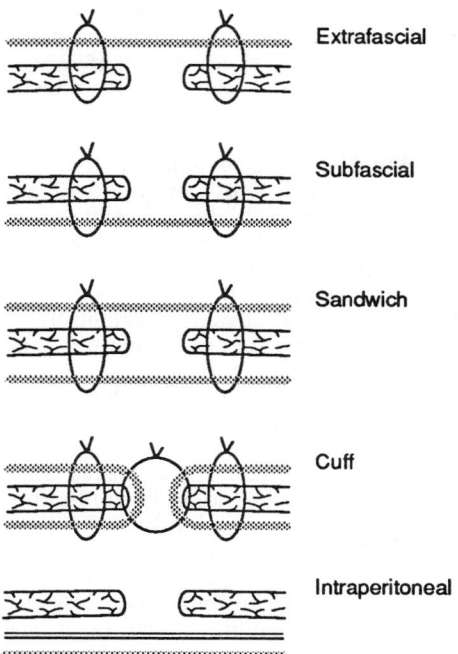

Figure 51.26. Various techniques for placing an abdominal wall prosthesis.

The wider tail is placed over the narrow one and held there with a hemostat. The cord is retracted downward and the upper edge of the patch is sutured to the internal oblique muscle and anterior rectus sheath, with care taken to avoid injury to the iliohypogastric nerve. This part of the repair is performed with upward retraction of the internal oblique, so that when it is released, there will be no tension on the repair. With a single polypropylene suture, the lower edges of the two tails are now fixed to the shelving margin of the inguinal ligament, so that a new, snug-fitting internal ring is created. Any excess prosthesis is trimmed, with 4 to 5 cm left lateral to the internal ring. The external oblique aponeurosis is closed to re-create the external ring. The wound is closed in layers.

During a 25-year period, investigators used the tension-free method to repair bilateral hernias in 2,953 patients (57). Postoperative pain was mild and the recovery period short. The recurrence rate was 0.1%. Repair of bilateral hernias via the laparoscopic approach has also yielded excellent results.

Femoral hernias can be repaired from a lower approach, in which a vertical incision is made over the femoral triangle in the upper thigh. The hernia is approached from below the inguinal ligament and reduced, and then the defect is closed by suturing the inguinal ligament to Cooper's ligament from below. With the Lichtenstein technique, a rolled plug of mesh can be inserted into the defect and sutured to the periphery of the inguinal ligament and Cooper's ligament (58). Alternatively, the repair can be carried out from above via an inguinal approach, as in the McVay repair. The posterior floor of the inguinal canal is dissected out, and Cooper's ligament is repaired after the hernia has been reduced. A third type of femoral hernia repair is the preperitoneal repair. Access to the preperitoneal space is gained through a midline abdominal incision. Femoral hernias are more common in women and often present with an acute episode of incarceration, intestinal obstruction, or strangulation, so that emergency surgery is necessary. It can be difficult to reduce the hernia at surgery, and is not uncommon to have to divide the inguinal ligament to obtain greater freedom to perform this reduction.

Another important factor contributing to the well-being of the patient after hernia is the use of local anesthesia (59, 60). Throughout the world, local anesthesia has become the standard method of anesthesia for this operation. When local anesthesia is used, the procedure can be carried out on an outpatient basis. The patient can walk immediately after the surgery and return to normal activities in a day. Hernias in high-risk patients can be safely repaired under local anesthesia.

Preperitoneal Approach

The preperitoneal space is situated between the transversalis fascia and the peritoneum. The transversus abdominis muscle and its aponeurosis and fascial coverings are probably the most important layer in the groin. The aim of hernia repairs should be to return this layer to normal. By strengthening the preperitoneal area, this goal can be achieved.

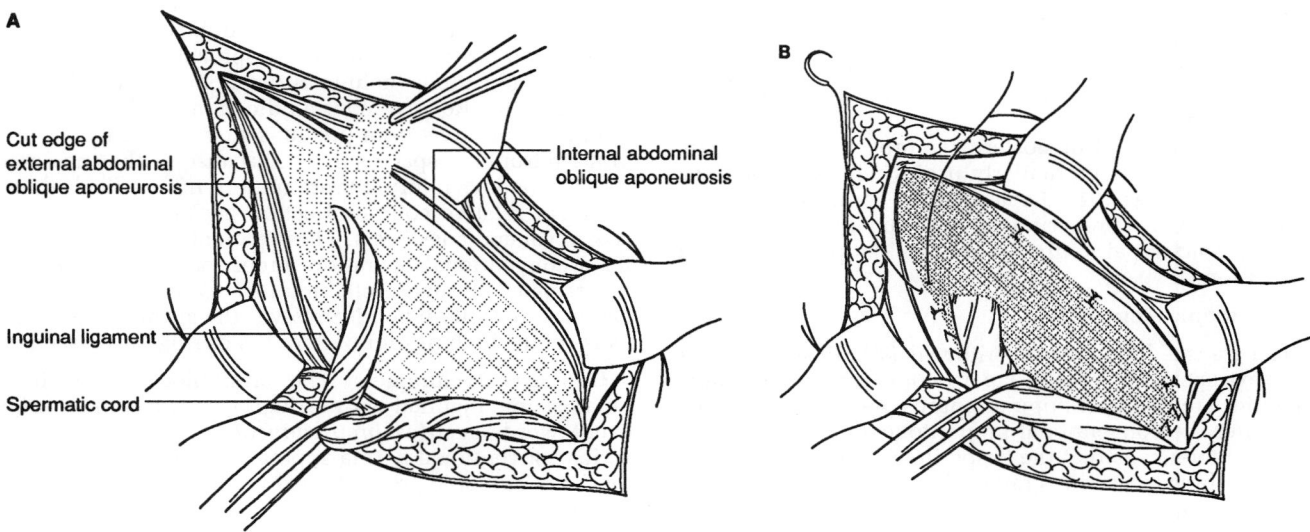

Figure 51.27. The Lichtenstein hernioplasty, showing placement of the mesh.

An operation may be performed through a lower midline incision, which gives one access to the preperitoneal space (38). The peritoneum can be dissected away from the undersurface of the transversalis fascia to expose the defect through which the hernia protrudes. Alternatively, a lateral rectus approach via a transverse incision can be used to expose the defect. A few centimeters above the pubic tubercle, the rectus sheath can be opened and the rectus muscle retracted medially (61). Access is then gained to the preperitoneal space, through which the repair is performed.

In 1983, investigators developed the concept of reinforcement of the preperitoneal layer in the lower abdomen by placing a large piece of mesh in this area (62). This can be done through a transverse lower abdominal incision (63–67). A large prosthesis is used that extends far beyond the margins of the myopectineal orifice and envelops the visceral sac. The mesh is held in place by intraabdominal pressure, which pushes outward toward the undersurface of the transversalis fascia. Later, as a consequence of connective tissue ingrowth, the mesh becomes incorporated in the body tissues, which further strengthens this layer. The mesh also adheres to the peritoneum, so that the peritoneum cannot protrude through the parietal defect. This technique works by preventing the peritoneum from bulging outward rather than by repairing abdominal wall defects. No sutures are placed in this method of hernia repair, and it is tension-free. Because the incision for a preperitoneal hernia repair is away from the groin area and directly accesses the preperitoneal space, dissection of the inguinal canal, spermatic cord, or sensory nerves of the groin is not performed. The complications involving these structures that occur with other hernia repairs are very rare with the preperitoneal repair. If the hernial sac is large, it is amputated or inverted beneath a pursestring suture to smooth the external surface of the visceral sac. The distal peritoneal sac is left in place, undissected and attached to the cord. With a sliding indirect hernia, the sac would have to be dissected away from the cord. The mesh is composed of multifilament fibers of Dacron, which is soft, elastic, supple, and rapidly integrated into tissue. Other meshes are not suitable because they are semirigid and buckle when bent in two directions.

In a bilateral repair, the chevron-shaped mesh is usually measured to be transversely 2 cm less than the distance between the anterior superior iliac spines and vertically the distance between the umbilicus and the symphysis pubis. The mesh is placed in the preperitoneal space so that it underlies the rectus muscle for a width of about 2 to 3 cm and extends this same distance above the level of the myopectineal orifice in all directions. The mesh is held in place by sutures attaching it to the undersurface of the abdominal wall.

The preperitoneal or posterior approach for the repair of groin hernias is particularly useful with very large or recurrent hernias (61). Laparoscopic hernioplasty is an extension of the preperitoneal concept. In many of the laparoscopic repairs, the prosthesis is placed in the preperitoneal space.

Laparoscopic Approach

The transabdominal preperitoneal (TAPP) and the totally extraperitoneal (TEP) laparoscopic inguinal herniorrhaphies are the most popular approaches. Both are modeled after the conventional preperitoneal operations. The major difference is that the preperitoneal space is entered through three trocar sites rather than through a large conventional incision. The ensuing radical dissection of the preperitoneal space with placement of a large prosthesis is similar to the conventional preperitoneal operation.

Laparoscopic versus Conventional Herniorrhaphy. The proponents of laparoscopic inguinal herniorrhaphy cite the following potential advantages (68–72): less postoperative discomfort and pain, reduced recovery time with an earlier return to full activity, easier repair of a recurrent hernia because it is performed in tissue that has not been previously dissected, ability to treat bilateral hernias concurrently, ability to perform a diagnostic laparoscopy simultaneously, highest possible ligation of the hernia sac, and improved cosmesis. In addition, it is felt that laparoscopic repair may be associated with fewer recurrences than conventional inguinal herniorrhaphy because of the mechanical advantage gained by placing the prosthesis in the preperitoneal space and the "tension-free" nature of the repair (73,74).

The laparoscopic approach also has disadvantages. These include complications related to the laparoscopy itself, such as bowel perforation and major vascular injury; potential for the development of adhesive complications at sites where the peritoneum has been breached or prosthetic material has been placed; need for general anesthesia; and increased cost because of the expensive equipment needed. On the other hand, the conventional operation can be performed under local anesthesia on an outpatient basis, with a minimal risk for intraabdominal injury and at lower cost.

In Table 51.4, 16 commonly cited prospective trials comparing laparoscopic and conventional hernia repair are summarized. All except one have shown a statistically significant advantage for laparoscopic repair over both tension and tension-free conventional repairs for one or more of the parameters studied. Despite these findings, many surgeons continue to feel that the potential risks associated with laparoscopy are greater than the benefits. The question will not likely be settled until the results of additional randomized, prospective trials are reported. Several such trials have been funded and are currently accruing patients.

Patient Selection. At the present time, all adult patients with inguinal hernias who are candidates for general anesthesia can be considered candidates for laparoscopic inguinal hernia repair. It is not clear that laparoscopic repair provides sufficient advantages for patients with uncomplicated inguinal hernias to outweigh the major disadvantages of the procedure, which include (a) laparoscopic accident, (b) bowel obstruction secondary to adhesions or an internal or ventral hernia, and (c) increased cost. Certain hernia types, such as those that are recurrent, bilateral, or otherwise complicated, are particularly suited for the laparoscopic approach.

Contraindications include intraabdominal infection and coagulopathy. Relative contraindications include intraabdominal adhesions from previous surgery, ascites, or previous retropubic space surgery, because of the increased risk for bladder injury. Severe underlying medical illness is also a relative contraindication because of the added risk of general anesthesia. These patients are better suited for a conventional operation under local anesthesia. An incarcerated sliding scrotal hernia is a relative contraindication, especially when it involves the sigmoid colon, because of the high risk for perforation during the dissection.

Operative Techniques. The terminology to describe a laparoscopic inguinal herniorrhaphy can be confusing because words such as *preperitoneal* are also used to describe conventional hernia approaches (104). In this chapter, a laparoscopic preperitoneal hernia repair, in which a laparoscopy is performed and the preperitoneal space is entered with a second incision in the peritoneum, is called a *transabdominal preperitoneal repair,* or TAPP re-

Table 51.4. COMPARATIVE TRIALS OF LAPAROSCOPIC AND OPEN INGUINAL HERNIA REPAIRS

Investigators, Year (reference)	Hernias (n) LH vs. OH	Intervention	Salient Features
Stoker et al., 1994 (127)	83 vs. 84	TAPP vs. Nylon darn	6 vs. 18 pain tablets Pain analogue score 1.8 vs. 3.1 Return to activity 14 vs. 28 days ↑ Cost
Payne et al., 1994 (128)	48 vs. 52	TAPP vs. Lichtenstein	Return to work 9 vs. 17 days ↑ Cost
Vogt et al., 1995 (129)	30 vs. 32	IPOM vs. tension-free	↓ Oral narcotics ↑ Return to normal activity Cost not mentioned
Lawrence et al., 1995 (130)	58 vs. 66	TAPP vs. nylon darn	Pain analogue scores better early No difference in return to work ↑ Complication rate ↑ Cost Better quality of life
Barkun et al., 1995 (131)	43 vs. 49	TAPP vs. various	↓ Postoperative narcotics Better quality of life at 1 month ↑ Satisfaction with LH ↑ Cost
Wright et al., 1996 (132)	67 vs. 64	Extra vs. Lichtenstein and Stoppa repair	↓ Pain scores ↓ Analgesia doses ↓ Wound complications
Kozol et al., 1997 (133)	30 vs. 32	TAPP vs. Bassini or McVay	↓ Pain at 24 and 48 hour with McGill pain and visual analogue pain scale score ↓ Pain medication
Maddern et al., 1994 (134)	42 vs. 44	TAPP vs. darn	↑ Discharge time Pain scores, activity levels, analgesia requirement and time to return to work not significantly different
Brooks, 1994 (135)	53 vs. 63	TAPP vs. tension-free (plug)	**Nonrandomized** ↑ Time ↑ Cost No difference in pain medication Earlier return to work
Millikan et al., 1994 (136)	75 vs. 51	TAPP vs. variety	**Nonrandomized** ↓ Time off work ↓ Pain medication ↓ Complication Hospital days better ↑ Cost
Cornell and Kerlabian, 1994 (137)	69 vs. 24	TAPP vs. ????	**Nonrandomized** Earlier return to activity at 14 days Earlier return to work in 3 weeks ↓ Pain ↑ Cost
Wilson et al., 1995 (138)	121 vs. 121	TAPP vs. Lichtenstein	**Nonrandomized** Earlier return to activity Earlier return to work No difference in analgesic requirements or pain scale
Leim et al., 1997 (139)	487 vs. 507	TAPP vs. Lichtenstein	↓ Incidence of wound abscesses ↑ Resumption of normal activity ↑ Return to work ↑ Resumption of athletic activities ↓ Recurrence rate
Wellwood et al., 1998 (140)	200 vs. 200	TEP vs. tension-free	↓ Pain score for first 2 weeks ↑ Functional scores ↑ Return to normal activity ↑ Patient satisfaction ↑ Cost
Johansson et al., 1999 (141)	613 total	TAPP vs. preperitoneal Mesh vs. conventional	↑ Resumption of normal activity ↑ Return to work ↑ Cost
MRC Group, 1999 (142)	468 vs. 460	TEP vs. mainly tension-free	↑ Resumption of normal activity ↓ Pain at 1 year ↑ Recurrence rate

IPOM, intraperitoneal onlay mesh repair; LH, laparoscopic hernia repair; OH, open hernia repair; TAPP, transabdominal preperitoneal repair; TEP, totally extraperitoneal repair.

pair. An inguinal hernia repair in which prosthetic material is placed intraperitoneally over the defect under laparoscopic guidance is referred to as an *intraperitoneal onlay mesh repair,* or IPOM repair. The third general type of laparoscopic approach is the *totally extraperitoneal laparoscopic repair,* or TEP repair. Laparoscopy, by definition, implies that the peritoneal cavity has been entered. To refer to this technique as *extraperitoneal* therefore represents a contradiction in terms. However, because a laparoscope and related instruments are used, it is fitting to discuss the extraperitoneal approach along with the other laparoscopic inguinal herniorrhaphies.

Transabdominal Preperitoneal Repair. The procedure is begun with a thorough diagnostic laparoscopy to rule out unrelated pathology and carefully inspect both myopectineal orifices. Two additional cannulae are placed just lateral to the rectus sheath on either side of the umbilicus (Fig. 51.28). For a unilateral hernia, a transverse incision is begun at the lateral side of the medial umbilical ligament and extended to open its lateral leaf to the anterior superior iliac spine. If the medial umbilical ligament appears to compromise exposure, it can be divided. Electrocautery is used to minimize bleeding from the remnants of the embryologic umbilical artery. A radical dissection of the preperitoneal space is then performed with mostly blunt dissection and generous use of electrocautery, as bleeding in this area is particularly troublesome if it interferes with illumination. The ipsilateral and contralateral pubic tubercles, the inferior epigastric vessels, Cooper's ligament, and the iliopubic tract are identified (Fig. 51.29). The cord structures are mobilized, and the peritoneal flap is dissected several centimeters proximal to the bifurcation of the vas deferens and the internal spermatic vessels.

Recurrences have been attributed to inadequate mobilization of the peritoneal flap, which does not allow the prosthesis to lie flat in this area. If small, an indirect sac is mobilized away from the cord structures and reduced. If large, the sac is divided at a convenient point distal to the internal ring and only the proximal portion is mobilized. A direct sac readily reduces during the preperitoneal dissection. An easily visible layer of fatty tissue separates the thinned out transversalis fascia lining the defect and the peritoneum.

A large piece of polypropylene mesh (at least 11×6 cm) is stapled in place, beginning at the contralateral pubic tubercle medially and extending onto the anterior abdominal wall superiorly at least 2 cm above the hernia defect, to the anterior superior iliac spine laterally, and to Cooper's ligament inferiorly. Most surgeons prefer to fasten the prosthesis with staples or tacks. Some surgeons feel fixation is not necessary at all when a large prosthesis is used that widely overlaps the entire myopectineal orifice. Staples or tacks are never placed below the iliopubic tract when lateral to the internal spermatic vessel because of the danger of damage to the important nerves in this area. Damage to these nerves results in neuralgia, such as was commonly observed in the developmental stages of lap-aroscopic inguinal herniorrhaphy, before the anatomy of the preperitoneal space was appreciated from a laparoscopic perspective. To decrease further the incidence of neuralgia, staples are placed horizontally for the superior border of the prosthesis to correspond to the direction of the more superficially located yet vulnerable ilioinguinal and iliohypogastric nerves. Laterally, staples are placed vertically, as this is the direction of the lateral cutaneous nerve of the thigh and the femoral branch of the genitofemoral nerve. The

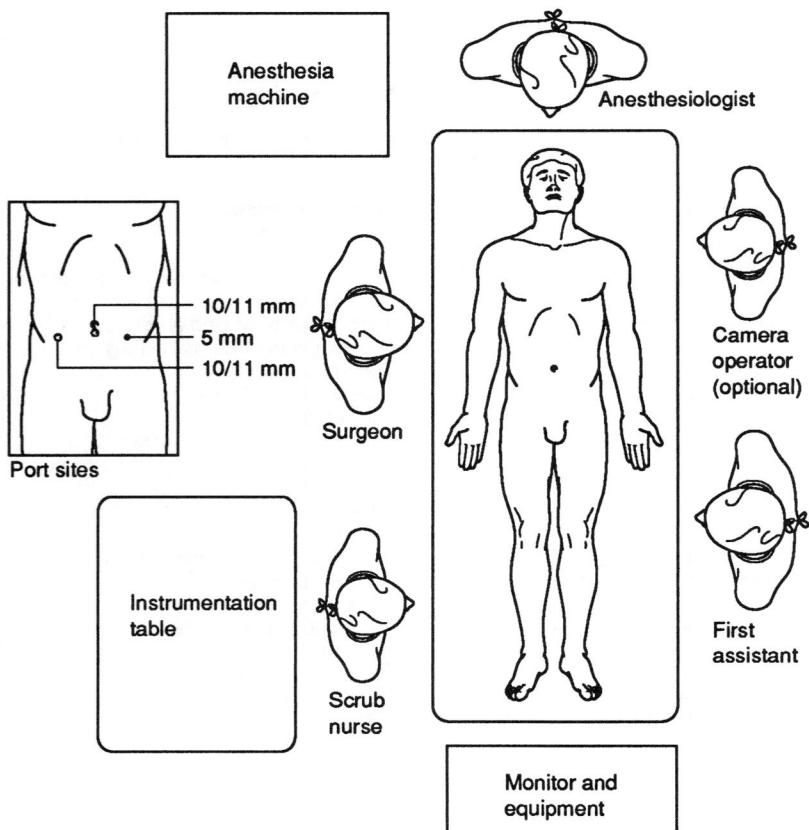

Figure 51.28. Typical operative setup and cannula site selection for a transabdominal preperitoneal *(TAPP)* laparoscopic inguinal herniorrhaphy.

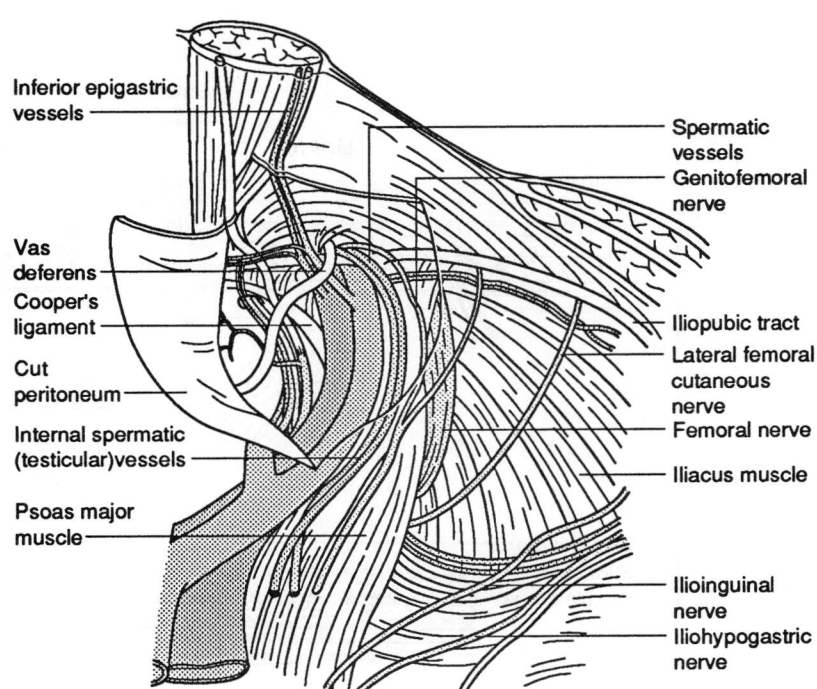

Figure 51.29. Important structures that must be identified after a preperitoneal dissection: inferior epigastric vessels, Cooper's ligament, spermatic vessels, vas deferens, iliopubic tract, genitofemoral nerve, femoral nerve, lateral femoral cutaneous nerve, ilioinguinal nerve, iliacus muscle, psoas major muscle.

last step is to cover the prosthesis with the inferior peritoneal flap.

For bilateral inguinal hernias, the same peritoneal incision and preperitoneal dissections are used. The symphysis pubis is completely exposed so that both preperitoneal dissections communicate with each other. This exposure allows the placement of one large prosthesis (at least 25 × 7.5 cm) that essentially covers the entire lower pelvis. By not incising the peritoneum between the two medial umbilical ligaments, one avoids the theoretical complication of dividing a patent urachus.

Totally "Extraperitoneal" Inguinal Herniorrhaphy. With extraperitoneal laparoscopic inguinal hernia repair, the peritoneal cavity is not intentionally violated (72). An incision is made at the umbilicus, as if one were planning to perform open laparoscopy. The rectus sheath is opened on one side and the rectus muscle is retracted laterally. Blunt dissection is then begun in the space between the rectus muscle and the posterior rectus sheath. The space is enlarged by placing a blunt instrument blindly or an operating laparoscope (a rigid laparoscope with a working channel). Once the space is large enough, two additional cannulae are placed in the midline, one approximately 5 cm above the symphysis pubis and the other midway between the umbilicus and the symphysis pubis. The dissection of the preperitoneal space is completed under direct vision. The rest of the operation is identical to the TAPP procedure, described above. Popular alternatives are to use a water- or air-filled balloon dissector to perform the preperitoneal dissection and to place the two accessory cannulae on either side of the umbilicus, as in the TAPP procedure, instead of in the midline.

The presumed advantages of the TEP procedure are that the inherent complications of entering the peritoneal cavity, such as intraabdominal organ injury or postoperative bowel obstruction secondary to adhesions or trocar site herniation, are avoided. However, the operative space is limited, and considerable experience is required to become familiar with the anatomy from this perspective. In addition, it is not yet clear whether inadvertent breaches in the peritoneal cavity that are difficult to visualize because of the direction of the optics might negate the potential benefits of this approach.

Intraperitoneal Onlay Mesh Technique. The development of the IPOM procedure was based on the concept that it should be possible to achieve the results of the TAPP procedure simply by placing the prosthesis one layer deep to the preperitoneal space directly onto the peritoneum. This could be accomplished laparoscopically and would eliminate the need for a radical preperitoneal dissection. Initial laparoscopy and accessory cannula placement are the same as in the TAPP procedure. A large piece of prosthetic material is introduced into the peritoneal cavity and secured in place with staples, tacks, or sutures. An attempt is made to use the same landmarks described above for the TAPP procedure. The main concern is development of the complications of intraperitoneal placement of a prosthesis in contact with intraabdominal organs. Some surgeons use the IPOM procedure for large direct hernias but add sutures that incorporate the mesh and entire thickness of the abdominal wall except for the skin and subcutaneous tissue. This is accomplished by making a small stab incision in the skin and then using a suture passer (Fig. 51.30) to place a suture through the musculofascial, peritoneal, and mesh layers. The suture passer is then withdrawn back to the subcutaneous tissue and redirected through the musculofascial, peritoneal, and mesh layers at a different angle. The free end of the suture within the peritoneal cavity is grasped with the suture passer, brought back into the subcutaneous tissue, and tied. The skin is then closed over the suture.

The IPOM technique appears to be effective for treating indirect inguinal hernias when it is performed by experienced surgeons. Reports of excessive recurrence rates may be related to training and patient selection (75). Simplicity makes this technique appealing. Nevertheless, IPOM must be considered an experimental operation because the prosthesis is placed in the peritoneal cavity in contact

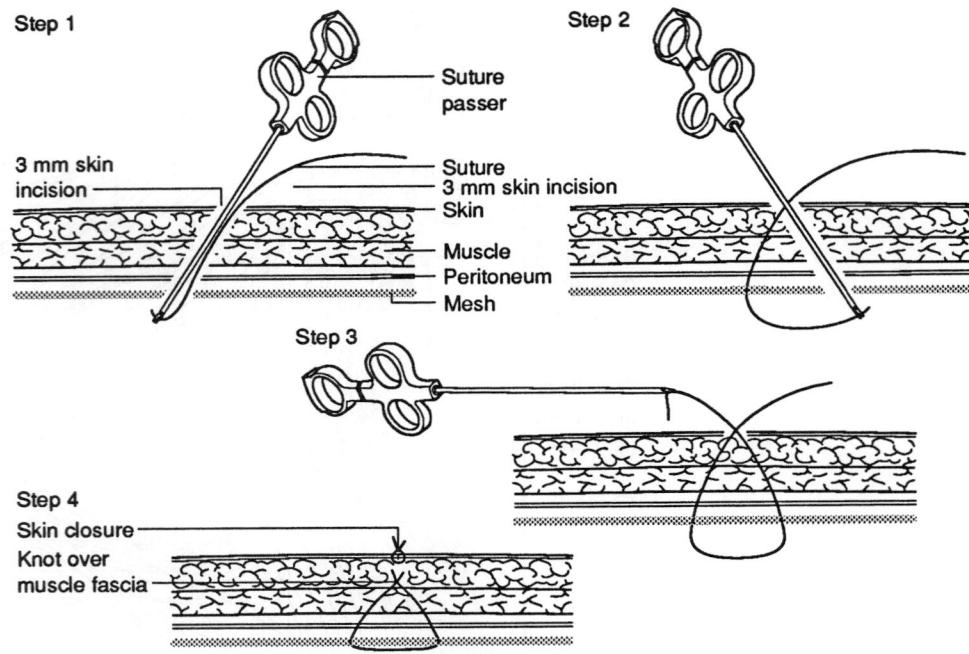

Figure 51.30. Fixation of prosthesis to the peritoneal surface of the abdominal wall with use of a suture passer. *Step 1:* The suture passer device with a heavy nonabsorbable suture is passed through a 3-mm stab incision in the skin at an oblique angle. The device and suture traverse the entire abdominal wall and then the prosthesis. Once the peritoneal cavity is entered, the suture is released and the passer is withdrawn back into the subcutaneous tissue. *Step 2:* The device is redirected at a different angle through the abdominal wall and prosthesis and the suture is grasped. *Step 3:* The suture is pulled out of the abdominal cavity so that the two free ends are extracorporeal. *Step 4:* The suture is tied with the knot resting on the fascia. The skin is then closed.

with intraabdominal organs. Until a completely inert prosthesis has been developed, IPOM should not be used in routine practice outside highly controlled trials.

Complications of Repair

The complications of groin hernia repair are many and varied (Table 51.5), but fortunately uncommon. The complications of inguinal herniorrhaphy can be categorized according to whether they are related to (a) the laparoscopy, (b) the patient, or (c) the herniorrhaphy. Except for the complications unique to laparoscopy, complications occur at similar rates in both laparoscopic and conventional procedures.

Complications Related to Laparoscopy

Vascular Injury. The most serious injuries occur to vessels that reside in the retroperitoneum (76,77). The risk for injury to vessels that requires operative intervention is 0.05% (78). The vessels most at risk are the distal aorta, common iliac arteries and veins, and inferior vena cava. Injuries to the renal vessels have also been reported. These vessels are fixed and may be penetrated even if the safety mechanisms of the needle or trocar are working properly. The mesenteric and omental vessels are also at risk, especially in the presence of adhesions. The epigastric arteries may be injured with secondary cannula placement.

Among vascular injuries requiring operative attention, 80% occur at the initial access (79). The most common agent in vascular injury is the insufflation needle. Placement of the initial trocar is the second most common cause of great-vessel injury and is more often catastrophic. Great-vessel injury is very unusual with the open technique.

When blood returns after placement of the insufflation needle, the needle should be pulled back and checked again for position, and insufflation should be started when the intraperitoneal position is confirmed. After the initial cannula has been placed, the retroperitoneum should be inspected for signs of injury. The indications for laparotomy and formal vascular repair in this setting are an expanding retroperitoneal hematoma, hemodynamic instability at any time during the operative or perioperative period, and active intraabdominal hemorrhage.

Vessel injuries caused by the trocar are usually more obvious and catastrophic. Because of the relatively large size of the trocar point, transmural injury is the rule rather than the exception. When an injury is recognized, the trocar and cannula should be left in place to tamponade the vessel and a formal vascular repair through a conventional laparotomy undertaken. The mortality associated with retroperitoneal injury secondary to trocar insertion ranges from 9% to 36%, even with rapid identification and repair. Mesenteric and omental vessel injuries should be treated as retroperitoneal vessel injuries. The indications for repair of these vessels are the same as for repair of the retroperitoneal vessels.

Most abdominal wall vascular complications occur during the placement of secondary cannulae. Usually, pressure can be applied to bleeding at the trocar site with the cannula. Occasionally, suture ligation is required, which has been simplified by the development of disposable "exit devices" designed to facilitate the placement of fascial sutures. Most of these complications can be avoided by placing the secondary trocars under direct vision.

Gas embolism may occur with intravascular insufflation (76,80). Gas embolism is an uncommon complication, unique to the needle insufflation technique, with an inci-

Table 51.5. COMPLICATIONS OF LAPAROSCOPIC HERNIORRHAPHY

Related to laparoscopy	Related to patient	Related to herniorrhaphy
Vascular injury	Urinary infection	Recurrence
Intraabdominal	Ileus	Neurologic
Retroperitoneal	Nausea and vomiting	Iliohypogastric
Abdominal wall	Aspiration pneumonia	Ilioinguinal
Gas embolism	Cardiovascular and respirator insufficiency	Genitofemoral
Visceral injury		Lateral cutaneous
Bowel perforation		Cord and testicular problems
Bladder perforation		Wound infection
Trocar site complications		Seroma
Hematoma		Hydrocele
Hernia		Hematoma
Wound infection		Wound
Keloid		Scrotal
Bowel obstruction		Retroperitoneal
Trocar or peritoneal closure site hernia		Osteitis pubis
Adhesions		Prosthetic complications
Diaphragmatic dysfunction		Contraction
Hypercapnia		Erosion
		Infection
		Rejection
		Pain

dence of 0.003%. Careful attention to tests confirming proper peritoneal needle placement will keep the incidence of this complication low.

Visceral Injury. Visceral injuries are uncommon, occurring in 0.05% to 0.4% of all laparoscopic procedures, but they have a mortality rate of 5%. The most common means of injury is the insufflation needle. Injuries caused by the needle usually do not require repair. A lateral tear injury to the bowel, especially in the presence of a fixed adhesion, requires correction. Quite often, the injury goes unnoticed at the time of insult, so that visceral injury is the most common cause of late morbidity and mortality associated with laparoscopic access. Patients typically present with peritonitis and sepsis 2 days to 1 week after surgery.

If the bowel is damaged by the initial trocar, transmural injury is probable. Because of its size, the trocar point often causes lateral tear injuries that require formal repair. If the skill of the laparoscopic surgeon is sufficient, the injury can be repaired laparoscopically. The tear may also require a mini-laparotomy or conventional laparotomy for repair.

Bowel injury is also possible during the open technique, during either initial entry into the peritoneum or placement of the stay sutures. The incidence of this complication is approximately 0.05% of its incidence in open access procedures. With the open procedure, it is more likely that the injury will be immediately obvious and repaired expeditiously.

Bladder injury with peritoneal access is rare but possible, usually as a result of a failure to decompress the bladder. Less commonly, injury is associated with a congenital bladder abnormality. Bladder injury has not been reported with the open access technique.

When bladder injury occurs, it is usually obvious. Urine is withdrawn into the syringe, or blood and gas are noticed in the urine if the patient is catheterized. If the insufflation needle is the culprit, the needle is left in place and a second attempt at access with a sterile needle can be made after decompression of the bladder is confirmed. If minor injury is confirmed, treatment is conservative, with postoperative decompression via an indwelling catheter. When the injury is caused by a trocar, formal bladder repair is usually necessary.

Complications at the Trocar Site. Complications of wounds at the trocar site are the most common abdominal wall problems. The formation of a hematoma is relatively uncommon and is caused by the disruption of small nutrient vessels of the abdominal wall muscle or preperitoneal fatty tissue. Careless introduction of secondary trocars can result in hematoma if the inferior epigastric vessels are lacerated. Hernia at the trocar site has become less common with the routine closure of any defect larger than 5 mm. Strict adherence to the principle of closing the umbilical fascial defect is likely to reduce the incidence of this complication.

Recent evidence suggests that umbilical wound infections occur at similar rates for open and closed insufflation (81). Unsightly scars, especially in patients with a tendency to keloid formation, have been observed at cannula insertion sites. Prominent scars may develop at sites where towel clips have been used to elevate the abdominal wall. Towel clips should not be used to elevate the skin of patients with a history of keloid scar formation.

Bowel obstruction is extremely uncommon with conventional groin herniorrhaphy, and its association with the laparoscopic approach is the most significant argument against the procedure. The complication was frequent in the developmental stages of the laparoscopic procedure because the need to close trocar sites larger than 5 mm at the fascial level was not understood (82). Inadequate peritoneal closure over the prosthesis, which allows bowel to migrate into the preperitoneal space, is also manifested by intestinal obstruction.

Diaphragmatic dysfunction causing phrenic nerve palsy has been reported with a variety of laparoscopic procedures; it is usually transient but has been known to require a short period of mechanical ventilation. Stretching during the pneumoperitoneum probably causes this complication. Hypercapnia is the result of inadequate compensatory ventilation, given the fact that in the vast majority of laparoscopic procedures, carbon dioxide is used as the insufflating agent.

Complications Related to the Patient

Urinary retention occurs in a significant number of patients after herniorrhaphy. Age and a history of urinary symptoms are predisposing factors. General anesthesia, overhydration with intravenous fluid, and opiates have also been implicated as predisposing factors. Treatment consists of repeated bladder catheterization until normal voiding resumes (106).

Ileus can be seen with either the conventional or the laparoscopic procedure but is more common with the latter. Treatment is symptomatic, and spontaneous resolution is the rule. Nasogastric decompression is occasionally needed.

Complications Related to the Herniorrhaphy

The recurrence rate has been reduced with the use of modern hernioplasty techniques. Although the recurrence rate for hernia repairs is less than 1% at the Shouldice Clinic, the recurrence rate has been slightly higher at other centers using this technique (84). Recurrence rates below 1% have uniformly been reported for tension-free repairs in which synthetic mesh is used. A 0.1% recurrence rate was reported in one study of 4,000 patients (32). Published studies of the Lichtenstein repair consistently demonstrate a recurrence rate of less than 1%. Investigators have reported a 9-year experience in almost 3,300 patients with mesh plug repairs (85). The recurrence rate with this method was 0.2%, and morbidity was minimal. The recurrence rates for laparoscopic repairs, when performed by experienced surgeons, are equally low (73, 86–105) (Table 51.6).

A hernial recurrence usually presents as a bulge with a cough impulse. The bulge might be either medial or lateral, depending on where the defect in the repair is situated. Recurrences are managed with the use of synthetic material as a patch. If the recurrence is complicated or large, it can be managed by placing a large piece of mesh in the preperitoneal space to cover the defect. Femoral hernias developing after previous inguinal hernia repairs are well recognized. The pectineal repair and the modification of the Lichtenstein repair in which the mesh is sutured to Cooper's ligament will prevent this complication.

Various neuralgias may develop after the incorporation of a nerve in staples or suture material during repair of the hernia (106). As evidenced by a recent prospective, randomized study, postoperative groin pain is often persistent and debilitating. At 1 year after surgery, 62.9% of patients had some degree of groin pain and 11.9% of those patients rated the pain as moderate to severe (107). At 2 years, the figures were 53.6% and 10.6%, respectively.

The nerves most commonly involved are the ilioinguinal nerve, the iliohypogastric nerve, both the genital and femoral branches of the genitofemoral nerve, and the lateral cutaneous nerve of the thigh (106). The ilioinguinal and iliohypogastric nerves are especially prone to injury during a conventional herniorrhaphy, whereas the other branches are most likely damaged during laparoscopy. The genital and femoral branches of the genitofemoral nerve and the lateral cutaneous nerve of the thigh are especially prone to injury when stapling is performed below the iliopubic tract lateral to the internal spermatic vessels. Femoral nerve injury is extremely rare. Pain and paresthesia in the nerve distribution are characteristic symptoms. Reassurance and conservative treatment with antiinflammatory medications and local nerve blocks are preferred

Table 51.6. NONCOMPARATIVE TRIALS OF LAPAROSCOPIC INGUINAL HERNIA REPAIR (SERIES WITH MORE THAN 100 REPAIRS)

Investigators (reference)	Technique	Recurrent hernias at enrollment (%)	Hernias (n)	Recurrence rate (%)	F/U (mo)
Arregui et al. (73)	TAPP/EXTRA	14	147	1.3	NA
Corbitt (86)	TAPP	12	100	0	18
Felix et al. (87)	TAPP	13	205	0	21
Felix et al. (88)	TAPP	14	733	0.3	24
Geis et al. (89)	TAPP	11	450	0.6	30
Hawasli (90)	TAPP plus plug and patch	10	143	1.4	7
Himpens (91)	TAPP	17	100	2	NA
Kald et al. (92)	TAPP	17	200	3.5	24
Kavic (93)	TAPP	10	244	1	34
Newman et al. (94)	TAPP	14	102	NA	1
Paget (95)	TAPP	15	222	1.8	18
Panton and Panton (96)	TAPP	18	106	0	12
Quilici et al. (97)	TAPP	5	173	0	NA
Ramshaw et al. (98)	TAPP	14	290	2.1	NA
	TEP	16	118	0.5	NA
Wheeler (99)	TAPP Mesh plus plug	5	135	0	18
Begin (100)	EXTRA	53	200	0.5	18
Ferzli and Kiel (101)	EXTRA/balloon CO_2/blunt	11	326	1.6	22
Voeller et al. (102)	EXTRA/balloon CO_2	12	365	0	15
Rubio (103)	IPOM	NA	120	48	0
Fitzgibbons et al. (104)	TAPP/EXTRA IPOM	14.5	867	4.5	34
Philips et al. (105)	TAPP/EXTRA IPOM Plug and patch Simple closure	1.6	3229	1.6	22

EXTRA, extraperitoneal mesh repair; IPOM, intraperitoneal onlay mesh repair; NA, information not available; TAPP, transabdominal preperitoneal repair.

initially, as symptoms frequently resolve spontaneously. When groin exploration is required, neurectomy and neuroma excision are performed. The results are often less than satisfactory.

Damage to the blood supply of the testicle can cause ischemic orchitis and testicular atrophy (108). Orchitis manifests as postoperative inflammation of the testicle developing within 1 to 2 days after surgery. The patient has a painfully enlarged testicle that is hard in consistency and associated with low-grade fever. Pain is severe and may last several weeks. Ischemic orchitis is caused by thrombosis of the veins draining the testicle after extensive dissection of the spermatic cord. The majority of patients with testicular problems as an immediate complication of herniorrhaphy recover without testicular atrophy. In one recent report, testicular atrophy developed in 19 patients among 52,583 primary inguinal hernia repairs (0.036%) and 33 patients among 7,169 recurrent inguinal hernia repairs (0.46%) (109). Although orchitis is more common after laparoscopic hernia repair, testicular atrophy is less common than with the open method. The management of a patient with ischemic orchitis is usually conservative. Doppler studies are performed to assess the arterial supply to the testis.

The vas deferens may be transected during herniorrhaphy. Anastomosis should be attempted immediately. In the dysejaculation syndrome, which develops after the vas is handled with a forceps, a fibrosis of varying severity develops throughout the muscular wall of the vas (109). This syndrome is characterized by searing, burning, painful sensations throughout the groin around the time of ejaculation. The incidence is approximately 0.04%.

Wound infection is a surprisingly unusual complication of groin herniorrhaphy. Seromas are common with the use of synthetic mesh in laparoscopic hernia repairs and are possibly related to the size of the mesh used. The fluid eventually resorbs spontaneously. Aspiration is performed for symptomatic relief only.

Bleeding can occur from the cremasteric, internal spermatic, or inferior epigastric vessels (106). Conservative treatment with reassurance is preferred. Evacuation is rarely required. Injuries to the deep circumflex artery, the corona mortis, or the external iliac vessels may result in a large retroperitoneal hematoma.

Because of the more liberal use of prosthetic material during conventional herniorrhaphy and its routine use in laparoscopy, a discussion of the complications related to foreign material is timely. The tissue response, which is variable from person to person, can be so intense that the prosthetic material is deformed by contraction. The development of intestinal obstruction or fistulization through erosion is possible if the prosthesis is in physical contact with the intestine (110,111). Local erosion into the cord structures has also been reported (112).

PERIUMBILICAL HERNIAS

Umbilical and paraumbilical hernias are caused by improper healing of the umbilical scar, which results in a defect in the fascia covered by skin. In infants, the fascial defect varies in size but is most commonly 1 to 2 cm. A large proportion of pediatric umbilical hernias heal spontaneously, and 80% of them close by the time the patient is 2 years old. Persistent umbilical hernias require surgery. In older patients, the onset is usually sudden and the defect is relatively small. An underlying cause of increased intraabdominal pressure, such as ascites or intraabdominal tumors, should be sought.

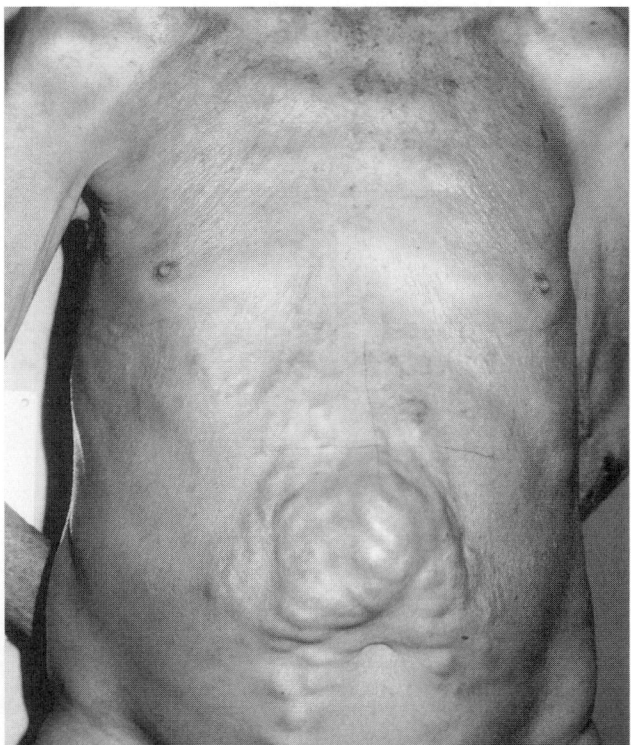

Figure 51.31. Caput medusae. Large periumbilical collaterals in a patient with portal hypertension.

The differential diagnosis of umbilical hernia includes the varicosities that extend radially from the umbilicus in persons with portal hypertension, the so-called caput medusae (Fig. 51.31). The varicosities have a bluish discoloration and fill when the patient is straining. A metastatic deposit of intraabdominal cancer at the umbilicus may mimic umbilical herniation. Cancer cells reach this area via lymphatics in the falciform ligament. Metastasis presents as a hard nodule, and biopsy is diagnostic. Other periumbilical masses that can be confused with an umbilical hernia include umbilical granulomas, omphalomesenteric duct remnant cysts, and urachal cysts.

The management of umbilical hernias is conservative in children up to the age of 2 years. In those who require surgery, the repair depends on the size of the hernia. The majority are small, and the defect can be closed by simple suture. A subumbilical semilunar incision is made. The sac of the hernia is opened and the contents reduced into the abdomen. The sac is then excised. An overlapping or waistcoat technique is used in which the upper edge of the linea alba overlaps the lower edge. Nonabsorbable sutures are used (Fig. 51.32). For larger hernias, particularly in adults, the sac may be dissected away from the undersurface of the skin of the umbilicus and reduced into the preperitoneal space. A prosthesis can then be used to bridge the fascial defect without contact with the intraabdominal viscera. The prosthesis is sutured circumferentially to the defect or to the undersurface of the posterior rectus sheath and the linea alba above the peritoneal closure. If it is not possible to keep the peritoneum intact beneath the defect, omentum should be tacked to the peritoneum circumferentially to isolate the abdominal viscera from the prosthesis.

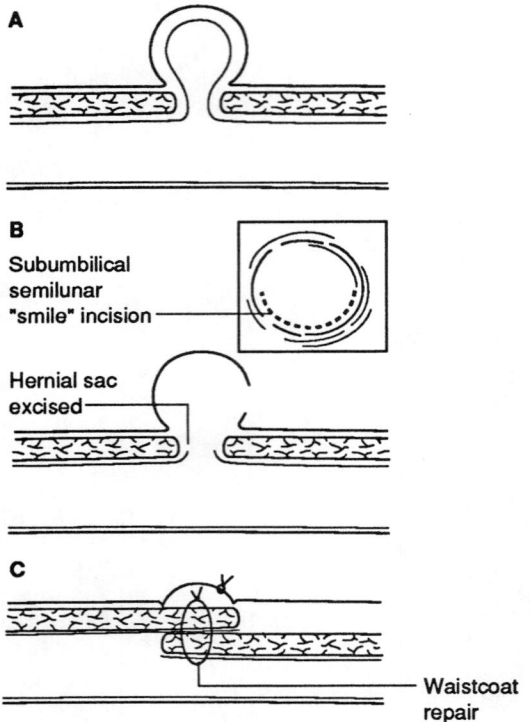

Figure 51.32. Repair of an umbilical hernia. *(A)* Diagram of longitudinal section through the hernia. *(B)* Subumbilical "smile" incision. The hernial sac is excised. *(C)* Waistcoat type of closure.

EPIGASTRIC HERNIAS

Epigastric hernias occur through a defect in the linea alba. In the majority of patients, only a single decussation of the fibers of the linea alba is present rather than the usual triple decussation (Fig. 51.6). The incidence of epigastric herniation reported varies from less than 1% to as high as 5%. Epigastric hernias are two to three times more common in men than in women. Twenty percent are multiple. Most are less than 1 cm and contain only incarcerated preperitoneal fat without a peritoneal sac. For this reason, epigastric hernias cannot be visualized with laparoscopy. Patients complain of a painful nodule in the upper midline. Repair by reduction of the preperitoneal fat and simple closure of the defect is curative. These hernias are prone to recur, with rates as high as 10%. Left untreated, an epigastric hernia can become large enough for a peritoneal sac to form, into which the intraabdominal contents can protrude. The sac is usually wide, and serious complications are not common.

In *diastasis recti,* the two rectus muscles are separated widely. The area of the linea alba is stretched and protrudes like a fin. Although diastasis recti is easily reducible and almost never produces complications, many patients find the defect unsightly and request treatment. Surgical therapy involves removal of a strip of the weakened linea alba and reapproximation. The alternative is a mesh repair.

INCISIONAL HERNIAS

Incisional hernias occur as a complication of prior surgery. These hernias can follow any type of abdominal surgery, regardless of the type of incision. The highest incidence is with midline and transverse incisions (113,

114), but hernias are well documented following paramedian, subcostal, appendectomy gridiron, and Pfannenstiel incisions. Poor surgical technique, rough handling of tissues, use of rapidly degraded absorbable suture materials, closure of the abdomen under tension, and infection of the wound are important causes of incisional hernias. Morbid obesity, cigarette smoking, pulmonary disease, and hypoalbuminemia have been incriminated as associated predisposing conditions. Many authorities believe that incisional hernias can be prevented by closing abdominal wounds with continuous running sutures and monofilament suture material. Sutures are placed 1 cm away from the edge and 1 cm apart from each other. The length of the suture should be four times the length of the wound to avoid excessive tension (115) (Fig. 51.33).

Repair of an incisional hernia depends on the size of the hernia. If the defect is solitary and 3 cm or less in size, primary closure with nonabsorbable suture material can be performed. For larger hernias or hernias with multiple small defects, primary closure results in unacceptably high recurrence rates. With large defects, the recurrence rate has been significantly reduced by using a tension-free mesh repair (116–119). When a hernia defect is bridged with mesh, attempts should be made to isolate the material from the intraabdominal viscera to prevent erosion with fistula formation or adhesive bowel obstruction. This can be accomplished with a peritoneal flap or omentum. When contact with intraabdominal organs cannot be avoided, e-PTFE should be considered.

Polytetrafluoroethylene is preferred by laparoscopic surgeons performing an incisional herniorrhaphy. In this procedure, the abdominal contents are reduced from the hernia defect under direct laparoscopic guidance. The number and location of the sites of trocar placement vary depending on the size and location of the hernia. The prosthesis is introduced through the largest cannula and positioned onto the peritoneum so that it widely overlaps the hernia defect. The prosthesis is secured to the anterior abdominal wall with staples, tacks, or sutures. A suture passer introduced through circumferentially located stab incisions is particularly useful for laparoscopic herniorrhaphy because it allows sutures to be placed through the prosthesis and the full thickness of the musculofascial elements of the abdominal wall. The sutures can be tied extracorporeally and then allowed to retract back into the subcutaneous tissue of the stab incisions. The skin is then closed over them (Fig. 51.30).

Alternatively, the posterior rectus sheath can be opened on each edge of the hernia defect and dissected away from the undersurface of the rectus muscles for a distance of 10 to 15 cm. The posterior rectus sheaths are then approximated to each other primarily. A large mesh prosthesis

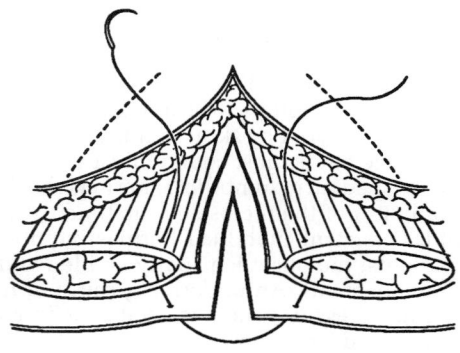

Figure 51.33. Mass closure of abdominal wall surgical wound.

(e-PTFE if the approximation of the posterior rectus sheath is inadequate) is then placed in this pocket outside the repaired posterior sheath but beneath the rectus muscles. The mesh is secured in this position with several sutures placed through small stab incisions at the periphery of the prosthesis with a suture passer and then tied in the subcutaneous tissue above the fascia.

Infection remains a major problem with prosthetic incisional hernia repairs. The incidence of infection is about 5%, and when infection occurs, healing can be delayed for a prolonged period. Factors leading to infection are preexisting infection or ulceration of the skin over the hernia, obesity, incarcerated or obstructed bowel within the hernia, and perforation of the bowel at the time of hernia repair. Seromas are common when a large prosthesis is required or flap dissection of the subcutaneous layer from the fascia has been extensive. Untreated seromas can become secondarily infected. Suction drains can be useful, but if left in place too long, they also result in infection of the prosthesis. Strategies to prevent and manage seromas are largely based on empiricism and personal opinion, as objective data are nearly absent. It is not always necessary to remove the mesh prosthesis in the presence of infection. A trial of local wound care after opening of the incision and débridement is warranted.

Several other factors contribute to the poor results obtained in repairing incisional hernias. These include preexisting comorbid conditions. Debilitation from cancer, morbid obesity, the use of steroids, and chemotherapy all influence results. In the past, incisional hernia repair was associated with a 30% to 40% recurrence rate; with modern tension-free repairs, the recurrence rate has been dramatically reduced (116–120).

PARASTOMAL HERNIAS

This incisional hernia is one of the most common complications of stoma formation. Studies designed with very careful follow-up suggest that a paracolostomy hernia develops in more than 50% of patients followed for longer than 5 years (121). The rate of herniation with small-bowel stomas is less than for colon stomas. Poor site selection or technical errors, such as making the fascial opening too large or placing a stoma in an incision, account for some of these hernias. Placing a stoma lateral to the rectus sheath is widely touted as a cause. Obesity, malnutrition, advanced age, collagen abnormalities, postoperative sepsis, abdominal distention, constipation, obstructive uropathy, steroid use, and chronic lung disease also contribute (122). Novel techniques for stomal reconstruction, such as extraperitoneal tunneling, have had little impact.

Fortunately, patients tolerate these hernias well, and life-threatening complications, such as bowel obstruction or strangulation, are rare. Fewer than 20% of patients with parastomal hernias have a complication that mandates repair (122). Routine repair is therefore not recommended. Table 51.7 lists possible indications.

The three general types of stomal hernia repair are (a) fascial repair, (b) stomal relocation, and (c) prosthetic repair. Fascial repair involves a local exploration around the stoma site, with primary closure of the defect. This approach should be considered of historical interest only. Stomal relocation produces better results than simple fascial repair. This approach is especially indicated in patients with other stomal problems, such as skin excoriation or suboptimal stomal construction. The use of a prosthesis with stomal relocation is not recommended because of the inherent danger of contamination.

Table 51.7. INDICATIONS FOR REPAIR OF A PARASTOMAL HERNIA

ABSOLUTE

Obstruction
Incarceration with strangulation

RELATIVE

Incarceration
Prolapse
Stenosis
Intractable dermatitis
Difficulty with appliance management
Large size
Cosmesis
Pain

Prosthetic repair is associated with the complications inherent in using a foreign body. Care must be taken to isolate the exit of the stoma from the abdominal wall from the surgical field to avoid infection of the prosthesis. The prosthesis can be placed extraperitoneally by making an incision around the stoma that is outside the periphery of the stomal appliance. Once the subcutaneous tissue is divided, dissection proceeds along the fascia until the hernia sac is identified and removed. The defect can be closed and an overlying prosthesis buttress sutured in place (Fig. 51.34). Alternatively, the fascial defect can be

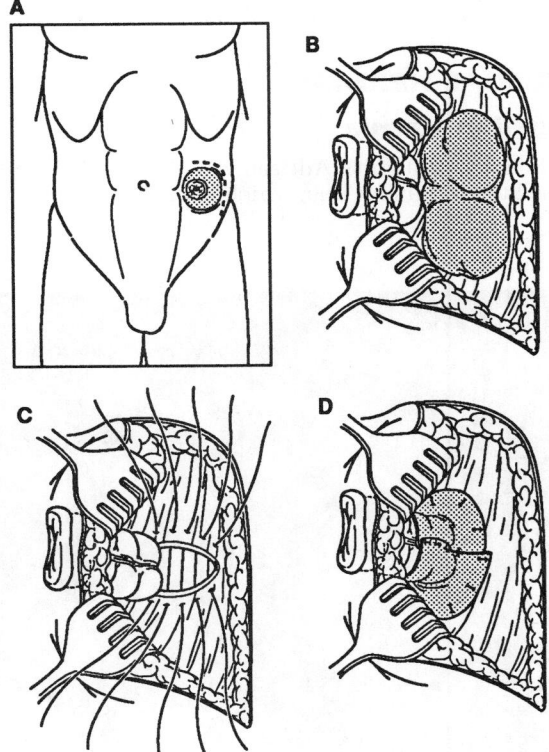

Figure 51.34. Repair of a parastomal hernia. *(A)* Incision around hernia. *(B)* Hernial sac is identified, the contents are reduced, and the peritoneum is closed. *(C)* The edges of the fascial defect are reapproximated. *(D)* The fascial repair is reinforced with polypropylene mesh, which is wrapped around the subcutaneous portion of the colon and sutured in place. (After Pearl RK. Parastomal hernias. *World J Surg* 1989;13:569–572.)

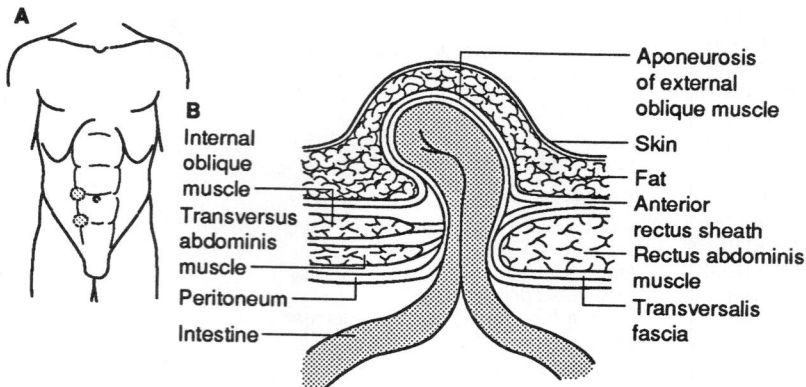

Figure 51.35. Spigelian hernia. *(A)* Usual site of occurrence. *(B)* Transverse section of abdominal wall showing site of defect.

bridged with the prosthesis for a "tension-free" repair. The extraperitoneal approach seems logical but can actually be technically demanding, as it is sometimes difficult to define the entire extent of the hernia defect. In addition, the undermining of subcutaneous tissue leads to seroma formation and eventual infection. An intraabdominal prosthetic repair has also been described that avoids the local complications of the extraperitoneal operation and incorporates the mechanical advantage of placing the prosthesis on the peritoneal side of the abdominal wall (123,124). Intraabdominal pressure then becomes a force that serves to fuse the prosthetic material to the abdominal wall instead of a factor in recurrence. The intraabdominal approach is particularly suited for laparoscopy, and several techniques have been described (125,126).

UNUSUAL HERNIAS

Spigelian Hernia

A Flemish anatomist, Adriaan van der Spieghel, first described the semilunar line, which is the lower limit of the posterior rectus sheath. A spigelian hernia protrudes through an area of weakness just lateral to the rectus sheath and just below this line (Fig. 51.35). The hernia is usually interparietal, rarely penetrating the external oblique fascia, and therefore can be difficult to appreciate. This is an unusual hernia; only 744 cases have been described in the literature, although the number may increase because this form of herniation is so easily diagnosed at laparoscopy. The usual presentation is a lower abdominal swelling just lateral to the border of the rectus muscle. Spigelian hernias often occur in elderly female patients. They are usually small, about 1 to 2 cm in diameter, although large hernias up to 14 cm in diameter have been described. Omentum and small or large bowel may enter the sac. Incarceration and strangulation are common complications of this hernia. Because the hernia is deep to the external oblique fascia, the clinical presentation may not be obvious. Pain and tenderness may be the only signs. Plain roentgenograms may show a bowel shadow in this area, and computed tomography can demonstrate the defect well. Treatment is operative repair. A transverse incision is centered over the mass. The external oblique

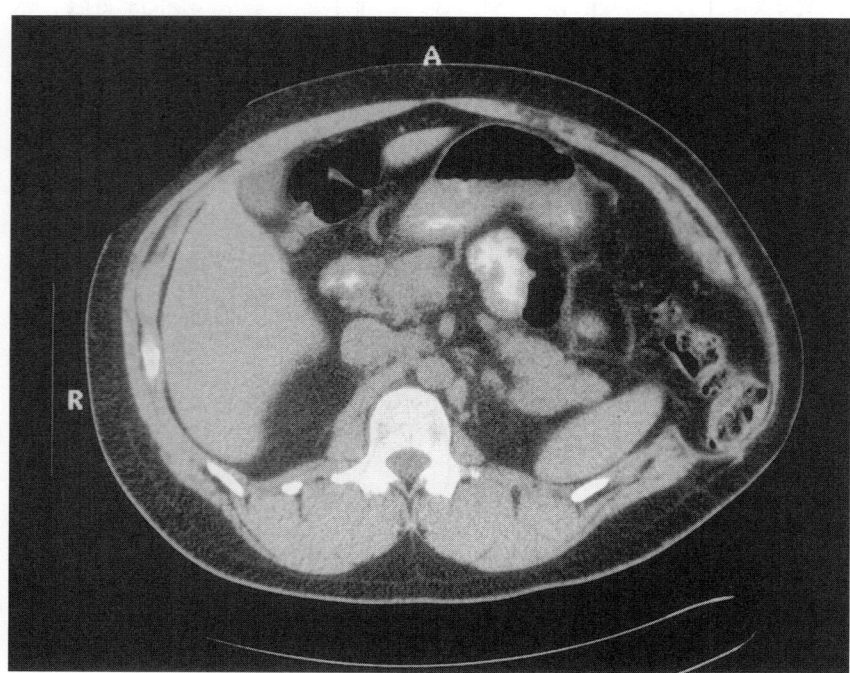

Figure 51.36. Computed tomogram of a left-sided lumbar hernia following nephrectomy for renal cell cancer.

aponeurosis is split to reveal the protrusion. If a large sac is present, it is divided and sutured. The aponeurotic defect is triangular, with its base at or near the lateral border of the rectus muscle. The defect is closed by joining the separated transversus and internal oblique layers. Recurrence is uncommon.

Lumbar Hernia

The lumbar region is the area bounded inferiorly by the iliac crest and superiorly by the 12th rib. Posteriorly, the boundary is the erector spinae group of muscles, and anteriorly, it is the posterior border of the external oblique muscle as it extends from the 12th rib to the iliac crest.

The three varieties of lumbar hernia are the following:

1. The *superior lumbar hernia of Grynfeltt*. The defect here is in a space between the latissimus dorsi, the serratus posterior inferior, and the posterior border of the internal oblique muscle.
2. The *inferior lumbar hernia of Petit*. This hernia occurs through a defect in the space bounded by the latissimus dorsi posteriorly, the iliac crest inferiorly, and the posterior border of the external oblique anteriorly.
3. *Secondary lumbar hernia*. This form develops as a result of trauma, mostly surgical (e.g., renal surgery; Fig. 51.36), or infection. Lumbar hernias were encountered relatively frequently in the past in cases of spinal tuberculosis with paraspinal abscesses.

These hernias require repair if they are large, and because of the size of the defect, synthetic mesh is used. For the inferior lumbar hernia, a rotation flap of fascia lata can be used (Fig. 51.37).

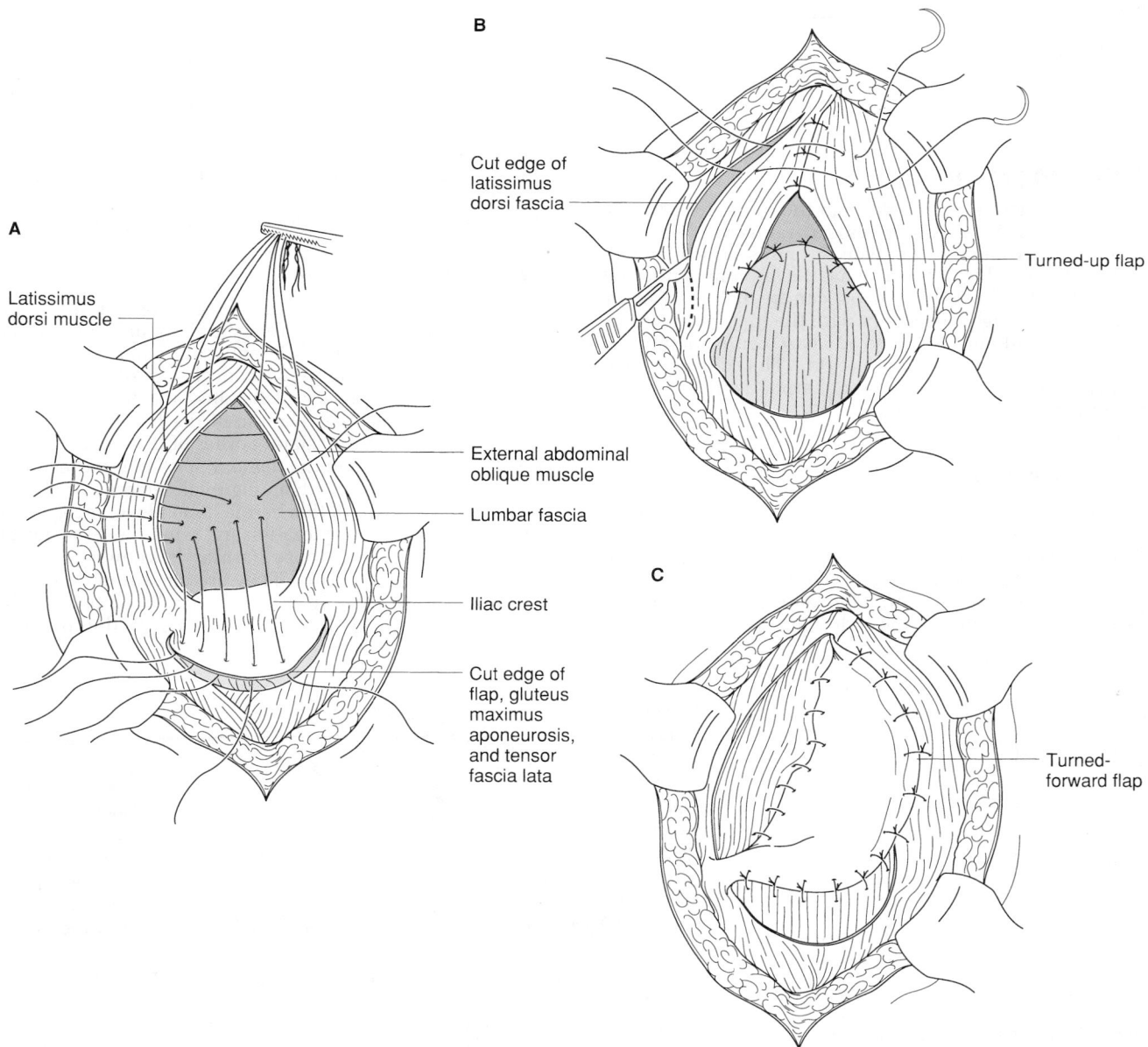

Figure 51.37. Sciatic hernias. (*A*) Suprapiriform. (*B*) Infrapiriform. (*C*) Subspinous.

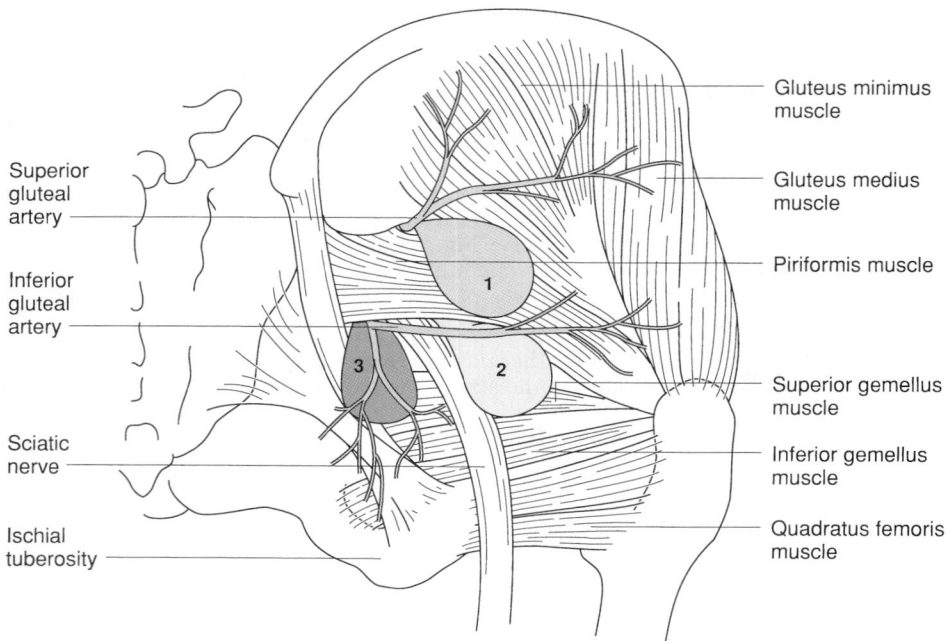

Figure 51.38. Technique of repair of inferior lumbar hernia.

Obturator Hernia

Obturator hernia occurs through the obturator canal accompanied by the obturator vessels and nerves. Obturator herniation is seen mostly in women and is associated with a laxity of the pelvic floor. The main symptom is intermittent pain. Occasionally, a mass can be palpated in the upper medial thigh, especially with the hip flexed and externally rotated and abducted. A mass can sometimes be palpated on vaginal examination. The defect is approached transperitoneally; the hernia is reduced and mesh placed over the defect.

Sciatic Hernia

A sciatic hernia is a protrusion of a peritoneal sac through the major or minor sciatic foramen (Fig. 51.38). These very rare hernias present with a swelling on the buttock. The sciatic nerve may be involved. A ureter can become obstructed if it is included with the herniated tissues. The treatment of these hernias is surgical. Both transperitoneal and transgluteal approaches have been described. A combination of the two is sometimes used. The defect usually requires a prosthetic mesh repair.

Supravesical Hernia

This hernia is anterior to the urinary bladder and forms when the integrity of the transversus abdominis muscle and the transversalis fascia fail, both of which insert into Cooper's ligament. The preperitoneal space is continuous with the retropubic space of Retzius, and the hernial sac protrudes into this area. The sac of the hernia is directed laterally, emerges at the lateral border of the rectus muscle, and presents in the inguinal, femoral, or obturator region. It can also be associated with an inguinal, femoral, or obturator hernia. Treatment of this hernia depends on recognizing it at the time of groin exploration and reinforcing the defect.

A second variety of these hernias is known as an internal supravesical hernia. They are classified according to whether they cross in front of, beside, or behind the bladder (Fig. 51.39). Bowel symptoms predominate in

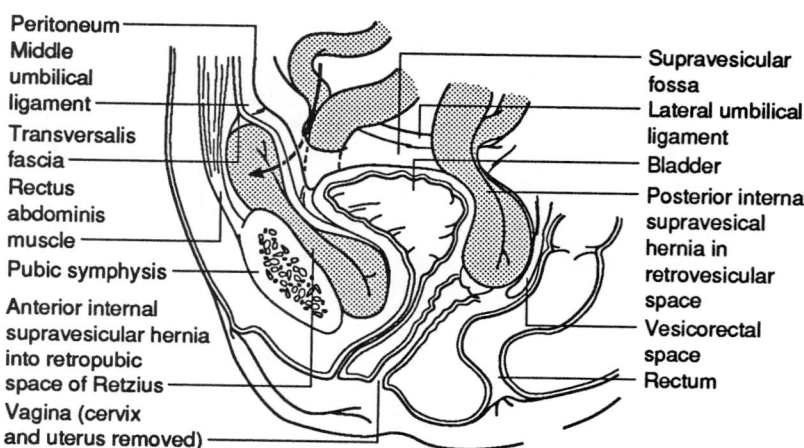

Figure 51.39. Internal supravesical hernias. (After Skandalakis JE. Internal and external supravesical hernia. *Am Surg* 1976;42:142, with permission.)

patients with these hernias, and urinary tract symptoms develop in up to 30%. The treatment is surgical, and a transperitoneal approach is used through a low midline incision. The hernias can usually be reduced without difficulty. The neck of the sac should be divided and closed.

Interparietal Hernia

This hernia is one in which the hernial sac lies between the layers of the abdominal wall. It may be either *preperitoneal* (between the peritoneum and the transversalis fascia) or *interstitial* (between the muscle layers of the abdominal wall). The majority are inguinal, in which case they are designated *inguinal interstitial* hernias. An *inguinal crural* hernia occurs when the sac passes behind the inguinal ligament in the region of the femoral ring.

The cause of these hernias appears to be related to congenital abnormalities; they have been associated with failure of the testis to descend, congenital pouches, and other abnormalities, such as absence of the cremaster and absence of the external abdominal ring.

The diagnosis of these hernias is difficult because no swelling of the abdominal wall is obvious unless the hernia is large. Pain is commonly the only symptom, and it is not unusual for patients to present with intestinal obstruction secondary to incarceration. Computed tomography, ultrasonography, and laparoscopy can be helpful in making the diagnosis. Not infrequently, the correct diagnosis is made only at operation. The defect is repaired according to the principles described for inguinal and incisional hernias.

Littre's Hernia

Littre's hernia is a groin hernia containing a Meckel's diverticulum. These hernias sometimes also contain the appendix. If the diverticulum is symptomatic or strangulated, then it is mandatory to resect it at the time of the hernia repair.

Perineal Hernia

These hernias are more common in older female patients and are related to a lax pelvic floor. They are termed *anterior* or *posterior* according to their relationship to the transversus perinei muscle. The anterior hernias usually present as a swelling in the labium or lateral vaginal wall. The posterior hernias present between the rectum and the ischial tuberosity. Surgical repair requires a transperitoneal approach, and if the opening is large, a prosthetic mesh repair is required.

Perivascular Hernia

These hernias present through defects between the inguinal ligament and the iliopubic bone. They are known by various eponyms according to their position. The hernia protruding through a defect in the lacunar ligament is *Laugier's hernia.* The hernia protruding through the pectineal fascia is *Cloquet's hernia.* The hernia extending anterior to the femoral vessels but behind the inguinal ligament is *Velpeau's hernia.* The hernia behind the vessels is *Serafini's hernia.* Lateral to the femoral artery are two hernias, the anterior one being *Hesselbach's hernia* and the more posterior one *Partridge's hernia* (Fig. 51.40).

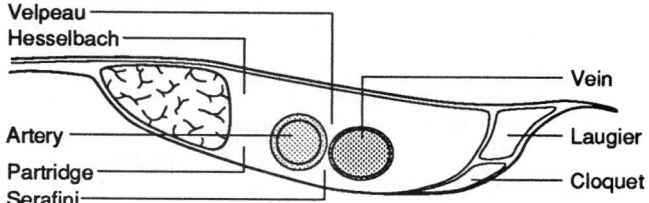

Figure 51.40. Perivascular hernias and their eponyms.

REFERENCES

1. Rutkow IM. Epidemiologic, economic, and sociologic aspects of hernia surgery in the United States in the 1990s. *Surg Clin North Am* 1998;78:941–951.
2. Whitely MS, Laws SA, Wise MH. Use of a hand-held Doppler to avoid abdominal wall vessels in laparoscopic surgery. *Ann R Coll Surg Engl* 1994;76:348–350.
3. Hurd WW, Bude RO, DeLancy OL, et al. The location of abdominal wall blood vessels in relationship to abdominal landmarks apparent at laparoscopy. *Am J Obstet Gynecol* 1994; 171:642–646.
4. Chatzipappas IK, Magos AL. A simple technique of securing inferior epigastric vessels and repairing the rectus sheath at laparoscopic surgery. *Obstet Gynecol* 1997;90: 304–306.
5. Green LS, Loughlin KR, Kavousi L. Management of epigastric vessel injury during laparoscopy. *J Endourol* 1992;6:99–101.
6. Hurd WW, Pearl ML, DeLancey OL, et al. Laparoscopic injury of abdominal wall blood vessels: a report of three cases. *Obstet Gynecol* 1993;82:673–676.
7. Hollingshead HW. The abdominal wall and inguinal region. *Anatomy for surgeons,* vol 2. New York: Hoeber-Harper, 1961:224–226.
8. Condon RE. The anatomy of the inguinal region and its relation to groin hernia. In: Nyhus LM, Condon RE, eds. *Hernia.* Philadelphia: JB Lippincott, 1995:31.
9. Milloy FJ, Anson BJ, McCaffee DK. The rectus abdominis muscle and the epigastric arteries. *Surg Gynecol Obstet* 1960; 110:293–302.
10. Rizk NN. A new description of the anterior abdominal wall in man and mammals. *J Anat* 1980;131:373–385.
11. Askar O. Patterns of midline decussation of the aponeurosis. *Ann R Coll Surg Engl* 1977;59:313.
12. Cooper A. The anatomy and surgical treatment of abdominal hernia. Philadelphia: Lee and Blanchard, 1804:26–27.
13. Zimmerman LM, Anson BJ. *Anatomy and surgery of hernia.* Baltimore: Williams & Wilkins, 1953:85–90.
14. Condon RE. Surgical anatomy of the transversus abdominis and transversalis fascia. *Ann Surg* 1971;173:1–5.
15. Read RC. Cooper's posterior lamina of transversalis fascia. *Surg Gynecol Obstet* 1992;174:426–434.
16. Colborn GL, Skandalakis JE. Laparoscopic inguinal anatomy. *Hernia* 1998;2:179–191.
17. Quinn TH, Ryberg A, Annibali R, et al. Anatomy of the anterior abdominal wall and deep inguinal region from the laparoscopic surgeon's perspective. In: Lansafame RJ, ed. *Prevention and management of complications in minimally invasive surgery.* New York: Igaku Shoin, 1996: 107–112.
18. Page DW, Gilroy A, Marks SC Jr. The iliopubic tract: an essential guide in teaching and performing groin hernia repairs. *Contemp Surg* 1996;49:219–222.
19. Gilroy A, Marks SC Jr, Quinfang L, et al. Anatomical characteristics of the iliopubic tract: implications for repair of inguinal hernias. *Clin Anat* 1992;5:255–263.
20. McVay CB, Anson BJ. Aponeurotic and fascial continuities in the abdomen, pelvis, and thigh. *Anat Rec* 1940;76:213–231.
21. Annibali R, Quinn TH, Fitzgibbons RJ Jr. Anatomy of the inguinal region from the laparoscopic perspective: critical areas for laparoscopic hernia repair. In: Bendavid R, ed. *Prostheses and abdominal wall hernias.* Austin, TX: Landes, 1994:82–103.

22. Urbanowicz Z. External structure of the genitofemoral nerve in postfetal life in man. *Folia Morphol (Warsz)* 1975;34:425–434.

23. Annibali R, Quinn TH, Fitzgibbons RJ Jr. Avoiding nerve injury during laparoscopic hernia repair: critical areas for staple placement. In: Arregui ME, Nagan RF, eds. *Inguinal hernia: advances or controversies?* Oxford: Radcliffe Medical, 1994:41–54.

24. Colborn GL, Skandalakis JE. Laparoscopic inguinal anatomy. *Hernia* 1998;2:179–191.

25. Gilroy AM, Hermey DC, Dibenedetto LM, et al. Variability of the obturator vessels. *Clin Anat* 1997;10:328–332.

26. Missankov AA, Asvat R, Maoba KI. Variation of the pubic vascular anastomoses in black South Africans. *Acta Anat* 1996;155:212–214.

27. Bendavid R. The space of Bogros and the deep inguinal venous circulation. *Surg Gynecol Obstet* 1992;174:356–357.

28. Flament JB, Visse CA, Palot JP. Tropic ulcers in giant incisional hernias—pathogenesis and treatment: a report of 33 cases. *Hernia* 1997;1:71–76.

29. Raynor RW, Deguercio LRM. The place of pneumoperitoneum in the repair of massive hernia. *World J Surg* 1989;13:581–585.

30. Bassini E. Nuovo metodo per la crura radicale dell'emia. *Atti Congr Ass Med Ital* 1889;2:179.

31. Rand Corporation. *Conceptualization and measurement of physiologic health of adults.* Santa Monica, CA: Rand Corporation, 1983:15.

32. Amid PK, Shulman AG, Lichtenstein IL. Open "tension-free" repair of inguinal hernias: the Lichtenstein technique. *Eur J Surg* 1996;162:447–453.

33. Amid PK, Shulman AG, Lichtenstein IL. Critical scrutiny of the open "tension-free" hernio-plasty. *Am J Surg* 1993;165:369–371.

34. Shulman AG, Amid PK, Lichtenstein IL. The safety of mesh repair for primary inguinal hernias: results of 3,019 operations from five diverse surgical sources. *Am Surg* 1992;58:255–257.

35. Wantz GE. Experience with the tension-free hernioplasty for primary inguinal hernias in men. *J Am Coll Surg* 1996;182:351–356.

36. Shulman AG, Amid PK, Lichtenstein IL. A survey of non-expert surgeons using the open tension-free mesh repair for primary inguinal hernias. *Int Surg* 1995;80:35–36.

37. Cheatle GL. An operation for the radical cure of inguinal and femoral hernia. *Br Med J* 1920;2:68.

38. Henry AK. Operation for femoral hernia by a midline extraperitoneal approach, with a preliminary note on the use of this route for reducible inguinal hernia. *Lancet* 1936;1:531.

39. Rignault DP. Properitoneal prosthetic inguinal hernioplasty through a Pfannenstiel approach. *Surg Gynecol Obstet* 1986;163:465.

40. Sparkman RS. Bilateral exploration in inguinal hernia in juvenile patients. *Surgery* 1962;51:393.

41. Rowe MI, Clatworthy HW. The other side of the pediatric hernia. *Surg Clin North Am* 1971;51:6.

42. Abrahamson J. Factors and mechanisms leading to recurrence. In: Bendavid R, ed. *Prostheses and abdominal wall hernias.* Austin, TX: Landes, 1994:138–170.

43. Read RC. The role of protease–antiprotease in the pathogenesis of hernia and abdominal aortic aneurysm in certain smokers. *Post Grad Gen Surg* 1992;14:161.

44. Metropolitan Life Insurance Company. Expectation of life and mortality rates at single years of age, by race and sex: United States, 1991. *Stat Bull Metrop Insur Co* 1996;75:16.

45. Neuhauser D. Elective inguinal herniorrhaphy versus truss in the elderly. In: Bunker JP, Barnes BA, Mosteller F, eds. *Costs, risks, and benefits of surgery.* New York: Oxford University Press, 1977:223–239.

46. Ponka JL. Surgical management of large bilateral indirect sliding inguinal hernias. *Am J Surg* 1966;112:52.

47. Williams JS, Hale HW. The advisability of inguinal herniorrhaphy in the elderly. *Surg Gynecol Obstet* 1966;122:100–104.

48. Nehme AE. Groin hernias in elderly patients: management and prognosis. *Am J Surg* 1983;146:257–260.

49. Tingwald GR, Cooperman M. Inguinal and femoral hernia repair in geriatric patients. *Surg Gynecol Obstet* 1982;154:704–706.

50. Rorbaek-Madsen M. Herniorrhaphy in patients aged 80 years or more: a prospective analysis of morbidity and mortality. *Eur J Surg* 1992;158:591–594.

51. Primatesta P. GMJ. Inguinal hernia repair: incidence of elective and emergency surgery, readmission, and mortality. *Int J Epidemiol* 1996;25:835–839.

52. Nilsson E, Kald A, Anderberg B, et al. Hernia surgery in a defined population: a prospective three-year audit. *Eur J Surg* 1997;163:823–829.

53. Cook TM, Britton DC, Craft TM, et al. An audit of hospital mortality after urgent and emergency surgery in the elderly. *Ann R Coll Surg Engl* 1997;79:361–367.

54. Rutkow IM, Robbins AW. Mesh plug hernia repair: a follow-up report. *Surgery* 1995;117:597–598.

55. Lichtenstein IL, Shulman AG, Amid PK, et al. The tension-free hernioplasty. *Am J Surg* 1989;157:188–193.

56. Amid PK, Shulman AG, Lichtenstein IL. The Lichtenstein open "tension-free" mesh repair of inguinal hernias. *Jpn J Surg* 1995;25:619–625.

57. Amid PK, Shulman AG, Lichtenstein IL. Simultaneous repair of bilateral inguinal hernias under local anesthesia. *Ann Surg* 1996;223:249–252.

58. Amid PK, Shulman AG, Lichtenstein IL. Femoral hernia resulting from inguinal herniorrhaphy: the "plug" repair. *Contemp Surg* 1991;39:19–24.

59. Amid PK, Shulman AG, Lichtenstein IL. Local anesthesia for inguinal hernia repair step-by-step procedure. *Ann Surg* 1994;220:735–737.

60. Kark AE, Kurzer MN, Belsham PA. Three thousand one hundred seventy-five primary inguinal hernia repairs: advantages of ambulatory open mesh repair using local anesthesia. *J Am Coll Surg* 1998;186:447–456.

61. Nyhus LM, Pollak R, Bombeck CT, et al. The preperitoneal approach and prosthetic buttress repair for recurrent hernia. *Ann Surg* 1988;208:733–737.

62. Wantz GE. The technique of giant prosthetic reinforcement of the visceral sac performed through an anterior groin incision. *Surg Gynecol Obstet* 1993;177:497.

63. Wantz GE. Giant prosthetic reinforcement of the visceral sac: the Stoppa groin hernia repair. *Surg Clin North Am* 1998;78:6 1075–1087.

64. Mathonnet M, Cubertafond P, Gainant A. Bilateral inguinal hernias: giant prosthetic reinforcement of the visceral sac. *Hernia* 1997;1:93–95.

65. Munshi IA, Wantz GE. Management of recurrent and perivascular femoral hernias by giant prosthetic reinforcement of the visceral sac. *J Am Coll Surg* 1996;182:417–422.

66. Hoffman HC, Vinton Traverso AL. Preperitoneal prosthetic herniorrhaphy: one surgeon's successful technique. *Arch Surg* 1993;128:964–970.

67. Champault G, Rizk N, Catheline JM, et al. Inguinal hernia repair: totally pre-peritoneal laparoscopic approach versus Stoppa operation—randomized trial: 100 cases. *Hernia* 1997;1:31–36.

68. Ger R, Mishrick A, Hurwitz J, et al. Management of groin hernias by laparoscopy. *World J Surg* 1993;17:46–50.

69. Fitzgibbons RJ Jr, Salerno GM, Filipi CJ, et al. A laparoscopic intraperitoneal onlay mesh technique for the repair of an indirect inguinal hernia [see comments]. *Ann Surg* 1994;219:144–156.

70. Johnson A. Laparoscopic surgery. *Lancet* 1997;349:631–635.

71. Filipi CJ, Fitzgibbons RJ Jr, Salerno GM, et al. Laparoscopic herniorrhaphy. *Surg Clin North Am* 1992;72:1109–1124.

72. McKernan JB, Laws HL. Laparoscopic repair of inguinal hernias using a totally extraperitoneal prosthetic approach. *Surg Endosc* 1993;7:26–28.

73. Arregui ME, Navarrete J, Davis CJ, et al. Laparoscopic inguinal herniorrhaphy: techniques and controversies. *Surg Clin North Am* 1993;73:513–527.

74. Spaw AT, Ennis BW, Spaw LP. Laparoscopic hernia repair: the anatomic basis. *J Laparoendosc Surg* 1991;1:269–277.

75. Kingsley D, Vogt DM, Nelson MT, et al. Laparoscopic intraperitoneal onlay inguinal herniorrhaphy. *Am J Surg* 1998; 176:548–553.

76. Crist DW, Gadacz TR. Complications of laparoscopic surgery. *Surg Clin North Am* 1993;73:265–289.

77. Baadsgaard SE, Bille S, Egeblad K. Major vascular injury during gynecologic laparoscopy. *Acta Obstet Gynecol Scand* 1989;68:283–285.

78. Mintz M. Risks and prophylaxis in laparoscopy: a survey of 100,000 cases. *J Reprod Med* 1977;18:269–327.

79. Nuzzo G, Giuliante F, Tebala GD, et al. Routine use of open technique in laparoscopic operations. *J Am Coll Surg* 1997; 184:58–62.

80. McMahon AJ, Baxter JN, O'Dwyer PJ. Preventing complications of laparoscopy. *Br J Surg* 1993;80:1592–1594.

81. Mayol J, Garcia-Aguilar J, Ortiz-Oshiro E, et al. Risks of the minimal access approach for laparoscopic surgery: multivariate analysis of morbidity related to umbilical trocar insertion. *World J Surg* 1997;21:529–533.

82. Patterson M, Walters D, Browder W. Postoperative bowel obstruction following laparoscopic surgery. *Am Surg* 1993;59: 656–657.

83. Mouton WG, Bessell JR, Otten KT, et al. Pain after laparoscopy. *Surg Endosc* 1999;13:445–448.

84. Bendavid R. The Shouldice technique: a cannon in hernia repair. *Can J Surg* 1997;40:199–205, 207.

85. Robbins AW, Rutkow IM. Mesh plug repair and groin hernia surgery. *Surg Clin North Am* 1998;78:1007–1023.

86. Corbitt JD Jr. Laparoscopic herniorrhaphy: a preperitoneal tension-free approach. *Surg Endosc* 1993;7:550–555.

87. Felix EL, Michas CA, McKnight RL. Laparoscopic herniorrhaphy: transabdominal preperitoneal floor repair. *Surg Endosc* 1994;8:100–103.

88. Felix EL, Michas CA, Gonzalez MH Jr. Laparoscopic hernioplasty: TAPP vs. TEP. *Surg Endosc* 1995;9:984–989.

89. Geis WP, Crafton WB, Novak MJ, et al. Laparoscopic herniorrhaphy: results and technical aspects in 450 consecutive procedures. *Surgery* 1993;114:765–772.

90. Hawasli A. Laparoscopic inguinal herniorrhaphy: classification and 1 year experience. *J Laparoendosc Surg* 1992;2: 137–143.

91. Himpens JM. Laparoscopic inguinal hernioplasty: repair with a conventional vs. a new self-expandable mesh [see comments]. *Surg Endosc* 1993;7:315–318.

92. Kald A, Smedh K, Anderberg B. Laparoscopic groin hernia repair: results of 200 consecutive herniorrhaphies. *Br J Surg* 1995;82:618–620.

93. Kavic MS. Laparoscopic hernia repair: three-year experience. *Surg Endosc* 1995;9:12–15.

94. Newman L III, Eubanks S, Mason E, et al. Is laparoscopic herniorrhaphy an effective alternative to open hernia repair? *J Laparoendosc Surg* 1993;3:121–128.

95. Paget GW. Laparoscopic inguinal herniorrhaphy: a personal audit of 222 hernia repairs [see comments]. *Med J Aust* 1994; 161:249–253.

96. Panton ON, Panton RJ. Laparoscopic hernia repair [see comments]. *Am J Surg* 1994;167:535–537.

97. Quilici PJ, Greaney EM Jr, Quilici J, et al. Laparoscopic inguinal hernia repair results: 131 cases. *Am Surg* 1993;59: 824–830.

98. Ramshaw BJ, Tucker JG, Mason EM, et al. A comparison of transabdominal preperitoneal (TAPP) and total extraperitoneal approach (TEPA) laparoscopic herniorrhaphies. *Am Surg* 1995;61:279–283.

99. Wheeler KH. Laparoscopic inguinal herniorrhaphy with mesh: an 18-month experience. *J Laparoendosc Surg* 1993;3: 345–350.

100. Begin GF. Laparoscopic extraperitoneal treatment of inguinal hernias in adults: a series of 200 cases. *Endosc Surg Allied Technol* 1993;1:204–206.

101. Ferzli G, Kiel T. Evolving techniques in endoscopic extraperitoneal herniorrhaphy. *Surg Endosc* 1995;9: 928–930.

102. Voeller GR, Mangiante EC Jr, Williams C. Totally preperitoneal laparoscopic inguinal herniorrhaphy using balloon dissection. *Surg Rounds* 1995;18:107–112.

103. Rubio PA. Laparoscopic intraperitoneal hernioplasty. *Int Surg* 1994;79:293–295.

104. Fitzgibbons RJ Jr, Camps J, Cornet DA, et al. Laparoscopic inguinal herniorrhaphy: results of a multicenter trial [see comments]. *Ann Surg* 1995;221:3–13.

105. Phillips EH, Arregui M, Carroll BJ, et al. Incidence of complications following laparoscopic hernioplasty. *Surg Endosc* 1995;9:16–21.

106. Condon RE, Nyhus LM. Complications of groin hernia. In: Condon RE, Nyhus LM, eds. *Hernia,* 4th ed. Philadelphia: JB Lippincott, 1995:269–282.

107. Cunningham J, Temple WJ, Mitchell P, et al. Cooperative hernia study: pain in the postrepair patient. *Ann Surg* 1996;224: 598–602.

108. Wantz GE. Testicular atrophy and chronic residual neuralgia as risks of inguinal hernioplasty. *Surg Clin North Am* 1993; 73:571–581.

109. Bendavid R. Complications of groin hernia surgery. *Surg Clin North Am* 1998;78:1089–1103.

110. Gray MR, Curtis JM, Elkington JS. Colovesical fistula after laparoscopic inguinal hernia repair. *Br J Surg* 1994;81: 1213–1214.

111. Miller K, Junger W. Ileocutaneous fistula formation following laparoscopic polypropylene mesh hernia repair. *Surg Endosc* 1997;11:772–773.

112. Silich RC, McSherry CK. Spermatic granuloma: an uncommon complication of the tension-free hernia repair. *Surg Endosc* 1996;10:537–539.

113. Ellis H, Bucknall TE. Abdominal incisions and their closure. *Curr Probl Surg* 1985;22:1–51.

114. Bucknall TE, Cox PJ, Ellis H. Burst abdomen and incisional hernia: a prospective study of 1,129 major laparotomies. *Br Med J* 1982;284:931–933.

115. Israelsson LA, Jonsson T, Knutsson A. Suture technique and wound healing in midline laparotomy incisions. *Eur J Surg* 1996;162:605–609.

116. Santora TA, Roslyn JJ. Incisional hernia. *Surg Clin North Am* 1993;73:557–570.

117. Makela JT, Kiviniemi H, Juvonen T, et al. Factors influencing dehiscence after midline laparotomy. *Am J Surg* 1995;170: 387–390.

118. Temudon T, Saidati M, Sarr MG. Repair of complex giant or recurrent ventral hernias by using tension-free intraparietal prosthetic mesh (Stoppa technique): lessons learned from our initial experience (50 patients). *Surgery* 1996;120: 738–744.

119. Bebawi MA, Moqtaderi F, Vijay V. Giant incisional hernia: staged repair using pneumoperitoneum and expanded polytetrafluoroethylene. *Am J Surg* 1997;63:375–381.

120. Sugerman HJ, Kellum JM, Reines HD, et al. Greater risk of incisional hernia with morbidly obese than steroid-dependent patients and low recurrence with prefascial polypropylene mesh. *Am J Surg* 1996;171:80–84.

121. Rubin MS, Schoetz DJ Jr, Matthews JB. Parastomal hernia: is stoma relocation superior to fascial repair? *Arch Surg* 1994; 129:413–418; discussion 418–419.

122. Pearl RK. Parastomal hernias. *World J Surg* 1989;13: 569–572.

123. Byers JM, Steinberg JB, Postier RG. Repair of parastomal hernias using polypropylene mesh. *Arch Surg* 1992;127: 1246–1247.

124. Sugarbaker PH. Peritoneal approach to prosthetic mesh repair of paraostomy hernias. *Ann Surg* 1985;201:344–346.

125. Bickel A, Shinkarevsky E, Eitan A. Laparoscopic repair of paracolostomy hernia. *J Laparoendosc Adv Surg Tech A* 1999;9:353–355.

126. Porcheron J, Payan B, Balique JG. Mesh repair of paracolostomy hernia by laparoscopy. *Surg Endosc* 1998;12: 1281.

127. Stoker DL, Spiegelhalter DJ, Singh R, et al. Laparoscopic versus open inguinal hernia repair: randomized prospective trial [see comments]. *Lancet* 1994;343:1243–1245.

128. Payne JH Jr, Grininger LM, Izawa MT, et al. Laparoscopic or open inguinal herniorrhaphy? A randomized prospective trial [see comments]. *Arch Surg* 1994;129:973–979.

129. Vogt DM, Curet MJ, Pitcher DE, et al. Preliminary results of

a prospective randomized trial of laparoscopic onlay versus conventional inguinal herniorrhaphy. *Am J Surg* 1995;169: 84–89.

130. Lawrence K, McWhinnie D, Goodwin A, et al. Randomized controlled trial of laparoscopic versus open repair of inguinal hernia: early results. *BMJ* 1995;311:981–985.

131. Barkun JS, Wexler MJ, Hinchey EJ, et al. Laparoscopic versus open inguinal herniorrhaphy: preliminary results of a randomized controlled trial. *Surgery* 1995;118:703–709.

132. Wright DM, Kennedy A, Baxter JN, et al. Early outcome after open versus extraperitoneal endoscopic tension-free hernioplasty: a randomized clinical trial. *Surgery* 1996;119: 552–557.

133. Kozol R, Lang PM, Kosir M, et al. A prospective, randomized study of open vs. laparoscopic inguinal hernia repair: an assessment of postoperative pain. *Arch Surg* 1997;132: 292–295.

134. Maddern GJ, Rudkin G, Bessell JR, et al. A comparison of laparoscopic and open hernia repair as a day surgical procedure. *Surg Endosc* 1994;8:1404–1408.

135. Brooks DC. A prospective comparison of laparoscopic and tension-free open herniorrhaphy. *Arch Surg* 1994;129: 361–366.

136. Millikan KW, Kosik ML, Doolas A. A prospective comparison of transabdominal preperitoneal laparoscopic hernia repair versus traditional open hernia repair in a university setting. *Surg Laparosc Endosc* 1994;4:247–253.

137. Cornell RB, Kerlakian GM. Early complications and outcomes of the current technique of transperitoneal laparoscopic herniorrhaphy and a comparison to the traditional open approach. *Am J Surg* 1994;168:275–279.

138. Wilson MS, Deans GT, Brough WA. Prospective trial comparing Lichtenstein with laparoscopic tension-free mesh repair of inguinal hernia. *Br J Surg* 1995;82:274–277.

139. Liem MS, van der Graaf Y, van Steensel CJ, et al. Comparison of conventional anterior surgery and laparoscopic surgery for inguinal-hernia repair. *N Engl J Med* 1997;29:336: 1541–1547.

140. Wellwood J, Sculpher MJ, Stoker D, et al. Randomised controlled trial of laparoscopic versus open mesh repair for inguinal hernia: outcome and cost. *BMJ* 1998;317:103–110.

141. Johansson B, Hallerback B, Glise H, et al. Laparoscopic mesh versus open preperitoneal mesh versus conventional technique for inguinal hernia repair: a randomized multicenter trial (SCUR Hernia Repair Study). *Ann Surg* 1999;230: 225–231.

142. Laparoscopic versus open repair of groin hernia: a randomized comparison: the MRC Laparoscopic Groin Hernia Trial Group. *Lancet* 1999;17:354(9174):185–190.

SURGERY: SCIENTIFIC PRINCIPLES AND PRACTICE, Third Edition, edited by Lazar J. Greenfield, Michael W. Mulholland, Keith T. Oldham, Gerald B. Zelenock, and Keith D. Lillemoe. Lippincott Williams & Wilkins Publishers, Philadelphia, © 2001.

CHAPTER 52

ACUTE ABDOMEN AND APPENDIX

JEFFREY B. MATTHEWS AND RICHARD A. HODIN

APPROACH TO THE PATIENT WITH ACUTE ABDOMINAL PAIN

Abdominal pain is one of the most frequent reasons for visits to physician offices and hospital emergency rooms and is a leading cause for hospital admission in the United States. Although most patients are found to have self-lim-

ited conditions of little consequence, a subset of patients with acute abdominal pain harbor serious intraabdominal or retroperitoneal disease that requires major surgical or medical intervention. It is this latter population to whom the term *acute abdomen* is commonly applied, although *abdominal emergency* might be more descriptive. The experienced clinician understands that the severity of the pain does not always correlate with the gravity of the situation, and that not all patients with the so-called acute abdomen require surgical intervention. Obtaining an early diagnosis, and in particular making an early distinction between conditions that require urgent operation and those best managed nonsurgically, is of paramount importance and must outweigh all other concerns. Evaluation by a surgical consultant and the performance of appropriate radiologic studies must proceed promptly regardless of the time of day and the disruption of normal routines and schedules (1).

In the vast majority of cases, a thorough history and physical examination will reveal the cause of the abdominal pain, or at least sufficiently narrow the possibilities to allow initial treatment decisions to be made (2). Important features to be elicited include the time and mode of onset of the illness, location of the pain, character of the pain, and associated symptoms and their relation to the pain (Table 52.1). Examination of the patient includes an assessment of general appearance and attitude in bed in addition to the abdominal examination itself (Table 52.2). The ability to group the symptoms and signs of acute abdominal pain and weigh their relative importance ("pattern recognition") perhaps best distinguishes the novice from the expert diagnostician in this setting. Blood tests may be complementary but are only occasionally of major importance in the initial evaluation. The same is generally true for radiologic studies, although in some circumstances, newer techniques of abdominal imaging do appear to enhance diagnostic accuracy. However, it cannot be overstated that an excessive reliance on tests can lead to unnecessary delay and must be avoided.

Most patients with acute abdominal pain evaluated in the emergency room setting do not require either hospital admission or surgical intervention (3). The most common causes of abdominal pain requiring admission include acute appendicitis, nonspecific abdominal pain, pain of urologic origin, intestinal obstruction, and biliary tract disease, depending on the population and geographic region considered (4). With the improvements in diagnostic imaging that have been made during the past few decades, more patients with acute abdominal pain can be assigned a specific diagnosis, and fewer instances of surgical disease are missed (5). The proportion of all patients evaluated for abdominal pain who are admitted to the hospital may also be declining.

Table 52.1. KEY HISTORICAL FEATURES IN ACUTE ABDOMINAL PAIN

Age
Time and mode of onset
Duration of symptoms
Character of pain
Location of pain and site(s) of radiation
Associated symptoms and their relation to pain
    Nausea or anorexia
    Vomiting
    Diarrhea or constipation
Menstrual history

Table 52.2. **EXAMINATION OF THE PATIENT WITH ACUTE ABDOMINAL PAIN**

GENERAL OBSERVATIONS

General appearance
Attitude in bed
Vital signs, including temperature

CHEST

Auscultation

ABDOMEN

Inspection (distention, localized swelling, hernia)
Percussion (tympany or dullness, tenderness, referred tenderness)
Palpation (muscle rigidity, tenderness, rebound pain, hyperesthesia)
Auscultation

PELVIS

Rectal examination (tenderness; presence of stool, occult blood, mass)
Bimanual examination (cervical motion tenderness, adnexal masses)
Obturator sign

BACK AND FLANKS

Percussion (costovertebral angle tenderness)
Iliopsoas sign

Embryologic and Physiologic Considerations

The developing gastrointestinal tract is divided into three regions based on blood supply and innervation, relationships that are maintained from embryonic to adult life. The foregut consists of the oropharynx, esophagus, stomach, proximal duodenum, pancreas, liver, biliary tract, and spleen. The midgut runs from the distal duodenum (ligament of Treitz) and includes the small intestine, appendix, cecum, ascending colon, and proximal two thirds of the transverse colon. The remainder of the colon and rectum make up the hindgut.

The intestinal tract itself, from the stomach to the distal sigmoid colon (with the exception of the duodenum), is covered by a layer of mesodermally derived visceral peritoneum. The liver, spleen, and gallbladder are largely covered by visceral peritoneum; the pancreas is located within the retroperitoneum. Although continuous with the parietal peritoneum that lines the abdominal cavity, the visceral peritoneum is supplied by autonomic (sympathetic and parasympathetic) nerves. In contrast, the parietal peritoneal layer has an entirely somatic innervation derived from spinal nerves. This difference accounts for the distinct character of the pain associated with irritation or inflammation of the parietal peritoneum, which is generally perceived as sharp, severe, and persistent; in contrast, painful stimuli involving the visceral peritoneum are

perceived as dull, cramping or aching, and poorly localized, and are often associated with nausea, diaphoresis, or both. The visceral peritoneum and its associated organs are insensitive to touching, pinching, cutting, burning, and electrical stimulation, but the sensation of pain from these sites can be induced by stretching, distention, or vigorous contraction against resistance. Additional painful stimuli to visceral organs include certain chemicals, ischemia, and inflammation. Visceral pain usually indicates the presence of significant intraabdominal disease but is not in itself an indication for surgical therapy. A transition from visceral to somatic pain implies extension of the underlying disease process to include the parietal peritoneum and often heralds the need for urgent operative intervention (e.g., acute appendicitis, intestinal obstruction with strangulation). However, somatic pain of intraabadominal origin should not be equated with an invariable need for operation (e.g., acute diverticulitis). In this regard, it is important to distinguish between localized somatic pain and diffuse somatic pain. Although conditions associated with localized peritonitis may require operation, the degree of urgency is far less than in diffuse peritonitis, which generally indicates a surgical emergency.

The tube of the central gut has a bilateral nerve supply, which accounts for the midline location of the visceral pain originating from these organs. Pain of foregut origin is usually perceived in the epigastrium, midgut pain in the periumbilical region, and hindgut pain in the hypogastrium. In contrast, pain originating in the bladder, prostate, uterus, ovaries, and fallopian tubes may be localized as pelvic or, occasionally, perineal. Pain originating in the abdominal wall musculature or parietal peritoneum is usually perceived in precise relation to the anatomic location of the stimulus because somatic pain nerve fibers enter the spinal cord ipsilaterally. The innervation of the anterior and lateral abdominal wall is from vertebral segments T-7 through L-1, whereas that of the posterior abdominal wall is from L-2 through L-5.

In addition to somatic and visceral pain, a third form of pain related to acute abdominal disorders is referred pain. Referred pain is perceived at a site removed from the anatomic location of the disease but in a region that shares a common embryonic origin. The most common example is radiation of the pain of biliary origin to the right subscapular region or right shoulder. This phenomenon reflects the fact that the phrenic nerve is derived from the fourth cervical nerve. Thus, irritation of the undersurface of the right hemidiaphragm, such as by an inflamed gallbladder or hepatic abscess, may induce pain or hyperesthesia in the skin distribution of the fourth cervical nerve. Similarly, splenic disease or injury, such as a rupture, may be perceived as pain in the left shoulder (Kehr's sign). Other examples of referred pain are listed in Table 52.3.

Inflammation of the parietal peritoneum leads to rigidity and tenderness of the overlying muscle groups, a phenomenon of great clinical significance in the diagnosis of

Table 52.3. **SITES OF REFERRED PAIN**

Site	Organ(s)	Common examples
Right subscapular or shoulder	Diaphragm, gallbladder, liver	Biliary colic, perforated ulcer, pneumoperitoneum
Left subscapular or shoulder	Diaphragm, spleen, stomach, tail of pancreas, splenic flexure	Splenic rupture, pancreatitis
Back	Pancreas, duodenum, aorta	Pancreatitis, ruptured AAA
Coccyx	Uterus, rectum	Uterine colic
Groin or genitalia	Kidney, ureter, iliac arteries	Ureterolithiasis

AAA, abdominal aortic aneurysm.

acute abdominal pain. These groups include not only the muscles of the anterior abdominal wall, such as the rectus abdominis, but also the diaphragm, psoas, quadratus lumborum, erector spinae, piriformis, and obturator internus. Thus, an inflamed retrocecal appendix overlying the right psoas muscle may produce spasm, reflected by the preference of the patient to maintain the right thigh in a flexed position; similarly, placing the patient on the left side and fully extending the right thigh may produce pain (psoas sign). Similarly, the presence of an inflamed appendix or periappendiceal abscess may be deduced by a positive finding in the so-called obturator test (pain on internal rotation of the right thigh). In contrast, irritation of the deep pelvic peritoneum is generally not associated with any overlying muscle group, which accounts for the striking lack of abdominal wall rigidity in cases of pelvic abscess from appendicitis or diverticulitis.

Differential Diagnosis

The sheer number of conditions that produce acute abdominal pain is overwhelming. However, the differential diagnosis can be narrowed substantially by anatomic considerations and an understanding of the general characteristics of the episode of pain.

It is useful to subdivide the abdomen into four quadrants and consider the conditions that cause abdominal pain localized to each region (Table 52.4). Pain that does not lateralize in this fashion can be characterized as epigastric, periumbilical, or hypogastric, and a relatively limited differential diagnosis can also be generated for each midline location (Table 52.5). Diffuse abdominal pain (Table 52.6) can be mild and not associated with significant physical findings, as in early acute appendicitis, or it can be severe and associated with generalized abdominal muscle rigidity, as in diffuse peritonitis.

The number of pathologic processes affecting the abdominal viscera that produce abdominal pain is limited, and each is associated with a characteristic evolution of clinical symptoms and signs (Table 52.7). *Obstruction* of a hollow viscus results in a form of pain, termed *colic,* that consists of a deep, nauseating ache. The pain may be cyclical, as in intestinal colic, or steady, as in biliary colic. *Inflammation* can be the result of bacterial infection and generally produces only mild pain until the process becomes transmural, at which point the resultant peritoneal

---

Table 52.4. PAIN LOCALIZING TO AN ABDOMINAL QUADRANT

RIGHT UPPER QUADRANT PAIN	LEFT UPPER QUADRANT PAIN
Biliary colic/cholecystitis	Splenic rupture
Cholangitis	Splenic infarction
Hepatic abscess	Splenomegaly
Hepatitis (toxic or viral)	Ruptured splenic artery aneurysm
Perihepatitis (FitzHugh-Curtis syndrome)	Gastritis
Hepatic congestion	Perforated gastric ulcer (phlegmonous gastritis)
Budd-Chiari syndrome	Jejunal diverticulitis
Hepatic tumor (primary or secondary)	Pancreatitis
Appendicitis	Diverticulitis (splenic flexure)
Perforated peptic ulcer	Perinephritis
Perinephritis	Pneumonia (left lower lobe)
Pneumonia (right lower lobe)	Pulmonary infarction
Pulmonary infarction	Pleuritis
Pleuritis	Pericarditis
Myocardial ischemia	Myocardial ischemia
Empyema	Empyema
Rib fracture	Rib fracture
Herpes zoster	Herpes zoster
RIGHT LOWER QUADRANT PAIN	**LEFT LOWER QUADRANT PAIN**
Appendicitis	Diverticulitis
Acute enterocolitis (viral or bacterial)	Appendicitis
Crohn's disease (ileitis)	Perforated colon cancer
Foreign body perforation	Intestinal obstruction
Right-sided diverticulitis	Crohn's colitis
Cecal diverticulitis	Ischemic colitis
Meckel's diverticulitis	Ruptured iliac artery aneurysm
Torsion of appendix epiploica	Ruptured ovarian cyst (including mittelschmerz)
Mesenteric adenitis	Ovarian torsion
Intestinal obstruction	Endometriosis
Perforated peptic ulcer	Salpingitis (pelvic inflammatory disease)
Pancreatitis	Ectopic pregnancy
Ruptured ovarian cyst (including mittelschmerz)	Renal or ureteral calculi
Ovarian torsion	Pyelonephritis
Endometriosis	Psoas abscess
Salpingitis (pelvic inflammatory disease)	Seminal vesiculitis
Ectopic pregnancy	Rectus sheath hematoma
Cholecystitis	Herpes zoster
Ruptured iliac artery aneurysm	
Renal or ureteral calculi	
Pyelonephritis	
Psoas abscess	
Seminal vesiculitis	
Rectus sheath hematoma	
Herpes zoster	

Table 52.5. MIDLINE ABDOMINAL PAIN

EPIGASTRIC

Peptic ulcer
Pancreatitis
Gastritis
Esophagitis
Mesenteric ischemia
Appendicitis (early)
Myocardial ischemia
Pericarditis
Cholecystitis

PERIUMBILICAL

Small-intestinal obstruction
Appendicitis
Pancreatitis
Mesenteric ischemia
Acute glaucoma

HYPOGASTRIC

Large-intestinal obstruction
Intussusception
Appendicitis
Diverticulitis
Enterocolitis
Ovarian torsion
Testicular torsion
Degeneration or torsion of uterine fibroid
Cystitis

Table 52.6. DIFFUSE ABDOMINAL PAIN

Early appendicitis
Perforated appendicitis
Perforated peptic ulcer
Perforated diverticulitis
Stercoral perforation of colon
Peritonitis (primary or secondary)
Pancreatitis
Mesenteric adenitis
Mesenteric ischemia
Ruptured abdominal aortic aneurysm
Diabetic coma
Tuberculous peritonitis
Food poisoning
Heavy metal poisoning
Acute porphyria
Sickle cell crisis
Acute leukemia

Table 52.7. PATHOLOGIC PROCESSES UNDERLYING ABDOMINAL PAIN

Process	Common examples
Obstruction	Intestinal colic, renal calculi, biliary colic
Inflammation	Enterocolitis, mesenteric adenitis
Perforation	Perforated peptic ulcer
Torsion	Ovarian torsion, sigmoid volvulus
Ischemia	Mesenteric artery thrombosis, splenic infarction

represents torsion and obstruction, whereas acute cholecystitis is initially caused by obstruction (of the cystic duct) but then progresses to transmural inflammation. It is not unusual for one process that initially causes pain to evolve into another (e.g., development of intestinal ischemia and infarction as a consequence of untreated adhesive obstruction).

Evaluation of the Patient with Abdominal Pain

It has been said that the most important diagnostic instrument available to the clinician is a chair, and this is perhaps nowhere more true than in the setting of the evaluation of a patient with acute abdominal pain. While eliciting the history, the clinician should take the opportunity to observe the patient's attitude in bed, the facial expression, particularly during paroxysms of pain, and the contour of the abdomen (2).

The course of the episode of illness should be retraced. The patient should be questioned about the exact time and mode of onset of the pain and also about any prodromic events that might have occurred in the hours or days after the patient was last subjectively at baseline health. The location and character of the pain, the direction of radiation of the pain, and changes in intensity or shifts in location over time are elicited. The presence of associated symptoms, in particular anorexia and vomiting, and their relation to the onset and evolution of pain are determined. Nausea and vomiting are usually caused either by severe irritation of the peritoneal or mesenteric nerves or by obstruction of a hollow viscus. The character and time of the most recent bowel movement or the occurrence of diarrhea is noted. The relevant past medical history is then documented in detail, with particular attention to prior episodes of similar pain, the presence of major digestive or other systemic disorders, and previous abdominal operations. Current medications are documented. Corticosteroid use or other conditions associated with immunosuppression may diminish the symptoms produced by inflammation and obscure a serious degree of intraabdominal disease. The presence of familial disorders or concurrent illness in family members or other contacts should be noted.

The age of the patient should be taken into account, as the differential diagnosis shifts considerably according to whether one is dealing with a pediatric or a geriatric patient. In women, a recent menstrual history is obtained and prior pregnancies noted. Gynecologic causes of acute abdominal pain to be considered include mittelschmerz or ruptured ovarian cyst, pelvic inflammatory disease, ectopic pregnancy, tuboovarian abscess (with or without rupture), and ovarian torsion.

As indicated above, the physical examination should begin with inspection of the patient's general appearance, attitude in bed, and facial expression. Unwillingness to change position may indicate underlying peritonitis; con-

irritation can cause localized somatic pain. *Perforation* or rupture of a hollow viscus or other structure (e.g., an ovarian cyst or a hepatic adenoma) typically results in pain of sudden onset that builds to maximum intensity within minutes to hours and produces signs of peritoneal irritation that are initially localized but may soon become generalized. *Torsion* may also produce a severe pain of sudden onset, but physical findings in the initial phase are usually limited to the site of torsion and do not become generalized. Finally, *ischemia* of a solid or hollow viscus produces a severe pain that is frequently described as out of proportion to the physical findings.

As a first step in the differential diagnosis, it is useful to assign an episode of abdominal pain tentatively to one of these pathologic processes and one of the locations previously described. These categories are of course not absolute because overlapping presentations are seen in a variety of conditions. For example, sigmoid volvulus simultaneously

versely, an inability to find a comfortable position may be seen in cases of ureteral colic resulting from nephrolithiasis. A patient with acute pancreatitis or mesenteric ischemia may prefer to lean forward. Intermittent grimacing may be observed in a patient with intestinal obstruction. Vital signs are measured. Cool, clammy skin or jaundice may be observed at this time.

Inspection of the abdomen reveals generalized distention or focal swelling. The presence of a hernia must be specifically excluded by direct examination of all hernial orifices and abdominal incisions. Auscultation of the abdomen may be performed next, although this only rarely provides valuable information. Auscultation of the chest, particularly the basilar regions, may reveal pneumonic consolidation that can simulate an acute abdominal process or may reveal a pleuritic rub. Gentle percussion of the abdomen helps distinguish gaseous distention from ascites; loss of dullness over the liver may indicate the presence of free intraperitoneal air, as in perforated duodenal ulcer. Tenderness to percussion, either localized or across the abdomen, suggests focal or diffuse peritonitis. Referred tenderness to percussion (pain perceived away from the site of percussion) is an extremely important finding that is essentially pathognomonic for peritonitis.

Palpation of the abdomen must be gentle. Rough or sudden deep palpation will frighten the patient, cause voluntary guarding, and hamper subsequent attempts to palpate the abdomen. Subtle muscle rigidity (involuntary guarding) or an intraabdominal mass is more likely to be detected by a gentle approach. It may be useful to ask the patient to flex the thighs during this phase of the examination. Areas of skin hyperesthesia may be noted during gentle palpation. Eliciting rebound tenderness rarely provides additional information beyond that obtained by careful percussion and palpation and is not recommended. The psoas and obturator tests may be performed next. In patients with a colostomy or ileostomy, direct examination of the stoma along with digitalization is important. The back is examined, with attention to the presence of spinal tenderness or tenderness in the costovertebral angle or flanks.

Examination of the pelvis is extremely important in most patients with abdominal pain. Suprapubic palpation may reveal an enlarged bladder or tenderness indicative of deeper disease. Digital rectal examination may reveal focal tenderness resulting from a periappendiceal or peridiverticular pelvic abscess. Anterior palpation may reveal the only evidence of pelvic peritonitis, particularly in male patients. A bimanual vaginoabdominal examination in female patients will reveal disease in the pouch of Douglas or involving the uterus, tubes, or ovaries.

Laboratory and Radiologic Examination

The common practice of ordering a "routine" panel of tests, even before evaluation by a physician, is wasteful of resources and may lead to unnecessary delays in diagnosis and treatment, particularly when normal values will lull care givers into a false sense of security. For example, the white blood cell count is notoriously normal in a substantial fraction of patients with serious intraabdominal disease and is frequently elevated in cases of nonsurgical disease (6). However, determination of the hematocrit and serum electrolyte and blood urea nitrogen levels may be useful to guide fluid resuscitation. Measurement of the serum amylase level and liver chemistries is usually indicated in patients with upper abdominal pain, but only rarely in those with lower abdominal pain. Although the liberal use of human chorionic gonadotropin testing may avoid a missed tubal pregnancy, its routine use in female patients with abdominal pain is not likely to be cost-effective. A urinalysis is frequently of value to screen for urologic causes of abdominal pain, but routine urine culture is unnecessary.

Plain radiographs of the abdomen are ordered far in excess of their usefulness in the evaluation of abdominal pain (7,8). Despite occasional positive findings (e.g., air–fluid levels, a fecalith, gallstones), plain films tend to be relatively nonspecific, complementing what is already obvious on history and examination, and rarely redirect therapeutic thinking. They are most helpful in patients with suspected ureteral calculus or intestinal obstruction. It is important to remember that the appearance of abdominal films is frequently normal or nondiagnostic in patients with strangulating obstruction. An upright chest film is the least expensive and perhaps best test to identify free intraperitoneal air.

An upper gastrointestinal series performed with water-soluble contrast is occasionally helpful in detecting ulcer perforation and determining whether such perforation is free or contained. A water-soluble contrast enema may be useful in cases of suspected large-bowel obstruction. Intravenous pyelography may be used to identify ureteral stones. All these studies, however, have been supplanted in many centers by computed tomography (CT), which, although somewhat more expensive, yields considerably more information of practical importance (9). CT is quite useful in patients with abdominal pain who do not require emergency surgery, particularly in delineating the cause and suggesting therapeutic strategy in patients with no prior history of abdominal disease (10). Arteriography may be useful in patients with suspected mesenteric ischemia, although CT angiography and magnetic resonance imaging are being increasingly applied in this situation. Ultrasonographic examination of the right upper quadrant may reveal gallstones, but it is important to remember that ultrasonographic signs of acute cholecystitis may be no more accurate than clinical examination findings. Ultrasonography in cases of lower abdominal pain may provide a more accurate diagnosis than can be derived from the clinical impression alone but is highly experience- and operator-dependent (11). A guiding principle in ordering radiologic tests is that the result should substantially influence plans for further testing or therapy. Redundant tests should be avoided.

Diagnostic laparoscopy may be appropriate in certain circumstances, especially the evaluation of acute lower abdominal pain in female patients. This has become a more attractive option as the techniques of therapeutic laparoscopy (e.g., appendectomy) have been refined (12–14). Nevertheless, laparoscopy requires a general anesthetic and should not be undertaken without due consideration.

Conditions Mimicking the Acute Abdomen

A variety of nonsurgical conditions may be associated with acute abdominal pain, including cardiovascular, respiratory, metabolic, and toxic conditions. For example, myocardial ischemia may produce epigastric pain, nausea, and vomiting that simulate acute cholecystitis; conversely, and perhaps more frequently, acute cholecystitis is mistaken for pain of cardiac origin. Abdominal wall injury, radiculopathy, and rectus sheath hematoma (the latter particularly in patients on anticoagulant therapy) may cause acute abdominal pain. Abdominal pain and vomiting may accompany influenza. Diabetic ketoacidosis and, rarely, blood dyscrasias such as acute porphyria or sickle cell hemolytic crisis may produce severe abdominal pain. Urologic disorders such as pyelonephritis or obstruction of the ureter, renal pelvis, or bladder outlet may be mistaken for intraabdominal disease. Urinalysis and renal ultrasonography may confirm the diagnosis. Testicular torsion can also be associated with severe abdominal pain.

Abdominal Pain in Special Circumstances

The evaluation of acute abdominal pain in children is particularly difficult. In neonates and infants, congenital causes such as midgut volvulus or pyloric stenosis must be considered, and entities such as intussusception and Meckel's diverticulitis are far more common in children than in adults. It may be impossible to obtain key historical information, and the physical examination may be difficult (15). The evaluation of older children is generally easier. It should be noted that anorexia may be absent in children with appendicitis or other important abdominal disease. Diarrhea as a manifestation of appendicitis is also frequent and may simulate acute infectious enterocolitis. Abdominal films may be more informative in pediatric than in adult patients. In certain instances, it may be appropriate to consider whether the child has been abused. Elderly patients can also present diagnostic difficulties, and if dementia is present, it may be impossible to elicit a meaningful history. In such patients, serious intraabdominal disease may present with few or subtle signs, and only minimal tenderness may be present on examination despite diffuse peritonitis. Laboratory values are frequently normal despite the presence of serious illness in this population (16). The majority of geriatric patients evaluated in the emergency setting are found to have significant disease requiring hospitalization (17).

Acute abdominal pain in immunosuppressed patients represents a particular diagnostic challenge (e.g., in the setting of organ transplantation, immunosuppressive therapy for autoimmune disorders, chemotherapy, and AIDS). Unusual infectious causes of acute abdominal pain, including cytomegalovirus (CMV), mycobacteria, protozoal species, and fungi, should be considered; these may all affect the gastrointestinal tract, gallbladder, liver, and pancreas. Perforation of the gastrointestinal tract in association with CMV infection, *Mycobacterium tuberculosis* or *M. intracellulare* infection, lymphoma, Kaposi's sarcoma, or corticosteroid use is seen in immunosuppressed patients. Acalculous cholecystitis should be considered in patients with AIDS and is often associated with *Cryptosporidium* or CMV infection. Splenic abscess resulting from infection with *Candida* or *Salmonella* may be a cause of left upper quadrant pain. Neutropenic enterocolitis is a common cause of abdominal pain and fever in patients with bone marrow suppression resulting from chemotherapy. In the transplant population, acute graft-versus-host disease should be considered. Abdominal pain in immunosuppressed patients is often treated nonoperatively, but vigilance must be maintained lest serious surgical disease be overlooked.

Acute abdominal pain after cardiac or major abdominal vascular surgery merits special mention because of the frequency of serious diagnoses that carry a particularly high mortality in this setting. Mesenteric or segmental colonic ischemia is commonly reported, as are acute colitis and cholecystitis (often acalculous). Acute pancreatitis associated with extracorporeal cardiopulmonary bypass occurs in about 2% of cases (18). Severe acute abdominal pain in hemodialysis patients is most commonly caused by mesenteric ischemia (19).

The diagnosis of abdominal pain in patients with spinal cord injury is particularly challenging. Mortality in this setting is high (about 10%), usually because of delayed diagnosis (20). Classic signs such as tenderness, guarding, and even fever are unreliable; more helpful are the presence of shoulder pain, abdominal distention, nausea, vomiting, and autonomic dysreflexia (21).

Finally, the evaluation of abdominal pain occurring during pregnancy involves additional considerations (22). Anatomic relationships may be distorted by the gravid uterus; in particular, the appendix is often displaced upward into the right upper quadrant. Nonsurgical causes of abdominal and pelvic pain are common. Physiologic alterations should be recognized in the interpretation of blood values; leukocytosis is frequently present during normal pregnancy. Although one should not hesitate to obtain radiologic tests when essential, unnecessary exposure to x-rays must be avoided. Ultrasonography is a particularly valuable diagnostic modality in pregnant patients.

APPENDIX

The clinical entity of appendiceal inflammation followed by perforation, abscess formation, and peritonitis was first described in 1889 by Reginald Fitz (23). Since that time, appendectomy has remained among the most common abdominal operations and, in fact, is the most common surgical procedure performed on an emergency basis in Western countries. Appendectomy remains the mainstay of treatment, but with the development of modern antibiotics and percutaneous drainage techniques, some cases are best managed nonoperatively. The morbidity and mortality associated with acute appendicitis have diminished with time, although because it usually affects young, healthy people, the overall effect on our work force remains significant. When not treated appropriately, appendicitis remains a potentially lethal condition. A case in point is that of the famous magician, Harry Houdini, who occasionally entertained by withstanding punches to the abdomen delivered by members of his audience. Unfortunately, Mr. Houdini performed this "act" while he had an appendiceal abscess and died several days later of diffuse peritonitis and sepsis, the abscess having been ruptured during one of the assaults (24).

Anatomy and Pathophysiology

The appendix is considered a vestigial organ with no known function in human beings. However, examination of the phylogenetic tree reveals that the appendix is absent from a number of carnivores, such as dogs, tigers, and lions, and surprisingly, progressive development of the appendix is noted in apes and as one ascends the primate scale (25). The appendix contains large amounts of lymphoid aggregates, similar to those within the Peyer's patches of gut-associated lymphoid tissue. Lymphoid nodules containing both B and T cells within the lamina propria differentiate the appendix from the adjacent colon (26). Because of this prominence of lymphoid tissue, some have hypothesized that the appendix may have an immune function, similar to that of the thymus or bursa of Fabricius, although no actual function has ever been documented. The appendiceal mucosa produces minimal amounts of fluid and digestive juices, so that it is unlikely to have any important exocrine function. Some associations have been made between the lack of an appendix and various disease states (inflammatory bowel disease), but a causal relationship remains unproven.

The appendix develops as an antimesenteric outpouching from the cecum and is first delineated during the fifth month of gestation. The position of the appendix can vary greatly. In almost two thirds of the population, the appendix is located in a retrocecal position, whereas in others it is located over the pelvic brim, occasionally descending to a position low in the pelvis. When the appendix occupies an unusual location, the diagnosis of appendicitis may be more difficult and contribute to delays in either presentation or diagnosis. The three taeniae coli of the ascending colon meet at the base of the appendix, with the anterior taenia serving as an important landmark. Following the taeniae can be a useful maneuver in identifying a difficult appendix at the time of operation. The appendix can vary in length from 2 to 20 cm, averaging approximately 9 cm. The blood supply of the appendix is from the appendicular artery, which is a branch of the ileocolic artery. Similarly, the lymphatic drainage follows that of the ileocolic nodes, and these are often hyperplastic in cases of acute appendicitis. The innervation of the appendix is derived from the autonomic nervous system. As in other visceral organs, no somatic pain fibers are found within the appendix. Therefore, early inflammation leads to poorly localized pain and is referred to the periumbilical region because the autonomic nerves follow the midgut embryologic origin. As the inflammation of appendicitis progresses, irritation of the surrounding parietal peritoneum results in the activation of somatic pain fibers and localization of symptoms and signs to the right lower quadrant.

In cross section, the appendix contains the same layers as the adjacent colon, including the mucosa, submucosa with prominent lymphoid tissue, circular and longitudinal muscle layers, and overlying serosa. Neurosecretory cells are located within the subepithelial layer and are the presumed source of carcinoid tumors, which are often found within the appendix.

The etiology of appendicitis remains somewhat unclear. In most patients, a luminal obstruction probably leads to bacterial overgrowth and increased luminal pressure, so that obstruction of venous outflow and then arterial inflow results in gangrene and eventual perforation. The cause of the luminal obstruction that initiates the process of appendicitis is postulated to involve lymphoid hyperplasia, a condition that is especially common in the teen years and correlates with the high incidence of appendicitis in this age group. It is felt that either viral or bacterial infections, such as shigellosis, salmonellosis, and infectious mononucleosis, can precede an episode of appendicitis and presumably initiate lymphoid hyperplasia and subsequent luminal obstruction.

In addition to lymphoid hyperplasia, fecaliths can cause appendiceal obstruction and subsequent appendicitis. It is thought that approximately 30% of cases of acute appendicitis in adults are linked to fecaliths. Fecaliths are thought to develop following the entrapment of vegetable matter, with subsequent deposition of mucus and eventual calcification. The "obstructive" model for appendicitis does not explain its development in all cases, however, because in some patients with appendicitis, the lumen appears to be patent on radiologic, gross, and histologic examination. The pathophysiology of these cases remains unclear.

Diagnosis

Early diagnosis remains the most important clinical goal in patients with suspected appendicitis. Although the mortality rates in modern series are well under 1%

Table 52.8. **TYPICAL SEQUENCE OF SYMPTOMS AND SIGNS OF ACUTE APPENDICITIS**

1. Periumbilical pain—vague, visceral, poorly localized
2. Anorexia, nausea, vomiting
3. Right lower quadrant pain and tenderness—localized
4. Fever
5. Leukocytosis

(27,28), the morbidity of patients with perforated appendicitis is much higher than that of nonperforated cases and is related to increased rates of wound infection and intraabdominal abscess formation, increased lengths of hospital stay, and delayed return to full activity (29).

By a thorough history and physical examination, experienced clinicians can accurately diagnose acute appendicitis in the majority of cases (2). A typical presentation (Table 52.8) is one of vague periumbilical pain (sometimes located more superiorly, in the epigastric region) followed by anorexia, nausea, or even frank vomiting. When vomiting occurs in appendicitis, it is usually of a limited nature; in contrast, vomiting is generally more severe in patients with viral gastroenteritis. The pain then shifts to the right lower quadrant region as the inflammatory process progresses and involves the overlying peritoneum. Eventually, fever ensues, followed by the development of leukocytosis. These clinical features are not entirely reliable, however. For example, not all patients become anorexic, so that an expression of hunger in a given patient should not necessarily deter one from surgical intervention for presumed acute appendicitis. Occasionally, patients have urinary symptoms, perhaps because of some inflammation adjacent to the ureter or bladder. Microscopic hematuria is quite common, and the clinician should not mistakenly consider the primary problem to be in the urinary tract. Intestinal function is usually unaffected in appendicitis, but some patients note diarrhea, perhaps related to the inflammation adjacent to the rectum or colon. Appendicitis can also be associated with adynamic ileus, which leads to constipation.

The physical examination findings generally most reliably indicate appendicitis. Except for young children and persons who are very elderly or otherwise neurologically impaired, patients with appendicitis have at least some degree of tenderness on palpation of the abdomen. In cases of an appendix located entirely within the pelvis, the tenderness on abdominal examination may be minimal, but on rectal examination the tenderness will be evident as the pelvic peritoneum is manipulated. Pelvic examination with cervical motion will also manipulate the pelvic peritoneum and elicit tenderness when an inflamed appendix is located within that region. Therefore, the finding of cervical motion tenderness does not necessarily indicate gynecologic pathology but rather is a nonspecific sign of inflammation in the pelvis.

Peritoneal irritation can be elicited on physical examination with the findings of percussion or rebound tenderness. Any movement, including coughing (Dunphy's sign), may cause increased pain. The most reliable indicator of peritoneal irritation, however, is involuntary guarding, a reflex contraction of the abdominal wall musculature overlying the inflamed peritoneum. This involuntary response is less likely to vary among individuals than are responses to external stimuli. Other physical signs (Table 52.9) associated with appendicitis include pain in the right lower quadrant during palpation of the left lower quadrant (Rovsing's sign), pain on internal rotation of the

Table 52.9. SIGNS ON PHYSICAL EXAMINATION SUGGESTIVE OF ACUTE APPENDICITIS

Sign	What it indicates	Description
Dunphy's	Inflammation involving the partial peritoneum	Increased pain with coughing or other movement
Rovsing's	Localized peritoneal inflammation in the right lower quadrant	Lower left quadrant palpation induces right lower quadrant pain
Obturator	Pelvic appendicitis	Pain on internal rotation of the right hip
Iliopsoas	Retrocecal appendicitis	Pain on extension of right hip

hip (obturator sign, suggesting a pelvic appendix), and pain on extension of the right hip (iliopsoas sign, typical of a retrocecal appendix).

In addition to the history and physical examination, a white blood cell count is usually obtained and in most patients will be elevated, although it may be in the normal range during the early stages. A very high white blood cell count (> 20,000/mL) suggests complicated appendicitis with either gangrene or perforation. A urinalysis can also be helpful to rule out pyelonephritis or nephrolithiasis. However, in pyelonephritis, the fever and white blood cell count will generally be much higher than in appendicitis, symptoms of dysuria will be present, and the tenderness is centered more in the flank or costovertebral angle region. Minimal pyuria, frequently seen in elderly women, should not deter one from the correct diagnosis of appendicitis. Although microscopic hematuria is common in appendicitis, gross hematuria is uncommon and may indicate the presence of a kidney stone. As a kidney stone passes down the urinary tract through the distal ureter, pain can often be referred to the right lower quadrant and occasionally down into the testicle. The pain is quite severe and entirely visceral in nature. Therefore, the signs of peritoneal irritation should not be found in a patient with nephrolithiasis. Other blood tests are generally not helpful and are not indicated in the patient with suspected appendicitis.

Plain abdominal radiographs are of little use in the patient with suspected appendicitis. Occasionally, calcified appendicolithiasis may be evident, but this is a rare event (~ 17%) and, in any case, does not really establish the diagnosis (30). Plain abdominal films can indicate the presence of mechanical bowel obstruction or free intraperitoneal air, but such conditions should rarely be confused with appendicitis.

Given the inherent limitations in establishing the diagnosis of acute appendicitis and the concern that a delay can result in perforation, with increased associated morbidity and possible mortality, a false appendectomy rate of approximately 20% has been considered acceptable. If the negative appendectomy rate is much higher than that, then one can question the diagnostic acumen of the clinicians involved. On the other hand, a negative appendectomy rate of less than 10% has been achieved in some centers (28). Clearly, clinical experience and expertise are important in establishing a correct diagnosis. In addition, in-hospital observation has been touted as an excellent way to follow patients closely and quickly intervene if abdominal pain, peritoneal irritation, or fever worsen. By using this approach, White et al. reported a negative appendectomy rate of 6% (31). Of course, if the negative appendectomy rate is low, one must be sure that cases of perforated appendix did not develop while patients were being observed in the hospital or after they were discharged from the emergency department.

To improve the diagnostic accuracy in patients with suspected appendicitis, other radiologic tests have been used. Ultrasonography has been reported to aid in the diagnosis of acute appendicitis (32,33) by demonstrating a so-called target lesion (i.e., a thick-walled, noncompressible luminal structure in the right lower quadrant). In more advanced cases, peritoneal fluid and even a frank abscess may be found. However, a number of large series (34,35) have shown ultrasonography to be unreliable, both in terms of sensitivity and specificity, so that it probably should not be used in the routine diagnosis of acute appendicitis. Ultrasonography may be helpful if it suggests a diagnosis other than appendicitis, especially gynecologic disease in women of menstrual age. It must be cautioned, however, that simple cysts of the ovary are common and usually nonpathologic. Therefore, the presence of an ovarian cyst does not weigh against the diagnosis of acute appendicitis. On the other hand, if ultrasonographic signs of a tuboovarian abscess, ovarian torsion, or even rare complications related to uterine fibroids are present, then the diagnosis of appendicitis may be excluded.

More recently, abdominal and pelvic CT has been used in the setting of suspected acute appendicitis (36,37) and appears to be more accurate than ultrasonography (38). Rao et al. (39) have suggested that the use of CT can lead to significant cost savings because a normal study result virtually excludes the diagnosis and obviates the need for (and costs of) in-hospital observation. CT should include thin cuts through the area of the appendix and the use of rectal contrast to distend the cecum and make the adjacent inflammatory changes more evident (Fig. 52.1). The role of CT in the diagnosis of appendicitis, however, remains controversial because in most patients an accurate diagnosis can be reached simply by history and physical examination. In the setting of early acute appendicitis, pathologic changes in the gross appearance of the appendix can be minimal, even with direct observation at the time of surgery, and may well be missed by all radiologic techniques. One advantage of CT, as of ultrasonography, may be the detection of disease other than acute appendicitis (40).

Barium enema has also been used in the past in an attempt to diagnose appendicitis (41). A failure of the appendix to fill has been associated with appendicitis, but up to 20% of normal appendices do not fill, and therefore the diagnosis cannot be accurately established with this criterion. Occasionally, in more advanced cases with abscess formation, a mass is seen compressing the adjacent cecum. However, such a finding would probably be better visualized on CT, which also provides the opportunity for percutaneous drainage. On occasion, barium enema can detect a colonic mucosal lesion, such as a neoplasm or a terminal ileal abnormality related to Crohn's disease, and so establish a diagnosis other than appendicitis. Overall, however, barium enema has little role in the modern management of suspected acute appendicitis.

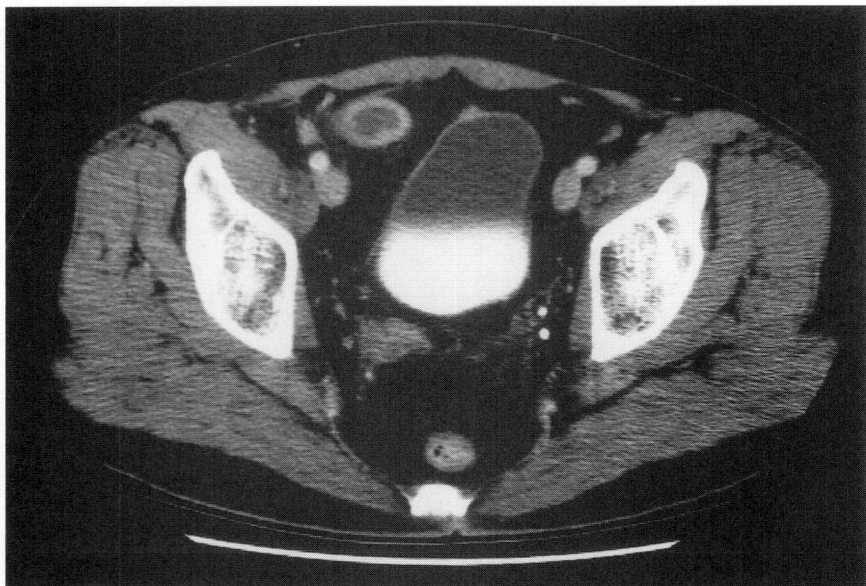

Figure 52.1. Acute appendicitis in a 53-year-old woman with fever and right lower quadrant pain and tenderness. Note the thick-walled, fluid-filled appendix with surrounding inflammation. A gangrenous appendix was found at operation.

Treatment

The standard treatment for suspected appendicitis is appendectomy via an incision in the right lower quadrant. In the classic McBurney incision, an oblique approach is employed; each of the three abdominal wall muscle layers is incised lateral to the rectus sheath. Ideally, the incision should follow Langer's skin lines to provide an optimal cosmetic result. The aponeurosis overlying the external oblique can be sharply incised and the remaining muscle layers split by retraction. The peritoneum is opened, the appendix is identified, and its blood supply is then ligated, usually from tip to base. Depending on the degree of surrounding inflammation and the duration of the illness, mobilization of the appendix may be difficult, and the lateral attachments of the cecum may have to be divided. The appendix itself is usually ligated with an absorbable suture and then inverted into the cecal wall through the use of a pursestring suture or Z-stitch. Inversion of the appendiceal stump has been advocated to prevent leakage and fistulization, but numerous reports have shown no difference in complication rates between inversion and simple ligation of the appendiceal stump (42). Following appendectomy, the peritoneal cavity should be irrigated and then the peritoneum and muscles should be closed in layered fashion, usually with absorbable sutures. The skin incision can generally be safely closed, although in grossly contaminated cases, one may consider delayed primary closure or simply healing by secondary intention. Intraperitoneal drains have not proved useful, even in cases of perforated appendicitis (43).

If a normal appendix is found at the time of laparotomy, other causes for the abdominal pain should be sought. The cecum and proximal ascending colon should be examined for right-sided diverticulitis, neoplasms, or other disease. The terminal ileum should be examined for Crohn's disease or acute ileitis, and at least 2 feet of the ileum proximal to the ileocecal valve should be inspected for the presence of a Meckel's diverticulum. If Crohn's disease is encountered, the appendix may be safely removed as long as the cecum and particularly the base of the appendix are not involved by the inflammatory process. If uncomplicated Crohn's inflammation is detected, ileal resection is not indicated, but in the case of a gross perforation or advanced Crohn's disease with obstruction, resection should be performed. Occasionally, sigmoid diverticulitis may be mistaken for acute appendicitis, especially when a redundant sigmoid colon reaches the right side of the abdomen. Finally, the fallopian tubes, ovaries, and uterus should be carefully examined in female patients.

Laparoscopy

The role of laparoscopy and laparoscopic appendectomy remains to be established. Many surgeons advocate diagnostic laparoscopy, especially for young women. Laparoscopy allows easy visualization of the pelvic organs and appendix and can establish the diagnosis of appendicitis or other processes (44,45). Laparoscopic appendectomy has gained substantial popularity. Generally, the laparoscope is inserted through a periumbilical incision and then additional trocars are placed, one in the right lower quadrant to grasp the appendix and another on the left side to dissect, ligate, and ultimately remove the appendix. An Endoloop (brand name) may be used to ligate the appendix, but this step has been simplified by the recent introduction of endoscopic stapling devices, which provide excellent hemostasis in the mesoappendix and allow closure of the appendiceal stump. Numerous series have compared laparoscopic with open appendectomy (46,47). As in many other minimally invasive procedures, a learning curve clearly exists and may explain the longer operative times in initial reports. With experience, however, operative times for the laparoscopic approach probably equal and may be superior to those of open appendectomy. Complication rates appear to be low and are probably no different for the laparoscopic and open techniques, although postoperative infections may be less common with laparoscopy. Laparoscopy may also be of benefit in regard to length of hospital stay and overall recovery. Most reports in the literature indicate that the length of stay is significantly reduced when the laparoscopic route is used, as is narcotic use and other parameters associated with postoperative morbidity (48). In a large retrospective series from the Beth Israel Deaconess Medical Center in Boston (28), laparoscopic appendectomy was found to be particularly valuable in cases of gangrenous or perforated appendicitis. For simple acute appendicitis, the hospital stay and recovery periods were short regardless of the operative approach. However, in more advanced cases, laparoscopy was associated with shorter hospital stays and faster recovery.

Appendiceal Mass

Some patients with appendicitis present at a relatively late stage (> 5 days). Although in most cases acute appendicitis progresses to perforation and diffuse peritonitis within the first few days of the illness, virtually forcing the patient to seek medical attention, occasionally an appendiceal perforation is contained by surrounding structures, including the omentum and adjacent bowel. Instead of diffuse peritonitis, a localized inflammatory mass or phlegmon develops in these patients, with or without a discrete abscess. The associated pain and other systemic signs are limited by this process, which may explain the delayed presentation. On examination, such patients usually have right lower quadrant abdominal pain and tenderness with a palpable mass or fullness, although overlying guarding of the abdominal wall musculature may obscure the mass. The key diagnostic feature to be recognized in these cases is the duration of the illness, as a walled-off appendiceal mass generally requires a minimum of 5 days to form. In such cases, CT may establish the diagnosis and allow for percutaneous drainage of the abscess (Fig. 52.2). In the acute setting, these patients are best treated nonoperatively because although the appendix can be removed, the risk for injury to adjacent structures, including the small bowel, is increased. The overall morbidity in these patients appears to be decreased by use of the nonoperative approach, with or without percutaneous drainage. Intravenous antibiotics are administered initially, and most of the patients respond within a 24- to 48-hour period, with a decrease in pain and fever. The patients can then be safely discharged on a course of oral antibiotics and a normal diet. The appendiceal inflammation generally subsides within 1 to 2 weeks. Antibiotics should be continued for a total of approximately 2 weeks.

It should be noted that fistulization from the cecum rarely develops in patients who have undergone percutaneous or open drainage of a periappendiceal abscess. Similarly, patients with perforated appendicitis almost always have pus within the peritoneal cavity, rather than actual enteric contents. These observations support the concept that most cases of appendicitis are associated with some obstruction of the lumen of the appendix. Following the successful nonoperative treatment of an appendiceal mass,

interval appendectomy should be considered. A period of approximately 8 weeks allows the inflammatory changes surrounding the appendix to resolve. Removal of the appendix after such a time period is generally safe and simple, although in rare circumstances, a significant amount of periappendiceal scar tissue and inflammation will persist. Whether or not to perform an interval appendectomy remains controversial. A number of investigators have examined the incidence of recurrent appendicitis following presentation with an appendiceal mass and successful nonoperative treatment. Based on a recurrence rate of approximately 10% (6 months to 13 years of follow-up), Ein and Shandling (49) suggested that interval appendectomy is not indicated in all patients. The incidence of recurrence may be higher in younger patients, and therefore the decision to perform the interval appendectomy should probably be individualized according to patient age. One must remember, however, especially in elderly patients, that the original diagnosis of appendicitis may have been mistaken, and it is important to rule out a cecal neoplasm in such patients if interval appendectomy is not performed.

More recently, interval laparoscopic appendectomy has been shown to be a safe and simple procedure, with a high degree of patient acceptance. The operation can generally be performed on an outpatient basis with minimal morbidity (50). Therefore, laparoscopy may have shifted the risk-to-benefit ratio in favor of interval appendectomy.

Antibiotic Therapy

Patients with acute appendicitis should be treated with perioperative broad-spectrum antibiotics directed against colonic flora, including gram-positive, gram-negative, and anaerobic organisms. Peritoneal cultures are generally not clinically helpful in the selection of the type of antibiotics (51). The optimal length of antibiotic therapy is not known. In simple cases of acute appendicitis, 24 hours or less is generally sufficient. However, in cases of perforated appendicitis, longer courses of antibiotics are generally used, approximately 5 to 7 days.

Recurrent Appendicitis

Rarely, a patient presents with recurrent episodes of presumed acute appendicitis. At each presentation, spontaneous resolution may occur, with or without the use of antibiotics. Such patients may eventually come to appendectomy, and it is only in retrospect that the previous

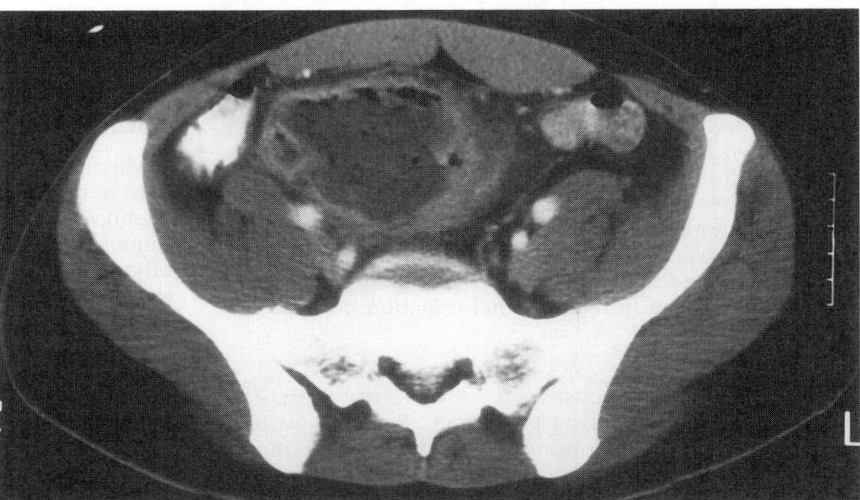

Figure 52.2. A 23-year-old man with right lower quadrant pain, fever, and leukocytosis of 2 weeks' duration. Note the large periappendiceal abscess containing gas. The patient was successfully treated with percutaneous drainage and antibiotics.

episodes are recognized to have been acute appendicitis. Recurrent appendicitis is occasionally termed *chronic appendicitis,* but this is probably a misnomer because the appendix is almost certainly not inflamed between episodes. Some patients present as outpatients for the evaluation of chronic or intermittent right lower quadrant pain, which raises the question of recurrent or chronic appendicitis. In this difficult scenario, clinical expertise is required to rule out causes other than appendicitis and determine whether surgery is indicated. In general, discrete episodes of right lower quadrant pain, especially if associated with fever or leukocytosis, are the best indicators of disease within the appendix, and these patients respond most favorably to appendectomy. In contrast, patients with chronic right lower quadrant pain recurring frequently or even daily, in the absence of associated fever, are unlikely to benefit from appendectomy.

Special Patient Populations

Children

The diagnosis of acute appendicitis is generally more difficult in young children than in adults (52). An accurate history may be difficult to obtain, and some of the signs of appendicitis, such as nausea, vomiting, and abdominal pain and tenderness, are often associated with extraabdominal processes (e.g., pneumonia, meningitis, otitis media). The difficulty of establishing an accurate diagnosis in children is the presumed reason for their higher perforation rate, reported to be as high as 50%. For this reason, the use of radiologic studies such as CT may be of particular benefit in children with suspected appendicitis.

Elderly Patients

Like elderly patients with a number of other disease entities, elderly patients with appendicitis tend to present later in the course of their illness and clearly have higher associated rates of morbidity and mortality (53). Perforation rates in elderly patients with appendicitis are quite high (> 50%). Elderly patients tend to have less subjective pain, fewer findings of peritonitis on examination, and a delayed leukocytosis. Therefore, the index of suspicion for an intraabdominal inflammatory/infectious process, including acute appendicitis, must be higher in elderly patients than in the general population.

Immunocompromised Patients

The patient with an impaired immune system who has abdominal pain represents a particularly challenging problem for the clinician (54). Patients with AIDS or who have been exposed to high-dose chemotherapy are susceptible to specific disease entities, including CMV-related bowel perforations and typhlitis (neutropenic colitis). Because these disease processes most commonly affect the terminal ileum and cecum, they can often be confused with acute appendicitis. CT can be particularly helpful in this setting to establish a definitive diagnosis, although in some cases the findings of pericecal inflammation are nonspecific. In general, regardless of the underlying disease process, surgery is indicated in the patient with spreading peritonitis or with systemic signs of sepsis related to an intraabdominal infection.

Pregnant Women

Appendicitis is the most frequent nonobstetric indication for laparotomy during pregnancy. Pregnant women often present with abdominal pain, particularly in the lower abdomen, which raises the possibility of appendicitis. A diagnosis can be difficult to establish, especially because abdominal pain, nausea, and vomiting are quite common in early pregnancy. The white blood cell count is slightly elevated in normal pregnancy, further complicating the diagnosis of appendicitis. In addition, as the uterus enlarges, the anatomic location of the appendix is shifted upward and the uterus may cover the appendix, so that the signs of peritoneal inflammation are diminished. Because of these complicating factors, the perforation rate of appendicitis during pregnancy is probably higher than that in the general population (55,56). Unfortunately, perforated appendicitis is also associated with a high rate of fetal mortality (> 30%), whereas the risk for fetal loss in simple acute appendicitis is in the range of 10%, and the risk to the mother is negligible. Therefore, it is best to be aggressive in recommending surgical exploration in pregnant women with suspected appendicitis, especially because a "negative" appendectomy is well tolerated, with minimal morbidity to mother and fetus. Numerous reports have indicated the safety of laparoscopy in the setting of pregnancy (57). However, in the third trimester, the enlarged uterus may limit the exposure and preclude a laparoscopic approach.

Appendiceal Neoplasms

Approximately 1% of all appendectomy specimens contain a neoplasm (58). The most common tumor is the carcinoid. Rare tumors of the appendix include benign and malignant mucoceles, adenocarcinoma, and adenocarcinoids.

Carcinoids

Approximately two thirds of all appendiceal neoplasms are carcinoids, tumors of neural crest origin and derived from enteroendocrine cells. Of all carcinoid tumors within the gastrointestinal tract, approximately half arise within the appendix. Carcinoid tumors of the appendix are usually found incidentally on pathologic examination of an inflamed appendix. These tumors have a characteristic firm yellow appearance and are often associated with a surrounding desmoplastic reaction. In regard to treatment and prognosis, the key feature is the size of the tumor. Most carcinoids are less than 1.5 cm in diameter, and these tumors are adequately treated by simple appendectomy. The chance of lymphatic or distant metastasis is essentially zero, and the chance for cure should be excellent. On the other hand, tumors that are 2 cm in size or larger begin to have metastatic potential. In such cases, a formal right hemicolectomy is generally indicated, and the prognosis remains quite good. Rarely, appendiceal carcinoids are associated with liver metastases, and in these cases the carcinoid syndrome may be present. The number and location of liver lesions, in addition to the associated symptoms, would dictate treatment in these cases (59,60).

Mucoceles

Mucoceles of the appendix can be caused by both benign and malignant disease, either cystadenomas or cystadenocarcinomas. These tumors obstruct the appendiceal lumen, so that a large mucin-filled structure develops, often with calcification in the wall. Such tumors can generally be diagnosed by CT.

Appendectomy is curative for benign cystadenomas, even if rupture has occurred with mucinous ascites. However, with rupture of a cystadenocarcinoma, peritoneal tumor implantation is possible and can lead to mucin secretion and a condition known as *pseudomyxoma peritonei.* The presence of mucin-secreting cellular elements in the peritoneal cavity distinguish this malignant condition from the benign cystadenoma rupture with simple mucinous ascites. No effective treatment is available for pseudomyxoma peritonei, and secondary complications can develop in these patients, including bowel obstruction and perforation. The neoplastic process tends to be fairly indolent (50% survival at 5 years), and repeated debulking procedures may be indicated (61).

Adenocarcinoma

Adenocarcinoma of the appendix is extremely rare and, like other appendiceal neoplasms, is generally found unexpectedly at the time of appendectomy. Unfortunately, up to one half of the patients have metastatic disease at the time of diagnosis, usually with peritoneal spread, presumably from rupture of the associated inflammatory process. The sequence of staging and treatment for appendiceal adenocarcinoma is similar to that for the more common colon carcinoma. Early lesions confined to the mucosa or submucosa (Dukes A) may be treated by simple appendectomy, as long as clear surgical margins are present. For Dukes B and C lesions, formal right hemicolectomy is required, with adjuvant therapy indicated similar to that given in colon carcinoma. Interestingly, appendiceal adenocarcinomas are associated with secondary tumors in up to 35% of patients, and most often these involve other areas of the gastrointestinal tract (62).

REFERENCES

1. Gill BD JJ. Cost-effective evaluation and management of the acute abdomen. *Surg Clin North Am* 1996;76:71–82.
2. Silen W. *Cope's early diagnosis of the acute abdomen,* 19th ed. New York: Oxford University Press, 1996.
3. Brewer BJ, Golden GT, Hitch DC, et al. Abdominal pain: an analysis of 1,000 consecutive cases in a university hospital emergency room. *Am J Surg* 1976;131:219–223.
4. Hawthorn IE. Abdominal pain as a cause of acute admission to hospital [see comments]. *J R Coll Surg Edinb* 1992;37:389–393.
5. Powers RD, Guertler AT. Abdominal pain in the ED: stability and change over 20 years. *Am J Emerg Med* 1995;13:301–303.
6. Nauta RJ, Magnant C. Observation versus operation for abdominal pain in the right lower quadrant: roles of the clinical examination and the leukocyte count. *Am J Surg* 1986;151:746–748.
7. McCook TA, Ravin CE, Rice RP. Abdominal radiography in the emergency department: a prospective analysis. *Ann Emerg Med* 1982;11:7–8.
8. Anyanwu AC, Moalypour SM. Are abdominal radiographs still overutilized in the assessment of acute abdominal pain? a district general hospital audit. *J R Coll Surg Edinb* 1998;43:267–270.
9. Gupta H, Dupuy DE. Advances in imaging of the acute abdomen. *Surg Clin North Am* 1997;77:1245–1263.
10. Siewert B, Raptopoulos V, Mueller MF, et al. Impact of CT on diagnosis and management of acute abdomen in patients initially treated without surgery. *AJR Am J Roentgenol* 1997;168:173–178.
11. Carrico CW, Fenton LZ, Taylor GA, et al. Impact of sonography on the diagnosis and treatment of acute lower abdominal pain in children and young adults. *AJR Am J Roentgenol* 1999;172:513–516.
12. Mutter D, Navez B, Gury JF, et al. Value of microlaparoscopy in the diagnosis of right iliac fossa pain. *Am J Surg* 1998;176:370–372.
13. Memon MA, Fitztgibbons RJ Jr. The role of minimal access surgery in the acute abdomen. *Surg Clin North Am* 1997;77:1333–1353.
14. Chung RS, Diaz JJ, Chari V. Efficacy of routine laparoscopy for the acute abdomen. *Surg Endosc* 1998;12:219–222.
15. Neblett WWd, Pietsch JB, Holcomb GW Jr. Acute abdominal conditions in children and adolescents. *Surg Clin North Am* 1988;68:415–430.
16. Potts FEt, Vukov LF. Utility of fever and leukocytosis in acute surgical abdomens in octogenarians and beyond. *J Gerontol A Biol Sci Med Sci* 1999;54:M55–M58.
17. Marco CA, Schoenfeld CN, Keyl PM, et al. Abdominal pain in geriatric emergency patients: variables associated with adverse outcomes. *Acad Emerg Med* 1998;5:1163–1168.
18. Simic O, Strathausen S, Hess W, et al. Incidence and prognosis of abdominal complications after cardiopulmonary bypass. *Cardiovasc Surg* 1999;7:419–424.
19. Bender JS, Ratner LE, Magnuson TH, et al. Acute abdomen in the hemodialysis patient population. *Surgery* 1995;117:494–497.
20. Sheridan R. Diagnosis of the acute abdomen in the neurologically stable spinal cord-injured patient: a case study. *J Clin Gastroenterol* 1992;15:325–328.
21. Bar-On Z, Ohry A. The acute abdomen in spinal cord injury individuals. *Paraplegia* 1995;33:704–706.
22. Tarraza HM, Moore RD. Gynecologic causes of the acute abdomen and the acute abdomen in pregnancy. *Surg Clin North Am* 1997;77:1371–1394.
23. Fitz R. Perforating inflammation of the vermiform appendix: with special reference to its early diagnosis and treatment. *Trans Assoc Am Physicians* 1886;1:107.
24. Silverman K. *Houdini: the career of Ehrich Weiss.* New York: HarperCollins, 1996.
25. Scott G. The primate caecum and appendix vermiformis: a comparative study. *J Anat* 1980;131:549–463.
26. Gray H. *Gray's anatomy,* 29th ed. Philadelphia: Lea & Febiger, 1973.
27. Styrud J, Eriksson S, Segelman J, et al. Diagnostic accuracy in 2,351 patients undergoing appendicectomy for suspected acute appendicitis: a retrospective study 1986–1993. *Dig Surg* 1999;16:39–44.
28. Nguyen DB, Silen W, Hodin RA. Appendectomy in the pre- and post-laparoscopic eras. *J Gastrointest Surg* 1999;3:67–73.
29. Hale DM, M, Pearl RH, Schutt DC, et al. Appendectomy: a contemporary appraisal. *Ann Surg* 1997;225:252–261.
30. Olutola PS. Plain film radiographic diagnosis of acute appendicitis: an evaluation of the signs. *Can Assoc Radiol J* 1988;39:254–256.
31. White JJ, Santillana M, Haller JA Jr. Intensive in-hospital observation: a safe way to decrease unnecessary appendectomy. *Am Surg* 1975;41:793–798.
32. Zielke ACH, Hasse C, Sitter H, et al. Influence of ultrasound on clinical decision making in acute appendicitis: a prospective study. *Eur J Surg* 1998;164:201–209.
33. Ooms HW, Koumans RK, Ho Kang You PJ, et al. Ultrasonography in the diagnosis of acute appendicitis. *Br J Surg* 1991;78:315–318.
34. Franke C, Bohner H, Yang Q, et al. Ultrasonography for diagnosis of acute appendicitis: results of a prospective multicenter trial—Acute Abdominal Pain Study Group. *World J Surg* 1999;23:141–146.
35. Wade DSSEM, Marrow SE, Balsara ZN, et al. Accuracy of ultrasound in the diagnosis of acute appendicitis compared with the surgeon's clinical impression. *Arch Surg* 1993;128:1039–1044; discussion 1044–1046.
36. Choi YH, Fischer E, Hoda SA, et al. Appendiceal CT in 140 cases: diagnostic criteria for acute and necrotizing appendicitis. *Clin Imaging* 1998;22:252–271.
37. Lane MJ, Katz DS, Ross BA, et al. Unenhanced helical CT for suspected acute appendicitis. *AJR Am J Roentgenol* 1997;168:405–409.
38. Balthazar EJ, Birnbaum BA, Yee J, et al. Acute appendicitis: CT and US correlation in 100 patients. *Radiology* 1994;190:31–35.
39. Rao PM, Rhea JT, Novelline RA, et al. Effect of computed tomography of the appendix on treatment of patients and use of hospital resources [see comments]. *N Engl J Med* 1998;338:141–146.
40. Shaff MI, Tarr RW, Partain CL, et al. Computed tomography and magnetic resonance imaging of the acute abdomen. *Surg Clin North Am* 1988;68:233–254.
41. Smith DE, Kirchmer NA, Stewart DR. Use of the barium enema in the diagnosis of acute appendicitis and its complications. *Am J Surg* 1979;138:829–834.
42. Street D, Bodai BI, Owens LJ, et al. Simple ligation vs. stump inversion in appendectomy. *Arch Surg* 1988;123:689–690.
43. Greenall MJ, Evans M, Pollack AV. Should you drain a perforated appendix? *Br J Surg* 1978;65:880–902.

44. Tytgat SH, Bakker XR, Butzelaar RM. Laparoscopic evaluation of patients with suspected acute appendicitis. *Surg Endosc* 1998;12:918–920.

45. Thorell A, Grondal S, Schedvins K, et al. Value of diagnostic laparoscopy in fertile women with suspected appendicitis [In Process Citation]. *Eur J Surg* 1999;165:751–754.

46. Chiarugi M, Buccianti P, Celona G, et al. Laparoscopic compared with open appendicectomy for acute appendicitis: a prospective study. *Eur J Surg* 1996;162:385–390.

47. Chung RS, Rowland DY, Li P, et al. A meta-analysis of randomized controlled trials of laparoscopic versus conventional appendectomy. *Am J Surg* 1999;177:250–256.

48. Sackier JM. Laparoscopy for acute appendicitis. *Semin Laparosc Surg* 1996;3:185–192.

49. Ein S, Schandling B. Is interval appendectomy necessary after rupture of an appendiceal mass? *J Pediatr Surg* 1996;31:849–850.

50. Nguyen DB, Silen W, Hodin RA. Interval appendectomy in the laparoscopic era. *J Gastrointest Surg* 1999;3:189–193.

51. Mosdell DM, Morris DM, Fry DE. Peritoneal cultures and antibiotic therapy in pediatric perforated appendicitis. *Am J Surg* 1994;167:313–316.

52. Neblett WW III, Pietsch JB, Holcomb GW Jr. Acute abdominal conditions in children and adolescents. *Surg Clin North Am* 1988;68:415–430.

53. Horattas MC, Guyton DP, Wu D. A reappraisal of appendicitis in the elderly. *Am J Surg* 1990;160:291–293.

54. Nylander WA Jr. The acute abdomen in the immunocompromised host. *Surg Clin North Am* 1988;68:457–470.

55. Tamir IL, Bongard FS, Klein SR. Acute appendicitis in the pregnant patient. *Am J Surg* 1990;160:571–575.

56. Horowitz MD, Gomez GA, Santiesteban R, et al. Acute appendicitis during pregnancy: diagnosis and management. *Arch Surg* 1985;120:1362–1367.

57. Nezhat FR, Tazuke S, Nezhat CH, et al. Laparoscopy during pregnancy: a literature review. *J Soc Laparoendosc Surg* 1997;1:17–27.

58. Connor SJ, Hanna GB, Frizelle FA. Appendiceal tumors: retrospective clinicopathologic analysis of appendiceal tumors from 7,970 appendectomies. *Dis Colon Rectum* 1998;41:75–80.

59. Moertal CG, Weiland LH, Nagorney DM, et al. Carcinoid tumor of the appendix: treatment and prognosis. *N Engl J Med* 1987;317:1699–1701.

60. Sandor A, Modlin IM. A retrospective analysis of 1,570 appendiceal carcinoids. *Am J Gastroenterol* 1998;93:422–428.

61. Smith JW, Kemeny N, Caldwell C, et al. *Pseudomyxoma peritonei* of appendiceal origin: the Memorial Sloan-Kettering Cancer Center experience. *Cancer* 1992;70:396–401.

62. Cortina R, McCormick J, Kolm P, et al. Management and prognosis of adenocarcinoma of the appendix. *Dis Colon Rectum* 1995;38:848–852.

SURGERY: SCIENTIFIC PRINCIPLES AND PRACTICE, Third Edition, edited by Lazar J. Greenfield, Michael W. Mulholland, Keith T. Oldham, Gerald B. Zelenock, and Keith D. Lillemoe. Lippincott Williams & Wilkins Publishers, Philadelphia, © 2001.

CHAPTER 53

SPLEEN

DOUGLAS L. FRAKER

The spleen has been a mysterious organ throughout surgical and medical history, and a clear understanding and appreciation of its function have been acquired only in the latter half of the 20th century. The reasons for this paucity of knowledge about the spleen are several: No obvious function of the spleen can be discerned from its anatomic structure or features; no clear relationships of gross pathology of the spleen to many of the diseases in which it is important are evident; and even at the present time, it is difficult to obtain a biopsy specimen of the spleen, so that the amount of tissue available for pathologic study is limited. The diseases (other than trauma) in which the spleen is important are generally of a hematologic or immunologic nature. Understanding the normal physiology and subsequent pathophysiology of the spleen is important in making surgical decisions regarding when to recommend splenectomy and whether a partial splenectomy is possible. During most of the history of medicine, the only surgical procedure applied to the spleen was splenectomy. Current variations of that procedure include laparoscopic splenectomy, partial splenectomy, and other spleen-preserving procedures. This chapter reviews the history of splenic surgery, the anatomy and physiology of the spleen, and the disease processes and operative techniques involving the spleen.

HISTORICAL BACKGROUND

The spleen has had a colorful history in that various functions have been ascribed to it by many prominent scientists throughout the ages (1) (Table 53.1). Even the origin of the English word *spleen* is unclear. It is thought to be derived from the Greek word *splen,* which may come from the Greek *splancknon* ("viscus") or *spaw* ("to draw"). Its dark purple–red color led ancients to believe that the spleen draws spoiled or bad parts of the blood to itself, an idea that predates one of the major roles of the spleen as a filtration device for senescent red blood cells. In ancient Greece, the spleen was thought to be the source of black bile, one of the four cardinal humors, related to melancholy (2). However, in the Talmud, other ancient authors wrote that the spleen is the seat of laughter, and that removal of the spleen would limit a person's capacity for mirth. The spleen was thought to be a source of discomfort, sometimes felt as "a stitch in the side" for athletes, and that if it were removed or ablated, an athlete would be able to run faster. Reports of the earliest procedures performed on the spleen indicate that runners in ancient Greece may have had their spleen ablated to improve their performance. This hypothesis was studied in an experimental model almost 2,000 years later at Johns Hopkins, in which splenectomized mice and control mice were evaluated for their ability to run a race, and the splenectomized mice were reported to be faster (2).

During the Renaissance, scientists began to question the various roles ascribed to the spleen. Paracelsus rejected the black bile theory and questioned whether the spleen has any meaningful role at all in the early 16th century. One of his students, Zaccarella, reportedly performed the first splenectomy in the year 1549 in Palermo, Italy, removing the enlarged spleen of a 24-year-old woman successfully (2) (Table 53.1). The organ was reportedly displayed in the town square after this landmark but unsubstantiated procedure. During that same era, Vesalius performed splenec-

Table 53.1. HISTORICAL MILESTONES IN SURGERY OF THE SPLEEN

1549	First reported splenectomy by Zaccarella in Italy
1826	First documented splenectomy by Quitterbaum in Germany
1865	First successful splenectomy by Paen in France
1892	First trauma splenectomy by Reigner in Germany
1911	Elective splenectomy for autoimmune hemolytic anemia
1916	Elective splenectomy for immune thrombocytopenic purpura
1952	First report of overwhelming post-splenectomy sepsis
1962	First report of splenic salvage procedure for trauma
1991	Laparoscopic splenectomy

tomies in mice and other animals and determined that the spleen is not essential to life, as he noted no clear changes following removal. The first authenticated splenectomy was performed in Germany in 1826 by Carl Frederick Quitterbaum in a patient with hypersplenism secondary to cirrhosis. This high-risk patient succumbed 6 hours after the procedure. The first successful operation in which the patient survived was performed by Jules Pean in France in 1865 for a large splenic cyst. The patient underwent surgery for what was thought to be an ovarian cystic mass, but it was found to arise from the inferior portion of the spleen; splenectomy was required for removal, and the patient survived. This early period of splenic surgery was characterized by a great deal of pessimism because of the high rate operative mortality, primarily from hemorrhage. A collective series published in 1877 reported 50 splenectomies, with a 70% overall mortality. By 1900, Bessel-Hagen reported 360 splenectomies, with a 40% mortality.

The 20th century brought technical advances in hemostasis and blood transfusion in addition to an understanding of the pathophysiology of splenic function (3). The spleen was identified as the site of red cell destruction in autoimmune hemolytic anemia by Micheli in 1911. In 1916, Paul Kaznelson, a Czech medical student, postulated that removal of the spleen would be a successful treatment of a patient with immune thrombocytic purpura (ITP). Throughout the 20th century, as the understanding of hematologic and immune disorders increased, the roles of splenectomy that are pertinent in modern day practice were clarified.

EMBRYOLOGY AND ANATOMY

The spleen develops from the mesoderm as an outpouching of the mesogastrium during the fifth week of gestation. Through the natural rotation of the gut during subsequent development, the spleen arrives at its typical position in the left upper quadrant of the abdomen (Fig. 53.1). In that location, the spleen relates to the diaphragm both superiorly and laterally, and it generally spans the 9th, 10th, and 11th ribs along the left middle to posterior axillary line. The ventral surface of the spleen relates to the greater curvature of the stomach and the tail of the pancreas. The tail of the pancreas touches the splenic capsule in 30% of individuals and is 1 cm away in 73%. The inferior pole relates to the left kidney posteriorly and the splenic flexure of the colon anteriorly.

The normal size of the spleen is approximately 13 x 7 x 4 cm. The typical weight of a spleen in a young adult is thought to be 150 to 200 g, which decreases to approximately 100 g in elderly persons (Fig. 53.2). The spleen must double in size, to the range of 300 to 400 g, to project below the costal margin so that the tip of the spleen can be palpated when a patient undergoing an abdominal examination inspires deeply. The weight assigned to the spleen in a definition of massive splenomegaly has been arbitrarily set at 1,500 g, or 10 times the average adult splenic weight.

The vascular anatomy of the spleen is rather straightforward (4). The splenic artery is one of the three major trunks, along with the left gastric artery and common hepatic artery, branching from the celiac axis (Fig. 53.3). This artery appears characteristically on celiac arteriograms as a serpentine structure with loops extending both superiorly and inferiorly. Several small pancreatic branches supply blood to the body and tail of the pancreas along the lengths of this vessel. The first major splenic branch, approximately 2 to 3 cm from the hilum, is called the *superior polar artery*. The main artery then divides into between three and five segmental branches that enter along the trabeculae of the spleen. Additional blood supply to the spleen comes from the left gastroepiploic artery via the short gastric vessels. When the spleen is massively enlarged, it may directly parasitize vessels from the omentum or mesentery of the splenic flexure of

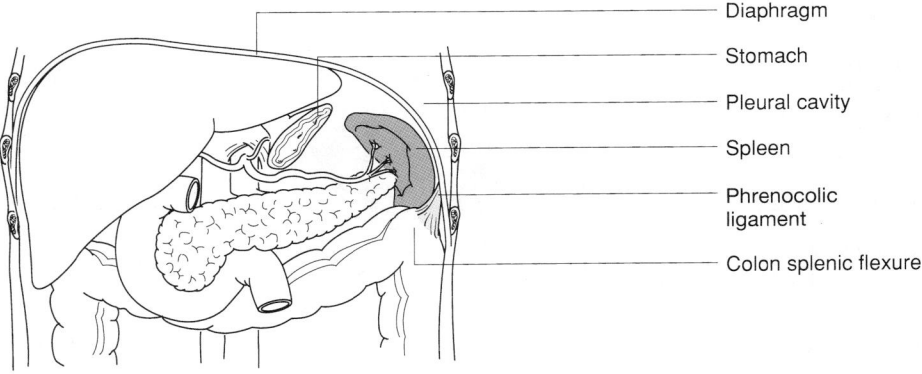

Diaphragm
Stomach
Pleural cavity
Spleen
Phrenocolic ligament
Colon splenic flexure

Visceral surface of spleen

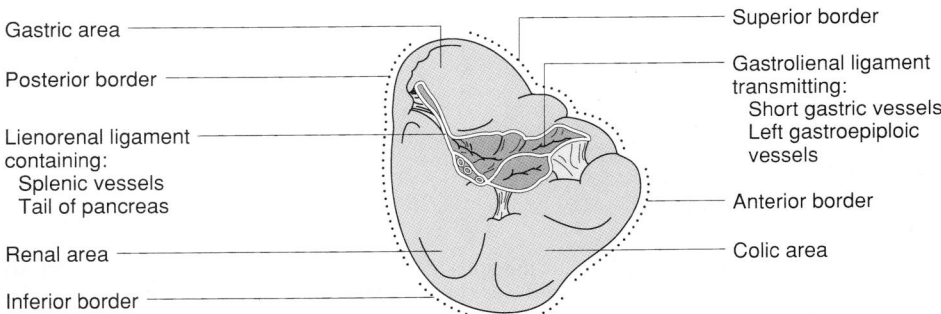

Gastric area
Posterior border
Lienorenal ligament containing:
 Splenic vessels
 Tail of pancreas
Renal area
Inferior border

Superior border
Gastrolienal ligament transmitting:
 Short gastric vessels
 Left gastroepiploic vessels
Anterior border
Colic area

Figure 53.1. Anatomic relation of the spleen to the liver, diaphragm, pancreas, colon, and kidney. The stomach is sectioned to illustrate the anatomic relations in situ.

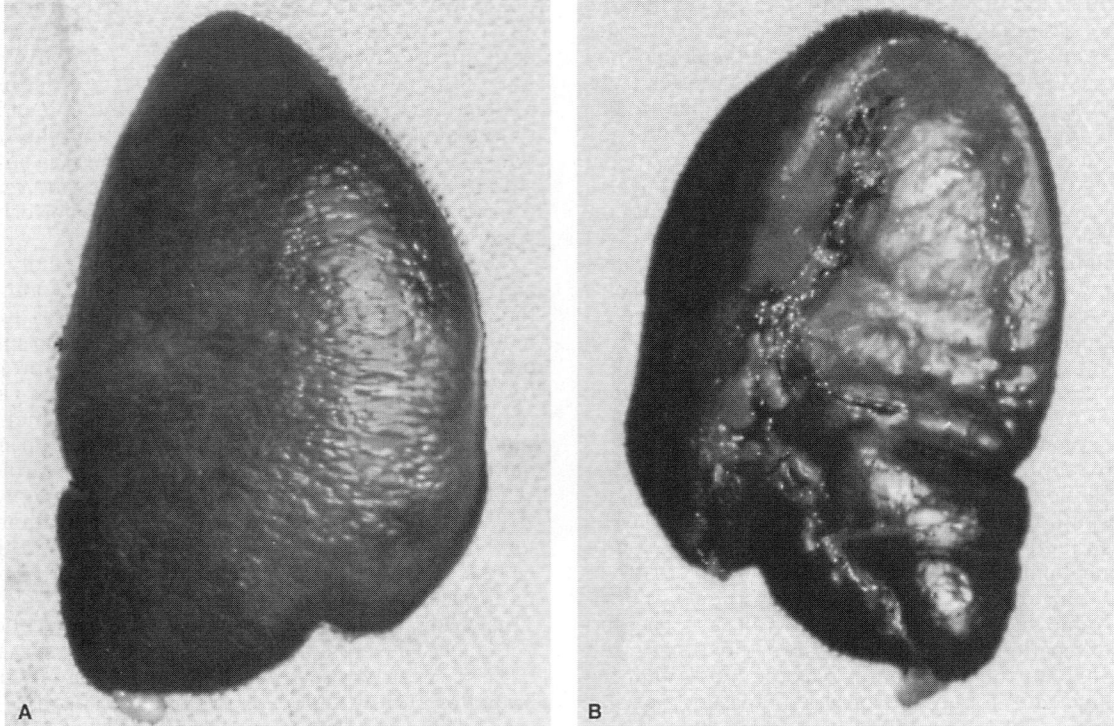

Figure 53.2. *(A)* The lateral or diaphragmatic surface of the spleen, with lobulated edge and glistening capsule. *(B)* The hilar surface of the spleen, with ligatures on the short gastric vessels cephalad and the hilar vessels caudad.

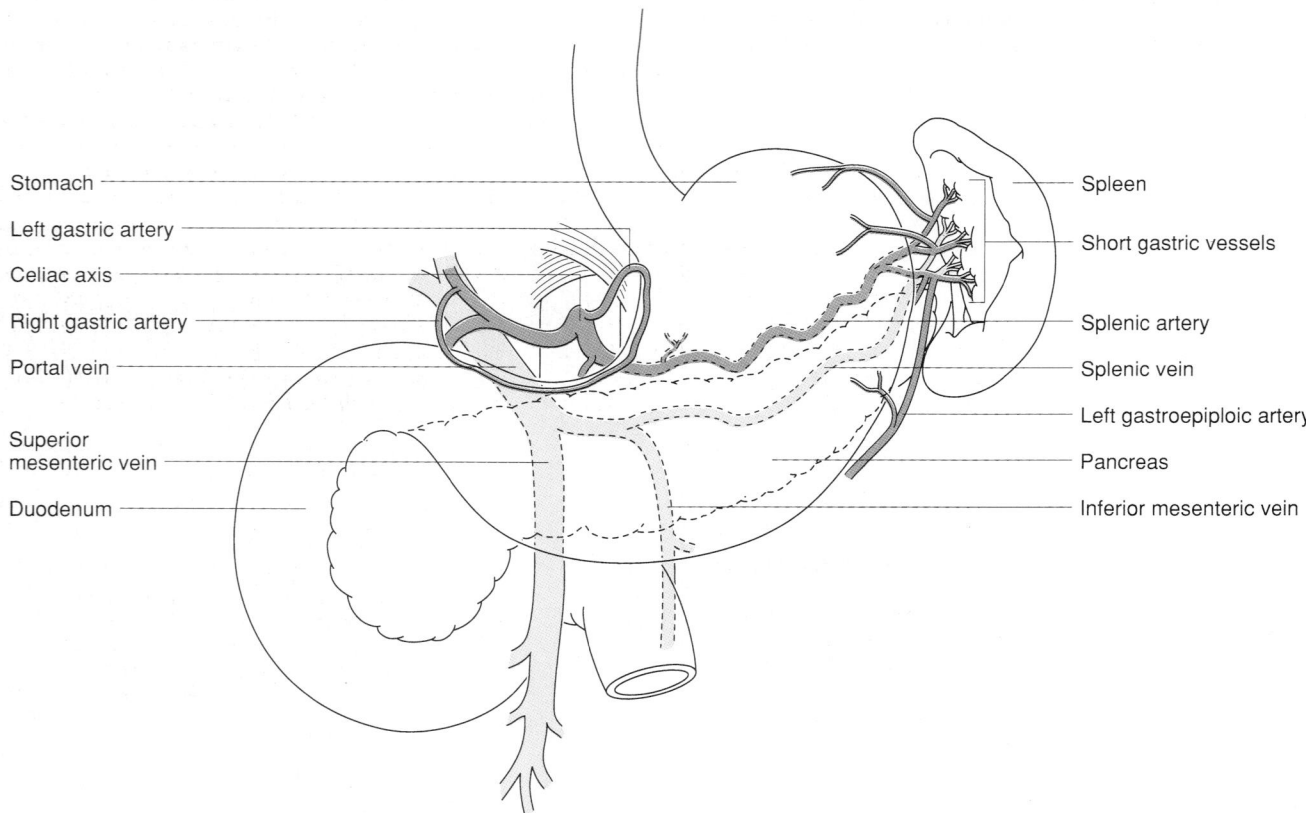

Figure 53.3. The arterial blood flow to the spleen is derived from the splenic artery, left gastroepiploic artery, and short gastric arteries (vasa brevia). The venous drainage into this portal vein is also shown.

the colon. The splenic artery generally travels outside the parenchyma of the pancreas just at its superior border, although loops that extend inferiorly may be completely covered by the posterior surface of the pancreas, and superior loops may be located well away from the pancreatic surface. These more cranial loops are optimally suited for the placement of ligatures to control bleeding from the splenic artery during procedures associated with significant thrombocytopenia or splenic enlargement. These areas generally have few pancreatic branches, and proximity to the splenic vein is avoided when it is located on the arterial loops inferiorly.

The splenic vein is formed by segmental venous branches that leave the trabeculae and coalesce in the hilum of the spleen (Fig. 53.3). The splenic vein is intimately associated with the posterior surface of the tail and body of the pancreas until its junction with the superior mesenteric vein to form the portal vein. The inferior mesenteric vein may join the splenic vein directly at several points along its course or at its junction with the superior mesenteric vein. Again, several pancreatic branches directly enter the splenic vein. The blood flow to the spleen in a typical adult is estimated to be 200 to 300 mL/min, or approximately 5% of the cardiac output (4).

The lymph node drainage generally follows the vasculature. The primary lymph nodes are located in the hilum of the spleen and also along the splenic artery at the superior border of the pancreas and along the short gastric vessels.

Several ligaments maintain the spleen in a fixed position in the left upper quadrant (4) (Fig. 53.4). Three of these ligaments are virtually always present (except in the condition of "wandering spleen") (5), and two are present to a variable extent, depending on the individual anatomy and the disease process. The first consistent ligament is the splenogastric ligament, which is a left-sided superior extension of the greater omentum along the proximal greater curvature of the stomach. Within this area, supplied by the left gastroepiploic vessels, are short gastric vessels that branch to the upper pole of the spleen and often provide the upper two thirds of the spleen with an alternative blood supply. The second and very important ligament is the splenorenal ligament, which runs parallel to the posterolateral border of the spleen and attaches this to the superior pole of Gerota's fascia on the left kidney. Division of the splenorenal ligament when the spleen is mobilized during splenectomy allows the spleen and tail of the pancreas to be reflected medially. The splenocolic ligament is short and may be avascular or have small blood vessels that extend from the inferior tip of the spleen to the splenic flexure of the colon. This ligament can be divided by cautery, or it may contain vessels that

must be controlled with ties or clips during mobilization of the splenic flexure of the colon.

Two ligaments that are variably present are the splenoomental attachments and the splenophrenic attachments (Fig. 53.4). The free part of the greater omentum may be variably associated with the splenic capsule along the inferior pole. Small vessels are often present that can be controlled by electrocautery. The splenoomental attachments may be absent or may be quite extensive over the lower pole of the spleen. These attachments to the omentum often lead to disruption of the capsule along the inferior pole, which results in bleeding; in cases of inadvertent injury, splenectomy is sometimes required for control. Before inferior traction is exerted on the omentum, during any procedure the extent of the attachments to the lower pole of the spleen should be investigated, and if present, they should be divided before more vigorous mobilization is undertaken. Ligaments may connect the spleen directly to the diaphragm; these are the splenophrenic ligaments. They typically are more numerous when the spleen is diseased or enlarged. They may be avascular or contain branches of vessels parasitized from the diaphragmatic blood supply, especially if the spleen is large.

The anatomy of the spleen itself is segmental; it is fed by arteries and drained by veins that leave via the trabeculae (6). The trabeculae are fibrous bands that attach to the splenic capsule. The parenchyma of the spleen between the trabeculae is divided into a small area of white pulp surrounding the arteries, a marginal zone, and the larger, predominant area of red pulp that comprises 75% of the splenic parenchyma. The capsule of the spleen is quite thin, comprising only a few cells layers. It consists of a single layer of mesothelium and several layers of fibroelastic tissue. In other mammals, but not in humans, variable amounts of smooth muscle may be found in the capsule. The smooth muscle allows contraction and mobilization of the circulating blood cells stored in the spleen. The trabecular arteries that enter the spleen as a continuation of the segmental arterial branches then give off perpendicular branches to form the central arteries (Fig. 53.5). Surrounding the central arteries is the periarterial lymphatic sheath, which is composed of T lymphocytes and follicles with B cells at various stages of development. During antigen stimulation, this area expands greatly with more mature and secondary follicles. The marginal zone is the borderline between the white pulp and the red pulp and contains a mixture of lymphatics and macrophages. The red pulp is made up of splenic cords with intervening areas called *splenic sinuses*. The splenic cords, also known as the *cords of Billroth*, are a meshwork of fibroblasts and a large number of mature macrophages.

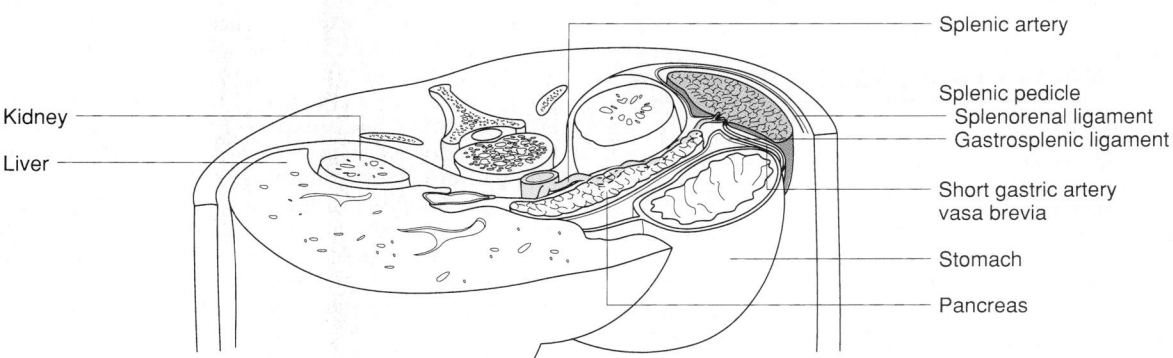

Figure 53.4. The relations of the spleen to the abdominal and retroperitoneal viscera are seen in a cross section of the left-facing torso.

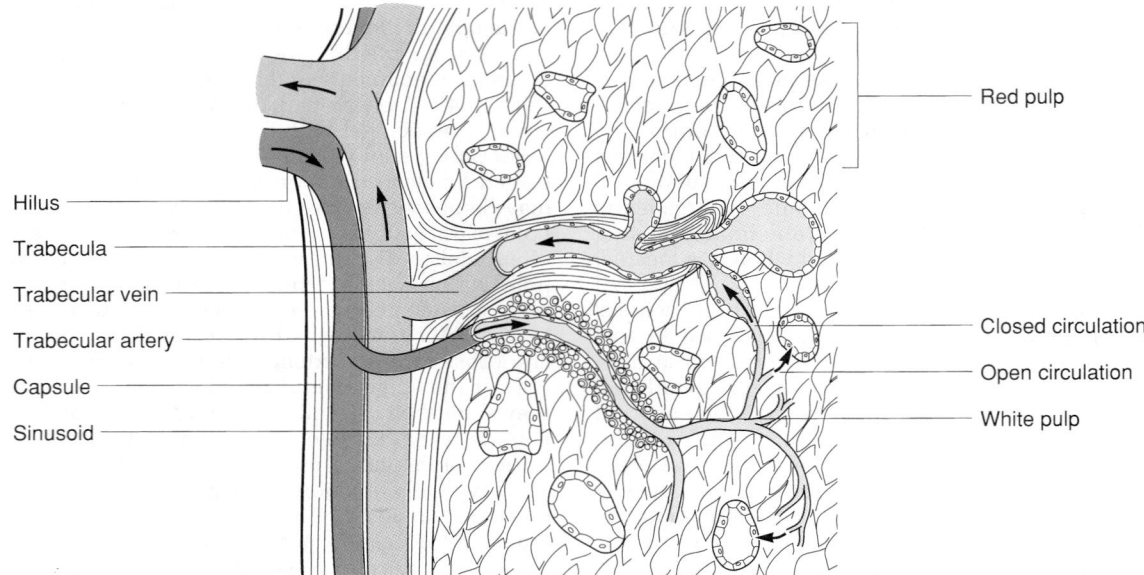

Figure 53.5. The splenic microanatomy, with depictions of both the open and closed circulations.

The splenic sinuses are an interconnective meshwork of fairly random red cell spaces that are thin-walled and generally filled with large numbers of erythrocytes.

Studies of blood flow show two alternative routes through the spleen: fast flow and slow flow. A small proportion of blood passes through the splenic arteries and returns rapidly to the splenic veins. This fast flow, in which plasma predominates and erythrocytes are fewer in number because of streaming, accounts for only 10% of the blood flow. A particularly large portion of the erythrocytes that enter the spleen travel through the highly fenestrated meshwork in the red pulp as part of the filtration process of the spleen. This slow path or slow flow comprises up to 90% of the splenic blood flow.

PHYSIOLOGY

The major functions of the spleen can be divided into two general categories: hematologic and immunologic (Table 53.2). In its hematologic functions, the spleen primarily is an organ functioning to destroy or clear circulating blood cell elements as a normal physiologic mechanism (7). This physiologic filtration function is increased in disease states that produce hypersplenism. The spleen may play a minor role in hematopoiesis and storage of blood cells, predominantly platelets. In its immunologic

---

Table 53.2. NORMAL FUNCTIONS OF THE SPLEEN

HEMATOLOGIC

Culling or destruction of senescent erythrocytes
Pitting or removal of cytoplasmic inclusions in erythrocytes
Reservoir for platelets and granulocytes
Hematopoiesis—during fetal life and in conditions associated with bone marrow destruction

IMMUNOLOGIC

Filtration and trapping of circulatory antigens
Lymphocyte stimulation and proliferation
Antibody production in germinal follicles
Production of opsonins: tuftsin and properdin

---

functions, the spleen relates to the vascular system in many of the same ways that the lymph nodes relate to the lymphatic system. The white pulp and marginal zones are most important in immunologic functioning, whereas the red pulp is primarily related to hematologic functioning. However, the macrophages that line the cords or fill the cords in the red pulp are clearly also important in immune surveillance of intravascular pathogens.

The primary hematologic function of the spleen is the removal of senescent erythrocytes or remodeling of abnormal red blood cells with various deformities. The average life span of a normal erythrocyte measured on clearance studies in humans is estimated to be approximately 120 days. It is also estimated that the spleen destroys approximately 100 billion erythrocytes daily in the red pulp (7). The process of removal or phagocytosis of erythrocytes or other blood cells is called *culling* (Table 53.2). As a consequence of the blood flow patterns of the spleen, an erythrocyte-laden fluid enters the sinuses of the red pulp. Here, slow flow through the sinusoid network with adjacent macrophage-filled cords creates an environment in which erythrocytes may become trapped and then phagocytized by the macrophages. The precise mechanism by which senescent red cells are identified for destruction in a normal physiologic environment is unclear. One hypothesis is that during the life span of an erythrocyte, either membranous elements or the total membrane material is lost, so that the red cells become less compliant and therefore are trapped in the mesh of the sinusoids. A second hypothesis is that specific cell surface marker molecules may either become more exposed or less available to allow identification of senescent cells targeted for destruction. The pathologic destruction of red cells occurs in diseases such as hereditary spherocytosis or elliptocytosis, in which a genetic defect causes abnormal red cell pliability, so that the passage of red cells through the red pulp is limited. Similarly, in sickle cell anemia, an alteration in red cell shape caused by genetically defective hemoglobin leads to destruction and clogging of the sinusoids. A second pathologic mechanism of an enlarged spleen, such as occurs in certain disease processes, increases the destruction of red cells; the removal of red cells is increased not because of red blood cell or hemoglobin abnormalities but because of an increase in red pulp volume. This condition is known as *hypersplenism*.

The second physiologic process involving circulating erythrocytes is remodeling or pitting, which is partial removal of the cell membrane typically associated with cytoplasmic inclusions. Erythrocytes containing a remnant of the cell nucleus pass more slowly through the splenic red pulp because of their large size (7). The nuclear remnant may be trapped while passing through a small space in the spleen; deformation of this solid particle is not possible, and the particle becomes pinched off in the process of pitting. Intracytoplasmic inclusions include Howell-Jolly bodies, which are nuclear remnants; Heinz bodies, which are denatured hemoglobin; and Pappenheimer bodies, which are iron granules.

The destruction of the other circulating cellular elements (platelets and leukocytes) is more within the realm of pathophysiology of the spleen than of normal physiologic function. The disease processes in which these cells are removed are related either to autoantibodies to cell surface elements or to hypersplenism. If either platelets or white blood cells become coated with antibodies, interaction of the Fc portion of the immunoglobulin with Fc receptors on macrophages in the splenic cords leads to phagocytosis of these cell types. In hypersplenism of various causes, a similar process of destruction may also occur, even without autoantibodies or defects in the cells, just because of an increase in splenic mass.

The spleen serves as a potential source for hematopoiesis of all cell types during gestation. In normal humans, very little if any production of red cells, granulocytes, or platelets is thought to occur, which is not true in other mammals. In the white pulp of the spleen there are germinal centers, in which amplification and production of reactive lymphocytes take place. The cords of the spleen are filled with macrophages, and throughout normal adult life, lymphocytes and macrophages may be produced in the spleen. In certain disease states, the spleen may acquire a capacity for erythropoiesis and myelopoiesis. The best example is agnogenic myeloid metaplasia. In this disease, the bone marrow is replaced with fibrotic scar, and a portion of the hematopoietic function of the marrow is taken over by the spleen, which is typically quite enlarged.

The final hematologic function of the spleen may be to serve as a reservoir of circulating cellular elements. In humans, the only significant cell type stored in the spleen is the platelet, and it is estimated that 30% of all platelets may reside in the spleen. This function may be more important in humans than in other mammals, particularly those with significant smooth muscle lining the capsule of the spleen, which allows contracture and expulsion of large numbers of stored cells as a physiologic response to injury.

The immunologic function of the spleen is primarily to generate an immune response to antigens that are identified and cleared from the blood system (Table 53.2). Opsonized antigens and particularly encapsulated microorganisms are important examples of target antigens trapped by the spleen. The spleen is an ideal environment for the generation of either a cellular or a humoral immune response. All the necessary cell types to stimulate an immune response are present, including phagocytic cells, dendritic cells, T cells, and B cells, which may form general follicles to generate specific antibody responses. These interactions primarily occur in the marginal zone in the white pulp, which can become quite enlarged and hypertrophied during antigen stimulation. These cellular components and the structure of the germinal follicles are essentially identical to those found in lymph node tissue, which also becomes enlarged during antigenic stimulation.

The spleen is also involved in nonspecific immune responses. It is the site of synthesis of properdin and tuftsin, both of which are opsonins. Tuftsin is a small peptide that binds to the surface of granulocytes and promotes phagocytic function by these cells. Properdin can initiate the alternate pathway of complement activation, which may be important in the destruction of abnormal cells or bacteria bound to antibodies. The spleen is not the only source of these nonspecific immune-enhancing proteins, and therefore splenectomy may lead to only a modest alteration in this function.

PATHOPHYSIOLOGY

Various characteristic responses with many common features fall under the broad categories of hyposplenism and hypersplenism. These features are related to the normal physiologic functions of the spleen and influence clinical decision making regarding the management of patients after splenectomy or the appropriateness of splenectomy. By far the most common cause of hyposplenism is surgical removal. Other explanations would be the unusual situation of a congenitally small or absent spleen or an acquired condition in which splenic tissue is destroyed, such as sickle cell anemia. Hypersplenism is the most frequent indication for elective splenectomy. Various causes of hypersplenism are typically neoplastic, but they may also be related to primary blood cell dysfunction or abnormalities or other conditions, such as portal hypertension secondary to cirrhosis or splenic vein thrombosis.

Hyposplenism or the changes seen after a splenectomy can be predicted according to the known functions of the spleen. Hematologic changes in the circulating cells can be predicted from the splenic functions of culling, pitting, and storing platelets (Table 53.3). Immunologic changes, which are important primarily in infants and young children, lead to the problem of overwhelming postsplenectomy sepsis.

The changes in circulating blood cells after splenectomy or in hyposplenism affect erythrocytes, leukocytes, and platelets. With time, the intracytoplasmic inclusions in red cells normally cleared by the spleen accumulate, resulting in the presence of Howell-Jolly bodies, Heinz bodies, and Pappenheimer bodies in addition to target cells with excess red blood cell membrane and occasionally increased numbers of circulating nucleated red blood cells or reticulocytes. Because the spleen is the organ of storage for a large proportion of the platelets, splenectomy often results in thrombocytosis, with platelet counts ranging between 500,000 and up to 1 million per cubic millimeter in

---

Table 53.3. HEMATOLOGIC EFFECTS OF SPLENECTOMY/HYPOSPLENIC CONDITION

ERYTHROCYTES

Howell-Jolly bodies (nuclear fragments)
Heinz bodies (hemoglobin deposits)
Pappenheimer bodies (iron deposits)
Target cells
Spur cells (acanthocytes)

PLATELETS

Transient thrombocytosis

LEUKOCYTES

Transient leukocytosis
Persistent lymphocytosis
Persistent monocytosis

some cases. This increased platelet count tends to be transient and may reflect the fact that the spleen, although a storage organ for platelets, may not be a primary area of platelet destruction after the typical half-life of 10 days. The immediate response in white cells after splenectomy is leukocytosis, again reflecting the storage of a large proportion of white cells in the spleen (8). Like the thrombocytosis, this effect is transient, but long-term increases in the proportion of circulating lymphocytes and monocytes may develop after splenectomy.

The changes in immune function seen in hyposplenism or after splenectomy result primarily in the phenomenon of overwhelming postsplenectomy sepsis. This was initially recognized as an important epidemiologic phenomenon in the early 1950s, and multiple studies of patients who have undergone splenectomy have defined key features of this increased susceptibility to infection. It is clear that the risk for postsplenectomy sepsis is inversely related to age. The younger the child, the greater the impact and the greater the risk for the development of overwhelming postsplenectomy sepsis (9). This feature has clinical implications, as elective splenectomy is not performed for patients with hereditary erythrocyte syndromes until after the age of 6 to 10. In adults, the risk for sepsis is still increased anywhere from 40% to 60% in comparison with persons with normal splenic function. Postsplenectomy septic episodes typically occur within the first 2 years after splenectomy in 80% of cases. In adults, the underlying reason for the splenectomy also relates to the incidence of sepsis. In cases of trauma, the instance of sepsis in a large series was 1.4%, whereas in cases of thalassemia, the incidence was 24.8%. Patients who are immunodeficient for any reason, such as malignancy or chemotherapy to treat Hodgkin's disease, are also at increased risk for sepsis. The mortality associated with postsplenectomy sepsis is between 50% and 60% in most series.

The organisms that account for infection are typically encapsulated. These may have special bacterial features that allow them to be opsonized and cleared from the circulation by the spleen, which makes them more dangerous in hyposplenic or splenectomized patients. The most common organism causing postsplenectomy sepsis is *Streptococcus pneumoniae*, which accounts for 50% of septic episodes in most series. In decreasing order of frequency, other bacteria associated with postsplenectomy sepsis are *Haemophilus influenzae*, *Neisseria meningitidis*, β-hemolytic streptococci, *Staphylococcus aureus*, *Escherichia coli*, and *Pseudomonas* species. The current recommendations for patients who are undergoing elective splenectomy include vaccination of persons susceptible to *Pneumococcus* strains (10,11) (Table 53.4). This is ideally performed 2 weeks before the operation if possible, but it should be done at any time preoperatively or even postoperatively if the patient has not been vaccinated. Choices of polyvalent vaccines include Pneumovax 23 and Pnu-Imune 23, both of which provide protection against virtually all common strains of *Pneumococcus*. For patients who are at particularly high risk because of immunosuppression, polyvalent

vaccines are also available against *Neisseria meningitidis* and *Haemophilus influenzae* type B. Patients under the age of 2 years and patients receiving chemotherapy for malignant disease may not be able to generate an immune response to vaccines, and they should be vaccinated after the age of 2 years or after chemotherapy has been discontinued, respectively. Finally, because of the risk for very rapid progression of sepsis in a postsplenectomy state, patients who have had splenectomy for any reason should wear a Medi-Alert bracelet.

HYPERSPLENISM

Hypersplenism is defined as an increase in splenic function that is manifested clinically by a decrease in one or more of the circulating blood elements. Specific criteria for hypersplenism are the following: (a) documented anemia, thrombocytopenia, or leukopenia; (b) a normal compensatory response by the bone marrow to correct the cytopenia; and (c) correction of the cytopenia by splenectomy. Some definitions of hypersplenism also include splenomegaly. If one considers an enlarged spleen to be a criterion for hypersplenism, then in some diseases or disorders related to abnormalities of the circulating blood cells, such as ITP or autoimmune hemolytic anemia, the criteria for hypersplenism are not fulfilled. In another approach to defining hypersplenism, disorders in which the spleen is normal anatomically and disease is related to abnormalities of the circulating cells are grouped together, and disorders in which the circulating cells are normal and the spleen is primarily altered, either anatomically or functionally, constitute another category (Table 53.5).

Table 53.4. GUIDELINES FOR PREVENTION OF POST-SPLENIC SEPSIS

- Vaccinate with polyvalent pneumococcal vaccine at least 10 to 14 days before splenectomy, if possible.
- For high-risk patients (immunosuppressed, children <10 years of age), meningococcal vaccine and Haemophilus influenzae vaccine.
- Antibiotic prophylaxis for children <5 years of age.
- Early antibiotic treatment for initial signs of infection.
- Medi-Alert bracelet.

Table 53.5. CAUSES OF HYPERSPLENISM

I. Primary diseases of blood cells; normal spleen
  A. Congenital
    i. Erythrocyte abnormalities
      a. Hereditary spherocytosis
      b. Hereditary elliptocytosis
      c. Glucose-6-phosphate dehydrogenase deficiency
      d. Pyruvate kinase deficiency
    ii. Hemoglobin abnormalities
      a. Thalessemia major
      b. Sickle cell anemia (eventually results in splenic infarction and hyposplenism)
    iii. Platelet abnormalities
      a. Wiskott-Aldrich syndrome
  B. Acquired
    i. Autoimmune hemolytic anemia
    ii. Autoimmune neutropenia—Felty's syndrome
    iii. Immune thrombocytopenic purpura
    iv. Thrombotic thrombocytopenic purpura
II. Primary disorders of the spleen
  A. Neoplastic
    i. Hairy cell leukemia
    ii. Chronic lymphocytic leukemia
    iii. Chronic myelogenous leukemia
    iv. Non-Hodgkin's lymphoma
  B. Cellular infiltration (hematopoiesis)
    i. Agnogenic myeloid metaplasia
    ii. Mastocytosis
    iii. Chédiak-Higashi syndrome
  C. Metabolic infiltration
    i. Gaucher's disease
    ii. Sarcoidosis
  D. Vascular
    i. Splenic vein thrombosis
    ii. Portal vein hypertension (cirrhosis)

Disorders associated with hypersplenism that are related to abnormalities of the circulating cells affect erythrocytes, platelets, and neutrophils (12). Diseases of the red blood cells may be either congenital or acquired, such as autoimmune hemolytic anemia. Similarly, the disorders of platelets and neutrophils are acquired autoimmune diseases. Hypersplenism associated with abnormalities of the spleen can be broadly divided into neoplastic disorders, in which the spleen is infiltrated and enlarged, typically by leukemic or lymphoma cells; hematopoietic disorders, in which the spleen is enlarged as a secondary site of hematopoiesis other than the bone marrow; metabolic or storage disorders, in which the spleen is enlarged when a metabolic deficiency results in the deposition of lipid (e.g., Gaucher's disease); and disorders of vascular enlargement, in which splenic vein pressures are increased by portal hypertension or splenic vein thrombosis. The pathophysiology of each of these diseases is discussed in the following sections, in addition to the indications for and benefits of splenectomy. Another problem associated with some of the conditions of hypersplenism is massive splenomegaly. The symptoms of some patients with splenomegaly may be caused primarily by the mass effect of the spleen. Early satiety and weight loss are the most important manifestations, but patients may experience generalized pain and bloating.

Disorders of Circulating Cells Associated with Hypersplenism

Hereditary Spherocytosis

Hereditary spherocytosis, also known as *congenital hemolytic jaundice* or *familial hemolytic anemia,* is an autosomal dominant disease. It is the most common of the congenital hemolytic anemias, affecting one in 5,000 persons. A variety of genetic defects in this syndrome primarily affect spectrin and ankyrin, which alter the binding of the cytoskeleton to the erythrocyte cellular membrane and cause a decrease in cellular plasticity with membrane loss. The shape of the erythrocyte is changed from a biconcave disk into a sphere, and the decreased membrane-to-volume ratio causes a lack of deformability that affects the passage of erythrocytes through channels of the splenic red pulp. Because of the delay in cell transit, adenosine triphosphate deprivation develops and results in increased cellular destruction. The condition is more frequent in whites than in African-Americans and is usually noted in childhood or adolescence. Because the disorder is inherited in an autosomal dominant pattern, patients can be screened and the diagnosis made at quite an early age.

The diagnosis is primarily made by evaluation of the red cell smear, which shows a large number of spherocytes. Spherocytes may also appear in autoimmune hemolytic anemias, but in hereditary spherocytosis, the Coombs' test result is negative and an osmotic fragility test may be performed, which is diagnostic. Also contributing to the diagnosis is a positive family history.

Patients with hereditary spherocytosis have mild to moderate anemia, splenomegaly, and jaundice. Intermittent flares of disease cause significantly increased rates of hemolysis, resulting in jaundice. Between 30% and 60% of patients have been reported to have pigmented gallstones secondary to the breakdown of hemoglobin.

The treatment for hereditary spherocytosis is splenectomy, which is indicated in virtually all patients. This treatment does not remove the spherocytes, but it relieves all symptoms. The major question involving management of these patients is the timing of splenectomy. Because of the increased incidence of overwhelming postsplenec-

tomy sepsis in very young children, it is usually recommended that patients wait until the age of at least 4 if not 6 years before undergoing splenectomy. For younger patients who are very symptomatic and require splenectomy, partial splenectomy has been reported to be beneficial in relieving the abdominal symptoms and the anemia and may be a useful alternative procedure until patients reach an age at which total splenectomy is safer (13,14). Patients should be assessed for gallstones at the time splenectomy is scheduled, and a laparoscopic cholecystectomy should be performed if stones are identified.

Hereditary Elliptocytosis

Hereditary elliptocytosis is related to hereditary spherocytosis, but the disease is not as severe. For patients with hereditary elliptocytosis who are symptomatic, virtually all the comments regarding the pathophysiology and treatment of hereditary spherocytosis can be applied. This disease is also inherited in an autosomal dominant pattern, and the defect is felt to affect spectrin. The predominant abnormality changes spectrin such that it exists as a dimer instead of tetramer, which is the normal structure. This change leads to an alteration in membrane plasticity, and as a result cells have the shape of an ellipse rather than a biconcave disk.

The signs and symptoms in this disease are much milder than in hereditary spherocytosis; only 10% of patients have clinical manifestations of anemia, splenomegaly, and in some cases jaundice. The treatment recommendation for symptomatic patients is again splenectomy, which may be performed with laparoscopic techniques. Cholecystectomy should also be performed if gallstones are present.

Hereditary Nonspherocytic Hemolytic Anemia

A heterogeneous group of rare hemolytic anemias are caused by inherited defects, primarily of enzymes involved in glycolysis. It is felt that these genetic defects may decrease cellular energy production, such that during passage through the red pulp of the spleen, cells do not have the ability to produce adenosine triphosphate in a relatively hypoxic environment, so that red cell destruction is increased. The most common subtypes in this group of hemolytic anemias are pyruvate kinase deficiency and glucose-6-phosphate dehydrogenase deficiency. Patients present with anemia, jaundice, increased reticulocytes, and possibly cholelithiasis. The differential diagnosis is based on the fact that the cells are not typically spherocytes and osmotic fragility is normal.

The primary treatment for these diseases is blood transfusion. In glucose-6-phosphate dehydrogenase deficiency, splenectomy is not thought to be beneficial, whereas it may reverse some of the symptoms associated with pyruvate kinase deficiency.

Thalassemia

Thalassemia is an autosomal dominant disease associated with a variety of structural defects in one of the globin chains. The disease is categorized as α-, β-, γ-, or δ-thalassemia, depending on which of the globin chains is defective. The vast majority of patients in North America have β-thalassemia. Thalassemia major, otherwise known as *Mediterranean anemia* or *Cooley's anemia,* is a homozygous expression of this genetic defect. Thalassemia minor is a heterozygous expression; these patients are only mildly symptomatic and are carriers for the more severe form of the disease.

The pathophysiologic basis of thalassemia major, or β-thalassemia, is the lack of normal production of beta-chain hemoglobin, which leads to a surplus of alpha-chain hemoglobin in adult patients. The excess globin chains precipitate in the cytoplasm and attach to the inner surfaces of cytoplasmic membranes, causing the cells to pass poorly through the splenic sinusoids. The intracellular inclusions then lead to increased destruction, and over time significant splenomegaly results from an increased clearance of red cells.

The diagnosis is made by identifying microcytic hypochromic anemia, with target cells and increased numbers of reticulocytes on the peripheral smear. Protein electrophoresis shows very low levels of hemoglobin A, with predominant amounts of the fetal hemoglobin, or hemoglobin F. α-Thalassemia is manifested as severe anemia within the first year of life. A decreased growth rate, enlargement of the head, splenomegaly, and hepatomegaly are the typical clinical findings.

The primary treatment for thalassemia major is frequent transfusions combined with iron chelation therapy. In some patients, significant splenomegaly may develop because of overload or hypertrophy resulting from from excess trapping of red cells. Patients may be referred for splenectomy if they have symptomatic splenomegaly or require massive and frequent transfusions. One report suggested that the annual number of episodes of transfusion is decreased from 18 to 4 after splenectomy. In general, if symptoms of massive splenomegaly are present, these will also resolve after splenectomy. As with other hematologic disorders in children, the recent trend has been toward partial splenectomy, particularly in children less than 4 or 5 years of age (15). This results in symptomatic improvement in between 1 and 2 years, with a recurrence of disease caused by hypertrophy of the residual splenic remnant (16).

Although splenectomy may be beneficial in terms of transfusion requirements and local symptoms, the typical cause of death in this disease is myocardial failure resulting from hemosiderin accumulation. Splenectomy does not alter this cardiac problem to any great extent.

Sickle Cell Anemia

Sickle cell anemia is a hereditary hemolytic anemia in which a genetic alteration leads to a single amino acid substitution in the beta chain of the hemoglobin molecule; valine replaces glutamic acid in the sixth amino acid position of the beta chain. Because of this substitution, the red blood cells of persons who are homozygous for sickle cell defect display a characteristic sickling and stiffening when they become hypoxic. The change in shape results in blockage in hypoxic areas, such as the red pulp of the spleen. Occasionally, sequestration crises occur, in which a portion of the blood volume becomes actively trapped or sequestered in the spleen. This pattern of change in red cell shape in relatively hypoxic areas can cause tissue infarction that is associated with bone and abdominal pain, hematuria, and priapism.

The incidence of homozygous disease, which occurs almost exclusively in blacks, is approximately 0.5%, but approximately 8% of African Americans are carriers of the sickle cell trait. Patients who have the combination of a sickle cell allele and a β-thalassemia allele manifest a similar disease process.

The clinical signs of the disease usually appear during the second 6 months of life; in early infancy, the patient is asymptomatic because of the presence of fetal hemoglobin. Patients may have acute crises with abdominal pain and bone pain in conjunction with significant anemia. During acute crises of splenic sequestration, the spleen may become massively enlarged, and an urgent decompressive splenectomy is required. Patients who do not require splenectomy to relieve splenic sequestration can be followed because progressive ischemic necrosis of large

areas of the spleen is part of the disease process, so that a shrunken organ and hyposplenism develop by early adolescence. Splenectomy is reserved for very young patients who have massive splenomegaly and sequestration crises early in life.

Wiskott-Aldrich Syndrome

Wiskott-Aldrich Syndrome is an X-linked disease characterized by thrombocytopenia, combined B- and T-cell deficiency, eczema, and a propensity for the development of other malignancies. The genetic defect in this disease is thought to be related to an abnormal adhesion molecule affecting immune cell interaction and platelet adhesion. Thrombocytopenia is the major problem in this rare disease, and most patients present with manifestations of poor clotting, bloody diarrhea, epistaxis, and petechiae at a young age. Platelet counts typically range between 20,000 and 40,000/mm^3, and the platelets are dysfunctional and small, comprising 25% to 50% of normal platelet volume. In this disease, the spleen sequesters platelets and partially degrades them, releasing "microplatelets" back into the circulation.

Splenectomy in the Wiskott-Aldrich syndrome was initially avoided because it was associated with a very difficult postoperative course characterized by severe and fatal infections resulting from the underlying immunodeficiency combined with the potential for overwhelming postsplenectomy infection. However, splenectomy does increase the number, size, and functioning of platelets and can lead to a decrease in bleeding in very symptomatic patients (17). The combination of splenectomy with antibiotic suppression, particularly in younger patients, may be beneficial. The optimal treatment for Wiskott-Aldrich syndrome is HLA-matched sibling bone marrow transplantation (18). However, splenectomy with antibiotics results in better survival than unmatched bone marrow transplantation. Patients who do not undergo bone marrow transplantation or splenectomy typically do not survive past the age of 5 years.

Autoimmune Hemolytic Anemia

Autoimmune hemolytic anemia or acquired hemolytic anemia develops when antibodies to red cell membrane proteins are produced and destroy red cells. The disease is more common in women than in men, with a female-to-male ratio of 2:1, and it typically presents after age 50. Patients have with acute symptoms of anemia, jaundice, and occasional fever. The spleen is enlarged in approximately half of patients. A positive direct Coombs' test result indicates antibody coating of the erythrocytes. Significant reticulocytosis and an increased indirect bilirubin in the serum are also present.

The disease is either idiopathic (in 40% to 50% of cases, in which no identified drug or infectious cause is identified) or secondary to infection or drug use. In the secondary cases, the most common infections are *Mycoplasma* pneumonia, viral infections, infectious mononucleosis, and AIDS. The condition can also develop in association with neoplastic diseases such as leukemia and lymphoma. The major drugs that cause secondary autoimmune hemolytic anemia are penicillin, quinidine, hydralazine, and methyldopa.

A second way in which autoimmune hemolytic anemia can be categorized is according to the presence of either cold or warm antibodies. Warm antibodies are predominantly immunoglobulin G (IgG), whereas cold antibodies are predominantly IgM. This distinction is quite important when splenectomy is being considered as a treatment. The spleen contains macrophages that bind the Fc portion of IgG. For this reason, in patients with warm antibody hemolytic anemia, the red pulp macrophages in the spleen are the primary source of destruction of red cells. However, because the spleen does not contain receptors to bind IgM, or cold antibodies, the red cells are not destroyed in the spleen in this form of hemolytic anemia. Rather, either IgM causes complement fixation, with destruction of red cells predominantly in the liver, or agglutination of red cells takes place in the peripheral circulation, as in the distal extremities, and peripheral red cell destruction leads to clinical manifestations similar to those of Raynaud's phenomenon. Splenectomy is not effective in patients with cold antibody hemolytic anemia.

The treatment of autoimmune hemolytic anemia initially consists of supportive therapy, such as blood transfusions. In patients who have disease secondary to an acute infection, such as *Mycoplasma* pneumonia, the disease may be self-limited. In cases of drug-induced hemolytic anemia, the offending agent is removed as quickly as possible. The initial form of treatment is typically high-dose corticosteroids, which induce a beneficial response in 75% of patients. If drug-induced disease recurs and the offending agent is removed, or if the acute infection resolves, long-term resolution may be achieved. Remission is sustained in only 25% of patients with idiopathic autoimmune hemolytic anemia after the administration of steroids. For patients with warm antibodies who relapse after steroid therapy or who are ineligible for steroid therapy, a splenectomy is very likely to be of benefit. In 80% of patients, the anemia is corrected by splenectomy. This response is felt to be almost certainly related to removal of the site of destruction of the erythrocytes, but it also may be a consequence of a decreased production of antibodies.

Autoimmune Neutropenia (Felty's Syndrome)

Splenomegaly and neutropenia develop in approximately 1% of patients with chronic rheumatoid arthritis. This triad of rheumatoid arthritis, neutropenia, and splenomegaly is known as *Felty's syndrome*. High levels of IgG have been identified on the surface of neutrophils, and evidence has been found of increased production of granulocytes in the bone marrow. Pathologic analysis of spleens removed from patients with Felty's syndrome shows a significant but proportional increase in the white pulp in comparison with spleens enlarged in other conditions (19). Examination under the microscope reveals an excess accumulation of neutrophils in both the T-cell zone and the white pulp, and also in the cords and sinuses of the red pulp.

This disease is characterized by recurrent infections secondary to neutropenia and dysfunction of the available neutrophils, which are coated with antineutrophil IgG. Recurrent infections and chronic leg ulcers are the predominant symptoms. Symptomatic patients should undergo splenectomy, and the neutropenia resolves in the vast majority of patients within 2 to 3 days. Even patients who do not have a significant increase in their neutrophil count derive some benefit because of improved neutrophil function (32).

Immune Thrombocytopenic Purpura

Immune thrombocytopenic purpura is characterized by the autoimmune destruction of platelets. The clinical manifestation of thrombocytopenia is bleeding (20). ITP occurs in an acute form and a chronic form. Acute ITP generally affects children under the age of 8 after a viral upper respiratory illness. The disease is usually self-limited and requires surgical intervention only in the case of intracranial bleeding. Chronic ITP accounts for the vast majority of cases considered for splenectomy. Like autoimmune hemolytic anemia, this disease may be either idiopathic or secondary to a lymphoproliferative disorder, a connective tissue disorder such as systemic lupus erythematosus, or exposure to drugs or bacteria. The diagnosis is usually made in persons in the fourth decade of life, and the disease affects women more commonly than men. As HIV became identified in the mid-1980s, it was noted that a disease virtually identical to ITP was developing in patients with AIDS (21). Clinical manifestations of the disease reflect low levels of platelets. In women, this may be manifested by an insidious onset of increased menstrual bleeding. As platelet counts continue to fall, the appearance of petechiae and spontaneous bleeding or the inability to form clot after a minor injury generally makes the diagnosis apparent.

The pathophysiology of ITP is the development of an IgG antibody to a platelet antigen. This is felt to be most commonly directed against the fibrinogen receptor (glycoprotein IIb/IIIa) (22). The spleen plays a predominant role in this disease; it may be the site of initial antibody production, it is almost certainly the site of continued antibody production, and in the majority of patients it is the primary site of platelet destruction. Because the targeted antigen (platelet) is an intravascular cell, and because the spleen stores large numbers of platelets, it is thought that the initial reaction to the platelet cell antigen may occur in the spleen. Studies of antibody levels have indicated that overall IgG production in spleens from patients with ITP is markedly increased over that in normal spleens. Similarly, after splenectomy, the amount of IgG antibody is somewhat decreased. The IgG antibody is not eliminated because helper T cells and plasma cells may be located in other areas, particularly the bone marrow, after prolonged immune stimulation.

The spleen is also the predominant site of platelet destruction. As noted above, the macrophages located in the cords of Billroth have receptors for the Fc portion of IgG and will bind and phagocytose the antibody-coated platelets.

For a patient to be considered to have ITP, the platelet count must be at least below 100,000/mm³, but typically patients do not become symptomatic unless platelet counts are below 50,000/mm³. Platelet counts in this disorder may drop to very low levels, well below 10,000/mm³ on occasion. Assays are now available to identify the IgG antiglobulin on the platelet surface and thereby verify the disease. Bone marrow analysis shows an increase in megakaryocyte production as a compensatory mechanism to the thrombocytopenia. In this disorder, splenomegaly is often absent, and the spleen may be somewhat smaller than is typical. Only 2% of patients with ITP have palpable spleens. For this reason, virtually no leukopenia or anemia is associated with ITP as a consequence of hypersplenism. Anemia may be present secondary to chronic blood loss.

The treatment of ITP includes standard measures to treat any ongoing bleeding, medical therapies designed to increase the platelet count, and splenectomy. Options for initial medical therapy include platelet transfusion, corticosteroids, gamma immunoglobulin, and the recently approved Rho(d) immunoglobulin (23). Platelet transfusions should be discouraged unless patients are actively bleeding because platelets rapidly become coated with IgG and are sequestered and destroyed in the spleen. High-dose corticosteroids produce an initial response in the majority of patients, but this is unfortunately not sustained. Approximately 75% of patients have an increase in their platelet count that is significant within 24 hours of the commencement of high-dose steroids (24). However, the remission is sustained in only 15% to 25% of patients with chronic ITP after steroid therapy.

A second-line treatment for chronic ITP has been the intravenous administration of IgG. This treatment takes only 3 to 5 days to produce an effect and generally does not put patients into complete remission. IgG may be a useful treatment to boost platelet counts before elective splenectomy to decrease the chance of intraoperative bleeding. The mechanism of action of gamma immunoglobulin is felt to be saturation of the Fc receptors on the splenic macrophages. The administered gamma globulin may coat red cells, and they may then provide a competitive interference such that platelet destruction is decreased. The newest available drug is the recently approved Rho(d) immunoglobulin, which specifically targets the Fc receptors. Initial experience indicates significant benefit in ITP, but the long-term role of this agent remains undetermined.

In the majority of patients, a sustained remission is not achieved with medical therapy, and an elective splenectomy is recommended for them. The reported complete remission rate after splenectomy ranges between 60% and 88% (25). In general, the platelet count returns to normal levels in approximately 75% of patients, and an additional 20% experience some improvement in their platelet counts to a safer level. Only 5% may have very significant persistent thrombocytopenia requiring additional therapy. The response to splenectomy is better in patients who are younger, with a shorter duration of disease and possibly an initial response to corticosteroids.

A recent study evaluated the role of indium-labeled platelets as a predictor for response to splenectomy in ITP (26). In this study, if the tagged platelets predominantly tracked to the spleen, a 96% complete remission was observed in patients under the age of 30, and a 91% complete remission in patients over the age of 30. If the tagged platelets tracked to the liver or elsewhere, the success rate was only an 8%. This test, the results of which are remarkably predictive, contrasts with earlier studies in which chromium-labeled platelets were used in a similar manner. The results of the earlier tests did not correlate with outcome.

One cause for a failed splenectomy for ITP would be residual splenic tissue, most commonly in the form of a missed accessory spleen but also in the form of splenosis. Both these problems are felt to have increased somewhat in the current era of laparoscopic splenectomy. Again, spleens in ITP are generally small and so are ideally suited for a laparoscopic approach. The incidence of accessory spleens identified in open procedures is in the range of 15% to 30%, whereas the incidence of accessory spleens reported in the laparoscopic approach is between zero and 15% (27). In a recent study, two of three patients in whom surgical splenectomy failed had accessory spleens that were missed at the time of the laparoscopic splenectomy. Reports have indicated that the use of indium-labeled platelets, particularly in conjunction with single-photon emission computed tomography (SPECT), precisely identified the location of accessory spleens and allowed subsequently successful removal. The second operation to remove the accessory spleen can generally also be accomplished with a laparoscopic approach.

Thrombotic Thrombocytopenic Purpura

Thrombotic thrombocytopenic purpura, or Moschcowitz's syndrome, is a poorly understood, much more virulent syndrome than ITP, of which thrombocytopenic purpura is only one manifestation. In this disease, arteries and capillaries throughout the body become occluded by hyaline membranes composed of a combination of platelets and fibrinogen. The classic pentad of symptoms reflects injury to various organs in this microvascular process. These include (a) thrombocytopenic purpura resulting from microvascular disease in the skin, (b) neurologic manifestations resulting from microvascular disease in the central nervous system, (c) renal failure or hematuria secondary to microvascular disease in the kidney, (d) microvascular hemolytic anemia secondary to the destruction of red cells traveling to damaged small vessels, and (e) fever. The precise etiology is unknown but may be related to an autoimmune response to endothelial cell antigen in small vessels. The therapeutic options for this disease include administration of fresh frozen plasma and plasmapheresis, high-dose corticosteroids, and antiplatelet drugs. The benefits derived from plasmapheresis would indicate that a toxic substance circulating in the plasma is a factor in this disorder, whereas the benefits of the administration of fresh frozen plasma would indicate a lack of some necessary substance that has yet to be identified. High-dose corticosteroids also provide some benefit. Aspirin and dipyridamole block platelet agglutination. A combination of these therapies now effects a significant reduction of symptoms in 70% of patients. In patients who fail to respond or who relapse, splenectomy has been performed with some success (28). The majority of long-term survivors with thrombotic thrombocytopenic purpura have undergone splenectomy, which implies that this organ plays a major role in the pathophysiology of this disease. The precise mechanism of splenic contribution is unclear. Mortality rates in the past have been as high as 90% to 95% for this disorder but are declining with aggressive treatment plans and a better understanding and diagnosis of this disorder.

Neoplastic Diseases Causing Hypersplenism

Splenectomy can play a role in the management of malignancies in any of three ways. The spleen may be the initial or sole site of primary or metastatic disease, in which case splenectomy is performed with a curative intent, as in the removal of other primary tumors. Splenectomy may be performed as a staging procedure, almost exclusively in Hodgkin's disease. Splenectomy also plays a role in the management of certain patients who have hypersplenism secondary to leukemia or lymphomas; splenectomy is indicated to relieve the symptoms of splenomegaly and the pancytopenias associated with secondary hypersplenism (29,30). The neoplastic disorders that cause hypersplenism are discussed here, and primary neoplastic diseases of the spleen and staging laparotomy are discussed later in the chapter. The malignancies in which splenectomy is or may be required are hairy cell leukemia, chronic lymphocytic leukemia, chronic myelogenous leukemia, and non-Hodgkin's lymphoma.

Hairy Cell Leukemia

Hairy cell leukemia is a low-grade lymphoproliferative disorder in which the characteristic appearance of "hairy cells" under light microscopy is caused by irregular filament projections from the cell surfaces. This leukemia is a B-lymphocyte tumor that infiltrates the bone marrow and spleen. Peripheral lymphadenopathy is almost entirely absent. The liver may or may not be enlarged. The disease is four times more common in men than in women, and the onset of disease is typically in the fifth or sixth decade of life.

The initial symptoms are most commonly either caused by the direct effects of splenomegaly or by pancytopenia secondary to hypersplenism (31) (Fig. 53.6). Patients may have early satiety or upper quadrant pain and a large, palpable spleen infiltrated with leukemic cells. The enlarged spleen often causes anemia with a transfusion require-

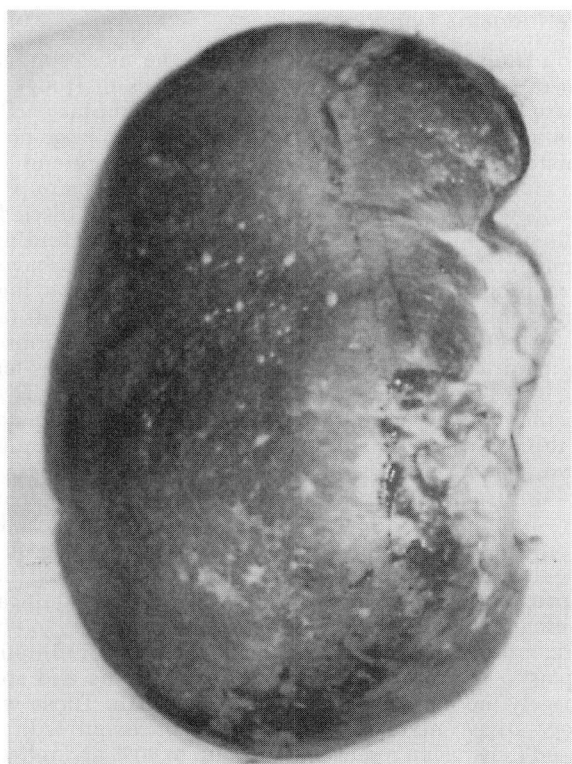

Figure 53.6. Spleen from a patient with hairy cell leukemia. Note the whitened anterior edge of the spleen and the white spots ("sugar coating") on the surface.

Table 53.6. **RAI STAGING FOR CHRONIC LYMPHOCYTIC LEUKEMIA**

Rai stage	Characteristic signs/symptoms
0	Lymphocyte count >50,000/mm^3
I	Lymphadenopathy
II	Splenomegaly/hepatomegaly
III	Hemoglobin <11 g/dL
IV	Platelets <100,000/mm^3

persplenism. The spleen often reaches a very large size, and patients may have symptoms secondary to the compressive effects of a large spleen on the stomach, with early satiety and pain (Fig. 53.7). The treatment for early-stage disease is either observation or treatment with nontoxic doses of alkylating agents such as chlorambucil or cyclophosphamide. A newer agent that is becoming a standard therapy is fludarabine. Medical therapy is never curative, and eventually the predominant symptoms are those of hypersplenism and splenomegaly. One strategy that has been employed, in particular for patients who are not operative candidates, is splenic radiation (33). Splenic radiation has decreased the size of the spleen, relieving symptoms caused by the mass effect, but it may entail complications of further thrombocytopenia and leukopenia.

Splenectomy is a highly successful treatment for both the pressure effects of splenomegaly and the cytopenias (34,35). Reports of an 85% resolution of thrombocytopenia and a 100% resolution of anemia have been published (36). The drawbacks of splenectomy in this situation are that the patients are typically elderly and debilitated from years of CLL and prior chemotherapy. In one series in which a prospective comparison was made

ment, thrombocytopenia with bleeding, and leukopenia with frequent infections. In the past, splenectomy was recommended as the primary treatment because the symptoms of splenomegaly resolved in virtually all patients, and cell counts initially improved in 80% to 90% of patients. However, the vast majority of patients relapsed, some after only 6 to 12 months, and only 40% to 50% of patients derived long-term relief from the cytopenias resulting from bone marrow replacement by hairy cell infiltrates.

In the past two decades, medical therapy, initially with recombinant interferon alfa, produced responses. Newer trials with purine analogues such as pentostatin (2-doxycoformycin) and 2-chlorodoxydenosine provided a beneficial nonsurgical therapy. A randomized trial comparing pentostatin with interferon alfa showed a complete response rate of 78% with pentostatin versus 11% with interferon alfa, and this has now become a first-line therapy (32). In the majority of these patients, significant benefit is sustained and splenectomy can be avoided. Of patients who are resistant to medical therapy, 5% to 10% can be offered splenectomy as a salvage therapy.

Chronic Lymphocytic Leukemia

Chronic lymphocytic leukemia (CLL) is the most common of all chronic leukemias. It affects men more than women, with a 2:1 predominance, and has a peak incidence in the sixth decade of life or later. This indolent disease presents with fatigue, lymphadenopathy, hepatosplenomegaly, and eventually anemia and thrombocytopenia. The disease may progress during a 5- to 10-year period. The Rai classification or staging system for CLL is shown in Table 53.6.

Patients in stage II or beyond by definition have splenomegaly, anemia, and thrombocytopenia secondary to hy-

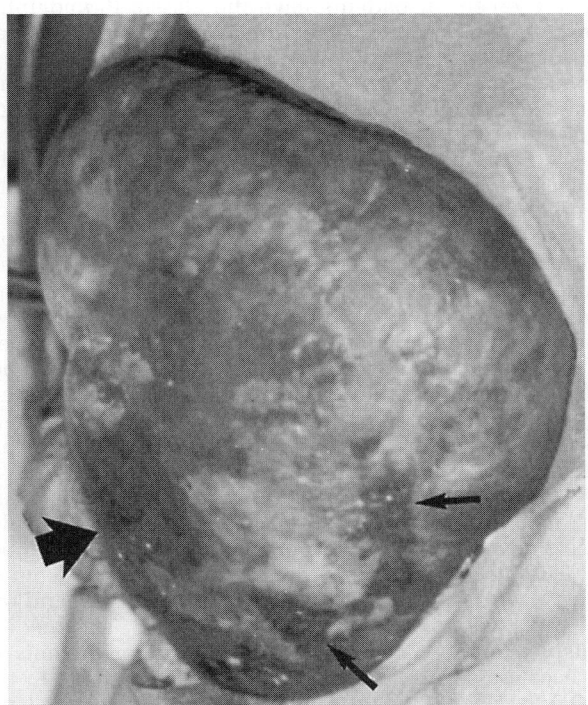

Figure 53.7. A massively enlarged, 2.2-kg spleen from a patient with chronic lymphocytic leukemia. Superficial areas of infarction are indicated by *thin arrows* and splenic infarction by the *thick arrow*.

between splenectomy and fludarabine for later-stage CLL, perioperative mortality in the splenectomy group was 9%, primarily as a result of sepsis (37). However, in this same study, highly significant improvements in thrombocytopenia and anemia were observed. Patients who are younger and have larger spleens tend to do better. In this comparative study, patients with Rai stage IV CLL had a 55% survival in the splenectomy arm and a 29% survival in the fludarabine arm. At present, splenectomy is recommended for patients who have failed medical therapy and have anemia with transfusion requirements, thrombocytopenia with bleeding, or compressive symptoms caused by splenomegaly.

Chronic Myelogenous Leukemia

In chronic myelogenous leukemia (CML), the cell of origin is a primitive hematopoietic cell. This primordial cell can differentiate into myeloid cell lines, erythroid cell lines, platelet cell lines, and possibly B-lymphoid and T-lymphoid cells. CML occurs more frequently in men, with a male-to-female ratio of 1.5:1, and like CLL it typically occurs in the sixth decade of life or later. This disease differs from CLL in that it invariably progresses from a chronic stage to an accelerated and then blast stage, whereas CLL generally remains indolent. The initial chronic phase may last anywhere between 1 and 5 years and is characterized by splenomegaly and constitutional symptoms of fatigue, abdominal fullness, and weight loss (38). In the accelerated phase, 15% of the circulating cells are relatively immature blast cells, and within 3 to 6 months the accelerated phase generally converts to the terminal blast phase, in which the blast cells fill the bone marrow and more than 30% of the circulating blood cells are leukocytes that may destroy other organs. Death from infection or bleeding invariably results after the blast crisis begins.

The diagnosis of CML is based on the identification of leukocytosis with myeloid differentiation and the presence of granulocytes filling the bone marrow spaces. Ninety percent of patients have the classic Philadelphia chromosome, which is a reciprocal translation between chromosomes 9 and 22. According to the results of randomized trials, no benefit is derived from delaying the accelerated and blast phases of the disease by performing a splenectomy during the chronic phase, although certain selected patients with significant hypersplenism or splenomegaly may obtain symptomatic relief during the chronic phase (39,40).

A recent study from M.D. Anderson reports their experience of splenectomy during the accelerated or blast phase of disease (41). Patients were referred for splenectomy to relieve symptoms of splenomegaly in 42% of cases, thrombocytopenia in 30% of cases, and both hypersplenism and thrombocytopenia in 9% of cases, and potentially to improve the results of chemotherapy by reducing hypersplenism in 19% of cases. The perioperative mortality in this series of 55 patients was 2%, with one patient death. A universal relief of symptoms related to splenomegaly was noted, in addition to a marked increase in platelet count and a decreased requirement for platelet transfusions in patients with preoperative thrombocytopenia. The median number of 6-month transfusion requirements decreased from 21 to 1 when both platelet and red cell transfusions were considered together. The median postsplenectomy survival was 19 months for patients in the accelerated phase and 6.5 months for patients in the blast phase. This report concludes that for selected patients in the later stages of CML with excessive transfusion requirements or severe symptoms of splenomegaly, splenectomy provides an objective benefit with relatively low morbidity.

Non-Hodgkin's Lymphoma

Non-Hodgkin's lymphoma (NHL) is the most common form of lymphoma; cases outnumber cases of Hodgkin's disease by a ratio of almost 6:1 in the United States. NHL is a much more heterogeneous disease, with a large range of histologic cell types defined by morphology and immunohistochemistry studies to differentiate subgroups of patients with the disease. The clinical courses of these different subgroups correlate with the microscopic findings. In general, diffuse or infiltrative NHL tends to have a worse prognosis than nodular NHL. The diffuse high-grade type occurs most commonly in younger patients (age < 35 years) or the very elderly. More aggressive forms of NHL tend to be T-cell lymphomas; the lower grades tend to be B-cell lymphomas. Unlike Hodgkin's disease, NHL at presentation is found in extranodal sites in approximately one third of cases, whereas two thirds of cases are limited to lymphadenopathy (42,43). In general, the disease is more diffuse at the time of presentation, so that treatment with combination chemotherapy is mandated. For this reason, the staging laparotomy classically used to stage Hodgkin's disease (see below) is not applicable in NHL.

Up to 80% of patients dying of NHL have significant splenic involvement, with splenomegaly secondary to lymphatic infiltration (44). As in patients with other infiltrative neoplastic diseases, symptoms of pancytopenia and splenomegaly are common in patients with NHL. Those who are operative candidates derive significant benefit, with decreased transfusion requirements in up to 80% and relief of gastric compression and pain associated with splenomegaly in the majority (45). As for the pancytopenias, the response is somewhat dependent on the reserve of bone marrow, which may have been heavily pretreated with chemotherapy or radiation therapy. No differential test is available to identify which patients have adequate marrow reserve, and the only means of assessment in this situation is whether a patient shows a response after splenectomy.

Cellular Infiltrative Processes Causing Hypersplenism

Hypersplenism may occur in the setting of general infiltrative processes, either infiltration of non-neoplastic cells or deposition of nonsoluble material. The principal condition associated with cellular infiltration is myeloid metaplasia, but hypersplenism also may occur in mastocytosis or Chédiak-Higashi syndrome. Metabolic storage diseases include Gaucher's disease and sarcoidosis.

Agnogenic Myeloid Metaplasia

Agnogenic myeloid metaplasia, or myelofibrosis with myeloid metaplasia, is a poorly understood disorder characterized by fibrotic replacement of the bone marrow compartment, extramedullary hematopoiesis, and massive splenomegaly (46). The pathophysiology of the disease is poorly understood but includes a nonclonal proliferation of fibroblasts to form a dense fibrous stroma that fills the marrow space and contributes to hepatosplenomegaly and lymphadenopathy. The fibrous proliferation may be under the control of secreted growth factors, such as transforming growth factor-β. Other myeloproliferative diseases include polycythemia vera and essential or idiopathic thrombocytosis.

The clinical symptoms and features of agnogenic myeloid metaplasia relate to anemia and splenomegaly via direct mass effects or hypersplenism. Patients tend to be in the fifth decade of life or older. They present with constitutional symptoms including weight loss, fatigue, and abdominal fullness and discomfort resulting from splenomegaly. Pain may be caused by splenic infarctions. Patients may present with bleeding resulting from thrombocytopenia. Hepatomegaly is present in 50% to 75% of patients, and splenomegaly in virtually all patients. The massively enlarged spleens in agnogenic myeloid metaplasia are often some of the largest by weight in most clinical series.

The combination of massive splenomegaly with increased blood flow through the enlarged spleen and hepatomegaly with fibrosis causing relative portal hypertension creates a unique situation in which some of the clinical symptoms may be similar to those of portal hypertension of other causes; patients may present with varices and ascites. The diagnosis is made by evaluating the peripheral blood smear, which shows immature red cells with poikilocytes and tear-shaped cells. Either thrombocytopenia or thrombocytosis with platelet counts above 1 million may be present. Similarly, either leukopenia or elevated white cell counts, as in CML, may be seen. Bone marrow biopsy often yields a dry tap because of fibrotic replacement of the marrow.

Treatment is generally targeted to the palliation of symptoms. Anemia and thrombocytopenia can be treated with transfusions. Alkylating agents and steroids are of some use, and in patients with thrombocytosis, hydroxyurea is of benefit. Splenectomy is indicated to relieve significant symptoms of hypersplenism or splenomegaly (47). Hypersplenism is manifested by anemia and thrombocytopenia, with bleeding and increased transfusion requirements. Patients with significant pain and early satiety caused by massively enlarged spleens may benefit from removal of the mass effect. Finally, agnogenic myeloid metaplasia is a unique situation in which splenectomy may relieve portal hypertension, as it will move a good portion of the increased blood flow through a fibrotic and enlarged liver and decrease variceal bleeding and possibly ascites.

It was initially debated whether loss of the spleen as a source of extramedullary hematopoiesis would be beneficial or harmful in this disease. The success rate in terms of correction of the cytopenias in agnogenic myeloid metaplasia is less than in hypersplenism secondary to neoplastic disease, discussed above. In a recent review of 223 patients from the Mayo Clinic with agnogenic myeloid metaplasia, the indications for splenectomy were transfusion-related anemia in 45%, mass effects of splenomegaly in 39%, portal hypertension in 11%, and thrombocytopenia in 5% (48). Anemia was corrected or transfusion requirements decreased in only 23% of patients, and a significant reduction in thrombocytopenia did not occur in any case. However, the symptoms of splenomegaly in the majority of patients and of portal hypertension in 50% of the patients were significantly improved. The operative mortality rate in this series was 9%.

The conclusions for agnogenic myeloid metaplasia are that in this chronic, poorly understood disorder, patients with significant pain or pressure effects caused by an enlarged spleen should undergo splenectomy for relief of symptoms. Blood transfusion requirements may be decreased somewhat, but because of the loss of extramedullary hematopoiesis and because of the fibrotic bone marrow, the benefits will not be prolonged in regard to these aspects of the disease.

Mastocytosis

Mastocytosis, or systemic mast cell disease, is a rare condition characterized by mast cell infiltration of a number of tissues, including the spleen (49). Mastocytosis occurs in an indolent form and in another form with an aggressive clinical course. For patients with indolent mastocytosis, splenectomy need not be considered. Aggressive mastocytosis is a hematologic disease with the characteristics of a malignant lymphoma. Splenomegaly may occur with subsequent hypersplenism, the most predominant manifestation in this syndrome being thrombocytopenia. In the subgroup of patients with aggressive disease and symptomatic hypersplenism, splenectomy improves platelet counts, and patients who undergo splenectomy have a longer median survival time than those with aggressive disease who do not (50).

Chédiak-Higashi Syndrome

Chédiak-Higashi syndrome is a rare autosomal recessive disease characterized by immunodeficiency with an increased susceptibility to bacterial and viral infections, recurrent fevers, nystagmus, and photophobia. In the majority of cases, widespread infiltration of tissues with histiocytes develops, as in lymphoma. Secondary hepatosplenomegaly with lymphadenopathy, leukopenia, and complications of bleeding occur in the accelerated phase of Chédiak-Higashi syndrome. The standard treatment includes chemotherapy, high-dose steroids, and ascorbic acid. The prognosis is poor. Patients with hypersplenism who can tolerate a procedure have been shown to benefit from splenectomy (51).

Metabolic Infiltration

Gaucher's Disease

Gaucher's disease is an autosomal recessive disorder characterized by a deficiency of the lysosomal hydrolase β-glucosidase, which is encoded by genome chromosome 1. Gaucher's disease is the most common lysosomal storage disease. β-Glucosidase typically degrades sphingolipids such as glucocerebroside. The incidence of this disorder is markedly increased in Ashkenazi Jews. Three subtypes are seen. Type I, the adult form, which comprises 99% of cases, was formerly treated by splenectomy. Because of the defect in the acid β-glucosidase, undegraded glycolipids accumulate, are taken up by the reticuloendothelial cells, and infiltrate the spleen, liver, and bone marrow. The most common symptoms of this disease relate to hypersplenism and the direct effects of massive splenomegaly. Thrombocytopenia with bleeding or anemia causing fatigue are the most common consequences of the hypersplenism. In addition, an extremely massive spleen may cause early satiety and weight loss secondary to gastric compression.

The diagnosis can be confirmed by measuring acid β-glucosidase activity in peripheral white blood cells or cultured fibroblasts. With cloning of the gene, patients can be screened by molecular techniques to identify carriers. Prenatal diagnosis is also available by amniocentesis.

In the past, treatment included supportive care with platelet and erythrocyte transfusions. Splenectomy was frequently performed in advanced cases, and a significant experience with partial splenectomy for this disease was developed in the early 1990s (52–54). The goals of a subtotal splenectomy are partially to prevent the complications of overwhelming postsplenectomy sepsis and partially to protect the lipid and bone marrow by leaving a residual splenic fragment for the continued deposition of lipid. Techniques were developed to perform partial splenectomy safely by leaving a small residual upper pole fragment vascularized by the short gastric vessels.

Recently, it has been established that enzyme replacement with purified placental acid β-glucosidase is safe and efficacious. When patients are given 30 to 60 U of enzyme per kilogram intravenously every other week, symptoms and signs are typically reversed. A recombinant β-glucosidase (alglucerase) is now available for therapy, and splenectomy has been replaced by medical management.

Sarcoidosis

Sarcoidosis is a granulomatous disease of unknown origin that can involve virtually any organ or area of the body. Pulmonary disease is most common, but autopsy studies have shown that the spleen is the second most common site of sarcoid deposits and is enlarged by noncaseating granulomas in 50% to 60% of patients. The majority of patients do not have splenomegaly, but when they do, as a result of significant granuloma formations, hypersplenism can develop. Also, patients with very bulky disease typically have the hypercalcemia of sarcoidosis. In this subgroup of patients, splenectomy is indicated as a curative procedure.

Splenic Vein Thrombosis

Splenic vein thrombosis is an unusual cause of upper gastrointestinal hemorrhage that can be cured by splenectomy. The pathophysiology of this disease is an isolated thrombosis in the splenic vein where it courses along the posterior pancreatic body and tail. The splenic venous outflow is then diverted to the short gastric vessels as collateral venous outflow channels. The increased flow in the short gastric veins causes an increase in pressure and dilation of the submucosal venous plexus, primarily in the gastric cardia and fundus, and the eventual development of gastric varices (55).

The cause of the splenic vein thrombosis does not involve any disease of the spleen but rather disease of the pancreas and possibly the stomach. Pancreatitis or pancreatic pseudocyst results in splenic vein thrombosis in more than 50% of patients in most series. Pancreatic carcinoma with direct invasion and infiltration of the splenic vein is the second most common cause. Other, unusual causes may be a penetrating gastric ulcer posteriorly or retroperitoneal fibrosis.

The diagnosis is made in patients with upper gastrointestinal bleeding in whom only gastric varices are detected on endoscopy. Because portal vein hypertension and cirrhosis of the liver are absent, esophageal varices do not develop. The spleen may or may not be enlarged, but again no other signs and symptoms of cirrhosis are seen. Definitive diagnosis in the past has been made by a celiac angiogram, which demonstrates an absence of the splenic vein and collateral flow via the gastric veins. Magnetic resonance angiography/venography and high-resolution ultrasonography may also be used to make the diagnosis.

Splenectomy is curative by removing blood flow through the splenic artery and spleen. The excess collateral flow is removed, and the venous hypertension and associated symptoms resolve. Whenever splenic vein thrombosis is diagnosed, even if the patient has not had an episode of bleeding, elective splenectomy should be performed as a prophylactic measure.

Patients with portal hypertension and cirrhosis have a complex of symptoms that include hypersplenism, splenomegaly, thrombocytopenia, and anemia. However, the operative risk associated with portal vein hypertension is excessive, and splenectomy is virtually never indicated in this setting.

INDICATIONS FOR SPLENECTOMY NOT RELATED TO HYPERSPLENISM

Occasionally, an elective or urgent splenectomy is indicated to treat a condition that is not associated with the signs and symptoms of hypersplenism discussed above. The most common indication in this category is splenic trauma with splenic rupture. Between 1960 and 1990,

elective splenectomy was frequently performed as part of a staging laparotomy for Hodgkin's disease, but since the development of different patterns of treatment and newer diagnostic techniques, splenectomy is less often indicated in this situation. Other unusual indications for splenectomy include primary splenic neoplasms and cysts, splenic abscesses, and splenic artery aneurysms.

Staging Laparotomy for Hodgkin's Disease

Hodgkin's disease is a malignant lymphoma characterized by the presence of a characteristic multinucleated cell identified as the Reed-Sternberg cell. The annual incidence of Hodgkin's disease in the United States is 8,000 cases, which is less than 20% of the incidence of NHL (56). A bimodal distribution is seen in terms of age, with peaks in the second and eighth decades of life. The pathologic classification of Hodgkin's disease comprises four subtypes: lymphocyte-predominant, nodular sclerosing, mixed cellularity, and lymphocyte-depleted. The lymphocyte-predominant and nodular sclerosing subtypes have a more favorable prognosis than the mixed cellularity and lymphocyte-depleted subtypes. However, in comparison with NHL and other malignancies, Hodgkin's disease has quite a good prognosis overall.

The typical presentation of Hodgkin's disease is painless lymphadenopathy. The cervical nodes are most frequently involved, in approximately two thirds of patients. In most series, the axillary nodes are the next most frequently involved (15% of cases); the inguinal and mediastinal lymph nodes are involved in 10% of patients. Extranodal disease is rarely the primary presentation in Hodgkin's disease, as it is in NHL. A constellation of general or constitutional symptoms affecting some patients with Hodgkin's disease are labeled *B symptoms*. These include fever, night sweats, weight loss, and pruritus. Patients with B symptoms generally have a less favorable prognosis than patients with disease of the same stage but no B symptoms.

The staging system typically used for Hodgkin's disease is the Ann Arbor system (56) (Table 53.7). It reflects the fact that Hodgkin's disease starting in nodal tissue generally spreads in an anatomic pattern from nodal group to nodal group. Stage I Hodgkin's disease involves a single nodal group. Stage II involves two contiguous nodal groups on the same side of the diaphragm. An example of stage II disease would be involvement of the cervical nodes and mediastinal sternal nodes. Another example would be involvement of the superficial inguinal nodes and deep inguinal/periaortic nodes. Stage III disease denotes involvement on both sides of the diaphragm, and in this situation, the spleen is considered as a lymph node. Stage IV disease includes involvement of one or more dis-

Table 53.7. ANN ARBOR STAGING SYSTEM FOR HODGKIN'S DISEASE

Stage	Description
I	Single nodal group involved
II	Two nodal groups on the same side of the diaphragm
III	Nodal and/or splenic involvement on both sides of the diaphragm
IV	Extranodal (E) involvement (e.g., liver, bone marrow, skin)
A	No constitutional symptoms
B	Constitutional symptoms of weight loss, fevers, night sweats, and pruritus

tinct extranodal organs, such as lung, bone, or skin. Within these four stages of Hodgkin's disease, patients are subcategorized as either A (for an absence of B symptoms) or B (for the presence of the constitutional symptoms described above).

Staging can be by clinical or pathologic assessment. Clinical assessment would include a physical examination and radiologic studies, typically computed tomography (CT) of the chest, abdomen, and pelvis and possibly lymphangiography. Lymphangiography is more sensitive than CT when correlated with pathologic staging to identify involved retroperitoneal lymph nodes, but it requires bilateral incisions on the feet and greater expertise in technique and interpretation. The sensitivity of lymphangiography is reported to be 90% and the sensitivity of CT in the range of 70% to 80% in the diagnosis of intraabdominal lymphadenopathy. The advantage of CT over lymphangiography is that it evaluates lymph nodes in areas not seen on lymphangiography, such as the mesentery, porta hepatis, and splenic hilum.

A standard part of pathologic staging between 1960 and 1990 was the staging laparotomy. This invasive procedure was performed because reports indicated that laparotomy altered the clinical stage of disease in approximately 35% of patients. Approximately 20% to 25% of patients were staged at a more advanced level after staging laparotomy, and approximately 10% to 15%, were staged at a lower clinical level based on laparotomy results. If the treatment of Hodgkin's disease depended on accurate staging (i.e., the treatment of early stages was different from the treatment of more advanced stages), then the staging laparotomy was essential in determining the proper therapeutic intervention for patients with Hodgkin's disease.

Staging laparotomy was performed via an upper abdominal midline incision. It included an exploration of the entire abdomen for any abnormal lymph nodes, including nodes identified by lymphography. Even if no abnormalities were found, multiple tissues were removed for pathologic assessment (Fig. 53.8). The spleen, bilobar hepatic wedge resections, bilobar hepatic core biopsies, and multiple lymph node samples were obtained. Lymph nodes were typically removed from the porta hepatis, celiac region, splenic hilum, periaortic region, and bowel mesentery. If any iliac lymph nodes were palpated, they were also removed. The spleen removed during a staging laparotomy for Hodgkin's disease is divided in thin sections with a thickness of 3 to 4 mm, and any suspect nodule, particularly in the white pulp, is examined microscopically for the presence of Hodgkin's disease. Another part of this operation in young women of childbearing age is a full oophoropexy. If pelvic irradiation along the nodal groups is planned, the ovarian pedicles are sutured to the uterus in the low midline position, so that they are out of the way of iliac lymph node chain radiation. They are also marked with a clip to be used when radiation fields are planned.

The use of staging laparotomy has decreased during the past 10 to 15 years for several reasons. The primary reason is that it does not alter the treatment of Hodgkin's dis-

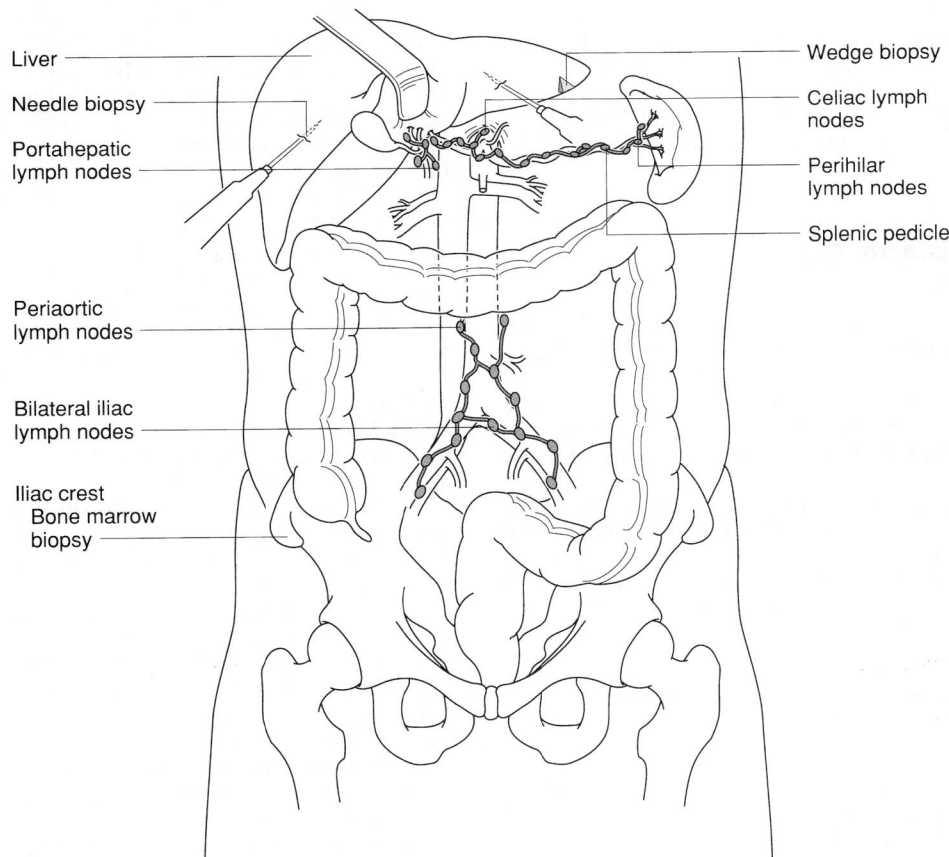

Figure 53.8. The tissues to be removed or to undergo biopsy in a staging laparotomy for Hodgkin's disease. Splenectomy, liver biopsy, and lymph node sampling in the specific sites are shown. Bone marrow biopsy can be performed if necessary.

ease based on results of recent clinical series. The treatment of patients with stages IB, IIB, IIIB, IVB, IIIA, and IVA Hodgkin's disease almost always involves systemic chemotherapy. Because systemic chemotherapy treats the whole patient, accurate pathologic staging has no effect on treatment decisions or outcome. The only patients who may theoretically benefit from staging laparotomy at present are those with stage IA or IIA Hodgkin's disease, who typically receive radiation therapy. Even in this subgroup of patients, the trend is not to perform a staging laparotomy. First, many oncologists use combination chemotherapy, even for early-stage disease. Second, for patients with stages IA and IIA disease treated with radiation alone, it has been demonstrated in several recent clinical series that the ultimate outcome is the same whether they undergo a staging laparotomy or are initially treated with radiation (57–59). The reason is that if these patients have a recurrence outside the radiation field during long-term follow-up, they can be salvaged with systemic chemotherapy. Third, a staging laparotomy is obviously a major abdominal operation with a potential for morbidity, and it delays the treatment of Hodgkin's disease typically between 4 and 6 weeks. Finally, data indicate that patients who survive Hodgkin's disease and undergo combination chemotherapy are at increased risk for the development of a secondary malignancy, primarily acute nonlymphocytic leukemia (60–62). In some series, the risk for the development of acute nonlymphocytic leukemia is increased up to 10-fold in patients who have undergone splenectomy as part of their staging work-up for Hodgkin's disease when they are compared with patients undergoing similar chemotherapy regimens without splenectomy. For all these reasons, this procedure, which accounted for a large number of the splenectomies performed in major tertiary referral centers and cancer centers, is rarely performed at the present time. The important feature to keep in mind when evaluating a patient with Hodgkin's disease is whether a staging laparotomy will lead to a definite change in the treatment plan for that person.

Primary Neoplasms/Cysts of the Spleen

As described above, splenectomy is often performed for hematologic malignancies, including multiple forms of leukemias and lymphoma, primarily to relieve symptoms of hypersplenism or splenomegaly or as a staging procedure. Splenectomy is infrequently indicated for primary neoplasms of the spleen, which are listed in Table 53.8.

Hemangioma is the most common benign primary neoplasm of the spleen. It is often an incidental finding and may be solitary or multiple. During operation, it can be identified from the surface as a more intensely bluish

purple area in comparison with the reddish purple color of the splenic parenchyma. Hemangiomas can be identified with excellent sensitivity and specificity by the characteristics on magnetic resonance imaging. It is unwise to perform a biopsy of a lesion that may be a splenic hemangioma. Hemangiomas of the spleen rarely cause symptoms, but massive hemangiomas either rupture spontaneously or make the spleen more susceptible to a traumatic rupture. In cases of massive hemangioma with capsular distention and pain, either a splenectomy or partial splenectomy may be indicated.

Hemangioendothelioma is a neoplasm that is thought to be slightly more aggressive than the typical benign hemangioma. It is thought to be pathologically an intermediate between benign hemangioma and malignant angiosarcoma. It is not considered to have metastatic potential and generally is an incidental finding. Larger lesions may cause symptoms or be notable for their size. Again, rupture, either spontaneous or after minor trauma, is the typical circumstance in which patients with these lesions undergo splenectomy.

Lymphangiomas also occur in the spleen but are much less common than hemangiomas. They may be multiple or solitary and can be identified by their lighter color and compressibility when seen during surgery.

Two mass lesions occurring in the spleen that are not true neoplasms are hamartomas and inflammatory pseudotumors. Hamartomas are focal abnormalities that develop in the spleen and other solid organs, such as the liver. Hamartomas contain normal cellular elements and are again non-neoplastic but have a random fibrotic organization. The major significance of hamartomas is that they are identified incidentally at laparotomy or are seen incidentally on CT performed for other reasons. Inflammatory pseudotumors are described in most organs and have also been described in the spleen. These sometimes are quite large with a wide variety of reactive cells. A subcategory of inflammatory pseudotumors of the spleen is related to mycobacterial infection, particularly in HIV-positive patients.

Cysts of the spleen are almost uniformly not related to parasitic infection. They are relatively common lesions, seen across all age groups, and may be multifocal. The diagnosis of splenic cysts can be ascertained by ultrasonography or CT. These benign lesions have no clinical significance unless they reach a large size. As discussed earlier in the section on the history of splenic surgery, the first reported case of a successful elective splenectomy was performed for a splenic cyst. This was an enormous cyst located at the tip of the spleen, thought likely to be an ovarian mass, but was found to arise from the spleen at laparotomy (Fig. 53.9). Today, a cyst enucleation or partial splenectomy would probably be performed for a large and symptomatic peripheral cystic lesion. An alternative approach is unroofing the cyst and leaving a portion of the cyst wall in place.

The only parasitic cysts involving the spleen are caused by *Echinococcus granulosus* or hydatid cysts. The ratio of echinococcal cysts in the spleen to those in the liver is approximately 30:1. The diagnosis should be suspected in patients in areas where echinococcal disease is common, such as New Zealand, Australia, and parts of the western United States. The complement fixation test is the most reliable serologic study for this organism. The treatment of echinococcal cysts is splenectomy. As with echinococcal cysts of the liver, it is of the utmost importance not to rupture the cyst and expose the patient to the scoleces. For large and peripheral cysts, in which risk for rupture is high, the contents of the cyst should be carefully aspirated and replaced with hypertonic saline solution (63).

Table 53.8. PRIMARY NEOPLASMS AND CYSTS OF THE SPLEEN

Hemangioma
Hemangioendothelioma
Lymphangioma
Pseudotumor
Mycobacterial pseudotumor
Hamartoma
Primary cyst
Echinococcal cyst

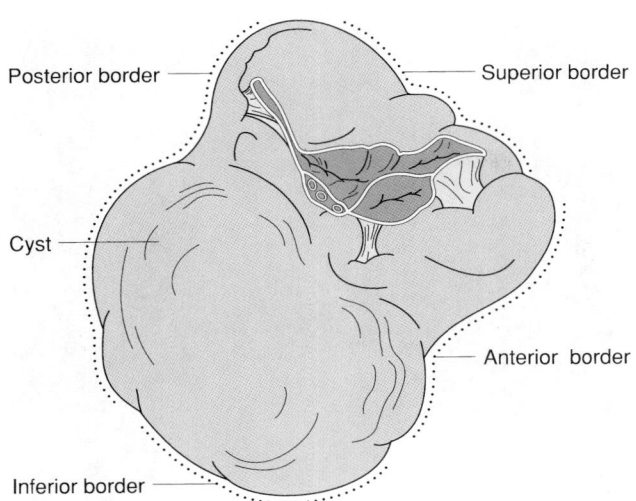

Figure 53.9. The visceral surface of a spleen with a true congenital splenic cyst.

Splenic Artery Aneurysm

Splenic artery aneurysm is uncommon, even though the splenic artery is the abdominal artery second most frequently affected by aneurysmal changes. Splenic aneurysms occur twice as often in women as in men. Patients can be divided into two distinct groups. First, aneurysms are manifestations of atherosclerosis in elderly persons. Second, an apparently congenital predisposition to form splenic artery aneurysms is found in young women. The risk for rupture of these aneurysms is increased during pregnancy. Inflammatory processes such as pancreatitis may involve the splenic artery and occasionally lead to aneurysm, but more frequently to acute bleeding.

Splenic artery aneurysms are typically asymptomatic and may be initially identified as a widened rim of calcification defining the aneurysm boundaries in the left upper quadrant. They may also be discovered as incidental findings on CT. If symptomatic, patients experience left upper quadrant pain, nausea, and vomiting. If the symptoms suggest impending aneurysmal rupture, urgent splenectomy with ligation of the splenic arteries is indicated.

When a calcified atherosclerotic splenic artery aneurysm is discovered in a patient over age 60 with no splenomegaly and no symptoms, surgical excision is not indicated, and the aneurysm can be followed to detect signs of enlargement. In younger patients in whom a symptomatic aneurysm is identified, particularly young women of childbearing age, an elective splenectomy is recommended to prevent rupture. A nonsurgical approach is to embolize the splenic artery in patients who are poor risks for open laparotomy (64).

Abscess of the Spleen

Splenic abscess is uncommon, but this is an important disease because it is associated with a significant mortality rate and can be cured by splenectomy (65). In most series, the mortality rate ranges between 40% and 100% (66). In the typical patient, the spleen has been seeded hematogenously by bacteria from a remote source, such as the heart (in endocarditis) or intravenous drugs. In some cases, infection spreads directly adjacent intraabdominal sources. Finally, splenic trauma treated conservatively may eventually result in an infected splenic hematoma. In 80% of cases, an additional source of infection is present in locations other than the spleen, and in only 20% of cases is the splenic abscess the sole source of sepsis identified. Enteric organisms account for two thirds of splenic abscesses, and staphylococci and streptococci for the remainder of cases.

Patients present with signs and symptoms of sepsis, including fever, malaise, and leukocytosis. When the spleen is the sole site of infection, significant left upper quadrant tenderness and guarding are seen. Abdominal roentgenograms may show gas in the spleen, and ultrasonography and CT with contrast are diagnostic, showing an abscess with a reactive rim.

The treatment of choice for patients who can undergo a laparotomy and who have the splenic abscess as an isolated or prominent component of septic syndrome is splenectomy. If the spleen is the only source of infection, removal of the spleen should be curative and result in recovery. If patients have multiple sites of infection or are too sick to undergo a laparotomy, percutaneous drainage may be attempted, but this is not as successful because of frequent spillage and assimilation of bacteria in the left upper quadrant of the abdomen.

Ectopic Spleen (Wandering Spleen)

Ectopic spleen, or so-called wandering spleen, is caused by either extreme laxity or absence of the normal ligaments that anchor the spleen in the left upper quadrant. The force of gravity causes the spleen to drop into the lower abdomen, either the right or left lower quadrant, attached by its vascular pedicle. Wandering spleen occurs 13 times more frequently in women than in men. The diagnosis can be made by a palpable lower abdominal mass confirmed by CT or nuclear imaging of the splenic tissue. An ectopic spleen typically causes symptoms when torsion of the pedicle results in acute ischemia and pain. If the torsion can be corrected and the spleen appears to be viable, the treatment is splenopexy, in which the spleen is tacked to its native position in the left upper quadrant. If the spleen appears infarcted, then a splenectomy must be performed.

Trauma of the Spleen

The spleen is the intraabdominal organ most frequently injured by blunt trauma in the United States, and in many institutions splenectomy remains the most common operative procedure performed on the spleen. The history of splenic surgery mirrors the history of surgery for trauma. In the ancient medical literature, the spleen often herniated through a flank wound, and partial splenectomy or total splenectomy of the herniated portions is described. The first documented splenectomy for penetrating trauma took place in San Francisco in 1816. It was performed by a British naval surgeon named O'Brien on a patient whose spleen protruded out of a knife wound (2). In the late 19th century, Theodor Billroth observed during an autopsy on a patient who had died of head trauma 5 days earlier that the amount of blood in the peritoneum from the fractured splenic capsule was minimal and predicted that these injuries might be managed non-operatively. Although during the earlier part of the 20th century splenic trauma was uniformly managed by complete splenectomy, Dr. Campos Christo of Brazil reported partial splenectomy and splenic salvage for both penetrating and blunt trauma in 1962 (2,3). Since this initial report, the ability to obtain repeated cross-sectional images coupled with a better understanding of splenic function and overwhelming postsplenectomy sepsis has led to the development of current management guidelines, in which lower-grade splenic injuries are managed nonoperatively and operative management is centered around splenic preservation when possible (67–69).

The most common blunt injuries leading to splenic rupture are associated with motor vehicle accidents and bicycle accidents, in which upper abdominal trauma may occur. Isolated splenic injury is manifested by tenderness in the left upper quadrant of the abdomen. Attention must be directed to the lower lateral left ribs, and focal tenderness over ribs 9 through 11 in that region should raise suspicion of possible splenic injury. Approximately 20% of cases of rib fracture can be demonstrated on radiographs. Patients may have referred pain to the left shoulder (Kehr's sign), particularly when they are placed in the Trendelenburg position and the upper abdomen is palpated. The spleen itself is rarely palpable, but when a left upper quadrant mass is palpable, it represents a contained hematoma or a subcapsular hematoma; this is known as Ballance's sign. Depending on the severity of the injury, patients may have no hemodynamic instability or be in frank hypovolemic shock. The grading system for splenic trauma is shown in Table 53.9.

Laboratory findings associated with splenic rupture would potentially include a decrease in hematocrit and hemoglobin, although initial assessment before volume resuscitation may show normal levels. After a short period of time, a leukocytosis in the range of 15,000 to 20,000/mm^3 often develops. Plain abdominal radiographs, in addition to left rib fractures, may show displacement or a corrugated appearance along the greater curvature of the stomach, caused by a hematoma infiltrating the gastrosplenic ligament (Fig. 53.10). Peritoneal lavage will reveal the presence of blood in the abdomen. The most important current diagnostic tool, particularly in patients with sufficient hemodynamic stability to be managed conservatively, is CT. Contrast CT will show the splenic contour and also the amount of extrasplenic blood (70) (Fig. 53.11).

Overall, blunt injuries account for most cases of splenic trauma, but the spleen is also susceptible to penetrating trauma, either in the retroperitoneum, lower thorax, or upper abdomen. Penetrating trauma of the thorax and upper abdomen poses less of a diagnostic dilemma because most of these patients undergo abdominal exploration for associated injuries. In some series, 90% to 100% of patients with penetrating trauma to the spleen have additional injuries, and 40% to 60% with blunt trauma have associated injuries.

The management of splenic injuries historically has been laparotomy with splenectomy. Since Christo introduced partial splenectomy and splenorrhaphy, in-

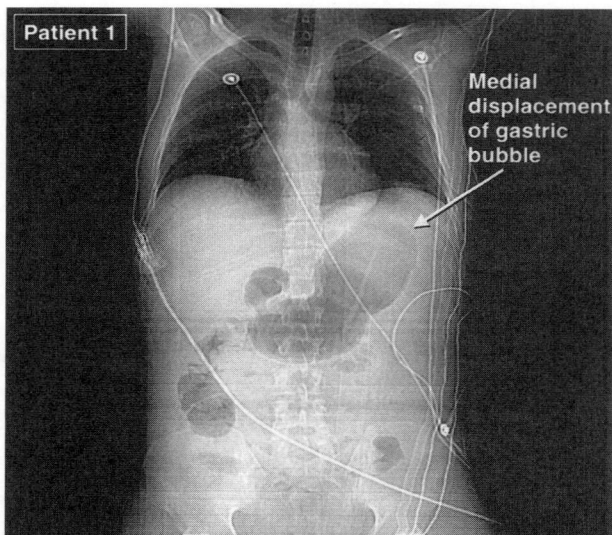

Figure 53.10. Abdominal film of a patient with a splenic rupture resulting from blunt trauma. A perisplenic hematoma displaces the greater curvature of the stomach medially. The scalloped appearance is indicative of blood in the gastrosplenic ligament. (Radiograph courtesy of Dr. C. William Schwab.)

creased attempts have been made during surgical procedures to repair or preserve part if not all of the spleen. The current trend in management is a nonoperative approach, with observation by serial CT scanning. Peritonitis, associated injuries requiring surgery, overall severity of injuries, evidence of hypovolemic shock and ongoing bleeding, and age are the primary factors considered in a decision regarding nonoperative versus operative management of blunt splenic injuries (71,72). If a patient has diffuse peritonitis or hypotension related to hypovolemic shock, urgent laparotomy is indicated. If the patient is hemodynamically stable and has no other injuries that require surgical management, the recom-

Table 53.9. SPLEEN INJURY SCALE

Grade	Laceration	Hemartoma
I	<1 cm in depth	Subcapsular <10% of surface
II	1 to 3 cm in depth not involving a trabecular vessel	Subcapsular 10%–50% of surface area or 5 cm in diameter
III	>3 cm depth or any depth involving a trabecular vessel	Subcapsular >50% of surface area or intraparenchymal
IV	Segmental or hilar vessel involvement	
V	Shattered spleen or hilar vessel disruption	

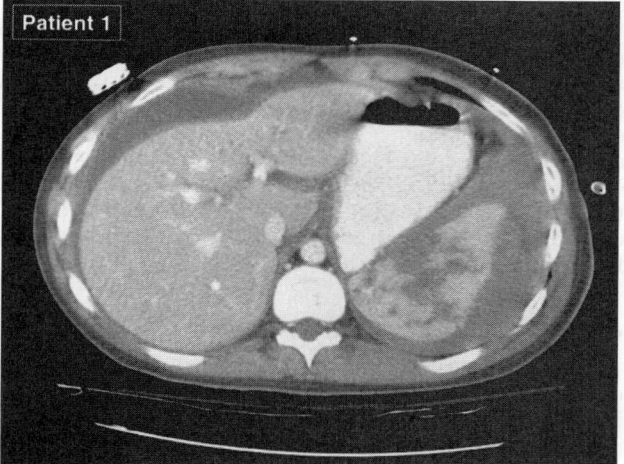

Figure 53.11. Contrast computed tomography in a patient with splenic rupture near the hilum. A considerable amount of blood is seen in the perisplenic fossa, in addition to free blood in the peritoneal cavity around the liver. (Radiograph courtesy of Dr. C. William Schwab.)

mendation is nonoperative observation. In some pediatric series, the vast majority of patients were candidates for nonoperative management. In other recent series of adult patients, approximately 30% to 50% of patients required urgent splenectomy because of associated injuries and ongoing bleeding (Fig. 53.12). Of the patients stable enough to undergo CT, 50% to 80% may be candidates for observation. Between 3% and 15% of patients selected for observation will ultimately require an operation for continued or recurrent bleeding.

The standard nonoperative management protocol would include very close observation in an intensive care unit or a similar monitored environment. Patients would undergo serial abdominal examinations and serial assessments of hemoglobin and hematocrit. If any change in status developed in which patients did remain somewhat stable, follow-up CT would be performed to detect any progressive or ongoing bleeding, demonstrated by an increased hemoperitoneum or expansion of splenic hematoma. With such conservative management, the majority of patients would avoid laparotomy for isolated splenic blunt trauma (73). In the past, delayed splenic rupture was thought to be caused by a capsular hematoma that subsequently liquefied; typically, 75% of these cases occurred within 2 weeks of the injury. However, delayed rupture may occur a month or up to several years after trauma. The recent approach of nonoperative management of splenic trauma supplemented by sequential CT has shown this phenomenon of delayed rupture to be a relatively rare event when patients are followed prospectively.

If patients are older or have associated injuries or ongoing blood loss, a laparotomy is appropriate for blunt splenic trauma. Again, the nature of the splenic injury is graded according to the degree of damage to the splenic parenchyma and the proximity to the splenic hilum and major blood vessels (Table 53.9). The principles of operative management would include stopping ongoing hemorrhage while preserving the maximal amount of viable splenic parenchyma. Nonviable or devascularized tissue must be débrided. Partial splenectomy has been popularized based on the concept of segmental blood supply via the trabecular arteries. A variety of approaches can be used to manage more minor, peripheral splenic trauma, including primary repair and mesh repair (Fig. 53.13). Various materials available for hemostasis, including microfibrillar collagen, Gelfoam, and fibrin glue sealants, have been utilized to control splenic hemorrhage. The argon beam coagulator is a very useful instrument for capsular tear or evulsions. Of note, all these techniques that are applied in patients with blunt trauma can be similarly applied in patients who sustain inadvertent trauma to the spleen during surgery on the splenic flexure of the colon, left kidney or adrenal gland, or stomach.

Recent series of blunt trauma to the spleen report an overall splenic salvage rate of 64%, with a 57% success rate in adults and a 96% success rate in children. Mortality from splenic injuries is usually caused by associated injuries or a delay in diagnosis or transport to a facility where appropriate procedures can be performed. In most series in which splenic trauma is involved, the overall mortality is approximately 10%, although it has been reported to be zero in some series and as high as 20% in others, again depending on associated injuries.

SPLENECTOMY

The elective operations currently available for the spleen are open splenectomy, laparoscopic splenectomy,

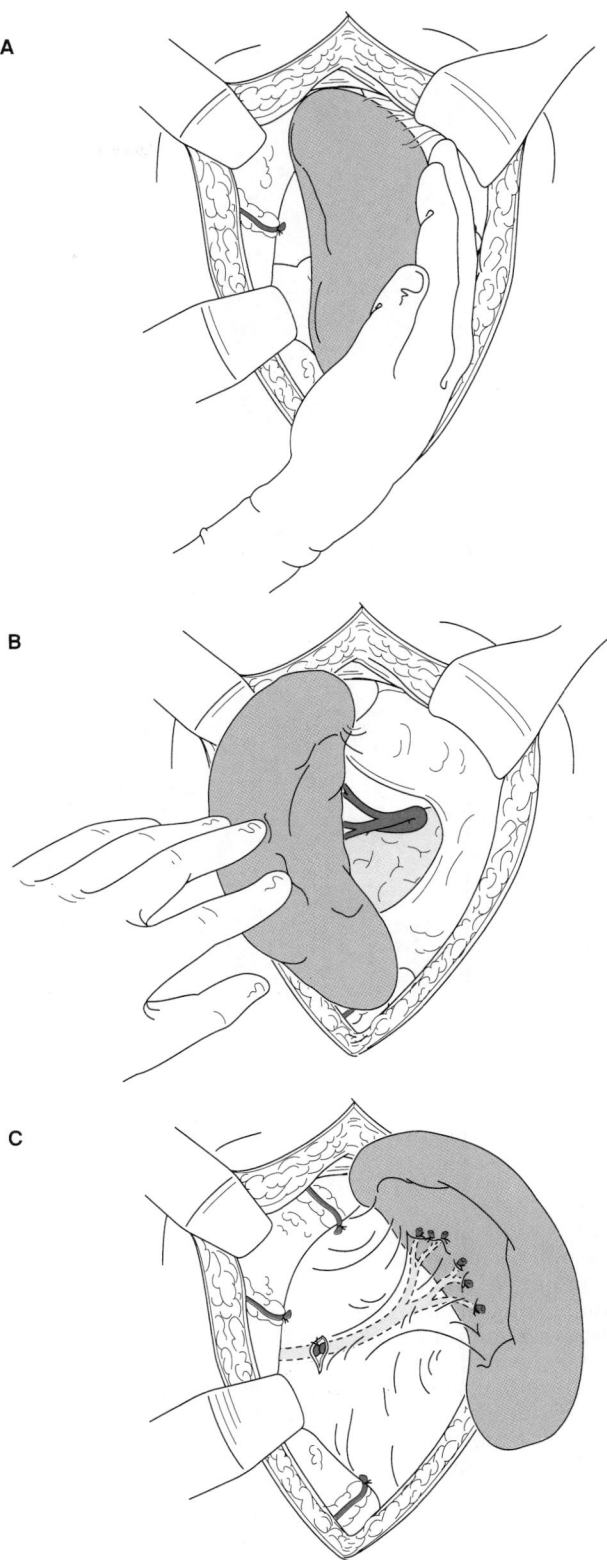

Figure 53.12. *(A,B)* A bleeding spleen can be mobilized rapidly in most patients by blunt dissection of the lateral attachments. *(C)* The splenic hilum can then be controlled quickly.

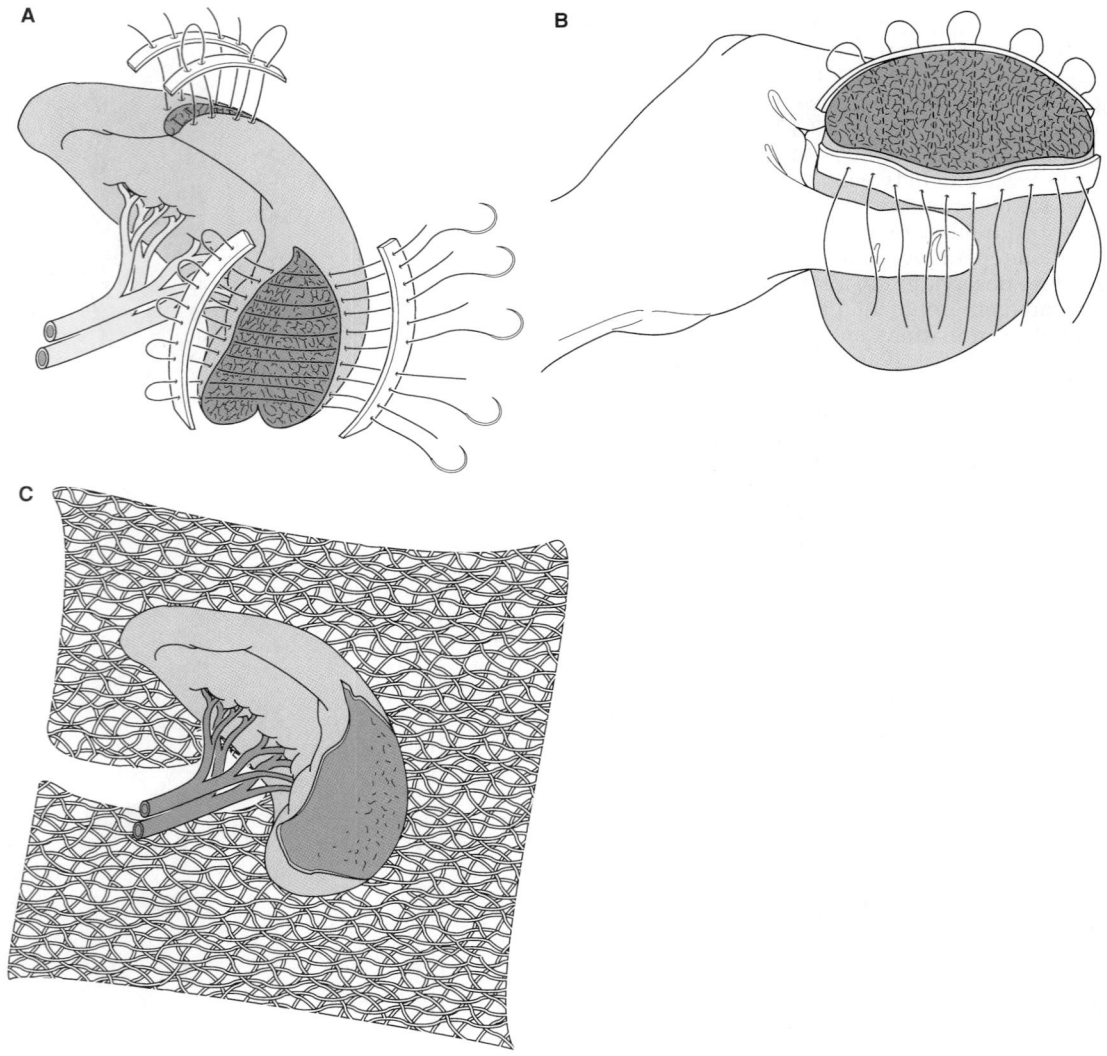

Figure 53.13. *(A)* Techniques to suture superficial splenic lacerations. *(B)* Technique to control bleeding after hemisplenectomy. The sutures can be interlocked. *(C)* A polyglycolic acid mesh sheet or mesh bag can be applied to a spleen from which the capsule has been stripped.

and partial splenectomy. Table 53.10 lists the indications for splenectomy and whether a partial splenectomy is appropriate. Certain principles apply to all patients undergoing elective splenectomy. First, all patients should receive appropriate preoperative vaccination with Pneumovax and possibly also vaccination against *Haemophilus influenzae* and *Neisseria meningitidis* 10 to 14 days before the procedure if possible. Patients must have appropriate blood products ready, as they are often anemic and thrombocytopenic because of hypersplenism, as described above.

The operative technique for open splenectomy involves either a midline abdominal or a left subcostal incision. For patients with massive splenomegaly, defined as a spleen weighing more than 1,500 g in adults and more than 1,000 g in children, a long midline incision should be used. The components of the splenectomy include division of the avascular lateral and posterior attachments to mobilize the spleen, ligation of the short gastric vessels separating the upper half of the spleen from the greater curvature of the stomach, and ligation of splenic hilar vessels in a controlled manner to avoid injury to the pancreatic tail. Al-

though one approach, especially for small spleens that are mobile, is to divide the lateral attachments initially, place packs in the left upper quadrant to elevate the spleen, and then proceed with the vascular dissection (Fig. 53.14), this should be discouraged, particularly if the patient is thrombocytopenic or has massive splenomegaly. In this situation, the surgeon should start by obtaining vascular control before manipulating the spleen and causing capsular rupture and significant blood loss.

The preferred operative approach in patients with splenomegaly (115) and hypersplenism is first to divide the attachments of the left lateral segment of the liver and retract this to the right side of the abdomen to expose the greater curvature of the stomach. Then, starting at the midportion of the greater curvature of the stomach, the branches of the left gastroepiploic artery and vein, including the short gastric vessels, are ligated sequentially and the stomach is completely dissociated from the superior portion of the spleen (Fig. 53.15). Through the window into the lesser sac created by dissecting the short gastric vessels, the splenic artery can be identified at variable locations along the superior border of the pancreas. A loop

Table 53.10. OPERATIVE INDICATIONS FOR SPLENECTOMY (TOTAL OR PARTIAL)

Disease	Splenectomy required	Partial splenectomy
Hereditary spherocytosis	Always	Yes
Hereditary elliptocytosis	Sometimes	Yes
Thalassemia	Sometimes	Yes
Sickle cell anemia	Rarely	No
Wiskott-Aldrich syndrome	Sometimes	No
Autoimmune hemolytic anemia	Usually	No
Autoimmune neutropenia	Sometimes	No
Immune thrombocytopenic purpura	Usually	No
Thrombotic thrombocytopenic purpura	Sometimes	No
Hairy cell leukemia	Rarely[a]	No
Chronic lymphocytic leukemia	Sometimes	No
Chronic myelogenous leukemia	Sometimes	No
Non-Hodgkin's lymphoma	Sometimes	No
Agnogenic myeloid metaplasia	Sometimes	Yes
Mastocytosis	Rarely	No
Gaucher's disease	Rarely[a]	Yes
Hodgkin's disease	Rarely[b]	No
Splenic vein thrombosis	Always	No
Splenic abscess	Usually	No
Splenic cyst	Rarely	Yes
Echinococcal cyst	Always	No

[a]Splenectomy rarely indicated in current practice because of effective medical therapy.
[b]Splenectomy rarely indicated because of change in current therapy.

of this tortuous artery is most safely ligated at its most superior or cranial portion, as at this point it is farthest from the splenic vein and also away from the pancreatic parenchyma. The artery may be simply ligated once or twice with heavy silk ties at that location and does not need to be divided. By dividing the short gastric arteries and ligating the main splenic artery, most if not all blood flow into the spleen is controlled before the spleen is even touched to be mobilized. If capsular disruption occurs, blood loss is greatly minimized. Following vascular control, the lateral and posterior attachments are divided and the spleen is elevated to near the level of the abdominal wall musculature ventrally. The splenic hilum can then be dissected by tying vessels in a controlled manner.

For patients with ITP, platelets should not be given until the spleen is removed or the arterial inflow is controlled because transfused platelets are cleared by the spleen in this disease. Similarly, in this disease and other diseases in which the spleen is the site of platelet or blood cell destruction, it is important to identify and remove accessory spleens. Most accessory spleens occur in the splenic hilum; they can also be found in the omentum, along the superior border of the pancreas, in the bowel mesentery, and in the pelvis in some situations. The incidence of accessory spleens in open splenectomy ranges between 15% and 30%.

The spleen can be approached reasonably well with a laparoscopic technique in this current era of minimally invasive or noninvasive surgical procedures. The approach to splenectomy includes positioning the patient with the left side up and dividing the lateral attachments of the spleen with electrocautery. The upper pole attachments can be divided with harmonic scalpel or electrocautery. The vascular supply to the spleen can then be safely divided with a laparoscopic vascular stapler or the harmonic scalpel for small vessels.

The surgeon's experience will dictate which patients are deemed eligible for laparoscopic splenectomy (74). Certainly, patients with ITP, in which splenomegaly is generally absent, and patients with hereditary erythrocyte disorders, in which the spleen is generally not enlarged, are outstanding candidates for this approach. Only very experienced laparoscopic surgeons should attempt to apply this technique in patients with an enlarged spleen, particularly patients with massive splenomegaly, and a laparoscopically assisted approach, in which a relatively large incision is made to remove the spleen, is more feasible.

Partial splenectomy can be performed based on the segmental blood supply to the spleen. The spleen is mobilized with good visualization. The inferior segmental arteries are generally ligated, and the artery and veins are ligated as a preliminary demarcation of blood flow to the spleen. The splenic parenchyma is then transected, and the cut to the surface can be controlled with the use of materials that induce coagulation or with the argon beam coagulator.

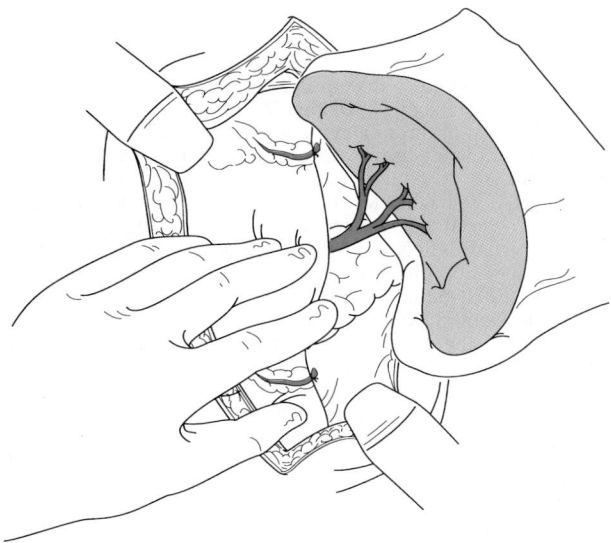

Figure 53.14. Lateral mobilization permits the spleen to reach the surface of a midline wound despite the presence of intact hilar vessels.

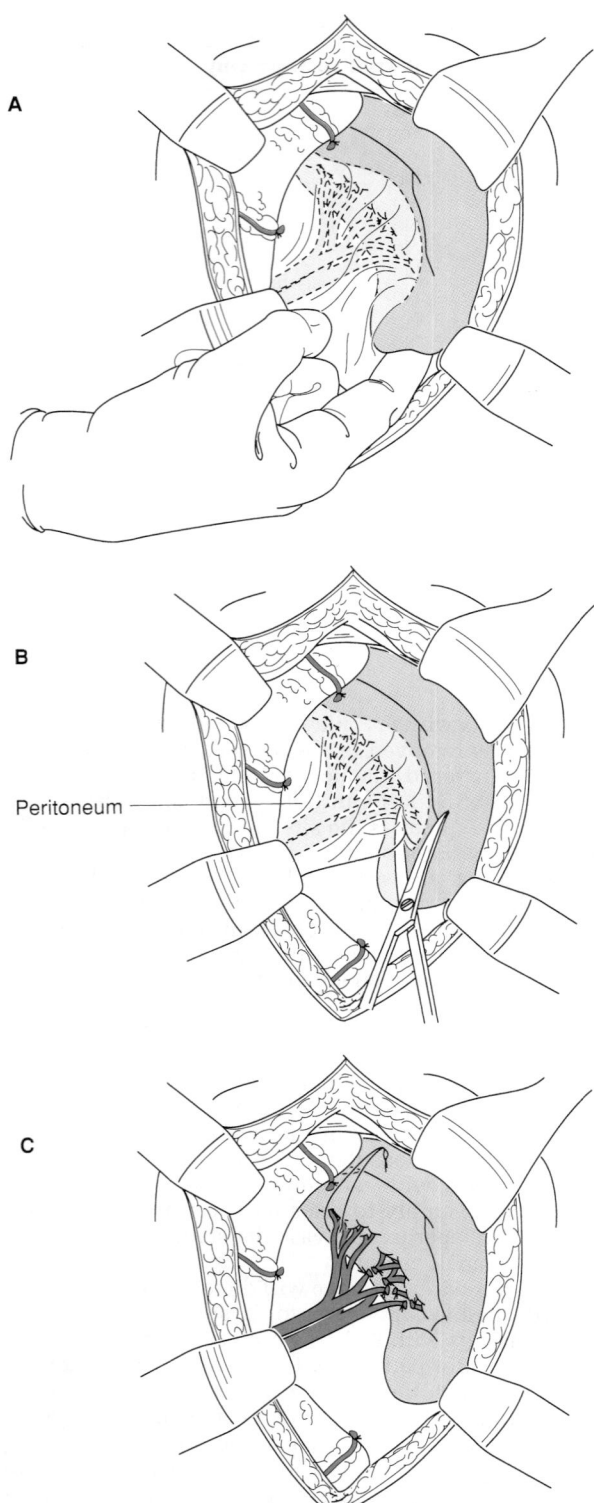

Figure 53.15. Technique for elective splenectomy. *(A)* The inferior pole is reflected laterally by the assistant's fingers to expose the lower edge of the hilar peritoneal envelope. *(B)* The hilar peritoneum is opened, inferiorly to superiorly in this case. *(C)* Individual vessels are identified and ligated with sutures.

REFERENCES

1. McClusky DA 3rd, Skandalakis LJ, Colborn GL, et al. Tribute to a triad: history of splenic anatomy, physiology, and surgery—part 1. *World J Surg* 1999;23:311–325.
2. Morgenstern L. A history of splenectomy. In: Hiatt JR, Phillips EH, Morgenstern L, eds. *Surgical diseases of the spleen.* Berlin: Springer-Verlag, 1997:3-22.
3. McClusky DA, Skandalakis LJ, Colborn GL, et al. Tribute to a triad: history of splenic anatomy, physiology, and surgery—part 2. *World J Surg* 1999;23-40.
4. Skandalakis PN, Colborn GL, Skandalakis LJ, et al. The surgical anatomy of the spleen. *Surg Clin North Am* 1993;73:747–768.
5. Desai DC, Hebra A, Davidoff AM, et al. Wandering spleen: a challenging diagnosis. *South Med J* 1997;90:439–443.
6. Liu DL, Xia S, Xu W, et al. Anatomy of vasculature of 850 spleen specimens and its application in partial splenectomy. *Surgery* 1996;120:574-581.
7. Rosse WF. The spleen as a filter. *N Engl J Med* 1987;317: 704–706.
8. Horowitz J, Leonard D, Smith J, et al. Postsplenectomy leukocytosis: physiologic or an indicator of infection? *Am Surg* 1992;58:387.
9. Lane PA. The spleen in children. *Curr Opin Pediatr* 1995;7: 36–41.
10. Lortan JE. Management of asplenic patients. *Br J Haematol* 1993;84:566–569.
11. Reid MM. Splenectomy, sepsis, immunisation, and guidelines. *Lancet* 1994;344:970–971.
12. Marble KR, Deckers PJ, Kern KA. Changing role of splenectomy for hematologic disease. *J Surg Oncol* 1993;52:169–171.
13. Tchernia G, Gauthier F, Mielot F, et al. Initial assessment of the beneficial effect of partial splenectomy in hereditary spherocytosis. *Blood* 1993;81:2014–2020.
14. Tchernia G, Bader-Meunier B, Berterottier P, et al. Effectiveness of partial splenectomy in hereditary spherocytosis. *Curr Opin Hematol* 1997;4:136–141.
15. Idowu O, Hayes-Jordan A. Partial splenectomy in children under 4 years of age with hemoglobinopathy. *J Pediatr Surg* 1998;33:1251–1253.
16. Al-Salem AH, al-Dabbous I, Bhamidibati P. The role of partial splenectomy in children with thalassemia. *Eur J Pediatr Surg* 1998;8:334–338.
17. Corash L, Shafer B, Blaese RM. Platelet-associated immunoglobulin, platelet size, and the effect of splenectomy in the Wiskott-Aldrich syndrome. *Blood* 1985;65:1439–1443.
18. Muller CA, Anderson KD, Blaese RM. Splenectomy and/or bone marrow transplantation in the management of the Wiskott-Aldrich syndrome: Long-term follow-up in 62 cases. *Blood* 1993;82:2961.
19. Van Krieken JHJM, Breedveld FC, de Velde J. The spleen in Felty's syndrome: a histological, morphometrical, and immunohistochemical study. *Eur J Haematol* 1988;40:58.
20. George JN, el-Harake MA, Raskob GE. Chronic idiopathic thrombocytopenic purpura. *N Engl J Med* 1994;331:1207–1211.
21. Ballem PJ, Belzberg A, Devine DV, et al. Kinetic studies of the mechanism of thrombocytopenia in patients with human immunodeficiency virus infection. *N Engl J Med* 1992;327: 1779–1784.
22. Beer JH, Rabaglio M, Berchtold P, et al. Autoantibodies against the platelet glycoproteins (GP) IIb/IIIa, Ia/IIa, and IV and partial deficiency in GPIV in a patient with a bleeding disorder and a defective platelet collagen interaction. *Blood* 1993;82:820–829.
23. Dan K, Gomi S, Kuramoto A, et al. A multicenter prospective study on the treatment of chronic idiopathic thrombocytopenic purpura. *Int J Hematol* 1992;55:287–292.
24. Andersen JC. Response of resistant idiopathic thrombocytopenic purpura to pulsed high-dose dexamethasone therapy. *N Engl J Med* 1994;330:1560–1564.
25. Sandler SG. The spleen and splenectomy in immune (idiopathic) thrombocytopenic purpura. *Semin Hematol* 2000;37: 10–12.
26. Najean Y, Rain JD, Billotey C. The site of destruction of autologous ^{111}In-labeled platelets and the efficiency of splenectomy in children and adults with idiopathic thrombocy-

topenic purpura: a study of 578 patients with 268 sple-nec-tomies. *Br J Haematol* 1997;97:547–550.

27. Targarona EM, Espert JJ, Balague C, et al. Residual splenic function after laparoscopic splenectomy: a clinical concern. *Arch Surg* 1998;133:56–60.

28. Wells AD, Majumdar G, Slater NG, et al. Role of splenectomy as a salvage procedure in thrombotic thrombocytopenic purpura. *Br J Surg* 1991;78:1389–1390.

29. Coad JE, Matutes E, Catovsky D. Splenectomy in lymphoproliferative disorders: a report on 70 cases and review of the literature. *Leuk Lymphoma* 1993;10:245–264.

30. Zhang B, Lewis SM.. The splenomegaly of myeloproliferative and lymphoproliferative disorders: splenic cellularity and vascularity. *Eur J Haematol* 1989;43:63–66.

31. Tallman MS, Hakimian D, Peterson L. Massive splenomegaly in hairy cell leukemia. *J Clin Oncol* 1998;16:1232–1233.

32. Grever M, Kopecky K, Foucar MK, et al. Randomized comparison of pentostatin versus interferon alpha-2a in previously untreated patients with hairy cell leukemia: an intergroup study. *J Clin Oncol* 1995;13:974–982.

33. Elliott MA, Tefferi A. Splenic irradiation in myelofibrosis with myeloid metaplasia: a review. *Blood Rev* 1999;13:163–170.

34. Delpero JR, Houvenaeghel G, Gastaut JA, et al. Splenectomy for hypersplenism in chronic lymphocytic leukemia and malignant non-Hodgkin's lymphoma. *Br J Surg* 1990;77:554–559.

35. Thiruvengadam R, Piedmonte M, Barcos M, et al. Splenectomy in advanced chronic lymphocytic leukemia. *Leukemia* 1990;4:758–760.

36. Neal TF Jr, Tefferi A, Witzig TE, et al. Splenectomy in advanced chronic lymphocytic leukemia: a single-institution experience with 50 patients. *Am J Med* 1992;93:435–440.

37. Seymour JF, Cusack JD, Lerner SA, et al. Case/control study of the role of splenectomy in chronic lymphocytic leukemia. *J Clin Oncol* 1997;15:52–60.

38. Savage DG, Szydlo RM, Goldman JM. Clinical features at diagnosis in 430 patients with chronic myeloid leukemia seen at a referral centre over a 16-year period. *Br J Haematol* 1997;96:111–116.

39. Hester JP, Waddell CC, Coltman CA, et al. Response of chronic myelogenous leukemia patients to COAP-splenectomy: a Southwest Oncology Group Study. *Cancer* 1984;54:1977–1982.

40. The Italian Cooperative Study on Chronic Myeloid Leukemia: results of a prospective randomized trial of early splenectomy in chronic myeloid leukemia. *Cancer* 1984;54:333–338.

41. Bouvet M, Babiera GV, Termuhlen PM, et al. Splenectomy in the accelerated or blastic phase of chronic myelogenous leukemia: a single-institution, 25-year experience. *Surgery* 1997;122:20–25.

42. Morel P, Dupriez B, Gosselin B, et al. Role of early splenectomy in malignant lymphomas with prominent splenic involvement (primary lymphomas of the spleen). A study of 59 cases. *Cancer* 1993;71:207–215.

43. Nair S, Shukla J, Chandy M. Non-Hodgkin's lymphoma presenting with prominent splenomegaly—clinicopathologic diversity in relationship to immunophenotype. *Acta Oncol* 1997;36:725–727.

44. Lehne G, Hannisdal E, Langholm R, et al. A 10-year experience with splenectomy in patients with malignant non-Hodgkin's lymphoma at the Norwegian Radium Hospital. *Cancer* 1994;74:933–939.

45. Brodsky J, Abcar A, Styler M. Splenectomy for non-Hodgkin's lymphoma. *Am J Clin Oncol* 1996;19:588–561.

46. Reilly JT. Pathogenesis of idiopathic myelofibrosis: present status and future directions. *Br J Haematol* 1994;88:1–8.

47. Barosi G, Ambrosetti A, Buratti A, et al. Splenectomy for patients with myelofibrosis with myeloid metaplasia: pretreatment variables and outcome prediction. *Leukemia* 1993;7:200–206.

48. Tefferi A, Mesa RA, Nagorney DM, et al. Splenectomy in myelofibrosis with myeloid metaplasia: a single-institution experience with 223 patients. *Blood* 2000;95:2226–2233.

49. Austen KF. Systemic mastocytosis. *N Engl J Med* 1992;326:639–640.

50. Friedman B, Darling G, Norton J, et al. Splenectomy in the management of systemic mast cell disease. *Surgery* 1990;107:94–100.

51. Harfi HA, Malik SA. Chédiak-Higashi syndrome: clinical, hematologic, and immunologic improvement after splenectomy. *Ann Allergy* 1992;69:147–150.

52. Cohen IJ, Katz K, Freud E, et al. Long-term follow-up of partial splenectomy in Gaucher's disease. *Am J Surg* 1992;164:345–347.

53. Morgenstern L, Verham R, Weinstein I, et al. Subtotal splenectomy for Gaucher's disease: a follow-up study. *Am Surg* 1993;59:860–865.

54. Zer M, Freud E. Subtotal splenectomy in Gaucher's disease: towards a definition of critical splenic mass. *Br J Surg* 1992;79:742–744.

55. Loftus JP, Nagorney DM, Ilstrup D, et al. Sinistral portal hypertension. Splenectomy or expectant management. *Ann Surg* 1993;217:35–40.

56. DeVita VT Jr, Hubbard SM. Hodgkin's disease. *N Engl J Med* 1993;328:560–565.

57. Blackwell EA, Joshua DE, McLaughlin AF, et al. Early supradiaphragmatic Hodgkin's disease. High-dose gallium scanning obviates the need for staging laparotomy. *Cancer* 1986;58:883.

58. Gospodarowicz MK, Sutcliffe SB, Clark RM, et al. Analysis of supradiaphragmatic clinical stage I and II Hodgkin's disease treated with radiation alone. *Int J Radiat Oncol Biol Phys* 1992;22:859.

59. Wasserman TH, Trenkner DA, Fineberg B, et al. Cure of early-stage Hodgkin's disease with subtotal nodal irradiation. *Cancer* 1991;68:1208.

60. Swerdlow AJ, Douglas AJ, Vaughan Hudson G, et al. Risk of second primary cancer after Hodgkin's disease in patients in the British National Lymphoma Investigation: relationships to host factors, histology, stage of Hodgkin's disease, and splenectomy. *Br J Cancer* 1993;68:1006–1011.

61. Tura S, Fiacchini M, Zinzanni PL, et al. Splenectomy and the increasing risk of secondary acute leukemia in Hodgkin's disease. *J Clin Oncol* 1993;11:925–930.

62. Linet MS, Yren O, Gridley G, et al. Risk of cancer following splenectomy. *Int J Cancer* 1996;66:611–616.

63. Manouras AJ, Nikolaou CC, Katergiannakis VA, et al. Spleen-sparing surgical treatment for echinococcosis of the spleen. *Br J Surg* 1997;84:1162.

64. Reidy JF, Rowe PH, Ellis FG. Splenic artery aneurysm embolisation—the preferred technique to surgery. *Clin Radiol* 1990;41:281–282.

65. Cohen MAA, Galera MJ, Ruiz M, et al. Splenic abscess. *World J Surg* 1990;14:513.

66. De Bree E, Tsiftsis D, Christodoulakis M, et al. Splenic abscess: a diagnostic and therapeutic challenge. *Acta Chir Belg* 1998;98:199–202.

67. Mangus RS, Mann NC, Worrall W, et al. Statewide variation in the treatment of patients hospitalized with spleen injury. *Arch Surg* 1999;134:1378–1384.

68. Morrell DG, Chang FC, Helmer SD. Changing trends in the management of splenic injury. *Am J Surg* 1995;170:686–689.

69. Williams MK, Young DH, Schiller WR. Trend toward nonoperative management of splenic injuries. *Am J Surg* 1990;160:588.

70. Gavant ML, Schurr M, Flick PA, et al. Predicting clinical outcome of nonsurgical management of blunt splenic injury: using CT to reveal abnormalities of splenic vasculature. *AJR Am J Roentgenol* 1997;168:207–212.

71. Villalba MR, Howells GA, Lucas RJ, et al. Nonoperative management of the adult ruptured spleen. *Arch Surg* 1990;125:836–838.

72. Smith JS Jr, Cooney RN, Mucha P Jr. Nonoperative management of the ruptured spleen: a revalidation of criteria. *Surgery* 1996;120:745–750.

73. Konstantakos AK, Barnoski AL, Plaisier BR, et al. Optimizing the management of blunt splenic injury in adults and children. *Surgery* 1999;126:805–812.

74. Lefor AT, Melvin WS, Bailey RW, et al. Laparoscopic splenectomy in the management of immune thrombocytopenia purpura. *Surgery* 1993;114:613–618.

SECTION J

SURGICAL ENDOCRINOLOGY

SURGERY: SCIENTIFIC PRINCIPLES AND PRACTICE, Third Edition, edited by
Lazar J. Greenfield, Michael W. Mulholland, Keith T. Oldham, Gerald B. Zelenock,
and Keith D. Lillemoe. Lippincott Williams & Wilkins Publishers, Philadelphia, © 2001.

CHAPTER 54

THYROID GLAND

ROBERT UDELSMAN

EMBRYOLOGY

The thyroid gland originates predominantly as a midline endodermal diverticulum that arises between the first and second pharyngeal pouches. Its site of origin in the region of the foramen cecum is recognizable at about the fourth week of gestation. The diverticulum grows and descends into the neck as a hollow cylinder of epithelial cells that passes ventral to the developing hyoid bone. The hollow cylinder consolidates during its caudal descent and develops into a bilobed organ. By the end of the seventh week, it has assumed a shieldlike shape and is located anterior to the developing trachea (1).

The duct through which the thyroid descended normally atrophies, and the original pharyngeal connection can be identified at the apex of the sulcus terminalis on the dorsum of the tongue as the foramen cecum. The two lobes remain connected by a narrow isthmus of thyroid tissue. Thyroid follicular cell function develops by the third month, when iodine trapping and thyroid hormone secretion begin (2).

The neural crest-derived calcitonin-secreting C cells develop from the ultimobranchial fourth pharyngeal pouches. They coalesce and migrate into the posterior aspect of the upper two thirds of the lateral thyroid lobes and assume positions scattered among the thyroid follicles.

Congenital Abnormalities

Congenital variations and abnormalities of the thyroid occur infrequently. Failure of thyroidal descent results in a lingual thyroid that is associated with agenesis of a eutopic thyroid gland. Therefore, a lingual thyroid is likely to represent the only functional thyroid tissue in an individual patient. A lingual thyroid may present as a mass in the base of the tongue that causes airway obstruction, dysphagia, or hemorrhage. The majority of patients with symptomatic lingual thyroid glands are treated by the administration of thyroid hormone, which results in the suppression of thyroid-stimulating hormone and subsequent atrophy of the lingual thyroid. Radioiodine therapy or surgical intervention is occasionally required for obstructive symptoms (3).

Thyroglossal duct cysts develop as a result of incomplete atrophy and involution of the thyroglossal duct.

They usually occur at or near the midline and are most commonly noted in infancy or childhood. They are often asymptomatic, although infection and spontaneous drainage can result in a chronically draining fistula. The diagnosis should be suspected in any patient with a midline or paramedian neck mass. The cysts elevate when the tongue is protruded and in some cases can be transilluminated. They are often lined by thyroid epithelium, which can give rise to thyroid carcinoma.

Surgical excision is the treatment of choice for thyroglossal cysts except when they are acutely infected, in which case drainage and staged resection is indicated. Surgical management of a thyroglossal duct cyst requires excision of the cyst in continuity with the central portion of the hyoid bone (4). Failure to excise the entire thyroglossal duct tract up to the foramen cecum is associated with recurrent cyst formation and the need for remedial surgery.

Thyroid carcinoma can arise in a thyroglossal cyst, and the cysts must be carefully examined histologically. These are usually papillary thyroid carcinomas, and local excision may be adequate in a subset of patients. However, in the setting of lymph node metastases, additional thyroid nodules, or the need to administer radioactive iodine, total thyroidectomy and possible lymph node dissection are indicated.

Ectopic thyroid tissue can be located in the neck or mediastinum. It occurs most commonly immediately inferior to the lower poles of the thyroid gland. This tissue may not have an anatomic connection to the thyroid gland. When located medial to the internal jugular veins in the central compartment of the neck, it may represent benign, sequestered thyroid nodules. However, when such nodules are located lateral to the internal jugular vein or in the carotid sheath, they represent metastatic thyroid carcinoma in cervical lymph nodes.

SURGICAL ANATOMY

The normal adult thyroid gland weighs between 15 and 25 g and is located in the lower neck. It extends from the cricoid cartilage and covers the anterior tracheal rings, wrapping around the anterolateral portion of the trachea. The thyroid gland consists of right and left lobes connected by the isthmus, which usually extends anterior to the second and third tracheal rings. Not uncommonly, a pyramidal lobe is present that ascends toward the hyoid bone, often from the upper portion of the isthmus, although it may extend from either the right or the left lobe superiorly. Occasionally, a fibrous band connects the body of the hyoid bone to the isthmus or pyramidal lobe, and when muscular, it is termed the *levator of the thyroid gland*. The posterior medial aspects of the thyroid lobes are attached to the cricoid cartilage by the ligament of Berry, which is also referred to as the *suspensory ligament of the thyroid* (2,5).

The thyroid gland is covered by a thin capsule of connective tissue and is divided into irregular masses by extensions

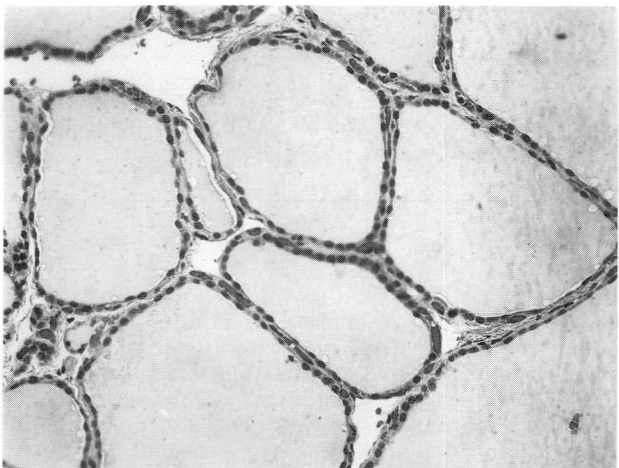

Figure 54.1. Normal thyroid histology. Thyroid follicles contain follicular cells surrounding intraluminal colloid. (Courtesy of Dr. William Westra, Department of Pathology, Johns Hopkins Hospital, Baltimore, MD.)

of this connective tissue into the thyroid parenchyma. The gland contains two major cell types, the thyroid follicular cells, which secrete thyroid hormone, and the parafollicular C cells, which secrete calcitonin. Thyroid epithelial cells form spherical groups of follicles that contain a semifluid viscous colloid material that is seen as a pink, amorphous fluid on routine histologic analysis. The follicles are arranged in groups to form glands that are each lined by a single layer of cubidal epithelium. Normal thyroid histology is demonstrated in Fig. 54.1. The parafollicular C cells are located predominantly in the upper two thirds of the thyroid lobe between the thyroid follicles.

Muscular Relationships

The thyroid gland is covered anteriorly by the sternothyroid muscle, which in turn is covered by the sternohyoid muscle (Fig. 54.2). Anterolaterally, the sternal head of the sternocleidomastoid muscle is present. Posterolaterally, the lateral thyroid lobes are bounded by the carotid sheaths.

Vascular Anatomy

The thyroid gland is highly vascular, each lobe supplied by two major groups of arteries and drained by three ve-

nous complexes (Fig. 54.3). The superior thyroid artery usually arises as the first branch of the external carotid artery near the bifurcation of the common carotid artery. It descends on the surface of the inferior pharyngeal constrictor muscle and divides into a dominant anterior and a smaller posterior branch at the upper portion of the lateral thyroid lobes. It is not uncommon for the external branch of the superior laryngeal nerve to be intimately associated with branches of the superior thyroid artery near the upper poles of the thyroid gland. The inferior thyroid artery arises from the thyrocervical trunk and ascends behind the carotid sheath, passing downward and medially to enter the midportion of the lateral thyroid lobes. The inferior thyroid artery is intimately associated with a recurrent laryngeal nerve, as described below. Occasionally, a thyroidea ima artery emanates directly from the innominate artery or the aorta and enters the lower surface of the isthmus or one of the thyroid lobes.

The thyroid gland is drained by three groups of veins. The superior thyroid veins form a complex at the apex of the thyroid lobes and drain into the internal jugular veins. The middle thyroid veins arise at the midportion of the lateral surface of the thyroid lobes and drain into the internal jugular veins. The inferior thyroid veins drain the inferior poles of the thyroid lobes and empty into the innominate or internal jugular veins.

Nerves

The recurrent laryngeal nerves are branches of the vagus and supply all the intrinsic muscles of the larynx with the exception of the cricothyroid muscle. The right recurrent laryngeal nerve arises from the vagus in front of the first portion of the right subclavian artery. It then passes around the subclavian artery and ascends obliquely on the right side of the trachea behind the common carotid artery (Fig. 54.4). As it ascends, it is intimately associated with the inferior thyroid artery and may cross in front of, behind, or between branches of this vessel (Fig. 54.5). On the left, the recurrent laryngeal nerve recurs around the arch of the aorta behind the attachment of the ligamentum arteriosum and ascends in the tracheoesophageal groove. It is also intimately associated with the inferior thyroid artery. The recurrent laryngeal nerves continue their superior ascent and pass posterior to the thyroid gland. They are not uncommonly embedded in the posterior aspect of the ligament of Berry (Fig. 54.6). Furthermore, the recurrent laryngeal nerves often have extralaryngeal branches that supply the esophagus and muscular fibers of the trachea in addition to the larynx. The recurrent laryngeal nerves enter the larynx behind the articulation of the infe-

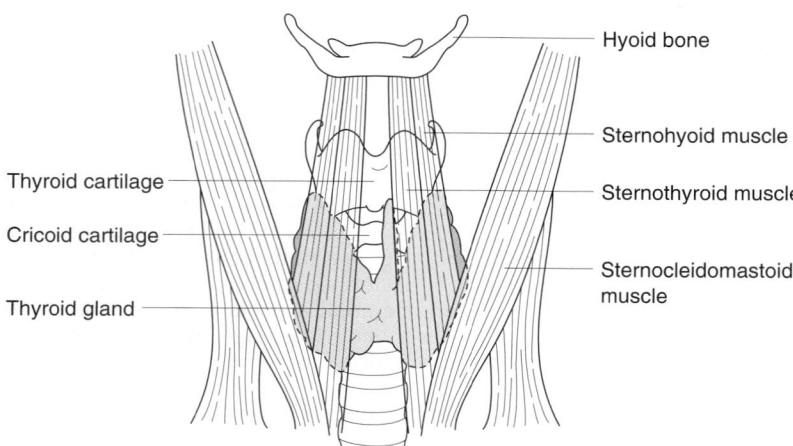

Hyoid bone

Sternohyoid muscle

Thyroid cartilage

Sternothyroid muscle

Cricoid cartilage

Sternocleidomastoid muscle

Thyroid gland

Figure 54.2. Muscular relationships to the thyroid gland.

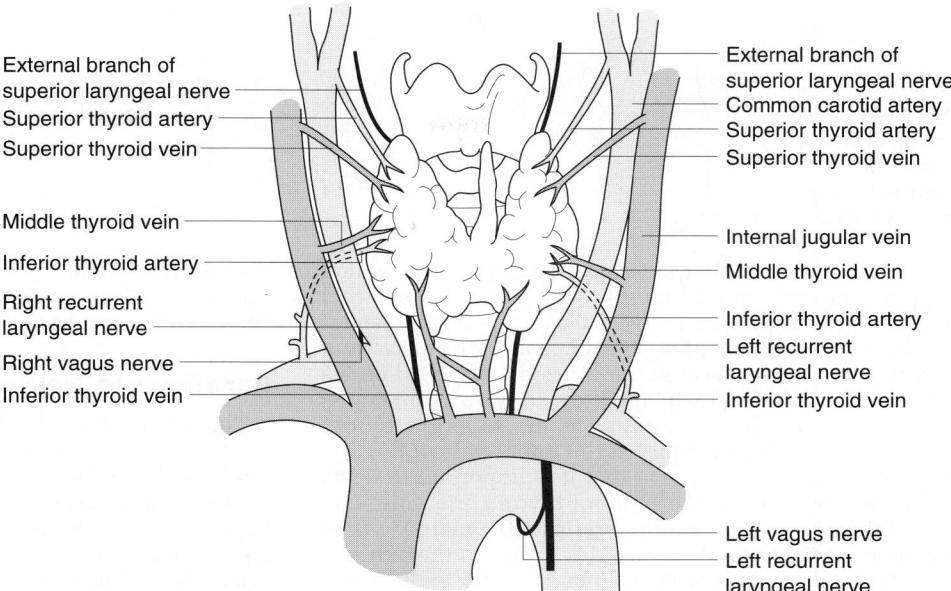

Figure 54.3. Vascular relationships to the thyroid gland.

rior cornu of the thyroid with the cricoid cartilage. The recurrent laryngeal nerves, in addition to supplying the muscles of the larynx, communicate with the internal laryngeal nerves supplying sensory nerves to the mucous membrane of the larynx. Injury to a recurrent laryngeal nerve results in paralysis of the ipsilateral vocal cord. The vocal cord becomes immobile, usually in the paramedian position. Unilateral vocal cord paresis can be minimally symptomatic but can also markedly alter the voice quality; if bilateral, it can severely compromise the airway.

It is important for the surgeon to be cognizant of anatomic variants of the recurrent laryngeal nerve. A nonrecurrent "recurrent laryngeal nerve" occurs on the right

in approximately 1% of persons (Fig. 54.4). In this case, the nerve arises from the vagus at the level of the cricoid cartilage and passes directly to the larynx. It is often closely associated with and parallel to the inferior thyroid artery and may be mistaken for an arterial branch. It is therefore subject to injury. A nonrecurrent nerve on the left is even more unusual. When present, it is usually associated with major vascular abnormalities involving a right-sided aortic arch or a retroesophageal aberrant left subclavian artery.

The bilateral superior laryngeal nerves arise from the inferior ganglion of the vagus and pass medial to the carotid arteries. They divide into a large sensory internal laryn-

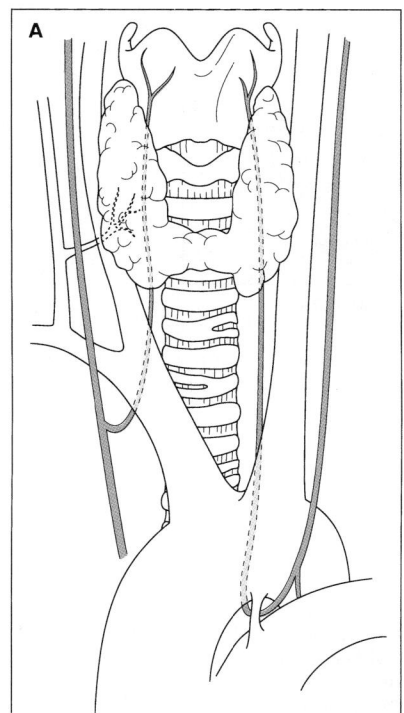
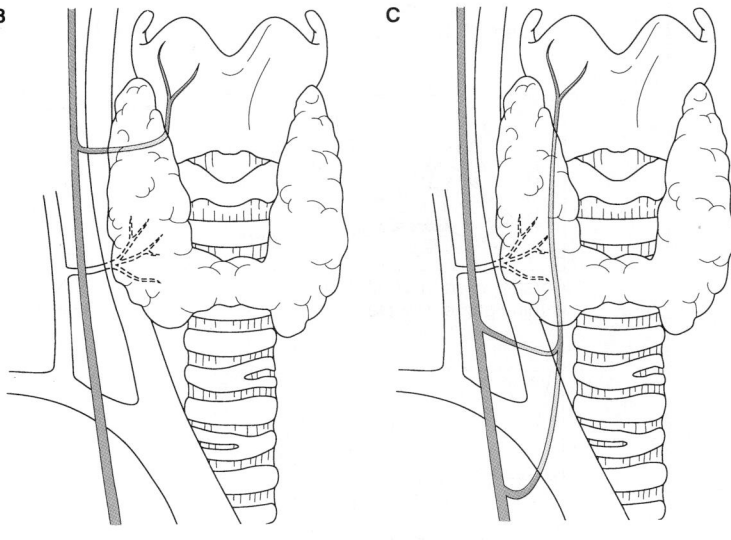

Figure 54.4. Relationships of the recurrent laryngeal nerve to the thyroid gland. *(A)* Normal course of right recurrent laryngeal nerve. *(B)* Nonrecurrent nerve from vagus. *(C)* Rare, nonrecurrent nerve and recurrent laryngeal nerve join to form a common distal nerve.

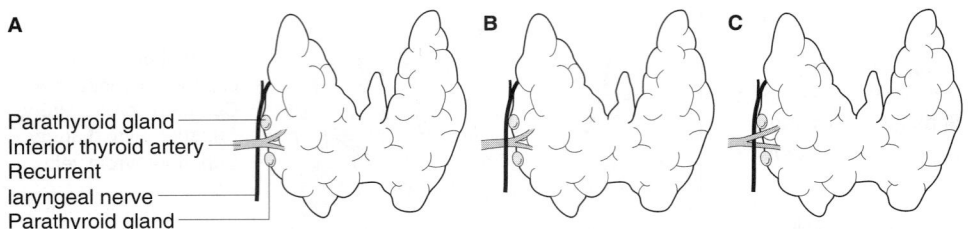

A

Parathyroid gland
Inferior thyroid artery
Recurrent
laryngeal nerve
Parathyroid gland

B

C

Figure 54.5. Relationship between recurrent laryngeal nerve and inferior thyroid artery. *(A)* Nerve posterior. *(B)* Nerve anterior. *(C)* Nerve between branches of artery.

geal nerve and a smaller external laryngeal nerve, which supplies the cricothyroid muscle (Fig. 54.3). The external branch of the superior laryngeal nerve lies on the lateral surface of the inferior pharyngeal constrictor muscle and descends medial to the superior thyroid artery as it enters the cricothyroid muscle. In approximately 15% of people, this nerve is in close proximity to the superior thyroid artery and is at risk for injury at the upper pole of the thyroid lobe. It is for this reason that it is important to ligate individual branches of the superior thyroid artery directly on the thyroid capsule and not to ligate the main trunk of the superior thyroid artery and risk injury to the external branch of the superior laryngeal nerve. Injury to the external branch of the superior laryngeal nerve results in paralysis of the cricothyroid muscle and an inability to tense the vocal cord. This results in an inability to reach and

sustain high-pitched notes and project one's voice, which can have devastating consequences for professional singers, speakers, and educators.

Parathyroid Relationships

The parathyroid glands are intimately associated with the thyroid gland and are at risk during thyroid surgery. The blood supply to the parathyroid glands is predominantly through a small terminal branch of the inferior thyroid artery (6). Occasionally, the superior thyroid artery also contributes a small branch. The terminal blood supply to the parathyroid glands is via a single end-artery; injury to this artery results in ischemic necrosis of the involved parathyroid gland. Furthermore, the inferior thyroid artery also supplies the thyroid gland. Therefore,

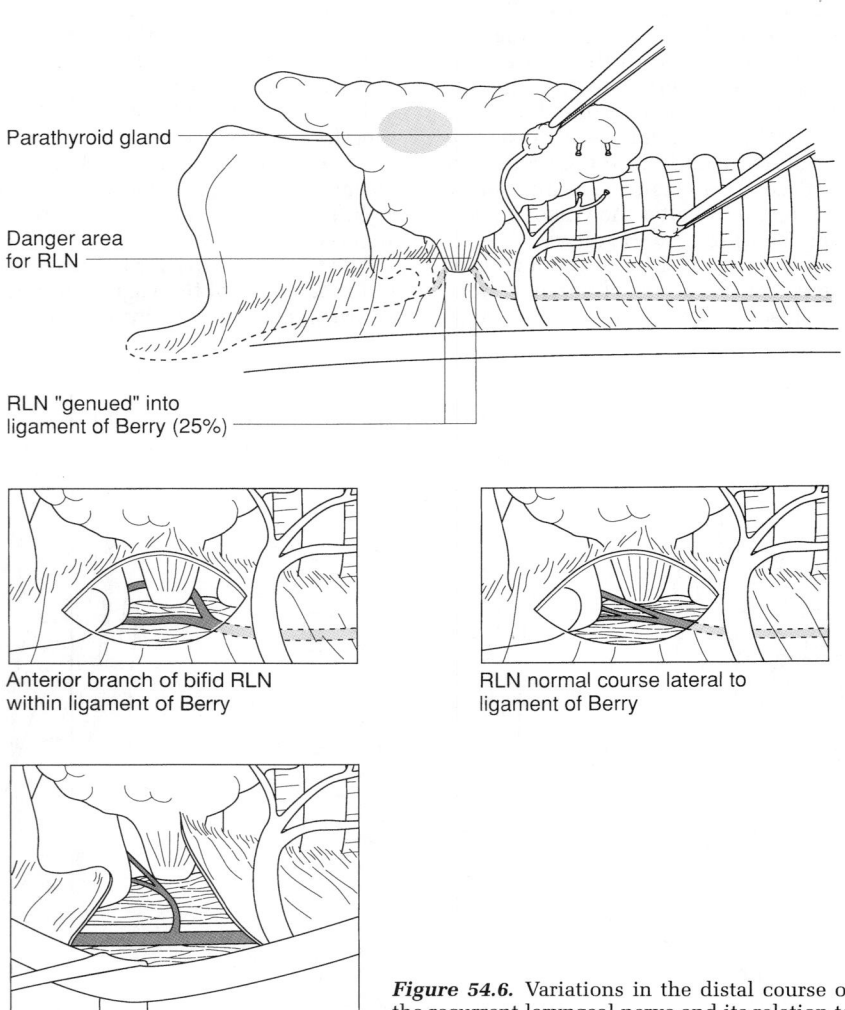

Parathyroid gland

Danger area
for RLN

RLN "genued" into
ligament of Berry (25%)

Anterior branch of bifid RLN
within ligament of Berry

RLN normal course lateral to
ligament of Berry

Non-RLN arising from vagus (1%)
on right side

Figure 54.6. Variations in the distal course of the recurrent laryngeal nerve and its relation to the posterior ligament of Berry of the thyroid gland. This is the region where the nerve is most at risk during thyroidectomy.

when mobilizing the parathyroid gland, the surgeon must be aware of the delicate nature of this end-arterial supply. When dissecting the parathyroid gland off the thyroid capsule, one must ligate terminal branches of the inferior thyroid artery distal to the parathyroid blood supply and not at the main trunk of the inferior thyroid artery. A close relationship also exists between the parathyroid glands and the junction between the inferior thyroid artery and the recurrent laryngeal nerve. Most parathyroid glands can be found within a 1-cm radius of this junction. The parathyroid glands can be supernumerary or ectopic.

Lymphatic Anatomy

The lymphatic drainage of the thyroid gland is extensive and multidirectional, characterized by intrathyroidal cross-communication between opposite lobes and the isthmus. Despite the extensive intrathyroidal communication, the pattern of lymphatic drainage is predictable, which is the basis for regional lymphadenectomy in the setting of thyroid cancer. The lymphatic drainage areas can be divided into two basic groups. The first, called the *central component* or *paraglandular space,* includes the prelaryngeal, pretracheal, and paratracheal lymph nodes in the tracheoesophageal grooves, in addition to the anterior superior mediastinal lymph nodes. For practical purposes, this area can be defined as extending from the hyoid bone superiorly to the left innominate vein inferiorly, and laterally to both carotid sheaths. The lymph nodes present in the midline immediately superior to the thyroid gland are often referred to as the *Delphian nodes*. The second area of lymphatic drainage is into the lateral and posterior neck zones. The lymphatic zones of the neck are divided into six regions, demonstrated in Fig. 54.7. Surgeons who operate on the thyroid gland must have a detailed knowledge of these lymphatic zones, as it is not uncommon to encounter metastatic disease in the central or lateral neck during thyroidectomy. This is particularly important for patients with medullary carcinoma of the thyroid, in whom extensive nodal dissections are performed routinely.

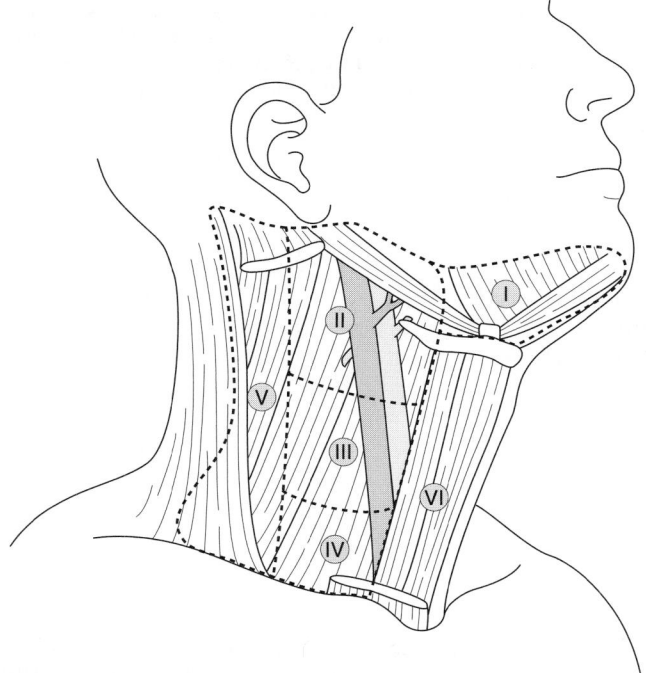

Figure 54.7. Lymphatic zones of the neck.

THYROID PHYSIOLOGY

Thyroid hormone production and release are under the control of the hypothalamic–pituitary–thyroid axis, as shown in Fig. 54.8. Thyrotropin-releasing hormone (TRH) produced within the hypothalamus traverses the infundibulum and then binds to receptors on the membranes of the thyrotrope cells in the anterior pituitary gland. Thyroid-stimulating hormone (TSH, thyrotropin), the major regulator of thyroid gland activity, is composed of alpha and beta subunits. The alpha subunit is identical to those in other glycoprotein hormones, including follicle-stimulating hormone (FSH), luteinizing hormone (LH), and human chorionic gonadotropin (hCG). TSH is released from the anterior pituitary gland into the peripheral circulation and then binds to a G-protein-coupled receptor on the surface of the thyroid cell (7).

Regulation of the hypothalamic–pituitary–thyroid axis is characterized by negative feedback of thyroid hormones on hypothalamic TRH production, TRH receptors on thyrotropes, and the synthesis and release of TSH. A pituitary deiodinase converts thyroxine (T_4) to triiodothyronine (T_3), which binds to the T_3 receptor. This in turn negatively regulates expression of the TSH beta and alpha subunit genes. Cyclic adenosine monophosphate (AMP) is the principal second messenger mediating TSH action, stimulating all steps in the synthesis and secretion of thyroid hormones.

The thyroid gland consists of two distinct functional units, the thyroid follicular cells, in which T_4 and T_3 are synthesized, and the parafollicular C cells, which produce calcitonin. The functional unit for thyroid hormone production is the thyroid follicle. The major steps of thyroid hormone synthesis and secretion are illustrated in Fig. 54.9. Iodine is normally ingested in food and water. In the United States, the daily iodine intake is approximately 200 to 500 µg, which is largely accounted for by iodized salt, bread with iodate preservatives, and milk products containing trace amounts of iodine disinfectants. The iodide is absorbed rapidly and is distributed to the extracellular compartment, which also receives iodide released from the thyroid. The daily dietary intake of iodine varies dramatically throughout the world. Although iodine deficiency is nonexistent in the United States, endemic goiter occurs when the daily iodine intake is less than 40 µg. When iodine deficiency is more severe (i.e., < 20 µg/d), cretinism can occur. Iodide is transported into the thyroid follicular cells by the sodium–iodide symporter (NIS) against both concentration and electrochemical gradients at the basal membrane. This energy-dependent process requires oxidative metabolism, phosphorylation, and the presence of TSH. Inorganic iodide is rapidly oxidized and covalently liked to tyrosine residues within the thyroid-specific protein thyroglobulin. This process occurs at the apical membrane and is catalyzed by thyroid peroxidase (TPO). The resulting iodotyrosines, monoiodotyrosine (MIT) and diiodotyrosine (DIT), are then coupled by an ester bond to form T_4 or T_3. The thyroid hormones remain covalently bound to thyroglobulin and are stored in the colloid within the lumen of the thyroid follicle.

The release of thyroid hormone is initiated by TSH, which stimulates the follicular cells to form pseudopodia at the apical membrane that endocytose thyroglobulin. The thyroid hormone–thyroglobulin complex undergoes hydrolysis, and T_4 and T_3 are released via the basement membrane into the peripheral circulation. Most of the thyroglobulin is retained within the follicular cells under normal conditions.

The normal daily thyroidal secretion rate of T_4 is approximately 70 to 90 µg, and that of T_3 is between 15 and

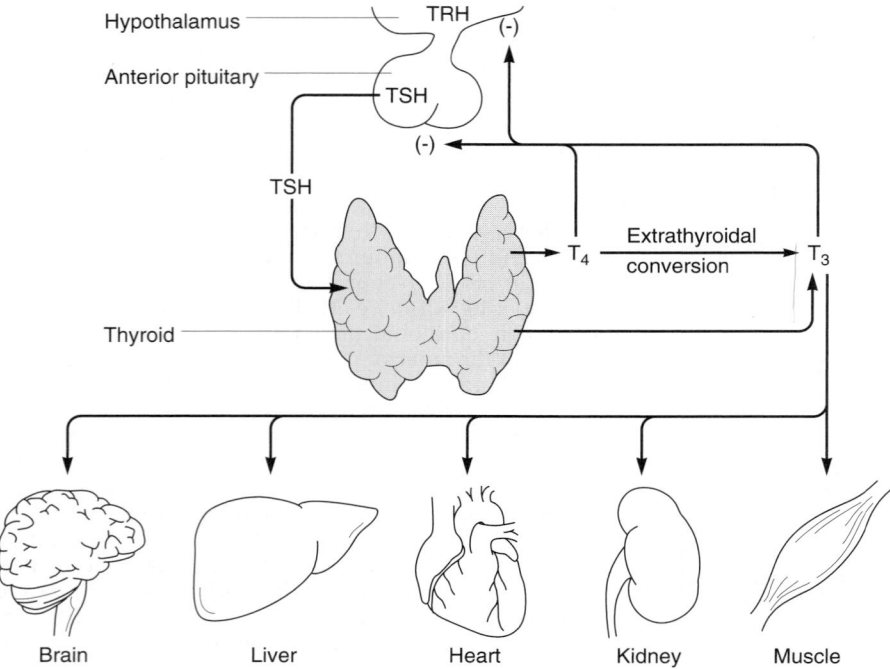

Figure ***54.8.*** Hypothalmic–pituitary–thyroid axis. *TRH,* thyrotropin-releasing hormone; *TSH,* thyroid-stimulating hormone; T_4, thyroxine; T_3, triiodothyronine.

30 µg. The thyroid gland is the only source of T_4, whereas most T_3 is produced by the extrathyroidal deiodination of T_4 in target tissues.

Peripheral Actions of Thyroid Hormone

Most (> 99.5%) of the thyroid hormones released into the circulation are bound to binding proteins in serum. These proteins include thyroxine-binding globulin, thyroxine-binding prealbumin, and albumin. The binding proteins act as reservoirs to maintain an equilibrium between bound and free thyroid hormones. The small amounts of free T_4 and T_3 are directly available for ligand–receptor interactions in the peripheral tissues. Changes in the concentration of serum binding proteins have marked effects on the total concentration of thyroid hormones. However, the levels of free thyroid hormones are maintained in a relatively constant range.

Thyroxine-binding globulin, the most abundant binding protein, is actually a glycoprotein synthesized in the liver. Its serum level is significantly increased in patients receiving exogenous estrogen and in pregnant women. In addition, chronic diseases and starvation may reduce the available binding proteins because hepatic synthesis is impaired. However, patients with nonthyroidal illness maintain relatively normal levels of free thyroid hormones. The circulating half-life of T_4 is approximately 7 days, and that of T_3 is 1 day.

Free T_4 and free T_3 enter peripheral target cells primarily by facilitated diffusion. Within the cells, T_4 is readily converted to T_3 by thyroxine 5′-deiodinases. Thyroid hormone actions are initiated by the interaction of T_3 with nuclear T_3 receptors. These receptors have been cloned, and

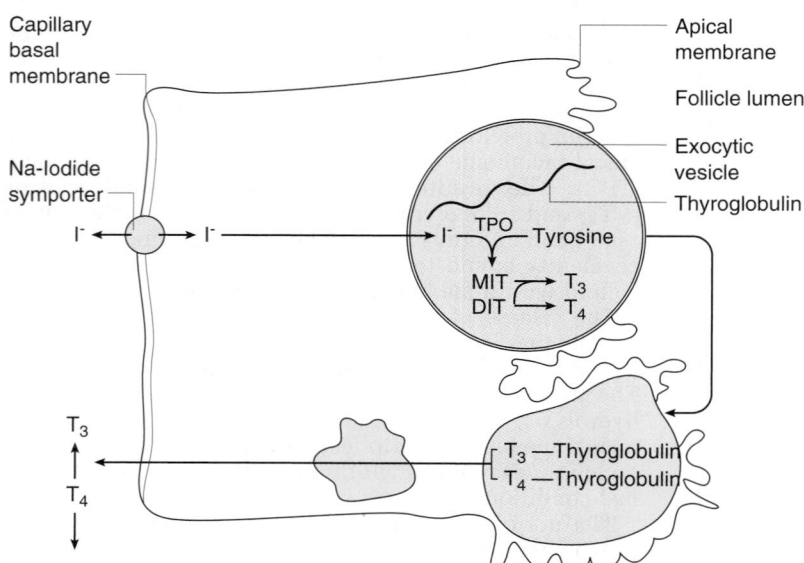

Figure 54.9. Thyroid hormone synthesis and secretion. *I^-,* iodide; *TPO,* thyroid peroxidase; *MIT,* monoiodotyrosine; *DIT,* diiodotyrosine; T_3, triiodothyronine; T_4, thyroxine.

many of the molecular mechanisms of thyroid hormone action have been elucidated (8). T_3 receptors contain three functional domains: a ligand-binding carboxyl terminal portion, a DNA-binding domain, and an amino terminal domain. The DNA-binding domain includes two "zinc fingers" that determine the specific DNA sequence to which the monomeric receptor binds. The specific DNA sequences that bind T_3 receptors determine which genes are stimulated or inhibited by T_3. Two T_3 receptor genes exist, termed *alpha* and *beta,* and tissue-specific expression of distinct subtypes occurs. The content of T_3 receptors is high in tissues such as pituitary and liver, which are exceedingly responsive to thyroid hormone (8).

Thyroid hormones modulate numerous metabolic responses and are required for normal growth and development (Fig. 54.8). They are intimately involved in thermogenic actions, modulation of catecholamine activities, protein synthesis, and carbohydrate and lipid metabolism. In addition, they reduce systemic vascular resistance and enhance cardiac contractility.

THYROID FUNCTION TESTS

A wide variety of blood-based thyroid function tests are available (9–13). A partial list and description of the most commonly used tests follows.

Thyroid-stimulating Hormone (Thyrotropin)

Normal serum TSH values range from 0.4 to 4.5 mIU/L. The highly sensitive TSH assay is the single most useful test to determine functional thyroid status. The so-called third-generation assay is capable of detecting TSH concentrations as low as 0.01 mU/L (14). In patients with hypothyroidism, insufficient thyroid hormone levels stimulate the pituitary gland to secrete TSH, which causes additional secretion of T_4 and T_3, which in turn inhibits additional TSH secretion. Older, second-generation TSH assays can detect concentrations only as low as 1.0 mU/L. This level of sensitivity is adequate to determine whether a patient is hypothyroid (elevated TSH) but cannot reliably distinguish between TSH concentrations in normal and hyperthyroid patients. It is therefore important to know the sensitivity of the TSH assay in a given institution.

Thyroxine

The total serum T_4 concentration is often determined by competitive protein-binding assays that measure the combined total of free and bound T_4. Most T_4 (> 99.97%) is bound to thyroxine-binding globulin, thyroxine-binding prealbumin, or albumin. Therefore, an increase in the serum proteins, particularly thyroxine-binding globulin, can cause an increase in the total T_4 concentration, which can be misinterpreted as thyrotoxicosis. Common causes of increased levels of thyroxine-binding globulin include pregnancy and exogenous administration of estrogen. Conditions that decrease the serum total T_4 concentration include the administration of anabolic steroids, inherited disorders, and the nephrotic syndrome. Despite these caveats, total serum T_4 concentrations are elevated in most patients with hyperthyroidism and decreased in patients with hypothyroidism.

Free Thyroxine

Measurement of the free T_4 concentration by radioimmunoassay and other methods avoids many of the potential pitfalls associated with total T_4 measurements. These tests are relatively sensitive, accurate, and expensive. The concentration of free T_4 in the blood is elevated in patients with hyperthyroidism.

Serum Total or Free Triiodothyronine

Serum total and free T_3 concentrations are generally elevated in patients with thyrotoxicosis. The total serum T_3 concentration reflects the sum of free and bound T_3 in the circulation. Therefore, an increase in serum binding proteins will cause an increase in the total T_3 concentration. Measurement of total or free serum T_3 is generally reserved for patients suspected of having toxicosis. It can be useful to detect rare cases of T_3 toxicosis and to assess the severity of hyperthyroidism.

Resin Uptake of Triiodothyronine

This test was designed to measure the effects of thyroid hormone-binding protein on serum thyroid hormone levels. It is usually performed in conjunction with measurement of total T_4. The T_3 resin uptake test measures the number of unoccupied protein binding sites for T_4. The test is performed by mixing radioactively tagged T_3 with serum, adding a resin, and then determining the amount of radioactively labeled T_3 that binds to the resin. The labeled T_3 will bind either to the resin or to the binding protein in the serum. If the patient has excess levels of thyroid hormone in the serum, thyroid hormone will already be bound to the binding proteins, and therefore more of the labeled T_3 will bind to the resin, resulting in a high reading. If the patient is hypothyroid, more serum protein binding sites are available for labeled T_3, and less T_3 will bind to the resin. The rate of resin uptake of T_3 is also be low in patients with excess thyroid hormone-binding proteins because their binding sites will bind radioactive T_3. The serum total T_4 and T_3 resin uptake should be evaluated simultaneously. If the resin uptake of both total T_4 and T_3 is high, or if the resin uptake of both is low, then thyroid hormone secretion is abnormal. If the uptake of both is decreased, the patient is hypothyroid. Discordance between the T_3 resin uptake and the total T_4 serum concentration suggests an abnormality in thyroid hormone-binding proteins. For example, the exogenous administration of estrogen results in elevated levels of thyroid hormone-binding globulins (low resin uptake of T_3) and elevated total serum T_4 concentrations.

Free Thyroxine Index

The free thyroxine index (FT$_4$I) is calculated by multiplying total serum T_4 by the resin uptake of T_3. It is designed to provide a single index that accounts for thyroxine-binding globulin levels. In cases of thyrotoxicosis, the FT$_4$I is high because the resin uptake of both total T_4 and T_3 is elevated. In contrast, patients who are euthyroid but have elevated levels of thyroxine-binding globulin (pregnancy or estrogen use) will have a normal FT$_4$I because the total T_4 is high but the resin uptake of T_3 is low.

Serum Antibodies

Patients with autoimmune thyroid diseases, including Graves' disease and Hashimoto's thyroiditis, often have detectable levels of serum antimicrosomal or antithyroglobulin antibodies.

Thyroid-stimulating Immunoglobulin

Measurement of thyroid-stimulating immunoglobulin is rarely required in the management of patients with Graves' disease.

Serum Thyroglobulin Concentration

Most thyroglobulin is retained within the thyroid gland. However, small amounts (5 to 25 ng/mL) can be detected in the circulation of normal persons. Thyroid disease, including thyroiditis, radiation injury, Graves' disease, and thyroid tumors (benign or malignant), can cause an increase in circulating thyroglobulin levels.

The main clinical use of serum thyroglobulin measurement is in the follow-up of patients with well-differentiated thyroid cancer. Patients who have undergone a total thyroidectomy or a subtotal thyroid resection and thyroid remnant ablation with radioactive iodine should have low or undetectable levels of serum thyroglobulin. A persistent rise in the serum thyroglobulin after ablative therapy is highly suggestive of recurrent thyroid cancer.

Approximately 20% of patients have antithyroglobulin antibodies that interfere with thyroglobulin measurement.

THYROID IMAGING

A variety of imaging procedures are available and have specific roles in the management of thyroid disease. Routine radiography of the neck not uncommonly demonstrates a cervical or mediastinal soft-tissue mass that may cause deviation of the airway. Additional thyroid-imaging studies were once obtained during the routine evaluation of dominant thyroid nodules. However, because of the availability and accuracy of fine-needle aspiration (FNA), the role of thyroid imaging has diminished. Imaging continues to play an important role in the evaluation of hyperperfusioning nodules and invasive lesions, and in the follow-up of thyroid cancer.

Imaging studies include ultrasonography, radionuclide scintigraphy, computed tomography (CT), magnetic resonance imaging (MRI), and positron emission tomography (PET).

Ultrasonography

Ultrasonography is a safe, noninvasive, sensitive, and innocuous technique that employs reflected sound waves to identify the size, shape, and density characteristics of thyroid nodules. It can differentiate solid from cystic lesions and can also demonstrate the presence of cervical lymphadenopathy. Nodules as small as 2 to 3 mm can be detected by high-resolution (5 to 10 MHz), real-time sonography. Thyroid ultrasonography cannot reliably distinguish between benign and malignant nodules. However, malignant nodules tend to be hypoechoic (63%) in comparison with the remainder of the thyroid parenchyma (15). Hyperechoic solid nodules are usually benign (96%) (16). Punctate calcifications within a nodule suggest psammoma bodies and raise the suspicion of papillary carcinoma (17). Simple cystic lesions that are smooth-walled, anechoic, and associated with acoustic enhancement are almost always benign (16). However, nodularity or mural projections within a thyroid cyst can be seen in papillary carcinoma.

Despite the ease and accuracy of thyroid ultrasonography for the detection of thyroid nodules, its lack of specificity limits its clinical utility. FNA of a dominant thyroid nodule obviates many of these limitations and is now widely considered to be the first-line diagnostic study.

Radionuclide Imaging

Radionuclide thyroid scintigraphy plays an important role in the management of thyroid disease and has the advantage of demonstrating thyroid function. The three most commonly used radionuclides for thyroid imaging are technetium pertechnetate Tc 99m (^{99m}TcO$_4$), iodine 123 (^{123}I), and iodine 131 (^{131}I).

Thyroid nodules in which the avidity for radionuclides is decreased in comparison with the normal thyroid tissue are termed *cold* and are malignant in up to 20% of cases. However, the majority of cold lesions represent degenerative nodules, colloid nodules, nonfunctioning adenomas, cysts, inflammatory nodules, or nonthyroid neoplasms. The finding of multiple nonfunctioning nodules further suggests benign disease.

A nodule in which the avidity for administered radioisotope is increased relative to the remainder of the thyroid gland is described as *hot*. A hot nodule is almost always benign, although rare cases of thyroid cancer have been reported in association with such nodules. A *warm* nodule concentrates the radioisotope to a similar degree as does the normal thyroid gland. Multiple hot or warm nodules can be seen in multinodular goiters.

Technetium Pertechnetate Tc 99m

Technetium pertechnetate Tc 99m is the most commonly employed thyroid imaging radionuclide (Fig. 54.10). The pertechnetate ions, similar to iodine, are trapped by the thyroid follicular cells via an active transport mechanism. However, organification does not occur, as it does with iodine. Advantages of pertechnetate scanning are that the entire study can be performed relatively easily during a single visit, little radiation is emitted, and a high-quality image can be obtained at a relatively low cost (17). Scanning with ^{99m}Tc-pertechnetate is useful in the evaluation of functional thyroid nodules. However, iodine-based scans are preferred for the evaluation of cold nodules and intrathoracic goiter and for dosimetry in the setting of thyroid cancer treatment.

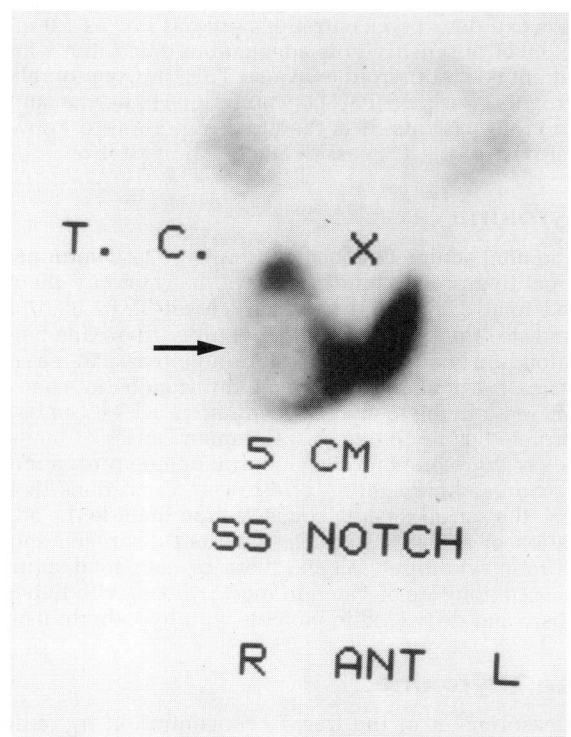

Figure 54.10. Technetium scan demonstrating a cold nodule *(arrow)* in the right lobe of the thyroid.

Iodine 123

A cyclotron is required to produce ^{123}I; furthermore, it has a relatively short half-life (13.2 hours), which increases its cost and decreases its availability. It is both trapped and organified by the thyroid gland and can therefore be used to assess thyroid functional status. [123]I delivers much less radiation than ^{131}I and produces images of good quality (17,18).

Iodine 131

Iodine 131 is readily available and is both trapped and organified by the thyroid gland. Its biologic behavior is similar to that of ^{123}I; however, it has a longer half-life (8.1 days) and produces a higher proportion of beta emissions, so that thyroid tissue receives a higher level of radiation exposure. It is mainly used for imaging after thyroidectomy and in the ablation of thyroid remnants and metastatic thyroid cancer. It is also used to treat Graves' disease.

Most well-differentiated thyroid cancers (approximately 85%) concentrate ^{131}I relative to the nonthyroidal cells. However, the efficiency of uptake in both primary and metastatic thyroid cancer is far less than that in normal thyroid tissue. Therefore, the ability to follow and treat patients with thyroid cancer is enhanced following total thyroidectomy and ^{131}I ablation of remnant thyroid tissue.

The majority of well-differentiated thyroid cancers trap [131]I. However, Hürthle cell cancers rarely trap ^{131}I, and medullary, anaplastic, and other poorly differentiated thyroid malignancies are, for the most part, ^{131}I-resistant. Thyroid lymphoma and nonthyroidal metastases to the thyroid do not trap [131]I.

Scanning after thyroidectomy in the setting of thyroid cancer has traditionally been performed 4 to 6 weeks postoperatively after the patient has maintained a low-iodine diet for 10 days. This interval is required to allow endogenous thyroid hormone to be metabolized; the resulting hypothyroid state stimulates pituitary TSH secretion. A 2- to

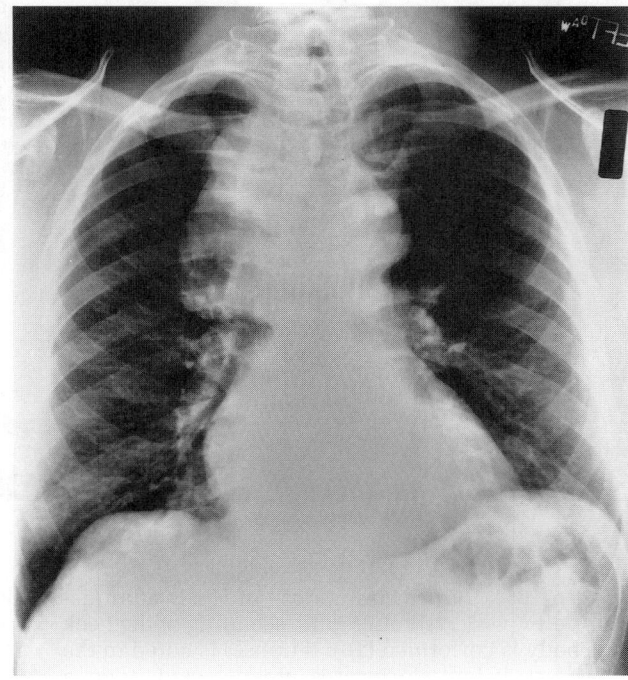

A

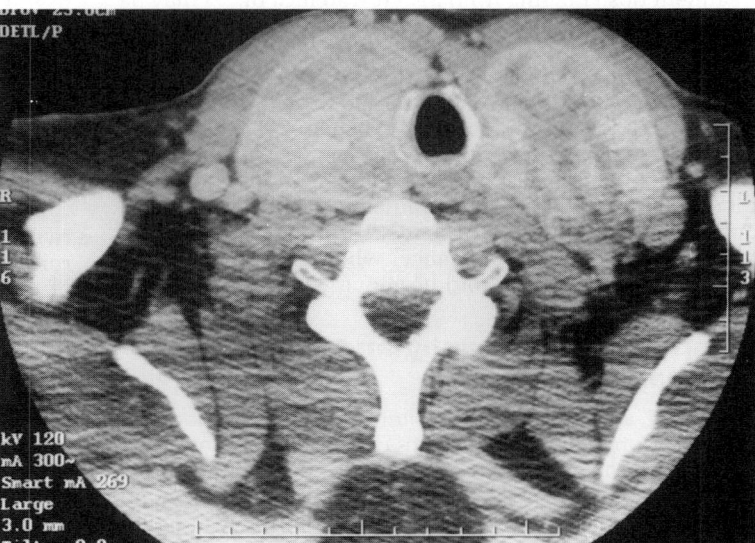

Figure 54.11. Substernal goiter on posteroanterior radiograph *(A)* and cervical goiter on computed tomogram *(B). (C)* Anterior mediastinal component. *(D)* Posterior mediastinal component. This goiter was extirpated by a cervical approach. *(continues)*

B

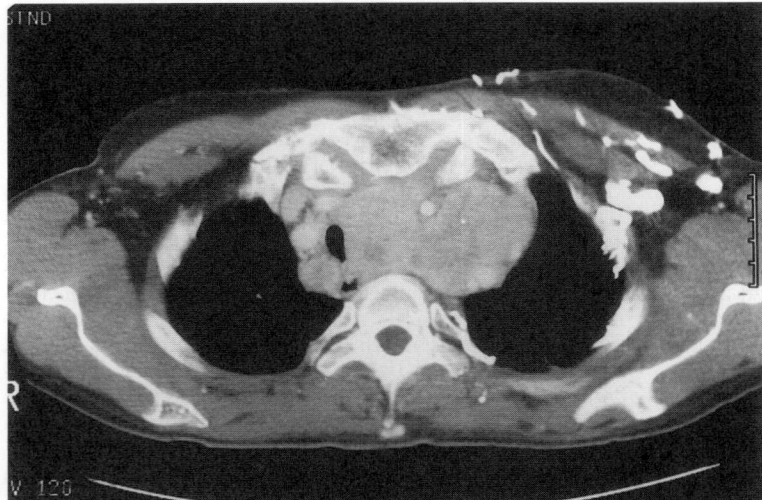

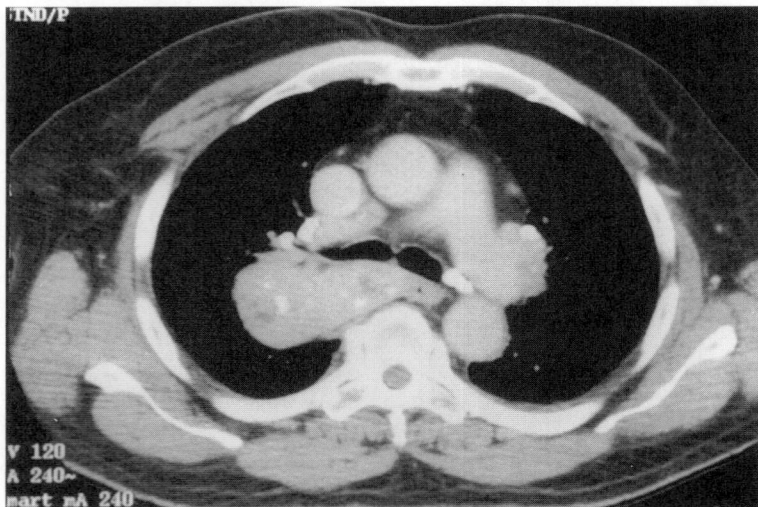

Figure 54.11. (Continued)

5-mCi (74- to 185-MBq) scanning dose of ¹³¹I is administered orally, after which scintigraphic scanning of the neck and whole body is performed (16). If uptake is noted in the thyroid bed or distant metastases are detected, then a treatment dose ranging from 29.9 to 150 mCi of ¹³¹I may be administered. Higher doses of ¹³¹I are occasionally used in conjunction with dosimetry protocols.

Recent clinical trials with recombinant TSH (rTSH) suggest that the traditional 6-week period of thyroid hormone withdrawal can be replaced by exogenous TSH stimulation (19). For patients with thyroid cancer who have undergone a total or near-total thyroidectomy followed by radioiodine ablation, rTSH-stimulated testing is a new option. In the future, rTSH may also prove efficacious to treat patients with thyroid cancer who cannot tolerate traditional protocols of thyroid hormone withdrawal.

Computed Tomography and Magnetic Resonance Imaging

Both CT and MRI yield anatomic information about the size, location, and characteristics of thyroid nodules. They also provide useful data about lymph node involvement, the extent of substernal involvement, and tracheal compression. They are not required for the routine evaluation of most thyroid nodules but are beneficial in the setting of local invasion and recurrent disease. The administration of iodinated contrast material can interfere with subsequent thyroid scanning and treatment with ¹³¹I.

Computed tomography is particularly useful for the evaluation of mediastinal goiters (Fig. 54.11). These lesions usually demonstrate anatomic continuity with the cervical thyroid and focal calcifications; they are relatively high in Hounsfield units and enhance after the administration of iodinated contrast.

FUNCTIONAL DISORDERS

Functional disorders of the thyroid gland fall into the two major categories of hyperthyroidism and hypothyroidism. Hypothyroidism is managed by the replacement of thyroid hormone and is not discussed in this chapter. Hyperthyroidism is caused by excess levels of circulating thyroid hormone. The causes of hyperthyroidism are numerous and include exogenous administration of thyroid hormone, subacute thyroiditis, postpartum thyroiditis, iodine-induced hyperthyroidism (Jod-Basedow syndrome), struma ovarii, and functional metastatic thyroid carcinoma. However, three major causes of hyperthyroidism may require surgical management: Graves' disease, toxic multinodular goiter, and an autonomously functioning toxic adenoma.

Graves' Disease

Graves' disease is an autoimmune disorder associated with a genetic predisposition, an increased incidence in women, and the presence of thyroid-stimulating immunoglobulins in addition to other tissue-specific antibodies (20,21). These antibodies bind to the thyroid follicular cell TSH receptor and stimulate thyroid hormone release. In addition, this autoimmune disease can affect the eyes and pretibial regions to cause exophthalmos and pretibial myxedema, respectively. The incidence of Graves' disease is five to seven times higher in female patients.

Patients often present with typical signs of thyrotoxicosis: heat intolerance, sweating, palpitations, tremor, hyperphagia, and thirst. On physical examination, the thyroid gland is generally diffusely enlarged, although it can be irregular. Ophthalmopathy may be the first manifestation of the disease, although it can develop simultaneously with the onset of hyperthyroidism. The spectrum of eye involvement is wide in patients with Graves' disease, ranging from subtle abnormalities that can be detected only with sophisticated measuring techniques to gross exophthalmos (22). Clinically significant ophthalmopathy requiring aggressive treatment occurs in only 5% of patients. The pathogenesis of the ophthalmopathy is not resolved, but it is associated with inflammation of the periorbital fibroblasts. Recently, an association has been established with heat shock protein 70 (23). Elderly patients with thyrotoxicosis often present with atrial fibrillation or congestive heart failure. In addition, these patients may present with the syndrome of apathetic thyrotoxicosis.

The diagnosis of Graves' disease is for the most part straightforward. The majority of patients have an enlarged thyroid gland and are noted to have elevated levels of T_4, T_3, or both. The uptake of radioactive iodine in the thyroid gland is uniformly increased, and uptake of ^{131}I generally shows a symmetrically enlarged gland. TSH levels are suppressed.

The three effective treatment modalities for Graves' disease are primary medical therapy, radioactive iodine treatment, and surgery. The selection of treatment depends on the age of the patient, severity of the disease, size of the goiter, coexistence of other indications for surgery, and the patient's preference. The selection is also influenced by the geographic locale of the patient, as prevailing treatments vary dramatically between the United States, Europe, and Asia.

The initial treatment in many patients involves the administration of antithyroid drugs to control thyrotoxicosis, and in a subset of the patients this may be the only treatment rendered. The agents of choice are thionamides, usually in the form of propylthiouracil or methimazole (Tapazole). Although these drugs can be used for extended periods of time, a small but significant risk (approximately 0.5%) for agranulocytosis, which can be life-threatening, exists. Furthermore, the drugs are associated with the long-term recurrence of thyrotoxicosis, which develops in an unpredictable manner. Therefore, most patients ultimately undergo one of the other two forms of treatment—radiotherapy or surgery.

Treatment with radioactive iodine is effective in Graves' disease and is not associated with a significant risk for subsequent radiation-induced oncogenesis (24). Nonetheless, endocrinologists are less likely to administer radioactive iodine to children. Furthermore, in Europe and notably in Japan, radioactive iodine treatment is less commonly used. Also, some patients in the United States are radiophobic and unwilling to accept radioactive iodine treatment. Patients are maintained or treated with antithyroid medications, or they can receive primary treatment with [131]I. However, during the 1- to 2-month delay between the administration of ^{131}I and definitive results, antithyroid medications must be continued. The effects of radioactive iodine are progressive, and virtually all patients eventually become hypothyroid.

An association has been demonstrated between the administration of radioactive iodine and a risk for exacerbation of Graves' ophthalmopathy (25). Although such exacerbation may be a consequence of the insidious development of hypothyroidism, this finding has dampened enthusiasm for ^{131}I treatment in some patients. The development of ophthalmopathy can be minimized by the administration of corticosteroids and the early administration of thyroxine during ^{131}I treatment (26,27).

Surgery is effective for controlling the hyperthyroidism associated with Graves' disease. It has no effect on the ophthalmopathy or other systemic manifestations of Graves' disease. In the past, the operation recommended for Graves' disease was a bilateral subtotal thyroidectomy. The theoretical basis of the operation was to preserve adequate thyroid tissue bilaterally to render the patient euthyroid. However, Graves' disease is characterized by remissions and exacerbations, and it is therefore impossible to determine the appropriate amount of thyroid tissue that should be retained. The performance of bilateral subtotal thyroidectomy was associated with an increased risk for recurrence requiring remedial therapy, usually in the form of radioactive iodine. Therefore, subtotal thyroidectomy for Grave's disease is now performed less frequently and has been abandoned in many major centers. Many authors now consider the optimal surgical treatment of Graves' disease to be a total or near-total thyroidectomy (28). The operative goal is to render patients permanently hypothyroid so that they will require life-long thyroid hormone replacement. This situation is far preferable to persistent or recurrent hyperthyroidism. It is important to recognize that patients with Graves' disease, especially after they undergo a total or near-total thyroidectomy, are at risk for transient hypocalcemia. This is caused by the combined effects of the operative procedure on the parathyroid glands and the preoperative condition of thyrotoxicosis, which in itself increases bone turnover. Nonetheless, these patients can be successfully treated, and the incidence of permanent hypoparathyroidism should be extraordinarily low.

Patients with hyperthyroidism should not undergo elective surgical therapy until clinical euthyroidism has been achieved. Under normal circumstances, this can be accomplished by the administration of thionamides, occasionally in combination with a β-adrenergic antagonist. In addition, iodine is often administered for approximately 2 weeks before surgery to decrease the vascularity of the thyroid gland. It is usually administered as saturated potassium iodide (50 mg per drop), with 1 drop given three times per day. It can also be administered in the form of Lugol solution (iodine plus potassium iodide, 6 mg of iodine per drop, 5 to 10 drops three times daily) (3). Patients may present with life-threatening thyrotoxicosis if, because of their thyrotoxicosis and social situation, they are unable to comply with a prescribed regimen of antithyroid medications. In such cases, thyrotoxicosis can be treated emergently with a combination of glucocorticoids, iopanoic acid (Telepaque), and β-adrenergic agents (29). Although this treatment does not normalize the TSH levels preoperatively, many patients can be brought to an acceptable state of euthyroidism within 5 days and then undergo thyroidectomy. The risk for thyroid storm when this regimen is used appears to be minimal. It has proved effective in making it possible to perform semiurgent thyroidectomy in patients who fail to take their antithyroid medications.

Toxic Multinodular Goiter

Patients with toxic multinodular goiters generally experience enlargement of their thyroid glands over a long period of time. These nodules have been associated with constitutive activation of the TSH receptor, which results in hyperfunction and hyperplasia. It is not unusual for one or more of the nodules to become autonomous and secrete thyroid hormone independently of TSH stimulation. Under these conditions, thyroid hormone levels rise progressively, and the patient is at risk for thyrotoxicosis. In addition, it is not unusual for physicians to administer thyroid hormone to patients with multinodular goiters in the hope of shrinking the nodules. If such patients already have a borderline elevation of their thyroid hormone levels, the additive effects of endogenous and exogenous thyroid hormone can result in thyrotoxicosis. Furthermore, thyrotoxicosis can be exacerbated in these patients following the administration of iodine containing contrast media, which results in the Jod-Basedow phenomenon. The symptoms of thyrotoxicosis are manifested by cardiac findings, particularly atrial fibrillation in elderly patients, tachycardia, congestive heart failure, or angina. In younger patients, one typically finds weight loss, anxiety, tremor, insomnia, and heat intolerance.

The treatment of hyperthyroidism is medical initially, usually with β-adrenergic antagonists and thionamides to control the clinical manifestations of thyrotoxicosis. The preferred long-term treatment is surgical resection. The optimal operation depends on the type of nodule. In the setting of bilateral, multiple nodules, a total or near-total thyroidectomy is indicated. If the patient has nodules predominantly on one side, then theoretically an ipsilateral thyroid lobectomy and isthmusectomy might be adequate. However, these patients are at risk for recurrent disease in the residual thyroid tissue.

Occasional patients are treated with radioactive iodine. However, patients with large, multinodular goiters, especially when they extend into the substernal location, are at risk for radiation-induced thyroiditis. This can rarely cause acute enlargement of the thyroid and airway compression.

Solitary Toxic Adenoma

Patients who present with thyrotoxicosis and a dominant thyroid nodule are likely to have a toxic thyroid adenoma. These patients generally have elevated T_4 or T_3 levels and a suppressed TSH level. In this setting, FNA occasionally confuses the clinical picture, as the cytology can show bizarre cells that may be misinterpreted as malignant. A hot nodule is almost never malignant. These autonomously functioning nodules suppress endogenous TSH and can cause hyperthyroidism. Demonstration on a thyroid scan of a single hot nodule and no uptake in the residual thyroid gland suggests that the normal thyroid tissue has been suppressed by excess secretion of thyroid hormone in the hyperfunctioning adenoma. Occasionally, these nodules secrete T_3 preferentially, and therefore the T_4 levels may be normal. Nodules that cause hyperthyroidism are generally larger than 3 cm in diameter. Autonomously functioning thyroid adenomas 3 or more cm in size can be expected to cause toxicosis in 20% of cases during the next 6 years. The treatment options include administration of ^{131}I or surgical resection. Surgery is generally recommended for younger patients with moderate-size to large nodules (30). Resection of the lobe containing the nodule preserves the contralateral lobe. In the vast majority of patients, preservation of a single lobe ensures adequate thyroid reserve to maintain normal thyroid homeostasis without thyroid hormone replacement.

THYROIDITIS

The term *thyroiditis* implies a benign, inflammatory disease of the thyroid gland. The most common form is chronic lymphocytic thyroiditis (Hashimoto's thyroiditis). Acute bacterial and also subacute thyroiditis can develop. Riedel's struma, which causes a fibrotic infiltrative process of the thyroid gland, develops rarely.

Hashimoto's Thyroiditis

Hashimoto's thyroiditis is a common autoimmune disease that results in diffuse enlargement of the thyroid gland. Although it can occur in any age group and in both sexes, it is most common in middle-aged women. A familial association has been noted between Hashimoto's thyroiditis and Graves' disease, which suggests a common genetic predisposition. Patients with Hashimoto's thyroiditis can present with euthyroidism, hypothyroidism, or rarely transient hyperthyroidism ("Hashitoxicosis"). Patients with Hashimoto's disease have a defective ability to organify trapped iodine. Eventually, the TSH secretion is increased as a result of hypothyroidism, and the TSH stimulates thyroid gland growth. These glands have a lymphocytic infiltrate and often become fibrotic. Goiters develop that can be asymmetric and contain dominant nodules. The goiter can obstruct the esophagus and trachea and can be confused with a thyroid cancer. Generally speaking, the thyroid glands in patients with Hashimoto's thyroiditis are firm and rubbery. The titers for antimicrosomal antibodies and antithyroglobulin are generally positive and can help establish the diagnosis. Patients in whom hypothyroidism develops are treated with thyroid hormone replacement in the hope of controlling the growth of the goiter. However, in a subset of these patients, the goiter enlarges progressively despite thyroid hormone suppression.

An increased incidence of lymphoma is associated with Hashimoto's thyroiditis. Therefore, a dominant nodule in the setting of Hashimoto's thyroiditis requires biopsy. If the suspicion of lymphoma is high, flow cytometry can be performed at the time of FNA. Unfortunately, the cytologic findings in the setting of Hashimoto's thyroiditis can be confusing, as intranuclear grooves and other findings may suggest papillary carcinoma of the thyroid.

Acute and Subacute Thyroiditis

Acute thyroiditis caused by bacterial or fungal infection of the thyroid gland is rare. The incidence appears to be increasing in immunocompromised hosts. The usual route of entry is through a thyroglossal duct cyst that becomes infected. In addition, infection can develop via a hematogenous route, particularly in drug addicts. Acute symptomatic thyroid enlargement may require urgent drainage.

Subacute thyroiditis (granulomatous thyroiditis, de Quervain's thyroiditis, or nonsuppurative thyroiditis) causes a painful thyroid gland, which has been associated with viral infection. It not uncommonly follows a history of upper respiratory infection and typically occurs in women. The pain may radiate to the upper neck, ears, or jaws. The thyroid gland is tender and diffusely enlarged, although it may be asymmetric. Clinical hyperthyroidism is present in 50% of patients, although biochemical hyperthyroidism can be demonstrated in virtually all cases (31). The disease is usually self-limited and can be treated with salicylates or glucocorticoids. In rare cases, surgery may be indicated to relieve chronic pain.

Riedel's Struma

In Riedel's struma, an enlarged thyroid gland with a woody or fibrous component is fixed to adjacent strap muscles or the carotid sheaths. The condition is extremely rare and is associated with other fibrotic diseases, particularly retroperitoneal fibrosis, sclerosing cholangitis, and fibrosing mediastinitis. These patients present a difficult clinical dilemma, as they may appear to have an undifferentiated thyroid carcinoma or lymphoma. The process can cause pain and compressive symptoms. The goal of surgical treatment is to establish a diagnosis by excision of adequate tissue for permanent histologic review.

NONTOXIC GOITER

Goiter or enlargement of the thyroid gland has been described since antiquity. The vast majority of these patients do not require surgical intervention. The goiters can range from small nodules to massive disease causing obstruction of the esophagus and airway. They can extend into the anterior or posterior mediastinum and cause the superior mediastinal syndrome. Approximately 80% of retrosternal goiters extend into the anterior and 20% into the posterior mediastinum. Most patients with multinodular goiters have normal thyroid hormone levels, and exogenous administration of thyroid hormone is often unsuccessful in reducing their size. One or more nodules within a multinodular goiter can become autonomous and produce excess thyroid hormone. This results in thyrotoxicosis and a suppressed serum level of TSH.

The major indications for surgical intervention are progressive enlargement and a need to rule out cancer. Surgical treatment is tailored to remove the goiters and protect the recurrent and superior laryngeal nerves and the parathyroid glands. Despite the massive size these goiters can attain in the mediastinum, they can almost always be resected by a cervical approach (Fig. 54.11).

SOLITARY OR DOMINANT THYROID NODULE

Thyroid nodules are common, with a prevalence of 4% to 7% in the United States. The vast majority are benign and do not require surgical treatment. However, 17,200 new cases of thyroid cancer occurred in the United States in 1990, and 1,200 deaths were attributed to thyroid cancer (32). The dilemma for physicians managing these patients is to develop a systematic approach to screen for those nodules that require surgical management and to reassure the vast majority of patients that they can be safely followed if they do not have evidence of malignancy. The routine evaluation of any patient with a thyroid nodule begins with a thorough history and physical examination. The physician should focus on eliciting a history of head and neck irradiation in childhood,

evaluating for possible familial types of thyroid cancer, and carefully examining the patient for evidence of local invasion or cervical adenopathy.

Clinical Evaluation

It is particularly important to elicit a history of irradiation to the head and neck in childhood. The importance of this history has been highlighted by the recent experience in Chernobyl. Although iodine deficiency is not a serious problem in the United States, persons who come from areas where iodine is deficient are at increased risk for the development of follicular (as opposed to papillary) carcinoma of the thyroid. Certain familial syndromes are associated with thyroid cancer. Medullary carcinoma of the thyroid occurs in three specific syndromes: multiple endocrine neoplasia type IIA (MEN-IIA), MEN-IIB, and familial medullary carcinoma of the thyroid (33) (Table 54.1). Less commonly, familial papillary carcinoma of the thyroid has been associated with Gardner's syndrome. Additional information to be elicited includes how long the nodule has been present and any associated pain, hoarseness, dysphagia, dyspnea, or hemoptysis. In addition, it is the obligation of the surgeon to rule out systemic disease that may affect the management of the patient during the perioperative period.

The physical examination is focused on the neck and the overall physiologic state of the patient. Nodules larger than 1 cm can usually be palpated, particularly if they are located anteriorly. The nodule should be examined carefully to assess size, consistency, extension, and fixation, and to determine whether it is single or multiple. The presence of cervical lymphadenopathy is extremely important, and normal cervical lymph nodes should be clinically differentiated from enlarged or firm cervical lymph nodes suggestive of metastatic disease. Lymphadenopathy resulting from thyroid cancer is particularly common in young patients. Certain nodules have characteristic findings on palpation; a rock-hard nodule with an irregular border can be highly suggestive of papillary carcinoma. Additional findings might suggest the presence of hyperthyroidism or clinically apparent hypothyroidism. A rapid pulse, tremor, exophthalmos, or dermatologic changes may be associated with Graves' disease. Routine examination of the vocal cords by indirect or direct laryngoscopy is an important aspect of the preoperative evaluation. Occult vocal cord dysfunction may be caused by thyroid cancer, previous neck surgery, or idiopathic vocal cord paresis. In the situation of anticipated surgical intervention, the presence of ipsilateral vocal cord paresis has significant ramifications.

Table 54.1. CLINICAL FEATURES OF SPORADIC AND GENETIC FORMS OF MEDULLARY THYROID CANCER

Disease	Endocrinopathies	Age at diagnosis	Virulence	Pathology
Sporadic	MTC	Varies	+++	Unifocal
MEN-IIA	MTC (100%)	1st–3rd decade	++	Multifocal
	Pheochromocytoma (42%)			Bilateral
	Hyperparathyroidism (35%)			
MEN-IIB	MTC (100%)	1st decade	++++	Multifocal
	Pheochromocytoma (50%)			Bilateral
	Mucosal ganglioneuromas (100%)			
	Marfanoid habitus			
Familial MTC	MTC	5th–6th decade	+	Multifocal
				Bilateral

MTC, medullary thyroid cancer; MEN, multiple endocrine neoplasia.
Modified from Chi DD, Moley JF. Medullary thyroid carcinoma: genetic advances, treatment recommendations, and the approach to the patient with persistent hypercalcitonemia. Surg Oncol Clin N Am 1998;7:683–706, with permission.

Fine-needle Aspiration

Fine-needle aspiration has revolutionized the evaluation of the thyroid nodule. It is by far the single most important preoperative diagnostic study. It has become routine, and its importance cannot be overemphasized. Expertise is required of both the aspirator and the interpreter of the aspirates. The technique is straightforward but should not be performed by the occasional aspirator whose specimens tend to be inadequate. An important adjunct in performing FNA is on-site cytologic review to determine specimen adequacy. The reported sensitivity of FNA in detecting malignancy ranges from 68% to 98%, and the specificity ranges 56% to 100% (34). If an FNA specimen is adequate, it can be categorized as benign, suspicious or indeterminate, or malignant. Approximately 75% of specimens are classified as benign, 25% as suspicious, and 5% malignant (35). Therefore, FNA allows the clinician to reassure the vast majority of patients that they most likely have a benign thyroid nodule. Such patients should not be discharged, as they require routine surveillance to detect any increase in the size of the nodule, with or without thyroid hormone suppression. Thyroid FNA can accurately diagnose papillary, medullary, and anaplastic thyroid cancer, in addition to thyroid lymphoma and metastatic carcinoma to the thyroid. FNA also has the ability to diagnose and treat cystic lesions of the thyroid gland. A thyroid cyst can be completely decompressed by FNA. Not uncommonly, however, a complex cyst is present. In this case, one must be concerned about the presence of thyroid cancer, particularly papillary carcinoma. Following FNA of a cyst, one should attempt to obtain samples of the wall of the cyst or any solid components to establish the diagnosis of malignancy. Cysts that completely resolve do not require additional therapy. Cysts that recur can be aspirated a second time. However, cysts that recur after two or more attempts at aspiration are unlikely to resolve with aspiration alone. Cyst have also been injected with alcohol as a treatment, but this technique is not commonly used in the United States (36).

Diagnostic Imaging Studies

In the past, a wide variety of imaging studies were used in the evaluation of thyroid nodules. These often included nuclear imaging and ultrasonographic examination. These studies are not required for the routine evaluation of the vast majority of patients with thyroid nodules. Nonetheless, it is not uncommon for patients to present to the surgeon with a thyroid nodule after having undergone one or several diagnostic imaging studies. In specific circumstances, imaging studies are appropriate, such as in the setting of a large nodule fixed to contiguous structures or vocal cord paresis. An anatomic imaging study of the neck, such as CT or MRI, can be useful in the evaluation of locally invasive thyroid tumors. It is important to avoid the preoperative administration of iodinated contrast material, as this can impair the postoperative administration of radioactive iodine. It is not unusual for patients to present with a thyroid scan demonstrating that the thyroid nodule is hypofunctioning or cold (Fig. 54.10). A cold nodule is consistent with thyroid cancer, and additional procedures are indicated. However, such a scan is also consistent with a benign solid or cystic nodule that could be diagnosed or even treated with FNA. Occasionally, a patient presents with a nodule and clinical signs of hyperthyroidism or with a suppressed serum TSH level. A thyroid scan is useful in this setting.

Thyroid ultrasonography is widely used and is an extraordinarily sensitive technique to determine the size, number, and location of thyroid nodules accurately. In fact, many endocrinologists now have ultrasonographic machines in their offices and use them as a routine part of the thyroid examination. There is little doubt that an ultrasonographic examination is far more sensitive than palpation; however, routine ultrasonography creates the dilemma of finding occult thyroid nodules or "thyroid incidentalomas" (37). A recent prospective North American study demonstrated the prevalence of asymptomatic thyroid nodules detected by ultrasonography to be 67% (38). These occult nodules are usually smaller than 1.5 cm and are almost always benign. Therefore, selective biopsy of only larger or enlarging nodules is recommended by some (37).

A wide variety of biochemical studies are available for the evaluation of thyroid nodules. For the most part, they are not useful in distinguishing benign from malignant lesions. However, the single most valuable biochemical study is the measurement of the serum TSH level. This test is a great aid in determining whether the patient is hyperthyroid or hypothyroid. Patients who are hyperthyroid have a suppressed serum TSH level because of endogenous thyroid hormone secretion by their nodule and do not need to undergo FNA. Hyperfunctioning thyroid nodules are almost never malignant, and FNA may yield follicular epithelial cells that can be difficult to discriminate cytologically. Therefore, a diagnostic biopsy in this setting may actually confuse the clinical picture.

Intraoperative Frozen Section Analysis

Intraoperative frozen section analysis of thyroidectomy specimens is accurate in diagnosing papillary, medullary, and anaplastic thyroid carcinoma, in addition to thyroid lymphoma and metastases to the thyroid gland (39). However, these diagnoses are usually established preoperatively. Although it was once commonly performed, the role of intraoperative frozen section analysis of the thyroid has diminished. When the diagnosis of thyroid cancer is clearly established on preoperative FNA, frozen section analysis is redundant and can prolong the operative procedure. On the other hand, if the FNA result is suggestive of but not diagnostic for papillary carcinoma of the thyroid, then intraoperative frozen section can be useful (40). Intraoperative frozen section analysis has also been advocated to guide the surgical management of follicular and Hürthle cell lesions of the thyroid. However, frozen section analysis in this situation is of virtually no diagnostic value because detection of the criterion for malignancy, which is capsular or vascular invasion, usually requires permanent histologic analysis. The majority of endocrine pathologists and surgeons believe that frozen section analysis rarely yields useful information in the setting of follicular and Hürthle cell lesions without gross capsular invasion (41).

Thyroid Hormone Suppression of Thyroid Nodules

In the past, it was widely recommended that patients with dominant thyroid nodules undergo thyroid suppression therapy in the hope that the nodules would shrink. This treatment modality is usually ineffective, and because of the widespread use of FNA, the routine use of thyroid suppression therapy is no longer advocated. Occasional patients, especially in the setting of an elevated or high-normal TSH level, may benefit from a time-limited trial of thyroid suppression therapy. Exogenous thyroid hormone is administered to maintain a suppressed but detectable level of TSH. Side effects of subclinical hyperthyroidism can occur, including bone loss and cardiac symptoms. These patients need to be followed carefully, as it is not uncommon for the normal thyroid parenchyma to regress while the nodule persists.

THYROID CARCINOMA

Thyroid cancer presents as a spectrum of disease ranging from well-differentiated tumors, in which the prognosis is excellent, to aggressive anaplastic thyroid cancer, in which rapid compromise and death are the expectation.

Occult thyroid cancer is not uncommon. In autopsy series performed for unrelated reasons, the prevalence of occult thyroid carcinoma ranges from 5% to 28%, which confirms that a large number of people harbor foci of microscopic carcinoma that are, for the most part, of no clinical significance (42). A female predominance of approximately 3:1 is noted. Although thyroid carcinoma can occur in any age group, it is more common after the age of 25 years, and its virulence increases significantly in elderly patients. The majority of patients present with an otherwise asymptomatic thyroid nodule, although local symptoms, including hoarseness, dysphagia, dyspnea, local neck pain, and cervical adenopathy, can occur (43).

The developing thyroid gland in the infant and child is particularly sensitive to the oncogenic effects of low-dose radiation. A linear relationship has been noted for the subsequent development of thyroid cancer following childhood exposure to external beam radiotherapy over a range of 5 to 1,000 cGy (44). In the past, these doses were achieved in children treated for tonsilar, thymic, or adenoid enlargement and for acne. Although childhood head and neck irradiation for benign conditions has for the most part been abandoned, the latency period of several decades has resulted in a population of elderly persons who are still at risk. In addition, nuclear accidents have and are likely to expose subsequent populations of children to the deleterious effects of ionizing radiation.

The common forms of thyroid cancer are summarized in Table 54.2 (45). The majority are derived from the follicular cells and include papillary, mixed papillary/follicular, follicular, Hürthle cell, and anaplastic cancers. Medullary carcinoma is derived from the calcitonin-producing C cells. Primary thyroid lymphoma and metastatic disease to the thyroid also occur. Well-differentiated thyroid cancers are papillary, follicular, mixed papillary/follicular, and

often Hürthle cell carcinomas of the thyroid. Some subtypes of papillary and follicular carcinomas histologically and biologically behave as poorly differentiated carcinomas. In addition, anaplastic carcinomas are always considered a poorly differentiated form of thyroid cancer. The biologic behavior of thyroid cancer is for the most part predictable based on the histology.

Histologic Subtypes of Thyroid Cancer

Papillary, Mixed Papillary/Follicular, and Follicular Variant of Papillary Carcinoma

Papillary and mixed papillary/follicular carcinoma of the thyroid are the most common thyroid malignancies, accounting for approximately 85% of all cases. The biologic behavior of mixed lesions is similar to that of pure papillary carcinoma and therefore they are discussed together (39). The follicular variant of papillary carcinoma, which has cytologic features similar to those of papillary carcinoma but on histologic examination appears to be a follicular lesion, also behaves clinically as a papillary carcinoma and is included in this section (46). Papillary carcinoma of the thyroid arises from the follicular cells and develops a papillary histologic architecture that is often associated with fibrosis, calcifications, squamous metaplasia, psammoma bodies, and lymphatic invasion. The cytologic findings, which are frequently diagnostic, include large, optically clear, overlapping nuclei. In addition, intranuclear grooves and inclusions and psammoma bodies are often present (34). Multicentricity is seen in 20% to 30% of the cases in which routine histologic sections are obtained. However, if whole-gland serial section is performed, the majority of patients demonstrate multicentric disease (47). Lymph node metastases are common, as demonstrated in the Japanese population, in which lymph node dissections are performed even for small papillary cancers (48). The significance of occult lymph node metastasis, however, is unclear. Distant metastases from well-differentiated papillary carcinoma are less common, occurring in approximately 5% of patients. The most common site is the lungs.

Approximately 10% of cases of papillary carcinoma of the thyroid develop in persons less than 20 years of age (49). Children are more likely to present with cervical node disease, which can dominate the clinical picture and mask a small, intrathyroidal primary cancer. Cervical node

Table 54.2. **THYROID CANCERS**

Type	Frequency	10-Year survival	Risk factors	Clinical factors
Follicular cell-derived				
Papillary	80%	92%	Radiation exposure	Younger onset, nodal spread (80%), multifocal (> 85%), bone metastases rare, ^{131}I-sensitive
Follicular	10%	72%	Radiation exposure, Iodine-deficient goiter	Older onset, hematogenous spread, bone metastases occur, ^{131}I-sensitive
Hürthle cell	1%	70%		Older onset, hematogenous spread, ^{131}I-resistant
Anaplastic	1%–2%	< 2%	Long-standing goiter Well-differentiated thyroid cancer	Much older onset, local, nodal, hematogenous spread. ^{131}I-resistant, rapid growth
C-cell derived				
Medullary	3%–5%	30%–50%	Genetic (20%) Sporadic (80%)	Nodal spread (65%), multifocal if genetic, ^{131}I-resistant
Lymphoma	1%	40%–50%	Hashimoto's thyroiditis	Nodal spread, sensitive to radiation and chemotherapy
Metastases	Rare	Varies	Previous carcinoma	Isolated metastases from renal cell tumors common

Modified from Kukora JS. Thyroid cancer. In: Cameron JL, ed. Current surgical therapy, 6th ed. St. Louis: Mosby, 1998: 593–598, with permission.

metastasis is found at the time of presentation in up to 90% of children, but in fewer adults (50). Extrathyroidal extension and pulmonary metastasis are also more common in children.

The classification of papillary carcinoma based on size continues to be somewhat controversial. In 1961, Woolner et al. (51) classified papillary carcinomas as occult, intrathyroidal, and extrathyroidal. Occult thyroid cancers are usually smaller than 1 cm, although some authors include cancers up to 1.5 cm in size. These are generally detected when the thyroid gland is removed for reasons other than thyroid cancer, as in thyroidectomy for Graves' disease. It is not uncommon to find occult lesions measuring 3 to 5 mm in size, and in this situation, the thyroid cancer is unlikely to affect the patient's life span. No clear consensus has been reached about the appropriate management of such patients. Most experienced physicians obtain an ultrasonographic examination of the residual thyroid tissue to determine if any nodules are present. In addition, the initial resected specimen should be examined for evidence of multicentricity. In the absence of multicentricity or contralateral residual thyroidal abnormalities, most patients can be managed with careful follow-up without completion thyroidectomy. These patients are often given thyroid hormone replacement to suppress TSH, a known trophic factor for both benign and malignant thyroid disease. However, no prospective studies have proved the effectiveness of this treatment.

Most clinically significant papillary carcinomas of the thyroid range between 1 and 4 cm in size and are usually contained within the thyroid parenchyma. In addition, cervical lymph node metastases are seen in approximately 30% of patients. Although lymph node metastases in most cancers are thought to portend a poor prognosis, this is not the case in papillary carcinoma of the thyroid.

Treatment of Papillary Carcinoma. The treatment of well-differentiated thyroid carcinomas consists of primary resection. This is followed by scanning with radioactive iodine to detect residual normal thyroid tissue in the thyroid bed and metastatic disease, and then treatment with radioactive iodine as appropriate. In addition, virtually all patients are placed on lifelong thyroid hormone to suppress pituitary TSH secretion. The extent of surgical resection for well-differentiated thyroid carcinoma has been debated, as is discussed elsewhere in this chapter. It is agreed that the minimal operation for a clinically significant papillary carcinoma of the thyroid is an ipsilateral thyroid lobectomy and isthmusectomy. Most endocrine surgeons and endocrinologists recommend a total or near-total thyroidectomy.

Patients who present with clinically significant nodal metastases should also undergo a lymph node dissection. This can be performed at the same time as a primary thyroid resection. Approximately 80% of metastases are found in the central compartment of the neck. Lymph nodes positive for cancer are unusual in the submental triangle. When disease is present in the lateral neck, a formal lymph node dissection is recommended. The technique described by Bocca et al. (52) preserves the sternocleidomastoid muscle, accessory nerve, and internal jugular vein. In addition, this operation has an acceptable cosmetic result. By removing both the thyroid cancer and normal thyroid tissue and nodal metastases, the postoperative use of radioactive iodine improves both the detection and treatment of metastatic disease. Furthermore, the ability to use serial thyroglobulin levels to detect recurrent disease is enhanced following complete thyroid ablation (53).

Aggressive forms of papillary carcinoma include tall cell, columnar, insular, and other poorly differentiated papillary carcinomas of the thyroid. These lesions behave aggressively and are associated with an increased risk for recurrence and metastatic disease. Surgical treatment is still required, and resection of adjoining structures, including strap muscles and portions of the esophagus and trachea, may be necessary.

Follicular Carcinoma

The incidence of follicular carcinoma of the thyroid is increased in regions in the world where iodine is deficient. These carcinomas demonstrate the formation of follicles on permanent histologic resection. A diagnosis of malignancy requires that either vascular or capsular invasion by tumor be demonstrated. On cytologic examination, a paucity of colloid is associated with an abundance of follicular cells (34). These lesions can be difficult to diagnose preoperatively because the results of FNA are generally consistent with a follicular neoplasm. Approximately 20% of all follicular neoplasms ultimately prove to be malignant; therefore, patients with this diagnosis generally undergo surgical exploration. Intraoperative frozen section analysis is also inherently insensitive; in the vast majority of patients, the frozen section confirms a follicular lesion but malignancy cannot be determined. Therefore, the diagnosis is deferred pending permanent histologic review. In a recent analysis of 120 consecutive patients, frozen section evaluation was of minimal diagnostic value for follicular thyroid lesions and rendered no additional information 87% of the time (41).

It has recently been appreciated that follicular carcinomas of the thyroid that demonstrate only minor capsular invasion and no vascular invasion have a relatively benign course. In a recent report, no deaths occurred in this group of patients (54).

Vascular invasion in follicular carcinoma of the thyroid, in addition to evidence of gross and multiple areas of capsular invasion, indicate more aggressive behavior. The surgeon or pathologist may readily identify areas of gross capsular invasion intraoperatively, and in this setting a frozen section of the selected area of the capsule can confirm the diagnosis. Multicentricity is uncommon. However, as in papillary carcinoma of the thyroid, recurrence and death are more frequent in older patients. Lymph node metastases are less common than in papillary carcinomas. Distant metastases to bone and lung are not unusual. In general, a total thyroidectomy is recommended for lesions larger than 4 cm, and in fact many recommend a total thyroidectomy for virtually all patients with a follicular carcinoma of the thyroid, regardless of size. The goal of surgery is to extirpate the tumor and increase the effectiveness of radioactive iodine postoperatively.

Hürthle Cell Carcinoma

Hürthle cell carcinoma is less common than follicular carcinoma and is often considered a subset of follicular carcinoma of the thyroid. It behaves more aggressively than other well-differentiated thyroid cancers, as evidenced by a higher incidence of metastasis and lower survival rate. In addition, avidity for ^{131}I is decreased. Accordingly, most surgeons recommend aggressive treatment for Hürthle cell carcinomas, usually in the form of total thyroidectomy. However, Hürthle cell carcinoma poses a diagnostic dilemma similar to that of follicular carcinoma due to the fact that it is inherently difficult to diagnose this lesion as malignant before or during surgery. Because a diagnosis of malignancy requires the demonstration of vascular or capsular invasion, cytologic analysis rarely renders a definitive diagnosis. Similarly, intraoperative frozen section often fails to yield useful information to the surgeon. However, a recent study of 57 consecutive patients who underwent resection for Hürthle cell neoplasms of the thyroid demonstrated a linear relationship between lesion size and incidence of malignancy (55). The chance of malignancy in Hürthle cell lesions larger than 4 cm was 65%, whereas the incidence of malignancy in tumors smaller than 1 cm was 17%. Therefore, it appears reasonable to advocate a one-stage total thyroidectomy for larger lesions if one is willing to accept that in a subset of these patients, a normal contralateral lobe will be removed in the setting of benign disease. This one-stage procedure obviates the need for a completion thyroidectomy if the permanent sections demonstrate malignancy. On the other hand, small Hürthle cell lesions are less likely to be malignant, and in this setting, thyroid lobectomy and isthmusectomy are indicated pending permanent histologic review. If the permanent histology is positive for Hürthle cell carcinoma, the surgeon is frequently asked to complete a total thyroidectomy and remove the contralateral lobe. Multicentricity is not common in Hürthle cell cancers, and the lesions tend to be resistant to radioactive iodine treatment. Therefore, the contralateral lobe is removed to improve the sensitivity of follow-up in the detection of recurrent disease. Once the contralateral lobe is removed, serial thyroid scans and thyroglobulin measurements become more sensitive in the detection of recurrence.

Medullary Carcinoma

Medullary thyroid cancer (MTC) is generally a slow-growing neuroendocrine tumor that originates from the parafollicular C cells. It comprises 3% to 5% of thyroid cancers. The majority (80%) of patients have sporadic MTC, whereas in 20%, MTC develops as a result of autosomal mutations in the *RET* protooncogene (56). *RET* protooncogene abnormalities are associated with MEN-IIA, MEN-IIB, and familial medullary thyroid cancer (FMTC) (Table 54.1). In the familial forms, an association is found between tumor aggressiveness and the specific syndrome. Patients with MEN-IIB have the most aggressive thyroid cancers, whereas FMTC is the least virulent. In general, MTC is more aggressive than papillary or follicular carcinoma of the thyroid. It metastasizes early to the perithyroidal lymph nodes, then to the lateral cervical lymph nodes and distant sites, especially the liver, lungs, and bones. Early detection and appropriate surgical treatment provide the only possibility for cure.

Patients with MTC generally present in either of two ways: a dominant sporadic thyroid nodule develops, or they present after family screening. Patients who present with a thyroid nodule usually undergo FNA. FNA in patients with MTC can be diagnostic, especially when the slides are assayed for calcitonin and carcinoembryonic antigen (CEA) immune reactivity. The diagnosis can be confirmed if serum calcitonin and CEA levels are obtained because both serum markers are invariably elevated in patients with palpable sporadic MTC. All patients with MTC should undergo screening for pheochromocytoma and hyperparathyroidism. Even in the setting of sporadic disease, the patient may represent an index case of familial disease and is therefore at risk for pheochromocytoma. If a pheochromocytoma is diagnosed, it is managed before the neck disease.

Up to 75% of patients with sporadic MTC presenting as palpable thyroid lesion have lymph node metastases (57). Therefore, the recommended treatment for these patients following screening for pheochromocytoma and hyperparathyroidism is a total thyroidectomy combined with a central lymph node dissection, in addition to an ipsilateral modified radical neck dissection. This is a formal undertaking designed to resect potential metastatic disease in the cervical lymph nodes. The most likely sites of metastatic disease are the tracheoesophageal grooves and the perithyroidal region. Because radioactive iodine therapy plays virtually no role in the initial management of these patients, the primary surgical treatment either effects a cure or leaves residual disease behind. Some advocate bilateral nodal dissection in the setting of sporadic disease because of the lack of available adjuncts and the fact that a surgeon can fail to detect the presence of bilateral metastatic disease. Furthermore, the surgeon's intraoperative assessment for nodal metastases is relatively insensitive (57).

Patients with familial forms of MTC can be detected via family screening programs, in which the children of affected members are assayed for abnormalities of the *RET* protooncogene. Wells et al. (58) demonstrated that DNA testing of patients at risk for familial forms of MTC can predict which are likely to benefit from prophylactic thyroidectomy. Theoretically, if disease in these children is detected at an early stage, curative resection is possible. This landmark contribution has revolutionized the management of patients with familial forms of MTC. Children in whom MEN-IIA is diagnosed should undergo thyroidectomy at around 5 or 6 years of age. A meticulous total thyroidectomy should be performed to remove all thyroid tissue. In addition, routine central neck dissection has been advocated for these patients; if the gross specimen demonstrates carcinoma, then an ipsilateral modified neck dissection should also be performed. However, the goal of surgery is to operate before carcinoma develops, when only C-cell hyperplasia is present. In this setting, lateral lymph node dissection does not appear to be indicated (58). Primary hyperparathyroidism also develops in patients with MEN-IIA. The hyperparathyroidism in MEN-IIA is distinct from the that in MEN-I. It is generally recommended that only enlarged parathyroid glands be removed, as the risk for recurrent disease and significant hyperparathyroidism does not justify total parathyroidectomy.

Patients with MEN-IIB have the most aggressive form of MCT. Characteristic are a marfanoid habitus, the development of bilateral pheochromocytomas, and autonomic neural system dysplasia manifested by ganglioneuromatosis throughout the gastrointestinal tract, especially notable in the lips. Because of the aggressive nature of MTC in MEN-IIB, it is recommended that these patients undergo thyroid resection, usually in conjunction with lymphadenectomy, as soon as the syndrome is recognized, preferably before 2 years of age (59).

Patients who have undergone primary resection for MTC not infrequently have persistently elevated serum calcitonin levels postoperatively. They are often asymptomatic, and their management is controversial. In most instances, these patients have undergone what in retrospect appears to have been inadequate primary neck surgery, and they might be considered for repeated neck exploration. The results of repeated aggressive neck dissection in this setting demonstrate that serum calcitonin levels are normalized in up 38% of carefully selected patients in short-term follow-up (60). However, a normal calcitonin level is not achieved in the majority of these patients despite remedial surgery. Furthermore, they often have occult distant metastases, most commonly in the liver. Therefore, if one contemplates remedial neck dissection in the setting of an elevated calcitonin level in an otherwise asymptomatic patient, formal screening should be performed for occult distant metastases. Standard imaging (CT or MRI) is insensitive for disease less than 1 cm in size. In the past, venous sampling of calcitonin levels from the liver was performed to rule out occult hepatic metastases. More recently, laparoscopic examination of the liver before neck dissection has been adopted (61). Metastatic

MTC to the liver can be seen as small granules on the surface, which can be sampled. If hepatic metastases are present and the cervical operation was planned for occult cervical nodal disease, then the lymphadenectomy is futile.

Patients also present with incurable metastatic disease that can cause local symptoms. They often live for decades despite significant tumor burdens, and meaningful palliation can be achieved through aggressive resection in the neck, mediastinum, and liver (62).

Adjuvant and other nonsurgical treatment of MTC has generally not been successful, although localized metastatic disease to the bone can be treated with external beam radiotherapy. Limited data suggest that external beam radiotherapy to the neck may be efficacious (63). The results of chemotherapy have, for the most part, been disappointing.

Anaplastic Carcinoma

Undifferentiated or anaplastic carcinoma of the thyroid has become increasingly rare in the United States. The cause of this decreased incidence is not clear but may be related to the increased use of dietary iodine and early management of follicular carcinoma of the thyroid. A subset of anaplastic thyroid carcinomas are derived from dedifferentiation of a follicular thyroid lesion. Patients generally present with a rapidly expanding neck mass, as demonstrated in Fig. 54.12. These tumors invade local structures, including the strap muscles, esophagus, trachea, and recurrent laryngeal nerves. It is unusual to extirpate these lesions, even with the most aggressive forms of therapy. It is essential to make an accurate diagnosis because in the past these lesions have been confused with MTC. The diagnosis can be established by cytologic techniques, although not infrequently core or open biopsy may be required. These patients often have airway compromise, and a surgical airway may be required. Patients are generally referred for radiation and chemotherapy protocols. It is not uncommon to see a significant response early in therapy, although tumor breakthrough should be anticipated.

Thyroid Lymphoma

Primary thyroid lymphoma generally presents as a rapidly enlarging neck mass. In this setting, FNA can be performed, which in conjunction with flow cytometry will demonstrate a monoclonal group of lymphocytes. However, in most situations, additional biopsy material will be required to establish the diagnosis of lymphoma accurately and obtain appropriate tumor markers. The primary treatment is usually radiotherapy and chemotherapy. One study demonstrated a complete remission in 88% of patients (64). Some authors have advocated surgical debulk-

ing; however, most studies have failed to demonstrate a benefit from surgical resection (64,65).

Metastatic Carcinoma to the Thyroid Gland

Metastatic disease to the thyroid gland is not uncommon in patients with primary extrathyroidal cancers. Autopsy series demonstrate a 1.9% to 24.2% incidence of metastatic disease to the thyroid gland in patients who die of extrathyroidal malignancies (66,67). The most common primary sites are the breast and lung. These patients, however, have widely disseminated disease, and their thyroid metastases are not often clinically significant. In contrast, clinically significant metastatic disease to the thyroid gland occurs in 5.7% to 7.5% of patients with extrathyroidal cancers (68). Isolated metastatic disease to the thyroid gland is most commonly from renal cell carcinoma, which accounts for approximately 50% of cases. Treatment of isolated metastatic disease to the thyroid gland is indicated in a subset of patients. A recent study demonstrated that following surgical resection, 60% of patients were alive and two patients were disease-free with a median follow-up of 5.2 years (69). The goal of surgery in the setting of metastatic disease is to remove all gross disease.

Staging of Thyroid Cancer

At least eight systems have been proposed and to a lesser or greater extent validated for the staging of thyroid cancer (70–77) (Table 54.3). None has been universally adopted, and the lack of a common staging system has impeded the development of multicenter trials and cross-institutional comparisons of thyroid cancer outcomes. In the absence of a universally accepted system, it is recommended that the TNM (tumor–node–metastasis) staging system, introduced by the International Union Against Cancer (UICC) and promoted by the American Joint Committee on Cancer (AJCC), the American Cancer Society (ACS), the National Cooperative Cancer Network (NCCN), and the American College of Surgeons (ACS), be adopted as the international staging system (77,78). The TNM system is presented in Table 54.4. Staging systems have confirmed that age above 40 or 50, increased extent of disease, presence of extrathyroidal extension, and increased size of the primary tumor are all predictive of more aggressive biologic activity in patients with well-differentiated thyroid carcinoma. Completeness of resection is also an important prognostic factor. In a recent follow-up study by Mazzaferri and Jhiang (74), advanced age, tumor size larger than 1.5 cm, presence of local invasion, and lymph node metastases were all independent risk factors for cancer death. Although the prognostic significance of lymph node metastases has been debated,

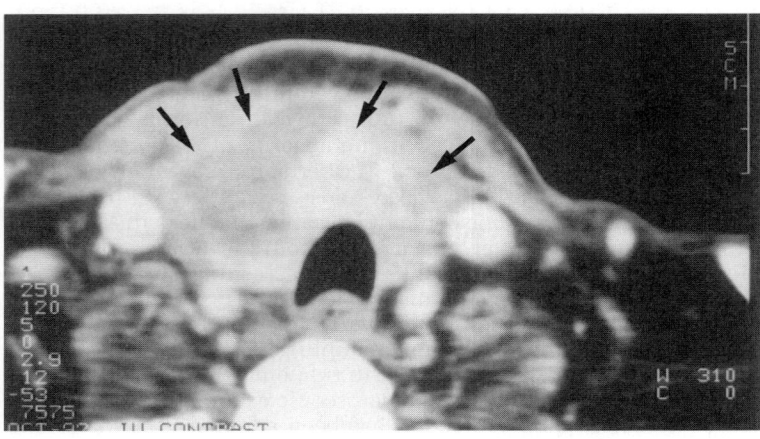

Figure 54.12. Anaplastic carcinoma of the thyroid *(arrows)* demonstrated on computed tomography. The normal tissue planes have been obliterated by the infiltrative cancer.

Table 54.3. **THYROID CANCER STAGING SYSTEMS**

System	Criteria	Reference
EORTC	Age, sex, cell type, invasion, metastases	70
AGES	**A**ge, **g**rade of tumor, **e**xtent, **s**ize	71
AMES	**A**ge, **m**etastases, **e**xtent, **s**ize	72
DAMES	**D**NA ploidy, **a**ge, **me**tastases, **s**ize	73
Ohio State	Size, cervical metastases, multiplicity, invasion, distant metastases	74
Sloan-Kettering	Age, histology, size, extension, metastases	75
NTCTS	Size, multifocality, invasion, differentiation, cervical metastases, extracervical metastases	76
TNM	Size, extension, nodal metastases, distant metastases	77

TNM, tumor–node–metastasis; EORTC, European Organization for Research and Treatment of Cancer; NTCTS, National Thyroid Cancer Treatment Cooperative Study.

they appear to be associated with a higher rate of recurrence and to have a minor or insignificant effect on survival. It is important to note that the interval between the first clinical manifestation of a tumor and the initiation of therapy directly correlated with cancer-specific mortality (74). Various authors have suggested that prognostic risk factors can be used preoperatively or intraoperatively to segregate patients into high- or low-risk groups (72,75). This concept is important if one accepts the premise that the ideal management of these patients varies according to

Table 54.4. **AJCC CLASSIFICATION SYSTEM FOR WELL-DIFFERENTIATED THYROID CANCER**

TNM CATEGORIES
Primary tumor (T)

TX	Primary tumor cannot be assessed
T0	No evidence of primary tumor
T1	Tumor ≤ 1 cm confined to the thyroid
T2	Tumor > 1 cm and < 4 cm confined to the thyroid
T3	Tumor > 4 cm confined to the thyroid
T4	Tumor of any size extending beyond the thyroid

Regional lymph nodes (N) (cervical and upper mediastinal)

NX	Regional lymph nodes cannot be assessed
N0	No regional lymph node metastasis
N1	Regional lymph node metastasis
N1a	Metastasis in ipsilateral cervical lymph node(s)
N1b	Metastasis in bilateral, midline, or contralateral cervical or mediastinal lymph node(s)

Distant metastasis (M)

MX	Presence of distant metastasis cannot be assessed
M0	No distant metastasis
M1	Distant metastasis

AJCC/UICC STAGE GROUPING
PAPILLARY OR FOLLICULAR
Under 45 years

Stage I	Any T	Any N	M0
Stage II	Any T	Any N	M1

45 Years and over

Stage I	T1	N0	M0
Stage II	T2	N0	M0
	T3	N0	M0
Stage III	T4	N0	M0
	Any T	N1	M0
Stage IV	Any T	Any N	M1

MEDULLARY

Stage I	T1	N0	M0
Stage II	T2	N0	M0
	T3	N0	M0
	T4	N0	M0
Stage III	Any T	N1	M0
Stage IV	Any T	Any N	M1

ANAPLASTIC

Stage IV	Any T	Any N	Any M

AJCC, American Joint Committee on Cancer; TNM, tumor–node–metastasis; UICC, International Union Against Cancer.

risk group analysis—specifically, the appropriate operation for well-differentiated carcinoma of the thyroid.

Issues Related to the Management of Thyroid Cancer

Thyroidectomy is the first and most important component of the management of papillary, follicular, medullary, and Hürthle cell carcinoma of the thyroid gland. The most controversial aspect of endocrine surgery is the extent of surgery that is appropriate for patients with well-differentiated thyroid carcinoma. Recommendations range from lobectomy and isthmusectomy on the ipsilateral side of the lesion to total extracapsular thyroidectomy for virtually all patients (79). Proponents of total thyroidectomy suggest that the operation can be performed with morbidity and mortality similar to those of a lesser procedure, and that removal of all thyroid tissue enhances the ability to diagnose and treat recurrent disease with radioactive iodine. Furthermore, the ability to measure serial serum thyroglobulin levels is improved once the thyroid gland has been removed or ablated with radioactive iodine. Arguments against routine total thyroidectomy suggest that removal of the entire thyroid gland provides no advantage for patients with well-differentiated thyroid carcinoma who are at low risk for recurrence. This argument is promulgated despite the fact that multicentricity is common in patients with papillary carcinoma of the thyroid (47). It has further been suggested that multicentricity is not necessarily clinically significant, and that the added risk of a total thyroidectomy cannot be justified in low-risk patients. It has also been postulated that thyroid lobectomy is adequate for patients with small, low-risk cancers, and that one could consider managing such patients without ^{131}I ablation or thyroid hormone suppression (80). The concept that thyroid hormone replacement or suppression is not necessary for a subset of patients with well-differentiated thyroid cancer is not accepted by most thyroid surgeons and endocrinologists. Therefore, because virtually all patients with thyroid cancer will receive lifelong thyroid hormone replacement, there is no logical reason to preserve thyroid tissue so long as a total or near-total thyroidectomy can be performed with complication rates similar to those associated with thyroid lobectomy.

The arguments for performing total thyroidectomy in the treatment of papillary thyroid carcinoma are listed in Table 54.5. Total thyroidectomy improves the feasibility of postoperative radioactive iodine ablation and has been shown to prolong survival and reduce recurrence rates (74,81–83). Because ^{131}I ablation depends on the amount of residual thyroid tissue remaining after surgery, total thyroidectomy lowers the dose of ^{131}I required (84). Serial serum thyroglobulin measurements have been shown to be the most sensitive marker for tumor recurrence, so it is

Table 54.5. RATIONALE FOR TOTAL THYROIDECTOMY IN THE TREATMENT OF PAPILLARY THYROID CANCER

Improves the ability to use ^{131}I ablative therapy postoperatively.
Lowers the dose of ^{131}I needed for ablative therapy.
Allows monitoring of recurrence with ^{131}I scans and serum thyroglobulin measurement.
Improves survival in subsets of patients.
Decreases recurrence rates.
Reduces the risk for development of pulmonary metastases.
Can be performed with the same morbidity and mortality as a unilateral procedure.
Decreases the small risk of a differentiated cancer becoming undifferentiated.

Modified from Chen H, Udelsman R. Papillary thyroid carcinoma: justification for total thyroidectomy and managmenet of lymph node metastases. Surg Oncol Clin North Am 1998;7:645, with permission.

logical to remove as much thyroid tissue as possible (85). Furthermore, the fact that ^{131}I scans can be used to diagnose and localize recurrent disease is significant because the probability of living with persistent disease or dying after treatment for recurrent thyroid cancer is lower in cases of ^{131}I-detected recurrence than in cases of clinically diagnosed recurrence (86). Furthermore, several studies have suggested that total or near-total thyroidectomy plus ^{131}I therapy improves survival in patients with well-differentiated thyroid cancer (74,81,87,88). In addition to Mazzaferri and Jhiang (74), De Groot et al. (81) reported that bilateral thyroid resections reduce tumor recurrence. Prevention of tumor recurrence is important because 50% of patients with recurrent tumors in the central neck ultimately die of their disease. In addition, total thyroidectomy plus ^{131}I therapy reduces the risk for development of distant metastases (89). Furthermore, several authors have reported that total thyroidectomy by an experienced thyroid surgeon can be performed with morbidity and mortality rates that are similar to those of thyroid lobectomy in the treatment of well-differentiated thyroid cancer (55,87,90,91).

To address the issue of the optimal treatment of well-differentiated thyroid cancer, a power analysis was performed analyzing the feasibility, scope, sample size, and length of follow-up required to determine the optimal operation for papillary carcinoma of the thyroid (92). The trial was designed to compare the endpoints of complications, recurrence, and cause-specific mortality. A trial comparing complications would be prohibitive because of the large population required, approximately 12,000 patients. A recurrence trial appears feasible based on sample size; approximately 360 to 800 patients would be required, with a 6- to 10-year follow-up. However, a recurrence trial would be severely compromised in the lobectomy arm, in that a unilateral lag-time bias would result from the impaired ability to detect recurrence in patients who have a thyroid lobe in situ. Therefore, a cause-specific mortality trial appears to be optimal. However, such a trial would require 3,100 patients (92).

The issue about total or less-than-total thyroidectomy in patients with well-differentiated thyroid will not be resolved in the absence of appropriate prospective trials. Nonetheless, it is important for all surgeons to remember that it is far better to leave a little bit of normal thyroid in situ, if necessary, than to have a little bit of normal recurrent laryngeal nerve ex vivo. A recent cross-sectional analysis of 5,800 patients who underwent thyroidectomy

during a 5-year period demonstrated a significant association between surgeon experience and complication rates and length of stay for thyroidectomy (93). Patients treated by high-volume surgeons, defined as those performing more than 100 thyroid procedures per year, had significantly shorter hospital stays and lower complication rates than did patients treated by low- or moderate-volume surgeons. Furthermore, the difference in outcomes was especially significant for patients with thyroid cancer, among whom those treated by high-volume surgeons had 60% fewer complications, despite the fact that they were more likely to have undergone a total thyroidectomy.

COMPLICATIONS OF THYROID SURGERY

Before the early 20th century, thyroid surgery was often associated with uncontrolled hemorrhage, thyroid storm, and infection. The introduction of controlled anesthesia, aseptic technique, and fine instruments in conjunction with the pioneering work of Kocher, Halsted, Lahey, and Crile brought about the current era of thyroid surgery, in which mortality is virtually nonexistent. However, three major complications of thyroid surgery remain: nerve injury, hemorrhage, and hypoparathyroidism. Hypothyroidism after thyroidectomy is an anticipated outcome when more than two thirds of the thyroid gland is resected.

Recurrent laryngeal nerve injury is, for the most part, preventable. It is impossible to determine the actual incidence of this event because occult injury may be unappreciated, and surgeons are inherently reluctant to report unfavorable results. Injury may occur via electrocautery, traction, ligation, suture entrapment, or localized hematoma. The injury may be transient, with spontaneous return of function within 6 months, or it may be permanent. The reported incidence of permanent recurrent laryngeal nerve paralysis ranges between zero and 4% for the nerves at risk (94). Injuries to the external branch of the superior laryngeal nerve can also occur and are often overlooked. The reported incidence appears to be about 1% (95).

Hypoparathyroidism following thyroidectomy can also be temporary or permanent. This should be more frequent when bilateral thyroid procedures are performed, yet even series of unilateral thyroid lobectomy report this complication. A detailed knowledge of the anatomy of the parathyroid glands and their vascular relationships is required to minimize this complication. The incidence of permanent hypoparathyroidism should be less than 2% after thyroid surgery (95,96).

Hematoma is a rare complication following thyroidectomy but has devastating consequences. An expanding hematoma in the neck can severely compromise the airway, and in the emergent situation, it may be necessary to open the wound at the bedside. Although anticoagulation and extensive surgery are predisposing factors, the complication of hematoma is related to surgical technique. Routine drainage of the operative field has not been documented to decrease its incidence (97).

SURGICAL APPROACH TO THE THYROID GLAND

Thyroid surgery must be performed in a meticulous, controlled fashion with exact hemostasis to prevent injury to the recurrent laryngeal nerve, external branch of the superior laryngeal nerve, and the parathyroid glands. Operative loupes can be of benefit during the surgery to protect both of these delicate structures and their blood supply.

Thyroid surgery is usually performed under general endotracheal anesthesia. However, cervical block anesthesia can be used and surgery can be performed in awake, conscious, but sedated patients (98). If a patient has a thyroid hormone disorder, it should be corrected before surgery.

The patient is placed in the reverse Trendelenberg position with an inflatable pillow behind the back to achieve moderate neck extension. The arms are carefully padded to prevent neurovascular injury and are placed at the sides. A Kocher incision is made approximately one or two fingerbreadths above the sternal notch. Subplatysmal flaps are elevated to the thyroid notch superiorly, laterally beyond the borders of the sternal heads of the sternocleidomastoid muscles, and inferiorly to the sternal notch. The anterior jugular veins can be preserved in almost all cases. The strap muscles are mobilized in the midline and distracted bilaterally. It is rarely necessary to transect the strap muscles. A self-retaining retractor can be quite useful in distracting both the skin and strap muscles. The thyroid gland is carefully examined for nodularity or associated lymphadenopathy. A thyroid lobectomy can be performed from any of several approaches, and in the past, many authors recommended early exposure of the recurrent laryngeal nerve. This is of theoretical advantage, however, there are practical limitations to this technique. Particularly in patients with large goiters, it can be difficult to expose the recurrent laryngeal nerve during the early phase of dissection, and attempts to do so can result in injury. It is often preferable to mobilize the upper pole through the potential space between the cricothyroid muscle and the upper pole of the thyroid gland.

Early mobilization of the pyramidal lobe is easily accomplished and is particularly important in patients suspected of having thyroid cancer or Graves' disease. A recurrent mass can develop in the midline in patients with Graves' disease as this tissue hypertrophies. In addition, in patients with thyroid carcinoma, the Delphian lymph nodes located above the thyroid gland should be removed. The superior pole of the thyroid gland can be approached via the avascular space between the cricothyroid muscle and the upper pole of the thyroid gland. This allows a medial approach to the superior pole vessels and early ligation of the vessels directly on the thyroid capsule. These vessels should be ligated close to the thyroid capsule to prevent injury to the external branch of the superior laryngeal nerve, which runs in proximity to the superior pole vessels in approximately 15% of patients. Once the superior pole has been mobilized, the inferior pole vessels can be mobilized carefully with preservation of the lower parathyroid gland, which is often located in or near the thyrothymic ligament. The thyroid lobe is then mobilized medially and the middle thyroid vein is ligated. This allows exposure and identification of the critical area at the junction of the inferior thyroid artery and the recurrent laryngeal nerve. It is extremely important to identify the branches of the inferior thyroid artery carefully, particularly in relation to the end-arteries supplying the parathyroid glands, and to delineate its relationship to the recurrent laryngeal nerve. As one approaches superiorly along the ligament of Berry, one needs to be particularly concerned about the recurrent laryngeal nerve, as this is a location where the nerve can be tethered and injured. It is not unusual for a portion of the thyroid gland, termed the *tubercle of Zuckerkandl*, to extend laterally over the recurrent laryngeal nerve. If necessary, it is far better to leave this small amount of normal thyroid tissue in situ than it is to injure the recurrent nerve in an attempt to remove every last vestige of normal thyroid tissue. One can transect the isthmus either early or late in the operation. If one

is performing a unilateral lobectomy, the isthmus is transected and the medial portion of the contralateral lobe is undersewn. In a bilateral resection, the same procedure is performed on the contralateral lobe. Many surgeons have advocated subtotal thyroidectomy, with a small remnant of thyroid tissue left in proximity to the inferior thyroid artery. However, it is frequently technically easier to perform a total thyroid lobectomy because the remnant can bleed, and sutures in this area can injure the recurrent laryngeal nerve.

Lymph nodes can be dissected at the time of thyroidectomy. Central lymph node dissection involves resection of the lymphatic tissue from the hyoid bone to the left innominate vein and bilaterally to the carotid sheaths. This dissection can result in injury to the parathyroid glands and the recurrent laryngeal nerves. A lateral dissection for clinically significantly enlarged lymph nodes can also be performed. For the most part, lymph node dissections are not performed in continuity with the thyroid. Some have advocated minimal procedures, "cherry picking," in which only enlarged lymph nodes are removed. However, it appears far preferable to perform a formal lymph node dissection, with preservation of the internal jugular vein, sternocleidomastoid muscle, accessory nerve, phrenic nerve, vagus nerve, brachial plexus, and greater auricular nerve. This is a formal undertaking that removes lymphatic tissue from zones II through V, as depicted in Fig. 54.7.

Large goiters can appear difficult to extract. However, these lesions can generally be removed easily via a cervical approach. Even very large goiters extending deep into the anterior or posterior mediastinum can be removed via a cervical approach, as demonstrated in Fig. 54.11. Nevertheless, in such cases, it is prudent to have the chest prepared in case a median sternotomy or, rarely, a lateral thoracotomy is required. For difficult lesions in the anterior superior mediastinum, a partial sternotomy up to the second interspace is a simple, well-tolerated approach that provides excellent exposure to the level of the carina.

THYROID MEDICATIONS

Medications to control thyrotoxicosis can be divided into five major groups, depicted in Table 54.6. The thionamide antithyroid medications include propylthiouracil, methimazole (Tapazole), and carbimazole (99). Both propylthiouracil and methimazole are readily available in the United States, whereas carbimazole, which is converted to methimazole, is used in the United Kingdom. These three drugs have a similar mode of action, with minor exceptions (100). They inhibit the synthesis of thyroid hormone by blocking the oxidation and organification of iodine and by blocking the coupling of iodotyrosine residues to form iodothyronines through competitive inhibition of the enzyme thyroid peroxidase. Although a decrease in thyroid hormone synthesis ultimately results in the depletion of intrathyroidal stores of iodinated thyroglobulin, a delay occurs between the administration of these drugs and the onset of their therapeutic action because large stores of intrathyroidal iodinated thyroglobulin are initially present. Propylthiouracil also inhibits the peripheral deiodination of T_4 to T_3; this action has theoretical advantages, and propylthiouracil consequently is often recommended for patients with thyroid storm. However, it has a circulating half-life of only 2 hours, whereas methimazole has a half-life of between 6 and 13 hours. Therefore, methimazole can be administered once per day, whereas propylthiouracil needs to be taken more often. Thionamide drugs do cross the placenta and are found in breast milk. However, they remain the treatment of choice

Table 54.6. ANTITHYROID MEDICATIONS

Class	Mechanism	Result
Thionamides PTU Methimazole (Tapazole) Carbimazole	Block iodine oxidation and organification Block iodotyrosine coupling PTU blocks periperal conversion of T_4 into T_3	Inhibit thyroid hormone synthesis and deplete stores of iodinated thyroglobulin
Ionic inhibitor Iodine	Inhibits organification, coupling, and release of thyroid hormone	Inhibits thyroid hormone secretion
Inhibitors of T_3 production PTU Oral cholecystographic agents-ipodate β-Adrenergic antagonists-propranolol Glucocorticoids	Inhibits extrathyroidal conversion of T_4 to T_3	Decrease available T_3 to bind to receptor
Inhibitors of periperal thyroid action β-adrenergic antagonists-propranolol	Ameliorate manifestations of hyperthyroidism	Decrease palpitations, diaphoresis, nervousness, tremor
Radiocative iodine ^{131}I ^{123}I	Trapped by thyroid, incorporated into iodoamino acids and deposited in colloid	Cytotoxic to thyroid follicular cells

PTU, propylthiouracil; T_4, tetraiodothyronine; T_3, triiodothyronine.

for women during pregnancy. Their side effects include fever and skin rash, which usually occur during the first few weeks or month of therapy. However, the potentially life-threatening complication of agranulocytosis can rarely occur with either agent; the incidence is approximately 0.44% for propylthiouracil and 0.12% for methimazole (101). Severe hepatotoxicity can also occur rarely (102).

Iodine has long been recognized as an antithyroid medication with short-term effects. It acts as an ionic inhibitor of thyroid hormone secretion, primarily by inhibiting thyroglobulin proteolysis. It also blocks organification and coupling within the thyroid gland. However, its major effect is the inhibition of thyroid hormone release (100). In addition, it appears to inhibit the ability of TSH and cyclic AMP to stimulate endocytosis of colloid. Iodine also decreases the vascularity of the thyroid gland. Most of its effect lasts for 10 to 14 days, after which escape occurs.

Several drugs act to inhibit the peripheral conversion of T_4 to T_3. These include propylthiouracil, oral cholecystographic agents, certain β-adrenergic blockers, and glucocorticoids (100,101). Because T_3 is the active form of thyroid hormone, the availability of T_3 to bind to thyroid hormone receptors is limited. The administration of β-adrenergic agents also relieves the peripheral manifestations of hyperthyroidism, including palpitations, diaphoresis, nervousness, and tremor.

The last form of antithyroid medication is radioactive iodine, usually administered in the form of ^{131}I. Radioactive iodine is readily trapped by the thyroid, incorporated into iodoamino acids, and deposited in the colloid, where it is in apposition to the thyroid follicular cells. Its beta emissions have a direct cytotoxic effect, causing follicular cell necrosis. Radioactive iodine causes minimal damage to surrounding nonthyroidal tissues and therefore has specific therapeutic efficacy. In low doses, it can be used for thyroid scanning, in moderate doses it can be used to treat hyperthyroidism, and in higher doses it can be used to destroy thyroid cancer.

REFERENCES

1. Boyd JD. Development of the thyroid and parathyroid glands and the thymus. *Ann R Coll Surg Engl* 1950;7:455.
2. Mansberger AR Jr, Wei JP. Surgical embryology and anatomy of the thyroid and parathyroid glands. *Surg Clin North Am* 1993;73:727.
3. Thompson NW. Thyroid gland. In: Greenfield LJ, Mulholland MW, Oldham KT, et al., eds. *Surgery: scientific principles and practice*, 2nd ed. Philadelphia: Lippincott–Raven, 1997:1283.
4. Sistrunk WE. Technique of removal of cysts and sinuses of the thyroglossal duct. *Surg Gynecol Obstet* 1928;46:109.
5. Skandalakis JE, Gray SW, Todd NW. The pharynx and its derivatives. *Embryology for surgeons*, 2nd ed. Baltimore: Williams & Wilkins, 1994:17.
6. Halsted WS, Evans HM. The parathyroid glandules: their blood supply and their preservation in operation upon the thyroid gland. *Ann Surg* 1907;44:489.
7. Brent GA. The molecular basis of thyroid hormone action. *N Engl J Med* 1994;331:847.
8. Lazar MA. Thyroid hormone receptors: multiple forms, multiple possibilities. *Endocr Rev* 1993;14:184.
9. Utiger RD. The thyroid: physiology, hyperthyroidism, hypothyroidism, and the painful thyroid. *Endocrinology and metabolism*, 2nd ed. New York: McGraw-Hill, 1988:389.
10. de los Santos ET, Mazzaferri EL. Thyroid function tests: guidelines for interpretation in common clinical disorders. *Postgrad Med* 1989;5:333.
11. Kaye TB. Thyroid function tests: application of newer methods. *Postgrad Med* 1993;94:81.
12. Kaplan MM. Clinical perspectives in the diagnosis of thyroid disease. *Clin Chem* 1999;45:1377.
13. Surks MI, Chopra IJ, Mariash CN, et al. American Thyroid Association guidelines for use of laboratory tests in thyroid disorders. *JAMA* 1990;263:1529.
14. Spencer CA, LoPresti JS, Patel A, et al. Applications of a new chemiluminometric thyrotropin assay to subnormal measurement. *J Clin Endocrinol Metab* 1990;70:453.
15. Naik KS, Bury RF. Imaging the thyroid. *Clin Radiol* 1998;53:630.
16. Freitas JE, Freitas AE. Thyroid and parathyroid imaging. *Semin Nucl Med* 1994;24:234.
17. Kaplan M. Clinical and laboratory assessment of thyroid abnormalities. *Med Clin North Am* 1985;69:863.
18. Sandler M, Patton J, Ossoff R. Recent advances in thyroid imaging. *Otolaryngol Clin North Am* 1990;23:251.
19. Ladenson PW, Braverman LE, Mazzaferri EL, et al. Comparison of recombinant human thyrotropin administration to thyroid hormone withdrawal for radioactive iodine scanning in patients with thyroid carcinoma. *N Engl J Med* 1997;337:888.
20. McDougall IR. Graves' disease: current concepts. *Med Clin North Am* 1991;75:79.
21. Feliciano DV. Everything you wanted to know about Graves' disease. *Am J Surg* 1992;164:404.
22. Burch HB, Wartofsky L. Graves' ophthalmopathy: current concepts regarding pathogenesis and management. *Endocr Rev* 1993;14:747.

23. Heufelder AE, Wenzel BE, Gorman CA, et al. Detection, cellular localization, and modulation of heat shock proteins in cultured fibroblasts from patients with extrathyroidal manifestations of Graves' disease. *J Clin Endocrinol Metab* 1991; 73:739.

24. Farrar JJ, Toft AD. Iodine-131 treatment of hyperthyroidism: current issues. *Clin Endocrinol* 1991;35:207.

25. Tallstedt L, Lundell G, Torring O, et al. Occurrence of ophthalmopathy after treatment for Graves' hyperthyroidism. *N Engl J Med* 1992;326:1733.

26. Bartalena L, Marcocci C, Bogazzi F, et al. Use of corticosteroids to prevent progression of Graves' ophthalmopathy after radioiodine therapy for hyperthyroidism. *N Engl J Med* 1989;321:1349.

27. Tallstedt L, Lundell G, Blomgren H, et al. Does early administration of thyroxine reduce the development of Graves' ophthalmopathy after radioiodine treatment? *Eur J Endocrinol* 1994;130:494.

28. Winsa B, Rastad J, Akerstrom G, et al. Retrospective evaluation of subtotal and total thyroidectomy in Graves' disease with and without endocrine ophthalmopathy. *Eur J Endocrinol* 1995;132:406.

29. Baeza A, Aguayo J, Barria M, et al. Rapid preoperative preparation in hyperthyroidism. *Clin Endocrinol* 1991;35:439.

30. O'Brien T, Gharib H, Suman VJ, et al. Treatment of toxic solitary thyroid nodules: surgery versus radioactive iodine. *Surgery* 1992;112:1116.

31. Christiansen NJB, Siersboek-Nielson K, Hansen JEM, et al. Serum thyroxine in the early phase of subacute thyroiditis. *Acta Endocrinol* 1970;64:359.

32. Landis SH, Murray T, Bolden S, et al. Cancer statistics 1998. *CA Cancer J Clin* 1998;48:6.

33. Chi DD, Moley JF. Medullary thyroid carcinoma: genetic advances, treatment recommendations, and the approach to the patient with persistent hypercalcitoninemia. *Surg Oncol Clin N Am* 1998;7:683.

34. Chen H, Nicol TL, Rosenthal DL, et al. The role of fine-needle aspiration in the evaluation of thyroid nodules. *Probl Gen Surg* 1997;14:1.

35. Gharib H, Goellner JR, Johnson DA. Fine-needle aspiration cytology of the thyroid: a 12-year experience with 11,000 biopsies. *Clin Lab Med* 1993;13:699.

36. Zingrillo M, Torlontano M, Chiarella R, et al. Percutaneous ethanol injection may be a definitive treatment for symptomatic thyroid cystic nodules not treatable by surgery: five-year follow-up study. *Thyroid* 1999;9:703.

37. Tan GH, Gharib H. Thyroid incidentalomas: management approaches to nonpalpable nodules discovered incidentally on thyroid imaging. *Ann Intern Med* 1997;126:22.

38. Ezzat S, Sarti DA, Cain DR, et al. Thyroid incidentalomas: prevalence by palpation and ultrasonography. *Arch Intern Med* 1994;154:1838.

39. Udelsman R, Chen H. The current management of thyroid cancer. *Adv Surg* 1999;33:1.

40. Chen H, Zeiger MA, Clark DP, et al. Papillary carcinoma of the thyroid: can operative management be based solely on fine-needle aspiration? *J Am Coll Surg* 1997;184:605.

41. Chen H, Nicol TL, Udelsman R. Follicular lesions of the thyroid: does frozen section evaluation alter operative management? *Ann Surg* 1995;222:101.

42. Harach HR, Franssila KO, Wasenius VM. Occult papillary carcinoma of the thyroid: a "normal" finding in Finland, a systemic autopsy study. *Cancer* 1985;56:531.

43. Mazzaferri EL. Management of a solitary thyroid nodule. *N Engl J Med* 1993;328:553.

44. Schneider AB. Radiation-induced thyroid tumors. *Endocrinol Metab Clin North Am* 1990;19:495.

45. Kukora JS. Thyroid cancer. *Current surgical therapy,* 6th ed. St. Louis: Mosby, 1998:593.

46. Tielens ET, Sherman SI, Hruban RH, et al. Follicular variant of papillary thyroid carcinoma: a clinicopathologic study. *Cancer* 1994;73:424.

47. Russell WO, Ibanez ML, Clark RL, et al. Thyroid carcinoma: classification, intraglandular dissemination, and clinicopathological study based upon whole organ sections of 80 glands. *Cancer* 1963;16:1425.

48. Noguchi S, Norguchi A, Murakama N. Papillary carcinoma

49. Patwardhan N, Cataldo T, Braverman LE. Surgical management of the patient with papillary cancer. *Surg Clin North Am* 1995;75:449.

50. Gorlin JB, Sallan SE. Thyroid cancer in childhood. *Endocrinol Metab Clin North Am* 1990;19:649.

51. Woolner LB, Beahrs OH, Black MB, et al. Classification and prognosis of thyroid carcinoma: a study of 885 cases observed in a thirty-year period. *Am J Surg* 1961;102:354.

52. Bocca E, Pignataro O, Sasaki CT. Functional neck dissection: a description of operative technique. *Arch Otolaryngol* 1980; 106:524.

53. Mazzaferri EL, Jhiang SM. Long-term impact of initial surgical and medical therapy on papillary and follicular thyroid cancer. *Am J Med* 1994;97:418.

54. Van Heerden JA, Hay ID, Goellner JR, et al. Follicular thyroid carcinoma with capsular invasion alone: a nonthreatening malignancy. *Surgery* 1992;112:1136.

55. Chen H, Nicol TL, Zeiger MA, et al. Hürthle cell neoplasms of the thyroid: are there factors predictive of malignancy? *Ann Surg* 1998;227:542.

56. Moley JF. Medullary thyroid cancer. *Surg Clin North Am* 1995;75:405.

57. Moley JF, DeBenedetti MK. Patterns of nodal metastases in palpable medullary thyroid carcinoma: recommendation for extent of node dissection. *Ann Surg* 1999;229:880.

58. Wells SA Jr, Chi DD, Toshima K, et al. Predictive DNA testing and prophylactic thyroidectomy in patients at risk for multiple endocrine neoplasia type 2A. *Ann Surg* 1994; 220:237.

59. Skinner MA, DeBenedetti MK, Moley JR, et al. Medullary thyroid carcinoma in children with multiple endocrine neoplasia types 2A and 2B. *J Pediatr Surg* 1996;31:177.

60. Moley, JF, Dilley WG, DeBenedetti MK. Improved results of cervical reoperation for medullary thyroid carcinoma. *Ann Surg* 1997;225:734.

61. Tung WS, Vesely TM, Moley JF. Laparoscopic detection of hepatic metastases in patients with residual or recurrent medullary thyroid cancer. *Surgery* 1995;118:1024.

62. Chen H, Roberts JR, Ball DW, et al. Effective long-term palliation of symptomatic incurable metastatic medullary thyroid cancer by operative resection. *Ann Surg* 1998;227:887.

63. Brierley J, Tsang R, Simpson WJ, et al. Medullary thyroid cancer: analysis of survival and prognostic factors and the role of radiation therapy in local control. *Thyroid* 1996;6:305.

64. Ryke CM, Grant CS, Habermann TM, et al. Non-Hodgkin's lymphoma of the thyroid: is more than biopsy necessary? *World J Surg* 1992;16:604.

65. Skarsgard ED, Connors JM, Robins RE. A current analysis of primary lymphoma of the thyroid. *Arch Surg* 1991;126:1194.

66. Abrams H, Spiro R, Goldstein N. Metastases in carcinoma: analysis of 1,000 autopsy cases. *Cancer* 1950;3:74.

67. Shimaoka K, Sokal J, Pickera J. Metastatic neoplasms in the thyroid gland. *Cancer* 1962;15:557.

68. Watts NB. Carcinoma metastatic to the thyroid: prevalence and diagnosis by fine-needle aspiration cytology. *Am J Med Sci* 1987;293:13.

69. Chen H, Nicol TL, Udelsman R. Clinically significant isolated metastatic disease to the thyroid gland. *World J Surg* 1999;23:177.

70. Byar DP, Green SB, Dor P, et al. A prognostic index for thyroid carcinoma: a study of the EORTC Thyroid Cancer Cooperative Group. *Eur J Cancer* 1979;15:1033.

71. Hay ID, Bergstralh EJ, Goellner JR, et al. Predicting outcome in papillary thyroid carcinoma: development of a reliable prognostic scoring system in a cohort of 1,779 patients surgically treated at one institution during 1940 through 1989. *Surgery* 1993;114:1050.

72. Cady B, Rossi R. An expanded view of risk-group definition in differentiated thyroid carcinoma. *Surgery* 1998;104:947.

73. Pasicka JL, Zedenius J, Auer G, et al. Addition of nuclear DNA content to the AMES risk-group classification for papillary thyroid cancer. *Surgery* 1992;112:1154.

74. Mazzaferri EL, Jhiang SM. Long-term impact of initial surgical and medical therapy on papillary and follicular thyroid cancer. *Am J Med* 1994;97:418.

75. Shah JP, Loree TR, Dharker D, et al. Prognostic factors in differentiated carcinoma of the thyroid gland. *Am J Surg* 1992; 164:658.

76. Sherman SI, Brierley JD, Sperling M, et al. Prospective multicenter study of thyroid carcinoma treatment: initial analysis of staging and outcome. *Cancer* 1998;83:1012.

77. Hermanek P, Sobin LH, eds. *TNM classification of malignant tumors,* 4th ed. International Union Against Cancer. New York: Springer-Verlag, 1967.

78. Beahrs OH, Henson DE, Hutter RVP, et al., eds. *Manual for staging of cancer,* 3rd ed. American Joint Commission on Cancer. Philadelphia: JB Lippincott, 1988.

79. Chen H, Udelsman R. Papillary thyroid carcinoma: justification for total thyroidectomy and management of lymph node metastases. *Surg Oncol Clin N Am* 1998;7:645.

80. Cady B, Rossi R, Silverman M, et al. Further evidence of the validity of risk-group definition in differentiated thyroid carcinoma. *Surgery* 1985;98:1171.

81. DeGroot LJ, Kaplan EL, McCortick M, et al. Natural history, treatment, and course of papillary thyroid carcinoma. *J Clin Endocrinol Metab* 1990;71:414.

82. Krishnamurthy GT, Blahd WH. Radiodine ^{131}I therapy in the management of thyroid cancer: a prospective study. *Cancer* 1977;40:195.

83. Samaan NA, Schultz PN, Hickey RC, et al. Well-differentiated thyroid carcinoma and the results of various modalities of treatment: a retrospective review of 1,599 patients. *J Clin Endocrinol Metab* 1992;75:714.

84. Maxon HR, Englaro EE, Thomas SR, et al. Radioiodine ^{131}I therapy for well-differentiated thyroid cancer: a quantitative radiation dosimetric approach—outcome and validation in 85 patients. *J Nucl Med* 1992;33:1132.

85. Ozata M, Suzuki S, Miyamoto T, et al. Serum thyroglobulin in the follow-up of patients with treated differentiated thyroid cancer. *J Clin Endocrinol Metab* 1994;79:98.

86. Coburn M, Teates D, Wanebo HJ. Recurrent thyroid cancer: role of surgery versus radioactive iodine. *Ann Surg* 1994; 219:587.

87. Clark OH. Total thyroidectomy: the treatment of choice for patients with differentiated thyroid cancer. *Ann Surg* 1982; 196:361.

88. Schlumberger M, Arcangioli O, Piekarski JD, et al. Detection and treatment of lung metastases of differentiated thyroid carcinoma in patients with normal chest x-rays. *J Nucl Med* 1988;29:1790.

89. Massin JP, Savoie JC, Garnier H, et al. Pulmonary metastases in differentiated thyroid carcinoma: study of 58 cases with implications for the primary tumor treatment. *Cancer* 1984; 53:982.

90. Attie JN, Moskowitz GW, Margouleff D, et al. Feasibility of total thyroidectomy in the treatment of thyroid carcinoma: postoperative radioactive iodine evaluation of 140 cases. *Am J Surg* 1979;138:555.

91. Thompson NW. Total thyroidectomy in the treatment of thyroid carcinoma. *Endocrine surgery update.* New York: Grune & Stratton, 1983:71.

92. Udelsman R, Lakatos E, Ladenson P. Optimal surgery for papillary carcinoma: the unresolved debate. *World J Surg* 1996;20:88.

93. Sosa JA, Bowman HM, Tielsch JM, et al. The importance of surgeon experience for clinical and economic outcomes from thyroidectomy. *Ann Surg* 1998;228:320.

94. Harness JK, Fung L, Thompson NW, et al. Total thyroidectomy: complications and technique. *World J Surg* 1986; 10:781.

95. Word PH, Berci G, Cacaterra TC. Superior laryngeal nerve paralysis: an often overlooked entity. *Trans Am Acad Ophthalmol Otolaryngol* 1977;84:78.

96. van Heerden JA, Grob MA, Grant CS. Early postoperative morbidity after surgical treatment of thyroid carcinoma. *Surgery* 1987;101:224.

97. Wihlborg O, Bergljung L, Martensson H. To drain or not to drain in thyroid surgery: a controlled clinical study. *Arch Surg* 1988;123:40.

98. Lo Gerfo PL, Kim LJ. Technique for regional anesthesia: thyroidectomy and parathyroidectomy. *Operative Techniques in General Surgery* 1999;1:95.

99. Cooper DS. Antithyroid drugs for the treatment of hyperthyroidism caused by Graves' disease. *Endocrinol Metab Clin North Am* 1998;27:225.

100. Haynes RC Jr. Thyroid and antithyroid drugs. In: *Goodman and Gilman's the pharmacological basis of therapeutics,* 8th ed. New York: Pergamon Press, 1990:1361.

101. Cooper DS, Goldminz D, Levin AA, et al. Agranulocytosis associated with antithyroid drugs. *Ann Intern Med* 1983;98: 26.

102. Liaw YF, Huang MJ, Fan KD, et al. Hepatic injury during propylthiouracil therapy in patients with hyperthyroidism. *Ann Intern Med* 1993;118:424.

SURGERY: SCIENTIFIC PRINCIPLES AND PRACTICE, Third Edition, edited by Lazar J. Greenfield, Michael W. Mulholland, Keith T. Oldham, Gerald B. Zelenock, and Keith D. Lillemoe. Lippincott Williams & Wilkins Publishers, Philadelphia, © 2001.

CHAPTER 55

PARATHYROID GLANDS

GERARD M. DOHERTY

ANATOMY

Typically, a person has four parathyroid glands—two superior and two inferior (1) (Fig. 55.1). The normal parathyroids are flat, ovoid, and red-brown to yellow. They measure 5 to 7 mm $\times$ 3 to 4 mm $\times$ 0.5 to 2 mm and weigh between 30 and 50 mg each. The lower glands are usually larger than the upper. The superior glands are most often embedded in the fat on the posterior surface of the upper thyroid lobe near the site where the recurrent laryngeal nerve enters the larynx. The inferior glands are usually more ventral and lie close to or within the portion of the thymus gland that extends from the inferior pole of the thyroid gland into the chest. Although this anatomy is fairly consistent, substantial variations from the norm can occur, and it is essential that the surgeon have a thorough understanding of these anatomic variations before beginning a neck exploration for hyperparathyroidism.

Variations in parathyroid anatomy are primarily caused by differences in patterns of embryogenesis. During the fourth and fifth weeks of fetal development, a series of four pharyngeal pouches develop (Fig. 55.2). The superior parathyroid actually arises from the fourth pharyngeal pouch in conjunction with the lateral thyroid, and the inferior gland arises from the third pouch along with the thymus. The derivatives of each pouch then migrate together so that the superior parathyroid usually remains in close association with the upper pole of the thyroid, although it may occasionally be loosely attached by a long vascular pedicle, migrating caudad along the esophagus into the posterior mediastinum. Occasionally, a gland may be totally embedded in the thyroid parenchyma. The inferior parathyroid descends with the thymus, but this migration is extremely variable. Inferior glands can be found anywhere from the pharynx to the mediastinum. Regardless of their location, they usually adhere to the thymus or are within the thyrothymic ligament. Supernumerary glands can be identified in up to 15% of patients, most often in association with the thymus. Autopsy studies suggest that four parathyroid glands are virtually always present.

The arterial supply to both the superior and inferior parathyroids is usually from the inferior thyroid artery, al-

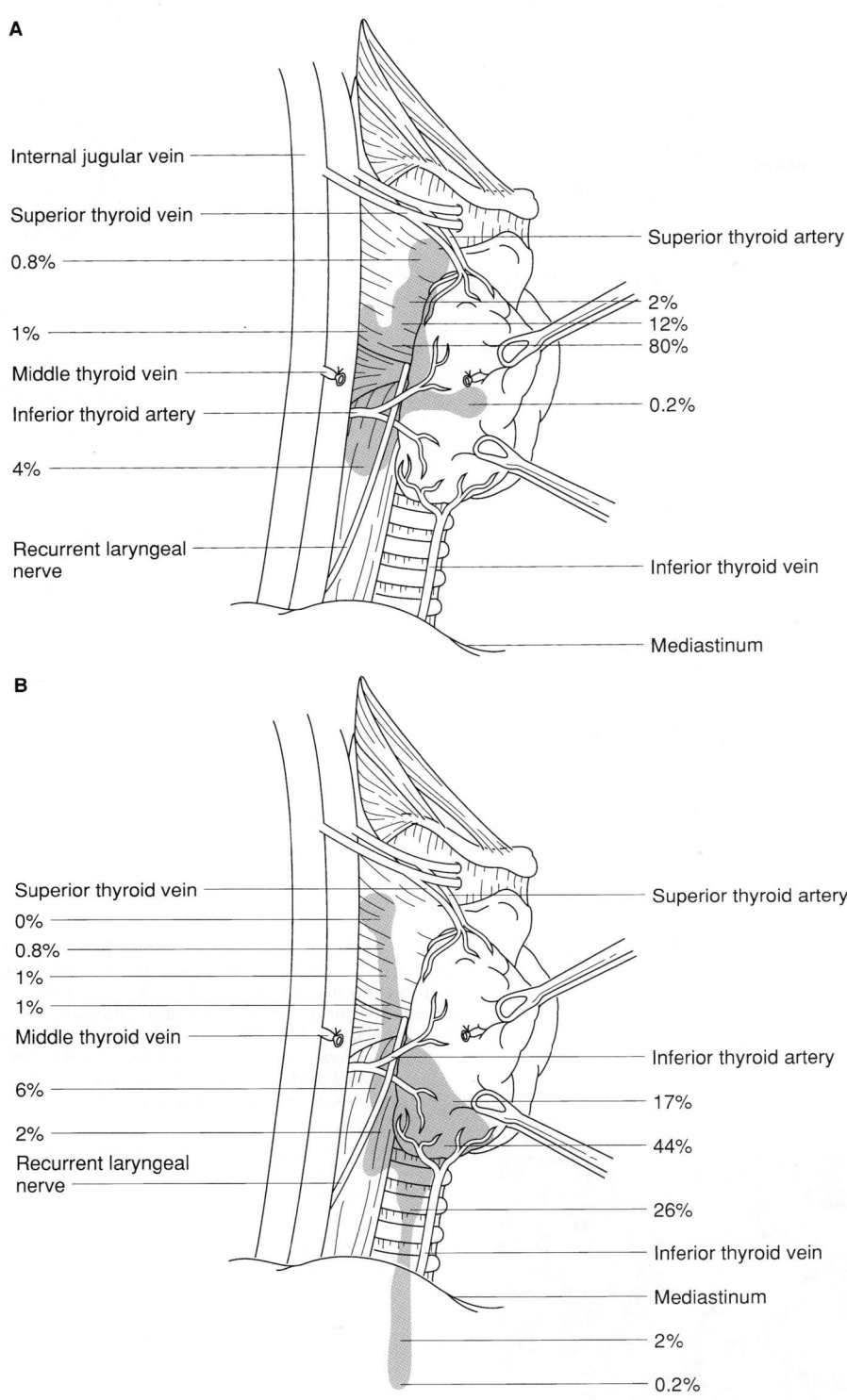

A

Internal jugular vein

Superior thyroid vein

0.8%

1%

Middle thyroid vein

Inferior thyroid artery

4%

Recurrent laryngeal
nerve

Superior thyroid artery

2%
12%
80%

0.2%

Inferior thyroid vein

Mediastinum

B

Superior thyroid vein

0%

0.8%

1%

1%

Middle thyroid vein

6%

2%

Recurrent laryngeal
nerve

Superior thyroid artery

Inferior thyroid artery

17%

44%

26%

Inferior thyroid vein

Mediastinum

2%

0.2%

Figure 55.1. Location of the superior *(A)* and inferior *(B)* parathyroid glands from 503 autopsy studies. The more common locations are indicated by the shaded areas. The numbers represent the percentage of glands found at each location. Typically, the glands were posterolateral to the thyroid and above or below the junction of the inferior thyroid artery with the recurrent laryngeal nerve. (After Akerstrom G, Malmaers J, Bergstrom R. Surgical anatomy of human parathyroid glands. *Surgery* 1984;95:14, with permission.)

though it may arise from the superior thyroid or thyroidea ima artery or from the rich anastomosis of vessels supplying the larynx, trachea, and esophagus. It has been suggested that a mediastinal parathyroid gland that descended during embryonic development usually receives its blood supply from either the internal mammary artery or small arteries within the thymus. In adults, however, an enlarged parathyroid gland that migrates into the mediastinum usually carries with it the corresponding branch

of the inferior thyroid artery. The inferior, middle, and superior thyroid veins, which drain the parathyroid glands, empty into the internal jugular vein or the innominate vein.

Histologically, the normal adult parathyroid is about half parenchyma and half stroma, including fat cells (Fig. 55.3). In children, the gland is almost entirely composed of parenchymal chief cells. Beginning at puberty, adipocytes appear, and with age, they occupy an increasing proportion

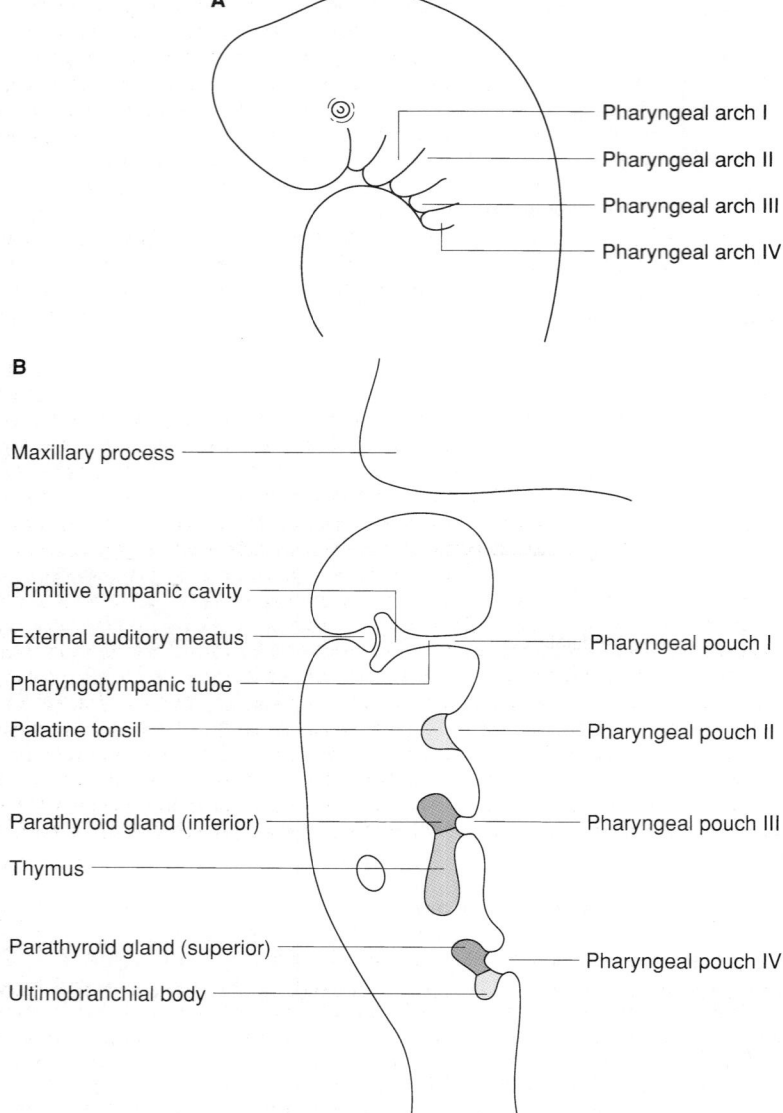

A

- Pharyngeal arch I
- Pharyngeal arch II
- Pharyngeal arch III
- Pharyngeal arch IV

B

- Maxillary process
- Primitive tympanic cavity
- External auditory meatus
- Pharyngotympanic tube
- Palatine tonsil
- Parathyroid gland (inferior)
- Thymus
- Parathyroid gland (superior)
- Ultimobranchial body

- Pharyngeal pouch I
- Pharyngeal pouch II
- Pharyngeal pouch III
- Pharyngeal pouch IV

Figure 55.2. *(A)* Pharyngeal arches in a 5-week embryo. The corresponding pouches extend from within the pharynx into each arch. *(B)* Schematic representation of the differentiating epithelium of the respective pharyngeal pouches. (After Langman J. *Medical embryology and human development: normal and abnormal.* Baltimore: Williams & Wilkins, 1975:262, with permission.)

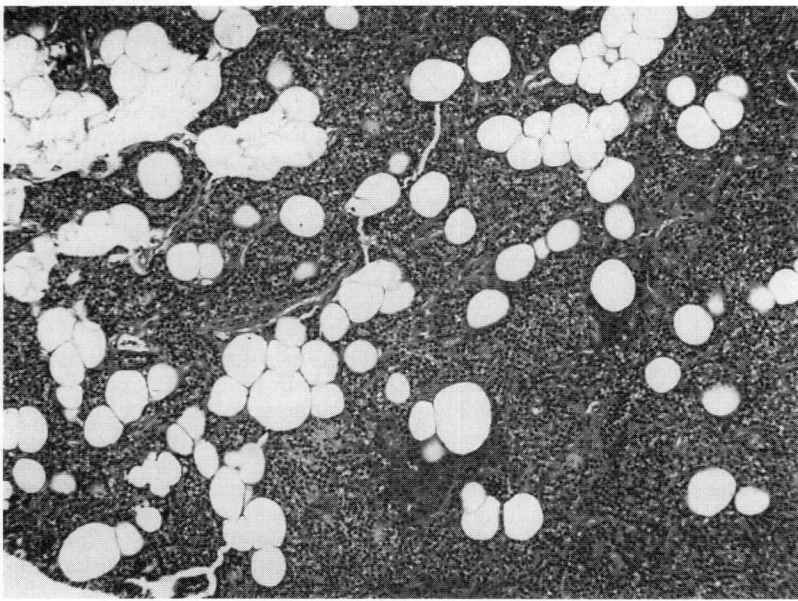

Figure 55.3. A normal adult parathyroid is composed of about half parenchyma and half fat. ×150.

of the gland. Also with increasing age, acidophilic, mitochondria-rich oxyphil cells are present in increasing numbers and are intermixed with the glycogen-laden, polygonal, water-clear cells. The functional significance of the various cell types remains unclear, although the water-clear cells and oxyphil cells are probably derived from the chief cells and secrete parathyroid hormone (PTH).

PHYSIOLOGY

The primary physiologic role of the parathyroid gland is the endocrine regulation of calcium and phosphate metabolism. Average daily exchanges of these ions from the gastrointestinal tract, bone, and kidney are shown in Fig. 55.4.

Calcium

Calcium ion plays a critical role in all biologic systems. It participates in enzymatic reactions and is a mediator in hormone metabolism. Calcium is intimately involved in the physiology of neurotransmission, muscle contraction, and blood coagulation. It is the major cation in bone and teeth. It represents about 2% of the average body weight, and almost all calcium is contained in the skeleton. The normal range of serum calcium is 9 to 10.5 mg/dL (4.5 to 5.2 mEq/L), and the daily variation in a normal person is generally less than 10%. About half of the total serum calcium is in an ionized, biologically active form; 40% is bound to serum protein, mainly albumin; and 10% forms compounds with organic ions, such as citrate. The total serum calcium concentration is a function of the serum protein content, and because hydrogen ion competes with calcium for the same binding sites on albumin, the body fluid pH is important. In general, for every change of 1 g/dL in the serum albumin level, a direct alteration of 0.8 mg/dL occurs in the serum calcium concentration. Almost all the physiologically important activity of calcium is represented by the unbound, or free, fraction.

Calcium is absorbed in its inorganic form from the duodenum and proximal jejunum. The rate of absorption is precisely regulated according to body calcium status. The calcium in the extracellular fluid is constantly being exchanged with that in the intracellular fluid, the exchangeable bone, and the glomerular filtrate. Calcium reabsorption by the kidney is closely related to that of sodium, and about 99% of the filtered load is reabsorbed under normal conditions.

Phosphate

Phosphate anion is also an integral component of most biologic systems. It is critical to the pathways of glycolysis and is the functional group for a number of high-energy transfer compounds, including adenosine triphosphate. It is also the major anion in crystalline bone. Normal levels of plasma phosphate range from 2.5 to 4.3 mg/dL, and the level varies inversely with the serum level of calcium. The relation is such that the product of plasma calcium and phosphate is constant and ranges between 30 and 40 mg/dL. When it increases above this level, a potential develops for the precipitation of calcium phosphate in body tissues.

In contrast to the percentage of calcium absorbed, the percentage of phosphate absorbed from the diet is relatively constant, and excretion usually provides the major mechanisms for regulating phosphate balance (Fig. 55.4). Unlike stores of calcium, the readily exchangeable soft-tissue stores of phosphate, such as those in muscle, are large.

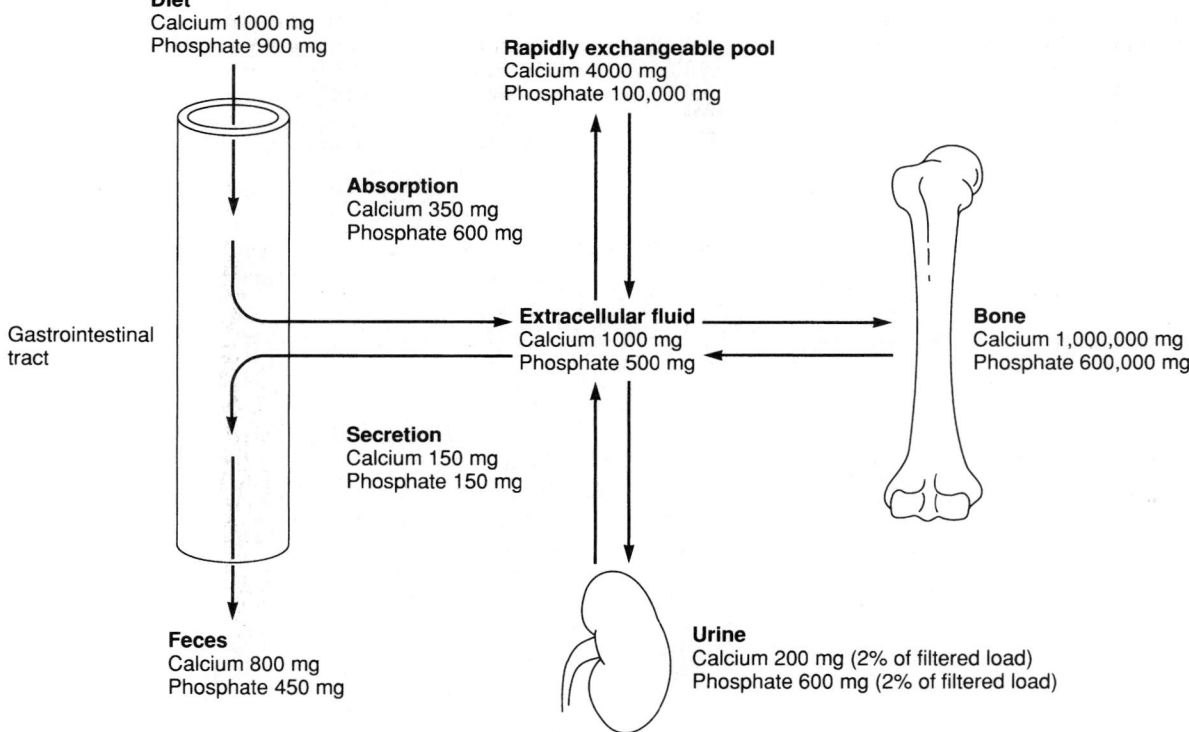

Figure 55.4. Average daily calcium and phosphate turnover in humans. (After Aurbach GD, Marx SJ, Spiegel AM, et al. Parathyroid hormone, calcitonin, and the calciferols. In: Wilson JD, Foster DW, eds. *Textbook of endocrinology,* 7th ed. Philadelphia: WB Saunders, 1985:1144, with permission.)

Table 55.1. HORMONAL REGULATION OF CALCIUM AND PHOSPHATE METABOLISM

	Parathyroid hormone	Vitamin D	Calcitonin
Gastrointestinal tract	No direct effect	Stimulates calcium and phosphate absorption	No direct effect
Skeleton	Stimulates calcium and phosphate resorption	Stimulates calcium and phosphate transport	Inhibits calcium and phosphate resorption
Kidneys	Stimulates calcium resorption Inhibits phosphate resorption	No direct effect	Inhibits calcium and phosphate resorption

Regulation of Calcium and Phosphate Metabolism

The maintenance of calcium and phosphate homeostasis depends on major contributions from three organ systems—the gastrointestinal tract, the skeleton, and the kidneys—with minor contributions from the skin and liver (2). The primary hormonal regulators of this metabolism are PTH, vitamin D, and calcitonin. The actions of each of these hormones in the organs are summarized in Table 55.1.

Parathyroid Hormone

Parathyroid hormone appears to be the single most important hormonal regulator of calcium and phosphate metabolism in humans. It has direct effects on the skeleton and kidney and indirect effects on the intestine, mediated through vitamin D. In target tissues, PTH binds first to membrane receptors, activating adenyl cyclase to generate cyclic adenosine monophosphate (cAMP), which in turn regulates other intracellular enzymes.

In bone, the effects of PTH are complex, stimulating both resorption and the formation of new bone. However, sustained elevations of PTH stimulate osteoclasts and inhibit osteoblasts. Osteocytes, in the matrix of cortical bone, may also act to reabsorb matrix in response to PTH, a process referred to as *osteocytic osteolysis*. Calcium and phosphate mobilization in response to PTH occurs in two phases. Initially, mineral is mobilized from areas of rapid equilibrium. This is followed by a more sustained release mediated by newly synthesized lysosomal and hydrolytic enzymes. In the kidney, PTH increases the reabsorption of extracellular fluid calcium at any given concentration, although excess secretion, because of hypercalcemia, increases the net daily amount of urinary calcium excretion. Reabsorption in the proximal tubule and loop of Henle is linked with sodium transport such that factors that alter sodium transport concomitantly alter calcium reabsorption. In contrast, reabsorption in the distal nephron is independent of sodium and directly influenced by PTH. PTH also increases phosphate excretion. This is accompanied by enhanced bicarbonate secretion. PTH probably has no direct effects on the gastrointestinal tract, although it does stimulate the hydroxylation of 25-hydroxyvitamin D to 1,25-dihydroxyvitamin D in the kidney. This activated metabolite enhances calcium and phosphate absorption from the gut.

Parathyroid hormone is synthesized initially as a precursor, prepro-PTH, that is sequentially cleaved in the parathyroid gland to pro-PTH and then to PTH (Fig. 55.5). Secretion of this 84-amino acid molecule is controlled by a negative feedback loop with extracellular fluid calcium. Most PTH is secreted in this form and then cleaved in the liver into N- and C-terminal fragments. The N-terminus contains most of the biologic activity and is rapidly degraded by the liver, whereas the inactive C-terminus is slowly metabolized by the kidney.

Vitamin D

Vitamin D acts at two major sites. It increases intestinal absorption of calcium and phosphate. In addition, in the skeleton, it promotes mineralization and enhances PTH-mediated mobilization of calcium and phosphate. It probably has no direct effect on the kidney.

Vitamin D_3, or cholecalciferol, is produced normally by the action of sunlight on 7-dehydrocholesterol in the skin (Fig. 55.6). It is then hydroxylated in the liver (25 position) and kidney (1 position) to form the active 1,25-dihydroxyvi-

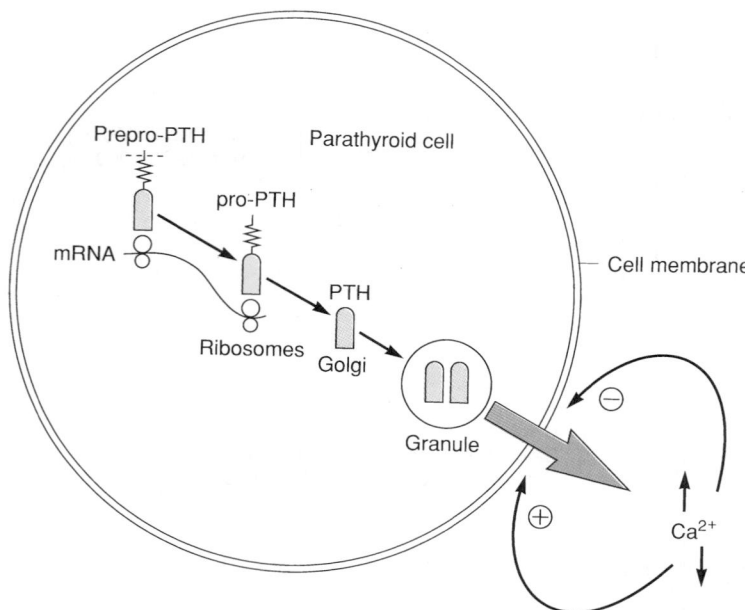

Figure 55.5. The parathyroid gland produces a precursor of parathyroid hormone *(PTH),* prepro-PTH, that is sequentially cleaved to pro-PTH and PTH. PTH secretion is controlled by the extracellular fluid volume. (After Klee GG, Kao PC, Heath H. Hypercalcemia. *Endocrinol Metab Clin North Am* 1988;17:573, with permission.)

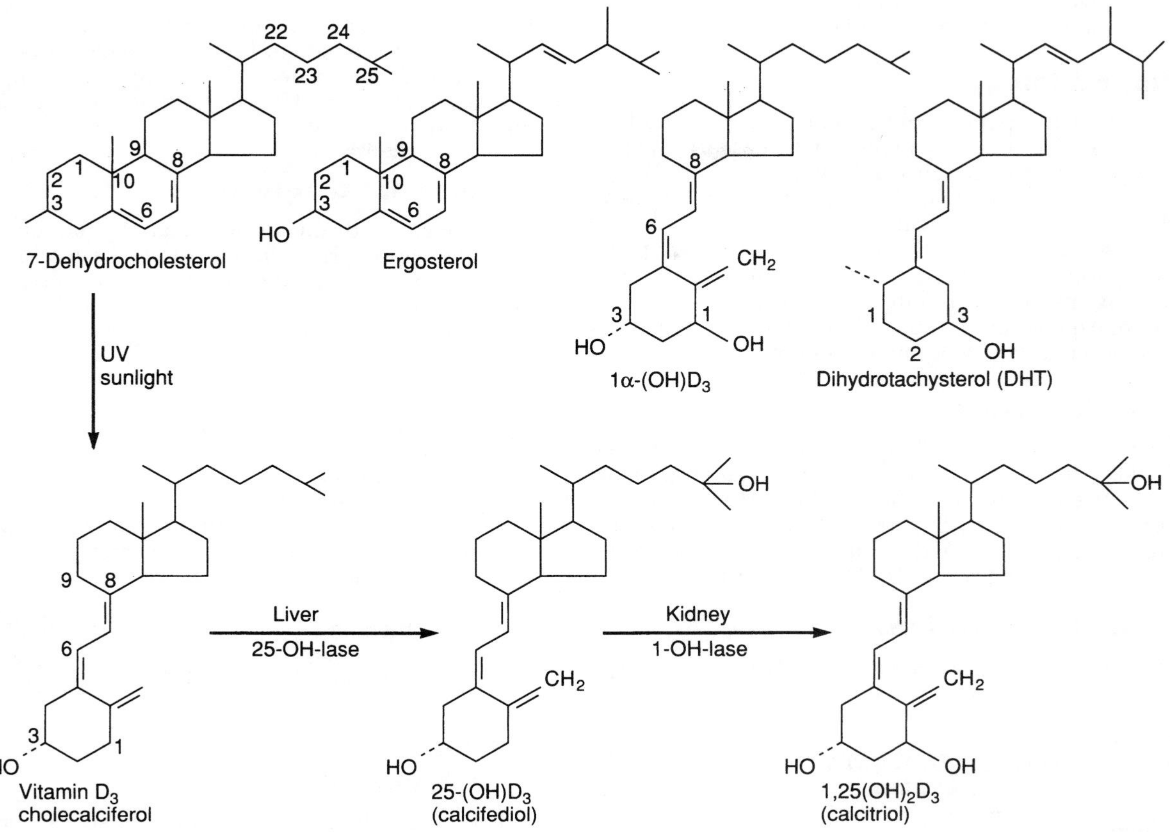

7-Dehydrocholesterol

Ergosterol

$1\alpha\text{-(OH)}D_3$

Dihydrotachysterol (DHT)

UV sunlight

Vitamin D$_3$
cholecalciferol

Liver
25-OH-lase

25-(OH)D$_3$
(calcifediol)

Kidney
1-OH-lase

1,25(OH)$_2$D$_3$
(calcitriol)

Figure 55.6. Synthesis of vitamin D$_3$. Ergosterol, 1-γ-hydroxyvitamin D$_3$, and dihydrotachysterol are synthetic preparations of vitamin D. (After Klee GG, Kao PC, Heath H. Hypercalcemia. *Endocrinol Metab Clin North Am* 1988;17:573, with permission.)

tamin D$_3$ (calcitriol). Vitamin D$_2$ is normally present in yeast and fungi but not in humans. It is the major pharmacologic source of vitamin D. Pharmaceutical preparations include vitamin D$_2$ (ergocalciferol), 25- hydroxycholecalciferol (calcifediol), and 1,25-dihydroxycholecalciferol (calcitriol). 1-Hydroxycholecalciferol and dihydrotachysterol are synthetic preparations that require only 25-hydroxylation for activity and so are useful for supplementation in patients with renal failure, who lack the 1-hydroxylase.

Calcitonin

Calcitonin is a 32-amino acid protein produced by the parafollicular C (calcitonin) cells of the thyroid. The C cells are embryologically derived from the neural crest and, in lower animals, are found in the ultimobranchial bodies, which are glandular structures derived from the lowest branchial pouch. In humans, these structures are incorporated into the superior and lateral aspects of the thyroid lobes.

Total thyroidectomy, with removal of all the C cells, is well tolerated, and it has been concluded that calcitonin is not essential for the normal control of calcium metabolism in adult humans. It does inhibit bone resorption and can produce hypocalcemia in experimental animals. It also increases urinary calcium and phosphate excretion. These effects appear to be mediated primarily through cAMP. Several secretagogues for calcitonin have been identified, including catecholamines, gastrin, and cholecystokinin, but the most potent appear to be calcium and pentagastrin.

Mineral Homeostasis

Under normal conditions, serum calcium and phosphate levels vary minimally during the course of the day. Regulation occurs primarily through PTH but also through a series of feedback loops involving vitamin D and calcitonin (Fig. 55.7). A fall in serum ionized calcium increases PTH secretion and stimulates the production of 1,25-dihydroxyvita-

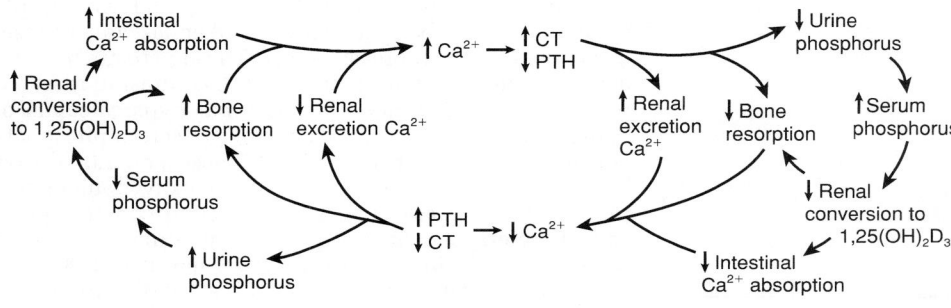

Figure 55.7. Feedback loops involved in the regulation of serum calcium and phosphorus. *PTH,* parathyroid hormone; *CT,* calcitonin.

min D$_3$. Conversely, increases in serum calcium inhibit PTH secretion and the formation of active calciferol.

Pathophysiology

Diseases of the parathyroid glands present almost exclusively as disorders of calcium metabolism. Hypercalcemia is the most common manifestation, and in the patient who presents with an elevated serum calcium level, the differential diagnosis can often be complex. A thorough understanding of both hypercalcemia and hypocalcemia is essential for the successful treatment of patients undergoing parathyroid surgery. Primary disorders of plasma phosphate are not usually related to surgical disease and are not discussed in detail here.

HYPERCALCEMIA

Hypercalcemia is a relatively common clinical problem (3). In the general population and in hospital outpatients, the incidence is between 0.1% and 0.5%. Most patients in this group have primary hyperparathyroidism. In contrast, hypercalcemia is identified in almost 5% of hospitalized patients, and nearly two thirds of them have a malignancy.

Clinical Manifestations

The symptoms of hypercalcemia are varied and nonspecific (Table 55.2). Severity is a function of both the magnitude and rapidity of onset of the hypercalcemia. Many of the manifestations are subtle and are evident only in retrospect, after the patient has been successfully treated for the cause of the elevated calcium. Specific symptoms and diagnostic tests are addressed in more detail in the section on hyperparathyroidism.

Differential Diagnosis

Although the diagnosis of primary hyperparathyroidism can, after appropriate investigation, be established with confidence in most patients, all causes of hypercalcemia must be considered and excluded. The multiple causes of hypercalcemia include the following:

Hyperparathyroidism
Malignancy
Vitamin A or D intoxication
Thiazide diuretics
Hyperthyroidism
Milk–alkali syndrome
Sarcoidosis and other granulomatous diseases
Familial hypocalciuric hypercalcemia
Immobilization
Paget's disease
Lithium therapy
Addisonian crisis
Idiopathic hypercalcemia of infancy

Etiology

Hyperparathyroidism

The diagnosis of hyperparathyroidism is discussed in detail below. Patients typically have elevated plasma concentrations of calcium and PTH, increased urinary excretion of calcium, and a low plasma concentration of phosphate.

Malignancy

Generally, patients with hypercalcemia and malignancy (humoral hypercalcemia of malignancy) can be divided into two groups (4). Patients with solid tumors, such as lung carcinoma (25% of all cases of humoral hypercalcemia of malignancy), breast carcinoma (20%), squamous cell carcinoma of the head, neck, esophagus, or female genital tract (19%), or renal cell cancer (8%), account for three fourths of all cases. Humoral hypercalcemia of malignancy in this setting generally presents late in the disease, with nearly all patients having known, or readily evident, malignancy. They have elevated levels of serum calcium, low levels of serum phosphorus, and elevated levels of urinary cAMP, consistent with increased parathyroid hormone activity, but serum PTH levels are normal or low. The hypercalcemia is now known to be caused by PTH-related protein (PTHrP), secreted by the tumor, rather than by the bony metastases that many of these patients have because of the advanced nature of their cancers. In the second group, accounting for one fourth of cases, are patients with hematologic malignancies, such as multiple myeloma, certain lymphomas and leukemias, and a subset of the patients with breast cancer. These patients have elevated levels of serum calcium, but in contrast to most patients with solid tumors and humoral hypercalcemia of malignancy, they have elevated levels of serum phosphate and low levels of urinary cAMP. These patients always have lytic bony lesions and histologically demonstrate increased osteoclast bone resorption adjacent to tumor cells. Formerly, a bone resorption-stimulating lymphokine secreted locally in and around the bone metastases was implicated as an osteoclast-activating factor. This osteoclast-activating activity is now thought to be an effect of

---

Table 55.2. CLINICAL FEATURES OF HYPERCALCEMIA

Neurologic
Lethargy
Confusion
Coma
Headache
Depression
Paranoia
Muscle weakness
Hyporeflexia
Incontinence
Memory loss
Hearing loss
Ataxia

Gastrointestinal
Constipation
Anorexia
Nausea and vomiting
Polydipsia
Weight loss
Pancreatitis
Peptic ulcer
Abdominal pain

Cardiovascular
ECG changes (short QT interval, widened T wave)
Bradycardia
Heart block
Hypertension

Renal
Polyuria
Uremia
Renal colic
Nephrocalcinosis

Other
Band keratopathy
Conjunctivitis
Change in vision
Pruritus
Thrombosis
Myalgia

ECG, electrocardiographic.

other known cytokines, mainly interleukin-1β and tumor necrosis factor-β (lymphotoxin). These cytokines promote local net bone resorption and thus produce hypercalcemia and hyperphosphatemia.

Vitamin D and Vitamin A Intoxication

When administered in excess, vitamins A and D can produce hypercalcemia. Affected patients tend to have normal or elevated serum phosphate levels associated with a low PTH level. Metastatic calcification may occur.

Thiazide Diuretics

Thiazides may increase serum calcium levels to a mild degree, primarily through hemoconcentration. Serum phosphate may also be depressed. It often takes several weeks for the hypercalcemia to resolve after the medication is discontinued.

Hyperthyroidism

Hyperthyroidism is associated with increased bone resorption. Often, the plasma PTH is low, and a history of other thyrotoxic symptoms can be elicited. The hypercalcemia usually resolves as the patient becomes euthyroid.

Milk–Alkali Syndrome

Typically, the milk–alkali syndrome occurs in patients with peptic ulcers who consume large quantities of milk and absorbable antacids. Usually, some degree of renal failure is present. PTH levels are low. This syndrome has become much less common with the increased use of nonabsorbable antacids and histamine (H_2)-receptor antagonists.

Sarcoidosis and Other Granulomatous Diseases

These syndromes are associated with hypersensitivity to vitamin D. Apparently, the granulomas can convert the inactive vitamin D to its active form. Patients have elevated plasma globulins and low PTH levels. The administration of large doses of cortisone for 10 days usually reduces the hypercalcemia. Biopsy of lymph nodes or the liver may confirm the diagnosis.

Familial Hypocalciuric Hypercalcemia

This disease is a generally asymptomatic, autosomal dominant condition characterized by mild to moderate hypercalcemia, hypocalciuria, and normal or only slightly elevated PTH levels. It develops in people heterozygous for a mutation in the calcium-sensing receptor (5). The mutation causes an increase in the set point for extracellular calcium concentration, so that the "normal" calcium level is higher in these people than in the normal population. No treatment is necessary, although people with this disease should receive genetic counseling. Neonatal severe hyperparathyroidism, which can be fatal, develops in children homozygous for mutations in this receptor. Treatment for neonates with this disease is controversial, but most benefit from early surgical management (6).

Immobilization

Immobilization produces hypercalcemia by increasing the ratio of bone resorption to bone formation. These patients can usually be distinguished by history, although on laboratory evaluation, they have elevated serum levels of calcium and phosphate and a decreased serum concentration of PTH. Often, hypercalciuria is present, which may lead to the development of renal stones. Treatment is early mobilization and forced diuresis.

Other Causes

A variety of other diseases may produce hypercalcemia. For example, Paget's disease (osteitis deformans) typically causes mild elevations in serum calcium. It can be diagnosed on the basis of the characteristic radiographic lesion. Adrenal insufficiency may be associated with hypercalcemia, although the symptoms are typically those of the primary abnormality. Lithium therapy appears to produce hypercalcemia by altering the parathyroid set point for inhibition by calcium. Idiopathic hypercalcemia of infancy is a rare disorder that is probably the result of hypersensitivity to vitamin D. It occurs in infants with mental retardation and is satisfactorily treated with glucocorticoids. Other causes include aluminum-induced renal osteomalacia and a host of analytic errors related to improper specimen collection with prolonged tourniquet times, tube contamination, and instrument drift.

Medical Treatment

Although the choice of therapy is tailored to the cause of the hypercalcemia, several general measures can prove effective (7).

For the patient with mild hypercalcemia, a decrease in dietary calcium is indicated. A reduction in intake of milk and other dairy products is suggested, along with discontinuation of thiazide diuretics and vitamin D preparations. Mobilization prevents bone demineralization and should be encouraged.

Patients with more marked hypercalcemia or severe symptoms should be admitted to the hospital for treatment, with careful observation and monitoring. In the patient with severe hyperparathyroidism, although the definitive therapy is surgical, it is unwise to proceed with neck exploration until the calcium has been reduced to near-normal levels. The mainstay of therapy is intravenous hydration, preferably with normal saline solution in sufficient quantities to maintain the urine output above 100 mL/h. These patients are often dehydrated before therapy, and fluid can be administered intravenously at a rate of 200 mL/h. Caution must be exercised in older patients, whose cardiac reserve may be marginal. This therapy exploits the parallel handling of calcium and sodium by the kidneys. The diuretic furosemide also increases sodium and calcium excretion but should not be used until the patient is well hydrated.

The end points of therapy are a decrease in the serum calcium level and a reduction of symptoms. Diuresis with saline solution is usually effective when the hypercalcemia results from hyperparathyroidism or a benign cause. In contrast, the hypercalcemia of malignancy may produce severe symptoms associated with extremely high serum calcium levels that are difficult to control. In this setting, a variety of other measures may be considered (Table 55.3). Some of the agents used to treat hypercalcemia cause significant toxicity, and close patient monitoring is required during treatment. Calcitonin is a fairly weak hypocalcemic agent, but it acts rapidly and appears to be associated with less toxicity than many of the other drugs. Salmon calcitonin appears to be the most potent preparation. Glucocorticoids may be particularly efficacious in patients with sarcoidosis and other granulomatous diseases. Mithramycin has proved useful in patients with hypercalcemia of malignancy, but it causes a cumulative toxicity (thrombocytopenia, hepatotoxicity, and nephrotoxicity). Biphosphonates appear to inhibit osteoclast activity directly. Disodium etidronate is the agent most commonly used. It is given intravenously and is particularly efficacious, although long-term use may be associated with significant osteomalacia. Prostaglandin synthetase inhibitors were initially considered useful, but their efficacy has proved to be limited. Intravenous phosphates and chelating agents have largely been abandoned because of their severe toxicity; however, oral phosphates may be beneficial in patients requiring prolonged therapy.

Table 55.3. TREATMENT OF HYPERCALCEMIA

Therapy of primary disease
Tumor resection (hypercalcemia of malignancy)
Parathyroidectomy (primary hyperparathyroidism)

Expansion of extracellular volume
Infusion of saline solution

Enhancement of urinary calcium excretion
Extracellular volume expansion
Loop diuretics (furosemide and ethacrynic acid)

Inhibition of bone resorption
Calcitonin
Glucocorticoids
Plicamycin (mithramycin)
Bisphosphonates
Gallium nitrate

Reduction of intestinal calcium absorption
Low-calcium diet
Glucocorticoids

Other
Dialysis
Mobilization
Oral phosphate
Estrogens or progestogens (postmenopausal women with primary
  hyperparathyroidism)
Chloroquine (sarcoidosis)

Modified from Attie MF. Treatment of hypercalcemia. Endocrinol Metab
  Clin North Am 1989;18:802, with permission.

Gallium nitrate is a promising agent for the potent inhibition of bone resorption; however, it can cause severe nephrotoxicity, and clinical experience with its use is still limited.

HYPOCALCEMIA

Hypocalcemia can occur as a consequence of various acquired and hereditary diseases (8). Generally, these disorders produce a deficiency or defect in the action of either PTH or vitamin D. It is most commonly a significant clinical problem after neck operation for thyroid disease. Vitamin D deficiency is associated with compensatory PTH excess. The end result is rickets in children or osteomalacia in adults.

Clinical Features

The major signs and symptoms of hypocalcemia are a direct consequence of the reduction in plasma levels of ionized calcium, which increases neuromuscular excitability (Table 55.4). The earliest clinical manifestations are numbness and tingling in the circumoral area, fingers, and toes. Mental symptoms are also common. Patients become anxious, depressed, and occasionally confused. Tetany may develop, characterized by carpopedal spasm, tonic–clonic convulsions, and laryngeal stridor. The magnitude of symptoms at any given plasma concentration of ionized calcium varies from patient to patient. On physical examination, contraction of the facial muscles is elicited by tapping anterior to the facial nerve (Chvostek's sign), although this sign may be positive in 10% of normal patients. Trousseau's sign is elicited by occluding blood flow to the forearm for 3 minutes. The development of carpal spasm indicates hypocalcemia, although the test is unpleasant and clinically impractical.

Table 55.4. CLINICAL FEATURES OF HYPOCALCEMIA

Neurologic
Circumoral paresthesia
Light-headedness
Depression
Anxiety
Confusion
Chvostek's sign
Trousseau's sign
Irritability
Laryngeal spasm
Seizures

Musculoskeletal
Tetany
Cramps
Involuntary twitching
Osteomalacia

Cardiovascular
ECG changes (prolonged QT interval, T-wave peaking)
Arrhythmia
Tachycardia, hypotension

Other
Lenticular cataracts

ECG, electrocardiographic.

Differential Diagnosis

The causes of hypocalcemia include the following:

Hypoparathyroidism
Vitamin D deficiency
Pseudohypoparathyroidism
Hypomagnesemia
Malabsorption
Pancreatitis
Hypoalbuminemia
Chelation of calcium
Osteoblastic metastases
Toxic shock syndrome
Hyperphosphatemia

The most common cause of hypocalcemia by far is excision of or damage to the parathyroid glands during thyroid surgery.

Etiology

Postoperative Hypoparathyroidism

Postoperative hypoparathyroidism commonly develops after total thyroidectomy for malignancy. Most patients undergoing operation on the thyroid experience some alteration in serum calcium, although they often are asymptomatic; the low calcium probably represents contusion or temporary alteration of the blood supply to the parathyroids. The hypocalcemia is usually transient and is not treated unless significant symptoms develop. Occasionally, in patients with preoperative hyperparathyroidism and significant bone disease, as evidenced by either radiographic changes or an elevation of the serum alkaline phosphatase level, a marked skeletal deposition of calcium and symptomatic hypocalcemia are present, so-called bone hunger. The plasma calcium usually reaches its nadir at 48 to 72 hours after surgery and then slowly returns to normal within 2 to 3 days. Occasionally, these patients may require calcium and vitamin D therapy for weeks or months after parathyroidectomy.

Idiopathic Hypoparathyroidism

A less common form of hypoparathyroidism is idiopathic lack of function. It occurs both sporadically and in families. In some cases, it develops as part of a polyglandular disorder and is thought to have an autoimmune basis. DiGeorge syndrome is a congenital disorder involving the branchial pouches that produces agenesis of the thymus and parathyroids. Hypoparathyroidism may also develop in newborns as a result of prenatal suppression of the fetal parathyroids as a consequence of maternal hypercalcemia. It is also common in otherwise normal but premature infants.

Vitamin D Deficiency

Vitamin D deficiency may occur as a result of dietary deficiency or lack of exposure to the sun. Likewise, renal disease produces a decrease in the 1-hydroxylase activity necessary for the formation of active vitamin D_3. The result is a decrease in calcium absorption and an increased secretion of PTH by the stimulated parathyroid glands. Osteomalacia, abnormal fractures, and the deformities of rickets may result.

Pseudohypoparathyroidism

Pseudohypoparathyroidism is a familial disease characterized by a rotund appearance, shortening of the extremities, and sometimes mental deficiency. The defect is not in PTH secretion; in fact, most patients have elevated plasma levels of PTH with evidence of increased bone resorption. Rather, the kidney is unresponsive to the hormone, and as a consequence, hypocalcemia and hyperphosphatemia develop. The deficit appears to be in the renal adenyl cyclase system.

Hypomagnesemia

This unusual deficit may result from chronic alcoholism, malabsorption, parenteral nutrition, or increased renal clearance during therapy with aminoglycosides. The deficit appears to block the physical response to PTH in addition to its release from the parathyroid gland.

Other Causes

In short-gut syndrome, after extensive small-bowel resection or bypass, vitamin D and calcium may be absorbed in insufficient quantities. In pancreatitis, the massive soft-tissue destruction and saponification that occur with hemorrhagic disease may sequester significant amounts of calcium in the retroperitoneum. Some undefined systemic factor also appears to contributes to hypocalcemia in these patients. Hypoalbuminemia causes a reduction in the total plasma calcium level, although the level of ionized calcium remains within the normal range and patients are asymptomatic. Circulatory substances, such as the citrate used to anticoagulate banked blood and radiographic contrast media, may bind to or form chelates with calcium. In patients with osteoblastic metastases, particularly associated with prostate carcinoma, hypocalcemia has been attributed to increased calcium flux into the lesions. Toxic shock syndrome is sometimes associated with hypocalcemia, but the mechanism has not been defined. Acute hyperphosphatemia, as a consequence of exogenous administration of phosphate or during the cytolytic chemotherapy of highly responsive tumors (e.g., Burkitt's lymphoma and acute lymphoblastic leukemia), may produce symptomatic hypocalcemia associated with soft-tissue calcification.

Treatment

The treatment of hypocalcemia can be summarized as follows:

1. Symptomatic hypocalcemia: oral calcium carbonate or intravenous calcium gluconate
2. Symptomatic tetany: intravenous calcium gluconate and diphenylhydantoin
3. Correction of hypomagnesemia: magnesium chloride
4. Vitamin D supplementation: ergocalciferol, calcifediol (liver disease), calcitriol (renal disease)
5. Long-term therapy: calcium carbonate; low-phosphate, low-oxalate diet; parathyroid grafting (immunosuppressed or cryopreserved autograft)

For acute symptomatic hypocalcemia, calcium should be administered intravenously. Calcium gluconate is less irritating to the veins and the calcium release is slower, without a risk for overcorrection. Usually, 20 to 30 mL of 10% solution is infused over a 15- to 20-minute period, and then 50 to 100 mL is administered over the next 12 hours in adults. Bicarbonate precipitates any calcium infused through the same intravenous line. Serum magnesium should always be measured, and hypomagnesemia should be corrected if present. In patients with convulsions from advanced tetany, diphenylhydantoin therapy may prove useful, but symptoms should never be allowed to progress to this point.

Long-term therapy is gauged on the basis of symptoms. In the postoperative patient, the continued stimulus of mild hypocalcemia to any remaining parathyroid tissue may prove useful. Concomitant therapy with calcium and vitamin D is effective in a timely fashion. A starting dose of 2 g of oral calcium carbonate per day in divided doses is usually well tolerated. Vitamin D can be administered as calcitriol, a synthetic vitamin D analogue. Most adults respond to a dose of 0.5 to 2.0 μg/d; reduced doses may be necessary for patients with renal dysfunction.

A low-phosphate, low-oxalate diet may also prove useful. Synthetic PTH is not yet available in sufficient quantities to make its use practical, and parathyroid allotransplantation is successful but requires immunosuppression therapy.

HYPERPARATHYROIDISM

Definitions

Like endocrine tumors, parathyroid neoplasms are usually recognized not because of physical enlargement but because of the peripheral effects of excess hormone. Although the distinction is somewhat artificial, primary hyperparathyroidism develops spontaneously, without apparent cause but possibly in response to exogenous stimuli. When the normal control of serum calcium is disturbed and the autonomous production of PTH is increased, the state is referred to as *primary hyperparathyroidism*. This category includes both benign single- and multiple-gland enlargements and the much rarer parathyroid carcinoma. In some cases, the disease is familial. In contrast, *secondary hyperparathyroidism* occurs when a defect in mineral homeostasis leads to a compensatory increase in parathyroid function. This occurs most commonly in response to renal disease but may also develop as a consequence of the hypocalcemia associated with some diseases of the gastrointestinal tract, bones, or other endocrine organs. Occasionally, with prolonged secondary stimulation, the hyperfunctioning glands are no longer physiologically responsive to an increase in ionized calcium. This rare, relatively autonomous state, referred to as *tertiary hyperparathyroidism,* develops most commonly after renal transplantation when the defect in calcium homeostasis is corrected.

Incidence

The advent in the 1970s of the widespread screening of serum calcium as part of automated multichannel analysis

Table 55.5. AGE- AND GENDER-SPECIFIC INCIDENCE OF PRIMARY HYPERPARATHYROIDISM

Age (y)	New cases per 100,000	
	Men	Women
< 39	5	8
40–50	26	104
> 60	92	189
Total	18	56

After Heath H III, Hodgson SF, Kennedy MA. Primary hyperthyroidism: incidence, morbidity, and potential economic impact in a community. N Engl J Med 1980;302:189, with permission.

has considerably altered our understanding of hyperparathyroidism. Before that time, primary hyperparathyroidism was thought to be a relatively rare condition. Most patients presented with symptoms of disease, usually renal stones or bony manifestations. Today, as a result of screening, most patients are asymptomatic or have only vague symptoms or signs that can be related to hyperparathyroidism (9,10). Occasionally, patients recognize that they had symptoms only after their well-being improves following parathyroidectomy. Incidence varies with both age and gender (Table 55.5), but hyperparathyroidism is believed to develop in about 50 to 100 people per 100,000 in the general population, with about 50,000 new cases occurring annually in the United States (11). Marked variations have been noted worldwide; the reasons for these differences remain unclear.

Etiology

The cause of primary hyperparathyroidism is not known. Although the sequence of progression from secondary to tertiary disease in response to chronic stimulation has a logical appeal, it is difficult to draw parallels with primary disease. Most patients with primary hyperparathyroidism have disease of a single rather than of multiple glands, which is not what might be predicted if an external stimulus were operative. Hyperparathyroidism is most common in postmenopausal women, the population group with the highest incidence of osteoporosis and the

most significant alterations in calcium and phosphate metabolism. Loss of renal function with aging is associated with elevations in PTH and decreases in phosphate clearance. It has been suggested but not demonstrated that a renal calcium leak, if sufficient, might result in a chronic calcium deficit stimulating the parathyroids.

Genetic studies of parathyroid adenomas have described an oncogene (PRAD1) that may be one step in the path to neoplasia in these tumors. Ongoing research indicates that overexpression of the normal PRAD1 gene, also known as *cyclin D1*, allows progression of the cell cycle from the G1 phase to the S phase, thus promoting cellular growth and division. PRAD1 is overexpressed in only a subset of parathyroid adenomas; further research may reveal other genetic alterations that contribute to the neoplastic growth (12,13).

Hyperparathyroidism occurs in several familial forms. It is a major component of the multiple endocrine neoplasia (MEN) syndromes types I and IIA. The parathyroid disease of these syndromes is multiglandular and transmitted in an autosomal dominant fashion. In other families, hyperparathyroidism is inherited in an autosomal dominant fashion without other manifestations of MEN-I or MEN-II; some have osseous abnormalities (tumor–jaw syndrome) and some apparently isolated disease.

Pathology

Single- versus Multiple-gland Disease

Although pathologic studies can usually distinguish parathyroid glands from other tissue, beyond this capacity, they may not prove useful. Intraoperative decisions frequently depend on recognizing disease of one or more parathyroid glands, and in this regard, the histologic description of adenoma or hyperplasia is generally unreliable in primary hyperparathyroidism.

Microscopically, the cell most commonly involved in primary hyperparathyroidism is the chief cell (14). Less frequently, the oxyphil cell is the predominant cell type. Diseased glands typically have an increase in the proportion of stromal cells and a reduction in the proportion of stromal fat. Single diseased glands, or adenomas, have been classically described with a predominance of chief cells centering in a single focus, with a compressed rim of surrounding normal tissue (Fig. 55.8). In contrast, parathy-

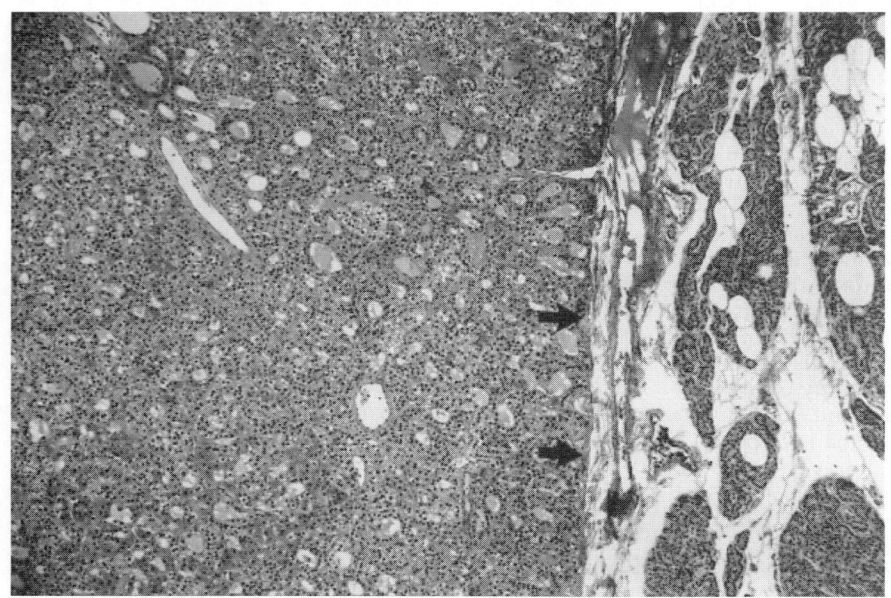

Figure 55.8. Classic histologic findings in parathyroid adenoma. A single focus of proliferating chief cells is surrounded by a compressed rim of normal parathyroid tissue *(arrows)* composed of half stroma and half fat. ×90.

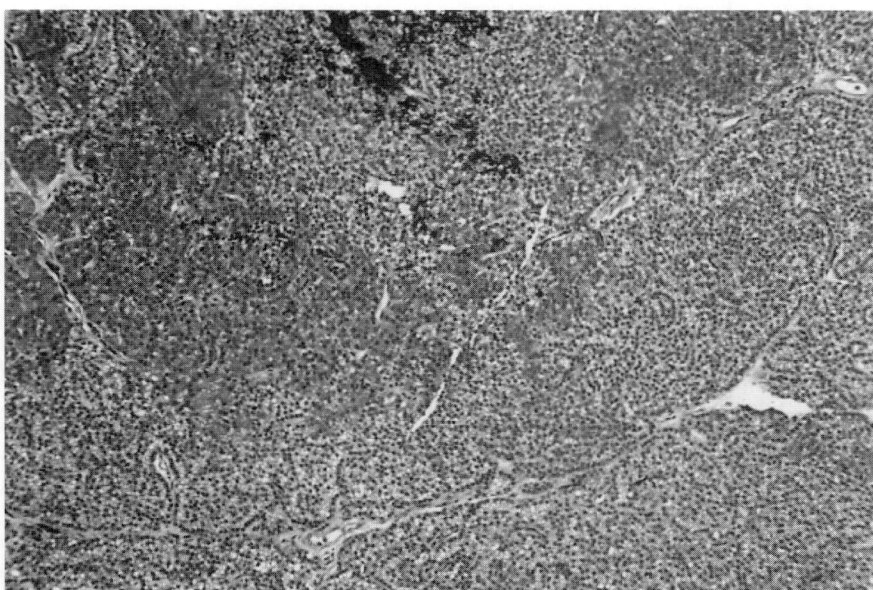

Figure 55.9. Classic findings in parathyroid hyperplasia consist of a diffuse proliferation of cells without any remaining normal gland. ×150.

roid hyperplasia has been characterized as a diffuse proliferation of clear cells in multiple glands, with little remaining normal tissue (Fig. 55.9). These criteria have proved to be totally unreliable. Patients with multiple-gland disease may have one gland that appears to be an adenoma and another that appears diffusely involved or even histologically normal with gross enlargement. Other methods of identifying normal glands, including staining of intracellular fat, measurement of glandular density, and flow cytometric analysis of cellular DNA content, have all been used with some reported success, although none provides unequivocal differentiation between normal and abnormal glands.

By far the most reliable index of abnormality is the determination of glandular enlargement by visual inspection. The incidence of single- and multiple-gland enlargement in 66 consecutive patients with hyperparathyroidism is shown in Table 55.6. The visual assessment and judgment of the experienced surgeon have proved to be the best basis for intraoperative decisions, although recent laboratory developments may change this. This approach requires that all four parathyroid glands be evaluated at the time of operation.

Carcinoma

Parathyroid carcinoma is a rare entity, and the histologic diagnosis can be exceedingly difficult. The surgeon may suspect the diagnosis when dense invasion and scarring are encountered, although this may be secondary to some other inflammatory disease in the neck. Pathologic criteria include marked mitotic activity, dense fibrous stroma, and

Table 55.6. **GLAND ENLARGEMENT IN 66 CONSECUTIVE PATIENTS WITH PRIMARY HYPERPARATHYROIDISM**

Pathology	No.	Percentage
Adenoma	50	76%
Double adenoma	4	6%
Hyperplasia	12	18%

From Lowney JK, Weber B, Johnson S, et al. Minimal incision parathyroidectomy: cure, cosmesis, and cost. World J Surg 2000;24: 1442–1445.

evidence of local invasion into the capsule or surrounding vessels. Malignant-appearing tumors, however, may pursue an apparently benign clinical course; the converse is less frequently true. An aneuploid pattern by flow cytometric analysis of tumor DNA content may help to distinguish carcinoma from atypical adenoma in borderline cases (15). The only reliable criteria of malignancy are metastases, most commonly to the lymph nodes, lung, or liver, and true local invasion.

Systemic Effects

The use of automated technology for determining serum calcium has changed not only the estimated incidence of hyperparathyroidism but also the usual mode of presentation (9). Before screening, three fourths of patients presented with renal disease, particularly nephrolithiasis; one third to one half had skeletal manifestations, and rare patients had both. Most recent series suggest that at least half of the patients in whom hyperparathyroidism is diagnosed do not have renal or osseous disease, and many are asymptomatic. Manifestations of the disease are protean but generally nonspecific, and they may be difficult to elicit in the history. A significant proportion of patients present without a readily quantifiable index of disease severity. This has created some controversy about the need for surgery in the asymptomatic and particularly the elderly or high-risk patient (10).

The earliest complaints are often the vague symptoms of hypercalcemia, as discussed previously. They vary with the magnitude of plasma calcium elevation and include muscle weakness, anorexia, nausea, constipation, polyuria, and polydipsia. These nonspecific symptoms may or may not cause the patient to seek medical attention (16). Some symptomatic patients have evidence of chronic disease involving the kidney or skeleton. Usually, only one of these systems is significantly involved in any individual patient. The treatment of hyperparathyroidism is designed to eliminate or halt the progression of the complications of the disease. Symptomatic patients can be divided into two groups. Members of the first group have renal manifestations, a slower onset of symptoms, and generally lower serum calcium concentrations. Patients in the second group have a more rapid onset of symptoms, higher serum calcium levels, and significant bone disease. No recognizable histologic or physiologic characteristics separate patients with renal disease from those with bone disease.

Renal Manifestations

Renal complications develop because the hypercalcemia leads to an increase in urinary calcium excretion and because PTH increases the excretion of phosphate and produces urinary alkalosis. Both these events predispose to stone formation. Urinary stones may be treated surgically or with lithotripsy, and subsequent definitive treatment of the hyperparathyroidism reduces the rate of re-formation. Nephrolithiasis develops in about 30% of patients. Of patients who present for the first time with renal colic, 5% to 10% are found to have primary hyperparathyroidism. Nephrocalcinosis (Fig. 55.10) represents calcification of the renal parenchyma and occurs in 5% to 10% of patients with hyperparathyroidism. It causes more significant renal damage than nephrolithiasis does. In general, the more severe the renal damage, the less likely it is that nephrocalcinosis will regress after parathyroidectomy.

The incidence of hypertension in hyperparathyroidism increases with the degree of renal impairment. Hypertension may be the most significant cause of the morbidity associated with hyperparathyroidism, but although a decrease in blood pressure has been demonstrated in some patients after parathyroidectomy, the correlation between the two conditions is not clear.

Skeletal Manifestations

Parathyroid bone disease in its most classic and severe form, osteitis fibrosa cystica, is seldom seen; however, 5% to 15% of patients present with significant symptoms of skeletal disease. Most commonly, these include bone pain and pathologic fractures.

Bone changes are often demonstrable on detailed plain radiographs of the hands (Fig. 55.11). Characteristically, subperiosteal resorption is evident on the radial aspect of the middle phalanx of the second or third finger. Because of tufting of the distal phalanges, clubbing may be evident on physical examination. Other findings that typically involve the skull and long bones include bone cysts, "brown" tumors (i.e., localized proliferations of osteoclasts), and diffuse demineralization or granularity.

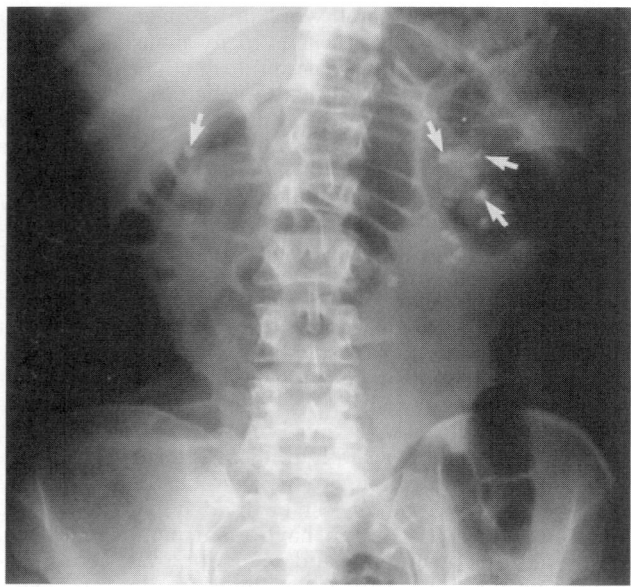

Figure 55.10. Abdominal film demonstrating nephrocalcinosis, or diffuse calcification of the renal parenchyma *(arrows)*.

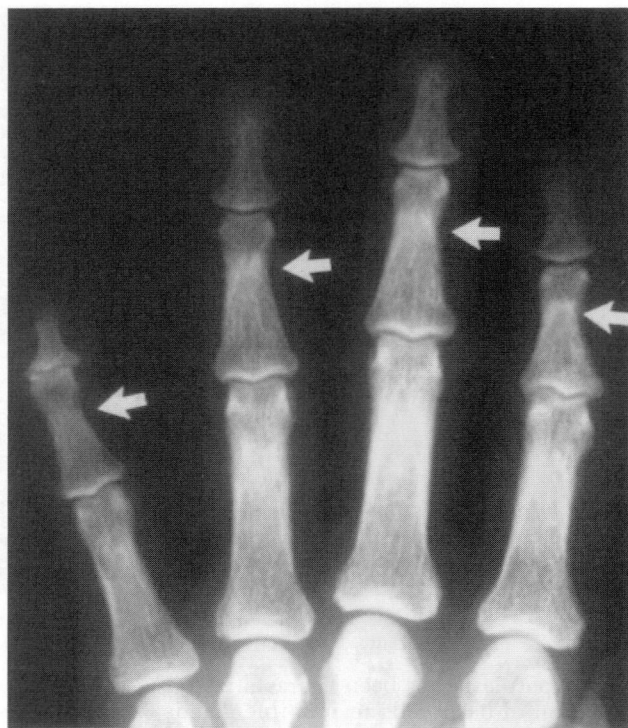

Figure 55.11. Magnification radiograph of the fingers in hyperparathyroidism. Subperiosteal cortical resorption *(arrows)* typically is most visible on the radial aspect of the middle phalanges.

More subtle bone loss can be detected by iliac crest bone biopsy or photon beam densitometry. The significance of mild derangements detectable only with such sophisticated technology has been questioned, and further studies are needed to determine the postoperative outcome of bone disease in patients with these presumably early manifestations of hyperparathyroidism.

Gastrointestinal Manifestations

Hypercalcemia is clearly associated with nonspecific gastrointestinal complaints, including nausea, vomiting, constipation, and anorexia, but attempts to demonstrate a definite relation between hyperparathyroidism and either peptic ulcer disease or pancreatitis remain unconvincing. Hypercalcemia stimulates gastric acid secretion experimentally and clinically and has been associated with pancreatitis. Therefore, a theoretic rationale for the complex of hyperparathyroidism and gastrointestinal symptoms does exist. The incidence of cholelithiasis also appears to be slightly increased in patients with hyperparathyroidism, presumably as a result of the higher concentrations of calcium in bile.

Neuromuscular Manifestations

Neurologic and muscular complaints are those of hypercalcemia in general. Fatigability and proximal muscle weakness are among the most debilitating. Atrophy of type II muscle fibers, consistent with a neuropathic and not a myopathic cause, has been demonstrated. Sensory complaints include dysesthesia, a reduced vibratory sense, and stocking–glove sensory deficits.

Psychological Manifestations

The emotional disturbances of hyperparathyroidism are often subtle and difficult to quantify. As with other forms of hypercalcemia, they range from depression or anxiety to psychosis and coma. Patients undergoing parathyroidectomy frequently experience a sense of well-being and relief from fatigue and dullness postoperatively, even they may have had no noticeable complaints preoperatively.

Other Manifestations

A variety of signs and symptoms of soft-tissue calcification have been described. Nonspecific arthralgia, particularly involving the proximal interphalangeal joints of the hands, is characteristic. The incidence of chondrocalcinosis is increased. Pruritus, vascular and cardiac calcification, and band keratopathy of the cornea have all been noted. Several reports have suggested an increased incidence of malignancy, but these remain unsubstantiated.

Diagnostic Investigations

Of the various clinical manifestations, only the skeletal changes of hyperparathyroidism are pathognomonic. Usually, the evaluation focuses on the differential diagnosis of an elevated serum calcium concentration, and the diagnosis is essentially one of exclusion, with other causes of hypercalcemia ruled out.

Physical Findings

Except in patients with the classic deformities of advanced bone disease, the physical examination is seldom helpful. Diseased parathyroids are infrequently palpable, except in patients with parathyroid carcinoma. A mass in the anterior neck in a patient with primary hyperparathyroidism is more commonly a thyroid nodule.

Calcium

Hypercalcemia is the single most important diagnostic finding; however, particularly in early or mild cases, serial analysis may show fluctuations in and out of the normal range. Coexistent hypoalbuminemia and acidosis may produce an apparently normal total serum calcium, even though the ionized fraction is actually elevated. Serum concentrations of ionized calcium may be helpful in the patient with intermittent or mild hypercalcemia.

Parathyroid Hormone

In the United States, PTH measurement has become an important method for establishing the diagnosis of hyper-

parathyroidism. Because of the heterogeneity of the various circulating forms of PTH, conflicting and confusing results were often obtained during the initial clinical experience with radioimmunoassays. The methodology continues to be refined, and most current assays are sufficiently sensitive, specific, and reliable that they can be recommended for wide clinical use. Intact hormone assays, as opposed to amino terminus or carboxyl terminus assays, appear to be the most dependable. The demonstration of an elevated plasma PTH concentration alone does not establish the diagnosis of hyperparathyroidism. In the setting of an inappropriately elevated serum calcium level, however, this finding is virtually diagnostic (Fig. 55.12).

Phosphate

Parathyroid hormone increases renal phosphate excretion and, in about half of patients, produces hypophosphatemia. In the presence of renal disease, however, the serum phosphate levels may be normal or significantly elevated.

Bicarbonate

Parathyroid hormone also increases bicarbonate excretion, so that a hyperchloremic metabolic acidosis may develop. It has been suggested that the finding of an elevated serum chloride-to-phosphate ratio may be helpful in the differential diagnosis of hypercalcemia. A ratio greater than 30 is considered highly suggestive of hyperparathyroidism.

Magnesium

Hypomagnesemia develops in 5% to 10% of patients. After parathyroidectomy, if both hypocalcemia and hypomagnesemia are present, it may be difficult to correct the calcium until the serum magnesium has been corrected.

Other Diagnostic Tests

A variety of special diagnostic tests are now available. None is more specific than the measurement of serum concentrations of calcium and PTH, although they may be useful in equivocal cases. For example, the 24-hour urinary calcium excretion is usually elevated in patients with hyperparathyroidism, although the finding is not specific for this disease. This test is helpful in identifying patients

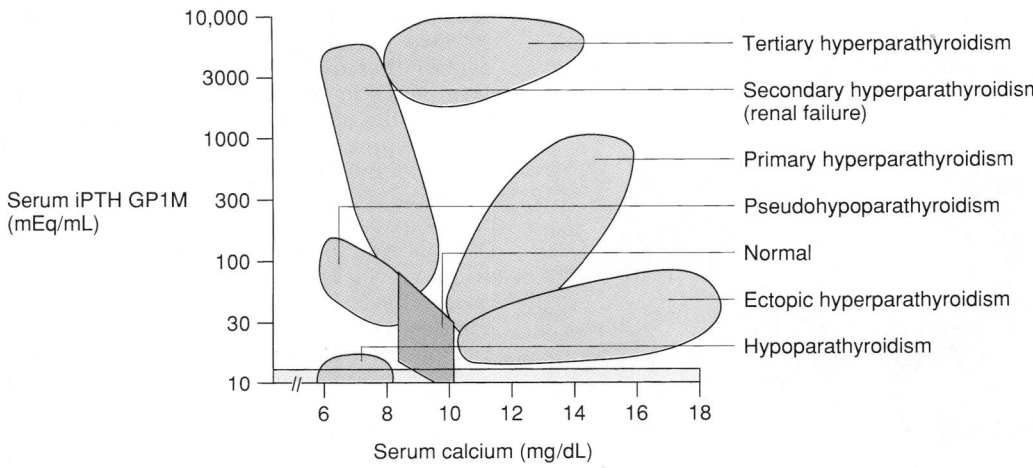

Figure 55.12. Relation between serum immunoreactive parathyroid hormone and serum calcium in patients with hypoparathyroidism, pseudohypoparathyroidism, ectopic hyperparathyroidism, and primary, secondary, and tertiary hyperparathyroidism. *GP1M,* guinea pig antiserum 1M. (After Clark OH, Way LW. Thyroid and parathyroid. In: Way LW, ed. *Current surgical diagnosis and treatment,* 8th ed. Norwalk, CT: Appleton & Lange, 1989:249, with permission.)

with familial hypercalcemic hypocalciuria, in whom the rate of urinary calcium excretion is low. Measurements of tubular reabsorption of phosphate below 30% suggest primary hyperparathyroidism. Urinary cAMP is generated specifically as a consequence of PTH activation of renal tubular adenyl cyclase. Increased urinary concentrations are identified in most patients with primary hyperparathyroidism. These measurements are rarely necessary because of the reliability of the intact PTH measurement.

Localization

Because of the ectopic location of some glands, the difficulty in differentiating single-gland from multiple-gland disease, and the fact that even the experienced endocrine surgeon occasionally has difficulty in identifying an abnormal gland, attempts have been made to localize enlarged glands preoperatively. In the hands of an experienced surgeon, however, the cure rate for hyperparathyroidism at the initial operation exceeds 95% with the conventional full neck exploration. However, three recent technologic developments have led surgeons to pursue alternatives to the full neck exploration. These innovations are (a) technetium 99m sestamibi scintigraphy, (b) intraoperative intact PTH measurement, and (c) videoscopic parathyroid exploration. Surgeons have used these technologies in various combinations to limit the extent of the neck exploration. All the current alternative strategies, however, depend on a preoperative parathyroid localization study to direct the exploration.

The study most frequently used for imaging previously unoperated patients is technetium 99m sestamibi scintigraphy (Fig. 55.13). Sestamibi scanning can identify the site of abnormal tissue in 75% to 80% of patients but has limitations in patients with small adenomas or multiple-gland disease. Sestamibi was originally developed for cardiac imaging. It also images parathyroid tissue on delayed scans and has been used recently for noninvasive parathyroid imaging. The use of a single nuclide with a short half-life and a high-energy profile has advantages in lateral, oblique, and three-dimensional imaging that technetium–thallium scanning, which was formerly used, does not provide.

In patients with persistent or recurrent hyperparathyroidism, preoperative imaging is important to guide the exploration. High-resolution real-time ultrasonography, computed tomography (CT), magnetic resonance imaging (MRI), and sestamibi scanning all appear to have comparable sensitivities of 50% to 60% (17–19). The results of these examinations may be less successful at centers without significant experience in their use. Ultrasonography is a more operator-dependent technique, and its use is lim-ited to evaluation of the neck. It is rapid and relatively inexpensive and can direct fine-needle aspiration for cytologic confirmation and immunoassay for PTH.

Computed tomography is more expensive but less operator-dependent than ultrasonography. It clearly is superior in identifying deeper structures and for examining the retrosternal mediastinum. MRI is considerably more expensive than CT and has not been shown to be superior. Most surgeons prefer to have results of two or more imaging tests that confirm an abnormality before exploration.

Treatment

Indications for Surgery

Recent reports have suggested that estrogen therapy, by reducing bone turnover and plasma calcium, may be useful in postmenopausal women with mild hyperparathyroidism. Generally, however, the only practical therapeutic option is surgery. Nephrolithiasis, bone disease, and neuromuscular symptoms all respond well to surgical intervention. In contrast, surgery in patients with renal failure, hypertension, and psychiatric symptoms is not so uniformly successful, although it benefits some patients and is usually indicated in all except those at highest risk. The question of how to manage the large group of patients with apparently asymptomatic disease requires particularly careful consideration.

Management of Asymptomatic Hyperparathyroidism

An increasing proportion of patients with the diagnosis of hyperparathyroidism are asymptomatic. The appropriate treatment for these patients remains controversial. Although little evidence indicates that irreversible complications, such as renal failure, eventually develop in patients with asymptomatic mild disease, the natural history of the disease remains incompletely defined. Many of the manifestations of this disease may go unrecognized until they are corrected surgically. Still unanswered is the question of how much asymptomatic disease may contribute to generalized osteopenia in this predominantly postmenopausal female population.

One study followed a group of 142 asymptomatic patients without operation (20). At the end of the 10-year study, more than 20% of the patients had required surgery for an increase in serum calcium to above 11 mg/dL or for specific complications attributable to the disease. Another 20% were lost to or declined follow-up. The remaining patients either died of unrelated causes or had persistent asymptomatic disease. The authors concluded that because of the large percentage (about 40%) of patients who either required operation or were lost to follow-up, they could not reliably recommend conservative management.

A more recent report detailed the 10-year natural history of 121 patients with asymptomatic hyperparathyroidism (10). Operation was recommended for those in whom symptoms or findings developed, according to the guidelines of the National Institutes of Health Consensus Conference (see below). During the monitoring period, indications for operation developed in 27% of the patients, and biochemical normalization and increased bone mass were observed in those who underwent surgery. However, although the patients who did not undergo operative correction continued to have biochemical abnormalities, renal stones or fractures did not develop in any of them. These data confirm the impression of most clinicians that mild hyperparathyroidism rarely takes a precipitously worsening clinical course, and so the risks and discomforts of management must remain appropriate to the disease.

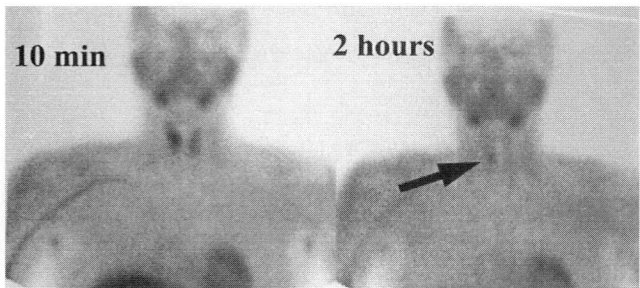

Figure 55.13. Technetium 99m sestamibi scan of a patient with a parathyroid adenoma. The radionuclide is present in both thyroid and parathyroid tissue on the 10-minute film; however, by 2 hours, the radionuclide has washed out of the thyroid and remains only in the right-sided parathyroid gland. This was a 794-mg right upper parathyroid adenoma *(arrow).*

In October 1990, a National Institutes of Health Consensus Development Conference reviewed the available evidence regarding the management of asymptomatic primary hyperparathyroidism; more recent data have not caused them to change their recommendations regarding the indications for intervention (21). The panel agreed that operation is the indicated treatment for all patients with symptoms; however, they recognized a subgroup of patients who have no symptoms attributable to hyperparathyroidism, and their conclusions included several indications for surgical intervention in these asymptomatic patients:

Markedly elevated serum calcium
History of an episode of life-threatening hypercalcemia
Reduced creatinine clearance
Presence of one or more kidney stones detected by abdominal radiography
Markedly elevated 24-hour urinary calcium excretion
Substantially reduced bone mass as determined by direct measurement

The panel mandated close (every 6 months) follow-up for those patients not treated by operation. In addition, they recommended surgery for cases in which medical surveillance is neither desirable nor suitable, such as when a patient requests surgery, consistent follow-up is unlikely, coexistent illness complicates management, or a patient is young (< 50 years old).

This remains an area of considerable controversy, and complete resolution of the question would require a randomized, controlled trial. The complication rate of operation by an experienced surgeon is very low. Within a short period, the financial cost of medical follow-up exceeds that of treatment by operation. Based on these considerations, most patients should undergo operation, and those who do not must be closely followed.

Principles of Surgical Correction

Although neck exploration for hyperparathyroidism may be straightforward, it sometimes becomes an arduous procedure requiring considerable patience because of the variability in both the location and the number of diseased glands. Persistent hyperparathyroidism and the necessity for reexploration can usually be avoided by a meticulous initial procedure. Reoperation is predictably more diffi-

cult than the initial operation, and the risks for damage to the recurrent laryngeal nerves and hypoparathyroidism are greater during reoperation.

It is essential that the surgeon be confident of the preoperative diagnosis and prospectively discuss the procedure with the patient. The potential complications of damage to either the recurrent laryngeal nerve or the superior laryngeal nerve and the development of hypocalcemia require discussion. Likewise, the possibility of an unsuccessful initial operation needs to be explained, and the patient should recognize that reexploration, including median sternotomy, may be required. Although alternatives to full neck exploration are often now applied, no patient should be explored by a surgeon who is unfamiliar with the principles and techniques of the conventional full neck exploration.

For a full neck exploration, the patient is placed under general anesthesia with a roll beneath the thoracic spine and with the neck extended. The neck is opened through a transverse incision overlying the thyroid isthmus, and the platysma is similarly divided. Superior and inferior flaps are developed. The strap muscles are separated in the midline and retracted laterally; division is unnecessary. One lobe of the thyroid is chosen and rotated medially. Important landmarks include the tracheoesophageal groove, the recurrent laryngeal nerve, the inferior and superior thyroid arteries, and the middle thyroid vein (Fig. 55.14). In most patients, the nerve lies in the tracheoesophageal groove or just laterally. Occasionally, it may be situated more anteriorly. Uncommonly, it may originate directly from the vagus without passing around the right subclavian artery. Both these variations make the recurrent nerve more susceptible to injury. The external branch of the superior laryngeal nerve, which innervates the cricothyroid muscle, usually lies medial to the superior thyroid vessels and should be carefully preserved.

Although in the past some have advocated unilateral exploration if a single enlarged gland and one normal gland are identified on the first side explored, most surgeons now agree that all four glands need to be identified at the initial exploration because of the possibility of multiple-gland disease, unless intraoperative PTH measurement is used to confirm removal of all pathologic parathyroid tissue. Supernumerary glands may be present and should be sought at the initial procedure. Although frozen section has not been helpful in differentiating diseased from nor-

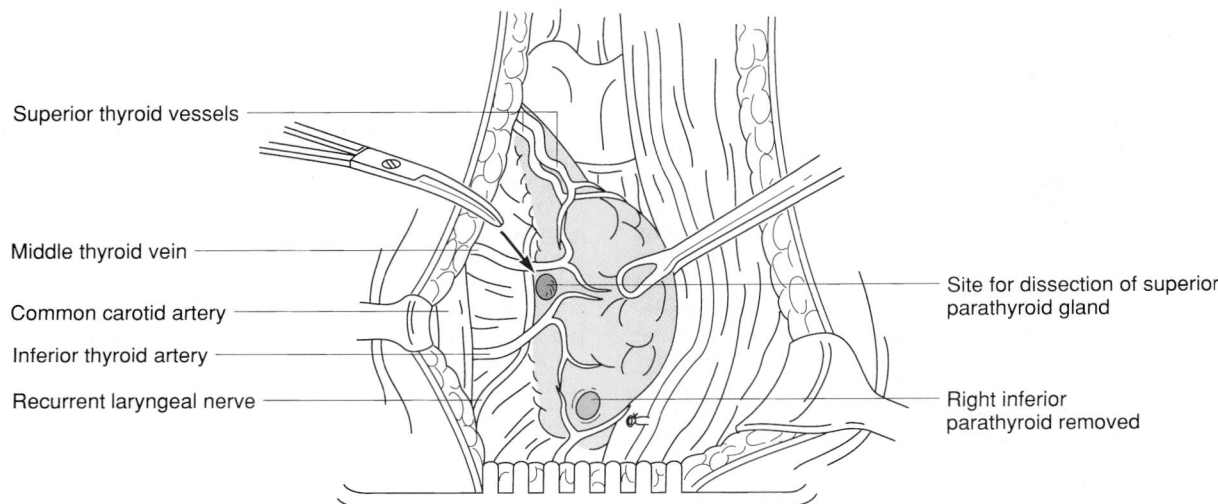

Figure 55.14. Lateral view of the right side of the neck after rotation of the thyroid lobe. The important anatomic landmarks are emphasized.

Superior thyroid vessels

Middle thyroid vein

Common carotid artery

Inferior thyroid artery

Recurrent laryngeal nerve

Site for dissection of superior parathyroid gland

Right inferior parathyroid removed

mal glands, it is generally reliable for confirming the presence or absence of parathyroid tissue. Small, thin biopsy specimens are sharply incised from the gland to be confirmed, with extreme care taken to avoid damaging its delicate blood supply. Most surgeons use frozen section selectively to confirm suspected abnormal parathyroid tissue or to document difficult or confusing situations (22).

The upper glands are usually located far dorsally on the surface of the thyroid lobe at the level of the upper two thirds of the gland. The lower glands are less constant and may be located anywhere from well above the thyroid to the anterior mediastinum. The lower glands are most typically in the region where the thyrothymic ligament attaches to the lower pole of the thyroid lobe. If the inferior glands cannot be localized, the thymic pedicle should be carefully examined and mobilized. Because of their common embryologic origin, the inferior gland is frequently associated with the thymic remnant. Parathyroid glands within the mediastinum sometimes can be removed by mobilizing the thymus through the cervical incision. If this is unsuccessful in identifying the parathyroid gland, the thyroid lobe on the side of the missing gland is mobilized and palpated. Intraoperative ultrasonographic examination may identify an intrathyroidal parathyroid gland. As a last resort, blind excision of the lobe may be indicated.

If after meticulous exploration of all these areas three or four parathyroid glands have been identified, none of which is enlarged, most surgeons would favor terminating the operation.

Extent of Resection

The operative procedure performed is based on the number of enlarged glands identified. In many instances, the pathologist cannot reliably distinguish diseased from normal glands based on frozen section, and this decision is based on the surgeon's experience and judgment. Traditionally, single-gland disease has been treated by simple excision, whereas any combination of two- or three-gland enlargement is treated by resecting the diseased tissue and leaving the normal glands in place. The question of whether two- or three-gland enlargement implies the presence of disease in all glands (hyperplasia) has not been resolved. If one gland is large and the remaining three are normal in size, resection of the single parathyroid cures virtually all patients. Of 76 patients with two- or three-gland disease treated by excising the large glands and leaving the normal glands, only eight (10.5%) had recurrent hypercalcemia, which tended to be mild (follow-up of 12 to 140 months postoperatively). This approach seems satisfactory in most patients (23).

Treating patients with four-gland disease has been more difficult. In many of these patients, the disease occurs as a component of one of the familial syndromes, particularly MEN-I. Patients with four-gland parathyroid hyperplasia can be treated by subtotal parathyroidectomy (removing three and a half glands) or by total parathyroidectomy with autotransplantation of some parathyroid tissue into the nondominant forearm. Both operations depend on meticulous identification of all parathyroid tissue for adequate results. The putative advantage of the subtotal parathyroidectomy is that it leaves the remaining parathyroid tissue with its native blood supply. Total parathyroidectomy has the advantage of removing all the abnormal parathyroid tissue from the neck and placing it in a site where reoperation for recurrent hyperparathyroidism is simpler. In either operation, parathyroid tissue should be viably cryopreserved to allow later autografting if the patient has persistent hypoparathyroidism postoperatively.

The reported incidence of recurrent hypercalcemia after subtotal parathyroidectomy for nonfamilial parathyroid hyperplasia is zero to 16%; the incidence of permanent hypoparathyroidism is 4% to 5%. In patients with MEN-I, however, the recurrence rate is 26% to 36% with long-term follow-up after subtotal parathyroidectomy (average time to recurrence is longer than 5 years). Total parathyroidectomy is associated with a similar risk for permanent hypoparathyroidism (5%) and a higher reported risk for recurrent hypercalcemia (familial, 64%; nonfamilial, 20%). Reoperation for recurrent hypercalcemia is greatly simplified by the approach of total parathyroidectomy with autotransplantation. Thus, given the current data, sporadic parathyroid hyperplasia can be acceptably treated by either operation. Our group has practiced with the philosophy that the substantial risk for recurrent hypercalcemia following either operation makes the option of total parathyroidectomy with autotransplantation preferable for patients with familial disease; however, the data to support this are not definitive.

Technique of Parathyroid Autotransplantation

Total parathyroidectomy is performed, and a parathyroid gland is sliced into 15 to 20 pieces and autografted into a forearm muscle bed. The sites are marked with silk sutures. This location permits easy subsequent access under local anesthesia if recurrent hypercalcemia develops. Function of the autograft is documented by normocalcemia, with the autograft as the only source of PTH, and by measuring higher concentrations of hormone in the antecubital vein draining the graft bed than in the corresponding vein in the opposite arm. Lack of function is unusual; hypoparathyroidism develops in about 5% of patients. Glands should also be viably frozen in dimethyl sulfoxide and serum. If in the postoperative period it becomes clear that the patient is aparathyroid, the cryopreserved tissue can be reimplanted under local anesthesia.

Special Situations

Persistent or Recurrent Hyperparathyroidism

Persistent hyperparathyroidism occurs in fewer than 5% of patients after exploration by an experienced surgeon. Most commonly, it is the result of a single diseased gland remaining in the neck or the mediastinum. Recurrent disease develops after an interval of normocalcemia and may be the result of regrowth of diseased tissue, implantation from a tumor broken at the initial procedure, or even recurrent parathyroid carcinoma.

In the evaluation of these patients, it is essential to document that the initial diagnosis was indeed correct. Familial hypocalciuric hypercalcemia should be ruled out by measuring urinary calcium excretion.

Reviewing the original operative notes and pathology reports may provide clues to the position of missed glands. The locations of parathyroid tumors not found at the initial operation but identified on subsequent exploration in one large series are shown in Fig. 55.15.

It is generally agreed that localization studies do have a place in the management of recurrent disease. Noninvasive methods are used first, and if these are unsuccessful in identifying the diseased gland, selective angiography and venous sampling for PTH are used. Selective angiography appears to be the most accurate technique, successfully localizing 50% to 80% of parathyroid glands that cannot be detected by any other modality. Venous sampling may also be helpful in some patients, although interpretation is often complicated by the collateralization that occurs postoperatively. Because it provides no direct

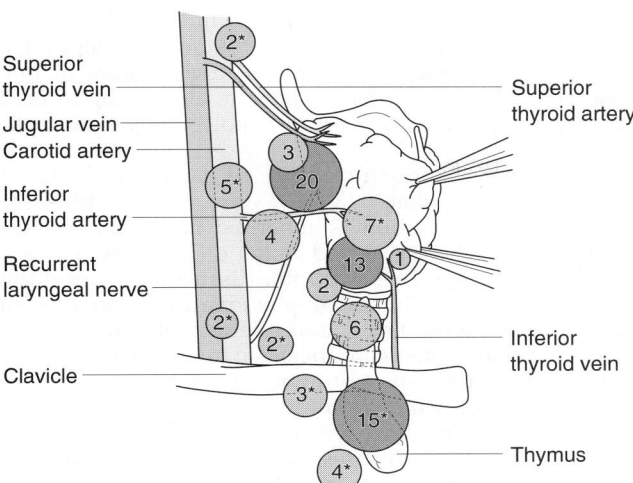

Superior thyroid vein

Jugular vein

Carotid artery

Inferior thyroid artery

Recurrent laryngeal nerve

Clavicle

Superior thyroid artery

Inferior thyroid vein

Thymus

Figure 55.15. Location of parathyroid tumors missed on initial exploration but identified on subsequent operation. (After Jaskowiak N, Norton JA, Alexander HR, et al. A prospective trial evaluating a standard approach to reoperation for missed parathyroid adenoma. *Ann Surg* 1996;224:308–320, with permission.)

image but indicates the side of the neck where the hyperfunctioning tissue is located, it may help to direct the exploration to one or the other side of the neck. Both these invasive radiographic techniques require considerable expertise. Transient cortical blindness, transverse myelitis, and cerebrovascular accidents have all been reported as complications of arteriography. Angiographic ablation of mediastinal parathyroid tissue with large doses of ionic contrast has been successful in selected patients. This technique may be used in some patients with mediastinal parathyroid adenomas who are at increased surgical risk and who have other functional parathyroid tissue remaining (24).

Surgical reexploration can be a difficult procedure. The neck should almost always be reexplored first. If the thymic remnant has not already been removed, it should be excised at this time. Two adjunctive techniques, intraoperative ultrasonography to locate glands and intraoperative measurement of PTH to document the adequacy of resection, may be useful in patients undergoing operation for persistent disease.

If the gland is not identified in the neck by means of the maneuvers described, the mediastinum is examined. Median sternotomy and exploration are necessary in only 1% to 2% of patients with hyperparathyroidism. Usually, a vertical incision is made from the center of the cervical incision to the xiphoid, and the sternum is divided. Successful transcervical mediastinal exploration is sometimes possible with use of the Cooper thymectomy retractor, a substernal retractor that permits more extensive mediastinal exploration and thymectomy through a cervical incision (25). Any remaining thymic tissue is first isolated and examined. Inferior parathyroids most commonly migrate into the anterior mediastinum. If the results of this exploration are negative, the area posterior and lateral to the trachea is then explored. The location of superior parathyroids may be as far posterior as the esophagus and as far superior as the pharynx.

Surgical reexploration is successful in experienced hands in 60% to 80% of cases. The incidence of complications is increased. Unilateral recurrent nerve injury occurs in 5% to 10% of patients postoperatively, and permanent hypoparathyroidism in 10% to 20% of patients.

Cryopreservation of excised tissue is an important component of the management of these patients, as it allows later autotransplantation if the patient becomes hypoparathyroid postoperatively. The risks of these complications must be clearly outweighed by the clinical improvement in patients with advanced disease. Reoperation in asymptomatic patients with mild disease is controversial.

Hypercalcemic Crisis

Occasionally, patients with hyperparathyroidism may become acutely hypercalcemic with severe symptoms. The pathogenesis appears to involve a vicious cycle of uncontrolled PTH secretion followed by hypercalcemia and secondary polyuria, dehydration, and reduced renal function, which exacerbate the hypercalcemia. Serum calcium concentrations may reach the range of 16 to 20 mg/dL, and the syndrome is manifested by rapidly developing muscle weakness, nausea and vomiting, lethargy, fatigue, and even coma. If the diagnosis of hyperparathyroidism is in question, ultrasonography or CT may help to identify the enlarged gland.

Definitive treatment involves resecting the diseased parathyroid tissue, which is almost always curative. Generally, however, it is safer to lower the serum calcium level before operation.

Hyperparathyroidism in Pregnancy

Hyperparathyroidism in pregnancy is a rare disorder that not only causes hypercalcemia in the mother but also is associated with increased morbidity and mortality rates in the fetus. Even the newborn is at risk for the development of tetany. The risk for fetal complications is higher if the hyperparathyroidism is left untreated. The mother should undergo operation in the second trimester.

Neonatal Hyperparathyroidism

Neonatal hyperparathyroidism occurs in infants who are homozygous for a mutation of the calcium-sensing receptor and is characterized by hypotonia, poor feeding, constipation, and respiratory distress (6). Each parent of these children is affected by familial hypocalciuric hypercalcemia. The 1-year survival rate in children with symptoms is less than 50%, and patients without symptoms appear to have significant bone disease. Total parathyroidectomy with autotransplantation is the treatment of choice (26).

Secondary Hyperparathyroidism

Secondary hyperparathyroidism develops as a consequence of chronic renal failure. Phosphate retention and hyperphosphatemia reduce the serum calcium levels. This effect is aggravated by the reduction in 1-hydroxylase activity in the kidney, necessary for the activation of vitamin D_3. The secondary increase in PTH levels to compensate for the hypocalcemic effects is exacerbated by aluminum accumulation in bone. Aluminum, present both in the dialysate water and in phosphate-binding medications, contributes to the osteomalacia (renal osteodystrophy) that develops in all these patients after several years of dialysis. Therapy includes controlling the hyperphosphatemia with dietary restriction and phosphate-binding gels, calcium supplementation orally and in the dialysate bath, correction of acidosis, administration of vitamin D sterol, and reduction in aluminum intake in both the dialysate and the diet. Therapy should be initiated carefully because metastatic soft-tissue calcification may occur. Indications for surgical therapy include persistent, symptomatic hypercalcemia that cannot be controlled medically, particularly in prospective renal transplant patients; bony pain and abnormal fractures; ectopic calcification; and intractable pruritus. Subtotal parathyroidectomy and total parathyroidectomy with heterotopic autotransplantation both appear to be acceptable options, although reexploration for recurrent disease is less complicated after total parathyroidectomy with autotransplantation. Parathyroidectomy can actually enhance aluminum deposition, so any excess should be corrected preoperatively through chelation.

Parathyroid Carcinoma

Parathyroid carcinoma is a rare condition, accounting for fewer than 1% of all cases of hyperparathyroidism. Histologic criteria remain controversial, and the diagnosis is securely made only on the basis of local invasion or distant metastases. In comparison with patients with benign disease, these patients tend to be somewhat younger and more symptomatic. In contrast to the marked female predominance in benign disease, the male-to-female ratio in carcinoma is equal. Serum calcium, PTH, and alkaline phosphatase levels are relatively more elevated, and patients often have an elevated level of human chorionic gonadotropin. Patients may have manifestations of both renal and bone disease. The affected gland is palpable in almost half of patients.

Initial treatment should include radical resection of the involved gland, ipsilateral thyroid lobe, and regional lymph nodes. Neither chemotherapy nor radiation therapy has shown any benefit. If the disease recurs, resection should be attempted because without treatment these patients usually succumb to uncontrolled hypercalcemia. The long-term prognosis is poor, and the opportunity for survival depends on complete initial resection (27).

MULTIPLE ENDOCRINE NEOPLASIA

Although these familial disorders are typically characterized by a predisposition to the development of tumors of multiple endocrine organs, the parathyroid is characteristically involved in two of them. The disorders are all inherited in an autosomal dominant fashion, and the tumors tend to be multicentric. The tumors may be benign or malignant and may occur metachronously or synchronously. MEN-I is characterized by the concurrence of parathyroid hyperplasia, pancreatic islet cell tumors, and pituitary adenomas. MEN-IIA consists of medullary thyroid carcinoma (MTC), pheochromocytoma, and parathyroid hyperplasia. MEN-2B includes MTC, pheochromocytoma, mucosal neuromas, and a distinctive marfanoid habitus. Together, these syndromes encompass much of the spectrum of endocrine neoplasia.

Pathogenesis

A unifying hypothesis for the MEN syndromes was offered by Pearse (28) based on both embryologic and cytochemical studies. He suggested that these tumors arise in cells that embryologically derive from the neural crest and are characterized by amine precursor uptake and decarboxylase activity (APUD cells). According to this theory, some defect in the development of the neural crest might explain the development of multicentric tumors in multiple organs. Although the theory could account for the development of MTC, pheochromocytomas, pituitary tumors, and the widespread nervous system hypertrophy of MEN-IIB, the endocrine cells of the parathyroid and pancreas do not appear to be of neural crest origin. Another unifying hypothesis, developed subsequently, whereby a tumor in one organ secretes endocrine products that secondarily stimulate neoplasia in other glands, has not been accepted. Although some evidence has suggested the presence of a mitogenic factor in the serum of patients with MEN-I, direct attempts to define the pathophysiology have not proved rewarding. As a result, investigators in this area have taken a different approach, attempting to map the diseased gene through modern molecular genetic techniques.

The genetic abnormality in MEN-I has been identified and described in detail (29,30). As a tumor-suppressor gene, the first mutation is inherited and becomes unmasked only when a second mutation, in some cases a deletion, develops in susceptible tissues. The resulting complete loss of the tumor suppressor allows neoplasia to develop. The occurrence of multiple second mutations explains the characteristic multicentric involvement of these diseases. Direct genetic testing is now available for some families with known mutations.

Mutations of the *RET* protooncogene are the cause of MEN-IIA (31,32). Genetic testing is now available to identify affected family members and provide the opportunity for early treatment of MTC in affected persons.

Clinical Features and Management of Multiple Endocrine Neoplasia Type I

Characteristically, MEN-I develops in the third and fourth decades, without any gender predilection (33). The gene is transmitted with nearly complete penetrance, and autopsy studies suggest that all three organs are affected in more than 90% of patients. The phenotype varies, however; more than 90% of patients have hyperparathyroidism, but evidence of islet cell neoplasms (30% to 80%) and pituitary tumors (15% to 50%) is less common. The cause of death in carriers of the MEN-I mutation is related to MEN-I in about 45% of patients and often caused by malignant islet cell or carcinoid tumors (34).

Parathyroid Disease

Hypercalcemia secondary to hyperparathyroidism is usually the first biochemical abnormality detected in MEN-I and represents the best screening study for members of affected kindreds until direct genetic screening is available. Many of these patients are asymptomatic and have relatively mild hypercalcemia. When symptoms do develop, they typically involve the urinary tract rather than the skeleton.

Typically, the patients have four-gland disease, which may be particularly difficult to manage. They are best treated with total parathyroidectomy and heterotopic autotransplantation (as noted earlier).

Pancreatic Tumors

In patients with pancreatic tumors, multicentric and diffuse hyperplasia of the pancreatic islets may occur in areas distant from any grossly evident tumor. The management of these tumors is controversial because although some patients have aggressive, malignant tumors, many patients have a fairly benign course. No reliable criteria are available to detect malignant tumors. Tumor size is often cited as a useful marker of prognosis, but substantial overlap has been noted between the sizes of primary benign and malignant tumors (35) (Fig. 55.16). Because of the difficulty in identifying the more aggressive subset, some authors have chosen a liberal policy of early operation to try to prevent metastasis and death (36,37). The detection of these tumors can also be diffiult; testing with meal stimulation can be used if an intervention plan supports the diagnosis at this early phase (38). Some evidence indicates that measuring serum concentrations of pancreatic polypeptide may provide a general screening measure for a variety of islet cell tumors (39). Pancreatic tumors are

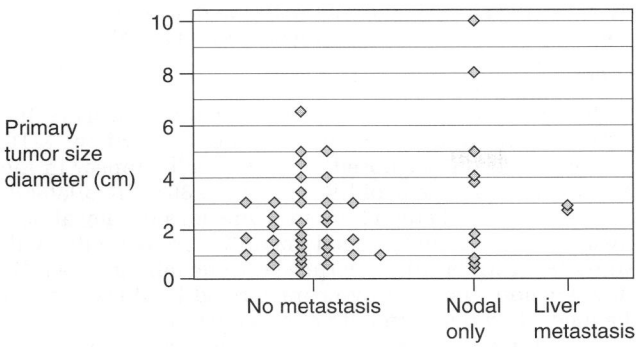

Figure 55.16. Scatter plot of largest primary tumor size versus metastatic status in 43 patients with pancreatic islet cell tumors associated with multiple endocrine neoplasia type I. Each point represents a single patient. Tumor size is not correlated with the presence of liver or lymph node metastases. (From Lowney JK, Frisella MM, Lairmore TC, et al. Islet cell tumor metastasis in multiple endocrine neoplasia type I: correlation with primary tumor size. *Surgery* 1998;124:1043–1049, with permission.)

typically multicentric and frequently malignant. Somatostatin receptor scintigraphy can be a useful imaging technique to demonstrate the extent of tumor (40) (Fig. 55.17).

Gastrinoma is the most common functional tumor in MEN-I; typically, a severe ulcer diathesis (Zollinger-Ellison syndrome) develops that is associated with secretory diarrhea. Serum gastrin levels are usually markedly elevated (> 100 pg/mL); when levels are equivocal (250 to 1,000 pg/mL), provocative testing with secretin (2 m/kg) may be useful. An absolute serum gastrin increase of 200 pg/mL is diagnostic. The primary tumors are often in the submucosa of the duodenal wall.

Biochemical cure of these gastrinomas is almost never possible, as it is in sporadic gastrinomas, although exploration can reduce the need for antisecretory medications and may reduce the risk for liver metastasis. H$_2$-receptor antagonists are often effective in controlling acid secretion, although very high doses may be necessary; the malignant disease is often indolent. In patients whose acid secretion is not controlled by H$_2$ blockers, omeprazole may be useful. Parietal cell vagotomy in this setting can re-

duce the amount of medications needed. Total gastrectomy is no longer ever necessary.

Insulinoma is the next most common pancreatic neoplasm. These tumors are usually small and multicentric. Patients present with a history of sweating, dizziness, confusion, and syncope, consistent with neuroglycopenia; these symptoms are relieved by consuming carbohydrates. The diagnosis is verified by documenting fasting hypoglycemia associated with inappropriately elevated plasma insulin levels. Preoperative tumor localization is usually achieved by a combination of CT and arteriography. Calcium is injected into various pancreatic arteries and plasma insulin levels in the hepatic vein plasma are measured to detect a gradient after the injection of specific pancreatic arteries.

Because the available medical therapy for insulinoma is limited, patients are treated operatively. Lesions in the tail of the gland can be enucleated if they are small; however, distal pancreatectomy carries little morbidity. Tumors of the head can usually be enucleated, so that pancreaticoduodenectomy can be avoided. In patients with malignant disease, metastases may respond to streptozocin. Diazoxide, verapamil, or octreotide may successfully reduce insulin secretion and control symptoms. A diet of complex carbohydrates can also help stabilize serum glucose levels in the hyperinsulinemic patient.

Other islet cell lesions occur only rarely in association with MEN-I.

Pituitary Adenomas

Prolactin-secreting tumors occur most commonly in this setting, although Cushing's disease or acromegaly develops in an occasional patient. Symptoms may result from compression of the optic chiasm, which produces bitemporal hemianopsia, or from prolactin excess, which produces amenorrhea and galactorrhea in female patients and hypogonadism in male patients.

Bromocriptine inhibits prolactin secretion and shrinks many prolactinomas. Refractory tumors and those producing other hormones can be managed by pituitary ablation or radiation.

Other Tumors

Multiple endocrine neoplasia type I is associated much less frequently with adrenocortical tumors and benign thyroid adenomas. Lipomas and carcinoid tumors may also occur.

Clinical Features and Management of Multiple Endocrine Neoplasia Type II

Like MEN-I, the MEN-II syndromes are inherited in an autosomal dominant fashion with complete penetrance but variable phenotype. Bilateral MTC occurs in every affected patient. More frequently than the other syndromes, MEN-IIB may arise as a new mutation that can be transmitted to subsequent generations.

Medullary Thyroid Carcinoma

Medullary thyroid carcinoma accounts for about 10% of all thyroid malignancies, and 20% of cases occur in the familial setting of MEN-IIA, MEN-IIB, or familial non-MEN MTC. It is usually the first tumor that develops in these patients and typically appears in the second or third decade. Tumors are virtually always bilateral and develop in multiple areas of the middle and upper portions of the thyroid lobe (Fig. 55.18). Occasionally, in young people, a diffuse proliferation of parafollicular C cells, termed *C-cell hyperplasia*, is present without frankly invasive carcinoma. This finding is highly suggestive of one of the fa-

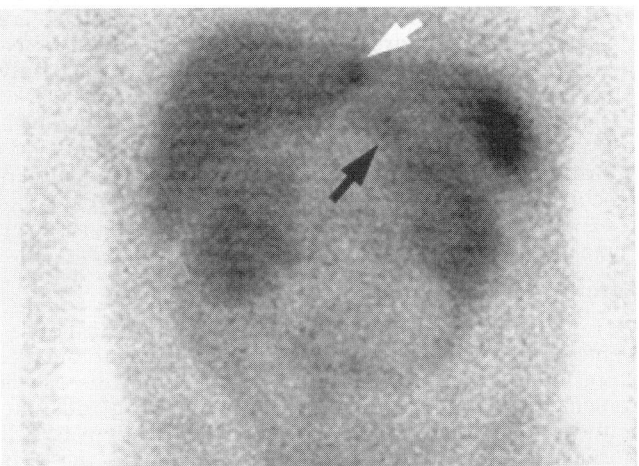

Figure 55.17. Somatostatin receptor scintigraphy in a patient with multiple endocrine neoplasia type I. This scintiscan detected an otherwise unrecognized metastasis to the left lateral segment of the liver *(white arrow),* which was resected along with the small primary tumor *(black arrow).*

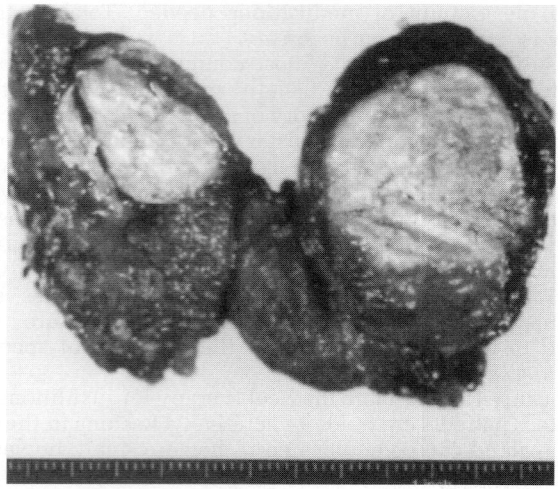

Figure 55.18. Primary medullary thyroid carcinoma from a total thyroidectomy specimen. The tumors are bilateral and centered in the upper pole.

milial MTC syndromes. Patients typically present with a neck mass and may have hoarseness, dysphagia, or palpable cervical adenopathy. MTC may produce a variety of hormones, including calcitonin, adrenocorticotropic hormone, prostaglandin, and serotonin. The hypercalcitoninemia is often asymptomatic, although severe diarrhea can develop.

By detecting minimal elevations of plasma calcitonin, it is possible to diagnose MTC at a clinically occult stage (41). Basal plasma calcitonin levels in normal subjects are in the range of 30 to 100 pg/mL. An increase to levels of 150 to 200 pg/mL occurs, however, after the administration of the potent secretagogues calcium and pentagastrin. The plasma calcitonin levels of patients with MTC show striking increases (> 1,000 pg/mL) after provocative testing, so that they can be identified readily. Patients with occult disease may have only minimally elevated basal calcitonin levels that increase in response to secretagogues. The combined infusion of calcium and pentagastrin was the most effective screening test for familial MTC before genetic testing became available. By means of provocative testing in kindred members at risk for disease, MTC was diagnosed at a preclinical stage, and a greater percentage of these patients were cured by surgical therapy. With genetic testing now available, prophylactic thyroidectomy to prevent the development of MTC is possible for all affected people (42).

Postoperatively, the presence of residual MTC can be readily detected by provocative testing. Recent reports have suggested that meticulous reoperation in patients with recurrent or persistently elevated plasma calcitonin levels postoperatively, including mediastinal dissection on occasion, can normalize elevated plasma calcitonin levels and apparently cure many of them (43). For the patient with unresectable metastases, few therapeutic options are available. Neither radiation nor chemotherapy is of significant benefit.

The clinical course of patients with the MEN-II syndromes is determined primarily by the status of their MTC. In the setting of MEN-IIA, the tumors are often indolent and survival prolonged, even in the presence of metastatic disease. By contrast, the tumors in patients with MEN-IIB occur at an earlier age and are generally more aggressive neoplasms. Patients may succumb to the disease at a young age. As a consequence of this aggres-

siveness, the size of kindreds with the disease is typically small, and usually only a few generations are affected.

Pheochromocytoma

Pheochromocytomas are usually detected during the initial screening or follow-up of patients in whom MTC has already been diagnosed. They typically appear in the second or third decade of life, and about 80% are bilateral. Usually, they are benign but multicentric, and they almost always arise in the adrenal medulla. In patients with MEN-IIA or MEN-IIB, hyperplasia of the adrenal medulla may develop first, grossly characterized by thickening of the medullary tissue in both adrenal glands.

Pheochromocytomas may be asymptomatic, but most commonly, patients have pounding frontal headaches, episodic diaphoresis, palpitations, or anxiety. Hypertension also occurs and is often episodic.

The diagnosis is made by measuring the urinary excretion of catecholamines and their metabolites. The best test is a 24-hour urine collection for total catecholamines, epinephrine, norepinephrine, metanephrine, and vanillylmandelic acid. Patients with MEN-IIA or MEN-IIB and MTC should be evaluated for pheochromocytoma before they undergo thyroidectomy. If a patient is found to have both lesions, adrenalectomy should be performed first, followed by neck exploration in 1 to 2 weeks. If urinary excretion rates are equivocal, CT of the abdomen can identify lesions 1 cm or larger, and sometimes hyperplasia is recognized. Scintigraphy withs ^{131}I-metaiodobenzylguanidine is based on the fact that this agent, which is similar to norepinephrine, is taken up and stored in neurotransmitter vesicles. Normal glands are not demonstrated, whereas about 90% of pheochromocytomas can be imaged. This test is particularly useful in identifying extraadrenal lesions. MRI is also sensitive for pheochromocytomas and has the advantage of allowing the differentiation of pheochromocytoma from benign adenoma based on T_2-weighted imaging characteristics.

Preoperatively, α-adrenergic blockade is induced with phenoxybenzamine. β-Adrenergic blockade with propranolol may be necessary if tachyarrhythmia subsequently develops, but it should not be initiated until after α-adrenergic blockade because of the risk for unopposed vasoconstriction ("unopposed-α effect"). Intraoperative hypertension is controlled with a vasodilator, such as sodium nitroprusside or phentolamine. The abdomen is explored through a bilateral subcostal incision or, more typically, with a laparoscope. Bilateral pheochromocytomas are treated by bilateral adrenalectomy. In patients with MEN-IIA or MEN-IIB and a unilateral pheochromocytoma, only the diseased adrenal gland is removed. In about 30% of patients treated in this manner, a tumor eventually develops in the opposite gland. In the remaining patients, this approach avoids the need for glucocorticoid and mineralocorticoid replacement and the risk for addisonian crisis (44). After unilateral adrenalectomy, patients are carefully screened at 6-month or 1-year intervals.

Parathyroid Disease

Hyperparathyroidism develops in about one third of patients with MEN-IIA, although it is usually asymptomatic. Occasionally, nephrolithiasis develops. Bone disease is unusual. Frequently, enlarged parathyroid glands are found at operation for MTC, although the patient is still normocalcemic. Multiglandular chief cell hyperplasia is the predominant histologic finding in MEN-IIA. Significant parathyroid disease rarely develops in MEN-IIB (45).

Total parathyroidectomy and heterotopic autotransplantation are performed in hypercalcemic patients with MEN-IIA. In normocalcemic patients with MEN-IIA undergoing thyroidectomy for MTC, a total parathyroidectomy and heterotopic autotransplantation are performed in one session to ensure that the complete thyroidectomy does not compromise the parathyroid blood supply and to avoid reoperation in the neck for subsequent hyperparathyroidism. Evidence suggests that these patients are more easily treated, with a lower incidence of recurrent hyperparathyroidism, than patients with MEN-I.

Nonendocrine Manifestations of Multiple Endocrine Neoplasia Type IIB

In addition to MTC and pheochromocytoma, marked abnormalities of the nervous and musculoskeletal systems develop in patients with MEN-IIB. The classic phenotype is characterized by thick lips and a thin, marfanoid habitus (Fig. 55.19A,B). The incidence of associated skeletal abnormalities is high; these include kyphosis, pectus excavatum, pes planus or cavus, and congenital dislocation of the hip. Diffuse autonomic nervous hypertrophy is another feature. Mucosal neuromas appear on the tongue (Fig. 55.19C), eyelids, lips, and pharynx. Slit-lamp examination may reveal hypertrophied corneal nerves. Ganglioneuromatosis develops in the submucosal and myenteric plexuses of the gastrointestinal tract. Constipation is common, and radiographic findings may suggest megacolon or Hirschsprung's disease.

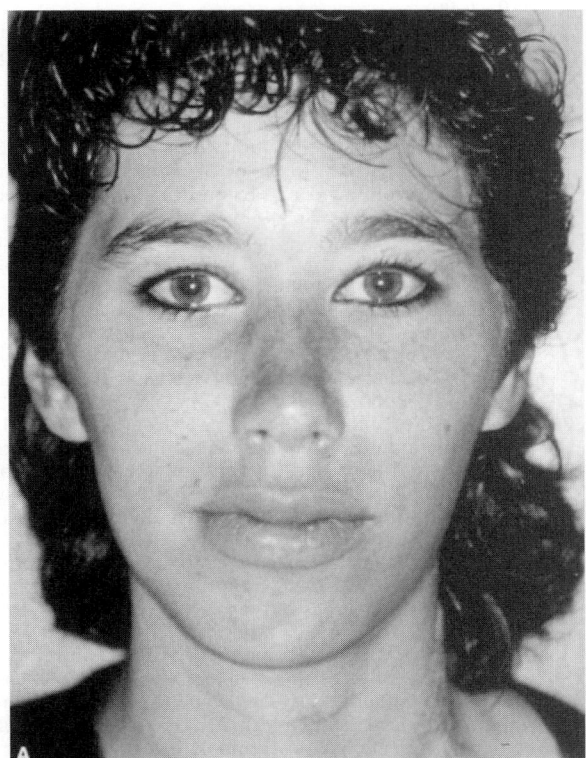
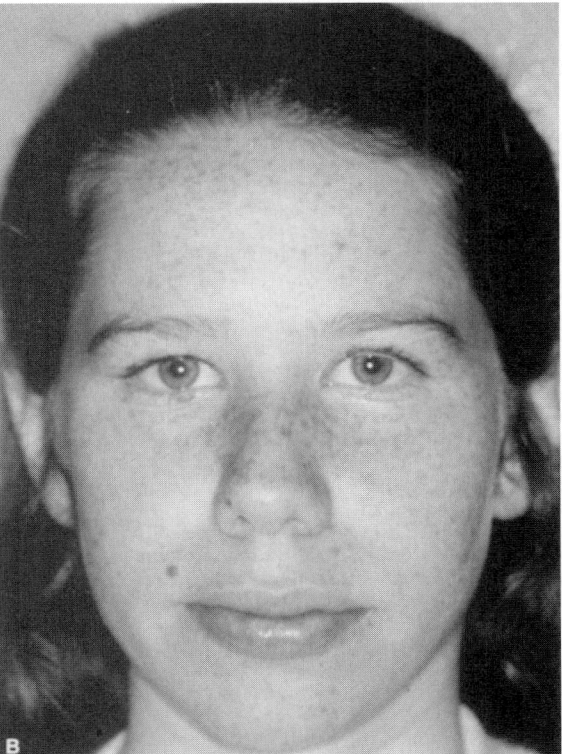
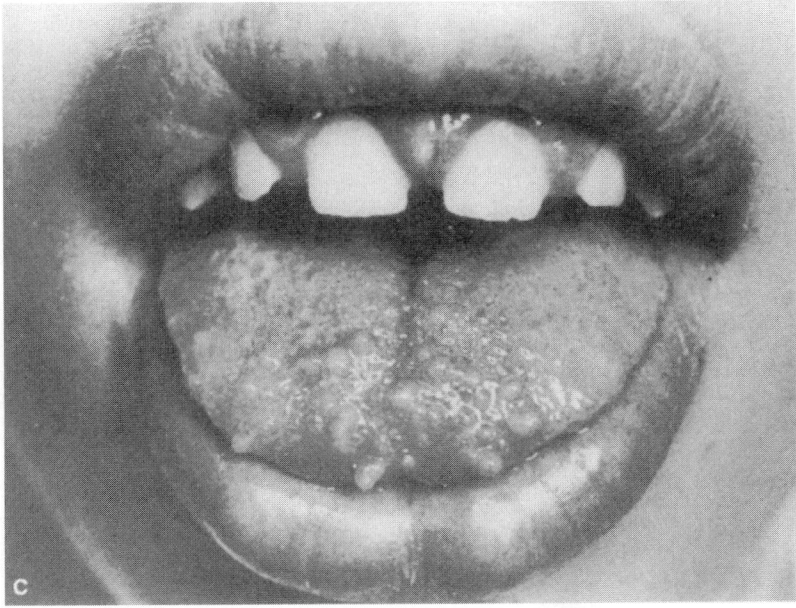

Figure 55.19. (A,B) Characteristic appearance of patients with multiple endocrine neoplasia type IIB, including thick lips. *(C)* Multiple mucosal neuromas on the tongue of a patient with MEN-IIB. (From Norton JA, Froome LC, Farrell FE, et al. Multiple endocrine neoplasia type 2b: the most aggressive form of medullary thyroid carcinoma. *Surg Clin North Am* 1979;59:109, with permission.)

REFERENCES

1. Akerstrom G, Malmaeus J, Bergstrom R. Surgical anatomy of human parathyroid glands. *Surgery* 1984;95:14–18.
2. Mallette LE. Regulation of blood calcium in humans. *Endocrinol Metab Clin North Am* 1989;18:601–610.
3. Nussbaum SR. Pathophysiology and management of severe hypercalcemia. *Endocrinol Metab Clin North Am* 1993;22:343–362.
4. Strewler GJ, Nissenson RA. Hypercalcemia in malignancy. *West J Med* 1990;153:635–640.
5. Pollak MR, Brown EM, Chou Y-HW, et al. Mutations in the human Ca-sensing receptor gene cause familial hypocalciuric hypercalcemia and neonatal severe hyperparathyroidism. *Cell* 1993;75:1297–1303.
6. Pollak MR, Chou Y-HW, Marx SJ, et al. Familial hypocalciuric hypercalcemia and neonatal severe hyperparathyroidism: effects of mutant gene dosage on phenotype. *J Clin Invest* 1994;93:1108–1112.
7. Bilezikian JP. Management of acute hypercalcemia. *N Engl J Med* 1992;326:1196–1203.
8. Tohme MF, Bilezikian JP. Hypocalcemic emergencies. *Endocrinol Metab Clin North Am* 1993;22:363–375.
9. Heath H. Clinical spectrum of primary hyperparathyroidism: evolution with changes in medical practice and technology. *J Bone Miner Res* 1991;6[Suppl 2]:S63–S70.
10. Silverberg SJ, Shane E, Jacobs TP, et al. A 10-year prospective study of primary hyperparathyroidism with or without parathyroid surgery. *N Engl J Med* 1999;341:1249–1255.
11. Heath H, Hodgson SF, Kennedy MA. Primary hyperparathyroidism: incidence, morbidity, and potential economic impact in a community. *N Engl J Med* 1980;302:189–193.
12. Arnold A. Molecular mechanisms of parathyroid neoplasia. *Endocrinol Metab Clin North Am* 1994;23:93–107.
13. Palanisamy N, Imanishi Y, Rao PH, et al. Novel chromosomal abnormalities identified by comparative genomic hybridization in parathyroid adenomas. *J Clin Endocrinol Metab* 1998;83:1766–1770.
14. Roth SI. Recent advances in parathyroid gland pathology. *Am J Med* 1994;50:612–622.
15. Levin KE, Chew KL, Ljung B-M, et al. Deoxyribonucleic acid cytometry helps identify parathyroid carcinomas. *J Clin Endocrinol Metab* 1994;67:779–784.
16. Wells SA, Leight GF, Ross A. Primary hyperparathyroidism. *Curr Probl Surg* 1980;17:398–467.
17. Miller DL, Doppman JL, Shawker TH, et al. Localization of parathyroid adenomas in patients who have undergone surgery. Part I. Noninvasive imaging methods. *Radiology* 1987;162:133–137.
18. Miller DL, Doppman JL, Krudy AG, et al. Localization of parathyroid adenomas in patients who have undergone surgery. Part II. Invasive procedures. *Radiology* 1987;162:138–141.
19. Weber CJ, Vansant J, Alazraki N, et al. Value of technetium 99m sestamibi iodine 123 imaging in reoperative parathyroid surgery. *Surgery* 1993;114:1011–1018.
20. Scholz DA, Purnell DC. Asymptomatic primary hyperparathyroidism: 10-year prospective study. *Mayo Clin Proc* 1981;56:473–478.
21. Potts JT Jr, Ackerman IP, Barker CF, et al. Diagnosis and management of asymptomatic primary hyperparathyroidism: consensus development conference statement. *Ann Intern Med* 1991;114:593–597.
22. Oertli D, Richter M, Kraenzlin M, et al. Parathyroidectomy in primary hyperparathyroidism: preoperative localization and routine biopsy of unaltered glands are not necessary. *Surgery* 1995;117:392–396.
23. Wells SA, Leight GS, Hensley M, et al. Hyperparathyroidism associated with the enlargement of two or three parathyroid glands. *Ann Surg* 1985;202:533–538.
24. Doherty GM, Doppman JL, Miller DL, et al. Results of a multidisciplinary strategy for management of mediastinal parathyroid adenoma as a cause of persistent primary hyperparathyroidism. *Ann Surg* 1992;215:101–106.
25. Wells SA Jr, Cooper JD. Closed mediastinal exploration in patients with persistent hyperparathyroidism. *Ann Surg* 1991;214:555–561.
26. Key LL, Thorne M, Pitzer B, et al. Management of neonatal hyperparathyroidism with parathyroidectomy and autotransplantation. *J Pediatr* 1990;116:923–926.
27. Wang C, Gaz RD. Natural history of parathyroid carcinoma: diagnosis, treatment, and results. *Am J Surg* 1985;149:522–527.
28. Pearse AGE. Common cytochemical and ultrastructural characteristics of cells producing polypeptide hormone (the APUD series) and their relevance to the thyroid and ultimobranchial C-cells and calcitonin. *Proc R Soc Lond (Biol)* 1968;170:71–80.
29. Chandrasekharappa SC, Guru SC, Manickam P, et al. Positional cloning of the gene for multiple endocrine neoplasia-type 1. *Science* 1997;276:404–407.
30. Mutch MG, Dilley WG, Sanjurjo F, et al. Germline mutations in the multiple endocrine neoplasia type 1 gene: evidence for frequent splicing defects. *Hum Mutat* 1999;13:175–185.
31. Mulligan LM, Kwok JBJ, Healey CS, et al. Germ-line mutation of the *RET* proto-oncogene in multiple endocrine neoplasia type 2A. *Nature* 1993;363:458–460.
32. Donis-Keller H, Dou S, Chi D, et al. Mutations in the *RET* proto-oncogene are associated with MEN 2A and FMTC. *Hum Mol Genet* 1993;2:851–856.
33. Skogseid B, Rastad J, Oberg K. Multiple endocrine neoplasia type 1: clinical features and screening. *Endocrinol Metab Clin North Am* 1994;23:1–18.
34. Doherty GM, Olson JA, Frisella MM, et al. Lethality of multiple endocrine neoplasia type 1. *World J Surg* 1998;22:581–586.
35. Lowney JK, Frisella MM, Lairmore TC, et al. Islet cell tumor metastasis in multiple endocrine neoplasia type I: correlation with primary tumor size. *Surgery* 1998;124:1043–1049.
36. Skogseid B, Oberg K, Eriksson B, et al. Surgery for asymptomatic pancreatic lesion in multiple endocrine neoplasia type 1. *World J Surg* 1996;20:872–877.
37. Skogseid B, Grama D, Rastad J, et al. Operative tumour yields obviate preoperative pancreatic tumor localization in multiple endocrine neoplasia type 1. *J Intern Med* 1995;238:281–288.
38. Skogseid B, Oberg K. Experience with multiple endocrine neoplasia type 1 screening. *J Intern Med* 1995;238:255–261.
39. Mutch MG, Frisella MM, DeBenedetti MK, et al. Pancreatic polypeptide is a useful plasma marker for radiographically evident pancreatic islet cell tumors in patients with multiple endocrine neoplasia type 1. *Surgery* 1997;122:1012–1020.
40. Yim JH, Siegel BA, DeBenedetti MK, et al. Prospective study of the utility of somatastatin receptor scintigraphy in the evaluation of patients with multiple endocrine neoplasia type I. *Surgery* 1998;124:1037–1042.
41. Cance WG, Wells SAJ. Multiple endocrine neoplasia type IIa. *Curr Probl Surg* 1985;22:1–112.
42. Wells SA Jr, Chi DD, Toshima K, et al. Predictive DNA testing and prophylactic thyroidectomy in patients at risk for multiple endocrine neoplasia type 2A. *Ann Surg* 1994;220:237–247.
43. Moley JF, Wells SA, Dilley WG, et al. Reoperation for recurrent or persistent medullary thyroid cancer. *Surgery* 1993;114:1090–1095.
44. Lairmore TC, Ball DW, Baylin SB, et al. Management of pheochromocytomas in patients with multiple endocrine neoplasia type 2 syndromes. *Ann Surg* 1993;217:595–603.
45. Herfarth K, Bartsch D, Doherty GM, et al. Surgical management of hyperparathyroidism in patients with multiple endocrine neoplasia type 2A. *Surgery* 1996;120:966–974.

SURGERY: SCIENTIFIC PRINCIPLES AND PRACTICE, Third Edition, edited by
Lazar J. Greenfield, Michael W. Mulholland, Keith T. Oldham, Gerald B. Zelenock,
and Keith D. Lillemoe. Lippincott Williams & Wilkins Publishers, Philadelphia, © 2001.

CHAPTER 56

ADRENAL GLANDS

H. H. NEWSOME, JR.

ANATOMY

Total Gland

The adrenal glands are paired structures located on each side of the body superior to the kidneys. They are flat and triangular structures, each weighing about 5 g. Three sets of adrenal arteries predominate—the *superior adrenal artery* is a branch of the inferior phrenic artery; the *middle adrenal artery* originates from the aorta on each side; and the *inferior adrenal artery* arises from each renal artery. Although some small random veins handle some effluent, most drainage is through a single, well-defined central vein, which empties into the renal vein on the left and into the vena cava on the right. Blood flow within the gland is predominantly from the cortex through the medulla into the central medullary venous system, forming the large adrenal vein. The adrenal gland is composed of two distinct regions. The outer, bright yellow, lipid-laden cortex gives the gland its characteristic external appearance. Sandwiched between the layers of the cortex is the thin, dark gray medulla. These features and relations are shown in Fig. 56.1 (1).

Adrenal Cortex

Embryology

The cortex is mesodermal in origin. It arises near the gonads on the adrenogenital ridge at about the fifth week of gestation. This location explains the bits of cortical tissue (adrenal rests) found in various sites, such as the ovaries, spermatic cords, and testes. Histologically, fetal zonation of the cortex disappears shortly after birth.

Microscopy

The fully developed cortex is organized into three distinct zones. The *zona glomerulosa* is found just under the fibrous, outer capsule of the gland and contains ovoid clusters of cells. This thin, indistinct layer is the site of production of the mineralocorticoid aldosterone. The middle layer, the *zona fasciculata,* is composed of cells in linear patterns arranged at right angles to the surface of the gland. The cells are full of lipid and are the source of the carbohydrate-active steroid cortisol and the adrenal sex steroids. The internal layer, the *zona reticularis,* lies adjacent to the medulla, and the cells are arranged in a more random, sheetlike pattern. The cells of the inner zone are lipid replete. They secrete cortisol, androgens, and estrogens, and they maintain cholesterol stores as a precursor for steroidogenesis. A schematic representation of these zones is shown in Fig. 56.2.

Adrenal Medulla

Embryology

The medulla is ectodermal in origin and is derived specifically from the neural crest. It is first seen in the 10-mm embryo and insinuates itself into the cluster of adrenocortical cells. The early cells from the neural crest are grouped into

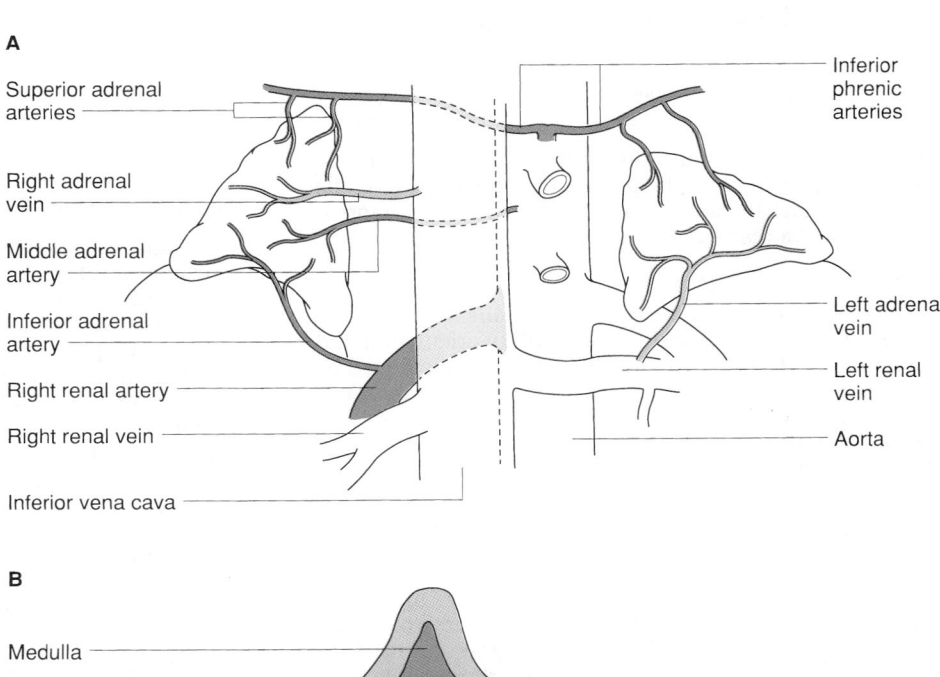

A

Superior adrenal arteries

Right adrenal vein

Middle adrenal artery

Inferior adrenal artery

Right renal artery

Right renal vein

Inferior vena cava

Inferior phrenic arteries

Left adrenal vein

Left renal vein

Aorta

B

Medulla

Cortex

Figure 56.1. *(A)* The arterial and venous anatomy of the right and left adrenal glands. *(B)* Division of the gland into the outer cortex and inner medulla.

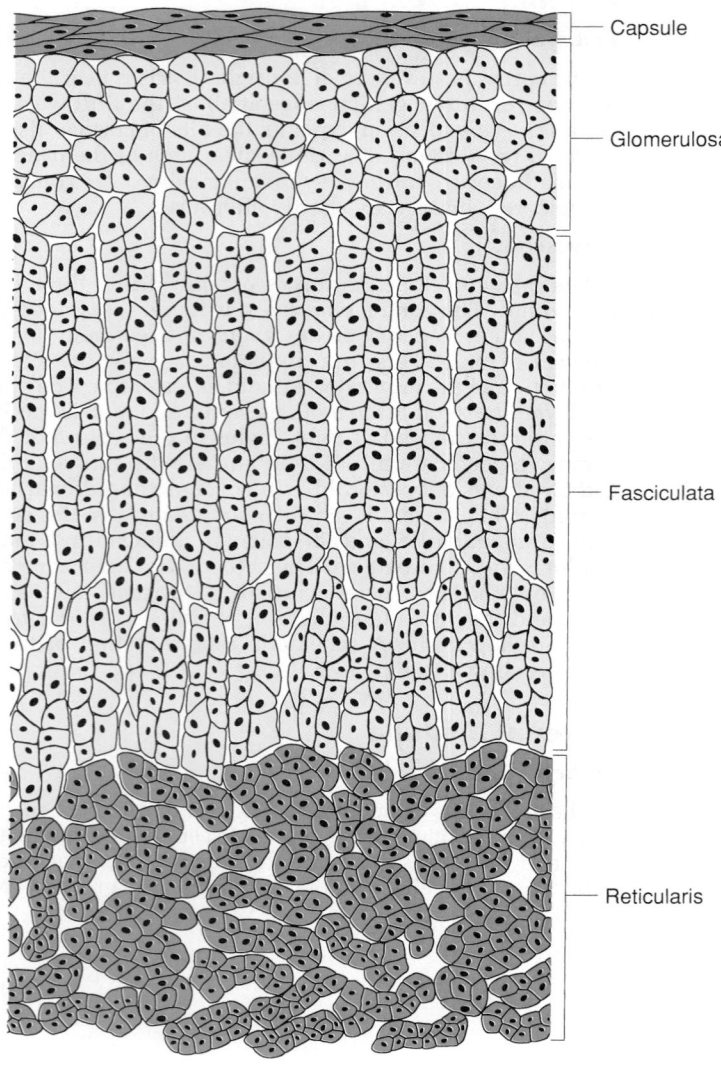

Capsule

Glomerulosa

Fasciculata

Reticularis

Medulla

Figure 56.2. Schematic representation of the microscopic anatomy of the adrenal cortex.

the *chromocell* system and the *neuronal system*. Both elements are represented in the population of adrenal medulla cells and explain the development of two distinct tumors—pheochromocytomas and neuroblastomas.

Microscopy

With light microscopy, the medullary cells appear as homogeneous sheets with nestlike or cordlike orientation and abundant cytoplasm. Their large nuclei are characterized by variation in size and shape and by the occasional presence of abnormal forms. Of clinical significance is their content of catecholamines and other substances, such as neuron-specific enolase and chromogranin. These substances help to identify tumors arising from the neural elements.

On electron microscopy, abundant secretory granules can be seen in the cytoplasm of medullary cells. Their presence is in contrast to the adrenocortical cells, in which a similar abundance of smooth endoplasmic reticulum, mitochondria, and Golgi complexes are seen, but few secretory granules are present. The medullary secretory granules containing epinephrine are slightly smaller than those containing norepinephrine and are more electron dense, with a loose-fitting membrane. The granules are carried to the periphery of the cell, where catecholamines and other contents are released by exocytosis into the surrounding milieu.

PHYSIOLOGY

Adrenocortical Secretion

Although the control of secretion of the major categories of corticosteroid products differs somewhat, the early steroidogenic pathway is common to all steroids (Fig. 56.3). Generally, however, cholesterol is converted to δ5-pregnenolone, progesterone, and 17-OH progesterone, and then either to the adrenal androgens or cortisol. Progesterone is converted to aldosterone by a different pathway. The amount of 17-ketosteroids (adrenal androgens) produced is 25 to 30 μg/d; 15 to 20 mg/d of the 17-hydroxysteroids (cortisol) is produced and 75 to 125 mg/d of aldosterone. As mentioned, aldosterone is produced primarily in the zona glomerulosa, whereas the 17-ketosteroids and 17-OH corticosteroids are produced in the zonae fasciculata and reticularis. The outer zone and the latter two inner zones are under separate regulatory mechanisms.

Control of Cortisol Secretion

The proximate stimulator of cortisol production is the peptide hormone adrenocorticotropic hormone (ACTH). It originates from the anterior pituitary gland and is regulated by corticotropin-releasing hormone (CRH). CRH

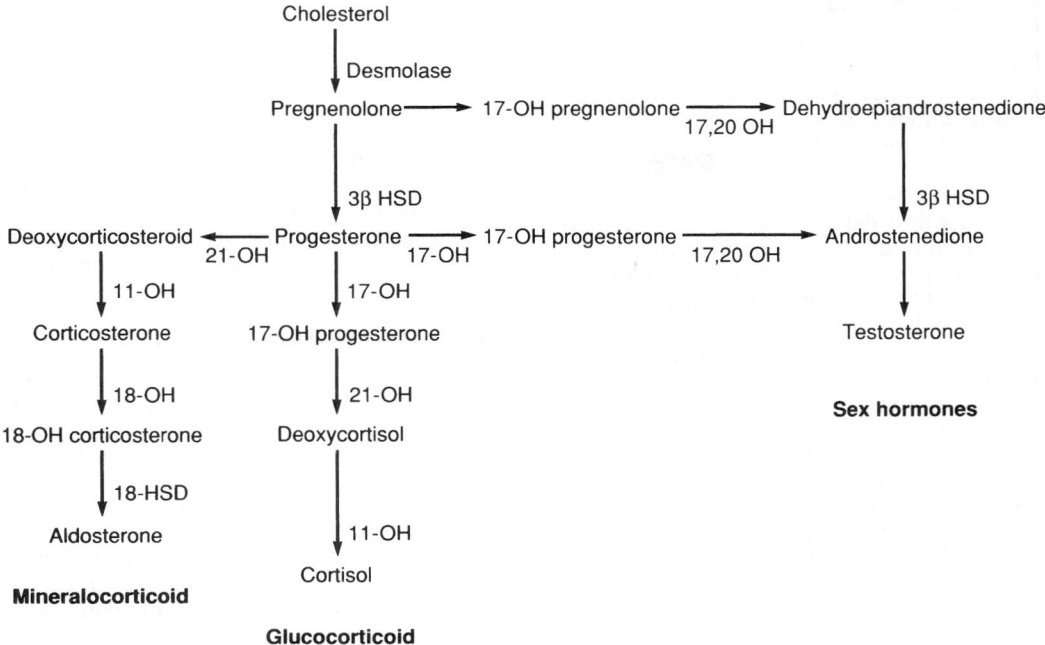

Figure 56.3. Steroidogenic pathways of the adrenal cortex. Sex hormones, mineralocorticoids, and glucocorticoids share the same initial synthetic steps.

is stored in the anterior hypothalamus and, on stimulation, is released into the pituitary portal system, where it reaches the anterior pituitary gland and releases ACTH. The stimulation of CRH is controlled by various neural influences. From the diurnal variation in CRH secretion, it is probable that intrinsic central nervous system influences are present. The increased cortisol production during fear or other emotional stress is another indicator of central nervous system regulation. On the other hand, the striking increase of cortisol secretion during pain and physical trauma attests to the importance of peripheral sensory pathways in stimulating cortisol production.

Release of CRH is under negative-feedback inhibition by cortisol. Although there is some evidence of a short-loop feedback of ACTH on CRH, both the slow and fast feedback by cortisol on the pituitary release mechanism are clinically noteworthy. Under normal circumstances, the set-point for negative-feedback inhibition of ACTH secretion is in the physiologic range of plasma cortisol concentrations. That is, a plasma cortisol concentration in the high-normal range of 15 to 20 µg/dL of plasma results in suppressed ACTH secretion and a consequent lowering of cortisol secretion by the adrenal cortex. Evidence also suggests that the fast feedback suppression, effected by acutely rising plasma cortisol concentrations, can suppress both CRH release and the response of ACTH to the stimulus of CRH. Considering the short half-life of plasma ACTH (measured in minutes) and its rapid onset of action compared with the longer plasma half-life of steroids and their slower onset of action, it is remarkable that this system can accomplish such fine homeostatic adjustment of plasma cortisol within a fairly narrow range. The feedback relations are shown in Fig. 56.4.

Clinically important examples of the slow feedback mechanism occur during chronic exogenous steroid administration for steroid-dependent diseases or during endogenous steroid excess from adrenocortical tumors. Under either circumstance, the pituitary adrenal axis is suppressed not only during the period of steroid excess but also for weeks and months after the steroid excess is corrected. The secretion of adrenal androgens, which are converted peripherally to estrogens, is basically controlled by the same mechanisms as cortisol secretion. This is distinct from the estrogens and androgens secreted by the gonads, which are regulated by a completely different set of pituitary peptides.

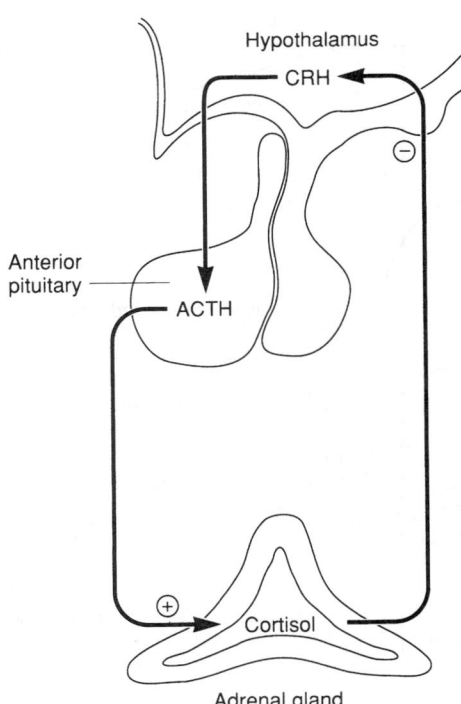

Figure 56.4. The feedback relations between the adrenal gland, the hypothalamus, and the anterior pituitary.

Control of Aldosterone Secretion

The primary proximate control of aldosterone secretion is by the octapeptide angiotensin II. The production of circulating angiotensin II begins with the action of a peptidase enzyme, renin, which is produced predominantly in the juxtaglomerular apparatus of the kidney, where it acts locally and where it is released into the system circulation. Both locally and when released, renin cleaves angiotensin I, a decapeptide derived from a large hepatic protein serving as renin substrate. Angiotensin I undergoes enzymatic cleavage in the lung to angiotensin II, which is the biologically active form of the peptide. Conversion of angiotensin I to angiotensin II is about 90% complete with one passage through the lung. The carboxypeptidase that is responsible for this cleavage is known as angiotensin-converting enzyme.

The rate of renin secretion is controlled by changes in the afferent arteriolar pressure in the renal cortex as well as by changes in sodium content in the renal tubule. These changes are sensed by the juxtaglomerular apparatus and by the macula densa. In general, a decrease in arterial pressure or in the sodium content of the renal tubule results in an increase in renin and angiotensin II production, with a subsequent increase in aldosterone secretion. Conversely, a sodium load, overhydration, or assumption of the supine position normally results in a decrease in renin and angiotensin production and a subsequent fall in aldosterone secretion.

At least two other factors influence aldosterone secretion. Aldosterone secretion is directly related to the serum potassium concentration. In view of aldosterone's ability to promote potassium excretion in the urine, it is not surprising that an increase in serum potassium directly stimulates aldosterone production, whereas a decrease in serum potassium has the opposite effect. Because of its early point of action in the steroidogenic pathway, ACTH also increases aldosterone secretion, although it is much less potent in this regard than in its stimulation of cortisol. The stimulatory effects of potassium and ACTH on aldosterone secretion can be overcome by angiotensin II stimulation. These concepts are summarized in Fig. 56.5.

Adrenomedullary Secretion

In reviewing the control of medullary secretion, it is useful to think of the adrenal medulla as a sympathetic ganglion. Instead of innervating postganglionic cells, the preganglionic sympathetic fibers innervate the secretory chromaffin cells. Stimulation of these cells increases the tyrosine hydroxylase activity and also moves the secretory granules to the surface of the cell, where exocytosis results in a discharge of the secretory product. The metabolic pathway in the medulla that culminates in catecholamine production is as follows. Tyrosine is converted to dihydroxyphenylalanine and then to dopamine as the immediate precursor to norepinephrine. Norepinephrine is converted to epinephrine. The various compound structures and enzyme names are shown in Fig. 56.6. A portion of the released norepinephrine and epinephrine is taken up again by the chromaffin cells, and part is released into the sys-

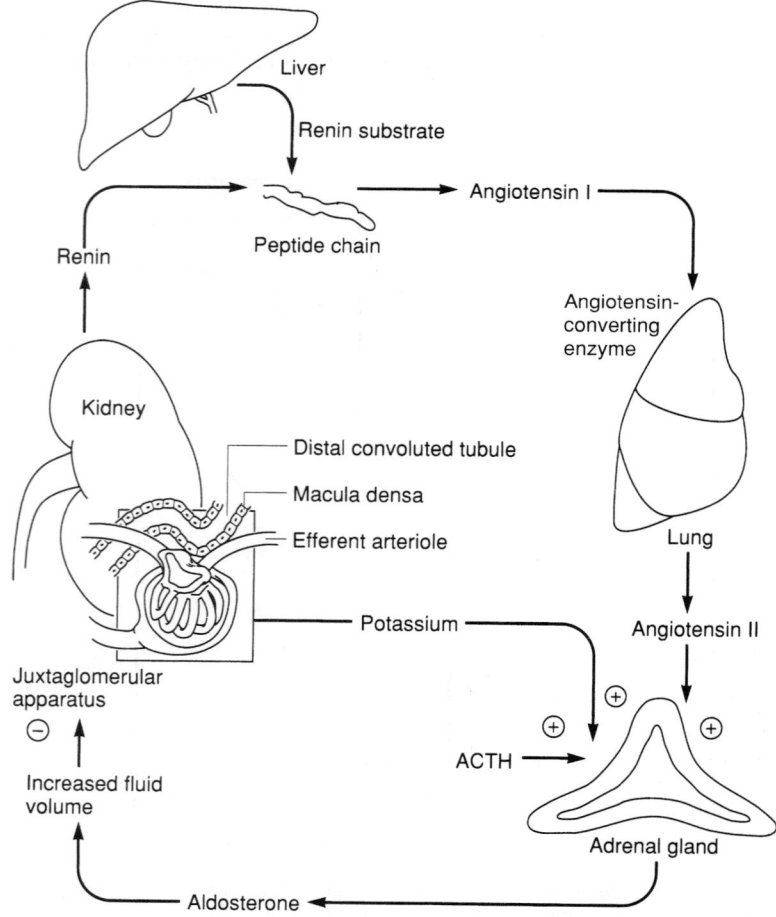

Figure 56.5. The relations of renin, angiotensin I, angiotensin II, and their anatomic sites of production and enzymatic conversion.

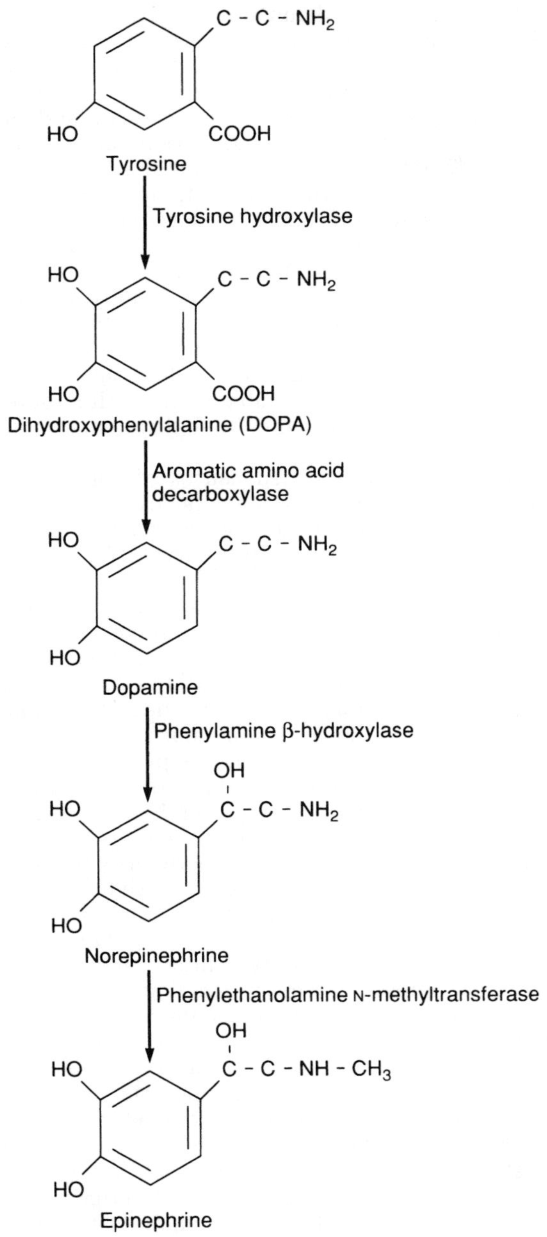

Figure 56.6. The enzymatic and structural relations on which the adrenal medullary synthesis of catecholomines depends.

temic circulation. In the systemic circulation, the catecholamines can undergo neuronal uptake and subsequent degradation, enzymatic degradation by other sites, or excretion in the urine. The catecholamines taken up by neurons are metabolized predominantly by monoamine oxidase, and they eventually yield vanillylmandelic acid (VMA). The enzyme, carboxy-o-methyl transferase, is responsible for the extraneuronal inactivation. The major metabolic product of this enzyme is normetanephrine for norepinephrine or metanephrine for epinephrine. Another fraction of the circulating catecholamines binds to tissue receptors for epinephrine and norepinephrine, and biologic effects are achieved. A small fraction is also excreted in the urine as free epinephrine and norepinephrine, which provides a useful way to diagnose pheochromocytomas.

In general, the factors that stimulate adrenal medullary secretion are those that increase sympathetic activity throughout the body. These include the assumption of an

upright position, pain, emotional stress, hypotension, cold, hypoglycemia, and many others. Two mechanisms diminish the stimulatory effects. One is feedback inhibition by norepinephrine on the presynaptic, preganglionic α_2-receptors. Stimulation of these receptors by norepinephrine decreases the release of acetylcholine. The second feedback mechanism is the suppression of tyrosine hydroxylase activity by high concentrations of norepinephrine. Because tyrosine hydroxylase is the rate-limiting enzyme in the synthetic pathway, increasing levels of the end product norepinephrine limit its own production through the effects on this short negative-feedback loop.

PATHOPHYSIOLOGY

For the surgeon concerned with the adrenal gland, functional pathology is heavily weighted toward tumor formation. Some of the other entities, however, such as steroidogenic enzymatic defects in congenital adrenal hyperplasia, are important and are considered here. In general, hormonal overproduction is the characteristic underlying problem. Before considering the clinical impact of these states, it is necessary to examine the effects of steroids and catecholamines on peripheral tissues.

Steroids

After secretion into the blood, most steroid molecules are bound to specific plasma proteins and are present only to a limited degree in unbound, or free, form. Except in unusual situations in which there is an excess of steroid-binding proteins, increased total circulating hormone accurately reflects increased secretion. This is usually seen with stress states, functioning tumors, or congenital adrenal hyperplasia.

The circulating unbound steroid molecules pass freely through the cellular membrane of the target cell, where they bind with a specific cytosolic receptor. After the receptor transforms, the receptor–steroid complex is translocated into the nucleus. In the nucleus, this complex directs new messenger RNA production and thus results in new biologic behavior of the target cell. The general schema of cytosolic receptor and nuclear signal transduction is common to all steroids. It is the distribution of receptors, specific for each of the steroids, among various cell populations that determines the differential effects of steroids among tissues. Cortisol, which is the key endogenous hormone for carbohydrate-active effects, has receptors in almost all tissues of the body. Androgenic and estrogenic receptors are somewhat more restricted in their distribution, with key cell populations in such organs as breast, prostate, and external genitalia, although effects of sex steroids can be demonstrated in some other cells, such as hepatocytes. The mineralocorticoids, such as aldosterone and deoxycorticosterone, have receptors with an even more limited distribution to target tissues, such as the renal tubule, salivary glands, and colonic mucosa.

Cortisol

Normal Effects. Of the many systemic effects of the glucocorticoids, most are probably related to their effect on intermediary metabolism. In this regard, perhaps the most important action is the effect of steroids on protein breakdown. A direct proteolytic effect of steroids has been suggested by several lines of evidence. The glucocorticoids release branched-chain and other amino acids from muscle. This release provides substrate for gluconeogenesis and is one of the several mechanisms by which steroids produce an increase in this process. The steroid-induced release of amino acids from muscle occurs even in the absence of insulin and is not simply an antiinsulin effect. In addition to the direct proteolytic effect on muscle, steroids accentuate the release of lactate from muscle. Both the lactate from muscle and the glycerol from fat cells released under the influence of epinephrine are additional precursors for gluconeogenesis. The glucocorticoids also have a direct effect on several of the gluconeogenetic hepatic enzymes, all of which promote hyperglycemia.

Gluconeogenesis is one of the two primary mechanisms whereby glucocorticoids promote hyperglycemia. On the other side of the equation, glucocorticoids effect a decrease in glucose use by peripheral tissues. First, there appears to be an inhibition of glucose transport into fat cells. Second, glucocorticoids appear to decrease insulin binding by insulin-sensitive tissues. Together, the decrease in peripheral use of glucose and the increased production of glucose primarily by gluconeogenesis explain the tendency toward hyperglycemia produced by glucocorticoids. The final aspect of glucocorticoid influence on substrate use is the apparent accentuation of lipolysis by these steroids. Both serum triglycerides and free fatty acids are increased. Such an effect is obviously countered by that of insulin on adipocytes. It is believed that the truncal obesity seen in steroid excess is related to the predominance of the lipogenic effect of insulin on these truncal adipocytes over the lipolytic effect of glucocorticoids. The opposite relation may hold true for the receptors in fat of the extremities and would explain the comparatively scant fat in these areas with steroid excess.

Glucocorticoids have effects specific to particular systems, including the gastrointestinal tract, the cardiovascular system, kidneys, and bone, and to specific processes, including the inflammatory response, immune function, and wound healing. The most notable effect in the gastrointestinal tract is a decrease in the rate of mucosal cell replication. In addition, decreased mucosal and pancreatic prostaglandin synthesis occurs. This may have important implications for the cytoprotective mechanisms in the stomach and for maintaining pancreatic acinar integrity in the face of various insults. In the cardiovascular system, glucocorticoids appear to produce an increased chronotropic and inotropic effect on the heart along with an increased peripheral vascular resistance. Receptors in the distal renal tubules respond to glucocorticoids by inducing increased tubular resorption of sodium. These are a different class of receptors from those mediating the more potent actions of aldosterone. In bone, there is a clear decrease in the rate of bone formation. This is probably secondary to delay in osteoblast development, resulting in qualitatively deficient protein constituents of the extracellular matrix.

Suppression of the inflammatory response by glucocorticoids is a particularly germane issue for surgical patients. The most obvious effect is the decrease of mononuclear cells in wounds. The function of these cells is also suppressed in terms of deficient chemotaxis and inadequate phagocytosis. Consequently, bacterial activity increases. Evidence is also accumulating that production of soluble mediators, important in the inflammatory process, may be suppressed in response to excess steroids.

Known steroidal effects on immune function are seen primarily in the behavior of cellular elements. There is a tendency to leukocytosis, eosinophilia, and lymphopenia. In higher ranges of steroid excess, there is a diminished response of lymphocytes to antigen stimulation. Finally, in wound healing, steroid-induced reductions in tensile strength are clearly demonstrable along with suppressed scar contraction and delayed epithelialization.

Cortisol Excess. The varied causes of cortisol excess produce clinical features that are collectively called *Cushing syndrome* (2). These include exogenous steroid administration, Cushing disease (pituitary ACTH excess), ectopic ACTH production, adrenal adenoma or carcinoma, micronodular pigmented hyperplasia, macronodular hyperplasia, and steroid-dependent adrenal hyperplasia. These entities are reviewed later in this chapter. Although treatments of these modalities differ, the clinical picture produced by the various causes is virtually the same and is clearly related to the cortisol actions mentioned previously. The peculiar fat distribution is probably related to the differential insulin and steroid receptors in various fat depositions in the body. Hyperglycemia is related to the decreased peripheral use of glucose as well as to increased gluconeogenesis. Muscle-wasting is primarily the result of direct steroidal effects on proteolysis. Abdominal striae and a tendency to poor wound healing can be related to suppression of both scar contraction and inflammatory response. Increased susceptibility to infection is also related to immunosuppression. The apparent increases in incidence of peptic ulcer disease and acute pancreatitis are related to the effects on the gastrointestinal tract. Sodium retention and the effects on the cardiovascular system contribute to hypertension. Osteoporosis and perhaps growth retardation in children are related in part to the steroidal effects on bone growth. Although the primary manifestations of adrenal disorders in children are those of sexual ambiguity and virilization, as described later, the delay in growth is a particularly notable feature in children with glucocorticoid excess. Some of the extensive effects of cortisol are outlined in Table 56.1.

Table 56.1. SYSTEMIC EFFECTS OF CORTISOL

Function	Normal amounts	Excessive amounts
Metabolic		
Protein	Proteolysis	Muscle wasting
Glucose	Gluconeogenesis	Hyperglycemia
Fat	Low-use peripheral lipolysis	Limb thinness
	Central lipogenesis	Truncal obesity
Gastrointestinal	Mucosal cells	Ulceration
	Prostaglandin	Pancreatitis(?)
Cardiovascular	Chronotropic, inotropic	Hypertension
	Vascular resistance	
Renal	Sodium resorption	Hypertension
Bone	Osteoblastic development	Osteoporosis
Inflammatory and immune	Circulating cells	Infection
	Soluble mediators	
	Antigen processing	
Wound healing	Fibroblasts	Striae
	Epithelial cells	Dehiscence

Androgens and Estrogens

Quantitatively, the major adrenal androgens are dehydroepiandrosterone, androstenedione, and testosterone. Androstenedione is the principal androgen converted in peripheral tissues to estrogens, and testosterone is the most potent masculinizing steroid on a per-weight basis.

Normal Effects. In adults, androgens have the obvious effect of deepening the voice, producing a male hair distribution, coarsening the skin, toughening and darkening facial hair, and promoting protein deposition in muscles. Estrogens have virtually opposite effects. Androgens in the fetus stimulate wolffian duct development and elongate the genital tubercle. They promote midline migration of the labial folds and a fusion of these folds to form the scrotum. To complete the transformation, the urethral opening migrates to the tip of the phallus. All these events are androgen-dependent. Since the ovary in the normal female fetus does not secrete androgens, the genital tubercle, labial folds, and urethral opening all remain in the normal female position in this circumstance. Excess androgen in the male fetus manifests itself only after birth, when masculinization and precocious puberty are in evidence. Excess androgen in the female fetus causes neonatal virilization, as is seen with congenital adrenal hyperplasia.

Excess Sex Steroids. In both the child and adult, excess androgen or estrogen production by the adrenal gland almost always arises from carcinoma. Androgen excess in the female, in addition to producing the masculinizing features already mentioned, results in clitoral hypertrophy and, in the adult, menstrual cessation. Androgen excesses are difficult to detect in adult men, but in children precocious puberty occurs. In the rare adrenal carcinoma producing estrogen, menstrual irregularities may be the only clinical manifestation in the female, whereas the male may experience disturbing loss of libido, enlarged breast tissue, and female distribution of hair.

Enzymatic defects in the steroidogenic pathway can produce the syndrome known as *congenital adrenal hyperplasia* (3). This syndrome presents predominantly in the neonatal period with sexual ambiguity. These enzymatic defects result in a lowered cortisol secretion, with consequent increased ACTH production and stimulation in the early steroidogenic pathway (Fig. 56.7). The specific enzyme defects present determine which clinical form the syndrome takes. The most common form is 21-hydroxylase deficiency. Both this defect and the 11β-hydroxylase deficiency result in excess androgen production in utero and masculinization with ambiguous genitalia in the female newborn. Masculinizing effects in the male may not be detected until precocious puberty is obvious. About 40% of patients with 21-hydroxylase deficiency have salt-wasting or sodium loss by urine, which, in males, may result in earlier detection than in those without salt-wasting. In the 11b-hydroxylase deficiency, there may also be hypertension because of excess secretion of deoxycorticosterone. In the 17-hydroxylase deficiency, hypertension caused by excess secretion of deoxycorticosterone and corticosterone occurs, and the testes may not secrete androgens, which may result in ambiguous female genitalia. In the female, ovarian failure to secrete estrogen prevents the appearance of secondary sex characteristics at the time of puberty. The 3-hydroxysteroid dehydrogenase deficiency is similar to the 21-hydroxylase deficiency, especially with regard to the salt-wasting variety, in that both mineralocorticoid and glucocorticoid synthesis may be decreased. In both the 21-hydroxylase deficiency and the 3-hydroxysteroid dehydrogenase deficiency, mild forms may not become obvious until later in childhood, when precocious puberty may draw attention to the excess androgen secretion.

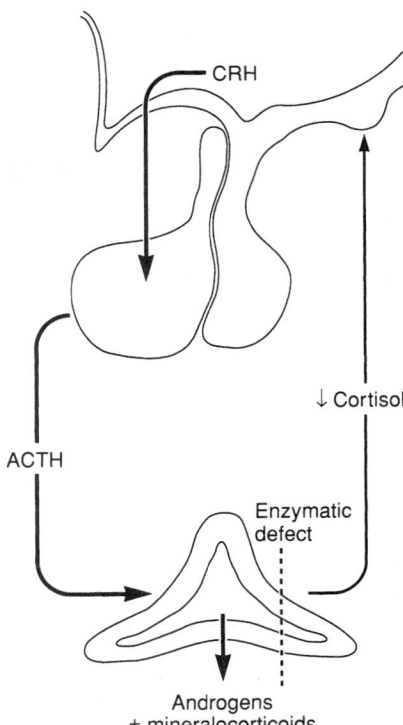

Figure 56.7. A variety of heritable enzymatic defects block the adrenal production of cortisol. This results in the loss of negative feedback to the hypothalamus with continued stimulation and excess production of androgens and possibly mineralocorticoids. The result is the congenital adrenal hyperplasia syndrome. The most common enzymatic deficiencies are 21-hydroxylase, 11β-hydroxylase, and 3β-hydroxysteroid dehydrogenase (Fig. 56.3).

Aldosterone

Normal Effects. Aldosterone is the primary mineralocorticoid in humans. It influences sodium, potassium, and hydrogen ion transport. Receptors for aldosterone are found in the parotid gland and colonic mucosa, but the principal site of action is the distal renal tubule. Aldosterone increases tubular sodium resorption and decreases sodium excretion and potassium resorption with kaliuresis. Aldosterone also increases secretion of hydrogen ion into the urine. Under normal conditions, aldosterone secretion is controlled by total body sodium and potassium content and is relatively constant around a physiologic set-point regardless of variations in intake. Excess sodium intake suppresses renin secretion, angiotensin formation, and aldosterone secretion. The deficit in aldosterone results in increased urinary sodium loss and excretion of the administered sodium load. Conversely, a negative sodium balance stimulates renin, angiotensin, and aldosterone secretion, with resorption of sodium from the urine. This results in conservation of sodium and prevention of further negative sodium balance. Aldosterone control also affords some protection from excess serum potassium levels in that hyperkalemia stimulates aldosterone secretion, which in turn promotes renal potassium loss and helps lower serum potassium levels.

Aldosterone Excess. Primary hyperaldosteronism occurs with certain abnormal adrenal entities, in which secretion is not only excessive but autonomous; that is, it does not suppress by the usual mechanisms. These adrenal entities are adenoma, primary hyperplasia of the zona glomerulosa, and adrenal carcinoma producing aldosterone (4). The rarity of adenomas that produce deoxy-

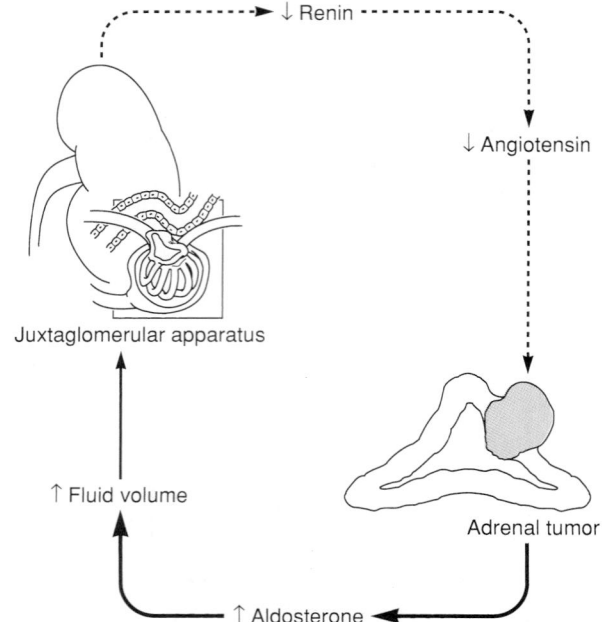

Figure 56.8. The physiologic consequences of primary hyperaldosteronism. The effects on the renin-angiotensin axis and intravascular volume are emphasized.

corticosterone precludes further mention here. Causes of secondary hyperaldosteronism are related to increased renin secretion, such as renal artery stenosis, congestive heart failure, and renal salt-wasting. Juxtaglomerular hyperplasia (Bartter syndrome) is a rare, nonhypertensive form of secondary hyperaldosteronism. These secondary, mainly nonsurgical, forms are not discussed here.

Primary hyperaldosteronism is characterized by mineralocorticoid hypersecretion, which promotes positive sodium balance secondary to stimulation of sodium resorption in the renal tubule (5). The autonomy of aldosterone secretion prevents suppression by the excess total body sodium and expanded fluid compartments. This positive sodium balance results in an excess volume of 2 to 3 L of saline before a new steady state of expanded extracellular fluid volume is reached. This new steady state is attributed to an escape phenomenon whereby a certain volume of positive sodium balance is tolerated, after which additional sodium intake is promptly excreted. Thus, normal fluid homeostasis is preserved. With the expanded extracellular volume or positive sodium balance of primary aldosteronism, renin secretion and angiotensin formation are suppressed (Fig. 56.8).

Another measurable hallmark of primary aldosteronism is hypokalemia. About 80% of patients with primary hy-

peraldosteronism have serum potassium levels of 3.5 mEq/L or less. If challenged with a saline load, up to 95% of patients exhibit hypokalemia and potassium excretion of more than 40 to 60 mEq/d in the urine because of an accentuated exchange of sodium for potassium in the renal tubule. In addition to hypernatremia and hypokalemia, metabolic alkalosis, due primarily to loss of hydrogen ions in the urine, is common. The increased tubular resorption of sodium, leading to the positive sodium balance, promotes hypertension. Hypokalemic nephropathy eventually leads to polyuria and nocturia. The hypokalemia further affects muscles by promoting weakness and paralysis. Hypokalemia also reduces β-cell insulin release, resulting in hypoinsulinemia and hyperglycemia. A summary of these events is given in Table 56.2.

Catecholamines

Normal Effects. The two major catecholamines, norepinephrine and epinephrine, mediate their effects through cellular membrane receptors. These receptors are found on many cell types, but their initial characterization was accomplished using smooth muscle. α-Receptors were found to be those that mediate contraction of smooth muscle, and β-receptors regulate relaxation. These were later characterized further into α_1- and α_2-receptors and β_1- and β_2-receptors. Several examples of β_1-receptor stimulation include increased inotropic and chronotropic responses in cardiac muscle, lipolytic effects in adipocytes, and a decrease in peripheral glucose use by most cells. Effects of β_2-receptors include relaxation of smooth muscle, especially that of the bronchus. Isoproterenol and epinephrine are well-known β-agonists. Effects of α_1-receptors are predominantly contraction of smooth muscle in peripheral vascular beds and in the uterus. α_2-Receptors mediate platelet aggregation and, on presynaptic neuronal terminals, suppress the release of norepinephrine or acetylcholine.

Both epinephrine and norepinephrine may have a-receptor effects, but the specific effects seem to depend both on the concentration of the catecholamines to which the receptors are exposed and the distribution of the various types of receptors within the tissues. For example, norepinephrine may have a β_2-receptor effect at high concentrations, whereas epinephrine exerts this effect at relatively low concentrations. On the other hand, white blood cells have a predominance of b-receptors and show little response to norepinephrine even at higher concentrations. Additional mechanisms modulate catecholamine effects. As the concentration of catecholamines increases, the receptor population decreases. This phenomenon is known as *down-regulation* and explains the relative insensitivity of a given tissue to catecholamines upon exposure to high concentrations (tachyphylaxis). With *up-regulation,* the number of receptors increases during the use of receptor antagonists or in the relative absence of catecholamines. This explains the increased sensitivity to catecholamines

Tubular action	Normal amounts	Excessive amounts
Increased resorption of sodium	Protects against low-volume states	Hypertension
		Positive sodium balance
		Hyporeninemia
Decreased resorption of potassium	Protects against hyperkalemia	Hypokalemia
		Metabolic alkalosis
		Hyperglycemia
		Nocturia, polyuria
		Muscle weakness

Table 56.2. **EFFECTS OF ALDOSTERONE SECRETION**

after surgical sympathectomy, for example. Another modulating mechanism is a change in adenyl cyclase activity as a postreceptor phenomenon. An excess of circulating thyroxine increases adenyl cyclase activity, which in turn increases cyclic adenosine monophosphate (cAMP) concentrations to amplify catecholamine activity. Thus, for a given a- or b-receptor number, sympathetic effects are amplified during a period of thyroxine excess.

Because of the wide distribution of catecholamine receptors, the effects achieved by catecholamines are predictably varied. The effects of catecholamines differ from those of steroids in at least two major ways. The onset of catecholamine action occurs within 1 or 2 minutes, as compared with 60 to 90 minutes for steroids. This difference reflects the quick mediation by membrane catecholamine receptors, whose changes are translated to the cAMP system. This contrasts with the slower mediation by cytosolic steroid receptors, which must be transported to the nucleus where changes are expressed through DNA and RNA synthesis. In part because of catecholamine's short plasma half-life, its effects tend to be short-lived. As mentioned, this rapid clearance is due to a combination of neuronal reuptake and the ubiquitous presence of the degradative catecholamine enzymes.

Catecholamine Excess. Pheochromocytomas are tumors primarily of the adrenal medulla (6,7). They are classified as functioning when they produce catecholamines, always autonomously and usually in great excess. Although some of these tumors produce only epinephrine or norepinephrine, most produce the two catecholamines in combination. The predictable clinical effects of this endogenous catecholamine outpouring include hypertension, tachycardia, nervousness, and sweating (Table 56.3). Dopamine is also produced in variable amounts, with clinical consequences that are unclear.

The secretory effects of these tumors tend to fall into three patterns. Patients may have sustained hypertension without episodic increases in blood pressure or any other signs of markedly excessive secretion. Patients may be predominantly normotensive with superimposed episodes of increased secretion manifested by tachycardia, hypertension, or flushing. Finally, patients may present with a combination of the two patterns, with sustained baseline hypertension and superimposed attacks of episodic hypertension. The episodes are best explained by changes in local blood flow since it is well documented that the tumors are not functionally innervated. A surge in blood flow in these tumors can wash out sinusoids rich in the catecholamines, producing a spike in circulating catecholamine concentrations. For patients with minimal clinical symptoms, it appears that released catecholamines are also taken up locally by the tumor and metabolized to their inactive products. For this reason, a large tumor may be relatively asymptomatic because its active products are metabolized mainly on site. This yields inactive metabolites, and few, if any, active products reach the systemic circulation. Diagnostic sensitivity can therefore be improved by measuring both the metabolites and the catecholamines in the urine. As implied, some pheochromocytomas apparently do not secrete active substances of any kind; these are termed *nonfunctioning*.

DIAGNOSTIC INVESTIGATIONS

Patients with functioning adrenal lesions usually come to the attention of the health care delivery system by virtue of an incidental finding such as hypertension or hypokalemia; changes in appearance, such as redistribution of fat or abdominal striae; or with other symptoms, such as palpitations or muscular weakness. The various symptoms and findings specific for the types of functioning adrenal tumors were outlined previously. Both functioning and nonfunctioning adrenal tumors come to the attention of physicians as incidental findings on radiologic scan as well as through the use of modern imaging techniques, including computed tomographic (CT) scans, ultrasound, and magnetic resonance imaging (MRI) of the abdomen. Therapeutic approaches to both functioning and nonfunctioning adrenal tumors are discussed in a subsequent section. Laboratory investigations used to determine the presence and type of functioning adrenal tumors and techniques used to determine their location are reviewed next.

Functional Assessment

The first diagnostic step in determining the functional state of an adrenal gland or lesion is to screen the urine or plasma for secretory products. The impetus for the screening is usually the presence of clinical findings or symptoms that suggest one of the various types of hyperfunctioning adrenal lesions, or it may simply be an incidental finding on an imaging test. Once hypersecretion is demonstrated, the specific type of pathology producing the syndrome must be determined with the aid of functional tests that manipulate the feedback mechanisms involved. In addition, relevant scanning and imaging tests can distinguish among the various types of lesions.

Hypercortisolism (Cushing Syndrome)

Screening Procedures. The simplest screening procedure for Cushing syndrome is the determination of plasma cortisol concentrations, preferably on multiple venous samplings. The sensitivity and specificity of this screening test is about 80% to 90%. The specificity can be increased by obtaining plasma samples at 8:00 A.M. and 6:00 P.M. Diurnal variation of plasma cortisol is lost both in adrenal tumor formation and in the hypercortisolism of pituitary origin (Cushing disease). The measurement of 17-OH corticosteroids in the urine is perhaps more sensitive than cortisol measurements in plasma, but urine collection is more complicated than plasma sampling. Measurement of urinary free cortisol is perhaps the most sensitive screening method of all. In equivocal cases, the low-dose dexamethasone suppression test can be used. Dexamethasone, by negative feedback, suppresses the hypothalamic–pituitary secretion of ACTH and consequently lowers both plasma cortisol and urinary 17-OH corticosteroid excretion. Administration of 2 mg of dexamethasone suppresses plasma cortisol and urinary 17-OH corticosteroid by at least half when compared with control values taken with a normal pituitary–adrenal axis. In Cushing disease, with the set-point of ACTH secretion higher than normal, low-dose dexamethasone is insufficient to suppress ACTH.

Table 56.3. CATECHOLAMINE EFFECTS

Receptor class	Normal amounts	Excessive amounts
β_1	Chronotropic, inotropic	Tachycardia
	Sweat glands	Sweating
	Decreased glucose use	Hyperglycemia
β_2	Smooth muscle relaxation	Hypotension
α_1	Smooth muscle contraction	Hypertension
	Gluconeogenesis	
	Glycogenolysis	Hyperglycemia
	Suppressed insulin effects	
α_2	††Smooth muscle contraction	Pallor

††Platelet aggregation

Determining the Cause. Once hypersecretion of cortisol has been established, confirmation of specific abnormalities is undertaken by manipulating the negative feedback loop for steroids on the hypothalamic–pituitary unit. High-dose dexamethasone is used for this. The classic version of the test consists of 2 mg of dexamethasone administered every 6 hours for 24 hours. Measurement of 24-hour 17-OH corticosteroid excretion is obtained for baseline values on the day before dexamethasone administration. This is then repeated on the day of dexamethasone administration. A normal response to overnight suppression is to lower the 17-OH corticosteroid excretion by more than half. In the case of Cushing disease, the hypothalamic steroid receptors that allow negative feedback are intact but are set at a higher point. In this case, the 17-OH corticosteroid secretion does decrease significantly after high-dose dexamethasone administration. The schema for Cushing disease is shown in Fig. 56.9. On the other hand, adrenal tumors, other causes of ectopic production of ACTH, and most cases of nodular hyperplasia do not respond to dexamethasone suppression with a decrease in steroid secretion. With an adrenal tumor, pituitary ACTH is already suppressed; therefore, dexamethasone cannot suppress it further (Fig. 56.10). With ectopic ACTH secretion, the tissue producing ACTH has no receptors for steroids, and negative feedback cannot be achieved. It is not clear why some cases of micronodular adrenal hyperplasia can be suppressed by dexamethasone. Because the classic dexamethasone suppression test uses cumbersome urinary measurements, an overnight test has been devised that uses a previous-day 8:00 A.M. plasma cortisol determination for control values and another sample taken at 8:00 the morning after the dexamethasone administration. The sensitivity and specificity of this simplified test are comparable to the classic form.

Potentially, the most helpful new test uses CRH to release ACTH and consequently to stimulate cortisol secretion. A standard dose of CRH is 1 µg/kg, or a maximum of 100 µg. The CRH is administered intravenously, and serial

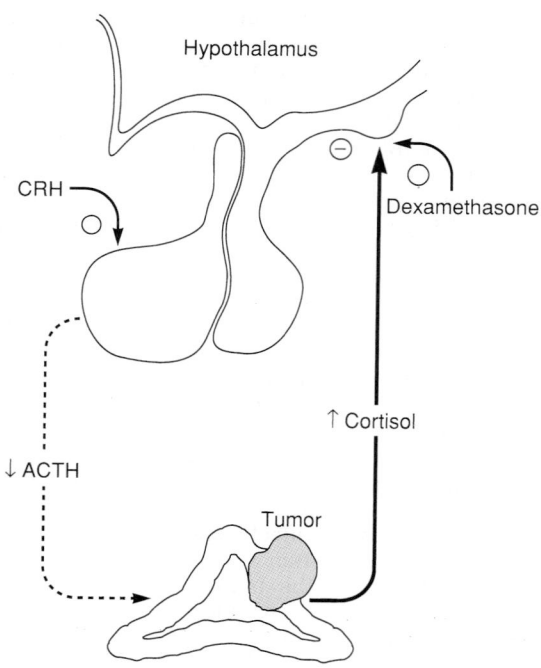

Figure 56.10. With a primary adrenal tumor producing hypercortisolism, pituitary ACTH is already maximally suppressed and dexamethasone produces no further decrease in output.

blood samples are obtained for about 3 hours after administration. The normal pituitary adrenal axis responds by a moderate increase in ACTH and cortisol. With Cushing disease, the ACTH and cortisol rise are accentuated. The overlap in results with this test for normal subjects and those with Cushing disease is not great. With adrenal autonomous production of cortisol (adrenal tumors or nodular hyperplasia) and with ectopic ACTH production, there is virtually no response to CRH. The diagnostic steps for Cushing syndrome are listed in Table 56.4.

Sex Steroid Excess

In adults, evidence of androgen excess is clinically apparent only in females. Although an ovarian source of androgen production must be sought in females, the predominant adrenal lesion is a cortical carcinoma. Male adults who become feminine are at high risk for having an adrenocortical carcinoma. In children, precocious puberty in males or virilization in females should point to the possibility of adrenal carcinoma. The differential diagnosis in children should include nonclassic or late 21-OH defi-

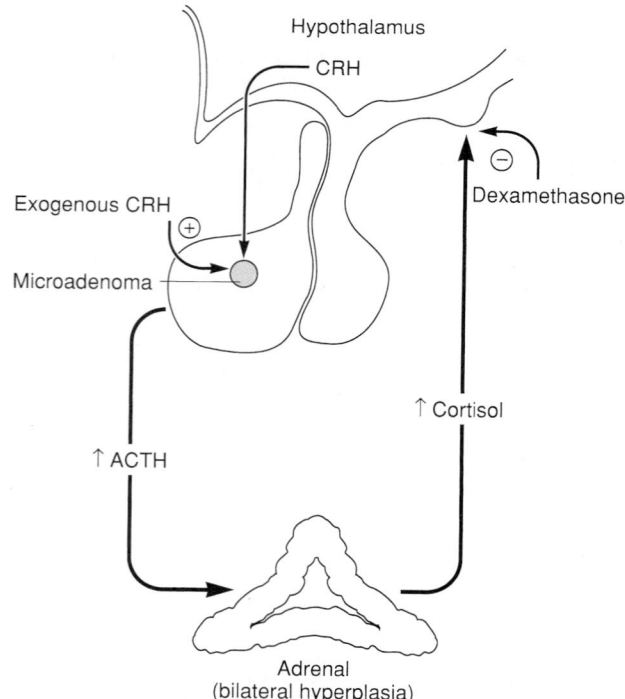

Figure 56.9. Cushing disease results from autonomous pituitary ACTH release. Dexamethasone does not suppress 17-OH corticosteroid production in patients with Cushing disease.

Table 56.4. **STEPS IN THE DIAGNOSIS OF CUSHING SYNDROME**

Screening tests
    Plasma cortisol—random and diurnal
    Urinary 17-OH corticosteroids
    Urinary free cortisol
    Overnight low-dose dexamethasone
Determining the cause
    Standard dexamethasone suppression
        Positive—pituitary cause
        Negative—adrenal or ectopic cause
    Corticotropin-releasing hormone stimulation
        Accentuated—pituitary cause
        No response—adrenal or ectopic cause
    Petrosal sinus sampling
        Lateralizing—pituitary cause
        Nonlateralizing—adrenal or ectopic cause

ciency, 11β-OH deficiency, and primary ovarian tumors. The screening test for an adrenal source of excessive sex steroids is measurement of urinary 17-ketosteroids. This is abnormally high in patients with an adrenal source. In the feminine male, urinary estrogens should be measured. The dexamethasone suppression test in children is a useful means to determine whether one is dealing with the autonomous secretion of 17-ketosteroids by a tumor or whether the suppressible steroid secretion suggests an enzymatic defect in the steroidogenic pathway.

Congenital adrenal hyperplasia is usually brought to the physician's attention because of ambiguous genitalia in the female at birth. About 90% of these cases involve 21-OH deficiency. Male patients may be recognized early since about two thirds of these cases have salt-wasting. In either sex, it is an important diagnosis to make early. In the female, there is the question of gender assignment. Usually, the assignment is female, regardless of genotype, and an early operation should be planned. The objectives are to correct the clitoral hypertrophy, to create an adequate vagina and introitus, and to perform whatever cosmetic revision of the labia is required. In either male or female, prompt treatment of the salt-wasting may be life-saving. The diagnostic measurement of choice in the case of 21-OH deficiency is that of 17-OH progesterone, whereas 11-deoxycortisol is the major steroid produced for 11b-hydroxylase deficiency. Any enzymatic defect can be detected by evaluating for excess of proximal intermediates (Fig. 56.3).

Hyperaldosteronism

For practical purposes, the best screening test in the hypertensive population for primary aldosteronism is the measurement of serum potassium levels. Since the prevalence of primary aldosteronism in the hypertensive population is less than 1 in 200 patients, it is not feasible to engage in more specific measurements in a screening program. When obtained with the patient in the fasting state and without any form of exercise or prolonged venostasis, the diagnostic sensitivity of this test for hypokalemia is close to 90%. Urinary potassium excretion above 30 mEq/24 h is confirmatory, especially when the serum potassium level is below 3.5 mEq/L. When there is borderline hypokalemia, salt supplementation at about 200 mEq/d can further improve the sensitivity of the screening test. Because there are so many other causes of hypertension and hypokalemia, the specificity of this test for hypokalemia is low, and further studies are required.

Determinations of urinary or plasma aldosterone and plasma renin are primary considerations in making a diagnosis of hyperaldosteronism. Taking 20 mg/24 h as the upper limit of normal, the sensitivity of a 24-hour urinary aldosterone measurement is up to 80%. When combined with a 3-day salt-supplemented diet, the sensitivity is increased to 95%. Measurement of plasma renin is also a reliable screening test for hyperaldosteronism. If plasma renin remains low when an upright position is assumed and during negative sodium balance, the likelihood of autonomous production of aldosterone is increased.

To confirm the diagnosis of primary aldosteronism, measurements must be made under special conditions that manipulate feedback control. The starting premise is that with primary aldosteronism, aldosterone values should be higher than in patients with other forms of hypertension, and these values cannot be lowered by various maneuvers that normally suppress aldosterone secretion. The infusion of 2,000 mL of normal saline over a 4-hour period normally suppresses plasma aldosterone to less than 10 ng/dL, but in primary aldosteronism it fails to suppress. The few false-positive results encountered with this test are typically associated with increased plasma renin activity, such as with renal artery stenosis. The captopril

test takes advantage of the fact that this agent blocks the conversion of angiotensin I to angiotensin II. The test is therefore similar in concept to the saline infusion test, except that angiotensin II levels are lowered by pharmacologic means rather than by volume expansion. Another outpatient test calculates the integrated plasma aldosterone concentrations over a 24-hour period. It is unclear whether this test has advantages over the others mentioned. In the equivocal case, the patient should be brought into the hospital for dietary control and prolonged observation. The patient can be subjected to a period of volume expansion to test the autonomous nature of the aldosterone hypersecretion. Alternatively, treatment with sodium restriction and diuretics tests whether suppression of renin activity is fixed. These considerations can be reviewed by referring to Figs. 56.5 and 56.8.

The problem of differentiating aldosterone-producing adenomas from hyperplasia of the zona glomerulosa remains. Because surgery is usually not effective in the latter situation, the differentiation is an important one. Although interest has been centered on localization procedures, several maneuvers can distinguish the two conditions. The first takes advantage of postural stimulation. Aldosterone and renin are measured at 8:00 A.M. after 2 hours in the recumbent position and again 2 to 4 hours later after quiet ambulation. With adenomas, plasma renin remains suppressed even on standing, and the plasma aldosterone tends to be lower on the second sampling because of decreasing ACTH levels as the morning progresses. Plasma renin activity is not as suppressed in patients with hyperplasia. The upright position produces postural response, which is a small increase in plasma renin activity, and plasma aldosterone consequently increases.

The second test is more promising and involves measuring an aldosterone precursor, 18-hydroxycorticosterone. For some unknown reason, this steroid is increased in patients with adenomas but remains in the normal range in those with hyperplasia. The 18-hydroxycorticosterone levels are above 100 µg/dL in virtually all patients with aldosterone-producing adenomas. An interesting subtype of primary adrenal hyperplasia is that which can be cured by surgery. These patients characteristically have elevated plasma 18-hydroxycorticosterone levels. Therefore, even if a patient with primary aldosteronism does not lateralize on CT or venous sampling, surgery may be curative in the presence of elevated 18-hydroxycorticosterone. Localization to distinguish aldosteronomas from hyperplasia is covered in the subsequent section. Table 56.5 provides a summary of screening and confirmation tests.

Table 56.5. STEPS IN THE DIAGNOSIS OF ALDOSTERONISM

Screening tests
    Serum potassium concentration—low
    Urinary potassium excretion—high
    Urinary aldosterone excretion—high
    Plasma renin—low
    Oral sodium loading
Confirming tests
    Plasma and urinary aldosterone
        Saline infusion
        Captopril
        Integrated plasma values
    Plasma renin
        Negative sodium balance
Tumor versus hyperplasia
    Upright posture—plasma aldosterone and renin levels
        Tumor—remain suppressed
        Hyperplasia—slight rise
    18-OH-corticosterone—high with tumor

Catecholamines

In a patient suspected of having a pheochromocytoma, the most efficient and sensitive means of screening is to measure the catecholamines or their metabolic products in the urine. The normal person excretes less than 100 μg/d of the catecholamines norepinephrine and epinephrine. Because of some overlap in values, specificity can be improved by using a normal range of up to 250 μg/d. Although 24-hour samples can reduce the possible episodic variations in catecholamine excretion, shorter sampling periods can be useful, especially if corrected for creatinine excretion. In general, creatinine also should be measured in all 24-hour samples to check for completeness of collection. Because of their stability and relative freedom from substances interfering with their measurement, the metanephrines are preferred by some centers. A value of greater than 1 mg/24 h is usually considered positive. Measurement of either the urinary catecholamines or the metanephrines usually yields a 95% detection sensitivity. A combination of the two is reported to have a greater than 98% sensitivity. The measurement of VMA can also be added for a virtual 100% sensitivity in the patient with an actively secreting pheochromocytoma. As mentioned, the clinical pattern in patients with pheochromocytoma is either sustained hypertension; sustained hypertension with episodes of increased blood pressure, tachycardia, or flushing; or, rarely, mostly normotensive, with infrequent and unpredictable episodes of hypertension. Timing of the collection is critical in patients who have only episodic hypersecretion. Urine collection should be started immediately after a suspected attack of hypertension.

With the advent of sensitive radioimmunoassays and high-pressure liquid chromatography for determining catecholamine levels in plasma, attention has turned to the use of these measurements. Fluctuations in plasma catecholamine concentrations are much greater than those in urinary excretion, even in normal subjects. As the upper limits of normal plasma values are increased to account for fluctuations, the specificity is improved but at the sacrifice of sensitivity. Conversely, by lowering upper limits of normal to 750 pg/mL for norepinephrine or 110 pg/mL for epinephrine (supine position), the sensitivity is raised to about 90%. The specificity is low in this circumstance, however, because of the overlap of normal spikes in catecholamine concentrations with those concentrations produced by minimally secreting pheochromocytomas. In spite of these shortcomings, plasma values are useful in other contexts. Measuring catecholamines in the plasma has made possible the clonidine suppression test. In patients without pheochromocytoma, clonidine suppresses high basal plasma concentrations into the normal range, whereas concentrations in patients with pheochromocytoma are not suppressed. Another use of plasma catecholamine measurement is in examining the ratio of 3,4-dihydroxyphenoglycol (DHPG) to norepinephrine in plasma. DHPG is released from the chromaffin cell and adrenergic neurons to a much greater extent than norepinephrine in pheochromocytoma patients compared with patients who have essential hypertension. A rare but important use of plasma catecholamine determinations is in patients who have elevated catecholamine levels on several occasions but negative CT scans. In this case, superior and inferior vena cava sampling with measurement of the plasma catecholamines at various points along the vessels can pinpoint the location of the tumor by showing a step-up in the catecholamine concentrations. The various urinary and plasma tests for determining the presence of a pheochromocytoma are as follows:

Urinary excretion
- Catecholamines
- Metanephrine, normetanephrine
- VMA
- Plasma epinephrine, norepinephrine
- Clonidine suppression test
- DHPG/norepinephrine ratio

In addition to the proper timing of urinary samples, several events, substances, and emotional states influence plasma and urinary catecholamine levels. Some of these are well-known events, whereas others relate to interfering substances that can falsely alter the assays, cause specific interferences with the assays, or affect catecholamine metabolism:

Endogenous release
- Pain
- Hypotension
- Hypoglycemia
- Psychic distress
- Drug withdrawal
- Surgery

Interfering drugs
- Catecholamines: calcium-channel blockers, captopril, α-agonists, β-blockers, α-blockers, methenamine mandelate
- VMA or metanephrine: clofibrate, nalidixic acid, methylglucamine
- Both catecholamines and metabolites: labetalol, levodopa, tricyclic antidepressants, phenothiazines, methyldopa, monoamine oxidase inhibitors

Localization Studies

Nonscintigraphic Studies

Although ultrasonography is the least expensive of the imaging procedures and is also able to distinguish solid from cystic lesions, its value is limited by the relative inaccessibility of the adrenal gland and by the small size of some of the adrenal lesions to be examined.

CT is the technique most commonly used to examine patients in whom adrenal abnormalities are suspected (8). In addition, because of the widespread use of abdominal CT, this method most often discovers the unsuspected adrenal tumors. CT reliably detects adrenal tumors greater than 1 cm in diameter (Fig. 56.11). The sensitivity of CT for tumors that are 1 cm in diameter is about 80%, and it

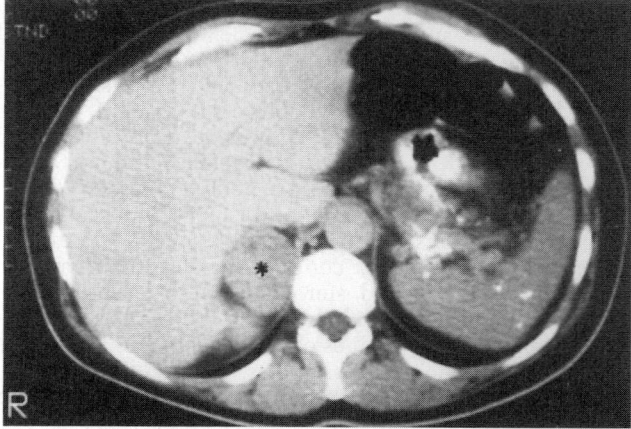

Figure 56.11. Abdominal computed tomography (CT) scan showing right adrenal tumor *(asterisk)*.

reaches 100% for tumors that are 3 to 4 cm. Although CT is noninvasive and reasonably sensitive, it is nonspecific. CT distinguishes cystic from solid adrenal abnormalities but does not distinguish functioning from nonfunctioning tumors, nor benign from malignant tumors, with any degree of reliability.

MRI has maintained a certain usefulness even after retrenchment from early optimistic predictions. It is more expensive and requires greater patient cooperation than CT, but it has greater versatility than CT because of the use of T_1- and T_2-weighted images. The relatively fast scanning time for the T_1-weighted images provides an increased sensitivity for identifying adrenal lesions in comparison with the T_2 sequences, which are more subject to motion artifact. In some cases, the T_2-weighted images can provide a differential diagnosis of adrenal lesions. The T_2-weighted images may distinguish such entities as metastatic or primary carcinoma and pheochromocytoma from adenomas, lipomas, myelolipomas, and cysts. On the T_2-weighted images, carcinomas generally have increased signal intensity, whereas the fat-laden adenomas and hyperplasia show decreased intensity. T_2-weighted images can provide adrenal/liver signal ratios that are higher for pheochromocytomas than for cortical adenomas or carcinomas. In a sense, MRI is complementary to CT in that the latter can better detect the lesion, whereas the former can distinguish one type of lesion from the other. In addition, MRI is probably better than CT for distinguishing anatomic relations and extent of involvement of surrounding tissues by carcinomas. A T_1-weighted MRI of a pelvic pheochromocytoma is shown in Fig. 56.12A. The same tumor is shown by CT scan in Fig. 56.12B.

Scintigraphic Imaging

Two radiopharmaceuticals have proved useful in imaging the adrenal gland. Adrenocortical lesions can be imaged by [131]I-6 ß-iodomethyl-19-norcholesterol, which is taken up as cholesterol in the adrenocortical steroidogenic pathway. The other agent is ^{131}I-methaiodobenzylguanidine (MIBG), a norepinephrine analogue. It indicates norepinephrine accumulation in storage vesicles and can detect sympathoadrenal tumors at any site in the body. NP-59 can accurately localize the adrenal cortex and any functioning tumors. NP-59 can distinguish adrenocortical hyperplasia from functioning adenomas or carcinomas. With the use of dexamethasone suppression, some cases of primary macronodular or micronodular adrenal hyperplasia, which do not suppress, can be distinguished from adrenal hyperplasia of pituitary origin, which does suppress. NP-59 has also been reported to distinguish unilateral aldosterone-producing tumors from bilateral hyperplasia of the zona glomerulosa in patients with primary hyperaldosteronism. Finally, in patients with incidentally discovered nonfunctioning adrenal tumors, NP-59 can separate adenomas, which ac-

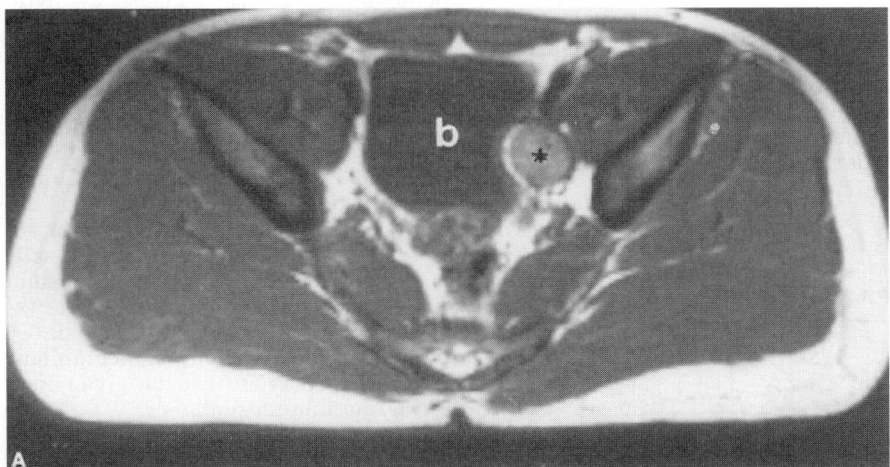

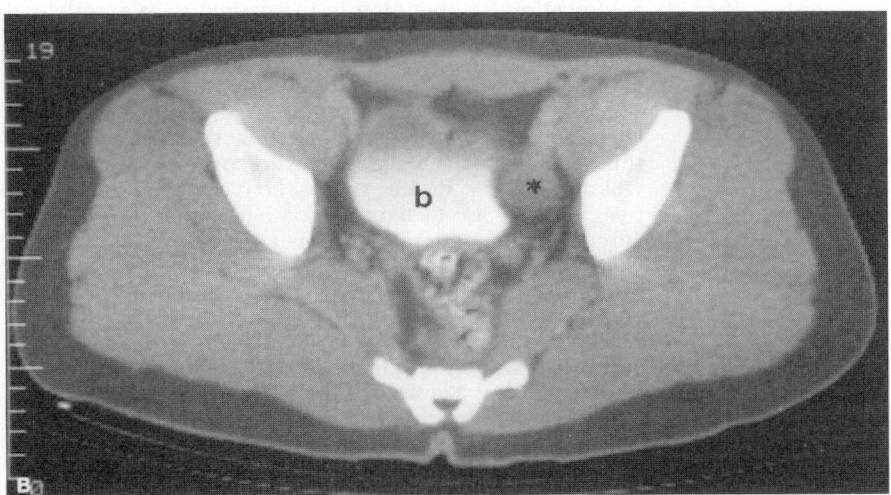

Figure 56.12. *(A)* T_1-weighted magnetic resonance imaging of a left pelvic pheochromocytoma *(asterisk)* compressing the bladder (b). *(B)* CT scan of the pelvis showing the left pelvic pheochromocytoma with bladder distortion *(asterisk)* as depicted in *A* (b).

cumulate the agent, from carcinomas, either primary or metastatic, which do not. MIBG is a useful agent in localizing pheochromocytomas throughout the body, especially when the tumors are multiple, extraadrenal, recurrent, or metastatic.

Invasive Localization Techniques

Arteriography, venography, and selective venous sampling became less popular as experience with the imaging techniques listed previously increased. Specific sampling of adrenal venous blood in primary aldosteronism and vena cava sampling in occult pheochromocytomas are still occasionally useful techniques. In addition to the disadvantages inherent in invasive procedures using intravascular contrast agents, arteriography is specifically dangerous in the study of patients with pheochromocytomas. The injection can cause a sudden rise in catecholamines and precipitate a hypertensive crisis. The same phenomenon has been reported with adrenal phlebography in pheochromocytomas, but the more common complication with this technique is disruption and bleeding of the adrenal venous system.

Localization Overview

In general, CT is the first choice for imaging because of its noninvasive nature, its ease in performance, and its sensitivity. In nonfunctioning tumors, some additional information can be derived concerning the nature of the lesion by using MRI. NP-59 scintigraphy is particularly useful in cases of Cushing syndrome and in hyperaldosteronism, and MIBG may be required in cases of pheochromocytoma in which multiple, extraadrenal, recurrent, or metastatic pheochromocytomas are suspected. Vena cava sampling of catecholamines may also be helpful in these patients. Finally, adrenal venous sampling is usually reserved for questionable cases of primary aldosteronism. A summary of these considerations is shown in Table 56.6.

Table 56.6. USE OF LOCALIZATION PROCEDURES

Procedure	Characteristics
Radiographic scans	
CT	Good first test; sensitive but not very specific
MR	Can identify some types of pathology and defines anatomy well; competes with scintigraphy in nonfunctioning tumors; lower sensitivity than CT; expensive
Scintigraphic scans	
NP-59	Adrenocortical imaging can distinguish unilateral from bilateral disease in most instances; dexamethasone can add specificity, potential for identifying carcinomas in nonfunctioning tumors
MIBG	Adrenal medulla imaging can supplement CT scan when extraadrenal, recurrent, or metastatic pheochromocytomas are suspected
Invasive studies	
Adrenal venous sampling	Greatest use in distinguishing adenoma from hyperplasia in primary aldosteronism; technically demanding; adrenal venography can cause hemorrhage
Vena cava sampling	Largely replaced by MIBG in search for extraadrenal pheochromocytomas
Arteriography	Can be dangerous with pheochromocytomas; largely replaced by noninvasive scanning

MIBG, metalodobenzylguanidine.

TREATMENT

Treatment of adrenal tumors is primarily surgical removal. The following sections describe the open, standard techniques, but in the next few years laparoscopic techniques will play a greater role (9). Although pharmaceutical agents are useful in preparing the patient for surgery or in palliating the patient with recurrent adrenal carcinoma, no agents render definitive therapy for adrenal tumors. Congenital adrenal hyperplasia is the only primary, hyperfunctioning adrenal syndrome that is amenable to medical therapy for definitive treatment.

Adrenal Hypercortisolism

Nonoperative Treatment

Functioning benign lesions of the adrenal cortex that are not ACTH dependent, such as adenomas or macronodular hyperplasia, respond to metyrapone and aminoglutethimide, which inhibit enzymes in the adrenal steroidogenic pathway. Both agents can effect a decrease in the production of cortisol when there is no increase in ACTH secondary to feedback stimulation by lowered cortisol levels. These drugs are not satisfactory long-term agents because of their high incidence of drug reactions, patient noncompliance, and continued growth of the lesions. They may be useful in patients whose surgery must be delayed. Although malignant, functioning, adrenocortical lesions should be debulked whenever possible, several chemotherapy agents offer adjunct therapy. The most noteworthy is mitotane (o,p,-DDD) (10). This is a cytolytic agent that has a 30% to 70% response rate in terms of decreasing steroid output. Unfortunately, patient survival is not affected. External irradiation and chemotherapy have not been effective for these malignant tumors.

As mentioned, nonoperative treatment is definitive therapy for congenital adrenal hyperplasia. Usually, 5 mg/d of cortisone acetate is sufficient in infants and is gradually increased to 25 to 35 mg/d in adults. For the salt-losing variety, intravenous steroid administration occasionally is required on an acute basis until the salt-losing tendency is brought under control by cortisone treatment. If a mineralocorticoid is required, oral 9α-fludrocortisone (Florinef) can be given in a dosage of 0.1 to 0.2 mg/d for an infant. In the occasional noncompliant patient, deoxycorticosterone pivalate can be given in a dosage of 12.5 to 25 mg/mo intramuscularly.

Operative Treatment

Indication for operation in the patient with a unilateral functioning adrenal tumor is clear. In the patient with a nonfunctioning adrenal tumor, the need for surgery is related to the size of the tumor and its rate of growth (11). There is consensus that a tumor larger than 6 cm should be removed. Some recommend that the acceptable size limit be 3 cm, especially when MRI suggests carcinoma or when functional studies suggest activity. When nonoperative therapy is elected, the patient should receive an adrenal scan 1, 3, and 6 months after the initial scan and yearly thereafter to assess growth of the lesion. If the tumor has grown, surgical removal is indicated. In bilateral functioning adrenocortical lesions, assessment of the pituitary–adrenal axis by dexamethasone suppression test and CRH stimulation must be done. If the pituitary is not implicated as the source of the hypercortisolism, bilateral adrenalectomy is indicated. In the case of nonfunctioning bilateral adrenal disease, the probability of metastasis to the adrenal gland is high. Image-guided needle biopsy may be the diagnostic approach of choice in that situation.

Preoperative preparation for adrenalectomy is straightforward. Other than the considerations of or preparation with enzyme inhibitors mentioned previously, the only specific issue is that of steroid replacement. It is best to treat patients prophylactically if there is any question about preexisting adrenal suppression or the possibility of adrenalectomy. At the start of the operation, 100 mg of hydrocortisone is administered intravenously and repeated in 4 hours.

The surgical approach is determined by the lateral position and size of the lesion. For small unilateral lesions, such as adenomas, a posterior approach through the bed of the 12th or 11th rib is preferred. An alternative extraperitoneal approach is through the flank, with the patient in the lateral decubitus position. The bilateral posterior approach is usually reserved for small, hyperplastic glands, such as in micronodular hyperplasia or hyperplasia of Cushing disease, in which pituitary treatment has failed. With transabdominal surgery, either unilateral subcostal or bilateral rooftop incisions are used for large adrenal tumors or macronodular hyperplasia, respectively. If the lesion proves to be a carcinoma growing into surrounding tissues, a thoracoabdominal approach may be necessary.

By far the most serious intraoperative complications are avulsion of the right adrenal gland from the inferior vena cava and a direct tear in the vena cava. The posterior approach is particularly hazardous in this regard because it is difficult to extricate a large tumor through the small posterior aperture. In addition, large tumors may be carcinomas, and the transabdominal approach allows for wide resection of lymph node–bearing areas and perhaps partial removal of attached surrounding structures. Other potential complications dependent on the incision include pneumothorax for the posterior approach and pancreatitis for the left abdominal approach.

The postoperative course involves tapering the exogenous steroid doses to maintenance levels in the case of bilateral adrenalectomy or to cessation in the case of unilateral adrenal removal. One simple regimen involves administering 100 mg of hydrocortisone intravenously every 6 hours during the first 48 hours. Some prefer alternating doses of intramuscular cortisone acetate in the event that intravenous access is lost. Provided that no intervening complications arise, the doses can be halved every 48 to 72 hours. In patients who have been exposed preoperatively to glucocorticoid excess, the maintenance dose may be as high as 100 mg/d for several months. Both high doses and normal maintenance of 35 to 50 mg/d can be given in the form of oral cortisone acetate as long as reliable alimentation and absorption have been achieved. It may be difficult to achieve normal maintenance dosages of 35 to 50 mg/d in many patients with Cushing syndrome without developing symptoms of steroid withdrawal. Also, the pituitary–adrenal axis remains suppressed for 6 to 12 months after operation, and even patients with normal contralateral adrenal glands cannot be taken off steroid replacement until after that time. Complications in the postoperative period include wound infection, pancreatitis, and thromboembolism. The latter complication has led some surgeons to prefer the preoperative placement of lower-extremity compression devices and their maintenance through the postoperative period. An alternative method is the use of low-dose heparin.

Hyperaldosteronism

Nonoperative Treatment

The only pharmaceutical agent that has practical benefit in this syndrome is spironolactone. This drug inhibits the sodium–potassium exchange in the distal tubule, normalizes serum potassium, and if tolerated for a period of time, can lower the blood pressure. Oral potassium chloride supplementation helps to correct the concomitant hypokalemia. Because of gynecomastia and other side effects, long-term spironolactone is problematic in some patients. Large doses of up 3 to 4 g/d may be required.

Operative Treatment

Primary aldosteronism due to an adrenal adenoma is best treated by surgically removing the adenoma. On the other hand, when the syndrome arises from adrenal hyperplasia, surgical removal of the adrenal gland is seldom curative. It is therefore essential that every effort be made to distinguish the two causes. Surgery is indicated only for adenomas or for those forms of hyperplasia that, on dynamic testing, behave as adenomas.

The important preoperative preparation is that of potassium replenishment. Correction of hypokalemia may be materially aided by the short-term use of spironolactone. Since the tumors are generally small and rarely malignant and hyperplasia is minimal, the unilateral or bilateral posterior approach is preferred. If bilateral adrenalectomy is anticipated, hydrocortisone should be administered as detailed above. Because these adenomas may be particularly small, it is necessary in some cases to thoroughly mobilize the adrenal gland and to examine it with bidigital palpation to assure an adequate examination. Pneumothorax and vena cava bleeding may occur as in other adrenalectomies, but the tissues are not as friable as those in chronic hypercortisolism. In addition, the lack of truncal obesity contributes to the comparative ease of surgery in primary hyperaldosteronism. Postoperatively, the patient usually experiences an uneventful recovery. Because of hyporeninemia, the remaining zona glomerulosa is usually temporarily suppressed, and a relative hypoaldosteronism may follow removal of an adenoma. Clinically, this is manifested by low blood pressure and hyperkalemia, which usually respond to the administration of a mineralocorticoid, such as fludrocortisone. Of course, bilateral adrenalectomy necessitates exogenous cortisol administration, which can usually be tapered to maintenance levels during the normal postoperative recovery period of 5 to 10 days.

Pheochromocytoma

Nonoperative Treatment

Nonoperative treatment of pheochromocytoma is generally unsatisfactory and entails pharmacologic blockade of the effects of catecholamines. Phenoxybenzamine and prazosin are two preferred agents that block the α-adrenergic effects of the catecholamines. The use of β-adrenergic blockers, such as labetalol, may be required in those patients with obvious b-adrenergic effects, such as resting pulse rates above 100 beats/min.

Operative Treatment

Because of the potential for wide swings in blood pressure and other effects of chronic catecholamine secretion, such as high blood glucose or cardiomyopathy, careful preoperative preparation is required in patients with these tumors (12). It is customary to institute α-adrenergic blockade 2 to 3 weeks before anticipated surgery. This controls the blood pressure for cardiovascular reasons and allows restoration of a decreased blood volume. It is the consensus that preoperative preparation in this manner makes the intraoperative treatment of the patient much more safe. In patients who require β-adrenergic blockade, it is essential to first establish good α-adrenergic blockade. These patients are especially prone to cardiac failure induced by β-adrenergic blockade because of the cardiomyopathy that may preexist. β-Adrenergic blockade in the cardiomyopathic patient, with failure to first reduce the afterload by a-adrenergic blockade, can precipitate cardiac failure. Many surgeons prefer having a pulmonary artery catheter in place before and during surgery because of the potential cardiovascular instability. Preoperative sedation appears to be important. The use of rectal thiopental sodium (Pentothal) or diazepam is efficacious, especially in children.

In the operating room, several preinduction maneuvers should be carried out. Although pulmonary artery monitoring is considered optional, it is essential that intraarterial blood pressure monitoring be done. With catecholamine excess, the peripheral pulse may disappear, and auditory monitoring of the blood pressure is impossible. A large array of pharmaceutical agents should be immediately available. These include agents that lower blood pressure, such as phentolamine (Regitine) or nitroprusside; b-adrenergic blockers, such as esmolol; antiarrhythmic agents, such as lidocaine; and blood-pressure support agents, such as norepinephrine, to counteract possible postoperative hypotension. Opinions vary as to the preferred anesthetic agents, but the principle of smooth induction is universally held. Most important are an anesthesiologist who has had experience with these tumors and an anesthetic regimen that is familiar to the user.

It is customary to approach these tumors by the transabdominal route, usually through a generous bilateral, subcostal rooftop incision. The rationale for this approach includes the significant incidence of bilateral, extraadrenal tumors and malignant tumors. As more experience is gained with imaging techniques, including MIBG, it may be possible to localize adrenal tumors exclusively to one side with sufficient accuracy so that a posterior approach in these situations would be justified. The two major technical principles in operation for these tumors are to minimize the manipulation of the tumor and to isolate and ligate the adrenal vein as soon as possible in the sequence of dissection. It is during the period of tumor manipulation that the anesthesiologist must be most alert in counteracting arrhythmia and high blood pressure with the agents noted. Once the tumor is removed, the blood pressure may fall precipitously. This can be counteracted immediately by instituting an α-adrenergic agonist, such as norepinephrine. A preexisting low blood volume may also contribute to hypotension, and transfusion of one or two units of blood may be considered. Conversely, failure to bring the blood pressure down at least to normal on removal of a pheochromocytoma should raise suspicion of a second pheochromocytoma or of metastases. A thorough intraabdominal search along the vertebral bodies, aorta, contralateral adrenal gland, and urinary bladder should be done before closure.

Postoperatively, once the hypotension is corrected, the patient usually has an uneventful recovery. When all functioning pheochromocytomas have been removed, normalization of blood pressure is achieved in virtually 100% of patients.

Nonfunctioning Adrenal Tumors

As mentioned previously, the indications for surgery in these tumors are a diameter greater than 6 cm, growth of the smaller tumors during a period of observation, or questions of functional status. Because carcinomas smaller than 6 cm have been reported, some clinicians prefer to re-

move any tumors larger than 3 cm. The principles of surgical approach are much the same as those for functioning tumors. Tumors larger than 5 to 6 cm are probably best approached by the flank or transabdominal routes. Smaller tumors with a low index of suspicion for malignancy can easily be removed through the posterior approach.

OUTCOMES

The prognosis for patients with benign functioning adrenal tumors is generally excellent. For patients with Cushing syndrome caused by benign lesions, such as pituitary adenomas, adrenal adenomas, or macronodular hyperplasia, the cure rate approximates 100%. This is in marked contrast to untreated Cushing syndrome patients, who have historically suffered a 50% 5-year mortality rate. The same good prognosis is true for treated adrenal adenomas secreting aldosterone or benign pheochromocytomas producing catecholamines. A notable exception in the benign diseases is hyperplasia of the zona glomerulosa, in which, for some unknown reason, surgical removal of the adrenal glands usually does not cure the hypertension. The prognosis for adrenocortical carcinoma is not good. The overall 5-year survival rate is 20% to 25% for these malignancies. When there is localized disease at the time of surgery, the 5-year survival may be higher, in the 40% to 50% range. The true prognosis in childhood is not clear, but the data suggest a 2-year survival rate of about 20%. In some instances, these early tumors were removed without benefit of exogenous steroid therapy. The precise 5-year survival rate of malignant pheochromocytomas is difficult to determine because of the rarity of these tumors and the propensity of the metastases to appear many years later. Also, some of these patients live a long time with their disease. Patients with previous pheochromocytomas should therefore be followed periodically for many years because of the possibility of late-appearing metastases. The follow-up regimen can be better determined when more useful criteria for distinguishing benign from malignant tumors are developed. The mitotic index and the determination of ploidy on the flow cytometer may help in this regard.

REFERENCES

1. Silverman ML, Lee AK. Anatomy and pathology of the adrenal glands. *Urol Clin North Am* 1989;16:417.
2. Perry RR, Nieman LK, Cutler GB, et al. Primary adrenal causes of Cushing's syndrome: diagnosis and surgical management. *Ann Surg* 1989;210:59.
3. New MI. Basic and clinical aspects of congenital adrenal hyperplasia. *J Steroid Biochem* 1987;27:1.
4. Merrell RC. Aldosterone-producing tumors (Conn's syndrome). *Semin Surg Oncol* 1990;6:66.
5. Gordon RD. Primary aldosteronism: a new understanding. *Med J Aust* 1993;158:729.
6. Sheps SG, Jiang NS, Klee GC, et al. Recent developments in the diagnosis and treatment of pheochromocytoma. *Mayo Clin Proc* 1990;65:88.
7. Bravo EL, Gifford RW. Pheochromocytoma. *Endocrinol Metab Clin North Am* 1993;22:329.
8. Lamki LM, Haynie TP. Role of adrenal imaging in surgical management. *J Surg Oncol* 1990;43:139.
9. Suzuki K, Kageyama S, Ueda D. Laparoscopic adrenalectomy: clinical experience with 12 cases. *J Urol* 1993;150:1099.
10. Wooten MD, King DK. Adrenal cortical carcinoma. *Cancer* 1993;72:3145.
11. Gajraj H, Young AE. Adrenal incidentaloma. *Br J Surg* 1993;80:422.
12. Pullerits J, Ein S, Balfe JW. Anaesthesia for phaeochromocytoma. *Can J Anaesth* 1988;35:526.

SURGERY: SCIENTIFIC PRINCIPLES AND PRACTICE, Third Edition, edited by
Lazar J. Greenfield, Michael W. Mulholland, Keith T. Oldham, Gerald B. Zelenock,
and Keith D. Lillemoe. Lippincott Williams & Wilkins Publishers, Philadelphia, © 2001.

CHAPTER 57

PITUITARY GLAND

WILLIAM F. CHANDLER AND RICARDO V. LLOYD

The pituitary gland, or hypophysis, is a remarkably complex way station in the connection between the brain and a wide range of organs throughout the body. The hypothalamus of the brain is the principal integrating organ for regulating the internal environment of the body, and the pituitary is its major link with the organs outside the nervous system. The pituitary has been called the master gland; even with advances in modern neuroendocrinology, it remains worthy of that description.

EMBRYOLOGY, ANATOMY, AND PHYSIOLOGY

To appreciate the gross and microscopic anatomy of this small but complex gland, it is important to review briefly the embryologic development of the hypophysis. By the fourth week, an evagination develops in the roof of the stomodeal depression that is lined by ectodermal cells of the cavity destined to become the pharynx (Fig. 57.1). This structure is known as *Rathke's pouch*. At the same time, a depression develops in the floor of the diencephalon; this is called the *infundibular process*. It too is lined with ectodermal cells. These are cells of the future diencephalic portion of the brain and therefore are more similar to the cells of central nervous system tissue. During a period of weeks, the two structures grow to meet each other—the infundibular process forming the neurohypophysis (pars neuralis) and Rathke's pouch forming the adenohypophysis (pars distalis). In lower animals, an intermediary lobe (pars intermedia) also forms, but in humans this is present only as a minor cleft. As the adenohypophysis enlarges, its upper portion (pars tuberalis) partially surrounds the stalk connecting the pituitary to the brain. Eventually, the connection between the adenohypophysis and the oral cavity disappears, but occasionally ectopic remnants of nonfunctioning pituitary cells, known as *pharyngeal pituitary tissue,* are left along its path.

In an adult, the dimensions of the hypophysis are $6 \times 9 \times 12$ mm, and it weighs about 0.6 g. It enlarges during pregnancy and weighs up to 1 g in multiparous women. The adenohypophysis constitutes 80% of the gland and contains the pars distalis, pars tuberalis, and the remnant of the pars intermedia. The pars distalis is the major functional portion of the adenohypophysis, and in this chapter, it is considered synonymous with the adenohypophysis, or anterior pituitary. The neurohypophysis, or posterior pituitary, is small and, according to its embryologic development, should be considered virtually as an extension of the hypothalamus of the brain.

The combined neurohypophysis and adenohypophysis are connected to the base of the brain by a common stalk (Fig. 57.2A). The stalk blends into the median eminence of the hypothalamus and serves to transport both hormone-rich portal blood to the adenohypophysis and nerve fibers to the neurohypophysis. The optic chiasm lies directly above the pituitary, just anterior to the stalk; thus, it is vulnerable to compression by a pituitary tumor. The supraoptic and paraventricular nuclei of the hypothalamus are depicted in Fig. 57.2A because they are the principal locations of cell bodies with axons directed toward the neurohypophysis.

The median eminence is where hormonal contributions from axons originating in various nuclei of the hypothalamus enter blood destined for the adenohypophysis (Fig. 57.2B). Blood reaches this region primarily through the superior hypophyseal artery and flows into gomitoli, which are small capillary plexuses within the median eminence through which hormones enter the blood. The blood then travels through the portal system to the adenohypophysis, where the hormones modulate the activity of secretory cells. These cells in turn secrete hormones into the general circulation to stimulate end-organs. This system comprises the following hormones:

1. Thyrotropin-releasing hormone (TRH) to stimulate the secretion of thyroid-stimulating hormone (TSH)
2. Corticotropin-releasing hormone to stimulate the release of adrenocorticotropic hormone (ACTH)
3. Growth hormone-releasing hormone to stimulate the secretion of growth hormone (GH)
4. Gonadotropin-releasing hormone to stimulate the secretion of luteinizing hormone (LH) and follicle-stimulating hormone (FSH)
5. Prolactin-inhibitory factor (dopamine) to inhibit the secretion of prolactin

Each of these hormonal combinations constitutes a feedback system in which the brain (hypothalamus) senses the level of end-organ hormone output and, in turn, positively

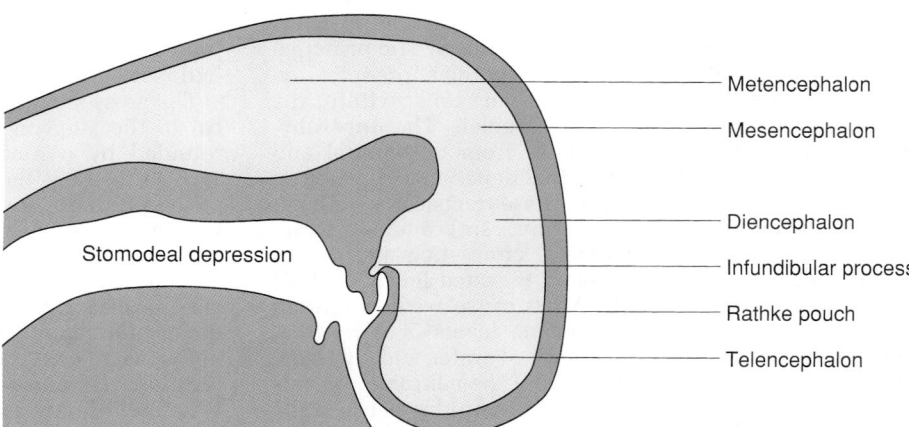

Figure 57.1. Diagram of a 4-week-old embryo illustrating how Rathke's pouch meets the infundibular process to form the anterior and posterior lobes, respectively, of the pituitary gland.

Metencephalon

Mesencephalon

Diencephalon

Infundibular process

Rathke pouch

Telencephalon

Stomodeal depression

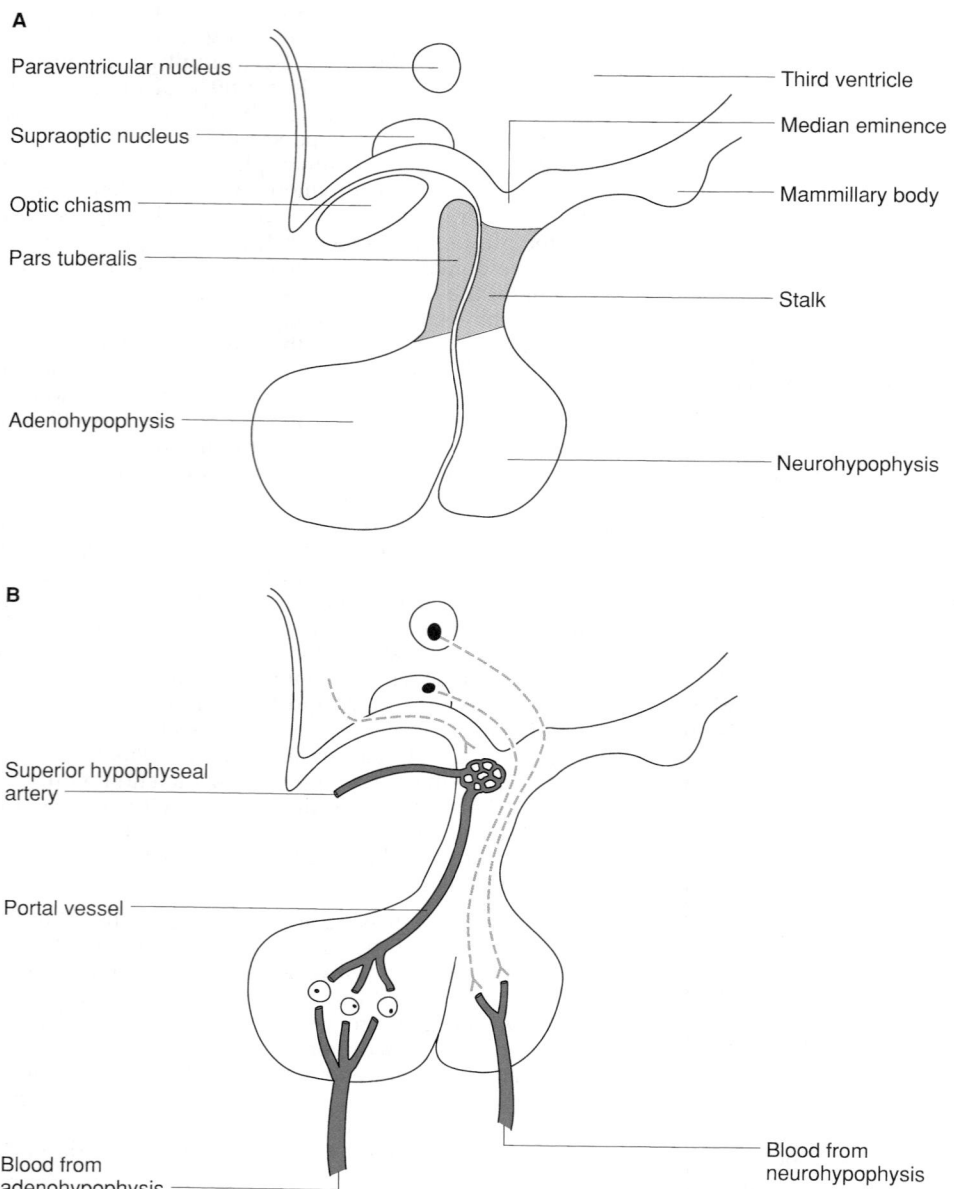

A

Paraventricular nucleus

Supraoptic nucleus

Optic chiasm

Pars tuberalis

Adenohypophysis

Third ventricle

Median eminence

Mammillary body

Stalk

Neurohypophysis

B

Superior hypophyseal artery

Portal vessel

Blood from adenohypophysis

Blood from neurohypophysis

Figure 57.2. *(A)* Schematic diagram of the pituitary and floor of the third ventricle as seen in a midline sagittal view. Anterior is to the left. *(B)* Physiology of hormone release. The adenohypophysis receives releasing hormones through a portal venous system, and the neurohypophysis receives hormones directly from hypothalamic nuclei by means of neurons.

or negatively adjusts the secretion of the various hypothalamic hormones into the portal system.

The neurohypophysis differs significantly from the adenohypophysis in that it does not receive controlling hormones by means of the portal system but rather by direct transport of hormones through nerve fibers. The principal input into the neurohypophysis is via the supraoptic–hypophyseal tract, which arises from cells within the supraoptic and paraventricular nuclei. The tuberohypophyseal tract, which originates from the central and posterior portions of the hypothalamus, also contributes input to the neurohypophysis. These tracts carry both antidiuretic hormone (ADH; vasopressin) and oxytocin. ADH is secreted into the general circulation and causes the kidneys to absorb free water. Elevated levels of ADH (syndrome of inappropriate ADH) cause water retention and hyponatremia, and inadequate levels of ADH (diabetes insipidus) cause excess loss of water and hypernatremia. Interestingly, surgical loss of the neurohypophysis does not usually result in diabetes insipidus because the stalk itself can still secrete ADH into the circulation. The

feedback mechanism to the brain for release of ADH is mainly serum osmolarity, with hyperosmolar conditions causing the release of ADH and retention of water. Blood volume also affects the release of ADH; thus, hemorrhage causes water retention. Oxytocin functions only during pregnancy and causes both uterine contractions and milk letdown within the breasts.

The gross surgical anatomy of the pituitary is also critical to the surgeon because the pituitary is closely surrounded by a number of important structures. Figure 57.3A illustrates the coronal cross section of the anatomy of the pituitary as seen from the front. The pituitary sits within the bony confines of the sella turcica ("Turkish saddle") and is bordered laterally by the cavernous sinuses (venous), inferiorly and anteriorly by the sphenoid sinus (air), posteriorly by the dorsum sellae, and superiorly by the membranous diaphragma sellae. The cavernous sinuses each contain the siphon region of the internal carotid artery and portions of cranial nerves III, IV, V, and VI, all within a venous plexus. The optic chiasm lies immediately above the diaphragma sellae. Directly below the

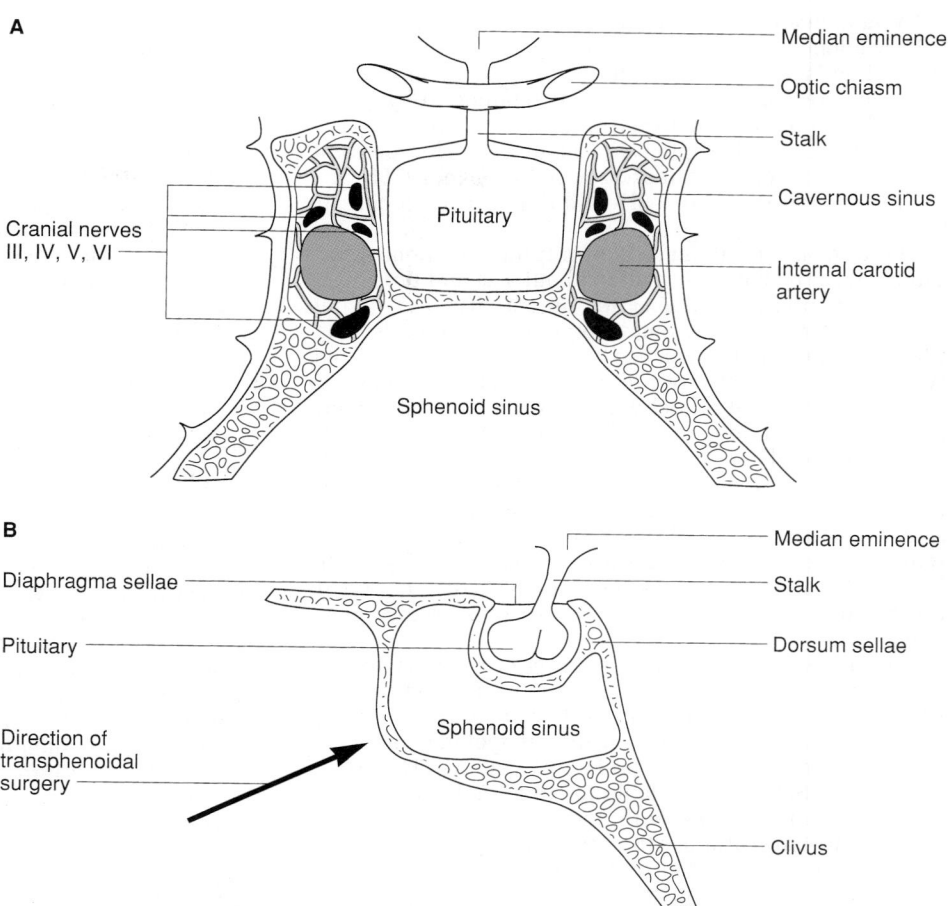

A

Median eminence

Optic chiasm

Stalk

Cavernous sinus

Pituitary

Cranial nerves
III, IV, V, VI

Internal carotid
artery

Sphenoid sinus

B

Median eminence

Diaphragma sellae

Stalk

Pituitary

Dorsum sellae

Direction of
transphenoidal
surgery

Sphenoid sinus

Clivus

Figure 57.3. *(A)* Mid-pituitary coronal view of parasellar region. The sphenoid sinus is below and the cavernous sinuses are lateral. *(B)* Midsagittal view of pituitary and surrounding bony structures. Note the approach for transsphenoidal surgery. Anterior is to the left.

anterior and inferior portions of the sella is the aerated sphenoid sinus. This is sufficiently large in 97% of patients to allow a transnasal, transsphenoidal surgical approach to the pituitary (Fig. 57.3B).

METHODS OF CELL ANALYSIS

Pituitary adenomas have been classified historically as acidophilic, basophilic, and chromophobic. Adenomas may show a variable staining pattern with conventional hematoxylin and eosin dyes, so it is difficult to classify adenomas based on these stains. For example, prolactinomas and sparsely granulated growth hormone adenomas may be acidophilic or chromophobic after hematoxylin and eosin staining (Table 57.1). Immunohistochemistry, ultrastructural studies, and in situ hybridization analyses for specific hormones are the most reliable methods of classifying pituitary adenomas today.

Table 57.1. FUNCTIONAL PITUITARY ADENOMAS: PATHOLOGIC FINDINGS

Adenoma type	Incidence (%)	Staining[a]	Immunoreactivity	Ultrastructure
PRL-secreting				
Sparsely granulated	28	C	PRL	Few SG 150–500 nm
				Misplaced exocytosis
Densely granulated	1	A	PRL	SG 400–1,200 nm
GH-secreting				
Sparsely granulated	5	C-A	GH	SG 300–600 nm
				Fibrous bodies
Densely granulated	5	A	GH	SG 100–250 nm
Mixed GH cell-PRL cell	5	A-C	GH, PRL	Variable pattern
Mixed GH cell-PRL cell	1	A	GH, PRL	SG 150–450 nm and 350–1,000 nm
ACTH-secreting	10	B	ACTH	SG 250–700 nm
				Prominent type I microfilaments
Gonadotrope cell	7–10	C-B	FSH, LH	SG 50–150 nm
				Distinct female pattern of honeycomb, golgi region
Thyrotrope cell	1	C-B	TSH	SG 50–250 nm

[a]Conventional H&E staining: A, acidophil; B, basophil; C, chromophobe.
ACTH, adrenocorticotropic hormone; FSH, follicle-stimulating hormone; GH, growth hormone; LH, luteinizing hormone; PRL, prolactin; SG, secretory granules; TSH, thyroid-stimulating hormone.

Other conventional stains that help in the analysis of pituitary adenomas include the reticulin stain, which helps to distinguish between pituitary hyperplasia and adenomas. The normal reticulin pattern is retained in hyperplasia and is similar to that seen in normal pituitary tissue, but it becomes disrupted in neoplasia. The periodic acid–Schiff reaction stains carbohydrates in ACTH-producing adenomas and in TSH- and FSH/LH-producing tumors.

The ultrastructural analysis of pituitary adenomas provides a great deal of information about size and type of secretory granules, cellular synthetic activity, and unique features of specific adenoma subtypes. For example, misplaced exocytosis is seen in prolactin-producing tumors, type I microfilaments are present in ACTH-producing tumors, and abundant mitochondria are characteristic of oncocytic null cell adenomas. The unique honeycomb pattern of the Golgi complex is a distinct morphologic feature of FSH/LH-producing adenomas in women (1). Because of the pleomorphism and variations in size that are typical of secretory granules, the classification of adenomas is more reliably based on immunohistochemical findings at the light microscopic and ultrastructural levels than on the ultrastructural morphologic appearance of secretory granules.

The immunohistochemical staining of pituitary adenomas with specific antibodies is a reliable method for classifying adenomas according to the hormones that are being produced (Fig. 57.4). Highly purified polyclonal and monoclonal antibodies against prolactin, GH, ACTH, FSH-β, LH-β, and TSH-β are available for immunohistochemical staining. Many studies with these antibodies have revealed that some pituitary tumors are composed of several cell types that produce various hormones (1). Ultrastructural immunohistochemistry provides a further degree of refinement in the classification and study of adenomas because the exact site of hormone storage in secretary granules and the subcellular sites of production and processing in the rough endoplasmic reticulum and Golgi regions can be visualized with this technique.

Some adenomas may not store specific hormones, so immunohistochemical staining may be weak or absent. Messenger ribonucleic acid (mRNA) is usually present in the cytoplasm of adenomas. The localization of mRNAs for specific protein hormones is becoming more widely used in the study and classification of pituitary adenomas. In situ hybridization studies have shown that many GH-producing adenomas in patients with acromegaly also express prolactin mRNA (2). In situ and Northern hybridization studies have contributed to the understanding of adenoma subtypes. For example, clinically silent GH adenomas express GH mRNA, although the protein that is produced does not cause acromegaly. Other studies have shown that null cell adenomas, which constitute up to 25% of pituitary neoplasms, commonly express the mRNA for gonadotropic hormones.

Although a great deal of information about the cell biology of pituitary adenomas has been gained through various methods of cell analysis, many gaps still remain in our knowledge of the biology of these neoplasms.

IMAGING OF THE PITUITARY AND PARASELLAR REGION

Modern, computerized imaging technology now provides remarkably detailed multiplanar images of the pituitary and parasellar structures. Magnetic resonance imaging (MRI) has evolved as the first choice for diagnostic imaging and is often the only test needed for a therapeutic decision to be made. With the intravenous infusion of a paramagnetic substance, such as gadolinium, MRI demonstrates intrasellar tumors as small as 5 mm and shows the growth pattern of larger tumors. It reveals the extent of suprasellar and sphenoid sinus extension, in addition to lateral extension into the cavernous sinuses (Fig. 57.5). Cysts and hemorrhage can be differentiated, as can blood flowing within an aneurysm.

Computed tomography (CT) also has a place in pituitary imaging and, if MRI is unavailable, may well suffice as the only mode of imaging. CT shows calcification better than MRI and thus is often helpful in imaging a craniopharyngioma. CT, even with intravenous contrast, cannot differentiate an aneurysm, so that MRI or angiography must be performed if this is suspected.

Plain skull radiographs are not needed if the diagnosis has been reached by CT or MRI, but they remain an important way to identify incidental lesions. A pituitary macroadenoma (> 10 mm) causes enlargement of the sella turcica, which can easily be observed on a plain lateral skull radiograph. If this finding is noted on a radiograph performed for any reason, such as trauma, a more detailed study, such as MRI or CT, should be obtained.

Angiography is performed only if an aneurysm is suspected or if a lesion is so large that occlusion or compression of the internal carotid artery is in question.

CLINICAL AND ENDOCRINE EVALUATION

General Clinical Signs and Symptoms

Patients with pituitary lesions may present with symptoms and signs related to a mass effect on the pituitary and its surrounding structures, hypersecretion of hormones by the lesion itself, or a combination of both. Tumors or other mass lesions are generally larger than 1 cm before they produce symptoms related to compression. As a lesion enlarges, it may cause a loss of function of the pituitary, usually manifested by a decrease in hormone secretion from the adenohypophysis. This may result in a loss of TSH and subsequent hypothyroidism. A decrease in ACTH results in Addison's disease, and a decrease in LH and FSH causes amenorrhea. A decline in GH is noted only in children with a loss of normal growth progress. The one ex-

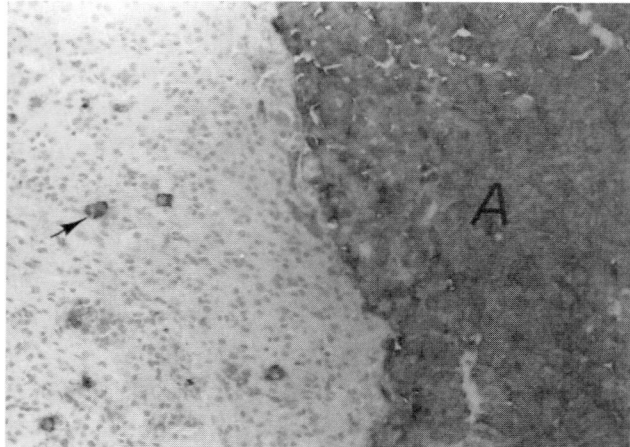

Figure 57.4. Immunohistochemical staining of an adrenocorticotropic hormone *(ACTH)*-producing adenoma *(A)* from a patient with Cushing's disease. The normal pituitary tissue on the left contains a few ACTH-positive cells *(arrow).* ×250.

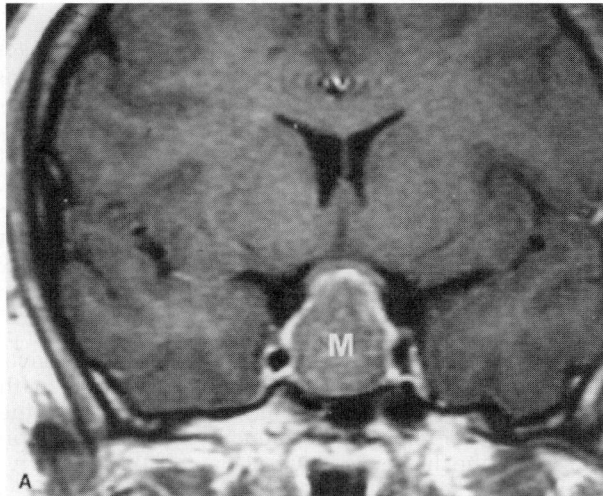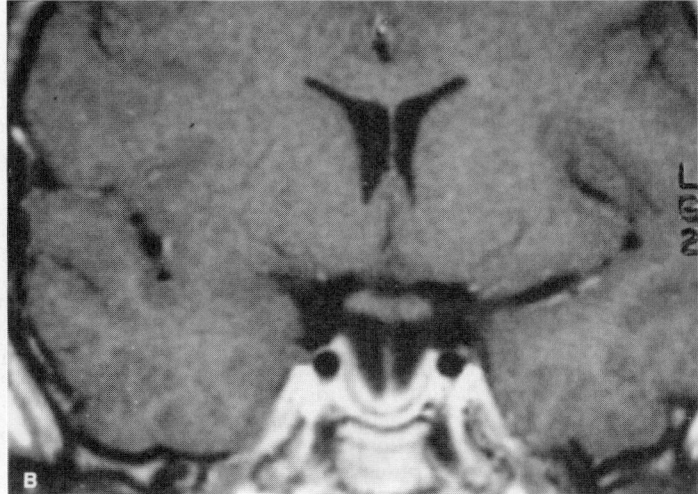

Figure 57.5. *(A)* Mid-pituitary coronal magnetic resonance imaging (MRI) shows a pituitary macroadenoma *(M)*. *(B)* Postoperative MRI demonstrates gross total resection of tumor with cerebrospinal fluid in the sella.

ception to this pattern is that generalized pituitary compression may cause a rise in prolactin levels because the activity of prolactin-inhibitory factor (dopamine) from the hypothalamus may be compromised by the compression. Generalized compression from within the sella rarely results in a loss of ADH from the neurohypophysis and subsequent diabetes insipidus. Lesions that originate in the region of the pituitary stalk, however, often present with early signs of diabetes insipidus. Symptoms related to a loss of pituitary function are usually insidious in onset, exception for those of sudden hemorrhage within the sella, or so-called pituitary apoplexy. Such hemorrhages are usually associated with a pituitary adenoma.

When mass lesions in the region of the pituitary enlarge, they may compress or invade nearby structures and cause symptoms unrelated to endocrine function. As tumors or other lesions grow laterally from the sella, they encounter the various contents of the cavernous sinuses. These include the third, fourth, first two divisions of the fifth, and sixth cranial nerves, in addition to the internal carotid artery. Compression of cranial nerves III, IV, or VI causes diplopia, and compression of cranial nerve V causes ipsilateral facial numbness. Invasion or constriction of the carotid may cause occlusion of this vessel, which in rare cases results in cerebral infarction. Upward growth of a tumor, which is relatively unrestricted, is much more common and often results in compression of the optic chiasm and loss of vision, typically a bitemporal hemianopsia. Extensive upward intracranial growth may compress the hypothalamus or the third ventricle and cause hydrocephalus. Rarely, intracranial extension results in cortical irritation and associated seizures. Downward growth of tumors into the sphenoid sinus is common but causes no clinical symptoms or signs.

The syndromes associated with hypersecretion of pituitary hormones are discussed at length later in this chapter. They include Cushing's disease (ACTH), acromegaly (GH), hyperprolactinemia (prolactin), and Nelson's syndrome (ACTH after adrenalectomy). Rare cases of TSH-secreting adenomas have been documented. Traditionally, pituitary adenomas have been divided into nonfunctioning and functioning tumors, but it has become clear through immunohistochemical studies that many nonfunctioning tumors are in fact endocrinologically active.

Although secreted hormones may not cause clinical symptoms or signs, they may serve as a marker for the presence of a tumor before and after treatment.

General Endocrine Evaluation

The extent of the endocrine evaluation of a patient with a pituitary lesion depends on the urgency of the situation (e.g., impaired vision) and whether a hypersecretory state is suspected. If time permits, a careful evaluation of the endocrine status is warranted, including testing of pituitary reserve. Although this is most critical after treatment, it is ideal to obtain a complete pretreatment evaluation for comparison. A pituitary endocrine evaluation should include baseline values for prolactin, GH, LH, FSH, testosterone (male), estrogen (female), cortisol, ACTH, electrolytes, and glucose. Thyroid function tests, including TSH, should be performed. Because baseline values may not reflect the ability of the pituitary to respond to stress, it is also important to test the reserve capacity of the pituitary. The most efficient way to do this is to administer insulin, to induce hypoglycemia, combined with TRH. Provided the patient has no contraindication to transient hypoglycemia (i.e., ischemic heart disease, cerebrovascular disease, or seizure disorder), insulin is given in a dose of 0.10 to 0.15 IU/kg, such that the serum glucose falls below 40 mg/dL. In the patient with normal pituitary function, transient hypoglycemia causes a rise in cortisol to above 20 µg/dL and a rise in GH to above 10 ng/mL. In patients with compromised ACTH or GH production, a response is not noted. The administration of TRH should normally cause a rise in both TSH and prolactin. If indicated, gonadotropin-releasing hormone may be administered to increase the gonadotropin levels (LH and FSH).

If urgent surgical decompression is indicated, the previously mentioned baseline values are obtained, and the patient is prepared for surgery with sufficient hydrocortisone to cover the possibility of inadequate cortisol reserve. Careful postoperative evaluation is then carried out to determine if long-term replacement therapy is needed. It should be stressed that if the patient receives postoperative radiation therapy, the status of the pituitary should be checked periodically during the following years because pituitary function may slowly decline after radiation exposure.

If diabetes insipidus is suspected, urine-specific gravity and serum sodium should be checked, and fluid intake and output should be carefully evaluated.

Cushing's Disease

Although the diagnosis of hypercortisolism (Cushing's syndrome) is often determined after physical examination by an astute physician, sometimes the physical manifestations are not obvious. Often, the precise cause of hypercortisolism is difficult to ascertain, even with detailed endocrine testing and imaging. The findings of Cushing's syndrome often include central obesity, hypertension, hirsutism, fatigue, easy bruising, striae, moonlike facies, dorsal fat pad, and often depression or other mental changes. Less common abnormalities include headache, osteoporosis, diabetes mellitus, galactorrhea, peripleural edema, and amenorrhea. Often, a patient presents without the classic cushingoid appearance and complains only of severe fatigue or depression.

The cause of hypercortisolism is an ACTH-secreting pituitary adenoma (Cushing's disease) in up to 80% of cases; the remainder are caused by an adrenocortical tumor or an ectopic neoplasm that secretes ACTH or corticotropin-releasing factor. Pituitary-dependent hypercortisolism is much more common in women (80%), and an ectopic cause is more common in men (80%). Thus, if an adult man presents with a rapid onset of Cushing's syndrome, particularly with weight loss, an ectopic neoplasm must be strongly considered. It should also be kept in mind that increased cortisol levels may be associated with primary depression, alcoholism, obesity, or drugs such as estrogens and phenytoin.

Because imaging studies are nondiagnostic in up to 60% of patients with pituitary disorders, the diagnosis is often based completely on the results of endocrine testing (3). Multiple measurements of cortisol and ACTH to evaluate the diurnal pattern are important but often misleading. They are mainly of value when clearly elevated. Urinary free cortisol excretion over 24 hours is an extremely important measurement. It is not elevated in patients who are obese or taking medications, but it is elevated in cases of depression or alcoholism. When the result of the overnight dexamethasone screening test (1 mg at 10:00 P.M.) is an 8:00 A.M. serum cortisol level below 5 μg/dL, hypercortisolism is rarely present. Generally, the cortisol level of patients with a pituitary cause of hypercortisolism is not suppressed with the low-dose dexamethasone test (0.5 mg given every 6 hours eight times) but is with the higher dose (2 mg every given 6 hours eight times). The cortisol level of patients with adrenal or ectopic disorders classically is not suppressed with either dose. Exceptions are seen with both these tests (Fig. 57.6).

When metyrapone is given, a rise in serum 11-deoxycortisol (or urinary 17-hydroxycortisol) is seen in normal patients or those with a pituitary disorder. Unfortunately, a positive response does not absolutely rule out an adrenal or ectopic source of hypercortisolism. The most specific diagnostic test for Cushing's disease is the measurement of ACTH levels in both inferior petrosal sinuses by transfemoral catheterization, along with simultaneous measurement of peripheral blood levels. This provides very convincing evidence for the existence of an ACTH-secreting pituitary tumor and even the laterality of the tumor (4). Inferior petrosal sinus sampling should be carried out in every case of suspected Cushing's disease when MRI results are not *definitive* for a tumor. If the results of standard endocrine testing are conclusive for hypercortisolism and indicate a pituitary source and if MRI clearly shows a tumor, then invasive petrosal sinus sampling is not necessary before surgery.

Acromegaly

Like Cushing's syndrome, acromegaly can be diagnosed clinically when patients present with advanced stages of the disease. The enlargement of the facial features and extremities may be subtle, and the presenting symptoms may be nonspecific headaches, fatigue, arthralgias, decreased libido, or amenorrhea. Patients often have hypertension, diabetes mellitus, and an early onset of atherosclerotic cardiovascular disease. It is critical that this disease be diagnosed and treated because the associated mortality rate is 50% above normal per decade beyond the age of 40 years. With rare exceptions, the cause of acromegaly is a GH-secreting pituitary adenoma. Like other functioning adenomas, the tumors may be either small or large and invasive. Patients with larger tumors may, of course, present with visual loss. Rarely, elevated GH levels are secondary to the production of GH-releasing hormone by an ectopic tumor.

The endocrine diagnosis now rests largely on serum levels of insulin-like growth factor-1 (IGF-1), also known as *somatomedin C,* because both normal and acromegalic patients may have GH levels below 5 ng/mL. Even though 90% of acromegalic patients have GH levels higher than 10 ng/mL, and although GH in a resting, nonstressed patient is normally below 5 ng/mL, both normal and acromegalic patients may have levels below 5 ng/mL. IGF-1, which mediates the effect of GH on peripheral tissues, should be measured in *all* circumstances in which acromegaly is suspected (Fig. 57.7). The cause of acromegaly is usually a GH-secreting pituitary adenoma, but rarely elevated GH levels are secondary to the production of GH-releasing hormone by an ectopic tumor.

Hyperprolactinemia

Because 60% to 70% of prolactin-secreting pituitary adenomas are microadenomas, most patients present with endocrine symptoms rather than local mass effects. Hyperprolactinemia in women usually causes amenorrhea and often galactorrhea; thus, young women have a reason to seek medical evaluation while the tumor is still at an early stage. Because men do not have these early warning signs, they almost invariably present with macroadenomas associated with loss of libido, infertility, or loss of vision. It should be kept in mind that the finding of amenorrhea or galactorrhea together with an elevated prolactin level does not always indicate the presence of a pituitary tumor. Table 57.2 lists other possible causes of hyperprolactinemia. Most important among these are renal failure, hypothyroidism, and the use of various drugs. Compression of the pituitary stalk by any type of mass lesion results in an increased secretion of prolactin. If the prolactin level is above 150 ng/mL, a pituitary tumor is almost invariably the cause, but microadenomas are often associated with prolactin levels below 100 ng/mL. The size of pituitary adenomas has been shown to correlate with the degree of prolactin elevation; levels may reach thousands of nanograms per milliliter. No reliable provocative tests are available to differentiate prolactinomas from other causes of hyperprolactinemia, so the diagnosis relies on ruling out other causes and imaging the adenoma (Fig. 57.8).

Nelson's Syndrome

In 1958, Nelson and colleagues (5) identified a syndrome of progressive hyperpigmentation, visual field loss, and amenorrhea associated with elevated ACTH levels related to a functional pituitary adenoma in a patient who had undergone bilateral adrenalectomy for hypercorti-

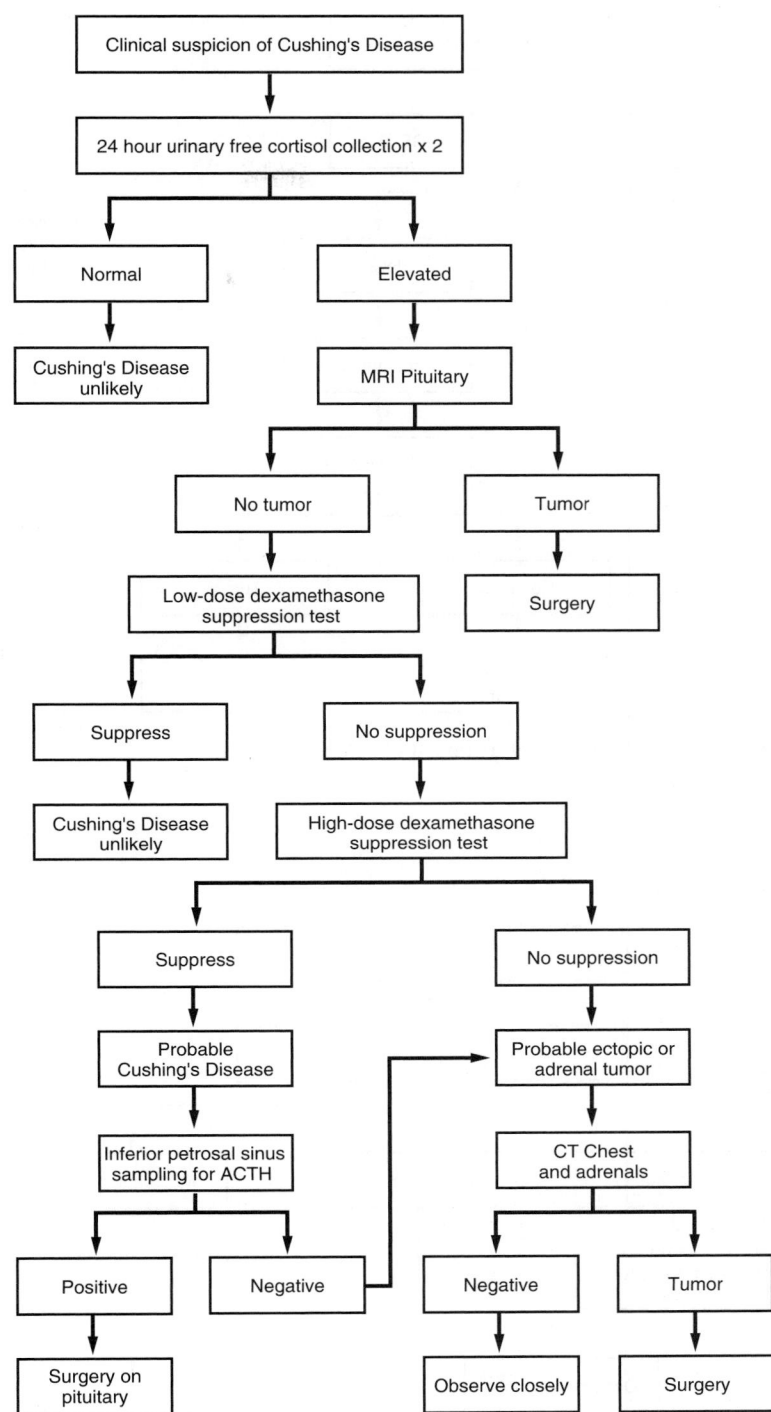

Figure 57.6. Work-up and treatment of Cushing's disease.

solism. This syndrome today generally represents a missed diagnosis of Cushing's disease that has been treated with adrenalectomy. Often, these tumors are aggressive or frankly malignant.

Differential Diagnosis

Table 57.3 lists the possible lesions that may occur within the sella or in the parasellar region. Pituitary adenomas head the list because they are the most common lesion in this region and constitute 8% to 10% of all brain tumors. Occasionally, they are cystic and confused with

other lesions. Craniopharyngiomas are the next most common tumor, and although more often suprasellar in location, they may be exclusively intrasellar. They are more common in children, but up to one third occur in adults. They are usually cystic and are calcified in 70% of children and 40% of adults. Meningiomas are also more commonly suprasellar and enhance strongly on CT and MRI. Germinomas, or so-called ectopic pinealomas, generally involve the pituitary stalk and often causes diabetes insipidus. It is a general principle that if a patient presents with diabetes insipidus, one should think of a lesion other than a pituitary adenoma. Metastatic malignancies, com-

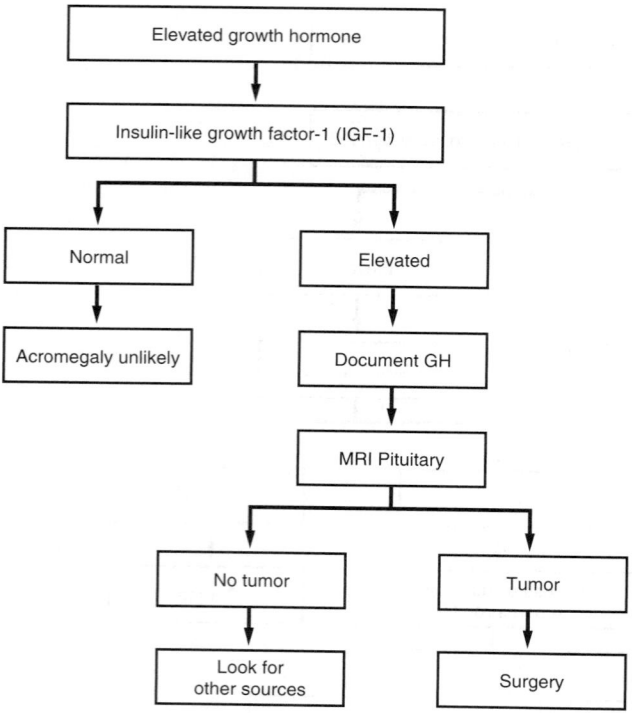

Figure 57.7. Work-up and treatment of acromegaly.

Table 57.2. CAUSES OF HYPERPROLACTINEMIA

Pituitary disease
  Prolactinoma
  Growth hormone-secreting adenoma
  Pituitary stalk section
  Empty sella syndrome
Hypothalamic disease
Tumors
Sarcoidosis
Radiation
Hypothyroidism
Chronic renal failure
Hepatic disease
Drugs
  Phenothiazines
  Tricyclic antidepressants
  Estrogen
  Opiates
  Reserpine
  Verapamil
  Others
Pregnancy
Stress

monly from lung and breast primary tumors, may be found in the pituitary, with 70% residing in the posterior pituitary. Optic nerve gliomas and hypothalamic gliomas may occasionally be confused with pituitary adenomas, as can the rare granular cell tumor (choristoma). Dermoids and epidermoids may occur within the sella, and fifth nerve neuromas may compress the sella.

Rathke's cysts are benign congenital remnants that develop within the sella and can cause a loss of pituitary func-

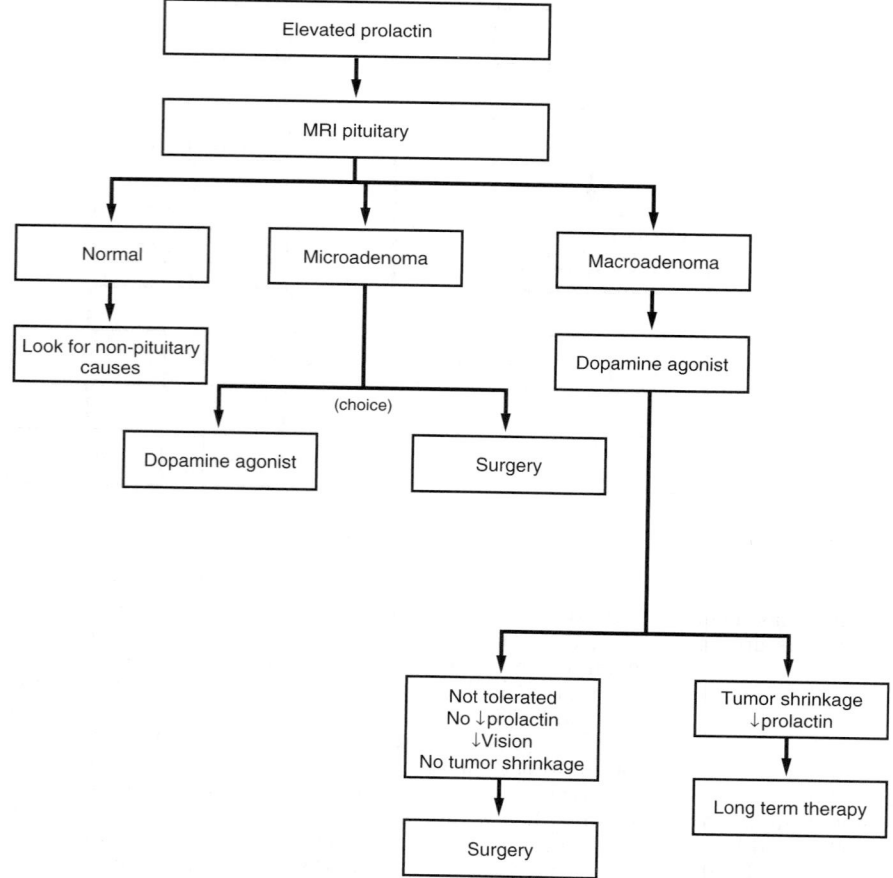

Figure 57.8. Diagnostic tests and treatment for hyperprolactinemia.

Table 57.3. DIFFERENTIAL DIAGNOSIS OF INTRASELLAR AND PARASELLAR LESIONS

Tumors
    Pituitary adenoma
    Craniopharyngioma
    Meningioma
    Lymphoma
    Germinoma
    Chordoma
    Granular cell tumor (choristoma)
    Neuroma (arising from cranial nerve V)
    Metastatic
    Optic nerve glioma
    Epidermoid
    Dermoid
    Infundibuloma
    Hypothalamic glioma
Cysts
    Rathke's cleft cyst
    Pituitary cyst
Inflammatory and granulomatous lesions
    Bacterial abscess
    Sarcoidosis
    Eosinophilic granuloma (histiocytosis X)
    Tuberculosis
    Mycoses
    Granulomatous hypophysitis
Aneurysm
Hamartoma
Empty sella syndrome
Pituitary apoplexy

tion by local compression. These can be confused on imaging studies with cystic adenomas or craniopharyngiomas, and biopsy and surgical decompression are required.

Inflammatory and granulomatous processes should also be kept in mind, including bacterial abscesses within the sella. Sarcoidosis may involve the pituitary or its stalk, as can the granulomas associated with histiocytosis X. Hamartomas may involve the pituitary stalk and hypothalamus and are impossible to differentiate from invasive gliomas on imaging studies.

Aneurysms, usually from the internal carotid arteries but occasionally from the basilar artery, may appear within the sella and must be ruled out preoperatively with MRI or angiography.

The empty-sella syndrome is generally an anatomic variation that rarely causes symptoms. If a patient with headaches or head trauma undergoes skull radiography or CT, an enlarged sella may be found. With high-resolution CT or MRI, usually the elongated stalk is seen to reach the sellar floor, so that a cystic lesion can be ruled out. A contrast cisternogram may be used to visualize cerebrospinal fluid within the sella if necessary.

Pituitary apoplexy occurs symptomatically only rarely but may cause a profound and emergent situation. Infarction and hemorrhage, usually in a pituitary adenoma, cause a sudden intrasellar expansion with severe headache and a rapid loss of pituitary function, resulting in hypotension. A sudden loss of vision and cranial nerve palsies may also develop. Treatment in severe cases involves the administration of steroids and surgical decompression of the sella.

TREATMENT AND RESULTS

The treatment of primary pituitary adenomas is generally surgical, although certain exceptions exist. Even with modern imaging techniques, the unequivocal diagnosis of an adenoma is not reached until tissue is obtained. As seen in Table 57.3, the list of possible parasellar lesions is extensive, and it is not within the scope of this chapter to delineate the specific treatment for each lesion. Along with surgical removal or decompression of pituitary adenomas, additional treatment in the form of radiation or medical therapy is often indicated. In addition to treatment directed at the primary lesion, it is critical to assess pituitary function thoroughly before and after treatment to decide whether hormone replacement is indicated.

More than 95% of pituitary adenomas can be approached by the transsphenoidal route. This is usually accomplished through a sublabial incision and a transseptal approach to the sphenoid. Once the sphenoid sinus has been entered, the operating microscope is brought in, and the anterior wall of the sella is carefully drilled away, and the dura surrounding the pituitary is identified. The dura is opened, and if a macroadenoma is present, the tumor is usually seen directly beneath the dura. If a microadenoma is present, the surgeon must carefully dissect around and often through the pituitary to identify the small tumor.

Contraindications to this approach, and therefore indications for a craniotomy, include the following: (a) massive suprasellar extension, (b) extensive lateral intracranial extension, and (c) the rare dumbbell-shaped tumor with a tight construction at the level of the diaphragma sellae. If a craniotomy is necessary, a right subfrontal approach to the optic nerve and chiasm is required; the tumor is removed in a piecemeal fashion with use of the operating microscope and microinstruments.

Nonfunctioning Adenomas

Because patients with nonfunctioning adenomas usually present with the effects of a mass lesion, these tumors are rarely microadenomas. Although their location can be either exclusively intrasellar or extensively intracranial, almost all these tumors are currently approached via the transsphenoidal route.

The three goals of surgery for nonfunctioning macroadenomas are the following: (a) establishment of a diagnosis, (b) decompression of surrounding structures, and (c) gross total removal of tumor tissue if possible. The first goal is usually accomplished easily, and although most tumors turn out to be adenomas, surprise findings are not unusual. Decompression is also usually accomplished readily because most tumors are soft and easily removed. Fewer than 5% of adenomas are so fibrous that decompression is difficult. Evidence of adequate decompression is the consistent finding that 75% to 80% of patients with visual field loss show recovery after transsphenoidal tumor removal (6). The third goal, total tumor resection, is much more difficult to accomplish with macroadenomas. It has been demonstrated that most macroadenomas (88% to 94%) invade at least the dura mater, and many grossly invade surrounding structures. Such invasion makes complete surgical resection impossible, and therefore these patients need to be followed indefinitely with high-quality imaging to monitor tumor progression or recurrence. Whereas it was once common practice to administer postoperative radiation to all macroadenomas, most neurosurgeons are now content to watch for progression with high-resolution imaging and reserve local radiation for that indication. Currently, no medical treatment is available for nonfunctional adenomas.

Cushing's Disease

Once it has been established that the cause of a patient's hypercortisolism is a pituitary lesion, the treatment of choice is transsphenoidal exploration of the pituitary. Only 40% of such patients have positive results on imaging studies, and therefore careful and systematic exploration of the sellar contents by an experienced pituitary surgeon is required in many cases (3). Microadenomas secreting ACTH may be very small and are often located deep within the gland itself. If a tumor is not evident when the dura is opened and all surfaces of the pituitary are examined, then incisions must be made into the gland and an internal exploration carried out. These microadenomas are usually in one lateral aspect of the pituitary gland, and the initial choice of which side to explore can be guided by the results of preoperative petrosal sinus sampling for ACTH levels, as described earlier. If no tumor is identified, then a decision must be made regarding whether to resect all or a portion of the gland. If the endocrine evidence is convincing for a pituitary origin and the patient has no desire to have children, then total hypophysectomy is warranted. If petrosal sinus sampling clearly indicates laterality of the ACTH secretion, then an appropriate hemiresection of the gland is carried out. Macroadenomas are treated with maximal tumor resection, but endocrine remission is, of course, more difficult to accomplish in these situations. Obviously, patients with adrenal or ectopic lesions are treated by resection of tumors in these locations. Microadenomas are the source of ACTH secretion in about 75% of patients (3,7,8). The postoperative remission rate in these patients is 88% to 96%, and the long-term recurrence rate appears to be no more than 5%. Therefore, selective microsurgical tumor resection in patients with microadenomas is clearly the current treatment of choice.

Some 10% to 20% of patients who undergo exploration have macroadenomas, and postoperative remission rates in these patients have been reported to be from 33% to 61% (3,7–10). Most of them require postoperative radiation therapy, which leads to remission in some of the surgical failures. Those whose tumors fail to remit after both surgery and radiation require either a surgical adrenalectomy or medical suppression of adrenal function. In a small percentage of patients who have undergone adrenalectomy, the pituitary tumors continue to grow and secrete ACTH (Nelson's syndrome).

Acromegaly

Like Cushing's disease, acromegaly is a condition that ultimately threatens life. For this reason, it must be treated aggressively, even at the expense of normal pituitary function. During the past two decades, a variety of medical, surgical, and radiation therapies have evolved that have proved effective in lowering GH levels. No single treatment is uniformly effective, and often a combination of treatments is necessary. The goals of treatment are to lower the circulating GH or somatomedin C levels to a normal range and to reduce the size of the mass lesion that is causing compression-related symptoms.

Unfortunately, only 20% to 34% of GH-secreting tumors are microadenomas, so that microsurgical tumor resection is less effective than in Cushing's disease. When a microadenoma is selectively removed transsphenoidally, endocrine remission may be expected in 80% to 88% of cases. When a macroadenoma is resected, immediate postoperative remission is reported in 30% to 68% of cases (11). Remission rates are inversely related to preoperative GH levels and the size and invasiveness of tumors. Preoperative treatment of macroadenomas with a somatostatin analogue may improve postoperative remission rates (12).

Radiation therapy has proved moderately effective, both as a primary mode of treatment and in conjunction with partial surgical resection. Proton beam heavy-particle therapy was reported in 510 patients, 428 of whom had been observed for 1 to 20 years (13). Analysis of these patients revealed a progressive fall in GH levels beginning immediately after treatment and continuing for up to 20 years. After 2 years, 47.5% of patients had GH levels below 10 ng/mL; at 4, 10, and 20 years, the rates were 65%, 87.5%, and 97.5%, respectively. If a GH level below 5 ng/mL is considered a cure, this level is achieved in 75% of patients at 10 years and 92.5% of patients at 20 years. Conventional radiation therapy provides comparable results (10-year posttreatment levels below 10 ng/mL in 81% and below 5 ng/mL in 69%). A recent review of our own patients, however, showed that after an average follow-up of 6.8 years, normalization of IGF-1 levels was attained in only 2 of 36 patients who received radiation (45 to 50 Gy) after surgical failure (14). The remaining 34 patients had persistently elevated IGF-1 levels (219 ± 26% of upper normal limit) despite plasma GH levels averaging 4.6 ± 1.1 µg/L. A recent report by Landolt et al. (15) suggests that stereotactic radiosurgery may be more effective than fractionated radiotherapy for persistant acromegaly after failed surgical treatment.

Bromocriptine, a dopamine receptor agonist, was shown to lower GH levels in 71% of 126 patients (16). Unfortunately, GH levels below 10 ng/mL were achieved in only 14% of patients in this study. A clinical response was achieved in up to 95% of acromegalic patients, and reduced somatomedin C levels were found in some patients with persistently elevated GH levels. Bromocriptine does not appear to be an effective primary treatment for acromegaly but may help to control GH and somatomedin C levels as an adjuvant therapy.

A somatostatin analogue recently used on an experimental basis has been demonstrated to reduce GH and somatomedin C levels significantly in most patients. This treatment provides only minimal tumor shrinkage, and GH levels rise again immediately after cessation of the drug. This drug may prove to be useful in preoperative treatment or surgical failure (12). The recurrence rate of GH-secreting tumors appears to be only 4% after successful surgery and less than 1% after radiation (15).

Given the variety of treatment modalities, a rational therapeutic approach is to resect tumors surgically when possible and to provide radiation therapy to those patients in whom a remission cannot be achieved. Somatostatin analogue is potentially useful as an adjuvant therapy in selected patients.

Prolactinomas

Prolactin-secreting adenomas are the most common functioning pituitary tumors but remain the most controversial with regard to treatment. The controversy exists because, unlike ACTH- or GH-secreting adenomas, prolactinomas can be treated medically with dopamine agonists, with reasonably good results. The treatment options include medical therapy, usually with bromocriptine; transsphenoidal surgical resection; radiation therapy; or, in some cases, no treatment. Because treatment considerations depend on tumor size, the treatments are discussed on that basis.

Macroadenomas

The goal in treating a patient with a large, prolactin-secreting adenoma is to decompress the optic pathways if they are involved and to reduce the prolactin levels to normal concentrations. Surgery is effective in improving vision in 80% of cases, but vision has also been reported to improve in patients treated with bromocriptine. The success of surgery in reducing prolactin levels to normal has generally been disappointing. The uniform finding of various investigators has been that the likelihood of normalizing prolactin levels is greatly reduced if the initial concentration is above 200 ng/mL or if the macroadenoma is larger than 10 mm.

The administration of bromocriptine to patients with macroadenomas reduces prolactin levels significantly in almost all instances, and reductions to normal ranges have been reported in more than 46% (17). In 90% of patients, the size of the tumor is decreased to some degree, and in many, the reduction is dramatic. However, with rare exceptions, the tumor returns to its original size once bromocriptine is stopped. It is recognized that up to 25% of patients with macroadenomas experience an increase in tumor size during pregnancy, whereas this is true in fewer than 1% of patients with microadenomas (17).

In patients with a mixture of prolactin-secreting and nonfunctioning tumors, the recurrence rate has been 21% at 10 years after radiation plus surgery, 29% with radiation alone, and 91% with only surgery (18). These data demonstrate the effectiveness of radiation therapy and the lack of effectiveness of surgery alone. The treating physician's obligation is to discuss in detail the treatment options with the patient and to decide on a specific course of action. A transsphenoidal debulking of the tumor is recommended, with remission achieved in up to 30% of patients. Usually, bromocriptine is used for 3 to 4 weeks preoperatively to reduce the size of the tumor. If a large, invasive tumor is encountered, postoperative radiation therapy is recommended. If remission is not achieved but the tumor is grossly removed, then bromocriptine alone is used postoperatively. Surgery is particularly recommended if subsequent pregnancy is desired because the tumor is likely to expand during pregnancy (off bromocriptine) and possibly jeopardize vision. Careful follow-up with CT or MRI is required for the lifetime of the patient because rapid tumor growth may occur. The recurrence rate of macroadenomas is from 25% to 75% within 5 years (18), so adjunctive therapy is clearly indicated if the postoperative prolactin level begins to rise.

Microadenomas

The surgical treatment of prolactin-secreting microadenomas results in postoperative remission in a much higher percentage of patients. Two large series reported remission in 77% (19) and 72% (20) of patients. In the latter report, 88% were in remission, with prolactin levels below 100 ng/mL, and only 50% had prolactin levels above 100 ng/mL. The incidence of new postoperative hypogonadism was only 1%. Others have reported an immediate postoperative remission rate of 81% without bromocriptine pretreatment but only a 33% rate with pretreatment (21). These data suggest that bromocriptine induces fibrosis within the tumor and that the lower remission rate is related to the fibrosis. Primary medical treatment is safe and effective but may lower the chance of long-term surgical cure by causing fibrosis. As in macroadenomas, long-term continued therapy is indicated because prolactin levels rapidly rise with cessation of dopamine agonists. Pregnancy is of less risk to the patient with a microadenoma because tumor expansion and visual loss are rare.

The recurrence rate in patients initially in remission after microsurgical tumor removal has been somewhat disappointing compared with the rates after removal of other functioning tumors. Recurrences have uniformly been found to be higher in patients with postoperative prolactin levels in the upper end of the normal range. Recurrence rates of 17% to 50% during 5 years have been reported. Radiation therapy does not play a role in the treatment of microadenomas unless they recur in an aggressive manner.

The approach to prolactin-secreting microadenomas that can be seen on imaging studies is to explain the medical and surgical options to the patient carefully. Surgery is offered as a primary option because it allows the possibility of long-term remission without continued medical therapy. In the final analysis, patients must make an educated choice between primary medical or surgical treatment.

Few objective data are available for surgical exploration in patients with presumed microadenomas. Unlike patients with Cushing's disease or acromegaly, most patients with hyperprolactinemia and normal findings on imaging studies have not undergone exploration. Once other causes of hyperprolactinemia have been ruled out, dopamine agonists are generally administered in an attempt to lower prolactin levels. These patients need to be followed carefully with imaging studies and measurement of prolactin levels. The incidence of subsequent development of obvious adenomas is unknown, but it appears to be as low as 5%.

REFERENCES

1. Kovacs K, Horvath E. Tumors of the pituitary gland. In: Hartmann WH, ed. *Atlas of tumor pathology,* series 2, fascicle 21. Washington, DC: Armed Forces Institute of Pathology, 1986: 192.
2. Lloyd RV, Cano M, Chandler WF, et al. Human growth hormone- and prolactin-secreting pituitary adenomas analyzed by in situ hybridization. *Am J Pathol* 1989;134:605.
3. Chandler WF, Schteingart DE, Lloyd RV, et al. Surgical treatment of Cushing's disease. *J Neurosurg* 1987;66:204.
4. Oldfield EH, Chrousos GP, Schulte HM, et al. Preoperative lateralization of ACTH-secreting pituitary microadenomas by bilateral and simultaneous inferior petrosal venous sinus sampling. *N Engl J Med* 1985;312:100–103.
5. Nelson DH, Meakin JW, Dealy JB, et al. ACTH-producing tumor of the pituitary gland. *N Engl J Med* 1958;259:161.
6. Ebersold MJ, Quast LM, Laws ER, et al. Long-term results in transsphenoidal removal of nonfunctioning pituitary adenomas. *J Neurosurg* 1986;64:713.
7. Boggan JE, Tyrrell JB, Wilson CB. Transsphenoidal microsurgical management of Cushing's disease. *J Neurosurg* 1983;59: 195.
8. Hardy J. Cushing's disease: 50 years later. *Can J Neurol Sci* 1982;9:375.
9. Kuwayama A, Kageyama N. Current management of Cushing's disease: part II. *Contemp Neurosurg* 1985;7:1.
10. Salassa RM, Laws ER, Carpenter PC, et al. Cushing's disease: 50 years later. *Trans Am Clin Climatol Assoc* 1982;94:122.
11. Tindall GT, Tindall SC. Transsphenoidal surgery for acromegaly: long-term results in 50 patients. In: Black PM, Zervas NT, Ridgeway EC, et al., eds. *Secretory tumors of the pituitary gland.* New York: Raven Press, 1984:175.
12. Barkan AL, Lloyd RV, Chandler WF, et al. Preoperative treatment of acromegaly with long-acting somatostatin: shrinkage of invasive pituitary macroadenomas and improved surgical remission rate. *J Clin Endocrinol Metab* 1988;67:1040.
13. Kliman B, Kjellberg RN, Swisher B, et al. Proton beam therapy of acromegaly: a 20-year experience. In: Black PM, Zervas NT, Ridgeway EC, et al., eds. *Secretory tumors of the pituitary gland.* New York: Raven Press, 1984:191.
14. Barkan AL, Halasz I, Dornfeld KJ, et al. Pituitary irradiation is ineffective in normalizing plasma insulin-like growth factor I in patients with acromegaly. *J Clin Endocrinol Metab* 1997;82: 3187–3191.
15. Landolt AM, Haller D, Lomas N, et al. Stereotactic radiosurgery for recurrent surgically treated acromegaly: comparison with fractionated radiotherapy. *J Neurosurg* 1998;88: 1002–1008.
16. Besser GM, Wass JAH. The medical management of acromegaly. In: Black PM, Zervas NT, Ridgeway EC, et al., eds. *Secretory tumors of the pituitary gland.* New York: Raven Press, 1984:155.
17. Thorner MO, Evans WS, Vance ML. Medical management of prolactinomas: I. In: Black PM, Servas NT, Ridgeway EC, et

al., eds. *Secretory tumors of the pituitary gland.* New York: Raven Press, 1984:53.

18. Sheline GE, Grossman A, Jones AE, et al. Radiation therapy for prolactinomas. In: Black PM, Zervas NI, Ridgeway EC, et al., eds. *Secretory tumors of the pituitary gland.* New York: Raven Press, 1984:93.

19. Hardy J. Transsphenoidal microsurgery of prolactinomas. In: Black PM, Zervas NT, Ridgeway EC, et al., eds. *Secretory tumors of the pituitary gland.* New York: Raven Press, 1984:73.

20. Randall RV, Laws ER, Abboud CF, et al. Transsphenoidal microsurgical treatment of prolactin-producing pituitary adenomas. *Mayo Clin Proc* 1983;58:108.

21. Landolt AM, Keller PJ, Froesch ER, et al. Bromocriptine: does it jeopardize the result of later surgery for prolactinomas? *Lancet* 1982;1:657.

SURGERY: SCIENTIFIC PRINCIPLES AND PRACTICE, Third Edition, edited by Lazar J. Greenfield, Michael W. Mulholland, Keith T. Oldham, Gerald B. Zelenock, and Keith D. Lillemoe. Lippincott Williams & Wilkins Publishers, Philadelphia, © 2001.

CHAPTER 58

BREAST
MONICA MORROW

ANATOMY

The adult female breast lies between the second and sixth ribs and between the sternal edge and the midaxillary line (Fig. 58.1). Breast tissue frequently extends into the axilla as the axillary tail of Spence. Posteriorly, the upper portion of the breast rests on the fascia of the pectoralis major muscle; inferolaterally, it is bounded by the fascia of the serratus anterior. Bands of fibrous tissue, known as *Cooper's ligaments,* extend from the fascia to the fibrous tissue of the dermis and support the breast. The size of the adult female breast varies widely among individuals, and considerable discrepancy in breast size may be seen between the breasts of an individual woman. This is rarely a sign of breast disease.

The breast is composed of skin, subcutaneous tissue, and breast tissue. The breast tissue includes both epithelial parenchymal elements and stroma. The epithelial component comprises about 10% to 15% of the breast mass, with the remainder being stroma. Each breast consists of 15 to 20 lobes of glandular tissue that are supported by a framework of fibrous connective tissue. The space between lobes is filled by adipose tissue. Variations in breast size are accounted for by differences in the amount of adipose tissue in the breast rather than the epithelial elements. Much of the epithelial tissue of the breast is found in the upper outer quadrant, which is why this is the most frequent site of both benign and malignant breast disease.

The lobes of the breast are subdivided into lobules, which are made up of branched tubuloalveolar glands. Each lobe ends in a lactiferous duct, 2 to 4 mm in diameter. Beneath the areola, the lactiferous ducts dilate into lactiferous sinuses and then open through a constricted orifice onto the nipple (Fig. 58.2).

The nipple is located over the fourth intercostal space in the nonpendulous breast and is surrounded by a circular, pigmented areola. Beneath the nipple and areola are bundles of radially arranged smooth-muscle fibers that are responsible for the erection of the nipple in response to a variety of stimuli. The nipple and areola contain sebaceous glands and apocrine sweat glands, but no hair follicles. In addition, the tubercles of Morgagni are nodular elevations formed by the openings of the Montgomery glands at the periphery of the areola. These glands are capable of secreting milk and are believed to represent an intermediate stage between sweat and mammary glands. The nipple and areolar region, as well as the remainder of the breast, is richly supplied with sensory innervation.

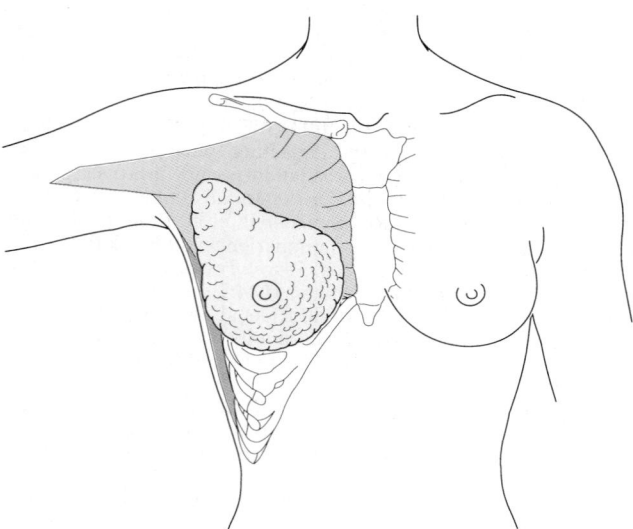

Figure 58.1. The adult female breast. The upper and medial portions of the breast rest on the pectoralis major muscle, and the inferolateral portion rests on the serratus anterior.

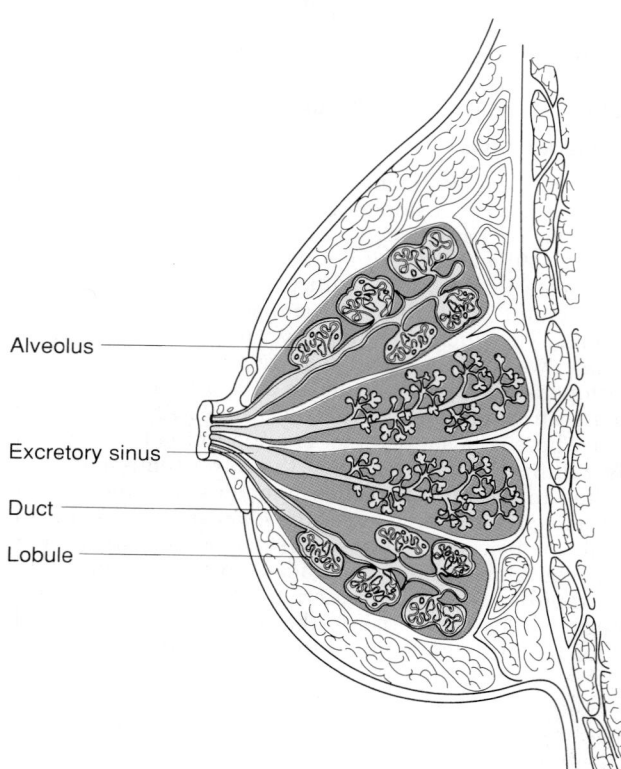

Alveolus

Excretory sinus

Duct

Lobule

Figure 58.2. The breast consists of 15 to 20 lobes of glandular tissue. Within each lobe, the lobules are composed of branched tubuloalveolar glands. Each lobule ends in a lactiferous duct. These ducts dilate into lactiferous sinuses beneath the nipple.

The blood supply of the breast is derived from the internal mammary and lateral thoracic arteries. The medial and central portions of the breast receive their major blood supply from anterior perforating branches of the internal mammary artery, and the upper outer quadrant is primarily supplied by the lateral thoracic artery. In general, the venous drainage of the breast follows the arterial supply.

Lymphatic Drainage

The lymphatics of the breast are thin-walled, valveless vessels that drain unidirectionally except when obstructed by inflammatory or neoplastic disease. The superficial subareolar lymphatic plexus drains primarily the skin of the breast and the nipple and areola, in addition to some of the central portion of the gland. This plexus is interconnected with the deep lymphatic plexus, which drains most of the breast parenchyma. Injections of radioactively labeled colloid have demonstrated that about 97% of the lymphatic flow from the breast drains directly into the axillary lymph nodes, with the remaining 3% draining into the internal mammary nodes (1). All quadrants of the breast drain into the internal mammary nodes. The hypothesis that all lymphatic flow in the breast drains initially into the subareolar plexus has been largely disproved by such studies.

The axillary space is bordered by the axillary vein superiorly, the latissimus dorsi laterally, and the serratus anterior medially (Fig. 58.3). The pectoralis major lies anterior to the axillary space, and the subscapularis comprises its posterior wall. Structures of clinical importance within this space include the long thoracic nerve, which innervates the serratus anterior; the thoracodorsal neurovascular bundle, which innervates and supplies blood to the latissimus dorsi; and the intercostobrachial nerves, which are sensory to the upper inner aspect of the arm.

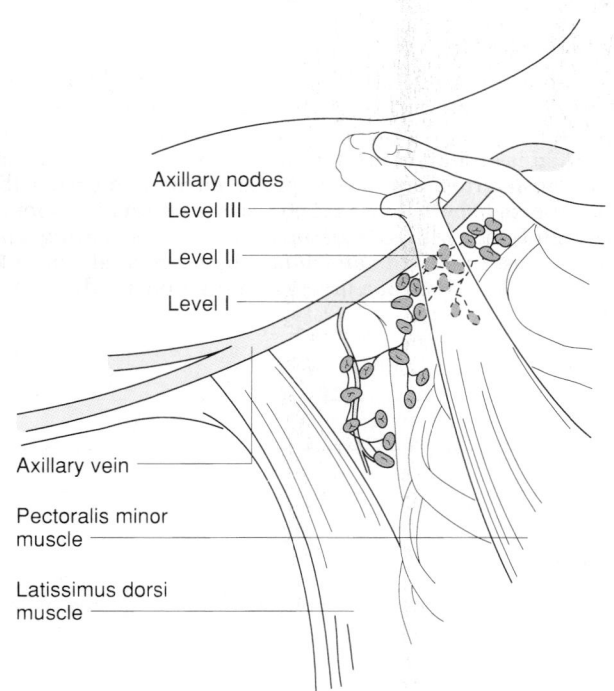

Figure 58.3. The axillary lymph nodes are divided into three levels by the pectoralis minor muscle. The level I nodes are inferior and lateral to the pectoralis minor, the level II nodes are below the axillary vein and behind the pectoralis minor, and the level III nodes are medial to the muscle against the chest wall.

The axillary nodes are embedded in fat and are variable in number. Surgeons have traditionally divided the axillary nodes into three levels: level I nodes, inferior and lateral to the pectoralis minor; level II nodes, behind the pectoralis minor and inferior to the axillary vein; and level III nodes, medial to the pectoralis minor and against the chest wall. The interpectoral (or Rotter's) nodes are located between the pectoralis major and minor muscles along the lateral pectoral nerve. Involvement of this node group in the absence of axillary metastases is extremely rare (2), and they are of limited clinical significance. The supraclavicular nodes are contiguous with the apex of the axilla. Metastatic involvement of this nodal group in the absence of extensive axillary disease is also uncommon, although direct lymphatic drainage to this node group is occasionally seen.

The internal mammary nodes are located in the first six intercostal spaces within 3 cm of the edge of the sternum. The highest concentration of internal mammary nodes is found in the first three intercostal spaces (3).

PHYSIOLOGY

Development of the Breast

Breast development is controlled by a large number of hormonal and biochemical factors. In the female, estrogens interact with the primordial breast bud to promote ductal development, whereas in the male, the interaction of androgen with the breast bud results in destruction of the epithelial component. In the female, ductal elongation and branching begin in puberty and are regulated by pituitary growth hormone, which may act through insulin-like growth factor I locally (4). In addition, the presence of estrogen and progesterone is required to stimulate DNA synthesis. This effect is believed to occur through both receptor-mediated and paracrine pathways.

Changes in breast size and shape begin at puberty and are secondary to growth of both the glandular and stromal elements of the breast. Russo and Russo (5) have described three types of breast lobules, related to a woman's parity and menopausal status. The type 1 (or virginal) lobule consists of a cluster of 11 alveolar buds around a terminal duct; it is the predominant lobule seen in nulliparous and postmenopausal women. Type 2 lobules contain an average of 47 alveolar buds, and type 3 lobules have 80, at which time they are referred to as *ductules* or *alveoli*. In parous women, type 3 lobules predominate, with a peak frequency in the early reproductive years until they begin to decline in the fourth decade of life. Cells within these lobules have been shown to proliferate at different rates, the rate being 10 times higher in type 1 than in type 3 lobules, and three times higher in type 1 than in type 2 lobules. The presence of estrogen receptor-α and the progesterone receptor within these lobules is directly proportional to the rate of cell proliferation (6). These differences in cell proliferation may explain some of the differences in breast cancer risk observed on the basis of parity and age at first birth (see section on breast cancer risk factors).

The cyclical increases in estrogen and progesterone that occur in the menstrual cycle also influence the gross and microscopic character of the breast. Many women experience increased breast fullness, nodularity, and sensitivity in the premenstrual period. During the follicular phase of the menstrual cycle (days 4 through 14), epithelial proliferation occurs, with epithelial sprouting and an increased mitotic rate. During the luteal phase of the cycle (days 15 through 28), when progestins predominate, proliferation is maximal, with ductal dilation and differentiation of the alveolar epithelial cells to secretory cells. This results in the formation of lipid droplets in the alveolar cells and some intraluminal secretion. With the onset of menstruation, secretory activity regresses secondary to epithelial apoptosis, or programmed cell death.

Pregnancy

Significant ductal, lobular, and alveolar growth occurs during pregnancy as a result of exposure to estrogen, progesterone, growth hormone, prolactin, and placental hormones. Clinically, this is manifested as breast enlargement, with associated dilation of the superficial veins and darkening of the nipple. At delivery, the breast may be three times the size of the nonlactating breast. Microscopically, lobular–alveolar differentiation to type 3 lobules begins in the first trimester, and the stromal elements of the breast are gradually replaced by the proliferating glandular epithelium. During the third trimester, terminal differentiation of the epithelium results in the development of secretory cells that are able to synthesize and secrete milk proteins. Oxytocin induces myoepithelial proliferation and differentiation (6).

Lactation and Involution

After delivery, the sudden fall in estrogen and progesterone levels results in lactation. Prolactin, in conjunction with growth hormone and insulin, induces the production and secretion of milk. Initially, colostrum, a sticky serous fluid rich in growth factors, is secreted, followed by milk. The secretion of milk is regulated by the pituitary production of oxytocin, which is released in response to neural reflexes activated by suckling.

Following weaning, the secretory activity of the lactogenic epithelium gradually decreases. Retained secretory products are removed by phagocytosis, although ruptured alveoli containing milk may be clinically manifested as galactoceles. Atrophy of glandular, ductal, and stromal elements results in a decrease in breast size. Withdrawal of the steroid hormones and growth factors of pregnancy and lactation results in apoptosis of the terminally differentiated secretory cells of the epithelial lumen. However, as previously noted, type 3 lobules persist.

Menopause

After menopause, the breast undergoes regression. Type 1 lobules predominate, as in the breasts of nulliparous women. Overall, involution of the ductal and glandular el-

ements of the breast occurs, and the breast becomes predominantly fat and stroma. With aging, a progressive decrease in the fat content and supporting stroma results in breast shrinkage and loss of contour.

EXAMINATION OF THE BREAST

A careful history is the initial step in a breast examination. Regardless of the presenting complaint, baseline information regarding menstrual status and breast cancer risk factors should be obtained. The basic elements of a breast history are listed in Table 58.1. In premenopausal women, knowing the date of the last menstrual period and the regularity of the cycle is useful in evaluating breast nodularity, pain, and cysts. Postmenopausal women should be questioned about the use of hormone replacement therapy, given that many benign breast problems are uncommon after menopause in the absence of exogenous hormones. Specific information about the patient's presenting complaint is then elicited. A breast lump is most often the clinical problem that causes women to seek treatment and remains the most common presentation of breast carcinoma. Today, many women present for a breast examination after an abnormality has been identified on a screening mammogram. Although the majority of these lesions are not clinically evident, a careful physical examination is an important part of the evaluation of a patient with an abnormal mammogram. Breast pain, a change in the size and shape of the breast, nipple discharge, and changes in the appearance of the skin are infrequent symptoms of carcinoma. The evaluation and management of these conditions are described in the section on clinical breast problems. For any breast complaint, the duration of the symptoms, their persistence over time, and their fluctuation with the menstrual cycle or relationship to exogenous estrogen should be ascertained.

Technique

A woman must be disrobed from the waist up for a complete breast examination. Although attention to modesty is appropriate and a gown or drape should be provided, inspection is an important part of the examination, and subtle abnormalities are best appreciated by comparing the appearance of both breasts. The breast examination should be performed with the patient in both the sitting and supine positions, and care should be taken at all times to be gentle. The steps of a breast examination are illustrated in Fig. 58.4.

Table 58.1. MEDICAL HISTORY OF A BREAST PROBLEM

General	Specific
Age at menarche	Onset
Number of pregnancies	Duration
Number of live births	Frequency
Age at first birth	Severity
Family history of breast cancer, including affected relative, age of onset, and presence of bilateral disease	Relationship to menstrual cycle or use of hormone replacement therapy
History of breast biopsies (and histologic diagnosis, if available)	
Premenopausal women	
Date of last menstrual period	
Length and regularity of cycles	
Use of oral contraceptives	
Postmenopausal women	
Date of menopause	
Use of hormone replacement therapy	

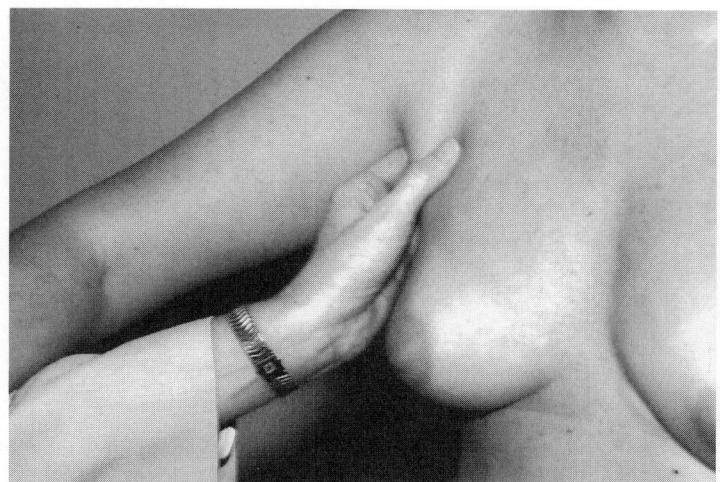

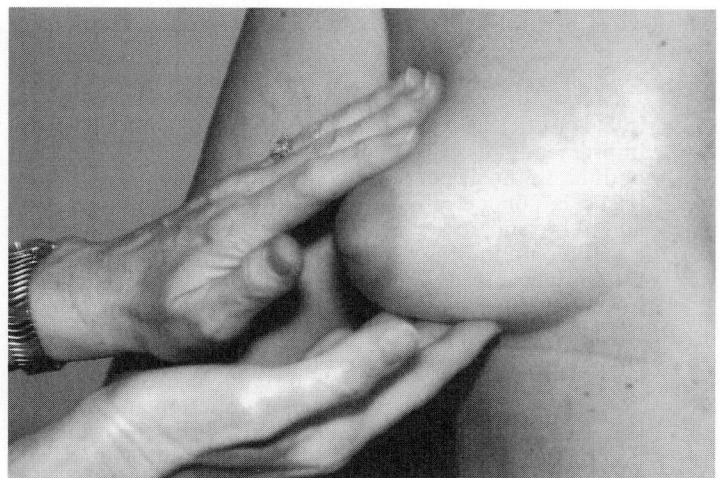

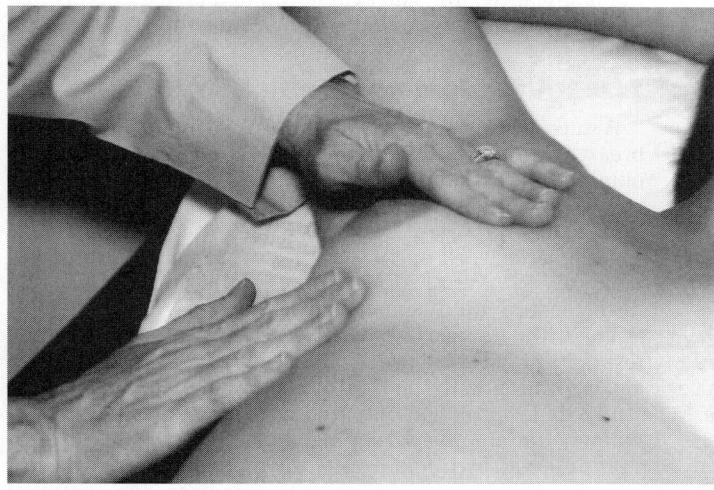

Figure 58.4. Breast examination. *(A)* The patient's ipsilateral arm is supported by the examiner to relax the pectoral muscle while the axillary nodes are examined. *(B)* Bimanual examination of the breast in the upright position. *(C)* Bimanual examination in the supine position with the arm raised over the head.

The breasts are initially inspected while the patient is in the sitting position with the arms relaxed. The size and shape of the breasts should be compared. If a discrepancy in size is noted, its chronicity should be determined. In many women, the breasts are not identical in size, and the finding of small discrepancies in size is rarely a sign of malignancy. Differences in breast size that are of recent onset or progressive in nature, however, may be caused by both benign and malignant tumors and require further evaluation (Fig. 58.5). Alterations in breast shape, in the absence of previous surgery, are of more concern. Superficially located tumors can cause bulges in the breast contour or retraction of the overlying skin. The skin retraction seen with superficial tumors may be caused by direct extension of tumor or fibrosis. Tumors deep within the substance of the breast that involve the fibrous septa (Cooper's

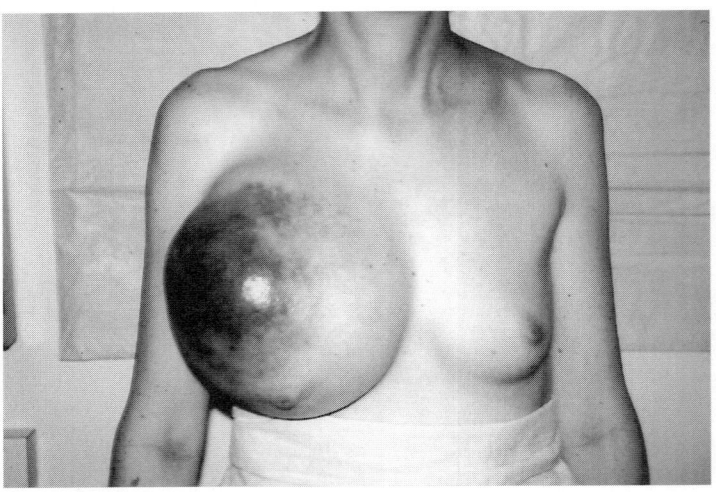

Figure 58.5. Breast asymmetry resulting from a benign phyllodes tumor. Skin changes are caused by pressure necrosis.

ligaments) can also cause retraction. Retraction is not itself a prognostic factor except when it is caused by the direct extension of tumor into the skin, and for this reason, it is not a part of the clinical staging of breast cancer (7). Although retraction is usually a sign of malignancy, benign lesions of the breast, such as granular cell tumors and fat necrosis, also cause retraction. Other benign causes of retraction include surgical biopsy and thrombophlebitis of the thoracoepigastric vein (Mondor's disease).

The skin of the breast and the nipples should also be carefully inspected. Edema of the skin of the breast *(peau d'orange),* when present, is usually extensive and readily apparent. Localized edema is frequently most prominent in the lower half of the breast and periareolar region and is most noticeable when the patient's arms are raised. Erythema is another sign of disease that is evident on inspection. It may be caused by cellulitis or abscess in the breast, but a diagnosis of inflammatory carcinoma should always be considered.

Examination of the nipples should include inspection for symmetry, retraction, and changes in the character of the skin. The new onset of nipple retraction should be regarded with a high index of suspicion, except when it occurs immediately after cessation of breast-feeding. Ulceration and eczematous changes of the nipple may be the first signs of Paget's disease.

After inspection with the arms relaxed, the patient should be asked to raise her arms to allow a more complete inspection of the lower half of the breasts. A final inspection is made with the hands on the hips and the pectoral muscles contracted.

The regional nodes are then examined with the patient upright. The size, character (soft, tender, firm), and number are assessed, and it should be noted whether the nodes are matted. The axillary nodes are most readily examined with the ipsilateral arm supported to relax the pectoral muscle (Fig. 58.4A). Bimanual examination of the breast is also carried out with the patient upright (Fig. 58.4B).

The breast examination is completed with the patient in the supine position and the ipsilateral arm raised above the head (Fig. 58.4C). The breast tissue is then systematically examined. Whether the examination is performed with a radial or a concentric circular search pattern is unimportant, provided that the entire breast is examined. The examination should extend superiorly to the clavicle, inferiorly to the lower rib cage, medially to the sternal border, and laterally to the midaxillary line.

One of the most difficult aspects of breast examination relates to the nodular, irregular texture of normal breasts in premenopausal women. Normal breasts tend to be most nodular in the upper outer quadrants, where the glandular tissue is concentrated, in the inframammary ridge area, and in the subareolar region. Generalized lumpiness is not a pathologic finding. Comparing the breasts is often helpful in determining whether a questionable area requires further evaluation. When the patient notices a mass that is not evident to the examiner, she should be asked to indicate the area of concern. If uncertainty remains regarding the significance of an area of nodular breast tissue in a premenopausal woman, a repeated examination at a different time during the menstrual cycle may clarify the issue. If a dominant mass is identified, it should be measured, and its location, mobility, and character should be described in the medical record. The evaluation of a breast mass is discussed in detail in the section on clinical breast problems.

Screening Mammography

A screening mammogram consists of two views of the breast (craniocaudal and mediolateral oblique), which are obtained in asymptomatic women in an effort to detect cancer in a preclinical state, when the likelihood of cure is higher. It is important that screening not be confused with a diagnostic work-up, which is performed to evaluate a woman with a clinical breast complaint and is discussed in the section on diagnostic imaging.

The ultimate measure of the effectiveness of a screening test is its effect on mortality. Eight randomized clinical trials, beginning with the Health Insurance Plan of New York study in 1963, have compared breast cancer mortality in women undergoing screening mammography at 1- to 2-year intervals with mortality in control populations. A 20% to 30% decrease in mortality has been demonstrated for screened women age 50 and older (8). The benefit of screening in women ages 40 to 49 has been controversial. Many of the trials were not designed to allow a separate analysis of women in this age group, and mortality benefits were often not apparent until after 8 years or more of follow-up. However, a metaanalysis of women ages 40 to 49 in the randomized trials suggests a 29% mortality reduction with screening in this age group (9).

The mortality reduction from screening is achieved by the identification of abnormalities that cannot be detected on physical examination. These include microcalcifications and masses smaller than 1 cm in size, the usual clinical limit of detection. In addition to reducing breast cancer mortality, the identification of smaller tumors increases the likelihood that a woman will be a candidate for breast-conserving surgery. In one study, only 10% of women with tumors 2 cm or less in size had contraindications to breast conservation, compared with 30% of women with tumors larger than 2 cm but less than 5 cm in size (10). Current screening recommendations are for annual mammography for women age 40 and older.

Screening mammography is a sensitive but nonspecific test, and only 20% to 30% of mammographically detected abnormalities that are examined further are found to be malignant. Biopsies for clinically occult, benign lesions represent the major induced cost of screening. The positive predictive value of a mammographic lesion varies with its appearance. For spiculated or stellate masses, the likelihood of malignancy is 75%; this falls to 20% for lobulated masses with slightly irregular margins and to 5% for well-circumscribed masses (Fig. 58.6). The classification of calcifications has proved to be even more difficult. Calcifications are analyzed based on their size, number, distribution, and morphology; those that are irregular in size and shape, particularly when they have a branching pattern suggestive of a ductal distribution, are most likely to be malignant (Fig. 58.7).

In an effort to standardize the reporting of mammographic abnormalities, the American College of Radiology has created a breast imaging reporting and data system (BI-RADS) (11). The BI-RADS classification is listed in Table 58.2. Category 3 lesions are those with a less than 2% probability of malignancy, and short-interval follow-up usually consists of repeated imaging studies at 6 months.

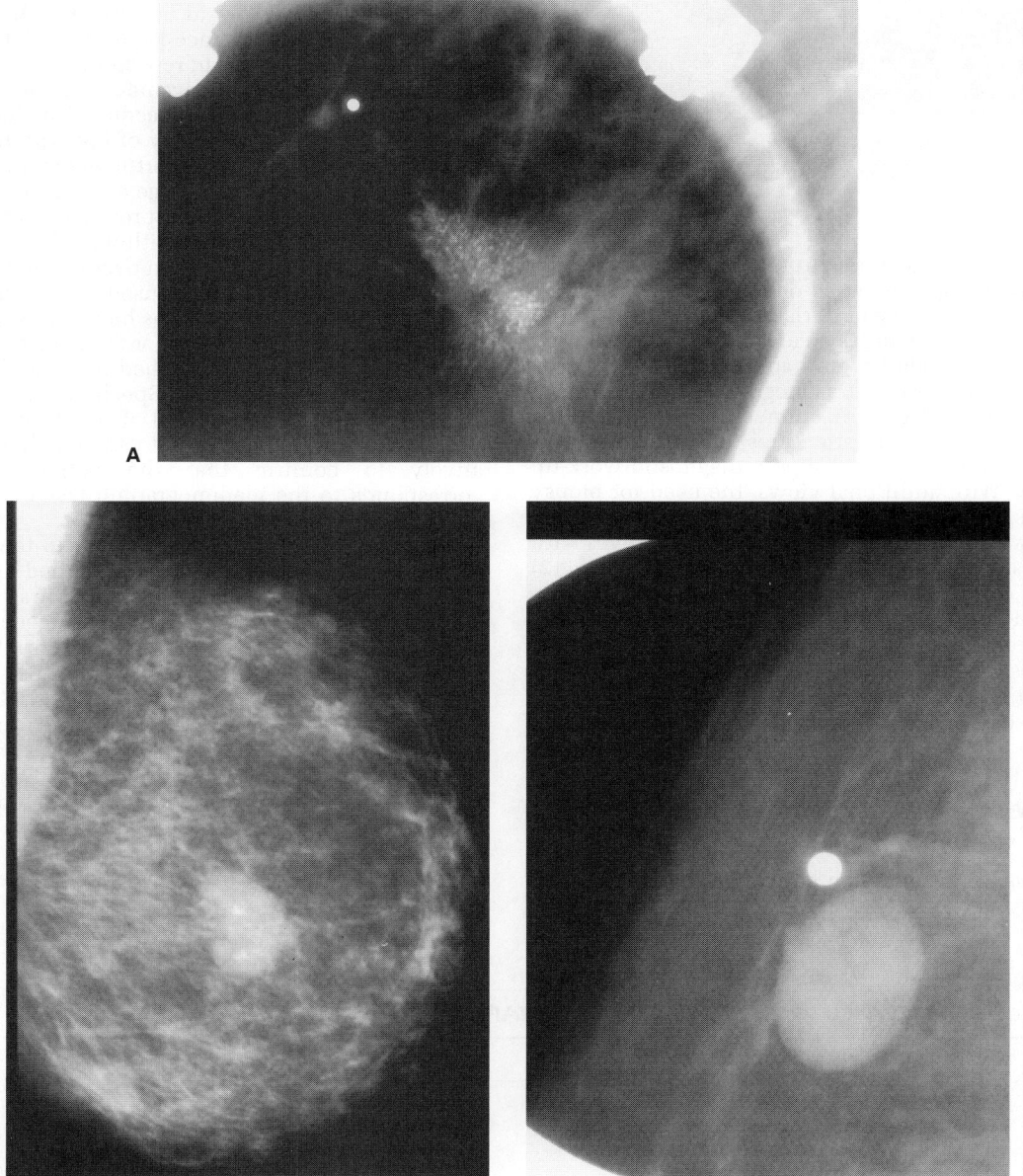

Figure 58.6. Mammographic masses. *(A)* Spiculated mass with calcifications. *(B)* Lobulated mass with indistinct posterior margin. *(C)* Well-circumscribed mass.

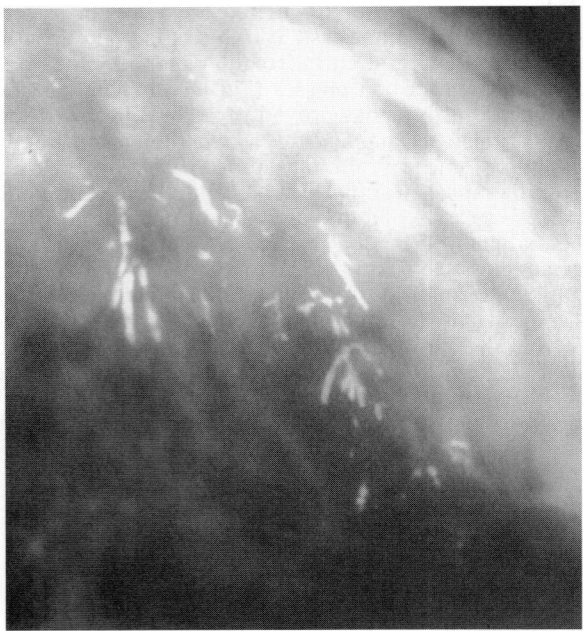

Figure 58.7. Microcalcifications. The branching, irregular appearance is classic for ductal carcinoma in situ.

Category 4 lesions range in risk from 2% to 50%, and a decision regarding biopsy is based on the appearance of the lesion and the patient's level of risk.

The BI-RADS also includes a category 0, which is used when analysis is incomplete and additional studies, such as magnification views or ultrasonography, are needed before a final BI-RADS classification can be assigned. In practice, the majority of abnormalities detected on screening mammography should undergo a diagnostic work-up before biopsy. With additional views, the need for biopsy of benign lesions is often avoided, as illustrated in Fig. 58.8, where what appears to be a mass lesion resolves with spot compression and magnification views. Sickles (12) reported that of 302 cases of calcifications felt to be equivocal (i.e., BI-RADS category 4) after a screening examination, 61% were shown to be benign on additional views. Even with lesions that are clearly malignant on a screening examination, additional views allow a better definition of the extent of the lesion for treatment planning.

Techniques of Biopsy for Lesions Detected on Screening

After a physical examination has confirmed that a mammographically detected abnormality is not clinically evident, a histologic diagnosis may be obtained by needle localization and excision or an image-guided core biopsy. For many years, needle localization with excision was the gold standard for the diagnosis of mammographic abnormalities. The advantages of this approach include the complete pathologic characterization of malignant lesions before local therapy is selected, and the ability of the diagnostic procedure to serve as the definitive lumpectomy in most cases. Disadvantages of this approach are related to the fact that the majority of mammographic abnormalities are benign. A surgical biopsy subjects patients to a small, but real, risk for discomfort and cosmetic deformity for no real benefit. In addition, failure to excise the mammographic abnormality is reported in 1% to 18% of cases, with most recent series reporting failure rates of 1% to 2%.

Accurate placement of the guide, a clear understanding by the surgeon of the relationship between the guide and the mammographic abnormality, and communication between the radiologist, surgeon, and pathologist are the most critical factors in the success of needle localization biopsies. The guide should be placed within 1 cm of the lesion. Any greater distance from the lesion is unacceptable and is an indication to reposition or replace the guide before surgery. Incision placement is another critical element in the success of the procedure. The incision should be placed at the point of entry of the wire into the breast only when the wire has a short course within the breast. When the wire traverses a large amount of the breast, the incision should be made just proximal to the area of disease and the wire identified within the breast parenchyma (Fig. 58.9). Placing the incision over the area of disease allows a smaller incision to be used and a single specimen to be removed, and it facilitates hemostasis. In addition, if repeated excision is required for the management of carcinoma, it is readily accomplished because the area of the tumor bed is clearly evident. Specimen radiography is essential to confirm the removal of calcifications and is appropriate for mass lesions that can be palpated intraoperatively to confirm that the palpable abnormality corresponds to the mammographic lesion that prompted the biopsy.

An alternative to excisional biopsy in the management of nonpalpable lesions is image-guided breast biopsy. Mass lesions can be sampled under ultrasonographic or stereotactic guidance; calcifications generally require stereotactic guidance. A comparison of the results of stereotactic core biopsy and surgical biopsy demonstrates concordance rates of 71% to 99% (13–16). Based on clinical experience, a number of circumstances in which a benign core biopsy should be followed by a surgical excision have been identified. These are listed in Table 58.3. The finding of atypical hyperplasia on a core biopsy is associated with carcinoma in 20% to 90% of cases (17). The majority of these are intraductal carcinomas, but approximately one third are invasive lesions. The use of large vacuum-assisted biopsy devices may reduce the incidence

---

Table 58.2. **BI-RADS CLASSIFICATION OF MAMMOGRAPHIC ABNORMALITIES**

Category	Assessment	Recommendation
1	Negative	Routine screening.
2	Benign finding	Routine screening.
3	Probably benign finding	Short-interval follow-up.
4	Suspicious abnormality	Definite probability of malignancy; consider biopsy.
5	Highly suggestive of malignancy	High probability of cancer; appropriate action should be taken.

BI-RADS, breast imaging reporting and data system.

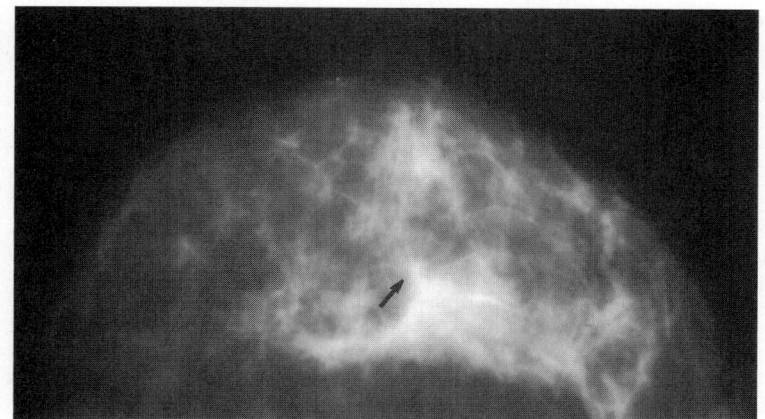

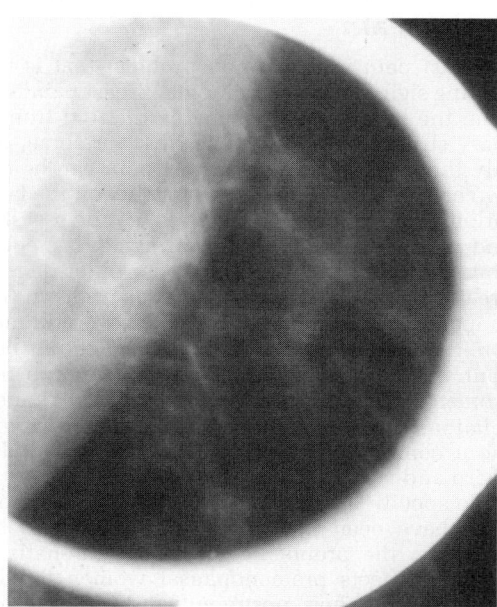

Figure 58.8. Work-up of abnormal screening mammogram. *(A)* Craniocaudal view showing an increased density with a slightly spiculated appearance *(arrow). (B)* Spot magnification view of the density demonstrating normal breast tissue.

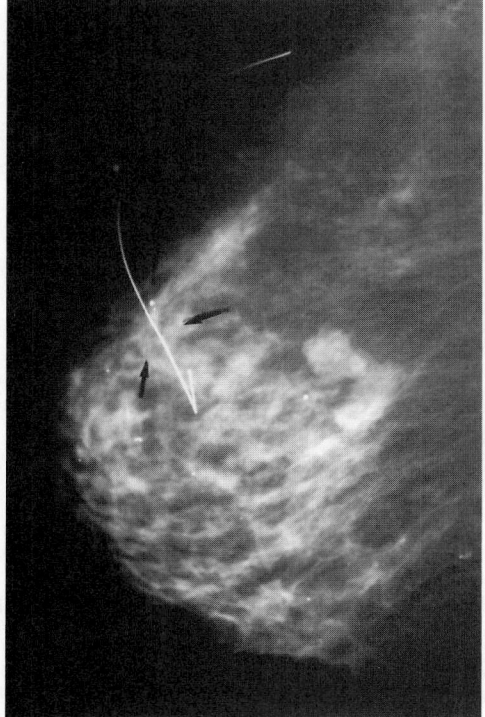

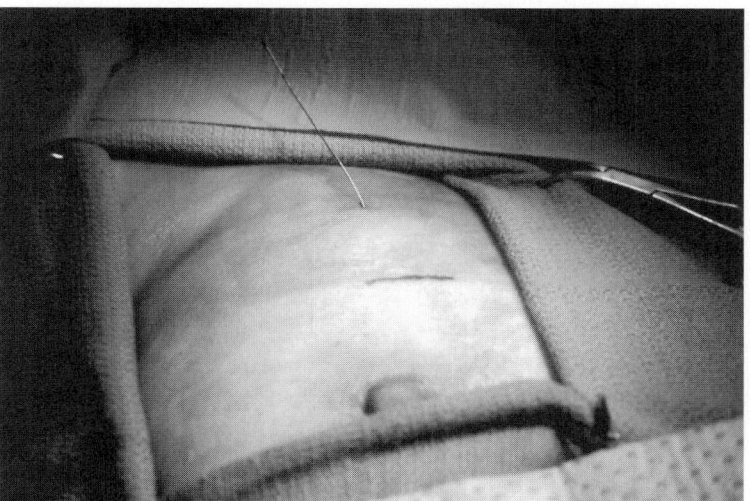

Figure 58.9. Incision placement for needle localization biopsy. *(A)* The mammogram demonstrates that the lesion *(arrow)* is inferior to the point of wire entry. *(B)* Incision placement inferior to wire entry to allow access to the lesion.

Table 58.3. **INDICATIONS FOR SURGICAL BIOPSY AFTER CORE BIOPSY**

Atypical ductal hyperplasia
Radial scar
Lack of concordance between appearance of mammographic lesion and histologic diagnosis
Nondiagnostic specimen (including absence of calcifications on specimen radiograph when biopsy is performed for calcifications)

of this problem. Similarly, radial scar has been found to be associated with coexistent carcinoma in 20% of cases. Lesions suspected of being radial scars are best approached initially with needle localization and excision.

Lack of concordance between the appearance of a mammographic abnormality and the histologic diagnosis obtained with core biopsy is an important indication for surgical biopsy. For example, the finding of a small amount of hyperplasia in a largely fatty specimen would not adequately explain a mass lesion seen on a mammogram. In addition, biopsies that reveal only fat, provide material insufficient for diagnosis, or lack calcifications on specimen radiography (if performed for that indication) must be repeated. An assessment of the cause of an insufficient sample (i.e., superficial location of the lesion, poor targeting, breast too thin for compression) will aid in determining if a repeated core biopsy is appropriate or if surgical excision is needed.

For most mammographic abnormalities, core biopsy is a more cost-effective, less morbid diagnostic technique than needle localization and excision. However, for highly suspect calcifications (BI-RADS category 5) that are suitable for lumpectomy, excision is often the preferred diagnostic approach because core biopsy does not reliably identify invasion and does not enhance the likelihood of achieving negative margins of resection with a single procedure (18,19). The clinical approach to a patient with a mammographic abnormality is summarized in Fig. 58.10.

CLINICAL BREAST PROBLEMS

Most breast complaints that cause a woman to seek medical attention are benign. The purpose of the evaluation of any breast problem is first to determine if it is caused by a benign or malignant condition. If the process is malignant, a prompt diagnosis with sufficient information to plan treatment is the goal. If the process is benign, reassurance and relief of troublesome symptoms are the goals. Clinical breast problems may be divided into the general categories of breast pain, nipple discharge, breast masses, and breast infections. Each is associated with different causes and a different risk for malignancy, and each is considered separately.

Breast Pain

Breast pain is a common problem that is rarely a presenting sign of breast carcinoma. Breast pain may originate from the breast itself or may be referred from extramammary structures, such as the ribs, vertebrae, or occasionally the teeth. Clinically, breast pain can be divided into two categories, cyclic and noncyclic, on the basis of its relationship to the menstrual cycle. Cyclic breast pain waxes and wanes with the menstrual cycle, is frequently bilateral, and often involves the upper outer quadrants of the breasts with radiation to the axillae or down the arms. Although the pain tends to be most severe immediately before the menses, it may persist throughout the month. In contrast, noncyclic pain occurs in postmenopausal women or, when seen in premenopausal women, bears no relationship to the menstrual cycle. Noncyclic pain is more commonly unilateral, localized, and described as sharp and stabbing or burning.

No specific hormonal abnormalities or histologic correlates have been identified in women with breast pain. However, the problem is clearly hormonally related because it affects premenopausal women much more frequently than their postmenopausal counterparts. Breast pain is often precipitated by hormonal change, and a history of menstrual irregularity, new medication, and emo-

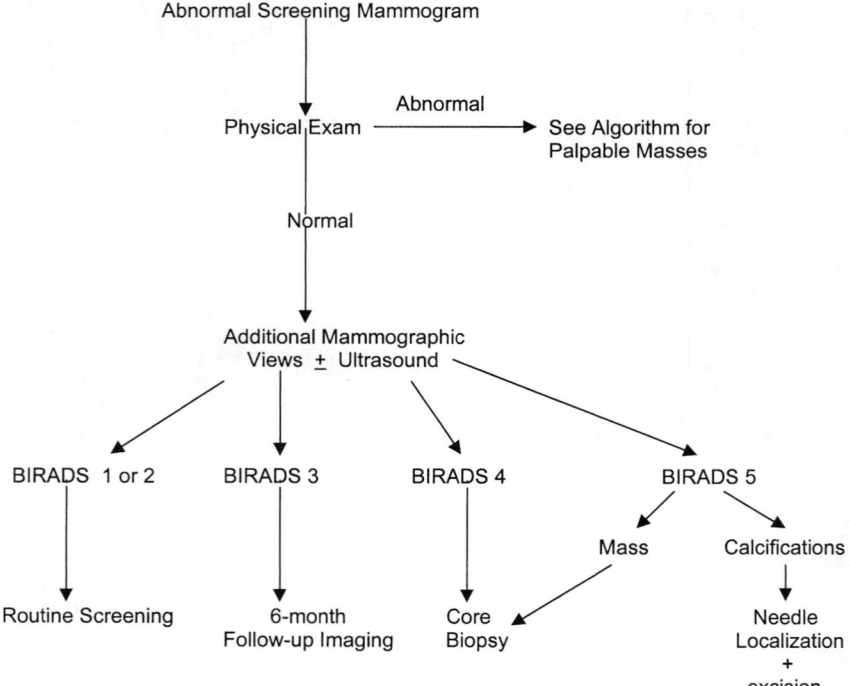

Figure 58.10. Algorithm for the management of mammographically detected breast lesions. A careful physical examination and a diagnostic imaging work-up must be performed before a decision is made about the need for biopsy. *BI-RADS,* breast imaging, reporting, and data system.

tional stress should be sought. In the evaluation, it is important to ascertain whether fear of an underlying cancer or the need for pain relief is the patient's primary concern. In almost all cases, fear of cancer predominates. A careful physical examination should be performed to exclude a specific cause of the pain. Noncyclic mastalgia is occasionally secondary to the presence of a fibroadenoma or cyst and may be relieved by treatment of the underlying lesion. In women age 35 and older, a mammogram is usually part of the evaluation of breast pain unless one has been obtained within the preceding year. In younger women, imaging is not usually necessary unless a palpable mass is present. In the vast majority of women with breast pain, examination and mammography demonstrate no evidence of breast disease. In these cases, reassurance that a malignancy is not the cause of the pain and a discussion of the normal physiology of the breast are usually all that is necessary. In the patient with persistent, localized pain, serial physical examinations should be carried out to exclude the presence of carcinoma.

Approximately 5% of patients have disabling breast pain requiring further treatment. The only drug approved by the Food and Drug Administration for the treatment of breast pain is the antigonadotropin danazol (Danocrine). Randomized controlled trials have demonstrated a response rate of approximately 50% for cyclical pain at doses of 100 to 400 mg (20). However, danazol is recommended only for the most severe, activity-limiting pain because of its side effects, which include menstrual irregularity, acne, weight gain, and hirsutism; these develop in approximately 20% of cases. Before they begin therapy with danazol, patients should be asked to document the frequency and severity of their pain on a daily basis for one to two menstrual cycles because the high spontaneous remission rate of breast pain makes evaluating the response to therapy difficult. Also suggested to be beneficial in the treatment of breast pain are vitamins E and B_6, diuretics, and avoidance of caffeine. However, controlled clinical trials have failed to demonstrate a reduction in symptoms with these measures (21–23). Evening primrose oil, which contains the long-chain fatty acid γ-linolenic acid, has also been proposed as therapy for cyclic breast pain, but clear evidence of its efficacy is lacking. Surgery should be avoided, even for apparently localized pain, as it rarely results in long-term pain relief.

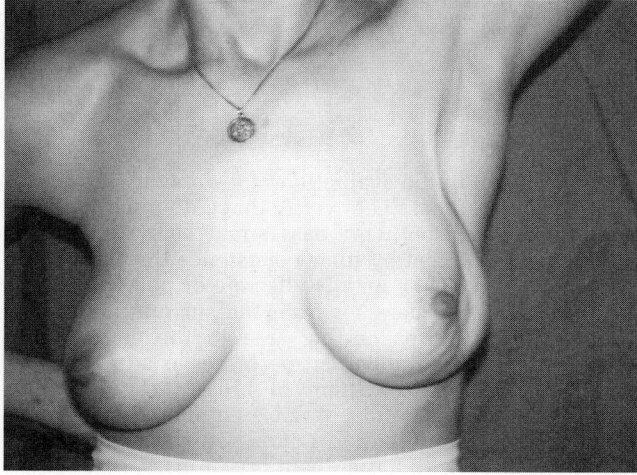

Figure 58.11. Mondor's disease. Thrombophlebitis of the thoracoepigastric vein causes retraction of the lateral portion of the breast, which crosses to the midline at the inferior areolar margin and is accompanied by a palpable cord.

Mondor's disease, or thrombophlebitis of the lateral thoracic or superior thoracoepigastric vein, is an uncommon cause of breast pain that is readily identified clinically by the presence of a tender subcutaneous cord in the lateral aspect of the breast. Skin retraction may be associated (Fig. 58.11), which raises concern about the presence of carcinoma. Mondor's disease may develop secondary to trauma, surgical procedures on the breast, such as biopsy or reduction mammoplasty, or breast irradiation. In approximately 50% of cases, no predisposing condition can be identified. Mondor's disease is occasionally seen in women with a nonpalpable breast cancer (24), and for this reason, a mammogram should be obtained in women age 35 and older who present with the condition. Mondor's disease resolves spontaneously and requires no specific therapy, although antiinflammatory agents may be used for pain relief.

Nipple Discharge

Evaluation

Nipple discharge is a common complaint, but an uncommon sign of breast carcinoma. Between 3% and 11% of women with carcinoma have an associated nipple discharge. Overall, in approximately 95% of women presenting with nipple discharge, the cause is benign. The likelihood that a nipple discharge is secondary to malignancy increases with age. In one study, 32% of women over the age of 60 who presented with nipple discharge and no mass had carcinoma, compared with 7% of women under age 60 with the same presentation (25). The initial step in the evaluation of nipple discharge is to determine whether it is physiologic or pathologic. Discharges are classified as pathologic if they are spontaneous and localized to one duct. Pathologic discharges may be bloody or serous and are almost always unilateral. In contrast, physiologic discharges occur only with nipple compression, frequently originate from multiple ducts, and are often bilateral. Fluid can be expressed from the nipples of approximately 80% of premenopausal women, and if the remainder of the breast examination is normal, patients with physiologic discharge should be advised to stop squeezing their nipples and be assured that no further therapy is needed. The clinical evaluation of a pathologic discharge should include testing the fluid for occult blood and identifying the quadrant of the breast from which the discharge originates. Although 70% to 85% of the discharges associated with carcinoma contain blood (26), a nonbloody discharge that meets the other criteria of a pathologic discharge is an indication for breast biopsy. Cytology is not usually useful in the evaluation of nipple discharge because the absence of malignant cells does not reliably exclude carcinoma, and positive cytologic findings do not differentiate between intraductal and invasive carcinoma. In one study, the sensitivity of nipple fluid cytology for the diagnosis of malignancy was only 46.5% (27).

As part of the evaluation of a pathologic discharge, a mammogram should be obtained to look for nonpalpable masses, calcifications, or dilated ducts. When a discharge is associated with a mass, the mass should be evaluated by biopsy. In the absence of a mass, a terminal duct excision should be performed. The role of galactography in the management of nipple discharge is controversial. Ductal lesions can be readily visualized in many women (Fig. 58.12), but biopsy is still required to determine whether they are benign or malignant, and a normal galactogram in a woman with a pathologic discharge does not reliably exclude the presence of significant ductal disease (28). Galactography may be useful in identifying lesions in the

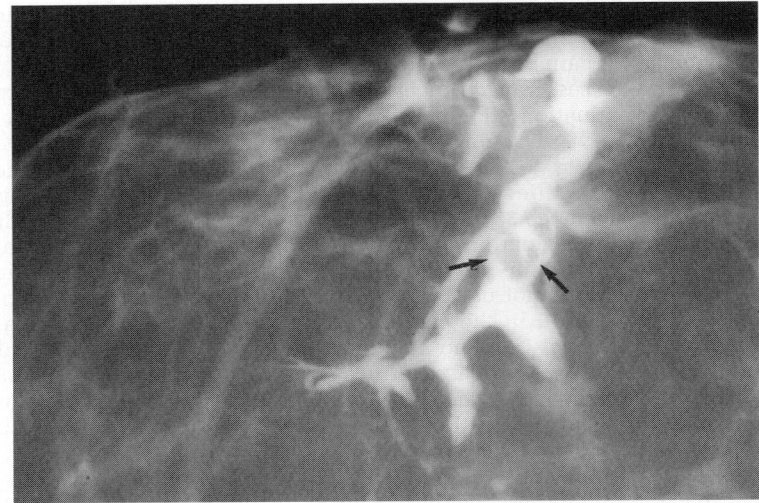

Figure 58.12. Ductogram. A large defect *(arrow)* represents an intraductal papilloma.

periphery of the breast that would not be removed with a standard terminal duct excision, and in minimizing the portion of the ductal system that is removed in women of childbearing age.

The evaluation of galactorrhea, defined as the nonpuerperal discharge of milky fluid from both nipples, differs significantly from that of other forms of nipple discharge. Galactorrhea is not a sign of primary breast pathology and should prompt a work-up to exclude an underlying endocrine disorder. It should be noted that milk may be intermittently secreted for as long as 2 years after breastfeeding has stopped, and this type of galactorrhea is not suggestive of endocrine disease. Galactorrhea may be secondary to a variety of amenorrhea syndromes that result in hyperprolactinemia. In addition, it may be secondary to hypothyroidism, pituitary adenoma, or chest trauma (including thoracotomy). A variety of medications, including oral contraceptives, phenothiazines, tricyclic antidepressants, metoclopramide, and reserpine, also cause galactorrhea. Persistent galactorrhea in a patient not taking any of these medications should be evaluated with measurement of the prolactin level. A persistently elevated prolactin level should prompt a search for a pituitary adenoma. Patients with galactorrhea and no evidence of an endocrine abnormality may be followed without intervention.

Etiology

The most common cause of pathologic discharge identified in surgical specimens is a solitary papilloma. These lesions, which develop in the major subareolar ducts, consist of an epithelial layer covering a fibrovascular stroma. They are attached to the duct wall by a stalk. Their location in the subareolar region makes them readily amenable to removal with a terminal duct excision. Peripheral papillomas are a distinctly different clinical entity, in which multiple papillomas develop in the peripheral ducts of the breast. These lesions rarely produce nipple discharge and are most likely to present as a palpable mass (29). Ductal ectasia may also cause nipple discharge, although this discharge is classically thick and cheesy, resembling "toothpaste." Ductal ectasia appears to be associated with aging, being most common in women age 50 and older. Nipple retraction may occur if the ducts are shortened and mimic carcinoma. The discharge of ductal ectasia is sometimes mistaken for an infectious process, but the ducts are usually sterile (30). Carcinoma is an uncommon cause of nipple discharge. When nipple discharge is the only presenting sign of malignancy, ductal carcinoma in situ is the most common cause. Invasive carcinoma presenting as discharge alone is rare.

Management

When a pathologic discharge has been identified, terminal duct excision, also called *microdochectomy,* is the appropriate management. Exceptions to this rule include women with a single, nonreproducible episode of discharge and normal mammographic findings and women with bloody nipple discharge during pregnancy.

Terminal duct excision is carried out through a circumareolar incision that includes no more than half of the circumference of the areola. It is critical that duct removal begin on the dermal surface of the nipple, as ductal disease often occurs in the proximal duct. Usually, a dilated duct can be visualized after the subareolar space has been entered and can be excised to a depth of 2 to 3 cm in the breast parenchyma. When the duct is transected distally, it should be carefully observed for discharge, which indicates that the ductal pathology is more distal in the breast. When no dilated duct is visualized, the entire central core of ductal tissue should be removed. No attempt to reapproximate the defect in the breast after terminal duct excision should be made, as this will often distort the breast contour. Patients should be warned that some nipple sensation may be lost after the procedure, in addition to the ability to breast-feed.

Breast Masses

Definition

The first step in the evaluation of a woman with a complaint of a breast mass is to verify that a dominant mass is actually present. Dominant masses may be cystic or solid and are characterized by their persistence throughout the menstrual cycle. They may be discrete or poorly defined, but they differ in character from the surrounding breast tissue and the corresponding area in the contralateral breast. Often, what the patient perceives as a breast mass is actually a normal variant of breast tissue. In premenopausal women, the normal glandular tissue of the breast is nodular, and patients often confuse such nodular glandular tissue with a dominant breast mass. Nodularity, particularly when it waxes and wanes during the menstrual cycle, is a physiologic process and not a predictor of breast disease. Morrow et al. (31) reviewed 605 women younger than 40 years of age who were referred for evaluation of a breast mass. Only 36% of the 484 masses detected by patient self-examination and 29% of the 121 masses detected by a primary care provider were confirmed surgically. The differential diagnosis of a palpable breast mass includes macrocyst, fibroadenoma, prominent areas of fibrocystic change, fat necrosis, and carcinoma.

Cysts

Cysts are a common cause of dominant breast masses, with a peak incidence in women in their 40s and perimenopausal years. Cysts are thought to result from cystic lobular involution; acini within the lobule distend to form microcysts, which in turn give rise to macrocysts. Clinically evident macrocysts are estimated to develop in 7% of Western women.

Cysts are usually well demarcated from the surrounding breast tissue, mobile, and firm. It is often difficult to distinguish a cystic from a solid lesion on physical examination, although cysts may fluctuate with the menstrual cycle, whereas solid lesions do not. Cystic lesions in postmenopausal women who are not on hormone replacement therapy are uncommon, and they should be regarded with a higher degree of suspicion than those found in premenopausal women because they may be secondary to ductal obstruction by a malignant lesion.

The initial step in the evaluation of a possible cyst is aspiration. If fluid is obtained that is not grossly bloody and the mass resolves completely, no further therapy other than a follow-up examination is needed. However, if the cystic fluid is bloody, the palpable abnormality does not resolve completely, or the same cyst recurs multiple times in a short time period, a biopsy to exclude the presence of a malignant lesion in the cyst wall is required. Cytologic examination of cyst fluid is of little value because intracystic carcinoma is rare and malignant cells are seen in fewer than 1% of cases (32). The presence of atypical cells, an indication for surgical biopsy, is not uncommon when cyst fluid is examined, and it may pose a dilemma when a patient's cyst has resolved with aspiration and the examination and mammographic findings are now normal.

Many patients present to the surgeon with a palpable mass and an ultrasonographic examination demonstrating that the mass is a simple cyst. If the cyst is symptomatic or alarming to the patient, it can be aspirated. Otherwise, because the diagnosis has been made, it can be left alone. Nonpalpable lesions which are proven to be simple cysts by ultrasonography do not require aspiration. The management of cystic lesions is summarized in Fig. 58.13. A dominant breast mass should not be dismissed as a cyst unless the diagnosis is confirmed by ultrasonography or cyst aspiration.

Solid Masses

Fibroadenomas. Fibroadenomas present most frequently in patients between the ages of 20 and 50 years. Their characteristic clinical presentation is that of a well-defined palpable mass that is rubbery in texture and mobile. Fibroadenomas are usually solitary, but they present as multiple lesions in 10% to 15% of cases. Although they have a characteristic clinical appearance, a clinical diagnosis of fibroadenoma is accurate in only one half to two thirds of cases (33). However, in women younger than age 20, fibroadenomas account for 75% of breast biopsies.

Fibroadenomas are thought to be the result of a minor aberration in the normal process of lobular development. Hormonal factors appear to be important in their growth, as evidenced by the clinical observation of the involution of fibroadenomas after menopause and their dramatic increase in size during pregnancy. In postmenopausal women receiving estrogen alone, fibroadenomas may increase in size relative to the surrounding breast parenchyma.

Sonographic criteria for the diagnosis of fibroadenoma include a round or oval, well-circumscribed, solid mass with homogeneous, low-level internal echoes and intermediate acoustic attenuation. However, as many as 30% of fibroadenomas lack these "classic" features.

In rare circumstances, fibroadenomas have been associated with carcinoma. More than 160 cases of associated cancers have been reported in the literature, including

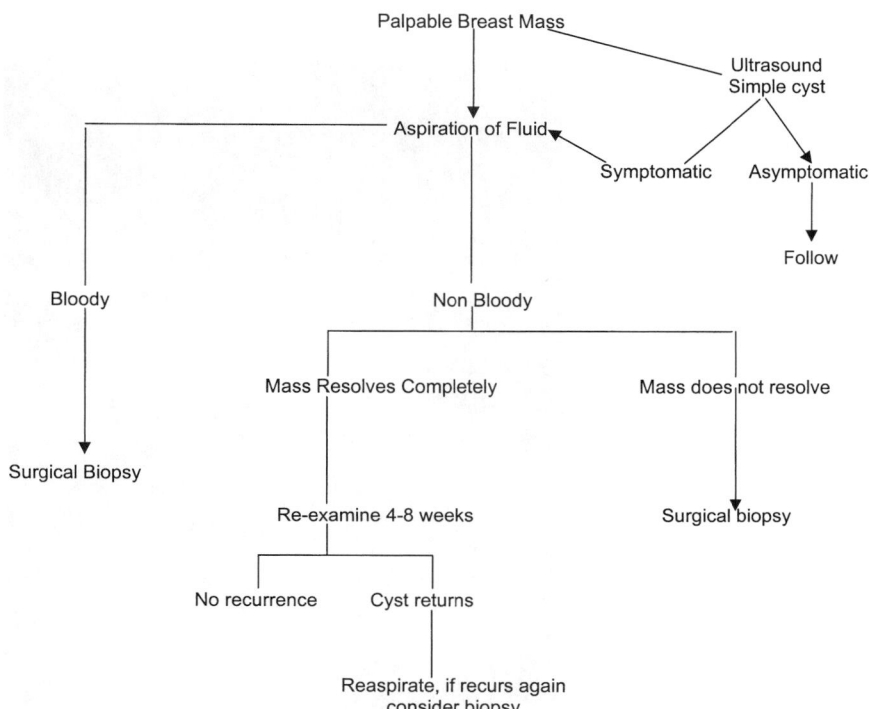

Figure 58.13. Algorithm for the management of cystic lesions. Bloody fluid on aspiration, failure of the mass to resolve completely, and prompt refilling of the same cyst are indications for surgical biopsy.

ductal carcinoma in situ and infiltrating lobular and ductal carcinomas. Historically, it has been widely accepted that fibroadenomas do not confer an increased breast cancer risk. However, four population-based retrospective studies have shown a small (relative risk of 1.3 to 1.9) but significant increased risk for breast cancer development that persists over time (34–37). This slight increase in risk should have no impact on the clinical management of fibroadenomas. Although fibroadenomas can be suspected on the basis of their characteristic clinical presentation, a final diagnosis cannot be made without histologic or cytologic confirmation.

Fibrocystic Disease. *Fibrocystic disease* is a common term that is used to describe a variety of benign breast disorders. It is not a clinically meaningful term because it encompasses a heterogeneous group of processes, some pathologic and some physiologic, with widely varying cancer risks. The cancer risks associated with benign breast disease are discussed in the section on breast cancer risk factors. The term *fibrocystic change* is not a synonym for lumpy breasts, and if used at all, it should be reserved for women in whom a breast biopsy has demonstrated one of the histologic components of fibrocystic change. Frequently, when a breast biopsy is performed for vague areas of nodularity that lack mammographic or ultrasonographic correlates, a fibrocystic process is the diagnosis.

Fat Necrosis. Fat necrosis in the breast may occur secondary to trauma, breast surgery, infection, or radiation therapy, although in approximately 50% of cases, no antecedent cause can be identified. Fat necrosis is seen most commonly in women with pendulous breasts and those who are overweight. It is clinically significant in that on both physical examination and mammography, it may be indistinguishable from carcinoma. The lesions of fat necrosis are typically firm, painless, and poorly defined. Because fat necrosis usually occurs in the superficial breast tissue, it may be accompanied by skin thickening, dimpling, or retraction. The mammographic findings of fat necrosis include spiculated masses, microcalcifications,

and architectural distortion. Only when the characteristic oil cyst, a circumscribed mass of mixed soft-tissue density and fat with a rim that is often calcified, is seen can an unequivocal diagnosis of fat necrosis be made radiographically (Fig. 58.14). In the absence of this finding or a clear history of trauma, biopsy is required to exclude the presence of malignancy.

Diagnostic Imaging. When a clinical abnormality has been identified in a woman over age 40, a diagnostic mammogram should be obtained before a histologic diagnosis is attempted. Imaging studies are used to define the extent of a potential malignancy and to identify nonpalpable masses or associated calcifications elsewhere in the ipsilateral or contralateral breast that might influence definitive therapy. The decision to perform a biopsy, however, is based on the clinical determination that a dominant mass is present, and nonvisualization of a mass on imaging studies should not dissuade the surgeon from performing a breast biopsy. Even in recent reports, between 9% and 22% of patients with palpable breast cancer had tumors that were not visible by mammography (38–40). Obtaining a diagnostic, rather than a screening, mammogram ensures that a marker will be placed on the area of palpable concern, so that the clinical and radiographic findings can be correlated. Identifying the site of a lesion also ensures that lesions at the periphery of the breast will be included on the film, which helps to eliminate one cause of false-negative mammograms. A diagnostic mammogram also includes magnification views of the lesion, which are useful in determining the extent of any associated calcifications.

The routine use of ultrasonography for the evaluation of solid palpable masses remains controversial. Studies of high-resolution ultrasonography have demonstrated that the technique is more accurate and sensitive and has a better negative predictive value than mammography alone (41). If follow-up of a clinically benign lesion is being considered, ultrasonography is a useful adjunct to mammography, as discussed in the section on the clinical approach to the patient with a solid breast mass. In the patient with a clinically suspect mass who will undergo biopsy regardless of the results of imaging studies, ultrasonography has

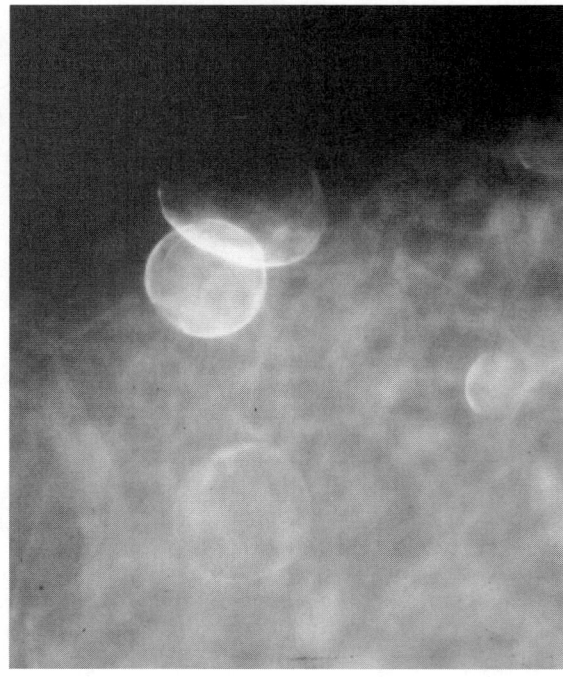

Figure 58.14. Oil cysts. The calcified rims of these cysts in a patient with a history of trauma are diagnostic.

been shown to provide a more accurate estimate of lesion size than mammography (42), and it may also identify satellite lesions not seen on mammography. Ultrasonography is also useful in the woman with a palpable mass that is not clearly seen on mammography; in such cases, it may help to define the extent of the lesion more completely than physical examination alone.

In women under age 40 presenting with a clinically unworrisome breast mass, the rationale for mammographic imaging is less compelling because carcinoma is uncommon and the density of the breasts often obscures mass lesions. Directed ultrasonography allows the presence of a true mass lesion to be confirmed when the significance of a physical finding is clinically uncertain (31). The presence of benign characteristics on ultrasonography also supports the use of a follow-up approach. In younger women with clinically suspect masses, mammography should be performed.

Other Imaging Studies. Magnetic resonance imaging (MRI) of the breast is increasingly being used for clinical breast imaging, although the lack of standardization of the procedure, the inability to sample lesions seen on MRI alone in most centers, and the high cost of MRI have limited its application. In addition, large-scale clinical trials to document its sensitivity and specificity have not been carried out. However, small studies suggest that MRI may be of value in determining the extent of a cancer within the breast (43), evaluating the response of a tumor to preoperative chemotherapy, and detecting recurrence in patients treated with breast-conserving therapy (44). The technique in which the differential uptake of gadolinium contrast is used to distinguish benign from malignant breast lesions has received a great deal of attention, but further work is required to demonstrate sufficient accuracy to avoid a tissue diagnosis. At present, the only routine clinical applications of MRI in most centers are to detect an implant rupture and to look for a primary breast tumor in patients presenting with axillary adenopathy caused by metastatic tumor from an unknown primary site (see section on occult primary tumor presenting with nodal metastases).

Nuclear imaging of breast lesions with technetium 99m sestamibi has also been studied. In a report of 389 patients, including 182 who had palpable abnormalities, sestamibi scanning identified 90% of the cancers, with a 3% false-negative rate and a 7% false-positive rate (45). However, a study of 31 nonpalpable lesions reported a sensitivity of only 29%, with a specificity of 83% (46). The effectiveness of sestamibi in identifying small mass lesions and calcifications is unclear, and its role in clinical breast management is undefined.

Positron emission tomography (PET) can be used not only to image breast abnormalities but also to assess their metabolic activity for diagnostic and prognostic purposes. At this time, its use remains experimental.

Biopsy Techniques for Solid Breast Masses. A variety of biopsy techniques are available to obtain a pathologic diagnosis of clinically evident breast masses. Each has advantages and disadvantages, and no single technique is applicable to all clinical circumstances.

Fine-needle Aspiration Biopsy. Fine-needle aspiration (FNA) cytology has a very high diagnostic accuracy rate in the hands of experienced clinicians and cytopathologists. In a review of 31,340 procedures (47), its sensitivity ranged from 65% to 98%. In most series, false-positive rates are less than 1%, false-negative rates are below 10%, and the incidence of insufficient specimens ranges from 4% to 13%. Small tumor size, fibrotic tumors, and certain histologic tumor types, such as infiltrating lobular, tubular, and cribriform carcinoma, have been associated with a higher likelihood of false-negative results. Most false-negative results are the consequence of sampling errors rather than misinterpretation by the cytopathologist, and in one series, physician experience was the factor that correlated best with a low rate of insufficient specimens (48).

The advantages of FNA include its simplicity and quickness, relatively low cost, and availability as an office procedure. In addition, associated morbidity is low, smears can be interpreted immediately, and patient discomfort is minimal. Results can be available in 24 hours, and because an unequivocal diagnosis of malignancy by FNA is reliable, treatment options can be discussed with the patient and definitive surgery can be performed without the need for a surgical biopsy. However, it is imperative that the surgeon be aware of the meaning of positive cytology at a particular institution, as the sensitivities of FNA at institutions that do not have access to an experienced cytopathologist may not be as high as those reported in the literature. A disadvantage of FNA is that it cannot distinguish invasive from intraductal carcinoma, so that overtreatment of gross ductal carcinoma in situ (DCIS) is possible. However, because fewer than 2% of palpable breast masses are pure DCIS, this is an infrequent problem. The other disadvantage of FNA is that a cytopathologist may not be available in all institutions. Because FNA does not provide histologic detail, pathologists are encouraged to stratify their malignant diagnoses into "definite" and "probable" malignancy, with only an unequivocal diagnosis of malignancy supporting definitive therapy. In the "probable" malignancy group, histologic confirmation is required to avoid false-positive results and also to recognize carcinomas in situ and low-grade carcinomas, which require special clinical management. Aspirates with insufficient cellular material for interpretation are an indication for a repeated FNA or an alternative type of biopsy. The management of breast lesions on the basis of FNA results is summarized in Table 58.4.

Core Needle Biopsy. Core needle biopsy is another office diagnostic technique that is rapid, inexpensive, and relatively painless. A core needle biopsy differs from FNA in that a core of tissue is obtained for histologic examination, so that a more detailed characterization of the lesion is possible and the adequacy of the specimen can be evaluated at the time of the biopsy. In addition, the material can be evaluated by any surgical pathologist. In one series in which the diagnostic accuracy of aspiration cytology was compared with core needle biopsy in 81 patients who had breast masses, aspiration cytology was diagnostic in 95% of cases, and core needle biopsy was diagnostic in 70% of the cases in which it was used (49). False-negative results occur when the needle is deflected into the surrounding fat by a hard tumor mass. In practice, the selection of the type of needle biopsy (FNA or core) often depends on the availability of a cytopathologist and the

---

Table 58.4. MANAGEMENT OF BREAST MASSES BASED ON FINE-NEEDLE ASPIRATION DIAGNOSIS

FNA diagnosis	Treatment
Malignant	Definitive therapy
Suspicious	Surgical biopsy
Atypia	Surgical biopsy
Benign	Possible observation[a]
Nondiagnostic	Repeated FNA or surgical biopsy

[a]See discussion in text on clinical approach to the patient with a solid breast mass.

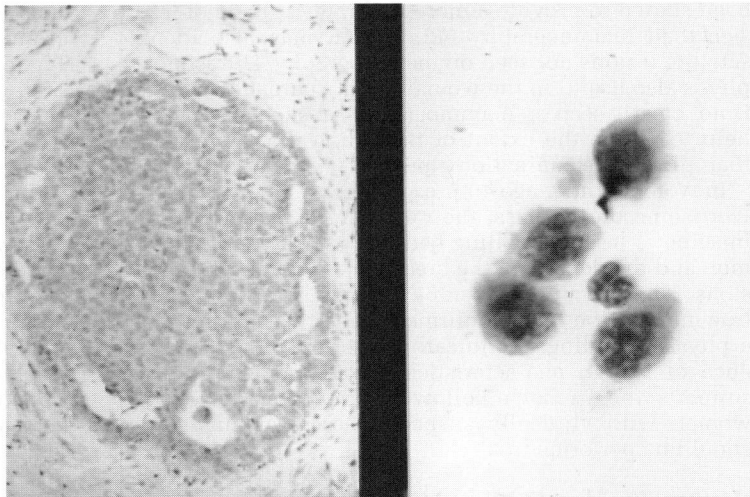

Figure 58.15. Comparison of fine-needle aspiration specimen and core needle biopsy specimen. Architectural detail is seen only in the core specimen.

surgeon's level of comfort with a cytologic diagnosis of malignancy without further histologic detail. The difference between an FNA specimen and a core needle specimen is illustrated in Fig. 58.15.

Excisional Biopsy. Excisional biopsy is the complete removal of a breast mass. It is definitive therapy for a benign breast mass and may also serve as a therapeutic lumpectomy if the specimen includes a margin of normal breast tissue around a malignant tumor. Kearney and Morrow (50) obtained negative margins with a conservative diagnostic lumpectomy in 161 of 173 (93.1%) consecutive patients. The adequacy of a biopsy specimen cannot be assessed unless the margins of the specimen are inked. The use of orienting sutures in two margins of the specimen makes it possible to identify which margin contains tumor should the excision be incomplete; as a result, less normal breast tissue has to be removed in a repeated excision. In this era of breast-conserving surgery, orientation and inking of excisional breast biopsy specimens should be routine practice.

Excisional biopsy is an outpatient procedure that can usually be carried out under local anesthesia with intravenous sedation as needed. Excisional biopsy is usually planned as a two-step procedure, (i.e., excisional biopsy with additional therapy at a later date if required). This allows for a detailed review of the pathology and a discussion of treatment options with the patient, in addition to consultation with a radiation oncologist or reconstructive surgeon as desired by the patient. Delays of up to 1 month from the time of diagnosis to definitive therapy have not been shown to affect prognosis (51); therefore, the two-step procedure is the preferred method of management.

Incisional Biopsy. Incisional biopsy is a diagnostic procedure reserved for masses that are too large to be completely excised. Today, the indications for incisional biopsy are few because FNA or core needle biopsy can be used to make a diagnosis of breast cancer with less morbidity and at lower cost. The widespread availability of immunohistochemistry allows hormone receptor status to be determined and tumor markers to be studied in core specimens or cytologic aspirates.

Clinical Approach to the Patient with a Solid Breast Mass. The accuracy of physical examination alone to detect carcinoma is limited because the clinical characteristics of benign and malignant masses are not absolute, and a clinical diagnosis is correct in only 60% to 85% of cases (49,52). The difficulty of distinguishing benign from malignant lesions is greatest in young women, and the use of

other studies to confirm the clinical diagnosis of a benign breast mass is essential before the patient is returned to routine follow-up.

The extent of the work-up necessary to exclude the presence of carcinoma varies with the degree of suspicion and the age of the patient. In the patient with a clinically suspect mass regardless of age, diagnostic mammography and ultrasonography should be performed before a histologic diagnosis is sought. A needle biopsy (either aspiration cytology or core biopsy) is the preferred initial method of making a diagnosis, for the reasons discussed in the preceding sections on fine-needle aspiration biopsy and core needle biopsy. If a diagnosis of malignancy is obtained, treatment options are discussed with the patient. If a diagnosis of cancer is not obtained, excisional biopsy is undertaken because of the known false-negative rates of both FNA and core biopsy. This approach is summarized in Fig. 58.16.

In the woman with a clinically benign mass, management varies somewhat with age (Fig. 58.17). In women under age 40, the first step is to determine if the patient wants the mass to be excised, regardless of the likelihood

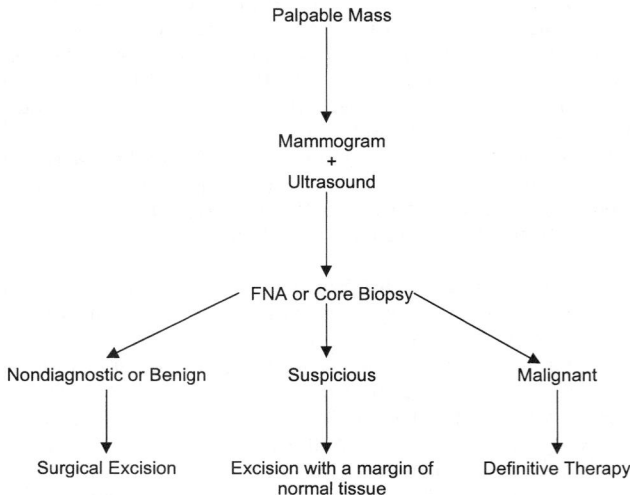

Figure 58.16. Algorithm for the management of the patient with a clinically indeterminate or suspect solid breast mass. In this circumstance, imaging studies are insufficient to exclude malignancy, and tissue sampling is required.

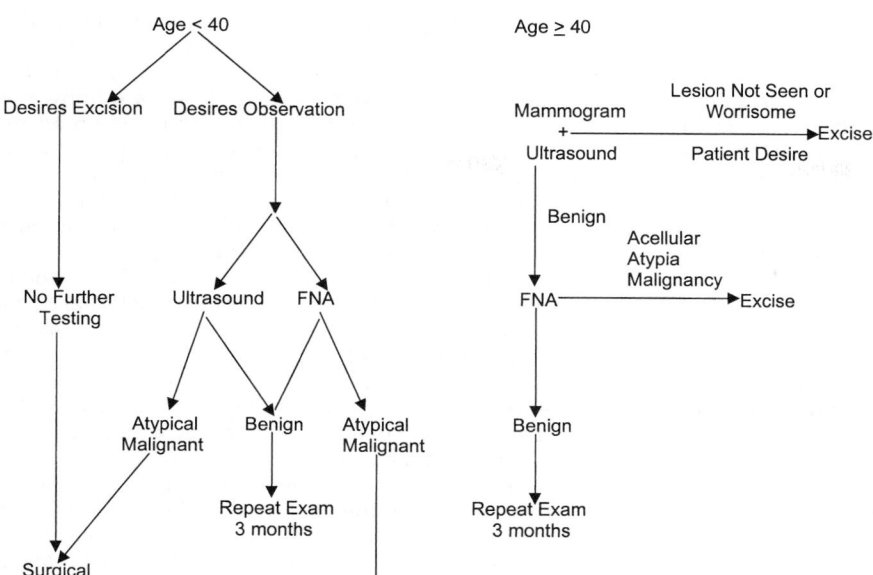

Figure 58.17. Algorithm for the management of clinically benign breast masses. The use of imaging studies varies according to age because carcinoma is infrequent in women under age 40.

of malignancy. If so, imaging studies are not indicated because of the low risk for carcinoma in this age group. For the patient who desires follow-up, ultrasonography and FNA should be performed. If both confirm that the lesion has benign features, clinical follow-up can be undertaken, with regular monitoring of the lesion for a period of 1 to 2 years to confirm that carcinoma is not present. The combination of clinical examination, FNA, and ultrasonography provides an accurate differentiation between benign and malignant lesions in 95% of cases (53). For this reason, in addition to the low risk for malignancy in this age group, follow-up is a safe approach.

In patients over age 40, mammography and ultrasonography should be obtained before a decision about the need for excision or follow-up is made. If follow-up is chosen, FNA is also performed. If the mass is visualized on mammography and appears benign, and if the FNA contains benign epithelial cells, the risk for carcinoma ranges from 0.6% to 3.4% (54,55). It must be emphasized that if any elements of the "triple test" cannot be evaluated (i.e., lesion not visualized on imaging studies, aspirate contains only blood and fat), these statistics do not apply. A follow-up approach to new breast lesions in women older than age 40 should be undertaken only by clinicians with experience in the management of breast disease, and patients must be advised of the small, but real, possibility of a delay in the diagnosis of breast carcinoma.

Breast Infections

Breast infections can be classified as lactating or nonlactating. Lactating infections are usually caused by *Staphylococcus aureus,* but they may be secondary to other skin flora. Infection is most common during the first 4 to 6 weeks of breast-feeding or during weaning and is thought to be caused by the proliferation of bacteria in poorly drained breast segments. The most common clinical presentation is cellulitis with fever, pain, redness, and swelling. Antibiotics are the first line of treatment, and breast-feeding should be continued to facilitate drainage of the engorged segment. Tetracycline, chloramphenicol, and ciprofloxacin should be avoided because they enter breast milk. If the infection fails to resolve, an abscess should be considered. When the breast skin is intact, re-

peated aspiration of the abscess combined with antibiotics is the preferred treatment (56). When the skin is thinned, a small incision will facilitate drainage.

In nonlactating women, periductal mastitis is the most common form of breast infection. This syndrome is characterized by periareolar inflammation, which is sometimes associated with a purulent nipple discharge. Periareolar abscess and mammary duct fistulae may develop secondary to this condition. Periductal mastitis usually affects premenopausal women. A number of studies have documented an association between smoking and recurrent periareolar abscess (57,58), although the mechanism by which cigarettes promote infection is unclear. Antibiotics that provide coverage for aerobic and anaerobic bacteria should be used in patients with periareolar inflammation without abscess formation. Abscesses can be treated with aspiration. For patients with recurrent episodes of infection, terminal duct excision is indicated.

Peripheral breast abscesses, which are less common than periareolar infections, should be treated with aspiration or incision and drainage. In any patient with a breast infection, the possibility of an underlying malignancy should be considered. A biopsy should be performed on any apparent "infection" that fails to respond to appropriate antibiotics and drainage to exclude the presence of an underlying carcinoma.

RISK FACTORS FOR BREAST CANCER

Breast cancer is the most common cancer in American women, and the second most common cause of cancer death. The disease is a major cause of cancer death in most industrialized nations. Approximately 180,000 cases of breast cancer and 44,000 breast cancer deaths occur annually in American women. Although the cause of breast cancer is unknown, many factors that increase the risk for the development of breast cancer have been identified. An understanding of breast cancer risk has assumed new importance for clinicians since the approval of tamoxifen for use to reduce breast cancer risk in high-risk women (see section on management of the high-risk woman). One of the difficulties in understanding risk arises from the different ways that risk is expressed. Risk may be described as a lifetime risk (the likelihood that breast cancer will develop in a woman if she lives to a given age, usually 70 to 90 years) or as an absolute risk within a given time interval (e.g., 2.5% during the next 5 years). Risk may also be expressed as a relative risk, a comparison of the incidence of disease in a population having a particular risk factor with the incidence in a population lacking that risk factor. Understanding the clinical implications of relative risk requires a knowledge of the absolute risk of breast cancer in the index population. For this reason, it is not a particularly useful way of discussing risk clinically. Risk information is best provided to patients as absolute risk within a given time period.

Age

The most common breast cancer risk factor is age. Half of a woman's lifetime risk for breast cancer development occurs after age 65. Between the ages of 35 to 55, the risk for breast cancer development is only 2.5%, and the risk for breast cancer death is only about one third of that (59). The incidence of breast cancer across age groups has been fairly stable. The perception of an epidemic of breast cancer in young women is the consequence of an increase in the number of young women at risk, which has resulted in an increase in the number of cases seen but no change in incidence. Breast cancer at a young age is more common in black women than in white women. At 40, the incidence curves cross, and the disease becomes more common in white women (60).

Family History

It is now recognized that two distinct types of risk are associated with a family history of breast carcinoma. Approximately 20% to 30% of women with breast cancer have a family history of the disease (61), but only 5% to 10% have an inherited mutation in a breast cancer susceptibility gene (62). Distinguishing between familial and true hereditary breast cancer is important because the level of risk associated with these conditions varies widely.

The majority of cases of genetic breast cancer are caused by mutations of BRCA1 and BRCA2. Mutations of either of these genes carry a lifetime risk for breast cancer development of 37% to 85% (62–64), a high risk of contralateral breast cancer, and an increased risk for ovarian cancer. Although the risk for ovarian cancer is elevated with mutations of both BRCA1 and BRCA2, it is greater in carriers of the BRCA1 mutation. The risk for prostate cancer is also increased in these families. These mutations can be inherited from both maternal and paternal relatives, and an increased risk for male breast cancer is noted in carriers of the BRCA2 mutation. These risks are summarized in Table 58.5. The carrier frequency of these mutations varies with the population under study. The frequency of BRCA1 mutations is between 1/500 and 1/800, and the frequency of BRCA2 mutations is lower in the general population.

However, in persons of Ashkenazi Jewish descent, two specific mutations of BRCA1 (185 del AG and 5382 ins C) and one BRCA2 mutation (6174 del T) are seen with a background frequency of 2.3% (64). These are known as *founder mutations,* thought to arise from common ancestry, and have been identified in other ethnic populations in Iceland, France, Russia, Holland, and Belgium.

Characteristics suggestive of mutations in BRCA1 or BRCA2 include having multiple relatives affected with breast or ovarian cancer, or both, with involvement of two or more generations in a pattern consistent with autosomal dominant inheritance. This can be through maternal or paternal relatives. Other suggestive features include a predominance of early-onset cancers and the occurrence of more than one primary cancer (such as breast and ovarian or bilateral breast). A typical pedigree is shown in Fig. 58.18. The likelihood of a mutation varies with family history, age, and ethnic ancestry. For example, in an Ashkenazi Jewish family with two cases of breast cancer and one case of ovarian cancer, the chance of a BRCA1 mutation is 75%, but in a non-Ashkenazi family with the same history, the probability is only 33% (65). Models have been developed to assist clinicians in estimating the probability of a mutation (65).

Genetic testing for mutations of BRCA1 and BRCA2 is now a commercially available option for women with a family history suggestive of a genetic mutation. Genetic testing should always be preceded by a counseling session in which the complexities of genetic testing and the potential emotional and financial ramifications of test results are discussed. The information obtained from testing will be maximized by first testing a family member affected with breast or ovarian cancer, or both. If the affected person does not carry a mutation, testing an unaffected relative is unlikely to be informative.

Other, infrequent genetic breast cancer syndromes include the Li-Fraumeni syndrome, Cowden's syndrome, and the Muir-Torre syndrome. The most common of these is the Li-Fraumeni syndrome, which is associated with mutations in the tumor-suppressor gene *p53*. Clinically, the Li-Fraumeni syndrome is an autosomal dominant condition characterized by soft-tissue sarcomas, osteosarcomas, brain tumors, leukemia, adrenocortical malignancies, and early-onset breast cancer (66).

For the majority of women with a family history of breast cancer that is not associated with an inherited mutation, the level of risk is much lower and rarely exceeds 30% (67).

Hormonal Factors

Numerous studies have linked breast cancer risk to age at menarche, menopause, and first pregnancy. The increased number of ovulatory cycles associated with early menarche, nulliparity, and late menopause appears to be

---

Table 58.5. ESTIMATED LIFETIME CANCER RISKS FOR BRCA1 AND BRCA2 MUTATIONS

Type of cancer	Risk in general population (%)	Risk in BRCA1 carrier (%)	Risk in BRCA2 carrier (%)
Breast cancer	12.5	55–85	37–85
Contralateral breast cancer	0.5–1/year	Up to 65	Similar to that for BRCA1
Male breast cancer	Very rare	Rare	Approximately 6
Ovarian cancer	1.4	15–60	15–27
Ovarian cancer after breast biopsy	2–3	30–55	Elevated

Modified from Isaacs C, Peshkin BN, Lerman C. Evaluation and management of women with a strong family history of breast cancer. In: Harris JR, Lippman ME, Morrow M, et al., eds. Diseases of the breast. Philadelphia: Lippincott Williams & Wilkins, 2000:241.

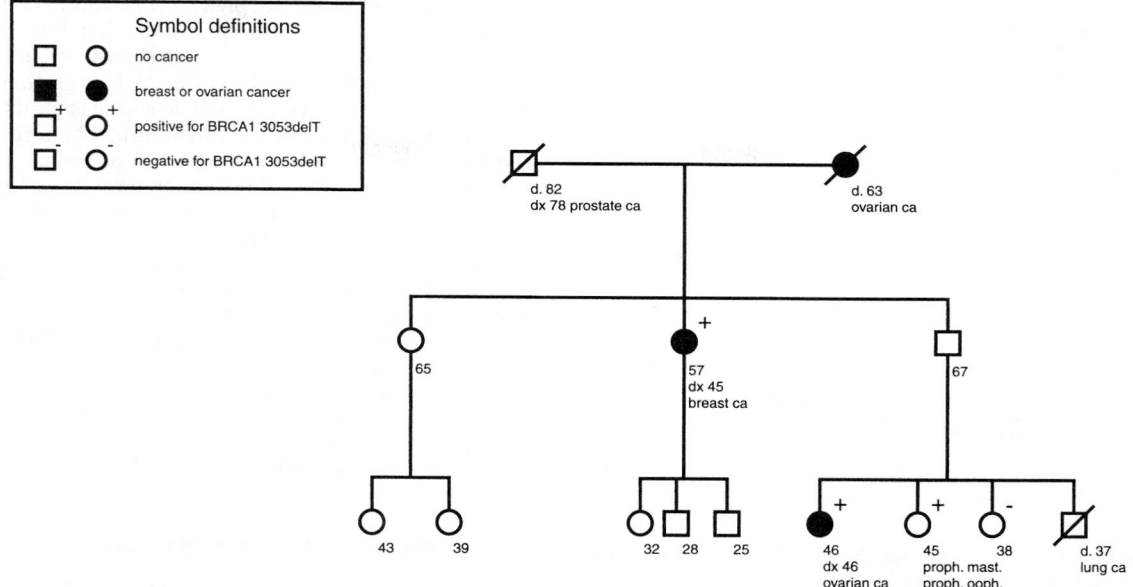

Figure 58.18. Pedigree of genetic breast cancer. The family illustrated in the pedigree carries a mutation of the *BRCA1* gene; multiple relatives are affected with breast and ovarian cancer.

the common mechanism of risk. Conversely, women who undergo bilateral oophorectomy before menopause are at decreased risk, with the magnitude of benefit increasing as the age at oophorectomy decreases. In general, hormonal risk factors are associated with relative risks in the range of 1.5 to 2.0. Studies of the effect of lactation on breast cancer risk have been inconclusive, but a long duration of lactation appears to reduce risk in premenopausal women (68). Postmenopausal obesity has also been shown to increase risk (69), perhaps through an increase in peripheral estrogen production, but this relationship has not been observed in premenopausal women.

The effects of both oral contraceptives and hormone replacement therapy on breast cancer risk have been extensively studied. Overall, no convincing evidence has been found of an increased risk in women who have ever used oral contraceptives. Estrogen replacement therapy, especially when used for longer than 5 years, appears to be associated with a small increase in breast cancer risk (70). A recent prospective study has suggested that the increase in risk is only for the subset of histologically favorable tumors, such as tubular and mucinous carcinomas (71).

Environmental Factors and Diet

Exposure to ionizing radiation, whether from a nuclear explosion or medical procedures, increases breast cancer risk. The level of risk varies with age at exposure, being greatest for exposures in childhood and adolescence, and minimal for exposures after age 40. Patients who were treated with mantle irradiation for Hodgkin's lymphoma in their adolescent or childhood years are the group at risk on the basis of radiation exposure most commonly encountered today (72).

Much attention has been devoted to the role of diet in breast cancer etiology. This link has been suggested by the large international variations in breast cancer incidence, and the observation that national per capita fat consumption correlates with breast cancer incidence. However, prospective studies of diet and breast cancer risk within the context of American diets fail to confirm this relation-

ship, at least for fat consumption within adult life (73,74). Stronger evidence exists to support an association between alcohol intake and breast cancer risk.

Benign Breast Disease

Benign breast lesions are classified as nonproliferative, proliferative, or proliferative with atypia (Table 58.6). Nonproliferative lesions, which are not associated with an increased risk for breast cancer development, account for approximately 70% of palpable breast masses (75). Proliferative lesions without atypia are associated with a small increase in breast cancer risk (relative risk of 1.5 to 2.0). Proliferative lesions with atypia are uncommon, comprising only 3.6% of palpable breast masses and 7% to 10% of nonpalpable abnormalities. Atypical lesions are associated with a relative risk of 4.0 to 5.0, which increases to 9.0 when they are found in a woman having a first-degree relative with breast cancer. However, as illustrated in Fig. 58.19, breast cancer will have developed at 15 years in only 10% of women with atypical hyperplasia alone.

Table 58.6. CLASSIFICATION OF BENIGN BREAST DISEASE

Nonproliferative: no increase in risk
  Cysts, micro or macro
  Ductal ectasia
  Fibroadenoma
  Mastitis
  Fibrosis
  Metaplasia, squamous or apocrine
  Mild hyperplasia
Proliferative: RR, 1.5–2.0
  Papilloma
  Sclerosing adenosis
  Hyperplasia, moderate or severe
Proliferative with atypia: RR, 4.5–5.0
  Atypical ductal hyperplasia
  Atypical lobular hyperplasia

RR, relative risk.

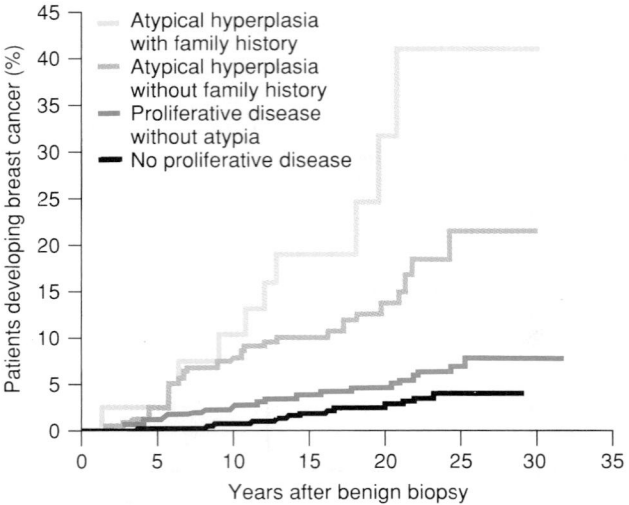

Figure 58.19. Cumulative risk for the development of invasive breast cancer after a biopsy for benign breast disease. Women with atypical hyperplasia (ductal or lobular type) are at a significantly increased risk for the development of breast cancer. (From Page DL, Dupont WD. Anatomic markers of human premalignancy and risk of breast cancer. *Cancer* 1990;66:1326, with permission.)

Lobular Carcinoma in Situ

In the past, lobular carcinoma in situ (LCIS) was thought to be a malignant lesion, but it is now accepted as a breast cancer risk factor. LCIS is predominantly found in premenopausal women and lacks both clinical and radiographic features. Women diagnosed with LCIS have a relative risk for breast cancer development ranging from 5.4 to 12 (76–83). This translates in most studies to a risk for breast cancer development of about 1% per year (Table 58.7). The risk is equal in both breasts and is unrelated to the amount of LCIS seen in the biopsy specimen. Infiltrating ductal carcinoma is the most common type of invasive carcinoma seen after a diagnosis of LCIS, although infiltrating lobular carcinoma is more frequent in women with LCIS than in the general population (76–82). The increased risk for breast cancer development after a diagnosis of LCIS persists indefinitely.

Clinical Assessment of Risk

Although many factors that increase breast cancer risk have been identified in studies of large populations, the majority of these have little meaning for the individual woman. A summary of the magnitude of risk associated

with known risk factors is provided in Table 58.8. No consensus has been reached regarding what level of risk is necessary to classify a woman as "high-risk." In addition, most women have a combination of factors that both increase and decrease risk, so that risk assessments based on a single risk factor are of dubious clinical benefit. A model based on the risk factors of age, age at menarche, age at first live birth, number of first-degree relatives with breast cancer, and number of prior breast biopsies was developed by Gail and colleagues (84). This model predicts risk over a defined time interval and allows comparison with an age-matched control population. The model has been shown to predict risk accurately in women undergoing annual mammographic screening, and it is a useful tool for counseling women who are concerned about their level of risk. It must be emphasized that this is not an appropriate model for women at risk on the basis of a strong family history of breast cancer or those with LCIS. A sample Gail model risk calculation is shown in Fig. 58.20.

Management of the High-risk Woman

Two strategies are available to reduce the risk for breast cancer in women at increased risk—prophylactic mastectomy and tamoxifen. Prophylactic mastectomy, which has been used for decades, clearly does not provide 100% protection against breast cancer development. Both subcutaneous and total (simple) mastectomies have been used for prevention, and the development of carcinoma in residual breast tissue has been reported after both types of surgery. The efficacy of prophylactic mastectomy in a group of high-risk women was defined in a study of 639 women from the Mayo Clinic (85). Patients were classified as being at moderate or high risk and were followed for a median of 14 years. Prophylactic mastectomy reduced the risk for breast cancer by 89.5% in the moderate-risk group, and by 90% to 94% in the high-risk group. Although prophylactic mastectomy is clearly effective for risk reduction, many women find it an unacceptably radical prevention option, particularly in the era of breast-conserving therapy for established carcinoma. Prophylactic mastectomy should be undertaken only after a complete risk assessment, consultation with a reconstructive surgeon, and a thorough discussion of management alternatives. Women should be advised of their level of risk and assisted in determining if that level of risk is unacceptable to them, rather than being told to undergo prophylactic surgery. When prophylactic mastectomy is performed, the procedure should be a simple mastectomy with removal of the nipple–areola complex, extended to the same anatomic limits as a therapeutic mastectomy. Patients undergoing prophylactic mastectomy are ideal candidates for a skin-sparing approach to facilitate immediate breast reconstruction (Fig. 58.21A).

Table 59.7. RISK FOR BREAST CANCER DEVELOPMENT AFTER LOBULAR CARCINOMA IN SITU

Study	No. patients	Invasive cancer (%)	Follow-up (y)	Relative risk
Haagensen et al. (76)	287	18	16.3	6.9
Rosen et al. (77)	99	12.5	24	9.0
Andersen (78)	47	26.4	15	12.0
Page et al. (79)	44	23	18	9.0
Salvadori et al. (80)	80	6.3	5	10.3
Ottesen et al. (81)	69	11.6	5	11.0
Bodian et al. (82)	236	26[a]	18	5.4
Fisher et al. (83)	182	33	5	—

[a]Includes intraductal and invasive cancer.

Table 58.8. MAGNITUDE OF KNOWN BREAST CANCER RISK FACTORS

Relative risk <2	Relative risk 2–4	Relative risk >4
Early menarche	Age >35 first birth	Gene mutation
Late menopause	First-degree relative with breast cancer	Lobular carcinoma in situ
Nulliparity	Radiation exposure	Atypical hyperplasia
Proliferative benign disease	Prior breast cancer	
Obesity		
Alcohol use		
Hormone replacement		

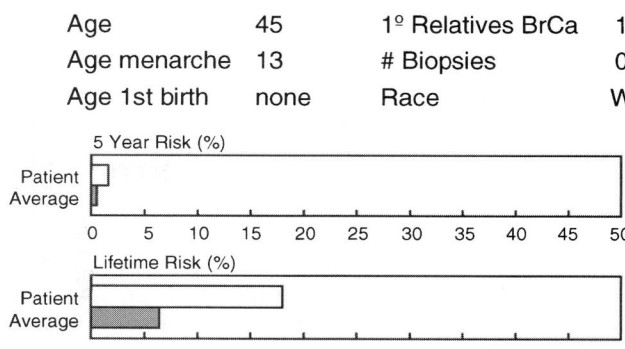

Age	45	1° Relatives BrCa	1
Age menarche	13	# Biopsies	0
Age 1st birth	none	Race	W

Figure 58.20. Breast cancer risk assessment according to the Gail model. This woman's 5-year risk for the development of breast cancer is 1.6%, and her lifetime risk is 18%.

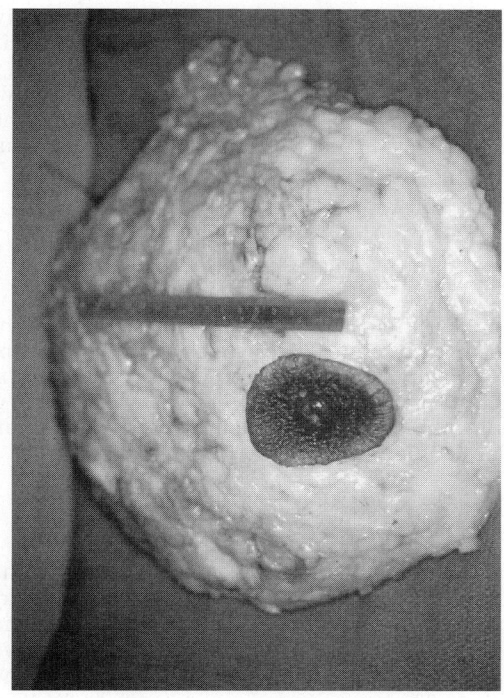

A

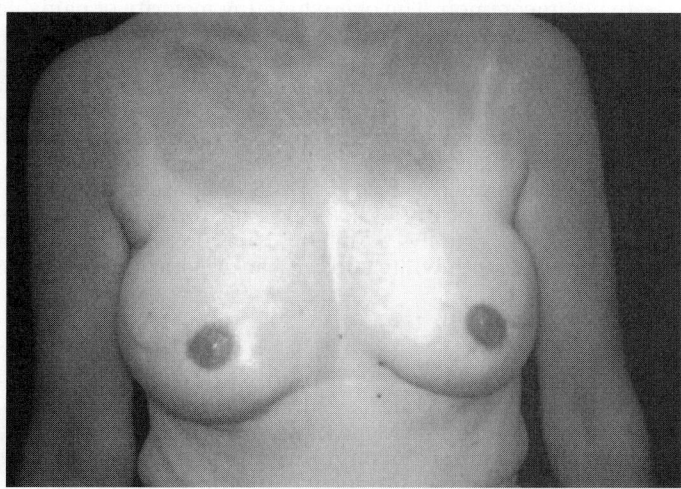

B

Figure 58.21. Skin-sparing mastectomy. *(A)* The only skin removed was the nipple–areola complex. *(B)* Cosmetic outcome after bilateral skin-sparing mastectomy and transverse rectus abdominis myocutaneous flap *(TRAM)* reconstruction.

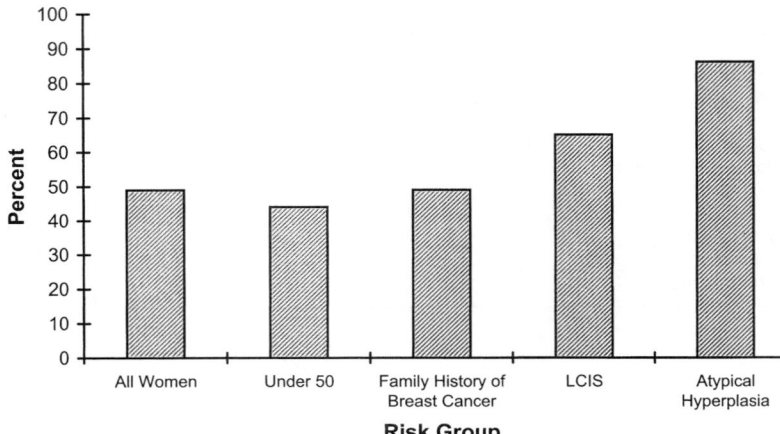

Reduction in Cancer Incidence by Risk Group

Figure 58.22. Tamoxifen for breast cancer prevention. Although tamoxifen was effective in all subgroups of high-risk women, particular benefit was seen in those at risk on the basis of lobular carcinoma in situ and atypical hyperplasia.

An alternative strategy for breast cancer prevention is tamoxifen. Tamoxifen has been used to treat established breast cancer for more than 20 years. Data from treatment trials, most recently updated in the 1998 Oxford Overview Analysis (86), demonstrated that women taking tamoxifen for 5 years had a 47% reduction in the incidence of contralateral breast cancer. This finding served as the impetus for the National Surgical Adjuvant Breast and Bowel Project (NSABP) P-1 prevention trial, in which 13,388 women at increased risk for breast cancer development were randomized to tamoxifen or placebo (83). Risk was defined by the Gail model (84). Women were eligible for study entry if they were age 60 or older, or if they were between the ages of 35 and 59 years and had a predicted 5-year breast cancer risk of 1.66% or more. After a median follow-up of 54.6 months, a 49% reduction in the risk for invasive cancer, and a 50% reduction in the risk for noninvasive cancer, were seen in the tamoxifen group (Fig. 58.22). The reduction occurred only in estrogen receptor-positive tumors. No change in the incidence of estrogen receptor-negative tumors was seen. Tamoxifen was found to be of benefit in all age groups, and in women at risk on the basis of a family history as well as those eligible for the study on the basis of other risk factors. A particular benefit was observed in women at risk on the basis of LCIS and atypical hyperplasia, in whom risk reductions of 65% and 86%, respectively, were seen (87). Postmenopausal women experienced a 19% reduction in the incidence of fractures, including a 45% reduction in hip fracture. This approached statistical significance.

The most common side effects of tamoxifen were hot flashes and vaginal discharge. Participants who took tamoxifen had a 2.5 times greater risk for endometrial carcinoma than those in the placebo group, and all the excess risk was seen in postmenopausal women. An increased risk for venous thrombosis, including pulmonary embolism, was also seen in the postmenopausal women taking tamoxifen. However, the rate of pulmonary embolism in these women was 1/1,000 annually. The presence of these competing risks emphasizes the need for a complete assessment of a woman's health status before a decision is made regarding the use of tamoxifen for prevention.

Raloxifene is an antiosteoporosis agent that also may be effective in reducing breast cancer incidence. Initial trials in 7,705 postmenopausal women demonstrated that in addition to maintaining bone density and reducing the risk for fracture, raloxifene reduced the incidence of invasive breast cancer by 66% (88). As in the tamoxifen trial, this effect was observed on the incidence of estrogen receptor-positive tumors only. However, only 40 patients with invasive breast cancers were included in this study, and the specific benefit of raloxifene in high-risk women is unknown. A prospective, randomized trial in 20,000 postmenopausal women at increased risk for breast cancer development [study of tamoxifen and raloxifene (STAR)] will directly compare the risks and benefits of tamoxifen and raloxifene.

DUCTAL CARCINOMA IN SITU

Ductal carcinoma in situ (DCIS), also known as *intraductal carcinoma,* is a distinct entity from LCIS, the other lesion classified as noninvasive breast cancer, with differences in both clinical presentation and biologic potential. DCIS is characterized by a proliferation of abnormal, presumably malignant epithelial cells that are confined within the basement membrane of the mammary ductal–lobular system (Fig. 58.23).

Presentation

Ductal carcinoma in situ has a variety of clinical presentations. In the past, DCIS was gross or palpable in most cases. Alternatively, it presented as a pathologic nipple discharge or Paget's disease of the nipple, or it was found incidentally when a biopsy was performed for another indication. These clinical presentations of DCIS are relatively uncommon. The overwhelming majority of palpable breast cancers are invasive carcinoma; fewer than 2% are DCIS. Today, clustered microcalcifications on a mammogram are the most frequent presentation of DCIS, although nonpalpable masses may also be DCIS. In many reports of biopsies performed for mammographic abnormalities, DCIS accounts for 30% to 50% of the malignancies identified. The number of cases of DCIS seen each year has increased dramatically as screening mammography has become more widely adopted. This increase has been observed in both white and African American women.

Pathology

Ductal carcinoma in situ has traditionally been classified on the basis of architectural pattern as comedo, cribriform, micropapillary, papillary, or solid. However, because a mixed architectural pattern is seen in as many as 30% to 60% of DCIS lesions, the utility of this classifica-

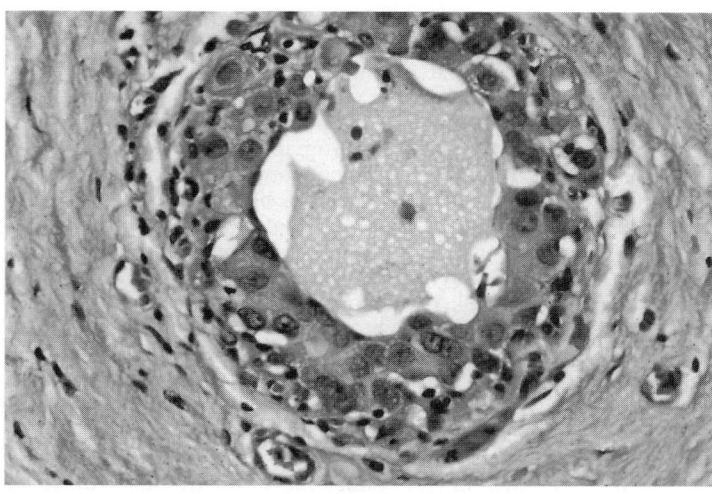

Figure 58.23. Photomicrograph of ductal carcinoma in situ. The abnormal cells do not cross the ductal basement membrane. The necrotic debris in the center of the duct is responsible for the calcification seen on mammography.

tion system is limited. Newer systems classify DCIS lesions on the basis of nuclear grade and necrosis, and usually recognize three groups of lesions of high, intermediate, and low grade (89). Multiple systems have been proposed, but their reproducibility and ability to predict the behavior of DCIS remain to be proved.

Management

Mastectomy, excision and irradiation (RT), and excision alone have all been proposed as management strategies for DCIS because of uncertainty about the natural history of the disease. Mastectomy is a curative treatment for approximately 98% of patients with DCIS, regardless of lesion size or grade (89,90). Treatment failure after mastectomy for DCIS is thought to a consequence of unrecognized invasive carcinoma; as many as 26% of patients undergoing mastectomy for DCIS are found to have invasive carcinoma that was not identified preoperatively (91). Invasive carcinoma is most frequently found in large, high-grade DCIS lesions.

Although mastectomy is an effective treatment for DCIS, it is a radical approach for a lesion that may not progress to invasive carcinoma during a patient's lifetime and is too small to be detected clinically. The use of breast-conserving therapy with excision and RT for invasive carcinoma (see section on local management of stages I and II breast cancer) has stimulated greater interest in the use of this approach for DCIS. No randomized trial has ever compared the treatment of DCIS by mastectomy with treatment by excision and RT. A large number of clinical studies have demonstrated that local recurrence is seen in 10% to 15% of cases after 10 years (89,90,92–94), and that approximately half of the local recurrences are invasive car-

cinoma. Deaths from DCIS are rare; 14 breast cancer deaths occurred in 814 patients followed for 8 years (93).

Other authors have suggested that DCIS can be treated by wide excision alone (95). The NSABP has addressed this issue in a prospective, randomized trial in which 818 patients with DCIS were randomized to excision alone or to excision plus RT (93,94). After 8 years of follow-up, the use of RT was found to reduce the risk for invasive breast recurrence from 13.4% to 3.9% ($p < .0001$) and to reduce the incidence of noninvasive recurrence from 13.4% to 8.2% ($p = .007$). In a more detailed pathologic analysis (94), the greatest benefits of RT were seen in the patients at highest risk for recurrence (those with comedo necrosis and uncertain margins), but even in the most favorable subgroup (absent or slight comedo necrosis, clear margins), the use of RT reduced the absolute incidence of breast recurrence by 7% at 8 years. The definition of negative margins used in this study was that tumor-filled ducts did not touch an inked surface. This has led to questions of whether this study adequately addresses the benefits of RT in a group of patients treated by wide excision (95).

Treatment selection for the patient with DCIS begins with a careful evaluation of the extent of the DCIS lesion by means of magnification mammography. Standard two-view mammography significantly underestimates the extent of well-differentiated DCIS (96). If the extent of the DCIS is too large relative to the patient's breast size to allow a cosmetically acceptable breast-conserving approach, the patient should be counseled about the options of mastectomy alone or mastectomy with immediate breast reconstruction. In patients with localized DCIS suitable for a breast-conserving approach, the decision regarding the need for RT should be made based on the estimated risk for recurrence and the patient's attitude toward

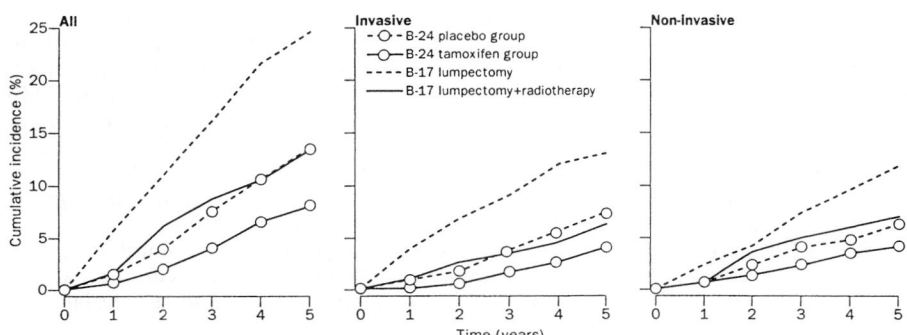

Figure 58.24. Benefits of radiation therapy and tamoxifen in ductal carcinoma in situ. The cumulative incidence of breast cancer events in the ipsilateral and contralateral breasts for patients treated in the National Surgical Adjuvant Breast and Bowel Project B-17 and B-24 trials is shown. The reduction in recurrence is greatest for patients receiving radiotherapy and tamoxifen.

risk. Patients with larger tumors, high-grade lesions, and close margins appear to derive the greatest benefit from RT. It also appears that younger women are at higher risk for recurrence than their older counterparts (97). However, even patients with small, low-grade lesions appear to benefit from RT (94), and it is in this low-risk subgroup that the patient's attitude toward risk becomes important.

Tamoxifen has been shown to be of benefit in reducing the risk for invasive carcinoma in patients with DCIS. In NSABP B-24 (97), 1,804 women with DCIS treated by excision and RT were randomized to tamoxifen or placebo for 5 years. A reduction in the incidence of all invasive breast cancer events (ipsilateral, contralateral, and distant) from 13.4% to 8.2% was seen with tamoxifen (p = .0009). The benefit of tamoxifen was observed in women over and under age 50 and in those with negative and positive margins. A benefit for tamoxifen was also observed whether or not comedo necrosis was present in the tumor. The effects of RT and tamoxifen in the NSABP B-17 and B-24 trials (93,97) are illustrated in Fig. 58.24. The decision to use RT, tamoxifen, or both in the patient with DCIS will depend on the patient's personal level of risk and attitude toward small benefits from therapeutic intervention, but both should be considered.

BIOLOGY AND NATURAL HISTORY OF BREAST CANCER

Breast cancer is a disease characterized by marked heterogeneity among patients and a long natural history. This is evident in the Middlesex Hospital series, in which Bloom et al. (98) reported the outcome of 250 patients with breast cancer observed without treatment between 1805 and 1933. Patients were generally admitted for advanced disease, with only 2% having stage II disease, 23% stage III, and 74% stage IV. Only 39% presented within 1 year of their first symptom. Despite this, 18% of patients receiving no treatment survived 5 years, and 4% survived 10 years. The mortality was constant over time, with approximately 25% of patients who were alive at the beginning of any given year dying during that year. In modern series, patients with varying annual hazards of death can also be identified, and these remain constant for at least 10 years after the diagnosis. For this reason, some have concluded that breast cancer is never cured, and that if death from other causes did not intervene, cancer eventually would recur in all patients. Although this may be true in the abstract, from a practical point of view, failures more than 20 years after treatment are rare, and many patients have a normal life expectancy after breast cancer treatment. The clinical variations in breast cancer are believed to reflect variable genetic changes that result in the disease.

The initial clinical understanding of breast cancer, as articulated by Halsted (99), was one of orderly disease progression, with a tumor beginning in the breast and spreading over time from the lowest to the highest axillary nodes, and then throughout the body via the lymphatic system. Halsted proposed *en bloc* extirpation of the primary tumor with a wide margin of normal tissue (i.e., the breast) and the draining lymphatics as the most likely strategy to cure breast cancer, based on the understanding of the biology of the disease at that time. Over time, it became clear that the majority of women with breast cancer were not cured by radical mastectomy. Of 1,640 women treated at Memorial Hospital from 1940 to 1943, only 13% survived for 30 years free of breast cancer (100). Recognition of this fact initially led to larger operations, such as the extended radical mastectomy to remove more of the lymphatic drainage of the breast. However, when these procedures failed to improve survival, a dramatic shift in thinking occurred. In the new disease paradigm, championed by Bernard Fisher (101), most breast cancer was considered to be systemic at the time of diagnosis, so that the extent of locoregional treatment would have little impact on survival from breast cancer. Acceptance of this concept led to the adoption of the modified radical mastectomy, and subsequently breast-conserving surgery, for the treatment of stages I and II breast cancer, in addition to the widespread use of adjuvant chemotherapy and hormonal therapy.

More recently, a spectrum hypothesis has been advanced suggesting that breast cancer exists in both a local and locoregional and in a systemic form, and that metastasis can occur during the clinical course of the disease (102). In this paradigm, effective locoregional treatment does contribute to survival. This concept is supported by studies demonstrating that the use of screening mammography reduces breast cancer mortality by 30% (8). If all breast cancers were systemic from their inception, early detection would have no impact on cancer mortality. The potential for locoregional treatment to affect survival has been emphasized in the recent studies of postmastectomy radiation therapy in node-positive breast cancer, in which a survival benefit was noted when chest wall and nodal irradiation were given (103–106). These studies are discussed in more detail in the section on postmastectomy radiotherapy. The spectrum theory suggests that treatment strategies should be tailored according to the characteristics of an individual patient's disease rather than based on the assumption that most breast cancers are systemic at the time of diagnosis. At present, treatment strategies can be selected only on the basis of clinically determined prognostic factors. Ultimately, as our understanding of the genetic changes that result in breast cancer improves, we may be able to identify those factors responsible for the metastatic as well as the locally invasive phenotype, and it will be possible to adjust the intensity of both local and systemic therapy according to the unique genetic profile of each tumor.

INVASIVE CARCINOMA

Pathology

Invasive carcinomas are defined as those in which tumor cells have crossed the basement membrane and have the biologic capability to metastasize. Any breast lesion that is surgically removed should be considered potentially malignant. Breast biopsy specimens should be oriented in the operating room and inked before sectioning so that the margin status can be assessed. The pathologic evaluation of a breast tumor should routinely include size, histologic type, grade, margin status, and hormone receptor status.

Histologic Type

Infiltrating ductal carcinoma is the most common type of breast carcinoma, accounting for 65% to 80% of all cases of breast cancer. These tumors are classically hard, irregular, grayish white lesions on gross inspection. Microscopically, they vary widely in appearance and often have features of other histologic subtypes of breast cancer, with areas of lobular, medullary, or tubular differentiation. For prognostic purposes, these mixed tumors are considered to be infiltrating ductal carcinomas.

Infiltrating lobular carcinoma is the second most frequently encountered subtype of invasive carcinoma. Approximately 10% of cancers are classified as lobular. Histologically, lobular cancers grow as a single file of malignant cells that tend to be arranged circumferentially around ducts and lobules. Because of this growth pattern, they are often difficult to recognize on clinical examination and mammography because they may not produce the distinctive mass lesions characteristic of infiltrating ductal carcinoma. Infiltrating lobular carcinoma has been said to have a rate of bilaterality as high as 30% to 50%. However, when patients with LCIS are excluded from consideration, the incidence of contralateral breast cancer in patients with infiltrating lobular carcinoma differs little from that in patients with ductal carcinoma. In one study of 4,748 patients, a contralateral cancer had developed after 5 years in 5.3% of patients with infiltrating lobular cancer, and in 4.0% of those with infiltrating ductal tumors (106). Thus, the routine use of bilateral mastectomy for patients with tumors of lobular histology cannot be justified. Lobular carcinoma is more likely to metastasize to the intraabdominal viscera, uterus, ovaries, and peritoneal surfaces than other histologic types of breast carcinoma. Most studies have found no difference in survival between patients with infiltrating ductal and those with lobular carcinoma after stratification for appropriate prognostic factors.

Favorable histologic subtypes of breast carcinoma include pure tubular and mucinous carcinoma. Tubular carcinomas form normal-appearing breast ductules or tubules. At least 75% of a tumor must be tubular to be classified in this subtype. Tubular carcinomas are uncommon, accounting for 2% or fewer of all cancers, although they are more frequent in women undergoing screening mammography. Their significance lies in their excellent prognosis. Nodal metastases are extremely rare in tubular carcinomas smaller than 1 cm, and even when nodal metastases do occur, the prognosis is much better than that for ductal or lobular carcinoma at the same stage. Mucinous or colloid carcinomas are also uncommon. They are characterized by relative acellularity and large pools of extracellular mucus. The prognosis is similar to that for tubular carcinoma. Medullary carcinoma is another variant of infiltrating ductal carcinoma with a favorable prognosis, although this is less well recognized than in tubular and mucinous tumors, perhaps because of the aggressive microscopic appearance of medullary carcinoma. The tumor cells have large pleomorphic nuclei and a high mitotic rate and are associated with an intense lymphoplasmacytic infiltrate. Grossly, the tumors are quite well circumscribed and may be mistaken for benign lesions. Medullary carcinomas are less likely to be associated with axillary nodal metastases than ductal or lobular carcinomas of the same size, and survival is also better. Other histologic types of breast cancer account for fewer than 2% of all cancers.

Grading Systems

The grade of a carcinoma is an estimate of differentiation. It may be histologic or nuclear. Nuclear grading is a cytologic assessment of the similarity of tumor nuclei to the nuclei of normal cells. The nuclear grade is usually reported as well differentiated, intermediate, or poorly differentiated. The histologic grade considers not only the cytologic differentiation but also the growth pattern of the carcinoma. The extent of tubule formation, nuclear hyperchromasia, and the mitotic index are assessed. In one of the most widely used systems, the Elston modification of the Scharf-Bloom-Richardson classification, each of these 3 elements is scored on a scale of 1 to 3, with a resultant classification of grade 1 (score of 3 to 5), grade 2 (score of 6 or 7), or grade 3 (score of 8 or 9) (107). Approximately

19% of the 2,000 cases reviewed by Elston and Ellis (107) were grade 1, 34% were grade 2, and 47% were grade 3.

Hormone Receptors

The concept of an estrogen receptor (ER) was described by Jensen and Jacobsen in 1962 (108), based on the observation that estrogens tagged with radioactive isotopes are preferentially concentrated in the estrogen target organs of animals (i.e., breast, uterus, vagina) and in human breast cancers. Subsequently, a second hormone receptor, the progesterone receptor (PR), was identified. ERs and PRs belong to a superfamily of nuclear hormone receptors that function as transcription factors when bound to their respective ligands. Approximately 70% of breast carcinomas are hormone receptor-positive; well-differentiated tumors and those occurring in older postmenopausal women have the highest rates of receptor positivity. Approximately 60% of patients with ER-positive tumors respond to endocrine therapy, but only 5% to 10% of patients with ER-negative tumors do so (109). In general, the ER status of a primary breast cancer is predictive of the ER status of any metastases, but in about 20% of ER-positive tumors, the metastases are ER-negative. It is now apparent that two subtypes of the ER exist, ER-α (the receptor identified by Jensen) and ER-β (110). At present, the functional significance of ER-β is uncertain. Tumor ER content was initially determined by a competitive binding assay, but this has been largely replaced by immunohistochemical techniques. Determination of hormone receptor status is a critical part of the pathologic analysis of breast tumors and is used to ascertain whether the patient is a candidate for hormonal therapy (see section on adjuvant systemic therapy).

Clinical Evaluation and Staging

The extent of the preoperative work-up should be guided by the clinical stage of the disease and the patient's symptoms. Patients with DCIS do not require screening for metastatic disease. Bone scans are frequently used as a preoperative screening test for patients with invasive cancer, but the incidence of occult bony metastases detected by scanning in patients with stage I or II disease is less than 5% (111). False-positive results are frequent, especially in older women. In contrast, bony metastases are identified by scanning in 20% to 25% of asymptomatic women with stage III disease, so that this a worthwhile screening procedure in patients with locally advanced breast cancer. The yield of screening liver scans is even lower than that of bone scanning, and the test is of little benefit in the preoperative evaluation of stage I and II breast cancer.

Serum tumor markers have not been shown to be of value preoperatively. Although carcinoembryonic antigen may be useful in monitoring response to therapy, it is infrequently elevated in primary breast cancer. In the study of Lee (112), only 3% of patients with stage I breast carcinoma and 6% with stage II disease had levels of carcinoembryonic antigen above 5 mg/mL. Other markers, such as sialomucin (e.g., CA 15-3, CA 549), are more commonly elevated in primary breast cancer, with abnormalities seen in 20% to 50% of patients. However, 20% of patients with benign breast disease have elevated levels of CA 15-3, and CA 15-3 is also elevated in benign gastrointestinal disease, so that the usefulness of this marker as a screening test is diminished (113,114).

Staging refers to the grouping of patients according to the extent of their disease. The stage is useful in (a) determining the choice of treatment for an individual patient,

(b) estimating prognosis, and (c) comparing the results of different treatment programs. Staging can be based on either clinical or pathologic findings.

Currently, the staging of cancer is determined by the American Joint Committee on Cancer (AJCC). The AJCC system is a clinical and pathologic staging system and is based on the TNM (tumor–node–metastasis) system..

The clinical stage is based on all the information available before the first definitive treatment is administered. This includes the findings from physical examination, imaging studies, operation, and pathologic examination of the breast or other tissues. The clinical stage is useful in selecting and evaluating therapy.

The pathologic stage (designated pTNM) is based on all the data used for clinical staging and surgical resection in addition to data derived from the pathologic examination of the primary carcinoma and axillary lymph nodes. A tumor cannot be evaluated for pathologic staging (pTX) if excision of the primary carcinoma reveals tumor in any margin of resection by gross pathologic examination. Regional nodes cannot be evaluated for pathologic staging (pNX) if the resection has not included the low axillary lymph nodes (level I). Metastatic nodules in the fat adjacent to the mammary carcinoma, without evidence of residual lymph node tissue, are considered regional lymph node metastases. The pathologic stage provides the most precise data to estimate the prognosis and calculate the end results. The current staging system is given in Table 58.9 (7).

Table 58.9. TNM CLASSIFICATION FOR BREAST CANCER STAGING

TNM definitions
Primary tumor
- TX   Primary tumor cannot be assessed
- T0   No evidence of primary tumor
- Tis   Carcinoma in situ or Paget's disease of the nipple with no tumor
- T1   Tumor 2 cm or smaller in greatest diameter
- T2   Tumor larger than 2 cm but not larger than 5 cm in greatest diameter
- T3   Tumor larger than 5 cm
- T4   Tumor of any size with direct extension to the chest wall (not including pectoral muscle) skin edema, skin ulceration, skin satellites, or inflammatory carcinoma

Regional lymph nodes
- NX   Nodes cannot be assessed
- N0   No lymph node metastases
- N1   Metastasis to movable ipsilateral axillary nodes
- N2   Metastasis to ipsilateral axillary nodes fixed to one another or to other structures
- N3   Metastases to ipsilateral internal mammary nodes

Distant metastases
- MX   Cannot be assessed
- M0   No distant metastasis
- M1   Distant metastasis (includes supraclavicular nodes)

Stage groupings

Stage 0	Tis	N0	M0
Stage I	T1	N0	M0
Stage IIA	T0	N1	M0
	T1	N1	M0
	T2	N0	M0
Stage IIB	T2	N1	M0
	T3	N0	M0
Stage IIIA	T0	N2	M0
	T1	N2	M0
	T2	N2	M0
	T3	N1	M0
	T3	N2	M0
Stage IIIB	T4	Any N	M0
	Any T	N3	M0
Stage IV	Any T	Any N	M1

Local Management of Stage I and Stage II Breast Cancer

The goal of the local therapy of breast cancer is to eradicate all clinically evident tumor in the breast and axillary lymph nodes. This can be accomplished with a modified radical mastectomy, a modified radical mastectomy with immediate breast reconstruction, or breast-conserving therapy (BCT), which consists of removal of the primary tumor with a margin of normal tissue and RT. Six modern prospective, randomized trials have compared mastectomy with BCT and have demonstrated no survival differences, even after long-term follow-up (115–120) (Table 58.10). In addition, no statistically significant differences were noted in local failure rates between procedures except in the National Cancer Institute trial (118), in which the extent of lumpectomy would now be considered inadequate. Mastectomy alone has never been compared with mastectomy and reconstruction in a randomized trial, but there is no reason to suspect that reconstruction would decrease survival. In the absence of survival differences, the role of the surgeon is to identify medical contraindications to the procedures and to counsel the patient regarding what is involved in each one.

Breast-conserving Therapy

For BCT to be successful, three conditions must be met: It must be possible to (a) reduce the tumor burden to a microscopic level likely to be controlled by irradiation, (b) safely deliver radiation therapy, and (c) promptly detect local recurrence. The contraindications to BCT arise logically from these conditions. In 1992, a joint committee of the American College of Surgeons, American College of Radiology, College of American Pathologists, and Society of Surgical Oncology developed guidelines for BCT. These were updated in 1997 and are listed in Table 58.11 (121).

The incidence of the contraindications to BCT in the breast cancer population determines the number of patients who advised to undergo mastectomy for medical reasons. Morrow et al. (10) reported a study in which a multidisciplinary team of physicians prospectively evaluated 456 patients with DCIS, clinical stage I breast cancer, or clinical stage II breast cancer between 1988 and 1991. Medical contraindications to breast preservation were present in only 26% of the patients, and the incidence and type of contraindications varied significantly by stage, with only 10% of stage I patients having contraindications to BCT.

In an effort to increase the number of patients eligible for breast conservation, the use of neoadjuvant chemotherapy to shrink the primary tumor before surgical therapy has been studied (122). In the largest randomized trial to date, NSABP protocol B-18, 1,523 patients with tumors of any size were randomized to receive four cycles of doxorubicin and cyclophosphamide either preoperatively or postoperatively (123). All patients over age 50 received tamoxifen. A reduction in tumor diameter of 50% was noted clinically in 80% of the patients, and in 37%, no tumor could be felt after chemotherapy. However, only one fourth of the patients thought to be complete responders had no tumor identified microscopically after surgery. Significant axillary down-staging also was observed, with pathologically negative nodes seen in 60% of the neoadjuvant group and in 42% of the postoperative adjuvant group (p < .001). Despite these impressive response rates, the rate of breast conservation increased by only 8%, from 60% to 68%. To date, neoadjuvant therapy has not been shown to improve survival in comparison with therapy given postoperatively.

In addition to the medical contraindications to BCT discussed above, patient desire is another indication for mas-

Table 58.10. SURVIVAL IN PROSPECTIVE RANDOMIZED TRIALS COMPARING BREAST-CONSERVING THERAPY WITH MASTECTOMY

Trial	Follow-up (y)	Overall survival		Local recurrence	
		BCT (%)	Mastectomy (%)	BCT (%)	Mastectomy (%)
Institut Gustave Roussy (115)	15	73	65	9	14
Milan I (116)	18	65	65	7	4
NSABP B06 (117)	12	63	59	10	8
NCI (118)	10	77	75	19	6
EORTC (119)	8	54	61	17	14
Danish (120)	6	79	82	3	4

BCT, breast-conserving therapy; EORTC, European Organization for Research and Treatment of Cancer; NCI, National Cancer Institute; NSABP, National Surgical Adjuvant Breast and Bowel Project.

tectomy. Not all women who are eligible for BCT opt for this therapy. In one study (122), 19% of eligible patients selected treatment with mastectomy, either alone or with immediate reconstruction. This decision was independent of age or race.

The amount of breast tissue to be resected in a lumpectomy in order to minimize the risk for local recurrence while optimizing the cosmetic appearance remains a major issue. The goal of surgery is to reduce the tumor burden to a microscopic level that is likely to be controlled with RT. In a study of mastectomy specimens in 264 patients in which serial sectioning and radiography were used, only 39% of specimens had no additional tumor beyond the primary tumor site (124). The likelihood of finding additional tumor was not related to the size of the primary tumor. Other studies have shown that the risk for residual tumor varies with the histology of the primary tumor, being lowest in pure infiltrating ductal carcinoma and highest in infiltrating ductal carcinoma with an extensive intraductal component (EIC); the risk in infiltrating lobular carcinoma falls between the other two (125). These studies indicate that the ideal balance between cosmesis and local failure is unlikely to be achieved by resecting the same amount of breast tissue in all patients. Magnification mammography is essential to identify the extent of the tissue that must be resected, and it allows large "quadrantectomy"-type resections to be reserved for patients with multifocal disease. With the use of physical examination and magnification mammography, the pa-

Table 58.11. CONTRAINDICATIONS TO BREAST-CONSERVING THERAPY IN INVASIVE CARCINOMA

Absolute contraindications
1. Two or more primary tumors in separate quadrants of the breast.
2. Persistent positive margins after reasonable surgical attempts.
3. Pregnancy is an absolute contraindication to the use of breast irradiation. When cancer is diagnosed in the third trimester, it may be possible to perform breast-conserving surgery and treat the patient with irradiation after delivery.
4. A history of prior therapeutic irradiation to the breast region that would result in re-treatment to an excessively high radiation dose.
5. Diffuse malignant-appearing microcalcifications.

Relative contraindications
1. A history of scleroderma or active systemic lupus erythematosus.
2. Extensive, gross, multifocal disease in the same quadrant. Studies in this area are not definitive.
3. Large tumor in a small breast that would result in cosmesis unacceptable to the patient.
4. Very large or pendulous breasts if reproducibility of patient setup and adequate dose homogeneity cannot be ensured.

tients who can undergo breast conservation can be identified with a success rate higher than 95% (126). The extent of surgical resection is the major determinant of cosmetic outcome, and approximately 90% of patients treated with conservative resection rate their cosmetic outcome as excellent or good (Fig. 58.25).

Local recurrence of tumor in the breast after BCT has been the subject of many studies. Local recurrence may be a consequence of inappropriate patient selection, inadequate surgery or RT, or biologic characteristics of the tumor. The presence of tumor at the margin of resection significantly increases the risk for local recurrence, as does the use of radiation doses to the whole breast of less than 4,500 to 5,000 cGy. Six randomized trials have attempted to identify a subgroup of patients with invasive carcinoma who do not require RT. All have shown a large reduction (average, 75%) in the rate of local recurrence with RT (127), and RT should be considered a standard part of BCT for invasive carcinoma. Patient factors, such as young age, have also been associated with an increased risk for local failure after BCT. However, young age has also been shown to increase rates of local failure after mastectomy, which indicates that young age is a prognostic factor rather than one that can be used to select therapy. In contrast, a family history of breast cancer does not increase local failure rates. Whether this is true for women with mutations of breast cancer predisposition genes is uncertain at this time. A number of tumor factors, such as size and involvement of axillary lymph nodes, which are strong predictors of the risk for distant recurrence, are not associated with the risk for recurrence in the breast. Histologic tumor type also is not a risk factor, and studies have shown that recurrence rates after excision of infiltrating lobular carcinoma to negative margins do not differ from those after excision of infiltrating ductal tumors. Most studies also indicate that histologic grade is not predictive of recurrence. Some studies have identified lymphatic invasion at the primary tumor site as a risk factor, but this has also been shown to be a risk factor for local recurrence after mastectomy.

An EIC, defined as the presence of intraductal carcinoma both within an infiltrating ductal carcinoma and in adjacent grossly normal breast tissue, was identified in older studies as a tumor feature strongly associated with an increased risk for local, but not distant, recurrence. This association was usually observed in studies in which limited surgical excisions were used and margins were not inked. More recent studies indicate that when EIC-positive tumors are excised to negative margins, local failure rates are similar to those seen with EIC-negative tumors (128). The presence of an EIC is best regarded as an indicator that the extent of disease may be greater than what is clinically appreciated. If negative margins are obtained, these patients are appropriate

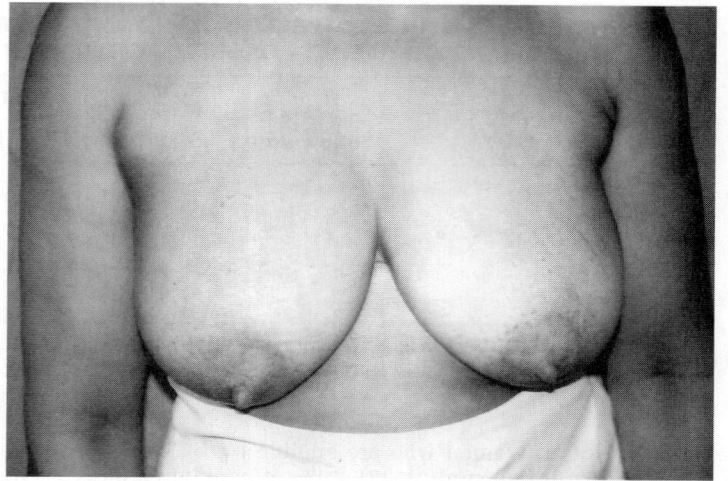

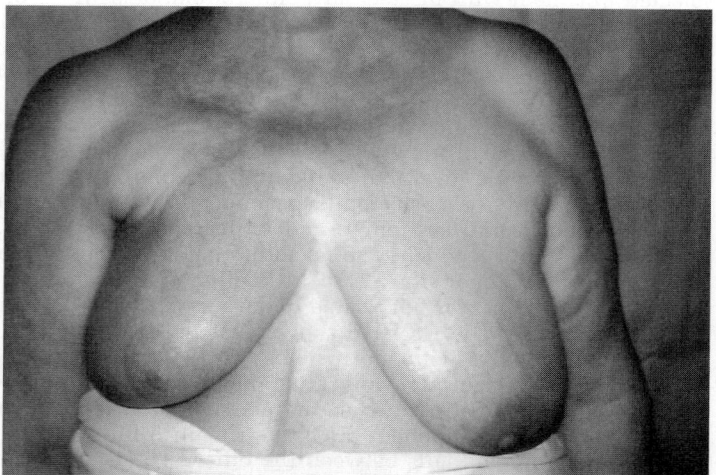

Figure 58.25. Cosmetic outcome after breast-conserving therapy with radiation. *(A)* Excellent cosmetic outcome. The treated breast *(left)* is identical to the untreated breast. *(B)* Fair cosmetic outcome. Significant shrinkage and loss of ptosis is evident in the treated right breast.

candidates for BCT. The use of adjuvant chemotherapy or tamoxifen in patients who have received breast RT reduces the risk for breast recurrence by approximately 50%. In modern series, local failure rates of 4% to 8% at 10 years are commonly reported in patients receiving RT plus systemic therapy. The information on factors associated with local recurrence suggests that two types of recurrences develop after BCT. One type of recurrence represents a heavy tumor burden in the breast that is not controlled by breast irradiation. This type of recurrence can be minimized by meticulous patient selection and attention to the technical details of surgery and irradiation. The other type of recurrence is a manifestation of a biologically aggressive tumor and represents a first site of metastatic disease. This type of recurrence is similar to the majority of chest wall recurrences seen after mastectomy.

Modified Radical Mastectomy

The term *modified radical mastectomy* encompasses several different operative procedures, depending on whether the pectoralis minor muscle is preserved, removed, or divided. In all the operations, the breast tissue and fascia of the pectoralis major muscle and some of the axillary lymph nodes are removed. Modified radical mastectomy is performed through an elliptical incision that encompasses the nipple–areola complex and the biopsy scar, if an open biopsy has been performed, in addition to the excess skin of the breast (Fig. 58.26). If the skin is needed for reconstruction, it can be preserved and exposure obtained through in-

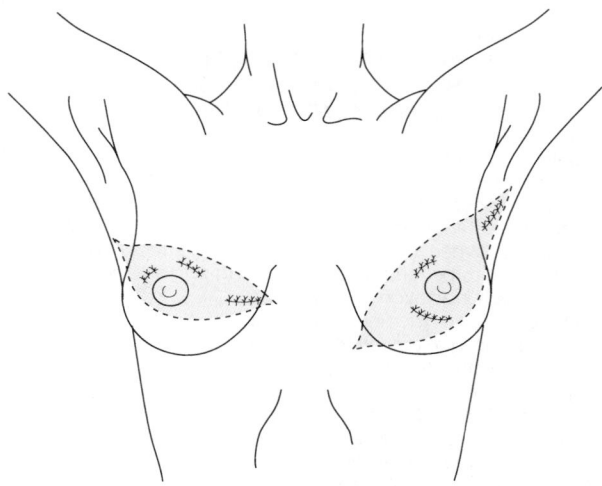

Figure 58.26. Incision placement for modified radical mastectomy. The incision should include the nipple–areola complex, biopsy scar, and excess skin of the breast.

cision rather than excision. Skin flaps are raised in the plane between the subcutaneous fat and the underlying breast tissue. To encompass all the breast tissue, the dissection should extend superiorly to the inferior border of the clavicle, medially to the lateral border of the sternum, inferiorly to the superior extent of the rectus sheath, and laterally to the latissimus dorsi. The fascia overlying the pectoralis major is the deep margin of resection, but it can be preserved when needed to facilitate reconstruction.

Mastectomy is an extremely safe operation. A review of the Surveillance, Epidemiology, and End Results (SEER) data for 10,056 patients treated between 1960 and 1973 reports a 30-day operative mortality of 0.35% (129). Early postoperative complications include wound infections, which tend to present as cellulitis and are seen in from 2% to 14% of cases (130). Open surgical biopsy before mastectomy (as opposed to a needle biopsy technique) has been shown to increase the rate of infection. Skin flap necrosis is relatively uncommon today. Factors associated with flap necrosis include vertical incisions, technical error with denuding of the subcutaneous fat from the flap, and closure under tension. Seromas form in 100% of patients and should be considered a side effect and not a complication. Extensive axillary nodal involvement is the strongest predictor of prolonged lymphatic drainage after mastectomy. Seroma formation can be minimized by leaving suction drains in place until their output is less than 40 mL/24 h rather than arbitrarily removing them on a predetermined day. Anesthesia of the chest wall is another side effect of mastectomy that patients should be informed of preoperatively.

Mastectomy and Immediate Reconstruction

The techniques of breast reconstruction have evolved dramatically during the past 30 years, and the switch from radical mastectomy to modified radical mastectomy has made immediate reconstruction an option for most women. Tissue expansion followed by removal of the expander and replacement with a permanent implant is the most common form of reconstruction in the United States. The advantage of this technique is that it adds little to the length of surgery or the time of recovery. Disadvantages include the need for a second surgical procedure routinely and the limitations in cosmetic outcome, particularly for women with large or pendulous breasts. However, these differences are minimized when a bra is worn (Fig. 58.27). In one study, 27.8% of women who underwent reconstruction with an expander or implant required surgery for complications, such as capsular contracture or implant deflation, or as part of a planned staged procedure by 5 years postoperatively (131). The anecdotal concerns regarding an association between silicone gel implants and connective tissue disease that were raised in the early 1990s have not been borne out by subsequent epidemiologic studies (132,133), but silicone gel implants continue to be available on an investigational basis only.

The alternative to implant reconstruction is the use of autologous tissue flaps. Both the transverse rectus abdominis myocutaneous flap (TRAM) and a latissimus dorsi flap have been used for reconstruction. These flaps have the advantage of allowing a more natural look and feel to the breasts than can be achieved with implants (Fig. 58.21B). The TRAM reconstruction has the added advantage of an abdominoplasty. However, both add significant time to the operative procedure, hospitalization, and recovery period, and they may not be suitable for patients with major comorbid conditions. In addition, in most women the latissimus flap does not provide enough tissue to create a breast mound, and an implant must be added.

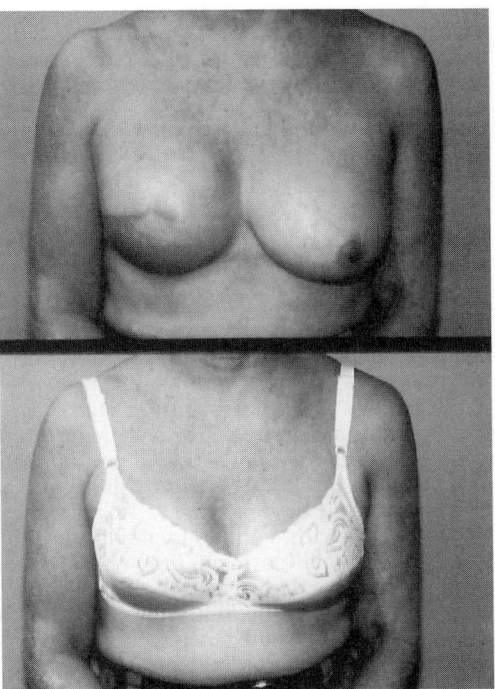

Figure 58.27. Breast reconstruction with tissue expanders. Although the breasts are not identical, this is not evident when a bra is worn.

The major oncologic issue in immediate reconstruction has been the incidence and detection of local recurrence. This has never been examined in a prospective randomized trial, but retrospective studies do not suggest an increase in the rate of local failure, even after skin-sparing mastectomies (134). The detection of local failure also does not appear to be altered by the presence of a reconstruction because the majority of chest wall failures occur in the skin or subcutaneous fat. A second issue is the use of immediate reconstruction in patients who will require postoperative RT. The incidence of implant loss and poor cosmetic outcome is clearly increased in patients who undergo postoperative RT. In contrast, TRAM flaps can be radiated with only minor fat necrosis and fibrosis and maintenance of a good cosmetic outcome (135). As the indications for postoperative RT are expanded (discussed below), the issue of the optimal method and timing of reconstruction assumes greater importance. One approach to the patient who is highly likely to require postoperative RT is to place an expander to allow skin preservation at the time of initial surgery. Once postoperative RT is completed, a decision to continue with the expander/implant or switch to a flap reconstruction can be made.

Management of the Axillary Nodes

Axillary dissection has been a part of the surgical management of breast cancer since the era of Halsted. Initially, axillary dissection was thought to be therapeutic. In the 1970s, when it was recognized that most women with axillary nodal metastases treated with local therapy alone died of breast cancer, axillary dissection came to be regarded as a staging procedure. In the 1990s, the increasing use of adjuvant systemic therapy for node-positive and node-negative breast cancer, the more frequent detection of small cancers associated with a low risk for nodal metastases, and an increased awareness of the morbidity of axillary dissection resulted in attempts to identify sub-

Table 58.12. INCIDENCE OF AXILLARY RECURRENCE IN RELATION TO NUMBER OF NODES REMOVED

Trial	Axillary recurrence (%) No. Nodes removed				
	0	<3	<5	>5	>10
Danish Breast Cancer Group (136)	19	10	5	3	—
NSABP (137)	21	—	12	0	—
Fowble et al. (138)	—	21	—	5	2

groups of patients who would not benefit from the procedure. In the majority of studies, tumor size was used to identify a low-risk subgroup. However, even for tumors smaller than 5 mm, the incidence of nodal metastases ranges from 3% to 12% (127). The only groups of patients reproducibly found to have a risk for axillary metastases below 5% are those with a single focus of microinvasion, with grade I tumors smaller than 5 mm, or with pure tubular carcinomas smaller than 1 cm. For the majority of patients with breast cancer, the axillary nodal status cannot be reliably predicted on the basis of the characteristics of the primary tumor. An alternative approach, which avoids axillary dissection when it will not change therapy, deprives the patient and physician of the prognostic information obtained from nodal status and places the patient at risk for local recurrence.

Axillary Dissection

The extent of axillary dissection has been defined on the basis of the number of nodes removed or their anatomic location. As discussed in the section on anatomy, the axilla is divided into three anatomic levels. Removal of the level I and II nodes accurately identifies metastases in 98% of patients because isolated metastases to level III are uncommon. A level I and II dissection is standard practice, with the removal of level III being reserved for patients with evidence of gross nodal involvement. Isolated axillary recurrence after a level I and II dissection is uncommon and is seen in fewer than 3% of patients undergoing BCT. The outcome of axillary surgery based on the number of nodes removed, often called *axillary sampling*, is more variable. It is often not possible to determine how many nodes are being removed intraoperatively. With random node removal, a clear relationship is noted between the number of nodes removed and the incidence of axillary failure (136–138), as shown in Table 58.12.

The increasing use of BCT, with its elimination of the morbidity caused by the loss of the breast, has focused attention on the sequelae of axillary dissection. Although major complications such as injury to the axillary vein and motor nerves of the axilla are rare, minor complications are much more common. These include numbness in the distribution of the intercostobrachial nerve, seen in 70% to 80% of patients unless the nerve is preserved, pain and weakness in 20% to 30% of patients 1 year after surgery, and lymphedema. The incidence of lymphedema is difficult to quantify because no standard definition of lymphedema is available and the frequency of lymphedema increases as the time from surgery increases. In a review of reports published in the 1990s (139), the incidence of lymphedema was found to range from 6% to 30%. The incidence of lymphedema is related to the extent of axillary dissection, being higher when level III is removed than when lesser dissections are performed. The radiation of an axillary field after surgical dissection significantly increases the risk for lymphedema. Beyond these two treatment-related factors, there is little agreement on which patient characteristics are associated with an increased risk for lymphedema.

Sentinel Node Biopsy

A sentinel lymph node is defined as the first lymph node that receives drainage from a cancer. The technique makes it possible to identify patients with axillary node involvement reliably by means of a low-morbidity operation, so that axillary dissection is limited to patients with nodal metastases who will benefit from the procedure. Lymphatic mapping can be performed with lymphazurin blue dye, colloids labeled with radioactive isotopes (usually technetium), or a combination of the two agents.

A number of studies have examined the ability to identify a sentinel node and the accuracy of the sentinel node in predicting the status of the remaining axillary nodes (140–146). These are summarized in Table 58.13. Regardless of the technique used, a sentinel node can be identified in 90% of patients and will predict the status of the remaining axillary nodes in more than 90% of cases. With experience, a number of contraindications to sentinel node biopsy have been identified. These are listed in Table 58.14. Lymph nodes that are filled with tumor may not take up the mapping agent and are a cause of false-negative results. Neither lymphazurin blue dye nor radiolabeled colloids are known to be safe in pregnant or lactating women. A major issue in sentinel node biopsy has been the amount of experience necessary to master the procedure, with several studies suggesting that 30 cases with completion of axillary dissection are necessary (147,148). Sentinel node biopsy also offers the pathologist the opportunity to perform a much more detailed study of the lymph node that is most likely to contain metastases than is possible when an entire axillary specimen containing 15 to 30 nodes is evaluated. With the use of multiple sections or immunohistochemistry, it is possible to identify tumor deposits in approximately 20% of nodes found to be "negative" with routine sectioning and hematoxylin and eosin staining. However, the prognostic sig-

Table 58.13. RESULTS OF LYMPHATIC MAPPING AND SENTINEL NODE BIOPSY

Study	No. patients	Technique	Sentinel node identified (%)	Sentinel node only metastasis (%)	False-negative rate (%)
Giuliano et al. (140)	174	B	66	38	12
Veronesi et al. (141)	163	R	98	38	5
Giuliano et al. (142)	107	B	94	67	0
Guenther et al. (143)	145	B	71	43	10
Borgstein et al. (144)	130	R	94	59	2
Krag et al. (145)	443	R	91	17	11
Veronesi et al. (146)	376	R, B + R	99	44	7

B, lymphazurin blue dye; R, radioactivity.

Table 58.14. CONTRAINDICATIONS TO SENTINEL NODE BIOPSY

Suspect palpable axillary adenopathy
Tumor >5 cm in size or locally advanced
Use of preoperative chemotherapy
Multicentric carcinoma
Pregnant or lactating patient

nificance of these micrometastases is uncertain. Prospective clinical trials being performed by the American College of Surgeons Oncology Group and the NSABP will determine whether immunohistochemistry of the sentinel node is a useful way to refine our ability to predict the risk for recurrence.

Postmastectomy Radiotherapy

The potential reasons for irradiating the chest wall and draining lymph node basins after mastectomy are twofold: first, to reduce the risk for locoregional recurrence of tumor, and second, to improve survival by eradicating residual locoregional disease that may be resistant to systemic chemotherapy. The risk for local failure after mastectomy is significant and is clearly related to the presence of axillary node metastases. Reported locoregional recurrence rates in randomized trials of mastectomy alone range from 4% to 26% (149). In patients with negative axillary nodes, local failure rates are usually less than 4%, and the risk increases as nodal involvement increases. An overview analysis of trials of RT after both mastectomy and BCT demonstrated that RT reduces the risk for local recurrence by approximately two thirds (150) but has no effect on survival. However, in older studies, a significant increase in late cardiac mortality was observed in patients who underwent radiation for left-sided cancers, which offset an apparent decrease in breast cancer mortality in the RT group.

Several recent studies have examined the use of RT in patients receiving adjuvant systemic therapy and have reported an improvement in survival with the addition of RT. The Danish Breast Cancer Group reported a randomized study of 1,708 premenopausal women with stage II or III breast cancer who received eight cycles of cyclophosphamide, methotrexate, and fluorouracil and were randomized to locoregional RT or no further treatment (103). After a median follow-up of 114 months, overall survival was 54% in the RT group versus 45% in the chemotherapy alone group (p < .01). A smaller trial of premenopausal women, from British Columbia, showed similar survival benefits (104). Further support for this concept comes from the Danish trial in postmenopausal women receiving tamoxifen, in which RT improved overall survival from 36% to 45% (p < .05) (105). To date, postmastectomy RT has been used primarily in patients with involvement of four or more axillary nodes to reduce the risk for locoregional recurrence. These studies suggest that RT should be considered in patients with involvement of one to three nodes to improve survival. However, because of concerns about the adequacy of the axillary surgery in the Danish studies, a large randomized trial is being performed in the United States in patients with involvement of one to three nodes to quantify better the benefits of RT in this subset.

Prognostic Factors

The clinical course of breast cancer varies from patient to patient. Prognostic factors can be used to predict the natural history of a tumor, usually in terms of disease-free or overall survival. Prognostic factors must be distinguished from predictive factors, which are associated with response to a particular therapy. Clinically, prognostic factors are used to determine which patients have such a favorable outcome after local therapy that adjuvant systemic therapy is not warranted. Although multiple prognostic factors have been described, those in standard use today include axillary lymph node status, tumor size, histologic subtype (discussed in the section on pathology), nuclear or histologic grade, and ER and PR status. Measurements of proliferation, such as S-phase fraction or Ki67, are more controversial but are used in many institutions.

The presence of metastases to the axillary nodes is the single most important prognostic factor in breast cancer. Although clinical studies usually divide patients into groups with negative nodes, one to three positive nodes, and four or more positive nodes, the number of involved nodes indicates the prognosis as a continuous variable (151). Efforts to predict nodal status by means of other factors have failed to identify reproducibly a subset of patients with a 95% chance of being node-positive or node-negative (152). Because node-positive patients are uniformly recognized as requiring adjuvant systemic therapy, most studies have concentrated on prognostic factors in node-negative patients. Tumor size is another strong predictor of outcome (153,154). Only 10% of patients or fewer with tumors 1 cm or less in size and negative axillary lymph nodes experience recurrence during long-term follow-up (153).

Tumor grade has also been shown to predict outcome in breast cancer. However, the availability of multiple grading systems, poor reproducibility among different observers unless specific guidelines are provided, and the failure of many pathologists to include a grade on the pathology report have limited its utility as a prognostic factor. Hormone receptor (ER and PR) status has long been recognized as a predictive factor for response to endocrine manipulations, such as tamoxifen or oophorectomy. In addition, studies have demonstrated that ER and PR are prognostic factors that are associated with increases in disease-free survival of about 10% at 5 years (155). ER and PR levels are strongly correlated with histologic grade and patient age and inversely correlated with measures of proliferation.

DNA cytometry allows the number of cells undergoing replication or cell synthesis (S phase) to be measured. The utility of flow cytometry in predicting outcome has been controversial, in large part because of the lack of methodologic standardization. A 1993 consensus conference (156) reviewed the published literature on flow cytometry and concluded that an increased S-phase fraction is clearly associated with an increased risk for breast cancer mortality. The S-phase fraction has been shown to correlate with the number of positive lymph nodes, tumor size, hormone receptor status, and patient age. An alternative method of determining the rate of cell proliferation is immunohistochemical staining for Ki67, a monoclonal antibody that is specific for a nuclear antigen in proliferating cells. Strong correlations between S-phase fraction and Ki67 have been reported by some, but not all, investigators. However, most studies investigating Ki67 have found a correlation with clinical outcome (157).

More recent studies of prognostic factors have focused on growth factor receptors such as epidermal growth factor receptor and *HER-2/neu*, tumor-suppressor genes such as *p53* and *nm23*, and angiogenesis. Most of these studies have involved relatively small numbers of patients and analyzed only a single prognostic factor. Significant methodologic issues regarding measurement also exist. Thus, the clinical utility of these factors remains uncertain.

Adjuvant Systemic Therapy

Adjuvant therapy is defined as the use of cytotoxic chemotherapy or endocrine therapy after the local treatment of breast cancer to kill clinically occult micrometastases. The risk for micrometastases is estimated based on prognostic factors, as they are not clinically detectable at the time of diagnosis. The initial trials of adjuvant systemic therapy were carried out in node-positive patients because it was recognized that an increased mortality is associated with axillary node metastases. Subsequently, the recognition that breast cancer death occurs in as many as 20% to 40% of node-negative breast cancer patients led to many trials of systemic treatment in that group.

The Early Breast Cancer Trialists Collaborative Group has conducted metaanalyses of the major prospective, randomized trials of chemotherapy, with the most recent analysis published in 1998 (158) (Table 58.15). After 15 years of follow-up, the overview analysis confirmed that adjuvant chemotherapy significantly reduces the risk for death in both node-positive and node-negative patients. The proportional risk reduction was equal for both groups. Benefit was seen in both premenopausal and postmenopausal women, and long-term polychemotherapy (≥ 12 months) was no better than short-term therapy (6 months). A small benefit was seen for anthracycline-based treatment (e.g., doxorubicin) versus cytoxan, methotrexate, and fluorouracil. These findings are summarized in Table 58.15. The proportional reduction in mortality must be translated into an absolute reduction to be meaningful for the individual patient. Thus, a 24% reduction in mortality for a patient with a 1-cm, node-negative tumor who has a 10% risk for death at 10 years corresponds to about a 2% benefit. The same proportional reduction in mortality for the patient with six positive nodes and a 75% risk for death at 10 years translates to a 30% benefit. In general, the benefit of chemotherapy was greatest in younger women, reducing the odds of death by 27% in those under 40 and by 8% in those ages 60 to 69. Newer agents that have been shown to be effective in breast cancer include the taxanes (paclitaxel and docetaxel), vinorelbine, and herceptin (an antibody against the c-*erb*-B-2 oncogene product). The role of these agents in adjuvant therapy is currently being defined. To date, studies of high-dose chemotherapy with stem cell support (bone marrow transplant) for high-risk patients in the adjuvant setting have failed to demonstrate a benefit for this treatment (159).

Tamoxifen is a nonsteroidal agent that exhibits site-specific estrogen agonist and antagonist properties (160). It was the first drug identified in the class of drugs now referred to as SERMs (selective estrogen receptor modula-

tors). Tamoxifen acts as an antiestrogen in the breast through competitive blockade of the estrogen receptor. In bones and lipids, tamoxifen acts as an estrogen agonist, preserving bone density and lowering blood cholesterol. Tamoxifen also acts as an agonist in the uterus, increasing the incidence of endometrial carcinoma (see section on management of the high-risk woman). A metaanalysis has been conducted of more than 37,000 patients in 55 trials of tamoxifen (161). The use of tamoxifen reduces the annual odds of breast cancer recurrence by 47% and the annual odds of death by 26%. Tamoxifen is beneficial in women of all ages, and 5 years of therapy is superior to treatment for shorter periods of time. The benefits of tamoxifen are limited to patients whose tumors express ERs, PRs, or both. The overview analysis (158,161) also demonstrates that combined therapy with chemotherapy and tamoxifen is superior to treatment with either agent alone in both premenopausal and postmenopausal women whose tumors are hormone receptor-positive. However, in postmenopausal women, the benefit from the addition of chemotherapy is quite modest and must be weighed against the toxicity of the treatment in the context of the patient's overall health status. Current recommendations for the use of adjuvant therapy in practice are shown in Table 58.16. These are intended as general guidelines because the individual attitudes of patients toward small benefits and treatment toxicities vary widely.

Special Problems

Breast Cancer in the Elderly

The incidence of breast cancer increases with age, and approximately 50% of cases in the United States are diagnosed in women age 65 and over. Therapy in the elderly should be based on physiologic, not chronologic, age. Mastectomy can be performed safely in the majority of older women, regardless of age. In the SEER report on mastectomy, the 30-day operative mortality rate was 0.39% for all ages, and 0.9% for the subgroup of women age 75 and older (129). Mastectomy is an excellent means of obtaining local control with a minimum number of outpatient visits, but many older women prefer BCT if offered this option. This is clearly a lesser operative procedure than a mastectomy, and several studies (162,163) suggest that local failure rates after BCT with RT are lower in women over age 65 than in their younger counterparts. Radiation toxicity has not been shown to vary with age, and treatment is generally well tolerated. However, daily visits for RT may be difficult for the elderly patient with limited mobility. When omission of breast irradiation in the treatment of an elderly patient is being considered, it is useful to remember than the majority of local failures occur in the first six postoperative years. The use of large, quadrantectomy-type excisions helps to minimize the risk for local recurrence, albeit at the expense of cosmesis.

In the elderly woman with significant comorbid conditions, tamoxifen has been studied as an alternative to conventional surgical treatment. In three randomized trials comparing tamoxifen alone versus some form of surgical therapy alone or with tamoxifen, no survival advantages were observed for surgical therapy (164–166). However, despite the fact that many of the surgical procedures utilized did not represent the best available therapy, significant improvements in local control were noted in the surgically treated woman. Response rates to primary tamoxifen treatment are high, but 12 months or more are often needed to achieve the best response, and with long-term follow-up, the risk for disease progression is significant (167). Because mastectomy or lumpectomy and radiotherapy are well tolerated by the majority of older women, there is no reason to

---

Table 58.15. OVERVIEW ANALYSIS OF CHEMOTHERAPY, 1998

Treatment	Reduction in annual odds	
	(Recurrence % ± SE)	Death (% ± SE)
Any multidrug chemotherapy	24 ± 2	15 ± 2
CMF	24 ± 3	14 ± 4
CMF + other cytotoxic agents	20 ± 2	15 ± 5
Non-CMF chemotherapy (i.e., anthracyclines)	25 ± 4	17 ± 4

CMF, cytoxan, methotrexate, 5-fluorouracil; SE, standard error.
From Early Breast Cancer Trialists' Collaborative Group. Polychemotherapy for early breast cancer: an overview of the randomized trials. Lancet 1998;352:930–942, with permission.

Table 58.16. RECOMMENDATIONS FOR ADJUVANT THERAPY

Patient group	Recommended treatment

Node-negative, low risk
  Tumor ≤1 cm
  Special histologic types
  1–2 cm, grade 1, or ER+ and low proliferation
	No treatment or tamoxifen if ER+

Node-negative, higher risk	
ER+	Tamoxifen or chemotherapy plus tamoxifen
ER–	Chemotherapy
Node-positive	
ER+	
Premenopausal	Chemotherapy plus tamoxifen
Postmenopausal	Chemotherapy plus tamoxifen or tamoxifen alone
ER–	Chemotherapy

ER+, estrogen receptor-positive; ER–, estrogen receptor-negative.

substitute tamoxifen as a routine treatment. However, for the elderly woman with a limited life span who is a poor operative risk because of comorbid conditions, tamoxifen represents a viable alternative as a primary therapy.

Breast Cancer in Pregnancy

Breast cancer occurring during pregnancy is relatively uncommon when all cases of breast cancer are considered. If only breast cancer patients in their childbearing years are evaluated, 7% to 14% are found to be pregnant at diagnosis (168). If pregnant women are used as a denominator, approximately 2.2 breast cancers per 10,000 pregnancies can be anticipated (169).

The clinical presentation of breast cancer during pregnancy is the same as in the nonpregnant patient, and a palpable mass is the most common symptom. Mammography is not particularly helpful in the evaluation of breast masses in pregnant women because of the increased density of the breast. Ultrasonography is often useful in distinguishing a true mass from the normal nodularity of pregnancy, but ultimately the decision about the need for biopsy should be made on the basis of the physical examination. Delay in the diagnosis of breast cancer during pregnancy remains a major problem, and most of this delay is physician-induced. Breast biopsy under local anesthesia is safe at any time during pregnancy and should be performed for any suspected mass.

The options for the local treatment of breast cancer during pregnancy are limited for the woman who wishes to continue her pregnancy. The use of irradiation during any trimester of pregnancy is contraindicated because of the inability to shield the fetus from internal radiation scatter. If breast cancer is diagnosed in the third trimester, lumpectomy and axillary dissection can be performed and radiation delayed until after delivery. The effect of longer delays in radiation to allow breast preservation is unknown and may be detrimental. Immediate reconstruction with tissue flaps is also contraindicated during pregnancy because of the risk to the fetus of a more prolonged anesthesia and increased blood loss, in addition to the inability to obtain symmetry with the postpartum breast. Thus, modified radical mastectomy remains the mainstay of the surgical therapy of breast cancer during pregnancy. Therapeutic abortion does not appear to play a role in the treatment of nonmetastatic breast carcinoma. A number of small, nonrandomized studies have failed to show a survival advantage associated with termination of pregnancy (170). Some patients may opt to terminate a pregnancy because of concerns about the long-term prognosis or the risk for fetal damage, but patients should not be advised that this is of therapeutic benefit.

Breast cancer during pregnancy is often thought to be a particularly aggressive disease with a poor prognosis. However, much of the poor prognosis seems to be secondary to advanced disease at the time of diagnosis. These women are generally too young to undergo regular mammographic screening before pregnancy, and even in recent series, more than 60% of patients with pregnancy-associated breast cancer had positive axillary nodes (170). After correction for age and tumor stage, some studies suggest that survival in women treated during pregnancy is similar to that in nonpregnant patients. However, a multiinstitutional study of 407 patients ages 20 to 29 at the time of cancer diagnosis found that the risk for cancer death in the 26 patients in whom the disease was diagnosed during pregnancy was almost three times higher than the risk for cancer death in those who had never been pregnant (171). A case–control study of 540 women treated at the Memorial Sloan-Kettering Cancer Center (172) and a population-based study from Denmark (173) also found a significant decrease in survival for women in whom breast cancer was diagnosed shortly after pregnancy.

Chemotherapy can be given to the pregnant breast cancer patient but is generally delayed until after the first trimester. Fetal malformation is seen in approximately 20% of patients treated during the first trimester, and this risk falls to about 2% for exposure in the second and third trimesters. However, some series have reported low birth weight in as many of 40% of infants exposed during pregnancy, and the long-term effects of chemotherapy exposure on growth, development, and cancer risk are largely unknown (170). The decision to treat any woman with chemotherapy during pregnancy depends on her risk for relapse and the woman's desire for treatment after a thorough discussion of the risks and benefits, and these decisions must be resolved on a case-by-case basis. When breast cancer is diagnosed in the third trimester, chemotherapy can usually be delayed until fetal maturity, when delivery can be induced. The effects of longer delays on the efficacy of chemotherapy is unknown. Tamoxifen is contraindicated in pregnant women.

Male Breast Cancer

Cancer of the male breast is an uncommon disease. Risk factors include a family history of breast cancer, mutations of the *BRCA2* gene, Klinefelter's syndrome, hepatic schistosomiasis, and radiation exposure. With the exception of the gynecomastia seen with Klinefelter's disease, gynecomastia does not seem to increase the risk for male breast cancer. The mean age of patients at presentation with male breast cancer is between 60 and 70 years, approximately 10 years older than that of women with the disease (174).

The typical presentation is a mass beneath the nipple–areola complex, and ulceration of the nipple is frequent. In contrast, isolated nipple discharge is uncommon. Approximately 80% of male breast cancers are hormone receptor-positive.

The most common local treatment for male breast carcinoma is mastectomy. Radical mastectomy is no longer the standard therapy, and when the tumor is not fixed to the pectoral muscle, a modified radical mastectomy can be performed. When muscle involvement is limited, the portion of the pectoralis to which the tumor is adherent can be excised. When extensive pectoral muscle invasion is present, radical mastectomy may be necessary, although the patient may also be approached with initial chemotherapy, as would a female breast cancer patient in this clinical scenario. BCT for male breast carcinoma is rarely feasible because of the small size of the breast and the central location of most tumors.

The survival rate of men with breast cancer is similar to that in women with disease of the same stage (175). As in women, axillary nodal status is the major predictor of outcome. The benefit of adjuvant systemic therapy in male breast cancer has not been evaluated in randomized clinical trials. However, the natural history of metastatic breast carcinoma in men is similar to that in postmenopausal women, as is the response to therapy, and this has influenced practice in the adjuvant setting. Because most male breast cancers contain hormone receptors, the largest adjuvant experience has been gained with hormonal therapy. The administration of tamoxifen to men with stage II or III disease resulted in a 55% 5-year survival, versus 28% in historical controls who received no systemic treatment (176). However, tamoxifen may not be as well tolerated in men as in women, and it frequently causes a loss of libido. In the absence of definitive studies in men, the use of adjuvant systemic therapy should be based on prognosis and hormone receptor status, and the guidelines for postmenopausal women should be followed. In the past, orchiectomy was the standard method of hormonal manipulation. A recent review found a 67% response rate to castration, which increased to 80% when only receptor-positive cancers were considered (177). Tamoxifen has a similar response rate and is increasingly used as the first-line hormonal therapy, with orchiectomy reserved for patients who have failed multiple other therapies.

Occult Primary Tumor Presenting with Nodal Metastases

Breast cancer presenting as metastatic disease in the axillary nodes with no evident tumor in the breast is uncommon, accounting for fewer than 1% of cases in most large series. Metastatic adenocarcinoma in axillary nodes may be secondary to a variety of primary cancers, but in women, breast cancer is by far the most common type. In the patient without historical or clinical evidence suggesting a primary tumor at another site, the radiologic evaluation should be confined to breast imaging and a chest radiograph. Examination of the nodal tissue for hormone receptors helps to confirm a breast primary if the tissue is hormone receptor-positive, but the breast cannot be excluded as the site of the primary tumor if the nodal tissue does not contain receptors.

The sensitivity of mammography in identifying occult lesions is low. In the majority of reports, fewer than one third of cases presenting with adenopathy had breast tumors identified by mammography. However, the majority of these cases were collected during long periods of time when the quality of imaging was not equal to that available today. Promising evidence suggests that MRI may be more accurate than conventional mammography in identi-

fying the location of the primary tumor in the breast in this clinical circumstance, and tumors not seen on mammography have been identified with screening ultrasonographic examinations (178).

Most women with axillary node metastases secondary to a presumed breast cancer are treated with mastectomy, and a breast carcinoma is identified during the pathologic evaluation in approximately 65% of these cases. The size of the occult tumors varies widely, with lesions as large as 6 cm reported. The availability of BCT for clinically evident primary tumors has stimulated interest in its use for occult tumors. Theoretical objections to this approach include the fact that the tumor burden in the breast may be extensive, even when the disease is clinically occult, and that it is not feasible to excise the primary or deliver a boost dose of radiation to the tumor bed. In several small studies, local recurrence rates after irradiation were in the 10% range at 5 years, which indicates that this therapy is acceptable. In contrast, studies in which the breast was observed without treatment indicate that evident breast cancers develop in close to 50% of patients within 5 years (179,180). Additional positive axillary nodes are frequent in this circumstance, so axillary dissection should be performed regardless of the method that is selected for managing the breast. The prognosis for patients with occult primary tumors is similar to that for patients with clinically evident tumors matched for the number of involved nodes, and adjuvant systemic therapy should be administered according to established guidelines for node-positive patients.

Locally Recurrent Breast Carcinoma

Local recurrence in the breast after BCT may be a consequence of inappropriate patient selection, poor surgical or radiotherapeutic technique, or tumor biology. When errors in technique and selection are excluded, local recurrence in the first two postoperative years is uncommon. From years 2 to 6, local recurrence develops at a constant rate, usually at or adjacent to the site of the original tumor. After year 6, most local recurrence develops in other quadrants of the breast, which suggests that these are new primary tumors rather than true local failures. This idea is supported by the observation that the risk for late recurrence in other quadrants of the breast, approximately 1% annually, is equal to the risk for development of a new contralateral breast carcinoma.

Most recurrences are in the breast parenchyma, with approximately 5% to 10% developing in the skin as diffuse inflammatory-type recurrences (181). Before further local therapy, an evaluation to exclude metastatic disease is appropriate because concomitant distant metastases are present in 5% to 10% of cases. In the absence of distant metastases, completion mastectomy has been the mainstay of therapy. Five-year relapse-free survival rates range from 60% to 79% after the procedure, and further chest wall recurrences are uncommon. Small experiences with further attempts at breast preservation by using excision alone or repeated irradiation of small areas of the breast after surgical excision have been reported, but larger numbers of patients and longer follow-up periods are needed to determine the role of these therapies. The role of adjuvant systemic therapy in the management of recurrence is not well defined. In patients who have not received prior systemic therapy, we use the same criteria for treatment that are used for patients with newly diagnosed cancer. Treatment decisions for patients who received adjuvant systemic therapy at the time of diagnosis are made on a case-by-case basis.

Local recurrence after mastectomy develops in a different time frame, and the predictors and outcome are differ-

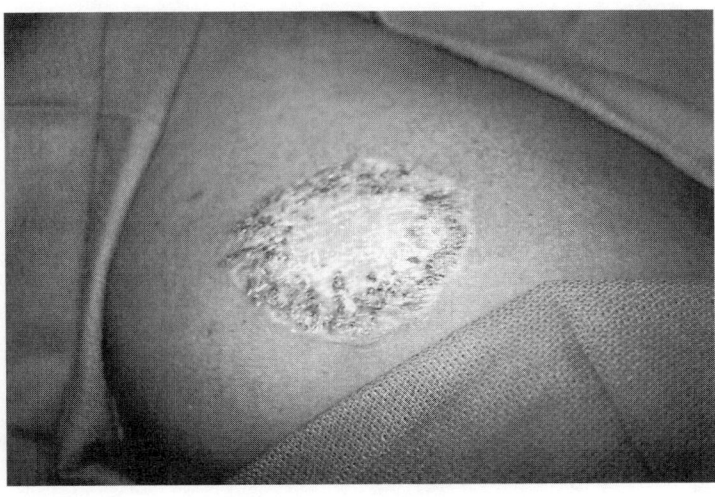

Figure 58.28. Paget's disease of the nipple. Depigmentation and desquamation of the nipple and areola are evident.

ent than for local recurrence after BCT. Approximately 75% of cases of local recurrence after mastectomy develop in the first three postoperative years, and about half of these are associated with the development of distant metastases at the time of local recurrence or within a few years. The number of axillary nodes containing metastasis is the best predictor of the risk for chest wall recurrence (148).

An evaluation for distant metastases is an essential part of the work-up of local recurrence after mastectomy. Small, localized recurrences are usually excised, but even with complete excision, RT should be administered to the chest wall because it is safe to assume that all the lymphatics are seeded with tumor. The supraclavicular space is usually included in the radiation field because these nodes are the second most frequent site of locoregional recurrence. The value of treating the axillary space and the internal mammary nodes is uncertain because clinical recurrence at these sites is uncommon. The value of additional systemic therapy for patients who have received postoperative adjuvant therapy is also uncertain.

Paget's Disease of the Nipple

Paget's disease of the nipple is a rare form of breast cancer characterized clinically by eczematoid changes of the nipple. Associated symptoms include itching, erythema, and nipple discharge (Fig. 58.28). Paget's disease is diagnosed histologically by the presence of large cells with pale cytoplasm and prominent nucleoli (Paget's cells) in-

volving the epidermis of the nipple. In 1874, Sir James Paget reported that this condition is invariably followed by cancer of the breast, usually within 1 year of diagnosis (182). In approximately half of women with Paget's disease, a breast mass is detected at presentation, and in most of the remainder, infiltrating or intraductal carcinoma is identified in the mastectomy specimen. The average age of women with Paget's disease does not differ from that of women with other forms of breast cancer, but symptoms are frequently present for 6 months or more before diagnosis.

Paget's disease has traditionally been treated with mastectomy. The reasons for this approach are the need to sacrifice the nipple–areola complex, the fact that subareolar ducts may be diffusely involved with tumor, and the observation that carcinoma may be found at a considerable distance from the nipple. A limited experience with breast-conserving procedures in the management of Paget's disease has been described. When therapeutic options are being considered in Paget's disease, it is helpful to think of the condition as DCIS involving the nipple that usually is associated with additional intraductal or invasive carcinoma in the underlying breast parenchyma. The extent of the underlying involvement determines the patient's suitability for BCT, and a detailed mammographic evaluation (including magnification views of the subareolar region) and histologic evaluation with margin assessment are essential components of this assessment. For patients with evidence of diffuse involvement or disease at a

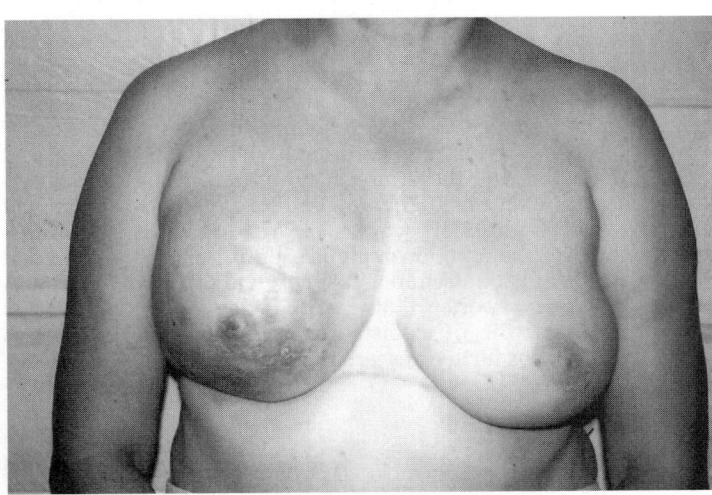

Figure 58.29. Locally advanced breast cancer. The breast is lifted and the upper half is bulging because of the large tumor. Distortion in the inferolateral contour is evident. The medial skin changes are caused by dermal tumor satellites.

distance from the nipple, mastectomy remains the standard therapy. In patients with disease localized to the subareolar area or the nipple–areola complex, BCT can be considered. This treatment requires removal of the entire nipple–areola complex and some of the underlying ductal region. In carefully selected patients, local failure rates with this approach appear to be similar to those reported for other breast carcinomas. The prognosis in Paget's disease is related to the stage of the disease and appears to be similar to that of women with other types of breast carcinoma. If invasive breast cancer is found, adjuvant systemic therapy should be administered according to the same guidelines used for other patients with invasive cancer.

Phyllodes Tumor

The term *phyllodes tumor* denotes a group of lesions of varying malignant potential, ranging from completely benign tumors to fully malignant sarcomas. (The previous name, *cystosarcoma phyllodes,* is now reserved for fully malignant lesions.) Clinically, phyllodes tumors are smooth, rounded, multinodular lesions that may be indistinguishable from fibroadenomas. Skin ulceration is seen with very large tumors, but this is usually caused by pressure necrosis rather than invasion of the skin by malignant cells (Fig. 58.5). Histologically, phyllodes tumor, like fibroadenoma, is composed of epithelial elements and a connective tissue stroma.

Phyllodes tumors are classified as benign, borderline, or malignant based on the nature of the tumor margins (pushing or infiltrative) and the presence of cellular atypia, mitotic activity, and overgrowth in the stroma. Which of these criteria is most important is a matter of disagreement, although most experts favor stromal overgrowth. The percentage of phyllodes tumors classified as malignant ranges from 23% to 50% (183,184). Axillary metastases are reported in fewer than 5% of cases but are a poor prognostic sign when present. Metastases more commonly follow the pattern seen with sarcomas (with the lung as the most common site) and histologically resemble sarcomas. Approximately 20% of phyllodes tumors recur locally if excised with no margin or a margin of a few millimeters of normal breast tissue. A wide excision with a 2-cm margin of normal breast tissue is appropriate therapy for benign and borderline phyllodes tumors unless they are so large that this is not cosmetically feasible. In the past, many authors have advocated mastectomy for the management of malignant phyllodes tumors. Because phyllodes tumors are not multicentric, there is no clear-cut biologic rationale for mastectomy, and the successful treatment of malignant phyllodes tumors with wide excision has been reported (185). The use of systemic therapy for malignant phyllodes tumors is based on the guidelines for treating sarcomas.

Other Cancers in the Breast

Sarcomas, lymphomas, and melanomas may all present as breast masses and are generally managed as recommended when they develop in other sites. Angiosarcoma is reported to involve the breast more frequently than other sites in the body. The tumors frequently grow rapidly and may be associated with a bluish discoloration of the skin. Bilateral disease is not uncommon. Angiosarcoma has traditionally been treated with mastectomy to clear margins. Axillary metastases are rare, and axillary dissection is not routinely indicated. The prognosis appears to be related to the grade of the lesion. No advantage has been proved for adjuvant RT or chemotherapy. Other sarcomas occur infrequently in the breast. Surgery is the primary therapy, and the decision to perform mastectomy or wide local excision is based on tumor size.

Melanoma arising from the skin of the breast is a more frequent finding in men than women. The diagnosis, treatment, and prognosis of melanoma arising in the breast are the same as for melanoma arising in other parts of the body. Mastectomy is not necessary for treatment of this lesion.

Primary breast lymphomas are rare and account for fewer than 1% of breast malignancies. They are believed to arise from intramammary lymph nodes or periductal and perilobular lymphoid tissue. Bilateral disease is seen in as many as 25% of patients. The diagnosis is usually made only after a biopsy, as neither the clinical nor the mammographic appearance of these lesions is diagnostic. Once the diagnosis of lymphoma is established, treatment with chemotherapy, RT, or both is used according to the disease stage and histologic subtype.

Locally Advanced Breast Cancer

The designation of *locally advanced breast cancer* includes T3 and T4 tumors, those with extensive axillary nodal involvement (N2), and inflammatory breast cancer (Fig. 58.29). Historical studies have demonstrated that for inflammatory carcinoma and tumors with evidence of skin involvement, chest wall fixation, or extensive axillary nodal disease, initial surgical therapy is associated with a high rate of locoregional recurrence and very poor 5-year survival, with treatment failure usually occurring within 2 years of diagnosis (186). For this reason, locally advanced breast cancer is now approached with a combination of chemotherapy, surgery, and RT. Multiple trials have reported the results of neoadjuvant chemotherapy in locally advanced breast cancer. With this approach, 60% to 80% of patients have a response (defined as a 50% reduction in the volume of tumor at the primary site), and 10% to 20% have a clinical complete response (187). However, only one half to two thirds of patients thought to have a complete response are found to have no residual tumor on pathologic examination. The extent of residual tumor after neoadjuvant chemotherapy is an important predictor of outcome in locally advanced breast cancer (188). Although induction chemotherapy is extremely effective in reducing tumor burden to allow a modified radical mastectomy with primary skin closure or breast conservation, no survival advantage has been demonstrated for the use of preoperative, as opposed to postoperative, chemotherapy in randomized trials. For patients with stage IIIB carcinoma, induction chemotherapy is the standard initial approach. After three to four cycles of treatment or maximal response, mastectomy or lumpectomy is undertaken. Depending on the extent of residual tumor, additional chemotherapy may be given postoperatively. After the completion of systemic therapy, chest wall RT is given to minimize the risk for local recurrence. For the patient with stage IIIA carcinoma that is operable by traditional criteria, the initial therapy can be surgery or chemotherapy. If the patient desires breast preservation, chemotherapy should be given in an effort to shrink the tumor. If not, mastectomy can be performed, with chemotherapy and RT given postoperatively in the traditional sequence. With modern combined-modality therapy, locoregional control can be maintained in 80% of patients, and 5-year survival rates of 50% to 80% have been reported (189–191). However, 50% of patients eventually die of metastatic disease, which underscores the need for further research in this area.

REFERENCES

1. Turner-Warwick R. The lymphatics of the breast. *Br J Surg* 1959;46:574.

2. Cody HS III, Egeli RA, Urban JA. Rotter's node metastases: therapeutic and prognostic considerations in early breast carcinoma. *Ann Surg* 1984;199:266–270.

3. Sacre R. Modern thoughts on lymph nodes in breast cancer. *Semin Surg Oncol* 1989;5:118–125.

4. Daniel CW, Silberstein GB. Development of the mammary gland. In: Neville MC, Daniel CW, eds. *The mammary gland.* New York: Plenum Publishing, 1987:3–10.

5. Russo J, Russo IH. Development of the human breast. In: *Encyclopedia of reproduction.* New York: Academic Press, 1998:3:71–76.

6. Dickson RB, Russo J. Biochemical control of breast development. In: Harris JR, Lippman ME, Morrow M, et al., eds. *Diseases of the breast.* Philadelphia: Lippincott Williams & Wilkins, 2000:303–318.

7. American Joint Committee on Cancer Staging. *Manual for staging of cancer,* 5th ed. Philadelphia: Lippincott–Raven Publishers, 1999:171–180.

8. Shapiro S. Screening: assessment of current studies. *Cancer* 1994;74:231–238.

9. Hendrick RE, Smith RA, Rutledge JH III, et al. Benefit of screening mammography in women aged 40–49: a new meta-analysis of randomized clinical trials. *J Natl Cancer Inst Monogr* 1997;22:87–92.

10. Morrow M, Bucci C, Rademaker A. Medical contraindications are not a major factor in the underutilization of breast-conserving therapy. *J Am Coll Surg* 1998;186:269–274.

11. American College of Radiology. *Breast imaging reporting and data system (BI-RADS),* 2nd ed. Reston, VA: American College of Radiology, 1995.

12. Sickles E. Further experience with microfocal spot magnification mammography in the assessment of clustered breast microcalcifications. *Radiology* 1980;137:9–14.

13. Dowlatshahi K, Yaremko MI, Kluskens LF, et al. Nonpalpable breast lesions: findings of stereotaxic needle-core biopsy and fine-needle aspiration cytology. *Radiology* 1991;183:745–750.

14. Parker SH, Lovin JD, Jobe WE, et al. Nonpalpable breast lesions: stereotactic automated large-core biopsies. *Radiology* 1991;180:403–407.

15. Parker SH, Burbank F, Jackman RJ, et al. Percutaneous large-core breast biopsy: a multi-institutional study. *Radiology* 1994;193:359–364.

16. Venta L. Image-guided breast biopsy. In: Harris JR, Lippman ME, Morrow M, et al., eds. *Diseases of the breast,* 2nd ed. Philadelphia: Lippincott Williams & Wilkins, 2000:149–164.

17. Liberman L, Cohen MA, Dershaw DD, et al. Atypical ductal hyperplasia diagnosed at stereotaxic core biopsy of breast lesions: an indication for surgical biopsy. *AJR Am J Roentgenol* 1995;164:1111–1113.

18. Liberman L, LaTrenta LR, Van Zee KJ, et al. Stereotactic core biopsy of calcifications highly suggestive of malignancy. *Radiology* 1997;203:673–677.

19. Morrow M, Venta L, Stinson T, et al. A prospective comparison of stereotactic core biopsy and surgical excision as diagnostic procedures for breast cancer patients. *Ann Surg* 2001 (in press).

20. Mansel RE, Wisbey JR, Hughes LE. Controlled trial of the antigonadotropin danazol in painful nodular benign breast disease. *Lancet* 1982;1:928–930.

21. Allen SS, Froberg DG. The effect of decreased caffeine consumption on benign proliferative breast disease: a randomized clinical trial. *Surgery* 1987;101:720–730.

22. Smallwood J, Ah-Kye D, Taylor I. Vitamin B_6 in the treatment of pre-menstrual mastalgia. *Br J Clin Pract* 1986;40:532–533.

23. London RS, Sundaram GS, Murphy L, et al. The effect of vitamin E on mammary dysplasia: a double-blind study. *Obstet Gynecol* 1985;65:104–106.

24. Catania S, Zurrida S, Veronesi P, et al. Mondor's disease and breast cancer. *Cancer* 1992;69:2267–2270.

25. Seltzer M, Perloff L, Kellye R, et al. The significance of age in patients with nipple discharge. *Surg Gynecol Obstet* 1979;131:519–522.

26. Murad T, Contesso G, Mouriesse H. Nipple discharge from the breast. *Ann Surg* 1989;195:250–264.

27. Groves AM, Carr M, Wadhera V, et al. An audit of cytology in the evaluation of nipple discharge: a retrospective study of 10 years' experience. *Breast* 1996;5:96–99.

28. Dawes LG, Bowen C, Venta LA, et al. Ductography for nipple discharge: no replacement for ductal excision. *Surgery* 1998;124:685–691.

29. Schnitt S, Connelly J. Pathology of benign breast disorders. In: Harris JR, Lippman ME, Morrow M, et al., eds. *Diseases of the breast,* 2nd ed. Philadelphia: Lippincott Williams & Wilkins, 2000:75–94.

30. Aitken RJ, Hood J, Going JJ, et al. Bacteriology of mammary duct ectasia. *Br J Surg* 1988;75:1041–1046.

31. Morrow M, Wong S, Venta L. The evaluation of breast masses in women younger than forty years of age. *Surgery* 1998;124:634–641.

32. Cowen PN, Benson EA. Cytological study of fluid from breast cysts. *Br J Surg* 1979;66:209–211.

33. Wilkinson S, Anderson TJ, Rifkind E, et al. Fibroadenoma of the breast: a follow-up of conservative management. *Br J Surg* 1989;76:390–391.

34. Dupont WD, Page DL, Parl FF, et al. Long-term risk of breast cancer in women with fibroadenoma. *N Engl J Med* 1994;331:10–15.

35. Dupont WD, Parl FF, Hartmann WH, et al. Breast cancer risk associated with proliferative breast disease and atypical hyperplasia. *Cancer* 1993;71:1258–1265.

36. London SJ, Connolly JL, Schnitt SJ, et al. A prospective study of benign breast disease and the risk of breast cancer. *JAMA* 1992;267:941–944.

37. McDivitt RW, Stevens JA, Lee NC, et al. Histologic types of benign breast disease and the risk for breast cancer. The Cancer and Steroid Hormone Study Group. *Cancer* 1992;69:1408–1414.

38. Feig SA, Shaber GS, Patchefsky A, et al. Analysis of clinically occult and mammographically occult breast tumors. *Am J Roentgenol* 1977;128:403–408.

39. Hollingsworth AB, Taylor LD, Rhodes DC. Establishing a histologic basis for false-negative mammograms. *Am J Surg* 1993;166:643–648.

40. Morrow M, Schmidt RA, Bucci C. Breast conservation for mammographically occult carcinoma. *Ann Surg* 1998;227:502–506.

41. Lister D, Evans AJ, Burrell HC, et al. The accuracy of breast ultrasound in the evaluation of clinically benign discrete, symptomatic breast lumps. *Clin Radiol* 1998;53:490–492.

42. Yang WT, Lam WW, Cheung H, et al. Sonographic, magnetic resonance imaging, and mammographic assessments of preoperative size of breast cancer. *J Ultrasound Med* 1997;16:791–797.

43. Orel SG, Schnall MD, Powell CM, et al. Staging of suspected breast cancer: effect of MR imaging and MR-guided biopsy. *Radiology* 1995;196:115–122.

44. Dao TH, Rahmouni A, Campana F, et al. Tumor recurrence versus fibrosis in the irradiated breast: differentiation with dynamic gadolinium-enhanced MR imaging. *Radiology* 1993;187:751–755.

45. Diggles L, Mena I, Khalkhali I. Technical aspects of prone-dependent breast scintimammography. *J Nucl Med Technol* 1994;22:165–170.

46. Kopans DB. Imaging analysis of breast lesions. In: Harris JR, Lippman ME, Morrow M, et al., eds. *Diseases of the breast,* 2nd ed. Philadelphia: Lippincott Williams & Wilkins, 2000:123–148.

47. Giard RW, Hermans J. The value of aspiration cytologic examination of the breast: a statistical review of the medical literature. *Cancer* 1992;69:2104–2110.

48. Barrows GH, Anderson TJ, Lamb JL, et al. Fine-needle aspiration of breast cancer: relationship of clinical factors to cytology results in 689 primary malignancies. *Cancer* 1986;58:1493–1498.

49. Shabot MM, Goldberg IM, Schick P, et al. Aspiration cytology is superior to Tru-Cut needle biopsy in establishing the diagnosis of clinically suspicious breast masses. *Ann Surg* 1982;196:122–126.

50. Kearney TJ, Morrow M. Effect of reexcision on the success of breast-conserving surgery. *Ann Surg Oncol* 1995;2:303–307.

51. Fisher ER, Sass R, Fisher B. Biologic considerations regarding the one and two step procedures in the management of patients with invasive carcinoma of the breast. *Surg Gynecol Obstet* 1985;161:245–249.

52. Layfield LJ, Glasgow BJ, Cramer H. Fine-needle aspiration in

the management of breast masses. *Pathol Annu* 1989;24: 23–62.

53. Greenberg R, Skornick Y, Kaplan O. Management of breast fibroadenomas. *J Gen Intern Med* 1998;13:640–645.

54. Bell DA, Hajdu SI, Urban JA, et al. Role of aspiration cytology in the diagnosis and management of mammary lesions in office practice. *Cancer* 1983;51:1182–1189.

55. Donegan WL. Evaluation of a palpable breast mass. *N Engl J Med* 1992;327:937–942.

56. Dixon JM. Repeated aspiration of breast abscesses in lactating women. *Br Med J* 1988;297:1517–1518.

57. Schafer P, Furrer C, Mermillod B. An association of cigarette smoking with recurrent subareolar breast abscess. *Int J Epidemiol* 1988;17:810–813.

58. Bundred NJ, Dover MS, Aluwihare N, et al. Smoking and periductal mastitis. *Br Med J* 1993;307:772–773.

59. Seidman H, Mushinski MH, Gelb SK, et al. Probabilities of eventually developing or dying of cancer—United States, 1985. *CA Cancer J Clin* 1985;35:36–56.

60. Slattery ML, Kerber RA. A comprehensive evaluation of family history and breast cancer risk: the Utah Population Database. *JAMA* 1993;270:1563–1568.

61. Claus EB, Risch NJ, Thompson WD. Age at onset as an indicator of familial risk of breast cancer. *Am J Epidemiol* 1990; 131:961–972.

62. Ford D, Easton DF, Stratton M, et al. Genetic heterogeneity and penetrance analysis of the *BRCA1* and *BRCA2* genes in breast cancer families: the Breast Cancer Linkage Consortium. *Am J Hum Genet* 1998;62:676–689.

63. Thorlacius S, Struewing JP, Hartge P, et al. Population-based study of risk of breast cancer in carriers of *BRCA2* mutation. *Lancet* 1998;352:1337–1339.

64. Struewing JP, Hartge P, Wacholder S, et al. The risk of cancer associated with specific mutations of *BRCA1* and *BRCA2* among Ashkenazi Jews. *N Engl J Med* 1997;336:1401–1408.

65. Shattuck-Eidens D, Oliphant A, McClure M, et al. *BRCA1* sequence analysis in women at high risk for susceptibility mutations: risk factor analysis and implications for genetic testing. *JAMA* 1997;278:1242–1250.

66. Hisada M, Garber JE, Fung CY, et al. Multiple primary cancers in families with Li-Fraumeni syndrome. *J Natl Cancer Inst* 1998;90:606–611.

67. Hoskins KF, Stopfer JE, Calzone KA, et al. Assessment and counseling for women with a family history of breast cancer: a guide for clinicians. *JAMA* 1995;273:577–585.

68. Newcomb PA, Storer BE, Longnecker MP, et al. Lactation and a reduced risk of premenopausal breast cancer. *N Engl J Med* 1994;330:81–87.

69. de Waard F, Baanders-van Halewijn EA. A prospective study in general practice on breast-cancer risk in postmenopausal women. *Int J Cancer* 1974;14:153–160.

70. Steinberg KK, Thacker SB, Smith SJ, et al. A meta-analysis of the effect of estrogen replacement therapy on the risk of breast cancer. *JAMA* 1991;265;1985–1990.

71. Gapstur SM, Morrow M, Sellers TA. Hormone replacement therapy and risk of breast cancer with a favorable histology: results of the Iowa Women's Health Study. *JAMA* 1999;281: 2091–2097.

72. Hancock SL, Tucker MA, Hoppe RT. Breast cancer after treatment of Hodgkin's disease. *J Natl Cancer Inst* 1993;85:25–31.

73. Hunter DJ, Spiegelman D, Adami HO, et al. Cohort studies of fat intake and the risk of breast cancer—a pooled analysis. *N Engl J Med* 1996;334:356–361.

74. Willett WC, Hunter DJ, Stampfer MJ, et al. Dietary fat and fiber in relation to risk of breast cancer: an 8-year follow-up. *JAMA* 1992;268:2037–2044.

75. Dupont WD, Page DL. Risk factors for breast cancer in women with proliferative breast disease. *N Engl J Med* 1985;312:146–151.

76. Haagensen CD, Bodian C, Haagensen DE. Lobular neoplasia (lobular carcinoma in situ) breast carcinoma: risk and detection. Haagensen CD, ed. Philadelphia: WB Saunders, 1981:238.

77. Rosen PP, Kosloff C, Lieberman PH, et al. Lobular carcinoma in situ of the breast: detailed analysis of 99 patients with average follow-up of 24 years. *Am J Surg Pathol* 1978;2:225–251.

78. Andersen JA. Lobular carcinoma in situ of the breast: an approach to rational treatment. *Cancer* 1977;39:2597–2602.

79. Page DL, Kidd TE Jr, Dupont WD, et al. Lobular neoplasia of the breast: higher risk for subsequent invasive cancer predicted by more extensive disease. *Hum Pathol* 1991;22: 1232–1239.

80. Salvadori B, Bartolic C, Zurrida S, et al. Risk of invasive cancer in women with lobular carcinoma in situ of the breast. *Eur J Cancer* 1991;27:35–37.

81. Ottesen GL, Graversen HP, Blichert-Toft M, et al. Lobular carcinoma in situ of the female breast: short-term results of a prospective nationwide study. *Am J Surg Pathol* 1993;17: 14–21.

82. Bodian CA, Perzin KH, Lattes R. Lobular neoplasia: long-term risk of breast cancer and relation to other factors. *Cancer* 1996;78:1024–1034.

83. Fisher B, Costantino JP, Wickerham DL, et al. Tamoxifen for prevention of breast cancer: report of the National Surgical Adjuvant Breast and Bowel Project P-1 study. *J Natl Cancer Inst* 1998;90:1371–1388.

84. Gail MH, Brinton LA, Byar DP, et al. Projecting individualized probabilities of developing breast cancer for white females who are being examined annually. *J Natl Cancer Inst* 1989;81:1879–1886.

85. Hartmann LC, Schaid DJ, Woods JE, et al. Efficacy of bilateral prophylactic mastectomy in women with a family history of breast cancer. *N Engl J Med* 1999;340:77–84.

86. Early Breast Cancer Trialists Collaborative Group. Tamoxifen for early breast cancer: an overview of the randomised trials. *Lancet* 1998;351:1451–1467.

87. Wickerham DL, Costantino J, Fisher B, et al. Average annual rates of invasive and noninvasive breast cancer by history of LCIS and atypical hyperplasia for participants in the BCPT. *Proc Am Soc Clin Oncol* 1998;18:87a(abst 327).

88. Cummings SR, Eckert S, Krueger KA, et al. The effect of raloxifene on risk of breast cancer in postmenopausal women: results from the MORE randomized trial—Multiple Outcomes of Raloxifene Evaluation. *JAMA* 1999;281: 2189–2197.

89. Morrow M, Schnitt SJ, Harris JR. Ductal carcinoma in situ and microinvasive carcinoma. In: Harris JR, Lippman ME, Morrow M, et al., eds. *Diseases of the breast,* 2nd ed. Philadelphia: Lippincott Williams & Wilkins, 2000:383–401.

90. Silverstein MJ. Van Nuys experience by treatment. In: Silverstein MJ, ed. *Ductal carcinoma in situ of the breast.* Baltimore: Williams & Wilkins, 1997:443.

91. Patchefsky AS, Schwartz GF, Finkelstein SD, et al. Heterogeneity of intraductal carcinoma of the breast. *Cancer* 1989; 63:731–741.

92. Solin LJ, Kurtz J, Fourquet A, et al. Fifteen-year results of breast-conserving surgery and definitive breast irradiation for the treatment of ductal carcinoma in situ of the breast. *J Clin Oncol* 1996;14:754–763.

93. Fisher B, Dignam J, Wolmark N, et al. Lumpectomy and radiation therapy for the treatment of intraductal breast cancer: findings from National Surgical Adjuvant Breast and Bowel Project B-17 study. *J Clin Oncol* 1998;16:441–452.

94. Fisher ER, Dignam J, Tan-Chiu E, et al. Pathologic findings from the National Surgical Adjuvant Breast Project (NSABP) eight-year update of protocol B-17: intraductal carcinoma. *Cancer* 1999;86:429–438.

95. Silverstein MJ, Lagios MD, Groshen S, et al. The influence of margin width on local control of ductal carcinoma in situ of the breast. *N Engl J Med* 1999;340:1455–1461.

96. Holland R, Hendricks JH, Verbeek AL, et al. Extent, distribution, and mammographic/histological correlations of breast ductal carcinoma in situ. *Lancet* 1990;335:519–522.

97. Fisher ER, Dignam J, Wolmark N, et al. Tamoxifen in treatment of intraductal breast cancer: National Surgical Adjuvant Breast and Bowel Project B-24 randomised clinical trial. *Lancet* 1999;353:1993–2000.

98. Bloom HJG, Richardson WW, Harries EJ. Natural history of untreated breast cancer (1805–1933). *Br Med J* 1962;2: 213–221.

99. Halsted WS. The results of radical operations for the cure of carcinoma of the breast. *Ann Surg* 1907;66:1–19.

100. Adair F, Berg J, Joubert L, et al. Long-term follow-up of breast cancer patients: the 30-year report. *Cancer* 1974;33: 1145–1150.

101. Fisher B. Laboratory and clinical research in breast cancer—a personal adventure: the David A. Karnofsky Memorial Lecture. *Cancer Res* 1980;40:3863–3874.

102. Hellman S. Karnofsky Memorial Lecture. Natural history of small breast cancers. *J Clin Oncol* 1994;12:2229–2234.

103. Overgaard M, Hansen PS, Overgaard J, et al. Postoperative radiotherapy in high-risk premenopausal women with breast cancer who receive adjuvant chemotherapy. *N Engl J Med* 1997;337:949–955.

104. Ragaz J, Jackson SM, Le N, et al. Adjuvant radiotherapy and chemotherapy in node-positive premenopausal women with breast cancer. *N Engl J Med* 1997;337:956–962.

105. Overgaard M, Jensen MB, Overgaard J, et al. Postoperative radiotherapy in high-risk postmenopausal breast-cancer patients given adjuvant tamoxifen: Danish Breast Cancer Cooperative Group DBCG 82c randomised trial. *Lancet* 1999; 353:1641–1648.

106. Broet P, de la Rochefordiere A, Scholl SM, et al. Contralateral breast cancer: annual incidence and risk parameters. *J Clin Oncol* 1995;13:1578–1583.

107. Elston CW, Ellis IO. Pathological prognostic factors in breast cancer. I. The value of histological grade in breast cancer: experience from a large study with long-term follow-up. *Histopathology* 1991;19:403–410.

108. Jensen CV, Jacobsen HI. Basic guides to the mechanism of estrogen action. *Recent Prog Horm Res* 1962;18:387.

109. McGuire W, Carbone P, Sears M, et al. Estrogen receptors in human breast cancer: an overview. In: McGuire W, Vollmer E, Carbone P, eds. *Estrogen receptors in human breast cancer.* New York: Raven Press, 1975:1–7.

110. Kuiper GG, Enmark E, Pelto-Huikko M, et al. Cloning of a novel receptor expressed in rat prostate and ovary. *Proc Natl Acad Sci USA* 1996;93:5925–5930.

111. Lee YT. Bone scanning in patients with early breast carcinoma: should it be a routine staging procedure? *Cancer* 1981;47:486–495.

112. Lee YT. Carcinoembryonic antigen as a monitor of recurrent breast cancer. *J Surg Oncol* 1982;20:109–114.

113. Kallioniemi OP, Oksa H, Aaran RK, et al. Serum CA 15-3 assay in the diagnosis and follow-up of breast cancer. *Br J Cancer* 1988;58:213–215.

114. Stearns V, Yamuchi H, Hayes DF. Circulating tumor markers in breast cancer: accepted utilities and novel prospects. *Breast Cancer Res Treat* 1998;52:239–245.

115. Arriagada R, Le MG, Rochard F, et al., for the Institute Gustave Roussy Breast Cancer Group. Conservative treatment versus mastectomy in early breast cancer: patterns of failure with 15 years of follow-up data. *J Clin Oncol* 1996;14: 1558–1564.

116. Veronesi U, Salvadori B, Luini A, et al. Breast conservation is a safe method in patients with small cancer of the breast: long-term results of three randomized trials on 1,993 patients. *Eur J Cancer* 1995;31A:1574–1579.

117. Fisher B, Anderson S, Redmond CK, et al. Reanalysis and results after 12 years of follow-up in a randomized clinical trial comparing total mastectomy with lumpectomy with or without irradiation in the treatment of breast cancer. *N Engl J Med* 1995;333:1456–1461.

118. Jacobson JA, Danforth DN, Cowan KH, et al. Ten-year results of a comparison of conservation with mastectomy in the treatment of stage I and II breast cancer. *N Engl J Med* 1995;332:907–911.

119. Van Dongen JA, Bartelink H, Fentiman IS, et al. Factors influencing local relapse and survival and results of salvage treatment after breast-conserving therapy in operable breast cancer: EORTC trial 1081, breast conservation compared with mastectomy in TNM stage I and II breast cancer. *Eur J Cancer* 1992;28A:801–805.

120. Blichert-Toft M, Rose C, Andersen JA, et al. Danish randomized trial comparing breast conservation therapy with mastectomy: six years of life-table analysis. *J Natl Cancer Inst Monogr* 1992;11:19–25.

121. Winchester DP, Cox JD. Standards for diagnosis and management of invasive breast cancer. *CA Cancer J Clin* 1998; 48:83–107.

122. Bonadonna G, Veronesi U, Brambilla C, et al. Primary chemotherapy to avoid mastectomy in tumors with diameters of three centimeters or more. *J Natl Cancer Inst* 1990;82: 1539–1545.

123. Fisher B, Bryant J, Wolmark N, et al. Effect of preoperative chemotherapy on the outcome of women with operable breast cancer. *J Clin Oncol* 1998;16:2672–2685.

124. Holland R, Veling S, Mravunac M, et al. Histologic multifocality of Tis, T1-2 breast carcinomas: implications for clinical trials of breast-conserving treatment. *Cancer* 1985;56: 979–990.

125. Schmidt-Ullrich RK, Wazer DE, DiPetrillo T, et al. Breast conservation therapy for early-stage breast carcinoma with outstanding 10-year locoregional control rates: a case for aggressive therapy to the tumor-bearing quadrant. *Int J Radiat Oncol Biol Phys* 1993;27:545–552.

126. Morrow M, Schmidt R, Hassett C. Patient selection for breast-conserving surgery with magnification mammography. *Surgery* 1995;118:621–626.

127. Morrow M, Harris JR. Local management of invasive breast cancer. In: Harris JR, Lippman ME, Morrow M, et al., eds. *Diseases of the breast,* 2nd ed. Philadelphia: Lippincott Williams & Wilkins, 2000:515–560.

128. Schnitt SJ, Abner A, Gelman R, et al. The relationship between microscopic margins of resection and the risk of local recurrence in breast cancer patients treated with conservative surgery and radiation therapy. *Cancer* 1994;74: 1746–1751.

129. Schneiderman MA, Axtell LM. Deaths among female patients with carcinoma of the breast treated by surgical procedure alone. *Surg Gynecol Obstet* 1979;148:193–196.

130. Platt R, Zucker JR, Zaleznik DF, et al. Prophylaxis against wound infection following herniorrhaphy or breast surgery. *J Infect Dis* 1992;166:556–560.

131. Gabriel SE, Woods JE, O'Fallon WM, et al. Complications leading to surgery after breast implantation. *N Engl J Med* 1997;336:677–682.

132. Perkins LL, Clark BD, Klein PJ, et al. A meta-analysis of breast implants and connective tissue disease. *Ann Plast Surg* 1995;35:561–570.

133. Sanchez-Guerrero J, Colditz GA, Karlson EW, et al. Silicone breast implants and the risk of connective-tissue diseases and symptoms. *N Engl J Med* 1995;332:1666–1670.

134. Kroll S, Ames F, Singletary S, et al. The oncologic risks of skin preservation at mastectomy when combined with immediate reconstruction of the breast. *Surg Gynecol Obstet* 1991;172:17–20.

135. Williams JK, Carlson GW, Bostwick J III, et al. The effects of radiation treatment after TRAM flap breast reconstruction. *Plast Reconstr Surg* 1997;100:1153–1160.

136. Graversen HP, Blichert-Toft M, Andersen JA, et al. Breast cancer: risk of axillary recurrence in node-negative patients following partial dissection of the axilla. *Eur J Surg Oncol* 1988;14:407–412.

137. Fisher B, Wolmark N, Bauer M, et al. The accuracy of clinical nodal staging and of limited axillary dissection as a determinant of histologic nodal status in carcinoma of the breast. *Surg Gynecol Obstet* 1981;152:765–772.

138. Fowble B, Solin LJ, Schultz DJ, et al. Frequency, sites of relapse, and outcome of regional node failures following conservative surgery and radiation for early breast cancer. *Int J Radiat Oncol Biol Phys* 1989;17:703–710.

139. Petrek JA, Heelan MC. Incidence of breast carcinoma-related lymphedema. *Cancer* 1998;83:2776–2781.

140. Giuliano AE, Kirgan DM, Guenther JM, et al. Lymphatic mapping and sentinel lymphadenectomy for breast cancer. *Ann Surg* 1994;220:391–401.

141. Veronesi U, Paganelli G, Galimberti V, et al. Sentinel-node biopsy to avoid axillary dissection in breast cancer with clinically negative lymph-nodes. *Lancet* 1997;349: 1864–1867.

142. Giuliano AE, Jones RC, Brennan M, et al. Sentinel lymphadenectomy in breast cancer. *J Clin Oncol* 1997;15: 2345–2350.

143. Guenther JM, Krishnamoorthy M, Tan LR. Sentinel lymphadenectomy for breast cancer in a community managed care setting. *Cancer J Sci Am* 1997;3:336–340.

144. Borgstein PJ, Pijpers R, Cormans EF, et al. Sentinel lymph node biopsy in breast cancer: guidelines and pitfalls of lym-

phoscintigraphy and gamma probe detection. *J Am Coll Surg* 1998;186:275–283.

145. Krag D, Weaver D, Ashikaga T, et al. The sentinel node in breast cancer: a multicenter validation study. *N Engl J Med* 1998;337:941–946.

146. Veronesi U, Paganelli G, Viale G, et al. Sentinel lymph node biopsy and axillary dissection in breast cancer: results in a large series. *J Natl Cancer Inst* 1999;91:368–373.

147. Morrow M, Rademaker AW, Bethke KP, et al. Learning sentinel node biopsy: results of a prospective randomized trial of two techniques. *Surgery* 1999;126:714–722.

148. Cody HS III, Hill AD, Tran KN, et al. Credentialing for breast lymphatic mapping: how many cases are enough? *Ann Surg* 1999;229:723–728.

149. Morrow M. Postmastectomy radiation therapy: a surgical perspective. *Semin Radiat Oncol* 1999;9:269–274.

150. Early Breast Cancer Trialists' Collaborative Group. Effects of radiotherapy and surgery in early breast cancer. *N Engl J Med* 1995;333:1444–1455.

151. Saez RA, McGuire WL, Clark GM. Prognostic factors in breast cancer. *Semin Surg Oncol* 1989;5:102–110.

152. Ravdin PM, De Laurentis M, Vendely T, et al. Prediction of axillary lymph node status in breast cancer patients by use of prognostic indicators. *J Natl Cancer Inst* 1994;86:1771–1775.

153. Rosen PR, Groshen S, Saigo PE, et al. A long-term follow-up study of survival in stage I (T1 N0 M0) and stage II (T1 N1 M0) breast carcinoma. *J Clin Oncol* 1989;7:355–366.

154. Quiet CA, Ferguson DJ, Weichselbaum RR, et al. Natural history of node-positive breast cancer: the curability of small cancers with a limited number of positive nodes. *J Clin Oncol* 1996;14:3105–3111.

155. Clark GM, McGuire WL. Steroid receptors and other prognostic factors in primary breast cancer. *Semin Oncol* 1988; 15:20–25.

156. Hedley DW, Clark GM, Cornelisse CJ, et al. Consensus review of the clinical utility of DNA cytometry in carcinoma of the breast: report of the DNA Cytometry Consensus Conference. *Cytometry* 1993;14:482–485.

157. Silvestrini R. Cell kinetics: prognostic and therapeutic implications in human tumours. *Cell Prolif* 1994;27:579–596.

158. Early Breast Cancer Trialists' Collaborative Group. Polychemotherapy for early breast cancer: an overview of the randomised trials. *Lancet* 1998;352:930–942.

159. Davidson N, Kennedy JM, Armstrong DK. Dose-intensive chemotherapy. In: Harris JR, Lippman ME, Morrow M, et al., eds. *Diseases of the breast,* 2nd ed. Philadelphia: Lippincott Williams & Wilkins, 2000:633–644.

160. Jordan VC, Morrow M. Tamoxifen, raloxifene, and the prevention of breast cancer. *Endocr Rev* 1999;20:253–278.

161. Early Breast Cancer Trialists' Collaborative Group. Tamoxifen for early breast cancer: an overview of the randomised trials. *Lancet* 1998;351:1451–1467.

162. Veronesi U, Salvadori B, Luini A, et al. Conservative treatment of early breast cancer: long-term results of 1,232 cases treated with quadrantectomy, axillary dissection, and radiotherapy. *Ann Surg* 1990;211:250–259.

163. Fourquet A, Campana F, Zafrani B, et al. Prognostic factors of breast recurrence in the conservative management of early breast cancer: a 25-year follow-up. *Int J Radiat Oncol Biol Phys* 1989;17:719–725.

164. Bates T, Riley DL, Houghton J, et al. Breast cancer in elderly women: a Cancer Research Campaign trial comparing treatment with tamoxifen and optimal surgery with tamoxifen alone. *Br J Surg* 1991;78:591–594.

165. Mustacchi G, Milani S, Pluchinotta A, et al. Tamoxifen or surgery plus tamoxifen as primary treatment for elderly patients with operable breast cancer: the G.R.E.T.A. Trial— Group for Research on Endocrine Therapy in the Elderly. *Anticancer Res* 1994;14:2197–2200.

166. Robertson JF, Ellis IO, Elston CW, et al. Mastectomy or tamoxifen as initial therapy for operable breast cancer in elderly patients: 5-year follow-up. *Eur J Clin Oncol* 1992;28A:908–910.

167. Margolese RG, Foster RS Jr. Tamoxifen as an alternative to surgical resection for selected geriatric patients with primary breast cancer. *Arch Surg* 1989;124:548–552.

168. Wallack MK, Wolf JA Jr, Bedwinck J, et al. Gestational carcinoma of the female breast. *Curr Probl Cancer* 1983;7:1–58.

169. Saunders CM, Baum M. Breast cancer and pregnancy: a review. *J R Soc Med* 1993;86:162–170.

170. Petrek JA, Moore A. Breast cancer treatment in pregnant or postpartum women and subsequent pregnancy in breast cancer survivors. In: Harris JR, Lippman ME, Morrow M, et al., eds. *Diseases of the breast,* 2nd ed. Philadelphia: Lippincott Williams & Wilkins, 2000:691–701.

171. Guinee VF, Olsson H, Moller T, et al. Effect of pregnancy on prognosis for young women with breast cancer. *Lancet* 1994; 343:1587–1589.

172. Olson SH, Zauber AG, Tang J, et al. Relation of time since last birth and parity to survival of young women with breast cancer. *Epidemiology* 1998;9:669–671.

173. Kroman N, Wohlfahrt J, Andersen KW, et al. Time since childbirth and prognosis in primary breast cancer: population-based study. *BMJ* 1997;315:851–855.

174. Thomas DB. Breast cancer in men. *Epidemiol Rev* 1993;15: 220–231.

175. Guinee VF, Olsson H, Moller T, et al. The prognosis of breast cancer in males: a report of 335 cases. *Cancer* 1993;71: 154–161.

176. Ribeiro G, Swindell R. Adjuvant tamoxifen for male breast cancer (MBC). *Br J Cancer* 1992;65:252–254.

177. Donegan WK, Redlich PN. Breast cancer in men. *Surg Clin North Am* 1996;76:343–363.

178. Morris EA, Schwartz LH, Dershaw DD, et al. MR imaging of the breast in patients with occult primary breast carcinoma. *Radiology* 1997;205:437–440.

179. Ellerbroek N, Holmes F, Singletary E, et al. Treatment of patients with isolated axillary nodal metastases from an occult primary carcinoma consistent with breast origin. *Cancer* 1990;66:1461–1467.

180. Merson M, Andreola S, Galimberti V, et al. Breast carcinoma presenting as axillary metastases without evidence of a primary tumor. *Cancer* 1992;70:504–508.

181. Gage I, Schnitt SJ, Recht A, et al. Skin recurrences after breast-conserving therapy for early-stage breast cancer. *J Clin Oncol* 1998;16:480–486.

182. Paget J. Disease of the mammary areola preceding cancer of the mammary gland. *St Bart Hosp Rep* 1874;10:79–89.

183. Salvadori B, Cusumano F, Del Bo R, et al. Surgical treatment of phyllodes tumors of the breast. *Cancer* 1989;63: 2532–2536.

184. Kessinger A, Foley JF, Lemon HM, et al. Metastatic cystosarcoma phyllodes: a case report and review of the literature. *J Surg Oncol* 1972;4:131–147.

185. Zissis C, Apostolikas N, Konstantinidou A, et al. The extent of surgery and prognosis of patients with phyllodes tumor of the breast. *Breast Cancer Res Treat* 1998;48:205–210.

186. Haagensen CD, Stout AP. Carcinoma of the breast. II. Criteria of operability. *Ann Surg* 1943;118:859–872.

187. Hortobagyi GN, Singletary SE, Stroul EA. Treatment of locally advanced and inflammatory breast cancer. In: Harris JR, Lippman ME, Morrow M, et al., eds. *Diseases of the breast,* 2nd ed. Philadelphia: Lippincott Williams & Wilkins, 2000:645–660.

188. Feldman LD, Hortobagyi GN, Buzdar AU, et al. Pathological assessment of response to induction chemotherapy in breast cancer. *Cancer Res* 1986;46:2578–2581.

189. Scholl SM, Fourquet A, Asselain B, et al. Neoadjuvant versus adjuvant chemotherapy in premenopausal patients with tumours considered too large for breast-conserving surgery: preliminary results of a randomised trial—S6. *Eur J Cancer* 1994;30A:645–652.

190. Rubens RD, Bartelink H, Engelsman E, et al. Locally advanced breast cancer: the contribution of cytotoxic and endocrine treatment to radiotherapy—an EORTC Breast Cancer Co-operative Group trial (10792). *Eur J Cancer Clin Oncol* 1989;25:667–678.

191. Buzdar AU, Singletary SE, Booser DJ, et al. Combined-modality treatment of stage III and inflammatory breast cancer—MD Anderson Cancer Center experience. *Surg Oncol Clin N Am* 1995;4:715–734.

SECTION K

THORAX

SURGERY: SCIENTIFIC PRINCIPLES AND PRACTICE, Third Edition, edited by
Lazar J. Greenfield, Michael W. Mulholland, Keith T. Oldham, Gerald B. Zelenock,
and Keith D. Lillemoe. Lippincott Williams & Wilkins Publishers, Philadelphia, © 2001.

CHAPTER 59

LUNG NEOPLASMS

JOCELYNE MARTIN AND VALERIE W. RUSCH

Primary and metastatic lung neoplasms are the most common diseases treated by thoracic surgeons. The clinical management of lung neoplasms, especially primary lung cancer, has evolved considerably during the past 20 years. Significant advances have been made in our understanding of the natural history of lung cancer and in the methods of selecting patients for surgical resection. The roles of both extended and limited pulmonary resection have been defined. Multimodality therapy has become increasingly important and requires that surgeons be able to select patients for adjuvant treatment and understand how to integrate surgical resection with radiation and chemotherapy. Molecular genetic techniques have begun to reveal the fundamental biology of lung cancer and offer the hope of newer, more effective treatments. This chapter emphasizes current information about tumor biology, multimodality therapy, and the rationale for surgical intervention in both primary and metastatic lung cancers.

INCIDENCE AND EPIDEMIOLOGY

It is estimated that 171,600 new cases of lung cancer were diagnosed in 1999 in the United States, making it the second most common malignancy in both men and women. However, the incidence of lung cancer, which rose steadily from the 1930s onward, has now started to decline. Since 1990, the incidence in men has decreased by 2.6% annually, and the incidence in women appears to be reaching a plateau.

Lung cancer is the leading cause of cancer-related deaths. Although lung cancer mortality rates in women are increasing by 1.7% annually, mortality rates for men decreased about 1.6% per year between 1990 and 1996. These incidence and mortality rates reflect the changing patterns of cigarette smoking among men and women. Because of an increase in smoking during the past 60 years, lung cancer recently surpassed breast cancer as the major cause of death in women. Decreasing lung cancer incidence and mortality rates in men have resulted from a decrease in smoking rates, particularly during the past 30 years. Unfortunately, if recent upward trends in smoking among adolescents are not reversed, lung cancer rates will rise again (1–3).

Cigarette smoking is the primary cause of lung cancer. More than 40 carcinogens have been identified among the constituents of cigarette smoke, including benzo[a]pyrene, nicotine, and several N-nitrosamines (4). Many components of tobacco smoke also function as carcinogens with other compounds (5). In addition, cigarette smoke contains radioactive components: the alpha emitters polonium 210 and lead 210 (6). Passive exposure to tobacco smoke also increases the risk of lung cancer. It is estimated that approximately one third of lung cancer cases occur in nonsmokers who live with smokers, and one fourth of cases in nonsmokers with general environmental exposure to cigarette smoke (7). The risk for lung cancer is directly related to the duration and intensity of exposure to tobacco smoke (8).

Occupational carcinogens associated with an increased risk for lung cancer include arsenic, chromium, nickel, copper, beryllium, vinyl chloride, benzene, uranium, radon, and asbestos (9,10). It is well-known that asbestos interacts synergistically with cigarette smoke; it is estimated that the risk for lung cancer in smokers exposed to asbestos is up to 92 times greater than that in the general nonsmoking population (11).

The role of poor intake of antioxidants and micronutrients in the development of lung cancer is still unclear. Two recent chemoprevention studies [Carotene and Retinol Efficiency Trial (CARET) and alpha tocopherol and beta-carotene (ATBC)] reported that β-carotene, administered at high doses, has a statistically significant and adverse effect on lung cancer incidence (12).

A genetic predisposition to lung cancer probably exists; lung cancer develops in only 20% of smokers, and it develops in some persons who have no known exposure to tobacco smoke or other carcinogens (9). Epidemiologic studies suggest an increased familial risk, most likely associated with the mendelian codominant inheritance of an autosomal gene, particularly in people in whom lung cancer develops before 50 years of age (13–15). This putative genetic abnormality is unidentified and requires investigation through genetic linkage studies. People in whom lung cancer develops may have genetic abnormalities that limit their ability to detoxify the carcinogens in tobacco smoke. Abnormalities of the cytochrome P-450 enzyme system may influence individual susceptibility to lung cancer (15).

Several diseases known to alter immune function are associated with an increased risk for lung cancer, including chronic lymphocytic leukemia (CLL), HIV infection, and AIDS (16). Recent analyses suggest that the risk for the development of primary lung cancer is increased 6.5-fold in patients with HIV infection and AIDS (17).

PATHOLOGIC CLASSIFICATION

Carcinomas of the lung are divided into two major categories: small cell lung cancer (SCLC) and non-small cell lung cancer (NSCLC). About 80% are NSCLCs, whereas 20% are SCLCs (18). The two types differ in their histology and clinical behavior, but occasional admixtures of small cell and non-small cell phenotypes in individual tumors suggest a common origin for all lung cancers. The possibil-

Table 59.1. HISTOLOGIC CLASSIFICATION OF LUNG TUMORS

WHO[a]	WPL-LCSG[b]

1. Squamous cell carcinoma
  Variants: 1.1 Papillary
        1.2 Clear cell
        1.3 Small cell
        1.4 Basaloid
	01 Carcinoma in situ
	
	10 Squamous cell carcinoma
	    11 Well-differentiated
	    12 Moderately differentiated
	    13 Poorly differentiated

2. Small cell carcinoma
  Variant: 2.1 Combined small cell carcinoma
	20 Small cell
	    21 Lymphocyte-like or oat cell
	    22 Intermediate

3. Adenocarcinoma
  3.1 Acinar adenocarcinoma
  3.2 Papillary adenocarcinoma
  3.3 Bronchioloalveolar carcinoma
  3.4 Solid carcinoma with mucin
  3.5 Adenocarcinoma with mixed subtypes
	30 Adenocarcinoma
	    31 Well-differentiated
	    32 Moderately differentiated
	    33 Poorly differentiated
	    34 Bronchiolar or alveolar

4. Large cell carcinoma
  Variants: 4.1 Large cell neuroendocrine carcinoma
        4.2 Others
	40 Large cell undifferentiated
	    41 Giant cell

5. Adenosquamous carcinoma
6. Carcinoma with pleomorphic, sarcomatoid, or sarcomatous elements
7. Carcinoid
  7.1 Typical
  7.2 Atypical
	50 Poorly differentiated carcinoma
	60 Bimulticomponent or multidifferentiated
	70 Carcinoid

8. Carcinoma of salivary gland type
  8.1 Mucoepidermoid carcinoma
  8.2 Adenoid cystic carcinoma
  8.3 Others
9. Unclassified
	80 Bronchial gland tumors
	    81 Adenoid cystic
	    82 Mucoepidermoid
	    83 Mixed tumors

[a]World Health Organization. Adapted from: Histological typing of lung tumours. Tumori 1981;67:253.
[b]Working Party for the Study of Lung Cancer. Modified by Lung Cancer Study Group, National Cancer Institute.

ity of this common origin is supported by the in vitro finding that c-*myc*– or N-*myc*–amplified SCLC cell lines undergo transition toward the NSCLC phenotype after insertion of an activated *ras* gene (14). NSCLCs are subdivided into squamous cell cancers, adenocarcinomas, and large cell cancers. The criteria for the histologic classification of lung tumors are shown in Tables 59.1 and 59.2.

Most squamous cell tumors arise centrally, in the main, lobar, or segmental bronchi, but one third occur in the small bronchi of lung tissue. In contrast, adenocarcinomas arise peripherally within the pulmonary parenchyma.

Table 59.2. HISTOLOGIC CRITERIA USED FOR DIAGNOSING COMMON LUNG NEOPLASMS[a]

Squamous cell carcinoma
Keratin formation, keratin pearl formation, intercellular junctions (bridges, processes) located between adjacent cells. These junctions are referred to as prickles or spines.

Adenocarcinoma
Definite gland formation or the presence of mucus production in a solid tumor, as determined by a mucosubstance special stain (e.g., PAS-D, mucicarmine).

Undifferentiated large cell carcinoma
Large cells with vesicular nuclei and prominent eosinophilic nucleoli; no evidence of squamous or glandular differentiation; negative for mucin stain.

Multicomponent tumor (mixed squamous cell and adenocarcinoma)
Tumors composed of more than one histologic type according to criteria defined above.

[a]Developed by the pathology section of the Lung Cancer Study Group. PAS-D, periodic acid–Schiff D.

During the past 20 years, a gradual shift in the incidence of non-small cell types has been noted, with adenocarcinomas overtaking squamous cell cancers as the most common type (18). This is probably related to the introduction of filter cigarettes; these have altered the chemical composition of smoke, lowering the concentration of aromatic benzopyrenes, which are associated with squamous cell carcinomas, and increasing the amounts of nitrosamines, which are known to cause adenocarcinomas. Filtered cigarettes also yield smaller smoke particles, which are more likely to be deposited in the pulmonary parenchyma than in the central airways (19).

The frequency of histologic cell types seen in the National Cancer Institute's Surveillance, Epidemiology, and End Results (SEER) program is shown in Table 59.3. Large cell cancers remain the least common form of NSCLC, and immunohistochemistry and electron microscopy allow

Table 59.3. FREQUENCY OF HISTOLOGIC CELL TYPES IN THE NATIONAL CANCER INSTITUTES SEER PROGRAM[a]

Cell type	Frequency (%)	
	1973–1983	1983–1987
Adenocarcinoma	28.0	31.5
Squamous cell carcinoma	32.3	29.4
Small cell carcinoma	16.1	17.8
Large cell carcinoma	6.2	9.2

[a]Based on results from 150,854 lung tumors reported to the SEER program. From Travis WD, Travis LB, Devesa SS. Lung cancer. Cancer 1995;75:191, with permission.
SEER: Surveillance, Epidemiology, and End Results.

some of these to be classified as poorly differentiated forms of either squamous cell carcinoma or adenocarcinoma. Bronchioloalveolar carcinoma, a subtype of adenocarcinoma, is characterized histologically by the growth of malignant cells along the walls of alveoli without destruction of the normal pulmonary architecture. Despite their uniform histologic appearance, bronchioloalveolar carcinomas vary in clinical behavior. They can present either as indolent, well-circumscribed, small, peripheral pulmonary nodules or as aggressive tumors with diffuse pneumonic involvement (20). Bronchioloalveolar carcinomas are more likely to be multifocal than the other types of NSCLC. Early-stage squamous cell cancers, adenocarcinomas, and large cell cancers differ somewhat in their clinical behavior, but up to 45% of non-small cell lung tumors show more than one of the three cell types, which again suggests a common origin for all lung cancers (21).

Small cell lung cancers are part of the larger family of neuroendocrine tumors that arise in many different areas of the body. In the lung and bronchial tree, neuroendocrine tumors comprise a spectrum ranging from well-differentiated and indolent typical carcinoid tumors, to the more aggressive atypical carcinoid tumors, to large cell neuroendocrine carcinomas, and finally to small cell cancers. Light microscopy permits the distinction between two subtypes of SCLC: oat cell carcinoma, a tumor composed of small, round uniform cells, and intermediate small cell cancer, which is composed of less regular, polygonal cells. These two categories are characterized respectively in SCLC cell lines as *classic* and *variant* subtypes. Classic cell lines express a panel of four biomarkers, including L-dopa decarboxylase, neuron-specific enolase, creatine kinase, and bombesin-like immunoreactivity. Variant cell lines express creatine kinase and low amounts of neuron-specific enolase, but not the other two markers. Variant cell lines also reveal amplification and expression of the oncogene c-*myc*, whereas classic cell lines do not. The variant cell line or intermediate form of small cell cancer is associated with a more malignant clinical course.

MOLECULAR BIOLOGY

Progress has been made in understanding the multiple-step process of lung carcinogenesis. The first phase, *initiation*, is the exposure of respiratory epithelium to carcinogens, such as cigarette smoke, that produce permanent alterations in cellular DNA. After the initiation phase, a wide variety of agents, such as growth factors, may produce tumor *promotion* and development of lung cancer. Oncogenes (*ras, myc, erb*-B-2) promote deregulation of cell growth when mutationally activated or overexpressed, whereas inactivation or deletion of tumor-suppressor genes (*p53, Rb,* 3p14-23) is required to produce malignant transformation. Mutation or deletion of both alleles of tumor-suppressor genes is usually required for cellular transformation to occur. These oncogenes encode a variety of proteins with functions that are critical to normal cellular proliferation and that are altered by genetic mutation (22).

The *ras* family of oncogenes (K-*ras*, H-*ras*, N-*ras*) becomes activated through point mutations of codon 12, 13, or 61. K-*ras* mutations occur in approximately 30% of adenocarcinomas but are rarely seen in squamous cell carcinomas and virtually never in SCLCs (23). K-*ras* point mutations are linked to smoking and account for 90% of all *ras* mutations in lung adenocarcinomas. Most of these mutations are G-T transversions in which normal glycine is substituted with either cysteine or valine. The presence of K-*ras* point mutations defines a subgroup of patients with lung adenocarcinoma in whom disease-free and overall survival rates are short despite radical resection and a small tumor load (24). Mutations of *ras* have not been reported in preneoplastic lesions in the lung, but their presence could be a biologic marker of early adenocarcinoma of the lung.

Members of the *myc* gene family (c-*myc*, L-*myc*, N-*myc*) encode nuclear phosphoproteins involved in the control of cell proliferation (25). Overexpression and amplification, particularly of the c-*myc* gene, are found in 10% to 25% of SCLCs and 4% to 10% of NSCLCs. It is not clear where in the sequential development of lung cancer *myc* plays a role.

The protein product p185 is encoded by *erb*-B-2 (*HER-2/neu*). It is highly expressed in more than one third of NSCLCs (especially in adenocarcinomas) and not seen in SCLCs (23,26). Overexpression of *erb*-B-2 correlates with a short survival in lung adenocarcinoma and may also be a marker for intrinsic multidrug resistance in NSCLC (27).

Abnormalities of *p53* are common genetic aberrations in lung cancer, occurring in more than 90% of SCLCs and more than 50% of NSCLCs, particularly squamous cell carcinoma (25,28). Mutations of *p53* are the most frequent genetic change found in solid tumors (29). Both K-*ras* point mutations and *p53* mutation and overexpression are linked to smoking. However, only 10% or fewer of NSCLCs are found to contain both *p53* abnormalities and K-*ras* mutations (30). A protein that controls the cell cycle and apoptosis (programmed cell death) is encoded by *p53* in response to DNA damage. The way in which alterations of the *p53* gene affect the clinical outcome of surgically treated patients with lung cancer is controversial (31). Structural and immunohistochemical abnormalities of *p53* were investigated in NSCLCs by the Lung Cancer Study Group (LCSG) (30). Of the 85 patients studied, 64% showed *p53* overexpression and 51% had mutant *p53* sequences in exons 5 to 8. However, the concordance rate between overexpression and mutation was only 67%, which suggests that several mechanisms contribute to *p53* overexpression. In this clinically well-defined cohort of patients for whom follow-up data were available, *p53* overexpression but not mutation was associated with a significantly worse overall survival. In another study, about 15% of patients with lung cancer were found to have antibodies specific for the protein encoded by *p53* in their sera. In SCLC, the development of antibodies was significantly associated with prolonged survival and good performance status (32). Mutation and overexpression of *p53* occur before lung cancer develops and have been identified in areas of high-grade bronchial dysplasia or carcinoma in situ (33,34). Mutations of *p53* in primary lung tumors are conserved in metastases developing from that tumor. Thus, the type of *p53* mutation might be used to discriminate between a new tumor, a second primary tumor, or a metastasis.

Another tumor-suppressor gene commonly inactivated in lung cancer is the *Rb* (retinoblastoma) gene located at chromosomal region 13q14. It encodes a nuclear phosphoprotein that regulates the G_1/S cell cycle. The protein encoded by *Rb* is abnormal in more than 90% of SCLCs and in about one third of primary NSCLCs of all histologic types. No clear correlation has been established between *Rb* inactivation and survival in patients with early-stage NSCLC (35).

One of the most prominent cytogenetic changes is the deletion of material from the short arm of chromosome 3 (3p14-23). This occurs in almost all small cell (> 90%) and many non-small cell (> 80%) cancers (23). The critical gene residing in this region has not yet been identified but is presumably a tumor-suppressor gene. Analyses have demonstrated allelic loss not only in invasive cancers but also as a very early change in preneoplastic respiratory epithelial lesions (hyperplasia, dysplasia, carcinoma in situ).

Many other genetic abnormalities are probably involved in lung carcinogenesis. Unlike the karyotypes in some hematologic malignancies, which are characterized by a single predominant chromosomal abnormality, karyotypes in NSCLC are complex, even in early-stage tumors. Of course, not all these chromosomal abnormalities necessarily reflect genetic changes that are biologically important.

Growth factors and their receptors also seem to play a role in lung tumorigenesis through autocrine or paracrine loops. For example, the epidermal growth factor receptor (EGFR) and one of its ligands, transforming growth factor-α (TGF-α), are thought to function as an autocrine loop in NSCLC, analogous to the well-characterized autocrine loop of gastrin-releasing peptide and its receptor in SCLC cell lines (36). Several immunohistochemical studies of EGFR and TGF-α suggest that these are overexpressed in primary tumors. One study examined the differential expression of EGFR and its ligands TGF-α, epidermal growth factor (EGF), and amphiregulin (AR) in primary NSCLCs and paired samples of benign lung tissue (37). EGF expression was not seen in either tumor or benign lung tissue. Overexpression of EGFR was found in 45% of tumors, whereas overexpression of TGF-α was seen in 61% of tumors and decreased expression of AR was seen in 63% of tumors. Differential expression of EGFR, TGF-α, and AR was not influenced by cell type and tumor stage and did not correlate with disease-free or overall survival. Thus, differential expression of EGFR and some of its ligands is a common event in NSCLC and probably promotes local tumor growth, but not tumor progression.

Primary tumors, even when histologically similar, manifest disparate cellular abnormalities. This suggests that different cellular pathways may lead to clinically similar outcomes. A better understanding the interplay between genetic changes in NSCLCs will provide insights into the mechanisms of tumor growth and progression. The precise sequence of molecular steps leading to the transformation of normal bronchial epithelial cells to metaplasia, dysplasia, carcinoma in situ, and invasive and metastatic cancer remains to be determined. The application of molecular techniques to the analysis of sputum samples and bronchial biopsy specimens may prove useful in the future in identifying persons at greater risk for the development of lung cancer, or it may provide prognostic information or detect occult disease (38). Furthermore, cancer-specific treatments could be designed to interfere with autocrine and paracrine growth loops.

NON-SMALL CELL LUNG CANCER

Non-small cell lung cancer is the most common lung neoplasm. Unfortunately, the mortality rate for this disease is very high, in direct proportion to its incidence, because approximately half of all patients present with disseminated disease, and another 20% present with disease that is too advanced locally to allow surgical resection. The recent improvements in chemotherapy and multimodality treatments for NSCLC have not been substantial enough to produce a significant effect on the overall mortality of this disease. Surgical resection remains the only curative form of treatment, and unfortunately, few patients are candidates for this approach.

Clinical Presentation

Signs and symptoms depend on the location of the tumor and locoregional or metastatic spread. Lung cancer is also occasionally associated with paraneoplastic syn-

Table 59.4. PARANEOPLASTIC SYNDROMES IN PATIENTS WITH LUNG CANCER

Endocrine	Hypercalcemia
	Cushing's syndrome
	Syndrome of inappropriate antidiuretic hormone
	Carcinoid syndrome
	Gynecomastia
	Hypercalcitoninemia
	Elevated growth hormone
	Elevated prolactin, FSH, LH
	Hypoglycemia
	Hyperthyroidism
Neurologic	Encephalopathy
	Subacute cerebellar degeneration
	Progressive multifocal leukoencephalopathy
	Peripheral neuropathy
	Polymyositis
	Autonomic neuropathy
	Eaton-Lambert syndrome
	Optic neuritis
Skeletal	Clubbing
	Pulmonary hypertrophic osteoarthropathy
Hematologic	Anemia
	Leukemoid reaction
	Thrombocytosis
	Thrombocytopenia
	Eosinophilia
	Pure red cell aplasia
	Leukoerythroblastosis
	Disseminated intravascular coagulation
Cutaneous	Hyperkeratosis
	Dermatomyositis
	Acanthosis nigricans
	Hyperpigmentation
	Erythema gyratum repens
	Hypertrichosis lanuginosa acquista
Other	Nephrotic syndrome
	Hypouricemia
	Secretion of VIP with diarrhea
	Hyperamylasemia
	Anorexia or cachexia

FSH, follicle-stimulating hormone; LH, luteinizing hormone; VIP, vasoactive intestinal peptide.
From Maddaus M, Ginsberg RJ. Diagnosis and staging. In: Pearson FG, Deslauriers J, Ginsberg RJ, et al., eds. Thoracic surgery. New York: Churchill Livingstone, 1995:671–690, with permission.

dromes. Many patients, however, are referred to a surgeon because of an asymptomatic nodule or mass discovered incidentally on a chest radiograph.

Centrally located tumors can cause cough, hemoptysis, atelectasis, or postobstructive pneumonia. When located peripherally, they may extend into the chest wall, spine, or brachial plexus and cause pain. One example of direct spread is Pancoast's syndrome, in which tumors of the superior sulcus are associated with lower brachial plexopathy, Horner's syndrome, and shoulder pain. Many patients present with systemic symptoms, such as weight loss, fatigue, and anorexia. Paraneoplastic syndromes are listed in Table 59.4. These conditions are not specific for lung cancer and may be found in small cell and non-small cell carcinomas in approximately 2% of patients.

Diagnosis

After a history and physical examination, studies are performed to obtain a diagnosis. When a nodule or a mass is discovered on a chest radiograph, old films are helpful for comparison. If the lesion has not grown in the past 2 years, it is likely to be benign. Radiographic characteristics, such as a smooth contour, dense homogeneous calci-

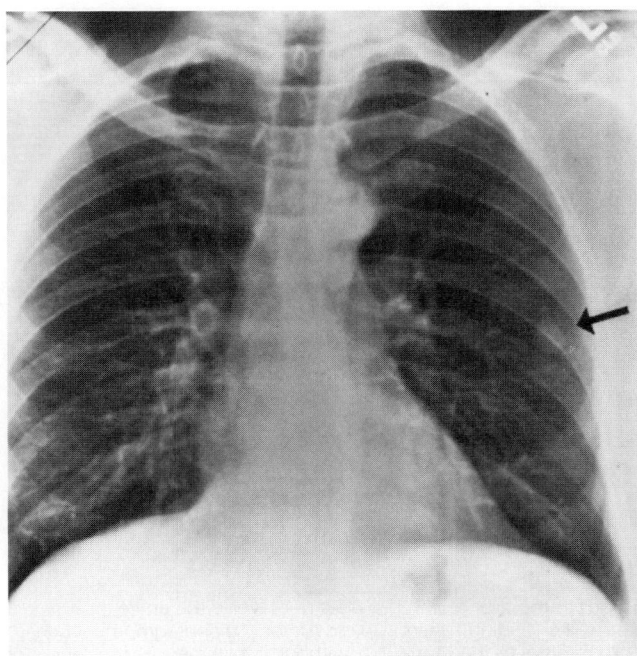

Figure 59.1. Smooth, well-circumscribed nodule of the left mid-lung field *(arrow)* that did not change on serial chest radiographs during a 2-year period. This is most likely a benign pulmonary nodule, perhaps a hamartoma.

fication, or "popcorn" calcification, suggest diseases other than lung cancer (Fig. 59.1). A tissue diagnosis can be established by bronchoscopy for centrally located lesions or by percutaneous needle aspiration for peripheral masses. Exploratory thoracotomy without a preoperative diagnosis is acceptable if the history and radiographic findings strongly suggest the possibility of lung cancer or if attempts to obtain a tissue diagnosis have failed and no evidence of distant disease is present. Videoscopically assisted thoracic surgery (VATS) with excisional biopsy is another diagnostic option and is considered the procedure of choice for suspect indeterminate nodules (39). An algorithm for the management of solitary pulmonary nodules is shown in Fig. 59.2.

Staging System

Non-small cell lung cancer is classified in four stages. The staging system and the descriptors for each TNM (tumor–node–metastasis) stage are outlined in Table 59.5. In June 1997, a revised system for staging lung cancer was published to replace the TNM system in use since 1986. The 1986 system had previously replaced the original 1977 American Joint Committee on Cancer (AJCC) staging system. It is important to be aware of these changes because lung cancer survival rates published before 1997 may differ from current survival figures simply because the older staging system has been used. The current TNM system is internationally accepted and more accurately identifies patient groups with similar prognoses and treatment options. It divides stages I and II into categories A and B, modifies stage IIIA (down-staging T3 N0 to stage IIB), and includes new rules for classifying multiple tumor nodules, called *satellite nodules* (40).

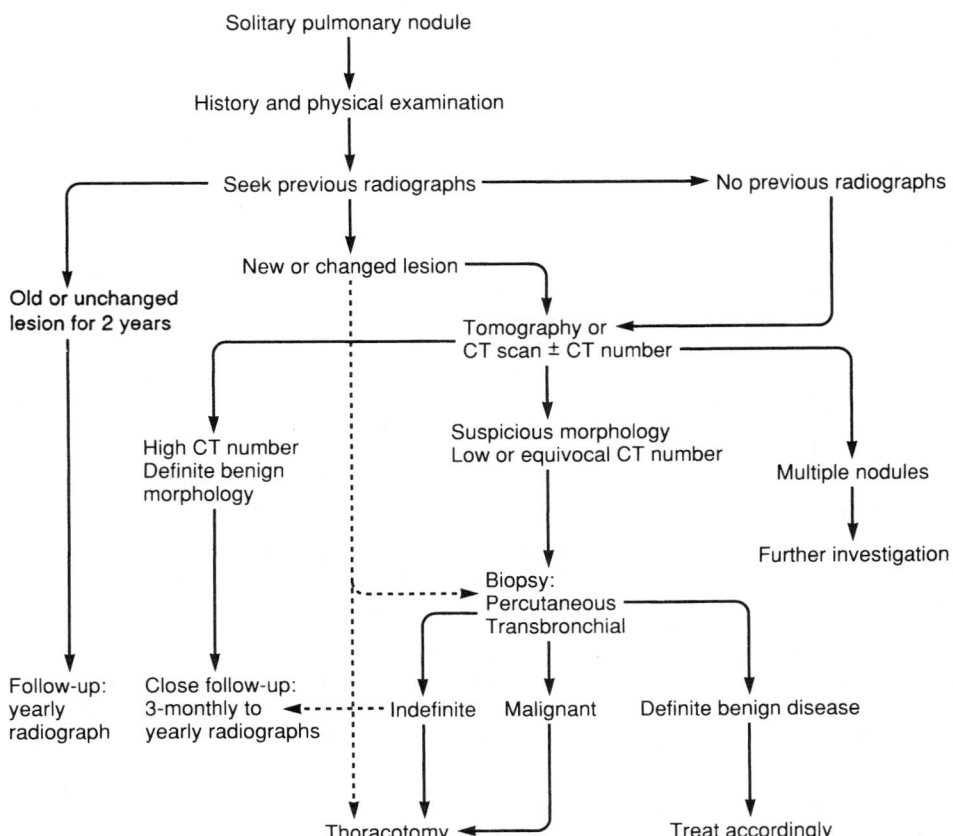

Figure 59.2. Algorithm for decision making in patients who present with a solitary pulmonary nodule.

Table 59.5. TNM CLASSIFICATION FOR STAGING SYSTEM OF NON-SMALL CELL LUNG CANCER

Stage	TNM status
IA	T1 N0 M0
IB	T2 N0 M0
IIA	T1 N1 M0
IIB	T2 N1 M0
	T3 N0 M0
IIIA	T3 N1 M0
	T1–3 N2 M0
IIIB	T4 Any N M0
	Any T N3 M0
IV	Any T any N M1

TNM definitions:

T **TX** Positive malignant cell, but primary tumor not visualized by imaging or bronchoscopy

T0 No evidence of primary tumor

Tis Carcinoma in situ

T1 Tumor ≤3 cm, surrounded by lung or visceral pleura, without bronchoscopic evidence of invasion more proximal than the lobar bronchus[a]

T2 Tumor with any of the following features of size or extent:
>3 cm in greatest dimension
Involves main bronchus, ≥2 cm distal to the carina
Invades the visceral pleura
Associated with atelectasis or obstructive pneumonitis that extends to the hilar region but does not involve the entire lung

T3 Tumor of any size that directly invades any of the following: chest wall (including superior sulcus tumors), diaphragm, mediastinal pleura, parietal pericardium; or tumor in the main bronchus <2 cm distal to the carina, but without involvement of the carina; or associated atelectasis or obstructive pneumonitis of the entire lung

T4 Tumor of any size that invades any of the following: mediastinum, heart, great vessels, trachea, esophagus, vertebral body, carina; or tumor with a malignant pleural or pericardial effusion, or with satellite tumor nodule(s) within the ipsilateral primary tumor lobe of the lung[b]

N **NX** Regional lymph nodes cannot be assessed

N0 No regional lymph node metastasis

N1 Metastasis to ipsilateral peribronchial and/or ipsilateral hilar lymph nodes, and involvement of intrapulmonary nodes by direct extension of the primary tumor

N2 Metastasis to ipsilateral mediastinal and/or subcarinal lymph node(s)

N3 Metastasis to contralateral mediastinal, contralateral hilar, ipsilateral or contralateral scalene, or supraclavicular lymph node(s)

M **MX** Presence of distant metastasis cannot be assessed

M0 No distant metastasis

M1 Distant metastasis present (including metastatic tumor nodule(s) in the ipsilateral non-primary tumor lobe(s) of the lung)

[a]The uncommon superficial tumor of any size with its invasive component limited to the bronchial wall that may extend proximal to the main bronchus is classified as T1.

[b]Most pleural effusions associated with lung cancer are caused by tumor. There are, however, some few patients in whom the pleural fluid (more than one specimen) is negative for tumor on cytopathologic examination and in whom the fluid is nonbloody and is not an exudate. In cases in which these elements and clinical judgment dictate that the effusion is not related to the tumor, the patient should be staged T1, T2, or T3, with effusion excluded as a staging element. Pericardial effusion is classified according to the same rules.

The nomenclature for nodal involvement (N status) is accompanied by a numbering system for lymph nodes, which are codified into lymph node maps. The most recent map for regional lymph node stations for lung cancer staging, adopted by the AJCC and the Union Internationale Contre le Cancer (UICC), is derived from previous Naruke and American Thoracic Society/Lung Cancer Study Group mapping systems (41) (Fig. 59.3).

Selection of Treatment

The selection of treatment for patients with NSCLC is based on the stage of the disease at diagnosis and on the patient's overall medical condition. Stage IV disease is treated primarily with chemotherapy. Stage IIIB disease is usually treated with chemotherapy and radiation. However, recent clinical trials suggest that the T4 tumor subset of stage IIIB may be appropriately treated by surgical resection after induction chemotherapy and radiation. In contrast, surgical resection is the treatment of choice for stages I and II. The most controversial area is the management of stage IIIA disease, especially N2 disease, for which surgical resection is occasionally the primary treatment but that is treated more often with a combination of chemotherapy, surgical resection, and radiation.

The aims of the initial evaluation of a patient with NSCLC are to determine whether distant metastatic disease is present and to assess the extent of intrathoracic disease. Common metastatic sites include the brain, supraclavicular nodes, contralateral lung, bones, liver, and adrenal glands. A thorough history and physical examination, combined with a plain chest radiograph and baseline laboratory data (complete blood cell count and measurement of serum sodium, calcium, alkaline phosphatase, and lactate dehydrogenase levels), may suggest the presence of metastatic disease. Abnormal findings are then investigated further with selected radionuclide, computed tomographic (CT), or magnetic resonance imaging (MRI) studies and by needle aspiration biopsy or open biopsy, if necessary, to determine the extent of disease.

If the initial clinical evaluation does not suggest the presence of distant disease, the extent of further evaluation by various scans is controversial. Some physicians always perform a complete metastatic work-up with CT of the chest and abdomen, CT or MRI of the brain, and a bone scan. CT of the chest and upper abdomen has become

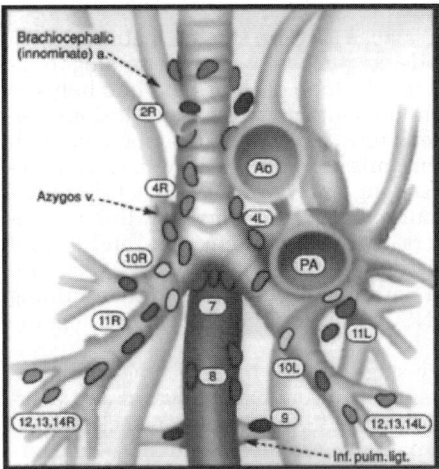 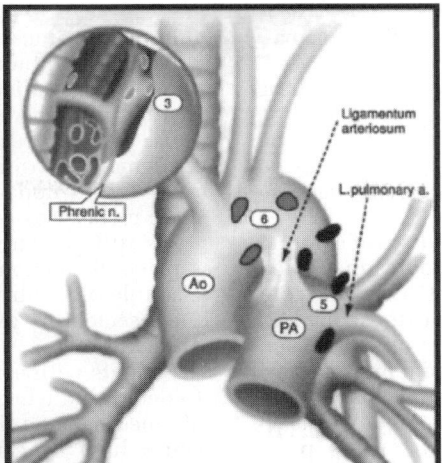

Nodal Station	Anatomic Landmarks
N2 nodes: All N2 nodes lie within the mediastinal pleural envelope	
1. Highest mediastinal nodes	Nodes lying above a horizontal line at the upper rim of the brachiocephalic (left innominate) vein where it ascends to the left, crossing in front of the trachea at its midline.
2. Upper paratracheal nodes	Nodes lying above a horizontal line drawn tangential to the upper margin of the aortic arch and below the inferior boundary of No. 1 nodes.
3. Prevascular and retrotracheal nodes	Prevascular and retrotracheal nodes may be designated 3A and 3P; midline nodes are considered to be ipsilateral.
4. Lower paratracheal nodes	The lower paratracheal nodes on the right lie to the right of the midline of the trachea between a horizontal line drawn tangential to the upper margin of the aortic arch and a line extending across the right main bronchus at the upper margin of the upper lobe bronchus, and contained within the mediastinal pleural envelope; the lower paratracheal nodes on the left lie to the left of the midline of the trachea between a horizontal line drawn tangential to the upper margin of the aortic arch and a line extending across the left main bronchus at the level of the upper margin of the left upper lobe bronchus, medial to the ligamentum arteriosum and contained within the mediastinal pleural envelope.
	Researchers may want to designate the lower paratracheal nodes as No. 4s (superior) and No. 4i (inferior) subsets for study purposes; the No. 4s nodes may be defined by a horizontal line extending across the trachea and drawn tangential to the cephalic border of the azygos vein; the No. 4i nodes may be defined by the lower boundary of No. 4s and the lower boundary of No. 4 as described above.
5. Subaortic (aortopulmonary window)	Subaortic nodes are lateral to the ligamentum arteriosum or the aorta or left pulmonary artery and proximal to the first branch of the left pulmonary artery and lie within the mediastinal pleural envelope.
6. Para-aortic nodes (ascending aorta or phrenic)	Nodes lying anterior and lateral to the ascending aorta and the aortic arch or the innominate artery, beneath a line tangential to the upper margin of the aortic arch.
7. Subcarinal nodes	Nodes lying caudal to the carina of the trachea but not associated with the lower lobe bronchi or arteries within the lung.
8. Paraesophageal nodes (below carina)	Nodes lying adjacent to the wall of the esophagus and to the right or left of the midline, excluding subcarinal nodes.
9. Pulmonary ligament nodes	Nodes lying within the pulmonary ligament, including those in the posterior wall and lower part of the inferior pulmonary vein.
N1 nodes: All N1 nodes lie distal to the mediastinal pleural reflection and within the visceral pleura	
10. Hilar nodes	The proximal lobar nodes, distal to the mediastinal pleural reflection and the nodes adjacent to the bronchus intermedius on the right; radiographically, the hilar shadow may be created by enlargement of both hilar and interlobar nodes.
11. Interlobar nodes	Nodes lying between the lobar bronchi.
12. Lobar nodes	Nodes adjacent to the distal lobar bronchi.
13. Segmental nodes	Nodes adjacent to the segmental bronchi.
14. Subsegmental nodes	Nodes around the subsegmental bronchi.

Figure 59.3. The Mountain-Dresler lymph node map. In this newer map, a stricter definition of the anatomic boundaries for each lymph node region facilitates correlation between findings at operation and findings on chest computed tomography. (From Mountain CF, Dresler CM. Regional lymph node classification for lung cancer staging. *Chest* 1997;111:1718, with permission.)

standard, as much to evaluate the extent of the primary tumor and the status of the mediastinal lymph nodes as to detect metastases in the ipsilateral or contralateral lung, liver, or adrenals. Additional scans in asymptomatic patients may detect the 5% to 10% of metastases that are occult, but these scans are not clearly cost-effective in patients with clinical stage I or II tumors who have no clinical indications of disease.

If no clinical evidence of extrathoracic disease is found, it is important to determine whether mediastinal nodal metastases (N2 or N3 disease) are present. This is accomplished by a combination of CT and mediastinoscopy (42). Mediastinal nodes 1 cm or less in diameter on CT are usually benign, with an associated risk for nodal metastases of less than 10% (43). Mediastinal nodes larger than 1.5 cm are often malignant but are sometimes enlarged because of underlying pulmonary disease or postobstructive pneumonia. Small (≤ 3 cm) peripheral tumors without associated mediastinal adenopathy on CT do not require mediastinoscopy (Fig. 59.4). Mediastinoscopy is indicated for centrally located tumors, for larger peripheral tumors, especially if the primary tumor is an adenocarcinoma or large cell cancer, and for any tumor with associated mediastinal adenopathy (Fig. 59.5). Most tumors are adequately staged by cervical mediastinoscopy, which allows access to the left and right paratracheal nodes, the right tracheobronchial angle nodes, and the subcarinal nodes. However, tumors of the left upper lobe drain primarily to the subaortic nodes. Complete mediastinal nodal staging requires either a combined cervical and parasternal approach (Chamberlain procedure) or an extended cervical mediastinoscopy, in which biopsy is performed on the subaortic nodes by passing the mediastinoscope over the aortic arch between the innominate and left carotid arteries (44). In the hands of experienced surgeons, mediastinoscopy carries virtually no mortality and minimal morbidity and fails to diagnose only the 10% of involved mediastinal nodes that are not technically accessible by this approach. Thus, mediastinoscopy is crucial to avoid a thoracotomy in patients with unresectable disease.

Magnetic resonance imaging of pulmonary lesions offers no improvement over CT except in the assessment of superior sulcus and paravertebral tumors, where it can define subclavian vessel, brachial plexus, or spinal cord invasion (42,45,46). Positron emission tomography with fluorodeoxyglucose may assist in staging patients with lung cancer. Fluorodeoxyglucose, a glucose analogue labeled with a radioactive isotope of fluorine, often helps to distinguish between benign and malignant lesions because of the increased glucose metabolism associated with malignancy. Positron emission tomography may complement CT in nodal staging and seems to detect extrathoracic metastases accurately (47,48). However, this modality is still not universally available, is costly, and cannot replace the anatomic definition provided by CT. The precise role of positron emission tomography in determining the resectability of NSCLC awaits the outcome of ongoing clinical trials.

Patients with early-stage NSCLC must also be evaluated to determine whether their pulmonary function and overall medical condition permit pulmonary resection. Because lung cancer patients are predominantly smokers older than 40 years of age, underlying coronary disease is common and is often a source of perioperative morbidity or mortality. The patient's cardiac status should be rigorously assessed if the history, physical examination, or baseline electrocardiogram suggests any cardiac dysfunction. Pulmonary function tests are performed to determine the patient's ability to tolerate pulmonary resection.

The details of pulmonary function testing as they relate to the risks of pulmonary resection are well covered in standard thoracic surgical texts and are not discussed in depth here. The forced expiratory volume in 1 second (FEV_1) is the most useful single parameter because most patients with lung cancer have chronic obstructive pulmonary disease. In general, pulmonary resection can be tolerated if the FEV_1 after resection is 800 mL/s or greater. Patients who have an initial FEV_1 of 2 L/s or more, or that is more than 50% of the value predicted for their age and size, can usually tolerate any form of pulmonary resection, including a pneumonectomy. Patients whose FEV_1 is less than 2 L/s should undergo a ventilation–perfusion lung scan to determine how much the area of planned pulmonary resection contributes to overall lung function. Sometimes, it contains primarily nonfunctional lung tissue, particularly if the tumor is centrally located. Patients with lung cancer may also have restrictive or interstitial lung disease because of occupational exposure to carcinogenic chemicals or dusts. This can be diagnosed by alterations in the total lung capacity, vital capacity, and diffu-

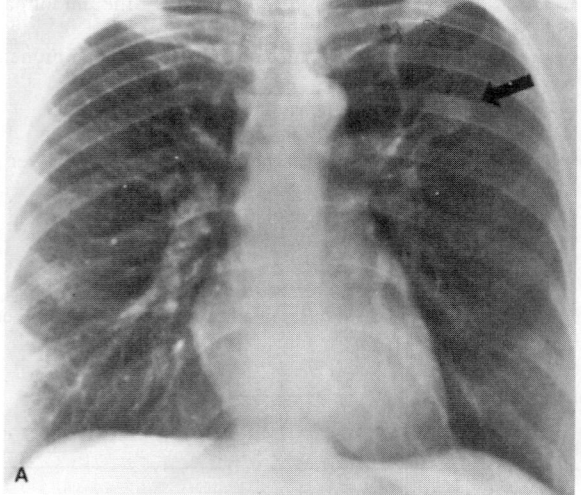
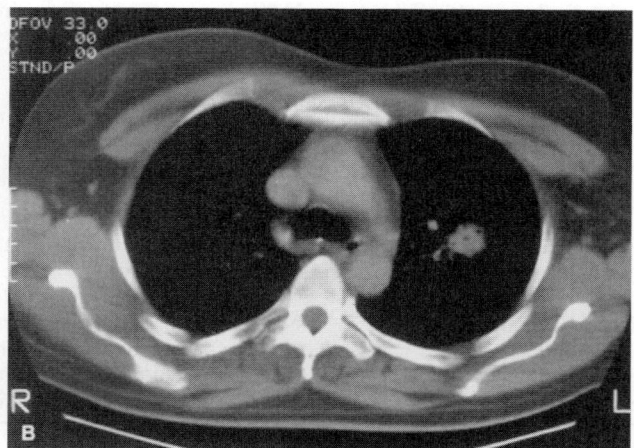

Figure 59.4. Solitary, irregular mass of the left upper lobe mass (*arrow*) diagnosed incidentally on a routine chest radiograph in a 50-year-old nonsmoking woman. Computed tomography of the chest confirmed the presence of the mass but did not demonstrate any mediastinal adenopathy. At exploratory thoracotomy, the patient had a T1 N0 adenocarcinoma.

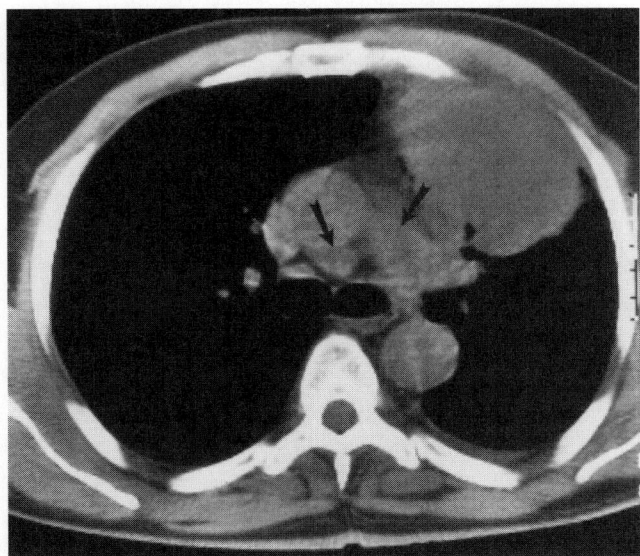

Figure 59.5. Computed tomogram *(CT)* from a patient with a huge squamous cell cancer of the left upper lobe. Mediastinal adenopathy was observed on CT in the aortopulmonary window and in the pretracheal regions *(arrows)*. Mediastinoscopy demonstrated enlarged but benign lymph nodes.

sion capacity (DLCO). Patients whose diffusion capacity is less than 50% of the predicted value should also have a quantitative ventilation–perfusion lung scan to calculate their diffusion capacity after resection. A value that is 35% of the predicted value after resection is usually a minimally acceptable value, beyond which the risk for respiratory failure becomes prohibitive. Baseline arterial blood gases mainly identify patients for whom the risk of pulmonary resection is prohibitively high because of resting hypercapnia. Resting hypoxemia may simply reflect the presence of a shunt or ventilation–perfusion mismatch caused by the tumor and is not usually helpful in selecting patients for pulmonary resection. However, a decrease in the arterial oxygen pressure during exercise is associated with an increased risk associated with resection because it usually reflects a diminished pulmonary vascular bed. Measurements of parameters such as the diffusion capacity are not routine in many pulmonary function laboratories. Unless the laboratory is specifically aware of what parameters need to be measured, patients may not be adequately evaluated. Surgeons must understand which tests should be ordered and know how to interpret them.

Patients who are smoking actively at the time of diagnosis should quit smoking. Patients are placed on intensive bronchodilator therapy and are treated with appropriate antibiotics if they have chronic bronchitis. These measures greatly reduce the risk for postoperative atelectasis or pneumonia. The ultimate benefits of smoking cessation, manifested by decreased sputum production and improved clearance of secretions, are not apparent for several months.

Surgical Resection of Stage I and Stage II Disease

Stage I and stage II NSCLCs are best treated by surgical resection. The goals of pulmonary resection in patients with lung cancer are to remove the primary tumor completely and stage it definitively. The details of surgical techniques and perioperative care are amply described in standard thoracic surgical texts and are not discussed

here. The extent of pulmonary resection is dictated by the location and size of the primary tumor and by whether the adjacent bronchopulmonary nodes are involved. Depending on these factors, a pneumonectomy, lobectomy, or bilobectomy is the appropriate operation and should provide microscopically negative vascular and bronchial margins. Several retrospective series suggest that a limited resection (wedge resection or segmentectomy) rather than a lobectomy may be adequate for some early-stage (T1 N0) tumors. However, a prospective, randomized trial by the North American LCSG has shown that limited resection is associated with a higher rate of local recurrence and poorer survival than lobectomy in patients with T1 N0 tumors (49).

A pneumonectomy can be performed with a mortality rate of less than 6%, a lobectomy with less than 3%, and a wedge resection or segmentectomy with 1% or less. The postoperative mortality rate is also age-related (50). The most common complications after resectional surgery are not technical failures of the operation but cardiopulmonary problems, especially supraventricular arrhythmias and respiratory failure (51).

If a tumor extends directly into the chest wall, diaphragm, or pericardium, an *en bloc* resection of the the adjacent involved structure should be performed with the pulmonary resection (52). Reconstruction is performed as necessary (Fig. 59.6). On the other hand, if extensive endobronchial involvement is present but no involvement of the surrounding vascular or lymphatic structures, the tumor can sometimes be completely removed by a lobectomy with segmental resection of the bronchus (sleeve resection), so that lung function is preserved.

The clinical staging of mediastinal nodes is inaccurate and should not be substituted for careful intraoperative staging by means of mediastinal nodal sampling or mediastinal lymph node dissection. Meticulous pathologic staging provides accurate prognostic information and allows appropriate decisions to be made regarding the use of postoperative adjuvant therapy. Complete *en bloc* mediastinal lymph node dissection is advocated by some groups as the most accurate means of staging. For right-sided tumors, this involves *en bloc* removal of the entire subcarinal packet of nodes and *en bloc* removal of all the paratracheal lymph nodes located between the trachea posteriorly, the superior vena cava anteriorly, the innominate artery superiorly, and the tracheobronchial angle inferiorly. For left-sided tumors, the dissection includes *en bloc* removal of the subcarinal nodes and the subaortic and periaortic nodes. If they are technically accessible, the left tracheobronchial angle nodes are also removed. Whether this extensive dissection results in more accurate staging than just sampling of lymph nodes from each one of these areas remains controversial and is the subject of an ongoing multiinstitutional clinical trial. No matter which method is chosen, each lymph node group must be identified by the surgeon and submitted with appropriately labeling to the pathologist. The standard nomenclature and numbering systems shown in Fig. 59.3 must be used.

Survival

The long-term survival after surgical resection for NSCLC is linked to the pathologic stage of disease. The overall 5-year survival rates are shown in Table 59.6. They range from 60% to 70% for stage I tumors, from 40% to 50% for stage II tumors, and from 15% to 30% for stage IIIA tumors. Nodal involvement has the strongest adverse influence on survival. Large peripheral tumors that extend directly into the chest wall without nodal involvement

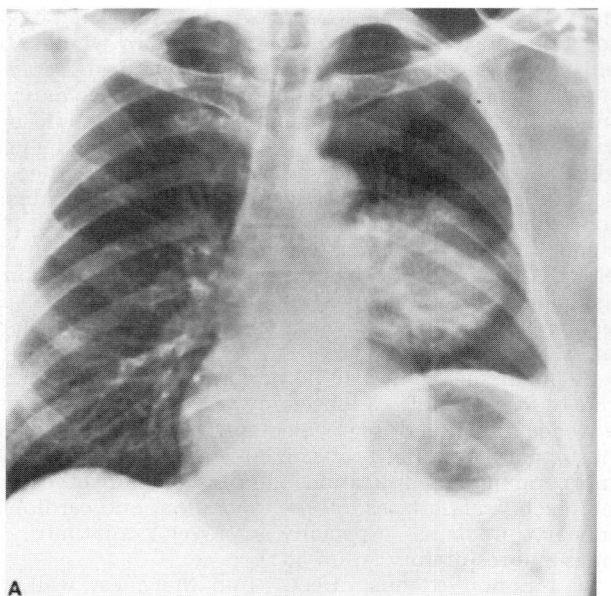
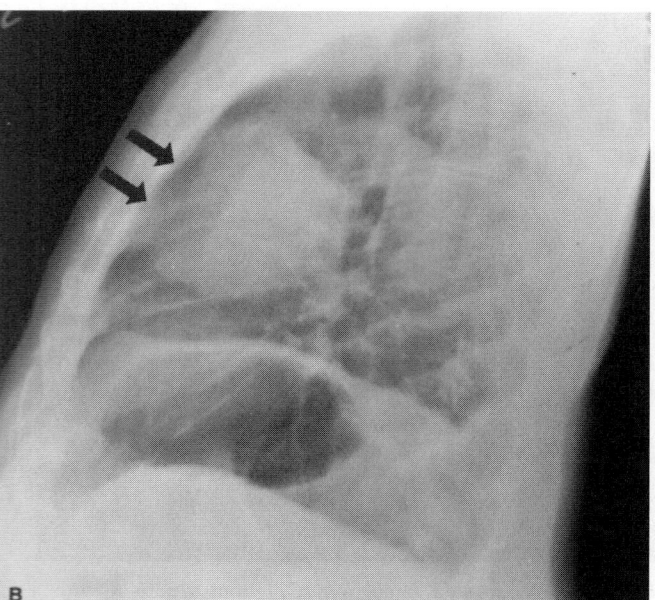
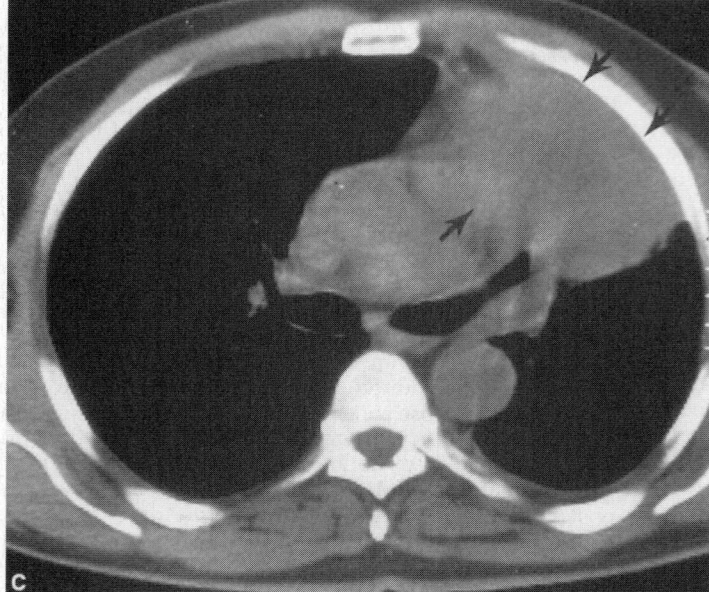

Figure 59.6. Imaging studies from the same patient as in Fig. 59.5. *(A)* Posteroanterior chest radiograph shows an elevated left hemidiaphragm, suggestive of phrenic nerve involvement by the mass. *(B)* Lateral chest radiograph shows extension of the mass to the anterior chest wall *(arrow)*. *(C)* Computed tomography suggests both pericardial and chest wall involvement *(arrows)*. At thoracotomy, the chest wall, phrenic nerve, and pericardium was found to be involved. All were resected *en bloc* with the tumor.

Table 59.6. **NEW STAGE DATA BASE: CUMULATIVE PERCENTAGE SURVIVING 5 YEARS BY CLINICAL AND SURGICAL TNM SUBSETS**

TNM subset	Clinical		Surgical	
	No. patients	Patients surviving (%)	No. patients	Patients surviving (%)
T1 N0 M0	687	61	511	67
T2 N0 M0	1,189	38	549	57
T1 N1 M0	29	34	76	55
T2 N1 M0	250	24	288	39
T3 N0 M0	107	22	87	38
T3 N1 M0	40	9	55	25
T1–3 N2 M0	471	13	344	23
T4 N0–2 M0	458	7	—	—
Any N3 M0	572	3	—	—
Any M1	1,427	1	—	—
TOTAL	5,230		1,910	

Adapted from Mountain CF. Revisions in the international system for staging lung cancer. Chest 1997;111:1710, with permission.

(T3 N0) are associated with a 5-year survival rate of 40% after complete resection, whereas involvement of hilar or mediastinal nodes is associated with only a 20% survival rate. The status of the primary tumor has a lesser but still important effect on survival. Within stage I, for instance, T1 N0 tumors are associated with a 5-year survival rate of 70%, substantially better than the 5-year survival rate of 60% associated with T2 N0 tumors.

Some series suggest that histology also affects survival. In stage I or II NSCLC, the North American LCSG consistently observed a better disease-free and overall survival for squamous cell cancer than for nonsquamous tumors (53). The influence of histology has not been reported in all series and is not seen in stage III and stage IV tumors. However, the T and N status and histology provide only a crude estimate of outcome. Within a given TNM category and histology, it is still impossible to discern which individual patients will experience relapse. A better understanding of lung cancer biology is needed to define which patients are truly at risk for recurrence.

Patterns of Recurrence

The predominant sites of relapse for all stages of NSCLC after surgical resection are distant metastases. Approximately 30% of recurrences are locoregional with tumors of both squamous and nonsquamous histology (54). For all stages of disease, the brain is the single most common site of relapse, and brain metastases occur more frequently with nonsquamous tumors. Other common metastatic sites include bone, ipsilateral or contralateral lung, liver, and the adrenal glands (54,55).

At least 60% of recurrences develop in the first 2 years after operation, and virtually all recurrences related to the original primary tumor occur within 5 years after surgery. Even the small proportion of patients with stage II or III disease who survive 5 years are likely to survive 10 years or more postoperatively. Most stage I patients, particularly those with T1 N0 tumors, do experience long-term survival. The North American LCSG followed 907 patients with T1 N0 tumors for a minimum of 5 years after operation (55). Recurrences of the original primary tumor were rare after 5 years, and after that time, the occurrence of new pulmonary cancers becomes the dominant problem. The risk for development of a second lung cancer in patients who survive resection of a NSCLC is approximately 2% to 3% per patient per year (56). Patients also face a consistent risk for the development of new, nonpulmonary primary cancers during the first 5 years after operation and thereafter. New, nonpulmonary malignancies develop in a wide variety of sites, but breast, colon, and prostate cancers are the most common (54).

These facts underscore the importance of long-term follow-up after resection of early-stage NSCLC. Traditionally, most thoracic oncologists see their lung cancer patients every 3 months during the first 2 years after operation, then every 6 months until 5 years after operation, and annually thereafter. There is no single way to detect recurrence, so follow-up includes a combination of history, physical examination, and serial chest radiographs. The cost-effectiveness of this approach is unproven (57), but clearly the primary physician following a patient should be aware of the risk for second primary tumors.

Adjuvant Therapy

The risk for recurrent disease, even after resection of early-stage NSCLC, has led to efforts to improve overall survival rates through the use of adjuvant therapy, even though no specific method is available to identify which patients will relapse. Various types of adjuvant therapy have been tested, including immunotherapy, radiation, chemotherapy, and combined chemotherapy and radiation.

In the early 1970s, a single-institution, nonrandomized study suggested that immunotherapy with intrapleural bacillus Calmette-Guérin (BCG) might improve survival after resection of stage I lung cancer. This prompted the North American LCSG to perform a large prospective, randomized trial comparing intrapleural BCG with placebo in patients with resected stage I NSCLC. Treatment was well tolerated, but no survival advantage was observed in the group of patients treated with BCG (58). Subsequently, the Ludwig Cancer Study Group performed a prospective, randomized, placebo-controlled trial of intrapleural *Corynebacterium parvum* in 475 patients after resection of stages I and II NSCLC. Adjuvant *Corynebacterium parvum* failed to improve survival and was associated with an increased number of side effects (59).

After these two trials, nonspecific adjuvant intrapleural immunotherapy was abandoned. However, several studies of systemic immunotherapy have been performed. Ratto et al. (59a) randomized 113 patients to receive either chemotherapy and radiation or adoptive immunotherapy with tumor infiltrating lymphocytes and interleukin-2 after resection of stage II or III NSCLC. Immunotherapy led to an improved 3-year survival. However, the results are not definitive because no true control arm was included in this trial, the number of patients accrued was small, and the patient population was heterogenous.

Radiation has been extensively evaluated as adjuvant therapy. Retrospective series suggesting that postoperative radiation potentially improves overall survival (60,61) led to randomized trials comparing adjuvant radiation with no further treatment after pulmonary resection (62–67). Although each of these studies randomized relatively small numbers of patients with tumors of various stages and histologic types, none showed a significant difference

Table 59.7. SUMMARY OF REPRESENTATIVE RANDOMIZED TRIALS COMPARING RADIATION WITH NO FURTHER TREATMENT AFTER SURGICAL RESECTION OF EARLY STAGE NON-SMALL CELL LUNG CANCER

Study (reference)	No. patients	NSCLC stages[a]	Radiation dose (Gy)	Overall survival difference
Van Houtte et al., 1980 (67)	224	I, II	60	NS
LCSG, 1986 (66)	210	II, IIIA	50	NS
Lafitte et al., 1996 (65)	132	IB	45–60	NS
MRC, 1996 (64)	308	II, IIIA	40 (15 fractions)	NS
Smolle-Juettner et al., 1996 (63)	155	I–IIIA	50–56	NS
Mayer et al., 1997 (62)	155	IA–IIIA	50–56	NS

[a]The stages are listed according to the 1997 international system for staging lung cancer (40).
LCSG, Lung Cancer Study Group; MRC, Medical Research Council; NS, not statistically significant; NSCLC, non-small cell lung cancer.

Table 59.8. SUMMARY OF REPRESENTATIVE RANDOMIZED TRIALS TESTING THE BENEFIT OF ADJUVANT CHEMOTHERAPY AFTER SURGICAL RESECTION OF EARLY-STAGE NON-SMALL CELL LUNG CANCER

Study (reference)	No. patients	NSCLC stages[a]	Chemotherapy agents	Overall survival difference
Hughes and Wiggins, 1962 (68)	1,002	Not stated	HN$_2$ vs. no Rx	NS
Slack, 1970 (69)	1,192	Not stated	HN$_2$ vs. no Rx	NS
Shields et al., 1977 (70)	417	Not stated	Cytoxan vs. Cytoxan + MTX	NS
Shields et al., 1982 (71)	865	Not stated	CCNU + hydroxyurea vs. no Rx	NS
Holmes et al., 1986 (154)	141	II, IIIA	CAP vs. immunotherapy	NS
Sadeghi et al., 1988 (155)	164	II, IIIA	CAP vs. RT + CAP	NS
Niiranen et al., 1992 (156)	110	IA–IIB	CAP vs. no Rx	NS
Feld et al., 1993 (73)	269	I–IIA	CAP vs. no Rx	NS
Ohta et al., 1993 (157)	209	IIB–IIIA	VP vs. no Rx	NS
Pisters et al., 1994 (82)	72	IIIA	VP + RT vs. RT	NS
Dautzenberg et al., 1995 (158)	267	I–IIIA	COPAC, RT vs. RT	NS
Wada et al., 1996 (75)	323	I–IIIA	VP, UFT vs. UFT vs. no Rx	$p = .053$
Keller et al., 1999 (74)	488	II, IIIA	EP + RT vs. RT	NS

[a]The stages are listed according to the 1997 international system for staging lung cancer (40).
CAP: cyclophosphamide, doxorubicin, cisplatin; CCNU, 1-(2-chlorethyl)-3-cyclohexyl-1 nitrosourea; COPAC: cyclophosphamide doxorubicin, cisplatin, vincristine, lomustine; Cytoxan, cyclophosphamide; EP: etoposide, cisplatin; HN$_2$, nitrogen mustard; MTX, methotrexate; NS, not significant; no Rx, no adjuvant treatment; RT, radiation; UFT, tegafur plus uracil; VP: vindesine, cisplatin.

in overall survival. Distant metastases remain the most common form of recurrent disease and are not affected by postoperative radiation to the mediastinum. However, several of these trials (62–64,66,67) showed that radiation significantly decreases the risk for locoregional recurrence in tumors of all histologic types (Table 59.7). Therefore, postoperative radiation may be appropriate adjuvant treatment for patients who are at high risk for locoregional recurrence, either because of bulky nodal disease or close margins.

Because distant metastases are the predominant mode of relapse after resection of early-stage NSCLC, multiple randomized trials, summarized in Table 59.8, have been performed to determine if postoperative adjuvant chemotherapy improves survival. The initial trials used chemotherapeutic agents now known to have no activity in NSCLC (68–71). However, since the 1970s, all chemotherapy regimens have been cisplatin-based. Despite the use of these more active regimens, no individual trial showed an improvement in overall survival. A metaanalysis of 9,387 patients entered into 52 randomized clinical trials showed a 5% survival benefit at 5 years for adjuvant cisplatin-based chemotherapy in comparison with surgery alone. Trials comparing adjuvant radiation with radiation plus chemotherapy showed an absolute survival benefit of 4% at 2 years in favor of the combined-modality treatment (72). The benefit of a cisplatin-based adjuvant chemotherapy remains modest, and for that reason, it is not accepted as routine treatment. One potential reason for this lack of efficacy is poor patient tolerance of cisplatin-based therapy in the postoperative setting. Several of these trials have shown that approximately half of all patients actually receive the full dose of chemotherapy planned (73,74). Intensive chemotherapy is probably better tolerated preoperatively, when patients are not recovering from a major operation.

The only recent trial suggesting that adjuvant chemotherapy confers a survival advantage was reported by Wada et al. (75). In this study, patients received UFT, a well-tolerated oral analogue of fluorouracil, for 1 year postoperatively. Although fluorouracil is not usually considered an active drug against NSCLC, the prolonged low-dose administration used in this trial appears to have a significant antitumor effect. A randomized trial to confirm these promising results is now being initiated in North America. However, at the current time, the routine use of adjuvant chemotherapy after the resection of stages I through IIIA NSCLC is not justified.

Treatment of Stage IIIA Disease

Role of Surgical Resection

The most controversial and complex part of the treatment of stage IIIA NSCLC is the management of patients with N2 disease. Reported 5-year survival rates after resection for N2 disease are usually 20% to 30% but range from zero to 40%. This variation reflects the extent of mediastinal nodal involvement, the T status of the primary tumor, and the ability to perform a complete resection. With respect to mediastinal nodal involvement, adverse prognostic factors include the presence of extracapsular nodal disease, multiple levels of involved lymph nodes, and superior mediastinal nodal metastases (76,77).

Historically, several series presented an inappropriately optimistic view of the benefit of surgical resection for N2 disease because they focused on highly selected groups of patients. The experience reported by Martini and Flehinger (78) from Memorial Sloan-Kettering Cancer Center places surgical resection for N2 disease in perspective because it examines the outcome of treatment of all patients with N2 disease, not just a small subset. From 1974 to 1981, a total of 1,598 patients with NSCLC were seen by the thoracic service, of whom 706 had mediastinal nodal metastases. Only 151 patients, or 21% of all patients with N2 disease, had technically complete resections of the primary tumor and all accessible mediastinal lymph nodes. The overall survival of these 151 patients was 29% at 5 years. Moreover, 33 of these 151 patients who had "clinical" N2 disease (mediastinal nodal involvement extensive enough to be visible on chest radiography or at bronchoscopy) had only an 8% survival rate at 3 years. Thus, only 16.7% of all patients potentially benefited in the long term from surgical resection. Overall survival was also influenced by the T status of the primary tumor; patients with T2 or T3 tumors fared significantly worse than those with T1 tumors. Based on these and other data, most surgeons consider for resective surgery only those patients who have a T1 or T2 primary tumor and single-level, intranodal N2 disease.

Two small randomized clinical trials further challenge the concept of surgical resection as the primary treatment for any patient with N2 disease. Rosell and colleagues (79) randomized 60 patients with stage IIIA NSCLC (16 of whom did not have N2 disease) to undergo surgical resection or to receive three cycles of cisplatin-based chemotherapy followed by surgical resection. The median survival of the patients who received preoperative chemotherapy was significantly longer (26 vs. 8 months) than the survival of patients who underwent only surgical resection. A study of similar design from the M. D. Anderson Cancer Center corroborated these results (80). Both trials were stopped early because of highly significant differences between the two study arms. These two studies suggest that it is appropriate to consider all patients with N2 disease diagnosed at mediastinoscopy for induction chemotherapy. Unfortunately, because pretreatment mediastinoscopy was not mandated in either trial, some patients who did not have N2 disease were included. The results of these trials are not universally accepted because of the small numbers of patients enrolled, the lack of systematic pretreatment staging, and the unusually poor survival of the patients in the control arms.

Rationale for Neoadjuvant Therapy

Although some patients with minimal N2 disease survive for long periods of time after surgical resection, most have more extensive nodal involvement and do not benefit from surgery as their primary treatment. Until the 1980s, the standard treatment for such patients was radiation. The reported survival rates after radiation are harder to interpret than those after surgical resection because most series include a mixture of stage IIIA and IIIB patients and do not define the precise extent of nodal involvement. Sequential trials by the Radiation Therapy Oncology Group showed that high-dose, continuous radiation yields the best chance of local control (81). Many attempts have been made to intensify radiation dose without increasing radiation side effects, either by altering radiation fractionation schemes or by using three-dimensional conformal treatment planning. On the whole, these efforts have led to minimal improvements in both local control and survival because most patients relapse in distant sites—just as they do after surgical resection. For this reason, postoperative chemotherapy has been used as adjuvant therapy to surgery and radiation therapy in patients with N2 disease. No benefit in survival has been shown (82). The poor long-term survival and the risk for distant metastatic disease prompted an investigation of neoadjuvant multimodality therapy for stage III NSCLC.

Early Trials of Neoadjuvant Therapy

The concept of preoperative therapy followed by surgical resection *(neoadjuvant therapy)* dates back to 1955, when Bromley and Szur (83) used radiation (at an average dose of 47 Gy) to treat 66 patients before surgical resection. At operation, no viable tumor was found in 29 of 62 (47%) patients, but 10 patients died of complications in the first month, and only two patients were alive 5 years after operation. At the time, the natural history of NSCLC was not well understood, the methods of staging before resection not very accurate, and the risk for distant metastases not fully recognized. Effective chemotherapy did not exist, and it was hoped that an approach that increased resectability might lead to better long-term survival. Thus, early neoadjuvant trials focused on the use of preoperative radiation.

Several subsequent studies further explored this approach (84). All these trials were flawed by a lack of pretreatment staging, by the use of widely varying amounts of radiation, and by excessively long intervals between irradiation and surgical resection. Nonetheless, it became apparent that aggressive local treatment did not improve long-term survival, even though radiation could sterilize tumor in a significant number of patients. The development of distant metastases in 50% to 80% of patients during or shortly after treatment underscored the need for systemic therapy in stage III NSCLC.

Recent Trials of Neoadjuvant Therapy

Chemotherapy is now the primary treatment for most patients with stage IIIA N2 disease, with surgical resection, radiation, or both being added to optimize control of locoregional disease. Many trials of neoadjuvant therapy have been performed. It is difficult to assess whether one neoadjuvant regimen is superior to others because of wide variations in the types of induction therapy and the eligibility criteria among trials. The initial neoadjuvant trials of induction chemotherapy were developed in the early 1980s, when less information about the natural history of stage III NSCLC was available, and therefore they included a heterogeneous patient population. Because of a better understanding of the natural history of early-stage lung cancer and the revision of the international staging system in 1986, recent trials were able to focus on more uniform patient populations, so that it has been easier to interpret trial results.

Although many different treatment regimens have been used in neoadjuvant trials, they can be grouped into three major categories: (a) chemoradiation without surgical resection, (b) chemotherapy followed by surgical resection, and (c) chemoradiation followed by surgical resection.

Trials of Chemoradiation without Surgical Resection

These trials cannot be equated with trials of neoadjuvant therapy that include surgical resection because patients entered into nonsurgical trials are staged clinically without the benefit of mediastinoscopy. Therefore, nonsurgical trials include a mix of patients with stage IIIA and IIIB cancers, and they may even include some patients with earlier-stage disease who are thought erroneously to have stage III disease because of benign mediastinal adenopathy diagnosed only by CT.

With the acceptance of chemotherapy and radiation as standard treatment, attention has focused recently on the optimal means to deliver both modalities. A study suggests that concurrent treatment is superior to sequential chemoradiotherapy. Furuse et al. (85) randomized 314 patients with stage III NSCLC to MVP (80 mg of cisplatin per square meter on day 1, 8 mg of mitomycin per square meter on days 1 and 29, and vindesine on days 1, 8, 29, and 36) with concurrent split-course radiation or to MVP followed by standard radiation. Patients who received concurrent treatment had a significantly better response and survival.

The results of several phase III randomized trials comparing radiation alone with either sequential or concurrent chemotherapy and radiation are shown in Table 59.9. These trials confirmed the feasibility of combined-modality treatment and overall have shown that patients receiving chemoradiation have a better survival than those receiving either standard fractionated or hyperfractionated radiation alone. In most studies, the addition of chemotherapy improved median survival from between 9 and 10 months to 14 months and 5-year survival from 5% to between 15% and 20%. The somewhat variable results among these trials are related to several factors, including differences in total radiation dose and method of administration (split vs. continuous course); differences in chemotherapy dose, espe-

Table 59.9. RESULTS OF PHASE III TRIALS COMPARING RADIOTHERAPY ALONE WITH CHEMORADIOTHERAPY FOR STAGE III NON-SMALL CELL LUNG CANCER

Investigators	No. patients	CT	RT (Gy)	Group	Median survival (mo)	Survival at 2-y (%)	p
Trials showing no advantage							
Trovo et al., 1990 (159)	111	CAMP	45 (seq)	CT-RT	11.7	17[a]	ND
				RT	10.0	19[a]	
Morton et al., 1991 (160)	114	MACC	60 (seq)	CT-RT	10.6	21	>.2
				RT	10.4	16	
Le Chevalier et al., 1991 (161)	353	VCPC	65 (seq)	CT-RT	12.0	21	.08
				RT	10.0	14	
Blanke et al., 1995 (162)	214	CDDP	60–65 (con)	CT-RT	10.0	18	.35
				RT	10.7	13	
Trials in favor of combined therapy							
Schaake-Konig et al., 1992 (163)	331	CDDP	55 (con)	CT daily-RT	—	26	.01
				CT wkly-RT	—	19	
				RT	—	13	
Jeremic et al., 1995 (164)	169	Carbo +VP-16	64.8 (con)	CT (wkly)-HXFRT	18	23[b]	.003
				CT (other wk)-HXFRT	13	16	
				HXFRT	8	6.6	
Dillman et al., 1990, 1996 (165,166)	155	CDDP +Vbl	60 (seq)	CT-RT	13.7	26	.01
				RT	9.6	13	
Sause et al., 1995, 1997 (167)	458	CDDP +Vbl	60 (seq)	CT-RT	13.6	31	.04
				HFXRT (69.6 Gy)	12.3	24	
				RT	11.4	20	

[a]From survival curve.
[b]Survival at 3 years.
CAMP: cyclophosphamide, doxorubicin, methotrexate, procarbazine; MACC: methotrexate, doxorubicin, cyclophosphamide, lomustine; VCPC: vindesine, cyclophosphamide, cisplatin, lomustine; CDDP, cisplatin; VP-16, etoposide; Vbl, vinblastine; ND, no difference; CT, chemotherapy; RT, radiotherapy; HFXRT, hyperfractionated radiation therapy; seq, sequential; con, concurrent.

cially with respect to cisplatin; and differences in patient selection based on staging criteria.

Trials of Neoadjuvant Therapy with Surgical Resection

These trials have used two different treatment strategies: induction chemotherapy alone or concurrent chemoradiation before surgical resection. The rationale for chemotherapy alone as induction treatment is that it potentially allows the use of a more intense dose and also the use of some drugs, such as mitomycin, that cannot be administered in conjunction with radiation. Proponents of this approach also believe that chemotherapy is as effective as induction treatment as combined chemoradiation, and that separating the two modalities allows irradiation to be used postoperatively, when a higher total dose can be given. Proponents of concurrent preoperative chemoradiation believe that this approach provides adequate systemic treatment of micrometastatic disease and more effective control of bulky primary and mediastinal tumors.

Neoadjuvant Trials of Chemotherapy Alone before Surgical Resection. One of the best-known early trials to demonstrate the feasibility of combining induction chemotherapy with subsequent pulmonary resection in patients with stage III NSCLC was developed by Martini et al. (86) at Memorial Sloan-Kettering Cancer Center. In 1984, they initiated a trial of high-dose, cisplatin-based (120 mg/m^2) chemotherapy followed by surgical resection for patients with clinical N2 disease. Vindesine or vinblastine and subsequently mitomycin were added to form the so-called MVP regimen. Postoperative radiation was given to patients who had persistent mediastinal nodal tumor at thoracotomy, and all patients received two additional cycles of chemotherapy postoperatively. In 136 patients treated from 1984 to 1991, the major response rate to induction chemotherapy was 77% (105/136), and the

complete resection rate was 65% (89/136). A complete pathologic response was noted in 19 patients (21%) at the time of resection. The overall survival at 5 years was 17%, and the median survival was 19 months, a distinct improvement over the historical survival for this group of patients. Seven treatment-related deaths (5%) occurred in this study, five of which were postoperative.

Two other groups, the Toronto group and the LCSG, performed confirmatory trials of MVP induction chemotherapy without postoperative radiation. All the patients in these two trials had N2 disease proven by mediastinoscopy, but the LCSG trial also included some patients staged as IIIB because they had T4 disease. In the Toronto trial, the overall response rate was 65% (25/39), and the complete resection rate was 46% (18/39). The overall 3-year survival was 26%, and the median survival was 18.6 months. The 15% (6/39) treatment-related mortality rate was related mainly to four patients who died during induction treatment of sepsis resulting from postobstructive pneumonia (87). The LCSG trial reported an overall response rate of 62% (16/26), a complete resection rate of 54% (14/26), and a treatment-related mortality of 15%. The actuarial survival rate at 4 years was 27%, and the median survival rate was 12 months (88).

A phase II trial of induction chemotherapy with two cycles of cisplatin (100 mg/m^2 on days 1 and 29) and vinblastine (5 mg/m^2 per week) without mitomycin followed by surgical resection for patients with mediastinoscopy-proven stage IIIA N2 disease was reported by the Cancer and Leukemia Group B (CALGB) in 1995 (89). In addition, two cycles of chemotherapy and 59.4 Gy of radiation were given postoperatively. Of the 74 patients entered into this trial, 63 (85%) had either an objective response or stable disease after induction therapy and underwent thoracotomy. Twenty-three patients (37% of thoracotomies, 31% of all patients) had a complete resection, and the operative mortality rate was 3.2%. The overall 3-year survival was

23%. The lower resectability rate in this trial than in the study performed at Memorial Sloan-Kettering potentially reflects both the multiinstitutional nature of this trial and the use of a less intensive chemotherapy regimen (primarily because of the omission of mitomycin). However, the overall long-term survival appears similar for the two trials.

Two small randomized trials, reported in 1994, compared surgical resection alone with cisplatin-based induction chemotherapy followed by surgery. Both studies demonstrated a significant overall survival benefit with the use of neoadjuvant chemotherapy (79,80). In the trial reported by Rosell et al. (79), 60 patients with stage III NSCLC were randomized to surgery alone or to three cycles of neoadjuvant chemotherapy (mitomycin, ifosfamide, cisplatin) followed by surgical resection. The median survival was significantly longer with the combined-modality therapy than with surgery alone (26 months vs. 8 months). Roth et al. (80) conducted a similar study in which 60 patients with pathologically determined N2 disease or unequivocal T3 disease were randomized to surgery alone or to three cycles of induction chemotherapy with cyclophosphamide, etoposide, and cisplatin followed by surgery and additional postoperative chemotherapy. Although the rates of complete resection were similar in both study arms (31% for surgery, 39% for combined modality), the median and 3-year overall survival rates were significantly better in the combined-modality arm (64 vs. 11 months and 56% vs. 15%, respectively). Several weaknesses in study design, including the small number of patients, the lack of uniform pretreatment staging, and the unusually poor survival of patients in the surgery-only arm, have raised doubts about the validity of the results of both of these trials. Unfortunately, it is unlikely that larger trials of similar design will be performed in the future to corroborate these results.

Other recent trials have either shown a trend toward improved survival after preoperative chemotherapy or have yielded equivocal results. Pass et al. (90) conducted a phase III trial in which 27 patients with biopsy-proven stage IIIA N2 disease were randomized to surgery plus postoperative mediastinal radiation (54 to 60 Gy) or to induction chemotherapy (two cycles of cisplatin and etoposide) followed by surgery with postoperative chemotherapy or radiation. The median survival in the induction chemotherapy group was 28.7 months, and it was 15.6 months in the surgery plus radiation group, but this difference was not statistically significant. In 1997, Elias et al. (91) reported a trial by the CALGB in which patients who had N2 disease proven by mediastinoscopy received either preoperative radiation or chemotherapy (etoposide and cisplatin) followed by surgical resection. The median survival rates were 23 months and 19 months, respectively. Unfortunately, the trial was terminated prematurely because of failure to meet accrual goals. A recent report confirmed the results of this trial with more mature data (92).

Trials of Induction Chemoradiation Followed by Surgical Resection. The second approach to combined-modality therapy and surgical resection for stage III NSCLC has been to combine chemotherapy and radiation preoperatively (Table 59.10). This strategy aims to control micrometastatic disease while utilizing the synergism of concurrent radiation and chemotherapy to reduce tumor bulk in the primary site and mediastinum. In one of the first trials of this type, performed by the LCSG, 39 patients with stage III NSCLC received three cycles of chemotherapy with cyclophosphamide, doxorubicin, and cisplatin (CAP) and 1,500 cGy of radiation in 300-cGy fractions given concurrently with cycles 2 and 3 of the chemotherapy. The overall response rate to induction therapy was 51% (20/39), and 33% (13/39) of patients had a complete resection at thoracotomy. However, the overall 2-year survival was only 8%, with a median survival of 11 months. No treatment-related deaths occurred (93).

The LCSG subsequently performed another phase II induction trial of cisplatin, 5-fluorouracil, and partially concurrent low-dose radiation (3,000 cGy in 15 fractions) in 85 patients with stage IIIA N2 or stage IIIB NSCLC (94). Although the cisplatin dose in this trial was higher than in the previous study (75 instead of 60 mg/m² per dose), the overall response rate and complete resection rates were similar (56% and 34%). The median survival was 13 months. Four of 54 patients (7%) died postoperatively.

Faber and colleagues (95) at Rush-Presbyterian performed two sequential phase II neoadjuvant trials of 5-fluorouracil and low-dose cisplatin (60 mg/m²) plus 4,000 cGy of split-course radiation administered concurrently with the four cycles of induction chemotherapy. The second group of 74 patients also received etoposide in addition to the cisplatin and 5-fluorouracil. Of the 130 patients entered into these trials, 85 were candidates for surgery after induction therapy, and 62 (73%) underwent thoracotomy. The complete resection rate was 68% (58/85), and the overall survival rate was 40% at 3 years, with a median survival of 22 months. The induction therapy was associated with significant toxicity, but only one treatment-related death occurred. The operative mortality rate was 5%

Table 59.10. RESULTS OF REPRESENTATIVE NEOADJUVANT TRIALS FOR STAGE III NON-SMALL CELL LUNG CANCER: INDUCTION CHEMORADIOTHERAPY 0FOLLOWED BY SURGICAL RESECTION

Study (reference)	No. patients	Chemotherapy	Radiotherapy (Gy)	Survival	
				Median (mo)	2 y (%)
Rush-Presbyterian, Faber et al., 1989 (95)	IIIA: 85 (including 19 N0)	CDDP (60 mg/m²) + 5-FU +/− VP-16 × 4	40(S), 20 fractions	21.7	40 (3 y)
LCSG, Weiden et al., 1991 (94)	IIIA, IIIB: 85	CDDP (75 mg/m²) + 5-FU × 2	30(C), 15 fractions	13	22ᵃ
CALGB, Strauss et al., 1992 (96)	IIIA: 41 (including 8 N0–1)	CDDP (100 mg/m²) + Vbl + 5-FU × 2	30(C), 15 fractions	15.5	30ᵃ
SWOG, Albain et al., 1995 (97)	IIIA, IIIB: 126	CDDP (50 mg/m² days 1 and 8) + VP-16 × 2	45(C), 30 fractions	13 (IIIA) 17 (IIIB)	37 (IIIA) 39 (IIIB)

ᵃFrom survival curve.
LCSG, Lung Cancer Study Group; CALGB, Cancer and Leukemia Group B; SWOG, Southwest Oncology Group; CDDP, cisplatin; Vbl, vinblastine; 5-FU, 5-fluorouracil; VP-16, etoposide; (C), continuous course; (S), split course.

(3/62). The excellent results of these trials may reflect the inclusion of some patients who did not have N2 disease but were considered at that time to have stage III NSCLC by virtue of T3 (chest wall) N0 tumor status.

A neoadjuvant trial of similar design was performed by the CALGB in which high-dose cisplatin (100 mg/m^2), vinblastine, and 5-fluorouracil were given with 3,000 cGy of continuous radiation in 15 fractions to patients with stage IIIA disease (96). The overall response rate was 51% (21/41), and the complete resection rate was 61% (25/41). The median survival was 15.5 months. Significant toxicity occurred, and treatment-related mortality was high at 15% (6/41).

The largest reported phase II neoadjuvant trial of concurrent chemotherapy and radiation was a multiinstitutional study performed by the Southwest Oncology Group (97). Both stage IIIA and stage IIIB patients were entered, although, notably, pathologic documentation of the initial tumor stage, usually by mediastinoscopy, was required. The induction regimen included two cycles of cisplatin (50 mg/m^2 on days 1 and 8) and etoposide with 4,500 cGy of concurrent radiation in 25 fractions. All patients underwent thoracotomy unless their disease progressed. The objective response rate to induction therapy in the 126 eligible patients was 59%. The resectability rates were 85% for the IIIA N2 group and 80% for the IIIB group. Nearly two thirds of the patients had no viable tumor or only minimal residual foci of tumor in their surgical specimens. The 3-year survival rate was 27% for the IIIA group and 24% for the IIIB group, with median survivals of 13 months and 17 months, respectively. The best predictor of survival after surgery was the absence of tumor in the mediastinal lymph nodes at surgery (3-year survival of 44%). The majority of recurrences were distant, and the brain was the single most common site. The operative mortality rate was 6%, and the overall treatment-related mortality was 10%. An important finding of this trial was that survival was the same for patients with stage IIIB NSCLC by virtue of T4 tumor status and patients with stage IIIA N2 disease. However, patients with N3 disease had a poor overall survival. Importantly, the long-term follow-up of this study shows that the survival rates at 3 years are sustained at 6 years (98).

Important differences between the Southwest Oncology Group trial and earlier neoadjuvant trials were the careful documentation of pretreatment stage, the use of a higher dose of continuous radiation (4,500 cGy rather than 3,000 cGy of continuous or 4,000 cGy of split-course radiation), and the fully concurrent manner in which the chemotherapy and radiation were administered. Attempts to intensify this therapeutic approach by increasing or accelerating the radiation have been associated with unacceptable toxicity. Two small single-institution trials illustrate this problem. Yashar et al. (99) treated 36 patients who had stage IIIA N2 disease with two cycles of cisplatin (25 mg/m^2 per day for 4 days) and etoposide and 55 Gy of concurrent radiation. All patients underwent exploratory thoracotomy, and 31 (86%) underwent resection, 27 with pneumonectomy. Although the overall 3-year survival rate was 34%, two operative deaths (5.6%) occurred, six patients required prolonged intubation because of postoperative adult respiratory distress syndrome (ARDS), and a bronchial stump leak developed in three patients.

In the second study, Fowler et al. (100) treated 13 patients who had stage IIIA N2 disease with two cycles of cisplatin (20 mg/m^2 per day for 4 days), 5-fluorouracil, and etoposide and 60 Gy of concurrent radiation in 30 fractions. Six patients then underwent lobectomy, and seven patients underwent pneumonectomy. The complication rate was unacceptably high; the adult respiratory distress syndrome (ARDS) developed in one of the lobectomy patients and in five of the seven pneumonectomy patients and was fatal in two patients. Bronchial stump leaks developed in three pneumonectomy patients, and one of them died. The trial was closed prematurely after 13 patients had been accrued because of the excessive morbidity and mortality. An additional 27 patients who received the same induction therapy but did not undergo thoracotomy tolerated the treatment without major problems.

Two additional recent trials have tested concurrent induction chemoradiation in stage III NSCLC. Milstein et al. (101) conducted a phase II trial in which 36 patients (10 with T3 N0 or T3 N1 disease and 11 with IIIB disease) received two cycles of cisplatin (25 mg/m^2) and etoposide plus concurrent radiation to 50 Gy during 28 sessions. Twenty-four patients (21 with IIIA and three with IIIB disease) underwent thoracotomy, with complete resection in 20 (86%). Three of the 21 IIIA patients had complete tumor sterilization. The overall survival at 2 years was 39% (57% for resectable patients and 15% for unresectable patients), and the median survival was 15 months. One death from sepsis occurred during the induction treatment, and two postoperative deaths resulted from ARDS and bronchopleural fistula. This attempt to intensify induction chemoradiation by increasing the dose of radiation was not successful.

Stimulated by the promising results of the Southwest Oncology Group 8805 trial for patients with T4 disease, Grunewald et al. (102) performed a phase II trial of similar design for stage IIIB T4 NSCLC. The induction regimen consisted of cisplatin (100 mg/m^2), 5-fluorouracil, and vinblastine with 45 Gy of concurrent hyperfractionated (twice daily) radiation. Of 25 patients enrolled, 16 were subsequently eligible for surgery, and 12 had complete surgical resection. No induction treatment-related or operative deaths occurred. This study confirms that complete resection after induction therapy is feasible in a significant number of stage IIIB T4 tumors, a subset of stage IIIB tumors previously considered inoperable under any circumstances. Further combined-modality studies are therefore appropriate in this select group of patients.

Only one study, reported by Fleck et al. (103) in abstract form, addresses the question of whether radiation augments the benefit of induction chemotherapy before surgical resection. This phase III trial involved 96 patients with N2 or T4 disease who were randomized to induction chemotherapy with MVP or to concurrent chemoradiation with cisplatin and 5-fluorouracil plus radiation to 30 Gy. Postoperatively, all patients received additional cisplatin and etoposide. The resection rate was significantly higher in the chemoradiation group (52% vs. 31%), as was 2-year disease-free survival (40% vs. 21%) and median survival (18 months vs. 12 months). Unfortunately, the definitive results of this trial have not been published in manuscript form.

Current Status of Neoadjuvant Therapy and Surgical Resection

Taken as a whole, neoadjuvant therapy trials have demonstrated the feasibility of induction chemotherapy and surgical resection for the treatment of stage III NSCLC. Most studies show improved rates of resectability and survival in comparison with the historical experience for surgical resection or radiation alone. However, the optimal treatment approach to these locally advanced tumors has not yet been fully defined, especially because neoadjuvant trials vary with respect to eligibility criteria, inclusion of both stage IIIA and stage IIIB tumors, accuracy of pretreatment staging, and type of induction regimens. Moreover, the response, resectability, and survival rates are not uniformly reported. In some cases, instead of reporting results as a percentage of the total number of patients entered into the study, the authors report resectability rates as a percentage of the patients with a radiographic response, and only the survival rates of patients who underwent resection are emphasized.

However, the potential toxicity of neoadjuvant regimens should not be overlooked. Induction regimens in which high-dose cisplatin ($\geq$ 100 mg/m²) or radiation doses of 4,000 to 4,500 cGy are used have been well tolerated, but radiation doses of 5,500 cGy or higher have been associated with an excessive risk for postoperative ARDS and bronchial stump leak. Good response rates have been achieved with newer chemotherapeutic agents, such as paclitaxel, docetaxel, gemcitabine, and carboplatin, and they are better tolerated by patients. Determining the contribution of these agents in combined-modality therapy will require further trials, especially as the major form of relapse continues to be distant metastatic disease.

Future Directions

In addition to new chemotherapeutic agents, new radiation techniques, such as hyperfractionated or accelerated schedules, also merit further exploration in neoadjuvant trials with concurrent chemotherapy. Rice et al. (104), from the Cleveland Clinic, conducted a study in which 45 patients with stage IIIA or IIIBceived induction cisplatin, paclitaxel, and 30 Gy of accelerated hyperfractionated radiation therapy (1.5-Gy fraction twice daily). Surgery was then performed approximately 4 weeks after induction. The overall response rate was 54%. Forty patients (89%) proceeded to surgery, and 32 patients (71%) underwent complete resection. Five complete pathologic remissions were seen. Fourteen patients overall were down-staged. The 2-year relapse-free survival rate was 47%, and the 2-year survival rate was 65%. No apparent therapy-related deaths occurred, but the toxicity was high, with 89% of patients experiencing significant mucitis and 20% experiencing esophagitis of grade 3 or worse.

Another new radiation technique is three-dimensional conformal therapy; higher radiation dosing (> 70 Gy) of the tumor is possible while surrounding normal lung is spared, so that the possibility of local control is improved (105).

The management of stage III NSCLC is complex and still evolving. Many trials indicate that resectability and survival rates are probably improved with the use of combined-modality therapy than with radiation or surgical resection alone. Regimens incorporating high-dose cisplatin with or without moderate-dose radiation have achieved the best results with acceptable levels of toxicity. Careful patient management leads to complete resection, and the operative risk is comparable with that of standard pulmonary resection. Very importantly, combined-modality treatment requires close collaboration among medical oncologists, radiation oncologists, surgeons, pulmonologists, and anesthesiologists. In the future, four key areas warrant further investigation: (a) The optimal combination and sequencing of newer, less toxic chemotherapeutic agents and a variety of new radiation techniques require further study. (b) An ongoing intergroup clinical trial in North America should determine whether neoadjuvant therapy including surgical resection is superior to nonsurgical treatment with chemotherapy and higher-dose radiation in patients with stage IIIA NSCLC. The National Cancer Institute has designated this study as a high-priority trial. Approximately 75% of the planned accrual of 512 patients has been reached, and it is of the utmost importance that this trial be completed to answer a pivotal question in the management of stage IIIA NSCLC. (c) Future clinical trials will need to determine whether concurrent chemoradiation is superior to chemotherapy alone as preoperative induction therapy. (d) Ongoing and future investigations of the molecular biologic features of tumors that dictate response to individual chemotherapeutic agents will allow a more individualized selection of induction treatment regimens and may in turn lead to improved long-term outcome.

NEUROENDOCRINE TUMORS

Neuroendocrine tumors of the lung constitute a varied group of lesions, ranging from tumors with low-grade malignant potential (typical carcinoid) to SCLC, which is among the most rapidly growing and aggressive of human tumors. Between those two extremes, atypical carcinoid and large cell neuroendocrine carcinoma have been defined (105).

Typical and Atypical Carcinoid Tumors

Carcinoid tumors, which are neoplasms with a low-grade malignant potential, comprise about 2% of lung tumors in the United States. They arise from neuroendocrine stem cells of the bronchial epithelium and are classified as either typical or atypical. Histologically, typical carcinoids consist of uniform polygonal cells with round nuclei and fine granular chromatin (Fig. 59.7). Mitotic figures are rare. Atypical carcinoids show increased mitotic activity, nuclear pleomorphism, areas of disorganization of the architecture, and tumor necrosis (107).

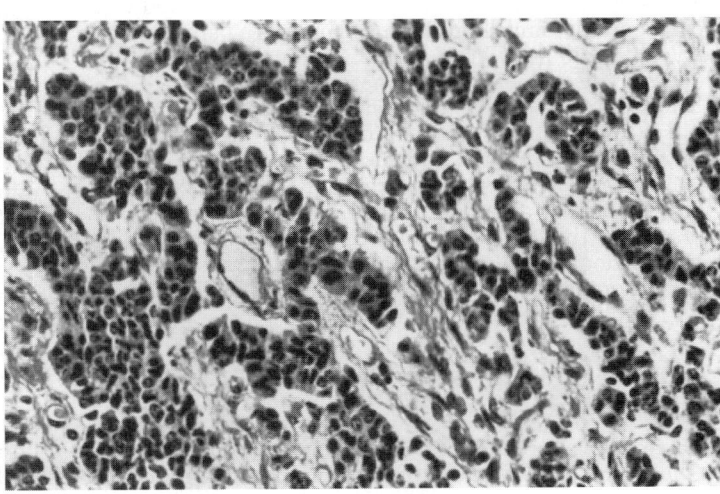

Figure 59.7. Photomicrograph of a typical carcinoid, with interlacing cords and masses of uniform cells. Vascular stroma is apparent.

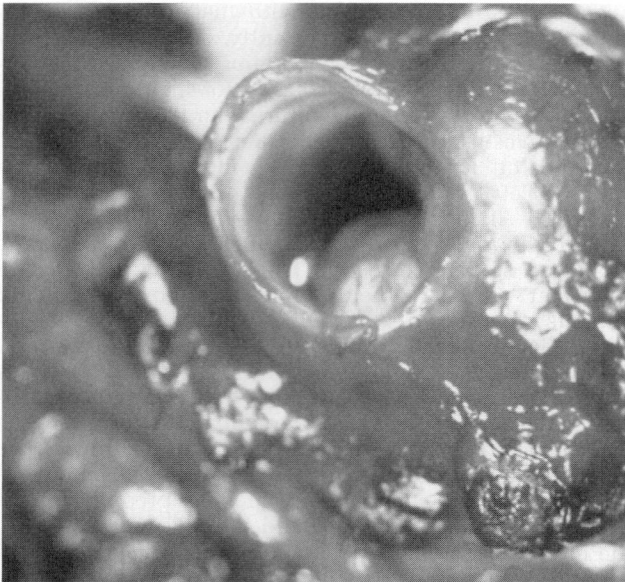

Figure 59.8. Bronchoscopic view of a carcinoid tumor.

Carcinoid tumors occur equally in both sexes and at a median age of 55 years. Half of patients present with pulmonary symptoms, including hemoptysis, dyspnea, and recurrent or persistent pneumonitis because 40% of lesions are centrally located in the main or lobar bronchi. The lesions may be diagnosed by bronchoscopy, appearing as pink or purple friable endobronchial masses covered by intact epithelium (Fig. 59.8). In the other half of patients, carcinoid tumors are diagnosed when radiologic abnormalities are detected on a chest roentgenogram as part of a routine examination (108).

Lymph node metastases occur in approximately 10% to 15% of patients at diagnosis but are more frequent in atypical carcinoids. The carcinoid syndrome is associated with bronchial carcinoids in only 2% of cases, usually in patients with metastatic disease, particularly of the liver. The most common sites of metastases are lung, bone, liver, adrenals, and brain (108).

The standard treatment of bronchial carcinoids is complete surgical resection, despite the presence of nodal involvement, with mediastinal lymph node sampling or dissection (109). Lobectomy is required in about 50% of patients. Lesser resections (segmentectomy, sleeve resection) are adequate for complete resection in about 20% of patients. Endoscopic resection is invariably associated with local recurrence and should be used only as a palliative maneuver in patients whose general medical condition precludes thoracotomy and pulmonary resection (108).

The long-term survival rate after surgical resection exceeds 90% in patients with typical carcinoids, even when hilar or mediastinal nodal metastases are present. In contrast, patients with atypical carcinoids have a 5-year survival rate of 60% after complete resection. The outcome is more closely linked to histology than to tumor size and location or nodal involvement. Recurrence is more frequent with tumors larger than 3 cm and in patients who present with lymph node metastases (108).

Large Cell Neuroendocrine Carcinomas

Large cell neuroendocrine carcinoma is characterized by the microscopic features of neuroendocrine tumors, but the tumor cells are large, have a high mitotic rate, and frequently show necrosis (106,107). According to Travis and colleagues (110–112), large cell neuroendocrine carcinomas are related to smoking, as is SCLC, and are also high-grade tumors, with 5- and 10-year survival rates of 27% and 9%, respectively, despite complete resection. Because this entity is fairly newly recognized (since 1991), few data are available concerning adjuvant therapy. For the time being, the management of large cell neuroendocrine carcinoma is identical to that of NSCLC.

Small Cell Lung Cancer

Small cell carcinoma of the lung has the most aggressive clinical course of any type of pulmonary tumor and is often widely disseminated by the time of diagnosis. In contrast to non-small cell tumors, these lesions are notably responsive to chemotherapy and are rarely within the domain of the surgeon. The staging system for SCLC was developed by the Veterans Administration Lung Cancer Staging Group and divides patients into those with limited and those with extensive disease. This distinction was first based on what could be encompassed by a tolerable radiation portal. After clarification by the International Association for the Study of Lung Cancer, limited disease includes patients with tumors confined to one hemithorax and regional lymph nodes (hilar, ipsilateral, and contralateral mediastinal nodes, and ipsilateral and contralateral supraclavicular nodes) and patients with ipsilateral pleural effusion, regardless of whether the cytology is positive or negative. On the other hand, pericardial and bilateral pulmonary involvement are considered as extensive disease (113).

Common sites of distant metastases are bone, liver, bone marrow, and the central nervous system, and therefore the metastatic evaluation includes a bone scan and CT of the chest, abdomen, and brain. Some oncologists also perform bone marrow biopsies, but because the marrow is the sole site of extensive disease in fewer than 5% of patients, biopsies are usually judged unnecessary (23). After the staging process, approximately 30% to 40% of patients are found to have limited disease.

For patients with limited disease, response rates of 85% to 90% and complete response rates of 50% to 60% can be expected with the combination of etoposide and cisplatin and radiation therapy (114,115). The median survival is 18 to 24 months, and the 2-year survival rates are 40% to 50% (5% more than before the use of radiation therapy) (116,117). In extensive SCLC treated with chemotherapy, response rates reach 75% to 85%, although complete response is seen in only 15% to 25% of patients. The median survival is between 7 to 11 months, with a 2-year survival near zero. The prognosis in SCLC depends primarily on the anatomic extent of disease, but after a review of prognostic variables in its 2,580-patient SCLC data base, the Southwest Oncology Group determined that the two-stage system should be extended into a four-stage system, with serum lactate dehydrogenase level, age, and pleural effusion used as additional staging criteria (118).

The small number of patients with SCLC seen by the surgeon represent fewer than 10% of all patients with SCLC. They have peripheral tumors with no nodal involvement or only hilar nodal involvement, which would be classified as T1–2 N0–1 tumors in the NSCLC staging system. In the past, such tumors were often diagnosed at exploratory thoracotomy for an asymptomatic coin lesion, but with the increasing use of diagnostic percutaneous needle aspiration, more patients with early-stage SCLC are now identified preoperatively. Such patients should be evaluated in conjunction with a medical oncologist, and surgical resection should be considered after distant disease has been excluded by a complete metastatic evaluation. For such cases, it has been suggested that the TNM classification be used in future trials and studies.

Retrospective series have demonstrated a 5-year survival rate of 50% after resection of T1 N0 or T2 N0 SCLC (119). Because of the propensity for small cell cancers to disseminate, adjuvant chemotherapy has traditionally been given to patients after surgical resection, even though, by virtue of the small numbers of patients available, no prospective, randomized trials have demonstrated whether this is of benefit. Relapse in the primary site, which is a problem for most patients with limited-stage SCLC, is distinctly uncommon after complete resection of these early tumors (120). Radiation therapy to the chest has been suggested after surgically complete resection, but because insufficient information is available in the literature and local relapse is uncommon, it cannot be considered a standard treatment (119).

Because the role of surgical resection in patients with mediastinal nodal involvement (N2 disease) is questionable, mediastinoscopy should be considered mandatory to exclude mediastinal nodal disease (121). This should ideally be performed separately from thoracotomy because it can be difficult for the pathologist to diagnose small cell cancer on a frozen section. The intraoperative management of SCLC is not significantly different from that of NSCLC, and an incomplete resection does not benefit the patient.

The addition of surgical resection after a response to induction chemotherapy has been proposed by some surgeons to cure a small number of patients with limited SCLC without mediastinal involvement (122). To date, the LCSG has performed the only prospective, randomized trial evaluating the role of surgery in limited SCLC (123). All patients enrolled in that study received chemotherapy, and those in whom at least a partial response was achieved were randomized to undergo or not undergo surgery. Because the survival rate was the same in both groups, this trial did not support the addition of pulmonary resection to the multimodality treatment of SCLC. Finally, the occurrence of a second primary lung carcinoma after treatment for SCLC is reported in the few patients with prolonged survival. It should not be assumed that the new tumor is of small cell histology, and these patients should be evaluated for the possibility of surgical resection (124). The average risk for the development of a second lung cancer in patients who survive SCLC is approximately 6% per patient per year (56).

BRONCHIAL GLAND CARCINOMAS

Bronchial gland carcinomas are rare primary tumors of the lung. They constitute about 1% of all lung neoplasms and 2% of the tumors for which surgical resection is performed. These tumors are also called *primary salivary gland-type tumors of the lung* because the tracheal and bronchial airway submucosa and the salivary glands contain serous and mucous glands that are histologically similar (125). Often, they are called *bronchial adenomas,* but this term is misleading because they are malignant. Care must be taken to separate these primary tumors from metastases of primitive salivary gland tumors (126). This group of carcinomas includes adenoid cystic carcinoma, mucoepidermoid carcinoma, and the even rarer mixed tumor (pleomorphic adenoma). The only truly benign tumors are mucous gland adenomas.

The symptomatology of these tumors is determined essentially by their location and size (126). Peripheral tumors, which are less frequent, are asymptomatic, generally presenting as a nodule on routine chest radiography. Proximally located tumors present with symptoms of bronchial irritation and obstruction, including cough, shortness of breath, hemoptysis, recurrent infection, wheezing, and stridor. Sometimes, patients have constitutional symptoms, such as weight loss and pain. On chest radiography, the nodule may again be seen, with pneumonia or atelectasis. Because of the slow growth of these tumors, signs and symptoms may develop over a period of years. Incompletely obstructing tumors frequently masquerade as asthma for prolonged periods of time. Smoking does not seem to be a risk factor for these tumors.

Peripheral tumors are diagnosed by percutaneous needle aspiration biopsy or at the time of thoracotomy. Tumors in major airways are diagnosed by bronchoscopy. Other studies, such as CT, are rarely required to make the diagnosis but may be of value in planning therapy.

Because most of these tumors do not metastasize, complete excision, with preservation of as much pulmonary tissue as possible, is the goal. Whenever possible, sleeve resections of main bronchi are performed to preserve pulmonary tissue.

Adenoid Cystic Carcinoma

Adenoid cystic carcinomas are slowly growing malignant tumors that arise from the submucosal glands of the trachea and main bronchi (Fig. 59.9). They have also been called *cylindromas, adenoid cystic basal cell carcinomas, adenomyoepitheliomas,* and *pseudoadenomatous basal cell carcinomas.* Adenoid cystic carcinomas behave much like the major and minor salivary gland tumors of the same name, to which they are microscopically identical. An important aspect of their clinical behavior is that they tend to spread in the submucosal plane along the perineural lymphatics, well beyond the obvious endoluminal component of the tumor. In a small biopsy specimen, it

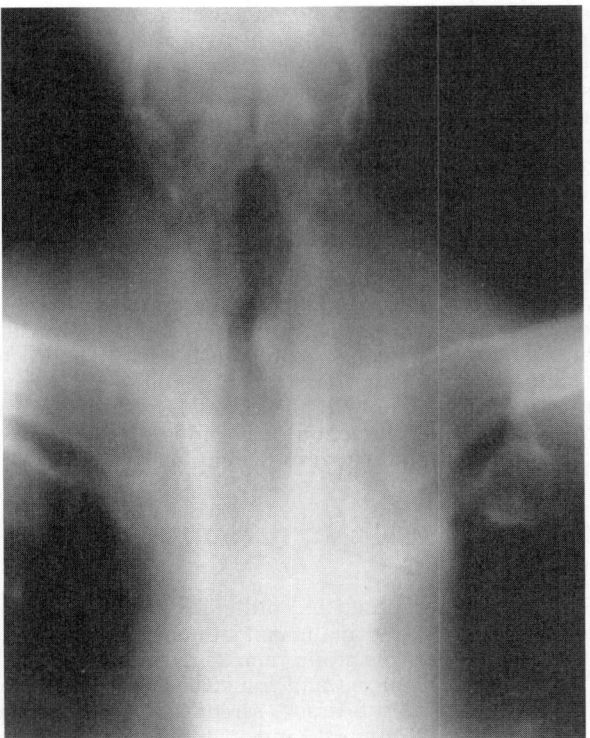

Figure 59.9. Tracheogram demonstrating airway obstruction by an adenoid cystic carcinoma of the upper trachea.

can be difficult to distinguish adenoid cystic carcinoma from a conventional adenocarcinoma. Immunohistochemical stains may help the pathologist differentiate the two by showing the presence of the myoepithelial cell immunophenotype in adenoid cystic carcinoma (126).

Whenever possible, total excision by tracheal resection or tracheobronchial resection is the treatment of choice (127). This is not always possible because of the extensive submucosal spread of tumor. In such cases, palliative resection may be necessary. Postoperative radiation is indicated because these tumors are radiation-sensitive.

When no surgical resection is feasible because of the extent of the lesion, a palliative treatment option is endoscopic laser removal followed by radiation (brachytherapy, external beam irradiation, or both).

When complete surgical resection is possible, the prognosis is excellent. However, because of the slow-growing nature of the tumor and its responsiveness to radiation, prolonged survival is possible even with incomplete resection or palliative measures. Patients frequently live 10 years or more with persistent disease, including pulmonary metastases. In such cases, repeated efforts at palliation are indicated.

Mucoepidermoid Carcinoma

Mucoepidermoid carcinomas may be of low- or high-grade malignancy and have the same microscopic appearance as mucoepidermoid tumors of salivary gland origin. These tumors also arise in the glandular submucosa, presenting as submucosal lesions. The distinction between low-grade and high-grade tumor is based on mitotic activity, cellular necrosis, and nuclear pleomorphism (125).

The principles of treatment of mucoepidermoid tumors are similar to those of carcinoid tumors. The more malignant variety must be treated as bronchogenic carcinoma. Some authors even think that adenosquamous carcinoma is the same entity as mucoepidermoid carcinoma, but arising in the periphery of the lung (125). The outlook for these tumors depends on the grade of malignancy and the stage of the disease. High-grade tumors have the same prognosis as bronchogenic carcinoma. Complete surgical resection is the mainstay of treatment. Mucoepidermoid tumors are too rare to permit an evaluation of combined-modality therapy for more aggressive, high-grade tumors (125).

Mucous Gland Adenoma

Mucous gland adenomas are rare submucosal tumors that arise from mucous glands. They are also known as *bronchial cysts* and *papillary cystadenomas*. Because of their totally benign behavior, they can usually be treated by endoscopic excision. Thoracotomy and surgical resection are indicated only if the distal lung has been destroyed by chronic infection or if endoscopic removal is technically contraindicated or incomplete.

OTHER MALIGNANT TUMORS OF THE LUNG

The lung is composed of epithelial, mesodermal, and endodermal cells, and malignant tumors may arise from any of these cells. This group represents fewer than 1% of all primary lung cancers and is usually subdivided into lymphoid tumors, soft-tissue sarcomas, mixed epithelial/mesenchymal tumors, and ectopic tissue tumors (128,129). Primary pulmonary lymphomas usually are excised for confirmatory diagnosis. Sarcomas arising from

soft tissue or large vessels are treated in a similar fashion to sarcomas occurring elsewhere. Treatment of the other rare tumors, including pulmonary blastomas, primary melanomas of the bronchus, and malignant teratomas, primarily involves complete surgical resection. Radiation and chemotherapy do not have well-defined roles in the treatment of any of these tumors but are occasionally used in particular situations.

SURGICAL RESECTION OF PULMONARY METASTASES

Historical Background

The first report of the resection of a pulmonary metastasis performed as a separate procedure is attributed to Divis in 1926. In North America, the most quoted case of lobectomy for a metastatic carcinoma was that performed by Barney and Churchill in 1939 (130). Their patient underwent a nephrectomy for an adenocarcinoma and was known to have a pulmonary mass. After the renal resection, the pulmonary tumor did not respond to radiation treatment and increased in size. They decided to explore surgically and resected the renal cell metastasis. The patient survived disease-free for more than 20 years.

From 1940 to the mid-1960s, pulmonary metastasectomy was performed infrequently and only in highly selected patients. A total of 169 pulmonary metastasis resections were performed on 165 patients at the Mayo Clinic from 1941 to 1959 (131). This large number of operations may reflect the high volume of cases seen at Mayo Clinic rather than the common use of surgical resection at that time. The first principles of pulmonary resection for metastatic disease were offered: complete removal of the primary disease, no evidence of recurrence or metastatic disease other than the lung lesion, and the patient in good general condition. Multiple lesions were not considered a contraindication to resection, but it was thought that bilateral disease indicated a poor prognosis and should not be resected. Surgeons were already convinced that the resection should be as conservative of lung function as possible.

Since then, experience from several institutions suggests that more liberal indications for pulmonary metastasectomy are appropriate (132). A striking example was the treatment of metastatic osteogenic sarcoma at Memorial Sloan-Kettering Cancer Center. From 1940 to 1965, only five such patients were treated surgically. During the same period, only 24 of 145 patients (17%) survived 5 years after resection of their primary tumors, and 118 of these patients (81%) died of pulmonary metastases. This experience prompted a more aggressive approach to the management of pulmonary metastases. Starting in 1965, a consecutive series of 22 patients with osteogenic sarcoma underwent pulmonary metastasectomy. Patients were considered for operation even if they had bilateral metastases or required multiple thoracotomies to remove all gross tumor. A total of 59 thoracotomies were performed in these 22 patients, with an overall 5-year survival rate of 32%. The dramatic improvement in survival in comparison with the historical experience strongly supported the aggressive use of pulmonary metastasectomy in these patients (133).

During the past 30 years, surgical resection has become a widely accepted treatment for certain pulmonary metastases; however, some of the criteria for patient selection remain controversial. In addition, advances in chemotherapy have changed the indications for surgical resection. With some cancers, pulmonary metastasectomy is performed to prolong life expectancy, whereas with others, it serves mainly to restage disease or to provide adjuvant treatment after initial chemotherapy. The role of pulmonary metastasectomy will undoubtedly continue to evolve as improvements in systemic treatment are made. This review provides a perspective on the approach to the surgical management of pulmonary metastases.

Clinical Presentation and Diagnosis

Metastases are asymptomatic 85% of the time and are usually detected on a routine chest radiograph. Patients who undergo resection of a primary tumor with a known tendency to metastasize to the lung should have a chest radiograph as part of their routine follow-up care. On a chest radiograph, metastases usually present as well-circumscribed, spherical solid masses with well-defined borders (Fig. 59.10). Cavitation is occasionally seen in large lesions with central necrosis, mostly squamous cell cancers. The distribution of lung metastases is predominantly subpleural or in the outer third of lung fields (134).

Metastases to the lung usually arise in the pulmonary parenchyma. Endobronchial metastases are uncommon but occur most typically with renal cell, colon, and breast cancers. Even with endobronchial metastases, half of patients are asymptomatic (135). More often, endobronchial disease represents an extension of contiguous parenchymal disease. The extent of endobronchial tumor can affect the approach to surgical resection. For these reasons, bronchoscopy should be performed before thoracotomy, especially if centrally located metastases are present.

Hilar or mediastinal nodal involvement sometimes accompanies pulmonary metastases. The determinants of nodal involvement and the prognostic and therapeutic implications remain poorly understood. Lymphangitic spread can occur with or without concomitant pulmonary nodules. This happens most frequently in breast cancer and produces a characteristic radiographic appearance of diffusely increased interstitial markings and a clinical presentation of severe dyspnea that is out of proportion to the radiographic findings.

When pulmonary metastases are thought to be present on a chest radiograph, CT should be performed to determine

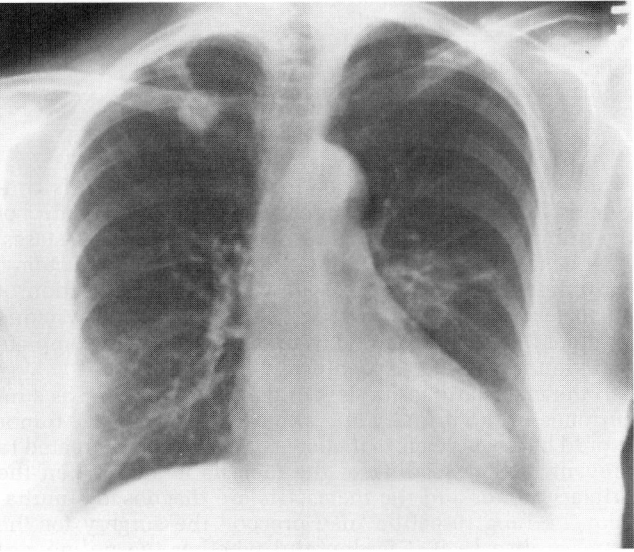

Figure 59.10. Chest radiograph of a patient with bilateral pulmonary metastases from endometrial cancer. The mass in the right upper lobe is well circumscribed and has the radiographic appearance typical of a metastasis.

their number, location, size, and potential resectability. Plain chest radiographs detect only lesions at least 9 mm in size. New lesions of this size seen on a chest radiograph in a patient already treated for a malignancy have a 90% chance of being malignant (136). Even though CT can identify lesions as small as 3 mm, it often underestimates the number of pulmonary metastases (Fig. 59.11). When radiologic and surgical findings are correlated, only 75% of malignant nodules are detected by CT. Fifteen percent of CT studies overestimate the number of lung metastases for an accurate radiologic assessment of 61% (137,138).

Patients who present with multiple pulmonary nodules in the setting of a previously treated malignancy rarely pose a diagnostic dilemma. Patients who present with solitary pulmonary nodules are more problematic. Generally, a solitary lesion is more likely to be a metastasis if the primary tumor was a sarcoma or a melanoma. If the primary tumor originated in the head, neck, or breast, it is more likely to be a new primary lung cancer (139). It has an equal chance of being a metastasis or a new primary if the initial tumor was of gastrointestinal or genitourinary origin. Percutaneous fine-needle aspiration biopsy usually yields a tissue diagnosis, but the necessity of a biopsy in the case of a solitary lesion is questionable. If the patient fits the criteria for resection, a biopsy of the lesion is best performed as an excisional biopsy. Because the findings on needle biopsy do not alter the recommendations for excision of a solitary lesion, this procedure should be undertaken only if the patient is not an operative candidate, if an alternative method of treatment is indicated, or if the patient requests that the diagnosis be established before consenting to surgery.

Criteria for Surgical Resection

The disease-free interval, number of metastatic nodules, and tumor doubling time have been used as criteria for the surgical resection of pulmonary metastases. Each of these remains controversial with respect to its effect on long-term outcome (140).

The disease-free interval is defined as the time from resection of the primary tumor to the diagnosis of metastases. The length of the disease-free interval is thought to be of prognostic significance and varies greatly among published reports from 7 months to 5 years (141).

The number of metastatic nodules resected has also been considered predictive of survival. In sarcomas, some have reported that the presence of four nodules is a significant breakpoint in survival; however, the significance of the number of nodules varies among reported series. Most consider the completeness of resection the best predictor of survival (142). Obviously, when a shower of numerous, tiny (1- to 2-mm) lesions is encountered, complete resection is not possible.

Tumor doubling time is a measure of the aggressiveness of tumor growth. The prognostic importance of tumor doubling time, however, is questioned because various doubling times, from 20 to 136 days, have been found to be significant in different studies (141). Many do not consider this a criterion for surgical resection. The disease-free interval, number of metastatic nodules, and tumor doubling time in fact reflect the intrinsic tumor biology.

In 1991, the International Registry of Lung Metastases was established. Five thousand two hundred six cases of pulmonary metastases were analyzed retrospectively with regard to prognostic variables (137). Multivariate analysis showed a better prognosis for patients with germ cell tumors, a disease-free interval of 36 months or more, a single metastasis, and complete resection. A simple system of classification into prognostic groups was designed (Table 59.11).

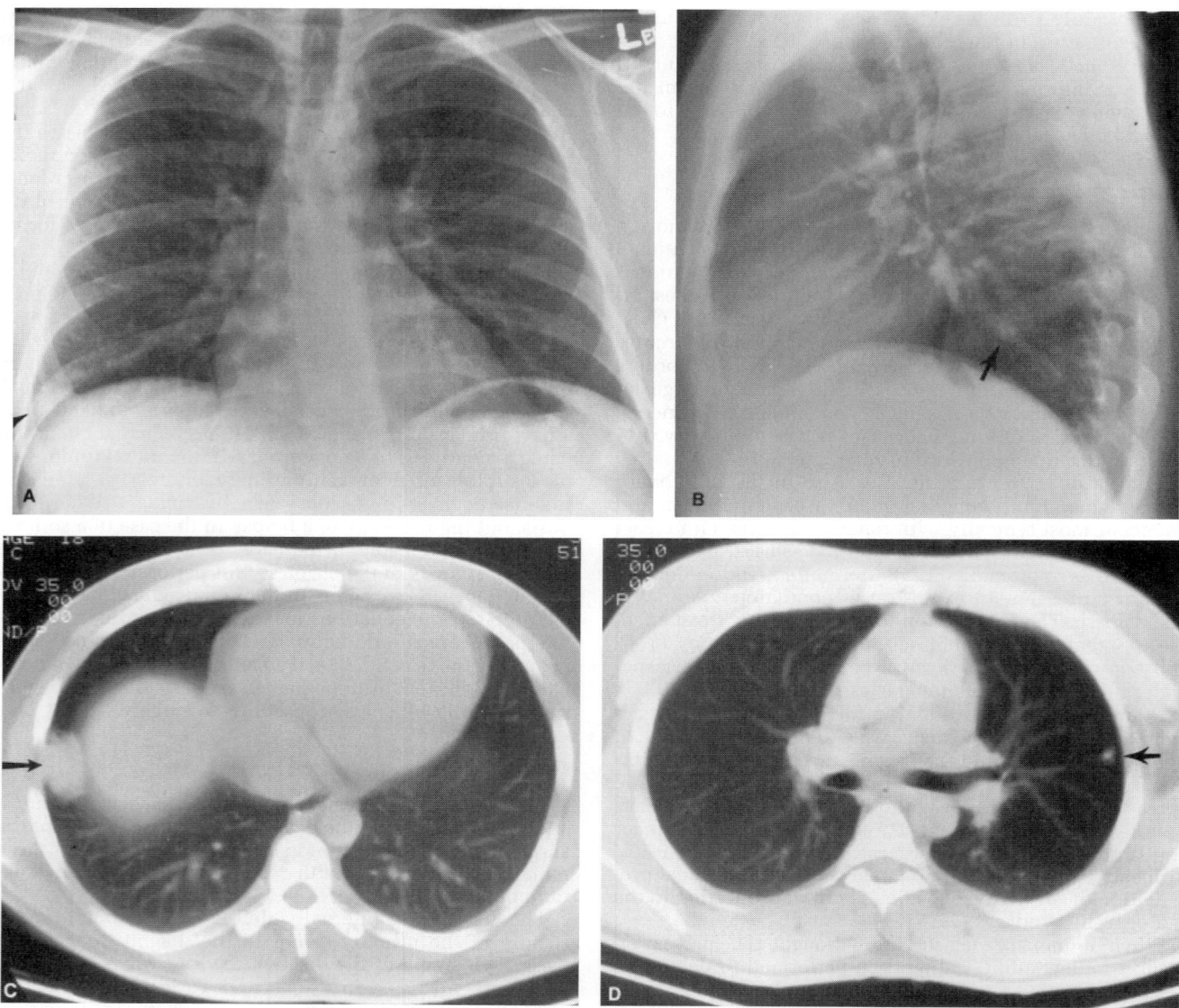

Figure 59.11. Imaging studies from a patient with metastatic embryonal rhabdomyosarcoma. Chest radiographs show a mass in the right lower lobe *(arrow, A)* that is best seen on the lateral view *(arrow, B)*. Computed tomography *(CT)* confirmed the presence of this mass *(arrow, C)* and showed an additional nodule in the left upper lobe *(arrow, D)*. At surgical exploration, however, multiple bilateral pulmonary metastases were found that measured less than 5 mm and therefore could not be seen on CT.

Table 59.11. SURVIVAL BY PROGNOSTIC GROUP: THE INTERNATIONAL REGISTRY OF LUNG METASTASES

Groups	Median survival (mo)
I. Resectable, no risk factor (DFI ≥36 mo and single metastasis)	61
II. Resectable, 1 risk factor (DFI <36 mo or multiple metastases)	34
III. Resectable, 2 risk factors (DFI >36 mo and multiple metastases)	24
IV. Unresectable	14

DFI, disease-free interval.
From Pastorino U, Buyse M, Friedel G, et al. Long-term results of lung metastasectomy: prognostic analyses based on 5,206 cases. J Thorac Cardiovasc Surg 1997;113:34–49.

Several guidelines must be met before a patient is considered for resection of pulmonary metastases: (a) control of the primary tumor, (b) absence of extrathoracic metastases, (c) a general medical condition that permits thoracotomy, (d) pulmonary function that allows complete resection of all metastases, and (e) a lack of more effective systemic treatment. Resection should be undertaken only if complete resection is considered technically feasible (143).

If the metastatic lesion is found at the same time as a recurrence of the primary site, the recurrent primary tumor should be treated before the metastatic disease is treated to prevent further seeding of the metastatic site. When the primary tumor and the metastasis are diagnosed simultaneously, lung resection may precede the surgery for the primary disease if it is doubtful whether the pulmonary disease can be completely resected, and immediate subsequent resection of the primary tumor is planned.

When a patient meets the criteria for resection of one or more pulmonary metastases, the natural history of the tumor and whether effective systemic therapy is available must be considered. Experience in breast cancer, testicular cancer, and osteogenic sarcoma illustrate this point (144). In contrast to metastatic sarcoma, which is usually confined to the lungs, metastatic breast cancer to the lungs signals the development of widely disseminated disease. Because effective systemic therapy is available for breast cancer, surgical resection of pulmonary metastases is rarely indicated.

The most striking example is the germ cell cancer. The advent of effective chemotherapy radically altered the management of pulmonary metastases of germ cell cancer and rendered an incurable disease curable. Chemotherapy is now the primary form of treatment. Surgical resection is reserved for patients who have a complete serologic response (normal levels of β-human chorionic gonadotropin and α-fetoprotein) with residual pulmonary lesions, evidence of persistent intrathoracic disease with elevated markers despite a full course of chemotherapy, or lesions that do not respond or progress with chemotherapy (145). Approximately one third of the resected pulmonary lesions contain viable tumor, one third contain fibrosis or necrosis, and one third are teratomas. Residual tumors are found mostly in patients with positive serologies, and the prognosis is usually not as good as when no residual disease is present. A teratoma is removed to prevent it from degenerating to a more malignant form of germ cell tumor and to avoid the potential complications of local tumor growth. Thus, surgical resection plays a strictly adjuvant role in the treatment of malignant germ cell tumors.

The development of more effective chemotherapy regimens for sarcomas, especially osteogenic sarcomas, has also altered the management of pulmonary metastases in this disease. Surgical resection is part of a multimodality treatment approach, but the manner in which chemotherapy and resection should be combined is less clear than in germ cell cancer. The timing of an operation in relation to chemotherapy depends on the number, size, and location of pulmonary metastases at diagnosis and on whether the patient has received any previous chemotherapy. Often, surgical resection is performed between cycles of chemotherapy, with the aim of controlling both gross and micrometastatic disease. This approach allows the sensitivity of the patient's tumor to chemotherapy to be assessed, and the advisability of continuing the regimen postoperatively can be determined. The thoracic surgeon should collaborate with the medical oncologist in planning a multidisciplinary treatment program for the patient with pulmonary metastases of sarcoma.

Preoperative Evaluation

The preoperative evaluation of the patient undergoing resection of pulmonary metastases is similar to that of the patient undergoing removal of a primary lung cancer. Tests pulmonary function, measurement of arterial blood gases, and, if necessary, ventilation–perfusion lung scanning are performed to be sure that the patient has sufficient reserve to tolerate complete resection of the metastases. The pulmonary function of patients who received chemotherapy may be substantially reduced. This is particularly true of patients treated with bleomycin and mitomycin, which can markedly diminish the diffusion capacity and occasionally and unpredictably cause an adult respiratory distress type of syndrome postoperatively. Maintaining patients on 35% or less inspired oxygen intraoperatively is thought to help prevent this complication.

Like patients with primary lung cancers, these patients should stop smoking. Patients who smoke actively up to the time of operation are at risk for postoperative atelectasis or pneumonia.

It is also important to assess the patient's general medical condition and cardiovascular status. Older patients may have underlying coronary artery disease that requires preoperative treatment and additional perioperative monitoring. The cardiac function of patients who previously received chemotherapy, especially doxorubicin, may be impaired. A preoperative radionuclide scan or echocardiogram should be performed to determine the left ventricular ejection fraction and assess whether intraoperative hemodynamic monitoring is necessary. Other drugs, such as cisplatin, can impair renal or neurologic function and may influence perioperative management.

If a patient has recently undergone chemotherapy, the timing of surgery should be planned after consultation with the medical oncologist, so that the operation is not performed when the patient is neutropenic or thrombocytopenic. Resumption of chemotherapy postoperatively should also be a joint decision between the surgeon and medical oncologist so that it does not compromise wound healing.

Surgical Technique

Two principles guide the approach to resecting pulmonary metastatic lesions: complete resection of disease and maximal sparing of functioning lung tissue. Wedge resections should be performed whenever possible. These can be carried out with staples, electrocautery, or laser. A lobectomy or even a pneumonectomy may be performed when wedge resection will not provide a complete resection. This may be necessary for recurrences (completion pneumonectomy), centrally located tumors, or multiple metastases (79,146).

Unilateral disease is approached by a standard anterolateral or posterolateral thoracotomy incision. Patients with bilateral pulmonary metastases should have a simultaneous resection of the bilateral lesions if technically feasible. This can be accomplished by a median sternotomy or a clamshell incision (bilateral anterior thoracotomy with transverse sternotomy). A clamshell incision provides better exposure to the posterior aspects of the lungs, particularly the left lower lobe, which is difficult to access by a median sternotomy (147). Bilateral pulmonary nodules may require sequential posterolateral thoracotomies

Table 59.12. HISTOLOGIC SUBTYPES FROM THE INTERNATIONAL REGISTRY OF LUNG METASTASES

Histologic groups	No. patients (%)	Subtypes
Carcinoma	2,260 (47)	Breast Lung Bowel Kidney Uterus Head and neck
Sarcoma	2,173 (45)	Osteosarcoma Other bone sarcomas Histiocytoma Leiomyosarcoma Synovial sarcoma Other soft-tissue sarcoma
Other types	328 (8)	Wilms' tumor Teratoma Embryonal carcinoma Other germ cell tumor Melanoma

From Pastorino U, Buyse M, Friedel G, et al. Long-term results of lung metatastasectomy: prognostic analyses based on 5,206 cases. J Thorac Cardiovasc Surg 1997;113:37–49, with permission.

Table 59.13. RESULTS OF PULMONARY RESECTIONS FOR METASTASES AT MEMORIAL SLOAN-KETTERING CANCER CENTER

	No. patients	Survival at 5 y (%)
Renal cell carcinoma (1980–1993) (168)		
Solitary metastasis	50	54
Head and neck cancer (1966–1995) (150)		
Squamous cell	41	34
Glandular tumors	36	64
Overall	83	50
Colorectal cancer (1965–1988) (169)		
Overall	144	44
Soft-tissue sarcoma (1982–1997) (170)[a]		
Complete resection	161	46
Incomplete resection	52	23
No resection	473	17
Unknown	33	—
Overall	719	25
Testicular germ cell tumors (1967–1995) (145)		
1967–1974	22	41
1975–1984	69	65
1984–1995	66	82
Overall	157	68

[a]Survival at 3 years.

if they are centrally located and good exposure of the hilar vessels is needed.

The role of VATS in the management of patients with isolated suspected pulmonary metastasis is clear when performed for diagnostic purposes. VATS wedge resection can be carried out with a high degree of success and minimal morbidity or inconvenience (148). However, the inability to palpate the entire lung adequately with the thoracoscope alone markedly impairs the surgeon's ability to determine whether all lesions have been resected when surgery is performed for metastatic disease. The value of VATS for the therapeutic resection of lung metastases is therefore questioned (138).

Results

Surgical resection remains the mainstay of treatment for pulmonary metastases from many solid tumors that cannot be treated effectively with chemotherapy. These include colon cancers, renal cell cancers, melanomas, head and neck tumors, and endometrial cancers. The histologic subtypes of the pulmonary metastases in the International Registry of Lung Metastases are listed in Table 59.12 (137).

Globally, the actuarial survival after complete metastasectomy is 36% at 5 years and 26% at 10 years (median survival of 35 months) (137). The experiences at Memorial Sloan-Kettering Cancer Center in the resection of pulmonary metastases from renal cell carcinoma, head and neck tumors, colorectal cancers, testicular germ cell tumors, and soft-tissue sarcoma are summarized in Table 59.13. These results again demonstrate that complete resection of metastatic disease is associated with prolonged survival in carefully selected patients. Furthermore, patients who are persistently free of disease at the primary tumor location but who have recurrent resectable metastatic disease of the lung also benefit from repeated surgery (148). Mortality rates of pulmonary metastasectomy do not differ from those of thoracic surgery performed for lung cancers, varying between 0.6% to 2% (132,145,150). The surgical removal of pulmonary metastases is widely accepted, but its role has changed as more effective chemotherapy has become available for some cancers. It is important that the surgeon un-

derstand the indications for operation, the potential side effects of initial chemotherapy, and the ways in which surgical resection should be integrated into the overall treatment plan for these patients.

BENIGN TUMORS OF THE LUNG

Benign tumors of the lung are rare neoplasms. Few series are found in the literature, but in a 10-year surgical review (1958 to 1968) from the Mayo Clinic, 130 patients were found to have benign tumors (151).

Like malignant tumors, benign tumors arising from epithelial, mesodermal, or endodermal cell lines can develop in the lung. They may present as endobronchial le-

Table 59.14. BENIGN TUMORS OF THE LUNG

Epithelial
Polyps
Papilloma
Mucous gland adenoma

Mesenchymal
Vessel
  Sclerosing hemangioma
  Lymphangioma
Nerve
  Granular cell tumor
  Neurilemoma
  Neurofibroma
Muscle
  Leiomyoma
Miscellaneous
  Hamartoma
  Teratoma
  Clear cell (sugar) tumor
Others
  Lipoma
  Chondroma
  Fibroma

Inflammatory pseudotumors
Plasma cell granuloma
Pulmonary hyalinizing granuloma

sions, but more commonly as peripheral nodules (152). Endobronchial tumors present with signs and symptoms related to airway obstruction or bleeding. Tumors arising in peripheral airways or within pulmonary parenchyma usually present as undiagnosed asymptomatic solitary pulmonary nodules. Types of benign lung tumors are listed in Table 59.14.

Hamartoma

The most frequent benign tumors are hamartomas, which represent 75% of benign lesions. They show a predilection for men (153). A hamartoma consists of an abnormal arrangement of normal cells. In the lung, the most frequent component is cartilage. A hamartoma usually presents as a solitary pulmonary nodule with an extremely slow growth pattern. Classically, the radiographic appearance is that of a well-circumscribed nodule that may contain popcorn calcification. If previous chest radiographs are available, these tumors are found to have been present for many years. Their growth pattern is variable but generally slow. These lesions can be diagnosed by CT if appropriate calcification is demonstrated. Needle aspiration is frequently diagnostic of a cartilaginous benign lesion.

Controversy exists regarding whether these lesions should be excised for pathologic diagnosis. Certainly, they do not require excision unless they are proximally located and cause symptoms related to endobronchial obstruction or unless carcinoma cannot be ruled out. If transthoracic needle aspiration biopsy confirms the presence of a hamartoma, many surgeons elect to follow patients with annual chest radiography rather than surgical excision. Occasionally, significant growth during follow-up necessitates excision.

Other Benign Tumors

Other benign tumors may present as endobronchial lesions (commonly fibromas, lipomas, chondromas, and granular cell myoblastomas). These tumors may be removed endoscopically, but frequently they also require surgical excision when the diagnosis is in doubt or when endoscopic excision has been incomplete. Peripheral tumors often are removed for diagnosis.

REFERENCES

1. American Cancer Society. *Cancer facts and figures—1999*. Atlanta: American Cancer Society, 1999.
2. Landis SH, Murray T, Bolden S, et al. Cancer statistics, 1998. *CA Cancer J Clin* 1998;48:6–29.
3. Wingo PA, Ries LAG, Giovino GA, et al. Annual report to the nation on the status of cancer, 1973–1996, with a special section on lung cancer and tobacco smoking. *J Natl Cancer Inst* 1999;91:675–690.
4. Dockery DW, Trichopoulos D. Risk of lung cancer from environmental exposures to tobacco smoke. *Cancer Causes Control* 1997;8:333–345.
5. Van Duuren BL, Goldschmidt BM. Brief communication: co-carcinogenic agents in tobacco carcinogenesis. *J Natl Cancer Inst* 1973;51:703–705.
6. Winters TH, Di Franza JR. Radioactivity in cigarette smoking. *N Engl J Med* 1982;306:364–365.
7. Wald NJ, Nanchahal K, Thompson SG, et al. Does breathing other people's tobacco smoke cause lung cancer? *Br Med J* 1986;293:1217–1222.
8. Doll R, Peto R. Cigarette smoking and bronchial carcinoma: dose and time relationships among regular smokers and lifelong non-smokers. *J Epidemiol Community Health* 1978;32:303–313.
9. Bonney GE. Interactions of genes, environment, and lifestyle in lung cancer development. *J Natl Cancer Inst* 1990;82:1236–1237.
10. Samet JM. Indoor radon and lung cancer: risky or not? *J Natl Cancer Inst* 1994;86:1813–1814.
11. Selikoff IJ, Hammond EC, Churg J. Asbestos exposure, smoking, and neoplasia. *J Am Med Assoc* 1968;204:106–112.
12. Goodman GE. Prevention of lung cancer. *Curr Opin Oncol* 1998;10:122–126.
13. Sellers TA, Bailey-Wilson JE, Elston RC, et al. Evidence for mendelian inheritance in the pathogenesis of lung cancer. *J Natl Cancer Inst* 1990;82:1272–1279.
14. Heighway J, Thatcher N, Cerny T, et al. Genetic predisposition to human lung cancer. *Br J Cancer* 1986;53:453–457.
15. Czerwinski M, McLemore TL, Gelboin HV, et al. Quantification of CYP2B7, CYP4B1, and CYPOR messenger RNAs in normal human lung and lung tumors. *Cancer Res* 1994;54:1085–1091.
16. Parekh K, Rusch V, Kris M. The clinical course of lung carcinoma in patients with chronic lymphocytic leukemia. *Cancer* 1999;86:1720–1723.
17. Parker MS, Leveno DM, Campbell TJ, et al. AIDS-related bronchogenic carcinoma: fact or fiction? *Chest* 1998;113:154–161.
18. Travis WD, Travis LB, Devesa SS. Lung cancer. *Cancer* 1995;75:191–202.
19. Wynder EL, Covey LS. Epidemiologic patterns in lung cancer by histologic type. *Eur J Cancer Clin Oncol* 1987;23:1491–1496.
20. Regnard J-F, Grunewald D, Spaggiari L, et al. Surgical treatment of hepatic and pulmonary metastases from colorectal cancers. *Ann Thorac Surg* 1998;66:214–219.
21. Roggli VL, Vollmer RT, Greenberg SD, et al. Lung cancer heterogeneity: a blinded and randomized study of 100 consecutive cases. *Hum Pathol* 1985;16:569–579.
22. Sabichi AL, Birrer MJ. The molecular biology of lung cancer: application to early detection and prevention. *Oncology* 1993;7:19–37.
23. Minna JD, Sekido Y, Fong KM, et al. Molecular biology of lung cancer. In: DeVita VT Jr, Hellman S, Rosenberg SA, eds. *Cancer: principles and practice of oncology*. Philadelphia: Lippincott–Raven Publishers, 1997:849–942.
24. Slebos RJC, Kibbelaar RE, Dalesio O, et al. K-*ras* oncogene activation as a prognostic marker in adenocarcinoma of the lung. *N Engl J Med* 1990;323:561–565.
25. Kalemkerian GP. Biology of lung cancer. *Curr Opin Oncol* 1994;6:147–155.
26. Weiner DB, Nordberg J, Robinson R, et al. Expression of the *neu* gene-encoded protein (p185^neu) in human non-small cell carcinomas of the lung. *Cancer Res* 1990;50:421–425.
27. Tsai C-M, Chang K-T, Perng R-P, et al. Correlation of intrinsic chemoresistance of non-small cell lung cancer cell lines with *HER-2/neu* gene expression but not with *ras* gene mutations. *J Natl Cancer Inst* 1993;85:897–901.
28. Chiba M, Takahashi Ta, Nau MM, et al. Mutations in the *p53* gene are frequent in primary, resected non-small cell lung cancer. *Oncogene* 1990;5:1603–1610.
29. Greenblatt MS, Bennett WP, Hollstein M, et al. Mutations in the *p53* tumor suppressor gene: clues to cancer etiology and molecular pathogenesis. *Cancer Res* 1994;54:4855–4878.
30. Carbone DP, Mitsudomi T, Chiba I, et al. p53 immunostaining positivity is associated with reduced survival and is imperfectly correlated with gene mutations in resected non-small cell lung cancer: a preliminary report of LCSG 871. *Chest* 1994;106[Suppl]:377S–381S.
31. Mitsudomi T. Correspondence–response. *J Natl Cancer Inst* 1994;86:802.
32. Minna JD. The molecular biology of lung cancer pathogenesis. *Chest* 1993;103:445S–456S.
33. Sozzi G, Miozzo M, Donghi R, et al. Deletions of 17p and *p53* mutations in preneoplastic lesions of the lung. *Cancer Res* 1992;52:6079–6082.
34. Lavigueur A, Maltby V, Mock D, et al. High incidence of lung, bone, and lymphoid tumors in transgenic mice overexpressing mutant alleles of the *p53* oncogene. *Mol Cell Biol* 1989;9:3982–3991.
35. Reissmann PT, Koga H, Takahashi R, et al. Inactivation of the retinoblastoma susceptibility gene in non–small-cell lung cancer. *Oncogene* 1993;8:1913–1919.
36. Cuttita F, Carney DN, Mulshine J. Bombesin-like peptides can function as autocrine growth factors in human small cell lung cancer. *Nature* 1985;316:823–826.

37. Rusch V, Baselga J, Cordon-Cardo C, et al. Differential expression of the epidermal growth factor receptor and its ligands in primary non-small cell lung cancers and adjacent benign lung. *Cancer Res* 1993;53:2379–2385.

38. Mountain CF. New prognostic factors in lung cancer: biologic prophets of cancer cell aggression. *Chest* 1995;108: 246–254.

39. Hazelrigg SR, Magee MJ, Cetindag IB. Video-assisted thoracic surgery for diagnosis of the solitary lung nodule. *Chest Surg Clin N Am* 1998;8:763–774.

40. Mountain CF. Revisions in the international system for staging lung cancer. *Chest* 1997;111:1710–1717.

41. Mountain CF, Dresler CM. Regional lymph node classification for lung cancer staging. *Chest* 1997;111:1718–1723.

42. Patterson GA, Ginsberg RJ, Poon PY, et al. A prospective evaluation of magnetic resonance imaging, computed tomography, and mediastinoscopy in the preoperative assessment of mediastinal node status in bronchogenic carcinoma. *J Thorac Cardiovasc Surg* 1987;94:679–684.

43. Lewis JW Jr, Pearlberg JL, Beute GH, et al. Can computed tomography of the chest stage lung cancer?—yes and no. *Ann Thorac Surg* 1990;49:591–596.

44. Ginsberg RJ, Rice TW, Goldberg M, et al. Extended cervical mediastinoscopy: a single staging procedure for bronchogenic carcinoma of the left upper lobe. *J Thorac Cardiovasc Surg* 1987;94:673–678.

45. Martini N, Heelan R, Westcott J, et al. Comparative merits of conventional, computed tomographic, and magnetic resonance imaging in assessing mediastinal involvement in surgically confirmed carcinoma. *J Thorac Cardiovasc Surg* 1985;90:639–648.

46. Moore EH, Templeton PA. Imaging the advancing frontier of lung cancer operability. *Semin Respir Med* 1992;13:293–307.

47. Steinert HC, Hauser M, Allemann F, et al. Non-small cell lung cancer: nodal staging with FDG PET versus CT with correlative lymph node mapping and sampling. *Radiology* 1997;202:441–446.

48. Weder W, Schmid RA, Bruchhaus H, et al. Detection of extrathoracic metastases by positron emission tomography in lung cancer. *Ann Thorac Surg* 1998;66:886–893.

49. The Lung Cancer Study Group, Ginsberg RJ, Rubinstein LV. Randomized trial of lobectomy versus limited resection for T1 N0 non-small cell lung cancer. *Ann Thorac Surg* 1995;60: 615–623.

50. Ginsberg RJ, Hill LD, Eagan RT, et al. Modern thirty-day operative mortality for surgical resections in lung cancer. *J Thorac Cardiovasc Surg* 1983;86:654–658.

51. Deslauriers J, Ginsberg RJ, Dubois P, et al. Current operative morbidity associated with elective surgical resection for lung cancer. *Can J Surg* 1989;32:335–339.

52. McCaughan BC, Martini N, Bains MS, et al. Chest wall invasion in carcinoma of the lung: therapeutic and prognostic implications. *J Thorac Cardiovasc Surg* 1985;89:836–841.

53. Feld R, Rubinstein LV, Weisenberger TH, et al. Sites of recurrence in resected stage I non-small cell lung cancer: a guide for future studies. *J Clin Oncol* 1984;2:1352–1358.

54. Martini N, Bains MS, Burt ME, et al. Incidence of local recurrence and second primary tumors in resected stage I lung cancer. *J Thorac Cardiovasc Surg* 1995;109:120–129.

55. Thomas P, Rubinstein L, The Lung Cancer Study Group. Cancer recurrence after resection: T1 N0 non-small cell lung cancer. *Ann Thorac Surg* 1990;49:242–247.

56. Johnson BE. Second lung cancers in patients after treatment for an initial lung cancer. *J Natl Cancer Inst* 1998;90:1335–1345.

57. Virgo KS, Naunheim KS, McKirgan LW, et al. Cost of patient follow-up after potentially curative lung cancer treatment. *J Thorac Cardiovasc Surg* 1996;112:356–363.

58. Mountain CF, Gail MH. Surgical adjuvant intrapleural BCG treatment for stage I non-small cell lung cancer: preliminary report of the National Cancer Institute Lung Cancer Study Group. *J Thorac Cardiovasc Surg* 1981;82:649–657.

59. Ludwig Lung Cancer Study Group. Adverse effect of intrapleural Corynebacterium parvum as adjuvant therapy in resected stage I and II non-small cell carcinoma of the lung. J Thorac Cardiovasc Surg 1985;89:842–847.

59a. Ratto GB, Melioli G, Zino P, et al. Immunotherapy with the use of tumor-infiltrating lymphocytes and interleukin-2 as adjuvant treatment in Stage III non-small cell lung cancer. *J Thorac Cardiovasc Surg* 1995;109:1212–1217.

60. Green N, Kurohara SS, George FWI, et al. Postresection irradiation for primary lung cancer. *Radiology* 1975;116: 405–407.

61. Sawyer TE, Bonner JA, Gould PM, et al. The impact of surgical adjuvant thoracic radiation therapy for patients with non-small cell lung carinoma with ipsilateral mediastinal lymph node involvement. *Cancer* 1997;80:1399–1408.

62. Mayer R, Smolle-Juettner F-M, Szolar D, et al. Postoperative radiotherapy in radically resected non-small cell lung cancer. *Chest* 1997;112:954–959.

63. Smolle-Juettner FM, Mayer R, Pinter H, et al. "Adjuvant" external radiation of the mediastinum in radically resected non-small cell lung cancer. *Eur J Cardiothorac Surg* 1996; 10:947–951.

64. Stephens RJ, Girling DJ, Bleehen NM, et al. The role of postoperative radiotherapy in non-small cell lung cancer: a multicentre randomised trial in patients with pathologically staged T1–2, N1–2, M0 disease. *Br J Cancer* 1996;74: 632–639.

65. Lafitte JJ, Ribet ME, Prévost BM, et al. Postresection irradiation for T2 N0 M0 non-small cell carcinoma: a prospective, randomized study. *Ann Thorac Surg* 1996;62:830–834.

66. The Lung Cancer Study Group. Effects of postoperative mediastinal radiation on completely resected stage II and stage III epidermoid cancer of the lung. *N Engl J Med* 1986;315: 1377–1381.

67. Van Houtte P, Rocmans P, Smets P, et al. Postoperative radiation therapy in lung cancer: a controlled trial after resection of curative design. *Int J Radiat Oncol Biol Phys* 1980;6: 983–986.

68. Hughes FA, Higgins G. Veterans Administration surgical adjuvant lung cancer chemotherapy study: present status. *J Thorac Cardiovasc Surg* 1962;44:295–304.

69. Slack NH. Bronchogenic carcinoma: nitrogen mustard as a surgical adjuvant and factors influencing survival. University Surgical Adjuvant Lung Project. *Cancer* 1970;25: 987–1002.

70. Shields TW, Humphrey EW, Eastridge CE, et al. Adjuvant cancer chemotherapy after resection of carcinoma of the lung. *Cancer* 1977;40:2057–2062.

71. Shields TW, Higgins GA Jr, Humphrey EW, et al. Prolonged intermittent adjuvant chemotherapy with CCNU and hydroxyurea after resection of carcinoma of the lung. *Cancer* 1982;50:1713–1721.

72. Stewart LA, Pignon JP, The Non-small Cell Lung Cancer Collaborative Group. Chemotherapy in non-small cell lung cancer: a meta-analysis using updated data on individual patients from 52 randomised clinical trials. *BMJ* 1995;311: 899–909.

73. Feld R, Rubinstein L, Thomas PA, et al. Adjuvant chemotherapy with cyclophosphamide, doxorubicin, and cisplatin in patients with completely resected stage I non-small-cell lung cancer. *J Natl Cancer Inst* 1993;85:299–306.

74. Keller SM, Adak S, Wagner H, et al. Prospective randomized trial of postoperative adjuvant therapy in patients with completely resected stages II and IIIA non-small cell lung cancer: an intergroup trial (E3590). *Proc Am Soc Clin Oncol* 1999; 18:465a(abst).

75. Wada H, Hitomi S, Teramatsu T, et al. Adjuvant chemotherapy after complete resection in non-small cell lung cancer. *J Clin Oncol* 1996;14:1048–1054.

76. Okada M, Tsubota N, Yoshimura M, et al. Prognosis of completely resected pN2 non-small cell lung carcinomas: what is the significant node that affects survival? *J Thorac Cardiovasc Surg* 1999;118:270–275.

77. Sagawa M, Sakurada A, Fujimura S, et al. Five-year survivors with resected pN2 non-small cell lung carcinoma. *Cancer* 1999;85:864–868.

78. Martini N, Flehinger BJ. The role of surgery in N2 lung cancer. *Surg Clin North Am* 1987;67:1037–1049.

79. Rosell R, Gómez-Codina J, Camps C, et al. A randomized trial comparing preoperative chemotherapy plus surgery with surgery alone in patients with non-small-cell lung cancer. *N Engl J Med* 1994;330:153–158.

80. Roth JA, Fossella F, Komaki R, et al. A randomized trial comparing perioperative chemotherapy and surgery with surgery alone in resectable stage IIIA non-small-cell lung cancer. *J Natl Cancer Inst* 1994;86:673–680.

81. Perez CA, Pajak TF, Rubin P, et al. Long-term observations of

the patterns of failure in patients with unresectable non-oat cell carcinoma of the lung treated with definitive radiotherapy. Report by the Radiation Therapy Oncology Group. *Cancer* 1987;59:1874–1881.

82. Pisters KMW, Kris MG, Gralla RJ, et al. Randomized trial comparing postoperative chemotherapy with vindesine and cisplatin plus thoracic irradiation with irradiation alone in stage III N2 non-small cell lung cancer. *J Surg Oncol* 1994; 56:236–241.

83. Bromley LL, Szur L. Combined radiotherapy and resection for carcinoma of the bronchus: experiences with 66 patients. *Lancet* 1955;2:937–941.

84. Payne DG. Pre-operative radiation therapy in non-small cell lung cancer of the lung. *Lung Cancer* 1991;7:47–56.

85. Furuse K, Kubota K, Kawahara M, et al. Phase II study of concurrent radiotherapy and chemotherapy for unresectable stage III non-small cell lung cancer. *J Clin Oncol* 1995;13: 869–875.

86. Martini N, Kris MG, Flehinger BJ, et al. Preoperative chemotherapy for stage IIIA N2 lung cancer: the Sloan-Kettering experience with 136 patients. *Ann Thorac Surg* 1993; 55:1365–1374.

87. Burkes RL, Ginsberg RJ, Shepherd FA, et al. Induction chemotherapy with mitomycin, vindesine, and cisplatin for stage III unresectable non-small cell lung cancer: results of the Toronto phase II trial. *J Clin Oncol* 1992;10:580–586.

88. Wagner H Jr, Lad T, Piantadosi S, et al. Randomized phase 2 evaluation of preoperative radiation therapy and preoperative chemotherapy with mitomycin, vinblastine, and cisplatin in patients with technically unresectable stage IIIA and IIIB non-small cell cancer of the lung. LCSG 881. *Chest* 1994;106[Suppl]:348S–354S.

89. Sugarbaker DJ, Herndon J, Kohman LJ, et al. Results of Cancer and Leukemia Group B protocol 8935: a multiinstitutional phase II trimodality trial for stage IIIA N2 non-small-cell lung cancer. *J Thorac Cardiovasc Surg* 1995;109:473–485.

90. Pass HI, Pogrebniak HW, Steinberg SM, et al. Randomized trial of neoadjuvant therapy for lung cancer: interim analysis. *Ann Thorac Surg* 1992;53:992–998.

91. Elias AD, Herndon J, Kumar P. A phase III comparison of "best local–regional therapy" with or without chemotherapy for stage IIIA, T1–3, N2. *Proc Am Soc Clin Oncol* 1997;16: 448a(abst).

92. Kumar P, Herndon J II, Elias AD, et al. Comparison of pre-operative thoracic radiation therapy to pre-operative chemotherapy in surgically staged IIIA N2 non-small cell lung cancer: initial results of Cancer and Leukemia Group B (CALGB) phase III protocol 9134. *Int J Radiat Oncol Biol Phys* 1997;39[2 Suppl 1]:195(abst).

93. Eagan RT, Ruud C, Lee RE, et al. Pilot study of induction therapy with cyclophosphamide, doxorubicin, and cisplatin (CAP) and chest irradiation prior to thoracotomy in initially inoperable stage III M0 non-small cell lung cancer. *Cancer Treat Rep* 1987;71:895–900.

94. Weiden PL, Piantadosi S, The Lung Cancer Study Group. Preoperative chemotherapy (cisplatin and fluorouracil) and radiation therapy in stage III non-small-cell lung cancer: a phase II study of the Lung Cancer Study Group. *J Natl Cancer Inst* 1991;83:266–272.

95. Faber LP, Kittle CF, Warren WH, et al. Preoperative chemotherapy and irradiation for stage III non-small cell lung cancer. *Ann Thorac Surg* 1989;47:669–677.

96. Strauss GM, Herndon JE, Sherman DD, et al. Neoadjuvant chemotherapy and radiotherapy followed by surgery in stage IIIA non-small-cell carcinoma of the lung: report of a Cancer and Leukemia Group B phase II study. *J Clin Oncol* 1992; 10:1237–1244.

97. Albain KS, Rusch VW, Crowley JJ, et al. Concurrent cisplatin/etoposide plus chest radiotherapy followed by surgery for stages IIIA N2 and IIIB non-small cell lung cancer: mature results of Southwest Oncology Group Phase II study 8805. *J Clin Oncol* 1995;13:1880–1892.

98. Albain K, Rusch V, Crowley J, et al. Long-term survival after concurrent cisplatin/etoposide (PE) plus chest radiotherapy (RT) followed by surgery in bulky stages IIIA N2 and IIIB non-small cell lung cancer (NSCLC): 6-year outcomes from Southwest Oncology Group study 8805. *Proc Am Soc Clin Oncol* 1999;18:467a(abst).

99. Yashar J, Weitberg AB, Glicksman AS, et al. Preoperative chemotherapy and radiation therapy for stage IIIa carcinoma of the lung. *Ann Thorac Surg* 1992;53:445–448.

100. Fowler WC, Langer CJ, Curran WJ Jr, et al. Postoperative complications after combined neoadjuvant treatment of lung cancer. *Ann Thorac Surg* 1993;55:986–989.

101. Milstein D, Kuten A, Saute M. Preoperative concurrent chemoradiotherapy for unresectable stage III non-small cell lung cancer. *Int J Radiat Oncol Biol Phys* 1996;34: 1125–1132.

102. Grunewald D, Le Chevalier T, Arrigada R. Surgical resection of stage IIIB non-small cell lung cancer after concomitant induction chemo-radiotherapy: preliminary results of a pilot study. *Proc Am Soc Clin Oncol* 1995;14:1057a(abst).

103. Fleck J, Camargo J, Godoy D, et al. Chemoradiation therapy versus chemotherapy alone as a neoadjuvant treatment for stage III non-small cell lung cancer: preliminary report of a phase III prospective randomized trial. *Proc Am Soc Clin Oncol* 1993;12:333(abst).

104. Rice TW, Adelstein DJ, Becker M. Stage III non-small cell lung cancer (NSCLC): short course multimodality treatment with accelerated fractionation radiation, concurrent cisplatin (DDP)/paclitaxel (TAX) chemotherapy and surgery. *Lung Cancer* 1997;18[Suppl 1]:A-245(abst).

105. Weil M, Roach M, Pickett B, et al. 3-D conformal radiotherapy in the sagittal plane for centrally located thoracic tumors. *Med Dosim* 1995;20:11–14.

106. Travis WD, Linnoila I, Tsokos MG, et al. Neuroendocrine tumors of the lung with proposed criteria for large-cell neuroendocrine carcinoma: an ultrastructural, immunohistochemical, and flow cytometric study of 35 cases. *Am J Surg Pathol* 1991;15:529–533.

107. Vuitch F, Sekido Y, Fong K, et al. Neuroendocrine tumors of the lung: pathology and molecular biology. *Chest Surg Clin N Am* 1997;7:21–47.

108. McCaughan BC, Martini N, Bains MS. Bronchial carcinoids: review of 124 cases. *J Thorac Cardiovasc Surg* 1985;89:8–17.

109. Martini N, Zaman MB, Bains MS, et al. Treatment and prognosis in bronchial carcinoids involving regional lymph nodes. *J Thorac Cardiovasc Surg* 1994;107:1–7.

110. Jiang S-X, Kameya T, Shoji M, et al. Large cell neuroendocrine carcinoma of the lung: a histologic and immunohistochemical study of 22 cases. *Am J Surg Pathol* 1998; 22:526–537.

111. Travis WD, Rush W, Flieder DB, et al. Survival analysis of 200 pulmonary neuroendocrine tumors with clarification of criteria for atypical carcinoid and its separation from typical carcinoid. *Am J Surg Pathol* 1998;22:934–944.

112. Travis WD. Classification of neuroendocrine tumors of the lung. Eighth World Conference on Lung Cancer, Dublin, 1997 (abst).

113. Stahel RA, Ginsberg R, Havermann K, et al. Staging and prognostic factors in small cell lung cancer: a consensus report. *Lung Cancer* 1989;5:119–126.

114. Shepherd FA. The role of chemotherapy in the treatment of small cell lung cancer. *Chest Surg Clin N Am* 1997;7:113–133.

115. National Cancer Institute. *Small cell lung cancer.* PDQ Treatment—Health Professionals, 1999 *(unpublished).*

116. Pignon JP, Arrigada R, Ihde DC, et al. A meta-analysis of thoracic radiotherapy for small-cell lung cancer. *N Engl J Med* 1992;327:1618–1624.

117. Warde P, Payne D. Does thoracic irradiation improve survival and local control in limited-stage small-cell carcinoma of the lung? a meta-analysis. *J Clin Oncol* 1992;10:890–895.

118. Albain KS, Crowley JJ, LeBlanc M, et al. Determinants of improved outcome in small-cell lung cancer: an analysis of the 2,580-patient Southwest Oncology Group data base. *J Clin Oncol* 1990;8:1563–1574.

119. Kreisman H, Wolkove N, Quoix E. Small cell lung cancer presenting as a solitary pulmonary nodule. *Chest* 1992;101: 225–231.

120. Shepherd FA, Evans WK, Feld R, et al. Adjuvant chemotherapy following surgical resection for small-cell carcinoma of the lung. *J Clin Oncol* 1988;6:832–838.

121. Shah SS, Thompson J, Goldstraw P. Results of operation without adjuvant therapy in the treatment of small cell lung cancer. *Ann Thorac Surg* 1992;54:498–501.

122. Shepherd FA, Ginsberg R, Patterson GA, et al. Is there ever a role for salvage operations in limited small-cell lung cancer? *J Thorac Cardiovasc Surg* 1991;101:196–200.

123. Lad T, Piantadosi S, Thomas P, et al. A prospective randomized trial to determine the benefit of surgical resection of residual disease following the response of small cell lung cancer to combination chemotherapy. *Chest* 1994;106:320S–323S.

124. Inoue H, Iwasaki M, Ogawa J-I, et al. Surgical resection of a second primary lung carcinoma in a survivor of small cell carcinoma. *Ann Thorac Surg* 1993;56:1160–1161.

125. Heitmiller RF, Mathisen DJ, Ferry JA, et al. Mucoepidermoid lung tumors. *Ann Thorac Surg* 1989;47:394–399.

126. Moran CA. Primary salivary gland-type tumors of the lung. *Semin Diagn Pathol* 1995;12:106–122.

127. Chin HW, DeMeester T, Chin RY, et al. Endobronchial adenoid cystic carcinoma. *Chest* 1991;100:1464–1465.

128. Berho M, Moran CA, Suster S. Malignant mixed epithelial/mesenchymal neoplasms of the lung. *Semin Diagn Pathol* 1995;12:123–139.

129. Miller DL. Rare pulmonary neoplasms. *Semin Respir Crit Care Med* 1997;18:405–415.

130. Barney JD, Churchill ED. Adenocarcinoma of the kidney with metastases to the lung cured by nephrectomy and lobectomy. *J Urol* 1939;42:269–276.

131. Clagett OT, Woolner LB. Surgical treatment of solitary metastatic pulmonary lesion. *Med Clin North Am* 1964; 48(4):939–943.

132. Mountain CF, McMurtrey MJ, Hermes KE. Surgery for pulmonary metastasis: a 20-year experience. *Ann Thorac Surg* 1984;38:323–330.

133. Martini N, Huvos AG, Miké V, et al. Multiple pulmonary resections in the treatment of osteogenic sarcoma. *Ann Thorac Surg* 1971;12:271–280.

134. Crow J, Slavin G, Kreel L. Pulmonary metastasis: a pathologic and radiologic study. *Cancer* 1981;47:2595–2602.

135. Heitmiller RF, Marasco MW, Hruban RH, et al. Endobronchial metastasis. *J Thorac Cardiovasc Surg* 1993;106:537–542.

136. Johnson H, Fantone J, Flye MW. Histological evaluation of the nodules resected in the treatment of pulmonary metastatic disease. *J Surg Oncol* 1982;21:1–4.

137. Pastorino U, Buyse M, Friedel G, et al. Long-term results of lung metastasectomy: prognostic analyses based on 5,206 cases. *J Thorac Cardiovasc Surg* 1997;113:37–49.

138. McCormack PM, Ginsberg KB, Bains MS, et al. Accuracy of lung imaging in metastases with implications for the role of thoracoscopy. *Ann Thorac Surg* 1993;56:863–866.

139. Deleyiannis FW-B, Thomas DB. Risk of lung cancer among patients with head and neck cancer. *Otolaryngol Head Neck Surg* 1997;116:630–636.

140. Robert JH, Ambrogi V, Mermillod B, et al. Factors influencing long-term survival after lung metastasectomy. *Ann Thorac Surg* 1997;63:777–784.

141. Rusch VW. Pulmonary metastasectomy: current indications. *Chest* 1995;107:322S–332S.

142. Girard P, Baldeyrou P, Le Chevalier T, et al. Surgery for pulmonary metastases: who are the 10-year survivors? *Cancer* 1994;74:2791–2797.

143. McCormack P. Surgical resection of pulmonary metastases. *Semin Surg Oncol* 1990;6:297–302.

144. La Quaglia MP. Osteosarcoma: specific tumor management and results. *Chest Surg Clin N Am* 1998;8:77–95.

145. Liu D, Abolhoda A, Burt ME, et al. Pulmonary metastasectomy for testicular germ cell tumors: a 28-year experience. *Ann Thorac Surg* 1998;66:1709–1714.

146. Putnam JB Jr, Suell DM, Natarajan G, et al. Extended resection of pulmonary metastases: is the risk justified? *Ann Thorac Surg* 1993;55:1440–1446.

147. Bains MS, Ginsberg RJ, Jones WG, et al. The clamshell incision: an improved approach to bilateral pulmonary and mediastinal tumor. *Ann Thorac Surg* 1994;58:30–33.

148. Liu H-P, Lin PJ, Hsieh M-J, et al. Application of thoracoscopy for lung metastases. *Chest* 1995;107:266–268.

149. Kandioler D, Krömer E, Tüchler H, et al. Long-term results after repeated surgical removal of pulmonary metastases. *Ann Thorac Surg* 1998;65:909–912.

150. Liu D, Labow DM, Dang N, et al. Pulmonary metastasectomy for head and neck cancers. *Ann Surg Oncol* 1999;6:572–578.

151. Arrigoni MG, Woolner LB, Bernatz PE, et al. Benign tumors of the lung: a ten-year surgical experience. *J Thorac Cardiovasc Surg* 1970;60:589–599.

152. Oldham HN Jr. Benign tumors of the lung and bronchus. *Surg Clin North Am* 1980;60:825–834.

153. Hansen CP, Holtveg H, Francis D, et al. Pulmonary hamartoma. *J Thorac Cardiovasc Surg* 1992;104:674–678.

154. Holmes EC, Gail M, The Lung Cancer Study Group. Surgical adjuvant therapy for stage II and stage III adenocarcinoma and large-cell undifferentiated carcinoma. *J Clin Oncol* 1986;4:710–715.

155. Sadeghi A, Payne D, Rubinstein L, et al. Combined modality treatment for resected advanced non-small cell lung cancer: local control and local recurrence. *Int J Radiat Oncol Biol Phys* 1988;15:89–97.

156. Niiranen A, Niitamo-Korhonen S, Kouri M, et al. Adjuvant chemotherapy after radical surgery for non-small cell lung cancer: a randomized study. *J Clin Oncol* 1992;10:1927–1932.

157. Ohta M, Tsuchiya R, Shimoyama M, et al. Adjuvant chemotherapy for completely resected stage III non-small-cell lung cancer: results of a randomized prospective study. *J Thorac Cardiovasc Surg* 1993;106:703–708.

158. Dautzenberg B, Chastang C, Arriagada R, et al. Adjuvant radiotherapy versus combined sequential chemotherapy followed by radiotherapy in the treatment of resected non-small cell lung carcinoma: a randomized trial of 267 patients. *Cancer* 1995;76:779–786.

159. Trovò MG, Minatel E, Veronesi A, et al. Combined radiotherapy and chemotherapy versus radiotherapy alone in locally advanced epidermoid bronchogenic carcinoma: a randomized study. *Cancer* 1990;65:400–404.

160. Morton RF, Jett JR, McGinnis WL, et al. Thoracic radiation therapy alone compared with combined chemoradiotherapy for locally unresectable non-small cell lung cancer: a randomized, phase III trial. *Ann Intern Med* 1991;115:681–686.

161. Le Chevalier T, Arriagada R, Quoix E, et al. Radiotherapy alone versus combined chemotherapy and radiotherapy in nonresectable non-small cell lung cancer: first analysis of a randomized trial in 353 patients. *J Natl Cancer Inst* 1991;83:417–423.

162. Blanke C, Ansari R, Mantravadi R, et al. Phase III trial of thoracic irradiation with or without cisplatin for locally advanced unresectable non-small cell lung cancer: a Hoosier Oncology Group protocol. *J Clin Oncol* 1995;13:1425–1429.

163. Schaake-Koning C, van den Bogaert W, Dalesio O, et al. Effects of concomitant cisplatin and radiotherapy on inoperable non-small cell lung cancer. *N Engl J Med* 1992;326:524–530.

164. Jeremic B, Shibamoto Y, Acimovic L, et al. Randomized trial of hyperfractionated radiation therapy with or without concurrent chemotherapy for stage III non-small cell lung cancer. *J Clin Oncol* 1995;13:452–458.

165. Dillman RO, Seagren SL, Propert KJ, et al. A randomized trial of induction chemotherapy plus high-dose radiation versus radiation alone in stage III non-small-cell lung cancer. *N Engl J Med* 1990;323:940–945.

166. Dillman RO, Herndon J, Seagren SL, et al. Improved survival in stage III non-small cell lung cancer: seven-year follow-up of Cancer and Leukemia Group B (CALGB) protocol 8433 trial. *J Natl Cancer Inst* 1996;88:1210–1215.

167. Sause WT, Scott C, Taylor S, et al. Radiation Therapy Oncology Group (RTOG) 88-08 and Eastern Cooperative Oncology Group (ECOG) 4588: preliminary results of a phase III trial in regionally advanced, unresectable non-small-cell lung cancer. *J Natl Cancer Inst* 1995;87:198–205; Komaki R, Scott CB, Sause WT, et al. Induction cisplatin/vinblastine and irradiation vs. irradiation in unresectable squamous cell lung cancer: failure patterns by cell type in RTOG 88-08/ECOG 4588. *Int J Radiat Oncol Biol Phys* 1997;39:537–544.

168. Kavolius JP, Mastorakos DP, Pavlovich C, et al. Resection of metastatic renal cell carcinoma. *J Clin Oncol* 1998;16:2261–2266.

169. McCormack PM, Burt ME, Bains MS, et al. Lung resection for colorectal metastases: 10-year results. *Arch Surg* 1992;127:1403–1406.

170. Billingsley KG, Burt ME, Jara E, et al. Pulmonary metastases from soft-tissue sarcoma. *Ann Surg* 1999;229:602–612.

SURGERY: SCIENTIFIC PRINCIPLES AND PRACTICE, Third Edition, edited by
Lazar J. Greenfield, Michael W. Mulholland, Keith T. Oldham, Gerald B. Zelenock,
and Keith D. Lillemoe. Lippincott Williams & Wilkins Publishers, Philadelphia, © 2001.

CHAPTER 60

CHEST WALL, PLEURA, MEDIASTINUM, AND NONNEOPLASTIC LUNG DISEASE

DAVID J. SUGARBAKER, LAMBROS ZELLOS, AND BEN D. DAVIS

ANATOMY OF THE CHEST WALL

The Bony Thorax

The bony thorax consists of 12 paired ribs, cartilage, thoracic vertebrae, the sternum, and the clavicles. This creates a noncollapsible, rigid structure that provides protection to organs of the chest and support for the upper extremities.

The first seven ribs are considered true ribs because they articulate directly with the sternum, while the remaining five ribs are considered false because they articulate with the cartilage above them. Additionally, ribs 11 and 12 are considered floating ribs in that they articulate only with the vertebrae (Fig. 60.1) (1). Each rib has a head, a neck, and a shaft. The head has two facets. The upper one is used for articulation with the upper vertebrae, while the lower one is used to articulate with its vertebrae creating the costovertebral joint. The costotransverse joint is formed by the facet tubercle of the neck and the transverse process of its vertebra (Fig. 60.2) (1). The shaft contains the costal groove at its inferior aspect, where the intercostal vein, artery, and nerve run. Procedures such as thoracentesis and chest tube placement should avoid the inferior aspect of the rib.

Three different muscles span the intercostal space (Fig. 60.3) (1). From innermost to outermost they are the transverse, the internal, and the external intercostal muscles. The neurovascular bundle lies beneath the internal intercostal muscle.

The sternum is flat and has three parts: the manubrium, body, and xiphoid bone. The sternum has a total length of 15 to 20 cm (Fig. 60.1B). The manubrium articulates with the clavicles and first costal cartilage at its superior aspect and with the body of the sternum at its inferior aspect forming the angle of Louis. On a plain chest x-ray the angle of Louis corresponds to the junction of the second rib anteriorly and the fourth thoracic vertebra posteriorly.

Blood Supply, Venous Drainage, and Lymphatics

The anterior and posterior intercostal arteries supply the intercostal space (Fig. 60.3). The first two posterior intercostal arteries arise from the subclavian artery while the remaining ones arise from the thoracic aorta. The anterior intercostal arteries are branches of the internal mammary arteries and they form an anastomosis with the posterior intercostal arteries.

The intercostal veins follow the course of the arteries along the inferior aspect of each rib and drain into the azygous and hemiazygous veins. The lymphatic drainage of the anterior part of the rib drains into the internal mammary nodes, while the lymphatics of the posterior part of the rib drain into the vertebral nodes and the thoracic duct.

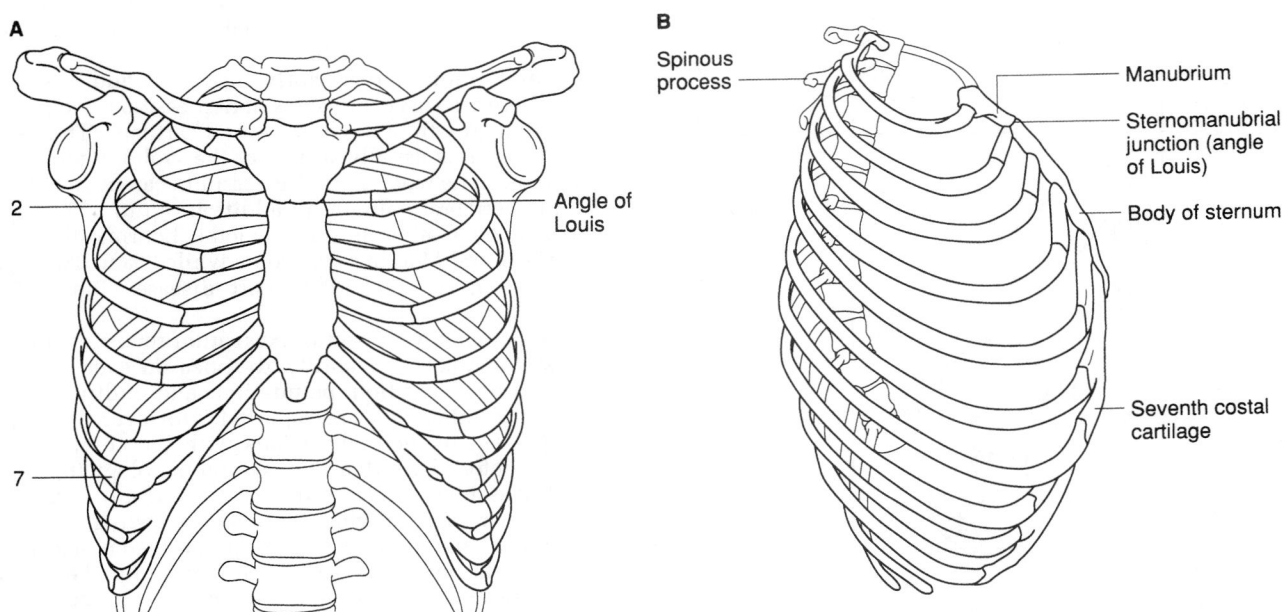

Figure 60.1. Skeletal support of the thorax. Anterior *(A)* and lateral *(B)* views. Note the anterior cartilaginous component of the upper 10 ribs, the fused costal cartilages of ribs 7 through 10, the location of the sternomanubrial junction (angle of Louis) at the level of the second rib, and the oblique course of the ribs laterally from posterior to anterior. (From Iannettoni MD, Orringer MB. Chest wall, pleura, mediastinum, and nonneoplastic lung disease. In: Greenfield LJ, Mulholland MW, Oldham KT, et al., eds. *Surgery: scientific principles and practice,* 2nd ed. Philadelphia: Lippincott–Raven, 1997:1440–1482, with permission.)

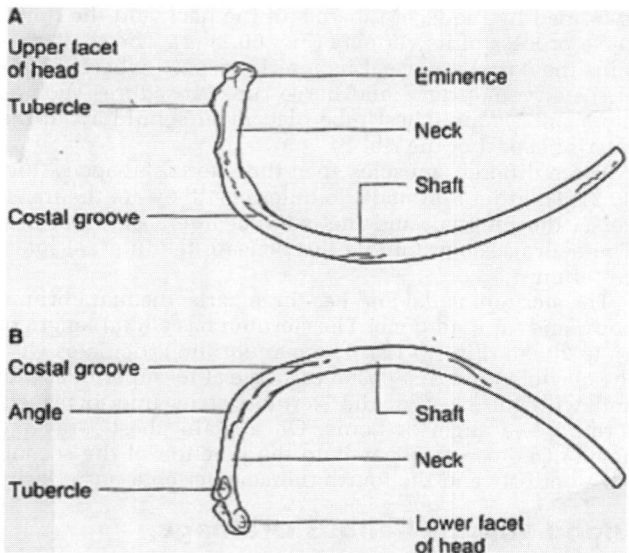

Figure 60.2. Anatomy of the rib as viewed from above *(A)* and *(B)*. (From Iannettoni MD, Orringer MB. Chest wall, pleura, mediastinum, and nonneoplastic lung disease. In: Greenfield LJ, Mulholland MW, Oldham KT, et al., eds. *Surgery: scientific principles and practice,* 2nd ed. Philadelphia: Lippincott–Raven, 1997: 1440–1482, with permission.)

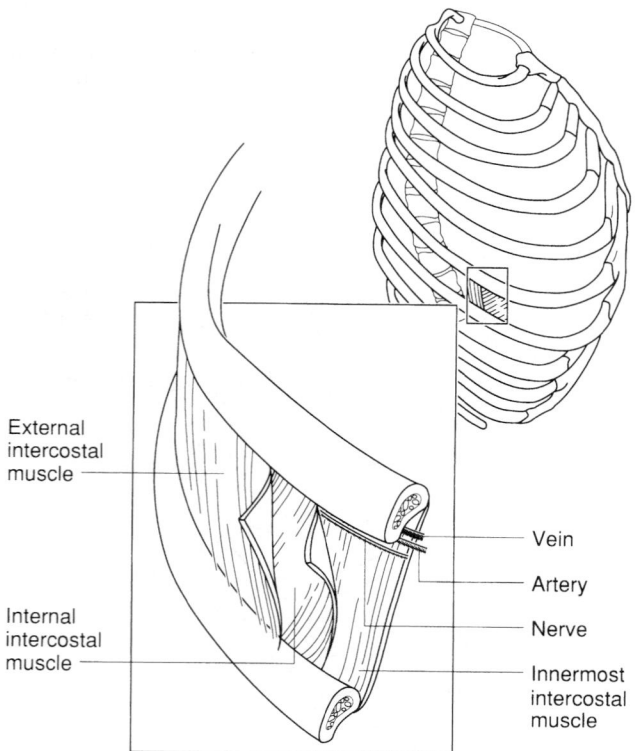

Figure 60.3. Anatomy of the intercostal space. The major intercostal muscles are the external and internal. The neurovascular bundle courses in the costal groove alone the inferior aspect of the rib. (From Iannettoni MD, Orringer MB. Chest wall, pleura, mediastinum, and nonneoplastic lung disease. In: Greenfield LJ, Mulholland MW, Oldham KT, et al., eds. *Surgery: scientific principles and practice,* 2nd ed. Philadelphia: Lippincott–Raven, 1997: 1440–1482, with permission.)

Musculature

Respiration

Despite its rigidity, the thorax can expand and contract allowing for movement of air and the process of respiration. Respiration is accomplished due to the motion of the anterior cartilaginous attachments of the true ribs to the sternum, along with the contraction of the intercostal muscles and the hemidiaphragms.

The muscles covering the bony thorax are divided into primary and secondary muscles of respiration. The diaphragm and the intercostal muscles constitute the primary respiratory muscles, while the secondary muscles are the latissimus, serratus, pectorals, trapezius, scalenes, and deltoid. The deltoid, pectoralis, and latissimus muscles help fixate the upper extremities and facilitate inspiration. In normal breathing, the diaphragm does about 75% of the total work of breathing while the intercostals do the remaining 25% of the work. During periods of respiratory distress, the secondary muscles are used as well. While inspiration is an active process, expiration is a passive one, facilitated by the elastic recoil of the lungs. Active expiration is accomplished with contraction of the abdominal muscles. (Figs. 60.4 and 60.5) (1).

CHEST WALL DEFORMITIES

A wide variety of chest wall abnormalities have been reported, most commonly involving the sternum. Most patients are asymptomatic. However, the most severe defects do cause cardiopulmonary compromise and are associated with other congenital malformations.

Depression Deformities/Pectus Excavatum

This is the most common chest wall deformity; it consists of sternal depression because of abnormalities of the lower costal cartilages and occurs in 1 out of 700 children (Fig. 60.6) (2). There is a 3.4:1 male to female ratio, and 37% occur in families with history of chest wall defects (4). The sternum is posteriorly displaced and often rotated. There are varying degrees of depression arising from differential growth of the lower costal cartilage. The deepest depression is usually seen near the xiphoid and it can be mild or, in its worst form, the sternum can be in contact with the vertebral column. In addition, up to 20% of patients may have other musculoskeletal abnormalities such as scoliosis and Marfan's syndrome while 2% to 3% of patients also have congenital heart disease (Table 60.1) (2,4,5).

Many patients with pectus excavatum report decreased exercise tolerance, fatigability, dyspnea on exertion, and sternal pain. In addition, palpitations and multiple respiratory tract infections are reported. However, most patients present to their physicians with the complaint of cosmetic deformity rather than symptomatology (6).

Cardiovascular and pulmonary work-up includes echocardiography, pulmonary function testing, exercise studies, and quantitative ventilation-perfusion scans (7). Decreased cardiac index, increased oxygen uptake at rest, and decreased stroke volume have been described. Also these hemodynamic changes were more pronounced when testing patients in the sitting instead of supine position. Various methods have been developed to objectively grade the severity of the defect based on measurements derived from lateral chest x-rays (8). One of these methods developed by Shamberger uses the ratio of two measured distances of the sternum from the vertebrae. These mea-

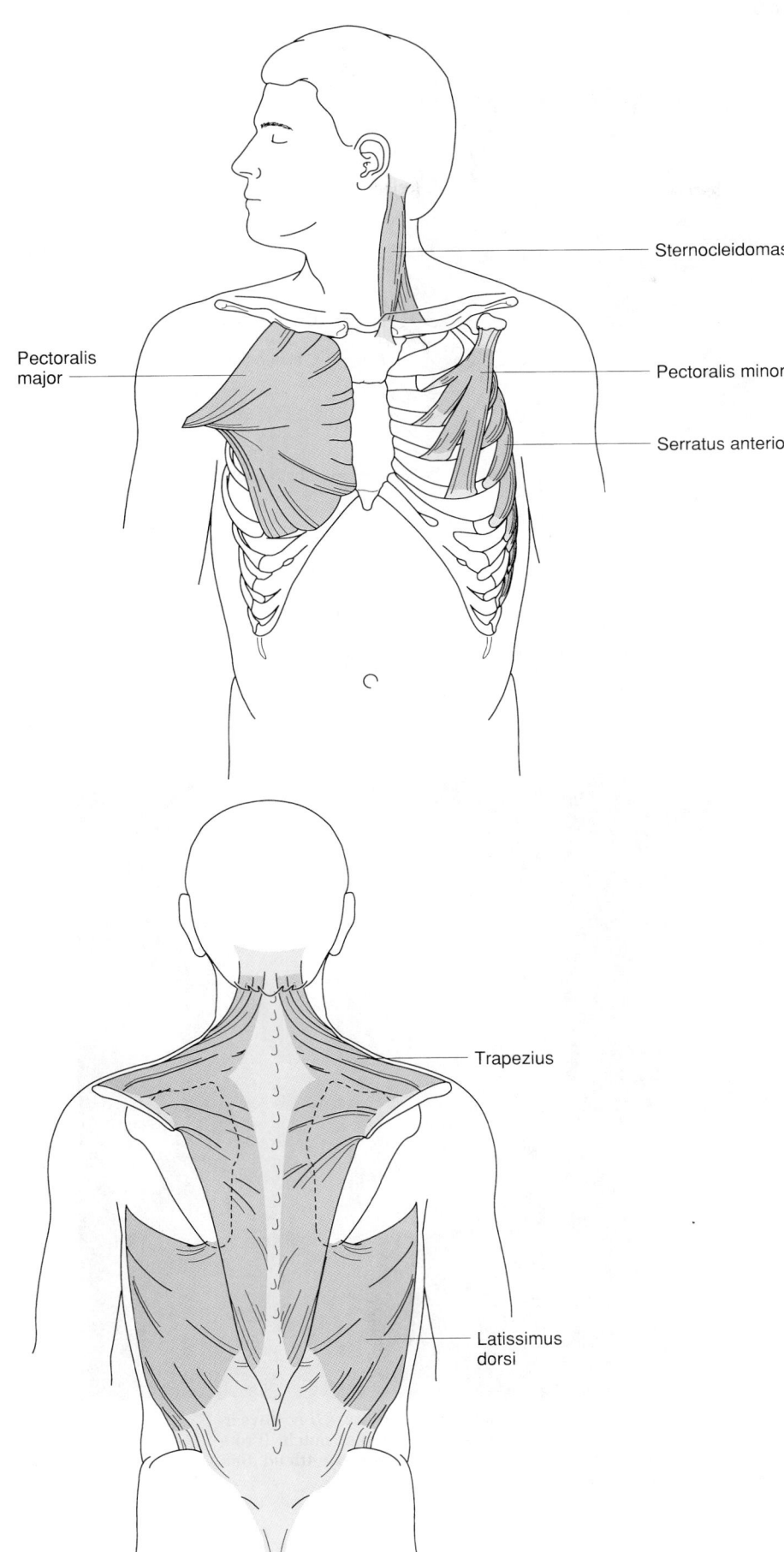

Sternocleidomast[...]

Pectoralis
major

Pectoralis minor

Serratus anterior

A

Trapezius

Latissimus
dorsi

B

Figure 60.4. Thoracic musculature. *(A)* Anterior view. *(B)* Posterior view. (From Iannettoni MD, Orringer MB. Chest wall, pleura, mediastinum, and nonneoplastic lung disease. In: Greenfield LJ, Mulholland MW, Oldham KT, et al., eds. *Surgery: scientific principles and practice,* 2nd ed. Philadelphia: Lippincott–Raven, 1997:1440–1482, with permission.)

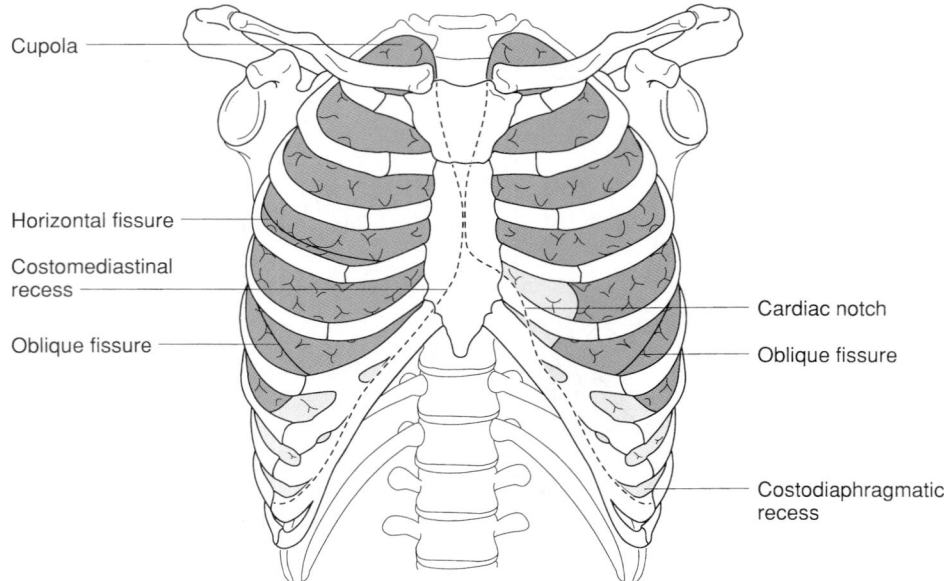

Figure 60.5. Topographic relations of the pleura to the chest wall. Laterally, the pleura extends to the level of the 11th to 12th ribs. The anterior reflection of the mediastinal and costal pleurae forms the costo-mediastinal recess, whereas the reflections of the costal and diaphragmatic pleurae form the costo-diaphragmatic recess. (From Iannettoni MD, Orringer MB. Chest wall, pleura, mediastinum, and nonneoplastic lung disease. In: Greenfield LJ, Mulholland MW, Oldham KT, et al., eds. *Surgery: scientific principles and practice,* 2nd ed. Philadelphia: Lippincott–Raven, 1997: 1440–1482, with permission.)

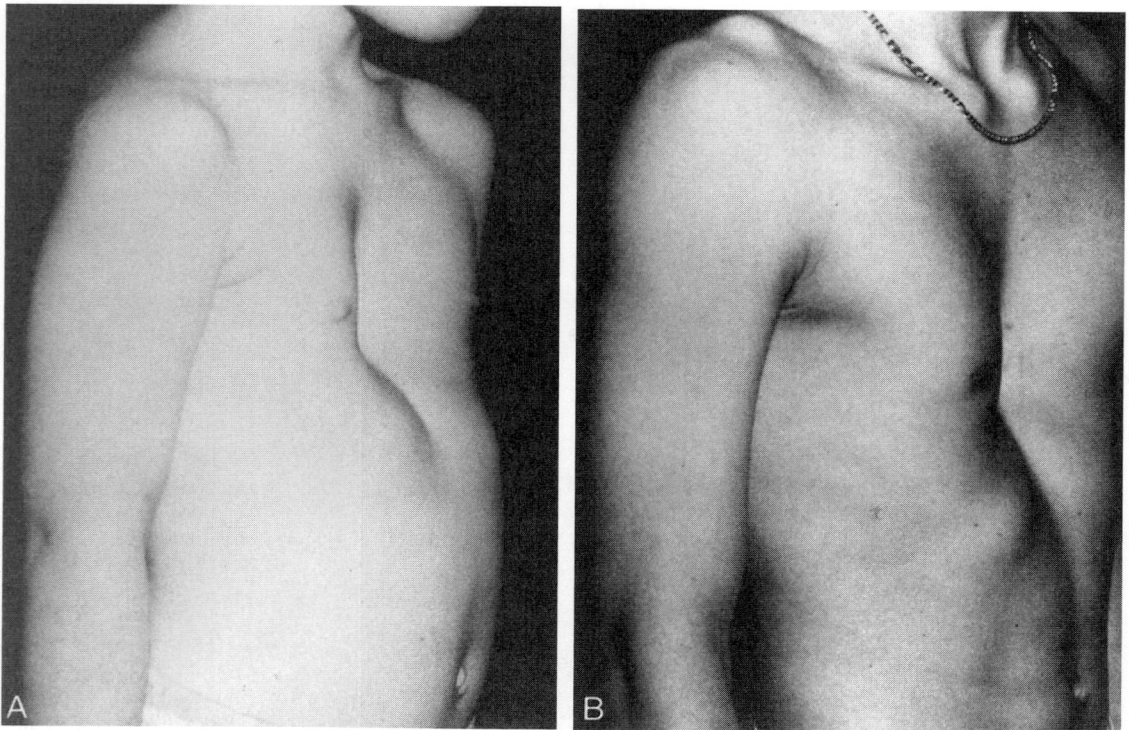

Figure 60.6. *(A)* A 4¹/₂-year-old girl with a symmetric pectus excavatum deformity. *(B)* A 16-year-old boy with pectus excavatum. Note that the depression extends to the sternal notch. (From Shamberger RC. Chest wall deformities. In: Shields TW, ed. *General thoracic surgery,* 4th ed. Baltimore: Williams & Wilkins, 1994:529–557, with permission.)

Table 60.1. MUSCULOSKELETAL ABNORMALITIES IDENTIFIED IN 130 OF 704 CASES OF PECTUS EXCAVATUM

Scoliosis	107
Kyphosis	4
Myopathy	3
Marfan's syndrome	2
Pierre Robin syndrome	2
Prune-belly syndrome	2
Neurofibromatosis	3
Cerebral palsy	4
Tuberous sclerosis	1
Congenital diaphragmatic hernia	2

From Shamberger RC, Welch KJ. Surgical repair of pectus excavatum. J Pediatr Surg 1988;23:615–622, with permission.

surements along with the angle of the sternum are used to develop a score. Usually these two distances are measured from the angle of Louis to the T3 vertebrae and from the xiphoid to the T9 vertebrae.

Operative correction should be undertaken to improve cosmesis, self-image, respiratory or cardiovascular compromise, and exercise tolerance. Repair should be ideally undertaken before adolescence (9). However, less than 15% of patients with pectus excavatum deformities undergo surgical repair. In Fonkalsrud and colleagues' (2) series of 375 pectus excavatum repairs, only 47% had their repair by age 11, and 10% were aged 20 years or older at the time of repair.

Since the Ochsner and DeBakey (10) series in 1939, various techniques have been developed to repair the pectus. Operative approaches can be classified into procedures that use no special support mechanism for sternal reconstruction and methods that use some type of support. Support can be either internal (vascularized and nonvascularized bone struts, metal struts, and Marlex) or external (11). The most popular approach currently involves transverse inframammary incision or a midline incision, exposure of the sternum and cartilages, subperichondrial resection of the cartilages, sternal osteotomy, and anterior displacement of the sternum with or without strut support. Another technique popularized in Japan involves 180-degree rotation of the sternum and cartilages while preserving the internal mammary arteries (12). One final technique popularized because of its simplicity involves placement of a subcutaneous silicone implant to correct the cosmetic defect but without correction of the sternal displacement and hence none of the hemodynamic benefits (13). Excellent results have been reported with each technique. The main postoperative complications are wound infection and a 1% incidence of pneumothorax. Over 90% of patients report excellent cosmetic results and improvement in cardiopulmonary function. The largest series reported recurrences of less than 10% (7,14,15). Nuss and colleagues (16) have reported on 42 patients (aged 15 months to 15 years) who underwent correction of their deformity by a minimally invasive technique. At a mean follow-up of 4.6 years, results are encouraging, and this technique has become preferred at a number of major centers.

Long-term follow-up is required, especially with regard to recurrences during the rapid growth phase of puberty that can dramatically alter the appearance of the chest wall. Fonkalsrud and Bustorff-Silva (17) reported on their experience with pectus repair in 23 adults aged 20 years and older who presented with poor exercise tolerance. Although the procedure was more difficult than when performed in younger patients, results were similar, with improved exercise tolerance and no recurrence.

Protrusion Deformities/Pectus Carinatum

Pectus carinatum (pigeon breast) is a anterior protrusion defect of the sternum and costal cartilages (Fig. 60.7) (3). Like pectus excavatum, this condition effects more males than females (3.6:1), but is less common than pectus excavatum by a ratio of 1:5 (18). This defect may not be apparent until the first decade of life. Similar to pectus excavatum, a familial predisposition is noted in 26% of cases and is associated with musculoskeletal defects such as scoliosis (15%) and congenital heart disease (18).

Protrusion deformities can be classified into three types. The most frequent type is the chondrogladiolar prominence variant (keel chest), which is an anterior displacement of the body of the sternum and symmetrical concavity of the costal cartilages. The sternum is elongated and the sterno-xiphoidal junction is prominent. The second

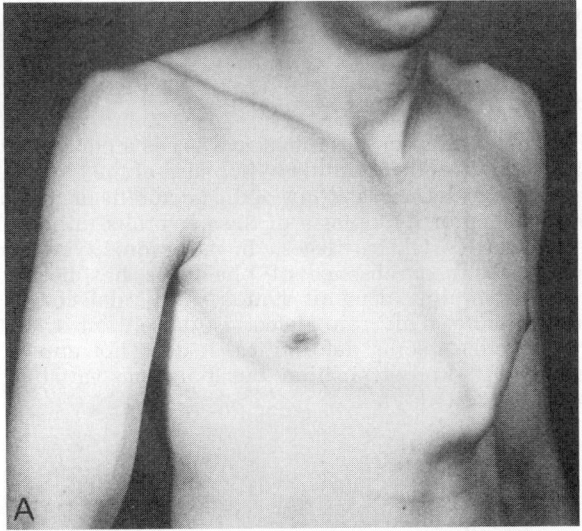

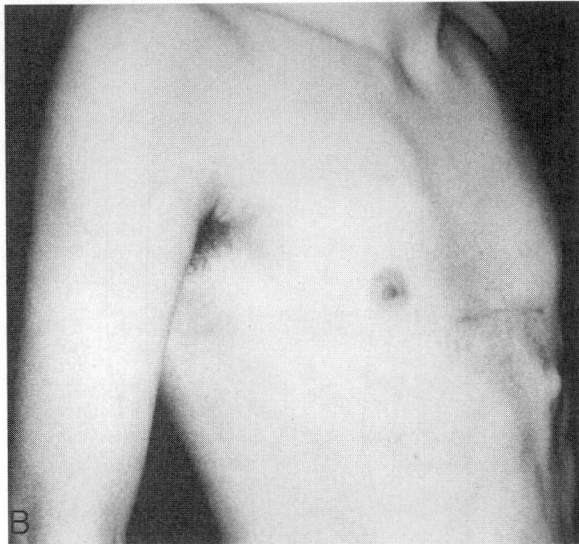

Figure 60.7. *(A)* Symmetric chondrogladiolar pectus carinatum in a 19-year-old man. *(B)* Postoperative photograph shows correction of the protruding sternum and costal cartilages. (From Shamberger RC. Chest wall deformities. In: Shields TW, ed. *General thoracic surgery,* 4th ed. Baltimore: Williams & Wilkins, 1994: 529–557, with permission.)

type is the lateral pectus carinatum. It occurs as a unilateral protrusion of the costal cartilages and is usually accompanied by sternal rotation about its long axis to the opposite side. The third and least common type is termed the pouter pigeon breast or chondromanubrial prominence and presents as an upper or chondromanubrial prominence with protrusion of the manubrium and depression of the sternal body.

Symptoms of pectus carinatum become more common as the patient ages and chest wall rigidity increases and include exertional dyspnea or cardiac arrhythmia. Evaluation of cardiopulmonary function includes pulmonary function tests, echocardiography, and exercise testing.

An operative technique similar to the one for excavatum repair is used via an inframammary transverse incision. The sternum and cartilage are exposed follow by subperichondrial resection of the cartilages. Sternal osteotomies may not be necessary except to correct sternal angulation (Fig. 60.8) (18). Postoperative complications are uncommon and include wound infection or dehiscence and pneumothorax. Most patients achieve excellent results with few recurrences.

Poland's Syndrome

Poland's syndrome described in 1841 is a constellation of abnormalities that include hypoplasia of the breast and subcutaneous tissues, absence of the pectoralis major muscles, absence or hypoplasia of the pectoralis minor, and absence of costal cartilages. In addition, syndactyly, brachydactyly, or absence of phalanges has been described. The clinical manifestation of this defect can be quite variable. This rare defect is present in 1:30,000 births. Unlike pectus deformities, it does not appear to have a familial predisposition, but it also has variable degrees of severity (19).

Most commonly this defect is repaired using a latissimus dorsi myocutaneous flap and with the addition of a breast implant in women. Three-dimensional computed tomography (CT) scan may assist in planning reconstructive procedures (Fig. 60.9) (3,20–25).

Sternal Clefts

The sternum starts to develop during the sixth week of gestation. The lateral plate mesoderm gives rise to the pectoralis muscles and the sternum. Migrating cells from lateral plate mesoderm start to migrate and eventually form two bands, one on either side of the midline that by the 10th week fuse to form the body of the sternum. The manubrium then starts to develop from primordia between the ventral ends of the clavicles. Abnormal fusion of the sternal band leads to cleft formation.

The superior sternal cleft has a **V** or **U** shape appearance that can extend to the fourth costal cartilage. This defect can be repaired by direct apposition of the two sternal bands after oblique chondrotomies. If the defect is broad enough, hypotension may occur during apposition and prosthetic material would have to be used to diminish the constriction of mediastinal structures (Fig. 60.10) (26).

Complete sternal clefts involve the entire sternum, but also are associated with a crescentic anterior diaphragmatic defect and diastasis recti, which results in free communication between the peritoneal and pericardial cavities. Repair is accomplished with approximation of the pericardium and recti muscles, and prosthetic material is used to cover the sternal gap.

Distal sternal clefts are the most extensive defects and are associated with Cantrell's pentalogy, which includes distal cleft in the sternum, omphalocele, diaphragmatic cleft, pericardial defect and congenital heart defect (ventricular septal defect, tetralogy of Fallot). Primary sternal closure can be accomplished (27–29).

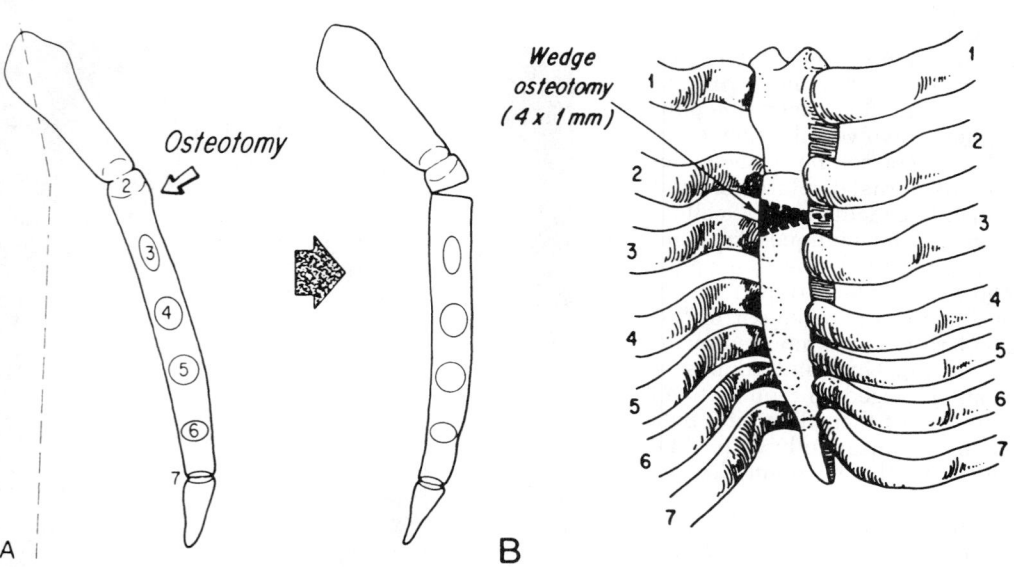

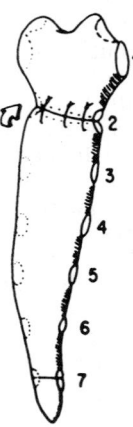

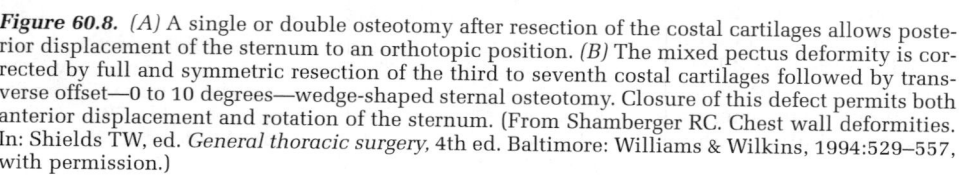

Figure 60.8. *(A)* A single or double osteotomy after resection of the costal cartilages allows posterior displacement of the sternum to an orthotopic position. *(B)* The mixed pectus deformity is corrected by full and symmetric resection of the third to seventh costal cartilages followed by transverse offset—0 to 10 degrees—wedge-shaped sternal osteotomy. Closure of this defect permits both anterior displacement and rotation of the sternum. (From Shamberger RC. Chest wall deformities. In: Shields TW, ed. *General thoracic surgery,* 4th ed. Baltimore: Williams & Wilkins, 1994:529–557, with permission.)

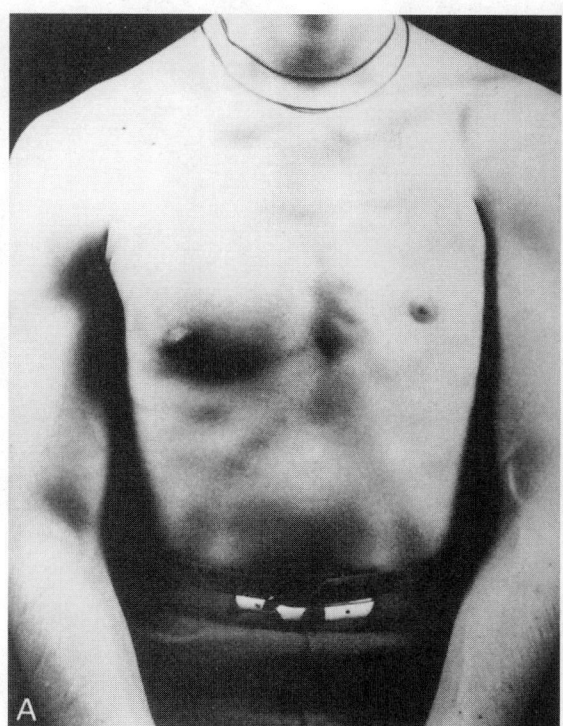

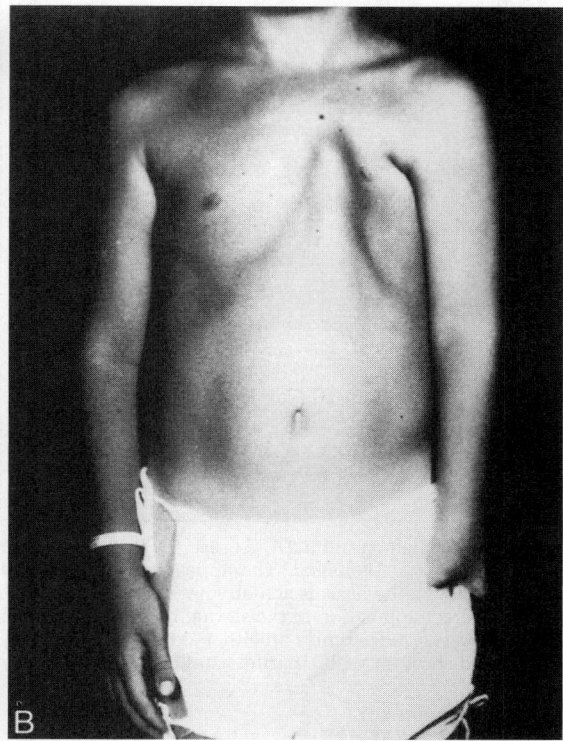

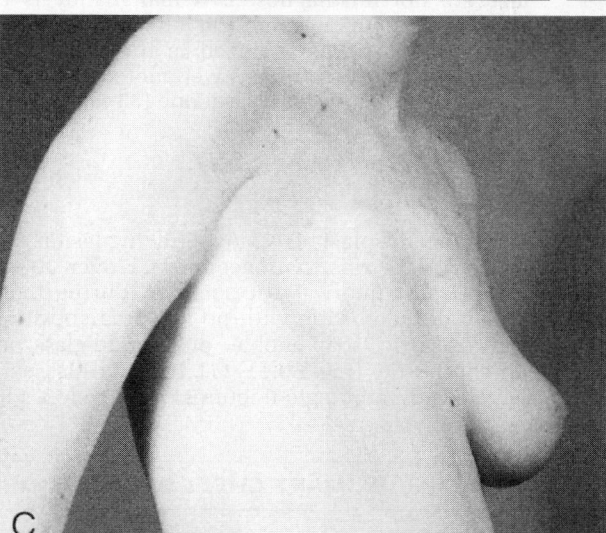

Figure 60.9. Muscular 15-year-old boy with loss of the left axillary fold, orthotopic sternum, and normal cartilages. He compensates adequately for loss of the pectoralis major and minor muscles. Surgery is not indicated in males with these findings. *(B)* An 8-year-old boy with Poland's syndrome. The pectoralis major and minor muscles and the serratus to the level of the fifth rib are absent. The boy has sternal obliquity and the third to fifth ribs are short, ending in points. The corresponding cartilages are absent. The endothoracic fascia lies beneath a thin layer of subcutaneous tissue. Note the hypoplastic nipple and ectromelia of the ipsilateral hand. *(C)* A 14-year-old girl with Poland's syndrome. Note the high position of the right nipple, amastia, sternal rotation, and depressed right anterior chest. The second to fourth ribs and cartilages were missing, reconstructed with rib grafts. Breast augmentation will be required at full growth. (From Shamberger RC. Chest wall deformities. In: Shields TW, ed. *General thoracic surgery,* 4th ed. Baltimore: Williams & Wilkins, 1994:529–557, with permission.)

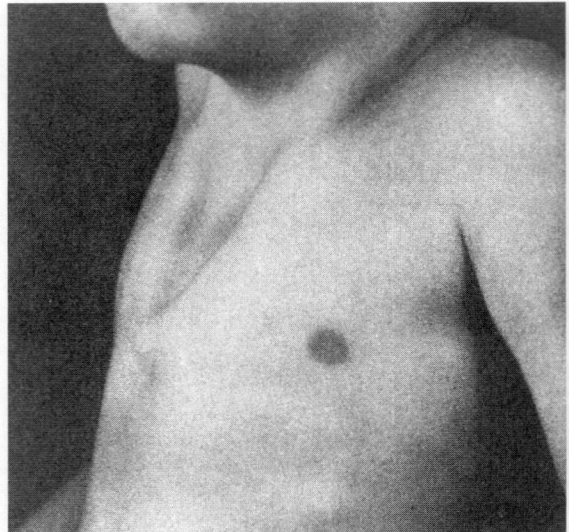 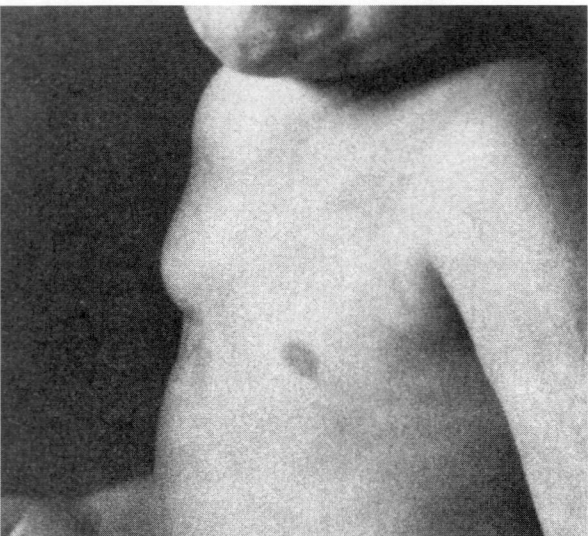

A   B

Figure 60.10. Cleft sternum. *(A)* At rest. *(B)* During forced expiration. Superior clefts of the sternum are variously V- or U-shaped. The appearance of the child as he cries explains the term "ectopia cordis," although the heart is actually not misplaced. In the newborn, defects of this kind can be corrected by direct apposition of the sternal halves. In this child, closure of the defect was made possible by sliding chondrotomies on either side. (From Sabiston DC Jr. The surgical management of congenital bifid sternum with a partial ectopia cordis. *J Thorac Surg* 1958;35:118, with permission.)

CHEST WALL TUMORS

Chest wall tumors are rare neoplasms. They can originate in the bone, cartilage, or soft tissues of the chest wall. Most arise in the ribs (85%) with the remainder arising from the scapula, sternum, and clavicle (30). These neoplasms can be classified as benign or malignant tumors of bone and soft tissue (Tables 60.2 and 60.3) (31) and as primary versus metastatic malignant tumors.

Metastatic tumors to the ribs are the most common malignant chest wall tumors, while primary bone tumors account for approximately 7% to 8% of all chest wall tumors.

Most chest wall tumors start as asymptomatic nodules that slowly enlarge and eventually cause pain. Pain signifies periosteal invasion and is more common with malignant tumors (32). Appropriate evaluation of these patients includes thorough history and physical examination, chest radiograph, CT scan and bone scan to rule out multiple lesions, as well as magnetic resonance imaging (MRI) to rule out neurovascular involvement.

Pathologic diagnosis is confirmed by an excisional rather than incisional biopsy so that low-grade malignan-cies are not misdiagnosed. If malignancy is confirmed, wide resection is needed. The effect of resection margins on recurrences was analyzed in the Mayo Clinic series. Twice as many recurrences were noted with a 2-cm resection margin than with a 4-cm one (33–35).

Benign Bone Lesions

Fibrous Dysplasia

Fibrous dysplasia is a slow-growing lesion of the lateral aspect of the ribs that accounts for over 30% of benign chest wall tumors. Most common during the third and fourth decade of life with no sex predisposition, it has a characteristic "soap bubble" or "ground glass" appearance on chest x-ray (Fig. 60.11) (1). It may cause pain as it enlarges, and pathologic fractures can develop. Fibrous dys-

Table 60.2. CLASSIFICATION OF CHEST WALL TUMORS

Primary neoplasms of chest wall
  Malignant
  Benign
Metastatic neoplasms to chest wall
  Sarcoma
  Carcinoma
Adjacent neoplasms with local invasion
  Lung
  Breast
  Pleura
Nonneoplastic disease
  Cyst
  Inflammation

From Pairolero P. Chest wall tumors. In: Shields TW, Locicero J, Ponn R, eds. *General thoracic surgery,* 5th ed. Philadelphia: Lippincott Williams & Wilkins, 2000:589–598, with permission.

Table 60.3. PRIMARY CHEST WALL TUMOR

Malignant
  Myeloma
  Malignant fibrous histiocytoma
  Chondrosarcoma
  Rhabdomyosarcoma
  Ewing's sarcoma
  Liposarcoma
  Neurofibrosarcoma
  Osteogenic sarcoma
  Hemangiosarcoma
  Leiomysarcoma
  Lymphoma
Benign
  Osteochondroma
  Chondroma
  Desmoid
  Fibrous dysplasia
  Lipoma
  Fibroma
  Neurilemoma

From Pairolero P. Chest wall tumors. In: Shields TW, Locicero J, Ponn R, eds. *General thoracic surgery,* 5th ed. Philadelphia: Lippincott Williams & Wilkins, 2000:589–598, with permission.

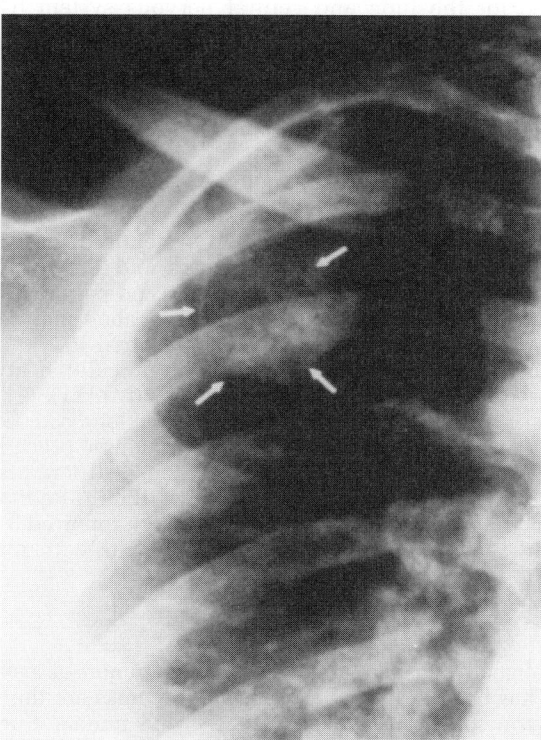

Figure 60.11. Fibrous dysplasia of the rib. Note the characteristic expansion and thinning of the cortex *(arrows)* and the central ground-glass appearance. (From Iannettoni MD, Orringer MB. Chest wall, pleura, mediastinum, and nonneoplastic lung disease. In: Greenfield LJ, Mulholland MW, Oldham KT, et al., eds. *Surgery: scientific principles and practice,* 2nd ed. Philadelphia: Lippincott–Raven, 1997:1440–1482, with permission.)

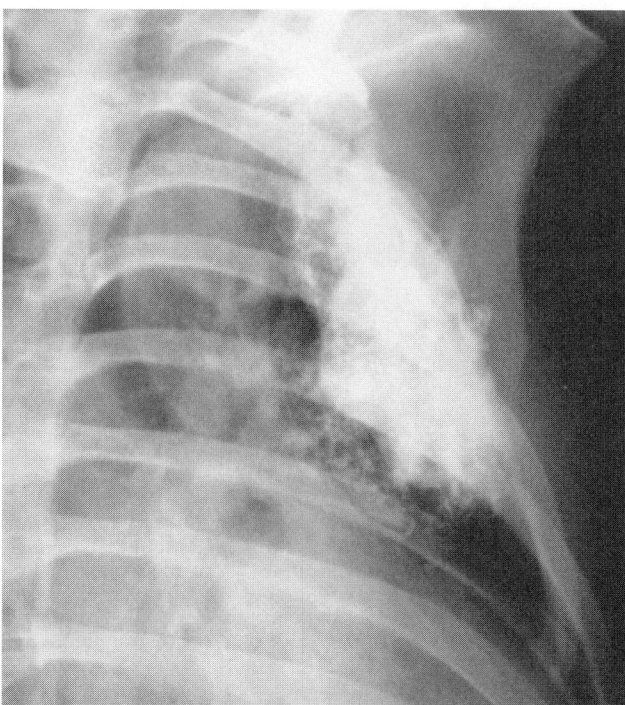

Figure 60.12. Osteochondroma of left second rib. The stippled calcification within the tumor and the intact cortex of the rib are characteristic. (From Iannettoni MD, Orringer MB. Chest wall, pleura, mediastinum, and nonneoplastic lung disease. In: Greenfield LJ, Mulholland MW, Oldham KT, et al., eds. *Surgery: scientific principles and practice,* 2nd ed. Philadelphia: Lippincott–Raven, 1997:1440–1482, with permission.)

plasia can also occur as part of Albright syndrome where the lesions are multiple and are associated with precocious puberty and skin pigmentation. Excision is indicated for symptom relief and to confirm the diagnosis.

Chondroma

Chondromas tend to occur during the second or third decade of life. They are also asymptomatic slow-growing tumors, but they tend to occur at the costochondral junction anteriorly. They have equal frequency in men and women and account for 15% to 20% of benign lesions of the chest wall. They can be divided into two types. The enchondroma arises in the medulla, while periosteal chondroma arises in the periosteum. Chondromas appear as lytic lesions with sclerotic margins on chest x-ray and are difficult to distinguish from chondrosarcomas either radiographically or histologically. Excisional biopsy is always recommended (36).

Osteochondroma

Osteochondromas present as a painless mass in young males (male to female ratio of 3:1). The mass originates from the cortex of the rib and has a characteristic appearance on a chest x-ray of a pedunculated bony mass capped with viable cartilage (Fig. 60.12) (1).

Familial osteochondromatosis is a variant that presents with multiple lesions. Resection is indicated for symptomatic and enlarging lesions. Recurrences are rare.

Eosinophilic Granuloma

This benign condition primarily affects men. Multiple lesions of skull and rib are common. On plain radiographs

they appear as expansile bone lesions. A solitary lesion can be excised, and radiotherapy is best for patients with multiple lesions.

Osteoid Osteomas

Osteoid osteomas are rare tumors that also affect men more frequently. They arise in the bony cortex of the rib or vertebral arches and tend to be symptomatic especially at night. A small, radiolucent nidus encircled by a sclerotic margin is frequently seen on chest x-ray. The entire rib should be resected for relief of symptoms.

Aneurysmal Bone Cysts

Aneurysmal bone cysts can arise as the result of chest wall trauma. They have a characteristic pattern of a "blowout" lytic lesion on chest x-ray. Symptomatic lesions should be excised.

Malignant Bone Lesions

Chondrosarcoma

Chondrosarcoma is the most common of the chest wall malignant tumors, accounting for 20% of such tumors. Usually seen after the fourth decade of life, these lesions can arise after local trauma to the chest or secondary to malignant degeneration of benign chondromas or osteochondromas. They tend to present as an anterior chest mass and usually involve the anterior costochondral junctions of the sternum (Fig. 60.13) (36,37). On chest x-ray, they tend to have a similar appearance to benign chondromas. Resection with wide margins of greater than 4 cm are needed. Five-year survival rates of 70% have been reported after complete excision (36,37).

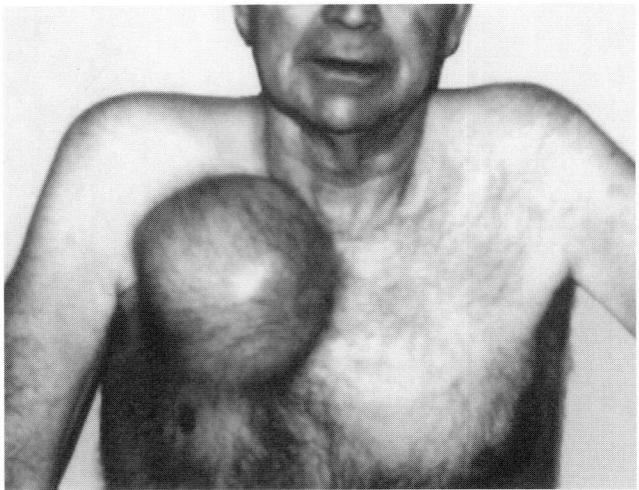

Figure 60.13. Large chondrosarcoma arising from the right anterior third costochondral junction. (From Iannettoni MD, Orringer MB. Chest wall, pleura, mediastinum, and nonneoplastic lung disease. In: Greenfield LJ, Mulholland MW, Oldham KT, et al., eds. *Surgery: scientific principles and practice,* 2nd ed. Philadelphia: Lippincott–Raven, 1997:1440–1482, with permission.)

Osteogenic Sarcoma

Although it is more common in the extremities, osteogenic sarcomas do occur in the ribs and account for 10% to 15% of malignant tumors. Chest radiographs reveal the characteristic "sunburst" pattern. Unlike chondrosarcomas, they tend to enlarge rapidly, and metastases are often present at initial evaluation. Chest and abdominal CT scan and bone scan are indicated for assessment of metastatic disease. Five-year survival following complete excision only can be as low as 20%, while survival after surgery and adjuvant chemotherapy rises to 60% (38).

Ewing's Sarcoma

Ewing's sarcoma is the third most common malignant chest wall tumor (5% to 10%). It occurs more frequently in children and young men and has 2:1 male to female ratio. Patients complain of intermittent pain, and often there is an inflammatory response with fever and leukocytosis. Chest radiographs show the characteristic "onion peel" appearance. Similar to osteogenic sarcoma, metastases are common at initial presentation, displaying a pref-

erence for the lung and central nervous system (CNS). Five-year survival has been improved to 50% using multimodality therapy treatment (surgery followed by chemotherapy and radiotherapy) (39–42).

Solitary Plasmacytoma

Solitary plasmacytoma is a rare tumor arising from plasma cells. Many believe that this is indicative of multiple myeloma, and often patients diagnosed with solitary plasmacytoma eventually develop systemic disease. Age at presentation is usually over 50 years, and there is a male predisposition. Symptoms of pain with no palpable mass are common. Patients usually have an abnormal serum protein electrophoresis, Bence-Jones protein in the urine and bone marrow aspiration demonstrate cellular atypia. Biopsy will confirm the diagnosis (Fig. 60.14) (1). A small solitary plasmacytoma should be completely resected. Whether to undertake extensive reconstructive procedures for this disease is controversial because differentiation from multiple myeloma can be quite difficult. Radiotherapy is the primary mode of therapy with a reported 5-year survival of 30%, although favorable results with radical excision have also been reported (43,44).

Soft Tissue Tumors

Malignant degeneration of most benign tumors of the chest wall has been described. Soft tissue sarcomas are the most common soft tissue malignant chest wall tumors. Surgical excision is the preferred mode of therapy. Biopsy establishes the diagnosis, and, similar to sarcomas at other sites, mitotic rate, cellular pleomorphism, and nuclear to cytoplasmic ratio are used to classify them as low or high grade. Resection with wide margins and reconstruction is indicated. Adjuvant chemoradiation protocols are routinely used.

Metastatic Tumors

Hematologic dissemination is the most common cause of metastatic disease to the chest wall. Often radiation therapy is used for palliation. Direct extension of breast and lung cancer to the chest wall is relatively common. In breast cancer, locoregional recurrence involving the chest wall can occur in over 10% of stage II lesions following mastectomy (45,46). Recurrences are treated with resection and adjuvant chemoradiotherapy.

Five percent of non–small-cell lung cancers (NSCLC) invade the chest wall. Complete resection and absence of nodal disease are associated with a favorable prognosis in

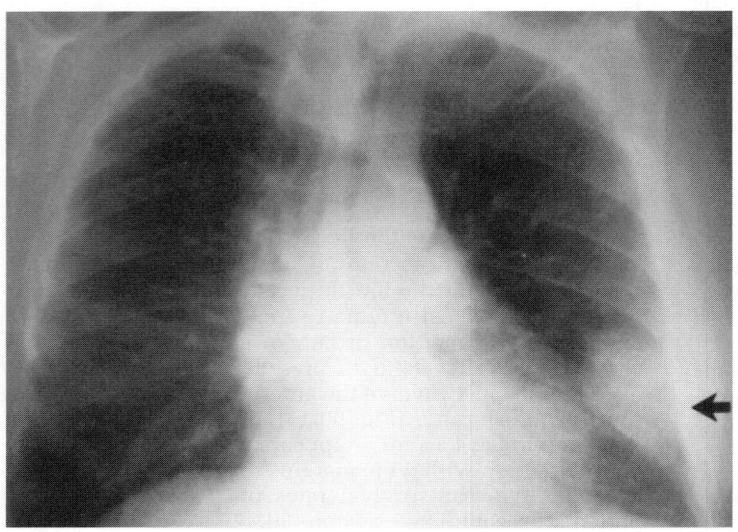

Figure 60.14. Plasmacytoma of the left seventh rib, showing characteristic cortical destruction and relatively large soft tissue component projecting into the chest. (From Iannettoni MD, Orringer MB. Chest wall, pleura, mediastinum, and nonneoplastic lung disease. In: Greenfield LJ, Mulholland MW, Oldham KT, et al., eds. *Surgery: scientific principles and practice,* 2nd ed. Philadelphia: Lippincott–Raven, 1997:1440–1482, with permission.)

these patients. Five-year survival of almost 60% has been reported for patients with chest wall invasion without lymph node involvement (T3 N0—stage IIB), while 5-year survival for patients with N1 and N2 disease is 35% and 7% to 16%, respectively (47–49).

In 1924, Pancoast (50) described the presentation of the posteroapical chest tumors that bear his name. These patients present with arm pain, atrophy of hand muscles, bone destruction, and Horner's syndrome. Nodal disease has a negative impact on survival. Surgery has produced a 30% 5-year survival in the subset of patients with no nodal disease (51–53). Most series using radiotherapy along with surgery have reported local control rates of 70% to 85% (54–57).

RECONSTRUCTION

The principal goals of chest wall reconstruction are protection of the intrathoracic organs, support of respiration by preventing paradoxical movement, and an acceptable cosmetic result without compromising an indicated cancer operation. To achieve these goals preoperative consultation with an experienced plastic surgeon is often crucial (Table 60.4) (31). Reconstruction of the chest wall involves two parts: the bony thorax and the soft tissues.

The bony thorax is reconstructed based on the size and location of the defect. If the size of the defect is less than 5 cm,

Table 60.4. CONSIDERATIONS FOR RECONSTRUCTION OF CHEST WALL DEFECTS

Location	General condition of patient
Size	Chemotherapy
Depth	Corticosteroid
Partial thickness	Chronic infection
Full thickness	Lifestyle and type of work
Duration	Prognosis
Condition of local tissue	
Irradiation	
Infection	
Residual tumor	
Scarring	

From Pairolero P. Chest wall tumors. In: Shields TW, Locicero J, Ponn R, eds. General thoracic surgery, 5th ed. Philadelphia: Lippincott Williams & Wilkins, 2000:589–598, with permission.

then no reconstruction is needed. If the defect is located posteriorly and deep to the scapula, then defects up to 10 cm in diameter do not need reconstruction. All other defects need repair. If reconstruction is needed, a variety of prosthetic materials are available such as Prolene mesh, Gore-Tex (W. L. Gore, Flagstaff, AZ), and methylmethacrylate-impregnated mesh (Fig. 60.15) (1). These can be anchored to the

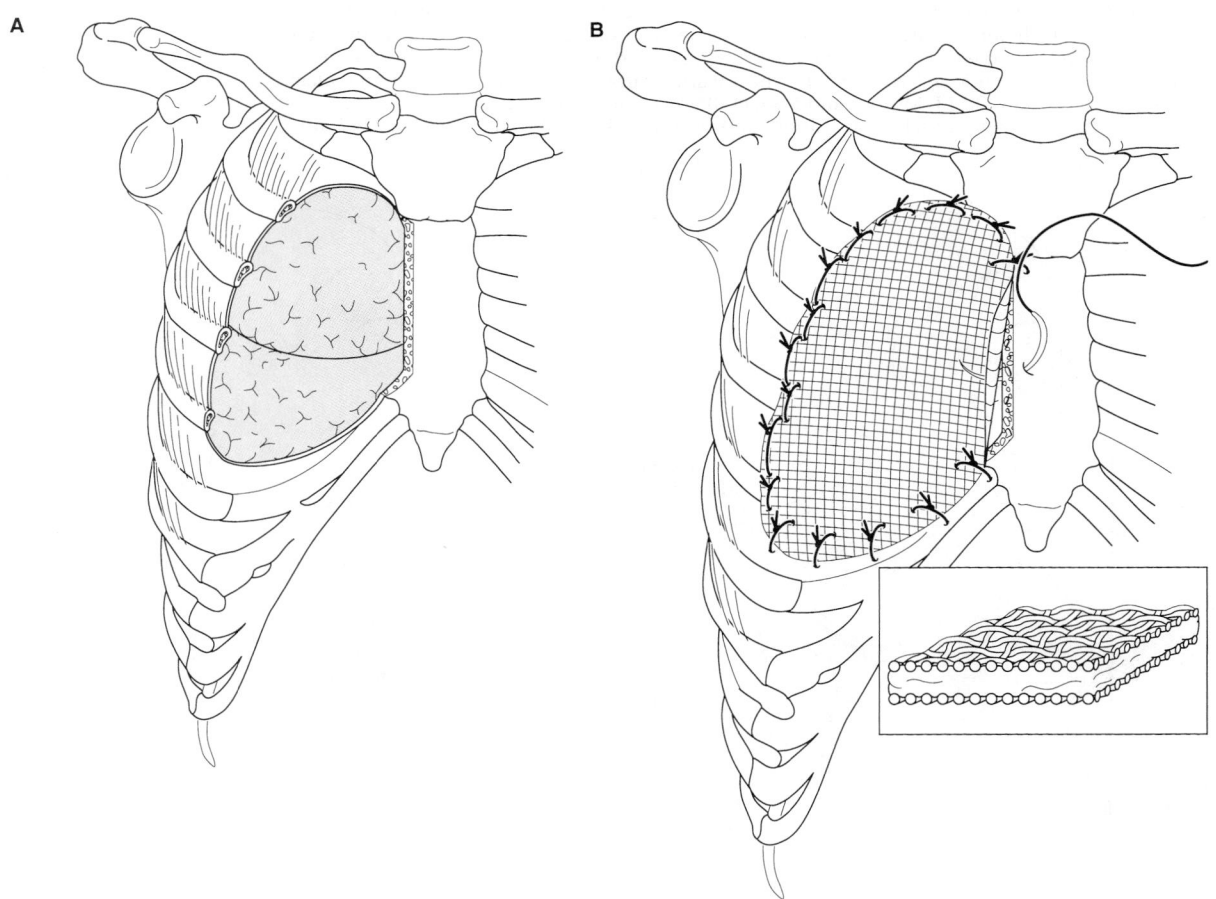

Figure 60.15. Marlex methylmethacrylate sandwich technique for chest wall reconstruction. *(A)* Upper anterior chest wall defect resulting from resection of ribs two to five and a portion of sternum. *(B)* Marlex methylmethacrylate prosthesis being sutured in place. Heavy, nonabsorbable sutures either encircling the ribs or passed through the sternum are used to anchor the prosthesis in place. *(Insert)* Detail of prosthesis showing sandwich of hardened methylmethacrylate between two sheets or Marlex. (From Iannettoni MD, Orringer MB. Chest wall, pleura, mediastinum, and nonneoplastic lung disease. In: Greenfield LJ, Mulholland MW, Oldham KT, et al., eds. *Surgery: scientific principles and practice,* 2nd ed. Philadelphia: Lippincott–Raven, 1997:1440–1482, with permission.)

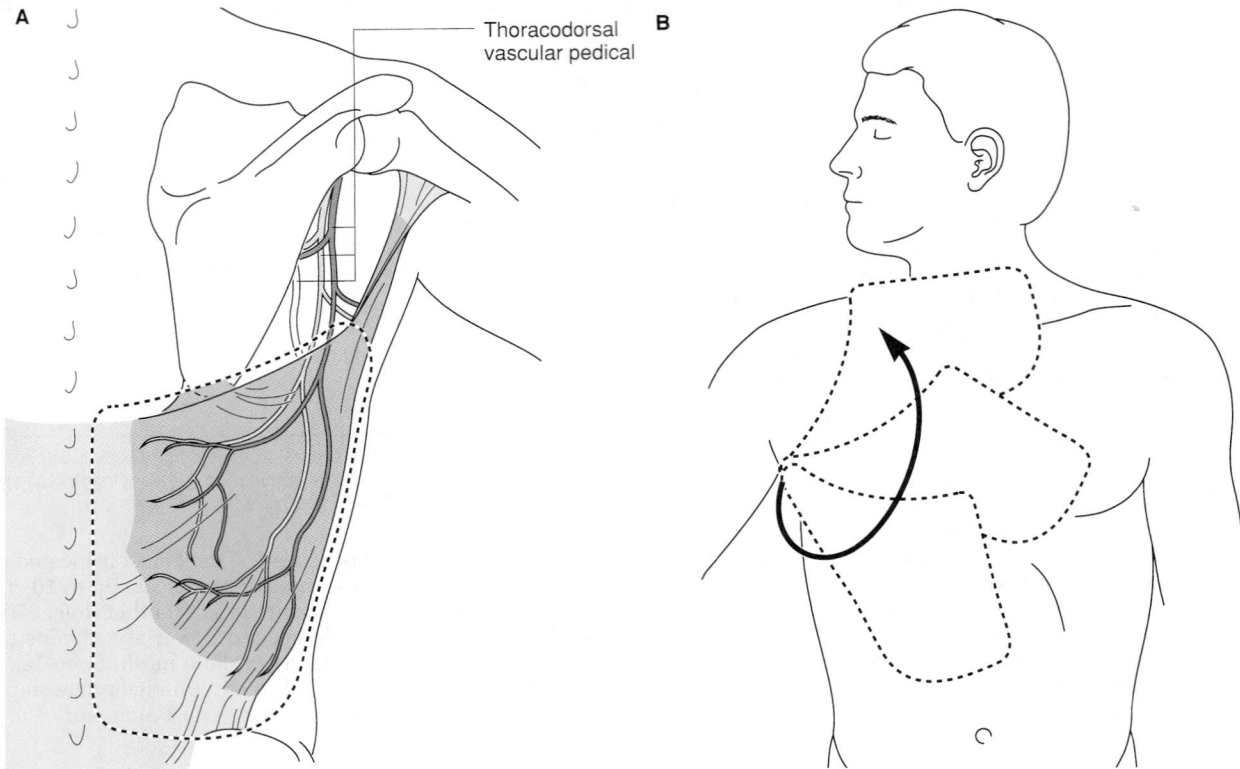

Figure 60.16. Latissimus dorsi muscle rotation flap for chest wall reconstruction. *(A)* Posterior view showing detachment of the origins of the muscle. The dominant blood supply, the thoracodorsal artery, is preserved. *(B)* Anterior view showing the extent to which the mobilized muscle reaches. (From Iannettoni MD, Orringer MB. Chest wall, pleura, mediastinum, and nonneoplastic lung disease. In: Greenfield LJ, Mulholland MW, Oldham KT, et al., eds. *Surgery: scientific principles and practice,* 2nd ed. Philadelphia: Lippincott–Raven, 1997:1440–1482, with permission.)

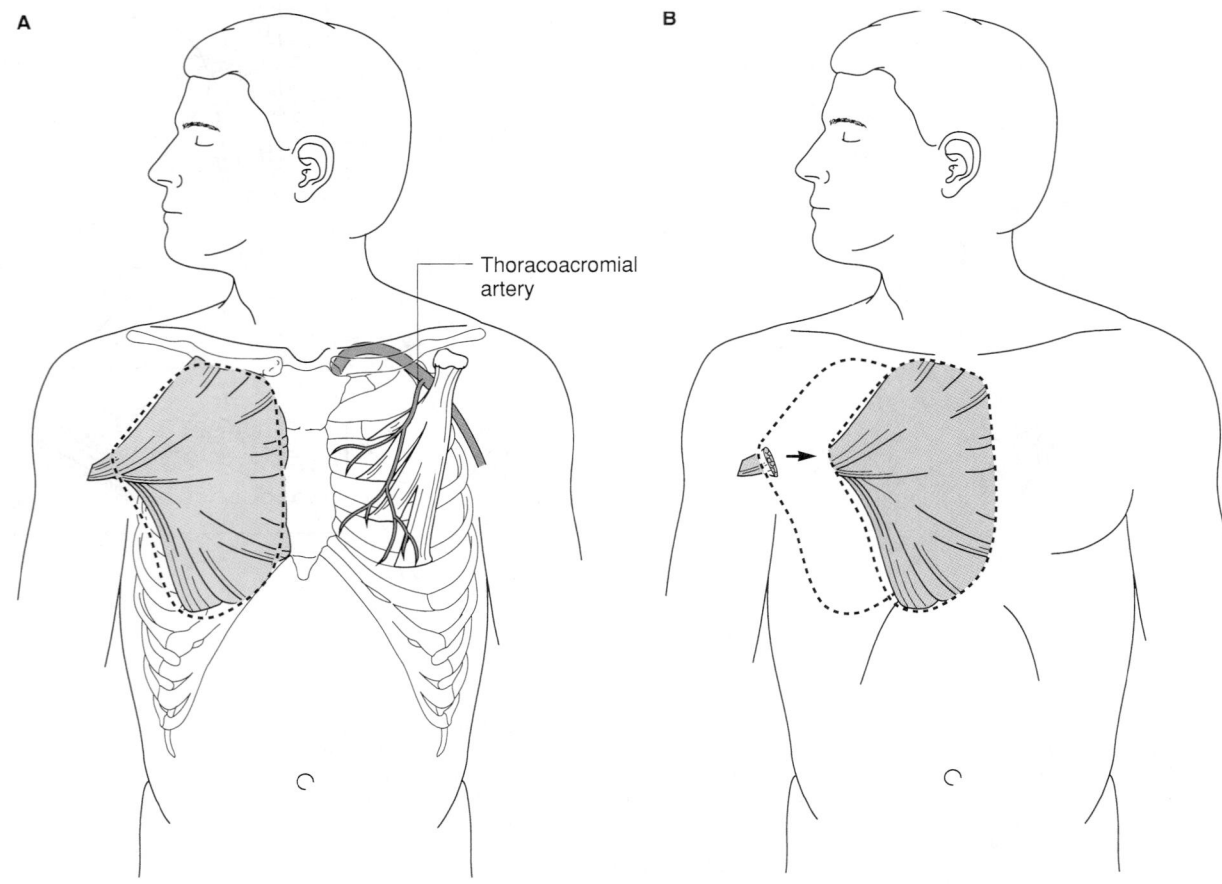

come the flap of choice for sternal defects (Fig. 60.17) (1). The rectus abdominis muscle is based on the internal mammary vessels and is mainly used for defects of the lower anterior chest wall and sternum (Fig. 60.18) (1). The external oblique and serratus anterior muscles can also be used, but offer less coverage than the other flaps. Other options include the omentum and free flaps such as tensor fascia lata, but free flaps are more complicated and the omentum does not provide adequate coverage of large defects (58–62).

THORACIC OUTLET SYNDROME

Thoracic outlet syndrome (Fig. 60.19) (63) refers to compression of neurovascular structures at the thoracic outlet. The neurovascular structures involved are the subclavian artery and vein, and the sympathetic and peripheral nerve components of the brachial plexus. The subclavian artery exits the chest behind the sternoclavicular joints, and, along with the trunks of the brachial plexus, it passes between the anterior and middle scalene muscles. Distal to the pectoralis tendon, the cords form the motor and sensory nerves of the upper extremity. The axillary vein courses posterior to the costocoracoid ligament and pectoralis minor tendon, eventually becoming the subclavian vein; it travels between the anterior scalene muscle and clavicle.

The neurovascular structures can be compressed at three anatomic sites: the interscalene triangle, the costoclavicular space, and the subcoracoid area. In addition numerous other factors such as cervical rib, scalene muscles, fibrous bands, spinal transverse processes, and trauma can cause compression (Table 60.5) (63–67).

The syndrome usually affects women. Neurologic complaints are more commonly seen than vascular ones, although a combination of both can also be present. Pain and paresthesias are the most common symptoms followed by motor weakness and possibly atrophy of thenar and hypothenar muscles secondary to ulnar nerve compression. Compression of median nerve results in index and middle finger paresthesias. Symptoms of vascular compromise include upper extremity claudication, coolness, and fatigue. Thrombosis and distal embolization are occasionally reported. Repetitive arm motion can in result in subclavian vein thrombosis, also known as Paget-Schroetter syndrome (68).

For diagnostic purposes, four clinical maneuvers are used to reproduce the symptoms of the patient with thoracic outlet syndrome: the Adson or scalene test (Fig. 60.20), the costoclavicular or military test (Fig. 60.21), the hyperabduction test (Fig. 60.22), and the Roos test (69). The Roos test involves abduction of the arm 90 degrees with external rotation of the shoulder while quickly opening and closing the fist for 3 minutes.

Plain radiographs are useful in detecting bony abnormalities. MRI can rule out cervical disease as the cause of the symptoms, whereas Doppler studies with provocative testing and angiogram may be needed to assess vascular involvement. Nerve conduction velocities are useful to determine the site of compression (70).

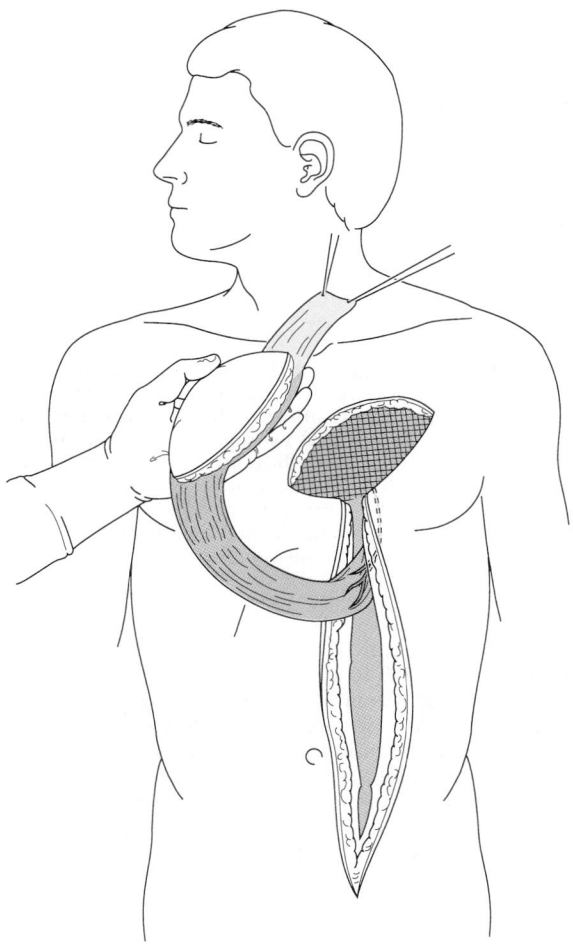

Figure 60.18. Rectus abdominis muscle rotation flap. Shown is the mobilization of the rectus abdominis muscle, which is based on the superior epigastric artery (the continuation of the internal thoracic artery), and rotation of the muscle and overlying skin to fill an anterior chest wall defect. (From Iannettoni MD, Orringer MB. Chest wall, pleura, mediastinum, and nonneoplastic lung disease. In: Greenfield LJ, Mulholland MW, Oldham KT, et al., eds. *Surgery: scientific principles and practice,* 2nd ed. Philadelphia: Lippincott–Raven, 1997:1440–1482, with permission.)

surrounding chest wall to provide stability and the necessary rigidity for protection and respiration. Drainage of the subcutaneous tissues and chest cavity depends on the type of mesh used and its permeability to fluid.

A variety of myocutaneous flaps have been developed. The latissimus dorsi flap, based on the thoracodorsal neurovascular supply, is the largest muscle of the thorax and hence can cover the largest defects (Fig. 60.16) (1). The pectoralis major flap, based on the thoracoacromial neurovascular supply, is the second largest muscle and has be-

Figure 60.17. Pectoralis major muscle rotation flap. *(A)* Mobilization of the flap by detaching the clavicular, sternal, and chest wall origins as well as the insertion of the muscle on the greater tubercle of the humerus. The dominant blood supply, the thoracoacromial artery, which arises from the axillary artery medial to the proximal border of the pectoralis minor muscle is shown on the left side, where the pectoralis major muscle has been removed. *(B)* Medial transposition of the muscle flap, preserving the thoracoacromial neurovascular bundle. (From Iannettoni MD, Orringer MB. Chest wall, pleura, mediastinum, and nonneoplastic lung disease. In: Greenfield LJ, Mulholland MW, Oldham KT, et al., eds. *Surgery: scientific principles and practice,* 2nd ed. Philadelphia: Lippincott–Raven, 1997:1440–1482, with permission.)

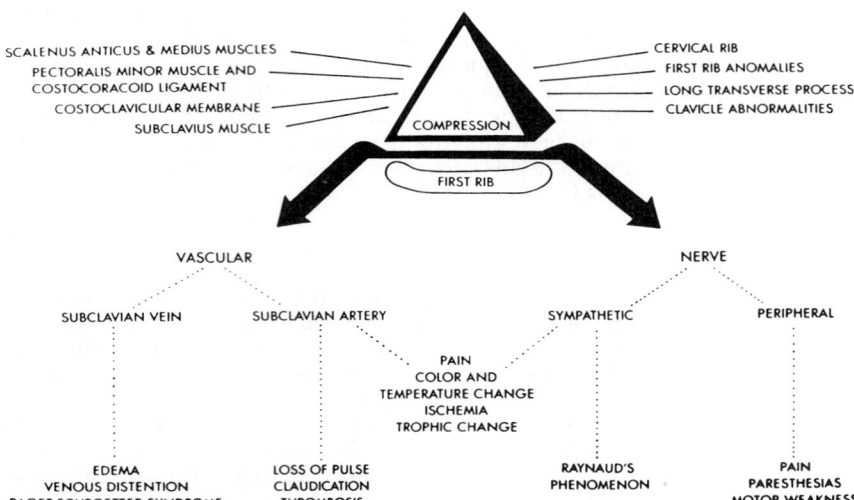

THORACIC OUTLET SYNDROME

Figure 60.19. Schematic diagram showing the relation of muscle, ligament, and bone abnormalities in the thoracic outlet that may compress neurovascular structures against the first rib. (From Urschel HC Jr, Razzuk MA. Thoracic outlet syndrome. In: Sabiston DC Jr, Spencer FC, eds. *Surgery of the chest.* Philadelphia: WB Saunders, 1990:536–553, with permission.)

Management

The vast majority of patients with thoracic outlet syndrome improve with physiotherapy such as posture training and stretching exercises (71,72). Indications for surgery include persistent symptoms and continuing neurovascular problems, such as delayed conduction velocities. In addition, persistent vascular lesions like stenosis of the subclavian artery or aneurysms are indications for surgery. The procedure of choice is the transaxillary resection of the first rib and cervical rib when present. This procedure has good cosmetic results with excellent relief

for neurologic symptoms. Recurrence of symptoms has been reported in 2% to 30% of patients usually secondary to excessive scar formation. Better results are reported in patients who are involved in nonlabor occupations (66,73–75). Complications include neurovascular injury, infection, incomplete resection of the cervical or first rib, and resection of the second rib instead of the first. Aneurysms of the subclavian artery can be addressed with saphenous or prosthetic graft bypass. Subclavian vein

Table 60.5.	**ETIOLOGIC FACTORS OF NEUROVASCULAR COMPRESSION SYNDROMES**

Anatomic
    Potential sites of neurovascular compression
        Interscalene triangle
        Costoclavicular space
        Subcoracoid area
Congenital
    Cervical rib and its fascial remnants
    Rudimentary first thoracic rib
    Scalene muscles
        Anterior
        Middle
        Minimus
    Adventitious fribrous bands
    Bifid clavicle
    Exostosis of first thoracic rib
    Enlarged transverse process of C7
    Omohyoid muscle
    Anomalous course of transverse cervical artery
    Brachial plexus postfixed
    Flat clavicle
Traumatic
    Fracture of clavicle
    Dislocation of head of humerus
    Crushing injury to upper thorax
    Sudden, unaccustomed muscular efforts involving shoulder girdle muscles
    Cervical spondylosis and injuries to cervical spine
Atherosclerosis

From Urschel HC Jr, Razzuk MA. Thoracic outlet syndrome. In: Sabiston DC Jr, Spencer FC, eds. Surgery of the chest. Philadelphia: WB Saunders, 1990:536–553, with permission.

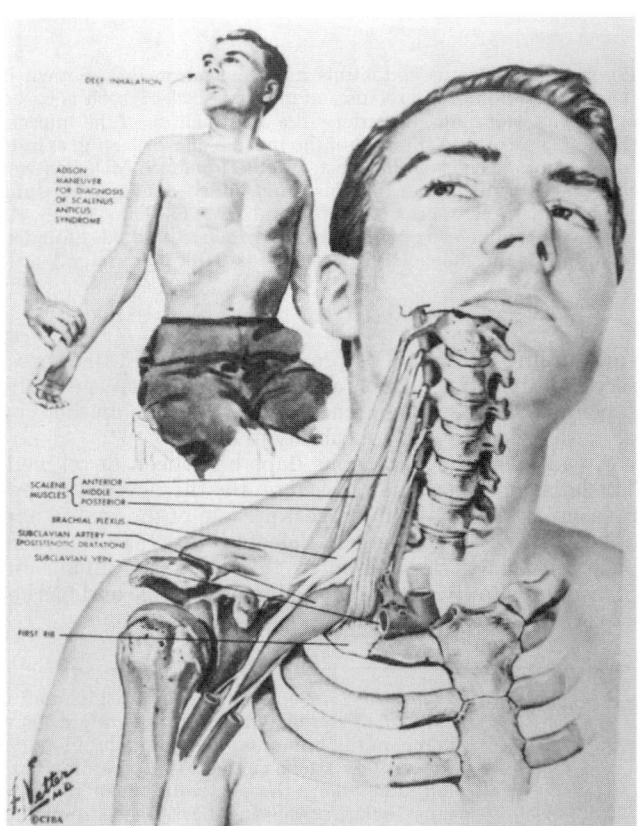

Figure 60.20. Adson's maneuver. Relation of scalene triangle to the neurovascular bundle. (From Netter FH. Clinical symposia. CIBA-GEIGY Corporation, 1971, with permission.)

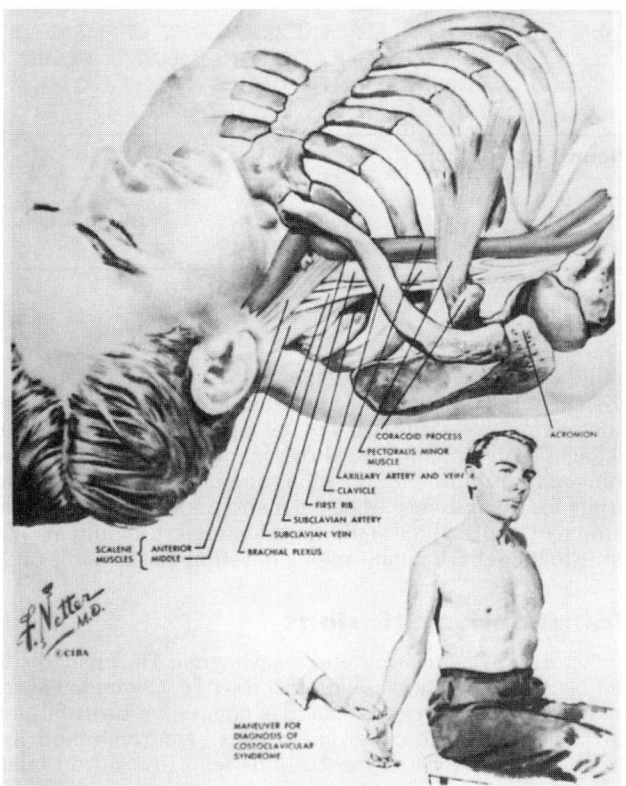

Figure 60.21. Costoclavicular maneuver (military position). Relation of costoclavicular space to neurovascular bundle. (From Netter FH. Clinical symposia. CIBA-GEIGY Corporation, 1971, with permission.)

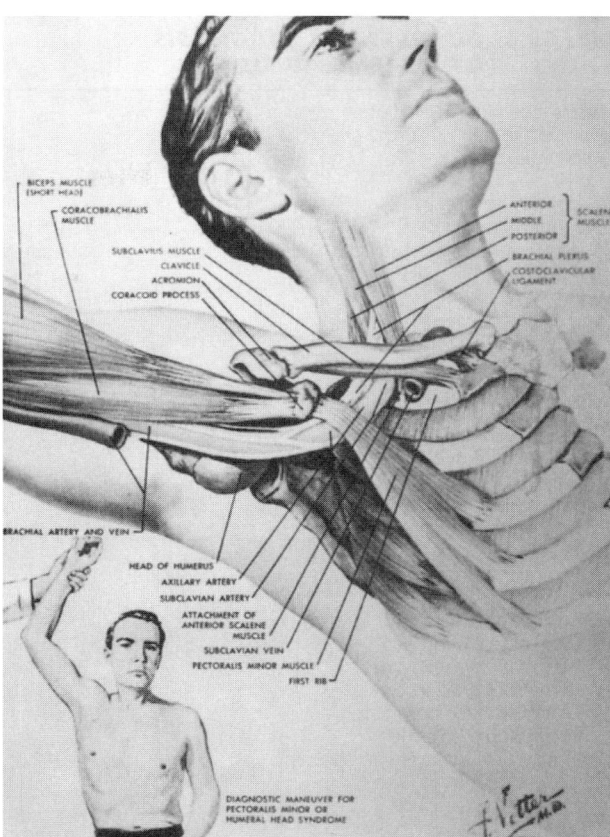

Figure 60.22. Hyperabduction maneuver. Relation of neurovascular bundle to pectoralis minor tendon, coracoid process, and humeral head (pulley effect). (From Netter FH. Clinical symposia. CIBA-GEIGY Corporation, 1971, with permission.)

thrombosis should be treated with thrombolytic agents followed by first rib resection.

PLEURA

Anatomy

The pleural space is a potential space between the visceral pleura that envelops the lung and the parietal pleura that lines the chest wall. A small amount of fluid secreted by the mesothelial cells of the pleura normally lubricates the two surfaces. The parietal pleura can be further subdivided into cervical, costal, mediastinal, and diaphragmatic components. The visceral pleura is intimately adherent to the lung and cannot be dissected off from pulmonary parenchyma. The parietal pleura receives its blood supply from the intercostal, internal mammary, superior phrenic, and anterior mediastinal arteries. The visceral pleura receives its blood supply via branches of the bronchial and pulmonary arteries. The venous drainage parallels the arterial branches for the parietal pleura, and for the visceral pleura drainage is into the pulmonary veins. The intercostal nerves innervate the costal and the peripheral parts of the diaphragm. The phrenic nerves innervate the remaining diaphragmatic and mediastinal pleura. The visceral pleura receives sympathetic and parasympathetic component, but it has no sensory component. The lymphatic drainage of the visceral pleura is directed toward the mediastinal lymph nodes, while the parietal pleura lymphatics drain into the regional nodes. Thus, the cervical pleura can drain into the axillary nodes, the costal pleura can drain into the intercostal and sternal nodes, the diaphragmatic pleura drains into the phrenic nodes, and the mediastinal pleura drains into the mediastinal nodes.

Pleural Effusions

Pleural effusion is an abnormal accumulation of fluid in the pleural space secondary to pleural or systemic disease. Normally only a small amount of fluid is present in the pleural space, although between 5 to 10 L of fluid is secreted daily by the parietal pleura and absorbed by the visceral pleura. Lymphatic drainage absorbs only 150 to 500 mL/d of this volume, but is responsible for protein absorption from the pleural space. Pleural effusions result from increased hydrostatic pressure in adjacent capillary beds, more negative intrapleural pressure, increased capillary permeability, decreased plasma oncotic pressure, and decreased or interrupted lymphatic drainage.

Pleural effusion can be asymptomatic or can present with pleuritic chest pain, dyspnea, and fever if secondary to an infectious process or with constant pain if secondary to malignancy.

The first sign of pleural effusion on an upright chest radiograph is blunting of the costophrenic angle; this requires more than 250 cc of fluid accumulation in order to show up on the radiograph. Larger amounts of fluid can be difficult to see on radiographs unless the patient is placed in the supine position. Lateral decubitus films can demonstrate these effusions in patients who cannot sit upright. Thoracentesis or tube thoracostomy are used for both diagnostic and therapeutic purposes.

Pleural effusions are either benign or malignant in origin and can be divided for diagnostic purposes into transudative or exudative categories. The distinction between transudates and exudates (Table 60.6) (1,76) is based on serum and pleural fluid ratios for lactate dehydrogenase (LDH) and pro-

Table 60.6. DIFFERENTIAL DIAGNOSIS OF PLEURAL EFFUSIONS

Transudative pleural effusions
  Congestive heart failure
  Pericardial disease
  Cirrhosis
  Nephrotic syndrome
  Peritoneal dialysis
  Superior vena cava obstruction
  Myxedema
  Pulmonary emboli
  Sarcoidosis
  Urinothorax
Exudative pleural effusions
  Neoplastic diseses
    Metastatic disease
    Mesothelioma
  Infectious diseases
    Bacterial infections
    Tuberculosis
    Fungal infections
    Viral infections
    Parasitic infections
  Pulmonary embolization
  Gastrointestinal disease
    Esophageal perforation
    Pancreatic disease
    Intraabdominal abscess
    Diaphragmatic hernia
    Postabdominal surgery
    Endoscopic variceal sclerotherapy
  Collagen vascular diseases
    Rheumatoid pleuritis
    Systemic lupus erythematosus
    Drug-induced lupus erythematosus
    Immunoblastic lymphadenopathy
    Sjögren syndrome
    Wegener granulomatosis
    Churg-Strauss syndrome
  Postcardiac injury syndrome
  Asbestos exposure
  Sarcoidosis
  Uremia
  Meigs' syndrome
  Yellow nail syndrome
  Drug-induced pleural disease
    Nitrofurantoin
    Dantrolene
    Methysergide
    Bromocriptine
    Procarbazine
    Amiodarone
  Trapped lung
  Radiotherapy
  Electric burns
  Urinary tract obstruction
  Iatrogenic injury
  Ovarian hyperstimulation syndrome
  Chylothorax
  Hemothorax

From Iannettoni MD, Orringer MB. Chest wall, pleura, mediastinum, and nonneoplastic lung disease. In: Greenfield LJ, Mulholland MW, Oldham KT, et al., eds. Surgery: scientific principles and practice, 2nd ed. Philadelphia: Lippincott–Raven, 1997:1440–1482, with permission.
Data from Light RW. The physiology of pleural fluid production and benign pleural effusion. In: Shields TW, eds. General thoracic surgery, 4th ed. Malvern, PA: Williams & Wilkins, 1994:676, with permission.

Table 60.7. CRITERIA FOR EXUDATIVE EFFUSIONS BASED ON RATIO OF PLEURAL FLUID PROTEIN AND LDH CONCENTRATIONS TO SERUM CONCENTRATION

Pleural Fluid/Serum

Protein/serum protein >0.5
LDH/serum LDH >0.6
Pleural LDH 1.67 times normal serum LDH

LDH, lactate dehydrogenase.

tein (Table 60.7). Transudative effusions form due to a change in the dynamics of pleural fluid absorption or secretion. Exudative effusions on the other hand result from changes in lymphatic vessel or pleural integrity and therefore are rich in protein. Effusions should also be tested routinely for the presence of bacteria and malignant cells. Measurement of pH, glucose, lipids, and amylase should also be done to help differentiate among the etiologies in Table 60.7.

Transudative Effusions

Transudative effusions tend to be benign. They usually do not become loculated and are free flowing. Common causes include systemic diseases such as congestive heart failure, cirrhosis, nephrotic syndrome, Meigs' syndrome, and hypoalbulinemia. Systemic conditions tend to result in bilateral effusions. Local processes that can cause transudative effusions include lobar collapse and pulmonary embolism. If these effusions remain untreated and become long-standing, they may develop exudative features. If an effusion is determined to be transudative, it can be treated usually by thoracentesis because of benign and treatable causes. Control of the systemic process that led to the effusion is of paramount importance to prevent fluid reaccumulation. If control of the systemic processes is suboptimal, which is often the case, then recurrent pleural effusions can be a problem. Repeat thoracentesis can be used, but the patient may need multiple treatments to control symptoms. Potential complications such as pneumothorax can be minimized with the use of ultrasound guidance at the time of drainage. However, loculations can eventually form with repeated thoracentesis from the pleural inflammatory response, and become infected secondarily. Alternatively, pleurodesis can be carried out via chest tube insertion or thoracoscopically by instilling doxycycline or talc into the pleural space. The resulting inflammation tends to obliterate the potential pleural space, and the effusion does not reaccumulate.

Exudative Effusions

The most common cause of exudative effusions is malignancy. Causes other than neoplastic disease include pulmonary infections that can result in empyemas, collagen vascular diseases, Dressler's syndrome, subdiaphragmatic intraperitoneal infections, and pulmonary infarction. The tumors most commonly involved with malignant pleural effusions are lung and breast cancer, lymphoma, ovarian, renal, and colon cancer.

Malignant Effusions

Most of these effusions are secondary to metastatic deposits on the pleura and malignant cells can be retrieved from the pleural fluid. Malignant effusions can also be caused by metastatic nodal treatment, causing lymphatic obstruction; thus these effusions can be free of malignant cells.

Small asymptomatic effusions do not require treatment once the diagnosis has been established. Symptomatic malignant effusions need intervention. This is best accomplished by addressing both the effusion and the neoplastic disease responsible for the effusion. Initially diagnostic and therapeutic thoracentesis should be used. Chemotherapy or irradiation can be used to treat the systemic malignancy. Radiotherapy is effective against many tumors causing lymphatic obstruction such as lymphoma, and lung and breast carcinomas. Radiation can take several weeks to relieve lymphatic obstruction and hence will not provide immediate symptomatic relief. Effusions that reaccumulate despite initial drainage and systemic therapy can be treated either by chest tube or thoracoscopic pleurodesis. Thoracoscopic pleurodesis has several advantages over that achieved with chest tube insertion. These include better distribution of the pleurodesing agent due to the ability to break up any loculations and to directly visualize the distribution. Also, biopsy of lesions can be done, if needed. Pleurodesis prevents recurrence of more than 90% of malignant effusions. Other management methods include pleuroperitoneal shunts in patients with recurrent effusions despite pleurodesis. Pleural and peritoneal catheters are inserted and connected to a valved pump chamber. The patient has to pump the chamber several times each day to decrease the effusion.

Complications of these interventions include pneumothorax, hemothorax, empyema, loculations, and lung entrapment due to inexpansile lung.

Empyema

Although empyema is not as common as during the preantibiotic era, it is still a disease that often requires surgical intervention. Empyema is an infection of the pleural space, most commonly secondary to a pneumonic infectious process. It can also occur because of mediastinal infections as in esophageal perforation, hematogenous spread due to sepsis from an infectious process at another site, or due to surgery or trauma. Common organisms isolated include a variety of anaerobic organisms, as well as streptococcal pneumococcus and other streptococcal organisms. Gram-negative organisms and fungi are also commonly isolated especially in trauma and immunosuppressed patients. Tuberculosis is seen more commonly in recent years due to the emergence of resistant strains and survival of a variety of patients who are immunocompromised. Cultures from patients who have been on antibiotics cultures may remain negative.

Empyemas are diagnosed with aspiration of pus from the pleural cavity, although not all empyemas will have this characteristic appearance. The aspirated fluid may be only cloudy. Diagnosis can be assisted by measuring the effusion pH, protein content, cell counts, LDH, glucose, and amylase, and with a Gram stain of the fluid.

Empyemas are classified into three phases: the exudative or acute phase, the fibrinopurulent or transitional phase, and the organizing or chronic phase. During the acute phase, the effusion has a low viscosity and cell count. The fibrinopurulent or transitional phase is characterized by increased viscosity and cellularity along with fibrin deposition on the pleural surfaces. The lung becomes less expandable, and loculations begin to form. During the organizing or chronic phase, there is ingrowth of capillaries and fibroblasts. At this stage the pleural fluid is viscous and composed mainly of sediment. There is pleural thickening, and the lung becomes entrapped. The chronic phase can be seen as early as 1 week after onset of symptoms. Symptoms start during the acute or transitional phase, and the patient complains of fever, cough, sputum production, chest pain, and sweats. Chest radiographs will demonstrate the pleural effusion, but CT scan will show the pleural effusion and the loculations. The extent of pleural thickening can be demonstrated on CT scan. Systemic therapy with antibiotics and drainage of the effusion is essential in all phases. Surgical intervention for drainage of the effusion varies according to the phase of the empyema.

Untreated empyema can decompress through the chest wall, it can involve the mediastinum, the pericardium, and the vertebrae, and result in CNS infections or in lung entrapment by the thick pleura.

Multiple procedures for open drainage procedures have been described. These include rib resection at the most dependent part of the effusion and thoracotomy with decortication depending on the patient's state of health and disease history.

Thoracentesis is the treatment of choice for acute-phase empyemas. The low-viscosity fluid of acute empyema can be drained in its entirety and the diagnosis verified.

If the fluid is too viscous for the small thoracentesis needles, then chest tube drainage of the effusion should be attempted. Chest tube drainage and antibiotics can be effective for acute- and transitional-phase empyemas. However, if significant loculations have already formed, then thoracostomy will also be ineffective, and operative drainage either open or via video-assisted thoracic surgery (VATS) is indicated. A trial of intrapleural fibrinolytic therapy can be tried prior to surgery. It can reduce the inflammatory peel and early loculations caused by fibrin. Fibrinolysis is less likely to be effective with more chronic empyemas. VATS has been shown to be effective for drainage of loculated effusions and for pleural débridement. Organized chronic empyemas, however, with extensive pleural thickening may be inadequately débrided with VATS, and open thoracotomy with decortication may be required for full lung expansion.

Wounds resulting from open pleural drainage can be packed open and managed like any other open wound. Management can be combined with chest tube drainage if visceral and parietal pleura are not adherent. A mobilized skin flap (an Eloesser flap) can be used to keep the cavity open. If the cavity is cleared of infection and systemic disease has been eradicated, then muscle flap closure can be used to obliterate the cavity (77–81).

Chylothorax

Chylothorax results when the contents of the thoracic duct accumulate into the pleural space. This accumulation can occur secondary to congenital causes, trauma (iatrogenic and otherwise), malignancies, infections, and thrombosis of the venous system (Table 60.8) (82).

Chylous fluid has high concentrations of fatty acids, cholesterol, and phospholipids, which gives chylous fluid its milky white color. The predominant cellular constituent is lymphocytes. Volume and content of fat within the chylous fluid varies with the composition of meals consumed. When the patient has not eaten for a few hours, chylous fluid will be clear.

The thoracic duct has a variable anatomic course. The most common anatomic relationship is found in approximately 50% of patients. The thoracic duct originates at the cisterna chyli between T10 and L3 and enters the chest through the aortic hiatus to the right of the aorta (Fig. 60.23) (82). It courses over the anterior surface of the vertebral bodies between the aorta and the azygous vein and posterior to the esophagus. At the level of the fifth thoracic vertebra the thoracic duct turns to the left as it passes posterior to the aortic arch. In the neck, it drains into the left jugulosubclavian junction. Two or more ducts can be present at any part of its course.

Table 60.8. ETIOLOGY OF CHYLOTHORAX

Congenital causes
   Atresia of the thoracic duct
   Thoracic duct-pleural fistual space
   Birth trauma
Traumatic causes
   Blunt
   Penetrating
   Surgery
      Cervical
         Excision of lymph nodes
         Radical dissection of the neck
      Thoracic
         Patent ductus arteriosus
         Coarctation of the aorta
         Vascular procedure reinvolving the origin of left subclavian
            artery
         Esophagectomy
         Sympathectomy
         Resection of thoracic aneurysm
         Resection of mediastinal tumors
         Left pneumonectomy
      Abdominal
         Sympathectomy
         Radical lymph node dissection
   Diagnostic procedures
      Translumbar arteriography
      Subclavian vein catheterization
      Left-sided heart catheterization
Neoplasms
Infections
   Tuberculous lymphadenitis
   Nonspecific mediastinitis
   Ascending lymphangitis
   Filariasis
Miscellaneous
   Venous thorombosis
      Left subclavian-jugular veins
      Superior vena cava
   Pulmonary lymphangiomatosis

From DeMeester TR, Lafontaine E. The pleura. In: Sabiston DC Jr, Spencer FC, eds. Surgery of the chest, 5th ed. Philadelphia: WB Saunders, 1990:456, with permission.

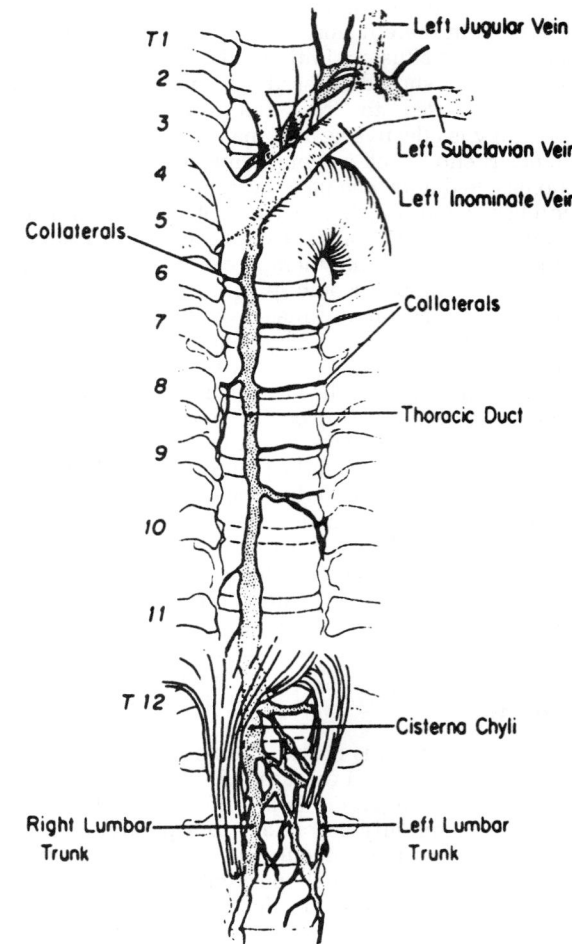

THORACIC DUCT

Figure 60.23. Schematic drawing of the most usual pattern and course of the thoracic duct. The single duct that enters the chest through the aortic hiatus between T12 and T10 is a relatively consistent finding and the usual site for surgical ligation. (From DeMeester TR, Lafontaine E. The pleura. In: Sabiston DC Jr, Spencer FC, eds. *Surgery of the chest,* 5th ed. Philadelphia: WB Saunders, 1990:444–497, with permission.)

The two most common causes of chylothorax are trauma and malignancy. Blunt trauma can result in chylothorax secondary to hyperextension of the spine and rupture of the duct, usually just above the diaphragm. Penetrating injury is usually associated with injuries of the aorta or esophagus. Iatrogenic trauma can occur during surgeries of the esophagus, aorta, and subclavian artery. Importantly, injury below the fifth thoracic vertebra most commonly results in right-sided chylothorax, while injury above this level results in left-sided chylothorax.

Both benign and malignant lesions can result in chylothorax. Malignant etiologies are responsible for more than half of nontraumatic effusions in adults. Thoracic and abdominal malignancies can invade the thoracic duct with rupture of the duct due to erosion or obstruction. The resulting effusions can be unilateral or bilateral. Lymphoma is the most common malignancy causing chylothorax. Of the benign lesions lymphangiomas, cystic hygromas and pulmonary lymphangiomatosis have most commonly been associated with chylous effusions.

Symptoms of chylothorax mimic those of other pleural effusions and include shortness of breath, chest pain, fatigue, and symptoms of the disease that caused the effusion such as an infectious or neoplastic disease. In addition, nutritional deficiencies can occur due to loss of fat, protein, and vitamins. Replacing the volume drained is essential to avoid volume depletion as well as to avoid nutritional deficiencies, which can present clinical challenges. Symptoms of pericardial tamponade can occur with chylous leaks into the pericardium.

Chylothorax is suspected when aspiration of the effusion reveals a milky type of effusion. Confirmation of a chylous effusion is aided by clearing of the effusion when fat is extracted; alternatively Sudan III stain can be used to confirm the presence of fat globules. The cell count reveals a predominance of lymphocytes, and this is quite helpful diagnostically. Triglyceride levels are very useful in diagnosing chylous effusion. Effusions with a triglyceride level greater that 110 mg/dL have a 99% chance of being chylous, while those with a level less than 50 mg/dL have only a 5% chance of being chylous. Administering cream to the patient and observing the change in the character of the drainage can confirm the diagnosis in certain patients.

The initial management of chylous effusions consists of lung reexpansion via chest tube drainage and nutritional support with volume replacement of the daily losses. A fat-free enteral diet with medium-chain triglycerides that are absorbed directly by the venous system can be used to decrease the output of the effusion. Intravenous alimentation can also result in an even further decrease in the daily output of the effusion. Nonoperative management can be attempted for up to 2 weeks.

Malignant causes of the effusion have to be addressed as well. Radiation is particularly useful for chylous effusions secondary to lymphomas. Surgical intervention has been advocated for effusions not responding to a 2-week trial of nonoperative management. Surgical approaches include pleuroperitoneal shunts, VATS or open thoracotomy with repair, fibrin glue application, or ligation of the thoracic duct. Operation at the same side as the effusion is usually preferred. Postoperative effusions are best approached with right-sided approaches with ligation of the duct above the diaphragm. Administration of cream preoperatively helps in identifying the site of the injury during surgery. Pleuroperitoneal shunts have been advocated to avoid the nutritional and immunologic sequelae of a chylous leak as well as to reduce hospital length of stay. The advent of VATS, however, has popularized earlier operative treatment for patients who do not appear to respond immediately to treatment. VATS thoracic duct clipping, pleurodesis, and fibrin glue application have all been described and may result in resolution of the effusion and hospital discharge within 10 days. Another technique that is described with increasing frequency in the management of chylothorax is the administration of somatostatin. Subcutaneous (SQ) injections of somatostatin along with the parenteral nutrition have been used with success to treat chylous effusions in patients who did not respond to initial parenteral nutrition. Percutaneous embolization of the thoracic duct has been attempted and has been successful in selected patients with demonstrable thoracic duct leak (83–85).

Pneumothorax

Pneumothorax is described as the presence of air in the chest, specifically the pleural space, resulting in compression of the lung (Fig. 60.24) (1). Pneumothoraces are either spontaneous or acquired. Spontaneous pneumothoraces can be further subdivided into primary or secondary. A primary spontaneous pneumothorax refers to pneumothoraces occurring in patients without known underlying pulmonary disease, while the secondary occurs in patients with a known predisposing process (86). Acquired pneumothoraces can occur as a complication of numerous procedures such as central venous access, thoracentesis, mechanical ventilation, surgery, or diagnostic lung biopsy (Table 60.9 (82).

Lung parenchyma injury with free egress of air into the pleural space results in loss of the negative intrapleural space that is needed for lung inflation. The lung begins to collapse with compromise of the ventilation resulting. Arterial hypoxemia can occur with 50% collapse of the lung due to the continuing perfusion of poorly ventilated lung. The extent of hypoxemia seen varies according to the underlying condition of the lung. Increasing positive intrapleural pressure is transmitted to mediastinal structures, and pressures as low as 15 to 20 cm H_2O can compromise venous return to the heart with decreasing cardiac output and hemodynamic collapse. These physiologic sequelae are collectively called tension pneumothorax. Failure to immediately address a tension pneumothorax results in death.

Patients with pneumothorax most commonly complain of chest pain, usually pleuritic. This can occur even with small pneumothoraces. Dyspnea is not usually seen in smaller pneumothoraces, but rather with larger pneumothoraces. Other symptoms such as orthopnea and cough with occasional hemoptysis are also seen.

The physical exam is usually normal with small pneumothoraces. With larger ones, decreased breath sounds are evident along with decreased chest wall motion. Percussion reveals hyperresonance. Cyanosis can be seen especially in patients with underlying lung disease. Subcutaneous emphysema can be present in patients with traumatic pneumothoraces.

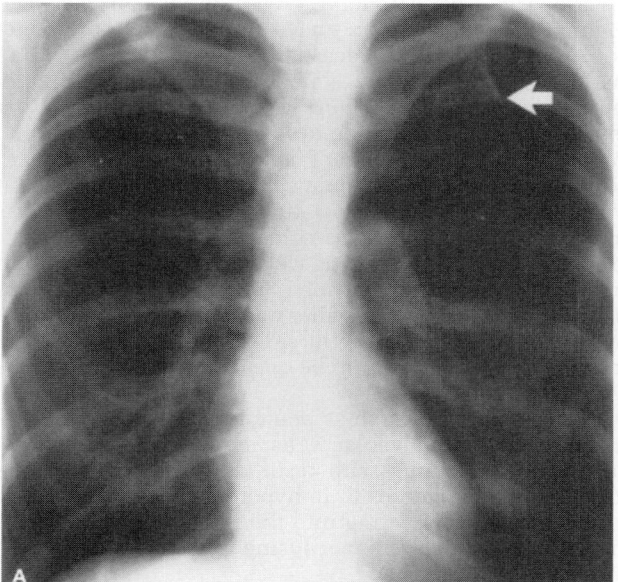
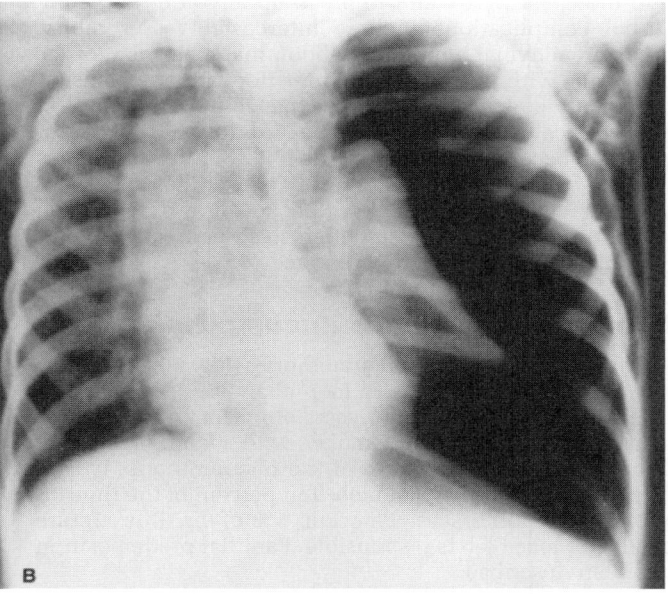

Figure 60.24. *(A)* Forty percent left-sided spontaneous pneumothorax *(arrow)*. *(B)* Progression of simple pneumothorax to a tension pneumothorax, showing the characteristic radiographic findings—virtual collapse of the entire involved lung, shift of the mediastinum to the contralateral side, and compression of the contralateral lung. Subcutaneous air dissecting along the left chest wall is also evident. (From Iannettoni MD, Orringer MB. Chest wall, pleura, mediastinum, and nonneoplastic lung disease. In: Greenfield LJ, Mulholland MW, Oldham KT, et al., eds. *Surgery: scientific principles and practice,* 2nd ed. Philadelphia: Lippincott–Raven, 1997:1440–1482, with permission.)

Table 60.9. CLASSIFICATION OF PNEUMOTHORAX

Spontaneous
  Primary: no underlying pathology
  Secondary: underlying pulmonary disorders
  Catamenial
  Neonatal
Traumatic
  Iatrogenic: thoracentesis, mechanical ventilation, central vein
    catheterization, postoperative
  Trauma: blunt, penetrating
Diagnostic
  Air-contrast study of pleuropulmonary pathology

From DeMeester TR, Lafontaine E. The pleura. In: Sabiston DC Jr, Spencer FC, eds. Surgery of the chest, 5th ed. Philadelphia: WB Saunders, 1990:456, with permission.

Posteroanterior (PA) chest radiographs can demonstrate the pneumothorax as a hyperlucent area with an absence of pulmonary markings. Depending on x-ray presentation, the pneumothoraces can be classified according to size into small (<20%), moderate (20% to 40%), and large (>40%). Displacement of the mediastinum and diaphragm signal the presence of tension pneumothorax. The PA radiograph may miss a large anterior pneumothorax. It can be readily seen, however, on lateral films. In addition, if a pneumothorax is suspected but not evident on PA and lateral films, an end expiratory film may facilitate the diagnosis. Patients with chronic obstructive pulmonary disease (COPD) may have apical bullae misdiagnosed as a pneumothorax due to a similar appearance on chest x-ray and resultant chest tube insertion into the bullae. Chest CT can be used to differentiate between these conditions.

Chest tube insertion to the apex of the hemithorax has been traditionally used for decompression of a pneumothorax and lung expansion. The usual approach is at the fourth, fifth, or sixth intercostal space in the midaxillary line. Digital palpation should be used to confirm entry into the chest cavity and to break up any adhesions. Potential complications include intercostal vessel injury, lung parenchymal injury, intraabdominal placement of the chest tube with visceral injury, infection, and reexpansion pulmonary edema after rapid reexpansion of the lung.

Needle catheter (thoracic vent aspiration) of pneumothoraces is becoming more popular (87). Similar principles to that of chest tube drainage apply except that the size of the catheter is much smaller. Special one-way Heimlich valves are also available so patients can be treated as outpatients after initial decompression.

Primary Spontaneous Pneumothorax

Primary spontaneous pneumothorax (Fig. 60.24) (1) is a disease of young adults with more than 85% of cases seen in patients younger than 40 years old. The typical patient is tall, thin, and perhaps a smoker, with a family history of pneumothoraces. The cause of the pneumothorax is rupture of a subpleural apical bleb. Ten percent of the time bilateral pneumothoraces can occur; 5% of the time rupture of a lower lobe bleb is responsible. Familial predisposition has been described.

Patients present with acute onset of chest pain that can subside within 24 hours despite persistence of the pneumothorax. Typical signs and symptoms of pneumothorax are present and include tachycardia, and decreased breath sounds if the pneumothorax is large enough. Chest radiographs confirm the diagnosis and chest CT can detect the blebs.

Treatment of primary spontaneous pneumothorax depends on its size and whether or not it is a first-time event. Healthy patients with small, first-time pneumothoraces have numerous options. They can be observed if minimally symptomatic, or they can have the pneumothorax decompressed by aspiration or chest tube insertion. If observation is chosen, a repeat chest film within 4 hours is needed to document progression. Reabsorption of air occurs at a rate of 1% to 2% per day. Persistent air leak occurs in fewer than 20% of patients.

With moderate-size pneumothoraces, aspiration or chest tube insertion is needed to ensure full reexpansion, whereas patients with a large-size pneumothorax should be decompressed with a chest tube. A review of 11 studies over 30 years comprising 1,242 patients treated for primary spontaneous pneumothorax with needle aspiration or chest tube insertion demonstrated a 30% recurrence rate (88). Patients who had a persistent leak or recurrence following initial aspiration had a 72% chance of recurrence.

Indications for surgery are persistent air leak, bilateral pneumothoraces, tension pneumothorax, recurrence, occupations involving acute environmental pressure changes (such as pilots and divers), and remote accessibility of medical care. The procedure of choice is VATS with stapling of the bleb responsible for the pneumothorax. Pleurodesis should be performed at the same time so that recurrences will be reduced, and if one does occur it will result in a small pneumothorax. Complications are prolonged air leak or recurrence from missed blebs, incomplete lung expansion, bleeding, or Horner's syndrome. Recurrence after VATS has been reported to be as low as 4% (89,90).

Secondary Spontaneous Pneumothorax

Secondary spontaneous pneumothorax occurs in patients who have underlying localized or generalized lung disease. These patients tend to be older, usually between 45 and 65 years of age, and have compromised lung function. Small pneumothoraces, therefore, can be symptomatic in this population. Numerous causes of secondary pneumothoraces exist. COPD is the most common; other common etiologies include cystic fibrosis and interstitial lung disease and infections (Table 60.10) (82). Malignant disease such as bronchogenic carcinoma can also present with a pneumothorax. Metastatic disease such as sarcomas and especially osteogenic sarcomas in children are known to predispose to this event as well. Catamenial pneumothorax occurs in women between 30 and 40 years old, usually within the first 3 days after onset of menses, and most commonly involves the right side. Pulmonary or pleural endometriosis is thought to be one of the etiologies of this type of pneumothorax.

A disease process such as pneumonia causes a progressive destruction of alveolar walls and decrease of the elastic recoil of the lung with resulting slow collapse. Obstructive disease can result in hyperexpansion of distal air spaces with air dissecting into the interstitial tissues, the hilum, and mediastinum, causing pneumomediastinum and pneumothorax.

Patients may present with sudden onset of dyspnea, cough, and chest pain. However, it may be difficult to distinguish these symptoms from an exacerbation of the underlying pulmonary disease. The size of the pneumothorax that results in significant symptoms depends on the severity of the underlying disease process and pulmonary function reserve that each patient may have. As with pri-

Table 60.10. CAUSES OF SECONDARY SPONTANEOUS PNEUMOTHORAX

Airway disease
  Bullous disease
  Chronic obstructive pulmonary disease
  Asthma
  Cyst (congenital)
  Cystic fibrosis
Interstitial disease
  Idiopathic pulmonary fibrosis
  Eosinophilic granuloma
  Sarcoidosis
  Tuberous sclerosis
  Collagen-vascular diseases
Infections
  Anaerobic pneumonia
  Staphylococcal pneumonia
  Gram-negative pneumonia
  Lung abscess
  Actinomycosis
  Nocardiosis
  Tuberculosis
  Atypical mycobacteria
Neoplasms
  Primary
  Metastatic
Other diseases
  Endometriosis
  Ehler-Danlos syndrome
  Pulmonary embolism
  Marfan's syndrome

From DeMeester TR, Lafontaine E. The pleura. In: Sabiston DC Jr, Spencer FC, eds. Surgery of the chest, 5th ed. Philadelphia: WB Saunders, 1990:456, with permission.

mary pneumothorax, tension pneumothorax can also occur in these patients with the aforementioned clinical signs and symptoms.

Chest radiographs are the first diagnostic test obtained. Both PA and lateral views should be obtained. Occasionally in patients with apical bullae, the diagnosis may be quite difficult to make and chest CT scan will be needed. Unlike patients with a primary pneumothorax, these patients are usually quite symptomatic and hypoxic. Observation is rarely a viable option. Patients can be treated with aspiration or chest tube insertion. Due to loss of elastic recoil, initial lung reexpansion may not be complete and may require more time to achieve than primary pneumothorax. Approximately two thirds of secondary pneumothoraces resolve within 1 week of chest tube drainage. Patients who have persistent air leaks or recurrent pneumothorax, patients with pneumonectomy and pneumothorax, and patients with continued pulmonary functional compromise despite chest tube drainage should undergo surgery.

Resections of bullae, pleurodesis, and parietal pleurectomy are the main goals of operative intervention. These goals can be achieved with open thoracotomy or VATS. VATS is preferable due to less postoperative compromise in these patients. Double-lumen intubation can be done in most of these patients. Resection of the bullae decreases the chance of a future pneumothorax, whereas pleurodesis decreases the chance that a recurrence will be of a significant size should one occur. Pleurodesis can be done via pleural abrasion, talc, or parietal pleurectomy. Although pleurodesis is not a contraindication to future lung transplantation, aggressive approaches such as parietal pleurectomy are best avoided. Patients who are not able to tolerate single-lung ventilation for VATS undergo open thoracotomy (90).

Mesothelioma

Mesothelioma is a rare and very aggressive, primary malignant pleural tumor. It originates from the mesothelial cells that line the parietal and visceral pleura. Approximately 3,000 new cases occur in the United States annually. The most significant risk factor for developing mesothelioma is exposure to asbestos. Other environmental risk factors have been reported such as exposure to other naturally occurring fibers, radiation exposure, and possibly simian virus 40 (SV 40) (Table 60.11) (91). Asbestos fibers are divided into amphibole (five types) and serpentine fibers. The amphibole fibers are most clearly associated with mesothelioma. Serpentine fibers are associated with lung cancer. While smoking and asbestos exposure have a synergistic effect in the development of lung cancer, there is no association of smoking with the development of mesothelioma. Before its ban in the U.S. in 1986, the industries that used asbestos included ship-

Table 60.11. NONASBESTOS CAUSES OF MESOTHELIOMA

Agent	Species Tumor Observed in or Induced in:
Naturally occurring mineral fibers	
Zeolites (eronite)	Human, rat
Minerals	
Nickel	Rat
Silica powder	Rat
Beryllium	Rat, ?human
Radiation	Human, rat
Organic chemicals	
Polyurethane, polysilicone	Rat
Sterigmatocystin (aflatoxin B1-related compound)	
Ethylene oxide	Rat
N-methyl-N-nitrosourea	Guinea pig
N-methyl-N-nitrosourethane	Mouse
3-Methylcholanthrene	Mouse
Methyl nitrosamine	Rat
1-Nitroso-5,6-dihydrouracil	Rat
Diethylstilbestrol	Monkey
Stilboestrol	Dog
3,4,5-Trimetholxycinnamaldehyde	Rat
Mineral oil	Human
Liquid paraffin	Human
Viruses	
MC 29 avian leukosis virus	Chicken
SV 40	Hamster
Chronic inflammation	
Recurrent lung infections	Human
Tuberculous pleuritis	Human
Recurrent diverticulitis	Human
Familial Mediterranean fever	Human
Nonspecific industrial exposure	
Shoe industry workers	Human
Petrochemical-oil industry workers	Human
Stone cutters	Human
Leather factory or textile workers	Human
Occupations involving exposure to copper, nickel, fiberglass, rubber or glass dust	Human
Cocarcinogens	
3-Methylcholanthrene-asbestos	Rat
Radiation-asbestos	Rat
N-methyl-N-nitrosourea-asbestos	Rat
Hereditary predisposition	Human

From Rusch VW. Diffuse malignant mesothelioma. In: Shields TW, LoCicero J III, Ponn RB, eds. General thoracic surgery, 5th ed. Philadelphia: Lippincott Williams & Wilkins, 2000:768, with permission.

Table 60.12. HISTOLOGIC CLASSIFICATION OF MESOTHELIOMA

Epithelial
   Tubulopapillary
   Epithelioid
   Glandular
   Large cell (giant cell)
   Small cell
   Adenoid-cystic
   Signet ring
Sarcomatoid (fibrous, sarcomatous, mesenchymal)
Mixed epithelial-sarcomatoid (biphasic)
Transitional
Desmoplastic
Localized fibrous mesothelioma

From Hammar SP, Bolen JW. Pleural neoplasms. In: Dail DH, Hammar SP, eds. Pulmonary pathology. New York: Springer, 1988:979, with permission.

building, construction, brake pad manufacturers, and others. Because these materials are still in use in making floor tiles, paint, and piping to car parts (92), shipping, construction, car repair, and railroad workers are still at risk for exposure, as are people living or working in buildings constructed before 1987. Worldwide exposure continues to be a serious concern.

The latency period between exposure and disease is quite long; the peak incidence for mesothelioma is during the sixth decade of life. Most cases are due to occupational exposure, and therefore mesothelioma is most common in men. Young patients have been seen with the disease including children of men who worked in occupations at risk.

Mesotheliomas can be classified based on the histologic type (Table 60.12) (93). The types seen are the epithelial, sarcomatous, or mixed. Epithelial histology is present in half of patients; mixed and sarcomatous histology follow in frequency. Mesothelioma can present as a localized or diffuse tumor, with diffuse tumors more common. Mesothelioma can be confused with metastatic adenocarcinoma. Immunohistochemistry and electron microscopy lead to a definitive diagnosis (Figs. 60.25 to 60.27) (94).

Mesotheliomas usually cause nonspecific symptoms in the early stages. These include chest pain and shortness of breath, usually due to the presence of a pleural effusion. Pleural effusion is present in the vast majority of patients at some point of their clinical course. Weight loss, fever, cough, hemoptysis, and anorexia are other signs and symptoms. Paraneoplastic syndromes such as hypoglycemia, hypercalcemia, and a syndrome of inappropriate antidiuretic hormone (ADH) have been occasionally reported.

Radiographically, pleural effusion is the most common sign of these tumors. If the disease is advanced, pleural thickening can be visible on chest radiograph. Chest CT scan or MRI are more sensitive in assessing pleural thickening and detecting pleural-based masses. Transdiaphragmatic involvement, neurovascular involvement, and mediastinal invasion are best assessed with MRI. Echocardiography can also assist in assessing pericardial involvement. Recently, positron-emission tomography (PET) scanning has been evaluated for assessment of metastatic disease and has been shown to be more sensitive than either CT or MRI.

Pleural fluid can be obtained for cytologic and cytogenetic analysis and yields a diagnosis of mesothelioma in half of the cases. Percutaneous pleural biopsy provides enough tissue for diagnosis in about one third of patients. The tissue sample obtained is usually not enough to perform immunohistochemistry, or necessary electron microscopy studies.

For biopsy, thoracoscopy has a diagnostic yield of more than 80% and does not commit the patient to a major procedure, while providing enough tissue for all the studies needed. In cases where the pleural space has been obliterated, thoracoscopy is not feasible and the procedure can be converted to an open biopsy. Half the patients are diagnosed within 8 weeks of onset of their symptoms if cytology is positive; however, if the cytology is negative, diagnosis is delayed, averaging 12 weeks from onset of symptoms.

Once diagnosis is confirmed, staging of the patient and treatment options present challenges in this disease. Several staging systems have been published, but are without universal acceptance. The commonly used staging systems include the Butchart (Table 60.13) (95),

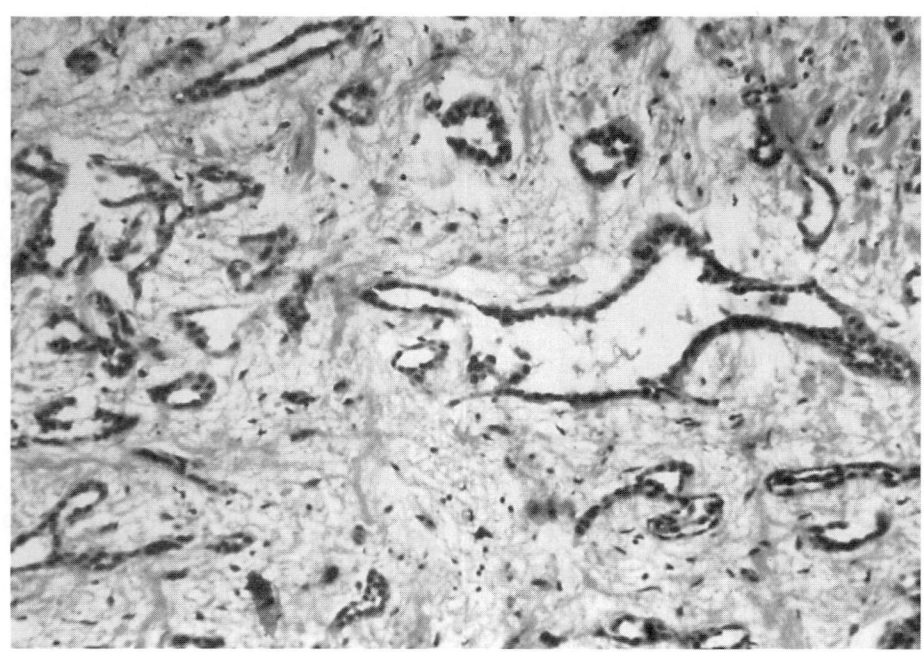

Figure 60.25. Histologic examination of a 54-year-old man with a history of asbestos exposure reveals epithelioid-type mesothelioma. (From Flores RM, Sugarbaker DJ. Malignant mesothelioma of the pleural space. *Ann Thorac Surg* 2000;70:306, with permission.)

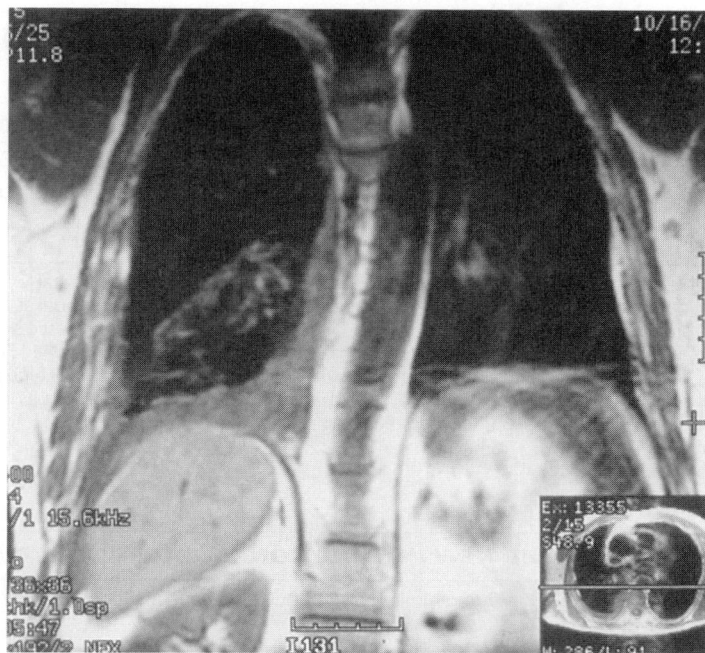

Figure 60.26. Magnetic resonance imaging of the patient in Fig. 60.25 shows a large amount of tumor within the pleural space and into the diaphragmatic sulcus with no evidence of extension outside the hemithorax. (From Flores RM, Sugarbaker DJ. Malignant mesothelioma of the pleural space. *Ann Thorac Surg* 2000;70:306, with permission.)

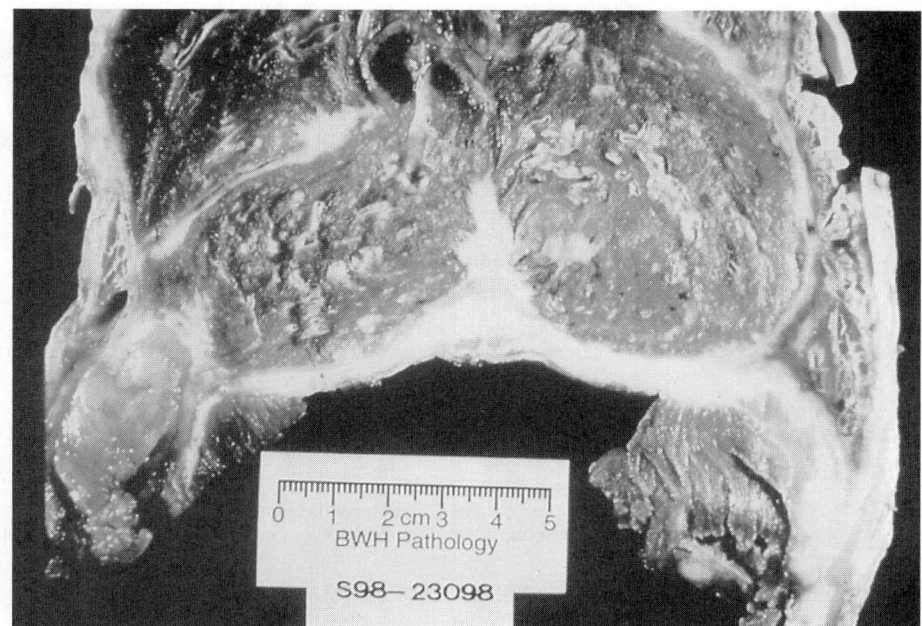

Figure 60.27. The gross pathologic specimen of the patient in Fig. 60.25 following extrapleural pneumonectomy demonstrates an intact pleural envelope, inferiorly diaphragmatic muscle fibers remain intact, and tumor present within the pleural space with lung parenchymal invasion. The patient went on to receive chemotherapy and radiation. (From Flores RM, Sugarbaker DJ. Malignant mesothelioma of the pleural space. *Ann Thorac Surg* 2000;70:306, with permission.)

Table 60.13. **THE BUTCHART STAGING SYSTEM**

Stage	Definition
I	Within the capsule of the parietal pleura: ipsilateral pleura, lung, pericardium, diaphragm
II	Invading chest wall or mediastinum: esophagus, heart, opposite pleura
	Positive lymph nodes within the chest
III	Through diaphragm to peritoneum; opposite pleura
	Positive lymph nodes outside the chest
IV	Distant blood-borne metastases

Modified from Butchart EG, Ashcroft T, Barnsley WC, et al. Pleuropneumonectomy in the management of diffuse malignant mesothelioma of the pleura: experience with 29 patients. Thorax 1976;31:15; with permission.

Table 60.14. **THE REVISED BRIGHAM AND WOMEN'S HOSPITAL STAGING SYSTEM**

Stage	Definition
I	Disease completely resected within the capsule of the parietal pleura without adenopathy: ipsilateral pleura, lung, pericardium, diaphragm, or chest-wall disease limited to previous biopsy sites.
II	All of stage I with positive resection margins and/or intrapleural adenopathy.
III	Local extension of disease into chest wall or mediastinum; heart, or through diaphragm, peritoneum; or with extrapleural lymph node involvement.
IV	Distant metastatic disease.

Note: Butchart stage II and III (95) patients are combined into stage III. Stage I represents resectable patients with negative nodes. Stage II patients are resectable but have positive nodal status.

From Sugarbaker DJ, Strauss GM, Lynch TJ, et al. Node status has prognostic significance in the multimodality therapy of diffuse, malignant mesothelioma. J Clin Oncol 1993;11:1172–1178; and Sugarbaker DJ, Flores RM, Jaklitsch MT, et al. Resection margins, extrapleural nodal status, and cell type determine postoperative long-term survival in trimodality therapy of malignant pleural mesothelioma; results in 183 patients. Thorac Cardiovasc Surg 1999;117:54–65, with permission.

Table 60.15. **THE NEW INTERNATIONAL STAGING SYSTEM (IMIG)**

T1	1a	Tumor limited to the ipsilateral parietal pleura, including mediastinal and diaphragmatic pleura; no involvement of the visceral pleura
	1b	Tumor involving the ipsilateral parietal pleura, including mediastinal and diaphragmatic pleura; scattered foci of tumor also involving the visceral pleura
T2		Tumor involving each of the ipsilateral pleural surfaces (parietal, mediastinal, diaphragmatic, and visceral pleura) with at least one of the following features: Involvement of diaphragmatic muscle Confluent visceral pleural tumor (including the fissures) or extension of tumor from visceral pleura into the underlying pulmonary parenchyma
T3		Locally advanced but potentially resectable tumor; tumor involving all of the ipsilateral pleural surfaces (parietal, mediastinal, diaphragmatic, and visceral pleura) with at least one of the following features: Involvement of the endothoracic fascia Extension into the mediastinal fat Solitary, completely resectable focus of tumor extending into the soft tissues of the chest wall Nontransmural involvement of the pericardium
T4		Locally advanced technically unresectable tumor; tumor involving all of the ipsilateral pleural surfaces (parietal, mediastinal, diaphragmatic, and visceral) with at least one of the following features: Diffuse extension or multifocal masses of tumor in the chest wall, with or without associated rib destruction Direct transdiaphragmatic extension of tumor to the peritoneum Direct extension of tumor to the contralateral pleura Direct extension of tumor to one or more mediastinal organs Direct extension of tumor into the spine Tumor extending through to the internal surface of the pericardium with or without a pericardial effusion; or tumor involving the myocardium

N—LYMPH NODES

NX	Regional lymph nodes cannot be assessed
N0	No regional lymph node metastases
N1	Metastases in the ipsilateral bronchopulmonary or hilar lymph nodes
N2	Metastases in the subcarinal or ipsilateral mediastinal lymph nodes, including the ipsilateral internal mammary nodes
N3	Metastases in the contralateral mediastinal, contralateral internal mammary, ipsilateral, or contralateral supraclavicular lymph nodes

M—METASTASES

MX	Presence of distant metastases cannot be assessed
M0	No distant metastasis
M1	Distant metastasis present

Stage	Description
I	
Ia	T1aN0M0
Ib	T1bN0M0
II	T2N0M0
III	Any T3M0
	Any N1M0
	Any N2M0
IV	Any T4
	Any N3
	Any M1

From Rusch VW, the International Mesothelioma Interest Group. A proposed new international TNM staging system for malignant pleural mesothelioma. Chest 1995;108:1122–1128, with permission.

Brigham and Women's Hospital (Table 60.14) (96,97), and the new International TNM Staging system (Table 60.15) (98) proposed by the International Mesothelioma Interest Group.

Treatment ranges from supportive care to multimodality therapy including aggressive surgery, chemotherapy, and radiotherapy. Survival with supportive care ranges from 4 to 12 months. Single-modality therapy has been ineffective whether it is radiation, chemotherapy, or surgery (99). Multimodality therapy that includes aggressive surgery has shown survival benefit in particular patients and some long-term survivors. The surgical procedures used in the management of mesothelioma include pleurodesis, pleurectomy with decortication, and extrapleural pneumonectomy (EPP). Surgery should be accompanied by chemotherapy and radiation in a multimodality setting. Cytoreductive surgery such as pleurectomy/decortication can provide palliation of the dyspnea secondary to lung encasement and chest wall pain. Pleurectomy with decortication followed by chemoradiation can result in a median survival as high as 21 months (100,101). In the authors' experience, EPP is the procedure of choice whenever feasible because it is the most effective cytoreductive surgery, and with experienced surgeons EPP has a mortality rate close to 4%. EPP includes the *en bloc* removal of the affected lung, diaphragm, pericardium, and parietal pleura. Approximately one quarter of the patients are candidates for EPP. Peritoneal invasion should be ruled out before undertaking EPP. EPP by itself does not offer a survival advantage. However, when followed by chemoradiation, long-term survival is reported.

Numerous independent predictors of survival have been demonstrated in patients treated with EPP in the multimodality setting. They include age less than 55, good performance status, epithelial histology, early stage disease, negative resection margins, and absence of lymph node involvement (97). Results in 183 patients treated over 17 years were reviewed at the Brigham and Women's Hospital. These patients underwent EPP with postoperative chemotherapy (carboplatin/paclitaxel) and radiation (55 Gy). This series reported a 5-year survival of 46% with a median survival of 51 months for the subset of patients who had epithelial-type tumors with negative resection margins and absence of nodal involvement (97).

For the patients who are not candidates for multimodality therapy with EPP, treatment options are being investigated; they include intracavitary chemotherapy, photodynamic therapy, and gene therapy (102–104).

MEDIASTINUM

Anatomy

The mediastinum is bound by the thoracic inlet, the parietal pleura laterally, the diaphragm inferiorly, the sternum anteriorly, and the vertebrae posteriorly. The mediastinum is arbitrarily divided into anterosuperior, middle, and posterior (Fig. 60.28) (1). The anterosuperior mediastinum is anterior to the pericardium and its reflection over the great vessels. The middle mediastinum is bound by the pericardial reflection. The posterior mediastinum is posterior to the pericardium and the pericardial reflection.

The anterosuperior mediastinum contains the thymus, the aortic arch and the great vessels, the upper trachea and upper esophagus, and lymphatics. Occasionally, ectopic parathyroid masses can be found here, arising be-

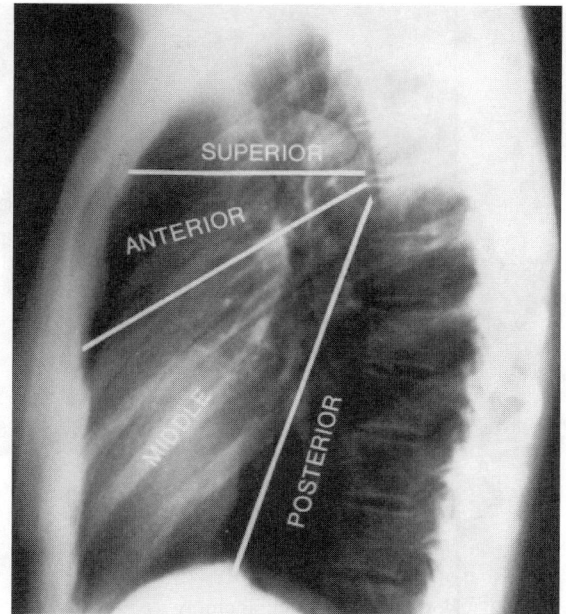

Figure 60.28. Compartments of the mediastinum. The superior and inferior mediastinum are separated by a line drawn from the sternomanubrial junction anteriorly on a lateral chest radiograph to the lower edge of the fourth vertebral body posteriorly. The inferior mediastinum is divided into anterior, middle, and posterior compartments by the pericardium. (From Iannettoni MD, Orringer MB. Chest wall, pleura, mediastinum, and nonneoplastic lung disease. In: Greenfield LJ, Mulholland MW, Oldham KT, et al., eds. *Surgery: scientific principles and practice,* 2nd ed. Philadelphia: Lippincott–Raven, 1997:1440–1482, with permission)

cause of the common embryologic origin with the thymus. The thyroid can also extend into this region when it enlarges. The middle mediastinum contains the heart, the pericardium, the tracheal bifurcation, the bronchi and their nodes, and the ascending aorta. The posterior mediastinum contains the esophagus, the thoracic duct, the azygous vein, the descending aorta, and the sympathetic, parasympathetic, and intercostals nerves (Table 60.16) (Fig. 60.29) (1,105).

Table 60.16. LOCATION OF PRIMARY MEDIASTINAL MASSES IN ADULTS AND CHILDREN

Location	Type of mass
Anterosuperior mediastinum	Thymoma
	Lymphoma
	Germ cell tumor
	Lymphangioma
	Hemangioma
	Lipoma
	Carcinoma
	Thyroid adenoma
	Parathyroid adenoma
Middle mediastinum	Pericardial cyst
	Bronchogenic cyst
	Lymphoma
Posterior mediastinum	Neurogenic tumor
	Enteric cyst

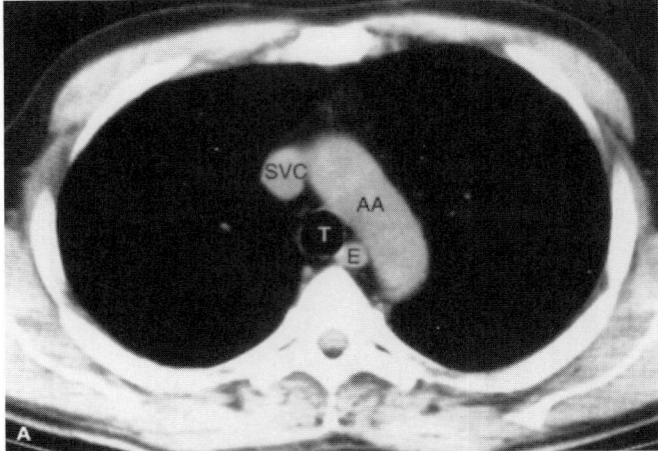

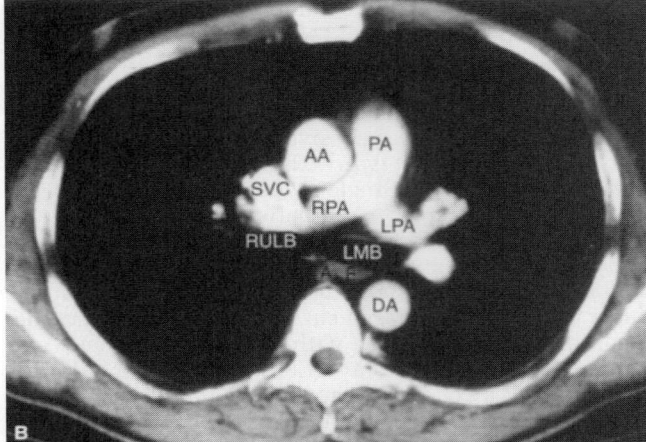

Figure 60.29. Normal mediastinal anatomy as shown with computed tomography (CT) scans. *(A)* Scan at level of the aortic arch and midtrachea. T, trachea; E, esophagus; AA, aortic arch; SVC, superior vena cava. *(B)* Scan at level of carina. RULB, right upper lobe bronchus; LMB, left mainstem bronchus; AA, ascending aorta; DA, descending aorta; A, azygos vein; E, esophagus; SVC, superior vena cava; PA, main pulmonary artery; LPA and RPA, left and right pulmonary arteries. *(C)* Scan at the level of the left atrium. LA, left atrium; RA, right atrium; LVOT, left ventricular outflow tract; RV, right ventricle; A, azygos vein; E, esophagus; DA, descending aorta. (From Iannettoni MD, Orringer MB. Chest wall, pleura, mediastinum, and nonneoplastic lung disease. In: Greenfield LJ, Mulholland MW, Oldham KT, et al., eds. *Surgery: scientific principles and practice,* 2nd ed. Philadelphia: Lippincott–Raven, 1997:1440–1482, with permisson.)

Mediastinal Masses

Epidemiology and Incidence

Numerous types of tumors can occur in the mediastinum. Tumor type varies by location and by patient age. When combining pediatric and adult populations, neurogenic tumors are the most common, followed by thymomas, cysts, and lymphomas. In the pediatric population, posterior mediastinal neurogenic tumors are more common, whereas in adults anterior mediastinal tumors predominate. In addition, the neurogenic tumors in children tend to be malignant (neuroblastomas), while the neuro-genic tumors in adults tend to be benign (106–108). In children, the most common mediastinal tumor is neuroblastoma followed by lymphoma and germ cell tumor. Other benign lesions can occur such as cysts of pericardial, aerodigestive, or thymic origin (109–116) (Table 60.17) (116).

Series reporting adult mediastinal masses show a distinctive histologic profile (117–122). The anterior mediastinal lesions are more common in adults, with thymomas most common, followed by lymphomas and germ cell tumors. One common feature of these tumors in both adults and children is the increasing incidence of malignancy. Series comparing patients from two different periods have shown that the incidence of malignancy has more than doubled in recent years without any clear etiology (123,124).

Symptoms and Signs

Symptoms at the time of diagnosis vary depending on the location and size of the mediastinal lesions (107,115,123). More than half of the lesions are symptomatic. Symptomatic lesions have a higher probability of malignancy. The patients' complaints may include chest pain, dyspnea and cough, dysphagia, hoarseness, Horner's syndrome, superior vena cava (SVC) syndrome, palpitations, malaise, weakness and weight loss, back pain, and signs of spinal cord compression. Some mediastinal tumors have endocrine activity that may cause symptoms of hyperthyroidism, hyperparathyroidism, hypoglycemia, or paroxysmal malignant hypertension suggestive of pheochromocytoma.

Table 60.17. MEDIASTINAL TUMORS IN CHILDREN

Type of tumor	Incidence reported in series (%)
Neurogenic	35
Lymphoma	25
Germ-cell	11
Primary malignancy	2
Cysts	
Mesenchymal	9
Bronchogenic	8
Enteric	4
Other	3
Pericardial	1

From Davis RD Jr, Oldham HN Jr, Sabiston DC Jr. The mediastinum. In: Sabiston DC Jr, Spencer FC, eds. Surgery of the chest, 5th ed. Philadelphia: WB Saunders, 1990:507, with permission.

Diagnostic Approach

Human chorionic gonadotropin (β-HCG) and a-fetoprotein (AFP) are useful diagnostic and monitoring serologic markers when a germ cell tumor is suspected. Seminomas do not produce these markers. Most masses can be seen on plain chest radiographs (125). If an esophageal duplication cyst is suspected, then a barium esophagogram will rule out communication with the esophagus. Chest CT scan will show the relationship of the mass to adjacent structures and better define its size and whether it is solid or cystic. MRI can provide additional information regarding neurovascular involvement and has largely replaced angiography in contemporary practice. In addition, MRI is used to assess intraspinal involvement of neurogenic tumors and has replaced CT myelograms (126–128). Radionucleotide scanning is useful for the diagnosis of endocrine tumors. Technetium or iodine scanning may help in the evaluation of potential thyroid and hyperparathyroid masses. Gallium scans are useful in tumors such as lymphomas and nonseminomatous germ cell tumors with an affinity for the isotopes. When mediastinal pheochromocytomas are suspected scanning with ^{131}I-metaiodobenzylguanidine (^{131}I-MIBG) is very useful in locating these extraadrenal paraganglionic tumors (129).

Biopsy of the lesion in question can be performed under CT or ultrasound guidance or with transbronchial biopsy (130–132).

Mediastinoscopy can be used in situations where a large tissue sample is needed for diagnosis as in the case of suspected lymphoma. Thoracoscopy is useful for lesions inaccessible by mediastinoscopy (133–135).

Anterior Mediastinal Masses

Thymoma

Thymoma is the most common adult tumor of the anterosuperior mediastinum. Thymoma can occur at any age, but is rare in children and most common between the ages of 40 and 60 years. It originates from thymic epithelial cells. Patients may complain of chest pain or dyspnea due to the mass effect of the tumor. Thymomas are associated with systemic syndromes such as myasthenia gravis, Cushing's syndrome, hyper- and hypogammaglobulinemia, systemic lupus erythromatosus, rheumatoid arthritis, megaesophagus, red blood cell aplasia, or granulomatous myocarditis (136). Differentiation of thymoma from lymphoma can be difficult (137).

Various classification systems have been proposed. Thymomas can be classified based on lymphocyte infiltration or resemblance to thymic medullary or cortical cells,

whereas the Masaoka staging system is used for staging (138–140). This staging system uses gross and microscopic invasion of capsule and adjacent structures to stage the thymomas (Table 60.18) (1,138).

Treatment. Complete surgical resection via median sternotomy is the treatment of choice for thymomas that do not have widespread dissemination (Fig. 60.30) (1). Other approaches such as transcervical resection have been described. However, complete excision of invasive

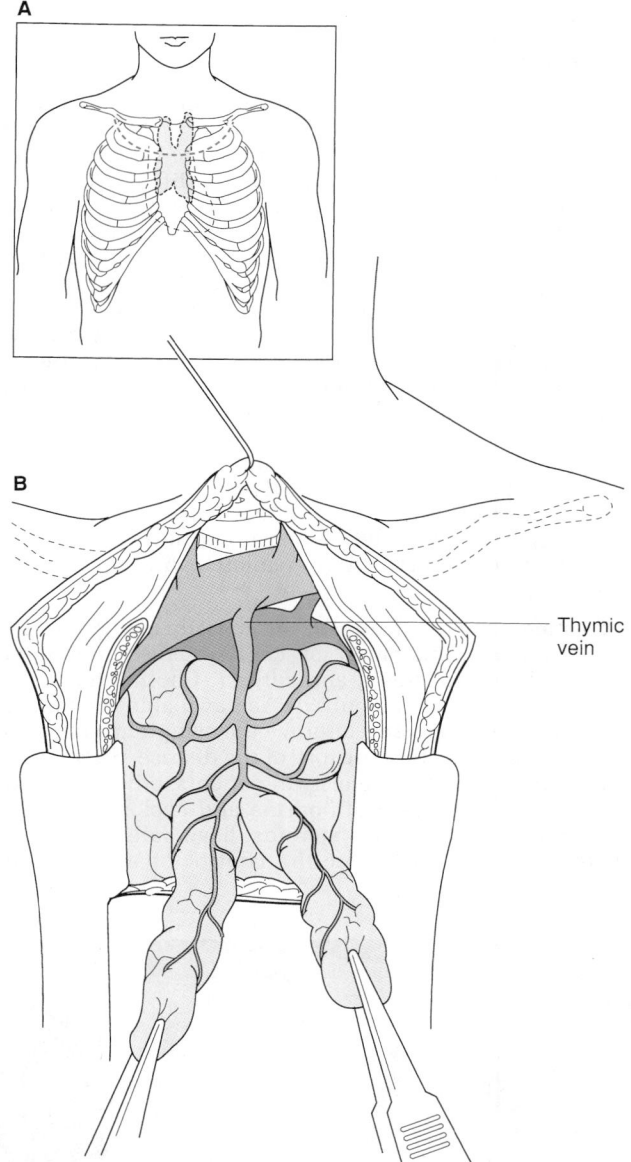

Figure 60.30. Technique of thymectomy. *(A)* Skin incision for partial sternotomy used to resect either a normal-sized thymus gland or one containing a small tumor. The incision placed over the sternomanubrial junction avoids a cervical scar and is more cosmetically appealing. After raising a skin and subcutaneous flap, the upper sternum is divided. *(B)* After the cervical extensions of the thymus glad are mobilized downward, the thymic vein is identified, ligated, and divided where it joins the innominate vein. (From Iannettoni MD, Orringer MB. Chest wall, pleura, mediastinum, and nonneoplastic lung disease. In: Greenfield LJ, Mulholland MW, Oldham KT, et al., eds. *Surgery: scientific principles and practice*, 2nd ed. Philadelphia: Lippincott–Raven, 1997:1440–1482, with permission.)

Table 60.18. **MASAOKA STAGING SYSTEM FOR THYMOMA**

Stage	Definition
I	Macroscopically, completely encapsulated; microscopically, no capsular invasion
IIA	Macroscopic invasion in surrounding fatty tissues or mediastinal pleura
IIB	Microscopic invasion into the capsule
III	Macroscopic invasion into a neighboring organ, such as pericardium, great vessels, or lung
IVA	Pleural or pericardial dissemination
IVB	Hematogenous or lymphogenous metastases

Adapted from Masaoka A, Monden Y, Nakahara K, et al. Follow-up study of thymomas with special references to their clinical stages. Cancer 1981;48:2485, with permission.

thymomas is best achieved via sternotomy. Local recurrence can occur secondary to tumor seeding (141,142).

Radiotherapy for invasive thymomas improves local control. Chemotherapy is used for disseminated thymomas (143–145).

The most common sites of recurrence are the lung, pleura, and mediastinum. For recurrent tumors, reexcision should be considered in addition to both chemotherapy and radiotherapy. Involvement of great vessels has a negative impact on survival (146). Survival correlates with stage. The 10-year survival rate for patients with stage I disease is approximately 85%; for those with stage II, 60% to 84%; for stage III, 21% to 77%; and 26% to 47% for stage IV-A patients (147–150).

Myasthenia Gravis

Myasthenia gravis is the most common syndrome associated with thymoma. It has a prevalence of 0.5 to 14.2 per 100,000 population. It is occurs more frequently in women, with a female to male ratio of 2:1 (151–153).

Autoantibodies to the acetylcholine receptors (AchRs) form, and complement activation is demonstrable. End plate destruction of the neuromuscular junction occurs. Fatigue and muscular weakness are the predominant symptoms. Facial muscles are most commonly involved. The patients can have ptosis, ophthalmoplegia, dysarthria, and dysphagia (154,155). Most patients with myasthenia gravis have thymic lymphoid hyperplasia; however only 10% have thymoma. The incidence of myasthenia gravis in patients with thymoma increases with age and can be as high as 80% over the age of 60 (156–158).

Diagnosis of myasthenia gravis is usually confirmed with the short-acting anticholinesterase edrophonium (tensilon) test. Any IV dose of tensilon results in improvement of muscle strength in patients with myasthenia gravis.

Treatment. The treatment of myasthenia gravis involves the administration of cholinesterase inhibitors, steroids, plasmapheresis, and surgery. Cholinesterase inhibitors increase the amount of Ach available at the neuromuscular junction and improve the symptoms, but they do not affect the natural history of the disease. Steroids induce remission in the majority of patients; other immunosuppressants such as azathioprine and cyclosporine can induce remission where steroids have failed. Plasmapheresis is very useful for the control of acute severe symptoms and for preoperative preparation. The benefits of plasmapheresis can last from weeks to months (159).

Thymectomy is associated with excellent clinical results and minimal morbidity, with up to 80% complete response. The chance of remission is best in young female patients who have a hyperplastic thymus and short duration of disease. Preoperative plasmapheresis facilitates perioperative management. Median sternotomy and transcervical and thoracoscopic approaches have been used for resection (160–166).

Lymphomas

Lymphoma can present with disease in the chest 10% of the time. It is the second most common tumor of the anterosuperior and middle mediastinum in adults and the most common one in children. It rarely occurs in the posterior mediastinum. Hodgkin's lymphoma of the nodular sclerosing type is most common (115,167). Symptoms include chest pain, dyspnea, cough, and systemic symptoms such as night sweats, fever, or weight loss. A large tissue sample may be needed to differentiate lymphoma from thymoma. Preoperative chest CT scan assists in the planning of the approach used for biopsy (168).

Treatment. Mediastinal lymphomas are treated primarily with radiation. For large tumors, adding chemotherapy can improve survival. Resection of mediastinal lymphomas is not necessary because chemoradiation can achieve excellent results (169–171).

Germ Cell Tumors

Primary germ cell tumors are the third most common anterosuperior mediastinal mass. Multiple types of germ cell tumors exist, including teratomas, teratocarcinoma, seminomas, embryonal cell carcinoma, choriocarcinoma, and endodermal sinus carcinoma. They arise from primordial germ cells that have migrated from the urogenital ridge. These tumors are not considered to be metastatic. However, scrotal evaluation with physical exam and sonogram is warranted to exclude a primary gonadal lesion (172–177).

Although benign germ cell tumors occur with equal frequency in males and females, 90% of malignant tumors occur in young males. The most common mediastinal germ cell tumor is the benign teratoma. Seminoma is the most common malignant tumor, making up 50% of malignant tumors, followed by teratocarcinoma (178–181).

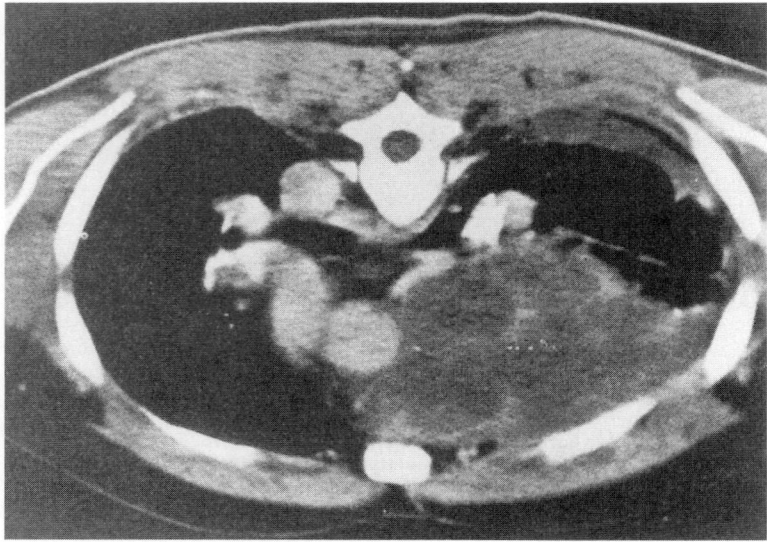

Figure 60.31. CT scan of a malignant nonseminomatous germ cell tumor of the anterior mediastinum reveals the inhomogeneous anterior mediastinal mass in contrast to the homogeneous density of a seminoma. Pleural effusion is also demonstrated in the right hemithorax. (From Shields TW. Primary lesions of the mediastinum and their investigation and treatment. In: Shields TW, ed. *General thoracic surgery.* Baltimore: Williams & Wilkins, 1994:1724–1769, with permission.)

Mediastinal Teratoma.   Most teratomas are benign tumors; approximately 10% are malignant. Dermoid cysts are the most common types of benign teratoma. They can contain hair, sweat glands, and sebaceous material (182). Surgery is the treatment of choice, with excellent long-term results. These lesions do not tend to recur if completely resected (183).

Seminoma.   Half of all malignant germ cell tumors are seminomas. CT scan of the chest, abdomen, and pelvis is required to evaluate the entire retroperitoneum and mediastinum. Serum β-HCG levels are elevated only in a minority of patients. Seminoma is a radiosensitive tumor and radiation is the primary treatment modality. In patients who have significant thoracic tumor burden or extrathoracic disease, the addition of chemotherapy improves remission rates. Surgery is reserved for patients with persistent masses after chemotherapy to determine the need for further treatment if viable tumor is still present (184–186).

Mediastinal Nonseminomatous Germ Cell Tumors

Nonseminomatous germ cell tumor of the mediastinum include malignant teratoma, embryonal cell carcinoma, choriocarcinoma, and endodermal tumors (Fig. 60.31) (187). These tumors produce AFP and β-HCG, which are elevated in some patients 90% of the time; they are useful markers for monitoring the adequacy of treatment and for surveillance. These lesions are more aggressive than seminomas and they are not radiosensitive. Chemotherapy is the primary treatment modality. Relapses and development of secondary hematologic malignancies are not uncommon (174,188).

Middle Mediastinal Masses

Mediastinal Cysts

These are the most common tumors of the middle mediastinum; they make up 20% of all mediastinal masses. The three most common in decreasing order are bronchogenic, pericardial, and enteric.

Bronchogenic Cysts.   Bronchogenic cysts are the most common type of the mediastinal cysts. They can be found either within the lung parenchyma or in the mediastinum near the carina and the major bronchi (Fig. 60.32) (187). They can produce symptoms secondary to extrinsic compression of the airways and cause stridor, chest pain, cough, and dyspnea. They are more likely to be symptomatic in children (189–193). CT scan confirms the diagnosis (192).

Treatment.   Symptomatic lesions should be excised. There are series supporting resection of asymptomatic lesions since many cysts eventually become symptomatic and resection of symptomatic lesions is associated with increased complications (193–196). In addition, malignancy is reported in these various congenital cystic malformations from lung, including bronchogenic cysts. Occasionally bronchogenic cysts can be very adherent to major bronchi or vessels, and complete resection may not be possible. Partial resection is associated with recurrence. Ethanol sclerosis has been reported as treatment for mediastinal cysts (189,197–199).

Pericardial Cysts.   Most common at the right pericardiophrenic angle, these cysts may communicate with the pericardium. They are usually filled with serous fluid and they are easily identified on CT scan (126,200). Resection is usually not required due to their characteristic appearance, lack of symptoms, and absence of malignant potential.

Enteric Cysts.   Enteric or duplication cysts or neuroenteric cysts when associated with vertebral anomalies usually have an inner lining of gastrointestinal epithelium. Esophageal lining is most common, although acid secreting gastric and intestinal epithelia are found as well (Fig. 60.33). These cysts are usually symptomatic in children and occasionally they can be multiple. A duplication of the alimentary tract may coexist. Most of them are found in the right chest. Patients present with symptoms like dysphagia secondary to a mass effect on the esophagus. Those cysts with acid-secreting gastric mucosa can bleed and acutely enlarge (201).

CT scan and endoscopic ultrasound have been used for diagnosis. Technetium scans show gastric mucosa and assist in localization. Surgical resection can yield esophageal muscle or mucosal defects requiring repair. Neuroenteric cysts can communicate with the dural space and can be associated with a variety of vertebral anomalies. Preoperative evaluation of the spinal column and dural anatomy via MRI is needed for an appropriately staged neurosurgical and thoracic approach if communication exists (109,202,203).

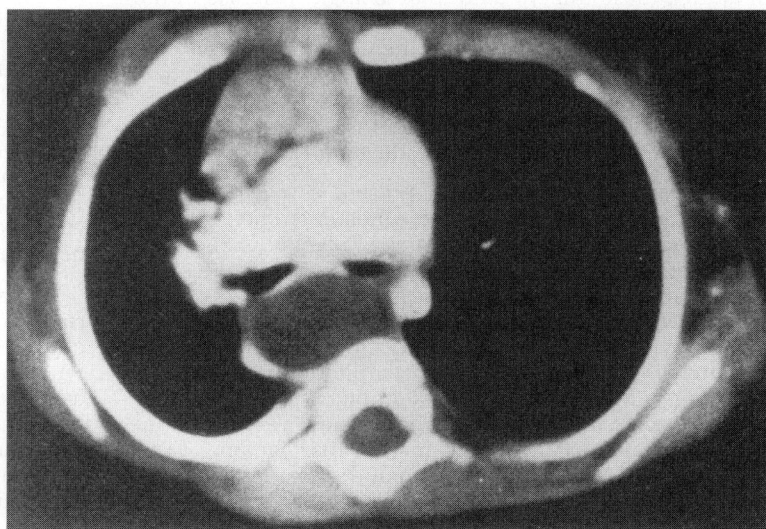

Figure 60.32. CT scan reveals a bronchogenic cyst located in the subcranial area with compression of the left mainstem bronchus with hyperinflation of the left lung and a mediastinal shift to the right. (From Shields TW. Primary lesions of the mediastinum and their investigation and treatment. In: Shields TW, ed. *General thoracic surgery*. Baltimore: Williams & Wilkins, 1994:1764–1769, with permission.)

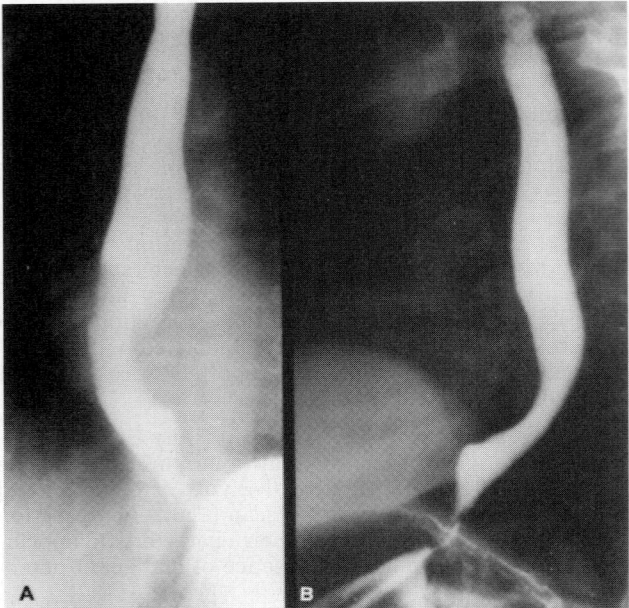

Figure 60.33. Barium esophagogram, posteroanterior *(A)* and lateral *(B)* views, showing an intramural esophageal duplication cyst. (From Iannettoni MD, Orringer MB. Chest wall, pleura, mediastinum, and nonneoplastic lung disease. In: Greenfield LJ, Mulholland MW, Oldham KT, et al., eds. *Surgery: scientific principles and practice,* 2nd ed. Philadelphia: Lippincott–Raven, 1997:1440–1482, with permission.)

Miscellaneous Cysts

Thymic and other nonspecific cysts can occur in the mediastinum. Thymic cysts are benign, but can be confused with cystic degeneration of thymomas, or if calcified with teratoma. Excision for diagnostic purposes can be performed (204). Chyle containing cysts, pancreatic pseudocysts, or cysts not otherwise specified can also occur (205,206).

Posterior Mediastinal Masses

Neurogenic Tumors

Neurogenic tumors are the most common neoplasms of the mediastinum, constituting 20% to 35% of all tumors. In adults, these tumors tend to be benign, whereas in the pediatric population they tend to be malignant. These tumors have multiple origins and include the nerve sheaths (neurilemomas, neurofibromas, and neurofibrosarcomas), the sympathetic ganglia (ganglioneuromas, ganglioneuroblastomas, and neuroblastomas), and the paraganglia cells (pheochromocytomas and chemodectomas).

Diagnosis. The tumors can present as asymptomatic masses incidentally found on diagnostic studies, or they can be symptomatic either because of mass effect and impingement on vital structures or due to systemic effects of hormonal activity. Mass effects can cause chest pain, back pain, dyspnea, Horner's syndrome, and Pancoast syndrome. Symptoms secondary to hormonal activity include hypertension, flushing, diarrhea palpitations, headaches, sweating, and abdominal distention. Vasoactive substances secreted include catecholamines, vasoactive intestinal peptide (VIP), and insulin-like factors. Catecholamine-secreting tumors include paragangliomas, pheochromocytomas, neuroblastomas, and ganglioneuromas. VIP-secreting tumors include neurofibromas, neu-

rofibrosarcomas, and ganglioneuromas. Insulin-like factor is secreted by neurofibrosarcomas (207). Dumbbell tumors extend into the spinal column; they compose 10% of neurogenic tumors. Sixty percent are symptomatic with back pain or radicular pain. Patients should undergo CT scan of the chest to better define the tumor and its relationship to adjacent structures. Neurovascular involvement is best assessed with MRI. Catecholamine metabolic products can be measured in the urine (208,209).

Nerve Sheath Tumors

Neurilemomas are the most common neurogenic tumors followed by the neurofibromas unless considering adults and children together. Neurilemomas are well-encapsulated tumors; neurofibromas are not. They are both slow-growing benign lesions. They tend to occur between the third and fifth decades of life and can be associated with von Recklinghausen disease. Symptoms are usually caused by pressure on the affected nerves. Both types of tumor can undergo malignant degeneration into neurofibrosarcomas. Neurofibrosarcomas are fast-growing tumors that can invade adjacent structures. Hypoglycemic episodes have been described secondary to insulin-like substances produced by these tumors (210).

Sympathetic Ganglia Tumors

This group of tumors is the second most common type of neurogenic mediastinal mass. These are most common in children and include benign and malignant lesions. Ganglioneuromas are benign, typically well-encapsulated elongated tumors. Ganglioneuroblastomas can occur as diffuse or composite subtypes. While the diffuse type generally behaves as a benign tumor, it can metastasize 5% of the time; the composite type has almost a 75% incidence of metastasis. Neuroblastomas generally occur in children and usually in a child under the age of 4. They can secrete a variety of hormonally active substances and produce a characteristic neurologic opsoclonus-polymyoclonus syndrome with cerebellar and truncal ataxia (211,212). Twenty percent of all neuroblastomas present within the thorax; the median age of the child at presentation with neuroblastoma is 11 months (207).

Paraganglionic Tumors

Paragangliomas are vascular and hormonally active tumors. They are the least common type of neurogenic tumors. Patients who have functional tumors present with headaches, hypertension, and palpitations. Although the tumor is most commonly found in the paravertebral area, it can also be found in the middle mediastinum. Ten percent of paragangliomas are multiple and are associated with the multiple endocrine neoplasm (MEN) syndrome (213). Chemodactomas are less likely to be functional. Malignancy is determined by the clinical course of the patient. Diagnosis of hormonally active lesions is confirmed with measurement of urine catecholamine metabolites. These lesions appear on CT scan as vascular tumors that enhance with IV contrast. The MIBG scan can detect most of these lesions when CT scan fails.

Treatment. Surgery is the treatment of choice for neurogenic mediastinal lesions. Preoperative management includes functional assessment of these lesions in patients with suggestive symptoms and evaluation for intraspinal extension. Catecholamine-secreting tumors should be managed preoperatively in a manner similar to adrenal pheochromocytomas. If a lesion is determined to have an intraspinal component, it should be resected first by the neurosurgeon followed by resection of the thoracic component by the thoracic team as a single stage procedure.

Thoracoscopic resections have also been performed (214–216). Complete surgical excision is essential; this may necessitate median sternotomy for middle mediastinal lesions. While patient prognosis is excellent for benign tumors, prognosis depends on staging for the neuroblastomas, with chemotherapy included in the treatment regimen for advanced stage tumors.

Mediastinal Infections

Mediastinitis is one of the most serious infections that a surgeon may have to manage. Multiple etiologies have been reported; these include esophageal perforations or postoperative esophageal anastomotic leaks, infections after median sternotomy for cardiac procedures, and extensions into the mediastinum of oropharyngeal, vertebral, pulmonary, or chest wall infections. Postoperative wound infections after cardiac procedures occur 2% of the time; they can range from a superficial cellulitis to severe sepsis with deep sternal and mediastinal involvement. Predisposing factors include diabetes, bilateral internal mammary artery harvesting, prolonged cardiopulmonary bypass and operative time, cardiogenic shock, and chest compressions during cardiopulmonary resuscitation.

Mediastinitis can present with fever, leukocytosis, sternal pain, chest pain, or neck pain depending on the initial site of the infection. Sternal instability may occur in patients with median sternotomy. Patients with esophageal-related infections secondary to cervical anastomotic leaks or trauma present with neck pain, wound drainage, and subcutaneous emphysema. Perforations from foreign bodies or diagnostic esophagoscopy tend to occur at the level of the cricopharyngeal muscle, whereas therapeutic dilation of strictures or achalasia occur at the site of intervention. Mediastinal esophageal perforations can cause chest pain, fever, and pleural effusion. On physical exam varying degrees of superficial neck and sternal cellulitis can be present. Subcutaneous emphysema from esophageal perforation or descending gas forming oropharyngeal infections can be present. Differentiation between superficial wound infections and deep mediastinal infections is facilitated with the use of CT scan. Confirmation of esophageal perforation is best with a water-soluble contrast esophagogram followed by barium esophagogram and esophagoscopy.

Treatment

Treatment of these infections varies from local wound care to extensive débridement and flap reconstruction. In superficial sternal infections or localized neck infections secondary to esophageal leaks, local wound care with incision and adequate drainage will suffice. In more extensive cases with deep mediastinal involvement, extensive débridement is necessary. All necrotic cartilage, sternal bone, and ribs have to be removed. Irrigation with antibiotics is helpful. The wound can be closed with the use of closed irrigation systems if débridement was adequate, or it can be left open for continuous irrigation and débridement. Pectoralis, rectus, or omental flaps can be used for obliteration of dead space.

Mediastinal granulomatous infections are chronic infections with multiple causes including all of the endemic mycoses, sarcoid, syphilis, tuberculosis, and lymphomas. In recent years, histoplasmosis has replaced tuberculosis as the most common cause of mediastinal granulomatous infection in the U.S. A sequela of mediastinal histoplasmosis is the development of mediastinal fibrosis. In one third of these patients, chronic granulomatous disease progressed to mediastinal fibrosis. In addition, airway compression and esophageal fistulas have been reported.

Mediastinal fibrosis is the most common benign cause of SVC syndrome. The use of antifungal agents does not result in regression of this fibrosis. The predominant finding at surgery is extensive and dense fibrotic reaction involving the mediastinal structures. Surgery has been performed to relieve airway compromise, repair esophageal fistulas, and reconstruct the SVC. Surgical excision of large or symptomatic granulomas is recommended to avoid these complications.

Superior Vena Cava (SVC) Syndrome

The SVC syndrome refers to compression, invasion, or occlusion of the SVC lumen. The causes vary and include benign, malignant, and iatrogenic etiologies. While benign disease was the main cause of this syndrome historically, malignant disease has become the most common etiology today representing about 90% of the cases (217–219). Iatrogenic causes of SVC syndrome commonly occur secondary to indwelling intravenous pacemaker and intravenous catheters (220).

Symptoms and Signs

Patients present with cough, and dyspnea on exertion; on physical exam there is facial and upper extremity edema with venous distention of the head face and chest wall. Symptoms may be minimal if the occlusion occurred gradually.

Malignant Etiology

Bronchogenic carcinoma is the most common malignant cause of SVC syndrome (75%), with 67% being non–small-cell and 33% small-cell histology. Lymphomas are the second most common malignant cause, followed by metastatic disease (221,222).

Benign Etiology

Multiple infectious diseases have been reported to cause the SVC syndrome, with *Histoplasmosis* the most common. Other causes of granulomatous reaction include blastomycosis, tuberculosis, nocardia infection, syphilis, actinomycosis, sarcoid tumors, and radiation therapy (223–225).

Diagnosis

The diagnosis of SVC syndrome begins with the physical exam and can be confirmed with contrast-enhanced CT or MRI; these have replaced other more invasive imaging methods (226,227). Histologic diagnosis can be obtained with CT-guided biopsies (228). Mediastinoscopy may be needed for adequate tissue sample when lymphoma is suspected.

Treatment

The average survival for untreated SVC syndrome is 7 months, but it is dependent on the etiology. Treatment consists of radiotherapy, chemotherapy, surgery, or thrombolysis specific to the etiology. Head elevation, diuretics, and O_2 are initial supportive measures. Radiotherapy is the most common treatment used, with excellent results in up to 90% of patients (229). Chemotherapy is used for malignancies known to respond, such as small-cell carcinomas or lymphomas (230,231). Other methods such as venous interposition grafting, replacement, bypass, thrombectomy, and thrombolysis have been used in patients who develop life-threatening symptoms (232,233). Thrombectomy and thrombolytic therapy have been used for catheter-induced syndromes, with the best results in patients who receive long-term anticoagulation and have the foreign body removed. Replacement or bypass of the vena cava has been more successful with autologous than prosthetic material (234–241).

TRACHEA

Anatomy

The adult trachea extends from the anterior border of the cricoid cartilage to the carinal spur, with an average length of 11 cm. It has between 18 and 22 cartilaginous rings or two rings per centimeter. The rings are C-shaped with the cartilaginous portion making up the anterior and lateral walls and the membranous portion making up the posterior wall. The blood supply of the trachea has multiple sources that interconnect along the lateral walls of the trachea. The cervical trachea receives its blood supply from the inferior thyroid artery branches and tracheoesophageal branches of the subclavian artery. The thoracic trachea has a more variable blood supply, and numerous arteries may contribute branches from sources such as the innominate, internal thoracic, subclavian, and intercostal arteries (Fig. 60.34) (242).

Tracheal Tumors

Tumors involving the trachea can be divided into intrinsic and extrinsic. Intrinsic tumors are either malignant or benign, with malignant being the most common. The benign tumors are divided into various subtypes including papillomas, chondromas, fibromas, hemangiomas, and miscellaneous lesion such as granular cell tumors, fibrous histiocytomas, glomus tumors, lipomas, leiomyomas, neurofibromas, and hamartomas.

The most common type of benign tumor is the papilloma, followed by chondroma, hamartoma, and fibroma.

Symptoms depend on the location of the tumors (distal vs. proximal) and include voice changes, cough, hemoptysis, and airway obstruction with stridor or shortness of breath. Some patients have no symptoms at all.

Benign

Papillomas. Papillomas are associated with the human papilloma viruses 6 and 11. They occur mainly in the larynx and have an irregular gross appearance. They can undergo malignant degeneration, especially in adults. Resection is indicated for lesions causing symptoms at any age and in adults to avoid malignancy. A variety of methods have been used, with laser resection increasing in popularity.

Chondromas. Chondromas originate from cartilage and tend to occur mainly in adults. They also have a tendency to recur, although not as commonly as papillomas. Surgical resection is the treatment of choice.

Hamartomas. Hamartomas also contain cartilage and in addition have epithelial and lymph tissue. They tend to be peripheral in location and hence tend to present as solitary nodules on chest radiograph. Resection is the treatment of choice because they cannot be differentiated from carcinoma without histology. These lesions rarely recur, and resections margins can be small.

Fibromas. Fibromas and fibrous histiocytomas tend to occur proximally, but unlike papillomas they have a smooth appearance. Resection can be accomplished bronchoscopically for fibromas, but fibrous histiocytomas have a tendency for recurrence, necessitating a complete surgical resection.

Hemangiomas. Hemangiomas can occur at any age but they represent the most common type of tracheal lesion in the pediatric population. They also have a female predilection. They tend to occur proximally, and, like other hemangiomas at other sites, they tend to enlarge and can cause threatening airway obstruction. Unlike other benign tracheal lesions, they do often regress spontaneously, and observation is the initial treatment. Biopsy is to be avoided because hemorrhage is a common sequela. Surgery is reserved for persistent lesions (243).

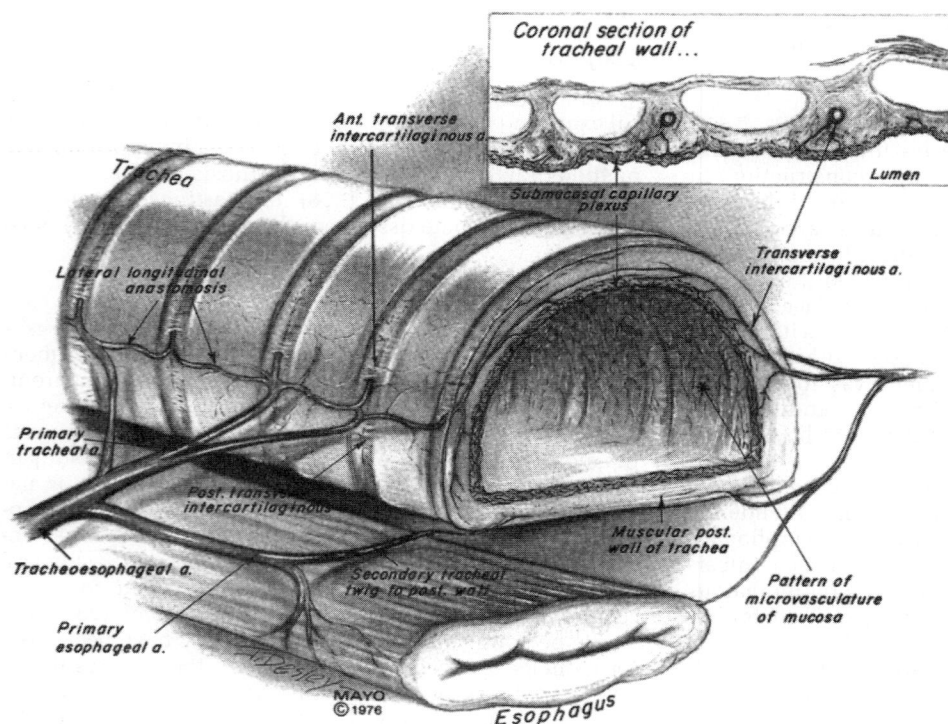

Figure 60.34. Semischematic view of the tracheal microscopical blood supply. Transverse intercartilaginous arteries derived from the lateral longitudinal anastomosis penetrate the soft tissues between each cartilage to supply a rich vascular network beneath the endotracheal mucosa. (From Salassa JR, Pearson BW, Payne WS, et al. Gross and microscopical blood supply of the trachea. *Ann Thorac Surg* 1977;24(2): 100–107, with permission.)

Malignant

Malignant tumors of the trachea are more common that benign tumors, but still represent only 1% to 2% of all lung carcinomas. Malignant tumors may be primary or secondary. Primary tumors typically are squamous cell, adenoid cystic, and carcinoid lesions. Multiple other types of primary tumors have been described, but these three types are the most common. Secondary malignant tumors include laryngeal, thyroid, lung, and esophageal cancer. Primary malignant tumors have similar clinical presentations to the benign lesions. Cough, hemoptysis, and airway obstruction are commonly seen. Biopsy establishes the diagnosis (Table 60.19) (244). Complete surgical resection is the treatment of choice for these primary tumors. Adjuvant chemoradiation is offered, although its role has not been established in randomized series due to the low number of accrued cases.

Squamous Cell Carcinoma. Squamous cell carcinoma of the trachea presents in a variety of ways, appearing as a single or multiple lesion fairly well localized to a superficially infiltrating lesion covering most of the trachea. Metastases to local nodes are seen in almost one third of the patients at presentation. It occurs more commonly in males, with a male to female ratio of 3:1.

Adenoid Cystic Carcinoma. Adenoid cystic carcinomas are slow-growing tumors that can also involve a significant part of the trachea. They have a tendency to grow submucosally and involve more of the trachea than is clinically evident. Metastases to regional nodes occur. This tumor has a tendency to displace rather than invade adjacent structures even when large. It occurs with equal frequency in males and females.

Table 60.19. HISTOLOGIC TYPES OF PRIMARY TRACHEAL TUMORS

Type	No. of patients
Benign	
Squamous papillomata	
Multiple	4
Solitary	1
Pleomorphic adenoma	2
Granular cell tumor	2
Fibrous histiocytoma	1
Leiomyoma	2
Chondroma	2
Chondroblastoma	1
Schwannoma	1
Paraganglioma	2
Hemangioendothelioma	1
Vascular malformation	2
Intermediate	
Carcinoid	10
Mucoepidermoid	4
Plexiform neurofibroma	1
Pseudosarcoma	1
Malignant	
Adenocarcinoma	1
Adenosquamous carcinoma	1
Small cell carcinoma	1
Atypical carcinoid	1
Melanoma	1
Chondrosarcoma	1
Spindle cell sarcoma	2
Rhabdomyosarcoma	1

From Grillo HC, Mathisen DJ. Primary tracheal tumors: treatment and results. Ann Thorac Surg 1990;49(1):69–77, with permission.

Carcinoids. Carcinoids tend to occur in more peripheral location than the other primary tumors, but proximal sites still represent the majority of lesions. Systemic symptoms of carcinoid such as flushing and diarrhea occur 10% of the time. For completely resected lesions, 5-year survival rates of up to 90% have been reported.

Secondary Malignant Tumors. Laryngeal, thyroid, lung, and esophageal cancer can involve the trachea by direct extension. Tracheoesophageal fistulas are more common with esophageal cancer, usually involving the left main bronchus, while the other carcinomas tend to present with obstruction or direct extension. Tracheal involvement usually indicates unresectable disease, with the notable exception of limited tracheal involvement and negative mediastinal lymph nodes. Palliation for thyroid and laryngeal carcinomas with tracheal extension can occasionally be achieved with resection.

Surgical Treatment

Surgical Airways

Surgical airways can be established either via tracheostomy (percutaneous or open) or cricothyroidotomy. The indications for a surgical airway are inability to control airway secretions with other methods, and need for chronic ventilatory support for respiratory failure for relief of upper airway obstruction.

Tracheostomy

Controversy exists regarding the timing of tracheostomy for chronic ventilatory support. Laryngeal complications of orotracheal intubation have been described as early as 2 to 5 days after intubation, hence early tracheostomy should be considered.

Multiple techniques of tracheostomy have been described. These have been performed via horizontal or vertical skin incisions, or cruciate, vertical, horizontal, or flap-creating tracheal incisions. No technique has proven superior. The important technical aspects of this procedure are placement of the tracheal incision over the second, third, or fourth tracheal rings but not lower; avoidance of a large tracheal incision; and limiting dilation of the incision to no more than the actual tube size. The larger the tracheal incision the greater the chance for tracheal stenosis. A low tracheal incision places the tracheotomy tube close to the innominate artery and increases the potential for tracheoinnominate fistula formation. Percutaneous tracheostomy has gained popularity in recent years. Reviews of the experience with this procedure show a tracheal stenosis rate of 1.6% to 6% (245,246).

Cricothyroidotomy

The main indication for cricothyroidotomy is the establishment of a surgical airway in an emergency situation. It is faster and easier to perform than tracheostomy because less dissection is needed, and it avoids the thyroid isthmus. A tube as large as 8 mm can be inserted through an incision in the cricothyroid membrane. With this procedure, there is greater chance for an injury to the vocal cords and for subglottic stenosis, which is a difficult problem to correct. Cricothyroidotomies should be converted to a tracheostomy when possible. This procedure should also be avoided in children younger than 12 years old.

Complications of Surgical Airways

The common complications of surgical airways are infection, hemorrhage, tracheal stenosis, and, rarely, tracheoesophageal fistulas.

Tracheostomies are typically colonized with both gram-positive and gram-negative organisms such as *Staphylococcus, Streptococcus,* and *Pseudomonas.* These organisms can cause cellulitis, tracheobronchitis, and pneumonitis. Meticulous skin care and stoma care is essential.

Early postoperative bleeding usually occurs from the divided thyroid isthmus. This can be controlled with epinephrine-soaked sponges. Late bleeding is usually secondary to granulation or tracheal erosions. The most

serious bleeding occurs from erosion of the cuff or the tip of the tube into the innominate artery. It is a particular risk with low-placed tracheostomies or a high artery. Immediate control of the bleeding is essential to prevent exsanguination. Repair of this fistula involves reconstruction of the artery without prosthetic materials and tracheal repair with or without resection (Fig. 60.35) (1).

Tracheoesophageal fistula can occur (Fig. 60.36) (247) with either orotracheal or tracheostomy tubes. Either the cuff or the tube tip can erode posterior into the esophagus.

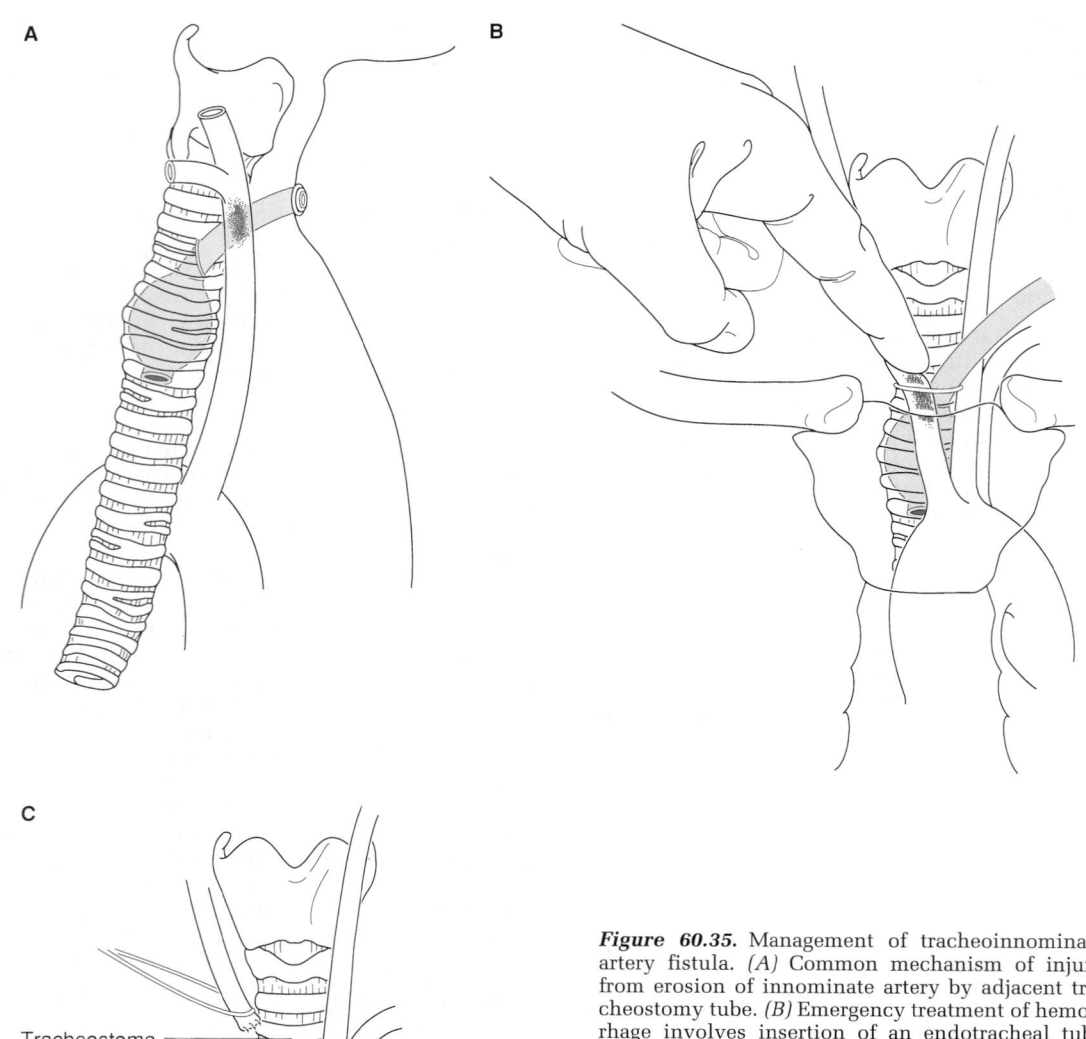

Tracheostoma

Figure 60.35. Management of tracheoinnominate artery fistula. *(A)* Common mechanism of injury from erosion of innominate artery by adjacent tracheostomy tube. *(B)* Emergency treatment of hemorrhage involves insertion of an endotracheal tube into the tracheostomy stoma, inflation of the cuff and downward and outward pressure on the fistula by the finger inserted through the tracheostomy incision to further tamponade the bleeding. *(C)* Through a partial upper sternal split, the segment of involved innominate artery is resected, and the oversewn ends covered with adjacent mediastinal fat or muscle. Tracheal resection is usually not necessary. A new tracheostomy tube may have to be inserted higher in the trachea or, if possible, the tracheostomy tube removed and the stoma covered with a sternohyoid muscle flap. (From Iannettoni MD, Orringer MB. Chest wall, pleura, mediastinum, and nonneoplastic lung disease. In: Greenfield LJ, Mulholland MW, Oldham KT, et al., eds. *Surgery: scientific principles and practice,* 2nd ed. Philadelphia: Lippincott–Raven, 1997:1440–1482, with permission.)

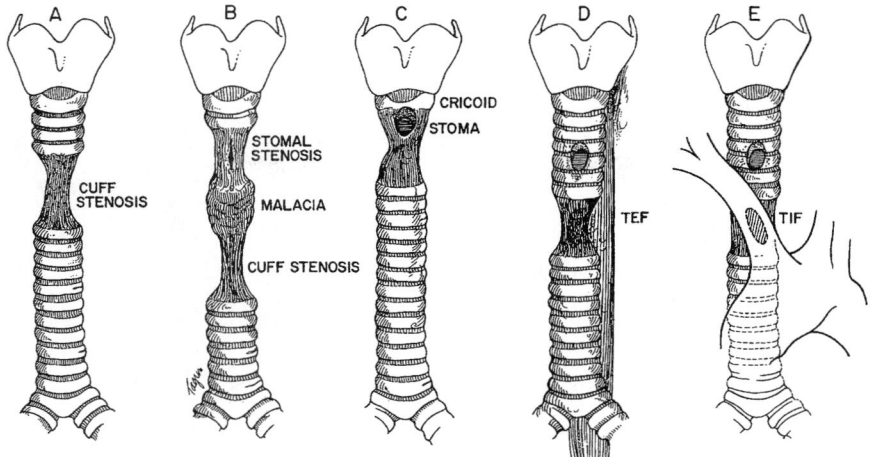

Figure 60.36. Diagrams of principal postintubation tracheal lesions. *(A)* Cuff stenosis from the cuff of an endotracheal tube. *(B)* Cuff stenosis from the cuff of a tracheostomy tube, usually lower in the trachea than that from an endotracheal tube. Stomal stenosis also occurs at the site of the tracheostomy itself. Malacia may occur either at the level of the cuff or in the segment between the stoma and the cuff stenosis. *(C)* Cuff stenosis at the site of a high tracheostomy stoma, which has eroded into the lower margin of the cricoid cartilage. In older patients, this may erode back further into the subglottic larynx, producing a laryngotracheal stenosis. A stoma placed in the cricothyroid membrane will, by definition, produce an intralaryngeal stenosis. *(D)* Tracheoesophageal fistula (TEF) produced by pressure of the cuff against the "party wall," often abetted by an indwelling firm nasogastric tube. *(E)* One type of tracheoinnominate fistula (TIF) as the result of a high pressure cuff erosion. The more common type, but also rare, is that seen with a low-placed tracheostomy stoma, which rests against the innominate artery itself. Not shown are the lesions that occur in the larynx as the result of endotracheal tubes. (From Grillo HC. Surgical treatment of postintubation tracheal injuries. *J Thorac Cardiovasc Surg* 1979;78:860, with permission.)

The unsupported weight of the ventilator tubing may contribute to this, as does a concomitant nasogastric tube in the esophagus. Signs include impaired ventilation and reflux of gastric contents into the tracheobronchial tree. The fistula should be controlled with a larger volume low-pressure cuff or by advancing the tube further. Any esophageal tube should be removed and a gastrostomy performed with definite correction when the patient no longer requires endotracheal intubation (Fig. 60.37). Tracheal stenosis occurs even with modern low-pressure cuffs if they are overinflated. The longer the period of endotracheal intubation, the higher the chance of such an injury. Large tracheal incisions for tracheostomy and hypotension have been implicated in the pathogenesis of this lesion.

Patients with tracheal stenosis can be asymptomatic early on, presenting years later with wheezing, dyspnea, or stridor, and be misdiagnosed with adult-onset asthma. In addition, segments of the trachea between the stoma and the cuff level can become malacic and collapse with respiratory effort. Treatment of tracheal stenosis involves tracheostomy at the site of the lesion to relieve airway obstruction and resection of the lesion with adequate mobilization to ensure a tension-free end-to-end anastomosis. The majority of patients in one large series achieved a satisfactory result (248).

LUNG INFECTIONS

Abscess

Since the advent of effective antibiotics beginning with the penicillins in the 1940s, many fewer pneumonic processes progress to abscess formation. Mortality rates of 30% and the residual chronic symptoms in 30% of pa-

tients prior to the introduction of the antibiotics have been greatly reduced. However, with the increasing incidence of solid organ transplantation requiring immunosuppression, bone marrow transplantation, cancer treatment, HIV infection, and other immune deficiencies, there is an increasing incidence of these abscesses with a different pathogenesis and microbiologic flora.

Pathogenesis

Lung abscesses occur as a result of aspiration of infected material from the oropharynx, usually in patients with altered mental status or suppressed cough reflexes. There is often poor oral hygiene and gingival disease. Liquefaction necrosis occurs by the proliferation of anaerobic bacteria, forming a necrotic cavity (Fig. 60.38) (1). Even though abscesses can occur in any part of the lung, there is a predilection for the posterior segment of the right upper lobe and the superior segment of the right lower lobe since these are the most dependent segments. Lung abscesses in immunocompromised patients are often hospital acquired; they tend to be multiple rather than single. *Staphylococcus* species, *Escherichia coli*, *Pseudomonas* species, and fungal organisms are all potential pathogens. If there is adequate communication between the bronchus and the abscess, the lesion can resolve with postural drainage, chest physiotherapy, and antibiotics. Inadequate communication results in incomplete drainage and chronic cavity formation.

Presentation

Typical symptoms are fever, cough, chest pain, occasional hemoptysis, and purulent sputum production. As the cavity erodes into adjacent bronchial segments, it may partially decompress with temporary improvement of

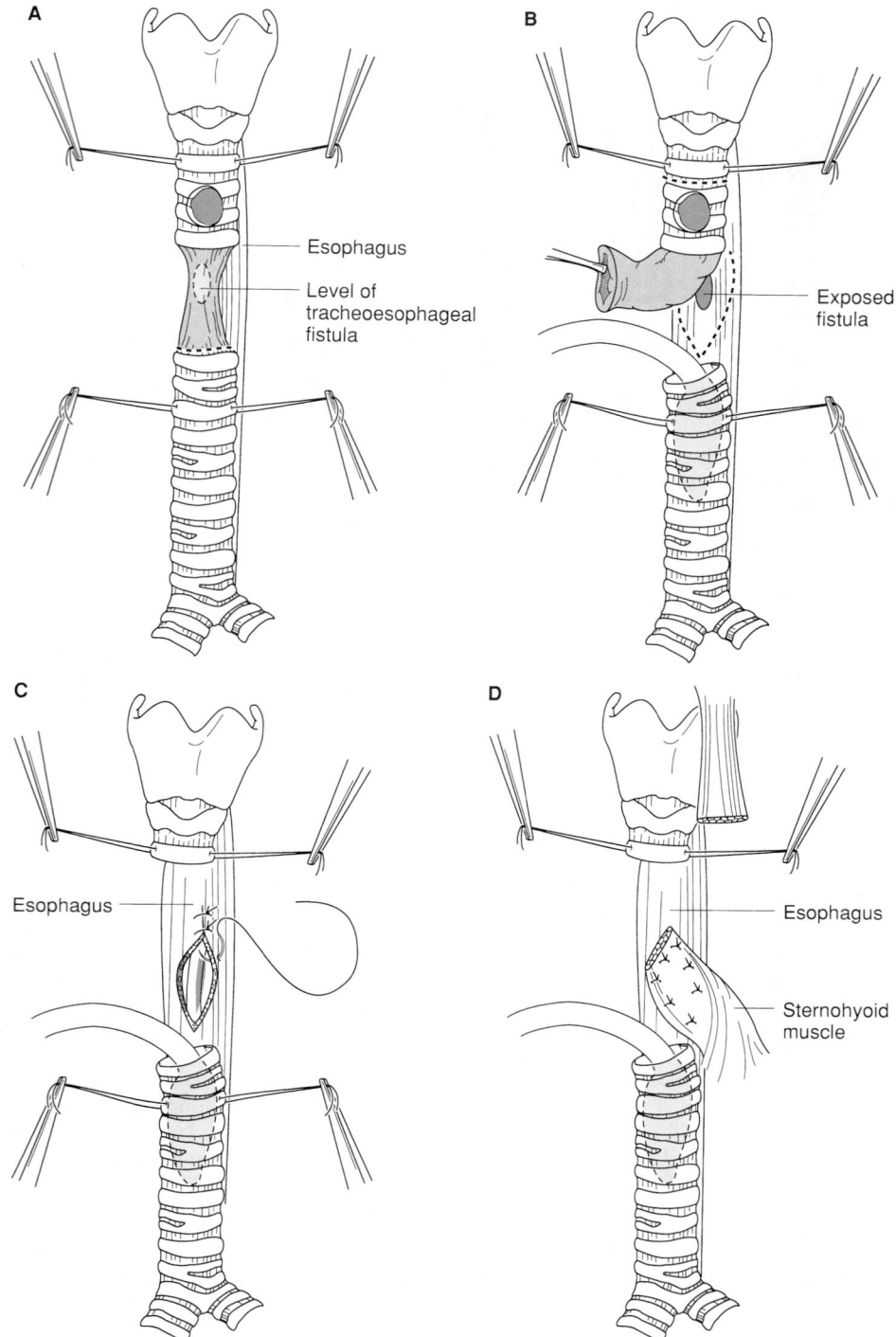

Figure 60.37. Management of postintubation tracheoesophageal fistula. *(A)* Only the length of damaged trachea to be resected (usually including the tracheostomy stoma) is circumferentially mobilized above and below the fistula to avoid devascularizing the remaining trachea. Stay sutures secure the trachea above and below this segment. *(B)* The trachea is transected, the distal trachea intubated across the field, and the fistula identified by elevating the damaged tracheal segment. *(C)* The stenotic tracheal segment is resected and closure of the esophageal fistula begun, being certain to invert the mucosa. A two-layered closure is completed. *(D)* After interposing the mobilized sternohyoid muscle and suturing it over the esophageal closure, an end-to-end tracheal anastomosis is performed. (From Iannettoni MD, Orringer MB. Chest wall, pleura, mediastinum, and nonneoplastic lung disease. In: Greenfield LJ, Mulholland MW, Oldham KT, et al., eds. *Surgery: scientific principles and practice,* 2nd ed. Philadelphia: Lippincott–Raven, 1997:1440–1482, with permission.)

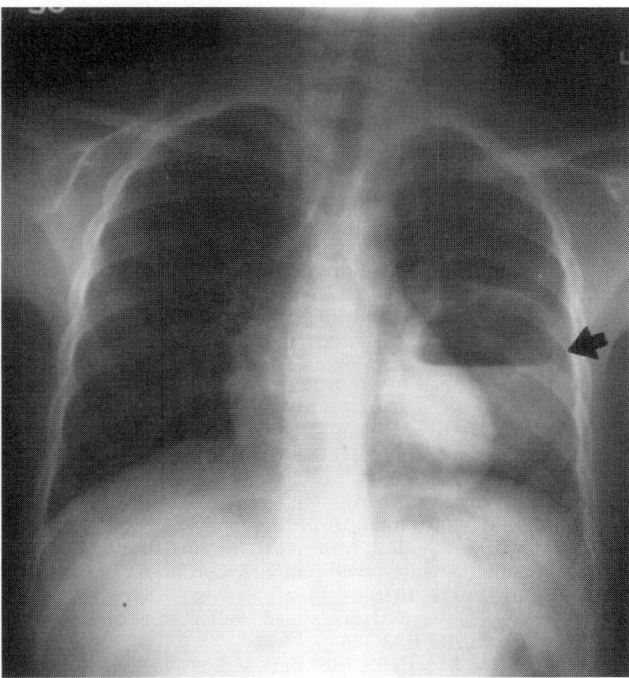

Figure 60.38. Chest roentgenogram showing a large abscess of the left lung with an air-fluid level *(arrow)*. (From Iannettoni MD, Orringer MB. Chest wall, pleura, mediastinum, and nonneoplastic lung disease. In: Greenfield LJ, Mulholland MW, Oldham KT, et al., eds. *Surgery: scientific principles and practice,* 2nd ed. Philadelphia: Lippincott–Raven, 1997:1440–1482, with permission.)

symptoms. As the new communication becomes occluded, the symptoms recur. Chest radiographs show consolidation early on with the characteristic air-fluid level in the upright chest x-ray as the disease progresses and establishes communication with a bronchus.

Treatment

Antibiotic therapy with efficacy against anaerobic organisms, postural drainage, and chest physiotherapy are the initial therapies. In immunocompromised patients broader coverage is needed. Bronchoscopy for cultures, drainage, and to rule out foreign bodies or neoplasm should be performed. This must include precautions to avoid contaminating the opposite lung. Operative treatment is reserved for patients who do not respond to antibiotics or in the setting of sepsis, a large residual abscess cavity, empyema, or bronchopleural fistula. Percutaneous aspiration of the cavity can be used for patients who are not candidates for an extensive pulmonary resection. The resultant bronchopleural fistula will heal if adequate drainage of the cavity is established. Mortality rates have decreased significantly compared to the preantibiotic era and are now less than 5%. Abscesses caused by opportunistic organisms have a higher mortality rate, reflecting the immunocompromised state of the patient.

Bronchiectasis

Bronchiectasis is an abnormal dilation of the distal bronchi that can be either congenital (Table 60.20) (249) or acquired. Seventy-five percent of the cases are acquired and occur as sequelae from chronic bacterial or viral infection. These infections result in obstruction of the distal airways from retained secretions and mucous plugs that lead to dilation and recurrent acute infection. Cystic fibro-

Table 60.20. **CAUSES OF BRONCHIECTASIS**

CONGENITAL

Cystic fibrosis
α_1 = antitrypsin deficiency
Kartagener syndrome
Intralobar bronchopulmonary sequestration
Congenital cystic bronchiectasis
Selective immunoglobulin A (IgA) deficiency
Congenital deficiency of bronchial cartilage
Primary hypogammaglobulinemia

ACQUIRED

Infection viral and bacterial
Bronchial obstruction
    Intrinsic—neoplasm, foreign body mucous plug
    Extrinsic—enlarged lymph nodes
Middle lobe syndrome
Scarring secondary to tuberculosis
Acquired hypogammaglobulinemia

From Bolman RM III, Wolfe WG. Bronchiectasis and pulmonary sequastration. Surg Clin North Am 1980;60(4):867–881, with permission.

sis is a common cause of acquired bronchiectosis. Multiple causes of congenital bronchiectasis exist. There are three types of bronchiectasis based on the gross appearance of the bronchi: varicose, cylindrical, and saccular, with varicose the most common. Most patients present with chronic foul sputum production, fever, and hemoptysis. CT scan and bronchoscopy are used for diagnosis, to rule out extrinsic lesions, and to obtain sputum specimens to guide antibiotic therapy.

Treatment

The treatment for bronchiectasis is mainly nonoperative and consists of antibiotics, chest physiotherapy, and postural drainage. Patients with multisegment disease tend to have more chronic disease and tend to respond less to either medical or surgical treatment. Surgery is reserved for those patients who do not respond after a prolonged course of antibiotics and nonoperative management. It is essential to localize the area to be resected preoperatively. Extensive resections such as pneumonectomy are rarely required in the modern era of antibiotics, but bilateral staged resections are occasionally needed. Double-lumen intubation is useful to avoid intraoperative spillage to the unaffected side (250).

REFERENCES

1. Iannettoni MD, Orringer MB. Chest wall, pleura, mediastinum, and nonneoplastic lung disease. In: Greenfield LJ, Mulholland MW, Oldham KT, et al., eds. *Surgery: scientific principles and practice,* 2nd ed. Philadelphia: Lippincott–Raven, 1997:1440–1482.
2. Fonkalsrud EW, Dunn JCY, Atkinson JB. Repair of pectus excavatum deformities: 30 years of experience with 375 patients. *Ann Surg* 2000;231(3):443–448.
3. Shamberger RC. Chest wall deformities. In: Shields TW, ed. *General thoracic surgery,* 4th ed. Baltimore: Williams & Wilkins, 1994:529–557.
4. Shamberger RC, Welch KJ. Surgical repair of pectus excavatum. *J Pediatr Surg* 1988;23:615–622.
5. Shamberger RC, Welch KJ, Castaneda AR, et al. Anterior chest wall deformities and congenital heart disease. *J Thorac Cardiovasc Surg* 1988;96:427.
6. Peterson RJ, Young WC Jr, Godwin JD, et al. Noninvasive assessment of exercise cardiac function before and after pectus excavatum repair. *J Thorac Cardiovasc Surg* 1985;90(2): 251–260.
7. Ellis DG. Chest wall deformities. *Pediatr Rev* 1989;11:147.

8. Shamberger RC. Congenital chest wall deformities. *Curr Probl Surg* 1996;33:471.

9. Shamberger RC, Welch KJ. Chest wall deformities. In: Ashcraft KW, Holder TM, eds. *Pediatric surgery*, 2nd ed. Philadelphia: WB Saunders, 1993:146.

10. Ochsner A, DeBakey M. Chone-chondrosternon: report of a case and review of the literature. *J Thorac Surg* 1939;8:469.

11. Robicsek F, Fokin A. Surgical correction of pectus excavatum and carinatum. *J Cardiovasc Surg* 1999;40:725–731.

12. Taguchi, TK, Mochizuki T, Nakagaki M, et al. A new plastic operation for pectus excavatum: sternal turnover surgical procedure with preserved internal mammary arteries. *Chest* 1975;67:606–608.

13. Sirensen JL. Subcutaneous silicone implants in pectus excavatum. *Scand J Plast Reconstr Surg* 1987;22:173.

14. Baue AE. Chest wall, pleura, lungs, and diaphragm. In: Davis JH, Drucker WR, Gann DS, et al., eds. *Clinical surgery*. St. Louis: Mosby, 1987:1190.

15. Kowalewski J, Brocki M, Zolynski K. Long-term observation in 68 patients operated on for pectus excavatum: surgical repair of funnel chest. *Ann Thorac Surg* 1999;67:821.

16. Nuss D, Kelly RE, Croitoru DP, et al. A 10-year review of minimally invasive technique for the correction of pectus excavatum. *J Pediatr Surg* 1998;33(4):545–552.

17. Fonkalsrud EW, Bustorff-Silva J. Repair of pectus excavatum and carinatum in adults. *Am J Surg* 1999;177:121–124.

18. Shamberger RC, Welch KJ. Surgical correction of pectus carinatum. *J Pediatr Surg* 1987;22:48.

19. Beiser GD, Epstein SE, Stampfer M, et al. Impairment of cardiac function in patients with pectus excavatum, with improvement after operative correction. *N Engl J Med* 1972;287:267.

20. Seyfer AE, Icochea R, Graeber GM. Poland's anomaly: natural history and long-term results of chest wall reconstruction in 33 patients. *Ann Surg* 1988;208(6):776–782.

21. Shamberger RC, Welch KJ, Upton J Jr. Surgical treatment of thoracic deformity in Poland's syndrome. *J Pediatr Surg* 1989;24:760.

22. Hurwitz DJ, Stofman G, Curtin H. Three-dimensional imaging of Poland's syndrome. *Plast Reconstr Surg* 1994;94(5):719–723.

23. Gatti JE. Poland's deformity reconstructions with a customized, extrasoft silicone prosthesis. *Ann Plast Surg* 1997;39(2):122–130.

24. Urschel HC Jr. Poland's syndrome. *Chest Surg Clin North Am* 2000;10(2):393–403.

25. Marks MW, Iacobucci J. Reconstruction of congenital chest wall deformities using solid silicone onlay prostheses. *Chest Surg Clin North Am* 2000;10(2):341–355.

26. Sabiston DC Jr. The surgical management of congenital bifid sternum with a partial ectopia cordis. *J Thorac Surg* 1958;35:118.

27. Cantrell JR, Haller JA, Ravitch MM. A syndrome of congenital defects involving the abdominal wall, sternum, diaphragm, pericardium, and heart. *Surg Gynecol Obstet* 1958;107:602.

28. Knox L, Tuggle D, Knott-Craig CJ. Repair of congenital sternal clefts in adolescence and infancy. *J Pediatr Surg* 1994;29(12):1513–1516.

29. Daum R, Zachariou Z. Total and superior sternal clefts in newborns: a simple technique for surgical correction. *J Pediatr Surg* 1999;34(3):408–411.

30. Anderson BO, Burt ME. Chest wall neoplasms and their management. *Ann Thorac Surg* 1994;58:1774.

31. Pairolero PC. Chest wall tumors. In: Shields TW, ed. *General thoracic surgery*, 4th ed. Baltimore: Williams & Wilkins, 1994:579–589.

32. Graeber GM, Jones DR, Pairolero PC. Primary neoplasms. In: Pearson FG, Deslauriers J, Ginsberg RJ, et al., eds. *Thoracic surgery*. New York: Churchill Livingston, 1995:1237.

33. King RM, Pairolero PC, Trastek VF, et al. Primary chest wall tumors: factors affecting survival. Ann Thorac Surg 1986;41:597–601.

34. Liptay MJ, Fry WA. Malignant bone tumors of the chest wall. *Semin Thorac Cardiovasc Surg* 1999;11(3):278–284.

35. Dang NC, Siegel SE, Phillips JD. Malignant chest wall tumors in children and young adults. *J Pediatr Surg* 1999;34(12):1773–1778.

36. Burt M, Fulton M, Wessner-Dunlap S, et al. Primary bony and cartilaginous sarcomas of the chest wall: results of therapy. *Ann Thorac Surg* 1992;54:226.

37. Somers J, Faber LP. Chondroma and chondrosarcoma. *Semin Thorac Cardiovasc Surg* 1999;11(3):270–277.

38. Douglas YI, Meuzelaar KJ, Van Der Lei B, et al. Osteosarcoma of the sternum. *Eur J Surg Oncol* 1997;23(1):90–91.

39. Miser JS, Kinsela TJ, Triche TJ, et al. Preliminary results of treatment of Ewing's sarcoma of bone in children and young adults: six months of intensive combined modality therapy without maintenance. *J Clin Oncol* 1988;6:484.

40. Schuck A, Hofmann J, Rube C, et al. Radiotherapy in Ewing's sarcoma and PNET of the chest wall: results of the trials CESS 81, CESS 86, and EICESS 92. *Int J Radiat Oncol Biol Phys* 1998;42(5):1001–1006.

41. Saenz NC, Hass DJ, Meyers P, et al. Pediatric chest wall: Ewing's sarcoma. *J Pediatr Surg* 2000;35(4):550–555.

42. Shamberger RC, LaQuaglia MP, Krailo MD, et al. Ewing sarcoma of the rib: results of an intergroup study with analysis of outcome by timing of resection. *J Thorac Cardiovasc Surg* 2000;119(6):1154–1161.

43. Faber LP, Somers J, Templeton AC. Chest wall tumors. *Curr Probl Surg* 1995;32(8):661–747.

44. Sabanathan S, Shah R, Mearns AJ. Surgical treatment of primary malignant chest wall tumours. *Eur J Cardiothorac Surg* 1997;11(6):1011–1016.

45. Pairolero PC, Arnold PG. Chest wall reconstruction. *Ann Thorac Surg* 1981;32:325.

46. McCormack PM, Bains MS, Burt ME, et al. Local recurrent mammary carcinoma failing multimodality therapy. *Arch Surg* 1989;124:158.

47. Patterson GA, Ilves R, Ginsberg RJ, et al. The value of adjuvant radiotherapy in pulmonary and chest wall resection for bronchogenic carcinoma. *Ann Thorac Surg* 1982;34:692.

48. Piehler JM, Pairolero PC, Weiland LH, et al. Bronchogenic carcinoma with chest wall invasion: factors affecting survival following *en bloc* resection. *Ann Thorac Surg* 1982;34:684.

49. McCaughan BC, Martini N, Bains MS, et al. Chest wall invasion in carcinoma of the lung: therapeutic and prognostic implications. *J Thorac Cardiovasc Surg* 1985;89:836.

50. Pancoast H. Importance of careful roentgen ray investigations of apical chest tumors. *JAMA* 1924;83:1407.

51. Paulson DL. Carcinomas of the superior pulmonary sulcus. *J Thorac Cardiovasc Surg* 1975;70:1095.

52. Hilaris BS, Martini N, Wong GY, et al. Treatment of superior sulcus tumor (Pancoast tumor). *Surg Clin North Am* 1987;67:9650.

53. Taylor LQ, Williams AJ, Santiago SM. Survival in patients with superior pulmonary sulcus tumors. *Respiration* 1992;59:27.

54. Wright CD, Moncure AC, Shepard JA, et al. Superior sulcus lung tumors: results of combined treatment (irradiation and radical resection). *J Thorac Cardiovasc Surg* 1987;94:69.

55. Neal CR, Amdur RJ, Mendenhall WM, et al. Pancoast tumor: radiation therapy alone versus preoperative radiation therapy and surgery. *Int J Radiat Oncol Biol Phys* 1991;21:651.

56. Jones DR, Detterbeck FC. Pancoast tumors of the lung. *Curr Opin Pulm Med* 1998;4(4):191–197.

57. Komaki R, Putnam JB Jr, Walsh G, et al. The management of superior sulcus tumors. *Semin Surg Oncol* 2000;18(2):152–164.

58. Mathes SJ. Chest wall reconstruction. *Clin Plast Surg* 1995;22:187.

59. Deschamps C, Tirnaksiz BM, Darbandi R, et al. Early and long-term results of prosthetic chest wall reconstruction. *J Thorac Cardiovasc Surg* 1999;117(3):588–591.

60. Pairolero PC. Extended resections for lung cancer: how far is too far? *Eur J Cardiothorac Surg* 1999;16(suppl 1):S48–S50.

61. Seyfer AE. Breast cancer invasion into the chest wall with resection and reconstruction. *Semin Thorac Cardiovasc Surg* 1999;11(3):285–292.

62. Lardinois D, Muller M, Furrer M, et al. Functional assessment of chest wall integrity after methylmethacrylate reconstruction. *Ann Thorac Surg* 2000;69(3):919–923.

63. Urschel HC Jr, Razzuk MA. Thoracic outlet syndrome. In: Sabiston DC Jr, Spencer FC, eds. *Surgery of the chest*. Philadelphia: WB Saunders, 1990:536–553.

64. Harding A, Silver D. Thoracic outlet syndrome. In: Sabiston DC Jr, ed. *Textbook of surgery: the biological basis of modern surgical practice,* 14th ed. Philadelphia: WB Saunders, 1991: 1757.

65. Urschel HC. Thoracic outlet syndromes. In: Baue AE, Geha AS, Hammond GL, et al., eds. *Glenn's thoracic and cardiovascular surgery,* 6th ed. Stamford, CT: Appleton & Lange, 1996:567.

66. Urschel HC, Razzuk M. Upper plexus thoracic outlet syndrome: optimal therapy. *Ann Thorac Surg* 1997;63:935.

67. Abe M, Ichinohe K, Nishida J. Diagnosis, treatment, and complications of thoracic outlet syndrome. *J Orthop Sci* 1999;4:66.

68. Mackinnon SE, Patterson GA, Novak CB. Thoracic outlet syndrome: a current overview. *Semin Thorac Cardiovasc Surg* 1996a;8:176.

69. Netter FH. Clinical symposia. CIBA-GEIGY Corporation, 1971.

70. Ryan GM. Thoracic outlet syndrome. *J Shoulder Elbow Surg* 1998;7:440.

71. Pang D, Wessel HB. Thoracic outlet syndrome. *Neurosurgery* 1988;22:105.

72. Novak CB. Conservative management of thoracic outlet syndrome. *Semin Thorac Cardiovasc Surg* 1996;8:201.

73. Mackinnon SE, Patterson AG. Supraclavicular first rib resection. *Semin Thorac Cardiovasc Surg* 1996;8:208.

74. Goff CD, Parent FN, Sato DT, et al. A comparison of surgery for neurogenic thoracic outlet syndrome between laborers and nonlaborers. *Am J Surg* 1998;176(2):215–218.

75. Urschel HC Jr, Razzuk MA. Neurovascular compression in the thoracic outlet: changing management over 50 years. *Ann Surg* 1998;228(4):609–617.

76. Light RW. The physiology of pleural fluid production and benign pleural effusion. In: Shields TW, ed. *General thoracic surgery,* 4th ed. Malvern, PA: Williams & Wilkins, 1994:676.

77. Jerjes-Sanchez C, Ramirez-Rivera A, Elijalde JJ, et al. Intrapleural fibrinolysis with streptokinase as an adjunctive treatment in hemothorax and empyema: a multicenter trial. *Chest* 1996;109(6):1514–1519.

78. Chin NK, Lim TK. Controlled trial of intrapleural streptokinase in the treatment of pleural empyema and complicated parapneumonic effusions. *Chest* 1997;111(2):275–279.

79. Wait MA, Sharma S, Hohn J, et al. A randomized trial of empyema therapy. *Chest* 1997;111(6):1548–1551.

80. Davies CW, Kearnry SE, Gleeson FV, et al. Predictors of outcome and long-term survival in patients with pleural infection. *Am J Respir Crit Care Med* 1999;160:1682–1687.

81. Huang HC, Chang HY, Chen CW, et al. Predicting factors for outcome of tube thoracostomy in complicated parapneumonic effusion for empyema. *Chest* 1999;115(3):751–756.

82. DeMeester TR, Lafontaine E. The pleura. In: Sabiston DC Jr, Spencer FC, eds. *Surgery of the chest,* 5th ed. Philadelphia: WB Saunders, 1990:444–497.

83. Rimensberger PC, Muller-Schenker B, Kalangos A, et al. Treatment of a persistent postoperative chylothorax with somatostatin. *Ann Thorac Surg* 1998;66:253–254.

84. Cope C, Salem R, Kaiser LR. Management of chylothorax by percutaneous catheterization and embolization of the thoracic duct: prospective trial. *J Vasc Intervent Radiol* 1999; 10(9):1248–1254.

85. Kelly RF, Shumway SJ. Conservative management of postoperative chylothorax using somatostatin. *Ann Thorac Surg* 2000;69:1944–1945.

86. Sassoon CS. The etiology and treatment of spontaneous pneumothorax. *Curr Opin Pulm Med* 1995;1:331–338.

87. Martin T, Fontana G, Olak J, et al. Use of pleural catheter for the management of simple pneumothorax. *Chest* 1996;110: 1169–1172.

88. Schramel FMNH, Postmus PE, Vanderschueren RGJRA. Current aspects of spontaneous pneumothorax. *Eur Respir J* 1997;10:1372–1379.

89. Cardillo G, Facciolo F, Giunti R, et al. Videothoracoscopic treatment of primary spontaneous pneumothorax: a 6-year experience. *Ann Thorac Surg* 2000;69:357–361; discussion 361–362.

90. Hatz RA, Kaps MF, Meimarakis G, et al. Long-term results after video-assisted thoracoscopic surgery for first-time and recurrent spontaneous pneumothorax. *Ann Thorac Surg* 2000;70(1):253–257.

91. Rusch VW. Diffuse malignant mesothelioma. In: Shields TW, LoCicero J III, Ponn RB, eds. *General thoracic surgery,* 5th ed. Philadelphia: Lippincott Williams & Wilkins, 2000:767–782.

92. Nicholson WJ, Perket G, Selikoff IJ. Occupational exposure to asbestos: population at risk and projected mortality—1980–2030. *Am J Ind Med* 1982;3:259–311.

93. Hammar SP, Bolen JW. Pleural neoplasms. In: Dail DH, Hammar SP, eds. *Pulmonary pathology.* New York: Springer, 1988:979.

94. Flores RM, Sugarbaker DJ. Malignant mesothelioma of the pleural space. *Ann Thorac Surg* 2000;70:306.

95. Butchart EG, Ashcroft T, Barnsley WC, et al. Pleuropneumonectomy in the management of diffuse malignant mesothelioma of the pleura: experience with 29 patients. *Thorax* 1976;31:15.

96. Sugarbaker DJ, Strauss GM, Lynch TJ, et al. Node status has prognostic significance in the multimodality therapy of diffuse, malignant mesothelioma. *J Clin Oncol* 1993;11: 1172–1178.

97. Sugarbaker DJ, Flores RM, Jaklitsch MT, et al. Resection margins, extrapleural nodal status, and cell type determine postoperative long-term survival in trimodality therapy of malignant pleural mesothelioma: results in 183 patients. *Thorac Cardiovasc Surg* 1999;117:54–65.

98. Rusch VW, The International Mesothelioma Interest Group. A proposed new international TNM staging system for malignant pleural mesothelioma. *Chest* 1995;108:1122–1128.

99. Taub RN, Antman KH. Chemotherapy for malignant mesothelioma. *Semin Thorac Cardiovasc Surg* 1997;9:361–366.

100. Wanebo JH, Martini N, Melamed MR, et al. Pleural mesothelioma. *Cancer* 1976;38:2481–2488.

101. Rusch VW. Pleurectomy/decortication in the setting of multimodality treatment for diffuse malignant pleural mesothelioma. *Semin Thorac Cardiovasc Surg* 1997;9:367–372.

102. Kaiser LR. New therapies in the treatment of malignant pleural mesothelioma. *Semin Thorac Cardiovasc Surg* 1997; 9:383–390.

103. Rusch VW, Venkatraman ES. Important prognostic factors in patients with malignant pleural mesothelioma managed surgically. *Ann Thorac Surg* 1999;68:1799–1804.

104. Jablons D. Positron emission tomography with F18-fluorodeoxyglucose in the staging and preoperative evaluation of malignant pleural mesothelioma. *J Thorac Cardiovasc Surg* 2000;120:128–133.

105. Esposito C, Romeo C. Surgical anatomy of the mediastinum. *Semin Pediatr Surg* 1999;8(2):50–53.

106. Heimburger IL, Battersby JS, Vellios F. Primary neoplasms of the mediastinum: a fifteen-year experience. *Arch Surg* 1963; 978–984.

107. Azanow KS, Pearl RH, Zurcher R, et al. Primary mediastinal masses: a comparison of adult and pediatric populations. *J Thorac Cardiovasc Surg* 1993;106:67–72.

108. Billmire DF. Germ cell, mesenchymal, and thymic tumors of the mediastinum. *Semin Pediatr Surg* 1999;8(2):85–91.

109. Heimburger IL, Battersby JS. Primary mediastinal tumors of childhood. *J Thorac Cardiovasc Surg* 1965;50–92.

110. Haller JA, Mazur DO, Morgan WM. Diagnosis and management of mediastinal masses in children. *J Thorac Cardiovasc Surg* 1969;58:385.

111. Grosfeld JL, Weinberg M, Kilmann JW, et al. Primary mediastinal neoplasms in infants and children. *Ann Thorac Surg* 1971;12:179.

112. Whittaker LD, Lynn HB. Mediastinal tumors and cysts in the pediatric patient. *Surg Clin North Am* 1973;53:893.

113. Pokorny WJ, Sherman JO. Mediastinal masses in infants and children. *J Thorac Cardiovasc Surg* 1974;68:689.

114. King RM, Telander RL, Smithson WA, et al. Primary mediastinal tumors in children. *J Pediatr Surg* 1982;17:512.

115. Davis RD, Oldham HN, Sabiston DC. Primary cysts and neoplasms of the mediastinum: recent changes in clinical presentation, methods or diagnosis, management and results. *Ann Thorac Surg* 1987;44:229–237.

116. Davis RD Jr, Oldham HN Jr, Sabiston DC Jr. The mediastinum. In: Sabiston DC Jr, Spencer FC, eds. *Surgery of the chest,* 5th ed. Philadelphia: WB Saunders, 1990:498–535.

117. Wychulis AR, Payne WS, Clagett OT, et al. Surgical treatment of mediastinal tumors. *J Thorac Cardiovasc Surg* 1971;62:379.

118. Rubush JL, Gardner IC, Boyd WK, et al. Mediastinal tumors: review of 186 cases. *J Thorac Cardiovasc Surg* 1973;65:216.

119. Lousta R, Koikkalainen K, Jyrala A, et al. Mediastinal tumors: a follow-up of 208 patients. *Scand J Thorac Cardiovasc Surg* 1978;12:258.

120. Nandi P, Wong KC, Mok CK, et al. Primary mediastinal tumours: review of 74 cases. *J R Coll Surg Edinb* 1980;25:460.

121. Ovum E, Birkeland S. Mediastinal tumors and cysts: a review of 191 cases. *Scand J Thorac Cardiovasc Surg* 1983;86:727.

122. Mullen B, Richardson JD. Primary anterior mediastinal tumors in children and adults. *Ann Thorac Surg* 1986;42:338–345.

123. Cohen AJ, Thompson L, Edwards FH, et al. Primary cysts and tumors of the mediastinum. *Ann Thorac Surg* 1991;41:378–386.

124. Whooley BP, Urschel JD, Antkowiak JG, et al. Primary tumors of the mediastinum. *J Surg Oncol* 1999;70(2):95–99.

125. Harris GJ, Harmon PK, Trinkel JK, et al. Standard biplane roentgenography is highly sensitive in documenting mediastinal masses. *Ann Thorac Surg* 1987;44:238.

126. Pugatch RD, Faling LJ, Robbins AH, et al. CT diagnosis of benign mediastinal abnormalities. *AJR* 1980;134:685.

127. VonSchulthess GK, McMurdok, Tscholakoff D, et al. Mediastinal masses: MR imaging. *Radiology* 1986;158:289.

128. Schamberger RC, Holzma RS, Griscow NT, et al. CT quantitation of tracheal cross-sectional area as a guide to the surgical and anesthetic management of children with anterior mediastinal masses. *J Pediatr Surg* 1991;26:138.

129. Shapiro B, Sisson J, Kalff V, et al. The location of a middle mediastinal pheochromocytoma. *J Thorac Cardiovasc Surg* 1984;87:814.

130. Helio A. Tumors in the mediastinum: US-guided histologic core core-needle biopsy. *Radiology* 1993;189:143.

131. D'Agostino HB, Sanchez RB, Laoide RM, et al. Anterior mediastinal lesions: transsternal biopsy with CT guidance work in progress. *Radiology* 1993;189:703.

132. Bressler EL, Kirkham JA. Mediastinal masses: alternative approaches to CT-guided needle biopsy. *Radiology* 1994;191:391–396.

133. Bonadies J, D'Agostino RS, Ruskis AF, et al. Outpatient mediastinoscopy. *J Thorac Cardiovasc Surg* 1993;106:686.

134. Mack M, Landreneau R. Thoracoscopy for the diseases of the mediastinum including thymectomy for myasthenia gravis. *Semin Laparosc Surg* 1996;3(4):245–252.

135. Roviaro G, Varoli F, Nucca O, et al. Videothoracoscopic approach to primary mediastinal pathology. *Chest* 2000;117(4):1179–1183.

136. Morgenthaler TI, Brown LR, Colby TV, et al. Thymoma. *Mayo Clin Proc* 1993;68:1110–1123.

137. Kohman LJ. Approach to the diagnosis and staging of mediastinal masses. *Chest* 1993;103(suppl):328–330.

138. Masaoka A, Monden Y, Nakahara K, et al. Follow-up study of thymomas with special references to their clinical stages. *Cancer* 1981;48:2485.

139. Kirchen T, Muller-Hermelink HK. New approaches to the diagnosis of thymic epithelial tumors. *Prog Surg Pathol* 1989;70:167–189.

140. Weide LG, Ulbright TM, Loehrer PJ, et al. Thymic carcinoma: a distinct clinical entity responsive to chemotherapy. *Cancer* 1993;71(4):1219–1223.

141. Nakahara K, Ohno K, Hashimoto J, et al. Thymoma: results with complete resection and adjuvant postoperative irradiation in 141 consecutive patients. *J Thorac Cardiovasc Surg* 1988;95:1041–1047.

142. Urgesi A, Monetti V, Ross G, et al. Role of radiation therapy in locally advanced thymoma. *Radiother Oncol* 1990;19:273–280.

143. Loeher PJ Sr, Perez CA, Roth LM, et al. Chemotherapy for advanced thymoma: preliminary results of an intergroup study. *Ann Intern Med* 1990;113:520–524.

144. Park HS, Shin DM, Lee JS, et al. Thymoma: a retrospective study of 87 cases. *Cancer* 1994;73(10):2491–2498.

145. Thomas CR, Wright CD, Loehrer PJ. Thymoma: state of the art. *J Clin Oncol* 1999;17(7):2280–2289.

146. Kirschner PA. Reoperation for thymoma: a report of 3 cases. *Ann Thorac Surg* 1990;49:550–554.

147. Gripp S, Hilgers K, Wurm R, et al. Thymoma: prognostic factors and treatment outcomes. *Cancer* 1998;83(8):1495–1503.

148. Langenfeld J, Graeber GM. Current management of thymoma. *Surg Oncol Clin North Am* 1999;8(2):327–339.

149. Okumura M, Miyoshi S, Takeuchi Y, et al. Results of surgical treatment of thymomas with special reference to the involved organs. *J Thorac Cardiovasc Surg* 1999;117(3):605–613.

150. Wilkins KB, Sheikh E, Green R, et al. Clinical and pathologic predictors of survival in patients with thymoma. *Ann Surg* 1999;230(4):562–572.

151. Treves TA, Rocca WA, Menoeghin F. Epidemiology of myasthenia gravis. In: Anderson DW, Schoenberg DG, eds. *Neuroepidemiology: a tribute to Bruce Schoenberg*. Boston: CRC Press, 1991:297.

152. Phillips LH, Torner JC. Has the natural history of myasthenia gravis changed over the past 40 years? An analysis of the epidemiological literature. *Neurology* 1993;43:A386.

153. Phillips LH. The epidemiology of myasthenia gravis. *Neurol Clin North Am* 1994;12:263–271.

154. Olanow CW, Wechsler AS, Roses AD. A prospective study of thymectomy and serum acetylcholine receptor antibodies in myasthenia gravis. *Ann Surg* 1982;196:113.

155. Maselli A. Pathophysiology of myasthenia gravis and Lambert Eaton syndrome. *Neurol Clin North Am* 1994;12:285–303.

156. Castleman B, Norris EH. The pathology of the thymus gland in myasthenia gravis: a study of 35 cases. *Medicine* 1949;28:27.

157. Hopkins LC. Clinical features of myasthenia gravis. *Neurol Clin North Am* 1994;12:243–261.

158. Trastek VF, Shields TW. Surgery of the thymus gland. In: Shields TW, ed. *General thoracic surgery*, 5th ed. Baltimore: Williams & Wilkins, 1994:1770–1801.

159. Saunders DB, Scoppetta C. The treatment of patients with myasthenia gravis. *Neurol Clin North Am* 1994;12:343–368.

160. Crucitti F, Doglietto GB, Bellanone R, et al. Effects of surgical treatment in thymoma with myasthenia gravis: our experience in 103 patients. *J Surg Oncol* 1992;50:43–46.

161. Nussbaum MS, Rosenthal GJ, Saunders KJ, et al. Management of myasthenia gravis by extended thymectomy with anterior mediastinal dissection. *Surgery* 1992;112(4):681–688.

162. Blossom GB, Erinstoff RM, Howells GA, et al. Thymoma for myasthenia gravis. *Arch Surg* 1993;128(8):855–862.

163. Sugarbaker DJ. Thoracoscopy in the management of anterior mediastinal masses. *Ann Thorac Surg* 1993;56:653–656.

164. Kirschner PA. Myasthenia gravis and other parathymic syndromes. *Chest Surg Clin North Am* 1994;2(1):183–201.

165. Frist WH, Thirumalai S, Doehring CB, et al. Thymectomy for the myasthenia gravis patient: factors influencing outcome. *Ann Thorac Surg* 1994;57:334–338.

166. Defilippi VJ, Richman DP, Ferguson MK. Transcervical thymectomy for myasthenia gravis. *Ann Thorac Surg* 1994;57:194–197.

167. Yellin A. Lymphoproliferative diseases. *Chest Surg Clin North Am* 1992;2:107–120.

168. Bonfiglio TA, Dvoretsky PM, Risciuli F, et al. Fine needle aspiration biopsy in the evaluation of lymphoreticular tumors of the thorax. *Acta Cytol* 1985;29:548.

169. Hope RT, Colemain CN, Cox RS, et al. The management of stage I-II Hodgkin's disease with irradiation alone or combined modality therapy: the Stanford experience. *Blood* 1982;59:455.

170. Glick RD, La Quaglia MP. Lymphomas of the anterior mediastinum. *Semin Pediatr Surg* 1999;8(2):69–77.

171. Suster S. Primary large cell lymphomas of the mediastinum. *Semin Diagn Pathol* 1999;16(1):51–64.

172. Luna MA, Johnson PE. Postmortem findings in testicular tumors. In: Johnson DE, ed. *Testicular tumors*. New York: Medical Examination, 1975.

173. Kuhn MW, Weissbach L. Localization, incidence, diagnosis, and treatment of extratesticular germ cell tumors. *Urol Int* 1985;40:166–172.

174. Nichols CR, Roth BJ, Heerema N, et al. Hematologic neoplasia associated with primary germ cell tumors. *N Engl J Med* 1990;322:1425–1429.

175. Nichols CR. Mediastinal germ cell tumors: clinical features and biologic correlates. *Chest* 1991;99:472–479.

176. Lakhoo BM, Drake DP. Mediastinal teratomas: review of 15 pediatric cases. *J Pediatr Surg* 1993;28:1161–1164.

177. Chaganti RSK, Rodriguez E, Mathew S. Origin of adult male mediastinal germ cell tumors. *Lancet* 1994;343:1130–1132.

178. Knapp RH, Hurt RD, Payne WS, et al. Malignant germ cell tumors of the mediastinum. *J Thorac Cardiovasc Surg* 1985; 89:82–89.

179. Dulmet EM, Macchiavini P, Suc B, et al. Germ cell tumors of the mediastinum: a 30 year experience. *Cancer* 1993;72: 1895–1901.

180. Gross PE, Schwartfeger L, Blackstein ME, et al. Extragonadal germ cell tumors: a 14 year Toronto experience. *Cancer* 1994;73:1971–1979.

181. Weidner N. Germ-cell tumors of the mediastinum. *Semin Diagn Pathol* 1999;16(1):42–50.

182. Mandelbaum I. Germ cell tumors of the mediastinum. *Chest Surg Clin North Am* 1992;2:203–211.

183. Lewis BD, Hurt RD, Payne WS, et al. Benign teratoma of the mediastinum. *J Thorac Cardiovasc Surg* 1983;86:727.

184. Jain KK, Bols GJ, Bains MS, et al. The treatment of extragonadal seminoma. *J Clin Oncol* 1984;2:820–827.

185. Loehrer PJ, Birch R, Williams SD, et al. Chemotherapy of metastatic seminoma: the Southern Cancer Study Group experience. *J Clin Oncol* 1987;5:1212–1220.

186. Motzer R, Bosl G, Heelan R, et al. Residual mass: an indication for further therapy in patients with advanced seminoma following systemic chemotherapy. *J Clin Oncol* 1987;5: 1065–1070.

187. Shields TW. Primary lesions of the mediastinum and their investigation and treatment. In: Shields TW, ed. *General thoracic surgery.* Baltimore: Williams & Wilkins, 1994:1724–1769.

188. Kantoff O. Surgical and medical management of germ cell tumors of the chest. *Chest* 1993;103:3315–3355.

189. Johnson SR, Adam A, Allison DJ, et al. Recurrent respiratory obstruction from a mediastinal bronchogenic cyst. *Thorax* 1992;47:660–662.

190. Patel SR, Meeker DP, Biscotti CV, et al. Preservation and management of bronchogenic cysts in the adult. *Chest* 1994;106:79–85.

191. Coran AG, Drongowski R. Congenital cystic disease of the tracheobronchial tree in infants and children: experience with 44 consecutive cases. *Arch Surg* 1994;129:521–527.

192. Haddon MJ, Bowen A. Bronchopulmonary and neurenteric forms of foregut anomalies: imaging for diagnosis and management. *Radiol Clin North Am* 1991;29:241–254.

193. Bolton JW, Shahian DM. Asymptomatic bronchogenic cysts: what is the best management? *Ann Thorac Surg* 1992;53: 1134–1137.

194. Hazelrigg SR, Landreneau RJ, Mack MJ, et al. Thoracoscopic resection of mediastinal cysts. *Ann Thorac Surg* 1993;56: 569–660.

195. Suen HC, Mathisen DJ, Grillo HC, et al. Surgical management and radiological characteristics of bronchogenic cysts. *Ann Thorac Surg* 1993;55:476–481.

196. Martinoid E, Pons F, Azorin J, et al. Thoracoscopic excision of mediastinal bronchogenic cysts: results in 20 cases. *Ann Thorac Surg* 2000;69(5):1525–1528.

197. Bennheim J, Griffel B, Versano S, et al. Mediastinal leiomyosarcoma in the wall of a bronchogenic cyst. *Arch Pathol Lab Med* 1980;104:221.

198. Read CA, Movont M, Varangelo R, et al. Recurrent bronchogenic cyst: an assessment for complete surgical excision. *Arch Surg* 1991;126:1306–1308.

199. Malde HM, Kedar RP, Chadda DJ. Ethanol sclerosis of a mediastinal cyst. *Can Assoc Radiol J* 1993;44:310–312.

200. Feigin DS, Fenoglis JJ, McAllister HA, et al. Pericardial cysts: a radiologic–pathologic correlation and review. *Diagn Radiol* 1977;125:15.

201. Whitaker JA, Deffenbaugh LD, Cooke AR. Esophageal duplication cyst. *Am J Gastroenterol* 1980;73:329.

202. D'Almeida AC, Steward DH Jr. Neuroenteric cysts: case report and literature review. *Neurosurgery* 1981;8:596.

203. Allen MS, Payne WS. Cystic foregut malformation in the mediastinum. *Chest Surg Clin North Am* 1992;2:89–106.

204. Rastegar H, Arger P, Harlan AH. Evaluation and therapy of mediastinal thymic cysts. *Ann Surg* 1980;46:236.

205. Furst H, Schmittenbecher PP, Dievemautt, et al. Mediastinal pancreatic pseudocyst. *Eur J CardioThorac Surg* 1992;6: 46–48.

206. Okabe K, Mivra K, Konish H, et al. Thoracic duct cyst of the mediastinum: case report. *Scand J Thorac Cardiovasc Surg* 1993;27:175–177.

207. Adams GA, Schochat SJ, Smith EI, et al. Thoracic neuroblastoma: a pediatric Oncology Group study. *J Pediatr Surg* 1993;28:372–378.

208. Ricci C, Rendina EA, Venuto F, et al. Diagnostic imaging and surgical treatment of dumbbell tumors of the mediastinum. *Ann Thorac Surg* 1990;50:586–589.

209. Moon WK, Jung-Gi I, Hau MC. Malignant schwannomas of the thorax: CT findings. *J Comp Assist Tomogr* 1993;17(2): 274–276.

210. Wain JC. Neurogenic tumors of the mediastinum. *Chest Surg Clin North Am* 1992;2(1):121–136.

211. Zajtchuk R, Bowen TD, Seyfer AD, et al. Intrathoracic ganglioneuroblastoma. *J Thorac Cardiovasc Surg* 1980;80: 605–612.

212. Joshi VV, Cantor AB, Altshuler G, et al. Age-linked prognostic categorization based on a new histologic grading system of neuroblastomas: a clinicopathologic study of 211 cases from the Pediatric Oncology Group. *Cancer* 1992;8:2197–2211.

213. Olson JL, Salyer WR. Mediastinal paragangliomas (aortic body tumors): a report of four cases and a review of the literature. *Cancer* 1978;41:2405–2412.

214. Alewari DE, Payne NS, Onofrio BM, et al. Dumbbell neurogenic tumors of the mediastinum. *Mayo Clin Proc* 1978;53:353.

215. Grillo HC, Ojemann RG, Scannell JG, et al. Combined approach to "dumbbell" intrathoracic and intraspinal neurogenic tumors. *Ann Thorac Surg* 1983;36:402.

216. Landreneau RJ, Dowling RD, Ferson PF. Thoracoscopic resection of a posterior mediastinal neurogenic tumor. *Chest* 1992;102(4):1288–1290.

217. McIntire FT, Sykes EM Jr. Obstruction of the superior vena cava: a review of the literature and report of two personal cases. *Ann Intern Med* 1949;30:925.

218. Lochridge SK, Knibble WP, Doty DB. Obstruction of the superior vena cava. *Surgery* 1979;85:14.

219. Parish JM, Marschke RF, Dines DE, et al. Etiologic considerations in superior vena cava syndrome. *Mayo Clin Proc* 1981;56:407.

220. Mazzetti H, Dussant A, Tentori C. Superior vena cava occlusion and/or syndrome related to pacemaker leads. *Am Heart J* 1993;125:831.

221. Perez CA, Presant CA, VanAmburg A. Management of superior vena cava syndrome. *Semin Oncol* 1978;5:123.

222. Nieto AF, Doty DB. Superior vena cava obstruction: clinical syndrome, etiology, and treatment. *Curr Probl Cancer* 1986; 10:441.

223. Mahajan V, Strimlan V, VanOrdstran HC, et al. Benign superior vena cava syndrome. *Chest* 1975;68:32.

224. Dines DE, Payne WS, Bernatz PE, et al. Mediastinal granuloma and fibrosing mediastinitis. *Chest* 1975;75:320.

225. Lagerstrom CF, Mitchell HG, Graham BS, et al. Chronic fibrosing mediastinitis and superior vena caval obstruction from blastomycosis. *Ann Thorac Surg* 1992;54:764.

226. Brown G, Husband JE. Mediastinal widening: a valuable radiographic sign of superior vena cava thrombosis. *Clin Radiol* 1993;47:415.

227. Kim JH, Kim HS, Chung SH. CT diagnosis of superior vena cava syndrome: importance of collateral vessels. *AJR* 1993; 161:539.

228. Ko J, Yang P, Yuan A, et al. Superior vena cava syndrome: rapid histologic diagnosis by ultrasound guided transthoracic needle aspiration biopsy. *Am J Respir Crit Care Med* 1994;149:783.

229. Abner A. Approach to the patient who presents with superior vena cava obstruction. *Chest* 1993;103:3945.

230. Kane RC, Cohen MH, Brader LE, et al. Superior vena cava obstruction due to small-cell anaplastic lung carcinoma. *JAMA* 1976;235:1717.

231. Perez-Soler R, McLaughlin P, Velasquez WS, et al. Clinical features and results of management of superior vena cava syndrome secondary to lymphoma. *J Clin Oncol* 1984;2:260.
232. Ferguson TB, Burford TH. Mediastinal granuloma: a 15 year experience. *Ann Thorac Surg* 1965;1:125.
233. Dodds GA, Harrison JK, O'Laughlin MO, et al. Relief of superior vena cava syndrome due to fibrosing mediastinitis using the Palmaz stent. *Chest* 1994;106:315.
234. Avasthi RB, Moghissi K. Malignant obstruction of the superior vena cava and its palliation: report of four cases. *J Thorac Cardiovasc Surg* 1977;74:244.
235. Doty DB, Doty JR, Jones KW. Bypass of superior vena cava: 15 years experience with spiral vein graft for obstruction of superior vena cava caused by benign disease. *J Thorac Cardiovasc Surg* 1990;99:889.
236. Dartevelle PG, Chapelier AR, Pastorino V, et al. Long-term follow-up after prosthetic replacement of the superior vena cava combined with resection of mediastinal–pulmonary malignant tumors. *J Thorac Cardiovasc Surg* 1991;102:259.
237. Moore WM Jr, Hollier LH, Pickett TK. Superior vena cava and central venous reconstruction. *Surgery* 1991;110:35.
238. Mathisen DJ, Grillo HC. Clinical manifestation of mediastinal fibrosis and histoplasmosis. *Ann Thorac Surg* 1992;54:1053–1058.
239. Roberts JR, Bueno R, Sugarbaker DJ. Multimodality treatment of malignant superior vena cava syndrome. *Chest* 1999;116(3):835–837.
240. Yim CD, Sane SS, Bjarnason H. Superior vena cava stenting. *Radiol Clin North Am* 2000;38(2):409–424.
241. Porte H, Metois D, Finzi L, et al. Superior vena cava syndrome of malignant origin: which procedure for which diagnosis? *Eur J Cardiothorac Surg* 2000;17(4):384–388.
242. Salassa JR, Pearson BW, Payne WS, et al. Gross and microscopical blood supply of the trachea. *Ann Thorac Surg* 1977;24(2):100–107.
243. Mathisen DJ. Tracheal tumors. *Chest Surg Clin North Am* 1996;6:875–898.
244. Grillo HC, Mathisen DJ. Primary tracheal tumors: treatment and results. *Ann Thorac Surg* 1990;49(1):69–77.
245. Kearney PA, Griffen MM, Ochoa JB, et al. A single-center 8-year experience with percutaneous dilational tracheostomy. *Ann Surg* 2000;231(5):701–709.
246. Norwood S, Vallina VL, Short K, et al. Incidence of tracheal stenosis and other late complications after percutaneous tracheostomy. *Ann Surg* 2000;232(2):233–241.
247. Grillo HC. Surgical treatment of postintubation tracheal injuries. *J Thorac Cardiovasc Surg* 1979;78:860.
248. Mathisen DJ. Surgery of the trachea. *Curr Prob Surg* 1998;35(6):455–542.
249. Bolman RM III, Wolfe WG. Bronchiectasis and bronchopulmonary sequestration. *Surg Clin North Am* 1980;60(4):867–881.
250. Johnson PC, Sarosi GA. The endemic mycoses: surgical considerations. *Semin Thorac Cardiovasc Surg* 1995;7(2):95–103. Review.

SECTION L

CARDIOVASCULAR SYSTEM

SURGERY: SCIENTIFIC PRINCIPLES AND PRACTICE, Third Edition, edited by
Lazar J. Greenfield, Michael W. Mulholland, Keith T. Oldham, Gerald B. Zelenock,
and Keith D. Lillemoe. Lippincott Williams & Wilkins Publishers, Philadelphia, © 2001.

CHAPTER 61

CONGENITAL HEART DISEASE AND CARDIAC TUMORS

RALPH S. MOSCA, JENNIFER C. HIRSCH, AND EDWARD L. BOVE

HISTORY

Cardiac surgery as a specialty is notable for the developments and rapid technical advances that have been made during the past few decades. Much of the original interest was focused on attempts to treat congenital heart defects associated with cyanosis and early mortality. The first successful treatment of a cyanotic lesion was the closure of a patent ductus arteriosus by Gross and Hubbard in 1938 (1). The description of the subclavian artery-to-pulmonary artery shunt by Blalock and Taussig in 1945 (2) opened the way to the palliation of many complex cyanotic lesions—most notably, tetralogy of Fallot. The 1950s represented the decade of greatest advances, which laid the foundation for the field of cardiac surgery. Lewis and Taufic in 1952 (3) performed the first open closure of an atrial septal defect by using surface hypothermia and inflow occlusion. In 1953, Gibbon (4) performed the first repair of an ASD with the use of a pump oxygenator that became the model for modern cardiopulmonary bypass. Next, Warden and colleagues (5) used controlled cross-circulation with an adult as the oxygenator during intracardiac repairs. Building on the work of Gibbon, Kirklin et al. (6) then published the first series of eight intracardiac operations performed at the Mayo Clinic with the use of cardiopulmonary bypass. With these landmark efforts, focused on congenital heart disease, the field of cardiac surgery was established.

ATRIAL SEPTAL DEFECT

The atrial and ventricular septa form between the third and sixth weeks of fetal development. After the paired heart tubes fuse into a single tube folded on itself, the distal portion of the tube causes an indentation to form in the roof of the common atrium. Near this portion of the roof, the septum primum arises and extends in a crescentic formation toward the atrioventricular (AV) junction. The gap remaining between the septum primum and the developing tissues of the AV junction is called the *ostium primum*. Before the septum primum fuses completely with the endocardial cushions, a series of fenestrations appear in the septum primum that coalesce into the ostium secundum.

During this coalescence, the septum secundum grows downward from the roof of the atrium, parallel to and to the right of the septum primum. The septum primum does not fuse but creates an oblique pathway, called the *foramen ovale*, from the right atrium to the left. After birth, the increase in left atrial pressure usually closes this pathway, so that separation of the atria becomes complete. Probe patency of the foramen ovale is commonly observed in normal persons (7).

An *atrial septal defect* (ASD) is a hole in the atrial septum (Fig. 61.1). ASDs are most commonly located in the central aspect of the septum and are referred to as *ostium secundum* or *fossa ovalis defects*. Ostium secundum defects account for more than 80% of all ASDs. These defects may range from a simple patent foramen ovale to a complete absence of the septum primum. In the latter condition, the orifice of the inferior vena cava may appear to connect directly with the left atrium. In 5% to 10% of patients, the defect occurs along the remnant of the right horn of the sinus venosus and is referred to as a *sinus venosus ASD*. Most often, this occurs adjacent to the superior vena cava and is associated with partial anomalous pulmonary venous return. The orifice of the superior vena cava appears to straddle the ASD, its posterior wall being continuous with the left atrium itself. Defects in the AV septum are commonly referred to as *ostium primum ASDs*. This actually represents a more complex form of atrial defect and is more properly referred to as the incomplete form of *AV septal defect* (AVSD). These are associated with abnormal mitral valve morphology. Coronary sinus defects occur when the coronary sinus is partially or completely unroofed in the left atrium. These defects result from a deficiency in the remnant of the left horn of the sinus venosus and allow communication between the right and left atria through the defect in the wall of the coronary sinus. One or more of the above types of ASDs may coexist.

Anomalies of pulmonary venous connection may be seen with ASDs, most commonly those of the sinus venosus type (8). In this condition, the pulmonary veins from the right upper and middle lobes enter the superior vena cava near its junction with the right atrium. Uncommonly, some or all of the right pulmonary veins may enter the right atrium directly, with or without an associated ASD. In a rare condition known as the *scimitar syndrome*, the right pulmonary vein courses inferiorly along the pericardial border and enters the heart in the region of the junction between the right atrium and the inferior vena cava. An ASD is frequently present. Scimitar syndrome is usually associated with a hypoplastic right lung that is supplied by an anomalous systemic artery originating from the abdominal aorta.

Atrial septal defects result in an increase in pulmonary blood flow secondary to left-to-right shunting through the defect. The flow of blood is directed from the left atrium to the right atrium because of the greater diastolic compliance and lower diastolic pressures in the right ventricle. When the pulmonary flow is twice that of the systemic

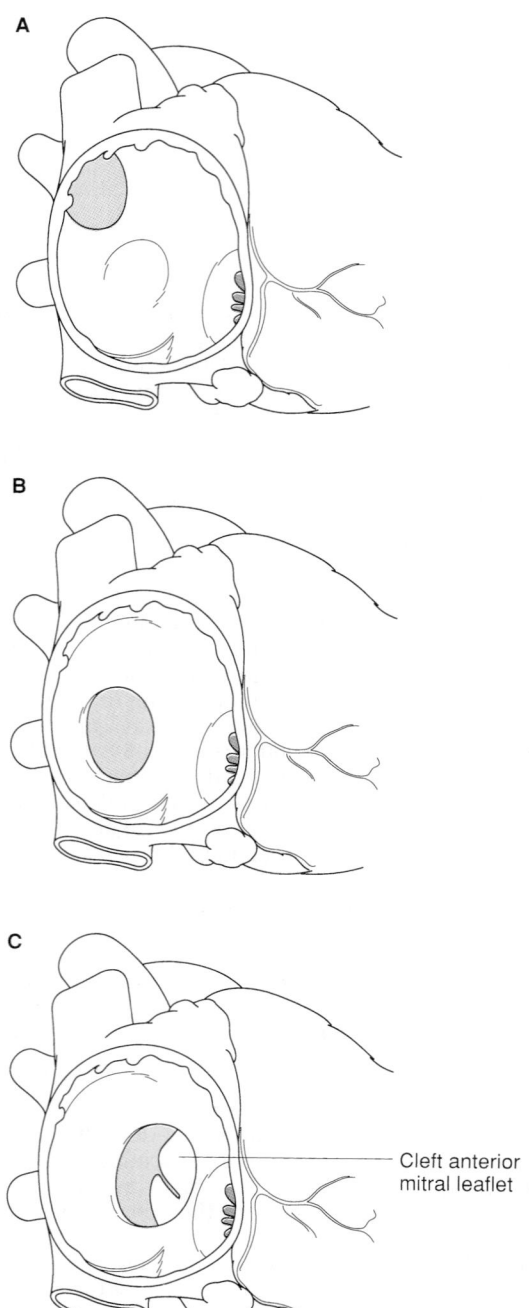

A

B

C

Cleft anterior
mitral leaflet

Figure 61.1. The anatomy of atrial septal defects. In the sinus venosus type *(A)*, the right upper and middle pulmonary veins frequently drain to the superior vena cava or right atrium. *(B)* Secundum defects generally occur as isolated lesions. *(C)* Primum defects are part of a more complex lesion and are best considered as incomplete atrioventricular septal defects.

circulation ($\dot{Q}_p/\dot{Q}_s$ ratio > 2), symptoms generally occur. Lesser degrees of shunting may be asymptomatic and remain so until late in life. The most common symptoms are fatigue, shortness of breath, and recurrent respiratory infections. Atrial dysrhythmias are common in adulthood. *Paradoxical embolism,* a term applied to systemic emboli that arise from the peripheral veins, is a rare complication of ASD. These emboli, which would normally go to the lungs, instead pass through the ASD to the systemic circulation.

The classic physical findings with large ASDs consist of a normal first heart sound and a wide, fixed splitting of the second heart sound. This results from the relatively fixed left-to-right shunt throughout all phases of the cardiac cycle. A soft ejection flow murmur across the pulmonary valve occurs as a result of the increased volume of flow. Additionally, a diastolic flow murmur may be audible across the tricuspid valve. A prominent right ventricular lift and increased intensity of the pulmonary component of the second sound may occur with pulmonary hypertension. Chest radiography demonstrates cardiomegaly, with enlargement of the right atrium, right ventricle, and pulmonary artery. The left atrium does not enlarge. The pulmonary vascular markings are increased. The electrocardiogram (ECG) shows right-axis deviation and an incomplete right bundle-branch block pattern. When right bundle-branch block is associated with a leftward or superior axis, an AVSD should be strongly suspected. Two-dimensional echocardiography is used to visualize the defect along with any associated anomalies of pulmonary venous return. Right ventricular volume overload with a flat or reversed septal motion is evidence of a significant volume of left-to-right shunting. Cardiac catheterization is rarely used today in isolated cases of ASD when two-dimensional Doppler echocardiography in addition to the other noninvasive evaluations demonstrate the classic findings. Cardiac catheterization may be important in assessing the quantity of left-to-right shunting and the degree of pulmonary hypertension in patients in whom the pulmonary vascular resistance is thought to be elevated. Although rare, the chronic left-to-right shunt from an ASD may produce pulmonary vascular occlusive disease later in life. When the $\dot{Q}_p/\dot{Q}_s$ ratio is less than 1.5 and the ratio of pulmonary to systemic vascular resistance (R_p/R_s) exceeds 0.7, advanced pulmonary occlusive disease may be present. An absolute pulmonary vascular resistance in excess of 10 to 12 Woods units per square meter (see VSD) indicates inoperability (9).

Any ASD with a significant left-to-right shunt producing volume overload should be closed surgically. This occurs with a $\dot{Q}_p/\dot{Q}_s$ ratio of approximately 1.5 or higher. The degree of left-to-right shunting tends to increase with advanced age as left ventricular dysfunction causes left ventricular compliance to decrease. Congestive heart failure (CHF), supraventricular dysrhythmias, and pulmonary hypertension occur with increasing frequency by the third to fourth decade of life in patients with large, untreated ASDs. Even smaller defects may be associated with paradoxical embolism, particularly during pregnancy. Elective repair is advised before school age in patients with moderate to large ASDs. Recently, some surgeons have proposed routine repair in infants and younger children. A recent review of 102 neonates (700 to 2,500 g) undergoing repair of simple and complex cardiac anomalies with the use of cardiopulmonary bypass demonstrated no intracerebral hemorrhages, no long-term neurologic sequelae, and a low operative mortality rate (10%), which correlated with the length of cardiopulmonary bypass and complexity of the repair. In addition, it was shown that growth after repair in this population followed the normal growth curves of weight-matched neonates without heart disease (10). It remains to be seen whether repair at this earlier age provides any significant advantage.

Atrial septal defects can be readily repaired with the use of standard techniques of cardiopulmonary bypass through a midline sternotomy approach. This approach has become well established, with minimal associated morbidity and a mortality rate of nearly zero. The focus has now been shifted to minimizing hospital stay and convalescence and maximizing the cosmetic result. This has led to the description of multiple alternative approaches, including right submammary incision with anterior thoracotomy, limited bilateral submammary incision with partial sternal split, trans-xiphoid window, and limited midline incision with partial sternal split. The morbidity and mortality of all these approaches are comparable with those of traditional approach; however, each has technical drawbacks. The submammary/thoracotomy approach increases the risk for phrenic nerve damage, mild breast and pectoral asymmetries (7.4%), and anesthetic and hyperesthetic areas involving the nipple–areolar complex (38.8%) (11,12). The trans-xiphoid window requires femoral cannulation, has limited exposure, and longer bypass times. Also, it is more difficult to de-air the heart (13). Some centers use thoracoscopic assistance in trans-xiphoid and submammary approaches, which adds further complexity to the procedure. A limited midline incision with a partial sternal split provides a cosmetically acceptable scar without limiting the exposure of mediastinal structures or increasing the complexity of the procedure with the use of ancillary equipment. This approach also can be easily extended to a full sternotomy should difficulty or unexpected anomalies be encountered (14).

The exact techniques for cannulation vary with the chosen approach. In general, the heart and pulmonary veins are carefully inspected to examine for anomalies of pulmonary venous connection or the presence of a left superior vena cava. Direct superior and inferior vena caval cannulation is used, and the core temperature is lowered to 32°C. Aortic cross-clamping with elective myocardial arrest by an infusion of cold cardioplegic solution is then performed. Alternatively, the aorta is left unclamped, and the heart is electively fibrillated to prevent the ejection of air during exposure of the ASD. A right atriotomy is made, and the atrial septum is carefully inspected. Closure of ostium secundum defects is accomplished either by direct suture or by the insertion of a patch. Care must be taken to identify all edges of the ASD accurately, particularly when the entire septum primum is absent. In these situations, the eustachian valve may be mistaken for the lower rim of the ASD and used in the repair, so that inferior vena caval blood is inadvertently diverted into the left atrium. Sinus venosus ASDs associated with partial anomalous pulmonary venous connection are repaired by inserting a patch, with redirection of the pulmonary veins behind the patch to the left atrium. Care must be taken not to obstruct the pulmonary veins or superior vena cava. Generally, the superior vena cava is dilated and provides ample room for inserting the patch. In some situations, one or more pulmonary veins may enter the superior vena cava far superiorly. When the abnormally connecting pulmonary vein represents part or all of the right upper lobe only, it may be best not to incorporate this vein in the repair to avoid creating an obstruction to venous return. The resultant left-to-right shunt generally has a $\dot{Q}_p/\dot{Q}_s$ ratio of less than 1.5 and should not cause problems later in life. The results for ASD closure are excellent. Morbidity is minimal, and convalescence is generally uncomplicated. Uncommonly, atrial arrhythmias or significant left atrial hypertension may occur soon after repair. The latter is caused by the noncompliant small left atrial chamber and generally resolves rapidly.

First performed in 1976 (15), transcatheter closure of ASDs with the use of various occlusion devices is increasing in popularity. Select types of ASDs, including patent foramen ovale, secundum defects, and certain fenestrated secundum defects, are amenable to device closure. Multiple devices have been introduced during the past two decades. A modification of the original umbrella device, the "clamshell" double umbrella, requires an 11F delivery sheath; it has demonstrated an 85% complete closure rate with no long-term complications. However, follow-up has revealed a rate of clinically silent arm fractures of up to 40% (16). The "angel wings" self-centering device requires an 11F to 13F introducing sheath; a 100% success rate has been achieved in patent foramen ovale, with a 4% risk for serious complications requiring surgical intervention (17). This device is difficult to reposition following deployment. Commonly used devices at the University of Michigan include the Sideris adjustable button device and the Amplatzer septal occlusion device. In a recent comparison trial, the Amplatzer device was easier to place and reposition after deployment (fluoroscopy time, 13.4 minutes vs. 23.7 minutes) and demonstrated a greater complete occlusion rate at 1 year (93% vs. 41%) (18). Complications reported to occur with transcatheter closure include air embolism (1% to 3%), thromboembolism from the device (1% to 2%), disturbed atrioventricular valve function (1% to 2%), systemic/pulmonary venous obstruction (1%), perforation of the atrium or aorta with hemopericardium (1% to 2%), atrial arrhythmias (1% to 3%), and malpositioning/embolization of the device requiring intervention (2% to 15%) (19). The minimally invasive nature and shorter period of convalescence associated with device closure are offset by the associated risks and variable rate of complete closure in comparison with the established surgical approach.

VENTRICULAR SEPTAL DEFECT

The ventricular septum forms in part from the endocardial cushions and in part from the relatively greater growth of the ventricles in comparison with the interventricular foramen. The spiral septation of the embryologic great arteries also contributes to septal formation. Ventricular septal defect (VSD) is a common anomaly; among congenital heart defects, only bicuspid aortic valve occurs more frequently. VSDs account for 20% to 25% of all cardiac lesions and are present in 2 of every 1,000 infants born alive. Although VSDs may occur in any portion of the ventricular septum, certain typical locations tend to predominate (Fig. 61.2). Most defects are single and are located high in the ventricular septum, just beneath the aortic valve. When the defects abut the tricuspid valve annulus, as is usually the case, they are called *perimembranous VSDs,* a term referring to the involvement of the membranous septum. The typical VSD, representing about 80% of all defects, is perimembranous and located in the infundibular septum, which is the portion of the septum separating the right and left ventricular outflow tracts. Defects located high in the infundibular septum, immediately beneath the pulmonary valve, are referred to as *supracristal, infundibular,* or *subarterial VSDs.* These defects account for about 5% to 10% of all VSDs. The infundibular septum may be extremely deficient or virtually absent in these defects, with little or no muscle separating the aortic and pulmonary valves. In about 5% of VSDs, the defect lies in the inlet septum beneath the septal leaflet of the tricuspid valve. These perimembranous inlet defects are also referred to as *AV canal-type defects.* The remaining VSDs have entirely muscular edges and are most commonly located in the apical muscular portion of the ventricular septum. These defects are often multiple and may be associated with additional perimembranous VSDs.

Associated lesions are common with VSDs, and the defect itself is often part of a more complex lesion. Prolapse of the aortic valve with aortic insufficiency may be caused by the VSD itself. This is more common with subpulmonic or supracristal defects. VSDs may be associated with ob-

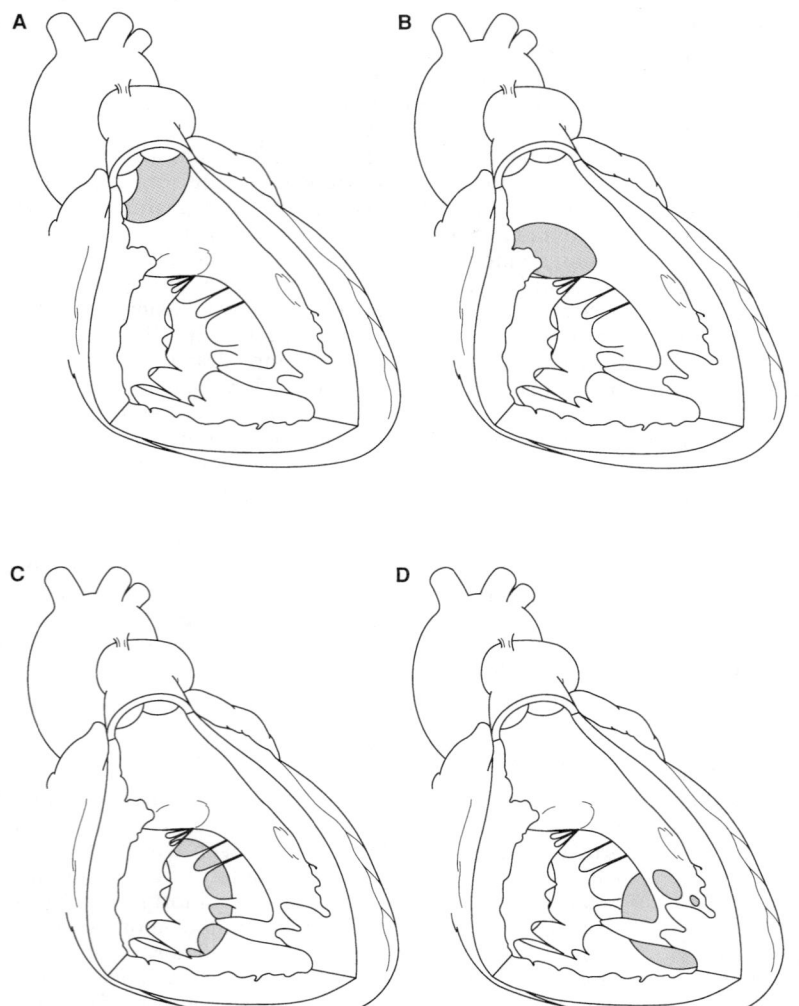

Figure 61.2. The anatomy of ventricular septal defects *(VSDs)* as seen through the right ventricle. *(A)* Subarterial VSDs, or high type, are generally bordered superiorly by the pulmonary valve annulus. *(B)* Perimembranous VSDs are most common, extending from the membranous septum into the infundibular septum. *(C)* Inlet defects are located predominantly beneath the septal leaflet of the tricuspid valve. *(D)* Muscular VSDs are situated away from the valves, toward the cardiac apex.

structive lesions of the left side of the heart, such as aortic stenosis, mitral stenosis, and coarctation.

Isolated VSDs result in left-to-right shunting with increased pulmonary blood flow. The hemodynamics and symptoms in patients with isolated VSDs depend on the size of the defect and the magnitude of the shunt. As the normally elevated pulmonary vascular resistance of the neonate falls during the first few weeks of life, the degree of left-to-right shunting increases and causes signs and symptoms of CHF. This generally occurs after the first 4 to 6 weeks of life in patients with large VSDs. Large, or nonrestrictive, VSDs are present when the defect size approximates the size of the aortic annulus, resulting in systemic or nearly systemic right ventricular pressure and a $\dot{Q}_p/\dot{Q}_s$ ratio generally in excess of 2.5 or 3. Moderately sized VSDs are restrictive, with the right ventricular pressure generally at about half of systemic levels or less. The $\dot{Q}_p/\dot{Q}_s$ ratio is 1.5 to 2.5. With small ventricular defects, right ventricular pressure remains normal, and the $\dot{Q}_p/\dot{Q}_s$ ratio is less than 1.5.

Large VSDs generally present at about 6 weeks to 2 months of age, when the normally elevated pulmonary vascular resistance falls, so that the left-to-right shunt increases. CHF is manifested by tachypnea, tachycardia, diaphoresis, poor feeding, and inadequate weight gain. About half of all VSDs discovered in infancy close spontaneously. Although this is less likely to occur with non-

restrictive defects, all VSDs are initially managed medically, with the administration of digoxin and diuretics to control symptoms of CHF. The increased pulmonary blood flow and pressure seen with moderate and large VSDs may lead to a gradual increase in pulmonary arterial resistance and the development of pulmonary vascular occlusive disease. The advanced changes of pulmonary vascular disease generally do not appear until the age of 2 years in patients with isolated, large VSDs. Histologically, these changes have been classified by Edwards (20). Grade 1 changes consist of medial hypertrophy alone, and grade 2 changes involve intimal proliferation. Grades 1 and 2 are considered reversible. More advanced findings consist of intimal fibrosis (grade 3) and lesions of progressive dilation, including arteriolar necrosis (grades 4 to 6). These advanced changes are not reversible.

The diagnosis of VSD may be made by two-dimensional echocardiography. The use of color flow imaging provides excellent anatomic information on the location, size, and number of VSDs. Associated lesions, such as aortic stenosis, coarctation, and mitral stenosis, can also be evaluated. Complete evaluation of the infant with a large VSD includes cardiac catheterization to assess pulmonary blood flow and pressure and pulmonary vascular resistance.

The most common indication for operative closure of large VSDs is CHF resulting in failure to thrive. Although this is uncommon during the first few months of life, operative repair is indicated when it occurs. By 6 months of age, the chances of spontaneous closure of large defects diminish, and pulmonary vascular resistance may be elevated. Pulmonary vascular resistance is calculated by using the following formula:

$$PVR = \frac{\text{mean } PAP - \text{mean } LAP}{\text{pulmonary blood flow}}$$

where *PVR* is the pulmonary vascular resistance, *PAP* is the pulmonary arterial pressure, and *LAP* is the left arterial pressure.

When the pressures are measured in millimeters of mercury and pulmonary flow is measured in liters per minute, the resulting value is expressed in Woods units (1 Woods unit = 80 dynes•s/cm^5). If the pulmonary vascular resistance remains below 4 U/m^2 of body surface area and the symptoms are minimal in the presence of a left-to-right shunt, repair can be deferred because spontaneous closure may still occur. Should failure to thrive or a significant elevation in pulmonary vascular resistance above 4 to 6 U/m^2 be present, operative repair is advised. In cases of elevated pulmonary vascular resistance, a more complete evaluation may be necessary to determine operability. An absolute pulmonary vascular resistance in excess of 10 to 12 U/m^2 is considered a contraindication to VSD closure. In these patients, the response of the pulmonary vascular resistance to pulmonary vasodilators such as tolazoline, isoproterenol, or oxygen may be used to assess whether the resistance remains fixed. The response to exercise may be helpful in older children. In favorable situations, a fall in pulmonary vascular resistance, associated with an increase in the $\dot{Q}_p/\dot{Q}_s$ ratio, indicates that operation remains advisable. If the $\dot{Q}_p/\dot{Q}_s$ ratio remains below 1.5, with an Rp/Rs ratio in excess of 0.6 to 0.7, operation is contraindicated. When this occurs, right-to-left shunting begins to develop, particularly with exercise, and the signs and symptoms of CHF are no longer apparent. VSD closure in these patients prevents the compensatory right-to-left shunting that is necessary to maintain cardiac output as pulmonary vascular resistance increases or systemic vascular resistance falls. Moderate defects that do not result in significant pulmonary artery hypertension or elevated pulmonary resistance can continue to be observed if symptoms are minimal. Even in these situations, surgical closure is indicated by 3 to 5 years of age because spontaneous defect closure is highly unlikely beyond that time.

In most cases, the surgical treatment of VSDs consists of primary repair with cardiopulmonary bypass. Most infants can be treated with the use of deep hypothermia and low-flow bypass at systemic temperatures of 20°C to 25°C. Cold cardioplegic solution is used to protect the heart. In some instances, a period of deep hypothermia and circulatory arrest may be used to facilitate exposure (21). Perimembranous VSDs may be adequately exposed and closed through a right atrial approach. Retraction on the leaflets of the tricuspid valve allows exposure of the margins of the defect. In rare situations, the superior margin of the defect may not be well visualized, and a right ventriculotomy may be necessary. The defect is closed with a patch in all cases, and great care must be taken to avoid injuring the conduction tissue that lies along the posterior and inferior rim of perimembranous infundibular defects. Inlet VSDs are also best approached through the tricuspid valve and right atrium. In some situations, the arrangement of the tricuspid valve tensor apparatus may interfere with accurate placement of the patch. In these cases, the base of the tricuspid valve can be detached 1 to 2 mm away from its annular attachment. Subpulmonary VSDs are best exposed through the pulmonary artery or right ventricle. Because these defects generally do not extend to the perimembranous region, the conduction tissue is remote from its edge. The superior margin of the defect is composed of the pulmonary valve itself, and suturing to the base of the leaflets is necessary to avoid injuring both the aortic and pulmonary valves. Muscular VSDs present a special problem and may need to be approached from the left ventricle. When viewed from the right ventricular side, these defects often appear multiple because the coarse trabeculations within the right ventricle make delineating the edges of the VSD nearly impossible. This is particularly true of anterior and apical muscular VSDs. In these situations, an apical left ventriculotomy is performed. The incision is carefully placed lateral to the anterior descending coronary artery and provides excellent exposure of the muscular septum. Defects often appear to be single from this view and can be closed with a single patch of prosthetic material (22).

In certain situations, repair is best delayed until the infant is older, in this circumstance, palliation with pulmonary artery banding is performed. Although rarely used today, pulmonary artery banding may be indicated for complex muscular VSDs that require left ventriculotomy in small infants, particularly those with the so-called Swiss cheese type of septum, in whom elimination of all residual shunting may be impossible. Removal of the pulmonary artery band and closure of the defects can then be performed by the age of 2 or 3 years.

The results for closure of isolated VSDs are excellent, even in infants. The hospital mortality rate approaches zero for uncomplicated defects. Young age, VSD location, and elevated pulmonary vascular resistance are no longer considered important risk factors. Major associated lesions may still adversely affect outcome. Although elevations in pulmonary vascular resistance do not increase operative mortality, late survival may be substantially reduced.

Given the complexity, associated morbidity, and high residual leak rate associated with the repair of multiple apical VSDs and also "Swiss cheese" muscular VSDs, several adjunctive methods have been devised to augment the standard surgical approaches. Leca et al. (23) reported the use of fibrin glue to close multiple muscular VSDs in 15 children. The fibrin glue is introduced into the defect with a dual injection device that allows the fibrin and thrombin to mix on being injected into the defect, with resultant immediate clot formation. The approach to the VSD was transatrial, transventricular, or via the pulmonary valve. The reported hospital mortality was 6%, with no long-term morbidity. All patients at 3-year follow-up had either no or trivial residual VSDs, and no patient required reoperation. These results are very encouraging in comparison with the results of a previously reported review of 29 cases of multiple muscular VSDs by Kirklin et al. (24), in which the mortality rate was 14% and the rate of reoperation for recurrence was 28%. Histologic examination of surgically produced VSDs in sheep subsequently repaired with fibrin glue reveals that the fibrin glue is reabsorbed and replaced with fibrosis and an endocardial covering (23). Device closure of apical and multiple muscular VSDs has also been reported. Two series described the use of the modified Rashkind double-umbrella device intraoperatively to close multiple muscular VSDs that were difficult to approach by conventional methods. Complete closure was noted in all patients at the time of follow-up (25,26).

AORTIC STENOSIS

Obstruction to left ventricular outflow can occur at multiple levels (Fig. 61.3). The most common obstruction is stenosis of the aortic valve, although the obstruction may also be located in the subvalvar or supravalvar areas. Val-

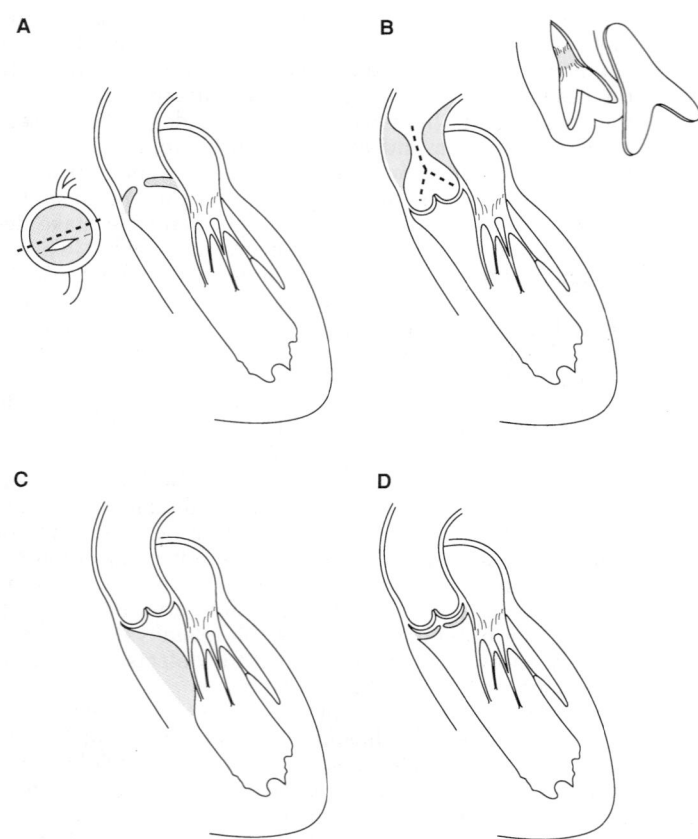

A

B

C

D

Figure 61.3. Anatomy of the types of congenital aortic stenosis. *(A)* Valvar aortic stenosis. *(B)* Supravalvar aortic stenosis and its repair *(inset)*. *(C)* Tunnel-type subvalvar aortic stenosis. *(D)* Membranous subvalvar aortic stenosis.

var aortic stenosis is secondary to various abnormalities of aortic valvar development, most commonly a bicuspid aortic valve with fusion of the commissures. A bicuspid aortic valve is estimated to occur in about 2% of the population. Less commonly, variable degrees of fusion along the commissures of a tricuspid valve may be found. In neonates, significant aortic stenosis is most often caused by a unicommissural valve. The most common lesions associated with aortic stenosis are coarctation of the aorta (COA), VSD, and mitral stenosis. Although valvar aortic stenosis may present at any age, the diagnosis is most often made in childhood with the finding of an asymptomatic murmur. In infancy, CHF may develop, but symptoms are distinctly uncommon beyond that age until adulthood is reached. Although rare in childhood, angina may occur when myocardial blood flow cannot adequately perfuse the hypertrophied and hypertensive ventricular muscle. In the neonate, angina may present as periodic episodes of inconsolable crying. The third classic symptom of aortic stenosis, syncope, results from an inability of the left ventricle to increase cardiac output through the fixed valvar orifice on demand, as during exercise.

The physical findings in patients with aortic stenosis include a reduced pulse volume, precordial thrill, and an ejection systolic murmur at the cardiac base that radiates into the neck. The presence of a systolic ejection click signifies that the stenosis is valvar. Severe stenosis may be accompanied by a fourth heart sound and paradoxical splitting of the second sound. Physical findings are notoriously unreliable in predicting the severity of the lesion. The chest radiograph is rarely helpful, and the appearance is often normal. The left ventricular apex may be prominent, and the ascending aorta dilated. The ECG usually shows left ventricular hypertrophy, but the tracing may

also be normal. Two-dimensional echocardiography is extremely useful in determining the site and severity of the lesion. The left ventricular outflow tract gradient can be estimated with Doppler techniques, and the Doppler findings correlate well with those of cardiac catheterization.

The neonate presenting with critical aortic stenosis and CHF requires urgent operative intervention. Many of these patients have extremely low cardiac output and metabolic acidosis. These conditions may be relieved by endotracheal intubation and inotropic support. An infusion of prostaglandin opens the ductus arteriosus or keeps it patent and stabilizes the systemic blood flow. Although symptoms are rare in children beyond infancy, intervention is indicated when any of the components of the classic triad of heart failure, angina, and syncope occur in association with a left ventricular outflow tract gradient of at least 50 mm Hg. Even in the absence of symptoms, a gradient in excess of 75 mm Hg is considered severe. Patients with aortic valve gradients between 50 and 75 mm Hg present a difficult dilemma. In the absence of symptoms, these patients should be carefully observed. An ECG that demonstrates left ventricular strain or ischemia, at rest or during exercise, is considered an indication for operation.

Relief of valvar aortic stenosis in infants and children is generally accomplished with standard techniques of cardiopulmonary bypass and direct exposure of the aortic valve. Fused commissures can then be incised to within 1 to 2 mm of the valve annulus. Careful assessment of valve morphology is essential to avoid dividing a false raphe and producing leaflet prolapse and severe aortic regurgitation. Increasingly, reports indicate that balloon dilation of the aortic valve is effective in reducing the gradient without producing regurgitation, even in neonates. For older children, balloon dilation is the procedure of choice, with operation reserved for those with more complex lesions or with annular hypoplasia. In neonates, the large catheters required for dilation have been associated with significant femoral arterial complications. The preferred approach is via the umbilical (27) or carotid (28) arteries. Alternatively, transventricular dilation through the left ventricular apex has proved effective, with or without normothermic cardiopulmonary bypass to support the circulation. This technique avoids the myocardial ischemia produced by aortic cross-clamping. Although the gradient is generally relieved satisfactorily, it is usually impossible to abolish the obstruction completely. A review of 30 patients undergoing transventricular dilation (TVD) versus balloon aortic valvuloplasty (BAV) at the University of Michigan demonstrated that both interventions provide adequate and equivalent relief of critical aortic stenosis. A decline in mean transvalvar gradients from 33.8 to 18.9 mm Hg (TVD) and from 42 to 15.9 mm Hg (BAV) was noted, with an associated improvement in the mean left ventricular ejection fraction from 39% to 47% (TVD) and from 51% to 67% (BAV). The mortality rates in the two groups were comparable: 9.5% (TVD) and 11.1% (BAV). The decision regarding the most appropriate method to use depends on the available medical expertise in addition to patient criteria, such as adequate arterial access and the presence of associated lesions requiring operative repair (29). Regardless of the approach chosen to treat critical aortic stenosis in the neonate, the goal is to relieve the obstruction without creating significant aortic insufficiency. All these treatments are palliative, and ultimately the patient will require an aortic valve replacement.

Aortic valve replacement for aortic stenosis in children has been viewed as a treatment of last resort because of the poor performance of valve substitutes, the inherent risks of long-term anticoagulation required with mechanical valves, and the rapid calcification and degeneration associated with pericardial and porcine bioprostheses. The use of human valve substitutes, such as aortic/pulmonary allografts and pulmonary autografts (Ross procedure), has significantly improved valve function and longevity. Thus, the emphasis has shifted to early operative intervention for recurrent critical aortic stenosis, before the irreversible depression of left ventricular function develops. Ross (30) first described transposition of the pulmonary valve into the aortic position with allograft reconstruction of the pulmonary outflow tract in 1967. Since that time, the safety and longevity of the Ross procedure have been well established, and it has become the procedure of choice for aortic valve replacement in children. A comparison study of aortic valve allograft versus the Ross procedure was undertaken by Jones and Lupinetti (31). They demonstrated that despite the added complexity and operative time required for the Ross procedure, the improved hemodynamics of the pulmonary autograft allowed rapid regression of left ventricular hypertrophy and normalization of left ventricular outflow tract velocities. Significant improvement in these parameters was not demonstrated in the allograft patients. The allografts are also prone to early degeneration in comparison with the pulmonary autografts. The Ross procedure should be the operation of choice for aortic valve replacement in children unless it is contraindicated because of concomitant disease (absence or disease of the pulmonary valve, Marfan syndrome). Pediatric patients with a significant size discrepancy between the pulmonary and aortic roots can undergo a Ross procedure with associated aortic root tailoring. In a review of 15 patients undergoing aortic root tailoring, patients had no residual aortic stenosis, no long-term morbidity, and no more than trace to 1+ aortic regurgitation (32).

Subvalvar aortic stenosis occurs beneath the aortic valve and may be discrete or diffuse. In the discrete type, a fibrous membrane is located immediately beneath the aortic valve leaflets. Anteriorly, the membrane is attached to the septum and posteriorly to the anterior leaflet of the mitral valve in the region of aortic–mitral continuity. Often, discrete subaortic stenosis represents a combination of a thick membrane and a localized muscular obstruction that form a fibromuscular collar in the left ventricular outflow tract. Although the aortic valve leaflets are generally normal in discrete subvalvar aortic stenosis, the turbulence beneath the valve usually results in leaflet thickening with aortic incompetence. In the diffuse form of subaortic stenosis, a long, tunnel-like obstruction beneath the valve may extend for a considerable distance toward the apex of the left ventricle.

Although the indications for operative intervention in subvalvar aortic stenosis are the same as those in valvar stenosis, the complexity of the lesion and the difficulty associated with relieving it must be considered in each individual patient. A left ventricular outflow tract gradient of 30 mm Hg in patients with discrete membranous subaortic stenosis is generally considered an adequate indication for operation. In these patients, resection of the membrane is generally uncomplicated and the results are favorable. Furthermore, the aortic insufficiency that accompanies this particular lesion is progressive and can be prevented by early resection of the membrane. Patients with diffuse, tunnel-like subaortic stenoses are far more difficult to treat and require more elaborate procedures. Tunnel subaortic stenosis associated with hypoplasia of the aortic valve annulus is best treated with an aortoventriculoplasty, as described by Konno et al. (33) and Rastan and Koncz (34). In this operation, the aortic valve annulus and the immediately adjacent septum are incised, and the incision is carried as far down toward the left ventricular apex as is necessary to relieve the subaortic narrowing. The resultant opening is closed with a patch to widen the area of stenosis, and the aortic valve is replaced with an allograft, autograft, or prosthesis. When the aortic valve annulus is adequate, the septal incision is confined to the immediate subvalvar area, and a patch is used to widen the left ventricular outflow tract without replacing the aortic valve.

Supravalvar aortic stenosis begins distal to the aortic valve; it also exists in either a discrete or diffuse form. The discrete form is localized to the immediate supravalvar area just above the aortic valve commissures. This produces an hourglass deformity of the ascending aorta. The intraluminal thickening results in adherence of the three leaflets of the aortic valve to the area of obstruction, which partially obstructs coronary flow during diastole ("cusp tuck"). This intramural thickening and fibrosis may extend into the orifices of the coronaries themselves and further impair coronary blood flow. Although the disease presents most commonly in the discrete or localized form, some patients have diffuse vascular abnormalities, with thickening of the aortic wall extending into the aortic arch and its branches.

The signs and symptoms of supravalvar aortic stenosis are similar to those in other forms of left ventricular outflow tract narrowing. Occasionally, supravalvar aortic stenosis may be associated with Williams syndrome, a constellation of elfin facies, mental retardation, and hypercalcemia. The diagnosis is established with cardiac catheterization and angiography, which are necessary to define accurately the extent of obstruction and any associated anomalies. The most common associated condition is peripheral pulmonary artery stenosis, which may be diffuse and severe.

Operation is indicated for patients with supravalvar aortic stenosis in which outflow tract gradients are higher than 50 mm Hg. At operation, a patch is placed across the area of obstruction along the ascending aorta and is extended deep into the noncoronary sinus of Valsalva. On occasion, it may be advisable to insert an upside-down, Y-shaped patch, with one limb of the Y extending into the noncoronary sinus of Valsalva and the other into the right coronary sinus to augment the narrowed supravalvar area in two places (35). In addition, the intramural tissue is generally resected by partial endarterectomy.

The results of surgery for the localized form of supravalvar aortic stenosis are generally good, with low operative mortality and excellent long-term survival. Obstruction is generally well relieved. The diffuse form of the disease is more difficult to treat, and recurrence is more likely. When diffuse, severe supravalvar pulmonary stenosis coexists, operative repair is far more hazardous and long-term results are poor.

TETRALOGY OF FALLOT

Tetralogy of Fallot is the most common congenital heart defect that results in cyanosis. In this condition, anterior displacement of the infundibular septum results in hypoplasia of the right ventricular outflow tract and pulmonary valve annulus. A large malalignment VSD with overriding of the aorta results. Right ventricular hypertrophy occurs secondary to the outflow tract obstruction. These are the four components of the tetralogy (Fig. 61.4). The anatomic hallmark of this condition is the anterior displacement of the infundibular septum, along with its leftward extension. The insertion of the infundibular septum is anterior to the anterior extension of the septal band, rather than between its anterior and posterior extensions. The pulmonary valve itself is stenotic in most cases and bicuspid in 58% of cases (36). The annulus of the pulmonary valve may be hypoplastic, as is frequently the case when the infundibular stenosis is severe. Abnormalities of pulmonary artery development are also common, with diffuse mild hypoplasia predominating. A branch pulmonary artery stenosis, more frequently of the left pulmonary artery at the region of the insertion of the ligamentum arteriosum, may also be seen. A unilateral pulmonary artery is rarely absent. When pulmonary valvar atresia accompanies the tetralogy of Fallot, pulmonary blood flow is then

supplied by multiple aorticopulmonary collaterals with or without a patent ductus arteriosus (PDA). These vessels generally originate from the upper descending thoracic aorta and traverse the mediastinum to reach the hilum of each lung. They join the true intralobar pulmonary arteries in the lung and are indistinguishable from these vessels histologically. In most patients, hemodynamically significant stenoses develop between the aortic origin and the intrapulmonary vessels. The VSD in tetralogy of Fallot is nonrestrictive. The defect is cradled between the anterior and posterior limbs of the septal band and most commonly extends to the annulus of the tricuspid valve and involves the membranous septum. The aortic arch may be on the right, crossing over the right main bronchus in 25% of patients with tetralogy of Fallot. The coronary arteries are usually normal, but in about 3% to 5% of patients, the anterior descending coronary originates from the right sinus of Valsalva and crosses over the right ventricular outflow tract to reach the interventricular groove. Other, uncommon associated anomalies include absence of the pulmonary valve, multiple VSDs, and complete AV canal defect.

Patients with tetralogy of Fallot present with cyanosis, the severity of which depends on the degree of right ventricular outflow tract obstruction. Frequently, the cyanosis is mild at birth and may be undetected for weeks or even months. In patients with severe hypoplasia of the pulmonary outflow tract and annulus, and those with pulmonary atresia, important cyanosis is present at birth or soon thereafter. Closure of the ductus arteriosus may unmask the cyanosis. In a few patients, the outflow tract obstruction may be so mild that the initial presentation is one of a large VSD with left-to-right shunting and CHF.

When the right ventricular outflow tract obstruction is predominantly located in the infundibulum and is muscular in nature, patients may be subject to cyanotic spells. These episodes are most commonly seen in tetralogy but also occur in patients with other types of cyanotic defects. The spells are characterized by aggravation of the cyanosis, labored breathing, and a fall in arterial blood pressure. These events may be triggered by anything that reduces systemic vascular resistance, from vigorous physical exertion to a warm bath or a fever. Other factors that can increase the right-to-left shunt and exacerbate cyanosis include hyperpnea, Valsalva's maneuver, tachycardia, and dehydration. Although most episodes resolve spontaneously in a few minutes, they may lead to seizures or death. Immediate treatment is directed toward relieving the hypoxia, reducing the right ventricular obstruction, and raising the systemic vascular resistance to reduce right-to-left shunting at the ventricular level. Supplemental oxygen, sedation with morphine, β-adrenergic blockers, and α-adrenergic agonists may help in this regard. The occurrence of cyanotic spells is an indication for surgical intervention.

Physical examination in patients with tetralogy of Fallot generally reveals some degree of cyanosis. Clubbing of the fingers and toes may be noted in older patients. The precordium is generally quiet, without thrill, and the second heart sound may seem to be single because of the soft pulmonic component. A mid-intensity systolic ejection murmur is present; the intensity may decrease with increasing degrees of outflow tract obstruction. Continuous murmurs may be audible over the back secondary to collaterals. CHF is rare and generally occurs only in the presence of large systemic-to-pulmonary collaterals or in the later stages of the disease, with associated ventricular failure or aortic incompetence. Chest radiography may demonstrate the classic boot-shaped heart, with a concave pulmonary outflow tract and an upward-tipped apex secondary to

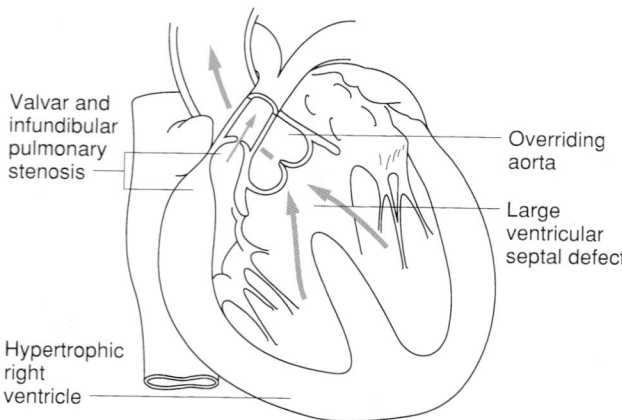

Figure 61.4. The four anatomic features of the tetralogy of Fallot. The primary morphologic abnormality, anterior and superior displacement of the infundibular septum, results in a malalignment ventricular septal defect, overriding of the aortic valve, and obstruction of the right ventricular outflow. Right ventricular hypertrophy is a secondary occurrence.

right ventricular hypertrophy. The heart size is generally normal, and the pulmonary vascular markings are decreased. A right aortic arch may be present. Two-dimensional echocardiography demonstrates the position and nature of the VSD, defines the nature of the outflow tract obstruction, and often can visualize the branch pulmonary arteries and proximal coronary arteries. For these reasons, echocardiography is often the only procedure required before surgery. Cardiac catheterization is occasionally necessary to outline the anatomy of the pulmonary arteries accurately, delineate multiple VSDs, and confirm the presence of important coronary abnormalities.

The most common indications for operative intervention include increasing cyanosis and the occurrence of cyanotic spells. Although spells may be treated with propranolol, more definitive surgical intervention is generally indicated. Important considerations for determining the type and timing of surgical repair include the size and distribution of the pulmonary arteries, coronary artery abnormalities, and right ventricle-to-pulmonary artery discontinuity. Although complete repair during infancy can be accomplished in most cases, certain anatomic features dictate that two-stage repair with preliminary shunting is optimal. The presence of an anomalous anterior coronary artery from the right coronary artery may limit the surgeon's ability to relieve pulmonary valvar hypoplasia with a transannular patch, and a conduit may be necessary. Although this can be inserted during infancy, repair may best be deferred until a larger conduit can be used. Conversely, when the pulmonary valve annulus is of adequate size and the infundibular stenosis is localized, repair can be accomplished in the neonate or infant, with ventriculotomy avoided entirely.

Severe pulmonary artery hypoplasia represents a relative contraindication to repair in infancy. In the past, patients with pulmonary atresia and multifocal pulmonary blood flow from aorticopulmonary collaterals were treated with preliminary shunting, ligation of collaterals, and unifocalization of nonconfluent branch pulmonary arteries. However, many of these patients were unable to undergo complete repair. For this reason, many centers now favor the early establishment of continuity between the right ventricle and pulmonary artery. This promotes uniform central pulmonary artery growth and allows the interventional cardiologist access to the branch pulmonary arteries for dilation, coil occlusion, and stenting. A team approach is often necessary to optimize the pulmonary vasculature for complete repair. Neonatal repair of tetralogy of Fallot with pulmonary atresia and multiple aorticopulmonary collaterals has been reported with good results. Among a group of 72 patients (mean age, 7.3 months), 93% underwent complete one-stage unifocalization, and in 64% of them, complete repair, including VSD closure, was accomplished at the initial procedure. Early mortality was 11%, with a 2-year actuarial survival of 95% (37). The basis for increased interest in early complete repair is the concern for morbidity associated with delayed or staged repairs, such as right ventricular dysfunction, failure to thrive, repeated pulmonary infections, and progressive derangement of the pulmonary and collateral vasculature. Emphasis is placed on unifocalization of all multiple aortopulmonary collateral arteries to the right and left pulmonary arteries through the use of extended end-to-side/side-to-side anastomoses with native tissue-to-tissue reconstruction. The objective is to use no or a minimal number of artificial conduits so that somatic growth is not impaired. With early unifocalization, normal flow can be restored to the entire pulmonary vascular bed to allow for optimal pulmonary vascular development.

When necessary, palliation is best accomplished with a modified Blalock-Taussig shunt (38), in which a Gore-Tex conduit is positioned between the undivided subclavian artery and ipsilateral pulmonary artery. Generally, a 4- or 5-mm shunt is used through a right thoracotomy. Patency rates are excellent; however, a small but real risk for pulmonary artery distortion is associated with the procedure.

Complete repair consists of VSD closure and relief of right ventricular outflow tract obstruction. The VSD is closed transatrially, and ventriculotomy is often avoided. Traction on the anterior and septal leaflets of the tricuspid valve generally affords excellent exposure, even in neonates. Relief of right ventricular outflow tract obstruction can involve division and resection of hypertrophic musculature, pulmonary valve commissurotomy, and patch enlargement of the outflow tract, which is extended across the annulus when necessary. Muscle resection can often be avoided entirely, particularly in neonates. The outflow tract is enlarged by incision of the anterior limb of the septal band, division of the hypertrophied parietal extensions of the infundibular septum, and relief of any other obstructing muscle bundles to the level of the moderator band. Pulmonary valve annular size can be assessed intraoperatively, and the postoperative right ventricle-to-left ventricle pressure ratio is predicted. If this ratio is less than 0.75, the annulus is left intact. If the outflow tract is judged to be deficient, pulmonary valve commissurotomy or a limited transannular patch may be needed. Only in cases of severe tubular infundibular stenosis is an extended right ventriculotomy warranted. The pulmonary valve regurgitation that results is well tolerated in the absence of tricuspid regurgitation, severe right ventricular dysfunction, significant residual VSD, or outflow tract obstruction. It is imperative to be certain that residual branch stenosis of either the right or left pulmonary artery is not present; otherwise, important outflow tract obstruction will remain distal to the outflow patch. In special circumstances, the insertion of a pulmonary valve prosthesis, generally a cryopreserved homograft, is indicated. These circumstances include severe pulmonary artery hypoplasia, absent pulmonary valve syndrome with aneurysmal pulmonary arteries in infancy, surgically inaccessible distal pulmonary artery stenosis, and unilateral absence of a pulmonary artery. Pulmonary regurgitation in these situations is poorly tolerated. The operative mortality rate is between 2% and 5%. Results for patients with tetralogy of Fallot and pulmonary atresia are not as good, particularly in the presence of multiple aortopulmonary collaterals. The long-term results of repair in which an extended ventriculotomy is avoided are likely to be excellent because the incidence of late right ventricular dysfunction and dysrhythmias is surely reduced (39).

It used to be thought that pulmonary insufficiency after repair of the right ventricular outflow obstruction was well tolerated in most patients. However, as long-term survival continues to improve, the role of pulmonary insufficiency in the impairment of right ventricular function is being recognized. In a follow-up of 74 patients with pulmonary insufficiency after tetralogy repair (all in New York Heart Association class I or II), 48 patients had right ventricular dysfunction on cardiac catheterization, with elevated end-diastolic volumes and depressed ejection fractions. Factors that correlated with right ventricular dysfunction included distal pulmonary artery stenosis, moderate pulmonary regurgitation, and a large or aneurysmal transannular outflow patch. Of the patients who went on to pulmonary valve replacement (42 of 48), 83% of those who underwent surgery within 2 years of their original repair had complete recovery of ventricular function on follow-up catheterization, whereas patients operated on more than 2 years after their original repair continued to demonstrate right ventricular dysfunction. Waiting for the appearance of symptoms as an indication for valve replacement may result in the development of irreversible ventricular dysfunction (40). The functional survival of homografts in the pulmonary position has been 84% at 10 years (41). Therefore, repair of pulmonary insufficiency should not be delayed if angiographic evidence of right ventricular dysfunction is found, even if the patient has no symptoms.

TRANSPOSITION OF THE GREAT ARTERIES

Transposition of the great arteries (TGA) is a congenital cardiac anomaly in which the aorta arises from the right ventricle and the pulmonary artery originates from the left ventricle (ventriculoarterial discordance; Fig. 61.5). In the form of transposition considered here, the connections between the atria and ventricles are normal (concordant). TGA is a relatively common cardiac anomaly and is the most common form of congenital heart disease presenting as cyanosis in the first week of life. The degree of cyanosis depends on the amount of mixing between the pulmonary and systemic circulations. In TGA, oxygenated pulmonary venous blood is returned to the lungs and desaturated systemic blood is returned to the body. Because the two circulations exist in parallel, some mixing between them must occur to allow oxygenated blood to reach the systemic circulation and the desaturated blood to reach the lungs. Mixing may occur at a number of levels, most commonly at the atrial level through an ASD or a patent foramen ovale. Often, a VSD or PDA serves as an additional site for cardiac mixing. In TGA, there can be no fixed shunt in one direction without an equal amount of blood passing in the other direction; otherwise, one circulation would eventually empty into the other. Therefore, the amount of desaturated blood reaching the lungs (effective pulmonary blood flow) must equal the amount of saturated blood reaching the aorta (effective systemic blood flow).

The newborn with TGA is noticeably cyanotic within hours of birth. As the ductus arteriosus closes, particularly in the face of a restrictive ASD, severe cyanosis occurs and may result in a metabolic acidosis. In the presence of a large VSD, cyanosis may be mild and go undetected for the first few weeks of life. When significant pulmonary stenosis is present, cyanosis may be profound, even with adequate mixing. In these cases, cyanosis is also caused by a decrease in absolute pulmonary blood flow.

The physical findings in the neonate with TGA and an intact ventricular septum are often unimpressive. Apart from cyanosis, no other clinical abnormalities may be found. The ECG is normal at birth, demonstrating the typical pattern of right ventricular dominance. Although the classic chest radiographic appearance of an egg on its side may be seen, this finding is often obscured by an enlarged thymic shadow. The abnormal ventriculoarterial connection is clearly seen on echocardiography, which demonstrates that the posterior great vessel arising from the left ventricle is a pulmonary artery that bifurcates soon after its origin. The anterior great vessel is the aorta and arises from the right ventricle. Associated lesions, including VSD, left ventricular outflow tract obstruction, and COA, may also be diagnosed. Although used less frequently, cardiac catheterization may be helpful to confirm the basic anatomy, discern associated lesions, define the coronary anatomy, and improve cardiac mixing by means of balloon atrial septostomy.

The infant with TGA and severe cyanosis requires prompt diagnosis and treatment to improve mixing and increase the arterial oxygen saturation. This is best accomplished either by early surgical repair or by balloon atrial septostomy, a technique developed by William Rashkind in 1966 (42). The procedure involves inserting a balloon-tipped catheter across the foramen ovale into the left atrium. Inflation and forcible withdrawal of the catheter tears the septum primum and enlarges the ASD. Mixing generally increases immediately, with a substantial increase in arterial oxygen saturation. In some situations, even the presence of an adequate atrial communication does not ensure adequate mixing, and the infant may remain severely cyanotic because of an associated left ventricular outflow tract obstruction or a failure of the elevated neonatal pulmonary vascular resistance to fall toward normal levels. In the latter situation, the compliance of both circulations remains about equal, and no mixing occurs across the ASD. An infusion of prostaglandin may help by increasing mixing at the level of the great vessels through the PDA and by decreasing pulmonary vascular resistance. Often, the infusion can then be weaned during the next few days as pulmonary vascular resistance decreases.

The definitive surgical treatment of patients with TGA has changed dramatically in the past decade with the advent of the arterial switch procedure. Before this procedure, repair of TGA was generally delayed until patients were at least 6 months of age. Historically, palliative procedures were often necessary to improve the systemic saturation before definitive repair. If balloon atrial septostomy failed to enlarge the ASD adequately, a Blalock-Hanlon septectomy was performed. Rarely used today, this operation is a method of surgically enlarging the ASD without cardiopulmonary bypass. In patients with large VSDs, significant CHF and pulmonary hypertension are present early in life. The main pulmonary artery may be banded to reduce distal pulmonary artery pressure and prevent the development of pulmonary vascular occlusive disease. Changes of pulmonary vascular disease may develop in about 25% of patients with hemodynamically large VSDs by 3 months of age; therefore, early reduction of pulmonary artery pressure is essential. Adjustment and positioning of the pulmonary artery band are critical for proper palliation. Too tight a band results in unacceptable cyanosis, whereas too loose a band does not adequately

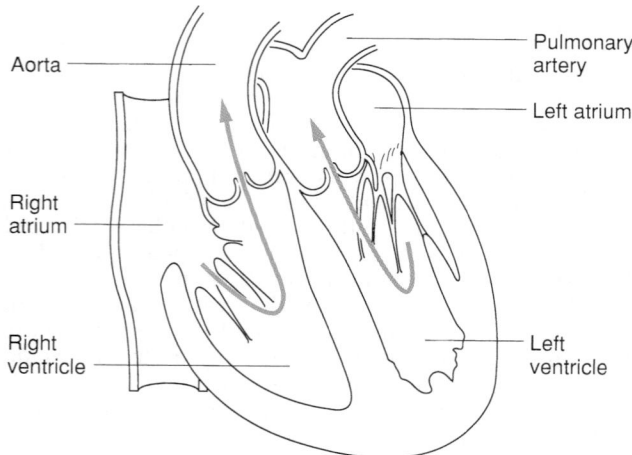

Figure 61.5. Anatomy of the most common type of transposition of the great arteries. The location of the ascending aorta is usually anterior to and to the right of the pulmonary artery.

reduce distal pulmonary arterial pressure. Migration of the pulmonary artery band distally may result in branch pulmonary artery stenosis, with excessive flow to one lung and diminished or absent flow to the other. If the band is placed too proximally, pulmonary valve function may be impaired and the valve distorted. For these reasons, pulmonary artery banding for uncomplicated cases of TGA is avoided. In those cases of transposition with severe left ventricular outflow tract obstruction, total pulmonary flow is reduced and systemic-to-pulmonary artery shunting is indicated. A classic or modified Blalock-Taussig shunt is used to increase pulmonary blood flow and allows postponement of definitive repair until a later age.

Until recently, definitive repair was achieved by redirecting venous inflow at the atrial level. First successfully performed by Senning in 1959, the operation was simplified by Mustard in 1964 (43) (Fig. 61.6). In both techniques, the atrial septum is repositioned such that superior and inferior vena caval blood drains to the mitral valve and then to the left ventricle and pulmonary artery. Pulmonary venous blood drains on the other side of the partition to the tricuspid valve and right ventricle. The right ventricle then ejects the oxygenated blood to the systemic circulation. The Mustard operation uses a large patch of pericardium or prosthetic material to create the intraatrial baffle. In the Senning procedure, the patient's atrial tissue is used, and little or no foreign material is necessary. Although physiologic repair at the atrial level is associated with a low operative mortality rate (< 5%), even in infants, a number of late problems have occurred. Obstruction to vena caval inflow, particularly at the junction of the superior vena cava and the right atrium, still occurs in about 5% of patients and may be considerably more common when the procedure is performed in an infant. Additionally, pulmonary venous obstruction may develop and is often difficult to repair. Perhaps because of the complex atrial suture lines, atrial dysrhythmias are common and occur in more than half of patients observed on a long-term basis. In addition, pacemakers may be necessary for troubling bradyarrhythmias in as many as 10% of these patients.

The most serious long-term complication of repair by either the Senning or Mustard technique has been right ventricular dysfunction. Right ventricular failure with an enlarged, poorly contractile chamber and secondary tricuspid regurgitation has been found in a significant number of these patients in long-term follow-up studies. The true incidence of significant right ventricular failure in these cases remains difficult to define and is clearly influenced by an earlier era of operation with different methods of myocardial protection and surgical technique. The fact that many of these infants underwent definitive repair after many months of significant cyanosis may also have influenced right ventricular function.

These long-term complications of atrial repair prompted a reexamination of direct arterial repair for transposing the great arteries. The "arterial switch" procedure, first successfully performed by Jatene in 1977, has become the optimal surgical procedure for infants with this condition (44). Current techniques have reduced the operative mortality to levels comparable with those of atrial repair. Additionally, because the operation is performed early in life, this approach has virtually eliminated the interim morbidity and mortality associated with postponement of surgery until at least 6 months of age. The operative technique involves transection of both great vessels and direct reanastomosis to reestablish ventriculoarterial concordance (Fig. 61.7). Additionally, the coronary arteries are removed from the anterior aorta and relocated to the posterior great vessel (neoaorta). The extensive experience gained with this procedure has confirmed that any variant of coronary artery anatomy can be successfully repaired, although certain unusual forms clearly impose a higher risk. Because most patients with TGA have an intact ventricular septum, left ventricular pressure falls early in life as pulmonary vascular resistance decreases. In this situation, it is essential that the arterial repair be performed within the first 2 to 3 weeks of life, while the left ventricle is still able to meet systemic workloads. In patients presenting later, the left ventricle can be retrained with a preliminary pulmonary artery banding and aorticopulmonary shunt followed by the definitive arterial repair. Although patients with large VSDs do not require early repair because of their decreased left ventricular pressure, experience has indicated that even in this subgroup, the operation must be performed within the first month of life, before secondary complications such as pulmonary hypertension, CHF, or infection develop.

Patients with fixed left ventricular outflow tract obstruction are not candidates for the arterial repair because

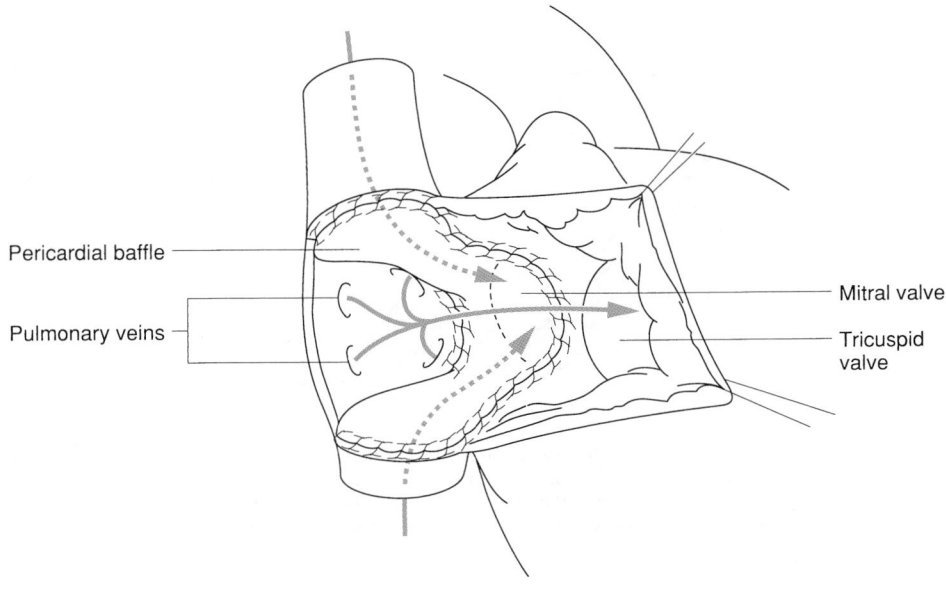

Figure 61.6. The Mustard operation for transposition of the great arteries. In this procedure, the atrial septum is excised and replaced with a pericardial baffle, so that pulmonary venous blood is redirected over the baffle to the tricuspid valve. Superior and inferior vena caval blood then drains to the mitral valve.

Pericardial baffle

Pulmonary veins

Mitral valve

Tricuspid valve

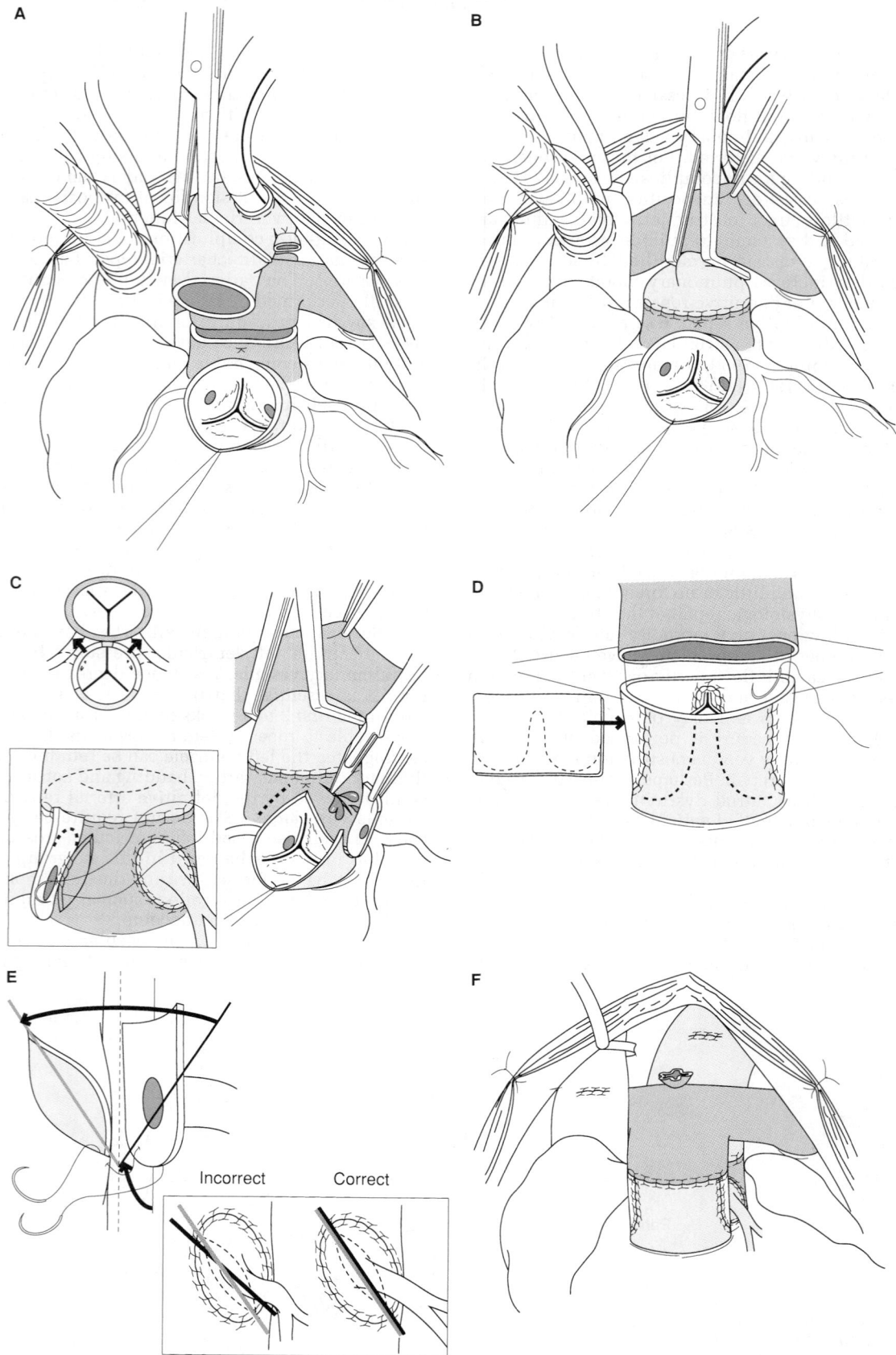

Figure 61.7. Arterial switch procedure for transposition of the great arteries. *(A)* Division of aorta and pulmonary artery. *(B)* LeCompte maneuver; posterior translocation of the aorta. *(C)* Mobilization of the coronary arteries. *(D)* Placement of pantaloon-shaped pericardial patch. *(E)* Proper alignment of the coronary arteries on the neoaorta. *(F)* Completed repair.

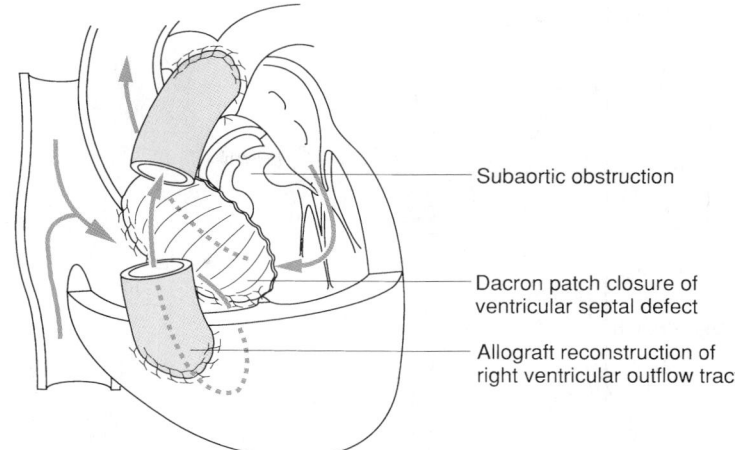

Figure 61.8. The Rastelli procedure for transposition of the great arteries with ventricular septal defect and pulmonary stenosis. A prosthetic patch placed within the right ventricle directs left ventricular blood through the defect to the aorta. The main pulmonary artery is ligated, and right ventricular blood then passes through a conduit to the distal pulmonary arteries.

Subaortic obstruction

Dacron patch closure of ventricular septal defect

Allograft reconstruction of right ventricular outflow tract

correction would result in systemic ventricular outflow tract obstruction. Most of these patients also have large VSDs. Palliation early in life with systemic-to-pulmonary artery shunting is preferred, and definitive repair is then postponed until the age of 3 to 5 years. At that time, the Rastelli procedure is performed, in which left ventricular blood is redirected through the VSD and to the anterior aorta by placement of an intraventricular patch (Fig. 61.8). The pulmonary artery is ligated, and right ventricle-to-distal pulmonary artery continuity is reestablished with a valve-bearing conduit.

DOUBLE-OUTLET RIGHT VENTRICLE

Double-outlet ventricle includes a variety of malformations in which, by 50% or more, both great arteries arise from one ventricle. Although double-outlet left ventricles occur, a far more common anomaly is the double-outlet right ventricle (DORV). A VSD is usually present in DORV, in addition to other defects, including discordant ventriculoarterial connections, valvar or subvalvar stenosis of the pulmonary artery and aortic outflow, and single ventricle.

The physiologic consequences of DORV vary depending on the associated defects. The three most critical factors determining the net effects on the circulation are the size of the VSD, the presence or absence of pulmonary stenosis, and the presence and degree of left-sided obstruction. As a result, DORV may clinically resemble an isolated VSD, tetralogy of Fallot, or TGA.

The size and location of the VSD are important considerations in planning operative management. The VSD may be primarily directed toward the aorta, toward the pulmonary artery, equally toward both arteries (doubly committed), or remote from both great vessels (noncommitted). The location of the VSD affects the direction of flow of oxygenated blood and thus affects the degree of cyanosis. VSDs in DORV seldom close spontaneously. This is fortunate, as closure would result in severe hemodynamic decompensation or death.

If the VSD is large and nonrestrictive, it can be closed with a tunnel-like patch that directs left ventricular flow into the aorta. A restrictive VSD must be enlarged to avoid creating subaortic stenosis. For patients with DORV and pulmonary stenosis, repair requires right ventricular outflow tract reconstruction with a patch or a valved allograft conduit, in addition to patch closure of the VSD.

Double-outlet right ventricle with transposition-type physiology may be treated by a variety of methods, depending on the specific anatomic details. With one approach, the VSD is patched to baffle left ventricular output into the pulmonary artery, and an atrial (Senning or Mustard) or arterial type of correction is then performed. A second approach requires construction of an intraventricular patch that connects the left ventricle to both great vessels, division of the pulmonary artery at its origin, and insertion of a conduit from the right ventricle to the distal pulmonary artery. In the Damus-Kaye-Stanzel operation, patch closure of the VSD and division of the pulmonary artery are performed. The proximal pulmonary artery is then anastomosed to the side of the ascending aorta. An extracardiac conduit is then placed from the right ventricle to the distal pulmonary artery. This approach may be particularly advantageous when the VSD is far removed from the aortic valve, so that making a direct connection is impossible.

TRUNCUS ARTERIOSUS

Truncus arteriosus is a rare anomaly that accounts for 0.4% to 4% of all cases of congenital heart disease. A single arterial vessel arises from the heart, overriding the ventricular septum and giving rise to the systemic, coronary, and pulmonary circulations. Two classification schemes have been proposed—one by Collett and Edwards (45) in 1949 and the other by Van Praagh and Van Praagh (46) in 1965 (Fig. 61.9). The Collett and Edwards classification focused on the origin of the pulmonary arteries from the common arterial trunk, as follows:

Type I: Common arterial trunk gives rise to a main pulmonary artery and the aorta.

Type II: Right and left pulmonary arteries arise directly and in close proximity from the posterior wall of the truncus.

Type III: Right and left pulmonary arteries arise from more widely separated orifices on the posterior truncal wall.

Type IV: Branch pulmonary arteries are absent. Pulmonary blood flow is derived from aorticopulmonary collaterals.

The system offered by Van Praagh and Van Praagh, a somewhat more surgically oriented scheme, is based on the presence or absence of a VSD, the degree of formation of the aorticopulmonary septum, and the status of the aortic arch:

Type A (with a VSD)
Type B (without a VSD)

1. The aorticopulmonary septum is partially developed (partially separate main pulmonary artery).

Collett and Edwards

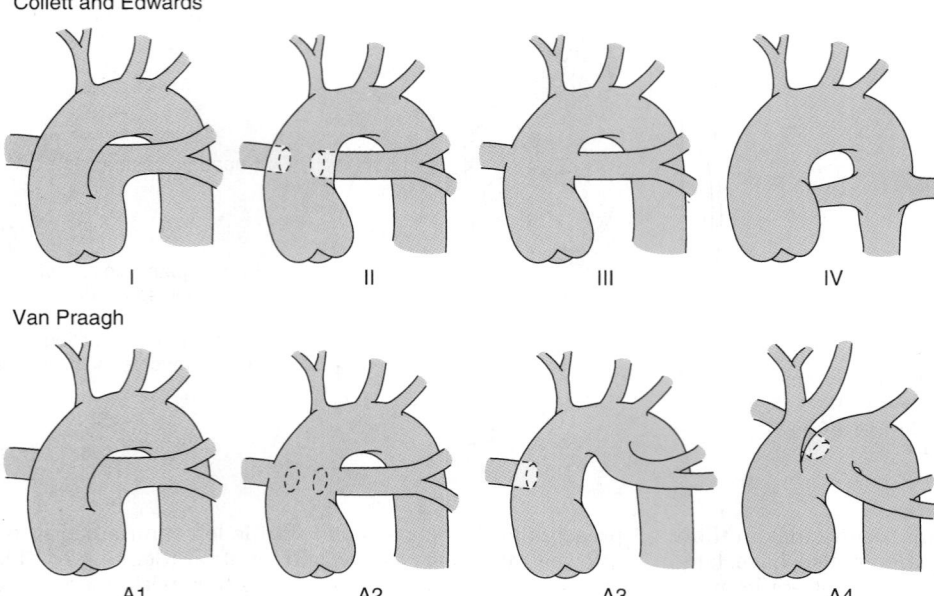

Van Praagh

Figure 61.9. Truncus arteriosus: classification schemes as described by Collett and Edwards (45) and by VanPraagh and VanPraagh (46). (From Hernanz-Schulman M, Fellows KE. Persistent truncus arteriosus: pathologic, diagnostic, and therapeutic considerations. *Semin Roentgenol* 1985; 20:121, with permission.)

2. The aorticopulmonary septum is absent (no main pulmonary artery segment); both branch pulmonary arteries arise from the common trunk.
3. Either branch pulmonary artery is absent.
4. Hypoplasia, coarctation, atresia, or absence of the aortic isthmus is associated with a large PDA.

Persistent truncus arteriosus is the result of failed development of the aorticopulmonary septum and subpulmonary infundibulum (conal septum). Normal septation leads to the development of both pulmonary and systemic outflow tracts, division of the semilunar valves, and formation of the aorta and pulmonary arteries. Failure of septation results in a VSD (absence of the infundibular septum), a single semilunar valve, and a single arterial trunk. Most cases are associated with a VSD reminiscent of the VSD associated with tetralogy of Fallot. However, in this anomaly, the superior margin of the defect is formed by the truncal valve. The truncal valve leaflets are generally dysmorphic, being thickened and fleshy, and their motion is often restricted. Leaflet number is highly variable, with about 65% tricuspid, 25% quadricuspid, and 9% bicuspid. As a result of these abnormally developed valve leaflets, about half of the patients present with some degree of truncal valve regurgitation. Truncal valve stenosis can be seen alone or in combination with regurgitation and is present in about one third of cases of truncus arteriosus. Significant obstruction is predicted by gradients of more than 30 mm Hg in the presence of normal cardiac output. The pulmonary arteries are usually of normal size and most often arise from the left posterolateral aspect of the truncal artery, often in close proximity to the truncal valve and ostium of the left coronary artery.

Associated lesions include patent foramen ovale, atrial septal defect (10%), persistent left superior vena cava (10%), and mitral valve anomalies (5%). Interrupted aortic arch (usually type B) occurs about 20% of the time, and a right aortic arch coexists in 25% to 35% of cases. Coronary artery abnormalities are common (50%) and can lead to coronary arterial injury during repair. Noncardiac anomalies are present in about 20% of cases and may contribute to death. In particular, the DiGeorge syndrome is often associated with truncus arteriosus, and screening of these infants is routine.

The anatomy of truncus arteriosus results in the obligatory mixing of systemic and pulmonary venous blood at the level of the VSD and truncal valve, which produces arterial saturations of 85% to 90%. The systemic arterial saturation depends on the volume of pulmonary blood flow, which in turn is determined by the pulmonary vascular resistance. As the pulmonary vascular resistance begins to fall, excessive pulmonary circulation ensues and leads to pulmonary congestion. This nonrestrictive left-to-right shunt may cause early development of irreversible pulmonary vascular obstructive disease.

The presence of truncal valve abnormalities poses further hemodynamic burdens. Truncal valve regurgitation leads to ventricular dilatation and low diastolic coronary perfusion pressures that can result in myocardial ischemia. Truncal valve stenosis promotes ventricular hypertrophy, increases the myocardial oxygen demand, and limits coronary and systemic perfusion, especially with the large volume of runoff into the pulmonary vascular bed.

Neonates with truncus arteriosus present with signs of CHF and collapsing peripheral pulses. Chest radiography shows marked cardiomegaly, pulmonary plethora, often with minimal thymus shadow, and a right aortic arch. The ECG most often depicts biventricular hypertrophy. Echocardiography is the diagnostic procedure of choice and can demonstrate the truncal vessel, the structure and function of the truncal valve, associated lesions such as interrupted aortic arch, and often the pulmonary arterial anatomy. Cardiac catheterization is not performed unless the anatomy is unclear, further information is needed about the status of the truncal valve, or the status of the pulmonary vasculature is unclear (i.e., infants older than 3 months at diagnosis).

The natural history of patients born with truncus arteriosus is early demise. More than 80% succumb by 1 year. Early death is caused by CHF. Survivors may do well for a period of time until the development of pulmonary vascular obstructive disease and Eisenmenger's syndrome. The ultimate treatment of truncus arteriosus is surgical therapy. Medical treatment is directed toward controlling CHF with fluid restriction, diuretics, digitalis, and afterload reduction. The onset of tachypnea can be used as a marker to identify declining pulmonary vascular resistance and the optimal timing for repair. Complete repair entails separating the pulmonary arteries from the truncus, repairing the resulting defect in the aorta, closing the ventricular septal defect, and restoring the continuity of the right ventricular outflow tract with an extra cardiac conduit. Severe truncal valve regurgitation requires truncal valve replacement, which is best done with a small, cryopreserved allograft. An associated interrupted aortic arch is repaired by constructing a primary end-to-end anastomosis of the distal ascending aorta with proximal augmentation if necessary.

The results of truncus arteriosus repair have improved greatly during the last two decades. Before the importance of early operation to avoid irreversible pulmonary vascular disease was appreciated, patients underwent repair at most institutions at an average age of 2 to 5 years. Most of them had pulmonary vascular disease, and mortality rates ranged from 25% to 88%. Ebert showed that repair in the first 6 months of life is not only possible but preferable, and he reported a mortality rate of 9% (46a). Results have improved in recent reports, with mortality rates for complicated neonatal repairs ranging from 11% to 20% (47,48). Aortic arch interruption, severe truncal valve regurgitation, coronary artery anomalies, and age older than 3 months are generally considered important risk factors. Primary repair promptly after presentation is the standard therapy for truncus arteriosus.

CORONARY ARTERY ANOMALIES

Anomalies of coronary artery anatomy are divided into three categories based on their functional significance. Abnormalities that are of no functional significance are usually detected as incidental findings on cardiac catheterization and occur in about 3 of 1,000 patients; however, such coronary artery anomalies may be associated with a frequency of atherosclerotic stenosis somewhat higher than expected. The most common example of this type of finding is the origin of the circumflex coronary artery from the right coronary sinus or as a branch of the right coronary artery.

The second type of coronary anomaly causes no intrinsic physiologic effects, but its presence in patients with other cardiac defects alters the surgical management. A common example is an abnormal course of the left anterior descending coronary artery in a patient with tetralogy of Fallot. This abnormal course occurs in 3% to 5% of patients with tetralogy and may prevent a right ventricular incision that might otherwise be performed as part of the operative repair.

The most important types of coronary artery anomalies are those that produce significant adverse effects on the myocardium. Coronary arteriovenous fistula is the most common major anomaly of the coronary circulation. In these defects, the coronary arteries arise normally from the aorta but connect with (in descending order of frequency) the right ventricle, right atrium (including the coronary sinus or the superior vena cava), pulmonary artery, left atrium, left ventricle, or bronchial veins. This produces a left-to-right shunt, which may result in symptoms of CHF. Angina, endocarditis, myocardial infarction, and, in infants, failure to thrive are other presenting manifestations (49). The diagnosis can be established by cardiac catheterization or by echocardiography and Doppler ultrasonography. Intraoperative echocardiographic and Doppler studies may help to localize the fistula.

The natural history of coronary artery fistulae has not been well defined. In light of the possible increase in size and predilection for the development of subacute bacterial endocarditis or rupture, most investigators recommend obliterating the fistula unless the shunt is insignificant ($\dot{Q}_p/\dot{Q}_s < 1.3$). Rare fistulae that are discrete and easily located can be closed without cardiopulmonary bypass. More commonly, operation requires opening the recipient cardiac chamber on bypass to identify and securely close all fistulous communications. Furthermore, obliterating the fistula may compromise coronary flow distal to it, and coronary artery bypass grafting may need to be performed to prevent myocardial ischemia.

The second most frequent clinically important coronary artery anomaly is origin of a coronary artery from the pulmonary artery. This abnormality is more often observed in the left coronary artery than in the right. The magnitude of physiologic derangement varies with the number of collaterals that form between the abnormal coronary artery and the normal vessels. In the postnatal period, as pulmonary vascular resistance falls, a decrease in the perfusion pressure in the distribution of the abnormal artery may result in a steal of blood from the normal coronary circulation into the low-pressure pulmonary artery. If the supply of collaterals from the right coronary artery is good and myocardial perfusion remains adequate, this condition may not present until later in life, when the diagnosis is established as part of an evaluation for a cardiac murmur. When the supply of collaterals from the opposite coronary vessel is poor, however, the resulting steal may cause myocardial ischemia. In the neonatal period, this may manifest as irritability, difficulty in feeding, ECG evidence of ischemia and infarction, and ischemic mitral regurgitation. Typically, symptoms first occur at about 6 weeks to 3 months of life. With this anomaly, angiography is usually required to establish the anatomic diagnosis, although echocardiography can often describe the origin and course of the coronary arteries. Surgical correction should be performed promptly when the condition is identified. The operative treatment used has varied with the age of the patient and the specifics of the coronary anatomy. When collaterals are extensive, simple ligation of the anomalous vessel at its origin has been used to eliminate the steal into the pulmonary circulation without impairing myocardial perfusion. Although this approach may be life-saving, particularly in the symptomatic infant, it results in a one-coronary artery system, leaving left coronary flow dependent on collaterals from the right. This situation often results in chronic ischemia later in life. Attempts at restoring a normal arterial supply with coronary artery bypass in which a saphenous vein, internal mammary artery, or subclavian artery is used have been successful. Bypass operations may be technically difficult in the diminutive vessels of an infant, and long-term patency is suboptimal, particularly when saphenous vein is used. The optimal surgical approach is to construct a direct connection between the aorta and the anomalous coronary artery, either by direct implantation or by the creation of a tunnel in the pulmonary artery. This technique has proved successful in neonates and has excellent long-term results (50).

A potentially dangerous abnormality exists when the left main coronary artery arises from the right coronary sinus and passes between the pulmonary artery and the aorta. Fatal complications may also occur when the right coronary artery arises from the left coronary sinus and passes between the great arteries, particularly when the right coronary is dominant. The precise pathophysiologic sequence by which these abnormalities cause death is the subject of debate. This condition often causes sudden death during vigorous physical exertion in young, healthy persons. It has therefore been suggested that an increase in aortic and pulmonary arterial pressure causes extrinsic compression of the coronary artery (the vascular vise). Others have observed that the orifice of these anomalous arteries is elliptic and have hypothesized that the increase in aortic diameter with increased cardiac output causes coronary obstruction by further narrowing the orifice. Regardless of the precise physiologic events, the diagnosis of this abnormality is an indication for operative treatment. Typically, coronary artery bypass with the internal mammary artery can be performed with a low operative risk.

PATENT DUCTUS ARTERIOSUS

Normally, pulmonary vascular resistance declines and pulmonary blood flow increases proportionally after birth. The resultant increase in arterial oxygen tension stimulates the closure of the ductus arteriosus. Closure may fail to occur because of the presence of other cardiac or pulmonary conditions associated with abnormally low levels of arterial oxygen, or it may be an isolated lesion. Isolated PDA is most frequently observed in premature infants. They typically are in respiratory distress, but it may be difficult to determine whether this is attributable to the PDA or to an immature pulmonary bed.

The administration of indomethacin can cause the ductus to close. Indomethacin works by inhibiting cyclooxygenase and diminishing the endogenous prostaglandins that contribute to ductal patency. Part of the effect of indomethacin may also be attributed to an increase in norepinephrine release, which in turn causes the richly innervated ductus to constrict. Indomethacin may adversely affect kidney and platelet function and is contraindicated in patients with sepsis, coagulopathy, intracranial hemorrhage, or hepatic dysfunction. The efficacy of indo-methacin is variable in babies weighing more than 1 kg. Operative closure can be performed safely in even the smallest neonates. Prophylactic surgical closure of the ductus arteriosus in extremely premature babies has been shown to reduce the risk for necrotizing enterocolitis (51). The improvement in pulmonary function is often dramatic, and rapid extubation of ventilator-dependent patients may be possible.

In older children, a PDA usually presents as an asymptomatic murmur—the classic "machinery" murmur—with or without a hyperdynamic precordium. Pharmacologic closure of the ductus is rarely successful beyond the neonatal period, and surgical closure is required. Operation is indicated for isolated PDA in virtually all cases to prevent the eventual development of pulmonary vascular changes and congestive failure. Even the small ductus that is hemodynamically insignificant should be closed to prevent the complications of endocarditis, which may be a consequence of abnormally turbulent blood flow in this area.

In virtually all infants and most older children, ductus closure is accomplished by ligation through a left thoracotomy. Some surgeons prefer to divide the ductus when it can be safely accomplished. In premature infants, closure can be accomplished with vascular hemoclips through a minithoracotomy. With careful definition of the anatomy—most importantly the recurrent laryngeal nerve—this procedure can be performed with an extremely low risk for complications. The mortality rate of the operation approaches zero.

Recent advances include thoracoscopic ligation and transcatheter closure. Transcatheter closure by the techniques of the Rashkind double umbrella is possible in older infants and children (52). Small PDAs can also be closed with coils. Although initial results have been encouraging, further follow-up is necessary to compare the results with those of the gold standard of surgical closure. Finally, thoracoscopic closure of PDAs has reached the clinical arena. Advances in pediatric fiberoptics and the improved smaller thoracoscopic equipment have made closure possible with acceptable initial results (53).

The rare adult with a PDA can pose difficult technical problems. Pulmonary artery pressures in these cases may be markedly elevated, and an aneurysm of the ductus may develop. The ductus in older persons is highly susceptible to calcification, which may make simple ligation hazardous. In other patients, recurrent episodes of endocarditis or endarteritis may have made the ductal tissue extremely friable. Safe operative division in some cases requires cardiopulmonary bypass with suture closure from within the pulmonary artery.

ATRIOVENTRICULAR SEPTAL DEFECT

Defects in the embryologic development of the endocardial cushions may result in a variety of morphologic abnormalities in the AV valves and the atrial and ventricular septa. These anomalies range from the ostium primum ASD to the complete AVSD (or AV canal defect), with a spectrum of intermediate forms. PDA and tetralogy of Fallot are occasionally seen in association with these defects. A high percentage of patients with abnormalities of the AV structures have Down syndrome.

Complete AVSD is an anomaly characterized by a common AV orifice, rather than separate mitral and tricuspid orifices, and a deficiency of endocardial cushion tissue, which results in an ASD and an inlet type of VSD. AVSDs are classified per Rastelli into the following three types according to the morphology of the anterior leaflet of the common AV valve:

Type A: The anterior bridging leaflet is divided and attached to the septum by multiple chordae.

Type B: The anterior bridging leaflet is attached to a papillary muscle in the right ventricle.

Type C: The anterior bridging leaflet is free-floating, with no attachments except to the valve annulus.

Despite the extremely abnormal supporting structures that are commonly found, the valves themselves are almost always competent.

Atrioventricular septal defect is rarely diagnosed in the neonatal period because the pulmonary vascular resistance remains elevated for longer than usual. The occasional patient with significant AV valve insufficiency may present as a newborn. Usually in the first 6 to 12 months of life, excessive pulmonary blood flow produces severe congestive failure, manifested by dyspnea, poor feeding, and delayed growth. Patients who present beyond the age of 2 or 3 years often have Eisenmenger's syndrome with irreversible pulmonary vascular disease.

Physical examination of patients with AVSDs demonstrates increased precordial activity and fixed splitting of the second heart sound. The chest radiograph in these patients shows increased pulmonary vascularity and cardiomegaly. The ECG shows right ventricular or biventricular hypertrophy.

Echocardiography provides an excellent assessment of the anatomy in AVSD and defines the presence or absence of valvular insufficiency. Echocardiography also provides important information about the relative sizes of the ventricles. Hypoplasia of one ventricle may dictate an alteration in the operative approach. Despite the proven value of echocardiography as a sole diagnostic modality in AVSD, many groups continue to recommend catheterization before operative intervention, primarily to evaluate pulmonary artery resistance, especially in patients with Down syndrome who are older than 6 months. If the pulmonary artery resistance is high, it is important to remeasure it while the child is breathing 100% oxygen. If the pulmonary resistance falls, it implies that much of the elevated resistance is dynamic and can be managed in the perioperative period by vigorous ventilation and supplemental oxygen. Markedly elevated pulmonary resistance (more than 8 to 10 Woods units) that does not respond to oxygen administration may in some cases contraindicate repair.

Operative treatment is almost always necessary as soon as symptoms are observed to prevent further clinical deterioration. Even in the absence of symptoms, operation is best performed before 6 months of age. Pulmonary artery banding, which permits delaying the repair until the child is larger, is no longer used today. This approach exposes the child to the risks of two operations, and the overall mortality exceeds that of primary repair in infancy.

Correcting AVSDs requires patch closure of both septal defects, with reattachment of the valve apparatus to the newly constructed septa. Separate atrial and ventricular patches or a single patch for both chambers can be used (54). During closure of the ventricular defect, the surgeon must carefully avoid injury to the conduction system, which passes along the posterior and inferior rim of the ventricular septum.

The success of the operation is highly dependent on the status of the pulmonary vascular resistance and the surgeon's ability to maintain competence of the mitral and tricuspid valves. Because the mitral valve usually has three component leaflets, much debate has focused on whether it should be made into a two-leaflet structure at operation by approximating the "cleft" between the two septal leaflets with sutures. Many surgeons believe that this separation is not a true cleft that should be closed, but is rather a commissure in a three-leaflet valve that should be preserved. Others believe that mitral competence is best preserved by closing the cleft and making the valve a two-leaflet structure. When important insufficiency is present, the location of the regurgitation must be precisely determined at operation to perform an accurate valvuloplasty.

The immediate operative results are good, especially if the patient is treated before the development of pulmonary vascular disease. Patients with severe preoperative valvar regurgitation, those with significant associated defects, and those with pulmonary vascular disease do not fare as well. Late reoperation sometimes is necessary because of problems with the mitral or tricuspid valve, but this should be rare if initial operative management is carried out precisely.

COARCTATION OF THE AORTA

Coarctation of the aorta is a narrowing that most commonly develops in the upper descending aorta just distal to the left subclavian artery. COA is thought to occur when this area contains ectopic tissue from the ductus arteriosus. As the ductus undergoes normal involution and closure, this ectopic tissue also constricts, leaving a luminal narrowing. Coarctations vary in the degree of luminal stenosis and the length of aorta affected. Typically, a shelflike projection of aortic media and intima is found at the area of tightest obstruction. COA may be associated with tubular hypoplasia of the more proximal aortic arch. Coarctation is associated with Turner's syndrome.

A prominent feature of COA is the extensive development of collateral arteries. These collaterals, which typically involve the internal mammary and intercostal arteries, produce many of the classic findings of COA.

Extensive flow through the collaterals causes pulsations under the ribs and near the scapula, bruits that may be heard diffusely over the chest wall, and the rib notching seen on chest radiography.

The most common cardiac anomaly found in association with COA is a bicuspid aortic valve, which may or may not be of clinical importance. VSDs and severe aortic stenosis may also be seen, particularly in highly symptomatic neonates.

In the newborn period, COA may present with profound CHF. The precordium is typically hyperdynamic, and a harsh murmur is audible over the left chest and back. Femoral pulses are diminished or undetectable. The onset of symptoms may coincide with closure of the ductus. Before ductal closure, differential cyanosis (pink upper body and cyanotic lower body) provides evidence that the lower body depends on ductal flow. Rib notching is not seen in this early period, although cardiomegaly is observed radiographically.

Older children are almost always asymptomatic. In these patients, the diagnosis is usually based on the presence of hypertension in the upper extremities with diminished or absent pulses in the lower extremities. The chest film generally shows rib notching and the typical "3" shadow in the aortic knob. Asymmetry of the rib notching may suggest anomalous origin or stenosis of a subclavian artery. In adults presenting with COA, severe hypertension and congestive failure may have developed. No single cause of hypertension in COA has been defined. Mechanical obstruction to ventricular ejection is one factor leading to an elevated arterial pressure. Hypoperfusion of the kidneys with resulting activation of the renin–angiotensin–aldosterone axis probably contributes to some degree. Abnormal aortic compliance, variable capacity of collateral vessels, and abnormal setting of baroreceptors have also been implicated in the pathogenesis of hypertension.

In many cases, COA can be diagnosed on physical examination alone. Echocardiography frequently can provide an excellent demonstration of the anatomy and estimate of the pressure gradient. Aortography with pressure measurement can be used when the diagnosis is unclear and permits definition of other possible cardiac anomalies. In adolescents and adults, the aortogram may be particularly useful to the surgeon in demonstrating the presence or absence of collaterals, which may influence the operative management.

In the neonate with COA and CHF, operative repair is performed as a life-saving measure. In older children, COA should be repaired to prevent the long-term sequelae of hypertension, heart failure, endocarditis, aortic rupture, and intracranial vascular lesions. Patients with COA and severe hypertension should undergo operation as early as possible. The earlier the operation is performed, the more likely the patient is to become normotensive.

The surgical technique varies with the patient's age and particular anatomy (55). Resection of the coarctation segment with direct end-to-end anastomosis is preferred when the anatomy is such that a direct anastomosis can be achieved without excessive tension. This method of repair removes all diseased tissue, particularly residual ductal tissue, which may contract and cause further narrowing if left behind. Absorbable sutures can be used to perform the reconstruction in the hope that growth of the aorta will not be compromised. The subclavian flap angioplasty is an alternative technique used to enlarge the narrowed portion of the aorta with viable arterial wall. The affected portion of the aorta is opened longitudinally and augmented with the adjacent subclavian artery. Blood flow to the left arm is subsequently provided by collateral vessels. Although growth and function of the arm almost always remain normal, long-term studies have demonstrated a slight discrepancy in limb length in some patients. Less commonly, reconstruction with a patch or an end-to-end interposition graft is performed. Many surgeons believe that patch reconstruction carries a high risk for the formation of aneurysm. These aneurysms do not occur on the patched side of the aorta but on the opposite wall.

One of the major intraoperative concerns during COA repair is the interruption of distal aortic blood flow, particularly to the spinal cord. The risk for paraplegia after this operation is low but increased in the absence of large collaterals. It is often advisable to place a femoral artery catheter to monitor arterial pressure in the lower body during the operative repair. If inadequate distal perfusion pressure is found, some method of providing additional flow to the lower body should be applied. We prefer partial cardiac bypass and use either the femoral artery or the distal thoracic aorta for arterial supply and the femoral vein or left atrium for venous return. This maintains blood flow to the spinal cord, kidneys, and other organs and assists in managing overall hemodynamics during aortic clamping and unclamping. Newborns with coarctation and large VSDs are at particularly high risk for hemodynamic instability. These patients are best treated by simultaneous VSD closure and coarctation repair with a median sternotomy and a short period of hypothermic circulatory arrest.

The treatment of patients after COA repair often focuses on controlling hypertension. Hypertension may be observed regardless of the degree of relief of anatomic obstruction, and the blood pressure may exceed preoperative levels. The pathogenesis of this so-called paradoxical hypertension is thought to be related to stimulation of sympathetic nerve fibers in the aortic wall. An infusion of sodium nitroprusside or intermittent administration of propranolol is usually effective in keeping the arterial pressure within an acceptable range (56).

Abdominal discomfort during this time may be a symptom of mesenteric arteritis, which is thought to develop when the restoration of pulsatile flow to the visceral vessels causes spasm and potential intestinal ischemia. This complication, which can be fatal, is almost completely preventable by proper control of blood pressure. In addition, it is advisable to forbid oral intake strictly until bowel function returns.

Some reports have described balloon dilation as an effective therapy for COA, although false aneurysms, dissection, and inadequate dilation have been problems with this technique and may complicate a subsequent operation. The application of balloon dilation appears to be more promising in the 7% to 10% of coarctations that recur after initial surgical repair. In such cases, because of the additional aortic wall mass from scarring and adhesions, this technique may be safer. The long-term results of coarctation repair are generally good, with the optimal technique in infants and children being resection with primary end-to-end anastomosis.

UNIVENTRICULAR HEART

In univentricular heart, a congenital anomaly, only one ventricular chamber is connected to the atria. To be classified as a ventricle, a chamber must receive at least half of an inlet valve. In the most common form of univentricular heart, both the mitral and tricuspid valves connect to a morphologic left ventricle (double-inlet left ventricle), which ejects blood through a hypoplastic outlet chamber and then to the aorta. The outlet chamber cannot be considered a ventricle, regardless of its size, because it does not receive an inlet valve. Univentricular hearts are frequently associated with malpositions of the great vessels and varying degrees of obstruction to the pulmonary blood flow. In double-inlet left ventricle, the aorta is usually anterior and to the left of the pulmonary artery.

The presentations of infants with univentricular heart are variable, depending on the status of the pulmonary blood flow (57). When the pulmonary flow is excessive, cyanosis may be mild, and the dominant feature is CHF. Pulmonary stenosis decreases the pulmonary blood flow, and the degree of cyanosis is then increased. Associated lesions may further complicate the picture, such as COA, subaortic stenosis, or a restrictive ASD. Patients with moderate pulmonary stenosis may achieve a well-balanced circulation with acceptable systemic oxygenation and normal pulmonary artery pressure. These patients may be symptom-free well into adolescence. Most patients, however, require intervention early in life to reduce pulmonary blood flow if excessive or to increase it in the presence of severe pulmonary stenosis. Pulmonary vascular obstructive disease develops early when pulmonary blood flow is excessive. With the possible exception of patients in whom the pulmonary and systemic blood flow is well balanced, the prognosis for patients with unoperated univentricular hearts is poor. More than half die early of CHF or dysrhythmias.

In the presence of excessive pulmonary blood flow and pulmonary hypertension, operation should be performed early in life to control pulmonary blood flow and prevent the development of pulmonary vascular occlusive disease. Options include pulmonary artery banding or division of the main pulmonary artery in conjunction with a controlled aorticopulmonary shunt. Pulmonary artery banding is a less complicated procedure; however, it is often difficult to adjust the pulmonary flow accurately, and too proximal or too distal a band can lead to distortion of the pulmonary artery, which further complicates later operations. Another option is division of the main pulmonary artery, side-to-side anastomosis with the native aorta, and a modified Blalock-Taussig shunt (modified Damus-Kaye-Stanzel procedure). This procedure more accurately limits the pulmonary blood flow and eliminates the possibility of subaortic obstruction, which can occur when the systemic blood flow depends on egress through a bulboventricular foramen. Pulmonary stenosis may be palliated by a systemic-to-pulmonary artery shunt procedure. We prefer a modified Blalock-Taussig shunt with a right thoracotomy in most patients. This procedure increases the systemic saturation, and the risk for causing excessive pulmonary blood flow or pulmonary artery distortion is minimal. In infants older than 4 to 6 months, a hemi-Fontan connection, in which the superior vena caval flow is directed into the pulmonary arteries, can be used to increase the effective pulmonary blood flow. This procedure maximizes pulmonary flow without causing a volume overload to the single ventricle. It is most commonly used as part of a complete atriopulmonary connection, often as a preliminary first stage.

The goal of surgical correction in patients with a univentricular heart is the total diversion of all vena caval blood directly into the pulmonary arteries (58). The Fontan procedure was first successfully performed in a patient with tricuspid atresia but has since evolved as an excellent way to establish physiologic repair for patients with more complex forms of univentricular heart. Although many modifications of the technique have been made, the best approach involves direct anastomosis of the right atrium and superior vena cava to the pulmonary artery without the use of a valve. Systemic and pulmonary venous blood flow is divided in the atrium by means of a prosthetic patch (i.e., lat-

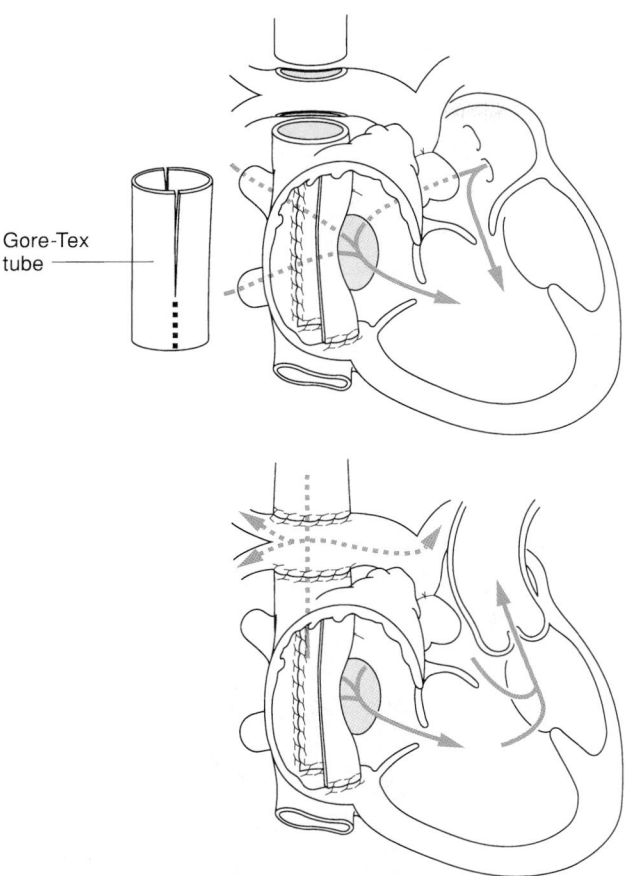

Figure 61.10. Total cavopulmonary connection for univentricular heart. The internal orifices of the superior and inferior venae cavae are connected in the right atrium with a patch cut from a Gore-Tex tube. The superior vena cava is divided just above its junction with the right atrium, and both ends are anastomosed to the right pulmonary artery. The main pulmonary artery is ligated.

eral tunnel technique). All pulmonary venous flow then empties into the ventricular chamber through the AV valves, while superior and inferior vena caval blood drains through the atriopulmonary anastomosis (Fig. 61.10). For the Fontan procedure to be performed with a low operative mortality and an acceptable functional result, certain criteria must be met. Normal pulmonary artery pressure (< 20 mm Hg) and pulmonary vascular resistance (< 2 Woods units) are the most important prerequisites. Additionally, it is essential that ventricular function and atrioventricular valve function be normal. Many of the criteria originally proposed, including normal cardiac rhythm, right atrial hypertrophy, normal systemic venous return, and age older than 4 years, are of little or no importance. Although the Fontan procedure cannot be considered a truly corrective operation, it offers benefits that cannot be equaled by those of any of the other palliative procedures. The major advantages include restoration of normal systemic oxygen saturation and reduction of ventricular volume overload. These benefits may well protect against later ventricular failure and the complications associated with long-standing cyanosis. The addition of a fixed-orifice right-to-left shunt (i.e., fenestrated Fontan), which preserves systemic output in the face of transient elevations in pulmonary vascular resistance, may help to reduce early postoperative morbidity (59).

Ventricular septation procedures have also been successfully performed in patients with univentricular hearts.

The subset of patients with a double-inlet left ventricle, anterior and leftward aorta, nonrestrictive outlet foramen, and mild or no pulmonary stenosis are best suited for septation. This anatomy allows placement of a relatively direct and straight prosthetic patch in the ventricle that separates the pulmonary and systemic circulations. The septation procedure has been associated with a relatively high morbidity, primarily related to complete heart block, so that its overall effectiveness is reduced. A few centers have continued to apply this procedure in carefully selected patients.

The operative risk for the Fontan procedure when all preoperative risk factors are within acceptable limits is 5% to 10%. Although the operation may be performed in patients who do not meet one or more of these criteria, the risk may increase substantially. The condition of survivors is significantly improved, and most attain a functional status of New York Heart Association class I or II. Although long-term results are encouraging, late complications may be seen. Continued surveillance for arrhythmias, CHF, protein-losing enteropathy, and hepatic dysfunction remains important.

HYPOPLASTIC LEFT-HEART SYNDROME

Hypoplastic left-heart syndrome comprises a spectrum of defects that can include aortic valve stenosis or atresia, mitral valve stenosis or atresia, and a severely underdeveloped left ventricle. The descending aorta is essentially a continuation of the ductus arteriosus, and the ascending aorta and aortic arch are a diminutive branch from this vessel. Initial management includes a prostaglandin infusion to maintain ductal patency and correction of metabolic acidosis. The patient may require intubation and ventilator adjustment to reduce supplemental oxygen and maintain a P_{CO_2} of about 40 mm Hg to avoid excessive pulmonary flow.

Alternative approaches to the treatment of this problem include cardiac transplantation and staged reconstructive surgery. Transplantation for hypoplastic left-heart syndrome is performed with essentially the same techniques that are standard for transplantation in older children and adults. At times, it is necessary to modify the procedure to accommodate the underdeveloped left atrium and relieve any possible obstruction to pulmonary venous drainage. In addition, it is almost always necessary to have a generous donor aortic arch that can be used to augment the tiny recipient arch. Results of transplantation in neonates have been excellent in centers with extensive experience in this area, and a 2-year survival as high as 70% has been reported (60). Because of the limited donor availability, however, up to 25% of these neonates die awaiting transplantation.

Immunosuppression is generally maintained with cyclosporin A, corticosteroids, and azathioprine, although corticosteroids have been eliminated by some groups. Antilymphocyte globulin may be given during the immediate postoperative period and as treatment for rejection. Myocardial biopsies are performed infrequently because of difficulty with access. Although transplantation remains a viable option, it is plagued by problems of infection, acute rejection, and the possibility of graft atherosclerosis.

Even if transplantation could be performed with perfect results, the limited supply of donor hearts necessitates reconstruction for a large number of babies with hypoplastic left-heart syndrome. The operation developed for first-stage palliation of this defect has permitted excellent growth and development (61) (Fig. 61.11). The Norwood procedure converts the pulmonary artery into the main

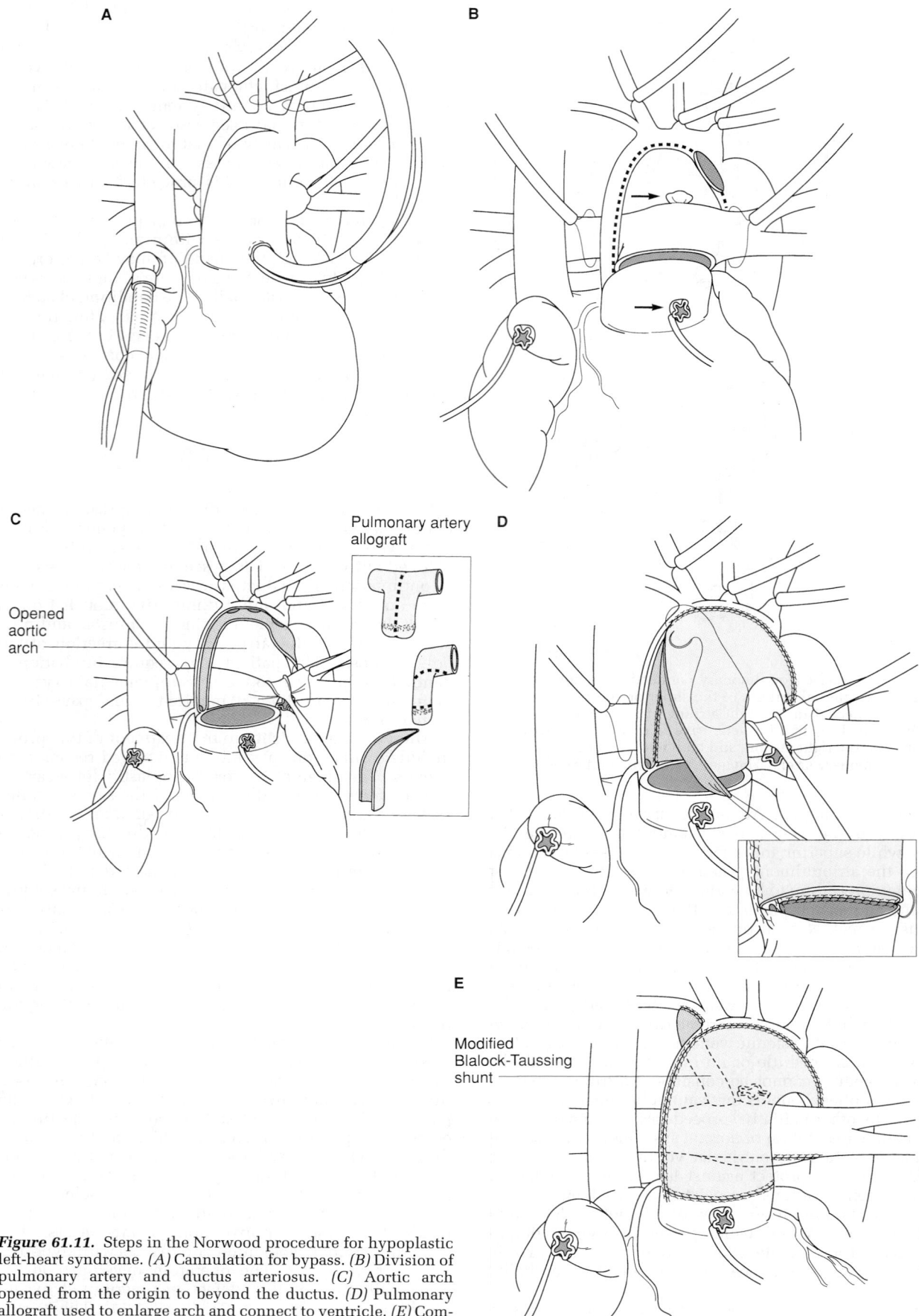

A

B

C

Pulmonary artery allograft

Opened aortic arch

D

E

Modified Blalock-Taussing shunt

Figure 61.11. Steps in the Norwood procedure for hypoplastic left-heart syndrome. *(A)* Cannulation for bypass. *(B)* Division of pulmonary artery and ductus arteriosus. *(C)* Aortic arch opened from the origin to beyond the ductus. *(D)* Pulmonary allograft used to enlarge arch and connect to ventricle. *(E)* Completed repair.

outlet for what is to be a functional single ventricle. The aortic arch is augmented with a large piece of allograft artery and anastomosed to the pulmonary root. The distal pulmonary arteries are separated from their origin and are supplied with blood through a systemic-to-pulmonary artery shunt. Critical elements of this operation include excising the interatrial septum, extending the arch augmentation beyond the ductus arteriosus, preserving coronary artery perfusion, and creating an appropriately sized aorticopulmonary shunt. Postoperatively, careful ventilator management is mandatory to help adjust pulmonary vascular resistance and maintain the proper balance of pulmonary and systemic blood flow. Subsequent reconstructive management of hypoplastic left-heart syndrome includes creation of a bidirectional superior vena cava–pulmonary artery anastomosis at about 6 months to 1 year of age, followed by completion of a modified Fontan reconstruction at about 18 months. In the latter operation, inferior vena caval blood is routed to the pulmonary artery, so that a physiologic repair is provided by diverting all systemic venous return directly to the lungs.

Survival after first-stage reconstruction for hypoplastic left-heart syndrome exceeds 80% in experienced centers (62). The use of an intermediate procedure in which the superior vena cava is transected and anastomosed to the undivided pulmonary artery is anticipated to improve late survival and reduce the risk of the Fontan procedure. Again, the bidirectional Glenn procedure or hemi-Fontan operation relieves the volume load on the ventricle while improving effective pulmonary blood flow. Although the reconstructive route entails three separate operations, when the results of primary transplantation include patients who die while waiting for donor organs, the short-term results of the replacement and reconstructive approaches are similar.

PRIMARY NEOPLASMS OF THE HEART AND PERICARDIUM

Primary tumors of the heart and pericardium are extremely rare. Metastatic lesions are 20 to 30 times more common. Among primary cardiac tumors, benign lesions predominate over malignant ones by a ratio of 3:1. The presentation of cardiac tumors may include congestive heart failure, angina, syncope, pulmonary hypertension, pulmonary or systemic emboli, arrhythmias, hemolysis, and a variety of systemic manifestations that may create a puzzling clinical picture.

Results of initial diagnostic studies in patients with cardiac neoplasms are rarely specific. Calcification of an occasional tumor may facilitate the roentgenographic diagnosis. ECG may show nonspecific chamber enlargement or rhythm disturbances. The diagnosis of these tumors has been greatly advanced in recent years by two-dimensional echocardiography, although distinguishing a tumor from thrombus may be difficult. Cardiac catheterization and angiography may be unable to identify the tumor by negative-contrast images. Furthermore, transseptal puncture to identify the most common cardiac tumors, located in the left atrium, may be hazardous because of the risk for systemic embolism.

The most common primary cardiac neoplasm is the myxoma. This may present in any cardiac chamber in patients of either sex at any age. Familial predilections to myxomas exist. Although some pathologists have argued that myxomas are really organized thrombi, most believe they are true neoplasms. More than 75% of myxomas arise in the left atrium, and 5% are multiple. Myxomas are most commonly attached to the fossa ovalis and are said never to arise from the cardiac valves. Myxomas are yellow-brown to pale gray gelatinous masses up to 15 cm in diameter. They rarely extend more deeply than the endocardium. Malignant degeneration is not thought to occur in myxomas, although their ability to recur after inadequate resection and their occasional multiplicity may cause one to suspect malignant behavior.

Because they commonly arise in the left atrium, patients with these lesions may present with symptoms typical of mitral valve disease, including murmurs, atrial arrhythmias, systemic emboli, and CHF. One striking symptom that should arouse suspicion of a myxoma is dyspnea that varies dramatically with posture, especially dyspnea that is aggravated by an upright position.

All myxomas should be resected because of their potential to cause CHF and stroke. At operation, the myxoma should be completely excised, including its base on the atrial septum. Often, a small patch is required to close the remaining ASD. A careful inspection of all cardiac chambers for possible undiagnosed tumors is a mandatory part of this procedure. The operative mortality rate approaches zero, and the long-term outlook is generally completely benign.

Rhabdomyoma is the most common cardiac tumor in infancy and childhood, usually presenting before the age of 1 year. Most are located in the left or right ventricle and often protrude into the ventricular lumen, where they may significantly obstruct blood flow. As many as half of these patients have tuberous sclerosis. On pathologic examination, these tumors are easily distinguished from the surrounding myocardium by their whitish yellow appearance. Intracavitary rhabdomyomas have been surgically excised with good relief of symptoms. Rarely, intramural tumors have been excised successfully. Most of these patients have a poor long-term prognosis.

Other benign tumors of the heart include papillary fibroelastomas, fibromas, and lipomas. Lambl's excrescence is considered by some to be a form of fibroelastoma. It is found most commonly on the lines of closure of valves but rarely causes valve dysfunction. Hemangiomas are the most common vascular tumors of the heart. Teratomas may arise from the base of the heart, attached to the root of the great vessels, and may undergo malignant degeneration.

The most common primary malignant neoplasm of the heart is the angiosarcoma. Most originate from the right atrium or pericardium and cause CHF. Operative excision is rarely possible by the time of presentation. Radiation and chemotherapy may provide some palliation, but few patients survive more than a year after diagnosis. Patients with other rare cardiac malignancies, such as rhabdomyosarcomas, mesotheliomas, fibrosarcomas, and osteosarcomas, have a similarly poor prognosis.

REFERENCES

1. Gross RE, Hubbard JP. Surgical ligation of a patent ductus arteriosus. *JAMA* 1939;112:729–731.
2. Blalock A, Taussig H. The surgical treatment of malformations of the heart in which there is pulmonary stenosis or pulmonary atresia. *JAMA* 1945;128:189.
3. Lewis FJ, Taufic M. Closure of atrial septal defects with the aid of hypothermia: experimental accomplishments and the report of one successful case. *Surgery* 1953;33:52–59.
4. Gibbon JH. Application of a mechanical heart–lung apparatus to cardiac surgery. *Minn Med* 1954;37:171.
5. Warden EH, Cohen M, Read RC, et al. Controlled cross-circulation for open intracardiac surgery: physiologic studies and results of creation and closure of ventricular septal defects. *J Thorac Surg* 1954;28:331–343.

6. Kirklin JW, DuShane JW, Patrick RT, et al. Intracardiac surgery with the aid of a mechanical pump-oxygenator system (Gibbon type): report of eight cases. *Proc Staff Meet Mayo Clin* 1955;30:201–206.

7. Garson A Jr, Bricker JT, McNamara DG, eds. *The science and practice of pediatric cardiology.* Philadelphia: Lea & Febiger, 1990:1143.

8. Yee ES, Turley K, Hsieh WR, et al. Infant total anomalous pulmonary venous connection: factors influencing timing of presentation and operative outcome. *Circulation* 1987;76[Suppl III]:83.

9. Steele PM, Fuster V, Cohen M, et al. Isolated atrial septal defect with pulmonary vascular obstructive disease: long-term follow-up and prediction of outcome after surgical correction. *Circulation* 1987;76:1037.

10. Reddy VM, McElhinney DB, Sagrado T, et al. Results of 102 cases of complete repair of congenital heart defects in patients weighing 700 to 2,500 grams. *J Thorac Cardiovasc Surg* 1999;117:324–331.

11. Dabritz S, Sachweh M, Walter M, et al. Closure of atrial septal defects via limited right anterolateral thoracotomy as a minimally invasive approach in female patients. *Eur J Cardiothorac Surg* 1999;15:18–23.

12. Dietl CA, Torres AR, Favalero RG. Right submammarian thoracotomy in female patients with atrial septal defects and anomalous pulmonary venous connections: comparison between the transpectoral and subpectoral approaches. *J Thorac Cardiovasc Surg* 1992;104:723–727.

13. Barbero-Marcial M, Tanamati C, Jatene MB, et al. Transxiphoid approach without median sternotomy for the repair of atrial septal defects. *Ann Thorac Surg* 1998;65:771–774.

14. Khan JH, McElhinney DB, Reddy M, et al. Repair of secundum atrial septal defect: limiting the incision without sacrificing exposure. *Ann Thorac Surg* 1998;66:1433–1435.

15. King TD, Mills NL. Secundum atrial septal defects: nonoperative closure during cardiac catheterization. *JAMA* 1976; 235:2506.

16. Perry S, van der Velde ME, Bridges ND, et al. Transcatheter closure of atrial and ventricular septal defects. *Herz* 1993; 18:135–142.

17. Rickers C, Hamm C, Stern T, et al. Percutaneous closure of secundum atrial septal defect with a new self-centering device ("angel wings"). *Heart* 1998;80:517–521.

18. Walsh K, Tofeig M, Kitchiner DJ, et al. Comparison of the Sideris and Amplatzer septal occlusion devices. *Am J Cardiol* 1999;83:933–936.

19. Rigby ML. The era of transcatheter closure of atrial septal defects [Editorial]. *Heart* 1999;81:227–228.

20. Edwards JE. Pulmonary hypertension of cardiac and pulmonary origins: pathologic aspects. *Prog Cardiovasc Dis* 1966;9:205.

21. Clarkson PM, MacArthur BA, Barratt-Boyes BG, et al. Developmental progress after cardiac surgery in infancy using hypothermia and circulatory arrest. *Circulation* 1980;62:855.

22. Doty DB, McGoon DC. Closure of perimembranous ventricular septal defect. *J Thorac Cardiovasc Surg* 1983;85:781.

23. Leca F, Karam J, Vouhe PR, et al. Surgical treatment of multiple ventricular septal defects using a biologic glue. *J Thorac Cardiovasc Surg* 1994;107:96–102.

24. Kirklin J, Castaneda A, Keane J, et al. Surgical management of multiple ventricular septal defects. *J Thorac Cardiovasc Surg* 1980;80:485–493.

25. Chaturvedi RR, Shore DF, Yacoub M, et al. Intraoperative apical ventricular septal defect closure using a modified Rashkind double umbrella. *Heart* 1996;76:367–369.

26. Murzi B, Bonanomi GL, Giusti S, et al. Surgical closure of muscular ventricular septal defects using double umbrella devices (intraoperative VSD device closure). *Eur J Cardiothorac Surg* 1997;12:450–455.

27. Beekman RH, Rocchini AP, Andes A. Balloon valvuloplasty for critical aortic stenosis in the newborn: influence of new catheter technology. *J Am Coll Cardiol* 1991;17:1172.

28. Fisher DR, Ettedgui JA, Park SC, et al. Carotid artery approach for balloon dilation of aortic valve stenosis in the neonate: a preliminary report. *J Am Coll Cardiol* 1990;15:1633.

29. Mosca RS, Iannettoni MD, Schwartz SM, et al. Critical aortic stenosis in the neonate: a comparison of balloon valvulo-

plasty and transventricular dilation. *J Thorac Cardiovasc Surg* 1995;109:147–154.

30. Ross DN. Replacement of aortic and mitral valves with a pulmonary aortograft. *Lancet* 1967;57:956–958.

31. Jones TK, Lupinetti FM. Comparison of Ross procedures and aortic valve allografts in children. *Ann Thorac Surg* 1998; 66:S170–S173.

32. Durham LA, desJardins SE, Mosca RS, et al. Ross procedure with aortic root tailoring for aortic valve replacement in the pediatric population. *Ann Thorac Surg* 1997;64:482–486.

33. Konno S, Imai Y, Iida Y, et al. A new method for prosthetic valve replacement in congenital aortic stenosis associated with hypoplasia of the aortic valve ring. *J Thorac Cardiovasc Surg* 1975;70:909.

34. Rastan H, Koncz J. Aortoventriculoplasty: a new technique for the treatment of left ventricular outflow tract obstruction. *J Thorac Cardiovasc Surg* 1976;71:920.

35. Doty DB, Polansky DB, Jenson CB. Supravalvar stenosis: repair by extended aortoplasty. *J Thorac Cardiovasc Surg* 1977;74:362–371.

36. Altrichter PM, Olson LJ, Edwards WD, et al. Surgical pathology of the pulmonary valve: a study of 116 cases spanning 15 years. *Mayo Clin Proc* 1989;64:1352–1360.

37. McElhinney DB, Reddy VM, Hanley FL. Tetralogy of Fallot with major aortopulmonary collaterals: early total repair. *Pediatr Cardiol* 1998;19:289–296.

38. Bove EL, Kohman L, Sereika S, et al. The modified Blalock-Taussig shunt: analysis of adequacy and duration of palliation. *Circulation* 1987;76[Suppl III]:19.

39. Walsh EP, Rockenmacher S, Keane JF, et al. Late results in patients with tetralogy of Fallot repaired during infancy. *Circulation* 1988;77:1062.

40. Ilbawi MN, Idriss FS, DeLeon SY, et al. Factors that exaggerate the deleterious effects of pulmonary insufficiency on the right ventricle after tetralogy repair. *J Thorac Cardiovasc Surg* 1987;93:36–44.

41. Ilbawi MN, Idriss FS, DeLeon SY, et al. Long-term results of porcine valve insertion for pulmonary regurgitation following repair of tetralogy of Fallot. *Ann Thorac Surg* 1986;41: 478–482.

42. Rashkind WJ. Historical aspects of surgery for congenital heart disease. *J Thorac Cardiovasc Surg* 1982;84:619.

43. Stark J, de Leval M, eds. *Surgery for congenital heart defects.* London: Grune & Stratton, 1983:331.

44. Norwood WI, Dobell AR, Freed MD, et al., and the Congenital Heart Surgeons' Society. Intermediate results of the arterial switch repair: a 20-institution study. *J Thorac Cardiovasc Surg* 1988;96:854.

45. Collett RW, Edwards JE. Persistent truncus arteriosus: a classification according to anatomic types. *Surg Clin North Am* 1949;29:1245.

46. Van Praagh R, Van Praagh S. The anatomy of common aorticopulmonary trunk (truncus arteriosus communis) and its embryologic implications: a study of 57 necropsy cases. *Am J Cardiol* 1965;16:406.

46a. Ebert PA, Turley K, Stanger P, et al. Surgical treatment of truncus arteriosus in the first 6 months of life. *Annals of Surgery* 1984;200(4):451–456.

47. Hanley FL, Heinemann MK, Jonas RA, et al. Repair of truncus arteriosus in the neonate. *J Thorac Cardiovasc Surg* 1993; 105:1047.

48. Bove EL, Lupinetti FM, Pridjian AK, et al. Results of a policy of primary repair of truncus arteriosus in the neonate. *J Thorac Cardiovasc Surg* 1993;105:1057.

49. Roberts WC. Major anomalies of coronary arterial origin seen in adulthood. *Am Heart J* 1986;111:941.

50. Kirklin JW, Barratt-Boyes BG. *Cardiac surgery.* New York: John Wiley & Sons, 1993:1179.

51. Cassady G, Crouse DT, Kirklin JW, et al. A randomized, controlled trial of very early prophylactic ligation of the ductus arteriosus in babies who weighed 1,000 g or less at birth. *N Engl J Med* 1989;320:1511.

52. Perry SB, Lock JE. Front loading of double umbrellas: improved delivery of umbrella devices. *Am J Cardiol* 1992;70:917.

53. Alvarez-Tostado RA, Millan MA, Tovar LA, et al. Thoracoscopic clipping and ligation of a patent ductus arteriosus. *Ann Thorac Surg* 1994;57:755.

54. Weintraub RG, Brawn WJ, Venables AW, et al. Two-patch repair of complete atrioventricular septal defect in the first year of life: results and sequential assessment of atrioventricular valve function. *J Thorac Cardiovasc Surg* 1990;99:320.

55. Arciniegas E, ed. *Pediatric cardiac surgery.* Chicago: Year Book, 1985:227.

56. Sealy WC. Paradoxical hypertension after repair of coarctation of the aorta: a review of its causes. *Ann Thorac Surg* 1990;50:323.

57. Hawkins JA, Thorne JK, Boucek MM, et al. Early and late results in pulmonary atresia and intact ventricular septum. *J Thorac Cardiovasc Surg* 1990;100:492.

58. Fontan F, Fernandez G, Costa F, et al. The size of the pulmonary arteries and the results of the Fontan operation. *J Thorac Cardiovasc Surg* 1989;98:711.

59. Laks H, Pearl JM, Haas G, et al. Advantages of an adjustable interatrial communication. *Ann Thorac Surg* 1991;52:1089.

60. Bailey LL, Gundry SR, Razzouk AJ, et al. Bless the babies: 115 late survivors of heart transplantation during the first year of life. The Loma Linda University Pediatric Heart Transplant Group. *J Thorac Cardiovasc Surg* 1993;105:805–814.

61. Pigott JD, Murphy JD, Barber G, et al. Palliative reconstructive surgery for hypoplastic left heart syndrome. *Ann Thorac Surg* 1988;45:122.

62. Iannettoni MD, Bove EL, Mosca RS, et al. Improving results with the first-stage reconstruction of hypoplastic left heart syndrome. *J Thorac Cardiovasc Surg* 1994;107:934.

SURGERY: SCIENTIFIC PRINCIPLES AND PRACTICE, Third Edition, edited by Lazar J. Greenfield, Michael W. Mulholland, Keith T. Oldham, Gerald B. Zelenock, and Keith D. Lillemoe. Lippincott Williams & Wilkins Publishers, Philadelphia, © 2001.

CHAPTER 62

VALVULAR HEART DISEASE

IVA A. SMOLENS AND STEVEN F. BOLLING

In 1953, with the introduction of the pump oxygenator by Gibbons, the first of many valvular operations was performed, but results, especially for valvular insufficiency, were often suboptimal. In 1963, the introduction of the Starr-Edwards ball-valve prosthesis marked the new era of valve surgery. Since then, many modifications and different forms of prosthetic heart valves have been developed, and today, more than 10,000 operations for valve repair or replacement are performed in the United States each year. During the past 15 years, significant improvements in the clinical outcome of patients with valvular heart disease have been achieved. It is impossible to attribute this success to any one specific factor; improvements in the noninvasive monitoring of ventricular function, improvements in prosthetic valves, advances in reconstructive techniques, and the development of guidelines for the timing of surgical intervention have all contributed to the improved prognosis for patients with valvular heart disease.

All forms of valvular heart disease place a hemodynamic burden on one or both ventricles, which may be initially tolerated as the cardiovascular system compensates for the overload. Eventually, however, the hemodynamic overload leads to left ventricular (LV) dysfunction and congestive heart failure, which ultimately may result in death.

VALVULAR ANATOMY

Proper valve function is one of the critical elements of efficient cardiac function. The aortic valve mechanism may be described as passive, whereas an active component of the mitral valve mechanism, which is papillary muscle contraction, facilitates leaflet alignment. The aortic valve has important anatomic relationships to the mitral valve, interventricular septum, and conduction system (Fig. 62.1).

The aortic valve is composed of three leaflets, which are semilunar. The attachments of the leaflets to the aorta are in one plane and are crescent-shaped. Although a normal aortic valve is described as having three leaflets that are equal in size, in 50% of the population, one leaflet is slightly larger than the others (1). No true aortic valve annulus exists; however, the surgical annulus of the aortic valve is situated at the junction between the ventricular chamber and the aorta. Its location is defined by the semilunar attachments to the aortic valve leaflets (2). The sinuses of Valsalva are defined as the areas situated between the aorta and the valve leaflet edge when the valve is open. The wall of the aorta in the sinuses is thinner than the wall of the distal aorta, and the aortic tissue balloons out at the sinuses (3).

The fibrous skeleton of the heart forms the posterior wall of the LV outflow tract. The right fibrous trigone is continuous with the membranous portion of the septum. It forms the central fibrous body that is located at the junction between the noncoronary and right coronary leaflets, through which the atrioventricular conduction tissue passes to the crest of the ventricular septum (2) (Fig. 62.2).

The mechanical properties of the aortic valve must allow the valve to open with a minimal transvalvar gradient and to close completely with minimal flow reversal. Under normal circumstances, the leaflets offer little or no obstruction to flow because the specific gravity of the leaflets is equal to that of blood (4). The mechanism responsible for the opening and closing of the valve is passive, responding to the pressure fluctuations of the cardiac cycle and the pressure differences between the LV and aorta.

In contrast to the aortic valve, the mitral valve is more complex. Mitral valve competence depends on the coordinated function of its components: the leaflets, annulus, papillary muscles, chordae tendineae, and the entire LV.

The mitral valve is the "inlet" to the LV. The mitral valve consists of two leaflets, the anterior (aortic) and posterior (mural) leaflets. The two leaflets are separated at the annulus by the posteromedial and anterolateral commissures. The anterior leaflet is semicircular and spans the distance between the two commissures. It is attached to the anterolateral wall of the LV in direct continuity with the fibrous skeleton of the heart and with the left and part of the noncoronary aortic valve leaflets (5,6). The posterior leaflet is rectangular in shape and is divided into three portions by clefts in the leaflet (7) (Fig. 62.3).

The mitral annulus represents the junction of the fibrous and muscular tissue that joins the left atrium and ventricle. The average human mitral annular cross-sectional area is 5 to 11 cm^2 (8). The annulus has two major collagenous structures: the right fibrous trigone (located at the intersection of the membranous septum, mitral and tricuspid valves, and aortic root) and the left fibrous trigone (located at the posterior junction of the mitral valve and left coronary leaflet of the aortic valve). During systole, the annulus assumes an elliptic shape and is able to contract and decrease in diameter, whereas in diastole it assumes a more circular shape (8). Annular flexibility allows for increased leaflet coaptation during systole and an increased annular orifice area during diastole. The flexibility of the anterior aspect of the annulus, which is in continuity with the fibrous skeleton of the heart, is limited, whereas the posterior aspect of the annulus, which is not attached to any rigid surrounding

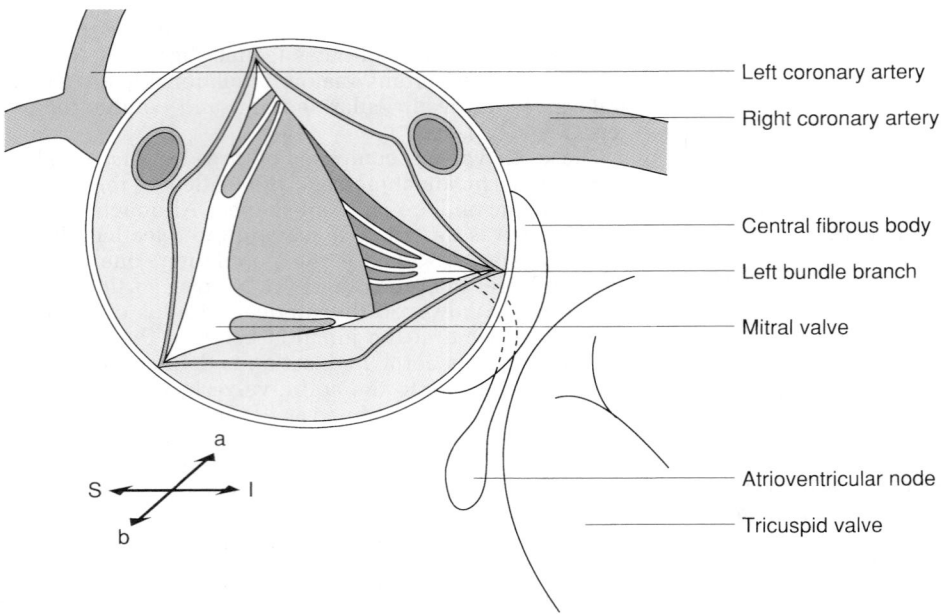

Figure 62.1. Schematic diagram of the anatomic relations of the aortic valve. The mitral valve is shown posterolaterally and the septum medially. (After Wilcox BR, Anderson RN. *Surgical anatomy of the heart.* New York: Raven Press, 1985.)

Labels for figure 62.1:
- Left coronary artery
- Right coronary artery
- Central fibrous body
- Left bundle branch
- Mitral valve
- Atrioventricular node
- Tricuspid valve

structures, is more flexible. In mitral regurgitation (MR), dilation typically occurs along the more flexible posterior aspect of the annulus.

The anterolateral and posteromedial papillary muscles arise directly from the apical portion and midportion of the ventricular wall and give rise to chordae tendineae that go to both leaflets (7). The anterolateral papillary muscle receives a dual blood supply, from the left anterior descending and from either a diagonal or marginal branch of the circumflex artery. In contrast, the posterolateral papillary muscle has a single blood supply, either from the right coronary or the circumflex artery, and is therefore more susceptible to ischemia and infarction (9,10). The posterior aspect of the LV wall and the papillary muscles together play a very important role in valvular competence and leaflet coaptation. The dynamics of both papillary muscles closely mimic the dynamics of the LV, and during LV contraction, the leaflets are pulled downward and together. The LV wall geometry and mechanics play a more significant role in valve competence than the papillary muscles alone. Dilation of the LV may alter the alignment and tension on the papillary muscles and thereby contribute to valvular incompetence.

The chordae tendineae are comprised of fibrous connective tissue and attach the leaflets to either the papillary muscles or the LV wall directly. The chordae are divided into three groups. The primary chordae attach directly to the free edge of the leaflet and ensure that the leaflets coapt without prolapse or flail. The secondary chordae are more prominent on the anterior leaflet, attach to the leaflet along the line of coaptation, and are important maintaining ventricular function. Tertiary chordae are present only on the posterior leaflet and attach directly to the ventricular wall or to the trabeculae carneae. In addition, commissural chordae arise directly from either of the papillary muscles and attach to both leaflets (11).

Maintenance of the chordal, annular, and subvalvar continuity and mitral geometric relationships is important in the preservation of overall ventricular function, and may be even more important in patients with compromised function. Secondary MR is observed in patients with either idiopathic or ischemic cardiomyopathy and can be caused by many factors. In patients with nonischemic dilated cardiomyopathy, in the absence of intrinsic mitral valve disease, MR is caused by a progressive dilation of the annular–ventricular apparatus, with altered ventricular geometry and subsequent loss of leaflet coaptation (12). In patients with ischemic cardiomyopathy, the mechanisms that contribute to MR are more complex. They may include a combination of both dilation of the annular–ventricular apparatus and LV wall–papillary muscle dysfunction, again with the net result being failure of leaflet coaptation (12). A large leaflet area is required for coaptation because the mitral leaflet area is two and a half times greater than the area of the mitral orifice. As more leaflet tissue is utilized for coverage of the enlarging orifice, a critical reduction in tissue available for coaptation is reached, such that leaflet coaptation becomes ineffective and a central regurgitant jet of functional or secondary insufficiency develops (12). Therefore, the dimensions of the mitral valve annulus are the most significant determinant of mitral valve coaptation, leaflet orifice area, and MR. The LV dimensions are less important in functional MR because chordal and papillary muscle length are not significantly altered in people with idiopathic cardiomyopathy with or without MR.

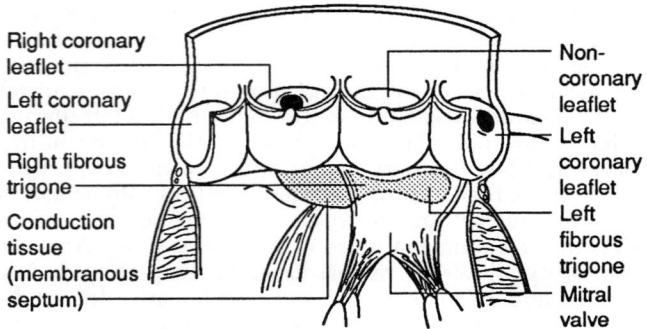

Labels for figure 62.2:
- Right coronary leaflet
- Left coronary leaflet
- Right fibrous trigone
- Conduction tissue (membranous septum)
- Noncoronary leaflet
- Left coronary leaflet
- Left fibrous trigone
- Mitral valve

Figure 62.2. Schematic diagram of the relationship of the aortic valve leaflets to the structures underlying the commissures.

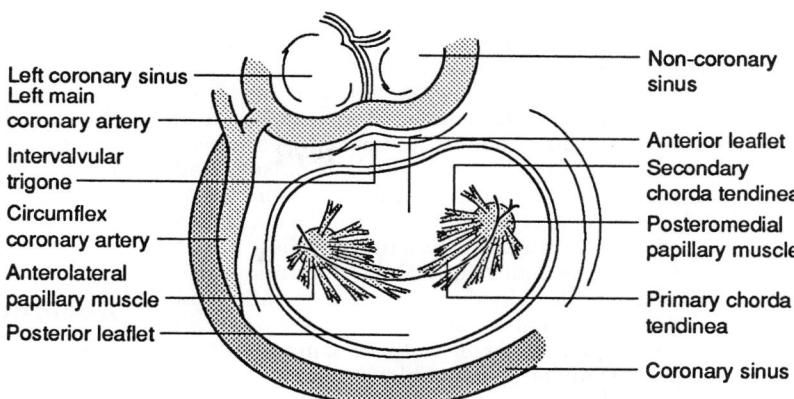

Figure 62.3. Important surgical anatomic features of the mitral valve and the closely related aortic valve, circumflex coronary artery, and coronary sinus.

DIAGNOSIS

The initial assessment of patients with valvular heart disease depends on a careful history and physical examination, which reveal information regarding the type of valvular disease and also provide an estimate of the severity, duration, and prognosis of the dysfunction. The history and physical examination findings are then supplemented by data obtained from chest roentgenography, 12-lead electrocardiography, echocardiography, and cardiac catheterization. Many now advocate surgical intervention without catheterization, so long as the patient does not have any risk factors for coronary artery disease, which impairs the reliability of the noninvasive procedures.

Physical Examination

Cardiac examination includes palpation and auscultation, with provocative maneuvers as appropriate. Examination of the peripheral arterial pulses, inspection of the jugular venous pattern, and a thorough search for systemic findings such as edema, ascites, or jaundice are all essential.

The classic midsystolic murmur of aortic stenosis (AS) is produced by turbulent, high-velocity flow across the narrowed aortic valve. This murmur is heard best at the base of the heart and usually radiates to both carotid arteries. A sustained, forceful, nondisplaced apical impulse may be palpable, produced by prolonged ventricular ejection through the stenotic valve. High-grade lesions can also be associated with palpable vibrations (thrills) resulting from transmission of the turbulent aortic flow.

Aortic insufficiency (AI) characteristically produces a hyperdynamic circulation with marked increases in systolic arterial pulse pressure. A high-pitched, decrescendo diastolic murmur that is best heard during expiration at the left sternal border is characteristic of AI. Acute AI may produce only a short diastolic murmur because rapid equalization of aortic and ventricular diastolic pressures limits the amount of regurgitant flow. Additionally, peripheral signs of low cardiac output, such as cold, vasoconstricted extremities, can be observed.

Mitral regurgitation, like AI, produces a hyperdynamic circulation. However, the peripheral findings of MR, unlike those of AI, are otherwise unremarkable. The cardiac auscultatory findings of MR include a widely split second heart sound, caused by early aortic valve closure. The holosystolic murmur of MR is a constant, blowing murmur heard best at the apex and usually radiating to the axilla. A diastolic murmur caused by diastolic reflow across the mitral valve can also be present. The midsystolic to late-systolic click murmur of mitral valve prolapse is more variable than the murmur of MR.

Mitral stenosis (MS) produces few peripheral signs on physical examination but many cardiac findings. Abrupt tensing of the fibrotic mitral valve produces the opening snap. Both the opening snap and the first heart sound are decreased as the valve becomes increasingly calcified and immobile. Presystolic accentuation is caused by the increased flow associated with atrial contraction and is therefore usually lost with the onset of atrial fibrillation. Rales are associated with the onset of pulmonary congestion.

Tricuspid regurgitation (TR) can be associated with a pulsatile liver, ascites, edema, right ventricular heave, and jugular venous distention. The pansystolic murmur of TR is localized more to the left lower sternal border.

Electrocardiogram

The 12-lead electrocardiogram is useful in assessing rhythm disturbances and specific chamber enlargement that can be associated with valvular disease. More often, the data obtained are nonspecific indicators of overall cardiac function. Increased QRS voltage associated with LV hypertrophy is a common finding associated with valvular heart disease. Atrial ectopic activity and atrial fibrillation are also common findings.

Imaging Techniques

Chest Roentgenogram

The routine posteroanterior and lateral chest roentgenograms provide relatively nonspecific information about cardiac chamber enlargement and pulmonary congestion that may be useful in assessing the physiologic impact of valvular heart disease. The ready availability and low expense of the chest roentgenogram make it a useful means of observing the patient with valvular heart disease despite the availability of more precise means of cardiac imaging, such as echocardiography.

Echocardiography

The practice of echocardiography rests on the principle that air, blood, and tissue reflect sound waves with different degrees of efficiency. The echo transducer transmits sound waves and receives reflected signals from the targeted structure. These reflected signals are then used to construct an image of the structure being scanned.

Cardiac echocardiography has revolutionized the diagnosis of valvular heart disease. M-mode and two-dimensional echocardiography allow real-time assessment of chamber size, wall thickness, and valve appearance and motion. Doppler echo with color Doppler overlay on the two-dimensional image now provides bedside physiologic data regarding blood flow across stenotic or regurgitant valves. Transesophageal echocardiography allows for even more accurate evaluation of valvular morphology.

In Doppler echocardiography, measurement of the velocity of red blood cells in a targeted area is based on Doppler principles. The two most commonly used formats are continuous-wave Doppler and gated, or pulsed, Doppler. Continuous-wave Doppler samples all sound waves returned along the course of the transducer beam. Instantaneous mean velocity and direction of blood flow are determined from the frequency shift of the returning signal. Pulsed Doppler samples blood velocity at a specific point along the beam course, known as the *sample volume.* Continuous-wave Doppler is lacking in that it cannot indicate where along the Doppler path the blood velocity is being reported. The chief disadvantage of pulsed Doppler is a phenomenon known as *aliasing,* which makes it difficult to measure high-speed blood velocities accurately. Continuous-wave Doppler is therefore most useful for measuring high-speed blood flow, such as that found in AS; pulsed Doppler is used to assess flow at a specific point. Modification of the Bernoulli principle, which relates velocity change to pressure drop across points of fixed resistance, allows the pressure gradients across a stenotic valve orifice to be quantified. Accurate correlation with subsequent catheterization data has been demonstrated. Assessment of regurgitant flow is less accurate. The severity of regurgitant flow can be determined qualitatively with pulsed Doppler by measuring how far the high-flow jet extends from the incompetent valve. Doppler techniques are especially applied in the assessment of TR because of the technical limitations of other studies.

Cardiac Catheterization

Cardiac catheterization may be used to obtain a wide range of intracardiac pressures and hemodynamic parameters (Table 62.1). The left side of the heart can be accessed by introducing catheters percutaneously through either the femoral or brachial artery. About 5% of severely stenotic aortic valves cannot be crossed with this retrograde approach. In these instances, a catheter can be passed from the venous circulation across the atrial septum to the left side of the heart. This technique is also useful in the presence of severe MR, when pulmonary capillary wedge pressure does not adequately estimate LV end-diastolic pressure, and in the presence of a tilting-disk aortic valve prosthesis.

Regurgitant lesions are graded qualitatively on a scale of 1+ to 4+ based on the injection of contrast upstream from the lesion in question; for example, an aortic root injection

is used to assess AI. Regurgitation of 1+ corresponds to a regurgitant fraction of about 20%, 2+ about 20% to 40%, 3+ between 40% and 60%, and 4+ more than 60%. Fractions exceeding 30% to 40% (≥ 2+) are considered hemodynamically significant. The most troublesome lesion in this regard is TR because no direct access to the right ventricle is technically feasible except across the valve itself. Artifactual TR can be caused when the catheter crosses the valve or when right ventricular injections induce ventricular ectopic activity.

Radionuclide Angiography

Radionuclide angiography yields visual and numeric data regarding cardiac function and valvular disease. With technetium 99m, forward flow can be measured in patients with regurgitation. Serial determinations of ventricular function with radionuclide cine-angiography are now a mainstay in the long-term follow-up of many patients with valvular heart disease.

AORTIC STENOSIS

In the adult population of the United States, the most common cause of AS is thickening (degeneration) of and deposition of calcium within the aortic leaflets (13,14) (Table 62.2). The overall impact of a lifetime of leaflet stress with each cardiac contraction causes shearing forces that may produce small deposits of calcium within the leaflets. This normal aging process can be accelerated by rheumatic heart disease. AS occurs more frequently in the presence of a congenitally bicuspid aortic valve, and in these instances, leaflet calcification can occur as early as between 20 and 30 years of age and may become symptomatic between the ages of 30 and 60. When the disease is acquired in a previously normal tricuspid valve, stenosis typically occurs in the sixth to eight decades of life. Whatever the etiology of the AS, the pathophysiologic consequences are the same.

Aortic stenosis may be defined as a point of resistance between the LV cavity and the aorta that prevents the proper ejection of blood. The area of the normal aortic valve orifice is approximately 3.0 to 4.0 cm². For any significant changes in the circulation to develop, the valve area must be reduced to one-fourth its normal size; once this occurs, the aortic valve becomes a point of fixed resistance in the LV outflow tract. Hemodynamic data have been used to grade the degree of AS as mild (> 1.5 cm²), moderate (1.0 to 1.5 cm²), or severe (≤ 1.0 cm²) (15). When AS is severe and cardiac output is normal, the mean transvalvar gradient generally exceeds 50 mm Hg, and this is a

Table 62.1. NORMAL CARDIAC HEMODYNAMIC PRESSURES AND VALVES

	Systolic	End-diastolic	Mean
Pressure (mm Hg)			
Right atrium			0–8
Right ventricle	15–30	0–8	
Pulmonary artery	15–30	3–12	9–16
Pulmonary artery wedge/left atrium			1–10
Left ventricle	100–140	3–12	
Aorta	100–140	60–90	70–105
Cardiac output index			
(L/min/m²)		2.6–4.2	
RESISTANCE (dynes s/cm²) (unit of measurement for resistance).			
Pulmonary		20–130	
Systemic		700–1600	

Modified from Grossman W, Barry WH. Cardiac catheterization. In: Braunwald E, ed. Heart disease: a textbook of cardiovascular medicine. Philadelphia: WB Saunders, 1988:287, with permission.

Table 62.2. CAUSES OF LEFT VENTRICULAR OUTFLOW TRACT OBSTRUCTION

Valvular (aortic stenosis)
Acquired
   Rheumatic disease
   Degenerative (fibrocalcific) disease
     Tricuspid valve
      Congenital bicuspid valve
   Infective endocarditis
   Other
Congenital
   Tricuspid valve with commissural fusion
   Unicuspid unicommissural valve
   Hypoplastic annulus
Supravalvular
Membranous
Hourglass
Hypoplastic
Subvalvular
Hypertrophic cardiomyopathy
Discrete (membranous) subaortic stenosis
Tunnel subaortic stenosis

rough cutoff for operative intervention. Some patients with severe AS may remain asymptomatic, whereas symptoms may develop in others with only moderate AS. Therapeutic decisions, particularly those related to surgical intervention, are based largely on the presence or absence of symptoms, not on the absolute valvar area or transvalvar gradient (15). A decrease in the effective orifice area progressively obstructs flow from the LV. Disturbance of the normal flow pattern through the outflow tract can contribute to further deterioration of valvular mechanical efficiency. In addition, ventricular adaptations to the increased resistance occur and can lead to ventricular dysfunction.

Because of the increased resistance created by the stenotic valve, the pressure is greater in the LV than in the aorta, and structural changes may develop within the ventricle over time. LV hypertrophy, the principal pathophysiologic consequence of AS, results in the development of a stiff LV because of the increase in wall thickness. With time, the hypertrophy affects both systolic and diastolic function and can be detrimental (16,17). LV systolic pressures increase as the degree of stenosis increases, and adequate cardiac output and normal systemic pressures are maintained until late in the course of AS. LV systolic pressures as high as 300 mm Hg can develop, and hypertrophic hearts can weigh as much as 500 to 700 g. Eventually, these alterations lead to a decrease in ventricular compliance, an increase in LV end-diastolic pressure, and pulmonary congestion. Diastolic dysfunction, one of the major causes of congestive heart failure, can occur in 15% to 40% of the cases. In AS, diastolic dysfunction may precede systolic dysfunction. Ultimately, the ventricular function in these patients is characterized by an afterload mismatch between the ventricle and the systemic circulation, which contributes to the development of congestive heart failure. Relief of the obstructive process may reverse these adverse ventricular adaptations (18).

The pressure difference that occurs across the aortic valve can be used to determine the degree of valvular stenosis. Echocardiography with Doppler examination of the aortic valve provides an accurate assessment of the transvalvar gradient and the area of the aortic valve. The product of the cross-sectional area and bloodstream velocity is flow, and as the bloodstream reaches a point of narrowing, the velocity must increase for flow to remain con-

stant. The increase in velocity can then be detected by the Doppler technique and be translated into a pressure gradient. The measured velocity can also be used in the continuity equation (based on the Bernoulli equation) to estimate aortic valve area. Echocardiographic assessment is also useful in determining the extent of LV hypertrophy (LV mass) and in estimating the LV ejection fraction (EF). Although the severity of AS can be measured accurately with noninvasive studies, many of the patients with AS are elderly and at risk for coronary disease; therefore, cardiac catheterization with coronary angiography is usually performed before valve replacement. From catheterization data, two techniques are utilized to assess the severity of AS; in the first, the pressure on both sides of the aortic valve is measured, and in the second technique, a pullback catheter is used to measure LV pressure and pressure above the aortic valve. The transvalvar pressure gradient can then be used in the Gorlin calculation of aortic valve area. As the transvalvar gradient increases, the correlation with degree of stenosis also increases (18).

The EF is the most commonly used index to measure LV systolic function. The EF is affected by both preload and afterload and therefore may not accurately indicate intrinsic ventricular contractility. Careful assessment of EF is needed to determine the severity of AS. Poor EF caused by afterload mismatch must be differentiated from poor EF caused by intrinsic myocardial disease.

The natural history of AS in the adult consists of a prolonged latent period in which the morbidity and mortality rates are low. The rate of progression of the stenotic lesion has been estimated in a number of studies, and the average rate of change is approximately 0.10 cm^2 annually. The systolic pressure gradient across the valve may increase by as much as 10 to 15 mm Hg per year (15). The progression of AS is thought to be more rapid in patients with degenerative calcific disease than in those with congenital or rheumatic disease. During this time, hypertrophy normalizes LV wall stress; however, symptoms ultimately develop as the stenosis progresses. The classic symptoms of AS are angina, syncope, and congestive heart failure. Most patients with moderate to severe AS are symptomatic. The average survival after the onset of angina is 4 to 5 years; after syncope, 2 to 3 years; and after congestive heart failure, 1 to 2 years (18,19) (Fig. 62.4). Symptomatic patients with significant uncorrected AS have 1-year and 2-year mortality rates of 25% and 50%, respectively (20). The majority of patients with AS succumb to heart failure. The risk for sudden death resulting from a ventricular arrhythmia in a truly asymptomatic patient with severe AS is not well defined but is approximately 1% to 2%. Aortic valve replacement for AS is clearly indicated in the symptomatic patient. However, it is not strictly indicated in the asymptomatic patient with severe AS to prevent sudden death (15).

Angina occurs in approximately 35% to 50% of patients with AS in the absence of coronary artery disease, and the risk for acute MI is increased in this population. In patients with hypertrophic hearts, the myocardial oxygen demand is increased by the increased muscle mass and high afterload, which ultimately lower the threshold for ischemia. Because coronary perfusion occurs predominantly during diastole, the increased intramyocardial pressure and LV end-diastolic pressure both present resistance to flow and reduce coronary flow reserve (21–23).

Syncope, which can occur in up to 25% of patients with symptomatic AS, is related to limitations in cardiac output and a decrease in cerebral perfusion. Syncope is usually associated with exertion, but its cause remains controversial. According to one theory, exercise induces a decrease in total peripheral resistance that goes uncompensated be-

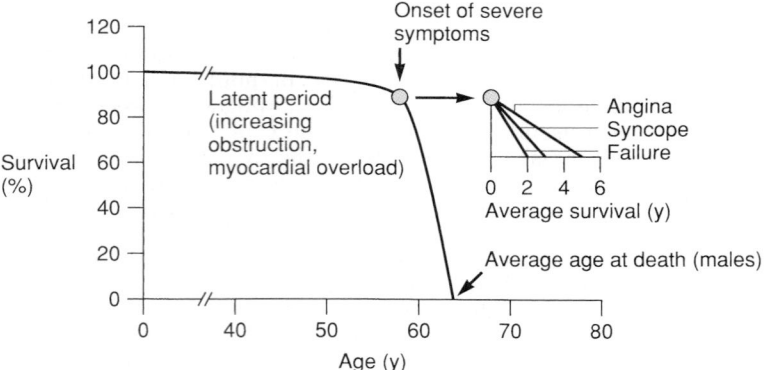

Figure 62.4. Natural history of aortic stenosis without surgical intervention.

cause the stenotic valve restricts cardiac output (23,24). Additional studies have indicated that the initial event in a syncopal episode is a drop in blood pressure, which is thought to arise secondary to an arrhythmia (18).

Symptoms of heart failure in AS may be caused by circulatory or myocardial failure (systolic or diastolic dysfunction). In circulatory failure, caused by a decrease in cardiac output, systemic acidosis can result from anaerobic metabolism. The lactic acidosis causes hyperventilation, which produces symptoms of dyspnea and fatigue. The cardiac output of patients with AS is fixed, and when systemic vasodilation occurs, arterial pressure decreases. Tachycardia is poorly tolerated in patients with AS because prolonged ejection times are required to maintain adequate flow through the stenotic valve. Eventually, an adequate pressure gradient across the stenotic valve can no longer be maintained, and LV failure ensues. Death occurs in 10% to 20% of patients secondary to heart failure.

No proven medical therapy is available for AS. The only effective means of relieving this mechanical obstruction to blood flow is aortic valve replacement. Although we can accurately determine the severity of AS, it is not the severity of the lesion that determines the optimal timing for surgical intervention. Rather, it is the presence of symptoms in combination with the severely stenotic valve that determines the timing of intervention.

Asymptomatic patients with AS should undergo a baseline two-dimensional echocardiogram with Doppler to confirm the presence of aortic disease; assess the transvalvar gradient; measure the area of the aortic valve; determine LV size, function, and degree of hypertrophy; and evaluate for any additional valvular disease. In some instances, the patient may need to undergo cardiac catheterization and coronary angiography if a discrepancy is noted between the clinical and echocardiographic findings, or if the patient is symptomatic and at risk for coronary artery disease (15).

Exercise testing in patients with AS has been discouraged because of concerns for safety and should not be used in patients who are symptomatic. The frequency of follow-up for the asymptomatic patient is determined by the severity of the stenotic lesion. Most patients with mild AS undergo an annual evaluation, but if symptoms develop, a prompt evaluation should be performed. Serial echocardiograms are helpful to assess changes in LV hypertrophy and function in addition to changes in valve area. Patients with severe AS should undergo at least an annual evaluation, those with moderate AS a serial study every 2 years, and those with mild AS, a study every 5 years (15).

About 75% of patients with symptomatic AS die within 3 years after the onset of symptoms unless their aortic valve is replaced (25). Typically, a gradient of more than 50 mm Hg or a valve area of less than 1.0 cm^2 indicates critical stenosis that is capable of causing symptoms and death. These are not absolute values; some patients with larger valve areas or smaller gradients may have symptoms related to the presence of AS and should undergo valve replacement. Aortic valve replacement in symptomatic patients with severe AS is indicated because an increased survival has been demonstrated in this population. Many of these patients have a depressed EF resulting from excess afterload, and in these patients, function improves following valve replacement. Asymptomatic patients with severe AS and LV dysfunction should also undergo aortic valve replacement. Relief of the obstruction reduces the LV afterload and may eventually lead to restoration of the contractile function. In asymptomatic patients with mild or moderate AS, the natural course may be benign, and these patients should be followed serially with noninvasive studies. A controversial group of patients with AS are those with a low EF and low transvalvar gradient. Studies in this population have shown a high operative mortality rate and persistence of symptoms, even after valve replacement (26,27). The criteria for deciding which patients in this group should undergo aortic valve replacement are in evolution. Some studies indicate that patients in this group may have a favorable outcome if both cardiac output and the gradient are increased with either inotropic stimulation or the administration of nitroprusside. Those patients who demonstrate an increase in cardiac output without an increase in transvalvar gradient may not benefit from valve replacement (28,29). In addition, patients with severe AS who are undergoing coronary revascularization should undergo simultaneous aortic valve replacement.

Balloon aortic valvotomy for acquired AS is now thought to be useful only for palliation. The rate of complications, including death, stroke, aortic rupture, AI, and vascular injury, is in excess of 10%. In addition, the mortality following this procedure is similar to that in the untreated population with AS (30). The procedure may be useful, however, in alleviating the symptoms of patients who are clearly not operative candidates because of other, precluding medical conditions. Balloon valvotomy has also been used successfully as a bridge to valve replacement in very sick patients.

AORTIC INSUFFICIENCY

Aortic insufficiency results from a failure of proper leaflet coaptation, caused either by an intrinsic leaflet abnormality or by distortion of the aortic root. Common causes of leaflet abnormalities that result in AI include infective endocarditis and rheumatic fever. Aortic root causes of AI include aortic annular ectasia, Marfan syndrome, aortic dissection, collagen vascular disease, and syphilis (Table 62.3). The causes of AI can be grouped ac-

Table 62.3. ETIOLOGY OF AORTIC INSUFFICIENCY

Cause	Pathology		
	Leaflet	Aortic root	Loss of commissural support
Common			
Rheumatic disease	+	−	−
Congenital disease	+	−	±
Endocarditis	+	−	±
Less common			
Syphilis	±	+	−
Connective tissue disease (e.g., Marfan syndrome)	+	+	−
Aortic dissection	−	+	+
Uncommon			
Trauma	+	+	+
Hypertension	±	±	±
Inflammatory disease (ankylosing spondylitis, Reiter's syndrome)	+	+	−

Modified from Greenberg BH. Acquired aortic valve disease. In: Greenberg BH, Murphy E, eds. Valvular heart disease. Littleton, MA: PSG Publishing, 1987:157, with permission.

cording to the structural components of the valve. Both calcific and rheumatic disease may prevent an inflexible valve from closing properly, or the leaflets may be destroyed, as in endocarditis. Enlargement of the aortic root with dilation of the commissures may cause the effective valve orifice to be greater than the surface area of the leaflets (31). Rheumatoid or degenerative diseases, collagen vascular diseases, and loss of commissural support resulting from acute aortic dissection can all produce an incompetent valve and similar hemodynamic consequences (32).

The inability of the valve leaflets to coapt fully leaves an effective opening between the aorta and the LV during diastole that allows a retrograde flow of ejected blood. The effective stroke volume is then less than the volume ejected, and both a volume and a pressure overload are produced in the LV. An eccentric hypertrophy of the LV results (the LV wall thickness increases in proportion to the increase in ventricular diameter), so that the ratio between wall thickness and chamber radius remains normal. The volume overload is caused by regurgitant flow, and the pressure overload is caused by the increased volume of blood ejected.

With increased diastolic loading and LV enlargement, the LV follows the law of Laplace, which states that the increase in LV wall tension is proportional to the increase in LV radius. This increase in wall tension produces a compensatory increase in the ratio of LV wall thickness to volume, and allows a normal amount of noncontractile systolic work to be performed. The degree of subendocardial ischemia and angina in patients with AI is therefore less than that in AS.

Aortic insufficiency, of all the valvular lesions, can cause the greatest increase in ventricular mass. LV chamber enlargement and hypertrophy allow for an increase in cardiac output and stroke volume in severe AI. The total cardiac output (not effective cardiac output) can be as high as 20 to 30 L/min in well-compensated chronic AI. A significant part of the volume returns to the heart as regurgitant flow, and the ejection fraction may remain normal.

The retrograde blood flow into the LV during diastole can cause dramatic decreases in systemic blood pressure and myocardial failure even before the onset of severe symptoms. Limitations in cardiac output produce symptoms of fatigue and weakness during the final stages of the disease. Cardiac failure ensues when the additional regurgitant volume cannot be ejected, LV end-diastolic pressure rises, and forward flow decreases.

Acute AI is seen in traumatic aortic injury, acute aortic dissection, and endocarditis. In acute AI, the LV does not have the opportunity to adapt to the increased volume load and therefore cannot accommodate the reversed blood flow. The regurgitant volume results in a rapid rise in LV end-diastolic and left atrial pressure, which is then transmitted back to the pulmonary circulation to produce fulminant pulmonary congestion. Overall, the hemodynamic effects of acute AI produce a state of low cardiac output or cardiovascular collapse, characterized by elevated end-diastolic ventricular pressure, tachycardia, peripheral vasoconstriction, and systemic hypotension (21,33).

Death from pulmonary edema, ventricular arrhythmias, electromechanical dissociation, and circulatory collapse is common in acute, severe AI. Early surgical intervention with aortic valve repair or replacement is advocated. Peripheral vasodilators (nitroprusside, dobutamine, and dopamine) can be used to augment forward flow and re-

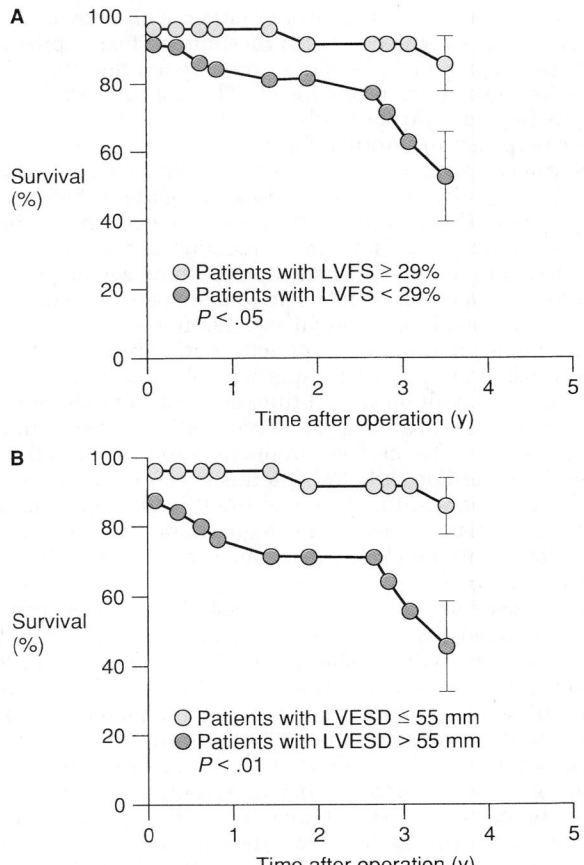

Figure 62.5. Survival after operation for aortic regurgitation as a function of left ventricular fractional shortening *(LVFS; A)* and left ventricular end-systolic diameter *(LVESD; B).* Both early and late survival are improved with improved LV function. (After Bonow RO, Rosing DR, Kent KM, et al. Timing of operation for chronic aortic regurgitation. *Am J Cardiol* 1982;50:325, with permission.)

Table 62.4. **MANAGEMENT OF AORTIC REGURGITATION**

Severity of aortic regurgitation	Symptoms	Left ventricular function	Management
Mild–moderate	No	Normal	No medical therapy
Severe	No	Normal	Vasodilator therapy
Severe	No	Depressed	Aortic valve replacement
Severe	Yes	Normal	Aortic valve replacement
Severe	Yes	Depressed	Aortic valve replacement
Severe	Severe	Severely depressed	Medical therapy followed by aortic valve replacement

duce LV end-diastolic pressures. They may be useful preoperatively (15). Intraaortic balloon counterpulsation is contraindicated because it further exacerbates AI.

Patients with chronic AI gradually adapt to the reversal of flow through the aortic orifice and are able to maintain an adequate EF. Eventually, EF and cardiac output decline and end-systolic volumes increase. The mechanism for the onset of the LV dysfunction is controversial and may be associated with inadequate hypertrophy with afterload mismatch or primary myocardial dysfunction. Once the symptoms of dyspnea, orthopnea, angina, and presyncope or syncope develop, the average survival is only 3 to 5 years (15,21).

Many patients with AI have angina; however, this occurs less frequently than in patients with AS. The oxygen demand in a heart with AI is very high because of the large stroke volumes and slightly increased ejection pressures, but the endocardium becomes ischemic with increased demand because of the decreased diastolic perfusion pressure (34). In the presence of stenotic coronary arteries, this effect may be even more pronounced. The use of vasodilating agents (sodium nitroprusside, hydralazine, nifedipine) has been proposed to improve forward stroke volume and decrease regurgitant volume in patients with chronic severe AI. Theoretically, these afterload-reducing agents facilitate a reduction in LV end-diastolic volume and wall stress, which results in the preservation of LV function and a decrease in LV mass. From a practical standpoint, these agents prolong the compensated phase in asymptomatic patients who have volume overload with normal systolic function (35).

In the evaluation of a patient with chronic AI, the echocardiogram plays an important role. End-systolic and end-diastolic volumes, wall thickness, EF, and shortening fraction can be measured. This information is useful in detecting irreversible changes in the LV and following the AI over time. Cardiac catheterization is used to determine the severity of the insufficiency and identify any concomitant coronary artery disease. The regurgitant volume can be calculated and the LV end-diastolic pressure directly measured (15,18).

In contrast to acute AI, compensated chronic AI can be well tolerated (36). Asymptomatic or minimally symptomatic patients with AI should be identified early and followed yearly with echocardiography to assess for a deterioration in LV function (EF < 40%), an increase in the end-systolic dimension (to > 55 mm), or decreases in fractional shortening (to < 30%), with the understanding that waiting for symptomatic decompensation may compromise the postoperative outcome. Proposed operative criteria for AI are ventricular decompensation, increased end-systolic LV diameter (> 55 mm), fractional shortening (< 30%), reduced ejection fraction (< 50%), and increased LV end-diastolic volume (35) (Fig. 62.5). The rate of sudden death averaged less than 0.2% per year (15,37,38). The rate of progression to symptoms or LV systolic dysfunction averaged 4.3% per year (15). An exercise tolerance test ensures that patients are not masking symptoms by limiting their own activity.

In patients with depressed LV function, symptoms tend to develop within 2 to 3 years, with an average rate of onset of more than 25% per year. Patients with normal systolic function who are symptomatic (New York Heart Association class III or IV heart failure, angina, or syncope) should undergo aortic valve replacement. Patients in New York Heart Association functional class II, III, or IV with mild to moderate LV dysfunction should also undergo aortic valve replacement. Patients with New York Heart Association class IV failure are at significantly higher operative risk because their systolic function is less likely to recover following valve replacement; however, valve replacement is a better alternative than medical management alone (15,35). Nonoperative management of patients with severe AI and abnormal LV function is associated with a 50% mortality at 1 year (39). Ideally, valve replacement should take place well before irreversible damage to the LV occurs (15,35) (Table 62.4).

MITRAL STENOSIS

Mitral stenosis is almost exclusively caused by rheumatic heart disease and tends to affect women more frequently. In developed countries, the incidence of rheumatic fever has declined steadily, and therefore the incidence of MS is reduced (Table 62.5). Causes of MS other than rheumatic fever include severe mitral annular and leaflet calcification, endocarditis, and congenital lesions (40,41). Both rheumatic fever and MS remain common in third world and developing countries. MS is a continuous, progressive disease, usually characterized by a slow, stable course and acceleration later in life. Typically, a long latent period elapses between an episode of rheumatic fever and the onset of symptoms. In asymptomatic patients, survival at 10 years is 80%, with 60% of the patients having no progression of symptoms. Once significant limiting symptoms occur, the 10-year survival rate is dismal, zero to 15%. Mortality in these patients is caused by heart failure (60% to 70%), systemic embolism (20% to 30%), pulmonary embolism (10%), and infection (1% to 5%) (15).

The area of the normal adult mitral valve is 4 to 5 cm². Reduction of this orifice area to less than 2.5 cm² repre-

Table 62.5. **CAUSES OF MITRAL STENOSIS**

Valvular
Rheumatic disease
Nonrheumatic disease
  Infective endocarditis
  Congenital mitral stenosis
  Single papillary muscle (parachute valve)
  Mitral annular calcification
Supravalvular
Myxoma
Left atrial thrombus
Other

sents mild MS. This is the point at which a transvalvar gradient first develops (Fig. 62.6). When the area of the orifice declines to 1 cm², the MS is considered critical, and the transvalvar gradient required to maintain a normal resting cardiac output is 20 mm Hg. This pressure gradient is transmitted through the pulmonary venous network and leads to pulmonary congestion. The transvalvar gradient can be exacerbated by any increase in cardiac output and transmitral flow. Thus, exercise, stress, infection, pregnancy, or atrial fibrillation with a rapid ventricular response often precipitate the first symptoms of dyspnea in patients with mild MS. Normal atrial contraction, as seen in sinus rhythm, augments diastolic filling of the ventricle by up to 30% in patients with MS. Loss of atrial augmentation, as seen in atrial fibrillation, which develops in 30% to 40% of patients with MS (15), results in at least a 20% decrease in cardiac output. The concomitant increase in heart rate associated with atrial fibrillation leads to further impaired filling of the left ventricle, decreased cardiac output, and increased left atrial pressure, which may result in acute pulmonary edema (42,43). Aggressive rate control with digoxin, beta blockers, or calcium channel blockers is warranted. An increased incidence of atrial fibrillation is correlated with increased age and left atrial dilation. The dilation of the atrium is associated with fibrosis and disorganization of the atrial fibers, which lead to disparate atrial conduction. Mural thrombi and thromboembolism are serious sequelae of MS and are directly related to the presence of atrial fibrillation. The emboli can enter the cerebral circulation, coronary arteries, and renal, splanchnic, or peripheral circulation, and multiple emboli can develop in up to 25% of cases (15,42,44). Anticoagulant therapy, therefore, is required in patients with chronic atrial fibrillation and MS.

Mitral stenosis is the most sparing of the left-sided valvar lesions in terms of ventricular function. The pathophysiologic signs and symptoms of MS are related to the pressure and stasis upstream from the point of valvar obstruction. In long-standing MS, pulmonary arterial pressures can exceed systemic pressures. At pressures above 70 mm Hg, impedance to outflow from the right side of the heart frequently results in right-sided failure, with right ventricular dilation, TR, and pulmonic insufficiency. Further decreases in preload in the left side of the heart result, and a syndrome of low cardiac output can develop.

Patients with MS typically have symptoms of left-sided heart failure: dyspnea on exertion, orthopnea, and paroxysmal nocturnal dyspnea. Less frequently, they exhibit hemoptysis, hoarseness, and symptoms of right-sided failure (42). Frequently, symptoms may not appear until atrial fibrillation develops or the patient becomes pregnant, and

then dyspnea and orthopnea become pronounced. Although the symptoms are those of left-sided ventricular failure, contractility of the LV is usually normal (45). In some instances, a reflexive increase in systemic vascular resistance and a decrease in EF may be noted. Right ventricular function is compromised by two mechanisms: (a) the afterload imposed on it by high left atrial pressure and (b) the development of secondary pulmonary vasoconstriction.

Echocardiography is the diagnostic tool of choice for assessing the severity of MS. The echocardiogram can be used to assess leaflet mobility, thickness, and calcification, subvalvar fusion, and the appearance of the commissures. In addition, the hemodynamic severity of the obstruction can be assessed with Doppler flow, and the valve area can be calculated (46). The mean transmitral gradient can be measured from the continuous-wave Doppler signal across the mitral valve, and this can be used to estimate the pulmonary artery systolic pressure.

For the asymptomatic patient, in sinus rhythm, with mild MS (valve area > 1.5 cm² and gradient < 5 mm Hg), prophylaxis against endocarditis is the only medical therapy indicated. These patients remain stable for many years. Yearly reevaluation and follow-up is recommended; however, a yearly echocardiogram is not warranted unless a change in symptoms occurs (15,21).

If the symptoms are mild or evidence is found that pulmonary hypertension is beginning, mechanical relief of the MS is indicated because further delay may worsen the prognosis (47). Percutaneous balloon valvotomy does provide good relief with prolonged benefits, unlike valvotomy in AS. Balloon valvotomy should not be utilized in the presence of heavy annular calcification, severe subvalvar distortion, atrial fibrillation or clot, and mild to moderate MR. In this instance, open commissurotomy, valve reconstruction, or mitral valve replacement improves survival and reduces symptoms (48,49). Some controversy still remains regarding the management of patients with MS who remain asymptomatic except for the presence of atrial fibrillation. Some advocate an appropriate operative intervention on the mitral valve in combination with the Cox maze procedure to ensure the maintenance of sinus rhythm postoperatively (50,51).

MITRAL REGURGITATION

The most common causes of MR are infective endocarditis, myxomatous degeneration of the mitral valve (mitral valve prolapse, or Barlow syndrome), collagen vascular disease, spontaneous rupture of the chordae tendineae, rheumatic fever, and ischemic disease. MR may also be secondary to cardiomyopathy (Table 62.6).

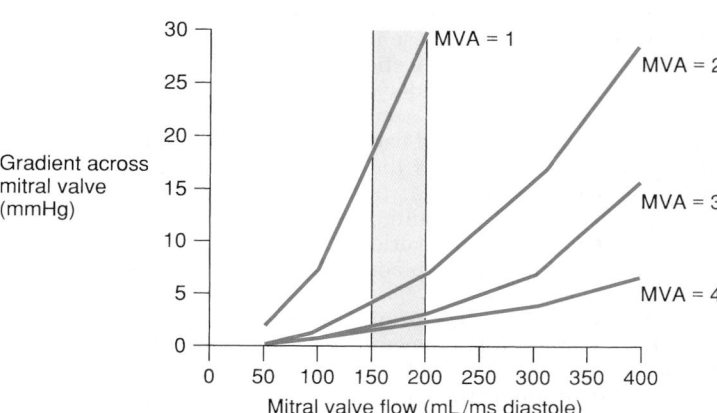

Figure 62.6. Mitral valve gradient as a function of mitral flow. *Blue area* represents normal transvalvular flow. Gradient increases exponentially with decreases in mitral valve area.

Table 62.6. CAUSES OF MITRAL REGURGITATION

Disorders of the mitral valve leaflets
Loss of contracture of valvular tissue
   Rheumatic fever
   Endocarditis
   Systemic lupus erythematosus
Congenital
   Cleft leaflet (isolated)
   Endocardial cushion defect
Connective tissue disorders
Other
Disorders of the mitral annulus
Calcification
Dilatation
Destruction
Disorders of the chordae tendineae
Rupture of the chordae tendineae
   Endocarditis
   Myocardial infarction
   Connective tissue disorder
   Other
Thickening or fusion of the chordae tendineae
Elongation of the chordae tendineae
Disorders of the papillary muscles
Dysfunction or rupture of papillary muscle
   Ischemia or infarction
   Endocarditis
   Inflammatory disorder
Malalignment
   Left ventricular dilatation
   Hypertrophic cardiomyopathy
   Infiltrative cardiomyopathy
Other

Modified from Silverman ME, Hurst JW. The mitral complex: clues to its afflictions. Cardiovasc Clin North Am 1973;5:35, with permission.

The primary pathophysiologic feature of MR is systolic unloading of the LV into the left atrium. With the onset of systole, LV pressure rises and exceeds the left atrial pressure long before it reaches the aortic root pressure. Therefore, more than half of the LV volume can be ejected through the incompetent mitral valve before the aortic valve has opened. MR leads to a cycle of continuing volume overload of the already dilated ventricle, progression of annular dilation, increased LV wall tension, progressive MR, and worsening CHF. The long-term survival of patients with MR refractory to medical therapy is poor. In a study of 28 patients with MR, cardiomyopathy, and an ejection fraction of less than 25%, the 1-year survival without transplantation was 46% (52).

The pathophysiology of acute severe MR from chordal rupture, endocarditis, blunt chest trauma, or myocardial infarction is different from that of chronic MR. In acute MR, the volume overload causes an increase in the end-diastolic volume and an increase in the LV preload. The afterload is reduced by the ejection of blood into the left atrium, and therefore the end-systolic volume is reduced. An acute increase in the EF occurs; however, because the stroke volume is regurgitated back into the left atrium, the volume of forward flow and the cardiac output are ultimately reduced. In addition, the acute increase in left atrial pressure can lead to pulmonary edema. In the acute setting, the hemodynamic overload often is not tolerated, and mitral valve repair or replacement must be performed on an urgent basis.

This is not the case in chronic and secondary MR, in which the compensatory changes occur slowly. In MR, the regurgitant volume ejected into the left atrium depends on the size of the mitral orifice, the ventricular-to-atrial pressure gradient, and the heart rate (53). In compensated

chronic MR, the regurgitant flow into the left atrium increases left atrial pressure and leads to atrial enlargement and an increase in compliance. Left atrial pressures rise during systole and decline in diastole. At end-diastole, the left atrial pressure remains mildly elevated, representing a flow gradient. In this setting, with only mild elevations in left atrial pressures, increases in pulmonary vascular resistance usually do not occur. The reduced impedance to LV emptying (afterload) allows the ventricle to adapt to the regurgitant volume by increasing total cardiac output to maintain an adequate forward output. The increases in LV preload, wall tension, diastolic volume, and stroke volume represent ventricular adaptations to severe MR. In compensated MR, the patient may remain asymptomatic, even with exercise, for years.

The prolonged volume overload eventually results in LV dysfunction and the transition to decompensated MR. As the LV begins to fail and end-systolic volumes increase, contractile dysfunction impairs ejection and end-systolic volume increases. The increase in preload eventually leads to LV dilation and a change in the shape of the ventricle from an ellipse to a sphere. Dilation of the ventricle causes an increase in the regurgitant fraction, a decrease in the forward stroke volume, and subsequent pulmonary congestion. The favorable loading conditions of MR tend to maintain the EF in the low normal range despite the presence of significant LV dysfunction. MR should be corrected before LV decompensation becomes advanced. With elimination of the regurgitant volume, the ventricle no longer has to expend excessive work on flow in the reverse direction. In severe myocardial dysfunction, the positive effects of elimination of regurgitant flow may be even more pronounced. In secondary MR, the ventricular mass also increases, and the degree of LV hypertrophy correlates with chamber dilation. The ratio of LV mass to LV end-diastolic volume remains normal. In the setting of decreased afterload, the EF may remain in the normal range, even in the presence of significantly impaired intrinsic LV contractility (54). Many of the commonly used indices of cardiac performance depend on both preload and afterload and therefore are not as reliable in the setting of MR. LV end-systolic volume is a better parameter, as it reflects changes in systolic ventricular function, is independent of preload, and varies directly with afterload (55).

Various interventions can alter the area of the regurgitant orifice. An increase in preload or afterload, or a decrease in contractility, results in dilation of the LV and an increase in the area of the regurgitant orifice. In a study of patients with severe CHF who were managed medically (with diuretics, nitrates, and agents to reduce afterload), the observed decrease in filling pressure and systemic vascular resistance led to a reduction in the MR associated with failure. This was attributed to a reduction in the area of the regurgitant orifice, which was related to the decrease in LV volume and annular distention (56). This complex relationship between mitral annular area and leaflet coaptation may explain why using an undersized annuloplasty ring to perform a "valvular" repair in patients with myopathy can represent a ventricular solution for a ventricular problem (Fig. 62.7).

Secondary MR also affects coronary flow characteristics. Coronary flow reserve is limited in patients with MR because of an increase in baseline coronary flow related to LV volume overload, hypertrophy, and preload (LV wall stress). The restricted coronary flow reserve improved following valve reconstruction because of a reduction in the baseline coronary flow and flow velocity once the LV preload, work, and mass were reduced (7).

In the setting of chronic CHF, cardiac reserve is depressed and a number of compensatory mechanisms are

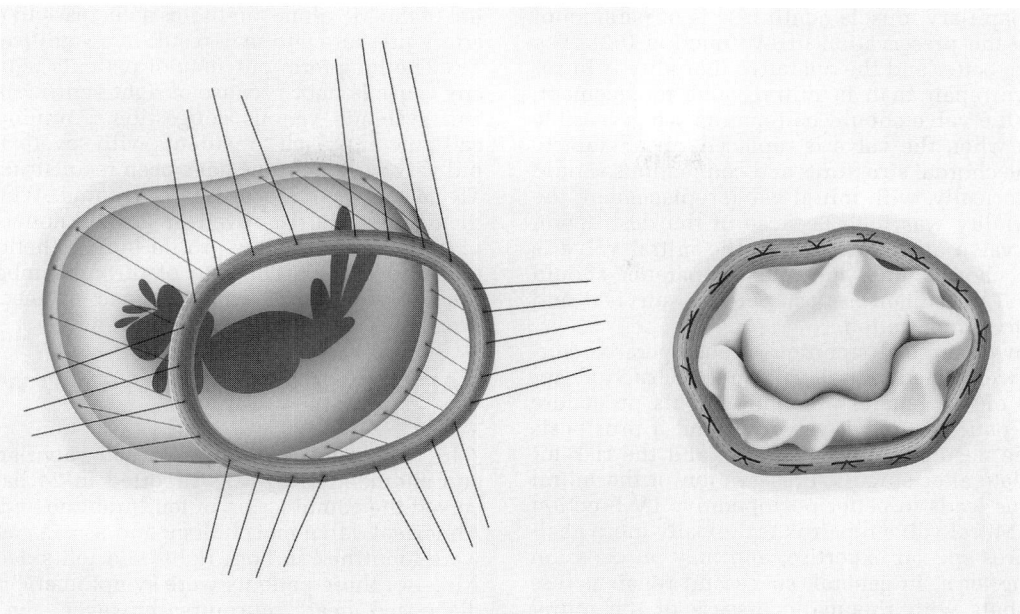

Figure 62.7. Mitral valve annuloplasty ring, used to overcorrect and undersize the mitral valve annulus.

activated. Some are responsible for the vasoconstriction seen in heart failure; these include stimulation and activation of the neuroendocrine and sympathetic nervous systems. Increases in circulating norepinephrine levels have been documented, and other studies have shown that proinflammatory cytokines [tumor necrosis factor-α (TNF-α), interleukin-1 (IL-1), IL-2, and IL-6] may be responsible for the myocardial depression in heart failure. TNF-α, which has been shown to be produced by the heart under stress, has negative inotropic effects, and it may play a role in the development of LV dysfunction, dilated cardiomyopathy, hypotension, and pulmonary edema, all of which can be seen in advanced CHF (57,58).

Chronic MR is compensated by eccentric cardiac hypertrophy, and cardiac enlargement becomes apparent on physical examination. Echocardiography can estimate left atrial and ventricular volume, EF, and the severity of regurgitation, and it may delineate the anatomic cause.

Transesophageal echocardiography is the study of choice to delineate the anatomic cause and severity of MR and can help direct successful repair of the valve. In MR, LV performance can best be gauged by the diameter to which the LV contracts at end-systole. Echocardiography can measure the end-systolic dimension, which is less dependent on preload than EF and can be used as a parameter of LV contractile function (59). When the end-systolic dimension exceeds 45 mm, the prognosis worsens (60). Therefore, patients should be referred for surgical intervention when mild symptoms develop, or if the EF is depressed (< 60%) or the end-systolic dimension exceeds 45 mm, even in the absence of symptoms. In patients with compromised right ventricular function, indicative of pulmonary hypertension, the prognosis is even worse (61).

Cardiac catheterization is necessary when a discrepancy is found between clinical and noninvasive findings. It is also performed when surgery is being planned to assess the extent and severity of coronary artery disease. Ventriculography provides an additional method to assess LV dilation and function and gauge the severity of MR. In addition, right-sided heart catheterization should be performed if pulmonary hypertension is a concern.

Asymptomatic patients with mild MR and no evidence of LV enlargement or dysfunction or of pulmonary hyperten-

sion should be reassessed yearly. Performance of echocardiography at that time is based on any evidence of clinical progression of regurgitation (15).

The management of asymptomatic patients with moderate to severe MR is somewhat controversial. Historically, this group of patients underwent echocardiography annually to assess for any changes in LV function, and surgical intervention was considered only with the onset of LV dysfunction. Today, with improved techniques of mitral valve reconstruction, earlier surgical intervention, before the onset of LV dysfunction, should be advocated (15).

Patients with acute severe MR are almost always symptomatic at presentation. The initial goal in management is to decrease the degree of MR and in turn increase forward flow and decrease pulmonary congestion. Reduction of ventricular preload with diuretics and nitrates relieves the pulmonary congestion. Preload and afterload reduction with vasodilators reduces MR by decreasing the gradient across the mitral valve. Inotropic agents can also be used to decrease the size of the regurgitant orifice by improving myocardial contractility. In addition, an intraaortic balloon pump can be effective as a temporizing measure before surgical intervention. No studies, however, have demonstrated that the use of agents to reduce afterload safely reduces or delays the need for surgery or improves outcomes. For patients with MR and preserved LV function in whom symptoms develop, surgical intervention is the most appropriate therapy. For those in whom atrial fibrillation develops, the heart rate should be aggressively controlled with digoxin, calcium channel blockers, or beta blockers; the risk for embolism is increased, although less so than in MS (15).

Patients who are asymptomatic or symptomatic with evidence of LV dysfunction (EF < 60% or end-systolic diameter > 45 mm) should also undergo operative intervention. Ideally, the EF should not be allowed to fall into the low normal range in patients with chronic MR before they undergo mitral valve surgery. Even in the face of advanced LV dysfunction, surgical intervention should still be performed, as symptoms are likely to improve and further deterioration of LV function can be prevented (15).

Two different operative interventions are performed for MR—mitral valve repair and mitral valve replacement. A number of studies have demonstrated that preservation of the annulus–papillary muscle continuity is of paramount importance to the preservation of LV function (62). The late outcome is better and the operative mortality is lower in mitral valve repair than in mitral valve replacement, and therefore the valve should be repaired when feasible (63–65). Even when the valve is replaced, an attempt to preserve all the chordal structures and connections should be made. Historically, with mitral valve replacement, the operative mortality was high because of the destruction of the mitral valve apparatus. When the mitral valve is replaced, the chordal and subvalvar apparatus should be preserved. This enhances postoperative survival and helps to preserve LV function.

With improved surgical techniques, postoperative survival after a well-timed mitral valve reconstruction approaches that of the general population. This procedure preserves the patient's native valve without a prosthesis and avoids the need for anticoagulation and the risk for valve failure late after surgery. Preservation of the mitral valve apparatus leads to better postoperative LV function and survival. Mitral valve repair is technically more challenging, requires special expertise, and may on occasion fail in the long term. In general, successful repair is less likely in patients with rheumatic disease of the mitral valve and severe annular calcification.

MITRAL VALVE PROLAPSE

Mitral valve prolapse (MVP), the most common form of valvular heart disease, occurs in 2% to 6% of the population. It often appears as a clinical entity without significant MR; however, it has become the most common cause of MR in the United States since the decline in rheumatic heart disease (53,66). The cause of MVP, defective fibroelastic connective tissue in the leaflets, chordae, and annulus, is likely congenital (67). MR develops in only 5% to 10% of patients with MVP (68). Moderate to severe MR may eventually result in LV dysfunction and the development of congestive heart failure. Pulmonary hypertension may develop with the onset of right ventricular failure.

Two-dimensional Doppler echocardiography is the most useful noninvasive test for defining MVP. Leaflet redundancy is often associated with an enlarged mitral annulus and elongated chordae tendineae. Patients with MVP who remain asymptomatic should be evaluated clinically every 3 to 5 years. Serial echocardiography is not necessary and should be performed only if cardiac symptoms develop. Antibiotic prophylaxis should be administered to these patients to prevent the development of infective endocarditis during procedures associated with bacteremia. Surgical intervention for MVP is reserved for those who progress to MR or in whom a flail leaflet develops secondary to a ruptured chorda. The majority of these valves are amenable to surgical repair (15).

TRICUSPID VALVE DYSFUNCTION

Tricuspid valve dysfunction can occur with anatomically normal or abnormal valves. The most common cause of tricuspid valve regurgitation is right ventricular enlargement with secondary dilation of the tricuspid annulus. Right ventricular systolic hypertension occurs in MS, pulmonic valve stenosis, and pulmonary hypertension. Right ventricular diastolic hypertension occurs in dilated cardiomyopathy and right ventricular failure of any cause.

Echocardiography is utilized to assess valve structure and motion by measuring annular size and identifying other abnormalities. Doppler imaging can assess the severity of TR, the right ventricular systolic pressure, and the diastolic gradient. In patients with severe MS and TR, re-

lief of the MS alone facilitates a decrease in the pulmonary artery pressure and may result in a significant decrease in TR. The long-term outcome of patients with severe TR of any cause is poor because of right ventricular dysfunction and systemic venous congestion. Annuloplasty is typically the approach to patients with severe TR. The tricuspid valve and chordae have been reconstructed in cases of TR caused by endocarditis or trauma. When the leaflets themselves are destroyed or grossly abnormal, valve replacement with a low-profile bioprosthetic valve is recommended (69). The rate of thromboembolic complications is very high with the use of mechanical valve prostheses in the tricuspid position (15).

VALVE DISEASE ASSOCIATED WITH ANORECTIC DRUGS

In 1997, an association between valvular heart disease and anorectic drugs was reported in 24 patients who received the combination of fenfluramine and phentermine. Abnormal valve morphology and associated regurgitation were identified in both right- and left-sided heart valves. All 24 of these patients were symptomatic and had newly diagnosed heart murmurs; however, the frequency of valvular pathology in asymptomatic patients receiving the drug combination could not be determined (70). The Food and Drug Administration has reported in echocardiographic prevalence surveys a 32% incidence of significant AI, MR, or both in patients who received the combination of fenfluramine and phentermine for 6 to 24 months. In light of these data, the drugs have been withdrawn from the market. From recent studies, it appears that the prevalence of significant valvar regurgitation is related to the duration of exposure to the drugs, and persons who were exposed for only a brief period of time have a much smaller risk. The Committee on the Management of Patients with Valvular Heart Disease recommends that all patients with a history of use of these agents should undergo a thorough physical examination. Echocardiography is reserved for those patients with symptoms, heart murmurs, or other physical evidence of cardiac involvement. Patients with clinical and echocardiographic evidence of valvar disease should then undergo directed treatment or further testing according to the specific lesion identified. Echocardiographic screening of patients who have used these agents but remain asymptomatic, without any evidence of cardiovascular disease, is not necessary. However, they should be monitored closely (15).

ENDOCARDITIS

Less than 50 years ago, endocarditis was uniformly fatal; however, during the last 40 years, with the discovery of new antibiotics, improvements in blood culture techniques, and the development of echocardiography and cardiopulmonary bypass for valve repair and replacement procedures, the mortality is now between 10% and 15%. The overall incidence of infective endocarditis is estimated to range from 1/100,000 to 6/100,000 annually (71).

Both diseased native heart valves and prosthetic heart valves are at increased risk for the development of endocarditis, but normal valves can also become infected. Preexisting heart disease has been discovered in a significant percentage of patients with endocarditis. In one recent study, of all patients with endocarditis, 24% had rheumatic heart disease, 23% had congenital abnormalities, and 32% had normal heart valves (72). A history of previous endocarditis is also a risk factor and was identified in 11% to 15% of patients (73). Endocarditis affects left-sided more frequently than right-sided valves. Right-sided endocarditis is often associated with intravenous drug use; tricuspid valve involvement was identified in 46% to 92% of patients with endocarditis associated with a history of drug abuse (74,75). Hypertrophic cardiomyopathy and MVP are also associated with an increased risk for endocarditis.

Endocarditis of diseased heart valves can be precipitated by anything that can cause a transient bacteremia. Associations of endocarditis with dental infection and procedures, surgery, endoscopy, intravenous catheterization, intravenous drug abuse, and infections of the skin, lungs, bowel, and urinary tract have been commonly reported. Endocarditis in previously diseased valves tends to run an indolent, subacute course, whereas endocarditis in previously normal valves is usually a fulminant process. *Staphylococcus aureus* and α-hemolytic streptococci *(Streptococcus viridans)* are the most commonly cultured organisms in this disease (73,75,76). α-Hemolytic streptococcal infection is most often associated with dental procedures. Infection with *S. aureus* is associated with a shorter time interval to diagnosis, greater morbidity, and a more virulent course. Enterococcal infections have been reported in 5% to 17% of the cases; gram-negative rod infections are rare, comprising 1% to 9% of the cases (75).

Prosthetic valve endocarditis, which comprises 15% to 30% of all cases of endocarditis, is reported to occur in 1% to 2% of all valve implants. Prosthetic valve endocarditis is associated with an overall higher mortality rate than native valve endocarditis (75,77). Prosthetic valve endocarditis that occurs in the early postoperative period (within the first 2 months) is frequently caused by Staphylococcus epidermidis, secondary to either a break in technique during the procedure or to skin contamination. Late-onset prosthetic valve endocarditis follows the profile of native valve endocarditis and is related to bacteremic seeding of the valve. Fungal infections tend to occur in patients with prosthetic valves who are immunocompromised or are intravenous drug users. Culture-negative endocarditis can be seen in patients who were given antibiotics before blood cultures were obtained and in patients with fungal infections or noninfective endocarditis, as in patients with systemic lupus erythematosus. The recommended antibiotic regimen in these cases is a full 6-week course of vancomycin and gentamycin (15).

The aortic and mitral valves are affected with almost equal frequency, and simultaneous involvement of both valves occurs in 5% to 15% of cases (77,71). Abscess formation is the most commonly reported perivalvar complication, occurring in 20% of cases, and is most often caused by *S. aureus*. Perivalvar involvement is most frequently reported with aortic valve infection. Other complications of endocarditis include leaflet tears, chordal rupture, aortic mycotic infections, conduction defects, sinus of Valsalva aneurysms, intrapericardial rupture with pyogenic pericarditis, and valve thrombosis. Fungal vegetations, because of their bulky size, can produce valvular stenosis.

Aortic valve disease remains the most common predisposing cause of aortic valve endocarditis. The proportion of rheumatic lesions has decreased from about 40% to 10% and has been replaced primarily by sclerotic lesions. Up to 20% of cases occur in patients with a bicuspid aortic valve (78). The aortic valve is the most common site of prosthetic valve endocarditis, in which staphylococci and gram-negative rods are most frequently responsible for the early form of infection, whereas streptococci and gram-negative rods are seen more frequently in late infection. In mitral valve endocarditis, the infection is primarily localized to the leaflet. Predisposing mitral valvular pathology includes annular calcification, chordal rupture, chordal shortening, and mitral stenosis. Extension beyond the valve into the annular tissue is common (79).

The clinical diagnosis of infective endocarditis requires a multifaceted approach. Physical examination, results of microbiology studies, laboratory testing, and invasive and noninvasive imaging procedures all aid in the diagnosis of infective endocarditis. The most common presenting symptoms are fever, fatigue, malaise, and dyspnea. Pyrexia, newly noted heart murmur, and microscopic hematuria are the most common clinical signs. Thirty percent of patients present with septic emboli, which can involve the spleen, kidneys, cerebral vasculature, and coronary system and cause ischemia. Septic emboli from tricuspid valve endocarditis can produce a picture of patchy infiltrates on chest radiographs. Blood cultures are the mainstay of diagnosis, and results are accurate in more than 90% of cases. False-negative results occur in patients with previous antibiotic treatment, intramyocardial abscess, or fungal infection.

Echocardiography is useful in the diagnosis of endocarditis and in detecting and characterizing the consequences of infection. These include vegetations on the valve leaflets, valvular regurgitation, ventricular dysfunction, abscess or aneurysm formation, leaflet perforation or destruction, fistula or shunt formation, and rupture of chordae. Echocardiography also plays a useful role in monitoring therapy and defining the need for and results of surgical intervention. Transesophageal is more accurate than transthoracic echocardiography in the detection of valvular vegetations (80). Two different sets of clinical criteria for the diagnosis of endocarditis have been established: the Von Reyn criteria (1981) and more recently the Duke criteria (1994), which take into account echocardiographic findings (81).

The mainstay of therapy for endocarditis is the appropriate administration of antibiotics, which must reach bactericidal levels for a period of 4 to 6 weeks. Factors associated with increased mortality and an increased risk for medical failure include older patient age, infection with *S. aureus*, the presence of emboli, and the degree of heart failure at presentation (77). Medical therapy is effective in sterilizing one third to two thirds of cases of prosthetic valve endocarditis. Continued medical therapy in the face of cardiac decompensation carries a mortality rate as high as 90%. The primary cause of death in endocarditis is congestive heart failure and AI.

Indications for surgical intervention in endocarditis include a new onset unmanageable congestive heart failure or cardiogenic shock secondary to treatable valvular heart disease with or without an established diagnosis of endocarditis. Surgical intervention should not be delayed in acute infective endocarditis when congestive heart failure ensues. Surgical intervention is not indicated if complications (severe embolic cerebral damage) or other comorbid conditions make recovery unlikely. Additional indications for surgical intervention in the hemodynamically stable patient with endocarditis include failure of antimicrobial therapy as demonstrated by cultures persistently positive for bacteria, valvular insufficiency, perivalvar abscess, and pericarditis. Fungal and gram-negative rod infections are associated with a very high failure rate of medical therapy, and therefore surgical intervention is often advocated earlier (15).

Aortic valve endocarditis is associated with the highest rate of complications, and surgical intervention is most often advocated. Treatment consists of excision of the infected valve, débridement of perivalvar abscess, and valve replacement, preferably with an aortic tissue allograft. In the surgical treatment of mitral valve endocarditis, repair rather than replacement of the mitral valve has demonstrated good functional results with a low risk for recurrent disease. Valvular repair techniques include anterior and posterior leaflet resection, leaflet patching, and direct suture. Pagani et al. (82) demonstrated that reconstructive techniques, including débridement of infected tissue, leafletoplasty, and implantation of a prosthetic annuloplasty ring, could be performed in this setting with low operative mortality and morbidity. Tricuspid valve endocarditis has been treated with valve excision alone; however, most patients should undergo valve repair and reconstruction, as long-term survivors of tricuspid valvectomy eventually require a tricuspid valve replacement (69).

Valve replacement in hemodynamically stable patients results in a favorable outcome in 80% to 95% of cases. A reinfection rate of 1% to 13% can be expected. David et al. (83) reported on 62 patients undergoing operative intervention for active endocarditis, with an operative mortality rate of zero for native valve endocarditis and 12.5% mortality for prosthetic valve endocarditis.

PROSTHETIC HEART VALVES

The development of prosthetic heart valves has changed the care of patients with valvular heart disease. A significant amount of progress has been made in the design and manufacturing of materials for both mechanical and biologic tissue valves. The characteristics of the ideal valve include adequate flow characteristics or hemodynamics, durability, biocompatibility, resistance to thrombosis, ease of insertion, and silence. A number of valve substitutes are available today for clinical use, and each type of prosthesis has its own inherent advantages and disadvantages. The two primary categories of prosthetic valves available today are mechanical valves and tissue (biologic) valves. The mechanical prostheses include caged-ball, tilting-disk, and bileaflet valves. The tissue valves include porcine (stented and stentless) and pericardial valves. In addition, allografts (tissue homografts) are available for use in both the aortic and mitral positions, and autografts (pulmonic valve) are available for the aortic position.

Mechanical Valve Substitutes

Despite the increasing age of patients undergoing valve replacement in the United States today and the trend toward implanting bioprostheses in older patients, mechanical valves still predominate in the United States.

The first successful mechanical prosthesis clinically implanted was the Starr-Edwards Silastic ball prosthesis (Fig. 62.8), which was the gold standard for more than 20 years. The performance of this valve is well documented (84). The Starr-Edwards valve is easy to implant, but it requires a generous amount of room for insertion because of the large size of the cage. Therefore, it is not utilized in patients with a small left ventricle or narrow aorta (85). The hemodynamics of the valve are adequate with the larger sizes, but the transvalvar gradients are consistently higher than those of the bileaflet and tilting-disk varieties of equal diameter (86). The thromboembolic rates with the Starr-Edwards valve are reported to be slightly higher than those with the bileaflet and tilting-disk valves used today. Durability statistics during long-term experience with this valve for up to 20 years have been excellent, but because of the higher transvalvar gradient and increased risk for thromboembolism, this valve is rarely used today.

In 1969, the Bjork-Shiley monostrut mechanical prosthesis was introduced (Fig. 62.9). This is a monoleaflet valve with a free-floating central tilting disk that is retained by a pair of struts. Hemodynamics with this valve are superior to those with the caged-ball valves (87), especially at the smaller sizes; however, the incidence of thromboembolic

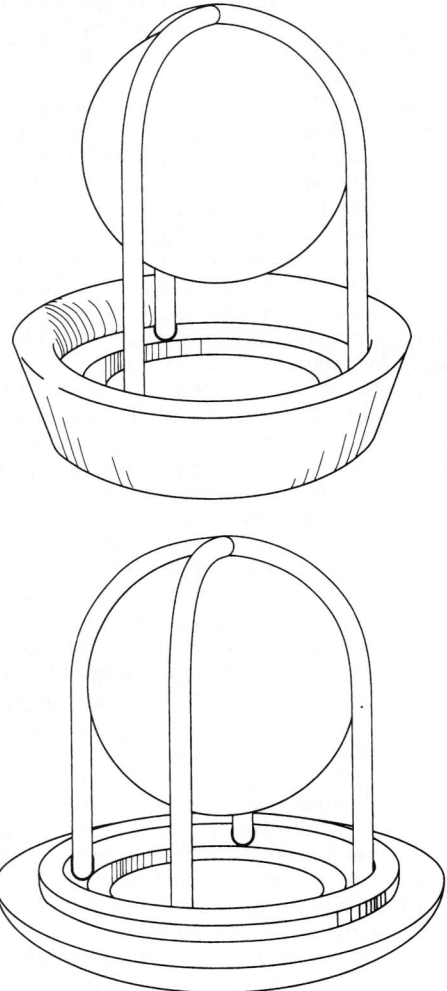

Figure 62.8. Starr-Edwards aortic caged-ball valve.

complications is similar to that with the Starr-Edwards valve (88). Valve thrombosis has occurred in a small percentage of patients, particularly in the mitral position. In 1976, in an attempt to improve the design of the valve, the original flat disk was made slightly convex–concave. Hemodynamics were better with this new valve, and thrombosis was virtually eliminated; however, a number of patients experienced the catastrophic complication of strut fracture and disk escape. This occurred more frequently with the larger valves and was more common with the 70-

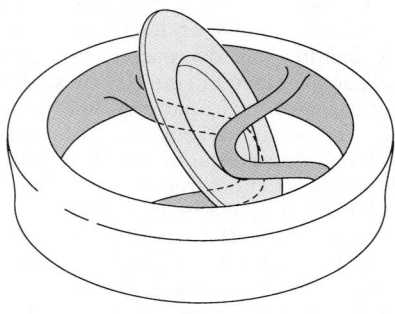

Figure 62.9. Bjork-Shiley tilting-disk valve.

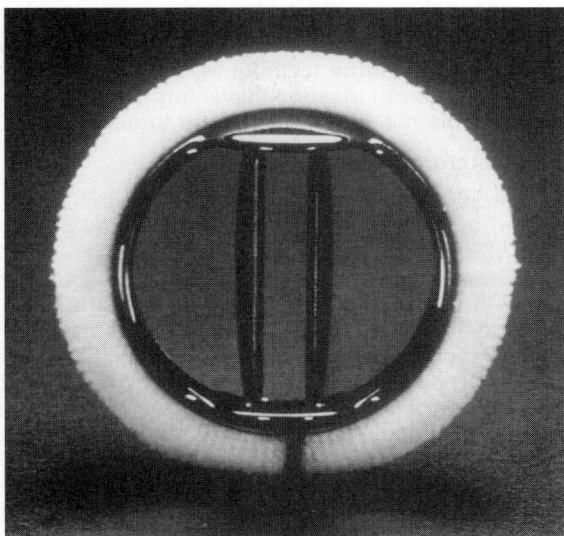

Figure 62.10. St. Jude bileaflet valve.

degree convex–concave valve. All convex–concave valves were recalled from the market in 1986 (89).

The St. Jude bileaflet valve was fist implanted clinically in 1977 (Fig. 62.10). This valve has two semicircular carbon disks that open to 85 degrees with a pivot mechanism, so the need for struts is eliminated. Hemodynamics are excellent, as the central leaflet opening provides for a large effective orifice area. The pressure gradients across these valves are the lowest for any of the mechanical prostheses (90). Thromboembolic rates (2% per patient-year) are similar to those associated with other mechanical valves. The St. Jude valve is less prone to the development of valve thrombosis than other tilting-disk valves, and in some instances only one leaflet may be involved in the thrombotic process, which allows time for reoperation before cardiovascular collapse develops (91). The durability of the valve is excellent, with a limited number of failures occurring at 10-year follow-up (92). Recently, St. Jude introduced a modification of the valve, which incorporated a Silzone coating into the sewing ring of the valve. Silzone, a silver-based material, was utilized to decrease the incidence of endocarditis and infection. Unfortunately, preliminary results demonstrated that these valves have a higher incidence of perivalvar leak, and so this valve product has been removed voluntarily from the market (93).

The CarboMedics prosthetic valve (Fig. 62.11) was first implanted in the United States in 1993. This is a bileaflet valve with two carbon-coated disks that open to 78 degrees. It is similar to the St. Jude valve; however, the design of the hinges and the mechanism of valve closure are different. The incidence of thrombosis and the transvalvar gradients with this valve are slightly higher than with the St. Jude valve. The incidence of thromboembolic complications is similar to that associated with the St. Jude valve, and no structural problems have been reported (94).

The Medtronic-Hall valve (Fig. 62.12) was first implanted clinically in 1977. This was a newly designed type of tilting-disk valve with a guiding rod placed through an opening in the center of the disk. The disk opens to a large angle, and so this valve has excellent flow characteristics, with hemodynamics similar to those of the St. Jude valve. Thromboembolic complication rates are similar to those of other tilting-disk prostheses. A small incidence of thrombotic occlusion has been noted, but the durability of the valve is excellent, with no structural failures reported to date (95).

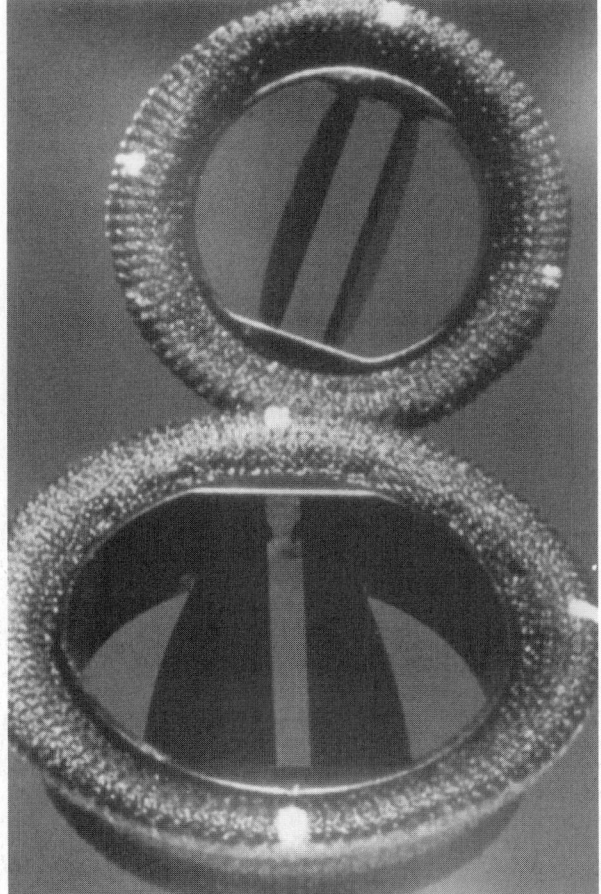

Figure 62.11. CarboMedics mechanical prosthesis.

All the mechanical valves share the advantage of long-term durability; however, the risk for thromboembolism and the risk for bleeding secondary to the need for anticoagulation are increased (96). The rates of thrombotic com-

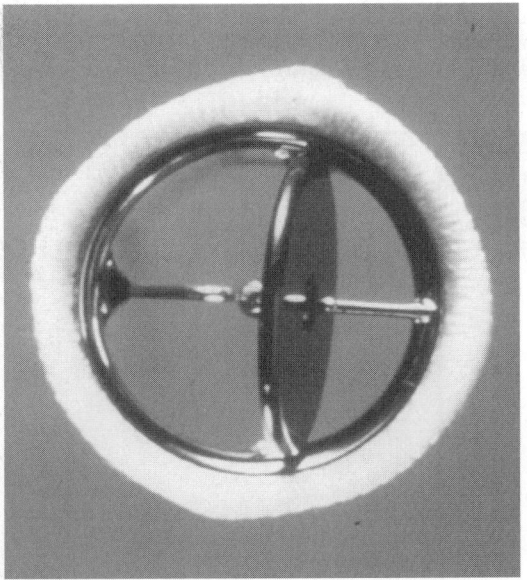

Figure 62.12. Medtronic-Hall mechanical prosthesis.

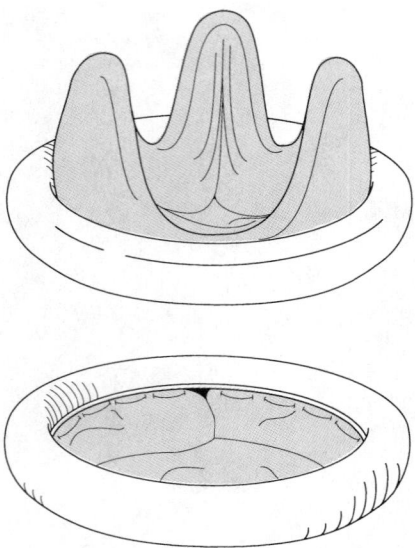

Figure 62.13. Carpentier-Edwards porcine bioprosthetic valve.

plications are low (< 1%) when anticoagulation is adequate. The incidence of thromboembolism in patients with adequate anticoagulation and a valve in the aortic position is 0.5% to 3% per patient-year, and for those with a valve in the mitral position, it is 0.5% to 5%. Anticoagulation-related bleeding remains one of the most common causes of valve-related morbidity (1% to 3% per patient-year) and mortality (0.1% to 0.5% per patient-year) (97).

Tissue Valves

Various tissue valves have been developed during the last 30 years, and most have proved unacceptable because of the rapidity with which they degenerate and become incompetent. In 1969, Carpentier et al. (98) introduced the use of glutaraldehyde for tissue valve preservation. Glutaraldehyde enhances the formation of collagen covalent cross-linkage bonds, increases tissue strength, renders the tissue nonviable, and reduces tissue antigenicity. One of the newer changes in the manufacture of tissue valves is based on the finding that fixation at pressures greater than 4 mm Hg causes severe alterations in the collagen fiber geometry that lead to earlier degeneration. Today, some of the manufacturers are using low-pressure or zero-pressure

fixation techniques, and preliminary long-term viability studies indicate better durability. Different fixation techniques, newer mounting techniques, and the addition of agents to retard calcification have improved the tissue valves now commercially available for implantation.

Porcine Heterograft Tissue Valves

The porcine heterograft tissue valves available for implantation today in the United States are the Carpentier-Edwards (Fig. 62.13) and Hancock valves (Fig. 62.14). Both of these valves are fixed with glutaraldehyde; however, they differ in strut design and construction. The effective orifice area of porcine aortic valves is limited by the presence of a shelf of myocardial tissue at the base of the right coronary cusp that is inherent in all porcine valves. The Carpentier-Edwards valve attempted to overcome this additional shelf of muscle tissue with the creation of an asymmetric stent. Overall, the average-sized and larger porcine heterograft valves have good hemodynamics; however, the smaller valves are associated with a significant gradient (99,100).

A significant advantage of these tissue valves is that anticoagulation is not needed. The thromboembolic complication rate is very low, but the risk does exist. The risk for thromboembolic complications is increased in patients with atrial fibrillation, an enlarged left atrium, a history of previous emboli, a left atrial clot, or significantly reduced LV function. These patients should be considered for anticoagulation therapy (100).

The main problem with the porcine heterograft tissue valve is tissue degeneration, and the risk for valve failure increases with time. The failure rate at 10 years is 70%, and this rate is accelerated in younger patients (101,102). Some of these durability issues may be resolved with the new, low-pressure fixation techniques.

Stentless Heterograft Valves

Stentless heterograft porcine valves are currently available for use in the aortic position (Figs. 62.15 and 62.16). The hemodynamics of these valves are excellent because the effective orifice area is larger than in stented tissue valves. Other demonstrated advantages are postoperative long-term ventricular remodeling, little early calcification, good early durability, and the lack of a need for anticoagulation. Stentless valves provide the same opportunities for implantation as allograft valves with use of the subcoronary technique or for complete root replacement (Medtronic Freestyle, Baxter Prima valves). Disadvantages

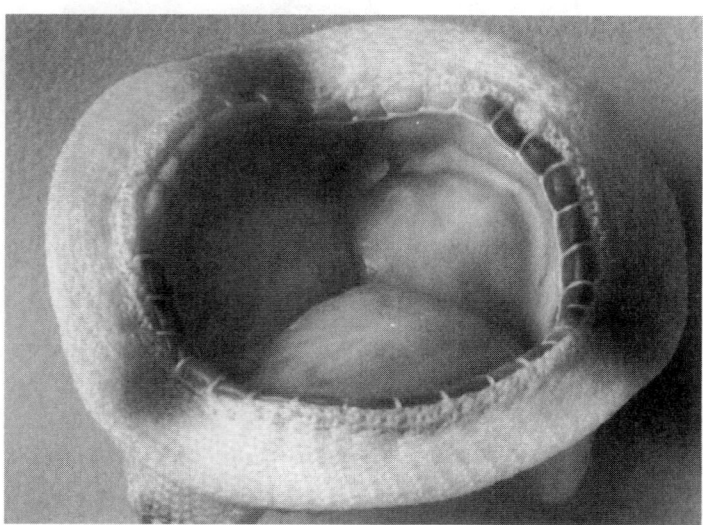

Figure 62.14. Hancock II porcine bioprosthesis.

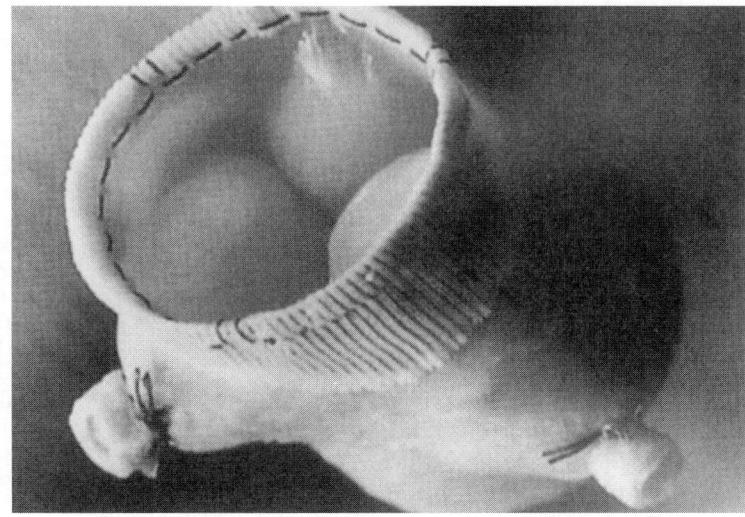

Figure 62.15. Medtronic Freestyle valve.

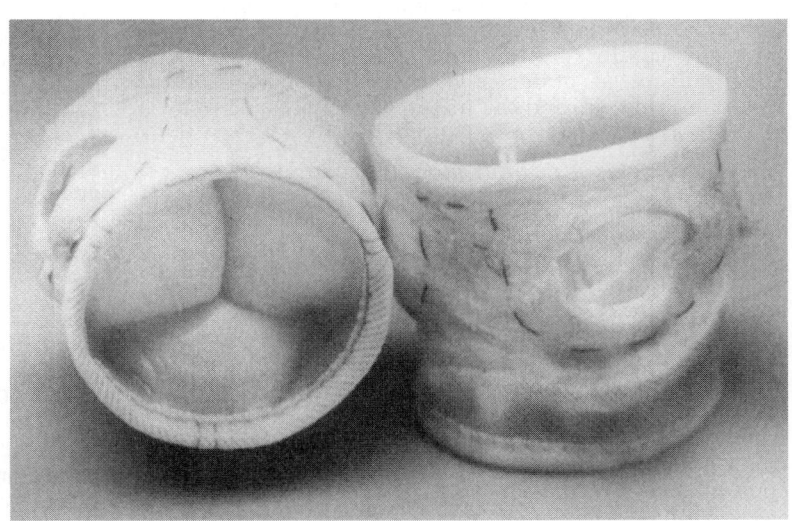

Figure 62.16. Baxter Prima valve.

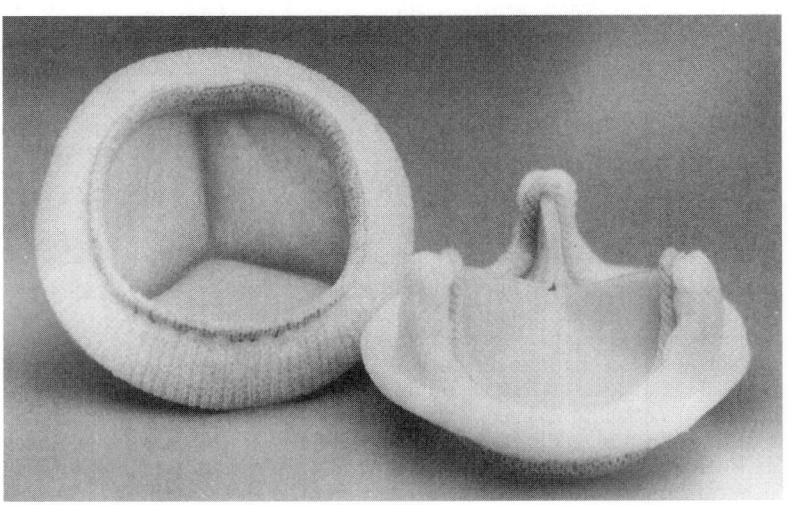

Figure 62.17. Carpentier-Edwards Perimont pericardial bioprosthesis.

of these newer valves are a steep learning curve for the surgeon in regard to implantation and a slightly longer cross-clamp time in comparison with stented valves (103).

Pericardial Bioprostheses

The original pericardial tissue valves were made of glutaraldehyde-preserved bovine pericardium, fashioned in a three-cusp valve mounted on a cloth-covered frame. These valves have a larger effective orifice area and therefore excellent hemodynamics, especially the smaller valves. For this reason, they are very attractive for use in patients with a small aortic root. In 1991, the Carpentier-Edwards pericardial bioprosthesis was introduced (Fig. 62.17). This valve has better hemodynamics than the porcine heterograft valves. Long-term durability studies are still being conducted (79).

Aortic Allografts

Aortic allografts have been used for aortic valve replacement since the 1960s. The valves are harvested and then cryopreserved with antibiotic solutions. Allografts are associated with very low thromboembolic complication rates and a very low incidence of endocarditis. Freedom from degeneration at 10 years is 95%. Indications for allograft use include contraindications to anticoagulation, a life expectancy longer than 10 years, native or prosthetic valve endocarditis, and abnormal aortic root morphology. The disadvantages of this valve are its limited availability and increased cost, and the increased technical complexity of insertion (104).

Pulmonary Valve Autograft (Ross Procedure)

In 1967, Ross introduced the pulmonary autograft for aortic root reconstruction and aortic valve replacement (104a). This procedure involves careful harvesting and transfer of the pulmonary valve and proximal pulmonary artery to the aortic position. The pulmonary valve autograft can be implanted as a free valve or as an entire root. A pulmonary allograft is then used to reestablish the continuity of the right ventricle and pulmonary artery. The autograft is used today primarily in infants and children, in whom growth of the pulmonary autograft has been documented (105). It is also used in selected young adults with contraindications for anticoagulation. Ross reported 339 cases, with 85% freedom from valve replacement at 20 years (106). Performance of this procedure requires significant technical expertise.

With all the tissue valves, the risk for thromboembolism is low, and anticoagulation is not usually required. Their durability is limited; at 6 to 7 years, the rate of freedom from valve failure in adults is 90% to 95%, and by 10 years it is approximately 70% to 80% (100,107). Embolic rates with tissue valves range from 0.2% to 3.8% per year for aortic valves and 0.3% to 5.1% for mitral valves (108). Failure rates are increased in younger patients.

Selection of a Valve Prosthesis

Selection of the appropriate valve prosthesis depends on the surgical procedure and patient factors (age, risk for anticoagulation, presence of infection).

Once the decision is made to replace a valve, it is important to evaluate the valve annulus carefully and choose the correct valve size for the patient. The overall objective of sizing is to use the largest valve size and design for the patient because prosthetic valve orifices are effectively smaller than their native counterparts. The size of the cavity of the chamber in which the valve is to be situated is also very important. In a narrow aortic root, a low-profile

valve is preferred. In the mitral position, the size of the LV chamber in systole should be considered because it must accommodate the prosthesis.

Among patient factors, age is critical in selecting the most appropriate prosthesis for insertion. Mechanical valves, with their increased durability relative to tissue valves, are preferred in younger patients. The current trend is toward the use of bioprosthetic valves in patients over the age of 70 and mechanical valves in younger patients (109). Anticoagulation is advisable for all mechanical valves in all positions, and therefore any contraindication to anticoagulation must be considered when a valve prosthesis is selected (87,108). Psychosocial factors are also important, as patient compliance with anticoagulation or the desire of a young woman to bear children should be considered. Although many factors need to be considered in selecting a valve prosthesis, some general guidelines can be stated. Bioprosthetic valves are recommended for patients who are older than 65 to 70 years or whose life expectancy is less than 10 years. Mechanical prosthetic valves are recommended for younger patients, those without contraindications to anticoagulation, and those with smaller aortic annuli.

ANTICOAGULATION

Anticoagulation in patients with diseased native valves or prosthetic valves is indicated when the risk for thromboembolism associated with these conditions exceeds the morbidity of hemorrhagic complications caused by the anticoagulant therapy. A second caveat of anticoagulant therapy is that lower rates of thromboembolism must be demonstrated with treatment.

Indications

Data from several large studies have stratified the relative risk for thromboembolism for specific valvular diseases. Rheumatic heart disease carries the highest risk for thromboembolism. Patients with mitral rheumatic disease have a 20% risk for the development of clinically significant emboli, and a 10% to 15% mortality rate without treatment (44). In patients with mitral valve disease in atrial fibrillation, the risk for thromboembolism is four to seven times greater than in similar patients in normal sinus rhythm. More specifically, in patients in atrial fibrillation with MS, the risk for thromboembolism is about a 50% greater than in patients with MR—31.5% versus

---

Table 62.7. ASSOCIATION OF THROMBOEMBOLISM WITH ATRIAL FIBRILLATION AND AGE IN PATIENTS WITH MITRAL VALVE DISEASE[a]

Age (y)	Sinus rhythm	Atrial fibrillation	Total
Mitral stenosis			
≤ 35	4.5	27.5	9.0
> 35	11.3	32.3	23.9
Total	7.9	31.5	19.0
Mitral regurgitation			
≤ 35	3.7	15.8	8.6
> 35	16.7	25.0	23.2
Total	7.6	22.2	16.7

[a]Incidence of thromboembolism in percentage of total patients studied.

Modified from Coulshed N, Epstein EJ, McKindrich CS, et al. Systemic embolisation in mitral valve disease. Br Heart J 1970;32:26, with permission.

Table 62.8. ANTICOAGULANT RECOMMENDATIONS

Indication	Recommended prothrombin time elevation with warfarin administration
Prosthetic heart valves	
Mechanical	1.5–2
Bioprosthetic	1.3–1.5 (3 mo postoperatively)
Native valve disease	
Rheumatic mitral valve	
Previous embolism	1.5–2 (1.3–1.5 after 1 y)
Atrial fibrillation	1.3–1.5
Dilated left atrium	1.3–1.5
(> 55 mm in diameter)	
Aortic valve disease	No treatment[a]
Mitral valve prolapse	No treatment[a]
Mitral annular calcification	No treatment[a]
Infective endocarditis	No treatment[a]
Atrial fibrillation	
Previous embolism	1.5–2 (1.3–1.5 after 1 y)
Mitral valve disease	1.3–1.5
Cardiomyopathy	
Dilated	1.3–1.5
Hypertrophic	1.3–1.5
Thyrotoxicosis	1.3–1.5[b]
Lone atrial fibrillation	No treatment[a]
Cardioversion	1.3–1.5[b]

[a]Unless other indications exist.
[b]Maintain therapy for 2 to 4 weeks after conversion to sinus rhythm.

22%, respectively (110) (Table 62.7). Although thromboemboli occur in only 8% of patients with MS or MR who are in sinus rhythm, patients in whom a single embolic event develops have a 30% to 65% chance of experiencing recurrent episodes, and more than half of these occur within 6 months. Patients with large atria (diameter > 55 mm) are at increased risk for the development of atrial fibrillation and therefore should be considered for prophylactic anticoagulation. In addition, advanced age and a decreased cardiac index are risk factors for thromboembolism. Anticoagulant therapy is therefore recommended for patients with atrial fibrillation and associated systemic emboli, mitral valve disease, and cardiomyopathy (111).

Lesions of the other valves carry a relatively low risk for embolism. Calcific emboli do not appear to be prevented by warfarin therapy. Anticoagulation is therefore not indicated for MVP, mitral annular calcification, or aortic valve disease without other risk factors. Emboli associated with endocarditis are usually not thrombotic in nature, and anticoagulation is not indicated for endocarditis unless other indications exist (e.g., prosthetic valve endocarditis).

Reliable data from randomized trials of anticoagulant therapy in patients with prosthetic heart valves are sporadic, but some specific recommendations are available (Table 62.8). Initial experiences with the Starr-Edwards ball valve showed an average embolic risk of 6% per year; the risk ranged up to 30% during the course of one study in which anticoagulants were not used. Anticoagulant therapy reduces this risk threefold to sixfold. The new generation of low-profile tilting-disk valves, although thought to be associated with a lower potential for thrombosis, still demonstrate thromboembolic rates without anticoagulation of up to 3% per year. Bioprosthetic tissue valves are associated with a low potential for thromboembolism, on the order of 2% per year. Half of all thromboembolic episodes in patients with tissue valves occur in the first 12 weeks after surgery. Lifelong anticoagulation is therefore recommended for all patients with mechanical valves, and an initial period of anticoagulation is recommended by some authors for patients with bioprosthetic valves to cover the early period of new intimal deposition. Antiplatelet therapy with either aspirin or dipyridamole (Persantine) may be an effective alternative treatment to lower the thromboembolic risk, but the data are not well supported. These agents may be useful as an adjunct to warfarin in cases in which single-drug therapy is ineffective in preventing embolic complications.

Summarizing all prosthetic valve data, Edmunds (112) concluded that the cumulative risk for thromboembolism for mechanical valves with anticoagulation and for bioprosthetic valves without anticoagulation was about equal, at 2% per year. Patients with mechanical valves who take anticoagulants assume an added risk for complications of bleeding, but 10% of patients with tissue valves in the aortic position, and up to 40% to 60% of patients with bioprosthetic mitral valves, eventually require warfarin anticoagulation, so that the benefits of the tissue prosthesis are partially negated.

Complications

Data derived from patients with prosthetic valves who are on warfarin therapy suggest a uniform risk for major episodes of bleeding of 1% to 2% per year, with a mortality rate of 0.17% per year for patients on anticoagulant therapy. Bleeding most commonly involves the central nervous, genitourinary, or gastrointestinal system, including the retroperitoneum. Fatal bleeding usually involves the central nervous system. Trauma is frequently an inciting cause. Previous recommendations that the prothrombin time be maintained at 2 to 2.5 times control appear to be excessive, and fewer complications of bleeding can be expected at the newly recommended levels of 1.3 to 1.5 times control for most patients (49,51,111,113).

Patients who have had an embolic cerebrovascular accident thought to be cardiac in origin should undergo urgent computed tomography of the brain. Anticoagulant therapy should be instituted immediately if the scan result is negative. If a large or hemorrhagic infarct is observed, therapy should be postponed for 1 week.

Few studies have addressed the management of patients requiring interruption of anticoagulation because of bleeding or because major surgery is planned. The authors believe that anticoagulation should be reversed by withholding warfarin for several days before the operation and allowing the prothrombin time to decrease to about 14 to 15 seconds. Therapy should be resumed 1 to 2 days postoperatively in low-risk patients. High-risk patients should be switched to heparin preoperatively once the prothrombin time reaches subtherapeutic levels. The heparin can be discontinued immediately before operation and resumed as soon as 12 hours postoperatively if operative bleeding is not an issue. Anticoagulation should be reversed rapidly with transfusions of fresh frozen plasma, if necessary. The administration of vitamin K makes subsequent warfarin therapy more difficult and should be avoided. The benefits of the use of aspirin through the perioperative period remain unconfirmed.

Contraindications

Anticoagulant therapy is specifically contraindicated for patients with a predisposition for bleeding secondary to systemic disease (e.g., active ulcer disease) or coagulopathy; it is also contraindicated for those likely to incur trauma through occupation or pastime, likely to be poorly compliant, or with a desire for future pregnancy.

Anticoagulation in the pregnant patient is a significant problem. Warfarin is a small molecule that readily crosses the placental barrier. The immature fetal liver is susceptible to the effects of warfarin, and a protracted hypocoagulable state develops. Levels of fetal clotting factors can take 2 to 3 weeks to return to normal after cessation of warfarin therapy. Warfarin is also a known fetal teratogen, especially when used during the first trimester. A fetal loss rate over 30% and a rate of premature labor over 50% have been reported with warfarin use during pregnancy (114). The use of warfarin late in pregnancy can produce fetal neurologic complications as a result of intracranial hemorrhage, and the trauma of delivery is a significant problem in this regard. Heparin is not transferred across the placental barrier but can produce fetal loss through placental hemorrhage. Conversely, the pregnant woman is in a hypercoagulable state, with elevated levels of clotting factors and decreased fibrinolytic activity. Cessation of anticoagulation during pregnancy can lead to an incidence of cerebral events as high as 25%. Antiplatelet agents are not as toxic to the fetus as warfarin but do not confer adequate protection to the mother.

The best solution to this problem is to use a bioprosthesis in patients wishing to become pregnant and administer antiplatelet agents during pregnancy. If an unforeseen pregnancy develops in a patient with a mechanical valve, a regimen of subcutaneous low-molecular-weight heparin is now advocated.

SUMMARY

The overall prognosis for patients with valvular heart disease has improved during the last 15 years. This can be attributed to a better understanding of the proper timing for surgical intervention, advances in the noninvasive assessment of the aortic and mitral valves, and improved surgical techniques for valve reconstruction and replacement. All these advances will be combined to improve the overall outlook for patients with valvular heart disease in the future.

REFERENCES

1. Silver MA, Roberts WC. Detailed anatomy of the normally functioning aortic valve in hearts of normal and increased weight. *Am J Cardiol* 1985;55:454.
2. Anderson RH, Devine WA, Ho SY, et al. The myth of the aortic annulus: the anatomy of the subaortic outflow tract. *Ann Thorac Surg* 1991;52:640.
3. Thubrikar MJ, Nolan SP, Aouad J, et al. Stress sharing between the sinus and leaflets of canine aortic valve. *Ann Thorac Surg* 1986;42:434.
4. Zimmerman J. The functional and surgical anatomy of the aortic valve. *Isr J Med Sci* 1969;5:862.
5. Davila JC, Plamer ET. The mitral valve: anatomy and pathology for the surgeon. *Arch Surg* 1962;84:174.
6. Walmsley R. Anatomy of human mitral valve in adult cadaver and comparative anatomy of the valve. *Br Heart J* 1978;40:351.
7. Ranganathan N, Lam JH, Wigle ED, et al. Morphology of the human mitral valve. II. The valve leaflets. *Circulation* 1970; 41:459.
8. Pollick C, Pitman M, Filly K, et al. Mitral and aortic valve orifice area in normal subjects and in patients with congestive cardiomyopathy: determination by two-dimensional echocardiography. *Am J Cardiol* 1982;49:1191.
9. Fenster MS, Feldman MD. Mitral regurgitation: an overview. *Curr Probl Cardiol* 1995;20:193.
10. Voci P, Bilotta F, Caretta Q, et al. Papillary muscle perfusion pattern: a hypothesis for ischemic papillary muscle dysfunction. *Circulation* 1995;91:1714.
11. Lam JH, Ranganathan N, Wigle ED, et al. Morphology of the human mitral valve. I. Chordae tendineae: a new classification. *Circulation* 1970;41:449.
12. Boltwood CM, Tei C, Wong M, et al. Quantitative echocardiography of the mitral complex in dilated cardiomyopathy: the mechanism of functional mitral regurgitation. *Circulation* 1983;68:498.
13. Passik CS, Ackermann DM, Pluth JR, et al. Temporal changes in the causes of aortic stenosis: a surgical pathologic study of 646 cases. *Mayo Clin Proc* 1987;62:119.
14. Waller B, Howard J, Fess S. Pathology of aortic valve stenosis and pure aortic regurgitation: a clinical morphologic assessment. *Clin Cardiol* 1994;17:85.
15. Bonow RO, Carabello B, de Leon AC, et al. ACC/AHA guidelines for the management of patients with valvular heart disease: executive summary. *J Heart Valve Dis* 1998;7:672.
16. Hess OM, Ritter M, Schneider J, et al. Diastolic stiffness and myocardial structure in aortic valve disease before and after valve replacement. *Circulation* 1984;69:855.
17. Huber D, Grimm J, Koch R, et al. Determinants of ejection performance in aortic stenosis. *Circulation* 1981;64:126.
18. Maier GW, Wechsler AS. Pathophysiology of aortic valve disease. In: Edmunds LH, ed. *Cardiac surgery in the adult.* New York: McGraw-Hill, 1997:835.
19. Lester SJ, Heilbron B, Gin K, et al. The natural history and rate of progression of aortic stenosis. *Chest* 1998;113:1109.
20. Chizner MA, Pearle DL, de Leon AC Jr. The natural history of aortic stenosis in adults. *Am Heart J* 1980;99:419.
21. Marcus ML, Doty DB, Hiratzka LF, et al. Decreased coronary reserve: a mechanism for angina pectoris in patients with aortic stenosis and normal coronary arteries. *N Engl J Med* 1982;307:1362.
22. Carabello BA, Crawford FA. Medical progress: valvular heart disease. *N Engl J Med* 1997;337:32.
23. Otto CM. Aortic stenosis: clinical evaluation and optimal timing of surgery. *Cardiol Clin* 1998;16:353.
24. Richards AM, Nicholls MG, Ikram H, et al. Syncope in aortic valvular stenosis. *Lancet* 1984;2:1113.
25. O'Keefe JH Jr, Vlietstra RE, Bailey KR, et al. Natural history of candidates for balloon aortic valvuloplasty. *Mayo Clin Proc* 1987;62:986.
26. Carabello BA, Green LH, Grossman W, et al. Hemodynamic determinants of prognosis of aortic valve replacement in critical aortic stenosis and advanced congestive heart failure. *Circulation* 1980;62:42.
27. Brogan WC III, Grayburn PA, Lange RA, et al. Prognosis after valve replacement in patients with severe aortic stenosis and low transvalvular pressure gradient. *J Am Coll Cardiol* 1993; 21:1657.
28. Cannon JD Jr, Zile MR, Crawford FA Jr, et al. Aortic valve resistance as an adjunct to the Gorlin formula in assessing the severity of aortic stenosis in symptomatic patients. *J Am Coll Cardiol* 1992;20:1517.
29. deFilippi CR, Willett DL, Brickner ME, et al. Usefulness of dobutamine echocardiography in distinguishing severe from nonsevere valvular aortic stenosis in patients with depressed left ventricular function and low transvalvular gradients. *Am J Cardiol* 1995;75:191.
30. Otto CM, Mickel MC, Kennedy JW, et al. Three-year outcome after balloon aortic valvuloplasty: insights into prognosis of valvular aortic stenosis. *Circulation* 1994;89:642.
31. Bellhouse BJ, Bellhouse F, Abbott JA, et al. Mechanism of valvular incompetence in aortic sinus dilatation. *Cardiovasc Res* 1973;7:490.
32. Carter JB, Sethi S, Lee GB, et al. Prolapse of semilunar cusps as causes of aortic insufficiency. *Circulation* 1971;43:922.
33. Mann T, McLaurin L, Grossman W, et al. Assessing the hemodynamic severity of acute aortic regurgitation due to infective endocarditis. *N Engl J Med* 1975;293:108.
34. Vinten-Johansen J, Weiss HR. Regional O_2 consumption in canine left ventricular myocardium in experimental acute aortic valvular insufficiency. *Cardiovasc Res* 1981;15:305.
35. Bonow RO. Chronic aortic regurgitation: role of medical therapy and optimal timing for surgery. *Cardiol Clin* 1998;16:449.
36. Goldschlager N, Pfeifer J, Cohn K, et al. The natural history of aortic regurgitation: a clinical and hemodynamic study. *Am J Med* 1973;54:577.
37. Henry WL, Bonow RO, Rosing DR, et al. Observations on the optimum time for operative intervention for aortic regurgitation. *Circulation* 1980;61:484.
38. Bonow RO, Lakatos E, Maron BJ, et al. Serial long-term as-

sessment of the natural history of asymptomatic patients with chronic aortic regurgitation and normal left ventricular systolic function. *Circulation* 1991;84:1625.

39. Aronow WS, Ahn C, Kronzon I, et al. Prognosis of patients with heart failure and unoperated severe aortic valvular regurgitation and relation to ejection fraction. *Am J Cardiol* 1994;74:286.

40. Waller BF, Howard J, Fess S. Pathology of mitral valve stenosis and pure mitral regurgitation, part I. *Clin Cardiol* 1994; 17:330.

41. Waller BF, Howard J, Fess S. Pathology of mitral valve stenosis and pure mitral regurgitation, part II. *Clin Cardiol* 1994; 17:395.

42. Wood P. An appreciation of mitral stenosis. *Br Med J* 1954; 1:1051.

43. Thompson ME, Shaver JA, Leon DF. Effect of tachycardia on atrial transport in mitral stenosis. *Am Heart J* 1977;94:297.

44. Neilson GH, Galea EG, Hossack KF. Thromboembolic complications of mitral valve disease. *Aust NZJ Med* 1978;8:372.

45. Gash AK, Carabello BA, Kent RL, et al. Left ventricular performance in patients with coexistent mitral stenosis and aortic insufficiency. *J Am Coll Cardiol* 1984;3:703.

46. Martin RP, Rakowski H, Kleiman JH, et al. Reliability and reproducibility of two-dimensional echocardiograph measurement of the stenotic mitral valve orifice area. *Am J Cardiol* 1979;43:560.

47. Carabello BA. Timing of surgery for mitral and aortic stenosis. *Cardiol Clin* 1991;9:229.

48. Reyes VP, Raju BS, Wynne J, et al. Percutaneous balloon valvuloplasty compared with open surgical commissurotomy for mitral stenosis. *N Engl J Med* 1994;331:961.

49. Wilkins GT, Weyman AE, Abascal VM, et al. Percutaneous balloon dilation of the mitral valve: an analysis of echocardiographic variables related to outcome and the mechanism of dilatation. *Br Heart J* 1988;60:299.

50. Kobayashi J, Kosakai Y, Isobe F, et al. Rationale of the Cox maze procedure for atrial fibrillation during redo mitral valve operations. *J Thorac Cardiovasc Surg* 1996;112:1216.

51. Kawaguchi AT, Kosakai Y, Sasako Y, et al. Risks and benefits of combined maze procedure for atrial fibrillation associated with organic heart disease. *J Am Coll Cardiol* 1996;28:985.

52. Stevenson LW, Fowler MB, Schroeder JS, et al. Poor survival of patients with idiopathic cardiomyopathy considered too well for transplantation. *Am J Med* 1987;83:871.

53. Fenster MS, Feldman MD. Mitral regurgitation: an overview. *Curr Probl Cardiol* 1995;20:193.

54. Starling MR, Kirsh MM, Montgomery DG, et al. Impaired left ventricular contractile function in patients with long-term mitral regurgitation and normal ejection fraction. *J Am Coll Cardiol* 1993;22:239.

55. Carabello BA, Williams H, Gash AK, et al. Hemodynamic predictors of outcome in patients undergoing valve replacement. *Circulation* 1986;74:1309.

56. Rosario LB, Stevenson LW, Solomon SD, et al. The mechanism of decrease in dynamic mitral regurgitation during heart failure treatment: importance of reduction in regurgitant orifice size. *J Am Coll Cardiol* 1998;32:1819.

57. Torre-Amione G, Kapadia S, Benedict C, et al. Proinflammatory cytokine levels in patients with depressed left ventricular ejection fraction: a report from the Studies of Left Ventricular Dysfunction (SOLVD). *J Am Coll Cardiol* 1996;27:1201.

58. Herrera-Garza EH, Stetson SJ, Cubillos-Garzon A, et al. Tumor necrosis factor-α: a mediator of disease progression in the failing human heart. *Chest* 1999;115:1170.

59. Carabello BA. Clinical assessment of systolic dysfunction. *ACC Curr J Rev* 1994;3:25.

60. Zile MR, Gaasch WH, Carroll JD, et al. Chronic mitral regurgitation: predictive value of preoperative echocardiographic indexes of left ventricular function and wall stress. *J Am Coll Cardiol* 1984;3:235.

61. Hochreiter C, Niles N, Devereux RB, et al. Mitral regurgitation: relationship of noninvasive descriptors of right and left ventricular performance to clinical and hemodynamic findings and to prognosis in medically and surgically treated patients. *Circulation* 1986;73:900.

62. David TE, Uden DE, Strauss HD. The importance of the mitral apparatus in left ventricular function after correction of mitral regurgitation. *Circulation* 1983;68(II):76.

63. Gallino A, Jenni R, Hurni R, et al. Early results after mitral valvuloplasty for pure mitral regurgitation. *Eur Heart J* 1987; 8:902.

64. Rankin JS, Feneley MP, Hickey MS, et al. A clinical comparison of mitral valve repair versus replacement in ischemic mitral regurgitation. *J Thorac Cadiovasc Surg* 1988;95:165.

65. Akins CW, Hilgenberg AD, Buckley MJ, et al. Mitral valve reconstruction versus replacement for degenerative or ischemic mitral regurgitation. *Ann Thorac Surg* 1994;58:668.

66. Olson LJ, Subramanian R, Ackermann DM, et al. Surgical pathology of the mitral valve: a study of 712 cases spanning 21 years. *Mayo Clin Proc* 1987;62:22.

67. Roberts WC, McIntosh CL, Wallace RB. Mechanisms of severe mitral regurgitation in mitral valve prolapse determined from analysis of operatively excised valves. *Am Heart J* 1987;113:1316.

68. Barlow JB, Pocock WA. Mitral valve prolapse, the specific billowing mitral leaflet syndrome, or an insignificant nonejection systolic click. *Am Heart J* 1979;97:277.

69. Sons H, Dausch W, Kuh JH. Tricuspid valve repair in rightsided endocarditis. *J Heart Valve Dis* 1997;6:636.

70. Connolly HM, Crary JL, McGoon MD, et al. Valvular heart disease associated with fenfluramine-phentermine. *N Engl J Med* 1997;337:581.

71. Hogevik H, Olaison L, Andersson R, et al. Epidemiologic aspects of infective endocarditis in an urban population: a 5-year prospective study. *Medicine* 1995;74:324.

72. Bayliss R, Clarke C, Oakley CM, et al. Incidence, mortality, and prevention of infective endocarditis. *J R Coll Physicians Lond* 1986;20:15.

73. Edmunds LH Jr, Clark RE, Cohn LH, et al. Guidelines for reporting morbidity and mortality after cardiac valvular operations. *Ann Thorac Surg* 1996;62:932.

74. Skehan JD, Murray M, Mills PG. Infective endocarditis: incidence and mortality in the North East Thames region. *Br Heart J* 1988;59:62.

75. Steusse DC, Vlessis AA. Epidemiology of native valve endocarditis. In: Vlessis AA, Bolling SF, eds. *Endocarditis: a multidisciplinary approach.* Armonk, NY: Futura Publishing, 1999:77.

76. Vlessis AA, Khaki A, Grunkemeier GL, et al. Risk, diagnosis, and management of prosthetic valve endocarditis: a review. *J Heart Valve Disease* 1997;6:443.

77. Vlessis AA, Hovaguimian H, Jaggers J, et al. Infective endocarditis: ten-year review of medical and surgical therapy. *Ann Thorac Surg* 1996;61:1217.

78. Aklog L, Gobezie R, Adams DH. Aortic valve endocarditis. In: Vlessis AA, Bolling SF, eds. *Endocarditis: a multidisciplinary approach.* Armonk, NY: Futura Publishing, 1999: 235.

79. Schwartz CF, Bolling SF. Mitral valve endocarditis. In: Vlessis AA, Bolling SF, eds. *Endocarditis: a multidisciplinary approach.* Armonk, NY: Futura Publishing, 1999:263.

80. Bach DS. Echocardiographic diagnosis and findings in infective endocarditis. In: Vlessis AA, Bolling SF, eds. *Endocarditis: a multidisciplinary approach.* Armonk, NY: Futura Publishing, 1999:135.

81. Armstrong WS, Shea M. Clinical diagnosis of infective endocarditis. In: Vlessis AA, Bolling SF, eds. *Endocarditis: a multidisciplinary approach.* Armonk, NY: Futura Publishing, 1999:107.

82. Pagani FD, Monaghan HL, Deeb GM, et al. Mitral valve reconstruction for active and healed endocarditis. *Circulation* 1996;94(II):133.

83. David TE, Bos J, Christakis GT, et al. Heart valve operations in patients with active infective endocarditis. *Ann Thorac Surg* 1990;49:701.

84. Cobanoglu A, Jamieson WR, Miller DC, et al. A tri-institutional comparison of tissue and mechanical valves using a patient-oriented definition of "treatment failure." *Ann Thorac Surg* 1987;43:245.

85. Pelletier L, Carrier M, Leclerc Y, et al. The Carpentier-Edwards pericardial bioprosthesis: clinical experience with 600 patients. *Ann Thorac Surg* 1995;60:S297.

86. Miller DC, Oyer PE, Mitchell RS, et al. Performance characteristics of the Starr-Edwards Model 1260 aortic valve prosthesis beyond ten years. *J Thorac Cardiovasc Surg* 1984;88: 193.

87. Bjork VO, Henze A. Ten years' experience with the Bjork-Shiley tilting disc valve. *J Thorac Cardiovasc Surg* 1979;78:331.
88. Borkon AM, Soule L, Baughman KL, et al. Ten-year analysis of the Bjork-Shiley standard aortic valve. *Ann Thorac Surg* 1987;43:39.
89. Hiratzka LF, Kouchoukos NT, Grunkemeier GL, et al. Outlet strut fracture of the Bjork-Shiley 60 degrees convexo-concave valve: current information and recommendations for patient care. *J Am Coll Cardiol* 1988;11:1130.
90. Czer LS, Matloff J, Chaux A, et al. A 6-year experience with the St. Jude Medical valve: hemodynamic performance, surgical results, biocompatibility, and follow-up. *J Am Coll Cardiol* 1985;6:904.
91. Czer LS, Chaux A, Matloff JM, et al. Ten-year experience with the St. Jude Medical valve for primary valve replacement. *J Thorac Cardiovasc Surg* 1990;100:44.
92. Crawford FA Jr, Kratz JM, Sade RM, et al. Aortic and mitral valve replacement with the St. Jude Medical prosthesis. *Ann Surg* 1984;199:753.
93. Company Press Release, St. Jude Medical, Inc. St. Jude Medical recalling heart valve products with Silzone coating. Monday, January 24, 2000.
94. Copeland JG III. An international experience with the CarboMedics prosthetic heart valve. *J Heart Dis* 1995;4:56.
95. Beaudet RL, Poirier NL, Doyle D, et al. The Medtronic-Hall cardiac valve: 7 1/2 years' clinical experience. *Ann Thorac Surg* 1986;42:644.
96. Akins CW. Results with mechanical cardiac valvular prostheses. *Ann Thorac Surg* 1995;60:1836.
97. Hammermeister KE, Henderson WG, Burchfiel CM, et al. Comparison of outcome after valve replacement with a bioprosthesis versus a mechanical prosthesis: initial 5-year results of a randomized trial. *J Am Coll Cardiol* 1987;10:719.
98. Carpentier A, Lemaigre G, Robert L, et al. Biological factors affecting long-term results of valvular heterografts. *J Thorac Cardiovasc Surg* 1969;58:467.
99. Chaitman BR, Bonan R, Lepage G, et al. Hemodynamic evaluation of the Carpentier-Edwards porcine xenograft. *Circulation* 1979;60:1170.
100. Wernly JA, Crawford MH. Choosing a prosthetic heart valve. *Cardiol Clin* 1998;16:491.
101. Edwards TJ, Livesey SA, Simpson IA, et al. Biological valves beyond fifteen years: the Wessex experience. *Ann Thorac Surg* 1995;60:S211.
102. Bernal JM, Rabasa JM, Lopez R, et al. Durability of the Carpentier-Edwards porcine bioprosthesis: role of age and valve position. *Ann Thorac Surg* 1995;60:S248.
103. Doty JR, Flores JH, Millar RC, et al. Aortic valve replacement with Medtronic Freestyle bioprosthesis: operative technique and results. *J Card Surg* 1998;13:208.
104. O'Brien MF, Stafford EG, Gardner MA, et al. Allograft aortic valve replacement: long-term follow-up. *Ann Thorac Surg* 1995;60:S65.
104a. Ross D. Homograft replacement of the aortic valve. *Br J Surg* 1967;54(10):842–843.
105. Elkins RC, Knott-Craig CJ, Ward KE, et al. Pulmonary autograft in children: realized growth potential. *Ann Thorac Surg* 1994;57:1387.
106. Ross D. The versatile homograft and autograft valve. *Ann Thorac Surg* 1989;48:S69.
107. Hammond GL, Geha AS, Kopf GS, et al. Biological versus mechanical valves: analysis of 1,116 valves inserted in 1,012 adult patients with a 4,818 patient-year and a 5,327 valve-year follow-up. *J Thorac Cardiovasc Surg* 1987;93:182.
108. Gohlke-Barwolf C, Acar J, Oakley C, et al. Guidelines for prevention of thromboembolic events in valvular heart disease. *Eur Heart J* 1995;16:1320.
109. Burr LH, Jamieson WR, Munro AI, et al. Porcine bioprosthesis in the elderly: clinical performance by age groups and valve positions. *Ann Thorac Surg* 1995;60:264.
110. Coulshed N, Epstein EJ, McKendrick CS, et al. Systemic embolism in mitral valve disease. *Br Heart J* 1970;32:26.
111. Levine HJ, Pauker SG, Eckman MK. Antithrombotic therapy in valvular heart disease. *Chest* 1995;108:360S.
112. Edmunds LH Jr. Thromboembolic complications of current cardiac valvular prostheses. *Ann Thorac Surg* 1982;34:96.
113. Stein PD, Kantrowitz A. Antithrombotic therapy in mechanical and biological prosthetic heart valves and saphenous vein bypass grafts. *Chest* 1989;95:107S.
114. Sareli P, England MJ, Berk MR, et al. Maternal and fetal sequelae of antocoagulation during pregnancy in patients with mechanical heart valve prostheses. *Am J Cardiol* 1989;63:1462.

SURGERY: SCIENTIFIC PRINCIPLES AND PRACTICE, Third Edition, edited by Lazar J. Greenfield, Michael W. Mulholland, Keith T. Oldham, Gerald B. Zelenock, and Keith D. Lillemoe. Lippincott Williams & Wilkins Publishers, Philadelphia, © 2001.

CHAPTER 63

ISCHEMIC HEART DISEASE

GLENN J.R. WHITMAN, VERDI J. DISESA, AND JAMIE BROWN

CORONARY CIRCULATION

Coronary Arteries

The right and left coronary arteries originate from the aorta just above the aortic valve cusps (Fig. 63.1). The orifices of the two arteries within the sinuses of Valsalva designate the right and left coronary cusps. The third aortic valve cusp is referred to as the *noncoronary cusp.*

The left main coronary artery travels posterolaterally to the left behind the pulmonary artery and divides (usually within 10 mm) into two main branches, the left anterior descending (LAD) coronary artery and the left circumflex coronary artery.

The LAD coronary artery emerges from behind the pulmonary artery to course anteriorly within the interventricular groove down to the cardiac apex, sometimes wrapping around it onto the posterior interventricular groove. The initial branches of the LAD coronary artery are usually the first diagonal, which takes off at an acute angle and runs over the anterolateral surface of the left ventricle, and the first septal perforator, which emerges at a right angle from the LAD artery and penetrates the interventricular septum. The continuation of the LAD artery may give off several more diagonal and septal branches. By means of this arborization, the LAD artery nourishes the anterior, anterolateral, septal, and apical walls of the left ventricle.

The circumflex coronary artery descends posteriorly from the left main coronary and runs within the posterior atrioventricular groove. In about 80% to 85% of persons, it terminates with branches to the posterolateral wall of the left ventricle. In the remainder, it extends to the crux of the heart and gives off the posterior descending artery (PDA), which runs in the posterior interventricular groove. The usual branches of the circumflex are referred to as *obtuse marginal branches* because they cover myocardium where, as seen in the left anterior oblique projection, the lateral wall and posterior wall of the heart form an angle of more than 90 degrees.

The right coronary artery descends in the right atrioventricular groove to the crux, where in 80% to 85% of cases it gives off the PDA, occasionally continuing and terminating as posterior left ventricular branches. The right ventricular free wall is fed by acute marginal branches from the right coronary artery, which feed the heart where (as seen in the left anterior oblique projection) it forms an

A

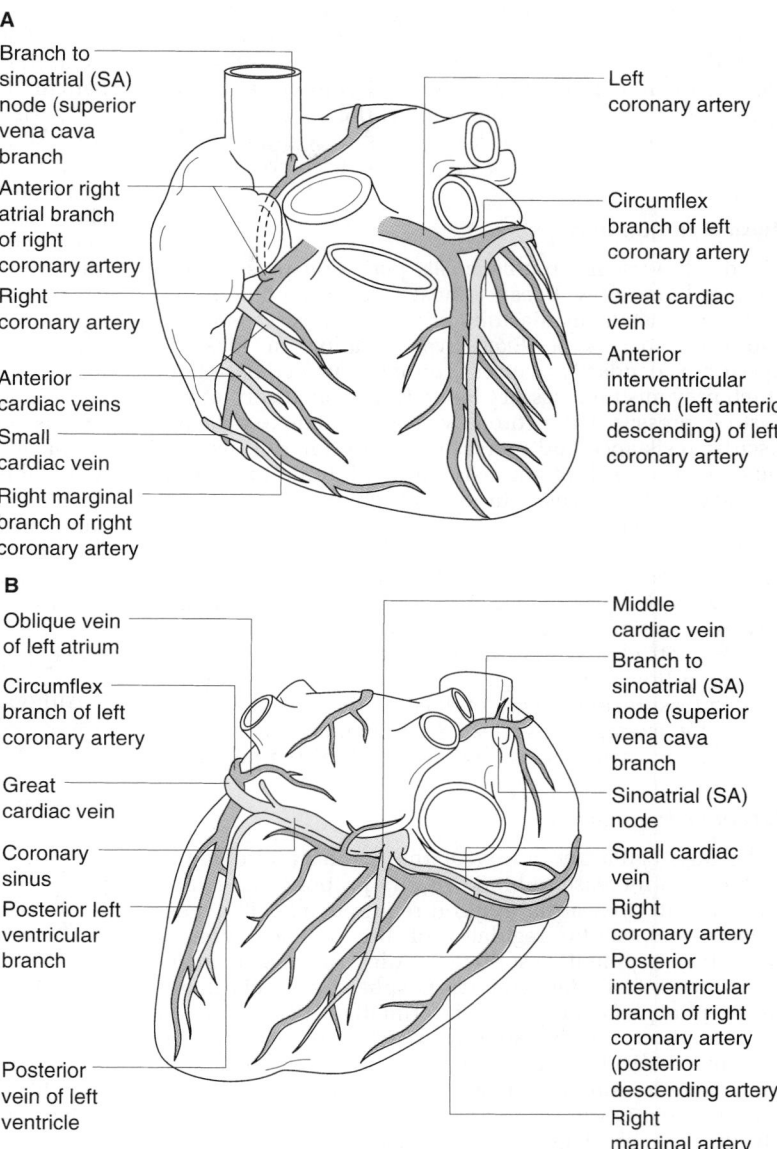

Branch to sinoatrial (SA) node (superior vena cava branch

Anterior right atrial branch of right coronary artery

Right coronary artery

Anterior cardiac veins

Small cardiac vein

Right marginal branch of right coronary artery

Left coronary artery

Circumflex branch of left coronary artery

Great cardiac vein

Anterior interventricular branch (left anterior descending) of left coronary artery

B

Oblique vein of left atrium

Circumflex branch of left coronary artery

Great cardiac vein

Coronary sinus

Posterior left ventricular branch

Posterior vein of left ventricle

Middle cardiac vein

Branch to sinoatrial (SA) node (superior vena cava branch

Sinoatrial (SA) node

Small cardiac vein

Right coronary artery

Posterior interventricular branch of right coronary artery (posterior descending artery)

Right marginal artery

Figure 63.1. Anatomy of the coronary arteries and cardiac veins. *(A)* Anterior view. The origin of the left main coronary artery is left lateral and somewhat posterior with respect to the aorta; it courses behind the pulmonary artery and then divides into the left anterior descending and circumflex coronary arteries. The origin of the right coronary artery is almost directly anterior, and it runs in the atrioventricular groove. *(B)* Posterior view. The great, middle, and small cardiac veins all come together at the level of the coronary sinus, which lies in the left inferior atrioventricular groove and empties into the right atrium.

angle of less than 90 degrees as it turns onto the diaphragm.

Whichever artery is responsible for supplying the PDA (i.e., the right coronary or left circumflex artery) determines whether the coronary circulation is *right dominant* or *left dominant.* The PDA gives off the atrioventricular nodal artery, and occlusion of this artery can result in heart block.

Cardiac Veins

The following three venous systems drain the coronary circulation:

1. The coronary sinus, located in the posterior atrioventricular groove, receives blood from the great, middle, and small cardiac veins and from the posterior veins of the left ventricle. It empties into the right atrium. The great cardiac vein ascends along the LAD artery in the interventricular groove and then turns posteriorly to follow the circumflex coronary artery to empty into the coronary sinus. The middle cardiac vein returns from the apex along the

posterior interventricular groove, and the small cardiac vein follows the right coronary artery. Both these veins empty at the level of the crux into the coronary sinus.

2. The thebesian veins are tiny venous orifices that drain the myocardium, emptying directly into any of the four chambers of the heart.

3. The anterior cardiac veins drain the right ventricular coronary system, traversing the right ventricular free wall and crossing the atrioventricular groove to empty directly into the right atrium or a correlating vein at its base.

Coronary Blood Flow

Perfusion of any organ provides oxygen and nutrients to support function. Every minute, the heart uses about 8 to 10 mL of oxygen per 100 g of myocardium. Given the fact that myocardial blood flow is 70 to 90 mL/min per 100 g and oxygen delivery is about 14 to 18 mL/min, myocardial oxygen extraction is high, and the oxygen content in the coronary sinus is only 4 to 6 mL/100 mL of blood. This corresponds to an oxygen pressure of about 20 mm Hg and a hemoglobin saturation of about 30%. Therefore, even at rest, the heart extracts oxygen maximally, and increased oxygen demand cannot be met by increased oxygen extraction. Rather, the coronary circulation has the ability to increase blood flow dramatically and must meet increased oxygen needs by increasing delivery (1).

Physical Regulation

Under the usual circumstances, perfusion pressure determines blood flow. Because most myocardial blood flow occurs in diastole, as diastolic pressure increases, so does myocardial perfusion. Excessive elevation in diastolic pressure secondarily causes coronary vasoconstriction, which prevents unnecessary blood flow. Conversely, at low diastolic pressures, the coronary arteries dilate to decrease vascular resistance and increase flow. Coronary flow may decrease as a result of coronary spasm, intramural clot, or coronary atherosclerosis. In general, clinically significant obstruction that limits flow occurs only with more than a two-thirds reduction in luminal diameter.

During systole, increased cavitary pressure compresses intramyocardial vessels and virtually eliminates forward flow. As mentioned, myocardial perfusion, particularly of the left ventricle, occurs during diastole, so that myocardial blood flow depends on coronary arterial patency, diastolic pressure, and length of diastole. That is why tachycardia, for example, can lead to ischemia, not only by increasing oxygen demand but also by limiting perfusion time.

Metabolic Regulation

The autoregulatory ability of the coronary circulation produces an increase in blood supply proportional to any increment in myocardial oxygen requirements. The most important metabolic regulator of this phenomenon is adenosine, a potent vasodilator. Adenosine is a breakdown product of adenosine triphosphate, a crucial high-energy phosphate metabolic intermediate (2). Increased myocardial oxygen demands increase adenosine triphosphate metabolism and directly cause an increase in adenosine concentration. This results in coronary vasodilation and increased oxygen delivery.

In general, prostaglandins produce decreases in coronary vascular resistance, but only thromboxane A_2 is thought to play a major role as a coronary vasoconstrictor. Thromboxane A_2 is released by platelets, particularly in the setting of angina and myocardial infarction (MI) (3).

Stimulation of the cardiac sympathetic nerves directly constricts the coronary arteries. This effect is usually overwhelmed by the autoregulatory vasodilator response to increased myocardial oxygen demand caused by sympathetic stimulation. Although acetylcholine, which is released by parasympathetic or vagal stimulation, produces coronary vasodilation directly, it lowers the heart rate and decreases contractility, so that oxygen requirements are diminished and vasoconstriction results.

CORONARY ATHEROSCLEROSIS

The Lesion

Although atherosclerotic plaques are not uniform within a person or throughout a population, certain common characteristics can be identified. In all cases, atherosclerosis represents a combination of smooth-muscle proliferation, formation by the smooth-muscle cells of tissue matrix consisting of collagen, elastin, and proteoglycans, and the accumulation of intracellular and extracellular lipid. The lesions characteristically occur within the intima, the innermost wall of the artery, and progress from benign "fatty-streak" lesions to complicated plaques.

As early as childhood, fatty-streak lesions consisting of lipid-laden macrophages and smooth-muscle cells line the arterial intima (Fig. 63.2). This process may occur in the aorta during the first decade of life, but coronary arterial lesions generally do not appear until the second or third decade of life. Fatty streaks are nonobstructive and frequently progress no further. In populations at risk, however, a whitish fibrous plaque may then develop. These lesions protrude into the arterial lumen and may obstruct. The subintimal proliferation of smooth-muscle cells is the factor most responsible for such protrusion. The fibrous surface of the lesion is the result of the buildup of connective tissue matrix and intracellular and extracellular lipid.

The advanced, complicated lesion develops from an aging fibrous plaque. The necrotic core of the plaque may enlarge and become calcified. Hemorrhage into the plaque can disrupt the smooth, fibrous surface, with resulting ulcerations that are thrombogenic. The organization of clot on the plaque surface increases the degree of protrusion into the arterial lumen and further decreases flow.

Risk Factors

Although the characteristics, locations, and severity of lesions in each person can vary, a number of established risk factors appear to predispose to atherosclerosis (4). These include advanced age, genetic predisposition, male sex, hypertension, diabetes mellitus, hyperlipidemia, and cigarette smoking. The presence of one risk factor increases the likelihood that the disease will develop at an earlier age, and the presence of more than one risk factor accelerates the process even further.

The association of aging with the development of atherosclerotic coronary disease is complex; many of the other risk factors, such as hypertension, hyperglycemia, and hyperlipidemia, are also associated with aging. Genetic factors play a major role, with direct effects on vascular endothelial biology and arterial wall structure. Indirectly, genetic factors predispose patients to risk factors with a genetic basis, such as hypertension, hyperlipidemia, and diabetes. Male sex is a well-documented major risk for the development of coronary disease. Men are three times more likely than women to have coronary disease, and angina or MI requiring treatment with bypass surgery occurs 10 years earlier in affected men than in women.

Hypertension

Although the mechanism is uncertain, high blood pressure exerts a profound influence on the development of ischemic heart disease. It has been suggested that the increase in heart stress at particular times may alter the vascular endothelium such that it is predisposed to fatty deposition and the development of plaque. The risk for coronary artery disease increases with increasing blood pressure; in middle-aged men with blood pressures higher than 160/95 mm Hg, the incidence of coronary disease is five times greater than in normotensive men. Control of hypertension decreases this risk, with the greatest benefit seen in patients whose diastolic blood pressure exceeds 105 mm Hg before treatment.

Diabetes Mellitus

A clear association is seen between diabetes mellitus and atherosclerosis. In both insulin-dependent and

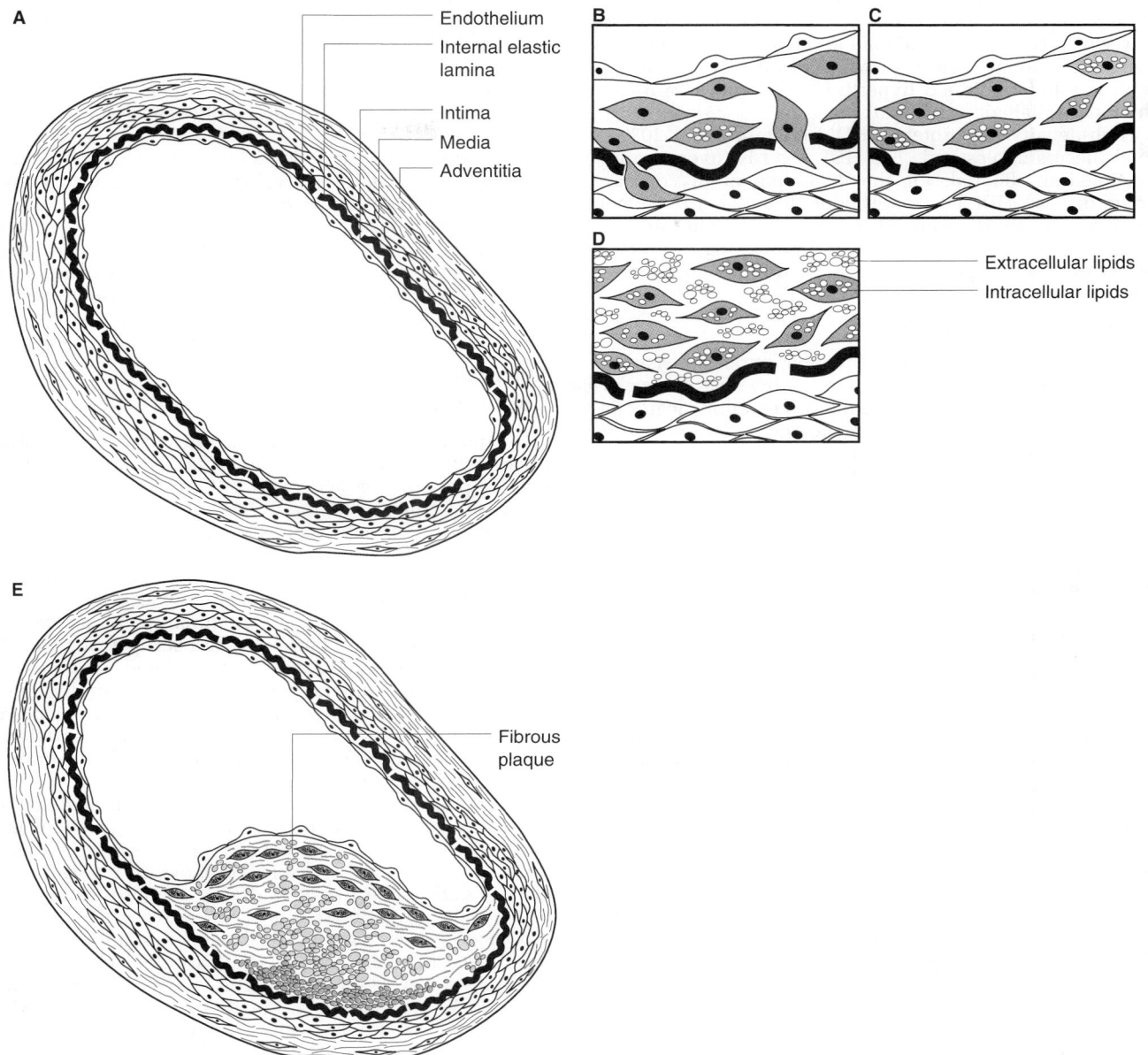

Figure 63.2. Developmental stages of the lesions of atherosclerosis. *(A)* The normal muscular artery consists of an internal intima with endothelium and internal elastic lamina. The smooth muscle of the vessel wall is in the media, and the thin adventitial layer contains connective tissue and the vasa vasorum. With age, the thickness and smooth-muscle cell content of the thin and sparsely muscled intima increase. *(B)* The first phase of an atherosclerotic lesion consists of focal thickening of the intima with smooth-muscle cells and extracellular matrix and an initial accumulation of intercellular lipid deposits. *(C)* Extracellular lipid may also develop. *(D)* Intercellular and extracellular lipid in the earliest phase is referred to as a *fatty streak*. *(E)* A fibrous plaque results as fibroblasts that cover the proliferating smooth-muscle cells laden with lipids and cell debris continue to accumulate. The lesion becomes more complex as continuing cell degeneration leads to an ingress of blood constituents and calcification. (After Glomset JA, Ross R. Atherosclerosis and the arterial smooth-muscle cells. *Science* 1973;180:1332, with permission.)

non–insulin-dependent diabetic patients, the risk for coronary artery disease is at least doubled, and the risk is even higher in patients with juvenile-onset diabetes and in diabetic women. Unfortunately, although hyperglycemia and atherosclerosis are strongly linked, rigorous control of elevated blood glucose concentrations by insulin does not appear to affect coronary mortality.

Hyperlipidemia

Both hypercholesterolemia and hypertriglyceridemia are important risk factors for coronary artery disease. The Lipid Research Clinics Trial (5) demonstrated a direct association between plasma lipoprotein levels, cholesterol levels, and morbidity and mortality from coronary artery disease. Furthermore, the risk in treated patients was decreased in direct proportion to the degree of cholesterol lowering. Hypertriglyceridemia appears to affect the incidence of coronary artery disease specifically in patients with familial combined hyperlipidemia, and accentuates the risk in diabetics and smokers.

High-density lipoproteins (HDL) contain about 20% of total plasma cholesterol. The HDL level is inversely proportional to the risk for the development of coronary artery disease. HDL levels are about 25% higher in women than in men, are raised by exercise and estrogens, and are decreased by androgens and cigarette smoking. High HDL levels offer some protection against the development of coronary artery disease.

Cigarette Smoking

Cigarette smoking is one of the most important risk factors for coronary artery disease. Smoking clearly accelerates the disease process, and smoking cessation clearly decreases the risk. In men who smoke one pack of cigarettes per day, the death rate from coronary artery disease is 70% higher and the incidence of the disease is three to five times greater than in nonsmokers. Cigarette smoking appears to potentiate other risk factors, such as hypertension and diabetes mellitus. Patients with these risk factors who also smoke manifest a severe increase in coronary artery disease mortality.

Prevention

Angina pectoris and MI are late manifestations of coronary artery disease. Because atherosclerosis, as evidenced by fatty streaks and early complicated lesions, has been found in men as early as the second decade of life, primary prevention of this disease must begin early. The importance of understanding the risk factors for coronary disease and eliminating or modifying those that can be controlled cannot be overemphasized.

Clinical Presentation

The clinical manifestations of ischemic heart disease result from an imbalance between coronary arterial blood flow, myocardial oxygen demands, and the capacity of the blood to transport oxygen. Atherosclerotic disease directly compromises coronary blood flow. When significant coronary obstructive disease is present, any of the three interrelated ischemic clinical syndromes can result—angina pectoris, MI, and ischemic cardiomyopathy.

The clinical presentation of coronary artery disease can take many forms. As many as 25% of patients who have positive results on exercise testing because of coronary occlusive disease have no clinical symptoms of typical angina pectoris. Similarly, some acute MIs are silent; patients may have electrocardiographic (ECG) or other evidence of past myocardial injury but no prior history of a clinical syndrome consistent with MI. In some patients, sudden death is the first and only manifestation of ischemic heart disease.

In another subset of patients without typical symptoms, progressive heart failure develops. Evaluation may show a diffuse loss of ventricular function associated with significant coronary obstruction. This entity is often referred to as *ischemic cardiomyopathy*. Patients who have had multiple symptomatic MIs and progress to severe heart failure resulting from the loss of ventricular muscle can be said to have ischemic cardiomyopathy.

Symptoms of Coronary Artery Disease

Symptomatic angina pectoris is the classic presentation of coronary artery disease. The typical description of angina is pressure or heaviness felt in the middle of the chest, sometimes radiating to the left shoulder and down the left arm. Patients typically clench their fists in the middle of the chest as they describe this discomfort. Other, less typical syndromes may signal the presence of significant coronary obstruction and myocardial ischemia. Patients may complain of abdominal pain, nausea, or belching. Other symptoms include back pain or pain in one or both shoulders, jaw pain, or hand heaviness or numbness. Stable angina pectoris is brought on by reproducible increases in myocardial demand for oxygen. Patients report that certain levels of activity, emotional stress, or excitement can trigger angina, which is promptly relieved by rest or relaxation.

The clinical presentations of patients with angina pectoris, therefore, vary considerably. The diagnosis of myocardial ischemia is suggested by the presence of angina pectoris but requires documentation of ECG changes of ischemia during chest pain or during exercise testing (Fig. 63.3). The differential diagnosis of angina includes esophagitis secondary to gastrointestinal reflux, peptic ulcer disease, biliary colic, visceral arterial ischemia, pericarditis, pleurisy, thoracic aortic dissection, and many musculoskeletal disorders. Furthermore, so-called angina equivalents develop in some patients with the onset of myocardial ischemia. These include shortness of breath caused by sudden reductions in ventricular contractility and compliance. Other patients have episodes of silent or asymptomatic myocardial ischemia, documented only by continuous ECG monitoring.

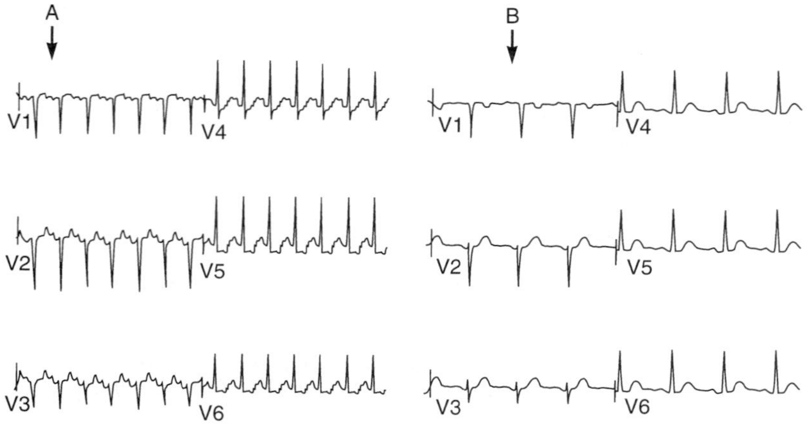

Figure 63.3. Electrocardiogram from a 60-year-old man during an exercise test showing the standard precordial leads, V_1 through V_6. *(A)* During exercise, depression of the ST segment and ischemia are seen in leads V_4 through V_6. *(B)* These resolve after exercise is stopped. (After Wagner GS. Ischemia due to increased myocardial demand. In: *Marriott's practical electrocardiography,* 9th ed. Baltimore: Williams & Wilkins, 1994, with permission.)

In unstable angina, these symptoms may occur at rest or when the patient is sleeping, and myocardial ischemia typically develops without demonstrable changes in myocardial oxygen demand. In these cases, the *supply* of blood to the myocardium may be so marginal that spontaneous coronary reactivity alone may lead to symptoms. The term *unstable angina* also is applied to patients with new-onset angina pectoris or a marked increase in the frequency or severity of episodes of angina pectoris after a stable period.

A less typical form of angina is Prinzmetal's or variant angina. This type of angina occurs at rest or during sleep. It is thought to result from coronary arterial spasm. Such spasm may be mediated by the autonomic nervous system or by local vasoconstrictive agents. It may also result from smooth-muscle irritation or contraction caused by adjacent plaques. Spasm is almost always associated with underlying fixed atherosclerotic disease. Patients may have ST-segment elevation, rather than the more typical ST-segment depression that occurs during episodes of classic angina.

Physicians often grade angina according to the Canadian Heart Association scheme. Class I patients do not have symptoms. Class II patients have angina on significant exertion. Class III patients have angina on mild exertion, and class IV patients have symptoms at rest. A similar classification from the New York Heart Association is used to describe the severity of heart failure. Patients in New York Heart Association class I have no symptoms of heart failure. Class II patients have symptoms on significant exertion. Class III patients have symptoms on mild exertion, such as during normal daily activities, and class IV patients have symptoms at rest.

Physical Examination Findings

Usually, no signs of coronary artery disease are detected during the physical examination, but evidence of associated conditions may be found. Peripheral vascular disease may be manifested by a loss of pulses or the presence of bruits in the carotid arteries, abdomen, or femoral arteries. Other signs, such as ocular xanthomas or hypertensive retinal changes, may provide corroborative evidence in patients at risk for coronary disease.

Diagnostic Studies

Laboratory studies may be useful for detecting cardiac risk factors, such as diabetes mellitus, hyperlipidemia, or hyperthyroidism. Anemia in the presence of subcritical or borderline coronary obstruction may precipitate angina; myocardial ischemia results from the reduced oxygen-carrying capacity of blood.

The ECG pattern is frequently normal but may reveal evidence of old MI. Typically, these changes include Q waves or loss of R-wave progression in the precordial leads. Chronic ST-segment and T-wave changes may be suggestive of underlying coronary disease but are not specific.

Stress testing may be useful for detecting the presence of coronary disease or assessing the functional significance of coronary lesions. In the standard test, a patient undergoes graded exercises on a treadmill with ECG monitoring. If signs or symptoms of angina pectoris develop in association with typical ischemic ECG changes, the test result is considered positive. The most diagnostic ECG changes are downward sloping ST-segment depressions. The accuracy of the test is reduced when the patient has underlying ECG abnormalities. Specificity may be improved if the test is combined with the administration of thallium. Thallium is a radioactive isotope that is distributed intracellularly,

like potassium. When thallium is injected during exercise, if coronary ischemia develops, the involved area of myocardium fails to take up thallium and a defect is apparent on a myocardial scan. As the patient recovers from exercise and the ischemia is relieved, the previous defect fills in. In patients who cannot exercise, thallium imaging can be performed after the administration of dipyridamole. Dipyridamole, a coronary vasodilator, may reveal areas of relative underperfusion, and a thallium defect appears on scanning, as with exercise testing. When exercise or the administration of dipyridamole is considered unsafe, a rest–rest thallium myocardial scan may reveal evidence of borderline regional myocardial perfusion. In this test, scanning is performed early after injection with thallium and again several hours later. A defect noted on the early scan that fills in later is considered a sign of significant coronary obstruction. A defect that never fills in on thallium scanning is a sign of irreversibly scarred, nonviable myocardium.

Coronary arteriography, which is an invasive diagnostic procedure, is the only way to make a definitive diagnosis of significant coronary obstruction. Coronary arteriography is indicated for patients with atypical presentations and borderline or normal stress test results in whom a definitive diagnosis of coronary artery disease is needed. When classic anginal symptoms and ECG changes make the diagnosis of coronary disease fairly certain, patients should not undergo coronary angiography unless they are refractory to medical therapy or are candidates for revascularization. Regardless of symptoms, patients suspected of having severe coronary artery disease, such as stenosis of the left main coronary artery or severe proximal three-vessel coronary disease, should undergo coronary arteriography to document their condition because of the survival benefits that accrue with revascularization. Diagnostic coronary arteriography is also indicated when cardiac surgery is being planned for patients with other cardiac disease, such as valvular heart disease, in whom concomitant coronary disease is suspected. Examples include patients with aortic stenosis who have angina as part of the presentation. Patients with valvular heart disease who do not have angina but nonetheless have risk factors for coronary disease should also undergo angiography before surgery. These include men older than 45 to 50 years with one or more risk factors for coronary disease.

Medical Management

The medical management of coronary artery disease includes the identification and reduction of controllable risk factors. Obviously, patients can do little about a genetic predisposition for the development of coronary obstructions. Control of risk factors by weight reduction, smoking cessation, blood pressure control, and limitation of dietary fats is sensible. Patients with hyperthyroidism or anemia, which may exacerbate anginal symptoms, should have these underlying conditions corrected.

The goal of all therapy for angina pectoris is to decrease the imbalance between the myocardial oxygen supply and demand. Most of the medications that are useful in angina pectoris are more effective in reducing myocardial oxygen demand than in increasing supply. *Nitroglycerin,* one of the most commonly used agents, primarily dilates venous capacitance vessels, but at higher doses, it may also cause systemic arterial dilation. Although nitrate compounds do not appear to increase coronary blood flow in the normal heart, these drugs may dilate the coronary arterioles to some extent, so that coronary collateral blood flow improves in patients with extensive atherosclerotic obstructive disease. The primary benefit of nitrates, however, appears to be that they reduce myocardial oxygen demand by reducing ventricular work. This is the consequence of a reduction in systemic vascular resistance and dilation of venous capacitance vessels, which lowers ventricular filling pressures, ventricular wall stress or tension, and contractile work.

β-*Adrenergic blockers* also reduce myocardial oxygen demand by decreasing both cardiac contractility and heart rate. These agents may also reduce blood pressure and systemic vascular resistance, and so further reduce the work of the heart. *Calcium channel blockers,* such as nifedipine and diltiazem, have more complex cardiac and vascular effects; these include a reduction in ventricular contractility, variable degrees of vasodilation, and possibly a direct protection of myocytes when these cells become hypoxic. Calcium channel blockers may be particularly effective in patients with a component of coronary vasospastic disease.

ACUTE MYOCARDIAL INFARCTION

Acute MI is the direct result of an interruption in the blood supply to the myocardium. It is not the result of increased myocardial oxygen demand, but rather of loss of oxygen supply. It usually occurs after a coronary artery thrombosis at the site of a significant stenosis over a complicated plaque. The clot may form as a result of plaque rupture or hemorrhage that incites thrombus formation, or it may be secondary to coronary spasm, which further reduces luminal diameter, markedly decreases flow, and leads to thrombosis. Although the acute event associated with MI is thrombosis, studies in which cardiac catheterization was used have shown that about 20% to 30% of culprit coronary arteries are patent again within a few days of infarction. This is more common in nontransmural than in transmural MIs (6).

One major determinant of the prognosis after acute MI is the amount of ventricular myocardium that undergoes necrosis. For post-MI patients with ejection fractions of more than 50%, the 3-year survival is nearly 90%, but when the ejection fraction falls below 37%, the 3-year survival rate is only 50% (Fig. 63.4). The loss of 25% of the ventricular myocardium leads to symptomatic cardiac dysfunction, whereas the acute loss of more than 40% is frequently associated with cardiogenic shock and death. Efforts to treat patients who are experiencing MI are therefore focused on decreasing myocardial loss by improving flow to the area at risk as quickly as possible. Interestingly, collateral vessels, although unable to meet myocardial oxygen requirements completely, may supply enough blood to

limit markedly the amount of myocardium lost. Thus, although well-developed collaterals may not prevent demand-induced angina, they may significantly diminish the loss of myocardium after an acute coronary occlusion.

Presentation

Pain is the most common presenting complaint in patients with MI. It is deep, visceral, and frequently described as heavy or crushing. However, pain is by no means universally present, and 20% to 25% of patients (most often diabetic or elderly patients) do not have symptoms. The combination of substernal chest pain lasting for more than 20 to 30 minutes and diaphoresis is strongly suggestive of MI. Interestingly, anterior MIs (usually involving the LAD coronary artery) result in sympathetic hyperactivity, with tachycardia and hypertension, whereas inferior MIs (involving the right coronary artery) frequently result in parasympathetic activity, with bradycardia and hypotension.

Diagnosis

The classic ECG picture of an acute MI is the development of Q waves and elevated, coved ST segments in leads reflecting the affected area (Fig. 63.5). Clinicians frequently characterize MIs by the associated ECG changes. Transmural infarctions usually cause Q waves, whereas subendocardial or nontransmural infarctions are characterized by transient ST-segment changes and evolving T-wave inversion, but not the development of Q waves. MIs are frequently referred to by these ECG changes and are called either *Q-wave* (transmural) or *non–Q-wave* (nontransmural or subendocardial) *infarctions.*

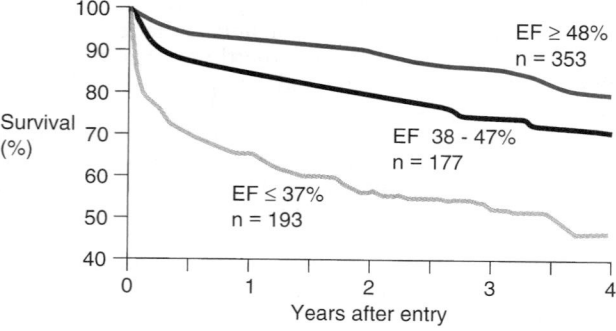

Figure 63.4. Survival of patients in the Multicenter Investigation on Limitation of Infarct Size. The probability of survival is reduced in patients with a poor ejection fraction at the time of admission for a myocardial infarction. (After Braunwald E. *Circulation* 1987;76[Suppl II]:406, with permission.)

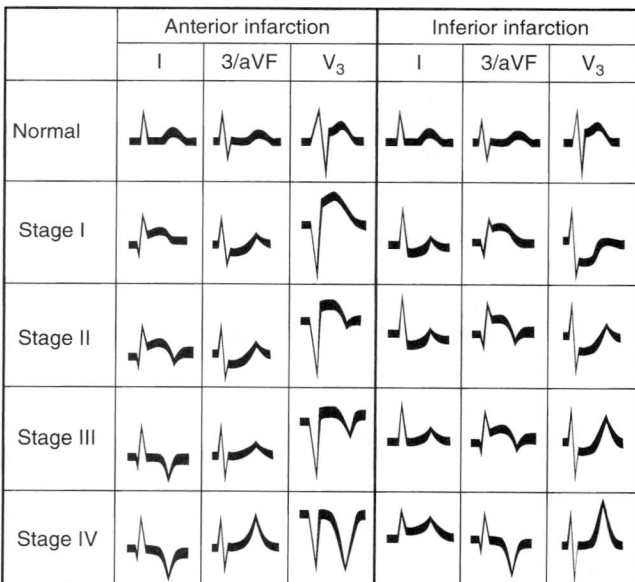

Figure 63.5. The pattern of evolution of the electrocardiogram in acute myocardial infarction. In the first stage, acute ST elevations are present in the leads reflecting the affected area of myocardium. Reciprocal ST depressions are seen in leads away from the site of the infarct. In stage 2, T-wave inversion begins, which deepens in stage 3. ST-segment elevations are no longer present. A Q wave may develop early, but Q waves are present by stage 4, and persistent T-wave inversions, which may be deep, are seen. (After Marriott HJL. Myocardial infarction. In: *Practical electrocardiography,* 7th ed. Baltimore: Williams & Wilkins, 1983:379, with permission.)

After MI, enzymes are released by necrotic myocytes in large enough quantities to be detected in the serum. As a result, enzyme elevations have become the sine qua non of the diagnosis of MI. In particular, serum levels of creatine kinase, a cardiac enzyme involved in high-energy phosphate metabolism, are increased after myocardial cell death and rise substantially within 8 to 24 hours, returning to normal within 1 to 2 days. Creatine kinase has several tissue-specific isoenzymes; the isoenzyme found specifically in cardiac tissue is denoted as CK-MB. Because creatine kinase is found in brain (CK-BB) and muscle (CK-MM) and can rise significantly after stroke, surgery, cardiac catheterization, or simply an intramuscular injection, it is crucial to measure the specific isoenzyme CK-MB when ruling out MI. Characteristic elevations of CK-MB occur in 95% of patients with clinically proven MI.

Medical Management

During the early phase of MI, it may not be clear whether the patient has unstable preinfarction angina or whether the symptoms indicate a process leading to irreversible myocardial injury. The ECG may be unrevealing, and cardiac isoenzymes may be unavailable. In this situation, oxygen should be administered, heart rhythm should be monitored, and lidocaine should be given to prevent ventricular fibrillation if warning arrhythmias occur. *Early evolving MI* is the term used to describe the condition of patients within 4 to 6 hours after the onset of continued chest pain. This state is important to recognize because ischemic myocardium may still be salvaged before irreversible necrosis develops.

The goal of initial treatment should be to control pain, most frequently with intravenous morphine. Reducing anxiety and pain may have a significant therapeutic effect by decreasing myocardial oxygen demand and limiting infarct size. Intravenous nitroglycerin, begun at a low dose of 0.2 mg/kg per minute to prevent the side effects of hypotension and headache, may diminish infarct size, prevent sudden death, and reduce the likelihood of congestive heart failure (7). The use of beta blockers is not uniformly agreed on, although they too have been shown to limit infarct size and decrease early mortality (8). Hypotension and bradyarrhythmias occur more frequently with beta blockers than with intravenous nitroglycerin. Giving them to patients with acute MI who have increased sympathetic tone, however, is probably a safe and beneficial practice. Unlike beta blockers, calcium channel blockers are of little benefit in the setting of acute MI (9).

Thrombolytic agents convert plasminogen to plasmin, a powerful thrombolysin. It was hypothesized that administration of thrombolytic agents would lead to the dissolution of coronary thrombi and reverse the process that leads to MI. In the late 1970s, a European trial of one thrombolytic agent, streptokinase, revealed a significant benefit when the drug was given within 12 hours of acute MI (10). Thrombolytic trials in the 1980s involving thousands of patients established the benefit of this approach, showing that thrombolysis reopens acutely occluded coronary arteries in most cases, restoring flow and reducing mortality (11).

Although initial thrombolytic trials involved intracoronary administration of the drugs, the cumbersome necessity for emergency cardiac catheterization led to investigations of systemic intravenous administration, which allows virtually immediate therapy in the setting of acute MI. Three intravenous thrombolytic agents have been approved by the Food and Drug Administration: streptokinase, recombinant tissue-type plasminogen activator (rTPA), and anisoylated plasminogen streptokinase activa-

tor complex (APSAC). The most widely used is streptokinase, which has been effective in several large trials (12) and is inexpensive. APSAC was developed to enable treating physicians to administer intravenous therapy as a bolus within a few minutes, with the effect maintained for a few hours, rather than as a continuous intravenous infusion, which is necessary with streptokinase and rTPA. However, results are not significantly better than with the other two drugs; furthermore, APSAC is expensive, and its prolonged half-life and thrombolytic effect can be a significant drawback rather than a benefit. Recombinant DNA techniques are used to produce rTPA, which is significantly more expensive than streptokinase. Although it generates less of a systemic fibrinolytic effect than either streptokinase or APSAC, its patency rates are higher (13).

Systemic intravenous thrombolytic therapy unquestionably decreases morbidity and mortality after MI. The earlier the treatment, the greater the impact, with the greatest benefit accruing in patients treated within 1 to 2 hours after the onset of symptoms (14). Furthermore, morbidity is decreased secondary to a reduction in arrhythmias and failure of ventricular power. Heparin and antiplatelet drugs such as aspirin provide an added benefit when combined with thrombolytic therapy, particularly in the case of rTPA, which has a short half-life and little antithrombin effect because it does not generate excessive amounts of fibrin degradation products.

Complications of thrombolytic therapy include allergic reactions in patients exposed to streptococci or streptokinase in the previous year; reactions occur in fewer than 2% of patients. Hemorrhage is a major problem with all lytic agents, commonly developing at a site of vascular access. Stroke occurs in fewer than 1% of patients but may be catastrophic because of its hemorrhagic nature. Bleeding and stroke occur most frequently in elderly, female, hypertensive, and small patients.

Indications for Mechanical Intervention

The use of thrombolytic therapy with early recanalization of the culprit vessel responsible for the MI has had a tremendous impact on the treatment and prognosis of patients experiencing acute MI. The issue then becomes whether anything more need be done acutely; despite reperfusion, significant residual stenoses remain. The Thrombolysis in Myocardial Infarction phase II trial compared elective catheterization and percutaneous transluminal coronary angioplasty (PTCA) within the first 2 days of lytic therapy for MI versus cardiac catheterization and PTCA only if ischemia developed later in the hospital course (15). The more invasive approach failed to provide a benefit with respect to early or late mortality and, in fact, increased risk significantly. Based on the results of this and other trials, cardiac catheterization and PTCA should be withheld in most patients who have no symptoms after thrombolytic therapy for an acute MI. A more invasive approach is justified in patients who exhibit residual ischemia during their hospital stay, either during convalescence or at a predischarge exercise stress test. PTCA may be appropriate, but if cardiac catheterization shows coronary artery disease in multiple vessels or anatomy more suitable for bypass than for PTCA, surgery should be carried out. The early and long-term results in patients operated on within 30 days of acute MI are excellent (16).

Postinfarction Angina

Chest pain recurs in 10% to 15% of patients after acute MI, a frequency that increases dramatically if thrombolytic therapy is used. In that situation, the incidence of angina after MI may be as high as 30% to 35%. Postinfarction angina is an indication that myocardial cells are ischemic, and it often occurs when a patient is at rest. This generally indicates that residual myocardial tissue at risk for infarct extension, a complication that can and should be avoided. After MI, the mortality rate may increase by 15% to as much as 40% if infarct extension occurs (17). In fact, infarct extension may be the most powerful predictor of mortality after MI; the average 1-year mortality increases from about 18% to 65% if infarct extension occurs. Thus, postinfarction angina is an indication for cardiac catheterization, with mechanical intervention, such as PTCA or coronary bypass surgery, if indicated. This is particularly relevant because the mortality rate associated with coronary bypass surgery after MI is extremely low, less than 4% in most advanced centers (16).

Cardiogenic Shock

The development of cardiogenic shock after MI is uncommon. In the multicenter investigation for the limitation of infarct size, cardiogenic shock developed in only 60 of 845 patients with acute MI (18). That group had a 65% mortality rate, whereas in the group in which shock did not develop, the mortality rate was only 4%. Infarct extension occurred in 23% of the shock group, and in 7% of the group without shock. More importantly, in 50% of patients, shock developed more than 24 hours after admission. Evaluation of these patients revealed that age above 65 years, ejection fraction below 35% on admission, a large MI as indicated by the magnitude of the CK-MB leak, a history of diabetes mellitus, and a history of previous MI are all risk factors for the development of shock. When three of these risk factors were present, the in-hospital mortality rate was 18%; when all five risk factors were present, the in-hospital mortality rate was 55% (18).

Animal studies have shown that even in the face of prolonged regional myocardial ischemia, intervention with emergency revascularization may decrease the amount of damage sustained by the myocardium. These studies have focused on ways to decrease energy expenditure during early reperfusion and ways to tailor the initial reperfusate so as to decrease cellular swelling, provide intermediary cellular metabolic substrates, and decrease oxidant injury. In this way, myocardial damage resulting from an ischemic insult can be drastically reduced (19). A prospective study has evaluated the effect on mortality of emergency coronary bypass surgery in patients in cardiogenic shock after MI (20). Emergency coronary bypass was performed on 80 consecutive patients in cardiogenic shock who were being maintained on vasopressors and intraaortic balloon pumps after MI. When surgery was performed within 18 hours of the onset of shock, the mortality rate was 7%; when surgery was performed after 18 hours, the mortality rate was 31%. This represents a definite improvement over the results of medical therapy (65% mortality) for this severe complication of MI. In centers capable of performing surgery of this kind, it may be the ideal approach to patients in shock after MI. These results, which have not been duplicated by other institutions, must be viewed as preliminary.

Ventricular Septal Defect

Ventricular septal defects occur in about 2% of patients after MI. In general, this complication develops at a time when the myocardium is at its weakest, about 3 to 5 days after MI. It is more common in anterior than in posterior MIs, and with medical treatment the associated mortality rate is more than 90%. At greatest risk for the development of this complication are elderly hypertensive women

with transmural infarction. Clinically, hypotension develops with congestive heart failure. Emergency cardiac catheterization reveals an oxygen step-up in the right ventricle, indicating a left-to-right shunt. Medical therapy involves decreasing the afterload as much as possible; an intraaortic balloon pump is invariably used, in addition to vasodilator therapy if possible. The preload is optimized, and surgery should be performed immediately. Previous approaches involved the stabilization of patients for a prolonged period in the hope that the infarcted area of myocardium would become firmer and hold sutures better. During the 3 weeks that were generally allowed for this process, however, irreversible failure of multiple organ systems frequently developed as a result of shock and sepsis. Early operation before complications occur appears to carry a much better survival rate. Surgical opinion now favors early intervention for this complication (21).

Acute Mitral Regurgitation

Papillary muscle rupture with acute mitral regurgitation occurs infrequently, in fewer than 2% of patients. Like ventricular septal defect, it develops between the third and fifth days, when infarcted myocardium is at its weakest. Posteroinferior MIs lead to this complication more frequently than anterior infarctions, almost certainly because the circumflex artery and PDA provide the most crucial blood supply to the papillary muscles. Clinically, this complication can present with signs and symptoms similar to those of a ventricular septal defect. A new murmur and symptoms of congestive heart failure with hypotension develop. The pulmonary capillary wedge pressure tracing, however, shows prominent V waves, and no right ventricular oxygen step-up occurs. Immediate medical therapy involves decreasing the afterload with an intraaortic balloon pump. Surgery, although it poses an added risk, leads to a better survival than continued medical therapy and decreases the mortality from more than 90% to less than 50%. Evidence has shown that if total mitral valve excision can be avoided and all or part of the subvalvular mitral apparatus saved, the mortality rate can be decreased even further, from 20% with mitral valve replacement to 5% if the mitral valve apparatus is preserved with either repair or replacement. Long-term survival is also improved. In one series, the 4-year survival rate was 89% in the group of patients in whom the mitral apparatus was conserved; it was 59% in the group of patients who underwent mitral valve replacement with total excision of the native valve (22).

Free Wall Rupture

Ventricular free wall rupture after MI occurs also at a time when the myocardium is at its weakest, between the third and sixth days after infarction. The incidence is not well known, but the medical mortality rate is exceedingly high (> than 90%). The benefits of surgical intervention are undocumented. A variety of case reports cite the dramatic rescue of some patients, but circumstances must be ideal. The free wall rupture must be small and contained, so that time is available for diagnosis and operative intervention. Most commonly, free wall rupture leads to death. In some cases, it is contained and may go unrecognized until a pseudoaneurysm develops, which is diagnosed at a later date.

MECHANICAL INTERVENTIONS

Catheter-based Coronary Revascularization

Percutaneous transluminal coronary angioplasty is a cardiac catheterization technique designed to reduce the degree of myocardial obstruction and improve regional coronary blood flow. In the mid-1970s, Gruentzig and Hoff designed a balloon dilation catheter for use in the coronary arteries and initiated this important treatment option for patients with ischemic heart disease. PTCA is performed in a standard cardiac catheterization laboratory. The technique is similar to coronary angiography. Under fluoroscopic guidance, a catheter is directed into the coronary artery to be treated. A guide wire is then placed across the obstructing lesion. A balloon catheter is passed over the guide wire and the balloon positioned in the midportion of the obstructing lesion. Under fluoroscopic control, the balloon is inflated to a pressure of 4 to 10 atmospheres for 20 to 60 seconds to reduce the degree of coronary obstruction. Balloon inflation may be repeated several times. It is unclear whether the beneficial effect of this treatment is compression or fracture of the plaque or fracture of the more pliable part of the coronary vessel circumference. After the balloon catheter is withdrawn, coronary angiography is undertaken immediately to assess the degree of dilation and to look for dilation-related complications, such as arterial dissection or acute thrombosis. Since the first successful coronary angioplasty was reported in 1977, the number of PTCA procedures has increased dramatically, to more than 400,000 cases per year in the United States.

In addition to transluminal angioplasty, several other techniques have been developed that can be applied in percutaneous catheter-based systems. These include the placement of intracoronary stents, which are wire mesh cylinders similar in design to the stents placed in other locations, including stenotic major vessels. The systems have been miniaturized so that they can be deployed in the coronary system. The results of initial, nonrandomized studies are encouraging in regard to rates of acute thrombosis and stent failure. Stents appear to be more effective for treating coronary dissections and abrupt vessel closures in the catheterization laboratory. On a long-term basis, the rates of restenosis appear to be lower with stents than with balloon angioplasty. Their long-term benefits are being evaluated. Atherectomy devices are useful in severely calcified coronary lesions in which inflation of a balloon is not effective. These are similar to high-speed rotating drill bits and literally drill a hole through obstructed and calcified coronary lesions over a guide wire. Multiple lasers have been developed for use in coronary revascularization. The results have been extremely varied to date, and as of yet, no laser has been accepted as a standard of care.

Indications

The indications for PTCA are the same as those for coronary artery bypass surgery, the main alternative revascularization technique. Patients with intractable symptoms and those with proximal coronary stenoses that place a large amount of myocardium at risk are potential candidates for angioplasty. The ideal lesion for angioplasty is a symmetric focal stenosis in an epicardial vessel. Long, asymmetric stenoses or those adjacent to bends in the artery or branch points are less likely to be treated successfully. In general, PTCA is contraindicated if significant disease is present in the left main coronary artery, the target coronary artery is less then 2 mm in luminal diameter, multiple significant obstructive lesions are present in the same artery, or the obstructive lesions are complex, such as those involving or straddling arterial bifurcations.

Complications

The primary risk of angioplasty is dissection of the coronary vessel with acute closure. This occurs in about 3% of cases and usually requires emergency coronary bypass surgery (23). MI may result but can be aborted by immediate surgical revascularization. Other risks are similar to those of coronary angiography and include cerebral vascular accident and local arterial trauma. Improvements in balloon catheter design and fabrication have enhanced the success rate of PTCA and made it possible to achieve more extensive dilation in patients with multiple-vessel or complex coronary artery disease. Also under development are atherectomy catheters, which incorporate tiny rotating blades to lyse atheromatous plaque, and catheters with laser tips, which vaporize intraluminal obstructions. Newer investigational devices also include coronary stents. These small, implantable, cylindric devices are designed to maintain patency of diseased arteries when more conventional balloon angioplasty is ineffective.

Results

Successful primary dilation of favorable coronary arterial obstructive lesions is accomplished in more than 90% of PTCA procedures, with an immediate complication rate of about 3%. The most significant long-term problem with PTCA is the high incidence of restenosis. Restenosis is probably the result of postdilation proliferation of intimal and smooth-muscle cells in response to the angioplasty. Restenosis rates of between 20% and 40% within the first 4 to 6 months after PTCA have been reported in patients with initially successful dilation for simple lesions (24). Restenosis rates as high as 60% have been reported for patients with complex lesions that required multiple dilations. Although redilation of recurrent stenotic lesions can be carried out successfully, many of these patients ultimately require bypass grafting.

In the 1990s, several large, randomized trials were completed that compared balloon angioplasty with coronary artery bypass surgery in the treatment of multiple-vessel coronary artery disease (24–32). As in most large, randomized clinical studies, large numbers of patients were screened, and a relative minority fulfilled the criteria for enrollment. In other words, the final patient cohort was highly selected. Nonetheless, the overall results of half a dozen of these studies in several thousand patients indicate that short- and intermediate-term results for angioplasty and surgery are similar. Mortality rates were the same for the two procedures, although patients treated with angioplasty tended to be discharged from the hospital sooner. Patients who underwent angioplasty also had a higher rates of repeated intervention and crossover to surgical intervention. In several subgroup analyses, patients with diabetes appeared to be treated best with coronary bypass grafting (29–31). Although initial reports of the use of stents, lasers, and atherectomy devices are encouraging, the results of large, randomized trials are still pending. Furthermore, even in single-vessel disease, including proximal high-grade LAD artery disease, it appears that intervention of some kind, whether revascularization by catheter-based techniques or by coronary artery bypass surgery, improves long-term outcomes (32).

Coronary Artery Bypass Surgery

Coronary artery bypass grafting (CABG) is among the most commonly applied major surgical operations in the United States, with more than 250,000 procedures performed yearly. The goals of CABG are identical to the goals of medical treatment and PTCA—to treat ischemic heart disease by relieving the imbalance of myocardial oxygen supply and demand. The indications for CABG versus medical treatment or PTCA in an individual patient may be controversial. Choosing the optimal therapy for a given patient necessitates weighing variables, such as the pattern of coronary artery obstruction, ventricular function, severity of symptoms, initial response to medical therapy, and presence of noncardiac disease. Patients require individual evaluation to determine the potential short- and long-term benefits of surgical revascularization versus medical treatment or less invasive angioplasty (25).

Indications

Patients are said to have *single-, double-,* or *triple-vessel* disease if significant atherosclerotic narrowing is present in one, two, or all three of the major arteries (i.e., LAD, circumflex, and right coronary arteries). In general, data from clinical trials and retrospective studies suggest that as the number of diseased major coronary arterial segments increases, the survival benefit of surgical therapy over medical therapy alone becomes greater (Table 63.1). This observation in general terms has been borne out by the three major prospective, randomized coronary bypass studies—the Coronary Artery Surgery Study (CASS) (34), the Veterans Administration Cooperative Study (51), and a European report (52) (see below). In patients with stable angina, the presence of severe, proximal, triple-vessel disease, especially in those with impaired left ventricular function, generally is an indication for surgical revascularization.

Another well-accepted indication for CABG is the presence of significant stenosis of the left main coronary artery (53). Both the Veterans Administration Cooperative Study (51) and the CASS (34) provide overwhelming evidence for improved survival with surgical treatment in patients with left main artery disease. Most cardiologists and cardiac surgeons also believe a surgical benefit exists for patients with normal or depressed left ventricular function and two-vessel disease associated with a high-grade proximal obstruction of the LAD artery (52). On the other hand, the need for surgery in patients with single- or double-vessel disease, without disabling symptoms or LAD artery involvement, has not been clearly established (31).

Above all, the most common indication for CABG continues to be the relief of disabling angina refractory to medical therapy. Bypass surgery reduces or eliminates angina in more than 90% of patients, and those patients with the most severe anginal syndromes derive the greatest benefit. The randomized studies (34,51,52) have provided strong evidence that CABG is more effective than medical treatment in relieving angina and improving the capacity for physical work and overall quality of life. Finally, the survival of patients with silent ischemia (i.e., patients without symptoms who have significant atherosclerotic disease and myocardial ischemia demonstrated by ECG changes, exercise stress testing, and coronary angiography) is improved after CABG.

Table 63.1. INDICATIONS FOR CORONARY BYPASS SURGERY

Anatomy
Left main coronary artery disease (53)
Triple-vessel disease involving the proximal left anterior descending coronary artery with normal or diminished ejection fraction
Double-vessel disease involving the proximal left anterior descending coronary artery with normal or diminished ejection fraction

Symptoms
Unstable (crescendo) angina
Postmyocardial infarction angina
Acute coronary occlusion after percutaneous transluminal coronary angioplasty
Symptoms unsuccessfully controlled with medical therapy
Controlled symptoms, but with unacceptable life-style

Patients with unstable angina are a heterogeneous group. In general, the occurrence of unstable (or crescendo) angina suggests that the patient is at risk for MI and death. These patients require aggressive medical therapy, including nitrates, β-adrenergic blockers, and calcium antagonists, in addition to heparin anticoagulation to forestall coronary arterial thrombosis. If the patient continues to experience unstable or rest angina despite maximal medical treatment, urgent coronary angiography is indicated in preparation for PTCA or surgery (31). Collective outcome data from several series of patients with unstable angina who underwent surgical revascularization demonstrated increased rates of perioperative MI, postoperative low cardiac output, and death in comparison with patients who underwent CABG for chronic stable angina. Nonetheless, patients with unstable angina had *late* outcomes after CABG similar to those of patients with chronic stable angina; relief of angina was excellent, the late MI rate was low, and, most importantly, long-term survival was similar.

Although the role of CABG in the setting of acute MI is not unequivocal, the development of recurrent angina early after infarction has become an accepted indication for operative intervention. These patients are at risk for infarct extension or for a second infarction. Even mild postinfarction angina mandates an aggressive response, with coronary angiography and consideration of revascularization (see above).

As mentioned, emergency CABG is necessary in the approximately 3% of patients in whom coronary occlusive complications develop during PTCA (23). Most of these occlusions result from coronary dissections proximal or distal to the site of dilation. Emergency CABG is indicated as soon as it is apparent that an acute coronary occlusion has developed, an event heralded by the onset of chest pain, ECG changes, and often hemodynamic instability. It is usually possible to verify the presence and nature of the acute coronary occlusion by immediate repeated coronary angiography, which allows the diagnosis to be confirmed.

In most cases of an evolving MI, the ischemic injury is somewhat attenuated and hemodynamic stability is better if intraaortic balloon counterpulsation is established promptly in the catheterization laboratory before the patient is transported to the operating room. If severe hemodynamic instability develops despite balloon pump support, portable cardiopulmonary bypass perfusion with femoral arterial and venous cannulation may provide sufficient stabilization so that the patient can be transported to the operating room. In general, these patients should be placed on cardiopulmonary bypass as quickly as possible to initiate cardioplegic arrest and myocardial cooling and prevent further extension of the infarction.

Standard Surgical Technique

In coronary artery surgery, the diseased coronary artery is bypassed by creating an alternative conduit to deliver blood beyond the coronary stenosis. Grafts are constructed by making an end-to-side anastomosis to the coronary artery distal to the obstruction. The proximal end of a vein graft is usually sutured end-to-side to the ascending aorta. When the aorta is diseased, the origin of the innominate artery is sometimes used. The vein most commonly used as a graft is the greater saphenous vein, although the lesser saphenous vein is sometimes employed. The cephalic vein from the arm may be used, but its long-term patency is extremely poor.

The use of arterial grafts has increased. The most commonly used arterial graft is the left internal mammary artery (IMA). It is used most often as a pedicle graft, with its origin at the subclavian artery retained. The distal end is anastomosed end-to-side to the coronary artery. The artery most commonly grafted with the left IMA is the left anterior descending coronary artery. When multiple arterial grafts are desired, the right IMA can be used either as a pedicle graft or as a free graft, with the proximal anastomosis made on the ascending aorta. More limited use has been made of the gastroepiploic artery, the radial artery, and the inferior epigastric artery. The main benefit of these arterial grafts is improved long-term patency. The actuarial probability of vein graft patency at 10 years is 50%. In contrast, the probability that the left IMA will be patent at 10 years is 90% to 95%. Also, evidence suggests that early mortality is reduced when at least one mammary artery graft is used.

To construct accurate anastomoses, a quiet, bloodless field is created in most cases with the use of cardiopulmonary bypass and cardioplegia for the purpose of arresting the heart (Fig. 63.6). With the patient on bypass and the heart empty, the distal ascending aorta is cross-clamped, and potassium cardioplegia solution is injected into the aortic root to cause nearly instantaneous cardiac arrest. Cardioplegic solution at a temperature of 4°C to 10°C induces rapid myocardial cooling along with cardiac arrest in diastole. In addition, many surgeons apply cold saline solution directly to the surface of the heart, either intermittently or continuously, to maintain the myocardial temperature between 10°C and 15°C during aortic cross-clamping. The most important components of cardioplegia are cold and potassium (usually 15 to 20 mEq/L),

which causes depolarization of the myocardial membrane and arrest of the heart in diastole. Myocardial temperatures of 10°C to 15°C decrease the metabolic rate of the heart by 80%, and arrest lowers the metabolic rate to as little as 5% of that of the normothermic, working heart.

A number of cardioplegia solutions are available, although the ones most commonly used are based on a dilute blood solution with potassium and often other additives. Some techniques employ initial warm induction of arrest followed by cold cardioplegia. A warm dose of cardioplegia before removal of the cross-clamp has been advocated. This may be particularly useful in patients with significant preoperative ischemic insults. Warm cardioplegia reperfusion supplies oxygen and substrates while maintaining diastolic arrest with the attendant decreases in metabolic demand. Some surgeons prefer to perform the entire operation with the patient and the heart kept warm while cardioplegia is administered continuously (54). The administration of cardioplegia is more commonly antegrade, with injection of the solution into the aortic root proximal to the cross-clamp. It has been shown that the retrograde administration of cardioplegia through a cannula placed in the coronary sinus can enhance myocardial protection because significant coronary arterial stenosis may prevent the homogenous delivery of cardioplegia, a problem avoided by the retrograde approach (56–58). The combination of antegrade and retrograde cardioplegia may be optimal in some cases. The retrograde cardioplegia

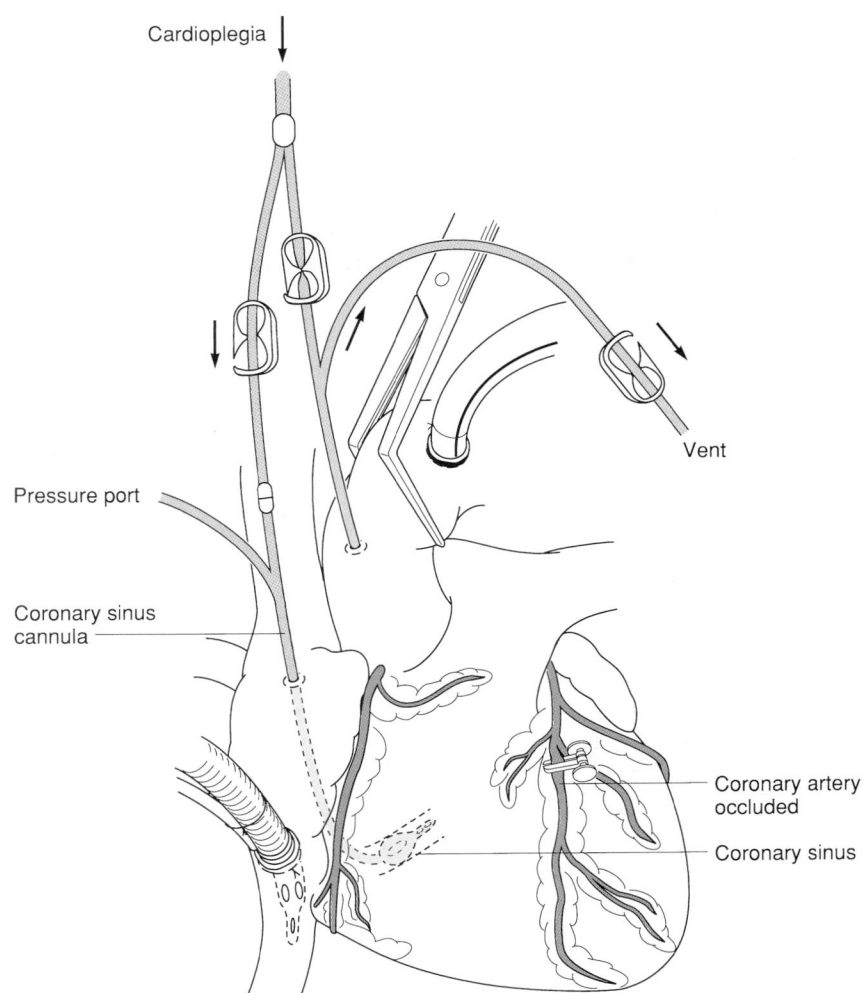

Cardioplegia

Pressure port

Coronary sinus cannula

Vent

Coronary artery occluded

Coronary sinus

Figure 63.6. Cardiac instrumentation for retrograde administration of cardioplegic solution through the coronary sinus. A catheter with an occlusive balloon tip has been placed within the coronary sinus through the right atrium. The cardioplegic solution can be administered through the coronary sinus or the aortic root (antegrade). A pressure-measuring side port on the coronary sinus catheter can be used to prevent excessive distention of the coronary venous system. (After Partington MT, et al. Studies of retrograde cardioplegia I. *J Thorac Cardiovasc Surg* 1989;97:613, with permission.)

technique is often applied in patients who have previously undergone CABG, in an effort to avoid the complication of atheromatous embolization in diseased bypass grafts (58). Retrograde cardioplegia is also helpful in the presence of significant aortic insufficiency.

Coronary artery bypass grafting is performed with the aid of optical magnification. Monofilament sutures are used by most surgeons, and specific techniques vary from a single continuous running anastomosis to multiple interrupted sutures. In addition to individual vein or mammary artery graft anastomoses to specific arterial branches, two or more distal anastomoses can be constructed from a single vein or mammary artery. These sequential grafts are especially favored when anastomoses are planned at multiple distal sites or when suitable conduit material is in short supply.

When the distal anastomoses are completed, the aortic clamp is released. After reperfusion is initiated, ventricular fibrillation often develops, but cardioversion is usually accomplished with a single, direct-current electric shock. If a partially occluding clamp is placed on the ascending aorta, the proximal aorta–saphenous vein graft anastomoses can be constructed as myocardial perfusion is maintained through the native circulation and the newly constructed mammary anastomoses (Fig. 63.7). In some cases, especially in reoperation, the proximal anastomoses are made during ischemic time with the cross-clamp still in place, so that the partially occluding clamp, which can be difficult to place and can cause atherosclerotic embolism in the presence of old grafts, is not needed.

When CABG is performed, if diffuse atherosclerotic changes are present or if the site chosen for a distal anastomosis is heavily diseased, the surgeon may need to perform an endarterectomy to allow for a more reliable graft-to-artery anastomosis. The data regarding the safety and efficacy of coronary endarterectomy are conflicting; endarterectomy sites are more prone to early thrombosis and reocclusion. Endarterectomy of the distal right coronary artery, the most common site for endarterectomy, appears to be safe and well tolerated, in part because the right coronary artery is often already nearly totally occluded.

Data comparing the long-term comparative value of endarterectomy of the LAD coronary artery versus grafting alone are not available. Endarterectomy should not be performed unless distal disease is so severe that it is necessary for distal flow. Because patients with diffuse distal disease are already likely to have a poor outcome, it has proved difficult to demonstrate a beneficial effect of coronary endarterectomy.

New and Future Techniques

In standard CABG, described above, a heart–lung machine and cardioplegia are used to achieve cardiac arrest and maintain a motionless, bloodless, operative field. Recently, the trend has been to perform CABG on the beating heart (35–46). It is ironic that the first coronary bypass procedures were performed on the beating heart. Now, however, with the development of epicardial stabilization devices and advances in technology, surgery performed on the beating heart is becoming commonplace. Kolessov (40), a Russian investigator, reported coronary bypass surgery on a beating heart in 1967, but since then, surgery on the beating heart has rarely been reported until recently. Off-pump coronary artery bypass surgery, as the name implies, is CABG performed on the beating heart. Minimal-access cardiac surgery is the use of an incision smaller than full median sternotomy for the purpose of cardiac surgery, which may include valve surgery in addition to CABG. Minimally invasive direct coronary artery bypass (MID CAB) has gained favor recently (41). Another term is *left anterior small thoracotomy* (LAST) for CABG (42,43). Clearly, the semantics and nomenclature can rapidly become confusing. To keep it simple, we refer to two separate entities. In the first, off-pump CABG, the heart–lung machine and the associated systemic inflammatory response are avoided. In the second, minimal access cardiac surgery, various incisions are used that are smaller than a standard sternotomy incision.

Off-pump heart surgery has been a recent trend. It is unclear how or why the trend began, but several factors have probably played a role. The standard technique of cardiopulmonary bypass is associated with a rate of stroke of 3% to 7%, and a temporary neurocognitive decline occurs in 65% of patients (31). Furthermore, the comorbid conditions, age, and noncardiac risk factors of patients undergoing coronary bypass grafting have been increasing in recent years. Finally, technologic advances have created devices that can be used to stabilize the epicardial surface of the heart and have advanced the wide applicability of off-pump surgery.

Cardiopulmonary bypass results in a systemic inflammatory response involving the activation of the complement system, inflammatory cytokines, monocytes, neutrophils, and platelets and the inhibition of the coagulation system (44–46). This total-body inflammatory response associated with cardiopulmonary bypass results in temporary organ dysfunction and tissue edema. Usually, these changes are inconsequential. However, if a patient is elderly or has a comorbid condition, such as severe emphysema, the cardiopulmonary bypass machine may mean the difference between a poor and a good outcome. Off-pump coronary bypass grafting is now considered appropriate for any patient with suitable anatomic features (coronary arteries of sufficient size and quality in approachable locations). Patients with preserved ventricular function and anterolateral diseased vessels requiring bypass are the best candidates. Patients who require more than three bypass grafts or intracardiac procedures, such as valve replacement, are not candidates.

The technique of off-pump coronary bypass involves stabilization of the epicardial surface with one of many

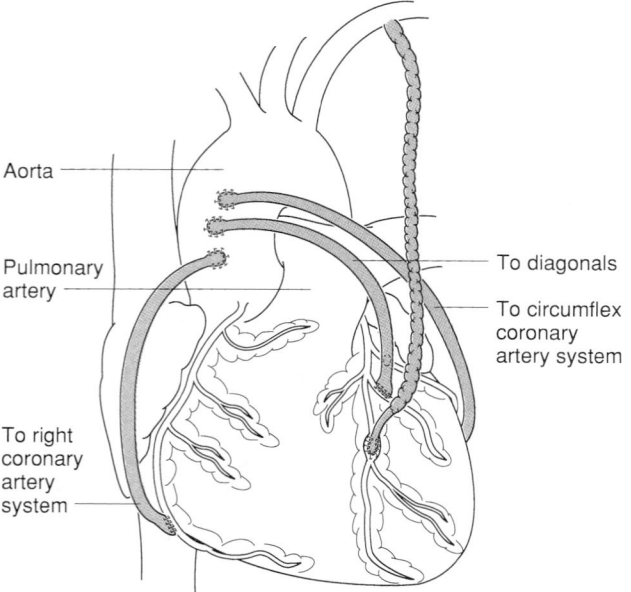

Aorta

Pulmonary artery

To right coronary artery system

To diagonals

To circumflex coronary artery system

Figure 63.7. Most patients require multiple-vessel grafting and typically have a combination of vein grafts and a mammary artery graft. The most common site for use of the left internal mammary artery is the left anterior descending artery.

devices. The devices fall into two categories—those that push and those that pull. The Octopus (Medtronic Corp.) stabilization system is used at the University of Maryland, where approximately 20% of operations are performed off-pump (Fig. 63.8). This is a suction system that latches onto the epicardial surface and stabilizes it without impinging on ventricular filling; therefore, hemodynamic parameters are maintained. Only half the dose of heparin used in conventional coronary bypass grafting is used with this system. Silastic tapes are used to encircle and occlude the coronary arteries while grafts are sewn in place. With the pericardium retracted and the apex of the heart tipped vertically, essentially all coronary arterial systems can be reached with this technique.

The outcomes for off-pump coronary bypass grafting have been excellent. Mortality rates are comparable with those of conventional CABG. The need for transfusion is reduced. Length of hospital stay is reduced by 1 to 2 days. Cost is reduced by approximately 40%. The neurocognitive decline seen after on-pump coronary bypass grafting appears to occur less often. This issue, however, is under investigation. Although complete revascularization can be performed off-pump, at present, 20% of patients referred for coronary bypass grafting are optimal candidates for this procedure. To date, results have been excellent, but longer follow-up is needed.

Minimal-access cardiac surgery has also been a recent trend (31). We are convinced that the size of the incision and whether the operation is performed on- or off-pump are two different issues, although they are often discussed together. Minimal-access incisions include partial sternotomies, small thoracotomies, and combined partial sternotomies and thoracotomies. Initial small series and reports indicate that these incisions can be used for both coronary bypass grafting and valve surgery. They appear to reduce patient discomfort and length of hospital stay. The overall risk of the procedure, however, remains the same. Minimal-access surgery has gained attention in the lay press and on the Internet. However, it is not yet accepted as standard practice.

In addition to direct procedures performed through smaller incisions, other new technologies have been applied in preliminary clinical series, such as the percutaneous institution of cardiopulmonary bypass, aortic cross-clamping, and administration of cardioplegia (the Heart-

port system) (47). Multiple institutions participated in the initial clinical trial. At present, results for the future appear promising, although it is both technically demanding and costly to institute cardiopulmonary bypass and cardiac arrest and perform the procedure percutaneously. This technique is currently considered investigational.

The use of videoscope- and robot-assisted heart surgery is under investigation (48–50). Advances in computer and robotic technologies have been used to improve image quality and reduce tremors and cardiac motion, so that it has become possible to create coronary artery anastomoses on the beating heart endoscopically. Such procedures have been demonstrated in the laboratory within a satisfactory time frame. The control console used by the surgeon can be placed at a site remote from the operative field. This technique, which is also investigational, combines the best of both worlds in that minimal-access surgery and off-pump techniques are applied together.

In summary, several new technologies and techniques for the treatment of coronary artery disease are on the horizon. Initial results, especially for off-pump surgery, appear promising. Off-pump surgery provides several advantages over the standard and well-tested technique of coronary artery bypass with use of a cardiopulmonary bypass machine. However, randomized trials demonstrating improved outcomes have not been completed to date. As always, time and careful analysis of patient outcomes will help us to choose appropriate therapies (Table 63.2).

Postoperative Management

Postoperative cardiac surgical management is based on hemodynamic monitoring in an intensive care unit setting. Arterial blood pressure, central venous pressure, pulmonary capillary wedge pressure, cardiac output, and urine output all provide valuable information regarding the adequacy of arterial circulation, tissue perfusion, and organ function, and these parameters should be followed closely. In addition, arterial blood gases, complete blood cell counts, electrolytes, and the ECG should be evaluated at regular intervals. A chest radiograph should be performed when the patient arrives in the intensive care unit to check for the position of the endotracheal tube, nasogastric tube, chest tubes, and Swan-Ganz catheter. Also, pleural effusion, pneumothorax, and mediastinal widening should be ruled out, and a follow-up chest film should be obtained 8 to 12 hours later. Mediastinal and chest tube drainage should be recorded hourly. Shed blood can be autotransfused to minimize the use of banked blood products. Patients should be weighed to assist in fluid management. In all patients, a capillary leak syndrome develops after cardiopulmonary bypass that results in fluid accumulation, and a marked increase in total body sodium with a weight gain of 5 to 10 kg is typical. After extubation, which is normally between 4 and 12 hours postoperatively, pulmonary toilet should be vigorous. Most patients who have undergone CABG can be transferred to a step-down unit on the day after surgery, where they are monitored for arrhythmias. Diuresis is begun gradually so that the weight returns to the preoperative level, and a regular diet is started. Early ambulation is desirable.

Common causes of reduced cardiac output in the early postoperative period are hypovolemia and an increase in

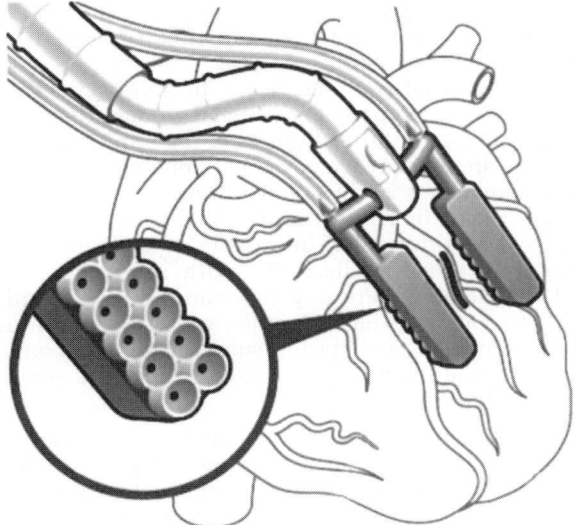

Figure 63.8. The Octopus epicardial stabilization device supplies suction to the surface of the heart and allows the surgeon to create a precise anastomosis on the beating heart.

Table 63.2. **COMPARISON OF OFF PUMP AND STANDARD CORONARY ARTERY BYPASS GRAFTING**

Cost, transfusion requirements and hospital stay are decreased by off-pump surgery T3, causes of low cardiac output.

systemic vascular resistance as a consequence of persistent hypothermia or increased circulating catecholamines. Arrhythmias, either bradycardia (secondary to resolving hypothermia), heart block (thought to be secondary to a transient but persistent effect of cardioplegia), or a supraventricular tachyarrhythmia (primarily atrial fibrillation), can also contribute to a low cardiac output. Management is more often directed at correcting such alterations than at increasing ventricular contractility. Patients are vigorously rewarmed, given adequate crystalloid or colloid solution to optimize cardiac filling pressures, and are often treated with a vasodilator, such as sodium nitroprusside, to maintain the mean blood pressure between 65 to 75 mm Hg in an effort to reduce systemic vascular resistance. Arrhythmias should be treated and bradycardia managed with atrial or atrioventricular pacing.

Low Cardiac Output. The causes of low cardiac output are listed in Table 63.3. If the calculated cardiac index is less than 2 L/min per square meter despite optimization of the heart rhythm, preload (cardiac filling pressures), and afterload (systemic vascular resistance), an inotropic agent may be indicated to enhance contractility. Poor ventricular contractility immediately after operation may be secondary to stunning from intraoperative ischemia or to preoperative ventricular dysfunction. Other correctable factors, such as poor oxygenation or persistent acidosis, may be responsible. If a low cardiac output continues after acidosis and inadequate oxygenation have been corrected, an inotropic drug is used. Appropriate first selections are β_1-agonists, such as dopamine, dobutamine, or epinephrine, a β-agonist that also has α-agonist activity.

If a postoperative patient remains in cardiogenic shock despite significant inotropic support, placement of an intraaortic balloon pump may be necessary. The balloon is inserted percutaneously into the femoral artery and positioned in the thoracic descending aorta. Balloon inflation and deflation are timed according to the ECG signals, with the balloon inflated during diastole and deflated during systole. Intraaortic balloon counterpulsation increases coronary artery perfusion because balloon inflation raises the intraaortic pressure during diastole, and active balloon deflation at the commencement of systole maximally decreases the afterload.

Rarely, if hemodynamic instability and shock continue despite the above aggressive measures, a left ventricular assist device should be considered. The cause of a persistently low cardiac output state should be pursued aggressively before this step is taken because persistent cardiac dysfunction may be a consequence of inadequate coronary revascularization, early graft occlusion, or an unrecognized intracardiac or valvular mechanical defect. Support with a left ventricular assist device is extremely labor-intensive and costly and should be considered only if myocardial failure is thought to be reversible or if the patient is a candidate for transplantation.

Table 63.3. **CAUSES OF LOW CARDIAC OUTPUT**

Inadequate preload
Excessive afterload
Poor ventricular contractility
Perioperative ischemia
Poor myocardial preservation
Arrhythmia
Severe acidosis
Tension pneumothorax
Tamponade

Bleeding. Platelet function and blood clotting factors are altered after cardiopulmonary bypass and may not normalize for up to 36 hours postoperatively. The average postoperative blood loss is 400 to 800 mL, and much of this shed blood can be reinfused. Continued bleeding at a rate faster than 200 mL/h for 4 hours or more postoperatively is considered excessive, and in these cases, specific abnormalities in coagulation should be corrected aggressively. It is simple and safe to give additional protamine to reverse residual heparin activity, but transfusion of platelets, fresh frozen plasma, or cryoprecipitate should be considered only if the results of coagulation studies indicate that they are needed. Reexploration is required if bleeding continues after correction of coagulopathy.

Tamponade. Cardiac tamponade is a potentially lethal cause of low cardiac output early after operation. Clinical features include a decreasing output in the presence of a narrowed pulse pressure, rising cardiac filling pressures, pulsus paradoxus, a widened mediastinal silhouette on chest film, and decreased urine output. These classic signs may be absent or equivocal. Sudden cessation of excessive bleeding should alert the physician to the possibility of tamponade. Transesophageal echocardiography can establish this diagnosis immediately and can assess ventricular function in addition to preload, an extremely useful parameter in treating the patient in shock.

Late cardiac tamponade can develop up to several weeks after operation and can be caused by hemopericardium or a transudative pericardial effusion. Presenting symptoms, which may be obvious but frequently are subtle, include lethargy, mild respiratory distress, nonspecific chest discomfort, fluid retention, and hepatomegaly. The diagnosis is made by echocardiography, and the tamponade nearly always can be managed successfully with either percutaneous or operative drainage.

Infection. The major wound complications after coronary artery surgery are sternal infection, dehiscence, and mediastinitis, problems that occur in 0.5% to 2% of patients. The wound infection rate is somewhat higher in patients who undergo bilateral mammary artery grafting, especially if they are elderly or diabetic. *Staphylococcus* species are the responsible organisms in most cases, and in an increasing number of these patients, the bacteria are methicillin-resistant. Risk factors associated with postoperative wound infections are a preoperative hospital stay of longer than 2 days, chronic obstructive pulmonary disease with prolonged ventilator support, the use of bilateral IMA grafts, and low cardiac output.

Sternal dehiscence and mediastinitis may occur even in the absence of an apparent superficial wound infection or drainage. Helpful clinical features of these initially occult infections are fever, elevated white blood cell count, and sternal tenderness or instability. Once the diagnosis is made, however, immediate mediastinal reexploration and aggressive débridement of infected bone and cartilage are necessary because mediastinitis with sepsis can cause rapid deterioration. Primary reclosure of the wound is sometimes possible, but it is often necessary to use pectoral or rectus muscle flaps for wound closure, not only to bring in a good blood supply but also to fill the void left by the débrided sternum.

Stroke. Cerebral vascular accident, or stroke, can be a devastating complication after bypass surgery. Stroke is usually caused by atherosclerotic emboli that frequently originate in the aorta and are loosened by cannulation, cross-clamping, or the construction of proximal anastomoses. Underlying cerebral vascular disease in conjunction with alterations in cerebral blood flow patterns resulting from cardiopulmonary bypass may also play a role. Strokes occur in 1% to 2% of low-risk patients after bypass surgery but in up to 10% of the elderly. The need to evaluate the extracranial cerebral circulation before bypass surgery is controversial. No data suggest that the investigation of asymptomatic carotid bruits and subsequent endarterectomy, if significant stenosis is found, reduce the incidence of stroke after bypass operation. In general, only symptomatic carotid stenoses should be addressed before bypass surgery. The issue of the timing of endarterectomy and CABG (i.e., whether they should be performed sequentially or as a combined procedure) is also controversial. If the carotid disease is asymptomatic, factors affecting the timing of coronary surgery usually take precedence.

Postpericardiotomy Syndrome. Postpericardiotomy syndrome is a delayed pericardial inflammatory reaction characterized by fever, anterior chest pain, and a pericardial friction rub. It occurs in up to 30% of cardiac surgery patients postoperatively. The syndrome is associated with the development of pericardial effusions, which rarely lead to cardiac tamponade. In addition, postpericardiotomy syndrome can result in mediastinal fibrosis and premature graft closure. Treatment with nonsteroidal antiinflammatory agents for 2 weeks or more usually eliminates the symptoms of postpericardiotomy syndrome, but corticosteroids may be required in patients with recurring episodes.

Risk Factors for Operative Mortality

The assessment and analysis of risk factors for operative mortality after coronary bypass surgery are important components of the preoperative evaluation of patients with coronary disease (Table 63.4). Furthermore, as an increasing number of interested parties scrutinize the results of bypass surgery, preoperative risk stratification is crucial. Among the many factors that affect outcome after CABG are the patient's state of general health and the potential for complete revascularization. Incomplete revascularization secondary to either severe distal coronary artery disease or inadequate conduits for bypass grafting is associated with a higher operative mortality rate and an uncertain long-term outcome. Likewise, patients with concurrent medical problems, such as cerebrovascular, pulmonary, or renal insufficiency, are much more likely to sustain additional complications during CABG and have a higher operative risk (59).

Poor ventricular function is among the most important factors increasing the mortality risk of bypass surgery. Operative risk also is increased when the patient requires additional operative intervention, such as valve repair or replacement. Furthermore, when ventricular function is not improved by bypass grafting or when mitral valve replacement or ventricular reconstruction is required because of

complications of previous infarction, the long-term outlook is noticeably worsened (59,63).

Several reports have documented increased morbidity and mortality in elderly patients undergoing CABG. In the CASS, the operative mortality rate in patients 70 years of age or older was nearly 8%, compared with an overall estimated mortality rate of about 3% in lower-risk, younger patients. An important observation made in elderly patients is that their increased mortality is the result of postoperative complications, such as stroke, respiratory failure, renal failure, or sepsis, and rather than cardiac failure. Although age is an incremental risk factor for early death after coronary bypass surgery, it is not a contraindication to surgery (59,60).

The influence of the patient's sex on surgical outcome is less clear, despite several reports suggesting a higher operative risk for women. In many of these studies, the women undergoing CABG were older, with a higher incidence of unstable angina, preoperative congestive heart failure, hypertension, and diabetes. Some reports have attributed the increased risk of bypass surgery in women to their smaller physical stature, with a correspondingly smaller coronary arterial bed and the technical limitations this poses. However, the higher risk for women is more likely a consequence of increased risk factors, such as advanced age and severity of the anginal syndrome (61).

Other factors that increase operative risk include renal insufficiency, diabetes mellitus, peripheral vascular disease, cerebral vascular disease, respiratory insufficiency, and obesity. Most of these conditions are also associated with premature or accelerated atherosclerosis and a high incidence of generalized cardiovascular disease secondary to hypertension, hyperlipidemia, and abnormal carbohydrate metabolism. The operative morbidity in patients with end-stage renal disease is increased, often as a result of bleeding and infection. Mortality is also increased. Patients with a functioning kidney transplant have a better outcome than patients requiring long-term hemodialysis.

Reoperative CABG has become increasingly more frequent during the past several years and accounts for an increasing proportion of all CABG procedures carried out in the United States. Reoperative surgery is associated with a higher operative mortality than primary bypass procedures. This is a consequence of the technical difficulty of the procedure, which results from pericardial adhesions and scar formation, and of the fact that patients who undergo reoperation are older and have more advanced coronary disease, and revascularization is more likely to be incomplete (62).

Long-term Outcomes

Controlled clinical trials have shown that surgical revascularization provides significant relief of anginal symptoms (33,55,64,65). Most series show initial elimination of angina in about 90% of patients, with about 70% of patients remaining free of cardiac events for 1 to 3 years. In one report, 67% of surviving patients were free of angina 20 years after surgery (63). Reoperation improved survival in patients with recurrent symptoms (62).

Several studies suggest that CABG may enhance ventricular function, both in the immediate postoperative period and late after surgery. Nonetheless, controversy continues regarding the long-term functional effects of bypass surgery, especially on systolic function, with some reports suggesting a deterioration in ventricular performance. In a few controlled clinical trials, functional improvement was documented both at rest and during exercise 8 months postoperatively. In addition, improvement in the left ventricular ejection fraction was demonstrated in one study and could be attributed to improved contractility in my-

---

Table 63.4. PREDICTION OF THE RISK FOR OPERATIVE MORTALITY[a]

	Low	Medium	High
Age	60 y	75 y	75 y
Gender	Male	Female	Female
Diabetes	No	Yes	Yes
Unstable angina	Yes	No	Yes
Ejection fraction	65%	35%	25%
Three-vessel disease	Yes	Yes	Yes
Operative incidence	First	First	Redo
Predicted mortality rate	0.8%	3.4%	12%

[a]Based on the Society of Thoracic Surgery National Cardiac Database Risk Stratification Algorithm.

ocardial regions that had been ischemic during exercise before surgery (66). Clinical improvement after coronary bypass surgery, including cessation of angina, stabilization of ventricular function, and, most importantly, enhanced survival, depends on short- and long-term graft patency. In a follow-up study that included postoperative coronary angiography, 82% of patients with at least one graft patent on the 1-year coronary angiogram were alive 12 years after surgery, compared with only 42% of the patients who had no patent grafts 1 year after operation. Vein graft occlusion within the first few months of surgery is almost certainly caused by poor blood flow, poor coronary arterial runoff, injury to the graft during preparation, or faulty surgical technique. Vein graft stenosis or graft failure within the first few years is associated with intimal hyperplasia, a process that is demonstrable angiographically in up to 75% of vein grafts after 1 year.

The overall occlusion rates for saphenous vein grafts are 5% to 20% during the first postoperative year, and 2% to 4% annually for the next 4 years; they reach 22% to 30% at 5 years and 50% at 10 years.

Use of the IMA graft has become increasingly favored because it greatly improves late patency. Patency rates for IMA grafts are 95% at 1 year, 94% at 8 years, and 85% or better at 10 years. This improved IMA graft patency has been reported for both pedicle and free IMA grafts. Excellent late IMA graft patency clearly correlates with increased patient survival, reduced symptom recurrence, and fewer reoperations. In a study from the Cleveland Clinic, where IMA grafts have been used extensively, 10-year survival rates in patients with saphenous vein grafts for single-, double-, and triple-vessel disease were 88%, 79.5%, and 71%, respectively, compared with 93.4%, 90%, and 82.6% in a comparable group of patients who had IMA grafts to the LAD artery (31,63).

About 90% of patients survive 5 years after a primary CABG, 80% survive 10 years, and about 58% survive 15 years. Use of the IMA graft improves long-term survival to 89% at 10 years. For all patients in the three major clinical trials, long-term surgical survival was 58% at 11 years in the Veterans Administration Study (51), 71% at 12 years in the European study (52), and 87% at 8 years in the CASS (34). At 5 years, 10% of the surgically treated patients in the CASS had died. One fourth of these deaths were sudden coronary, 47% were not sudden but of cardiac cause, and 28% were noncardiac deaths. In the European trial, the 5-year surgical survival rate in patients with stable angina and good left ventricular function was 92%; this decreased to 71% at 12 years. Medical therapy in a matched group of patients resulted in 83% survival at 5 years and 67% at 12 years. The difference between medical and surgical therapy at 12 years is still significant, but of less magnitude, possibly because of the fact that the patients received only saphenous vein grafts. Better long-term survival should result from mammary grafting, which is now universally performed.

About one in seven patients who had vein grafts required reoperation after 15 years, twice the reoperation rate of patients who received at least one mammary artery bypass. As mentioned earlier, patients who undergo reoperation have at least double the operative risk of primary elective CABG patients because the operation is technically more difficult, the patients' average age is higher, and atherosclerotic disease is more advanced. In addition, long-term results after reoperation are poorer because of these factors and because revascularization may not be as complete. Symptom relief is usually of shorter duration.

Principles Derived from Cooperative Studies

Although the clearest indication for a mechanical intervention such as PTCA or CABG is unstable angina on max-imal medical therapy, improvement in long-term survival in certain anatomic patterns of coronary disease provides another indication for bypass surgery. The three prospective, randomized trials comparing coronary bypass with medical therapy were carried out in the 1970s. Both surgical and medical management of coronary artery disease have improved dramatically since that time. For example, the use of IMA grafts was negligible during the time period of these studies, as was the use of PTCA and platelet-inhibiting drugs. Nonetheless, important principles derived by these studies still shape the clinical approach to coronary artery disease.

Veterans Administration Cooperative Study. The Veterans Administration Cooperative Study (27) randomly assigned 686 male patients (average age, 50 years) to initial medical versus surgical therapy. All patients had medically stable angina, single-vessel disease or worse, and an ejection fraction of more than 30%. Despite a much higher operative mortality rate than was acceptable, even at that time, the study revealed a tremendous benefit derived from surgery for patients with left main artery disease (51). In these patients, the 3-year survival rate was 93% in the surgery group and 68% in the medical group. Furthermore, patients with a history of hypertension, previous MI, abnormal resting ECG, and increasingly severe symptoms (high clinical risk), in addition to patients with three-vessel disease and decreased left ventricular function (high anatomic risk), fared significantly better with surgery.

European Coronary Surgery Study. The European Coronary Surgery Study (52) examined only men younger than 65 years who had mild to moderate angina, normal left ventricular function, and at least two-vessel disease. At 8 years of follow-up, surgery improved survival in the population as a whole (89% vs. 80%), in patients with three-vessel disease (92% vs. 77%), and in patients with two-vessel disease involving the proximal LAD artery (90% vs. 79%). Immediate surgery provided no benefit in single-vessel disease, even if it involved the proximal LAD artery (but the IMA was not used).

Coronary Artery Surgery Study. The CASS was a prospective, randomized study (34) carried out between 1975 and 1979 in the United States in men and women younger than 65 years who had symptoms no more severe than mild angina. At 10 years of follow-up, the group as a whole had derived no benefit from surgery. In patients with an ejection fraction between 30% and 50%, however, surgery conferred an increased survival (79% vs. 61%). Furthermore, in the observational studies that were part of this project, surgery provided a survival advantage in all patients with three-vessel disease, but patients who had the more severe anatomic disease with the worst ventricular function benefitted the most. Although it appears that surgery provides the greatest benefit to those with left ventricular dysfunction, congestive heart failure is a major determinant of *poor* surgical outcome. When heart failure, not angina, is the predominant symptom, surgery yields a poor result. Pulmonary rales, use of diuretics and digitalis, and an enlarged heart are predictors of increased operative risk (59). Nonetheless, in patients with significant angina, although left ventricular dysfunction increases the surgical risk and decreases long-term survival, bypass surgery bestows the greatest benefit in terms of improved long-term survival.

Transplantation versus High-risk Coronary Bypass Surgery

Patients with severely impaired ventricular function may be referred for bypass surgery when severe associated coronary obstructions are detected. Often, it is difficult to decide whether the patient who is at severely increased risk because of ventricular dysfunction is a candidate for bypass surgery, or whether transplantation should be pursued. In patients with ischemic but viable myocardium, ventricular function may improve after bypass surgery once adequate blood flow is restored. The term *hibernating myocardium* has been used to describe ventricular dysfunction secondary to inadequate coronary flow even in the absence of ECG changes or anginal symptoms (66). The term *ischemic cardiomyopathy* implies irreversible myocardial dysfunction associated with extensive myocyte necrosis and infarction. Surgical revascularization improves the contractile function of hibernating muscle, whereas little functional benefit is derived from revascularization in ischemic cardiomyopathy if the myocardium is extensively scarred or infarcted.

In deciding whether to recommend transplantation or bypass surgery to a patient at high risk because of severely depressed left ventricular function, it is therefore important to determine the viability of the myocardium. Anginal symptoms suggestive of reversible ischemia are often a useful indicator of viable myocardium that would benefit from revascularization. Patients whose only symptom is heart failure should be approached with caution. Myocardial viability may be assessed better with positron emission tomography, but this is not widely available. Some cardiologists and surgeons find it useful to perform thallium scanning, either during exercise, with dipyridamole, or at rest, to assess myocardial viability. Muscle that takes up thallium (early or late) is presumed to be viable. Radionuclide scanning provides data with which to estimate the potential for improved ventricular function after revascularization in patients with coronary obstructive disease and significant left ventricular dysfunction because it can identify poorly functioning but viable ischemic areas. A thallium defect during exercise or even at rest that subsequently fills on the delayed images is evidence that viable myocardium is present despite poor function. In a patient with these findings, especially if angina is present, bypass surgery rather than transplantation is generally indicated if operable coronary disease is present. The postoperative outcome in these patients is acceptable, and left ventricular function is usually improved. In patients with congestive heart failure and no evidence of reversible ischemia, bypass surgery entails a high risk and provides little benefit, and transplantation should be considered.

REFERENCES

1. Messer JV, Wagman RJ, Levine HJ, et al. Patterns of myocardial oxygen extraction during rest and exercise. *J Clin Invest* 1962;41:725.
2. Berne RM. The role of adenosine in the regulation of coronary blood flow. *Circ Res* 1980;47:807.
3. Robertson RM, Robertson D, Roberts LJ, et al. Thromboxane A₂ in vasotonic angina pectoris. *N Engl J Med* 1981;304:998.
4. McGill H. Risk factors for atherosclerosis. *Adv Exp Med Biol* 1977;104:273.
5. The Lipid Research Clinics Program. The Lipid Research Clinics Coronary Primary Prevention Trial results. II. The relationship of reduction in incidence of coronary heart disease to cholesterol lowering. *JAMA* 1984;251:365.
6. DeWood MA, Spores J, Notske R, et al. Prevalence of total coronary occlusion during the early hours of transmural myocardial infarction. *N Engl J Med* 198;303:897.
7. Flaherty JT, Becker LC, Bulkley BH, et al. A randomized prospective trial of intravenous nitroglycerin in patients with acute myocardial infarction. *Circulation* 1976;54:766.
8. Herlitz J, Elmfeldt D, Hjalmarson A, et al. Effect of metoprolol on indirect signs of the size and severity of acute myocardial infarction. *Am J Cardiol* 1983;51:1282.
9. Yusuf S, Held P, Fuberg C. Update of effects of calcium antagonists in myocardial infarction or angina in light of the second Danish verapamil infarction trial (DAVIT-II) and other recent studies. *Am J Cardiol* 1991;67:1295.
10. European Cooperative Study Group for Streptokinase Treatment in Acute Myocardial Infarction. Streptokinase in acute myocardial infarction. *N Engl J Med* 1979;301:797.
11. Fry ETA, Sobel BE. Coronary thrombosis. In: Zipes DP, Rowlands DJ, eds. *Progress in cardiology,* vol 2. Philadelphia: Lea & Febiger, 1990:199.
12. Yusuf S, Collins R, Peto R, et al. Intravenous and intracoronary fibrinolytic therapy in acute myocardial infarction: overview of results on mortality, reinfarction and side effects from 33 randomized control trials. *Eur Heart J* 1985;6:556.
13. White HD, Rivers JT, Maslowski AH, et al. Effect of intravenous streptokinase as compared with that of tissue plasminogen activator on left ventricular function after first myocardial infarction. *N Engl J Med* 1989;320:817.
14. Tiefenbrunn AJ, Sobel BE. The impact of coronary thrombolysis on myocardial infarction. *Fibrinolysis* 1989;3:1.
15. TIMI Study Group. Comparison of invasive and conservative strategies after treatment with intravenous tissue plasminogen activator in acute myocardial infarction: results of the Thrombolysis in Myocardial Infarction (TIMI) phase II trial. *N Engl J Med* 1989;320:618.
16. Naunheim KS, Kessler KA, Kanter KR, et al. Coronary artery bypass for recent infarction: predictors of mortality. *Circulation* 1988;78[Suppl I]:1–122.
17. Maisel AS, Ahnve S, Gilpin E, et al. Prognosis after extension of myocardial infarct: the role of W wave on non-Q wave infarction. *Circulation* 1985;71:211.
18. Hands ME, Rutherford JD, Muller JE, et al. The in-hospital development of cardiogenic shock after myocardial infarction: incidence, predictors of occurrence, outcome, and prognosis factors. *J Am Coll Cardiol* 1989;14:40.
19. Allen BS, Okamoto F, Buckberg GD, et al. Studies of controlled reperfusion after ischemia. XIII. Reperfusion conditions: critical importance of total ventricular decompression during regional reperfusion. *J Thorac Cardiovasc Surg* 1986;92:605.
20. Allen BS, Rosenkranz E, Buckberg GD, et al. Studies on prolonged acute regional ischemia. IV. Myocardial infarction with left ventricular failure. *J Thorac Cardiovasc Surg* 1989;98:691.
21. Daggett WM, Buckely MR, Akins CW, et al. Improved results of surgical management of postinfarction ventricular septal rupture. *Ann Surg* 1982;196:269.
22. David TE, Ho WL. The effect of preservation of chordae tendineae on mitral valve replacement for postinfarction mitral regurgitation. *Circulation* 1986;74[Suppl I]:116.
23. Green MA, Gray LA Jr, Slater AD, et al. Emergency aortocoronary bypass after failed angioplasty. *Ann Thorac Surg* 1991;51:194.
24. King SB III, Talley JD. Coronary arteriography and percutaneous transluminal coronary angioplasty: changing patterns of use and results. *Circulation* 1989;79[Suppl I]:19.
25. Pocock SJ, Henderson RA, Rickards AF, et al. Meta-analysis of randomised trials comparing coronary angioplasty with bypass surgery. *Lancet* 1995;346:1184–1189.
26. King SB III, Lembo NJ, Weintraub WS, et al. A randomized trial comparing coronary angioplasty with coronary bypass surgery. *N Engl J Med* 1994;331:1044–1050.
27. Hamm CW, Reimers J, Ischinger T, et al. A randomized study of coronary angioplasty compared with bypass surgery in patients with symptomatic multivessel coronary disease. *N Engl J Med* 1994;331:1037–1043.
28. Alderman EL, Andrews K, Bost J, et al. The Bypass Angioplasty Revascularization Investigation (BARI) Investigations: comparison of coronary bypass surgery with angioplasty in patients with multivessel disease. *N Engl J Med* 1996;335:217–225.
29. Barsness GW, Peterson ED, Obman EM, et al. Relationship between diabetes mellitus and long-term survival after coronary bypass and angioplasty. *Circulation* 1997;97:2551–2556.
30. Weintraub WS, Stein B, Kosinski A, et al. Outcome of coronary bypass surgery versus coronary angioplasty in diabetic patients with multivessel coronary artery disease. *J Am Coll Cardiol* 1998;31:10–19.

31. Eagle KA, Guyton RA, Davidoff R, et al. ACC/AHA guidelines for coronary artery bypass graft surgery: executive summary and recommendations—a report of the American College of Cardiology/American Heart Association task force on practice guidelines (committee to revise the 1991 guidelines for coronary artery bypass graft surgery). *Circulation* 1999;100: 1464–1480.

32. Jones RH, Kesler D, Phillips HR III, et al. Long-term survival benefits of coronary artery bypass grafting and percutaneous transluminal angioplasty in patients with coronary artery disease. *J Thorac Cardiovasc Surg* 1996;111:1013–1025.

33. Nwasokwa ON, Koss JR, Friedman GH, et al. Bypass surgery for chronic stable angina: predictors of survival benefit and strategy for patient selection. *Ann Intern Med* 1991;114:1035.

34. Myers WO, Marshfield WI, Gersh BJ, et al. Medical versus early surgical therapy in patients with triple-vessel disease and mild angina pectoris: a CASS registry study of survival. *Ann Thorac Surg* 1987;44:471.

35. Benetti FJ, Naselli G, Wood M, et al. Direct myocardial revascularization without extracorporeal circulation: experience in 700 patients. *Chest* 1991;100:312–316.

36. Benetti FJ, Ballester C, Sani G, et al. Video-assisted coronary bypass surgery. *J Cardiovasc Surg* 1995;10:620–625.

37. Westaby S. Coronary surgery without cardiopulmonary bypass. *Br Heart J* 1995;73:203–205.

38. Grundeman PF, Borst C, van Herwaarden JA, et al. Hemodynamic changes during displacement of the beating heart by the Utrecht Octopus method. *Ann Thorac Surg* 1997;63: S88–S92.

39. Wan S, LeClerc JL, Vincent JL. Inflammatory response to cardiovascular bypass: mechanisms involved and possible therapeutic strategies. *Chest* 1997;112:676–692.

40. Kolessov VI. Mammary artery–coronary artery anastomosis as method of treatment for angina pectoris. *J Thorac Cardiovasc Surg* 1967;54:535–544.

41. Subramanian VA. Less invasive arterial CABG on a beating heart. *Ann Thorac Surg* 1997;63:S68–S71.

42. Calafiore AM, Di Giammarco G, Teodori G, et al. Left anterior descending coronary artery grafting via left anterior small thoracotomy without cardiopulmonary bypass. *Ann Thorac Surg* 1996;61:1658–1663.

43. Lloyd CT, Calafiore AM, Wilde P, et al. Integrated left anterior small thoracotomy and angioplasty for coronary artery revascularization. *Ann Thorac Surg* 1999;68:908–912.

44. Wan S, Izzat MB, Lee TW, et al. Avoiding cardiopulmonary bypass in multivessel CABG reduces cytokine response and myocardial injury. *Ann Thorac Surg* 1999;68:52–57.

45. Struber M, Cremer JT, Gohrbandt B, et al. Human cytokine responses to coronary artery bypass grafting with and without cardiopulmonary bypass. *Ann Thorac Surg* 1999;68: 1330–1335.

46. Downing SW, Edmunds LH. Release of vasoactive substances during cardiopulmonary bypass. *Ann Thorac Surg* 1992;54: 1236–1243.

47. Stevens JH, Burdon TA, Peters WS, et al. Port access coronary artery bypass grafting: a proposed surgical method. *J Thorac Cardiovasc Surg* 1996;111:567–573.

48. Stephenson ER Jr, Ducko ST, Sankholkar S, et al. Computer-assisted endoscopic coronary artery bypass anastomoses: a chronic animal study. *Ann Thorac Surg* 1999;68:838–843.

49. Shennib H, Bastawisy A, Mack MJ, et al. Computer-assisted telemanipulation: an enabling technology for endoscopic coronary artery bypass. *Ann Thorac Surg* 1998;66:1060–1063.

50. Stephenson ER Jr, Sankholkar S, Ducko CT, et al. Robotically assisted microsurgery for endoscopic coronary artery bypass grafting. *Ann Thorac Surg* 1998;66:1064–1067.

51. Detre KM, Takaro T, Hultgren H, et al., and the study participants. Long-term mortality and morbidity results of the Veterans Administration randomized trial of coronary artery bypass surgery. *Circulation* 1985;72[Suppl V]:84.

52. Varnauskas E, and the European Coronary Surgery Study Group. Twelve-year follow-up of survival in the randomized European Coronary Surgery Study. *N Engl J Med* 1988;319: 332.

53. Takaro T, Pifarre R, Fish R. Left main coronary artery disease. *Prog Cardiovasc Dis* 1985;28:229.

54. Akins CW. Controversies in myocardial revascularization:

coronary artery surgery for single-vessel disease. *Semin Thorac Cardiovasc Surg* 1994;6:109.

55. Hammermeister KE, Morrison DA. Coronary bypass surgery for stable angina and unstable angina pectoris. *Cardiol Clin* 1991;9:133.

56. Gundry SR, Wang N, Bann D, et al. Retrograde continuous warm blood cardioplegia: maintenance of myocardial homeostasis in humans. *Ann Thorac Surg* 1993;55:358.

57. Noyez L, van Son JA, van der Werf T, et al. Retrograde versus antegrade delivery of cardioplegic solution in myocardial revascularization: a clinical trial in patients with three-vessel coronary disease who underwent myocardial revascularization with extensive use of the internal mammary artery. *J Thorac Cardiovasc Surg* 1993;105:854.

58. Rosengart TK, Krieger K, Lang SJ, et al. Reoperative coronary artery bypass surgery: improved preservation of myocardial function with retrograde cardioplegia. *Circulation* 1993;88 [Suppl II]:330.

59. Grover FL, Johnson RR, Marshall G, et al. Factors predictive of operative mortality among coronary artery bypass subsets. *Ann Thorac Surg* 1993;56:1296.

60. Smith JM, Rath R, Feldman DJ, et al. Coronary artery bypass grafting in the elderly: changing trends and results. *J Cardiovasc Surg* 1992;33:468.

61. Barbir M, Lazem F, Ilsley C, et al. Coronary artery surgery in women compared with men: analysis of coronary risk factors and in-hospital mortality in a single centre. *Br Heart J* 1994:71:408.

62. Lytle BW, Loop FD, Taylor PC, et al. The effect of coronary reoperation on the survival of patients with stenoses in saphenous vein bypass grafts to coronary arteries. *J Thorac Cardiovasc Surg* 1993;105:605.

63. Lawrie GM, Morris GC Jr, Earle N. Long-term results of coronary bypass surgery: analysis of 1,698 patients followed 15 to 20 years. *Ann Surg* 1991;213:355.

64. Myers WO, Schaff HV, Gersh BJ, et al. Improved survival of surgically treated patients with triple vessel coronary disease and severe angina pectoris. *J Thorac Cardiovasc Surg* 1989; 98:487.

65. Nwasokwa ON, Koss JR, Friedman GH, et al. Bypass surgery for chronic stable angina: predictors of survival benefit and strategy for patient selection. *Ann Intern Med* 1991;114:1035.

66. Braunwald E, Rutherford JD. Reversible ischemic left ventricular dysfunction: evidence for the hibernating myocardium. *J Am Coll Cardiol* 1986;8:1467.

SURGERY: SCIENTIFIC PRINCIPLES AND PRACTICE, Third Edition, edited by Lazar J. Greenfield, Michael W. Mulholland, Keith T. Oldham, Gerald B. Zelenock, and Keith D. Lillemoe. Lippincott Williams & Wilkins Publishers, Philadelphia, © 2001.

CHAPTER 64

MECHANICAL CIRCULATORY SUPPORT

FRANCIS D. PAGANI AND KEITH D. AARONSON

The spectrum of mechanical circulatory support has changed dramatically since the time when Denton Cooley first implanted an orthotopic cardiac prosthesis as a bridge to heart transplantation (1) and William DeVries first implanted a total artificial heart as a permanent replacement for a failing native heart (2). Since then, numerous technologic advances and rigorous scientific investigations have dramatically improved the availability, durability, and safety of mechanical cardiac support devices.

Mechanical circulatory support is indicated when the heart can no longer pump blood and supply oxygen to meet the needs of the body. "A variety of devices, ranging from the widely available intraaortic balloon pump (IABP) to the sophisticated permanent total artificial heart, are used to treat patients with failing hearts. The appropriate support system is always that device that can provide the best potential results in the simplest possible manner" (3).

INDICATIONS: SELECTION OF PATIENTS AND DEVICES

Reasonable judgment is required to determine who requires intervention with mechanical circulatory support, as no absolute hemodynamic criteria indicate when to initiate support. However, several guidelines are followed: evidence of cardiogenic shock, manifested by a cardiac index below 1.8 L/min/M^2; systolic blood pressure below 90 mm Hg; pulmonary capillary wedge pressure or left atrial pressure above 20 mm Hg; right atrial pressure above 20 mm Hg; and evidence of poor tissue perfusion, reflected by oliguria, mental status changes, and cool extremities, despite the maximal administration of pharmacologic therapy. The patient's history and the overall clinical setting also need to be considered in the decision to initiate mechanical circulatory support. When patients reach this degree of hemodynamic compromise, the risk for death is substantial (4). A more subtle indication to initiate mechanical circulatory support may be progressive organ dysfunction despite inotropic therapy in a patient with chronically low cardiac output who is awaiting heart transplantation, even though the hemodynamic parameters may not have changed significantly. In addition, patients who cannot tolerate inotropic therapy because of refractory ventricular arrhythmias or who have life-threatening coronary disease and unstable angina not amenable to revascularization and are therefore at risk for imminent death (hours, days, or weeks) may be considered for mechanical circulatory support if they do not meet hemodynamic criteria.

Patient selection is perhaps the single most crucial factor in determining outcome after mechanical circulatory support has been initiated. Patients should not be considered for mechanical circulatory support if they have any significant contraindication to such support or to heart transplantation, or if they are unlikely to be weaned from circulatory support once it has been initiated. Contraindications to the initiation of mechanical circulatory support include irreversible renal, hepatic, or respiratory failure; sepsis; and significant neurologic deficit. Severe obstructive or restrictive pulmonary disease is also a contraindication to mechanical circulatory support. Perioperative hypoxia as a result of significant underlying lung disease can contribute to pulmonary vasoconstriction with right-sided circulatory failure. Often, patients with severe pulmonary disease have an elevated pulmonary vascular resistance that is fixed (not responsive to pulmonary artery vasodilators). Such fixed pulmonary vascular resistance represents a contraindication to heart transplantation. Moderate elevations in pulmonary vascular resistance can be encountered in patients in cardiogenic shock and do not preclude the successful use of mechanical circulatory support if reversibility (lowering) of the pulmonary vascular resistance is documented during therapy with inotropic agents or pulmonary vasodilators. Acute renal failure requiring dialysis is a relative contraindication to initiating mechanical circulatory support. In the setting of cardiogenic shock with acute renal failure, establishing normal hemodynamics with mechanical circulatory support may resolve the renal failure in a relatively short period of time. Thus, the degree and duration of cardiogenic shock, along with the patient's baseline renal function,

must be considered in estimating the probability of recovery of renal function. This is important in considering whether the patient will be a transplant candidate or not, in the event that native heart function does not recover while the patient is mechanically supported. Similarly, hepatic congestion can resolve and synthetic functions of the liver recover after the institution of mechanical circulatory support. Portal hypertension or liver cirrhosis is an absolute contraindication to initiating mechanical circulatory support. Risk stratification models have supported the observation that patients with progressive multiple-organ failure do poorly following intervention with mechanical circulatory support (5).

In addition to the degree of organ dysfunction, age correlates with survival in patients placed on mechanical circulatory support. Age can represent an absolute contraindication to the initiation of mechanical support if the patient is unlikely to be weaned and is too old to qualify for heart transplantation. Data from the American Society for Artificial Organs–International Society for Heart and Lung Transplantation (ASAIO–ISHLT) registry have demonstrated that the survival of patients older than 70 years on mechanical circulatory support is decreased (6). The probability of weaning from mechanical circulatory support is not affected by age (6).

The timing of the initiation of mechanical circulatory support is also crucial to outcome. In the setting of postcardiotomy shock, data from the Abiomed BVS 5000 registry demonstrate that a delay of longer than 6 hours in initiating mechanical circulatory support after the initial weaning from cardiopulmonary bypass is associated with a significant decrease in survival from 44% to 14% (7,8). A delay in instituting mechanical circulatory support also increases the need for biventricular support, as opposed to just univentricular support. Patients requiring biventricular support have decreased survival (6,7,9). As the severity of illness and organ dysfunction increases, patients are more likely to require biventricular support (10,11). An episode of cardiac arrest before the initiation of mechanical circulatory support significantly reduces survival from 47% to 7% (7,8).

Selection of the appropriate mechanical circulatory device is also critical to successful outcome and depends on a number of factors (Table 64.1). These include the following: underlying cause of circulatory failure, duration of support required, whether biventricular or univentricular support is required, whether combined cardiac and pulmonary failure

---

Table 64.1. CONSIDERATIONS IN INSTITUTING MECHANICAL CIRCULATORY SUPPORT

What is the likelihood of reversing the myocardial injury?
What is the probable duration of support needed?
What is the urgency of the need for support (minutes, hours, days)? (e.g., cardiac arrest vs. advanced heart failure)
To what degree is myocardial performance impaired?
What degree of circulatory support and device invasiveness is needed? (e.g., IABP vs. LVAD)
Is univentricular or biventricular support needed? (Right-sided heart failure indicated by right atrial pressure >20 mm Hg, severe tricuspid regurgitation, hepatic failure, coagulopathy, renal dysfunction)
Is cardiac or cardiopulmonary support needed?
What is the patient's size?
What device will offer the patient the greatest degree of mobility and potential for rehabilitation during circulatory support?
What are the current FDA-approved indications for this device?

IABP, intraaortic balloon pump; *LVAD,* left ventricular assist device; *FDA,* Food and Drug Administration.

Table 64.2. **CURRENT BODY SURFACE AREA LIMITATIONS FOR MECHANICAL CIRCULATORY SUPPORT DEVICES**

Device	BSA limitation (M²)
HeartMate LVAD	1.5
Thoratec VAS	0.8–1.0
Abiomed BVS 5000	0.8–1.0
Abiomed TAH	1.7
CardioWest TAH	
Novacor LVAS	1.5

LVAD, left ventricular assist device; VAS, ventricular assist system; BVS, biventricular support; TAH, total artificial heart; LVAS, left ventricular assist system.

is present, size of the patient (Table 64.2), intended use of the device, and the current Food and Drug Administration restrictions and regulations for use of a particular device (Table 64.3). Consideration of all these factors helps define the end point of therapy, which may be bridge to recovery, bridge to heart transplant, or, in the near future, "destination therapy" (permanent device placement) (12–14).

Currently, mechanical circulatory support is beneficial in two groups of patients, and devices have been approved by the Food and Drug Administration specifically for them. The first group comprises patients who have sustained reversible myocardial injury and in whom myocardial function is reasonably expected to recover after a short period of support (generally < 2 weeks). Possibly reversible forms of myocardial injury include acute myocardial infarction, acute viral myocarditis, and postcardiotomy shock with failure to be weaned from cardiopulmonary bypass. Under these circumstances, several types of devices can be utilized, including IABPs, extracorporeal ventricular assist devices (either pulsatile or nonpulsatile), and extracorporeal membrane oxygenation (ECMO). The second group of patients comprises those in whom myocardial function is unlikely to recover (long-standing ischemic, valvular, or idiopathic end-stage heart failure, severe acute myocardial infarction) and who require mechanical circulatory support as a bridge to heart transplantation. Long-term circulatory support devices that are implantable, allowing for greater patient mobility, rehabilitation, and discharge to home, are more appropriate under these circumstances.

In the near future, two additional groups of patients will likely be considered for mechanical circulatory support. These include patients in whom long-term support (weeks to months) is required for ventricular remodeling and recovery from various types of cardiomyopathies, and those in whom permanent device support is being considered as destination therapy, an alternative to heart transplantation or medical therapy. Anecdotal observations from the cumulative experience with long-term circulatory support for bridge to heart transplant and recent small clinical studies have demonstrated that long-term circulatory support (weeks to months), associated with sustained mechanical unloading of the left ventricle, can improve the myocardial function of patients thought to have irreversible, dilated, end-stage cardiomyopathies (15–18). Several studies have demonstrated that long-term mechanical circulatory support can restore ventricular geometry (19–21); improve myocyte function, orientation, and size (16,22–26); reduce myocyte apoptosis (27); reduce myocardial cytokine gene and protein expression (28,29); reverse abnormal neurohormonal patterns associated with advanced heart failure (30,31); and improve myocardial mitochondrial function (32). These observations have led clinicians to consider mechanical circulatory support, either alone or in conjunction with other future possible therapies (gene therapy, myocyte implantation), as a potential modality to reverse end-stage cardiomyopathy. Whether these observations will hold up under future rigorous experimental scrutiny remains unknown at this time.

Table 64.3. **CLASSIFICATION AND INDICATIONS OF MECHANICAL CIRCULATORY SUPPORT DEVICES**

Pump type	Intended duration of support*	FDA status	Indications or potential uses
Intraaortic balloon pump	Short-term	Approved	Cardiogenic shock.
Extracorporeal nonpulsatile			Respiratory failure (ECMO); postcardiotomy
ECMO	Short-term	Approved	failure to wean; cardiogenic shock secondary to
Centrifugal pumps	Short-term	Approved	myocardial infarction or acute myocarditis; right-sided support following LVAD implant.
Extracorporeal pulsatile			Postcardiotomy failure to wean; cardiogenic shock
Thoratec VAS	Short- or long-term	Approved	Secondary to myocardial infarction or acute
Abiomed BVS 5000	Short-term	Approved	myocarditis; right-sided support following LVAD implant; bridge to heart transplantation (Thoratec only).
Implantable pulsatile			Bridge to transplantation, bridge to recovery.
HeartMate IP-1000 LVAD	Long-term	Approved	
HeartMate VE LVAS	Long-term	Approved	
Novacor LVAS	Long-term	Approved	
LionHeart LVAS	Long-term	Investigative	
HeartSaver LVAD	Long-term	Investigative	
Implantable nonpulsatile			Bridge to transplantation, bridge to recovery, destination therapy.
HeartMate II	Long-term	Investigative	
HeartMate III	Long-term	Investigative	
DeBakey/NASA LVAD	Long-term	Investigative	
Jarvik 2000	Long-term	Investigative	
Total artificial heart			Bridge to transplantation, destination therapy (Abiomed TAH, Sarns/Penn State).
CardioWest	Long-term	Investigative	
Abiomed TAH	Long-term	Investigative	
Sarns/Penn State	Long-term	Investigative	

*Short-term ≤ 2 weeks; long-term > 2 weeks.
ECMO, extracorporeal membrane oxygenation; LVAD, left ventricular assist device; LVAS, left ventricular assist system; BVS, biventricular support; TAH, total artificial heart.

Permanent circulatory support, or destination therapy, is currently under investigation (14). The Randomized Evaluation of Mechanical Assistance for the Treatment of Congestive Heart Failure (REMATCH) is the first prospective, randomized medical trial to compare the use of permanent mechanical circulatory support (HeartMate VE LVAS, Thermo Cardiosystems, Woburn, MA) versus optimal medical management in patients with advanced congestive heart failure who are not candidates for heart transplantation. Outcomes evaluated in the trial include overall survival, quality of life, and cost-effectiveness of care. Results of this trial should be available in the year 2001.

OTHER IMPORTANT MEDICAL CONSIDERATIONS IN INSTITUTING MECHANICAL CIRCULATORY SUPPORT

Valvular Heart Disease

Abnormalities of the cardiac valves have important adverse consequences in patients being considered for mechanical circulatory support and may require repair or replacement if successful mechanical circulatory support is to be initiated or weaning from support achieved.

Mild to moderate aortic stenosis in the absence of insufficiency is not a contraindication to the placement of a ventricular assist device. Severe aortic stenosis should be corrected before placement of a ventricular assist device, preferably with a bioprosthetic or homograft valve, to facilitate future weaning or optimize native heart function in the event of device failure. The presence of even mild or moderate aortic insufficiency can have a significant impact on the effectiveness of ventricular assist devices. In cases in which left ventricular assistance is initiated with left atrial-to-aortic cannulation, aortic insufficiency results in left ventricular distention in the presence of significant left ventricular dysfunction. Left ventricular distention adversely affects subendocardial blood flow and can ultimately prevent weaning from circulatory support. In cases in which left ventricular assistance is initiated with devices that require left ventricular apical-to-aortic cannulation, reductions in left ventricular pressure elicited by mechanical assistance increase the pressure gradient across the aortic valve and increase the degree of aortic insufficiency. Thus, blood pumped into the aortic root by the device flows backward across the incompetent aortic valve (aortic insufficiency), thereby decreasing net forward flow and compromising end-organ perfusion. Even mild or moderate aortic insufficiency may become severe with the initiation of mechanical support with a left ventricular assist device (LVAD) because the elevated left ventricular end-diastolic pressure is significantly reduced by emptying of the left ventricular cavity by the device and the aortic root pressure is elevated above baseline because of device flow. The significance of the regurgitant volume of blood can easily be determined by measuring cardiac output with a thermodilution catheter and comparing it with device flow. In cases in which device flow exceeds the cardiac output, measured by thermodilution technique, by more than 2 L/min, the volume of regurgitation is considered significant. In addition, the presence of significant aortic insufficiency can be confirmed by echocardiography. Patients with a mechanical valve prosthesis in the aortic valve position should have the mechanical valve replaced with a bioprosthetic valve before the institution of left ventricular assistance. During complete unloading of the left ventricle by an LVAD, the aortic valve may not open and would therefore be prone to thrombus formation.

Patients with significant preexisting mitral stenosis at the time device support is initiated may require correction of the valvular problem before the device is implanted, depending on the device selected and the site of cannulation. In the setting of significant mitral stenosis, left ventricular filling is impaired. With LVADs that require apical ventriculotomy for cannula placement for ventricular drainage, device filling may be limited because of the mitral stenosis. This problem can be circumvented either by choosing a device that can utilize left atrial drainage or by correcting the underlying valvular disease (mitral valve repair or replacement with a bioprosthetic valve). Mitral regurgitation does not affect the filling of an LVAD. In situations in which weaning from mechanical circulatory support may be feasible, correction of the mitral disease, either stenosis or regurgitation, is necessary to optimize cardiac function.

Adequate function of the right side of the heart is extremely important to maintain LVAD flow in the early postoperative period in patients on univentricular support. Severe tricuspid regurgitation can significantly impair the forward flow of blood on the right side, particularly in cases of high pulmonary vascular resistance. Further, severe tricuspid regurgitation contributes to elevated central venous pressure, hepatic congestion, and renal dysfunction. Severe tricuspid regurgitation may be present preoperatively in the setting of volume overload and biventricular failure, or it may develop following the institution of LVAD support as a consequence of right ventricular dilation resulting from a leftward shift of the interventricular septum (33–35). If severe tricuspid regurgitation is present during the initiation of LVAD support, tricuspid valve repair should be performed to improve right ventricular performance.

Coronary Artery Disease

Patients with significant obstructive coronary artery disease or those in postcardiotomy shock following failed coronary bypass operations may continue to experience angina during mechanical circulatory support. Generally, coronary artery disease does not cause adverse hemodynamic consequences during the period of device support. However, the presence of obstructive coronary disease with ongoing ischemia may limit the degree of myocardial recovery and significantly affect the ability to be weaned from device support.

Perioperative ischemia of the right ventricle may be of hemodynamic significance during the institution of LVAD support. If right ventricular ischemia causes myocardial stunning or infarction during or soon after implantation of an LVAD, subsequent right-sided circulatory failure can result in decreased flow to the LVAD. In patients who have undergone coronary bypass surgery and are candidates for mechanical circulatory support, patent bypass grafts, particularly to the right coronary artery or left anterior descending coronary artery, should be preserved to reduce the risk for perioperative right-sided circulatory failure and arrhythmias. In selected cases, it may be important to perform a coronary artery bypass to the right coronary artery or left anterior descending coronary artery systems to optimize functioning of the right side of the heart in the perioperative period if significant obstructive coronary lesions amenable to bypass are present in the distribution of these arteries.

Arrhythmias

Atrial and ventricular arrhythmias are common in patients with cardiogenic shock and underlying ischemic heart disease or idiopathic cardiomyopathies. The arrhythmias generally persist in the immediate postoperative period and subsequently resolve with time as the hemodynamic condition of the patient improves and inotropic therapy is withdrawn. In some patients, the arrhythmia persists because of underlying disease (e.g., giant cell myocarditis). Severe ventricular arrhythmias have traditionally been thought to be a contraindication to univentricular support. However, recent experience has revealed that the hemodynamic consequences in patients in whom these arrhythmias develop in the late postoperative period are generally not life-threatening (36,37). In the absence of pulmonary hypertension and elevated pulmonary vascular resistance in the postoperative period, adequate LVAD flows are maintained during ventricular fibrillation. This situation is analogous to a Fontan (systemic vein to pulmonary artery) circulation. In the early perioperative period, some patients with refractory ventricular arrhythmias may require biventricular support until the pulmonary vasculature resistance drops and a Fontan circulation is tolerated. The addition of right ventricular support for hemodynamic compromise secondary to refractory ventricular arrhythmia is unusual. In situations in which weaning from mechanical support is feasible or planned, elimination of the ventricular arrhythmias with antiarrhythmic therapy is essential.

Atrial fibrillation and flutter hinder right ventricular filling but are reasonably well tolerated in recipients of ventricular assist devices. Early electric or pharmacologic cardioversion is indicated to avoid thrombus formation and improve exercise tolerance. Anticoagulation is indicated in patients with persistent atrial or ventricular arrhythmias to prevent thrombus formation (even in those with devices for which anticoagulation is otherwise unnecessary).

Intracardiac Shunts

Potential intracardiac shunts, such as a patent foramen ovale or atrial septal defect, should be closed at the time of initiation of left ventricular assistance to prevent right-to-left shunting. These anomalies should be identified before surgery by means of transesophageal echocardiography (38). During the initiation of left ventricular assistance, left atrial pressure is reduced below right atrial pressure. This gradient causes shunting of deoxygenated blood from the right atrium into the left, which results in significant systemic hypoxemia. When a patent foramen ovale or atrial septal defect has been missed, treatment includes administering pulmonary vasodilators and inotropic agents to decrease the shunt by improving function in the right side of the heart and lowering right atrial pressure. If significant hypoxia persists, reoperation to close the anomaly is required.

MANAGEMENT OF COMPLICATIONS OF MECHANICAL CIRCULATORY SUPPORT

Bleeding, right-sided circulatory failure, air embolism, and progressive multiple-organ failure are the most frequent complications that occur in the early postoperative period following the initiation of mechanical circulatory support. Complications most common in the late postoperative period include infection, thromboembolism, and device failure.

Bleeding

Bleeding is a frequent early complication in patients supported by mechanical assist devices and generally requires reoperation in the early postoperative period. Risk factors for bleeding include preoperative hepatic congestion and failure, poor preoperative nutritional status, prolonged cardiopulmonary bypass times, extensive surgical dissection, reoperative surgery, multiple cannulation sites, decreased platelet function, and induction of fibrinolysis as a result of contact with biomaterial surfaces during cardiopulmonary bypass and implantation of mechanical circulatory support devices. In the early experience of mechanical circulatory support, about 50% of patients required reoperation for bleeding. The risk for major hemorrhage has decreased substantially with the use of the serine protease inhibitor aprotinin and the supplemental administration of vitamin K before operation (39,40). Meticulous surgical technique is also an important factor to reduce hemorrhagic complications.

Right-sided Circulatory Failure

Right-sided circulatory failure occurs in approximately 10% to 20% of patients supported by left ventricular assistance. The causes of right-sided circulatory failure are multiple and include primary disease within the pulmonary vascular bed, right ventricle, or both. Factors contributing to right-sided circulatory failure include impaired right ventricular function as a result of intraoperative air embolism, myocardial stunning as a result of poor intraoperative myocardial protection, ischemia and infarction resulting from coronary artery disease, arrhythmias, volume loading, and alteration of right ventricular septal geometry induced by left ventricular unloading. Several studies have demonstrated that factors such as elevated central venous pressure, a transpulmonary gradient higher than 16 mm Hg, an acute decrease in pulmonary artery pressures of 10 mm Hg or more at the onset of LVAD support, preoperative pulmonary edema, and the need for perioperative transfusions all increase the requirement for right ventricular mechanical support following LVAD implantation (5,11,41). Multiple perioperative transfusions elicit the expression and release of numerous inflammatory cytokines, including interleukin-1β, interleukin-6, and tumor necrosis factor-α (TNF-α) (42). TNF-α can induce pulmonary hypertension, and its effect can be mediated by a platelet-activating factor, a potent vasoconstrictor of the pulmonary circulation (43). Acute unloading of the left ventricle by mechanical assistance may cause a leftward shift of the septum, which increases right ventricular volume loading and reduces its function (33,34). The negative consequences of this phenomenon may be offset by the reduction in pulmonary artery pressures and right ventricular afterload achieved by device-mediated left ventricular decompression (33,34). Hemodynamic stability can be attained with isolated mechanical left ventricular support in about 90% of patients without the need for right ventricular assistance, even in patients with substantial right ventricular dysfunction, if effective replacement of left-sided heart function and aggressive treatment of pulmonary hypertension are carried out. More recently, the improved perioperative management of patients with elevated pulmonary vascular resistance, including the use of inhaled nitric oxide, a specific, potent pulmonary vasodilator, in combination with milrinone, isoproterenol, or dobutamine, has significantly reduced the need for placement of a right ventricular assist device (44–46). In patients with markedly elevated central venous pressure, multiple-organ failure, and severe right ventricular dysfunction with low pulmonary artery pressures, early biventricular support may be indicated.

Thromboembolism and Anticoagulation

The occurrence of thromboembolic events following mechanical circulatory support is variable and depends on a number of factors, including the type of device, duration of support, location and number of cannulation sites, and the presence of prosthetic valves within the heart. Overall, approximately 20% to 30% of patients receiving mechanical circulatory support experience a thromboembolic event. The rate of thromboembolic events has been reduced by the more aggressive use of antiplatelet therapy in conjunction with warfarin, improvements in device design, and the more frequent use of left ventricular apical rather than left atrial cannulation. In patients supported for short periods only, anticoagulation is usually achieved with heparin and antiplatelet therapy. Longer-term support usually requires a transition to warfarin and antiplatelet therapy with most, but not all, devices.

The single most significant technologic advance in preventing thromboembolic events in patients on long-term left ventricular assistance has been the use of textured blood-contacting surfaces within the devices. This technology has been applied in the HeartMate series of implantable LVADs (47,48). The interior surfaces of these LVADs have been textured with the use of sintered titanium microspheres on the rigid metallic surfaces and integrally textured polyurethane on the movable diaphragm (Fig. 64.1). This design feature permits a uniform autologous tissue lining to be established on all blood-contacting surfaces of the pump, so that thrombus formation and bacterial colonization are minimized. The tightly adherent fibrin–cellular matrix, once mature, contains macrophages, mesenchymal cells, endothelial cells, and other blood components. This densely adherent neointima eliminates direct contact between the device and blood elements, thereby substantially reducing the risk for peripheral embolization. In a recent multicenter study, the total thromboembolic event rate for patients supported on the HeartMate device was 0.01 per patient-month of device use among 223 patients supported for a total of 531 patient-months (49). Most thromboembolic events occur either perioperatively in association with air emboli or remotely from the time of device implantation in association with device infection, particularly fungal infection. Patients supported with the HeartMate LVAD require an-

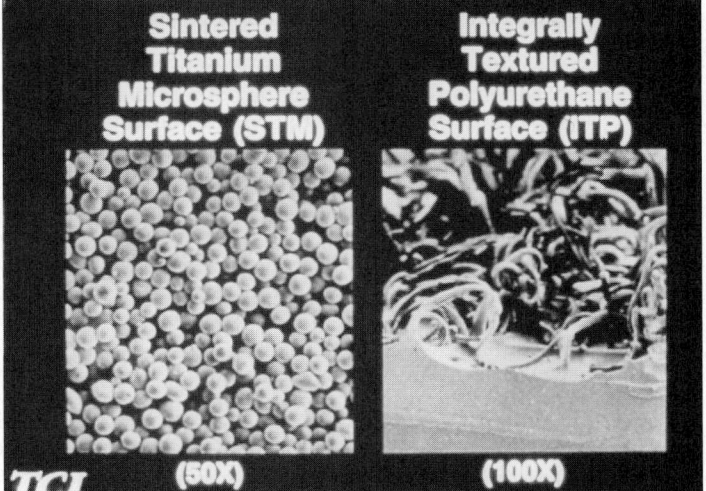

A

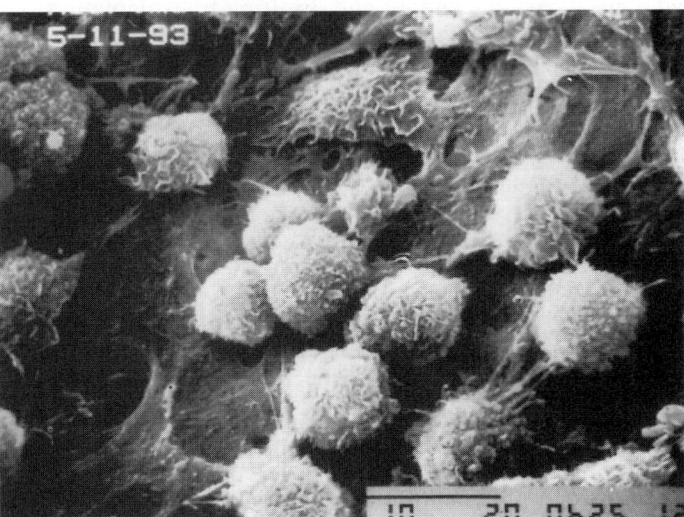

B

Figure 64.1. Sintered titanium microsphere surface and integrally textured polyurethane surface incorporated in the HeartMate LVAS. (Photograph courtesy of Betty Silverstein Russell, Senior Vice President, Thermo Cardiosystems, Woburn, MA.)

Table 64.4. ANTICOAGULATION REQUIREMENTS FOR MECHANICAL CIRCULATORY SUPPORT DEVICES

Device	Anticoagulation protocol
Centrifugal (BioMedicus, St. Jude, Sarns)	Heparin/antiplatelet therapy
ECMO	Heparin
Abiomed BVS 5000	Heparin/antiplatelet therapy
CardioWest TAH	Heparin/antiplatelet therapy followed by Coumadin/antiplatelet therapy for long-term support
Thoratec VAS	Heparin/antiplatelet therapy followed by Coumadin/antiplatelet therapy for long-term support
Novacor LVAS	Heparin/antiplatelet therapy followed by Coumadin/antiplatelet therapy for long-term support
HeartMate LVAD	Antiplatelet therapy

ECMO, extracorporeal membrane oxygenation; BVS, biventricular support; TAH, total artificial heart; LVAS, left ventricular assist system; LVAD, left ventricular assist device.

tiplatelet therapy with aspirin alone, but they do not require systemic anticoagulation with heparin or warfarin, as do patients with other forms of mechanical circulatory support (Table 64.4).

Infection

Infections can be device-related [e.g., device endocarditis, drive line or cannula site infection, pocket infection (infection external to an implanted device)] or non–device-related (e.g., pneumonia, urinary tract infection). The incidence of early nosocomial non–device-related or device-related infections in patients undergoing mechanical circulatory support is approximately 30% to 40% in many series and is related to the acuteness of illness in this population of patients (50–58). Mortality tends to be higher in patients with persistent or recurrent sepsis or with device-related infections than in patients without such complications (54). Prolonged hospitalization, immobilization, endotracheal intubation, poor nutritional status, diabetes, obesity, indwelling catheters, intravascular lines, transcutaneous cannulae, and broad-spectrum antibiotic therapy all contribute to the high incidence of nosocomial infections. Device-related infections can sometimes be successfully treated with antibiotic suppression and device exchange or removal. Infections involving the preperitoneal pocket (subfascial space created for device placement) surrounding implantable LVADs require more aggressive treatment, including open drainage, débridement, and rerouting of the drive line through a fresh exit site. However, patients who are device-dependent and awaiting transplantation generally cannot tolerate device removal as a therapeutic option to eradicate the infection. Antibiotic suppression and transplantation remain the only chance for cure of device-related infections in some instances. Fortunately, these infections do not generally preclude heart transplantation, and transplant outcomes and survival are generally not significantly affected in this situation (54).

In patients on long-term (> 2 weeks) mechanical circulatory support, infection remains the single most significant obstacle to successful outcome. Recent data have demonstrated significant immune system derangements in patients maintained on long-term mechanical circulatory support that are secondary to patient–device interactions. These data suggest that LVAD implantation is accompanied by progressive defects in cellular immunity; these seem to be the result of an aberrant state of T-cell activation involving the CD95 (FAS) pathway and activation-induced cell death of CD4-positive T cells (59,60). These defects of cellular immunity predispose recipients of LVADs to fungal and other systemic infections (59,61).

Sensitization to HLA Antigens

Recent evidence has demonstrated that prominent B-cell activation develops in recipients of long-term mechanical circulatory support, evidenced by the heightened production of anti-HLA and antiphospholipid antibodies. The incidence of antibody development to HLA class I or II antibodies may be as high as 80% (62). This enhanced B-cell reactivity is thought to be secondary to activation-induced cell death of CD4-positive T cells, as noted above (59).

The presence of preformed lymphocytotoxic antibodies reactive against donor lymphocytes in recipient serum detected in a routine cross-match is considered a significant obstacle to successful solid organ transplantation. The presence of preformed lymphocytotoxic antibodies is associated with a high incidence of humoral allograft rejection, early graft failure, and poorer patient survival (63,64). These antibodies are primarily directed against donor major histocompatability complex (MHC) class I HLA antigens constitutively expressed by the allograft endothelium; nonactivated endothelium does not express MHC class II HLA antigens. Consequently, the risk for early graft failure (i.e., within the first 24 to 48 hours) is significantly higher in the presence of a positive cross-match with donor T lymphocytes, which in the absence of activation express only MHC class I antigens, than with donor B lymphocytes, which strongly express both MHC class I and class II antigens. In addition, the real risk for early graft failure after a positive cross-match appears to reside in the immunoglobulin G fraction of donor-specific antibodies. An immunoglobulin M-positive cross-match can result from the presence of antilymphocytic autoantibodies, which do not specifically react with donor HLA allotypes, so that their presence generally does not lead to early graft failure.

Device Malfunction

As with any mechanical device, malfunction is an anticipated occurrence. The types and severity of device malfunctions vary between devices. Many devices have built-in backup systems that, in the event of catastrophic device failure, provide support to the patient. Also, most patients supported by an LVAD have enough residual left ventricular function to help sustain them until corrective measures can be taken. Device malfunctions in total artificial hearts are more problematic, as no native heart is available to provide hemodynamic support in the event of a total device failure. Stringent quality control measures in fabrication and testing and very low mechanical failure rates are therefore even more essential with total artificial hearts.

CONSIDERATIONS IN WEANING PATIENTS FROM MECHANICAL CIRCULATORY SUPPORT

A number of factors must be considered when patients are weaned from mechanical circulatory support. First and foremost is the consideration of any pathologic abnormalities of the heart, such as valvular disease or severe coronary disease, that has not been addressed and corrected. If the underlying condition that has caused the patient to require mechanical circulatory support is not corrected, then the chances of weaning from mechanical circulatory support will be negligible. Cardiac tamponade must also be excluded. Bleeding is a major early complication of mechanical circulatory support, and reoperation for cardiac tamponade and bleeding is frequent. Transesophageal echocardiography may not reliably identify cardiac tamponade in the early postoperative period. Thus, a high index of suspicion and a low threshold for reoperation are critical to rule out tamponade. Volume status, preload and afterload, cardiac rhythm, and degree of inotropic support should be optimized for weaning. Noncardiac causes can contribute to failure in weaning from mechanical circulatory support. Pulmonary edema, elevated pulmonary vascular resistance, acute respiratory distress syndrome, and pneumonia may hinder right ventricular function.

Once a patient's status has been optimized, weaning from mechanical circulatory support with the use of transesophageal echocardiography is ideal. As device flows are reduced, transesophageal echocardiography provides information on ventricular filling and performance and valve function. If patients can maintain satisfactory hemodynamics with a reduction of pump flow, they can be considered for weaning. In the setting of biventricular support, it is important that device flows on the right side be reduced before left-sided device flows are turned down to prevent pulmonary edema in the event of inadequate left ventricular function. As device flows are reduced, native heart function begins to support the circulation, and monitoring of the systemic arterial waveform demonstrates native heart contractions in synchronization with the electrocardiogram.

If hemodynamics are unsatisfactory during the weaning trial, the patient will require continued support and subsequent weaning trials. In situations in which weaning from mechanical circulatory support is not possible, patients should be evaluated for heart transplantation and bridged to a mechanical device with long-term support capabilities when feasible.

MECHANICAL CIRCULATORY SUPPORT DEVICES

Intraaortic Balloon Pump

The IABP was first introduced in 1962 by Moulopolous and colleagues (65). The first clinical use of the IABP was reported in 1968 by Kantrowitz et al. (66), who described the use of the pump in three patients suffering from postinfarction cardiogenic shock refractory to medical therapy. Since that time, the IABP has become one of the simplest, most affordable, and most utilized circulatory assist devices available to support patients in cardiogenic shock (Fig. 64.2). The IABP can be inserted percutaneously and may augment cardiac output by as much as 10% to 25% depending on a number of factors, including balloon size, patient size, degree of aortic compliance, cardiac rhythm, blood pressure, and IABP settings and timing. The greatest increase in cardiac output is seen in patients with ischemic cardiomyopathy, in whom enhanced coronary perfusion leads to improved cardiac contractility. The IABP has become a standard in coronary care and cardiac surgery centers for the treatment of left ventricular dysfunction and cardiogenic shock that is refractory to medical management.

The concept underlying the IABP is that the area under the arterial pressure trace (time–tension index) is an indirect estimation of the oxygen consumption of the heart, and that decreasing the area during systole by reducing afterload effectively supports the failing heart. Claus and colleagues (67) described a device that lowered the time–tension index by withdrawing blood from the arterial tree just before ventricular systole and returning it to the circulation in diastole. In 1962, Moulopolous and associates (65) described a catheter-based balloon producing hemodynamic effects similar to those of the Harken pump, but without an extracorporeal pump. Moulopolous passed a balloon into the aorta that inflated during ventricular diastole, thereby augmenting diastolic blood pressure. Deflation just before ejection effectively decreased the afterload of the heart and thus the work of the heart during systole.

The major hemodynamic effects of the IABP are a decrease in left ventricular afterload and an increase in coronary artery perfusion pressure. Cardiac output improves as a result of enhanced myocardial contractility by an increase in coronary blood flow and a reduction in afterload and preload. The IABP is positioned with the tip of the balloon lying just distal to the left subclavian artery. The balloon should fill the aorta so that during the inflation cycle it nearly occludes the vessel. In adults, balloon volumes of 30 to 40 mL are optimal. Inflation should be timed to coincide with closure of the aortic valve, which is identified by the dicrotic notch on the aortic blood pressure tracing (Fig. 64.3). Deflation should occur as late as possible to maintain the duration of augmented diastolic blood pressure but before the aortic valve opens and the ventricle ejects. Deflation is timed to occur with the onset of the electrocardiographic R wave. A regular heart rate with an easily identified R wave or a good arterial pulse tracing with a discrete aortic dicrotic notch optimizes performance of the IABP. Current balloon pumps are triggered off the electrocardiographic R wave or the arterial pressure tracing. During tachycardia, the IABP is usually timed to inflate every other beat. In unstable patients, obtaining a regular rhythm or regularly paced rhythm optimizes proper timing of the IABP.

The IABP can be inserted into the common femoral artery either percutaneously by using a modified Seldinger technique or by surgical cut-down. A cut-down is generally performed during cardiopulmonary bypass when the arterial pulse is absent as a consequence of the nonpulsatile flow. During insertion, a guide wire is introduced into the femoral artery, then the dilating catheters and the balloon. After passage of the flexible guide wire, the soft-tissue tract and vessel are progressively dilated until an appropriately sized sheath can be inserted. Sheathless IABP catheters are available. Next, the furled catheter (standard size 9.5F, 40-mL balloon) is passed proximally until its tip rests in the thoracic aorta just distal to the left subclavian artery. When the common femoral or iliac arteries cannot be used because of occlusive disease and an inability to advance the guide wire, the axillary artery, exposed below the middle third of the clavicle, can be used as an entry site. Alternatively, in situations of postcardiotomy failure to wean, the ascending aorta can be utilized as an insertion site. Fluoroscopy or trans-

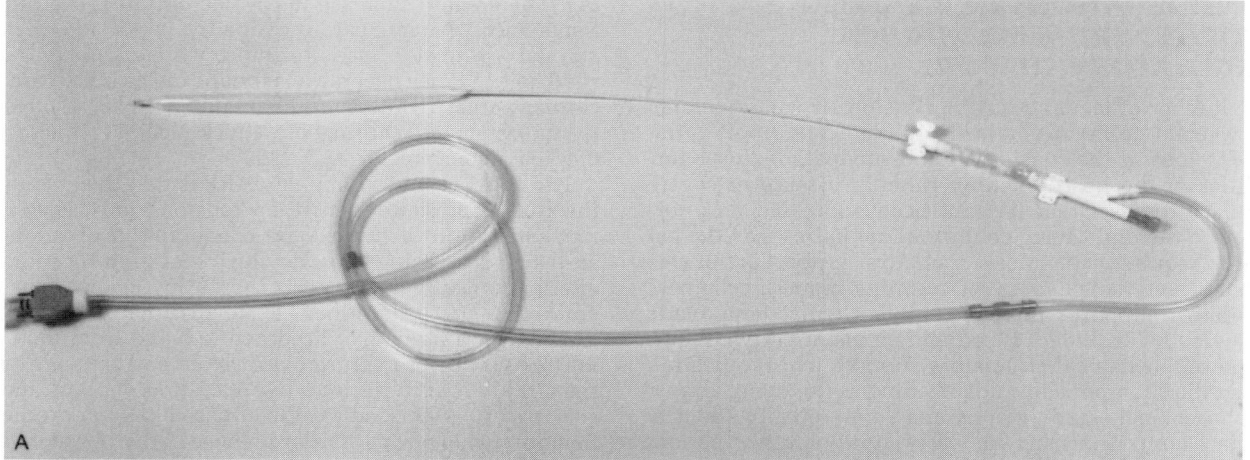

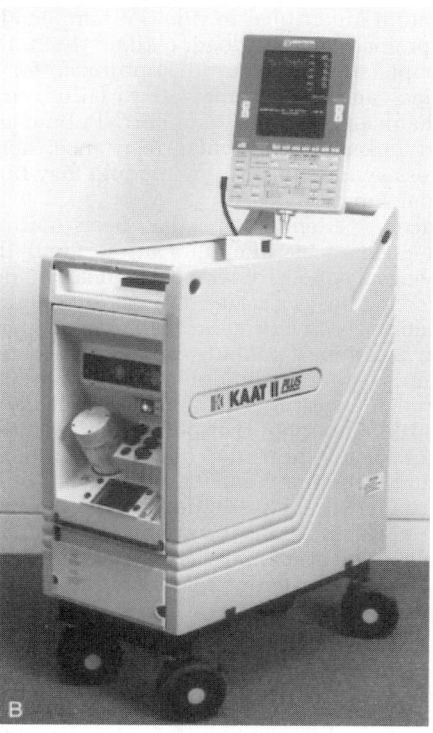

Figure 64.2. Intraaortic balloon pump. *(A)* A catheter-mounted balloon is typically inserted into the thoracic aorta through a percutaneous insertion in the groin. *(B)* Console for the intraaortic balloon pump.

esophageal echocardiography should be utilized to ensure proper positioning of the guide wire. The balloon should be positioned so that it does not occlude the left subclavian artery during inflation. Heparin is recommended if the IABP will remain in place for more than 24 hours. Weaning from the IABP entails observing the clinical response to reducing the ratio of assisted heart beats to total beats from 1:1 to 1:3 or 1:4. At the time of removal of the IABP, every effort should be made to flush out any thrombus as the balloon catheter is removed. Hemostasis should be obtained by application of direct pressure to the entry site for at least 30 to 45 minutes. Removal of the IABP placed through a cut-down on the femoral artery may require repair of that artery and concomitant embolectomy if signs of ischemia of the lower extremity are present.

Complications of use of the IABP include leg ischemia, balloon rupture, thrombosis within the balloon, sepsis, in-

fection at the insertion site, bleeding, false aneurysm, lymph fistula, femoral neuropathy, vessel perforation with hemorrhage, and aortic dissection resulting from catheter passage below the intima. Depending on the extent of peripheral vascular disease, the balloon can occlude major branches of the aorta and elicit ischemia of the tissues supplied by those vessels. Examples of this scenario include intestinal "angina" caused by occlusion of the mesenteric vessels, and upper extremity symptoms when the balloon impinges on the left subclavian artery. Female sex, peripheral vascular disease, diabetes, smoking, advanced age, obesity, and cardiogenic shock are risk factors for the development of leg ischemia. Balloon rupture is usually indicated by the appearance of blood within the balloon catheter. Leg ischemia, balloon rupture, and sepsis are indications for removal of the IABP. If the patient is balloon-dependent, a replacement balloon can be inserted

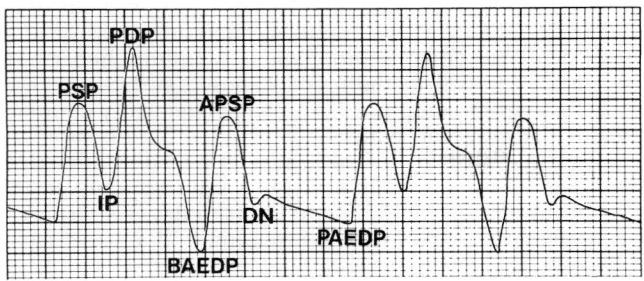

Figure 64.3. Aortic pressure tracing during intraaortic balloon pump support. Balloon counterpulsation is occurring after every other heartbeat (1:2 counterpulsation). With correct timing, balloon inflation *(IP)* begins immediately after aortic valve closure, signaled by the dicrotic notch *(DN)*. In contrast to what occurs in unassisted ejection, the pump augments diastolic blood flow by increasing peak aortic pressure during diastole *(PDP)*. Balloon deflation before systole decreases the ventricular afterload, with lower aortic end-diastolic pressure *(BAEDP vs. PAEDP)* and lower peak systolic pressure *(APSP vs. PSP)*. (Courtesy of St. Jude Medical, Cardiac Assist Division, Chelmsford, MA.)

in a new site. The IABP has several disadvantages. In the best of circumstances, cardiac output is augmented by 25%; in comparison, LVADs can augment baseline cardiac output threefold to fivefold. The IABP offers no significant support to the right side of the heart. Mobilization and ambulation of the patient are limited while the IABP is being utilized.

Extracorporeal Nonpulsatile Devices

Extracorporeal Membrane Oxygenation

Extracorporeal membrane oxygenation (ECMO) is a temporary form of mechanical circulatory support that provides circulatory assistance in addition to oxygenation and carbon dioxide removal from the blood (68–70). The ECMO circuit is similar in concept to the cardiopulmonary bypass routinely used in the operating room for cardiac procedures. However, with ECMO, safe application for extended periods of time (days) has required certain modifications, particularly the inclusion of membrane oxygenators. The first successful use of prolonged ECMO was reported by Hill et al. in 1972 (71). Subsequently, ECMO has been used for an increasing number of indications, including neonatal, pediatric, and adult respiratory support and postcardiotomy support, and as a bridge to placement of an LVAD or heart and lung transplantation.

Extracorporeal membrane oxygenation supports the circulation by unloading the right ventricle and draining blood from the venous circulation, oxygenating it, then returning it to the arterial circulation at physiologic perfusion pressures. ECMO does not unload the left ventricle, although the left ventricular preload is reduced by the decreased pulmonary venous return. In patients with severe left ventricular dysfunction, the use of an IABP helps reduce left ventricular afterload during systole and improves myocardial contractility. The use of the IABP and inotropic therapy can maintain sufficient cardiac contractility to prevent stasis within the ventricle, where clot formation is possible (72). If left ventricular function is so severely reduced that ejection is absent, an atrial septostomy can be performed to vent pulmonary venous return. Alternatively, a left-sided vent can be connected to the venous line to relieve ventricular distention. It is important during ECMO support to maintain some degree of pulmonary

blood flow to prevent thrombosis. Additionally, it is important to continue ventilation of the lungs to maintain the oxygen saturation of the blood ejected from the left ventricle above 90%. Poorly oxygenated blood ejected from the left ventricle will perfuse the coronary arteries and further damage the already injured heart. Venovenous ECMO, unlike venoarterial ECMO, maintains flow through the heart. Venoarterial ECMO is used primarily for cardiac or cardiorespiratory support, whereas venovenous ECMO is used for pulmonary support.

Current ECMO circuits typically comprise a centrifugal pump with either a hollow fiber or membrane oxygenator, oxygen blender, pump console, heat exchanger, and pump cart. A roller pump is used by some centers. Cannulation for ECMO is extremely variable and depends on the clinical situation and whether a venoarterial or venovenous circuit is desired. In emergent situations, when institution of mechanical circulatory support is needed within minutes (acute cardiac or respiratory arrest), percutaneous cannulation of the femoral vein and artery can be performed. In less urgent situations, cut-down on the internal jugular and carotid artery or respective femoral vessels can be performed. In cases of postcardiotomy failure in the operating room, venous access can be obtained by insertion of the cannula in the right atrium and arterial outflow obtained by cannulation of the ascending aorta.

Extracorporeal membrane oxygenation is usually continued for several days to weeks, and during this time, patients are given vigorous diuresis or undergo continuous veno-venous hemofiltration (CVVH) to remove excess third-space fluid. Right and left atrial pressures and pump flows are monitored, and mixed venous saturations are maintained above 75%, which is an accurate reflection of the adequacy of systemic flows. A sudden decrease in venous drainage is usually manifested by chugging of the venous lines, with wide respiratory fluctuations and flow. Causes include hypovolemia, cannula kinking or malposition, pneumothorax, and pericardial tamponade. Centrifugal pumps are afterload-sensitive, and kinking of the inflow cannula will result in a decreased flow.

Although the results of ECMO are very encouraging, its use is associated with significant side effects, including bleeding, stroke, infection, hematologic abnormalities, and initiation of a whole-body inflammatory response that occurs in response to circulatory bypass. Complement activation through the alternative pathway is a well-documented response to hemodialysis and cardiopulmonary bypass. Circulating C3a and C5a lead to neutrophil adherence, aggregation, and activation; activated neutrophils in turn release free radicals, proteases, and arachidonic acid metabolites that, among other things, damage the integrity of cellular membranes. Additionally, the complexity of ECMO requires continuous intensive care unit monitoring by skilled personnel.

Centrifugal Pumps

Centrifugal pumps are extracorporeal systems that provide short-term mechanical circulatory support (73,74) (Fig. 64.4). The systems are easy to operate, widely available, disposable, and relatively inexpensive in comparison with most other forms of mechanical circulatory assist. These systems are most commonly used in cardiopulmonary bypass to support open-heart operations. Thus, an extensive knowledge base on the use of these devices has accumulated. Worldwide, numerous centrifugal pumps are available or are in development for clinical use. However, in the United States, only three centrifugal pumps were commercially available until recently. All are disposable, cost less than $200.00 per unit, and are relatively simple to operate. The Sarns centrifugal pump (3M

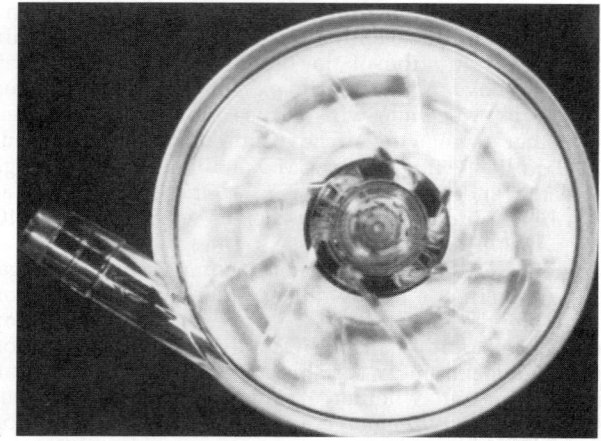

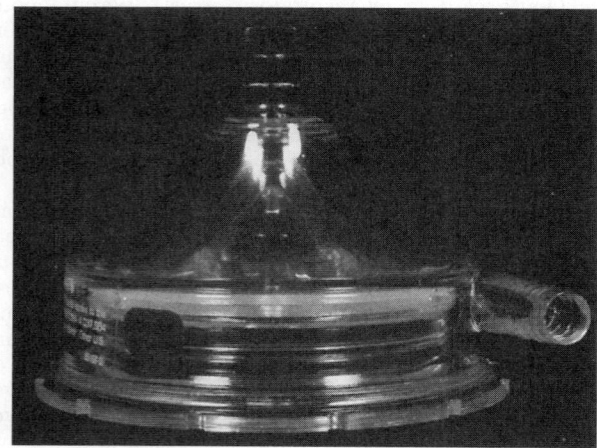

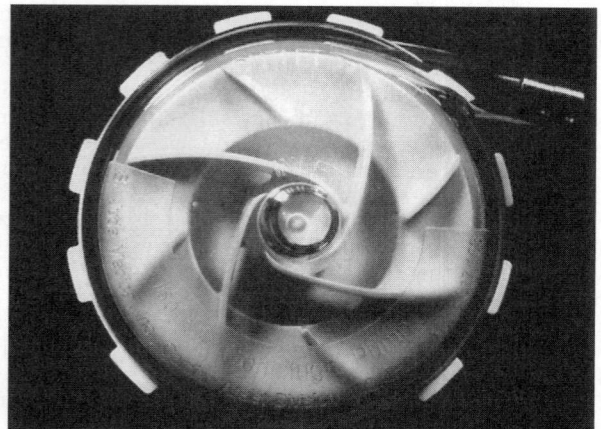

Figure 64.4. *(A)* Sarns centrifugal pump head. *(B)* BioMedicus BioPump centrifugal pump head. *(C)* St. Jude Medical Lifestream centrifugal pump head.

Health Care, Ann Arbor, MI) uses a spinning impeller system to impart a rotary motion to incoming perfusate. The St. Jude Medical Lifestream centrifugal pump (St. Jude Medical, Cardiac Assist Division, Chelmsford, MA) employs a curved vane design and angled egress blood flow path that purports to minimize turbulence, decrease hemolysis, and reduce periods of flow stasis. The Bio-Medicus BioPump centrifugal pump head, manufactured and marketed by Medtronic BioMedicus (Eden Prairie, MN), consists of valveless rotator cones that impart a cir-

cular motion to incoming blood according to viscous drag and constrained vortex principles generating pressure and flow. With the Carmeda BioMedicus BioPump, heparin is covalently bonded to the blood exposed surfaces. These four disposable pump heads can be magnetically coupled to an electric motor, which is controlled by a computerized console. Control of flow is accomplished by adjusting the revolutions per minute of the spinning pump head. Short-term (generally limited to hours to days) ventricular or pulmonary support can be provided with a centrifugal pump. It can be used for femoral–femoral bypass, conventional cardiopulmonary bypass, left ventricular assistance, right ventricular assistance, and ECMO.

The most common use of the centrifugal pump, other than for conventional cardiopulmonary bypass in open-heart procedures, is for the management of postcardiotomy failure and cardiogenic shock. Postcardiotomy cardiac failure occurs in 2% to 6% of patients undergoing cardiac procedures (73). One percent require mechanical support in addition to the IABP pump for counterpulsation. In a voluntary registry reporting the use of the centrifugal pump as a right, left, or biventricular assist device, approximately 25% of patients were weaned from the device and eventually discharged (75). The centrifugal pump can be used to provide left, right, or biventricular assistance. Cannulation for left ventricular assistance is most commonly performed through the right superior pulmonary vein into the left atrium with return into the ascending aorta. Right ventricular assistance is provided by cannulation of the right atrium and pulmonary artery. The pulmonary artery catheter is either placed through the right ventricle and threaded through the pulmonary valve or inserted directly into the pulmonary artery. Cannulae are secured in place with two pursestring pledgeted sutures and tourniquets.

Extracorporeal Pulsatile Devices

Thoratec VAS

The Thoratec VAS (Thoratec Laboratories, Pleasonton, CA) is a paracorporeal, pneumatically powered, pulsatile system configured for univentricular or biventricular support that consists of a seamless polyurethane blood sac contained within a rigid polycarbonate housing (76–78) (Fig. 64.5). An external drive console sends pressurized air to the pump, which compresses the blood sac and causes blood to be ejected. Bjork-Shiley concavoconvex tilting-disk valves within the inflow and outflow conduits ensure unidirectional blood flow. The device has a stroke volume of approximately 65 mL and a maximum output of 7 L/min. For left ventricular support, the pump inflow cannula can be placed in the left ventricular apex or the left atrium, and the pump outflow conduit is anastomosed to the ascending aorta. For right ventricular support, a large-bore cannula is placed in the right atrium, and the outflow conduit is sewn to the main pulmonary artery. When biventricular support is needed, right pump flow is adjusted so that it is less than left pump flow to prevent excessive pulmonary congestion. After the cannulae have been externalized subcostally, the inflow and outflow cannulae are connected to the pump(s), which reside externally on the anterior surface of the abdomen. During the support period, anticoagulation with dextran, heparin, warfarin, and dipyridamole is required. Patients may be ambulatory, but their mobility is limited by the size of the drive console and the paracorporeal position of the pump(s). The Thoratec VAS can be operated in fixed-rate, volume, or synchronous mode. Volume mode is preferred because it maximizes support of the cardiac output. In the

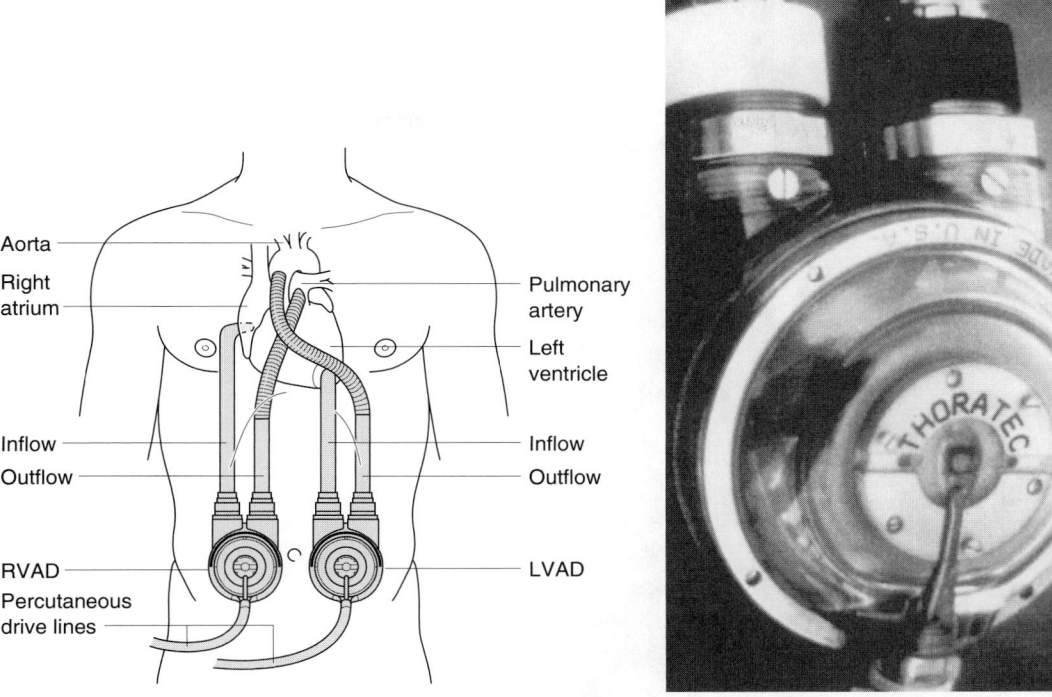

Figure 64.5. *(A)* Thoratec VAS. *(B)* The Thoratec VAS in the biventricular support configuration. *RVAD*, right ventricular assist device. *LVAD*, left ventricular assist device.

synchronous mode, the pump empties when triggered by the R wave obtained from the patient's electrocardiogram. In this mode, weaning may be achieved by adjusting the device rate to a heart rate ratio in the range of 1:1 to 1:3. Synchronous mode is intended for weaning patients from support. Although the console can function automatically to achieve maximum pump flows, the operator must adjust the systolic driving pressure and diastolic vacuum pressure. The Food and Drug Administration has approved the Thoratec VAS for use as a bridge to recovery and a bridge to transplantation. New system designs that are currently being tested include a small, portable drive console that will enhance patient mobility and permit discharge from the hospital (78).

Abiomed BVS 5000

The Abiomed BVS 5000 (Abiomed, Danvers, MA) support system is an automated ventricular support device intended to provide complete temporary support of the left and/or right side of the heart (78,79) (Fig. 64.6). The Abiomed BVS 5000 has been approved by the Food and Drug Administration for short-term mechanical circulatory support as a bridge to recovery in cases of cardiogenic shock resulting from postcardiotomy failure to wean, acute myocarditis, and myocardial infarction. Positioned externally, this pulsatile system simulates normal physiologic mechanical cardiac function. A microprocessor-based drive console is used to supply power to a disposable, pneumatically driven, two-chambered blood pump that supports one side of the heart. Left atrial blood inflow is returned to the ascending aorta, and right atrial inflow is returned to the pulmonary artery. Transthoracic cannulae are used to connect the external system with the patient. Each blood pump consists of two Angioflex polyurethane atrioventricle-like chambers (Fig. 64.7). Trileaflet polyurethane valves are strategically positioned to separate (a) atrial and ventricular bladders and (b) ventricular blad-

ders and outflow cannulae. One or two disposable blood pumps are operated by a single console, which automatically adjusts the beat rate and systolic-to-diastolic ratio based on compressed air flow into and out of the external system. The pump is placed at the bedside, and blood is drained from the patient's left or right atrium by gravity, without the use of vacuum pressure, into the top of the pump. It returns to the patient's aorta or pulmonary artery from the bottom of the pump. Filling of the blood pump chambers can be regulated by adjusting the height of the blood pump relative to the patient's heart. The blood pump is a dual-chamber device that incorporates an atrial (filling) chamber and a ventricular (pumping) chamber. Unidirectional flow is ensured by two trileaflet polyurethane valves fabricated from Angioflex, a biomaterial. The duration of pump systole and the duration of diastole are calculated automatically by the microprocessor to optimize pump filling and maintain a stroke volume of 83 mL. The console drives and adjusts the left and right sides independently of each other. System controls are essentially limited to "on" and "off."

Implantable Left Ventricular Assist Devices

HeartMate IP-1000 LVAD and HeartMate VE LVAS

The HeartMate LVAD is an implantable, pulsatile LVAD designed for long-term circulatory support. It has been approved by the Food and Drug Administration as a bridge to heart transplantation (13,80–82) (Fig. 64.8). The unique feature of this device is that the blood-contacting surfaces of the pump are textured with sintered titanium spheres on the rigid surface and integrally textured polyurethane on the movable surfaces to encourage the deposition of circulating cells (see earlier section on thromboembolism

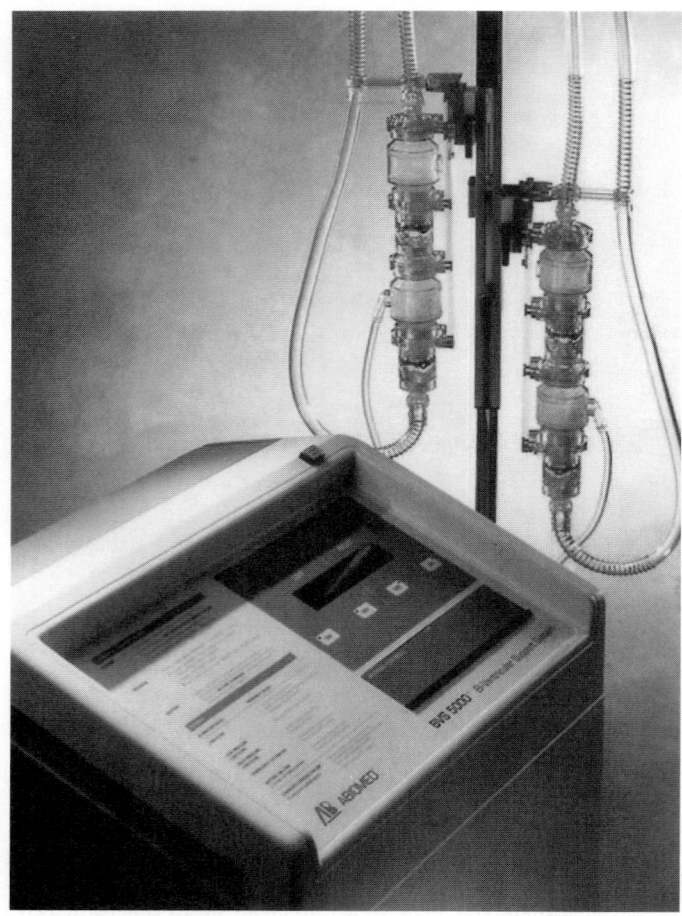

A

Figure 64.6. Abiomed BVS 5000 biventricular assist device. The drive console with blood pumps is shown.

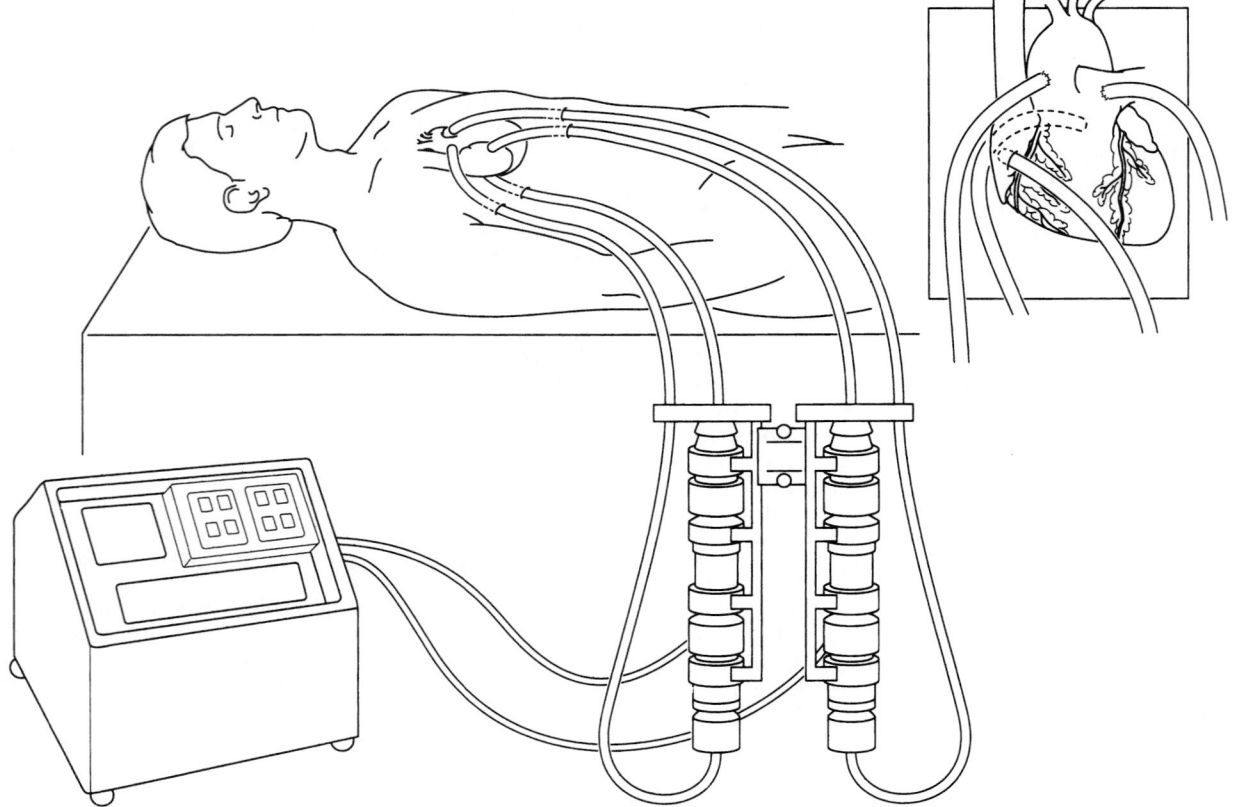

B

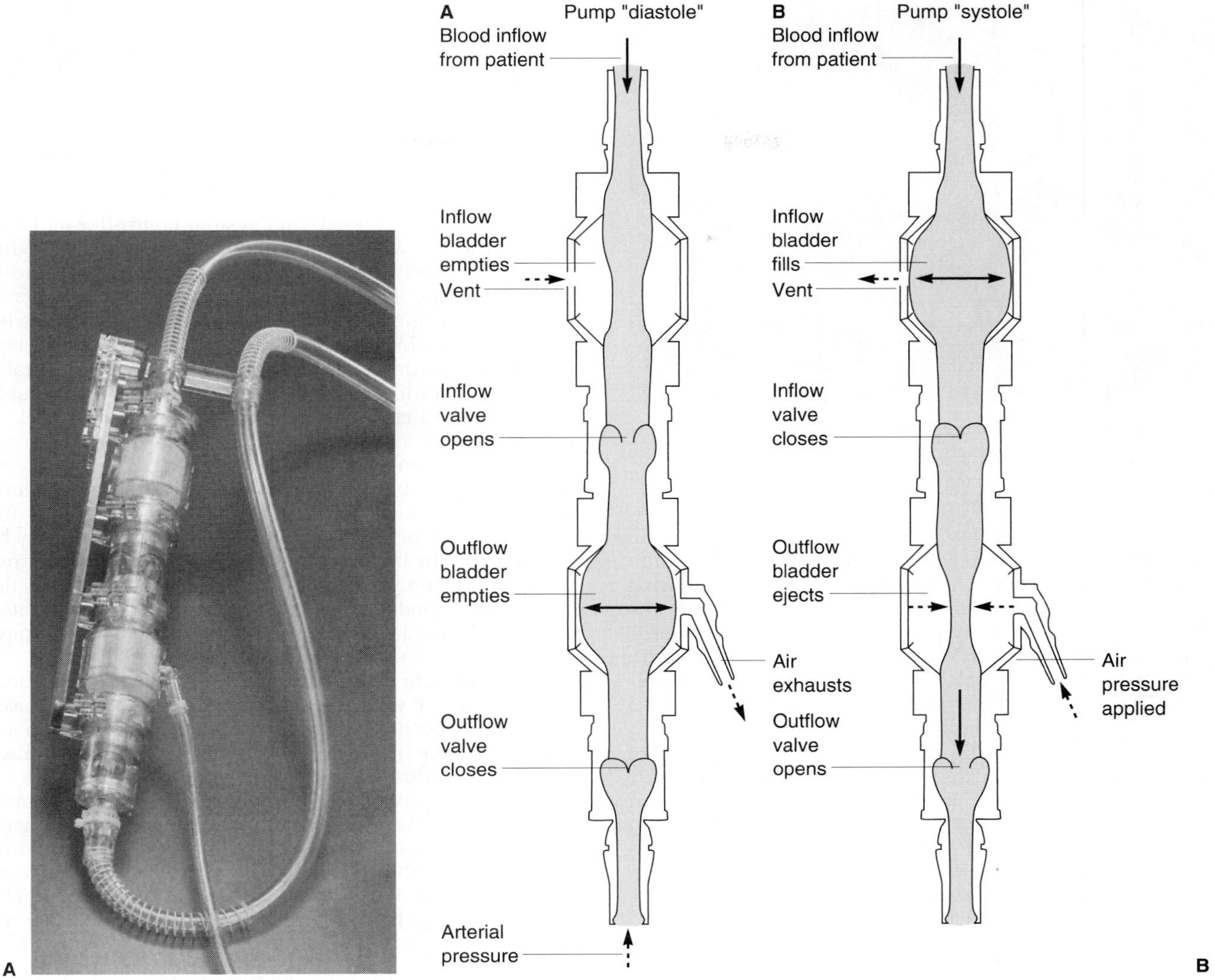

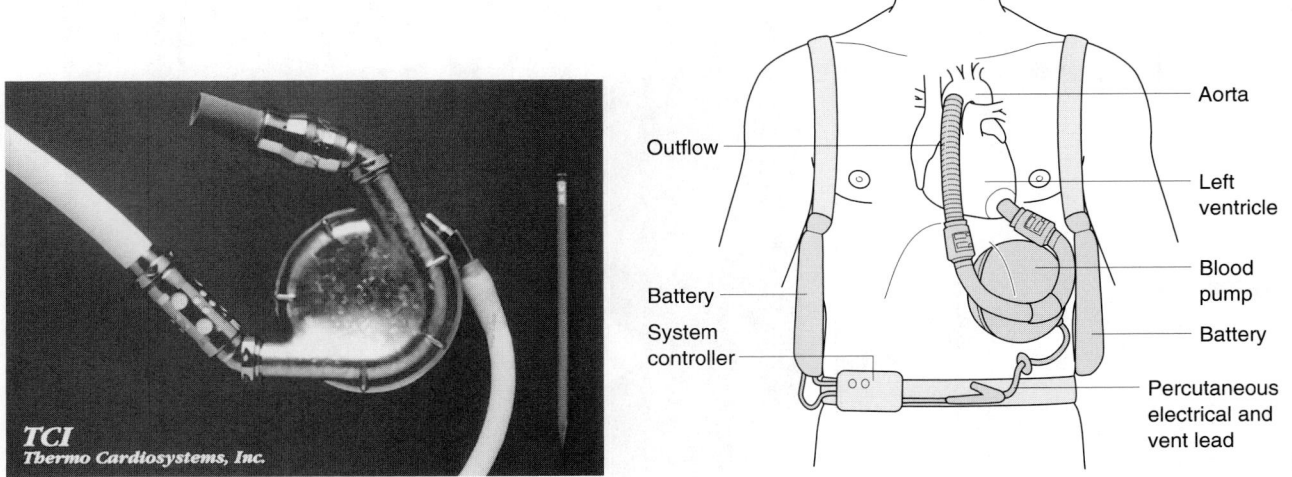

A Pump "diastole"
Blood inflow from patient

Inflow bladder empties
Vent

Inflow valve opens

Outflow bladder empties

Outflow valve closes

Arterial pressure

B Pump "systole"
Blood inflow from patient

Inflow bladder fills
Vent

Inflow valve closes

Outflow bladder ejects

Air exhausts

Outflow valve opens

Air pressure applied

Figure 64.7. *(A)* Abiomed blood pump. *(B)* Mechanism of Abiomed blood pump action.

Outflow

Battery

System controller

Aorta

Left ventricle

Blood pump

Battery

Percutaneous electrical and vent lead

TCI
Thermo Cardiosystems, Inc.

Figure 64.8. The Thermo Cardiosystems HeartMate VE LVAS.

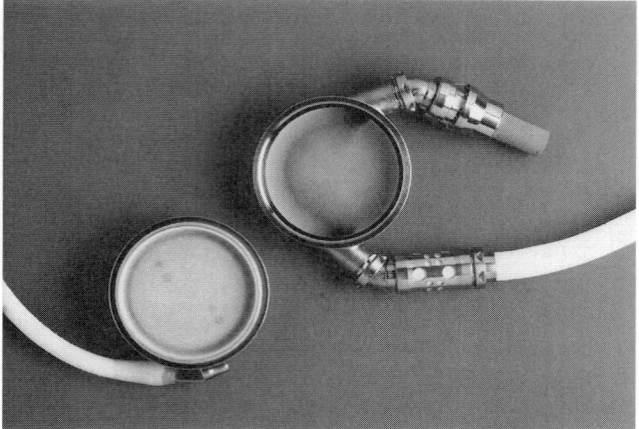

Figure 64.9. Illustration of the Thermo Cardiosystems HeartMate VE LVAS, showing the textured surfaces of the metal housing and diaphragm.

and anticoagulation) (Figs. 64.1 and 64.9). In addition to the unique surface design, the pusher plate of the pump moves the diaphragm in a way that creates a wandering vortex in the blood chamber. This feature prevents the stagnation of blood in any part of the chamber. Presently, two versions of the HeartMate are in clinical use: a pneumatic version (IP-1000 LVAD) and a vented electric version (VE LVAS). The HeartMate blood pump consists of a flexible polyurethane diaphragm within a ridged outer titanium alloy housing. The inflow and outflow conduits of the HeartMate device each contain a 25-mm porcine valve within a titanium cage to ensure unidirectional blood flow. The outflow conduit is extended by a 20-mm woven Dacron graft. With the IP-1000 LVAD, a mobile 75-lb external drive console emits pulses of air that propel the flexible diaphragm of the pump upward, pressurize the blood chamber, and cause blood to flow into the aorta (Fig.

64.10). A more portable drive console that enhances patient mobility and permits discharge from the hospital is currently in clinical testing. With the VE LVAS, diaphragm movement and blood ejection depend on an electric motor positioned below the diaphragm (Fig. 64.11). The electric rotary motor within the titanium housing drives a cam up and down (translational movement) to move the diaphragm. An external vent equalizes the air pressure and permits emergency pneumatic actuation in the event of electrical failure. The external system controller and batteries in the VE LVAS are small and lightweight, allowing the patient nearly unlimited mobility. The drive line is covered with a polyester velour that promotes tissue bonding and anchoring to the skin and reduces the risk for infection. The VE LVAS is powered by two rechargeable batteries that provide 4 to 6 hours of charge; they are usually worn in a shoulder holster, vest, or belt. The wearable electric devices currently available have external backup mechanisms to continue support without the need for reoperation in case of failure of the device. If the device should fail, the native heart is able to provide systemic support until the device can be examined. Because the electronic control unit is outside the body, it can easily be repaired should failure of the software, chip, or electronics occur (Fig. 64.12). Finally, if the motor device fails, the single pusher plate device can be pneumatically activated with a hand-held portable pump or with the 75-lb pneumatic console that operates the IP-1000 model.

The HeartMate is implanted through an extended median sternotomy with the aid of cardiopulmonary bypass. The pump is positioned below the left hemidiaphragm, either within the peritoneal cavity or in a preperitoneal pocket. The inflow tube crosses the diaphragm and is inserted in the apex of the left ventricle. A 20-mm Dacron outflow graft exits from the pocket, crosses the diaphragm, and is anastomosed to the ascending aorta. The drive line is externalized through the right or left abdominal wall and connected to the external power and control unit. The maximum pump flow is 11.6 L/min for the IP-1000 LVAD

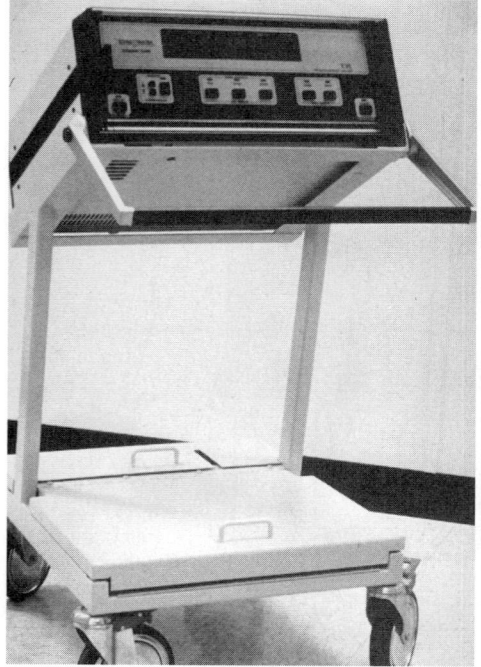

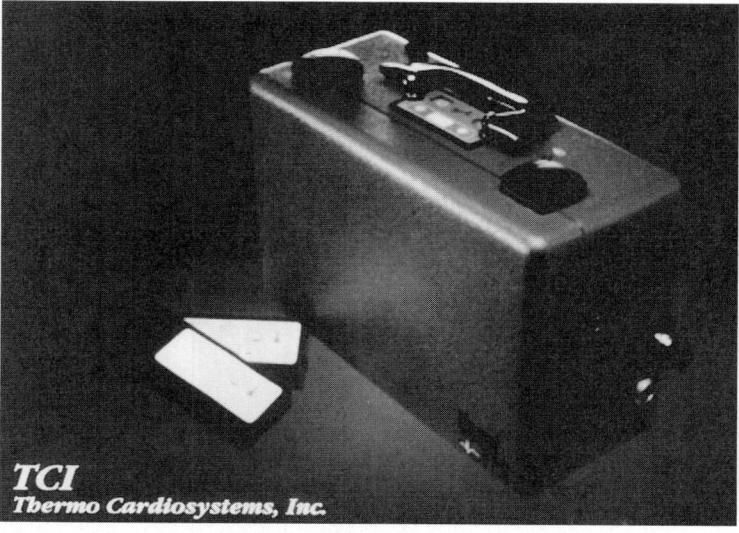

A   B

Figure 64.10. *(A)* The pneumatic drive console for the HeartMate IP LVAD. *(B)* The portable pneumatic driver for the HeartMate IP LVAD.

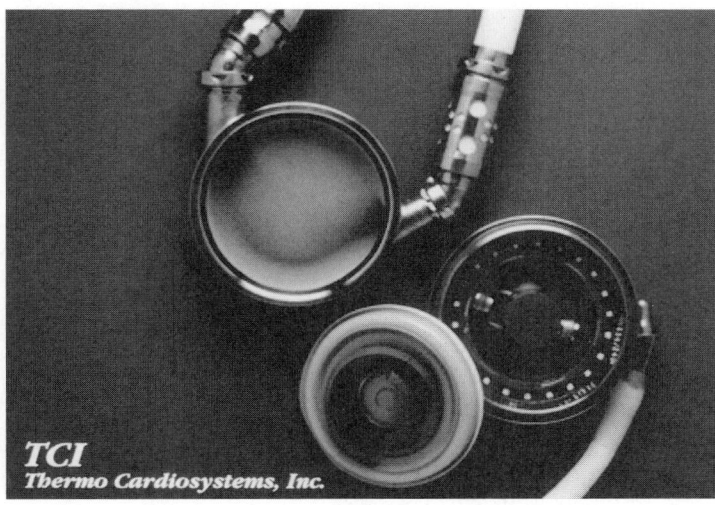

Figure 64.11. Illustration of the HeartMate VE LVAS, showing the internal rotary motor that drives the movable diaphragm.

and 9.6 L/min for the VE LVAS. The HeartMate device can be operated either in a fixed-rate mode or, more often, in an automatic mode that more closely resembles normal physiologic conditions. In the automatic mode, the device ejects when the pump is 90% full or when it senses a decreased rate of filling. As the patient's activity increases, the pump fills faster and the rate (or stroke volume) automatically increases, so that pump output increases. With a decrease in activity, pump filling and output decrease. Because the aortic valve rarely opens when the heart is fully supported by an LVAD, pump output is synonymous with cardiac output. During normal operation, the pump completely unloads the left ventricle and supports cardiac output at physiologic levels. Because of the portability and ease of operation of the HeartMate VE LVAS, patients can be discharged to await heart transplantation outside the hospital.

Novacor LVAS

The Novacor LVAS is a portable, implantable device designed for long-term circulatory support (83–85) (Fig. 64.13). It differs significantly from the HeartMate in its mode of pump actuation. Additionally, its blood-contacting surfaces are smooth. During pump systole, two opposing pusher plates compress a seamless polyurethane blood sac to cause ejection of blood. Unidirectional flow is ensured by the use of 21-mm bioprosthetic valved conduits at the inlet and outlet orifices. The device produces a maximum stroke volume of 70 mL and is monitored by an external drive console. An internal solenoid converts the electric energy from the console to mechanical energy, compressing the pusher plates and pressurizing the pump sac for blood ejection. A percutaneous lead contains the necessary electrical wires and a vent to transfer air. In 1993, the Novacor LVAS was converted from a console-operated system into a wearable system to enhance patient mobility. The wearable system eliminates the need for a bulky console by incorporating a compact controller and rechargeable power packs that are worn on the patient's belt. The wearable system is designed for out-of-hospital use and can be monitored with a bedside monitor. The Novacor LVAS is implanted through an extended median sternotomy. The pump is positioned in the abdominal wall just anterior to the posterior rectus sheath between the left iliac crest and the costal margin. Cardiopulmonary bypass support is necessary during placement of the left ventricular apical inflow conduit and anastomosis of the outflow graft to the ascending aorta. A percutaneous drive line is brought out through the right lateral abdominal wall and is connected to the cable from the controller. The external controller provides power and allows control and monitoring of the pump. The system can be operated in either a fixed-rate, synchronous, or fill-to-empty mode. The synchronized mode maximizes cardiac unloading. In this mode, an electrocardiographic signal causes pump diastole to correspond with cardiac systole, so that the heart

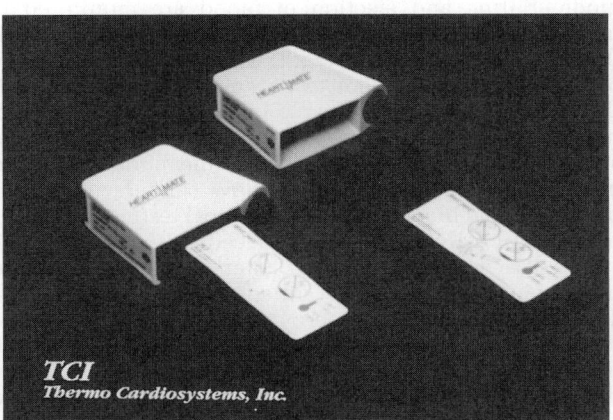

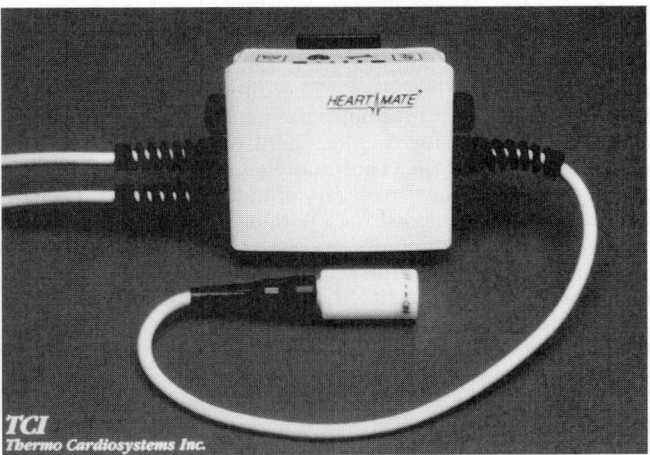

Figure 64.12. The computer controller for the HeartMate VE LVAS *(A)* with power source *(B)*.

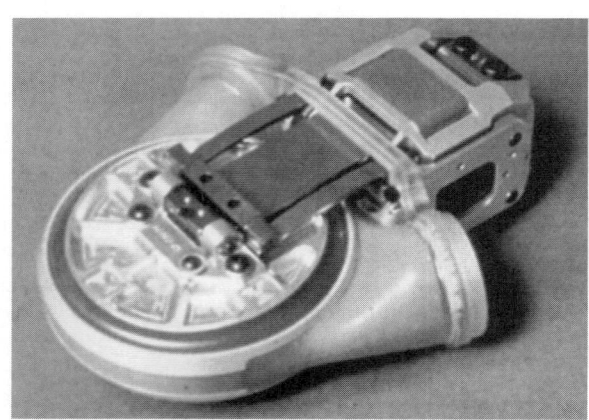

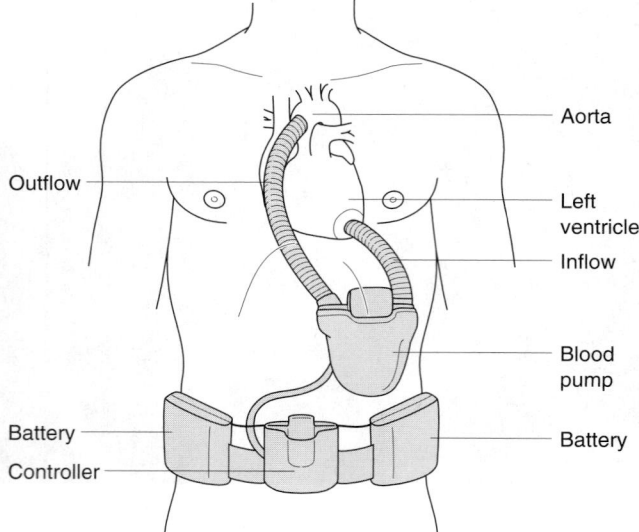

Figure 64.13. *(A)* The Baxter Novacor LVAS.

can fill the pump with little effort. Alternatively, pump output may be maximized by means of the fill-to-empty mode, in which the pumping rate is adjusted automatically depending on the filling rate of the pump. Thirdly, the system can be operated in a fixed-rate mode, in which the operator sets a constant pumping rate. During device use, anticoagulation with heparin and later with warfarin and antiplatelet therapy is necessary to prevent thromboembolism. During long-term support, ambulatory patients can be discharged and live outside the hospital while awaiting a suitable donor heart. The Novacor LVAS is approved by the Food and Drug Administration for use as a bridge to heart transplantation.

LionHeart LVD2000 LVAS

The Arrow/Penn State LionHeart LVD2000 LVAS (Fig. 64.14) is a completely implantable device that has been under development at Pennsylvania State University for more than 15 years with the collaborative research efforts of Arrow International (Reading, PA) (3). The LionHeart device was designed to operate without percutaneous wires or vents, so that the patient needs to carry only a rechargeable, extracorporeal battery pack. A roller screw mechanism moves the titanium pusher plate of the pump back and forth to permit ejection and passive filling of a 70-mL blood sac. The seamless blood sacs are solution-cast from segmented polyurethane. Delrin tilting-disk valves ensure a unidirectional blood flow. An intrathoracic compliance chamber and implanted controller/backup batter are included. The flexible intrathoracic compliance chamber eliminates the need for percutaneous venting and allows for displacement of the actuating air during device diastole. The chamber is in contact with lung tissue, which in turn is in contact with atmospheric pressures, so that the need for a percutaneous vent is eliminated. The transcutaneous energy transmission system (TETS) is used to power the brushless direct current motor of the pump and to modify the algorithm of the internal controller if desired. The TETS transfers power from an external source across intact skin and tissue to the device by means of electromagnetic induction. This is accomplished with a pair of wire coils, one implanted subcutaneously and one located directly over the implanted coil on the skin surface. By selecting an appropriate operating frequency and coil geometry, a coupling coefficient suit-

able for power transfer across intact skin and tissue can be obtained. System telemetry takes place by means of an implanted radio frequency transmitter. The pump is placed in the preperitoneal position, and cannulae pass into the mediastinum through the diaphragm. The system is currently undergoing long-term feasibility trials in animals.

HeartSaver LVAD

The HeartSaver LVAD is based on an electrohydraulic actuating mechanism. It consists of a compact implantable unit with a blood pump volume-displacement chamber, energy converter, and internal electronic module. These components are encapsulated together and shaped to permit intrathoracic positioning (86) (Fig. 64.15). The implantable unit has a total displacement volume of 480 mL and a weight of 680 g. The unit consists of a 70-mL blood chamber with a flexible polyurethane diaphragm within a rigid housing. The silicone-based hydraulic fluid is pumped during systole through the energy converter, which consists of a bidirectional brushless direct current motor, a bladed impeller, and a bladed housing. The hydraulic fluid actuates the flexible blood chamber diaphragm, which ejects blood from the chamber. The blood chamber fills passively during diastole, with the hydraulic fluid returning to the volume-displacement chamber through a one-way valve. Diastolic filling may be augmented with reversal of the motor in the active filling mode. Filling and ejection of blood are monitored by means of Hall effect sensors and a magnet embedded in the blood-pumping diaphragm, which allow the position of the flexing diaphragm to be determined dynamically throughout the pumping cycle by the internal electronic module. Mechanical valves (Medtronic-Hall extended side tilting disk, Medtronic, Minneapolis, MN) are mounted in the inflow and outflow cannulae to ensure unidirectional blood flow. Once clinical testing begins, the mechanical valves will be replaced with bioprosthetic valves (Carpentier-Edwards, Baxter Healthcare Corporation, Irvine, CA) to reduce anticoagulation requirements. To eliminate the need for percutaneous venting, a volume-displacement chamber is integrated into the implantable unit. This allows for the displacement of the actuating hydraulic fluid during device diastole. It consists of an integrated hydraulic fluid chamber with a flexible diaphragm. The flexible diaphragm is in contact with lung tissue,

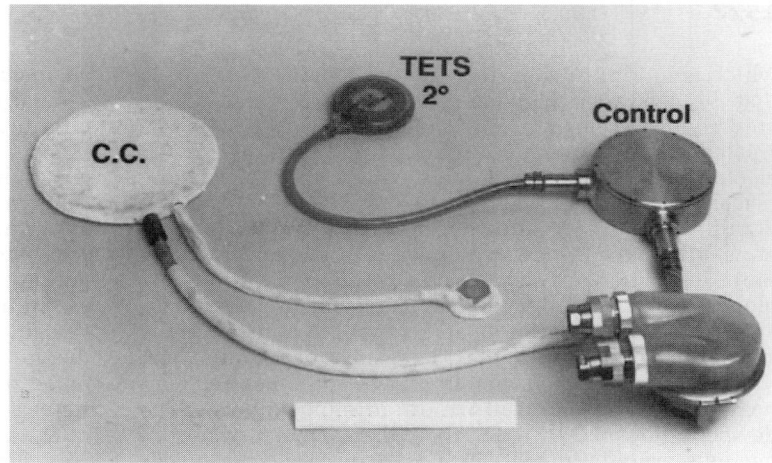

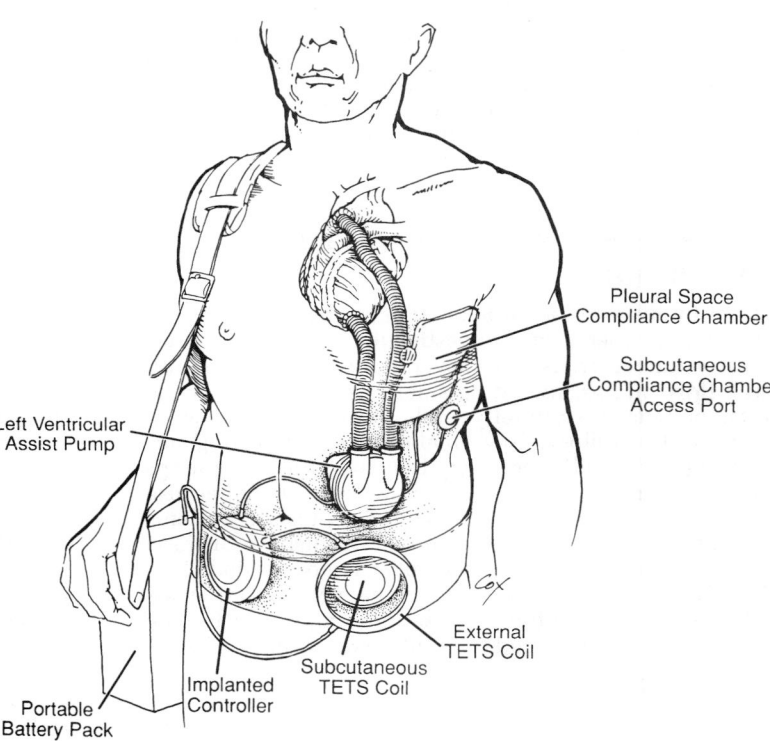

Figure 64.14. The Penn State/Arrow LionHeart LVAS.

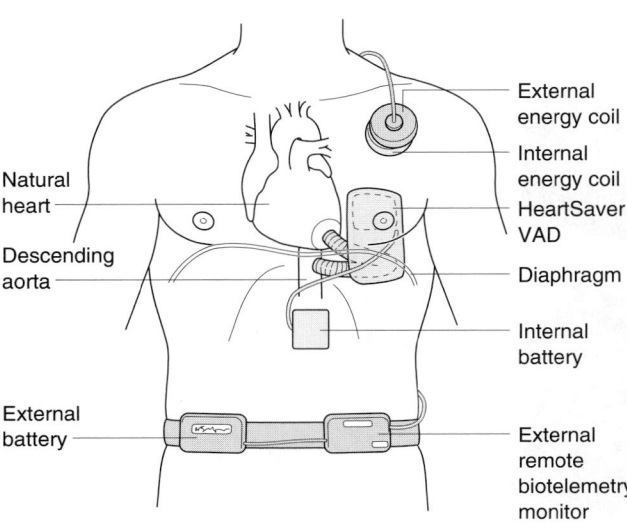

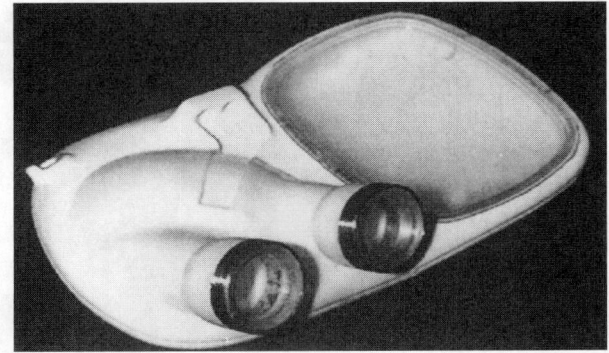

Figure 64.15. The HeartSaver LVAD.

which is in turn in contact with atmospheric pressure, so that the need for a percutaneous vent is eliminated. The volume-displacement chamber also permits heat to be dissipated from the internal electronic module. The internal electronic module is mounted within the volume-displacement chamber surrounded by the actuating hydraulic fluid, which allows excess heat generated to be transferred over the entire surface area of the implanted unit. Heat is transferred across the blood diaphragm to the bloodstream, across the volume-displacement chamber diaphragm to the lung tissue, and across the housing to the surrounding tissue. With these large areas of potential heat transfer, local hot spots are eliminated and operating temperatures can be kept well within physiologic limits. The device is powered by a TETS, so that percutaneous connections are eliminated. The TETS performs two major functions: It provides operating power from an external power source to the implanted device, and it provides power to recharge the implanted battery, which is used as a backup power supply. The implanted battery also makes it possible for the patient to bathe, shower, swim, and participate in other activities unencumbered by any external components.

Implantable, Nonpulsatile/Axial Flow Pumps

Continuous-flow or impeller pumps that are currently undergoing experimental investigation in animal studies or early human trials offer several advantages over pulsatile flow pumps, including smaller size, fewer moving parts, enhanced simplicity and durability, absence of valves to direct blood flow, smaller blood-contacting surfaces, and reduced energy requirements. Smaller pumps can be designed based on axial flow technology because the large blood chambers necessary with pulsatile systems are eliminated. An additional important feature of these pumps is that a compliance chamber is not needed. This feature obviates the problem of internal compensation, associated with conventional pulsatile pumps, that to date has significantly hindered total internalization.

HeartMate II

The HeartMate II is a small integrated pump–motor assembly that connects into the circulatory system through an apical cannula that draws blood flow from the left ventricular apex through an inlet orifice and an outflow cannula that is anastomosed to the ascending aorta (87,88) (Fig. 64.16). The pump is placed below the left costal margin under the left rectus abdominal muscle. The inflow cannula exits the left ventricular apex and crosses the diaphragm in the costophrenic angle, entering the subrectus pocket under the left rib margin to attach to the pump. The outflow cannula is tunneled back under the sternum to the ascending aorta. The pump consists of a 12-mm-diameter straight duct, and 14-mm-diameter grafts are used for both the inlet and outlet cannulae. On entering the pump, blood passes through inlet stator vanes. After exiting the stator vanes, the blood flow is energized by the pump rotor, which imparts tangential velocity and kinetic energy. Blood leaving the rotor then passes through a set of exit stator vanes that turn and diffuse the stream velocity; kinetic energy is recovered in the process. The net action results in the generation of a net pressure rise across the pump. Torque required to drive the pump rotor is developed by an integral electric motor. The 12-mm-diameter duct of the pump is actually a thin-walled tube that passes through the bore of the coil windings of the motor. The rotor of the motor is a permanent magnet located in the hub of the rotor of the pump. The location of the pump rotor in the tube is such that the motor magnet is in the proper position with respect to the coils, which is at the center line of the axis of the windings, and centered longitudinally with respect to the length of the coil. Excitation current sequentially transmitted to the coils creates a spinning magnetic field, thereby imparting torque and angular velocity to the motor magnet. The pump rotor spins on two bearings located at either end. Both bearings react against radial and axial thrust forces. The stationary element of each bearing is located in the hub of the respective inlet and outlet stators; the bearings themselves are similar to standard ball–cup jewel bearings. The outer boundaries of the adjacent static and moving surfaces of the bearings are washed directly by the main blood flow. Under normal operation, inlet pressure to the axial flow pump is cyclic and varies with systole/diastole of the left ventricle. Pressures developed within the left ventricle during systole depend on cardiac contractility and the overall flow demand of the patient. In the clinical situation of compromised cardiac contractility, with the pump operating at some nominal speed, systolic contractions of the heart

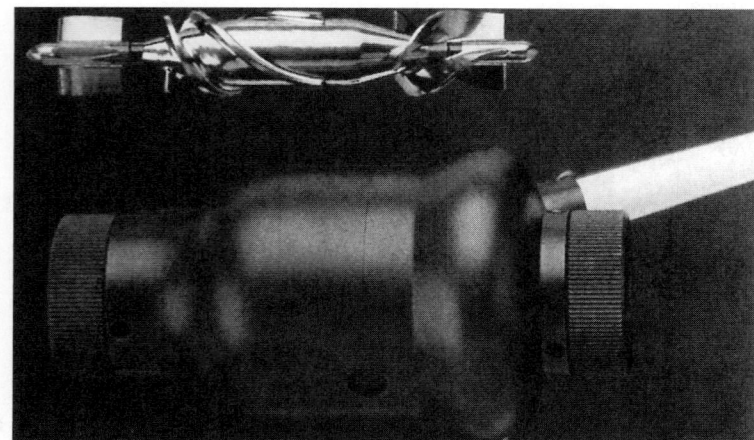
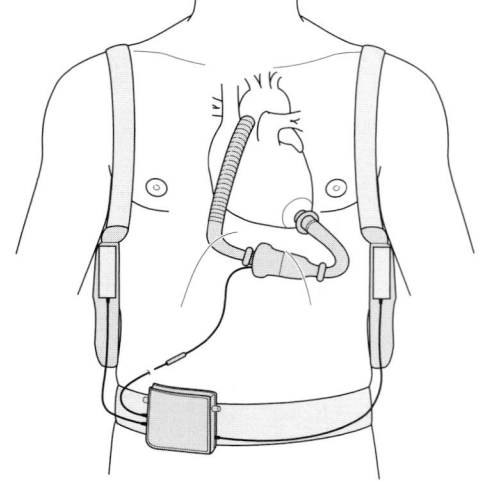

A   B

Figure 64.16. The Thermo Cardiosystems HeartMate II.

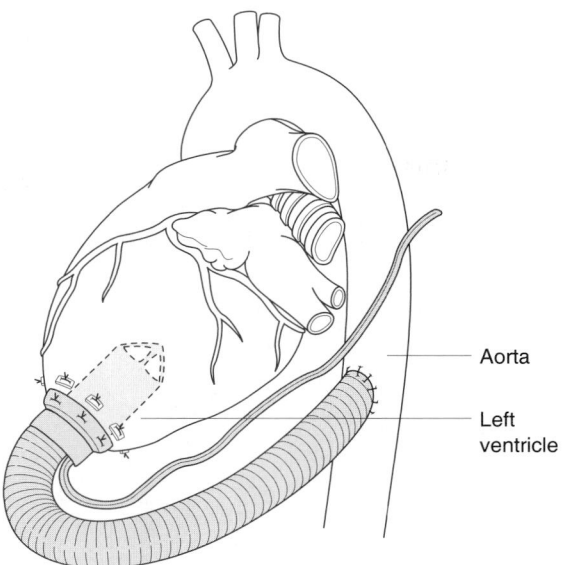

Figure 64.17. The Jarvik 2000 LVAD.

generate a pressure rise at the pump inlet; during diastole, this is followed by a fall in inlet pressures to their lowest level. A changing differential pressure across the pump results, which in turn causes a corresponding fluctuation of flow to the aorta. Thus, under most circumstances, the rotary pump generates some pulsatility. Totally nonpulsatile flow occurs if the heart is in fibrillation, a state that cannot be tolerated on a long-term basis, or if the pump is operated at too high a speed or negative inflow pressure causes left ventricular collapse. Testing of the HeartMate II in humans will begin in the year 2000.

Jarvik 2000

The Jarvik 2000 heart is a compact axial flow impeller pump (89,89) (Fig. 64.17). The outflow orifice of the pump is attached to a Dacron graft for anastomosis to the descending thoracic aorta. The Jarivk 2000 pump is inserted

through a cuff sewn into the apex of the left ventricle. The current adult version of the Jarvik 2000 measures 2.5 cm in diameter and 5.5 cm in length, with a weight of 85 g and a displacement volume of 25 mL. The pediatric iteration of the device measures 1.4 cm in diameter and 5 cm in length, with a weight of 18 g and displacement volume of 5 mL. The pump rotor contains the permanent magnet of a brushless direct current motor and mounts the impeller blades. A titanium shell accommodates the rotor and suspends it at each end by tiny, blood-immersed ceramic bearings. The adult pump functions at speeds of 8,000 to 12,000 rpm, achieving a blood flow of up to 8 L/min. The pediatric version of the Jarvik 2000 achieves pump flows of up to 3 L/min. Noise and hemolysis are minimal with each device. Percutaneous power is delivered from external batteries via a controller unit. Internal electrical wires are brought via the left pleural cavity to the apex of the chest and then subcutaneously across the neck to the base of the skull, where a percutaneous titanium pedestal transmits fine electrical wires through the skin of the scalp. The Jarvik 2000 LVAD is currently undergoing testing in humans.

DeBakey/NASA LVAD

The DeBakey/NASA LVAD is an axial flow pump that measures approximately 86 mm long and 25 mm wide (about the size of an AA battery) (91–93) (Fig. 64.18). It weighs 95 g and has a displacement of 15 mL. Within the flow tube, the components consist of an inducer–impeller (the only moving part), a fixed-flow straightener that acts as the front-bearing support for the inducer–impeller, and a fixed rear diffuser that provides the rear bearing of the inducer–impeller. The diffuser retards the highly tangential blood flow velocity by redirecting it axially, an action that results in fluid pressure build. Rare earth magnets, which are embedded in the blades of the impeller, act as the rotor of the brushless motor, causing it to spin in a magnetic field. This pump can produce a flow of 5 to 6 L/min against a pressure of 100 mm Hg at about 10,000 rpm and requires less than 10 W of power. Extensive computational analyses of fluid dynamics were performed jointly with NASA–Ames Research Center to optimize the

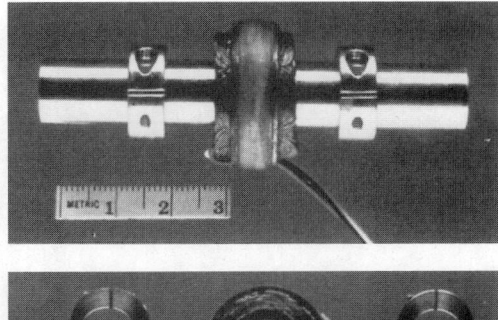

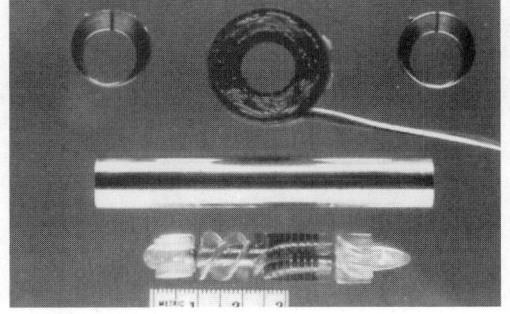

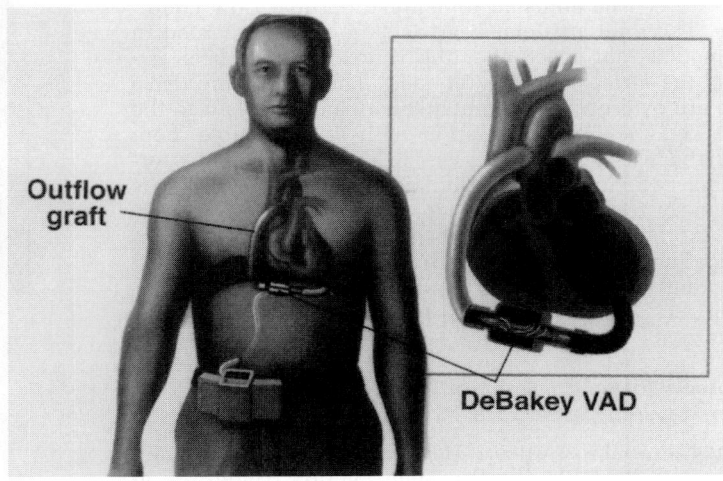

A

B

Figure 64.18. The DeBakey/NASA LVAD.

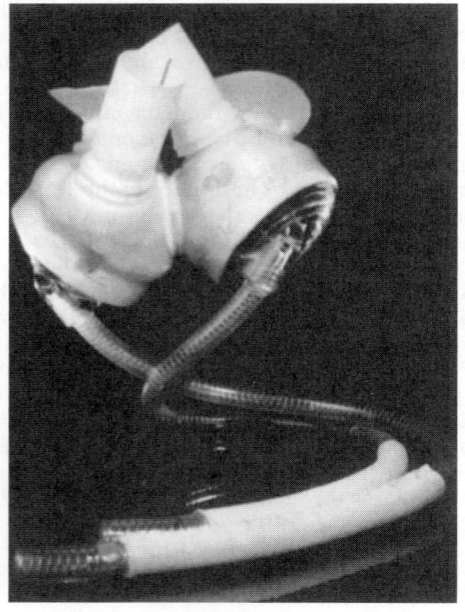
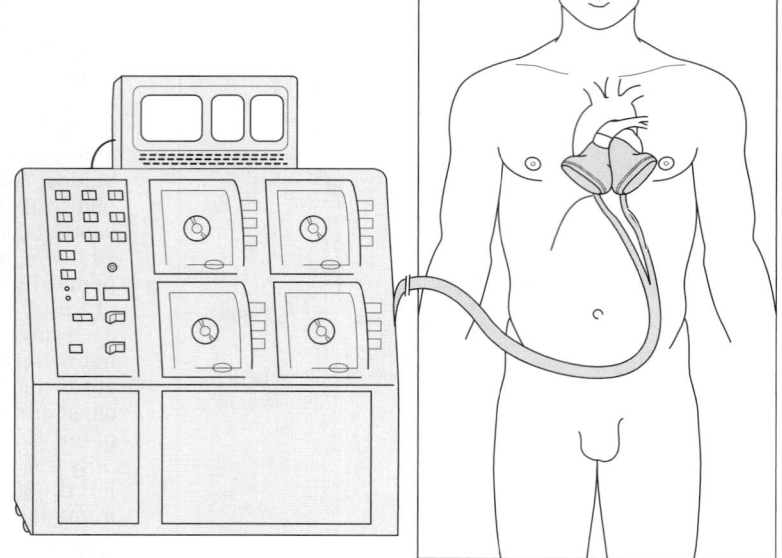

Figure 64.19. The CardioWest total artificial heart.

hydraulic performance and minimize hemolysis of the pump. The DeBakey/NASA LVAD is currently under investigation in human trials.

Total Artificial Hearts

CardioWest C-70 Total Artificial Heart

The CardioWest C-70 total artificial heart (CardioWest Technologies, Tucson, AZ), formerly called the *Jarvik* or *Symbion total artificial heart,* is a pulsatile biventricular cardiac replacement system (94,95) (Fig. 64.19). The rigid polyurethane pump contains a smooth, flexible polyurethane diaphragm that separates the blood and air chambers. Two Medtronic-Hall mechanical valves located at the inflow and outflow orifices ensure unidirectional blood flow. Compressed air from the external drive console moves the diaphragm upward, pressurizing the blood chamber and causing ejection of blood. The pump has a maximum stroke volume of 70 mL and a maximum flow rate of 15 L/min, although the average flow rate is less than 8 L/min. Pump rate, duration of systole, and driving pressure can be adjusted to achieve optimal flow conditions. The total artificial heart is surgically implanted in the mediastinal space after the ventricles have been excised; the atrial cuffs are retained. The pneumatic drive lines are externalized percutaneously and attached to the drive console. Anticoagulation with dipyridamole, heparin, and warfarin is necessary to prevent thrombus formation. Patients may be ambulatory, but their mobility is frequently restricted by the large drive console. The CardioWest total artificial heart is currently under clinical investigation at selected institutions in the United States. It is currently being used only as a bridge to heart transplantation. A portable driver is being developed to allow greater patient mobility.

Abiomed Total Replacement Heart and Penn State/3M Sarns Total Artificial Heart

The National Institutes of Health artificial heart program was initiated in 1964 by President Lyndon B. Johnson at the suggestion of Dr. Michael DeBakey. The original goal of the program was to develop a fully implantable long-term artificial heart. However, because of technology limitations, the program shifted its focus to the development of LVADs. Toward the latter part of the 1980s, the National Heart, Lung, and Blood Institute initiated a program for the specific development of an untethered, fully implantable total artificial heart, intended for long-term use. The goal was to create a device with no percutaneous lines that would be responsive to the varying circulatory demands of everyday activities and offer the recipient a reasonable quality of life. The total artificial heart was to be capable of supplying an output of 8 L/min from each ventricle, given physiologic preloads and afterloads. Biocompatibility of the device and durability for 5 years were additional objectives. In 1993, four research teams were

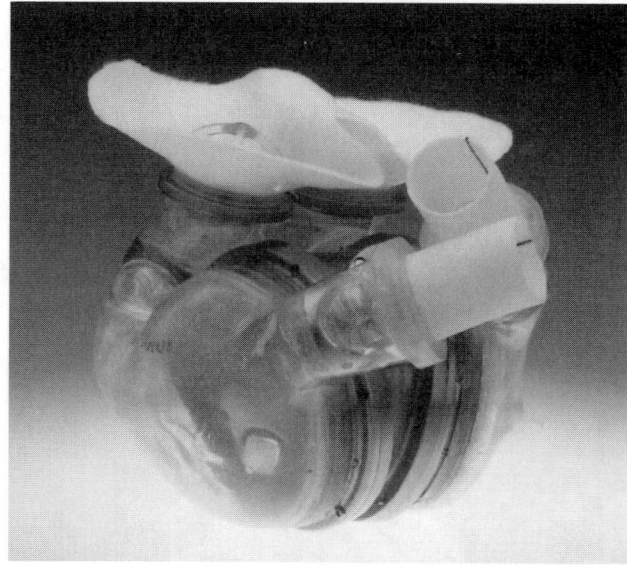

Figure 64.20. The Abiomed total replacement heart.

awarded contracts. In September of 1996, the National Institutes of Health announced the recipients of the final preclinical total artificial heart program contract; these included research teams from Abiomed/Texas Heart Institute and Pennsylvania State University/3M Sarns (96). Under this contract, initial systems were designed and modifications have been implemented on the basis of extensive in vitro and in vivo testing. The National Heart, Lung, and Blood Institute is continuing careful oversight throughout the term of the project. The current phase of this project will fund two groups for 4 years of testing of device readiness and long-term in vivo analysis. During this time, the final system configurations must demon-

strate flawless in vitro performance for at least 2 years in addition to failure-free performance in animals for 3 to 5 months. Application to the Food and Drug Administration for an Investigational Device Exemption should follow completion of the second phase. Initial human use may be as early as 2001.

Both the Abiomed (Fig. 64.20) and Penn State/Sarns (Fig. 64.21) total artificial heart systems are orthotopically positioned blood pumps that alternately eject blood into the pulmonary and systemic vasculature. Both systems use brushless direct current motors that are powered by TETS. Implanted nickel–cadmium batteries can also drive the systems in case the external coils detach. In the Penn State

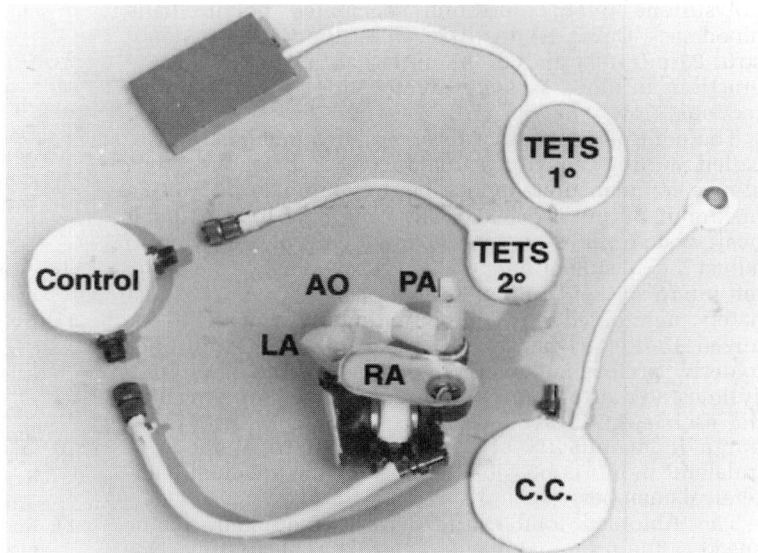

A

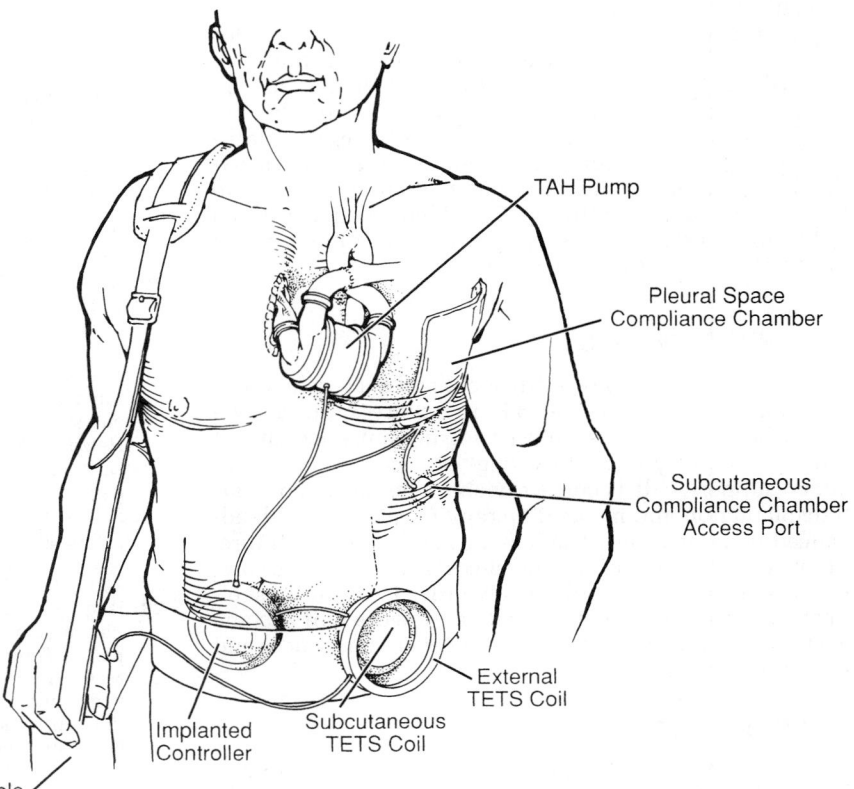

B

Figure 64.21. The Penn State/ Sarns total artificial heart.

total artificial heart, a roller screw fixed at either end to circular pusher plates rotates to allow the pusher plates to compress blood sacs and alternately create left- or right-sided systole and diastole. The Abiomed total artificial heart shifts hydraulic fluid to pump blood in a one-to-one fashion. A unidirectional centrifugal pump combined with a rotating valve transmits hydraulic fluid against one of the diaphragms of the pump while simultaneously withdrawing fluid from the contralateral side. In this fashion, the pumps are alternately filled with and emptied of blood.

The Abiomed total artificial heart is cast from a solution of proprietary polyetherurethane and then externally reinforced to provide rigidity. The system incorporates 24-mL polyetherurethane trileaflet valves in both the inlet and outlet orifices. In the Penn State total artificial heart, rigid polysulfone pumps surround segmented polyurethane blood sacs. Delrin tilting-disk valves (Bjork-Shiley Monostrut 27-mL inlet and 25-mL outlet) are positioned at the junctions of blood sacs and pump ports to ensure unidirectional flow.

The control schemes of these systems demonstrate so-called Starling behavior, so that increases in venous return elicit a commensurate increase in left pump output until a maximum output is reached. The Penn State total artificial heart system relies on an implanted control algorithm to adjust the diastolic time period and speed of systole of the left pump so that complete filling of the left pump is just barely maintained while the pumping rate remains maximized. Hall effect (magnetic) sensors allow the controller to derive preload and afterload parameters, the duration of systole and diastole, and the speed of pump emptying during each ejection cycle. Passive diastolic filling of one pump independently of the ejection speed of the contralateral pump is possible because of the attached compliance chamber.

The Abiomed total artificial heart modulates motor speed as the principal way to control cardiac output. Optimal pumping rate is made a function of right atrial pressure, inferred from transducer-measured pressure readings within the right hydraulic chamber. Compensation for right and left flow imbalances depends on a flexible, 20-mL hydraulic chamber positioned against the left atrium. This compliance chamber, in continuity with the hydraulic chamber of the right pump, exerts negative feedback on right pump filling. As left atrial pressure rises, hydraulic fluid shifts into the right hydraulic chamber to limit passive diastolic filling of the blood chamber of the right pump. Less blood is then delivered to the left side until left atrial pressure decreases.

FUTURE DIRECTIONS

Recent rapid technologic advances and successful clinical applications of mechanical circulatory support have made the future of this field promising but uncertain. It now appears very likely that long-term mechanical circulatory support will become a viable alternative to heart transplantation and medical therapy for patients with advanced congestive heart failure in the immediate future. Because of the technologic advances, it is difficult to predict which devices will ultimately prove to be the most efficacious. It is likely that a variety of devices will become available for use, depending on clinical circumstances and patient characteristics.

REFERENCES

1. Cooley DA, Liotta D, Hallman GL, et al. Orthotopic cardiac prosthesis for two-staged cardiac replacement. *Am J Cardiol* 1969;24:723.
2. DeVries WC, Anterson JL, Joyce LD, et al. Clinical use of the total artificial heart. *N Engl J Med* 1984;310:273–278.
3. Sapirstein JS, Pierce WS. Mechanical circulatory support. In: Greenfield LJ, Mulholland MW, Oldham KT, et al., eds. *Surgery: scientific principles and practice*, 2nd ed. Philadelphia: Lippincott–Raven Publishers, 1997:1550–1565.
4. Norman JC, Cooley DA, Igo SR, et al. Prognostic indices for survival during postcardiotomy intra-aortic balloon pumping. *J Thorac Cardiovasc Surg* 1977;74:709–720.
5. Oz MC, Goldstein DJ, Pepino P, et al. Screening scale predicts patients successfully receiving long-term implantable left ventricular assist devices. *Circulation* 1995;92[Suppl II]:II-169–II-173.
6. Pae WE. Ventricular assist devices and total artificial hearts: an ASAIO–ISHLT registry experience. *Ann Thorac Surg* 1993;55:295–298.
7. Guyton RA, Schonberger J, Everts P, et al. Postcardiotomy shock: clinical evaluation of the BVS 5000 biventricular support system. *Ann Thorac Surg* 1993;56:346–356.
8. Jett GK. Postcardiotomy support with ventricular assist devices: selection of recipients. *Semin Thorac Cardiovasc Surg* 1994;6:136–139.
9. Pennington DG, Merjavy JP, Swartz MT, et al. The importance of biventricular failure in patients with postoperative cardiogenic shock. *Ann Thorac Surg* 1985;39:16–26.
10. Farrar DJ, Hill JD, Pennington DG, et al. Preoperative and postoperative comparison of patients with univentricular and biventricular support with the Thoratec ventricular assist device as a bridge to cardiac transplantation. *J Thorac Cardiovasc Surg* 1997;113:202–209.
11. Kormos RL, Gasior TA, Kawai A, et al. Transplant candidate's clinical status rather than right ventricular function defines the need for univentricular versus biventricular support. *J Thorac Cardiovasc Surgery* 1996;111:773–783.
12. Catanese KA, Goldstein DJ, Williams DL, et al. *Ann Thorac Surg* 1996;62:646–653.
13. McCarthy PM. HeartMate implantable left ventricular assist device: bridge to transplantation and future applications. *Ann Thorac Surg* 1995;59:S46–S51.
14. Rose EA, Moskowitz AJ, Packer M, et al. The REMATCH trial: rationale, design, and end points. *Ann Thorac Surg* 1999;67:723–730.
15. Frazier OH, Myers TJ. Left ventricular assist system as a bridge to myocardial recovery. *Ann Thorac Surg* 1999;68:734–741.
16. Dipla K, Mattiello JA, Jeevanandam V, et al. Myocyte recovery after mechanical circulatory support in humans with end-stage heart failure. *Circulation* 1998;97:2316–2322.
17. Mueller J, Wallukat G, Weng Y-G, et al. Weaning from mechanical cardiac support in patients with idiopathic dilated cardiomyopathy. *Circulation* 1997;96:542–549.
18. Westaby S, Jin XY, Katsumata T, et al. Mechanical support in dilated cardiomyopathy: signs of early left ventricular recovery. *Ann Thorac Surg* 1997;64:1303–1308.
19. Levin HR, Oz MC, Chen JM, et al. Reversal of chronic ventricular dilation in patients with end-stage cardiomyopathy by prolonged mechanical unloading. *Circulation* 1995;91:2717–2720.
20. Nakatani T, Sasako Y, Kobayashi J, et al. Recovery of cardiac function by long-term left ventricular support in patients with end-stage cardiomyopathy. *ASAIO J* 1998;44:M516–M520.
21. Hetzer R, Muller J, Weng Y, et al. Cardiac recovery in dilated cardiomyopathy by unloading with a left ventricular assist device. *Ann Thorac Surg* 1999;68:742–749.
22. Scheinin SA, Capek P, Radovencevic B, et al. The effect of prolonged left ventricular support on myocardial histopathology in patients with end-stage cardiomyopathy. *ASAIO J* 1992;38:M271–M274.
23. Jacquet L, Zerbe T, Stein KL, et al. Evolution of human cardiac myocyte dimension during prolonged mechanical support. *J Thorac Cardiovasc Surg* 1991;101:256–259.
24. McCarthy PM, Nakatani S, Vargo R, et al. Structural and left ventricular histologic changes after implantable LVAD insertion. *Ann Thorac Surg* 1995;59:609–613.
25. Nakatani S, McCarthy PM, Kottke-Marchant K, et al. Left ventricular echocardiographic and histologic changes: impact of chronic unloading by an implantable ventricular assist device. *J Am Coll Cardiol* 1996;27:894–901.

26. Zafeiridis A, Jeevanandam V, Houser SR, et al. Regression of cellular hypertrophy after left ventricular assist device support. *Circulation* 1998;98:656–662.

27. Milting H, Bartling B, Schumann H, et al. Altered levels of mRNA of apoptosis-mediating genes after mid-term mechanical ventricular support in dilative cardiomyopathy—first results of the Halle Assist Induced Recovery Study (HAIR). *Thorac Cardiovasc Surg* 1999;47:48–50.

28. Altemose GT, Gritsus V, Jeevanandam V, et al. Altered myocardial phenotype after mechanical support in human beings with advanced cardiomyopathy. *J Heart Lung Transplant* 1997;16:765–773.

29. Torre-Amione G, Stetson SJ, Youker KA, et al. Decreased expression of tumor necrosis factor-alpha in failing human myocardium after mechanical circulatory support: a potential mechanism for cardiac recovery. *Circulation* 1999;100:1189–1193.

30. James KB, McCarthy PM, Thomas JD, et al. Effect of the implantable left ventricular assist device on neuroendocrine activation in heart failure. *Circulation* 1995;92[Suppl II]:II-191–II-195.

31. Delgado R III, Radovancevic B, Massin EK, et al. Neurohormonal changes after implantation of a left ventricular assist system. *ASAIO J* 1998;44:299–302.

32. Lee SH, Doliba N, Osbakken M, et al. Improvement of myocardial mitochondrial function after hemodynamic support with left ventricular assist devices in patients with heart failure. *J Thorac Cardiovasc Surgery* 1998;116:344–349.

33. Santamore WP, Gray LA. Left ventricular contributions of right ventricular systolic function during LVAD support. *Ann Thorac Surg* 1996;61:350–356.

34. Pavie A, Leger P. Physiology of univentricular versus biventricular support. *Ann Thorac Surgery* 1996;61:347–349.

35. Mandarino WA, Winowich S, Gorcsan J, et al. Right ventricular performance and left ventricular assist device filling. *Ann Thoracic Surg* 1997;63:1044–1049.

36. Aria H, Swartz MT, Pennington DG, et al. Importance of ventricular arrhythmias in bridge patients with ventricular assist devices. *ASAIO Trans* 1991;37:M427–M428.

37. Oz MC, Rose EA, Slater JP, et al. Malignant ventricular arrhythmias are well tolerated in patients receiving long-term left ventricular devices. *J Am Coll Cardiol* 1994;24:1688–1691.

38. Shapiro GC, Leibowitz DW, Oz MC, et al. Diagnosis of patent foramen ovale with transesophageal echocardiography in a patient supported with a left ventricular assist device. *J Heart Lung Transplant* 1995;14:594–597.

39. Goldstein DJ, Seldomridge JA, Chen JM, et al. Use of aprotinin in LVAD recipients reduces blood loss, blood use, and perioperative mortality. *Ann Thorac Surg* 1995;59:1063–1068.

40. Kaplon RJ, Gillinov AM, Smedira NG, et al. Vitamin K reduces bleeding in left ventricular assist device recipients. *J Heart Lung Transplant* 1999;18:346–350.

41. Nakatani S, Thomas JD, Savage RM, et al. Prediction of right ventricular dysfunction after left ventricular assist device implantation. *Circulation* 1996;94[9 Suppl]:II-216–II-221.

42. Shenkar R, Coulson WF, Abraham E. Hemorrhage and resuscitation induce alterations in cytokine expression and the development of acute lung injury. *Am J Respir Cell Mol Biol* 1994;10:290–297.

43. Horvath CJ, Ferro TJ, Jesmok G, et al. Recombinant tumor necrosis factor increases pulmonary vascular permeability independent of neutrophils. *Proc Natl Acad Sci U S A* 1988;85:9219–9223.

44. Argenziano M, Choudhri AF, Moazami N, et al. Randomized, double-blind trial of inhaled nitric oxide in LVAD recipients with pulmonary hypertension. *Ann Thorac Surg* 1998;65:340–345.

45. Salamonsen RF, Kaye D, Esmore DS. Inhalation of nitric oxide provides selective pulmonary vasodilation, aiding mechanical cardiac assist with the Thoratec left ventricular assist device. *Anaesth Intensive Care* 1994;22:209–210.

46. Hare JM, Shernan SK, Body SC, et al. Influence of inhaled nitric oxide on systemic flow and ventricular filling pressure in patients receiving mechanical circulatory assistance. *Circulation* 1997;95:2250–2253.

47. Rose EA, Levin HR, Oz MC, et al. Artificial circulatory support with textured interior surfaces: a counterintuitive approach to minimizing thromboembolism. *Circulation* 1994;90 [Suppl II]:II-87–II-91.

48. Rafii S, Oz MC, Seldomridge JA, et al. Characterization of hematopoietic cells arising on the textured surface of left ventricular assist devices. *Ann Thorac Surg* 1995;60:1627–1632.

49. Slater JP, Rose EA, Levin HR, et al. Low thromboembolic risk without anticoagulation using advanced-design left ventricular assist devices. *Ann Thorac Surg* 1996;62:1321–1327.

50. Holman WL, Fix RJ, Foley BA, et al. Management of wound and left ventricular assist device pocket infection. *Ann Thorac Surg* 1999;68:1080–1082.

51. McKellar SH, Allred BD, Marks JD, et al. Treatment of infected left ventricular assist device using antibiotic-impregnated beads. *Ann Thorac Surg* 1999;67:554–555.

52. Arabia FA, Copeland JG, Smith RG, et al. Infections with the CardioWest total artificial heart. *ASAIO J* 1998;44:M336–M339.

53. Argenziano M, Catanese KA, Moazami N, et al. The influence of infection on survival and successful transplantation in patients with left ventricular assist devices. *J Heart Lung Transplant* 1997;16:822–831.

54. Hermann M, Weyand M, Greshake B, et al. Left ventricular assist device infection is associated with increased mortality but is not a contraindication to transplantation. *Circulation* 1997;95:814–817.

55. Fischer SA, Trenholme GM, Costanzo MR, et al. Infectious complications in left ventricular assist device recipients. *Clin Infect Dis* 1997;24:18–23.

56. Springer WE, Wasler A, Radovancevic B, et al. Retrospective analysis of infection in patients undergoing support with left ventricular assist systems. *ASAIO J* 1996;42:M763–M765.

57. McCarthy PM, Schmitt SK, Vargo RL, et al. Implantable LVAD infections: implications for permanent use of the device. *Ann Thorac Surg* 1996;61:359–365.

58. Holman EL, Murrah CP, Ferguson ER, et al. Infections during extended circulatory support: University of Alabama at Birmingham experience 1989 to 1994. *Ann Thorac Surg* 1996;61:366–371.

59. Ankersmit HJ, Tugulea S, Spanier T, et al. Activation-induced T-cell death and immune dysfunction after implantation of left ventricular assist device. *Lancet* 1999;354:550–555.

60. Deng MC, Erren M, Tjan TD, et al. Left ventricular assist system support is associated with persistent inflammation and temporary immunosuppression. *Thorac Cardiovasc Surg* 1999;47[Suppl 2]:326–331.

61. Goldstein DJ, el-Amir NG, Ashton RC, et al. Fungal infections in left ventricular assist device recipients: incidence, prophylaxis, and treatment. *ASAIO J* 1995;41:873–875.

62. Nader M, Itescu S, Williams MR, et al. Platelet transfusions are associated with the development of anti-major histocompatibility complex class I antibodies in patients with ventricular assist support. *J Heart Lung Transplant* 1998;17:876–880.

63. Itescu S, Tung TC, Burke EM, et al. Preformed IgG antibodies against major histocompatibility complex class II antigens are major risk factors for high-grade cellular rejection in recipients of heart transplantation. *Circulation* 1998;98:786–793.

64. Kobashigawa JA, Sabad A, Drinkwater D, et al. Pretransplant panel reactive-antibody screens: are they truly a marker for poor outcome after cardiac transplantation? *Circulation* 1996;94:II-294–II-297.

65. Moulopolous SD, Topaz S, Kolff WJ. Diastolic balloon pumping (with carbon dioxide) in the aorta: a mechanical assistance to the failing circulation. *Am Heart J* 1962;63:669.

66. Kantrowitz A, Tjonneland S, Freed PS, et al. Initial clinical experience with intraaortic balloon pumping in cardiogenic shock. *JAMA* 1968;203:135.

67. Claus RH, Birtwell WC, Albertal G, et al. Assisted circulation, the arterial counterpulsator. *J Thorac Cardiovasc Surg* 1961;41:447.

68. Muehrcke DD, McCarthy PM, Stewart RW, et al. Extracorporeal membrane oxygenation for postcardiotomy cardiogenic shock. *Ann Thorac Surg* 1996;61:684–691.

69. Smedira NG, Wudel JH, Hlozek CC, et al. Venovenous extracorporeal life support for patients after cardiotomy. *ASAIO J* 1997;43:M444–M446.

70. McGovern GJ, Magovern JA, Benckart DH, et al. Extracorporeal membrane oxygenation—preliminary results in patients

with postcardiotomy cardiogenic shock. *Ann Thorac Surg* 1994;57:1462–1467.

71. Hill JD, O'Brien TG, Murray JJ, et al. Extracorporeal oxygenation for acute post-traumatic respiratory failure. *N Engl J Med* 1972;286:629–634.

72. Bavaria JE, Furukawa S, Kreiner G. Effect of circulatory assist devices on stunned myocardium. *Ann Thorac Surg* 1990;49:123–128.

73. Noon GP, Lafuente JA, Irwin S. Acute and temporary ventricular support with BioMedicus centrifugal pump. *Ann Thorac Surg* 1999;68:650–654.

74. Curtis JJ, Walls JT, Wagner-Mann CC, et al. Centrifugal pumps: description of devices and surgical techniques. *Ann Thorac Surg* 1999;68:666–671.

75. Mehta SM, Aufiero TX, Pae WE, et al. Results of mechanical ventricular assistance for the treatment of postcardiotomy cardiogenic shock. *ASAIO J* 1996;42:211–218.

76. McBride LR, Naunheim KS, Fiore AC, et al. Clinical experience with 111 Thoractec ventricular assist devices. *Ann Thorac Surg* 1999;67:1233–1238.

77. El-Banayosy A, Korfer R, Arusoglu L, et al. Bridging to cardiac transplantation with the Thoratec ventricular assist device. *Thorac Cardiovasc Surg* 1999;47[Suppl 2]:307–310.

78. Farrar DJ, Buck KE, Coulter JH, et al. Portable pneumatic biventricular driver for the Thoratec ventricular assist device. *ASAIO J* 1997;43:M631–M634.

79. Gray LA, Champsaur GG. The BVS 5000 biventricular assist device: the worldwide registry experience. *ASAIO J* 1994;40:M460–M464.

80. Oz MC, Argenziano M, Catanese KA, et al. Bridge experience with long-term implantable left ventricular assist device. *Circulation* 1997;95:1844–1852.

81. Frazier OH, Myers TJ, Radovancevic B. The HeartMate left ventricular assist systems—overview and 12-year experience. *Tex Heart Inst J* 1998;25:265–271.

82. McCarthy PM, Smedira NO, Vargo RL, et al. One hundred patients with the HeartMate left ventricular assist device: evolving concepts and technology. *J Thorac Cardiovasc Surg* 1998;115:904–912.

83. Robbins RC, Oyer PE. Bridge to transplant with the Novacor left ventricular assist system. *Ann Thorac Surg* 1999;68:695–697.

84. El-Banayosy A, Deng M, Loisance DY, et al. The European experience of Novacor left ventricular assist (LVAS) therapy as a bridge to transplant: a retrospective multi-centre study. *Eur J Cardiothorac Surg* 1999;15:835–841.

85. Murali S. Mechanical circulatory support with the Novacor LVAS: world-wide clinical results. *Thorac Cardiovasc Surg* 1999;47[Suppl 2]:321–325.

86. Mussivand T, Hendry PJ, Masters RG, et al. Progress with the HeartSaver ventricular assist device. *Ann Thorac Surg* 1999;68:785–789.

87. Thomas DC, Butler KC, Taylor LP, et al. Progress on development of the Nimbus–University of Pittsburgh axial flow left ventricular assist system. *ASAIO J* 1998;44:M521–M524.

88. Butler KC, Dow JJ, Litwak P, et al. Development of the Nimbus/University of Pittsburgh innovative ventricular assist system. *Ann Thorac Surg* 1999;68:790–794.

89. Westaby S, Katsumata T, Evans R, et al. The Jarvik 2000 Oxford System: increasing the scope of mechanical circulatory support. *J Thorac Cardiovasc Surg* 1997;114:467–474.

90. Westaby S, Katsumata T, Houel R, et al. Jarvik 2000 Heart: potential for bridge to myocyte recovery. *Circulation* 1998;98:1568–1574.

91. DeBakey ME. Development of a ventricular assist device. *Artif Organs* 1997;21:1149–1153.

92. DeBakey ME. A miniature implantable axial flow ventricular assist device. *Ann Thorac Surg* 1999;68:637–640.

93. Fossum TW, Morley D, Benkowski R, et al. Chronic survival of calves implanted with the DeBakey ventricular assist device. *Artif Organs* 1999;23:802–806.

94. Arabia FA, Copeland JG, Pavie A, et al. Implantation technique for the CardioWest total artificial heart. *Ann Thorac Surg* 1999;68:698–704.

95. Copeland JG, Pavie A, Duveau D, et al. Bridge to transplantation with the CardioWest total artificial heart: the international experience 1993–1995. *J Heart Lung Transplant* 1996;15:94–99.

96. Nose Y. Final stretch for the totally implantable TAH [editorial]. *Artif Organs* 1997;21:89–90.

SURGERY: SCIENTIFIC PRINCIPLES AND PRACTICE, Third Edition, edited by Lazar J. Greenfield, Michael W. Mulholland, Keith T. Oldham, Gerald B. Zelenock, and Keith D. Lillemoe. Lippincott Williams & Wilkins Publishers, Philadelphia, © 2001.

CHAPTER 65

PERICARDIUM

SCOTT M. BRADLEY

EMBRYOLOGY AND ANATOMY

The pericardium forms during the fifth week of gestation, when the two pleuropericardial membranes fuse with each other and the root of the lungs to divide the primitive thoracic cavity into the pericardial cavity and the pleural spaces (1). The pleuropericardial membranes contain the cardinal veins and phrenic nerves, and in the adult they form the fibrous pericardium. After development, the serous pericardium, consisting of a single layer of mesothelial cells, lines the fibrous pericardium. Together, the serous pericardium and fibrous pericardium comprise the parietal pericardium. The visceral pericardium, or epicardium, covers the heart and intrapericardial great vessels. The phrenic nerves lie in the parietal pericardium. For this reason, diaphragmatic paralysis can complicate operations on the pericardium. The pericardium superiorly merges with the adventitia of the great vessels, and inferiorly it is attached to the central tendon of the diaphragm. The oblique sinus is a blind cul-de-sac located behind the left atrium, and the transverse sinus is a tubular space situated between the aorta and main pulmonary artery anteriorly, and the right and left atria posteriorly (Fig. 65.1). The vascular supply of the pericardium is from the internal thoracic arteries via the pericardiophrenic branches, and from the descending aorta. Venous drainage is to the internal thoracic veins and azygous system. Lymphatic drainage is to the local bronchial and tracheal nodes, and to the thoracic duct. Innervation is by the sympathetic trunks and the phrenic and vagus nerves. The pericardium normally contains 15 to 50 mL of serous fluid. This fluid is an ultrafiltrate of plasma with a protein content lower than that of plasma (2).

NORMAL PHYSIOLOGY

Not all the functions of the pericardium are well understood, and people can do well with a congenital absence or after surgical removal of the pericardium. Structural functions appear to include mechanically protecting and anchoring the heart, preventing acute cardiac distention, and serving as a barrier to infection (2). The pericardium contributes to diastolic coupling of the ventricles. Diastolic coupling links pressure rises in the right ventricle to those in the left ventricle, so that movement of the two ventricles is coordinated along their respective Starling curves. The pericardium also functions as an absorptive surface, transmitting fluid to both the thoracic duct system and the pleural spaces. Regulatory functions include controlling the blood pressure and heart rate via mechanoreceptors. Pericardial fluid exhibits fibrinolytic activity, which prevents intrapericardial blood from clotting.

Pericardial disease produces characteristic changes in hemodynamics and systemic venous pulsations. Normal intrapericardial pressure is essentially the same as pleural pressure, and at end-expiration it is about 2 mm Hg below

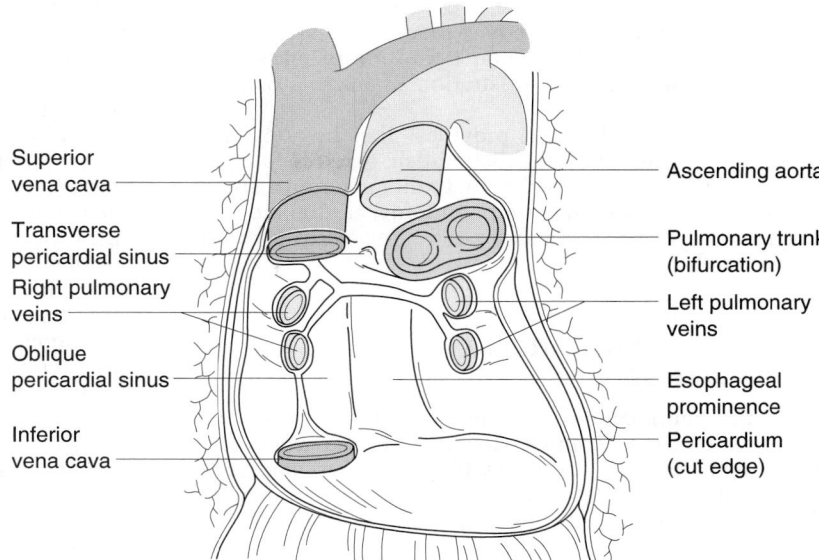

Figure 65.1. Diagrammatic illustration of the pericardial attachments to the great vessels and pulmonary veins, after the heart has been removed. The transverse sinus is a free space behind the aorta and main pulmonary artery. The oblique sinus lies behind the left atrium. (From Harken AH, Hammond GL, Edmunds LH Jr. Pericardial diseases. In: Edmunds LH Jr, ed. *Cardiac surgery in the adult.* New York: McGraw-Hill, 1997:1304, with permission.)

atmospheric pressure. During inspiration, pericardial pressure decreases slightly. The normal hemodynamic effect of inspiration is to increase right-sided venous return, right ventricular preload, right ventricular stroke volume, pulmonary arterial flow, and pulmonary vascular bed capacity. Inspiration decreases pleural pressure and pericardial pressure. Pooling of blood in the lungs causes a decrease in pulmonary capillary wedge pressure, left-sided venous return, left ventricular stroke volume, systemic arterial pressure, and aortic flow. The decrease in arterial pressure seen during normal inspiration is less than 10 mm Hg. Increased right ventricular filling during inspiration also causes a leftward shift of the interventricular septum, which further decreases left ventricular volume and stroke volume.

Normal jugular venous pulsations show three positive pulse waves, the a, c, and v waves, and two negative waves, the x and y descents (Fig. 65.2). The a wave results from normal atrial contraction. Its peak corresponds to S_4. The c wave is caused by the bulging of the atrioventricular valve into the atrium during isovolumic ventricular systole. It begins at S_1. The x descent (systolic collapse) is caused by downward displacement of the base of the heart during ventricular systole and atrial relaxation. Its lowest point is in midsystole. The v wave is caused by passive atrial filling from the venae cavae and occurs just after S_2. The y descent (diastolic collapse) follows the opening of the atrioventricular valve and subsequent passive ventricular filling. The effects of respiration are that during inspiration, with decreasing intrathoracic pressure, the x descent is lower than the y descent. During expiration, with more positive intrathoracic pressure and lower systemic venous return, the y descent is equal to or lower than the x descent.

DIAGNOSTIC STUDIES

The electrocardiogram is usually nonspecific but can contribute to the diagnosis of pericardial disease. QRS voltage may be decreased in the presence of a large pericardial effusion. Electrocardiographic changes in pericarditis typically evolve through four stages, which are believed to be caused by a generalized superficial myocarditis: (a) diffuse ST-segment elevation in all leads except aVR and V_1, without reciprocal depression; (b) normalization of ST segments with flattening of T waves; (c) T-wave inversion; and (d) normalization of T waves. Progression through the first three stages takes several days, whereas the fourth stage occurs weeks or months later (3).

The chest radiograph may show pericardial calcifications in chronic constrictive pericarditis, especially if caused by tuberculosis. The cardiac silhouette may be enlarged or irregular in the presence of effusion, cyst, or tumor. In the presence of a large pericardial effusion, the cardiac silhouette takes on the shape of a water bottle. Pneumopericardium may also be seen on a chest radiograph.

The echocardiogram is the most useful noninvasive modality in pericardial disease. Echocardiography (either transthoracic or transesophageal) can demonstrate structural changes in the pericardium, including effusion, thickening, and masses, in addition to accompanying cardiac disease. It is extremely sensitive for pericardial fluid, being able to detect as little as 15 mL. Echocardiography can also demonstrate the functional changes caused by pericardial disease and can help to differentiate between tamponade, constriction, and restriction. It is very helpful in guiding pericardiocentesis.

Computed tomography (CT) and magnetic resonance imaging (MRI) are occasionally useful to define pericardial

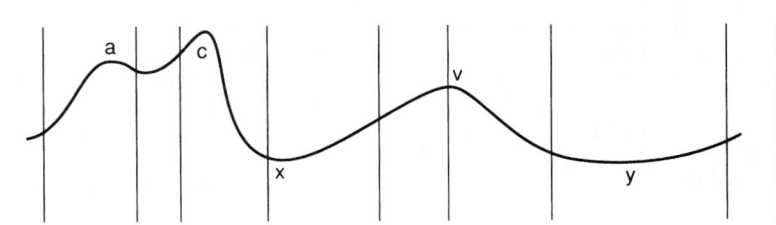

Figure 65.2. The jugular venous pulse contour. (From Berne RM, Levy MN. *Cardiovascular physiology,* 5th ed. St. Louis: Mosby, 1986: 66, with permission.)

masses and thickening (4). CT provides a better definition of calcification and is more expedient in an unstable patient. MRI can provide a better definition of masses and does not require the administration of intravenous contrast.

Cardiac catheterization provides the hemodynamic pressure tracings that can distinguish between tamponade, constriction, and restriction. Catheterization also provides an opportunity to perform endomyocardial biopsy to diagnose myocardial disease, including restrictive cardiomyopathy.

CARDIAC (PERICARDIAL) TAMPONADE

Cardiac tamponade can be defined as hemodynamically significant cardiac compression that results when accumulating pericardial contents (effusion, blood, pus, gas, or tumor) evoke and defeat compensatory mechanisms (3). Cardiac compression by the contents of the pericardial space prevents adequate filling of the heart, decreases stroke volume and cardiac output, and increases systemic and pulmonary venous pressures. The occurrence of tamponade is dependent on both the volume and rate of accumulation of pericardial contents. The rapid accumulation of a small amount of pericardial fluid (100 to 200 mL in an adult) may produce acute tamponade, whereas liters of fluid may accumulate slowly in a chronic effusion before tamponade occurs. Cardiac tamponade results when the pericardial pressure rises to 20 to 30 mm Hg. Cardiac filling pressures (namely, right and left atrial, pulmonary arterial diastolic and wedge, and right and left ventricular end-diastolic pressures) become equal to one another and to the pericardial pressure. Right atrial pressure in tamponade is usually 15 to 35 mm Hg. However, with accompanying hypovolemia, such as occurs during postoperative bleeding or traumatic tamponade, central venous pressures may be lower.

Cardiac tamponade can be associated with neoplastic disease, any of the causes of pericarditis (see below), or intrapericardial bleeding resulting from anticoagulation, procedures, surgery, or trauma. The trauma may be either penetrating or blunt. Tamponade may result from myocardial rupture during myocardial infarction, or aortic rupture secondary to aneurysmal disease or dissection. Clinical findings in tamponade include dyspnea and tachycardia. The three classic signs of acute tamponade (Beck's acute cardiac compression triad) are (a) falling arterial pressure, (b) rising venous pressure, and (c) a small, quiet heart. In actuality, the systemic blood pressure may be low, normal, or even elevated in patients with chronic hypertension. Blood pressure is more likely to be normal when pericardial fluid has accumulated gradually, and low in acute tamponade. The neck veins are typically distended, and peripheral cyanosis, particularly in the face, reflects venous congestion. However, venous distention may be minimal or absent with accompanying hypovolemia. The heart sounds may also be normal rather than faint.

Tamponade produces characteristic changes in the jugular venous pulsations: the x descent (systolic collapse) remains, whereas the y descent (diastolic collapse) disappears (5). With tamponade, a fall in systolic blood pressure of more than 10 mm Hg typically occurs during inspiration ("pulsus paradoxus"). Pulsus paradoxus may be absent in cases of left ventricular dysfunction, atrial septal defect, or regional (postoperative) tamponade. It may also be absent in a patient receiving positive-pressure ventilation. Causes of pulsus paradoxus other than tamponade

include chronic obstructive pulmonary disease, asthma, pulmonary embolism, right ventricular heart failure or infarction, obesity, and tense ascites.

Echocardiography can be very useful in the diagnosis of cardiac tamponade. It may reveal the presence of pericardial fluid. More specific echocardiographic signs of tamponade include right atrial compression, right ventricular diastolic collapse, and abnormal inspiratory decreases in left ventricular dimensions, mitral valve excursion, and mitral valve inflow. Localized atrial compression (usually postoperative) may cause tamponade without these characteristic echocardiographic features.

Cardiac tamponade is definitively diagnosed only when the removal of pericardial fluid improves the clinical picture. Removal of as little as a few milliliters of fluid may result in a significant improvement in cardiac output. When tamponade causes systemic blood pressure to fall, emergency pericardiocentesis is indicated. Needle pericardiocentesis with hemodynamic monitoring and echocardiographic guidance is optimal. Placement of a drainage catheter into the pericardial space over a guide wire (Seldinger technique) can provide ongoing fluid drainage and allow the rate of fluid accumulation to be monitored. Surgical drainage (placement of a pericardiostomy tube via a subxiphoid approach, creation of a pericardial window, or pericardial resection) is an alternative when pericardiocentesis fails or tamponade recurs.

Postoperative Cardiac Tamponade

Tamponade after cardiac surgery can occur in the absence of many or all of the classic signs of tamponade. Accompanying hypovolemia may limit the absolute rise in filling pressures, and positive-pressure ventilation may mask pulsus paradoxus. Tamponade should always be included in the differential diagnosis of low cardiac output after any closed or open heart operation. It should be particularly suspected in the presence of rising filling pressures and falling systemic blood pressure, urine output, and cardiac output that are poorly responsive to volume loading, inotropic agents, vasopressors, and diuretics. Mediastinal chest tube drainage that abruptly increases or ceases is highly suggestive. Chest radiography may show an enlarged cardiac silhouette or more subtle findings, such as a shift of epicardial markers (e.g., temporary pacemaking wires) away from the edge of the pericardium. However, postoperative tamponade may result from the accumulation of relatively small amounts of intrapericardial blood, and the chest radiograph is most often not helpful. Echocardiography is less sensitive for intrapericardial blood than for serous fluid. More specific echocardiographic signs of tamponade may be absent if clotted intrapericardial blood causes localized atrial compression. Reexploration of the chest is the only definitive method of diagnosing acute postoperative tamponade and is indicated in any patient with low cardiac output of unclear origin. Late postoperative tamponade typically occurs in patients on anticoagulants and may present insidiously.

PERICARDIAL CONSTRICTION

Pericardial constriction occurs when the heart is constrained by a thickened, fibrotic pericardium. The pericardial space may be obliterated or may contain effusion (effusive constrictive pericarditis). Constrictive pericarditis typically progresses over months to years. The clinical picture may include dyspnea, orthopnea, cough, fatigue, pleural effusions, abdominal swelling and discomfort, hepatomegaly, ascites, peripheral edema, fatigue, and pulsus paradoxus. Kussmaul's sign is an increase in jugular venous distention with inspiration. Electrocardiograpic changes of low voltage and nonspecific T-wave changes may be seen. Up to 25% of patients will have atrial fibrillation or flutter. Fibrotic obstruction of the right ventricular outflow tract may produce an electrocardiographic pattern of right ventricular hypertrophy. Chest radiography shows a normal heart size and clear lung fields. Pericardial calcification is essentially pathognomonic but is present in only about 40% of cases. Echocardiography shows small ventricles with good systolic function. Ventricular expansion shows an abrupt halt during diastole. The inferior vena cava is dilated. Doppler interrogation may show an abnormal inspiratory increase in tricuspid flow and a decrease in mitral flow. Patients with effusive constrictive pericarditis are more likely to have cardiomegaly on the chest roentgenogram and pericardial fluid on the echocardiogram. Beck's chronic cardiac compression triad consists of (a) high venous pressure, (b) ascites, and (c) a small, quiet heart.

Unlike cardiac tamponade, pericardial constriction produces no restriction of early diastolic filling, but a sudden restriction in late diastole (5). During the rapid ventricular filling of early diastole, the limit of ventricular distensibility is quickly reached. Late diastolic restriction produces an early diastolic dip, followed by a rapid increase and plateau (square root sign) in the right ventricular pressure tracing (Fig. 65.3). Jugular venous pulsations show prominent x and y descents, with a y descent (diastolic collapse) that is deeper and more rapid than normal. The right atrial pressure, pulmonary arterial diastolic and wedge pressures, and both right and left ventricular end-diastolic pressures are elevated (15 to 30 mm Hg) and within 5 mm Hg of one another. In effusive constrictive pericarditis, right atrial and ventricular pressure tracings more closely resemble those seen in tamponade: a deep x descent and small y descent in the right atrium, and no early diastolic dip in the right ventricle. Once the pericardial fluid is removed, the pressure tracings revert to those of constrictive pericarditis, with prominent x and y descents in the atrium and a prominent early diastolic dip in the ventricle.

Constriction may be a late result of any type of acute pericarditis. Other causes include mediastinal irradiation, cardiac surgery, amyloidosis, scleroderma, hemochromatosis, neoplastic disease, and sarcoidosis. The diagnosis of constrictive pericarditis is made by the typical clinical and hemodynamic findings in the presence of pericardial thickening (at least 4 mm by CT or MRI). Differentiation between pericardial constriction and restrictive cardiomyopathy may be difficult. Patients with restrictive cardiomyopathy do not have pericardial thickening. They are also more likely to have impaired systolic ventricular function, mitral and tricuspid regurgitation, left-sided pressures higher than right-sided pressures, slower filling in early and mid-diastole, and left and right ventricular pressures that move in the same, rather than opposite, directions with inspiration (6). Constriction

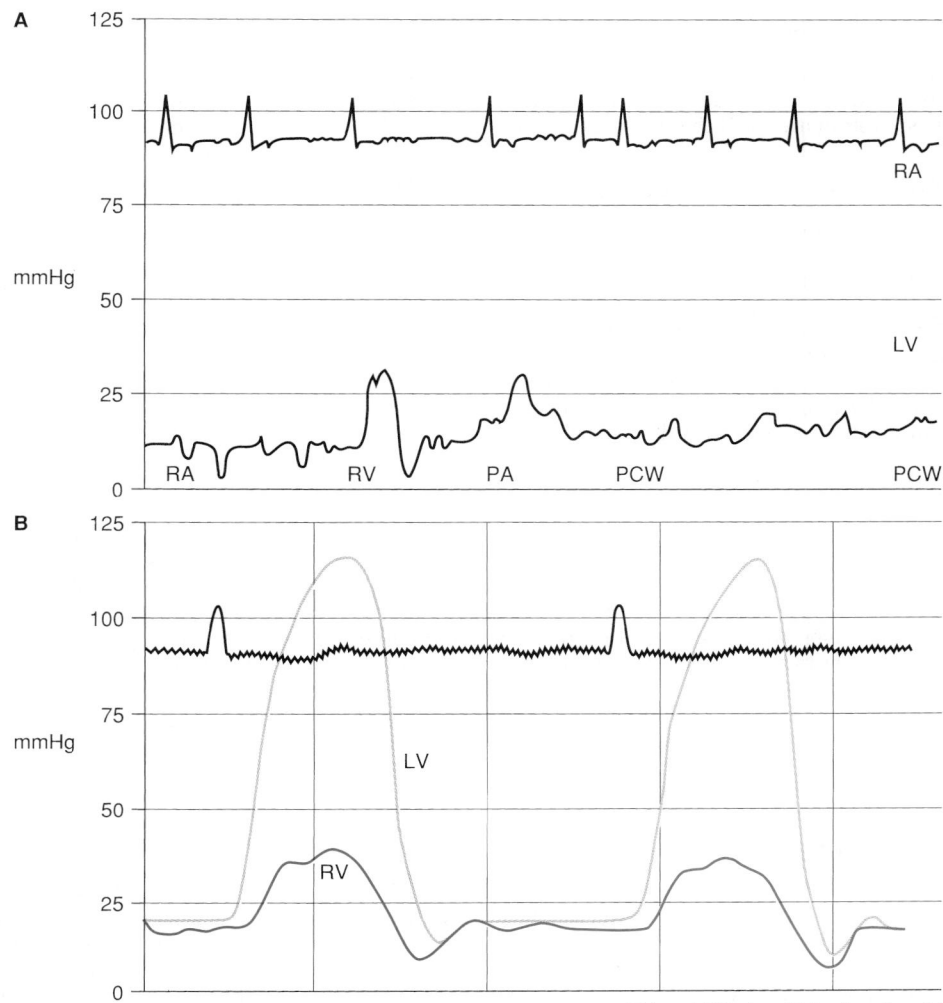

Figure 65.3. Pressure recordings from a patient with constrictive pericarditis. *(A)* The right atrial *(RA)* tracing shows an elevated mean pressure and a prominent y descent. The right ventricular *(RV)* tracing exhibits the dip and plateau pattern (square root sign). The RA, RV diastolic, pulmonary artery *(PA)* diastolic, pulmonary capillary wedge *(PCW)*, and left ventricular *(LV)* diastolic pressures are equalized. *(B)* The RV and LV diastolic pressures increase and are equalized after the administration of 500 mL of saline solution. (From Brockington GM, Zebede J, Pandian NG. Constrictive pericarditis. *Cardiol Clin* 1990;8:649, with permission.)

with accompanying ascites and peripheral edema may also be confused with primary liver disease (e.g., Budd-Chiari syndrome or cirrhosis) or other causes of right-sided heart failure. In some cases, biopsy of the pericardium, myocardium, or both may be necessary to make the appropriate diagnosis. The definitive treatment of constrictive pericarditis is pericardiectomy (see below).

CONGENITAL ABNORMALITIES

Congenital deficiency of the pericardium may be complete, but it is more often partial and left-sided. Such a deficiency is more common in male patients. Partial absence is usually asymptomatic. However, herniation of the right atrium, right ventricle, and right lung have been reported in association with right-sided partial defects. CT and MRI can demonstrate pericardial defects. Symptomatic herniation can be treated by completion pericardiectomy or patch closure of the pericardial defect with bovine pericardium or polytetrafluoroethylene (fabric). Congenital total absence is also usually asymptomatic and an incidental finding at operation or autopsy.

Pericardial cysts range from 1 to 15 cm in size. Most occur at the right cardiophrenic angle, are asymptomatic, and are noticed on chest radiographs performed for other reasons. On rare occasions, pericardial cysts may cause mediastinal compression with respiratory or hemodynamic collapse in neonates. Diagnosis can be confirmed by CT, which shows a cyst adjacent to the pericardium that contains homogeneous fluid with the density of water. The differential diagnosis of a pericardial cyst includes foramen of Morgagni hernia, bronchogenic cyst, lipoma, and other homogeneous neoplasms of the mediastinum. Surgical removal should be undertaken if the cyst increases in size or is symptomatic, or if the diagnosis is in doubt.

NEOPLASTIC PERICARDIAL DISEASE

Primary neoplasms of the pericardium are rare. Malignant tumors include sarcomas, teratomas, and mesotheliomas; benign tumors include fibromas, lipomas, hemangiomas, lymphangiomas, leiomyomas, and neurofibromas. Primary malignancies of the mediastinum, lung, or esophagus may directly extend to the pericardium. Metastatic neoplasm is the most common source of neoplastic pericardial disease and remains the most common cause of pericardial effusion. Cardiac involvement is found in 5% to 10% of patients dying of cancer (85% of the lesions are pericardial). Metastatic lung cancer, breast cancer, lymphoma, leukemia, and melanoma are the most common. Many cases present as cardiac tamponade. Diagnosis is by echocardiography, CT or MRI, and aspiration of pericardial fluid to identify tumor cells. The results of cytologic analysis of pericardial fluid may be negative in 20% to 50% of cases, and pericardial biopsy then may be helpful in establishing a diagnosis. Treatment can include radiotherapy, direct instillation of antineoplastic agents into the pericardium, and tube drainage for relief of effusion and tamponade. Sclerosing agents such as doxycycline can also provide good control of malignant pericardial effusions.

PERICARDITIS

The term *pericarditis* includes any inflammatory or infectious process affecting the pericardium. Pericarditis has a wide range of causes and may be either acute or chronic in course. The clinical picture of acute pericarditis may mimic, and must be differentiated from, myocardial ischemia and infarction. The predominant symptom of acute pericarditis is chest pain. Like angina pectoris, the pain is precordial or retrosternal and may radiate to the left shoulder and arm. Unlike angina, chest pain resulting from pericarditis is typically pleuritic in nature and can last for a period of days. The pain is worsened by deep breathing, lying down, or turning, and it is relieved by sitting up or leaning forward. Fever, which is usually low-grade, may be seen, along with nonspecific symptoms such as anorexia. Dyspnea and syncope may occur. Physical examination may reveal a diphasic (systolic and diastolic) pericardial friction rub that is scratchy or creaky in nature. The electrocardiogram may show the characteristic four-stage progression discussed above. In contrast, the electrocardiographic changes seen with myocardial ischemia are less generalized, ST-segment elevation is accompanied by reciprocal ST-depression, and pathologic Q waves develop. In patients with pericarditis, echocardiography can reveal pericardial fluid and diagnose cardiac tamponade. The symptoms of chronic pericarditis usually reflect either pericardial constriction or cardiac tamponade secondary to pericardial effusion.

Idiopathic and Viral Pericarditis

Other than neoplastic disease, idiopathic or nonspecific pericarditis is the most common cause of pericardial effusion. The symptoms are caused by acute pericardial inflammation or pericardial effusion. Chest pain, fever, and nonspecific malaise are common. Cardiac tamponade occurs rarely. The erythrocyte sedimentation rate is typically elevated. A viral source can be definitively identified in only a minority (15% to 20%) of cases. The most common viral pathogens are coxsackievirus, echovirus, adenovirus, and influenza virus. Treatment is with nonsteroidal antiinflammatory drugs or aspirin. Corticosteroids may be used as second-line therapy. Pericardiocentesis, surgical drainage, or pericardiectomy may be necessary for cases unresponsive to medical therapy or cases with constriction.

Uremic Pericarditis

Pericarditis may occur in up to 50% of patients with untreated renal disease and 20% of patients undergoing hemodialysis. It is less common in those undergoing peritoneal dialysis. The exact pathogenesis remains unclear, and occurrence is not directly related to the levels of blood urea nitrogen and creatinine. Chest pain is less common than in idiopathic pericarditis, so that a delay in diagnosis is common. Treatment is with increased dialysis, nonsteroidal antiinflammatory drugs, and, if necessary, corticosteroids. Pericardiocentesis or surgical drainage may be necessary for effusions that are hemodynamically significant or unresponsive to medical therapy. The pericardial fluid is usually bloody. Pericardiectomy is reserved for continued reaccumulation of fluid or late constriction.

Purulent Pericarditis

Bacteria may enter the pericardium by direct injury, extension from contiguous pneumonia or peritonitis, or hematogenous or lymphatic spread during sepsis. Clinical findings are chest pain, fever, and elevation of the white blood cell count. Inciting organisms in adults are *Staphylococcus* and gram-negative bacteria. In children, *Staphylococcus* and *Haemophilus influenzae* are typical. Less commonly, fungal or nocardial infection may involve the pericardium, by lymphatic spread or direct extension. Treatment is by pericardiocentesis (both diagnostic and therapeutic) and antibiotics. Surgical drainage with a pericardial tube or even pericardiectomy may be necessary for cases with thick, purulent drainage (often seen with *H. influenzae*) or recalcitrant cases.

Parasitic pericarditis is rare. Amebic infection may occur by intrapericardial rupture of a liver abscess and can result in tamponade. Echinococcal pericarditis is caused by rupture of a myocardial cyst into the pericardium. The clinical results range from localized pericardial inflammation to rapid cyst multiplication with cardiac compromise.

Tuberculous Pericarditis

Pericarditis may be seen in 1% to 2% of cases of tuberculosis. In countries where pulmonary tuberculosis has declined, tuberculous pericarditis is also uncommon. However, pericarditis caused by atypical organisms *(Mycobacterium avium* or *Mycobacterium intracellulare)* may be seen in immunocompromised patients. In nonindustrialized countries, tuberculous pericarditis remains common. Organisms usually reach the pericardium by hematogenous spread, although lymphatic spread and direct extension from neighboring lymph nodes or the lung are also possible. Four stages of tuberculous pericarditis are recognized: fibrinous, effusive (nonconstrictive), fibrous (nonconstrictive), and fibrous (constrictive, calcific). Diagnosis is by staining or culture of pericardial fluid or tissue (pericardial biopsy). Treatment is by multidrug antituberculous chemotherapy and pericardiocentesis. Corticosteroids are generally of no benefit (7,8). Open pericardial drainage should be avoided. The development of pericardial constriction is prevented by early diagnosis, closed drainage, and chemotherapy. If late constriction does develop, pericardiectomy may be necessary.

AIDS

Up to 20% of AIDS patients may have pericardial effusions. Pericarditis may be associated with tuberculosis and other mycobacterial infections, lymphoma, and Kaposi's sarcoma. The inflammation may also be nonspecific.

Dressler's Syndrome and Postpericardiotomy Syndrome

Pericarditis occurs during the evolution of acute myocardial infarction in 3% to 5% of patients (Dressler's syndrome) (9). A similar syndrome occurs in 10% to 40% of patients undergoing cardiac surgery, and it may also be seen after blunt or penetrating cardiac trauma and permanent placement of a pacemaker. Symptoms are chest pain, fever, and malaise. A pericardial friction rub is generally present. Laboratory studies show lymphocytosis and elevation of the erythrocyte sedimentation rate. Pericardial effusion and tamponade may develop. The syndrome typically develops 10 days to 2 months after cardiac surgery. The pathogenesis of Dressler's syndrome and postpericardiotomy syndrome is thought to involve an inflammatory reaction to intrapericardial blood, viral activation, or antimyocardial autoantibodies. Treatment is with nonsteroidal antiinflammatory drugs, aspirin, and occasionally steroids. Pericardiocentesis or pericardiectomy may be required for symptomatic effusion, recurrent effusion, or late pericardial constriction.

Vasculitis, Connective Tissue Disease, and Drugs

Pericarditis may be seen in patients with acute rheumatic fever, rheumatoid arthritis, systemic lupus erythematosus, scleroderma, Wegener's granulomatosis, polyarteritis nodosa, dermatomyositis, ankylosing spondylitis, Reiter's syndrome, Behçet's disease, and familial Mediterranean fever. Large pericardial effusions may be seen in acute rheumatic fever and rheumatoid arthritis. Treatment is by management of the underlying disease and appropriate approaches to effusion or tamponade. A variety of drugs have been implicated in pericarditis, including procainamide, hydralazine, dantrolene, methysergide, and cromolyn sodium.

PERICARDIOCENTESIS

Pericardiocentesis may be used for both diagnostic and therapeutic purposes. Diagnostic pericardiocentesis is indicated for a newly discovered pericardial effusion if the clinical picture suggests an infectious or neoplastic cause. In this setting, the results of pericardiocentesis guide subsequent therapy. Diagnostic pericardiocentesis may also be useful in the setting of a persistent or unresolved effusion. Therapeutic pericardiocentesis is indicated in the clinical setting of acute cardiac tamponade.

Pericardiocentesis is optimally performed in the cardiac catheterization laboratory so that the hemodynamic response can be monitored. Echocardiography is very useful for directing pericardiocentesis and for monitoring the successful evacuation of pericardial contents. With the use of local anesthesia and sterile technique, a long needle (16- to 22-gauge, depending on the patient's size and anticipated viscosity of the pericardial fluid) attached to a syringe is introduced into the pericardial space. The most common approach is subxiphoid, with the needle inserted just to the left of the xiphoid process and aimed posteriorly at a 45-degree angle toward the patient's left shoulder or midscapular area (Fig. 65.4). If echocardiography shows the distribution of the effusion to be mainly anterior, rather than inferior, a parasternal approach may be used instead. The needle is introduced 1 to 2 cm to the left of the sternum, in the fourth or fifth intercostal space, and directed posteriorly at a 90-degree angle to the body. With either approach, the needle is slowly advanced until fluid is aspirated. An electrocardiographic lead may be attached to the needle to monitor for an "injury current" (negative deflection of the QRS complex), which indicates contact with the epicardium. However, with echocardiographic guidance, this is now rarely used. If the pericardiocentesis is diagnostic, aspirated fluid is sent for bacteriologic, chemical, hematologic, and cytologic analysis, and the needle is removed. If ongoing drainage of pericardial fluid is desired, a guide wire can be passed through the needle and a soft drainage catheter with multiple holes introduced by the Seldinger technique.

Potential complications of pericardiocentesis include puncture or laceration of the heart or coronary arteries, lung, and upper abdominal organs. Arrhythmias are also possible, although they are usually self-limited and resolve when the needle is withdrawn. Echocardiography is quite effective in showing the location of the pericardial fluid and whether the needle is within the pericardial space, so that the likelihood of complications is reduced. Pericardiocentesis and drainage via a small tube may be ineffective if a pericardial effusion is made highly viscous by the presence of pus, as in purulent pericarditis, or blood, as after surgery. Open surgical drainage may be required in such cases.

The pericardial fluid obtained through pericardiocentesis can be diagnostic of a variety of pericardial disorders. Neoplastic pericardial disease is diagnosed by cytologic studies. Gram's stain and cultures reveal the source of purulent pericarditis. Tuberculous pericarditis is diagnosed

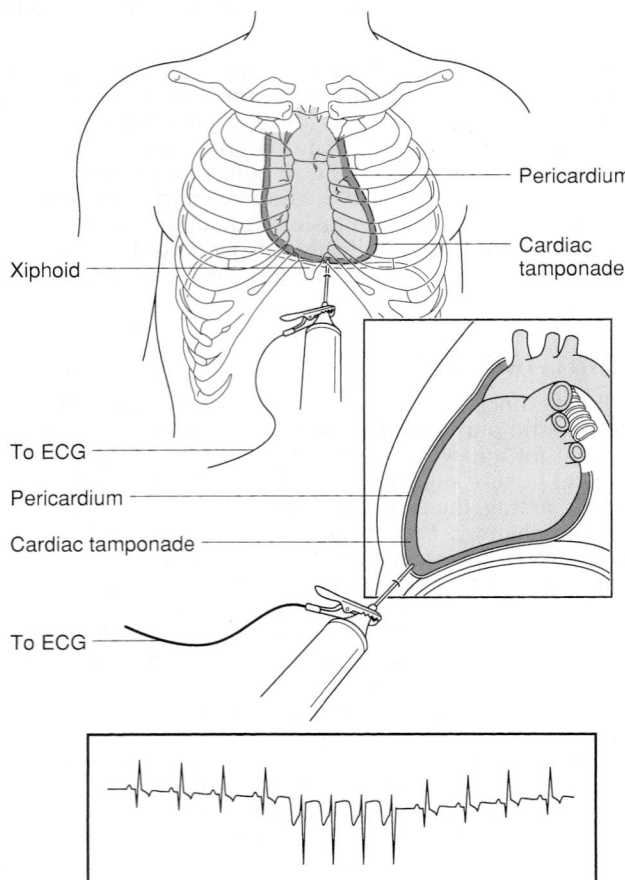

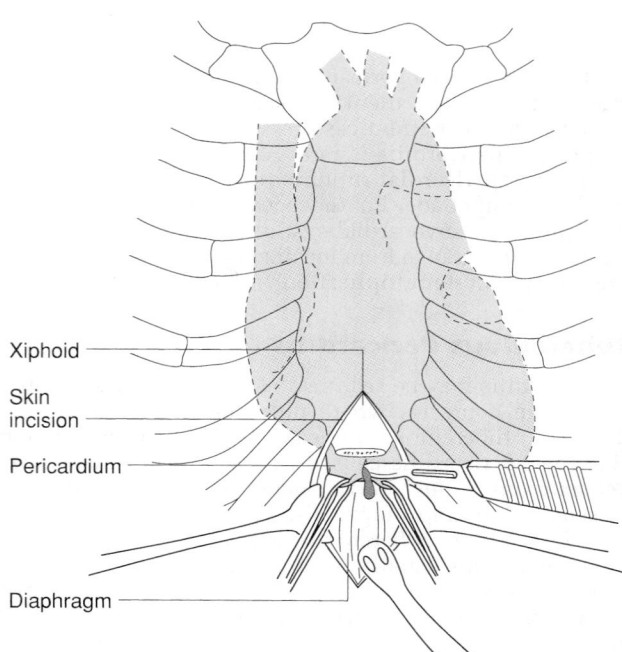

Figure 65.5. Open pericardial biopsy or drainage. The xiphoid is exposed through a midline incision and either retracted or removed. Limited exposure to the pericardium is achieved. (From Hood RM. *Techniques in general thoracic surgery.* Philadelphia: WB Saunders, 1985:58, with permission.)

Figure 65.4. Pericardiocentesis. The needle is inserted to the left of the xiphoid and directed toward the left shoulder or midscapular area posteriorly at a 45-degree angle. An electrocardiographic lead may be attached to the needle, and the negative deflection of the QRS complex represents contact with the epicardium. (From Ebert PA, Najafi H. In: Sabiston DC Jr, Spencer FC, eds. *Gibbon's surgery of the chest,* 5th ed. Philadelphia: WB Saunders, 1990:1234, with permission.)

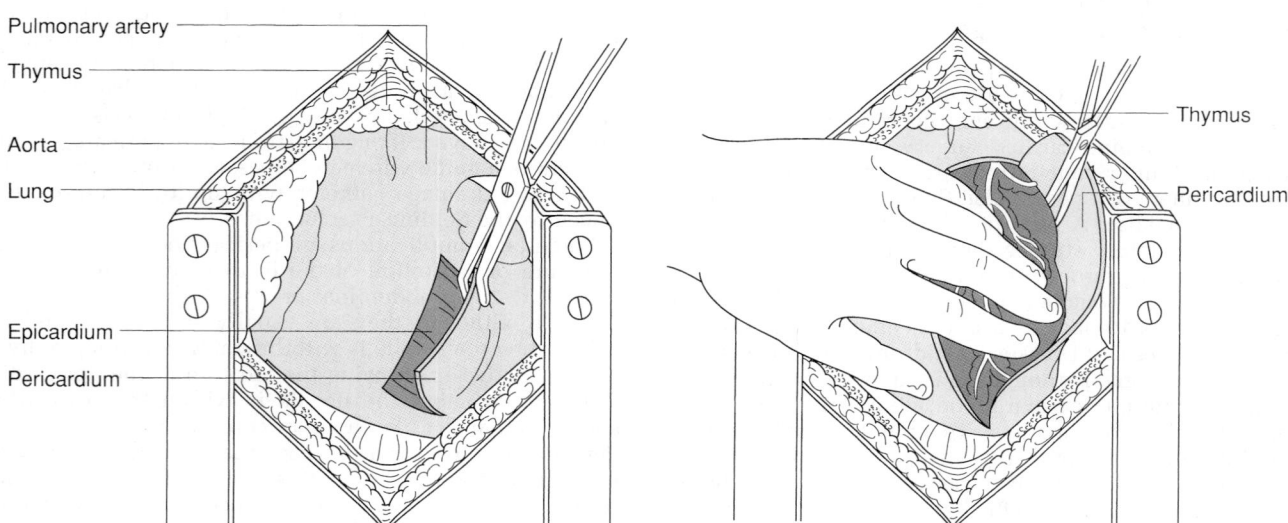

Figure 65.6. Pericardiectomy via a median sternotomy. *(A)* The pericardium is incised and a dissection plane established between the fibrous pericardium and the epicardium. *(B)* The heart is retracted to the right so that complete pericardiectomy from one phrenic nerve to the other can be achieved. (From Ebert PA, Najafi H. In: Sabiston DC Jr, Spencer FC, eds. *Gibbon's surgery of the chest,* 5th ed. Philadelphia: WB Saunders, 1990:1242, with permission.)

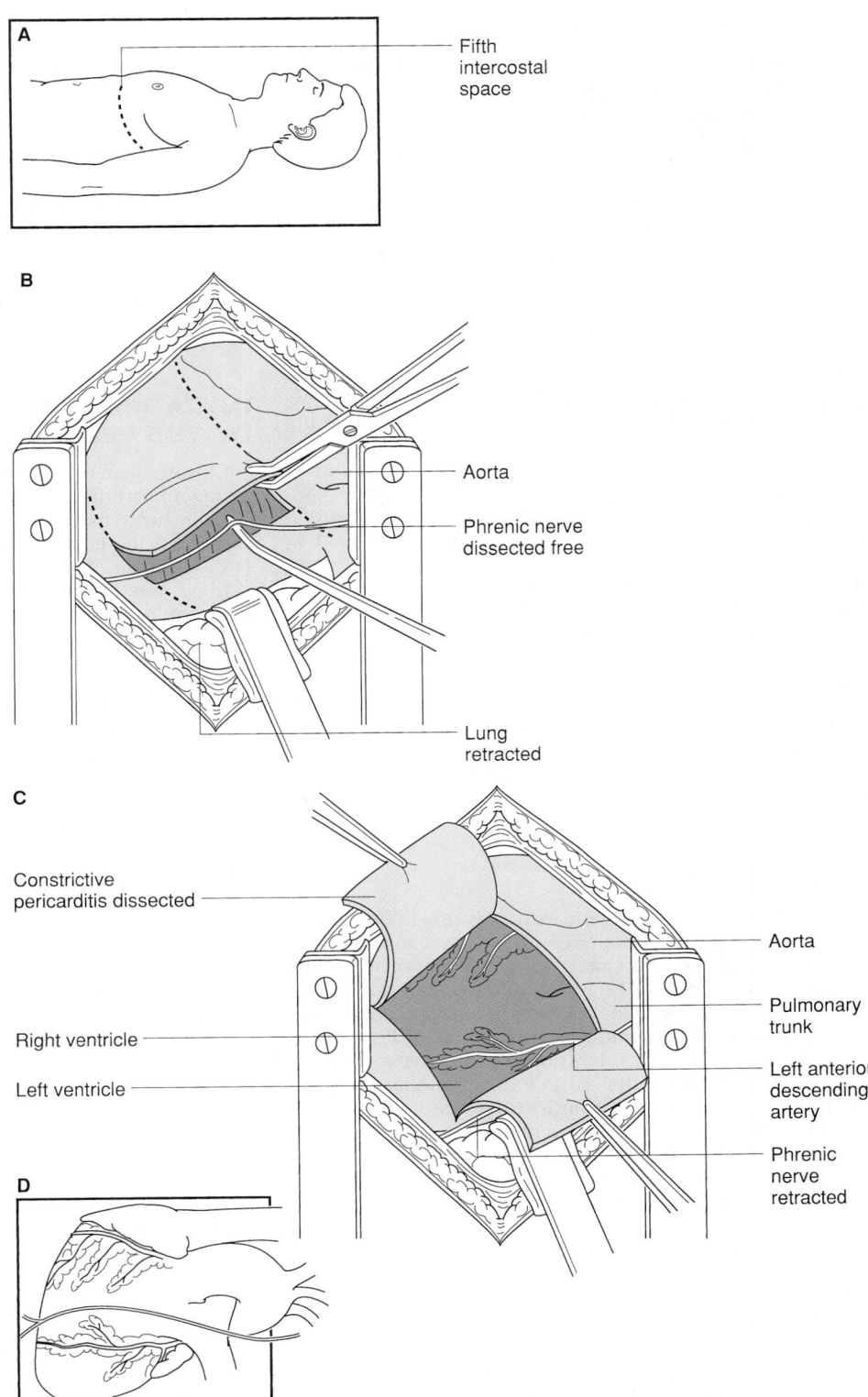

Figure 65.7. Pericardiectomy via an anterolateral left thoracotomy in the fifth intercostal space. The appropriate dissection plane is established and the phrenic nerve mobilized (usually on a 2- to 3-cm pedicle of pericardium) to allow removal of the posterolateral pericardium overlying the left ventricle. (From Kirklin JW, Barratt-Boyes BG. *Cardiac surgery.* New York: John Wiley & Sons, 1986:1438, with permission.)

by the presence of acid-fast bacilli in the pericardium. Uremic pericarditis is characterized by bloody pericardial fluid. Rheumatic pericarditis is marked by fluid high in protein and leukocytes and low in glucose. Pericardial fluid in myxedema, tuberculosis, or rheumatoid arthritis may contain cholesterol crystals. Pericardial fluid in systemic lupus erythematosus has a high protein content, a normal to low glucose level, and a low complement level;

lupus cells may be seen. Viral or nonspecific pericarditis is diagnosed by excluding other causes.

PERICARDIAL BIOPSY AND SURGICAL DRAINAGE

Pericardial biopsy may be required to establish a diagnosis if pericardiocentesis is unsuccessful or unrevealing.

This is particularly common in cases of neoplastic pericardial disease and tuberculous pericarditis. Biopsy may be via a subxiphoid approach under local or general anesthesia, or via an anterior thoracotomy under general anesthesia. A small incision is made, the pericardium grasped with a clamp, and a small piece excised for pathologic examination (Fig. 65.5). Any fluid present is sent for analysis, and if indicated, a tube may be placed in the pericardium for ongoing drainage. If the approach is via anterior thoracotomy, the pericardium is left open to drain into the left pleural space, and a pleural chest tube is placed.

Open surgical drainage may be necessary if a pericardial effusion is viscous (purulent or bloody), recurrent, or recalcitrant. A subxiphoid approach allows placement of a pericardiostomy tube and excision of a pericardial specimen for analysis. With this approach, contamination of the pleural spaces is avoided, which may be desirable in cases of purulent pericarditis. It may be better to deal with a chronic effusion, particularly if malignant, via an anterior thoracotomy. A large segment of pericardium is excised, and the effusion is left to drain into the left pleural space. Such partial pericardial resection is also termed a *pericardial window*.

General anesthesia in the presence of pericardial compression may be poorly tolerated. The induction of anesthesia removes many of the patient's compensatory mechanisms and produces a precipitous fall in blood pressure. Preinduction pericardiocentesis and volume loading may prevent this response. Patients undergoing anesthesia for the drainage of pericardial fluid that is causing hemodynamic compromise should be prepared and draped, with the surgeon gowned and gloved, before anesthesia is induced.

PERICARDIECTOMY

Surgical removal of the pericardium is most commonly performed for constrictive pericarditis. It may also be performed for chronic malignant effusions or recalcitrant pericardial effusion resulting from other causes and unresponsive to less aggressive measures. The approach is via median sternotomy or anterior thoracotomy (Figs. 65.6 and 65.7). Resection aided by thoracoscopy has also been reported, with good results (10). Cardiopulmonary bypass may be used for safety if the pericardial dissection is particularly difficult, or for hemodynamic support if extensive cardiac manipulation is required. However, its use is associated with an increased risk for bleeding, and it should be used only if necessary. The anterior thoracotomy approach is more traditional and allows resection of the pericardium over the left ventricle with minimal cardiac manipulation. However, the use of cardiopulmonary bypass generally requires femoral cannulation, with its attendant risks. Because of its familiarity, the median sternotomy approach is more commonly used today (11). It allows relatively easy institution of cardiopulmonary bypass via the chest. However, with the sternal approach, more extensive cardiac manipulation is required to reach the pericardium overlying the left ventricle. The recommended technical approach is to resect the pericardium overlying the left ventricle before that over the right, to avoid unimpeded pumping of the right ventricle in the presence of a still constricted left ventricle, which can result in pulmonary edema. In practice, especially when the procedure is carried out via a sternotomy, this sequence of resection may not be feasible. Regardless of approach, pericardium should be removed from phrenic nerve to phrenic nerve anteriorly, and also posterior to the left phrenic nerve.

Operative mortality for pericardiectomy is closely related to the patient's preoperative status (12). In the extensive experience of the Mayo Clinic, mortality was 1% for patients in preoperative New York Heart Association class I or II, 10% for those in class III, and 46% for those in class IV (13). Most cases (70%) of operative mortality were the consequence of low cardiac output. Operative survivors fared well, with 5- and 15-year survivals of 84% and 71%, respectively; 99% of late survivors were in New York Heart Association class I or II. Patients with constriction secondary to radiation treatment may also have a worse outlook, perhaps because of accompanying radiation-induced myocardial injury.

INTRAOPERATIVE CLOSURE OF THE PERICARDIUM

Closure of an otherwise normal pericardium at the end of an open heart operation may have the advantage of separating the heart from the sternum and of facilitating sternal reentry in the event of reoperation via median sternotomy (14). However, it may have the disadvantage of depressing cardiac function in the early postoperative period. In one study of 10 patients after cardiac valve replacement, pericardial closure (with the sternum still open) produced significant decreases in mean stroke volume (from 72 to 51 mL) and cardiac output (from 5.1 to 3.7 L/min) (15). In the same 10 patients, cardiac function was measured before and after the pericardium was reopened (by removing a sliding pericardial suture) with the chest closed. Reopening the pericardium resulted in increases in mean stroke volume (from 53 to 67 mL) and cardiac output (from 4.1 to 5.3 L/min). Thus, closure of the pericardium after an open heart operation should be avoided in patients whose cardiac function is already compromised, and perhaps in all cases.

REFERENCES

1. Sadler TW. *Langman's medical embryology*, 7th ed. Baltimore: Williams & Wilkins, 1995:154–167.
2. Spodick DH. Macrophysiology, microphysiology, and anatomy of the pericardium: a synopsis. *Am Heart J* 1992;124:1046–1051.
3. Spodick DH. The normal and diseased pericardium: current concepts of pericardial physiology, diagnosis, and treatment. *J Am Coll Cardiol* 1983;1:240–251.
4. Moncada R, Kotler MN, Churchill RJ, et al. Multimodality approach to pericardial imaging. *Cardiovasc Clin* 1986;17:409–441.
5. Shabetai R, Fowler NO, Gunteroth WG. The hemodynamics of cardiac tamponade and constrictive pericarditis. *Am J Cardiol* 1970;26:480–487.
6. Hatle LK, Appleton CP, Popp RL. Differentiation of constrictive pericarditis and restrictive cardiomyopathy by Doppler echocardiography. *Circulation* 1989;79:357–370.
7. Quale JM, Lipschik GY, Henrich AE. Management of tuberculous pericarditis. *Ann Thorac Surg* 1987;43:653–655.
8. Sagrista-Sauleda J, Permanyer-Miralda G, Soler-Soler J. Tuberculous pericarditis: ten-year experience with a prospective protocol for diagnosis and treatment. *J Am Coll Cardiol* 1988;11:724–728.
9. Dressler W. A post-myocardial infarction syndrome: preliminary report of a complication resembling idiopathic recurrent, benign pericarditis. *JAMA* 1956;160:1379–1383.
10. Hazelrigg SR, Mack MJ, Landreneau RJ, et al. Thoracoscopic pericardiectomy for effusive pericardial disease. *Ann Thorac Surg* 1993;56:792–795.
11. DeValeria PA, Baumgartner WA, Casale AS, et al. Current indications, risks, and outcome after pericardiectomy. *Ann Thorac Surg* 1991;52:219–224.

12. Seifert FC, Miller DC, Oesterle SN, et al. Surgical treatment of constrictive pericarditis: analysis of outcome and diagnostic error. *Circulation* 1985;72[Suppl II]:II-264–II-273.

13. McCaughan BC, Schaff HV, Piehler JM, et al. Early and late results of pericardiectomy for constrictive pericarditis. *J Thorac Cardiovasc Surg* 1985;89:340–350.

14. Rao V, Komeda M, Weisel RD, et al. Should the pericardium be closed routinely after heart operations? *Ann Thorac Surg* 1999;67:484–488.

15. Hunter S, Smith GH, Angelini GD. Adverse hemodynamic effects of pericardial closure soon after open heart operation. *Ann Thorac Surg* 1992;53:425–429.

SURGERY: SCIENTIFIC PRINCIPLES AND PRACTICE, Third Edition, edited by
Lazar J. Greenfield, Michael W. Mulholland, Keith T. Oldham, Gerald B. Zelenock,
and Keith D. Lillemoe. Lippincott Williams & Wilkins Publishers, Philadelphia, © 2001.

CHAPTER 66

ATHEROSCLEROSIS AND THE PATHOGENESIS OF OCCLUSIVE DISEASE

ANTON N. SIDAWY, SUBODH ARORA,
AND ALEXANDER W. CLOWES

Atherosclerosis is a disease of the intima of large arteries that causes luminal narrowing, thrombosis, and occlusion associated with ischemia of the end-organ. Throughout much of its course, the disease is not detectable. Thrombosis, including vascular occlusion and embolism, produces clinical events of importance, such as myocardial infarction, stroke, and ischemic gangrene of the extremities. The widespread prevalence of lesions in the arteries of asymptomatic people, the chronicity of the process, the suddenness of the terminal vascular events, and the lack of a single etiologic factor make it impossible to provide a simple explanation for atherogenesis and atherosclerosis progression. In fact, atherosclerosis might be considered a form of nonspecific adaptation on the part of large blood vessels to a variety of harmful stimuli, the clinical consequences of which, or what we might call the true disease process, appear only when the compensatory mechanisms are overwhelmed.

In this chapter, we describe the factors that influence the structure of normal arteries and that may also play a role in the development of atherosclerotic plaque.

NORMAL STRUCTURE OF BLOOD VESSELS

Normal arteries and veins, both large and small, are formed from endothelium, smooth muscle, and extracellular matrix synthesized by the vascular wall cells. The vascular wall is invariably organized into layers (Fig. 66.1). The intima, defined as the part of the wall between the blood and the internal elastic lamina, is composed of a monolayer of endothelium at the luminal surface and may overlie one

This chapter is based in part on Clowes AW. Theories of atherosclerosis. In: White RA, ed. *Atherosclerosis and arteriosclerosis: human pathology and experimental animal methods and models.* Boca Raton, FL: CRC Press, 1989:3.

or more layers of smooth muscle. The media, lying beneath the intima, constitutes the bulk of the vessel and contains smooth-muscle cells arranged in layers and dispersed in a matrix composed of elastin, collagen, and proteoglycan. The adventitia lies outside the external elastic lamina and forms the outer coat. It is composed of loose connective tissue, fibroblasts, capillaries, neural fibers, and occasional leukocytes. In very large arteries with more than 28 elastic layers, a microvasculature (vasa vasorum) penetrates the media from the adventitial side and provides an alternative nutrient supply to the flux from the luminal surface (1). In thickened, atherosclerotic vessels, the vasa vasorum are extensive and penetrate into the diseased intima (2,3).

In the fetus, the vessel wall is derived from mesoderm. A brief review of this process is of interest, as many aspects of wound healing and atherogenesis in adult vessels represent a recapitulation of the fetal program of angiogenesis. The earliest vascular primordia in the embryo are isolated "hemangioblasts" that display endothelial and hematopoietic immunologic markers (4,5). The hemangioblasts cluster and form cords and later tubes, which become the major vascular conduits. Some of the clusters become blood islands, the precursors of hematopoietic tissues. These structures sprout, grow, and remodel to form the primitive vascular system (6).

Endothelial cells probably play a central role in the organization and building of vascular structures. They are derived from the hemangioblasts, organize at sites of later vessel development, and are followed by local mesenchymal cells, which form the outer layers of the emerging blood vessels. The mesenchymal cells are the precursors of smooth-muscle cells and fibroblasts. Once associated with the vessel wall, many of these cells begin to express smooth muscle-specific α-actin. This pattern of endothelial invasion followed by smooth-muscle recruitment is reactivated in later life during angiogenesis in the presence of tumors and in wounds undergoing repair.

The adult form of blood vessels appears to be established by birth. In large vessels, the number of elastic and smooth-muscle layers remains constant, although increases in wall mass result from smooth-muscle proliferation and matrix synthesis (7,8). The vascular architecture is probably genetically determined because alterations in animal size by hormonal manipulations (e.g., excess growth hormone) are associated with increased wall mass but no change in the number of cell layers (9). It is likely that the primitive endothelial cell regulates wall architecture, as it is involved in the recruitment of the corresponding primitive smooth-muscle cell. As we shall see, these activities of the endothelial cell in the embryo presage its role in determining vascular diameter and mass in normal and diseased adult arteries.

These observations on the embryologic origin of vascular wall cells and the development of blood vessels provide many insights into vascular wall organization and function

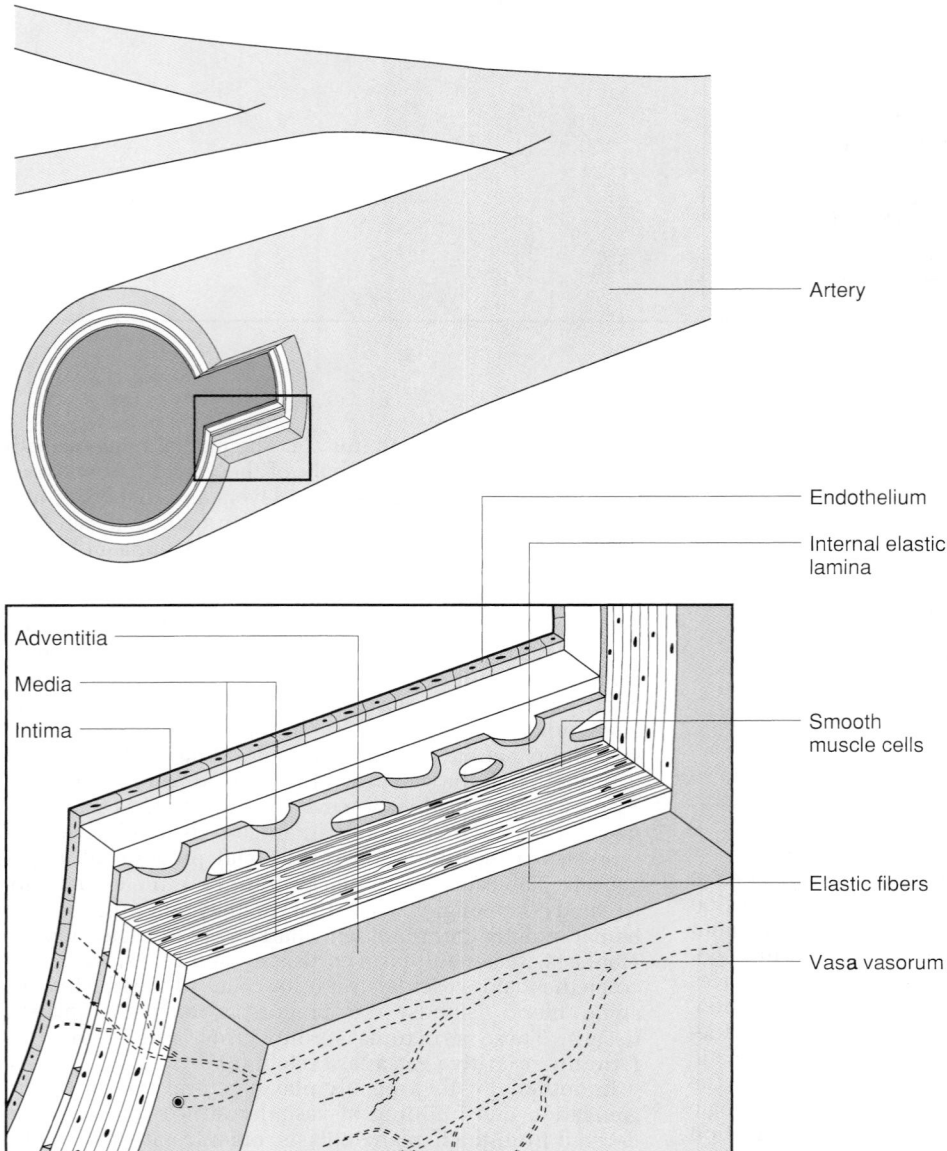

— Artery

— Endothelium

— Internal elastic lamina

Adventitia

Media

Intima

— Smooth muscle cells

— Elastic fibers

— Vasa vasorum

Figure 66.1. The arterial wall is made up of multiple layers (intima, media, and adventitia) that vary in composition, depending on the artery.

in the adult and raise numerous questions for which we have few answers. What determines the initial organization of the hemangioblasts (the primitive endothelium)? Are they tracking some kind of predetermined scaffolding? What are the signals that regulate the proliferation of these cells? How do they go about recruiting the primitive smooth-muscle cells? How do the endothelial cells then regulate the number and function of smooth-muscle cells? Does the molecular language of endothelial cell–smooth-muscle cell discourse extend to other types of cell interactions (e.g., between leukocytes or platelets and vascular wall cells)? In the last decade, we have begun to realize how complex the answers to these questions are and to develop a rudimentary understanding of how vascular cells interact in normal and disease states. In the next section, we review some of the recent evidence that vascular wall function and structure depend absolutely on cell–cell interactions.

REGULATION OF LUMINAL AREA

The preceding description of the usual arterial wall anatomy provides no clue to how a vessel adjusts its mass and dimensions in response to external stimuli (hypertension, increased blood flow, vascular injury) or to how it maintains a nonthrombogenic state at the luminal surface. For this, we must consider the array of possible physiologic functions of the wall and its cellular components under normal and abnormal conditions.

Blood vessels, both large and small, become larger during growth and development. They also enlarge to compensate for an increase in blood flow (or more appropriately an increase in blood flow velocity) (Fig. 66.2). A particularly striking example of this mechanism is found in an artery proximal to an arteriovenous fistula; if the fistula is not treated, the artery can become frankly aneurysmal (10). Similarly, the velocity of blood flow increases in a stenotic vessel at the point of luminal narrowing. When the stenosis is caused by intimal thickening or atherosclerotic plaque, the vessel dilates at the site of the lesion. For example, a diseased coronary vessel dilates and can maintain the correct luminal dimensions despite changes in wall structure so long as the intimal lesion does not occupy more than 40% of the area inside the internal elastic lamina (Fig. 66.3) (11). At this point, pathologic narrowing

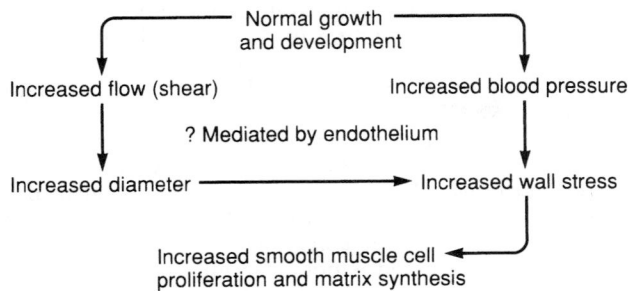

Figure 66.2. Changes in blood flow and pressure can have profound effects on arterial wall structure. In part, the response to hemodynamic changes may be mediated by the endothelium. (After Clowes AW. Theories of atherosclerosis. In: White RA, ed. *Atherosclerosis and arteriosclerosis: human pathology and experimental animal methods and models.* Boca Raton, FL: CRC Press, 1989:3, with permission.)

begins to take place. Why vessels should dilate in each of these instances when the velocity of flow increases has not been determined. One possibility is that the cells in the wall, particularly the endothelium, are somehow capable of sensing changes in blood velocity and shear and can translate this biomechanical information into biochemical signals that then regulate the contractile state of the artery (12–15). The effect of shear stress on the regulation of arterial motility is described in further detail later in this section. Endothelial cell secretory products play a critical role in smooth-muscle cell function (16). They secrete vasodilating (prostaglandins I_2 and E_2, adenosine, nitric oxide) and vasoconstricting (endothelin) substances.

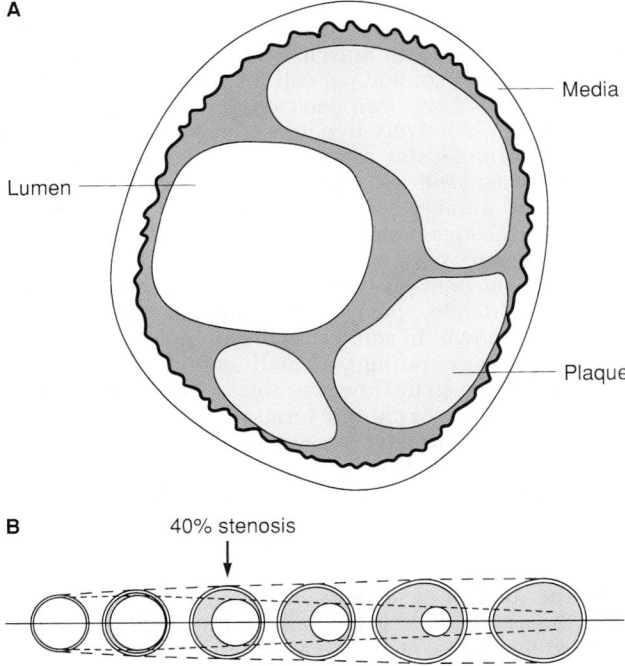

Figure 66.3. *(A)* Coronary arteries dilate as atherosclerotic plaques form and maintain normal luminal dimensions *(A).* Luminal narrowing begins only after the plaque occupies more than 40% of the cross-sectional area within the internal elastic lamina and bulges outward at sites of medial atrophy. *(B)* The course of lesion formation and luminal narrowing. (From Glagov S, Weisenberg E, Zarins CK, et al. Compensatory enlargement of human atherosclerotic coronary arteries. *N Engl J Med* 1987;316:1371–1375, with permission.)

Where endothelium is damaged or absent, adherent platelets release the vasoconstrictor thromboxane A_2.

Nitric oxide, previously called *endothelium-dependent relaxing factor,* is an important regulator in normal and diseased vessels (17). It is a short-acting substance that is derived from the metabolic breakdown of arginine (18–20). A number of factors stimulate endothelial cells to secrete nitric oxide, including thrombin, acetylcholine, brady kinin, serotonin, and products of platelet release. Hence, when the endothelium is present and functional, neighboring thrombotic events are likely to cause vasodilation; when the endothelium is absent or dysfunctional, these same factors cause vasoconstriction. Moreover, when the endothelium is missing, the vessel does not respond normally to changes in blood flow, either in the short or long term (21). Changes in blood flow affect wall mass (22–24). In this regard, it is interesting to note that various factors that affect smooth-muscle contraction or relaxation also modulate growth (nitric oxide, endothelin, thrombin, prostaglandins) (25–29). These observations may be the first preliminary evidence that transient signals affecting the diameter of vessels may have, in the long term, more permanent effects on wall structure. Certain pathologic conditions in which endothelium is either missing or abnormal are associated with acute and chronic vasospasm; it is quite possible that the acute problems of atypical angina (coronary vasospasm) and cerebral vasospasm after cerebral hemorrhage are manifestations of abnormal endothelial function and decreased nitric oxide (30). A relationship has been noted between shear stress exerted on the arterial lumen, the production of nitric oxide, and the development of atherosclerosis. Normal shear stress in arteries (usually > 15 dyne/cm^2) is protective, whereas low levels of shear stress (< 4 dyne/cm^2) induce the formation of atherosclerotic lesions (31). In addition, Malek and colleagues (32) have found that increases in shear stress lead to an increase in the expression of endothelial nitric oxide synthase (eNOS) mRNA, an increase in nitric oxide production, and vasodilation. Areas of low shear stress in the arterial tree, such as the carotid bifurcation, are foci for the formation of atherosclerotic lesions (31).

Endothelial dysfunction underlies and is the earliest change in the development and progression of atherosclerosis. The role of endothelial dysfunction has been emphasized recently. It probably begins in childhood and extends through clinical events later in life. Most studies have shown that endothelial function is impaired very early in the development of atherosclerosis, before the appearance of visible lesions. Clear evidence of endothelial dysfunction has been found in the children of parents with genetic defects of lipid transport and in children living with smokers. As these children grow, endothelial dysfunction becomes more pronounced and remains after atherosclerosis is established (33). It is present in numerous conditions associated with an increased risk for cardiovascular disease, including hypertension, hypercholesterolemia, cigarette smoking, diabetes mellitus, and estrogen deficiency in postmenopausal women (34).

The endothelium is very active. Endothelial cells have the ability to transduce signals from blood and chemicals and convert them into actions in the underlying vessel wall. The surface of the endothelial cell has a wide variety of receptors, including those for shear stress, oxidized low-density lipoproteins (LDLs), and inflammatory mediators, to name a few. Through these receptors, the endothelial cells orchestrate actions that affect not only the endothelium but also the entire vascular wall. In disease states, such actions include adverse changes in vascular tone, the proliferation of smooth-muscle cells to result in hypertrophy, and the recruitment and adhesion of mononuclear cells, which are early steps in the development and progression of atherosclerosis. One of the most important defenses of the endothelium in maintaining vascular health is nitric oxide, which has been shown to inhibit the expression of receptors for substances implicated in the development of atherosclerosis, such as oxidized LDL, inflammatory mediators, and angiotensin II (35). The chief role of nitric oxide in reversing pathologic changes appears to be its ability to counteract oxidative stress, a common pathogenic pathway for most major risk factors for atherosclerosis. The classic atherosclerotic risk factors, such as hypertension, smoking, and hyperlipidemia, all act at the endothelial level by increasing oxidative stress, which inactivates nitric oxide and upsets the balance between endogenous vasodilators and vasoconstrictors, growth promoters and growth inhibitors, antiinflammatory and proinflammatory mediators, and other factors important to endothelial function and vascular health (36).

The normal endothelium functions in an inhibitory mode, maintaining a relaxed vascular tone and inhibiting smooth-muscle cell growth, platelet and leukocyte adhesion and aggregation, and thrombosis. In hypertensive, hypercholesterolemic, and diabetic patients, endothelial dysfunction has been associated with a decreased production or decreased activity of nitric oxide (37). Endothelial dysfunction is associated with most of the known risk factors for atherosclerosis and cardiovascular disease and may contribute to the development of such disease. This concept has important clinical implications, especially in terms of preventive strategies.

Angiotensin-converting enzyme (ACE) acts both to produce angiotensin II, a potent vasoconstrictor, from angiotensin I and to degrade bradykinin. Angiotensin II is highly atherogenic, stimulating the synthesis of various growth and chemotactic factors and promoting the generation of superoxide anions that degrade nitric oxide. In contrast, bradykinin is a vasodilator that exerts its effect via nitric oxide. Within the endothelium, excess angiotensin II is not only a vasoconstrictor but also a promoter of smooth-muscle cell proliferation and a potent stimulator of inflammatory mediators, such as tissue necrosis factor. All these processes can be inhibited or reversed by ACE inhibitor therapy, which decreases the level of angiotensin II and inhibits the degradation of bradykinin. ACE inhibitors prevent not only the adverse effects of hypertension but also the effects of oxidative stress from other mechanisms. Clinical trials have shown that 6 months of ACE inhibition therapy, with quinapril, is associated with a significant improvement in endothelial function in normotensive patients who have coronary artery disease (38). ACE inhibition at the tissue level appears to be critical to prevent oxidative stress within the endothelium. This is the reason why tissue-avid ACE inhibitors like quinapril may have advantages over other drugs in their class. The restoration of endothelial function by means of ACE inhibitors has become an attractive therapeutic target.

REGULATION OF MEDIAL AND INTIMAL THICKENING

Earlier, we observed that for embryonic vessels to form, primitive endothelial cells must migrate and become aligned and then recruit smooth-muscle precursors from the surrounding mesenchyme. Because endothelial cells grow as a monolayer, they can proliferate only when the vascular structure is enlarging in circumference, during vascular elongation (angiogenesis), or when injured endothelium is being replaced. Massive denudation and endothelial loss are not normal events and probably occur only during pathologic degeneration of the intima or during surgical instrumentation of the vessel. In any event, endothelial proliferation does not contribute significantly to an increase in wall mass. Smooth-muscle cell proliferation does.

Under several circumstances, vessels of adult animals respond by becoming thicker. In hypertensive animals and humans, arteries exhibit medial thickening, whereas after endothelial denudation or in the presence of hypercholesterolemia, the intima thickens (39,40). Exactly how these responses are regulated is not clear, although it is certain that in each instance, the proliferation of smooth-muscle cells and accumulation of extracellular matrix are important components. In addition, in hypercholesterolemic subjects, the accumulation of lipid and lipid-filled macrophages contributes to the intimal lesion (41).

Vessel wall mass is largely determined by the accumulation of smooth-muscle cells and matrix synthesized by smooth-muscle cells. Hence, we need to consider how the number of smooth-muscle cells is regulated (42). Under normal circumstances, smooth-muscle cells proliferate in the vessels of young animals and enter a quiescent state at maturity. For example, smooth-muscle cells in adult rat carotid artery do not increase in number and turn over at a daily rate of 0.06% (43). In animal models of disease, these cells can readily be stimulated to enter the growth cycle by the induction of hypertension or by direct vascular injury. As we shall see, the observations made in these models provide us with insights into possible mechanisms for the initiation and progression of vascular disease in humans.

Although the effect of hypertension is greatest in the small "resistance" vessels, large arteries are in fact equally affected. In response to increased pressure, the wall thickens (39,44). Morphometric studies have shown that this increase is largely a medial process and involves all components of the vessel wall, including the mass of smooth-muscle cells and matrix. In some forms of hypertension, the number of smooth-muscle cells increases, whereas in others, the DNA content per cell increases. Tetraploid and octaploid cells have been detected. In venous grafts transposed from a relatively hypotensive venous environment into the normotensive arterial circulation, an increase in wall thickness and a corresponding increase in smooth-muscle cell number have been observed (45). In each instance, the change in pressure affects the mass of cells and associated matrix.

How a change in pressure might induce smooth-muscle cells to proliferate, change their ploidy, or synthesize matrix is not known. In some circumstances (e.g., severe hypertension, vein grafting), a small amount of endothelial loss can be detected. However, this is not a usual feature in more moderate or chronic forms of hypertension. Leung and associates (46) have suggested that increased tension and stretch have a direct effect on matrix protein synthesis, but not on cell proliferation. Alternatively, increased wall tension might affect the endothelium, and the endothelium might in turn secrete factors regulating smooth-muscle mass.

Of the models of smooth-muscle growth in vivo, perhaps the best studied is the balloon injury model first developed by Clowes et al. (43) and Baumgartner and Studer (47). In this model, smooth-muscle proliferation is stimulated by the passage of an inflated balloon catheter along an artery. The artery is at once stretched and denuded of its endothelium. Immediately thereafter, platelets begin to adhere to the wall wherever endothelium is missing; they then spread and degranulate. In most situations, endothelial denudation and platelet adherence are followed 1 to 2 days later by the onset of medial smooth-muscle proliferation. In the ballooned rat carotid (Fig. 66.4), this response

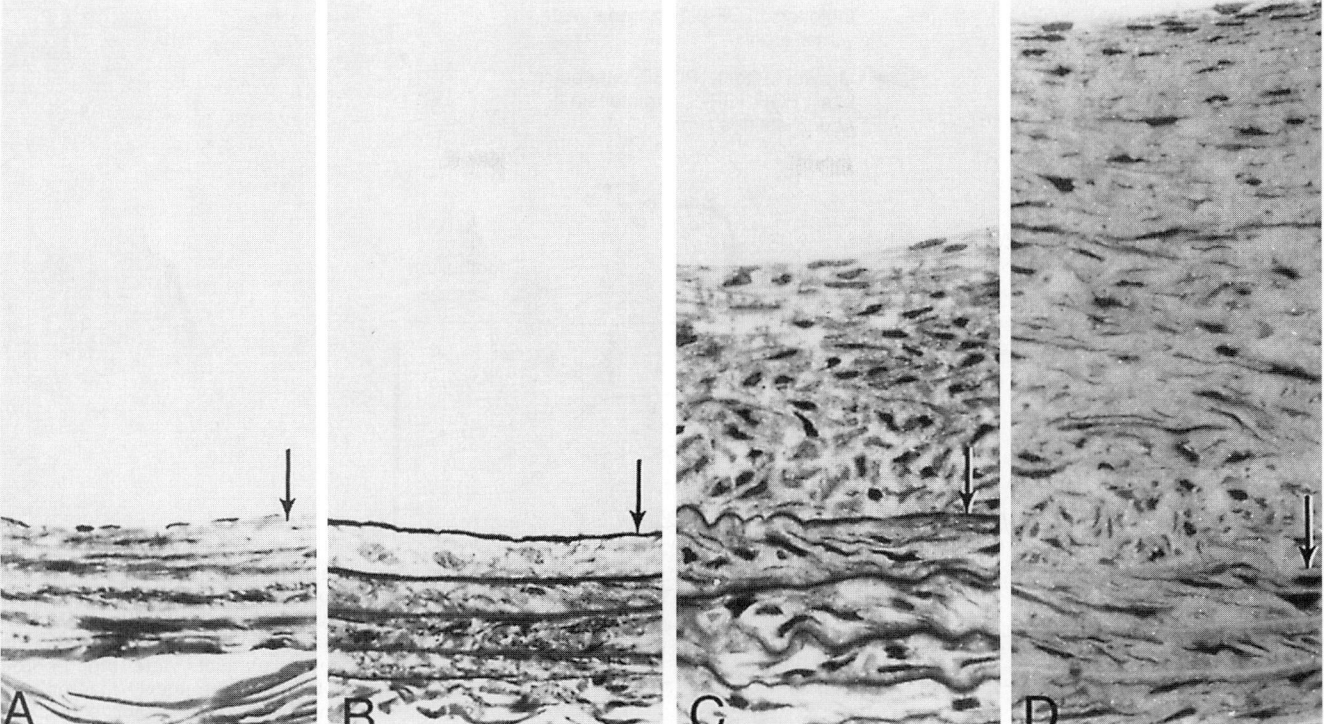

Figure 66.4. Substantial intimal thickening develops in elastic arteries injured by the passage of a balloon embolectomy catheter. In this series of histologic cross-sections of rat carotid artery before *(A)* and after ballooning *(B–D)*, the endothelium is stripped away and the inner layer of medial smooth-muscle cells is damaged *(B)*. By 2 weeks *(C)*, the intima is thickened by the migration and proliferation of smooth-muscle cells derived from the media. The mass of cells does not change significantly after this time; nevertheless, the intima is thicker at 3 months *(D)* because of matrix synthesis and accumulation. (From Clowes AW, Reidy MA, Clowes MM. Kinetics of cellular proliferation after arterial injury. I. Smooth-muscle growth in the absence of endothelium. *Lab Invest* 1983;49:327–333, with permission.)

can be most dramatic, with a three-logarithmic increase in the thymidine labeling index (a measure of proliferation). This early proliferation in the media does not lead to an increase in wall thickness; the wall thickens only after smooth-muscle cells migrate from the media and proliferate in the intima. In normal animals, this process continues for a period of time and subsides spontaneously whether or not endothelium reappears at the luminal surface. The intimal mass is further increased by the accumulation of extracellular matrix synthesized by the smooth-muscle cells (48).

A link between smooth-muscle proliferation and earlier platelet granule release has been proposed. Among the proteins released are several growth factors, including platelet-derived growth factor (PDGF), transforming growth factor-β (TGF-β), and an epidermal growth factor-like protein (49). Where these granule proteins go after being released from the platelets is not known. One hypothesis suggests that these factors accumulate in the artery wall and stimulate subsequent smooth-muscle growth (40). This hypothesis (the reaction-to-injury hypothesis) was first proposed many decades ago as a general mechanism for atherogenesis and has been refined in view of recent information. Although the theory is attractive, it is based on rather slim evidence mainly derived from experiments in thrombocytopenic animals (50). Injured arteries in these animals show very little intimal thickening.

The hypothesis that the decrease in intimal thickening in the injured arteries of thrombocytopenic animals is attributable to a decreased proliferation of smooth-muscle cells has proved to be incorrect (51). In the ballooned rat carotid model, even though intimal thickening is diminished in thrombocytopenic animals, smooth-muscle proliferation and early cell cycle gene expression are the same as in controls. The interpretation of these findings is that platelet products play a role in the movement of smooth-muscle cells from one vascular compartment to the next (media to intima) but do not affect the initiation of proliferation. Whether platelet factors can influence the growth of intimal smooth muscle has yet to be determined.

Although little is known of what starts or stops the process of intimal thickening, several observations are interesting and perhaps important when we consider the current theories of atherosclerosis. The first is that the surface of the injured artery accumulates a single layer of platelets. Fibrin and microthrombi are seen at the luminal surface only when the artery is reinjured after an intimal thickening has formed, or in small craters in association with adherent macrophages in hypercholesterolemic animals (52–55). Active, fulminant thrombosis is not a usual feature of injured vessels; when it occurs, it must represent a major aberration of vessel function. Secondly, in models demonstrating early reendothelialization or partial deendothelialization without medial injury, intimal thickening does not develop, although one or two rounds of medial smooth-muscle proliferation can occur (56). This result suggests that endothelium may play a role in suppressing smooth-muscle growth and migration from the media to the intima. We know that smooth-muscle growth inhibitors can be extracted from the vessel wall, that en-

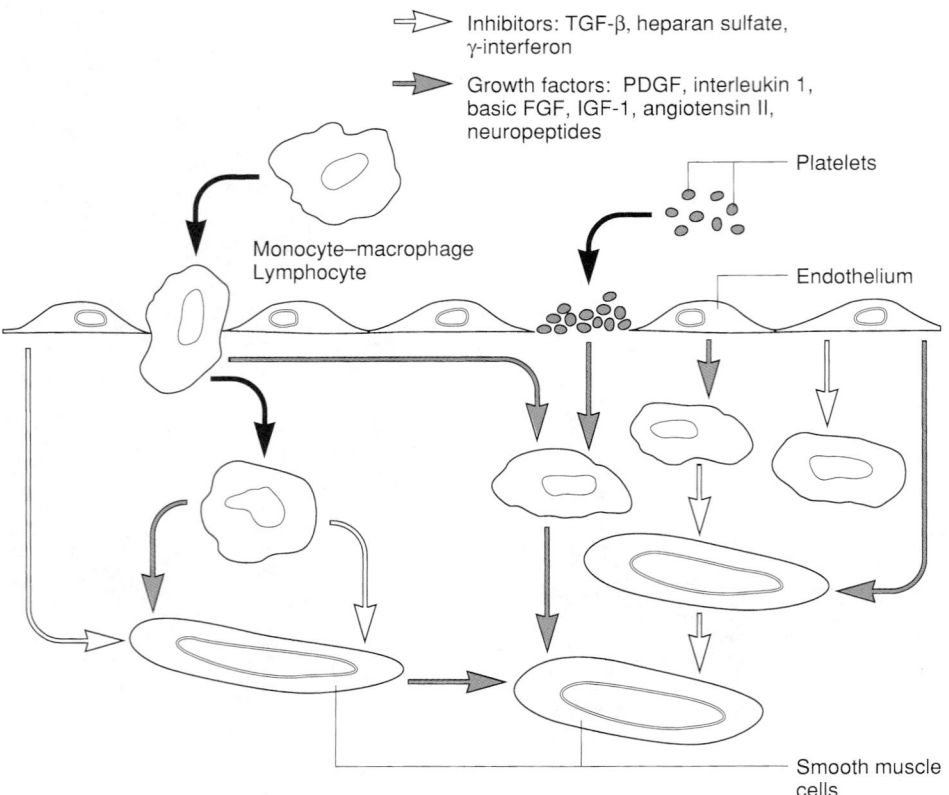

Figure 66.5. Diagram depicts the complexity of the interactions between vascular wall cells (endothelium and smooth-muscle cells), platelets, and blood-borne leukocytes (monocyte/macrophage and lymphocyte). Each cell is capable of synthesizing and releasing several smooth-muscle growth factors and inhibitors.

dothelium can synthesize a heparin-like molecule that inhibits smooth-muscle cell growth in vitro, and that heparin itself can suppress both the proliferation and migration of smooth-muscle cells in vitro and in vivo (57). Taken together, these findings suggest that the endothelium can inhibit smooth-muscle proliferation, and that the quiescent state of smooth-muscle cells in the normal arteries of adult animals may be actively maintained rather than attributable to the lack of growth factors (Fig. 66.5).

REGULATION OF SMOOTH-MUSCLE GROWTH

Platelets have long been considered the major source of mitogen for proliferating smooth muscle. However, smooth-muscle cells are able to proliferate in injured and hypertensive arteries when platelets are absent. If platelet factors are not important, what, then, is the stimulus for smooth-muscle growth? Three alternatives are (a) growth factors from vascular wall cells or resident leukocytes, (b) exogenous neuroendocrine factors, and (c) loss of local inhibitors of smooth-muscle proliferation. All three mechanisms may be important. Let us consider the first alternative. It is of some interest that when a rat carotid is denuded of endothelium with a balloon catheter, a substantial fraction of the medial smooth-muscle cells proliferate (about 20% to 30%), but when denudation is accomplished with a fine nylon wire, very little proliferation is noted (about 2% to 4%) (58). These procedures differ only in regard to the degree to which the media is damaged. Ballooning destroys 20% of the medial smooth muscle in addition to the endothelium, whereas passage of the nylon wire destroys only the endothelium. The observations become more interesting if we note that cultured cells, when damaged, release substances that promote growth (59,60), predominantly fibroblast growth factors (61,62). These factors have been found in a wide variety of tissues and cell types and are synthesized by endothelium and smooth-muscle cells. They are distinguished from other polypeptide mitogens by their ability to bind strongly to heparin. Furthermore, both acidic and basic fibroblast growth factors are potent smooth-muscle mitogens in vitro. Finally, fibroblast growth factors can bind to heparin-like molecules, so that released fibroblast growth factors may readily be "stored" in the heparan sulfate proteoglycan-containing matrix at sites of cell death (63). The experiments of Lindner and Reidy (64,65) provide strong evidence to support the conclusion that basic fibroblast growth factor is an important growth factor for the first wave of proliferation in balloon-injured rat carotid artery. This mechanism of tissue repair is probably quite relevant to the development of the fibrous cap in advanced atherosclerotic lesions. At these sites, toxic oxidized lipids accumulate, and injury and necrosis are clearly evident (41). The release of cellular fibroblast growth factor could provide the stimulus for smooth-muscle proliferation in the overlying fibrous cap.

Because cell death is not necessarily a prominent feature of growing tissues, other means for controlling smooth-muscle proliferation must exist. Not only do smooth-muscle cells respond to factors from dead cells, platelets (PDGF, TGF-β, epidermal growth factor-like molecules), and plasma (thrombin, lipoproteins, insulin-like growth factor-1), they also synthesize and respond to their own secreted factors (42). Both endothelial and smooth-muscle cells as well as macrophages are potential sources of mitogen. In addition to fibroblast growth factors, these cell types synthesize and secrete PDGF, interleukin-1 (IL-1), TGF-β, and insulin-like growth factor-1.

Platelet-derived growth factor in particular has been studied in some detail (66). The original studies of PDGF stemmed from the observation that serum prepared from whole blood contains substantially more growth-promoting activity than serum prepared from plasma. These findings led to the discovery of PDGF, a basic dimeric protein with a molecular weight of approximately 30,000. It is transported in the blood in the alpha granule of the platelet and is released along with other alpha-granule proteins. PDGF is by itself extremely potent and is active as a smooth-muscle mitogen in trace amounts (nanograms per milliliter). It also exhibits a range of other activities on smooth muscle and other types of cells (stimulates smooth-muscle migration and contraction, and matrix synthesis), although it is not a mitogen for endothelium. When placed in a wound chamber in vivo, it induces a granulation tissue response (67).

An important development in the field of growth factor research in the last decade was the demonstration that the structure of the gene for PDGF is nearly identical to that of the oncogene v-*sis,* a gene associated with cellular transformation by the simian sarcoma virus (68,69). This discovery, coupled with the finding that a variety of cells, including normal cells, synthesize and secrete active PDGF, raises the possibility that normal wound healing and malignant, unscheduled growth of tumor cells may have striking similarities with subtle differences in gene regulation. It also led to a search for growth factors in vascular wall cells. We now have solid evidence that endothelium, smooth-muscle cells, and leukocytes, including macrophages, can express the PDGF gene (c-*sis* or PDGF B chain) in vitro and in vivo (66). PDGF research is complicated by the observation that PDGF is not a single molecule but is either a heterodimer or homodimer of two isoforms, PDGF A and PDGF B. The cellular receptors are also dimers of two isoforms, alpha and beta, such that PDGF B binds to both alpha and beta, but PDGF A binds only to the alpha form of the receptor. The implications of this complexity of growth factor and receptor expression have yet to be understood. At present, we know that human platelets transport mainly PDGF AB, whereas cultured smooth-muscle cells from human plaque, baboon graft intima, and rat intima thickened in response to injury express mainly PDGF A-chain mRNA. This observation is probably not an artifact of cell culture because the primary lesions from which the cells are derived contain relatively large amounts of PDGF A-chain mRNA. Macrophages in atherosclerotic lesions express PDGF B protein. What role PDGF plays in wall function remains to be determined. It is not clear how the expression of the protein is regulated, nor is it clear whether regulation also occurs at the level of receptor expression. These findings suggest the intriguing possibility that vascular wall cells as well as platelets are a source of growth factors in the artery wall, and that through the endogenous production of growth factors they may be able to regulate their own growth (autocrine control) or the growth of neighbors (paracrine control). Alternatively, PDGF may control some function other than proliferation. At least after injury and in atherosclerotic mouse arteries, PDGF may act as a chemoattractant and regulate the movement of smooth-muscle cells from the media into the intima or from the wall into the overlying thrombus (70,71). The PDGF signaling pathway in smooth-muscle cell migration differs from that in proliferation (72).

Another alternative for regulation, in addition to factors from the blood and the cells themselves, is neuroendocrine control of smooth-muscle growth (73,74). Several neurotransmitters affect smooth-muscle hypertrophy and proliferation (serotonin, neurokinin A, substance K, substance P). Furthermore, sympathectomy or inhibitors of sympathetic nerve function inhibit the increase in DNA observed in the media of developing arteries and arteries subjected to hypertension (75,76). In injury models, prazosin (an α_1 antagonist) and cilazapril (an ACE inhibitor)

both inhibit intimal thickening (77,78). These recent observations provide some support for the possibility that neuroendocrine factors also influence intimal smooth-muscle proliferation.

Although smooth-muscle mass may be determined in large measure by the presence or absence of growth factors (i.e., positive effectors of growth), smooth-muscle mass may also be influenced by endogenous inhibitors. Growth may be viewed as release from quiescence. Earlier, we pointed out that endothelial regeneration in injured arteries is associated with cessation of underlying intimal smooth-muscle growth. On the other hand, in healing vascular grafts, intimal smooth-muscle cells proliferate only underneath the newly formed endothelial surface (79). These observations are in parallel with those from studies of endothelial and smooth-muscle cells in culture demonstrating that vascular wall cells can synthesize and secrete both inhibitors and promoters of smooth-muscle growth (13). The growth-promoting factors have already been described. Both cell types also synthesize heparan sulfate, which, when released from the larger proteoglycan, can inhibit the growth of cultured smooth-muscle cells (80,81). Both cell types synthesize and secrete a TGF-β precursor (82), and TGF-β can be found in the arterial wall after injury (83). The precursor molecule can then be activated. In general, TGF-β acts as an inhibitor, although at times it can promote smooth-muscle growth. Antibody to TGF-β administered to rats suppresses injury-induced intimal thickening (84).

Other growth inhibitors may be released in vivo by leukocytes present in the vascular wall. Although this mechanism is not important for the regulation of mass in normal artery, it is probably very important in diseased vessels. Large numbers of macrophages and lymphocytes are found in atherosclerotic plaque. Hansson et al. (85) have shown that resident T cells secrete interferon-γ (INF-γ) and induce the expression of class II major histocompatibility antigens. INF-γ also inhibits smooth-muscle growth in culture, and a significant population of I_a-positive, growth-inhibited, intimal smooth-muscle cells is present in the injured rat carotid (86). Although smooth-muscle cells account for the bulk of the intimal thickening, 1% or fewer of the intimal cells are T cells. Because I_a expression is absolutely dependent on the presence of INF-γ, these observations strongly support the view that INF-γ is an endogenous regulator of intimal smooth-muscle growth. A recent study of the effects of INF-γ refutes this conclusion and suggests that it may at times promotes smooth-muscle cell growth (87). Finally, the growth of vascular wall cells may be regulated not only by secreted soluble factors but also by direct cell–cell contact. This inhibitory mechanism is very important for endothelium and perhaps less so for smooth-muscle cells.

Growth factors exert their effects via specific receptors located in cell membranes. Most growth factors receptors belong to a family of peptide receptors called *receptor tyrosine kinases.* The function of a growth factor can be endocrine, paracrine, or autocrine in nature. Function is said to be "endocrine" when the growth factor is released into the circulation and becomes active after attaching to receptors located on cells in a distant organ. A growth factor functions in a "paracrine" manner when it acts on cells located in the vicinity of the cells that secrete it. A growth factor can also affect the same cell that secretes it in an "autocrine" manner. In each of these situations, the growth factor interacts with its own specific receptors located on distant cells, adjacent cells, or the same cells that secreted it. The paracrine and autocrine functions are important in case of arterial injury. When endothelial cells and smooth-muscle cells are injured, they secrete growth factors, such as PDGF, that bind to receptors on the same or adjacent cells. The result is smooth-muscle cell proliferation and migration and the development of intimal hyperplasia (40).

Once a growth factor binds to the extracellular domain of its receptor, the kinase function becomes activated and phosphorylates specific cytoplasmic substrates to activate pathways required for the function of the growth factor. The actions of various growth factor receptors involve specific substrates, and the same growth factor may interact with a different substrate depending on the ultimate function required—cell division, motion, or differentiation. Therefore, the most important events in signal transduction take place in the cytoplasm of the cell (88). Triggered by growth factor attachment, the intracellular domains interact on a molecular level. Then, intracellular protein molecules belonging to various protein families bind to specific sites along the intracellular cytoplasmic domain of the phosphorylated receptor. These proteins carry specific recognition sites that allow a certain family of proteins to bind to a specific area of the intracellular domain. In this way, various cellular signaling pathways are activated. Each pathway controls a specific function of the growth factor. The recognition sites found on the cellular proteins are called *src homology-2* and *src homology-3 domains*. In addition, the src homology-2 and src homology-3 phosphorylated sites of the proteins serve to bind them to other cellular proteins that belong to the signaling cascade. Proteins that are involved in these pathways include guanosine triphosphatase-activating protein, phospholipase C, and phosphatidylinositol-3 kinase-binding protein. These cascades of phosphorylation and specific protein binding eventually lead to a specific function of the growth factor; the function may be one of differentiation, proliferation, cell shape changes, or motility (89).

The signaling pathways or cascades rely on protein phosphorylation for transmission of the signal to the nucleus and gene activation. One of these pathways is the Ras pathway. Once the growth factor attaches to its receptor, the receptor undergoes phosphorylation. Ras, a protein that attaches to the cytoplasmic aspect of the cellular membrane, undergoes phosphorylation and activates Raf-1 protein, which indirectly phosphorylates mitogen-activated protein kinase. Mitogen-activated protein kinase phosphorylates transcription factors inside the nucleus (e.g., Myc, jun) that stimulate gene activity (89). The Jak-STAT pathway is another important signaling pathway (90,91). STATs (signal transducers and activators of transcription) are families of proteins that have been found to undergo phosphorylation by Jaks, kinase enzymes activated in response to growth factor–receptor interaction. The two pathways to the nucleus, Ras and Jak-STAT, may intersect to cause gene activation. It is believed that mitogen-activated protein kinase from the Ras pathway enhances STAT activity by inducing additional phosphorylation (92).

Direct cell-to-cell communication and the presence of gap junctions have been demonstrated in monolayers of endothelium (93) and in mixed-cell populations between endothelium and smooth muscle (94). The significance of these direct links has not been defined, although a recent study has demonstrated that cultured pericytes or smooth-muscle cells can inhibit endothelial growth when the cells are in contact with one another. In vivo capillary endothelial cells appear to grow when pericytes are absent and to stop growing when the pericytes reappear. Endothelial cells can also regulate each other's growth. Plasma membrane preparations from the epithelium of confluent large vessels actively inhibit growing endothelial cells (95). The intercellular links may help to regulate endothelial proliferation and endothelium-mediated vascular relaxation in collateral vessels by propagating signals from one cell to the next upstream from a large-vessel occlusion. Direct cell-to-cell communication may also provide a mechanism for local response in a vessel without the release and wide dissemination of potent vasoactive or growth-regulatory substances.

In summary, the size of a vessel wall depends on the mass of cells and matrix. Because smooth-muscle cells and associated matrix proteins make up the bulk of the tissue, an understanding of the regulation of smooth-muscle growth during development and in disease is extremely important. Smooth-muscle cell number and distribution are affected by growth factors from the blood (particularly from platelets and leukocytes), growth factors and inhibitors from the vascular wall cells themselves, and neuroendocrine factors, particularly from sympathetic nerves in the vessel wall. Smooth-muscle quiescence in normal adult artery may be maintained by heparin-like inhibitors synthesized by vascular wall cells or by the absence of growth factor. The initiation of growth may be the consequence of a shift in the balance of these negative and positive stimuli (Fig. 66.5). For example, any condition causing injury of vascular wall cells or inducing an influx of macrophages would be expected to set up a favorable environment for smooth-muscle growth. Hypercholesterolemia, a significant risk factor for atherosclerosis, is associated with macrophage migration and the accumulation of toxic, oxidized LDL in susceptible large arteries. The release of endogenous fibroblast growth factor from dying foam cells and the release of other growth factors (possibly PDGF) from stimulated endothelium, smooth-muscle cells, and macrophages may increase the local concentration of growth-promoting activity. Smooth-muscle cells would be expected to respond by proliferating and migrating into the intima; if collections of these cells have been left in the intima after the completion of fetal development, they might be even more responsive. These factors might also regulate the traffic of other leukocytes (macrophages, T cells) in and out of the wall, and the activated cells would in turn amplify or retard the initial smooth-muscle response by producing growth factors or inhibitors. The extent and complexity of these interactions between the cells of the vessel wall and the blood have yet to be unraveled.

REGULATION OF THE ANTICOAGULATED STATE

Blood does not clot in normal arteries, even when flow is stopped for prolonged periods of time. On the other hand, endothelial injury or loss provokes a dramatic thrombotic response. These observations define the importance of the endothelial layer in the maintenance of the anticoagulated state (96,97). Studies performed primarily on cultured cells have demonstrated that endothelial cells possess an array of anticoagulant and antithrombotic functions, and it is certain that many of these are of importance in vivo. Endothelial cells also have several procoagulant functions, and the balance between procoagulant and anticoagulant functions is regulated by signals from the blood and from neighboring cells.

On the anticoagulant side of the balance, the endothelium synthesizes a membrane-associated heparan sulfate that, like heparin, increases the affinity of antithrombin III for thrombin (98). Because this interaction requires the binding of heparan sulfate to antithrombin III, the complex must be active at the level of the endothelial surface. Heparan–antithrombin III then rapidly inactivates circulating thrombin and other activated serine proteases in the clotting cascade, including factors VII, IX, and X. Thus, endothelium-derived heparan sulfate can act to impede two aspects of the injury response: the activation of the clotting cascade and the stimulation of smooth-muscle proliferation, which we referred to earlier. In addition, endothelial cells can inhibit clotting by means of the protein C pathway (99). Endothelium synthesizes and secretes a protein, thrombomodulin, that in turn is bound to a surface receptor. The receptor–thrombomodulin complex binds thrombin and in so doing inactivates the proteolytic activity for fibrinogen. The thrombomodulin–thrombin complex activates protein C, and the activated protein C binds to protein S on the endothelial surface. The protein C–protein S complex can then inactivate factor Va to inhibit the clotting cascade. The importance of this pathway is amply demonstrated in homozygous protein C-deficient patients, in whom spontaneous thrombosis develops. Finally, endothelial cells can inhibit platelet adhesion and aggregation through the synthesis of prostaglandin I_2 and can degrade formed fibrin by activating plasminogen to plasmin.

On the procoagulant side, endothelial cells synthesize and secrete tissue factor, platelet-activating factor, a plasminogen activator inhibitor, and von Willebrand's factor, and they express a number of receptors for factors of the clotting cascade (96). When the cells are exposed to a variety of inflammatory mediators derived from the blood or from resident macrophages [e.g., endotoxin, IL-1, tumor necrosis factor (TNF)], endothelial cells respond by changing the balance of their anticoagulant and procoagulant activities to favor coagulation. Furthermore, the cells synthesize and express IL-1, which may possibly affect underlying smooth-muscle cells (100). At present, these conclusions are largely based on in vitro experiments; although they relate mainly to the microvasculature, they also may prove important in large vessels, in view of the recent evidence that not only macrophages but also other populations of lymphocytes are present in atherosclerotic plaque. Furthermore, the ability of the vascular wall cells to maintain the anticoagulant state at the luminal surface must have a direct bearing on the thrombotic complications associated with end-stage atherosclerosis.

LESIONS OF ATHEROSCLROSIS

Atherosclerosis is a disease of the intima characterized by the accumulation of smooth-muscle cells and lipid (100,101). The earliest lesion appears to be a local accumulation of lipid in the vessel wall, located either in the extracellular matrix or inside "foam cells" (lipid-filled smooth-muscle cells or macrophages). The relationship between the so-called fatty streak (Fig. 66.6), made up of foam cells, and the pathologic process of atherosclerosis, comprising the formation of fibrous plaque and a complicated lesion, has been the subject of some debate (102). Fatty streaks are found even in young children. Although atherosclerosis has a predilection for certain countries, the extent of fatty streaks of the aorta and coronary arteries in young people is about the same in countries with low mortality rates from heart attack as in countries with high rates. The lipid streaks have been found to be just as common in female as in male subjects, although atherosclerosis is more prevalent in males. Finally, even though lipid streaks are distributed throughout the aorta, end-stage disease is mostly confined to the abdominal segment. Hence, if the fatty streak is the precursor of the more advanced lesion, then either a selection process is at work or the whole concept is wrong. The issue remains unresolved.

An alternative precursor of the atherosclerotic plaque is the intimal cell mass (103,104). These focal accumulations of smooth-muscle cells are frequently found in the vessels of children in locations where fibrous plaques later develop. In fat-fed swine, the intimal cell masses enlarge and become atherosclerotic (105). Although the concept of the intimal cell mass as the initial lesion is attractive, it entails several problems. First, this initial lesion is present in people throughout the world regardless of their eventual risk for atherosclerosis. Secondly, as a general rule, a gradual thickening of the intima occurs throughout the arterial tree as part of the aging process; this has little to do with atherosclerosis. Finally, it has been difficult to find animal models of atherosclerotic change in intimal masses, whereas the formation of fibrous–fatty lesions from fatty streaks has been rather easily modeled by cholesterol feeding in a number of species. For these reasons, support for the intimal cell mass as the initial lesion has not achieved wide acceptance.

Whatever the initial lesion may be in atherosclerosis, it is widely agreed that the lesions characteristic of late atherosclerosis are the fibrous and the complicated plaques. The fibrous plaque is characterized by a thick fibrous luminal cap containing smooth-muscle cells and leukocytes overlying a central core of necrotic debris and lipid (the "atheroma"). Animal studies have suggested that either denudation or nondenuding injury may be present at the surface of the endothelium (54). The functional state of the endothelial and smooth-muscle cells and leukocytes in these lesions is not known. Macrophages, by becoming "foamy," clearly play a role in the metabolism of lipid; activated macrophages also secrete a range of factors that modulate the metabolism and growth of vascular wall cells, and they proliferate locally in lesions (106,107). Other leukocytes, particularly T lymphocytes, are also present; because some adjacent smooth-muscle cells express the class II antigen HLA-DR, they must be exposed to INF-γ, presumably derived from the neighboring T cells (108). In addition to inducing the expression of HLA-DR, INF-γ inhibits smooth-muscle proliferation. Hence, in the advanced atherosclerotic lesion, these leukocytes may play a critical role in regulating smooth-muscle proliferation and accumulation (109,110).

The complicated lesion of atherosclerosis is a fibrous plaque with the additional features of ulceration, luminal thrombosis, calcification, and wall hemorrhage (Fig. 66.6). It is the source of the thromboembolic activities associated with symptomatic disease. Why a fibrous lesion evolves into a complicated plaque is not understood. This process may be accelerated by such risk factors as hypertension, whereas atherogenesis may be affected more by hypercholesterolemia and cigarette smoking. More importantly, the arrival of inflammatory cells and release of potent mediators of inflammation must play a role in the development of the complicated lesion. Earlier, we pointed out that growth factors for smooth muscle not only are liberated from platelets but also are synthesized and secreted by macrophages and the vascular wall cells themselves. In addition, potent cytokines, such as IL-1, TNF, and INF-γ, alter the growth and metabolism of the vascular wall cells. In particular, the balance of anticoagulation–coagulation at the surface of the endothelium may be shifted away from anticoagulation toward coagulation. In the plaque, large amounts of tissue factor and plasminogen activator-1 are present (111–113). These changes, in addition to frank endothelial desquamation (in response to injurious agents, including oxidized LDL, homocystinemia, tobacco products), may promote thrombosis in the vessel, an event that is decidedly unusual in normal vessels. Small accretions of thrombus with subsequent fibrotic remodeling, together with hemorrhage from new blood vessels forming in the ischemic central region of the plaque, may account for the rela-

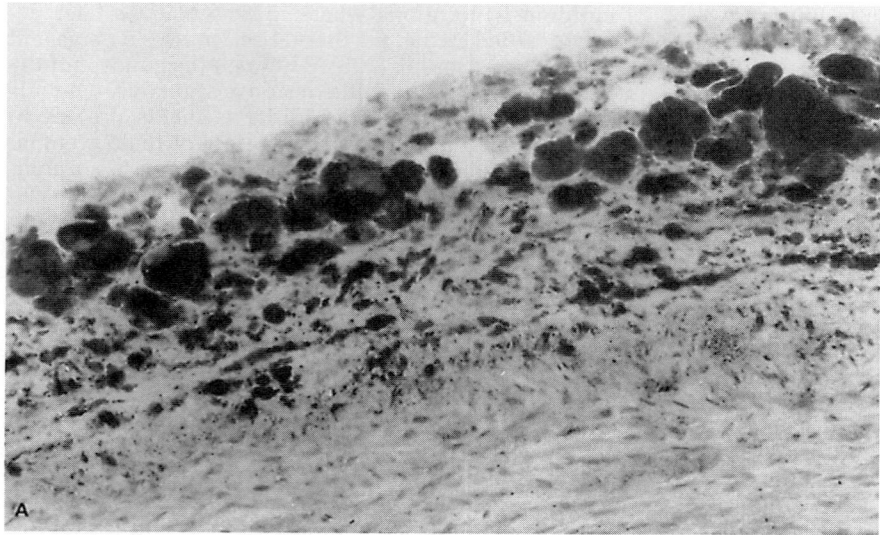

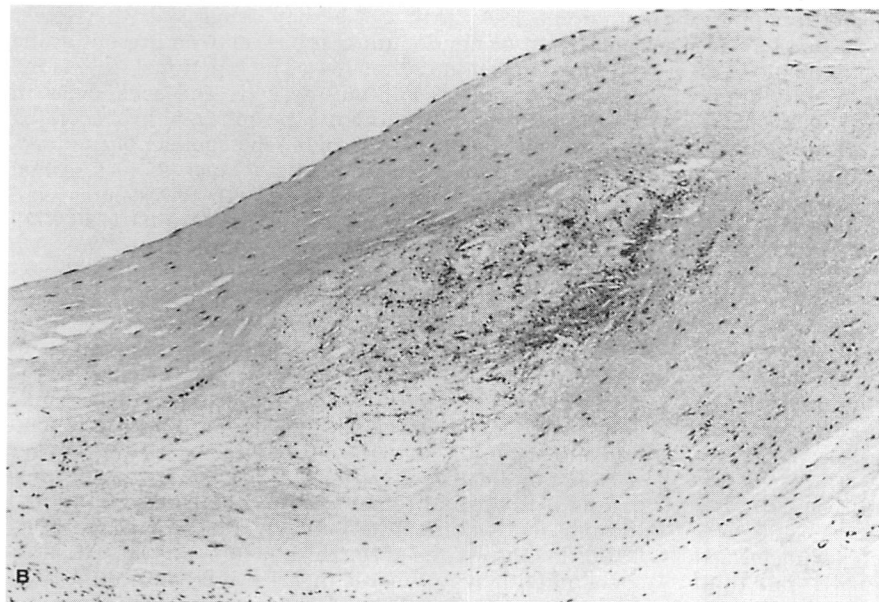

Figure 66.6. Histologic cross sections of a fatty streak containing foam cells stained with oil red O *(A)* and atherosclerotic plaque with a fibrous cap *(B)*. (Courtesy of David Gordon, M.D., Department of Pathology, University of Washington School of Medicine, Seattle, WA.)

tively rapid increase in plaque size and luminal narrowing that has been observed in some arterial beds.

THEORIES OF ATHEROSCLEROSIS

We have summarized some of the information on vascular wall structure and function that may be relevant to general theories of atherosclerosis. From the preceding discussion, it should be evident that an artery is not just an inert, nonthrombogenic conduit for blood; rather, it is an organ with a structure and function that are very carefully modulated by interactions between vascular wall cells themselves and between vascular wall cells and blood. Bearing this in mind, we can reexamine the prevailing theories of atherosclerosis.

During the last century, a number of theories have been advanced to explain how atherosclerosis evolves. In reality, these theories attempt to account for one or more aspects of the disease and are therefore not mutually exclusive. Much of the controversy regarding these theories has to do with individual opinions concerning which aspect of atherosclerosis is most important.

Lipid-insudation Hypothesis

Perhaps the oldest hypothesis, the "lipid-insudation" hypothesis, states that lipid in the atherosclerotic lesion is derived from lipoproteins in the blood (41,114); it therefore links the risk factor of hypercholesterolemia directly to the development of the plaque foam cell, the atheroma, and eventually the complicated lesion. Good evidence now is available demonstrating that lipid in the plaque comes from the blood; substantial evidence also correlates the degree of hypercholesterolemia (particularly elevations of LDL cholesterol) with the degree of atherosclerosis, both in humans and in animal models. When animals are made hyperlipidemic, the initial change is a migration of macrophages through the endothelium into the subintima and media. These cells then engorge the lipids carried into the wall by lipoproteins to form foam cells. The foam cells presumably secrete chemoattractants, growth factors, and cytokines, which trigger complex events that lead to the formation of an atherosclerotic plaque (115). The most important study to demonstrate that an elevated blood cholesterol level is a risk factor for coronary artery disease and hence atherosclerosis is the Framingham study. When a large group of healthy men and women were studied, it was found that the risk for the development of clinically evident coronary artery disease is related to cholesterol levels (116). Although a high level of LDL cholesterol is an important risk factor for atherosclerosis, epidemiologic studies have shown that levels of apolipoprotein B (the primary protein constituent of LDL), very low-density lipoprotein (VLDL), and chylomicrons correlate more accurately with the risk for atherosclerosis. Particles resembling VLDL and intermediate LDL have been identified within atherosclerotic plaque (117). High-density lipoproteins (HDLs) oppose the deposition of cholesterol by transporting cholesterol to the liver. Thus, low levels of HDL correlate with an increased risk for atherosclerosis and high levels of HDL are protective. The lipid-insudation theory states that the lipid in atherosclerotic lesion is derived from lipoproteins in the blood (41,118). The earliest lesions induced by elevated plasma cholesterol levels are the fatty streaks, which contain an impressive accumulation of lipids. For a considerable period of time, it was thought that the lipid-containing foam cells were derived from smooth-muscle cells, but considerable evidence now indicates that most of these cells originate from circulating monocytes/macrophages and that only a fraction represent cholesterol-laden smooth-muscle cells. Although not all fatty streaks become fibrous plaques, results from the Pathological Determinants of Atherosclerosis in Youth program have shown that atherosclerosis commences as a fatty streak that progresses to the complicated lesion—namely, the fibrous plaque (119).

It is still unclear how the monocytes penetrate the endothelium to reach the subendothelial space. The endothelial injury hypothesis postulates that endothelial denudation makes this penetration possible, but a number of experimental studies have failed to show any damage to the endothelium over the fatty streaks. Once in the subendothelial space of the intima, the monocytes take up lipoprotein cholesterol to become foam cells. Denudation of endothelial cells probably occurs later in the development of the lesion and exposes the underlying foam cells. Brown and colleagues (120), however, showed that even the highest concentration of LDL could not induce the accumulation of cholesterol in monocytes/macrophages or in smooth-muscle cells, the precursors of arterial foam cells. Thus, it is not circulating LDL that causes lipid to accumulate in the monocytes/macrophages; rather, it is oxidized LDL, which is taken up avidly by the macrophages. Oxidized LDL is more atherogenic than native LDL, and in animal models, antioxidant compounds can slow the rate of atherosclerotic lesion progression by 50% or more (121). A good deal of epidemiologic evidence correlates a high intake of antioxidant vitamins with a decreased risk for coronary artery disease in humans (122). Several clinical trials of antioxidant vitamins are in progress, and the results should be available in a few years.

Regarding the role of genetic background in the development and progression of atherosclerosis, Dansky and colleagues (123) have demonstrated that expression of the human apo A-I transgene on the apo E-deficient background increases HDL cholesterol levels and greatly diminishes the formation of fatty streak lesions. They have also shown that increases in apo A-I and HDL cholesterol inhibit foam cell formation in apo E-deficient/human apo A-I transgenic mice at a stage following lipid deposition, endothelial activation, and monocyte adherence, without increases in HDL-associated paraoxonase.

The role of "statins" in delaying the progression of the atherosclerotic lesion has been investigated. Several studies, such as the Coronary Primary Prevention Trial and the Helsinki Heart Study, have shown a relation between a reduction in the lipoprotein profile and a reduction in cardiac events (124,125). In the first study, a 20% reduction in LDL cholesterol yielded a reduction of more than 30% in coronary events, and in the second study, gemfibrozil reduced LDL cholesterol by 8% and triglycerides by more than 35% and effected a 15% increase in HDL and a 34% reduction in coronary events.

The discovery of the statin group of drugs (simvastatin, lovastatin, and others) was a major advance in the pharmacologic management of hypercholesterolemia. The statins are analogues of hepatic hydroxymethylglutaryl coenzyme A (HMG CoA) reductase; therefore, they block its action and inhibit the synthesis of cholesterol. Statins are highly effective agents for the primary and secondary prevention of coronary artery disease. Although the lowering of cholesterol, especially LDL cholesterol, appears to be the most important mechanism underlying the beneficial effects of statins, other effects, including an improvement in endothelial function, may also play an important role. The inhibition of cholesterol synthesis increases hepatic expression of the LDL receptor and leads to an increased clearance of circulating LDL. Several studies have shown that lipid-lowering statin therapy achieves a reduction in cardiovascular events and mortality from cardiac events (126). These studies also have demonstrated a reduction in the incidence of stroke, which is relatively weakly associated with cholesterol levels. Simvastatin and lovastatin have been shown to reduce vascular injury after experimental stroke in a rodent model, independently of lipid changes (127). The precise mechanism by which statins reduce the risk for atherosclerosis warrants further study, and such knowledge may revolutionize preventive intervention.

Encrustation Hypothesis

Like the lipid-insudation hypothesis, the encrustation hypothesis focuses on one aspect of the disease (128). This hypothesis proposes that plaque initiation and progression are the consequence of repeated cycles of thrombosis and remodeling. However, autopsy studies of vessels of children and experiments in cholesterol-fed animals have shown that thrombosis is not the initial event in atherogenesis; in fact, thrombosis appears to be a feature of advanced disease. Hence, this hypothesis is applicable only to the problem of plaque progression. Furthermore, it does not explain how lipid and smooth-muscle cells accumulate in the lesion.

Reaction-to-injury Hypothesis

This hypothesis attempts to explain how smooth-muscle growth is regulated in atherogenesis (40). As originally proposed, it stated that the initial event is some form of injury to the endothelium. In regions denuded of endothelium, platelets adhere and release growth factors; these growth factors accumulate in the wall and stimulate medial smooth-muscle proliferation and migration into the intima. As discussed above, this theory is based on the observation that platelets carry potent smooth-muscle mitogens in their granules and that the injury-induced arterial lesion closely resembles the fibrous cap found in atherosclerotic plaque. A modified version of this theory suggests that injuries to the endothelium that do not produce denudation may also cause smooth-muscle growth by stimulating damaged endothelium to synthesize and release growth factors. Alternatively, monocytes may be attracted to the zone of injury; the monocyte/macrophage may then be activated and start to elaborate growth-promoting activity. The reaction-to-injury hypothesis suggests a possible mechanism for the accumulation of connective tissue cells and matrix; it fails to provide an explanation for lipid accumulation or the monoclonal nature of the advanced atherosclerotic plaque.

Monoclonal Hypothesis

This hypothesis focuses on smooth-muscle accumulation in the lesion (129). It states that the cells of any particular plaque are likely to arise as a clone from a single progenitor smooth-muscle cell. The hypothesis is based on the observation that individual plaques in female humans heterozygous for the X-linked marker glucose-6-phosphate (G-6-PD) dehydrogenase frequently exhibit one but not both of the G-6-PD isotypes. At a certain moment in time, single cells may be stimulated to enter the growth cycle and undergo several rounds of division; the formation of a monoclonal lesion is the result. The mechanism of cell activation leading to such lesions is not yet evident; the only other known monoclonal cell masses in humans are neoplasms (e.g., leiomyomas). The suggestion that carcinogens or possibly viruses are possible etiologic agents might explain the link between cigarette smoking and atherosclerosis. An alternative to carcinogenesis as an explanation for monoclonality is the possibility of activation of a susceptible population of stem cells (130). Smooth-muscle cells might have a limited replicative capacity, and only a small population of stem cells in the wall might be capable of responding to growth factors. Whatever the mechanism of activation, any theory attempting to explain how smooth-muscle cells accumulate in atherosclerotic plaque must take into account this observation of monoclonality.

Intimal Cell Mass Hypothesis

This hypothesis was mentioned earlier and states that an accumulation of intimal smooth-muscle cells is one of the two possible initial lesions in atherosclerosis (103, 104). Small accumulations of smooth-muscle cells are found in children at sites where atherosclerosis later develops. How they happen to get there is unclear, nor is it evident why they are susceptible to atherogenic stimuli. It could be that these cells are primordial rests and really are a form of stem cell capable of responding to external mitogenic stimuli. Because intimal cell masses are found in the vessels of children throughout the world regardless of the prevalence of atherosclerosis, it is likely that the atherosclerotic change is largely determined by extrinsic risk factors, such as hypercholesterolemia.

Infection Hypothesis

Although the role of infection in the development of atherosclerosis has been debated for many years, only recently has it has been emphasized by a panel convened by the National Heart, Lung, and Blood Institute (131). The expert panel examined the evidence linking infection to the development of the atherosclerotic process, in particular the role of cytomegalovirus (CMV) and *Chlamydia pneumoniae*. The panel described seroepidemiologic evidence and reports localizing these infectious agents to human plaque. In addition, they examined the results of studies aiming to show cause and effect between CMV and *C. pneumoniae* and the development of atherosclerotic lesions in animal models.

Cytomegalovirus belongs to the herpesvirus family, which also includes the Epstein-Barr virus. Melnick and colleagues (132) found significantly higher titers of CMV antibodies in patients undergoing coronary artery bypass surgery (70%) than in matched controls (43%). Atherosclerosis is more likely to develop after cardiac transplantation in recipients with prior CMV exposure, evidenced by increased serum levels of CMV immunoglobulin G antibodies, than in patients without prior exposure to CMV (133). CMV infection has been associated with recurrence of stenosis following coronary angioplasty (134). In addition, CMV has been implicated in the development of carotid atherosclerosis. CMV antigens have been isolated from carotid plaque, and increased CMV antibody titers are associated with carotid intimal and medial thickening (135). Although it has been difficult to culture viral particles from atherosclerotic lesions, this by itself does not constitute strong evidence against the role of CMV infection in atherosclerosis; it is possible that the virus triggers infection without persisting in the tissue (131,132,136).

Three species of *Chlamydia,* which are gram-negative bacteria, are known to cause human disease. *C. pneumoniae* causes upper respiratory infections. *C. pneumoniae* organisms have been isolated in atherosclerotic plaque from both carotid and coronary arteries (137,138). In a rabbit model, infection with *C. pneumoniae* has been shown to accelerate the formation of the atherosclerotic lesion. In addition, treatment with azithromycin prevented the formation of the lesion (139). To gain insight into the mechanism by which *C. pneumoniae* infection affects the process of atherogenesis, Kol and colleagues (140,141) analyzed atherosclerotic plaque to detect the presence of chlamydial heat shock protein 60 (HSP 60). Studying plaque from human carotid atherosclerotic arteries, these investigators found that chlamydial and human HSP 60 co-localize within macrophages in atherosclerotic lesions. They showed that both chlamydial and human HSP 60 induce the production of TNF-α and matrix metalloproteinase (MMP) by macrophages. They concluded that by inducing the production of such factors by macrophages, chlamydial HSP 60 may represent the mechanism by which infection with *C. pneumoniae* promotes atherosclerosis (140). In addition, the same investigators showed that chlamydial and human HSP 60 activate human endothelial cells, smooth-muscle cells, and macrophages to secrete various factors (e.g., E-selectin, intercellular adhesion molecule-1, vascular cell adhesion molecule-1) important in the pathophysiology of atherosclerosis (141).

More work needs to be done to establish definitively the relationship between these and other agents and atherosclerosis. Establishing the role of infectious agents in the development of atherosclerosis is very important because a role for antiinfective agents, such as known antibiotics, might be indicated in preventing or slowing the atherosclerotic process.

Inflammatory and Immune Hypothesis

Mediators of inflammation, such as cytokines and growth factors, have been found in atherosclerotic plaque. These mediators, which are involved in the synthesis and degradation of collagen by vascular smooth-muscle cells, include TGF-β and INF-γ (142). IL-2 receptors are markers suggesting the activation of T lymphocytes, and INF-γ is produced and secreted by activated T lymphocytes (143).

The involvement of macrophages and T lymphocytes in atherogenesis suggests an immune in addition to an inflammatory response. The lymphocytes found in atherosclerotic lesions are polyclonal, which indicates that these cells do not develop in response to a single antigen. Several different subclasses of T lymphocytes have been identified in atherosclerotic plaque, including both CD4 (helper-inducer) and CD8 (cytotoxic) T cells (144). In addition, the development of accelerated coronary artery atherosclerosis, a unique variant of atherosclerosis, in transplanted hearts suggests an immunologic basis. The lesions in transplanted hearts involve the entire coronary tree and contain all the cellular elements characteristic of atherosclerosis; in addition, T lymphocytes and macrophages are more numerous than in typical atherosclerotic lesions (145). Heterotopic heart transplants and arterial interposition grafts have been used to produce arterial lesions in mouse transplant models that resemble transplant arteriosclerosis (146,147).

Activation of the complement system is an important step in the immune process that causes the deposition of immune complexes in the arterial wall or precipitates the binding of specific antibodies to antigens found in vascular tissues. Cholesterol particles are potent activators of the complement system (148). Activation of the complement system results in the production of proinflammatory molecules and the terminal membrane attack complex, which has been known to stimulate the production of cytokines (e.g., TNF-α and IL-8) and growth factors (e.g., basic fibroblast growth factor and PDGF) by vascular smooth-muscle and endothelial cells (148). The membrane attack complex has been identified in atherosclerotic lesions, particularly fibrous plaque (149).

Most complications related to atherosclerotic lesions may be a consequence of plaque disruption or rupture. Plaque disruption exposes circulating blood to the lipid core, with subsequent formation of thrombus (Fig. 66.7) and acute arterial occlusion (150,151). Plaque stability is very important in preventing plaque rupture. Stability is provided by the integrity of the extracellular matrix within the plaque. Plaque instability is related to the degree of inflammation because inflammatory cells produce cytokines that decrease the production of collagen or increase its

degradation (152). Therefore, the balance between the production of matrix metalloproteinases (MMPs), which degrade collagen, and the production of tissue inhibitors of metalloproteinases (TIMPs) regulates plaque stability (153). The expression of both MMPs and TIMPs can be demonstrated in atheromas. TIMPs have been found in macrophages within plaques (153). Inflammatory cytokines such as IL-1 and TNF can induce the expression of MMPs by macrophages (154). In addition, INF-γ produced by T lymphocytes decreases collagen synthesis, which in turn leads to weakening of the plaque extracellular matrix and rupture (155). Interestingly, lipid-lowering strategies have been shown to decrease the number of macrophages in plaque and the expression of MMP-1, thereby increasing collagen production and retention and plaque stability (156,154).

Each of these hypotheses attempts to explain one or more aspects of atherogenesis. We might reasonably conclude that each is applicable at a different time during lesion development (Fig. 66.8). Susceptibility to atherosclerosis might be determined by both intrinsic (number of intimal masses) and extrinsic (hypercholesterolemia, hypertension, diabetes, cigarette smoking) factors. The initial event might be the accumulation of lipid by insudation in regions of increased susceptibility. This would lead to the production of macrophage chemotactic factors and an influx of monocytes from the blood, which together with smooth-muscle cells would sequester lipid and become foam cells. LDL oxidized in the wall and other extrinsic injurious agents could produce some degree of endothelial injury and perhaps at later times even limited denudation. Growth factors might then be released from the endothelium, activated macrophages and other leukocytes, smooth-muscle cells, and adherent platelets; these growth factors could then stimulate the proliferation and migration of susceptible smooth-muscle cells to form isolated

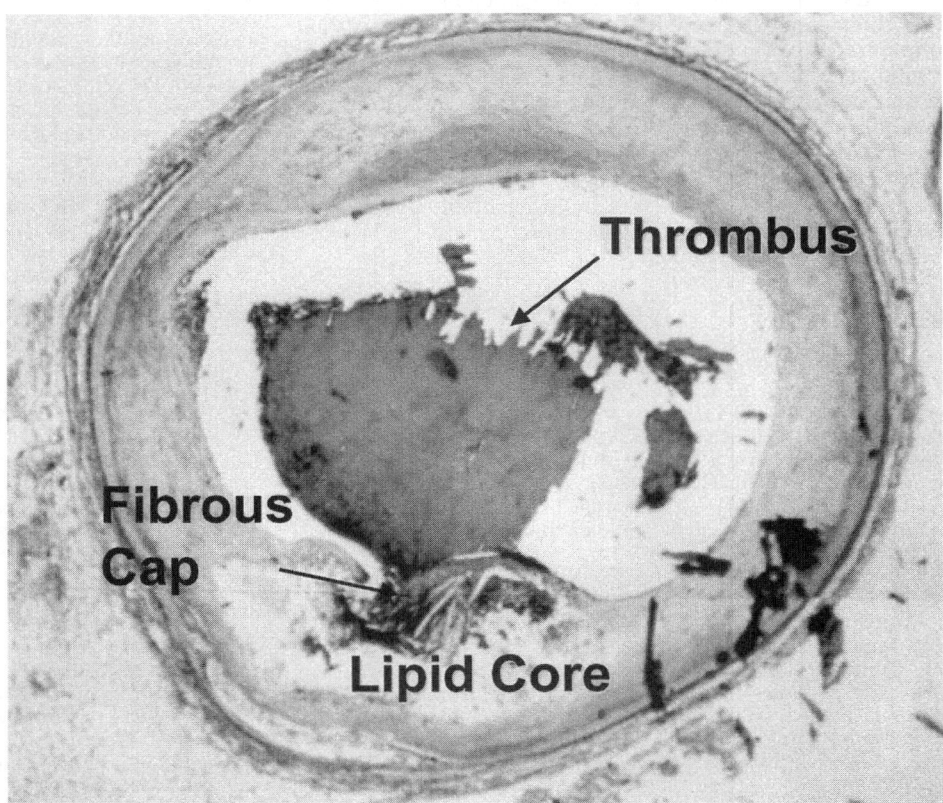

Figure 66.7. Plaque cap rupture exposing lipid core of the atheroma and leading to thrombus formation. (Courtesy of Dr. Maria de Lourdes Higuchi, Department of Pathology, University of Sao Paulo, Brazil. Also published in Libby P, Simon D. Thrombosis and atherosclerosis. In: Colman RW, Hirsh J, Marder VJ, et al., eds. *Hemostasis and thrombosis: basic principles and clinical practice,* 4th ed. Philadelphia: Lippincott Williams & Wilkins, 2000, with permssion).

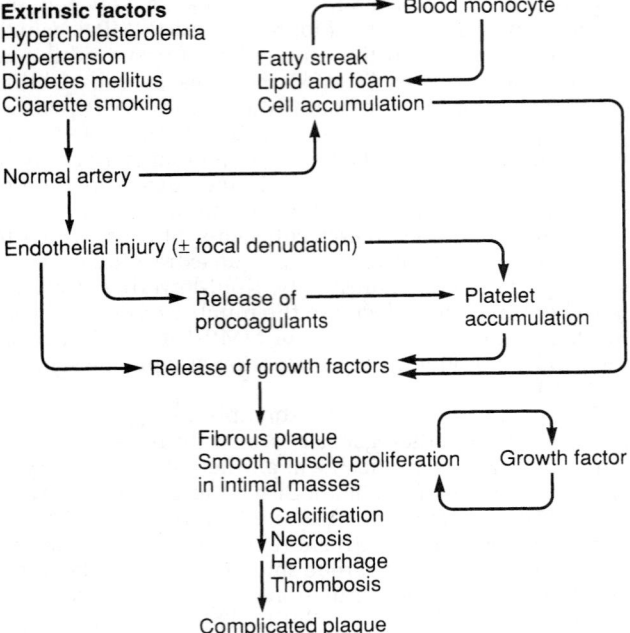

Figure 66.8. Atherogenesis and progression of atherosclerosis are probably the consequence of multiple factors acting on the arterial wall. (Reprinted from Clowes AW. Theories of atherosclerosis. In: White RA, ed. *Atherosclerosis and arteriosclerosis: human pathology and experimental animal methods and models.* Boca Raton, FL: CRC Press, 1989:3, with permission.)

smooth-muscle clones and fibrous lesions. Further production of matrix by the smooth-muscle cells would permit the continued accumulation of lipid. Like a growing tumor, these lesions would enlarge and ischemic cores would develop, thereby inducing an angiogenic response. The thickened plaque with its necrotic lipid core (the atheroma) might not be able to withstand the rigors of continued arterial pulsation, and hemorrhage might develop within the lesion as a consequence of shearing forces exerted on new capillaries. Breakdown of the surface and a change in the coagulation function of the endothelium would render the plaque more thrombogenic. Such changes would lead to the terminal thrombotic event, the hallmark of all ischemic complications in atherosclerotic patients.

REFERENCES

1. Wolinsky H, Glagov S. Nature of species differences in the medial distribution of aortic vasa vasorum in mammals. *Circ Res* 1967;20:409–421.
2. Heistad DD, Armstrong ML. Blood flow through vasa vasorum of coronary arteries in atherosclerotic monkeys. *Arteriosclerosis* 1986;6:326–331.
3. Barger AC, Beeuwkes R III, Lainey LL, et al. Hypothesis: vasa vasorum and neovascularization of human coronary arteries. *N Engl J Med* 1984;310:175–177.
4. Coffin JD, Poole TJ. Embryonic vascular development: immunohistochemical identification of the origin and subsequent morphogenesis of the major vessel primordia in quail embryos. *Development* 1988;102:735–748.
5. Pardanaud L, Altmann C, Kitos P, et al. Vasculogenesis in the early quail blastodisc as studied with a monoclonal antibody recognizing endothelial cells. *Development* 1987;100:339–349.
6. Le Douarin NM. Cell migrations in embryos. *Cell* 1984;38:353–360.
7. Wolinsky H, Glagov S. A lamellar unit of aortic medial structure and function in mammals. *Circ Res* 1967;20:99–111.
8. Wolinsky H, Glagov S. Structural basis for the static mechanical properties of the aortic media. *Circ Res* 1964;14:400–413.
9. Dilley RJ, Schwartz SM. Vascular remodeling in the growth hormone transgenic mouse. *Circ Res* 1989;65:1233–1240.
10. Zarins CK, Zatina MA, Giddens DP, et al. Shear stress regulation of artery lumen diameter in experimental atherogenesis. *J Vasc Surg* 1987;5:413–420.
11. Glagov S, Weisenberg E, Zarins CK, et al. Compensatory enlargement of human atherosclerotic coronary arteries. *N Engl J Med* 1987;316:1371–1375.
12. Frangos JA, Eskin SG, McIntire LV, et al. Flow effect on prostacyclin production by cultured human endothelial cells. *Science* 1985;227:1477–1479.
13. Gibbons GH, Dzau VJ. The emerging concept of vascular remodeling. *N Engl J Med* 1994;330:1431–1438.
14. Davies PF, Tripathi SC. Mechanical stress mechanisms and the cell: an endothelial paradigm. *Circ Res* 1993;72:239–245.
15. Resnick N, Collins T, Atkinson W, et al. Platelet-derived growth factor B chain promoter contains a *cis*-acting fluid shear stress-responsive element. *Proc Natl Acad Sci USA* 1993;90:4591–4595.
16. Vanhoutte PM. The endothelium—modulator of vascular smooth-muscle tone. *N Engl J Med* 1988;319:512–513.
17. Furchgott RF. Role of endothelium in responses of vascular smooth muscle. *Circ Res* 1983;53:557–573.
18. Ignarro LJ, Buga GM, Wood KS, et al. Endothelium-derived relaxing factor produced and released from artery and vein is nitric oxide. *Proc Natl Acad Sci USA* 1987;84:9265–9269.
19. Palmer RMJ, Ferrige AG, Moncada S. Nitric oxide release accounts for the biological activity of endothelium-derived relaxing factor. *Nature* 1987;327:524–526.
20. Ignarro LJ. Biological actions and properties of endothelium-derived nitric oxide formed and released from artery and vein. *Circ Res* 1989;65:1–21.
21. Langille BL, O'Donnell F. Reductions in arterial diameter produced by chronic decreases in blood flow are endothelium-dependent. *Science* 1986;231:405–407.
22. Kohler TR, Jawien A. Flow affects development of intimal hyperplasia after arterial injury in rats. *Arterioscler Thromb* 1992;12:963–971.
23. Kohler TR, Kirkman TR, Kraiss LW, et al. Increased blood flow inhibits neointimal hyperplasia in endothelialized vascular grafts. *Circ Res* 1991;69:1557–1565.
24. Geary RL, Kohler TR, Vergel S, et al. Time course of flow-induced smooth muscle cell proliferation and intimal thickening in endothelialized baboon vascular grafts. *Circ Res* 1994;74:14–23.
25. Shultz PJ, Knauss TC, Mené P, et al. Mitogenic signals for thrombin in mesangial cells: regulation of phospholipase C and PDGF genes. *Am J Physiol* 1989;257:F366–F374.
26. Bobik A, Grooms A, Millar JA, et al. Growth factor activity of endothelin on vascular smooth muscle. *Am J Physiol Cell Physiol* 1990;258:C408–C415.
27. Libby P, Warner SJC, Friedman GB. Interleukin 1: a mitogen for human vascular smooth muscle cells that induces the release of growth-inhibitory prostanoids. *J Clin Invest* 1988;81:487–498.
28. Nakaki T, Nakayama M, Yamamoto S, et al. Endothelin-mediated stimulation of DNA synthesis in vascular smooth muscle cells. *Biochem Biophys Res Commun* 1989;158:880–883.
29. Garg UC, Hassid A. Nitric oxide-generating vasodilators and 8-bromo-cyclic guanosine monophosphate inhibit mitogenesis and proliferation of cultured rat vascular smooth muscle cells. *J Clin Invest* 1989;83:1774–1777.
30. Freiman PC, Mitchell GG, Heistad DD, et al. Atherosclerosis impairs endothelium-dependent vascular relaxation to acetylcholine and thrombin in primates. *Circ Res* 1986;58:783–789.
31. Malek AM, Alper SL, Izumo S. Hemodynamic shear stress and its role in atherosclerosis. *JAMA* 1999;282:2035–2042.
32. Malek AM, Izumo S, Alper SL. Modulation by pathophysiological stimuli of the shear stress-induced upregulation of endothelial nitric oxide synthase expression in endothelial cells. *Neurosurgery* 1999;45:334–344.

33. Stary HC, Chandler AB, Dinsmore RE, et al. A definition of advanced types of atherosclerotic lesions and a histological classification of atherosclerosis—a report from the Committee on Vascular Lesions of the Council on Arteriosclerosis, American Heart Association. *Circulation* 1995;92: 1355–1374.

34. Celermajer DS, Sorensen KE, Gooch VM, et al. Non-invasive detection of endothelial dysfunction in children and adults at risk of atherosclerosis. *Lancet* 1992;340:1111–1115.

35. Zeiher AM, Fisslthaler B, Schray-Utz B, et al. Nitric oxide modulates the expression of monocyte chemoattractant protein 1 in cultured human endothelial cells. *Circ Res* 1995;76: 980–986.

36. Griendling KK, Alexander RW. Oxidative stress and cardiovascular disease [editorial; comment]. *Circulation* 1997;96: 3264–3265.

37. Vane JR, Anggard Ee, Botting RM. Regulatory functions of the vascular endothelium. *N Engl J Med* 1990;323:27–36.

38. Mancini GB, Henry GC, Macaya C, et al. Angiotensin-converting enzyme inhibition with quinapril improves endothelial vasomotor dysfunction in patients with coronary artery disease: the TREND (Trial on Reversing ENdothelial Dysfunction) study [see comments] [published erratum appears in *Circulation* 1996;94:1490]. *Circulation* 1996;94:258–265.

39. Wolinsky H. Long-term effects of hypertension on the rat aortic wall and their relation to concurrent aging changes: morphological and chemical studies. *Circ Res* 1972;30: 301–309.

40. Ross R. Pathogenesis of atherosclerosis—an update. *N Engl J Med* 1986;314:488–500.

41. Steinberg D, Parthasarathy S, Carew TE, et al. Modifications of low-density lipoprotein that increase its atherogenicity. *N Engl J Med* 1989;320:915–924.

42. Schwartz SM, Campbell GR, Campbell JH. Replication of smooth muscle cells in vascular disease. *Circ Res* 1986;58: 427–444.

43. Clowes AW, Reidy MA, Clowes MM. Kinetics of cellular proliferation after arterial injury. I. Smooth muscle growth in the absence of endothelium. *Lab Invest* 1983;49:327–333.

44. Owens GK. Control of hypertrophic versus hyperplastic growth of vascular smooth muscle cells. *Am J Physiol* 1989; 257:H1755–H1765.

45. Zwolak RM, Adams MC, Clowes AW. Kinetics of vein graft hyperplasia: association with tangential stress. *J Vasc Surg* 1987;5:126–136.

46. Leung DY, Glagov S, Mathews MB. Cyclic stretching stimulates synthesis of matrix components by arterial smooth muscle cells in vitro. *Science* 1976;191:475–477.

47. Baumgartner HR, Studer A. Consequences of vessel catheterization in normal and hypercholesterolemic rabbits. *Pathol Microbiol* 1966;29:393–405.

48. Kumagai H, Suzuki H, Matsukawa S, et al. Captopril therapy following percutaneous transluminal angioplasty for bilateral renal artery stenosis. *Arch Intern Med* 1989;149: 1973–1976.

49. Bowen-Pope DF, Ross R, Seifert RA. Locally acting growth factors for vascular smooth muscle cells: endogenous synthesis and release from platelets. *Circulation* 1985;72: 735–740.

50. Friedman RJ, Stemerman MB, Wenz B, et al. The effect of thrombocytopenia on experimental atherosclerotic lesion formation in rabbits: smooth muscle cell proliferation and re-endothelialization. *J Clin Invest* 1977;60:1191–1201.

51. Fingerle J, Johnson R, Clowes AW, et al. Role of platelets in smooth muscle cell proliferation and migration after vascular injury in rat carotid artery. *Proc Natl Acad Sci USA* 1989;86:8412–8416.

52. Groves HM, Kinlough-Rathbone RL, Richardson M, et al. Thrombin generation and fibrin formation following injury to rabbit neointima: studies of vessel wall reactivity and platelet survival. *Lab Invest* 1982;46:605–612.

53. Hatton MWC, Moar SL, Richardson M. Deendothelialization in vivo initiates a thrombogenic reaction at the rabbit aorta surface: correlation of uptake of fibrinogen and antithrombin III with thrombin generation by the exposed subendothelium. *Am J Pathol* 1989;135:499–508.

54. Faggiotto A, Ross R. Studies of hypercholesterolemia in the nonhuman primate. II. Fatty streak conversion to fibrous plaque. *Arteriosclerosis* 1984;4:341–356.

55. Faggiotto A, Ross R, Harker L. Studies of hypercholesterolemia in nonhuman primate. I. Changes that lead to fatty streak formation. *Arteriosclerosis* 1984;4:323–340.

56. Reidy MA. A reassessment of endothelial injury and arterial lesion formation. *Lab Invest* 1985;53:513–520.

57. Clowes AW, Clowes MM. Regulation of smooth muscle proliferation by heparin in vitro and in vivo. *Int Angiol* 1987;6: 45–51.

58. Clowes AW, Clowes MM, Fingerle J, et al. Regulation of smooth muscle cell growth in injured artery. *J Cardiovasc Pharmacol* 1989;14[Suppl 6]:S12–S15.

59. Gajdusek CM, Schwartz SM. Comparison of intracellular and extracellular mitogen activity. *J Cell Physiol* 1984;121: 316–322.

60. Gajdusek CM, Carbon S. Injury-induced release of basic fibroblast growth factor from bovine aortic endothelium. *J Cell Physiol* 1989;139:570–579.

61. Burgess WH, Maciag T. The heparin binding (fibroblast) growth factor family of proteins. *Annu Rev Biochem* 1989; 58:575–606.

62. Gospodarowicz D, Neufeld G, Schwiegerer L. Fibroblast growth factor: structural and biological properties. *J Cell Physiol* 1987;[Suppl 5]:15–26.

63. Vlodavsky I, Folkman J, Sullivan R, et al. Endothelial cell-derived basic fibroblast growth factor: synthesis and deposition into subendothelial extracellular matrix. *Proc Natl Acad Sci USA* 1987;84:2292–2296.

64. Lindner V, Lappi DA, Baird A, et al. Role of basic fibroblast growth factor in vascular lesion formation. *Circ Res* 1991; 68:106–113.

65. Lindner V, Reidy MA. Proliferation of smooth muscle cells after vascular injury is inhibited by an antibody against basic fibroblast growth factor. *Proc Natl Acad Sci USA* 1991;88: 3739–3743.

66. Raines EW, Bowen-Pope DF, Ross R. Platelet-derived growth factor. In: Sporn MB, Roberts AB, eds. *Handbook of experimental pharmacology: peptide growth factors and their receptors.* Heidelberg: Springer-Verlag, 1989.

67. Sprugel KH, McPherson JM, Clowes AW, et al. Effects of growth factors in vivo. I. Cell ingrowth into porous subcutaneous chambers. *Am J Pathol* 1987;129:601–613.

68. Doolittle RF, Hunkapillar MW, Hood LE, et al. Simian sarcoma virus oncgene, v-*sis,* is derived from the gene (or genes) encoding a platelet-derived growth factor. *Science* 1983;221:275–277.

69. Waterfield MD, Scrace GT, Whittle N, et al. Platelet-derived growth factor is structurally related to the putative transforming protein p28-sis of simian sarcoma virus. *Nature* 1983;304:35–39.

70. Ferns GAA, Raines EW, Sprugel KH, et al. Inhibition of neointimal smooth muscle accumulation after angioplasty by an antibody to PDGF. *Science* 1991;253:1129–1132.

71. Jawien A, Bowen-Pope DF, Lindner V, et al. Platelet-derived growth factor promotes smooth muscle migration and intimal thickening in a rat model of balloon angioplasty. *J Clin Invest* 1992;89:507–511.

72. Bornfeldt KE, Raines EW, Graves LM, et al. Platelet-derived growth factor: distinct signal transduction pathways associated with migration versus proliferation. *Ann N Y Acad Sci* 1995;766:416–430.

73. Blaes N, Boissel JP. Growth-stimulating effect of catecholamines on rat aortic smooth muscle cells in culture. *J Cell Physiol* 1983;116:167–172.

74. Dalsgaard CJ, Hultgardh-Nilsson A, Haegerstrand A, et al. Neuropeptides as growth factors: possible roles in human disease. *Regul Pept* 1989;25:1–9.

75. Bevan RD. Trophic effects of peripheral adrenergic nerves on vascular structure. *Hypertension* 1984;6:III-19–III-26.

76. Bevan RD, Tsuru H. Functional and structural changes in the rabbit ear artery after sympathetic denervation. *Circ Res* 1981;49:478–485.

77. Powell JS, Clozel JP, Muller RKM, et al. Inhibitors of angiotensin-converting enzyme prevent myointimal proliferation after vascular injury. *Science* 1989;245:186–188.

78. Jackson CL, Bush RC, Bowyer DE. Inhibitory effect of cal-

cium antagonists on balloon catheter-induced arterial smooth muscle cell proliferation and lesion size. *Atherosclerosis* 1988;69:115–122.

79. Clowes AW, Reidy MA. Mechanisms of graft failure: the role of cellular proliferation. *Ann N Y Acad Sci* 1987;516:673–678.

80. Fritze LMS, Reilly CF, Rosenberg RD. An antiproliferative heparan sulfate species produced by postconfluent smooth muscle cells. *J Cell Biol* 1985;100:1041–1049.

81. Castellot JJ Jr, Addonizio ML, Rosenberg R, et al. Cultured endothelial cells produce a heparin-like inhibitor of smooth muscle cell growth. *J Cell Biol* 1981;90:372–379.

82. Antonelli-Orlidge A, Saunders KB, Smith SR, et al. An activated form of transforming growth factor-β is produced by co-cultures of endothelial cells and pericytes. *Proc Natl Acad Sci USA* 1989;86:4544–4548.

83. Majesky MW, Lindner V, Twardzik DR, et al. Production of transforming growth factor-β₁ during repair of arterial injury. *J Clin Invest* 1991;88:904–910.

84. Wolf YG, Rasmussen LM, Ruoslahti E. Antibodies against transforming growth factor-β₁ suppress intimal hyperplasia in a rat model. *J Clin Invest* 1994;93:1172–1178.

85. Hansson GK, Jonasson L, Seifert PS, et al. Immune mechanisms in atherosclerosis. *Arteriosclerosis* 1989;9:567–578.

86. Hansson GK, Jonasson L, Holm J, et al. Gamma interferon regulates vascular smooth muscle proliferation and Iₐ expression in vitro and in vivo. *Circ Res* 1988;63:712–719.

87. Tellides G, Tereb DA, Kirkiles-Smith NC, et al. Interferon-gamma elicits arteriosclerosis in the absence of leukocytes. *Nature* 2000;403:207–211.

88. Aaronson SA. Growth factors and cancer. *Science* 1991;254:1146–1151.

89. Brugge JS. New intracellular targets for therapeutic drug design. *Science* 1993;260.

90. Schindler C, Shuai K, Prezioso VR, et al. Interferon-dependent tyrosine phosphorylation of a latent cytoplasmic transcription factor. *Science* 1992;257:809–813.

91. Zhong Z, Wen Z, Darnell JE. Stat3: a stat family member activated by tyrosine phosphorylation in response to epidermal growth factor and interleukin. *Science* 1994;264:95–98.

92. Baringa M. Two major signaling pathways meet at MAP-kinase. *Science* 1995;269:1673.

93. Larson DM, Haudenschild CC, Beyer EC. Gap junction messenger RNA expression by vascular wall cells. *Circ Res* 1990;66:1074–1080.

94. Orlidge A, D'Amore PA. Inhibition of capillary endothelial cell growth by pericytes and smooth muscle cells. *J Cell Biol* 1987;105:1455–1462.

95. Heimark RL, Schwartz SM. The role of membrane–membrane interactions in the regulation of endothelial cell growth. *J Cell Biol* 1985;100:1934–1940.

96. Hawiger JJ. Hemostasis, bleeding, and thromboembolic complications of trauma and infection. In: Clowes GHA Jr, ed. *Trauma, sepsis, and shock: the physiological basis of therapy.* New York: Marcel Dekker, 1988:123–159.

97. Rodgers GM. Hemostatic properties of normal and perturbed vascular cells. *FASEB J* 1990;2:116–123.

98. Marcum J, McKenney J, Rosenberg R. The acceleration of thrombin–antithrombin III complex formation in rat hindquarters via heparin-like molecules bound to endothelium. *J Clin Invest* 1984;74:341–350.

99. Esmon CT. The roles of protein C and thrombomodulin in the regulation of blood coagulation. *J Biol Chem* 1989;264:4743–4746.

100. Cotran RS, Kumar V, Robbins SL. *Pathologic basis of disease.* Philadelphia: WB Saunders, 1989:553–595.

101. Benditt EP, Gown AM. Atheroma: the artery wall and the environment. *Int Rev Exp Pathol* 1980;21:55–118.

102. McGill HC Jr. Persistent problems in the pathogenesis of atherosclerosis. *Arteriosclerosis* 1984;4:443–451.

103. Velican C, Velican D. Intimal thickening in developing coronary arteries and its relevance to atherosclerotic involvement. *Atherosclerosis* 1976;23:345–355.

104. Velican C, Velican D. The precursors of coronary atherosclerotic plaques in subjects up to 40 years old. *Atherosclerosis* 1980;37:33–46.

105. Thomas WA, Kim DN. Atherosclerosis as a hyperplastic and/or neoplastic process. *Lab Invest* 1983;48:245–255.

106. Gordon D, Reidy MA, Benditt EP, et al. Cell proliferation in human coronary arteries. *Proc Natl Acad Sci USA* 1990;87:4600–4604.

107. O'Brien ER, Alpers CE, Stewart DK, et al. Proliferation in primary and restenotic coronary atherectomy tissue: implications for antiproliferative therapy. *Circ Res* 1993;73:223–231.

108. Jonasson L, Holm J, Skalli O, et al. Expression of class II transplantation antigens on vascular smooth muscle cells in human atherosclerosis. *J Clin Invest* 1985;76:125–131.

109. Stemme S, Rymo L, Hansson GK. Polyclonal origin of T lymphocytes in human atherosclerotic plaques. *Lab Invest* 1991;65:654–660.

110. Sharrett AR, Patsch W, Sorlie PD, et al. Associations of lipoprotein cholesterols, apolipoproteins A-I and B, and triglycerides with carotid atherosclerosis and coronary heart disease: the Atherosclerosis Risk In Communities (ARIC) study. *Arterioscler Thromb* 1994;14:1098–1104.

111. Wilcox JN, Smith KM, Schwartz SM, et al. Localization of tissue factor in the normal vessel wall and in the atherosclerotic plaque. *Proc Natl Acad Sci USA* 1989;86:2839–2843.

112. Schneiderman J, Sawdey MS, Keeton MR, et al. Increased type 1 plasminogen activator inhibitor gene expression in atherosclerotic human arteries. *Proc Natl Acad Sci USA* 1992;89:6998–7002.

113. Lupu F, Bergonzelli GE, Heim DA, et al. Localization and production of plasminogen activator inhibitor-1 in human healthy and atherosclerotic arteries. *Arterioscler Thromb* 1993;13:1090–1100.

114. Page JH. Atherosclerosis: an introduction. *Circulation* 1954;10:1–27.

115. Masuda J, Ross R. Atherogenesis during low-level hypercholesterolemia in the nonhuman primate. I. Fatty streak formation. *Arteriosclerosis* 1990;10:164–177.

116. Castelli WP. Epidemiology of coronary heart disease: the Framingham study. *Am J Med* 1984;76:4–12.

117. Rapp JH, Harris HW, Hamilton RL, et al. Particle size distribution of lipoproteins from human atherosclerotic plaque: a preliminary report. *J Vasc Surg* 1989;9:81–88.

118. Breslow JL. Insights into lipoprotein metabolism from studies in transgenic mice. *Annu Rev Physiol* 1994;56:797–810.

119. Strong JP, Malcom GT, Oalmann MC, et al. The PDAY study: natural history, risk factors, and pathobiology—pathobiological determinants of atherosclerosis in youth. *Ann N Y Acad Sci* 1997;811:226–237; discussion 235–237.

120. Brown MS, Basu SK, Falck JR, et al. The scavenger cell pathway for lipoprotein degradation: specificity of the binding site that mediates the uptake of negatively-charged LDL by macrophages. *J Supramol Struct* 1980;13:67–81.

121. Steinberg D. A critical look at the evidence for the oxidation of LDL in atherogenesis. *Atherosclerosis* 1997;131[Suppl]:S5–S7.

122. Rimm EB, Stampfer MJ. The role of antioxidants in preventive cardiology. *Curr Opin Cardiol* 1997;12:188–194.

123. Dansky HM, Charlton SA, Barlow CB, et al. Apo A-I inhibits foam cell formation in apo E-deficient mice after monocyte adherence to endothelium. *J Clin Invest* 1999;104:31–39.

124. Lipid Research Clinics Program [letter]. *JAMA* 1984;252:2545–2548.

125. Frick MH, Elo O, Haapa K, et al. Helsinki Heart Study: primary prevention trial with gemfibrozil in middle-aged men with dyslipidemia—safety of treatment, changes in risk factors, and incidence of coronary heart disease. *N Engl J Med* 1987;317:1237–1245.

126. Randomised trial of cholesterol lowering in 4,444 patients with coronary heart disease: the Scandinavian Simvastatin Survival Study (4S) [see comments]. *Lancet* 1994;344:1383–1389.

127. Endres M, Laufs U, Huang Z, et al. Stroke protection by 3-hydroxy-3-methylglutaryl (HMG)-CoA reductase inhibitors mediated by endothelial nitric oxide synthase. *Proc Natl Acad Sci USA* 1998;95:8880–8885.

128. Duguid JB. Thrombosis as a factor in the pathogenesis of aortic atherosclerosis. *J Pathol Bacteriol* 1948;60:57.

129. Benezra M, Vlodavsky I, Ishai-Michaeli R, et al. Thrombin-induced release of active basic fibroblast growth factor–heparan sulfate complexes from subendothelial extracellular matrix. *Blood* 1993;81:3324–3331.

130. Schwartz SM, Reidy MA, Clowes AW. Kinetics of atherosclerosis: a stem cell model. *Ann N Y Acad Sci* 1985;454: 292–304.

131. Libby P, Egan D, Skarlatos S. Roles of infectious agents in atherosclerosis and restenosis: an assessment of the evidence and need for future research. *Circulation* 1997;96: 4095–4103.

132. Melnick JL, Adam E, DeBakey ME. Cytomegalovirus and atherosclerosis. *Eur Heart J* 1993;14[Suppl K]:30–38.

133. Grattan MT, Moreno-Cabral CE, Starnes VA, et al. Cytomegalovirus infection is associated with cardiac allograft rejection and atherosclerosis. *JAMA* 1989;261:3561–3566.

134. Epstein SE, Speir E, Zhou YF, et al. The role of infection in restenosis and atherosclerosis: focus on cytomegalovirus. *Lancet* 1996;348[Suppl 1]:S13–S17.

135. Nieto FJ, Adam E, Sorlie P, et al. Cohort study of cytomegalovirus infection as a risk factor for carotid intimal–medial thickening: a measure of subclinical atherosclerosis [see comments]. *Circulation* 1996;94:922–927.

136. Galloway DA, McDougall JK. The oncogenic potential of herpes simplex viruses: evidence for a "hit-and-run" mechanism. *Nature* 1983;302:21–24.

137. Grayston JT, Kuo CC, Coulson AS, et al. *Chlamydia pneumoniae* (TWAR) in atherosclerosis of the carotid artery [see comments]. *Circulation* 1995;92:3397–3400.

138. Kuo CC, Shor A, Campbell LA, et al. Demonstration of *Chlamydia pneumoniae* in atherosclerotic lesions of coronary arteries. *J Infect Dis* 1993;167:841–849.

139. Muhlestein JB, Anderson JL, Hammond EH, et al. Infection with *Chlamydia pneumoniae* accelerates the development of atherosclerosis and treatment with azithromycin prevents it in a rabbit model. *Circulation* 1998;97:633–636.

140. Kol A, Bourcier T, Lichtman AH, et al. Chlamydial and human heat shock protein 60s activate human vascular endothelium, smooth muscle cells, and macrophages. *J Clin Invest* 1999;103:571–577.

141. Kol A, Sukhova GK, Lichtman AH, et al. Chlamydial heat shock protein 60 localizes in human atheroma and regulates macrophage tumor necrosis factor-alpha and matrix metalloproteinase expression. *Circulation* 1998;98:300–307.

142. Amento EP, Ehsani N, Palmer H, et al. Cytokines and growth factors positively and negatively regulate interstitial collagen gene expression in human vascular smooth muscle cells. *Arterioscler Thromb* 1991;11:1223–1230.

143. Hansson GK, Holm J, Jonasson L. Detection of activated T lymphocytes in the human atherosclerotic plaque. *Am J Pathol* 1989;135:169–175.

144. Libby P, Hansson GK. Involvement of the immune system in human atherogenesis: current knowledge and unanswered questions. *Lab Invest* 1991;64:5–15.

145. Salomon RN, Hughes CC, Schoen FJ, et al. Human coronary transplantation-associated arteriosclerosis: evidence for a chronic immune reaction to activated graft endothelial cells. *Am J Pathol* 1991;138:791–798.

146. Russell PS, Chase CM, Winn HJ, et al. Coronary atherosclerosis in transplanted mouse hearts. I. Time course and immunogenetic and immunopathological considerations. *Am J Pathol* 1994;144:260–274.

147. Shi C, Russell ME, Bianchi C, et al. Murine model of accelerated transplant arteriosclerosis. *Circ Res* 1994;75: 199–207.

148. Torzewski J, Bowyer DE, Waltenberger J, et al. Processes in atherogenesis: complement activation. *Atherosclerosis* 1997; 132:131–138.

149. Rus HG, Niculescu F, Constantinescu E, et al. Immunoelectron-microscopic localization of the terminal C5b-9 complement complex in human atherosclerotic fibrous plaque. *Atherosclerosis* 1986;61:35–42.

150. Richardson PD, Davies MJ, Born GV. Influence of plaque configuration and stress distribution on fissuring of coronary atherosclerotic plaques [see comments]. *Lancet* 1989;2: 941–944.

151. Cheng GC, Loree HM, Kamm RD, et al. Distribution of circumferential stress in ruptured and stable atherosclerotic lesions: a structural analysis with histopathological correlation. *Circulation* 1993;87:1179–1187.

152. Kinlay S, Selwyn AP, Libby P, et al. Inflammation, the endothelium, and the acute coronary syndromes. *J Cardiovasc Pharmacol* 1998;32[Suppl 3]:S62–S66.

153. Fabunmi RP, Sukhova GK, Sugiyama S, et al. Expression of tissue inhibitor of metalloproteinases-3 in human atheroma and regulation in lesion-associated cells: a potential protective mechanism in plaque stability. *Circ Res* 1998;83: 270–278.

154. Libby P, Aikawa M. New insights into plaque stabilisation by lipid lowering. *Drugs* 1998;56[Suppl 1]:9–13.

155. Libby P, Schoenbeck U, Mach F, et al. Current concepts in cardiovascular pathology: the role of LDL cholesterol in plaque rupture and stabilization. *Am J Med* 1998;104: 14S–18S.

156. Aikawa M, Rabkin E, Okada Y, et al. Lipid lowering by diet reduces matrix metalloproteinase activity and increases collagen content of rabbit atheroma—a potential mechanism of lesion stabilization. *Circulation* 1998;97:2433–2444.

SURGERY: SCIENTIFIC PRINCIPLES AND PRACTICE, Third Edition, edited by Lazar J. Greenfield, Michael W. Mulholland, Keith T. Oldham, Gerald B. Zelenock, and Keith D. Lillemoe. Lippincott Williams & Wilkins Publishers, Philadelphia, © 2001.

CHAPTER 67

NONATHEROSCLEROTIC VASCULAR DISEASE

GREGORY J. LANDRY, LLOYD M. TAYLOR, JR., AND JOHN M. PORTER

Arteriosclerosis is responsible for most arterial abnormalities encountered by practicing vascular surgeons. This disease process is sufficiently common that the clinical importance of the various nonatherosclerotic causes of arterial pathologic processes might not be immediately apparent. Despite their relative rarity, nonatherosclerotic diseases constitute an important component of vascular surgery. Detailed knowledge of these conditions is essential both to provide requisite surgical treatment and to permit the vascular surgeon to act as a consultation resource, because many internal medicine specialists routinely turn to vascular surgeons for information concerning optimal treatment of nonatherosclerotic vascular diseases.

This chapter discusses the major nonatherosclerotic causes of arterial disease. Other nonatherosclerotic vascular conditions, such as compression and entrapment syndromes, vascular infections, and congenital vascular malformations, are discussed in later chapters.

FIBROMUSCULAR DYSPLASIA

Fibromuscular dysplasia (FMD) is the descriptive term applied to an abnormality characterized by multiple areas of eccentric arterial stenosis alternating with segments of arterial dilation. The angiographic appearance of involved arteries, frequently described as a string of beads, is unmistakable (Fig. 67.1). FMD is thought to be an arterial developmental abnormality, although the cause remains obscure. Multiple stenoses in sequence, as seen in Fig. 67.1, are usually present; rarely, FMD causes a single focal stenosis. FMD most frequently involves the renal artery. The carotid and iliac arteries are the next most frequently affected. Mesenteric, subclavian, vertebral, axillary, forearm, and coronary arteries have been reported as rarely occurring sites of FMD involvement. Over 90% of cases

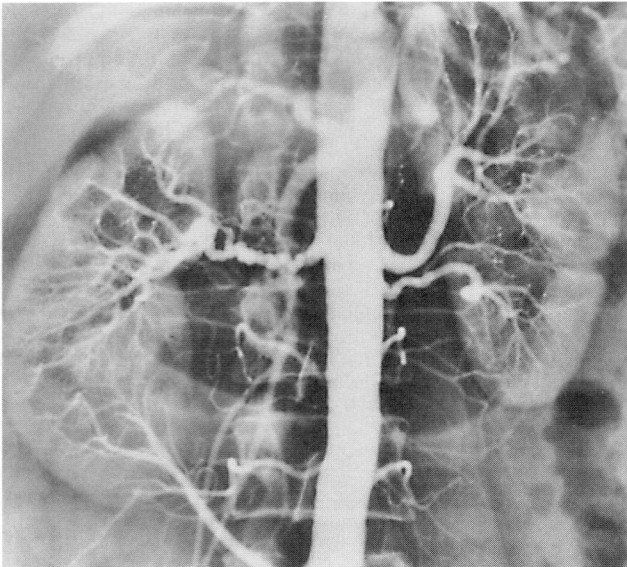

Figure 67.1. Fibromuscular dysplasia involving the right renal artery in a young woman with hypertension. Some changes of fibromuscular dysplasia are also seen in the left segmental renal artery. (From Porter JM, Taylor LM Jr, Harris EJ Jr. Nonatherosclerotic vascular disease. In: Moore WS, ed. *Vascular surgery: a comprehensive review.* Philadelphia: WB Saunders, 1994:111, with permission.)

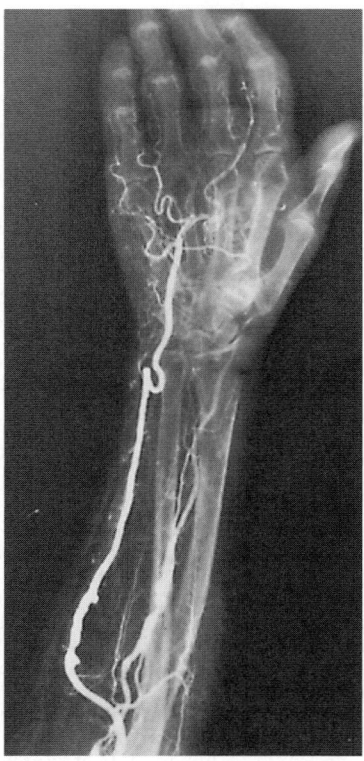

Figure 67.2. Arteriogram showing multiple localized stenotic and aneurysmal formations in a patient with advanced fibromuscular dysplasia of radial and ulnar arteries. (From Edwards JM, Antonius JI, Porter JM. Critical hand ischemia caused by forearm fibromuscular dysplasia. *J Vasc Surg* 1985;2:459, with permission.)

occur in female patients, and 80% of the renal artery involvement is on the right side.

The clinical findings of FMD are related to the vascular bed involved and are indistinguishable from those caused by atherosclerotic obstructive disease. As is true of atherosclerotic disease, many patients with documented FMD who have no symptoms have been identified. Hypertension caused by renal artery stenosis and transient cerebral ischemic attacks caused by internal carotid artery stenosis are the two most frequently encountered clinical syndromes associated with FMD.

Four distinct variants of FMD are recognized based on differences in histologic appearance—intimal fibroplasia, medial fibroplasia, medial hyperplasia, and perimedial dysplasia (1). Medial fibroplasia is the most common renal arterial pathologic type of FMD, accounting for 85% of cases, with perimedial dysplasia accounting for 10%. Differentiation of the pathologic groups is determined by the layer of the vessel wall involved, as well as by the predominant tissue involved in the dysplastic segment. With medial fibroplasia, infiltration of the media with increased amounts of fibrous connective tissue, collagen, and glycosaminoglycans is seen. Medial hyperplasia is characterized by increased numbers of medial smooth muscle cells; these medial smooth muscle cells define the proliferative changes seen in FMD. Although the cause of FMD is unknown, a number of theories have received varied support, including hormonal imbalance, primarily estrogenic; embryologic maldevelopment; immunologic phenomena; injury from arterial stretching; and abnormal distribution of the vasa vasorum with secondary mural ischemia.

Surgical treatment of FMD is indicated primarily for symptomatic arterial stenoses. Most authorities have not recommended treatment of asymptomatic stenoses; this is particularly true of internal carotid artery FMD, for which the natural history of untreated asymptomatic stenosis is unknown, in contrast to the situation with atherosclerosis. Surgical treatment of symptomatic carotid artery FMD has resulted in excellent long-term stroke-free survival rates

(2). Results of surgical management of children with renovascular FMD have also been encouraging (3). True, false, or dissecting aneurysms can occur in areas of FMD and may be amenable to surgical management. An example of a rare case involving radial and ulnar artery aneurysms resulting from FMD is seen in Fig. 67.2. Surgical treatment methods include arterial dilatation, arterial patch angioplasty, and interposition arterial bypass grafting using autogenous or prosthetic materials. Transluminal balloon angioplasty has given satisfactory short-term results in treatment of FMD lesions of the main renal artery (4), particularly in younger patients with milder hypertension of a shorter duration (5). Balloon angioplasty has been applied infrequently to the treatment of carotid artery FMD because of appropriate concern about the risk of embolization associated with the procedure.

BUERGER'S DISEASE

Buerger's disease, also known as *thromboangiitis obliterans,* is a clinical syndrome characterized by the occurrence of extensive segmental thrombotic occlusions of small and medium arteries in the lower and, frequently, upper extremities, accompanied by a prominent arterial wall inflammatory cell infiltration (6). The arterial involvement is often sufficiently severe to produce gangrene and tissue loss. Buerger's disease is clinically and pathologically distinct from immune arteritis and atherosclerosis. Despite the severe nature of the arterial involvement, life expectancy of patients with Buerger's disease does not differ significantly from that of age-matched control subjects, indicating an absence of primary coronary arterial involvement. Buerger's disease occurs frequently in Asia, but is infrequently encountered in North America. The reason for this striking geographic variance is unknown.

Affected patients are predominantly young male smokers who present with distal limb ischemia, often accompanied by digital (toe or finger) gangrene. Although men are more frequently affected, women represented up to 20% of the patients reported in several North American series. Between 40% and 50% of patients with Buerger's disease have a clear history of superficial migratory thrombophlebitis, Raynaud's syndrome, or both. Although cerebral, coronary, and visceral arterial involvement with Buerger's disease have been reported, in most patients the disease is limited to extremity vessels distal to the elbow and knee. There have been occasional reports, both arteriographically and pathologically, of iliac artery involvement. In North America, 50% of patients with Buerger's disease have symptoms confined to the lower extremities, 30% to 40% have symptomatic involvement of both the upper and lower extremities, whereas only 10% of patients have symptomatic involvement confined to the upper extremities (7).

The acute pathologic lesion of Buerger's disease is a non-necrotizing panarteritis associated with intraluminal thrombus. In contrast to both atherosclerosis and immune arteritis, the internal elastic lamina remains intact in Buerger's disease. Both T- and B-cell-mediated activation of macrophages or dendritic cells in the intima have been implicated in the pathogenesis of Buerger's disease (8). The chronic phase of Buerger's disease includes a decline in hypercellularity with the production of perivascular fibrosis and frequent recanalization of the luminal thrombus. Adjacent veins and nerves are frequently involved in the perivascular inflammatory process. Although the cause of Buerger's disease remains unknown, the association with heavy tobacco use has been universal.

Diagnostic criteria for Buerger's disease based on clinical, pathologic, and arteriographic criteria have been established as follows (7):

Major Criteria

Onset of distal extremity ischemic symptoms before age 45 years
Tobacco use
Exclusion of:
    Proximal embolic sources
    Trauma and local lesions
    Autoimmune disease
    Hypercoagulable state
    Atherosclerosis
    Atherosclerotic risk factors (diabetes, hypertension, hyperlipidemia)
No evidence of arterial disease proximal to popliteal or distal brachial arteries
Objective documentation of distal occlusive disease by either plethysmography, histopathology, or arteriography

Minor Criteria

Migratory superficial phlebitis
Raynaud's syndrome
Upper extremity involvement
Instep claudication

The major criteria are essential to diagnosis, whereas the minor criteria are supportive.

Vascular laboratory testing for Buerger's disease consists of digit (finger and toe) plethysmography, combined with segmental proximal limb pressures and Doppler analogue waveform recording. Plethysmographic evidence of digital arterial obstruction in all four extremities, combined with normal proximal vessels, is sufficient evidence of intrinsic small artery obstructive disease, and arteriography is not required. Patients with unilateral digital plethysmographic abnormalities should undergo arteriography to rule out proximal arterial lesions as an embolic source of this distal digital ischemia. Arteriography is also advised for patients with vascular laboratory findings that localize the disease to the distal feet and toes, in the presence of normal hand and finger plethysmography, to rule out a proximal arterial embolic source for the ischemia.

Although not pathognomonic, characteristic arteriographic findings have been shown to occur repeatedly in Buerger's disease. The arterial tree appears normal proximal to the popliteal and distal brachial levels. Distally, there is an abrupt transition to occlusion, which is most often segmental rather than diffuse. Extensive digital, palmar, and plantar arterial occlusions are common. The collaterals have a characteristic arteriographic appearance, termed *corkscrew collaterals* (Fig. 67.3).

Treatment of Buerger's disease is most importantly centered on achieving abstinence from tobacco use. If successful, patients usually experience remarkable improvement in symptoms, despite extensive small artery occlusive disease. In our experience, no patient has sustained further tissue loss after cessation of smoking. We and others have noted that Buerger's disease undergoes remissions and relapses that correlate with cessation and resumption of tobacco use (7).

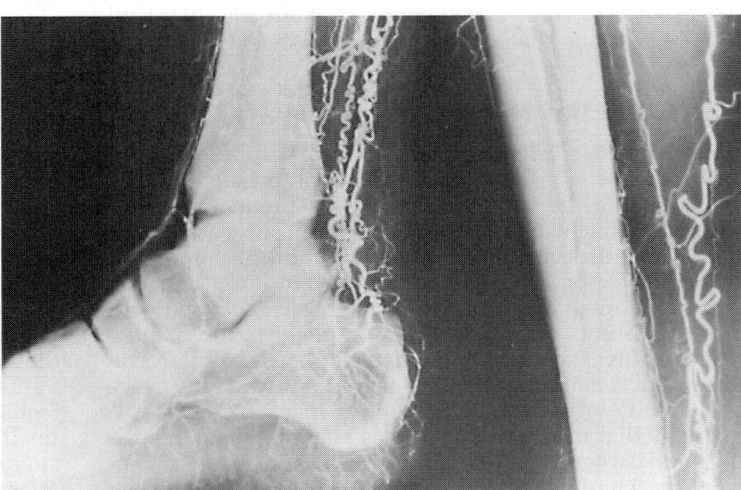

Figure 67.3. Typical arteriogram of patient with Buerger's disease showing abrupt occlusion of proximal normal tibial vessel and characteristic corkscrew collaterals. (From Mills JL, Taylor LM Jr, Porter JM. Buerger disease in the modern era. *Am J Surg* 1987;154:123, with permission.)

Management of upper extremity Buerger's disease consists of minor local débridement of ischemic segments, including partial excisions of exposed phalangeal bone combined with simple soap and water scrubs of ischemic ulcers, together with antibiotics as indicated by culture results. Although regional surgical sympathectomy has been recommended in this setting, we find no convincing evidence in support of this operation and do not recommend it in the treatment of Buerger's disease. Major tissue loss is rare in upper extremity Buerger's disease and is virtually unknown if patients successfully stop smoking.

In marked contrast to upper extremity disease, lower extremity involvement with Buerger's disease often leads to limb loss, with major leg amputation rates of 12% to 31% over 5 to 10 years reported in several large series (9). Thirty-one percent of our patients with Buerger's disease required leg amputations (7). Occasionally, patients with Buerger's disease have arteriographically patent distal arterial segments in the calf and foot, suggesting the possibility of arterial bypass grafting. Japanese data suggest that acceptable primary (49%) and secondary (63%) 5-year patency rates can be achieved in lower extremity bypasses, including inframalleolar bypasses, in patients with Buerger's disease (10). Bypass procedures may be considered in patients with Buerger's disease if a patent distal vessel can be identified with arteriography.

Although several medications have been advocated in the medical treatment of Buerger's disease, including steroids, prostaglandin E_1, vasodilators, hemorrheologic agents, anticoagulants, and antiplatelet agents, no agent has been proven efficacious. A randomized European trial comparing the oral prostacyclin analogue, iloprost, with placebo did demonstrate improved pain control with iloprost, but no improvement in wound healing (11). Preliminary results of gene therapy with intramuscular injection of vascular endothelial growth factor have been promising in promoting ulcer healing (12). Based on mechanism of action, we use nifedipine, pentoxifylline, and aspirin for patients with Buerger's disease, although none of these agents has been subjected to a randomized, controlled clinical trial in this setting.

DISEASES AFFECTING THE ARTERIAL MEDIA

Collagen, elastin, and smooth muscle are found in the arterial media and are responsible for both the strength and resilience of normal arteries. A variety of conditions that affect the amount, strength, or stability of collagen and elastin are surgically important. These conditions all have in common the presence of medial defects.

Cystic Medial Necrosis

In the 1930s, Erdheim (13) described a pathologic condition characterized by uniform hyaline degeneration of the arterial media with replacement by a mucoid-appearing basophilic substance that was clinically associated with aortic dissection. Subsequently, multiple reports of aortic dissection, spontaneous arterial rupture, and disseminated aneurysm formation have been associated with this condition, which Erdheim termed *cystic medial necrosis*. Investigations have identified metabolic aberrations with specific biochemical abnormalities as the cause of the pathologic changes present in many patients with cystic medial necrosis. Syndromes affecting the composition and structure of collagen and elastin and the mucopolysaccharides of the ground substance have been identified. Marfan syndrome, Ehlers-Danlos syndrome, and neurofibromatosis can each present with the typical arterial lesions of cystic medial necrosis, with its associated pathologic findings.

Most patients identified with cystic medial necrosis have a clinical syndrome characterized by a heritable disorder of collagen metabolism, the most frequent of which have been Marfan syndrome and Ehlers-Danlos syndrome. The most common clinical manifestation of cystic medial necrosis is aortic dissection, with spontaneous arterial rupture and diffuse aneurysm formation occurring less frequently. Cystic medial necrosis has also been implicated as a cause of abdominal aortic aneurysms in children (14).

Marfan Syndrome

Marfan syndrome is a heterogeneous disorder characterized clinically and biochemically by ocular abnormalities (myopia and lens dislocation), skeletal disproportion (tall stature, chest wall deformities, arachnodactyly, scoliosis), and cardiovascular abnormalities (mitral valve prolapse, aortic dissection with aortic aneurysm formation). Marfan first noted the orthopedic abnormalities of the syndrome in the late 19th century. The ocular abnormalities were identified in the 1940s, and the cardiovascular abnormalities were described by McKusik in the 1950s (15).

Inheritance of Marfan syndrome is by an autosomal dominant pattern. Mutations in the fibrillin gene on chromosome 15 are thought to be causative. Both a reduction in fibrillin formation and abnormalities in the fibrillin molecule have been identified (16). A number of conditions have been recognized that share some features of Marfan syndrome but have different natural histories. These include homocystinuria (discussed later); contractural arachnodactyly, which is a disorder distinguished by joint stiffness rather than laxity; and the mitral valve prolapse syndrome, a syndrome sharing many of the skeletal abnormalities of Marfan syndrome without ocular manifestations or the propensity for aortic dissection.

In almost all patients with Marfan syndrome, a predictable dilation of the aortic root develops, leading to the development of an ascending aortic aneurysm (Fig. 67.4) that can progress to the development of aortic valvular incompetence. A smaller percentage of patients have mitral valve prolapse and mitral insufficiency. Untreated, the life expectancy of a patient with Marfan syndrome is approximately 40 years, with 95% of deaths related to cardiovascular complications. The most frequent causes of death are aortic insufficiency and ascending aortic dissection and rupture.

Both medical and surgical interventions have been proposed for prophylaxis against aortic dissection and aortic insufficiency. The medical regimens are centered around the use of β-adrenergic blockers in a regimen designed to decrease the force of cardiac contraction and reduce blood pressure, potentially protecting the weakened ascending aorta (17,18).

The surgical treatment has usually consisted of replacement of the ascending aorta and aortic valve with a composite graft. It is recommended that elective repair be performed before either severe aortic insufficiency compromises left ventricular function or the ascending aortic diameter has reached 55 to 60 mm, at which point the risk of dissection and rupture increases. With modern surgical techniques and uncomplicated aneurysm replacement, the life expectancy of these patients can be improved considerably, with low morbidity and operative mortality rates (19–21).

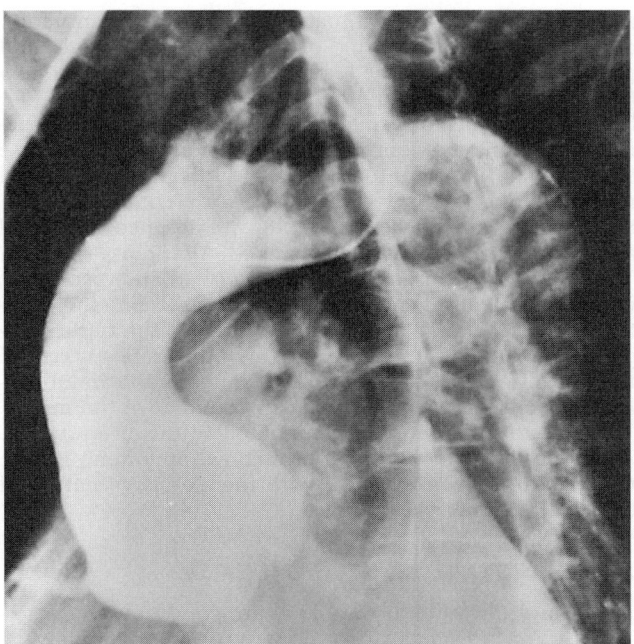

Figure 67.4. Aortogram of a patient with Marfan syndrome showing marked dilation of aortic root and aortic valvular insufficiency. (From Porter JM, Taylor LM Jr, Harris EJ Jr. Nonatherosclerotic vascular disease. In: Moore WS, ed. *Vascular surgery: a comprehensive review.* Philadelphia: WB Saunders, 1994:136, with permission.)

Ehlers-Danlos Syndrome

Ehlers-Danlos syndrome is a heterogeneous group of generalized connective tissue disorders, first clearly described by von Meekeren in 1682, characterized by hyperextensible skin, hypermobile joints, fragile tissues, and a bleeding diathesis primarily related to fragile vessels. Detailed genetic and biochemical studies have defined more than 10 types of Ehlers-Danlos syndrome, each with variable signs, symptoms, and patterns of inheritance. For certain types of Ehlers-Danlos syndrome, definable molecular defects have been characterized. It is important to identify correctly the various types because the natural histories differ among them.

Three types of Ehlers-Danlos syndrome—types I, III, and IV—frequently have arterial complications, with type IV, the vascular or ecchymotic type, being most important to the vascular surgeon. Although first recognized as a distinct entity in 1967, the biochemical lesion of Ehlers-Danlos syndrome type IV, which results in abnormalities in the structure, synthesis, and secretion of type III procollagen, was not identified until 1975 (22). These patients produce little or no type III collagen, which is of major structural importance in vessels, viscera, and skin. Clinical features, although not uniformly expressed, consist of a thin, translucent skin, easy bruisability, and venous varicosities.

The major vascular complication of Ehlers-Danlos syndrome is arterial rupture, although aneurysm formation (Fig. 67.5) and acute aortic dissection also occur. Spontaneous arterial rupture can lead to stroke, intraabdominal or intrathoracic bleeding, or compartment syndromes in the extremities. The most common site of spontaneous arterial rupture is the abdominal cavity, with smaller visceral arteries more frequently involved than the aorta. Repair of the ruptured vessels is difficult because of their extreme friability, although successful repairs have been reported (23), emphasizing atraumatic vascular control,

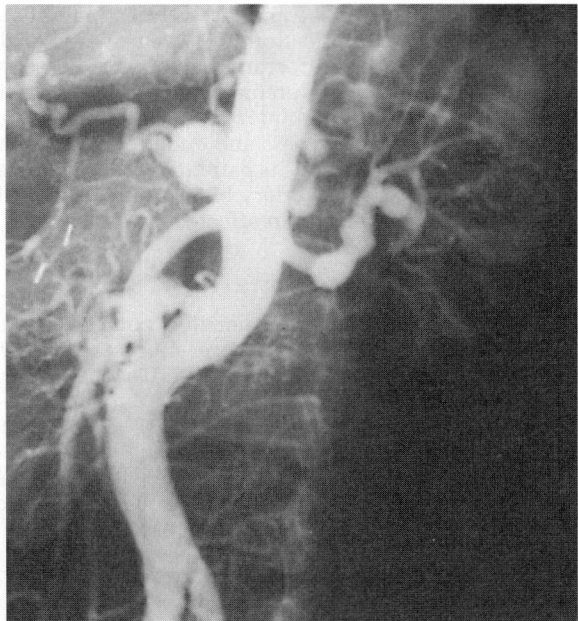

Figure 67.5. Celiac and renal artery aneurysms in a patient with Ehlers-Danlos syndrome type III.

gentle dissection, and vessel ligation with plication pledgets. Experienced surgeons advise against arteriography because of increased risk of vessel laceration and hemorrhage (23). Whenever possible, treatment of spontaneous arterial rupture in patients with Ehlers-Danlos syndrome type IV should be nonoperative, consisting of compression and transfusion. If unsuccessful, the operative objective should be ligation to control hemorrhage. If tissue loss would result, arterial reconstruction can be attempted (24).

Most patients with Ehlers-Danlos syndrome type IV have shortened life spans compared with their unaffected siblings. Death typically occurs in the third or fourth decade, and survival beyond 50 years of age is unusual.

Pseudoxanthoma Elasticum

Pseudoxanthoma elasticum is a group of genetically heterogeneous disorders involving elastic fibers whose basic pathogenetic abnormality remains unknown. Clinical manifestations of the disorder most frequently involve the skin, eyes, and arteries. Pseudoxanthoma elasticum derives its name from the characteristic yellow xanthoma-like cutaneous papules and the loose, baggy skin identified in intertriginous areas such as the axillae, antecubital fossae, and groins. Most patients with pseudoxanthoma elasticum have stenoses or occlusions of the peripheral, cerebral, or coronary arteries, separately or in combination. The basic pathologic change in the arterial wall is the replacement of normal medial elastic fibers by calcium deposits. Clinically, the diminished arterial elasticity and resultant resistance to distention is expressed as weak or absent pulses, which have characteristic plethysmographic tracings (25). Plain radiographs often identify vascular calcifications in young patients at low risk for the development of atherosclerosis.

Arterial occlusive disease occurs at an early age, usually before the end of the fourth decade. Hypertension is another common manifestation of pseudoxanthoma elasticum. Diffuse arterial elastin degeneration can also involve the visceral arteries, and gastrointestinal hemorrhage is a common complication (26). Neurovascular disease is characterized by intracranial aneurysms and cerebral ischemia caused by premature arterial occlusive disease (27). Standard techniques of vascular surgery, including autogenous vein bypass and endarterectomy, have been successfully performed in patients with pseudoxanthoma elasticum. Coronary artery bypass surgery has also been successfully performed in affected patients.

Arteria Magna Syndrome

Arteria magna syndrome is a peculiar condition of the aorta and iliofemoral arteries that presents as diffuse arterial elongation, dilation, and tortuosity. Leriche (28) was the first to describe the clinical, angiographic, and operative findings of this arteriopathy in 1943; he termed the condition *dolicho et mega-artere*. Subsequently, numerous reports have described this syndrome with terms such as *arteriomegaly* and *arteria dolicho et magna*. These descriptive terms have been applied to a broad spectrum of findings, ranging from generalized ectasia to contiguous aneurysms from the thoracic aorta to the popliteal trifurcation (29).

Although the condition was initially thought to be a variant of atherosclerosis, more recent pathologic analysis has suggested the arterial media of these patients are devoid of the usual elastic tissues (30). Characteristic arteriographic findings include arterial widening and tortuosity, markedly diminished arterial flow velocities with delayed distal arterial filling, and the presence of multiple aneurysms (Fig. 67.6). Lawrence et al. reported a 36% familial incidence among first-degree relatives (31).

Clinical management of patients with arteria magna is centered on detection of aneurysms and replacement using standard vascular surgical techniques. Aneurysms

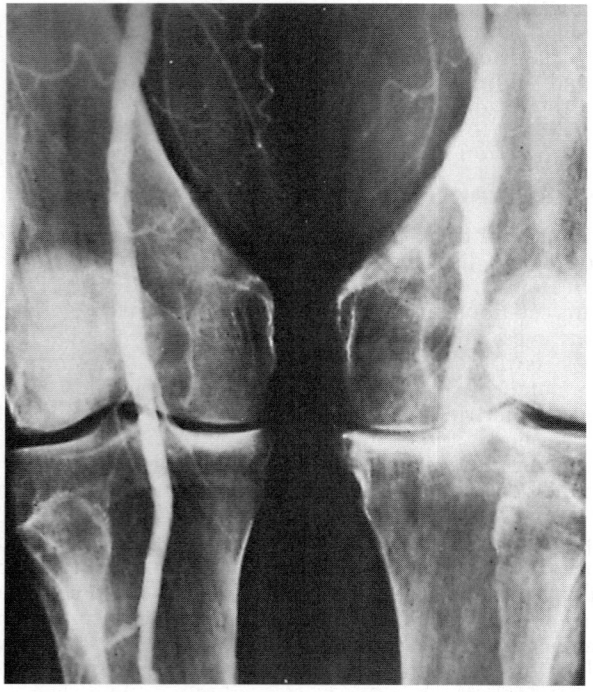

Figure 67.6. Popliteal artery aneurysm in a patient with the arteria magna syndrome. (From Porter JM, Taylor LM Jr, Harris EJ Jr. Nonatherosclerotic vascular disease. In: Moore WS, ed. *Vascular surgery: a comprehensive review*. Philadelphia: WB Saunders, 1994:137, with permission.)

are detected using a combination of physical examination and ultrasound screening of abdominal, femoral, and popliteal sites. Localized aneurysms reaching 2 to 2.5 times the size of the parent artery should be replaced. Embolisms of intraaneurysmal thrombus and thrombotic arterial occlusions are common complications of this diffuse aneurysmal disease and are also an indication for arterial replacement. Coronary artery disease is common in patients with arteria magna, despite the absence of typical arterial occlusive disease elsewhere (32).

The relation of arteria magna to typical atherosclerosis is uncertain. Pathologically, aneurysms associated with arteria magna have an appearance similar to the typical degenerative aneurysm. The histologic appearance is one of fragmentation of the internal elastic membrane and a profound decrease in the elastic tissue content of the media. There is no inflammatory component in the arterial wall. Although intimal atheromatous changes are often present, they are minimal compared with the extensive nature of the medial changes.

ADVENTITIAL CYSTIC DISEASE

Adventitial cystic disease is a rare condition characterized by the presence of single or multiple synovial-like cysts in the subadventitial layer of the arterial wall, with resultant arterial stenosis. These mucin-filled cysts are similar to ganglion cysts. The disease is most often bilateral, usually affects men, and has a median age of presentation of 40 years (33).

Adventitial cystic disease was initially described by Atkins and Key in 1947, with the first report of successful operative management 7 years later. Although the popliteal artery is by far the most frequently affected artery (33), adventitial cystic disease has been described in the femoral, brachial, radial and ulnar arteries, branches of the popliteal arteries, and popliteal vein.

Three etiologic theories have been proposed: (a) repeated arterial microtrauma; (b) the presence within the arterial wall of mucin-secreting cell rests derived embryologically from the synovial anlage of the adjacent joint; and (c) the development of true ganglia in the adventitia, arising from an adjacent joint capsule or tendon sheath (34). The frequent presence of a direct communication from the arterial cyst to the adjacent bony joint supports the latter hypothesis.

Adventitial cystic disease, along with Buerger's disease and popliteal entrapment syndrome, should be considered in any young patient complaining of intermittent claudication. Further examination rarely detects a palpable cyst, and the stigmata of generalized arterial insufficiency are not present. Palpable pulse alterations depending on knee flexion or extension have been described, presumably resulting from variable luminal compression, depending on position, but this finding is so nonspecific as to be without value in diagnosis. Diagnosis is possible using ultrasonography, computed tomographic scanning, and magnetic resonance imaging. More recently, intravascular ultrasound has emerged as a helpful imaging modality (35). Classically, arteriograms demonstrate a scimitar sign of luminal encroachment by the cyst (Fig. 67.7) in a normally placed vessel with no other signs of occlusive disease (36).

Several methods of treatment of adventitial cystic disease have been described. When the vessel is not occluded, simple cyst excision, enucleation, or aspiration are acceptable therapies, although there is a 10% recurrence rate. In 30% of patients, there is occlusion of the involved vessel. Resection of the occluded segment with the cystic mass and primary end-to-end anastomosis has

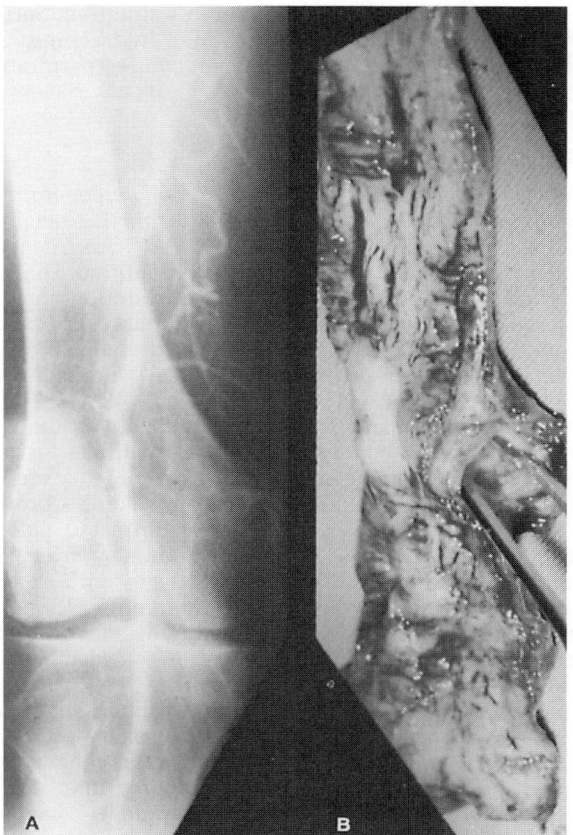

Figure 67.7. Arteriogram *(A)* and operative photograph *(B)* of adventitial cyst of popliteal artery.

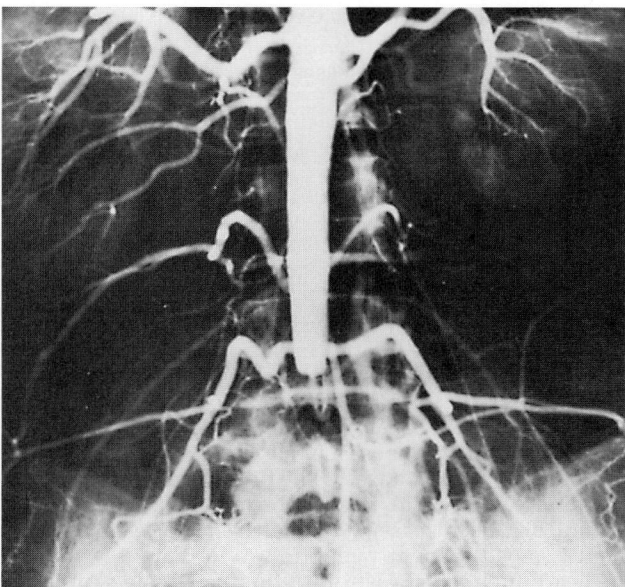

Figure 67.8. Radiation arteritis: abrupt occlusion of normal distal aorta. (From Porter JM, Taylor LM Jr, Harris EJ Jr. Nonatherosclerotic vascular disease. In: Moore WS, ed. *Vascular surgery: a comprehensive review.* Philadelphia: WB Saunders, 1994:122, with permission.)

been reported, but interposition grafting is usually required and is best accomplished using autogenous saphenous vein (37). Several reported attempts at percutaneous transluminal angioplasty have been unsuccessful. Ultrasound- and computed tomography-guided aspirations of popliteal artery cysts have been reported (38,39). Although early results have been good, no long term follow-up is available.

RADIATION-INDUCED ARTERIAL INJURY

Arterial injury resulting from tumoricidal external beam irradiation in the treatment of regional malignancy is well recognized. Radiation-induced arterial injury has been classified into three pathologic forms. The first type, occurring early in the posttreatment period, is characterized by an intense arterial inflammatory reaction with endothelial sloughing and luminal thrombosis. The second type, developing from 1 to 10 years after radiation therapy, apparently represents the healing phase of the arterial inflammatory response to radiation injury, and consists of intense fibrosis and scar formation within the arterial wall, resulting in areas of arterial stenosis (Fig. 67.8). The third type, developing from 2 to 30 years after radiation therapy, represents accelerated atherosclerosis. The arterial plaque is typically indistinguishable from nonirradiated atherosclerotic plaques.

Most experience with radiation-induced arterial injury has involved the carotid artery (40), although visceral and extremity arterial involvement has also been described. Vascular surgery on these irradiated arteries can

be performed with standard techniques. Prosthetic and autogenous bypass grafts, as well as endarterectomy, have been performed satisfactorily (41). Late graft infections occurring 2 to 5 years after surgery have been described (42). Currently, there is no defined role for endovascular treatment of radiation-induced arterial disease (43).

IMMUNE ARTERITIS

The terms *arteritis* and *vasculitis* properly apply only to necrotizing transmural inflammation of the arterial wall and not to perivascular round cell infiltrates that can be seen in such conditions as livedo reticularis, eczema, cutaneous drug reactions, and Buerger's disease. Substantial evidence indicates that most, if not all, immune vasculitis is associated with the deposition of antigen–antibody immune complexes on the endothelium followed by the production of arterial wall damage. Complement components bind these exposed antigen–antibody complexes, activating the complement cascade. This in turn results in chemotaxis of polymorphonuclear leukocytes, and these leukocytes infiltrate the arterial wall. Leukocyte lysosomal enzymes, including elastase and collagenase, are released within the arterial wall and appear to be the primary cause of the arterial wall necrosis. Thrombosis, aneurysm formation, hemorrhage, and arterial occlusion can all follow or accompany the transmural arterial enzymatic injury (44). Cell-mediated immune injury can also contribute to the arterial wall damage, yet considerably less information exists about this mechanism. A suggested classification of the immune arteritides of surgical interest follows:

Polyarteritis Nodosa (PAN) Group (Medium Muscular Arteries)

Classic PAN
Kawasaki's disease
Cogan's syndrome
Behçet's syndrome

Hypersensitivity Angiitis Group (Small Arteries)

Hypersensitivity angiitis
Arteritis of collagen diseases
Mixed cryoglobulinemia
Arteritis of malignancy

Giant Cell Arteritis (Large Arteries)

Temporal arteritis
Takayasu's arteritis

Polyarteritis Nodosa

Polyarteritis nodosa is a systemic disease characterized by focal necrotizing arterial inflammatory lesions involving primarily small and medium-sized muscular arteries. There is a 2 : 1 male/female incidence for this disease process, with the peak incidence in the fifth decade. Aneurysm formation associated with inflammatory destruction of the media was a key finding in the original description of PAN and is still considered a characteristic feature of this disease. Although renal arterial involvement is most frequently reported in PAN, involvement of the heart, lung, liver, gastrointestinal tract, and skin is also recognized (Fig. 67.9). Major lower extremity arterial involvement has been reported. Medical treatment has centered around steroids with or without plasma exchange or cyclophosphamide (45). Interferon alpha and antiviral agents have been used to treat PAN associated with hepatitis B. Amazingly, aneurysms associated with PAN have been shown to regress with steroid therapy as assessed by serial arteriograms (46).

Arteriographic evaluation of patients with PAN has suggested that the presence of an abnormal arteriogram identifies a subset of patients who exhibit more serious disease manifestations (47). It has been suggested that prognosis can be predicted at the time of presentation based on the absence or presence of creatinemia, proteinuria, cardiomyopathy, and gastrointestinal or central nervous system involvement. Five-year mortality rates with none, one, or more than two of these signs were 12%, 26%, and 46%, respectively (48). Specific vascular complications of PAN include aneurysm rupture and arterial stenosis or thrombosis with resulting ischemia. Spontaneous rupture of a PAN visceral arterial aneurysm has been well described and usually presents as a surgical emergency because of associated intraperitoneal or retroperitoneal hemorrhage. Interventional radiologic techniques have been successfully used to occlude bleeding vessels in this situation. Serious gastrointestinal surgical complications in ischemic segments are frequent, including hemorrhage, perforation, and segmental gangrene (49).

Kawasaki's Disease

Kawasaki's disease, also known as *mucocutaneous lymph node syndrome,* is a form of arteritis that occurs in infants and children and is similar to PAN. An infectious etiology is suspected but has not been identified. Diagnostic criteria include a fever of five days' duration and four of the following: (a) nonexudative conjunctival injection, (b) oral lesions, (c) peripheral edema or desquamation, (d) polymorphous rash, or (e) acute cervical lymphadenopathy (50).

Although arterial involvement is widespread, the most striking feature of Kawasaki's disease is diffuse fusiform and saccular aneurysm formation of the coronary and occasionally brachiocephalic arteries (Fig. 67.10). Coronary artery involvement occurs in 25% of untreated patients during the acute phase (51). Although coronary artery rupture can occur, these children usually succumb to acute cardiac arrhythmias or myocardial infarctions. Treatment during the acute phase with acetylsalicylic acid and intravenous immunoglobulin has been shown to decrease the incidence of coronary complications.

As with adult PAN, the role of the vascular surgeon in Kawasaki's disease remains unclear. Coronary artery bypass surgery and coronary aneurysmectomy have been successfully performed in several patients. Internal thoracic arterial grafts have been demonstrated to have improved patency (77% vs. 46%) and reduced late cardiac death rates (1% vs. 3%) at 7 years compared with saphenous vein grafts in a recent multicenter study (52).

Cogan's Syndrome

Cogan's syndrome is a rare condition consisting of non-syphilitic interstitial keratitis associated with vestibuloauditory symptoms (53). Cogan's syndrome is a disease predominantly of young adults, with the mean age of onset in the third decade. The vasculitic component of the disease, present in a minority of patients, is predominantly an aortitis. Aortitis with subsequent development of clinically significant aortic insufficiency occurs in 10% of patients with Cogan's syndrome.

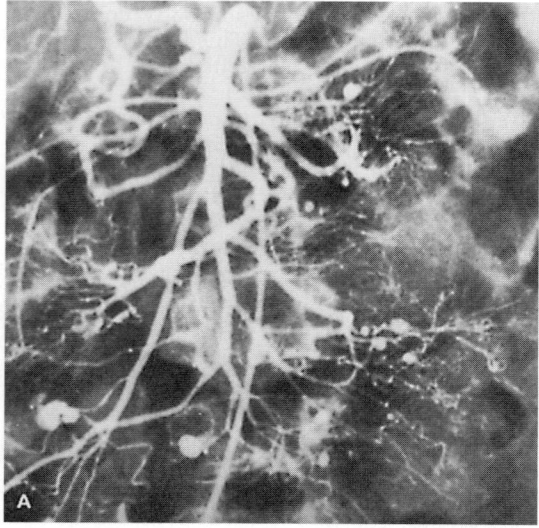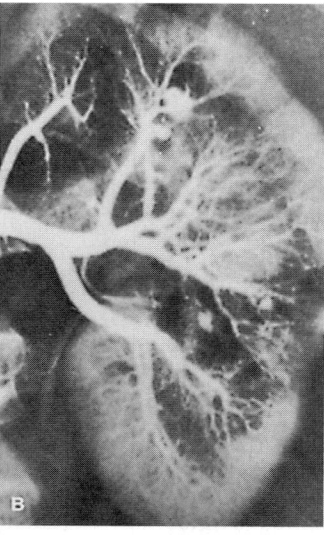

Figure 67.9. Arteriogram showing typical aneurysm formation in medium-sized visceral *(A)* and renal *(B)* arteries in a patient with polyarteritis nodosa. (From Porter JM, Taylor LM Jr, Harris EJ Jr. Nonatherosclerotic vascular disease. In: Moore WS, ed. *Vascular surgery: a comprehensive review.* Philadelphia: WB Saunders, 1994:111, with permission.)

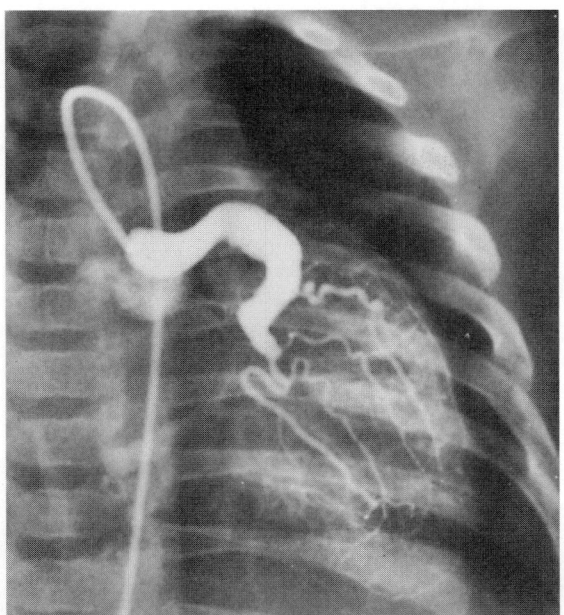

Figure 67.10. Selective coronary arteriogram showing typical aneurysm in a child with Kawasaki's disease.

Daily administration of high-dose corticosteroids has been successful in reversing both the visual and auditory stigmata of Cogan's syndrome and is indicated when aortitis is present. Aortic valve replacement, in the presence of compromised hemodynamic function, has been performed successfully. Long-term prognosis is excellent for Cogan's syndrome in the absence of aortic valve involvement (54).

Behçet's Disease

In 1937, Behçet described three patients with iritis and associated oral and genital mucocutaneous ulcerations, and this association has subsequently become known as *Behçet's disease.* The underlying pathologic lesion is a vasculitis, with venous thrombotic lesions occurring more frequently than arterial lesions. Lower extremity superficial or deep venous thrombosis occurs in 12% to 27% of patients (55). The arterial component consists of occlusive and aneurysmal lesions. When present, the aneurysmal lesions portend mortality rates of up to 20%.

As noted, the predominant pathologic lesion in Behçet's disease is a nonspecific panarteritis. Thickening of the endothelium is sometimes seen, whereas disorganization of the elastic fibers in the media and perivascular infiltration by monocytes or lymphocytes are frequently observed. The perivascular infiltration is often associated with luminal thrombosis. The lesions can lead to aneurysmal or occlusive disease, although occlusions are rarely encountered. Aneurysms have been described in numerous locations, including the carotid, subclavian, iliac, femoral, and popliteal arteries, with the aorta as the most frequent site of aneurysm formation. Because of vascular wall disruption and associated fragility of these vessels, aneurysms frequently recur at anastomotic sites after resection with interposition grafting (56). Arterial puncture can lead to the development of pseudoaneurysms in Behçet's disease, rendering diagnostic arteriography hazardous. The arterial aneurysms have a high probability of recurrence elsewhere after repair, frequently necessitating numerous surgical interventions. Unfortunately, interposition bypass

grafts have a high incidence of thrombosis in addition to their propensity to development of anastomotic pseudoaneurysms, with long-term graft patency the exception rather than the norm (57). The use of an aortic endograft in a patient with Behçet's disease has been described (58).

This systemic disease largely affects the populations of the Mediterranean area and Japan, suggesting an environmental or genetic factor. Both bacterial and viral infectious causes have been proposed, although definitive evidence is lacking for the implication of any infectious agent in the cause of Behçet's disease (59). Autoimmune dysfunction is the likely cause of this condition. Several investigators have identified circulating immune complexes in patients with Behçet's disease and have suggested some component of autoimmunity as causative in the vascular changes identified in this diffuse vasculitis. Immune complexes and complement have been demonstrated in the arterial wall and surrounding tissues. The activation of complement in the vascular wall can lead to destruction of the media and subsequent aneurysm formation. An alternate hypothesis implicates vasculitis of the vasa vasorum as the cause of large artery destruction (56).

Behçet's disease might also have a genetic component because there is an increased incidence of the human leukocyte antigen (HLA) B5 in patients with this condition. Specific HLA genetic markers have been identified with the various common clinical subtypes of Behçet disease: HLA-B5 is associated with ocular symptoms, HLA-B27 is associated with arthritic symptoms, and HLA-B12 is associated with the presence of mucocutaneous lesions.

Azathioprine, thalidomide, colchicine, and interferon alpha have been used with some success for nonarterial symptoms, as have corticosteroids. Although corticosteroids can suppress symptoms, especially arthritic and ophthalmic symptoms, they do not alter the progression or course of the underlying disease (60). Reports of corticosteroid prevention of pseudoaneurysm recurrence must therefore be viewed cautiously. Although no uniformly satisfactory therapy exists for Behçet disease, early diagnosis and aggressive reconstructive management of identified arterial aneurysms has provided long-term limb salvage despite arterial graft complications (59).

Hypersensitivity Angiitis Group

The term *hypersensitivity angiitis group* incorporates a large and heterogeneous group of clinical syndromes characterized by involvement of small arteries in the vasculitic process. The arteritides of this group include classic hypersensitivity angiitis, arteritis of collagen vascular disease, mixed cryoglobulinemia arteritis, and arteritis associated with malignancy. Involved arteries exhibit a thickened basement membrane, swelling of the collagenous and elastic connective tissues, and fragmentation of the elastic fibers. The end result of these conditions is vascular occlusion, which can lead to regional ischemia. This process appears to result from the deposition of immune complexes in the small arteries. In certain of these conditions, the inciting antigen can be identified, such as a drug or chemical, a virus, or a tumor antigen.

The clinical syndromes typically associated with this group of diseases include skin rash, fever, and evidence of organ dysfunction, none of which specifically concerns the vascular surgeon. Vascular surgeons might be called on to evaluate certain patients presenting with arterial involvement substantially limited to the hands and fingers. Plethysmography and arteriography typically identify widespread palmar and digital arterial occlusions, which are frequently associated with digital ischemia.

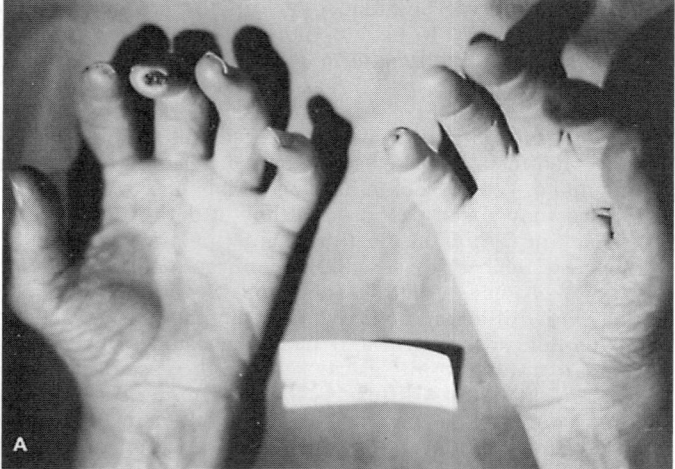
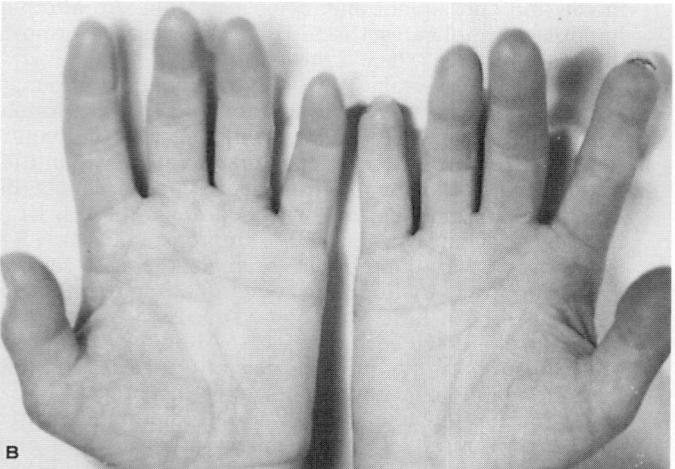
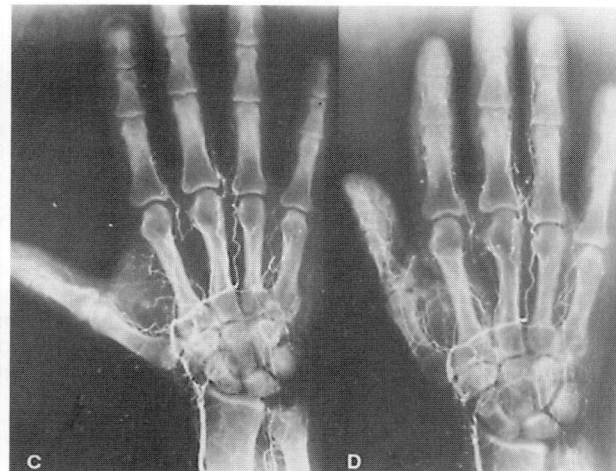

Figure 67.11. *(A)* Hands of a patient with systemic lupus erythematosus and multiple ischemic finger ulcers. *(B)* Same patient with healed ulcers after 2 months of conservative therapy. *(C)* Arteriogram of same patient, demonstrating extensive palmar and digital arterial occlusions. *(D)* Arteriogram showing formation of collaterals.

Our own interest in patients with upper extremity digital ischemia is ongoing, and we have collected detailed clinical and serologic data from more than 150 patients with digital ischemic ulceration. Although certain of these patients have clinically manifested autoimmune disorders, a significant number have no serologic evidence of autoimmune disease, have no clinical evidence of any systemic disease process, and have presented only with the acute onset of hand arterial occlusion and finger ischemia (61). Each of these patients showed extensive occlusion of the palmar and digital arteries on arteriography. We have had success with a conservative program of local wound care and limited débridement in healing the ischemic lesions (Fig. 67.11). Anecdotally, we have observed symptomatic improvement in a number of these patients after initiation of calcium channel blockers or pentoxifylline.

Giant Cell Arteritis Group

Two easily distinguishable clinical disease patterns occur within the giant cell arteritis group: (a) temporal arteritis, or systemic giant cell arteritis; and (b) Takayasu's arteritis. Numerous similarities exist between these two conditions, suggesting to some that these two diseases might represent different expressions of the same disease process. Both conditions consist of localized periarteritis with inflammatory mononuclear infiltrates and giant cells, along with disruption and fragmentation of the elastic fibers of the arterial wall.

Temporal Arteritis

Temporal arteritis, or systemic giant cell arteritis, is predominantly a disease of white women, usually occurring after 55 years of age. This condition is a systemic disease process characterized by chronic inflammation of the aorta and its major branches. The most frequent presenting complaint is headache. Polymyalgia rheumatica, a condition associated with severe pain in the pelvic and shoulder girdles, is often identified in these patients.

Although systemic giant cell arteritis can affect any large artery of the body, the branches of the carotid artery are most frequently involved. The onset of the disease is heralded by a febrile myalgic process, usually involving the back, shoulder, and pelvic regions. The most characteristic complaint is severe pain along the course of the temporal artery, frequently bilateral, accompanied by tenderness and nodularity of the artery with overlying skin erythema. Temporal artery biopsy remains the gold standard diagnostic test, but may be supplanted by color-flow duplex examination of the temporal artery, in which the presence of a dark halo around the temporal artery is a highly specific finding (62).

Visual alterations are severe and occur in over 50% of patients. The disturbances can be secondary to either ischemic optic or retrobulbar neuritis, or occlusion of the central retinal artery. Up to 40% of patients with symptomatic giant cell arteritis experience a permanent partial or complete loss of vision (63) that can be prevented by early steroid administration. Systemic giant cell arteritis can cause aneurysms or stenoses of the aorta and its main branches. Thoracic aortic aneurysms and aortic dissections have been reported, and surgical replacement of these lesions has been successful.

Some have speculated that early high-dose corticosteroid therapy minimizes the likelihood of aortic lesions, although convincing evidence of this hypothesis is unavailable. The clinical effectiveness of corticosteroid therapy is uniform in that laboratory findings often improve and the patient's constitutional symptoms resolve or improve. Microscopic evaluation of surgical specimens pretreated with steroids fails to identify any effect of steroid therapy on the arterial pathologic features of this disease. Some authors suggest that corticosteroid therapy might increase the chance of aneurysmal rupture (64). We and others believe that surgical procedures in this disease fail in a high percentage of patients unless accompanied by high-dose steroid administration (65).

The angiographic features most suggestive of giant cell arteritis include long segments of smooth stenosis interspersed with normal segments, smoothly tapered occlusions, absence of irregular plaques and ulcerations, and distribution of these abnormalities among the subclavian, axillary, and brachial arteries (Fig. 67.12).

Takayasu's Arteritis

Takayasu's arteritis is a rare primary arteritis of unknown cause that frequently affects the aorta, its major branches, and the pulmonary artery. It occurs predominantly in female patients, with the age of onset between 3 and 35 years. Takayasu's arteritis can produce stenosis, occlusion, dilation, or aneurysm formation of the involved artery. Elastic fibers in the arterial wall are involved in an intense periarteritis, characterized by a granulomatous inflammatory process with mononuclear cell infiltration and the formation of multinucleated giant cells.

Although more common in Asia, the disease has a worldwide distribution. Patients present with symptoms of cerebral, visceral, or extremity ischemia. The clinical course of Takayasu's arteritis has been described as having two stages. The initial stage is characterized by nonspecific symptoms of fever, myalgia, and anorexia. The second stage can follow closely and consists of a pulseless phase with multiple arterial occlusions and cardiovascular symptoms depending on disease location (66). Hypertension is common and might be due to aortic coarctation or renal artery stenosis. Neurologic symptoms can result from hypertension or from central nervous system ischemia associated with large artery stenosis or occlusion. Coronary artery involvement is rare in Takayasu's disease. The cardiac pathologic process most frequently found is nonspecific and appears to result from heart failure associated with systemic and pulmonary hypertension.

Takayasu's disease has been divided into four types, characterized by the pattern of cardiovascular involvement. Type I is limited to involvement of the aortic arch and arch vessels and occurs in 8.4% of patients. Type II involves the descending thoracic and abdominal aorta and accounts for 11.2% of cases. Type III is the most common, involves the arch vessels and the abdominal aorta and its branches, and accounts for 65.4% of cases. Type IV primarily involves the pulmonary arteries with or without the other types and accounts for 15% of patients (67). Stenosis is the most common angiographic finding in the aorta and its branches, whereas occlusion is the most common pulmonary angiographic finding.

The role of surgery in Takayasu's arteritis remains uncertain because no studies have compared operative with nonoperative therapy in a controlled fashion. Surgery has been widely performed, and some conclusions are possible. Endarterectomy has resulted in early failure and usually is not recommended. Successful management requires bypass graft implantation into disease-free arterial segments and continuation of corticosteroid therapy (68) (Fig. 67.13). Percutaneous transluminal angioplasty has provided variable results with no proven long-term efficacy, often requiring several attempts to reduce the stenosis significantly. Successful surgical correction of pulmonary arterial stenosis has been reported. Available information suggests a conservative surgical approach to these patients, although the risk of stroke is sufficiently great that some have recommended prophylactic repair of high-grade brachioce-

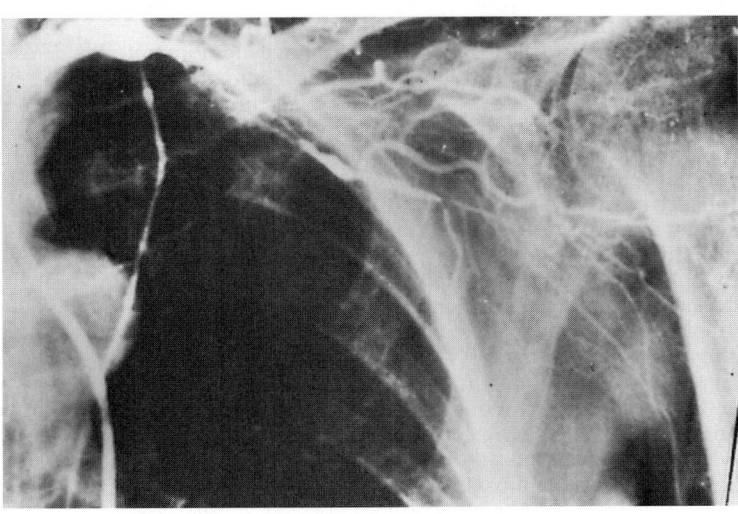

Figure 67.12. Typical tapered stenosis of left axillary artery in giant cell arteritis.

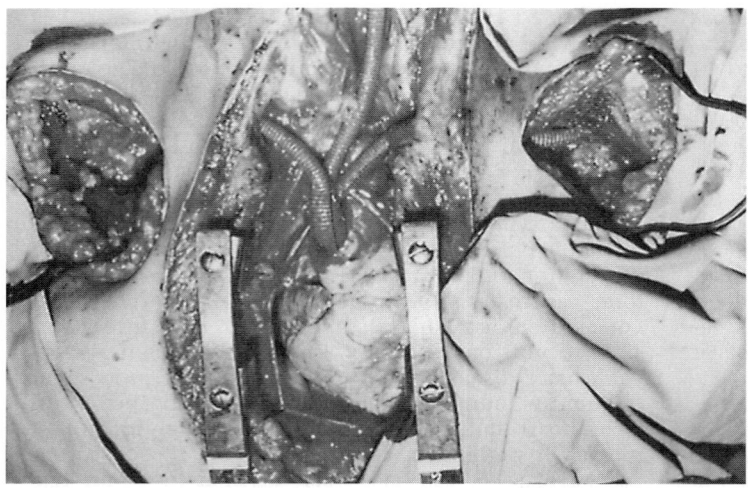

Figure 67.13. Extensive bypass from ascending aorta to left carotid and both axillary arteries in a patient with Takayasu's arteritis.

phalic stenoses. Corticosteroid therapy is the key to successful management. Surgical reconstruction has a selective role and produces acceptable long-term relief of symptoms.

HOMOCYSTEINEMIA AND HOMOCYSTINURIA

Homocystinuria, an inborn error of metabolism in which homocysteine accumulates abnormally in plasma and tissues and is excreted in large quantities in the urine, was first described in 1962. Patients with the disorder have multiple abnormalities, including ectopia lentis, mental retardation, rapidly progressive arteriosclerotic vascular disease, and thromboembolic disorders. Three specific enzyme deficiencies responsible for inherited homocystinuria have been identified: (a) cystathionine synthetase, (b) homocysteine methyltransferase, and (c) methylene tetrahydrofolate reductase. These enzymes require the cofactors pyridoxine, folate, and cobalamin. Deficiencies of any of these cofactors can also cause elevated homocysteine levels. Regardless of the primary cause, all forms of homocysteine accumulation in humans have been associated with atherosclerosis, frequently complicated by thrombosis (69). The arteriosclerotic plaques identified in homocystinura are typical fibrous plaques. Microscopic evaluations reveal medial hypertrophy, elaboration of extracellular matrix and collagen, and degeneration and destruction of the elastic laminae. Lipid deposition in the plaques is characteristically absent (70).

Although multiple clinical studies have demonstrated the association between homocystinuria and premature atherosclerosis and thrombosis, the exact mechanism of homocysteine-induced atherogenesis and thrombosis is not known. Accumulation of homocysteine leads to the production of homocysteine thiolactone by the liver, and this reduced thiol has been implicated as the toxic substance in homocysteinemic atherogenesis. In vitro, homocysteine induces endothelial cell desquamation, promotes oxidation of low-density lipoproteins, increases monocyte adhesions to the vessel wall, and stimulates platelet aggregation. Elevated levels of homocysteine have been shown to enhance factor V activity, decrease protein C activation, diminish fibrinolysis, and increase tissue factor activity, thereby reducing the antithrombotic properties of endothelial cells. The precise in vivo mechanism by which homocysteine might induce acceleration of atherosclerosis and thrombosis remains to be defined.

Homocysteine exists in human plasma in at least three forms: as the mixed disulfide homocysteine–cysteine, as free homocysteine, and as protein-bound homocysteine. Men have higher levels of plasma homocysteine than women, and premenopausal women have lower levels than postmenopausal women.

Evidence has accumulated that mildly elevated levels of plasma homocysteine are associated with symptomatic atherosclerotic disease. Boers and colleagues (71) detected a heterozygous trait they termed *homocysteinemia* in 14 of 70 patients with premature atherosclerotic vascular disease. These investigators performed an oral methionine loading test to aid in the detection of elevated plasma homocysteine in high-risk groups. Kang and associates (72) simplified the investigations when they demonstrated elevated levels of protein-bound homocysteine in patients with coronary artery disease without any requirements for oral methionine loading.

Our own ongoing evaluation of patients with peripheral vascular disease has confirmed elevated total plasma homocysteine levels when compared with age- and sex-matched control subjects (73). Elevated homocysteine levels were also associated with an increased incidence of death and progression of cardiovascular disease in patients with lower extremity disease and cerebrovascular disease (74). Investigators have attempted to lower these supranormal plasma homocysteine levels through alteration of the homocysteine–methionine pathways with pharmacologic doses of the cofactors for these enzymatic pathways (75), namely, folic acid, pyridoxine, vitamin B_{12}, and cobalamin. Although reduction in the plasma homocysteine levels was observed with this therapy, no investigation has established any clinical benefit from this therapy. Intuitively, one would expect clinical improvement or at least cessation of disease progression once the toxic homocysteine levels declined. Serial evaluation of the progression of peripheral vascular disease in groups randomized to treatment and nontreatment is necessary to answer this question; until then, the anecdotal reports appear encouraging.

HYPERVISCOSITY SYNDROMES

Multiple conditions characterized by an increase in the blood viscosity can cause arterial or venous thromboembolism. These are classified as *hyperviscosity syndromes,* and can be divided into two categories (76). The first group includes pathophysiologic conditions in which a primary blood abnormality causes an increase in the formed elements of the blood, such as the myeloproliferative disorders. The second group includes pathologic conditions that elevate serum proteins, such as myeloma, benign monoclonal gammopathy, macroglobulinemia, cryoglobulinemia, and neoplasia. In our clinical experience, hyperviscosity syndromes result in thrombosis most frequently in the venous system, next most often in the small peripheral arteries (i.e., hands and fingers), and least often in the major arteries.

Treatment of these hyperviscosity syndromes is directed at correction of the underlying disorders, with appropriate anticoagulation therapy as needed. Vascular surgery procedures are rarely required in these patients.

REFERENCES

1. Stanley JC, Gewertz BL, Bove EL, et al. Arterial fibrodysplasia, histopathologic character, and current etiologic concepts. *Arch Surg* 1978;110:561.
2. Chiche L, Bahnini A, Koskas F, et al. Occlusive fibromuscular disease of arteries supplying the brain: results of surgical treatment. *Ann Vasc Surg* 1997;11:496.
3. O'Neill JA Jr. Long-term outcome with surgical treatment of renovascular hypertension. *J Pediatr Surg* 1998;33:106.
4. Mahler F, Probst PN, Haertel M, et al. Lasting improvement of renovascular hypertension by transluminal dilation of atherosclerotic and non-atherosclerotic renal artery stenosis: a follow-up study. *Circulation* 1982;65:611.
5. Davidson RA, Barri Y, Wilcox CS. Predictors of cure of hypertension in fibromuscular renovascular disease. *Am J Kidney Dis* 1996;28:334.
6. Buerger L. Thromboangiitis obliterans: a study of the vascular lesions leading to presenile spontaneous gangrene. *Am J Med Sci* 1908;136:567.
7. Mills JM, Porter JM. Buerger's disease: a review and update. *Semin Vasc Surg* 1993;6:14.
8. Kobayashi M, Ito M, Nakagawa A, et al. Immunohistochemical analysis of arterial wall cellular infiltration in Buerger's disease. *J Vasc Surg* 1999;29:451.
9. Borner C, Heidrich H. Long-term follow-up of thromboangiitis obliterans. *Vasa* 1998;27:80.
10. Sasajima T, Kubo Y, Inaba M, et al. Role of infrainguinal bypass in Buerger's disease: an eighteen-year experience. *Eur J Vasc Endovasc Surg* 1997;13:186.
11. Verstraete M, et al. Oral iloprost in the treatment of thromboangiitis obliterans (Buerger's disease): a double-blind, randomised, placebo-controlled trial. The European TAO Study Group. *Eur J Vasc Endovasc Surg* 1998;15:300.
12. Isner JM, Baumgartner I, Rauh G, et al. Treatment of thromboangiitis obliterans (Buerger's disease) by intramuscular gene transfer of vascular endothelial growth factor: preliminary clinical results. *J Vasc Surg* 1998;28:964.
13. Erdheim J. Medionecrosis aortae idiopathica cystica. *Virchows Arch [A]* 1930;276:187.
14. Millar AJW, Gilbert RD, Brown RA, et al. Abdominal aortic aneurysms in children. *J Pediatr Surg* 1996;31:1624.
15. McKusick VA. *Heritable disorders of connective tissue,* 4th ed. St. Louis: Mosby, 1972:61.
16. Aoyama T, Francke U, Dietz HC, et al. Quantitative differences in biosynthesis and extracellular deposition of fibrillin in cultured fibroblasts distinguish five groups of Marfan syndrome patients and suggest distinct pathogenetic mechanisms. *J Clin Invest* 1994;94:130.
17. Pyeritz RE. Propranolol retards aortic root dilatation in the Marfan syndrome. *Circulation* 1983;68[Suppl III]:365.
18. Shores J, Berger KR, Murphy EA, et al. Progression of aortic dilatation and the benefit of long-term β-adrenergic blockade in Marfan's syndrome. *N Engl J Med* 1994;330:1335.
19. Smith JA, Fann JI, Miller C, et al. Surgical management of aortic dissection in patients with the Marfan syndrome. *Circulation* 1994;90:11235.
20. Coselli JS, LeMaire SA, Büket S. Marfan syndrome: the variability and outcome of operative management. *J Vasc Surg* 1995;21:432.
21. Gott VL, Cameron DE, Pyeritz RE, et al. Composite graft repair of Marfan aneurysm of the ascending aorta: results in 150 patients. *J Card Surg* 1994;9:482.
22. Pope FM, Martin GR, Liechtenstein JR, et al. Patients with Ehlers-Danlos syndrome type IV lack type III collagen. *Proc Natl Acad Sci USA* 1975;72:1314.
23. Hunter GC, Malone JM, Moore WS. Vascular manifestations in patients with Ehlers-Danlos syndrome. *Arch Surg* 1982;117:495.
24. Bergqvist D. Ehlers-Danlos type IV syndrome: a review from a vascular surgical point of view. *Eur J Surg* 1996;162:163.
25. Carlborg U. Studies of circulatory disturbances, pulse wave velocity, and pressure pulses in large arteries in cases of pseudoxanthoma elasticum and angioid streaks. *Acta Med Scand Suppl* 1944;151:1.
26. Carter DJ, Vince FP, Woodward DAK. Arterial surgery in pseudoxanthoma elasticum. *Postgrad Med J* 1976;52:291.
27. Schievink WI, Michels VV, Piepgras DG. Neurovascular manifestations of heritable connective tissue diseases: a review. *Stroke* 1994;25:889.
28. Leriche R. Dilation pathologique des arteres es en dehors des aneurysmes vie tissulaire des arteres. *Presse Med* 1942;50:641.
29. Rabinov K, Simon M, Sears J. Diffuse arteriectasis of the aorta, iliac, femoral, and popliteal arteries. *Vasc Dis* 1966;3:122.
30. Thomas ML. Arteriomegaly. *Br J Surg* 1971;58:690.
31. Lawrence PF, Wallis C, Dobrin PB, et al. Peripheral aneurysms and arteriomegaly: is there a familial pattern? *J Vasc Surg* 1998;28:599.
32. Hollier LH, Stanson AW, Gloviczki P, et al. Arteriomegaly: classification and morbid implications of diffuse aneurysmal disease. *Surgery* 1983;93:700.
33. Flannigan DP, Burnham SJ, Goodreau JJ, et al. Summary of cases of adventitial cystic disease of the popliteal artery. *Ann Surg* 1979;189:165.
34. Savage PEA. Arterial cystic degeneration. *Postgrad Med J* 1972;48:603.
35. Koppensteiner R, Katzenschlager R, Ahmadi A, et al. Demonstration of cystic adventitial disease by intravascular ultrasound imaging. *J Vasc Surg* 1996;23:534.
36. MacFarlane R, Livesey SA, Pollard S, et al. Cystic adventitial arterial disease. *Br J Surg* 1987;74:89.
37. Tsolakis IA, Walvatne CS, Caldwell MD. Cystic adventitial disease of the popliteal artery: diagnosis and treatment. *Eur J Vasc Endovasc Surg* 1998;15:188.
38. Deutsch AL, Hyde J, Miller SM, et al. Cystic adventitial degeneration of the popliteal artery: CT demonstration and directed percutaneous therapy. *AJR Am J Roentgenol* 1985;145:117.
39. Do DD, Braunschweig M, Baumgartner I, et al. Adventitial cystic disease of the popliteal artery: percutaneous US-guided aspiration. *Radiology* 1997;203:743.
40. Francfort JW, Gallagher JF, Penman E, et al. Surgery for radiation-induced symptomatic atherosclerosis. *Ann Vasc Surg* 1989;3:14.
41. Andros G, Schneider PA, Harris RW, et al. Management of arterial occlusive disease following radiation therapy. *Cardiovasc Surg* 1996;4:135.
42. Phillips GR III, Peer RM, Upson JE, et al. Late complications of revascularization for radiation-induced arterial disease. *J Vasc Surg* 1992;16:921.
43. Saliou C, Julia P, Feito B, et al. Radiation-induced arterial disease of the lower limb. *Ann Vasc Surg* 1997;11:173
44. Lie JT. The classification and diagnosis of vasculitis in large and medium-sized blood vessels. *Pathol Ann* 1987;22:125.
45. Allen NB, Bressler PB. Diagnosis and treatment of systemic and cutaneous necrotizing vasculitis syndromes. *Med Clin North Am* 1997;8:243.
46. Robins JM, Bookstein JJ. Regressing aneurysms in periarteritis nodosa. *Radiology* 1972;104:39.
47. Ewald EA, Griffin D, McCune WJ. Correlation of angiographic abnormalities with disease manifestations and disease severity in polyarteritis nodosa. *J Rheumatol* 1987;14:952.
48. Guillevin L, Lhote F, Gayraud M, et al. Prognostic factors in polyarteritis nodosa and Churg-Strauss syndrome: a prospective study in 342 patients. *Medicine (Baltimore)* 1996;75:17.

49. Cabal E, Holtz S. Polyarteritis as a cause of intestinal hemorrhage. *Gastroenterology* 1971;61:99.

50. Barron KS, Shulman ST, Rowley A, et al. Report of the National Institutes of Health workshop on Kawasaki disease. *J Rheumatol* 1999;26:170.

51. Laupland KB, Dele Davies H. Epidemiology, etiology, and management of Kawasaki disease: state of the art. *Pediatr Cardiol* 1999;20:177.

52. Kitamura S, Kameda Y, Seki T, et al. Long-term outcome of myocardial revascularization in patients with Kawasaki coronary artery disease: A multicenter cooperative study. *J Thorac Cardiovasc Surg* 1994;107:663.

53. Cogan DG. Syndrome of non-syphilitic interstitial keratitis and vestibuloauditory symptoms. *Arch Ophthalmol* 1945;33:144.

54. Haynes BF, Kaiser-Kupfer MI, Mason P, et al. Cogan syndrome: studies in thirteen patients, long-term follow-up, and a review of the literature. *Medicine (Baltimore)* 1980;59:426.

55. Chajek T, Fainaru M. Behçet's disease: report of 41 cases and a review of the literature. *Medicine (Baltimore)* 1975;54:179.

56. Bartlett ST, McCarthy WJ, Palmer AS, et al. Multiple aneurysms in Behçet's disease. *Arch Surg* 1988;123:1004.

57. Jenkins AAL, MacPherson AIS, Nolan B, et al. Peripheral aneurysms in Behçet's disease. *Br J Surg* 1976;63:199.

58. Vasseur MA, Haulon S, Beregi JP, et al. Endovascular treatment of abdominal aneurysmal aortitis in Behçet's disease. *J Vasc Surg* 1998;27:974.

59. Sezer FN. Further investigations of the virus of Behçet's disease. *Am J Ophthalmol* 1956;41:41.

60. O'Duffy JD, Lehner T, Barnes CG. Summary of the Third International Conference on Behçet's Disease. *J Rheumatol* 1983;10:154.

61. Porter JM, Taylor LM. Small artery disease of the upper extremity. *World J Surg* 1983;7:326.

62. Schmidt WA, Kraft HE, Vorpahl K, et al. Color duplex ultrasonography in the diagnosis of temporal arteritis. *N Engl J Med* 1997;337:1336.

63. Hollenhorst RW, Brown JR, Wagener HP, et al. Neurologic aspects of temporal arteritis. *Neurology* 1960;10:490.

64. Takagi A, Kajiura N, Tada Y, et al. Surgical treatment of non-specific inflammatory arterial aneurysms. *J Cardiovasc Surg* 1986;27:117.

65. Rivers SP, Baur GM, Inahara T, et al. Arm ischemia secondary to giant cell arteritis. *Am J Surg* 1982;143:554.

66. Hall S, Barr W, Lie TE, et al. Takayasu arteritis: a study of 32 North American patients. *Medicine* 1985;64:89.

67. Lupi-Herrera E, Sanchez-Torres G, Marcustiamer J, et al. Takayasu's arteritis: clinical study of 107 cases. *Am Heart J* 1977;93:94.

68. Robbs JV, Abdool-Carrim ATO, Kadwa AM. Arterial reconstruction for non-specific arteritis (Takayasu's disease): medium to long term results. *Eur J Vasc Surg* 1994;8:401.

69. McCully KS. Homocysteine theory of atherosclerosis: development and current status. *Atheroscler Rev* 1983;11:157.

70. McCully KS. Vascular pathology of homocysteinemia: implications for the pathogenesis of atherosclerosis. *Am J Pathol* 1969;56:111.

71. Boers GHJ, Smals AGH, Trijbels FJM, et al. Heterozygosity for homocysteinuria in premature peripheral and cerebral occlusive arterial disease. *N Engl J Med* 1985;313:709.

72. Kang SS, Wong PWK, Cook HY, et al. Protein-bound homocysteine: a possible risk factor for coronary artery disease. *J Clin Invest* 1986;77:1482.

73. Harris EJ Jr, Taylor LM Jr, Malinow MR, et al. The association between elevated plasma homocysteine and symptomatic peripheral arterial disease. *Surg Forum* 1989;40:307.

74. Taylor LM Jr, Moneta GL, Sexton GJ, et al. Prospective blinded study of the relationship between plasma homocysteine and progression of symptomatic peripheral arterial disease. *J Vasc Surg* 1999;29:8.

75. Olszewski AJ, Szostak WB, Bialkowska M, et al. Reduction of plasma lipid and homocysteine levels by pyridoxine, folate, cobalamin, choline, riboflavin, and troxerutin in atherosclerosis. *Atherosclerosis* 1989;75:1.

76. Forconi S, Pieragalli M, Guerrini C, et al. Primary and secondary blood hyperviscosity syndromes, and syndromes associated with blood hyperviscosity. *Drugs* 1987;33[Suppl]:19.

SURGERY: SCIENTIFIC PRINCIPLES AND PRACTICE, Third Edition, edited by Lazar J. Greenfield, Michael W. Mulholland, Keith T. Oldham, Gerald B. Zelenock, and Keith D. Lillemoe. Lippincott Williams & Wilkins Publishers, Philadelphia, © 2001.

CHAPTER 68

PERIPHERAL ARTERIAL EMBOLISM

LOUIS M. MESSINA AND RAJABRATA SARKAR

ACUTE ARTERIAL EMBOLISM

Source and Etiology

Between 80% and 90% of acute arterial emboli originate in the heart (1–4). Of the remaining emboli, the site of origin of half is never identified, and the remainder arise from a variety of uncommon sites (Fig. 68.1). These uncommon sites include arterial aneurysms, most commonly infrarenal aortic and popliteal aneurysms, as well as subclavian aneurysms secondary to thoracic outlet obstruction. Peripheral arterial atherosclerotic plaques can also be the source of macroemboli. Other uncommon sources of arterial emboli include sites of vascular trauma (both iatrogenic and civilian), malignant tumors, and areas of venous thrombosis that result in paradoxical embolus (i.e., venous emboli passing through a patent foramen ovale into the arterial circulation). Emboli from these uncommon sources occur more frequently in younger patients (5).

Although thrombus can develop on the endothelial surfaces of the heart as a result of a variety of underlying diseases, two thirds arise secondary to atrial fibrillation. In this circumstance, thrombus forms on the endocardial surface of the fibrillating atrium, especially in the large left atrial appendage. Historically, rheumatic heart disease was the most common underlying heart disease responsible for atrial fibrillation; more recently, ischemic heart disease has become the most common cause of atrial fibrillation (1). Other heart diseases that have been implicated in the development of endocardial thrombus formation are acute myocardial infarction, cardiomyopathy, congestive heart failure, and prosthetic heart valves. Rare sources of intracardiac emboli include subacute bacterial endocarditis and cardiac tumors, principally atrial myxomas.

As the relative frequency of rheumatic heart disease has diminished and that of ischemic heart disease has increased as the most common underlying heart disease causing intracardiac thrombus formation, a change in the clinical profile of the patients presenting with acute arterial embolism has been documented. Patients who have rheumatic heart disease tend to be younger, and the ratio of women to men in this group is 2 : 1. Patients who have atrial fibrillation secondary to atherosclerotic ischemic heart disease are older, and the ratio of women to men is approximately 1 : 1. Nonetheless, atrial fibrillation of any origin carries a significant risk for peripheral arterial embolism.

A better understanding of the risk of thromboembolic complications and their prevention in patients with nonrheumatic atrial fibrillation has more recently developed (6). Chronic atrial fibrillation carries an annual risk of significant thromboembolic complications of 3% to 6%. In these studies, paroxysmal atrial fibrillation has a lower risk of thromboembolic complications than does chronic atrial fibrillation. In addition, patients with chronic atrial fibrillation have a higher prevalence of silent cerebral infarction. A disagreement exists among various retrospec-

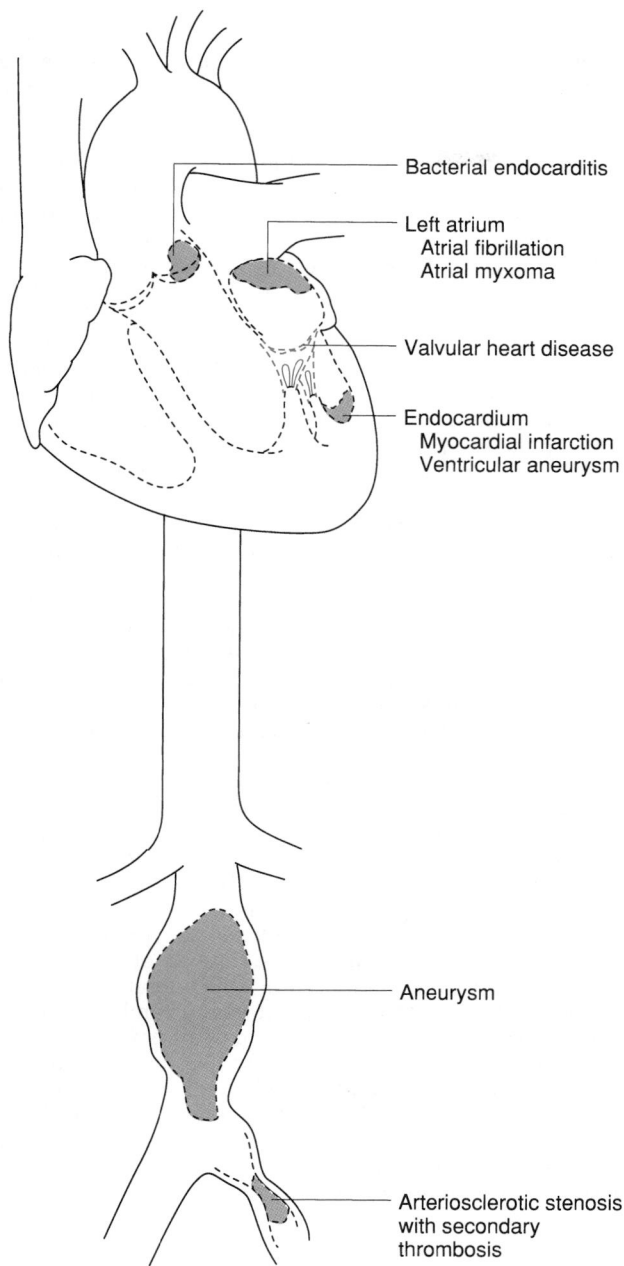

Figure 68.1. Common sources of arterial emboli.

patients with atrial fibrillation by 68% without a significant increase in the risk of major bleeding complications (8). Aspirin was consistently less effective. One of these studies showed that the incidence of thromboembolic complications was approximately 80% lower in the groups receiving either aspirin or warfarin than in the placebo group (event rates were 1.6% per year in the two active treatment arms of warfarin and aspirin and 8.3% per year in the placebo arm). These studies indicate that chronic anticoagulation therapy with warfarin and possibly with aspirin is effective in reducing the risk of stroke and other systemic complications of acute arterial emboli.

The second most common underlying disease process responsible for the development of thrombus on the endocardium is acute myocardial infarction (9). In a study of 1,277 patients who had acute transmural myocardial infarction, 22 patients had 30 episodes of systemic arterial embolism (10). Postmortem autopsy studies show an even higher, often clinically silent incidence of peripheral arterial embolism after acute myocardial infarction. In most patients, the myocardial infarction is anterolateral in location and accompanied by congestive heart failure. The mortality rate is 55% after the embolism. The risk of emboli after acute myocardial infarction is not indefinite because most emboli occur within 6 weeks of the infarction. Anticoagulation has been shown to reduce the clinical incidence of systemic arterial embolism after acute myocardial infarction. A more recent multicenter, randomized, double-blind, placebo-controlled trial of subcutaneous dalteparin showed a 63% reduction of left ventricular thrombus formation after acute anterior infarction, but at an increased risk of hemorrhagic complications (11).

Ventricular aneurysm formation, a complication of acute myocardial infarction, can also be a source of arterial emboli. Approximately half of left ventricular aneurysms are found at the time of surgery to have mural thrombus (12). Clinically apparent arterial embolism occurs in 5% of patients who have ventricular aneurysms after acute myocardial infarction. Cardiomyopathies and congestive heart failure are other, less common causes of mural thrombus formation as a source of peripheral arterial emboli.

Various cardiac arrhythmias have been associated with the occurrence of peripheral arterial embolism, particularly the bradycardia–tachycardia arrhythmia, the so-called sick sinus syndrome. A 16% incidence of embolism was found in patients suffering from chronic sinoatrial disorders, whereas only 1.3% of age-matched controls with complete heart block developed peripheral arterial embolism (13). Patients with idiopathic or alcoholic cardiomyopathy also have a relatively high incidence of arterial embolism.

Uncommon cardiac sources of peripheral arterial embolism include bacterial endocarditis, prosthetic heart valves, and cardiac atrial myxomas. In patients suffering from bacterial endocarditis, valvular vegetations fragment and embolize into the arterial circulation, usually obstructing small arteries such as the palmar or plantar arches or the digit arteries. Arterial embolism remains the most common potentially serious complication of bacterial endocarditis. Emboli occur in 15% to 35% of such patients. The vessels of the cerebral circulation are affected most often by acute embolism secondary to bacterial endocarditis. Finally, mitral stenosis, even in the absence of atrial fibrillation can result in systemic embolism. For this reason, anticoagulation is recommended in patients with mitral stenosis and left atrial thrombus (14).

Prosthetic heart valves can become an important source of arterial emboli. The mitral valve is a more common source of emboli than aortic valves. Approximately 25%

tive studies concerning the importance of cardiovascular risk factors for the development of thromboembolic complications in people who have chronic atrial fibrillation. One study showed that a previous myocardial infarction was a significant risk factor for the development of future thromboembolic complications (7). In contrast, age, sex, heart failure, chest pain, hypertensive heart disease, diabetes, systolic and diastolic high blood pressure, smoking, relative heart volume, and left atrial size were not significant risk factors.

Studies have also shown for the first time that drug therapy can reduce significantly the incidence of thromboembolic complications in people with chronic, nonrheumatic atrial fibrillation. In five randomized trials, warfarin reduced the risk of stroke and cardiovascular mortality in

of patients who have emboli due to prosthetic valves have more than one embolic event. In addition, over 80% of these emboli lodge in the cerebral circulation, and approximately 10% of these are fatal. Finally, cardiac tumor fragments from an atrial myxoma or an angiosarcoma can also embolize. Because the initial clinical presentation of bacterial endocarditis or atrial myxomas is often an acute arterial embolism, this reinforces the necessity of sending specimens of acute emboli for microscopic analysis and culture after they are removed during surgical embolectomy.

Emboli can also arise from the surface of atherosclerotic plaques (Fig. 68.2). Atherosclerotic plaques give rise to both macroscopic and microscopic emboli. Microscopic emboli are often referred to as *atheroemboli*. Because the natural history, clinical manifestations, and management of microscopic atheroembolism differ substantially from those of macroemboli composed entirely of thrombus and plaque, they are discussed as a separate entity at the end from this chapter. Macroemboli have been identified with increasing frequency to originate from thoracic aortic plaque or ulcers (15,16). Primary treatment is directed toward thromboendarterectomy of the thoracic aortic lesion.

Arterial aneurysms are an important noncardiac source of peripheral arterial embolism. Thrombus forms along the dilated portion of the artery, and increasing layers of thrombus formation occur as the aneurysm enlarges. Fragments of this laminated thrombus can break loose and obstruct the downstream arterial circulation. The most common arterial aneurysms associated with peripheral arterial embolism are infrarenal abdominal aortic, femoral artery, and popliteal artery aneurysms. Arterial embolism is a common complication of popliteal aneurysms, occurring in approximately 25% of symptomatic patients (17). These embolic events are often clinically silent and are detected only after complete obstruction of the outflow arteries of the popliteal artery occurs. Embolism from true femoral artery aneurysms is less frequent, occurring in 5% to 10% of patients. Finally, subclavian artery aneurysms that develop as a consequence of thoracic outlet obstruction or atherosclerosis can give rise to peripheral embolism in up to 33% of patients.

Trauma, both civilian and iatrogenic, is an increasingly important cause of peripheral arterial embolism. Gunshot injuries, particularly those to the thorax, can result in the entry of a bullet into the heart or great vessels and then subsequent embolism downstream from the point of arterial entry. This injury is usually identified on the basis of the clinical manifestations of a distal vessel obstruction. After a bullet embolus is identified, it is most important to locate the vascular site at which the bullet entered the vascular tree. The site of entry of the bullet is usually a more life-threatening injury than is the ischemia that develops downstream from the level of the bullet obstruction.

Iatrogenic trauma in the form of operative manipulation or as a consequence of diagnostic and therapeutic vascular catheterization is an important cause of trauma-related arterial embolism. These emboli usually arise from thrombus that forms on the surface of catheters, particularly those that have been indwelling for long periods. These thrombi often obstruct the digital arteries of the hand or foot. In addition to thrombus formation on the catheters, the catheters themselves can fracture and embolize.

Portions of malignant tumors can fragment and embolize into the arterial circulation. Most commonly, these involve primary or metastatic tumors within the lung (18) (Fig. 68.3). Embolism of lung tumor fragments occurs during surgical manipulation of the tumor or in the immediate postoperative period. These emboli are usually identified in the early postoperative period. Patients with malignant tumor embolism have a good short-term outlook if the emboli are diagnosed and treated promptly.

Finally, arterial embolism can arise from a site of venous thrombosis, the so-called paradoxical embolus. Most commonly, an embolus arises from a site of venous thrombosis and passes through a patent foramen ovale, an atrial septal defect, a patent ductus arteriosus, or a pulmonary arteriovenous fistula. The most common intracardiac defect through which a venous embolus passes to the arterial circulation is a "probe-patent" foramen ovalis. This defect is common but usually results in a small left-to-right shunt because left atrial pressure normally exceeds right atrial pressure. After a patient experiences pulmonary embolism, pulmonary and right ventricular hypertension can occur. Under these circumstances, right atrial pressure can greatly exceed left atrial pressure. This interatrial pressure gradient facilitates the passage of venous emboli into the arterial circulation. Thus, paradoxical emboli usually occur in patients who have already had clinical manifestations of acute pulmonary embolism or chronic pulmonary hypertension. Paradoxical embolism should be suspected when patients have acute arterial embolism in the absence of any of the well defined conditions predisposing to arterial embolism.

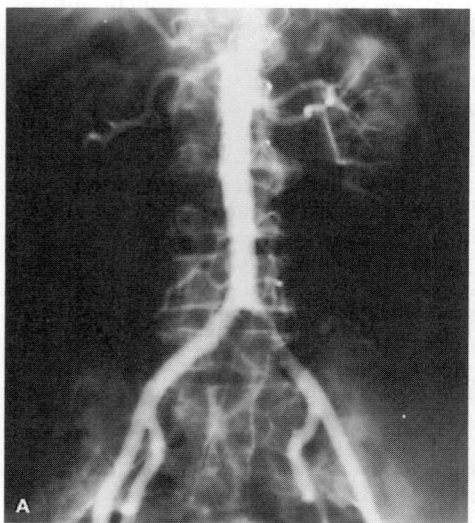
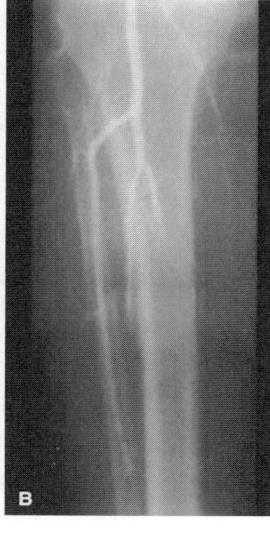

Figure 68.2. *(A)* A thrombus can be seen on the surface of the atherosclerotic plaque in the left common iliac artery. *(B)* Left lower extremity angiogram in the same patient shows occlusion of the anterior tibial, peroneal, and posterior tibial arteries by macroatheroembolus.

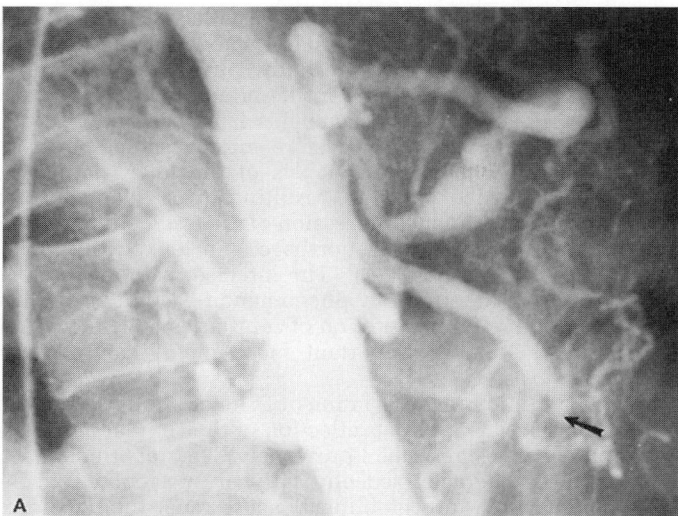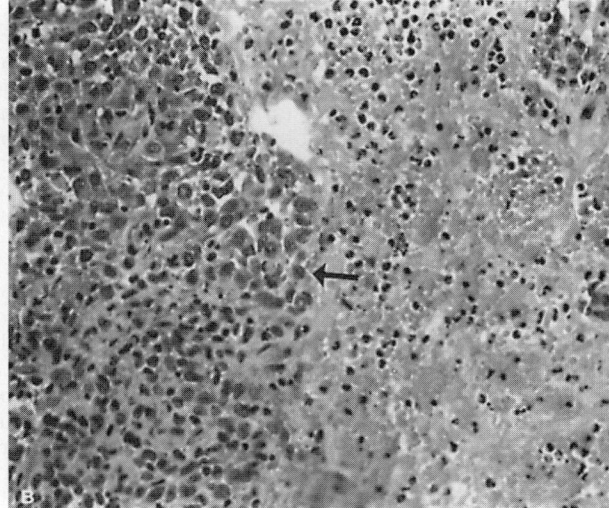

Figure 68.3. *(A)* Arteriogram of a patient who had abdominal pain and acidosis 48 hours after resection of a primary lung tumor. A tumor embolus caused acute occlusion of the superior mesenteric artery at the origins of the middle colic and inferior pancreaticoduodenal arteries. *(B)* Photomicrograph of a tumor embolus, showing poorly differentiated carcinoma *(arrow)* surrounded by organizing thrombus. Hematoxylin–eosin, ×40. *(B* courtesy of B. Markey, M.D., Department of Pathology, University of Michigan Medical School, Ann Arbor, MI.)

Distribution

Arterial emboli do not distribute in the arterial circulation proportionate to the flow rate of a particular artery. Other factors influence their distribution in the arterial tree, including the size and density of the embolus, the arterial diameter, the arterial branch angle, and the shape of arterial bifurcations. A number of factors make it difficult to estimate precisely the distribution of arterial emboli in the arterial circulation, largely because of difficulties in identifying the mechanisms of cerebral infarction. For example, some authors suggest that up to half of arterial emboli go to the cerebral circulation (19). The frequency of cerebral embolism differs with the type of underlying heart disease. Patients who have rheumatic heart disease complicated by mitral valve disease and atrial fibrillation are at higher risk for development of cerebral embolism and clinical strokes than are patients with the other types of underlying heart disease.

Significant differences exist between autopsy reports of the distribution of arterial emboli and reports based on emboli that are detected clinically. This discrepancy between the incidence and distribution of arterial emboli found at autopsy and those identified on the basis of their clinical manifestations is particularly true for renal emboli. One large study found an autopsy incidence of 1.4% of renal infarction secondary to renal embolism (20). The diagnosis of acute renal embolism was made in less than 1% of these cases before the patient died. Finally, up to 11% of patients who have arterial embolism present with multiple synchronous arterial occlusions (4).

Most arterial emboli lodge at arterial bifurcations, where there is a sudden change in arterial diameter. Excluding carotid embolism, 80% to 90% of all arterial emboli lodge at the bifurcations of large arteries in the upper or lower extremity (4,19) (Fig. 68.4). Approximately 15% of arterial emboli lodge in the upper extremity, 10% in the visceral vessels of the abdomen, and the remainder at the aortic bifurcation or in its more distal branches. The common femoral artery is the most typical site for an arterial embolus to lodge. The next most common site is the aortic bifurcation and the iliac arteries. Arterial em-

boli lodge in the popliteal arteries in approximately 10% to 20% of patients. In the upper extremity, three fourths of arterial emboli lodge at the level of the brachial artery. The axillary artery is the site of obstruction in approximately 20%; the remainder lodge in the subclavian, radial, or ulnar arteries.

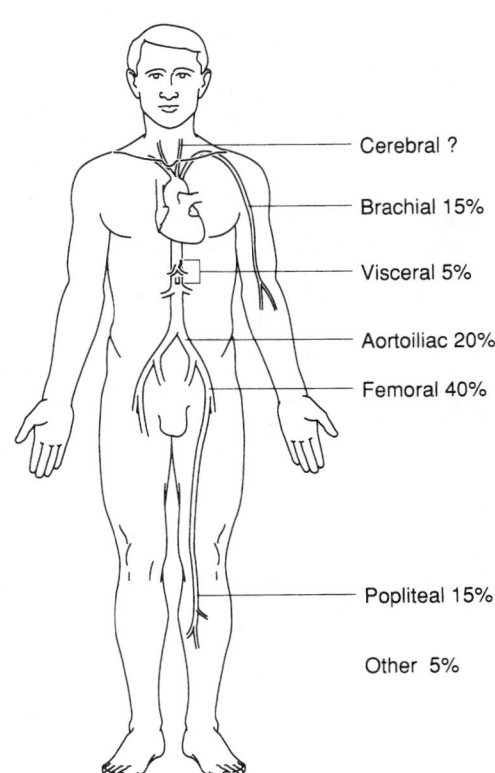

Figure 68.4. Approximate distribution of arterial emboli based on pooled data.

Pathophysiology

The pathophysiologic process of acute limb ischemia secondary to arterial embolism primarily reflects changes that occur in the skeletal muscle secondary to ischemia and subsequently, after embolectomy, during reperfusion. Although skeletal muscle constitutes 40% of the total body mass and clinical syndromes involving skeletal muscle ischemia occur commonly, little work has been done until recently to clarify the pathophysiologic process of skeletal muscle ischemia. Experimental work in both humans and animals shows that skeletal muscle is more tolerant of ischemia than other organs. Skeletal muscle's tolerance to ischemia is due to its low resting metabolic rate, high levels of alternative energy sources such as phosphocreatine and glycogen, its capacity for anaerobic glycolysis, the tolerance of certain subpopulations of its mitochondria to ischemia, and, finally, its capacity to regenerate even after periods of severe ischemia (21). Another important facet of the pathophysiology of skeletal muscle ischemia is the development of the no-reflow phenomenon, that is, the inability to restore perfusion after ischemia.

The extent of skeletal muscle necrosis is a function of the duration and severity of the ischemia, the metabolic rate of the muscle, and the type and duration of reperfusion (21). Under resting conditions and normothermia, skeletal muscle can tolerate 1 to 3 hours of ischemia. The first detectable ultrastructural changes are those of mitochondrial swelling, and a decrease of glycogen granules in the muscle fibers, intramuscular nerves, and nerve endings of the motor end plate. After long periods of ischemia, irreversible histologic changes occur, including disappearance of the Z-line, disruption of the cell membrane, and vacuolization of the muscle mitochondria. After periods of ischemia greater than 6 hours, autolysis of the muscle fibers occurs.

The low resting energy requirements and the phosphocreatine and glycogen stores enhance the tolerance of skeletal muscle to ischemia. Adenosine triphosphate (ATP) levels are maintained at a fairly constant level for up to 3 hours of ischemia. During the ischemic period, ATP levels are constantly replenished by the phosphocreatine-mediated rephosphorylation of adenosine diphosphate. Phosphocreatine stores then become exhausted at approximately 3 hours of ischemia. In addition, skeletal muscles that have a high glycogen content can maintain anaerobic glycolysis in the absence of blood flow for up to 6 hours. The linear decline in glycogen levels is paralleled by an increase in lactate levels and thus a decrease in pH. These high lactate levels and the low pH level have a deleterious effect on skeletal muscle membrane integrity. High lactate and low pH levels are associated with a loss of potential across the cellular membranes, resulting in an inability of the cell to maintain proper ionic concentration gradients (22).

During reperfusion of skeletal muscle that has been ischemic for 4 hours or less, there is a rapid restoration of ATP levels in the first 15 minutes, with normalization of levels by 3 hours (23). Phosphocreatine levels return to normal 30 minutes after reperfusion. Glycogen returns to preischemic levels after 3 hours of reperfusion. In contrast, when ischemia lasts longer than 7 hours, on reperfusion there is no resynthesis of ATP or phosphocreatine, and there is no metabolic recovery of the muscle. During this reperfusion period, because there is a loss of cell membrane integrity, extensive edema formation occurs intracellularly and interstitially. In addition, a release of intracellular electrolytes and enzymes into the circulation occurs, particularly potassium, lactic acid, and myoglobin.

The inability to restore microvascular perfusion during reperfusion of ischemic tissue is known as the *no-reflow phenomenon* (24). The no-reflow phenomenon has been identified experimentally in the brain, heart, kidney, and adrenal gland. Four mechanisms have been advanced to explain the inability to restore microvascular perfusion during reperfusion: thrombosis of the microcirculation; endothelial cell swelling, resulting in capillary obstruction; extravascular compression of the microcirculation by interstitial edema or hemorrhage; and leukocyte obstruction of capillaries (21). The precise pathophysiologic process of the no-reflow phenomenon has not been elucidated; however, obstruction of capillaries by leukocytes is probably a more important mechanism than capillary thrombosis.

The clinical manifestations of skeletal muscle reperfusion injury are a direct reflection of the cellular and metabolic changes described previously. This reperfusion syndrome is characterized clinically by metabolic acidosis, hyperkalemia, myoglobinuria, acute renal tubular necrosis, and muscle edema. The metabolic acidosis, hyperkalemia, and myoglobinuria result from the release of intracellular ions and proteins of skeletal myocytes into the systemic circulation. Both the release of these intracellular constituents and the muscle edema are the consequence of the ischemic injury to the cell membrane. The other clinical manifestations of this reperfusion syndrome are acute tubular necrosis and compartment syndrome. Acute tubular necrosis results from the precipitation of myoglobulin in the renal tubules. Compartment syndromes are caused by compression of nerves, arteries, and veins in the fascial compartments of the lower extremity. Because these compartments have a finite volume, as muscle edema increases, eventual neurovascular compression occurs.

Clinical Manifestations

Sudden occlusion of a peripheral artery by an acute embolus results in unmistakable signs and symptoms of acute limb ischemia, often referred to as the five "Ps" of acute limb ischemia:

- Pain
- Pallor
- Pulselessness
- Paresthesia
- Paralysis

These signs and symptoms occur in a characteristic distribution that usually permits accurate localization of the arterial embolus on the basis of physical examination alone.

The pain that occurs as a result of acute arterial occlusion is usually of such sudden onset and severity that the patient can remember precisely its time of onset. The pain is most often described as a severe, deep pain, well localized and unremitting. The pain does not dissipate until there is restoration of arterial circulation or irreversible ischemic injury to the sensory nerves. Paresthesias usually appear early after the arterial occlusion and reflect the increased sensitivity of sensory nerves to ischemia. Because small nerve fibers have a relatively increased sensitivity to ischemia, the first loss of sensation is that of light touch (25). Sensation to deep pain, pressure, and temperature is usually well preserved until late after the acute arterial occlusion. The paresthesia and diminished sensation are not in the cutaneous nerves but rather in a so-called stocking or glovelike distribution. Pallor of the limb appears immediately after the onset of ischemia and is a result of diminished skin blood flow because of the arterial obstruction, as well as reflex vasoconstriction as a secondary response to the tissue ischemia. Although some weakness of the involved extremity can be present early after the onset of ischemia, paralysis of any muscle group is a late feature. In addition to these physical signs, the limb is invariably cool, with the temperature changes becoming greater in the areas more distal to the arterial occlusion. All of these signs and symptoms of acute ischemia progress as the duration of ischemia increases. Eventually, signs of irreversible limb ischemia occur. These signs include loss of sensation or near-complete anesthesia of the involved extremity, and rigor mortis when pallor progresses to diffuse mottling of the skin and the muscles become firm and involuntary contraction develops. The latter findings usually suggest that attempts at restoration of flow in the arterial circulation cannot save the leg and may result in life-threatening complications secondary to reperfusion injury. Complete examination of the patient usually reveals the presence of an acute atrial arrhythmia, most commonly atrial fibrillation. There is no antecedent history of peripheral vascular occlusive disease (i.e., no claudication or rest pain). Physical examination of the contralateral limb usually shows normal pulses and no signs of acute or chronic ischemia.

The clinical manifestations of acute arterial embolism are influenced by a number of factors, including the level and duration of arterial occlusion, the adequacy of collateral circulation, the extent of preexisting arterial occlusive disease, the general condition of the patient, the presence or absence of synchronous arterial emboli, and, finally, the metabolic consequences of the tissue ischemia. Seven to 27% (26,27) of patients with acute arterial embolism have no signs or symptoms of arterial occlusion, whereas in others there is an onset of signs and symptoms so gradual that some patients present days and weeks after the embolic occlusion.

When signs and symptoms of acute limb ischemia are present, clinical manifestations usually permit precise localization of the embolus (Fig. 68.5). This is based on the level of absent pulses as well as the level of changes in skin temperature and color. The change in skin temperature is the most sensitive sign of ischemia and is found one skeletal segment below the level of arterial obstruction. Changes in skin color, which initially are usually either a pale yellow or lemon-yellow color, occur one to two skeletal segments below the level of arterial obstruction. Thus, acute occlusion of the distal infrarenal aorta, a so-called saddle embolus, is manifested by the absence of femoral pulses bilaterally, a decrease in skin temperature starting at the level of the upper thigh, and changes in skin color beginning at the level of the knee. Occlusion of the common femoral artery is manifested by a decrease in skin temperature at the level of the lower thigh and a change in skin color starting at the level of the midcalf. Finally, a popliteal occlusion is manifested by a change in skin temperature beginning in the upper calf and a change in skin color beginning at the level of the ankle. The changes in

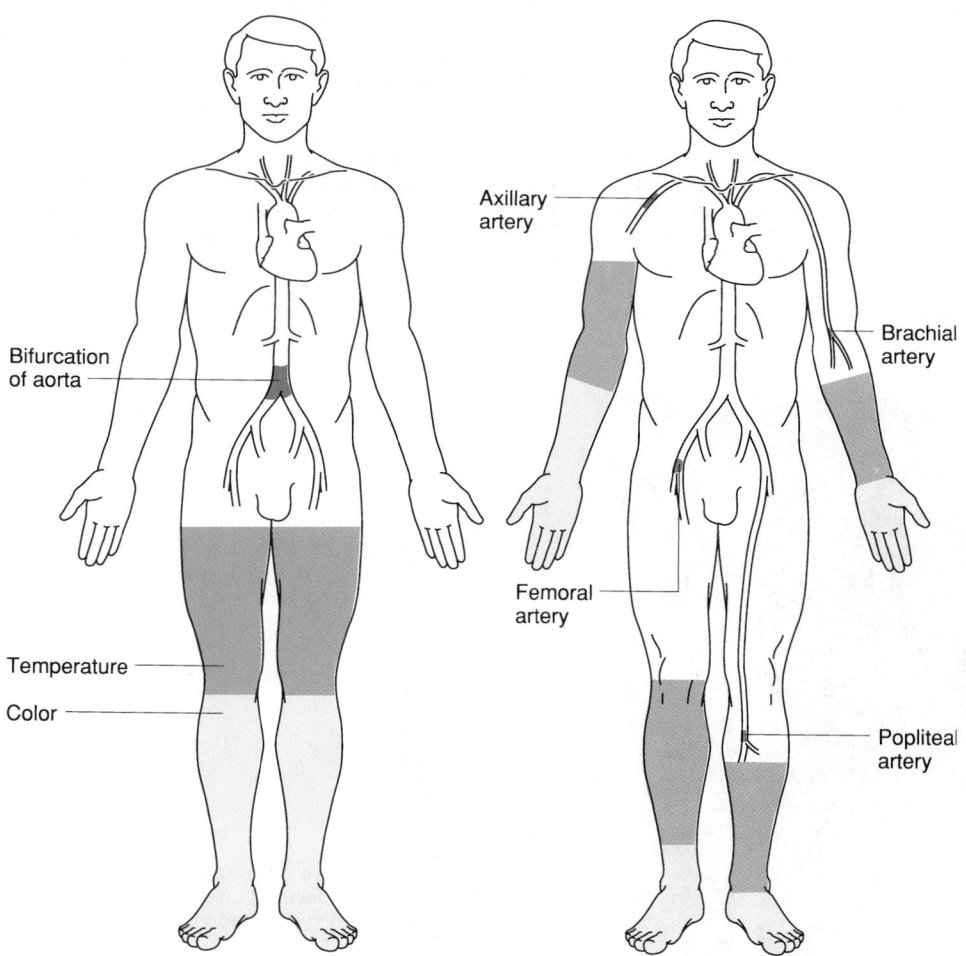

Figure 68.5. The location of an acute arterial embolus can usually be determined precisely based on physical examination of the patient.

skin temperature and color become more pronounced in areas that are progressively distal to the level of arterial occlusion. A similar relation between the location of the arterial embolus and the changes in skin temperature and color is observed in the upper extremity.

Other factors that influence the clinical manifestations and accurate diagnosis of acute arterial embolism are the general condition of the patient, the presence of synchronous arterial embolism, and the metabolic consequences of the tissue ischemia. Many patients with acute arterial embolism have other severe underlying medical illnesses. Common concurrent illnesses are acute congestive heart failure complicated by peripheral edema, acute myocardial infarction, chronic obstructive pulmonary disease, and pneumonia. The general debility of the patient and the presence of concurrent systemic illness can obscure the signs and symptoms of acute limb ischemia, thus preventing rapid diagnosis and treatment. Because up to 20% of patients with acute arterial embolism have multiple synchronous emboli, the clinical manifestations of one of the arterial occlusions can obscure the clinical manifestations of another synchronous lesion. This is particularly true of acute cerebral or visceral embolism occurring in patients with acute limb ischemia. There also can be multiple systemic complications because of the metabolic consequences of tissue ischemia. These include the development of systemic acidosis, renal failure, and altered mental status.

There is a subgroup of patients who present for evaluation weeks or months after the embolic event. Most of these patients have evidence of subacute limb ischemia that is not consistent with acute embolic occlusion or chronic occlusive disease. Rather, these patients present with a history of a sudden onset of calf claudication or ischemic limb pain. Less commonly, they are referred for evaluation for presumptive diagnosis of acute deep venous thrombosis. The diagnosis of acute arterial embolism is usually made after arteriography discloses findings consistent with embolic occlusion. Although a significant period has elapsed since the onset of their symptoms, these patients can still undergo successful embolectomy in most cases. Thus, recognition of this subacute clinical picture is important in the consideration of any patient who presents with atypical features of either acute or chronic limb ischemia.

TABLE 68.1. CLINICAL DISTINCTIONS BETWEEN ACUTE ARTERIAL EMBOLISM AND ACUTE ARTERIAL THROMBOSIS

Embolism	Thrombosis
Arrhythmia	No arrhythmia
Sudden onset	Sudden onset
No prior claudication or rest pain	History of claudication or rest pain
Normal contralateral pulses	Contralateral pulses absent
No physical findings of chronic limb ischemia	Physical findings of chronic limb ischemia

Differential Diagnosis

The differential diagnosis of acute limb ischemia includes acute arterial embolism, acute arterial thrombosis, acute aortic dissection, acute venous thrombosis, and arterial spasm. This differential diagnosis is particularly appropriate for consideration in the elderly patient who has generalized atherosclerosis, has no cardiac arrhythmia or acute myocardial infarction, and presents with acute limb ischemia, or in the younger patient who presents with acute limb ischemia and has no cardiac abnormalities.

The most important distinction to make in this differential diagnosis of acute limb ischemia is between acute arterial embolism and acute arterial thrombosis (Table 68.1). The diagnosis of acute arterial embolism is favored when the patient presents with the sudden onset of severe pain, has physical findings consistent with acute ischemia, has no prior history of claudication or rest pain, and when the contralateral extremity has a normal arterial pulse examination. Clinical features that favor the diagnosis of acute arterial thrombosis are a prior history of claudication or rest pain or prior vascular reconstruction, evidence of generalized atherosclerotic occlusive disease, and physical signs of chronic limb ischemia. These signs of chronic ischemia include absence of leg pulses, diminished hair growth, thinning of the skin, thickening of the nails, and the presence of chronic ulceration. In addition, for the same level of arterial occlusion, the signs and symptoms

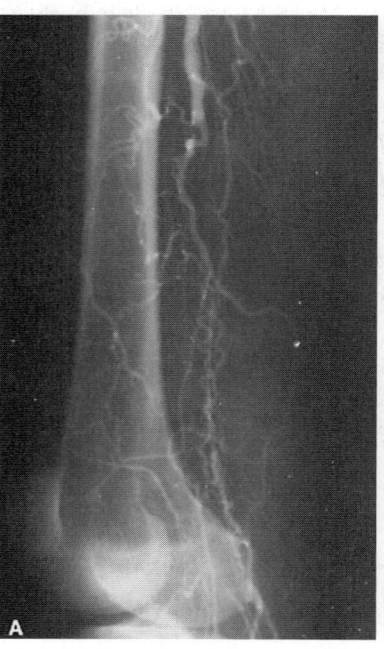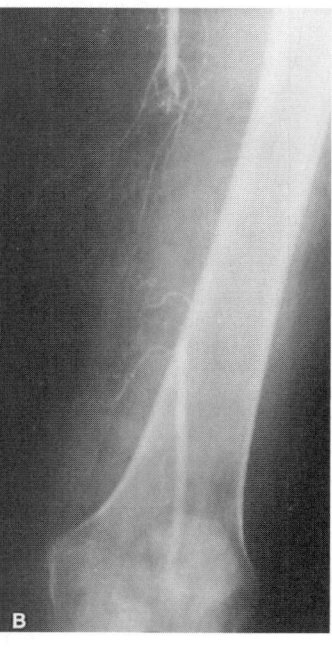

Figure 68.6. (A) Angiogram showing a chronic superficial femoral artery thrombosis. Large, preexisting collateral vessels are visible, some of which have a corkscrew appearance. (B) Angiogram showing an acute superficial femoral artery embolus. Collaterals are absent, there is a sharp cutoff above the occlusion, and luminal defects show the tail of the obstructing embolus.

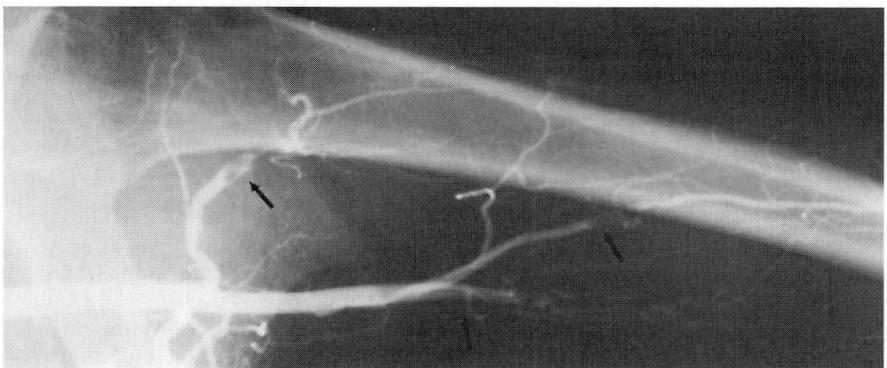

Figure 68.7. Left upper extremity angiogram showing acute embolic occlusion of the brachial artery. The thrombus is obstructing branches of the brachial artery, further reducing arterial inflow to the distal extremity.

of limb ischemia are usually less than those anticipated in patients with preexisting occlusive disease who have an acute thrombosis. Despite these distinguishing features between acute embolic and acute thrombotic occlusion, a correct diagnosis often requires angiography (Figs. 68.6 and 68.7), and occasionally the correct diagnosis can be made only at the time of surgical exploration of the vessel. Although it is frequently assumed that the clinical distinction between these entities is clear-cut, studies suggest that the presence of atrial fibrillation is the only reliable clinical sign to distinguish between acute thrombosis and acute embolism (28).

Management

The diagnosis of acute arterial embolism can be established confidently on the basis of a careful history and physical examination in most patients. Patients who present with the classic signs of acute limb ischemia and have a readily identifiable cardiac abnormality such as atrial fibrillation or acute myocardial infarction need no further evaluation. When the diagnosis is in doubt, particularly if there is a serious question between acute arterial embolism and acute arterial thrombosis, angiography should be used. The first step in the management of patients with acute limb ischemia is immediate heparinization. Heparin prevents proximal and distal propagation of thrombus, maintains patency of collateral vessels, and in addition can have a beneficial effect by reducing the extent of ischemic injury (29). Although variability is seen among patients, most patients cannot tolerate more than 4 to 6 hours of acute limb ischemia before serious nerve and muscle injury occurs. Thus, prompt diagnosis and expeditious evaluation and treatment are necessary to preserve limb function.

The cornerstone of treatment of acute arterial embolism is thromboembolectomy using arterial embolectomy catheters. Because the perioperative morbidity and mortality rates for this operation remain high, poor-risk patients such as those who have had an acute myocardial infarction and who are unstable for transport or who have intractable, severe congestive heart failure should be considered for nonoperative treatment with the use of heparin (30).

Although the ease of catheter embolectomy makes such an option appear of little value, treatment of arterial embolism by catheter embolectomy has the highest morbidity and mortality rate of any vascular operation except for the treatment of ruptured aortic aneurysms. This reflects the seriousness of the underlying illnesses that are found in patients experiencing acute arterial embolism. Some have advocated percutaneous catheter suction embolectomy for high-risk patients. This form of therapy has met with some initial limited success.

The technique of catheter embolectomy is a simple one, but this operation still requires careful planning and execution. After prompt heparinization, all patients should be prepared adequately for the operating room by placing a Foley catheter and arterial and central venous pressure catheters as indicated by the patient's condition. In high-risk patients, cardiac status should be optimized, particularly control of arrhythmias or congestive heart failure. The clinician should always bear in mind the possibility of synchronous embolism, particularly embolism to the viscera, which may not initially be associated with clear signs and symptoms of visceral ischemia.

Catheter embolectomy is undertaken through an artery that provides easy access to the embolus and has a low likelihood of postoperative thrombosis. Most commonly, catheter embolectomy is done through the common femoral artery. Most aortic, iliac, superficial femoral, and popliteal artery occlusions can be managed successfully through this vessel. After the common femoral artery is exposed and proximal and distal control is obtained, a longitudinal or transverse arteriotomy is made. The transverse arteriotomy is preferred in patients with small arteries so that closure of the arteriotomy does not narrow the vessel. Because acute and chronic complications can occur as a result of injudicious use of embolectomy catheters, catheters should always be passed gently. Catheters are first passed distally until the arterial tree is free of all clot, and then the profunda and proximal aortoiliac vessels are cleared of emboli. When an infrarenal aortic bifurcation occlusion occurs, bilateral femoral artery incisions are used. When severe ischemia of prolonged duration is present, it may be helpful to vent the first 300 to 500 mL of venous outflow into a cell saver (31). This technique conserves red blood cells and reduces the metabolic consequences of reperfusing a severely ischemic limb. At times, the serum potassium levels are so elevated that they cause cardiac arrest. In addition, the vein parallel to the site of arterial embolectomy should be inspected for venous thrombosis, and venous thrombectomy should be undertaken when clot is found.

When the duration of ischemia has exceeded 4 hours, serious consideration should be given to the use of four-compartment fasciotomy. The consequences of reperfusion of ischemic skeletal muscle are not manifested fully until 12 to 24 hours after operation. Except in patients with congestive heart failure, edema is rarely present at the time of the initial operation. At the completion of the embolectomy, long fasciotomy incisions through relatively small skin incisions can prevent the development of compartment syndrome.

Before leaving the operating room, the patient must have adequate arterial circulation to maintain limb viability and function. This usually can be ascertained adequately by a hand-held continuous-wave Doppler probe evaluation of the pedal pulses. When the viability of the extremity is threatened or when there are poor Doppler signals in the distal extremity, intraoperative arteriography or angioscopy should be performed. Retrieving thrombus from the tibial vessels can be difficult from the common femoral artery. Under these circumstances, passing multiple catheters simultaneously permits separate catheterization of the different tibial vessels. Normally, catheters passed from the common femoral artery toward the foot tend to enter the tibial–peroneal trunk. Leaving the catheter that has passed through the peroneal artery to the level of the ankle in place and then passing a second catheter may allow entry of the second catheter into the posterior tibial artery, and very rarely the anterior tibial artery.

When residual thrombus exists below the popliteal artery, the options are to make a second incision over the popliteal artery or to use intraoperative thrombolytic therapy. Thrombolytic therapy has been shown to be of value in patients with irretrievable clot in small vessels. Angiography is necessary to define the position of the clots so that the catheter can be placed as close to the clot as possible. Thrombolytic therapy is then undertaken for 30 minutes. Concerns remain about the use of fibrinolytic therapy in patients with arterial embolism because lytic therapy can precipitate the release of more emboli, which can have life-threatening consequences.

Upper extremity emboli are treated in a fashion similar to that for emboli of the lower extremity. An incision can often be made directly over the level of arterial occlusion. This usually involves the axillary or proximal brachial artery. It is frequently necessary to expose the brachial artery bifurcation to catheterize the radial and ulnar arteries selectively. Special care should be taken when thrombectomizing the subclavian or axillary artery so that no clot is dislodged into the common carotid artery or vertebral arteries.

After surgery, these patients require careful and close monitoring. They typically have multiple severe underlying medical illnesses and are at risk for complications associated with reperfusion of an ischemic limb (Table 68.2). Thus, the ischemic skeletal muscle can undergo rhabdomyolysis, which results in release of myoglobin into the circulation. Myoglobin can precipitate in the renal tubules, leading to renal tubular obstruction and acute renal failure. In addition, there is loss of capillary membrane integrity resulting in extensive transudation of fluids and electrolytes. This can lead to a compartment syndrome whereby the increased compartment pressures cause neurovascular compression. In addition, there can be severe hyperkalemia and lactic acidosis. These complications can be minimized by the use of fasciotomy, adequate hydration, the administration of mannitol to maintain a renal diuresis, and intravenous sodium bicarbonate sufficient to alkalinize the urine. Alkalinization of the urine reduces the extent of myoglobin precipitation in the renal tubules. Insulin and glucose given intravenously may be necessary for extreme or sudden elevations in serum potassium levels. Heparin is reinstituted 6 to 12 hours after surgery because of a significant incidence of recurrent embolism.

Results

The results of treatment of patients with acute arterial embolism depend on the location of the embolus, the duration and severity of ischemia, and the seriousness of underlying cardiac and pulmonary disease. In spite of the development of the arterial embolectomy catheter by Fogarty, which has greatly simplified the removal of arterial emboli, and despite significant improvements in the perioperative management of acutely ill patients, there has been only modest improvement in morbidity and mortality rates with widespread use of arterial embolectomy. This may reflect the overwhelming impact of the often severe underlying cardiac and pulmonary disease in these patients at the time of the acute arterial embolism. Reports of the results of treatment of patients with acute arterial embolism consistently show a high postoperative mortality rate, ranging between 7.5% and 34% (1,30–36). Amputations are required in approximately 15% of patients after embolectomy.

The major causes of morbidity after arterial embolectomy are myocardial complications, pulmonary complications including pneumonia and pulmonary embolism, renal failure, and synchronous or recurrent arterial emboli. More than half of the deaths after arterial embolectomy are due to myocardial complications (32,35). This is particularly true in patients who present with acute myocardial infarction, ventricular aneurysms, or arrhythmias secondary to atherosclerotic heart disease. The second most common cause of death is pulmonary failure due to either pneumonia or pulmonary embolism. In some series, pulmonary embolism is the second most common cause of death (26). In fact, many instances of pneumonia are thought to be due to underlying pulmonary infarction. This is supported by the study by Darling and associates (19), which showed that 9 of 76 patients who underwent autopsy study after treatment for arterial embolism had pulmonary embolism; in half of these patients, it was the main cause of death. This significant incidence of pulmonary embolism reflects the propensity of these patients to development of deep venous thrombosis, which is estimated to occur in 7% to 27% of patients after arterial embolectomy (27,37).

Other important causes of mortality after arterial embolectomy are renal failure and the cumulative effects of multiple emboli. Acute renal failure is estimated to occur in approximately 11% of patients after arterial embolectomy (33). The mortality rate from acute renal failure after arterial embolectomy is approximately 50%. Finally, an important cause of mortality after arterial embolectomy is the occurrence of synchronous or recurrent arterial embolism. Patients who present with multiple arterial emboli have a substantially increased mortality rate of approximately three times that for patients who present with a single embolus to a limb vessel (4,19,38) (Fig. 68.8). This increased mortality rate is often due to the failure to diagnose a visceral embolus in patients presenting with acute limb ischemia.

Complications and limb loss after arterial embolectomy of the upper extremity are lower than those after embolectomy of the lower extremity (39–42). Mortality rates remain between 10% and 12%, and amputation rates remain at approximately 7%. In addition, although many of the

TABLE 68.2. MANAGEMENT OF SKELETAL MUSCLE REPERFUSION SYNDROME

Clinical manifestation	Treatment
Lactic acidosis	Sodium bicarbonate
Hyperkalemia	Insulin and glucose
Myoglobinuria or acute tubular necrosis	Alkalinization of urine to prevent precipitation of myoglobin in renal tubules
Muscle edema or compartment syndrome	Fasciotomy

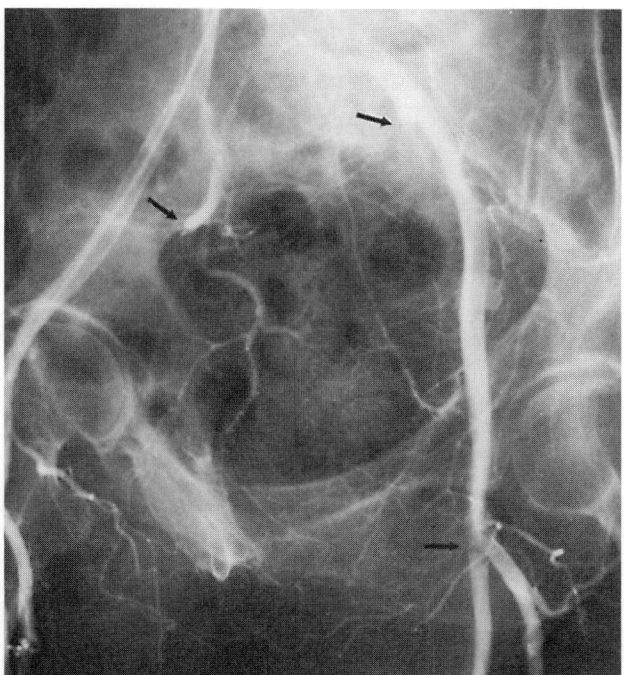

Figure 68.8. Oblique iliac angiogram showing embolic occlusion of the distal right internal iliac artery, the origin of the left internal iliac artery, and the common femoral artery. The patient was also found to have an acute superior mesenteric artery occlusion.

patients do not undergo amputation, as many as one third have a residual severe disability (42). Because of a general impression of reduced mortality and amputation rates in patients with upper extremity arterial embolism, some have advocated nonoperative therapy for many of these patients; nevertheless, Ricotta and associates (41) report a nearly threefold increase in mortality rates in patients treated nonoperatively.

Although the limb salvage rate after arterial embolectomy is usually 85% to 90%, when patients require amputation it most often is at the above-knee level (32,43). In view of the high level of amputation and the frequent presence of severe underlying cardiac disease, most of these patients never ambulate independently again. Amputation rates after arterial embolectomy and mortality rates are both frequently related to the level and duration of arterial occlusion, but many studies do not show a constant relation between these variables. Initially, mortality and amputation rates increase with increasing durations of ischemia up to 24 hours after the onset of occlusion. After that, patients presenting more than 24 hours after their initial event often have lower mortality and amputation rates. This so-called harvesting effect is due to the fact that patients presenting days or weeks after the arterial embolism represent a group who survived the early critical period because they have better native collateral circulation as well as less severe underlying cardiac disease. Thus, timeliness of revascularization remains an important goal in the treatment of patients who have acute arterial embolism, but the most important variables in terms of outcome are the duration and severity of the underlying ischemia.

Recurrence of arterial embolism has an important influence on mortality and limb salvage during the immediate postoperative period, as well as on the long-term prognosis of these patients (1,4,19,44,45). Recurrence rates in patients not receiving anticoagulation vary from 28% to

45.5% (4,19). The incidence of recurrent embolism appears to be more frequent in patients presenting with acute atrial fibrillation than in patients who present with other cardiac abnormalities, such as acute myocardial infarction (19). In addition, 31% to 82% of recurrences happen during the initial hospitalization (44,45). Recurrent embolism has a clear and direct impact on mortality. Mortality rates in general double after each recurrence and are as high as 50% after the third embolic event.

Anticoagulation with heparin or warfarin has been shown convincingly to reduce the rate of recurrent embolism, as well as associated limb loss and mortality. Although heparin reduces the recurrence rate by at least 50% in most studies, significant recurrent embolism occurs even in patients receiving anticoagulation.

Patients receiving anticoagulation after arterial embolectomy had a reduction in early mortality rates in one series, from 51% in untreated patients to 5% in those receiving anticoagulation (32). In addition, the late survival rate was improved from 12% in the untreated patients to 43% in those receiving anticoagulation. Anticoagulation has also been shown to reduce the need for amputation from 38% to 10% in patients treated conservatively without operation (34). In addition, the amputation rate in patients who underwent embolectomy was reduced from 39% to 7% by the addition of anticoagulation in the immediate postoperative period. Most reports show a low complication rate associated with anticoagulation in the immediate postoperative period. On the basis of these results, most patients who have arterial embolism should receive lifelong anticoagulation. Some recommend short-term therapy in those who have arterial embolism after an acute myocardial infarction. Patients with acute myocardial infarction usually are at significant risk for development of arterial embolism for only a short period after the acute infarction. In addition, anticoagulation is probably not necessary for people who have embolism from extracardiac sources, particularly those in whom this source is removed.

Specific complications can occur as a result of the use of balloon catheters in the treatment of arterial embolism. Intimal injury is common after the use of balloon embolectomy catheters. In most patients, this injury is minor and heals spontaneously. Other acute injuries include arterial perforation, vessel wall disruption, the development of arteriovenous fistulae, pseudoaneurysm formation, and the development of arterial stenoses (46). Diffuse arterial narrowing secondary to intimal hyperplasia has been identified increasingly as a delayed complication of balloon catheter embolectomy (46,47) and occurs with increased frequency in women. Excessive shear forces are important in the development of a number of these complications. It is recommended that the physician use the smallest catheter that is effective. Important technical points include never passing the catheter against resistance and never withdrawing it under excessive tension. Although complete embolectomy is important, repetitive passing of the catheter increases the incidence of complications (48).

ATHEROEMBOLISM

Atheroembolism results from the release of cholesterol-rich atheromatous debris from ulcerated atherosclerotic plaques. Most atheroemboli are composed of cholesterol crystals that typically obstruct 200- to 900-μm arterioles. A minority of these emboli are macroemboli that cause large vessel occlusion. Perhaps the most familiar clinical syndrome of atheroembolism is the blue toe syndrome, in which there is obstruction of the digital arteries of the toes. Atheroembolism can have protean clinical manifestations (Fig. 68.9 and Table 68.3), and the diagnosis of atheroembolism is made most frequently at autopsy. Atheroembolism can produce a clinical picture of multisystem organ failure resembling acute polyarteritis nodosa or other acute systemic vasculitides characterized by acute or subacute renal failure, cerebral infarction, retinal embolism, gastrointestinal hemorrhage, pancreatitis, myocardial infarction, and livedo reticularis.

Atheroembolism can occur by at least three mechanisms. It can occur spontaneously, sometimes as a consequence of coughing, tenesmus, or lifting. It can be precipitated by surgical manipulation of the aorta or its major branches. Finally, atheroembolism can be induced by catheter manipulation during angiography.

The true incidence and clinical consequences of atheroembolism remain a matter of conjecture. Florey (49) is responsible for stimulating modern interest in atheroembolism. During an autopsy of a man with extensive aortic atherosclerosis, he first documented atheroembolism to the kidneys, spleen, pancreas, and thyroid. He then reviewed the autopsy findings in 267 patients who had significant aortic atherosclerosis and found a 3.4% incidence of atheroembolism. In patients with advanced degenerative atherosclerosis, the incidence was as high as 12.3%. In a later study by Handler (50) of 77 consecutive autopsies of patients who died with severe atherosclerosis, an incidence of 8.6% was found. This study was also the first to call attention to the relation between renal atheroembolism and the onset of severe episodic hypertension and subacute renal failure. Thurlbeck and Castleman (51) found a 77% incidence of atheroembolism to the kidneys in an autopsy study of 22 patients who died after aortic reconstruction during the 1950s at Massachusetts General

TABLE 68.3. LABORATORY ABNORMALITIES ASSOCIATED WITH MULTIPLE CHOLESTEROL EMBOLI

Elevated erythrocyte sedimentation rate
Eosinophilia
Leukocytosis
Abnormal urinalysis—proteinuria, hematuria, albuminuria, granular or hyaline casts
Elevated amylase
Elevated creatinine phosphokinase, aldolase
Azotemia
Findings of disseminated intravascular coagulopathy (rare)
Biopsy of skin, muscle, or kidney—cholesterol clefts in small arteries

From Kalter DC, Rudolph A, McGavran M. Livedo reticularis due to multiple cholesterol emboli. J Am Acad Dermatol 1985;13:235.

Hospital. A similarly high incidence of atheroembolism was found at autopsy in patients dying with unruptured aortic aneurysms. There was no evidence of atheroembolism in age-matched control subjects who had minimal atherosclerosis. Studies of necropsies on all patients older than 60 years of age showed that the overall incidence of atheroembolism was 0.8% (52). Most patients were men whose average age was 76.7 years; 100% had hypertension. In each case of documented atheroembolism, the aorta showed advanced atherosclerosis, sometimes associated with aneurysmal degeneration.

Pathophysiology

Atheroembolism results from the sudden rupture of an atherosclerotic plaque, resulting in showers of cholesterol-rich atheromatous debris into the distal arterial circulation. Depending on the size and concentration of particles, these emboli can either pass through the microcirculation or obstruct a microvessel. Most episodes of atheroembolism probably do not result in any detectable clinical sequelae. When the mass of embolus is large, tissue infarction occurs. Cholesterol microemboli can be identified histologically as biconvex, needle-shaped clefts in the arterial lumen (Fig. 68.10). The birefringent crystals themselves are dissolved during the fixation process unless special techniques are used to preserve them. Thus, in routine fixation procedures, the examiner sees the shape of the space they occupied, rather than the crystals themselves. These microemboli are found jammed at the arterial bifurcations with red cells and fibrin adherent to their surface. Typically, the obstructed arteriole is 100 to 900 μm in diameter (average, 200 μm). At this early stage, the emboli project irregularly into the lumen of the microvessels and have a jagged shape with sharp outlines. Evidence of an acute inflammatory response is found. Intermediate stages are characterized by endothelial and fibroplastic proliferation, an occasional giant cell reaction, and a perivascular lymphocytic infiltration. The surface of the embolus appears smooth and is partially covered with a neoendothelium. The emboli gradually become incorporated into the vessel wall, and eventually an obliterative endarteritis, including intimal and medial thickening and fibrosis, occurs. Cholesterol crystals that have penetrated through the microvessel walls incite a perivascular granulomatous inflammation. Occasionally, a necrotizing angiitis similar to polyarteritis nodosa is present. Both in vitro and in vivo studies have shown that atherosclerotic plaques, particularly ulcerated plaques in which crystalline cholesterol is exposed to circulating plasma, provoke a complement-mediated neutrophil aggregation and

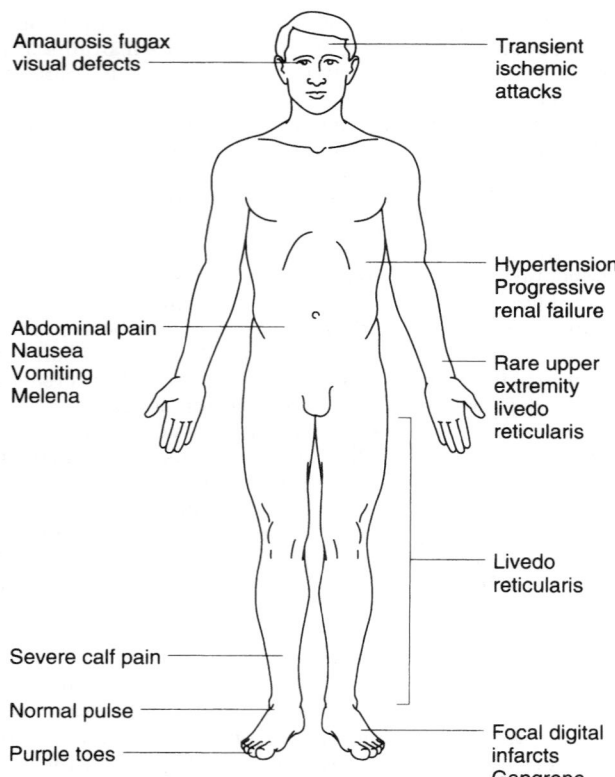

Figure 68.9. Clinical manifestations of multiple cholesterol emboli. (After Kalter DC, Rudolph A, McGavran M. Livedo reticularis due to multiple cholesterol emboli. *J Am Acad Dermatol* 1985;13:235.)

Amaurosis fugax visual defects
Transient ischemic attacks
Hypertension Progressive renal failure
Abdominal pain Nausea Vomiting Melena
Rare upper extremity livedo reticularis
Livedo reticularis
Severe calf pain
Normal pulse
Purple toes
Focal digital infarcts Gangrene

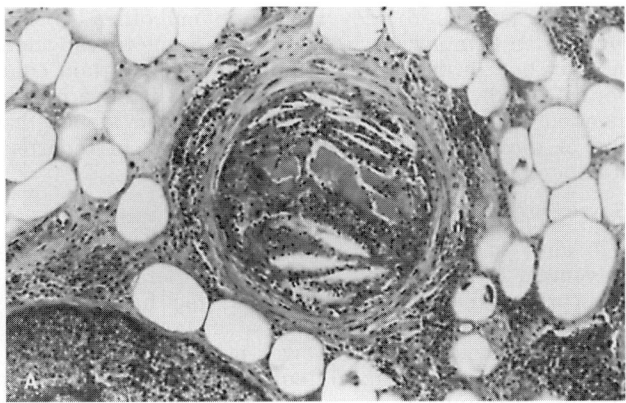

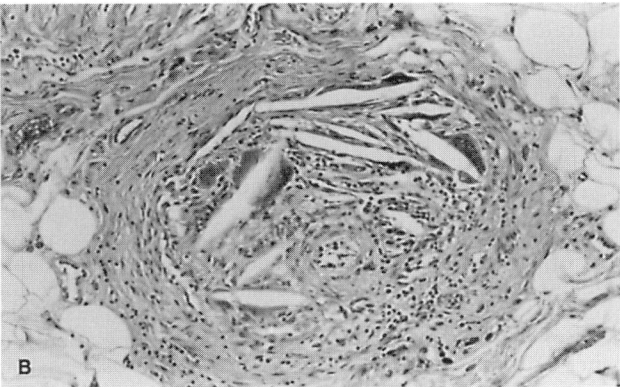

Figure 68.10. *(A)* Fresh atheroembolism. Cholesterol crystals *(clear spaces)* and amorphous debris from a distant atherosclerotic plaque largely occlude this small arterial branch in the colon. Hematoxylin–eosin, ×235. *(B)* Old atheroembolism. Much of the embolus has been organized, but cholesterol crystals remain, with an associated giant cell reaction. Hematoxylin–eosin, ×235. (Courtesy of J. Abrams, M.D., Department of Pathology, University of Michigan Medical School, Ann Arbor, MI.)

inflammatory vasculitis (53). Patients with cholesterol embolism syndrome have been shown to have high levels of activated complement cofactors. In addition, it causes aggregation of normal neutrophils, possibly sharing a common mechanism with other causes of vasculitis.

Specific Clinical Syndromes

Arterial Catheter-related Atheroembolism

Atheroembolism can be a serious complication of angiography that is undertaken for diagnostic or therapeutic indications. The frequency of atheroembolism during angiography is unknown. Undoubtedly, many episodes of atheroembolism are asymptomatic. When clinically significant episodes of atheroembolism do occur, they often are not identified correctly because of failure to recognize the clinical syndrome. Thus, the larger and more rigid catheters used for balloon angioplasty have greater potential for dislodging cholesterol emboli. In addition, transfemoral catheterization is associated with a higher incidence of complications than transbrachial catheterization because of the necessity for the transfemoral catheters to traverse the diseased abdominal aorta.

In a retrospective study of autopsy findings of patients who died soon after coronary angiography, it was found that approximately 30% had evidence of atheroembolism (54). In a series of 70 aged-matched control subjects who

had diffuse atherosclerosis but had not undergone angiography, the incidence of atheroembolism was only 4.3%. Thus, this study confirms the suspicion that cholesterol embolism is common during angiography. Because of a delay in the appearance of complications after angiography, a true appreciation of the clinical significance of these complications has not occurred.

A variety of clinical manifestations can be seen after atheroembolism during angiography, but the most commonly involved organ is the kidney. Other common signs of atheroembolism in these patients include the appearance of livedo reticularis and digital infarction in the feet. When diffuse atheroembolism occurs, a clinical picture of episodic or sustained hypertension, fever, and eosinophilia can be seen. The diagnosis of renal cholesterol embolism after angiography can be difficult. The overall incidence of nephrotoxicity after angiography is approximately 2% in nonazotemic patients and 33% in azotemic patients. The patterns of nephrotoxicity in contrast-induced renal failure and in renal atheroembolism are different. Contrast-induced nephrotoxicity is usually apparent by elevation of the serum creatinine level within 48 hours of angiography, which reaches its peak 1 week after angiography and usually returns to baseline levels after several weeks in most patients. In contrast, acute renal failure after renal atheroembolism often occurs over a more prolonged time. In most cases, it is usually not clinically detectable until 1 to 4 weeks after angiography, and then it often pursues a downhill course over the next several weeks (55). There is no effective therapy for any form of atheroembolism; however, it is important to distinguish between the two forms of renal failure after angiography to provide an accurate prognosis for the patient, and to limit any future angiographic procedures in these patients.

Lower Extremity Atheroembolism

Lower extremity atheroembolism is manifested by sharply demarcated areas of focal ischemia of the lower leg or foot, typically in the toes (Fig. 68.9). Livedo reticularis can be seen to a variable extent, sometimes extending from the umbilicus to the feet. Thigh and calf myalgias are common and are secondary to atheroembolism of the muscle. The areas of focal ischemia are usually characterized by purplish discoloration of the skin and surrounding petechial hemorrhages (Fig. 68.11). These lesions together represent the so-called blue toe syndrome. Characteristically, these lesions are intensely painful. The areas of bluish discoloration sometimes resemble localized bruising and often are misdiagnosed by both patients and physicians unfamiliar with the syndrome. Pedal pulses may or may not be present.

Atheroembolism of the lower extremities can also result in large vessel obstruction, producing a clinical picture that is indistinguishable from emboli of cardiac origin (Fig. 68.3). Usually the diagnosis is not made until the time of inspection of the embolus. Although the immediate clinical course after atheromatous macroembolism is the same as that for patients after embolism of cardiac thrombus, these patients must undergo angiography to identify the responsible plaque.

The natural history of microembolism of the extremities is one of repetitive events if left untreated (56). More than half of the patients have additional complications. Nearly 40% of patients with atheroembolism of an extremity experience some degree of tissue loss. Major amputations are necessary in approximately 25% of patients. Long-term follow-up shows that up to 20% of these patients die within 1 year of their event. This high mortality rate underlies the severity of the diffuse atherosclerosis in these patients. Because of this poor outlook for patients experi-

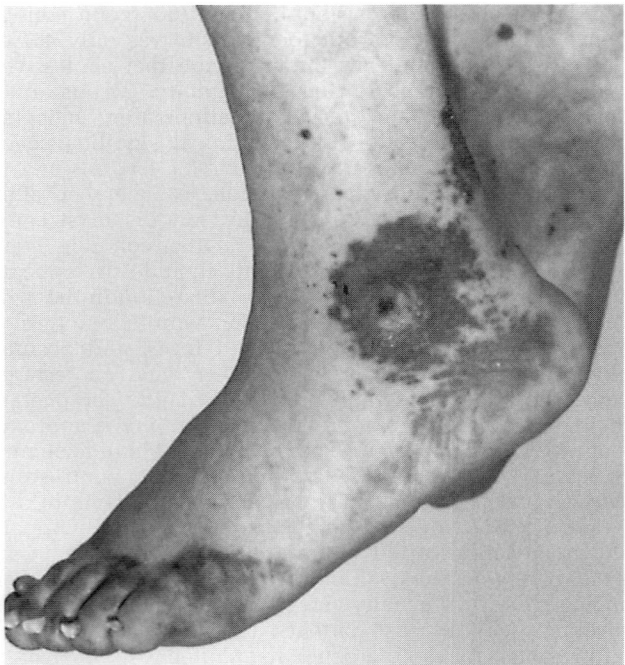

Figure 68.11. Feet of a patient with spontaneous atheroembolism. Well circumscribed areas of skin discoloration and petechial hemorrhages are visible.

encing extremity atheroembolism, they should undergo prompt arteriography to delineate possible sources of the emboli. It is important to obtain lateral and oblique films of the aorta and its branches because many of these lesions are subtle, located on the lateral or posterior walls of the arteries. Although early reports identified aortic lesions, specifically aortic aneurysms, as the most common source of atheroembolism, more recent reports show that the most common source of embolism has been stenotic or ulcerated lesions, or both, of the distal superficial femoral artery (57,58). In addition, many of these patients have vascular occlusive disease on angiography, which is consistent with reports that show that approximately half have abnormal pulses. Thus, the emboli can readily pass through collaterals around chronic occlusions of large vessels.

Treatment of arterial lesions identified by arteriography as responsible for the emboli is removal of the lesion by endarterectomy or excision of the diseased portion of the vessel. When these techniques cannot be used, bypass and exclusion of the lesion is an alternative approach. Occasionally there are proximal and distal lesions identified by angiography that could be potentially embologenic. Usually, the lesion that appears more ulcerated and thus more likely to be an embolic source is removed, or, if there are no distinguishing features between multiple lesions, the more distal lesions are removed. Lumbar sympathectomy can be valuable as an adjunctive measure to relieve the cutaneous ischemia, particularly in those patients in whom the arterial source cannot be identified or removed.

There is no effective drug therapy for atheroembolism. Dextran, intraarterial vasodilators, and sympathetic blockers have been used without clear benefit. Some have advocated anticoagulation in these patients. The evidence is contradictory in that there are many reports in which these lesions developed in patients soon after the institution of warfarin therapy for some other purpose. Thus, warfarin itself has been implicated as an etiologic or pre-

cipitating factor in the development of embolism by causing sudden hemorrhage into a plaque. Some investigators believe that fibrin platelet emboli are an important component of atheroembolism and on this basis have recommended antiplatelet therapy. There is no evidence that any of these drugs reduces the incidence of recurrent atheroembolism.

Gastrointestinal Microembolism

In view of the predominance of abdominal organ involvement in most autopsy studies of atheroembolism, it is surprising that the gastrointestinal tract has been mentioned relatively infrequently as a separate clinical syndrome. The stomach, small bowel, pancreas, and gallbladder have been affected most frequently by atheroembolism to the gastrointestinal tract. Pathologic studies have shown that atheroembolism usually causes occlusion of multiple submucosal arterioles, which leads to variable degrees of mucosal ischemia. Transmural necrosis of the gut wall can develop, or there can be a pattern of diffuse ulceration. These ulcers undergo cycles of healing and breakdown. Eventually, some ulcers become contracted and fibrotic.

The most common clinical manifestations of atheroembolism to the gastrointestinal tract are diffuse abdominal pain, paralytic ileus, bleeding, and, rarely, small bowel obstruction. Atheroembolism has been implicated as a cause of pancreatitis in patients who have normal biliary and pancreatic ducts. Autopsy studies have shown a correlation between the intensity of the parenchymal evidence of pancreatitis and the degree of associated atherosclerosis in the aorta. Atheroembolism has also been implicated as a cause of perforation of the intestine and gallbladder. Finally, some have drawn an association between cholesterol embolism and the development of angiodysplasia. Cholesterol crystals have been found in areas of angiodysplasia, suggesting that there may be a causal relation. According to this hypothesis, the angiodysplasia is thought to occur as a response of the microvessels to ischemia. In addition, atheroembolism has been implicated as the linking mechanism in patients who are known to have aortic stenosis and gastrointestinal bleeding secondary to angiodysplasia of the right colon (59). Biopsy in one of these patients showed, in addition to cholesterol emboli and granuloma formation, subepithelial ectasia of vessels and epithelial atrophy. No effective treatment for atheroembolism to the gastrointestinal tract, other than resection of the involved portion, has been developed. Most reports of patients with gastrointestinal involvement secondary to atheroembolism have been autopsy studies.

Coronary Atheroembolism

Atheroembolism of the coronary arteries can cause acute myocardial infarction. It has been reported to occur during cardiopulmonary resuscitation, after strenuous exercise, and, more recently, as a cause of perioperative myocardial infarction during coronary artery bypass grafting. As in other parts of the arterial circulation, atheroembolism results from plaque rupture and the release of cholesterol crystals and other atheromatous debris into the circulation. Histologically, there are areas of arteriolar obstruction. There is an inflammatory response in the vessel walls that is characterized in its later stages by eosinophilic infiltration. The vasculitis is attributed to a hypersensitivity reaction to noncholesterol constituents of atheroma. In patients dying of acute myocardial infarction secondary to coronary atheroembolism, different-aged microinfarcts are found in the myocardium, thus confirming the episodic nature of these emboli before the terminal infarction. In addition, atheroembolism has been shown to be an important cause of perioperative myocardial infarction after coronary artery bypass grafting. In one report, 13 fatal cases of perioperative myocardial infarction after coronary artery bypassing were thought to be secondary to intraoperative atheromatous embolism during manipulation of vein grafts (60). In somewhat less than half the cases, the emboli originated from ulcerations of the aortic root rather than the proximal coronary artery. The overall incidence of perioperative myocardial infarction secondary to atheroembolism is approximately 0.22% during redo coronary artery bypass grafting. This increased risk of coronary atheroembolism during cardiac surgery was identified in patients who had severe graft atherosclerosis, rather than in patients who had intimal hyperplasia as a cause of recurrent graft stenosis. To minimize this complication, it has been recommended that the distal vein graft be ligated as early as possible during redo operations.

Renal Atheroembolism

The most frequent organ affected by atheroembolism is the kidney. It is estimated by autopsy studies that renal atheroembolism is found in up to 4% of patients who have minimal aortic atherosclerosis and in 15% of those who have severe aortic atherosclerosis. Histologically, there is extensive occlusion of the arcuate and interlobar arteries, and there can be hyalinization of glomeruli. Variable degrees of inflammatory response in vessel walls, as well as around cholesterol that is outside of vessel walls, can be seen. Renal atheroembolism can be a complication of angiography, it can be a result of manipulation of the aorta or its branches during surgery, or it can occur as a spontaneous event. The clinical picture can be one of acute, subacute, or chronic renal failure. Typically, a patient presents with a recent onset of episodic hypertension or an exacerbation of preexisting hypertension. In a minority of patients, renal atheroemboli do not cause hypertension. An elevated erythrocyte sedimentation rate, peripheral eosinophilia, and urine containing increased protein, white blood cells, and red blood cells can be seen. In general, the prognosis for patients with renal failure secondary to atheroembolism has been poor; only a few cases of reversal of renal failure and survival have been reported. The diagnosis is suspected by identifying predisposing factors of the patients who present with subacute renal failure. Renal biopsy can be performed to confirm the diagnosis. Some have recommended punch biopsy of any skin lesion suspect for atheroembolism. In the event that the patient recovers from the renal failure, under appropriate clinical circumstances angiography should be done to see if the offending lesion can be removed. For others, management involves appropriate use of dialysis and the treatment of hypertension.

Diffuse Atheroembolism

Diffuse atheroembolism results from showers of cholesterol emboli sufficient to obstruct the microcirculation of multiple organs. Diffuse atheroembolism can mimic many other illnesses, especially polyarteritis nodosa. Many cases of diffuse atheroembolism are misdiagnosed as systemic necrotizing vasculitis, and its true incidence remains unknown. Diffuse atheroembolism is not a rare finding in autopsy studies of patients with severe atherosclerotic disease of the aorta. This syndrome is typically found in patients in the sixth and seventh decades of life who have other manifestations of atherosclerosis. Common signs and symptoms are abdominal pain, lower extremity pain, livedo reticularis, blue toes, neurologic dysfunction, melena, and azotemia. Acute or chronic renal failure can be present. Laboratory studies show an elevated erythrocyte sedimentation rate, hematuria, thrombocytopenia, and depletion of complement. The differential diagnosis includes infectious etiologies, especially bacterial endocarditis, disseminated neoplasm, and vasculitis. Diagnosis is made on clinical suspicion of the syndrome as well as on biopsy of the skin, muscle, or kidney. Angiography should be considered with great caution because this can induce further complications. Again, there is no specific treatment for this disorder. The aortic atherosclerosis is usually diffuse, extending over the thoracic and abdominal aorta. Thoracoabdominal aortic resection is often required. The prognosis of patients with atheroembolism is dismal. The mean interval of survival to death was an average of 2.2 months among 53 patients reported in the literature. In one series, all patients were dead within 6 months of diagnosis (61).

REFERENCES

1. Abbott WM, Maloney RD, McCabe CC, et al. Arterial embolism: a 44-year perspective. *Am J Surg* 1982;143:460.
2. Stallone RJ, Blaisdell FW, Caferata HT, et al. Analysis of morbidity and mortality from arterial embolectomy. *Surgery* 1969;65:207.
3. MacGowan WAL, Mooneeram R. A review of 174 patients with arterial embolism. *Br J Surg* 1973;60:694.
4. Elliott JP Jr, Hageman JH, Szilagyi E, et al. Arterial embolization: problems of source, multiplicity, recurrence, and delayed treatment. *Surgery* 1980;88:833.
5. AbuRahma AF, Richmond BK, Robinson PA. Etiology of peripheral arterial thromboembolism in young patients. *Am J Surg* 1998;176:158.
6. Petersen P. Thromboembolic complications in atrial fibrillation. *Stroke* 1990;21:4.
7. Petersen P, Boysen G, Godtfredsen J, et al. Placebo-controlled, randomised trial of warfarin and aspirin for prevention of thromboembolic complications in chronic atrial fibrillation: the Copenhagen AFASK Study. *Lancet* 1989;1:175.
8. Risk factors for stroke and efficacy of antithrombotic therapy in atrial fibrillation: pooled data from five randomized controlled trials. *Arch Intern Med* 1994;154:1449.
9. Arvan S. Mural thrombi in coronary artery disease: recent advances in pathogenesis, diagnosis, and approaches to treatment. *Arch Intern Med* 1984;144:113.
10. Puletti M, Cusmano E, Testa MG, et al. Incidence of systemic thromboembolic lesions in acute myocardial infarction. *Clin Cardiol* 1986;9:331.
11. Kontny F, Dale J, Abildgaard U, et al. Randomized trial of low molecular weight heparin (dalteparin) in prevention of left ventricular thrombus formation and arterial embolism after acute anterior myocardial infarction: the Fragmin in Acute Myocardial Infarction (FRAMI) study. *J Am Coll Cardiol* 1997;30:962.
12. Reeder GS, Lengyel M, Tajik AJ, et al. Mural thrombus in left ventricular aneurysm: incidence, role of angiography, and relation between anticoagulation and embolization. *Mayo Clin Proc* 1981;56:77.
13. Fairfax AJ, Lambert CD, Leatham A. Systemic embolism in chronic sinoatrial disorder. *N Engl J Med* 1976;295:190.
14. Chiang CW, Lo SK, Ko YS, et al. Predictors of systemic embolism in patients with mitral stenosis: a prospective study. *Ann Intern Med* 1998;128:885.
15. Blackshear JL, Pearce LA, Hart RG, et al. Aortic plaque in atrial fibrillation: prevalence, predictors, and thromboembolic implications. *Stroke* 1999;30:834.
16. Lau LD, Blanchard DG, Hye RJ. Diagnosis and management of patients with peripheral macroemboli from thoracic aortic pathology. *Ann Vasc Surg* 1999;11:348.
17. Vermillion BD, Kimins SA, Pace WG, et al. A review of 147 popliteal aneurysms with long-term follow-up. *Surgery* 1981;90:1009.
18. Prioleau PG, Katzenstein AA. Major peripheral arterial occlusion due to malignant tumor embolism: histologic recognition and surgical management. *Cancer* 1978;42:2009.
19. Darling RC, Austen WG, Linton RR. Arterial embolism. *Surg Gynecol Obstet* 1967;124:106.

20. Hoxie HJ, Coggin CB. Renal infarction: statistical study of 205 cases and detailed report of unusual case. *Arch Intern Med* 1949;65:587.

21. Messina LM, Faulkner JA. The skeletal muscle. In: Zelenock GB, D'Alecy LG, Fantone JC, et al., eds. *Clinical ischemic syndromes*. St. Louis: Mosby, 1990:457.

22. Haberg H. Intracellular pH during ischemia in skeletal muscle: relationship to membrane potential, extracellular pH, tissue lactic acid, and TNP. *Pflugers Arch* 1985;404:342.

23. Harris K, Walker PM, Mickle AG, et al. Metabolic response of skeletal muscle to ischemia. *Am J Physiol* 1986;250:H213.

24. Messina LM. In vivo assessment of microvascular injury after reperfusion of ischemic anterior tibialis of the hamster. *Surg Res* 1990;48:615.

25. Chin AK, Fogarty TJ. Management of arterial emboli: gleanings from 20 years of experience. *Postgrad Med* 1987;81:271.

26. Haimovici H. Arterial embolism. In: Haimovici H, ed. *The surgical management of vascular diseases*. Philadelphia: JB Lippincott, 1970:71.

27. Eastcott HHG. Embolism. In: Eastcott HGG, ed. *Arterial surgery*, 2nd ed. Philadelphia: JB Lippincott, 1973:258.

28. Cambria RP, Abbott WM. Acute arterial thrombosis of the lower extremity: its natural history contrasted with arterial embolism. *Arch Surg* 1984;119:784.

29. Wright JG, Kerr JC, Valeri R, et al. Heparin decreases ischemia-reperfusion injury in isolated canine gracilis muscle. *Arch Surg* 1988;123:470.

30. Blaisdell FW, Steele M, Allen RE. Management of acute lower extremity arterial ischemia due to embolism and thrombosis. *Surgery* 1978;84:822.

31. Tawes RL, Harris EJ, Brown WH, et al. Arterial thromboembolism: a 20-year perspective. *Arch Surg* 1985;120:595.

32. Takolander R, Lannerstad O, Bergqvist D. Peripheral arterial embolectomy, risks, and results. *Acta Chir Scand* 1988;154:567.

33. Bugge M, Jelnes R, Arendrup H, et al. Arterial embolism of the legs and follow-up study of 252 patients. *Ann Chir Gynaecol* 1985;74:137.

34. Baxter-Smith D, Ashton F, Slaney G. Peripheral arterial embolism: a 20-year review. *J Cardiovasc Surg* 1988;29:453.

35. Murie JA, Mathieson M. Arterial embolectomy in the leg: results in a referral hospital. *J Cardiovasc Surg* 1987;28:184.

36. Surowiec SM, Isiklar H, Sreeram S, et al. Acute occlusion of the abdominal aorta. *Am J Surg* 1998;176:193.

37. Fogarty TJ. Arterial embolism. In: Dale A, ed. *Management of arterial occlusive disease*. Chicago: Yearbook Medical, 1971:329.

38. Jivegard L, Holm J, Schersten T. Acute limb ischemia due to arterial embolism or thrombosis: influence of limb ischemia versus pre-existing cardiac disease on postoperative mortality rate. *J Cardiovasc Surg* 1988;29:32.

39. Banis JC Jr, Rich N, Col MC, et al. Ischemia of the upper extremity due to noncardiac emboli. *Am J Surg* 1977;134:131.

40. Kretz JG, Weiss E, Limuris A, et al. Arterial emboli of the upper extremity: a persisting problem. *J Cardiovasc Surg* 1984;25:233.

41. Ricotta JJ, Scudder PA, McAndrew JA, et al. Management of acute ischemia of the upper extremity. *Am J Surg* 1983;145:661.

42. Baird RJ, Lajos TZ. Emboli of the arm. *Ann Surg* 1964;160:905.

43. Hight DW, Tilney NL, Couch NP. Changing clinical trends in patients with peripheral arterial emboli. *Surgery* 1976;79:172.

44. Green RM, DeWeese JA, Rob CG. Arterial embolectomy before and after the Fogarty catheter. *Surgery* 1975;77:24.

45. Silvers LW, Royster TS, Mulcare RJ. Peripheral arterial emboli and factors in their recurrence rate. *Ann Surg* 1980;192:232.

46. Schwarcz TH, Dobrin PB, Mrkvicka R, et al. Balloon embolectomy catheter-induced arterial injury: a comparison of four catheters. *J Vasc Surg* 1990;11:382.

47. Bowles CR, Olcott CW, Pakter RL, et al. Diffuse arterial narrowing as a result of intimal proliferation: a delayed complication with the Fogarty catheter. *J Vasc Surg* 1988;7:487.

48. Dobrin PB. Mechanisms and prevention of arterial injuries caused by balloon embolectomy. *Surgery* 1989;106:457.

49. Florey CM. Arterial occlusions produced by emboli from eroded aortic atheromatous plaques. *Am J Pathol* 1945;21:549.

50. Handler FP. Clinical and pathologic significance of atheromatous embolization, with emphasis on an etiology of renal hypertension. *Am J Med* 1956;20:366.

51. Thurlbeck WM, Castleman B. Atheromatous emboli to the kidneys after aortic surgery. *N Engl J Med* 1957;257:442.

52. Kealy WF. Atheroembolism. *J Clin Pathol* 1978;31:984.

53. Hammerschmidt DE, Greenberg CS, Yamada O, et al. Cholesterol and atheroma lipids activate complement and stimulate granulocytes: a possible mechanism for amplification of ischemic injury in atherosclerotic states. *J Lab Clin Med* 1981;98:68.

54. Ramirez G, O'Neill WM, Lambert R, et al. Cholesterol embolization: a complication of angiography. *Arch Intern Med* 1978;138:1430.

55. Smith MC, Ghose MK, Henry AR. The clinical spectrum of renal cholesterol embolization. *Am J Med* 1981;71:174.

56. Wingo JP, Nix ML, Greenfield LJ, et al. The blue toe syndrome: hemodynamics and therapeutic correlates outcome. *J Vasc Surg* 1986;3:475.

57. Mehigan JT, Stoney RJ. Lower extremity atheromatous embolization. *Am J Surg* 1976;132:163.

58. Karmody AM, Popwers SR, Monaco VJ, et al. "Blue toe" syndrome. *Arch Surg* 1976;111:1263.

59. Bank S, Aftalion B, Anfang C, et al. Acquired angiodysplasia as a cause of gastric hemorrhage: a possible consequence of cholesterol embolization. *Am J Gastroenterol* 1983;78:206.

60. Keon WJ, Heggtveit HA, Leduc J. Perioperative myocardial infarction caused by atheroembolism. *J Thorac Cardiovasc Surg* 1982;84:849.

61. Kaufman JL, Stark K, Brolin RB. Disseminated atheroembolism from extensive degenerative atherosclerosis of the aorta. *Surgery* 1987;102:63.

SURGERY: SCIENTIFIC PRINCIPLES AND PRACTICE, Third Edition, edited by Lazar J. Greenfield, Michael W. Mulholland, Keith T. Oldham, Gerald B. Zelenock, and Keith D. Lillemoe. Lippincott Williams & Wilkins Publishers, Philadelphia, © 2001.

CHAPTER 69

ARTERIAL COMPRESSION SYNDROMES

LLOYD A. JACOBS

Extrinsic compression of vascular structures can produce ischemic injury and ultimately cellular death, leading to organ or extremity dysfunction or loss. Vascular compression syndromes are a heterogeneous group of clinical entities, including some that are poorly described and others whose very existence is controversial. Some are well described and well understood but are uncommon or rare. Still others, such as closed compartment syndromes, are common and important to recognize because they profoundly affect clinical outcomes.

Anomalous muscle, tendinous slips, and congenital osseous abnormalities all can produce extrinsic compression of vascular structures, as can acquired conditions such as osteophytes, various cystic structures, benign and malignant tumors, and a host of other conditions. No catalogue of vascular compression syndromes can be exhaustive because the compressing structures can occur in unpredictable patterns. Representative vascular compression syndromes include the thoracic outlet syndrome (TOS), vertebral artery compression syndrome, popliteal artery entrapment syndromes, and vascular compression syndromes caused by increased soft tissue pressure in a closed compartment.

THORACIC OUTLET SYNDROMES

Thoracic outlet syndrome occurs when upper extremity neurovascular structures are impinged on by bones or ligaments in the anatomically complex and congested thoracic outlet or in the costal clavicular space (Fig. 69.1). Such compression is usually due to distinct congenital or acquired abnormalities, but occasionally typical symptoms of TOS occur without any demonstrable abnormality (1–4). Skeletal abnormalities such as a cervical rib, an elongated C-7 transverse process, congenital anomalies of the scalene muscles, or abnormal fibromuscular bands can contribute. Acquired lesions such as excessive callus formation or deformity from a clavicular fracture can also produce TOS. Finally, cervical trauma such as the whiplash deceleration injury can be associated with symptoms of TOS. At times, a demonstrable anatomic abnormality may not be apparent or is extremely subtle. An atypically located scalene tubercle, a hypertrophied or overly broad insertion of the anterior scalene muscle, and a fibrotic, foreshortened scalene muscle can all contribute to TOS (Fig. 69.2). A hypoplastic or anomalous first thoracic rib can also set the stage for TOS. Many patients with TOS have multiple anomalies. A small group of patients has been described in whom compression of the axillary artery by the humeral head developed during the subluxation that occurs during some athletic activities.

Thoracic outlet syndrome has been such classified as arterial TOS, venous TOS, and neurogenic TOS. Irritation of the brachial plexus is by far the most common presentation of TOS and produces symptoms that are classified in accordance with the nerves and nerve roots involved. Compression of the lower portion of the brachial plexus produces symptoms in the ulnar nerve distribution, whereas compression of the upper portion of the brachial plexus is more likely to produce symptoms in the distribution of the radial nerve. Occasionally, both distributions are involved and there may be associated neck, back, anterior chest, and posterior paraspinous symptoms as well.

Venous compression can produce an acute axillary or subclavian vein thrombosis. A chronic picture has also been described that is characterized by intermittent venous obstruction with an increase in upper extremity volume and cyanosis associated with particular movements. The acute complication has been related to periods of strenuous physical activity and is sometimes termed *effort thrombosis*. As this term implies, thrombosis is often preceded by unusually strenuous activity. Acute thrombosis causes pain, cyanosis, and edema and can lead to chronic upper extremity venous insufficiency or, uncommonly, can cause pulmonary embolism. The acute symptoms lessen as compensatory circulation is established.

Arterial complications of thoracic outlet obstruction are the least common of the types outlined earlier but have the

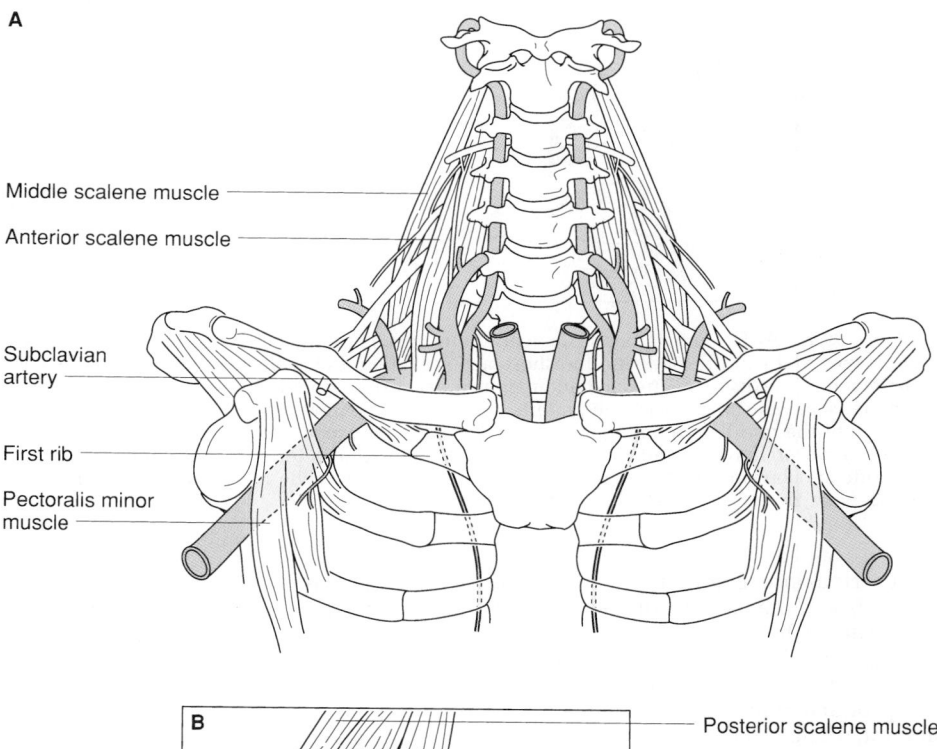

A

Middle scalene muscle

Anterior scalene muscle

Subclavian artery

First rib

Pectoralis minor muscle

B

Posterior scalene muscle

Middle scalene muscle

Anterior scalene muscle

Subclavian artery

Subclavian vein

First rib

Figure 69.1. The normal anatomy of the thoracic outlet in anteroposterior *(A)* and oblique *(B)* views. The brachial plexus and subclavian artery traverse the narrow triangle formed by the anterior and middle scalene muscles and the first rib. The subclavian vein lies anteriorly. (After Zelenock GB. Nonpenetrating subclavian artery injuries. *Arch Surg* 1985;120:685, with permission.)

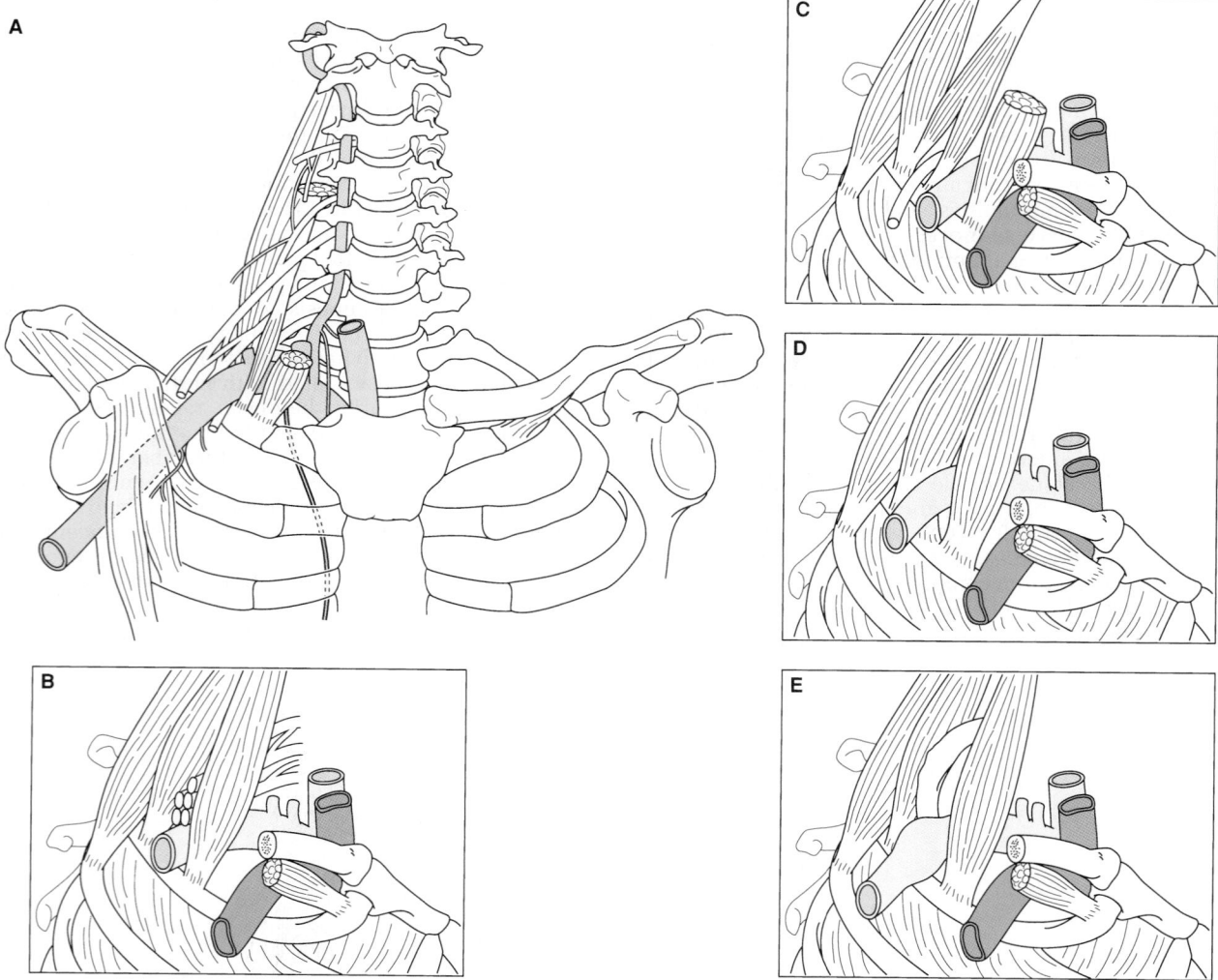

Figure 69.2. *(A)* The anomalous scalene minimus muscle can irritate lower brachial plexus trunks. *(B)* Hypertrophied, fibrosed, and foreshortened scalene muscles elevate the first rib and compress the brachial plexus. *(C)* Unnamed anomalous muscle slips from either the anterior or middle scalene muscle can cause a variable pattern of nerve root compression. *(D)* A broad insertion of the tendon of the middle scalene muscle along the superior aspect of the first rib. *(E)* An anomalous cervical rib or fibrous band is the most common cause of arterial compression. Note the poststenotic subclavian artery aneurysm (see Fig. 69.3). (After Wylie EJ. *Manual of vascular surgery,* vol 2. New York: Springer-Verlag, 1986, with permission.)

most serious prognostic implications (Fig. 69.3). Approximately 5% of the patients operated on for TOS have symptoms related to arterial compression. Long-standing and repeated compressive trauma to the subclavian artery can lead to arterial injury with intimal abnormalities, which can produce stenosis or thrombosis. Alternatively, poststenotic dilatation or even aneurysm can occur and can be complicated by embolism or thrombosis. Distal microembolism can produce Raynaud-like phenomena, petechiae, or necrosis of the fingertips. On occasion, the poststenotic dilatation can become significantly aneurysmal, and a pulsatile supraclavicular mass can be the presenting complaint. Arterial complications are almost always secondary to long-standing compression, usually by a bony abnormality, most commonly in the costoscalene passage and somewhat less frequently in the costoclavicular passage of the artery (1).

In the group of patients with TOS who manifest arterial compression, cervical ribs are common. A complete cervi-

cal rib articulates anteriorly to the superior aspect of the first thoracic rib, usually just behind the insertion of the anterior scalene muscle. Incomplete short cervical ribs can be free floating but invariably are associated with a dense fibrous band that follows the same anatomic course as a complete cervical rib. They have been demonstrated to cause arterial compression. Congenital anomalies of the first thoracic rib are also frequently associated with arterial complications. The most common abnormality is an incomplete first thoracic rib with articulation of its anterior end to the superior aspect of the second thoracic rib. In this situation, the first thoracic rib may be mobile and readily moved by the anterior scalene muscle. Uncommon abnormalities in this area include a bifid first rib or an abnormal tubercle of the first thoracic rib, which can cause compression of the subclavian artery. Congenital bands can also cause arterial compression in this area.

Physical examination findings in patients with acute arterial or venous thrombosis should be obvious. For the for-

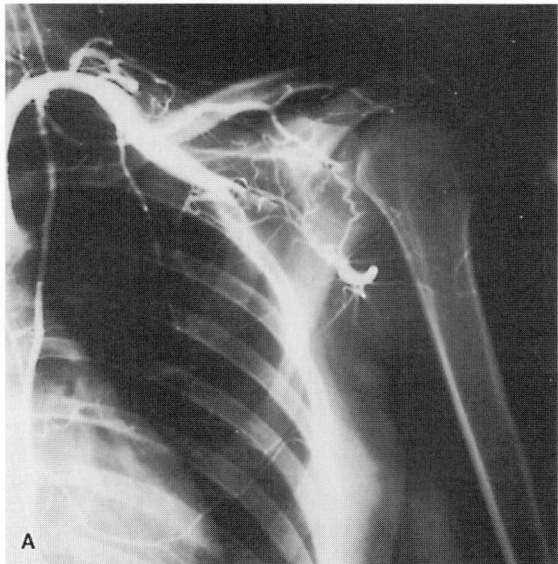

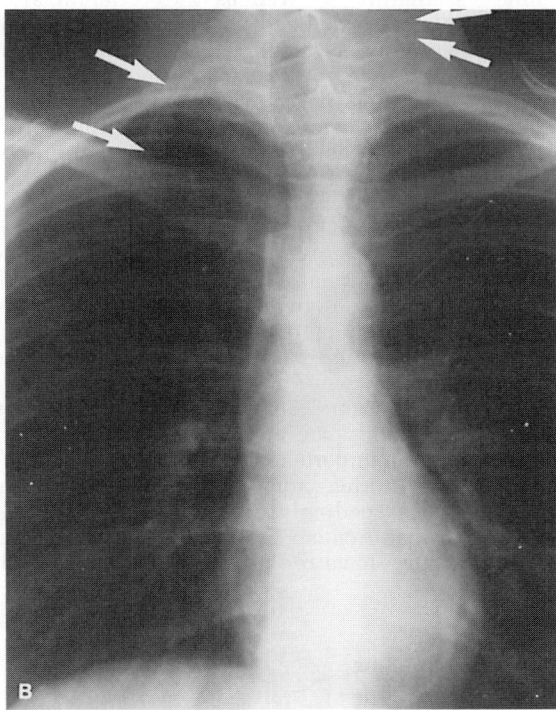

Figure 69.3. *(A)* Upper extremity arteriography demonstrating thromboembolic occlusion of the left axillary artery, the brachial artery, and all forearm arteries (radial, ulnar, and interosseous) as a result of an anomalous cervical rib and a resultant poststenotic subclavian artery aneurysm. *(B)* Immediate postoperative view demonstrating the resected left cervical rib. Also readily seen is a prominent right cervical rib. The resected left subclavian artery aneurysm, which was reconstructed with autogenous saphenous vein, is not seen.

mer, diminished pulses and a pale or mottled, cool extremity that fatigues rapidly with exercise should strongly suggest the diagnosis. At times, the upper extremity arterial insufficiency can be even more advanced. In acute venous obstruction, a swollen, tender, congested, and plethoric arm is pathognomonic. A pattern of collateral veins may be apparent across the anterior chest. Unfortunately, TOS most commonly presents with a long pro-

dromic history characterized by intermittent and vague but progressive neurologic symptoms, making diagnosis difficult. These symptoms include pain, paresthesias, and weakness in the neck, shoulder, or hand that may have been exacerbated by certain activities, postures, or unusual exercise. Neurologic examination can be entirely negative or can reveal weakness or atrophy of the triceps or the intrinsic hand muscles. Direct palpation in the supraclavicular fossa or axilla can reproduce the symptoms, as can provocative positioning such as Adson's maneuver, although the latter may not be particularly sensitive or specific.

Many tests have been used to aid in the early diagnosis of TOS. Standard chest roentgenograms and cervical and upper thoracic spine, clavicle, and shoulder films are often obtained. Such plain radiographic studies, in anteroposterior and lateral projections, can display a cervical rib or an abnormal first thoracic rib. Nonunion or hypertrophic callus formation from a clavicular fracture can also be present. Myelograms, electromyograms, nerve conduction studies, computed tomography (CT), magnetic resonance imaging, and somatosensory evoked potentials have all been used in the diagnosis of TOS (2). These diagnostic tests are seldom definitive, and none has achieved widespread acceptance. They are often most helpful in excluding other causes of the patient's symptoms.

Arterial lesions resulting from TOS are most definitively diagnosed with arteriography. Selective injection of the appropriate subclavian artery is performed, but adequate visualization may require multiple views and subtraction techniques as well as positional maneuvers. Even minor intimal lesions can produce microembolism, and any lesion in this area should be considered significant. Diagnosis is easy when sizable impingements are associated with an abnormal first thoracic rib or cervical rib. In such cases, poststenotic dilatation may be obvious and may have progressed to aneurysmal proportions. The presence of mural thrombus in an aneurysm or associated with an intimal lesion is of considerable significance and dictates early surgical intervention. Occasionally, complete thrombosis of the vessel is seen, and arteriography can be helpful in demonstrating distal embolic occlusions.

Treatment of arterial complications of TOS is always surgical. Emergent operation occasionally is required because of the presence of upper extremity ischemia, continued embolism, or free-floating thrombus in the area. Operation must deal with the underlying arterial compression as well as the complications of aneurysm formation or thromboembolism. Intraarterial thrombolytic therapy followed by definitive operative repair has been used in an attempt to deal with the troublesome distal small vessel thromboses and emboli that have proved difficult for standard surgical approaches.

Several surgical approaches have been advocated for decompressing the thoracic outlet. The transaxillary and anterolateral thoracic approaches provide effective neurologic and venous decompression through a cosmetically acceptable and relatively hidden incision. Arterial complications of TOS are always best dealt with through the supraclavicular approach, and many surgeons prefer this approach for all TOS procedures. Occasionally, a transclavicular approach can be used when excision of the clavicle is in order because of malunion or excessive callus formation. The goal of thoracic outlet decompression is attained by transection or resection of the anterior scalene muscle and excision of the first thoracic rib. Arterial aneurysms should be resected, as should an area of artery that shows arteriographic evidence of mural thrombosis or intimal ulceration. Standard arterial reconstructions with saphenous vein or prosthetic conduits are used. Balloon catheter embolectomy may be required during these procedures, and when microembolism has been part of the clinical presentation, upper extremity sympathectomy is sometimes advocated. Intraoperative infusion of urokinase has been reported to be successful in clearing multiple small vessel occlusions.

Current therapy for upper extremity venous thrombosis consists of lytic therapy delivered directly into the clot, which is best accomplished by a special catheter that allows a pulse spray of the agent into the clot, followed by heparin anticoagulation. Once flow is reestablished, interval, elective decompression of the thoracic outlet is often indicated.

Results of treatment of the arterial complications of TOS are usually good. However, when distal embolism is diffuse or gangrene is found at presentation, the results are predictably poor, and permanent forearm deformities can result. Amputations are occasionally required. Likewise, treatment of venous complications of TOS usually is successful. Unfortunately, when the operation is performed solely on the basis of patient symptoms, the uncertainties of clinical presentation and the lack of a confirmatory diagnostic test produce results that are not uniformly ideal. In properly selected patients, elimination or improvement of symptoms is achieved in about 85% of cases.

VERTEBRAL ARTERY COMPRESSION

The vertebral artery arises from the subclavian artery and courses cephalad in the neck. It enters the C-6 transverse process and exits the C-2 transverse process (Fig. 69.4A). Occasionally, an abnormally low entry at the level of C-7 is found and is associated with an increased likelihood of the vertebral artery being compressed by tendinous structures in the low neck. Osteophytic spurring and subluxation of the cervical vertebra are common and can result in chronic repeated compression (Fig. 69.4B). Repeated trauma to the vessel can cause intimal lesions or a permanent and nonexpandable cicatricial narrowing. In extreme cases, complete occlusion of the vertebral artery can be seen.

Vertebral artery compression can cause vertebrobasilar insufficiency (5,6), although isolated symptomatic vertebral artery compression is rare. Often, a combination of arteriosclerotic lesions and compression is seen in patients whose symptoms are produced by positional changes of the head and neck. In such cases, one vertebral artery can be occluded by atherosclerotic disease and the other subject to compression on rotation of the head. The symptoms of vertebral basilar insufficiency, whatever the cause, can be vague. Dizziness, vertigo, and paresthesias are fairly commonly reported but are easily confused with other syndromes. Classic drop attacks, in which muscle tone is lost but consciousness is maintained, are uncommon. Alternating or unilateral paresis has also been reported but is likewise uncommon. Because the nonspecific symptoms of vertebral basilar insufficiency are easily confused with symptoms of other origins, the investigation of patients with symptoms of vertebral basilar insufficiency should be systematic and methodical. Efforts to rule out orthostatic and drug-induced hypotension, middle ear labyrinthine disease, and cardiac causes of the patient's symptoms should be undertaken.

Arteriographic study of vertebrobasilar insufficiency requires an evaluation of the entire cerebral vasculature but is indicated only after careful exclusion of other causes of the patient's symptoms. Both the carotids and the intracranial vasculature, as well as the vertebral system, must be completely visualized. Atherosclerotic lesions of the vertebral artery or at other sites in the vertebral system are the most common findings at arteriography, and diffuse extracranial cerebrovascular disease is also common. Evidence of an extrinsic compression of the vertebral artery may require special views and orientations, subtraction techniques, and maneuvers to reproduce the patient's symptoms.

Treatment of symptomatic extrinsic compression of the vertebral artery is operative when symptoms are compelling or when there is any objective evidence of posterior circulation emboli. Relief of the extrinsic compression may require resection of osteophytes, unroofing of the transverse process foramina, or transection of musculotendinous bands associated with the cervical muscles. In the event of an abnormal change in the vertebral artery serving as an embolic source, standard vascular reconstruction should be undertaken.

Osteophytes and other bony abnormalities of the cervical vertebra are exceedingly common, yet symptoms of vertebrobasilar insufficiency are vague, and operations on the vertebral artery have the potential to be overused. In

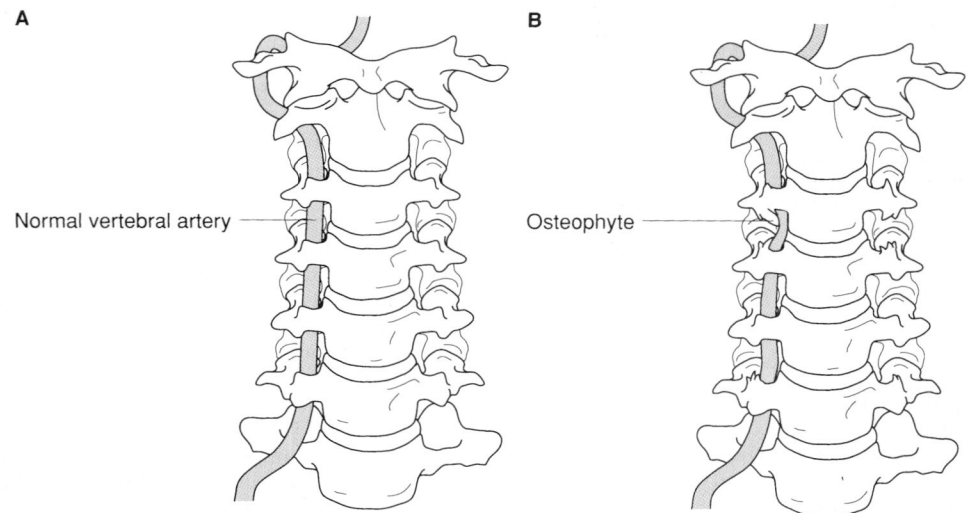

A

B

Normal vertebral artery

Osteophyte

Figure 69.4. *(A)* A normal vertebral artery lying in the vertebral canal. *(B)* A large osteophyte compresses the vertebral artery at the level of C-3. Rotation or flexion–extension can exacerbate the compression.

carefully selected patients, judicious operative therapy produces excellent results.

MEDIAN ARCUATE LIGAMENT SYNDROME

Intestinal angina, a syndrome of intermittent intestinal ischemia, may be produced by compression of the celiac axis by the median arcuate ligament (7).

The celiac axis arises from the midline of the aorta, ventrally, and is encased by periarterial neural tissue. Furthermore, the median arcuate ligament of the diaphragm may press directly on the celiac or indirectly on the periarterial neural tissue. In either case, a typical radiographic picture is produced, an example of which is shown in Fig. 69.5. The clinical presentation for patients with median arcuate ligament syndrome consists of cramping abdominal pain, usually epigastric, and often occurring 20 to 30 minutes after eating. This pain syndrome is, however, more variable and considerably more vague than that seen in patients with arteriosclerotic stenosis or occlusion of both the celiac axis and the superior mesenteric artery. Furthermore, the latter patients invariably have weight loss, whereas patients with isolated celiac axis compression often do not. Indeed, the patient whose magnetic resonance image is shown (Fig. 69.5) denied all symptoms, including weight loss and pain. The variability of this pain pattern has led to poor patient selection for operation and then to poor outcomes. Indeed, some authors have questioned whether this compression syndrome ever produces symptoms or whether it ever requires operation. A consensus of vascular surgeons, however, believe that when weight loss is present or when symptoms are persistent and reproducible after food ingestion that surgery is indicated. The operative treatment consists of division of the left crus of the diaphragm and clearing of the aorta, celiac axis, and superior mesenteric artery origin of the fascia and neurogenic tissue that encases them. Operative results in carefully selected patients are good, but pain persistence has been reported.

POPLITEAL ARTERY ENTRAPMENT SYNDROME

The popliteal artery entrapment syndrome is an uncommon problem and usually presents as unilateral calf claudication in a young person (8–10).

Some investigations have suggested, however, that even normal, well muscled young people may intermittently occlude their popliteal arteries under strenuous muscle exertion (11). Popliteal artery entrapment is most commonly seen in male patients, with a male-to-female ratio of approximately 15 : 1, and tends to occur more frequently in heavily muscled people.

Calf claudication is by nature episodic, but patients can frequently relate the onset of symptoms to a specific and intense exercise such as running. During this phase, the artery presumably is compressed intermittently, producing claudication. A more acute phase is entered when repeated trauma damages the intima or when scar tissue envelops the artery and arterial thrombosis occurs. In these cases, acute ischemia of the lower limb develops and the patient can present with a pulseless, cold, painful, and paralyzed extremity.

Patients with popliteal artery entrapment syndrome usually lack the risk factors and secondary signs of atherosclerotic occlusive disease. Those with entrapment but without an occluded popliteal artery frequently have normal foot pulses. These pulses may disappear on passive dorsiflexion of the foot or active plantar flexion against resistance. The sensitivity of this portion of the physical examination can be enhanced by the detection of a decreased Doppler signal or by decreased ankle pressures under similar circumstances in the noninvasive vascular laboratory. An occasional associated popliteal aneurysm is found, presumably a result of the progression of longstanding poststenotic dilatation.

The popliteal artery entrapment syndrome usually is associated with a distinct congenital anomaly that was first described more than a century ago. Normally, the popliteal artery passes through the adductor canal and traverses the popliteal space between the medial and lateral heads of the gastrocnemius muscle (Fig. 69.6). Congenital variations of the popliteal artery have been classified into four types (Fig. 69.7). In type I, the popliteal artery deviates medially around the normally located medial head of the gastrocnemius muscle. In type II, the medial head of the gastrocnemius arises from an abnormally lateral position on the femoral condyles so that the popliteal artery descends in a nearly normal course but is still impinged on by the abnormal origin of that muscular head. In type III, the popliteal artery passes through the medial head of the gastrocnemius or between the normal medial head and an accessory muscle slip that originates more laterally. In type IV, the popliteal artery is entrapped by the popliteus muscle, or occasionally the artery is impinged on by a fibromuscular band arising more laterally and joining the gastrocnemius fascia. Other anomalies have been described, and classifications including as many as 10 variants have been given. Schemes recognizing displacement

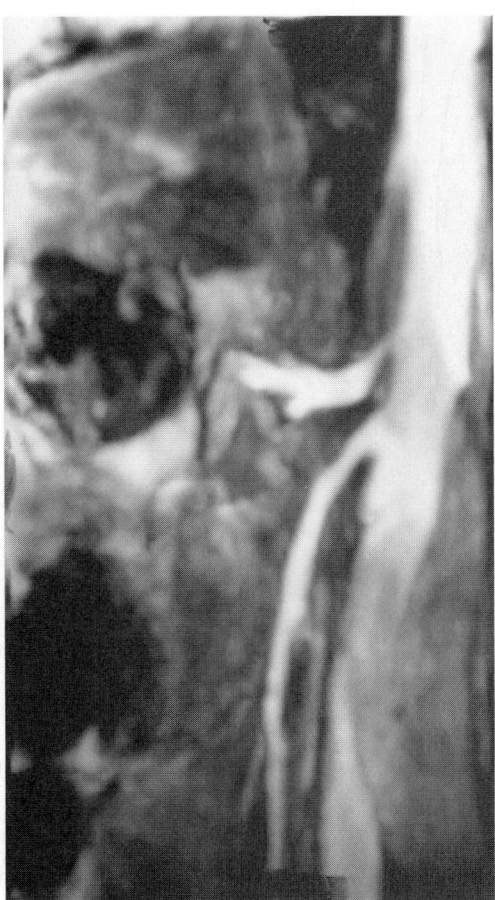

Figure 69.5. Magnetic resonance image of a lateral view of celiac axis compression by the median arcuate ligament. Note the poststenotic dilatation.

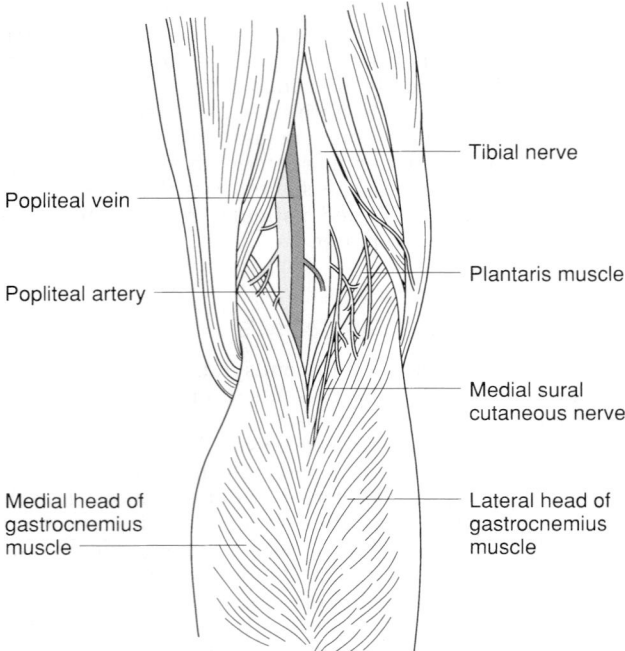

Figure 69.6. The normal anatomy of the popliteal fossa. The popliteal artery and vein and the tibial nerve lie between the medial and lateral heads of the gastrocnemius. The peroneal nerve courses lateral to the head of the gastrocnemius and the head of the fibula.

and impingement of the popliteal vein and nerve have also been reported. Popliteal entrapment by the soleus and plantaris tendons has been described. A single case suggestive of popliteal artery compression by hypertrophied calf musculature has been reported. Whatever the precise anatomy, popliteal artery entrapment syndrome should be recognized as an uncommon but important cause of lower extremity arterial occlusive symptoms in healthy young men.

Computed tomography scans of the popliteal fossa have been reported to be of value in the diagnosis of popliteal artery abnormalities and, in the hands of a skilled radiographer, may give detailed information about the origin of the head of the gastrocnemius muscle. More experience with the CT scan is necessary before this approach can be considered routine, and the definitive diagnostic procedure in this syndrome is arteriography. Arteriography should be performed bilaterally, because the anomaly is frequently found in the asymptomatic leg as well. In the appropriate setting, medial deviation of the popliteal artery, occlusion of the popliteal artery, and stenosis with poststenotic dilatation may confirm the popliteal artery entrapment syndrome.

Popliteal artery entrapment syndrome should be treated surgically whether the symptoms are minimal or extreme. The grave prognosis and high incidence of limb loss for acute popliteal artery occlusion warrant an aggressive posture even with minimal or absent symptoms.

Either a posterior or medial approach to the popliteal artery is acceptable. The posterior approach allows clear

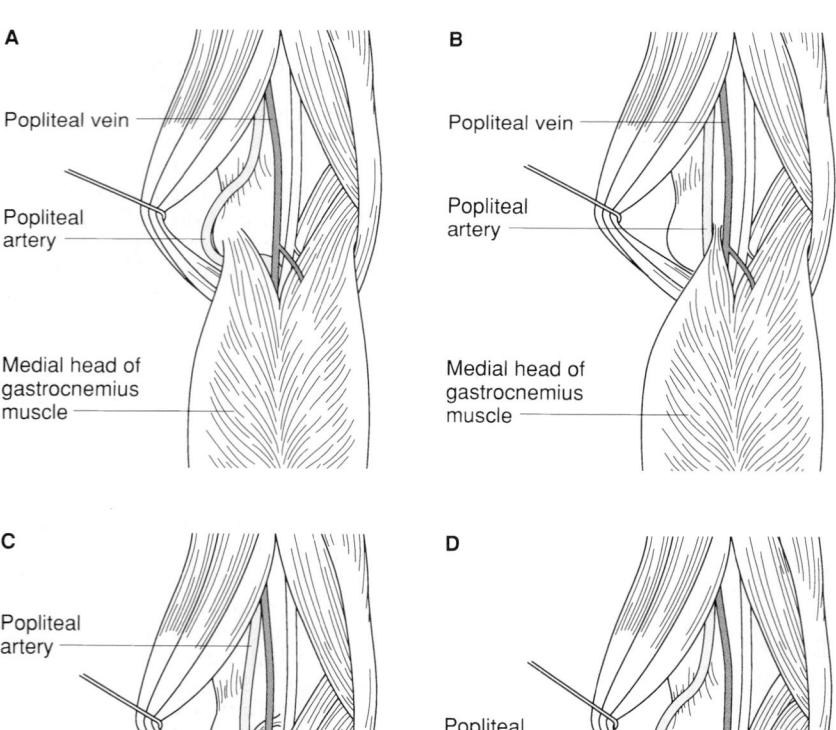

Figure 69.7. (A) Posterior view of right popliteal fossa. Normally located medial head of gastrocnemius with deviant medial pathway of popliteal artery (type I). (B) In the type II anomaly, an abnormally lateral origin of the medial head of the gastrocnemius muscle places traction on an otherwise normally placed popliteal artery. (C) An accessory slip of the gastrocnemius muscle compressing the popliteal artery. (D) Medial deviation of the popliteal artery and compression by the popliteus muscle. (After Whelan TJ. Popliteal artery entrapment. In: Rutherford RB, ed. *Vascular surgery,* 3rd ed. Philadelphia: WB Saunders, 1989, with permission.)

visualization of the precise relation between the medial head of the gastrocnemius muscle and the popliteal artery and helps in the recognition of type II, III, and IV anomalies. Most vascular surgeons are more familiar with the medial approach; however, in the case of an occluded vessel, particularly when the occlusion extends distally to the popliteal trifurcation, the medial approach is technically superior. Transection of the compressing portion of the medial head of the gastrocnemius or fascial band relieves the entrapment and is all that is required in most cases. When intimal thickening has been demonstrated or when stenosis or occlusion has occurred, reconstructive arterial surgery must be performed, using autogenous saphenous vein in most cases. Most surgeons make no attempt to reconstruct the medial head of the gastrocnemius muscle, although reattachment in a normal relation to the popliteal artery can be undertaken. Little or no loss of muscle function occurs with either approach. The results of operation for early popliteal artery entrapment syndrome are in general excellent. When arterial thrombosis has occurred, the overall result depends most on the degree of ischemic compromise of the limb.

ADVENTITIAL CYSTIC DISEASE OF THE POPLITEAL ARTERY

Adventitial cystic disease of the popliteal artery, like popliteal artery entrapment syndrome, causes intermittent claudication in young, physically active patients and can result in debilitating symptoms and irreversible damage if occlusion of the vessel ensues. Like other arterial compression syndromes, this disease entity is rare, and its precise pathophysiologic process is not known (Fig. 69.8). Analysis of the cyst fluid in one reported case led to the suggestion that the contents were of synovial origin (12), but this view is not widely held. A more likely hypothesis is that the cysts are due to abnormal embryonic development (13). Pulses may be normal in the foot, particularly at rest. The diagnosis of adventitial cystic disease of the popliteal artery has been improved by the use of CT scans of the popliteal space. More recently, the diagnosis has been adequately made by magnetic resonance imaging (14). In addition, CT scanning can help distinguish between popliteal artery entrapment syndrome and a Baker's or synovial cyst in the popliteal space. Arteriography may therefore be reserved for cases in which there is a question

of distal embolism or thrombosis of the artery. Uncomplicated adventitial cysts of the popliteal artery may be difficult to visualize angiographically, particularly when presented en face. Lateral projection typically demonstrates a smooth indentation into the column of dye and is noteworthy for the lack of atherosclerotic lesions.

Treatment of adventitial cystic disease of the popliteal artery that has become symptomatic is operative. Percutaneous transluminal angioplasty has been attempted, but the results usually have not been satisfactory. Cyst aspiration has not been particularly successful. At operation, the artery and the cystic area should be exposed. The cyst itself can be unilocular or multilocular, and occasionally adventitial cysts appear to contain old blood. The cyst should be incised and its contents removed. This usually completes the operation. Cicatricial stenosis of the artery, poststenotic dilatation, or thrombosis may necessitate further procedures. Treatment results in early, nonoccluded cases have been uniformly good. When thrombosis has occurred and has progressed distally, the results depend on the degree of ischemia on presentation.

COMPARTMENT SYNDROMES

Compartment syndromes are encountered when increased tissue pressure in a limited anatomic space compromises circulation (15–18). These syndromes usually occur because of the increasing volume of the compartment's contents, but occasionally because the capacity of the compartment is reduced by application of a tight plaster cast or by a tight fascial closure during surgery. Compartment syndromes can also be produced by hemorrhage into a closed compartment in association with bleeding disorders, anticoagulant therapy, trauma, or aneurysm rupture. The most common and important compartment syndromes occur in relation to interruption and subsequent restoration of blood flow to an extremity made ischemic by an embolism, thrombus, trauma, or unusual prolonged positioning (15). The hyperperfusion and edema that follow ischemic injury doubtless contribute to the development of intracompartmental swelling (16,17). Swelling of tissue in ischemic and reperfused limbs can be documented by weight gain of the limb and is due to increased interstitial fluid and intracellular swelling.

The clinical manifestations of compartment syndromes include throbbing and unrelenting pain and the loss of neuromuscular function. The forearm and the leg are the most frequent sites of compression. Because each compartment of the forearm and leg contains at least one major peripheral nerve, careful examination of the hand or foot may disclose neurologic deficits. Subtle sensory changes or paresthesias are often observed before the development of clear-cut signs of ischemia. Movement or stretching of the involved muscle by passive motion of the wrist or ankle usually exacerbates pain. Objective signs include a tense, tender, or swollen compartment on direct palpation, and subcutaneous edema or hematoma (Fig. 69.9A,B). Distal pulses may be weak, but capillary or venous compression usually precedes the cessation of arterial inflow, and significant tissue damage can occur before intracompartmental pressure exceeds arterial perfusion pressure (Fig. 69.9C). Paralysis of the involved musculature suggests that the compression is advanced.

The most important aspect of the diagnosis of this syndrome is careful repeated clinical evaluations of the involved limb. All patients with major trauma or crush injury should have repetitive neurovascular examinations for 48 to 72 hours after injury. During the postoperative period after embolectomy or prolonged reconstructive vascular surgery, similar repetitive examinations are in order.

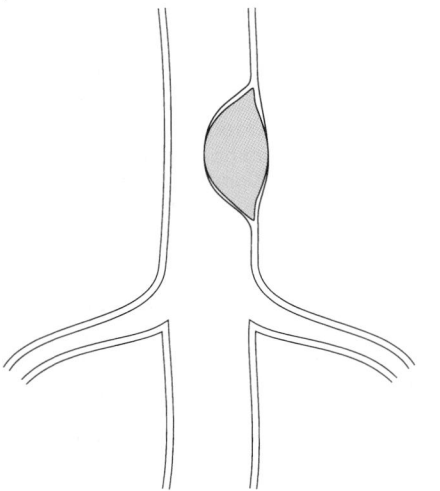

Figure 69.8. Adventitial cystic disease of the popliteal artery causes luminal compromise.

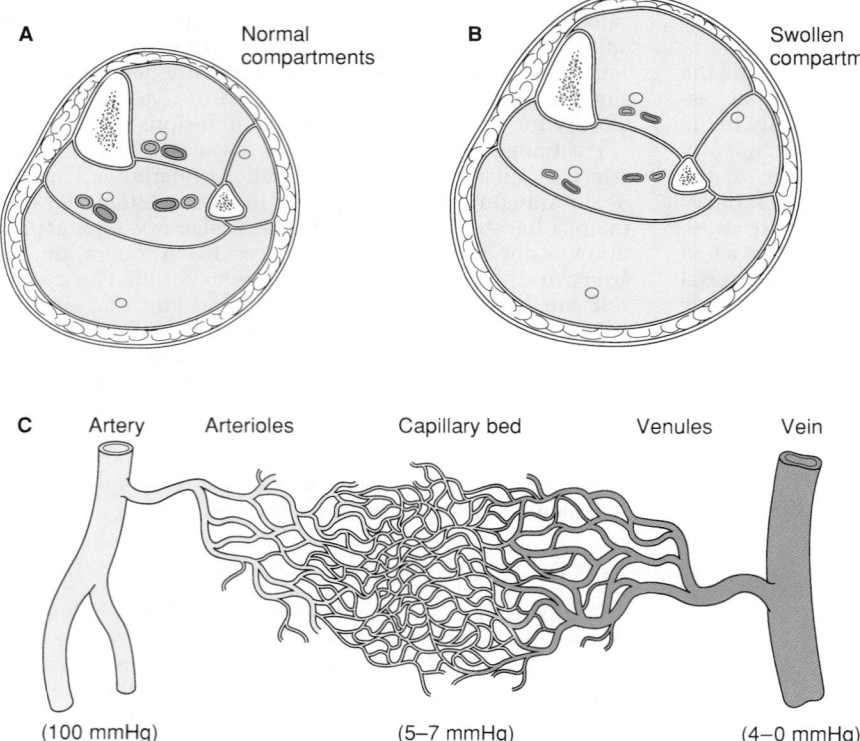

Figure 69.9. *(A)* Compartments of the leg at midcalf. The anterior, lateral, and both the deep and superficial posterior compartments contain major nerves. *(B)* When cellular swelling and interstitial edema develop in the fixed confines of the various compartments, pressure necrosis of the compartment's contents may result. The tissue most sensitive to ischemia is the peripheral nerve. *(C)* As compartment pressures rise to 20 to 40 mm Hg, obstruction to flow occurs first at the capillary–venule level. Profound ischemia may then result despite normal distal arterial pulses. (After Mubarak SJ, Hargens AR. *Compartment syndromes and Volkmann's contracture.* Philadelphia: WB Saunders, 1981, with permission.)

In most cases, such clinical examination is adequate to make the diagnosis of compression in an appropriate time frame. In an unconscious patient, many surgeons prefer intermittent or continuous measurement of intracompartmental pressures (17). Such compartmental pressure monitoring is the subject of some controversy; some surgeons believe it makes no important contribution to the clinical management of patients with the potential for compartment syndromes (18).

Several methods of measuring intracompartmental pressure have been described. These range from simple measurements with a central venous manometer to the use of recently developed, solid-state pressure transducers small enough to be inserted into the appropriate compartment on a catheter tip. Two other catheter methods are commonly used. The Wick technique uses a catheter kept open with strands of polyglycolic acid suture and a continuous electronic pressure sensor. Others have described a small catheter using a continuous slow infusion and electronic monitoring of the pressure developed by that infusion. Compartmental pressures are normally in the range of 10 mm Hg. Pressures exceeding 20 mm Hg are considered abnormal, and those exceeding 40 mm Hg are dangerous and require decompression.

Fasciotomy is the preferred operative therapy for compartment syndrome involving the forearm or leg. The leg is composed of four compartments, each nonexpandable and delineated by thick fascia (Fig. 69.9A). The four compartments of the lower extremity include both a deep and a superficial posterior compartment, a lateral compartment, and an anterior compartment. Decompression of all four compartments is the goal. Fibulectomy accomplishes this end, although this operation has been largely supplanted by less extensive procedures. The anterior and lateral compartments should be decompressed through an anterior lateral incision, and the posterior compartments decompressed through a posteromedial incision. These longitudinal incisions are usually left open for delayed

primary closure or skin grafting when the edema subsides. An appropriate rehabilitative program is of utmost importance.

Another important compartment syndrome occurs when excessive intraabdominal pressure develops in a tightly closed postoperative abdomen. This may result from bleeding or from edema of the viscera. At sufficiently high pressure, caval return of blood may be impeded and cardiac output may fall precipitously. Renal failure may ensue as a result of underperfusion added to direct pressure on the renal parenchyma. Multisystem organ failure may be avoided only by timely return to the operating room for decompression. Abdominal compartment syndrome may require leaving the abdomen open, or closed with a gusset of appropriate material.

Ankle and foot fasciotomy, as an adjunct to leg fasciotomies, is undertaken when continued foot swelling and tenseness over the medial aspect of the proximal foot are encountered (19). The foot can be decompressed through incisions over the dorsum of the foot and ankle, with incisions in the dorsal deep aponeurosis over the metatarsal spaces and an incision through the distal portion of the inferior extensor retinaculum. A longitudinal incision along the medial and inferior border of the foot allows decompression of the plantar compartment. Ankle and foot fasciotomies appear to be valuable in prolonged reconstructive vascular procedures for arteriosclerotic disease.

Most compartment syndromes in the forearm are adequately decompressed by a single long volar incision from the antecubital fossa to the proximal palm. Carpal tunnel release is usually included in this procedure, and occasionally a second incision directly over the dorsal compartment of the forearm is necessary. These incisions, like those in the lower extremity, are left open for delayed primary closure or skin grafting as appropriate.

Results of fasciotomy depend on the underlying disease. Severe atherosclerosis, excessively delayed revascularization, or extensive trauma can preclude limb salvage despite fasciotomy. Furthermore, an unpredictable number of patients with compartment syndrome have a slow, progressive course of skeletal muscle death with ultimate shrinkage and fibrosis of the muscle despite adequate and timely compartment decompression, resulting in the classic Volkmann's contracture. The goal of fasciotomy is a functional extremity. Despite the extensive incisions involved and the frequent need for delayed primary closure or skin grafting, the cosmetic results are acceptable.

OTHER COMPRESSION SYNDROMES

Diverse processes such as retroperitoneal fibrosis, Baker's cysts, and primary or metastatic neoplasms have all been reported to cause compression of nearby vascular structures. An exhaustive catalogue of these syndromes is not possible. One example is involvement of the carotid bifurcation by metastatic head and neck cancer. In the treatment of selected patients with extensive laryngeal or oropharyngeal cancer, resection and reconstruction of the carotid artery can be used in concert with radical excision of the malignancy. In one report, 15 patients were treated with reconstruction or simple ligation for advanced neck cancer. Two of these patients had immediate postoperative strokes, and there was one postoperative death. Seven patients were believed to be free of cancer more than 1 year after operation. These data suggest that in selected cases, malignancies compressing adjacent arteries can reasonably be treated by radical excision and concomitant reconstructive vascular surgical techniques.

REFERENCES

1. Cormier JM, Amrane M, Ward A, et al. Arterial complications of the thoracic outlet syndrome: fifty-five operative cases. *J Vasc Surg* 1989;9:778.
2. Machleder HI, Moll F, Nuwer M, et al. Somatosensory evoked potentials in the assessment of thoracic outlet compression syndrome. *J Vasc Surg* 1987;6:177.
3. Roos DB. Thoracic outlet nerve compression. In: Rutherford RB, ed. *Vascular surgery,* 3rd ed. Philadelphia: WB Saunders, 1989.
4. Wylie EJ, Stoney RJ, Ehrenfeld WK, et al., eds. *Manual of vascular surgery,* vol 2. New York: Springer-Verlag, 1986.
5. Bauer RB. Mechanical compression of the vertebral arteries. In: Berguer R, Bauer RB, eds. *Vertebrobasilar arterial occlusive disease: medical and surgical management.* New York: Raven Press, 1984:45.
6. Berguer R, Caplan LR. *Vertebrobasilar arterial disease.* St. Louis: Quality Medical, 1992.
7. Dunbar JD, Molner W, Berma FF, et al. Compression of the celiac trunk and abdominal angina. *AJR Am J Roentgenol* 1965;95:731–744.
8. Collins PS, McDonald PT, Lim RC. Popliteal artery entrapment: an evolving syndrome. *J Vasc Surg* 1989;10:484.
9. Williams LR, Flinn WR, McCarthy WJ, et al. Popliteal artery entrapment: diagnosis by computed tomography. *J Vasc Surg* 1986;3:360.
10. Whelan TJ. Popliteal artery entrapment. In: Rutherford RB, ed. *Vascular surgery,* 3rd ed. Philadelphia: WB Saunders, 1989.
11. Hoffmann U, Vetter J, Rainoni L, et al. Popliteal artery compression and force of active plantar flexion in young healthy volunteers. *J Vasc Surg* 1997;26:281–287.
12. Jay GD, Ross FL, Mason RA, et al. Clinical and chemical characterization of an adventitial popliteal cyst. *J Vasc Surg* 1989; 9:448.
13. Levien LJ, Benn CA. Adventitial cystic disease: a unifying hypotheses. *J Vasc Surg* 1998;28:193–205.
14. Crolla RMPH, Steyling JF, Hennipman A, et al. A case of cystic adventitial disease of the popliteal artery demonstrated by magnetic resonance imaging. *J Vasc Surg* 1993;18:1052–1055.
15. Khalil IM. Bilateral compartmental syndrome after prolonged surgery in the lithotomy position. *J Vasc Surg* 1987;5:879.
16. Forrest I, Lindsay T, Romaschin A, et al. The rate and distribution of muscle blood flow after prolonged ischemia. *J Vasc Surg* 1989;10:83.
17. Mubarak SJ, Hargens AR. *Compartment syndromes and Volkmann's contracture.* Philadelphia: WB Saunders, 1981.
18. Skillman JJ, Dohlman LE, Gerhart TN, et al. Compartmental pressure monitoring after arterial reconstruction lacks clinical relevance. *J Vasc Surg* 1986;3:871.
19. Ascer E, Strauch B, Calligaro KD, et al. Ankle and foot fasciotomy: an adjunctive technique to optimize limb salvage after revascularization for acute ischemia. *J Vasc Surg* 1989;9:594.

SURGERY: SCIENTIFIC PRINCIPLES AND PRACTICE, Third Edition, edited by Lazar J. Greenfield, Michael W. Mulholland, Keith T. Oldham, Gerald B. Zelenock, and Keith D. Lillemoe. Lippincott Williams & Wilkins Publishers, Philadelphia, © 2001.

CHAPTER 70

ARTERIAL HEMODYNAMICS

MARK F. FILLINGER AND JACK L. CRONENWETT

An understanding of hemodynamic principles is essential to the functional success of contemporary vascular surgery. These principles are used to guide the diagnostic evaluation, plan an appropriate intervention, and monitor the outcome. The evaluation of hemodynamics in vivo was once confined to physical examination and measurement of blood pressure. Now, sophisticated noninvasive techniques make it possible to measure blood flow velocity, and hemodynamic principles, formerly relegated to textbook status, are applied daily in the evaluation and management of vascular disease. This chapter summarizes the aspects of arterial hemodynamics most commonly applied in vascular surgery. A more detailed discussion can be found in many comprehensive monographs, especially the superb text by Strandness and Sumner (1–6).

ARTERIAL STRUCTURE AND FUNCTION

The arterial wall is composed primarily of endothelial cells, smooth-muscle cells, collagen, and elastin. These basic elements are organized into three recognizable layers of the vessel wall: intima, media, and adventitia. The intima is composed mostly of endothelial cells and the internal elastic lamina, with few of the other elements intervening. The media carries most of the tensile load and is thus primarily composed of collagen, elastin, and smooth-muscle cells arranged in bundles oriented along the lines of greatest tension (circumferentially). The adventitia consists primarily of fibrous connective tissue, vasa vasorum for nutrient supply to the outer layers of larger arteries, and nerve fibers that regulate the tone of medial smooth-muscle cells. The adventitia generally carries little of the tensile load. When the adventitia does perform a significant support function (e.g., in the proximal visceral arteries), collagen and elastin fibers are more abundant.

Although the media is responsible for much of the structural integrity of the arterial wall, the elements making up the media are strongly influenced by endothelial cells in the intima. The endothelium is much more than an antithrombotic barrier interacting with platelets to promote hemostasis at a site of physical injury. Endothelial cells also produce cell adhesion molecules that are important in local inflammatory responses of the arterial wall. The most important hemodynamic function of endothelial cells, however, is to interact with smooth-muscle cells to regulate acute and chronic luminal diameter (7–9). Endothelial cells respond to luminal shear stress (the tangential drag force on the endothelial surface caused by the friction of blood flow), and they secrete a number of biologic mediators that maintain shear stress within a narrow range. Mediators of acute vasodilation include nitric oxide and prostaglandins; endothelin and angiotensin II are among the mediators of acute contraction. When changes in shear stress are chronic, these biologic mediators can produce structural changes in the arterial wall. For example, the production of platelet-derived growth factor by endothelial cells subjected to low shear rates results in the migration and proliferation of smooth-muscle cells. Functionally, the interactions of endothelial and smooth-muscle cells allow arteries (and vein grafts placed in an arterial environment) (10) to accommodate acute and chronic changes in blood flow, and they optimize the hemostatic and inflammatory mechanisms affected by shear rates.

The hemodynamic forces to which vessels adapt are not limited to shear stress. The artery wall is subject to a number of hemodynamic stresses, and its structure must accommodate all of them (Fig. 70.1). These stresses (described in detail later) are primarily controlled by intraluminal blood pressure, blood flow velocity, arterial diameter, and wall thickness. Just as the arterial diameter responds to changes in shear stress, the thickness of the arterial wall and the elements within it are regulated to normalize wall tension. Interestingly, the circumferential and longitudinal stresses within the arterial wall are not identical for any given blood pressure (Fig. 70.1). The structure of the wall, however, makes it *anisotropic*—that is, the wall is stronger circumferentially than it is longitudinally (11). Tethering of the arteries in situ affects longitudinal stiffness and prevents excessive motion. Acute changes in circumferential wall stiffness are primarily controlled by smooth-muscle contraction or relaxation (6).

Acute and chronic adaptation to hemodynamic stress allows arteries to accommodate changes in blood flow and pressure to a remarkable degree. For example, the arterial system must accommodate fivefold changes in cardiac output between rest and exercise and must alter distribution according to different metabolic demands. Not surprisingly, wall composition varies from central to more peripheral arteries to accomplish specific functions (2,3) (Fig. 70.2). Although the three layers of the arterial wall have different functions, most of the variation occurs in

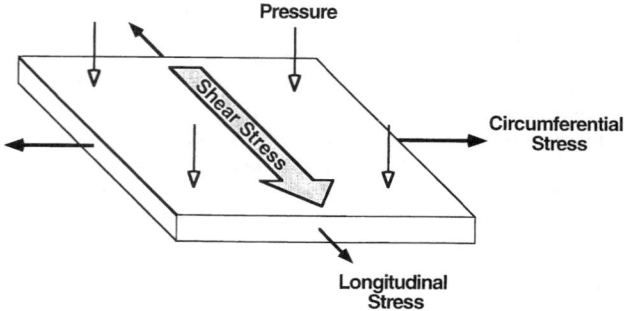

Figure 70.1. Stresses exerted on the arterial wall. Circumferential stress = $\tau_{circ} = Pr/\delta$; longitudinal stress = $\tau_{long} = Pr/2\delta$; shear stress = $\tau_w = 4\eta Q/(Pr^3)$, where P = pressure (intraluminal blood pressure), r = internal radius of the artery, δ = wall thickness, η = viscosity, and $\dot{Q}$ = volumetric blood flow rate. Details are presented later in the chapter.

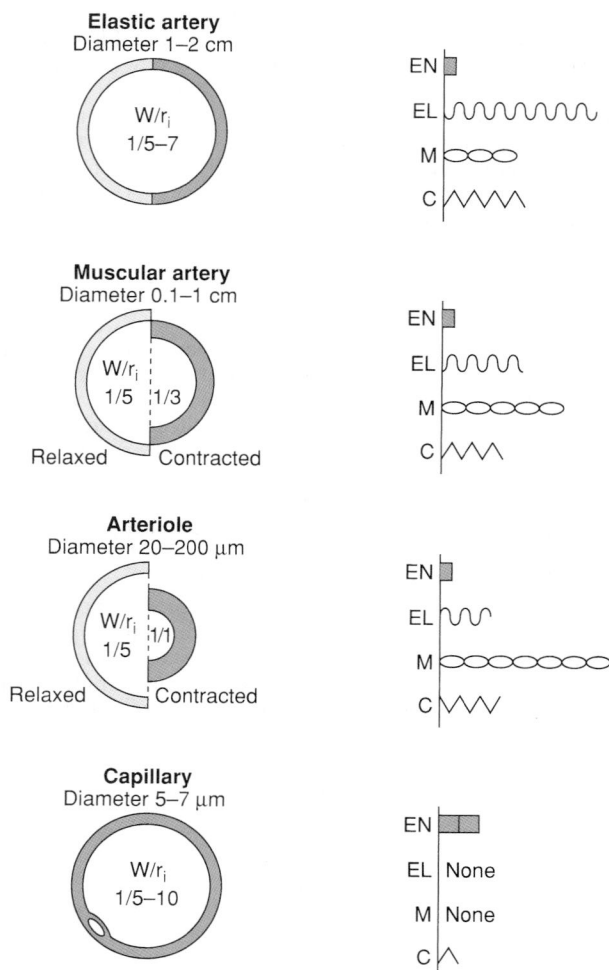

Figure 70.2. Approximate wall composition and relation between wall thickness (W) and internal radius (r_i) in large elastic arteries, medium muscular arteries, arterioles, and capillaries. *EN*, endothelium; *EL*, elastin; *M*, smooth muscle; *C*, collagen. (After Folkow B, Neil E. *Circulation*. New York: Oxford University Press, 1971, with permission.)

the media. Collagen is primarily responsible for wall strength and increases in proportion to artery diameter. Elastin, which is five to 10 times more deformable than rubber, provides stretch to artery walls and also increases with arterial size. The elastin-to-collagen ratio determines the relative distensibility (compliance) of arteries. Compliance is higher in large central arteries, in which it buffers the changes in systemic pressure that occur during the cardiac cycle by allowing expansion during systolic ejection and recoil during diastolic relaxation. As the elastin content and distensibility decrease in more peripheral arteries, the content of smooth muscle, the active component of the arterial wall, increases. In medium to large muscular arteries (5 to 10 mm in diameter), resting smooth-muscle tone does not contribute significantly to peripheral resistance but does decrease arterial compliance. By stiffening these arteries, resting smooth-muscle tone augments systolic pressure and increases the propagation rate of pulse waves. In small muscular arteries, arterioles, and precapillary sphincters, smooth-muscle tone is the primary determinant of total peripheral resistance, regional blood flow, and the regulation of flow within the microcirculation. Arterioles and precapillary sphincters are well suited to regulate peripheral resistance and capillary perfusion because of their high ratio of wall thickness to lumen diameter, which causes maximal lumen constriction with minimal muscle shortening.

Although luminal diameter rapidly decreases from central to peripheral arteries (i.e., the aorta, 2.5 cm in diameter, is 1,000 times larger than arterioles, 25 µm in diameter), the total cross-sectional area increases in the arteriolar and capillary bed as a result of an even more rapid increase in the number of these vascular channels. In fact, the cross-sectional area of arterioles is estimated to be 50 times that of the aorta, and the cross-sectional area of capillaries is 800 times that of the aorta (2). This geometry permits rapid blood flow in large central arteries with a high mean velocity (20 to 30 cm/s in the aorta), but extremely slow blood flow in capillaries with a low mean velocity (0.5 to 1 mm/s). The inverse relation observed between cross-sectional area and blood velocity is well suited to the distributional function of central arteries and the exchange function of capillaries. The need for a large capillary bed is illustrated by the volume flow through a single 8-µm-diameter capillary; 15 months would be required for 1 mL of blood flowing at a velocity of 0.5 mm/s to traverse the capillary.

CONTROL OF BLOOD FLOW

Local Control

Vascular smooth muscle has an intrinsic tone that is responsible for maintaining partial vascular constriction in the absence of external stimuli. Blood flow remains relatively constant in most organs despite wide changes in perfusion pressure. Two theories of local control mechanisms have been proposed to explain this autoregulation (2,3,12). The myogenic theory states that vascular smooth muscle contracts in response to stretch caused by increases in intravascular pressure and relaxes in response to decreased stretch when perfusion pressure falls. This direct feedback loop stabilizes organ blood flow by adjusting arteriolar smooth-muscle tone to changes in perfusion pressure. The metabolic theory states that tissue blood flow parallels metabolic activity. If the demands of tissue metabolism exceed the blood supply, certain metabolic by-products accumulate and cause precapillary resistance vessels to dilate. The increased flow resulting from the decreased resistance then removes the vasodilating metabolites and restores baseline vascular smooth-muscle tone. Factors that have been implicated in metabolic autoregulation include Po_2, Pco_2, pH, adenosine, lactate, potassium, and inorganic phosphate (12). It is likely that these factors act in concert to produce metabolic vasodilation in response to reduced blood flow, poor systemic oxygen delivery, or increased metabolite production.

The myogenic and metabolic mechanisms of vascular control probably have complementary roles, not only in autoregulation but also during active (exercise) and reactive (postocclusive) hyperemia. In the extreme case of transient arterial occlusion, loss of myogenic tone (because of decreased stretch pressure) and accumulation of vasodilating metabolites results in reactive hyperemia, the nearly maximal but transient increase in blood flow that occurs when blood flow is reestablished. The increase in blood flow subsides as metabolites are cleared and myogenic tone restored by perfusion pressure, so that the duration and degree of reactive hyperemia are proportional to the duration and severity of ischemia.

Nervous System Control

The sympathetic nervous system has primary neural control of vascular smooth-muscle tone (12). Sympathetic adrenergic nerves function primarily by releasing norepinephrine, which stimulates α-adrenergic receptors to produce smooth-muscle contraction and vasoconstriction. Basal sympathetic tone is responsible for only 15% to 20% of total vascular resistance, most of which is a consequence of intrinsic myogenic activity (or intrinsic smooth-muscle tone). Basal intrinsic arterial tone varies considerably among different organs. It is high in skeletal muscle and other tissues that have a wide range of metabolic rates but low in organs, such as kidney or brain, that have more stable metabolic rates and flow demands. The density of sympathetic innervation of vascular smooth muscle also varies in different organs, ranging from few fibers in cerebral or coronary arteries to dense innervation in cutaneous arterioles. The density of innervation influences the sensitivity of an organ to sympathetic vasoconstriction. This sensitivity is maximal in the skin, where sympathetic discharge can nearly stop cutaneous blood flow during the fight-or-flight reflex.

Organs also differ in the sensitivity of their vascular smooth muscle to the vasoconstrictor effects of sympathetic innervation and the vasodilator effects of local metabolites. An important example is the difference in sensitivity of precapillary and postcapillary sphincter muscles. Postcapillary sphincter mechanisms are more sensitive to sympathetic innervation than to local metabolic effects, whereas precapillary sphincters respond primarily to accumulating local metabolites and function independently of sympathetic discharge. Although changes in postcapillary sphincter resistance do not contribute significantly to the total resistance of the peripheral circulation, small changes in postcapillary contraction cause large changes in the precapillary-to-postcapillary pressure gradient. This gradient is important for regulating the capillary filtration coefficient and thus the tendency to accumulate peripheral edematous fluids or absorb tissue fluids, which is under subtle sympathetic control.

The cortical–hypothalamic–medullary axis of the central nervous system control controls sympathetic nerve discharge. The sympathetic activity that arises from the medullary cardiovascular center is significantly influenced by stretch receptors in the carotid sinus, aortic arch, thyrocervical junction, and cardiopulmonary vascular bed. These stretch receptors are in turn influenced by arterial blood pressure and degree of vascular filling (blood volume). For example, deformation and stretch of carotid sinus receptors stimulates the carotid sinus nerve, a branch of the glossopharyngeal nerve, which excites inhibitor neurons in the medial depressor area of the medulla. This provides negative feedback, or inhibition, of sympathetic activity arising from the medullary cardiovascular center. In addition, bradycardia results from vagal nerve stimulation. Stretch receptors are sensitive to stretch or vascular dilation, as their name suggests, but not to changes in arterial pressure. Thus, in a normal artery, an increase in arterial pressure increases the stretch of the arterial wall, so that the stretch receptor is stimulated. In an artery that cannot expand (e.g., a calcified artery in an atherosclerotic patient), an increase in arterial pressure does not stimulate this receptor. Removal of the arterial calcification, as during carotid endarterectomy, may expose the adventitial stretch receptor to intense stimulation. This can result in a significant inhibition of sympathetic discharge and an increase in vagal stimulation, which result in hypotension and bradycardia.

Local Humoral Control

Many humoral substances also affect vascular smooth-muscle tone. Epinephrine, norepinephrine, vasopressin, angiotensin, serotonin, prostaglandins, histamine, and plasma kinins participate in the control of vascular smooth-muscle tone under certain circumstances and in specific organ beds (12). Epinephrine has different, organ-specific effects based on the predominance of α- or β-adrenergic receptors. Its alpha effect causes vasoconstriction in kidney, skin, and intestine, whereas its beta effect causes vasodilation in the myocardium, skeletal muscle, and liver. These effects are generally minimal in comparison with the effect of sympathetic stimulation on blood flow regulation.

Humoral substances, such as nitric oxide, endothelin, and prostaglandins, play an important role in the regulation of vascular tone in response to hemodynamic stress. In particular, inhibition of nitric oxide greatly enhances the myogenic response of vasoconstriction to increased blood flow.

Flow-related Control

Blood flow is an important regulator of acute and chronic arterial diameter. Flow-related shear stress causes numerous biologic effects in endothelial cells. Some effects, such as the activation of potassium channels, occur within milliseconds (7). Other acute responses to shear include effects on endothelium-derived relaxing factor (nitric oxide), prostaglandins, adenylate cyclase, and neurotransmitters (7). Chronic changes include transcriptional control of endothelin and platelet-derived growth factor, and also remodeling of the vascular wall through changes in the production of collagen and proliferation of smooth-muscle cells. This explains how the diameter (and blood flow capacity) of more proximal feeder arteries increases or decreases in response to changes in blood flow requirements at the end-organ.

ARTERIAL PRESSURE AND ENERGY

Determinants of the Arterial Pressure Curve

Blood pressure can be directly measured with an intraarterial catheter and a pressure transducer. It is more frequently measured noninvasively with a sphygmomanometer and a stethoscope or a Doppler ultrasonographic device. Although it is simple to measure, systemic arterial pressure is the result of a complex interaction between the cardiac pump, aortic valve, compliance of large central arteries, peripheral vascular resistance, and total vascular volume. The pressure wave that is transmitted after systolic contraction is a result not only of the stroke volume of the heart but also of the compliance (distensibility) of the aorta and proximal arteries. The expansion of large central arteries tends to reduce systolic pressure, whereas subsequent contraction helps sustain diastolic pressure. The compliance of large-diameter arteries can be reduced by the contraction of smooth muscle in the walls of these vessels. Thus, sympathetic nervous system-mediated vasoconstriction during exercise causes an increase in pulse pressure (the difference between systolic and diastolic pressure) through a decrease in aortic expansion, which results in the propagation of a larger systolic pressure wave. Systolic hypertension is also produced in geriatric patients with calcified and poorly compliant arterial walls.

As arterial pressure waves generated by cardiac contraction proceed peripherally, a gradual increase in the pulse pressure amplitude develops in addition to a qualitative change in the shape of both pressure and flow waves. This is primarily a consequence of the reflection of pulse waves as they strike the high-resistance segments of the peripheral circulation—the distal arterioles and points of arterial branching. The reflection of pulse waves results in a ret-

rograde flow of each wave, which then interacts with the next prograde pressure wave. The sum of these pressure waves results in an amplification of the systolic pressure as each pressure wave proceeds peripherally. The influence of arteriolar resistance is significant but variable, as it depends on the state of peripheral vasoconstriction. Major arterial branch points also contribute significant (and constant) resistance for pulse-wave reflection because the sum of the cross-sectional areas of the branches (A2) is less than the area of the proximal artery (A1). Wave reflections at a bifurcation are minimal when the ratio of A2 to A1 is 1.15 (i.e., when the total branch area is slightly greater than the parent artery). At the human aortoiliac bifurcation, this value is approached only during infancy (1.11). In the adult aorta, even without atheromatous disease, the ratio becomes progressively smaller, reaching 0.75 in patients between 40 and 50 years of age (1) and resulting in a significant reflection of the amplitude of each pulse wave (26%). Although the effect of this reflection is attenuated by the viscoelastic arterial system during retrograde flow, it effectively increases the pressure in the distal abdominal aorta, a factor that may contribute to the tendency for aneurysms to form at this site. Pulse-wave reflection is also responsible for the periods of retrograde flow in peripheral arteries seen immediately after the primary pulse wave has passed, a phenomenon augmented by peripheral vasoconstriction (with increased wave reflection) and decreased by vasodilation (with diminished resistance and decreased wave reflection).

Pressure and Energy

Blood pressure is commonly considered to be the driving force that controls the movement of blood from the heart to various body regions. A more precise and useful concept is that blood flow is controlled by energy gradients, to which arterial pressure makes the largest contribution. Total energy within the circulation is the sum of potential energy (PE) and kinetic energy (KE), with PE representing the greater portion of total energy during normal blood flow [pressure (mm Hg) = 1,330 dyne/cm^2]. PE is the sum of intraarterial pressure and gravitational energy. Intraarterial pressure results primarily from the pressure caused by cardiac contraction (P_c); the weight of the column of blood between the heart and the point of pressure measurement provides a hydrostatic contribution. Hydrostatic pressure is defined as follows:

$$\text{hydrostatic pressure} = P_H = -\rho g h$$

where

ρ = density of blood (1.056 g/cm^3)
g = acceleration of gravity (980 cm/s^2)
h = height (cm) *above* a fixed reference point (atrium) to the point of pressure measurement
(This is important to note because if the height is measured by convention *below* the fixed reference point, the equation becomes $P_H = +\rho g h$.)

Thus, if the point of measurement is below the atrium, then hydrostatic pressure is additive to the pressure resulting from cardiac contraction. In the legs of an erect human, this position represents a pressure increase (in the neck, it is a pressure decrease). Gravitational PE derives from the ability of blood to do work based on its position relative to another location and is calculated with the term $+\rho g h$. In the human body, the two most relevant points for determining the height, h, in this equation are the atrium and the feet. When the above units are used, PE is then expressed as follows:

$$PE \text{ (erg/cm}^3) = P_c + P_H + \rho g h = P + \rho g h \qquad [1]$$

As blood moves from the heart to the feet in the erect position, it gains hydrostatic pressure but loses gravitational energy. Thus, arterial pressure measured at the ankle in an upright person is significantly increased by hydrostatic pressure because of the added weight of the upright column of blood. Total *PE* is unchanged because it is reduced by an equivalent amount as a result of the loss of gravitational *PE*. Thus, no net change in the total driving force (energy) occurs between the erect and the supine position despite changes in measured arterial pressure. This explains the apparent paradox of blood flowing against a major pressure gradient, as it does between the heart and the feet in the erect position (Fig. 70.3A).

Kinetic energy derives from the ability of flowing blood to perform work based on its velocity. In a nonpulsatile flow system with rigid tubing and a newtonian fluid (see later section on viscosity and laminar blood flow), *KE* is defined as follows:

$$KE \ (\text{erg/cm}^3) = 1/2\rho v^2 \qquad [2]$$

where
ρ = density of fluid
v = mean velocity (cm/s)

This definition of *KE* is valid in an ideal system, but in the human arterial system, it significantly underestimates energy losses resulting from the pulsatile nature of blood flow, the non-newtonian characteristics of blood, and many alterations in geometry (e.g., those caused by atherosclerotic disease). For the purpose of discussion, this formula is useful because it indicates that the total energy of flowing blood is derived in large part from the characteristics of its velocity and, hence, flow rate.

Energy in the Ideal System

Bernoulli first characterized the flow of a newtonian fluid in a frictionless system in which total energy remains constant (3). Because total energy is equal to *PE* + *KE*, Bernoulli stated that total energy at point A is equal to total energy at point B, or

$$PE_A + KE_A = PE_B + KE_B \qquad [3]$$

In a horizontal tube, which eliminates gravitational effects (i.e., $\rho gh_A = \rho gh_B$), this formula can be expanded by using Eq.1 and Eq. 2 and rewritten as the one-dimensional Bernoulli formula, which relates pressure and velocity:

$$P_A + 1/2\rho v_A^2 = P_B + 1/2\rho v_B^2 \qquad [4]$$

This equation explains another apparent paradox, the flow of fluid from a low-pressure to high-pressure region, which results from the conversion of kinetic energy to potential energy in an enlarging tube (Fig. 70.3B). A clinical example is an aortic aneurysm in which an increase in vessel diameter from 2 to 6 cm results in a predicted nine-fold decrease in fluid velocity to maintain constant flow:

$$\dot{Q} = v \cdot A = v \cdot \pi r^2 \qquad [5]$$

where
$\dot{Q}$ = flow
v = velocity
A = tube area
r = tube radius

KE thus decreases 81-fold (proportional to v^2), and *PE* must increase by an equivalent amount to maintain constant energy in this system. This translates into a small increase in pressure (about 1 mm Hg) and emphasizes the predominant contribution of *PE* rather than *KE* to blood flow in

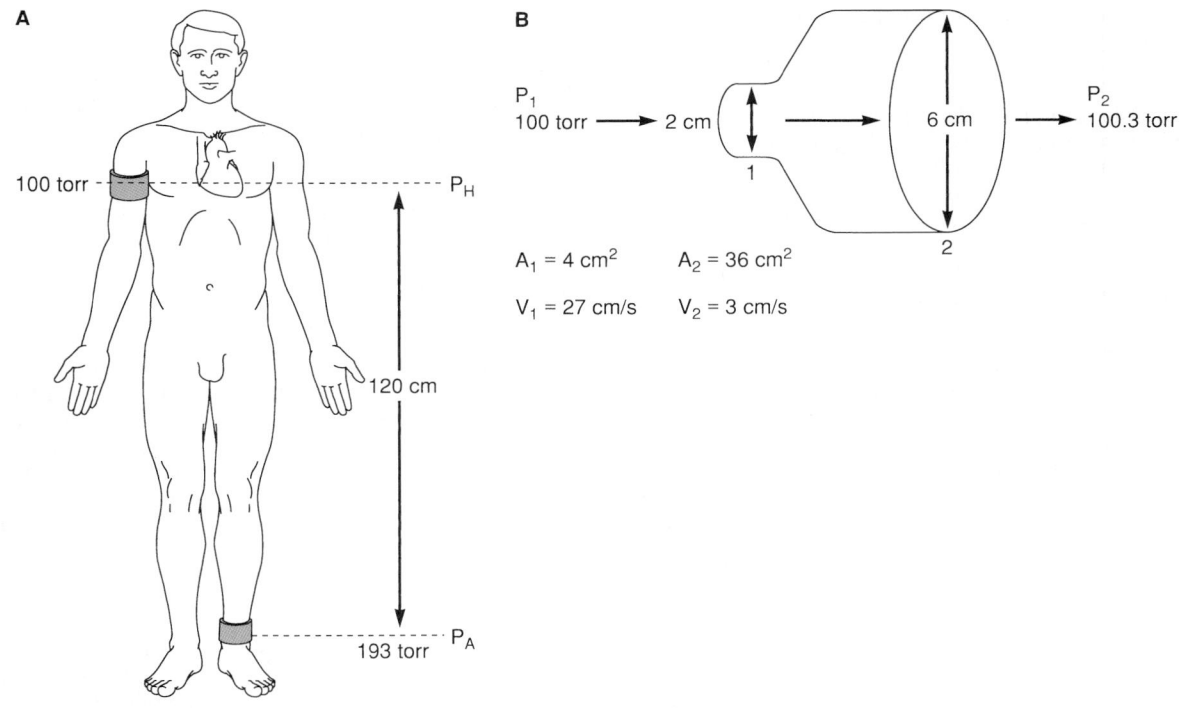

Figure 70.3. *(A)* Effect of gravity on intravascular pressure measured in an erect subject. Pressure at the ankle (P_A) is increased substantially in comparison with pressure at the heart level (P_H) as a result of the weight of the erect column of blood [$P_A = P_H + \rho\gamma h = P_H + (\rho g)\ (120 \text{ cm})$]. *(B)* Effect of luminal expansion on intravascular pressure resulting from conversion of kinetic energy to potential energy as velocity decreases to maintain constant flow. Effect is minimal in a tube with dimensions similar to those of a 6-cm-diameter aortic aneurysm. (After Sumner DS. Essential hemodynamic principles. In: Rutherford RB, ed. *Vascular surgery,* 3rd ed. Philadelphia: WB Saunders, 1989, with permission.)

most cases. In a real aneurysm, even this small increase in pressure is probably eliminated because of the energy lost through flow turbulence at the aneurysm orifice.

ARTERIAL FLOW AND ENERGY LOSS

Measurement

Although arterial blood flow rather than pressure is of ultimate importance for tissue perfusion, flow is more difficult to measure (1). Most blood flow transducers actually measure instantaneous velocity and calculate the volumetric flow based on vessel diameter. Electromagnetic flow probes detect the voltage generated by charged particles as blood flows through the electromagnetic field created by the probe. Because this technique requires direct access to an artery, it is sometimes useful during surgery but is more often used in experimental laboratories. Clinically, blood flow in an individual artery is usually measured with an ultrasonic flowmeter based on the Doppler effect. This technique relies on the shift in the frequency of sound waves that occurs when the distance between the sound wave generator and reflector is changing. A Doppler probe detects the shift in frequency of returning versus emitted sound waves, which is proportional to the velocity of blood from which the sound waves reflect.

More complex duplex ultrasonographic machines calculate the volume in addition to the velocity of blood because they measure artery diameter with B-mode ultrasound. Arterial flow to an entire limb can also be determined by plethysmography (volume measurement). Plethysmographs detect changes in limb volume after venous occlusion by measuring electrical impedance, the stretch of external wires around the limb (strain gauges), or even fluid displacement. After brief inflation of a proximal pneumatic cuff above venous pressure, the immediate increase in volume in a distal extremity is proportional to the total arterial inflow, expressed as flow per volume of tissue measured by the plethysmograph. Cardiac output is frequently measured by thermodilution techniques according to the Fick principle. Originally based on oxygen consumption, this method calculates flow according to the rate of dilution of a rapidly injected indicator (e.g., indocyanin green or cold saline solution). Arterial flow can also be measured according to the rate of tissue uptake of radionuclide-labeled microspheres or the clearance of locally injected, diffusible radiolabeled materials. These latter techniques are generally used only in research applications.

Viscosity and Laminar Blood Flow

Sir Isaac Newton recognized that friction developed between the layers of a flowing fluid, and he defined viscosity as the lack of slipperiness between adjacent laminae (4). In an ideal fluid with no viscosity (i.e., no internal friction between layers) flowing in a frictionless conduit, all fluid particles would travel at the same velocity, and the velocity profile would be flat (Fig. 70.4A). In a real system, the development of cohesive attraction forces between the

conduit wall and the fluid in contact with the wall prevents the outermost, infinitesimally thin layer of fluid from moving. Although some molecular exchange occurs between the outermost fluid layer and the inner fluid layers, the outermost fluid layer does not actually move or slip along the conduit wall. Because a net fluid movement takes place within the conduit, it follows that a velocity gradient must exist across the conduit, with the maximal velocity attained at the greatest distance from the conduit wall, the axial center of the tube. From this center toward the conduit wall, the velocity of each lamina of fluid decreases progressively. Zero velocity is reached at the conduit wall, which results in a parabolic profile for the laminar flow of real liquids (Fig. 70.4B).

Real arteries are not smooth, straight tubes, however. Atherosclerotic plaques, branches, and vessel curvature, together with pulsatile flow, cause a significant departure from the parabolic velocity profile of laminar flow. Disturbances in blood flow result in a disruption of the parallel streamlines characteristic of laminar flow and may produce turbulence. In truly turbulent flow, fluid particles move randomly, and an instantaneous "snapshot" of the fluid velocity vectors would appear chaotic (Fig. 70.4C). When averaged over time, this turbulent flow produces a mean velocity profile similar to that of laminar flow, only much more blunted (Fig. 70.4D). The conditions of physiologic blood flow are generally too stable for true turbulence. Flow disturbances do occur, but they tend to dampen out over short distances and are more accurately termed *disturbed flow* rather than *turbulence*. In common usage, however, these terms are often applied interchangeably.

In an analysis of blood flow, it is best to start with the more straightforward equations related to laminar flow. The stress or force (F) per unit area (A) required to overcome the friction between adjacent fluid layers is defined as shear stress (τ) (3,4), where

$$\tau \ (\text{dyne/cm}^2) = F/A \qquad [6]$$

Shear rate (D) is defined as the velocity gradient (dv) that develops between fluid layers divided by the distance, or radius (dr), between adjacent layers:

$$D \ (\text{s}^{-1}) = dv/dr \qquad [7]$$

Thus, shear rate is proportional to velocity. Viscosity (η) is measured in poise, after Poiseuille, or dyne/s^{-1}/cm^2. Viscosity is precisely defined as the ratio of shear stress to shear rate, expressed as follows:

$$\eta = \tau/D = (F \cdot dr)/(A \cdot dv) \qquad [8]$$

Expressed more simply, viscosity is the tangential force required to maintain a constant velocity between two adjacent laminae with area (A) and distance (dr) constant. Commonly, viscosity is conceptualized as the thickness of a liquid (e.g., oil has a greater viscosity than water). In reality, viscosity is difficult to measure and depends on the temperature of the fluid. Its value in the actual circulation probably differs from that in vitro. Approximate values for viscosity in centipoise (cP) at 37°C are the following:

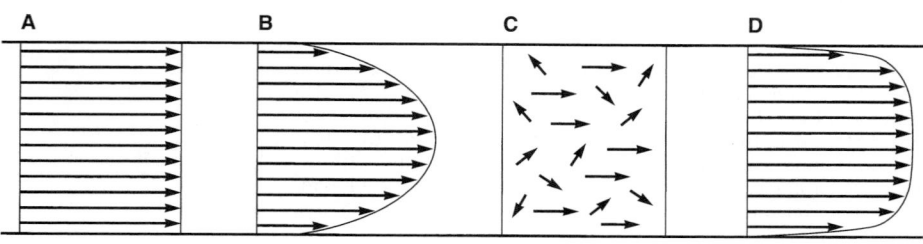

Figure 70.4. (A) Flat velocity profile of an ideal fluid (zero viscosity) in a straight, rigid tube. (B) Parabolic laminar flow profile of a real, newtonian fluid. (C) Turbulent flow of a real fluid at a high Reynolds number. Velocity vectors at any moment in time are random. (D) Time-averaged velocity profile for turbulent flow is blunted in comparison with that for laminar flow.

water, 0.69 cP; plasma, 1.1 to 1.8 cP; blood, 3 to 5 cP (at high shear rate) (3).

A newtonian fluid (e.g., water) is one in which viscosity is constant despite changes in velocity (shear rate) (2,3). Although plasma may be considered newtonian in behavior, blood may not, primarily because of the presence of red blood cells. At low shear rates, red blood cells aggregate and increase the viscosity, particularly in the presence of large plasma proteins such as fibrinogen. At high shear rates, red blood cells are drawn into the central, high-velocity portion of the flow pattern, so that viscosity is reduced. Thus, blood viscosity depends primarily on its shear rate (e.g., velocity), the hematocrit, and the plasma protein concentration. The hematocrit, or packed cell volume, is proportional to the logarithm of viscosity (η), so that at 40% packed cell volume, $\eta = 4$ cP; at 20%, $\eta = 2.2$ cP; and at 60%, $\eta = 8$ cP (3). Thus, elevations in the hematocrit above 45% cause disproportionately large increases in viscosity.

Despite these non-newtonian characteristics, the behavior of physiologic blood flow is often newtonian. Red blood cell aggregation at low shear rates has been found to have little or no effect in vessels in which shear can be measured in vivo (6). The effect of red blood cells at high shear rates is important only when the particle size is large in relation to the vessel. Thus, the effect of red blood cells is not measurable until the luminal diameter drops below 1 mm; it becomes marked when the lumen decreases to 100 to 200 μm (6). In these very small arteries, the reduction in viscosity is crucial to decreasing the resistance to blood flow. The shear stress that typically defines tube flow is that of wall shear. For laminar flow in a newtonian fluid:

$$\tau = 4\eta \dot{Q}/\pi r^3$$

where
τ = shear stress
η = viscosity
$\dot{Q}$ = volumetric rate of blood flow
r = internal radius of the artery

Viscous Energy Loss

As a real fluid flows through a rigid, straight tube, energy is lost in proportion to fluid viscosity as heat generated by friction between layers of the fluid (4). The details of this relation were empirically determined by Poiseuille in 1846. Using a series of glass microcapillary tubes, Poiseuille derived the relation between pressure and flow in this steady flow system as follows:

$$\Delta P = \dot{Q} \cdot 8L\eta/\pi r^4 \qquad [9]$$

where
ΔP = pressure gradient between two points
$\dot{Q}$ = flow
L = tube length between the points
η = coefficient of viscosity
r = tube radius

The latter term in this formula ($8L\eta/\pi r^4$) represents the resistance to flow in this system according to the generalized hemodynamic formula, pressure = flow × resistance:

$$P = \dot{Q}R \qquad [10]$$

This equation is analogous to Ohm's law of electrical circuits, which states that electromotive force (voltage) = current × resistance ($E = IR$). Because vascular resistance cannot be directly measured, it is calculated from direct measurements of pressure (P) and flow ($\dot{Q}$) according to the relation $R = P/\dot{Q}$. Accordingly, resistance is expressed as mm Hg/cm³/min and is defined as a *peripheral resistance unit* for simplicity. The units of mm Hg/cm³/s are expressed in standard resistance units of dyne/s⁻¹/cm⁵.

Poiseuille's equation reveals that resistance to a steady flow of newtonian fluid in a straight, rigid tube is proportional to tube length and fluid viscosity but inversely proportional to the fourth power of the tube radius. Poiseuille's law cannot be used to analyze these variables precisely in the human circulatory system because of the non-newtonian characteristics of blood, the pulsatile nature of arterial flow, and the tapering and elliptic cross section of nonrigid blood vessels. In general, Poiseuille's equation underestimates resistance, so that a higher mean flow than appropriate is calculated for a given pressure gradient. This formula, however, qualitatively illustrates the important hemodynamic principle that vascular resistance (and viscous energy loss) depends far more on small changes in vessel diameter (r^4) than on changes in vessel length or blood viscosity. In a horizontal system (which eliminates gravitational effects), Eqs. 1, 5, and 9 indicate that *PE* lost as a result of viscous effects may be considered as follows:

$$PE = \dot{Q} \cdot 8L\eta/\pi r^4 = v \cdot 8L\eta/r^2 \qquad [11]$$

Inertial Energy Loss

Although Poiseuille stated that changes of pressure in straight tubes are proportional to changes of flow ($\Delta P \propto \Delta Q$), he realized that at high flow rates, larger pressure gradients result than can be predicted by his formula. It remained for Osborn Reynolds in 1883 to characterize these additional energy losses and attribute them to flow turbulence (2). Reynolds injected dye into the axial stream of a long, rigid, cylindric tube and showed that turbulence disrupts the laminar flow pattern of parallel streamlines when the flow rate reaches a certain critical value. From these experiments, he derived the following formula:

$$Re = \rho D v/\eta \qquad [12]$$

where
Re = a dimensionless number (Reynolds number)
ρ = fluid density (g/cm³)
D = diameter (cm)
v = fluid velocity (cm/s)
η = viscosity (cP)

In steady (nonpulsatile) flow, v is taken to be the mean cross-sectional fluid velocity, whereas in pulsatile systems, the peak Reynolds number (calculated according to the cross-sectional velocity at peak flow) is often used. Reynolds demonstrated that in long, straight, rigid tubes, turbulence occurs when Re exceeds 2,000 during steady flow (referred to as the *critical Reynolds number*). Turbulence within an artery may result in an audible noise, or bruit, as a result of vibration of the arterial wall. Severe wall vibration in superficial arteries can be palpated as a thrill. Reynolds' observation indicates that turbulence is more likely with increased velocity and decreased viscosity. The former explains the frequent association of bruits with arterial stenoses; blood velocity increases markedly as it flows through the stenosis. Viscosity may be decreased sufficiently in patients with severe anemia to produce turbulence and a bruit in an otherwise normal artery. Furthermore, the Reynolds number predicts the lack of turbulence observed in arterioles and capillaries, in which velocities are low and vessel diameters are minimal.

Like Poiseuille's formula, the critical value of the Reynolds number cannot be exactly applied to the arterial circulation because of the assumptions inherent in its derivation. In the human arterial system, the Reynolds number does not exceed 2,000 except in the ascending aorta. The classic value for the critical Reynolds number, however, was derived for steady flow in straight, smooth, rigid, cylindric tubes. The critical Reynolds number depends on a number of factors, including the roughness of the conduit walls, the shape of the conduit, and the presence of discontinuities, such as branches or step-offs. It can vary from 100 to 50,000 (depending on inlet, conduit, and flow characteristics) (13). In the arterial circulation, pulsatile flow, compliant vessels, arterial branching, wall irregularities, stenoses, and the non-newtonian characteristics of blood all affect the critical Reynolds number at which turbulence occurs. The Reynolds number is a useful parameter, however, and in the absence of pathologic lesions, severely disturbed flow is associated only with cardiac valves and the ascending aorta (6). Physiologic values of the Reynolds number predict that most disturbances will dampen out quickly in arterial blood flow, and this is usually the case. This situation is more appropriately characterized as disturbed flow rather than true, fully developed turbulence, although many use the terms interchangeably.

In addition to viscous energy losses (Eq. 11), real fluids lose inertial (kinetic) energy as a result of changes in velocity that cause turbulence or flow disturbance (Eq. 2). Because velocity is a vector quantity, pulsatile blood flow and altered arterial geometry result in complex velocity directional changes. These are virtually impossible to measure in vivo, so energy losses cannot be accurately calculated. Inertial energy losses are directly proportional to the second power of velocity (Eq. 2), whereas viscous energy losses are proportional to the first power of velocity (Eq. 11). Thus, at low flow velocities, viscous forces predominate, and pressure gradients are more linearly proportional to flow (i.e., Poiseuille's law). At high flow velocities, inertial energy losses predominate because of the rapidly increasing magnitude of v^2. As predicted by Reynolds, turbulence occurs beyond a certain critical velocity and imparts significantly greater energy loss than that predicted by Poiseuille's formula for viscous energy losses alone.

Local Effects of Turbulent Flow

Changes in geometry at an arterial bifurcation result in altered velocity vectors that create subtle but important local turbulence or disturbed flow (1,4). These effects have been studied in clear glass tubes and specially prepared arteries in which flow streaming and turbulence can be observed by injecting colored dyes. During normal laminar flow, a boundary layer of fluid with essentially zero velocity exists at the fluid–vessel interface because of the viscous properties discussed earlier. At a bifurcation, where the direction of flow changes suddenly, local pressure gradients develop and the laminar velocity profile changes, being skewed with higher velocities toward the central flow divider. This results in a new region of zero velocity separated from the arterial wall, termed *boundary layer separation* (Fig. 70.5). Flow between this boundary layer and the arterial wall remains low or stagnant until more typical laminar flow is reestablished downstream from the bifurcation (*boundary layer separation* is not synonymous with *turbulence*). This region of low flow (and low shear stress) at the site of boundary layer separation has been shown to correspond to the region of the carotid artery bifurcation where atherosclerosis develops and is predominant (14). Conversely, the flow divider, the site of high shear stress, is not usually the site of atherosclerosis. This has led to speculation that an increase in particle residence time, which occurs at sites of boundary layer separation, may accelerate atherosclerosis because of the more prolonged contact of the arterial wall with bloodborne stimulants derived from platelets and other blood elements. As discussed previously, low shear is also a stimulus for endothelial cells to increase the production of biologic mediators that induce narrowing of the vessel lumen through vasoconstriction, proliferation of smooth-muscle cells, and production of extracellular matrix (7).

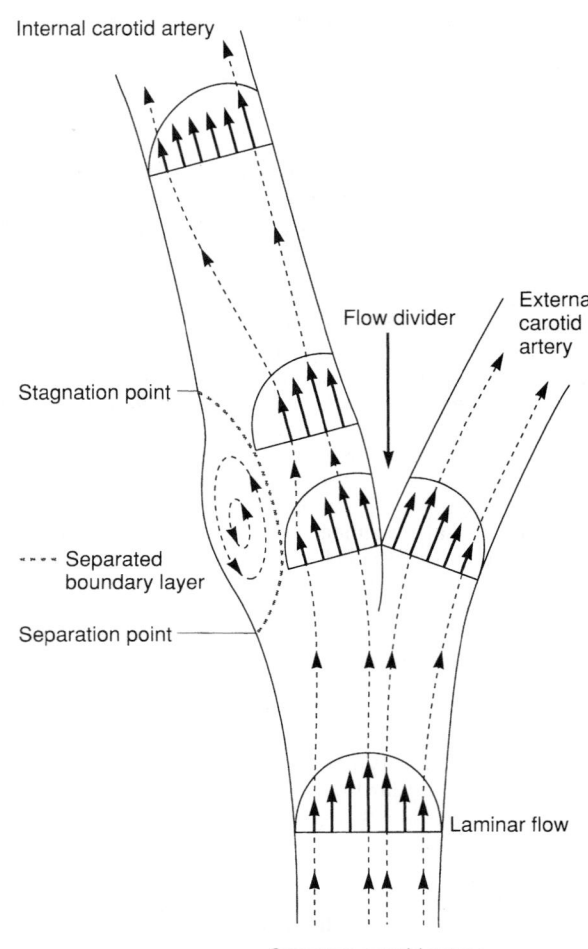

Figure 70.5. Alteration in flow at the human carotid artery bifurcation results in boundary layer separation and stagnant flow along the outer wall of the internal carotid artery. This corresponds to the region where atherosclerotic plaque develops. (After Zarins CK, Giddens DP, Bharaduaj BK, et al. Carotid bifurcation atheroscleroses: quantitative correlation of platelet localization with flow velocity profiles and wall shear stress. *Circ Res* 1983;53:502, with permission.)

ARTERIAL STENOSIS

Energy Loss

Atherosclerotic occlusive disease primarily affects the circulation through energy loss at arterial stenoses or occlusions. As blood flow encounters a fixed stenosis within an artery, its velocity must increase across the stenosis to maintain constant flow (Eq. 5). This is a consequence of conservation of mass and the fact that blood is an essentially incompressible fluid. Inertial energy is lost when the velocity changes at the entrance and exit of the stenosis (4,5). Considerably less flow disturbance results at the convergence of a stenosis than at its divergence, although precise calculations of energy loss depend on factors such as abruptness of tapering, roughness, and tortuosity, which are practically impossible to measure in vivo. For practical considerations, the inertial energy losses at a stenosis are proportional to the second power of the change in velocity (Δv^2), as predicted by Eq. 2. Because the change in velocity is inversely proportional to the second power of the change in radius $(1/\Delta r^2$; Eq. 5), it follows that inertial energy lost at an arterial stenosis is inversely proportional to the fourth

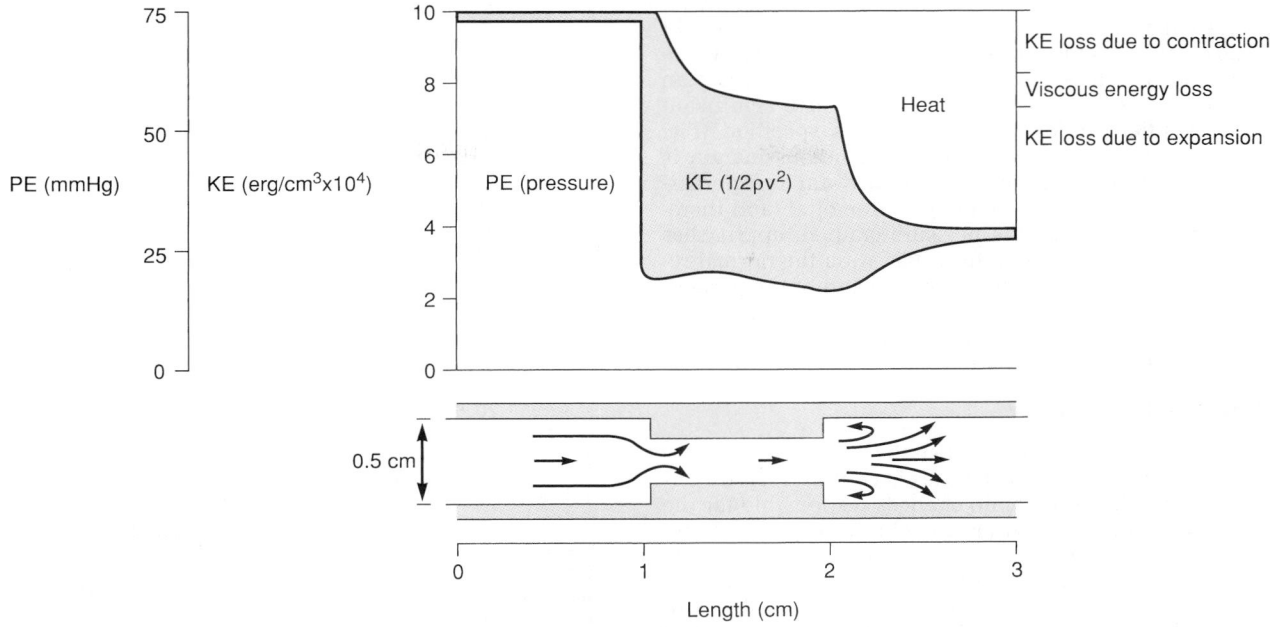

Figure 70.6. Losses of kinetic energy and potential energy resulting from blood passing through a fixed stenosis under steady flow conditions. Most energy is lost at the stenosis exit, with little loss of viscous energy. (After Sumner DS. Essential hemodynamic principles. In: Rutherford RB, ed. *Vascular surgery,* 3rd ed. Philadelphia: WB Saunders, 1989, with permission.)

power of the change in radius ($1/\Delta r^4$). Although Poiseuille's law was derived for long, straight tubes rather than short arterial stenoses, it provides a useful approximation of the viscous energy lost at an arterial stenosis, which is also proportional to $1/\Delta r^4$ (Eq. 9). These estimates of inertial and viscous energy lost at an arterial stenosis predict that a 50%

reduction in luminal diameter will cause at least a 16-fold energy loss. Inertial effects (turbulence), which depend on v^2, contribute significantly more to this energy loss than do viscous effects, which depend on v (Fig. 70.6). At the exit of a stenosis, the loss of *KE* resulting from turbulence has been estimated as follows:

$$\Delta P = k\rho(v_s - v_e)^2/2 \qquad [13]$$

where
k depends on the exact geometric configuration
v_s = velocity in the stenosis
v_e = velocity after the stenosis
ρ = fluid density

This formula can be rewritten as

$$\Delta P = kv^2[(r/r_s)^2 - 1]^2 \qquad [14]$$

where
v = velocity after the stenosis
r = radius of the uninvolved artery
r_s = radius of the stenosis

This formula emphasizes that the energy lost at an arterial stenosis is proportional to the fourth power of the change in radius and the second power of the velocity within the normal artery. This illustrates that the energy lost at any fixed stenosis increases exponentially with increasing blood flow or velocity (Fig. 70.7).

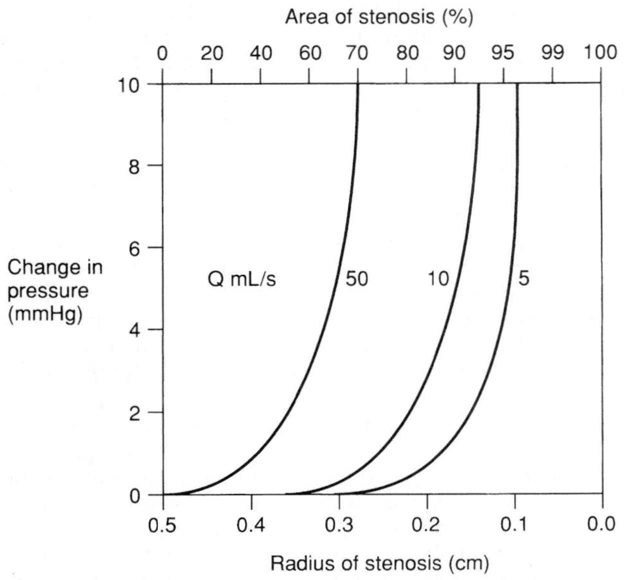

Critical Stenosis

Experimental studies have investigated the above relation between blood flow and pressure lost at an arterial stenosis to determine the clinical significance of varying degrees of stenosis. A pressure gradient or reduction in flow does not occur until a rather significant arterial stenosis is reached, usually a 75% to 90% reduction of the cross-sectional area, which corresponds to a 50% to 70% reduction in diameter, if one assumes that the stenosis is symmetric (1,15). An arterial stenosis is termed *critical* when it reduces distal pressure or flow. The point at which this hap-

Figure 70.7. The effect of increasing the rate of blood flow ($\dot{Q}$) on inertial energy loss (expressed as change in pressure) at the exit of a stenosis in a tube with a radius of 0.5 cm. At a low rate of flow, a larger stenosis is required to reduce pressure. The curves demonstrate the exponential effect of stenosis radius ($1/r^4$) on pressure loss at any given flow. Calculations are based on Eq. 14. (After Sumner DS. Essential hemodynamic principles. In: Rutherford RB, ed. *Vascular surgery,* 3rd ed. Philadelphia: WB Saunders, 1989, with permission.)

pens depends on the blood flow (velocity) within the artery. A stenosis that is not critical at a lower rate of flow might become critical at a higher rate of flow (hence the term *subcritical stenosis*). It is impossible to predict that a certain percentage of arterial stenosis will result in a significant pressure gradient unless the flow rate is specified (Fig. 70.7). Under normal circumstances, a generous margin is incorporated into the size of large and medium transport arteries, which results in such a large value of r^4 (and therefore low resistance) that the pressure gradient approaches zero regardless of the rate of flow. Based on the normal relation between artery size and flow demand of the particular organ supplied, a flow-limiting stenosis generally occurs in the clinical setting at about a 50% reduction in diameter and becomes exponentially worse beyond that point.

Subcritical Stenosis

The fact that arterial an stenosis becomes increasingly significant at higher flow velocities is central to an understanding of the hemodynamic changes responsible for the symptoms of peripheral arterial occlusive disease. A stenosis that is subcritical during resting conditions (low blood flow) may become critical during the increased blood flow associated with exercise. This is easily conceptualized with the general formula $P = \dot{Q}R$ (Eq. 10). If flow ($\dot{Q}$) increases across a fixed stenosis, or resistance (R), the pressure gradient across the stenosis (P) must increase accordingly. This results in a reduced distal blood pressure, which limits the increase in blood flow that would otherwise occur to meet the increased metabolic demands of exercise. Inadequate blood flow then leads to metabolite accumulation and pain (claudication). Only when exercise stops is the resting blood flow sufficient to remove accumulated metabolites and relieve pain.

If an arterial stenosis in a lower extremity is subcritical during resting conditions, the systolic cuff pressure measured at the ankle demonstrates no gradient in comparison with the central arterial pressure (commonly estimated by the brachial artery pressure, hence the term *ankle–brachial index*). The reduction in distal blood pressure that results from the increased flow across a subcritical stenosis can be used to detect such a stenosis. Immediately after or during exercise, the ankle–brachial index decreases in proportion to the reduction in blood flow and returns gradually to normal after cessation of exercise (Fig. 70.8). This principle is used clinically to detect subcritical stenoses and to verify the presence of early arterial occlusive disease in patients who manifest symptoms of claudication but do not have a reduced resting blood pressure. Exercise hyperemia is induced by having the patient walk at a fixed rate and grade on a treadmill until symptoms of claudication develop. Then distal (ankle) pressures are measured and compared with arm and resting ankle pressures. An increase in blood flow across a suspected subcritical stenosis can also be induced with reactive hyperemia. Transient arterial occlusion in the extremity is created by inflating a cuff for 3 to 5 minutes at the thigh or upper calf; as a result, the arterioles distal to the cuff dilate. The resulting decrease in peripheral resistance causes a sudden increase in flow after cuff release, during which the ankle pressure is measured. In patients with subcritical stenoses, ankle or femoral pulses are often normal or only slightly reduced at rest. These pulses may actually disappear during and immediately after exercise because of the reduction in pressure that occurs as flow increases across the proximal stenoses.

Multiple Stenoses

Because atherosclerotic occlusive disease is a diffuse process, it is unlikely that an isolated arterial stenosis will

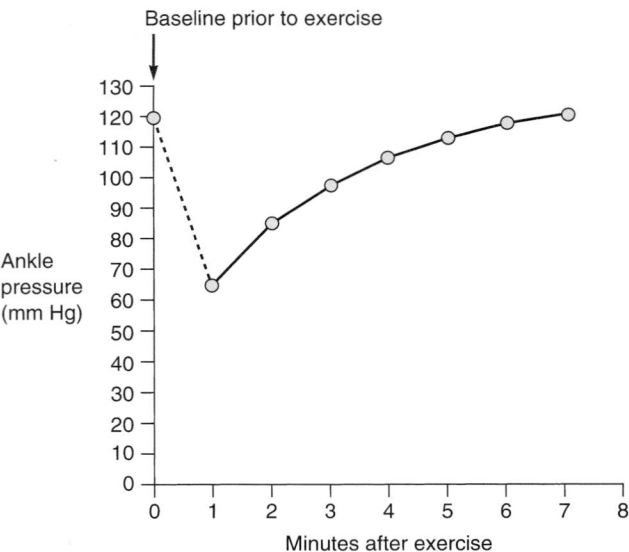

Baseline prior to exercise

Figure 70.8. Decrease in blood pressure at the ankle during exercise reveals the presence of a stenosis that is subcritical at rest. This type of plot is obtained with a treadmill exercise test.

occur but rather that multiple sequential stenoses will eventually develop. Theoretically, resistances in series are additive:

$$R_T = R_1 + R_2 + R_3 \qquad [15]$$

Resistances in parallel (e.g., in collateral vascular beds) are additive as an inverse function:

$$1/R_T = 1/R_1 + 1/R_2 + 1/R_3 \qquad [16]$$

Multiple factors, such as the distance between stenoses, the Reynolds number, the contour and severity of the stenoses, and other intervening geometric variables prevent an exact calculation of the contribution of sequential stenoses in a real arterial system. Experimental results indicate that multiple sequential stenoses generally have an additive effect, although each subsequent stenosis contributes less resistance (15). In practice, the single most critical stenosis largely determines any limitation of blood flow. Multiple subcritical stenoses can produce the effect of a single critical stenosis.

It is clinically expedient to divide the lower extremity into three major subsegments—the aortoiliac, femoropopliteal, and distal (below the knee) circulations. Frequently, significant stenoses occur in more than one of these segments, so that the influences on distal arterial pressure are complex. It is important to determine the hemodynamic significance of stenoses in each of these areas to reconstruct arterial occlusive disease optimally and achieve maximal clinical effects with minimal intervention. Although arteriography provides an anatomic representation of atherosclerotic disease, it is frequently impossible to measure the severity of stenoses accurately because of irregularities in their geometry and three-dimensional asymmetry that confounds single-plane or even biplane arteriography. For these reasons, the measurement of segmental pressure gradients in the lower extremity, by placing blood pressure cuffs at different levels, is an important part of the clinical evaluation.

It is possible to illustrate the effect of sequential stenoses on segmental pressures in the lower extremity by assuming fixed arterial resistances (stenoses) without changes in collateral blood flow (Fig. 70.9). Aortoiliac and superficial femoral artery stenoses result in progressive

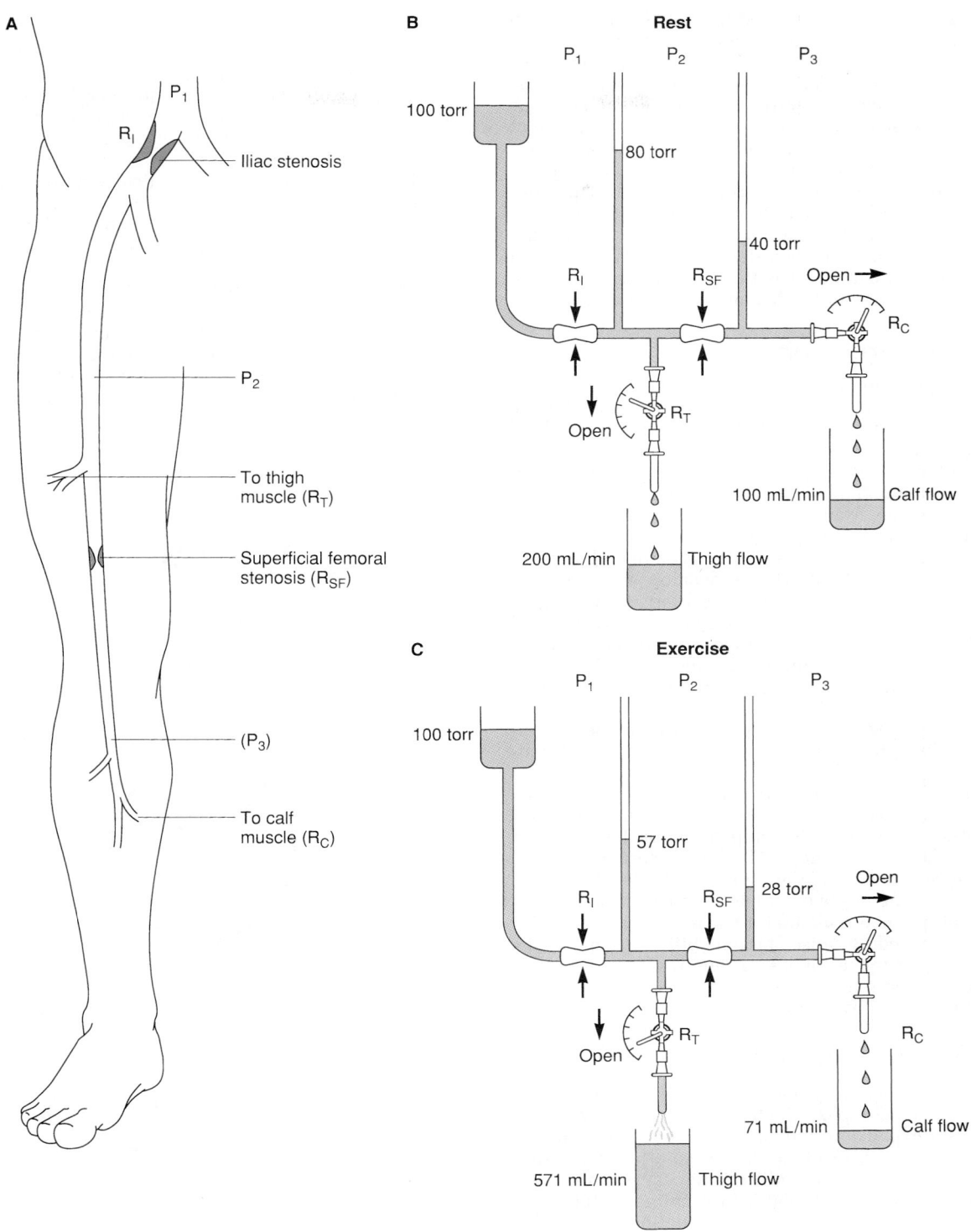

Figure 70.9. *(A)* Atherosclerosis producing stenoses in the common iliac and superficial femoral arteries with fixed resistance values (R_I and R_{SF}). Arterioles in the thigh and calf muscle control muscle flow with variable resistance values (R_T and R_C). Intravascular pressure is measured at points shown (P_1, P_2, P_3). *(B)* Hydraulic model illustrating the effect of iliac and superficial femoral artery stenoses on resting thigh and calf muscle flow. Pressure reduction across R_I results in diminished P_2, which forces decreased R_C to provide sufficient calf muscle flow. *(C)* Exercise causes a decrease in R_T, which increases thigh muscle flow across fixed R_I and results in even lower P_2. This causes a reduction in calf muscle flow because R_C is already maximally reduced (dilated) and pressure at P_2 cannot overcome fixed R_{SF}. The calculation is based on Eq. 10. (After Sumner DS. Essential hemodynamic principles. In: Rutherford RB, ed. *Vascular surgery,* 3rd ed. Philadelphia: WB Saunders, 1989, with permission.)

pressure decrements because resting flow is maintained in the extremity by compensatory increases in peripheral vasodilation. During exercise, peripheral resistance is further decreased by the dilation of arterioles in skeletal muscle to augment flow, as required by local metabolism. The resulting increase in flow causes a larger pressure gradient across the first (proximal) fixed stenosis in the aortoiliac segment, so that the pressure "head" seen by the superficial femoral system is even further reduced. This ultimately results in inadequate flow to the calf muscles despite maximal vasodilation, so that calf claudication occurs. This distal watershed depletion explains the calf claudication that can occur with aortoiliac occlusive disease before buttock and thigh claudication develops.

Collateral Circulation

Assessment of an arterial stenosis by measuring the resultant pressure gradient is further complicated by the presence of collateral arteries that may augment blood flow around a major stenosis or occlusion. Blood flows through collateral arteries when an energy gradient develops across a stenosis in a major artery, which induces flow through collaterals from the proximal, higher-energy level to the distal, lower-energy level (16). Chronically, this leads to dilation and perhaps proliferation of collateral arteries. Because collateral arteries develop as a result of limitation of flow through the major artery, they are generally maximally dilated and represent a relatively fixed resistance. The presence of an effective collateral circulation, however, limits the effect of a major arterial stenosis. In reality, clinical pressure and flow measurements cannot separate the contribution of flow across the stenosis and the collateral flow. Instead, they determine the overall flow reduction and pressure gradient in affected extremities.

Because collateral arteries are considerably smaller than the primary diseased vessel, a much larger number of collateral vessels is required to compensate for the change in resistance caused by stenosis of a large artery. Resistance is an inverse function of the radius to the fourth power; therefore, to compensate completely for a 50% stenosis in a 0.5-cm artery, 625 collateral arteries 1 mm in diameter would be required. Because of the inability to achieve this compensation, surgical bypass or endovascular intervention becomes necessary to restore the original diameter of the conduit and relieve symptoms.

ARTERIAL ANEURYSMS

Although the factors responsible for the development of an aneurysm are complex, the hemodynamic contribution to aneurysm expansion and rupture is well defined. Expansion occurs as a result of tangential stress (τ) within the wall of an aneurysm, and rupture occurs when τ exceeds the wall tensile strength. In a cylindric tube, circumferential wall tensile stress (τ_c) is defined by the following equation:

$$\tau_c = P \cdot r/\delta \qquad [17]$$

where
P = pressure
r = internal radius
δ = wall thickness

This is a modification of LaPlace's law for cylinders of negligible thickness, expressed as

$$T = P \cdot r \qquad [18]$$

In a sphere, circumferential wall tensile stress is defined by the formula

$$\tau_c = P \cdot r/2\delta \qquad [19]$$

According to these formulas, increases in arterial blood pressure and aneurysm size (radius) are linearly proportional to the wall tensile stress and, therefore, to the risk for aneurysm expansion and rupture. Conversely, aneurysm wall thickness is inversely proportional to wall stress, so that thinner aneurysms are more prone to rupture (Fig. 70.10). These mathematically derived risk factors for aneurysm rupture, hypertension, and aneurysm size have been confirmed by clinical observation (17). Unfortunately, the wall thickness (and strength) of real aneurysms cannot be accurately measured in vivo at present. Of interest is the predicted difference between wall stress in a fusiform versus a saccular aneurysm. Fusiform aneurysms are best approximated by cylinders, whereas saccular aneurysms are more analogous to spheres. A comparison of Eqs. 17 and 19 predicts that saccular aneurysms will experience about half the circumferential wall stress

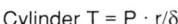

Cylinder T = P · r/δ

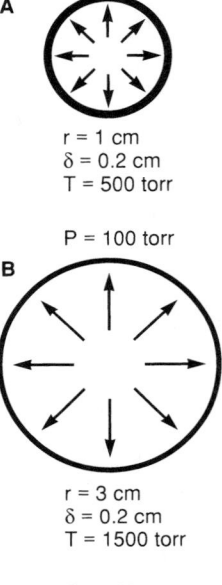

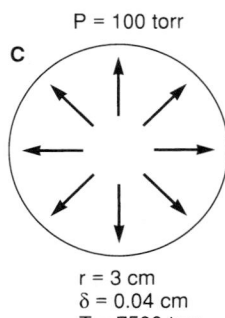

Figure 70.10. Cross-sectional views of cylinders representing normal-diameter infrarenal aorta *(A)* and 6-cm-diameter aortic aneurysms *(B,C)* to demonstrate the effect of radius (*r*) and wall thickness (δ) on circumferential wall stress (*T*; τc elsewhere in chapter) at constant pressure (*r* = 100 torr). Expansion of a 2-cm-diameter cylinder *(A)* to a 6-cm-diameter cylinder with no change in wall thickness *(B)* increases wall tensile stress sixfold. If expansion occurs without an increase in wall mass, wall thinning occurs *(C)* and results in even greater tensile stress within the wall.

of a fusiform aneurysm. These analogies are oversimplifications, however, because real aneurysms have complex shapes.

A more accurate method to estimate aneurysm wall stress uses finite element analysis. This mathematical technique breaks a structure down into small components, so that the equations relating pressure and stress can be solved by high-powered computers. Initially, this work was performed on theoretical symmetric shapes to simplify the analysis (18). The technique predicts a greater circumferential stress in cylindric than in spherical aneurysms, although longitudinal stress is equivalent. Furthermore, the tensile stress in an aneurysm wall is inversely related to the size of the native (proximal) aorta if wall thinning occurs during aneurysm expansion. In theory, the wall stress developing in a 6-cm aneurysm arising from a 1-cm aorta might be three to four times greater than the wall stress developing in a 6-cm aneurysm arising from a 3-cm aorta. Interestingly, data have been obtained suggesting that thickness is not the primary factor in aneurysm wall stress. Based on wall thickness data from 60 abdominal aortic aneurysms, it appears that the effect of thickness on maximum wall stress is small relative to the effect of shape and diameter over an appropriate clinical range (unpublished data). This is probably because the initial aortic diameter does not vary a great deal in a typical patient with an abdominal aortic aneurysm. The role of wall thickness may also be lessened when a stimulus to increase wall thickness as the aortic diameter increases partially compensates for the increase in stress.

Of course, applying the aforementioned equations and techniques to theoretical shapes and diameters does not allow the risk for aneurysm rupture to be calculated for individual patients. More recently, finite element analysis has been performed on three-dimensional reconstructions of computed tomographic data from actual patients (19). By means of sophisticated computational techniques, the wall stress for an abdominal aortic aneurysm can be mapped onto a three-dimensional reconstruction of the aneurysm (Fig. 70.11) (see color insert following page 1190). This technique is still investigational, but results suggest that the area subjected to the greatest stress in an abdominal aortic aneurysm is typically posterolateral, which is the most common site for rupture in autopsy studies and clinical series. Our own (unpublished) data, derived by using this technique to study abdominal aortic aneurysms in vivo, suggest that shape is a key factor in determining the risk for wall stress and rupture in abdominal aortic aneurysms. The effect of shape appears to be at least as important as the effect of diameter and blood pressure on wall stress in aneurysms. Ultimately, this type of analysis may replace estimates of rupture risk based on diameter alone.

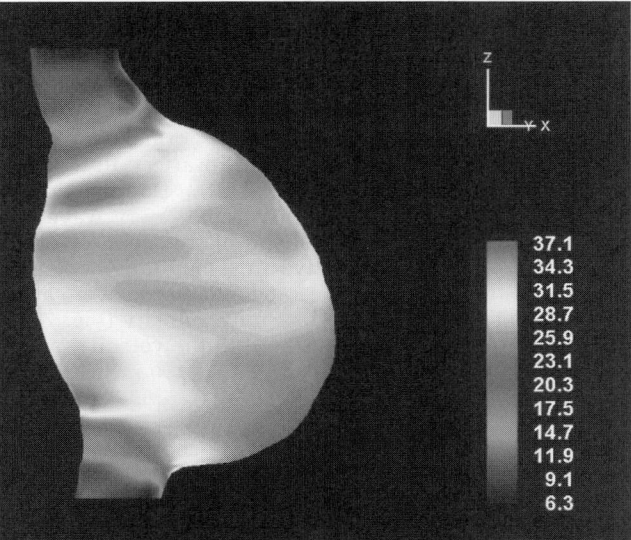

Figure 70.11. Wall stress distribution in an actual abdominal aortic aneurysm. *Colors* represent levels of tensile stress within the aortic wall at that location (correlation of color and stress level is displayed in the *bar* on the right). A three-dimensional reconstruction of the aneurysm was generated from computed tomographic data and transformed into the wall stress distribution by means of finite element analysis and the patient's blood pressure values (see text). This is a lateral view (see three-dimensional framework, upper right). Note that the highest levels of stress are not at the maximal diameter but along the posterolateral wall, where ruptures most commonly occur in clinical experience and autopsy series. Thus, stresses induced by the shape of the abdominal aortic aneurysm appear to be at least as important as the stresses induced by diameter alone.

REFERENCES

1. Strandness DE, Sumner DS. *Hemodynamics for surgeons.* New York: Grune & Stratton, 1975.
2. Folkow B, Neil E. *Circulation.* New York: Oxford University Press, 1971.
3. Burton AC. *Physiology and biophysics of the circulation,* 2nd ed. Chicago: Year Book, 1972.
4. Daugherty RL, Franzini JB. *Fluid mechanics with engineering application,* 7th ed. New York: McGraw-Hill, 1977.
5. Sumner DS. Essential hemodynamic principles. In: Rutherford RB, ed. *Vascular surgery,* 3rd ed. Philadelphia: WB Saunders, 1989.
6. Nichols WW, O'Rourke MF. *McDonald's blood flow in arteries,* 3rd ed. Philadelphia: Lea & Febiger, 1990.
7. Davies PF, Robotewskyj A, Griem ML, et al. Hemodynamic forces and vascular cell communication in arteries. *Arch Pathol Lab Med* 1992;116:1301.
8. Giddens DP, Zarins CK, Glagov S. Response of arteries to near-wall fluid dynamic behavior. *Appl Mech Rev* 1990;43: S96.
9. Langille BL, O'Donnell F. Reductions in arterial diameter produced by chronic decreases in blood flow are endothelium-dependent. *Science* 1986;231:405.
10. Fillinger MF, Cronenwett JL, Besso S, et al. Vein adaptation to the hemodynamic environment of infrainguinal grafts. *J Vasc Surg* 1994;19:970.
11. Dobrin PB. Biaxial anisotropy of dog carotid artery. *J Biomech* 1986;19:351.
12. McGrath MA, Verhaeghe RH, Shepard JT. The physiology of limb blood flow. In: Jaergens JL, Spittel JA Jr, Fairbairn JF II, eds. *Peripheral vascular diseases.* Philadelphia: WB Saunders, 1980:83.
13. Whitmore RL. The flow of fluids. In: Whitmore RL, ed. *Rheology of the circulation.* New York: Pergamon Press, 1968:37.
14. Zarins CK, Giddens DP, Bharaduaj BK, et al. Carotid bifurcation atheroscleroses: quantitative correlation of platelet localization with flow velocity profiles and wall shear stress. *Circ Res* 1983;53:502.
15. Karayannacos PE, Talukder N, Nerem RM, et al. The role of multiple noncritical arterial stenoses in the pathogenesis of ischemia. *J Thorac Cardiovasc Surg* 1977;73:458.
16. Strandness DE Jr. *Collateral circulation in clinical surgery.* Philadelphia: WB Saunders, 1969.
17. Cronenwett JL, Sargent SK, Wall MH, et al. Variables that affect the expansion rate and outcome of small abdominal aortic aneurysms. *J Vasc Surg* 1990;11:260.
18. Stringfellow MM, Lawrence PF, Stringfellow RG. The influence of aorta-aneurysm geometry upon stress in the aneurysm wall. *J Surg Res* 1987;42:425.
19. Raghavan ML, Vorp DA, Webster MW. Ex vivo biomechanical behavior of abdominal aortic aneurysm: assessment using a new mathematical model. *Ann Biomed Eng* 1996;24:573–582.

SURGERY: SCIENTIFIC PRINCIPLES AND PRACTICE, Third Edition, edited by
Lazar J. Greenfield, Michael W. Mulholland, Keith T. Oldham, Gerald B. Zelenock,
and Keith D. Lillemoe. Lippincott Williams & Wilkins Publishers, Philadelphia, © 2001.

CHAPTER 71

VASCULAR LABORATORY TESTING FOR ARTERIAL DISEASE

HUGH G. BEEBE AND SERGIO X. SALLES-CUNHA

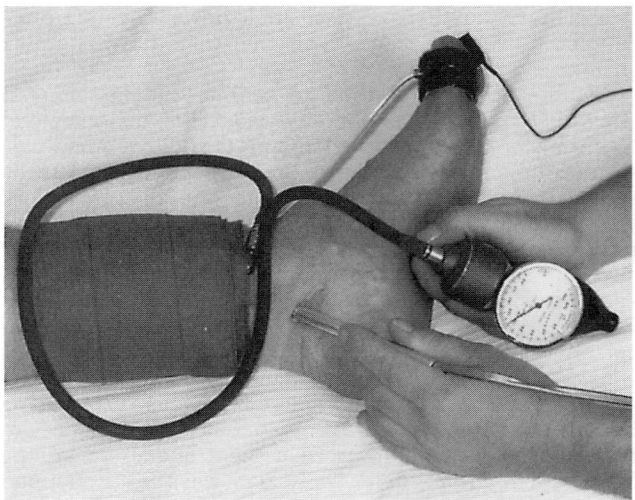

Figure 71.1. A continuous-wave (CW) Doppler ultrasound probe, aimed at the posterior tibial artery, detects arterial flow signals. A pneumatic cuff wrapped around the ankle or toe is used to measure ankle or toe pressures. Toe pulses are detected with a photoplethysmograph.

Noninvasive arterial testing performed in the vascular laboratory has several important clinical functions. It may reveal unsuspected arterial disease or help clarify the relative importance of coexisting conditions. Laboratory testing provides objective documentation to establish treatment qualification thresholds of severity or a basis for serial follow-up. Because modern vascular diagnostic laboratories have achieved high levels of effectiveness in quantifying pathophysiology and useful graphic display of pathologic anatomy, noninvasive arterial testing is increasingly used as a sufficient, stand-alone evaluation before surgical procedures. Thus, the role of the vascular laboratory is of central importance to clinical decision making and for long-term guidance in managing a chronic disease state.

BASIC NONINVASIVE TESTS: HOW DO WE USE THEM?

Noninvasive arterial testing has two distinct but complementary components: physiologic evaluation and anatomic imaging. Physiologic evaluation describes the overall status of an arterial segment and includes blood pressure, blood flow, and skin temperature or oxygen gradient measurements (1–3). Improvement resulting from treatment or degeneration caused by disease progression can be quantified. The condition of individual arteries, however, is poorly defined by physiologic testing. Anatomic imaging allows further interrogation of the arterial lumen by providing a graphic representation of any abnormalities present (1,4,5). The combination of physiologic testing, sometimes using challenge–response perturbations to heighten sensitivity, and anatomic imaging is often needed for a complete and clinically useful description.

Physiologic Methods

Continuous-wave Doppler

Continuous-wave (CW) Doppler detects blood flow waveforms of arteries insonated with an ultrasound probe (Fig. 71.1). The probe has two transducers: one transmits and the other receives ultrasound continuously. The common range of peripheral Doppler ultrasound frequencies is 2 to 10 MHz (1 MHz = 1,000,000 oscillations per second). The incident ultrasound wave is reflected back by moving red blood cells with a frequency shift that is proportional to blood velocity in the direction of insonation. Placing the ultrasound probe perpendicular to the artery results in a poor waveform signal. The probe must be angulated in search of an optimal signal. The strongest flow signal is obtained if the blood is moving parallel to the ultrasound beam. The Doppler frequency shift is in the audio range,

20 Hz to 20 kHz, allowing for auscultation of the arterial blood flow signal.

Continuous-wave Doppler is recommended as a first approach for extremity arterial evaluation and is commonly used as a pulse detector during systolic pressure measurements. The Doppler waveform is analyzed qualitatively. The normal Doppler waveform varies according to the artery being studied. For example, a leg artery Doppler waveform is triphasic with a rapid, steep upslope during systole followed by a secondary reverse waveform and a third, small antegrade waveform (Fig. 71.2). These oscillations result from a combination of reflected and elastic recoil waves. The internal carotid artery Doppler waveform, however, is different owing to the continuous, low-resistance, diastolic run-off available under normal conditions. Figure 71.3 shows an internal carotid artery flow waveform, most commonly detected with the Doppler duplex technique described later. Normal renal artery waveform also has diastolic flow. The shape of the Doppler waveform gives valuable qualitative information. A common example is the damped appearance distal to severe arterial stenosis showing reduced systolic velocity (Fig. 71.2). In the region of critical stenosis itself, the velocity is usually markedly increased.

Pressure Measurements

The hemodynamic effects of arterial occlusive disease are commonly quantified with noninvasive systolic pressure measurements (6). These determinations can be performed at various levels with pneumatic cuffs applied to the arm, upper and lower thigh, below the knee, ankle, foot, or toe (Fig. 71.1). The cuff is inflated to suprasystolic pressures and then deflated slowly. Systolic pressure is determined once a distal flow signal, usually detected with a CW Doppler probe, reappears. Systolic pressures can also be determined during slow cuff inflation, but the exact end point may not be as discrete or easy to detect.

Ankle systolic pressure is compared with the higher of the right or left arm systolic pressure for calculation of the ankle–arm or ankle–brachial index (ABI). Normally, systolic pressures in the lower extremity are equal to or slightly higher than arm pressures. A drop in pressure from one level to the other or compared with the same

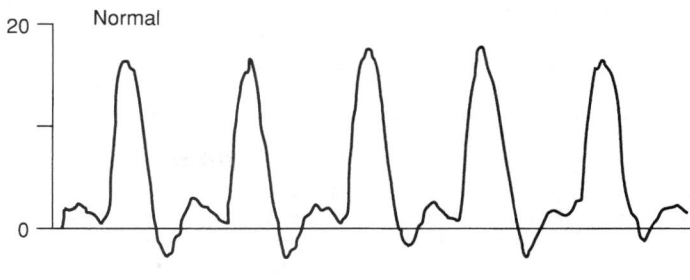

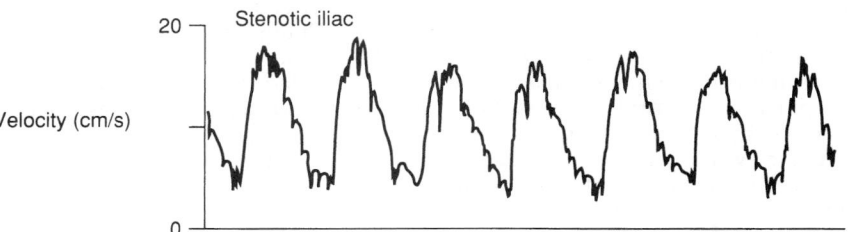

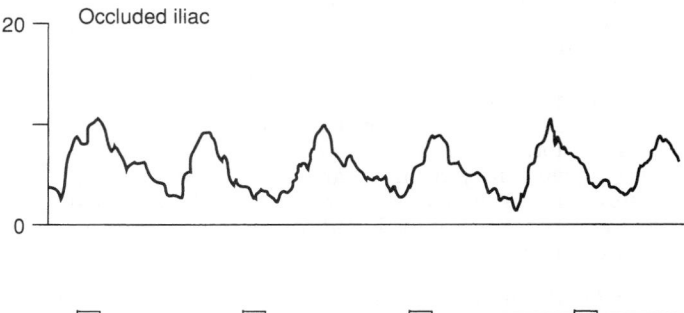

Figure 71.2. Analogue recordings of Doppler signals obtained from the common femoral artery of a normal subject, a patient with an iliac artery stenosis, and a patient with occlusion of the iliac artery. (After Strandness DE Jr, Sumner DS. *Hemodynamics for surgeons.* New York: Grune & Stratton, 1975:257.)

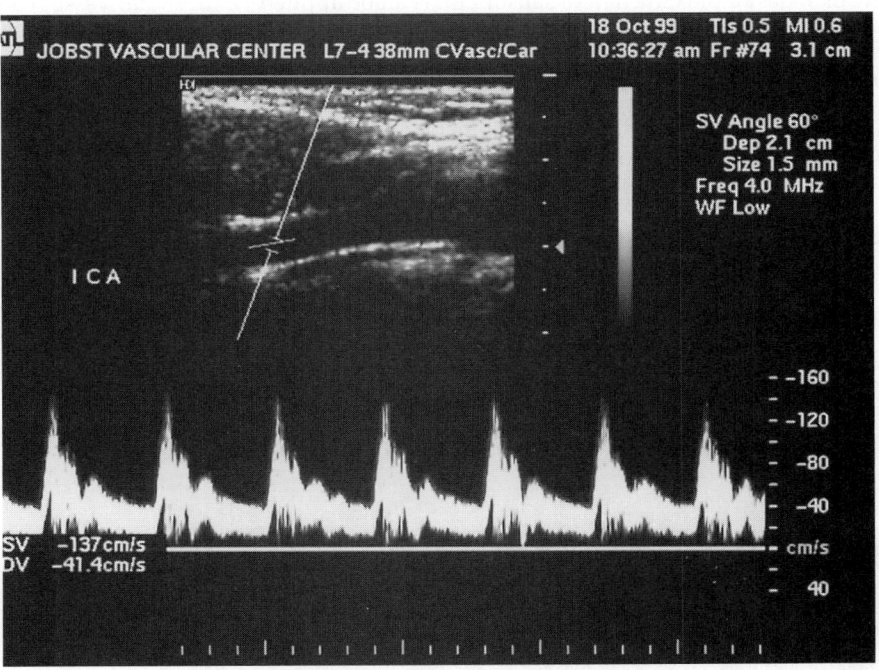

Figure 71.3. Normal internal carotid artery velocity spectral waveform obtained with duplex Doppler ultrasound. Placement of velocity sample volume is guided by B-mode imaging.

level in the opposite leg indicates presence of occlusive disease. Usually, if the posterior and anterior tibial pressures are different, the highest ABI is used for interpretation of disease severity. We recommend that both posterior tibial and anterior tibial ABIs be considered in the interpretation of distal ischemia. Normal ABIs are in the 1.0 to 1.2 range, and a level below 0.9 is abnormal. An ABI less than 0.5 suggests severe arterial ischemia. Toe pressures are usually 20% less than ankle pressures. Normal toe–brachial indices are in the 0.7 to 0.9 range. A toe–brachial index less than 0.4 suggests severe ischemia.

Postexercise measurements of ankle pressure enhance sensitivity to detect and quantify peripheral arterial occlusive disease. This test is most commonly performed in claudicants with normal ankle pressures at rest. Standard exercise is treadmill walking at 5 mph and 2% incline. Toe raises or reactive hyperemia have been used as satisfactory and practical substitutes for treadmill testing in the clinic. Reactive hyperemia follows release of arterial flow obstruction with a cuff wrapped around the thigh or upper calf, inflated to suprasystolic pressures for 2 to 5 minutes. Immediately after exercise, toe raises, or release of cuff pressure, ankle pressures drop proportionately to the severity of obstructive arterial disease and the reduction of outflow resistance. Recovery time until ankle pressures return to baseline is also a function of disease severity.

Cuff width must be at least 20% larger than limb diameter to avoid falsely elevated measurements. A common artifact causing falsely elevated leg arterial pressures is arterial wall calcification, often present in patients with long-standing diabetes. This occurs because the pneumatic cuff must exert higher pressure to occlude the noncompliant arterial wall of these patients. Failure to take this into account may result in an erroneous conclusion that arterial occlusive disease is not present. Thus, a good practice is to obtain great toe blood pressure measurement in patients with diabetes whose ABI is greater than 0.6.

Air Plethysmography

Plethysmography records pulse volume changes (7). A pneumatic cuff is wrapped around the limb, and changes in limb volume, caused by arterial pulsations, are transmitted to the cuff. An electronic transducer detects pressure changes in the cuff. These sensor cuffs can be applied to the thigh, calf, ankle, foot, and digits. As the obstructive arterial disease progresses, waveforms distal to the obstruction are altered (Fig. 71.4). First the waveform dicrotic notch disappears, then the amplitude diminishes, the pulse becomes rounded, the upslope takes longer, and the downslope bows away from the baseline. Finally, the amplitude flattens out in the presence of severe arterial occlusive disease.

Photoplethysmography

Photoplethysmography uses a light sensor, in contact with the skin, to detect arterial pulsations (Fig. 71.1). Re-

flected light spectrum changes caused by systolic red blood cell surges in skin vessels are detected. Photoplethysmography is used primarily for digital pulse examinations and for toe pressure measurement. Changes in arterial pulse recording as disease progresses are similar to those detected by air plethysmography, described in the previous section.

Transcutaneous Oxygen Tension

Oxygen pressure can be measured transcutaneously with a noninvasive transducer applied to the skin (8). This measurement depends on blood flow delivered to the region, oxygen extraction from the blood, and oxygen diffusion to and through the skin. Transcutaneous oxygen tension ($TcPO_2$) measurement is performed at the dorsum of the foot or other ischemic area of interest. To normalize for variations in arterial PO_2, cardiac output, and age-related changes, foot $TcPO_2$ is compared with central area $TcPO_2$, usually measured from a well perfused infraclavicular region. Foot $TcPO_2$ is usually 90% of infraclavicular $TcPO_2$, in the range of 60 mm Hg. With severe ischemia, foot $TcPO_2$ level drops to 20 mm Hg or less and is often unrecordable. Attempts have been made to enhance clinical utility of $TcPO_2$ measurements by obtaining values before and after various perturbations such as supplemental inspired oxygen or changes in limb dependency. It is often true that abnormal physiologic response to a stimulus is a more sensitive indicator of disease state than absolute values, but because $TcPO_2$ is clinically useful only in severe ischemia, the resting state level is usually used.

Thermometry

A few laboratories measure digital skin temperature with an infrared thermometer to standardize peripheral hemodynamic measurements. Toe pressures and limb flow rates can be significantly altered by changes in peripheral temperature. By performing such measurements within a narrow range of digital skin temperatures, such as 28°C to 30°C, measurement reproducibility is improved.

Pulsed-wave Doppler

If two or more vessels are insonated with CW Doppler, their flow signals are mixed together. Flow from each individual vessel cannot be identified. Commonly, the flow signals from adjacent arteries and veins are superimposed. With pulsed-wave Doppler, each vessel can be interrogated individually. This technique is used primarily with duplex ultrasound imaging, a technique described later.

Velocity Spectral Waveform

Blood velocities vary within an artery, especially in areas of turbulent blood flow. By placing a pulsed-wave Doppler sample volume at various locations inside the artery, a spectrum of velocities can be detected. Normally, a narrow range of high velocities concentrates in the center of the artery while low velocities occur near the wall (Fig. 71.5A).

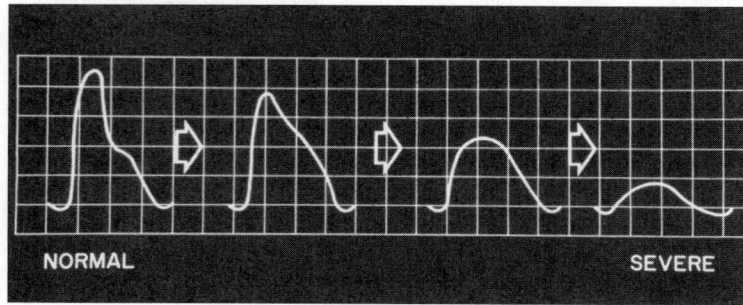

NORMAL   SEVERE

Figure 71.4. Arterial pulse volume recorded with a pneumatic cuff wrapped around a limb segment. Alterations in waveforms correspond to severity of disease.

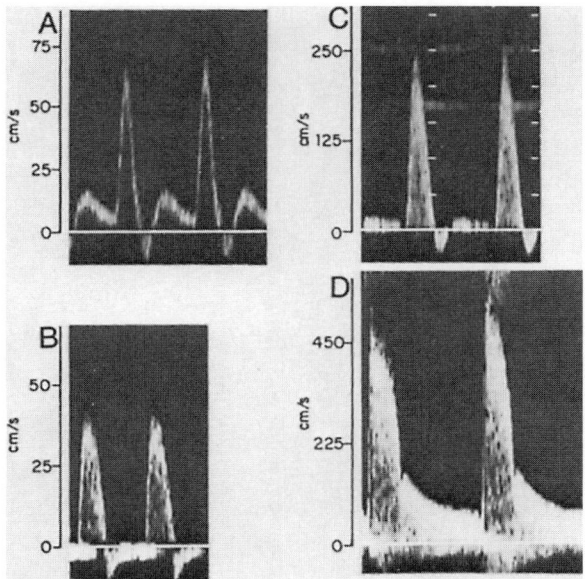

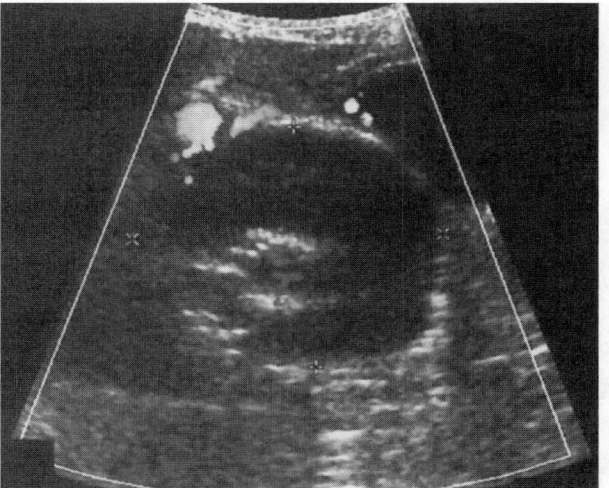

Figure 71.6. B-mode ultrasound image of an abdominal aortic aneurysm treated with a bifurcated endovascular prosthesis.

Figure 71.5. Spectral analysis of Doppler flow signals: *(A)* normal, *(B)* 1% to 19% stenosis, *(C)* 20% to 49% stenosis, and *(D)* 50% to 99% stenosis. (After Kohler TR, Nance DR, Cramer MM, et al. Duplex scanning for diagnosis of aortoiliac and femoropopliteal disease: a prospective study. *Circulation* 1987;76:1075, with permission.)

When a plaque develops, velocity spectral broadening representing a wider range of velocities is detected (Fig. 71.5B). As the stenosis progresses, velocity at the site of stenosis increases (Fig. 71.5C,D). This technique is used primarily with duplex ultrasound imaging, described later.

Flowmetry

Blood flow can be measured by several methods and has an intrinsic appeal because, in the final analysis, it is volume of blood delivered to tissue that is the most important function of circulation (9). Blood pressure is easy to measure but reveals little about flow volume. Reasons that blood flow data are not common in the vascular laboratory include the use of measurement methods that are complex and difficult and, most important, the greater variability and range of blood flow values compared with blood pressure measurements. Venous occlusion plethysmography, electromagnetic, magnetic resonance, and duplex Doppler ultrasound techniques have been used to measure volumetric flow rates noninvasively. When venous outflow is occluded using a low-pressure cuff, limb volume increase per unit time is proportional to arterial inflow. Electromagnetic flowmetry has been used accurately to record arterial blood flow invasively through individual arteries for over 30 years. Noninvasive electromagnetic and magnetic resonance flowmetry, however, require expensive, dedicated equipment and advanced operator skills that have prevented general use. Today, duplex Doppler ultrasound is most often used to measure arterial flow. Volumetric blood flow rate is estimated by multiplying average Doppler velocity and vessel area. The area is often estimated from diameter measurements performed on the B-mode ultrasound image.

Imaging Methods

B-mode Ultrasound Imaging

An image of anatomic structures is created by using reflection and diffusion of ultrasound beams (Fig. 71.6). The traditional image in gray scale depicts a range of pixels from black to white as echo amplitude increases from weak to strong. Transducer probes with linear arrays of a few hundred crystals create rectangular images. Linear arrays are used primarily for carotid and peripheral arterial evaluations (Figs. 71.3, 71.7). Curvilinear arrays or sector probes create pie-shaped images and are used primarily for abdominal scans (Fig. 71.6).

High-frequency ultrasound transducers yield relatively higher-resolution B-mode images than those of lower-frequency transducers. In contrast, the ability to penetrate through tissue into deep structures of the body is better with low- than with high-frequency transducers. Therefore, a compromise exists between the high resolution obtained with high-frequency ultrasound and the deep penetration obtained with low-frequency ultrasound. Deep abdominal studies are performed with frequencies around 3 MHz, whereas carotid and peripheral studies use 5 to 10 MHz.

Duplex Ultrasound

Imaging alone fails to determine if an artery is patent or occluded. This differentiation is made by detection of arterial blood flow. Traditionally, blood flow velocity measurements have been used to determine the degree of arterial stenosis. Duplex ultrasound is the dual technique that provides an image of the blood vessel as well as flow velocity information (Figs. 71.3, 71.8). Pulsed-wave Doppler provides velocity data from a sample selected within the arterial lumen with B-mode image guidance. Short pulse waves are transmitted intermittently and repetitively. In the time interval between these transmitting pulses, the transducer receives reflected ultrasound signals. By processing Doppler ultrasound flow signals at different time intervals between pulse transmission and echo reception, blood flow velocities are detected and calculated within defined regions of the arterial lumen.

A shift in the frequency (ΔF) of the transmitted ultrasound signal is caused when the signal strikes a moving object (blood flow). When it returns by reflection off the moving bloodstream to the ultrasound probe, now in the receiving mode, velocity (V) can be determined by the Doppler equation:

$$V = \frac{1}{2}\ (\Delta F/F_t)\ c/\cos\theta$$

where F_t is the transmitted frequency, c is the speed of ultrasound in tissue, and θ is the angle between the ultra-

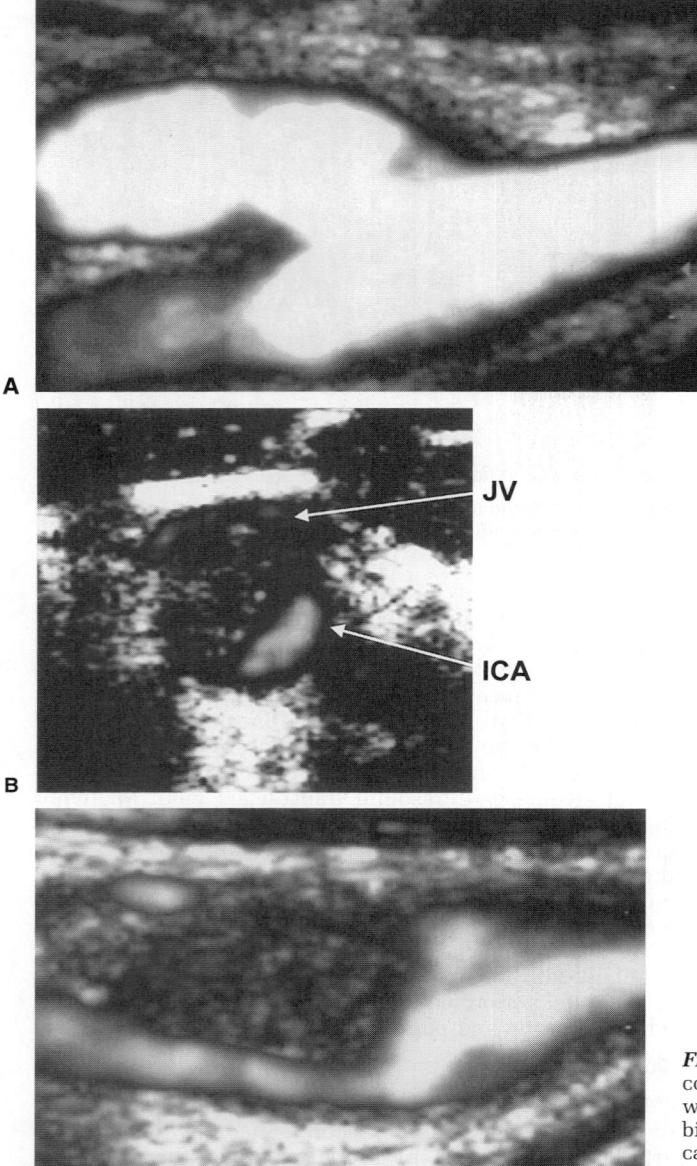

Figure 71.7. Carotid ultrasound imaging. Black-and-white print of a color picture showing a B-mode image and vessel lumina obtained with power Doppler. *(A)* Normal, longitudinal section of the carotid bifurcation. *(B)* Transverse section through the proximal internal carotid artery showing 75% lumen reduction. A compressed jugular vein (JV) is shown above the obstructed internal carotid artery (ICA). *(C)* Longitudinal section corresponding to Fig. 71.7B.

sound beam and the direction of flow. This angle of insonation is estimated by the operator. For this purpose, the Doppler cursor is placed parallel to the vessel wall. A recommended angle of insonation is 60 degrees. A common error is to place the Doppler cursor at 60 degrees but not parallel to the arterial wall. Angles greater than 60 degrees are not recommended. Because the cosine of a 90-degree angle is zero, Doppler frequency shifts cannot be measured when the insonation angle is exactly perpendicular to blood flow.

Absolute and relative values of peak–systolic velocity (PSV) and end-diastolic velocity (EDV) have been used to quantitate degrees of stenosis. Normal velocities are often below 100 cm/s. Severe carotid stenosis, for example, is suspected if the PSV is greater than 250 or 300 cm/s, the EDV is greater than 100, 120, or 140 cm/s, or if the internal/common carotid PSV ratio is greater than 2.5 or 4.0 (1,5,10). For bypass graft or peripheral arterial stenosis, doubling or tripling of the PSV at the stenotic site, relative to the prestenotic or poststenotic region, has been used as a criterion for severe stenosis. This criterion ratio may be valid for the primary stenosis but is inaccurate for evaluation of stenoses in series. Severe stenosis velocity threshold criteria are instrument dependent and must be determined individually for each instrument (10).

Color Flow

Color flow, or color Doppler, expands the amount of flow information obtained and the way the information is presented. Color flow provides velocity-related information to a larger area of the vessel, as opposed to duplex, which provides flow information limited to a small sample volume. Color flow is rarely used as a stand-alone diagnostic technique. Typically, color flow is combined with Doppler and B-mode imaging, thus providing "triplex" ultrasound, an extension of the duplex combination of Doppler and B-mode that is widely available and used in vascular laboratories today.

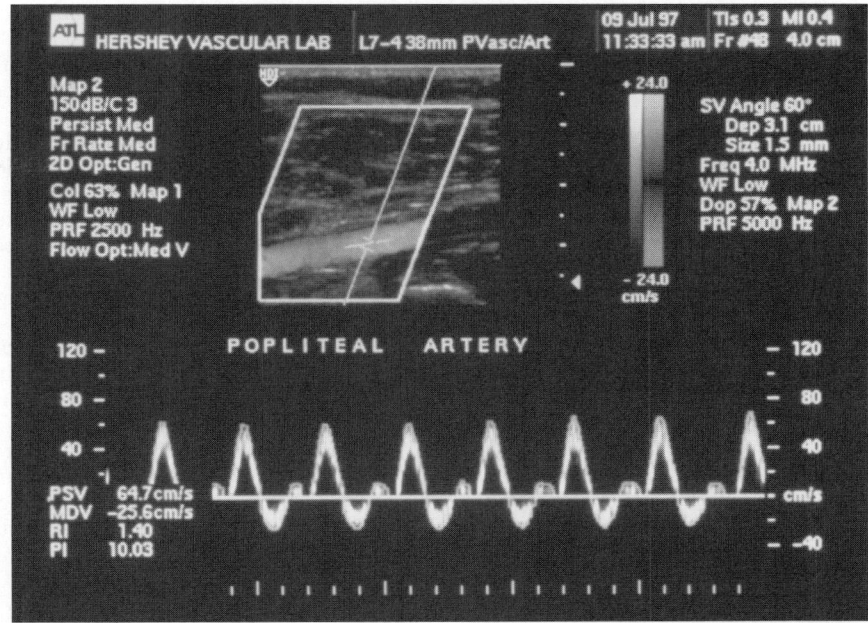

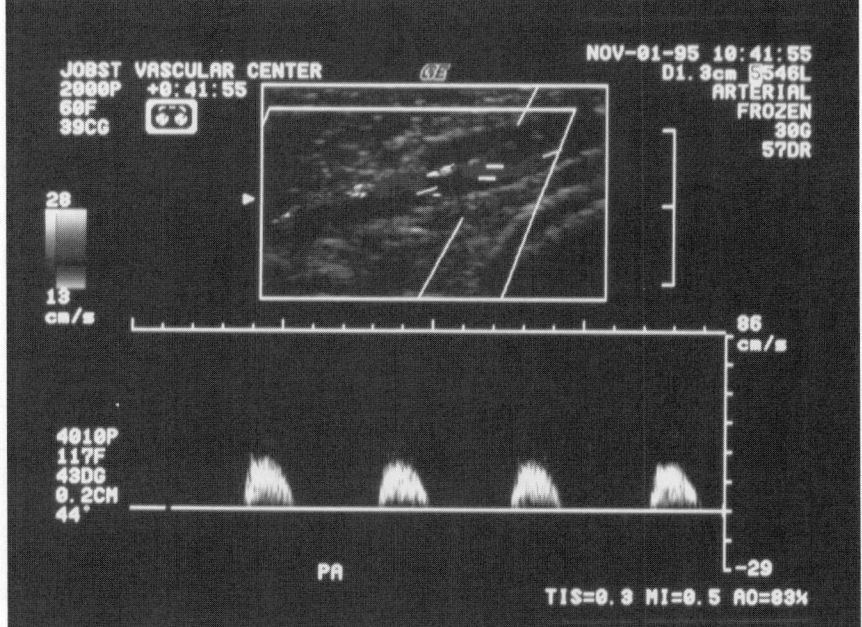

Figure 71.8. Black-and-white representation of a color print. *(A)* Duplex ultrasound scan of normal popliteal artery showing the anatomic image of the vessel with placement of sample volume for simultaneous recording of a normal, triphasic velocity spectral waveform. *(B)* Duplex ultrasound scan of abnormal popliteal artery. Note damped appearance of velocity waveforms distal to superficial femoral artery occlusion.

Color flow imaging superimposes, in real time, a flow map on the B-mode image. Each pixel in the image is processed for the presence, direction, and speed of movement or flow. If there is no movement (i.e., no change in Doppler frequency), the signal is represented by B-mode gray scale according to echo strength. If movement or blood flow is present, it is assigned a different color value depending on velocity and direction relative to the transducer position. Typically, flow toward the transducer is displayed in red scale, and flow away from the transducer is processed in blue scale. Note that color selection is arbitrary and that any colors can be selected to display the flow activity.

Color flow has improved localization of high-velocity flow jets at stenotic sites, detection of a patent, narrow arterial lumen otherwise thought to be occluded by duplex ultrasound, and visualization of tortuous arteries (Fig. 71.9).

Analysis of turbulence by color flow can also be done, but it is often misconstrued. Changes in color may be due to turbulence, normal changes in flow direction relative to the ultrasound probe, or aliasing due to the use of small velocity scales. *Aliasing* describes a velocity increase beyond the upper limit of the velocity scale, with the image changing color from red to blue or vice versa. Interpretation of color patterns, therefore, must include analysis of color flow scale, flow direction, and anatomic patterns.

Power Doppler

Power Doppler ultrasound is used to create a type of ultrasound image that is analogous to an arteriogram. Blood flow is displayed without regard to direction to create an easily seen, single-color image of the blood flow lumen. Tortuosity, turbulence, and aliasing in Doppler color flow may produce complicated color schemes. Similar to color

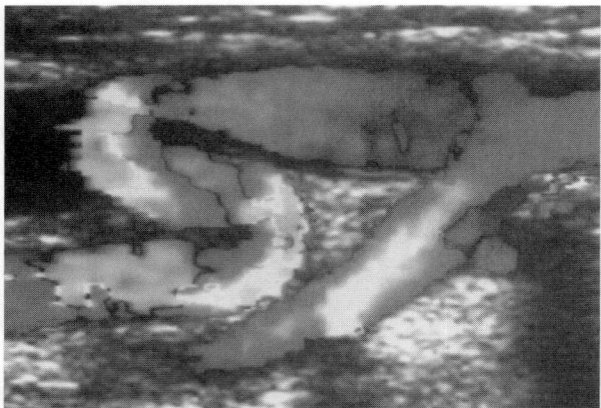

Figure 71.9. This image of a tortuous internal carotid artery, shown in black and white, was originally detected with color flow. This technique improves perception of continuous flow through the unusual, tortuous anatomy.

flow, pixel color is proportional to speed of movement. Power Doppler may improve sensitivity of blood vessel interrogation in small arteries, arteries with low flow, and flow within calcified plaques (Fig. 71.10).

New Imaging Developments

Several new imaging modalities are being tested in vascular applications.

Harmonic imaging. Traditional B-mode imaging relies on echoes detected at the same frequency of the transmitted ultrasound signal. Image resolution may be improved by processing multiple harmonics of the original frequency.

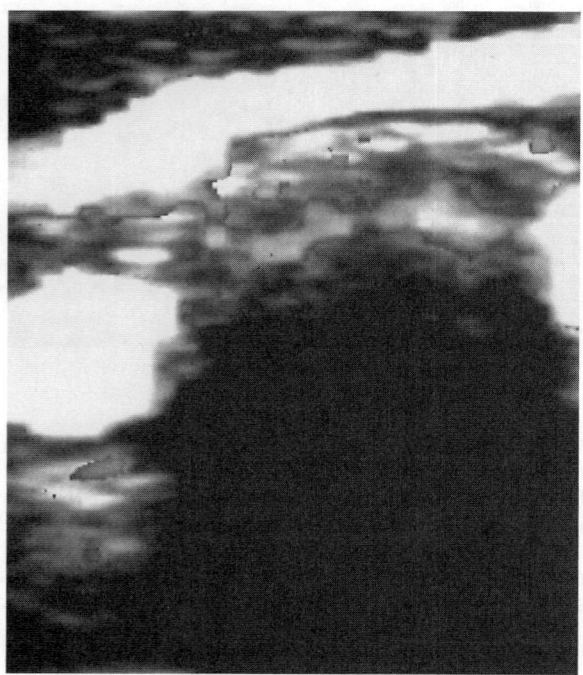

Figure 71.10. Increased sensitivity of power Doppler permitted visualization of a narrow lumen inside a calcified plaque. Blockage of the ultrasound beam's propagation by the calcified tissue did not permit visualization of the deeper vessel wall or detection of Doppler flow waveforms at the site of maximum stenosis. (After Beebe HG, Salles-Cunha SX, Scissons RP, et al. Carotid arterial ultrasound scan imaging: a direct approach to stenosis measurement. *J Vasc Surg* 1999;29:843, with permission.)

Extended field of view. A limitation of ultrasonography is its small field of view. Overall interpretation of a wide region is often difficult to document. This new technique composes ultrasound images to present a longer, broader B-mode or color flow image. The ultrasonic field of view is extended from a few centimeters to images longer than 50 cm.

Tissue Doppler. Special Doppler techniques can be applied to detect stronger, slower echoes of moving tissue compared with weaker, faster movement of red blood cells. This technique developed for cardiac muscle imaging is now being investigated in vascular applications.

B-mode colorization. Modern technology allows for B-mode imaging to be displayed in other colors besides gray. For certain individuals, imaging contrast or sensitivity may be enhanced by orange, blue, or other colored backgrounds. This technique may enhance detection of small or unusual arterial anatomy.

Contrast imaging. Ultrasound contrast agents contain materials, such as microbubbles of gas, that heighten ultrasound reflectivity. Contrast agents can be injected into the circulation to strengthen the ultrasound echo received and improve sensitivity. This is particularly useful in regions of low-velocity or low-volume flow such as the cortex of the kidney. Velocity waveforms are also enhanced and measurements of maximum PSV are higher than with standard duplex techniques.

B-flow. Instead of detecting blood motion as in color flow, the B-flow technique detects a characteristic ultrasound echo pattern of a particular volume of blood cells. This ultrasonic blood cell pattern is followed pixel by pixel in the B-mode image, creating the perception of blood movement, or flow in the vessel. This technique may compete with color flow or power Doppler in the future.

Pulsatile flow imaging. Under conditions of multiple vessels with variable flow in multiple directions, it is often difficult to separate arteries from veins. In other applications, the degree of arterial flow pulsatility related to abnormal peripheral resistance may provide useful information. A new technique to map only pulsatile flow may improve arterial hemodynamic evaluation of abdominal organs, malformations, and unusual vascular anatomy.

CLINICAL APPLICATIONS

Extracranial Cerebrovascular Evaluation

Carotid ultrasonography is recommended most often for patients with transient symptoms of cerebral ischemia, those found to have cervical bruits, for high-risk asymptomatic patients, or before major cardiac or abdominal surgery. The cervical carotid and vertebral arteries are primarily investigated with duplex or color flow ultrasonography. The examination may also include evaluation of the subclavian arteries and bilateral arm blood pressure measurements. The basic protocol includes transverse and longitudinal imaging from the proximal common carotid artery to the most distally accessible portions of the internal and external carotid arteries (Figs. 71.3, 71.7A–C). Using duplex ultrasound to document the anatomic site of sampling, PSV and EDV measurements are performed. A moderate stenosis, at least greater than 50% diameter reduction, is suspected if the PSV exceeds 125 cm/s. Severe stenosis is suspected if the EDV exceeds 100 cm/s or the PSV exceeds 250 cm/s. Other criteria have been proposed, as discussed previously. Therefore, each laboratory must validate its own criteria.

The feasibility of measuring carotid stenosis reliably from color flow-aided B-mode ultrasound images has been reported (11). We recommend that transverse pictures at the location of the most severe stenosis be used as the best descriptor of residual lumen, extent of disease, and carotid artery size. With a longitudinal scan, measurements can be confirmed, and the length and location of carotid plaque are delineated in the neck. Velocity estimations of carotid stenosis should confirm the stenosis estimates determined by B-mode images. Otherwise, valid explanations for mismatch should be investigated. These may include velocity increase due to tortuosity, kinking, or contralateral carotid occlusion. Cardiac disease may result in low carotid velocities even in the presence of severe stenosis. Plaque calcification with shadowing may limit the ultrasound test to velocity measurements obtained from other sites near the stenosis.

Ultrasound has excellent positive predictive value for severe carotid stenosis and negative predictive value for mild, minimal, or lack of disease (11). Unfortunately, estimations of moderate disease in the 50% to 70% range and of occlusion by ultrasonography, arteriography, or magnetic resonance are all not completely reliable. The reasons for this center around a large number of clinically significant artifacts, errors, and limitations that are inherent and specific to each imaging method. Multiple testing may have to be considered based on examination quality, clinical signs and symptoms, potential risk of stroke, or other medical findings. Carotid endarterectomy follow-up with bilateral testing is often recommended annually, but this is controversial. Restenosis is rare, but disease in the contralateral side may eventually progress in a significant number of patients. The documentation of the anatomic result of a vascular surgical procedure that was intended to correct an anatomic problem (endarterectomy of carotid stenosis) is an excellent idea that is threatened by the intense pressures to reduce medical cost in the modern era.

Transcranial Doppler

A limited number of investigators have used transcranial Doppler (TCD) to evaluate collateral cerebral circulation in severely stenosed or occluded internal carotid arteries. During either carotid endarterectomy or endovascular stenting, intraoperative TCD has been used to monitor cerebral circulation and to detect both air and particle emboli. Diagnosis of vasospasm, arteriovenous malformation, aneurysms, and cerebral death are other applications of TCD (12).

Modern TCD uses color flow ultrasound imaging with velocity spectral analysis. Ultrasound frequencies of 2 to 3 MHz are used for depth penetration through an aperture or through thin sections of cranial bone. The circle of Willis and its related arterial network can be visualized from several anatomic windows. The middle and anterior cerebral arteries are insonated through the temporal and orbital windows, respectively. The vertebral and basilar arteries are examined through the foramen magnum.

Upper Extremity Arterial Evaluation

Clinical assessment is often complemented by physiologic evaluation as a means of functional quantification (13). Bilateral arm blood pressure determinations are normally considered part of the clinical vascular examination.

Essential physiologic evaluation could be limited to finger and wrist pressures at the radial and ulnar arteries

with calculation of finger and wrist–arm systolic pressure ratios. If the arterial abnormality is bilateral and involves the subclavian–axillary arteries, ankle pressure could substitute for arm pressure as a reference. Examination for vasospasm often includes manometry and photoplethysmography of all five digits repeated after contralateral or ipsilateral hand immersion in iced water. We prefer to insert the hand in cold water and then add ice until pulses disappear. Water and finger temperature before immersion and at the time of pulse disappearance provide additional information. Recovery time after pulse disappearance is indicative of disease severity. Examination for thoracic outlet syndrome is best performed with the arm in a position that causes signs or symptoms. An often-used stress position of abduction and external rotation mimics the throwing position of a baseball pitcher. The hand is raised as if a baseball is being thrown while the head is forcefully rotated to the opposite side. However, it is common for asymptomatic, normal subjects to occlude the subclavian or axillary artery with this maneuver.

Preoperative ultrasound imaging includes evaluation of the subclavian, axillary, brachial, ulnar, radial, palmar arch, and finger arteries. Imaging is complemented by waveform analysis. Atherosclerotic, traumatic, and arteritic obstructions, true and false aneurysms, thrombosis, and embolization are all usefully evaluated with ultrasound imaging.

Dialysis Access

Arterial and venous systems of the upper extremity can be evaluated before vascular procedures to provide hemodialysis access. Adequacy of brachial and radial arterial inflow with triphasic waveforms, standard diameters, and lack of obstructive disease are investigated with pressure measurements and ultrasound imaging. The arterial examination is complemented with ultrasonic imaging evaluation of patency and size of cephalic and basilic veins, and adequacy of venous outflow. Evaluation of the lower extremity follows a similar protocol.

Dialysis access follow-up includes measurement of blood flow rate and duplex ultrasound scanning. Thrombosis, stenosis at the venous or arterial anastomosis, stenosis at mid-graft or the access vein, aneurysms and dilatations, hematomas, arteriovenous fistulae, and graft incorporation are detected in transverse, oblique, and longitudinal ultrasound images and with velocity measurements. Digital arterial steal, which may follow surgical creation of an arteriovenous short circuit, is documented with finger pressures. Usually the finger–brachial index is decreased to 0.6 to 0.8 in the presence of a dialysis access arteriovenous fistula. If this index decreases to below 0.5, digital ischemia is suspected.

Dialysis grafts originating at the brachial artery normally have a flow rate of 800 to 1,000 mL/min. Radiocephalic arteriovenous fistulae normally have flow rates of 400 to 500 mL/min. Higher flow rates are not unusual, but rates above 2 L/min may result in cardiac overload. Flow rates decreased to abnormally low values (i.e., <200 mL/min for a radiocephalic fistula) or a drop in flow rates greater than 30% between measurements performed on different occasions suggests the presence of occlusive disease.

Abdominal Arterial Evaluation

Aortic aneurysmosis, renal artery stenosis, celiac–mesenteric artery stenosis, and aortoiliac artery stenosis are common lesions evaluated with duplex ultrasound (14). Duplex ultrasound provides a readily available and less expensive method reliably to evaluate the arterial physiology and anatomy of the abdomen. Visceral ultrasound examination begins with forceful recommendations to the patient to avoid food and liquid intake for at least 10 hours before the test. Efforts to generate ultrasound images of blood vessels with the abdominal cavity containing gas-filled intestines are flawed because the gas prevents transmission of the ultrasound signal. Anti-gas medication may be necessary; the recommended dosage is every 6 hours for 2 days before the examination. A mild laxative is also recommended the evening before the examination. For patient comfort, breakfast should be very limited. Tests are usually scheduled in the morning.

Transverse and longitudinal B-mode ultrasound images of aortic aneurysms are obtained to size the aneurysm, rule out suprarenal aortic involvement, and investigate potential iliac artery aneurysm. The abdominal aorta and the iliac arteries are evaluated with duplex ultrasound in patients with ischemic symptoms who are candidates for a therapeutic procedure. The imaging examination should be preceded by ankle pressure measurements at rest or after a stress test such as treadmill walking exercise. Duplex ultrasound imaging with velocity measurements locates and quantifies iliac stenoses and occlusions. Usually a two- to threefold increase in PSV occurs at the site of a severe stenosis. This criterion varies for different instruments and often cannot be applied to multiple stenoses in series. Documentation of the stenosis in transverse and longitudinal color flow-aided B-mode images is recommended. The current limitations of ultrasonography are too great to overcome to obtain the detailed diameter, length, angulation, and other measurements needed before endovascular procedures.

Quantification of renal artery stenosis is based on the ratio of renal artery to aortic PSV, kidney size, and velocity waveforms of the kidney arteries (15). A PSV ratio greater than 3.5, a 1- to 2-cm reduction in kidney size, or monophasic waveforms in kidney arteries suggests severe renal artery stenosis. Unfortunately, high-level accuracy depends on extensive experience and often time-consuming examinations. Accessory renal arteries are frequently missed. Duplex scanning has been recommended as the initial screening method when a renovascular cause of hypertension is suspected and for monitoring renal artery reconstructions.

Celiac trunk, proximal hepatic and splenic artery, and superior mesenteric artery duplex evaluation is performed in patients with mesenteric ischemia (5,14). The inferior mesenteric artery can sometimes be evaluated in lean patients. PSVs and velocity ratios measured at and near the stenotic site are often used as diagnostic criteria for stenosis severity. Measurements and decision criteria, however, are instrument and laboratory dependent. Data from the literature cannot be indiscriminately applied without quality control and confirmation by individual laboratories. Often, however, patients with severe symptoms have occluded segments of the celiac–mesenteric arteries with extensive collateralization. This abnormal anatomy results in extensive examination times and incomplete ultrasound examination results. Conversely, patients with mild or intermittent symptomatology may have negative tests at rest. A stress test after food intake can be performed, usually based on evaluation of superior mesenteric artery flow velocity waveforms. The diastolic component of preprandial blood flow is minimal or absent, but it normally increases significantly after food intake.

Follow-up of visceral arterial percutaneous transluminal angioplasty, stenting, or bypass grafting with noninvasive ultrasonography is recommended. Bypasses to the iliac or femoral artery are long lasting, and regular ultrasound follow-up examinations are not common because

serial ABI measurement offers a readily available, indirect substitute method.

Lower Extremity Arterial Evaluation

Noninvasive, quantitative evaluation of the ischemic lower extremity starts with ankle pressure measurements. Medicare guidelines state that the ankle–brachial systolic pressure index should be part of a regular clinical vascular evaluation (16). In the vascular laboratory, toe pressure determinations replace or complement ankle pressure measurements in patients with arterial calcification or atherosclerosis of the foot arteries, particularly in patients with diabetes. As the next step after distal pressure measurements, we recommend qualitative segmental flow waveform evaluation. During ankle pressure measurements at the posterior and anterior tibial or dorsal pedal arteries, flow velocity waveforms are recorded with a CW Doppler or a duplex ultrasound scanner. Segmental flow velocity waveforms are then recorded with duplex ultrasonography at the common femoral, mid-superficial femoral, and popliteal arteries. Screening for femoropopliteal stenosis can be performed quickly with ultrasound color flow imaging while the probe is moved from one position to another along the arterial segments. This physiologic evaluation is greater than 80% accurate with regard to location and severity of iliac, femoral, or tibial arterial occlusive disease, but provides only preliminary information to guide the clinician in further decisions (17). Segmental velocity waveform analysis has proven more informative than measurements of segmental pressures at the thigh and upper calf level (17). Segmental arterial blood pressure measurements are redundant, ineffective, misleading on occasion, somewhat painful, and take longer than duplex waveform recording. Laboratories that do not have acces to duplex ultrasound scanners may have to obtain segmental flow waveforms using CW Doppler or air plethysmography. Duplex ultrasound, however, is so valuable that it has become the main focus of all modern vascular laboratories.

Medicare regulations may restrict conditions for reimbursement of lower extremity duplex ultrasound arterial mapping if arteriography is planned routinely (16). Therefore, detailed arterial mapping must be performed primarily as an attempt to avoid or limit the scope and extent of arteriography (18). Patients have been selected for percutaneous transluminal angioplasty or stenting based on ultrasound mapping as a replacement for diagnostic arteriography. There are a few reports of successful surgical bypass revascularization extending to popliteal and even tibial arteries performed without preoperative arteriography, based solely on duplex arterial mapping (19). Besides the inherent advantages of low cost and lack of morbidity, ultrasound imaging can select normal or less calcified arterial segments for anastomotic sites, and may show patency of arteries with low, reversed, or no flow, often not visualized with standard arteriography. Inadequate laboratory personnel training, long test duration, and poor visualization due to arterial calcification with shadowing, deep vessel location in large limbs, or certain types of edema limit effectiveness of ultrasound arterial mapping. The test duration can be shortened if it is limited to identifying sites for proximal and distal anastomoses (20). Extensive documentation of the segment to be bypassed, as commonly done to mimic arteriography, is unnecessary. Scanning down the groin and thigh to the first severe obstruction and up the foot and leg to the last obstruction may be sufficient. Discrepancies between ultrasonography, arteriography, and magnetic resonance imaging exist, but vascular surgeon preferences for anastomotic sites may be the most significant variable (21). Knowing the preferences of the vascular surgeon who is going to perform the operation is essential for effective scanning. Leg or arm vein mapping can follow arterial mapping to complete a preoperative study.

Because a graft surveillance program can be effective in preserving patency, bypass graft follow-up by ultrasound should be scheduled routinely every 3 months in the first postoperative year, two times in the second year, and yearly thereafter. Three types of abnormal flow findings can be observed: (a) graft with low flow, (b) decreased flow between consecutive studies, and (c) significantly increased velocities at a stenotic site. A mid-graft PSV below 45 cm/s has been used as a criterion for low flow in popliteal and tibial bypass grafts. Low flow is often caused by poor cardiac performance or arrhythmias. A drop in velocity greater than 20% or 30% in serial studies is significant, and its cause should be closely evaluated. A two- to threefold increase in PSV at a stenotic site suggests severe stenosis that should be repaired. Velocity criteria are instrument/laboratory dependent and may not be applicable to multiple serial stenoses. Additional documentation using transverse and longitudinal high-quality color flow/B-mode images is recommended.

REFERENCES

1. Beebe HG, Salles-Cunha S. Rational use of the vascular diagnostic laboratory. *Probl Gen Surg* 1994;11:527–541.
2. Sumner DS, Thiele BL. The vascular laboratory. In: Rutherford R, ed. *Vascular surgery,* 4th ed. Philadelphia: WB Saunders, 1995:45–64.
3. Zierler RE, Sumner DS. Physiologic assessment of peripheral arterial occlusive disease. In: Rutherford R, ed. *Vascular surgery,* 4th ed. Philadelphia: WB Saunders, 1995:65–117.
4. Salles-Cunha S, Andros G. *Atlas of duplex ultrasonography: essential images of the peripheral vascular system.* Pasadena, CA: Appleton and Davis, 1988:190.
5. Strandness DE Jr. *Duplex scanning in vascular disorders,* 2nd ed. New York: Raven Press, 1993.
6. Carter SA. Role of pressure measurements. In: Bernstein EF, ed. *Vascular diagnosis,* 4th ed. St. Louis: Mosby, 1993:486–512.
7. Raines JK. The pulse volume recorder in peripheral arterial disease. In: Bernstein EF, ed. *Vascular diagnosis,* 4th ed. St. Louis: Mosby, 1993:534–543.
8. Fronek A. Clinical experience with transcutaneous PO_2 and PCO_2 measurements. In: Bernstein EF, ed. *Vascular diagnosis,* 4th ed. St. Louis: Mosby, 1993:620–625.
9. Salles-Cunha SX, Beebe HG. Magnetic resonance blood flowmetry: a review. *J Vasc Technology* 1994;18:141–147.
10. Howard G, Baker WH, Chambless LE, et al. An approach for the use of Doppler ultrasound as a screening tool for hemodynamically significant stenosis (despite heterogeneity of Doppler performance): a multicenter experience. Asymptomatic Carotid Atherosclerosis Study Investigators. *Stroke* 1996;27:1951–1957.
11. Beebe HG, Salles-Cunha SX, Scissons RP, et al. Carotid arterial ultrasound scan imaging: a direct approach to stenosis measurement. *J Vasc Surg* 1999;29:838–844.
12. Aaslid R. *Transcranial Doppler sonography.* New York: Springer-Verlag, 1986.
13. Edwards JM, Porter JM. Evaluation of upper extremity ischemia. In: Bernstein EF, ed. *Vascular diagnosis,* 4th ed. St. Louis: Mosby, 1993:630–640.
14. Special Issue devoted to the Abdominal Vasculature. *J Vasc Technology* 1995;19:233–338.
15. Hansen KJ, Tribble RW, Reavis SW, et al. Renal duplex sonography: evaluation of clinical utility. *J Vasc Surg* 1990;12:227–236.
16. Medicare Newsletter. *Revised medical policies: noninvasive vascular testing.* Columbus, OH: Nationwide Mutual Insurance Company, 1999:19–25.
17. Gale SS, Scissons RP, Salles-Cunha SX, et al. Lower extremity arterial evaluation: are segmental arterial blood pressures worthwhile? *J Vasc Surg* 1998;27:831–838.
18. Salles-Cunha SX, Andros G. Preoperative duplex scanning prior to infrainguinal revascularization. *Surg Clin North Am* 1990;70:41–59.
19. Mazzariol F, Ascher E, Salles-Cunha SX, et al. Values and limitations of duplex ultrasonography as the sole imaging method of preoperative evaluation for popliteal and infrapopliteal bypasses. *Ann Vasc Surg* 1999;13:1–10.
20. Salles-Cunha SX. Arterial ultrasound imaging prior to infrainguinal revascularization. *Vasc Ultrasound Today* 1999;4:129–148.
21. Kohler TR, Andros G, Porter JM, et al. Can duplex scanning replace arteriography for lower extremity arterial disease? *Ann Vasc Surg* 1990;4:280–287.

SURGERY: SCIENTIFIC PRINCIPLES AND PRACTICE, Third Edition, edited by Lazar J. Greenfield, Michael W. Mulholland, Keith T. Oldham, Gerald B. Zelenock, and Keith D. Lillemoe. Lippincott Williams & Wilkins Publishers, Philadelphia, © 2001.

CHAPTER 72

DIAGNOSTIC ANGIOGRAPHY

DAVID M. WILLIAMS AND KYUNG J. CHO

Angiography is the study of blood vessels. In conventional percutaneous angiography, radiographs are made as blood is mixed with contrast medium injected through a catheter that has been selectively placed in an artery or vein. When the lumina of vessels become visible as branching columns of contrast medium, subtle inferences can be made about the vessels themselves, their surroundings, and the organs or tumors they supply. Transcatheter angiography (hereafter called *angiography,* unqualified by a technical modifier) is unrivaled in its global, high-resolution demonstration of vascular anatomy and remains the gold standard by which newer vascular imaging modalities such as computed tomographic (CT) and magnetic resonance (MR) angiography are judged. Angiography is used to demonstrate vascular anatomy, identify abnormalities of the vascular wall and lumen, and guide interventional vascular radiologic procedures.

ANGIOGRAPHIC TECHNIQUE

The percutaneous catheterization technique pioneered by Seldinger in 1953 provides vascular access for most diagnostic and therapeutic angiographic procedures (1). The percutaneous transfemoral route is the preferred approach for most diagnostic and therapeutic procedures (2). The transaxillary or transbrachial route is used when it offers a mechanical advantage for selective catheterization of aortic branches or when severe aortoiliac disease precludes the transfemoral approach. When severe occlusive disease, a recent surgical procedure, or local infection precludes catheterization of the femoral or brachial arteries, the translumbar route may be used for evaluation of the aorta and arteries of the lower extremities. This route limits the options for selective aortic branch injections.

After the route of catheterization is chosen, the puncture site is determined by palpation. In the absence of a palpable pulse, fluoroscopically visualized bone landmarks or Doppler ultrasound may assist in puncturing the nonpalpable artery. The artery is punctured with a quick thrust of an 18- or 19-gauge needle (20- or 21-gauge for children). The needle is slowly withdrawn, and, after pulsatile arterial blood return is observed, a guide wire is advanced through the needle into the artery. The needle is replaced over the wire by a catheter with a preformed tip, and the wire is removed. In general, central (e.g., aortic) injections of contrast medium are made before selective injections, especially when ostial lesions are a concern or when a global view of arterial anatomy is desired. Aortic injections are made with a pigtail catheter, which has an end hole that allows the catheter to track over a guide wire. A preformed terminal pigtail-shaped curve prevents intimal laceration during catheter recoil, and multiple side holes are distributed symmetrically around the shaft just proximal to the pigtail to achieve radially uniform contrast injection. Aortic branch artery injections are made after the pigtail catheter is exchanged for one with an end hole and tip conforming to the proximal course of the artery of interest.

Contrast medium is introduced into the artery by a power injector at a rate sufficient to replace blood for several cardiac cycles. The blood flow rate in the artery is estimated by fluoroscopic observation of a hand injection of contrast medium. Underinjection of contrast medium results in dilution of the contrast by blood and poor filling of the arterial bed of interest. Overinjection results in reflux of contrast medium into the aorta or adjacent branch arteries and visualization of irrelevant or potentially confusing vessels. In the adult, typical iodinated contrast injection rates are 25 to 35 mL/s for 2 seconds in the thoracic aorta and 6 to 8 mL/s for 1.5 seconds in the renal artery. In general, filming or image recording proceeds rapidly during the arterial phase at the onset of contrast injection and more slowly during the capillary and venous phases. In the thoracic aorta, typical filming sequences are three exposures per second for 3 or 4 seconds (no capillary or venous phase); in the renal artery, typical sequences are two per second for 3 seconds, one per second for 3 seconds, and one every other second for 6 seconds.

DIGITAL ANGIOGRAPHY

Conventional (film, screen-based) angiography combines high-spatial-resolution vascular imaging with sturdy and simple equipment, but is rapidly being replaced by digital angiography. Certain clinical questions can be resolved without the high-resolution imaging of film, such as graft patency, presence of an arteriovenous fistula, and pattern of arterial branching as a reference for guide wire or catheter placement. In digital angiography, image recording is on an image intensifier rather than on film, at the sacrifice of high spatial resolution. The intensifier image is electronically read and stored on a computer disk. An image recorded before the injection of contrast medium can be used as a mask and subtracted, in real time, from images recorded as the contrast bolus passes through the circulatory bed of interest. Simple translations of the mask can be performed after the study to reduce small misregistration artifacts from cardiac, respiratory, and peristaltic motion. The accumulation of multiple masks allows the angiographer to choose the best mask (in place of the initial default mask) to subtract from a given postcontrast image. The images demonstrating the pertinent arterial and venous anatomy are recorded on film.

When used in the subtraction mode, digital angiography provides high visual contrast resolution, which may re-

duce the amount of iodinated contrast medium required for an angiogram and even allows the use of carbon dioxide gas as a contrast medium (see later). Digital angiography provides images promptly, streamlining the conduct of vascular interventional procedures, and reduces film costs because only images showing the pertinent anatomy are transferred to film (usually multiple images on a single sheet of film). Digital subtraction angiography (DSA) with an intravenous injection of contrast medium is technically simple. When used to demonstrate arteries, however, it requires the injection of a large volume of contrast medium (40 to 50 mL) into the vena cava or right atrium and sacrifices the selectivity of the intraarterial examination. DSA with a peripheral venous injection is useful for studying venous abnormalities such as subclavian vein thrombosis or the venous side of dialysis fistulae. DSA with an intraarterial injection of contrast medium uses smaller volumes of contrast medium to produce angiograms and is superior in quality to intravenous DSA. Intraarterial DSA can be performed with small-bore catheters (3F to 4F); in conventional angiography, larger-bore catheters must be used. The significant disadvantages of digital angiography compared with film or screen angiography are its inferior spatial resolution and its motion-induced misregistration artifact.

Because of the widespread use of digital angiography, misregistration artifacts should be thoroughly understood. They are caused by slight differences in the position of internal organs between the times of the acquisition of the mask image and of the contrast-filled image. Peristalsis, cardiac and arterial pulsation, and diaphragmatic motion all contribute to these artifacts, which can simulate vessels, tumor blush, or contrast extravasation. Subtle findings on digital angiography, therefore, should be confirmed on nonsubtracted images.

HELICAL COMPUTED TOMOGRAPHIC ANGIOGRAPHY

In conventional CT, contiguous axial images are obtained by alternating table movement and rotation of the x-ray tube or detector gantry. In helical CT, table movement and rotation of the x-ray tube or detector are continuous, so that the path traced by the x-ray beam on a cylindrical patient is a helix rather than a series of circles. Eliminating the delays required for table movement allows the acquisition of many slices in a single breath hold. With proper timing of the contrast injection, initiation of data acquisition, and choice of slice thickness and table speed, images can be obtained during peak arterial opacification. After image reconstruction, the vascular system is displayed by computer interaction using contrast thresholds, regions of interest, and other picture-processing tools. There is a trade-off between the resolution of the image (how small a vessel can be reliably detected) and the volume imaged (how long a segment of the aorta is included). Helical CT angiography (CTA) seems reliable for visualizing the aorta and the first- and second-order vessels. Selection of the proper imaging protocol requires clear communication of the clinical question to be answered. Indications for helical CTA include preoperative evaluation of thoracic and abdominal aortic disease; in some institutions, this study has already replaced conventional aortography. Helical CTA evaluation of prospective renal donors and the screening of patients with normal renal function for renovascular hypertension are promising and under investigation at many institutions (3) (Fig. 72.1).

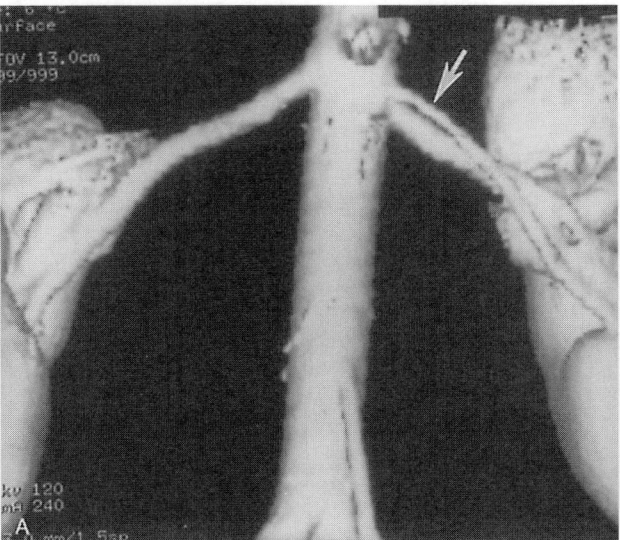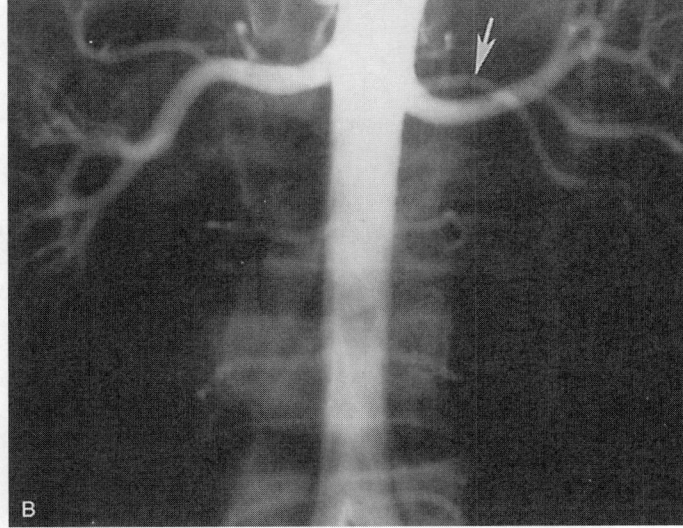

Figure 72.1. Helical computed tomographic *(A)* and conventional transcatheter *(B)* abdominal aortograms in a prospective renal donor. Both images demonstrate renal artery anatomy, including an accessory left renal artery *(arrows)*. (Courtesy of Joel F. Platt, M.D., University of Michigan Hospitals, Ann Arbor, MI.)

MAGNETIC RESONANCE ANGIOGRAPHY

Magnetic resonance imaging has revolutionized musculoskeletal radiology and neuroradiology. Using the same basic technology and exploiting motion-sensitive pulse sequences, MR angiography provides an unparalleled noninvasive demonstration of vascular anatomy. Cardiac and respiratory artifacts have been reduced by electrocardiographic gating of data acquisition and by adding compensatory pulses to the imaging train. Patient compliance with the requirements of immobility and breath holding can be enhanced with intravenous sedation, hyperventilation with oxygen-rich air, and verbal encouragement. Imaging of the arterial system is significantly improved by carefully coordinating the intravenous injection of an MR contrast agent with data acquisition. With careful attention to detail, impressive demonstration of the aorta and first-order branches is feasible, even in patients unable to hold their breath (Fig. 72.2). As in helical CT, there is a trade-off between resolution (the smallest vessel imaged) and the patient volume surveyed. The indications for MR angiography include the diagnosis and preoperative evaluation of thoracic aortic disease, abdominal aortic aneurysms, adult renovascular hypertension, and carotid artery disease. On the venous side, MR angiography is useful to evaluate deep venous thrombosis involving the portal, iliocaval, and lower extremity venous systems (4–6). Contraindications to MR angiography include pacemakers and certain metallic devices adjacent to easily traumatized critical structures such as the eye and brain.

CONTRAST MEDIA

The contrast medium used for conventional angiography is a viscous, water-soluble, radiopaque liquid that is injected at the time of the angiogram. The radiopacity is due to the high content of iodine; hence, this class of contrast materials is called *iodinated*. There are two general classes of iodinated contrast agents—the conventional high-osmolality ionic agents, which dissociate into a radiopaque anion and a cation, and the newer, low-osmolality nonionic agents. Examples of the ionic agents are sodium methylglucamine diatrizoate and methylglucamine iothalamate; examples of the nonionic agents are iohexol and iopamidol. Sodium methylglucamine ioxaglate is an example of an ionic, low-osmolality agent. The high-osmolality agents are associated with direct cardiac and renal toxicity, idiosyncratic anaphylactoid reactions, and an uncomfortable tissue response (e.g., coughing during pulmonary artery injection and pain during injection of arteries supplying the body wall or extremities). The nonionic agents appear safer in every respect, although they have shown no overwhelming advantage in patients with renal failure (7–9).

Carbon dioxide gas is also a suitable contrast agent for many peripheral applications (10). Because of its inherent biocompatibility, it is especially useful in patients with a history of a severe contrast reaction and in those with renal failure. Its low viscosity permits the use of small-bore catheters, but its high compressibility makes it difficult to achieve uniform injection rates without the use of a special injector, which is not yet commercially available in the United States. It has been used safely as a contrast agent for abdominal aortography and lower extremity arteriography, for inferior vena cavography to guide placement of vena cava filters, and for venous opacification to guide placement of venous access devices such as Hickman catheters. It has not been used for thoracic aortography because of the potential risk of neurologic complications. Carbon dioxide angiography must be performed with the use of DSA (Fig. 72.3).

Contrast materials for MR angiography are typically gadolinium-based compounds. These are expensive, but patent expiration may reduce their cost in the near future. They are less nephrotoxic than the iodinated contrast materials used in catheter-based angiography or CT. For MR angiographic applications, the volumes of contrast material (20 to 60 mL) required for an adequate MR signal from blood are relatively small; therefore, the risk of fluid overload is reduced compared with conventional angiography, which re-

(text continues on page 1618)

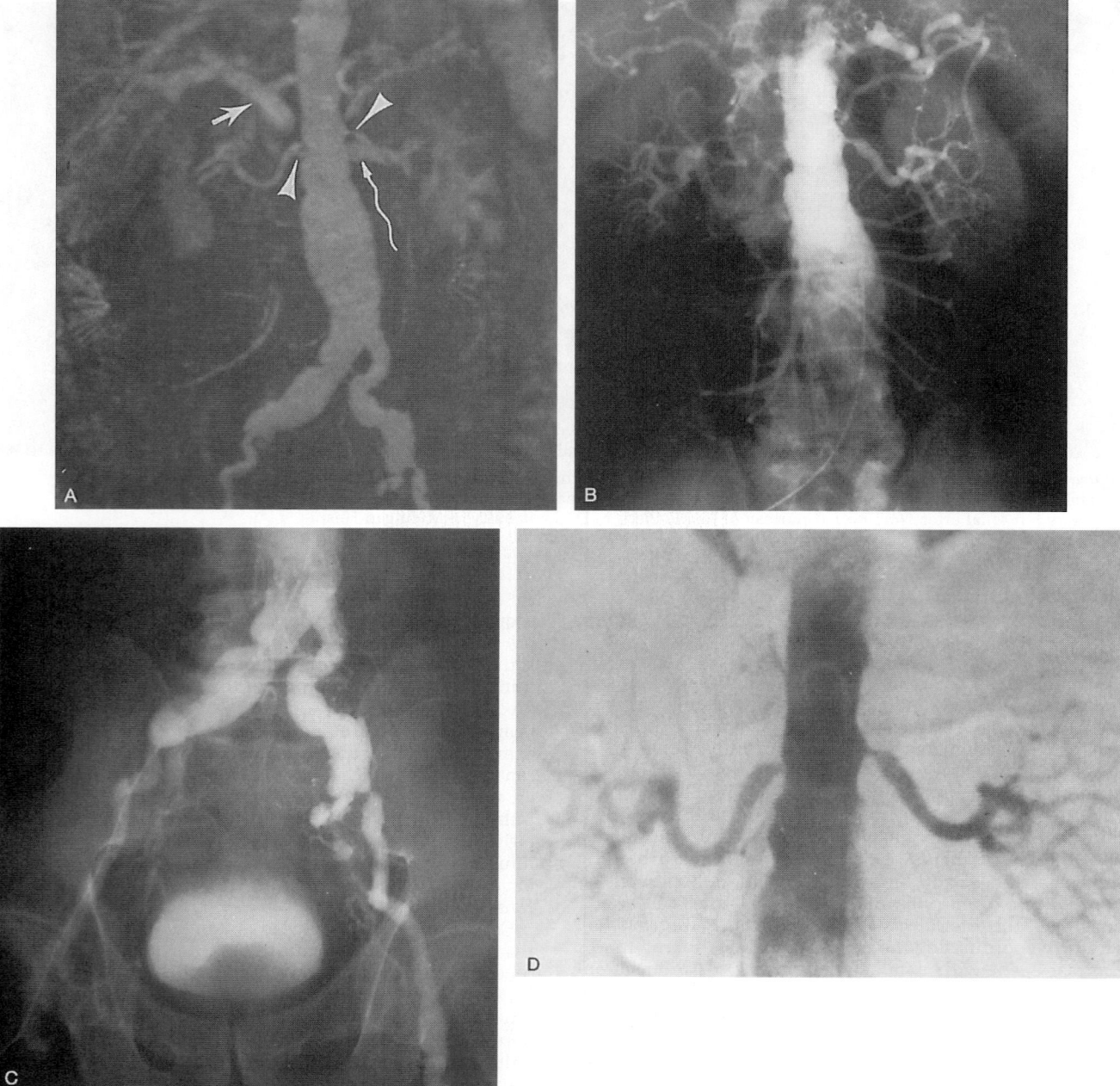

Figure 72.2. *(A)* Gadolinium-enhanced magnetic resonance (MR) abdominal aortogram shows, in a coronal reconstruction, an infrarenal aortic aneurysm with proximal stenoses involving bilateral single renal arteries *(arrowheads)*. Iliac artery aneurysms are also present. The celiac and superior mesenteric artery origins were demonstrated on a sagittal reconstruction of the dataset (not shown). Gadolinium has reached the portal *(straight arrow)* and left renal *(wavy arrow)* veins, but in this instance the study is not compromised. *(B and C)* Transcatheter aortography (using three injections) confirms the extent of the aneurysm. *(D)* Digital subtraction angiography with rapid image acquisition rate confirms the renal artery anatomy. *(E)* In another patient, gadolinium-enhanced MR abdominal aortogram shows the celiac and superior mesenteric origins *(arrowheads)* in profile. At the level of the left renal vein *(straight arrow)*, an infrarenal aortic aneurysm buckles anteriorly; other reconstructions showed that the aneurysm extended to the bifurcation (not shown). Mural thrombus is apparent anteriorly and posteriorly *(open arrows)*. *(F)* Conventional aortogram confirms visceral artery anatomy, but the caudal extent of the aneurysm is poorly opacified, even on later films in this sequence, because of contrast medium layering in the dependent posterior aspect of the aorta. *(A to D* from Prince M, Narasimham D, Stanley J, et al. Gadolinium-enhanced magnetic resonance angiography of abdominal aortic aneurysms. *J Vasc Surg* 1995;21:656; *E* and *F* from Prince M. Gadolinium-enhanced MR aortography. *Radiology* 1994;191:155. Courtesy of Martin R. Prince, M.D., University of Michigan Hospitals, Ann Arbor, MI.) *(continues)*

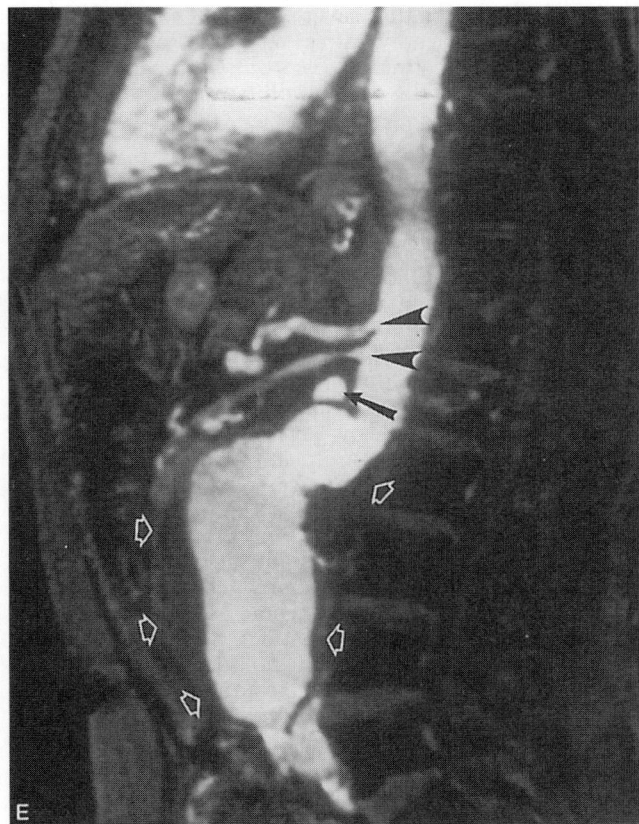
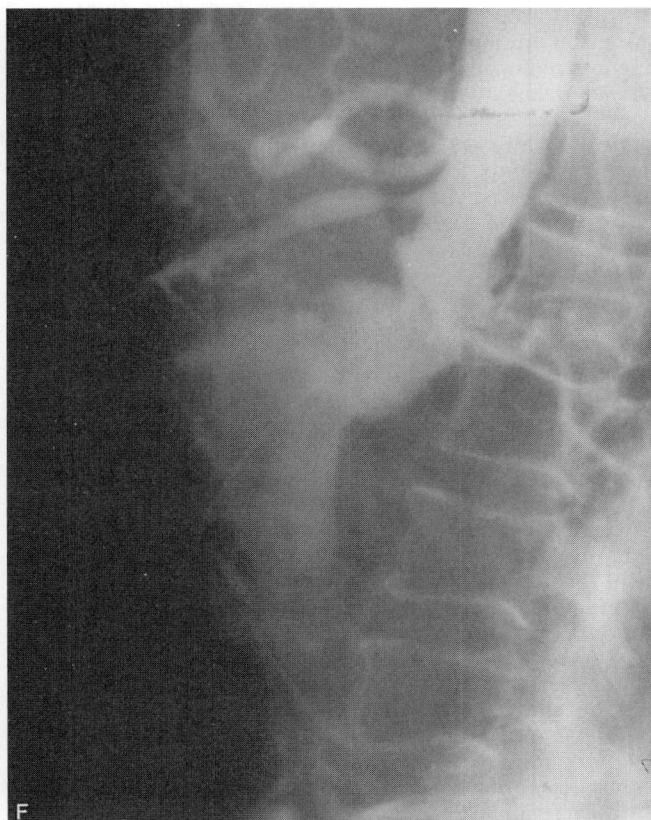

Figure 72.2. *(Continued)*

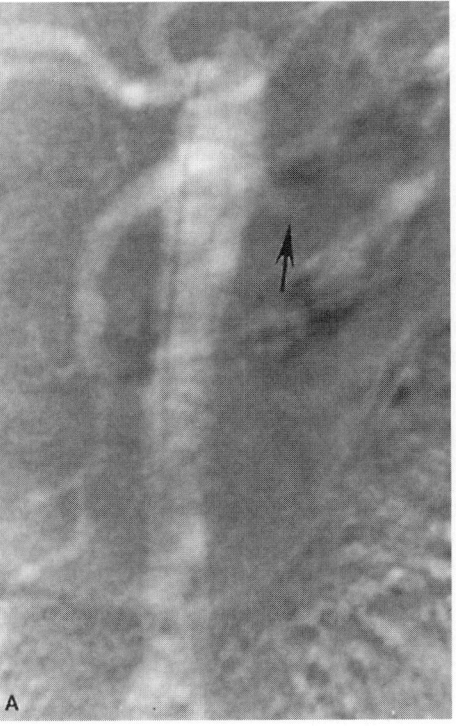
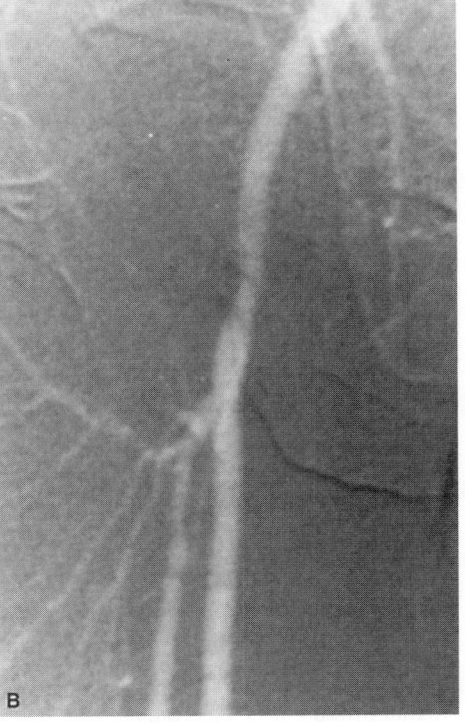

Figure 72.3. Carbon dioxide gas used as a contrast medium. A lumbar aortogram *(A)* and right common femoral arteriogram *(B)* were made during hand injection of carbon dioxide gas using digital subtraction angiography. The renal and lumbar arteries, which course posteriorly, usually are not filled by the buoyant gas with the patient in the supine position. The left renal artery is incompletely opacified *(arrow)*.

quires 100 to 200 mL of hyperosmolar liquid. Because of the reduced nephrotoxicity of these agents, and despite their being less radiopaque than the conventional iodinated contrast materials, these MR contrast agents have been used off-label for direct arterial injection in patients with renal compromise or allergy to iodinated contrast materials. In nonobese patients who are cooperative and have minimal bowel gas, these agents can provide diagnostically adequate arteriography and guide interventional procedures.

COMPLICATIONS

The overall rate of serious complications with diagnostic angiography is less than 5% (2). The complications of angiography occur at the puncture site, in conjunction with catheterizing and injecting the selected vessel, or in association with the contrast medium. Puncture site complications include hematomas, dissections, pseudoaneurysms, arteriovenous fistulae, thrombosis, and, when applicable, graft infection. The frequency and severity of these complications depend on the experience of the angiographer, the attention to postprocedure hemostasis, the size of the catheter or sheath, the choice of puncture site, the number of catheter exchanges, and the duration of the procedure. Patients with uncontrolled hypertension, obesity, severe atherosclerosis, precariously compensated renal or cardiac disease, spasm-prone vessels, or poor coagulation status are at increased risk of complications. Several percutaneous devices have become available to close the puncture site with a collagen plug or transmural sutures. Assuming they gain wide acceptance, these closure devices may decrease puncture site complications, allow high-risk patients to remain anticoagulated after removal of endovascular devices, and reduce the duration of postprocedure medical monitoring in outpatients (11).

Catheterization and injection complications include arterial dissection, perforation, and embolism (including stroke). The risks depend on the experience of the angiographer, anatomic variations affecting the ease of selective catheterization, the vessel catheterized, and intrinsic arterial disease. Thus, embolic stroke is associated with catheter manipulation or contrast injection in the aortic arch or brachiocephalic arteries. The gravity of a given complication such as arterial dissection or thrombosis depends on the vessel involved and the integrity of collaterals. For example, celiac artery dissection is usually well tolerated, but superior mesenteric artery (SMA) dissection may require urgent surgical repair.

The complications related to the administration of contrast medium include renal failure, fluid overload and congestive heart failure, transverse myelitis, and anaphylactoid reactions. These complications can be minimized by adequate hydration of the patient, careful catheter placement, and the appropriate use of a steroid preparation (e.g., 32 mg of oral methylprednisolone 12 and 2 hours before the procedure) or nonionic contrast medium, or both (12,13).

As a result of improvements in catheter and guide wire technology, the complication rate of diagnostic angiography has been reduced. Small-diameter (3F and 4F) catheters have fewer puncture site complications and have made outpatient arteriograms a routine procedure in low-risk patients. Coaxial catheter systems and guide wires with excellent torque control and atraumatic radiopaque tips facilitate superselective catheterization for both diagnostic and therapeutic angiography.

CONTRAINDICATIONS

There are no absolute contraindications to angiography. Relative contraindications include severe hypertension, poor coagulation status, severe renal or cardiac failure, and a history of severe contrast reaction. Reversible medical conditions affecting the risks of the procedure should be corrected before the angiographic procedure.

OUTPATIENT ANGIOGRAPHY

Outpatient angiography is a safe procedure and a realistic option for elective procedures in many patients (14). The use of small-bore catheters, postprocedure patient monitoring for 4 to 6 hours by radiology nursing staff, and discharge of the patient to attendant care by a family member or friend minimize the risk of puncture site hematomas. Intraarterial DSA and hydration with intravenous or oral fluids reduce the nephrotoxicity of the contrast medium. In selected patients, uncomplicated procedures such as angioplasty may be appropriate on an outpatient basis (15). Communication between the surgery and angiography departments well in advance of the procedure is desirable to ensure that the patient is properly prepared for the examination. Such preparation includes review of the clinical history and screening laboratory tests, the appropriate use of prophylactic antibiotics, preprocedure hydration, and arrangements for observed care after discharge from the outpatient facility. Alternative contrast agents such as carbon dioxide and gadolinium-based agents and percutaneous closure devices may allow outpatient procedures to be performed on patients at increased risk for puncture site complications or renal failure (see Complications, earlier). Otherwise, these patients should probably undergo angiography as inpatients.

FUTURE DEVELOPMENTS

Helical CT and MRI have had a significant impact on conventional diagnostic angiography. In general, both studies provide accurate anatomic detail of the aorta and vena cava and their first- to third-order branches. In the study of these large vessels, the role of angiography is increasingly limited to the hemodynamic evaluation of vascular lesions and the guidance of endovascular therapy. Conventional angiography retains a strong role in the diagnosis of medium- and small-vessel disease. During complicated interventional procedures, conventional angiography and fluoroscopy are used in conjunction with intravascular ultrasound and angioscopy. In interventional angiography, stent grafts have revolutionized the treatment of aortic disease, although the ideal combination of stent, cover, fixation device, and delivery system has yet to be found. Long-term follow-up on these devices is lacking. All stents and possibly stent grafts are plagued by restenosis at the transition zone between the stented and unstented vessel wall. Effective therapy for neointimal hyperplasia is required before these devices can be used for routine treatment rather than just for salvage-type procedures.

VASCULAR ANATOMY AND IMPLICATIONS

Although a detailed description of the vascular anatomy of individual organs is beyond the scope of this chapter, a brief discussion of vascular anatomy is important for both the performance and interpretation of angiograms.

Thoracic Aorta

Thoracic aortography is indicated for the study of congenital anomalies and acquired diseases of the thoracic aorta and its major branches (e.g., aneurysm, dissection, traumatic laceration, aortic valvular disease, and aortic arch syndrome). Catheter-based aortography is performed with use of the right posterior oblique, anteroposterior, and lateral projections, with injection of contrast medium into the aortic root. Helical CT or MR aortography are performed with intravenous injections of iodinated or gadolinium-based contrast media, respectively. Thoracic aortography should demonstrate the thoracic aorta from the aortic root to the level of the diaphragm, the innominate artery, and the subclavian, common carotid, and vertebral arteries. Other branches of the thoracic aorta, which usually require selective catheterization for visualization, are the bronchial and intercostal arteries and the anterior radiculomedullary artery. The bronchial arteries arise from the ventral surface of the upper part of the thoracic aorta or from the upper intercostal arteries between the fifth and seventh thoracic vertebrae. They become dilated in a variety of conditions, including pulmonary thromboembolism, chronic inflammatory disease of the lung, and congenital heart diseases associated with a decrease in pulmonary artery blood flow. Because the anterior radiculomedullary artery (artery of Adamkiewicz) may arise anywhere from the descending thoracic and proximal lumbar aorta, extreme care should be exercised to avoid spinal cord injury during bronchial and intercostal angiography. Precautions include the use of nonionic contrast medium, scrupulous care not to wedge the catheter in the bronchial or intercostal artery during contrast injection, prompt removal of the catheter from the artery after injection, and meticulous inspection of diagnostic arteriograms for the characteristic appearance of the spinal artery.

Abdominal Aorta

Abdominal aortography is performed to demonstrate the abdominal aorta and its branches, including the celiac, mesenteric, renal, lumbar, and iliac arteries. The celiac artery and SMA arise from the ventral surface of the aorta

proximal to the renal arteries between the 12th thoracic body and the 1st lumbar vertebral body. Thus, lateral aortography (Fig. 72.4) in catheter-based studies, or reconstruction in the sagittal plane of three-dimensional helical CTA or MR angiography datasets, is needed to visualize their origins in profile.

The renal arteries arise from the lateral margins of the aorta below the origin of the SMA, and their orifices are seen by aortograms obtained in the anteroposterior and slight left anterior oblique projections. Each kidney usually has a single renal artery. In approximately 20% to 30% of cases, more than one renal artery supplies a kidney (Fig. 72.5). The supplementary renal arteries are usually smaller than the main renal artery and may arise from anywhere between the 11th thoracic vertebral body and the iliac arteries. It is important to identify the origins of supplementary arteries before surgery for aortic aneurysm, aortoiliac occlusive disease, and renal artery stenosis. The arterial supply of ectopic and fused kidneys is variable in the origin, number, and course of renal arteries, and multiple injections of contrast may be necessary for complete evaluation. The lumbar arteries are ordinarily small and supply the body wall, retroperitoneum, paravertebral muscles, and spine. They provide collateral flow to the pelvis and lower extremities in the presence of aortoiliac occlusive disease. Supplemental collateral flow to the lower trunk can also develop from the subclavian artery by way of the internal mammary artery and from the axillary artery by way of the lateral thoracic artery.

Pelvic Arteries

Pelvic arteriography is indicated for suspected abnormalities of the common, external, internal iliac, and femoral arteries and as part of the arteriographic study of the lower extremities. Contrast material is injected into the distal abdominal aorta. Optimal evaluation of the bifurcations of the common iliac and femoral arteries requires oblique pelvic arteriograms. Selective catheterization of the branches of the internal iliac artery is done for visual-

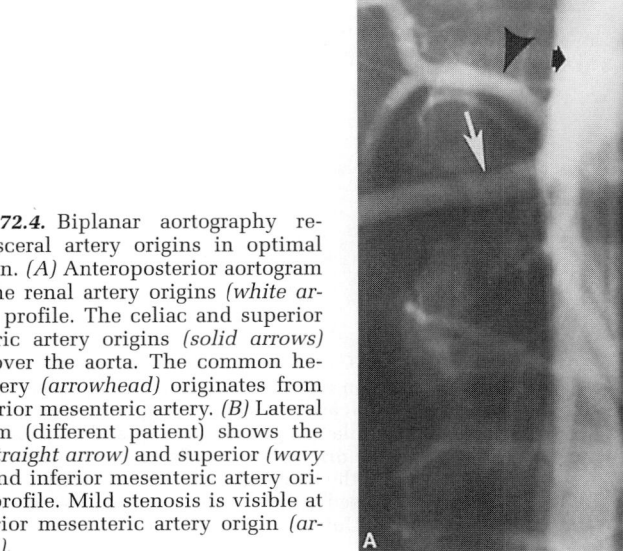
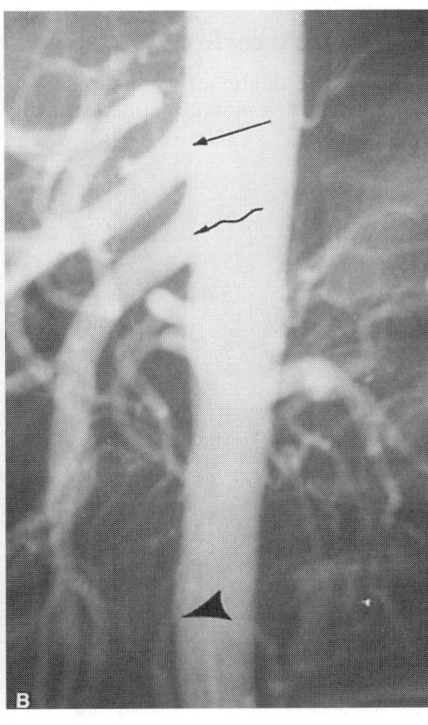

Figure 72.4. Biplanar aortography reveals visceral artery origins in optimal projection. *(A)* Anteroposterior aortogram shows the renal artery origins *(white arrows)* in profile. The celiac and superior mesenteric artery origins *(solid arrows)* project over the aorta. The common hepatic artery *(arrowhead)* originates from the superior mesenteric artery. *(B)* Lateral aortogram (different patient) shows the celiac *(straight arrow)* and superior *(wavy arrow)* and inferior mesenteric artery origins in profile. Mild stenosis is visible at the inferior mesenteric artery origin *(arrowhead).*

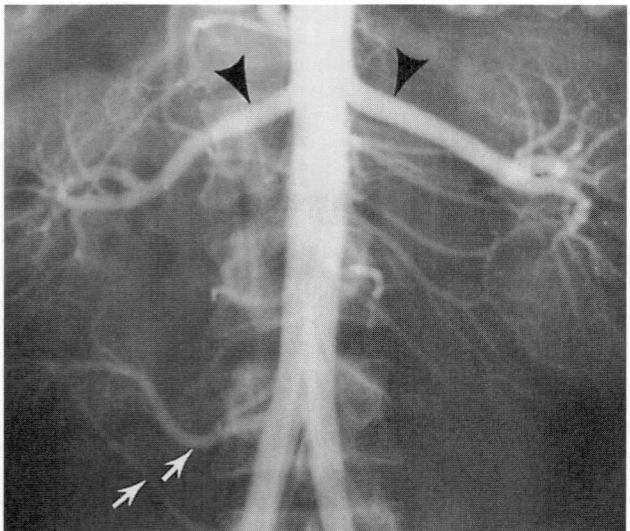

Figure 72.5. Multiple renal arteries. Lumbar aortogram shows normal right and left main renal arteries *(arrowheads)*. In addition, two accessory right lower pole arteries arise from the aortic bifurcation and mid-portion of the right common iliac artery *(white arrows)*. Multiple jejunal arteries arising from the superior mesenteric artery are seen below the level of the left renal artery.

ization of the penile arteries in the work-up of impotence and for embolization in pelvic neoplasms and hemorrhage. Proximal embolization of the branches of the internal iliac artery with particulate materials can be performed safely because of the availability of abundant collateral circulation. Liquid materials, such as alcohol, sclerosing agents, and tissue adhesives, usually are not used because of the potential for tissue necrosis and sciatic nerve paralysis. Anastomoses of the external and internal iliac arteries with their contralateral mates and with branches of the lumbar and deep femoral arteries allow collateral reconstitution of major pelvic vessels in the event of proximal occlusive disease.

Visceral Arteries

The three major arteries supplying the abdominal visceral organs are the celiac artery, SMA, and inferior mesenteric artery (IMA). Celiac artery and SMA angiography are routinely performed for any suspected abnormalities of the gastrointestinal tract, liver, pancreas, and mesentery, including tumors, aneurysms, cysts, occlusive disease, and bleeding. Knowledge of the many normal variants in arterial anatomy of abdominal organs is crucial to planning surgical procedures.

In standard anatomy, the celiac artery divides into the splenic and common hepatic arteries after giving rise to the left gastric artery (Fig. 72.6). The inferior phrenic and dorsal pancreatic arteries may also arise from the celiac axis. The common hepatic artery divides into the right, middle, and left hepatic arteries distal to the origin of the gastroduodenal artery. The right hepatic artery divides into the anterior and posterior segmental arteries, which further subdivide into superior and inferior subsegmental branches. The middle hepatic artery arises from the right, proper, or left hepatic arteries and supplies blood to the medial segment of the left lobe of the liver. The left hepatic artery divides into two subsegmental branches.

In approximately half of the population, the liver receives blood from aberrant hepatic arteries. The aberrant hepatic artery may be a lobar (or replaced) hepatic artery or a segmental (accessory) hepatic artery. At least 10 basic types of hepatic artery variations have been demonstrated angiographically or in dissection studies of human cadavers. Both replaced (10% incidence) and accessory (5% incidence) right hepatic arteries usually originate from the SMA, but in rare cases they arise from other branches of the celiac artery and SMA (Fig. 72.7). Most replaced (12% incidence) and accessory (12% incidence) left hepatic arteries originate from the left gastric artery. Thus, the left gastric artery should be visualized to determine the presence of an aberrant left hepatic artery. The left gastric artery usually originates from the ventral surface of the celiac axis distal to the origin of the inferior phrenic artery and gives rise to mural branches to the stomach while coursing along the lesser curvature of the stomach. In 3% of cases, the left gastric artery has an aberrant origin from the aorta. Because the left gastric artery freely anastomoses with the right gastric, short gastric, and gastroepiploic arteries, embolization of its branches can be performed safely to control arterial bleeding from the stomach. The gastroduodenal artery usually arises from the hepatic artery but may have an aberrant origin from other branches of the celiac artery or SMA. It supplies blood to the duodenum and pancreas

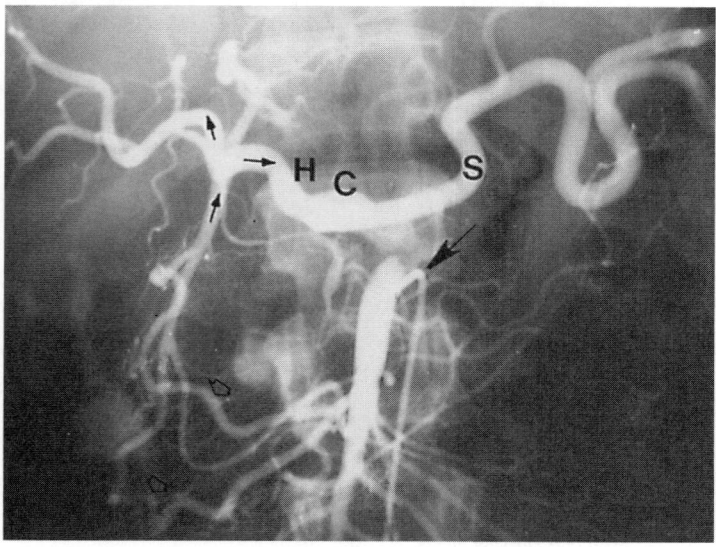

Figure 72.6. Celiac occlusion (C). Superior mesenteric artery injection (catheter, *large arrow*) fills the hepatic (H) and splenic (S) arteries from the superior mesenteric artery through the enlarged gastroduodenal and pancreatic arcade arteries *(open arrows)*. Blood flows in the gastroduodenal artery toward the liver and in the common hepatic artery toward the spleen *(small arrows)*. (Courtesy of James Andrews, M.D., University of Michigan Hospitals, Ann Arbor, MI.)

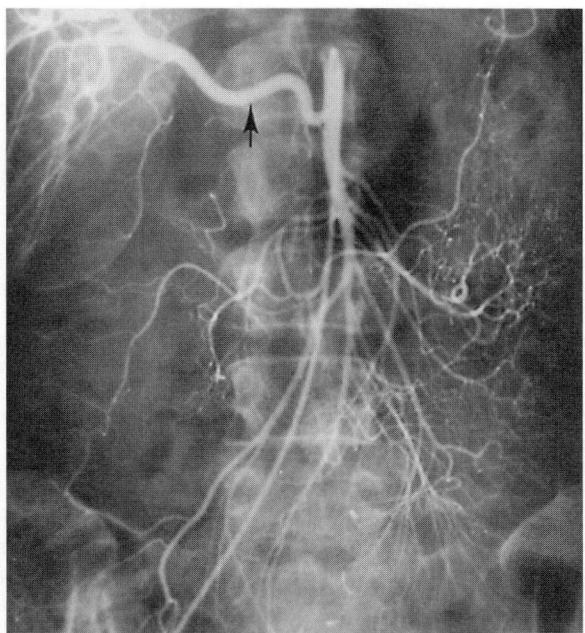

Figure 72.7. Replaced right hepatic artery. The right hepatic artery *(arrow)* originates from the superior mesenteric artery. (Courtesy of James Andrews, M.D., University of Michigan Hospitals, Ann Arbor, MI.)

pancreatic arcade arteries are the main collateral pathways in celiac artery and SMA occlusion (Fig. 72.6). When angiography is performed for the diagnosis and embolization of duodenal bleeding, injections into both the celiac artery and SMA are necessary to complete the examination.

The dorsal pancreatic artery may arise from the splenic artery, celiac artery, hepatic artery, or SMA. It usually divides into the transverse and anastomotic branches immediately after its origin. These branches in turn anastomose with the branches of the pancreatic arcade and splenic arteries. While coursing along the pancreas, the splenic artery gives rise to numerous branches to the pancreas, the most important of which are the pancreatica magna and caudal pancreatic arteries.

The SMA runs posterior to the pancreas after its origin from the ventral surface of the aorta between the celiac and renal arteries. It then gives rise to jejunal, ileal, and colic branches (Fig. 72.8). Occasionally, the dorsal pancreatic and retroportal arteries arise from the main trunk of the SMA proximal to the origin of the middle colic artery. The middle colic artery arises from the ventral surface of the SMA at or distal to the origin of the first jejunal artery and divides into the right and left branches, which anastomose with the right colic, ileocolic, and left colic arteries by way of the arc of Riolan and the marginal artery of Drummond. The IMA originates from the anterolateral surface of the aorta between the left renal artery and the aortic bifurcation. It divides into the sigmoidal and superior hemorrhoidal arteries after giving rise to its first branch, the left colic artery (Fig. 72.9). The superior hemorrhoidal artery anastomoses with the middle and inferior hemorrhoidal arteries of the internal iliac artery and provides collateral blood flow to the lower extremities when there is aortic and iliac occlusion.

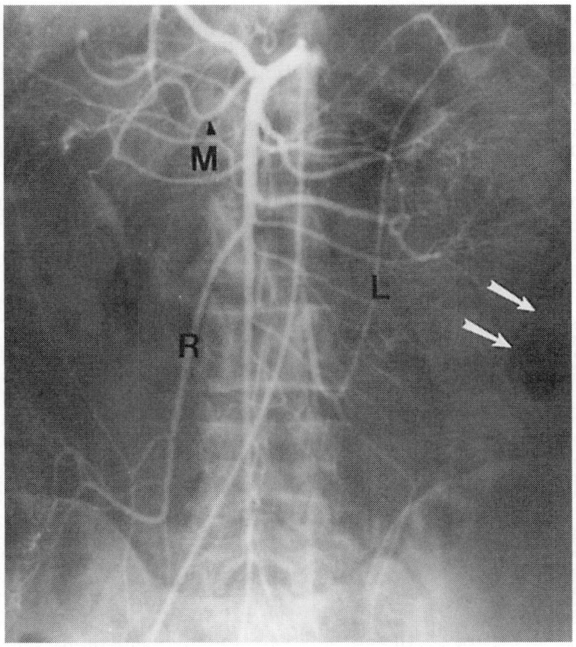

through the anterior and posterior pancreatic arcade arteries and to the stomach through the gastroepiploic artery. The anterior and posterior arcade arteries anastomose with the inferior pancreaticoduodenal artery, arising either separately or as a common trunk with the first jejunal artery from the SMA. The gastroduodenal and

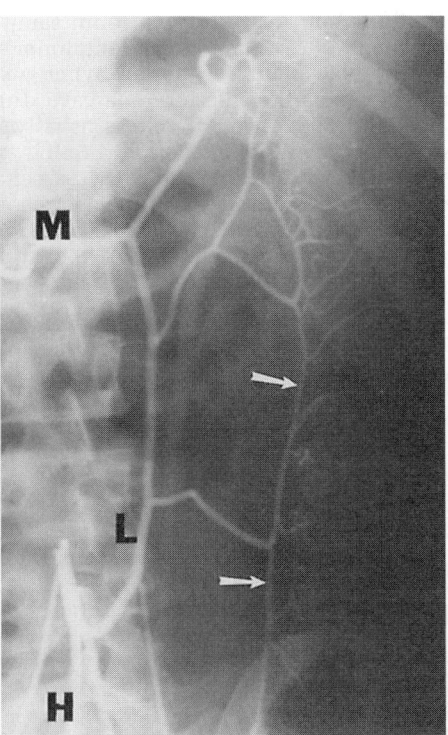

Figure 72.8. Superior mesenteric arteriogram demonstrates right (R), middle (M), and left (L) colic arteries. The marginal artery of Drummond *(arrows)* can be seen adjacent to the gas-filled descending colon. The common hepatic artery originates from the superior mesenteric artery.

Figure 72.9. Inferior mesenteric arteriogram demonstrates the left colic (L), middle colic (M), and superior hemorrhoidal (H) arteries and the marginal artery of Drummond *(arrows).*

Visceral Veins

The portal venous system can be demonstrated by injection of contrast medium into the celiac artery, splenic artery, and SMA. Earlier techniques such as splenoportography and umbilical vein cannulation are rarely used for opacification of the portal venous system. Percutaneous transhepatic portal vein catheterization is an alternative approach in the evaluation of the portal vein and its hemodynamics; it provides access to the coronary vein for embolization of bleeding esophageal varices (Fig. 72.10).

The portal vein commences at the junction of the splenic and superior mesenteric veins. It runs anterior to the inferior vena cava toward the porta hepatis, where it divides into the right and left portal branches. In normal conditions, the blood in the portal vein and its tributaries (i.e., the coronary and inferior mesenteric veins) flows toward the liver. Reversal of blood flow in any of the portal venous tributaries indicates the presence of portosystemic collaterals induced by portal hypertension. Angiography continues to play a major role in the evaluation of patients with portal hypertension before and after a portosystemic shunt procedure.

The hepatic veins lie between hepatic segments or lobes and join the inferior vena cava either separately or as a single trunk, just before the right atrium. The hepatic veins can be catheterized through the femoral, jugular, or peripheral arm veins. In the presence of a postsinusoidal block such as alcoholic cirrhosis, manometry through a catheter wedged in the hepatic vein reflects portal vein pressure. Hepatic venography is indicated for evaluation of the hepatic venous drainage pattern before hepatic resection for liver tumor or hepatic venoocclusive disease. Wedged hepatic venography is useful for visualizing the portal vein when indirect portography (after intraarterial injection of contrast medium) has failed to do so.

The renal veins, usually one from each kidney, join the inferior vena cava. Knowledge of both normal and variant anatomy is important for renal vein renin sampling, preoperative evaluation of a renal transplant donor, and splenorenal shunt placement for portal hypertension. The right renal vein joins the inferior vena cava directly and may be multiple. The left renal vein is usually joined by the adrenal and gonadal veins before running anterior to the aorta and joining the inferior vena cava. Rarely, the renal vein may run behind the aorta (retroaortic renal vein), or both preaortic and retroaortic renal veins may exist together (circumaortic renal vein).

Arteries of the Upper Extremities

Upper extremity arteriography is indicated for the study of suspected arterial abnormalities of the shoulder, arm, forearm, and hand. The study usually begins with arch aortography using standard cut-film technique or DSA to demonstrate the innominate and subclavian arteries, followed by selective injections into the axillary artery to see the brachial, ulnar, radial, and digital arteries.

The brachial artery gives off the deep brachial artery and divides into the ulnar, radial, and interosseous arteries below the level of the neck of the radius. In approximately 10% of cases, the bifurcation arises in the upper arm or even from the axillary artery; this variation can be confused with an arterial occlusion if the injection of contrast material is distal to the aberrant origin. The deep brachial artery provides the main collateral flow to the arm in the presence of brachial artery occlusion.

In the forearm, the ulnar artery gives rise to the common interosseous artery (which divides into the anterior and posterior interosseous arteries) and the anterior and posterior ulnar recurrent arteries. The radial artery supplies a recurrent artery near the elbow as well as muscular branches distally. The median artery is an embryologic remnant that can originate from the proximal ulnar, radial, or interosseous arteries and normally runs with the median nerve.

Terminology of palmar arch arterial anatomy varies among authors and is not discussed here (16,17). Digital angiography is usually performed with the injection of a vasodilator such as tolazoline (usual dose, 25 to 50 mg) before contrast injection. Magnification filming is useful for identifying the distal ulnar and radial artery contributions to the wrist and hand circulation through the superficial and deep palmar arches. Arteries are usually opacified as far distally as the fingertip plexus. The radial, ulnar, and digital arteries anastomose with each other through the palmar arches.

Arteries of the Lower Extremities

Lower extremity arteriography is indicated for suspected arterial abnormalities in the thigh, calf, and foot. In patients at risk for arteriosclerotic occlusive disease, arteriography is usually preceded by abdominal aortography and pelvic arteriography. Both extremities can be studied simultaneously by injecting contrast material into the distal abdominal aorta and recording the image with conventional film or DSA. In some circumstances, such as evalu-

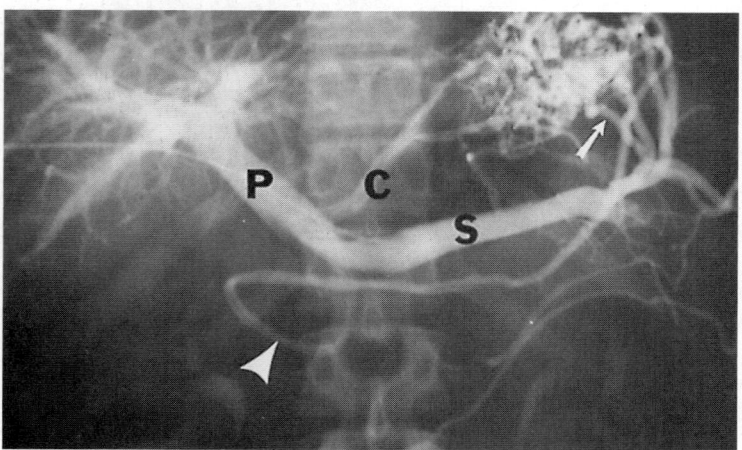

Figure 72.10. Transhepatic splenic venography demonstrates splenic (S), portal (P), and coronary (C), or left gastric, veins. The gastrocolic trunk *(arrowhead)* and short gastric veins *(arrow)* are also demonstrated. All these veins are normally demonstrated during the venous phase of celiac angiography.

ation of distal anatomy for placement of a free flap, a single-leg outflow study is performed with an injection into the external iliac artery from either the ipsilateral or contralateral femoral artery approach. In patients with poor cardiac output, significant aneurysmal disease, or multilevel occlusive disease, visualization of distal calf vessels and the plantar arch is often poor with aortic injections of contrast medium. Visualization of these vessels is crucial when surgical bypass for limb salvage is contemplated, and it can be enhanced by augmenting distal flow (by intraarterial vasodilators, postischemic hyperemia, or contrast injection distal to an occlusion balloon) or by using DSA.

The common femoral artery bifurcates into the deep and superficial femoral arteries several centimeters distal to the inguinal ligament. In most patients, the bifurcation is best seen on the ipsilateral anterior oblique projection. Angiographically, the superficial femoral artery courses in a medial and anterior direction, and the deep femoral artery courses in a lateral and posterior direction. Numerous communications between branches of the deep femoral and internal iliac arteries above and the genicular branches below emphasize the importance of the deep femoral artery in reconstituting lower extremity outflow in the presence of aortoiliac or femoropopliteal occlusive disease. The superficial femoral artery continues at the adductor hiatus as the popliteal artery. Major branches of the popliteal artery include the "trifurcation" branches (peroneal and anterior and posterior tibial arteries) and the genicular complex with its important anastomoses with

the deep femoral artery above and the recurrent tibial branches below. The posterior tibial artery terminates in the foot as the lateral and medial plantar arteries. The anterior tibial artery continues at the foot as the dorsalis pedis, whose terminal deep plantar branch connects with the lateral plantar artery to form the plantar arch. Two distal branches of the peroneal artery, the anterior and posterior perforating branches, anastomose with the anterior and posterior tibial arteries and are important sources of collateral blood flow when occlusive disease affects these vessels. The arteries of the distal calf and foot are best seen in the lateral projection.

NORMAL VARIATIONS SIMULATING DISEASE

Anatomic variations and artifacts of the angiographic procedure can simulate arterial occlusions, arterial encasement, and parenchymal perfusion defects. Such confusion can be minimized by knowledge of the normal variations in arterial anatomy and common artifacts encountered during angiography. Failure to fill the expected arterial pattern of an organ or limb may be due to arterial occlusion or to an avascular mass, but it may also result from a contrast injection that fails to fill aberrant or accessory arteries. Catheter- and guide wire-induced spasm can mimic neoplastic encasement; thus, selective catheterization should be preceded by proximal arterial injections to demonstrate true arterial narrowing (Fig. 72.11). For example, aortogra-

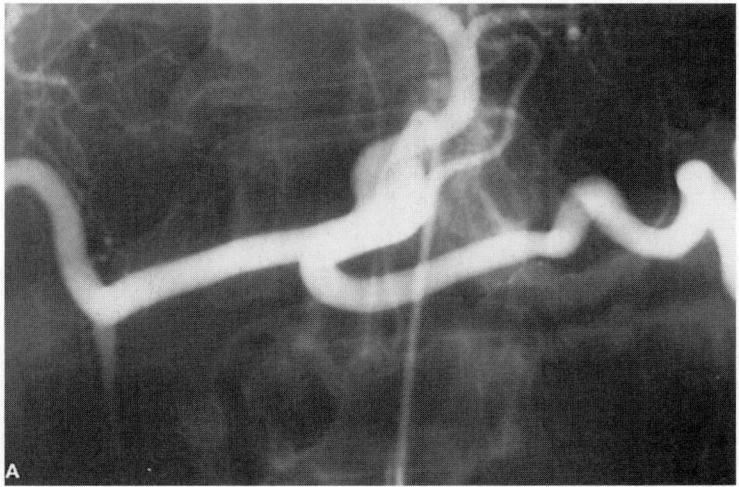
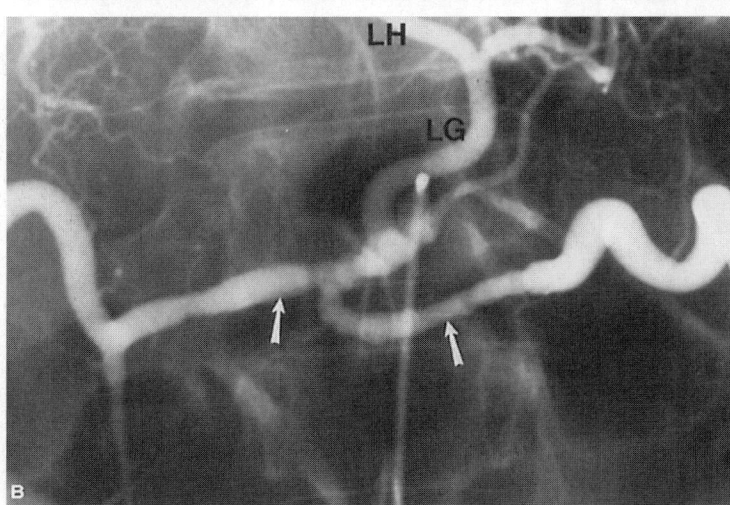

Figure 72.11. Guide wire-induced arterial spasm in a patient with pancreatitis. Celiac arteriograms made before *(A)* and after *(B)* catheterization of the splenic artery. Irregular narrowing of the splenic and common hepatic arteries *(arrows in B)* can be seen, mimicking tumor encasement. The left hepatic artery (LH) originates from the left gastric artery (LG).

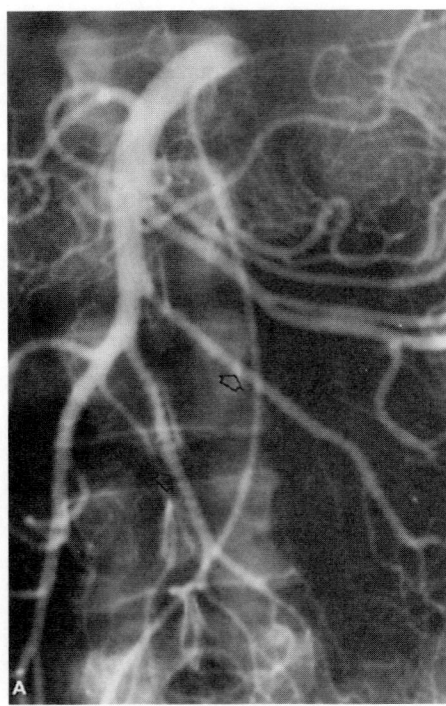
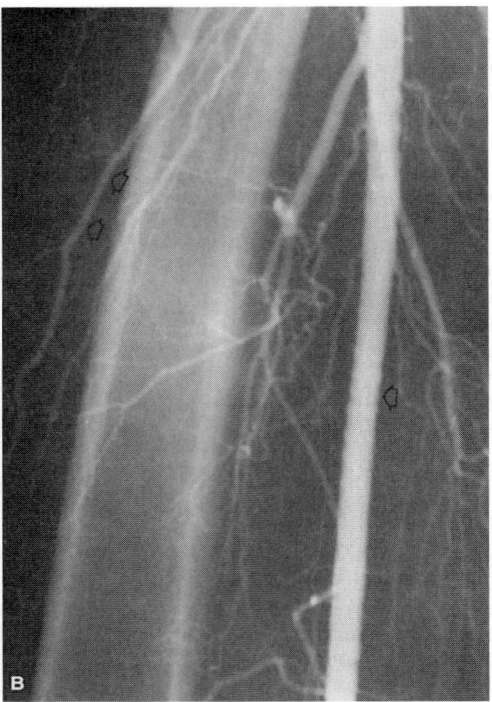

Figure 72.12. Arterial standing waves. Smooth, repetitive bands of mild narrowing *(open arrows)* are demonstrated in branches of the superior mesenteric *(A)* and superficial femoral *(B)* arteries during contrast injection.

phy should precede renal arteriography, and celiac arteriography should precede gastroduodenal arteriography. Contrast injection occasionally demonstrates an ill-understood phenomenon called *standing waves,* in which the arterial lumen is distinguished by smooth, regular, alternating bands of mild narrowing and expansion (Fig. 72.12). This condition can be distinguished from drug-induced (Fig. 72.13) or hypovolemic vasoconstriction and from ar-

terial fibrodysplasia (Fig. 72.27A) by the monotonous regularity of the alternating bands. The high specific gravity of contrast material compared with blood contributes to incomplete mixing of the contrast during injection, especially at the head and tail of the contrast bolus. When mixing is incomplete, contrast material tends to pool along the dependent surface of large vessels such as the aorta or along the mural surface of small arteries. This layering of

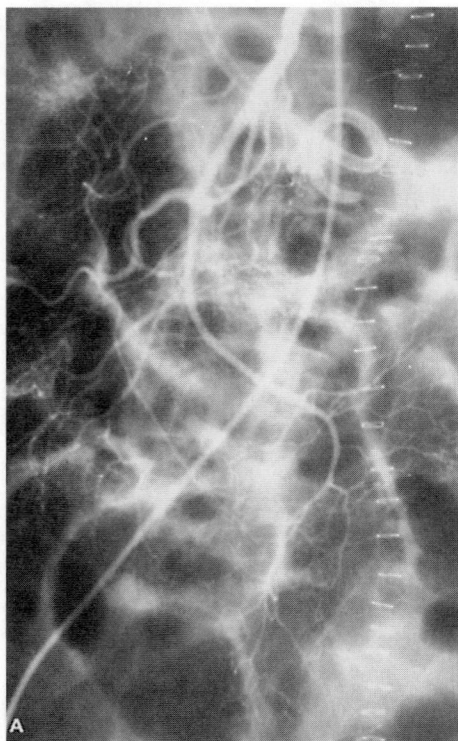
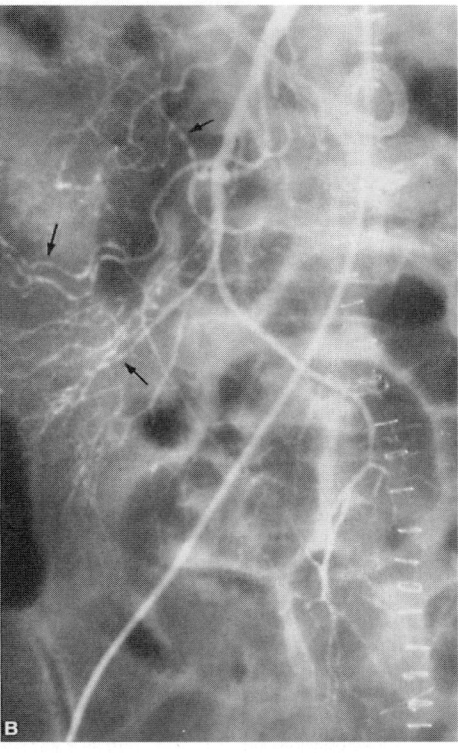

Figure 72.13. Vasopressin-induced arterial spasm in a woman with gastrointestinal bleeding and multiple vascular ectasias in the small bowel. *(A)* Celiac and superior mesenteric arteriograms show no vascular abnormalities. *(B)* A second mesenteric arteriogram after 12 hours of vasopressin infusion into the superior mesenteric artery (0.2 IU/min) shows diffuse arterial vasoconstriction. Multiple focal vasodilated segments *(small arrows)* reflect uneven response to vasopressin.

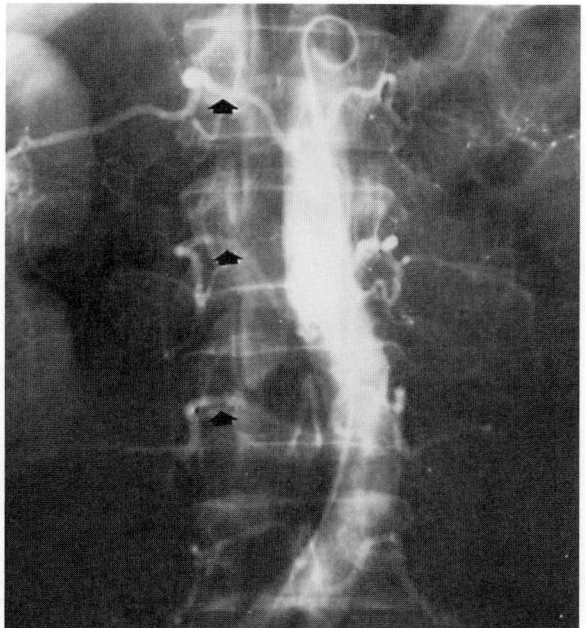

Figure 72.14. Dependent layering of contrast material. Late arterial phase of a lumbar aortogram demonstrates contrast material pooling along the posterior surface of the aorta in a patient in the supine position. Contrast material continues to fill lumbar arteries *(arrows)* after it has cleared from renal and mesenteric branches.

contrast is responsible for visualization of lumbar arteries on abdominal aortograms after visceral and renal arteries have cleared (Fig. 72.14). In small arteries, the mural layering of contrast material with nonopacified blood flowing in the center of the lumen can simulate an embolus (Fig. 72.15).

DIAGNOSTIC ANGIOGRAPHY: INDICATIONS AND FINDINGS

Hemorrhage and ischemia, real or threatened, are the indications for most diagnostic angiography. Other indications include the demonstration of vascular anatomy before surgical or transcatheter intervention and venous thromboembolism. Hemorrhage, except in association with catastrophes such as a ruptured aneurysm, is an indication for both diagnostic and therapeutic angiography and is discussed in the next section. The clinical presentation of ischemia depends on the organ involved and includes stroke, angina, renovascular hypertension, mesenteric ischemia, and limb claudication. Neurologic and cardiac disease are not discussed in this chapter. The prototypical ischemic diseases are macroemboli and nonaneurysmal atherosclerosis. Although aneurysms, arterial fibrodysplasia, dissection, arteritis, and trauma may present as ischemic disease (or as hemorrhage), the angiographic findings and work-up of the primary disease are distinct enough to merit separate discussion.

Macroembolism

Most macroemboli involving the abdominal viscera or the extremities are cardiac in origin and present as one of the acute ischemic syndromes. The indications for angiography in acute ischemia are to document the cause of acute occlusion (e.g., arterial emboli), to show arterial anatomy proximal and distal to significant occlusions, and to demonstrate associated or incidental disease. If emboli are documented, angiography should search for an aortic or arterial source such as an aneurysm or atherosclerotic plaque or ulcer (Fig. 72.16). The search for a cardiac source of emboli requires echocardiography. The appropriateness of intraarterial lytic therapy should be considered at the time of diagnostic angiography. If no emboli are found, other causes of acute ischemia should be considered, including mesenteric arterial spasm or in situ thrombosis secondary to a low flow state. Dissection and trauma

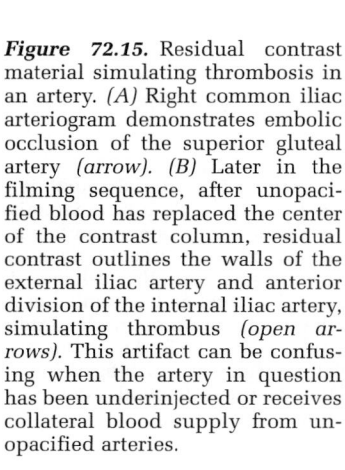

Figure 72.15. Residual contrast material simulating thrombosis in an artery. *(A)* Right common iliac arteriogram demonstrates embolic occlusion of the superior gluteal artery *(arrow)*. *(B)* Later in the filming sequence, after unopacified blood has replaced the center of the contrast column, residual contrast outlines the walls of the external iliac artery and anterior division of the internal iliac artery, simulating thrombus *(open arrows)*. This artifact can be confusing when the artery in question has been underinjected or receives collateral blood supply from unopacified arteries.

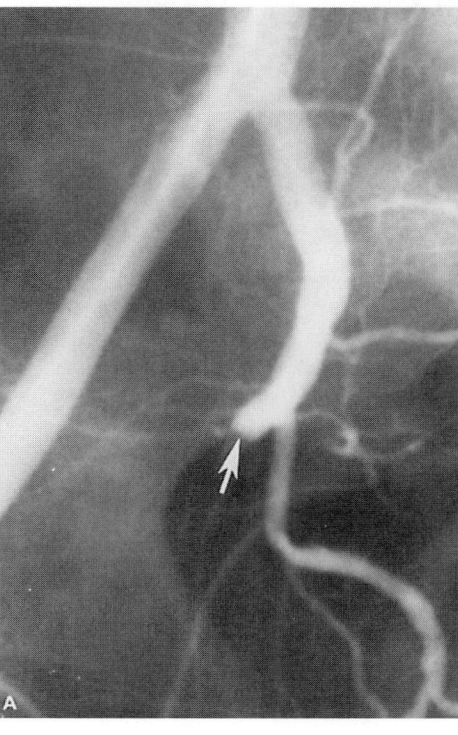

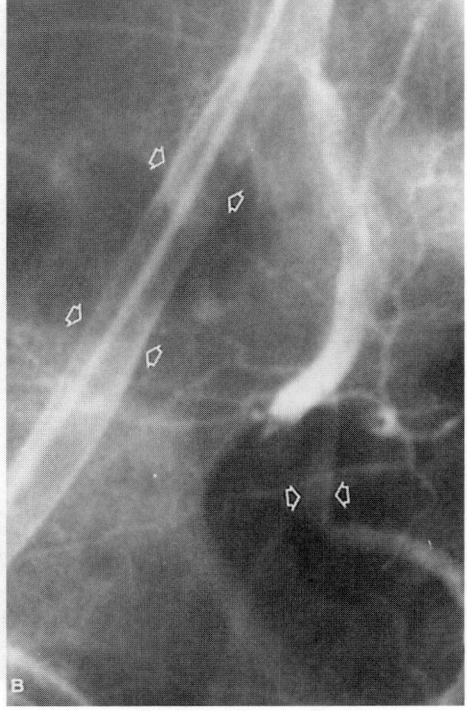

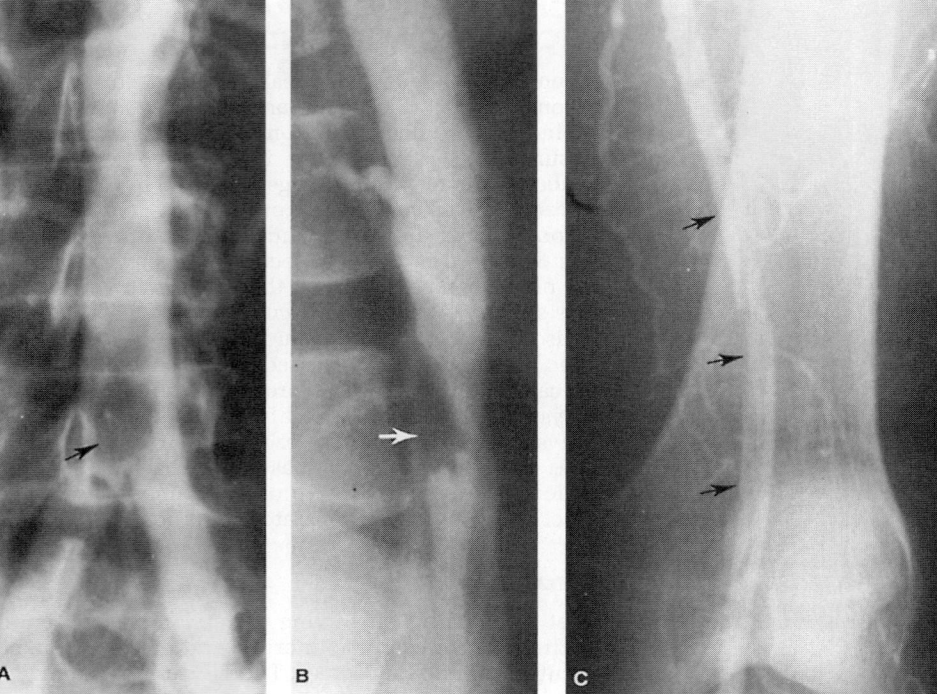

Figure 72.16. Recurrent lower extremity macroemboli from an atherosclerotic plaque in a man with recurrent lower extremity emboli, in whom surgical embolectomy failed to restore peripheral pulses. Biplanar aortogram shows a large, irregular posterior plaque *(arrow)* at the aortic bifurcation, subtle on the frontal film *(A)* but evident on the lateral film *(B)*. *(C)* A detail from the lower extremity outflow study shows extensive thromboemboli *(arrows)* in the left popliteal artery.

may also cause acute ischemia but are usually suggested by the clinical history.

Contrast medium surrounding the leading or trailing edge of an arterial clot indicates acute occlusion, either embolic or thrombotic (Figs. 72.17 and 72.18). It may be impossible to distinguish between acute embolism and in situ thrombosis unless multiple sites of acute occlusion due to random embolism are demonstrated. The distinc-

tion between acute and chronic occlusion is usually based on the size of the collaterals bridging the occlusion; they are small when the occlusion is acute and large when long-standing.

If the patient history and presentation suggest embolic disease, the angiographic work-up includes thoracic and biplane abdominal aortography to search for a source of emboli, and selective arteriography tailored to the clinical

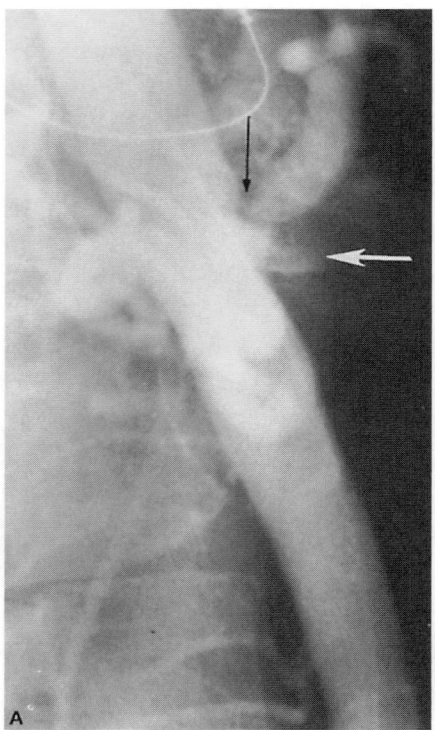
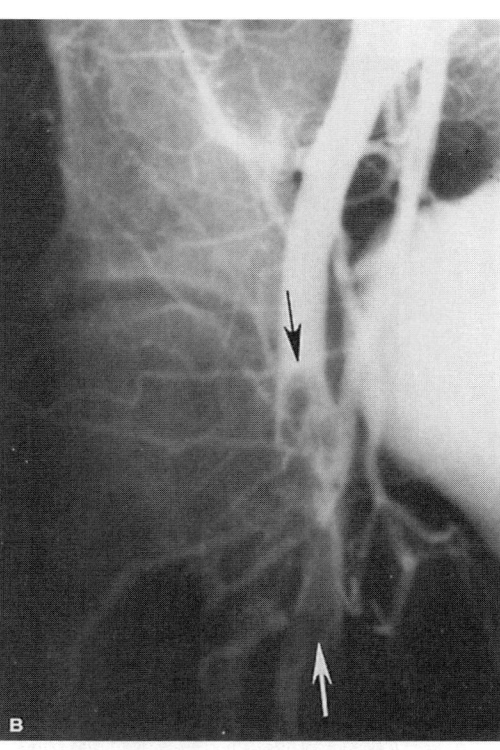

Figure 72.17. Arterial emboli in a woman with right lower extremity ischemia. *(A)* Lateral aortogram shows median arcuate ligament compression on the celiac axis *(black arrow)* and an embolus in the superior mesenteric artery *(white arrow)*. *(B)* An embolus is also visible at the bifurcation of the common femoral artery *(arrows)*.

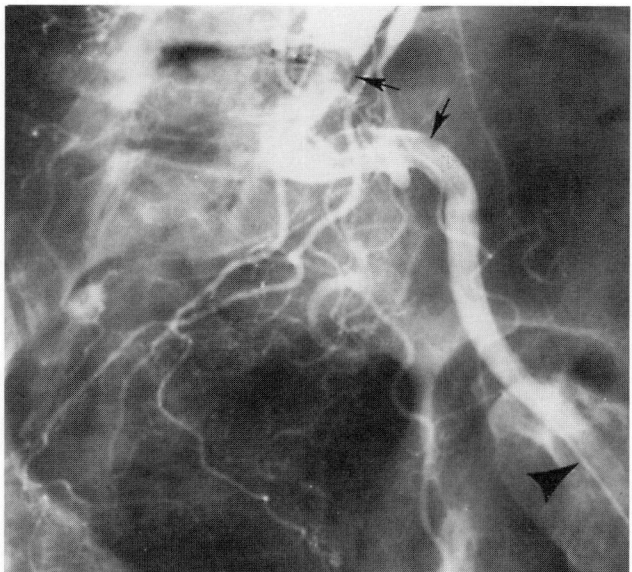

Figure 72.18. Aortic saddle embolism in a man in atrial fibrillation presenting with acute right leg pain. Pelvic arteriogram shows an acute saddle embolus *(arrows)* at the aortic bifurcation, extending into the left common iliac artery and occluding the right common iliac artery. Despite the large amount of thrombus in the left common iliac artery, the left femoral pulse was palpable, allowing the transfemoral approach for catheter access *(arrowhead).*

problem (e.g., mesenteric, renal, lower extremity, and so forth).

Nonaneurysmal Atherosclerosis: Renal, Mesenteric, and Peripheral

Atherosclerosis is a progressive, systemic disease primarily affecting large and medium-sized arteries. The ischemic syndrome varies with the organ involved and disease severity. Renal arteriosclerosis may present as hypertension or renal failure; mesenteric ischemia as postprandial epigastric pain, weight loss, and bowel infarction; and peripheral occlusive disease as claudication, rest pain, and gangrene.

The purposes of angiography are to document hemodynamically significant occlusive disease, to show the arterial anatomy of the donor and receptor sites of a prospective revascularization graft, and to demonstrate associated or incidental disease. Advances in helical CT and MR aortography have resulted in widespread acceptance of these studies as reliable screens for disease in the abdominal aorta and proximal trunks of the celiac artery, SMA, and renal artery. Frequently, when catheter-based angiography is undertaken, a general knowledge of the underlying pathologic process is already available. The roles of catheter-based angiography include to confirm, when necessary, the significance of noninvasive findings and to attempt endovascular treatment of the offending lesion. The appropriateness of transcatheter interventional procedures such as percutaneous angioplasty should be discussed before the time of diagnostic angiography.

Atherosclerosis is characterized angiographically by ulcers (pocket-like collections of contrast communicating with the arterial lumen), irregular or smooth narrowing

and occlusions of large and medium-sized arteries, and the presence of collaterals. Atherosclerotic stenoses may be confused with neoplastic encasement or arterial fibrodysplasia (see later). Angiographic features of stenoses favoring atherosclerosis are eccentricity, calcification, a tendency to involve the ostium or branch points, evidence of atherosclerosis in other vessels, and normal associated veins. An arterial stenosis is considered significant when associated with bridging collaterals, poststenotic dilatation, a pressure gradient exceeding 10 mm Hg, or, in the appropriate clinical setting, ipsilateral renal vein renin hypersecretion (18–20). Stenoses of questionable hemodynamic significance during baseline blood flow should be reassessed after augmenting flow by pharmacologic or physiologic stimulation such as vasoactive drugs or postischemic hyperemia (21). Vasospasm (diffuse narrowing of an arterial bed) may be distinguished from severe diffuse arteriosclerotic narrowing by its involvement of collaterals and branch arteries in the affected distribution, which are relatively spared in arteriosclerosis. Vasospasm is not a prominent finding on angiograms of atherosclerosis and should suggest drug toxicity (e.g., ergot, digitalis), Raynaud's phenomenon, cellulitis or compartment syndrome, heavy smoking, or other conditions with increased vascular tone. The angiographic findings and work-up of arteriosclerotic occlusive disease vary with the duration of the occlusion and the organ system involved.

Renovascular occlusive disease resulting in hypertension or renal failure is most commonly due to atherosclerosis (Fig. 72.19). Other causes include arterial fibrodysplasia, abdominal or thoracic aortic coarctation, neurofibromatosis, aortic dissection, and trauma. The indication for angiography is to document a hemodynamically adequate conduit from the aortic root to the renal parenchyma. If aortic coarctation or arterial stenoses are present, angiography should document their hemodynamic significance and demonstrate vascular anatomy necessary for planning a revascularization or angioplasty procedure. In an older adult, an abdominal aortogram that demonstrates all renal artery origins in profile along the aorta or iliac artery is usually sufficient to rule out a surgically correctable stenosis. In children and young adults, hypertension may be due to renal artery branch stenoses that could require selective renal artery injections with magnification filming for convincing documentation. Alternatively, hypertension may be due to aortic coarctation. Revascularization in the presence of densely calcified or severely ulcerated aortic and iliac vessels may require use of the splenic or hepatic–gastroduodenal artery. Consequently, a lateral aortogram must be obtained to rule out celiac artery stenosis.

Mesenteric ischemia may be acute or chronic, occlusive or nonocclusive (22). Biplane aortography demonstrates the celiac artery and SMA origins. It is useful in documenting proximal stenosis or embolic occlusion and in demonstrating mesenteric collateral flow. Selective injections into the celiac artery, SMA, and IMA may be necessary to demonstrate distal emboli, branch occlusions, or unsuspected neoplasm mimicking ischemic bowel disease. The mesenteric injection rates should be large enough to document patency of the mesenteric and portal veins. Acute embolic occlusion appears as a filling defect in the contrast column, usually at branch points. The angiogram in nonocclusive mesenteric ischemia may show diffuse vasoconstriction of the SMA and its branches (often drug related) with slowing of blood flow and decreased contrast accumulation in the bowel wall, or it may

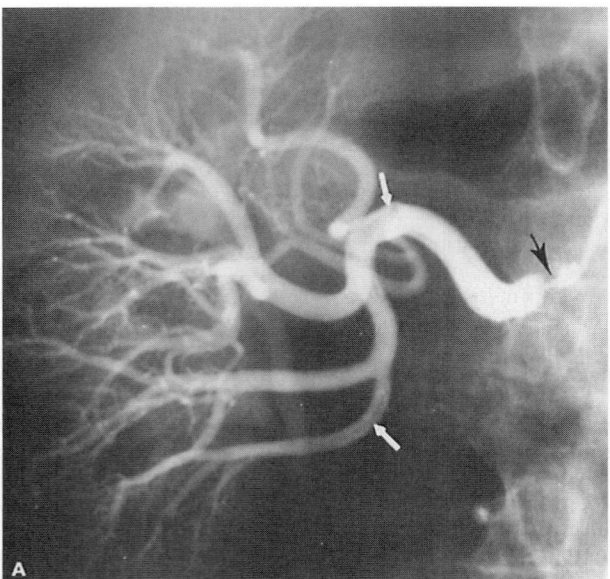
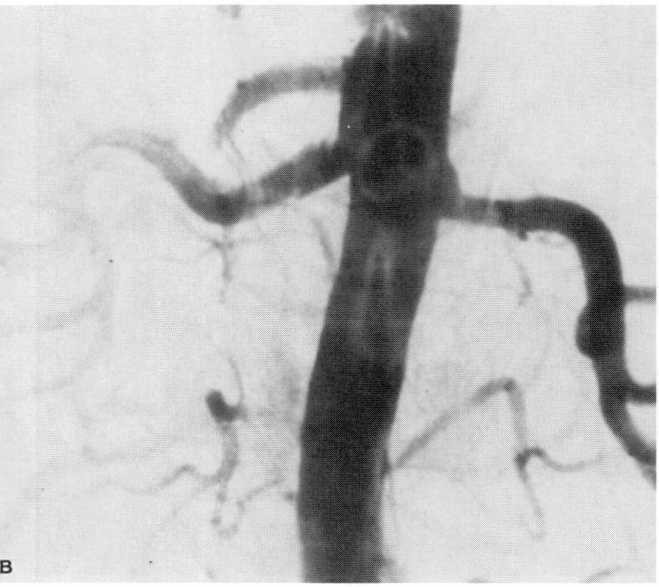

Figure 72.19. Atherosclerotic renal artery stenosis. *(A)* Right renal arteriogram shows a tight concentric proximal stenosis of the renal artery *(black arrow)*. The linear filling defects in the main renal artery and its segmental branches *(white arrows)* represent flow defects caused by unopacified blood flowing retrograde from nonparenchymal renal artery branches. The presence of collateral flow to the kidney indicates that the stenosis is hemodynamically significant. *(B)* Lumbar aortogram after percutaneous angioplasty shows significant improvement in the caliber of the arterial lumen.

be distressingly normal (Fig. 72.20). Isolated celiac artery or SMA occlusion is common and usually asymptomatic because of abundant, short (and therefore low-resistance) peripancreatic collaterals (Fig. 72.6). Proximal SMA stenosis may also be relieved by collateral supply from the IMA through the left colic to middle colic anastomosis. In general, at least two of the three visceral arteries must be occluded or significantly narrowed before mesenteric ischemia develops. The angiogram should document collateral supply reconstituting the bowel at risk; such collaterals are usually sparse and long compared with those in simple celiac stenosis.

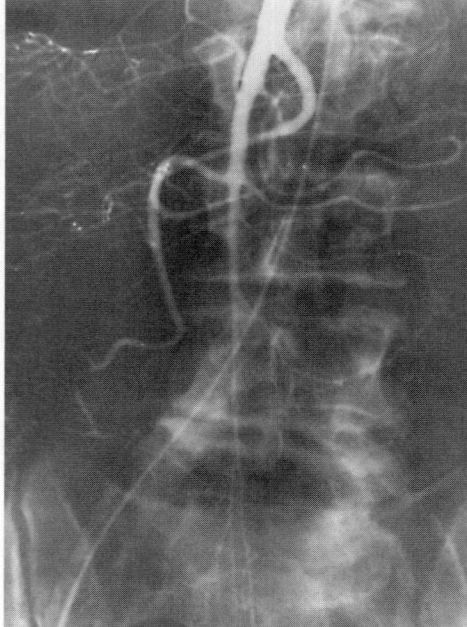
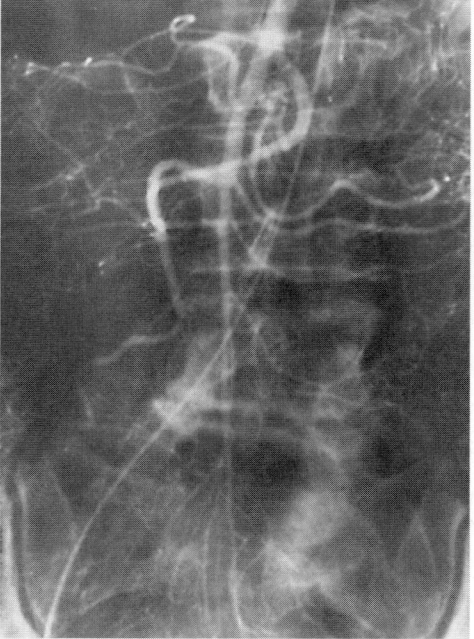

Figure 72.20. Nonocclusive mesenteric ischemia. *(A, left)* Superior mesenteric angiogram shows diffuse arterial vasoconstriction without occlusion. *(B, right)* A second arteriogram after injection of 50 mg of tolazoline into the superior mesenteric artery shows decreased vasoconstriction.

Lower extremity ischemia can be documented noninvasively by blood pressure measurements and pulse waveforms. Angiography is reserved for planning surgical or percutaneous revascularization procedures and demonstrates the distribution of disease, the distribution of relatively healthy arteries (necessary for planning surgical bypass procedures), and the status of collaterals. A complete study consists of an aortogram to demonstrate renal artery anatomy and distal aortic disease, one or both oblique pelvic arteriograms to display the iliac and femoral artery bifurcations, and a lower extremity outflow study to demonstrate thigh and calf vessels. Visualization of distal calf vessels may be technically difficult, especially in the presence of severe proximal disease. If a femoral to distal tibial or peroneal bypass is contemplated, additional studies, including occlusive angiography or DSA, may be used to demonstrate the optimal site for the distal graft anastomosis.

Aneurysmal Disease

A number of diseases or conditions interact with the arterial system and result in aneurysm formation. The size and distribution of aneurysms vary with the underlying disease. For example, atherosclerosis typically causes aneurysms along the aorta and its proximal branches, whereas polyarteritis nodosa may result in microaneurysms along the small branches of the renal and visceral arteries. Aneurysms and pseudoaneurysms may present as slowly growing asymptomatic masses or as masses of indeterminate or rapid growth with symptoms due to intermittent bleeding or impending rupture. The indication for angiography is to demonstrate the exact origin of the aneurysm and its relation to nearby critical normal vessels (Figs. 72.21 and 72.22). Safe and effective deployment of stent grafts requires an accurate depiction of aneurysm dimensions, the location of critical aortic branch origins,

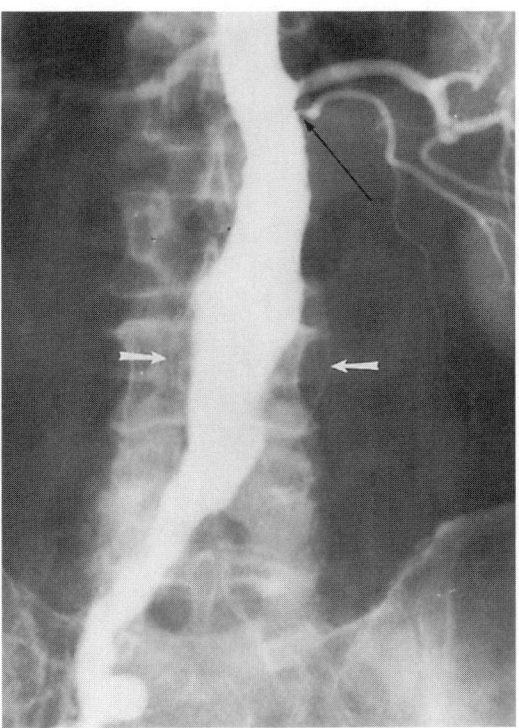

Figure 72.21. Abdominal aortic aneurysm in a 67-year-old man. Lumbar aortogram demonstrates an infrarenal aortic aneurysm. The opacified lumen underestimates the true diameter of the aneurysm, here outlined by a shell of intimal calcification *(white arrows)*. The orifice of the accessory lower pole left renal artery is narrowed *(black arrow)*.

Figure 72.22. Abdominal aortic aneurysm in a 74-year-old man. *(A)* Lumbar aortogram shows subtle widening of the infrarenal aortic lumen *(wavy arrows)*. Renal and superior mesenteric artery branches are normal, but infrarenal aortic branches are apparently missing. *(B)* A later film shows filling of lumbar *(arrows)* and inferior mesenteric *(arrowheads)* arteries through collaterals as a result of occlusion of these vessels by mural thrombus in the aneurysm.

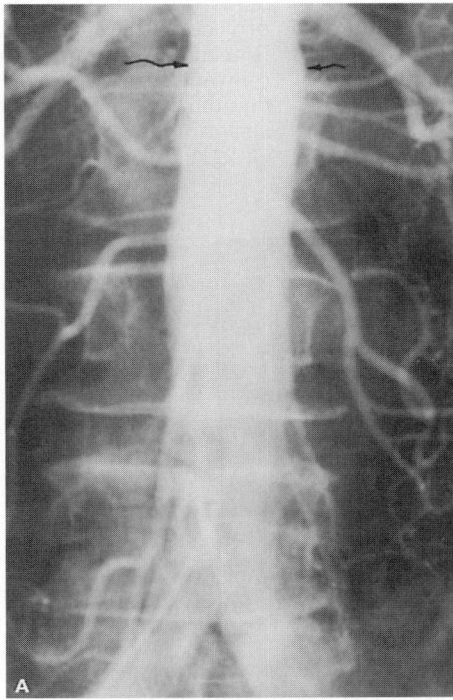
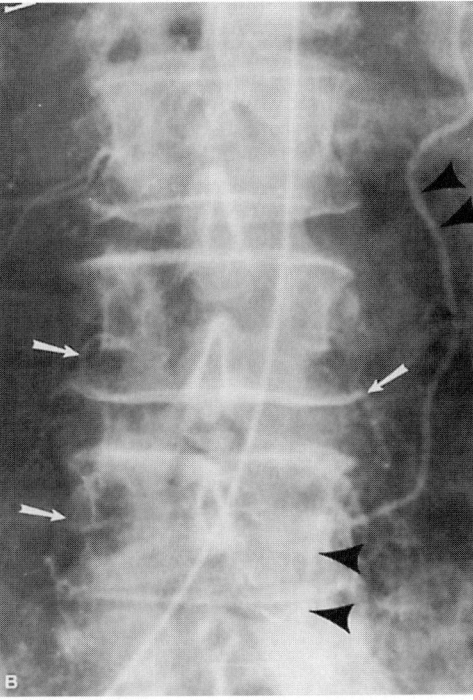

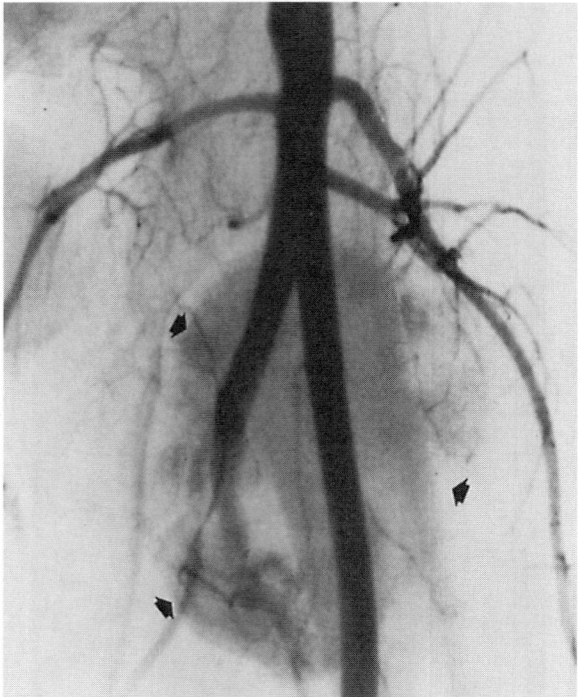

Figure 72.23. Mycotic pseudoaneurysm. Left common femoral arteriogram shows a saccular pseudoaneurysm *(arrows)* originating from the deep femoral artery.

and the length of the aneurysm "necks" between the margins of the aneurysm and branch vessel origins. Other relevant information includes the presence of inflammatory or mycotic aneurysms and aneurysmal rupture. Three-dimensional rendering of aneurysms and periaortic inflammatory changes are best seen with CT. Mycotic aneurysms have no distinctive angiographic appearance other than an unusual location and configuration (Fig. 72.23; see Fig. 72.31C). Rupture of an atherosclerotic thoracic or abdominal aortic aneurysm is an indication for emergent surgical intervention. The patient is usually too unstable to undergo angiography, which in any case is less sensitive than CT in demonstrating the periaortic hematoma. In intermittent hemorrhage, by definition, the mural defect has re-

sealed and the lumen is intact; the angiogram can only suggest the site of rupture when asymmetric, nipple-like projections of contrast extend radially from the principal axis of the vessel.

Angiographically, aneurysms appear as dilatations in the arterial lumen. With extensive mural thrombus, the caliber of the lumen may be normal, and the presence of the aneurysm may only be inferred from mural calcification or stereotypic thrombosis of arterial branches such as lumbar arteries.

Large degenerative aneurysms of the thoracic and abdominal aorta may distort the axis of the aorta and dilute the injected bolus of contrast medium. Additional contrast injections or filming projection may be required to demonstrate branch artery anatomy. The angiogram, then, is a compromise between a thorough anatomic study and the contrast medium load. In current practice, for planning of open aortic reconstruction as well as endovascular treatment with covered stents, helical CT and MR aortography have largely replaced catheter-based aortography. The roles of conventional aortography include confirming the lengths of aortic and iliac dimensions critical to endograft planning, such as the distance between renal arteries and the aneurysmal segment of aorta, between the renal arteries and the aortic bifurcation, and between the aortic and iliac bifurcations. It is also used for the treating renal artery stenosis, embolizing small accessory renal arteries arising from within the aneurysm, and occluding internal iliac artery trunks when the endograft must be extended into the external iliac artery. The thoracic aortogram should demonstrate the coronary and brachiocephalic artery origins. The abdominal aortogram should demonstrate the visceral and renal artery origins, with specific attention focused on multiple renal arteries. Thoracic aortic aneurysms are studied from the aortic root to the diaphragm; abdominal aneurysms are studied from the diaphragm to the inguinal ligaments. If infrainguinal arterial disease is suspected clinically, an arterial runoff study is obtained.

Renal or visceral artery aneurysms are studied with selective injections of the parent artery, often in multiple projections. Angiography should demonstrate the relation of the aneurysms to nearby branch arteries. When relevant, the adequacy of collateral arteries should be demonstrated in sufficient detail to plan surgical reconstruction or resection or percutaneous embolization (Fig. 72.24).

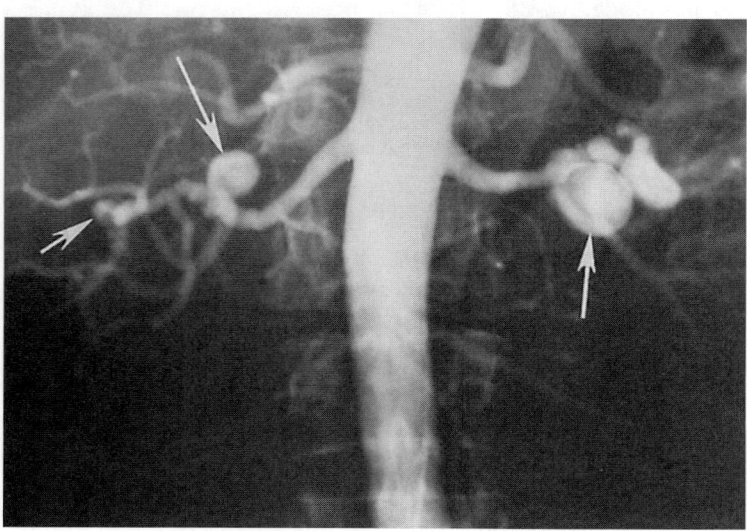

Figure 72.24. Renal artery aneurysms. Lumbar aortogram in a normotensive woman demonstrates multiple bilateral renal artery aneurysms *(arrows)* associated with renal arterial fibrodysplastic disease.

Arterial Dissections

Dissections can occur as spontaneous intramural hematomas (in the presence of medial arterial disease) or as the result of intimal trauma (usually iatrogenic). Spontaneous dissections are most common in the thoracic aorta and represent a surgical or medical emergency (Fig. 72.25). In the typical aortic dissection, the normal (or true) lumen communicates by way of the intimal tear with an intramedial (or false) lumen. The tear is usually several centimeters above the aortic valve or just distal to the subclavian artery. As the false lumen spirals longitudinally both antegrade and retrograde in the aorta, normal aortic branches may be spared, occluded, or sheared from their true lumen origins. The false lumen expands because of its thin and fragile outer wall, and the true lumen collapses. The diagnosis of aortic dissection and its classification with respect to involvement of the ascending aorta are usually established by transesophageal echocardiography, CT, or MR angiography. The indications for transcatheter aortography are to resolve equivocal or discordant findings by cross-sectional imaging tests, to evaluate the hemodynamic significance of branch vessel compromise by the dissection, and to plan and perform endovascular treatment of ischemic and aneurysmal complications of dissection. The angiographic appearance of aortic dissection depends on the site of contrast injection and the vagaries of the dissection in a given patient. If the injection is upstream from the intimal tear or a reentry point, it fills the true and false lumina, usually at different rates, and outlines the intervening septum as a linear filling defect in the contrast column. If the injection is remote from a transseptal communication and fills a single lumen, the margins of the lumen are variable, smoothly scalloped as the septum is seen in profile, and normal or possibly aneurysmal elsewhere. Aortic dissection is frequently complicated by branch artery occlusion. Involvement of aortic branches is best demonstrated by cross-sectional imaging such as helical CT, MR aortography, or intravascular ultrasound. There are two mechanisms of branch artery obstruction, based on the relation of the dissection flap to the branch artery origin. In static ob-struction, the dissection flap intersects, and possibly enters, the branch artery origin. In dynamic obstruction, the dissection flap spares the vessel origin but instead prolapses across the vessel origin like a washcloth over a bathtub drain (23). Manometry in the aortic true and false lumina and in branch arteries distal to reentry tears may help determine the hemodynamic significance of a given branch artery stenosis.

The angiographic work-up of dissections in the renal or visceral arteries is analogous to the work-up of occlusive and aneurysmal disease. Angiography should document the hemodynamic significance of arterial narrowing, the extent of the dissection, the relation of the dissection to nearby normal branches, and the integrity of the collateral circulation. Dissections in these medium-sized arteries appear as long, smooth narrowings of the artery, with smooth sigmoid contour changes or socklike dead ends reflecting the spiral course of the dissection, which usually terminates at a branch point of the parent artery. A double lumen is not always seen.

Occasionally, an atherosclerotic ulcer penetrates the media and results in intramedial dissection (24). This penetrating ulcer may be associated with a pseudoaneurysm or a false lumen and may simulate a classic dissection clinically. The dissecting hematoma or pseudoaneurysm of the penetrating aortic ulcer tends to originate in the distal thoracic aorta.

Iatrogenic dissections result from the intraarterial manipulation of guide wires or catheters, percutaneous angioplasties, and cannulation of the aorta during bypass (Fig. 72.26). The significance of these dissections depends on the vessel involved, the status of the collateral circulation, and the direction of dissection with respect to blood flow. Celiac artery dissection is usually well tolerated because of the immediate recruitment of collateral blood supply (through the pancreatic arcades) and because of the dual blood supply to the liver. SMA dissection extending beyond the origins of the first jejunal and middle colic arteries requires surgical intervention. Retrograde iliac artery dissection (such as that caused by subintimal passage of a guide wire) usually heals spontaneously and re-

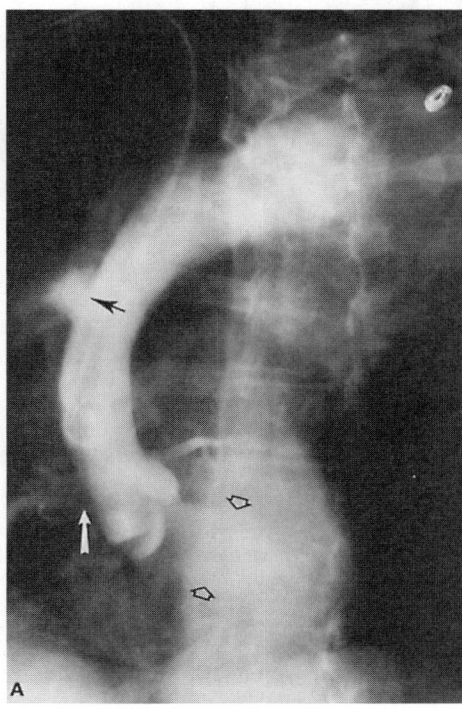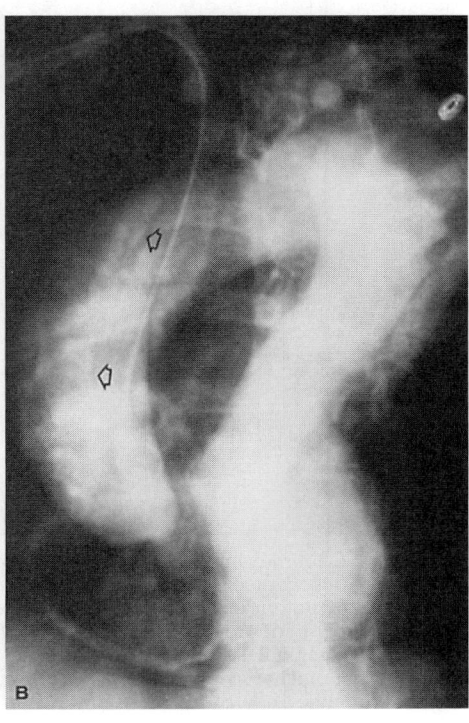

Figure 72.25. Type I aortic dissection in an 86-year-old hypertensive woman with acute onset of back pain. *(A)* Arch aortogram, performed from a right brachial artery approach, shows early opacification of the true lumen. The jet of contrast material is opacifying the intimal tear that initiated the dissection *(black arrow)*. The false lumen extends retrograde, compressing the ascending aorta along its right lateral margin, narrowing the origin of the right coronary artery *(white arrow)*, and undermining the aortic valve leaflets with secondary aortic insufficiency *(open arrows)*. *(B)* A few seconds later, the entire false lumen is opacified, and the dissection septum appears as a radiolucent line *(open arrows)* between the false and true lumina. The dissection extends into the descending aorta with involvement of the innominate artery.

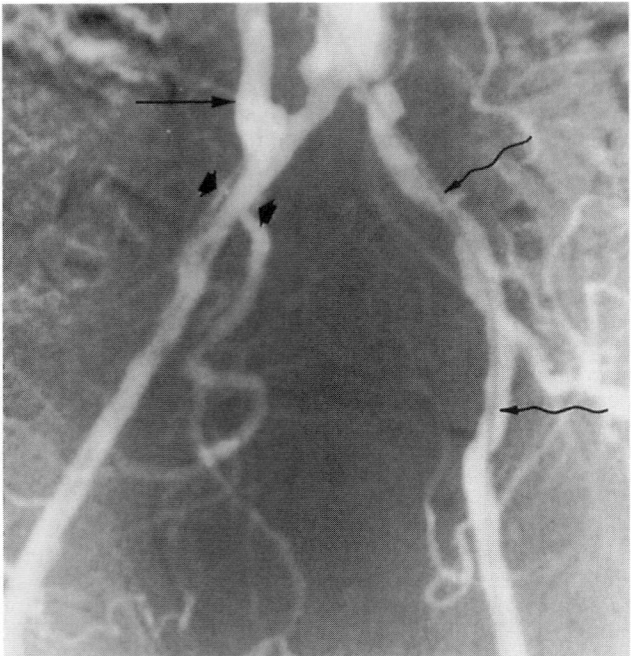

Figure 72.26. Iatrogenic dissection in a 70-year-old woman with cholesterol emboli after cardiac catheterization. Pelvic arteriogram performed with digital subtraction angiography demonstrates a linear collection of contrast medium outside the arterial lumen, representing a dissection. The dissection extends into the common iliac artery *(solid arrows),* stopping short of the origin of the iliorenal bypass graft *(straight arrow).* The linear filling defect in the left iliac artery *(wavy arrows)* is produced by the angiographic catheter.

mains asymptomatic unless blood flow is significantly altered. Flow-limiting dissections in the iliac, renal, or mesenteric arteries can sometimes be treated by the use of intravascular prostheses such as the Palmaz stent or Wallstent (Fig. 72.42).

Arterial Fibrodysplasia

Arterial fibrodysplasia is a disease of medium-sized muscular arteries that is of uncertain etiology, although retrospective reviews have documented significant associations with cigarette smoking, a history of hypertension, human leukocyte antigen type, and female sex. Arterial fibrodysplasia most commonly affects the renal, carotid, and external iliac arteries but may be found in the coronary, vertebral, mesenteric, and brachial arteries as well. Histologic classification of the disease is based on the type and distribution of dysplastic material in the arterial wall (25). The accumulation and proliferation of this material can result in narrowing of the arterial lumen or weakening of the arterial wall and loss of elastic material, which may result in secondary dissection or widening of the lumen and even aneurysm formation. The patients present with organ-related symptoms associated with arterial stenoses, dissections, or aneurysms. These symptoms include hypertension, stroke, and claudication. Angiography is directed at the presenting symptoms, and the indications for angiography parallel those for atherosclerosis, aneurysms, and dissections. The histologic changes lead to an angiographic appearance of arterial fibrodysplasia that is easily distinguished from atherosclerosis, except when the disease is focal or in an unusual location. The classic angiographic appearance of arterial fibrodysplasia is the "string of beads" appearance of medial fibroplasia, the most common histologic type of the disease (Figs. 72.27 and 72.28).

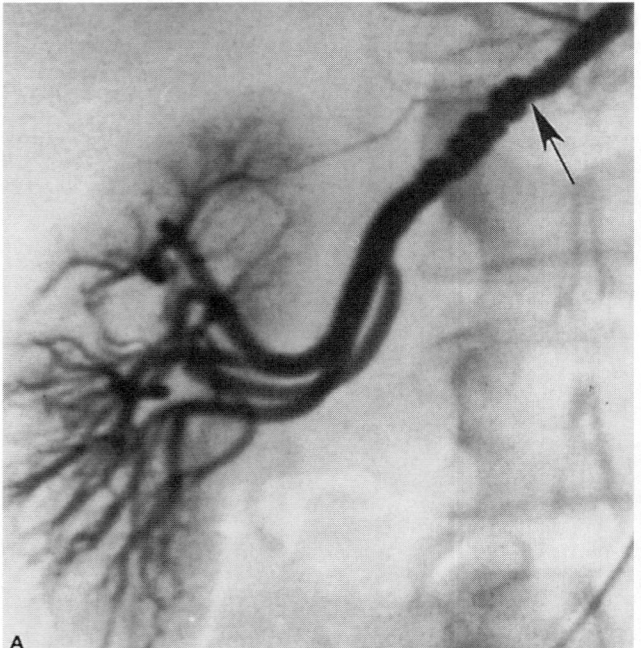
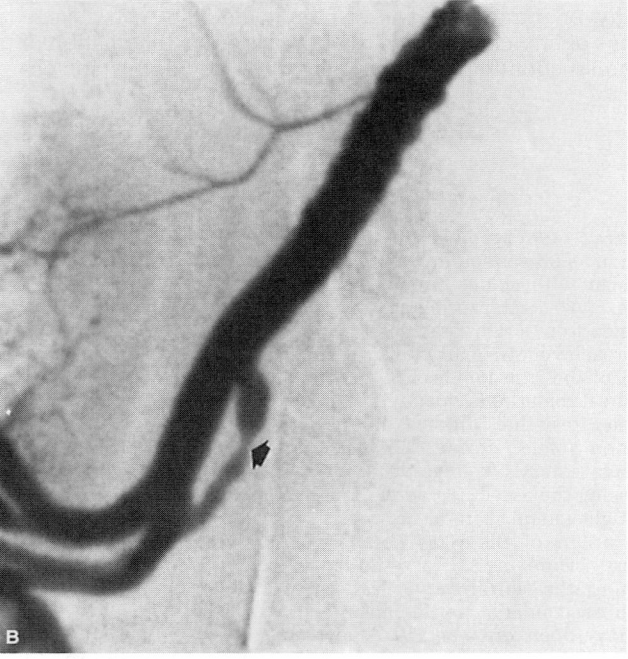

Figure 72.27. Fibrodysplasia of the renal artery in a 51-year-old hypertensive woman. *(A)* Digital subtraction angiogram of the right renal artery shows a ptotic kidney with alternating bands of narrowing and dilatation in the middle third of the main renal artery *(arrow),* in the so-called string-of-beads configuration of medial fibroplasia. *(B)* A second arteriogram made after percutaneous transluminal angioplasty shows improvement in the arterial lumen. Irregularity in the small branch of the renal artery *(solid arrow)* represents transient guide wire-induced spasm. (Courtesy of James Shields, M.D., St Joseph Mercy Hospital, Ann Arbor, MI.)

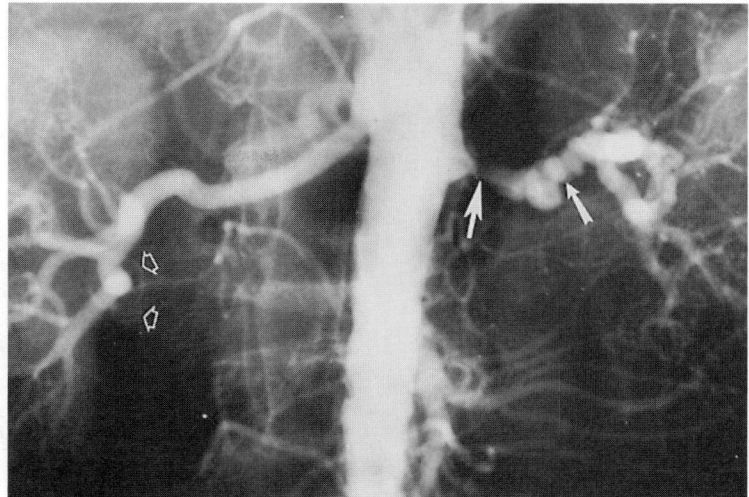

Figure 72.28. Concurrent atherosclerotic and dysplastic renal artery stenoses in a 60-year-old hypertensive woman. Lumbar aortogram shows smooth, concentric narrowing of the proximal left renal artery *(large arrow)* and alternating constrictions and aneurysmal dilations in the distal main renal artery *(small arrow)*. A calcified bilobed aneurysm involves the right renal artery *(open arrows)*.

Angiographic findings in renal arteries that favor fibro-dysplasia include the following:

- Long, smooth narrowing
- Long, irregular, beaded narrowing often with associated poststenotic dilatation or large aneurysms
- Discrete, weblike stenoses
- Spontaneous dissections
- Involvement of the middle and distal thirds of the main trunk that often extends into segmental arteries (26).

These findings are typical of the disease in other arteries as well.

Arteritis

Inflammatory arteritis becomes a surgical problem in the presence of arterial insufficiency syndromes, hemorrhage, or threatened tissue loss. The indication for angiography in inflammatory arteritis is to determine the extent of disease and demonstrate the status of the proximal and distal circulation for a prospective vascular reconstruction procedure. At times, angiography is helpful in the primary diagnosis of an inflammatory arteritis. The angiogram may demonstrate diffuse spasm or microaneurysms in active disease. Arterial stenoses, occlusions, and prominent collaterals may be present in active or quiescent disease. The vessels involved range in size from the aorta and pulmonary arteries in Takayasu's arteritis to the renal interlobar arteries of necrotizing arteritis. Small-caliber vessels found on muscle or skin biopsy are too small to be seen by standard angiographic techniques.

Trauma

Blunt and penetrating trauma can result in acute ischemia or hemorrhage, either immediate or delayed. Deceleration injuries (e.g., motor vehicle accidents, falls) are associated with injuries to the thoracic aorta or brachiocephalic vessels. Penetrating wounds are associated with vascular injuries along the track of the foreign body (e.g., knife, low-speed bullets). Shock waves radiated through tissue by high-speed missiles may injure vessels remote from the missile track. The role of angiography is to demonstrate the extent of the arterial injury and the status of the proximal and distal normal circulation. Angiographic findings include pseudoaneurysm, arterial or venous occlusions, arteriovenous fistulae, and contrast ex-travasation indicating active hemorrhage. The work-up for traumatic occlusive disease parallels that of the preceding discussions. Certain traumatic vascular injuries warrant specific comments.

Aortic rupture is best demonstrated by thoracic aortography in the right posterior oblique projection. The most common site of rupture is at the level of the ligamentum arteriosum, at the transition between the relatively immobile descending aorta and the relatively mobile arch (Figs. 72.29 and 72.30). The diagnosis of a subtle injury is occasionally difficult in the presence of an unusual ductus diverticulum or atherosclerotic plaque (Fig. 72.31). Multiple views of the aorta may be helpful in clarifying the unusual

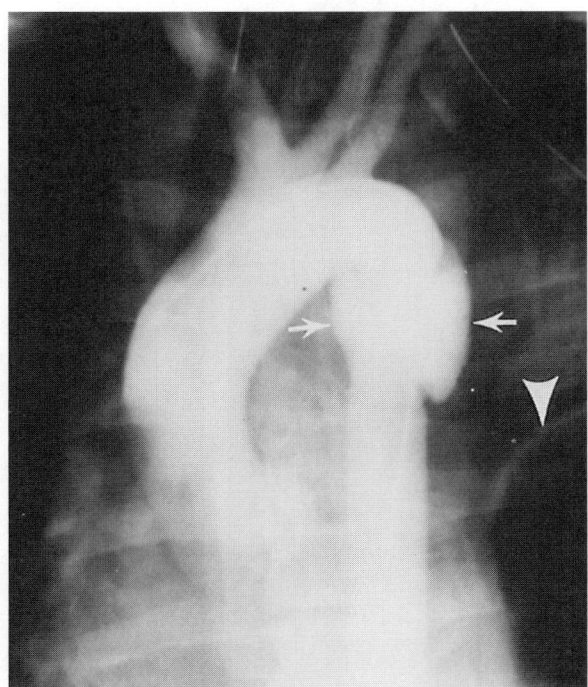

Figure 72.29. Traumatic thoracic aortic rupture in a 30-year-old man involved in a motor vehicle accident. Arch aortogram shows a contained rupture of the proximal descending aorta *(arrows)*, just distal to the origin of the left subclavian artery. A ruptured left hemidiaphragm with herniation of the stomach *(arrowhead)* is visible.

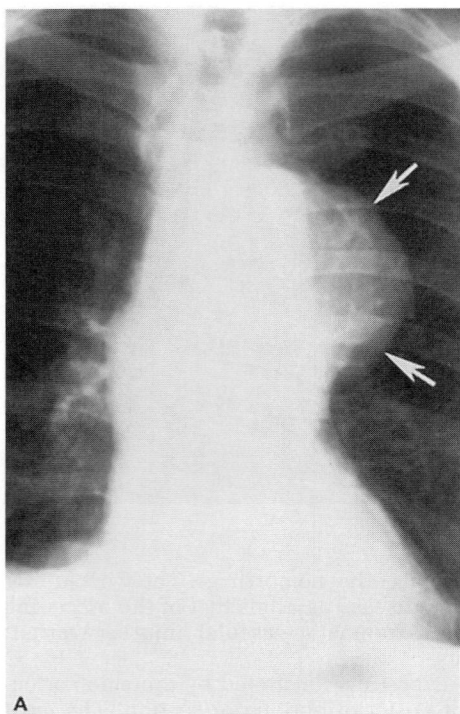
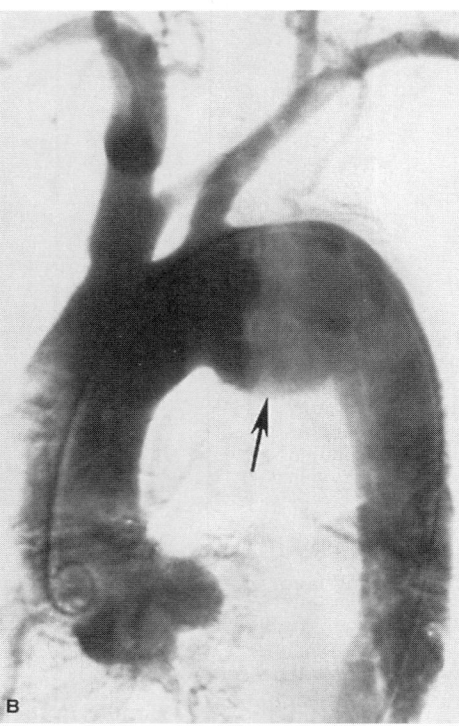

Figure 72.30. Posttraumatic chronic aortic pseudoaneurysm in a 71-year-old man with a 6-week history of increasing hoarseness. *(A)* Chest film shows localized enlargement of the aortic knob *(arrows)*. *(B)* Arch aortogram in the right posterior oblique position shows focal dilatation of the thoracic aorta just distal to the left subclavian artery *(arrow)*. The rupture was successfully repaired surgically.

normal variant. Other sites of cardiovascular decelerating injury are the aortic root, the aorta at the level of the diaphragm, and the proximal innominate artery. Although helical CT is accurate in diagnosing contained traumatic aortic rupture, it is less sensitive than conventional aortography in demonstrating less severe intimal injuries. Furthermore, adequate demonstration of the traumatic tear with respect to the brachiocephalic artery origins may require three-dimensional reconstruction of the raw data.

The thoracic aortogram is followed routinely by supine radiographs of the abdomen to evaluate the kidneys and bladder. If renal injury is suspected, an abdominal aortogram is obtained (Fig. 72.32).

In the angiographic work-up of arterial injury in the extremities, therapeutic considerations may require extension of the diagnostic examination. For example, if occlusive therapy is contemplated (either surgical ligation or transcatheter embolism), the status of the collateral circu-

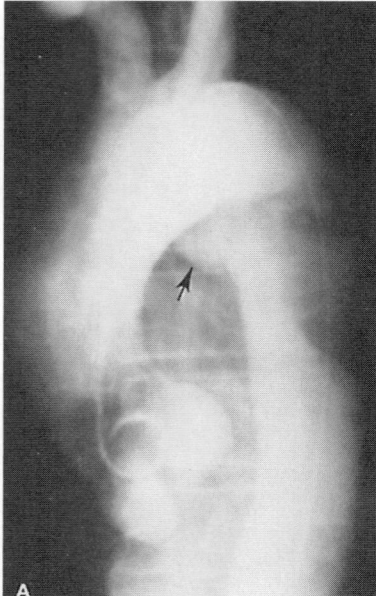
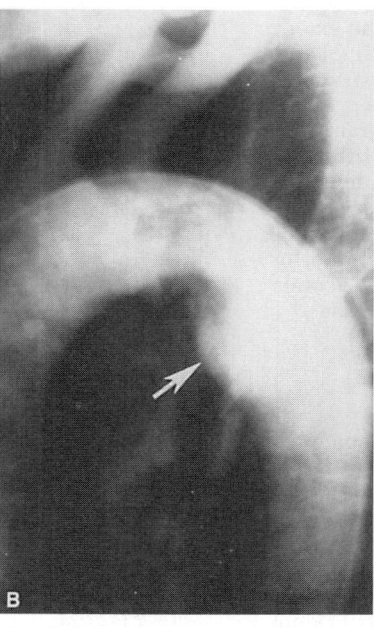
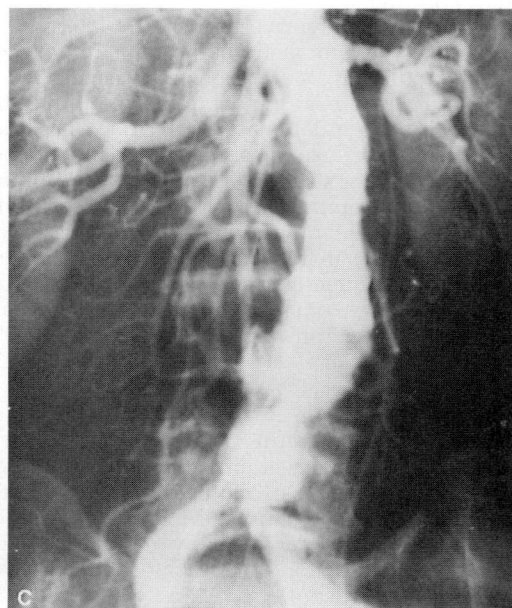

Figure 72.31. Prominent ductus bump simulating a posttraumatic aortic pseudoaneurysm in a man with septic peripheral emboli. *(A* and *B)* Biplanar arch aortograms show focal bulging from the anteromedial surface of the descending aorta at the ligamentum arteriosum *(arrow)*. *(C)* Abdominal aortogram shows an irregular infrarenal aneurysm with mural debris. At exploration, the thoracic aorta was normal, and a mycotic abdominal aortic aneurysm was resected. Angiographically, this mycotic aneurysm cannot be distinguished from a bland atherosclerotic aneurysm.

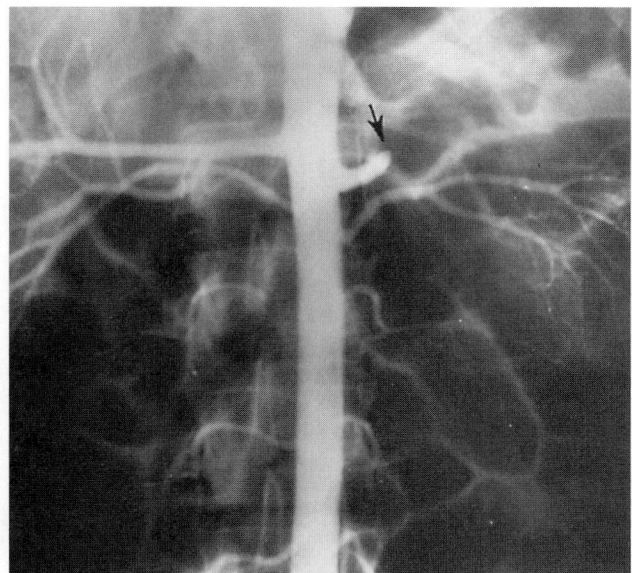

Figure 72.32. Traumatic renal artery occlusion in a 20-year-old male victim of a motor vehicle accident. Abnormal nephrogram was demonstrated on an abdominal film obtained after arch aortography. A subsequent lumbar aortogram confirmed left renal artery occlusion *(arrow)*. The lower pole artery, fortuitously originating separately from the aorta, is irregular and deformed secondary to a retroperitoneal hematoma.

lation and the arterial bed distal to the arterial injury should be carefully evaluated before intervention.

Hemangiomas and Vascular Malformations

Hemangiomas and vascular malformations constitute a spectrum of neoplasms and congenital vascular dys-

plasias, including capillary, venous, and arteriovenous lesions (27,28). Angiography is used to identify and describe the arterial supply to the lesion and nearby normal structures. In the extremities, venography is often performed in addition to arteriography to demonstrate the deep veins. This is done because some malformations in the limbs are associated with deep-vein abnormalities and because the relation between the venous component of the lesion and the deep veins is important if sclerotherapy is to be used. CT and MR imaging (MRI) are useful in demonstrating the three-dimensional relation between the malformation or hemangioma and the normal structures.

Angiographic findings in an arteriovenous malformation consist of tortuous and enlarged feeding arteries, a nidus of innumerable small arteries, and large draining veins (Fig. 72.33). When rapid flow throughout the malformation is demonstrated, venography is not indicated. In a venous malformation, the arterial phase of the angiogram may be normal. Veins are large and tortuous with slow flow; occasionally, large venous lakes are present. The venous malformation is best studied by closed-system venography or by direct injection of contrast material into the malformation (Fig. 72.34). No persistent tissue stain is present after contrast injections in arteries supplying pure venous or arteriovenous malformations. The arteries supplying and the veins draining a capillary hemangioma may be normal or mildly enlarged. Selective injection of contrast into feeding arteries results in a dense and persistent tumor stain.

Neoplasm

In the past, angiography was performed to identify and stage neoplasms and inflammatory masses. Since the early 1980s, tests that are more sensitive than angiography in these diagnostic applications have been developed, including CT, ultrasound, and MRI. Angiography is usually performed after CT or MRI has defined the location of the primary tumor, the presence of metastases, or both. Angiography no longer has a prominent role in the diagnosis

Figure 72.33. Arteriovenous malformation in a 50-year-old schizophrenic woman. Cardiac output measured 16 L/min. *(A)* The arterial phase of the pelvic angiogram shows gross asymmetry of the common iliac arteries, with a massively dilated left internal iliac artery supplying a large nidus of innumerable small arteries *(arrows)*. Other arterial injections documented contributions from the left external, deep femoral, and right internal iliac arteries. *(B)* A large tangle of tortuous veins *(arrows)* empties into dilated left iliac veins.

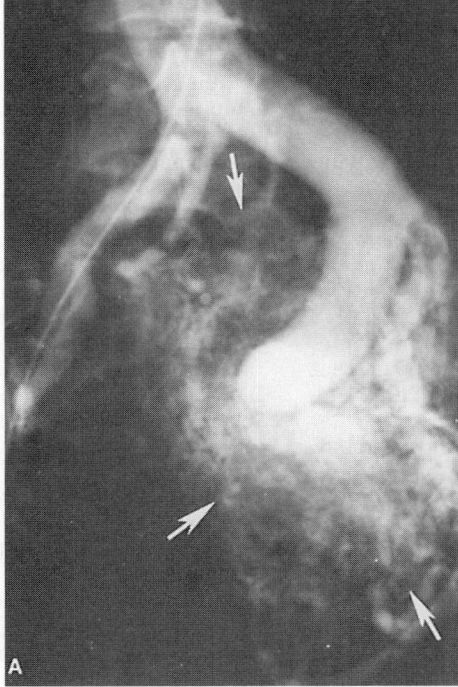

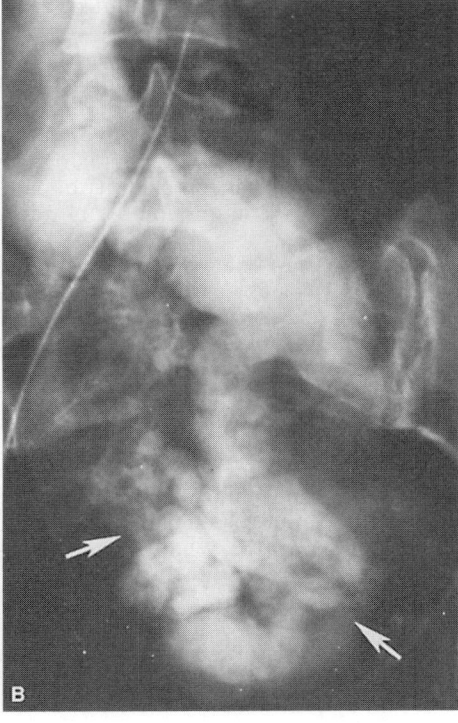

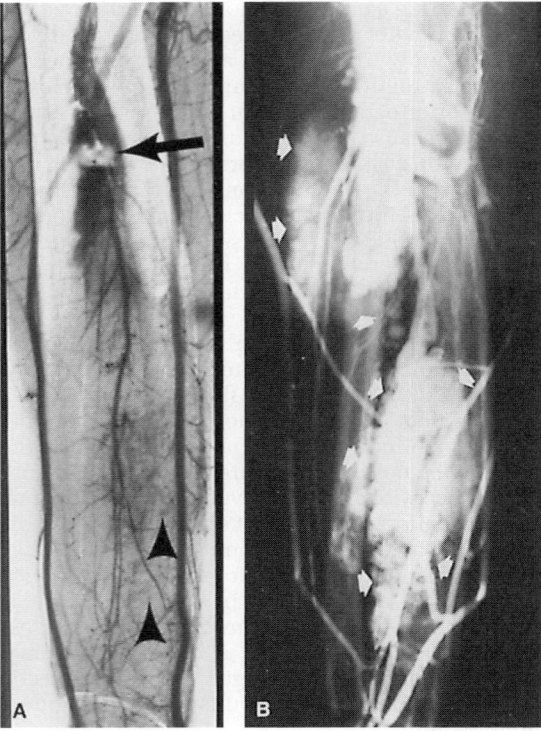

Figure 72.34. Venous angioma in a 19-year-old woman with symptoms of recurrent right forearm venous thrombosis and a mass noticed at age 6 years. *(A)* Photographic subtraction of the capillary phase of the forearm arteriogram shows normal radial, ulnar, interosseous, and muscular arteries; faint, scattered punctate areas of contrast pooling *(arrowheads);* and draining vein containing thrombus *(arrow).* (B) A closed-system venogram provides much better documentation of the component of the angioma *(solid arrows).*

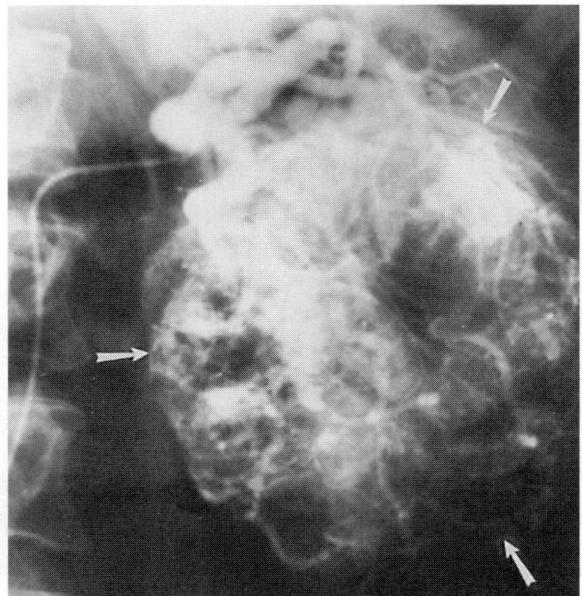

Figure 72.35. Tumor neovascularity in a 52-year-old man with a hypernephroma. Left renal arteriogram demonstrates a large hypervascular tumor in the lower pole of the left kidney *(arrows)* with abundant neovascularity and intense contrast accumulation (tumor stain).

of tumors, although it is more sensitive than cross-sectional studies in the demonstration of small (5-mm) hypervascular tumors and is useful in the study of large tumors growing at the interface of two abdominal structures (e.g., the mesentery and omentum, or liver and adrenal gland). Angiography is commonly used to provide a vascular road map before resection of abdominal neoplasms, especially in the pancreas and liver; to document vascular invasion by nonresectable tumors; to answer specific clinical questions such as resectability of pancreatic or hepatic masses; and in conjunction with transcatheter chemotherapy.

Neoplasms are characterized angiographically as avascular, hypovascular, or hypervascular, depending on the number and size of tumor vessels and on the intensity of contrast medium stain in the tumor (tumor blush) relative to surrounding normal tissue. Tumor vessels are somewhat disorderly and meandering compared with normal parenchymal branches, which branch systematically. The contour of tumor vessels may be smooth, somewhat beaded in appearance, or highly irregular and serrated. Early or intense venous opacification is common with hypervascular tumors such as hepatomas, hypernephromas, and leiomyomas (Fig. 72.35).

Postsurgical Follow-up

Angiography is often performed after a surgical procedure to establish a vascular baseline (after a revascularization procedure), to rule out a surgical complication (after

transplantation, revascularization, or shunt surgery), or to demonstrate progression of disease (Fig. 72.36). Vascular complications consist of stenoses, occlusions, dissections, pseudoaneurysms, and arteriovenous fistulae. The angiographic work-up proceeds as in the earlier discussions, except that the examination may be tailored on the basis of the clinical signs, the surgeon's impression of a specific complication, and the known preoperative anatomy. In addition, multiple views may be necessary to observe vascular anastomoses in profile to exclude arterial strictures (especially after renal revascularization or transplant surgery).

Peripheral Venous Disease

Venography is the most accurate means of diagnosing deep-vein thrombosis and incompetent lower extremity venous valves. It is also the best way to demonstrate venous anatomy in certain vascular malformations or hemangiomas, or before dialysis shunt construction or venous reconstructive procedures. When injections are in a peripheral vein, venography can demonstrate deep and superficial veins of the extremity. Inferior vena cavography is usually performed by the percutaneous transfemoral venous approach. For the diagnosis of deep-vein thrombosis (when the display of global venous anatomy is of secondary interest), conventional contrast venography has been largely replaced by duplex (Doppler and B-mode imaging) or color flow ultrasonography for the extremities and MR venography for the iliocaval, portal, and renal systems.

Lower extremity ascending venography requires injection of contrast medium in a dorsal foot vein with the leg relaxed and dependent (29). In an adult patient, 100 mL of 43% contrast medium fills deep and superficial veins from the foot to the inguinal ligament. Visualization of the external and common iliac veins and the caudal inferior vena cava can be enhanced by maneuvers that evacuate the contrast medium from the calf, such as weight bearing.

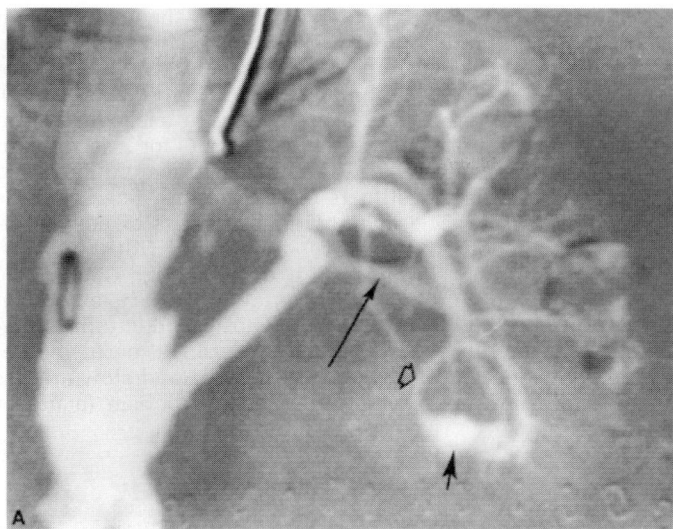
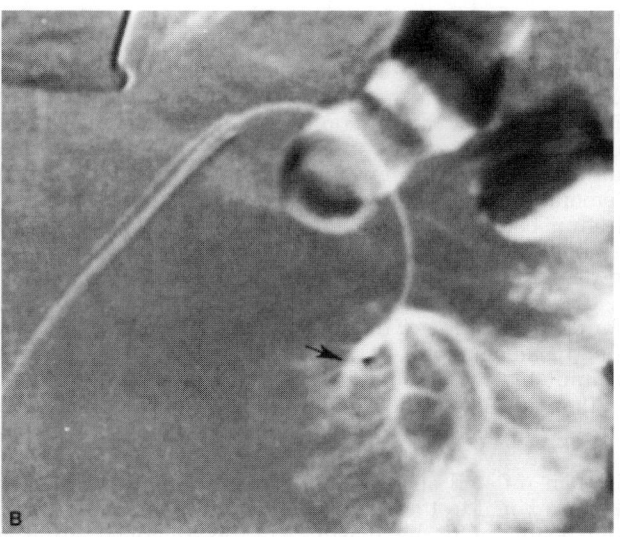

Figure 72.36. Postoperative renal artery pseudoaneurysm with an arteriovenous fistula in a woman with hematuria 1 day after a left aortorenal revascularization procedure. *(A)* Lumbar aortogram with digital subtraction angiography demonstrates a lower-pole pseudoaneurysm *(short arrow)* supplied by a normal-sized segmental artery *(open arrow).* Early venous filling is present *(long arrow).* The segmental artery supplying the pseudoaneurysm was subselectively catheterized with a 3F coaxial catheter system and embolized with polyvinyl alcohol (Ivalon) particles. *(B)* A segmental arteriogram after embolization shows successful occlusion of the pseudoaneurysm *(arrow),* with sparing of the adjacent arteries.

Acute deep-vein thrombosis appears as a castlike filling defect in the contrast column in the deep veins (Fig. 72.37A). Acute thrombosis may be so extensive that contrast does not enter the deep system. Absence of deep-vein filling in acute deep-vein thrombosis is distinguished from that in chronic deep-vein thrombosis by the size of the superficial veins and venous collaterals; they are small when accompanying acute disease and large when accompanying chronic disease. In the patient with chronic deep-

vein thrombosis, venography demonstrates linear or web-like intraluminal filling defects representing organized thrombus, occluded deep veins with large collaterals, or, rarely, no abnormality (Fig. 72.37B).

Lower extremity descending venography is performed to evaluate the competence of the valves in the saphenous, femoral, and popliteal veins. The study can be performed by retrograde catheterization of the opposite femoral vein and manipulation of the catheter tip across the iliac con-

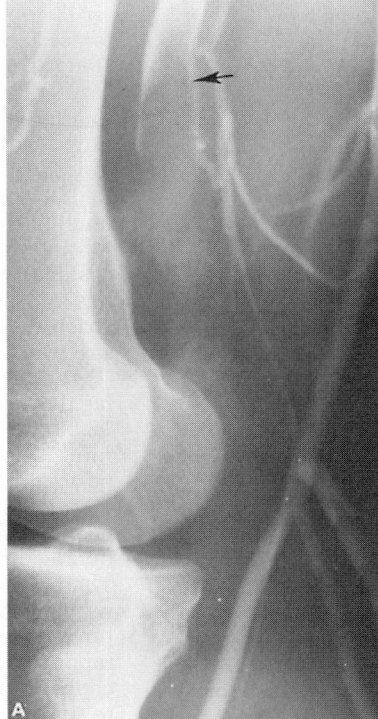
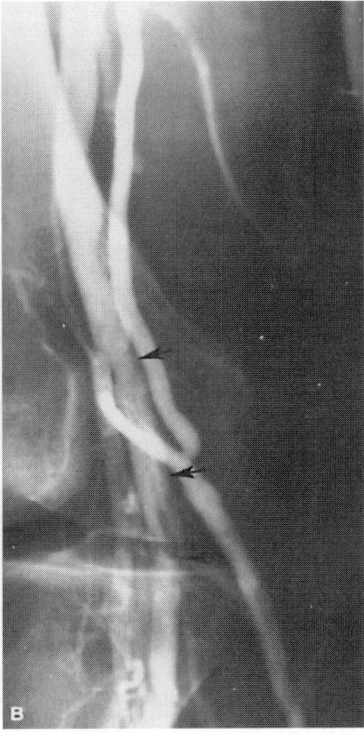

Figure 72.37. Acute and chronic deep venous thrombosis in a 19-year-old man who presented with acute right calf swelling. *(A)* An ascending leg venogram shows acute thrombus in the popliteal vein. The patient was examined 25 months later for right calf pain. *(B)* A second venogram shows recanalization of the popliteal vein with residual linear filling defects *(arrows),* representing organized clot. No valves are seen in this segment of popliteal vein.

fluence into the external iliac vein on the side of interest. If the femoral vein cannot be punctured, venous access may be obtained by use of an antecubital vein puncture. Contrast medium is then injected at the level of the inguinal ligament under fluoroscopic observation as the patient breathes quietly or performs the Valsalva maneuver. Reflux in the greater saphenous, deep femoral, and superficial femoral veins is assessed and graded from 0 (no reflux) to 4 (reflux below the knee) (30). A global view of venous anatomy (necessary if a venous bypass or valvuloplasty procedure is planned) requires ascending venography.

Closed-system extremity venography may be required for demonstration of the full extent of a venous malformation or hemangioma (31,32). A vein distal to the lesion is cannulated with a soft angiocatheter. A tight elastic wrap is then applied to the limb beginning at the angiocatheter. It is wrapped proximally, compressing the lesion and evacuating venous blood centrally. A blood pressure cuff is then inflated above systolic pressure (250 to 300 mm Hg) proximal to the lesion, preventing arterial refilling of the lesion, and the elastic wrap is removed. Contrast medium is then injected during fluoroscopic observation of the limb. The closed-system venogram demonstrates contrast filling in the capillary and venous components of a malformation or hemangioma as well as deep and superficial venous anatomy of the limb distal to the blood pressure cuff (Fig. 72.34B).

Pulmonary Embolism

The diagnosis of pulmonary embolism often requires confirmation by pulmonary angiography because of the low specificity of ventilation–perfusion scans in certain clinical settings. In addition to documenting the presence of pulmonary emboli, angiography can demonstrate an alternative pathologic process that explains abnormalities on chest radiographs or ventilation–perfusion scans. Pul-

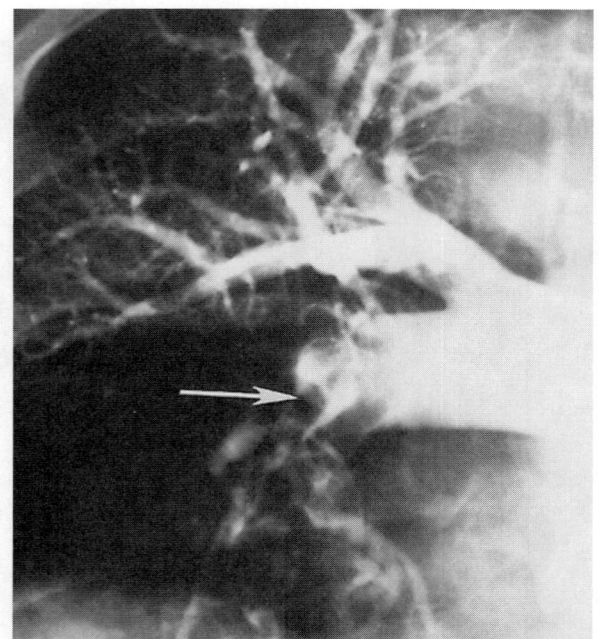

Figure 72.38. Acute pulmonary embolism in a 39-year-old man with a renal transplant. A selective right pulmonary arteriogram shows a large saddle embolus in the right main pulmonary artery with occlusion of the middle lobe arteries and a cast of thrombus *(arrow)* in the lower lobe arteries.

monary artery injections are preceded by the measurement of pulmonary artery pressures because the risk of sudden cardiac decompensation is increased in the presence of right ventricular or pulmonary artery hypertension (33). When mean pulmonary artery pressure exceeds 40 mm Hg, the injection rate (ordinarily 25 mL/s for 2 seconds in a main pulmonary artery) is reduced to match decreased pulmonary flow as estimated at fluoroscopy (e.g., 16 mL/s for 3 seconds). The angiographic findings of acute pulmonary embolism consist of intraarterial filling defects, arterial cutoffs, and perfusion defects (Fig. 72.38). The angiographic findings of chronic pulmonary embolism are intraluminal webs, arterial stenoses and cutoffs, collateral reconstitution of occluded vessels, and perfusion defects. Arterial cutoffs, perfusion defects, and slow arterial flow are nonspecific for pulmonary embolism (acute or chronic).

INTERVENTIONAL ANGIOGRAPHY

A large number of percutaneous therapeutic options for acute or chronic occlusive disease, active or intermittent hemorrhage, and neoplasm are available, and others are under investigation. Transcatheter therapy should be considered in appropriate clinical circumstances when diagnostic angiography is undertaken because the mechanical constraints of the therapeutic catheter system affect the choice of puncture site and because thorough pretherapy evaluation may require additional diagnostic injections.

Angioplasty

Percutaneous transluminal angioplasty (PTA) is generally accepted as a safe and technically simple nonsurgical alternative for the treatment of certain arterial and venous occlusive lesions. The hemodynamic significance of the lesion in question should be established before proceeding with an interventional procedure, as discussed previously in the section on nonaneurysmal atherosclerosis. PTA requires crossing the stenosis or occlusion with a guide wire. After the intraluminal position of the guide wire is confirmed, the balloon (chosen so that the inflated diameter is approximately 20% greater than the normal diameter of the vessel) is advanced over the wire across the stenosis or occlusion and inflated. Balloon inflation is observed at fluoroscopy. Adequate dilation is assessed by intraarterial manometry, ankle–brachial pressure indices, or improvement in the luminal diameter of the vessel as judged by post-PTA angiography. PTA is often performed for femoropopliteal (Fig. 72.39), iliac (Fig. 72.40), and renal occlusive lesions. It is less commonly performed for infrapopliteal, mesenteric, and aortic lesions, and only occasionally for subclavian and carotid lesions (34,35). PTA has also been performed for renal transplant anastomotic strictures, renal or limb revascularization anastomotic strictures, dialysis graft stenoses, and venous stenoses (Fig. 72.41). The ideal PTA lesion is the renal fibromuscular dysplastic lesion without associated aneurysms (Fig. 72.29), or concentric, nonostial, noncalcified atherosclerotic lesions. Complications of PTA include thrombosis, perforation, dissection, and distal embolism.

Late failures of PTA are due to restenosis at the PTA site or progression of disease. Percutaneous approaches to reducing the restenosis rate have not shown proven benefits. These approaches include physically stenting the lesion with meshlike prostheses (36). Intravascular stents are approved for use in the iliac arteries, but there are numerous reports of their use in the aorta and visceral and brachiocephalic arteries. The indications for their use include restenosis at a site of angioplasty, elastic recoil of a lesion

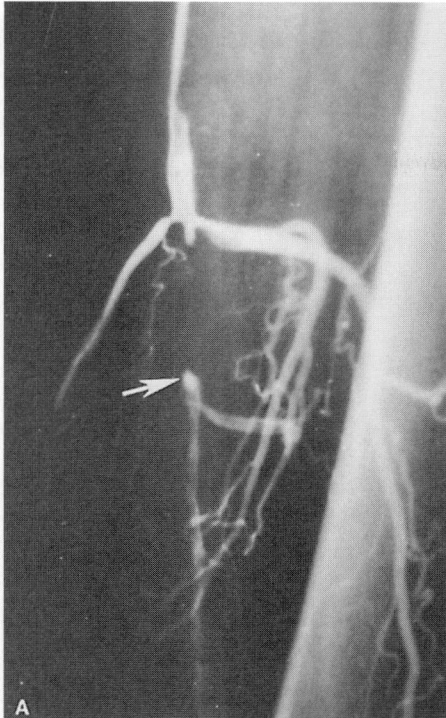
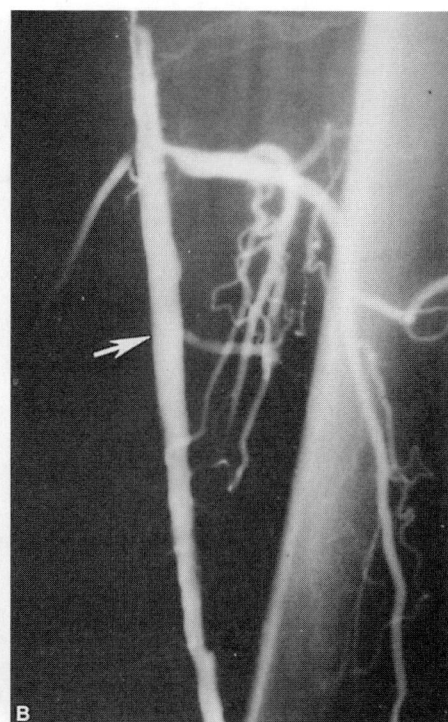

Figure 72.39. Percutaneous transluminal angioplasty of a superficial femoral artery occlusion in a 60-year-old man with claudication. Superficial femoral arteriograms before *(A)* and after *(B)* recanalization and angioplasty of a distal superficial femoral artery occlusion. The caliber of the popliteal artery *(arrow)* is increased after inflow has been improved.

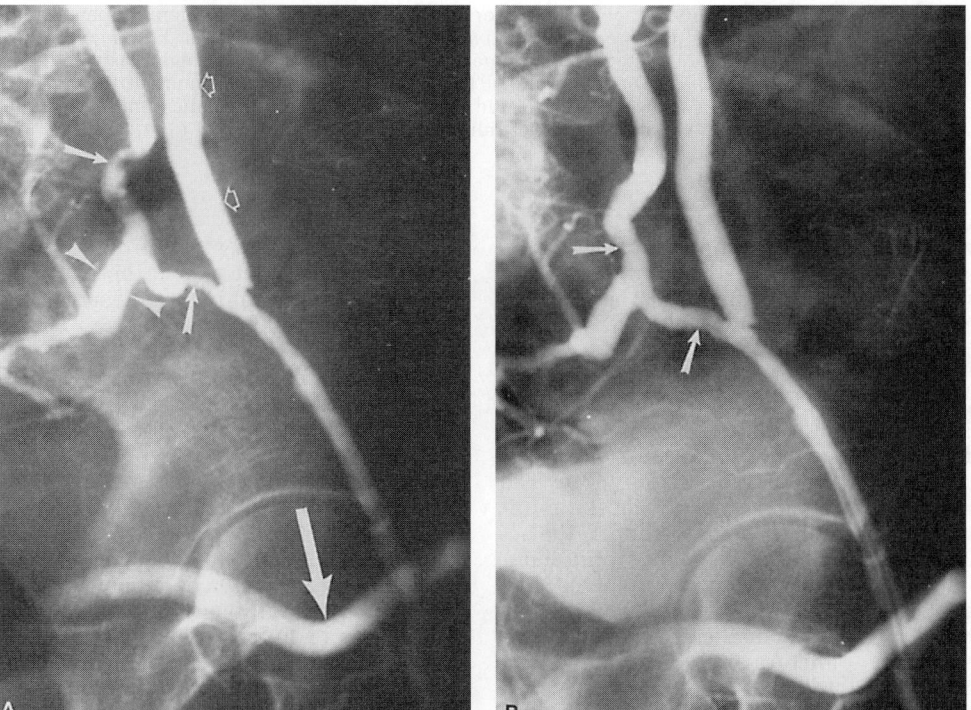

Figure 72.40. Percutaneous transluminal angioplasty of the iliac arteries in a man with right buttock claudication after aorto-left external iliac bypass and left-to-right femorofemoral bypass. *(A)* Lumbar aortogram shows a patent aortoiliac graft *(open arrows)* in continuity with the mid-external iliac artery and the femorofemoral graft *(large arrow)*. The graft did not fill the right pelvis, which was perfused by transpelvic collaterals from the left internal iliac artery *(arrowheads)*. Tight stenoses in the common iliac and proximal external iliac arteries *(small arrows)* limit internal iliac perfusion. *(B)* Both stenoses responded to percutaneous angioplasty *(arrows)*, and buttock claudication resolved.

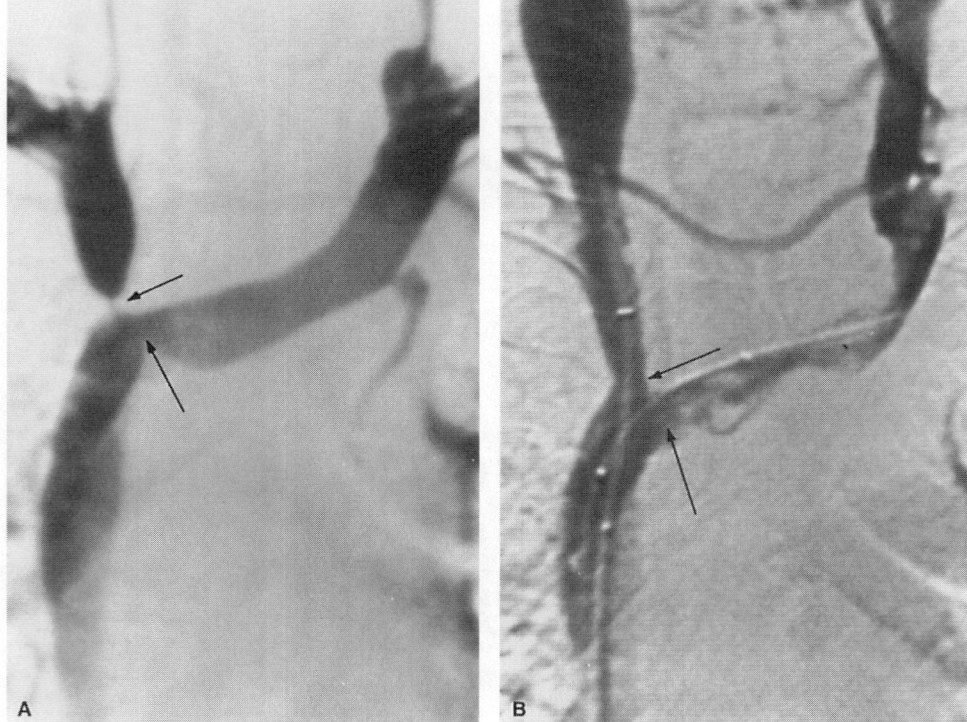

Figure 72.41. Percutaneous transluminal angioplasty (PTA) of brachiocephalic vein strictures in a 70-year-old woman with superior vena cava syndrome after radiation for breast cancer. Computed tomography scans (not shown) showed no tumor in the mediastinum. *(A)* Bilateral upper extremity venogram demonstrates strictures of the right and left brachiocephalic veins at their confluence *(arrows)*. The strictures were dilated by simultaneous inflation of two 10-mm angioplasty balloons, one across each stricture. *(B)* Venogram after PTA shows improved appearance of the brachiocephalic vein confluence *(arrows)*. Pressure gradients from the brachiocephalic vein to the superior vena cava were improved from 27 cm of saline to 2 cm on the right and from 21 to 4 cm on the left.

that just underwent angioplasty, and flow-limiting dissection at a site of angioplasty or other arterial injury (37,38) (Fig. 72.42). Lesions of the external iliac artery or proximal main renal artery are frequently stented without a trial of unassisted balloon angioplasty.

Thrombolytic Therapy

Embolic or thrombotic occlusion of vascular conduits can often be managed by thrombolytic therapy (39). The success of such therapy (measured by clot lysis and minimal complications) depends on the composition of the occlusive material (thrombus vs. atheroembolus), the duration of occlusion, the vascular structure involved, the thrombolytic agent, and the route and duration of infusion. Complications of thrombolytic therapy include hemorrhage (remote or at the puncture site), distal embolism, and reperfusion injury. Clot lysis depends on surface interaction between the thrombus and the lytic agent. Lysis may be enhanced (shortening infusion time and perhaps decreasing hemorrhagic complications) by increasing the plasma concentration of the lytic agent at the plasma–clot interface and maximizing the molecular interface at which it may act. Numerous strategies have been described to enhance clot lysis, including transcatheter delivery of the lytic agent at the leading (upstream) edge of the clot or within the clot, the use of coaxial catheters with simultaneous proximal and distal infusion of the lytic agent within the clot, and breaking up the clot with a guide wire or with high-pressure radial sprays of a lytic agent. Be-

cause of potentially catastrophic hemorrhagic complications, transcatheter lytic therapy requires close observation of the patient in the intensive care unit and scrupulous angiographic monitoring with respect to the remaining clot burden.

Diagnostic angiography should precede lytic therapy to define vascular anatomy, and it should follow lytic therapy to identify the cause of arterial occlusion or graft failure (Fig. 72.43). Judicious choice of the initial puncture site (based on the patient's symptoms and, if known, the arterial and bypass anatomy) may greatly simplify placement of the infusion catheter in the occluded conduit and the subsequent percutaneous management of the underlying cause of occlusion. Acute embolic occlusion of a vessel presents additional considerations. Emboli are often multiple, precluding efficient lysis even when they are accessible by catheter. Emboli may be composed of organized material less susceptible to lytic agents. The symptomatic embolus in the leg may mask a more serious embolus in the bowel or kidney, and a cardiac source of emboli may shower additional emboli during the lytic state.

Agents commonly used for lytic therapy include urokinase, streptokinase, and tissue plasminogen activator, which are reviewed in detail elsewhere (40,41). Until recently, urokinase was the lytic agent of choice for peripheral arterial and graft occlusions. Because of concerns of risk of viral contamination, urokinase was taken off the market. Two third-generation lytic agents are available in the United States, reteplase and alteplase. As

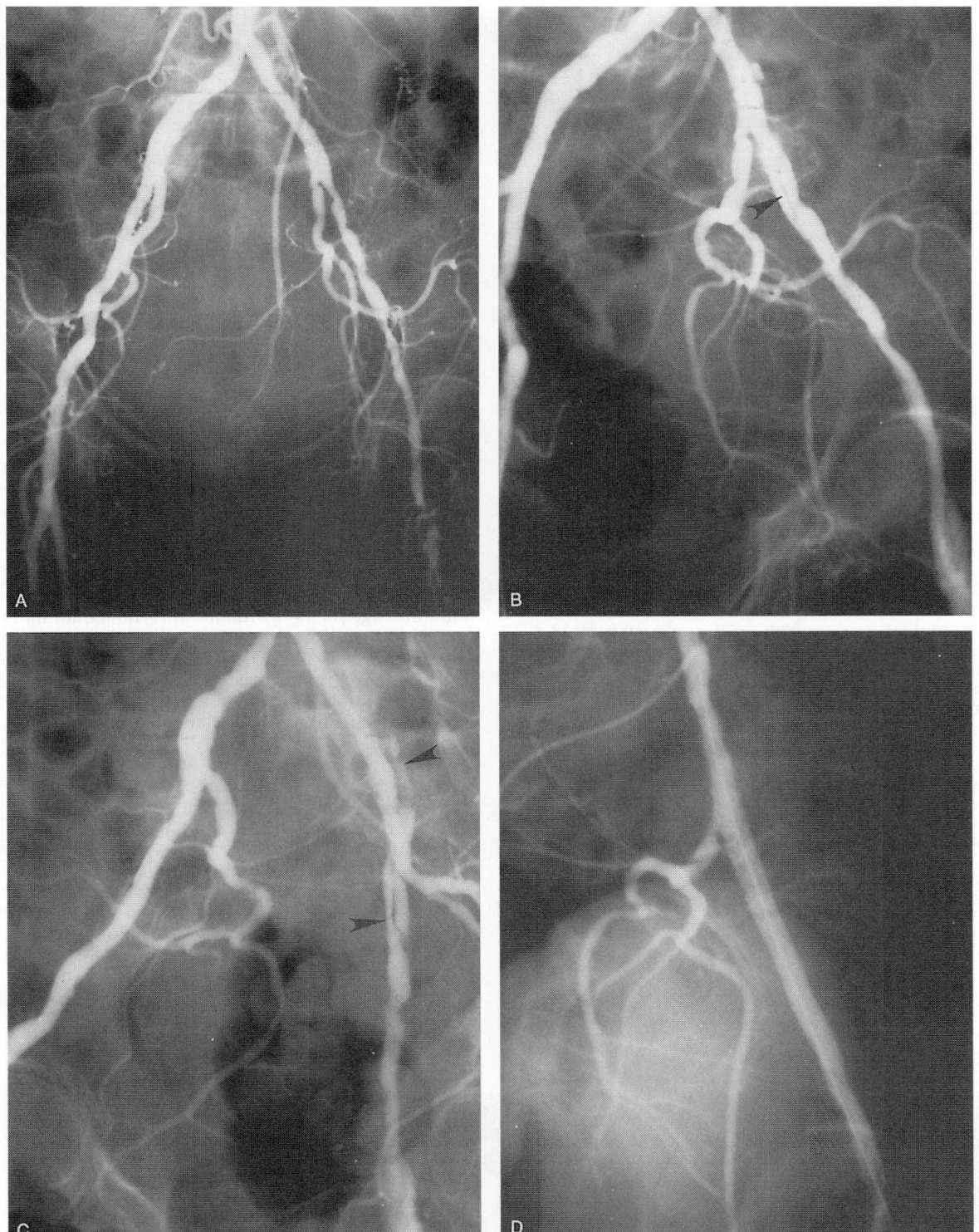

Figure 72.42. Serial pelvic arteriograms in a patient with left lower extremity occlusive disease. *(A)* Initial outflow study shows moderate external iliac artery occlusive disease. The superficial femoral artery was occluded. Inflow was judged to be adequate, and the patient underwent a femoropopliteal bypass graft. Several days after the operation, the left ankle–brachial index reverted to the preoperative level. *(B and C)* Postoperative oblique pelvic arteriograms show a dissection involving the external iliac artery *(arrowheads)* and reflecting a Fogarty catheter-induced injury sustained during the surgical procedure. The femoropopliteal graft is occluded as a result of compromised inflow. With fluoroscopic guidance and injections of contrast from the right transfemoral catheter, the left femoral artery was punctured between the endarterectomized hood of the femoropopliteal graft and the inguinal ligament. The dissected segment of artery was then paved with Palmaz stents tapering from 7 to 6 mm in diameter. *(D)* After stent deployment, left common iliac artery injection shows unobstructed flow; the aortofemoral pressure gradient was ablated. Distal flow was restored by operative thrombectomy of the graft.

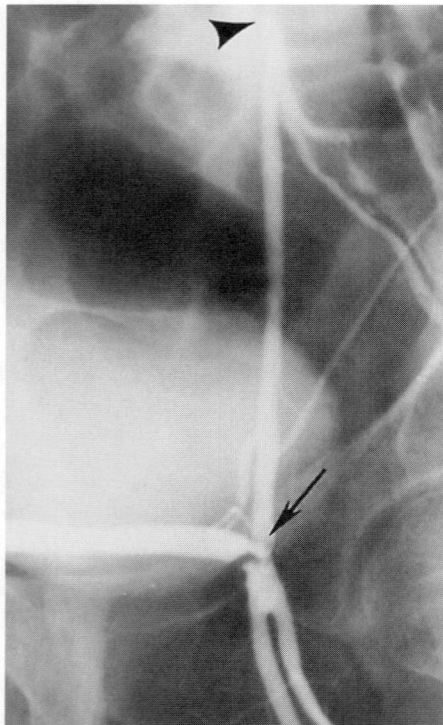

Figure 72.43. Lytic therapy with urokinase. A 50-year-old man presented with occluded right axillofemoral and right-to-left femorofemoral bypass grafts. With use of a right brachial artery approach, flow in the axillofemoral graft was reestablished after 12 hours of urokinase infusion at 2,000 IU/min. With use of a right femoral artery approach, flow in the femorofemoral graft was reestablished after 6 hours of urokinase infusion at 2,000 IU/min through a catheter with the tip just distal to the graft origin. Angiogram made at the termination of the procedure shows narrowing of the distal graft lumen and a filling defect in the left common femoral artery *(arrow)*. Because of the angle of the graft insertion site (nearly 90 degrees) and the filling defect above and below the anastomosis, this lesion is not suitable for angioplasty or atherectomy from the right femoral approach. A mound of intimal hyperplasia was removed during surgical revision of the anastomosis. The left internal iliac artery fills through retrograde flow in the external iliac artery *(arrowhead)*.

of this writing, there is no consensus on drug infusion strategy with respect to infusion rates, duration, and use of concomitant anticoagulation or antiplatelet agents. The concomitant use of heparin (300 to 500 IU/h) may be necessary when a long segment of catheter is exposed upstream from the lytic agent in a low-flow conduit. Close clinical monitoring of the patient, laboratory determination of coagulation status, and frequent angiographic inspection of progress are important to avoid complications and maintain the necessary surface contact between the catheter tip and the remaining thrombus. The infusion is terminated when complete recanalization of the vessel is achieved, as long as no complication supervenes. If an underlying lesion is discovered, appropriate endovascular or open surgical treatment is undertaken.

Embolotherapy

Transcatheter delivery of embolic agents has proved useful in managing life-threatening hemorrhage and in certain devascularization procedures. With the use of steerable guide wires and coaxial catheter systems, superselective catheterization of vessels as small as 1 mm in diameter is possible. Two clinical considerations guide the choice of embolic materials—the level of occlusion required, either proximal (corresponding to surgical ligation) or distal, and the duration of occlusion desired (either permanent or temporary). A variety of embolic agents is available for the combination best suited to the clinical problem and to the proximity of accessible vessels in the area of interest (42,43). As with other interventional procedures, embolotherapy should be preceded by thorough diagnostic angiography to document the pertinent vascular anatomy and predict the hemodynamic effect of embolization with respect to target organ infarction, recanalization of vessels, and recruitment of collaterals (Fig. 72.44). Indications for embolotherapy include treatment of gastrointestinal (Fig. 72.45) or traumatic (Fig. 72.46) hemorrhage (44,45), management of vascular malformations and arteriovenous fistulae (46–48), and tumor therapy (devascularization or vascular redistribution to optimize perfusion therapy) (49,50). The principal complications of embolotherapy (in addition to those of selective angiography) include abscess formation and infarction of normal tissue due to

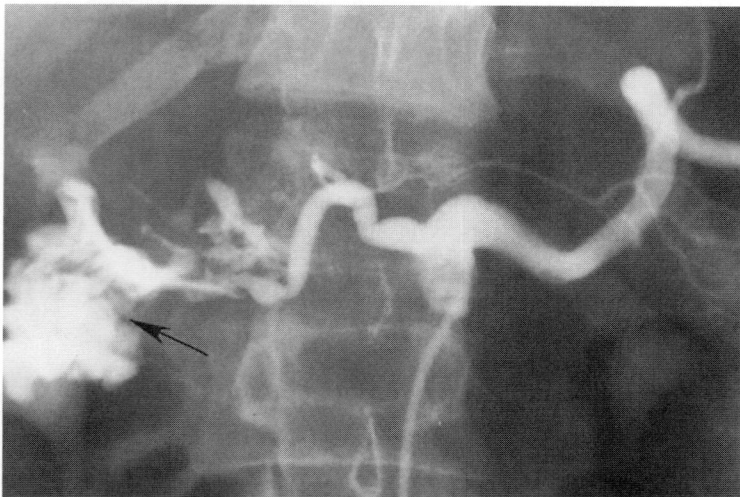

Figure 72.44. A 31-year-old man with a peptic ulcer and a previous vagotomy, antrectomy, and Billroth II procedure presented with massive upper gastrointestinal bleeding. Selective celiac arteriogram shows contrast extravasation into the second portion of the duodenum *(arrow)*. Celiac stenosis was present, and retrograde flow in the common hepatic artery (temporarily reversed by the power injection of contrast) precluded safe transcatheter embolization of the bleeding artery. (Courtesy of James Andrews, M.D., University of Michigan Hospitals, Ann Arbor, MI.)

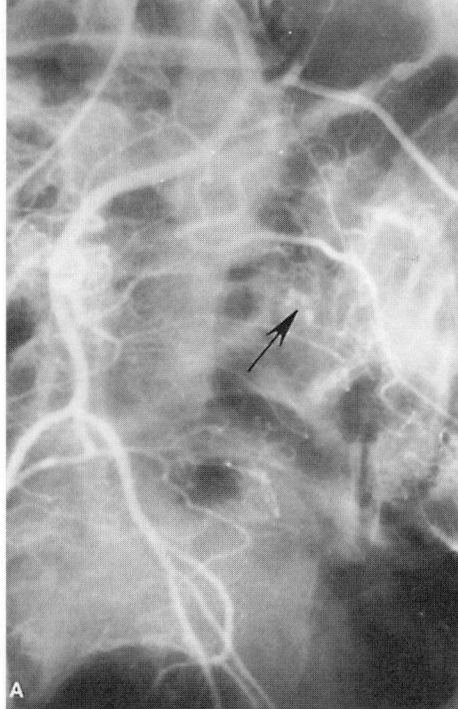
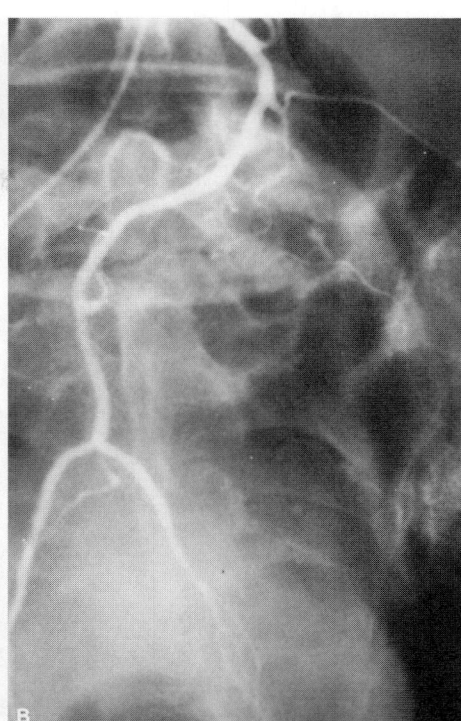

Figure 72.45. Lower gastrointestinal bleeding. A 72-year-old man presented with hematochezia after endoscopic polypectomy. *(A)* Inferior mesenteric arteriogram shows extravasation of contrast from a sigmoidal branch. *(B)* A second arteriogram after a 30-minute infusion of vasopressin at 0.2 IU/min shows arrest of the bleeding and marked constriction of all sigmoidal and rectal branches. Superselective embolotherapy would have been indicated if the hemorrhage had failed to respond to vasopressin.

inadvertent reflux of embolic material. A postinfarction syndrome of fever, pain, and leukocytosis may follow extensive embolic procedures in solid organs (48). Antibiotic coverage depends on the immune status of the patient, the level of occlusion, and the amount and type of tissue infarcted.

Caval Interruption

The indications for caval interruption procedures are discussed in Chapter 91. Placement of an inferior vena cava filter should be preceded by cavography to identify inferior vena cava anomalies and anatomic variations in the renal veins (Fig. 72.47). Percutaneous placement of caval filters is best accomplished through the right femoral or internal jugular approach.

Transjugular Intrahepatic Portosystemic Shunt

In the transjugular intrahepatic portosystemic shunt (TIPS) procedure, an 8- to 12-mm conduit between intrahepatic portal and hepatic venous branches (usually the right hepatic and right portal veins) is created through a percutaneous transjugular approach and buttressed open with intravascular stents (51,52). Indica-

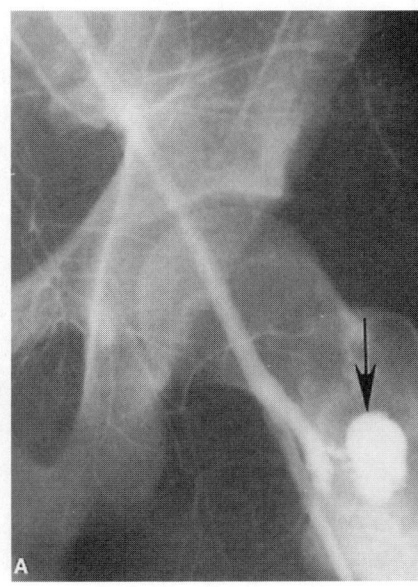
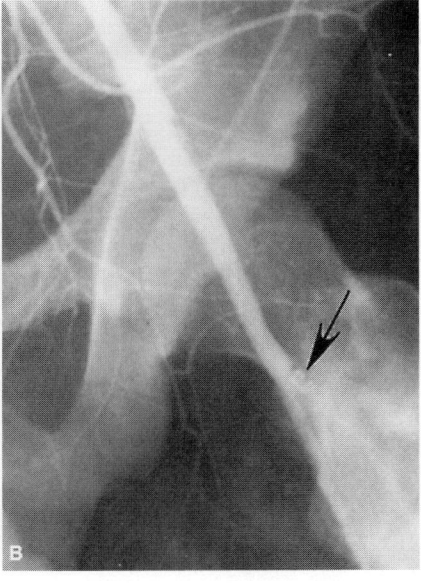

Figure 72.46. Posttraumatic hemorrhage. A 17-year-old man presented with an enlarging left groin hematoma after a gunshot wound. *(A)* Left pelvic arteriogram shows extravasation of contrast medium *(arrow)* from the deep femoral artery. The deep femoral artery was selectively catheterized from the right femoral artery approach and occluded with Gelfoam pledgets and two 3-mm Gianturco steel coils. *(B)* Pelvic arteriogram after embolization shows the coil in the proximal deep femoral artery with arrest of the bleeding. The superficial femoral artery remains patent.

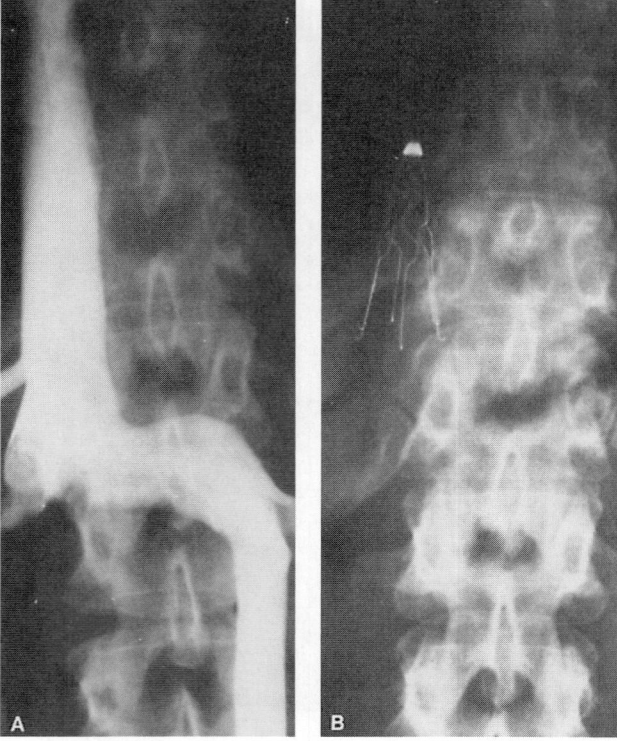

Figure 72.47. Suprarenal Greenfield filter placement through the left inferior vena cava. *(A)* Vena cavogram demonstrates a left-sided inferior vena cava joining the left renal vein and suprarenal cava. A 24F carrier was advanced into the suprarenal cava with use of the percutaneous left transfemoral approach. *(B)* Abdominal film after filter placement shows the filter in satisfactory position.

tions for TIPS construction include variceal bleeding unresponsive to medical and endoscopic therapy (sclerotherapy or banding), recurrent variceal bleeding that has failed endoscopic therapy, and intractable ascites. Technical success rates are approximately 80% to 90%. Restenosis of the TIPS, usually at the hepatic venous end, occurs in approximately 60% of patients by 6 months. This usually responds to repeat angioplasty and stenting. Because the TIPS requires relatively vigilant follow-up and angiographic maintenance, its role in terms of surgical portosystemic shunting in the management of the stable patient with good liver function requires further study.

Miscellaneous Interventional Procedures

Percutaneous retrieval of catheter fragments in the arterial or venous system is usually straightforward (Fig. 72.48). The use of a Check-Flo sheath at the puncture site facilitates atraumatic removal of the snared fragment.

Indwelling central venous access devices (peripherally inserted central catheters, Hickman catheters, or subcutaneous ports) may be placed with the help of fluoroscopic guidance for localization of the venous entry (e.g., brachial vein or the infrarenal inferior vena cava), for optimal catheter placement in the right atrium or superior vena cava–atrium junction, and for guidance across chronic thromboses or venous strictures (53). Venous access procedures are preceded by diagnostic venography to ensure venous patency.

Percutaneous treatment of the ischemic complications of aortic dissection has been described. These procedures include fenestration of the aortic septum, internal stenting of the aortic true lumen or affected branch arteries, and placement of a stent–graft across the entry tear in the dissection flap (54,55).

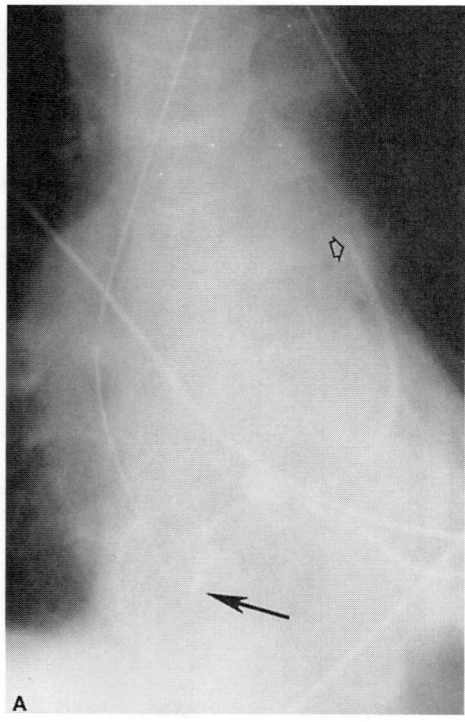
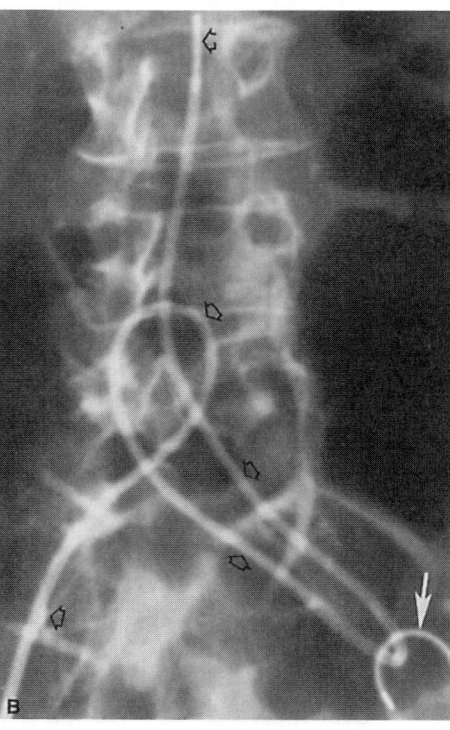

Figure 72.48. Knotted Swan-Ganz catheter. *(A)* Chest film shows an overhand loop *(arrow)* in the shaft of a right transfemoral Swan-Ganz catheter. The catheter tip is in the main pulmonary artery *(open arrow);* the knot is in the right atrium. *(B)* From the right groin, the catheter knot was retracted into the iliac vein confluence, where the knot *(open arrows)* was engaged and teased loose by a left transfemoral catheter *(arrow).*

REFERENCES

1. Seldinger S. Catheter replacement of needle in percutaneous arteriography: new technique. *Acta Radiol* 1953;39:368.
2. Hessel S, Adams D, Abrams H. Complications of angiography. *Radiology* 1981;138:273.
3. Rubin G, Dake M, Semba C. Current status of three-dimensional spiral CT scanning for imaging the vasculature. *Radiol Clin North Am* 1995;33:51.
4. Edelman R. MR angiography: present and future. *AJR Am J Roentgenol* 1993;161:1.
5. Prince M. Gadolinium-enhanced MR aortography. *Radiology* 1994;191:155.
6. Prince M, Narasimham D, Stanley J, et al. Gadolinium-enhanced magnetic resonance angiography of abdominal aortic aneurysms. *J Vasc Surg* 1995;21:656.
7. Dawson P. Chemotoxicity of contrast media and clinical adverse effects: a review. *Invest Radiol* 1985;20:S84.
8. Palmer F. The RACR survey of intravenous contrast media reactions: final report. *Aust Radiol* 1988;32:426.
9. Katayama H, Yamaguchi K, Kozuka T, et al. Adverse reactions to ionic and nonionic contrast media. *Radiology* 1990;175:621.
10. Hawkins I. Carbon dioxide digital subtraction arteriography. *AJR Am J Roentgenol* 1982;139:19.
11. Chamberlin JR, Lardi AB, McKeever LS, et al. Use of vascular sealing devices (VasoSeal and Perclose) versus manual compression (Femostop) in transcatheter coronary interventions requiring abciximab (ReoPro). *Catheter Cardiovasc Intervent* 1999;47:143.
12. Eisenberg R, Bank W, Hedgcock M. Renal failure after major angiography can be avoided with hydration. *AJR Am J Roentgenol* 1981;136:859.
13. Lasser E, Berry C, Talner L, et al. Pretreatment with corticosteroids to alleviate reactions to intravenous contrast material. *N Engl J Med* 1987;317:845.
14. Block P, Ockene I, Goldberg R, et al. A prospective randomized trial of outpatient versus inpatient cardiac catheterization. *N Engl J Med* 1988;319:1251.
15. Rogers W, Kraft M. Outpatient angioplasty. *Radiology* 1990;174:753.
16. Coleman S, Anson B. Arterial patterns in the hand based upon a study of 650 specimens. *Surg Gynecol Obstet* 1961;113:409.
17. Lippert H, Pabst R. *Arterial variations in man.* New York: Springer-Verlag, 1985:121.
18. Stanley J, Whitehouse W. Occlusive and aneurysmal disease of the renal arterial circulation. *Dis Mon* 1984;30:7.
19. Neiman H, Bergan J, Yao J, et al. Hemodynamic assessment of transluminal angioplasty for lower extremity ischemia. *Radiology* 1982;143:639.
20. Mannick J. Evaluation of chronic lower-extremity ischemia. *N Engl J Med* 1983;309:841.
21. Bookstein J, Ernst C. Vasodilatory and vasoconstrictive pharmacoangiographic manipulation of renal collateral flow. *Radiology* 1973;108:55.
22. Boley S, Brandt L, Veith F. Ischemic disorders of the intestines. *Curr Probl Surg* 1978;15:1.
23. Williams DM, Lee DY, Hamilton BH, et al. The dissected aorta. Part III. Anatomy and radiologic diagnosis of branch-vessel compromise. *Radiology* 1997;203:37.
24. Stanson A, Kazmier F, Hollier L, et al. Penetrating atherosclerotic ulcers of the thoracic aorta: natural history and clinicopathologic correlations. *Ann Vasc Surg* 1986;1:15.
25. Stanley J, Gewertz B, Bove E, et al. Arterial fibrodysplasia: histopathologic character and current etiologic concepts. *Arch Surg* 1975;110:561.
26. Bookstein J, Abrams H, Buenger R, et al. Radiologic aspects of renovascular hypertension: I. aims and methods of the radiology study group. *JAMA* 1972;220:1218.
27. Mulliken J, Glowacki J. Hemangiomas and vascular malformations in infants and children: a classification based on endothelial characteristics. *Plast Reconstr Surg* 1982;69:412.
28. Burrows P, Mulliken J, Fellows K, et al. Childhood hemangiomas and vascular malformations: angiographic differentiation. *AJR Am J Roentgenol* 1983;141:483.
29. Rabinov K, Paulin S. Roentgen diagnosis of venous thrombosis in the leg. *Arch Surg* 1972;104:134.
30. Ackroyd J, Thomas M, Browse N. Deep vein reflux: an assessment by descending phlebography. *Br J Surg* 1986;73:31.
31. Geiser J, Eversmann W. Closed system venography in the evaluation of upper extremity hemangiomas. *J Hand Surg* 1978A;3:173.
32. Braun S, Moore A, Mills S, et al. Closed-system venography in the evaluation of angiodysplastic lesions of the extremities. *AJR Am J Roentgenol* 1983;141:1307.
33. Mills S, Jackson D, Older R, et al. The incidence, etiologies and avoidance of complications of pulmonary angiography in a large series. *Radiology* 1980;136:295.
34. Becker G, Katzen B, Dake M. Noncoronary angioplasty. *Radiology* 1989;170:921.
35. Casarella W. Noncoronary angioplasty. *Curr Probl Cardiol* 1986;11:138.
36. Waller B. "Crackers, breakers, stretchers, drillers, scrapers, shavers, burners, welders and melters": the future treatment of atherosclerotic coronary artery disease? A clinical-morphologic assessment. *J Am Coll Cardiol* 1989;13:969.
37. Becker G. Intravascular stent: general principles and status of lower-extremity arterial applications. *Circulation* 1991;83 [Suppl I]:122.
38. Martin E. Percutaneous therapy in the management of aortoiliac disease. *Semin Vasc Surg* 1994;7:17.
39. Motarjeme A. Thrombolytic therapy in arterial occlusion and graft thrombosis. *Semin Vasc Surg* 1989;2:155.
40. Marder V, Sherry S. Thrombolytic therapy: current status, part 1. *N Engl J Med* 1988;318:1512.
41. Marder V, Sherry S. Thrombolytic therapy: current status, part 2. *N Engl J Med* 1988;318:1585.
42. Kunstlinger F, Brunelle F, Chaumont P, et al. Vascular occlusive agents. *AJR Am J Roentgenol* 1981;136:151.
43. Amplatz K, Coleman C. Therapeutic embolization of thorax and abdomen. *Semin Intervent Radiol* 1984;1:95.
44. Ben-Menachem Y. Logic and logistics of radiography, angiography, and angiographic intervention in massive blunt trauma. *Radiol Clin North Am* 1981;19:9.
45. Keller F. Nonoperative management of gastrointestinal hemorrhage. *Semin Intervent Radiol* 1988;5:1.
46. Gomes A, Mali W, Oppenheim W. Embolization therapy in the management of congenital arteriovenous malformations. *Radiology* 1982;144:41.
47. Yakes W, Haas D, Parker S, et al. Symptomatic vascular malformations: ethanol embolotherapy. *Radiology* 1989;170:1059.
48. White R, Lynch-Nyhan A, Terry P, et al. Pulmonary arteriovenous malformations: techniques and long-term outcome of embolotherapy. *Radiology* 1988;169:663.
49. Wallace S, Chuang V, Swanson D. Embolization of renal carcinoma: experience with 100 patients. *Radiology* 1981;138:563.
50. Chuang V, Wallace S. Hepatic arterial redistribution for intra-arterial infusion of hepatic neoplasms. *Radiology* 1980;135:295.
51. Kerlan R, LaBerge J, Gordon R, et al. Transjugular intrahepatic portosystemic shunts: current status. *AJR Am J Roentgenol* 1995;164:1059.
52. Coldwell D, Ring E, Rees C, et al. Multicenter investigation of the role of transjugular intrahepatic portosystemic shunt in management of portal hypertension. *Radiology* 1995;196:335.
53. Andrews J, Walker-Andrews S, Ensminger W. Long-term central venous access with a peripherally placed subcutaneous infusion port: initial results. *Radiology* 1990;176:45.
54. Williams DM, Lee DY, Hamilton BH, et al. The dissected aorta: percutaneous treatment of ischemic complications—principles and results. *J Vasc Intervent Radiol* 1997;8:605.
55. Dake MD, Kato N, Mitchell RS, et al. Endovascular stent-graft placement for the treatment of acute aortic dissection. *N Engl J Med* 1999;340:1546.

SURGERY: SCIENTIFIC PRINCIPLES AND PRACTICE, Third Edition, edited by
Lazar J. Greenfield, Michael W. Mulholland, Keith T. Oldham, Gerald B. Zelenock,
and Keith D. Lillemoe. Lippincott Williams & Wilkins Publishers, Philadelphia, © 2001.

CHAPTER 73

VASCULAR INFECTIONS

G. PATRICK CLAGETT

Vascular infections are among the most challenging and difficult problems encountered by vascular surgeons. Patients are often elderly, frail, desperately ill with multiple medical comorbid conditions, and unable to tolerate the extensive, complex operations usually required to treat the problem. Medical treatment based on specific antibiotic therapy is rarely successful when used alone, and complete resection and excision of all infected vascular structures are usually necessary to eradicate infection. Immediate restoration of blood flow to critical vascular beds by alternate anatomic routes or with replacement vascular conduits that minimize the risk for recurrent infection present additional challenges that tax the skill and ingenuity of vascular surgeons. Despite a great deal of progress in the treatment of vascular infections, morbidity and mortality remain among the highest associated with vascular conditions (1–3).

VASCULAR PROSTHETIC INFECTIONS

Pathogenesis

Vascular prostheses are foreign bodies that can be primarily infected by contamination at the time of placement or secondarily infected after implantation by hematogenous, lymphatic, or contiguous spread of microorganisms. The overall incidence of clinically overt prosthetic infection varies according to anatomic site. Aortic prostheses confined to the abdominal or thoracic cavity rarely become infected; the incidence ranges from 0.5% to 2% (2). The incidence is higher, from 2% to 6%, in proximal or distal anastomotic sites at the femoral level (e.g., aortofemoral or femoral–popliteal bypasses) (4). Several features of the femoral area predispose to infectious complications. The groin is a relatively dirty area that is difficult to clean, and incisions placed in the groin are prone to infection and healing problems. Vertical groin incisions cut obliquely across the inguinal crease, tend to gape, and in obese patients they lie buried in moist folds of skin. Furthermore, superficial inguinal lymph nodes are usually transected during exposure of the common femoral artery, and if they are not ligated, they will bathe a vascular prosthesis in lymph fluid that may contain bacteria. Potential sources of prosthetic contamination in this circumstance include open, infected ischemic ulcers of a lower extremity, gangrenous toes, and wounds in any other area drained by the inguinal lymphatics, such as the perineum and perianal area. Another factor implicating the groin wound in the etiology of vascular prosthetic infections is transient local ischemia during placement of an aortic cross-clamp, which may render the wound more susceptible to infection.

Most authorities agree that the majority of vascular prosthetic infections are initiated at the time of operation (2,3,5). Although direct proof of this tenet is difficult to obtain, the prevalence of *Staphylococcus epidermidis* among offending organisms suggests that skin contamination with the patient's own flora is an important mechanism (6,7). The presence of *Staphylococcus aureus* and other nosocomially acquired bacteria is also common and points to environmental sources of contamination. Other intraoperative sources of contamination include intestinal flora when the gastrointestinal tract is entered or operations such as cholecystectomy are performed concomitantly. Laminated thrombus lining the wall of aneurysms has been implicated as a source of contamination and, when cultured, yields bacteria in about 10% of specimens. *S. epidermidis* is the most common isolate (8,9).

Postoperative sources of vascular prosthetic infection include wound complications, urinary tract infections, and invasive line sepsis. Early and late hematogenous seeding of prostheses can occur during transient bacteremia associated with remote, noncontiguous infections or dental procedures.

Although bacteria are most often cultured from infected arterial prostheses, other, less common microorganisms, such as fungi, *Mycoplasma,* and *Mycobacterium,* have been encountered. *S. epidermidis* is the most common pathogen reported in modern series and outnumbers *S. aureus* in infections two to one. Gram-negative and polymicrobial infections are being increasingly encountered but remain less prevalent than gram-positive infections. In many cases, negative cultures are reported despite convincing local evidence of infection, including a nonincorporated prosthesis surrounded by grossly purulent fluid (10). These cases are most likely caused by *S. epidermidis* or other low-virulence organisms that are exposed to perioperative antibiotics at the time of sampling and require fastidious microbiologic techniques for growth. Sonication of infected prosthetic material, growth in tryptic soy broth, and prolonged incubation for several days have been reported to increase the yield of cultures positive for *S. epidermidis* (11).

The presence of a foreign body, such as an implanted device, increases the risk for infection. Early investigations documented that it takes only 10^2 *S. aureus* organisms to cause an abscess at the site of a suture but 10^6 organisms to cause an infection in normal skin. The explanations of why foreign materials are prone to infection involve physicochemical properties of the material, impairment of host defenses, and special properties of bacteria that facilitate their growth in the presence of a biomaterial (12). The biologic reaction to an implanted vascular prosthesis comprises an acute inflammatory response in the early stages that progresses to formation of a fibrous capsule or tissue growth into porous materials. Neutrophils rapidly become associated with any implanted biomaterial in vivo, become prematurely activated by contact with the material, and rapidly lose the capacity to become activated in response to subsequent stimuli, such as the presence of bacteria. Neutrophils in contact with biomaterials rapidly lose their ability to produce superoxide and other reactive oxygen species and become relatively impotent in their microbicidal activity (13,14). In a sense, the biomaterial becomes a massive "decoy" that averts and diverts the ability of neutrophils to respond normally to bacteria in the microenvironment. In addition, neutrophil products released in these circumstances may promote dysfunction of new neutrophils entering the microenvironment (15).

Vascular prosthetic biomaterials may vary in their susceptibility to infection by different microorganisms. Highly textured or rough-surfaced biomaterials, such as textiles manufactured from Dacron (woven or knitted), are more prone to bacterial adherence than smooth-surfaced biomaterials, such as expanded polytetrafluoroethylene (ePTFE) or polyurethane (16). In vivo, adherence of platelets, plasma proteins, and other blood constituents and varying conditions of shear may dramatically alter the responses of different biomaterials to microorganisms, and all biomaterials remain susceptible to infection (17,18).

The principal organism responsible for infections of all implanted medical devices, including vascular prostheses, is *S. epidermidis.* The organism is a ubiquitous skin commensural of relatively slow growth and low virulence. It causes chronic infections with local manifestations but little or no systemic toxicity. Pivotal in the pathogenesis of *S. epidermidis* infection is the production of multilayered biofilms composed of exopolysaccharides, usually referred to as *slime.* The elaboration of biofilms takes place following the adherence of *S. epidermidis* to biomaterials and usually occurs when organisms adhere to one another in microcolonies (19). Both adherence of organisms to polymer surfaces and to each other (cell–cell adhesion) is mediated by capsular polysaccharide adhesins (19,20). Mutant bacteria that do not produce adhesins lack cell–cell adhesion and do not produce biofilms (21). Once elaborated, biofilms form a protective shield that allows continued bacterial growth in relatively hostile environments. Bacterial nutrients and metabolic wastes freely traverse the polysaccharide biofilm but antibiotics do not. Biofilms also alter inflammatory changes, impair host defenses, and promote tenacious adherence of microbial colonies to the biomaterial (22). *S. epidermidis* infections tend to be persistent and refractory to antibiotics, and the implant must be removed to clear the infection.

Once established, bacterial infection spreads throughout a vascular prosthesis and eventually involves anastomotic sites. The eventual destruction of vascular tissue leads to the formation of an anastomotic false aneurysm. The first manifestation of a vascular prosthetic infection is often an anastomotic false aneurysm or its most frequent complication, prosthetic limb thrombosis in the case of an aortobifemoral bypass. When the false aneurysm involves the aortic anastomosis, rupture into the duodenum may occur and produce an aortoduodenal fistula with catastrophic hemorrhage. Although all microorganisms producing vascular prosthetic infections are associated with false aneurysms, they vary in their propensity to destroy vascular tissue. Gram-negative organisms, such as *Pseudomonas aeruginosa, Proteus* species, and *Escherichia coli,* are particularly notorious for their ability to digest vascular tissue (23). These organisms elaborate elastase and alkaline protease, which break down elastin, collagen, fibronectin, and fibrin. In addition to causing vascular disruption and the formation of false aneurysms, many bacteria produce substances that are highly thrombogenic and may induce the thrombosis that is the first manifestation of a vascular prosthetic infection.

Clinical Presentation

The clinical presentations of vascular prosthetic infections can be protean and subtle, so that the diagnosis is difficult. The tempo and severity of the clinical manifestations often depend on the microorganism. A patient whose infection is caused by a virulent organism, such as *S. aureus, P. aeruginosa,* or *E. coli,* presents with systemic signs of sepsis. As an example, a patient with a vascular prosthesis who has persistent fever, chills, and an elevated white blood cell count with a left shift should be suspected of having a vascular prosthetic infection. Virulent microorganisms also tend to cause earlier manifestations of infection, with the interval between implantation of the prosthesis and diagnosis of infection often being months. Very early prosthetic

infections, diagnosed within weeks of implantation, are most often associated with wound infections that involve the vascular prostheses by contiguous spread.

In contrast, patients with infection caused by a low-virulence organism, such as *S. epidermidis,* present later, often years after placement (7). Systemic signs and symptoms are usually mild or absent. These patients most often present with local manifestations, such as a chronic groin sinus that discharges small amounts of pus, a chronic wound infection exposing the prosthesis, femoral anastomotic false aneurysm, or aortofemoral bypass limb thrombosis. They may have low-grade fever and mild constitutional symptoms, but overt systemic signs of sepsis are absent. The white blood cell count is usually normal or only mildly elevated, but the erythrocyte sedimentation rate is often abnormal. A patient presenting with a femoral anastomotic false aneurysm or limb thrombosis who has an elevated erythrocyte sedimentation rate should be suspected of having a vascular prosthetic infection.

Patients presenting with massive gastrointestinal hemorrhage from an aortoduodenal or aortoenteric fistula frequently have had lesser episodes of bleeding hours to days before the major episode. These are often referred to as "herald" or "sentinel" episodes of bleeding and offer a window of opportunity for diagnosis and management that may avert exsanguinating hemorrhage. Any patient with an intraabdominal vascular prosthesis who has an episode of upper or lower gastrointestinal bleeding should be suspected of having an underlying aortoenteric fistula, and an expeditious work-up is important. Chronic gastrointestinal bleeding can also occur in patients with an aortoenteric fistula but is more often associated with an enteric erosion. This condition, often referred to as *graft–enteric erosion,* differs from aortoenteric fistula in that the body or limb of the vascular prosthesis erodes into bowel and the aortic suture line is not involved. This produces chronic bleeding from the eroded bowel mucosa, analogous to bleeding from an ulcer, and patients may present with chronic anemia. The diagnosis should be suspected in a patient with an intraabdominal vascular prosthesis who has anemia, stool positive for occult blood on guaiac testing, and fever.

An increasingly recognized manifestation of aortofemoral and aortoiliac prosthetic infections is hydroureteronephrosis. This can develop if the ureter becomes obstructed as a result of periprosthetic inflammation and may be bilateral or unilateral, depending on the extent of infection. It is unusual for hydroureteronephrosis to be the initial manifestation of vascular prosthetic infection because the urologic condition is usually asymptomatic. This complication most often is noted during the work-up of a patient with an infected vascular prosthesis who presents with other symptoms, such as a groin sinus or gastrointestinal bleeding.

Diagnosis

Because the manifestations of vascular prosthetic infections are so varied and subtle and because the consequences of a missed diagnosis may be lethal, imaging tests are important (24). The types of imaging and other diagnostic tests used are based on the clinical presentation. Computed tomography (CT) has long been the mainstay of diagnostic imaging for suspected vascular prosthetic infection. CT findings suggestive of infection include ectopic gas, periprosthetic fluid, loss of tissue planes, periprosthetic inflammatory changes, thickening of adjacent bowel, hydroureteronephrosis, and anastomotic false aneurysm (25) (Fig. 73.1). These findings are most specific and useful for late infections. During the immediate pe-

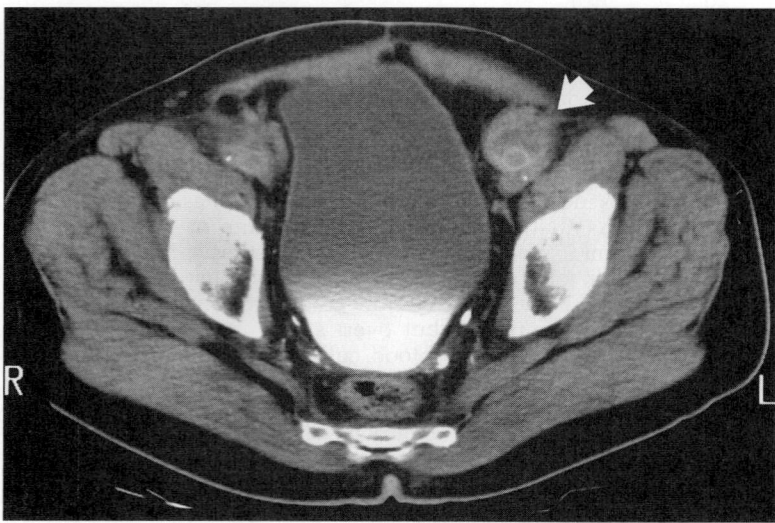

Figure 73.1. Computed tomogram of lower pelvis demonstrating fluid and an enhancing ring around the left limb of an aortobifemoral bypass *(arrow).*

riod following implantation, periprosthetic fluid, air, and inflammatory changes may be present for 2 to 3 months. After 3 months, postoperative hematoma and gas should resolve and tissue planes return to normal (26).

Magnetic resonance imaging (MRI) has provided an alternative to CT for cross-sectional imaging. In addition to demonstrating the same features seen on CT (periprosthetic air, fluid, and structural abnormalities), MRI is particularly helpful in assessing periprosthetic inflammatory changes. These are seen as high-intensity signals on T_2-weighted images in the tissues surrounding the prosthesis and accurately portray tissue edema (27) (Fig. 73.2). Such images can be particularly helpful in assessing the extent of infection, which may determine the operative approach. For example, in a patient with an infection localized to a single, distal limb of an aortobifemoral bypass, removal of the entire prosthesis may not be required for adequate treatment of the infection.

Radionuclide scanning has also been used in the diagnosis of vascular prosthetic infections. Scintigraphy with the use of autologous white blood cells labeled with indium oxine In 111 is the most common technique currently used, although the use of white cells labeled with gallium 67, technetium, and other isotopes has also been reported (28,29). In addition, scintigraphy based on labeled human immunoglobulin G has been used and may

be more sensitive than scintigraphy with white blood cells (30). A problem with all scintigraphic methods in diagnosing vascular prosthetic infections is a lack of specificity caused by uptake in other organs or tissues that may be contiguous. In addition, faint or no uptake in the presence of limited or low-virulence infection can result in false-negative results. Scintigraphy is most helpful when occult prosthetic infection is suspected. An example would be a patient with a vascular prosthesis presenting with a fever of unknown origin or a complex of other nonspecific symptoms in whom white blood cell scintigraphy "lights up" the prosthesis.

Arteriography is of limited usefulness in the diagnosis of vascular prosthetic infection but it may, on occasion, demonstrate an aortic false aneurysm or even active leakage of contrast into the bowel lumen, which is pathognomonic for aortoenteric fistula. Arteriography is helpful in planning reconstruction after removal of the prosthesis and is most useful in late infection, when the vascular anatomy may have been altered by progressive occlusive disease.

In patients presenting with gastrointestinal bleeding and suspected aortoenteric fistula, complete upper gastrointestinal endoscopy with visualization of the third and fourth portions of the duodenum, the most common site of fistula, is necessary. Even if this study is incomplete, with

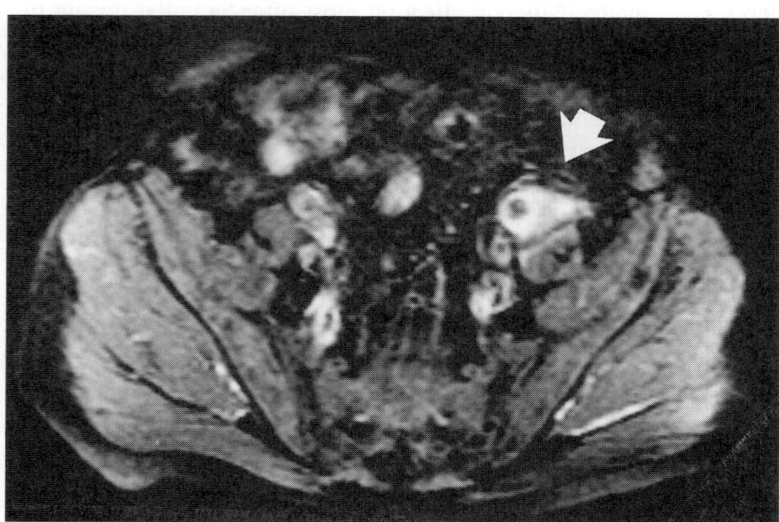

Figure 73.2. Magnetic resonance image of the lower pelvis of the patient in Fig. 73.1. The *arrow* points to high-intensity signals on a T_2-weighted image, characteristic of inflammation and tissue edema.

inability to visualize the distal duodenum or the finding of gastrointestinal lesions (e.g., chronic peptic ulcer) that are not actively bleeding, an aortoenteric fistula may still be present. Continued, unexplained bleeding mandates operative exploration to rule out aortoenteric fistula. At the time of operation, the duodenum, proximal jejunum, and any other bowel in contact with a vascular prosthesis must be dissected free to make or exclude this diagnosis.

Treatment

The primary goal of treatment is to save life and limb, and this is best accomplished by eradicating infection and maintaining adequate circulation to portions of the body perfused by the infected prosthesis. Secondary goals include minimizing morbidity, restoring normal function, and maintaining long-term function without the need for repeated intervention and risk of amputation.

These goals are best achieved by excision of all infected prosthetic material and vascular tissues combined with appropriate arterial reconstruction. The currently favored methods of arterial reconstruction for aortic prosthetic infection include extraanatomic bypass (31–44) and in situ replacement with the use of autogenous superficial femoral popliteal veins (45–47), arterial allografts (48–51), and vascular prostheses that are often treated or soaked in antibiotic solutions (52–56). Pooled outcome data from contemporary series reported since 1985 are presented in Table 73.1. Direct comparisons of these data to judge the relative success of the various approaches is difficult because of the heterogeneity of patients with different degrees of illness and different comorbid conditions in the reported series. All of these approaches are valid and useful depending on patient-specific characteristics and circumstances. It is a mistake to think that a single surgical approach is applicable to all patients with this condition. These complicated and multifaceted patients with varying degrees of illness require individualized attention. The pros and cons of each approach are also outlined in Table 73.1.

Extraanatomic bypass, usually involving an axillofemoral bypass, is an excellent choice for infected aortoiliac reconstructions in which femoral sites are free of sepsis and arterial runoff is good (Fig. 73.3). It is also possibly less of a physiologic insult than other procedures, particularly when the operations can be staged so that extraanatomic bypass precedes removal of the infected aortic prosthesis by a period of days (32). This approach has the advantage of preserving lower extremity blood flow during removal of the aortic prosthesis, so that ischemic time is minimized. Unfortunately, the durability of an extraanatomic bypass is limited in patients with multilevel occlusive disease and poor runoff. Most patients with infected aortic prostheses have an aortobifemoral bypass, and extraanatomic bypass in such patients usually requires bilateral axillofemoral procedures with distal anastomoses to diseased and small profunda femoral or popliteal arteries. These are disadvantaged reconstructions with poor long-term patency despite the administration of antithrombotic agents. They are prone to sudden thrombotic occlusion without warning, and amputation rates are high, even after thrombectomy and multiple revisions. In one large series, one third of patients required major amputation during long-term follow-up (33). In addition, reinfection of the extraanatomic bypass prosthesis occurs in 10% to 20% of patients, and this condition is often lethal. A final problem with extraanatomic bypass is continuing infection at the site of aortic closure, or aortic "stump." Although an infrequent occurrence (< 10% of cases), aortic stump blowout is almost always fatal.

Dissatisfaction with the long-term patency of extraanatomic bypass led to the development of in situ autogenous venous reconstruction (45–47). Early experiences were with greater saphenous veins, but the use of superficial femoropopliteal veins rapidly evolved because of their large caliber and superior patency (45) (Figs. 73.4 and 73.5). This reconstruction is most applicable in patients with extensive occlusive disease and poor runoff, a circumstance in which the patency of an autogenous venous reconstruction would theoretically be better than the patency of a prosthetic bypass. The situation is analogous to the use of vein grafts in femoropopliteal and distal bypasses because of their superior patency in comparison with prosthetic conduits. This advantage has been realized, with excellent 5-year cumulative rates of 85% for primary patency and 100% for secondary/assisted patency in superficial femoropopliteal vein aortofemoral reconstructions (47). Long-term amputation rates have been reported to be correspondingly low.

The principal disadvantage of using superficial femoropopliteal veins for aortofemoral reconstruction is that the procedure is technically demanding and long. The lower extremity ischemic time is longer than with other approaches but can be minimized by using a two-team approach and carefully sequencing the procedure to shorten aortic cross-clamp time. To minimize open body cavity exposure and lower extremity ischemia, the operation is carried out in the following order: (a) Dissect superficial femoropopliteal veins and leave in situ until needed, (b) isolate and control femoral vessels, (c) enter abdomen and obtain aortic control, (d) remove infected prosthesis, and (e) perform reconstruction with superficial femoropopliteal veins (57).

Lower extremity venous morbidity is also a potential drawback to harvesting the superficial femoropopliteal veins. However, venous morbidity has been surprisingly infrequent and mild (46,47). The benign course following removal of the superficial femoropopliteal veins is a consequence of several compensating mechanisms (58). First, the junction of the profunda femoral and common femoral veins is carefully preserved after disconnection of the proximal superficial femoral vein to allow unimpeded drainage via the profunda system. Second, several anatomic collateral connections are found between the remaining distal popliteal vein and the profunda system, and many of these collaterals enlarge to accommodate the increase in volume flow following removal of the superficial femoropopliteal vein. Finally, the valves in the tibial veins and collateral circuits remain functional, so that distal venous reflux does not occur.

A final concern is that placing superficial femoropopliteal veins in an infected field may lead to reinfection and disruption. Experience with this approach has documented that these vein grafts resist gram-positive, gram-negative, and fungal infections, and disruption of anastomoses has been rare. Long-term aneurysmal degeneration has also been studied for up to 8 years after placement of these vein grafts and has not occurred (47).

In situ allograft replacement has been reported with varying degrees of success (48–51). Acute and delayed aortic allograft disruption has been reported and is a distinct limitation of using allografts in infected fields (50,59). In addition, long-term deterioration leading to thrombosis and aneurysmal degeneration has been reported. Ready availability of allograft material is another limitation of this approach in situations in which emergency or urgent operations are often required.

Replacement of the infected aortic prosthesis with a new prosthesis has also been reported (52–56). Most often, the new prosthesis is soaked in an antibiotic solution, usu-

Table 73.1. **TREATMENT OF AORTIC PROSTHETIC INFECTIONS**[a]

	References	No. patients	Mortality (range) (%)	Major amputation (range) (%)	Aortic disruption (%)	Reinfection (%)	Five-year primary patency (%)	Advantages	Disadvantages
Extraanatomic bypass	31–44	515	20.6 (5.0–40.6)	13.6 (0–15.6)	8.9	12.0	61.8	Procedure can be staged. Less physiologic stress.	Poor patency, high long-term amputation rate. Potential for reinfection of bypass and aortic stump blowout. Thrombectomy, revision often required.
In situ superficial femoral–popliteal vein replacement	46,47	59	8.9 (6.7–9.8)	5.3 (4.9–6.7)	0	0	84	Autogenous reconstruction, resists infection. Good patency, low long-term amputation rate. Low rate of secondary procedures to maintain patency.	Complex procedure. Long ischemia time.
In situ allograft replacement	48–51	224	18.8 (8.3–24.0)	1.3 (0–3.0)	4.0	4.0	?	Expeditious procedure. No aortic stump.	Reinfection. Allograft deterioration. Unavailability of allografts.
In situ prosthetic replacement	52–56	77	14.3 (8.0–21.7)	0	0	15.3	?	Expeditious procedure. No aortic stump.	Reinfection rate high and unpredictable.

[a]Pooled data from major series reported since 1985.

In situ prosthetic and allograft reconstructions may be most useful in very ill and unstable patients and in those with actively bleeding aortoenteric fistulae. Expeditious in situ replacement in these circumstances can be lifesaving and may be used as a "bridge" procedure, with definitive reconstruction (extraanatomic or superficial femoropopliteal vein) carried out at a later date when the patient has been rendered fit for such a reconstruction.

Conservative approaches that do not involve removal of the infected prosthesis have also been reported (60–63). These are based on aggressive drainage and débridement of infected tissues; intensive, culture-specific antibiotic therapy; meticulous wound care to achieve coverage of exposed prosthetic material; and coverage of exposed prosthetic material with muscle flaps. Conservative approaches are most appropriately used when infection is extracavitary and limited in extent, systemic signs of sepsis are absent, the virulence of the infecting organisms is low, and anastomotic sites are uninvolved (63). Like those who have undergone in situ prosthetic replacement, these patients require close follow-up and indefinite oral antibiotic treatment.

If an infection involves only one limb of a bifurcated aortic prosthesis, the limb is usually resected (11,64–67). Revascularization is often carried out via obturator bypass or another prosthetic reconstruction performed in a clean field. Autogenous superficial femoropopliteal or greater saphenous veins have also been used for this purpose (67). It is important that the extent of infection be assessed with imaging studies in addition to direct visual inspection. In the case of a unilateral femoral infection of an aortofemoral bypass, the general approach is to begin the operation by inspecting the intraabdominal portion of the prosthesis. If the infection grossly involves the main body of the bifurcated prosthesis, complete removal is necessary. If the suspected limb is well incorporated and free of gross infection, division of the limb, closure of the tunnel, and obturator or other extraanatomic bypass are performed. The final portion of this operation is removal of the infected limb from below, with care taken to prevent cross-contamination of other, freshly placed incisions that have been closed.

Infection of Femoropopliteal/Distal Prosthetic Bypasses

In general, the management principles for infected infrainguinal prosthetic bypasses are similar to those for in-

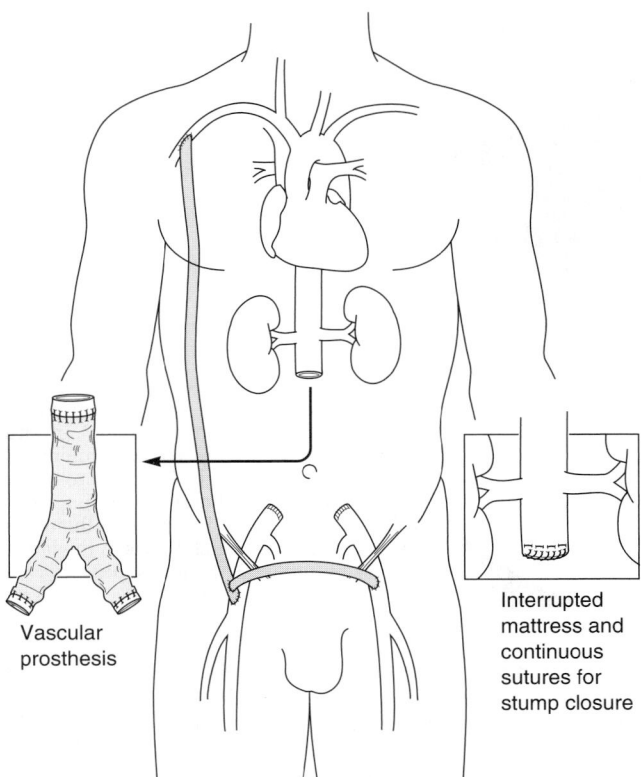

Figure 73.3. Standard treatment for an infected aortic vascular prosthesis. An axillobifemoral bypass is performed first. A few days later, the infected aortic prosthesis is removed and the aortic stump is carefully oversewn, as illustrated. This operation is most useful in patients with infected aortoiliac prostheses who have femoral areas free of infection and good runoff.

Vascular prosthesis

Interrupted mattress and continuous sutures for stump closure

ally rifampin, before implantation (55,56). This approach is most often successful in patients with limited infections of low virulence following aggressive débridement of all infected vascular and surrounding tissues to create a clean field. Despite these precautions, the potential for reinfection is a serious drawback (41), and patients treated in this manner require close and vigilant follow-up with frequent imaging studies, such as CT or MRI. They also are usually treated with lifelong oral antibiotics.

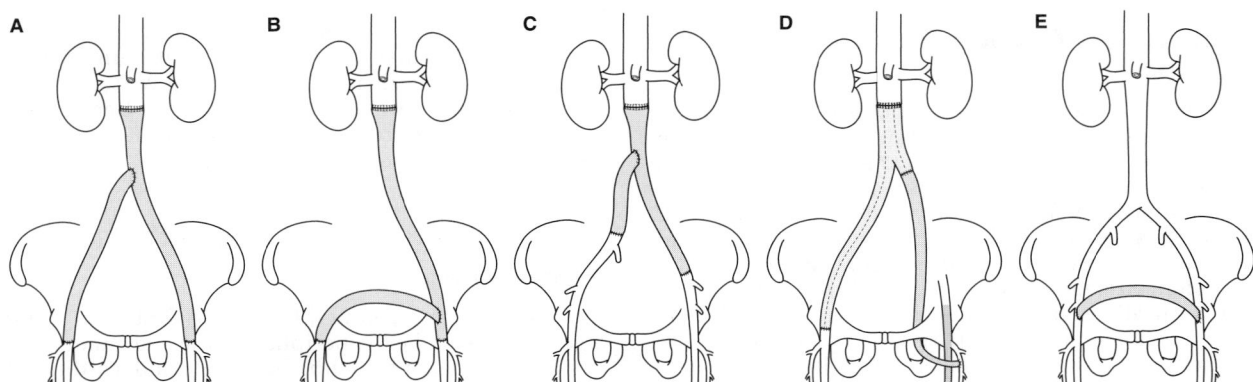

Figure 73.4. Use of the superficial femoropopliteal vein in multiple reconstructions after removal of an infected vascular prosthesis. *(A)* Standard aortobifemoral replacement in situ. *(B)* Left aortofemoral bypass in situ with left-to-right femoral crossover bypass. *(C)* Aortoiliac reconstruction in situ. *(D)* Unilateral transobturator aorta profunda bypass. *(E)* Femoral crossover bypass.

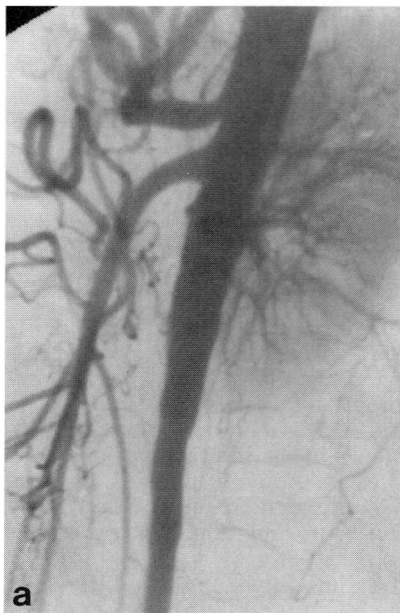
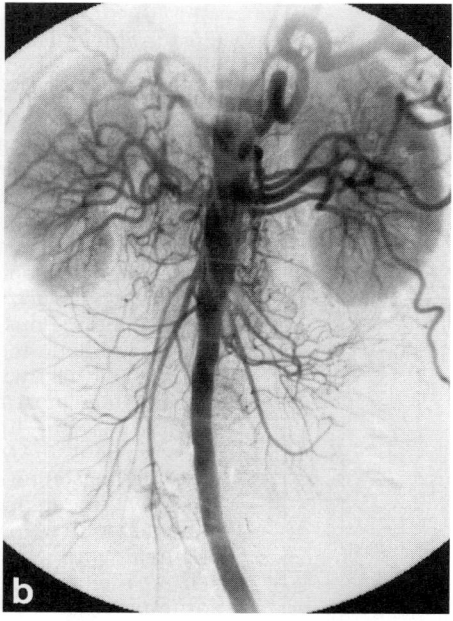

Figure 73.5. Lateral *(A)* and anteroposterior *(B)* arteriogram of a superficial femoropopliteal vein replacement in situ after removal of an infected aortobifemoral bypass. The left-to-right femoral crossover bypass with superficial femoropopliteal vein is not shown. The figure illustrates the excellent size match between the large-caliber superficial femoropopliteal vein and the infrarenal aorta.

fected aortic prostheses. Excision of all infected prosthetic material and creation of a new bypass through clean tissue planes are optimal (68). Venous autografts are preferable to vascular prostheses because of the low risk for reinfection. Unfortunately, many of these patients have limited sources of adequate vein for a new vein graft bypass. Additionally, because of the limited anatomic area, cross-contamination and infection of a new prosthetic conduit are probable. The overall mortality of patients undergoing operations for infected prosthetic infrainguinal bypasses approaches 20% and may be higher in those undergoing limb salvage procedures (68,69). These considerations have led some experts to recommend excision of the infected prosthesis and amputation in circumstances in which the limb remains in jeopardy after removal of the infected prosthesis. The rate of major amputation is approximately 40% (68,69). If assessment with Doppler ultrasonography indicates that the limb remains viable (audible arterial signals present at the ankle level), removal of the infected prosthesis with vein patch closure of anastomotic sites is preferred. If only a limited portion of the prosthesis is involved, nonresectional, conservative measures have been successfully used (60,70). Results with this approach are best when virulence of the infection is low, sepsis is absent, and anastomoses are free of infection.

Prevention of Vascular Prosthetic Infections

The benefit of short-term antibiotic prophylaxis in preventing wound infections after vascular surgery has been demonstrated in randomized trials (71–73). Most often, a first-generation cephalosporin is administered intravenously shortly before operation, during operation if blood loss is extensive or the operation is prolonged, and 2 hours after operation. Recent evidence suggests that a more prolonged course, for up to 4 to 5 days after operation or until all invasive lines have been removed, may provide additional protection (74). When patients have infected ischemic lesions of a lower extremity, culture-specific antibiotics should be administered perioperatively. Also, the use of more specific prophylactic antibiotic therapy should be considered in hospitals where certain organisms are prevalent, especially when exposure is increased by prolonged preoperative hospitalization.

Attention to intraoperative factors is also important in preventing vascular prosthetic infections. Patients undergoing repeated and emergency operations are especially prone to wound infections and present additional risks. Meticulous attention to hemostasis and avoidance of wound hematomas and seromas that can become secondarily infected are important surgical tenets that are often difficult to achieve in patients given anticoagulants during the operation and who are also taking antithrombotic agents, such as aspirin or clopidogrel. If possible, these agents should be discontinued 1 week before the operation. Ligation and control of the femoral lymphatics are also probably important technical features in preventing vascular prosthetic infections. Electrocautery of lymphatic tissue leads to coagulation necrosis of lymphatic vessels but does not prevent extravasation of lymph fluid. Patients undergoing aortic operations are prone to intraoperative hypothermia, and this condition has been shown to impair neutrophil function and increase the incidence of postoperative wound infection (75). Maintenance of normal body temperature should be the goal during major vascular operations. Additional procedures on the gastrointestinal or biliary tract that may result in intraoperative contamination of a vascular prosthesis should be avoided unless the additional procedure is deemed necessary to avoid life-threatening postoperative complications. Hematogenous seeding of a vascular prosthesis is a continuing risk for as long as the prosthesis is in place. Dental work, procedures on the gastrointestinal and genitourinary tracts, and angiographic procedures should be carried out with the patient protected by antibiotic prophylaxis.

INFECTED (MYCOTIC) ANEURYSMS

Pathogenesis

In the late 19th century, Osler (76) first used the term *mycotic* to describe the peripheral, infected aneurysms occurring in patients with bacterial endocarditis. The beaded gross appearance of the multiple aneurysms in these patients resembled a fungus growth, hence the term *mycotic*. However, he delineated the pathogenesis to be destruction of the arterial wall subsequent to embolism with bacteria-laden material from the heart. In the era before antibiotics, the presence of such lesions indicated a malignant form of endocarditis because death was inevitable.

Mycotic aneurysms, as described by Osler, are now rare, and a more comprehensive term is *infected aneurysm* or *microbial arteritis* (77). Infected aneurysms include preexisting aneurysms that are secondarily infected by hematogenous or contiguous spread, infections of the arterial wall that subsequently cause aneurysmal degeneration, and contaminated false aneurysms resulting from direct trauma to the arterial wall (78). Currently, fewer than 10% of infected aneurysms are caused by bacterial endocarditis (79).

It is difficult to infect the normal arterial wall during bacteremia, but such a mechanism has been postulated in severely immunocompromised patients. Special risk factors for microbial arteritis include long-term steroid use, chemotherapy for malignancy, severe alcoholism, chronic renal failure, and extensive radiation therapy (80,81). Such infections may be initiated by the hematogenous spread of bacteria through the vasa vasorum. Much more common is the infection of abnormal arterial walls with irregular luminal surfaces, to which microorganisms attach during bacteremia (77). Arterial wall defects and irregularities associated with infected aneurysms include atherosclerotic plaque, degenerative arterial aneurysms, and congenital abnormalities such as aortic coarctation and patent ductus arteriosus. Host compromise, malnutrition, and advanced age are also seen in many of these patients. Contiguous spread of infection is common in infected aortic aneurysms and is seen in such conditions as spinal osteomyelitis, pancreatitis, and retroperitoneal abscess associated with diverticulitis and other gastrointestinal and severe urinary infections (77). Trauma is becoming an increasingly common mechanism by which infected aneurysms develop; bacteria are introduced at the time of intraarterial drug injection with contaminated needles (drug abuse) (82) or the placement of arterial catheters for diagnostic and therapeutic interventions or for monitoring. Almost all infected arterial aneurysms associated with trauma are false aneurysms in which arterial wall continuity is lost.

In reports of infected preexisting aortic aneurysms, gram-positive organisms predominate over gram-negative organisms and are present in about 60% of cases (77,83). Of these, *Staphylococcus* species are the most prevalent, with *S. aureus* being the most commonly encountered overall. Streptococci are also etiologic agents, with *Streptococcus viridans* being the most common subtype. In iatrogenic arterial infections associated with indwelling arterial catheters, methicillin-resistant *S. aureus* and other nosocomial organisms are being seen with increasing frequency.

Salmonella is the most prevalent organism associated with infection of a non-aneurysmal aorta (77,81,83,84). The diseased, plaque-ridden aorta has a unique susceptibility to *Salmonella* infections. *S. choleraesuis* and *S. enteritidis*, especially the subtype *S. typhimurium,* account for more than half of reported cases of *Salmonella* aortitis (77).

Gram-negative arterial infections are much more virulent than gram-positive infections, and arteries infected with gram-negative organisms are much more prone to rupture. Gram-negative organisms such as *Pseudomonas aeruginosa* can elaborate alkaline proteinase and a variety of elastases that cause vascular wall necrosis (23). In addition, many bacteria, both gram-positive and gram-negative, produce collagenases (85–87). Bacteria can also upregulate collagenases and metalloproteinases in the inflammatory cells associated with aneurysms (87). Recent interest has centered on neutrophil elastase in the pathogenesis of aneurysms (88). According to this view,

bacteria may play an indirect role, acting principally through the recruitment of acute inflammatory cells, which subsequently release neutrophil elastase.

Once the arterial wall is infected, rapid, focal, and progressive deterioration occurs. The process results in the characteristic saccular or multiloculated appearance of these aneurysms and often leads to locally contained rupture and the formation of a false aneurysm. In aortas without a preexisting aneurysm, infected aneurysms tend to occur in the posterior wall of the suprarenal or supraceliac aorta (77,80,81). When a preexisting aortic aneurysm becomes secondarily infected, the infrarenal location is the most common site (83,89,90).

Clinical Presentation

The clinical presentation of an infected aneurysm depends on the virulence of the organism, the anatomic location, and the duration of infection. *Salmonella* aortic infections may present after a febrile gastrointestinal illness. The presence of a tender abdominal aortic aneurysm in such a patient in association with continued fever and positive blood cultures strongly suggests this diagnosis. Infection of a preexisting aortic aneurysm may present as fever of unknown origin, malaise, or back and flank pain. Such patients are frequently debilitated, malnourished, and immunocompromised as the result of chronic illness, and the presence of an aortic aneurysm and positive blood cultures in this setting should arouse suspicion of an infected aneurysm. Chronic osteomyelitis or other retroperitoneal infectious processes contiguous to the aorta may also be present.

Infected aortic aneurysms are prone to rupture, even when small (83,84). They may have been unsuspected before rupturing, and the diagnosis of infection may not be obvious at the time of emergency operation (89). The diagnosis should be entertained in a patient presenting with a ruptured aortic aneurysm who has a fever and an elevated white blood cell count, especially when the aneurysm is small (< 5 cm in diameter). At operation, additional clues include the presence of chronically inflamed retroperitoneal tissues with indistinct dissection planes and a focal aneurysm with relatively normal aorta above and below the site. Gram's stains of smears from involved tissues and thrombus may be diagnostic, and cultures should be obtained even if the results of Gram's stains are negative.

In contrast to aortic and other central aneurysms, peripheral infected aneurysms are usually readily apparent and the diagnosis obvious. A painful, cellulitic, warm pulsatile mass over a major artery in a febrile patient is a common clinical presentation (82). An elevated white blood cell count and positive blood cultures are usual. The patient may have a history of drug abuse, and inadvertent or deliberate arterial injection with a contaminated needle should be suspected (82). The common femoral artery is the most common site, and a prior history of arterial catheterization or the presence of an indwelling angiographic catheter or sheath for endovascular procedures is being increasingly seen. Many of these procedures require repeated angiography and manipulation during prolonged periods, and femoral arterial sheaths or catheters are left in place for access. This increases the opportunity for arterial infection, and the risk is proportional to catheter residence time.

Diagnosis

Infected aortic aneurysms can be difficult to diagnose. Leukocytosis is sensitive but not specific for an infected

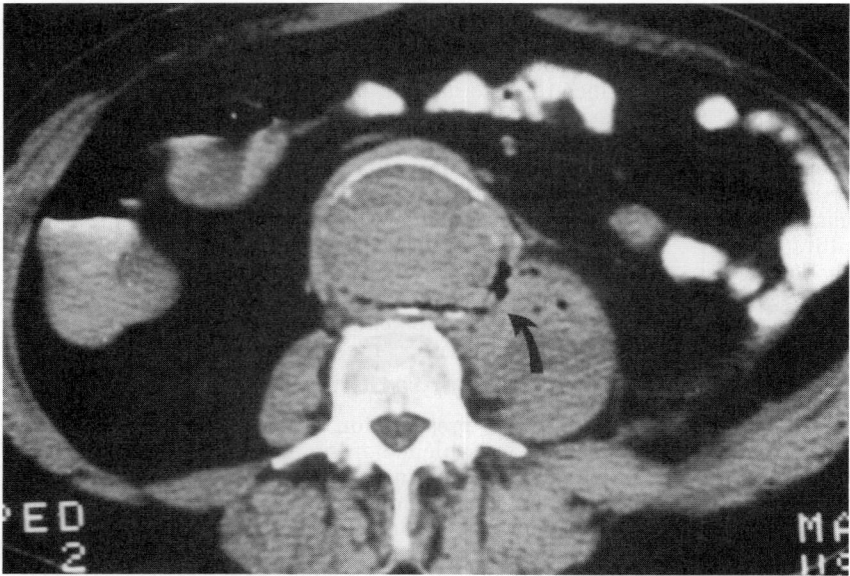

Figure 73.6. Computed tomogram of an infected aortic aneurysm. Gas *(arrow)* is present within the aorta and adjacent soft tissue.

aneurysm. Blood cultures are important but may be negative in as many as 50% of patients with an infected aortic aneurysm (77). Positive blood cultures in the presence of an abdominal aortic aneurysm should be considered evidence of an infected aneurysm until they are proven otherwise.

Radiologic studies are useful in confirming the diagnosis; CT and aortography are the most important tests (84). MRI may also be helpful. CT and MRI will demonstrate the aneurysm and may show perivascular retroperitoneal inflammation and edema. A contained rupture may be present and suggests the diagnosis. The presence of periaortic air along with inflammatory changes is diagnostic (Fig. 73.6). Arteriography may aid in the diagnosis but is most useful in planning arterial reconstruction. A saccular aneurysm in an otherwise normal-appearing vessel or a multilobulated aneurysm strongly suggests the presence of aortic infection (77) (Fig. 73.7).

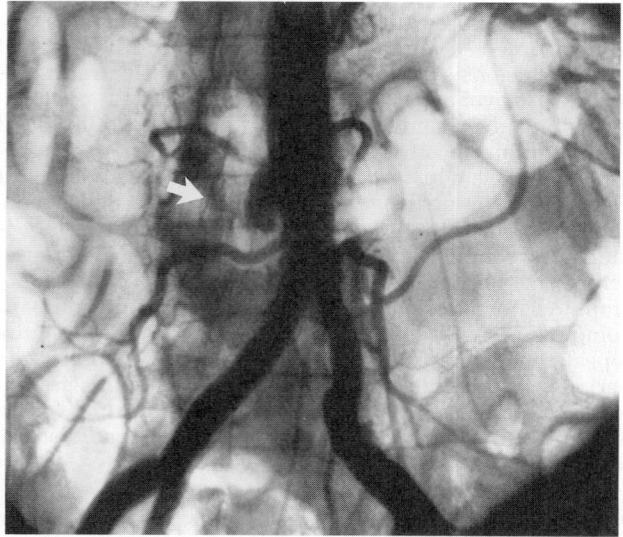

Figure 73.7. Arteriogram demonstrating a focal, saccular aneurysm *(arrow)* in an otherwise relatively normal infrarenal aorta.

Treatment

Although culture-specific antibiotic therapy is important in the treatment of an infected aneurysm, surgical therapy is almost always necessary and lifesaving. Antibiotic therapy is started preoperatively and continued for at least 6 weeks after operation (80). Surgical treatment must be expeditious because of the risk for aneurysm rupture and death. Reports of rupture of an infected aneurysm during prolonged antibiotic therapy in an attempt to sterilize the aneurysm reinforce the urgency of expeditious operation (77).

The principles of treatment of an infected aneurysm are similar to those of surgical therapy of an infected arterial prosthesis: eradication of infection by resection of the infected aneurysm and surrounding tissues, and creation of a new bypass to restore circulation. Most authorities favor creating a new bypass through clean tissues. For infected aortoiliac aneurysms, axillofemoral bypass is most commonly performed (79,81,84,89,92). For infected femoral aneurysms, an obturator bypass from the common iliac to the distal superficial femoral artery with a vascular prosthesis or vein graft routed through the obturator foramen successfully avoids the infected groin and restores distal circulation (82) (Fig. 73.8).

Prosthetic reconstruction in situ has been successfully used for infected aortic aneurysms when gross purulence is absent and contamination is minimal (80,83,90,92). It is especially appropriate in patients with an aortic aneurysm that ruptures into the overlying duodenum, a condition usually referred to as *primary aortoduodenal fistula.* Contamination is minimal in this condition, and long-term results with prosthetic reconstruction in situ are good (83,92,93). Patients treated in this manner require close follow-up because of the risk for recurrent infection, and most should be treated with lifelong oral antibiotics. Prosthetic reconstruction in situ is usually necessary for unstable patients with ruptured, infected aortic aneurysms (83). Extraanatomic bypass is not feasible in this circumstance because of the prolonged lower extremity ischemia time, especially when hypotension has been present. Overall mortality for patients with an infected aortic aneurysm is approximately 25% and is higher when rupture is present (77).

A promising new approach involves harvesting superficial femoral popliteal veins to reconstruct the aortoiliac

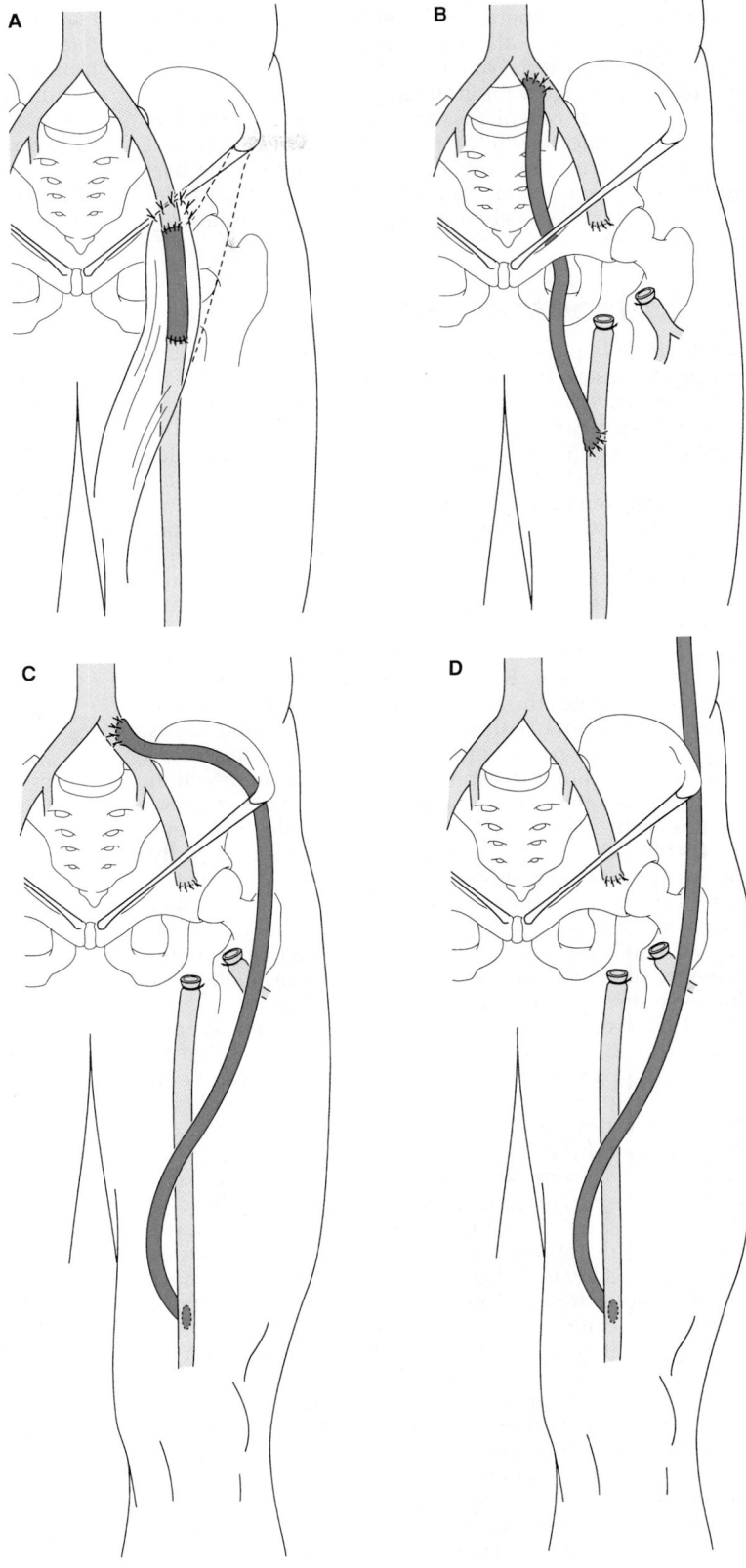

Figure 73.8. Methods of femoral artery reconstruction after excision and ligation of a femoral mycotic aneurysm. *(A)* Interposition vein autograft with sartorius muscle flap coverage. *(B)* Obturator bypass. *(C)* Lateral femoral bypass. *(D)* Unilateral axillofemoral bypass. (From Reddy DJ, Smith RF, Elliott JP Jr, et al. Infected femoral artery false aneurysms in drug addicts: evolution of selective vascular reconstruction. *J Vasc Surg* 1986;3:718, with permission.)

system after resection of an infected aneurysm and débridement of retroperitoneal tissues (47) (Fig. 73.8). These vein grafts have also been used to replace infected common femoral arterial aneurysms associated with drug abuse (82). The large vein grafts appear to be resistant to infection by most organisms, and disruption when they are placed in infected fields has not been reported. Because of the additional operative time required for harvesting veins, reconstruction in situ with superficial femoral popliteal veins should be performed in relatively stable patients.

SEPTIC THROMBOPHLEBITIS

Septic thrombophlebitis most commonly involves upper extremity and neck veins after the insertion of intravenous catheters and needles or intravenous drug abuse. However, venous thrombi can become secondarily infected during bacteremia or contiguity with areas of infection. Examples of contiguous infection include pelvic septic thrombophlebitis developing after obstetric infection (94), internal jugular thrombophlebitis associated with severe pharyngitis and peritonsillar abscess (95), and visceral thrombophlebitis stemming from appendicitis. *S. aureus* is the most common organism cultured from patients with peripheral septic thrombophlebitis, and gram-negative and polymicrobial infections are common when a contiguous infection is the cause. Regardless of the source, infected thrombus propagates throughout the lumen of the involved vein, and septicemia with high spiking fevers and chills quickly develops. An intense perivascular inflammatory response accompanies the spread of intraluminal infection and is clinically manifest by marked edema, pain, tenderness, and erythema overlying the involved vein. *S. aureus* and other virulent organisms infecting clot can rapidly form an intravascular abscess. In this circumstance, the lumen of the vein becomes a "closed space," and excision or surgical drainage is necessary to treat the infection. Propagation of the infected clot can also give rise to septic pulmonary embolism resulting in pneumonia, metastatic pulmonary abscess, and septic pleural effusion.

The clinical diagnosis is readily apparent when peripheral veins in the extremities are involved. In addition to pain, swelling, and redness along the course of the vein, pus may be expressed at the site of catheter or needle insertion. When deep or central veins are involved, the diagnosis is more difficult. These patients may present with clinical signs of severe sepsis and occasionally with complications of septic pulmonary embolism. CT or MRI can be particularly helpful and may demonstrate enlarged, dilated veins with intravenous thrombus and perivascular inflammatory changes. These imaging modalities are most useful for septic thrombophlebitis involving iliofemoral, caval, axillary–subclavian, and pelvic veins.

The treatment of septic thrombophlebitis depends on its anatomic location. Along with antibiotic therapy, excision of a superficial vein in an extremity is curative (96–98). One must take care to remove the entire length of involved vein to eradicate infection. When deep veins of an extremity or central veins of the chest or pelvis are involved, vein excision is difficult and associated with large losses of blood and severe morbidity. The mainstays of therapy for septic deep or central vein thrombophlebitis are intensive antibiotic therapy and heparin anticoagulation to halt the thrombotic process and prevent embolism (99). Therapy may have to be continued for 2 to 3 weeks and is successful in most cases. If it is not successful and sepsis continues despite medical therapy, surgical intervention is indicated. Venous thrombectomy and vein excision have been reported to be successful in cases refractory to medical therapy (94). When thrombectomy of the iliocaval system is undertaken, placement of a stainless steel caval filtration device (Greenfield filter) for protection against pulmonary embolism may be advisable (100). Sepsis does not preclude placement of these devices. In advanced cases in which abscess forms within large veins that cannot be subjected to thrombectomy because of organization of thrombus and vein scarring, abscess drainage and débridement are indicated.

REFERENCES

1. Balas P. An overview of aortofemoral graft infection. *Eur J Vasc Endovasc Surg* 1997;14[Suppl A]:3–4.
2. Kearney RA, Eisen HJ, Wolf JE. Nonvalvular infections of the cardiovascular system. *Ann Intern Med* 1994;121:219–230.
3. O'Brien T, Collin J. Prosthetic vascular graft infection. *Br J Surg* 1992;79:1262–1267.
4. Lorentzen JE, Nielsen OM, Arendrup H, et al. Vascular graft infection: an analysis of sixty-two graft infections in 2,411 consecutively implanted synthetic vascular grafts. *Surgery* 1985;98:81–86.
5. Seabrook GR. Pathobiology of graft infections. *Semin Vasc Surg* 1990;3:81–88.
6. Bandyk DF, Berni GA, Thiele BL, et al. Aortofemoral graft infection due to *Staphylococcus epidermidis*. *Arch Surg* 1984;119:102–108.
7. Jones L, Braithwaite BD, Davies B, et al. Mechanism of late prosthetic vascular graft infection. *Cardiovasc Surg* 1997;5:486–489.
8. Schwartz JA, Powell TW, Burnham SJ, et al. Culture of abdominal aortic aneurysm contents. *Arch Surg* 1987;122:777–780.
9. Ernst CB, Campbell HC, Daugherty ME, et al. Incidence and significance of intra-operative bacterial cultures during abdominal aortic aneurysmectomy. *Ann Surg* 1977;185:626–633.
10. Padberg FT Jr, Smith SM, Eng RHK. Accuracy of disincorporation for identification of vascular graft infection. *Arch Surg* 1995;130:183–187.
11. Bandyk DF, Bergamini TM, Kinney EV, et al. In situ replacement of vascular prostheses infected by bacterial biofilms. *J Vasc Surg* 1991;13:575–583.
12. Merritt K, Hitchins VM, Neale AR. Tissue colonization from implantable biomaterials with low numbers of bacteria. *J Biomed Mater Res* 1999;44:261–265.
13. Kaplan SS, Basford RE, Jeong MH, et al. Mechanisms of biomaterial-induced superoxide release by neutrophils. *J Biomed Mater Res* 1994;28:377–386.
14. Kaplan SS, Basford RE, Jeong MH, et al. Biomaterial–neutrophil interactions: dysregulation of oxidative functions of fresh neutrophils induced by prior neutrophil–biomaterial interaction. *J Biomed Mater Res* 1996;30:67–75.
15. Kaplan SS, Heine RP, Simmons RL. Defensins impair phagocytic killing by neutrophils in biomaterials-related infection. *Infect Immun* 1999;67:1640–1645.
16. Brunstedt MR, Sapatnekar S, Rubin KR, et al. Bacterial/blood/material interactions. I. Injected and preseeded slime-forming *Staphylococcus epidermidis* in flowing blood with biomaterials. *J Biomed Mater Res* 1995;29:455–466.
17. Wang I, Anderson JM, Jacobs MR, et al. Adhesion of *Staphylococcus epidermidis* to biomedical polymers: contributions of surface thermodynamics and hemodynamic shear conditions. *J Biomed Mater Res* 1995;29:485–493.
18. Shive MS, Hasan SM, Anderson JM. Shear stress effects on bacterial adhesion, leukocyte adhesion, and leukocyte oxidative capacity on a polyetherurethane. *J Biomed Mater Res* 1999;46:511–519.
19. Veenstra GC, Cremers FFM, van Dijk H, et al. Ultrastructural organization and regulation of a biomaterial adhesion of *Staphylococcus epidermidis*. *J Bacteriol* 1996;178:537–541.
20. Mack D, Riedewald J, Rohde H, et al. Essential functional role of the polysaccharide intercellular adhesion of *Staphylococcus epidermidis* in hemagglutination. *Infect Immun* 1999;67:1004–1008.

21. Rupp ME, Ulphani JS, Fey PD, et al. Characterization of the importance of polysaccharide intercellular adhesin/hemagglutinin of *Staphylococcus epidermidis* in the pathogenesis of biomaterial-based infection in a mouse foreign body infection model. *Infect Immun* 1999;67:2627–2632.

22. Henke PK, Bergamini TM, Watson AL, et al. Bacterial products primarily mediate fibroblast inhibition in biomaterial infection. *J Surg Res* 1998;74:17–22.

23. Geary KJ, Tomkiewicz ZM, Harrison HN, et al. Differential effects of a gram-negative and a gram-positive infection on autogenous and prosthetic grafts. *J Vasc Surg* 1990;11:339–347.

24. Modrall JG, Clagett GP. The role of imaging techniques in evaluating possible graft infections. *Semin Vasc Surg* 1999; 12:339–347.

25. Low RN, Wall SD, Jeffrey RB, et al. Aortoenteric fistula and perigraft infection: evaluation with CT. *Radiology* 1990;175: 157–162.

26. Qvafordt PG, Reilly LM, Mark AS, et al. Computerized tomographic assessment of graft incorporation after reconstruction. *Am J Surg* 1985;150:227–231.

27. Auffermann W, Olofsson PA, Rabahie GN, et al. Incorporation versus infection of retroperitoneal aortic grafts: MR imaging features. *Radiology* 1989;172:359–362.

28. Brunner MC, Mitchell RS, Baldwin JC, et al. Prosthetic graft infection: limitations of indium white blood cell scanning. *J Vasc Surg* 1986;3:42–48.

29. Fiorani P, Speziale F, Rizzo L, et al. Detection of aortic graft infection with leukocytes labeled with technetium 99m-hexametazime. *J Vasc Surg* 1993;17:87–96.

30. LaMuraglia GM, Fischman AJ, Strauss HW, et al. Utility of the indium 111-labeled human immunoglobulin G scan for the detection of focal vascular graft infection. *J Vasc Surg* 1989;10:20–28.

31. O'Hara PJ, Hertzer NR, Beven EG, et al. Surgical management of infected abdominal aortic grafts: review of a 25-year experience. *J Vasc Surg* 1986;2:725–731.

32. Reilly LM, Stoney RJ, Goldstone J, et al. Improved management of aortic graft infection: the influence of operation sequence and staging. *J Vasc Surg* 1987;5:421–431.

33. Quinones-Baldrich WJ, Hernandez JJ, Moore WS. Long-term results following surgical management of aortic graft infection. *Arch Surg* 1991;126:507–511.

34. Ricotta JJ, Faggioli GL, Stella A, et al. Total excision and extra-anatomic bypass for aortic graft infection. *Am J Surg* 1991;162:145–149.

35. Leather RP, Darling RC III, Chang BB, et al. Retroperitoneal in-line aortic bypass for treatment of infected infrarenal aortic grafts. *Surg Gynecol Obstet* 1992;175:491–494.

36. Olah A, Vogt M, Laske A, et al. Axillo-femoral bypass and simultaneous removal of the aorto-femoral vascular infection site: is the procedure safe? *Eur J Vasc Surg* 1992;6:252–254.

37. Bacourt F, Koskas F, and the French University Association for Research in Surgery. Axillobifemoral bypass and aortic exclusion for vascular septic lesions: a multicenter retrospective study of 98 cases. *Ann Vasc Surg* 1992;6:119–126.

38. Lehnert T, Gruber HP, Maeder N, et al. Management of primary aortic graft infection by extra-anatomic bypass reconstruction. *Eur J Vasc Surg* 1993;7:301–307.

39. Sharp WJ, Hoballah JJ, Mohan CR, et al. The management of the infected aortic prosthesis: a current decade of experience. *J Vasc Surg* 1994;19:844–850.

40. Kuestner LM, Reilly LM, Jicha DL, et al. Secondary aortoenteric fistula: contemporary outcome with use of extraanatomic bypass and infected graft excision. *J Vasc Surg* 1995;21:184–196.

41. Hannon RJ, Wolfe JHN, Mansfield AO. Aortic prosthetic infection: 50 patients treated by radical or local surgery. *Br J Surg* 1996;83:654–658.

42. Schmitt DD, Seabrook GR, Bandyk DF, et al. Graft excision and extraanatomic revascularization: the treatment of choice for the septic aortic prosthesis. *J Cardiovasc Surg* 1990;31: 327–332.

43. Bunt TJ. Vascular graft infections: a personal experience. *Cardiovasc Surg* 1993;1:489–492.

44. Yeager RA, Taylor LM, Moneta GL, et al. Improved results with conventional management of infrarenal aortic infection. *J Vasc Surg* 1999;30:76–83.

45. Clagett GP, Bowers BL, Lopez-Viego MA, et al. Creation of a neo-aortoiliac system from lower extremity deep and superficial veins. *Ann Surg* 1993;218:239–249.

46. Nevelsteen A, Lacroix H, Suy R. Autogenous reconstruction with the lower extremity deep veins: an alternative treatment of prosthetic infection after reconstructive surgery for aortoiliac disease. *J Vasc Surg* 1995;22:129–134.

47. Clagett GP, Valentine RJ, Hagino RT. Autogenous aortoiliac/femoral reconstruction from superficial femoral-popliteal veins: feasibility and durability. *J Vasc Surg* 1997;25: 255–270.

48. Kieffer E, Bahnini A, Koskas F, et al. In situ allograft replacement of infected infrarenal aortic prosthetic grafts: results in forty-three patients. *J Vasc Surg* 1993;17:349–356.

49. Vogt PR, Pfammatter T, Schlumph R, et al. In situ repair of aortobronchial, aortoesophageal, and aortoenteric fistulae with cryopreserved aortic homografts. *J Vasc Surg* 1997;26: 11–17.

50. Ruotolo C, Plissonnier D, Bahnini A, et al. In situ arterial allografts: a new treatment for aortic prosthetic infection. *Eur J Vasc Endovasc Surg* 1997;14[Suppl A]:102–107.

51. Nevelsteen A, Feryn T, Lacroix H, et al. Experience with cryopreserved arterial allografts in the treatment of prosthetic graft infections. *Cardiovasc Surg* 1998;4:378–383.

52. Chiesa R, Astore S, Piccolo G, et al. Fresh and cryopreserved arterial homografts in the treatment of prosthetic graft infections: experience of the Italian Collaborative Vascular Homograft Group. *Ann Vasc Surg* 1998;12:457–462.

53. Walker WE, Cooley DA, Duncan JM, et al. The management of aortoduodenal fistula by in situ replacement of the infected abdominal aortic graft. *Ann Surg* 1987;205:727–732.

54. Speziale F, Rizzo L, Sbarigia E, et al. Bacterial and clinical criteria relating to the outcome of patients undergoing in situ replacement of infected abdominal aortic grafts. *Eur J Vasc Endovasc Surg* 1997;13:127–133.

55. Hayes PD, Nasim A, London NJM, et al. In situ replacement of infected aortic grafts with rifampicin-bonded prostheses: the Leicester experience (1992 to 1998). *J Vasc Surg* 1999;30:92–98.

56. Young RM, Cherry KJ Jr, Davis PM, et al. The results of in situ prosthetic replacement for infected aortic grafts. *Am J Surg* 1999;178:136–140.

57. Clagett GP. Treatment of aortic graft infection. In: Ernst CB, Stanley JC, eds. *Current therapy in vascular surgery*, 4th ed. Philadelphia: Mosby 2001;422–428.

58. Wells JK, Hagino RT, Bargmann KM, et al. Venous morbidity after superficial femoral–popliteal vein harvest. *J Vasc Surg* 1999;29:282–291.

59. Koskas F, Plissonnier D, Bahnini A, et al. In situ arterial allografting for aortoiliac graft infection: a 6-year experience. *Cardiovasc Surg* 1996;4:495–499.

60. Calligaro KD, Veith FJ, Schwartz ML, et al. Selective preservation of infected prosthetic arterial grafts: analysis of a 20-year experience with 120 extracavitary infected grafts. *Ann Surg* 1994;220:461–471.

61. Morris GE, Friend PJ, Vassallo DJ, et al. Antibiotic irrigation and conservative surgery for major aortic graft infection. *J Vasc Surg* 1994;20:88–95.

62. Belair M, Soulez G, Oliva VL, et al. Aortic graft infection: the value of percutaneous drainage. *Am J Radiol* 1998;171: 119–124.

63. Calligaro KD, Veith FJ. Graft-preserving methods for managing aortofemoral prosthetic graft infection. *Eur J Vasc Endovasc Surg* 1997;14[Suppl A]:38–42.

64. Becquemin JP, Qvarfordt P, Kron J, et al. Aortic graft infection: is there a place for partial graft removal? *Eur J Vasc Endovasc Surg* 1997;14[Suppl A]:53–58.

65. Miller JH. Partial replacement of an infected arterial graft by a new prosthetic polytetrafluoroethylene segment: a new therapeutic option. *J Vasc Surg* 1993;17:546–558.

66. Towne JB, Seabrook GR, Bandyk D, et al. In situ replacement of arterial prosthesis infected by bacterial biofilms: long-term follow-up. *J Vasc Surg* 1994;19:226–235.

67. Sladen JG, Chen JC, Reid JDS. An aggressive local approach to vascular graft infection. *Am J Surg* 1998;176:222–225.

68. Mertens RA, O'Hara PJ, Hertzer NR, et al. Surgical management of infrainguinal arterial prosthetic graft infections: re-

view of a thirty-five year experience. *J Vasc Surg* 1995;21: 782–791.

69. Kikta MJ, Goodson SF, Bishara RA, et al. Mortality and limb loss with infected infrainguinal bypass grafts. *J Vasc Surg* 1987;5:566–571.

70. Cherry KJ, Roland CF, Pairolero PC, et al. Infected femorodistal bypass: is graft removal mandatory? *J Vasc Surg* 1992;15: 295–303.

71. Kaiser AB, Clayson KR, Mulherin JL, et al. Antibiotic prophylaxis in vascular surgery. *Ann Surg* 1978;188:283–288.

72. Pitt HA, Postier RG, MacGowan WAL, et al. Prophylactic antibiotics in vascular surgery: topical, systemic, or both? *Ann Surg* 1980;192:356–364.

73. Hasselgren P, Ivarsson L, Risberg B, et al. Effects of prophylactic antibiotics in vascular surgery: a prospective, randomized, double-blind study. *Ann Surg* 1984;200:86–92.

74. Hall JC, Christiansen KJ, Goodman M, et al. Duration of antimicrobial prophylaxis in vascular surgery. *Am J Surg* 1998; 175:87–90.

75. Kurz A, Sessler DL, Lenhardt R, and the Study of Wound Infection and Temperature Group. Perioperative normothermia to reduce the incidence of surgical wound infection and shorten hospitalization. *N Engl J Med* 1996;334:1209–1215.

76. Osler W. The Gulstonian lectures on malignant endocarditis. *Br Med J* 1885;1:467–470.

77. Reddy DJ, Ernst CB. Infected aortic aneurysms: recognition and management. *Semin Vasc Surg* 1988;1:174–181.

78. Patel S, Johnston KW. Classification and management of mycotic aneurysms. *Surg Gynecol Obstet* 1977;144:691–694.

79. Dean RH, Waterhouse G, Meacham PW, et al. Mycotic embolism and embolomycotic aneurysms. *Ann Surg* 1986;204: 300–307.

80. Chan FY, Crawford ES, Coselli JS, et al. In situ prosthetic graft replacement for mycotic aneurysm of the aorta. *Ann Thorac Surg* 1989;47:193–203.

81. Oz MC, Brener BJ, Buda JA, et al. A ten-year experience with bacterial aortitis. *J Vasc Surg* 1989;10:439–449.

82. Benjamin ME, Cohn EJ, Purtill WA, et al. Arterial reconstruction with deep leg veins for the treatment of mycotic aneurysms. *J Vasc Surg* 1999;30:1004–1015.

83. Fichelle JM, Tabet G, Cormier P, et al. Infected infrarenal aortic aneurysms: when is in situ reconstruction safe? *J Vasc Surg* 1993;17:635–645.

84. Gomes MN, Choyke PL, Wallace RB. Infected aortic aneurysms: a changing entity. *Ann Surg* 1992;215:435–442.

85. McGregor JA, Lawellin D, Franco-Buff A, et al. Protease production by microorganisms associated with reproductive tract infection. *Am J Obstet Gynecol* 1986;154:109–114.

86. Tilson MD, Newman KM. Proteolytic mechanisms in the pathogenesis of aortic aneurysms. In: Yao JST, Pearce WH, eds. *Aneurysms: new findings and treatments.* Norwalk, CT: Appleton & Lange, 1994:3–10.

87. Pierce RA, Sandefur S, Doyle GA, et al. Monocytic cell type-specific transcriptional induction of collagenase. *J Clin Invest* 1996;97:1890–1899.

88. Buckmaster MJ, Curci JA, Murray PR, et al. Source of elastin-degrading enzymes in mycotic aortic aneurysms: bacteria or host inflammatory response? *Cardiovasc Surg* 1999;7:16–26.

89. Reddy DJ, Shepard AD, Evans JR, et al. Management of infected aortoiliac aneurysms. *Arch Surg* 1991;126:873–879.

90. Sessa C, Farah I, Voirin L, et al. Infected aneurysms of the infrarenal abdominal aorta: diagnostic criteria and therapeutic strategy. *Ann Vasc Surg* 1997;11:453–463.

91. Moneta GL, Taylor LM Jr, Yeager RA, et al. Surgical treatment of infected aortic aneurysm. *Am J Surg* 1998;175:396–399.

92. Robinson JA, Johansen K. Aortic sepsis: is there a role for in situ graft reconstruction? *J Vasc Surg* 1991;13:677–684.

93. Daugherty M, Shearer GG, Ernst CB. Primary aortoduodenal fistula: extraanatomic vascular reconstruction not required for successful management. *Surgery* 1979;86:399–401.

94. Kniemeyer HW, Grabitz K, Buhl R, et al. Surgical treatment of septic deep venous thrombosis. *Surgery* 1995;118:49–53.

95. Bach MC, Roediger JH, Rinder HM. Septic anaerobic jugular phlebitis with pulmonary embolism: problems in management. *Rev Infect Dis* 1988;10:424–427.

96. Leonard JD, Printen KJ. Thrombophlebitis in the elderly. *Am Surg* 1980;46:441.

97. Munster AM. Septic thrombophlebitis: a surgical disorder. *JAMA* 1974;230:1010.

98. Pruitt BA Jr, McManus WF, Kim SH, et al. Diagnosis and treatment of cannula-related intravenous sepsis in burn patients. *Ann Surg* 1980;191:546.

99. Ang AK, Brown OW. Septic deep vein thrombosis. *J Vasc Surg* 1986;4:563–566.

100. Hoffman MJ, Greenfield LJ. Central venous septic thrombosis managed by superior vena cava Greenfield filter and venous thrombectomy: a case report. *J Vasc Surg* 1986;4: 606–611.

SURGERY: SCIENTIFIC PRINCIPLES AND PRACTICE, Third Edition, edited by Lazar J. Greenfield, Michael W. Mulholland, Keith T. Oldham, Gerald B. Zelenock, and Keith D. Lillemoe. Lippincott Williams & Wilkins Publishers, Philadelphia, © 2001.

CHAPTER 74

BASIC ENDOVASCULAR CONSIDERATIONS AND SURGICAL TECHNIQUES

MICHAEL J. ROHRER AND KIM J. HODGSON

The Portuguese neurologist Moniz (1) is credited with being the first to perform contrast arteriography. In 1927, he injected sodium iodide by direct puncture into the carotid arteries. In 1953, Seldinger (2) described the use of coaxial guide wires to gain access to the vascular system. This technique, which bears his name, won him a Nobel Prize and provided the foundation for the development of most of the endovascular techniques in use today. Radiologic vascular imaging, however, was limited to diagnostic use until Dotter and Judkins (3) performed the first arterial dilation in 1964. They used a series of graduated dilators, introduced percutaneously and guided under radiologic imaging, to dilate a superficial femoral artery stenosis. Since that date, exponential growth in the numbers of diagnostic and therapeutic procedures performed by means of endovascular techniques has been fueled by the development of high-pressure–low-compliance balloons and various types of stents to manage both early and late complications of balloon angioplasty. Other devices have been designed to facilitate the extraction of thrombus from occluded vessels, and pharmacologic research has produced several drugs, operating through a variety of pathways, that have proved effective in lysing thrombus. Advances in fiberoptic technology and optical miniaturization paved the way for the development of angioscopy, while research in physics led to the development of ultrasonic probes that could image the inner surface of the arterial wall. These initially diagnostic modalities are now being used therapeutically; for example, coils can be delivered through an angioscope to occlude in situ vein graft branches, and intravascular ultrasonography guides the placement of vena caval filters and endografts.

The minimally invasive nature of endovascular techniques to treat occlusive and aneurysmal disease makes them very attractive alternatives to traditional operative reconstructions. In addition to the obvious patient preference for less invasive, less painful, and less disabling interventions, there exists the opportunity to realize cost savings through the decreased utilization of expensive inpatient hospital resources. Therefore, it is the responsibility of the vascular surgeon, who is often the only adequately trained vascular specialist involved, to evaluate the patient before intervention, define the indications for intervention, perform the endovascular or surgical procedure, and provide timely and responsible follow-up.

By virtue of their surgical training, vascular and general surgeons are thoroughly familiar with the pathology, natural history, and operative management of peripheral vascular diseases; however, to be able to perform endovascular procedures, they must acquire expertise in the fields of radiologic imaging and radiation safety, catheter and guide wire skills, familiarity with the techniques of balloon angioplasty and stent placement, and familiarity with the uses of intravascular ultrasonography, angioscopy, and thrombolytic drugs. At the moment, because of the relatively large delivery systems in use, a combination of endovascular and operative skills is needed to perform aortic endografting. However, future refinements in endograft devices and puncture closure devices may render surgical vascular access unnecessary and so diminish the role of vascular surgeons in these procedures. With the addition of the above-mentioned skills to their armamentarium, vascular surgeons will continue to play a role in the treatment of vascular diseases, and will also be able to offer comprehensive diagnostic and therapeutic care to patients with peripheral vascular disease. In this way, they will be able to make objective treatment decisions, free of the bias inherently present when the controlling physician is able perform only some of the available therapeutic procedures.

FUNDAMENTALS OF RADIOLOGIC IMAGING

Despite significant advances in less invasive methods of imaging the vascular system, such as duplex ultrasonography and magnetic resonance angiography, contrast arteriography remains the definitive method of imaging the arterial anatomy. Although it is an invasive technique, arteriography continues to be the imaging modality most commonly used to plan both operative and endovascular reconstructions. Because it provides a high level of image resolution and the opportunity for definitive and rapid feedback after interventions, contrast arteriography is the cornerstone of almost all endovascular interventions.

Generating Images

Traditionally, contrast angiography has been performed by placing a sheet of radiographic film between an anatomic region of interest and a source of x-rays while a radiopaque contrast agent is injected into the vessel to be studied. Although surgeons frequently perform "single-shot" completion arteriograms to evaluate newly created bypass grafts, comprehensive diagnostic angiography requires that a series of images be recorded while the contrast agent passes through the vessel of interest. To achieve this with the use of individual sheets of film, a mechanism is needed to move a series of films under the anatomic area of interest as it is exposed to x-rays, a technique referred to as *cut-film angiography.* Such rapid-sequence film changers can transport up to 30 individual films at a rate of six films per second. Although the anatomic resolution of these images is excellent, the films must be developed before the series of images can be viewed. Furthermore, a comprehensive diagnostic angiogram can easily generate dozens of sheets of film, only a few of which optimally characterize the pathologic region of interest, with the remainder representing a considerable

waste of resources. Other methods of recording angiographic images during contrast flow in vessels of interest include videoradiography, in which the fluoroscopic images are recorded on videotape for later review, and cineradiography, which involves the recording of radiographic images on motion picture film. Although this method may be advantageous for imaging the constantly moving heart during cardiac catheterization, it is less practical for imaging peripheral vessels, for which static images on stationary film have historically been the display medium of choice.

Advances in computer image processing have led to the development of digital subtraction angiography, a recording technique in which the fluoroscopic image is amplified and digitized; subsequent processing after angiography then enhances the quality of images obtained at the areas of interest. In perhaps the most powerful of these methods, the radiodensities of the surrounding tissues and vessel wall are *subtracted* from the images obtained after a contrast agent has been injected into the lumen of a vessel.

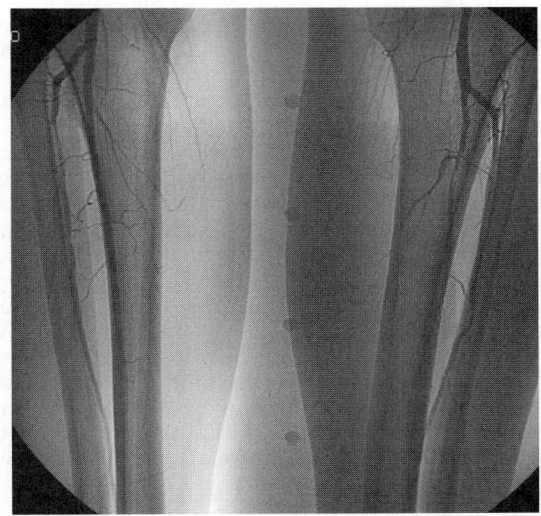

A

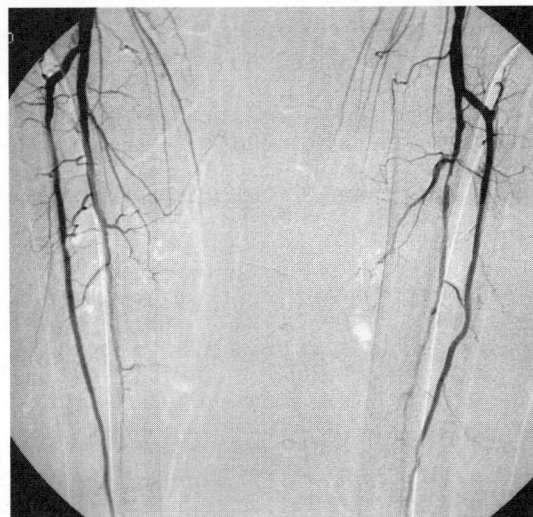

B

Figure 74.1. *(A)* Standard (nonsubtracted) angiogram of the trifurcation region. Overlying bone compromises visualization of the peroneal and anterior tibial arteries. *(B)* Identical view in digital subtraction mode. When background structures are digitally "subtracted" from the picture, the quality of the vascular image is enhanced.

Table 74.1. COMMONLY USED CONTRAST AGENTS AND THEIR PROPERTIES

Contrast agent	Manufacturer	Type	Iodine content (mg/mL)	Osmolality (mOsm/kg)
Conray 60	Mallinckrodt	Ionic	282	1,539
Isovue-300	Bracco Diagnostics	Non-ionic	300	524
Omnipaque 300	Nycomed	Non-ionic	300	672
Optiray 320	Mallinckrodt	Non-ionic	320	702
Renografin-60	Bracco Diagnostics	Ionic	292	1,549
Visipaque 320	Nycomed	Non-ionic	320	290

The computer algorithm digitally "subtracts" the pixels of the first image of the series (the "mask" image) from the subsequent images. This technique has the effect of visually eliminating background structures from the image and so enhances the quality of the vascular image (Fig. 74.1). However, for the quality of images obtained with digital subtraction techniques to be optimal, movement must be minimal between the time that the mask image is acquired and the time that the image of the vessel of interest with contrast opacification is acquired. Fortunately, most image processing systems allow any image of the series to be designated as the mask image, so that the undesirable consequences of movement occurring before the contrast agent reaches the vessel can be minimized by selecting as a new mask image one that was obtained after the movement occurred but before the contrast agent arrived.

Other useful digital postprocessing techniques include the use of pixel shifting, whereby the mask image is moved subtly over the contrast-enhanced image to realign the two and eliminate the image-degrading effect of movement. View tracing, in which early and late images are digitally combined to display a single image with complete opacification of the vessels of interest, can be valuable when transit time through the area being filmed is slow. In the technique of road mapping, an arteriographic image is displayed on the fluoroscopic monitor, with simultaneous superimposition of a real-time image showing the movement of endovascular devices within the vessel; this technique facilitates the passage of catheters or guide wires through complex vascular anatomy.

Contrast Agents

For intravascular anatomic imaging to be effective, an agent with a radiodensity different from that of the adjacent soft tissue must be injected into the vessels of interest at the time of the radiographic exposure. Typically, the radiodensity of the contrast agents used is greater than that of the surrounding tissues, usually because of the presence of radiodense iodine atoms. Vascular imaging can also be performed with an agent that is less radiopaque than the adjacent soft tissues, typically a gaseous agent. Although air is less radiodense than blood and soft tissue, its poor solubility in blood results in distal vascular occlusive problems, so that air is unsuitable as a contrast agent. The high solubility of carbon dioxide, however, allows it to be used successfully as an intravascular contrast agent. Unfortunately, carbon dioxide angiograms often lack sufficient clinical detail to be useful routinely, but they may be of value in the limited group of patients with severely compromised renal function, in whom the nephrotoxicity associated with iodinated contrast materials is a serious concern.

The angiographic contrast agents commercially available today are radiopaque by virtue of the presence of iodine atoms attached to one or more benzene rings. Conventional agents are compounds of one fully substituted benzene ring acting as an anion and a cationic component

(hence the designation "ionic" contrast agents) consisting of either sodium, methylglucamine, or a combination of the two. In solution, these contrast agents dissociate, so that their osmolality is doubled. More recently developed contrast agents have a non-ionic formulation and therefore do not dissociate in solution. The result is a high concentration of iodine atoms and therefore an effective contrast agent without the high osmolality that is responsible for much of the toxicity of the traditional contrast agents. Common, commercially available contrast agents and their properties are listed in Table 74.1.

RISKS OF ARTERIOGRAPHY

The safety of arteriography has been well documented during many years of use, but because of the invasive nature of the study and the exposure to iodinated contest agents, a small but real risk for significant complications exists. A mortality rate associated with aortography has been reported at 0.025%. Deaths have been caused by arterial dissection, aneurysm rupture, vasovagal and heart-related problems, neurologic complications, and renal failure [4]. The risk for complications is related to the site of vascular access; the incidence of complications requiring therapeutic intervention has been reported at 1.7%, 2.9%, 3.3%, and 7% after transfemoral, translumbar, axillary, and brachial artery punctures, respectively [4,5].

Technical Complications

The most common complication after angiography is bleeding at the arteriographic puncture site. Bleeding is more likely to occur in hypertensive patients, those undergoing therapeutic interventions (probably because of the need to place larger sheaths to insert appropriate endovascular hardware), and those taking anticoagulants or who have recently received thrombolytic agents [6]. Although small hematomas are commonplace, the need for intervention to address ongoing bleeding or false aneurysms occurs in fewer than 2% of patients. New developments in agents and devices to seal arterial puncture sites show promise to reduce this risk even further and perhaps allow the percutaneous use of endovascular devices that otherwise would require direct arterial access. Other potential technical complications include atheroembolization and the creation of arterial dissections. Although the latter can often be addressed in an endovascular procedure, the success of endovascular extraction of emboli or thrombolysis depends greatly on the size, nature, and age of the emboli.

Systemic Toxicity of Iodinated Contrast Agents

The most common side effects of contrast injection are nausea, vomiting, and discomfort, often described as an unpleasant sensation of warmth, in the distribution of the contrast infusion. This sensation can, at times, be frankly painful and is very closely related to the osmolality of the contrast agent and the extent to which it was diluted before infusion. Although uncommon, serious allergic reactions to iodinated contrast agents can be life-threatening. The relative rarity of such an occurrence is evidenced by the low incidence of contrast media complications during cardiac catheterization: 0.23%, with one death occurring in 55,000 contrast exposures (7). Contrast agents can also trigger the release of histamine, which is responsible for the development of symptoms ranging from urticaria to cardiopulmonary arrest. Although some of these reactions are mediated by immunoglobulin E antibodies and are therefore true anaphylactic reactions (7,8), most are anaphylactoid in origin (7). Nevertheless, histamine release, complement activation, and activation of other mediators produce a clinical presentation indistinguishable from true anaphylaxis (7).

The treatment of contrast-induced anaphylactoid reactions depends on the type and severity of the reaction. Minor reactions such as urticaria may be watched for signs of progression and treated with diphenhydramine (Benedryl) for symptomatic relief (7). Severe anaphylactoid reactions may necessitate endotracheal intubation and mechanical ventilation to support respiration, in addition to the infusion of large volumes of crystalloid to treat the associated hypotension. Epinephrine may also be required to support the blood pressure and treat the bronchoconstriction associated with severe reactions (7).

Clinical risk factors for the occurrence of systemic side effects during iodinated contrast injection include the following:

- History of reactions to contrast
- Asthma
- Other allergies to drugs and substances
- Anxiety

The administration of corticosteroids (100 mg of hydrocortisone intravenously or 32 mg of methylprednisolone orally, 12 and/or 2 hours prior) and diphenhydramine (Benadryl) before the injection of contrast media has proved effective at decreasing the rates of new and recurrent contrast-related side effects (7,9,10). In a multiinstitutional prospective, randomized study, 6,763 patients received 32 mg of methylprednisolone or placebo 12 and 2 hours before contrast exposure. Patients receiving two doses of steroids before receiving contrast had fewer reactions of all types ($p < .05$), although a single dose of methylprednisolone was sufficient to prevent minor hives and urticaria ($p < .055$) (10). Although the use of non-ionic, low-osmolality contrast agents does not eliminate these risks entirely, Katayama (11) demonstrated a reduction in the rates of all adverse reactions (from 0.22% to 0.04%) in patients receiving intravenous non-ionic, low-osmolality agents in comparison with those receiving ionic, high-osmolality agents. It has also been shown that the incidence of allergy-like reactions can be reduced by the use of the more expensive non-ionic contrast agents (8). Although it seems intuitively obvious that the procedure should be aborted in the setting of a major contrast-mediated reaction, at least some authors have recommended completing the diagnostic study if the patient can be stabilized because histamine stores should be relatively depleted (7).

Organ-specific Toxicity of Iodinated Contrast Agents

All presently available contrast agents are cleared from the body by glomerular filtration, with no appreciable tubular reabsorption. Although numerous risk factors for the development of renal failure after contrast exposure have been proposed, only the presence of preexisting renal dysfunction has been directly correlated with the development of this complication (12). Therefore, in patients with normal renal function, contrast infusion need not be limited for fear of causing contrast-related renal failure. However, in patients with diminished renal function or disorders associated with a hyperosmolar state (e.g., multiple myeloma), the contrast volume should be minimized and the adequacy of hydration and urine flow ascertained before elective angiography is undertaken. Another form of contrast-related toxicity that is less well recognized is a consequence of the effect of contrast on the cardiac conduction system, myocardial contractility, and coronary artery tone (13). This effect is generally manifested by a fall in heart rate and blood pressure and can be minimized by the use of a low-osmolality agent (13). Contrast agents of all types also cause red blood cells to aggregate and can lead to clot formation and possible emboli-related organ ischemia, obviously of great concern during cerebral and arch angiography.

Radiation Safety

Exposure of the patient and operator to ionizing radiation is an unavoidable aspect of angiographic and endovascular procedures. The requisite close proximity of the operator to the source of x-rays during fluoroscopically guided guide wire and catheter manipulation makes fluoroscopy the single greatest source of occupational radiation exposure in medicine today (13). As procedures have become more complex (e.g., endoluminal aortic grafting, angioplasty, stent placement, thrombolytic procedures), fluoroscopic times have increased substantially, and therefore the risk for excessive radiation exposure has increased for the patient, endovascular therapist, and support staff in the room.

The two approaches for limiting exposure to radiation are (a) minimizing the use of radiation and (b) shielding the operator from exposure. The simplest means of reducing radiation exposure to both the patient and the endovascular team is the judicious use of fluoroscopy during imaging procedures. Unless it is necessary to observe motion, fluoroscopy need not be in use and exposure to x-rays need not be incurred. Furthermore, when rectangular areas of interest, such as the extremities, are being imaged, it is possible to narrow the field of view to the area of interest (collimation); this not only reduces radiation output but often improves image quality. Lastly, fluoroscopic frame rates and power can be reduced to diminish radiation output, although image quality often suffers or the fluoroscopic motion becomes somewhat "choppy."

Lead aprons and thyroid shields are universally used by the operator and the endovascular team to shield the most radiation-sensitive organs: the thyroid, gonads, breasts, and bone marrow. It has been well documented that the thickness of lead aprons is the only variable that significantly affects the degree of radiation exposure recorded on monitoring badges worn beneath the aprons. The best protection is provided by aprons with a 1.0-mm layer of lead in front (14). Many endovascular therapists who perform large numbers of procedures wear leaded glasses with side shields during endovascular procedures to minimize the risk for cataract formation associated with exposure to radiation (13).

ANCILLARY ENDOVASCULAR DIAGNOSTIC IMAGING TECHNIQUES

Angioscopy

During angioscopy, the luminal surface of vascular structures can be visualized from remote access sites through the use of fiberoptic scopes that range in diameter from 0.8 to 3.3 mm, so that fairly small-diameter blood vessels can be inspected. Larger angioscopes with multiple lumina make it possible to administer clear crystalloid fluids under pressure to clear blood from the vascular lumen and perform an endovascular inspection. Additional lumina allow guide wires to be passed to facilitate selective vascular cannulation and the use of snares and valvulotomes to perform endovascular interventions. Originally, angioscopy, like endoscopy, required the operator to look through the end of the angioscope. In modern angioscopy, the angioscope is coupled to a video camera and the image is projected on monitors, so that the image is magnified and the entire operative team can review images.

Angioscopy has been utilized as a clinical adjunct to assess the completeness of thrombus removal during thrombectomy and embolectomy of native arteries and grafts, to monitor venous valve lysis in in situ or orthograde vein bypass grafts, to ascertain the completeness of venous valve lysis, and to inspect femoral venous valvular reconstructions (15,16). When used to guide in situ vein graft valve lysis, the angioscope is typically introduced from the proximal end of the vein graft being examined, and a retrograde cutting valvulotome is introduced through the distal end of the vein graft or a distal side branch (17,18). The valve cusps are serially lysed in a proximal to distal direction, with visual confirmation of effective valve lysis. Recent technologic advances also permit the embolization of side-branch veins under direct visualization through the angioscope during in situ bypass graft preparation (Fig. 74.2). The primary factor limiting the utility of this approach is the size of the vein, which must be large enough to accommodate an angioscope without trauma to the vein graft itself (17,18).

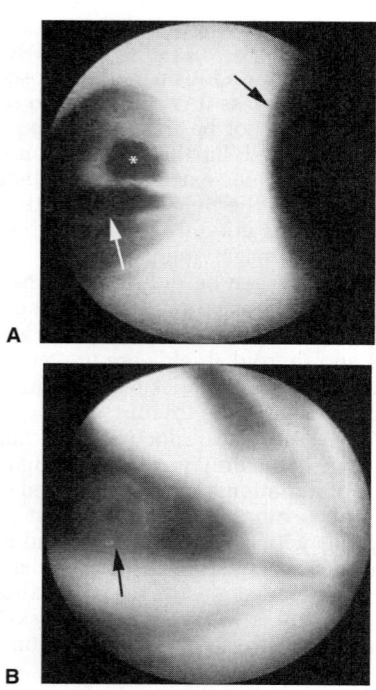

Figure 74.2. *(A)* Angioscopic view of the lumen of an in situ saphenous vein showing a side-branch vein valve with blood behind it *(white arrow).* The main lumen of vein is indicated by the *black arrow,* and the *asterisk* marks a hole in the valve created by the tip of the coil embolization catheter during coil deployment. *(B)* Close-up view of an embolization coil that has been deposited behind the valve in the side-branch vein *(arrow).*

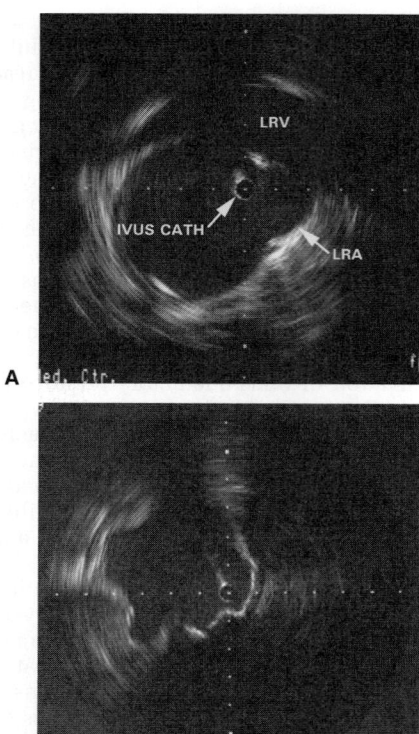

Figure 74.3. *(A)* Intravascular ultrasonographic *(IVUS)* image of the abdominal aorta demonstrates the overlying left renal vein *(LRV)* and origin of the left renal artery *(LRA).* *(B)* IVUS image of the neck of an abdominal aortic aneurysm demonstrates marked irregularity of the wall, which could make it difficult to attain a hemostatic seal with aortic endografting.

Intravascular Ultrasonography

The development of high-frequency ultrasonographic probes incorporated into small catheters that can be introduced transluminally has made it possible to perform intravascular ultrasonographic (IVUS) examinations (Fig. 74.3). The images produced are cross sections of the vessel, but advanced processing systems have been developed to generate three-dimensional images from these axial slices. The tissue-penetrating capability of the high-frequency (typically 12.5- to 50-MHz) transducers employed is limited, but the transducers are able to provide fine morphologic detail of the blood vessel anatomy, including the eccentricity and other features of arterial plaque and the technical results of balloon angioplasty and stent deployment (19,20). IVUS is also useful for the precise sizing of vessels, to aid in the selection of appropriately sized angioplasty balloons, stents, and aortic aneurysm endografts (21). Unlike angioscopes, IVUS catheters are able to image the vascular walls in a flowing blood field and can be used in any procedure provided a 5F to 9F catheter can be inserted.

GAINING AND MAINTAINING VASCULAR ACCESS

Percutaneous Cannulation Techniques

All endovascular procedures begin with gaining access to the vascular system in question and conclude with efforts to seal that source of access after removal of all endovascular devices. This discussion is limited to arterial access sites and techniques because they are by far the most common. However, the techniques and access sites used in the venous system are generally similar. The initial arterial puncture for endovascular procedures can be created by either of two standard techniques. In the "single-wall" puncture technique, a bevel-tipped hollow needle is used that is large enough to accommodate a 0.035-in guide wire. The needle is advanced toward the palpable pulse until the anterior wall of the vessel is punctured and pulsatile blood return is noted. A J-tipped wire is then advanced through the needle into the lumen of the vessel. The course of the wire is imaged fluoroscopically to ensure its smooth passage and minimize the risk that the wire will dissect between the arterial layers. Once the wire has been successfully inserted, the needle is withdrawn from the guide wire and a sheath is advanced over the guide wire to maintain the intraarterial position.

A "double-wall" puncture technique uses a two-component system that incorporates a blunt-tipped hollow needle and a sharp, beveled stylet that projects beyond the end of the blunt needle. This entry technique deliberately involves puncturing both the anterior and posterior walls of the artery, with the end of the needle left outside and behind the punctured vessel. The stylet is then removed, and the blunt needle is withdrawn until pulsatile bleeding is noted through the lumen of the needle. A J-tipped guide wire is then inserted under fluoroscopic guidance, as in the single-needle technique, and a sheath is placed over the guide wire. Although in theory the double-wall puncture technique can minimize the risk for a subsequent guide wire dissection, the increased risk for bleeding from the second wall puncture may outweigh any speculated benefit. Generally, the choice of puncture technique depends on personal preference rather than any well-defined benefit.

Vascular Access Sites

Access to the arterial system for angiography and endovascular interventions is generally achieved through one of three approaches:

- Retrograde common femoral puncture
- Antegrade common femoral puncture
- Retrograde axillary or brachial puncture

The choice of approach is based on the patient's symptoms, physical findings, noninvasive vascular findings, and relative risk for complications. Because the arterial puncture and initial sheath placement comprise the most uncontrolled part of the procedure (by virtue of the fact that no angiographic visualization of the target vessel has yet been performed), it is generally advisable to puncture the side opposite the symptoms (Fig. 74.4). Access to the venous system is typically gained through the jugular or common femoral veins by means of standard approaches familiar to all surgeons. Dialysis access grafts are commonly punctured directly for radiologic imaging and interventions.

Once the site of intended needle insertion has been ascertained, the skin and subcutaneous tissue should be injected with lidocaine (1%), and a small skin nick can be made with the tip of a No. 11 scalpel blade. The appropriate entry needle is used to puncture the artery. Once pulsatile blood return is noted, a J-tipped wire can be advanced through the entry needle and advanced under fluoroscopic guidance. If resistance is met when the wire is advanced or the wire "hangs up" or becomes kinked or damaged, it is best to replace it. Although plastic-coated hydrophilic guide wires (Turemo Glide Wire, Boston Sci-

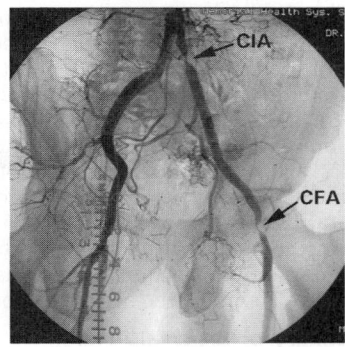

Figure 74.4. Diagnostic angiography, performed via a right retrograde femoral approach in a patient with claudication of the left lower extremity and a diminished left femoral pulse, demonstrates stenoses of both the left common iliac artery *(CIA)* and left common femoral artery *(CFA)*. Had the procedure been performed through a left retrograde femoral puncture, it is highly likely that the puncture would have been complicated by plaque in the common femoral artery.

entific, Natick, Massachusetts) may be used to negotiate tortuous or diseased vessels, they should *never* be inserted though an entry needle because the plastic hydrophilic coating may be shaved off by the sharp bevel of the needle (22,23). The standard Teflon coating found on a number of guide wires does not appear to cause this problem.

Retrograde Common Femoral Artery

The retrograde common femoral artery puncture is the most common approach used for angiography because of the relatively large size of the artery, ease of accessibility, and the fact that it can be readily compressed against the underlying osseous structures to achieve hemostasis after the procedure. Care must be taken to puncture the artery at a point no more than several centimeters distal to the inguinal ligament. More proximal punctures, above the inguinal ligament, can be complicated by the development of retroperitoneal hematomas because it is difficult to compress the puncture site above the inguinal ligament effectively after the endovascular hardware has been removed. Puncture sites below the femoral bifurcation can be complicated by thrombosis and ischemia in the extremity because of the smaller diameter of the superficial femoral artery and the propensity for plaque formation at the femoral bifurcation, or by bleeding from a deep femoral artery puncture because of the difficulty of compressing the deeply positioned puncture site. When the femoral pulse is weak or absent, a puncture site at the fluoroscopic landmark 1 cm lateral to the most medial portion of the femoral head is likely to be successful (24).

Antegrade Common Femoral Artery

The antegrade common femoral artery puncture is a useful approach for the management of lesions of the ipsilateral middle to distal superficial femoral artery and popliteal artery, but it is more technically challenging because access to the common femoral artery is frequently hindered by a large abdomen. Once the arterial puncture has been made, a guide wire is advanced and its course observed fluoroscopically. The wire must be seen to follow the expected course of the superficial femoral artery before the sheath is advanced over the wire to avoid having to remove an introducer sheath inadvertently placed in the deep femoral artery. Alternatively, contrast can be injected through the entry needle, or a small (4F) dilator can be advanced over the initially placed guide wire to maintain access and allow for contrast injection to determine the exact location of the dilator tip and its point of entry into the vascular system. The latter factor determines whether a catheter in the deep femoral artery can be retracted into the common femoral artery and readvanced into the superficial femoral artery, or whether the puncture is simply too low and must be abandoned. Once access to the superficial femoral artery has been obtained, the issues of whether to cross the lesion with a guide wire and perform the intended intervention become analogous to those involved in the more standard retrograde femoral approach.

Retrograde Axillary or Brachial Artery

Bilateral occlusive disease of the iliac arteries can preclude access to the more proximal arterial circulation for diagnostic and therapeutic interventions. Alternative access for catheterization of the proximal vessels can be obtained through either an axillary artery or a brachial artery approach. Although the presence of significant proximal subclavian occlusive disease is more common on the left than on the right, access from the left upper extremity is preferred for several reasons. First, it is technically more difficult to direct guide wires and catheters into the descending thoracic aorta from the right, especially when the innominate artery arises low on the ascending aorta. Secondly, an approach to the aorta through the right upper extremity requires traversing the innominate artery with catheters and guide wires, as a result of which embolic material can travel to the right carotid territory and cause a stroke. A comparison of the pulses and blood pressures in the two upper extremities can direct a rational decision regarding which upper extremity can be most advantageously used for access in the proposed study.

In addition to the technical difficulties of directing catheter and guide wire placement through an upper extremity, complications are more common with this route of arterial access. Thrombotic occlusion of the brachial artery is more likely because of the smaller caliber of the artery in comparison with the common femoral artery or even the more proximal axillary artery. The axillary artery puncture site has the disadvantage that even a small amount of hemorrhage from the puncture site can compress the brachial plexus within the axillary sheath. Axillary sheath hematomas can cause severe pain and neuropraxia in the upper extremity, even in the absence of clinical findings of an arm hematoma. Therefore, when severe pain in the extremity develops after axillary artery cannulation, even in the absence of other sensory or motor deficits, exploration is mandatory to control hemorrhage and decompress the brachial plexus.

Management of the Puncture Site

The most common method for managing the puncture site after removal of endovascular devices is simple manual compression over the punctured vessel for 15 to 30 minutes, with inspection to be sure that all bleeding has ceased when pressure is released. Mechanical devices resembling C-clamps are available to maintain pressure over the puncture site but are only partially effective and variably tolerated by patients. Patients are generally required to lie flat and relatively still for 4 to 6 hours before they are allowed to ambulate or go home. Recently, a number of agents and devices to facilitate puncture site closure have appeared on the market. Some variations rely on the placement of a hemostatic plug on top of the artery, whereas others actually place sutures in the puncture site to seal it. The purported advantage of these devices has been a reduction in the length of compression and bed rest, leading to earlier discharge and possibly a reduced rate of significant hematoma formation. Whether or not the use of these devices translates into reduced hospital costs is debatable when the cost of the devices themselves and the relatively low rate of significant puncture site complications are considered.

ENDOVASCULAR HARDWARE

Introducer Sheaths

If a straightforward diagnostic study is planned and multiple catheter and guide wire exchanges are not likely to be necessary, the size of the arterial puncture can be minimized by inserting a full-length guide wire into the vessel at the time of initial puncture and advancing the diagnostic catheter over that guide wire without the use of a sheath. If a more complex study is anticipated, likely requiring multiple catheter and guide wire exchanges, one should use a sheath to maintain access to the artery between exchanges of endovascular devices. This minimizes the risk for arterial trauma associated with each catheter–guide wire exchange and the risk for extravasation of blood during exchanges, which may compromise subsequent compression of the puncture site. An arterial sheath is sized in French units according to its inner diameter (one French unit equals a diameter of 0.33 mm), and the sheaths come in a wide variety of luminal diameters and lengths. A typical diagnostic angiogram is performed through a 4F to 5F catheter, which requires a sheath of at least the same size because a catheter is sized according to its outer diameter. The passage of an angioplasty balloon with a diameter larger than 7 mm or of most arterial stents typically requires a 7F to 10F sheath to accommodate the larger diameters of these devices.

Guide Wires

Despite differences in materials, shape, and stiffness, all guide wires serve the same purpose: to facilitate the atraumatic positioning of catheters in particular locations by providing guidance and support for the catheter being advanced over them. Standard guide wires are constructed of two different wire components. A stiff inner wire, called a *mandrel,* provides stiffness to the shaft of the wire, which is needed for the catheter to track over the wire. Although the guide wire shaft may be relatively stiff, the tip is typically made softer to provide an atraumatic leading end that is less likely to cause vessel dissection or perforation. In addition to the inner mandrel, an outer wrap on the wire, frequently made of stainless steel, is responsible for some of the handling characteristics of the wire. Most wires have some type of antifriction coating to facilitate passage through the vascular system and subsequent catheter exchanges. One such coating, the hydrophilic coating on the Turemo "Glide Wire," renders the wire extremely slippery when wet and is useful to facilitate passage of the wire through tortuous arteries or tight stenoses. However, the very low coefficient of friction of this guide wire increases the risk for inadvertent dissection, and therefore these wires must be passed with utmost care.

Guide wires are available in two general lengths. The standard length is 145 to 180 cm, and guide wires in this range are useful for the routine passage of catheters into the abdominal aorta. Although their relatively short length makes them convenient to use, one loses the flexibility to exchange catheters while maintaining a position across a lesion if the area of concern is more than 25 to 30 cm from the point of vascular access. This problem can be readily addressed by the use of more cumbersome but versatile

Diagnostic Catheters

Diagnostic catheters serve three general functions. Most commonly, catheters are utilized to inject radiopaque contrast material selectively into the vessels of interest to generate diagnostic images, or to direct a guide wire into a vessel in preparation for subsequent catheterization. Selectively positioned catheters can also be utilized to deliver pharmacologic agents or embolic material. Finally, catheters can be used to obtain blood samples selectively, as in the measurement of renal vein renin levels.

Catheters vary in shape, size, length, stiffness, tip design, torque response, antifriction properties, radiopacity, and the number of holes at the end through which contrast material can be injected. Catheters with a length of 65 cm are typically used in the abdominal aorta, and 100-cm catheters are used for aortic arch and carotid angiography. In contrast to introducer sheaths, which are sized according to their inner diameter, diagnostic catheters are sized according to their outside diameter. The inner diameter of the catheter therefore depends on the wall thickness and is important because it determines which size guide wires are to be used.

The most important characteristic of a catheter is its shape. Commonly used selective catheters and their applications are listed in Table 74.2 and illustrated in Fig. 74.6. Once the catheter is positioned within the vessel, its intrinsic shape is used to facilitate cannulation of the arterial branch points of interest for selective contrast injection, coil embolization, or whatever other procedure is planned. Catheters with multiple side holes are useful for the rapid injection of large amounts of contrast within a brief period of time, typically in large vessels such as the aorta and vena cava. Furthermore, the use of multiple side holes attenuates the "jet" effect of contrast on the vessel wall, which would be greater if power injection were performed through a single hole and could injure the vessel wall. End-hole catheters are useful for the low-pressure injection of contrast into selectively cannulated arteries or the delivery of coils or other embolic material.

A catheter that has a curve with a radius smaller than that of the blood vessel in which it is placed is said to be *self-forming,* in that it assumes its predetermined shape in the vessel once the guide wire is removed. Such catheters are the easiest to use and are suitable for the selective cannulation of a number of branch vessels. In some situations, most commonly aortic arch branch catheterization, catheters with a larger radius are needed, so that the catheter must be "manually formed" into its predetermined shape. This maneuver is typically accomplished by engaging the tip of the catheter in a side branch or softly pressing the catheter tip against the wall of the vessel while advancing the shaft of the catheter, so that the catheter essentially folds over on itself. Such maneuvers are associated with a potential risk for atheroembolization; when possible, they should be performed in the descending thoracic aorta rather than the ascending aorta, for obvious reasons.

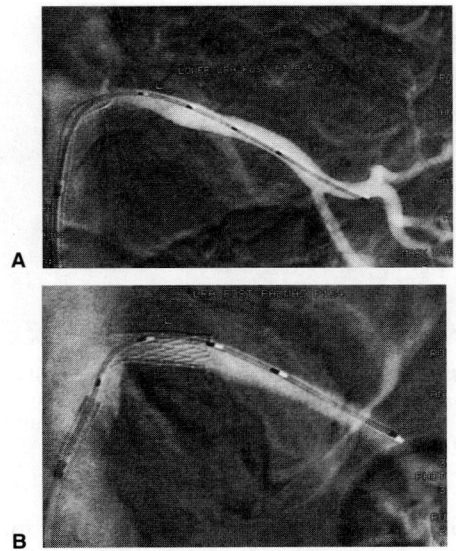

Figure 74.5. *(A)* Angiogram of the left renal artery. The calibrated guide wire, in place, was used to measure the diameter of the vessel for proper balloon and stent selection. *(B)* Completion of angiogram after placement of a Palmaz stent.

exchange-length wires, which are typically 240 to 300 cm long.

The diameter of a guide wire is traditionally expressed in fractions of an inch. The diameter of a standard guide wire is generally 0.035 or 0.038 in, although commercially available diameters range from 0.012 to 0.052 in. Smaller wires are advantageous because they can be used with small catheters, but they may not provide adequate tracking support in all situations or for relatively stiff devices. Larger wires provide more stiffness, which can make it easier to track catheters and endovascular hardware. In general, the larger-diameter, 0.035-in guide wires are used for most peripheral endovascular work except in the tibial region, where small-vessel balloon catheters are required. These most often accommodate a guide wire no larger than 0.18 in.

Guide wire tips come in three general shapes: straight, J-tipped, and angled. Many guide wire tips can be custom-shaped by pinching them between the fingers to achieve the exact shape necessary for the particular application. Some guide wire tips, particularly small-vessel guide wires, are made of radiodense platinum to improve their fluoroscopic visibility. Other special features found on some guide wires include radiopaque calibration markers, which facilitate endovascular measurements of length and diameter (Fig. 74.5). Lastly, some guide wires have a removable core that basically allows the guide wire to be used as a very small catheter—a feature that is clinically useful for the delivery of thrombolytic agents into small vessels.

Table 74.2. COMMONLY USED ANGIOGRAPHIC CATHETERS AND THEIR USES

Catheter name	Type	Primary use(s)
Pigtail and tennis racquet	Self-forming	Abdominal and arch aortography
Internal mammary	Self-forming	Crossing from one iliac artery to the other
Cobra	Self-forming	Cannulating renal and mesenteric artery branches
Simmons	Manually forming	Subclavian and carotid cannulation
Multipurpose	Self-forming	Directing guide wires, blood sampling

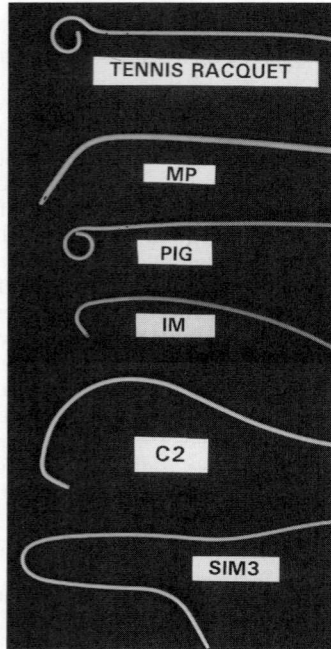

Figure 74.6. Commonly used diagnostic catheters.

Guiding Catheters

Guiding catheters have a large diameter and are usually preshaped into one of the self-forming curves, through which balloon catheters, stents, or other interventional devices are passed; in essence, such a catheter is a long, shaped introducer sheath (Fig. 74.7). Guiding catheters differ from introducer sheaths, however, in that the latter are equipped with hemostatic seals and side ports for injection; these features are not present on guiding catheters. Consequently, guiding catheters require the use of a *Y-adapter,* which serves as a hemostatic seal to prevent blood loss from the lumen of the guiding catheter while instruments are passed through it. A guiding catheter facilitates the passage of a catheter to a site of intervention; in addition, contrast can be injected through the lumen of the catheter, even when the balloon- or stent-loaded catheter is in place across the lesion of interest, to guide

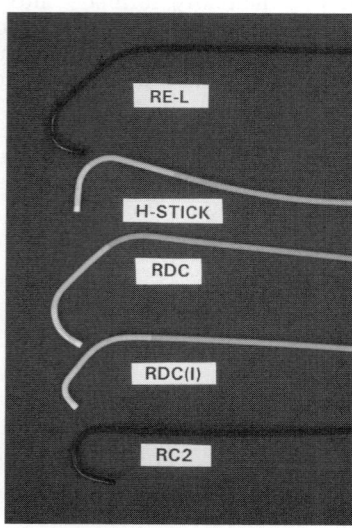

Figure 74.7. Commonly used guiding catheters.

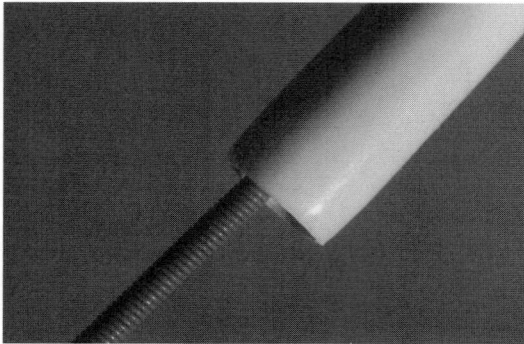

Figure 74.8. Photograph of the tip of an 8F guiding catheter with a standard 0.035-in guide wire in place demonstrates the step-off, which can snag and traumatize plaque during advancement if care is not taken.

the final placement of the device. Furthermore, following intervention, it is possible to inject contrast through the lumen of the guiding catheter to assess the final result before the balloon is removed, so that any necessary final balloon "touch-up" can be immediately performed.

Because the lumen of the guiding catheter must be large enough to accommodate the diameter of the balloon or stent to be used, the use of a guiding catheter requires the placement of a larger introducer sheath at the site of arterial access. Like diagnostic catheters, guiding catheters are sized in French units according to their outside diameter, which indicates the smallest sheath through which they will fit. Also of obvious importance is the inside (luminal) diameter of the guiding catheter, which determines the largest device that can be passed through it and how much additional channel is available for injection of contrast. Although some guiding catheters come with a tapered obturator, analogous to the tapered dilator typically found on introducer sheaths, most do not, so that a considerable step-off is left between the guide wire and the guiding catheter; this can snag atheromatous plaque and tissue at vascular bifurcations and thereby injure the vessel (Fig. 74.8). Consequently, a guide catheter, especially one without a tapering dilator, must be observed fluoroscopically while it is being advanced to the area of interest.

Angioplasty Balloons

Relevant characteristics of angioplasty balloons include the balloon construction material, length of the catheter extending beyond the end of the balloon, and length of the "shoulders" of the balloon (the part of the balloon at each end that does not attain the rated balloon diameter because of its tapering attachment to the shaft of the catheter). Early balloons were constructed of polyvinyl chloride, which was overly compliant and had a low burst strength. Contemporary balloon catheters, however, are made of less compliant materials, such as polyester or Dacron. Some catheters have an attached hydrophilic coating to minimize friction when the balloon is advanced through stenoses or guiding catheters. The drawback to such a coating is that it becomes difficult to secure balloon-expandable stents to the angioplasty balloon, so that the risk that the stent will become dislodged during advancement to the intended site of deployment is increased. Consequently, when it is necessary to mount a stent on a coated balloon, one should make a diligent effort to remove as much of the the hydrophilic coating as possible by rubbing the balloon vigorously with a gauze sponge before the stent is mounted.

Available angioplasty balloon sizes range from 1.5 to 5 mm in 0.5-mm increments, and from 6 to 18 mm in 1.0-mm increments. With the advent of endoluminal aortic grafting, balloons with even larger diameters are likely to appear soon. Ideally, the balloon diameter should be about 10% larger than the size of the "normal" artery adjacent to the lesion to be dilated. Balloon lengths vary between manufacturers, but lengths of 2.0, 4.0, and 10.0-cm are generally available. Ideally, balloon length is selected to dilate a lesion with a single positioning of the balloon catheter, but it is sometimes necessary to perform overlapping dilations to cover an entire lesion. The use of overlapping dilations may be desirable when a longer balloon would dilate far beyond the area of disease or over a branch vessel, in which case dissection and occlusion of the branch vessel might occur, or when a vessel is particularly tortuous and straightening it during balloon inflation might result in vascular injury.

Stents

Numerous stents are commercially available, but all stents can be classified into two broad categories: balloon-expandable stents and those that are self-expanding on retraction of an outer, constraining covering. The Palmaz stent, the prototypic balloon-expandable stent, is deployed after being mounted on an angioplasty balloon for delivery to the intended site. In general, these stents are relatively short and have very little longitudinal flexibility, but they exert a strong radial force. The Wallstent (Boston Scientific) is the prototypic self-expanding stent. In general, these stents have better longitudinal flexibility and therefore can adapt better to curved vessels. Furthermore, their more flexible delivery system makes it possible to advance longer stents through tortuous vessels, or from a contralateral femoral approach to the intended site of deployment. These stents spontaneously expand to their unconstrained size once the delivery system confining them is withdrawn. The self-expanding property of these stents is based on either of two mechanisms. The Wallstent expands by virtue of its stainless steel braid construction. Other stents, such as the Smart Stent (Cordis, Warren, NJ), are constructed of the thermal memory metal Nitinol, an alloy of nickel and titanium. Stents can be fabricated from this pliable metal in specific shapes and sizes and compressed into relatively small delivery devices (7F to 10F) for transport to the intended location. Once released at body temperature, the stent assumes its predesigned size and shape.

Stent Grafts

Stent grafts are essentially fabric grafts placed within the vascular lumen; stents are used to attach them to the vessel wall (Fig. 74.9). Currently, two such devices have been approved by the Food and Drug Administration, both of which are designed to treat abdominal aortic aneurysms. A number of other aortic endografts are presently in trial; they integrate many features of the approved grafts with a variety of other modifications designed to enhance performance. Although a detailed discussion of aortic endografting is beyond the scope of this chapter, major variations in endograft design relate to the following: fabric used for the graft (presently either polytetrafluoroethylene or Dacron), material used for the stent (presently either Nitinol or stainless steel), unibody versus modular construction, presence or absence of uncovered stent beyond the fabric at the aortic end for suprarenal endograft fixation, and use of stents throughout the length of the graft or only at the attachment sites. Mechanisms of

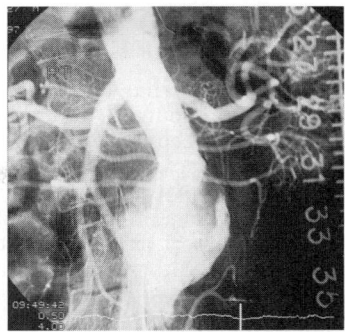
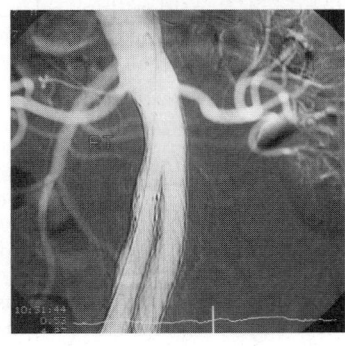

Figure 74.9. *(A)* Angiogram of an abdominal aortic aneurysm obtained before endografting. *(B)* Angiogram of an abdominal aortic aneurysm obtained after grafting with the AneuRx device.

deployment of various endografts also differ substantially, the ultimate goal being to design an efficacious endograft that can be inserted percutaneously. Whether this will be accomplished by creating smaller endograft delivery systems or by designing better closure devices remains to be seen.

Perhaps the most significant difference between the two presently approved endografts, however, pertains to their mechanism of vessel wall "attachment." With the AneuRx aortic endograft (Medtronic Arterial Vascular Engineering, Santa Rosa, CA), fixation of the graft at its intended location is accomplished through the friction provided by the radial force of the stent on the aortic wall. Because the stents are of the self-expanding Nitinol variety, the endograft can be oversized to create a constant outward force on the vessel wall to provide fixation and a hemostatic seal. These grafts are currently available in diameters ranging from 20 to 28 mm, with a modular bifurcated design that permits the customized assembly of components chosen to adapt the stent graft to an individual patient's anatomy. Because the largest endograft is 28 mm and 10% to 20% oversizing is recommended, aortic neck diameters must be less than 26 mm. Full-length stent support minimizes kinking and twisting of the endograft limbs.

The Ancure aortic endograft (Guidant, Menlo Park, CA) provides an alternate mode of fixation, in which radially aligned stainless steel hooks are embedded in the vessel wall by a balloon at the time of deployment. As with the AneuRx endograft, no bare stent extends beyond the graft fabric, so fixation occurs in the immediate infrarenal segment of the aorta. Another difference is that the "stents" are present only at the proximal and distal attachment sites of the bifurcated unibody graft. This configuration has led to a considerable incidence of twisting and kinking of the endograft limbs, such that supplemental stenting of the limbs has become almost routine.

OVERVIEW OF BASIC ENDOVASCULAR TECHNIQUES

Every procedure is somewhat unique, but certain sequences of steps are common to all, and failure of any one of them can doom the procedure. For example, although obtaining initial vascular access is conceptually simple, as described above, it can prove humbling at times to even the most experienced endovascular therapist, yet the procedure clearly cannot be performed unless this is accomplished. Even more than with surgical revascularization procedures, correct sequencing of the maneuvers is critical to optimize the chance for success and minimize the risk for complications. Considerations relevant to the fundamental therapeutic procedures of balloon angioplasty and stenting are summarized below.

Balloon Angioplasty

Once the lesion to be treated has been identified by appropriate imaging, the next step is to define the best approach to gain access to the lesion. A guide wire is selected based on the performance characteristics previously described and manipulated across the lesion under fluoroscopic guidance. A J-tipped guide wire is least likely to injure the artery of interest or create a dissection. However, the standard 3-mm-radius guide wire may have too large a profile to cross a tight or tortuous lesion. Alternatives include smaller (1.5-mm radius) J-tipped guide wires or straight or angled wires with floppy tips (Benson, Wholey, or Turemo). The hydrophilic coating of the Turemo wire reduces friction so much that care must be taken that the guide wire does not create a dissection.

Occasionally, wires with floppy tips require more support, and a diagnostic catheter with an appropriate shape can be advanced to within 1 to 2 cm of the end of the wire to "stiffen" the shaft of the guide wire. This technique is frequently used when complete occlusions are traversed; in such cases the guide wire is often pushed through the plaque/thrombus rather than "navigated" through a stenosis. Not surprisingly, crossing of the occluded segment often occurs in a subintimal plane. Reentry of the guide wire into the lumen of the vessel must be confirmed to ensure that the anticipated arterial dilation will reestablish continuity of the flow channel rather than extend and enlarge an area of iatrogenic arterial dissection. When an angled or J-tipped wire is used to cross the lesion, reentry into the vessel lumen can be documented by spinning the wire and observing the free rotation of the tip in its angled or J-form. Alternatively, a small diagnostic catheter can be advanced over the wire to maintain the lesion crossing, and a small amount of contrast can be injected to confirm that the distal end of the catheter has reentered the lumen of the vessel on the other side of the occlusion.

After a lesion has been crossed with a wire and the intraluminal position of the wire beyond the stenosis has been ascertained, the selected angioplasty balloon can be prepared for use. Typically, syringe-mediated suction is applied to the end of the catheter, and half-strength contrast in the syringe is drawn back into the balloon inflation channel after suction is released. This removes most air from the system and minimizes the risk for air embolization should the balloon rupture, and it also reduces the overall size or "profile" of the balloon for easier passage through the sheath, vascular system, and, of course, the stenosis. Balloons are typically inflated with a syringe, with or without a pressure-monitoring device. Usually, half-strength iodinated contrast is used for balloon inflation so that the radiopaque balloon profile can be ob-

served. Half-strength contrast allows for adequate balloon imaging during inflation; higher concentrations of contrast are so viscous that inflation and deflation times may be excessive. Worse yet, achieving full balloon deflation may prove impossible, so that balloon withdrawal is complicated substantially.

The anatomic results of balloon dilation can be assessed by numerous means. Most commonly, angiography in multiple planes is used to confirm a technically satisfactory result of balloon dilation. IVUS has also been used successfully to identify residual areas of stenosis or segments of arterial dissection. Pressure measurements across the dilated lesion should demonstrate that the area of hemodynamically significant stenosis has been eliminated. In general, a balloon dilation procedure is considered to be successful if angiography or IVUS shows a residual stenosis of less than 30% after the procedure has been completed (24). Alternatively, no blood pressure gradient should be observed across the dilated lesion, although a pressure differential of less than 5 to 10 mm Hg is probably not clinically significant. Small gradients may be demonstrated to be hemodynamically significant after pharmacologic measures have been taken to lower distal arterial resistance. The injection of either 100 to 200 µg of nitroglycerin or 20 mg of papaverine lowers the outflow resistance, increases flow across the lesion of interest, and potentially unmasks the hemodynamic effect of a residual area of stenosis.

Intravascular Stent Deployment

After dilation with an appropriately sized balloon has been completed, a residual stenosis of more than 30%, a significant pressure gradient at rest or with pharmacologic provocation, or a large arterial dissection can often be managed by deploying an arterial stent (Fig. 74.10). Presently, only two stents have been approved by the Food and Drug Administration for use in the peripheral vascular system, and they have been approved only for use in the iliac arteries. However, "off-label" uses of stents are commonplace; for example, iliac stents are used in locations other than the iliac vessels, and stents approved for use in the the biliary tree are deployed in peripheral arteries and veins. These practices reflect the investment required to receive Food and Drug Administration approval for a given indication more than it does the performance characteristics of a given stent in the vascular system. As discussed above, stent designs and deployment procedures vary widely, and a detailed review of specific deployment characteristics is beyond the scope of this chapter. Nonetheless, a few general technical considerations are mentioned.

The precise deployment of a stent requires a thorough understanding of both the mechanism of deployment and the characteristics of the stent itself. Balloon-expanded stents and most Nitinol stents shorten only modestly on deployment, whereas the Wallstent shortens appreciably. Consequently, predicting exact ultimate coverage is more challenging with the latter stent. However, the Wallstent can be recaptured before complete deployment, so that some last-minute repositioning is possible if it appears to be needed. All self-expanding stents are housed in delivery systems that constrain the stent by covering it with a retractable outer sheath. Therefore, the stent is protected from becoming dislodged during passage through the vascular system, and the vascular wall is protected from being injured by the stent. This is not the case with available balloon-expanded stents; therefore, they must be advanced into position within a prepositioned sheath or guiding catheter.

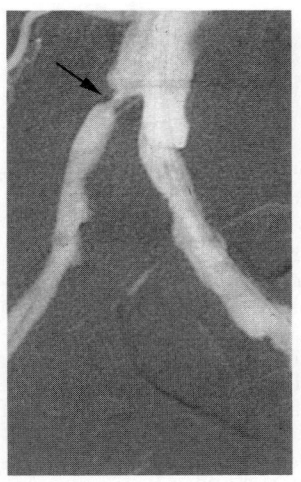 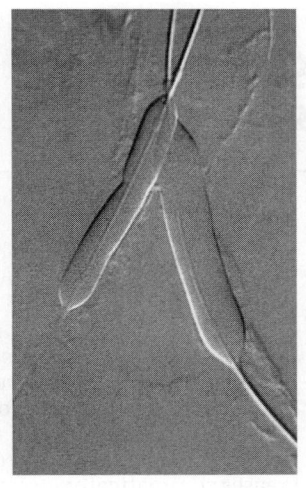 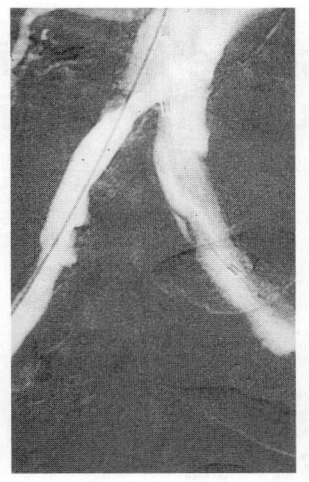 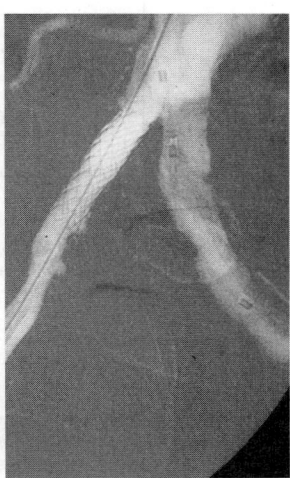

A   B   C   D

Figure 74.10. *(A)* High-grade stenosis of the proximal right common iliac artery *(arrow)* in a patient with claudication of the right lower extremity. *(B)* The kissing balloon technique, shown here, is required because of the proximity of the stenosis to the aortic bifurcation. *(C)* Residual stenosis exceeding 30% with an associated pressure gradient after angioplasty. *(D)* Residual stenosis and pressure gradient resolved after placement of a stent.

SUMMARY

Although rooted in the diagnosis of vascular disorders, endovascular techniques have evolved to become therapeutically useful in an ever-increasing number of vascular disorders. Although they have traditionally been considered the domain of interventional radiologists, an increasing number of vascular surgeons have become proficient in applying these techniques, which require that radiologic imaging and catheter/guide wire skills be combined with surgical evaluation and management skills. Although not a component of vascular surgical training in the past, endovascular training is now a requirement for all vascular fellowships. Mastery of these techniques expands the armamentarium of the vascular surgeon, and they can frequently be used to simplify and facilitate many standard surgical procedures. Ultimately, the vascular surgeon who acquires endovascular skills is more well-rounded and capable than one who does not, being able to perform both percutaneous and operative procedures.

REFERENCES

1. Moniz E. L'encéphalographie arterielle, son importance dans la localization des tumeurs cérébrales. *Rev Neurol* 1931;2:646.
2. Seldinger SI. Catheter replacement of the needle in percutaneous arteriography. *Acta Radiol* 1953;39:368–376.
3. Dotter C, Judkins MP. Transluminal treatment of arteriosclerotic obstruction: description of a new technique and preliminary report of its application. *Circulation* 1964;30:654–670.
4. Hessel SJ, Adams DF. Complications of angiography. *Radiology* 1981;138:271–281.
5. Grollman JH Jr, Marcus R. Transbrachial arteriography: techniques and complications. *Cardiovasc Intervent Radiol* 1988; 11:32–35.
6. Waugh JR, Sacharias N. Angiographic complications in the DSA era. *Radiology* 1992;182:243–246.
7. Goss JE, Chambers CE, Heupler FA Jr. Systemic anaphylactoid reactions to iodinated contrast media during cardiac catheterization procedures: guidelines for prevention, diagnosis, and treatment. Laboratory Performance Standards Committee of the Society for Cardiac Angiography and Interventions. *Cathet Cardiovasc Diagn* 1995;34:99–104.
8. Laroche D, Namour F, Lefrancois C, et al. Anaphylactoid and anaphylactic reactions to iodinated contrast material. *Allergy* 1999;54:13–16.
9. Greenberger PA, Patterson R, Tapio CM. Prophylaxis against repeated radiocontrast media reactions in 857 cases: adverse experience with cimetidine and safety of beta-adrenergic antagonists. *Arch Intern Med* 1985;145:2197–2200.
10. Lasser EC, Berry CC, Talner LB, et al. Pretreatment with corticosteroids to alleviate reactions to intravenous contrast material. *N Engl J Med* 1987;317:845–849.
11. Katayama H, Yamaguchi K, Kozuka T, et al. Adverse reactions to ionic and nonionic contrast media: a report from the Japanese Committee on the safety of contrast media. *Radiology* 1990;175:621–628.
12. Parfrey PS, Griffiths SM, Barrett BJ, et al. Contrast material-induced renal failure in patients with diabetes mellitus, renal insufficiency, or both: a prospective controlled study. *N Engl J Med* 1989;320:143–149.
13. Hodgson KJ. Principles of arteriography. In: Rutherford RB, ed. *Vascular surgery,* 5th ed. Philadelphia: WB Saunders, 1999:286–302.
14. Marx MV, Niklason L, Mauger EA. Occupational radiation exposure to interventional radiologists: a prospective study. *J Vasc Interv Radiol* 1992;3:597–606.
15. Welch HJ, McLaughlin RL, O'Donnell TF Jr. Femoral vein valvuloplasty: intraoperative angioscopic evaluation and hemodynamic improvement. *J Vasc Surg* 1992;16:694–700.
16. Pevec WC. Angioscopy in vascular surgery: the state of the art. *Ann Vasc Surg* 1996;10:66–75.
17. Rosenthal D, Arous EJ, Friedman SG, et al. Endovascular-assisted versus conventional in situ saphenous vein bypass grafting: cumulative patency, limb salvage, and cost results in a 39-month multicenter study. *J Vasc Surg* 2000;31:60–68.
18. Clair DG, Golden MA, Mannick JA, et al. Randomized prospective study of angioscopically assisted in situ saphenous vein grafting. *J Vasc Surg* 1994;19:992–999.
19. Nishanian G, Kopchok GE, Donayre CE, et al. The impact of intravascular ultrasound (IVUS) on endovascular interventions. *Semin Vasc Surg* 1999;12:285–299.
20. Cavaye DM, White RA, Kopchok GE, et al. Intravascular ultrasound imaging: the new standard for guidance and assessment of endovascular interventions? *J Clin Lasers Med Surg* 1992;10:349–353.
21. Wilson EP, White RA. Intravascular ultrasound. *Surg Clin North Am* 1998;78:561–574.
22. Reagan K, Matsumoto AH, Teitelbaum GP. Comparision of the hydrophilic guidewire in double- and single-wall entry needles: potential hazards. *Cathet Cardiovasc Diagn* 1991;24 205–208.
23. Kim JK, Kang HK. Percutaneous retrieval of the peeled-off plastic coating from a guide wire [Letter]. *J Vasc Interv Radiol* 1994;5:657–658.
24. Hodgson KJ. Fundamental techniques in endovascular surgery. In: Rutherford RB, ed. *Vascular surgery,* 5th ed. Philadelphia: WB Saunders, 2000:499–526.

Occlusive Disease Involving Specific Vascular Territories

SURGERY: SCIENTIFIC PRINCIPLES AND PRACTICE, Third Edition, edited by
Lazar J. Greenfield, Michael W. Mulholland, Keith T. Oldham, Gerald B. Zelenock,
and Keith D. Lillemoe. Lippincott Williams & Wilkins Publishers, Philadelphia, © 2001.

CHAPTER 75

CEREBROVASCULAR OCCLUSIVE DISEASE

LOUIS M. MESSINA, RAJABRATA SARKAR,
AND GERALD B. ZELENOCK

Cerebrovascular disease encompasses a variety of clinical disorders of the extracranial cerebral arteries that can cause transient cerebral ischemia or stroke. In the past, most causes of stroke were considered untreatable. However, significant advances in the surgical treatment of extracranial cerebrovascular disease have contributed greatly to reducing the mortality associated with stroke.

The first carotid endarterectomy took place in 1954. By 1984, carotid endarterectomy had become the most frequently performed vascular surgical procedure and the third most frequently performed operation in the United States. Nonetheless, much controversy surrounded the operation owing to the publication of a number of clinical reports showing a wide variability in mortality and morbidity rates after carotid endarterectomy, so that many questioned its efficacy. Recently, prospective, randomized studies comparing the efficacy of carotid endarterectomy plus optimal medical treatment with optimal medical treatment alone have been published and have established unambiguously the efficacy of carotid endarterectomy in the management of cerebrovascular disease.

This chapter reviews the epidemiology, anatomy, pathophysiology, diagnosis, and treatment of cerebrovascular disease of the extracranial arteries.

EPIDEMIOLOGY

Stroke remains the third most common cause of death in the United States, and atherosclerotic occlusive disease of the extracranial portion of the carotid artery is the most common cause of stroke. Stroke is a devastating illness in every respect. Five hundred thousand people suffer strokes each year, and of these, 200,000 die as a consequence of stroke (Fig. 75.1). Of the remaining patients who survive stroke, two thirds are disabled, and one third require prolonged hospitalization because of residual disability (Table 75.1). The disability caused by stroke is greater than that associated with other ischemic disorders, such as myocardial infarction. Neurologic deficits resulting in paralysis, blindness, and aphasia compromise the stroke victim's ability to perform many normal daily functions and live a satisfying existence. The cumulative public health cost for the disabilities caused by strokes are enormous, exceeding $16 trillion a year (1).

Although the incidence of stroke in the general population is declining, the prevalence is increasing. The decrease in the incidence of stroke is thought to reflect the improved management of risk factors for stroke, particularly hypertension. Because the U.S. population is aging, however, the prevalence remains high and is increasing. The effect of an aging population on the incidence of stroke is illustrated by the fact that in the general population, the incidence of stroke is 195/100,000, but it increases dramatically, to 1,440/100,000, in persons between 75 to 84 years old. Thus, stroke, owing to its frequency in the population and its personal and financial costs, will remain an exceedingly important public health issue in the years to come.

ANATOMY

The embryonic derivation of the blood supply to the brain is complex (Fig. 75.2). This rich blood supply reflects the high oxygen requirement of neural tissue. Although the brain constitutes only 2% of the total body weight, it takes up 17% of the cardiac output and 20% of the available oxygen supply (2). A clinical implication of

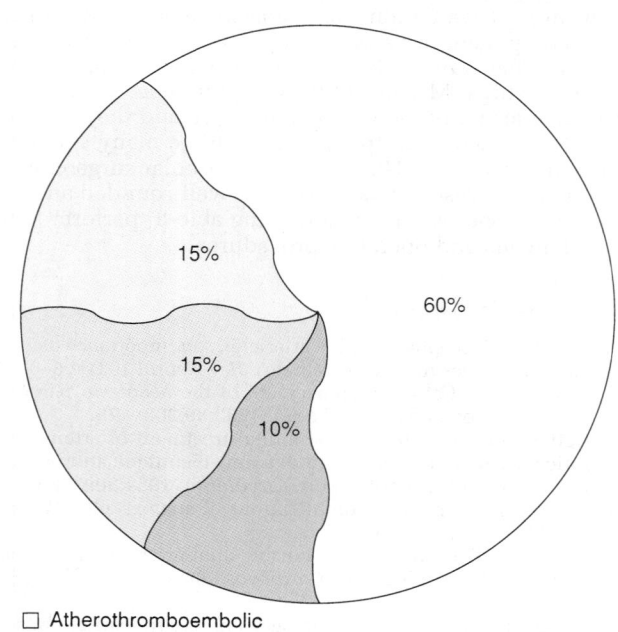

☐ Atherothromboembolic
☐ Cardiocerebral embolic
☐ Hemorrhagic—subarachnoid, intracerebral
▨ Other

Figure 75.1. The precise distribution of the causes of stroke varies among reports, but the most common causes are atherothromboembolic events originating in the extracranial arteries, heart, and intraparenchymal or subarachnoid hemorrhage. (After Zelenock GB, D'Alecy LG. The brain. In: Zelenock GB, D'Alecy LG, Fantone JC III, et al., eds. *Clinical ischemic syndrome mechanisms and consequences of tissue injury.* St. Louis: Mosby, 1990:353, with permission.)

Table 75.1. RESIDUAL DISABILITY IN 119 STROKE SURVIVORS: FRAMINGHAM STUDY

Disability level	Occurrence (%)
Institutionalized	16
Dependent in self-care activities	31
Dependent for mobility	20
Dependent for vocational activity	71
Decreased socialization	62

Adapted from Gresham GE, Fitzpatric TE, Wolf PA, et al. Residual disability in stroke survivors: the Framingham study. *N Engl J Med* 1975;293:954, with permission.

the high oxygen requirements of neural tissue is that the tissue can become necrotic within minutes of a loss of arterial circulation.

In adults, the ascending aorta rises from the left ventricle and courses anteriorly in the mediastinum. The branches of aortic arch are the brachiocephalic (innominate) artery, the left common carotid artery, and the left subclavian artery. These arteries supply blood to the head and neck, both upper extremities, and the proximal trunk. The aortic arch crosses the upper mediastinum obliquely from a right anterior to a left posterior position. The brachiocephalic artery is the first and most anterior branch of the aortic arch. Beneath the head of the right clavicle, the brachiocephalic artery bifurcates to form the right subclavian artery and the right common carotid artery. It is because of this anterior position that the brachiocephalic artery is accessible for reconstruction through a median sternotomy. The left common carotid artery arises within 1 cm of the brachiocephalic artery and courses posteriorly into the left side of the base of the neck. In 10% of the normal population, the left common carotid artery arises directly from the brachiocephalic artery. Finally, the left subclavian artery arises from a posterior location at the distal end of the aortic arch. Because of its distal and posterior location, it is not easily reached through a median sternotomy and is best approached through a high left anterior or anterolateral thoracotomy.

The brain is supplied by the paired internal carotid arteries anteriorly and the vertebral arteries posteriorly (Fig. 75.3). Under normal conditions, the paired internal carotid arteries supply about 80% to 90% of the total cerebral blood flow, and the paired vertebral arteries supply 10% to 20% of the total cerebral flow. The common carotid artery bifurcates at the level of the angle of the mandibles into the internal and external carotid arteries. The branches of the external carotid artery include the ascending pharyngeal artery, which supplies the hypopharynx and oropharynx, and the superior thyroid, lingual, occipital, and posterior auricular arteries. Its terminal branches are the internal maxillary and superior temporal arteries.

The internal carotid artery can be divided into four segments: cervical, intrapetrosal, intracavernous, and supraclinoid. The cervical, extracranial portion of the internal carotid artery has no branches. The intracavernous and supraclinoid portions are referred to clinically as the *carotid siphon.* The first major branch of the internal carotid artery is the ophthalmic artery. The supraclinoid portion of the internal carotid artery gives rise to the major

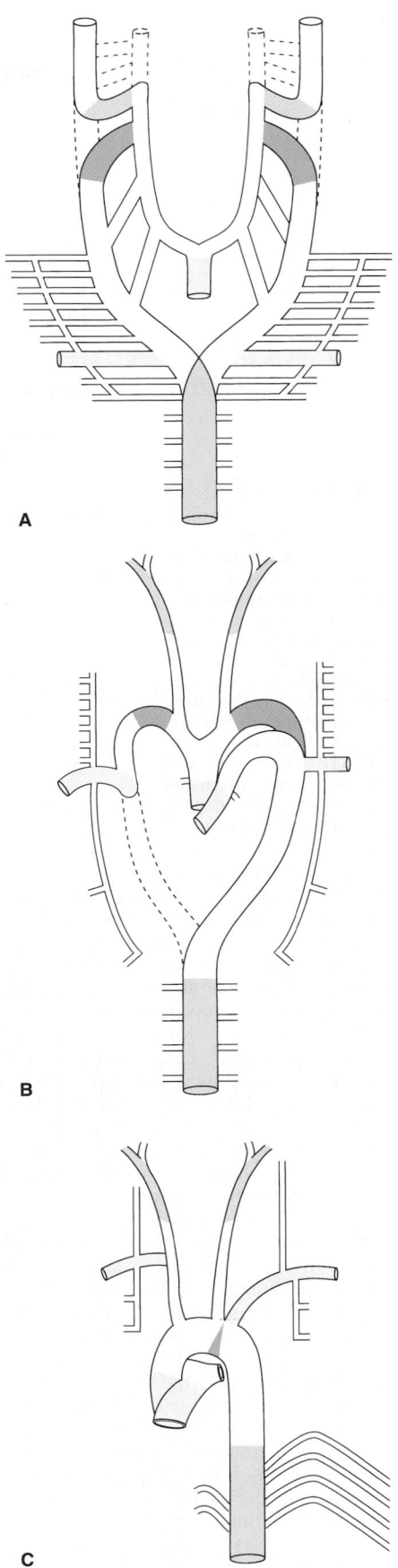

Figure 75.2. Development of the great arteries. *(A)* Fifth week. *(B)* Seventh week. *(C)* Ninth week. (After Barry A. The aortic arch derivatives in the human adult. *Anat Rec* 1951;111:221, with permission.)

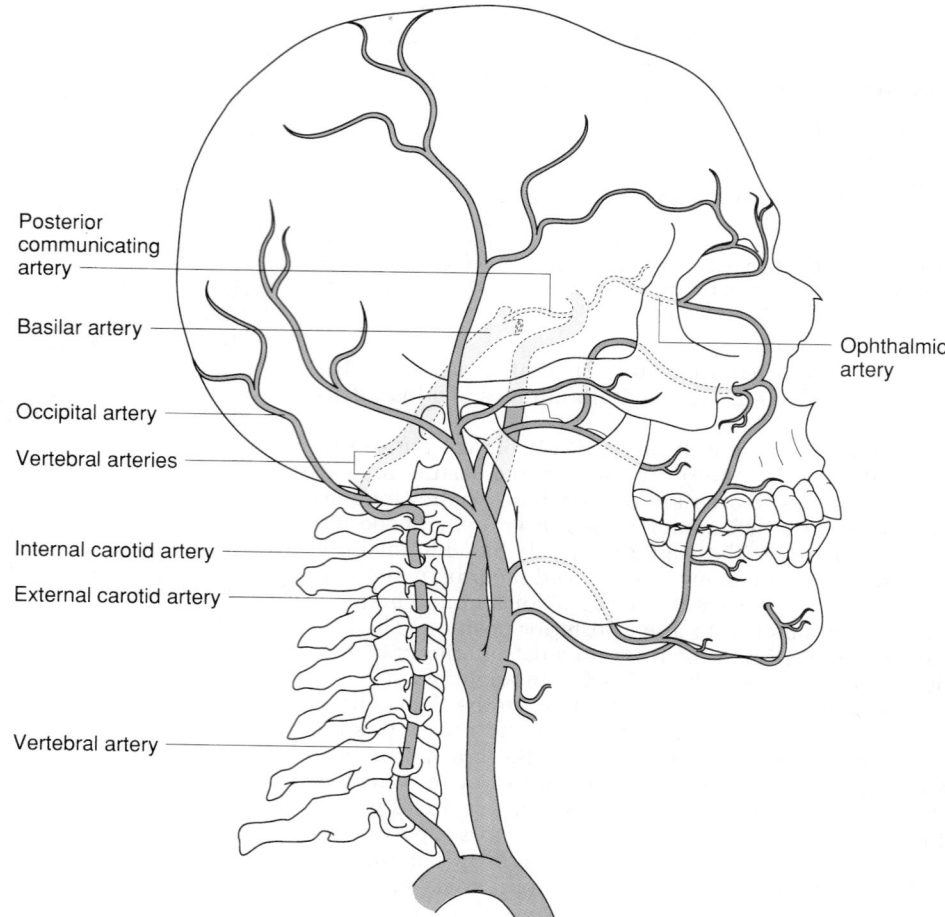

Figure 75.3. The paired carotid and vertebral arteries supply blood to the brain. Extensive extracranial collaterals between the external carotid and vertebral systems allow for antegrade perfusion when a proximal occlusion develops in either vessel. Likewise, periorbital collaterals allow for retrograde flow through the ophthalmic artery to the internal carotid artery in the presence of a cervical internal carotid artery occlusion. Extensive side-to-side collaterals are found between the right and left external carotid arteries and right and left vertebral arteries.

branches of the internal carotid artery, including the ophthalmic, posterior communicating, and anterior choroidal arteries. Eventually, the internal carotid artery bifurcates into its terminal branches, the anterior cerebral and middle cerebral arteries. The anterior communicating artery joins the comparable vessel from the contralateral hemisphere, whereas the posterior communicating artery provides anterior–posterior communication between the carotid system and the ipsilateral posterior cerebral branches of the basilar artery. Together, these branches form the circle of Willis (Fig. 75.4). Variations in the anatomy of the circle of Willis occur in 50% to 80% of the normal population. About 15% of the population have no anastomoses between the anterior and the posterior cerebral circulations, and as many as 35% lack the anastomotic channels between the anterior and posterior circulations or between the right and left hemispheric circulations. A deficiency of this collateral pathway has important clinical consequences when one of the four major cerebral arteries becomes occluded.

The vertebral arteries arise from the first portion of the subclavian artery and enter the transverse cervical process at the level of the sixth cervical vertebra and ascend in the transverse foramen, eventually piercing the posterior allantoid–occipital membrane and coursing into the posterior fascia through the foramen magnum. The vertebral arteries course along the lateral border of the medulla and unite to form the basilar artery. The extracranial portion of the vertebral artery has segmental spinal and muscular branches. The basilar artery terminates as the right and left posterior cerebral arteries, from which arise the posterior communicating arteries of the circle of Willis.

A number of clinically important collateral pathways exist between cerebral arteries. These collaterals become significant sources of arterial flow to the brain when arterial occlusive disease develops in one of the four major arteries supplying blood to the brain. Branches of the exter-

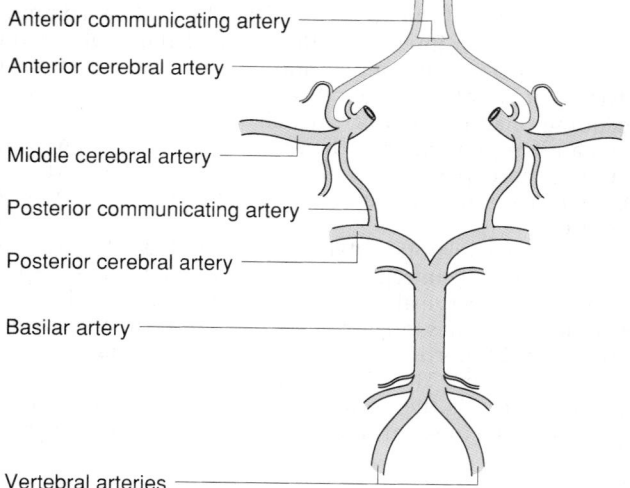

Figure 75.4. The circle of Willis is a highly efficient intracranial collateral network; however, multiple important variations occur, and an incomplete circle producing an isolated hemisphere is not uncommon.

nal carotid artery, particularly the facial, internal maxillary, and superficial temporal arteries, may anastomose with the infraorbital and supraorbital arteries. These anastomotic networks become important sources of blood flow into the intracranial portions of the internal carotid artery when a hemodynamic stenosis develops at the carotid bifurcation in the cervical portion of the internal carotid artery. Communication between these branches of the external carotid artery and the ophthalmic artery, a branch of internal carotid artery, is the most important of the collateral networks. The collateral pathway can be identified angiographically or by means of a directional Doppler probe. Similarly, the vertebral artery gives off numerous muscular branches in the neck. If the proximal vertebral artery becomes occluded, collateral branches from the external carotid artery may anastomose to the distal vertebral artery by way of these branches. In addition, if the common carotid artery becomes occluded, blood may flow from the vertebral artery through the external carotid artery branches into the internal carotid artery, so that antegrade blood flow in the internal carotid artery is maintained. Finally, branches of the left and right external carotid arteries may anastomose freely across the face.

PATHOPHYSIOLOGY

Although stroke has many causes (Tables 75.2 and 75.3), most are the result of a few distinct pathologic processes. Atherosclerosis remains the most common cause of stroke in adults. Less common pathologic processes include aneurysms of the internal carotid artery; anatomic abnormalities, including coils, which are loops or gentle curves in the internal carotid artery; and kinks, in which acute bends in the internal carotid artery cause the carotid artery to fold up on itself. Fibromuscular dysplasia is a vessel wall abnormality that occurs typically in women 30 to 50 years of age and involves the cervical internal carotid artery distal to the carotid bifurcation (3,4). Fibromuscular dysplasia is usually subdivided into four categories: intimal fibroplasia, medial fibroplasia, medial hyperplasia, and perimedial dysplasia. In its most common form, the internal carotid artery becomes alternatingly thickened and thinned and acquires a beaded appearance on angiography. Stroke can be the result of emboli or a low-flow state. Fibromuscular disease can affect a number of arteries systematically and is also associated with congenital intracranial aneurysms. Another disorder that occurs more commonly in women is Takayasu's arteritis. This inflammatory arteritis can affect any branch of the aorta or pulmonary arteries. When this entity causes symptoms and signs of cerebrovascular insufficiency, it usually affects the three branches of the aortic arch. Temporal arteritis, a condition typically seen in the elderly, most commonly affects muscular arteries, such as the superficial temporal artery, and is characterized clinically by headache, monocular visual symptoms, low-grade fever, and tenderness of the superficial femoral artery. If left untreated, it can result in permanent blindness.

Both spontaneous arterial dissections and aneurysms can affect the intracranial portion of the carotid artery, al-

---

Table 75.2. CAUSES OF CEREBRAL ISCHEMIA AND INFARCTION

ISCHEMIC
Atherothromboembolic
High-grade stenoses and occlusions
Emboli
Plaque
Platelet–fibrin debris
Intraplaque hemorrhage

Cardioembolic
Arrhythmias (atrial fibrillation, other arrhythmias)
Myocardial infarction with mural thrombus
Mitral valve prolapse, calcified annulus
Rheumatic heart disease (valvular, nonvalvular)
Prosthetic heart valves
Other (myopathy, atrial myxoma, subacute
  bacterial endocarditis, paradoxic emboli)

Systemic
Cardiac arrest and resuscitation
Profound shock
Cardiopulmonary bypass

Venous thromboses
Dural venous sinuses
Bilateral jugular vein occlusions

Miscellaneous causes
Lacunar infarcts
Lipohyalinosis
Fibrinoid necrosis
Charcot-Bouchard aneurysms
Migraine and vasospasm
Diabetes
Moyamoya
Kawasaki syndrome
Amyloid degeneration
Fibromuscular disease
Giant cell arteritis

Spontaneous dissections
Trauma (extracranial cerebral vessels)
  Blunt
  Penetrating
Hypercoagulable states
Binswanger's encephalopathy
Substance abuse

HEMORRHAGIC
Intraparenchymal hemorrhage
Hypertensive encephalopathy
Amyloid angiography
Arteriovenous malformation
Trauma

Subarachnoid hemorrhage
Berry aneurysms
Arteriovenous malformation
Trauma

EXTRACRANIAL
Atherosclerosis
  Great vessels
  Carotid artery
Fibromuscular dysplasia
Trauma
Aortic aneurysms
  Dissecting
  Atherosclerotic
  Traumatic
Takayasu's panarteritis
Temporal arteritis
Carotid dissections
  Spontaneous
  Trauma-associated
Carotid aneurysms

Modified from Zelenock GB. The brain. In: Clinical ischemic syndromes: mechanisms and consequences of tissue injury. St. Louis: Mosby, 1990:350, with permission.

Table 75.3. CLASSIFICATION OF SYMPTOMS

Hemispheric
Contralateral hemiparesis
Contralateral paresthesias or hemisensory changes
Ipsilateral monocular visual changes
Aphasia

Nonhemispheric
Vertigo
Ataxia
Diplopia
Bilateral visual symptoms
Shifting pareses or paresthesias
Drop attacks
Dysarthria
Syncope
Dizziness
Light-headedness
Decreased mentation
Headache
Personality change
Tinnitus
Seizures

---

though these are rare (5). Spontaneous dissection of the internal carotid artery usually originates just distal to the carotid bifurcation and reenters at the most distal aspect of the extracranial portion of the internal carotid artery. Spontaneous dissection can occur as a result of fibromuscular dysplasia. False aneurysms of the carotid artery are also uncommon and most often are caused by a traction injury to the internal carotid artery at the base of the skull associated with forceful flexion and extension of the neck. Spontaneous dissections and aneurysms of the internal carotid artery are most frequently complicated by thromboembolic events causing transient ischemia or stroke.

Atherosclerosis is the pathologic process most often responsible for symptoms of cerebrovascular insufficiency. The cause of atherosclerosis in the cerebral arterial circulation or in any portion of the systemic arterial circulation remains incompletely understood (6). Clinically, atherosclerosis tends to be a segmental disease; it usually develops at areas of local turbulence, such as vessel bifurcations, and causes focal vessel wall injury. Thus, the origins of the great vessels at the aortic arch or their proximal cervical bifurcations are involved frequently. Typically, the common carotid artery is spared. The carotid bifurcation is the most common location of atherosclerotic lesions in the cerebral circulation. The predilection of atherosclerosis for the carotid bulb is thought to be a consequence of the turbulent blood flow at the carotid bifurcation, which results in areas of *low* shear stress and increased particle residence time. Grossly, the atherosclerotic plaque is thickest at the carotid bifurcation and extends 2 cm into the distal internal carotid artery. The plaque occupies the media and intima, sparing the outer media and adventitia. Usually, the plaque tapers from the media into the normal intima. Such tapering often permits a smooth surface after endarterectomy. Finally, atherosclerotic stenosis can develop at the origins of the anterior and middle cerebral arteries, but these lesions are significantly less common than those found in the cervical portion of the internal carotid artery.

Atherosclerotic plaque at the carotid bifurcation, as at other locations in the systemic arterial circulation, initially appears as a *fatty streak,* which is largely an intimal lesion characterized by fat deposition and some mononuclear and foam cell infiltration. Fatty streaks do not cause hemodynamically significant stenoses of the vessel, and not all fatty streaks develop into complex plaques. As the

plaques increase in size, ulceration or intraplaque hemorrhage may occur intermittently; both processes can result in thrombosis or embolism. Mature atherosclerotic plaques are characterized by endothelial cell damage and denudation, intimal hyperplasia secondary to smooth-muscle cell proliferation, and then a gradual deposition of collagen matrix and extensive intracellular and extracellular lipid accumulation. Mature atherosclerotic plaques are usually covered by a *fibrous cap.* Disruption of the fibrous cap is often the precipitating event that causes a plaque to become symptomatic. The disruption of a fibrous cap can be secondary to a number of processes, including progressive growth of the atherosclerotic lesion, an increase in blood flow velocity and shear stress, hemorrhage into the plaque, or rupture of the vasa vasorum. Loss of a fibrous cap secondary to intraplaque hemorrhage or surface disruption by mechanical forces results in a loss of endothelial cell coverage, so that the underlying necrotic core of the plaque is exposed to the circulating blood. These changes promote platelet deposition and thrombus formation on the ulcerated surface. The disruption of a mature, complex plaque may then result in stroke following the embolization of atheromatous debris or platelet–fibrin aggregates (Figs. 75.5 and 75.6). Alternatively, thrombosis of the artery can result in ischemic necrosis when collateral blood flow is insufficient.

Some of these pathologic changes can be revealed by carotid duplex scanning. A mature plaque that is hard and calcified is highly echogenic, whereas a mature plaque complicated by intraplaque hemorrhage or loss of the fibrotic cap is normally anechoic, in which case it is called *soft plaque.* Some prospective studies have shown a correlation between the presence of soft plaque and transient ischemia and stroke, whereas the presence of hard, calcified plaque is characterized by a lack of associated symptoms.

The tendency of atherosclerosis to develop at the carotid bifurcation is most likely the consequence of a variety of hemodynamic changes (7). Atherosclerotic plaques tend to occur along the outer wall, not the inner wall, of the carotid bifurcation, and they often spare or involve only the most proximal portion of the external carotid artery. At the outer wall of the carotid bifurcation, disruption of normal laminar blood flow results in flow separation, flow stasis, increased particle residence time, and increased oscillations in shear stress—that is, alternating areas of high and low shear stress. The clinical risk factors for the development of carotid artery atherosclerotic lesions are the same as those for coronary artery disease and include age, hypertension, diabetes mellitus, hyperlipidemia, hypercoagulable states, positive family history, and tobacco use. A strong correlation between carotid plaque and elevated plasma homocysteine levels has been identified (8).

Stroke secondary to cerebrovascular disease can occur by either of two distinct mechanisms—ischemia associated with a low-flow state or embolism. Cerebral ischemia in a low-flow state is the consequence of the development of hemodynamically significant stenoses involving multiple cerebral arteries or of stenosis in an artery supplying a vascular territory with a poor collateral network. Although the earliest reports linking stroke and extracranial carotid occlusive disease were published in the 19th century, it was not until the 1950s that Fisher and colleagues (9) and Milliken (10) established the correlation between extracranial carotid artery occlusive disease and stroke. These investigators showed that most strokes associated with carotid artery occlusive disease are caused by cholesterol or platelet–fibrin emboli that dislodge from atherosclerotic plaques within the extracranial carotid artery and subsequently occlude distal branches of the internal

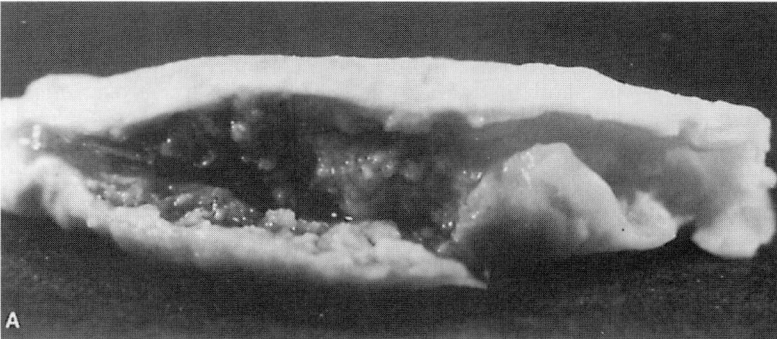

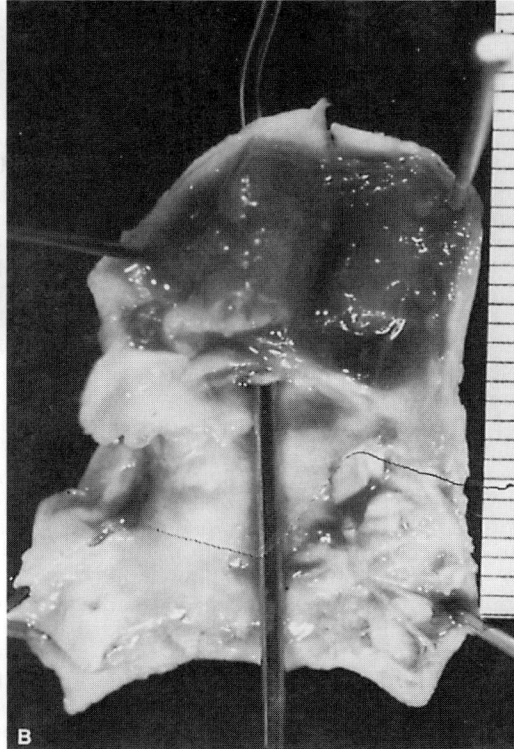

Figure 75.5. Endarterectomy specimens. *(A)* The thickened atherosclerotic plaque is almost totally occluded by intraluminal thrombus. This patient had symptoms of repeated embolism. *(B)* Hemorrhage is seen within the plaque, not in the lumen. If this hemorrhagic plaque excavates into the lumen, an ulceration will form.

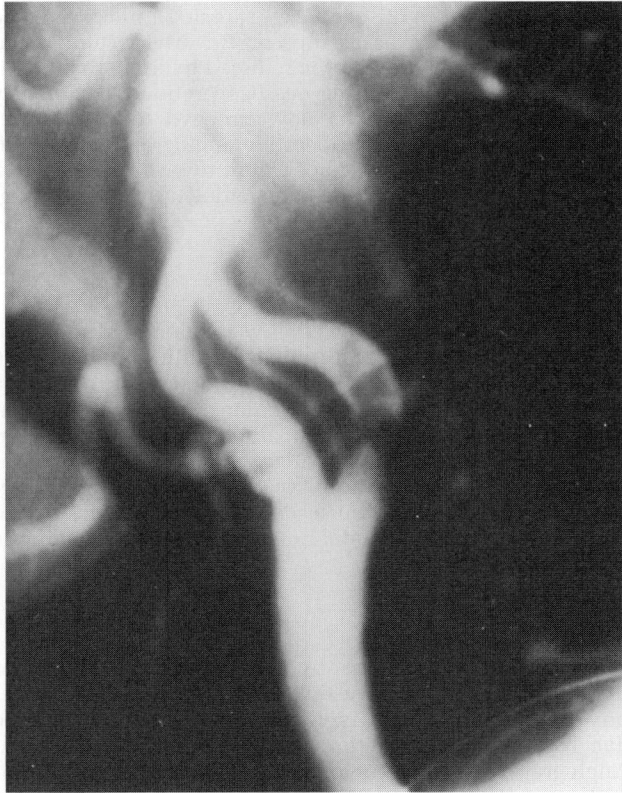

Figure 75.6. An isolated atherosclerotic lesion at the origin of the internal carotid artery. Free-floating intraluminal thrombus can be seen distal to the atherosclerotic plaque in this patient with crescendo transient ischemic attacks.

carotid artery. Their hypothesis differed substantially from the conventional dogma that most strokes were caused by cerebral ischemia secondary to reduced cerebral perfusion. One way in which this hypothesis was established was by the identification of *Hollenhorst plaques,* which are platelet–fibrin aggregates or cholesterol crystals obstructing branches of the retinal artery (11).

CLINICAL PRESENTATION

The most common clinical presentations of cerebrovascular occlusive disease are transient ischemic attack (TIA) and hemispheric stroke. Cerebrovascular disease resulting in atheroembolism or thrombosis accounts for up to 60% of cerebral infarctions (Fig. 75.1). A TIA is the sudden onset of a focal neurologic deficit that resolves completely within 24 hours of onset. It can be manifested as a transient hemispheric ischemic attack or as transient mononuclear blindness. A transient hemispheric attack presents clinically as contralateral motor and sensory deficits or as a purely motor or purely sensory deficit. The specific clinical presentation depends on the anatomic location of the area of cerebral ischemia. Transient mononuclear blindness, also known as *amaurosis fugax,* is a transient loss of vision secondary to mechanical obstruction of a branch of the retinal artery by either a cholesterol crystal or a Hollenhorst plaque (10). In most patients examined immediately after an episode of amaurosis fugax, however, the retinal circulation is found to be normal. When ischemia occurs transiently in the distal distribution of the posterior circulation of the brain, it causes transient *vertebrobasilar insufficiency.* This can present as binocular visual loss; *drop attacks,* in which the patient does not lose consciousness but collapses to the floor; dysarthria; vertigo; dysphasia; incoordination; and other signs of cerebellar insufficiency. The differential diagnosis of TIA includes cerebral tumor, hypoglycemia, hyponatremia, hypercalcemia, and hepatic or renal failure. In addition, vasospasm, particularly that associated with migraine headache, can present as transient ischemia. A significant clinical finding in patients with TIA secondary to atheromatous emboli is that the TIA is usually short, lasting less than 15 minutes. Although the distinction between a TIA and a completed stroke is sharply defined, serial computed tomography (CT) in patients with TIAs has shown that as many as 25% have had strokes in the area corresponding to the distribution of their symptoms (12).

A stroke is an acute neurologic deficit that lasts more than 24 hours. Like TIAs, most strokes are the result of embolic occlusion of a branch of the middle cerebral artery by atheromatous debris or a platelet–fibrin aggregate. Alternatively, a minority of strokes occur after internal carotid artery occlusion and subsequent cerebral infarction in a "watershed" distribution secondary to low flow. The watershed areas are located at the border areas between the anterior and posterior cerebral circulation, typically between the superior parietal and posterior temporooccipital lobes of the ipsilateral hemisphere. When strokes occur in this area, they are characterized clinically by a contralateral sensorimotor deficit that is more pronounced in the proximal than in the distal limb, a prominent visual field defect, aphasia, and features of partial inattention (13).

Stroke in the distribution of the anterior cerebral artery is characterized by weakness or paralysis in the contralateral limbs, numbness and tingling in the contralateral limbs, sparing of the face, dyspraxia, and abnormalities of higher cerebral function secondary to frontal lobe involvement. The latter is manifested by the presence of a grasp reflex, behavior disorder, poor concentration, and slowness of response. Strokes in the distribution of the middle cerebral artery are characterized by sensorimotor deficits in the contralateral limbs and homonymous hemianopsia. If the dominant hemisphere is involved, aphasia may be present. Strokes in the distribution of the anterior choroidal artery are characterized by contralateral hemiplegia, hypesthesia, and homonymous hemianopsia. Anterior circulation strokes should be distinguished clinically from lacunar strokes and vertebrobasilar strokes. Lacunar strokes are usually characterized by pure motor or sensory dysfunction in the contralateral limb in patients with hypertension. The term *lacunar,* derived from the Latin word for "hole" or "cavity," refers to the appearance of infarcted tissue within the substance of the brain on gross examination. The pathophysiologic basis of lacunar strokes is usually disease of small (200-μm) arterioles. Pathologically, lamellae of lipohyalinosis are often found. Finally, patients with vertebrobasilar strokes present with ipsilateral cranial nerve deficits, contralateral sensorimotor deficits, and signs of cerebellar insufficiency, including ataxia, vertigo, nystagmus, diplopia, and drop attacks. Symptoms of global cerebral ischemia can be difficult to distinguish from those of vertebrobasilar dysfunction.

DIAGNOSIS

Despite the development of various sophisticated diagnostic technologies, the clinical diagnosis of patients with symptomatic cerebrovascular occlusive disease remains centered on the careful performance of a neurologic examination before any of these diagnostic studies are obtained. Of paramount importance is to establish the distinction between a focal and a nonfocal neurologic deficit, such as dizziness. The history and physical examination should localize the area of cerebral ischemia responsible for the neurologic deficit. The neurologic examination of the patient should be complemented by a more complete physical examination to determine the presence of vascular occlusive disease in either the coronary or peripheral arteries, and to define other risk factors for stroke, such as acute arrhythmia.

A wide variety of noninvasive and invasive diagnostic studies can be performed to determine the causes and effects of stroke. In color-flow duplex scanning, real-time B-mode ultrasonography and color-enhanced pulsed Doppler flow measurements are used to determine the extent of carotid stenosis with reliable sensitivity and specificity (14,15) (Figs. 75.7 and 75.8) (see color insert following page 1190). Real-time B-mode imaging permits the localization of disease and determination of the presence or absence of calcification within plaque. Determination of the extent of stenosis is based largely on velocity criteria. In the Doppler technique, a predetermined ultrasonic frequency is transmitted. The emitted sound frequency is then reflected by moving red blood cells within a vessel back to a receiver crystal within the probe. The *Doppler effect,* which is the delay between the emission and reception of the ultrasonic frequency, is proportional to the velocity of the red cells. As stenosis increasingly obliterates the lumen of a vessel, the velocity of the blood flow must increase in the area of stenosis so that the total volume of flow remains constant within the vessel. Thus, velocity correlates with the extent of stenosis (Fig. 75.7). Typically, the internal carotid artery velocity profile is one of low resistance characterized by significant blood flow during diastole. Low-resistance velocity profiles also are typical of the hepatic and renal arteries. In contrast, the external carotid artery reflects a signal typical of a high-resistance, muscular artery, such as the common femoral artery, in which little blood flow occurs during diastole.

Performing and interpreting a carotid duplex scan requires considerable skill and experience. Duplex scanning is most accurate in assessing carotid artery stenoses in which the luminal diameter is reduced by more than 50%. Color-flow duplex scanning has been refined sufficiently such that some clinicians now proceed to carotid endarterectomy without preoperative angiography. As mentioned earlier, the presence of calcium within the carotid wall, indicated by increased echogenicity, may be of prognostic significance.

Transcranial Doppler

In transcranial Doppler, a low-frequency directional Doppler probe is focused through the thin temporal bone on the anterior, middle, and posterior cerebral arteries. Transcranial Doppler is of particular clinical value in patients with vasospasm after subarachnoid hemorrhage. In patients with cerebrovascular disease, transcranial Doppler complements duplex scanning by identifying significant intraarterial stenoses and revealing patterns of collateral flow. Transcranial color-flow duplex imaging is also available.

Angiography

Some consider angiography to be the gold standard for the diagnosis of cerebrovascular disease. During angiography, the arterial system is visualized after a radiopaque dye has been injected through an intraarterial catheter. Angiography remains the only method that allows a complete and detailed visualization of both the intracranial and extracranial arterial circulations. Nonetheless, angiography remains painful for the patient and poses serious inherent risks; these include dye allergy, renal toxicity (par-

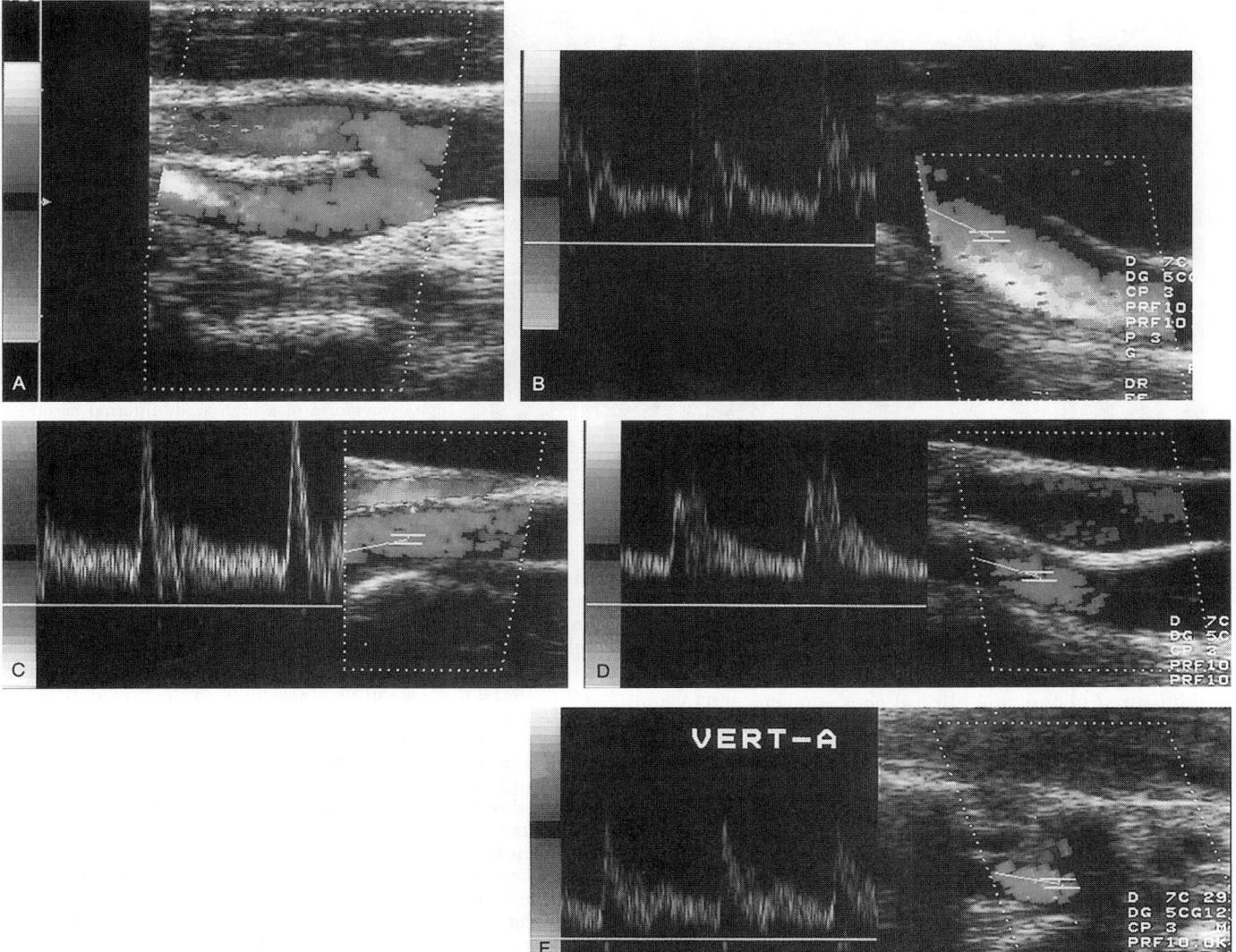

Figure 75.7. *(A)* Color-flow duplex scan showing a normal carotid artery bifurcation, the external carotid artery, and the internal carotid artery. *(B to D)* Duplex B-mode and analogue waveform of the common carotid artery *(B)*, external carotid artery *(C)*, and internal carotid artery *(D)*. There is a typical high-resistance waveform of the external carotid artery, which has reversal of flow in early diastole and minimal diastolic flow. In contrast, the internal carotid artery has a classic low-resistance waveform characterized by continuous flow throughout diastole. *(E)* Color-flow duplex image and analogue waveform of the vertebral artery.

ticularly in patients with diabetes mellitus), chronic renal insufficiency, and neurologic complications such as stroke (2% to 4% of patients). Digital subtraction angiography has reduced the need for selective carotid artery catheterization and so has reduced the risk for neurologic complications.

Computed Tomography and Magnetic Resonance Imaging

Computed tomography of the brain is a valuable test for patients with TIAs or stroke. Contrast-enhanced scans that assess density changes and the presence of edema or mass effect can determine the location and extent of a stroke and can rule out other conditions. CT of the brain distinguishes accurately between cerebral hemorrhage and infarction. Hemorrhage is associated with areas of increased

density on CT, whereas infarction is associated with areas of decreased density that do not appear until at least 8 hours after the stroke has occurred.

Magnetic resonance imaging (MRI) and MR angiography are highly sensitive techniques for the evaluation of patients with symptomatic cerebrovascular disease. MRI is more sensitive than CT in detecting an acute stroke. MRI can detect a stroke immediately after the infarction has occurred, whereas CT cannot. Cerebral hemorrhage, however, is less well identified by MRI than by CT. MR angiography, which is evolving rapidly, permits evaluation of both the extracranial and intracranial cerebral circulations. The precision of MR angiography in determining the extent of stenosis, although improving rapidly, remains inferior to that achieved by conventional angiography. Nonetheless, MR angiography probably will play an increasingly important role in the diagnostic evaluation of patients with cerebrovascular disease.

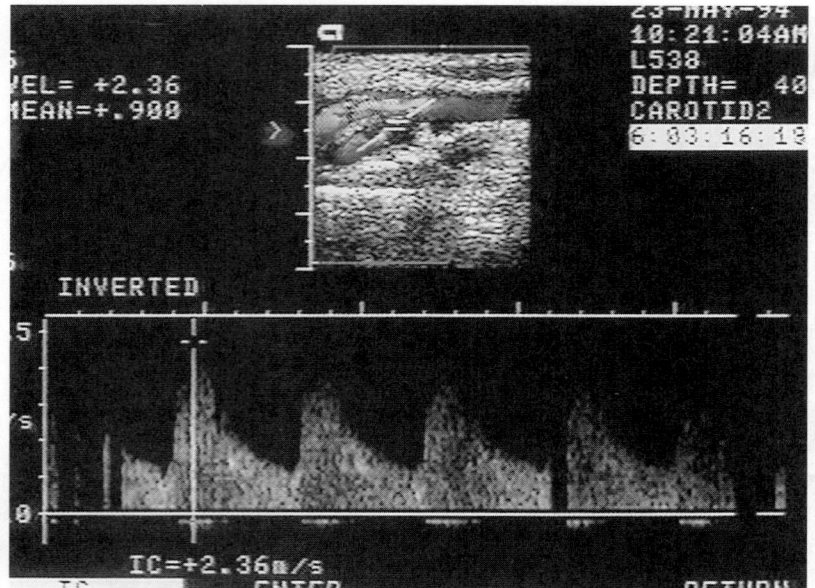

Figure 75.8. Color-flow duplex scan and analogue waveform of a high-grade internal carotid artery stenosis. Note acoustic shadowing in the region of the stenosis caused by calcification of the artery wall. Doppler taken at midstream of the jet of flow through the stenosis shows marked elevation of the peak systolic velocity (236 cm/s).

NATURAL HISTORY OF CAROTID ARTERY OCCLUSIVE DISEASE

Symptomatic Disease

Although many studies have been undertaken to define the natural history and clinical consequences of TIA and stroke, a variety of methodologic problems have limited the conclusions that can be drawn from these studies. Despite limitations, it is clear that the risk for stroke is substantial after a carotid territory TIA or stroke. In community-based studies, the risk for stroke in the first 3 years after a TIA varied from 12% to 17% (16,17). In hospital-based studies, the risk for stroke following a TIA varied from 10% to 30% after the first year, and then patients had a 6% risk for stroke each year for the subsequent 5 years. The cumulative risk for stroke after a TIA at 5 years was 30% to 50%. More important is the very high mortality rate secondary to coronary artery disease; one third of the patients died within 5 years after TIA, usually of coronary occlusive disease. The natural history of ischemic stroke is ominous. The initial stroke carries a 20% to 30% hospital mortality rate. The risk for recurrent stroke is high, ranging from 5% to 40%, and 30% of these are fatal (18,19).

Asymptomatic Disease

Because only 10% of patients who experience a stroke from any cause have had an antecedent TIA, a clear definition of the natural history of asymptomatic carotid artery disease is of significant clinical importance. Much of the early literature that addressed this issue studied asymptomatic carotid *bruits,* which are relatively common and have been reported to occur in about 5% of the population older than 50 years (20). Unfortunately, carotid bruits do not always arise from significant carotid artery stenosis; they can represent radiation of cardiac murmurs or denote the presence of mild carotid artery disease associated with calcification of the arterial wall. In fact, the poor correlation between the presence of a bruit and stenosis is illustrated by the fact that only 23% of patients identified to have bruits on physical examination have a significant (> 50%) carotid stenosis (21). With the wide availability of relatively inexpensive but accurate noninvasive studies to determine the presence and degree of carotid artery stenosis, a carotid bruit is of little significance in regard to a patient's neurologic prognosis. A carotid bruit, however, remains a significant predictor of symptomatic, life-threatening coronary artery disease.

The development of carotid duplex ultrasonography has permitted a more accurate assessment of the prevalence of asymptomatic carotid stenosis in older and high-risk populations. The prevalence of internal carotid artery stenosis is 30% in patients older than 50 years; however, the prevalence of carotid stenosis in which the luminal diameter is reduced by more than 50% is only 3.7%, and only 0.9% of patients have a reduction in diameter of more than 80%.

Studies of the natural history of patients with asymptomatic carotid artery stenosis do not provide a clear and definitive estimate of their risk for stroke. Studies do show, however, that the risk for stroke appears to be proportional to the degree of stenosis in that the patients at highest risk are those in whose luminal diameter is reduced by more than 80%. In addition, in studies that employed serial carotid duplex scanning, the degree of stenosis progressed in 85% of patients during follow-up. For patients found to have a stenosis of 75% to 80%, the risk for stroke varied from 18% and 46% (21,22).

An important clinical question is whether severe but asymptomatic carotid artery stenosis increases the risk for stroke in patients who undergo a major surgical procedure, such as coronary artery bypass grafting or peripheral vascular surgery. With noncardiac surgery, most studies have found that the perioperative risk for stroke is not increased, but when patients are followed carefully, a high neurologic complication rate can be identified (23). Most studies specifically addressing the issue of perioperative stroke after coronary artery bypass grafting have found that unilateral asymptomatic high-grade stenosis does not increase the risk for stroke (24–27). However, it is recommended that prophylactic repair be considered when bilateral asymptomatic high-grade stenosis is present.

MANAGEMENT

Medical Treatment

Both asymptomatic and symptomatic carotid artery occlusive disease is virtually always caused by atherosclerosis, a systemic disease. As with symptomatic atherosclerosis in other parts of the systemic arterial circulation, it is important to make every effort to modify risk factors to prevent progression of disease. The most important risk factor for stroke that should be controlled is hypertension. In addition, cessation of smoking, management of lipid disorders, attainment of ideal body weight, and regular exercise should be undertaken. No drug therapy has been shown to reduce the risk for stroke in patients with asymptomatic carotid artery occlusive disease. A number of studies have examined the role of antiplatelet drugs and anticoagulation therapy to reduce the risk for stroke in patients after TIA or stroke (1). No study has provided definitive evidence that systemic anticoagulation reduces the risk for stroke in patients with significant carotid artery occlusive disease who have experienced a TIA and stroke. The efficacy of aspirin in preventing stroke is also controversial. Aspirin, by reducing platelet adhesion and aggregation, has been shown to reduce morbidity and mortality from symptomatic coronary artery occlusive disease. When the end points of stroke and death are combined, a number of studies have shown a benefit in patients treated with aspirin. A number of serious methodologic criticisms of these studies have been made, however, and a metaanalysis of the prospective placebo-controlled trials of antiplatelet and anticoagulant therapies concluded that therapeutic benefit for either treatment could not be established and that anticoagulants probably have an adverse effect (28).

Surgical Treatment

The major indications for reconstruction of the cerebrovascular arteries are hemispheric TIA, stroke that leaves minimal residual neurologic deficits, and high-grade asymptomatic carotid artery stenosis. Less common indications include global cerebral ischemia, which usually occurs when three of the four major cerebral arteries are affected by hemodynamically significant stenosis. Such patients should undergo an extensive evaluation to detect other possible causes of their global symptoms, such as cardiac arrhythmia and middle ear abnormalities.

Technique of Carotid Endarterectomy

Although carotid endarterectomy has been performed for more than 40 years and is the most common vascular operation, certain aspects of this procedure still vary, particularly the type of anesthesia administered and the methods used to determine the adequacy of cerebral perfusion during transient internal carotid artery occlusion. Anesthesia during carotid endarterectomy can be either general endotracheal anesthesia, regional cervical block, or local anesthesia. Proponents of general anesthesia argue that the the operation is safer when performed on a motionless patient, and that it allows for more direct control of hemodynamic variables. In addition, general anesthesia reduces the cerebral metabolic rate and therefore may increase the threshold for ischemia. Proponents of regional or local anesthesia believe that these techniques minimize the risk for perioperative myocardial infarction associated with general anesthesia and make possible a more accurate assessment of the adequacy of cerebral perfusion during the period of transient internal carotid occlusion.

Surgical exposure of the carotid artery can be achieved through an incision along the medial border of the sternocleidomastoid muscle or by an oblique transverse incision through a skin crease. During dissection and mobilization of the common carotid artery and its branches, it is important to proceed with gentle dissection and minimal manipulation of the carotid bulb to prevent the embolization of atherosclerotic plaque. After the administration of systemic heparin, the carotid artery is occluded,

and a lateral arteriotomy is made from just proximal to the plaque in the common carotid artery to just beyond the distal extent of the plaque in the internal carotid artery (Fig. 75.9). The feasibility of carotid endarterectomy is based on the unique location of arterial atherosclerotic plaque, which occupies the intima and media and usually spares the adventitia of the involved arterial wall. In addition, atherosclerotic plaque is segmental in nature and tapers from within the deep media into the intima of the diseased artery distally. The cleavage plane for the endarterectomy is chosen at the thickest portion of the plaque, usually in the carotid bulb. This plane is then extended proximally and circumferentially, and the proximal plaque is transected. As the endarterectomy is extended toward the internal carotid artery, it is important to identify the transition zone of the plaque from within the deep media to the intima. This usually allows the plaque to be feathered distally, with a naturally molded arterial wall left in the internal carotid artery distally. The operation is completed by performing an eversion endarterectomy of the portion of the plaque that extends into the proximal external carotid artery. The plaque in the external carotid artery usually ends at the first bifurcation of this artery. At completion of the endarterectomy, any loose fragments of artery wall are removed, and if any residual shelf or loose intima is noted distally, tacking sutures are placed to prevent a flap from being raised during restoration of blood flow. The carotid arteriotomy is closed with a running suture, and if the internal carotid artery is small, a patch angioplasty can be performed (Fig. 75.9).

Some surgeons believe that patch angioplasty should be performed routinely after carotid endarterectomy to reduce the incidence of recurrent carotid stenosis, and this practice is supported by follow-up data from the Asymptomatic Carotid Atherosclerosis Study (ACAS), in which the use of a patch lowered the risk for restenosis from 21% to 7% (29). An objective technique to determine the patency of the endarterectomy should be undertaken at completion of the procedure: continuous-wave Doppler assessment, B-mode ultrasonography, or intraoperative arteriography. The patient should be monitored carefully for the first 12 to 24 hours after endarterectomy to evaluate hemodynamic stability and monitor neurologic status. Most patients tolerate this procedure well and can be discharged 24 to 72 hours after the operation.

Depending on the surgeon's preference, a variety of methods can be used to monitor the adequacy of cerebral perfusion during the period of internal carotid artery occlusion. These include neurologic assessment of the awake patient under local or regional cervical block, assessment of the internal carotid artery back pressure in the anesthetized patient, or continuous bilateral electroencephalographic monitoring. Pulse oximetry may also provide an estimation of the adequacy of collateral flow during carotid clamping. Cerebral protection during carotid cross-clamping involves optimal maintenance of systemic hemodynamics. The placement of shunt during the period of carotid clamping is essential in some patients. Some surgeons use shunts in all patients, whereas others shunt selectively based on the previously mentioned monitoring criteria. In large series, results do not vary between practitioners who never shunt, those who always shunt, and those who shunt selectively. Avoidance of elevated glucose levels during carotid clamping and pharmacologic therapy are other effective methods of cerebral protection.

Complications of Carotid Endarterectomy

Neurologic Complications. Stroke can occur during or after carotid endarterectomy secondary to a variety of

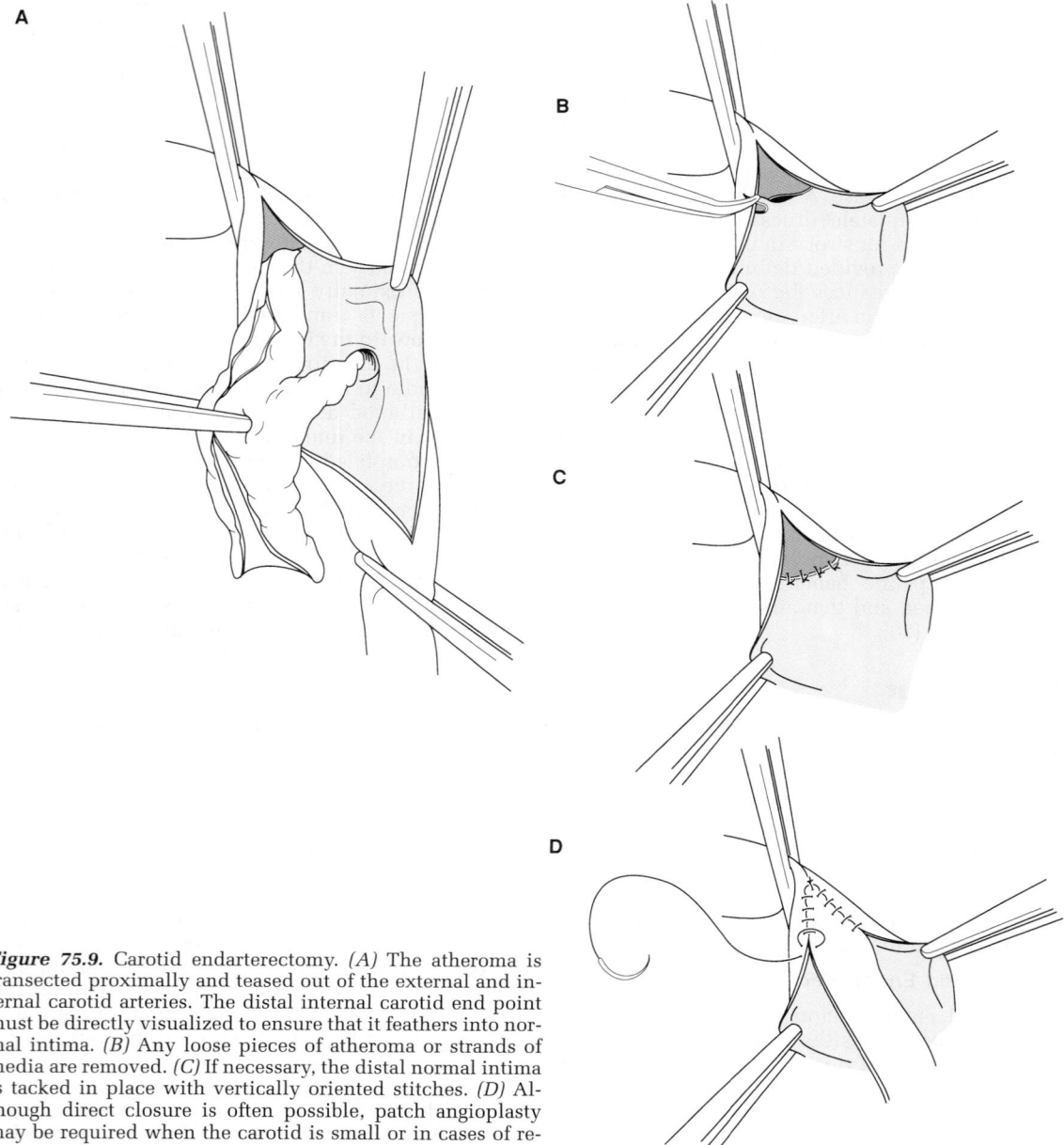

Figure 75.9. Carotid endarterectomy. *(A)* The atheroma is transected proximally and teased out of the external and internal carotid arteries. The distal internal carotid end point must be directly visualized to ensure that it feathers into normal intima. *(B)* Any loose pieces of atheroma or strands of media are removed. *(C)* If necessary, the distal normal intima is tacked in place with vertically oriented stitches. *(D)* Although direct closure is often possible, patch angioplasty may be required when the carotid is small or in cases of reoperation.

mechanisms, including inadequacy of collateral blood flow to the brain during temporary internal carotid artery occlusion, embolization during dissection of the carotid artery, or embolism or thrombosis of the reconstruction during the early postoperative period. Thrombosis after carotid endarterectomy usually is a result of sudden intimal dissection secondary to a loose flap or an inadequate distal endarterectomy end point. Embolization after carotid endarterectomy is usually secondary to the formation of platelet aggregates on the surface of the endarterectomized vessel. Finally, stroke can be caused by intracerebral hemorrhage, which appears to be more common in patients with multiple-vessel involvement preoperatively. It tends to occur on the second or third postoperative day.

Postoperative cranial nerve dysfunction can develop in up to 39% of patients undergoing carotid endarterectomy (30). Only 60% of these injuries produce clinical symptoms, such as hoarseness, difficulty in swallowing, or a change in speech patterns. Common cranial nerve injuries are to the recurrent laryngeal nerve, causing hoarseness; the hypoglossal nerve, causing the tongue to deviate toward the side of the injury; and the superior laryngeal nerve, causing the voice to become fatigued easily. Less common is injury of the marginal mandibular nerve, which results in drooping of the nasolabial fold ipsilateral to the injury. Also vulnerable to injury are the great auricular nerve, spinal accessory nerve, and glossopharyngeal nerve.

Most cranial nerve injuries resolve completely within 6 months after the operation. Particularly important are bilateral injuries, which may occur after bilateral endarterectomy. All patients who undergo carotid endarterectomy should have a careful cranial nerve examination before and after the operation. In patients undergoing second-stage contralateral carotid endarterectomies, it is common to perform preoperative indirect laryngoscopy to assess the vocal cord ipsilateral to the previous operation. A patient who sustains a bilateral recurrent laryngeal nerve injury may require an emergency tracheostomy.

Non-neurologic Complications. Carotid endarterectomy may result in a number of non-neurologic complications. Significant hemorrhage occurs after carotid endarterectomy in about 1% to 5% of patients. A somewhat higher rate of postoperative hemorrhage is noted in patients who receive aspirin perioperatively. Patients may also experience episodes of hypertension and hypotension (31). Hypotension and bradycardia occur secondary to increased baroreceptor reflex activity during dissection of the carotid artery or stimulation of the sinus nerve after removal of a rigid atheromatous plaque. Hypertension may develop if the carotid sinus nerve is interrupted, either by transection or a change in arterial wall compliance. Episodes of severe hypertension or hypotension are associated with an increased risk for neurologic deficits (31). Finally, myocardial infarction remains the most common cause of morbidity and mortality not related to stroke after carotid endarterectomy. Death from myocardial infarction accounted for 20% to 100% of all deaths after carotid endarterectomy (32). Myocardial infarction is also the most common cause of late death in patients who have undergone prior carotid endarterectomy. The 10-year cumulative survival rate after carotid endarterectomy in patients with coronary artery disease who underwent coronary artery bypass grafting before carotid endarterectomy was 55%, but it was only 32% in patients whose disease remained uncorrected (33).

Recurrent carotid stenosis is a relatively common but infrequently serious complication after carotid endarterectomy (Fig. 75.10). Residual or recurrent carotid artery stenosis can be detected in up to 30% of patients undergoing careful postoperative surveillance with carotid duplex scanning; however, fewer than 3% of patients experience symptomatic recurrence. Two forms of recurrent disease have been identified (34). Carotid stenosis that recurs within 6 months of the initial endarterectomy usually is secondary to intimal hyperplasia, characterized by the proliferation of vascular smooth muscle and an increase in matrix deposition. When stenosis recurs 2 years or more after endarterectomy, recurrent atherosclerosis is usually found at the time of reoperation. The risk for recurrent carotid stenosis has been documented to be higher in women and in patients with hypercholesterolemia.

Efficacy of Carotid Endarterectomy in the Prevention of Stroke

In the past, the efficacy of carotid endarterectomy in preventing stroke in patients with carotid stenosis was the subject of considerable controversy. The controversy arose in part from wide variations (1% to 24.4%) in the reported rates of stroke after carotid endarterectomy (35). In response to this controversy, a number of prospective, randomized studies examining the efficacy of carotid endarterectomy were undertaken. Three studies have established unambiguously the efficacy of carotid endarterectomy in preventing stroke in symptomatic patients with carotid stenosis (36–38) (Table 75.4).

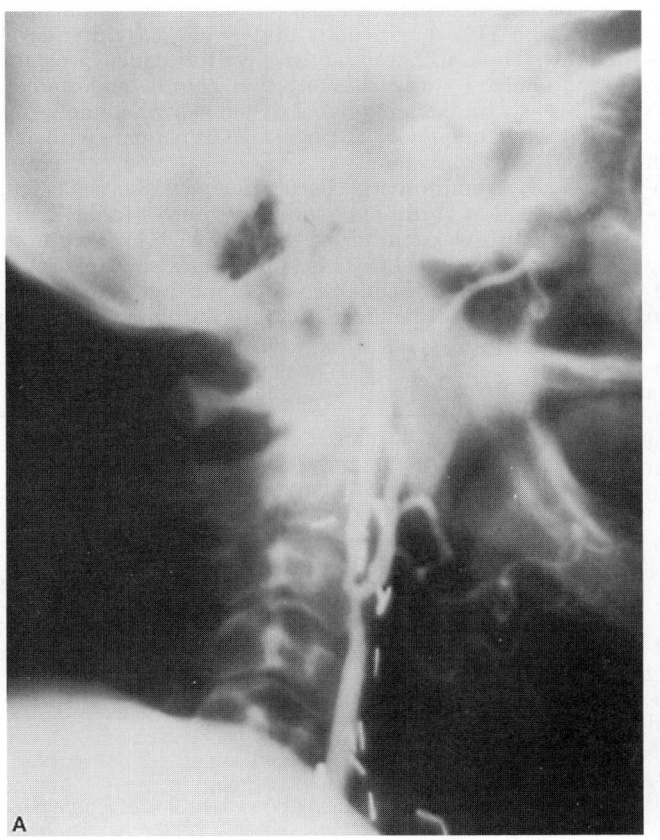
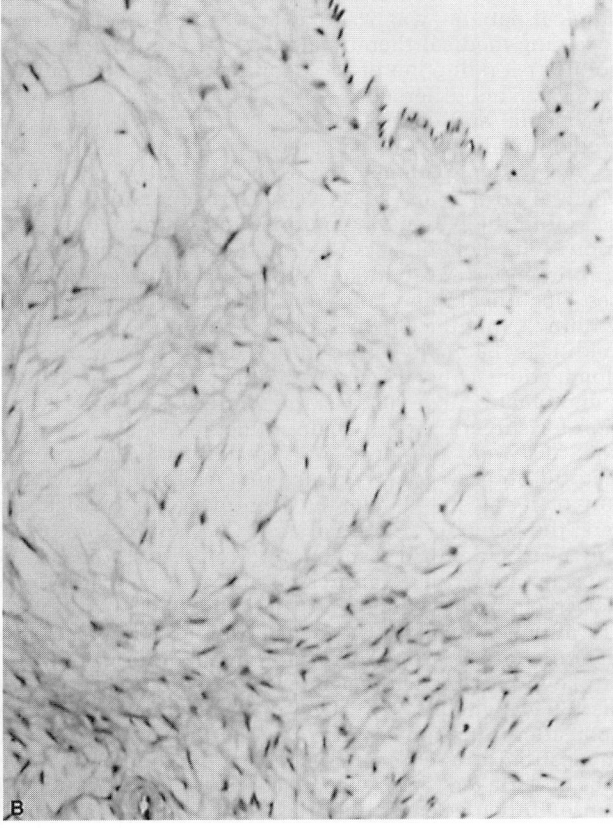

Figure 75.10. *(A)* Angiogram showing recurrent carotid stenosis. *(B)* This fibrous hyperplastic lesion was excised at operation.

Table 75.4. OUTCOME OF CLINICAL TRIALS OF CAROTID ENDARTERECTOMY IN PATIENTS WITH SYMPTOMATIC HIGH-GRADE CAROTID ARTERY STENOSIS

Study	Mean follow-up	Ipsilateral stroke rate (%)		Risk reduction (%)	
		Surgical	Nonsurgical	Absolute	Relative
NASCET	2 y	9[a]	26[b]	17	65
ECST	3 y	12.3[a]	21.9[b]	9.6	56
VA CSP 2309		7[a]	19.4[b]	11.7	63

[a]Significantly different from nonsurgery, p < .05.
[b]Included episodes of crescendo transient ischemic attack in addition to stroke as major end point of study.
NASCET, North American Symptomatic Carotid Endarterectomy Trial; ECST, European Carotid Surgery Trial; VA CSP, VA Cooperative Study.

In the first of these studies published, the North American Symptomatic Carotid Endarterectomy Trial (NASCET), patients were randomized to the best available medical management or to an experimental group that received the best medical management plus carotid endarterectomy (36). The patients were stratified according to degree of stenosis, 30% to 69% and 70% to 99%. Although the study was to include a 5-year follow-up, in February 1991, the Data Monitoring Board found a difference in treatment that was considered beyond the preapproved stop points for the trial. Thus, after only 18 months, a clinical alert was issued by the National Institutes of Health indicating that carotid endarterectomy is highly beneficial in patients with recent hemispheric or retinal TIA or nondisabling stroke and an ipsilateral high-grade carotid stenosis (70% to 99%). The conclusion was based on an interim analysis of 328 patients undergoing carotid endarterectomy and 331 receiving best medical therapy alone. At 18 months, the incidence of stroke in the surgical patients was 9%, and it was 26% in the patients receiving medical therapy alone. This represented an absolute risk reduction of 17% and a relative risk reduction of 65%. This difference is one of the largest between experimental and control groups in a prospective, randomized clinical trial. An even greater risk reduction was seen in the group of patients who experienced major or fatal ipsilateral stroke; an 81% relative risk reduction was observed in the patients who underwent carotid endarterectomy. The benefit accruing to the patients undergoing carotid endarterectomy held up under all subgroup analyses. Of clinical importance, the benefit of surgery was seen within 3 months of operation. The implication of this finding is that many of the strokes occurred soon after randomization. Thus, when a patient is identified as having a symptomatic high-grade carotid artery stenosis, evaluation for surgery should begin immediately. The results of NASCET were supported in a second trial, the European Carotid Surgery Trial, and also in a trial undertaken at 16 university-affiliated Veterans Administration medical centers, the Veterans Administration Cooperative Study 309. The nearly identical results found in these studies further substantiated the significant efficacy of carotid endarterectomy in symptomatic patients (37,38).

A number of studies have also been undertaken to evaluate the efficacy of carotid endarterectomy in preventing stroke in patients with asymptomatic carotid artery stenosis (39–41) (Table 75.5). One of the studies was aborted soon after initiation because of a high rate of postoperative myocardial infarction. A second study, the CASANOVA, was undertaken in Europe and completed in 1988 (39). Because of the design of this trial, the results did not clarify the appropriate management of patients with high-grade asymptomatic stenosis; all patients with a reduction in luminal diameter of more than 90% were excluded from randomization. The Veterans Administration Asymptomatic Carotid Stenosis Trial was a multicenter prospective, randomized trial in which 440 patients who had asymptomatic carotid stenosis of 50% or more were randomized to carotid endarterectomy plus aspirin or aspirin alone (40). When the primary end point of this study was examined, a benefit for the patients who underwent carotid endarterectomy was identified. At the time of analysis, 8% of the patients undergoing carotid endarterectomy experienced a TIA or stroke, whereas 20.6% of patients who received aspirin alone experienced a neurologic complication, a statistically significant difference. When the patients who experienced TIA were excluded and only the patients who experienced ipsilateral stroke were examined, no significant difference between the two groups was identified. The latter finding is not surprising because once patients in the nonsurgical group experienced a TIA, they usually underwent carotid endarterectomy. Thus, this was the first well-designed prospective, randomized study showing that carotid endarterectomy plus aspirin is more effective than aspirin alone in reducing the frequency of TIA or stroke in patients with asymptomatic carotid stenosis.

The Asymptomatic Carotid Artery Stenosis Trial, a prospective study sponsored by the National Institutes of Health, was similar to the NASCET for symptomatic carotid stenosis (41). This study was also interrupted because of a significant benefit identified in patients undergoing carotid endarterectomy. Patients with asympto-

Table 75.5. OUTCOME OF CLINICAL TRIALS OF CAROTID ENDARTERECTOMY IN PATIENTS WITH ASYMPTOMATIC CAROTID STENOSIS

Study	Rate of ipsilateral neurologic events (%)		Risk reduction (%)	
	Surgical	Nonsurgical	Absolute	Relative
VA CSP[a]	8[c]	20.6	12.6	38
ACAS[b]	4.8[c]	10.6	5.8	55

[a]Transient ischemic attacks and stroke were end points.
[b]Stroke was only end point.
[c]p ≤ .05 compared with nonsurgical group.
VA CSP, Veterans Administration Cooperative Studies Program (carotid stenosis ≥50%); ACAS, Asymptomatic Carotid Artery Study (carotid stenosis ≥60%).

matic stenosis of 60% or more were randomized to either carotid endarterectomy and aspirin or aspirin alone. At the time the study was interrupted, a relative reduction in the stroke rate of 50% had been observed in patients undergoing carotid endarterectomy. The benefit was much greater in men than in women. In this study, stroke was used as the primary end point. This group has now unequivocally demonstrated the effectiveness of carotid endarterectomy in good-risk patients with high-grade stenosis.

These prospective, randomized studies established the role of carotid endarterectomy in preventing stroke in patients with both symptomatic and asymptomatic high-grade carotid artery stenosis. All the patients in these studies were carefully selected as being good risks, and the complication rates of the surgeons performing the operations were extremely low. For patients to benefit from this operation, it must be performed by experienced surgeons with a record of very low complication rates.

External Carotid Endarterectomy

External carotid endarterectomy is recommended for patients with ipsilateral internal carotid artery occlusion and clinical evidence of retinal or hemispheric TIA or stroke. Many of them have a large cul-de-sac in the proximal internal carotid artery that may serve as a source of emboli (Fig. 75.11). These are relatively uncommon clini-

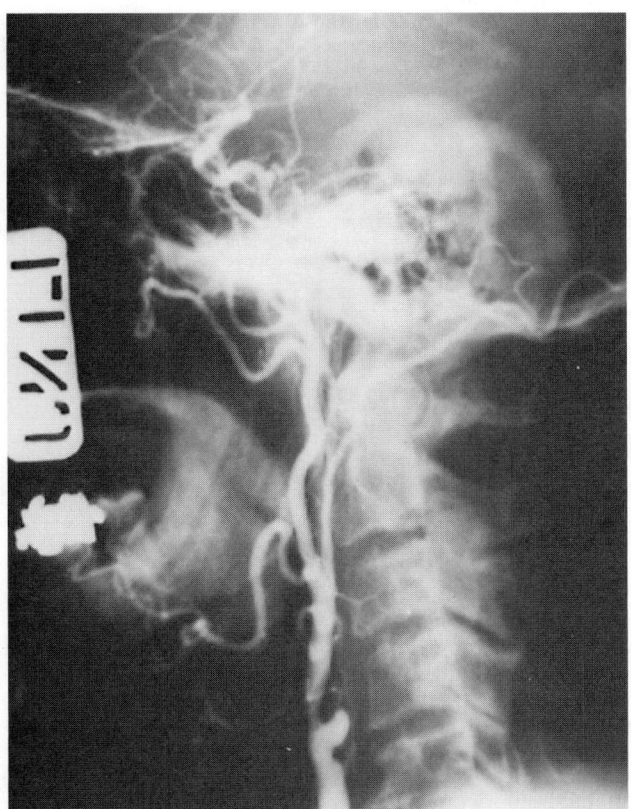

Figure 75.11. A totally occluded internal carotid artery with a residual stump may be a source of emboli. Note the periorbital collateral circulation.

cal occurrences, but external carotid endarterectomy has been shown to be safe and effective in such patients.

Direct Aortic Arch Reconstruction

Atherosclerotic lesions at the origin of the great vessels can result in TIA or stroke. Most commonly involved are the brachiocephalic and left common carotid arteries. When such lesions are identified, they can be repaired by direct reconstruction through a median sternotomy. For patients with lesions of the brachiocephalic artery, the options of endarterectomy or aortobrachiocephalic bypass grafting with a synthetic graft are available. Often, it is necessary to undertake revascularization of both the brachiocephalic and left common carotid arteries. Despite the complexity of these operations, they are in general attended by low complication rates and a neurologic morbidity rate of 2% or less.

Vertebral Artery Reconstruction

Atherosclerosis at the origin of the vertebral arteries can become symptomatic, causing TIA or stroke in the posterior cerebral circulation. When appropriate indications exist, a variety of techniques are available for reconstruction of the vertebral arteries. Vertebral artery endarterectomy can be undertaken through an arteriotomy in the subclavian artery. Alternatively, the vertebral artery can be ligated at its origin and replanted into a normal ipsilateral common carotid artery. Less commonly, distal vertebral artery reconstructions are accomplished with a carotid–vertebral bypass in which saphenous vein is used.

Nonanatomic Bypass

Patients with atherosclerotic stenosis at the origin of the aortic arch vessels may present with not only neurologic symptoms but also symptoms related to ischemia of the upper extremities. For patients who are not candidates for direct aortic arch reconstruction, a variety of alternative, nonanatomic bypasses can be undertaken, such as subclavian–carotid, carotid–subclavian, axillary–axillary, carotid–carotid, and even femoral–axillary bypass. Some have suggested that the patency of synthetic Dacron grafts is superior to that of saphenous vein grafts. Saphenous vein grafts are preferred by some surgeons, however, owing to a theoretically lower rate of platelet embolization. Most of these nonanatomic reconstructions have good long-term patency rates.

Endovascular Therapy

As experience with angioplasty and stenting in other peripheral arteries increases, the application of these techniques to atherosclerosis and restenosis of the carotid artery has been examined. Although the possibility of embolic stroke resulting from angioplasty of a friable and complex atherosclerotic lesion is concerning, initial experience with angioplasty and stenting has been associated with periprocedural stroke and death rates of 7.9% in a high-risk population of patients (42). The clinical benefits of this less invasive approach are obvious, although questions remain regarding the efficacy of angioplasty in preventing later strokes. The safety and efficacy of angioplasty and stenting in comparison with that of carotid endarterectomy will be determined in forthcoming multicenter propective, randomized clinical trials.

REFERENCES

1. Marshall RS, Mohr JP. Current management of ischaemic stroke. *J Neurol Neurosurg Psychiatry* 1993;56:6.
2. Carpenter MB. Blood supply of the central nervous system. In: *Core text of neuroanatomy.* Baltimore: Williams & Wilkins, 1974:231.
3. Stanley JC, Gerwertz BL, Bove EL, et al. Arterial fibrodysplasia, histopathological character, and current etiologic concepts. *Arch Surg* 1975;11:561.
4. Effeney DJ, Ehrenfeld WK, Stoney RJ, et al. Why operate on carotid fibromuscular dysplasia? *Arch Surg* 1980;115:1261.
5. Ehrenfeld WK, Wylie EJ. Spontaneous dissection of the internal carotid artery. *Arch Surg* 1976;111:1294.
6. Ross R. The pathogenesis of atherosclerosis: a perspective for the 1990s. *Nature* 1993;362:801.
7. Zarins CK. Pathology of carotid atherosclerosis. In: Ernst CB, Stanley JC, eds. *Current therapy in vascular surgery,* 2nd ed. Philadelphia: BC Decker, 1991:1.
8. Selhub J, Jaques PF, Bostom AG, et al. Association between plasma homocysteine concentrations and extracranial carotid artery stenosis. *N Engl J Med* 1995;332:286.
9. Fisher CM, Pritchard JE, Mathews WH. Arteriosclerosis of the carotid arteries. *Circulation* 1952;6:457.
10. Milliken CH. The pathogenesis of transient focal cerebral ischemia. *Circulation* 1965;32:438.
11. Hollenhorst RW. Significance of bright plaques in the retinal arteries. *JAMA* 1961;178:23.
12. Norris JW, Zhu CA. Silent stroke and carotid stenosis. *Stroke* 1992;23:483.
13. Mohr JP, Barnett HJM. Classification of ischemia strokes. In: Barnett HJM, Mohr JP, Stein BM, et al., eds. *Stroke: pathophysiology, diagnosis, and management.* New York: Churchill Livingstone, 1986:281.
14. Moneta GL, Edwards JM, Chitwood RW, et al. Correlation of North American Symptomatic Carotid Endarterectomy Trial (NASCET) angiographic definition of 70% to 99% internal carotid artery stenosis with duplex scanning. *J Vasc Surg* 1993;17:152.
15. Londrey GL, Spadone DP, Hodgson, et al. Does color flow imaging improve the accuracy of duplex carotid evaluation? *J Vasc Surg* 1991;13:659.
16. Friedman GD, Wilson WS, Mosier JM, et al. Transient ischemic attacks in a community. *JAMA* 1969;210:1428.
17. Whisnant JP, Matsumoto N, Elveback LR. Transient cerebral ischemic attacks in a community. *Mayo Clin Proc* 1973;48:194.
18. Matsumoto N, Whisnant JP, Kurland LT, et al. Natural history of stroke in Rochester, Minnesota, 1955 through 1969: an extension of a previous study, 1945 through 1954. *Stroke* 1973;4:20.
19. Bardin JA, Bernstein EF, Humbert PB, et al. Is carotid endarterectomy beneficial in prevention of recurrent stroke? *Arch Surg* 1982;117:1401.
20. Mohr JP. Asymptomatic carotid artery disease. *Stroke* 1982;13:431.
21. Chambers BR, Norris JW. Outcome in patients with asymptomatic neck bruits. *N Engl J Med* 1986;315:860.
22. Roederer GO, Langlois YE, Jager KA, et al. The natural history of carotid arterial disease in asymptomatic patients with cervical bruits. *Stroke* 1984;15:605.
23. Barnes RW, Marzalek PB. Asymptomatic carotid disease in the cardiovascular surgical patient: is prophylactic endarterectomy necessary? *Stroke* 1981;12:497.
24. Brener BJ, Brief DK, Alpert J, et al. The risk of stroke in patients with asymptomatic carotid stenosis undergoing cardiac surgery: a follow-up study. *J Vasc Surg* 1987;5:269.
25. Breslau PJ, Fell G, Ivey TD, et al. Carotid arterial disease in patients undergoing coronary artery bypass operations. *J Thorac Cardiovasc Surg* 1981;82:765.
26. Ivey TD, Strandness DJ Jr, Williams DB, et al. Management of patients with carotid bruit undergoing cardiopulmonary bypass. *J Thorac Cardiovasc Surg* 1984;87:183.
27. McCann RL. Surgical management of carotid artery atherosclerotic disease. *South Med J* 1993;86:2S23.
28. Ramirez-Lassepas M, Cipolle RJ. Medical treatment of transient ischemic attacks: does it influence mortality? *Stroke* 1988;19:397.
29. Moore WS, Kempczinski RF, Nelson JJ, et al. Recurrent carotid stenosis: results of the Asymptomatic Carotid Atherosclerosis Study. *Stroke* 1998;29:2018.
30. Hertzer NR. Postoperative management and complications of extracranial carotid reconstruction. In: Rutherford RM, ed. *Vascular surgery.* Philadelphia: WB Saunders, 1984:1300.
31. Bove EL, Fry WJ, Gross WS, et al. Hypotension and hypertension as consequences of baroreceptor dysfunction following carotid endarterectomy. *Surgery* 1979;85:633.
32. O'Donnell TF, Callow AD, Willett C, et al. The impact of coronary artery disease on carotid endarterectomy. *Ann Surg* 1983;198:705.
33. Hertzer NR, Arison R. Cumulative stroke and survival ten years after carotid endarterectomy. *J Vasc Surg* 1985;2:661.
34. Stoney RJ, String ST. Recurrent carotid stenosis. *Surgery* 1976;80:705.
35. Easton JP, Sherman DG. Stroke and mortality rate in carotid endarterectomy: 228 consecutive operations. *Stroke* 1977;8:565.
36. North American Symptomatic Carotid Endarterectomy Trial Collaborators. Beneficial effect of carotid endarterectomy in symptomatic patients with high-graft carotid stenosis. *N Engl J Med* 1991;325:445.
37. European Carotid Surgery Trialists' Collaborative Group. MRC European Carotid Surgery Trial: interim results for symptomatic patients with severe (70%–99%) or with mild (0%–29%) carotid stenosis. *Lancet* 1991;337:1235.
38. Mayberg MR, Wilson SE, Yatsu F, et al., for the Veterans Affairs Cooperative Studies Program 309 Trialist Group. Carotid endarterectomy and prevention of cerebral ischemia in symptomatic carotid stenosis. *JAMA* 1991;266:3289.
39. The CASANOVA Study Group. Carotid surgery vs. medical therapy in asymptomatic carotid stenosis. *N Engl J Med* 1993;328:221.
40. Hobson RW II, Weiss DG, Fields WS, et al. Efficacy of carotid endarterectomy for asymptomatic carotid stenosis. *N Engl J Med* 1993;328:221.
41. Executive Committee for the Asymptomatic Carotid Atherosclerosis Study. Endarterectomy for asymptomatic carotid artery stenosis. *JAMA* 1995;273:1421.
42. Yadav JS, Roubin GS, Iyer S, et al. Elective stenting of the extracranial carotid arteries. *Circulation* 1997;95:376.

SURGERY: SCIENTIFIC PRINCIPLES AND PRACTICE, Third Edition, edited by Lazar J. Greenfield, Michael W. Mulholland, Keith T. Oldham, Gerald B. Zelenock, and Keith D. Lillemoe. Lippincott Williams & Wilkins Publishers, Philadelphia, © 2001.

CHAPTER 76

UPPER EXTREMITY OCCLUSIVE DISEASE

JAMES S. T. YAO

A wide spectrum of arterial occlusive diseases in an upper extremity can cause ischemic symptoms. An accurate diagnosis requires a thorough history, careful physical examination, and the liberal use of ancillary tests. Appropriate surgical treatment depends on the location of the occlusive lesion and the nature of the underlying occlusive process. In general, proximal lesions involving the subclavian, axillary, and brachial arteries are more amenable to reconstructive surgery.

HISTORY TAKING

Taking an appropriate history is the most important initial step in the work-up of a patient with upper extremity

Table 76.1. CONDITIONS AND RISKS FOR UPPER EXTREMITY ISCHEMIA

Occupational injury	**Medical conditions**
Vibration syndrome	Atherosclerosis
Pneumatic tools	Arteritis
Chain saws	Collagen disease
Grinders	Scleroderma
Electrical burns	Rheumatic arteritis
Hypothenar hammer syndrome	Systemic lupus erythematosus
Mechanical work or auto repair	Dermatomyositis
Lathe operation	Allergic necrotizing arteritis
Carpentry	Takayasu's disease
Electrical work	Giant cell arteritis
Occupational acroosteolysis—polyvinylchloride exposure	Blood dyscrasias
Athletic activities	Cold agglutinins
Thoracic outlet compression	Cryoglobulins
Baseball pitching	Polycythemia vera
Kayaking	Behçet's syndrome
Weight lifting	Antiphospholipid syndrome
Rowing	Thoracic outlet syndrome
Butterfly swimming	Congenital arterial wall defects
Golfing	Pseudoxanthoma elasticum
Hand ischemia	Ehlers-Danlos syndrome
Baseball catching	Fibromuscular dysplasia
Frisbee	Iatrogenic injury
Karate	Arterial blood gas and pressure monitoring
Handball	Cardiac catheterization
Pharmacologic history	Arteriography
Ergot poisoning	Frostbite
Beta blockers	Renal transplantation and related problems
Drug abuse, cocaine use	Azotemic arteriopathy
Cytotoxic drugs	Hemodialysis shunts
Dopamine overdose	Radiation
	Breast carcinoma
	Hodgkin's disease
	Aneurysms of the upper extremity

ischemia. In addition to a careful delineation of the patient's symptoms, an appropriate inquiry should include occupational, pharmacologic, and athletic risks and a pertinent medical history. Table 76.1 lists conditions and activities that can be related to the development of upper extremity ischemic symptoms.

SYMPTOMS

The presenting symptoms of upper extremity occlusive disease include evidence of arterial emboli, Raynaud's phenomenon, pain, and exercise-related forearm fatigue. Embolic symptoms include gangrene of the tips of the fingers, petechiae of the skin, splinter hemorrhages of the nail bed, and livedo reticularis. The term *Raynaud's phenomenon* refers to episodic digital color changes provoked by stimuli such as cold or emotion. The digits first exhibit pallor, then cyanosis, and then a reactive hyperemia. The pathophysiology of the color changes from white to blue to red is thought to be digital ischemia (resulting from vasospasm), followed by desaturation of hemoglobin (which produces cyanosis), and then by a reactive hyperemia. Raynaud's phenomenon should not be confused with Raynaud's disease. The former is a secondary process, whereas the latter is a primary disease without a known cause. The diagnosis of primary Raynaud's disease is made only after all the etiologic factors listed in Table 76.1 have been excluded and after symptoms persist for at least 2 years in the absence of other conditions that might be causal. Raynaud's phenomenon secondary to an underlying cause can be unilateral or bilateral. In patients with unilateral Raynaud's phenomenon, organic arterial occlusive disease should be suspected. In contrast, bilateral symptoms are often the consequence of a systemic disease that causes vasospasm. The precise classification of pri-

mary and secondary Raynaud's phenomenon is often difficult, and the terminology is imprecise. Many physicians prefer to use the term *Raynaud's syndrome* to characterize all patients with episodic vasospastic disease of the hands. Raynaud's phenomenon should also be distinguished from acrocyanosis, a disorder characterized by painless, persistent, diffuse cyanosis of the fingers and hands.

CLINICAL EXAMINATION

The physical examination should include an examination of the thoracic outlet and the entire upper extremity. Palpation of the supraclavicular region may help to detect the presence of a subclavian aneurysm or a cervical rib. Auscultation of the subclavian artery with the stethoscope placed just below the midclavicular region and listening for a bruit with the patient's arm placed in a neutral position (or abduction) and external rotation (or hyperabduction) help to establish the diagnosis of thoracic outlet compression to the artery. Pulse palpation begins with the subclavian artery in the supraclavicular fossa and continues with the axillary artery under the armpit, the brachial artery at the upper arm and elbow, and the radial and ulnar arteries at the wrist level. A decreased or absent pulse in any site other than the supraclavicular fossa indicates major artery occlusion. Conversely, a readily palpable pulse in the supraclavicular fossa can represent a subclavian artery aneurysm.

Examination of the hand is not complete unless an Allen test is performed. The examiner stands beside or facing the subject. The radial and ulnar arteries of one wrist are compressed by the examiner's fingers. The subject is asked to open and close the hand rapidly for 1 minute to empty blood out of the hand and then to extend the fingers quickly. The radial or the ulnar artery is released, and the hand is observed for capillary refilling and return of color. The test result is judged normal if refilling of the hand is complete within a short period (< 6 seconds). Any portion of the hand that does not blush is an indication of incomplete continuity of the arch. Hyperextension of the fingers must be avoided because it produces a false-positive result. In addition to the Allen test, examination of the hand must include palpation of the palm for a pulsatile mass or excess scar tissue. Assessment of the patency of digital arteries by palpation is often difficult and unreliable. Upper extremity digital capillary refill is nearly instantaneous in normal subjects.

NONINVASIVE TESTING

Several noninvasive tests, including plethysmography, transcutaneous Doppler examination, and duplex scan, are available for the objective evaluation of patients with upper extremity ischemia (1). Of these, the Doppler examination is the most straightforward and consists of audible signal interpretation, waveform recording with spectral analysis, and systolic pressure measurements. Bilateral examinations should be performed for comparative purposes. Because many of the diseases affecting the hand are symmetric, the asymptomatic hand often will have significant disease (2). This is especially true in patients with systemic disease causing hand ischemia.

Because both the axillary and brachial arteries are superficial vessels, they are amenable to Doppler examination. Any change from normal signals (triphasic) to abnormal signals (monophasic) indicates the presence of an occlusive lesion. Distal to the elbow, arterial signals are more difficult to obtain. At the wrist, both the radial and ulnar arteries become superficially situated once again. Palpation of the ulnar artery can be difficult, and Doppler examination is helpful in determining the patency of this artery. In the hand, Doppler examination of the palmar arches is performed best at the midthenar and hypothenar regions. The common digital vessels should be examined at the base of the fingers where they divide into the proper digital arteries, which lie along the shaft of the proximal phalanx of each finger. Waveform recording is useful in both analysis and record keeping.

For segmental upper extremity pressures, a pneumatic cuff is placed at the upper arm, as in routine blood pressure recording. The brachial artery blood pressure reflects the pressure in all proximal arteries, and the value should be within 10 to 20 mm Hg of that in the opposite extremity. A greater difference signifies innominate, subclavian, axillary, or brachial stenosis. If brachial artery occlusion is suspected, a pressure cuff is applied to the forearm and the pressure recorded in a similar manner, with the radial artery used for signal detection. A pressure drop of 20 to 30 mm Hg signifies an obstruction distal to the brachial artery. For finger pressure measurement, a 2.5-cm cuff is placed at the base of the finger, and the return of Doppler signals after cuff deflation is monitored at the fingertip. An arterial occlusion distal to the palmar arch is defined by a pressure gradient between the fingers of more than 15 mm Hg or a wrist-to-digit difference of 30 mm Hg.

The Doppler technique is of particular value in determining palmar arch patency in a patient who is unconscious or uncooperative in performing an Allen test. Before arterial line placement, this simple test may help to avoid hand ischemia. In the modified Allen test, the Doppler probe is placed over the radial artery while the ulnar artery is compressed. If the signal disappears, the arch depends on the ulnar artery for supply. If the signal remains strong, the arch is complete. A similar maneuver is repeated over the ulnar artery while the radial artery is compressed.

The plethysmograph is used to record finger pulse contours for analysis and to differentiate between a normal state and obstructive or vasospastic disease (1). The duplex scan is helpful in establishing the diagnosis of aneurysm.

LABORATORY TESTING

In severe bilateral hand ischemia, a systemic cause of the arterial lesions should be sought. Laboratory tests include serologic, immunologic, and hematologic studies to help establish the diagnosis.

  Erythrocyte sedimentation rate
  Rheumatoid factor
  Antinuclear antibody
  Immunoglobulin electrophoresis
  Cryoglobulins
  Cold agglutinins
  VDRL (Venereal Disease Research Laboratory) test
  Complement (C3, C4)
  Anticardiolipin antibody
  Blood cell counts

The erythrocyte sedimentation rate remains a useful screening test to aid in the diagnosis of various forms of arteritis. A positive antinuclear antibody test result suggests connective tissue disease or other arteritides. When the antinuclear antibody titer is abnormal, immunofluorescent pattern analysis of antibodies can help to establish the diagnosis of various connective tissue disorders. The speckled pattern antibody is more specific for systemic lupus erythematosus. A nucleolar pattern suggests scleroderma. A positive anticardiolipin antibody is diagnostic for antiphospholipid syndrome, which is characterized by thromboembolic events in young adults (3).

RADIOLOGIC TESTING

A combination of laboratory and radiologic testing may be needed to establish the proper diagnosis of systemic disease. The radiologic examination includes soft-tissue radiography of the hand, chest roentgenography, esophageal barium swallow and motility test, and arteriography. The soft-tissue radiograph of the hand may reveal calcinosis, which is diagnostic for the CREST (calcinosis cutis, Raynaud's phenomenon, esophageal motility disorder, sclerodactyly, and telangiectasia) syndrome, or diffuse calcified arteries in diabetic or azotemic arteriopathy (Fig. 76.1). The chest film is essential to detect bony anomalies of the thoracic outlet, such as cervical ribs (Fig. 76.2), anomalous first ribs, and healed fractures of the first rib or clavicle. Pulmonary fibrosis on the chest film is another indication of systemic sclerosis.

Arteriography is useful in defining the vascular anatomy of the hand and calculating the degree of peripheral ischemia. In the investigation of upper extremity ischemia, arteriography must include all arteries from the aortic arch to the hand (4). The liberal use of subtraction techniques, multiple views, and magnification films should provide proper detail. In addition to the state of the inflow arteries, the anatomic characteristics of the palmar arches may aid in determining the degree of hand ischemia. The anatomic variability of the upper extremity arteries, especially the palmar arches (superficial and deep), is well known (5), and incomplete palmar arches play a significant role in ischemic disease and contribute to digital ischemia. In general, the deep palmar arch is formed primarily by the terminal part of the radial artery, and the superficial arch by the ulnar artery. According to the manner in which the contributing arteries join, arches

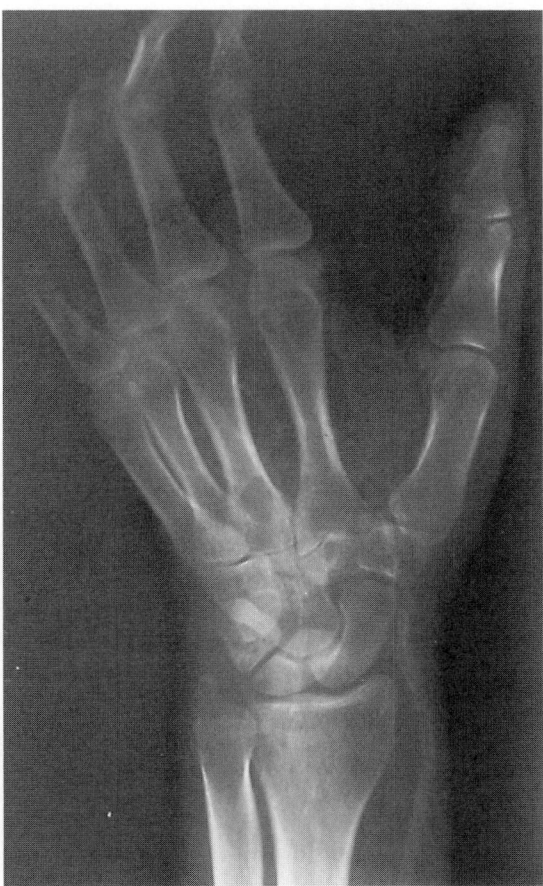

Figure 76.1. Typical appearance of azotemic arteriopathy (calciphylaxis) in a diabetic patient with a renal transplant. All the digital arteries are distinctly seen on plain film. The radial artery has a "pipe stem" appearance. An arteriogram shows multiple digital artery occlusions. (From Yao JST. Arterial surgery of the upper extremity. In: Haimovici H, Callow AD, DePalma RG, et al., eds. *Vascular surgery: principles and techniques,* 3rd ed. Norwalk, CT: Appleton & Lange, 1989:863, with permission.)

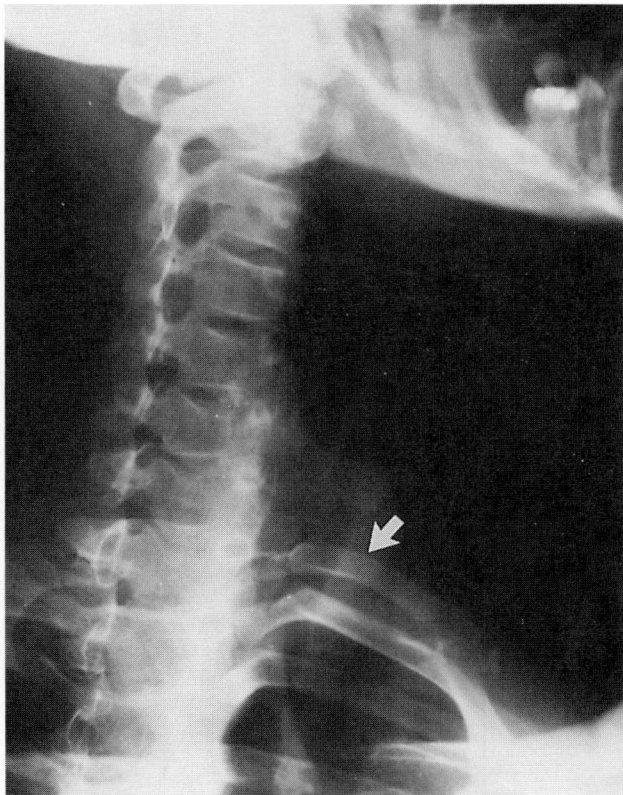

Figure 76.2. Cervical rib *(arrow)* in a patient with subclavian aneurysm caused by thoracic outlet compression.

are categorized as complete or incomplete. In a study of 500 hand arteriograms, the deep palmar arch appeared complete in 95.2% of cases (6). The finding is similar to that reported in an earlier study in which classic techniques of anatomic dissection were used (5). Because the ulnar artery predominates in supplying blood to the hand, the completeness of the superficial palmar arch is the determining factor in hand ischemia. In contrast to the deep arch, the superficial palmar arch exhibits many variations (Fig. 76.3). Six types of complete arch are known; however, a complete superficial palmar arch was seen in only 42.4% of cases in the angiographic study (6). In contrast, the anatomic dissection study found a complete superficial arch in 78.5% of cases (5). Such discrepancies are important and undoubtedly are related to the methods used. Arteriographic studies allow a substantially better visualization of arteries of small caliber and an increased recognition of luminal obstruction contributing to the incomplete arch. The angiographic studies, however, were performed in patients with symptoms. Thus, a higher frequency of incomplete arches might be expected.

DIAGNOSIS

The diagnosis of large-artery occlusion is usually not difficult, and a careful pulse examination often helps to establish it. In distal arterial lesions causing hand or finger ischemia, the use of noninvasive testing to detect digital artery occlusion helps to distinguish Raynaud's phenomenon from Raynaud's disease. The diagnosis of primary Raynaud's disease should not be made until secondary causes of Raynaud's phenomenon have been eliminated. Furthermore, because the onset of Raynaud's phenomenon may precede other manifestations of underlying systemic disease by many years, the diagnosis of Raynaud's disease is usually not made until 2 years have elapsed with no appearance of systemic disease. If this strict criterion is followed, most patients will be found to have Raynaud's phenomenon (secondary) rather than Raynaud's disease (primary).

The diagnosis is facilitated by classifying arterial lesions according to proximal or distal sites of involvement. Proximal lesions are those involving arteries above the elbow, and distal lesions are those involving arteries below the elbow, predominantly in the wrist and hand.

Proximal Arterial Lesions

Atherosclerosis is the most common cause of upper extremity occlusive lesions. The most common site of involvement is the first part of the subclavian artery, and the innominate artery is also a common site of disease. Lesions include total occlusion with or without associated steal phenomena, high-grade stenoses, and ulcerating plaques causing distal embolism.

Forms of arteritis producing upper extremity ischemic symptoms include such diverse processes as Takayasu's arteritis, giant cell arteritis, temporal arteritis, and polymyalgia rheumatica. Takayasu's arteritis is a nonspecific inflammatory process of unknown cause that seg-

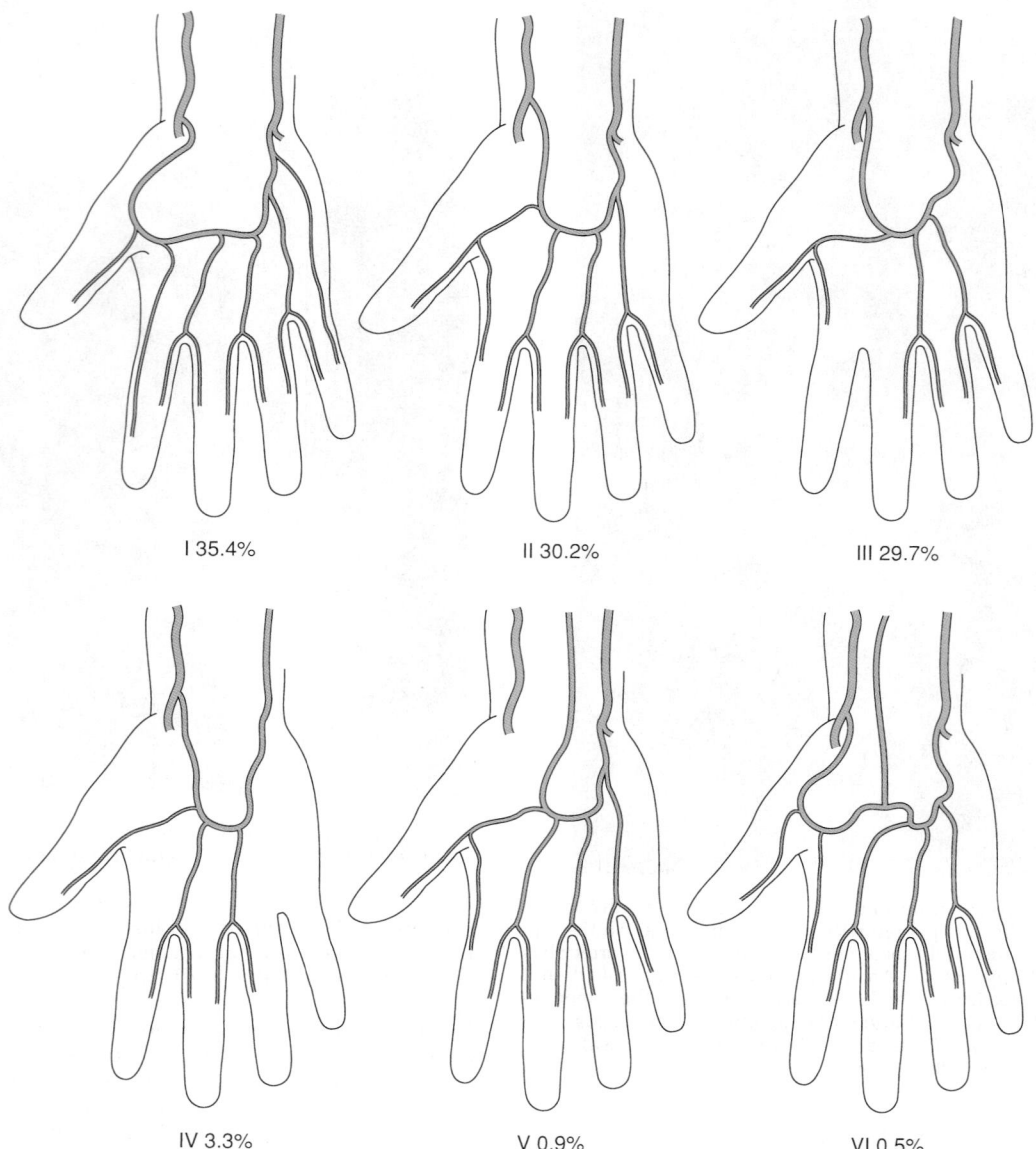

I 35.4% II 30.2% III 29.7%

IV 3.3% V 0.9% VI 0.5%

Figure 76.3. Different types of complete superficial palmar arch found on 500 hand arteriograms. (After Janevski BK. *Angiography of the upper extremity.* Amsterdam: Martinus Nijhoff, 1982, with permission.)

mentally affects the aorta and its main branches. The disease process can involve the carotid, subclavian, axillary, and pulmonary arteries and is noted most often in young women from 10 to 30 years of age.

The most frequently recognized clinical features of giant cell arteritis (cranial, temporal, and granulomatous arteritis) are related to involvement of the cranial arteries. In temporal arteritis and polymyalgia rheumatica, the subclavian or axillary arteries are common sites of involvement. In addition to upper extremity ischemic symptoms, patients with arteritis often present with fever, malaise, headache, and joint pain. The erythrocyte sedimentation rate is often elevated. The results of some serologic tests can also be positive, but none of the tests are sufficiently sensitive or specific for findings to be considered diagnostic.

Arteriographic examination in patients with upper extremity occlusive symptoms is often diagnostic. The in-

volvement of multiple arteries and a well-developed network of collaterals are characteristic of Takayasu's disease; the pulmonary artery is affected in more than 45% of patients. Characteristic arteriographic findings in giant cell arteritis include long segments of smooth arterial stenosis alternating with areas of normal or increased caliber, smoothly tapered occlusions, and the absence of irregular plaques and ulcerations (Fig. 76.4).

Thoracic outlet syndrome is by far the most common condition producing upper extremity vascular complications in young adults. Possible sites of compression include the costoclavicular space, formed by the first thoracic rib and clavicle; the interscalene triangle; the angle between the insertion of the pectoralis minor tendon and the coracoid process in the axilla; and the head of the humerus in extreme external rotation. Thoracic outlet compression may be caused by bony anomalies, such as a cervical rib or an abnormal first thoracic rib, or it may be

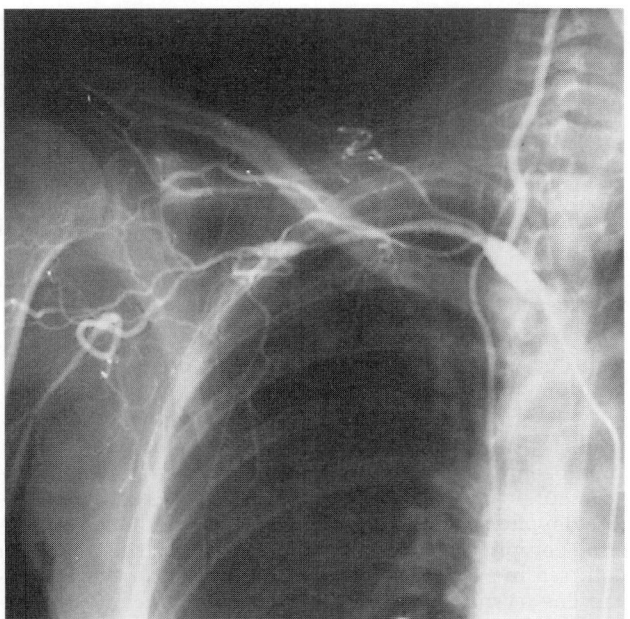

Figure 76.4. Characteristic long, segmental narrowing of the subclavian artery in a patient with giant cell arteritis. (From Yao JST. Arterial surgery of the upper extremity. In: Haimovici H, Callow AD, DePalma RG, et al., eds. *Vascular surgery: principles and techniques,* 3rd ed. Norwalk, CT: Appleton & Lange, 1989:858, with permission.)

cause digital gangrene or severe hand ischemia. Aneurysm formation is not confined to the subclavian or axillary arteries; repetitive trauma to branch arteries, such as the posterior circumflex humeral artery, has been reported to lead to aneurysm formation in baseball pitchers and volleyball players (7,8). In such persons, Raynaud's phenomenon is often an initial complaint and is often unilateral. Neurologic symptoms and upper extremity venous thrombotic complications are more common presentations of thoracic outlet syndrome than are arterial complications, but the latter are more threatening to limb and function and are always an urgent indication for arteriography.

Distal Arterial Lesions

Several collagen vascular disorders produce ischemia of the distal upper extremity, including scleroderma, rheumatoid arthritis, systemic lupus erythematosus, polyarteritis nodosa, and dermatomyositis. All cause systemic symptoms and present with upper extremity symptoms ranging from Raynaud's phenomenon to gangrene of the digits. Extensive involvement of the palmar arches or digital arteries is common (Fig. 76.6).

Buerger's disease (thromboangiitis obliterans) was first described in 1879, but its existence as a distinct entity is still questionable. It was initially described in male patients of Mediterranean origin who presented with digital gangrene but no occlusion of the larger arteries; however, contemporary practice recognizes that men and women of

secondary to hypertrophy of the anterior scalene muscle. Although a cervical rib is found in 0.5% to 1% of the population, fewer than 10% of such persons have symptoms of neurovascular compression (Fig. 76.5). Arterial complications include aneurysm formation, post-stenotic dilation, thrombosis, and distal embolism. The latter can

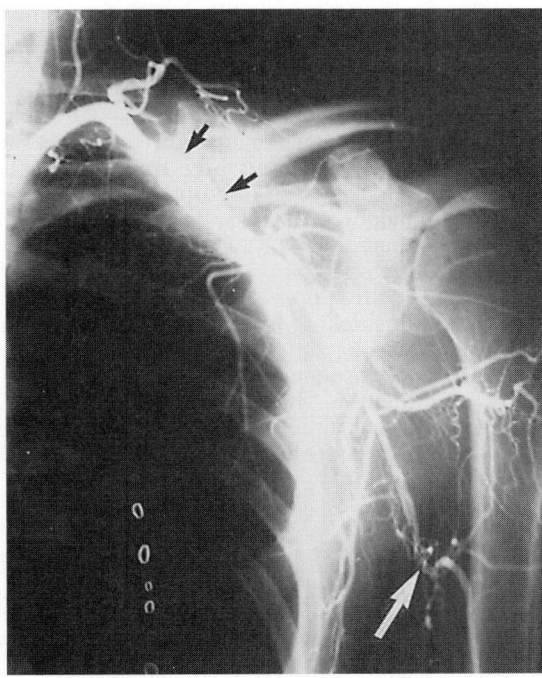

Figure 76.5. Arteriogram in a patient with subclavian aneurysm *(black arrows)* caused by a cervical rib. Multiple distal arterial occlusions have developed as a result of embolism *(white arrow).*

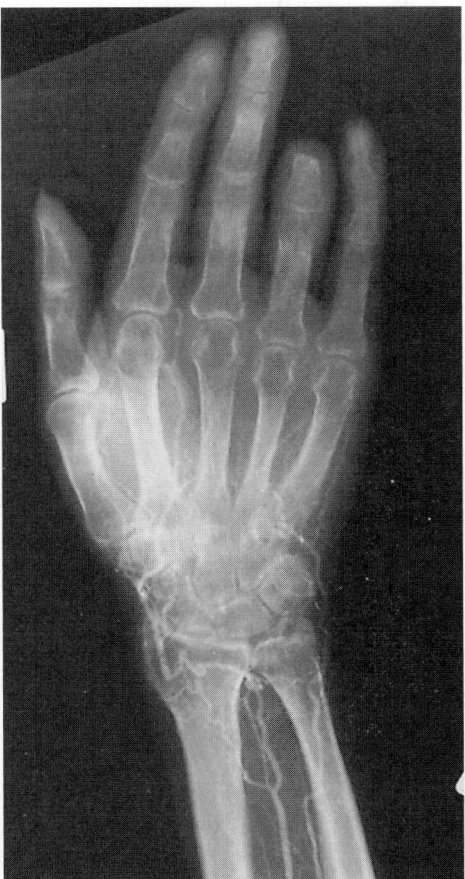

Figure 76.6. Arteriogram of a patient with scleroderma and digital gangrene. Extensive small-artery occlusion involves the palmar arch and digital arteries.

many ethnic backgrounds can be affected. A persistent characteristic of the disease is a strong association with heavy smoking of a particularly addictive nature. The diagnosis of Buerger's disease is based on histologic evidence of the involvement of both arteries and veins. Venous involvement can be manifested clinically as migrating phlebitis. Characteristic arteriographic findings are occlusion of the small arteries of the digits and the presence of abundant collaterals. The typical corkscrew appearance of the collaterals and lack of the large-vessel plaques characteristic of atherosclerosis are strongly suggestive of Buerger's disease. Like the symptomatic hand, the asymptomatic hand may demonstrate digital artery occlusions.

Polycythemia vera, cryoglobulinemia, and the presence of cold agglutinins are the most common forms of blood dyscrasia associated with occlusion of the arteries of the hand. Occlusion of the small arteries is generally thought to be caused by local thrombosis or embolism. Specific immunologic and blood tests help to establish the diagnosis.

Catheter injuries to the radial and brachial arteries have become more common because of the increasing use of diagnostic and therapeutic procedures involving catheterization. These are especially troublesome when an incomplete palmar arch is not recognized before placement of a catheter in the radial artery. Gangrene or severe ischemia can result from the injury.

Vibration syndrome, characterized by blanching and numbness of the hands after the use of pneumatic drills, is a well-recognized clinical entity causing hand ischemia. The so-called vibratory white finger is a form of occupational trauma. Repetitive trauma to the digital arteries that initially causes spasm but ultimately causes thrombosis and permanent occlusion is believed to be the primary factor responsible for ischemic symptoms.

Hypothenar hammer syndrome is another form of occupational trauma, commonly seen in mechanics and carpenters. The mechanism of injury is the repetitive use of the palm of the hand in activities that involve pounding, pushing, or twisting. The anatomic location of the ulnar artery at the area of hypothenar eminence makes it vulnerable to stress. When this area is repeatedly traumatized, ulnar artery occlusion or aneurysm formation can result (Fig. 76.7). Digital artery occlusion is a consequence of embolism from the injured artery.

Calciphylactic arteriopathy (heavily calcified arteries) in patients with diabetes or chronic renal failure can lead to gangrene or severe ischemia of the hand. So-called azotemic arteriopathy (calciphylaxis) is characterized by calcification of the media of the digital arteries, which produces a "pipe stem" pattern on plain film.

TREATMENT

The treatment of upper extremity ischemic vascular disorders is directed toward the underlying cause. Stenosis or embologenic lesions of proximal large vessels usually require surgical therapy. The type of reconstructive procedure depends on the nature and location of the lesion. Arterial complications of thoracic outlet obstruction often require a bypass procedure after resection of the subclavian aneurysm and removal of the cervical rib (9). A bypass graft with autogenous vein (saphenous or cephalic) often relieves occlusion of the brachial artery and its major branches (10–12). A short segmental occlusion of either the radial or ulnar artery is best treated by thrombectomy or endarterectomy with a vein patch. An aneurysm in the hand can be resected and continuity restored by end-to-end anastomosis or an interposed vein graft.

The results of bypass grafting in the upper extremity are rather similar to those of lower extremity revascularization—that is, proximal grafts fare better than distal grafts. In a recent report, the overall 5-year patency was 52.2% in 43 patients (13). The patency rate for anastomosis proximal to the brachial artery bifurcation was better than that for more distal placement (61.9% vs. 34.8%). Major amputation is not often required, even after graft occlusion, as it is in lower extremity surgery.

Steroid therapy may be needed if arteritis is causing systemic symptoms. Iatrogenic drug-induced ischemia must be treated by cessation of the drug. Dramatic improvement can occur in patients with ergot poisoning.

Distal lesions with occlusion at or distal to the palmar arch are unlikely to be amenable to direct surgical treatment. In these patients, conservative treatment with the use of a calcium blocker (e.g., nifedipine) may reduce the severity and frequency of attacks. A host of medications have been recommended (14). Unfortunately, none has proved consistently effective.

In all patients with upper extremity ischemia of any cause, cessation of smoking is an important step. Many of the constituents of tobacco smoke cause adverse vascular effects, particularly vasoconstriction, and this effect seems especially prominent in the upper extremity. Likewise, general protective measures, such as avoiding exposure to cold temperatures and mechanical trauma, have beneficial effects when scrupulously applied.

REFERENCES

1. Sumner DS. Noninvasive assessment of upper extremity ischemia. In: Bergan JJ, Yao JST, eds. *Evaluation and treatment of upper and lower extremity circulatory disorders.* Orlando, FL: Grune & Stratton, 1984:75.
2. Erlandson EE, Forrest ME, Shields JJ, et al. Discriminant arteriographic criteria in the management of forearm and hand ischemia. *Surgery* 1981;90:1025.
3. Love PE, Santoro SA. Antiphospholipid antibodies: anticardiolipin and the lupus anticoagulant in systemic lupus ery-

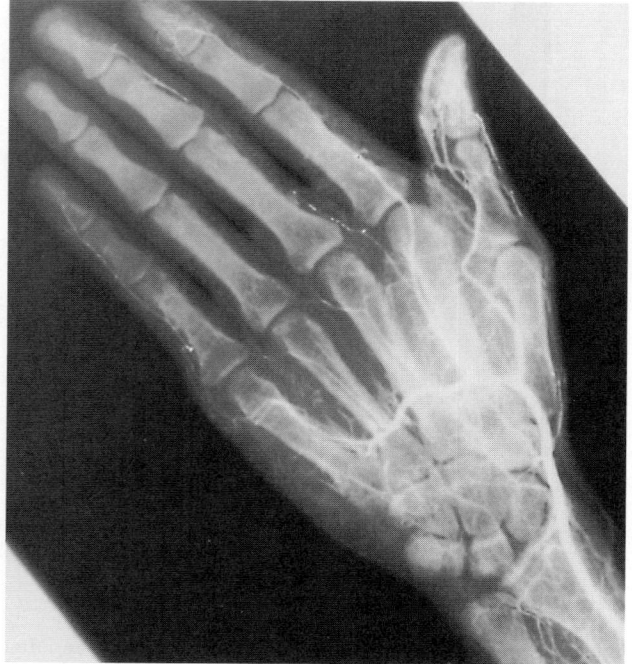

Figure 76.7. Occlusion of the ulnar artery over the hamate bone in a patient with hypothenar hammer syndrome.

thematosus (SLE) and in non-SLE disorders. *Ann Intern Med* 1990;112:682.

4. Yao JST, Bergan JJ, Neiman HL. Arteriography for upper extremity and digital ischemia. In: Neiman HL, Yao JST, eds. *Angiography of vascular disease.* New York: Churchill Livingstone, 1985:353.

5. Coleman SS, Ansun BJ. Arterial patterns in the hand based upon a study of 650 specimens. *Surg Gynecol Obstet* 1961; 113:409.

6. Janevski BK. *Angiography of the upper extremity.* Amsterdam: Martinus Nijhoff, 1982.

7. Durham JR, Yao JST, Pearce WH, et al. Arterial injuries in the thoracic outlet syndrome. *J Vasc Surg* 1995;21:57.

8. Yao JST. Upper extremity ischemia in athletes. *Semin Vasc Surg* 1998;2:96–105.

9. Yao JST, Flinn WR, McCarthy WJ, et al. Upper extremity revascularization. In: Bergan JJ, Yao JST, eds. *Techniques in arterial surgery.* Philadelphia: WB Saunders, 1990:328.

10. Garrett HE, Morris GC, Howell FJ, et al. Revascularization of the upper extremity with autogenous vein bypass graft. *Arch Surg* 1965;91:751.

11. Whitehouse WM Jr, Zelenock GB, Wakefield TN, et al. Arterial bypass grafts for upper extremity ischemia. *J Vasc Surg* 1986;3:569.

12. McCarthy WJ, Flinn WR, Yao JST, et al. Result of bypass grafting for upper limb ischemia. *J Vasc Surg* 1986;3:741.

13. Mesh CL, Yao JST. Upper extremity bypass: five-year follow-up. In: Yao JST, Pearce WH, eds. *Long-term results in vascular surgery.* Norwalk, CT: Appleton & Lange, 1993:353.

14. Porter JM, Rivers SP. Management of Raynaud's syndrome. In: Bergan JJ, Yao JST, eds. *Evaluation and treatment of upper and lower extremity circulatory disorders.* Orlando, FL: Grune & Stratton, 1984:181.

SURGERY: SCIENTIFIC PRINCIPLES AND PRACTICE, Third Edition, edited by Lazar J. Greenfield, Michael W. Mulholland, Keith T. Oldham, Gerald B. Zelenock, and Keith D. Lillemoe. Lippincott Williams & Wilkins Publishers, Philadelphia, © 2001.

CHAPTER 77

VISCERAL OCCLUSIVE DISEASE

GERALD B. ZELENOCK

The relatively complex functions of the abdominal viscera are subserved by a circulation uniquely adapted for absorbing and distributing nutrients. As organogenesis proceeds in fetal development, the primitive dual arterial supply to the abdominal viscera changes such that the ventral anastomosis disappears and the paired segmental vitelline arteries fuse. The 10th arterial pair form the celiac trunk; the 13th, the superior mesenteric artery (SMA); and the 21st or 22nd, the inferior mesenteric artery (IMA) (Fig. 77.1). Variations in the persistence or regression of parts of the primitive ventral anastomosis result in anatomic variations and recognized patterns of collateral circulation. A common celiac–mesenteric trunk, replaced hepatic branches from the celiac artery to the SMA, and a persistent ventral anastomosis producing an arch of Bühler are common anatomic variations that are important to surgeons.

VASCULAR ANATOMY OF THE ABDOMINAL VISCERA

The vascular anatomy of the abdominal viscera follows well-described patterns. The celiac artery typically gives rise to three branches: the splenic, common hepatic, and left gastric arteries (Fig. 77.2). In addition, it gives rise to the inferior phrenic arteries in about 55% of the population. The splenic artery originates from the celiac artery distal to the origin of the left gastric artery. The splenic artery is closely associated with the pancreas and provides arterial input to the spleen, pancreas (dorsal pancreatic artery, transverse pancreatic artery, great pancreatic artery, caudal pancreatic artery, and other small, unnamed pancreatic branches), and stomach by way of the short gastric and left gastroepiploic arteries. The common hepatic artery divides into the gastroduodenal and proper hepatic arteries. Through its proper hepatic branch, it typically gives rise to both the right and left hepatic arteries. In about 25% of the population, the left hepatic artery is derived from the left gastric artery. In about 15% to 20% of the population, the right hepatic artery has a replaced origin from the SMA. This replaced state may be either complete or partial. The arterial blood supply to the middle lobe of the liver is typically from the right hepatic artery. The left hepatic artery supplies the lateral and medial segments of the left lobe, and in almost half of the population, it also contributes blood supply to the middle hepatic lobe. The proper hepatic artery is the origin of the right gastric artery, supplying the distal lesser curvature of the stomach. The gastroduodenal artery is a branch of the common hepatic artery, with several constant branches: the anterior and posterior pancreaticoduodenal arcades and the right gastroepiploic artery. Other, highly variable branches of the gastroduodenal artery occur. The gastroduodenal artery is an important source of large-vessel collateral circulation in the event of occlusion or stenosis of either the celiac artery or SMA.

The SMA originates from the anterior surface of the aorta within 1 to 2 cm of the celiac trunk (Figs. 77.2 and 77.3). The SMA passes behind the pancreas and above the fourth portion of the duodenum. The vessel provides arterial blood supply to the pancreas through the inferior pancreaticoduodenal artery, to most of the small intestine through jejunal and ileal branches, and to the ascending and right half of the transverse colon through its ileocolic, right colic, and middle colic branches. Extensive large-vessel anastomotic arcades occur among the 10 to 20 jejunal and ileal arteries. In addition, well-defined anastomoses between the main branches of the SMA and IMA in the region of the splenic flexure have significant implications for surgeons.

The IMA arises 5 to 6 cm distal to the SMA, typically supplying the left half of the transverse colon and the entire descending colon through the left colic artery (Fig. 77.3). The IMA gives off a variable number of sigmoid branches and terminates as the paired superior hemorrhoidal arteries. Important SMA-to-IMA anastomoses course between the middle colic and left colic arteries in the region of the splenic flexure and between the superior hemorrhoidal artery and internal iliac branches supplying the pelvis. The marginal artery of Drummond and the arch of Riolan are discrete branch vessels capable of significant enlargement, and they are important sources of collateral blood supply in the face of occlusion or stenosis of the proximal visceral vessels (Fig. 77.4).

The venous anatomy of the gastrointestinal tract tends to parallel the arterial blood supply and drains into the portal venous system perfusing the liver. The inferior mesenteric vein drains into the splenic vein. The anastomosis of the splenic vein with the superior mesenteric vein forms the origin of the portal vein. The portal vein subdivides into right and left portal veins and by repetitive subdivision supplies the liver parenchyma. Hepatic venous blood is drained by right, middle, and left hepatic

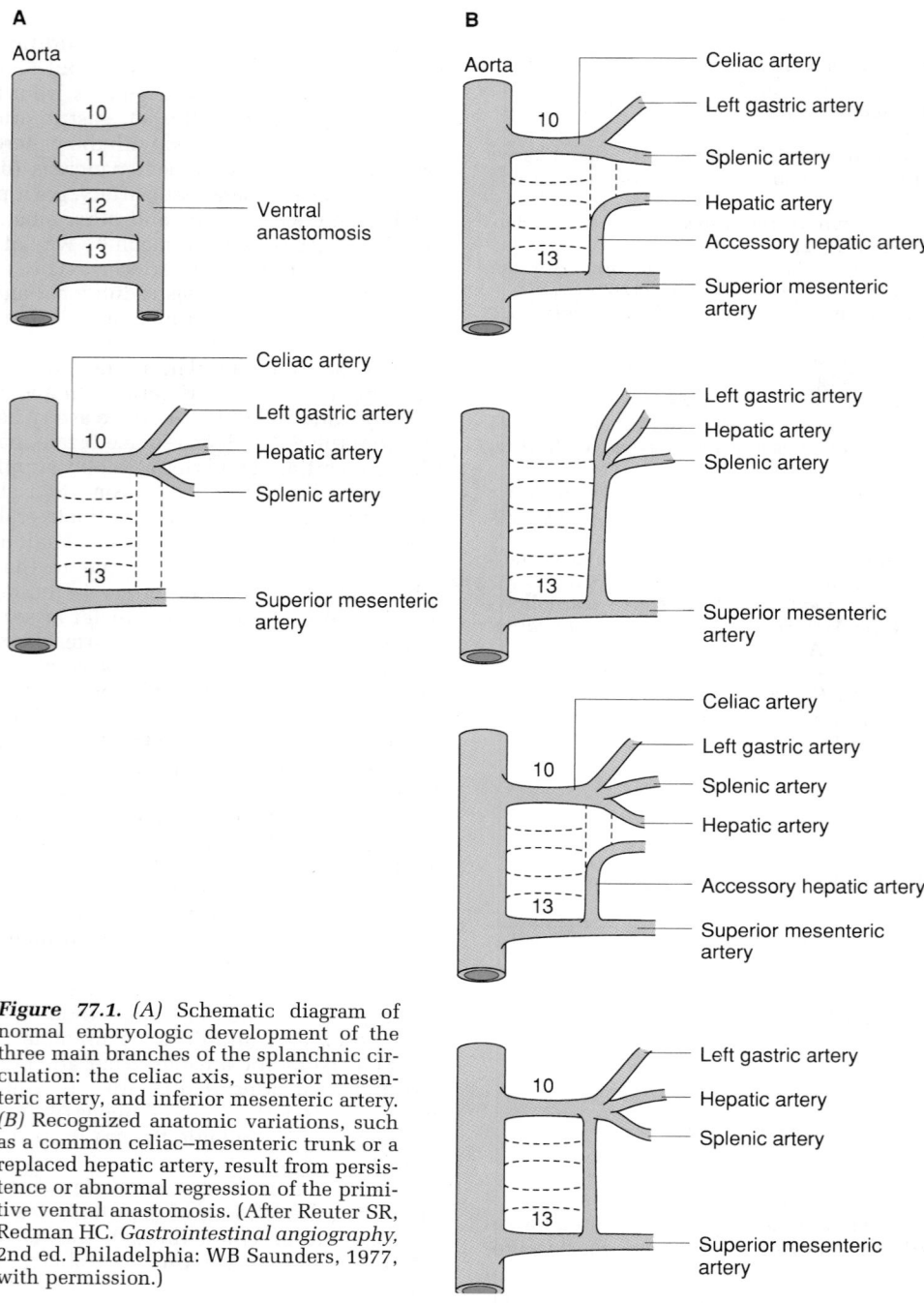

A

B

Figure 77.1. (*A*) Schematic diagram of normal embryologic development of the three main branches of the splanchnic circulation: the celiac axis, superior mesenteric artery, and inferior mesenteric artery. (*B*) Recognized anatomic variations, such as a common celiac–mesenteric trunk or a replaced hepatic artery, result from persistence or abnormal regression of the primitive ventral anastomosis. (After Reuter SR, Redman HC. *Gastrointestinal angiography*, 2nd ed. Philadelphia: WB Saunders, 1977, with permission.)

Figure 77.2. The celiac artery distributes blood to the stomach, duodenum, pancreas, liver, and spleen; in addition, the gastroduodenal artery and pancreaticoduodenal arcades provide important collateral flow between the celiac and superior mesenteric arteries. The superior mesenteric artery is retropancreatic but crosses anteriorly to the fourth portion of the duodenum. It supplies blood to the duodenum and head of the pancreas, jejunum, ileum, ascending colon, and right half of the transverse colon (Fig. 77.3). Large anastomotic arcades course between the jejunal and ileal branches.

veins, which enter the vena cava. Portal–systemic anastomoses are common and are of considerable importance in the presence of portal hypertension.

Extensive visceral–visceral and visceral–systemic collaterals, in addition to the "redundancy" built into the system by normal anatomic patterns, afford a measure of protection from vascular occlusion (Fig. 77.5). Virtually every visceral organ has multiple sources of blood supply and outlets for venous drainage. Further, the extensive collateral circulation is enhanced by the arcade arrangement and by frequently encountered collateral patterns. The left and right gastric and right and left gastroepiploic blood vessels, the anterior–posterior and superior–inferior pancreaticoduodenal arcades, and the anastomosis between the middle and left colic arteries are almost invariably observed. Furthermore, visceral–systemic collaterals, such as occur between the IMA and the hypogastric artery or between the celiac axis and the systemic vessels by way of phrenic, esophageal, and intercostal arteries, are well described. An extensive intramural plexus and the specialized circulation within the mucosa and tip of the villus allow the intestinal circulation to perform its physiologic function but also account for the unique vulnerability of the mucosal tip.

A variety of techniques in humans and experimental studies have been used to quantify intestinal blood flow. Electromagnetic flow meters, indicator dilution techniques, microspheres, aminopyrine, inert gases, pulsed Doppler ultrasonographic flow meters, and angiographic techniques such as spillover and video dilution all have

been applied to the measurement of intestinal blood flow. With the use of such techniques, typical large-vessel intestinal blood flow in humans has been estimated to be between 500 and 1,200 mL/min, or about 10% to 20% of the cardiac output. Recent advances in noninvasive vascular diagnostic technology allow visualization and volume flow determinations within the celiac artery and SMA. Duplex scanning, combining Doppler blood flow velocity determinations with B-mode ultrasonography, allows precise measurement of cross-sectional areas and enables calculation of volumetric flows (Fig. 77.6) (see color insert following page 1190). Such technology is useful in diagnosing intestinal vascular disorders and also makes possible repetitive physiologic investigations in humans without resort to the operative implantation of flow transducers or intraarterial injection of dyes and tracers. Baseline flow in fasted human subjects and the response to standard meals are shown in Table 77.1. *Changes in celiac artery blood flow occur with all meal types; however, they are not significant,* whereas significant increases in SMA blood flow occur 20 to 30 minutes after the ingestion of food that persist for up to 90 minutes after ingestion. The earliest maximal blood flow response occurs after ingestion of a carbohydrate meal, whereas the largest overall increase in blood flow occurs after ingestion of a mixed meal containing carbohydrate, protein, and fat. A better definition of the factors involved in the regulation of intestinal blood flow under physiologic and pathologic conditions should become possible as investigations proceed.

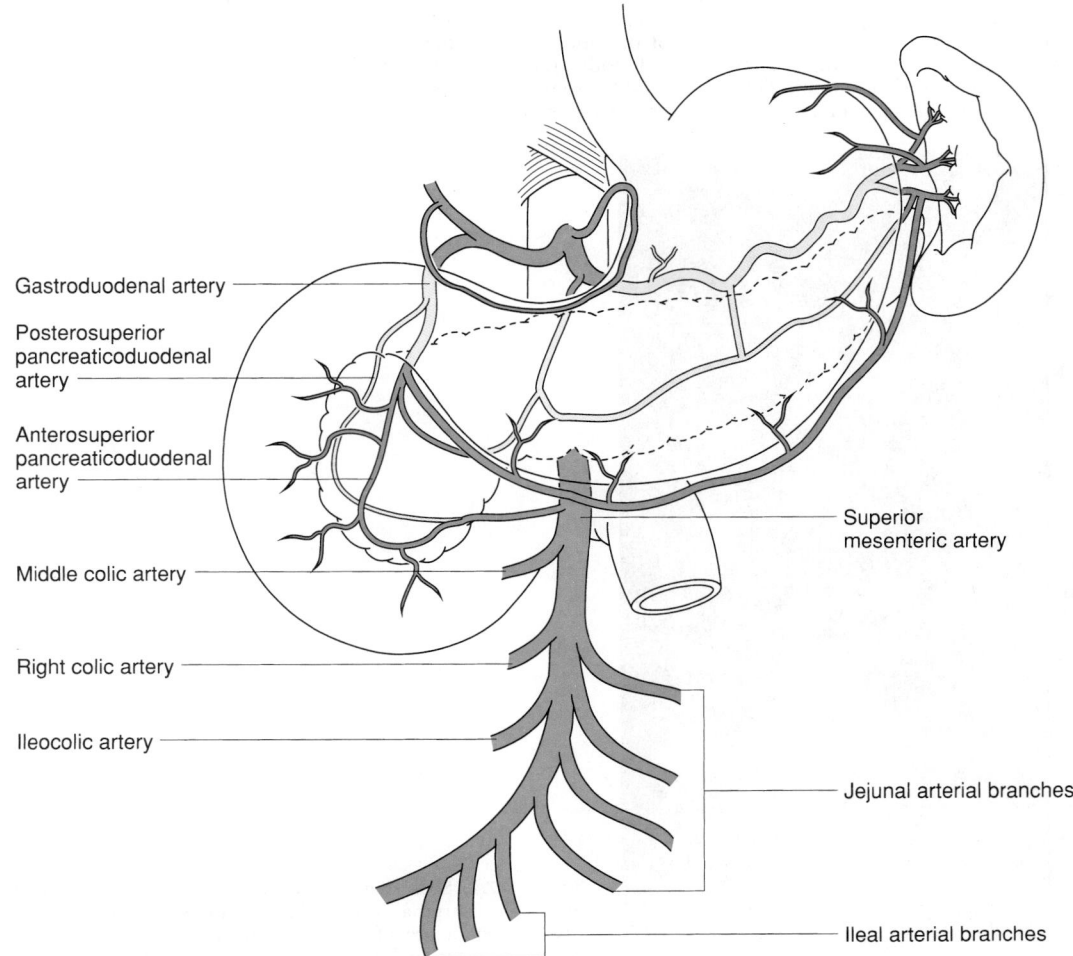

Gastroduodenal artery

Posterosuperior pancreaticoduodenal artery

Anterosuperior pancreaticoduodenal artery

Middle colic artery

Right colic artery

Ileocolic artery

Superior mesenteric artery

Jejunal arterial branches

Ileal arterial branches

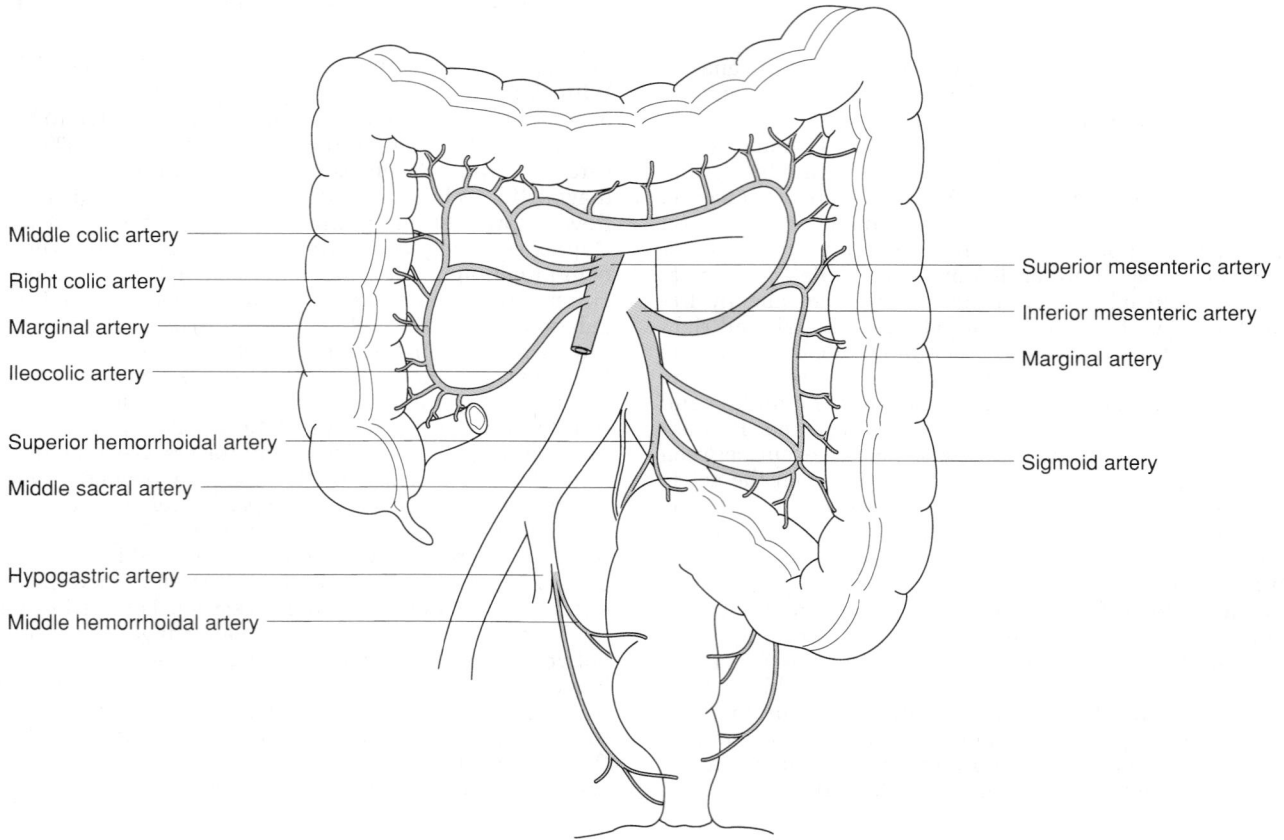

Middle colic artery
Right colic artery
Marginal artery
Ileocolic artery

Superior hemorrhoidal artery
Middle sacral artery

Hypogastric artery
Middle hemorrhoidal artery

Superior mesenteric artery
Inferior mesenteric artery
Marginal artery

Sigmoid artery

Figure 77.3. The inferior mesenteric artery *(IMA)* supplies blood to the left half of the transverse colon and the entire descending colon, including the sigmoid colon and rectum (via sigmoid and superior hemorrhoidal branches). The left branch of the middle colic artery, from the superior mesenteric artery, and the ascending portion of the left colic artery, from the IMA, form a collateral network in the region of the splenic flexure. The IMA serves as an important source of collateral blood supply when the proximal two visceral vessels are occluded.

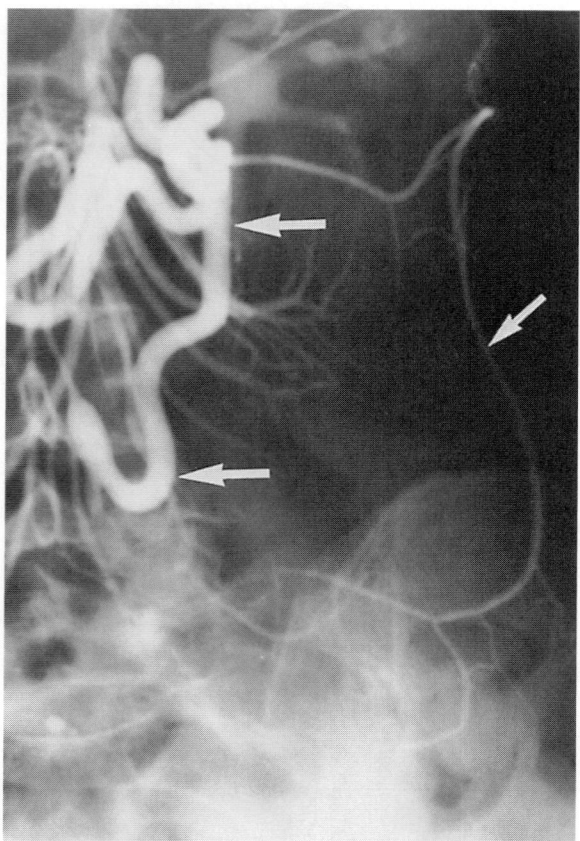

Figure 77.4. Selective inferior mesenteric artery angiography demonstrates the marginal artery of Drummond and the larger, more functionally important arc of Riolan, or central anastomotic artery. (From Zelenock GB. Splanchnic arteriosclerotic disease and intestinal angina. *Arch Surg* 1980;115:497, with permission.)

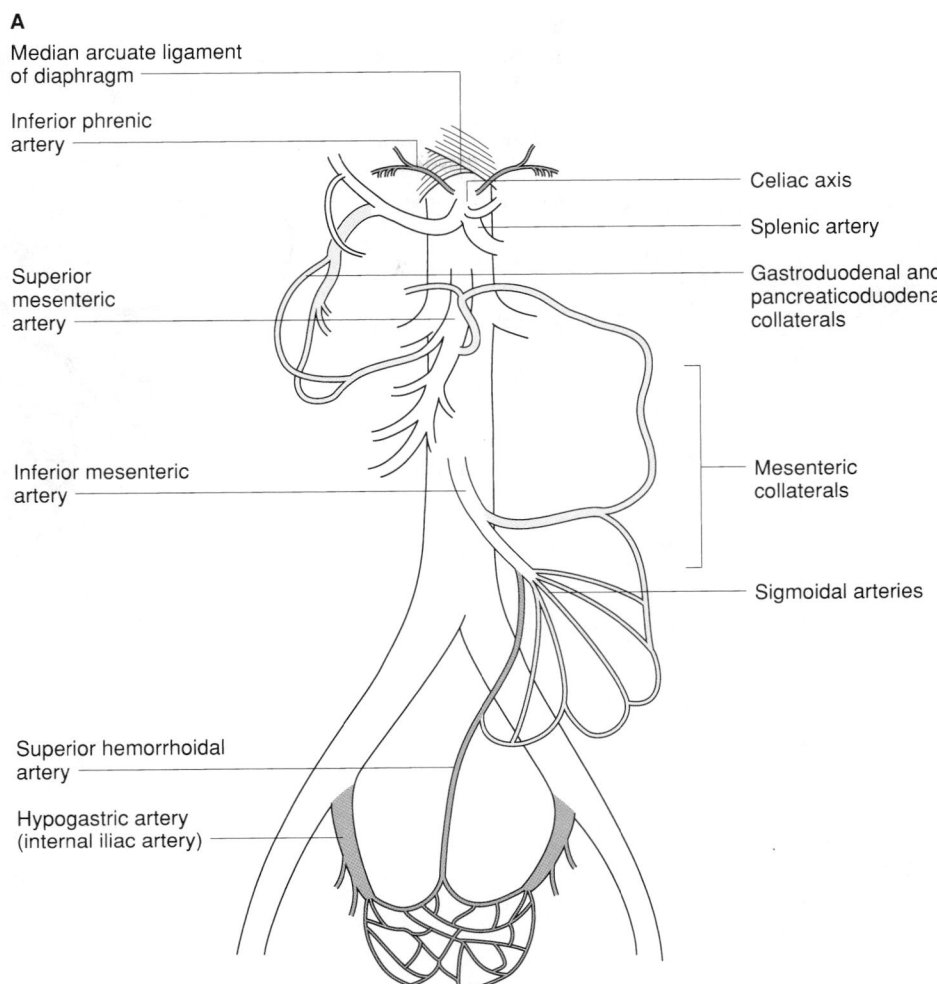

A

Median arcuate ligament of diaphragm

Inferior phrenic artery

Superior mesenteric artery

Inferior mesenteric artery

Superior hemorrhoidal artery

Hypogastric artery (internal iliac artery)

Celiac axis

Splenic artery

Gastroduodenal and pancreaticoduodenal collaterals

Mesenteric collaterals

Sigmoidal arteries

Figure 77.5. *(A)* The collateral circulation to the intestine occurs at several levels. Well-recognized visceral–visceral and visceral–parietal collateral branches and anastomoses are important. The unnamed intestinal arcades *(B)* and the intramural anastomoses *(C)* are effective short-segment collaterals. *(continues)*

Within the wall of the intestine, most blood flow is to the mucosa. This tissue, representing 50% of the mass of the intestine, receives about 75% of the resting blood flow. The muscular and serosal layers of the intestine receive the remaining 25%. Control of blood flow in the splanchnic circulation is affected by the sympathetic nervous system and also by metabolic, myogenic, and extrinsic factors. The stimulation of sympathetic nerves increases vascular tone and decreases splanchnic blood flow. Parasympathetic nerve fibers appear to have little direct effect on blood flow. Numerous intrinsic hormonal regulators (e.g., secretin, gastrin, cholecystokinin, glucagon, and vasoactive intestinal peptide), in addition to substances such as histamine, serotonin, bradykinin, and the prostaglandins, may play important physiologic roles in the regulation of blood flow. Circulating hormones and regulatory substances (e.g., epinephrine, norepinephrine, and angiotensin) and many commonly used pharmaceuticals may also have important effects on the splanchnic circulation (Table 77.2).

PATHOPHYSIOLOGY OF ISCHEMIC INJURY

The general pathophysiology of ischemic injury is more fully discussed elsewhere. Within the gut, in addition to the issues of ischemia and reperfusion, which are common to all ischemic events, the potential for bacterial translocation and toxin and mediator absorption is associated with other significant adverse effects. These adverse effects may exacerbate local (intestinal) injury and may also have important indirect systemic effects, including myocardial depression and increased capillary permeability with edema formation and organ dysfunction. Loss of the intestinal mucosa, which normally functions as a barrier to prevent the luminal transfer of bacteria, endotoxin, and cytokines, is noted in multiple clinical conditions, including shock, burns, major trauma, and multiple-organ failure. A loss of mucosal barrier function is clearly present in the visceral ischemic syndromes. Three important factors predisposing to a loss of intestinal mucosal barrier function have been proposed: (a) physical disruption of the mucosa, (b) a change in the normal intestinal microflora (usually resulting from treatment with broad-spectrum antibiotics), and (c) impairment of host immune defenses. The first two are invariably present in patients with visceral ischemia, and the third is often demonstrably present in patients with significant weight loss and associated malnutrition. The repair of locally damaged mucosa and enhancement of host defenses appear to be facilitated by early enteral feeding, by specific nutrients (e.g., glutamine), and perhaps by growth factors and gut trophic hormones.

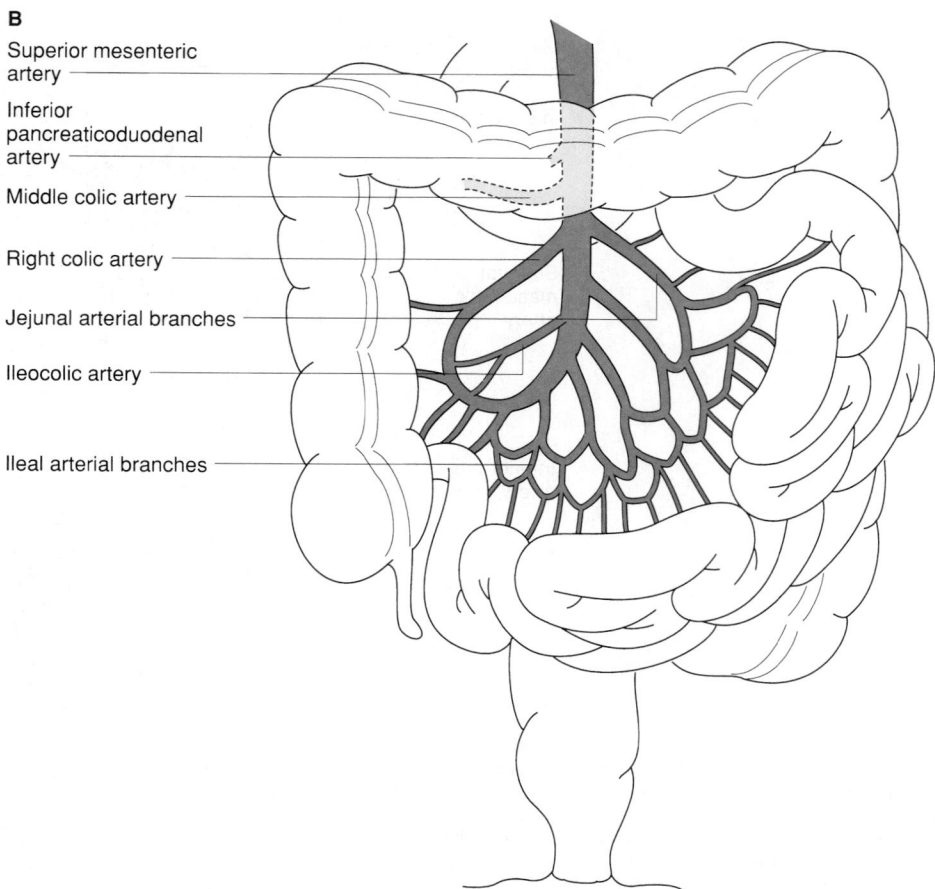

B

Superior mesenteric artery

Inferior pancreaticoduodenal artery

Middle colic artery

Right colic artery

Jejunal arterial branches

Ileocolic artery

Ileal arterial branches

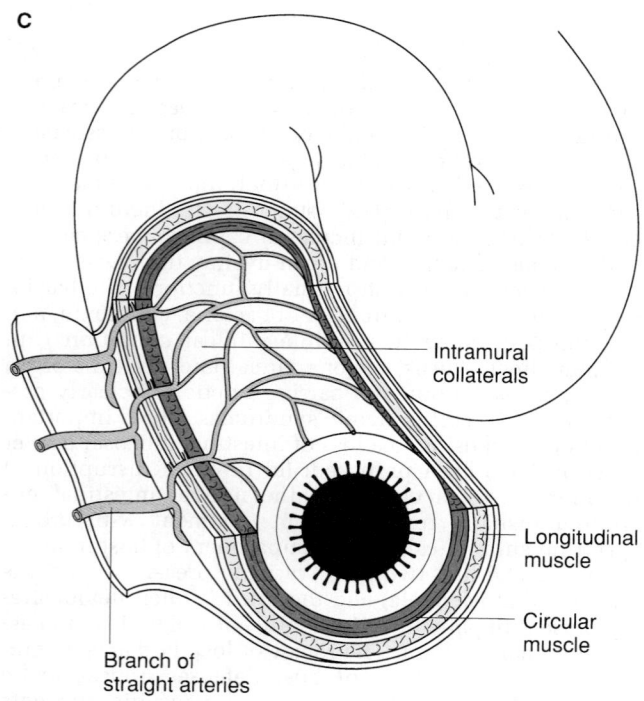

C

Intramural collaterals

Longitudinal muscle

Circular muscle

Branch of straight arteries

Figure 77.5. *(Continued)*

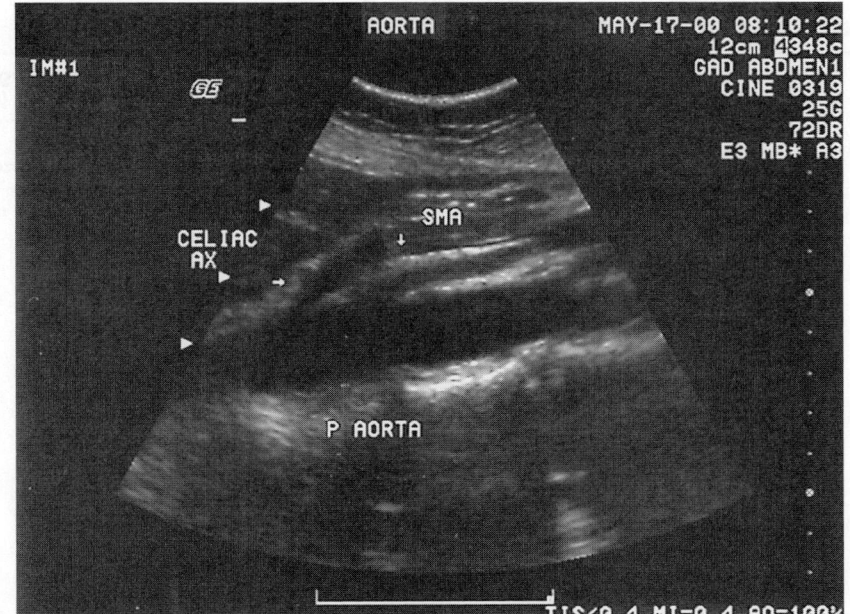

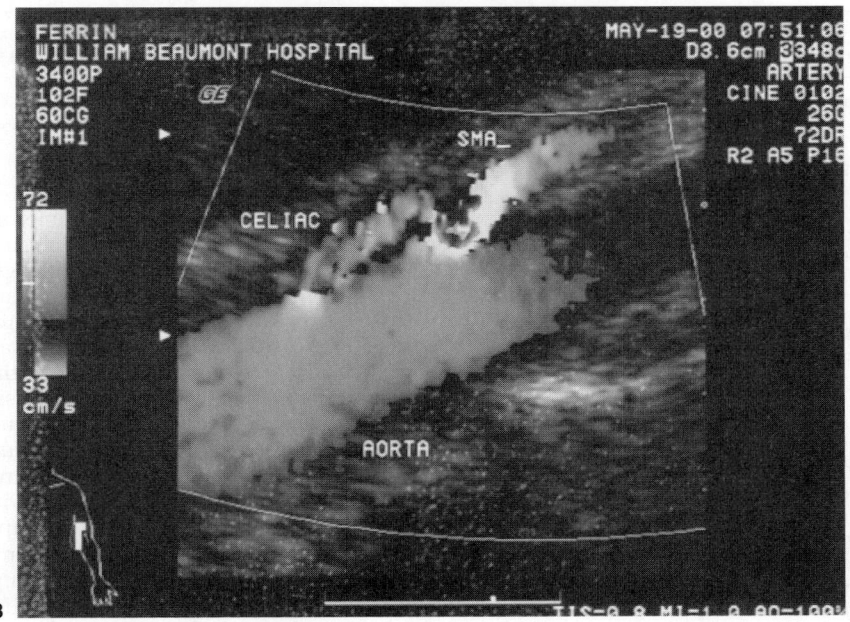

Figure 77.6. *(A)* Duplex scan of the aorta and celiac and superior mesenteric arteries. Vessel diameter, flow velocity, calculated volumetric blood flow, spectral analysis, and the response to physiologic stimuli allow a precise assessment of the visceral circulation. (Courtesy of Dr. Phillip Bendick, William Beaumont Hospital, Royal Oak, MI.) *(B)* Color-flow Doppler scanning allows rapid identification of flow disturbances. (Courtesy of Dr. Phillip Bendick.)

Table 77.1. DUPLEX MEASUREMENT OF INTESTINAL BLOOD FLOW

Vessel	Average diameter (range)	Characteristics on duplex scan	Calculated fasting volume flow (mL/min)	Calculated volume flow change from fasting by type of meal[a] (%)					
				Mixed	Cholesterol	Fat	Protein	Mannitol	Water
Celiac artery	0.66 cm (0.4–0.8 cm)	Continuous forward flow; no reverse flow: end-diastolic velocity about one-third peak systolic velocity No significant changes with meals	1,083 ± 75	18 ± 4	1 ± 4	10 ± 8	21 ± 6	37 ± 19	14 ± 5
Superior mesenteric artery	0.59 cm (0.44–0.68 cm)	Early diastolic flow reversal; forward diastolic flow; end-diastolic velocity about zero After eating, loss of reverse flow and increased peak systolic and end-diastolic velocities noted	538 ± 37	164 ± 30	118 ± 23	117 ± 25	78 ± 15	48 ± 11	24 ± 8

[a]Calculated volume flow changes that occurred after meals were not significantly increased in the celiac artery but were significantly increased with all meals except water in the superior mesenteric artery.
From Moneta GL, Taylor DC, Heiton WS, et al. Duplex ultrasound measurement of postprandial intestinal blood flow: effect of meal composition. Gastroenterology 1988;95:1294, with permission.

Table 77.2. EFFECTS OF VARIOUS SUBSTANCES ON MESENTERIC CIRCULATION AND MOTOR ACTIVITY

Substance	Intestinal blood flow	Intestinal O₂ uptake	Intestinal motility
Acetylcholine	Increase	Increase	Increase
Adenosine	Increase	Variable	—
Angiotensin II	Decrease	—	Increase
Bradykinin	Variable	—	Increase
Ca²⁺, high levels	Decrease	—	Increase
Ca²⁺ antagonists	Increase	—	Decrease
Dopamine	Variable	Decrease	—
Epinephrine	Variable	Variable	—
Gastrin	Increase	Increase	Increase
Glucagon	Increase	Increase	Decrease
Histamine	Increase	Increase	Increase
Isoproterenol	Increase	Variable	—
K⁺ high levels	Decrease	—	Increase
Mg²⁺	Increase	—	—
Nitroprusside	Increase	—	—
Norepinephrine	Decrease	Decrease	—
Papaverine	Increase	No change	—
PGE₁	Increase	Increase	—
PGF₂ₐ	Decrease	Variable	Increase
PGI₂	Increase	—	—
Secretin	Variable	No change	—
Serotonin	Variable	Variable	Variable
Somatostatin	Decrease	—	Decrease
Vasopressin	Decrease	Decrease	Variable
Vasoactive intestinal polypeptide	Increase	Increase	—

PG, prostaglandin.
From Wakefield TW, Stanley JC. The intestine. In: Zelenock G8, D'Alecy LG, Schlafer M, et al., eds. Clinical ischemic syndromes: mechanisms and consequences of tissue injury. St. Louis: Mosby, 1990, with permission.

CLINICAL SYNDROMES

The visceral ischemic syndromes are most conveniently considered as acute or chronic (subacute), according to their clinical presentation. Acute visceral ischemic syndromes include mesenteric embolism, mesenteric thrombosis, low-flow nonocclusive mesenteric ischemia, and iatrogenic ischemia. These are always serious and potentially life-threatening events; the mortality attending such processes is typically in excess of 70%. *Visceral ischemia severe enough to cause intestinal infarction is three times as lethal as myocardial infarction and five times as lethal as a brain infarct.* Chronic, or subacute, visceral ischemic syndromes include visceral angina, mesenteric venous thrombosis, and perhaps the median arcuate ligament syndrome. The designation of "chronic" visceral ischemia is questioned by some and is perhaps a misnomer because even when the clinical presentation is chronic, the underlying pathophysiology is characterized by repetitive, nearly critical ischemic events. The traditional designations are used in this chapter, but the severity of the ischemic process and the precarious and profoundly threatening nature of chronic visceral ischemia are recognized.

Acute Visceral Ischemic Syndromes

Mesenteric Embolism

Mesenteric embolism accounts for about half of cases of acute mesenteric ischemia. Typically, the embolus arises from a cardiac source. Classically, atrial fibrillation or a myocardial infarction with mural thrombus formation is the source of the embolus, but virtually any arrhythmia or anatomic cardiac defect may result in a mesenteric embolus. Embolism of intracardiac tumor, such as an atrial myxoma or a paradoxic embolus, are *other possible causes but uncommon.*

Acute mesenteric embolism tends to cause the sudden onset of severe epigastric or midabdominal pain, which is followed promptly by evacuation of the gut, either through emesis or explosive diarrhea. Typically, the patient feels well before the onset of pain and can often precisely pinpoint the onset of pain. Fully 25% of patients have had previous embolic events. The general physical examination may indicate the underlying cardiac disorder. An *irregularly* irregular rhythm indicating atrial fibrillation, the classic murmur of mitral stenosis, or an enlarged heart all support the diagnosis. The abdominal examination may reveal signs of an acute abdomen, or the findings may be normal. Slight to moderate abdominal distention is common. Bowel sounds are highly variable, as are findings on palpation. A well-recognized presentation of acute mesenteric insufficiency is severe abdominal complaints out of proportion to the physical findings. Peritoneal signs or blood in the stool are late and ominous signs, implying severe ischemia with infarction.

No laboratory tests are pathognomonic. An electrocardiogram may confirm cardiac abnormalities, suspected from the history and physical examination, or an echocardiogram or ultrasonography may demonstrate mural thrombus. Such tests are helpful but not diagnostic. Standard hematology and biochemical evaluation are unrewarding early in the clinical course. Late evaluation may demonstrate hemoconcentration, acidosis, leukocytosis, and serum phosphorus or transaminase elevations. None of these abnormalities need be present, even with a major mesenteric embolus. None is sufficiently sensitive or specific to confirm the diagnosis. The diagnosis depends on clinical suspicion followed by characteristic angiographic findings. Emboli tend to lodge at branch points of the SMA. In this regard, the origin of the SMA is typically spared, and the lodging point is close to the origin of the inferior pancreaticoduodenal artery or the middle colic artery (Fig. 77.7).

After diagnosis, the patient is heparinized, volume-resuscitated, and taken emergently to the operating room. Prophylactic antibiotics and full hemodynamic monitoring are required. The SMA is approached beneath the transverse mesocolon. Proximal and distal control are obtained, and Fogarty catheter embolectomy through either a transverse or longitudinal arteriotomy is performed. Patch closure of the SMA is not usually required with a transverse arteriotomy, but it is used if the SMA is small or a longitudinal incision has been made. In most instances, this approach should result in prompt return of the visceral blood flow. Intestinal viability is assessed. After restoration of blood flow, an important consideration is the possibility of multiple emboli lodging in distal branches of the SMA.

Mesenteric Thrombosis

Mesenteric thrombosis is a common cause of acute visceral ischemia. The presentation is that of an acute intestinal catastrophe, with the progressive development of severe midabdominal pain. Acute symptoms may be superimposed on a background of chronic intestinal angina or may occur without antecedent symptoms. Usually, the onset is less abrupt than with SMA embolus. If the patient has a history of postprandial abdominal pain, substantial weight loss is common. The weight loss typically results from a fear of eating, which precipitates the pain. A his-

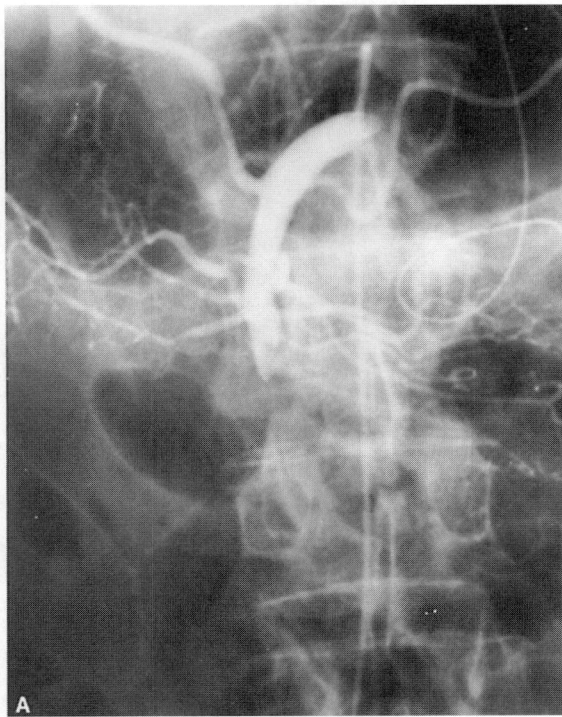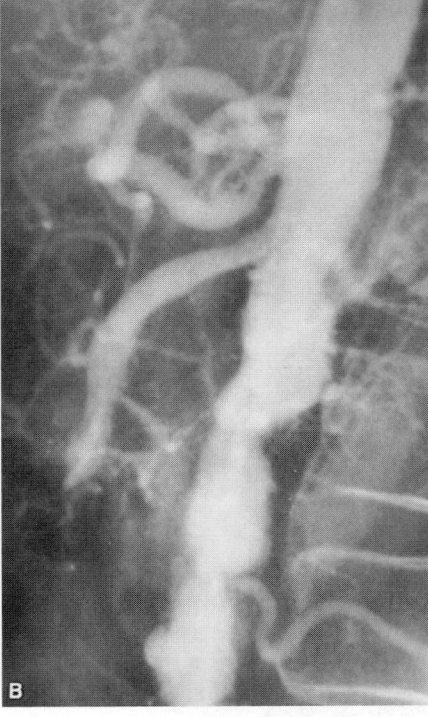

Figure 77.7. *(A)* Anteroposterior view of a typical superior mesenteric artery *(SMA)* embolus lodged distal to the origin of the middle colic artery and first jejunal branches of the SMA. The pattern of injury typically spares the first few inches of the jejunum and the colon distal to the midtransverse portion. *(B)* Lateral aortogram demonstrates embolus with sparing of proximal SMA. This pattern is distinct from SMA thrombosis.

tory compatible with motility disturbances causing symptoms such as nausea, diarrhea, or constipation is much more common than malabsorption syndromes. Often, the patient has undergone an extensive diagnostic evaluation to rule out the possibility of an underlying gastrointestinal malignancy.

Urgent visceral angiography is required for diagnosis and involves lateral aortography in addition to standard anteroposterior views (Fig. 77.8). The occlusive process is always more widespread than may be apparent on angiography. Multiple-branch stenoses and occlusions within the intestinal arcades are not well demonstrated on standard arteriography.

Reperfusion of the visceral circulation is a major priority. Until recently, mesenteric thrombosis has been an urgent indication for operation. However, in these acutely ill patients, recent massive weight loss with attendant nutritional, wound-healing, and immunologic compromise makes a major operative procedure extraordinarily hazardous. Reperfusion to maintain intestinal viability temporarily may sometimes be accomplished by infusion of thrombolytic agents or other angioplastic techniques, and if the blood flow is restored successfully, vigorous hyperalimentation allows optimization of the patient's condition and an elective surgical procedure. The latter approach is not often used in clinical practice and is never appropriate when frankly necrotic bowel requiring resection is a consideration. Used selectively, however, this combined approach has potential benefit.

Operations for acute mesenteric thrombosis must be individualized. Emergent revascularization procedures ideally should parallel those used to treat chronic visceral ischemia. Contemporary opinion favors multiple-vessel revascularization and the use of short antegrade conduits (prosthetic or vein) whenever possible. Nevertheless, in the acute setting, a variety of alternative surgical techniques, including single-vessel revascularization and the use of vein and retrograde conduits, have resulted in survival and are appropriate in certain circumstances. In the presence of frankly necrotic bowel requiring resection, autogenous conduits are always preferred.

Low-flow Nonocclusive Mesenteric Ischemia

Low-flow nonocclusive mesenteric ischemia seems to have diminished in frequency and severity in recent years. Vasoconstriction in mesenteric blood vessels is the underlying mechanism most commonly cited as the cause of low-flow nonocclusive ischemia. This vasoconstriction occurs in response to diminished cardiac output, shock, hypovolemia, dehydration, and the use of medications known to diminish splanchnic blood flow. Virtually all vasoconstrictors and many inotropic agents have been implicated. Other drugs may also have significant effects on intestinal blood flow (Table 77.2). The diagnosis is typically suspected in critically ill patients receiving intensive care, often with unstable hemodynamics secondary to shock, congestive heart failure, cardiac arrhythmia, recent myocardial infarction, or valvular insufficiency. These problems often coexist with renal or hepatic disease. Evidence of gastrointestinal bleeding may be present, or guaiac-positive secretions noted in nasogastric aspirates. Diagnosis in these instances may require angiography (Fig. 77.9). Because no definitive surgical therapy is available other than resection of necrotic intestine, the focus of in-

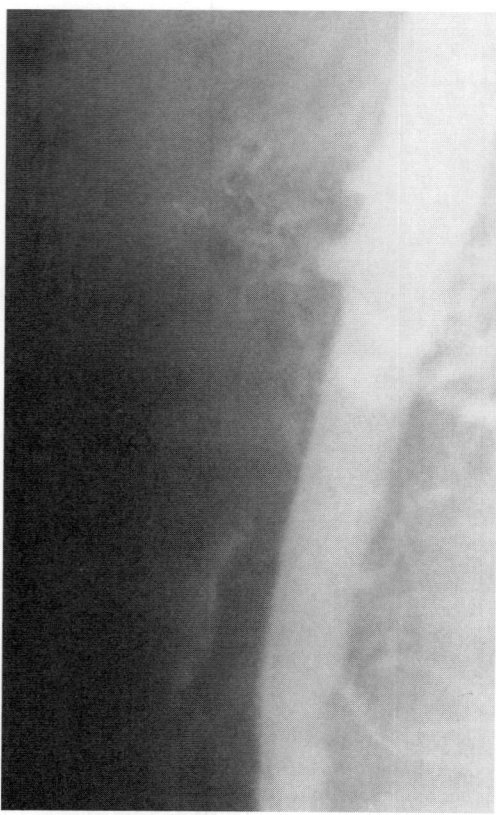

Figure 77.8. Lateral aortogram demonstrating acute celiac and superior mesenteric artery thrombosis, which results in widespread necrosis of the abdominal viscera.

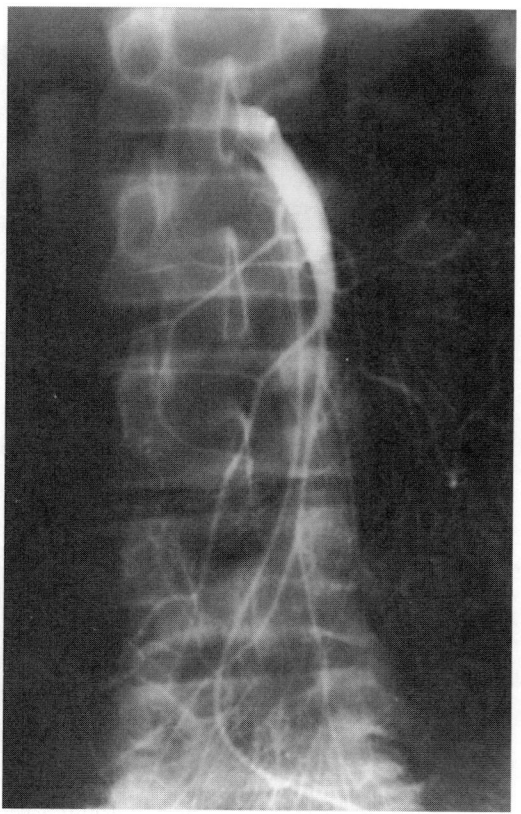

Figure 77.9. Low-flow nonocclusive ischemia causes profound vasoconstriction within the mesenteric arcades. This may be sufficient to cause mucosal necrosis or transmural infarction if not relieved.

tervention is on pharmacologic support of the circulation with relief of splanchnic vasoconstriction. Treatments include optimizing hemodynamic and volume status, correcting contributing medical conditions, and eliminating (when possible) adverse pharmacologic agents. Under some circumstances, infusion of vasodilators is appropriate. Papaverine (30 to 60 mg/h) is used by some groups, but selective intraarterial infusion is required to avoid systemic hypotension. Glucagon (2 to 4 mg/h), which selectively increases splanchnic blood flow, may be given by peripheral venous infusion and has positive inotropic effects; it may therefore be more suitable in some settings.

Iatrogenic Visceral Ischemia

Iatrogenic visceral ischemia can occur after operations or diagnostic procedures or with the use of certain pharmacologic agents. Digitalis preparations clearly decrease intestinal blood flow, as do ergotamines and virtually all pressor agents. Diagnostic or therapeutic angiography may cause iatrogenic visceral ischemia as a consequence of embolization, and selective mesenteric angiography has the potential to cause intimal flap formation or dissection.

Aortic aneurysm resection is the prototypic surgical procedure associated with iatrogenic intestinal ischemia. Its potential for compromising the colonic and occasionally the intestinal circulation is underappreciated, and compromise may occur with or without ligation of the IMA. Intestinal ischemia is more common with ruptured aneurysms, when occlusive and aneurysmal disease coexist, and when important collateral vessels are compromised by the aortic procedure (Fig. 77.10). After aneurysm

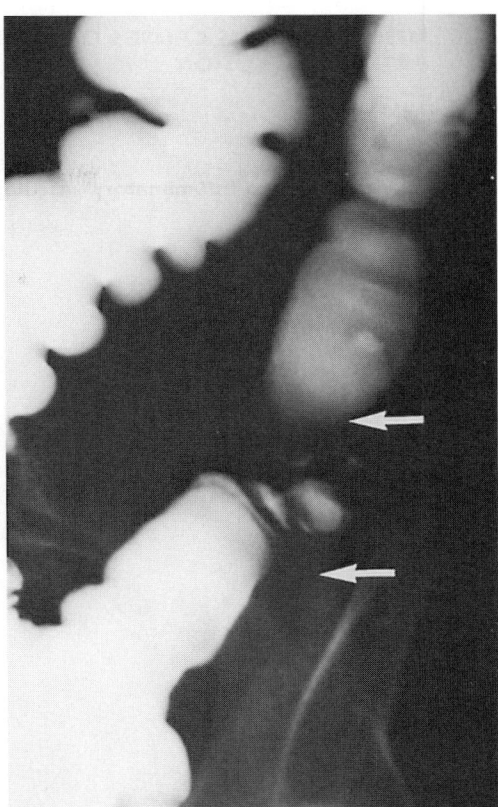

Figure 77.11. Stricture formation resulting from sigmoid colon ischemia after repair of a ruptured aortic aneurysm. A loss of haustrations is seen through the descending colon and the fixed narrowing in the midportion of the sigmoid colon *(arrows)*.

repair, colonic ischemia is clinically apparent in 1% to 2% of cases and has been detected endoscopically in upward of 6% to 8% of cases. Patients present with diarrhea, and the stool is often bloody or *guaiac-positive*. When hemorrhagic diarrhea occurs, immediate colonoscopy is indicated. If the ischemia is confined to the mucosa and submucosa and subsequently heals, the patient typically survives but strictures form (Fig. 77.11). If the ischemia is more profound and transmural infarction occurs, resection is required, and the mortality rate approaches 60%. The incidence of colonic ischemia after aortic surgery can be decreased by aggressive colonic and pelvic revascularization. Other operative procedures, such as extensive resections for gastrointestinal and genitourinary cancer, also can compromise intestinal blood flow.

Miscellaneous Causes of Acute Visceral Ischemia

Acute visceral ischemia can occur with an aortic dissection, traumatic injuries, inflammatory arteriopathy, or vasculitis (Table 77.3). The clinical presentation in each instance usually depends on the underlying cause, with superimposed symptoms of abdominal distention, an acute abdomen, or gastrointestinal bleeding. The diagnosis depends on recognizing the potential for intestinal ischemia and often is confirmed by angiography. The treatment in these instances must be highly individualized. Branch revascularization in the setting of acute aortic dissection is essential when ischemia is profound. Likewise, traumatic injuries require acute surgical intervention. Inflammatory arteriopathy and vasculitis, however, require treatment of the underlying medical condition, with oper-

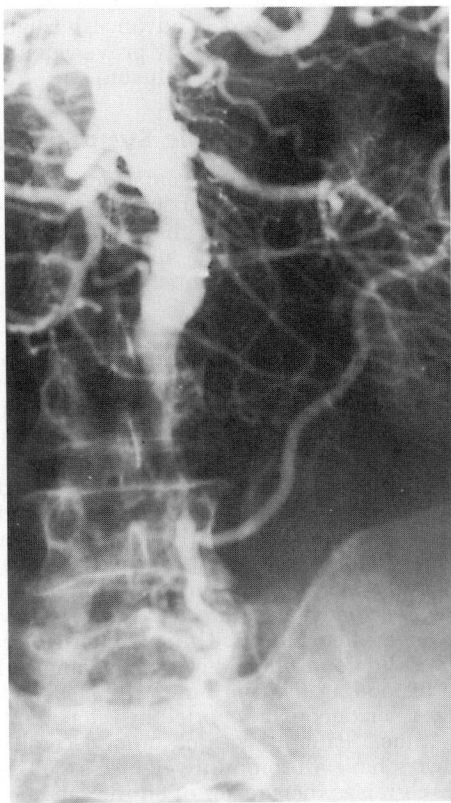

Figure 77.10. The multiple causes of iatrogenic visceral ischemia include medications, diagnostic and therapeutic angiographic procedures, and surgical procedures. A common surgical cause is aortic aneurysm resection. Coexistent aneurysmal and occlusive disease, seen in this aortogram, identify a patient at high risk.

Table 77.3. MISCELLANEOUS CAUSES OF VISCERAL ARTERY OCCLUSION

Mechanical causes
Aortic dissection
Blunt and penetrating trauma

Collagen vascular disease and inflammatory vasculopathy
Polyarteritis
Dermatomyositis
Rheumatoid arthritis
Sjögren's syndrome
Henoch-Schönlein purpura
Essential mixed cryoglobulinemia
Wegener's granulomatosis
Giant cell arteritis
Hepatitis B-associated antigens
Typhoid
Inflammatory bowel disease

Localized injury
Cholesterol embolism
Radiation
Enteric-coated potassium salts

Systemic vasculopathy
Diabetes mellitus
Polycythemia vera
Köhlmeier-Degos syndrome

Reactive vasculopathy
Estrogen–progesterone compounds
Pheochromocytoma
Carcinoid syndrome
Ergotism
Buerger's disease
Associated with renal vascular hypertension or accelerated phase of malignant hypertension

Table 77.4. TECHNIQUES FOR ASSESSING INTESTINAL VIABILITY

Commonly used
Clinical assessment
Intraoperative Doppler
Fluorescein dye or Wood lamp

Infrequently used
Surface oximetry
Laser Doppler
Radiolabeled microspheres
Ultrasonography of intestinal wall
Intraluminal tonometry
Electronic contractility monitor

Second-look procedures
Surgery
Laparoscopy or peritoneoscopy

Second-look Procedures

If large segments of ischemic small intestine are resected, the potential exists for the development of short-gut syndrome, a condition in which insufficient intestinal mucosal surface remains for adequate nutrient absorption. A dilemma then exists in dealing with damaged but potentially viable intestine. In this specialized circumstance, a second-look procedure may be beneficial. Contemporary clinical practice is to leave all definitely viable and marginally viable intestine and resect only unequivocally necrotic tissue. At the original operation, the decision for a planned second-look surgical procedure is made, and the patient is prepared for a return to the operating room in 24 to 48 hours to evaluate further the status of the intestine. Innovative technical advances, such as laparoscopy and peritoneoscopy, may prove valuable in this setting but have not been fully evaluated.

Chronic Visceral Ischemic Syndromes

The chronic, or subacute, presentations of visceral occlusive disease include visceral angina, mesenteric venous thrombosis, and possibly the median arcuate ligament syndrome. Although some authorities question the latter, the first two are well established.

Visceral Angina

Visceral angina secondary to arteriosclerotic occlusive disease of the splanchnic trunks causes midepigastric pain 30 to 45 minutes after eating. The responsible anatomic lesions usually involve the origins of at least two of the three visceral vessels (Fig. 77.12), but the occlusive process also is relatively widespread throughout the mesenteric arcades. The patient is typically either atherosclerotic or relatively young (usually a woman) with an extensive cigarette-smoking habit. In the latter case, a proliferative overflow of adjacent aortic intima into the origins of the visceral vessels develops. Affected patients have "food fear" and have often modified their pattern of eating so they avoid solid food altogether or consume only small quantities of food at any one time. This small-meal syndrome may be erroneously reported by the patient as "eating all the time." Patients with chronic visceral ischemia almost always have a profound weight loss (11 kg on average), which raises the specter of an intraabdominal malignancy. Weight loss represents avoidance of food secondary to pain rather than a malabsorption problem. Many times, an extensive series of gastrointestinal contrast studies, endoscopies, and scans has been undertaken and

ation reserved for resection of clearly nonviable segments of bowel.

Recognition of Intestinal Viability

Any acute intervention for visceral occlusive disease raises the issues of intraoperative recognition of viability, the appropriate limits to resection, and consideration of a second-look procedure. Distinguishing between viable and nonviable intestine might seem straightforward, but it is not. When critical lengths of intestine are compromised, decisions regarding how much to resect are of paramount importance. Clinical parameters of color, spontaneous peristalsis, and palpable pulses are not sensitive or specific enough to provide a basis for precise and confident clinical decisions. A variety of techniques to assess intestinal viability have been described. These range from straightforward but relatively insensitive to more sensitive but cumbersome or complex, requiring technologies not regularly available at the time an acute problem develops (Table 77.4). Commonly used techniques are not necessarily sensitive or specific, nor do they directly assess viability or reversibility of injury. They do have the advantage of ready availability and ease of application. The infrequently used techniques often are cumbersome, relatively unavailable, and not yet widely accepted in clinical practice.

By far the most common adjunctive technique to aid in clinical decisions regarding the margin of resection is Doppler ultrasonography. Although Doppler detects blood flow signals, and does not necessarily determine viability, it is frequently applied because of its ease of use and availability. Fluorescein dye or Wood lamp analysis is also frequently used.

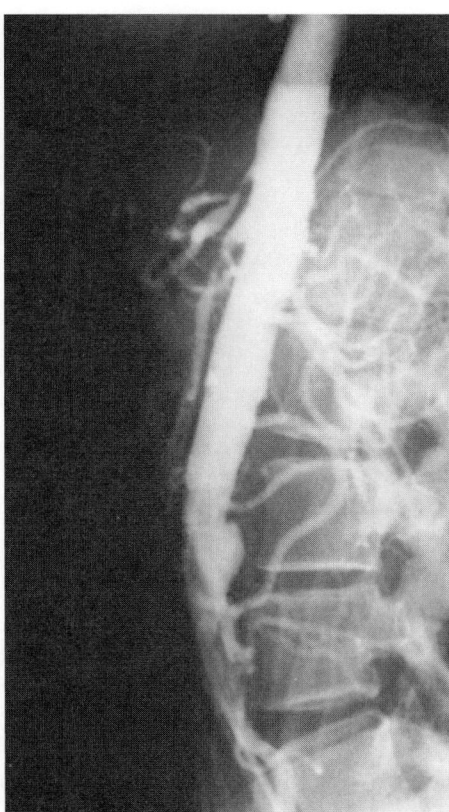

Figure 77.12. High-grade stenoses of the celiac and superior mesenteric arteries are apparent in this lateral aortogram. (From Zelenock GB. Splanchnic arteriosclerotic disease and intestinal angina. *Arch Surg* 1980;115:497, with permission.)

yielded normal results. Occasionally, nonproductive exploratory laparotomies are noted in the history, and an *erroneous diagnosis of anorexia nervosa* has been made.

The progression from symptoms to infarction is unpredictable. Many patients with intestinal infarction are discovered, in retrospect, to have had preexisting symptoms of visceral angina. Although delayed recognition is the rule, diagnostic and therapeutic interventions must proceed expeditiously because progress from symptomatic visceral angina to visceral thrombosis with transmural infarction is attended by an 80% mortality rate.

Aortography, including both anteroposterior and lateral views, confirms the clinical suspicion (Fig. 77.13). Multiple proximal vascular trunks are either totally occluded or exhibit a high-grade, hemodynamically significant stenosis. In some clinical series, 85% of the potential sites within the celiac, *superior mesenteric,* and *inferior mesenteric arteries* were totally occluded or severely stenosed. Although diseased, the IMA frequently serves as the major source of intestinal blood supply.

Confidence is developing in the ability of the noninvasive vascular diagnostic laboratory to image the celiac and mesenteric blood vessels. Expeditious screening of patients with postprandial pain and weight loss may enable a more timely diagnosis. *In patients with postprandial abdominal pain and weight loss who have normal findings on conventional diagnostic studies, intestinal vascular disease must be considered. At the least, duplex scanning of the aorta and visceral vessels should be undertaken. Magnetic resonance angiography, conventional angiography, or both can then be used as appropriate.*

Elective but relatively urgent intestinal revascularization is standard therapy. Multiple-vessel revascularization with short, antegrade conduits of either autogenous saphenous vein or prosthetic material are favored (Fig. 77.14). A variety of techniques, however, have resulted in long-term relief of symptoms and may be appropriate in some circumstances (Fig. 77.15). Endarterectomy through a trapdoor aortotomy is appropriate after thoracoabdominal exposure (Figs. 77.16 and 77.17) and is particularly effective when multiple proximal intestinal arterial stenoses or occlusions and concomitant renal artery lesions are present. In certain settings, a percutaneous angioplastic procedure may suffice, but long-term follow-up and collected series of patients treated in this fashion are lacking.

Mesenteric Venous Thrombosis

Mesenteric venous thrombosis is most often subacute in its presentation. A vague prodrome of crampy abdominal pain, abdominal distention, nausea, and malaise may occur for a few days to several weeks. Alternatively, in the presence of widespread and major venous occlusions, the presentation may be more acute. Mesenteric venous thrombosis may be secondary to an underlying condition or may present without a recognized cause. Associated conditions include intraabdominal inflammatory processes, peritonitis, portal hypertension, hypercoagulable states, and the use of oral contraceptives. Plain films reveal edema of the bowel wall. The venous phase of a selective mesenteric arteriogram may reveal the thrombus, and *computed tomography may demonstrate thrombus within the portal vein or the superior mesenteric vein. The markedly increased use of abdominal computed tomography has led to an increased recognition of mesenteric venous thrombosis.* In *many* instances, the diagnosis is made intraoperatively. At exploration, a bloody ascites may be present. The intestine appears dusky and feels thick and rubbery. Arterial pulses are palpable in the mesentery. The small mesenteric veins feel cordlike and exude clot when cut. Surgical therapy consists of resection of nonviable intestine, occasional large-vessel venous thrombectomy, and the use of anticoagulants. Correction of any predisposing cause and an investigation to detect hypercoagulable states, such as deficiency of antithrombin III and proteins C and S and the presence of *factor V Leiden anticardiolipin antibodies* (the lupus anticoagulant), are always appropriate. *In cases of primary mesenteric venous thrombosis,* postoperative anticoagulant therapy is continued indefinitely because venous thrombosis recurs in 30% to 40% of untreated patients; anticoagulation reduces this incidence to 3% to 5%. *In cases secondary to a treatable cause,* relatively short-term anticoagulation similar to that used for deep venous thrombosis is appropriate.

Median Arcuate Ligament Syndrome

Median arcuate ligament syndrome is controversial. Symptoms include postprandial abdominal pain but may or may not represent visceral ischemia. An alternative pathophysiologic mechanism may be irritation of neural tissue overlying the origin of the celiac artery. Patients typically present with abdominal pain, and in the course of their evaluation, arteriography demonstrates a significant compression of the celiac axis by the median arcuate ligament of the diaphragm (Fig. 77.18). Other visceral vessels seldom show involvement with an occlusive process. Lysis of the overlying median arcuate ligament and surrounding neural tissue affords relief of symptoms in many instances, provided alternative causes of the symptoms have been thoroughly and exhaustively evaluated.

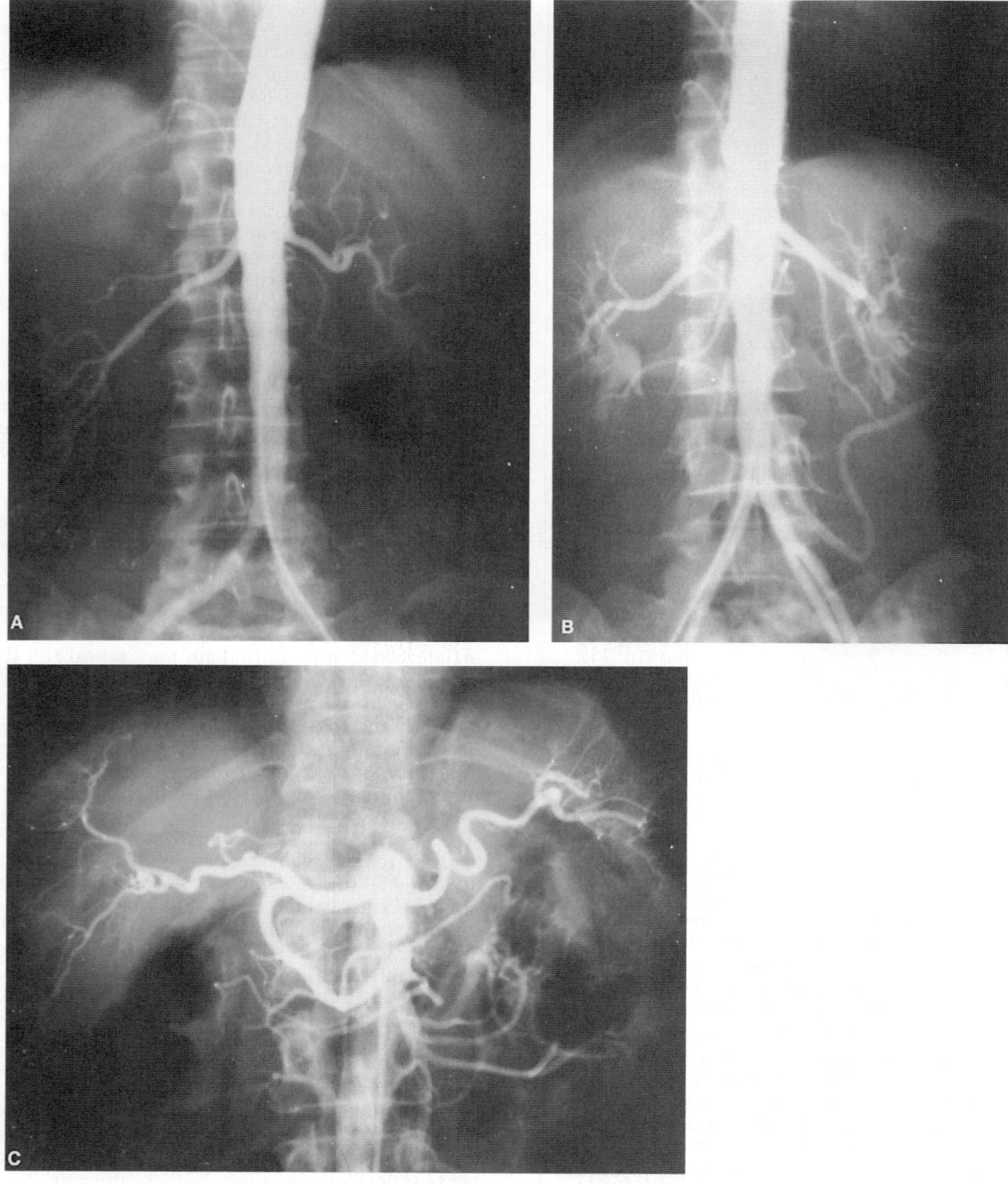

Figure 77.13. Chronic visceral ischemia produces visceral angina when multiple occlusions of major splanchnic blood vessels are present. Lack of apparent intestinal blood flow *(A)* and an unusually prominent inferior mesenteric artery *(B)* are angiographic signs of chronic visceral ischemia. Selective celiac injection *(C)* also fills the superior mesenteric artery distribution secondary to occlusions of the proximal superior and inferior mesenteric arteries.

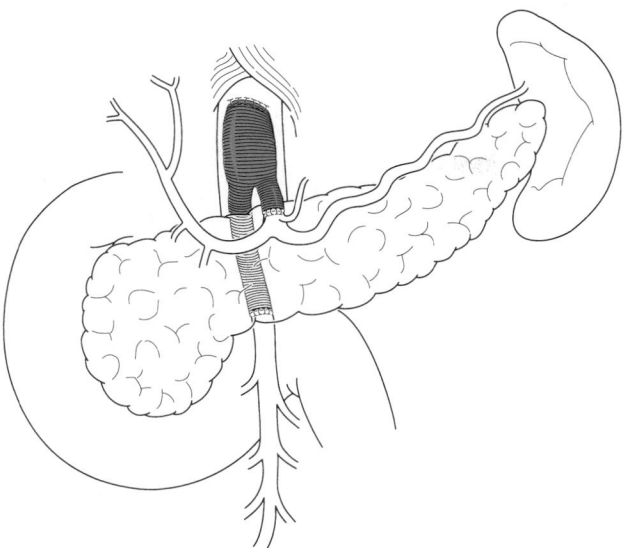

Figure 77.14. Bypass grafts to the visceral vessels may originate from the supraceliac aorta. Short antegrade conduits and multiple-vessel revascularization are favored.

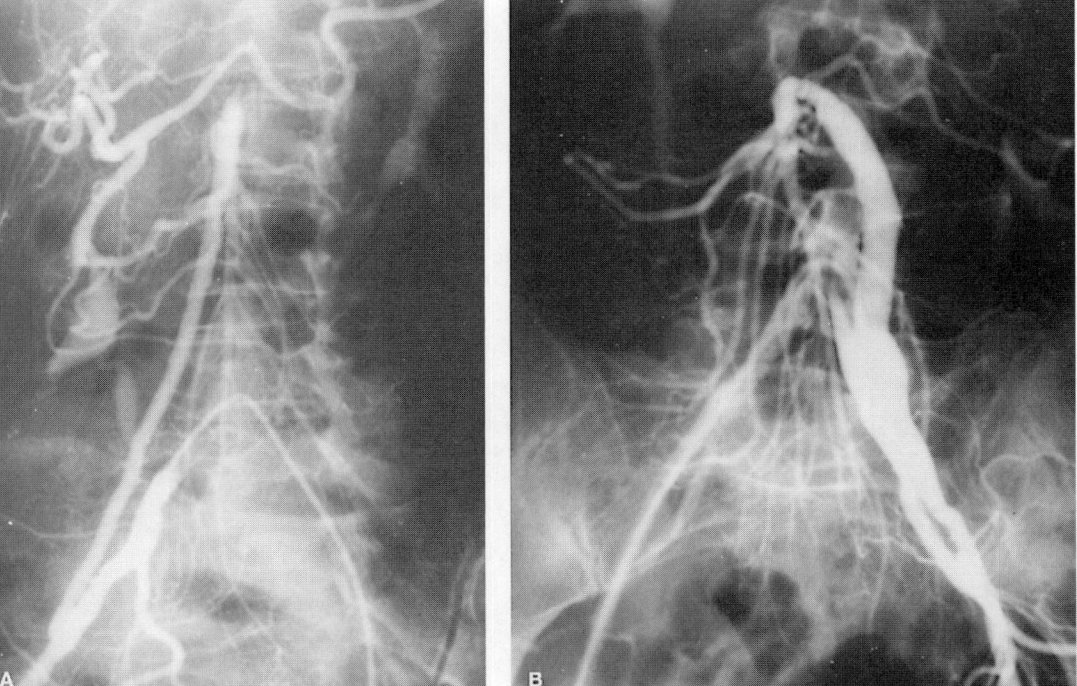

Figure 77.15. Retrograde conduits are an alternative bypass, and even single-vessel revascularization may provide effective long-term relief of symptoms in selected circumstances. *(A)* Retrograde right external iliac artery to superior mesenteric artery *(SMA)* vein graft. Filling is excellent throughout the distribution of the SMA and in the branches of the celiac artery as a result of collateral flow through the gastroduodenal artery. *(B)* A left common iliac artery–SMA bypass.

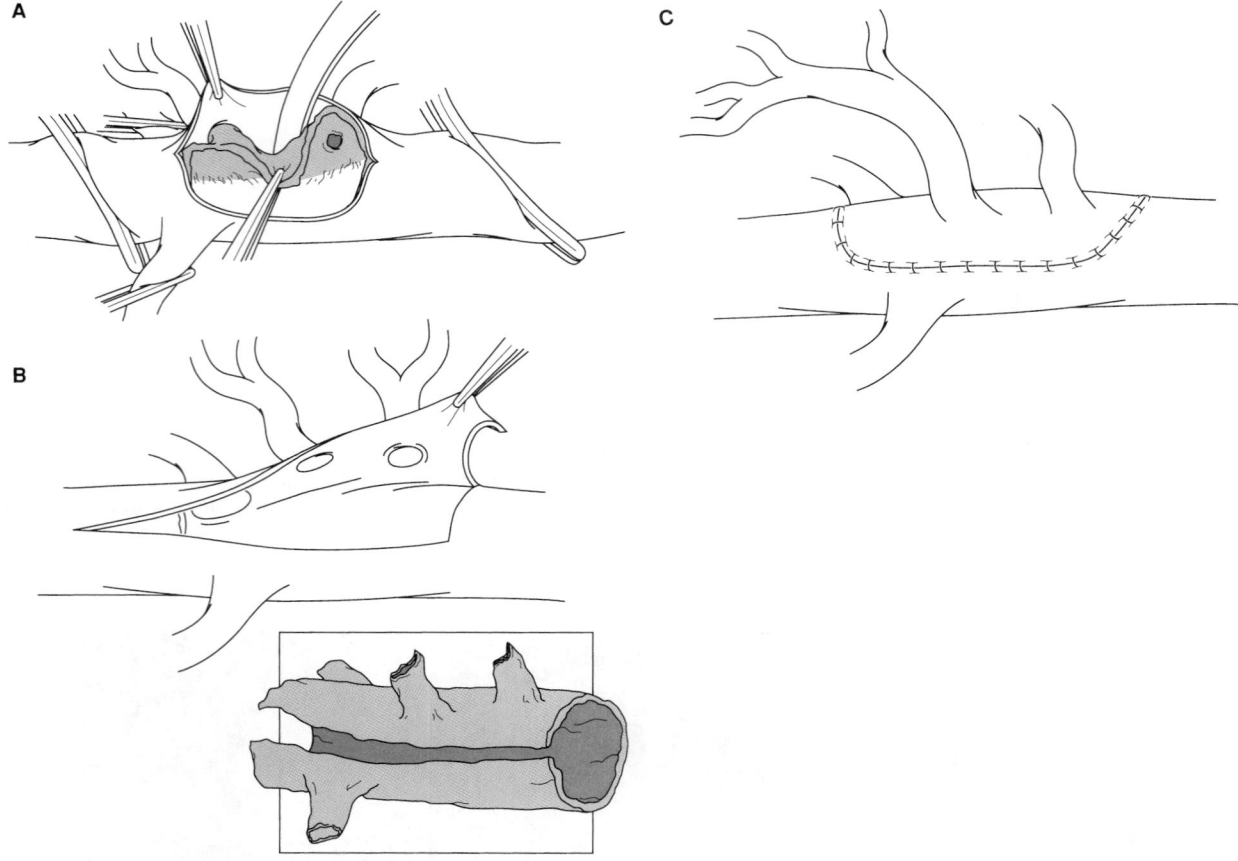

Figure 77.16. Endarterectomy of the celiac and superior mesenteric arteries is performed through a longitudinal trapdoor aortotomy. (After Wylie EJ. *Manual of vascular surgery,* vol 1. New York: Springer-Verlag, 1980, with permission.)

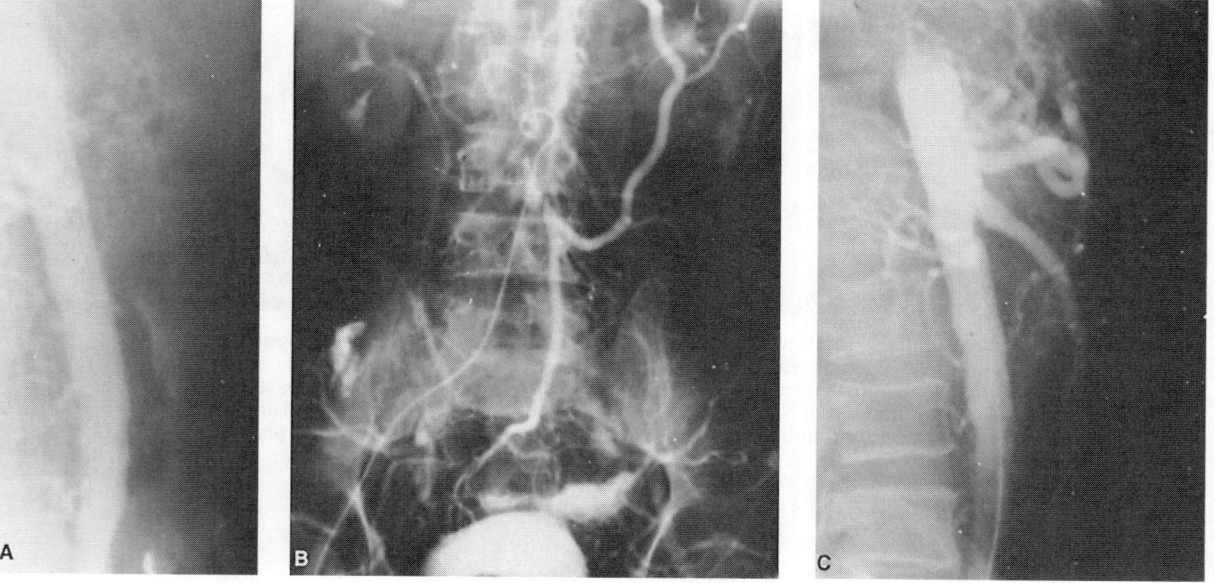

Figure 77.17. *(A)* Preoperative lateral aortogram demonstrates total occlusion of the celiac and superior mesenteric arteries. *(B)* Anteroposterior view with selective injection demonstrates large inferior-to-superior mesenteric artery collateral flow. *(C)* Postoperative angiography demonstrates widely patent celiac and superior mesenteric arteries after transaortic endarterectomy.

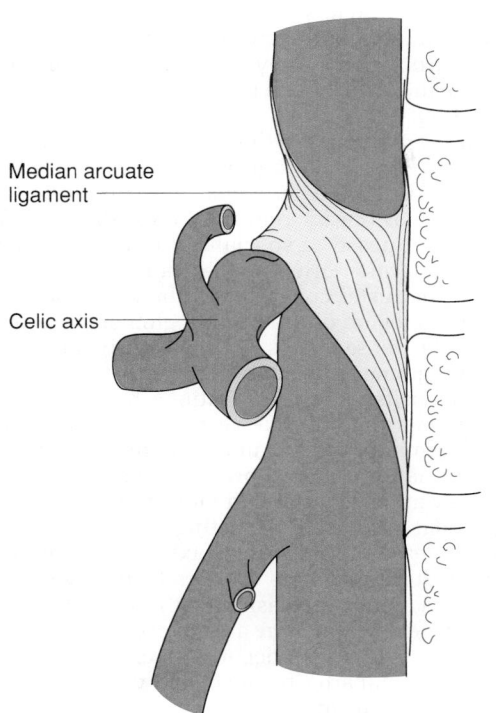

Median arcuate ligament

Celic axis

Figure 77.18. The median arcuate ligament syndrome is controversial, but the anatomic structure is very real. This firm, fibrous connection between the crura of the diaphragm is extraordinarily strong and may significantly narrow the celiac axis.

CONCLUSION

The acute and chronic visceral ischemic syndromes may be dramatic or pedestrian in presentation. Unattended, they are associated with substantial mortality and morbidity. Prompt recognition of the clinical syndromes, early and liberal use of diagnostic angiography, urgent or emergent operative intervention, vigorous resuscitation, and ancillary pharmacologic support offer the best chance for patient survival.

BIBLIOGRAPHY

Ballard J, Stone W, Hallett J, et al. A critical analysis of adjuvant techniques used to assess bowel viability in acute mesenteric ischemia. *Am Surg* 1993;59:309–311.

Beebe H, MacFarlane S, Raker E. Supraceliac aortomesenteric bypass for intestinal ischemia. *J Vasc Surg* 1987;5:749–754.

Boley SJ, Borden EB. Acute mesenteric vascular disease. In: Wilson SE, Veith FJ, Hobson RW, et al., eds. *Vascular surgery: principles and practice.* New York: McGraw-Hill, 1987.

Brolin RE, Semmlow JL, Sehonanda A, et al. Comparison of five methods of assessment of intestinal viability. *Surg Gynecol Obstet* 1989;168:6.

Burkart D, Johnson C, Reading C, et al. MR measurement of mesenteric venous flow: prospective evaluation in healthy volunteers and patients with suspected chronic mesenteric ischemia. *Radiology* 1995;194:801–806.

Cronenwett JL, Ayad M, Kazmer A. Effects of intravenous glucagon on the survival of rats after acute occlusive mesenteric ischemia. *J Surg Res* 1985;38:445.

Deitch EA. The role of intestinal barrier failure and bacterial translocation in the development of systemic infection and multiple organ failure. *Arch Surg* 1990;125:403.

Garcia JG, Rollan CM, Enriquez MAR, et al. Improved survival in intestinal ischemia by allopurinol not related to xanthine-oxidase inhibition. *J Surg Res* 1990;48:144.

Gentile A, Moneta G, Taylor L, et al. Isolated bypass to the superior mesenteric artery for intestinal ischemia. *Arch Surg* 1994;129:926–932.

Harward T, Brooks D, Flynn T, et al. Multiple organ dysfunction after mesenteric artery revascularization. *J Vasc Surg* 1993; 18:459–469.

Jamieson W, DeRose G, Harris K, et al. Myocardial and circulatory performance during the ischemic phase of superior mesenteric artery occlusion. *Can J Surg* 1993;36:435–439.

Kazmers A. Operative management of chronic mesenteric ischemia. *Ann Vasc Surg* 1998;12:299–308.

Landreneau RJ, Fry WJ. The right colon as a target organ of nonocclusive mesenteric ischemia. *Arch Surg* 1990;125:591.

Levy PJ, Krausz MM, Manny J. Acute mesenteric ischemia: improved results—a retrospective analysis of ninety-two patients. *Surgery* 1990;107:372.

Levy PJ, Krausz MM, Manny J. The role of second-look procedures in improving survival time for patients with mesenteric venous thrombosis. *Surg Gynecol Obstet* 1990; 170:287.

McShane M, Proctor A, Spencer P, et al. Mesenteric angioplasty for chronic intestinal ischemia. *Eur J Vasc Surg* 1992;6:333–336.

Mesh CL, Gewertz BL. The effect of hemodilution on blood flow regulation in normal and post-ischemic intestine. *J Surg Res* 1990;48:183.

Moneta G, Lee R, Yeager R, et al. Mesenteric duplex scanning: a blinded prospective study. *J Vasc Surg* 1993;17:79–86.

Moneta GL, Taylor DC, Helton WS, et al. Duplex ultrasound measurement of postprandial intestinal blood flow: effect of meal composition. *Gastroenterology* 1988;95:1294.

Oshima A, Kitajama M, Sakai N, et al. Does glucagon improve the viability of ischemic intestine? *J Surg Res* 1990;49:524.

Pargger H, Staender S, Studer W, et al. Occlusive mesenteric ischemia and its effects on jejunal intramucosal pH, mesenteric oxygen consumption, and oxygen tensions from surfaces of the jejunum in anesthetized pigs. *Intensive Care Med* 1997;23:91–99.

Park PO, Haglund U, Bulkley GB, et al. The sequence of development of intestinal tissue injury after strangulation ischemia and reperfusion. *Surgery* 1990;107:574.

Reuter SR, Redman HC. *Gastrointestinal angiography,* 2nd ed. Philadelphia: WB Saunders, 1971.

Rutherford R, Taylor L, eds. Mesenteric ischemia. *Semin Vasc Surg* 1990;3:141–205.

Stoney RJ, Reilly LM, Ehrenfeld WK. Chronic mesenteric ischemia and surgery for chronic visceral ischemia. In: Wilson SE, Veith FJ, Hobson RW, et al., eds. *Vascular surgery: principles and practice.* New York: McGraw-Hill, 1987.

Stoney RJ, Schneider PA. Technical aspects of visceral arterial revascularization. In: Bergan JJ, Yao JST, eds. *Techniques in arterial surgery.* Philadelphia: WB Saunders, 1990.

Taylor LM Jr. Mesenteric ischemia. *Semin Vasc Surg* 1990;3:141.

Thompson JS, Bragg LE, West WW. Serum enzyme levels during intestinal ischemia. *Ann Surg* 1990;211:369.

Zelenock GB, Graham LM, Whitehouse WM Jr, et al. Splanchnic arteriosclerotic disease and intestinal angina. *Arch Surg* 1980;115:497.

Zelenock GB, Strodel WE, Knol JA, et al. A prospective study of clinically and endoscopically documented colonic ischemia in 100 patients undergoing aortic reconstructive surgery with aggressive colonic and direct pelvic revascularization, compared with historic controls. *Surgery* 1989;106:771.

SURGERY: SCIENTIFIC PRINCIPLES AND PRACTICE, Third Edition, edited by
Lazar J. Greenfield, Michael W. Mulholland, Keith T. Oldham, Gerald B. Zelenock,
and Keith D. Lillemoe. Lippincott Williams & Wilkins Publishers, Philadelphia, © 2001.

CHAPTER 78

RENAL ARTERY OCCLUSIVE DISEASE

JAMES C. STANLEY AND GILBERT R. UPCHURCH, JR.

Renovascular hypertension secondary to renal artery occlusive disease is the most common form of surgically correctable hypertension. Systemic blood pressure elevations in these patients follow reductions in renal perfusion with activation of the renin–angiotensin system. Although this physiologic response tends to restore the renal artery perfusion pressures toward normal, it does so in a pathologic manner by producing hypertension in the systemic circulation.

PATHOPHYSIOLOGY OF RENOVASCULAR HYPERTENSION

The physiologic basis of renovascular hypertension is relatively well defined. This form of hypertension was first recognized more than 60 years ago by Goldblatt and associates (1), who produced sustained hypertension in dogs by gradually reducing renal artery blood flow with an externally controlled vascular clamp. Subsequent studies have discounted the importance of renal ischemia *per se* as the cause of renovascular hypertension, with other hemodynamic signals, particularly a decrease in mean renal artery perfusion pressure, appearing essential to an increase in renin release. An 80% reduction in renal artery

cross-sectional area, so-called critical stenosis, induces a pressure gradient sufficient to cause an increased release of renin from the kidney. Renin and its effects on angiotensin and aldosterone account for renovascular hypertension (Fig. 78.1).

Renin is produced by the juxtaglomerular apparatus of the kidney. This anatomic area consists of a variety of cells, including *myoepitheloid* or *granular cells,* located on the wall of the afferent arterioles; the *macula densa,* which is composed of specialized tubular epithelial cells in the glomerular hilus at the transition of the loop of Henle to the distal convoluted tubule; and *lacis cells,* located in the region of the efferent glomerular arteriole and the macula densa. Lacis cells are intimately associated with the glomerulus and are anatomically similar to mesangial cells. The interrelations between the macula densa, glomerular arteriole vasomotion, and renal tubular function are important in understanding renin kinetics.

The regulation of renin production and its release from the kidney at the cellular and molecular level are complex (2–4). Renal baroreceptors, acting as stretch receptors, affect the release of renin from juxtaglomerular cells. Activation of these receptors appears to involve the calcium ion, with evidence increasing that renin release and intracellular levels of calcium are inversely related. Alternatively, renin release can occur with changes in pressure at the afferent renal arteriole level and with changes in renal interstitial volume and pressure.

Renin is a proteolytic enzyme, active at a neutral pH on its only known substrate, angiotensinogen. The renin gene is located on chromosome 1 (5) (Figs. 78.2 and 78.3). This gene is composed of nine exons and an additional miniexon, interrupted by eight introns (6). Transcription of the renin gene to renin mRNA is followed by its translation into a preprorenin molecule with a molecular weight of 45 kd (7). Subsequent cleavage and glycosylation of this molecule in the rough endoplasmic reticulum produce prorenin, which has a molecular weight of 47 kd.

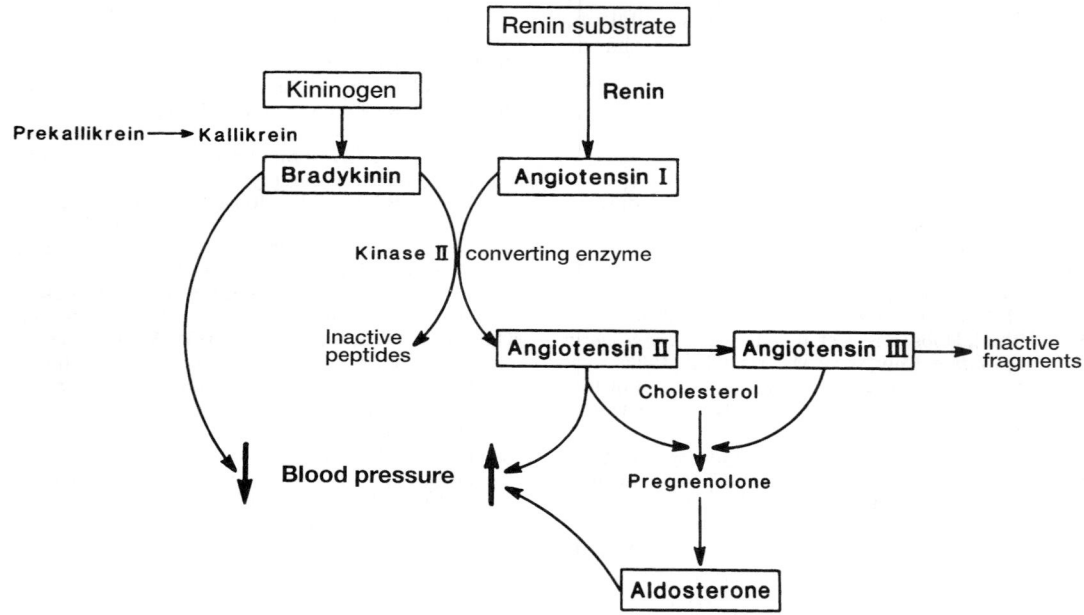

Figure 78.1. Renin–angiotensin system: interrelation with aldosterone and bradykinin in the regulation of blood pressure. (After Stanley JC, Graham LM, Whitehouse WM Jr. Renovascular hypertension. In: Miller TA, ed. *Physiologic basis of modern surgical care,* 2nd ed. St. Louis: Quality Medical, 1998:918, with permission.)

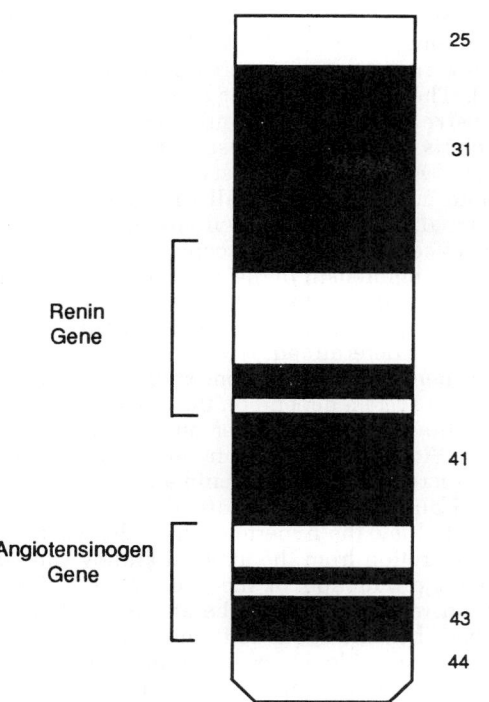

Figure 78.2. Chromosome 1 contains both the human renin and angiotensinogen genes.

Prorenin is transferred into the Golgi complex, where it is secreted and processed to active renin. Renin is a single-chain polypeptide with a molecular weight of about 38 kd (8). It is stored as granules within the juxtaglomerular cells and, in some instances, as granules within the arteriolar wall.

Renin has a half-life of 20 to 30 minutes. Under the usual circumstances of normal sodium balance, the sum of renin activity measured in both renal veins is about 48% greater than that in the infrarenal vena cava or peripheral arterial and venous circulations (9). The renin levels in the peripheral circulation appear to be maintained in a steady state because of this relatively constant 48% contribution of renin from the kidneys. The liver is the primary site for the removal and clearance of renin (10). Extrarenal renin or renin-like enzymes (isorenins) exist in the submaxillary salivary gland, uterus, placenta, and brain, but no evidence has been found that these substances are functionally important in elevating blood pressure.

The biochemistry of the renin–angiotensin system has been well defined (Fig. 78.4). The primary, if not sole, function of renin is the hydrolysis of renin substrate (a circulating peptide known as *angiotensinogen*) to form angiotensin I. Angiotensinogen is an α_2-globulin produced in the liver that has a molecular weight of 60 kd. The gene for angiotensinogen is located on chromosome 1 and is composed of five exons and four introns (11,12) (Figs. 78.2 and

78.5). The nucleotides coding for the angiotensin I peptide are located within the second exon. Expression of the angiotensinogen gene is subject to a variety of physiologic and pathophysiologic stimuli, including steroid hormones, angiotensin II, salt loading, and various drugs. Angiotensinogen itself has no vasoactive properties.

Angiotensin I, a decapeptide produced by the renin–renin substrate reaction, has little vasoactivity. It does exert an effect on the adrenal medulla, the sympathetic and central nervous systems, and the renal arterioles. Angiotensin II is formed when two C-terminus peptides are cleaved from angiotensin I by angiotensin-converting enzyme (ACE), a carboxypeptidase. Angiotensin II, an octapeptide, represents the vasoconstrictive element of renovascular hypertension. Although angiotensin II stimulates the hepatic production of renin substrate, in normal subjects, it has a continuous negative feedback effect on the renal release of renin (13). Angiotensin II has a half-life of about 4 minutes (14). Angiotensin III, a heptapeptide, is produced with the aminopeptidase cleavage of angiotensin II to I-desaspartyl angiotensin II. Angiotensin III is known to inhibit angiotensin II, but its most relevant effect is to increase aldosterone synthesis. Nevertheless, angiotensin III has little biologic activity of physiologic importance.

Aldosterone is secreted from the zona glomerulosa of the adrenal cortex and represents the volume element of renovascular hypertension. The biosynthesis of this mineralocorticoid includes the cleavage of a side-chain of cholesterol to form pregnenolone. This step is facilitated by both angiotensin II and angiotensin III. Aldosterone increases renal conservation of sodium and water, with a subsequent extracellular fluid volume expansion and an eventual increase in blood pressure.

Angiotensin-converting enzyme (dipeptidylcarboxypeptidase) is a zinc metallopeptidase responsible for producing angiotensin II from angiotensin I by removing C-terminus peptides from angiotensin I. The molecular weight of ACE is 150,000 to 180,000 kd. The ACE gene has been mapped to chromosome 17 in humans (15,16). The highest concentration of ACE is found in the endothelium of the pulmonary circulation. Conversion of angiotensin I to angiotensin II, at physiologic concentrations, occurs in a single passage through the lungs (17). ACE has been found at lower levels in the blood and kidney and in other vascular beds. ACE is also important in the metabolism of the vasodepressor bradykinin. At least two enzymes appear to inactivate bradykinin. The first is kinase I, which acts by cleaving the C-terminus arginine of bradykinin. The second, kinase II, acts by cleaving the C-terminus dipeptide group Phe-Arg. Kinase II and ACE appear to be similar in that they have nearly identical substrate specificities, cofactor requirements, and antigenic specificities (18).

The most common means of determining plasma renin activity is to measure angiotensin I generation with a modified radioimmunoassay. Renin activity is expressed as the hourly amount of angiotensin I generated per volume of plasma assayed. The assay involves two phases: (a) an incubation of plasma to generate angiotensin I, and (b) the actual radioimmunoassay of generated angiotensin I. Vari-

Figure 78.3. Human renin gene, consisting of nine exons and eight introns and a miniexon comprising nine base pairs *(5a)* of unknown function located between exons 5 and 6. This gene is about 12.18 kb long. The coding sequence *(black boxes)* is contained in the second to eighth exons and in portions of the first and ninth exons.

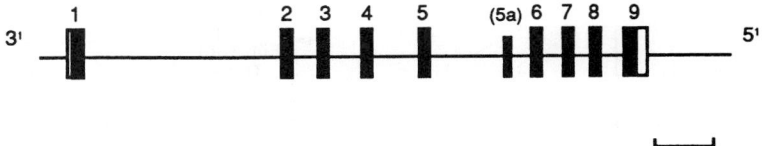

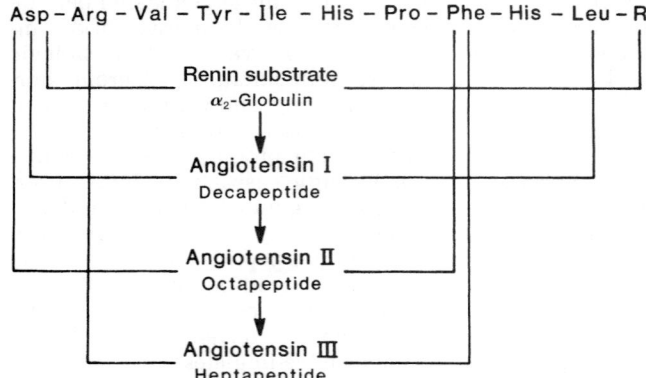

Figure 78.4. Biochemical composition of renin substrate and the angiotensins. (After Stanley JC, Graham LM. Renovascular hypertension. In: Miller TA, ed. *Physiologic basis of modern surgical care,* 2nd ed. St. Louis: Quality Medical, 1998:918, with permission.)

ations in assay techniques among laboratories often make interlaboratory comparisons difficult. Renin secretion is calculated as the renal arteriovenous difference in renin activity multiplied by renal plasma flow and is expressed as nanograms per milliliter per hour.

The actions of angiotensin on cardiac activity, vascular smooth-muscle reactivity, and sodium and water metabolism contribute to an increase in arterial pressure (Fig. 78.6). The most important consequence of renal artery occlusive disease is the production of angiotensin II, which is one of the most potent pressor substances known. Angiotensin II acts directly on the arteriolar smooth muscle of nearly all vascular beds; the splanchnic, renal, and cutaneous circulations are most sensitive to its effects. Despite an acceptance of the central importance of angiotensin in the generation of renovascular hypertension, the exact role of cellular or locally secreted renin and generated angiotensin in this clinical setting remains undetermined.

The hemodynamic responses to an activated renin–angiotensin system depend on the rate of alterations in renal blood flow and on whether one or both kidneys are affected. Acute reductions in renal blood flow result in rapid increases in plasma renin and blood pressure. In the case of unilateral renovascular disease with a normal opposite kidney, the hypertension is characterized by renin hypersecretion from the affected kidney and suppression of renin production in the contralateral kidney (19,20). Sodium retention within the affected kidney is counterbalanced by continuous sodium excretion from the normal contralateral kidney, resulting in relative intravascular volume depletion. This vasoconstrictive form of hyperten-

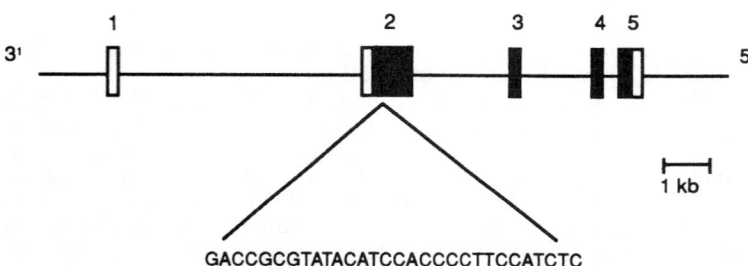

GACCGCGTATACATCCACCCCTTCCATCTC

Figure 78.5. Human angiotensinogen gene, which consists of five exons and four introns. This gene is about 14.55 kb long. The coding sequence *(black boxes)* for angiotensinogen is contained in the second to fifth exons. The second exon contains the coding sequence for angiotensin I.

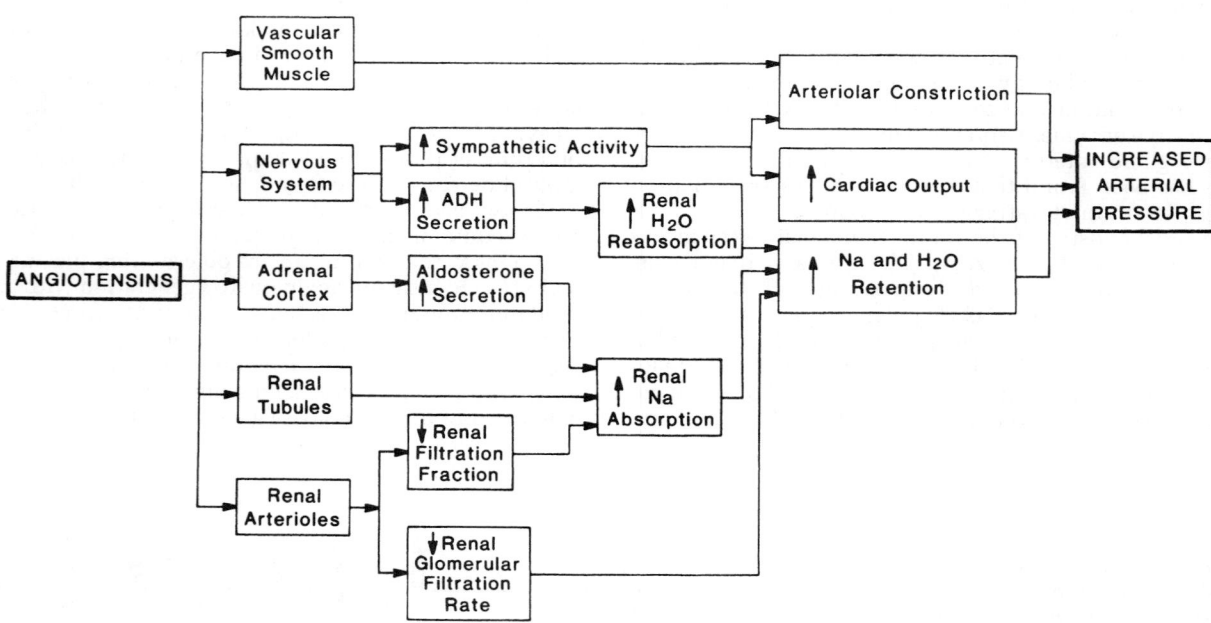

Figure 78.6. Effects of angiotensins contributing to increased arterial pressure. (After Stanley JC, Graham LM. Renovascular hypertension. In: Miller TA, ed. *Physiologic basis of modern surgical care,* 2nd ed. St. Louis: Quality Medical, 1998:918, with permission.)

sion is angiotensin II-dependent and responds to ACE inhibitors.

Pathophysiologic alterations in the case of bilateral renovascular disease, or unilateral disease of a solitary kidney, are related to changes other than vasoconstriction. Angiotensin II causes sodium retention, diminutions in glomerular filtration, stimulation of aldosterone production, and stimulation of norepinephrine release from the adrenergic nervous system. In chronic bilateral renovascular hypertension or unilateral renovascular hypertension in patients with only one kidney, sodium retention accounts for late reductions in renin secretion, although it is possible that absolute renin activity is abnormally high with regard to the existing sodium balance. Blood pressure elevations do not appear as dependent on the renin–angiotensin system in sodium-replete chronic renovascular hypertension. In this setting, ACE inhibitors are more effective in reducing elevated blood pressures with sodium depletion (21).

PATHOLOGY OF RENAL ARTERY OCCLUSIVE DISEASE

Different macrovascular occlusive diseases affect the renal arterial circulation. The most common, arteriosclerosis and arterial fibrodysplasia, have been well characterized in recent decades (22). Developmental renal artery

narrowings are also a rare cause of renovascular hypertension, and although uncommon, renal artery emboli, spontaneous dissections, and traumatic occlusions are occasionally associated with acute renin-mediated hypertension.

Arteriosclerosis

Arteriosclerotic renal artery occlusive disease accounts for about 95% of reported cases of renovascular hypertension (Fig. 78.7). This type of renovascular hypertension may be even more common because most reported experiences are surgical series that exclude many older patients who are not operative candidates. Arteriosclerotic renovascular disease most commonly presents during the sixth decade of life. Men are affected twice as often as women. Although arteriosclerotic renal artery stenotic disease affects nearly half of the elderly population to some degree, it is not always associated with elevated blood pressures. Many of these patients have occlusive disease of the coronary, cerebral, mesenteric, or peripheral vessels (23–26), particularly those who are black, in whom extrarenal arteriosclerotic vascular disease tends to be severe (27).

Arteriosclerotic renal artery occlusive disease characteristically affects the proximal third of the vessel in the form of eccentric or concentric stenoses. In nearly 80% of cases, these lesions occur as spillover of diffuse aortic atherosclerosis. Arteriosclerotic renal artery lesions are bilateral

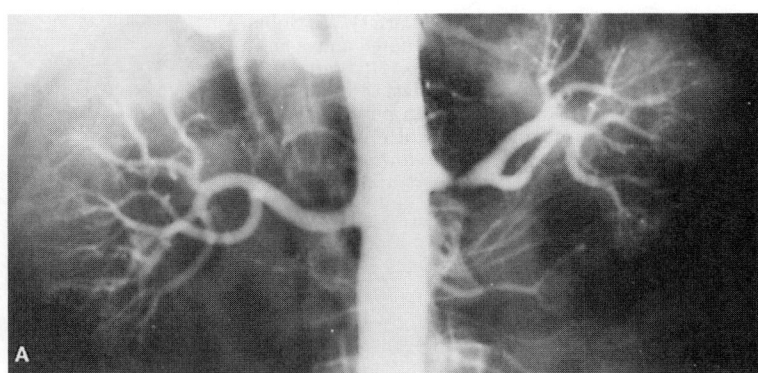

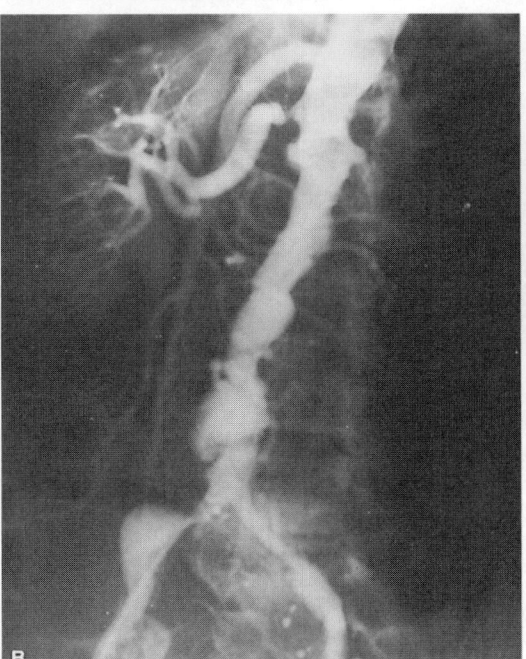

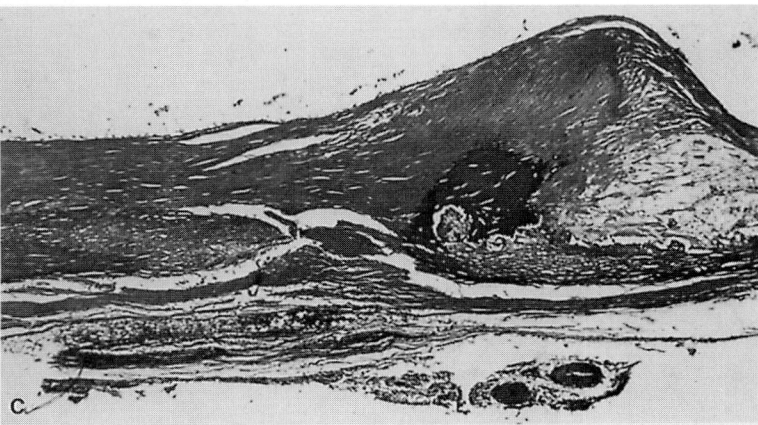

Figure 78.7. Renal artery arteriosclerosis. *(A)* Intrinsic focal lesion of proximal renal artery. *(B)* Severe aortic spillover disease affecting renal artery orifice and entire abdominal aorta. *(C)* Complicated renal artery plaque with collections of cholesterol, extensive fibrosis, and calcification. H&E, ×60. (Parts A and C from Stanley JC. Morphologic, histopathologic, and clinical characteristics of renovascular fibrodysplasia and arteriosclerosis. In: Bergan JJ, Yao JST, eds. *Surgery of the aorta and its body branches.* New York: Grune & Stratton, 1979:355, with permission. Part B from Stanley JC, Graham LM. Renovascular hypertension. In: Miller TA, ed. *Physiologic basis of modern surgical care*, 2nd ed. St. Louis: Quality Medical, 1998:918, with permission.)

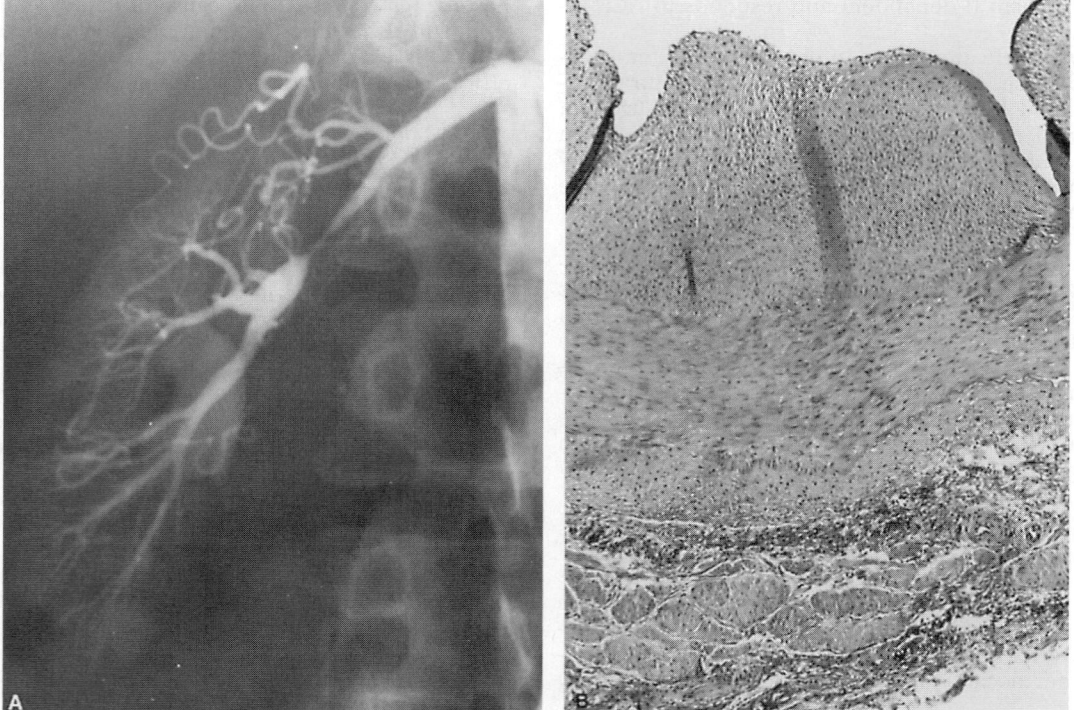

Figure 78.8. Intimal fibroplasia. *(A)* Focal stenosis of midportion of main renal artery. *(B)* Subendothelial mesenchymal cells within a loose fibrous connective tissue matrix are noted above an intact internal elastic lamina, normal media, and normal adventitial tissues. H&E, ×120. (Part A from Stanley JC, Fry WJ. Renovascular hypertension secondary to arterial fibrodysplasia in adults: criteria for operation and results of surgical therapy. *Arch Surg* 1975;110:922, with permission. Part B from Stanley JC. Morphologic, histopathologic, and clinical characteristics of renovascular fibrodysplasia and arteriosclerosis. In: Bergan JJ, Yao JST, eds. *Surgery of the aorta and its body branches.* New York: Grune & Stratton, 1979:355, with permission.)

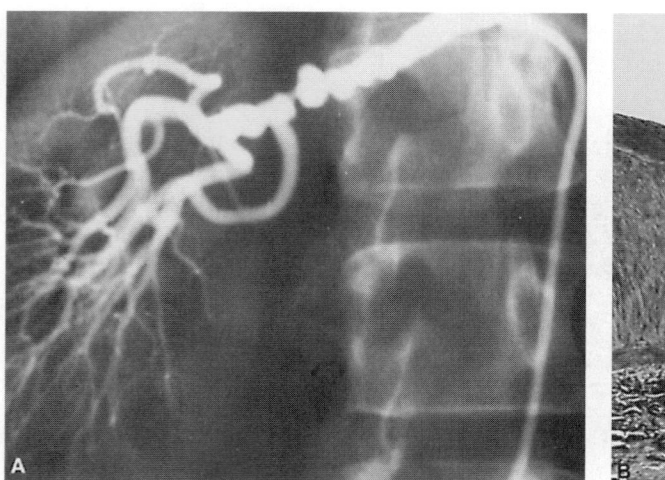
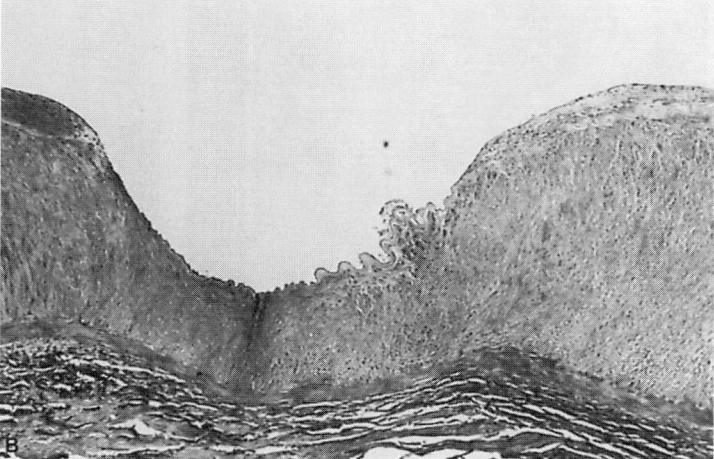

Figure 78.9. Medial fibroplasia. *(A)* Serial stenoses alternate with mural aneurysms to produce a "string-of-beads" appearance in the middle and distal portions of the main renal artery. *(B)* Diffuse form of medial fibroplasia exhibits regions of excess fibroproliferation with intervening areas of medial thinning. Masson stain, ×60, longitudinal section. (From Stanley JC. Morphologic, histopathologic, and clinical characteristics of renovascular fibrodysplasia and arteriosclerosis. In: Bergan JJ, Yao JST, eds. *Surgery of the aorta and its body branches.* New York: Grune & Stratton, 1979:355, with permission.)

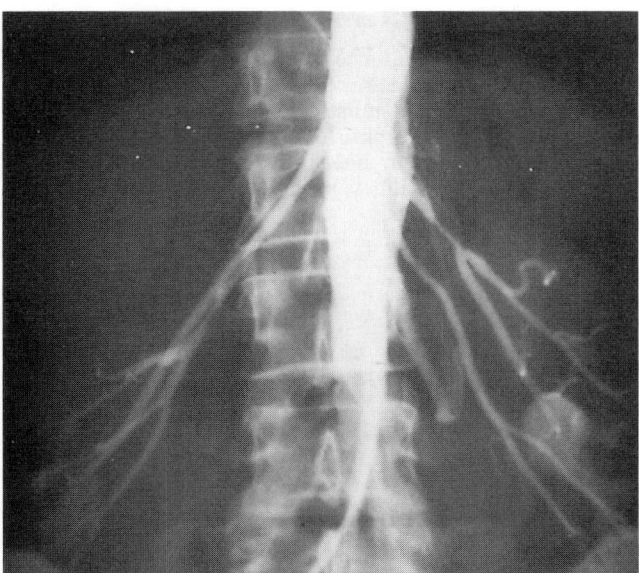

Figure 78.10. Medial fibrodysplasia, manifested as irregular narrowings to ptotic kidneys, affecting the midportions of the main renal arteries, which appear stretched during upright aortography. (From Stanley JC, Wakefield TW. Arterial fibrodysplasia. In: Rutherford RB, ed. *Vascular Surgery,* 5th ed. Philadelphia: WB Saunders, 2000:387, with permission.)

in three fourths of patients. When unilateral, these lesions affect the right and left renal arteries with equal frequency, although the left renal artery often appears more severely diseased. Intimal and medial accumulations of cholesterol-laden foam cells and fibrous tissue

are typical of these lesions. Necrosis, hemorrhage, calcification, and luminal thrombus are characteristic of complicated atherosclerotic plaques associated with more advanced disease.

Arterial Fibrodysplasia

Arterial fibrodysplasia is the second most common type of renal artery disease, accounting for about 5% of reported cases of renovascular hypertension. Dysplastic renal artery stenoses represent a heterogenous group of lesions. They are classified by the specific pathologic process and vessel wall region most affected. Included among these lesions are intimal fibroplasia, medial fibroplasia, and perimedial dysplasia (28,29). The last two entities appear to be a continuum of the same disease process. Each category has certain characteristic features deserving individual comment.

Intimal fibroplasia accounts for about 5% of all dysplastic renal artery stenoses (29) (Fig. 78.8). These lesions occur in children and young adults more often than in the elderly, and they affect both sexes equally. The cause of primary intimal fibroplasia is unknown but may be related to persistent embryonic myointimal cushions. Secondary intimal fibroplasia has been attributed to flow disturbances, blunt abdominal trauma during childhood, and previous arteritis, such as occurs with rubella. Progression of intimal fibroplasia may cause turbulent blood flow and an accelerated fibroproliferative response that rapidly compromises the arterial lumen.

Intimal fibroplasia usually presents as a smooth, focal stenosis of the distal main renal artery. In some patients, these lesions produce long, tubular stenoses, and in rare cases, they present as webs affecting segmental arteries. Proximal ostial lesions most often represent the secondary

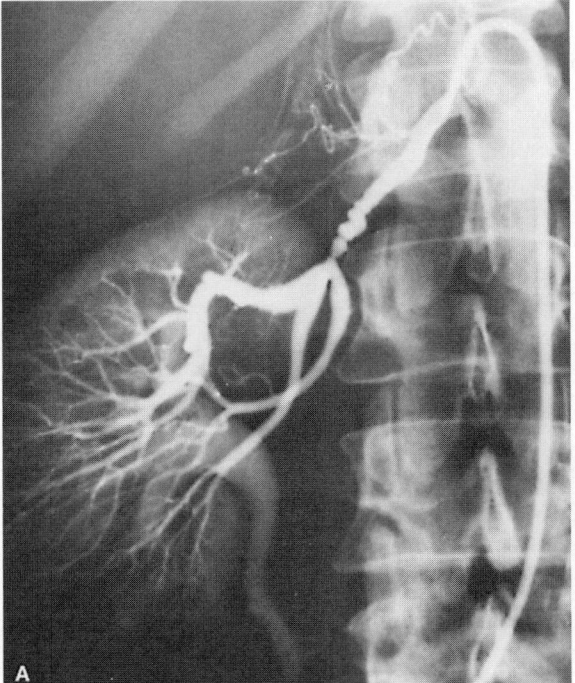
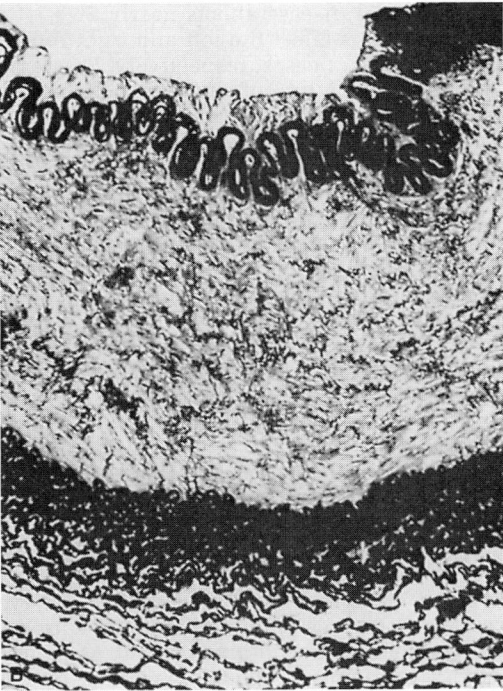

Figure 78.11. Perimedial dysplasia. *(A)* Multiple stenoses without mural aneurysms in the midportion of the renal artery are characteristic of these lesions. *(B)* The lesions represent excessive accumulations of elastic tissue at the medial–adventitial junction. Verhoeff stain, ×120. (From Stanley JC. Morphologic, histopathologic, and clinical characteristics of renovascular fibrodysplasia and arteriosclerosis. In: Bergan JJ, Yao JST, eds. *Surgery of the aorta and its body branches.* New York, Grune & Stratton, 1979:355, with permission.)

form of this disease, associated with abdominal aortic hypoplasia and coarctation (30,31). Subendothelial accumulations of irregularly arranged mesenchymal cells surrounded by loose fibrous connective tissue are typical of all intimal fibrodysplastic lesions (28). The internal elastic lamina is usually intact, but partial fragmentation may occur. Medial and adventitial structures are normal in primary intimal fibrodysplasia.

Medial fibroplasia is the most commonly diagnosed dysplastic renal artery disease, accounting for 85% of these lesions (29) (Fig. 78.9). Medial fibroplasia is invariably found in women, with encounters in men being anecdotal. The clinical presentation of this disease is most common in persons between 25 and 45 years of age. Medial fibroplasia appears to be a systemic arteriopathy, with the internal carotid and external iliac arteries being the extrarenal vessels most often affected. The cause of medial fibroplasia remains poorly understood but appears to be associated with the modification of smooth muscle to myofibroblasts secondary to estrogenic stimuli during the reproductive years, unusual traction forces on affected vessels, and mural ischemia resulting from impairment of vasa vasorum blood flow (28). The physical forces contributing to medial fibroplasia may be attributed to ptotic kidneys and stretching of the renal arteries (Fig. 78.10). The fact that renal ptosis occurs more often in women than in men may explain the almost unique involvement of the renal artery with medial fibroplasia in women.

The morphologic appearance of medial dysplasia ranges from a solitary stenosis to multiple constrictions with intervening mural dilations affecting the middle and distal main renal artery. The latter are responsible for the classic "string-of-beads" appearance of this lesion. Actual macrovascular aneurysms occurring at branchings affect nearly 13% of patients with arterial fibrodysplasia (32), but these are an unusual cause of a hypertensive state (33). Stenotic disease of segmental branches occurs in about 25% of cases. Bilateral disease affects nearly 60% of patients. Unilateral lesions affect the left and right renal arteries in 10% and 30% of cases, respectively. Progression of disease occurs in about 20% of patients and is most evident among premenopausal women.

Gradations in medial fibroplasia can be seen, including diffuse and peripheral forms of the disease in the same vessel (28). Diffuse medial fibroplasia is typified by severe disorganization of medial smooth-muscle cells, which appear to be transformed to myofibroblasts (34). These latter secretory cells generate accumulations of ground substances that encroach on the vessel lumen. The stenoses often alternate with areas of medial thinning and mural dilations. In peripheral medial fibroplasia, the fibroproliferative process is limited to the outer portion of the media and stenoses are less severe than those occurring in diffuse disease.

Perimedial dysplasia accounts for nearly 10% of dysplastic renal artery stenotic disease (29) (Fig. 78.11). These lesions invariably occur in women, usually between the ages of 30 and 50 years. Perimedial dysplasia is bilateral in 20% of patients and appears to be more progressive than medial fibrodysplasia. Perimedial dysplasia is characterized by solitary or multiple constrictions, without intervening dilations. Most stenoses involve the distal main renal artery, without segmental branch involvement. Certain histologic features are common to both perimedial dysplasia and medial fibroplasia, and they may represent different manifestations of the same pathologic entity. Although unusual accumulations of elastic tissue in inner adventitial regions are the most prominent abnormality in perimedial dysplasia, increases in medial ground substances may also accompany this type of dysplastic disease (28).

Developmental Renal Artery Disease

Developmental renal artery stenoses are a rare cause of renovascular hypertension (29–31) (Fig. 78.12). These lesions are encountered most often in children and young adults. About 40% of children with renovascular hypertension are thought to have developmental renal artery stenoses (35,36). Similarly, nearly 20% of adults with inti-

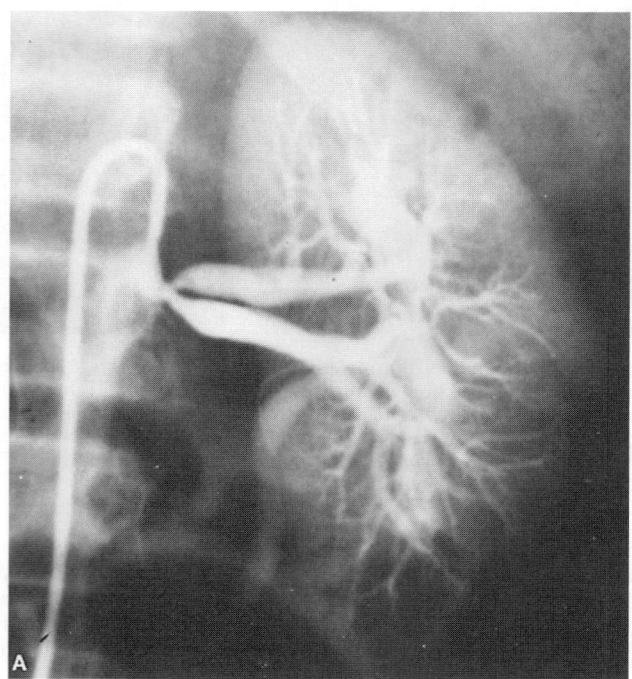

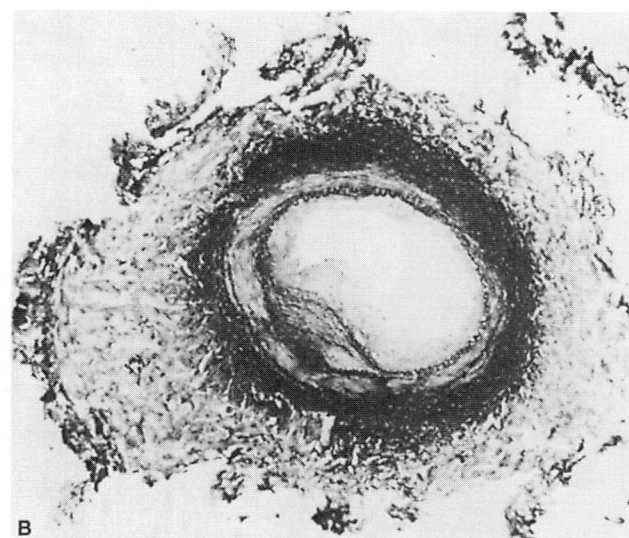

Figure 78.12. Developmental renal artery stenoses. *(A)* Proximal vessel stenosis in a patient with neurofibromatosis and infrarenal aortic hypoplasia. *(B)* Fragmentation and duplication of the internal elastic lamina and deficient medial tissues characterize these lesions. Intimal fibroplasia encroaches on the vessel lumen, which is less than 1 mm in diameter. Adventitial elastic tissues appear excessive. Movat stain, ×100. (Part A from Stanley JC, Fry WJ. Pediatric renal artery occlusive disease and renovascular hypertension: etiology, diagnosis, and operative treatment. *Arch Surg* 1981;116:669, with permission. Part B from Stanley JC, Graham LM, Whitehouse WM Jr, et al. Developmental occlusive disease of the abdominal aorta and the splanchnic and renal arteries. *Am J Surg* 1981;142:190, with permission.)

mal fibroplastic renal artery disease have stenoses that can be attributed to developmental defects. Both sexes are affected equally. These stenotic lesions, which represent true hypoplasia of the renal artery, exhibit an external hourglass appearance. Developmental lesions usually occur at the aortic origin of the artery. Sparse medial tissue, intimal fibroplasia, fragmentation and duplication of the internal elastic lamina, and disproportionate excesses in adventitial elastic tissue are the most common histologic abnormalities in these diminutive vessels (29,31).

Developmental renal artery narrowings may be attributed to certain embryonic events occurring as the two fetal dorsal aortas fuse and all but one of their lateral branches to the kidney regress (30). Abnormal transition of mesenchyme to medial smooth muscle at that time, or later impairment of its growth, can cause both aortic and renovascular anomalies. Vessels to the mesonephros within mesenchymal tissue around the two dorsal aortas are replaced during fetal growth by a more cephalic group of vessels to the metanephros. A solitary artery to each kidney evolves from these arteries in 75% of people because of an obligate hemodynamic advantage over adjacent channels. Flow changes in the region where single central renal arteries usually arise may afford coexisting polar arteries hemodynamic advantages that ensure their persistence. Supporting such a hypothesis concerning the cause

of developmental lesions is the fact that multiple stenotic renal arteries are found in up to 70% of patients with central abdominal aortic coarctation or hypoplasia (30,31).

CLINICAL FEATURES OF RENOVASCULAR HYPERTENSION

The frequency of renovascular hypertension among patients who have diastolic blood pressures higher than 100 mm Hg is about 2%. It is much more common in patients with relatively more severe elevations of diastolic blood pressure; as many as 5% of such patients are found to have a renovascular cause of their hypertension.

Findings suggestive of renovascular hypertension include systolic and diastolic upper abdominal bruits, initial diastolic blood pressures greater than 115 mm Hg, a sudden worsening of mild to moderate essential hypertension, development of hypertension during childhood, and rapid onset of high blood pressure after the age of 50 years. Hypertension resistant to drug therapy and malignant hypertension are also more likely to represent this form of secondary hypertension. Similarly, patients whose renal function deteriorates while they are receiving multiple antihypertensive drugs, especially ACE inhibitors, may have underlying renal artery stenotic disease. The costs and errors associated with indiscriminate evaluations for this

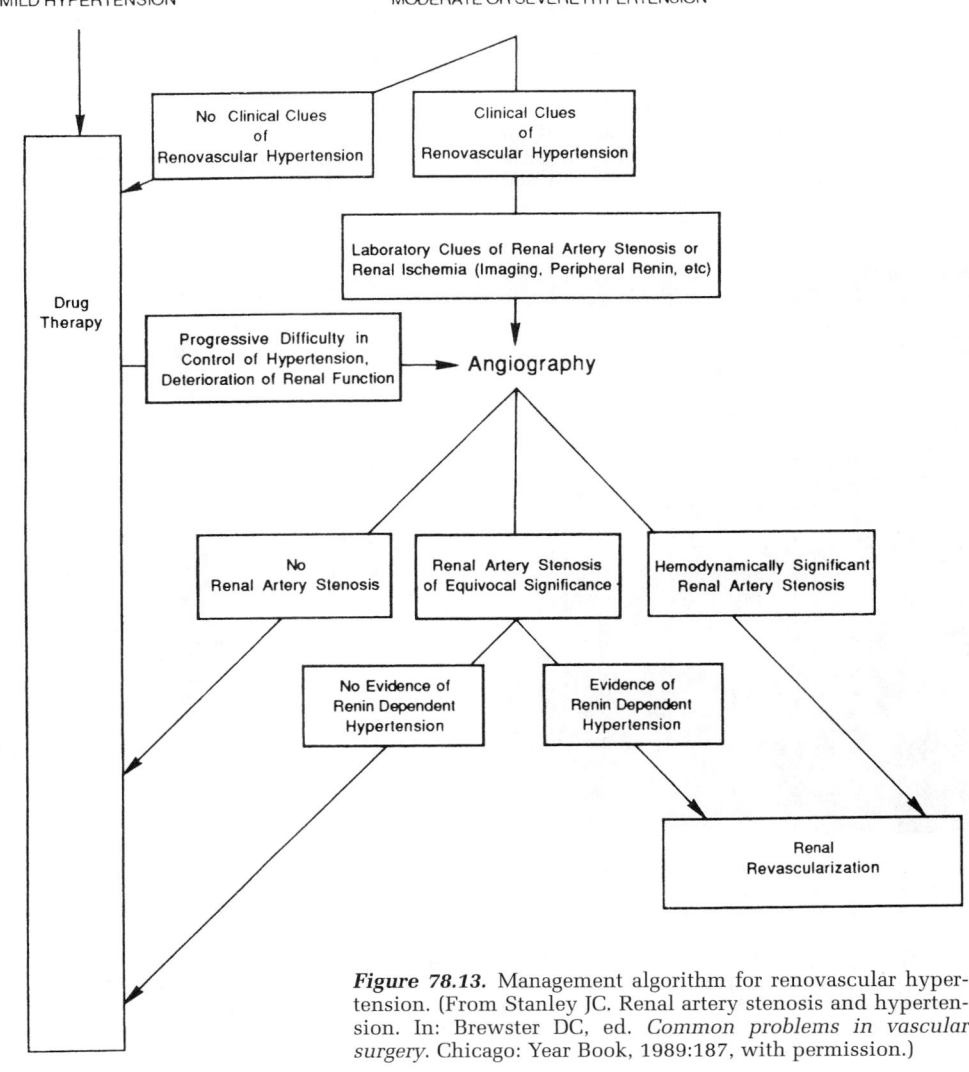

Figure 78.13. Management algorithm for renovascular hypertension. (From Stanley JC. Renal artery stenosis and hypertension. In: Brewster DC, ed. *Common problems in vascular surgery.* Chicago: Year Book, 1989:187, with permission.)

form of hypertension are prohibitive (37). A decision algorithm based on the presenting degree of hypertension and the presence or absence of clinical and laboratory evidence of renovascular hypertension is necessary in contemporary practice (Fig. 78.13).

DIAGNOSIS OF RENAL ARTERY STENOSIS AND SECONDARY HYPERTENSION

Most diagnostic and prognostic tests for renovascular hypertension assess either the anatomic stenosis or derangements of renal function attributed to the stenosis. The usefulness and limitations of these tests become relevant in the proper selection of patients for surgical intervention (37).

Conventional arteriography was central to the evaluation of patients in the past when renovascular hypertension was suspected. Oblique aortography and multiple-plane selective renal arteriography have improved the recognition of the morphologic character and extent of renal artery stenoses in this disease entity. The presence of collateral vessels circumventing a renal artery stenosis is evidence of the hemodynamic importance of this lesion. A pressure gradient of about 10 mm Hg is necessary for collateral vessel development, and the same degree of pressure change is associated with activation of the renin system. Thus, the functional importance of an otherwise benign-appearing stenosis is established when collateral vessels are evident (Fig. 78.14). Intraarterial digital substraction angiography is a useful modification of conventional studies in assessing the presence of renal artery stenotic disease. The latter makes it possible to use smaller quantities of contrast agents than are required for conventional arteriography or intravenous digital substraction arteriography, so that the potential for contrast-induced nephrotoxicity is less. This is of particular rele-

vance in patients with compromised renal function. Sequential helical (spiral) computed tomography (CT) is often of use in assessing coexistent renal artery and aortic disease, but it does carry a risk for contrast-induced nephrotoxicity and is rarely the diagnostic study of choice in assessing a patient for renovascular hypertension.

Magnetic resonance angiography, especially with breath-hold techniques and gadolinium enhancement, provides high-resolution images of diseased renal arteries (38–40). Further refinements in the use of magnetic resonance angiography to assess patients suspected of having renovascular hypertension will undoubtedly evolve. Its noninvasiveness and lack of nephrotoxicity make it an attractive diagnostic test.

Deep abdominal renal artery ultrasonography may identify hemodynamically significant renal artery narrowings by directly imaging the renal arteries and characterizing flow velocity patterns through these vessels (41,42). The existence of a stenosis is established when peak systolic velocities are in the range of 180 to 200 cm/s and the ratio of these velocities to those in the aorta approaches 3.5. Unfortunately, ultrasonography does not detect renal artery stenoses in which the luminal cross section is narrowed by more than 60%. Failure to identify a main renal artery in the absence of any parenchymal flow signal suggests main renal artery occlusion. Failure to recognize an occluded accessory or segmental renal artery, however, results in false-negative findings with this technology.

Assessment of renin activity in peripheral and renal venous blood is a recognized means of detecting functionally

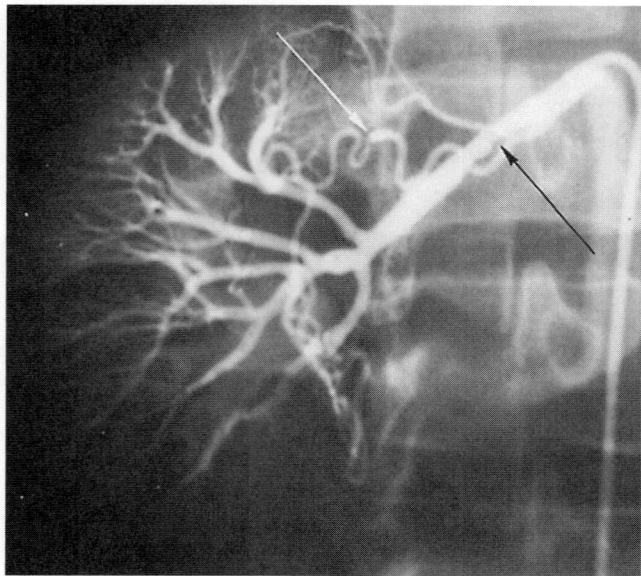

Figure 78.14. Arteriogram of a benign-appearing stenosis *(black arrow)* associated with a large collateral vessel *(white arrow)* circumventing the lesion defines the hemodynamic significance of the stenosis and underscores its functional importance. (From Stanley JC, Graham LM, Whitehouse WM Jr. Limitations and errors of diagnostic and prognostic investigations in renovascular hypertension. In: Bernhard VM, Towne JM, eds. *Complications in vascular surgery.* Orlando, FL: Grune & Stratton, 1984:213, with permission.)

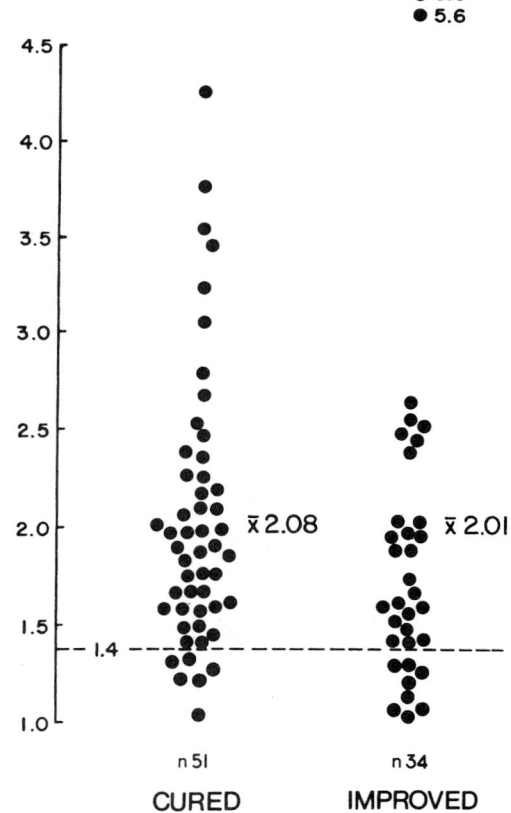

Figure 78.15. The limited diagnostic and prognostic value of renal vein renin ratios. (From Stanley JC, Gewertz BL, Fry WJ. Renal:systemic renin indices and renal vein renin ratios as prognostic indicators in remedial renovascular hypertension. *J Surg Res* 1976;20:149, with permission.)

important renal artery disease. Renin assays in peripheral blood may not be useful unless they are related to sodium balance. A more common practice is to assess renal vein renin activity. The renin–angiotensin system should be stimulated before sampling to reduce interpretive errors of data that may otherwise result from minimal fluctuations in nonstimulated basal renin activity. In most adults, this is accomplished by limiting sodium intake to 20 mEq/d and administering a diuretic for 3 days before testing. Renin-suppressing drugs, such as beta blockers, are discontinued whenever possible. Blood samples for renin assays should be obtained with the patient tilted to an upright position. The role of ACE inhibitors in stimulating renin release and improving test results remains to be defined further in patients with renovascular hypertension. Renin activity is usually reported as either a ratio or index.

The *renal vein renin ratio* (RVRR) is calculated by dividing the renin activity in venous blood from the affected kidney by that from the contralateral kidney. An RVRR above 1.48 is indicative of functionally important renovascular stenotic disease (19,20). Because this test compares one kidney with another, it may not be useful in patients with bilateral disease if both kidneys exhibit elevated but equal degrees of abnormally high renin secretion. This is believed to be the case in the 15% of patients benefiting from operation in whom the RVRR is less than 1.48 (Fig. 78.15).

The *renal–systemic renin index* (RSRI) is calculated by subtracting systemic renin activity from individual renal vein renin activity and dividing the remainder by systemic renin activity (19). It is an expression of renin release from an individual kidney. In patients who have essential but not renovascular hypertension, the renal vein renin activity in each kidney is usually 24% higher than the systemic activity (9). Thus, the total activity of both kidneys is usually 48% higher than the systemic activity. This figure of 48% represents a steady state of renal renin release.

In renovascular hypertension, the RSRI of the affected kidney is above 24%. In mild degrees of renal artery disease, an increase in ipsilateral renin release is normally balanced by suppression of the renin production in the contralateral kidney, with a drop in its RSRI to below 24%. In bilateral renal artery disease, this servomechanism may be lost, and the autonomous release of renin from both kidneys may cause the sum of the individual RSRIs to be considerably higher than 48%. Renin production then exceeds the capacity of normal hepatic degradation, and a hyperreninemic form of hypertension evolves.

The usefulness of ischemic kidney renin hypersecretion (RSRI > 48%) and contralateral kidney renin suppression (RSRI < 24%, approaching zero) as a means of discriminating between expected cured and improved operative outcomes has been well established (19,20,43) (Fig. 78.16). The prognostic accuracy of the RSRI appears limited in that nearly 8% of patients who are cured do not exhibit contralateral renin suppression (43). Renin secretion from the nonoperated kidney must be suppressed if a cure is to be expected. Although the RSRI represents an important refinement in the use of renin data in managing renovascular hypertensive patients, these data must be applied cautiously in clinical decision making.

Hypertensive urography is not a good diagnostic test for renovascular hypertension because of its limited sensitivity (44). Bilateral or segmental disease often interferes with the recognition of gross differences in contrast excretion between the two kidneys. Nevertheless, rapid-sequence urog-

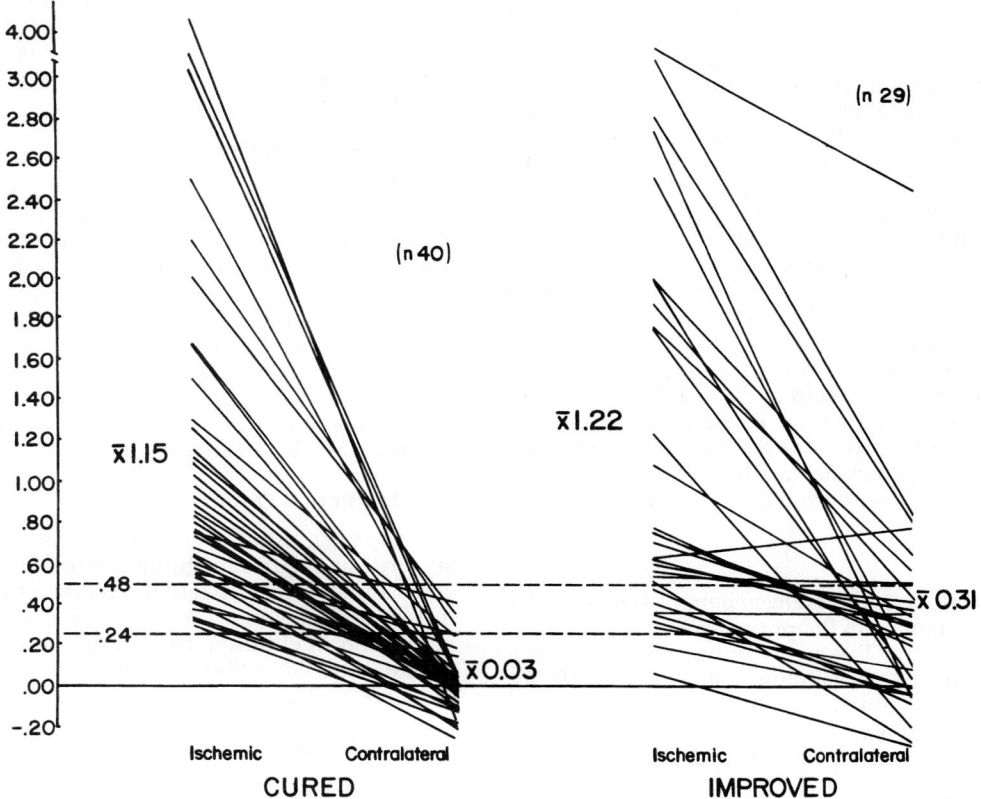

Figure 78.16. The prognostic usefulness of renal–systemic renin indices. (From Stanley JC, Fry WJ. Surgical treatment of renovascular hypertension. *Arch Surg* 1977;112:1291, with permission.)

raphy may contribute to a diagnosis of renovascular hypertension in the following circumstances: (a) The appearance of contrast within the collecting system of the affected kidney is delayed by at least 1 minute in comparison with its appearance in the contralateral kidney; (b) a discrepancy in renal length exists, with the right kidney being 2 cm shorter than the left or the left being 1.5 cm shorter than the right; and (c) a hyperconcentration of contrast in the collecting system of the affected kidney is evident on late radiographs. Ureteral or pelvic irregularities secondary to the presence of large collateral vessels may accompany the aforementioned urographic findings. In a large series of patients with proven renovascular hypertension, findings on urography were abnormal in 27% of children, 48% of adults with arterial fibrodysplastic disease, and about 72% of adults with atherosclerotic lesions (45). Thus, the continued use of hypertensive urography as a diagnostic or prognostic test for renovascular hypertension appears unjustified.

Isotopic renography allows both renal imaging and analysis of the washout curve of a number of radioactive tracers. The most common compounds used for these studies include ^{99m}Tc-DTPA (diethylenetriamine pentaacetic acid), ^{123}I- or ^{131}I-orthoidohippurate, ^{99m}Tc-MAG3, ^{99m}Tc-DMSA (dimercaptosuccinic acid), and ^{99m}Tc-glucoheptonate. The studies provide an assessment of renal blood flow and excretory function. Unfortunately, different states of hydration and intrarenal vascular resistance often contribute to flow abnormalities and false-positive results in nonrenovascular hypertensives. The specificity and sensitivity of these studies are both about 75%. Administration of ACE inhibitors improves the sensitivity and specificity by blocking the compensatory change in glomerular filtration, causing it to fall in the affected kidney. This modified technology has not been widely adopted, although some view ACE inhibitor-modified studies to be of greater value (46). Renal perfusion–excretion ratios and more sophisticated computer analyses offer a potential means of increasing the predictive value of radionuclide screening for renovascular hypertension.

Split renal function studies were among the earliest tests used in evaluating patients with suspected renovascular hypertension (47). These studies necessitate the placement of a ureteral catheter to sample urine from each kidney. The two studies used most widely are (a) the Howard test, which documents reduced urine volume in addition to increased sodium and creatinine concentrations in urine from the affected kidney, and (b) the Stamey test, which reveals a smaller volume of urine and a greater concentration of paraaminohippurate in urine from the affected kidney. A liberalization of the diagnostic criteria for split renal function studies has been proposed with a constant lateralization to the affected kidney, evident by a 25% decrease in urine volume and a 15% increase in creatinine concentration. The diagnostic sensitivity when these criteria are used is improved, but an appreciable number of patients without renovascular hypertension have positive results.

TREATMENT

Therapeutic results in the management of renovascular hypertension often relate to the proper execution of an appropriate intervention. Treatment options include drug therapy, percutaneous transluminal angioplasty (PTA), transcatheter renal ablation, arterial reconstructive surgery, and nephrectomy.

Drug Therapy

Antihypertensive drugs are often successful in the initial management of patients with renovascular hyperten-

sion. Beta blockers, such as propranolol and atenolol, are commonly used as first-line therapy. Refractory hypertension, especially that resulting from bilateral disease or unilateral lesions with contralateral parenchymal disease, may respond to the addition of a thiazide diuretic, although with impaired renal function, the use of a loop diuretic such as furosemide is more effective. ACE inhibitors, such as captopril and enalapril, have proved to be the most effective drugs in treating renovascular hypertension. Unfortunately, ACE inhibitors may have a deleterious effect on renal function by critically decreasing the intrarenal blood pressure and altering intrarenal autoregulation. Certainly, ACE inhibitors should be used cautiously when the entire renal parenchymal mass is at risk, such as in renovascular hypertensive patients who have bilateral disease or a solitary kidney. The use of angiotensin receptor blockers has not been well defined in this subgroup of hypertensive patients. Because stenotic disease of the renal artery often progresses with concomitant loss of renal mass and function, a definitive means of restoring normal renal blood flow may be a more logical therapy than drug treatment once a diagnosis of renovascular hypertension has been established.

Percutaneous Transluminal Angioplasty

In 1978, Gruntzig and colleagues (48) were the first to report the use of PTA in the management renovascular hypertension. The minimally invasive nature of renal artery PTA offers certain advantages over operative intervention. Most renal artery stenoses can be traversed with a guide wire and subsequently dilated with or without a stent; morbidity and mortality are minimal. To justify PTA, the physiologic and hemodynamic significance of the renal artery stenosis should be documented before endovascular therapy is initiated. In particular, the patient should have adequate renal cortical reserve to recover renal function after the intervention.

Arterial Fibrodysplasia

Patients with renal artery fibrodysplasia derive more benefit and incur fewer complications following renal PTA than patients with other forms of renovascular disease. Medial dysplastic stenoses are most amenable to PTA, and PTA is often considered primary therapy for lesions limited to the main renal artery. Excellent early technical and clinical results usually follow renal artery PTA in these patients (49–52). Similarly, such patients have experienced excellent long-term clinical results, with a primary patency rate of 87% after more than 3 years of follow-up (53) (Table 78.1).

Developmental Disease

In contrast, ostial lesions associated with developmental aortic anomalies in children represent true hypoplastic vessels that are less likely to be dilated successfully (57). In like fashion, less common causes of renovascular hypertension in children, including arteritis, William's syndrome, and neurofibromatosis, do not respond well to renal artery PTA.

Arteriosclerosis

The presence of aortic spillover arteriosclerosis versus isolated renal artery arteriosclerosis has an important effect on long-term clinical results. PTA alone, without adjunctive stent placement, has resulted in a technical suc-

Table 78.1. PERCUTANEOUS TRANSLUMINAL ANGIOPLASTY FOR FIBRODYSPLASTIC RENOVASCULAR HYPERTENSION

Institution (ref.)	No. patients	Mean follow-up (mo)	Postprocedural blood pressure response (%)[a]		
			Cured	Improved	Failed
Mayo Clinic (49)	105	43	22	41	37
University of Virginia (53)	66	39	39	59	2
University Hospital, Zurich, Switzerland (54)	28	15	50	39	11
University of Florida (55)	23	6	52	22	26
University Hospitals, Leuven, Belgium (56)	22	26	95	—	5
Hospital Broussais, Paris (50)	20	19	68	16	15

[a]Outcomes defined in reports from individual institutions.

cess rate of only 70% to 80% in patients with arteriosclerotic renovascular disease. The treatment of ostial spillover lesions by PTA alone has had a technical success rate of only 30% to 50%. These latter stenoses often manifest excessive recoil, and many exhibit acute dissections. Because of the high rates of early restenosis after PTA, stenting of atherosclerotic lesions is considered appropriate in many patients. Results following renal artery stenting for atherosclerotic disease vary depending on outcome definitions and the indication for intervention, yet many studies have demonstrated good long-term technical results (Table 78.2). For example, when Palmaz stents were placed in 64 renal arteries in 59 patients, the 2-year secondary patency rate was 92% (61). Others have documented 5-year primary and secondary patency rates of 84% and 92%, respectively (59). In treating hypertension, long-term benefits have been reported in 52% to 78% of patients (Table 78.2). PTA with stenting for progressive ischemic nephropathy is not as effective at reversing renal failure. In these cases, benefits appear to be related to the degree and duration of ischemic nephropathy before PTA, with patients having a serum creatinine level below 2 mg/dL demonstrating the best response.

Complications accompanying renal artery PTA for either atherosclerotic or fibrodysplastic disease are uncommon, with severe complications developing in only a small percentage of cases (64). Intimal disruption occurs more often with dilation of the proximal renal artery, where vessel elasticity is greater and medial disruption is less likely. Medial tears are more common with dilation of the distal renal artery, where vessel elasticity is less.

Surgery following failed renal artery PTA is much more hazardous than primary surgery alone (65), being associated with a much higher incidence of emergent repair and nephrectomy. Blood pressure benefits after a failed renal artery PTA that necessitates secondary operation are significantly lower, being 57% after reoperation versus 89% for a primary operation (65).

Arterial Reconstructive Surgery

The operative treatment of patients with renovascular occlusive disease has become relatively well defined (66–73). It is important that the primary revascularization procedure be successful. This is underscored by the fact that nephrectomy accompanies nearly half of the reoperations for failed initial reconstructions (74). Careful preoperative assessment of extrarenal occlusive disease in patients with arteriosclerotic renovascular disease is mandatory to ensure the patient's ability to undergo complex renal artery surgery (23–27). Operative details vary when patients with the various subcategories of renal artery disease are treated (73).

Aortorenal bypass in adults with arteriosclerotic and fibrodysplastic occlusive disease is most often performed with the use of autologous reversed saphenous vein (Fig. 78.17). Dacron or expanded polytetrafluoroethylene conduits may also be used in reconstructing these vessels. Because vein grafts in children often become aneurysmal (35,36,75), autologous hypogastric artery grafts and direct aortic reimplantations of the renal artery are favored in children (Figs. 78.18 and 78.19).

Table 78.2. PERCUTANEOUS TRANSLUMINAL ANGIOPLASTY WITH STENT PLACEMENT FOR ARTERIOSCLEROTIC RENOVASCULAR DISEASE

Institution (ref.)	No. patients	Stents	Indication		Mean follow-up (mo)	Postprocedural blood pressure response (%)[a]		
			Hypertension	Renal insufficiency		Cured	Improved	Failed
Dorros-Feuer Foundation (58)	76	92	76	48	6	6	46	48
University Hospital, Freiburg, Germany (59)	68	74	68	29	27	16	62	22
Ochsner Clinic (60)	66	88	66		19	2	64	34
Polyclinique D'Essey (61)	59	64	59	10	14	19	57	24
Hotel-Dieu de Montreal (62)	33	35	33	17	13	6	61	33
University of Texas Health Center (multicenter study) (63)	28	28	28	14	7	11	48	36

[a]Outcomes defined in reports from individual institutions.

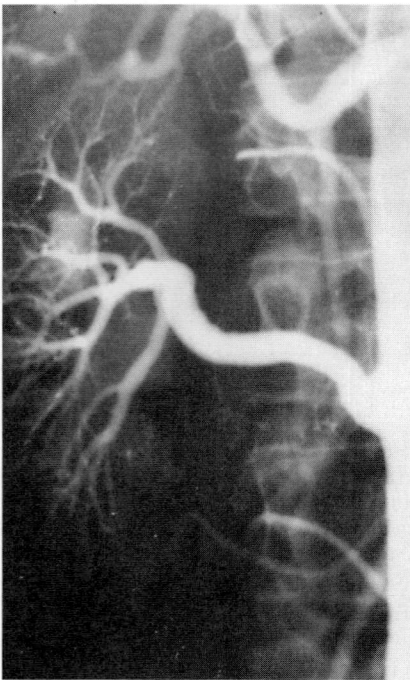

Figure 78.17. Autogenous saphenous vein aortorenal graft. (From Stanley JC, Graham LM. Renovascular hypertension. In: Miller DC, Roon AJ, eds. *Diagnosis and management of peripheral vascular disease.* Menlo Park, CA: Addison Wesley, 1981, with permission.)

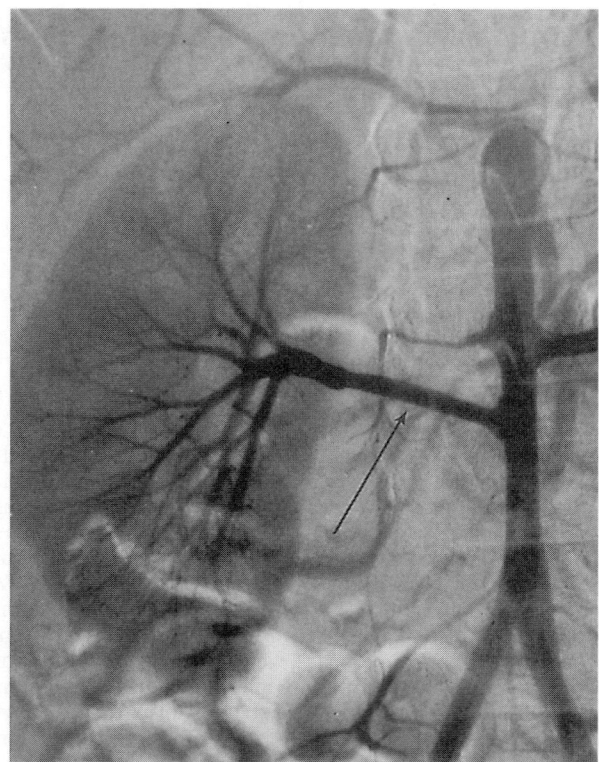

Figure 78.18. Autogenous iliac artery aortorenal graft in a child. (From Stanley JC, Zelenock GB, Messina LM, et al. Pediatric renovascular hypertension: a thirty-year experience of operative treatment. *J Vasc Surg* 1995;21:212, with permission.)

Nonanatomic bypass procedures are important in treating many patients with renovascular hypertension (76–79). The hepatic artery or iliac arteries may be used as sites of origin for bypass grafts to the renal artery, especially when a graft originating from the aorta would entail unacceptable risks (77). Use of the splenic artery in situ for a left-sided splenorenal bypass is appropriate in adults, but only after it has been ascertained that this vessel and the celiac trunk are free of stenotic disease (78,80). Splenorenal bypasses are not recommended in children because of the possibility of a celiac artery growth arrest

that may not be evident at the time of reconstruction but that may evolve later.

Ex vivo renal artery reconstruction is an alternative means of treating selected cases of renovascular hypertension, especially those involving revascularization of multiple second- or third-order segmental branches (69,81,82). Most renal artery reconstructions can be successfully performed in situ. Disadvantages of ex vivo reconstructions include the necessity to cool the kidney, longer operating

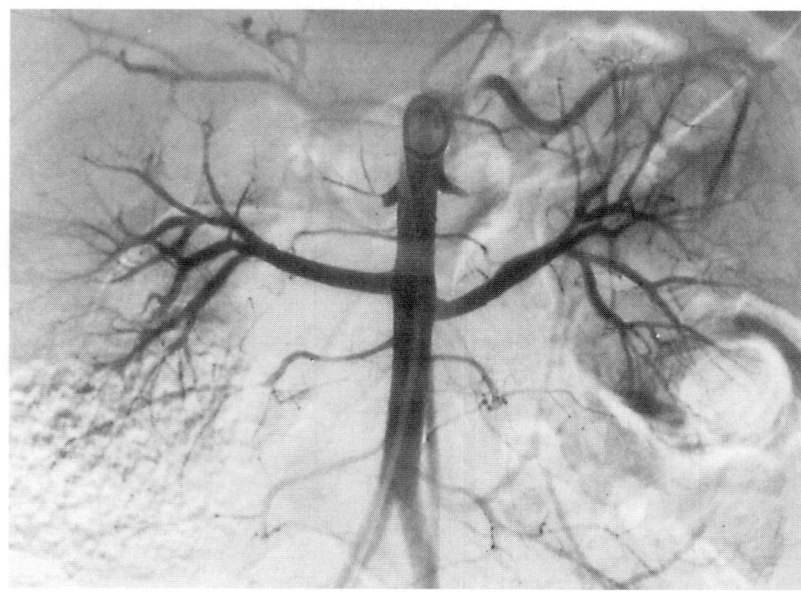

Figure 78.19. Aortic reimplantation of main renal arteries beyond orificial stenoses in a child. (From Stanley JC, Zelenock GB, Messina LM, et al. Pediatric renovascular hypertension: a thirty-year experience of operative treatment. *J Vasc Surg* 1995; 21:212, with permission.)

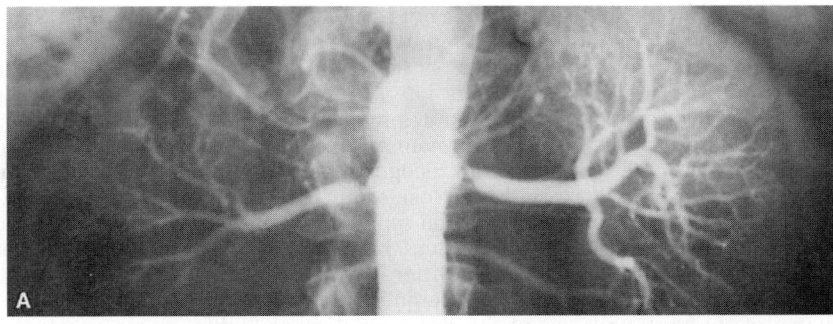
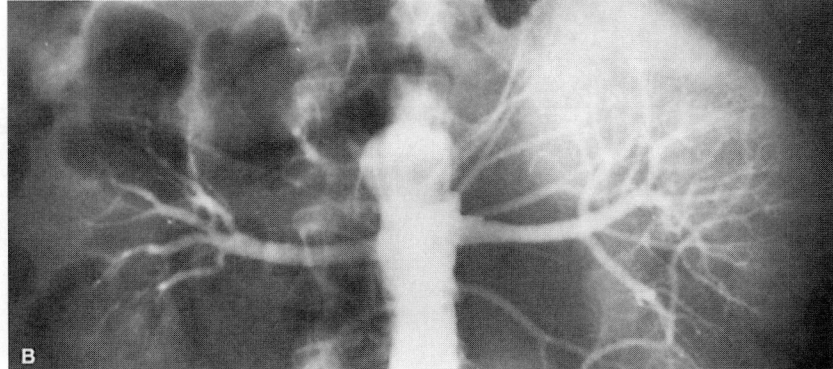

Figure 78.20. Transaortic bilateral renal artery endarterectomy. Preoperative *(A)* and postoperative *(B)* aortography. (From Stanley JC, Messina LM, Wakefield TW, et al. Renal artery reconstruction. In: Bergan JJ, Yao JST, eds. *Techniques in arterial surgery.* Philadelphia: WB Saunders, 1990:247, with permission.)

times, and perhaps most important, the disruption of preexisting collateral channels.

Operative arterial dilation, alone or in conjunction with a bypass procedure, is useful in the treatment of fibrous intraparenchymal stenotic disease. In this setting, sequentially larger metal dilators, which increase in size by 0.5-mm increments, are advanced through a transverse arteriotomy in the main renal artery after heparin anticoagulation. The dilators must be advanced with care so that the vessel is not excessively dilated and the intima fractured.

Endarterectomy is often the preferred means of treating proximal renal artery arteriosclerotic disease (68,73, 83–85). The two techniques most often used are (a) transaortic renal endarterectomy through an axial aortotomy or the transected infrarenal aorta, and (b) direct renal artery endarterectomy. The extent of aortic and renal artery disease, in addition to the need to perform coexistent aortic reconstructive surgery, dictates which of these procedures is most appropriate. In most cases, a linear aortotomy is begun just to the left of the superior mesenteric artery and extended in the midline to below the renal arteries. The diseased aortic intimal and medial tissues are elevated, and with gentle traction, the renal artery atheroma is extracted. This type of endarterectomy is particularly useful in treating bilateral disease (Fig. 78.20) or disease in multiple renal arteries. Extensive plaque of the more distal renal artery, especially when bifurcations are involved, may be better treated by a direct renal artery arteriotomy and endarterectomy with a patch-graft closure.

Results of Operative Therapy

Renal preservation and the maintenance of renal function are important in assessing clinical experiences

Table 78.3. RESULTS OF SURGICAL TREATMENT OF RENOVASCULAR HYPERTENSION IN SPECIFIC PATIENT SUBGROUPS, UNIVERSITY OF MICHIGAN EXPERIENCE

| | | Postoperative status[a] | | | |
Subgroup	No. patients	Cure rate (%)	Improvement rate (%)	Failure rate (%)	Operative mortality rate (%)
Pediatric disease	34	85	12	3	0
Arterial fibrodysplasia	144	55	39	6	0
Arteriosclerosis					
Focal renal artery disease	64	33	58	9	0
Overt extrarenal disease	71	25	47	28	8.5

[a]Represents outcome of 405 operations (346 primary, 59 secondary), including initial nephrectomy in 17 patients.

Cure: Blood pressures 150/90 mm Hg or less for a minimum of 6 months postoperatively, during which time no antihypertensive medications administered. Improvement: Normotensive while on drug therapy, or diastolic blood pressures between 90 and 100 mm Hg but at least 15% lower than preoperative levels. Failure: Diastolic blood pressures above 90 mm Hg but less than 15% lower than preoperative levels or above 110 mm Hg. Lower pressure standards were used in evaluating children.

From Stanley JC, Whitehouse WM Jr, Graham LM, et al. Operative therapy of renovascular hypertension. Br J Surg 1982;63[Suppl]:S63, with permission.

(86–93). Nephrectomy usually does not offer as much benefit as revascularization (92). Even when nephrectomy provides good results, the patient is left at considerable risk if contralateral disease occurs later. Cumulative primary and secondary nephrectomy rates in any given practice should not exceed 10%. Improvement in renal function after revascularization is well recognized and is most likely to occur in patients with arteriosclerotic disease and a relatively sudden onset of impaired renal function.

The surgical treatment of renovascular hypertension affords excellent outcomes (70–72). Differences among most individual experiences reflect differences in the prevalence of the various types of renovascular disease (Table 78.3). A salutary outcome in children with renovascular hypertension is most likely after normal renal blood flow has been restored (Table 78.4). Arterial fibrodysplastic renovascular hypertension (Table 78.5) is more likely to benefit from operation than is arteriosclerotic renovascular hypertension (Table 78.6). This is probably a reflection of coexistent essential hypertension in older patients with arteriosclerotic disease. Arteriosclerotic renovascular hypertension occurs in two subgroups of patients: (a) those with focal renal artery disease whose only clinical manifestation of arteriosclerosis is secondary hypertension, and (b) those with clinically overt extrarenal arteriosclerosis affecting the aorta or the coronary, carotid, or periph-

Table 78.4. RENOVASCULAR HYPERTENSION IN CHILDREN

Institution	No. patients	Operative outcome (%)			Surgical mortality rate (%)
		Cured	Improved	Failed	
University of Michigan	57	79	19	2	0
Cleveland Clinic	27	59	18.5	18.5	4
University of California, Los Angeles	26	84.5	7.5	4	4
Vanderbilt University	21	68	24	8	0
University of Pennsylvania	17	76.5	23.5	0	0
Argentinian Institute, Buenos Aires	15	53	13	27	7
University of California, San Francisco	14	86	7	0	7

Modified from Stanley JC. The evolution of surgery for renovascular occlusive disease. Cardiovasc Surg 1994;2:195, with permission.

Table 78.5. FIBRODYSPLASTIC RENOVASCULAR HYPERTENSION IN ADULTS

Institution	No. patients	Operative outcome (%)			Surgical mortality rate (%)
		Cured	Improved	Failed	
University of Michigan	144	55	39	6	0
Baylor College of Medicine	113	43	24	33	0
Cleveland Clinic	92	58	31	11	Unstated
University of California, San Francisco	77	66	32	1.3	0
Mayo Clinic	63	66	24	10	Unstated
University Hospital Leiden, The Netherlands	53	53	34	13	2
Vanderbilt University	44	72	24	4	2.3
Columbia University	42	76	14	10	Unstated
Bowman Gray	40	33	57	10	0
University of Lund, Malmö, Sweden	40	66	24	10	0

Modified from Stanley JC. The evolution of surgery for renovascular occlusive disease. Cardiovasc Surg 1994;2:195, with permission.

Table 78.6. ARTERIOSCLEROTIC RENOVASCULAR HYPERTENSION IN ADULTS

Institution	No. patients	Operative outcome (%)			Surgical mortality rate (%)
		Cured	Improved	Failed	
Baylor College of Medicine	360	34	31	35	2.5
Bowman Gray	152	15	75	10	1.3
University of Michigan	135	29	52	19	4.4
University of California, San Francisco	84	39	23	38	2.4
Cleveland Clinic	78	40	51	9	2
Columbia University	67	58	21	21	Unstated
University of Lund, Malmö, Sweden	66	49	24	27	0.9
Hospital Aiguelongue, Montpellier, France	65	45	40	15	1.1
Vanderbilt University	63	50	45	5	9

Modified from Stanley JC. The evolution of surgery for renovascular occlusive disease. Cardiovasc Surg 1994;2:195, with permission.

eral vessels. Severity and duration of hypertension, age, and sex in these two subgroups are similar, yet the surgical outcome in regard to lowering blood pressure is worse in patients with overt extrarenal arteriosclerotic disease. Salutary outcomes justify surgical intervention in properly selected patients with renovascular hypertension.

REFERENCES

1. Goldblatt H, Lynch J, Hanzal RF, et al. Studies on experimental hypertension. I. The production of persistent elevation of systolic blood pressure by means of renal ischemia. *J Exp Med* 1934;59:347.
2. Hackentahl E, Paul M, Ganten D, et al. Morphology, physiology, and molecular biology of renin secretion. *Physiol Rev* 1990;70:1067.
3. Lynch KR, Peach MJ. Molecular biology of angiotensinogen. *Hypertension* 1991;17:263.
4. Morris BJ. Molecular biology of renin. I. Gene and protein structure, synthesis, and processing. *J Hypertens* 1992;10:209.
5. Griffiths LR, Board PG, Zwi MB, et al. The B subunit of coagulation factor VIII is linked to renin and the Duffy blood group to α-spectrin on human chromosome 1. *Hum Hered* 1989;39:107.
6. Hobart PM, Fogliano M, O'Connor BA, et al. Human renin gene: structure and sequence analysis. *Proc Natl Acad Sci USA* 1984;81:5026.
7. Pratt RE, Ouellette AJ, Dzau VJ. Biosynthesis of renin: multiplicity of active and intermediate forms. *Proc Natl Acad Sci USA* 1983;80:6809.
8. Pratt RE, Carleton JE, Richie JP, et al. Human renin biosynthesis and secretion in normal and ischemic kidneys. *Proc Natl Acad Sci USA* 1987;84:7837.
9. Sealey JE, Buhler FR, Laragh JH, et al. The physiology of renin secretion in essential hypertension: estimation of renin secretion rate and renal plasma flow from peripheral and renal vein renin levels. *Am J Med* 1973;55:391.
10. Schneider EG, Davis JO, Baumber JS, et al. The hepatic metabolism of renin and aldosterone: a review with new observations on the hepatic clearance of renin. *Circ Res* 1970;26/27[Suppl 1]:175.
11. Gaillard-Sanchez I, Mattei MG, Clauser E, et al. Assignment by in situ hybridization of the angiotensinogen gene to chromosome band 1qr, the same region as the human renin gene. *Hum Genet* 1990;84:341.
12. Fukamizu A, Takahashi S, Seo MS, et al. Structure and expression of the human angiotensinogen gene. *J Biol Chem* 1990;265:7576.
13. Samuels AI, Miller ED Jr, Fray JCS, et al. Renin–angiotensin antagonists and the regulation of blood pressure. *Fed Proc* 1976;35:2512.
14. Semple PF, Boyd AS, Dawes PM, et al. Angiotensin II and its heptapeptide (2), hexapeptide (3), and pentapeptide (4) metabolites in arterial and venous blood of man. *Circ Res* 1976;39:671.
15. Hubert C, Houot AM, Corvol P, et al. Structure of the angiotensin I-converting enzyme gene. *J Biol Chem* 1991;15:377.
16. Mattei MG, Hubert C, Alhene-Gelas F, et al. Angiotensin-I converting enzyme is on chromosome 17. *Cytogenet Cell Genet* 1989;51:1041.
17. Oparil S, Tregear GW, Koerner TJ, et al. Mechanism of pulmonary conversion of angiotensin I to II in the dog. *Circ Res* 1971;29:682.
18. Oshima G, Gecse A, Erdos EG. Angiotensin I-converting enzyme of the kidney cortex. *Biochim Biophys Acta* 1974;350:26.
19. Stanley JC, Gewertz BL, Fry WJ. Renal:systemic renin indices and renal vein renin ratios as prognostic indicators in remedial renovascular hypertension. *J Surg Res* 1976;20:149.
20. Vaughan ED Jr, Buhler FR, Laragh JH, et al. Renovascular hypertension: renin measurements to indicate hypersecretion and contralateral suppression, estimate renal plasma flow, and score for surgical curability. *Am J Med* 1973;55:402.
21. Gavras H, Brunner HR, Vaughan ED Jr, et al. Angiotensin–sodium interaction in blood pressure maintenance of renal hypertensive and normotensive rats. *Science* 1973;180:1369.
22. Stanley JC. Pathologic basis of macrovascular renal artery disease. In: Stanley JC, Ernst CB, Fry WJ, eds. *Renovascular hypertension*. Philadelphia: WB Saunders, 1984:46.
23. Louie J, Isaacson JA, Zierler RE, et al. Prevalence of carotid and lower extremity arterial disease in patients with renal artery stenosis. *Am J Hypertens* 1994;7:436.
24. Missouris CG, Buckenham T, Cappuccio FP, et al. Renal artery stenosis: a common and important problem in patients with peripheral vascular disease. *Am J Med* 1994;96:10.
25. Valentine RJ, Clagett GP, Miller GL, et al. The coronary risk of unsuspected renal artery stenosis. *J Vasc Surg* 1993;18:433.
26. Valentine RJ, Martin JD, Myers SI, et al. Asymptomatic celiac and superior mesenteric artery stenoses are more prevalent among patients with unsuspected renal artery stenoses. *J Vasc Surg* 1991;14:195.
27. Novick AC, Zaki S, Goldfarb D, et al. Epidemiologic and clinical comparison of renal artery stenosis in black patients and white patients. *J Vasc Surg* 1994;20:1.
28. Stanley JC, Gewertz BL, Bove EL, et al. Arterial fibrodysplasia: histopathologic character and current etiologic concepts. *Arch Surg* 1975;110:551.
29. Stanley JC, Wakefield TW. Arterial fibrodysplasia. In: Rutherford RB, ed. *Vascular surgery,* 5th ed. Philadelphia: WB Saunders, 2000:387.
30. Graham LM, Zelenock GB, Erlandson EE, et al. Abdominal aortic coarctation and segmental hypoplasia. *Surgery* 1979;86:519.
31. Stanley JC, Graham LM, Whitehouse WM Jr, et al. Developmental occlusive disease of the abdominal aorta and the splanchnic and renal arteries. *Am J Surg* 1981;142:190.
32. Stanley JC, Fry WJ. Renovascular hypertension secondary to arterial fibrodysplasia in adults. *Arch Surg* 1975;110:922.
33. Stanley JC, Rhodes EL, Gewertz BL, et al. Renal artery aneurysms: significance of macroaneurysms exclusive of dissections and fibrodysplastic mural dilations. *Arch Surg* 1975;110:1327.
34. Sottiurai V, Fry WJ, Stanley JC. Ultrastructure of smooth muscle, myofibroblasts, and fibroblasts in human arterial dysplasia. *Arch Surg* 1978;113:1280.
35. Stanley JC, Fry WJ. Pediatric renal artery occlusive disease and renovascular hypertension: etiology, diagnosis, and operative treatment. *Arch Surg* 1981;116:669.
36. Stanley JC, Zelenock GB, Messina LM, et al. Pediatric renovascular hypertension: a thirty-year experience of operative treatment. *J Vasc Surg* 1995;21:212.
37. Stanley JC, Graham LM, Whitehouse WM Jr. Limitations and errors of diagnostic and prognostic investigations in renovascular hypertension. In: Bernhard VM, Towne JM, eds. *Complications in vascular surgery*. Orlando, FL: Grune & Stratton, 1984:213.
38. Hertz SM, Holland GA, Baum RA, et al. Evaluation of renal artery stenosis by magnetic resonance angiography. *Am J Surg* 1994;168:140.
39. Kent KC, Edelman RR, Kim D, et al. Magnetic resonance imaging: a reliable test for the evaluation of proximal atherosclerotic renal arterial stenosis. *J Vasc Surg* 1991;13:311.
40. Prince MR, Narasimham DL, Stanley JC, et al. Breath-hold 3D gadolinium MRA: new developments for imaging the abdominal aorta and its major branches. *Radiology* 1995;197:785.
41. Hansen KM, Tribble RW, Reavis SW, et al. Renal duplex sonography: evaluation of clinical utility. *J Vasc Surg* 1990;12:227.
42. Kohler TR, Zierler RE, Martin RL, et al. Noninvasive diagnosis of renal artery stenosis by ultrasonic duplex scanning. *J Vasc Surg* 1986;4:450.
43. Stanley JC, Fry WJ. Surgical treatment of renovascular hypertension. *Arch Surg* 1977;112:1291.
44. Thornbury JR, Stanley JC, Fryback DG. Hypertensive urogram: a nondiscriminatory test for renovascular hypertension. *Am J Roentgenol* 1982;138:43.
45. Stanley JC, Whitehouse WM Jr, Graham LM, et al. Operative

therapy of renovascular hypertension. *Br J Surg* 1982;63 [Suppl]:S63.

46. Meier GH, Sumpio B, Setaro FJ, et al. Captopril renal scintigraphy: a new standard for predicting outcome after renal revascularization. *J Vasc Surg* 1993;17:280.

47. Dean RH, Rhamy RK. Split renal function studies in renovascular hypertension. In: Stanley JC, Ernst CB, Fry WJ, eds. *Renovascular hypertension.* Philadelphia: WB Saunders, 1984: 135.

48. Gruntzig A, Vetter W, Meier B, et al. Treatment of renovascular hypertension with percutaneous transluminal dilatation of a renal artery stenosis. *Lancet* 1978;1:801.

49. Bonelli FS, Mckusick MA, Textor SC, et al. Renal artery angioplasty: technical results and clinical outcome in 320 patients. *Mayo Clin Proc* 1995;70:1041.

50. Cluzel P, Raynaud B, Beyssen B, et al. Stenoses of renal branch arteries in fibromuscular dysplasia: results of percutaneous transluminal angioplasty. *Radiology* 1994;193:227.

51. Sos TA, Pickering TG, Sniderman K, et al. Percutaneous transluminal renal angioplasty in renovascular hypertension due to atheroma or fibromuscular dysplasia. *N Engl J Med* 1983;309:274.

52. Tegtmeyer CJ, Kellum CD, Ayers C. Percutaneous transluminal angioplasty of the renal artery: results and long-term follow-up. *Radiology* 1984;153:77.

53. Tegtmeyer CJ, Selby JB, Hartwell GD, et al. Results and complications of angioplasty in fibromuscular disease. *Circulation* 1991;83[Suppl 2]:1155.

54. Luscher TF, Keller HM, Imhoff HG, et al. Fibromuscular hyperplasia: extension of the disease and therapeutic outcome—results of the University Hospital Zurich Cooperative Study on Fibromuscular Hyperplasia. *Nephron* 1986;44 [Suppl 1]:109.

55. Davidson R, Barri Y, Wilcox CS. Predictors of cure of hypertension in fibromuscular renovascular disease. *Am J Kidney Dis* 1996;28:334.

56. Baert AL, Wilms G, Amery A, et al. Percutaneous transluminal renal angioplasty: initial results and long-term follow-up in 202 patients. *Cardiovasc Intervent Radiol* 1990;13:22.

57. Martin EC, Diamond NG, Casarella WJ. Percutaneous transluminal angioplasty in nonatherosclerotic disease. *Radiology* 1980;135:27.

58. Dorros G, Jaff M, Jain A, et al. Follow-up of primary Palmaz-Schatz stent placement for atherosclerotic renal artery stenosis. *Am J Cardiol* 1995;75:1051.

59. Blum U, Krumme B, Flugel P, et al. Treatment of ostial renal artery stenoses with vascular endoprostheses after unsuccessful balloon angioplasty. *N Engl J Med* 1997;336:459.

60. Harjai K, Khosla S, Shaw D, et al. Effect of gender on outcomes following renal artery stent placement for renovascular hypertension. *Cathet Cardiovasc Diagn* 1997;42:381.

61. Henry M, Amor M, Henry I, et al. Stent placement in the renal artery: three-year experience with the Palmaz stent. *J Vasc Intervent Radiol* 1996;7:343–350.

62. Boisclair C, Therasse E, Oliva VL, et al. Treatment of renal angioplasty failure by percutaneous renal artery stenting with Palmaz stents: midterm technical and clinical results. *AJR Am J Roentgenol* 1997;168:245–251.

63. Rees CR, Palmaz JC, Becker GJ, et al. Palmaz stent in atherosclerotic stenoses involving the ostia of the renal arteries: preliminary report of a multicenter study. *Radiology* 1991;181: 507.

64. Dorros G, Jaff M, Mathiak L, et al. Four-year follow-up of Palmaz-Schatz stent revascularization as treatment for renal artery stenosis. *Circulation* 1998;98:642.

65. Wong JM, Hansen KJ, Oskin TC, et al. Surgery after failed percutaneous renal artery angioplasty. *J Vasc Surg* 1999;30: 468.

66. Anderson CA, Hansen KJ, Benjamin ME, et al. Renal artery fibromuscular dysplasia: results of current surgical therapy. *J Vasc Surg* 1995;22:207.

67. Cambria RP, Brewster DC, L'Italien G, et al. Simultaneous aortic and renal artery reconstruction: evolution of an eighteen-year experience. *J Vasc Surg* 1994;21:916.

68. Hansen KJ, Starr SM, Sands RE, et al. Contemporary surgical management of renovascular disease. *J Vasc Surg* 1992;16: 319.

69. Murray SP, Kent KC, Salvatierra O, et al. Complex branch renovascular disease: management options and late results. *J Vasc Surg* 1994;20:338.

70. Stanley JC. The evolution of surgery for renovascular occlusive disease. *Cardiovasc Surg* 1994;2:195.

71. Stanley JC. Surgical treatment of renovascular hypertension. *Am J Surg* 1997;174:102.

72. Stanley JC, Ernst CB, Fry WJ. Surgical treatment of renovascular hypertension: results in specific patient subgroups. In: *Renovascular hypertension.* Stanley JC, Ernst CB, Fry WJ, eds. Philadelphia: WB Saunders, 1984:363.

73. Stanley JC, Messina LM, Wakefield TW, et al. Renal artery reconstruction. In: Bergan JJ, Yao JST, eds. *Techniques in arterial surgery.* Philadelphia: WB Saunders, 1990:247.

74. Stanley JC, Whitehouse WM Jr, Zelenock GB, et al. Reoperation for complications of renal artery reconstructive surgery undertaken for treatment of renovascular hypertension. *J Vasc Surg* 1985;2:133.

75. Stanley JC, Ernst CB, Fry WJ. Fate of 100 aortorenal vein grafts: characteristics of late graft expansion, aneurysmal dilatation, and stenosis. *Surgery* 1973;74:931.

76. Cambria RP, Brewster DC, L'Italien GJ, et al. The durability of different reconstructive techniques for atherosclerotic renal artery disease. *J Vasc Surg* 1994;20:76.

77. Chibaro EA, Libertino JA, Novick AC. Use of the hepatic circulation for renal revascularization. *Ann Surg* 1984;199:406.

78. Khauli RB, Novick AC, Ziegelbaum M. Splenorenal bypass in the treatment of renal artery stenosis: experience with 69 cases. *J Vasc Surg* 1985;2:547.

79. Novick AC, Stewart R, Hodge EE, et al. Use of the thoracic aorta for renal arterial reconstruction. *J Vasc Surg* 1994;19: 605.

80. Moncure AC, Brewster DC, Darling RC, et al. Use of the splenic and hepatic arteries for renal revascularization. *J Vasc Surg* 1986;3:196.

81. Brekke IB, Sodal G, Jakobsen A, et al. Fibromuscular renal artery disease treated by extracorporeal vascular reconstruction and renal autotransplantation: short- and long-term results. *Eur J Vasc Surg* 1992;6:471.

82. van Bockel JH, van den Akker PJ, Chang PC, et al. Extracorporeal renal artery reconstruction for renovascular hypertension. *J Vasc Surg* 1991;13:101.

83. Dougherty MJ, Hallett JW Jr, Naessens J, et al. Renal endarterectomy vs. bypass for combined aortic and renal reconstruction: is there a difference in clinical outcome? *Ann Vasc Surg* 1995;9:87.

84. McNeil JW, String ST, Pfeiffer RB Jr. Concomitant renal endarterectomy and aortic reconstruction. *J Vasc Surg* 1994;20: 331.

85. Stoney RJ, Messina LM, Goldstone J, et al. Renal endarterectomy through the transected aorta: a new technique for combined aortorenal arteriosclerosis—a preliminary report. *J Vasc Surg* 1989;9:224.

86. Dean RH, Lawson JD, Hollifield JW. Revascularization of the poorly functioning kidney. *Surgery* 1979;85:44.

87. Dean RH, Shack RB, Rhamy RK, et al. The effect of renal revascularization on kidney function. *J Surg Res* 1977;22: 443.

88. Hallett JW Jr, Textor SC, Kos PB, et al. Advanced renovascular hypertension and renal insufficiency: trends in medical comorbidity and surgical approach from 1970 to 1993. *J Vasc Surg* 1995;21:750.

89. Hansen KJ, Thomason RB, Craven TE, et al. Surgical management of dialysis-dependent ischemic nephropathy. *J Vasc Surg* 1995;21:197.

90. Jacobson HR. Ischemic renal disease: an overlooked clinical entity? *Kidney Int* 1988;34:729.

91. Jamieson GG, Clarkson AR, Woodroffe AJ, et al. Reconstructive renal vascular surgery for chronic renal failure. *Br J Surg* 1984;71:338.

92. Oskin TC, Hansen KJ, Deitch JS, et al. Chronic renal artery occlusion: nephrectomy versus revascularization. *J Vasc Surg* 1999;29:140.

93. Whitehouse WM Jr, Kazmers A, Zelenock GB, et al. Chronic total renal artery occlusions: effects of treatment on secondary hypertension and renal function. *Surgery* 1981;89: 753.

SURGERY: SCIENTIFIC PRINCIPLES AND PRACTICE, Third Edition, edited by
Lazar J. Greenfield, Michael W. Mulholland, Keith T. Oldham, Gerald B. Zelenock,
and Keith D. Lillemoe. Lippincott Williams & Wilkins Publishers, Philadelphia, © 2001.

CHAPTER 79

AORTOILIAC DISEASE

DANIEL J. REDDY, ALEXANDER D. SHEPARD,
AND IRAKLIS I. PIPINOS

Atherosclerotic occlusive disease of the aorta and iliac arteries is one of the most common problems encountered by vascular surgeons. Alone or in combination with more common femoropopliteal/tibial occlusive disease, it is the most frequent cause of chronic lower extremity arterial insufficiency. Because a greater number of muscle groups are affected by aortoiliac atherosclerosis than by infrainguinal disease, the resulting symptoms may be particularly disabling. The treatment of symptomatic aortoiliac disease also represents one of the major success stories of modern vascular surgery. Since the first reconstructive procedures on the abdominal aorta were performed nearly five decades ago, treatment has undergone significant progress. Advances in noninvasive vascular diagnosis, arteriography, preoperative assessment, and anesthesia and critical care in addition to those in surgical technique have contributed to improved outcomes. Reconstructive procedures for aortoiliac disease have become routine, with low perioperative morbidity and mortality and excellent early and long-term outcomes. The excellent durability of such reconstructions is undoubtedly in large part related to the large caliber and high flow rates of the vessels involved.

Depending on the pattern of the occlusive process and patient risk, a variety of revascularization techniques are currently available. Selection of a patient-specific treatment strategy from an increasing array of alternatives, although challenging, frequently will alleviate symptoms, avoid an amputation, and prevent or reverse organ dysfunction.

ANATOMY

The arteries supplying blood to the lower extremities are frequently divided into abdominal, or "inflow," arteries (the aorta and iliac arteries) and infrainguinal, or "outflow," arteries (the femoropopliteal/tibial arteries). The aorta enters the abdomen from the chest through the aortic hiatus, located between the 12th thoracic and first lumbar vertebrae, and ends at the level of the fourth lumbar vertebra, where it bifurcates into the right and left common iliac arteries. This terminal bifurcation roughly corresponds to the level of the umbilicus. Each common iliac artery curves posteriorly into the sacral hollow and divides into an internal and an external iliac branch. The external iliac then curves anteriorly and continues along the psoas muscle under the inguinal ligament to become the common femoral artery, which in turn bifurcates into the superficial and deep (profunda) femoral arteries. The internal iliac (hypogastric) artery follows the curve of the pelvic side wall and branches repeatedly to supply the pelvic viscera and gluteal musculature (Fig. 79.1).

The branches of the abdominal aorta can be divided in three groups: (a) Three unpaired arteries to the gut arise from its anterior wall; the celiac trunk supplies the foregut, the superior mesenteric artery supplies the midgut, and the inferior mesenteric perfuses the hindgut. (b) Arteries to the three paired genitourinary glands arise

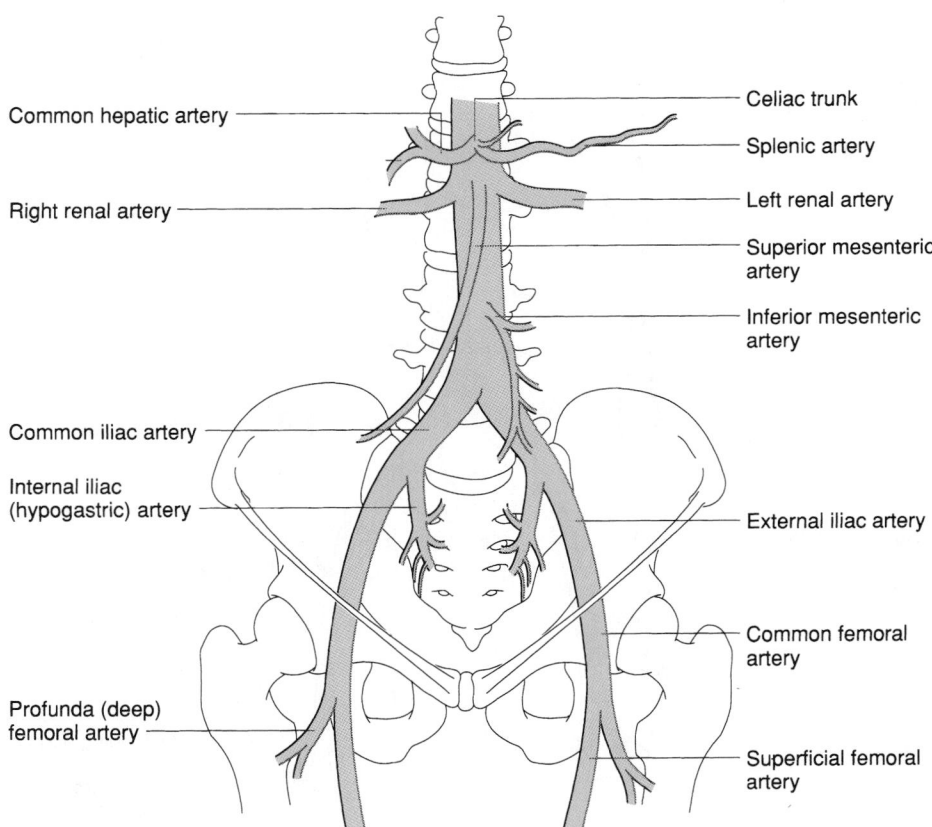

Figure 79.1. Anatomy of the abdominal aorta and iliac arteries.

close together from the lateral wall of the aorta—the adrenal, renal, and gonadal branches. (c) Branches to the "roof" and walls of the abdominal cavity include the phrenic, lumbar, and median sacral arteries. These branches assume varying degrees of importance in the formation of collateral perfusion channels around occlusive lesions in the aorta and iliac arteries.

Because the abdominal aorta and its iliac branches are retroperitoneal structures coursing through the deepest portions of the abdominal cavity, a sophisticated operative technique is required to expose them. The proximal (suprarenal) abdominal aorta is rendered particularly inaccessible by the overlying stomach, pancreas, and colon. Fortunately, occlusive lesions of this portion of the aorta are relatively uncommon in comparison with those of the distal (infrarenal) aorta. The crossing left renal vein serves as a useful surgical landmark defining the usual boundary between these two segments of the abdominal aorta. Although transabdominal exposure of the infrarenal aorta is fairly routine, it requires reflection of the transverse colon superiorly and of the small bowel and its mesentery and distal duodenum to the right. The iliac bifurcations can also be difficult to expose because of their location deep in the pelvis; in addition, the bifurcation of the left iliac artery lies directly behind the sigmoid colon.

PATHOPHYSIOLOGY

Although atherosclerosis is a generalized disease, the earliest and most severe lesions tend to occur at arterial bifurcations and in areas of relative fixation, where the disruption of normal laminar flow is greatest. The aortic bi-

furcation is in fact the location where the earliest atherosclerotic changes are first noted in most young adults. In persons predisposed to the development of more advanced disease, plaque gradually extends proximally into the infrarenal aorta and distally into the common iliac arteries, usually along the posterior wall first. With progressive worsening of the occlusive process, hemodynamic alterations lead to the enlargement of a network of auxiliary or collateral channels around the involved segments. Important collateral arterial pathways around the aortic bifurcation and common iliac segments are the following: (a) intercostal and lumbar arteries to circumflex iliac and iliolumbar arteries, (b) superior to inferior epigastric arteries, and (c) superior and inferior mesenteric arteries to rectal and internal pudendal arteries. Collateral pathways around occlusive lesions of the external iliac arteries include the hypogastric-to-circumflex femoral channels (Figs. 79.2 and 79.3).

With slowly developing occlusive lesions, this collateral network is usually sufficient to provide enough blood flow to meet the resting metabolic needs of the lower extremities. However, these channels do not have the capacity to increase blood flow to the levels necessary to meet the exercise demands of the leg musculature. *Claudication* (from the Latin verb *claudicare,* "to limp") is the term used to denote the characteristic exercise-induced, cramping pain in the muscles of the lower extremity that results. With acute arterial occlusions and multiple-level disease (occlusive disease in both the aortoiliac and infrainguinal segments), collateral pathways may be inadequate to meet even the basal metabolic needs of nonexercising tissue. The outcome is critical limb ischemia associated with

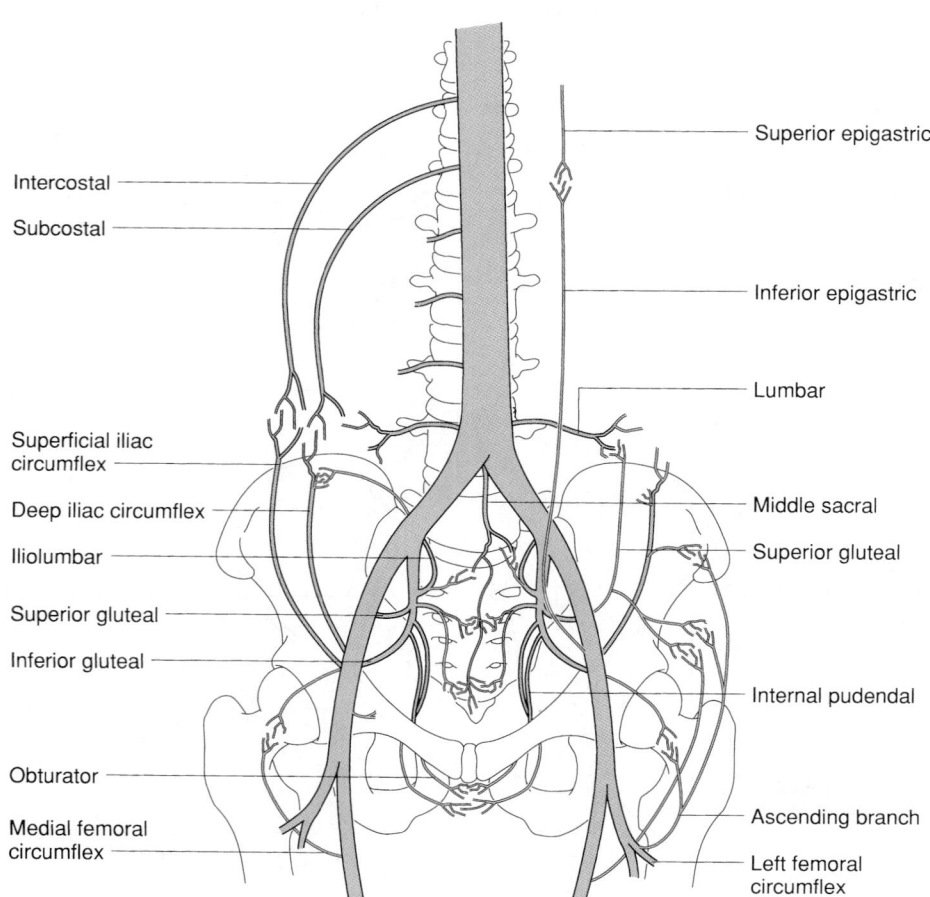

Intercostal
Subcostal
Superficial iliac circumflex
Deep iliac circumflex
Iliolumbar
Superior gluteal
Inferior gluteal
Obturator
Medial femoral circumflex

Superior epigastric
Inferior epigastric
Lumbar
Middle sacral
Superior gluteal
Internal pudendal
Ascending branch
Left femoral circumflex

Figure 79.2. Major pathways of parietal–visceral collateral circulation in aortoiliac occlusive disease.

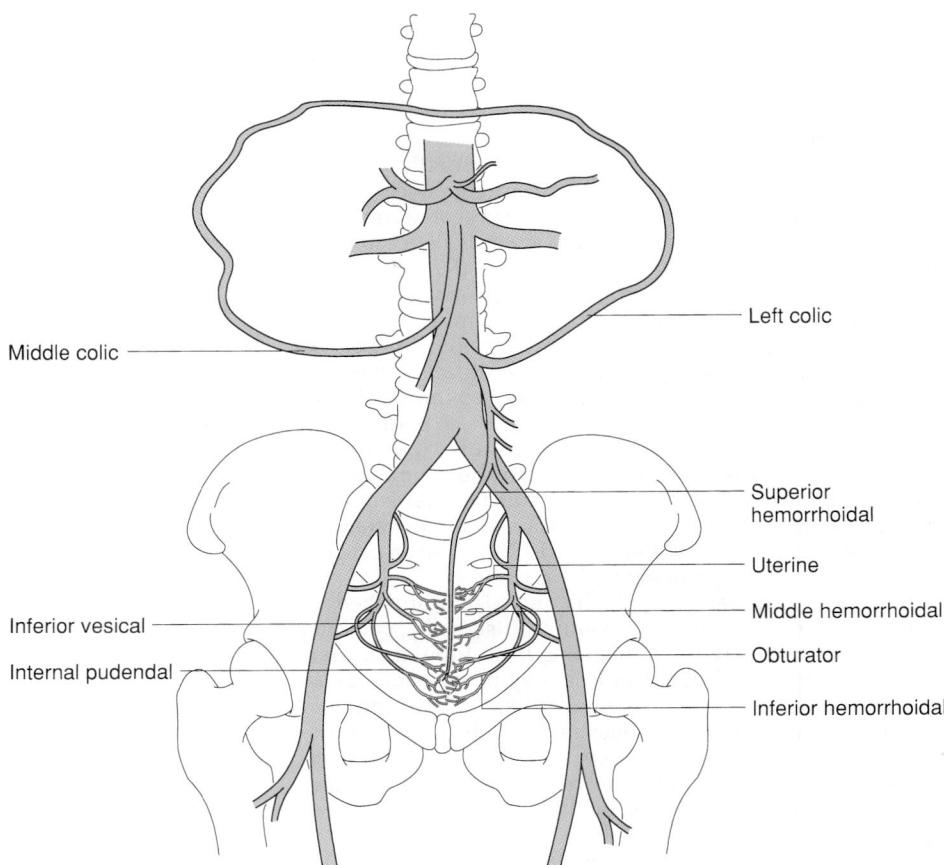

Middle colic

Left colic

Superior hemorrhoidal

Uterine

Middle hemorrhoidal

Inferior vesical

Obturator

Internal pudendal

Inferior hemorrhoidal

Figure 79.3. Major visceral collateral network available to compensate for occlusive aortoiliac disease.

pain at rest, tissue loss (gangrene, nonhealing ulceration), and threatened limb viability.

PRESENTATION

The risk factors for aortoiliac occlusive disease are those for atherosclerosis in general—smoking, hypertension, lipid abnormalities, diabetes mellitus, male sex, older age, and genetic predisposition. Smoking appears to be a particularly important risk factor for the development of lower extremity atherosclerotic occlusive disease (1). Patients with symptoms of aortoiliac occlusive disease usu-

ally present in their 50s and 60s, whereas patients with symptoms of infrainguinal disease are generally in their 70s (2). Patients with critical limb ischemia secondary to multiple-level disease are also generally in this older age group.

Claudication is the most common presenting symptom of patients with significant aortoiliac disease. Induced by ambulation and quickly relieved by rest, claudication is usually described as a cramping pain, tiredness, or easy fatigability of the involved muscle groups. Although patients with aortoiliac disease classically present with claudication of the thighs, hips, and buttocks, a significant mi-

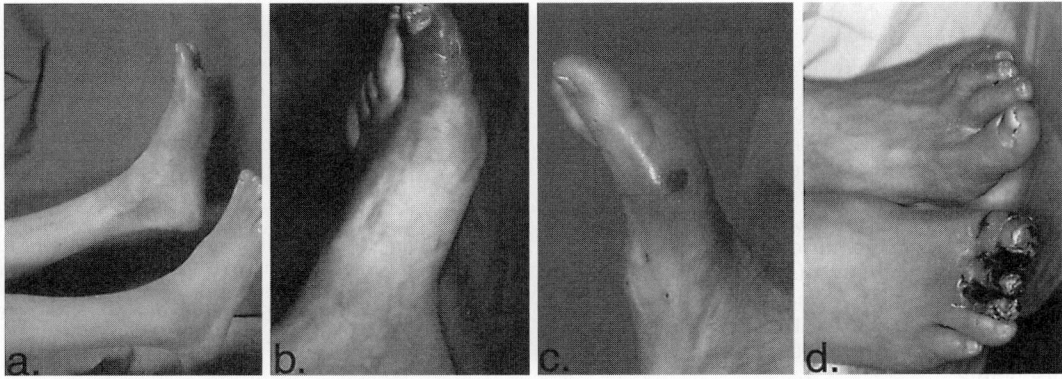

Figure 79.4. Clinical manifestations of critical limb ischemia. *(A)* Patient with ischemic rest pain. Note the absence of hair on the atrophic shiny skin of the feet and the rubor at dependency. *(B)* First-toe ischemia and dermal discoloration of blue-toe syndrome. *(C)* Ischemic ulceration. *(D)* Digital gangrene.

nority may complain of only calf claudication. Erectile dysfunction in men secondary to reduced hypogastric perfusion is another common complaint. The combination of bilateral lower extremity claudication, atrophy of the leg muscles, impotence, and diminished or absent femoral pulses is known as *Leriche's syndrome,* after the French physician who first described these classic manifestations of aortoiliac disease (3). Critical limb ischemia associated with rest pain or tissue loss may be a manifestation of aortoiliac occlusive disease but almost always occurs in combination with more distal femoropopliteal disease (Fig. 79.4). In the absence of infrainguinal disease, aortoiliac collaterals are almost always able to maintain adequate resting tissue perfusion. An exception to this rule is atheroembolic disease, or "blue toe" syndrome. Degenerative plaque(s) in the aortoiliac (or any proximal arterial) segment can ulcerate or rupture to release platelet microthrombi and atheromatous debris into the arterial lumen. Downstream embolization into the microcirculation of the lower extremities can produce digital ischemia and gangrene and dermal discoloration in a characteristic reticular pattern (livedo reticularis) (Fig. 79.4). Such patients usually have palpable pedal pulses.

Physical examination typically reveals diminished or absent femoral pulses. Severely diseased, calcified femoral arteries may be palpable as firm, tubular masses. Normal femoral and distal pulses may be palpable, however, even in the presence of hemodynamically significant aortoiliac stenoses. Such pulses rapidly disappear following ambulation as the increased flow demands of the exercising leg muscles lead to lowered peripheral vascular resistance. Bruits heard over the lower abdomen or groins suggest the presence of turbulent flow resulting from occlusive plaque. Patients with long-standing aortoiliac atherosclerosis may have disuse atrophy of the lower extremity musculature. Other common signs of lower extremity arterial occlusive disease include trophic changes, such as hair loss on the legs or toes and thin shiny skin on the feet, in addition to rubor on limb dependency coupled with pallor on elevation. Such chronic advanced changes in addition to gangrene and nonhealing ulceration(s) are unusual in the absence of multiple-level disease.

Different patterns of aortoiliac disease have been identified on preoperative arteriographic studies (4) (Fig. 79.5). Disease confined to the distal infrarenal aorta and common iliac arteries, classified as type I, accounts for only 10% of patients with inflow disease. Patients with type I disease are younger and more frequently female than patients with other forms of aortoiliac disease, and they usually present with complaints of disabling claudication in the buttocks, hips, and thighs (5). Such localized disease may be amenable to endarterectomy or percutaneous transluminal angioplasty. More extensive disease is the rule; atherosclerotic plaque extends distally into the external iliac artery and not infrequently to the common femoral bifurcation in more than 80% of patients. In somewhat less than half this group, no significant occlusive disease is present in the femoropopliteal/tibial segments (type II disease) (Fig. 79.6). Such patients experience worse claudication than persons with more localized, type I disease. In the remaining patients, occlusive disease in the aortoiliac segment is combined with femoropopliteal/tibial disease (type III disease) (Fig. 79.7). As outlined previously, patients with such multiple-level disease are usually older than those in the other two groups and more frequently present with symptoms of critical limb ischemia.

In all three groups, the atherosclerotic process progresses unpredictably, but the end result in a small percentage of patients (approximately 5% to 6% in our experience) is occlusion of the terminal infrarenal aorta with

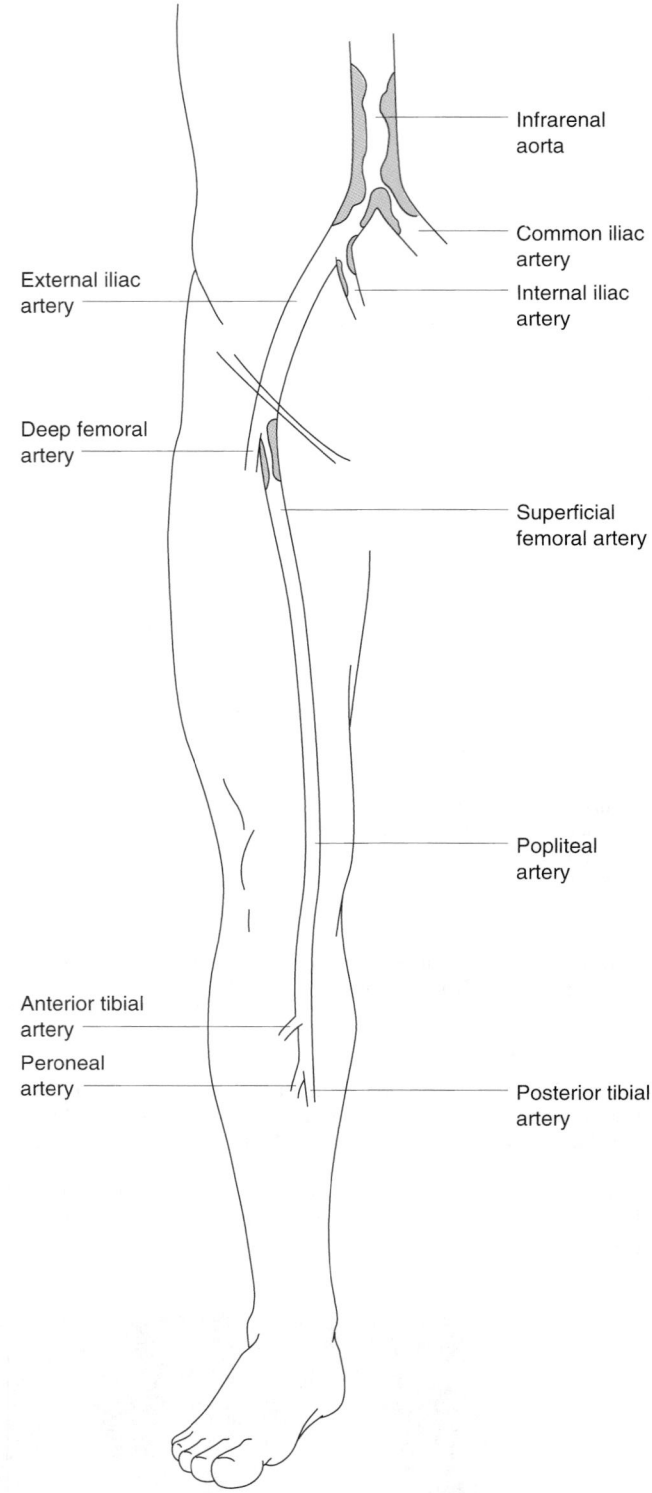

Figure 79.5. Common sites of arteriosclerotic lesions in aortoiliofemoral occlusive disease. Although often a generalized process, partially segmental distribution of major disease, most prominent at arterial bifurcations, usually allows surgical revascularization.

propagation of clot proximally to the levels of the renal arteries (Fig. 79.8). In the absence of significant renal artery stenoses, propagation proximally to the renal arteries is an unusual event. One other pattern worthy of mention is aortoiliac hypoplasia, an uncommon variant usually encountered in young to middle-aged women who smoke cigarettes. The infrarenal aorta and iliac arteries are unusually small in caliber and hence prone to significant narrowing, even with modest disease. Operative treatment in such patients can be particularly challenging.

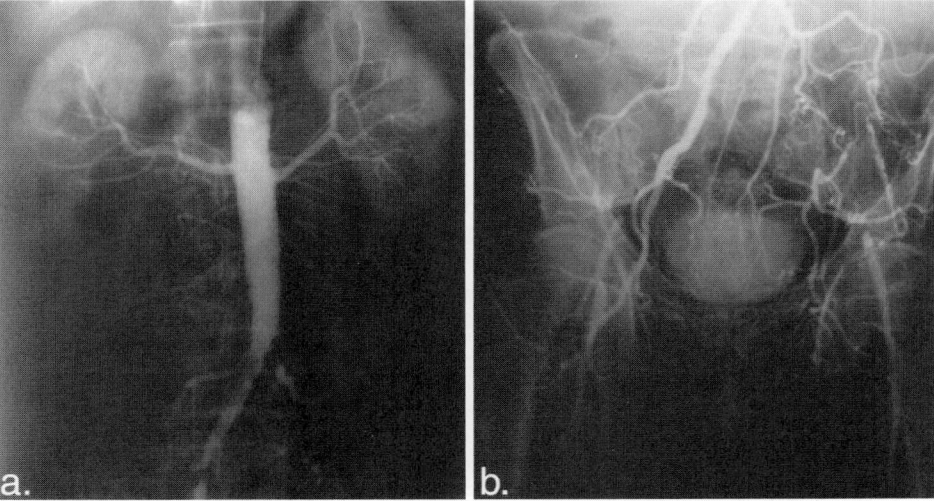

Figure 79.6. Abdominal aortogram demonstrating type II disease. Left common and external iliac occlusion can be seen, with reconstitution of the ipsilateral internal iliac and common femoral arteries through visceral and lumbar collaterals. The right external iliac artery is also occluded, and the right common femoral artery is reconstituted through right hypogastric-to-circumflex femoral channels.

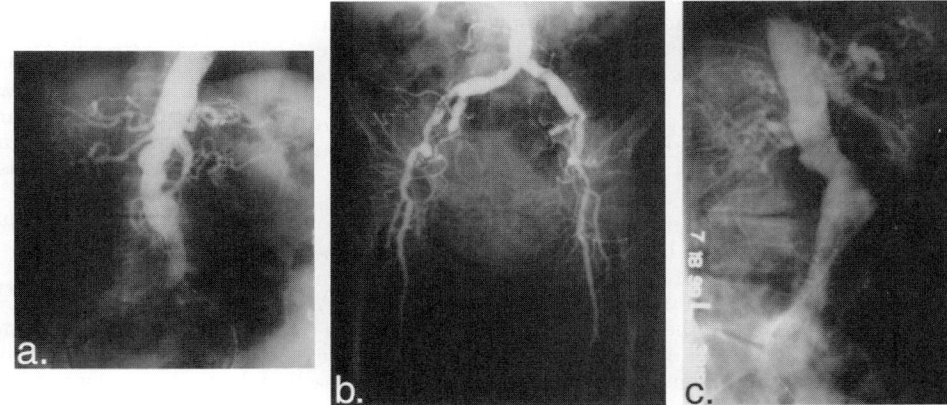

Figure 79.7. Abdominal aortogram demonstrating type III disease. *(A)* Note the extensive atherosclerotic disease producing both ulcerated plaques and aneurysmal degeneration in the aorta and common iliac arteries bilaterally. *(B)* Preocclusive stenoses in the proximal right external and internal iliac arteries and in the left internal iliac artery. The superficial femoral arteries are occluded bilaterally.

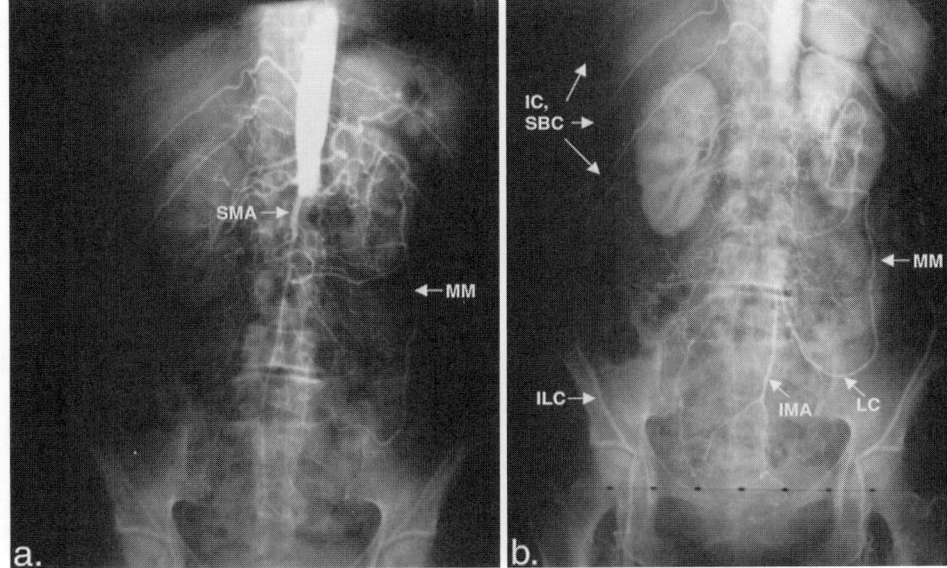

Figure 79.8. Abdominal aortogram demonstrating juxtarenal aortic occlusion and an extensive collateral network reconstituting the femoral arterial segments. *(A) SMA,* superior mesenteric artery; *MM,* meandering mesenteric. *(B) IC,* intercostal; *SBC,* subcostal; *ILC,* iliac circumflex; *IMA,* inferior mesenteric artery; *LC,* left colic; *MM,* meandering mesenteric.

EVALUATION

In the overwhelming majority of cases, a diagnosis of significant aortoiliac occlusive disease can be made on the basis of the history and physical examination alone. A clinical diagnosis can and should be supplemented by noninvasive vascular testing. Such testing provides valuable information to the treating clinician by confirming the presence of disease and objectively documenting the degree of ischemia and the arterial segment(s) involved. A baseline is established according to which the patient can be followed and interventions planned. Treatment results can be assessed by repeated testing. Such information is particularly useful in a patient with an equivocal history or pulse examination. Arteriography can then be reserved for those patients considered suitable candidates for operative or endovascular (catheter-based) intervention.

Segmental Pressure Measurements

Measurement of the systolic arterial pressures at different levels of the lower extremity with a hand-held, pencil-sized, continuous-wave Doppler flow probe is the simplest and most useful noninvasive method to assess arterial occlusive disease. The ratio of the ankle systolic pressure to the brachial systolic pressure is the ankle–brachial index (ABI), or pressure ratio, and is a good indicator of the degree of ischemia present. With the Doppler probe used as an ultrasonic stethoscope, the systolic pressures in the dorsalis pedis and posterior tibial artery are measured at the ankle, and each of these values is then the numerator of a simple fraction in which the higher of the two brachial pressures is the denominator. Normal ABIs are generally equal to or slightly greater than 1. Patients with claudication usually have ABIs ranging from 0.5 to 0.9, whereas patients with rest pain and tissue loss have ABIs of less than 0.5.

Determination of limb systolic pressures at different locations (with the "four-cuff" technique, pressures are measured at the upper thigh, lower thigh, calf, and ankle) provides information about which arterial segment(s) are involved with occlusive disease (Figs. 79.9 and 79.10). A pressure drop of more than 20 mm Hg between consecutive levels is indicative of significant disease within the intervening arterial segment. A reduced upper thigh pressure signifies occlusive disease in the aortoiliac or common femoral segments.

In patients with extensive calcification in the walls of the tibial arteries (as is frequently seen in diabetes mellitus or end-stage renal disease), the ankle pressures may not be interpretable because the vessels are too "stiff" to be compressed by the externally applied cuff. In this situation, the pressure in the digital arteries of the great toe can be measured because these small vessels are generally spared calcification. A toe pressure of less than 30 mm Hg indicates severe ischemia. Inspection of the Doppler-derived arterial waveforms can provide additional information when tibial vessels are incompressible.

Patients with claudication occasionally have normal or nearly normal ABIs. As described previously, in such cases the arterial stenosis is not severe enough to cause a pressure drop while the limb is at rest but does produce a hemodynamic effect under conditions of higher rates of flow, as during exercise. Higher rates of flow through a moderately stenotic segment increase the energy lost at the site, so that a significant distal pressure drop results. Exercise stress testing can be used to evaluate patients suspected of having such disease. ABIs are measured before and after a treadmill exercise protocol; a drop of 15% or more in the ABI following exercise is indicative of hemodynamically significant occlusive disease.

Duplex Scanning

Duplex scanning of the aorta and iliac arteries has been advocated by some as a more precise noninvasive diagnostic tool (6). Some authorities have even suggested that duplex scanning can be used to plan therapeutic interventions without the need for arteriography. Imaging of the abdominal arteries, however, is difficult because of their deep retroperitoneal and pelvic locations. Many patients are not candidates for such studies because of body habitus and overlying bowel gas, and even in experienced hands, this procedure is quite time-consuming. These problems have limited the widespread use of this modality.

Differential Diagnosis

The diagnosis of aortoiliac disease is usually straightforward, but occasional diagnostic confusion may arise when other causes of lower extremity pain are present. Irritation of lumbosacral nerve roots by spinal stenosis or intervertebral disk herniation may cause buttock and leg

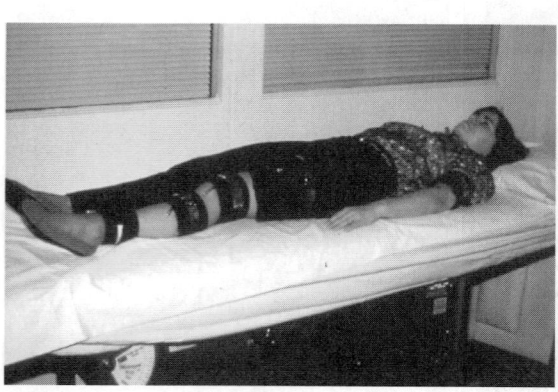
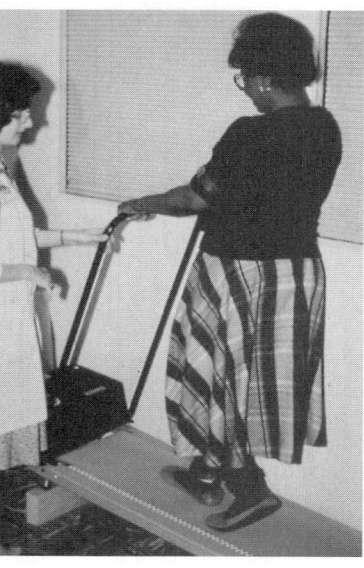

Figure 79.9. Noninvasive testing to evaluate lower extremity ischemia. *(left)* Segmental pressure measurements with cuffs placed at the upper thigh, lower thigh, calf, and ankle. *(right)* Stress testing with treadmill ergometry.

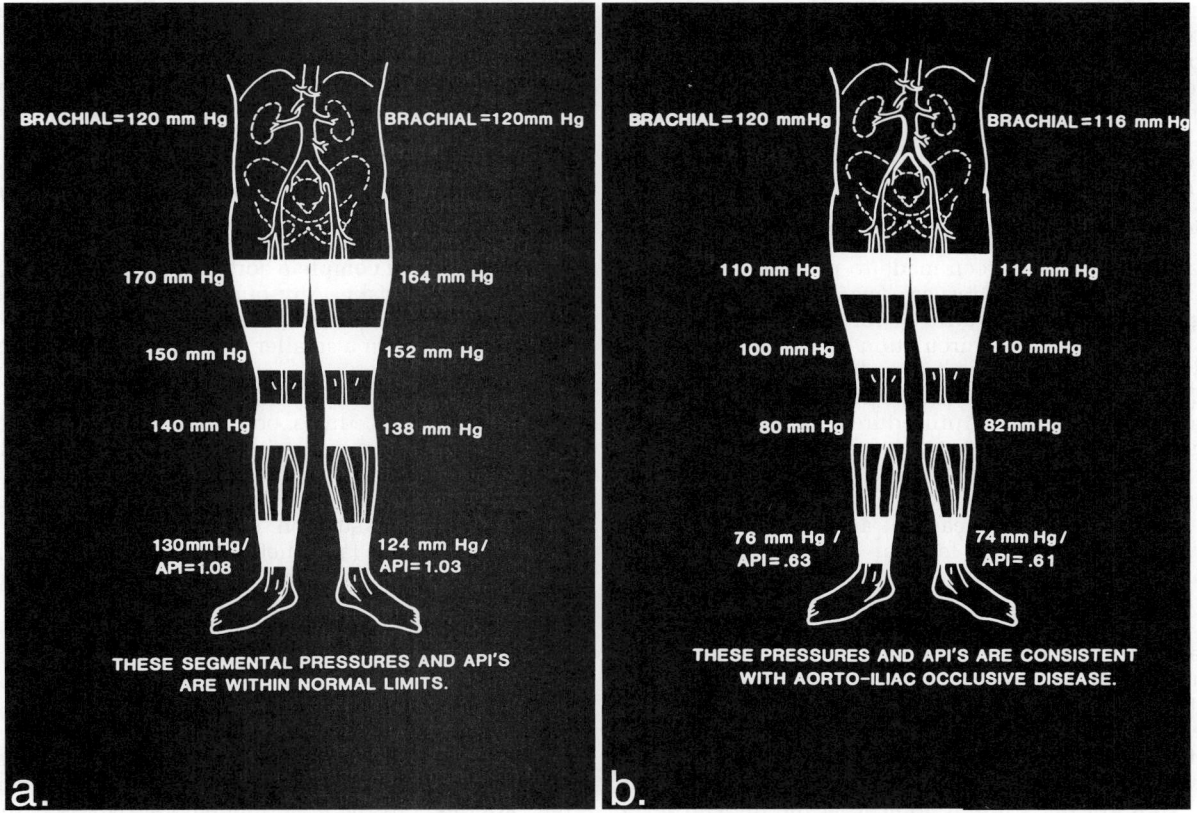

Figure 79.10. Segmental pressure measurements typical of *(A)* normal and *(B)* aortoiliac occlusive disease.

pain that is associated with activity. However, such symptoms ("neurogenic claudication") usually cannot be reproduced at the same level of activity and frequently occur when the patient is standing, so that the patient must sit or lie down to obtain relief. In addition, the pain is usually in a classic sciatic distribution. Degenerative arthritis of the hip joints may produce similar buttock, hip, and referred thigh pain. The physical examination typically reveals pain directly over the hip joint that is exacerbated by movement of the joint. Peripheral neuropathy, particularly that associated with diabetes mellitus, may masquerade as ischemic rest pain. In all these situations, segmental limb pressure measurements with or without stress testing can be extremely helpful in determining the contribution of arterial occlusive disease to the patient's symptoms.

TREATMENT

The aims of therapy in aortoiliac occlusive disease are to relieve symptoms and, in cases of critical limb ischemia, prevent limb loss. Medical therapy should be instituted in all patients with symptomatic disease but is obviously insufficient as sole therapy in patients with limb-threatening ischemia.

Medical Therapy

Risk factor modification, including smoking cessation and the follow-up and treatment of diabetes mellitus, systemic arterial hypertension, and hyperlipidemia should be an important component of primary care for all these patients (7). Although control of these factors will not reverse the atherosclerotic process, it may limit the progression of disease. Furthermore, some data indicate that

smoking cessation lessens the severity of symptoms in many patients. Also, a daily exercise program of regular walking may improve collateral development and increase the anaerobic tolerance of ischemic skeletal muscle. Finally, pharmacotherapy with medications such as pentoxifylline and cilostazol can be a valuable adjunct in selected patients (8,9). Although the mechanisms of action of these agents are unclear, both have effected a modest but significant reduction in claudication symptoms in controlled trials. Some form of platelet inhibition, usually with aspirin, should also be considered for all patients. Although no specific data have demonstrated that antiplatelet therapy is helpful in the treatment of lower extremity arterial occlusive disease, abundant evidence has shown it to be beneficial in the treatment of atherosclerotic occlusive disease in other vascular territories (e.g., coronary and cerebral vessels).

Revascularization

Indications for Revascularization

Revascularization is clearly indicated in patients with critical limb ischemia; without intervention, the vast majority progress to limb loss in a fairly short period of time. Patients with significant or repetitive atheroembolism from an aortoiliac source represent another group who clearly benefit from operative therapy. Removal or bypass of the culprit lesion(s) eliminates the risk for further macroembolism and microembolism. The treatment for patients with claudication secondary to aortoiliac occlusive disease remains somewhat controversial and must be individualized. Patients with mild to moderate symptoms can be treated medically with quite satisfactory results.

Patients with severe, disabling, lifestyle-limiting symptoms of claudication can benefit from revascularization therapy. The current safety and long-term durability of direct aortic reconstruction make this approach acceptable even for older, higher-risk patients with significant symptoms. For patients who cannot tolerate such procedures, a variety of other methods of revascularization are available that have had good long-term success rates.

Arteriography

Once a decision has been made to proceed with revascularization therapy, contrast arteriography, either cut film or digital subtraction, is utilized for a detailed anatomic evaluation of the arterial circulation of the lower extremities. Such information is necessary to choose the most appropriate method of revascularization (operative or endovascular) and plan the procedure. Biplane abdominal aortography with demonstration of the arterial tree below the inguinal ligament ("runoff") is required. This procedure is most commonly performed from the femoral artery with the best pulse by means of a retrograde Seldinger technique. When neither femoral artery is available, a transaxillary or translumbar approach provides good access. Anteroposterior views of the aortoiliofemoral segments demonstrate the extent of the occlusive process and the pattern of collateral formation. Oblique views of the iliac and femoral arteries are frequently necessary to document posterior wall plaque and stenoses at the origins of the deep femoral arteries. Lateral aortography provides information about the origins of the visceral arteries, whereas anteroposterior views demonstrate the renal arteries. Views of the "runoff" to at least the midcalf level are required to assess the degree of associated occlusive disease; in cases of critical limb ischemia, visualization of the pedal circulation is usually necessary.

Occasionally, the hemodynamic effect of a stenosis or series of stenoses along an iliac arterial segment may be difficult to determine, even with oblique views. When the significance of a stenosis remains in question, pressures proximal and distal to the lesion(s) can be measured. A drop of more than 5 to 10 mm Hg across the stenosis is indicative of a hemodynamically significant lesion. For borderline cases, distal pressure measurements can be obtained before and after interarterial injection of a vasodilator, such as tolazoline (Priscoline), to simulate the hyperemic hemodynamics of exercise. A pressure drop of 20 mm Hg or more during hyperdynamic flow is considered to indicate hemodynamic significance.

The information supplied by arteriography is crucial to the success of a revascularization procedure. In addition to providing a detailed "road map" of the exact arterial segments involved and the pathology present, arteriography identifies associated anatomic variations (e.g., accessory renal arteries) and aortic wall characteristics (e.g., extensive calcification, ulcerated plaque), which may alter the operative approach and the conduct of the procedure. For example, an operating surgeon who knows that the aortic wall just below the renal arteries is heavily diseased with ulcerated plaque may decide to control the aorta at a more proximal level rather than risk dislodging atheromatous debris with standard infrarenal aortic clamping. Similarly, documented occlusive lesions in the visceral or renal arteries (e.g., a patent inferior mesenteric artery with a large "meandering mesenteric artery") may best be addressed at the time of aortic reconstruction or require particular attention to avoid complications.

The major risks of arteriography, allergic reactions and contrast-induced renal dysfunction, have been greatly reduced during the last several years by the introduction of newer non-ionic contrast agents and recognition of the importance of adequate hydration before the procedure. Nevertheless, interest has been increasing in the use of magnetic resonance (MR) imaging to avoid these and other complications of angiography. Unfortunately, current MR angiography technology, although promising, does not provide sufficient detail or accuracy to supplant traditional angiography in the evaluation of aortoiliac occlusive disease (10). We currently utilize MR angiography in patients with moderately severe renal dysfunction (serum creatinine ≥ 3.0 mg/dL), for whom the burden of radioactive contrast in a complete aortogram with runoff study is considered too risky. Any questions remaining after MR angiography can be answered by a more focused arteriographic study with a smaller load of radioactive contrast.

Choice of Revascularization Technique

A variety of procedures, both endovascular and surgical, are available for revascularization of the patient with aortoiliac occlusive disease. Selection depends on a number of factors, including the pattern of the occlusive process, patient risk, and surgeon experience. Commonly used techniques include (a) catheter-based balloon dilation with or without luminal stenting, (b) aortoiliac endarterectomy, (c) arterial reconstruction with an anatomically placed bypass prosthesis (aortofemoral or iliofemoral), and (d) arterial reconstruction with a remote or extraanatomically placed bypass prosthesis (axillofemoral/bifemoral, femorofemoral, thoracofemoral). Catheter-based techniques are best suited for focal lesions of the common iliac arteries. Endarterectomy is limited to good-risk patients with focal occlusive disease at the aortic bifurcation and common iliac arteries. Prosthetic aortobifemoral bypass is the procedure of choice for most patients with advanced, extensive aortoiliac involvement and is considered the gold standard technique for aortoiliac revascularization. Axillofemoral/bifemoral bypass is reserved for the small subpopulation of patients in whom standard direct aortic reconstruction is considered too risky, either for medical reasons (usually severe pulmonary or cardiac disease) or technical reasons (aortic reoperations, multiple prior abdominal procedures with dense adhesions, prior abdominal irradiation, prosthetic graft infections). The descending thoracic aorta can be considered as an alternative arterial source for the construction of a thoracofemoral bypass in good-risk patients with a "hostile" abdomen (11). Femorofemoral or iliofemoral bypass can be used in poor-risk patients with diffuse unilateral iliac disease or bilateral iliac involvement when the stenosis in one of the iliac arteries can be appropriately treated by balloon angioplasty with or without intraluminal stenting.

Preoperative Evaluation

The evaluation of patients for whom aortoiliac reconstruction is being considered should include a careful assessment of overall operative risk. Age *per se* is not a contraindication to a standard direct aortic reconstruction, if it is needed. A "lesser" procedure of more limited durability, however, may provide a similarly excellent outcome in a patient with reduced life expectancy. Patients with significant aortoiliac disease may have atherosclerotic occlusive disease in other vascular territories (e.g., coronary, cerebral) that affects their operative risk. The detection and treatment of significant coronary artery disease is particularly important because myocardial infarction is the leading cause of both perioperative and late mortality (12). More than 50% of patients with aortoiliac occlusive disease have clinical or electrocardiographic evidence of coronary disease (13). Selected patients may require cardiac catheterization and even occasional coronary angioplasty or bypass grafting before undergoing

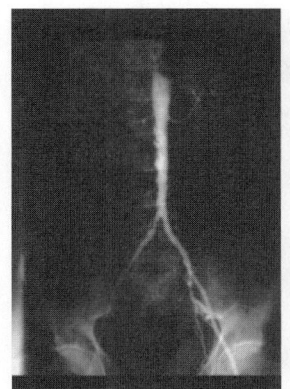 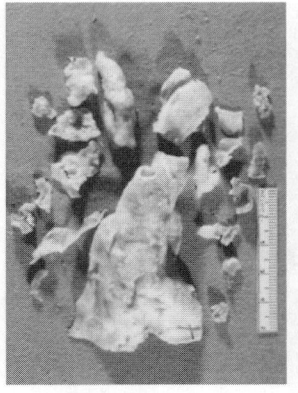 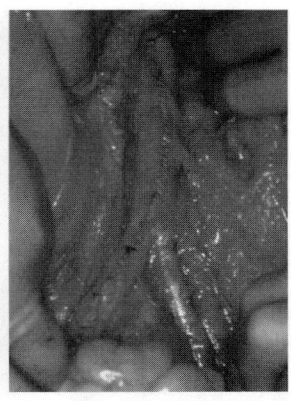

A **B** **C**

Figure 79.11. *(A)* Preoperative angiogram revealing diffuse infrarenal aorta atherosclerosis with severe right common iliac stenosis and right internal iliac occlusion (type I disease). *(B)* Atherosclerotic plaque is removed. *(C)* Long arteriotomy over the entire length of the infrarenal aorta and right common iliac artery is closed after the endarterectomy is complete.

aortic reconstruction. Pulmonary and renal function should also be routinely assessed because of the higher mortality associated with postoperative dysfunction of these organ systems.

Endovascular Treatment

Since the very first transarterial dilation procedures, percutaneous transluminal angioplasty (PTA) has become the standard and in some cases the preferred therapy for iliac artery occlusive disease. Like operative reconstruction, PTA at this site is likely to be successful because of the large caliber of the vessels and high rates of flow in the aortoiliac segment. The best results are obtained with short, focal, nonocclusive lesions in the common iliac arteries. Occlusions, stenoses longer than 10 cm, and external iliac lesions respond less favorably (14). Initial success rates as high as 80% to 90% and long-term patency rates of 70% to 80% have been reported. Complications (thrombosis, dissection, perforation, and distal embolism) in experienced hands are uncommon and can frequently be remedied with intraluminal stenting or thrombolytic therapy. Stents have made it possible to apply angioplasty in a larger number of lesions (e.g., longer occlusions) and may improve long-term patency rates by reducing rates of restenosis (15). In our practice, approximately 20% to 25% of patients presenting with lesions in the aortoiliac segment can be effectively treated with iliac PTA with or without stenting. This technique is particularly useful in high-risk patients, those with critical ischemia secondary to multiple-level disease, and patients in whom iliac PTA can be combined with an infrainguinal bypass for limb salvage. Even in good-risk patients with focal iliac disease,

however, PTA may be the preferred initial approach, with surgical intervention reserved for failures. If the presence of an appropriate lesion is suspected, PTA should be considered at the same time that the diagnostic arteriogram is performed.

In the most recent development in the endovascular treatment of aortoiliac occlusive disease, stented prosthetic grafts are placed in the diseased iliac segment through an open femoral artery cutdown. Early results are encouraging but far too preliminary to determine the eventual role of this new technique (16).

Endarterectomy

Endarterectomy was more commonly performed in the era before prosthetic graft conduits were developed. Currently, direct arterial repair is reserved for the management of focal atheroocclusive disease (type I) limited to the distal aorta and common iliac arteries (Figs. 79.11 and 79.12). When performed for this specific indication , aortoiliac endarterectomy can produce excellent long-term results, similar to those of aortofemoral grafting. Endarterectomy is less well suited for disease extending in the external iliac arteries and is to be avoided when aneurysmal degeneration complicates the primary atheroocclusive aortoiliac process.

The aorta and common iliac arteries are exposed and vascular control is secured. During dissection, care is taken to preserve the autonomic nerves overlying the aortic bifurcation so that normal sexual function is not disturbed. The patient is then heparinized and atraumatic occlusion clamps or tapes are applied. Arteriotomies are made over the aorta and the common iliac arteries to ex-

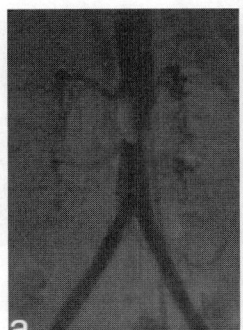 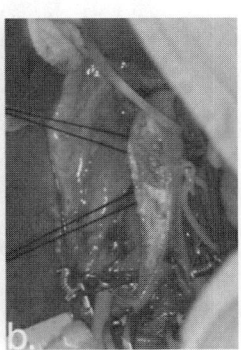 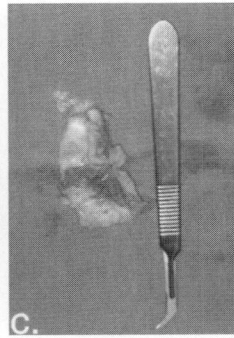 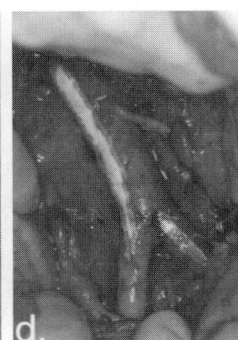

Figure 79.12. *(A)* Preoperative angiogram demonstrates severe stenosis of the infrarenal aorta with mild stenosis bilaterally at the origin of the common iliac arteries (type I disease). *(B)* Long arteriotomy over the infrarenal aorta and proximal right common iliac artery reveals advanced ulcerated luminal disease. A second, separate arteriotomy over the left common iliac artery was also created to approach plaque in that vessel. *(C)* Aortic component of the atherosclerotic plaque. *(D)* The two arteriotomies are closed, and polytetrafluoroethylene patches are used for angioplasty.

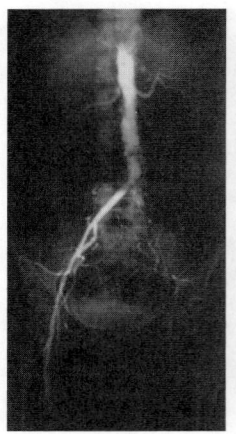
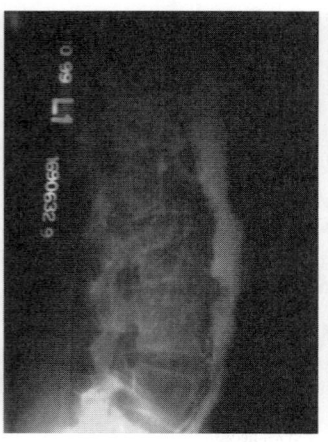
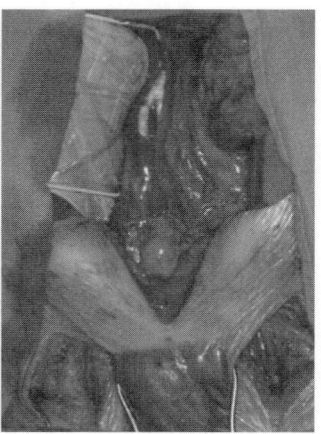

A **B** **C**

Figure 79.13. *(A,B)* Preoperative biplane aortogram demonstrates advanced preocclusive disease of the infrarenal aorta and its bifurcation with occlusion of the left common and external iliac arteries (type II disease). *(C)* Patient was treated with placement of an aortobifemoral prosthesis. The short shaft and limbs of the prosthesis are in a retroperitoneal location and are partially covered with a layer of posterior parietal peritoneum. The two groin incisions are kept open to display the anastomoses of the two limbs to the common femoral arteries.

pose the diseased lumen. The atherosclerotic plaque, along with the overlying intima and inner portion of the involved media, is removed. Good "breakoff" points for the removed plaques are needed to prevent postoperative thrombosis that results from the formation of an occluding flap of retained atheroma. The arteriotomies are closed by direct suture or with patch angioplasty, depending on vessel caliber.

Aortofemoral Prosthesis

Aortofemoral bypass is the most durable and reliable of all treatment options, for which reason it is the reference standard for the reconstruction of advanced aortoiliac occlusive disease (Figs. 79.13 and 79.14). The operative sequence starts with exposure of the abdominal aortic seg-

ment between the renal and inferior mesenteric arteries by means of appropriate retroperitoneal dissection and cephalad mobilization of the fourth portion of the duodenum and the left renal vein. Care is taken during dissection to avoid injury to the lumbar veins. Moreover, gentle handling of the dissected segment may lessen the risk for atheroembolism during the operation. The common, su-

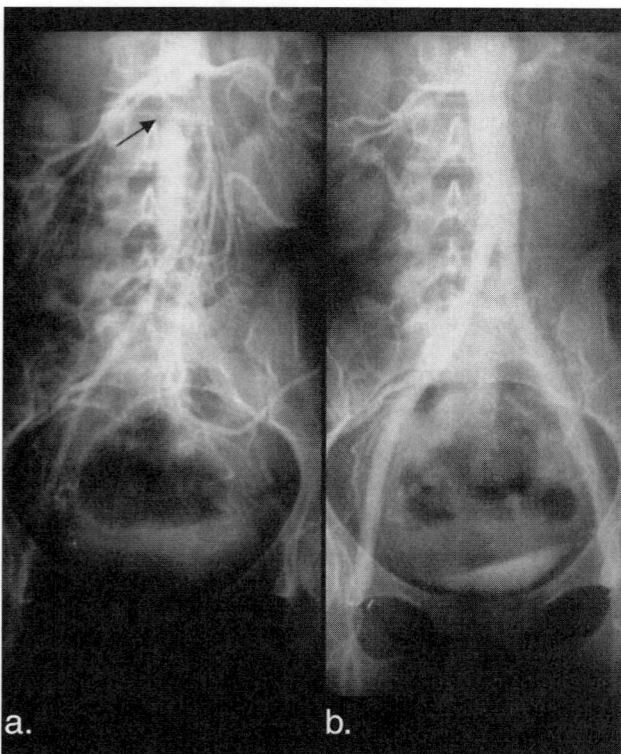

a.   b.

Figure 79.14. *(A)* Preoperative aortogram demonstrates advanced preocclusive disease of the infrarenal aorta and its bifurcation with occlusion of the left common and external iliac arteries (type II disease). *(B)* Aortography after placement of an aortobifemoral prosthesis.

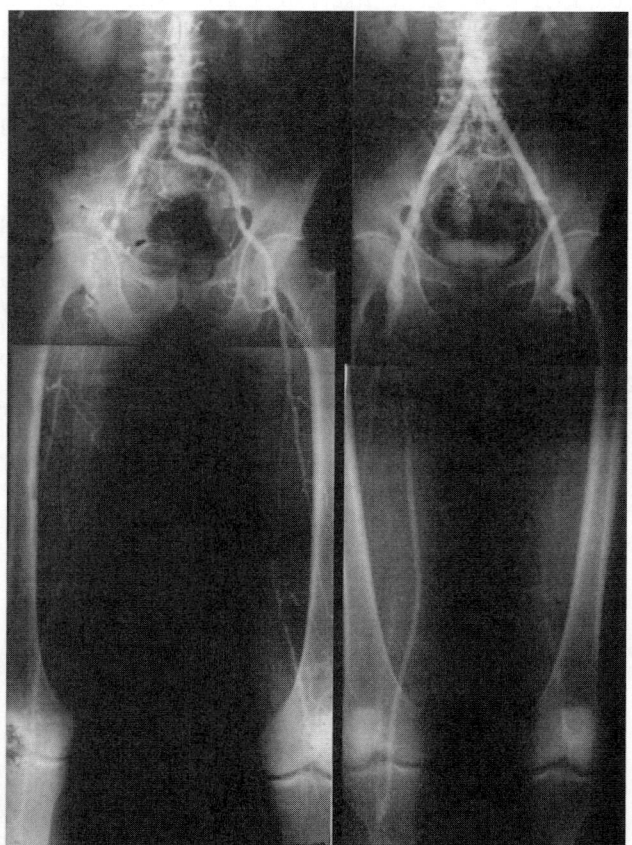

Figure 79.15. This diabetic patient presented with gangrene of the right first and second toes. Preoperative angiogram *(left)* revealed aortic bifurcation disease, right external iliac and superficial femoral arterial occlusion, and reconstitution of a heavily diseased right deep femoral artery. On the left, occlusion of the superficial femoral artery is seen, with a patent left deep femoral artery supplying the left leg (multiple-level type III disease). The patient underwent an aortobifemoral bypass with a concomitant right femoral-to-below knee popliteal bypass *(right)* to bring pulsatile flow to the diseased forefoot.

perficial, and deep femoral arteries are secured through separate groin incisions. Retroperitoneal tunnels are then developed between the exposed infrarenal aorta and the groins by means of blunt dissection. Care is taken to avoid injury to the bowel, particularly the rectosigmoid on the left. The tunnels are directed posterior to the ureter to avoid postoperative obstructive uropathy from graft limb compression of the ureter. A prosthesis of the appropriate size (polytetrafluoroethylene or Dacron) is selected, and the patient is heparinized. With an occluding clamp below the renal arteries and another just above the inferior mesenteric artery, the proximal anastomosis is performed

as either an end-to-end or end-to-side graft to the aorta. The end-to-side technique has been found to be just as good, depending on the pattern of occlusive lesions and opportunity to perfuse the internal iliac arteries. The proximal anastomosis is placed as close to the renal arteries as practical to prevent future compromise of the bypass resulting from progression of atherosclerosis in the remaining infrarenal cuff. The limbs of the prosthesis are then delivered through the retroperitoneal tunnels into the groins. The distal anastomoses are performed to the common femoral arteries and may be carried into the deep femoral arteries as needed. The technique for distal femoral anas-

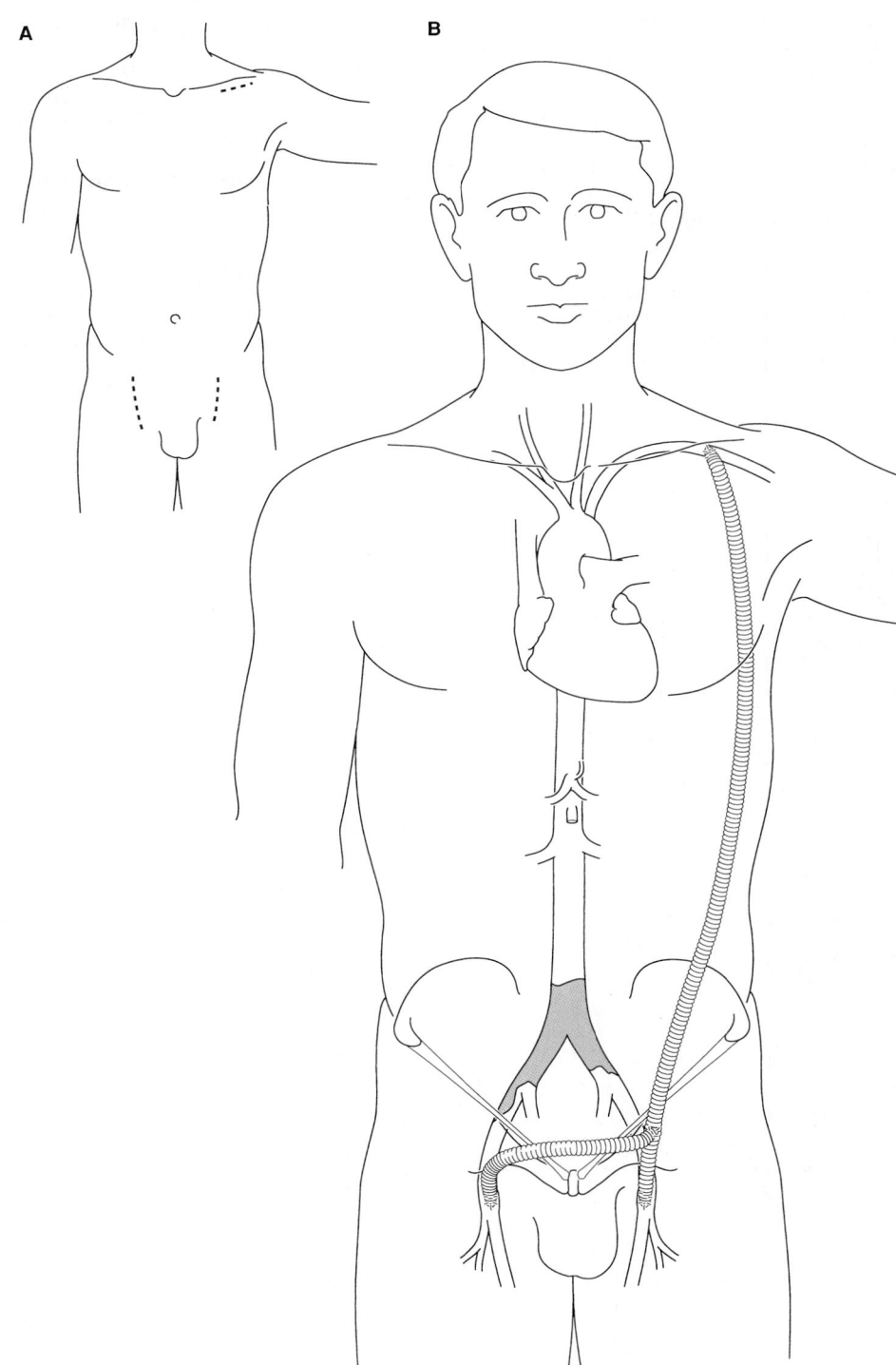

Figure 79.16. A unilateral axillary to upsilateral femoral artery bypass graft is supplemented with a cross-femoral-to-femoral artery bypass graft limb. This extraanatomic graft is frequently implanted on the right (although the artist's depiction shows the left) to allow unimpeded access to the thoraco-abdominal aorta when necessary.

tomosis is chosen to ensure adequate graft outflow, particularly if superficial femoral artery disease is present. In the patient with tissue loss secondary to type III or multiple-level aortoiliac disease associated with occluded superficial femoral arteries and compromised deep collaterals, concomitant distal reconstruction should rarely be required (Fig. 79.15).

Aortofemoral bypass has excellent 5- and 10-year graft patency rates of approximately 85% and 75%, respectively. Perioperative morbidity and mortality are reported to be below 10% and 5%, respectively, in many centers (12,17).

Axillofemoral Prosthesis

Axillofemoral extraanatomic reconstruction has been utilized for revascularization in poor-risk patients or those with a hostile abdomen and has been reported to be an acceptable alternative to aortofemoral prosthesis. The axillary artery supplying the arm with the higher systolic blood pressure is usually chosen as the inflow vessel. The operative sequence starts with exposure of the most proximal part of the axillary artery through an infraclavicular incision and splitting of the pectoralis major muscle between its sternal and clavicular heads. The common, superficial, and deep femoral arteries are then dissected through groin incisions. The axillary or long limb of an externally supported polytetrafluoroethylene graft is then advanced behind the pectoralis major muscle and through a subcutaneous tunnel in the anterior axillary line connecting the axillary artery and the ipsilateral groin. Next,

a crossfemoral-to-femoral limb of the graft is delivered through a subcutaneous suprapubic tunnel connecting the two groins. An anastomosis between the proximal axillary artery and the prosthesis is constructed in an end-graft to side-of-artery fashion. The graft is positioned parallel to the axillary artery and behind the pectoral muscles for the first 10 cm, before it enters the subcutaneous channel along the anterior axillary line. Following this plan seems to minimize traction on the anastomosis during arm movement and reduces the incidence of anastomotic disruption. The distal anastomoses are performed to the common femoral arteries and may be carried over or onto the deep femoral arteries to ensure adequate graft outflow (Fig. 79.16).

The reported 5-year patency of the axillofemoral graft varies widely (30% to 80%) but is generally accepted to be lower than the patency of an aortofemoral prosthesis. The axillobifemoral bypass should therefore be reserved for patients with bilateral advanced aortoiliac disease who are either poor surgical risks or have a hostile abdomen (18).

Other Prosthetic Reconstructions

For high-risk patients with diffuse advanced disease limited to one iliac artery, unilateral femorofemoral or iliofemoral bypass may be employed to revascularize the ischemic extremity. If the contralateral iliac artery is normal or bears a lesion that is well treated by angioplasty/stenting, crossfemoral-to-femoral artery bypass is worthy of consideration. Iliofemoral bypass has a modest graft patency advantage over femorofemoral bypass (70% vs.

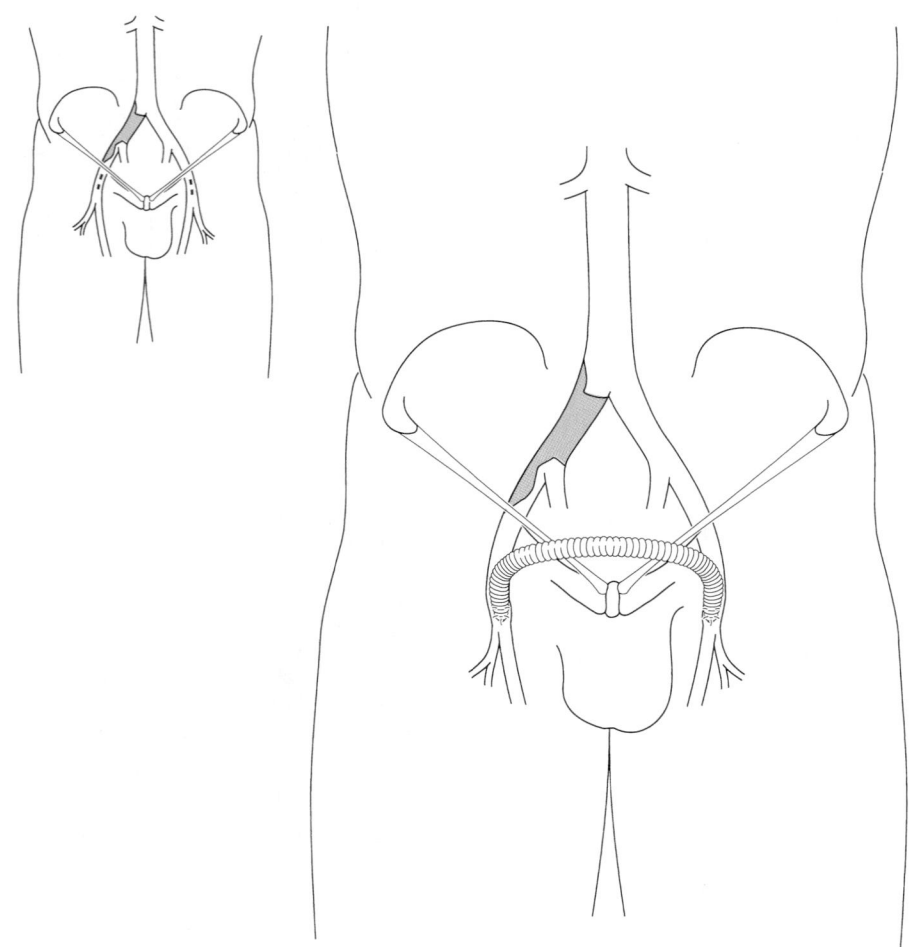

Figure 79.17. The crossfemoral-to-femoral artery bypass graft is well tolerated and can be performed with the patient under regional anesthesia.

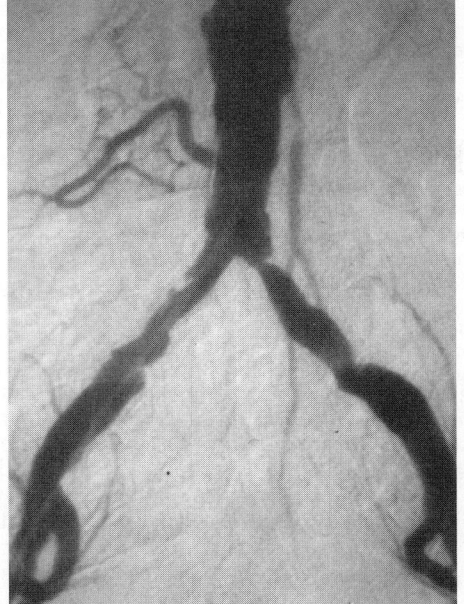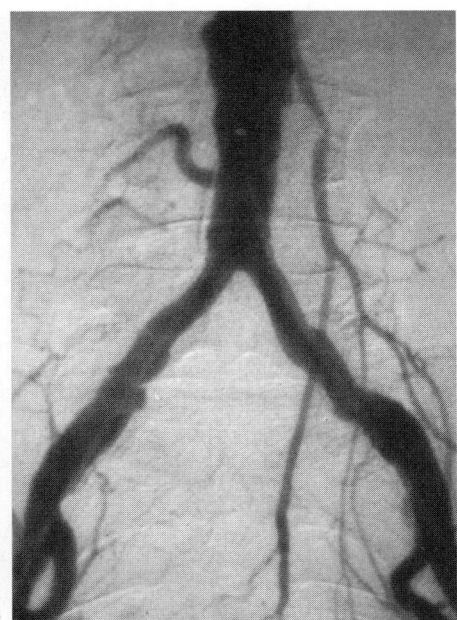

Figure 79.18. *(A)* Preoperative angiogram revealing severe focal proximal stenoses bilaterally in the common iliac arteries (type I disease). *(B)* Angioplasty was performed bilaterally with excellent immediate results.

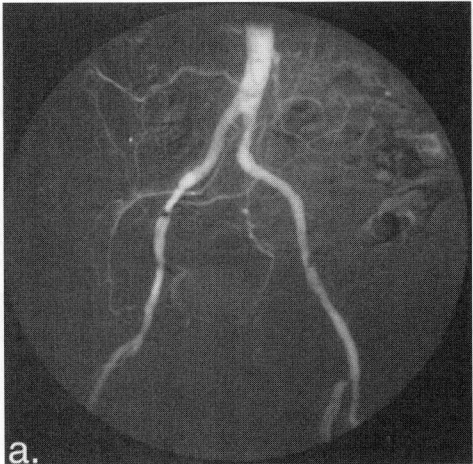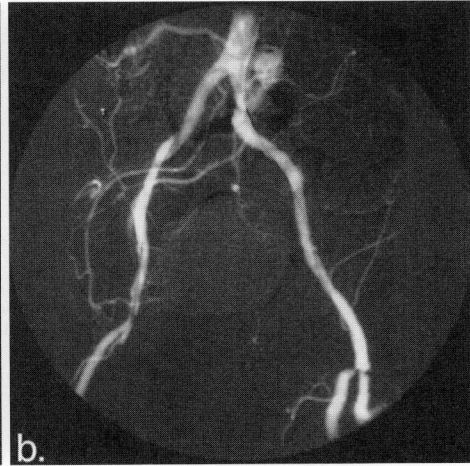

Figure 79.19. *(A)* Preoperative angiogram revealing severe focal stenoses in the external iliac arteries bilaterally and occluded internal iliac arteries. *(B)* Angioplasty and stenting were performed bilaterally on the external iliac arteries with good immediate results.

60%, respectively), but the main advantage is avoidance of a second groin incision and its associated complications. Femorofemoral bypasses are reserved for patients with occluded or heavily diseased common iliac arteries, in whom iliofemoral bypass is not advisable (Fig. 79.17).

Angioplasty and Stenting

Since its introduction in 1963 by Dotter (19), the technique of intraluminal arterial dilation has evolved through various refinements and become more frequently applied. In a prospective, randomized trial comparing angioplasty and operative repair in the treatment of claudication (functional ischemia) secondary to iliac occlusive disease, operations produced successful outcomes at 3 years in 81% of the patients, versus 62% for angioplasty. When angioplasty was used to treat either functional or critical limb ischemia secondary to iliac occlusive disease, an overall success rate of 50% at 3 years was achieved (13). The same study identified four variables predictive of success. Specifically, angioplasty results were best when (a) performed for claudication, (b) limited to a common iliac lesion, (c) applied for stenosis rather than occlusion, and (d) good distal runoff was present. The results of angioplasty are suboptimal in cases with a residual pressure

gradient, extensive plaque dissection, or significant recoil and residual stenosis, and the results can be improved by adding intraluminal stenting. In these cases, stenting may produce an incremental 10% improvement in the result of long-term angioplasty alone. Based on these findings, catheter-based interventions are currently reserved for the treatment of symptomatic short-segment stenoses of the common iliac arteries, either as primary treatment or as an adjunct to crossfemoral-to-femoral or femoral-to-distal graft reconstructions (Figs. 79.18 and 79.19).

REFERENCES

1. Kannel WB, Shurtleff D. The Framingham study: cigarettes and the development of intermittent claudication. *Geriatrics* 1973;28:61–68.
2. Hughson WG, Mann JI, Garrod A. Intermittent claudication: prevalence and risk factors. *Br Med J* 1978;1:1379–1381.
3. Leriche R, Morel A. The syndrome of thrombotic obliteration of the aortic bifurcation. *Ann Surg* 1948;127:193–206.
4. DeBakey ME, Lawrie GM, Glaeser DH. Patterns of atherosclerosis and their surgical significance. *Ann Surg* 1985;201:115–131.
5. Brewster DC, Darling RC. Optimal methods of aortoiliac reconstruction. *Surgery* 1978;84:739.
6. Kohler TR, Nance DR, Cramer MM, et al. Duplex scanning for

diagnosis of aortoiliac and femoropopliteal disease: a prospective study. *Circulation* 1987;76:1074–1080.

7. Girolami GB, Bernardi E, Prins MH, et al. Treatment of intermittent claudication with physical training, smoking cessation, pentoxifylline, or nafronyl: a meta-analysis. *Arch Intern Med* 1999;159:337–345.

8. Porter JM, Cutler BS, Lee BY, et al. Pentoxifylline efficacy in the treatment of intermittent claudication: multicenter controlled double-blind trial with objective assessment of chronic occlusive arterial disease patients. *Am Heart J* 1982;104:66–72.

9. Money SR, Herd JA, Isaacsohn JL, et al. Effects of cilostazol on walking distances in patients with intermittent claudication caused by peripheral vascular disease. *J Vasc Surg* 1998;27:267–275.

10. Haney TF, Debatin JF, Leung DA, et al. Evaluation of the aortoiliac and renal arteries: comparison of breath-hold, contrast-enhanced, three-dimensional MR angiography with conventional angiography. *Radiology* 1997;204:357–362.

11. Passman MA, Farber MA, Criado E, et al. Descending thoracic aortoiliofemoral artery bypass grafting: a role for primary revascularization for aortoiliac occlusive disease? *J Vasc Surg* 1999;29:249–258.

12. Szilagyi DE, Elliott JP Jr, Smith RF, et al. A thirty-year survey of the reconstructive surgical treatment of aortoiliac occlusive disease. *J Vasc Surg* 1986;3:421–436.

13. Hertzer NR, Young JR, Kramer JR, et al. Routine coronary angiography prior to elective aortic reconstruction: results of selective myocardial revascularization in patients with peripheral vascular disease. *Arch Surg* 1979;114:1336–1344.

14. Johnston KW, Rae M, Hogg-Johnston SA, et al. Five-year results of a prospective study of percutaneous transluminal angioplasty. *Ann Surg* 1987;206:403–413.

15. Henry M, Amor M, Ethevenot G, et al. Palmaz stent placement in iliac and femoropopliteal arteries: primary and secondary patency in 310 patients with 2- to 4-year follow-up. *Radiology* 1995;197:167.

16. Rutherford RB. Options in the surgical management of aortoiliac occlusive disease: a changing perspective. *Cardiovasc Surg* 1999;7:5–12.

17. Brewster DC. Current controversies in the management of aortoiliac occlusive disease. *J Vasc Surg* 1997;25:365–379.

18. Passman MA, Taylor LM, Moneta GL, et al. Comparison of axillofemoral and aortofemoral bypass for aortoiliac occlusive disease. *J Vasc Surg* 1996;23:263–269; discussion 269–271.

19. Dotter C, Judkins M. Transluminal treatment of arteriosclerotic obstruction: description of a new technic and a preliminary report of its application. *Circulation* 1964;30:654–670.

SURGERY: SCIENTIFIC PRINCIPLES AND PRACTICE, Third Edition, edited by Lazar J. Greenfield, Michael W. Mulholland, Keith T. Oldham, Gerald B. Zelenock, and Keith D. Lillemoe. Lippincott Williams & Wilkins Publishers, Philadelphia, © 2001.

CHAPTER 80

FEMOROPOPLITEAL AND INFRAPOPLITEAL OCCLUSIVE DISEASE

CAROL PROSS AND JULIE ANN FREISCHLAG

As the age of the population in the United States increases, the prevalence of lower extremity ischemia secondary to atherosclerosis is increasing. The American lifestyle contributes to the development and progression of this disease. Increasing evidence supports the fact that appropriate diet, exercise, and smoking cessation can prevent or delay the onset of vascular disease. However, despite education by physicians and the media, many patients continue to maintain habits that put them at high risk for the development of atherosclerosis. In addition, the role of predisposing factors such as diabetes and genetics are not clearly understood, and lower extremity ischemia develops in many patients without clearly identified risk factors. With the advent of new radiologic and operative technologies, the physician has a large array of interventions to offer. As therapeutic options have increased, so has the knowledge of risks, benefits, and indications. Physicians must be equipped with this knowledge to be able to treat the patient with lower extremity ischemia more effectively.

ANATOMY

The abdominal aorta divides at the fourth lumbar vertebra to give rise to the right and left common iliac arteries (Fig. 80.1). Each common iliac artery divides to form an internal and external iliac artery. The external iliac artery lies along the wall of the pelvis, and as it passes the inguinal ligament into the femoral triangle, it becomes the common femoral artery. The femoral triangle is bordered by the inguinal ligament superiorly, the sartorius muscle laterally, and the adductor longus muscle medially. The floor is made up of the iliacus, psoas major, and pectineus muscles. The femoral sheath courses through this triangle with its contents, the femoral nerve, common femoral artery, and femoral vein, laterally to medially.

The common femoral artery provides most of the blood to the lower extremity, although some collaterals are derived from the internal iliac artery. About 3 cm past the inguinal ligament, the common femoral artery divides to form the deep femoral artery laterally and posteriorly and the superficial femoral artery medially. The deep femoral artery gives off the medial and lateral circumflex arteries and three perforating arteries before terminating in the fourth perforating artery. Through these, the deep femoral artery provides most of the blood supply to the thigh muscles. Collaterals are found between these vessels and branches supplied by the internal iliac artery.

The superficial femoral artery travels deep to the sartorius muscle and then through the adductor (Hunter's) canal, where it becomes the popliteal artery. The superficial femoral artery gives off the descending genicular arteries. The popliteal artery exits the canal and travels posteriorly between the lateral and medial gastrocnemius heads. It gives off the superior lateral and medial genicular and inferior lateral and medial genicular arteries. These geniculate arteries form a complex collateral circulation at the knee with the descending branch of the lateral circumflex artery and branches of the anterior tibial artery.

Below the knee, the popliteal artery divides into the anterior tibial artery laterally and the posterior tibial–peroneal trunk medially. This trunk immediately divides into the posterior tibial artery medially and the peroneal artery laterally. These three arteries supply blood to the lower leg and foot. The anterior tibial artery begins at the lower border of the popliteal muscle and passes between the two heads of the tibialis posterior muscle and then through the interosseous membrane, where it courses alongside the deep peroneal nerve in the anterior compartment. It gives off the anterior and posterior tibial recurrent, fibular, anterior medial and anterior lateral malleolar, and muscular branches. It then passes the ankle joint, where it becomes the dorsalis pedis artery.

The posterior tibial artery lies posterior to the tibia and continues posteriorly to the medial malleolus and into the foot. It gives off the posterior medial malleolar, communicating, medial calcaneal, and muscular branches, and then in the foot it gives off the medial and lateral plantar arteries.

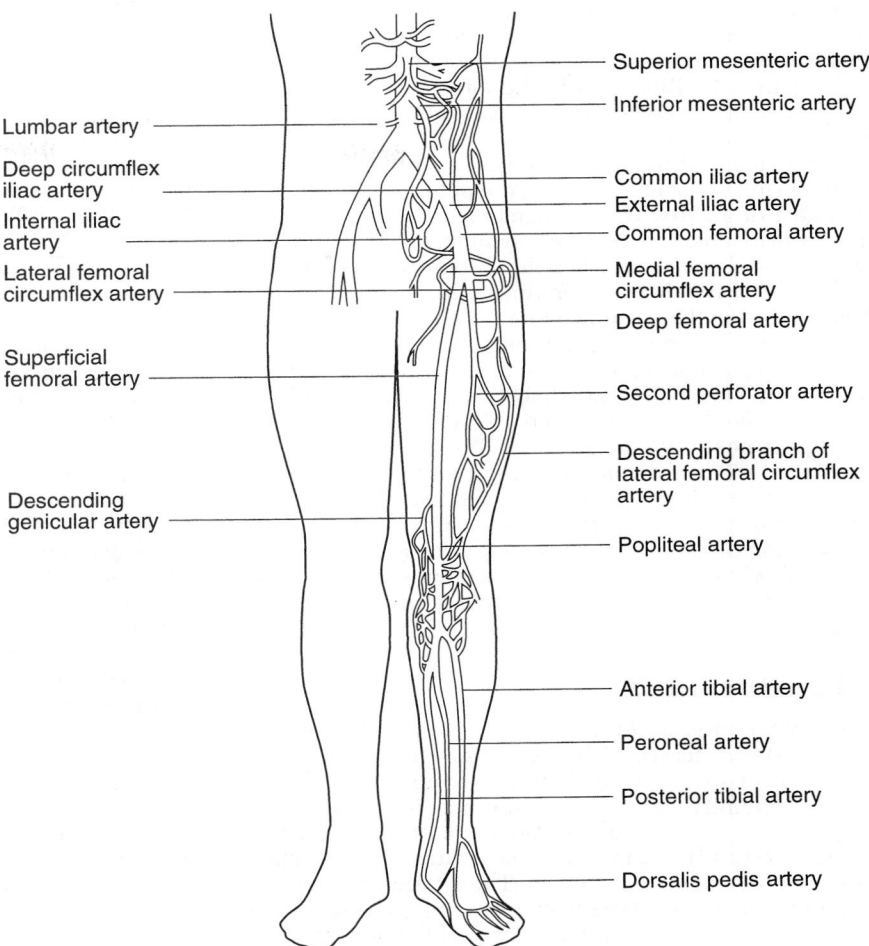

Figure 80.1. Arterial anatomy of the lower extremity. Note the well-developed collateral network around each joint.

The peroneal artery lies between the tibialis posterior and flexor hallucis longus muscles. It gives rise to the perforating, communicating, lateral calcaneal, muscular, and nutrient branches. These various branches of the anterior and posterior tibial and peroneal arteries form multiple collaterals around the ankle joint and in the foot.

PATHOLOGY AND PATHOPHYSIOLOGY

Multiple causes of lower extremity ischemia are recognized, but by far the most predominant is atherosclerotic disease. Other causes include arteritis, antiphospholipid syndrome, popliteal aneurysms, adventitial cystic disease, popliteal artery entrapment, and trauma.

The favorable anatomy of the lower extremity helps to prevent progressive ischemia. The collateral circulation allows for blood flow to all areas of the lower extremity in the face of localized occlusive disease. Also, through complex neurohumoral control, the muscle arterial resistance can be decreased to allow a large increase in blood flow. This is physiologic during exercise and compensatory during ischemia. However, as occlusive disease progresses, it usually involves multiple sites in the lower extremity vasculature. The first symptoms are noted by the patient during exercise because the leg is no longer able to increase blood delivery in the normal fashion. Claudication, which is reproducible lower extremity muscle pain on walking that is relieved by rest, develops. The site of pain depends on the arteries involved but in general is one level distal to the site of occlusion. Most commonly, it includes the calf.

As ischemic disease progresses, blood flow is also decreased at rest. When the decrease limits normal metabolic function, a level of critical ischemia is reached. With critical ischemia, the patient experiences rest pain and wounds are unable to heal, so that the patient is predisposed to infection, gangrene, and limb loss (Fig. 80.2). Those with gan-

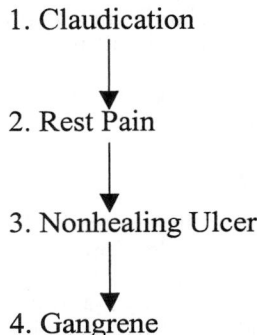

1. Claudication

2. Rest Pain

3. Nonhealing Ulcer

4. Gangrene

Figure 80.2. Levels of ischemia. As the blood supply decreases with arterial disease, a patient can be expected to progress through the various levels of ischemia. In claudication, the blood supply is unable to meet increased requirements during exercise. As ischemia advances to rest pain, the blood supply is further limited and unable to meet baseline needs at rest. With nonhealing ulcers, the blood supply is minimal and unable to provide the nutrients necessary for healing. Once the extremity progresses to gangrene, the blood supply is minimal and unable to maintain the life of the limb.

grene and infection require emergent hospitalization, antibiotics, debridement, and revascularization. Otherwise, limb loss will occur within the next few weeks.

Rest pain initially begins in the forefoot (metatarsalgia) and toes and progresses proximally. Patients often notice a beneficial effect of gravity on their arterial blood flow. They complain of night pain and may let their legs hang over the side of the bed in a dependent fashion to increase the effect of gravity, which augments minimal perfusion and decreases pain. Conversely, symptoms of rest pain are provoked and worsened when the extremity is elevated. In patients with rest pain, ulcerations and infection usually develop during the ensuing 6 months and lead to amputation if no revascularization has been undertaken.

It should be noted that ischemic disease does not always progress. In fact, 75% of nondiabetic patients with mild to moderate claudication have no worsening of symptoms during the next 5 years, and only 5% to 7% require amputation (1). Thus, when evaluating a patient with claudication, the physician should limit the use of procedures; all are associated with a risk for mortality, and they may increase the limb threat. A clear judgment should be made regarding whether an intervention is required according to the degree that the patient's life-style is inhibited by the inability to walk.

Atherosclerosis

Atherosclerosis is the number one cause of lower extremity arterial disease. Atherosclerosis affects the arteries of the lower extremity frequently, whereas those of the upper extremity are rarely affected. The superficial femoral artery is the most frequent site of of multiple lesions, specifically in the area of the adductor canal, where early stenosis most often occurs. The arteries of the lower extremity are more subject to changes in flow velocity, depending on exercise, than other areas of the body, and the hydrostatic pressure is higher in these vessels. A lack of exercise may favor plaque formation as a consequence of lower flow rates. It has been postulated that because the adductor canal region of the superficial femoral artery is unable to dilate, intimal plaque causes a greater degree of constriction and thus hemodynamic effects that may lead to the development of atherosclerosis.

Atherogenesis, marked by the initiation and progression of processes followed by healing and remodeling, is not continuous. Thus, atherosclerosis may not always lead to stenosis or clinically significant complications. Why the disease progresses in some and not in others is still unknown. Much research is devoted to inhibiting progression and promoting regression by manipulating various predisposing factors.

Predisposing Factors

As with all vascular disease, multiple factors have been identified that affect the development and progression of atherosclerosis and thus arterial disease leading to ischemia of the lower extremity (Table 80.1). Heredity plays a role through both identified genetic diseases and less clearly identified mechanisms. Thus, a detailed family history of peripheral vascular disease, cardiac disease, cerebrovascular disease, and other stigmata of atherosclerosis can be helpful in identifying patients at risk for the development and progression of atherosclerosis.

Tobacco use, especially cigarette smoking, is the number one preventable cause of peripheral vascular disease. It is known to promote atherosclerosis. Multiple factors have been identified within tobacco smoke that play a role in atherogenesis and peripheral vascular disease via hemato-

Table 80.1. SELECTED RISK FACTORS FOR ATHEROSCLEROSIS

Diabetes
Smoking
Hypertension
Genetics
Obesity
Hypercholesterolemia
Hyperlipidemia

logic, neurohormonal, metabolic, hemodynamic, genetic, and biochemical pathways. Cessation of smoking can halt progression of disease and has been shown to lead to regression over time. In fact, in one study, 11.4% of patients with claudication who continued to smoke required amputation, whereas none of those who quit smoking required amputation (2).

Buerger's disease (thromboangiitis obliterans), which affects small vessels of the hands and feet, is a rare cause of lower extremity ischemia in the United States, being more common in the Middle and Far East. It is a chronic inflammation of the neurovascular bundle that leads to blood vessel thrombosis and fibrosis. Buerger's disease usually affects men in the third and fourth decades and is always associated with tobacco use. Cessation of smoking stops progression of the disease.

Diabetes mellitus predisposes a person to the development of atherosclerotic disease. In the diabetic patient, atherogenesis occurs at a younger age and progresses at a faster rate than in the nondiabetic. Diabetic atherosclerosis affects the distal leg arteries more than the aorta and iliac arteries. Involvement of small vessels is often noted in diabetics. In combination with diabetic peripheral neuropathy, such involvement increases the frequency of foot lesions, infection, and limb threat. The evaluation of lower extremity vascular disease in diabetic patients is often complicated by the presence of calcific medial sclerosis, which prevents the accurate measurement of ankle pressures because the vessels cannot be compressed. Toe pressures can often be substituted to determine the severity of disease.

Hypercholesterolemia, hyperlipidemia, obesity, and hypertension have been shown to be predisposing factors for atherosclerosis and lower extremity ischemic disease. These conditions can be familial or specific to the individual patient. Dietary and drug therapies can lessen the progression of atherosclerosis in patients with these problems.

Hypercoagulable states may contribute to the development of peripheral vascular disease, although arterial thrombosis is much less common than venous thrombosis. When arterial thrombosis does occur, it predominantly affects patients over the age of 50 years with other risk factors. Thrombi develop at sites of vessel injury where shear stress is elevated. Histologically, they are composed mostly of platelets, and disorders of platelet function and the vessel wall predispose a patient to arterial thrombosis. Disease processes include homocystinuria, abnormalities of lipoprotein(a), and fibromuscular dysplasia. A hypercoagulable state should be suspected in a patient with recurrent venous thromboembolism; unexplained thromboembolism before the age of 45 years; intraperitoneal, retroperitoneal, or cerebral thrombosis; diffuse cutaneous microvascular thrombosis; or a family history of thrombosis.

PATIENT EVALUATION

A detailed, problem-oriented history and physical examination are vital in the evaluation of lower extremity ischemia (Tables 80.2 and 80.3). Patients usually present

Table 80.2. **HISTORY**

I. Present illness
  A. Pain
    1. Type (claudication versus rest pain)
    2. Location
    3. Dependency versus elevation
  B. Nonhealing ulcers
  C. Infection
II. Past medical history
  A. Diabetes mellitus
  B. Cardiac history
  C. Hypertension
  D. Coagulopathic disorders/hypercoagulable states
  E. Hypercholesterolemia/hyperlipidemia
III. Social history
  A. Smoking
  B. Activity level
IV. Family history
  A. Peripheral vascular disease
  B. Coagulopathy disorders/hypercoagulable states
  C. Cardiac disease
  D. Stroke

with specific complaints characteristic of peripheral vascular disease, and the history often suggests the diagnosis before the physical examination or any additional studies are performed. Pain is the most common complaint. The characteristics of the pain can indicate the urgency of the problem and the risk for limb loss or infection. Chronic ischemic complaints are usually either claudication or rest pain. In diabetic patients, peripheral neuropathy may decrease or even eliminate pain, and the chief complaint may be one of nonhealing ulcers, infection, or dry or even wet gangrene. Peripheral neuropathy can also cause a severe, burning dysesthesia that can be hard to differentiate from ischemic pain. However, the pain of peripheral neuropathy is usually constant and is present in a stocking distribution over both lower legs. In addition, neuropathic pain often involves the hands and upper extremities (stocking–glove distribution).

The location of pain also assists in the diagnosis. The pain of claudication is usually one level distal to the oc-

Table 80.3. **PHYSICAL EXAMINATION**

I. Appearance
  A. Color
    1. Pallor
    2. Dependent rubor
  B. Hair growth
  C. Muscle mass
  D. Deformities/lesions: location
  E. Nail thickening
  F. Skin appearance
II. Touch
  A. Temperature
  B. Capillary refill
  C. Tenderness
  D. Elevation
III. Pulses
  A. Femoral
  B. Popliteal
  C. Dorsum pedis
  D. Posterior tibial
IV. Stethoscope for bruits
V. Other vascular disease
  A. Carotid examination
  B. Abdominal examination
  C. Cardiac examination
VI. Other nonvascular systems for preoperative evaluation

clusion. Thus, an occlusion of the superficial femoral artery may cause calf claudication. Proximal disease may influence a distal lesion and make it hemodynamically significant; for example, distal symptoms may be caused by aortoiliac disease.

Ischemic rest pain is often nocturnal. It usually involves the distal foot and progresses proximally. Proximal rest pain is rare without distal pain. Patients often describe sleeping with legs off the bed or in a recliner, rubbing the foot, or walking to decrease pain. While the "five *ps*" (pain, paresthesia, pallor, paralysis, and pulselessness) of acute ischemia are helpful in the evaluation of infrainguinal ischemia, they are not always evident in the patient with chronic lower extremity ischemia.

A careful cardiac history is important in the patient with suspected peripheral vascular disease. Cardiac disease in itself is a risk factor for lower extremity ischemia, and because atherosclerosis is a systemic disease, some coronary occlusive disease is found in almost all patients with lower extremity atherosclerosis. Also, as the median age of the population increases, the prevalence and extent of coronary artery disease will increase. This coexistence of coronary and peripheral vascular disease is important; a frequent complication during coronary bypass is symptomatic lower extremity ischemia. The complications of interventions for peripheral artery disease account for 70% of the associated morbidity and mortality. It is therefore important for the cardiac surgeon to evaluate the patient for peripheral artery disease and the vascular surgeon to evaluate the patient for coronary artery disease before intervention is undertaken.

The past medical history and family history should focus on diseases predisposing to ischemia. The social history should include an inquiry about tobacco use and the patient's normal activity level.

During the physical examination, a full vascular examination should be performed because vascular disease can present in multiple areas at once (Table 80.3). Special attention should be given to the heart and aorta as possible sources of emboli, especially if blue-toe syndrome is noted (see Chapter 79). A bilateral examination of the lower extremities should be performed, and the two extremities should be compared and any differences noted. The examiner should assess the extremities for color (pallor or dependent rubor, a purplish erythema in the distal lower extremity during dependency that decreases on elevation in advanced ischemia), hair growth, muscle mass, deformities, and lesions. Decreased hair growth is one of the first signs of ischemia. Nail thickening may be noted. More advanced ischemic changes include skin atrophy or shine. Muscle wasting is often late, and unless it is unilateral, it may be difficult to identify. Ischemic lesions are very painful and tend to occur distally or on the dorsum of the foot. In contrast, the ulcers of venous stasis are usually on the lower third of the leg or over bony prominences and are not very painful. Neurotrophic ulcers tend to form under callus or at pressure points. On touch, temperature, capillary refill, and tenderness should be noted. Elevation of the lower extremity can result in the development of pallor, and dependency can cause the erythema of dependent rubor, seen in advanced ischemia, to return. Finally, the pulses should be examined for strength and bilateral equality. Specifically, the femoral, popliteal, dorsal pedal, and posterior tibial pulses should be examined. A hand-held Doppler probe can be used if the pulse is too weak to be palpated. Listening with a stethoscope for potential bruits can also aid in the detection of a suspected stenosis and can easily be done over the carotid and common femoral arteries and the abdomen.

By the end of the history and physical examination, a diagnosis can usually be reached. The level of stenosis can also be appreciated by a diminished or absent pulse just beyond the level of the lesion. Ischemia can be categorized as critical or noncritical. Further evaluation can then serve multiple purposes by confirming the level of stenosis, providing baseline values with which to detect progression or regression of disease, and indicating the appropriateness of operative treatment options.

Noninvasive Techniques

The Doppler examination can be used in infrainguinal occlusive disease to evaluate the blood supply of the lower extremity, confirm the presence of disease, and obtain a base measurement from which the evolution of disease and response to therapy can be monitored (see Chapters 71 and 79). In itself, it does not provide a precise measurement of the extent of disease; rather, it is a semiquantitative assessment of circulation in the lower extremity.

The ankle–brachial index (ABI) can easily be determined with the Doppler technique (Fig. 80.3). The ABI is a rough evaluation of blood flow and has been useful in predicting the likelihood of wound healing. In a study by Barnes et al. (3), amputations healed in all patients with an ABI above 70%, whereas healing did not occur in 25% of those with an ABI below 70%. Advantages in obtaining this test are that it is simple and inexpensive and can be performed at the bedside or in the vascular laboratory. It is an excellent means to evaluate and monitor claudication. It is not very specific and does not define the anatomy. Results in the diabetic patient are often unreliable because of abnormal wall calcification and noncompressibility. Toe pressures may be more reliable than the ABI in diabetic patients. A pneumatic or photoplethysmographic cuff is used to measure toe pressures. In normal persons, toe pressures are roughly 5 to 10 mm Hg lower than arm pressures. Rest pain usually develops below 20 to 30 mm Hg, although ischemic ulcers are usually present at somewhat higher levels.

Additional information can be obtained by measuring pressures at various levels of the lower extremity. In this way, the location of a lesion can be approximated because gradients of more than 20 mm Hg are diagnostic of a hemodynamically significant lesion.

Duplex ultrasonography can be used to examine vessels from the distal aorta to the tibial branches. This modality measures the velocity of blood flow through the arteries and provides additional information on flow as well as ultrasonographic images of the vessels themselves. With advances in technology and more sophisticated ultrasonographic machines, this technique has improved such that its specificity and sensitivity in the diagnosis of lesions occluding the vascular lumen by more than 50% are in the 90% range (4).

When peripheral vascular occlusive disease is suspected despite relatively normal resting ABI values, an exercise stress test can be performed. An increase in blood flow velocity through a fixed stenosis causes additional energy to be lost because of turbulence and the amplified hemodynamic effects of such lesions. If a cardiac condition or other circumstances preclude an exercise stress test, one can administer a reactive hyperemia stress test to the same end.

At present, magnetic resonance angiography is of limited use in the lower extremity. In a patient who is a poor candidate for conventional angiography, magnetic resonance angiography may be an alternate choice.

Invasive Techniques

Angiography is the gold standard for evaluating lower extremity ischemic disease. It can visualize blood flow from the aorta to the distal foot arteries and defines the location and extent of arterial disease (see Chapter 72).

Before a surgical bypass is undertaken, clear and precise anatomic knowledge from an arteriogram is vital. The aorta and iliac arteries must be evaluated because disease in these areas may amplify the distal symptoms and influence the planned procedure. A runoff study to the level of the ankle or plantar arch is usually performed. Hemodynamically significant lesions are identified by a reduction in the cross-sectional area of 75% or more or a 50% decrease in diameter. Reactive hyperemia or pharmacologic angiography can increase blood flow and improve the study results.

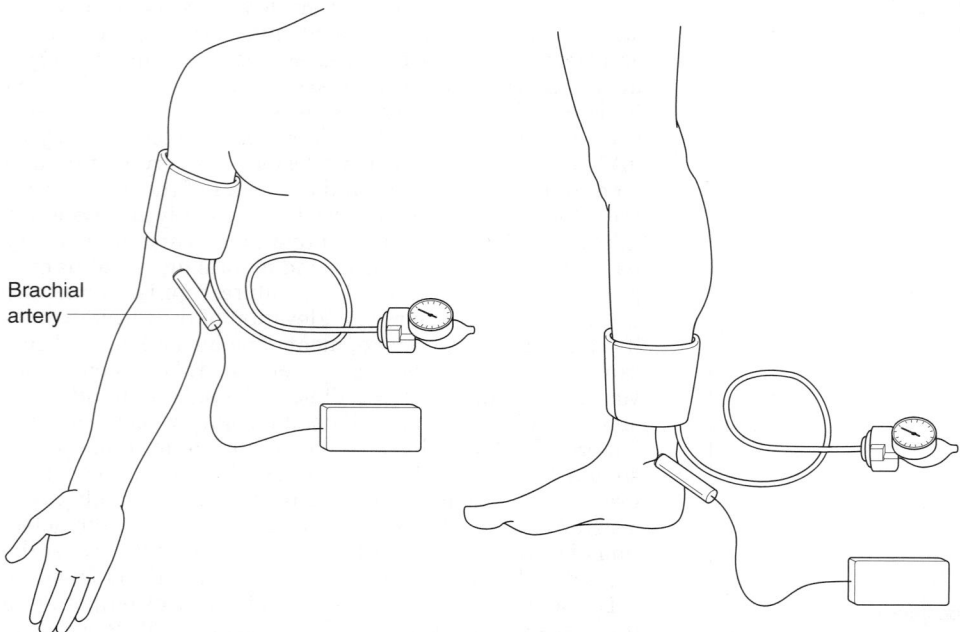

Brachial artery

Figure 80.3. Measurement of the ankle–brachial index. The systolic blood pressure is determined at the ankle and at the brachial artery. For each leg, the blood pressure is determined at the posterior tibial artery and the anterior tibial/dorsalis pedis artery. A simple ratio between the ankle pressure(s) and the highest (*either right or left*) brachial pressure is then constructed. Measurement of the ankle–brachial index is a quick, noninvasive test that can be performed at the bedside to estimate blood flow in the lower extremity.

To visualize the entire lower extremity arterial tree properly, a substantial dye load and multiple exposures are necessary. In the patient with renal insufficiency, this can be problematic. Other risks include contrast hypersensitivity and local and distal complications. The risk for contrast hypersensitivity is less than 3%, and the rate of local puncture site complications (e.g., bleeding, hematoma, thrombosis, pseudoaneurysm, and the creation of an arteriovenous fistula between the artery and vein at the puncture site) is less than 1% to 2%. The risk for local thrombosis with limb-threatening ischemia is less than 1%. Distal complications can also develop, including embolism with subsequent thromboses, which can also lead to limb threat and loss.

Although angiography is an important and vital part of the evaluation of the presurgical vascular patient, it carries real risk. Thus, careful thought is necessary before arteriography is attempted, and if intervention is not planned, angiography should not be performed. This is especially true in claudication. Conservative management of claudication does not include angiography.

TREATMENT

It is important to differentiate between infrainguinal disease that is causing claudication and limiting activity and infrainguinal disease that is threatening a limb. When limb-threatening ischemia is present, surgical intervention must be considered. In claudication, on the other hand, surgical intervention should be used only in those patients whose life-style is significantly compromised. The inability to work or carry out the normal activities of daily living is a reasonable indication for intervention in good-risk patients. In patients at high risk for operative morbidity, however, alternate strategies or less risky operations may be warranted. When a treatment plan is chosen, the patient's overall health, ways of using the extremity, and coexisting disease processes must be considered.

Conservative Therapy

Optimal control of all modifiable atherosclerotic risk factors, such as hypertension, lipid disorders, and diabetes, is desirable. All patients with peripheral vascular disease should be strongly urged to stop smoking. This alone is the most effective treatment for claudication. Quick and Cotton (5) noted significant improvement in the ABI and distance walked (mean improvement of 214 to 300 m) when patients with claudication stopped smoking. In the study of Jurgens et al. (2), 11.4% of patients with claudication who continued to smoke required amputation, whereas none of those who quit smoking required amputation.

Patients should also be urged to begin a walking program. They often misinterpret their pain as a sign of impending damage and so decrease their activity level; they must be encouraged not to do this. Formal walking programs have been shown to increase the overall distance that patients can walk before pain begins. Various studies have shown the increase in distance walked to be between 80% and 234%. Creasy et al. (6) showed the long-term benefits of exercise programs to be greater than those of angioplasty. Walking programs might, in theory, increase the number of collateral vessels and so increase blood delivery and relieve claudication, but this has never been shown to be the case, and ABI values do not increase. The alternative explanation for the increase in distances walked is an improvement in muscular oxygen extraction and metabolic efficiency.

Foot care in the diabetic patient is of vital importance in preventing the complications of peripheral vascular disease. Diabetic patients are predisposed to the development of foot lesions because of peripheral neuropathy, poor wound healing, and an increased susceptibility to infection. These factors are all compounded by poor blood flow. In addition to the early recognition and treatment of lesions, prevention is essential; patients must wear suitable shoes and examine their feet regularly. Regular visits to a podiatrist are helpful.

Optimal control of blood glucose in diabetic patients lessens the progression of peripheral vascular disease. Regular exercise and dietary adjustments to decrease elevated cholesterol levels and promote weight loss also slow the progression of disease in diabetics and nondiabetics alike.

Many of the above recommendations and treatments entail basic life-style changes, and good compliance is required for optimal effect. Programs for smoking cessation, support groups, and counseling by dietitians may help the patient to make the necessary changes.

Pharmacologic Therapy

Various drug therapies are being used in the treatment of lower extremity ischemia. Of note are hemorrheologic, antiplatelet, and metabolic enhancing agents.

Hemorrheologic drugs work on the basis that a decrease in viscosity will result in an increase in blood flow, as per Poiseulle's law. Red blood cell mass and fibrinogen are the major determinants of viscosity in vivo. Ernst et al. (7) showed a reduction in claudication with a decrease in hematocrit. Therapeutic anemia is impractical in most cases but should be considered in polycythemia. A decrease in viscosity can also be achieved through pharmacologic means. If cessation of smoking and a walking program do not adequately relieve symptoms of claudication, a trial of pentoxifylline may be undertaken. Pentoxifylline is a theobromine derivative that has been shown to increase blood filtration and decrease platelet aggregation and plasma fibrinogen in vitro. In vivo, it increases blood flow in the lower extremity and increases muscle oxygen tension. In various trials, pentoxifylline relieved symptoms of claudication and enabled patients to increase their walking distance, although fewer than half of them doubled their walking distance. It has also been suggested that pentoxifylline promotes healing of ulcers. Side effects include dizziness and gastrointestinal complaints, especially nausea.

Cilostazol is a drug recently approved for the treatment of claudication. It is a phosphodiesterase inhibitor that suppresses platelet aggregation and also acts as a direct vasodilator. In a prospective, randomized trial that included 77 patients, the mean distance that patients could walk before the onset of claudication increased by 58%, and the increase in maximum distance walked was 63% (8). Further study of this drug in larger groups of patients with claudication are needed to confirm efficacy.

Antiplatelet agents include aspirin, nonsteroidal antiinflammatory drugs, calcium channel blockers, prostaglandins, ticlopidine, and thromboxane synthetase inhibitors. The most frequently used of these is aspirin. Aspirin blocks the production of thromboxane A_2, which is a stimulus of platelet aggregation. Unlike the effects of other nonsteroidal antiinflammatory drugs, those of aspirin are irreversible. Although no direct benefit on lower extremity ischemia is known, aspirin has been shown to increase survival by reducing the incidence of myocardial infarction and stroke in patients with atherosclerotic disease (9).

Thromboxane synthetase inhibitors are vasodilators, and they inhibit platelet aggregation via a slightly different mechanism. Ticlopidine inhibits adenosine diphosphate receptors. It has been shown to decrease blood viscosity and may function via hemorrheologic effects. It has not been shown to relieve symptoms of claudication in clinical trials.

Metabolic enhancing agents enhance the metabolism of ischemic muscle. Carnitine is under investigation as a potential therapy for claudication. Carnitine acts to facilitate the entry of pyruvate into the citric acid cycle. Thus, it decreases lactate and increases adenosine triphosphate. Ischemic muscle is relatively deficient in carnitine, so that it is inefficient during anaerobic metabolism. Brevetti et al. (10) demonstrated an increase in walking distance in patients with claudication. Further trials are under way.

Endovascular Therapy

Discrete stenotic lesions and acute thrombosis are amenable to endovascular therapy. Discrete lesions of the superficial and deep femoral arteries have been successfully treated with percutaneous transluminal angioplasty (PTA). In this technique, a catheter is inserted into the artery, usually via an ipsilateral or contralateral femoral artery approach. The catheter is equipped with a balloon that can be inflated at the site of the lesion. The balloon causes the atherosclerotic intima to rupture and stretches the media. Increased blood flow allows for continued patency. PTA can be complicated by neointimal hyperplasia, which can lead to partial or total reocclusion. The atherosclerotic lesion can also re-form over time.

Success rates for PTA of the femoropopliteal arteries are about 85% (11), and a 5-year patency rate of 52% was noted by Rutherford et al. (12). The use of stents to maintain patency distal to the iliac artery has actually proved to decrease patency and at this time is not warranted. The success of PTA depends on patient selection. Because it carries a complication risk of about 4%, it should be reserved for patients in whom this risk is warranted; therefore, many patients with claudication are not candidates. Patients who are candidates for standard surgical therapy are potential candidates for PTA. The best results are observed in those with short focal lesions. The size of the vessel also must be taken into account; initial success rates are higher in larger vessels. Good runoff is important for patency. Thus, distal disease increases the risk for restenosis and failure, and the consequences would be devastating if acute thrombosis were to occur during the procedure.

In high-risk surgical patients with longer or multiple lesions, PTA may be a better alternative, even though success rates will be lower. PTA has also been used successfully as an adjunct to surgery to improve inflow for a more distal bypass and outflow for a more proximal bypass. Stenosis in bypass grafts is also amenable to PTA. Recently, PTA has been used to treat tibial artery stenosis and occlusion. Although results are not as yet well quantified, it is anticipated that patency and success rates will be lower than those for PTA in the femoropopliteal region.

Percutaneous transluminal angioplasty offers several potential advantages. Hospital stay and expense are lessened, although the procedure may have to be repeated. Morbidity and mortality are less for PTA than for surgery. The risks of PTA are similar to those of angiography and include bleeding, thrombosis, infection, pseudoaneurysm or arteriovenous fistula formation, and distal embolization and possible thrombus formation. These are particularly important to consider when PTA is planned for a patient with non–limb-threatening ischemia.

In the event of acute lower extremity ischemia, an immediate angiogram is optimal and fibrinolytic therapy may be warranted. The currently used fibrinolytic agents include streptokinase, urokinase, and tissue plasminogen activator. Other agents are being developed. Fibrinolytic agents function by stimulating the conversion of plasminogen to plasmin and thus triggering lysis of clot. In fibrinolytic therapy, a catheter is inserted into the clot and the fibrinolytic agent is infused into the clot during the ensuing hours along with heparin.

Complications of fibrinolytic therapy are similar to those of PTA, but hemorrhage is the major complication and patients must be monitored closely. An advantage of PTA is that it does not activate plasminogen outside the clot and so has less of a systemic effect. Streptokinase carries a risk for allergy and anaphylaxis, and hypothermia develops in one third of patients who receive streptokinase. Fever develops in only 2% to 3% of patients treated with urokinase. Contraindications to fibrinolytic therapy include a central nervous system ischemic or hemorrhagic event, history of bleeding or a coagulopathy, surgery within the previous 2 weeks, open wounds, and severe hypertension.

Surgical Intervention

The patient with peripheral vascular disease virtually always has multiple other medical problems. These should be optimized before surgery. Cardiac disease is almost universal, and the preoperative work-up should include an expert cardiac evaluation—even when cardiac disease is asymptomatic. Sepsis is a relative contraindication to bypass, and if urgent treatment is necessary, aggressive debridement or amputation may be necessary. In the nonambulatory patient, bypass surgery is rarely warranted, and amputation may be preferred.

A clear evaluation of the patient's anatomy is necessary before surgical intervention, and traditionally this required an angiogram. Recently, however, some surgeons have been using duplex scanning alone or with intraoperative angiography to identify anatomy for surgical intervention. The surgical options are then thromboendarterectomy, bypass, or amputation.

Thromboendarterectomy was a common technique for femoropopliteal disease in the 1950s and 1960s. This procedure is similar to carotid endarterectomy; a longitudinal incision is made in the artery, and the plaque, intima, and inner media are removed. The artery is then closed with a vein or prosthetic patch. With the advent of vein graft bypasses, endarterectomy was mostly abandoned. Darling and Linton (13) compared saphenous vein graft bypass with extended endarterectomy and found 5-year patency rates of 72% and 32%, respectively (13). The patency rate for endarterectomy increases with shorter, more discrete lesions and with larger arteries. The operation requires less time than bypass, and the surgical risk is less. Endarterectomy is still used for short, discrete lesions of the common femoral, superficial femoral, deep femoral, and popliteal arteries, especially in high-risk patients.

Infrainguinal bypass is the gold standard in the treatment of peripheral vascular disease (Fig. 80.4). It is indicated for the patient with critical ischemia and, in specific instances, the patient with claudication. Before a bypass is performed for claudication, both the physician and the patient must be certain that the disease is truly incapacitating and limits the activities of daily living, that conservative and medical management have been unsuccessful, and that the mortality risk and threat of limb loss as a complication of surgery are worth the possible relief of symptoms. It must be remembered that claudication progresses

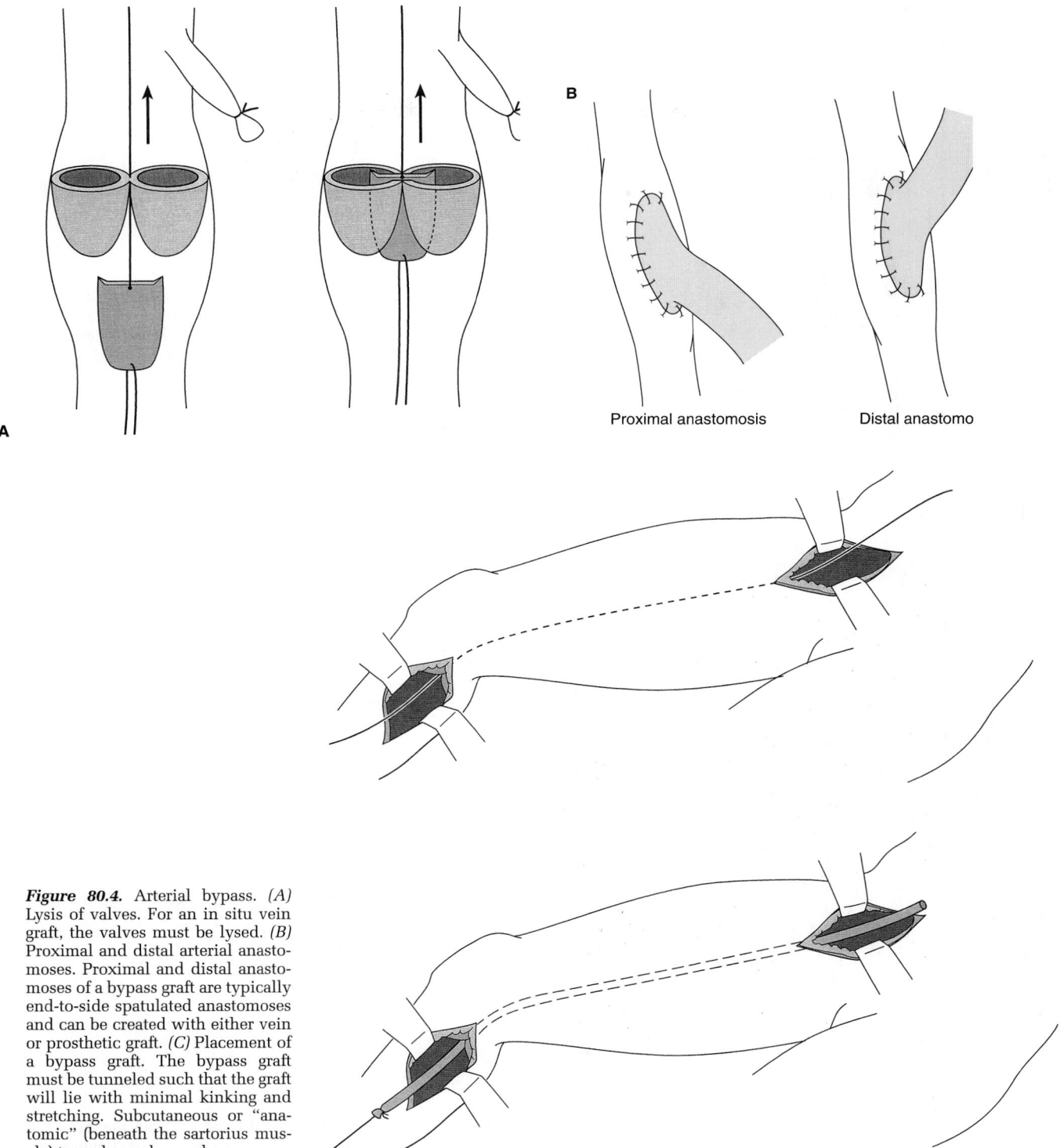

Proximal anastomosis   Distal anastomo

A

B

C

Figure 80.4. Arterial bypass. *(A)* Lysis of valves. For an in situ vein graft, the valves must be lysed. *(B)* Proximal and distal arterial anastomoses. Proximal and distal anastomoses of a bypass graft are typically end-to-side spatulated anastomoses and can be created with either vein or prosthetic graft. *(C)* Placement of a bypass graft. The bypass graft must be tunneled such that the graft will lie with minimal kinking and stretching. Subcutaneous or "anatomic" (beneath the sartorius muscle) tunnels can be used.

to critical ischemia and limb loss in relatively few cases, and that all interventions in the peripheral circulation can be complicated by limb loss.

Before surgery, a clear delineation of the patient's anatomy must be obtained. This is usually accomplished with an angiogram. It is important to identify the critical stenoses that must be bypassed, and the inflow and outflow of blood must be good for the graft to remain patent.

A bypass graft can in theory start and end at any site along the arterial tree (Fig. 80.5), and various generaliza-

tions can be made regarding patency rates. Patency rates are better in shorter, large-caliber vein grafts placed in vascular beds with higher rates of flow; thus, relatively proximal grafts, grafts that do not pass the knee, and vein grafts rather than artificial grafts are preferred. Frequently performed procedures include femoral-to-popliteal above-the-knee and below-the-knee bypass, and femoral- or popliteal-to-distal bypass.

Bypass can be accomplished with saphenous or other vein, or with an artificial graft. However, femoral- or

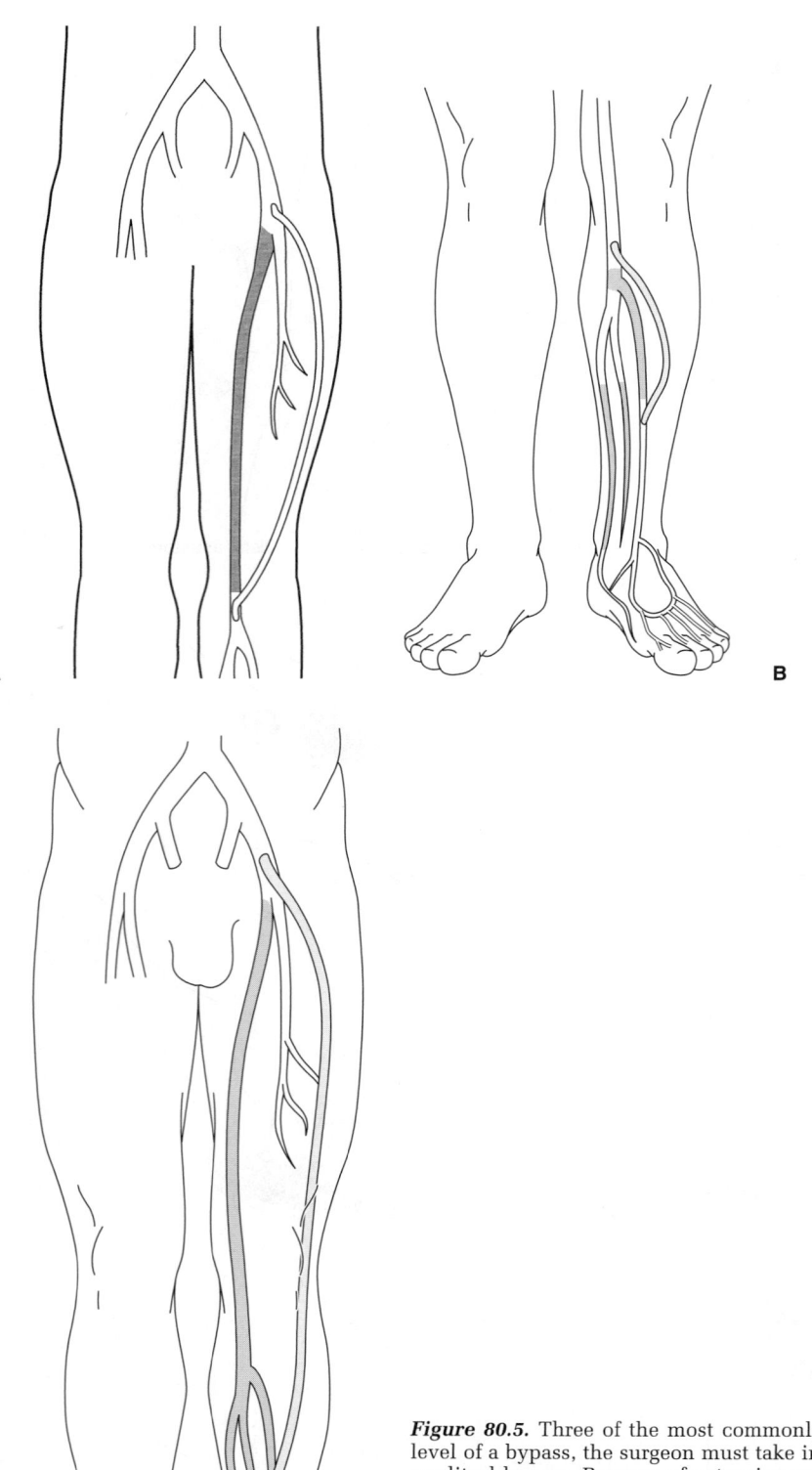

Figure 80.5. Three of the most commonly used types of arterial bypass. When planning the level of a bypass, the surgeon must take into account the level of the stenosis. *(A)* Femoral-to-popliteal bypass. Because of extensive superficial femoral artery and popliteal artery disease extending below the knee, the distal anastomosis is performed at an infrapopliteal site. If the disease were less distal, an above-the-knee femoral-to-popliteal artery bypass would be a better choice. *(B)* Popliteal-to-anterior tibial bypass. If the occlusive process is confined to the region of the knee (as commonly occurs in diabetes), the superficial femoral artery or popliteal artery can serve as the site of origin for a distal bypass. *(C)* Femoral-to-posterior tibial bypass. Long bypass from common femoral artery to below-the-knee posterior tibial artery. Such bypasses can be carried to the level of the ankle and occasionally beyond.

popliteal-to-distal bypasses are almost exclusively performed with the vein because the combined effects of lower flow rate and smaller diameter decrease the patency of artificial grafts to an impractical level. When a femoral-to-popliteal bypass is performed, autogenous vein grafts are still preferred; however, multiple other uses of the vein, including coronary artery bypass and future distal bypass, may make artificial graft a reasonable choice in some cases.

Saphenous vein grafts can be either in situ or reversed. In situ saphenous vein grafts are left in place in the patient's leg, all valves are cut to allow for unimpeded blood flow through the vein, and all branches are ligated. The vein is anastomosed to the artery proximally and distally. In the reversed saphenous vein graft, the vein is removed from the body and all branches are ligated. The valves are not cut, and the graft is reversed and tunneled under the tissue and attached to the artery proximally and distally.

Following a revascularization procedure, an intraoperative evaluation of patency is important. This can be accomplished via angiography, angioscopy, or duplex scan. It is also important to document pulses postoperatively as a reference for further evaluation and postoperative management.

The complications of bypass surgery are significant. Many are the consequence of multiple comorbid conditions in patients with peripheral vascular disease. Perioperative mortality has been reported to be between 2% and 5%, depending on patient selection, and cardiac complications are the most frequent. Perioperative myocardial infarction rates have been reported as 3%, and if silent and unnoticed myocardial infarctions are included, they may be as high as 10% to 15% (14). Other complications include hemorrhage, hematoma, thrombosis, infection, and edema. Donaldson et al. (15) documented graft thrombosis in 2% to 7% of procedures within the first 30 days.

When bypass surgery carries a very high risk, or when a patient is not ambulatory or has unreconstructable anatomy, irreversible tissue compromise, or invasive infection, an amputation may be the best treatment. An important issue in selecting the level of amputation is the need to remove all painful, infected, and necrotic tissue. In addition, a level must be chosen that offers a good chance of healing, rehabilitation, and use of a prosthetic device.

The most common amputation procedures for patients with peripheral vascular disease are toe, ray, and transmetatarsal amputations for disease confined to the forefoot. Below-knee and above-knee amputation and occasionally a Symes amputation are used in patients with more extensive disease. Various methods to estimate blood flow are used in planning the level of amputation, including the ABI or pressure measurements, skin temperature, and transcutaneous oxygen measurements.

Rehabilitation is important to all patients. It may be straightforward, or considerable effort may be required to enable use of a prosthesis. Many patients with severe peripheral vascular disease have limited muscle mass and poor exercise tolerance, which make the use of a prosthesis difficult. Ambulation with a below-knee prosthesis requires 40% more energy and with an above-knee prosthesis 70% more energy than normal gait (16). Although often quoted as higher, mortality from below-knee amputation

has been shown to be 6%, and from above-knee amputation it is 11%. The difference can be accounted for by a difference in comorbidity (17). Immediate and later death is usually caused by cardiac disease. Life tables show that 50% of elderly persons who undergo a lower extremity amputation die within 3 years.

As the population of the United States ages, the prevalence of atherosclerosis and peripheral vascular disease will increase. Physicians must be prepared to recognize and diagnose peripheral vascular occlusive disease and employ a spectrum of treatment options, ranging from risk factor modification to actual reconstruction, to manage these patients optimally.

REFERENCES

1. Imparato AM, Kim GE, Davidson T, et al. Intermittent claudication: its natural course. *Surgery* 1975;78:795–799.
2. Jurgens IL, Barker NW, Hines EA. Arteriosclerosis obliterans: a review of 520 cases with special reference to pathogenic and prognostic factors. *Circulation* 1960;21:188–197.
3. Barnes RW, Shanik GD, Slaymaker EF. An index of healing in below-knee amputation: leg blood pressure by Doppler ultrasound. *Surgery* 1976;79:13–20.
4. Kohler TR, Nance DR, Cramer MM, et al. Duplex scanning for the diagnosis of aortoiliac and femoropopliteal disease: a prospective study. *Circulation* 1987;76:1074–1080.
5. Quick CRG, Cotton LT. The measured effect of stopping smoking on intermittent claudication. *Br J Surg* 1982;69[Suppl]: 524–526.
6. Creasy TS, McMillan PJ, Fletcher EW, et al. Is percutaneous transluminal angioplasty better than exercise for claudication? Preliminary results from a prospective randomized trial. *Eur J Vasc Endovasc Surg* 1990;4:135–140.
7. Ernst E, Matrai A, Kollar L. Placebo-controlled double-blind study of hemodilution in peripheral arterial disease. *Lancet* 1987;1:1449–1451.
8. Dawson DL, Cutler BS, Meissner MH, et al. Cilostazol has beneficial effects in the treatment of intermittent claudication. *Circulation* 1988;98:678–686.
9. Antiplatelet Trialists' Collaboration. Secondary prevention of vascular disease by prolonged antiplatelet treatment. *Br Med J* 1988;296:320–331.
10. Brevetti G, Chiariello M, Ferulano G, et al. Increases in walking distance in patients treated with L-carnitine: a double-blind, cross-over study. *Circulation* 1988;77:767–773.
11. Krepel VM, Van Andel GJ, Van Erp WF, et al. Percutaneous transluminal angioplasty of the femoropopliteal artery: initial and long-term results. *Radiology* 1985;156:325–328.
12. Rutherford RB, Durham J. Percutaneous balloon angioplasty for arteriosclerosis obliterans: long-term results. In: Yao JST, Pearce WH, eds. *Technologies in vascular surgery.* Philadelphia: WB Saunders, 1992:329–345.
13. Darling RC, Linton RR. Durability of femoropopliteal reconstruction. *Am J Surg* 1972;123:472–479.
14. Yeager RA. Basic data related to cardiac testing and cardiac risk associated with vascular surgery. *Ann Vasc Surg* 1990;4: 193–197.
15. Donaldson MC, Mannick JA, Whittemore AD. Causes of primary graft failure after in situ saphenous vein bypass grafting. *J Vasc Surg* 1992;15:113–120.
16. Waters RL, Perry J, Antonelli D, et al. Energy cost of walking amputees: the influence of level of amputation. *J Bone Joint Surg Am* 1976;58:42–46.
    Bodily RC, Burgess EM. Contralateral limb and patient survival after leg amputation. *Am J Surg* 1983;146:280–282.

SURGERY: SCIENTIFIC PRINCIPLES AND PRACTICE, Third Edition, edited by Lazar J. Greenfield, Michael W. Mulholland, Keith T. Oldham, Gerald B. Zelenock, and Keith D. Lillemoe. Lippincott Williams & Wilkins Publishers, Philadelphia, © 2001.

CHAPTER 81

LOWER EXTREMITY AMPUTATION

JOSEPH GIGLIA

More than 115,000 lower extremity amputations are performed in the United States each year, and vascular and general surgeons are involved in most of these (Table 81.1). The goal of amputation surgery is to maintain maximal function of the patient, not necessarily maximal length of the limb. The clinical judgment and experience of the surgeon have been shown to be of key importance to a successful outcome (1).

INDICATIONS

The vast majority of lower extremity amputations are performed because of complications of diabetes or arterial insufficiency (Table 81.2). Chronic infection and trauma account for less than 10% of the total number. Miscellaneous indications include neuroma, frostbite, malignancy, chronic pain, arterial embolization, venous insufficiency, and cryoglobulinemia (2).

Elective lower extremity amputation in diabetic and dysvascular patients is indicated for gangrene (dry gangrene), gangrene with infection (wet gangrene), unremitting and unreconstructable rest pain, and nonhealing ulcers. The goal of the operation is to remove all nonviable tissue, relieve ischemic rest pain, ensure primary wound healing, and facilitate rehabilitation. Elective amputation should be performed only after an evaluation for revascularization and a potential limb salvage procedure by a surgeon capable of performing the procedure. Veith and colleagues (3) reported that 96% of their patients who underwent lower extremity arteriorgraphy for limb-threatening infrainguinal arteriosclerosis were candidates for arterial reconstruction. However, not all patients are candidates for arteriography, including those with nonfunctional limbs, fixed-joint contractures, insensate feet, extensive gangrene, and incapacitating organic brain injury.

Emergent amputation is indicated in the face of uncontrolled or ascending infection. In the case of uncontrolled sepsis, it can even be a life-saving maneuver. A diabetic patient with a foot abscess is a surgical emergency. Frequently, incision and drainage with or without a toe re-

Table 81.1. TOTAL AMPUTATIONS EACH YEAR IN THE UNITED STATES

Type of amputation	No.	Percentage
Phalangeal	36,800	32
Foot	11,500	10
Below-knee	33,350	29
Above-knee	33,350	29
Total	115,000	100

From Frang RD, Tayor LM, Porter JM. Amputations. In: Porter JM, Taylor LM, eds. Basic data underlying clinical decision making in vascular surgery. St. Louis: Quality Medical, 1994:153, with permission.

Table 81.2. INDICATIONS FOR LOWER EXTREMITY AMPUTATION

Indication	Percentage
Complications of diabetes mellitus	60–80
Nondiabetic infection with ischemia	15–25
Ischemia without infection	5–10
Chronic osteomyelitis	3–5
Trauma	2–5
Miscellaneous (neuroma, frostbite, tumor, pain, nonhealing wound)	5–10

From Malone JM. Lower extremity amputation. In: Moore WS, ed. Vascular surgery: a comprehensive review. Philadelphia: WB Saunders, 1993:810, with permission.

section or a combined toe and metatarsal resection is sufficient to control the acute problem. If the process has extended proximal to the foot, an open (guillotine) amputation of the leg is indicated. An above-knee amputation is indicated in patients with infection involving the entire leg, a fixed-knee contracture, or a nonfunctional limb.

Primary amputation is occasionally indicated in cases of treatment for lower extremity trauma. Both penetrating and blunt injuries of the lower extremities are frequently associated with vascular, nerve, bone, and extensive soft-tissue injuries. A decision for treatment with primary amputation is extremely difficult and requires extensive clinical judgment and multidisciplinary input. Relevant factors include the severity of the injury, the overall clinical status, and the ultimate rehabilitation potential of the patient. Several treatment guidelines have been developed. Lange (4) recommends primary amputation for open tibial fractures with associated vascular injuries if the posterior tibial nerve is disrupted in an adult or if warm ischemia lasts longer than 6 hours in a crush injury. Additionally, this author suggests that primary amputation is relatively indicated in patients with multiple trauma, severe ipsilateral foot injuries, and an expected protracted postoperative course. Johansen and colleagues (5) devised a mangled extremity severity score to predict the need for amputation based on the extent of skeletal or soft-tissue damage and limb ischemia, presence of shock, and age.

EVALUATION OF POTENTIAL FOR REVASCULARIZATION

Modern vascular surgery techniques allow successful limb salvage in situations in which it was not previously possible. All patients who present for possible lower extremity amputation should be considered for revascularization by a surgeon fully capable of providing such care. The evaluation may require only a thorough history and physical examination if an obvious contraindication to revascularization is noted (e.g., nonfunctional limb or severe organic brain syndrome). Conversely, contrast angiography with selected lower extremity injections may be necessary to define fully the patient's anatomy and suitability for reconstruction. Even if high-quality contrast angiography cannot visualize an adequate target vessel, successful limb salvage can be obtained with a pedal bypass if duplex examination identifies a preserved dorsalis pedis artery.

Upper extremity vein (6) and cryopreserved cadaver vein (7) have increased the options for conduit in limb salvage situations. Prosthetic grafts with vein cuffs provide an alternative method when appropriate autogenous conduit is not available (8,9). An operation for limb salvage should seldom be denied *only* for lack of conduit.

Revascularization is often performed in conjunction with a limited amputation, either simultaneously or as a staged procedure. This allows management of the acute problem of sepsis and the underlying chronic ischemia. In extreme cases, a limited amputation can be combined with revascularization and a tissue transfer (free or rotational flap) to achieve limb salvage (10,11).

CHOICE OF LEVEL OF AMPUTATION

General Considerations

The choice of amputation level depends on the indication for the procedure, condition of the patient, and rehabilitation potential of the patient. The most common amputation levels are illustrated in Fig. 81.1. Because most amputations are performed for the complications of diabetes or arterial insufficiency, the selected level must allow the removal of all nonviable and painful tissue, allow primary healing, and maximize rehabilitation po-

tential. Selection of the amputation level for malignant disease depends on the biologic characteristics of the neoplasm and is not discussed further here.

The general medical condition and rehabilitation potential of the patient are important factors when one is deciding to proceed with amputation and in selecting the appropriate level. If the patient has been ambulatory and independent preoperatively, the level at which the likelihood that function will be maintained is greatest should be selected. If the patient is not ambulatory or has significant comorbid conditions, the primary wound healing rate should be the determining factor.

Specific Situations

Aggressive attempts at limb salvage with a distal amputation level are not indicated for patients who are unlikely to ambulate with a prosthesis (12). For example, patients with fixed-joint contractures greater than 15 degrees at the knee or 10 degrees at the hip are unlikely to ambulate with a prosthesis. Below-knee amputations are relatively contraindicated in patients with paraplegia because flexion contractures at the knee can lead to stump ulceration.

Energy Requirement

The energy required to ambulate following a lower extremity amputation increases with the level of amputation. The more proximal the amputation, the less likely it is that the patient will be able to ambulate postoperatively. Table 81.3 illustrates the increased energy costs of common lower extremity amputations. In clinical practice, the most significant increase is between a below-knee and an above-knee amputation. Ambulation on an above-knee prosthesis requires the use of muscle groups poorly suited for that purpose. These increased energy costs are minor issues for young trauma or cancer patients; however, they represent a considerable obstacle for the older diabetic or dysvascular patient.

Clinical Assessment

The primary preoperative consideration for wound healing is the status of the skin and muscle blood flow. Operative technique, the patient's nutritional status, and the presence of infection also affect wound healing. An experienced surgeon can accurately predict whether a below-knee amputation will heal based on clinical judgment in approximately 80% of cases (13). A palpable pulse at the level immediately proximal to the proposed amputation essentially ensures healing (14); however, the converse is not true. Noninvasive arterial testing is the most common adjunctive test used to predict healing at a specific amputation level. However, its usefulness is limited when medial sclerosis prevents vessel compression, a

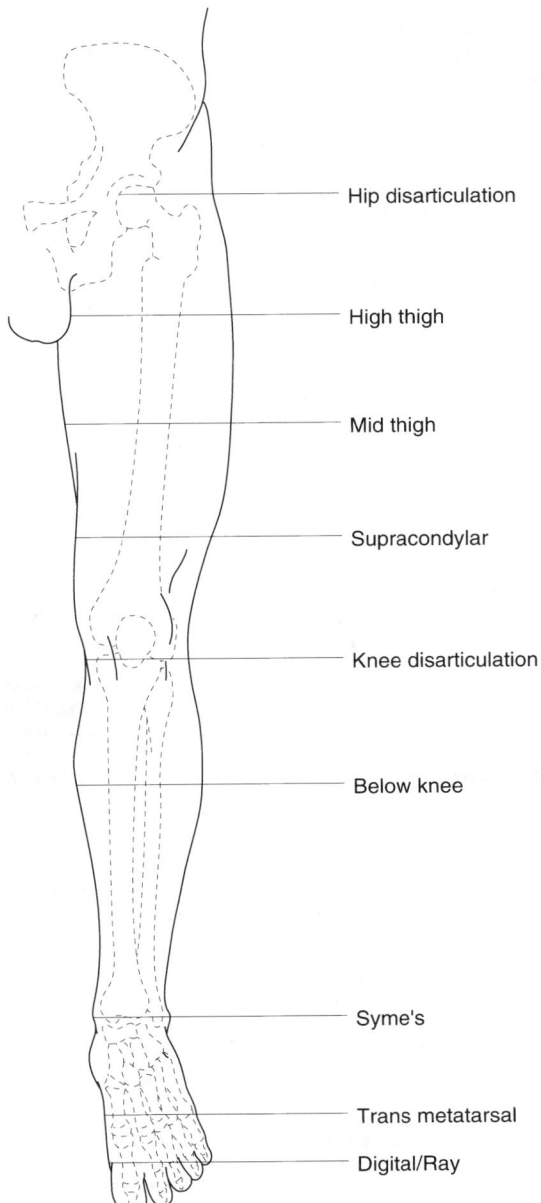

Figure 81.1. Common amputation levels for the lower extremity.

Hip disarticulation

High thigh

Mid thigh

Supracondylar

Knee disarticulation

Below knee

Syme's

Trans metatarsal

Digital/Ray

Table 81.3. **REHABILITATION ENERGY COST OF AMPUTATION AT VARIOUS LEVELS**

Amputation level	Energy cost
Digital or ray	Minimal (except first ray)
Transmetatarsal	Minimal during normal walking
Below-knee	30%–60% increase in energy required for ambulation
Above-knee	60%–100% increase in energy required for ambulation
Hip disarticulation	100%–110% increase in energy required for ambulation

Table 81.4. PREOPERATIVE LEVEL SELECTION: TOE AMPUTATION

Selection criteria	Successful healing, primary and secondary per total
Empiric	86/115 (75%)
Presence of pedal pulses	357/365 (98%)
Doppler toe pressure >30 mm[a]	47/60 (78%)
Doppler ankle pressure >35 mm[a]	44/46 (96%)
Photoplethysmographic digit or [a]TMA pressure >20 mm	20/20 (100%)
^{133}Xe skin blood flow >2.6 mL/100 g of tissue/min	5/6 (83%)

[a]Systolic pressure (mm Hg).
TMA, transmetatarsal.
From Durham JR. Lower extremity amputation levels: indications, methods of determining appropriate level, technique, prognosis. In: Rutherford RB, ed. Vascular surgery, 3rd ed. Philadelphia: WB Saunders, 1989:1693, with permission.

condition common in diabetic patients. Because the digital vessels are often spared from this process, digital pressure readings may be helpful in this setting.

A variety of nuclear medicine techniques have been used to assess skin perfusion at the proposed amputation level (15,16); however, reproducibility among centers is lacking. Fluorescein skin blood flow measurements did not correlate with amputation healing in a blinded study

Table 81.5. PREOPERATIVE LEVEL SELECTION: FOOT AND FOREFOOT AMPUTATION

Selection criteria	Successful healing, primary and secondary per total
Empiric	11/24 (46%)
	36/50 (72%)
Doppler ankle systolic pressure	
<40 mm Hg	5/9 (56%)
>40 mm Hg	20/60 (33%)
40–60 mm Hg	4/5 (80%)
>50 mm Hg	14/21 (66%)
>60 mm Hg	68/91 (75%)
>70 mm Hg	70/93 (75%)
Doppler toe systolic pressure >30 mm Hg	4/5 (80%)
Doppler ankle–brachial pressure index	
>0.45 (nondiabetic)	
>0.50 (diabetic)	58/60 (97%)
Photoplethysmographic toe systolic pressure	
>55 mm Hg	14/14 (100%)
>45 and <55 mm Hg	2/8 (25%)
<45 mm Hg	0/8 (0%)
Fiberoptic fluorometry (dye fluorescence index >44)	18/20 (90%)
Laser Doppler velocimetry	2/6 (33%)
^{125}I-iodopyrine skin blood flow	
>8 mL/100 g of tissue/min	18/18 (100%)
^{133}Xe skin blood flow >2.6 mL/100 g of tissue/min	23/25 (92%)
Transcutaneous Po$_2$	
>10 mm (or a >10-mm increase on FIo$_2$ = 1.0)	6/8 (75%)
>28 mm Hg	3/3 (100%)
Transcutaneous Pco$_2$ <40 mm Hg	3/3 (100%)

From Durham JR. Lower extremity amputation levels: indications, methods of determining appropriate level, technique, prognosis. In: Rutherford RB, ed. Vascular surgery, 3rd ed. Philadelphia: WB Saunders, 1989:1695, with permission.

Table 81.6. PREOPERATIVE LEVEL SELECTION: BELOW-KNEE AMPUTATION

Selection criteria	Successful healing, primary and secondary per total
Empiric	794/974 (82%)
Doppler ankle systolic pressure >30 mm Hg	66/70 (94%)
Doppler calf systolic pressure	
>50 mm Hg	36/36 (100%)
>68 mm Hg	96/97 (99%)
Doppler thigh systolic pressure	
>100 mm Hg	31/31 (100%)
>80 mm Hg	104/113 (92%)
Fluorescein dye	24/30 (80%)
Fiberoptic fluorometry (dye fluorescence index >44)	12/12 (100%)
Laser Doppler velocimetry	8/8 (100%)
Skin perfusion pressure	
^{99m}Tc-pertechnetate	24/26 (92%)
^{131}I- or ^{125}I-antipyrine >30 mm	60/62 (97%)
Photoelectric skin perfusion pressure >20 mm	60/71 (85%)
^{133}Xe skin blood flow	
Epicutaneous >0.9 mL/100 g of tissue/min	14/15 (93%)
Intradermal >2.4 mL/100 g of tissue/min	83/89 (93%)
Intradermal >1 mL/100 g of tissue/min	11/12 (92%)
Transcutaneous Po$_2$ = 0	0/3 (0%)
>10 mm Hg (or >10-mm increase on FIo$_2$ = 1.0)	76/80 (95%)
>10 and <40 mm Hg	5/7 (71%)
>20 mm Hg	25/26 (96%)
>35 mm Hg	51/51 (100%)
Transcutaneous Po$_2$ index >0.59	17/17 (100%)
Transcutaneous Pco$_2$ <40 mm Hg	7/8 (88%)

From Durham JR. Lower extremity amputation levels: indications, methods of determining appropriate level, technique, prognosis. In: Rutherford RB, ed. Vascular surgery, 3rd ed. Philadelphia: WB Saunders, 1989:1700, with permission.

Table 81.7. PREOPERATIVE LEVEL SELECTION: ABOVE-KNEE AMPUTATION

Selection criteria	Successful healing, primary and secondary per total
Empiric	390/430 (91%)
Fiberoptic fluorometry (dye fluorescence index >44)	6/7 (86%)
Laser Doppler velocimetry	6/6 (100%)
Photoelectric skin perfusion pressure >21 mm	19/19 (100%)
Skin perfusion pressure (^{131}I- or ^{125}I-antipyrine)	44/48 (92%)
^{133}Xe skin blood flow intradermal >2.6 mL/100 g of tissue/min	20/20 (100%)
Transcutaneous Po$_2$	
>10 mm (or 10-mm increase on FIo$_2$ = 1.0)	15/23 (65%)
>20 mm	12/12 (100%)
>23 mm	2/2 (100%)
>35 mm	21/24 (88%)
Transcutaneous Pco$_2$ <38 mm	5/5 (100%)

From Durham JR. Lower extremity amputation levels: indications, methods of determining appropriate level, technique, prognosis. In: Rutherford RB, ed. Vascular surgery, 3rd ed. Philadelphia: WB Saunders, 1989:1707, with permission.

(17). Transcutaneous oxygen measurement has been shown to predict primary healing; however, the technique is not widely used (18,19). Laser Doppler velocimetry (20), photoplethysmography (21), thermography (22), and pulse volume recordings (23) have all been applied with mixed results. Tables 81.4 through 81.7 summarize the results of various preoperative tests to predict wound healing for toe, foot and forefoot, below-knee, and above-knee amputations, respectively.

OPERATIVE TECHNIQUE

General Considerations

Diabetic patients who present with sepsis require adequate fluid resuscitation, broad-spectrum antibiotics (including anaerobic coverage), and an emergent operation. Although maintenance of limb length and function is a worthy goal, control of sepsis and wide débridement of all nonviable tissue are essential and potentially life-saving. All patients require atraumatic handling of tissue. The placement of forceps on the skin edge is to be avoided whenever possible. Excessive skin flaps and dead space predispose to complications of wound healing. Amputations performed in the face of active infection are kept open and treated with dressing changes, but delayed primary closure can be considered in cases in which perfusion is intact and the infection controlled.

Postoperatively, the amputation stump is elevated to minimize tissue edema and promote healing. Ambulation is delayed until healing is certain. This sedentary patient population requires effective prophylaxis against deep venous thrombosis.

Digital and Ray Amputations

Digital amputations are indicated for gangrene or osteomyelitis localized to areas distal to the middle phalanx. The technique is illustrated in Fig. 81.2A. A circumferential skin incision is made over the distal end of the proximal phalanx and carried down to bone. Nerves and tendons are transected under tension and allowed to retract. The proximal phalanx is divided with bone shears, and the transected end is smoothed with a Rongeur. Alternatively, a pneumatic reciprocating saw can be used, although this is rarely necessary. The wound is closed in layers. The patient is kept at bed rest for several days.

A ray amputation is indicated when the disease process extends to the digital crease. The technique is similar to a digital amputation and is illustrated in Fig. 81.2B. A cir-

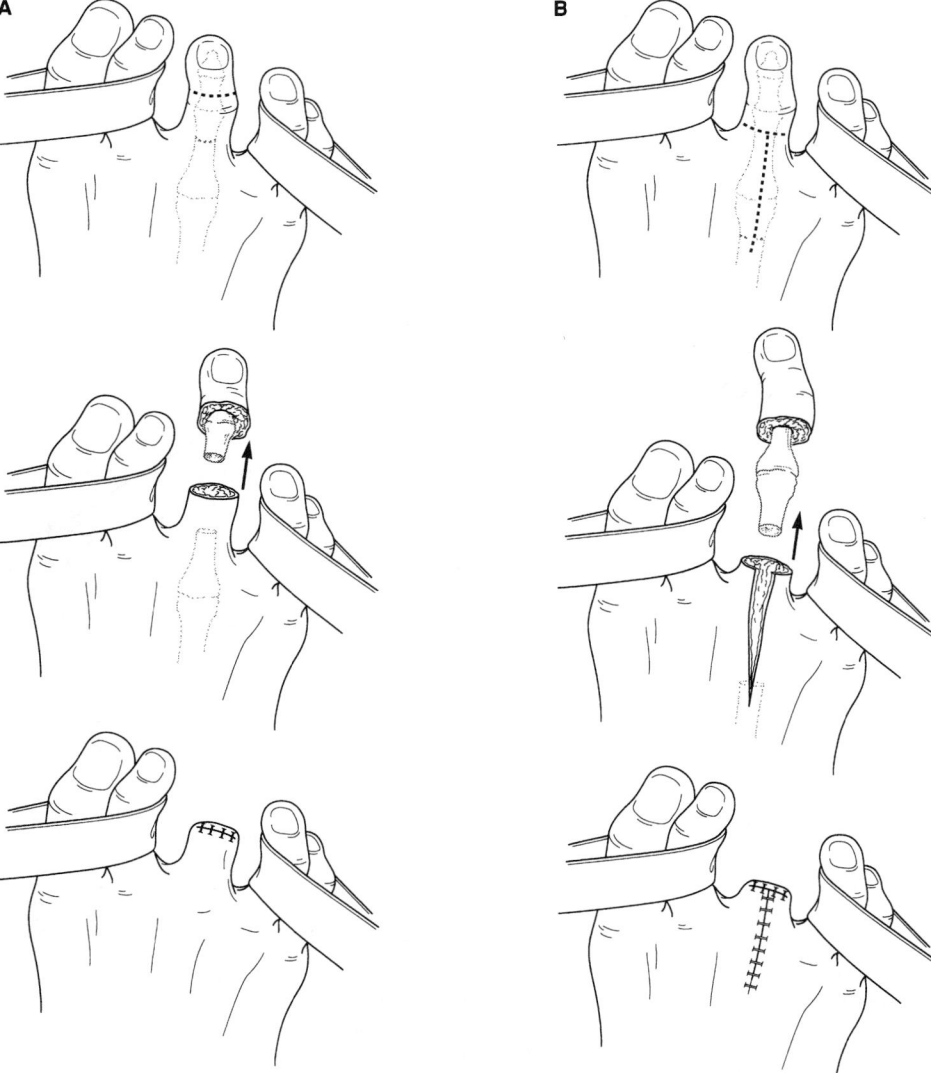

Figure 81.2. *(A)* Digital amputation. A circumferential skin incision is made proximal to the gangrenous process. The proximal phalanx is transected and the soft tissue approximated. *(B)* Metatarsal head resection (ray amputation). A racquet-shaped skin incision is made with the circular component extending circumferentially around the digit and the longitudinal component extending proximal to the metatarsal head. The metatarsal is transected proximal to the head and the soft tissue approximated.

cumfrential incision is made at the base of the involved toe and extended proximally on the dorsum of the foot over the metatarsal. The incision is extended to bone. The periostium is cleared circumferentially, and the bone is transected at a level that will allow tension-free closure of the wound. In the case of the first or fifth toe, the incision is extended on the medial or lateral aspect of the foot, respectively.

In selected cases of neuropathic ulcers, the metatarsal head can be resected, with the toe left intact. A dorsal longitudinal incision is made over the metatarsal bone, and a counterincision is made at the region of the ulcer on the plantar aspect of the foot. The distal portion of the metatarsal and the metatarsal head are then resected. The wound is packed in a through-and-through fashion until significant healing has occurred.

Transmetatarsal Amputation

Transmetatarsal amputation maintains a patient's ability to ambulate without the aid of a prosthesis and is indicated when the gangrenous or infectious process involves multiple digits or the forefoot. It is contraindicated when the underlying process extends to the proposed skin incision or the plantar aspect of the foot is affected. In the latter situation, an open amputation through the metatarsal bones can be performed. The wound is allowed to close secondarily or covered with a skin graft. Unfortunately, thin skin grafts in this position are prone to breakdown secondary to the pressure related to ambulation. The technique is demonstrated in Fig. 81.3. A skin incision is made on the dorsum of the foot immediately proximal to the metatarsal heads and extended medially and laterally to a point midway between the plantar and dorsal surfaces. The plantar incision is made along the digital crease and extended diagonally medially and laterally to connect to the dorsal incision. The dorsal incision is deepened to the periostium, which is cleared with a small periostial elevator. The metatarsal bones are transected 0.5 mm proximal to the dorsal skin incision. The plantar flap is fashioned by continuing the dissection just superficial to the metatarsal heads. Care is taken to maintain plantar flap thickness. The nerves and tendons are transected sharply under tension and allowed to retract. The plantar flap is rotated anteriorly and assessed for length. Excess tissue is excised sharply, and the deep tissue is approximated with

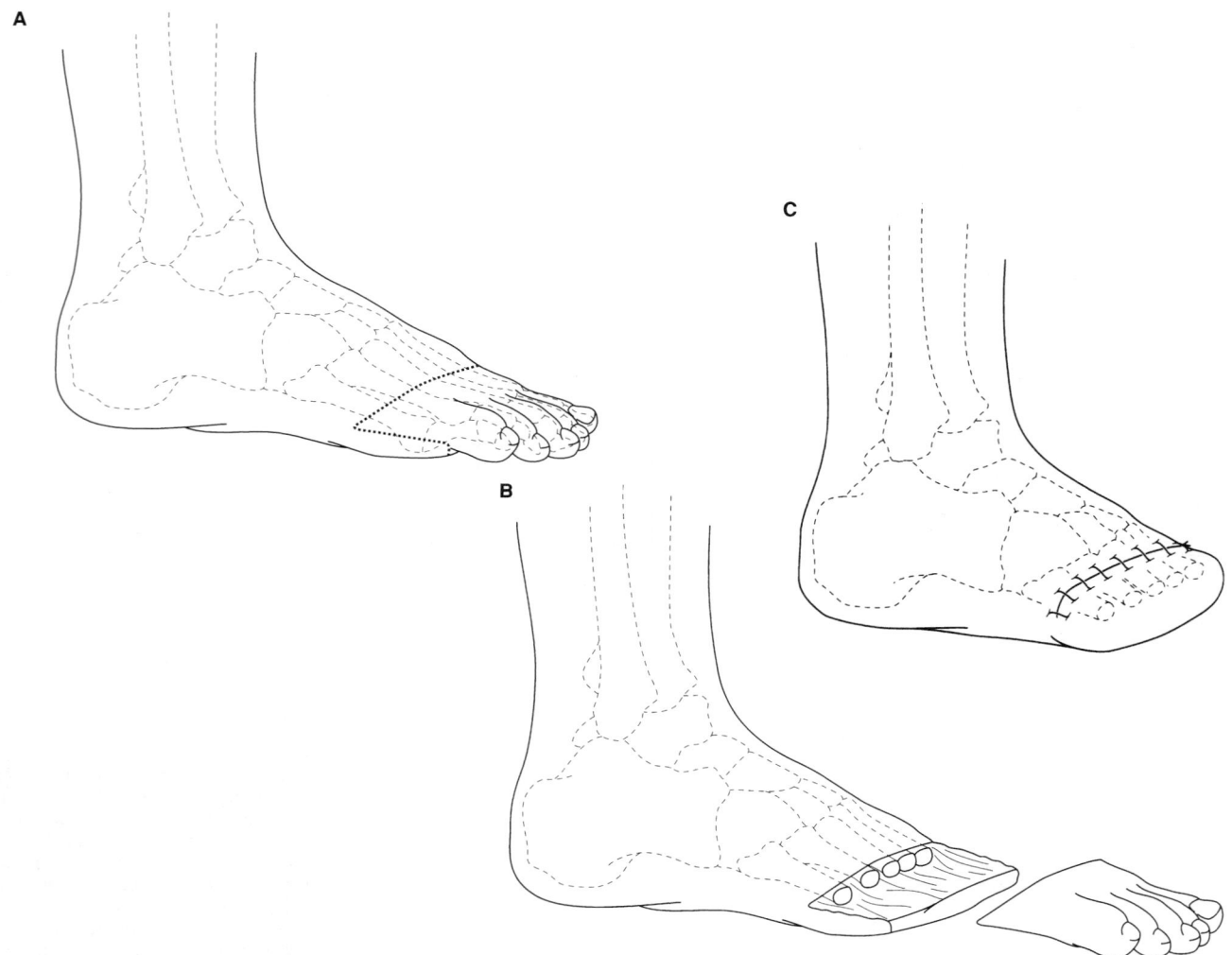

Figure 81.3. *(A)* The skin incision for the transmetatarsal amputation is made on the dorsum of the foot immediately proximal to the metatarsal heads and on the plantar surface within the digital crease. *(B)* The metatarsal heads are transected proximal to the skin incision and separated from the plantar soft-tissue flap along a plane adjacent to the bone. *(C)* The plantar soft-tissue flap is rotated anteriorly and approximated.

absorbable suture. The skin is closed without tension with monofilament suture.

Ambulation is delayed for 1 month to allow adherence of the plantar flap. Either a soft dressing or a short leg cast can be used for a postoperative dressing.

Syme Amputation

The Syme amputation is an uncommon foot amputation that preserves limb length and the epiphyseal growth plates and allows ambulation without a prosthesis. It is indicated in cases of extensive foot trauma. It is relatively contraindicated for patients with neurotrophic sensory changes and in dysvascular patients.

The procedure can be performed in one or two stages, as illustrated in Fig. 81.4. When a Syme amputation is performed in two stages, the stump is less bulky and therefore more easily fitted with a prosthesis and visually more appealing.

The initial steps for both procedures are identical except that the skin incision for the two-stage procedure is located 1.5 cm more distally. The skin incision for the one-stage procedure extends from the medial to the lateral malleolus in the horizontal and vertical planes. The dorsal incision is extended to the bone, and the tendons are transected under tension. The anterior tibial artery is identified, divided, and suture-ligated. The dissection is carried into the tibiotalar joint space as the foot is forcibly plantarflexed. The ligaments are transected and the talus is dislocated. The plantar aspect of the incision is deepened to the calcaneus, and the calcaneus is sharply dissected from the plantar fascia. The plantar fascia is densely adherent, and care must be taken to prevent damage to the heel pad, especially at the level of the Achilles tendon. The posterior tibial artery must be preserved, as it perfuses the heel pad. The foot is then removed. The two procedures differ from this point forward.

In the one-stage procedure, the medial and lateral malleoli are transected flush with the tibiotalar joint space, and the heel pad is rotated over the ends of the tibia and fibula. The deep fascial layers are approximated with absorbable suture, and the skin is closed with monofilament suture.

In the two-stage procedure, the heel pad is similarly positioned, and the wound is closed without further bone transection. After 6 weeks, elliptic incisions are made over the medial and lateral malleoli, and the distal ends of the tibia and fibula are transected flush with the ankle joint. In addition, the distal flares of the tibia and fibula are transected to create the rectangular stump of the two-stage procedure. The wound is closed in a similar fashion.

With both procedures, weight bearing is delayed for at least 4 weeks to allow heel pad fixation. A soft dressing or a short leg cast can be used.

Below-knee Amputation

The complications of diabetes and arterial insufficiency constitute most of the indications for a below-knee amputation. Table 81.8 outlines the criteria used to decide between a below-knee and an above-knee amputation in this setting.

The most common technique, in which a long posterior flap is utilized, is illustrated in Fig. 81.5. When gangrene, wounds, or incisions preclude the use of a posterior flap, equal anteroposterior or sagittal flaps can be used; however, the posterior flap is associated with the highest incidence of primary healing and is thus preferred whenever possible. This higher rate of healing presumably reflects the fact that the posteriorly located gastrocnemius and soleus muscles are supplied by the sural arteries, which originate proximal to the knee.

The proposed skin incision is drawn on the leg with a marker. The tibia should be transected 10 cm distal to the tibial tuberosity, and the anterior aspect of the skin incision should be 1 cm distal to the site selected for the tibial transection. The anterior incision is extended medially and laterally. The length of the anterior incision should equal two thirds of the circumference of the leg at the proposed level of the tibial transection. The incision is then extended longitudinally along the medial and lateral aspects of the leg. The length of the longitudinal incisions should equal one third of the circumference of the leg at the level of the tibial transection. Distally, the medial and lateral incisions are connected posteriorly. Curving the distal corners of the posterior flap prevents the accumulation of redundant tissue at the medial and lateral aspects of the completed amputation. The skin incisions should be down to the fascia to allow separation of the skin edges. This step decreases the chance of inadvertent injury to the posterior flap later in the procedure. The greater and lesser saphenous veins may be transected and ligated.

The anterior aspect of the incision is deepened through the periostium of the tibia. The muscles of the anterior compartment are divided at the level of the skin incision, and the anterior tibial neurovascular bundle is identified and ligated. The proximal tibia is circumferentially cleared of periosteum and transected 1 cm proximal to the skin incision. The anterior aspect of the tibia is cut on a 45-degree bevel. The fibula is cleared and transected 1 cm proximal to the transected tibia. The bones are divided with either a power-driven reciprocating saw or a manual saw. Regardless, care must be taken to avoid trauma to the anterior skin flap.

The posterior tibial and peroneal neurovascular bundles are identified and ligated. The tibia is retracted anteriorly, and the posterior musculature is divided along the plane of the longitudinal skin incisions with an amputation knife. Extreme caution must be taken to avoid injury to the skin edges of the posterior flap during this step. Often, a scalpel is needed to complete the division of the gastrocnemius tendon distally. The specimen is removed, and manual compression achieves temporary hemostasis while the remaining vascular structures are identified and ligated. The nerve is retracted distally, ligated, transected, and allowed to retract. The posterior flap is rotated anteriorly to assess thickness and length. Frequently, the musculature needs to be debulked to allow a tension-free closure. Rough edges of the bones are filed smooth and the wound is irrigated. Bone wax is not used. The end of the tibia is covered and stabilized with absorbable 2-0 sutures placed medially, laterally, and anteriorly. The fascia is closed with absorbable suture, and the skin is closed with monofilament suture or staples.

The below-knee amputation can be shortened if required by the infectious or gangrenous process. Although not ideal, a short below-knee amputation is functionally superior to an above-knee amputation. In the extreme case, the tibia can be transected at the level of the tibial tuberosity and the stump can still be fitted with a prosthesis. If a below-knee amputation is necessary at this level, the biceps tendon and collateral ligament should sutured to the tibia, the common peroneal nerve should be transected above the knee, and the fibula should be removed.

In the face of extensive foot infection, an open (guillotine) amputation should be performed as the first part of a staged procedure. A circumferential incision is made in the distal leg just proximal to the malleoli. The fascia is divided, and the tibia and fibula are dissected free. The bones are divided at the level of the skin incision. All major neurovascular bundles are ligated, and the remaining soft tissue is divided to complete the amputation. Sev-

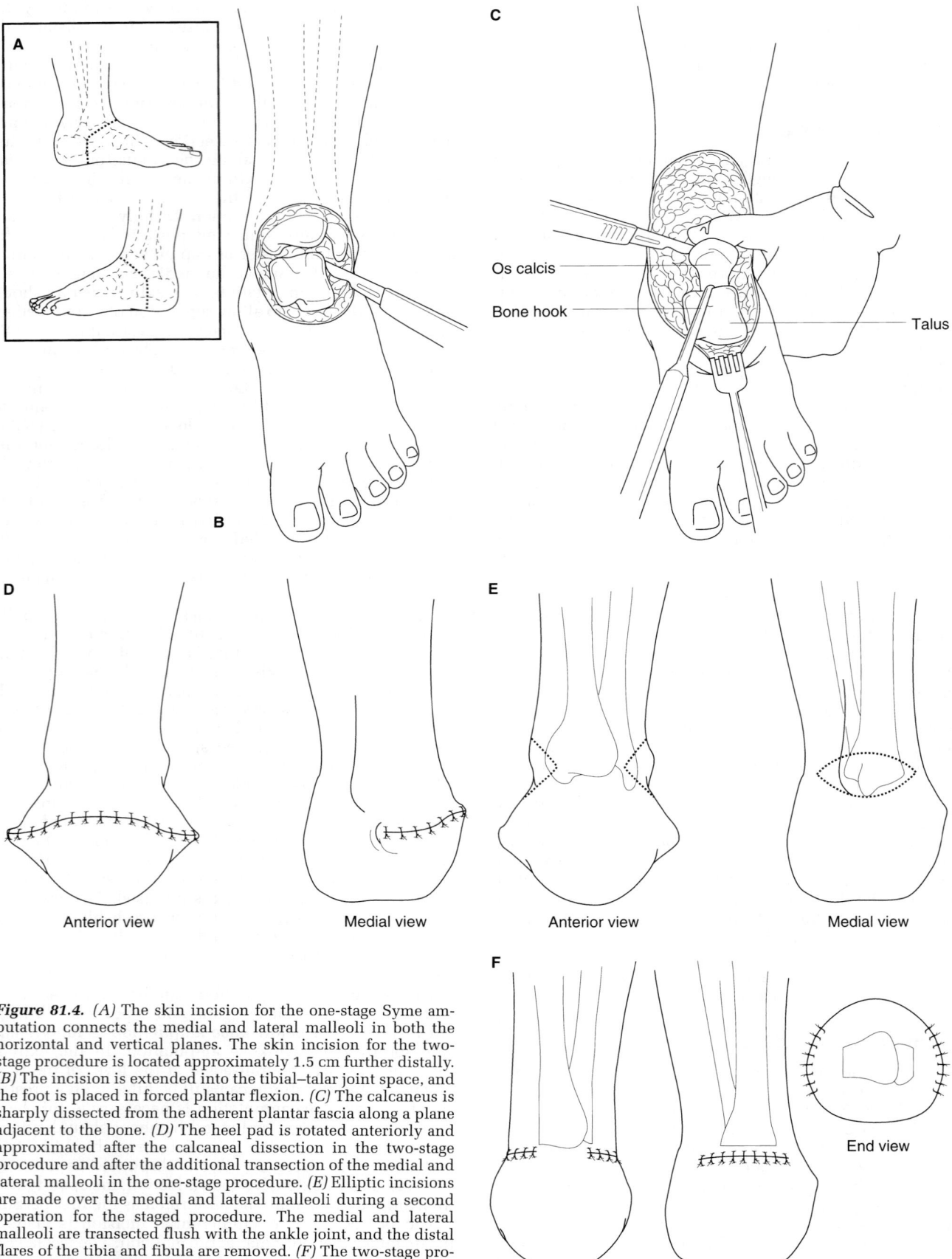

Figure 81.4. *(A)* The skin incision for the one-stage Syme amputation connects the medial and lateral malleoli in both the horizontal and vertical planes. The skin incision for the two-stage procedure is located approximately 1.5 cm further distally. *(B)* The incision is extended into the tibial–talar joint space, and the foot is placed in forced plantar flexion. *(C)* The calcaneus is sharply dissected from the adherent plantar fascia along a plane adjacent to the bone. *(D)* The heel pad is rotated anteriorly and approximated after the calcaneal dissection in the two-stage procedure and after the additional transection of the medial and lateral malleoli in the one-stage procedure. *(E)* Elliptic incisions are made over the medial and lateral malleoli during a second operation for the staged procedure. The medial and lateral malleoli are transected flush with the ankle joint, and the distal flares of the tibia and fibula are removed. *(F)* The two-stage procedure results in a less bulbous, more cosmetically acceptable residual limb.

Table 81.8. AMPUTATION MORTALITY

Category	Percentage	Number
Below-knee	2	25/1,200
Above-knee	9	54/609
Diabetic vs. nondiabetic	No difference	
After amputation revision	5.5	12/218

From Frang RD, Taylor LM, Porter JM. Amputations. In: Porter JM, Taylor LM, eds. Basic data underlying clinical decision making in vascular surgery. St. Louis: Quality Medical, 1994:154, with permission.

eral sutures are placed through the skin and underlying fascia to prevent retraction. The wound is left open and dressed, and a definitive below-knee amputation is delayed until the infectious process has resolved

Rarely, a patient may require an emergent amputation yet have overwhelming medical problems that preclude any operative intervention. As a temporizing maneuver, a tourniquet is placed proximal to the infectious or gangrenous process, and the extremity is packed in dry ice. This prevents the systemic release of muscle degradation products and allows the required procedure to be delayed while the patient's condition is stabilized.

Although soft dressings are most often used following a below-knee amputation, rigid dressings have several re-

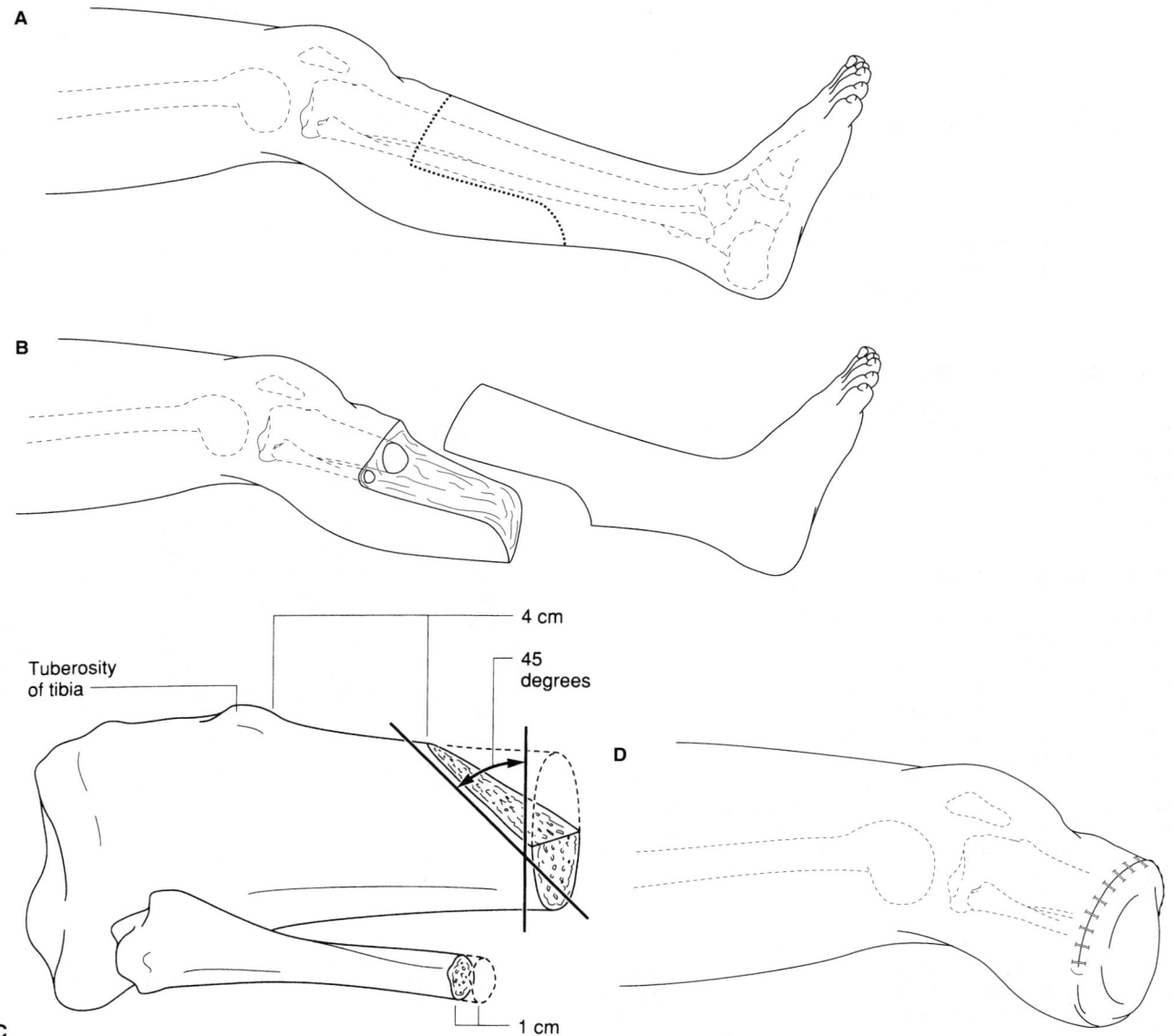

Figure 81.5. (A) The skin incision for a below-knee amputation based on a posterior flap is made 11 cm distal to the tibial tuberosity and extended medially and laterally to the midpoint of the calf. The length of the posterior flap is about 2 cm longer than the diameter of the calf at the point of the proximal incision. (B) The tibia is transected 1 cm proximal to the skin incision. The fibula is transected an additional 1 cm proximal to the level of the tibial transection, and the posterior calf muscles are incised along the plane of the skin incision. (C) The anterior aspect of the tibia is beveled at an angle of about 45 degrees, and the bone edges are filed. (D) The posterior flap is rotated anteriorly and approximated.

ported advantages, including stump protection, stump molding, prevention of edema, acceleration of wound healing, better patient comfort, and prevention of contractures. Additionally, they afford the potential for an immediate-fit prosthesis.

Above-knee Amputation

An above-knee amputation is indicated for patients with a fixed-knee contracture or a nonfunctional limb who require an amputation.

Typically, a transverse fish-mouth incision is made in the lower thigh. Care is taken to carry the initial skin incision to the subcutaneous tissue. This step decreases the likelihood of inadvertent injury to the posterior skin flap during transection of the posterior muscle groups. The dissection is carried down to the femur, which is cleared by means of a periostial elevator to a level 2 to 3 cm proximal to the skin incision. The superficial femoral artery is dissected free and suture-ligated. The bone is transected with a reciprocating or manual saw, and the posterior muscle flap is divided with an amputation knife. Manual compression with a laparotomy pad on the newly divided stump will control hemorrhage while vessels are identified and ligated or electrocoagulated.

Alternative incisions can be made to accommodate surgical wounds. Most above-knee amputation wounds heal even when the femoral pulse is nonpalpable. More proximal thigh amputations are performed when arterial perfusion is in question.

Hip Disarticulation

Lower extremity amputation at the level of the hip is an uncommon operation. The indications include malignancy, trauma, infection, and rarely the complications of arterial insufficiency. Hip disarticulation performed for an ischemic above-knee amputation is often associated with complications in the absence of revascularization.

Other Lower Extremity Amputations

Two additional midfoot amputations have been well described. Although these are not often indicated in the dysvascular patient, they may have a role in selected cases (24). A Lisfranc amputation is performed at the tarsometatarsal joint level and may be an option if soft-tissue coverage is inadequate for a transmetatarsal amputation (25). A Chopart amputation is performed at the level of the calcaneocuboid and talonavicular bones. A modified Chopart amputation includes a percutaneous heel cord lengthening (26). Knee disarticulation is a useful amputation for patients with immature growth plates. It is superior to an above-knee amputation, allowing end weight bearing and providing improved proprioception and prosthetic control. The required prosthesis is bulky and less cosmetically appealing than that used with a below-knee amputation. The technique is well described (27). Rotationplasty is an uncommon procedure performed primarily for the treatment of osteogenic sarcoma of the thigh (28). It involves nerve-sparing resection of the femur and knee, 180-degree rotation of the leg, and reattachment of the leg. This results in a functional, sensate foot that can easily be fitted with a prosthesis.

COMPLICATIONS

Mortality

Operative mortality depends on the indication for the procedure and the level of amputation. Mortality rates for major lower extremity amputations in dysvascular and diabetic patients have been reported between zero and 35% (29). Combined mortality rates from multiple series are shown in Table 81.8 (30). Cardiovascular causes account for two thirds of these deaths, with myocardial infarction responsible for one third (30).

Long-term survival following amputation in the dysvascular population is shown in Table 81.9. The 5-year survival is only 37%, compared with 85% for age-matched controls (31).

Deep Venous Thrombosis and Pulmonary Embolism

The incidence of deep venous thrombosis following lower extremity amputation ranges from 4% to 38% (32–34). Prophylactic measures, including subcutaneous heparin, early mobilization, and pneumatic compression devices, are mandatory.

Stump Complications

Stump complications include failure to heal, infection, hematoma, contractures, ulceration, phantom pain, and trauma. Although most amputations heal primarily, a small percentage do not. Amputation at a more proximal level usually is successful. Postoperative infections complicate 12% to 28% of all amputations, with the percentage higher in cases performed for infection (35). Local wound care with drainage, débridement and dressing changes, and systemic antibiotics should be instituted. Wound hematomas are best treated by prevention. Meticulous hemostasis and the avoidance of subcutaneous cavities decrease the incidence of hematoma. Closed-suction drains are inadequate to drain blood and have been reported to increase the incidence of wound infection. Hematomas should be treated in the operating room with evacuation, irrigation, and closure of the wound. An infected hematoma should be treated as an abscess.

Joint contractures complicate 1% to 3% of all amputations (29,31). These contractures can develop rapidly postoperatively and are best treated by prevention. Rehabilitation specialists and physical therapists should evaluate patients preoperatively, and active and passive range-of-motion exercises should be initiated immediately postoperatively. Adequate pain medication, ideally with patient-controlled or epidural anesthesia, is crucial (36,37). Pillows and bed positions that result in hip flexion, knee flexion, or both are to be strictly avoided.

Ulcers are prone to develop over bony prominences. Poorly fitting prostheses or shoes are the most common causes. Diabetic patients with peripheral neuropathy are especially prone to the development of ulcers following toe and limited foot amputations. They can also form on

Table 81.9. SURVIVAL AFTER AMPUTATION FOR ISCHEMIA

Time (y)	Survival rate (%)
1	75
2	60
3	50
4	45
5	37

From Frang RD, Taylor LM, Porter JM. Amputations. In: Porter JM, Taylor LM, eds. *Basic data underlying clinical decision making in vascular surgery.* St. Louis: Quality Medical, 1994:155, with permission.

the anterior aspect of above-knee amputations secondary to the disproportional contraction of the hip flexors relative to the hip extensors. Local wound care and bed rest usually result in healing if the ulcer is superficial. Deep skin ulcers with involvement of the soft tissue and the underlying bone are more complicated. They often suggest borderline perfusion of the stump, and formal revision to a higher level is required for definitive treatment.

Neuromas are regenerative nerve tissue that form in response to transection. They can cause pain if trapped in the fibrous scar or if irritated by a prosthesis. Proximal nerve division under tension during the original operation decreases the incidence of this complication. Symptomatic neuromas should be treated with proximal resection of the nerve because local excision of the neuroma is rarely adequate.

Some element of phantom extremity pain occurs in nearly all amputations (38), although these complaints are not always directed to the treating surgeon. It is necessary to describe these common symptoms to the patient and specifically inquire about their presence. The pain is disabling in 5% to 30% (39) of patients surveyed. Currently, the pain is felt to be a component of a central pain syndrome and unrelated to either a neuroma or the perception of an intact extremity. Although no universally effective treatment is available, Malone (29) has reported a low incidence with an aggressive rehabilitation program, including immediate fitting of a prosthesis. Recently, electroconvulsive therapy has been suggested as an effective treatment for refractory cases of phantom pain (40).

Trauma to a limb following an amputation can convert a healed amputation to a nonhealing wound, so that a more proximal amputation is required. Perioperatively, patients with a below-knee amputation have to be observed closely to prevent them from attempting ambulation. Diabetic patients with retinopathy should not walk barefoot following toe and foot amputations because of the risk that minor trauma may lead to a major problem in wound healing.

Additional Amputation

The incidence of future amputation in dysvascular patients is significant. In the report of Little and colleagues (41), a more proximal amputation was required in 75% of all dysvascular patients within 3.5 years after toe amputation. The incidence of contralateral limb loss in dysvascular and diabetic patients has been reported between 15% to 33% at 5 years after a major lower extremity amputation (42). These dismal figures reflect the systemic nature of the underlying diseases and underscore the importance of appropriate foot care, patient education, close follow-up, and early intervention (43). Recent work suggests that a concerted multidisciplinary approach can dramatically decrease the incidence of initial and subsequent lower extremity amputation (44).

Special Situations

In selected cases, hyperbaric oxygen therapy can provide benefit in treating nonhealing amputation sites. Patients require a thorough evaluation of their cardiopulmonary status before such treatment is initiated. In addition, the treating vascular surgeon has to determine that revascularization is completed or is not indicated. Patients may benefit from treatment if a substantial increase in transcutaneous oxygen pressure ($TcPo_2$) occurs near the wound with administration of 100% oxygen. Daily treatments are typically continued for 30 days. Platelet-derived growth factor [becaplermin (Regranex)] has recently been approved for use in the United States and has been effec-

tive in the management of diabetic foot ulcers and following open foot amputations or débridements. The wound must be clear of all necrotic tissue before the initiation of therapy.

REHABILITATION AND MANAGEMENT OF PROSTHESES

General Considerations

Rehabilitation needs to be individualized. For some patients, successful rehabilitation means ambulation on a prosthesis and resumption of an independent life-style. For others, success may mean being able to pivot on the contralateral limb and assist with transfer.

Ambulating with a prosthesis depends on the physiologic status of the patient. Table 81.3 illustrates the dramatic increase in energy requirement that occurs as the level of the amputation rises. As expected, the chance of ambulating on a prosthesis decreases as the amputation level rises. The percentage of diabetic and dysvascular patients who are able to ambulate with amputations at various levels is illustrated in Table 81.10. In addition, the likelihood of ambulating postoperatively is inversely related to the patient's age and length of the rehabilitation process (45).

Specific Considerations

Digital and Ray Amputations

All patients who were ambulatory preoperatively should be able to achieve their preoperative functional status following a digital or ray amputation. The first digit and metatarsal head are important for weight bearing and for power. A shoe orthosis should effectively compensate for these functions with limited training.

The most important component of postoperative rehabilitation for patients following a digital or ray amputation is education. The rate of repeated amputation (other toe, more proximal level, contralateral limb) is extremely high. Several studies have indicated that the rate of repeated amputation is diminished with a coordinated education program (46,47).

Transmetatarsal Amputation

A transmetatarsal amputation does not increase the energy requirement of ambulation; therefore, postoperative ambulation is expected following successful healing. The absence of the toes and metatarsal heads results in the loss of some forward thrust during the push-off phase of ambulation. This deficit can be overcome with either a steel-

Table 81.10. AMBULATION AFTER LOWER EXTREMITY AMPUTATION FOR DIABETES OR OCCLUSIVE DISEASE

Amputation level	Postoperative ambulation (%)
Digit or ray	100
Transmetatarsal	100
Syme amputation	90–100
Below-knee	75
Above-knee	39
Hip disarticulation	<10

From Frang RD, Taylor LM, Porter JM. Amputations. In: Porter JM, Taylor LM, eds. *Basic data underlying clinical decision making in vascular surgery.* St. Louis: Quality Medical, 1994:155, with permission.

shank or a rigid, roller-soled shoe. The void in the distal part of the shoe is filled with an insert.

Syme Amputation

The prognosis for return to bipedal ambulation following a Syme amputation is excellent. The required energy expenditure is only 10% more than baseline (48). A significant advantage of this amputation is the ability to ambulate on the stump with only a cup slipper. Even though this activity is permitted only on a limited basis in the home, it is much more convenient for the patient, especially when arising at night. For routine activity, the patient uses a prosthesis consisting of a nonmotion foot attached to a leg shaft. The shaft has a cutout on the medial aspect to allow passage of the flared distal end of the stump. The configuration of the distal end of the stump results in a bulbous ankle, which is less aesthetically pleasing then the typical below-knee prosthesis.

Below-knee Amputation

The rehabilitation potential following a below-knee amputation is very good. Even when the indication for amputation is arterial insufficiency, approximately 75% of patients are able to ambulate with a prosthesis (30). Multiple design options are available; however, the patellar tendon and the medial and lateral tibial flares are the weight-bearing surfaces for most prostheses. A variety of foot designs are possible that permit extension, flexion, rotation, and energy storage.

Above-knee Amputation

Ambulation on an above-knee prosthesis is achieved by fewer than 40% of patients with arterial insufficiency (30). In this patient population, the rate of ambulation on bilateral above-knee prostheses is less than 10% (49). Most above-knee prostheses use the ischial tuberosity as the primary weight-bearing surface and are secured by either a belt or a suction socket. For younger patients, a suction socket works well. Patients with groin scars from previous revascularization attempts may benefit from a belt mechanism. The knee design depends on the patient's general condition and thigh strength. A knee that engages during the stance phase of gait is more stable and is frequently used in older patients.

REFERENCES

1. Falstie-Jensen N, Christensen K. A model for prediction of failure in amputation of the lower limb. *Dan Med Bull* 1990;37:283.
2. Sanmugarajah J, Hussain S, Schwartz J, et al. Monoclonal cryoglobulinemia with extensive gangrene of all four extremities—a case report. *Angiology* 2000;51:431–434.
3. Veith F, Gupta S, Samson R, et al. Progress in limb salvage by reconstructive arterial surgery combined with new or improved adjunctive procedures. *Ann Surg* 1981;194:386.
4. Lange R. Limb reconstruction versus amputation: decision making in massive lower extremity trauma. *Clin Orthop* 1989 (Jun);92–99.
5. Johansen K, Daines M, Howey T, et al. Objective criteria accurately predict amputation following lower extremity trauma. *J Trauma* 1990;30:568–572; discussion 572–573.
6. Harwood T, Coe E, Flynn T, et al. The use of arm vein conduits during infrageniculate arterial bypass. *J Vasc Surg* 1992;16:420–423.
7. Leseche G, Penna C, Bouttier S, et al. Femorodistal bypass using cryopreserved venous allografts for limb salvage. *Ann Vasc Surg* 1997;11:230–236.
8. Raptis S, Miller J. Influence of vein cuff on polytetrafluoroethylene grafts for primary femoropopliteal bypass. *Br J Surg* 1995;82:478–491.
9. Stonebridge P, Prescott R, Ruckley C, et al. Randomised trial comparing polytetrafluoroethylene graft patients with and without Miller cuff. *Br J Surg* 1995;2:555–556.
10. Lepantalo M, Tukiainen E. Combined vascular reconstruction and microvascular muscle flap transfer for salvage of ischaemic legs with major tissue loss and wound complications. *Eur J Vasc Endovasc Surg* 1996;12:65–69.
11. Briggs S, Banis JJ, Kaebnick H, et al. Distal revascularization and microvascular free tissue transfer: an alternative to amputation in ischemic lesions of the lower extremity. *J Vasc Surg* 1985;2:806–811.
12. Biancari F, Kantonen I, Alback A, et al. Limits of infrapopliteal bypass surgery for critical leg ischemia: when not to reconstruct. *World J Surg* 2000;24:727–733.
13. Keagy B, Schwartz J, Kolb M, et al. Lower extremity amputation: the control series. *J Vasc Surg* 1986;4:321–326.
14. Dwars B, Van Ben Broek T, Ravwerda J, et al. Criteria for reliable selection of the lowest level of amputation in peripheral vascular disease. *J Vasc Surg* 1992;15:536.
15. Avci S, Musdal Y. Skin blood flow level and stump healing in ischemic amputations. *Orthopedics* 2000;23:33–36.
16. Moore W. Determination of amputation level: measurement of skin blood flow with xenon-133 clearance. *Arch Surg* 1973; 107:798.
17. Burnham S, Wagner W, Keagy B, et al. Objective measurement of limb perfusion by dermal fluorometry: a criterion for healing of below knee amputation. *Arch Surg* 1990;125:513.
18. Malone J, Anderson G, Halka S, et al. Prospective comparison of noninvasive techniques for amputation level selection. *Am J Surg* 1987;154:179.
19. Misuri A, Lucertini G, Nanni A, et al. Predictive value of transcutaneous oximetry for selection of the amputation level. *J Cardiovasc Surg* 2000;41:83–87.
20. Holloway G, Watkins B. Laser Doppler measurement of cutaneous blood flow. *J Invest Dermatol* 1977;69:300.
21. Schwartz J, Schuler J, O'Connor R, et al. Predictive value of distal perfusion pressure in the healing of amputation of the digits and forefoot. *Surg Gynecol Obstet* 1982;154:865.
22. Golbranson F, Yu E, Gelberman R. The use of skin temperature determinations in lower extremity amputation level selection. *Foot Ankle* 1982;3:170–172.
23. Gibbons G, Wheelock F, Hoar C, et al. Predicting success of forefoot amputations in diabetics by noninvasive testing. *Arch Surg* 1979;114:1034.
24. Chang B, Bock D, Jacobs R, et al. Increased limb salvage by the use of unconventional foot amputations. *J Vasc Surg* 1994;19:341–349.
25. Roach J, Deutsch A, McFarlane D. Resurrection of the amputations of Lisfranc and Chopart for diabetic gangrene. *Arch Surg* 1987;122:931–934.
26. Leiberman J, Jacobs R, Goldstock L, et al. Chopart amputation with percutaneous heel cord lengthening. *Clin Orthop* 1993;292:245–249.
27. Burgess E. Disarticulation of the knee: a modified technique. *Arch Surg* 1977;112:1250.
28. Merkel K, Gebhardt M, Springfield D. Rotationplasty as a reconstructive operation after tumor resection. *Clin Orthop* 1991;270:231–236.
29. Malone J. Lower extremity amputation. In: Moore W, ed. *Vascular surgery: a comprehensive review.* Philadelphia: WB Saunders, 1993:809.
30. Frang R, Taylor L, Porter J. Amputations. In: Porter J, Taylor L, eds. *Basic data underlying clinical decision making in vascular surgery.* St. Louis: Quality Medical, 1994:153.
31. Roon A, Moore W. Below-knee amputations: a modern approach. *Am J Surg* 1977;134:153.
32. Williams J, Britt L, Eades T, et al. Pulmonary embolism after amputation of the lower extremity. *Surg Gyn Obst* 1975;140:246–248.
33. Yeager R, Moneta G, Edwards J, et al. Deep vein thrombosis associated with lower extremity amputation. *J Vasc Surg* 1995;22:612–615.
34. Burke B, Kumar R, Vickers V, et al. Deep vein thrombosis after lower limb amputation. *Am J Phys Med Rehabil* 2000;79:145–149.
35. Fisher DJ, Clagett G, Fry R, et al. One-stage versus two-stage amputation for wet gangrene of the lower extremity: a randomized study. *J Vasc Surg* 1988;8:428–433.
36. Enneking F, Morey T. Continuous postoperative infusion of a regional anesthetic after an amputation of the lower extremity: a randomized clinical trial [letter; comment]. *J Bone Joint Surg* 1997;79:1752–1753.
37. Pinzur M, Garla P, Pluth T, et al. Continuous postoperative in-

fusion of a regional anesthetic after an amputation of the lower extremity: a randomized clinical trial [see comments]. *J Bone Joint Surg* 1996;78:1501–1505.

38. Iacono R, Linford J, Sandyk R. Pain management after lower extremity amputation. *Neurosurgery* 1987;20:496–500.

39. Sherman R, Sherman C, Parker L. Chronic phantom and stump pain among American veterans: results of a survey. *Pain* 1984;18:83.

40. Rasmussen K, Rummans T. Electroconvulsive therapy for phantom limb pain. *Pain* 2000;85:297–299.

41. Little J, Stephen M, Zylstra P. Amputation of the toes for vascular disease: fate of the affected leg. *Lancet* 1976;2:1318.

42. Whitehouse F, Jurgensen C, Block M. The later life of the diabetic amputee: another look at the fate of the second leg. *Diabetes* 1968;17:520.

43. Powell T, Burnham S, Johnson GJ. Second leg ischemia: lower extremity bypass versus amputation in patients with contralateral lower extremity amputation. *Am Surg* 1984;50:577–580.

44. Van Gils C, Wheeler L, Mellstrom M, et al. Amputation prevention by vascular surgery and podiatry collaboration in high-risk diabetic and nondiabetic patients: the Operation Desert Foot experience. *Diabetes Care* 1999;22:678–683.

45. Harris W. Lower-extremity amputation in elderly patients. *Can J Surg* 1987;30:315.

46. Bild D, Selby J, Sinnock P, et al. Lower-extremity amputation in people with diabetes: epidemiology and prevention. *Diabetes Care* 1989;12:24–31.

47. Del Aguila M, Reiber G, Koepsell T. How does provider and patient awareness of high-risk status for lower-extremity amputation influence foot-care practice? *Diabetes Care* 1994;17:1050–1054.

48. Waters R, Perry J, Antonelli D, et al. Energy cost of walking amputees: the influence of level of amputation. *J Bone Joint Surg* 1976;58A:42.

49. Malone J. Above the knee amputation and hip disarticulation. In: Ernest CB, ed. *Current therapy in vascular surgery*, 2nd ed. Philadelphia: BC Decker, 1991:699.

Aneurysmal Disease

SURGERY: SCIENTIFIC PRINCIPLES AND PRACTICE, Third Edition, edited by Lazar J. Greenfield, Michael W. Mulholland, Keith T. Oldham, Gerald B. Zelenock, and Keith D. Lillemoe. Lippincott Williams & Wilkins Publishers, Philadelphia, © 2001.

CHAPTER 82

PATHOGENESIS OF ANEURYSMS

B. TIMOTHY BAXTER AND ALEX ESQUIVEL

An aneurysm is a permanent, localized dilation of a blood vessel. The Committee for Reporting Standards of the major North American vascular societies has put forth a more precise definition of an aneurysm as a 50% increase in the diameter of a vessel in comparison with its expected normal diameter (1). Aneurysms can occur in any segment of the arterial tree, including cerebral vessels, the aorta (thoracic and abdominal), peripheral vessels (iliac, femoral, and popliteal), and various others. The intracranial circulation is the most common site of aneurysm formation. The most common location for extracranial aneurysms is the infrarenal aorta. Each year, approximately 15,000 deaths in the United States are attributed to abdominal aortic aneurysm (2). Although this disease is thought to affect approximately 2% of the general population based on ultrasonographic screening studies, it primarily affects elderly persons, who comprise a rapidly growing segment of our population.

In 1804, Scarpa (3) attributed abdominal aortic aneurysm to atherosclerotic degeneration based on the large amounts of plaque in such aneurysms. Since that time, most authors have ascribed aneurysm pathogenesis to atherosclerosis. Despite a decrease in the rate of coronary artery disease and stroke, the incidence of aneurysm development appears to have increased (4,5). In a study by Lillienfeld et al. (6), the incidence of abdominal aortic aneurysm was found to have increased sevenfold during a 30-year period. This increase is thought to be in part a consequence of better de-

tection, but the study also found that the true incidence of symptomatic aneurysms had doubled. Repair by interposition grafting with a synthetic graft is the only proven therapy for abdominal aortic aneurysm, and 40,000 patients undergo elective repair each year in the United States alone (2). This number will substantially increase as 79 million baby boomers reach their 60s and 70s. When performed as an emergency for rupture, surgical repair is associated with a mortality rate of approximately 50%. Even elective repair is not without significant risk to the elderly patient in terms of both morbidity and mortality. Indeed, a statewide survey in Michigan found the mortality rate for elective aneurysmorrhaphy to exceed 5% (7). The increasing size of the population at risk, the increased incidence among this group, and the significant mortality rates associated with rupture and both elective and emergent repair are sobering statistics. They underscore the increasing impact this common disorder will have in the next decade.

Although less invasive options are currently being explored, the fundamental treatment of abdominal aortic aneurysm has changed very little in the past 35 years. Encouragingly, the past decade has seen some important progress in building a foundation for understanding the pathogenesis of the disease. Basic scientists from many disciplines have contributed to a detailed description of the disease in terms of its histologic, biochemical, and genetic characteristics. This work provides a springboard for an even greater challenge: to define the factors that initiate and promote aortic dilation, identify patients in whom these factors are present, and offer such patients an intervention that will alter the natural history of their disease.

The pathogenesis of abdominal aortic aneurysm is complex and undoubtedly multifactorial. Although aortic aneurysms are strongly associated with systemic atherosclerosis (8,9), and although many of the same risk factors known to promote atherosclerosis are predisposing factors for aortic aneurysm (10), aneurysms develop in only a small percentage of patients with atherosclerosis of the distal aorta (11). The familial tendency to aneurysm formation strongly suggests a genetic component, but its late onset obscures a clear pattern of heritability (12,13). The aneurysm process itself appears focal, and yet evidence of systemic arterial changes has also been found (14–16).

One approach to elucidate the pathogenesis of aneurysms is to study aneurysmal tissue and compare it with normal aorta and also with aorta affected by atherosclerosis but not aneurysmal dilation. Differences in cellular composition, matrix macromolecule content, or proteolytic activity between these specimens help to identify factors uniquely associated with aneurysms and provide clues to pathogenesis. This approach to the study of aneurysm pathogenesis provides us with important information about factors that may promote the growth of an existing aneurysm, and, importantly, it provides a fundamental descriptive foundation on which more sophisticated methods of research, such as genetic analysis and the study of animal models, can be based.

Another method employed in the investigation of aneurysm pathogenesis is to study the disease process as it is induced in an animal model. A reproducible animal model allows for careful analysis and manipulation of potentially important etiologic factors in the early stages of the process. This approach can be a powerful tool in elucidating the molecular and cellular mechanisms responsible for aortic dilation, but only if the model recapitulates human disease. A diverse variety of experimental methods can induce arterial dilation, including mechanical or chemical injury (17,18), long-term dietary manipulations (19–22), and inhibition of post-translational processing of matrix macromolecules (23,24). As our understanding of the genetic basis of aneurysm formation becomes more clearly defined, transgenic animal studies will likely play an important role in clarifying the particular genes of interest.

ROLE OF ATHEROSCLEROSIS

As previously mentioned, atherosclerosis has been thought to play a key role in aortic aneurysm development because of the strong clinical and histopathologic association between the two disease processes. Aortic aneurysms tend to localize to the infrarenal aorta, a site also prone to the development of atherosclerosis (25). Furthermore, "atherosclerotic" plaque is present in the aneurysm wall (25) and also at remote sites, such as the coronary arteries (8). Furthermore, the two diseases share various risk factors, such as smoking, hypertension, and hypercholesterolemia (10). Although it has been argued that atherosclerosis in the aneurysm segment is a response to the aortic dilation rather than its cause (26), the strength of the association suggests that, at a minimum, atherosclerosis is a permissive factor required for aneurysm development.

Although clinical observations strongly implicate atherosclerosis in the genesis of abdominal aortic aneurysm, evidence from animal studies has been less compelling. In two separate reports of squirrel monkeys that were fed an atherogenic diet for 9 to 79 months, severe atherosclerosis developed in all, but aneurysms develop in only 1.5% (13 of 833) (20,21). Similarly, DePalma et al. (19) reported a single aneurysm among five dogs fed an atherogenic diet for 60 months. Zarins et al. (22) reported a higher incidence of aneurysms (10%) in cynomolgus monkeys fed an atherogenic diet followed by a regression diet with cholestyramine for 16 to 24 months. This work suggests that plaque regression could play a role in aneurysm formation. Of note, these experimental aneurysms tended to be diverse in location and favored the thoracic aorta, in contrast to human aortic aneurysmal disease. Nevertheless, the studies suggest that chronic atherosclerosis may be a prerequisite for aneurysm formation and that plaque regression may also contribute. The fact that chronic atherosclerosis results in aneurysm formation in only a small percentage of animals (or patients) indicates that other factors must also be important.

MATRIX CHANGES IN ABDOMINAL AORTIC ANEURYSM

The aorta is the largest of the elastic arteries, performing two important functions. It acts as a conduit, transporting blood from the heart to the rest of the body, and it reduces the cardiac workload by absorbing energy as blood is ejected from the heart. These functions require that the aortic wall possess both tensile strength and elasticity, properties conferred largely by the matrix proteins collagen and elastin. These proteins are synthesized and maintained by the resident mesenchymal cells in a highly regulated fashion designed to maintain the functional integrity of the vascular wall.

Collagen is an important component of both the normal lamellar structure of the aortic media and the surrounding fibrous adventitia (27). The fiber-forming collagens, especially types I and III, are the predominant collagen types in the aorta (28). Together, these collagens primarily impart tensile strength (29), but they also contribute to the extensile properties of the aorta (30). Given their critical role in maintaining the structural integrity of the vascular wall, the relationship between these collagen types in patients with aneurysms in comparison with the relationship in normal controls has been studied extensively (31–33).

Although the ratio of collagen types I and III does not appear to be altered in the diseased aorta, the expression of both types is increased in aneurysm tissue in comparison with normal tissue or aortas affected by atherosclerotic occlusive disease (34–36). By in situ hybridization, the increased expression localizes to three areas in the aortic wall: (a) adventitial fibroblasts, (b) medial smooth-muscle cells adjacent to inflammatory infiltrates, and (c) transformed myofibroblasts within the plaque (37). Expression of these collagens in abdominal aortic aneurysm is regulated by a soluble tissue factor (38), with synthesis of the fiber-forming collagens normally regulated at the level of transcription (39). The increased procollagen expression is translated into collagen protein, as the mass of this protein in the aneurysm has been shown to increase progressively with increasing aneurysm size (38). However, it is unclear whether the increase in collagen production is compensatory or pathogenic in abdominal aortic aneurysm. Several mutations in type III collagen have been linked to late-onset abdominal aortic aneurysm (33,40). A systematic search for other fibrillar collagen mutations in 50 cases of adult-onset abdominal aortic aneurysm did not identify another structurally significant mutation (41).

Elastin is another important component of the vascular wall matrix and is responsible for the viscous and elastic properties of the aorta (42). Amorphous tropoelastin is arranged on a scaffold of microfibrillar proteins to form the elastin fibers of the medial lamellae (43). By forming stable cross-links, these fibers become highly resistant to proteolytic degradation and have a half-life measured in decades (44). Tropoelastin synthesis, unlike the synthesis of fibrillar collagens, is regulated post-transcriptionally by destabilization of the mRNA, which occurs in the perinatal period (45). It has been suggested that little elastin is synthesized in the aorta after birth. Certainly, no evidence for the synthesis of new elastin fibers beyond the perinatal period has been found, and it is true that the number of elastin lamellae is not increased with growth. However, we have observed that the mass of elastin in the adult thoracic aorta is twice that found in the thoracic aorta of the

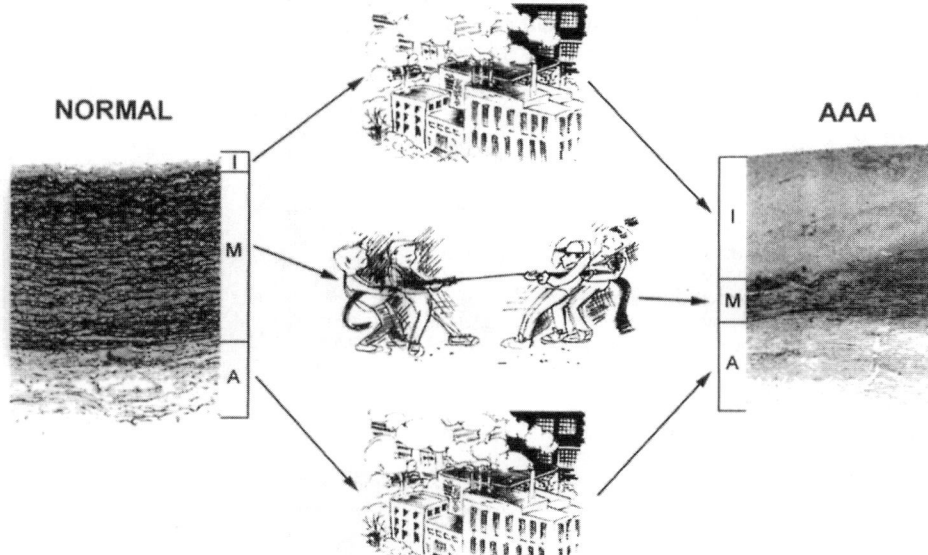

Figure 82.1. Changes in the aorta associated with aneurysm formation. In a diseased aorta, most of the metabolic activity occurs in the intima *(I)* and adventitia *(A),* where collagen is deposited during aortic dilation. The elastic fibers of the media *(M)* are stretched and attenuated, and their structural role is diminished under constant pressure. The progressive remodeling of collagen in the adventitia leads to growth and eventual failure (rupture) of the aortic wall. (From Rehm JP, Baxter BT. The formation of aneurysms. *Semin Vasc Surg* 1998; 11:193–202, with permission.)

child. Thus, some organized low levels of elastin synthesis after birth appear likely to add to existing fibers. This idea is consistent with findings on electron micrographs of normal aorta, which show medial smooth-muscle cells adjacent to the elastin fibers (46), and with the detection of low levels of elastin mRNA in the adult aorta (35). Two fibrillin mutations have been found in association with abdominal aortic aneurysm (47). Given the strong association of fibrillin with elastin, and the markedly higher levels of elastin in the proximal compared with the distal aorta, it seems quite unlikely that fibrillin or elastin mutations would be manifested primarily in the distal aorta. So, despite the considerable work done in this area, no mutations of the major aortic connective tissue proteins have been found that could account for the high frequency of adult-onset abdominal aortic aneurysm.

One of the most striking histologic features of aneurysmal tissue is the fragmentation of the medial lamellae and decreased concentration of elastin (31,48) (Fig. 82.1). Several studies have compared tropoelastin expression and elastin content in normal, atherosclerotic, and aneurysmal aorta. Elastin mRNA levels in adult tissue are very low, and by Northern blot analysis, no detectable differences in expression are seen between normal tissue and abdominal aortic aneurysm tissue (35). However, two separate studies have shown that the absolute mass of elastin is increased in the aneurysmal aorta in comparison with normal aorta (38,49). The apparent discrepancy between this observation and the marked decrease in elastin staining of abdominal aortic aneurysm tissue may relate to poor uptake of the elastin stain by the newly synthesized, unorganized elastin fibrils, and to a general redistribution of the elastin over a larger aortic diameter. Any increase in elastin does not keep pace with aortic expansion, and its concentration is markedly decreased relative to that of collagen (31,38).

Although it seems logical to assume that these changes in elastin content and architecture noted in aneurysm tissue play a causal role in pathogenesis, similar changes are also present in the nondilated but severely atherosclerotic aorta (aortic occlusive disease) (50). This observation suggests that the changes could be the result, rather than the cause, of the disease. Work in animal models, however, provides evidence that the changes in elastin metabolism may in fact be pathogenic and has fueled considerable investigation into the role of proteolysis in the genesis of abdominal aortic aneurysm.

PROTEOLYSIS IN ABDOMINAL AORTIC ANEURYSM

The role of collagenolytic and elastolytic enzymes found in aneurysm tissue has been the subject of a number of important studies. Table 82.1 summarizes the discoveries made during the past two decades of study of proteolytic enzymes contributing to abdominal aortic aneurysm. Busuttil et al. (51) and Cannon and Read (52) were the first to report increased elastolytic activity in abdominal aortic aneurysm. Enzymes for which elastin is a substrate include the serine proteases, neutrophil elastase, and the matrix metalloproteinases (MMPs), which include 92-kd gelatinase (MMP-9), 72-kd gelatinase (MMP-2), matrilysin (MMP-8), and macrophage metalloelastase (MMP-12). The MMPs are a family of endopeptidases that can degrade all components of extracellular matrix. The crystal structure of MMP-2 has recently been elucidated (53) (Fig. 82.2). Both of the gelatinases (MMP-2 and MMP-9) effectively degrade elastin and type IV collagen, and MMP-2 has been shown to have true collagenolytic activity (54). Cohen et al. (55) have performed extensive studies of neutrophil elastase and reported that peripheral neutrophils from patients with abdominal aortic aneurysm exhibit increased neutrophil elastase activity. They have also shown that smooth-muscle cells from abdominal aortic aneurysm explants secrete increased amounts of proteolytic enzymes in response to stimulation by elastin degradation products (56). This work does suggest increased proteolytic enzyme production by circulating neutrophils from patients with abdominal aortic aneurysm and by abdominal aortic aneurysm smooth-muscle cells. Although neutrophils are not seen in significant numbers in advanced aneurysmal tissue, this observation does not preclude their potential role in the initiation of the disease process.

Several of the MMPs have been identified in abdominal aortic aneurysm tissue, including MMP-1, MMP-2, MMP-3, MMP-9, and MMP-12. Herron et al. (57) and Newman and colleagues (58), using gelatin zymography, have demonstrated increased activity of the 92-kd gelatinase in abdominal aortic aneurysm tissue homogenates in comparison with homogenates from normal tissue. Thompson

Table 82.1. **COLLAGENOLYTIC/ELASTOLYTIC ACTIVITY IN ANEURYSMAL TISSUE**

Authors (ref.)	Sample	Method	Findings	No. AOD specimens
Busuttil et al., 1980 (78)	Tissue homogenate	Colorimetric collagenase assay	Collagenase activity AAA > AOD	5
Busuttil et al., 1982 (51)	Tissue colorimetric homogenate	Colorimetric elastase assay	Elastase activity AAA > AOD	9
Manashi et al., 1987 (79)	Tissue homogenate	Radiolabeled collagenase assay	Collagenase AAA + AOD	6
Cohen et al., 1988 (55)	Tissue homogenate	Colorimetric elastase assay	Elastase AAA > AOD	12
Cohen et al., 1992 (56)	Tissue homogenate	Elastase assay	Elastase AAA > AOD = CON	10
Herron et al., 1991 (57)	Tissue homogenate	Zymography Radiolabeled substrate release	MMP-9 AAA > CON	0
Vine and Powell, 1991 (60)	Tissue homogenate	Zymography Radiolabeled substrate release	Gelatinase collagenase AAA > CON AAA ≅ AOD	8
Webster et al., 1991 (80)	Tissue homogenate	Colorimetric collagenase assay	Collagenase activity AAA > CON or AOD	2
Newman et al., 1994 (110)	Tissue homogenate	Zymography Immunoblot	MMP-9 AAA > CON	3
Thompson et al., 1995 (59)	Conditioned media (72 h)	Zymography ELISA	MMP-2 no difference	10
McMillan et al., 1995 (61)	Tissue RNA	Northern blot	MMP-9 mRNA AAA > normal AAA ≅ AOD	8
McMillan et al., 1995 (67)	Tissue RNA	Northern blot	MMP-2 mRNA AAA > AOD > normal	9
Patel et al., 1996 (65)	Cultured SMC Conditioned media	Substrate assays Zymography Immunoblot	MMP-2, MMP-9 AAA > AOD > CON	4
Li et al., 1996 (69)	Tissue homogenate	Zymography Immunoblot Immunohistochemistry	MMP-2 AOD > CON (no AAA)	8
Sakalihasan et al., 1996 (111)	Tissue homogenate	Zymography Substrate assay	MMP-9 AAA > CON Activated MMP-2 AAA > CON	0
Knox et al., 1997 (112)	Tissue	In situ zymography Immunohistochemistry	AOD = AAA	7
Davis et al., 1998 (63)	Tissue	Zymography Immunoblot	MMP-2 ↑AAA active MMP-2↑	7
Curci et al., 1998 (76)	Tissue	Zymography	MMP-12↑	3

AAA, abdominal aortic aneurysm; AOD, aortic occlusive disease; CON, control; SMC, smooth-muscle cells; MMP, matrix metalloproteinase; ELISA, enzyme-linked immunosorbent assay.

et al. (59) examined conditioned media from explant cultures of normal, aortic occlusive disease, and abdominal aortic aneurysm tissue and showed that aneurysm explants produce more MMP-9 than either normal or aortic occlusive disease controls. This conclusion was further supported by immunohistochemical tissue analysis. However, a study by Vine and Powell (60), in which a radioactively labeled gelatin substrate was used, found a significant amount of gelatinase activity around 92 kd (MMP-9), but found no significant difference in gelatinase activity (measured as micrograms per hour per milligram of protein) between abdominal aortic aneurysm (13.3 ± 3.3) and aortic occlusive disease (10.9 ± 1.8). Similarly, studies of tissue RNA by McMillan et al. (61) reported an increased expression of MMP-9 in diseased aorta in comparison with normal aorta, but they found no differences in MMP-9 mRNA between the two disease states of abdominal aortic aneurysm and aortic occlusive disease. However, McMillan and Pearce (62) did identify increased circulating levels of MMP-9 in patients with abdominal aortic aneurysm in comparison with patients with aortic occlusive disease, making this a potentially important serum marker for aneurysmal disease. This theme has been reiterated in many of the studies listed in Table 82.1.

Because of the prominence of MMP-9 in both aortic occlusive disease and abdominal aortic aneurysm, a number of studies have addressed the cellular source of this protease. Macrophages are believed to be the primary source of MMP-9 in abdominal aortic aneurysm (59,63), but good evidence is available to suggest that smooth-muscle cells may also be a source of this enzyme. The normal aorta appears to express MMP-9 in the absence of invading inflammatory cells (61,64), and smooth-muscle cells derived from abdominal aortic aneurysm secrete MMP-9 in culture (65). In addition, cultured aneurysmal smooth-muscle cells demonstrate an increased expression of metalloproteinases in response to proinflammatory cytokines (66). Because the smooth-muscle cell phenotype may change dramatically under culture conditions, these studies should be interpreted with some caution.

Although much attention has been focused on the role of MMP-9 in aneurysm pathogenesis, recent work suggests that MMP-2 may have a greater potential to regulate the matrix than other proteinases. MMP-2 is the only proteinase capable of degrading not just elastin but also fibrous collagen. It has been shown that degradation of the fibrous collagen of the adventitia is essential for the development of abdominal aortic aneurysm. Furthermore, the primary source of MMP-2 is the same mesenchymal cells that produce elastin and collagen—in the media, smooth-muscle cells, and in the adventitia, fibroblasts (67). Moreover, MMP-2 is a more potent elastase than MMP-9 (68). Like those of MMP-9, tissue levels of MMP-2 appear to be increased in aorta in both disease states, abdominal aortic aneurysm and aortic occlusive disease, in comparison with normal aorta (69,70). In media conditioned by explant cultures from both abdominal aortic aneurysm and aortic occlusive disease, Thompson et al. (59) found no difference in MMP-2. However, Freestone et al. (70) reported an increase in MMP-2 in small aneurysms in comparison with aortic occlusive disease controls, and McMillan et al. (67) found an increase in MMP-2 mRNA in abdominal aortic aneurysm in comparison with aortic occlusive disease controls. Davis et al. (63) reported that a far greater proportion of the abdominal aortic aneurysm MMP-2 is in the active 62-kd form and that it is tightly

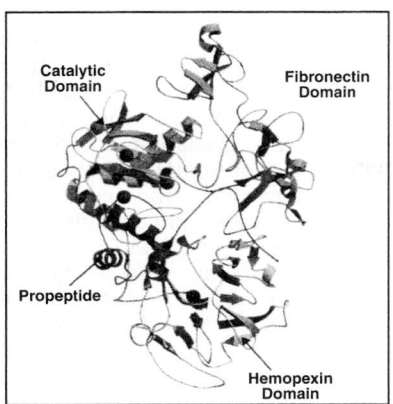

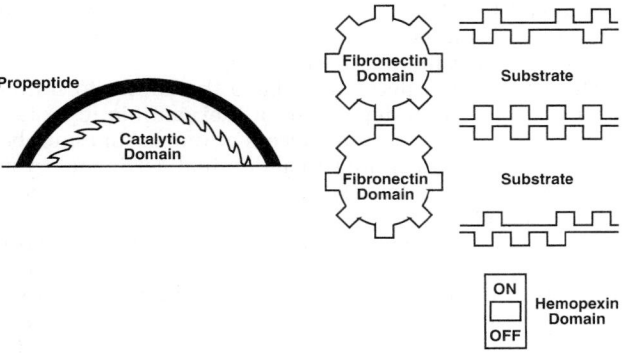

Figure 82.2. Matrix metalloproteinase *(MMP)* functional domains. The structure of pro-MMP-2 was recently derived by means of x-ray crystallography. (Reprinted from Morgunova E, Tuuttila A, Bergmann U, et al. Structure of human pro-matrix metalloproteinase-2: activation mechanism revealed. *Science* 1999;284:1667–1670, with permission.) A schematic shows the relationship and role of each functional domain. The propeptide acts as a guard, keeping the active site covered until its activity is required. Removal of the propeptide by membrane-bound MMPs results in the active 62-kd form of MMP-2. The fibronectin domains "grab" the substrate. The three-dimensional structure around the active site and the fibronectin-binding sites confer specificity because only substrates with the appropriate conformation and with corresponding fibronectin-binding domains can be bound. The catalytic domain performs the cleavage. The hemopexin domain helps to confer specificity by contributing to the three-dimensional structure of the active site. Additionally, it can be thought of as an on/off switch because it is the tissue inhibitor of metalloproteinases *(TIMP)*-binding site. TIMP inactivates MMP. (Reprinted from Lewis K, Rehm JP, Baxter BT. Molecular demolition: the role of metalloproteinase in arterial disease. *Adv Vasc Surg* 2000;197–213.)

bound to its matrix substrate, findings that lend additional support for a direct role in matrix destruction.

Like other MMPs, MMP-2 is secreted as a latent proenzyme (72 kd) that must be cleaved to its active, 62-kd form. Some MMPs are activated by serine proteinases, but MMP-2 cannot be activated by this pathway (71). MMP-2 is uniquely activated on the cell surface by a newly recognized family of membrane-bound or membrane-type (MT) MMPs (72–74). Five different MT-MMPs have been identified and are designated MT1-MMP through MT5-MMP. All were identified by homology screening of cDNA libraries and placed in the MT-MMP family because of their putative transmembrane domains (74). They form a distinct MT subclass of the MMP family, as all other MMPs are secreted in a soluble form. In this subclass, only MT1-MMP has been well characterized. MT1-MMP appears to

play a central role in MMP-2 activation in vascular smooth-muscle cells. Tissue inhibitor of metalloproteinases (TIMP)-2 has been found to be a cofactor required for MT1-MMP activation of MMP-2 at precise, relatively low molar concentrations.

The most convincing data to date indicating that MMPs may cause abdominal aortic aneurysm were recently reported in a study by Allaire et al. (75) of a xenotransplantation model of an acellular guinea pig aorta into a rat infrarenal aorta. The aortic lumen was coated with rat smooth-muscle cells retrovirally transfected with the *TIMP1* gene. This model mimics human abdominal aortic aneurysm in the up-regulation of MMP-9 and activation of MMP-2. TIMP-1 overexpression blocked activity of MMP-9 and blocked activation of MMP-2 and therefore inhibited aneurysm formation. The exact mechanism of inhibition of MMP-2 activation is not clear because high local concentrations of TIMP-2 (not TIMP-1) are required to block MT1-MMP activation of MMP-2. Therefore, these studies suggest a possible role for MMP-9 and MMP-2 in the early development of abdominal aortic aneurysm.

Matrix metalloproteinase-12, also known as *macrophage elastase,* is a 54-kd proenzyme that is converted into an active, 22-kd enzyme capable of degrading elastin. Two articles suggest that it could have a role in abdominal aortic aneurysm formation. Curci et al. (76) have shown that MMP-12 is present in the media of abdominal aortic aneurysm tissue. Importantly, the macrophage product appears to have a high affinity for elastin fibers, as it localizes to residual elastin fibers in aneurysms. Additional data supporting the involvement of MMP-12 in abdominal aortic aneurysm have been provided by Carmeliet et al. (77). Although not consistently, aneurysms occasionally develop in the apolipoprotein E knockout mouse. In their study, Carmeliet and colleagues showed that MMP-12, activated by the serine protease plasmin, accounts for the most of the elastolytic activity in this model. Their findings suggest a potentially important role for MMP-12 in abdominal aortic aneurysm pathogenesis and progression.

Although significant work has focused on characterizing the elastolytic activity of abdominal aortic aneurysm, other studies have focused on collagen proteolysis. Busuttil and colleagues (78) provided the initial evidence of increased collagenolytic activity in the aneurysmal aorta. Extending this observation, Manashi and colleagues (79) demonstrated low levels of true collagenase activity in aneurysm tissue collected at elective repair, with higher levels noted in specimens from ruptured aneurysms. Interestingly, Webster et al. (80) demonstrated increased collagenolytic activity in pulverized and lyophilized abdominal aortic aneurysm tissues in comparison with occlusive or normal aorta. They were unable to prove the identity of the specific collagenase involved. Similarly, Irizarry et al. (81) demonstrated an increase in MMP-1 in abdominal aortic aneurysm tissue in comparison with normal or aortic occlusive disease tissue, and this finding was corroborated in a second report from the same group (58). Meanwhile, Herron et al. (57) were unable to confirm the presence of MMP-1 in abdominal aortic aneurysm tissue with the use of a monospecific antibody to rabbit collagenase, but Vine and Powell (60) demonstrated MMP-1 to be present in all of 10 aneurysm homogenates, only 3 of 8 aortic occlusive disease homogenates, and none of their normal aorta homogenates by immunoblot analysis. With the recent development and characterization of a knockout mouse for a membrane-bound MMP, MT1-MMP, this MMP has been shown to play a pivotal role in collagen degradation (82).

The cellular source and synthetic regulation of MMP-1 have been the subject of considerable investigation. MMP-

1 is made by macrophages, but Welgus et al. (83) showed that mesenchymal cells produce significantly more MMP-1 than macrophages, and that the expression of this enzyme is up-regulated by inflammatory mediators (84). Keen et al. (66) demonstrated that both platelet-derived growth factor and interleukin-1β up-regulate MMP expression in cultured aortic smooth-muscle cells. The intracellular signaling events associated with this up-regulation appear to involve both protein kinase C and tyrosine kinase (85). The arachidonic acid metabolite prostaglandin E$_2$ has also been identified as an important regulator of the MMPs (84).

ROLE OF INFLAMMATION

It is well-known that inflammatory cells are capable of elaborating proteolytic enzymes in addition to cytokines that modulate the expression of matrix proteins and proteolytic enzymes by resident mesenchymal cells. Inflammation is a prominent feature of both abdominal aortic aneurysm and aortic occlusive disease, with infiltrating macrophages and lymphocytes scattered throughout the intima/plaque and adventitia (86). Although the inflammatory infiltrates in abdominal aortic aneurysm and aortic occlusive disease are similar, they differ in two subtle but important ways: (a) The lymphocytes in aortic occlusive disease are predominantly T cells, whereas both T cells and B cells have been identified in abdominal aortic aneurysm tissue (86,87); (b) adventitial and outer medial inflammation is seen only in more advanced stages of aortic occlusive disease (88,89), but it is consistent feature of abdominal aortic aneurysm. Indeed, the entity called *inflammatory aneurysm* appears to represent the extreme on a continuum of periadventitial inflammation found in all abdominal aortic aneurysms (86). Clinical experience in aortic endarterectomy performed for aortic occlusive disease suggests that this involvement of the outer media and, importantly, the adventitia may be a critical factor in aneurysm formation. The fact that aortic endarterectomy, in which the entire media is removed, is rarely followed by aneurysm formation demonstrates the ability of the aortic adventitia to maintain dimensional stability. Thus, the fibrous collagen of the adventitia must also undergo matrix destruction for an aneurysm to develop, and the distinct distribution of the inflammatory infiltrate to this location in aneurysms is thought to play a crucial etiologic role.

The fact that the prominent inflammatory response associated with aneurysms includes B lymphocytes (86) and also contains relatively large amounts of immunoglobulin (87) and complement (90) suggests an autoimmune component to abdominal aortic aneurysms. In support of this thesis, Tilson (91) has identified a matrix protein that is immunoreactive with the immunoglobulin G isolated from the aneurysm wall. Initial characterization of this putative autoantigen demonstrates homology with elastin-associated microfibrils. In addition, studies are in progress to determine whether an association exists between abdominal aortic aneurysm and class II major histocompatibility locus DR4, which has a known association with another common autoimmune disease, rheumatoid arthritis (92).

Two experimental aneurysm models lend strong support to the theory that the inflammation noted in abdominal aortic aneurysm plays an etiologic role. Gertz et al. (17) found that aneurysms can be created reliably in the rabbit carotid artery by applying calcium chloride to the adventitia. This produces a transmural chemical injury that is associated with the same type of periadventitial lymphocytic infiltrate that is found in human abdominal aortic aneurysm. Importantly, aneurysm formation occurred only after the inflammatory response was present. Longo et al. (93) have ex-

tended this model to the mouse aorta. Similarly, Anidjar et al. (18) have shown that elastase infusion under supraphysiologic pressures produces aneurysms in the rat aorta. The theoretic basis for this model was direct elastin degradation, but in fact the dilation corresponded temporally not with the early elastin degradation, but rather with the ensuing inflammatory response (94). This suggests that the inflammation and inflammatory mediators occurring in response to chemical and mechanical injury produce the aneurysm rather than direct elastolysis.

More recent work suggests that the role of inflammatory cells in the pathogenesis of abdominal aortic aneurysm may be related to their ability to regulate proteolysis. Additional characterization of the elastase infusion model first described by Anidjar has shown that the inflammatory cell infiltration is accompanied by an increase in the gelatinases, MMP-2 and MMP-9 (95). Holmes et al. (96) have investigated the role of the inflammatory cascade in this model by blocking arachidonic acid metabolite production with indomethacin to inhibit both MMP production and aneurysm formation.

The tetracycline derivatives have the ability to inhibit MMPs, a property independent of their antibiotic moiety. They have been used with success clinically in a number of diseases that are similar to abdominal aortic aneurysm in that chronic inflammatory infiltrates are associated with local matrix destruction. The extensive work of Golub et al. (97) demonstrated the efficacy of doxycycline in treating periodontal disease, a finding that correlates with local inhibitory effects on MMPs. Inhibition occurs at relatively low doses (40 mg/d), likely because of high rates of local uptake by the inflamed gingiva. Whether this might also be true in the aorta is not known, although given the marked inflammation and neovascularity, it would not be surprising. Because this low dose of doxycycline has little antibiotic activity, the side effects should be reduced. Yu et al. (98) have demonstrated inhibition of osteoarthritis by doxycycline treatment in an animal model. Petrinec et al. (95) have shown that doxycycline inhibits aneurysm formation in the rat elastase model of aneurysms. They demonstrated that both MMP-2 and MMP-9 levels are decreased in the aortic tissue of doxycycline-treated rats. These findings correlated with relative preservation of the media. Curci et al. (76) have shown that a short preoperative course of doxycycline decreases MMP levels in aneurysm tissue. These studies provide supportive evidence for a role of MMPs in abdominal aortic aneurysm. However, doxycycline may have various effects in addition to its MMP inhibitory ability, so its exact mechanism of action in blocking aneurysm formation can only be inferred.

GENETIC BASIS FOR ABDOMINAL AORTIC ANEURYSM

Although clinicians treating large numbers of patients with abdominal aortic aneurysm were undoubtedly aware of clusters of aneurysms within families, Clifton (99) was the first to describe three affected siblings. Data supporting this observation did not appear until 7 years later, when Tilson and Seashore (100) in one publication and Norrgard et al. (101) in another described 50 and 87 families, respectively, with more than one affected member. Although important in verifying the familial clustering of abdominal aortic aneurysm, these studies did not investigate aneurysm incidence in comparison with a control group. This was done by Johansen and Koepsell (102) in 1986, who reported an incidence of abdominal aortic aneurysm of 19% among first-degree relatives of matched

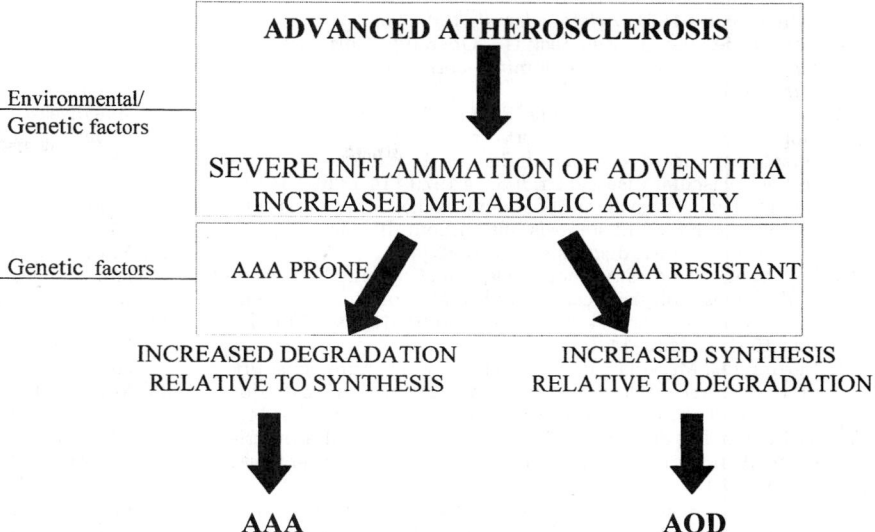

Figure 82.3. Pathogenesis of abdominal aortic aneurysm *(AAA)*. Schematic diagram of the proposed mechanism of interaction between environmental and genetic factors that results in the development of AAA. *AOD,* atherosclerotic occlusive disease. (From Rehm JP, Baxter BT. The formation of aneurysms. *Semin Vasc Surg* 1998;11:193–202, with permission.)

controls. This marked difference in incidence provided the strongest evidence to date of the potential significance of genetic factors in abdominal aortic aneurysm. Subsequently, two other studies reported remarkably similar rates of abdominal aortic aneurysm (15% and 16%) in first-degree family members (103,104).

Although these studies identified the familial tendency to abdominal aortic aneurysm, they did not use genetic models in an attempt to determine the inheritance of abdominal aortic aneurysm. Based on simple observation, Tilson and Seashore (100) suggested that the mode of transmission might be linked to the X chromosome. Powell et al. (105) analyzed normal persons and patients with aortic occlusive disease or abdominal aortic aneurysm and found an increased frequency of the haptoglobin α^1 allele in those with abdominal aortic aneurysm. They suggested that the inheritance of abdominal aortic aneurysm is multifactorial and not likely related to a single gene. However, two of the more conclusive studies (12,13) to date have used segregation analysis of large pedigrees, and both have concluded that the genetic transmission of abdominal aortic aneurysm is best explained by a single gene rather than by multiple factors. These studies do not agree on whether the gene is recessively (12) or dominantly (13) inherited. To summarize, the data published during the past 20 years have clearly demonstrated that a susceptibility to abdominal aortic aneurysm is inherited and that it is likely related to a single gene.

In searching for a gene that might explain abdominal aortic aneurysm, considerable work has focused on the genes regulating matrix protein metabolism. Thoracic aneurysms often present as part of a well-defined matrix disorder, such as Marfan syndrome (106). Abdominal aortic aneurysms, on the other hand, are rarely associated with known connective tissue abnormalities, although evidence has been found of systemic vascular abnormalities, including generalized matrix changes throughout the aorta (107), dilation and elongation of other arteries (14–16), and aneurysm formation at remote sites, such as the popliteal artery (108,109). Except for rare cases of collagen and fibrillin mutations, no known mutations in matrix proteins account for most abdominal aortic aneurysms. Given the apparently significant role of the inflammatory process in the pathogenesis of abdominal aortic aneurysm, a better understanding of the genes regulating the relationship between inflammatory cells and the mesenchy-

mal cells of the vascular wall may prove helpful in elucidating a genetic basis for this disease.

CONCLUSION

The past decade has seen significant strides in defining the pathogenesis of abdominal aortic aneurysm as the expertise of researchers from a broad range of scientific backgrounds has been brought to bear on the disease. Enhanced by the convergence of matrix biochemistry, cell biology, and immunology, this work is providing important new insight into how matrix metabolism is regulated in the diseased aorta. A schematic illustrating the interaction of these factors in aneurysm pathogenesis is shown in Fig. 82.3. As we have learned during the evolution of treatments for other pathologic processes, the most effective pharmacologic therapies are designed with a thorough understanding of the pathophysiology of the disease. We are quickly developing that understanding as we move from the descriptive research of the past decade to the current work defining the various complex interactions that result in the formation of an aortic aneurysm. Given the progress of this past decade, we can expect the next decade to bring clinical trials of antiinflammatory medications and protease inhibitors designed to prevent the formation of aneurysms or inhibit the growth of existing aneurysms.

REFERENCES

1. Johnston KW, Rutherford RB, Tilson MD, et al. Suggested standards for reporting on arterial aneurysms. Subcommittee on Reporting Standards for Arterial Aneurysms, Ad Hoc Committee on Reporting Standards, Society for Vascular Surgery and North American Chapter, International Society for Cardiovascular Surgery [see comments]. *J Vasc Surg* 1991;13:452–458.
2. Graves E. Detailed diagnosis and procedures, National Hospital Discharge Survey, 1988. *Vital Health Stat 13* 1991:107:91.
3. Scarpa A. *Treatise on the anatomy, pathology, and surgical treatment of aneurysm, with engravings.* Translated from the Italian by John Henry Wishart, FRCS, Edinburgh, 1808.
4. Bickerstaff LK, Hollier LH, Van Peenen HJ, et al. Abdominal aortic aneurysm repair combined with a second surgical procedure—morbidity and mortality. *Surgery* 1984;95:487–491.
5. Melton LJD, Bickerstaff LK, Hollier LH, et al. Changing incidence of abdominal aortic aneurysms: a population-based study. *Am J Epidemiol* 1984;120:379–386.
6. Lillienfeld D, Gunderson P, Sprafka J, et al. The epidemiol-

ogy of abdominal aortic aneurysm: mortality trends in the United States 1951. *Arteriosclerosis* 1987;7:637.

7. Katz DJ, Stanley JC, Zelenock GB. Operative mortality rates for intact and ruptured abdominal aortic aneurysm. *J Vasc Surg* 1994;19:804–815.

8. Hertzer NR, Young JR, Kramer JR, et al. Routine coronary angiography prior to elective aortic reconstruction: results of selective myocardial revascularization in patients with peripheral vascular disease. *Arch Surg* 1979;114:1336–1344.

9. Kang S. Higher prevalence of abdominal aortic aneurysms in patients with carotid stenosis but without diabetes. *Surgery* 1999;126:687–691; discussion 691–692.

10. Burchfiel CM, Laws A, Benfante R, et al. Combined effects of HDL cholesterol, triglyceride, and total cholesterol concentrations on 18-year risk of atherosclerotic disease. *Circulation* 1995;92:1430–1436.

11. Darling RC, Messina CR, Brewster DC, et al. Autopsy study of unoperated abdominal aortic aneurysms: the case for early resection. *Circulation* 1977;56[3 Suppl]:II-161–II-164.

12. Majumder PP, St Jean PL, Ferrell RE, et al. On the inheritance of abdominal aortic aneurysm. *Am J Hum Genet* 1991; 48:164–170.

13. Verloes A, Sakalihasan N, Koulischer L, et al. Aneurysms of the abdominal aorta: familial and genetic aspects in three hundred thirteen pedigrees. *J Vasc Surg* 1995;21:646–655.

14. Makherjee D, Mayberry J, Inahara T, et al. The relationship of the abdominal aortic aneurysm to the tortuous internal carotid artery. *Arch Surg* 1989;124:955–956.

15. Tilson MD, Dang C. Generalized arteriomegaly: a possible predisposition to the formation of abdominal aortic aneurysms. *Arch Surg* 1981;116:1030–1032.

16. Ward A. A generalized dilating diathesis? *Arch Surg* 1992; 127:990–991.

17. Gertz SD, Kurgan A, Eisenberg D. Aneurysm of the rabbit common carotid artery induced by periarterial application of calcium chloride in vivo. *J Clin Invest* 1988;81:649–656.

18. Anidjar S, Salzmann JL, Gentric D, et al. Elastase-induced experimental aneurysms in rats. *Circulation* 1990;82:973–981.

19. DePalma R, Koletshy S, Bellon E, et al. Failure of regression of atherosclerosis in dogs with moderate cholesterolemia. *Atherosclerosis* 1977;27:297–310.

20. Manilow M, Maruffo C, Perley A. Experimental atherosclerosis in squirrel monkeys *(Saimiri sciurea)*. *J Pathol Bacteriol* 1966;82:491–510.

21. Strickland HL, Bond MG. Aneurysms in a large colony of squirrel monkeys *(Saimiri sciureus)*. *Lab Anim Sci* 1983;33: 589–592.

22. Zarins CK, Xu CP, Glagov S. Aneurysmal enlargement of the aorta during regression of experimental atherosclerosis [see comments]. *J Vasc Surg* 1992;15:90–98; discussion 99–101.

23. Boucek R, Gunja-Smith Z, Noble N, et al. Modulation by propranolol of the lysyl cross-links in aortic elastin and collagen of the aneurysm-prone turkey. *Biochem Pharmacol* 1983;32:275–280.

24. Rowe DW, McGoodwin EB, Martin GR, et al. Decreased lysyl oxidase activity in the aneurysm-prone mottled mouse. *J Biol Chem* 1977;252:939–942.

25. Zarins C, Glagov S. *Artery wall pathology in atherosclerosis*, 5th ed. Philadelphia: WB Saunders, 2000:313–330.

26. Tilson M. Aortic aneurysms and atherosclerosis. *Circulation* 1995;92:378–379.

27. Glagov S. *Hemodynamic risk factors: mechanical stress, mural architecture, medial nutrition, and the vulnerability of arteries to atherosclerosis*. Baltimore: Williams & Wilkins, 1972.

28. Barnes MJ. Collagens in atherosclerosis. *Coll Relat Res* 1985;5:65–97.

29. Dobrin P, Baker WH, Gley WC. Elastolytic and collagenolytic studies of arteries. *Arch Surg* 1984;119:405–409.

30. Oxlund H, Andreassen T. The role of hyaluronic acid, collagen, and elastin in the mechanical properties of connective tissue. *J Anat* 1980;131:611–620.

31. Rizzo RJ, McCarthy WJ, Dixit SN, et al. Collagen types and matrix protein content in human abdominal aortic aneurysms. *J Vasc Surg* 1989;10:365–373.

32. Powell J, Adamson J, MacSweeney S, et al. Influence of type III collagen genotype on aortic diameter and disease. *Br J Surg* 1993;80:1246–1248.

33. Deak SB, Ricotta JJ, Mariani TJ, et al. Abnormalities in the biosynthesis of type III procollagen in cultured skin fibroblasts from two patients with multiple aneurysms. *Matrix* 1992;12:92–100.

34. McGee GS, Baxter BT, Shively VP, et al. Aneurysm or occlusive disease—factors determining the clinical course of atherosclerosis of the infrarenal aorta. *Surgery* 1991;110:370–375; discussion 375–376.

35. Mesh CL, Baxter BT, Pearce WH, et al. Collagen and elastin gene expression in aortic aneurysms. *Surgery* 1992;112: 256–261; discussion 261–262.

36. Minion DJ, Wang Y, Lynch TG, et al. Soluble factors modulate changes in collagen gene expression in abdominal aortic aneurysms. *Surgery* 1993;114:252–257.

37. Hunter GC, Smyth SH, Aguirre ML, et al. Incidence and histologic characteristics of blebs in patients with abdominal aortic aneurysms. *J Vasc Surg* 1996;24:93–101.

38. Minion DJ, Davis VA, Nejezchleb PA, et al. Elastin is increased in abdominal aortic aneurysms. *J Surg Res* 1994;57: 443–446.

39. De Wet W, Chu M, Prockop D. The mRNAs for the pro-alpha (I) chains of type I procollagen are translated at the same rate in normal human fibroblasts and in fibroblasts from two variants of osteogenesis imperfecta with altered steady state ratios of the two mRNAs. *J Biol Chem* 1983;258:14385–14389.

40. Kontusaari S, Tromp G, Kuivaniemi H, et al. A mutation in the gene for type III procollagen (COL3A1) in a family with aortic aneurysms. *J Clin Invest* 1990;86:1465–1473.

41. Tromp G, Wu Y, Prockop DJ, et al. Sequencing of cDNA from 50 unrelated patients reveals that mutations in the triple-helical domain of type III procollagen are an infrequent cause of aortic aneurysms. *J Clin Invest* 1993;91:2539–2545.

42. Boucek R. *Contributions of elastin and collagen organization to passive mechanical properties of arterial tissue*. Boca Raton, FL: CRC Press, 1988.

43. Mecham R, Broekelmann T, Davis E, et al. Elastic fibre assembly: macromolecular interactions. *Ciba Foundation Symposium* 1995;192:172–181; discussion 181–184.

44. Shapiro S, Endicott S, Province M, et al. Marked longevity of human lung parenchymal elastic fibers deduced from prevalence of D-aspartate and nuclear weapons-related radiocarbon. *J Clin Invest* 1991;87:1828–1834.

45. Parks W, Secrist W, Wu L, et al. Developmental regulation of tropoelastin isoforms. *J Biol Chem* 1988;282:226–232.

46. Baxter B, Halloran B. Matrix protein metabolism in abdominal aortic aneurysms. *Aneurysms: new findings and treatment*. Norwalk, CT: Appleton & Lange, 1994:25–34.

47. Dietz H. New insights into the genetic basis of aortic aneurysms. *Monogr Pathol* 1995;37:144–155.

48. Baxter BT, McGee GS, Shively VP, et al. Elastin content, cross-links, and mRNA in normal and aneurysmal human aorta. *J Vasc Surg* 1992;16:192–200.

49. Sumner DS, Hokanson DE, Strandness DE Jr. Stress–strain characteristics and collagen elastin content of abdominal aortic aneurysms. *Surg Gynecol Obstet* 1970;130:459–466.

50. Glagov S. Morphology of collagen and elastin fibers in atherosclerotic lesions. *Adv Exp Med Biol* 1977;82:767–773.

51. Busuttil R, Rinderbriecht H, Flecher A, et al. Elastase activity: the role of elastase in aortic aneurysm formation. *J Surg Res* 1982;32:214–217.

52. Cannon D, Read R. Elastolytic activity in patients with aortic aneurysms. *Ann Thorac Surg* 1982;34:5–10.

53. Morgunova E, Tuuttila A, Bergmann U, et al. Structure of human pro-matrix metalloproteinase-2: activation mechanism revealed. *Science* 1999;284:1667–1670.

54. Aimes RT, Quigley JP. Matrix metalloproteinase-2 is an interstitial collagenase. *J Biol Chem* 1995;270:5872–5876.

55. Cohen JR, Mandell C, Chang JB, et al. Elastin metabolism of the infrarenal aorta. *J Vasc Surg* 1988;7:210–214.

56. Cohen J, Sarfati I, Danna D, et al. Smooth muscle cell elastase, atherosclerosis, and abdominal aortic aneurysms. *Ann Surg* 1992;216:327–332.

57. Herron GS, Unemori E, Wong M, et al. Connective tissue proteinases and inhibitors in abdominal aortic aneurysms: involvement of the vasa vasorum in the pathogenesis of aortic aneurysms. *Arterioscler Thromb* 1991;11:1667–1677.

58. Newman KM, Malon AM, Shin RD, et al. Matrix metallopro-

teinases in abdominal aortic aneurysm: characterization, purification, and their possible sources. *Connect Tissue Res* 1994;30:265–276.

59. Thompson RW, Holmes DR, Mertens RA, et al. Production and localization of 92-kilodalton gelatinase in abdominal aortic aneurysms: an elastolytic metalloproteinase expressed by aneurysm-infiltrating macrophages. *J Clin Invest* 1995;96: 318–326.

60. Vine N, Powell JT. Metalloproteinases in degenerative aortic disease. *Clin Sci (Lond)* 1991;81:233–239.

61. McMillan WD, Patterson BK, Keen RR, et al. In situ localization and quantification of mRNA for 92-kD type IV collagenase and its inhibitor in aneurysmal, occlusive, and normal aorta. *Arterioscler Thromb Vasc Biol* 1995;15:1139–1144.

62. McMillan WD, Pearce WH. Increased plasma levels of MMP-9 are associated with abdominal aortic aneurysms. *J Vasc Surg* 1999;122–127.

63. Davis V, Persidskaia R, Baca-Regen L, et al. Matrix metalloproteinase-2 production and its binding to the matrix are increased in abdominal aortic aneurysms. *Arterioscler Thromb Vasc Biol* 1998;18:1625–1633.

64. Newman KM, Jean-Claude J, Li H, et al. Cellular localization of matrix metalloproteinases in the abdominal aortic aneurysm wall. *J Vasc Surg* 1994;20:814–820.

65. Patel MI, Melrose J, Ghosh P, et al. Increased synthesis of matrix metalloproteinases by aortic smooth muscle cells is implicated in the etiopathogenesis of abdominal aortic aneurysms. *J Vasc Surg* 1996;24:82–92.

66. Keen RR, Nolan K, Cipollone M, et al. Interleukin-1 beta induces differential gene expression in aortic smooth muscle cells. *J Vasc Surg* 1994;20:774–784; discussion 784–786.

67. McMillan WD, Patterson BK, Keen RR, et al. In situ localization and quantification of seventy-two–kilodalton type IV collagenase in aneurysmal, occlusive, and normal aorta. *J Vasc Surg* 1995;22:295–305.

68. Murphy G, Cockett MI, Ward RV, et al. Matrix metalloproteinase degradation of elastin, type IV collagen, and proteoglycan: a quantitative comparison of the activities of 95-kDa and 72-kDa gelatinases, stromelysins-1 and -2 and punctuated metalloproteinase (PUMP). *Biochem J* 1991;277(Pt 1): 277–279.

69. Li Z, Li L, Zielke HR, et al. Increased expression of 72-kd type IV collagenase (MMP-2) in human aortic atherosclerotic lesions. *Am J Pathol* 1996;148:121–128.

70. Freestone T, Turner RJ, Coady A, et al. Inflammation and matrix metalloproteinases in the enlarging abdominal aortic aneurysm. *Arterioscler Thromb Vasc Biol* 1995;15: 1145–1151.

71. Atkinson SJ, Crabbe T, Cowell S, et al. Intermolecular autolytic cleavage can contribute to the activation of progelatinase A by cell membranes. *J Biol Chem* 1995;270: 30479–30485.

72. Sato H, Kinoshita T, Takino T, et al. Activation of a recombinant membrane type 1-matrix metalloproteinase (MT1-MMP) by furin and its interaction with tissue inhibitor of metalloproteinases (TIMP)-2. *FEBS Lett* 1996;393:101–104.

73. Takino T, Sato H, Shinagawa A, et al. Identification of the second membrane-type matrix metalloproteinase (MT-MMP-2) gene from a human placenta cDNA library: MT-MMPs form a unique membrane-type subclass in the MMP family. *J Biol Chem* 1995;270:23013–23020.

74. Shofuda K, Yasumitsu H, Nishihashi A, et al. Expression of three membrane-type matrix metalloproteinases (MT-MMPs) in rat vascular smooth muscle cells and characterization of MT3-MMPs with and without transmembrane domain. *J Biol Chem* 1997;272:9749–9754.

75. Allaire E, Forough R, Clowes M, et al. Local overexpression of TIMP-1 prevents aortic aneurysm degeneration and rupture in a rat model. *J Clin Invest* 1998;102:1413–1420.

76. Curci JA, Liao S, Huffman MD, et al. Expression and localization of macrophage elastase (matrix metalloproteinase-12) in abdominal aortic aneurysms. *J Clin Invest* 1998;102: 1900–1910.

77. Carmeliet P, Moons L, Lijnen R, et al. Urokinase-generated plasmin activates matrix metalloproteinases during aneurysm formation. *Nat Genet* 1997;17:439–444.

78. Busuttil RW, Abou-Zamzam AM, Machleder HI. Collagenase

79. activity of the human aorta: a comparison of patients with and without abdominal aortic aneurysms. *Arch Surg* 1980; 115:1373–1378.

79. Manashi S, Campa J, Greenhalgh R, et al. Collagen in abdominal aortic aneurysms: typing, content, and degradation. *J Vasc Surg* 1987;6:578–582.

80. Webster MW, McAuley CE, Steed DL, et al. Collagen stability and collagenolytic activity in the normal and aneurysmal human abdominal aorta. *Am J Surg* 1991;161:635–638.

81. Irizarry E, Newman KM, Gandhi R, et al. Demonstration of interstitial collagenase in abdominal aortic aneurysm disease. *J Surg Res* 1993;54:571–574.

82. Holmbeck K, Blanco P, Caterina J, et al. MT1-MMP-deficient mice develop dwarfism, osteopenia, arthritis, and connective tissue disease due to inadequate collagen turnover. *Cell* 1999;99:81–92.

83. Welgus H, et al. Neutral metalloproteinases produced by human mononuclear phagocytes: enzyme profile, regulation, and expression during cellular development. *J Clin Invest* 1990;86:1496–1502.

84. Pentland A, Shapiro S, Welgus H. Agonist-induced expression of tissue inhibitor of metalloproteinases and metalloproteinases by human macrophages is regulated by endogenous prostaglandin E$_2$ synthesis. *J Invest Dermatol* 1995;104: 52–57.

85. Sudbeck BD, Parks WC, Welgus HG, et al. Collagen-stimulated induction of keratinocyte collagenase is mediated via tyrosine kinase and protein kinase C activities. *J Biol Chem* 1994;269:30022–30029.

86. Koch AE, Haines GK, Rizzo RJ, et al. Human abdominal aortic aneurysms: immunophenotypic analysis suggesting an immune-mediated response. *Am J Pathol* 1990;137:1199–1213.

87. Brophy CM, Reilly JM, Smith GJW, et al. The role of inflammation in nonspecific abdominal aortic aneurysm disease. *Ann Vasc Surg* 1991;5:229–233.

88. Parums D, Mitchinson M. Autoallergy in atherosclerosis. *Pathology* 1985;146:245A(abst).

89. Ross R. The pathogenesis of atherosclerosis: a perspective for the 1990s. *Nature* 1993;362:801–809.

90. Capella JF, Paik DC, Yin NX, et al. Complement activation and subclassification of tissue immunoglobulin G in the abdominal aortic aneurysm. *J Surg Res* 1996;65:31–33.

91. Tilson MD. Similarities of an autoantigen in aneurysmal disease of the human abdominal aorta to a 36-kDa microfibril-associated bovine aortic glycoprotein. *Biochem Biophys Res Commun* 1995;213:40–43.

92. Weynard C, Hicok D, Goronzy J. The influence of HLA-DRB1 gene on the disease severity in rheumatoid arthritis. *Ann Intern Med* 1982;117:801–806.

93. Longo G, Rehm J, Mayhan W, et al. Calcium chloride-induced experimental aneurysms in mice. *Surg Forum* 1999; L:450–451.

94. Anidjar S, Dobrin P, Eichorst M, et al. Correlation of inflammatory infiltrate with the enlargement of experimental aortic aneurysms. *J Vasc Surg* 1992;16:139–147.

95. Petrinec D, Liao S, Holmes DR, et al. Doxycycline inhibition of aneurysmal degeneration in an elastase-induced rat model of abdominal aortic aneurysm: preservation of aortic elastin associated with suppressed production of 92-kD gelatinase. *J Vasc Surg* 1996;23:336–346.

96. Holmes DR, Petrinec D, Wester W, et al. Indomethacin prevents elastase-induced abdominal aortic aneurysms in the rat. *J Surg Res* 1996;63:305–309.

97. Golub LM, et al. Minocycline reduces gingival collagenolytic activity during diabetes: preliminary observations and a proposed new mechanism of action. *J Periodontal Res* 1983;18:516–526.

98. Yu LP Jr, Smith GN Jr, Brandt KD, et al. Reduction of the severity of canine osteoarthritis by prophylactic treatment with oral doxycycline [see comments]. *Arthritis Rheum* 1992;35:1150–1159.

99. Clifton MA. Familial abdominal aortic aneurysms. *Br J Surg* 1977;64:765–766.

100. Tilson M, Seashore M. Human genetics of abdominal aortic aneurysm. *Surg Gynecol Obstet* 1984;158:129–132.

101. Norrgard O, Rais O, Angquist K. Familial occurrence of abdominal aortic aneurysm. *Surgery* 1987;95:650–656.

102. Johansen K, Koepsell T. Familial tendency of abdominal aortic aneurysms. *JAMA* 1986;256:1934–1936.
103. Darling RC, Brewster DC, Darling RC, et al. Are familial abdominal aortic aneurysms different? *J Vasc Surg* 1989;10:39–43.
104. Webster MW, Ferrell RE, St. Jean PL, et al. Ultrasound screening of first-degree relatives of patients with an abdominal aortic aneurysm. *J Vasc Surg* 1991;13:9–13; discussion 13–14.
105. Powell J, Greenhalgh RM. Genetic variation on chromosome 16 is associated with abdominal aortic aneurysm. *Clin Sci* 1990;78:13–16.
106. Dietz H. Molecular biology of Marfan syndrome. *J Vasc Surg* 1992;15:927–928.
107. Baxter BT, Davis VA, Minion DJ, et al. Abdominal aortic aneurysms are associated with altered matrix proteins of the nonaneurysmal aortic segments. *J Vasc Surg* 1994;19:797–802; discussion 803.
108. Vermilion BD, Kimmins SA, Pace WG, et al. A review of one hundred forty-seven popliteal aneurysms with long-term follow-up. *Surgery* 1981;90:1009–1014.
109. Bouhoutsos J, Martin P. Popliteal aneurysm: a review of 116 cases. *Br J Surg* 1974;61:469–475.
110. Newman KM, Ogata Y, Malon AM, et al. Identification of matrix metalloproteinases 3 (stromelysin-1) and 9. *Arterioscler Thromb* 1994;14:1315–1320.
111. Sakalihasan N, Delveene P, Husgens BV, et al. Activated forms of MMP-2 and MMP-9 in abdominal aortic aneurysms. *J Vasc Surg* 1996;24:127–133.
112. Knox JB, Sukhova GK, Whittemore AD, et al. Evidence for altered balance between matrix metalloproteinases and their inhibitors in human aortic diseases. *Circulation* 1997;95:205–212.

SURGERY: SCIENTIFIC PRINCIPLES AND PRACTICE, Third Edition, edited by Lazar J. Greenfield, Michael W. Mulholland, Keith T. Oldham, Gerald B. Zelenock, and Keith D. Lillemoe. Lippincott Williams & Wilkins Publishers, Philadelphia, © 2001.

CHAPTER 83

EXTRACRANIAL CAROTID, INNOMINATE, SUBCLAVIAN, AND AXILLARY ARTERY ANEURYSMS

JOHN W. HALLETT, JR., AND TODD E. RASMUSSEN

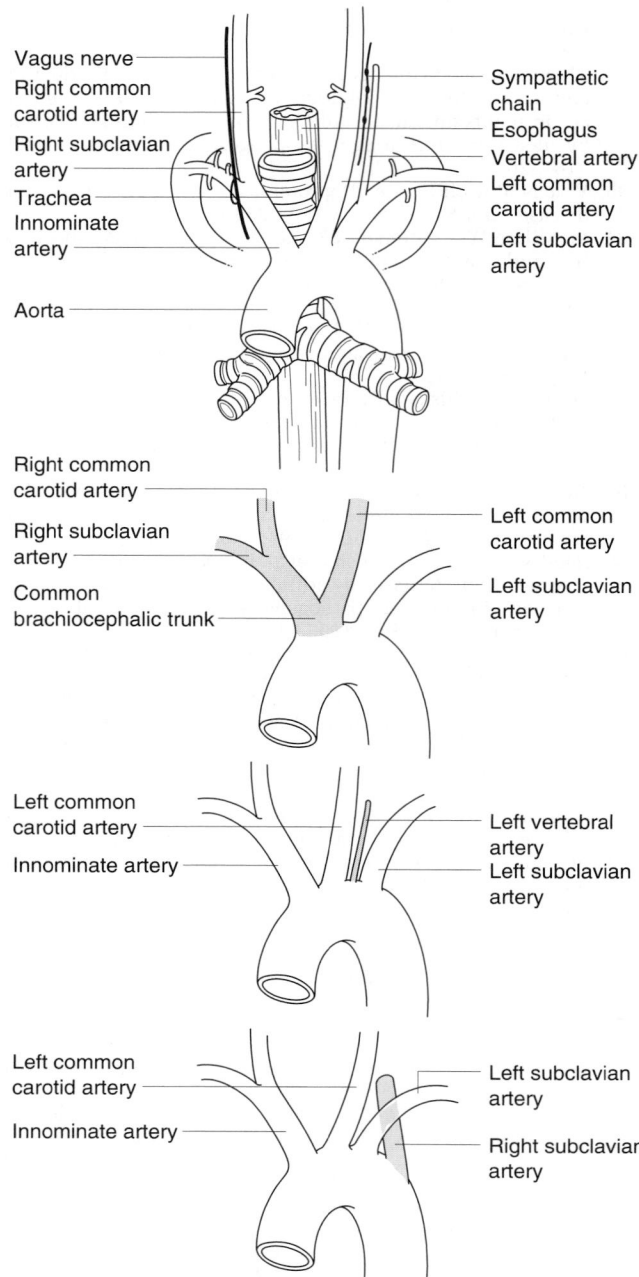

Figure 83.1. *Top:* Normal anatomy of the aortic arch, present in 80% of people. *Bottom:* The three most common anatomic variations. *1.* Common origin of left common carotid artery and brachiocephalic trunk. *2.* Anomalous origin of the left vertebral artery. *3.* Anomalous origin of right subclavian artery.

Aneurysms of the innominate, extracranial carotid, subclavian, and axillary arteries are rare in comparison with other types of peripheral aneurysms. They account for fewer than 5% of all aneurysms (1). Nonetheless, their recognition and management present several unique challenges for the surgeon. Their causes are diverse. They generally present as a thromboembolic event; rarely do they rupture. Exposure and repair of these aneurysms can be problematic, testing the judgment and skill of the most experienced surgeon.

ANATOMIC CONSIDERATIONS

During embryologic development, the aortic arch and brachiocephalic arteries evolve from paired dorsal aortae, which lie on either side of the trachea proximally and fuse in the thorax. The normal sequence of aortic arch branches is present in 80% of the population (Fig. 83.1). In approximately 10% of patients, the brachiocephalic trunk and left common carotid artery have a common origin from the aortic arch. An origin of the left vertebral artery from the aortic arch between the left common carotid artery and the left subclavian artery occurs in about 6% of people. A less common aberration, found in 1 of every 200 autopsies, is an anomalous origin of the right subclavian artery (2) (Fig. 83.1). As the aberrant right subclavian artery courses toward the right upper extremity, its position is retroesophageal in 80% of patients, between the trachea and the esophagus in 15%, and anterior to the trachea in 5% (3,4). In addition to arterial abnormalities, extraneous cervical and malformed first ribs are associated with subclavian aneurysms related to thoracic outlet syndrome (5,6).

PREVALENCE OF BRACHIOCEPHALIC ANEURYSMS

Various clinical studies have emphasized the rarity of brachiocephalic aneurysms. They account for approximately 2% of all peripheral aneurysms and for fewer than 1% of all surgically treated peripheral aneurysms. In a 40-year review from the Mayo Clinic, the most common type of brachiocephalic aneurysm was subclavian (56%), followed by extracranial carotid (34%) and innominate aneurysms (10%) (7) (Fig. 83.2). More specifically, approximately 250 carotid endarterectomies for occlusive disease are performed for every one carotid artery aneurysm repair (8,9).

ETIOLOGY

Unlike atherosclerosis, which is highly prevalent in aortic, iliac, and femoropopliteal aneurysms, the causes of brachiocephalic aneurysms are more diverse. In many ways, the pathogenesis is specific to the brachiocephalic artery. Both true and false aneurysms play etiologic roles, and their relative prevalence depends on the local practice. For example, busy trauma centers more frequently report false aneurysms from blunt and penetrating trauma. Tertiary medical centers have larger series of brachiocephalic aneurysms related to atherosclerosis, thoracic outlet syndrome, and degenerative arterial dysplasias (1,10).

Innominate Artery

Isolated innominate artery aneurysms are extraordinarily rare. Most are associated with atherosclerosis, hypertension, and a history of smoking. A few others are mycotic (7).

Carotid Artery

Only one third of carotid artery aneurysms appear to be related to atherosclerosis, and these usually occur at the carotid bifurcation. The other two thirds usually involve the internal carotid artery and are evenly distributed among cases of fibromuscular dysplasia, spontaneous dissection, congenital abnormalities, and trauma (9,11,12). Post-endarterectomy pseudoaneurysm is another type of carotid aneurysm that has become more prevalent with the increased use of carotid artery patching (13).

Subclavian Artery

Proximal subclavian artery aneurysms are usually atherosclerotic. They account for fewer than half of all subclavian artery aneurysms. A more prevalent cause of subclavian artery aneurysm is thoracic outlet compression and chronic injury of the artery caused by an abnormal cervical or first rib (5,6,14). Although less common, an aberrant artery is another cause of subclavian aneurysm. Like other congenitally persistent arteries, an aberrant subclavian artery is prone to aneurysmal degeneration (3,4,15).

Axillary Artery

Extensive reviews of aneurysms in the axillary–subclavian region reveal that the vast majority involve the subclavian artery (88%), whereas solitary axillary artery aneurysms are much less common (12%) (16,17). In elderly patients, atherosclerosis is the cause of solitary axillary artery aneurysms. In younger patients, some type of trauma, such as the use of a crutch, precedes most cases of axillary artery aneurysm (16,17).

CLINICAL FEATURES

Several general clinical features distinguish brachiocephalic aneurysms from other peripheral arterial aneurysms (1). First, brachiocephalic aneurysms are detected over a much wider age range. Although the mean age of patients is about 50 years, the range extends from the second to the ninth decade of life. Like lower extremity aneurysms, atherosclerotic brachiocephalic aneurysms usually occur in the sixth or seventh decade of life. In contrast, subclavian artery aneurysms related to thoracic outlet compression and internal carotid artery aneurysms caused by fibromuscular disease occur in patients in their third or fourth decade of life.

Second, the sex distribution is variable and depends on aneurysm location. Proximal innominate, subclavian, and common carotid aneurysms are at least twice as common in men. Distal subclavian artery aneurysms related to thoracic outlet syndrome and internal carotid aneurysms caused by fibromuscular disease are observed predominantly in women (1,6).

Third, brachiocephalic aneurysms are much more likely to be symptomatic at presentation than are peripheral femoral or popliteal aneurysms. In fact, two thirds of patients with brachiocephalic aneurysms are symptomatic at recognition (7).

Finally, brachiocephalic atherosclerotic aneurysms are commonly associated with other aneurysms (7–9). In one fourth to one half of patients, an additional aneurysm is present or develops later (10,16). In addition to these general clinical features, aneurysms in each anatomic brachiocephalic region have some unique clinical features.

Innominate Artery Aneurysm

Innominate artery aneurysms are symptomatic in more than one half of patients and are associated with three basic clinical presentations: (a) local compressive symptoms of regional nervous or venous structures, (b) tran-

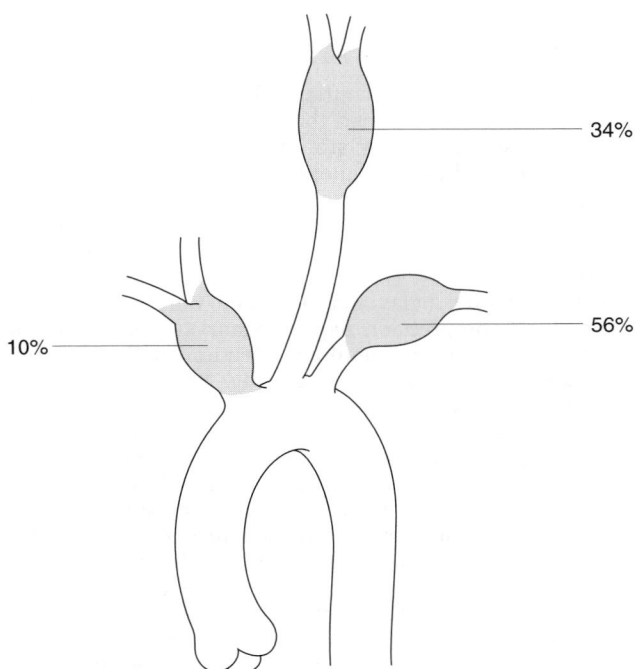

Figure 83.2. Relative frequencies of brachiocephalic aneurysms in 73 patients.

34%

56%

10%

sient ischemic attacks or strokes resulting from thromboembolism, or (c) upper extremity ischemia. Because these lesions usually lie behind the sternum, they may not be palpable (10). However, a large pulsatile and expansive supraclavicular mass should arouse suspicion of an innominate artery aneurysm.

Subclavian Artery Aneurysm

Subclavian artery aneurysms are related most commonly to thoracic outlet compression. Many patients have an abnormal cervical rib (6). Frequently, they present with digital embolization. Recognition of the offending arterial aneurysm or ulcerative plaque is often delayed because it is hidden behind the clavicle. Other manifestations of subclavian artery aneurysms include supraclavicular or shoulder pain, shoulder and arm paresthesias, and upper extremity claudication following aneurysm thrombosis (14,16,18). Subclavian artery aneurysms rarely rupture, but large, proximal intrathoracic atherosclerotic aneurysms are more prone to this event.

Aberrant Subclavian Artery Aneurysm

Aberrant subclavian artery aneurysms occur more often in men and may present over a wide age range. Various clinical presentations include esophageal or tracheal compression; obstruction of the venous outflow of the head, neck, and upper extremities; thromboembolism; and rupture. The most common symptom is dysphagia, which has been termed *dysphagia lusoria* (1,4,15). In general, one third of patients present with dysphagia and another third with dyspnea and respiratory problems; the remainder are asymptomatic (4). These aneurysms are more likely to rupture than most other brachiocephalic aneurysms, and rupture is the clinical outcome in approximately 10% to 15% of such patients (15).

Carotid Artery Aneurysm

Approximately 70% of carotid artery aneurysms involve the internal carotid artery, and the remaining 30% affect the carotid bifurcation. Their main risk is thromboembolic (12). The risk for transient ischemic attack or stroke depends on associated stenosis and thrombus formation in the aneurysm (11). Other symptoms associated with carotid artery aneurysms include cranial nerve dysfunction, neck or ear pain, and headache (7,19).

Axillary Artery Aneurysm

Isolated axillary artery aneurysms generally present with thromboembolic complications. Acute thrombosis often precipitates a vascular emergency (16). Distal thrombus propagation or thromboembolism may cause severe hand ischemia.

DIAGNOSIS AND EVALUATION

The sternum and clavicles prevent palpation of most innominate or proximal subclavian artery aneurysms. Even carotid artery aneurysms may lie deep in the neck and not be palpable until they are large. Cervical common carotid aneurysms must be differentiated from enlarged lymph nodes, head or neck malignancies, and carotid body tumors (1,13). In elderly, hypertensive women, the proximal right common carotid artery may be tortuous and easily mistaken for an aneurysm.

Initial diagnostic tests depend on the clinical presentation of the patient. Computed tomography of the chest, supraclavicular fossa, and neck is usually definitive. Duplex ultrasonography can detect carotid artery aneurysms and most subclavian or axillary aneurysms. Arteriography with views of the aortic arch, great vessels, and intracranial circulation is essential for diagnosis and planning treatment (1,19) (Fig. 83.3). Recently, time-gated gadolinium-enhanced magnetic resonance imaging has provided diagnostic and therapeutic information for many patients (20).

SURGICAL OR ENDOVASCULAR TREATMENT

Surgical resection with arterial reconstruction is indicated for most patients with brachiocephalic aneurysms. Although endovascular stent grafts have been placed percutaneously to treat isolated cases of brachiocephalic aneurysms, their safety and durability remain controversial (21–23). Asymptomatic brachiocephalic aneurysms in patients with poor health or adverse anatomic situations are usually observed. Each type of aneurysm presents its own unique therapeutic challenge.

Innominate Artery Aneurysm

Isolated innominate artery aneurysms are approached through a median sternotomy, with extension of the incision into the neck or right supraclavicular region as needed (Fig. 83.4A, approach No. 1). They are generally replaced with an 8- to 10-mm single-limb prosthetic distal aorta–innominate artery graft (Fig. 83.5A). The need to shunt rarely arises during these reconstructions, but intraoperative electroencephalography or measurement of common carotid stump pressures is a useful adjunct to determine the adequacy of collateral cerebral blood flow. If the innominate artery aneurysm is infected, direct in-line reconstruction with autogenous material, such as arterial homografts, internal iliac or superficial femoral arteries, or superficial femoral veins, can be performed.

Subclavian Artery Aneurysm

Proximal intrathoracic atherosclerotic subclavian artery aneurysms are approached through a median sternotomy, with extension of the incision into the right supraclavicular area for right-sided aneurysms (24) (Fig. 83.4A, approach No. 1). Isolated left intrathoracic subclavian artery aneurysms are best approached through a left posterolateral thoracotomy. A synthetic graft is generally necessary for reconstruction (24).

Patients with subclavian artery aneurysms related to thoracic outlet compression require aneurysm resection, graft replacement, and concomitant resection of the abnormal cervical or anomalous first rib (Fig. 83.5B). This reconstruction can generally be accomplished through two incisions, one supraclavicular and one infraclavicular (Fig. 83.4A, approach No. 3). Occasionally, transaxillary incision is necessary for adequate removal of an offending first rib. An alternative is a single incision with resection of the clavicle. This approach provides excellent exposure but does leave the patient with some cosmetic deformity and occasionally shoulder discomfort. The subclavian artery can be replaced with saphenous vein, hypogastric artery, or a synthetic graft, depending on the size of the artery (Fig. 83.5B).

Axillary artery aneurysms are generally exposed through a subpectoral and medial upper arm incision (Fig. 83.4B). An interposition vein graft is generally appropriate.

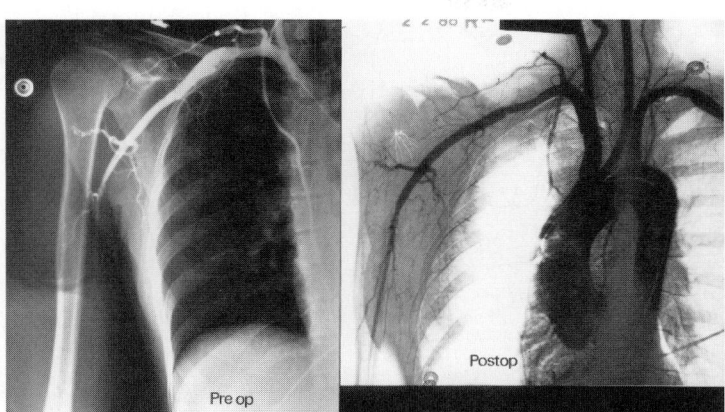

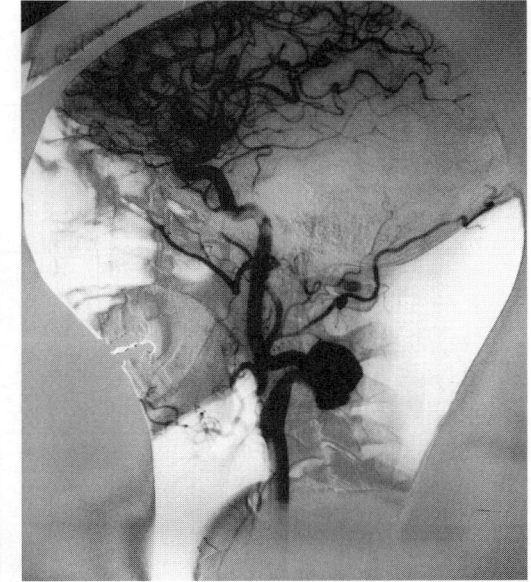

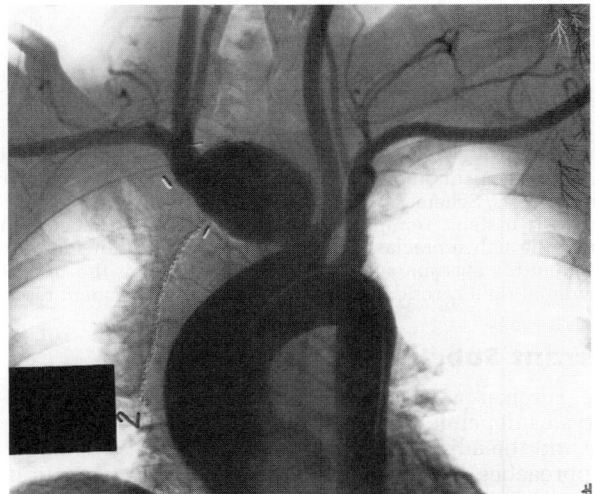

Figure 83.3. *(A)* Arteriography of subclavian artery aneurysm preoperatively and postoperatively. *(B)* Arteriography of carotid artery aneurysm. *(C)* Arteriography of innominate artery aneurysm.

Figure 83.4. *(A)* Approach No. 1: Median sternotomy with extension into cervical or right supraclavicular incision as approach to innominate artery aneurysm. Approach No. 2: Cervical incision as approach to carotid artery aneurysm. Approach No. 3: Supraclavicular incision to proximal portion of right subclavian artery and infraclavicular incision to middle and distal portions of subclavian artery. *(B)* Approach No. 4: Surgical incision to approach distal subclavian or axillary artery aneurysm. Patient's arm is away from side. Note that the medial extent can become the infraclavicular incision in approach No. 3 if more proximal exposure is necessary.

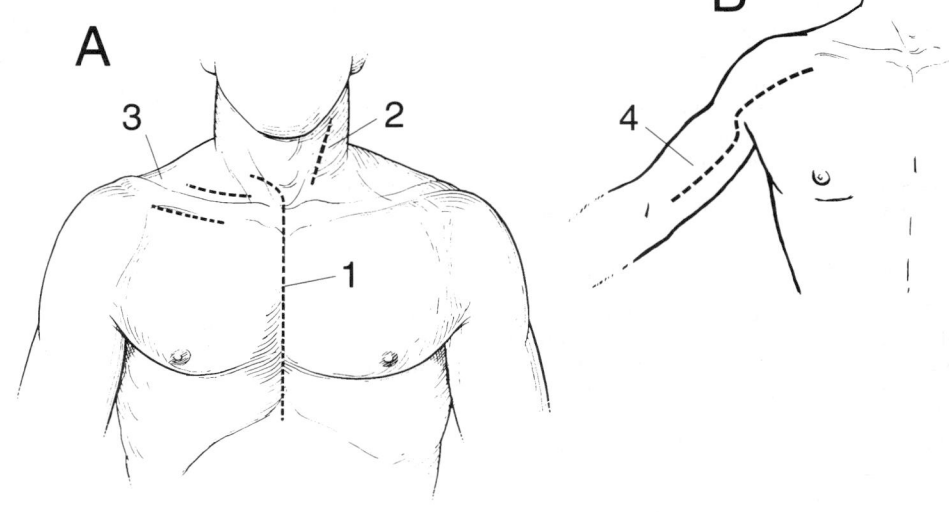

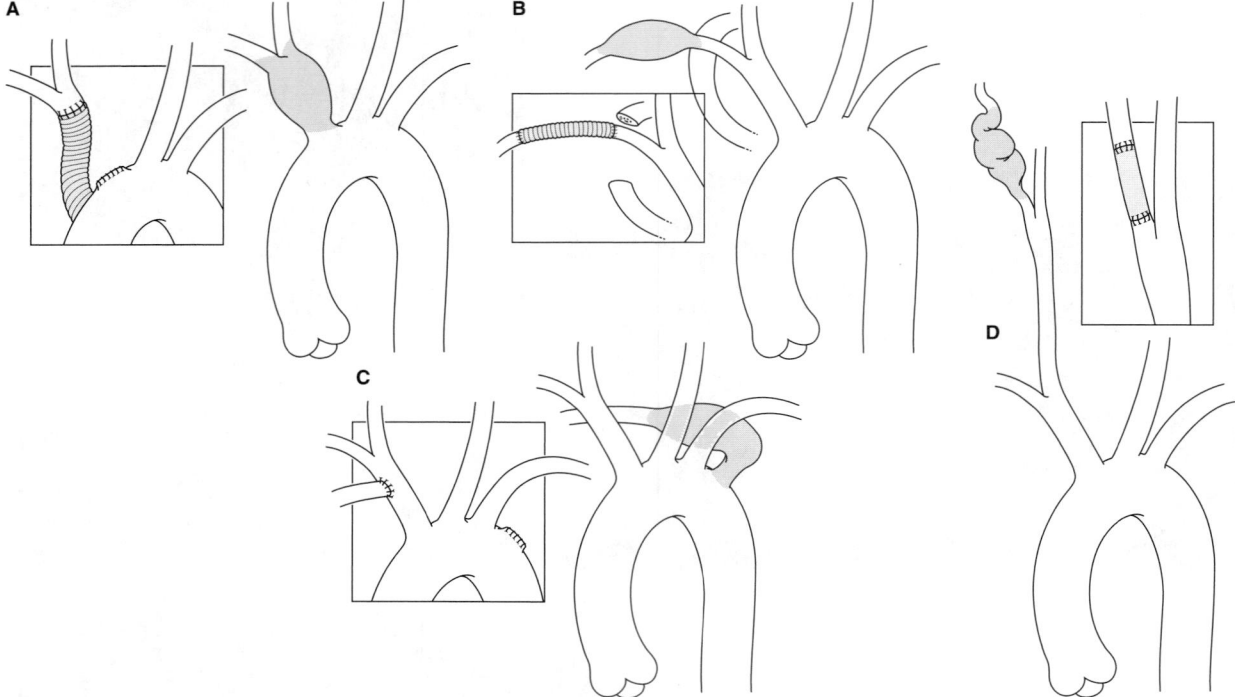

Figure 83.5. *(A)* Schematic representation of aneurysm resection and graft replacement for an innominate artery aneurysm. *(B)* Schematic representation of subclavian artery aneurysm resection, graft replacement, and rib resection for subclavian artery aneurysm related to thoracic outlet obstruction. *(C)* Schematic representation of an aberrant right subclavian artery aneurysm. Repair involves two steps: reimplantation of normal distal subclavian artery into right common carotid artery through supraclavicular approach, followed by left posterolateral thoracotomy to obliterate origin of the aberrant subclavian artery and repair the aorta. *(D)* Schematic representation of extracranial right carotid artery aneurysm with subsequent resection and interposition grafting.

Aberrant Subclavian Aneurysm

The surgical approach to aberrant subclavian artery aneurysms depends on the pathology of both the aberrant artery and the adjacent aorta. Although a variety of surgical approaches have been described, a single operation performed in two stages is most common (4). Initially, a supraclavicular approach is used to reimplant the normal distal subclavian artery into the ipsilateral right common carotid artery. A posterolateral thoracotomy is then performed to obliterate the origin of the aberrant artery and repair the aorta (Fig. 83.5C). The proximal aberrant subclavian artery may be associated with a large, conical duct of Kommerell, which makes aortic control more difficult. In such patients, aortic cross-clamping is generally necessary for safe repair. Although simple cross-clamping with thoracic aortic repair may be possible in 50% of such patients, the remaining patients may require cardiopulmonary bypass or hypothermic circulatory arrest (4).

Carotid Artery Aneurysm

Repair of a common carotid artery aneurysm is accomplished by aneurysm resection or endoaneurysmorrhaphy combined with either primary end-to-end anastomosis or an interposition prosthetic or autogenous graft (Fig. 83.5D). A standard cervical neck incision along the anterior border of the sternocleidomastoid muscle is suitable for aneurysms at the bifurcation or proximal internal carotid artery (Fig. 83.4A, approach No. 2). Exposure of high cervical internal carotid aneurysms is more difficult and may be facilitated by adjuncts such as nasotracheal intubation with or without subluxation of the jaw, mobiliza-

tion of the parotid gland, and division of the posterior belly of the digastric muscle, styloid mandibular ligament, and styloid process (25). Distal carotid control in high cervical aneurysms may require an aneurysm clip, the bulb tip of a shunt, or an indwelling small-balloon occlusion catheter. In reported cases, the distal internal carotid artery has been ligated, and an extracranial–intracranial bypass has been performed to the middle cerebral artery or its M2 segment (25).

OUTCOME OF SURGICAL THERAPY

Elective repair of brachiocephalic aneurysms is associated with a mortality of zero to 8% (6,7,12). Most deaths occur in patients undergoing simultaneous cardiovascular procedures, such as coronary revascularization or aortic arch reconstruction (1). The risk for stroke depends on the type of aneurysm. Perioperative neurologic deficits are more common in patients with atherosclerotic carotid artery aneurysms than in those with aneurysms that are not atherosclerotic (10% to 15% vs. 5%). Most surgical series report a neurologic complication rate higher than that for routine carotid endarterectomy. For high carotid artery aneurysms, cranial nerve injury is problematic and affects as many as 15% of patients (12,13). Glossopharyngeal nerve injury is considered the most morbid, as a permanent gastrostomy is occasionally required.

LATE SURVIVAL

All factors considered, the late survival for patients with brachiocephalic arterial aneurysms is favorable. In a large

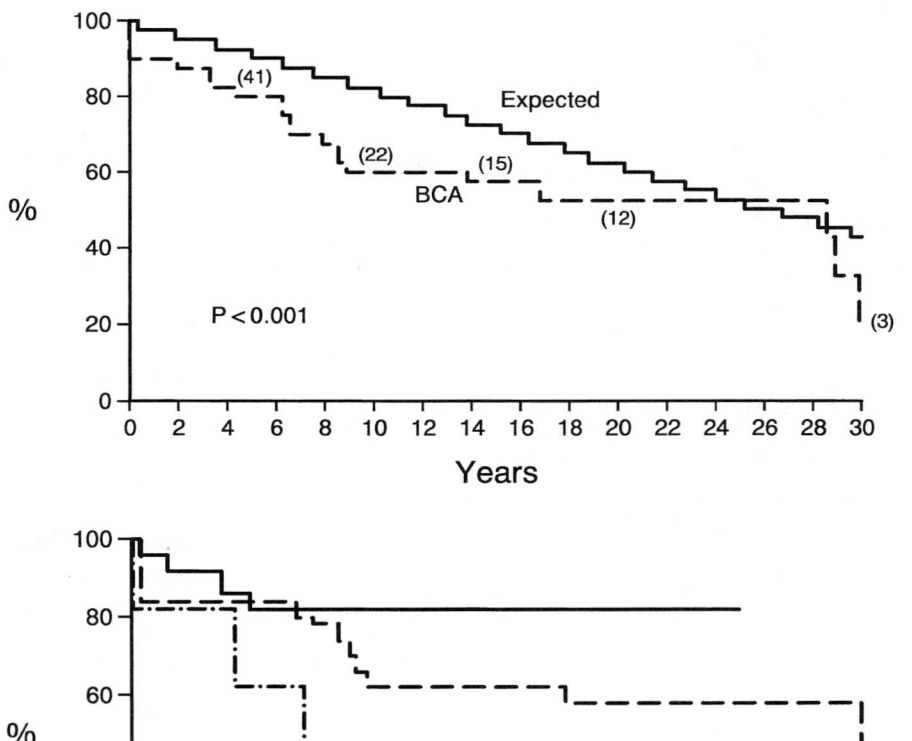

Figure 83.6. (A) Survival of 73 patients with brachiocephalic aneurysms in comparison with expected survival adjusted for age, sex, and year of operation. (B) Survival for each group of brachiocephalic aneurysms. (From Bower TC, Pairolero PC, Hallett JW Jr, et al. Brachiocephalic aneurysm: the case for early recognition and repair. *Ann Vasc Surg* 1991;5:125–132, with permission.)

series from the Mayo Clinic, 5- and 10-year survival rates were 81% and 61%, respectively (7) (Fig. 83.6A). Aneurysm location affects late survival. Patients who undergo repair of carotid artery aneurysms have a 10-year survival of 80%, which is no different from that of age- and sex-matched controls (Fig. 83.6B). However, patients with atherosclerotic subclavian artery aneurysms have a significantly shorter survival than matched controls (7). This difference is generally related to associated cardiovascular morbidity.

ENDOVASCULAR THERAPY

Recently, endovascular approaches have been reported for brachiocephalic aneurysms. These have included a combination of embolization and stent grafts. They have generally been reserved for patients who are not good surgical candidates (e.g., irradiated fields, multiple previous operations, or areas anatomically difficult to approach surgically). Although successful in some cases, embolization and early stent thrombosis have been problematic (21–23). In general, endovascular therapy should be reserved for patients who are not surgical candidates.

REFERENCES

1. Bower TC. Aneurysms of the great vessels and their branches. *Semin Vasc Surg* 1996;9:134–146.
2. Bosniak MA. An analysis of some anatomic–roentgenologic aspects of the brachiocephalic vessels. *Am J Roentgenol* 1964; 91:1222.
3. Stone WM, Brewster DC, Moncure AC, et al. Aberrant right subclavian artery: varied presentations and management options. *J Vasc Surg* 1990;11:812–817.
4. Kieffer E, Bahnini A, Koskas F. Aberrant subclavian artery: surgical treatment in thirty-three adult patients. *J Vasc Surg* 1994;19:100–111.
5. Hood DB, Kuehne J, Yellin AE, et al. Vascular complications of thoracic outlet syndrome. *Am Surg* 1997;63:913–917.
6. Nehler MR, Taylor LM Jr, Moneta GL, et al. Upper extremity ischemia from subclavian artery aneurysm caused by bony abnormalities of the thoracic outlet. *Arch Surg* 1997;132: 527–532.
7. Bower TC, Pairolero PC, Hallett JW Jr, et al. Brachiocephalic aneurysm: the case for early recognition and repair. *Ann Vasc Surg* 1991;5:125–132.
8. Painter TA, Hertzer NR, Beven EG, et al. Extracranial carotid aneurysms: report of six cases and review of the literature. *J Vasc Surg* 1985;2:312–318.
9. Zwolak RM, Whitehouse WM Jr, Knake JE, et al. Atherosclerotic extracranial carotid artery aneurysms. *J Vasc Surg* 1984; 1:415–422.
10. Brewster DC, Moncure AC, Darling RC, et al. Innominate artery lesions: problems encountered and lessons learned. *J Vasc Surg* 1985;2:99–112.
11. Schievink WI, Piepgras DG, McGaffrey TV, et al. Surgical treatment of extracranial internal carotid artery dissecting aneurysms. *Neurosurgery* 1994;35:809–816.
12. Moreau P, Albat B, Thevenet A. Surgical treatment of extracranial internal carotid artery aneurysms. *Ann Vasc Surg* 1994;8:409–416.

13. Faggioli GL, Freyrie A, Stella A, et al. Extracranial internal carotid artery aneurysms: results of a surgical series with long-term follow-up. *J Vasc Surg* 1996;23:578–595.

14. Cormier JM, Amrane M, Ward A, et al. Arterial complications of the thoracic outlet syndrome: fifty-five operative cases. *J Vasc Surg* 1989;9:778–787.

15. Kiernan PD, Dearani J, Byrne WD, et al. Aneurysm of an aberrant right subclavian artery: case report and review of the literature. *Mayo Clin Proc* 1993;68:468–474.

16. Pairolero PC, Walls JT, Payne WS, et al. Subclavian–axillary artery aneurysms. *Surgery* 1981;90:757–763.

17. Abbott WM, Darling RC. Axillary artery aneurysms secondary to crutch trauma. *Am J Surg* 1973;125:515–520.

18. Dougherty MJ, Calligaro KD, Savarese RP, et al. Atherosclerotic aneurysm of the intrathoracic subclavian artery: a case report and review of the literature. *J Vasc Surg* 1995;21:521–529.

19. Coffin O, Maiza D, Galateau-Salle F, et al. Results of surgical management of internal carotid artery aneurysm by the cervical approach. *Ann Vasc Surg* 1997;11:482–490.

20. Laitt RD, Thompson JF, Goddard P, et al. Subclavian artery aneurysm: the role of magnetic resonance imaging. *Cardiovasc Surg* 1994;2:612–614.

21. May J, White G, Waugh R, et al. Transluminal placement of a prosthetic graft–stent device for treatment of subclavian artery aneurysm. *J Vasc Surg* 1993;18:1056–1059.

22. Beregi JP, Prat A, Willoteaux S, et al. Covered stents in the treatment of peripheral arterial aneurysms: procedural results and midterm follow-up. *Cardiovasc Intervent Radiol* 1999;22:13–19.

23. Parodi JC, Schonholz C, Ferreira LM, et al. Endovascular stent–graft treatment of traumatic arterial lesions. *Ann Vasc Surg* 1999;13:121–129.

24. Coselli JS, Crawford ES. Surgical treatment of aneurysms of the intrathoracic segment of the subclavian artery. *Chest* 1987;91:704–708.

25. Sundt TM Jr, Pearson BW, Piepgras DG, et al. Surgical management of aneurysms of the distal extracranial internal carotid artery. *J Neurosurg* 1986;64:169–182.

SURGERY: SCIENTIFIC PRINCIPLES AND PRACTICE, Third Edition, edited by Lazar J. Greenfield, Michael W. Mulholland, Keith T. Oldham, Gerald B. Zelenock, and Keith D. Lillemoe. Lippincott Williams & Wilkins Publishers, Philadelphia, © 2001.

CHAPTER 84

THORACIC AORTIC ANEURYSMS

R. SCOTT MITCHELL

The incidence of aneurysmal disease of the thoracic aorta appears to be increasing. Whether this reflects an actual increase in incidence, an increase in the number of cases detected through improved diagnostic modalities, or an increasing population at risk remains unknown. True aneurysmal dilation of the aorta involves all three layers of the arterial wall (intima, media, and adventitia) and can be fusiform or saccular. In false aneurysms, conversely, an intimal disruption is contained only by adventitial layers and surrounding reactive fibrosis. Arteriosclerotic aneurysms typically demonstrate degenerative changes within the aortic media, whereas intrinsic abnormalities of connective tissue account for the degenerative aneurysms found in Marfan's syndrome and Ehlers-Danlos syndrome, in which all parts of the aorta, including the sinuses of Valsalva, are involved. These entities are to be differentiated from aortic dissections, in which an intimal tear creates a high-pressure entry point into the subadventitial layer, which can then propagate proximally and distally and possibly lead to rupture or branch vessel compromise. In a patient with Marfan's syndrome, the risk for aortic dissection appears directly related to the extent of aneurysmal dilation of the aortic root.

The development of cardiopulmonary bypass and synthetic graft materials has allowed tremendous progress to be made in the management of these life-threatening disorders. DeBakey and Cooley (1) pioneered many of the techniques that have been accepted and refined by surgeons throughout the world. The use of new graft materials (including aortic homografts), composite valve–graft conduits, new suture materials, modern techniques of cardiopulmonary bypass, and more effective methods of myocardial and cerebral protection has allowed acceptable survival after surgical treatment of even the most severe disease of the thoracic aorta.

ARTERIOSCLEROTIC ANEURYSMS

Only slightly less common than abdominal aortic aneurysms, aneurysmal disease of the thoracic aorta is increasingly detected in aging populations with associated hypertension and chronic obstructive lung disease. Most commonly, these aneurysms are asymptomatic and are discovered on routine chest radiographs or during evaluation for another medical problem. Men are affected more commonly than women, in a ratio of 3:1, and the descending aorta is more commonly involved than the ascending aorta. A positive family history for many patients with thoracic aortic aneurysms raises the question of whether these aneurysms, like their abdominal aortic counterparts, may have a genetic basis.

Once aneurysmal dilation of the aorta has begun, it tends to progress. Whether this represents a gradual but constant increase in size or episodic incremental increases is unknown, but both appear likely. Concomitant hypertension contributes to continued expansion in two ways; increased radial pressure results in increased wall tension, and ongoing damage to the structural integrity of the aortic wall develops through accelerated arteriosclerotic change. Unlike the classic natural history studies of abdominal aortic aneurysms (2), no such studies exist for aneurysms of the thoracic aorta. However, in a series of more than 600 patients with thoracic aneurysms described before operative repair was possible, 66% of patients died as a result of their aneurysms. A 1980 study reinforced the dismal outcome of patients managed nonoperatively after discovery of a large thoracic aneurysm (3). The high rupture rates for aneurysms larger than 10 cm in diameter and for symptomatic aneurysms were alarming. The mean survival after diagnosis was only 2.6 years, and only 20% of patients survived 5 years. Aneurysm rupture accounted for 40% of deaths, with an additional 30% resulting from other cardiovascular causes. A more recent population-based study from Olmstead County, Minnesota, confirms that an absolute increase in the incidence of thoracic aneurysms has occurred, and also suggests that the natural history may be more benign. From the 1970s to the 1980s, the incidence appeared to increase from 3 to approximately 10 cases per 100,000 person-years. The cumulative risk for rupture at 5 years continues to depend on the size of the aneurysm at the time of diagnosis. The risk with aneurysms measuring less than 4 cm in diameter is less than 5%; it increases to approximately 16% for aneurysms between 4 and 6 cm, and to 31% for aneurysms larger than 6 cm (4). These figures represent a significant improvement over the overall survival of 19% noted in the earlier studies. Additionally, although women comprise about 50% of the aneurysm population, and although their aneurysms are diagnosed on average 12 to 13 years later in life, women account for almost 80% of ruptures. Thus, it may be prudent to normalize aneurysm size to body surface area, as suggested by McDonald et al. of the Cleveland Clinic (5). Signs and symptoms of rapid expansion, including hemoptysis, hematemesis, hoarseness, stridor, and an increase in chest pain, warrant surgical intervention. We also favor repair for thoracic aortic aneurysms larger than 7 cm in diameter, for those with a diameter more than twice that of the normal adjacent aorta, and for aneurysms that rapidly increase in size.

Several new diagnostic modalities allow much closer monitoring and detection of thoracic aneurysms than was previously possible. Although the routine biplane diagnostic chest radiograph can alert the clinician to the presence of an aneurysm (Fig. 84.1), the cross-sectional images available through computed tomography (CT) and magnetic resonance imaging (MRI) allow much more accurate sizing of the aneurysm and can differentiate between aneurysmal chronic dissections and true arteriosclerotic or degenerative aneurysms. This differentiation is important because chronic dissections tend to be more extensive, and their operative repair is more complex. Once an aneurysm is suspected, imaging of the entire thoracic and abdominal aorta must be performed because multiple aneurysms are found in as many as 40% of patients. Because angiography delineates only the aortic lumen within the laminated thrombus, it can seriously underestimate aneurysm size and extent; thus, it is only of minimal usefulness for ongoing clinical assessment.

Operative Management

Once the need for operation has been determined and cardiac evaluation has been completed, aneurysm replacement with an interposition graft during cardiopulmonary bypass is the treatment of choice. Proper anesthetic management of these patients is critical and requires arterial, central venous, and pulmonary arterial pressure monitoring, urinary catheterization, and double-lumen endotracheal intubation. Additionally, large-volume intravenous infusion lines and central infusion ports for vasoactive drugs are essential. Transesophageal echocardiography has also been extremely helpful in assessing regional wall motion and intravascular volume status intraoperatively. Within the operative field, blood-scavenging systems are extensively used to reduce the need for donor bank blood. Collagen-coated woven double-velour Dacron grafts and monofilament suture allow for a more hemostatic repair and minimize tearing of the fragile aortic wall.

Repair of an ascending aortic aneurysm is accomplished through a median sternotomy by replacing the diseased aorta from the sinotubular ridge to the level of the innominate artery and, if necessary, the transverse aortic arch. Cardiopulmonary bypass is established through bicaval atrial cannulation and femoral artery cannulation, with either pulmonary artery or left atrial venting. Myocardial protection is achieved by infusion of crystalloid or blood cardioplegia into the coronary ostia and retrograde into the coronary sinus, usually with use of a cooling jacket for local hypothermia. Surgical judgment is important in deciding the extent of repair because generalized aortic ectasia can coexist with more extensive focal aneurysmal disease. Operative morbidity, the patient's physiologic age, and expectations for longevity are all-important in determining the extent of operative repair (Fig. 84.2). The development of full-thickness cuffs for proximal and distal anastomoses eliminates concerns regarding inadequate tissue bites and the subsequent problems with hemostasis and false-aneurysm formation that can result from use of the inclusion technique. Management of the degenerative aneurysms of Marfan's disease and of aortic dissections requires additional technical considerations and is covered separately. After rewarming is accomplished, all air is removed from the left side of the heart and graft, and the aortic cross-clamp is removed. After a sufficient period of resuscitation, with continuous venting of the ascending aorta for entrapped air, the patient is weaned from cardiopulmonary bypass. Avoidance of postoperative hypertension is critical to prevent excessive bleeding or anastomotic disruption.

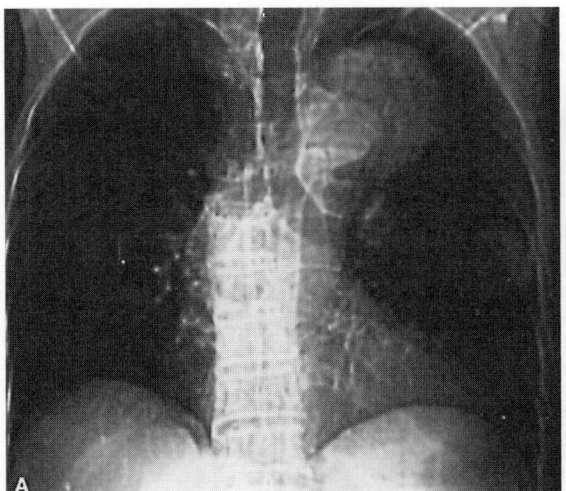
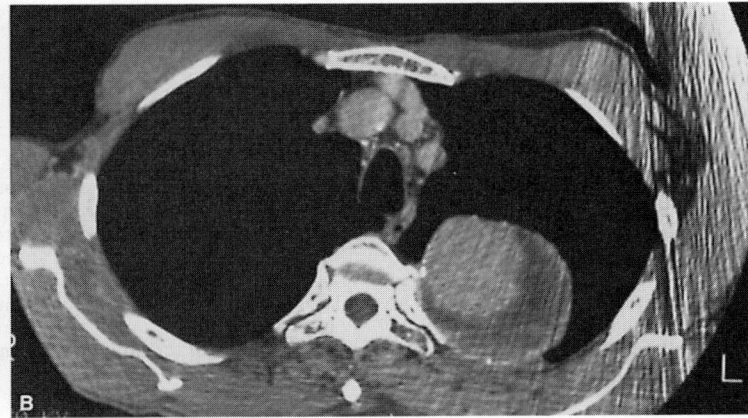

Figure 84.1. *(A)* Large, asymptomatic aneurysm of the descending thoracic aorta discovered incidentally on routine chest radiograph. A peripheral left upper zone pulmonary mass is also apparent. *(B)* Computed tomography of the thorax allows precise determination of aneurysm size and location and frequently obviates the need for angiography.

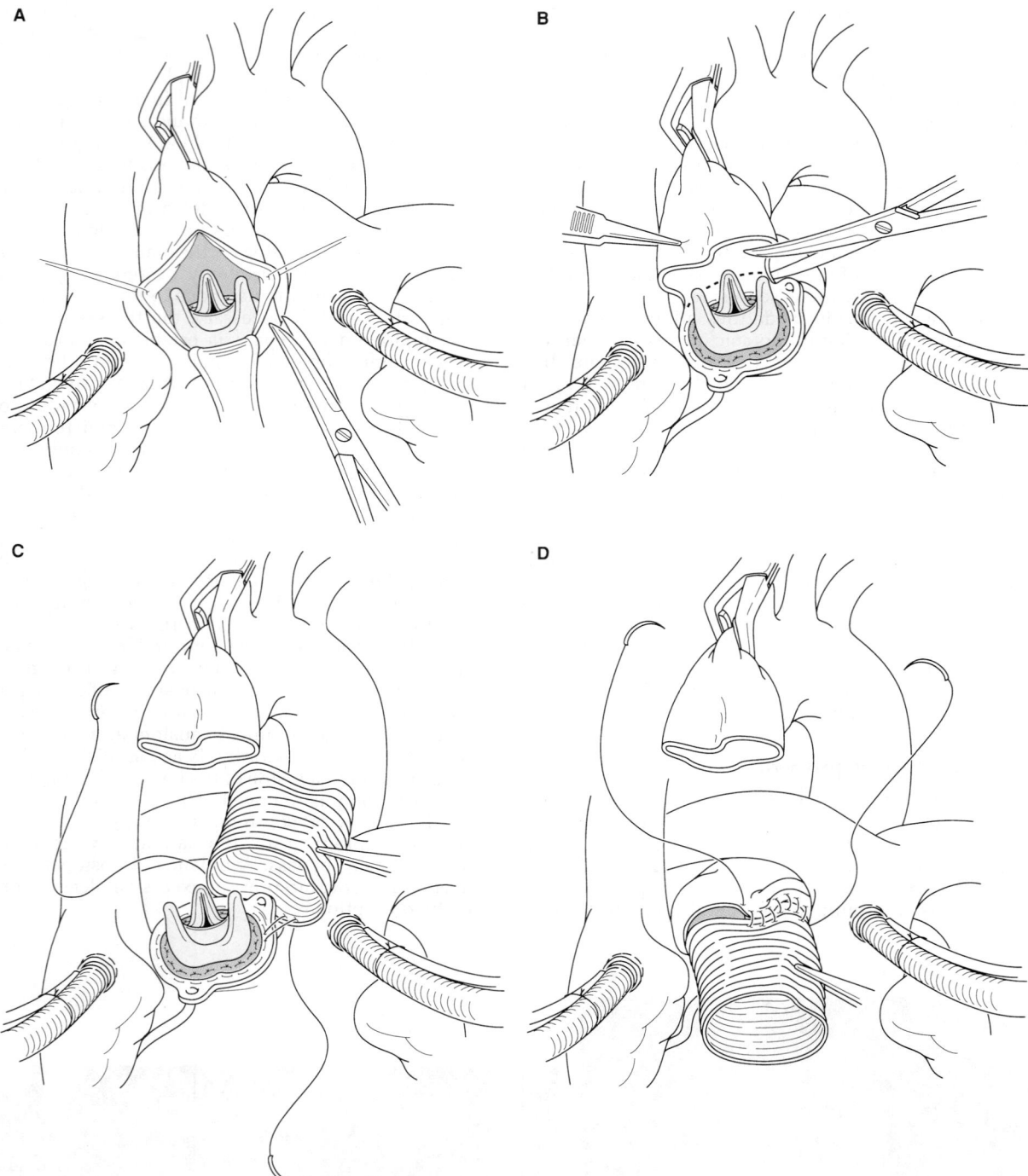

Figure 84.2. *(A)* Operative repair of ascending aortic aneurysm without degenerative aortic disease. Valve replacement, if indicated, is performed after cardiac arrest with cardioplegia and during continuous topical hypothermia. *(B)* A full-thickness cuff of proximal aorta is developed by meticulous dissection of the aorta off the pulmonary artery, and the aorta is transected just distal to the coronary ostia. *(C)* The posterior suture line begins to the left of the left main coronary ostium and proceeds rightward over the ostium. Meticulous hemostasis is mandatory because repair sutures in this area can narrow the left main coronary artery. *(D)* Completion of the posterior suture line demonstrates the exposure attained by extensive mobilization of the aorta and pulmonary artery. *(continues)*

E

F

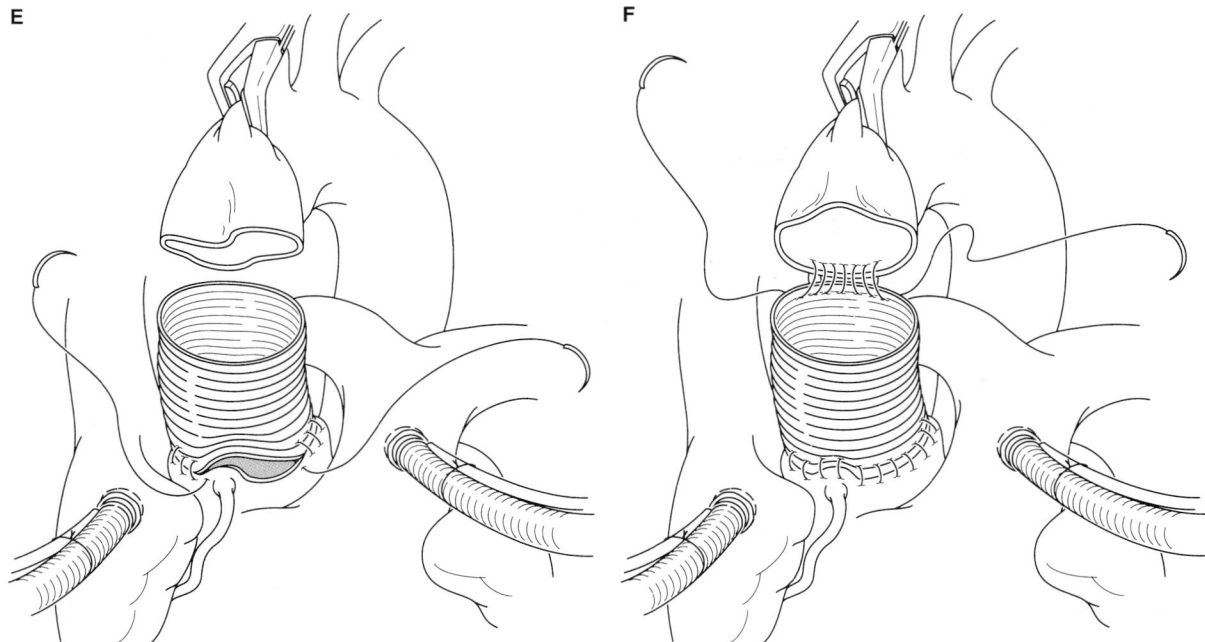

Figure 84.2. *(Continued) (E)* The anterior suture line may compromise the right coronary artery in the atrioventricular groove. *(F)* Careful measurement of graft length ensures a tension-free distal anastomosis. (After Frist WH, Miller DC. Repair of ascending aortic aneurysms and dissections. *J Card Surg* 1986;1:33, with permission.)

Operations on the transverse aortic arch are usually performed with profound hypothermic circulatory arrest and retrograde cerebral venous perfusion. Alternatively, separate arterial cannulation of a single nondiseased arch vessel and lesser degrees of hypothermia have been used. As techniques of myocardial preservation and cerebral protection improve, aggressive repairs of complex arch problems are associated with decreased morbidity and improved long-term survival.

Operative repair of descending thoracic aneurysms is performed through a left posterolateral thoracotomy with a double-lumen endotracheal tube in place. When left atrial–bifemoral bypass with a centrifugal pump and minimal heparinization is used, proximal aortic control is usually attained just distal to the left common carotid artery after mobilization of both phrenic and vagus nerves. Large aneurysms adherent to the chest wall or lung parenchyma can be left incompletely dissected until proximal and distal control is attained and cardiopulmonary bypass is established. After cross-clamping distally and proximally, full-thickness cuffs of aorta are fashioned, and an interposition graft is sutured in place. Although the necessity for bypass remains controversial, we believe that its use allows distal perfusion and more optimal management of preload, with minimal adverse effects of heparinization. Although proponents of the clamp-and-sew technique emphasize its simplicity, freedom from complications of anticoagulation, and generally good results, cross-clamp times in excess of 30 minutes are associated with an increased risk for paraplegia, a dreaded complication of operations on the distal thoracic aorta (6).

Bypass techniques in which heparin-bonded shunts are used, although they avoid the bleeding complications of full-dose heparin, may deliver variable and inadequate flows for distal perfusion. Left atrium-to-femoral artery partial bypass with a centrifugal pump and minimal heparinization is an attractive alternative to the full heparinization required for partial (venoarterial) cardiopulmonary bypass. No single technique, however, obviates the possibility of postoperative paraplegia. Multiple adjunctive techniques have been explored, both clinically and in the laboratory, in an effort to protect the spinal cord, including monitoring of evoked potentials, perfusion of cord with cooled blood, drainage of spinal fluid to lower intrathecal pressure, the use of neuroprotective agents, the use of local and systemic hypothermia, reimplantation of critical intercostal vessels, and administration of corticosteroids. Although all these adjuncts can lessen the incidence of paraplegia, none confers absolute protection. Research continues in an effort to prevent this complication.

Multivariate analysis of preoperative variables has been attempted in an effort to identify significant clinical predictors of early and late mortality for all aneurysms of the ascending and descending aorta (7). The operative mortality rate for ascending aneurysm repair was 7%, with a range of 5% to 15% reported in large series in the literature. Only emergency operation and age over 62 years were independent predictors of increased mortality. For aneurysms of the descending aorta, the operative mortality rate was 17%, and it correlated significantly with emergency operation and preoperative congestive heart failure. The survival rate after 10 years for this group was about 50% (Fig. 84.3), which reflects diffuse involvement with arteriosclerotic cardiovascular disease. Thirty percent of patients suffered late deaths from myocardial failure, cerebrovascular accidents, or aneurysm rupture. For all patients, the possibility of late survival was significantly diminished by increased age at the time of operation and by the preoperative presence of congestive heart failure and renal dysfunction.

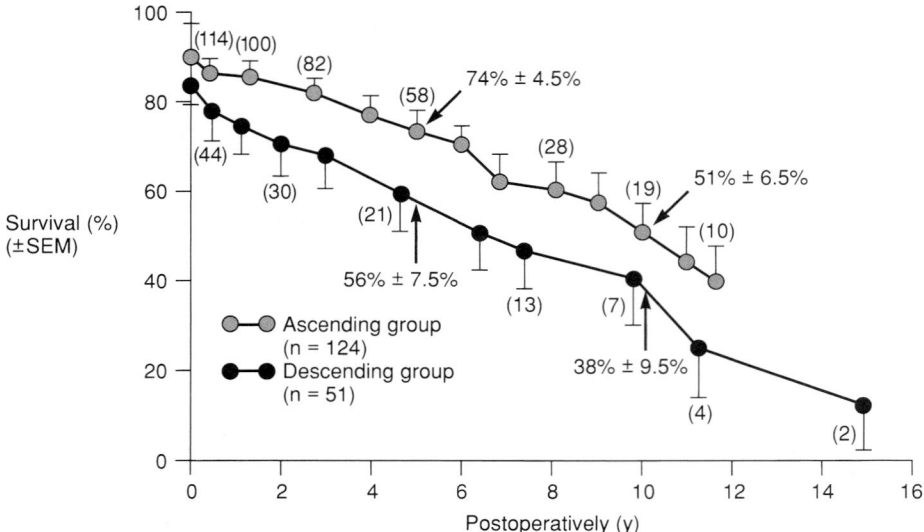

Figure 84.3. Actuarial survival curves for patients with thoracic aortic aneurysms treated operatively. (After Moreno-Cabral CE, Miller DC, Mitchell RS, et al. Degenerative and atherosclerotic aneurysms of the thoracic aorta. *J Thorac Cardiovasc Surg* 1984;88: 1025, with permission.)

DEGENERATIVE ANEURYSMS

Aneurysms classified as degenerative are those thought to be secondary to the defective formation of collagen, the fibrous ground substance that is the main constituent of skin, tendons, ligaments, and blood vessels. Although these genetic defects are being elucidated, the actual molecular defect remains unknown. In Marfan's syndrome, which is an autosomal dominant disorder with variable clinical presentations, specific abnormalities of fibrillin, the main component of extracellular microfibrils, have been detected. The defective gene FBN1, located on the long arm of chromosome 15, is responsible for the abnormal fibrillin. Quantitative analysis of fibrillin synthesis in these patients has allowed the differentiation of four phenotypes with varying clinical manifestations. It has also allowed fibrillin abnormalities to be identified in pa-

tients in whom the clinical diagnosis of Marfan's syndrome cannot be made. Further elucidation of these defects may allow the identification, by genetic screening, of a patient population having a propensity for aneurysm formation without the clinical stigmata of Marfan's syndrome or Ehlers-Danlos syndrome. Further clarification of the abnormal synthesis, secretion, and matrix deposition of fibrillin in these syndromes will be available shortly. These abnormalities are diffuse, and they involve not only the entire aorta, including the coronary sinuses, but also the cardiac valvular tissues. In contrast to arteriosclerotic aneurysmal disease, the aortic aneurysms found in patients with Marfan's syndrome begin at the level of the aortic annulus and involve the coronary sinuses in addition to the supracoronary aorta, so that replacement of the entire aortic root is required. Because these changes may not be obvious on serial diagnostic

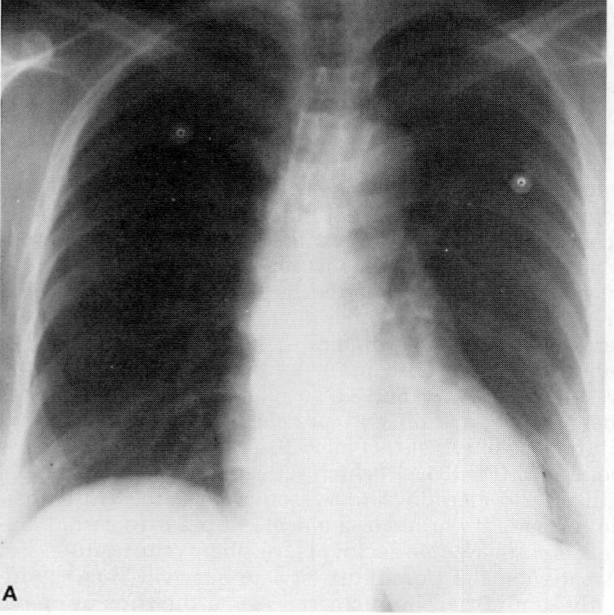
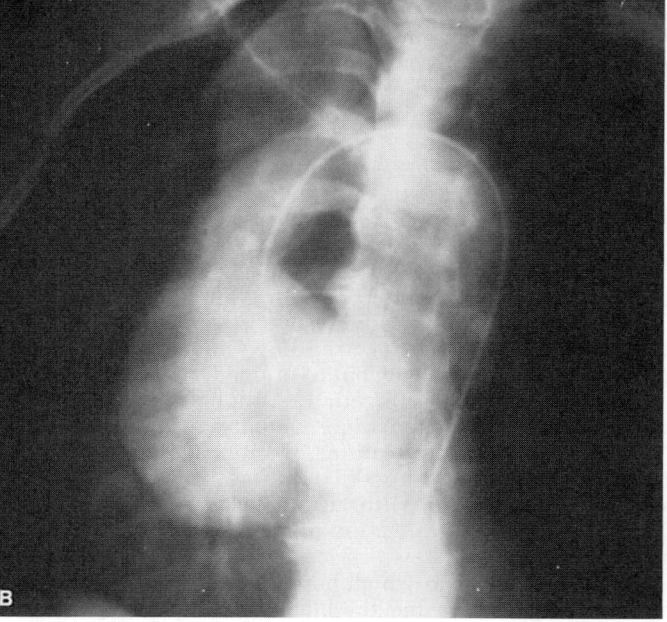

Figure 84.3. (*A*) Dilation of the proximal aorta may be hidden by mediastinal structures on routine posteroanterior chest radiograph. (*B*) Aortography reveals dilation of the entire ascending aorta, including the coronary sinuses, as well as aortic regurgitation.

chest radiographs (Fig. 84.4), echocardiography, CT, or MRI may be required for serial evaluation.

In patients with the obvious stigmata of Marfan's syndrome (i.e., long extremities, hyperextendable joints, ectopic lenses, and pectus deformity of the sternum), the diagnosis may be straightforward. In a significant number of patients, however, the diagnosis may not be obvious. The criteria from the Johns Hopkins registry have been used to identify patients with Marfan's syndrome (8). Patients were considered to have the syndrome if they had an affected family member or had evidence of lens dislocation, aortic insufficiency, or musculoskeletal involvement. Historically, the severely diminished longevity of both male and female patients with Marfan's syndrome has been graphically illustrated, with fewer than half of them surviving past the age of 45 years. Cardiac deaths account for more than 90% of early deaths of known cause, and 75% of these deaths are secondary to aortic root dilation or aortic dissections and their complications.

These dismal statistics prompted recommendations for prophylactic replacement of the aortic root before rupture or dissection, despite its known attendant morbidity and mortality. The direct relation between increasing aortic root size and the propensity for both rupture and dissection supports prophylactic aortic root replacement for aneurysmal dilation larger than 6 cm. As surgical results improve and the durability of these repairs is documented, these criteria may be revised downward so that prophylactic repair can be accomplished early and the morbidity associated with the long-term management of aneurysmal dilation in chronic aortic dissections involving the entire aorta can be avoided.

Operative Management

Methods of surgical repair of the aorta in Marfan's syndrome have evolved during the past two decades. Initially, the supracoronary aorta was replaced, with separate aortic valve replacement, and surgical results were acceptable. Long-term follow-up, however, demonstrated progressive aneurysmal dilation of the aortic sinuses, which frequently necessitated a difficult second operation for replacement of the entire aortic root. Because of the known involvement of the aortic sinuses, a second procedure evolved, the Bentall procedure. In this operation, of a valved conduit is sewn directly onto the aortic annulus, with the coronary ostia sewn to the ascending graft in a side-to-side fashion. Late follow-up of this procedure, however, revealed a disturbingly high incidence of false-aneurysm formation at the coronary anastomoses secondary to either poor integrity of the aorta or tension on the anastomoses. Most surgeons now advocate repair by means of a valved conduit and circumferential dissection of the coronary ostia with buttons of aortic tissue. These buttons are then anastomosed to the ascending graft in an end-to-side fashion and are frequently buttressed with a circular felt pledget (Fig. 84.5). The distal anastomosis is performed to the completely transected aorta proximal to the innominate artery.

In some patients, particularly those with lesser degrees of aneurysm formation, the coronary ostia may not have migrated cephalad sufficiently to allow reattachment to the valved conduit. The use of a U-shaped loop of synthetic graft material anastomosed end to end to the coronary ostia and then end to side to the ascending graft (Carbol modification) allows coronary perfusion (Fig. 84.6). Great care must be taken with this repair to avoid kinking, with resultant insufficient coronary blood flow. Improved techniques of myocardial protection and the use of valved conduits have resulted in an operative mortality rate of less than 5%, and long-term durability is promising.

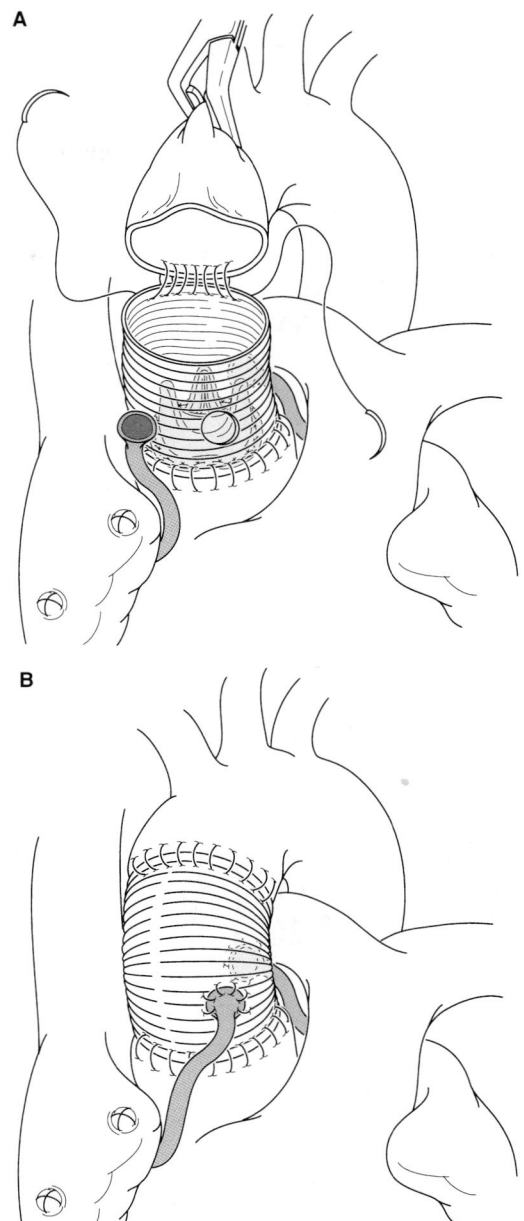

Figure 84.5. *(A)* Replacement of the aortic root is accomplished with a valved conduit anastomosed directly to the aortic annulus. The left coronary anastomosis is already complete, performed as an end-to-side anastomosis of a full-thickness aortic button before completion of the distal anastomosis. The full-thickness right coronary anastomosis is completed after the distal anastomosis to allow proper positioning without torsion or tension. *(B)* The completed repair, with reimplanted right and left coronary anastomoses. Circular Teflon felt bolsters may be necessary if the aortic tissues are unduly friable. (After Frist WH, Miller DC. Repair of ascending aortic aneurysms and dissections. *J Card Surg* 1986;1:33, with permission.)

Long-term follow-up from several centers indicates that prophylactic replacement of the dilated aortic root decreases the complications of aortic root dissection in patients with Marfan's syndrome. Historically, these patients have had a 50% mortality rate at 8 years after operation, although this is still a significant improvement over the untreated natural history of Marfan's syndrome. Further-

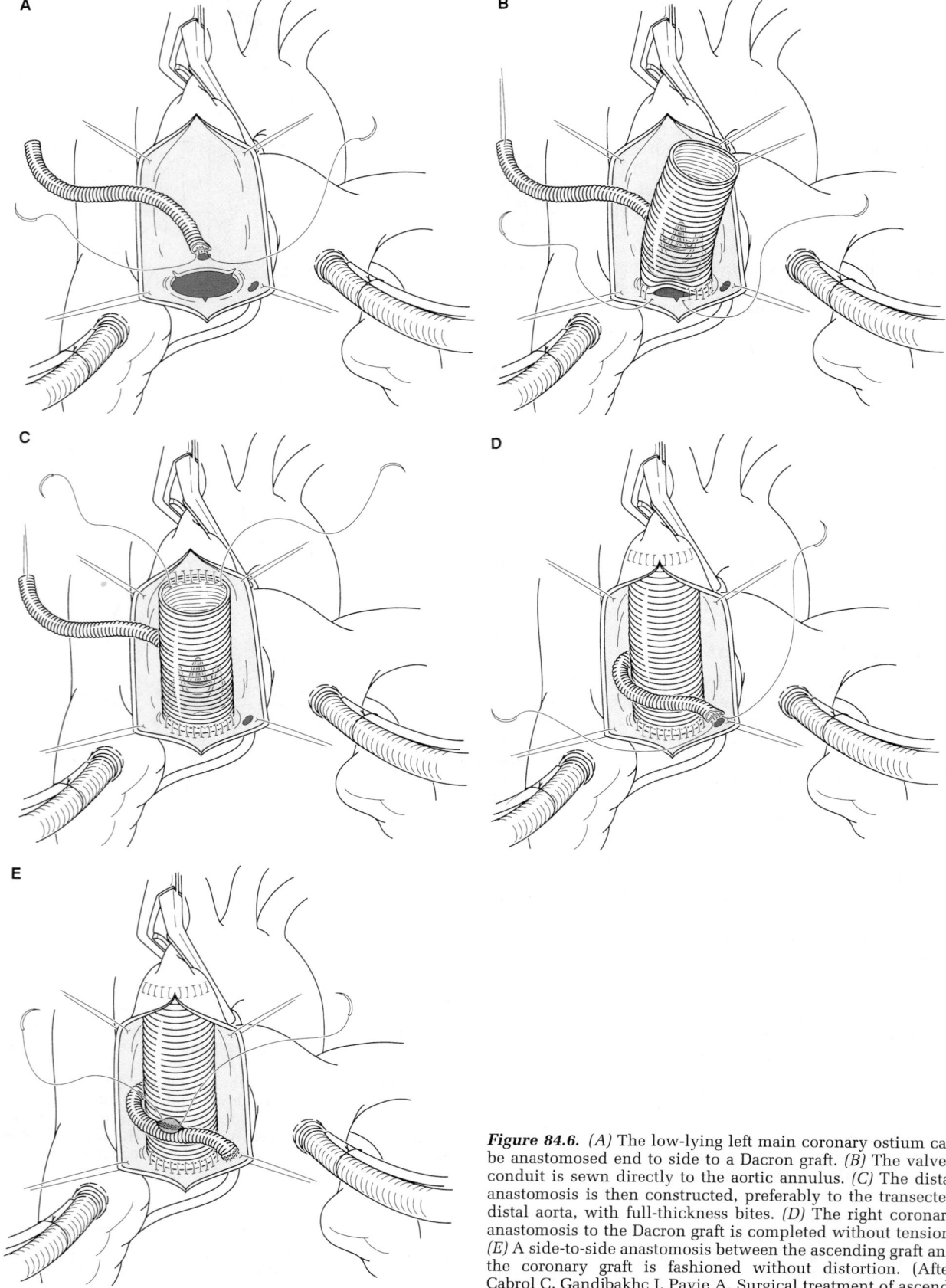

Figure 84.6. *(A)* The low-lying left main coronary ostium can be anastomosed end to side to a Dacron graft. *(B)* The valved conduit is sewn directly to the aortic annulus. *(C)* The distal anastomosis is then constructed, preferably to the transected distal aorta, with full-thickness bites. *(D)* The right coronary anastomosis to the Dacron graft is completed without tension. *(E)* A side-to-side anastomosis between the ascending graft and the coronary graft is fashioned without distortion. (After Cabrol C, Gandjbakhc I, Pavie A. Surgical treatment of ascending aortic pathology. *J Card Surg* 1988;3:167, with permission.)

more, these patients are still subject to complications in other segments of the aorta, particularly if they have had an aortic dissection preoperatively. Most of these problems are remediable by surgical techniques, however, and aggressive follow-up is advocated so that problem areas can be repaired or replaced before a new catastrophic event occurs. Both dramatic progress in understanding the syndrome and the development of surgical approaches to the marfanoid aorta have made it possible to attenuate a morbid natural history to a significant degree.

AORTIC DISSECTIONS

Acute dissection of the thoracic aorta remains the most frequent catastrophe involving the aorta, with an incidence almost double that of ruptured abdominal aortic aneurysm. Failure to diagnose this entity probably accounts, at least in part, for the lack of appreciation of its prevalence. Most commonly affected are middle-aged and elderly men with coexistent hypertension, although younger women, particularly during the third trimester of pregnancy, can also be affected, as can patients with Marfan's disease.

Classification

Multiple classification systems from various institutions have been promulgated, based primarily on anatomic features. Involvement of the ascending aorta remains the most important single feature of acute dissections because this alone predicts unfavorable clinical behavior. Neither the exact location of the primary tear nor the distal extent of the dissection correlates as significantly with subsequent clinical behavior. Therefore, classification schemes should be based on anatomic features as they relate to clinical behavior or management. Thus, Stanford type A, Massachusetts General proximal, University of Alabama ascending, and DeBakey type 1 all connote involvement of the ascending aorta, whereas Stanford type B, Massachusetts General distal, University of Alabama descending, and DeBakey type 3 denote dissections not involving the ascending aorta (Figs. 84.7 and 84.8).

Acute aortic dissection can present with protean signs and symptoms, mimicking other more common illnesses. Typically, affected patients experience the sudden onset of severe, sharp retrosternal or intrascapular pain, which may then migrate. Occasionally, it is entirely silent, the diagnosis becoming apparent only after the onset of a secondary effect, such as congestive heart failure subsequent to aortic regurgitation or limb ischemia caused by arterial occlusion. A high index of suspicion for seemingly unrelated signs and symptoms remains the key to timely diagnosis, which is critical to avoid the 1% to 2% *per hour* mortality rate during the first 24 to 48 hours after acute dissection of the ascending aorta. When ascending dissection is not diagnosed, the mortality rate approaches 90% at 3 months; the prognosis for type B or descending dissections is somewhat less ominous. Unfortunately, even in the modern era, as many as one third of cases may go undiagnosed.

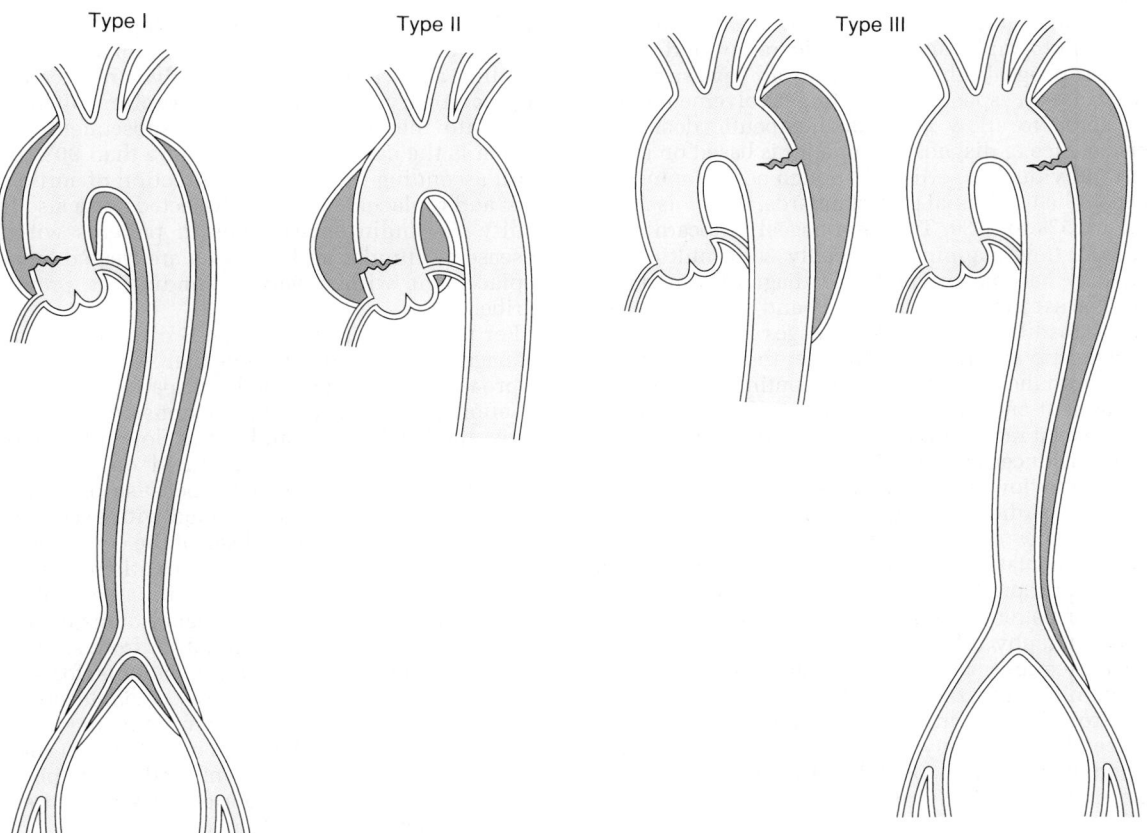

Figure 84.7. Classification scheme of DeBakey for aortic dissections. Three types are depicted, according to the site of tear and extent of dissection. (After DeBakey ME, McCollum CH, Crawford ES, et al. Dissection and dissecting aneurysms of the aorta: twenty-year follow-up of five hundred twenty-seven patients treated surgically. *Surgery* 1982;92:1118, with permission.)

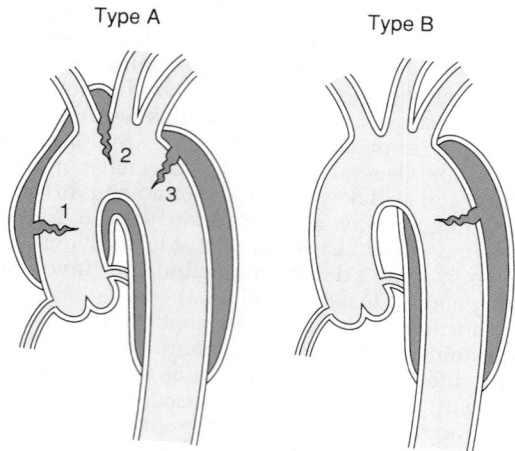

Figure 84.8. Stanford classification of aortic dissections based on the presence or absence of involvement of the ascending aorta. *Numbers* indicate possible locations of the primary intimal tear. (After Miller DC, Stinson EB, Oyer PE, et al. Operative treatment of aortic dissections. *J Thorac Cardiovasc Surg* 1979;78:365, with permission.)

Diagnosis

A careful history and physical examination can produce subtle clues to suggest the diagnosis; a new murmur of aortic regurgitation or an absent pulse can provoke the critical further evaluation.

The single best definitive diagnostic technique remains unclear. Given the critical importance of early diagnosis and treatment, however, the best diagnostic test may be the one most rapidly available. Contrast-enhanced dynamic CT, MRI, biplane aortography and cine-angiography, and multiplanar transesophageal echocardiography all have sufficient diagnostic accuracy, especially regarding involvement of the ascending aorta, to allow accurate therapeutic decisions. The precise choice of diagnostic modality is based on availability and individual expertise. Although aortography and CT have been the traditional gold standards, their false-negative rates are 5% to 10%. Transesophageal echocardiography with color-flow mapping, especially with multiplanar capability, may become the preferred diagnostic modality (Fig. 84.9). The ascending aorta is easily and clearly imaged, and a flap is readily detected. Advantages include a high level of diagnostic accuracy and the fact that the machine can be brought to the patient, allowing continuous monitoring and treatment and avoiding transport of a critically ill patient to a distant radiology suite. If ascending repair is required, the transducer can be left in place and used to ascertain retrograde flow in the transverse arch during bypass and to monitor cardiac segmental wall motion and aortic valve function after repair. Because of the constraints on medical instrumentation within a strong magnetic field, MRI is more appropriate for the evaluation and long-term management of patients with chronic dissection. Intravascular ultrasonography offers dramatic diagnostic capabilities, but it also requires patient transport to a radiology suite.

Hemodynamic stabilization, with particular attention paid to control of hypertension to levels just adequate for maintenance of cerebral, myocardial, and renal perfusion, is the immediate goal of medical therapy. Blunting the rate of pressure increase ($\Delta P/\Delta T$) is also advocated. Although the intravenous titration of sodium nitroprusside has been the traditional pharmacologic therapy of choice, intravenous esmolol more effectively reduces the aortic and left ventricular hyperdynamic state and may allow a stable interval during which a definitive diagnosis can be attained and appropriate therapy instituted.

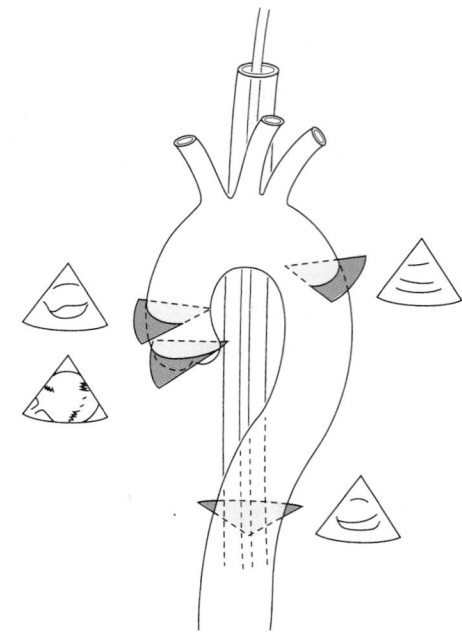

Figure 84.9. Transesophageal two-dimensional echocardiography with color-flow mapping accurately detects an intimal flap in the ascending, transverse, and descending aorta. (After Erbel RB, Borner N, Steller D, et al. Detection of aortic dissection by transesophageal echocardiography. *Br Heart J* 1987;58:45, with permission.)

After stabilization and diagnosis, appropriate treatment should be directed toward correcting the life-threatening aspects of the dissection. For dissections involving the ascending aorta (type A), this involves replacement of the supracoronary aorta to prevent rupture of the proximal root into the pericardium with subsequent tamponade, which is the cause of death in more than 90% of patients with ascending dissections. Correction of aortic regurgitation and replacement of the dissected aorta also limit morbidity. Ascending dissections in patients with Marfan's disease or annular aortic ectasia are treated by aortic root replacement with a valved conduit, as previously described.

For patients with acute type B dissections, the optimal management is more controversial. An aggressive surgical approach for younger, good-risk patients is advocated in an effort to prevent proximal extension of the dissection, resect the intimal tear, and direct flow into the distal true lumen. Surgical therapy instituted only after failure of medical management, usually because of limb, renal, or mesenteric ischemia, is associated with excessive morbidity and mortality. In an analysis of the combined Duke and Stanford databases, about 22% of patients with acute descending dissections presented with a compelling indication for surgical repair. The presence of major concomitant disease excluded an additional 37% from surgical consideration. Of the remaining 40% of patients, for whom either surgical or medical therapy was a viable option, multivariate analysis failed to detect any treatment-related benefit for either early or late survival. The fact that only advanced age was an independent predictor of poor outcome after a surgical repair supports a bias toward surgical repair in young, healthy patients.

Operative Management

The ascending aorta is approached through a median sternotomy, and cardiopulmonary bypass is achieved by bicaval atrial cannulation and femoral arterial cannulation into the true arterial lumen. Cardiopulmonary bypass with full heparinization is established, and the left ventricle is vented. The latter is especially important in cases with significant aortic regurgitation. Rapid cooling to 15°C is commenced, with the use of atraumatic clamping of the midportion of the ascending aorta if left ventricular distention occurs after the onset of fibrillation (Fig. 84.10). Myocardial protection is achieved with retrograde coronary sinus perfusion and a hypothermia blanket. After a

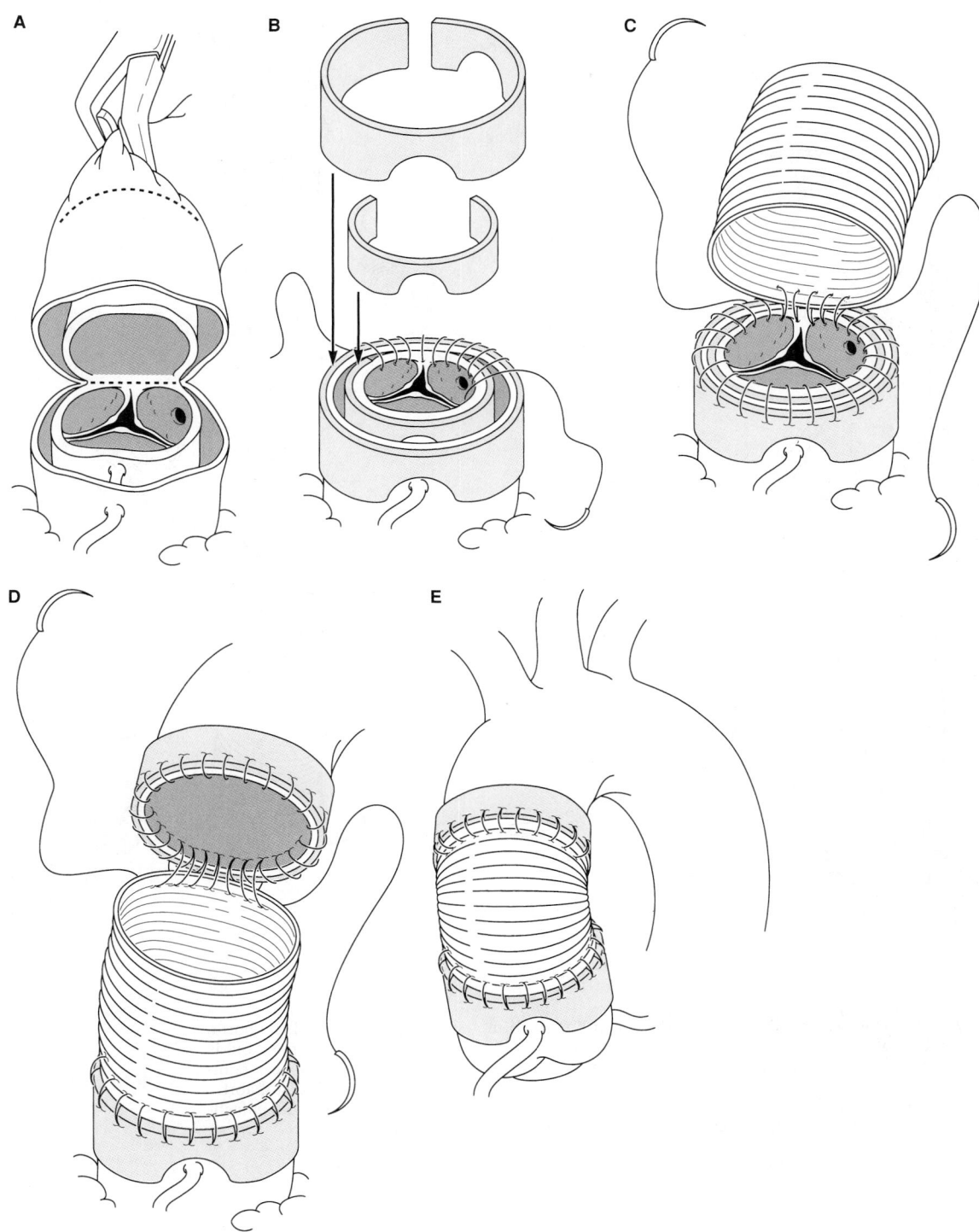

Figure 84.10. *(A)* Acute aortic dissection involving the ascending aorta. The false lumen, septum, and involvement of the right coronary are apparent. *(B)* A strip of Teflon felt is carefully tailored to obliterate the false lumen between the intima and adventitia that extends proximally to the aortic annulus. A second layer of felt can be used as an adventitial support if the vessel is particularly fragile. *(C)* With the native aortic valve preserved, the proximal anastomosis is constructed end to end with full-thickness bites. *(D)* The distal false lumen is similarly obliterated, and a full-thickness anastomosis is constructed end to end. *(E)* Completed repair after ascending aortic dissection.

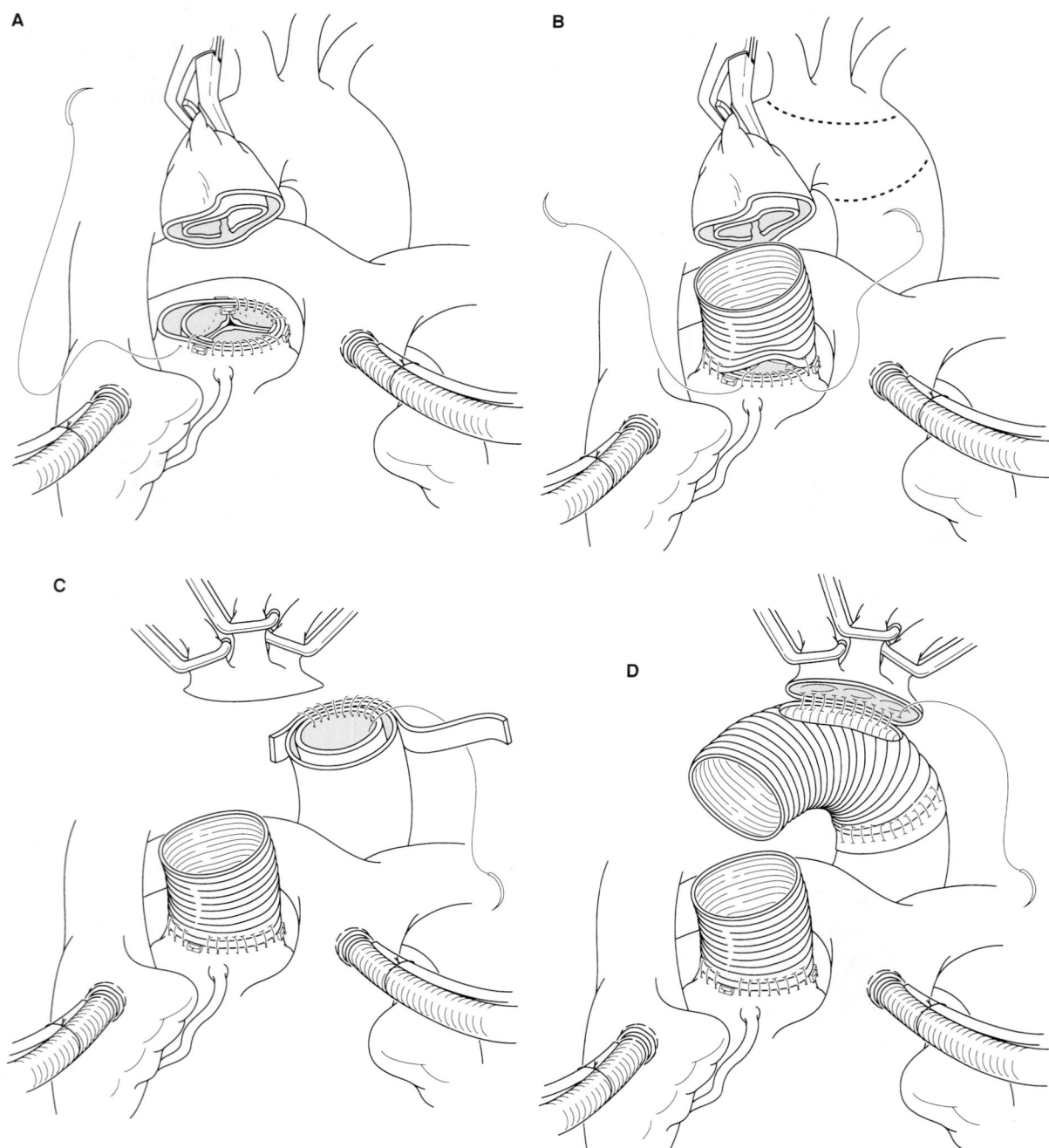

Figure 84.11. *(A)* Repair of dissection of the ascending portion and transverse arch of the aorta. Administration of cardioplegia and repair of the ascending dissection, with aortic resuspension, is completed with the cross-clamp in place. *(B)* Ascending graft is sutured in place while core cooling continues. *(C)* During a period of profound hypothermic circulatory arrest (18°C), distal aortic repair is accomplished, and a button of aorta containing the origin of the cerebral vessels is fashioned. *(D)* Distal graft anastomosis and aortic button are completed. *(continues)*

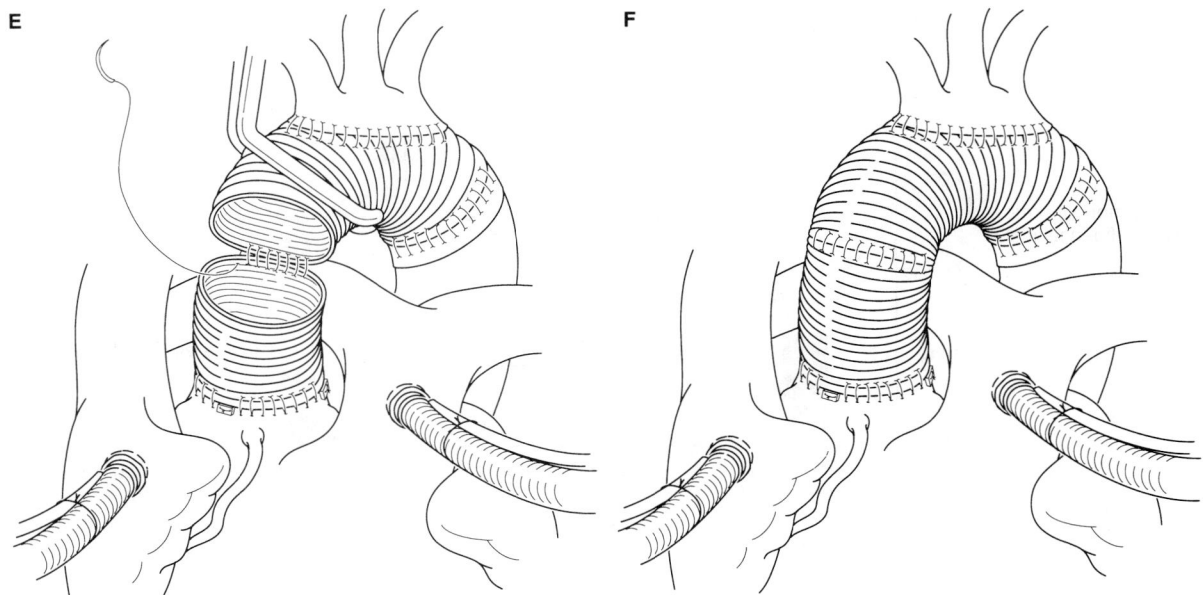

Figure 84.11. *(Continued)* *(E)* Cross-clamp is placed proximally, rewarming is instituted, and proximal and distal grafts are joined. *(F)* Completed repair before decannulation. (After Griepp RB, Stinson EB, Hollingsworth, JF, et al. Prosthetic replacement of the aortic arch. *J Thorac Cardiovasc Surg* 1975; 70:1051, with permission.)

core and tympanic membrane temperature of 15°C is attained, circulatory arrest is instituted, the cross-clamp removed, and the distal aorta assessed regarding the extent of dissection and presence of arch tear to determine the site of distal anastomosis. The distal aorta is then fashioned so as to allow a full-thickness end-to-end anastomosis buttressed by Teflon felt strips. Usually, this requires only 20 to 25 minutes of circulatory arrest time, after which circulatory support and rewarming can commence. Retrograde cerebral perfusion is used to flush air and particulate debris from the brachiocephalic vessels and to provide some additional cerebral protection. The distal graft is then clamped just proximal to the anastomosis, and the arterial perfusion is repositioned into the distal graft to allow antegrade perfusion. The proximal anastomosis and any aortic valve repairs are then accomplished during this subsequent period of systemic rewarming. Absolute surgical hemostasis is mandatory to avoid a cascading coagulopathy or the late development of false aneurysms.

Surgical repair of descending dissections is accomplished through a left posterolateral thoracotomy with an interposition graft of woven Dacron. Access for cardiopulmonary bypass is established through cannulation of the femoral artery and the left atrial appendage, and proximal control of the aorta is obtained just distal to the left carotid artery. Only a short segment of aorta, the most severely affected, is resected, unless a known single intimal tear is present more distally. After intimal and adventitial continuity has been reestablished with an interposed medial layer of Teflon felt, the interposition graft is sewn carefully to full-thickness cuffs, and the patient is immediately weaned from cardiopulmonary bypass.

Patients with tears of the transverse arch represent a small (5%) but perplexing proportion of acute dissections. Medical management alone is associated with substantial mortality. Concomitant surgical repair with either an ascending or descending dissection can double the operative mortality. Nevertheless, given the adverse affect of the unresected arch tear on both short- and long-term survival,

arch replacement under profound hypothermic circulatory rest may be justified in young, otherwise healthy patients who would sustain the greatest long-term benefit (Fig. 84.11).

Results of Surgical Therapy

Despite continued improvements in surgical technique, operative mortality remains high for this complex problem (9). In the most recent Stanford analysis (Fig. 84.12), the operative risk was 7% ± 5% for type A dissections, with preoperative renal failure, tamponade, and renal or visceral ischemia heralding a poor outcome. For patients with acute type B dissections, older age, aortic rupture, and renal or visceral ischemia were independent predictors of perioperative death.

The 5-year actuarial survival rate for discharged patients was relatively good, 78% ± 6% for type A dissections. For type B dissections, the actuarial 5-year survival rate for discharged patients was 80% ± 12%, and significantly, the survival rate at 10 years was no different from that of an age- and sex-matched population.

Given the frequent complications of aneurysmal disease elsewhere in the thoracic and abdominal aorta, long-term follow-up and aggressive medical therapy are critical for patients after acute dissections. Operative procedures remain palliative at best, designed only to curtail lethal complications. CT or MRI should be performed on a regular basis indefinitely to detect progressive aneurysmal dilation and allow timely elective repair. In a 20-year follow-up, aortic rupture accounted for nearly one third of late deaths, a situation that clearly can be improved. Progressive dilation of the false lumen of chronic aortic dissections (Fig. 84.13) should be managed like other aneurysmal diseases of the thoracic aorta.

The clinical presentation of penetrating atherosclerotic ulcers of the thoracic aorta can closely mimic that of acute aortic dissection or rupturing aneurysm of the thoracic aorta (10). Evaluation of these patients may demonstrate only a localized area of subintimal hemorrhage along the

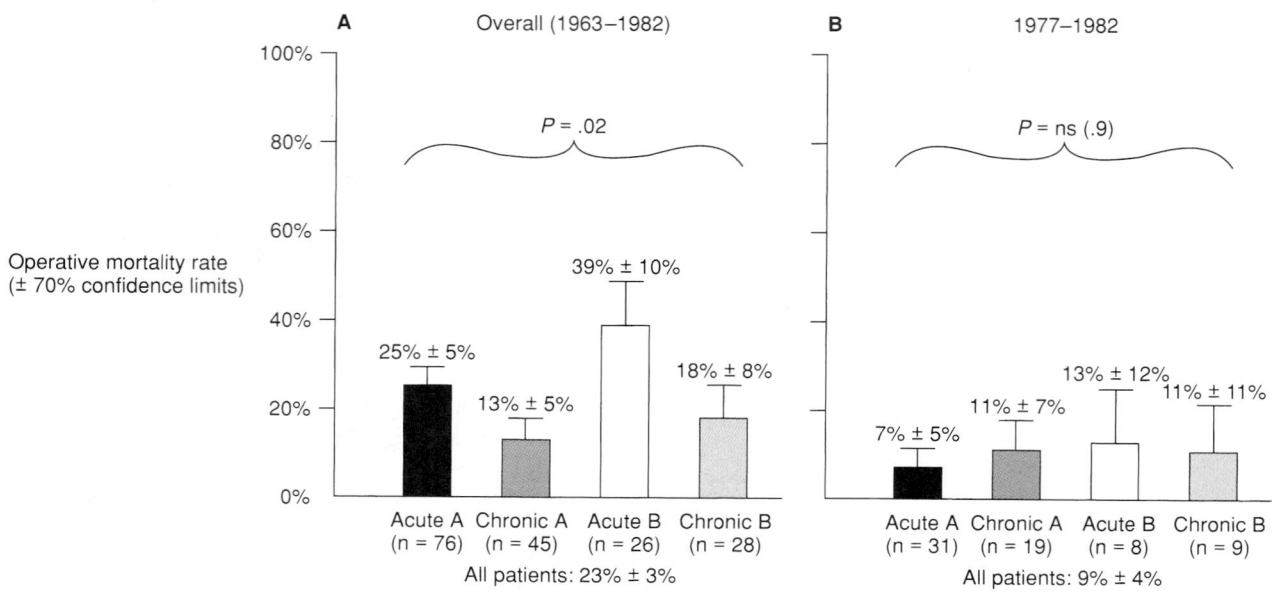

Figure 84.12. *(A)* Operative mortality rates for aortic dissection between 1963 and 1982. *(B)* The operative mortality rate was reduced by almost 50% in the more recent interval between 1977 and 1982. (After Frist WH, Miller DC. Ascending aortic aneurysms and dissections. *J Cardiac Surg* 1986;1:50, with permission.)

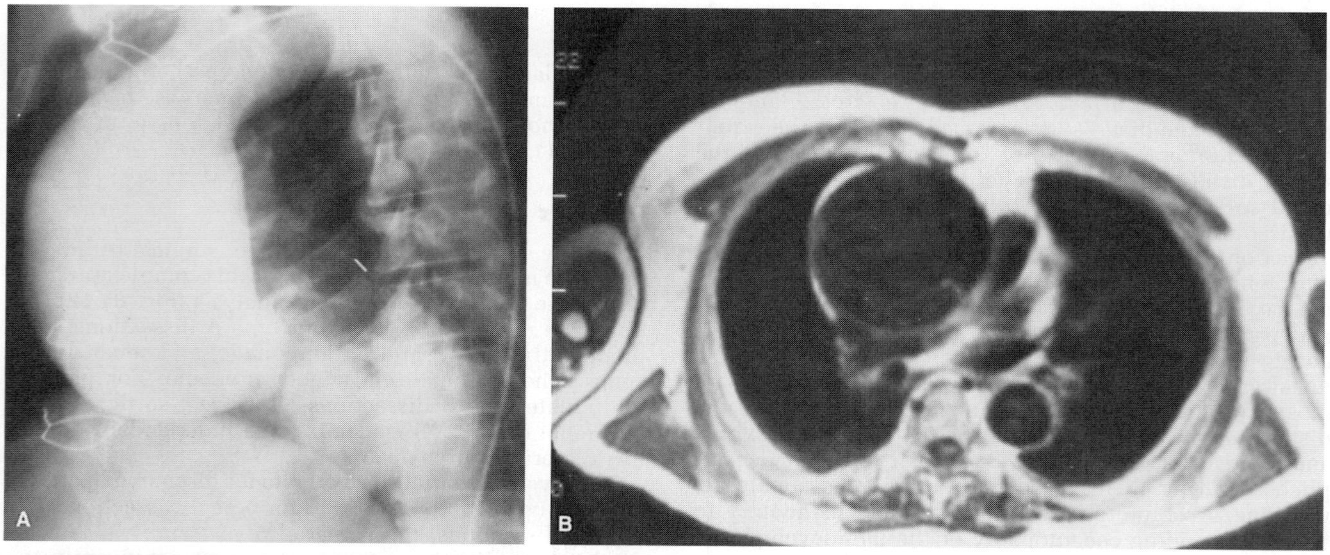

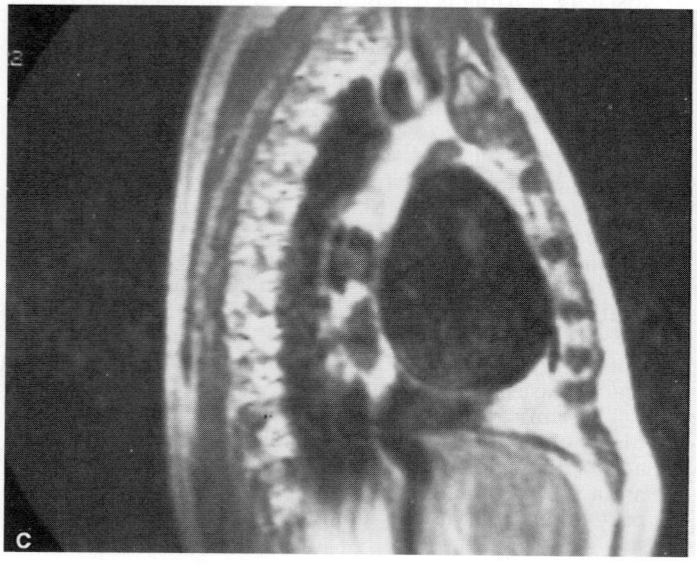

Figure 84.13. *(A)* Progressive aneurysmal dilation of a chronic aortic dissection that developed soon after coronary artery bypass grafting 7 years earlier. *(B,C)* Magnetic resonance imaging demonstrates a huge aneurysm of the ascending aorta eroding into the posterior table of the sternum, potentially complicating reoperation.

thoracic aorta, with an enhancing subadventitial layer on MRI. Although the long-term sequelae of this entity remain unknown, we have been impressed with the rapid progression to aneurysmal dilation in the short term and therefore recommend careful aggressive follow-up and surgical repair for any patient with continued pain or evidence of enlargement.

MISCELLANEOUS CONDITIONS

Trauma is perhaps the most common cause of nondegenerative disease affecting the thoracic aorta. Whether the apparent increase in incidence of thoracic aortic injuries represents a real increase in injuries secondary to high-speed vehicular trauma or an increase in diagnoses incidental to the increased use of CT in cases of blunt trauma is unknown. Regardless, during sudden deceleration, the untethered aortic arch and descending aorta can flex anteriorly so that the aorta is stretched against the ligamentum, with a resultant partial or complete circumferential intimal disruption. For the 10% to 20% of patients who survive this acute event, the rupture is partially contained by the aortic adventitia and pleurae, but the risk for subsequent hemorrhage is ongoing; thus, early diagnosis is essential.

The diagnosis should be suspected in any patient with a history of sudden deceleration and a severe chest injury or other evidence of thoracic trauma, such as multiple posterior rib fractures, thoracic spine fractures, or fracture of the scapula. Remarkably, aortic transection can be present in patients with a history of sudden deceleration who have no other signs of chest trauma. Given the rapidly lethal nature of the undiagnosed injury, suggestive clinical or radiographic findings should prompt further investigation. The subsequent diagnostic test remains problematic. Many imaging techniques, including biplane aortography or cine-angiography, dynamic contrast-enhanced CT, MRI, and intravascular ultrasonography, have demonstrated adequate sensitivity in experienced hands. These techniques, however, all require transfer from the emergency department, with loss of monitoring capabilities and the ongoing potential for hemodynamic instability or catastrophic hemorrhage. OmniPlane transesophageal echocardiography may allow adequate visualization of the distal transverse arch. This technique is advantageous because the equipment is transportable to the emergency department and because rapid data acquisition is possible.

After the initial evaluation and stabilization, the first priority is recognition and management of all life-threatening injuries, including intracranial or intraabdominal trauma. In the patient with multiple trauma, mature judgment regarding priorities for diagnostic studies and the sequence of therapeutic interventions is required. If the patient is stable and the initial evaluation indicates the necessity for abdominal or cranial CT, the patient should be expediently transported to the radiography suite, where rapid-sequence, contrast-enhanced CT of the thorax, abdomen, or brain can be performed. If no other injuries are suspected, efforts focus on the aortic injury, and the choice of aortography or cross-sectional CT can be made on the basis of local expertise and ready availability.

Operative exposure is gained through a left posterolateral thoracotomy, and control of the proximal aorta is obtained. This can be proximal to the left subclavian artery in patients with minimal mediastinal hematoma, or access can be gained more proximally by opening the pericardium if a large mediastinal hematoma is encountered. After satisfactory proximal and distal control, repair is accomplished either by direct suture anastomosis or with an interposition graft. Significant controversy continues regarding the optimal method for maintaining distal perfu-

sion. The clamp-and-sew technique has been advocated, which avoids the complications of heparinization and complex bypass procedures. Others have recommended a heparin-bonded shunt, which avoids systemic heparinization but results in inconstant shunt flows. Femorofemoral cardiopulmonary bypass offers excellent organ perfusion and control of proximal hypertension but requires full heparinization, which can be a significant hazard for patients with multiple trauma, especially those with intracranial involvement. Perhaps most attractive is a bypass from the left atrium to the femoral artery with use of a centrifugal pump and minimal heparinization; bypass without heparin is becoming a reality with the advent of heparin-bonded bypass circuits.

No technique confers complete protection from the dreaded complication of postoperative paraplegia. In general, if repair can be accomplished in under 30 minutes, the clamp-and-sew technique is appropriate. However, a trend has been noted toward an increased incidence of spinal cord injury with cross-clamp times in excess of 30 minutes (Fig. 84.14). A 1988 review of a 15-year experience emphasized the priority of repair and observed that increasing age is the only significant adverse factor for postoperative survival. Typically, if the patient reaches the operating room in stable condition, a successful procedure can be performed in most cases. Of patients who reach the hospital alive, however, 30% to 50% die before definitive therapy, which emphasizes the need for a rapid and complete evaluation.

Mycotic aneurysms, although unusual, can result from endocarditis, bacteremic seeding of existing aneurysms, contiguous pleural and mediastinal infections, or contaminated intravenous injections. In general, the essential nature of the brachiocephalic and visceral vessels precludes resection and extraanatomic bypass. Intensive preoperative antibiotic therapy, combined with extensive surgical débridement, in situ grafting, and long-term antibiotic therapy, especially for distal thoracic aneurysms and thoracoabdominal aneurysms infected with *Salmonella* organisms, may allow long-term survival. For infections arising in the ascending aorta or ascending grafts contaminated by mediastinitis, débridement, graft replacement, and a vascularized omental wrap may confer more protection than transposed muscle flaps alone (11). Early diagnosis, isolation of the infective organism, institution of appropriate antibiotic therapy, and débridement and repair of the infection before the aneurysm ruptures are essential to any realistic hope for success.

Aneurysms of the ductus diverticulum have been reported in a small number of patients, usually presenting as

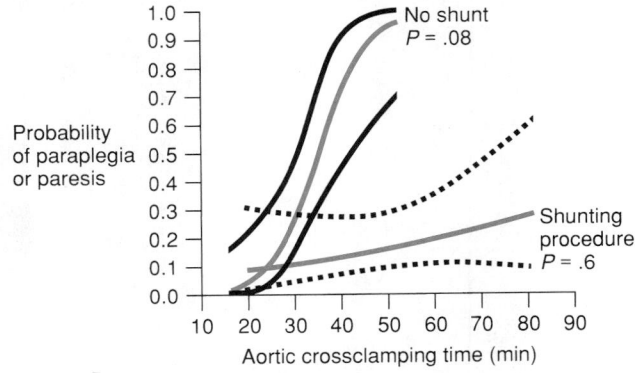

Figure 84.14. The probability of spinal cord dysfunction appears to be directly related to aortic cross-clamp time. (After Katz NM, Blackstone EH, Kirklin JW, et al. Incremental risk factors for spinal cord injury following operation for acute traumatic aortic transection. *J Thorac Cardiovasc Surg* 1981;81:669, with permission.)

an asymptomatic mass in the aortopulmonary window on an incidental chest radiograph. Hoarseness has been a presenting complaint in a significant number of patients, secondary to stretching of the recurrent laryngeal nerve. Erosion into the esophagus or bronchus can provoke life-threatening hemorrhage.

Contrast-enhanced CT or MRI confirms the diagnosis in most patients and allows planning of the operative approach. Aortography adds little additional information, especially if the aneurysm lumen is thrombosed. Because of the relatively narrow aneurysm neck, repair frequently can be accomplished by Dacron patch closure on cardiopulmonary bypass. Although repair can be accomplished through a median sternotomy, superior exposure can be attained through a left lateral thoracotomy if a concomitant cardiac procedure is not needed. Generalized atherosclerosis and obstructive pulmonary disease may limit long-term survival in these patients.

Finally, the recent introduction of minimally invasive endovascular techniques holds great promise for the management of descending thoracic aneurysms and dissections (12). Self-expanding stents covered with nonporous graft material (Fig. 84.15) have been introduced through femoral cutdowns, advanced and positioned under fluoroscopic guidance, and then deployed within the aortic lumen to exclude the aneurysm sac from the circulation. Success depends on an adequate proximal and distal neck of at least 2 cm to allow for secure fixation.

Although this technology remains investigational, experience with more than 200 patients does allow some perspectives (13). Distal access must accommodate a 24F (outer diameter) sheath and dilator to pass over a superstiff guidewire. The landing zones can extend proximally to within 2 cm of the left common carotid artery if the left subclavian artery has been previously transposed, and distally to within 2 cm of the celiac axis. Aortic segments free of aneurysm and devoid of mural thrombus are essential for adequate fixation. Important morbidity can occur during the procedure, including cerebral atheroembolism resulting from device manipulation within a diseased aortic arch segment. More peripheral atheroembolism has not been a significant feature.

Endoleaks, resulting from failure to achieve a hemostatic seal at either attachment site, remain the "Achilles heel" of this technology; they allow the aneurysm sac to remain pressurized, with an ongoing risk for rupture. Whether supplemental endovascular techniques, such as coiling or thrombin injection, can reduce such risk remains unknown. Other complications have included renal insufficiency, perhaps a result of contrast nephrotoxicity exacerbated by unrecognized atheroembolism, worsened respiratory failure, and myocardial infarction. Interestingly, paraplegia occurred in only three patients, two of whom underwent simultaneous abdominal aneurysm repair and one of whom had previously undergone abdominal aneurysm repair. In no patient without abdominal aneurysm repair was paraplegia noted, regardless of intentional coverage of all intercostal arteries between T-7 and T-12. Late endoleaks were noted at proximal implantation sites in the distal arch, where the descending thoracic aorta angles sharply caudally and distally as it follows a serpentine course into the diaphragmatic crura. Many of these difficulties may be surmounted by the newer, more flexible, second-generation endografts. Longer-term follow-up will be necessary before their true efficacy can be established. However, for the elderly, high-risk patient (Fig. 84.16), total aneurysm exclusion and rapid recovery can be very impressive.

Finally, endograft technologies may have significant applications in the management of patients with aortic dissections. Although the medical management of acute type B dissections is frequently successful (14), the management of patients presenting with visceral ischemia is more problematic. Williams et al. (15) have categorized these arterial malperfusion syndromes as secondary to dynamic or static mechanisms. Indeed, true-lumen collapse (Fig. 84.17) has proved recalcitrant to many reperfusion strategies, and late aneurysmal dilation of the large false lumen has complicated the long-term management of these patients. Recent experience by Dake et al. (16) and Nienaber et al. (17) has demonstrated healing of the proximal dissection in four patents after coverage of the primary intimal tear in the proximal descending thoracic aorta. Similarly, malperfusion syndromes secondary to dynamic obstruction (n = 22) were reversed in all patients (Fig. 84.18), and false-lumen

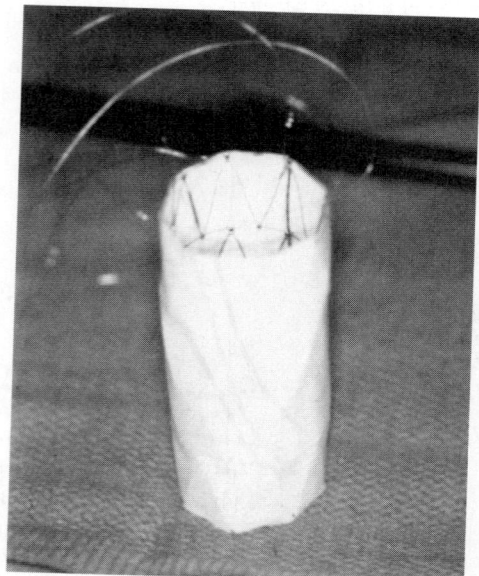

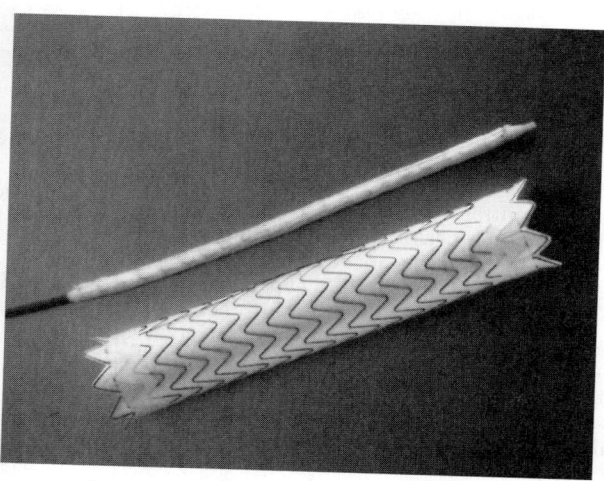

A

B

Figure 84.15. (A) First-generation endograft constructed from self-expanding "Z" stents wired together and covered by a woven Dacron graft. (B) Second-generation graft, in which a temperature-sensitive Nitinol exoskeleton supports a Gortex thin-walled graft.

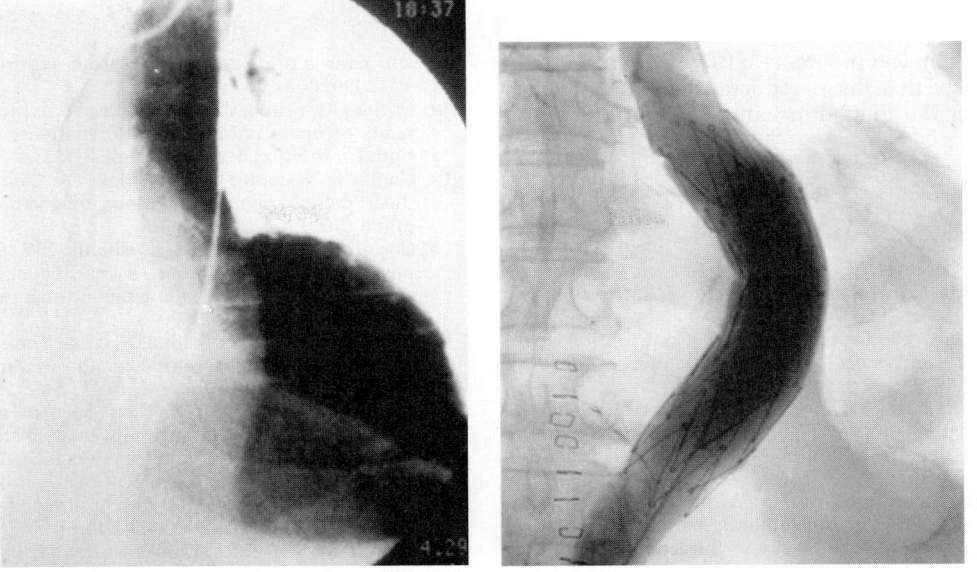

Figure 84.16. *(A)* Preoperative angiogram showing a large (10-cm) aneurysm of the descending thoracic aorta. *(B)* Complete exclusion of aneurysm sac filling by a transfemorally placed endograft.

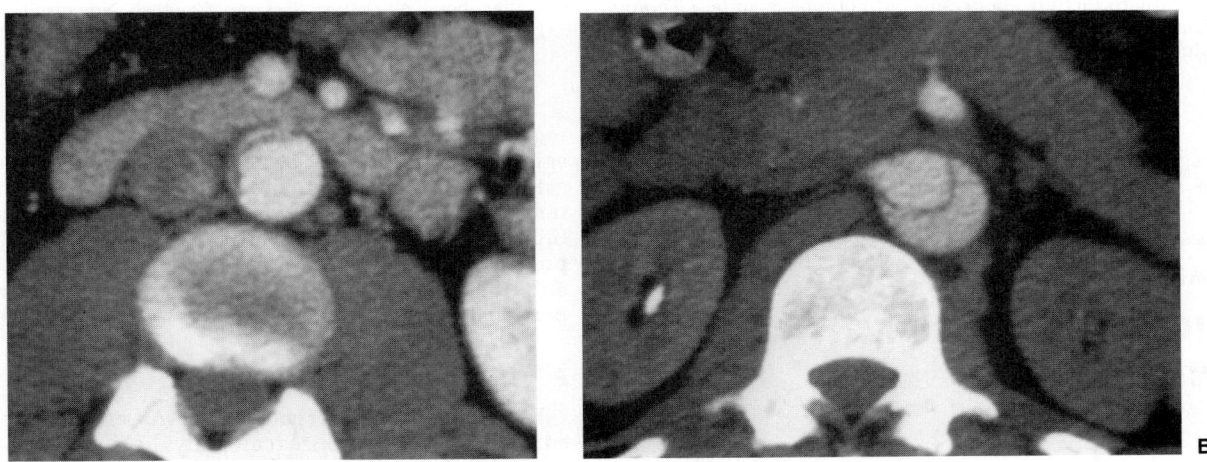

Figure 84.17. *(A)* Typical true-lumen collapse in an acute type B dissection, with resultant malperfusion of the right renal and iliac arteries. *(B)* Endograft coverage of the primary intimal tear in the proximal descending thoracic aorta markedly improves flow in the true lumen and restores flow to the renal and iliac arteries.

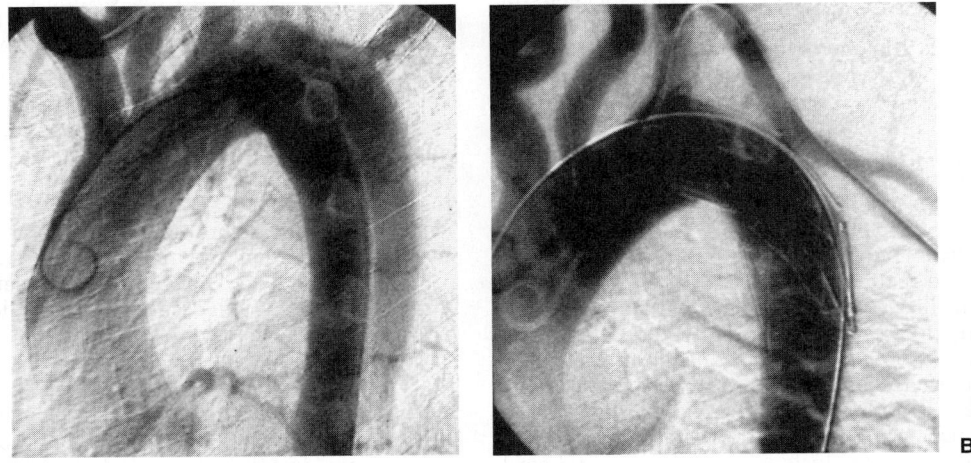

Figure 84.18. *(A)* Dual-lumen aorta after acute type B aortic dissection. *(B)* Magnetic resonance angiograms demonstrating resolution of dual-lumen aorta after endograft coverage of primary intimal tear.

thrombosis was achieved in 79% (15/19) of patients. It is an exciting possibility that these endograft technologies may significantly alter the long-term natural history of type B dissections.

REFERENCES

1. DeBakey ME, Cooley DA. Successful resection of aneurysm of thoracic aorta and replacement by graft. *JAMA* 1953;152:673.
2. Szilagyi DE, Smith RF, DeRusso FJ, et al. Contribution of abdominal aortic aneurysmectomy to prolongation of life. *Ann Surg* 1966;164:678.
3. Pressler V, McNamara JJ. Thoracic aortic aneurysm. *J Thorac Cardiovasc Surg* 1980;79:486.
4. Clouse WD, Hallett JW, Schaff HV, et al. Improved prognosis of thoracic aortic aneurysms. *JAMA* 1998;280:1926–1929.
5. McDonald ML, Smedira NG, Lytle BW, et al. Aortic rupture after aortic valve surgery in women. Abstract presented at AATS, (American Assoc. of Thoracic Surgeons) April 1999, New Orleans.
6. Cartier R, Orszulak TA, Pairolero PC, et al. Circulatory support during cross-clamping of the descending thoracic aorta. *J Thorac Cardiovasc Surg* 1990;99:1038.
7. Moreno-Cabral CE, Miller DC, Mitchell RS, et al. Degenerative and atherosclerotic aneurysms of the thoracic aorta. *J Thorac Cardiovasc Surg* 1984;88:1020.
8. Murdoch JL, Walker BA, Halpern BL, et al. Life expectancy and causes of death in the Marfan syndrome. *N Engl J Med* 1972;286:804.
9. Miller DC, Mitchell RS, Oyer PE, et al. Independent determinants of operative mortality for patients with aortic dissection. *Circulation* 1984;70[Suppl I]:153.
10. Cooke JP, Kazmier FJ, Orszulak TA. The penetrating aortic ulcer: pathologic manifestations, diagnosis, and management. *Mayo Clin Proc* 1988;63:718.
11. Coselli JS, Crawford ES, Williams TW, et al. Treatment of postoperative infection of ascending aorta and transverse arch, including use of viable omentum and muscle flaps. *Ann Thorac Surg* 1990;50:868.
12. Dake MD, Miller DC, Semba CR, et al. Transluminal placement of endovascular stent grafts for the treatment of descending thoracic aortic dissections. *N Engl J Med* 1997;336:1320.
13. Mitchell RS, Miller DC, Dake MD, et al. Thoracic aortic aneurysm repair with an endovascular stent graft: the "first generation." *Ann Thorac Surg* 1999;67:1971–1974.
14. Glower DID, Fann JI, Speier RH, et al. Comparison of medical and surgical therapy for uncomplicated descending aortic dissection. *Circulation* 1990;82[Suppl IV]:IV-39–IV-46.
15. Williams DM, Lee DY, Hamilton BH, et al. The dissected aorta: part III. Anatomy and radiologic diagnosis of branch vessel compromise. *Radiology* 1997;203:37–44.
16. Dake MD, Kato FN, Mitchell RS, et al. Endovascular stent graft placement for the treatment of acute aortic dissection. *N Engl J Med* 1999;340:1546–1552.
17. Nienaber CA, Fattori R, Lund G, et al. Nonsurgical reconstruction of thoracic aortic dissection by stent graft placement. *N Engl J Med* 1999;340:1539–1545.

SURGERY: SCIENTIFIC PRINCIPLES AND PRACTICE, Third Edition, edited by Lazar J. Greenfield, Michael W. Mulholland, Keith T. Oldham, Gerald B. Zelenock, and Keith D. Lillemoe. Lippincott Williams & Wilkins Publishers, Philadelphia, © 2001.

CHAPTER 85

THORACOABDOMINAL ANEURYSMS

C. W. ACHER AND M. M. WYNN

The goal of this chapter is to illustrate a comprehensive approach to the diagnosis and treatment of thoracoabdominal aneurysms, and to provide the reader with insight regarding how patients should be selected for treatment and with some understanding of why treatment succeeds or fails.

Aortic aneurysms that involve the descending thoracic and abdominal aorta are designated as *thoracoabdominal aortic aneurysms* (TAAAs). As with other aortic aneurysms, the primary risk to the patient is rupture and death as the aneurysm enlarges. Since 1956, when the feasibility of repairing these complex aneurysms was first reported, they have continued to pose a major challenge to surgeons who treat aortic disease (1). The repair of a TAAA is difficult for several reasons. The visceral and renal vessels are involved and require reattachment in most cases. Also, the vessels are often diseased, so that endarterectomy or bypass is necessary to reestablish normal blood flow. The aortic occlusion required for repair subjects the patient's heart, lungs, liver, intestines, and kidneys to extreme physiologic stress, which can lead to cardiac, pulmonary, renal, and hepatic failure in addition to severe coagulopathies and metabolic acidosis. Stroke of the spinal cord resulting from the interruption of blood flow from the thoracic and upper abdominal aorta can result in permanent paralysis of the lower extremities. The challenge of managing all these complex issues successfully requires dedicated anesthesiologists and surgeons with specialized training and experience who work as a team to obtain optimal results. However, even with a specialized team approach, significant morbidity and mortality of 10% to 50%, depending on patient mix (acute and elective proportions), are reported.

EPIDEMIOLOGY

Fortunately for our species, TAAAs are relatively uncommon. The incidence can only be inferred because screening data from the general population are lacking. Infrarenal abdominal aortic aneurysms occur in approximately 5% of the male population over 60 years of age, but only about 1% have aneurysms larger than 4 cm in diameter. A male-to-female ratio of 4:1 or 5:1 has been noted (2). Approximately 40,000 to 50,000 infrarenal aneurysms are repaired annually in the United States, with 20% of these ruptured at the time of repair (3). Fewer than 1,000 TAAAs are repaired yearly in the United States; however, they are less likely to be treated surgically because of perceived operative risks. Extrapolation from these data would place the incidence at approximately 0.02% of the adult population, which is about 5% of the incidence reported for thoracic aortic aneurysms, including dissections of the ascending and descending aorta (4). Unlike the sex ratio for infrarenal aortic aneurysms, which predominate in elderly men, the male-to-female ratio for TAAAs is 1.5:1. A bimodal age distribution represents occurrence in younger patients with a variety of vasculopathies.

ETIOLOGY

The development of aortic aneurysms in humans is multifactorial, depending on complex interactions that lead to a spectrum of clinical presentations defined by age of onset and extent of aortic involvement. However, evidence is growing that the root cause of a predisposition to extensive aneurysm development and aortic dissection is a defect of the fibrillin gene located on chromosome 15 (5–7). Although this defect has been clearly defined in such disorders as Marfan syndrome, genetic polymorphism at these or other sites involved in the production of matrix structure proteins may lay the foundation for the many phenotypes that are seen clinically. Genetic polymorphism may also account for the variable effects of predisposing environmental factors such as smoking, physiologic factors such as hypertension and chronic obstructive pulmonary disease, and autoimmune factors in the pathogenesis of aortic aneurysms (8–10).

PATHOPHYSIOLOGY, NATURAL HISTORY, AND SYMPTOMS

Structurally, a gradation of abnormalities is seen in the wall of the aorta from younger (marfanoid) to older patients (11,12). Younger patients generally have soft, nonatherosclerotic aortic walls characterized by relatively few or fragmented elastin layers, cystic medial necrosis, and abnormal collagen, which lead to weakened aortic walls that expand under normal physiologic conditions. Older patients (> 60 years) tend to have aortic walls that are stiff with calcified plaque; ulceration, intimal and medial destruction, and hyperplasia and fibrosis associated with the arterial degenerative plaques commonly seen in the advanced atherosclerosis of aging are typical features. These age-related differences are also seen in patients with aortic dissection leading to the development of TAAA. In our experience of more than 300 patients, 76% had degenerative (atherosclerotic) disease, 18% had nonspecific medial degeneration with or without dissection, and 2.5% had mycotic disease. Disease processes such as Marfan syndrome, lupus erythematosis, and Takayasu's arteritis were found in the remaining 3% (Fig. 85.1).

The result of a weakened aortic wall is gradual expansion from a vessel of normal diameter through ectasia to aneurysmal size, which is arbitrarily defined as a diameter more than 1.5 times normal. It is helpful to think of normal as a range rather than a fixed number. Large-scale screening of aortic size (diameter) has been performed only for the infrarenal aorta, the mean diameter of which is 1.5 cm; 95% are less than 2.5 cm in diameter (13). However, the normal range for the thoracoabdominal aorta can be inferred from these data, with the understanding that the more proximal aorta is normally slightly larger (by as much as 0.5 to 0.75 cm in the ascending aorta) than the infrarenal aorta. From a practical standpoint, this normal range makes the absolute diameter hard to use except at larger diameters (> 3 cm), so comparing the aneurysmal aorta with a more proximal "normal" aortic segment is a reasonable compromise in definition.

The important concept is that as the aorta enlarges, the wall tension increases according to Laplace's law and eventually exceeds the aortic wall tensile strength; aortic rupture is the result. The growth rate of TAAAs is comparable with that of infrarenal aneurysms. Enlargement from 4 cm to 6 cm occurs at an average rate of about 0.4 cm/y, with larger aneurysms expanding more rapidly and smaller aneurysms expanding less rapidly (14,15). It is clear that the natural history of aortic aneurysms is to increase in diameter and at some point rupture if the patient does not die first of other causes (16). Death from other causes is more likely to occur in elderly patients (approximately 40% of elderly patients with aneurysms die of other cardiovascular events or malignancies before their aneurysm ruptures), whereas in younger patients, aortic disease is the greatest risk for mortality.

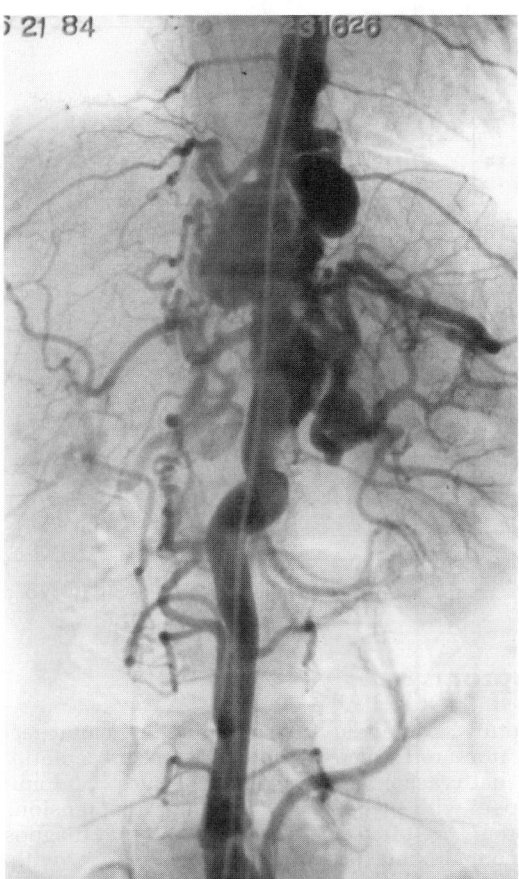

Figure 85.1. A patient with Takayasu's arteritis has a series of complex aneurysms and arterial occlusions requiring a Crawford type 4 replacement with visceral and renal reconstruction.

The diameter at which rupture will occur cannot be predicted for any individual patient because of a myriad of other relevant factors, such as blood pressure, aortic diameter, and wall thickness. However, if we examine the data critically, adverse events for fusiform aneurysms are uncommon at diameters of less than 5 cm and significantly more frequent at diameters of more than 6 cm. So-called saccular aneurysms are less predictable. In our experience with 135 ruptured aneurysms in which the diameter was known at the time of rupture, the mean size was 8 cm for infrarenal aortic aneurysms and 8.2 cm for TAAAs. Event frequency increased as diameter increased (Fig. 85.2).

Classification

The Crawford classification of TAAAs is the most widely accepted and is based on the extent of aortic involvement or replacement (Fig. 85.3). The late E. Stanley Crawford was one of the pivotal figures in the treatment of TAAAs from the mid-1970s to his death in 1993. He dominated the field with his vast experience, his ability to reduce morbidity in comparison with other centers treating this disease, and his classification of the risk for paraplegia associated with repair. Crawford type 2 aneurysms have twice the risk for paraplegia as type 1 aneurysms and 10 times the risk as type 4 aneurysms. For any group of patients, the risk for paralysis doubles with rupture or dissection (17,18).

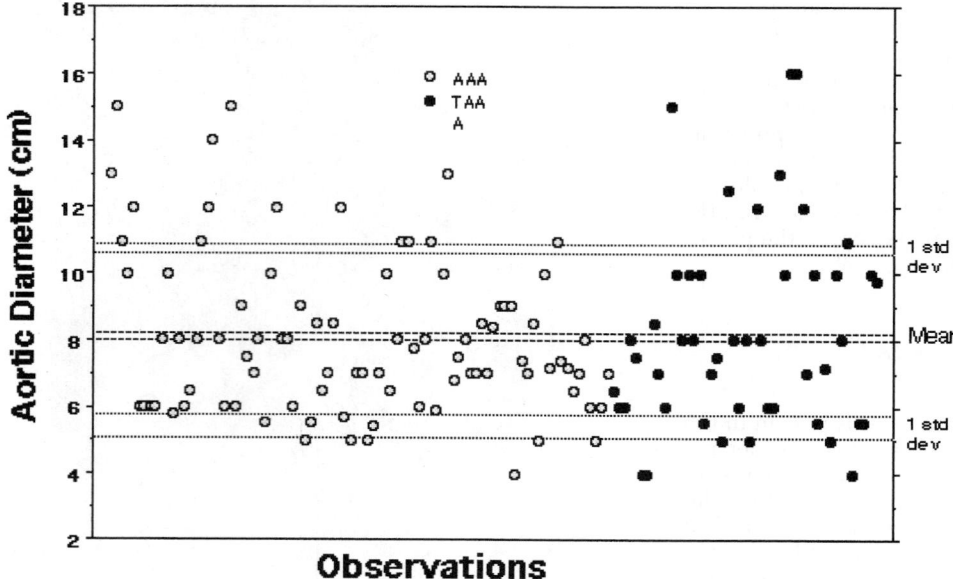

Figure 85.2. A scatter plot of aortic diameters in 135 patients with acute (rupture, contained rupture, or dissection) aortic aneurysms. Eighty-one had infrarenal aneurysms and 54 had thoracoabdominal aneurysms. The mean size and relative distribution of sizes at the time of rupture are very similar. Of the 135 patients, only four had aneurysms less than 5 cm in diameter, and three of these were mycotic. Of the acute events, 12% occurred in 5 to 6-cm aneurysms, and 85% of the ruptures occurred in aneurysms larger than 6 cm.

Symptoms

Rupture, contained rupture, plaque hemorrhage, and dissection are the most common acute presentations and are usually accompanied by severe chest, abdominal, or back pain with severe hypertension or hypotension. These symptoms are often misinterpreted, so that diagnosis and treatment are delayed in many patients. Fever with sepsis from aortic infections may also cause saccular aneurysms; thoracoabdominal aortic replacement is required because of extensive endovascular infection with aortic wall destruction. Patients with nonacute disease may present with a variety of symptoms, and many patients have no symptoms.

As a TAAA increases in diameter, adjacent structures may be compressed or stretched. Stretching of the recurrent laryngeal nerve leads to hoarseness, which may be acute in onset if expansion is rapid. Mechanical compres-

sion of the trachea or bronchus may cause respiratory distress, bronchoconstriction, or obstructive pneumonia (Fig. 85.4). Inflammatory changes in the aortic wall (inflammatory aneurysm) or shear size can lead to anorexia with significant weight loss and lassitude or uremia from ureteral obstruction. Esophageal compression by a large, pulsatile aneurysm may present as dysphagia with weight loss and simulate upper gastrointestinal pathology. Nonspecific back, chest, or abdominal pain may be the only symptom of an expanding TAAA and can easily be overlooked or attributed to other causes. Uncommonly, a TAAA may erode into a visceral structure, such as the esophagus or small intestine, and present as gastrointestinal bleeding. The patient usually dies, either of exsanguinating hemorrhage (often preceded by a sentinel, less severe hemorrhage) or of the consequences of placement of a synthetic graft in an infected field in an attempt at repair. However, 60% of elective patients have no symptoms before diagnosis.

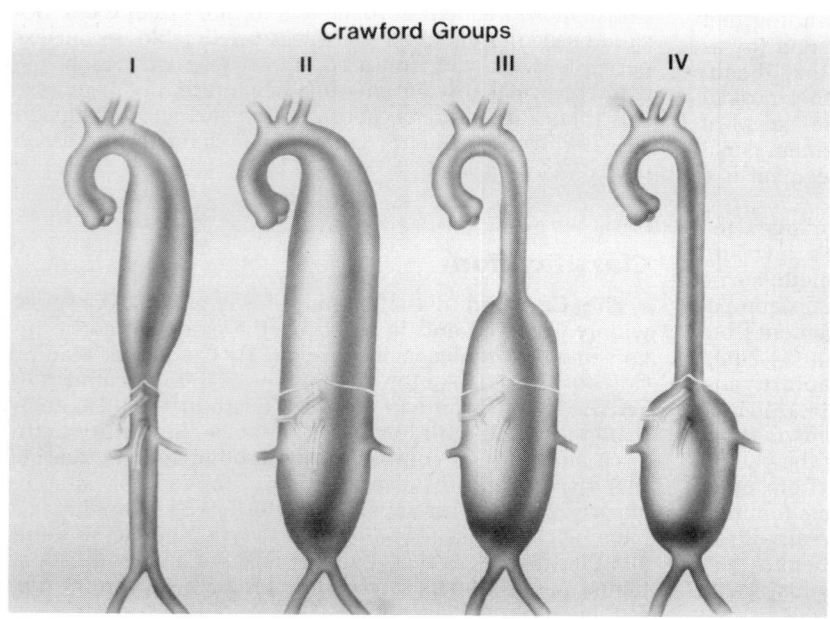

Figure 85.3. Dr. E. Stanley Crawford classified thoracoabdominal aneurysms by the extent of aortic involvement, which correlated with paraplegia risk during repair. Crawford type 1 involves most of the descending thoracic aorta and upper abdominal aorta, not including the renal arteries. Type 2 involves most of the descending thoracic and abdominal aorta inclusive of the visceral and renal vessels. Type 3 involves the distal half of the descending thoracic and most of the abdominal aorta. Type 4 involves just the abdominal aorta, including the visceral vessels. The risk for paralysis associated with type 2 aneurysms is twice that of type 1 aneurysms, four times that of type 3 aneurysms, and 10 times that of type 4 aneurysms.

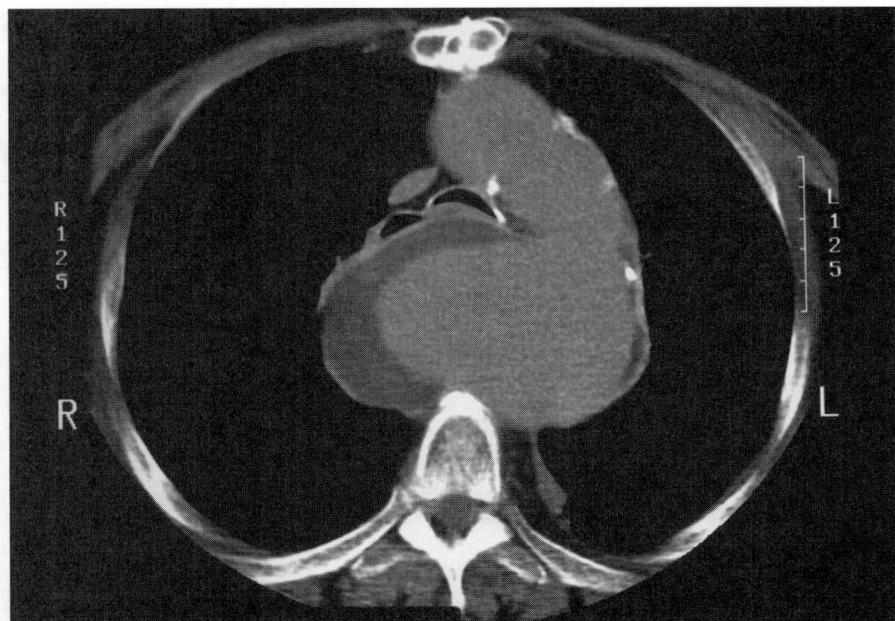

Figure 85.4. Computed tomogram of a large Crawford type 2 thoracoabdominal aneurysm. The patient, who had underlying chronic obstructive pulmonary disease, presented with respiratory failure resulting from airway compression. It was relieved by aneurysm repair.

DIAGNOSIS AND IMAGING

The diagnosis of nonacute or acute TAAAs is usually serendipitous and haphazard because of low incidence and nonspecific symptoms. The physical examination gives few clues to the presence of a TAAA unless the abdominal portion is large and palpable, in which case an infrarenal aneurysm is usually suspected until more extensive diagnostic tests are performed. Imaging with abdominal ultrasonography, chest roentgenography, computed tomography (CT), magnetic resonance imaging (MRI), magnetic resonance angiography (MRA), or transesophageal echocardiography usually provides the first clue to the presence of an extensive TAAA (Fig. 85.5). Similarly, acute symptoms are many times misinterpreted until an imaging study identifies a large aneurysm.

Because of recent advances in technology, MRA and spiral computed axial tomography (CAT) with three-dimensional reconstruction have replaced riskier conventional arteriography as the primary imaging techniques for TAAAs in most large medical centers (Fig. 85.6). MRA with an accompanying aortic MRI is the safest procedure because a nephrotoxic contrast agent is unnecessary and image resolution has improved significantly with newer machines and software (Fig. 85.7). Transesophageal or transthoracic echocardiography in our experience (contrary to some reports) is poor at anatomic localization of TAAAs and identification of acute disease. TAAA imaging should provide information regarding aneurysm size, extent, branch vessel (renal, superior mesenteric artery, celiac) location (aberrant anatomy), and pathology (stenosis, occlusion, aneurysm).

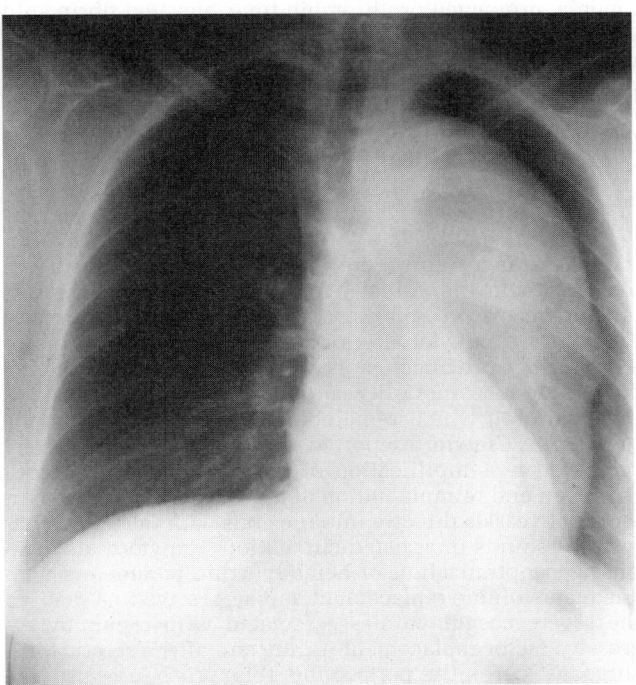

Figure 85.5. Chest roentgenogram of a 65-year-old woman with a large thoracoabdominal aneurysm filling most of the left side of the thorax. The patient presented with crescendo angina from three-vessel coronary disease, and her aneurysm was not diagnosed until this chest film was obtained. Retrospectively, she had had chronic interscapular back pain for the previous 2 years. The aneurysm, which measured 15 cm, escaped detection for years as it slowly enlarged. At surgery, the aneurysm was seen to have a very thick wall, which allowed it to reach such a large size.

SURGICAL RISK ASSESSMENT AND ASSOCIATED DISEASES

Patients with TAAAs commonly have diseases affecting a variety of other organ systems, and the risk for and incidence of multiple-system disease (cardiac, pulmonary, renal, cerebral vascular, peripheral vascular, malignancy) increases with age. Assessment of the cardiac, pulmonary, and renal systems is most important in determining operative risk. No magic formula or number can determine whether a patient is an operative candidate or not, and ultimately the surgeon, anesthesiologist, and patient must decide together whether the risk is warranted. However, some general guidelines can be established. Patients with ischemic heart disease and angina should be evaluated with coronary arteriography for possible coronary artery

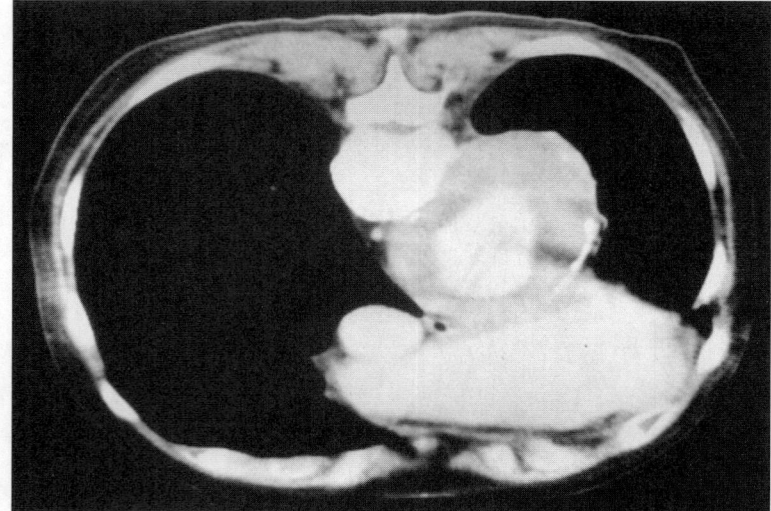

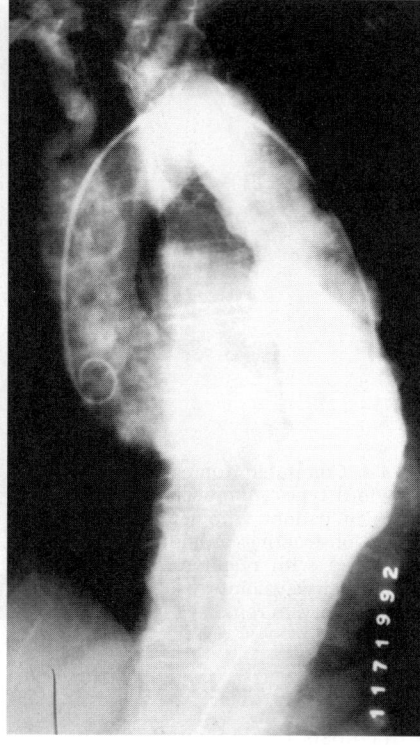

Figure 85.6. (A) Computed tomogram of a large Crawford type 2 thoracoabdominal aneurysm. Iodinated contrast enhances the luminal flow channel surrounded by laminated thrombus, not seen in the arteriogram (B) from the same patient. Arteriography or other flow contrast imaging techniques, such as three-dimensional reconstructed computed tomography or magnetic resonance angiography, are unreliable in measuring aneurysm diameter.

revascularization before undergoing aneurysm repair. Similarly, patients with symptomatic valve disease may require correction before aneurysm repair. A reduced ejection fraction (< 30%) with angina almost guarantees an extremely high mortality risk and is a contraindication to surgery, whereas a reduced ejection fraction in a well-compensated patient without myocardium at risk (no angina, no reperfusion ischemia on thallium cardiac perfusion scans) is usually an acceptable risk with proper anesthetic and surgical management. Patients with severely compromised pulmonary function [forced expiratory volume in 1 second (FEV$_1$) < 1.5 L but > 0.80 L; < 30% of predicted value and/or on supplemental oxygen) are at significantly increased risk for lethal pulmonary complications or prolonged ventilator dependence in the replacement of Crawford types 1, 2, and 3 aneurysms, but they may do quite well in the repair of a type 4 aneurysm because of the lower level of the thoracotomy (eighth intercostal space as opposed to the fifth or sixth). Surgery is probably contraindicated for patients with an FEV$_1$ of less than 0.80 L. Other factors may also play a significant role in determining pulmonary risk. Obesity may severely compromise weaning from a ventilator, and at any given level of pulmonary function, the patient's negative inspiratory force (NIF < 25 mm Hg) and vital capacity (VC < 30%) may reflect lung mechanics unsuitable for surgery, or gas exchange may be compromised (carbon dioxide retention with hypoxia) (19). Renal function is less of an issue than cardiac and pulmonary function because patients can undergo dialysis to manage fluid overload and their condition may improve in some cases with surgical revascularization, but poor renal function is a marker for advanced generalized atherosclerosis and reduced organism vigor. Age is another risk factor that is hard to quantify but has to be considered because overall vitality and the reserve to deal with stress decrease with advancing age. In our experience, at any given age, women tend to be more physically fit than men, especially over the age of 80. Other factors, such as underlying liver disease (cirrhosis)

and preexisting coagulopathy, can also be important. Some large aneurysms are associated with a consumptive diffuse intravascular coagulopathy marked by thrombocytopenia, prolonged prothrombin time, elevated fibrin split products, and reduced thrombin levels. Diffuse intravascular coagulopathy can usually be managed with factor replacement, but even if it is cured by aneurysm repair, it may contribute to significant perioperative bleeding and morbidity.

SURGERY

DeBakey reported in 1956 that the first attempts to repair these aneurysms were complex, requiring aneurysm excisions and individual bypasses to the visceral, renal, and intercostal vessels. In addition, surface cooling and temporary shunts for afterload reduction and distal perfusion during aortic occlusion were used with minimal success to reduce mortality and morbidity (paralysis and renal failure), which remained in excess of 40%. In the mid-1970s, Crawford reported that outcomes were greatly improved by simplification of the surgery; he used graft inclusion and reimplantation of the visceral, renal, and intercostal vessels directly into the graft with Carrel patches without shunts or assisted circulation. Crawford also emphasized optimization of hemodynamic parameters with adequate volume replacement and aggressive treatment of the severe coagulopathies associated with repair by aggressive factor replacement during and after surgery. Most surgeons currently performing this procedure use the Crawford template technique; however, considerable debate continues regarding the methods used to prevent such morbidities as spinal cord ischemia and renal failure. In this section, we describe the basic Crawford technique of graft inclusion and then detail some of the different modifications used to reduce morbidity and mortality. In addition, attention is given to the anesthetic management of these patients, which is as important as the surgical details in reducing morbidity.

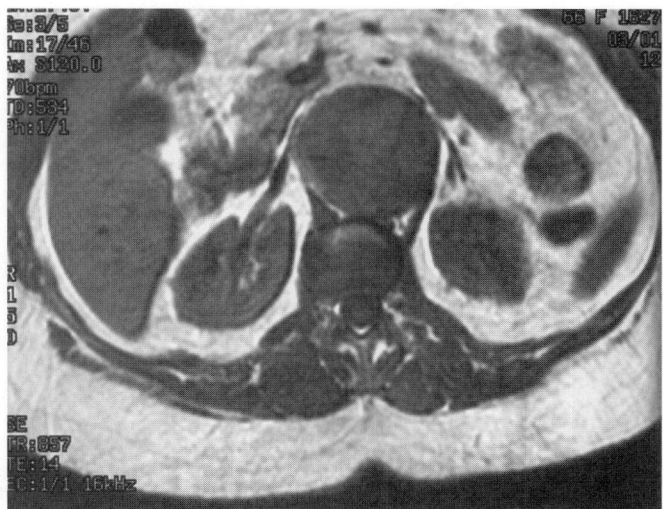

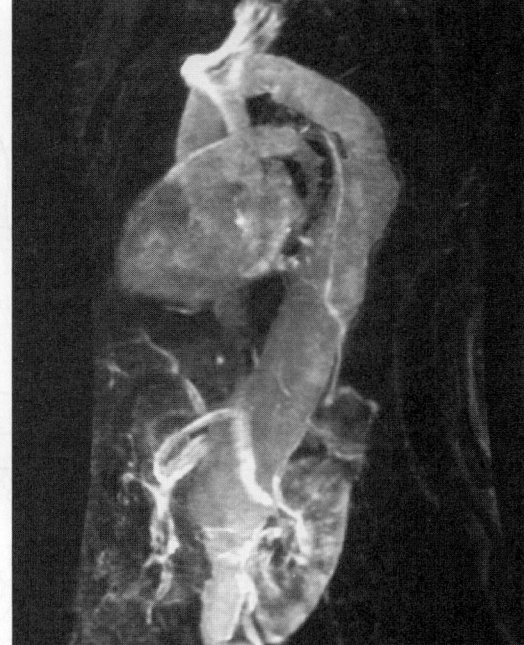

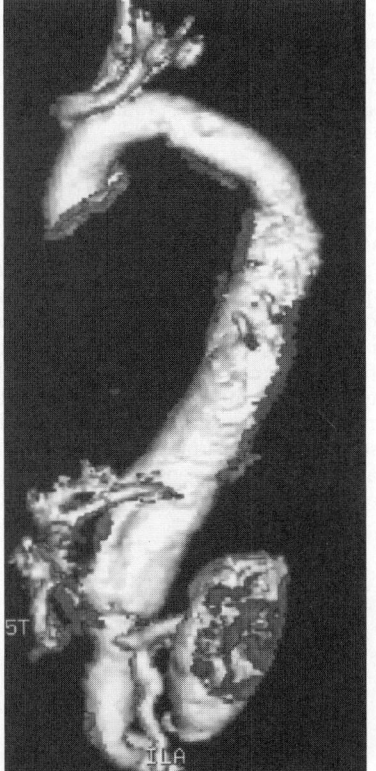

Figure 85.7. With the recent advances in magnetic resonance imaging *(MRI)* and angiography *(MRA),* it is possible in most cases to avoid conventional arteriography and computed tomography, which have associated risks of contrast nephrotoxicity and arterial injury and embolism (arteriography). *(A–C)* MRI, MRA, and three-dimensional MRA reconstruction of a Crawford type 2 thoracoabdominal aneurysm in a patient with a previous infrarenal aneurysm repair. In addition to branch vessel anatomy, renal volume and blood flow can be measured with MR technology.

Patient Preparation

Before surgery, the bowel is prepared with GoLYTELY. The patient showers the night before and the morning of surgery with an antibacterial scrub. The morning of surgery, electroencephalographic leads are placed before the patient is transported to the operating room.

Operative Technique

In this section, we describe our operative technique in some detail to demonstrate the complexity of these repairs (20). In the final section, on results, adjuncts for spinal cord protection and organ perfusion are discussed in further detail.

After the patient is transported to the operating room, a drain for cerebral spinal fluid (CSF) is placed under fluo-roscopy. Such drainage controls CSF pressure, which increases after aortic occlusion, and decreases spinal cord perfusion pressure. A functional drain is very important for spinal cord protection. If bloody CSF is encountered when the spinal drain is placed, the surgery may be aborted because of the risk for subarachnoid hemorrhage. Before the patient is positioned for surgery, the anesthesiologist places an arterial line in the right radial artery because the aortic clamp may be placed between the left carotid and subclavian arteries. A thermal Swan-Ganz catheter to monitor body temperature, volume status, and cardiac function is placed, in addition to at least two-large bore intravenous catheters for rapid volume replacement. We use an endotracheal tube with a double lumen or bronchial blocker to collapse the left lung and thereby reduce interference in the thoracic cavity during aneurysm repair. A Foley catheter is placed to measure urine output.

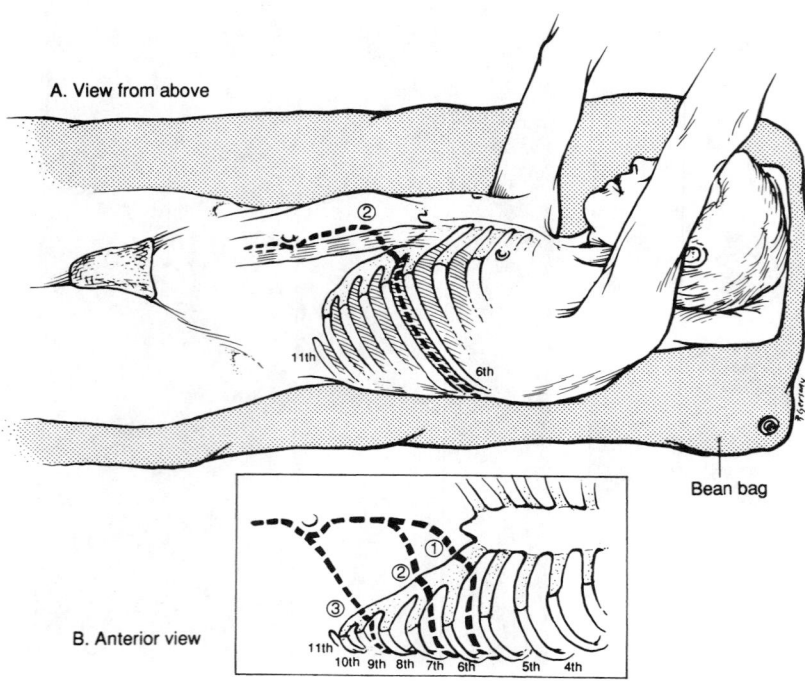

A. View from above

11th

6th

Bean bag

B. Anterior view

11th 10th 9th 8th 7th 6th 5th 4th

Figure 85.8. The intercostal level of the incision is determined by the extent of aortic replacement. Crawford type 2 aneurysms are exposed through the fifth or sixth intercostal space, whereas Crawford type 4 aneurysms can be exposed through the eight or ninth space. (Reprinted from Acher CW, Wynn MM. Technique of thoracoabdominal aneurysm repair. *Ann Vasc Surg* 1999;9:585–595, with permission.)

The patient is then placed in the left lateral decubitus position, and the chest and abdomen are prepared and draped for a thoracoabdominal incision. The intercostal level of incision is determined by extent of aorta to be replaced, with a fifth intercostal incision used for aneurysms arising proximate to the left subclavian artery and the eighth or ninth intercostal space used when only the abdominal aorta is involved (Fig. 85.8). The thoracic incision is carried to the midline (linea alba) and then caudad along the midline. After access to the thoracic and abdominal cavities has been gained, the spleen, left side of the colon, pancreas, and left kidney are mobilized off the retroperitoneum by incising along the lateral peritoneal reflection and medially through Gerota's fascia, which surrounds the kidney. The diaphragm is then incised to its aortic hiatus (Fig. 85.9). The periaortic lymphatics that are encountered along the lateral posterior portion of the aorta are divided with a cautery or between ligatures. Usually, a large lumbar vein drains into the left renal vein; this is ligated, with the adrenal and gonadal vein left intact. In a small number of patients, the left renal vein is retroaortic and should be divided between vascular clamps just before aortic occlusion and then reanastomosed after reestablishment of arterial continuity. The left renal artery is usually exposed as

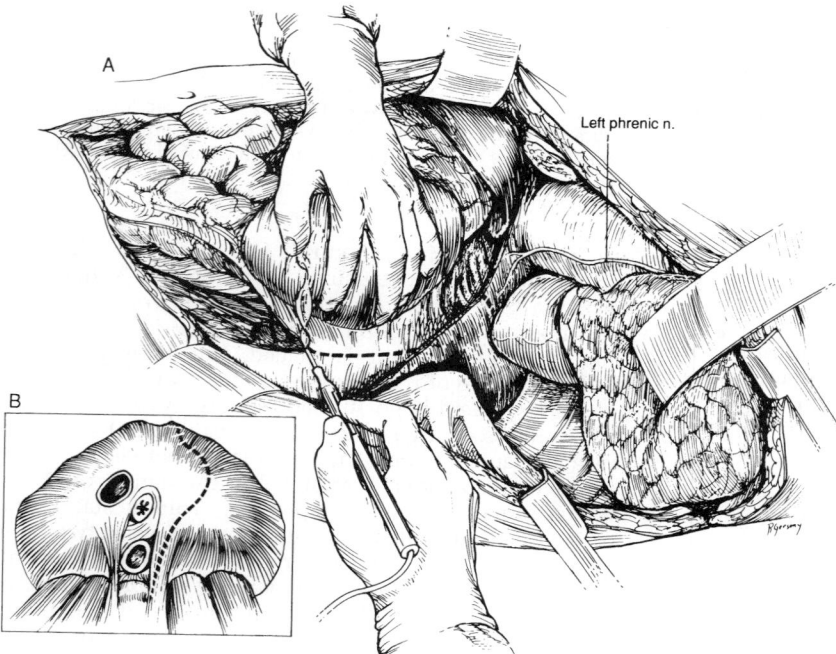

A

Left phrenic n.

B

Figure 85.9. The spleen, pancreas, left side of the colon, and left kidney are mobilized off the retroperitoneum to expose the aorta. The diaphragm is incised through the aortic hiatus, with care taken to avoid the phrenic innervation of the diaphragm. (Reprinted from Acher CW, Wynn MM. Technique of thoracoabdominal aneurysm repair. *Ann Vasc Surg* 1999;9:585–595, with permission.)

a reference landmark, but it is not necessary to expose the celiac and superior mesenteric arteries in most patients unless extended endarterectomy or bypass is required. For greater access to the iliac arteries, the inferior mesenteric artery can be divided. This is safe to do if it is chronically occluded, but if patent, preservation and reattachment of the artery may be required to avoid ischemia of the sigmoid colon and rectum.

Before dissection is begun for proximal aortic control, the left lung is collapsed with a bronchial blocker unless the repair involves just the abdominal aorta (Crawford type 4). Dissection of the aorta for proximal control may involve division of the ligamentum arteriosum just distal to the left subclavian artery, with care taken not to injure the aorta or pulmonary artery. The phrenic nerve should be identified to avoid injury, which is more likely to occur when control of the aorta is gained between the left carotid and left subclavian arteries. Injury of the vagus nerve with its recurrent laryngeal branch is sometimes impossible to avoid, depending on the level of the aortic clamp, proximal anastomosis, or exposure of the aorta. However, the vagus nerve can be cut distal to the origin of the recurrent laryngeal nerve for additional mobilization and recurrent nerve preservation, which should be attempted whenever possible. Through such extensive incision and dissection, the entire descending thoracic and abdominal aorta can be exposed (Fig. 85.10).

Before aortic cross-clamping is undertaken, the anesthesiologist lowers the body temperature to below 34°C and maximizes the cardiac index with afterload reduction, volume replacement, and administration of inotropic agents. The CSF is drained slowly to keep the CSF pressure below 6 mm Hg. The anesthesiologist also lowers the blood pressure with a beta blockade (esmolol), nitroglycerin, amrinone, and, just before aortic occlusion, thiopental, the dose of which is determined by electroencephalographic burst suppression. Close communication and coordination between the anesthesiologist and surgeon are essential so that the surgeon knows when to cross-clamp the aorta.

When all the parameters measured are within acceptable zones, the aorta is slowly cross-clamped during 30 to 60 seconds to allow the heart to accommodate to aortic occlusion because the entire cardiac output may be directed to the innominate and left carotid arteries with a high cross-clamp. Significant afterload reduction is required to keep cardiac strain within acceptable limits.

After proximal aortic occlusion, a second aortic clamp (sequential clamping) may be placed to minimize blood loss during the proximal anastomosis. This may be especially important in younger patients, those with chronic dissections, or patients with Marfan syndrome who have many open, back-bleeding intercostal vessels, which can lead to exsanguination if uncontrolled. The aorta is opened, and any open intercostal or lumbar vessels are immediately oversewn to increase perfusion pressure in the collateral vascular bed and therefore spinal cord perfusion pressure. If the visceral vessels are visible, they are occluded with Fogarty balloon catheters, as are the renal vessels after perfusion with 400 to 500 mL of cold perfusion solution (lactated Ringer's solution at 4°C with 12.5 g of mannitol and 1,000 U of heparin per liter). Renal perfusion may further lower the body temperature 2°C. The proximal anastomosis is then created with a running prolene suture line that may be reinforced with Teflon or Dacron pledgets if the wall is thin, weak, or disrupted, as in aortic dissection. After the suture line is tested for hemostasis, the clamp is placed on the aortic graft to allow perfusion of any intercostal vessels occluded by the clamp. The visceral and renal vessels are then reattached from inside the aneurysm (graft inclusion) with use of a Carrel patch sewn to a window cut in the graft (Fig. 85.11). If the visceral and renal vessels are not too far from each other, multiple vessels can be included in one patch, the most common arrangement being the celiac artery, superior mesenteric artery, and a renal artery in one patch and the remaining renal artery in a separate patch. Occasionally, the vessels may be spaced so that an individual anastomosis is required for each vessel. About 35% of the time, endarterectomy for occlusive disease of these branch vessels is required before reattachment, and if endarterectomy is not technically possible or the result is unsatisfactory, a bypass may be required. After the renal artery

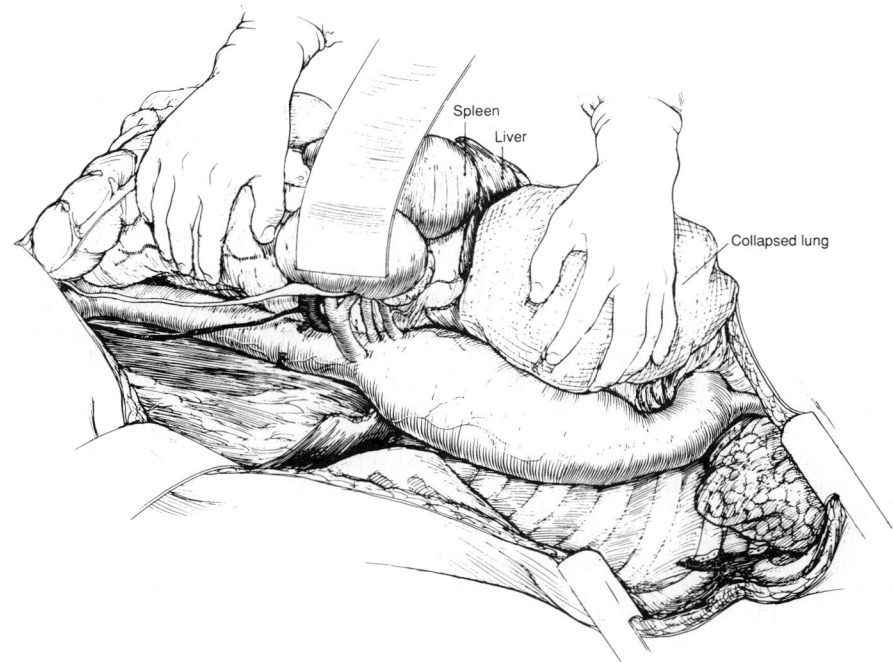

Figure 85.10. Through an extensive thoracoabdominal incision, the entire descending thoracic and abdominal aorta is exposed in preparation for aneurysm repair in this patient with a Crawford type 1 aneurysm. (Reprinted from Acher CW, Wynn MM. Technique of thoracoabdominal aneurysm repair. *Ann Vasc Surg* 1999;9:585–595, with permission.)

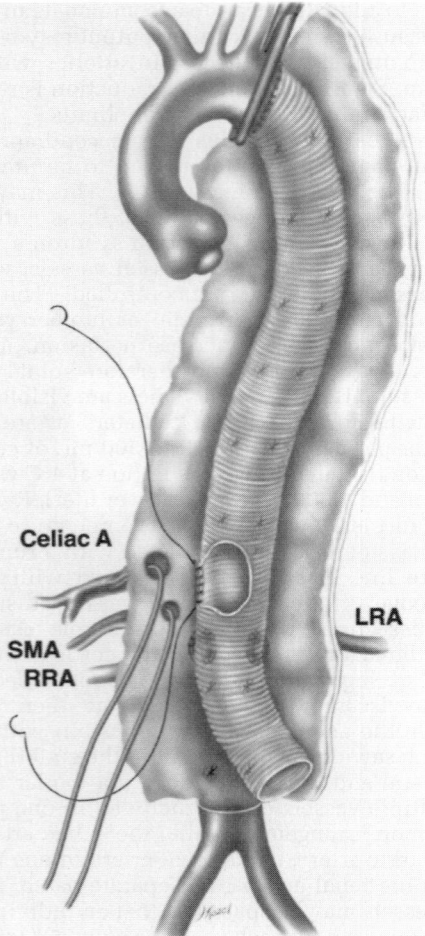

Figure 85.11. After the aorta is clamped proximal to the aneurysm, the aneurysm is opened and the visceral and renal vessels are reattached to the aortic graft with Carrel patches that include various combinations of these vessels, depending on how far they are spaced from each other. In this patient, the celiac and superior mesenteric arteries are on one Carrel patch, and the renal arteries are attached separately.

reattachment is completed, the graft is flushed to remove clots and debris and then clamped below the renal arteries to reestablish blood flow to the viscera and kidneys with removal of the balloon occlusion catheters. The mean time to complete these anastomoses after aortic occlusion is 46 minutes. This portion of the surgery is very focused, and great concentration and precision are required to minimize organ ischemic time. After blood flow to the kidneys and viscera has been reestablished, it is evaluated with a Doppler probe and palpation of the vessels. Intravenous indigo carmine is administered, and the time to appearance in the urine is noted. This is an indication that the kidneys are perfused adequately and functioning. The left lung can be reinflated at this point in the surgery if necessary for oxygenation.

The aortic graft is then sutured to the distal aorta at its bifurcation into the iliac arteries. Endarterectomy of the distal aortic plate may be required because of calcification. A bifurcated graft may have to be sutured to the long tube graft used for the upper aortic reconstruction if iliac artery replacement is necessary for occlusive or aneurysmal disease. After adequate hemostasis has been confirmed, the aneurysm sac is closed over the graft with a running suture; The thoracoabdominal incision is then closed, with a

chest tube for the thorax and a flat suction drain for the retroperitoneum to minimize retroperitoneal fluid and blood collection. The average skin-to-skin surgery time is 3.8 hours, with 95% of procedures lasting between 2.5 and 5 hours.

During the aortic reconstruction, the anesthesiologist monitors and replaces lost blood. The volume of blood lost can be up to 5 L in some patients but averages about 1,500 mL. A high-speed cell saver is used to scavenge the patient's blood and thereby minimize the need for banked blood. In addition, the anesthesiologist monitors and maximizes cardiac index and oxygenation, which tend to deteriorate during aortic occlusion. The CSF pressure is controlled by continuous drainage of CSF, which averages 110 mL. Because of the metabolic acidosis that develops with end-organ ischemia, a bicarbonate drip is required. With the reestablishment of blood flow, hypotension is treated with aggressive fluid replacement and inotropic agents for depressed cardiac function. A large portion of the initial volume replacement is with coagulation factors in the form of fresh frozen plasma pooled in liter bags. Platelets are also given in most cases to aid in hemostasis. If the patient's temperature has dropped to below 32°C, intracavitary warming with warm saline solution may be necessary in addition to an increase in ambient temperature and blood warmers.

Postoperative Care

During the immediate postoperative period (first 48 hours), the primary tasks are monitoring and optimizing cardiac, pulmonary, and renal function, protecting the spinal cord, and correcting the usual coagulopathy of repair.

The cardiac index should be optimized to more than 2 L/m^2 for normal perfusion of end-organs such as the kidneys and spinal cord, and intravenous fluids may have to be administered at a rate of 300 to 400 mL/h to maintain optimal preload and intravascular volume because of postoperative diuresis and third spacing. The average volume replacement for the first 24 hours, including intraoperative time, is 10 L. Vasodilation and beta blockade with nitroglycerin and esmolol are used to keep the blood pressure under control and reduce systemic vascular resistance and cardiac work. Vasodilators like nitroprusside and hydralazine are not used because of their demonstrated negative effects on myocardial, renal, and spinal cord blood flow. Dopamine is infused at 2 μg/kg per hour to optimize renal perfusion.

Historically, coagulopathy resulting from blood loss and diffuse intravascular coagulation has been a source of major morbidity but can be avoided with aggressive coagulation factor replacement, both intraoperatively and postoperatively. Factor replacement with fresh frozen plasma is expectant, with the administration of large volumes of 6 to 20 U (1 to 3 L) intraoperatively and 75 mL/h for 24 hours postoperatively. The postoperative infusion is to compensate for liver dysfunction resulting from the ischemic time of repair and reperfusion with transient decrease in factor production. The goal is to maintain a normal international normalized ratio and partial thromboplastin time. Consumptive thrombocytopenia on the graft surface occurs for several days postoperatively, but platelet transfusions are required only if bleeding develops or if the platelet count falls below 30,000 to 40,000/mm^3.

The CSF pressure is monitored, and CSF is drained for 24 hours to keep the pressure below 6 to 10 mm Hg. Naloxone is infused intravenously at 1 microgram/kg per hour for 48 hours for spinal cord protection. The patient usually has a core temperature of 33° to 34°C when the procedure is finished. The patient is allowed to warm slowly without thermal blankets or bear huggers to minimize rapid peripheral vascular dilation that may shunt blood away from the spinal cord. Postoperative analgesia is with 25 to 50 mg of meperidine (Demerol) per hour until the neurologic findings are normal, and then hydromorphone (Dilaudid) can be given. Morphine is never used because it is the most β-endorphin-like analgesic, and endorphins may have a negative effect on spinal cord blood flow. Sequential venous compression of the lower extremities is used to minimize deep venous thrombosis and pulmonary embolism.

RESULTS

In discussing patient outcomes, it is not enough to look at survival alone. Because of the devastating complications of paraplegia and renal failure, as well as death, the personal price of survival in terms of quality of life has to be considered. In attempting to understand the reasons for failure to achieve optimal outcomes, it can be misleading to look at just the incidence of complications without analyzing some of the factors that increase the risks for them. In our own efforts to understand the risk factors for complications, we have used multivariate analysis of our own data and mathematically modeled outcomes from the surgical literature. This discussion of outcomes attempts to clarify objectively why we fail in our treatment of these complex cases.

Lower Extremity Paralysis

Probably no complication is more frustrating and difficult to experience, understand, and discuss than lower extremity paralysis resulting from thoracic or thoracoabdominal aneurysm repair. Part of this difficulty derives from the fact that paralysis is so capricious, sparing most patients but striking others who have what appear to be identical aneurysms and clinical presentations. It is clear from clinical reports that a more extensive aortic replacement and an acute presentation (rupture or dissection) increase the risk for paralysis, with Crawford type 2 aneurysms having about twice the risk of Crawford type 1, type 3 about half the risk of type 1, and type 4 about half the risk of type 3 (21). In patients presenting with acute rupture or dissection, the risk for paralysis is two or more times greater than that in patients treated electively with the same extent of replacement. Paralysis can be complete (paraplegia) or partial (paraparesis), and can be immediate or delayed by hours or days. In a very few patients, paralysis is completely or partially reversible. The anatomic paradigm to explain paraplegia was developed and published by Adams and Van Geertruyden in 1956 (22). They described the desegmentation of the spinal cord circulation with phylogenetic progression to primates, in which continuous anterior spinal arteries supplemented by a few radicular arteries from the thoracic and upper abdominal aorta augment flow to the anterior spinal artery. Interruption of blood flow to these radicular arteries, either temporarily or permanently, causes spinal cord stroke and paraplegia. The largest and most important of the radicular arteries is the arteria magna radicularis, or artery of Adamkeiwitz. Adam's paradigm made clear that collateral blood flow is a major factor in cord preservation during aortic occlusion. Therefore, the logical solution would be to perfuse and reimplant the radicular arteries during repair, and for the last quarter of a century, that is what surgeons have attempted to do. However, this approach to preventing paralysis was never validated experimentally

and has been unsuccessful in thoracoabdominal aortic replacement (23–25). The experimental literature did validate other interventions that appeared to provide significant protection to the spinal cord by extending the permissible aortic occlusion time for repair. CSF drainage and systemic or regional hypothermia have been the most effective of these interventions (26–35). Other experimentally validated factors may be beneficial in spinal cord preservation, such as the avoidance of anemia, hypoxia, and proximal or systemic hypotension (36,37). High-dose steroids, endorphins, and excitatory receptor antagonists are beneficial experimentally and, we believe, clinically (38–42). Deleterious factors have also been validated experimentally. Nitroprusside for blood pressure control during aortic occlusion has a negative effect on spinal cord blood flow, and this effect is strong enough to negate the protective effects of CSF drainage (43–45). Normothermia or hyperthermia can significantly shorten allowable aortic occlusion times. What is clear from the experimental and clinical work is that the risk for paralysis is not just a consequence of the anatomy of spinal cord circulation but rather of a complex interaction of competing and overlapping effects that can augment each other or cancel each other in determining the eventual outcome.

To study the clinical benefits of the various strategies for spinal cord protection more objectively, we modeled paraplegia risk mathematically. The model contains factors for acuity and dissection and uses Crawford's groups to represent extent of replacement, with a risk coefficient determined for each group (46). With this model, we have studied 5,000 patients in 41 clinical reports for the actual versus estimated number of deficits (Table 85.1, Fig. 85.12A). The model has been extremely accurate in accounting for 95% of the variability between clinical reports. What this model demonstrates is that most of the variation in paralysis incidence between reports can be accounted for by extent of replacement and clinical presentation, so that what appear to be large differences in paralysis rates do not exist when Crawford aneurysm type and clinical presentation are accounted for. So whether a surgeon uses a Gott shunt or an atrial–femoral bypass for retrograde perfusion of the aorta and its branches, or tries to identify the arteria magna radicularis with arteriography and somatosensory evoked potentials or just blindly reimplants open intercostal vessels, the results are the same and predictable. The model also demonstrates that strategies based on experimentally validated interventions, such as hypothermia and CSF drainage, yield better results than the traditional methods of using intercostal reimplantation with or without assisted circulation.

In developing our operative and anesthetic protocols, we demonstrated that the effect of CSF drainage and endorphin receptor blockade is additive, providing a level of spinal cord protection that is greater than that obtained with either treatment alone (47). In addition, we have identified cardiac function as a major factor in paralysis risk, along with extent of aortic replacement and clinical presentation. Core temperature at the time of aortic occlusion is also important, but less important than cardiac function. The predictive model confirms our own analysis that with our present protocol of moderate hypothermia, CSF drainage, endorphin receptor blockade, and elimination of deleterious drugs like nitroprusside, we have reduced paralysis risk in elective patients by 90% and in acute patients by 80% (48). Cambria et al. (31) have achieved similar results by using epidural cooling with assisted circulation to the visceral and renal arteries. Fehrenbacher et al. (49) have had similar results with a different method of regional cooling, and Kouchoukos and Rokkas (50) have reduced the mortality associated with hypothermic circulatory arrest to make it a tenable strategy for

Table 85.1. DEFICIT RISK AND MORTALITY OF THORACOABDOMINAL ANEURYSMS

Technique	No. series	C1	C2	C3	C4	TA	Total	Acute	Est D	Actual	A/E D	Acute	Est M	Actual	A/E M
AFB	20	232	196	152	61	408	1,049	197	126	127	1.01	86	107	109	1.02
AFBHA	5	55	67	21	9	119	271	92	44	19	0.43	12	28	35	1.25
CSFD	5	43	55	44	82	4	228	47	32	16	0.5	21	26	49	1.88
CSFDN	1	24	50	21	33	22	150	58	31	5	0.16	53	42	8	0.19
CSFDP	5	109	151	100	70	4	434	89	70	31	0.44	22	47	39	0.83
EPIDC	1	32	15	33			80	33	16	3	0.19	6	11	8	0.73
XCLMP	16	616	725	661	632	103	2,737	653	418	409	0.98	345	388	363	0.94
Total		**1,111**	**1,259**	**1,032**	**887**	**660**	**4,949**	**1,169**	**737**	**610**		**545**	**649**	**611**	

C1, Crawford type 1; AFB, atrial femoral bypass; AFBHA, atrial femoral bypass with hypothermic arrest; CSFD, cerebral spinal fluid drainage; CSFDN, cerebral spinal fluid drainage with intravenous naloxone; CSFDP, cerebral spinal fluid drainage with atrial femoral bypass; EPIDC, epidural cooling; XCLMP, cross-clamping with adjuncts (Crawford technique); Est D, estimated deficit; Est M, estimated mortality.
A/E is the actual to estimated ratio.

cord protection. Also, Jacobs et al. (51) have achieved dramatically improved results with CSF drainage, motor evoked potentials, and endarterectomy and reimplantation of chronically occluded thoracic intercostal arteries (51). All these clinical experiments are based on experimentally validated methods of spinal cord protection.

Mortality rates in clinical reports average about 12%. However, when mortality is modeled according to the variables of acuity and estimated paralysis, 85% of the variation can be accounted for (Fig. 85.12B). Therefore, like paralysis, the percentage of mortality is not a good measure of relative mortality. Ninety percent of our mor-

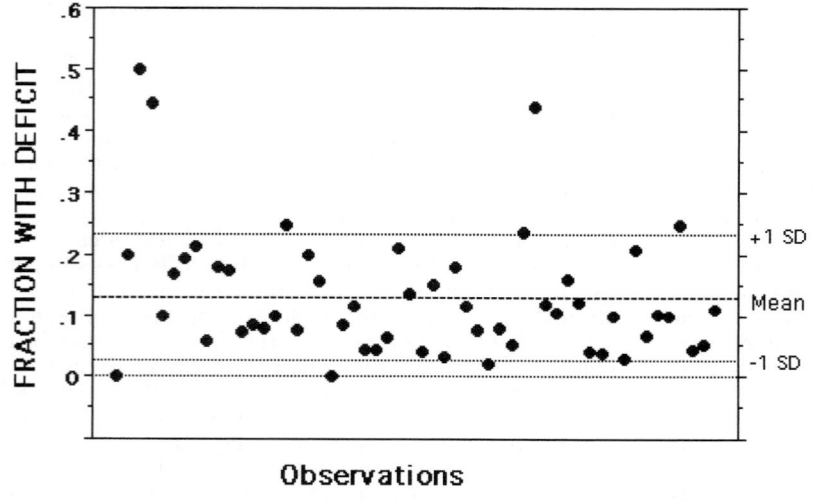

A   Observations

Figure 85.12. Scatter plots of actual versus estimated number of lower extremity neurologic deficits *(A)* and deaths *(B)* with regression lines and confidence intervals in clinical reports from a total of approximately 5,000 patients. Modeling these outcomes explains most of the differences between clinical series.

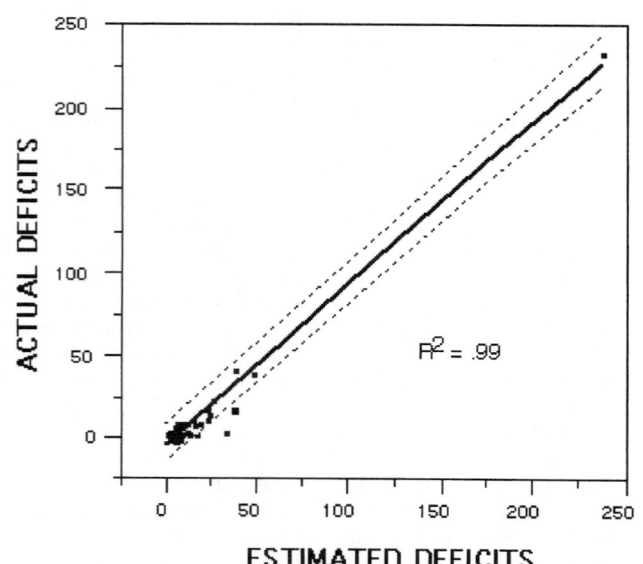

B

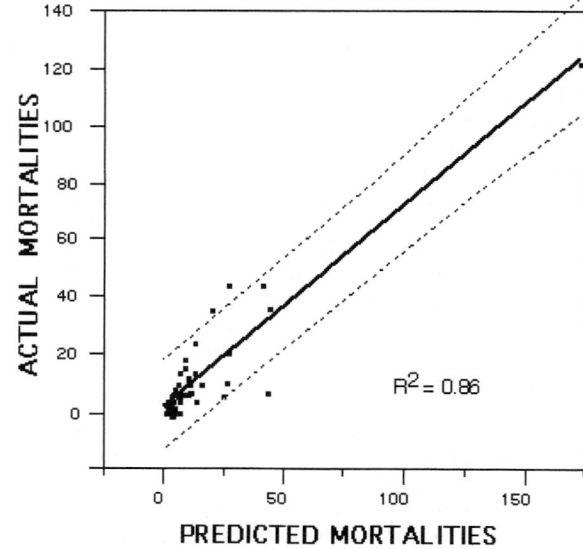

C

Table 85.2. CAUSES OF OPERATIVE DEATH

Cause of death	No. (%)
Cardiac	3 (14.28)
Cerebrovascular accident	2 (9.52)
Gastrointestinal bleeding	1 (4.76)
Multisystem failure	7 (33.33)
Rupture with cardiac arrest	8 (38.10)
Total	21

Table 85.3. OTHER COMPLICATIONS

Complications	No.	Percentage
Renal failure	16	7.37
Cerebrovascular accident	10	4.61
Recurrent nerve injury	8	3.69
Sepsis	7	3.23
Wound infection	7	3.23
Arrhythmia	6	2.76
Coagulopathy	6	2.76
Pulmonary embolus	6	2.76
Femoral embolus	5	2.30
Colitis	4	1.84
Ischemic bowel	4	1.84
Myocardial infarction	4	1.84
Gastrointestinal bleeding	2	0.92
Pancreatitis	2	0.92
Phrenic nerve injury	2	0.92
DTs	1	0.46

talities occurred in patients requiring acute care, and the primary causes of death were rupture with cardiac arrest and multiple-system failure (Table 85.2). Our elective mortality rate was 1.9% (2 of 127). Other than acuity, age, preoperative renal function, cardiac function, and paraplegia were significant factors; however, age, acuity, and preoperative renal function were the most important of these in a multivariate model. No patient over the age of 75 with a preoperative creatinine level above 2.8 mg/dL who presented acutely survived in our experience. A third of the deaths were from multiple-system failure, which usually was precipitated by shock, myocardial infarction, or gram-negative pneumonia.

Other Measures of Outcome

In most clinical series, dialysis-dependent renal failure occurs in 6% to 10% of patients. The reasons for this are not clear but are assumed to be poor preoperative renal function, ischemia of prolonged occlusion time, embolization, shock, and technical difficulties at surgery. Godet et al. (52), reporting on 474 patients, identified only age and preoperative renal function as independent predictors of the need for dialysis (52). Although renal cooling may be beneficial in renal preservation, attempts to perfuse the kidneys continuously during the time of aortic occlusion have had mixed results (53–55). Twenty-five percent of our patients had elevated serum creatinine levels preoperatively (> 1.5 mg/dL), which indicate some degree of renal failure. This was the only significant factor that correlated with poor renal function (13 of 217, or 7%) or the need for dialysis (4 of 210, or 2%) postoperatively. Patients who underwent renal revascularization for renal artery stenosis had significantly improved function in comparison with patients without revascularization.

Pulmonary complications that prolonged hospitalization occurred in 14% (31 of 217) of our patients. Of 31 patients, 18 had pneumonia and 13 had respiratory failure resulting from poor pulmonary capacity or acute respiratory distress syndrome. Pulmonary complications were much more likely to occur in paraplegic patients (41% vs. 14%) and patients with less strength or more advanced pulmonary disease. It has been our experience that gram-negative pneumonia is difficult to treat and can lead to multiple-system failure and death; however, pulmonary complications were not risk factors for operative mortality. Other complications are listed in Table 85.3. Acute patients had twice the number of complications as elective patients (75% vs. 34%).

In summarizing our own and others' experience in treating patients with these complex aneurysms, it is clear that in selected centers, significant reductions in death and paralysis following treatment have been made in the last 10 years. These improved outcomes, however, still must be weighed against continued failures when patients are advised about their options for treatment. This is especially true in the very elderly (> 80 years old), who may have little to gain in longevity or quality of life and are at

higher risk for mortal complications. From a surgeon's perspective and personal experience with patients and their families, no worse end to life is possible for an elderly patient than to die of multiple-system failure in an intensive care unit as a result of surgical treatment meant to prolong a functional and useful life.

REFERENCES

1. DeBakey ME, et al. Surgical considerations in the treatment of aneurysms of the thoracoabdominal aorta. *Ann Surg* 1965; 162:650–662.
2. Lederle FA, et al. Prevalence and associations of abdominal aortic aneurysm detected through screening. Aneurysm Detection and Management (ADAM) Veterans Affairs Cooperative Study Group. *Ann Intern Med* 1997;126:441–449.
3. Lederle FA, Parenti CM, Chute EP. Ruptured abdominal aortic aneurysm: the internist as diagnostician. *Am J Med* 1994; 96:163–167.
4. Bickerstaff LK, et al. Thoracic aortic aneurysms: a population-based study. *Surgery* 1982;92:1103–1108.
5. Furthmayr H, Francke U. Ascending aortic aneurysm with or without features of Marfan syndrome and other fibrillinopathies: new insights. *Semin Thorac Cardiovasc Surg* 1997;9:191–205.
6. Kielty CM, Shuttleworth CA. Fibrillin-containing microfibrils: structure and function in health and disease. *Int J Biochem Cell Biol* 1995;27:747–760.
7. Milewicz DM. Identification of defects in the fibrillin gene and protein in individuals with the Marfan syndrome and related disorders. *Tex Heart Inst J* 1994;21:22–29.
8. Tilson MD, Roberts MP. Molecular diversity in the abdominal aortic aneurysm phenotype. *Arch Surg* 1988;123:1202–1206.
9. Tilson MD, Newman K. Rationale for molecular approaches to the etiology of abdominal aortic aneurysm disease. *J Vasc Surg* 1992;15:924–925.
10. Tilson MD, et al. A genetic basis for autoimmune manifestations in the abdominal aortic aneurysm resides in the MHC class II locus DR-beta-1. *Ann N Y Acad Sci* 1996;800: 208–215.
11. Limet R, et al. Pathogenesis of abdominal aortic aneurysm (AAA) formation. *Acta Chir Belg* 1998;98:195–198.
12. Grange JJ, Davis V, Baxter BT. Pathogenesis of abdominal aortic aneurysm: an update and look toward the future. *Cardiovasc Surg* 1997;5:256–265.
13. Lederle FA. Relationship of age, gender, race, and body size to infrarenal aortic diameter. The Aneurysm Detection and Management (ADAM) Veterans Affairs Cooperative Study Investigators. *J Vasc Surg* 1997;26:595–601.
14. Cambria RA, et al. Outcome and expansion rate of 57 thoracoabdominal aortic aneurysms managed nonoperatively. *Am J Surg* 1995;170:213–217.
15. Dapunt OE, et al. The natural history of thoracic aortic

aneurysms. *J Thorac Cardiovasc Surg* 1994;107:1323–1332; discussion 1332–1333.

16. Juvonen T, et al. Prospective study of the natural history of thoracic aortic aneurysms. *Ann Thorac Surg* 1997;63: 1533–1544.

17. Svensson LG, et al. Experience with 1,509 patients undergoing thoracoabdominal aortic operations. *J Vasc Surg* 1993;17: 357–368; discussion 368–370.

18. Crawford ES, et al. Progress in treatment of thoracoabdominal and abdominal aortic aneurysms involving celiac, superior mesenteric, and renal arteries. *Ann Surg* 1978;188:404–422.

19. Svensson LG, et al. A prospective study of respiratory failure after high-risk surgery on the thoracoabdominal aorta. *J Vasc Surg* 1991;14:271–282.

20. Acher CW, Wynn MM. Technique of thoracoabdominal aneurysm repair. *Ann Vasc Surg* 1995;9:585–595.

21. Crawford ES, et al. Thoracoabdominal aortic aneurysms: preoperative and intraoperative factors determining immediate and long-term results of operations in 605 patients. *J Vasc Surg* 1986;3:389–404.

22. Adams H, Van Geertruyden H. Neurologic complications of aortic surgery. *Ann Surg* 1956;144:574–610.

23. Lowell RC, et al. Failure of selective shunting to intercostal arteries to prevent spinal cord ischemia during experimental thoracoabdominal aortic occlusion. *Int Angiol* 1992;11: 281–288.

24. Griepp RB, et al. Looking for the artery of Adamkiewicz: a quest to minimize paraplegia after operations for aneurysms of the descending thoracic and thoracoabdominal aorta. *J Thorac Cardiovasc Surg* 1996;112:1202–1223; discussion 1213–1215.

25. Acher CW, Heisey DM. Regarding "Importance of intercostal artery reattachment during thoracoabdominal aortic aneurysm repair" [Letter]. *J Vasc Surg* 1998;28:570–571.

26. Miyamoto K, et al. A new and simple method of preventing spinal cord damage following temporary occlusion of the thoracic aorta by draining cerebral spinal fluid. *J Cardiovasc Surg* 1960;1:188–197.

27. Svensson LG, et al. Cross-clamping of the thoracic aorta: influence of aortic shunts, laminectomy, papaverine, calcium channel blocker, allopurinol, and superoxide dismutase on spinal cord blood flow and paraplegia in baboons. *Ann Surg* 1986;204:38–47.

28. Bower TC, et al. Effects of thoracic aortic occlusion and cerebrospinal fluid drainage on regional spinal cord blood flow in dogs: correlation with neurologic outcome. *J Vasc Surg* 1989; 9:135–144.

29. Safi HJ, et al. Cerebral spinal fluid drainage and distal aortic perfusion decrease the incidence of neurological deficit—the results of 343 descending and thoracoabdominal aortic aneurysm repairs. *Eur J Vasc Endovasc Surg* 1997;14: 118–124.

30. Baraka A. Influence of surface cooling and rewarming on whole-body oxygen supply–demand balance. *Br J Anaesth* 1994;73:418–420.

31. Cambria RP, et al. Clinical experience with epidural cooling for spinal cord protection during thoracic and thoracoabdominal aneurysm repair. *J Vasc Surg* 1997;25:234–241; discussion 241–243.

32. Berguer R, et al. Selective deep hypothermia of the spinal cord prevents paraplegia after aortic cross-clamping in the dog model. *J Vasc Surg* 1992;15:62–71; discussion 71–72.

33. Kouchoukos NT. Hypothermic circulatory arrest and hypothermic perfusion for extensive disease of the thoracic and thoracoabdominal aorta. *Jpn J Thorac Cardiovasc Surg* 1999; 47:1–5.

34. Kieffer E, et al. Hypothermic circulatory arrest for thoracic aneurysmectomy through left-sided thoracotomy. *J Vasc Surg* 1994;19:457–464.

35. Rokkas CK, et al. Profound systemic hypothermia protects the spinal cord in a primate model of spinal cord ischemia. *J Thorac Cardiovasc Surg* 1993;106:1024–1035.

36. Wisselink W, et al. Ischemia–reperfusion injury of the spinal cord: the influence of normovolemic hemodilution and gradual reperfusion. *Cardiovasc Surg* 1995;3:399–404.

37. Taira Y, Marsala M. Effect of proximal arterial perfusion pressure on function, spinal cord blood flow, and histopathologic changes after increasing intervals of aortic occlusion in the rat. *Stroke* 1996;27:1850–1858.

38. Woloszyn TT, et al. Cerebrospinal fluid drainage and steroids provide better spinal cord protection during aortic cross-clamping than does either treatment alone. *Ann Thorac Surg* 1990;49:78–82; discussion 83.

39. Craenen G, et al. The role of excitatory amino acids in hypothermic injury to mammalian spinal cord neurons. *J Neurotrauma* 1996;13:809–818.

40. Faden A, Jacobs T, Zivin J. Comparison of naloxone and a δ-selective antagonist in experimental spinal stroke. *Life Sci* 1983;33:707–710.

41. Zabramski JM, et al. Naloxone therapy during focal cerebral ischemia evaluation in a primate model. *Stroke* 1984;15: 621–626.

42. Acher C, Wynn M. Naloxone and spinal fluid drainage as adjuncts in the surgical treatment of thoracoabdominal aneurysms. *Surgery* 1990;108:755–762.

43. Cernaianu AC, et al. Effect of sodium nitroprusside on paraplegia during cross-clamping of the thoracic aorta [see comments]. *Ann Thorac Surg* 1993;56:1035–1037; discussion 1038.

44. Gelman S, et al. Regional blood flow during cross-clamping of the thoracic aorta and infusion of sodium nitroprusside. *J Thorac Cardiovasc Surg* 1983;85:287–291.

45. Woloszyn TT, et al. Cerebrospinal fluid drainage does not counteract the negative effect of sodium nitroprusside on spinal cord perfusion pressure during aortic cross-clamping. *Curr Surg* 1989;46:489–492.

46. Acher CW, et al. Combined use of cerebral spinal fluid drainage and naloxone reduces the risk of paraplegia in thoracoabdominal aneurysm repair. *J Vasc Surg* 1994;19: 236–246; discussion 247–248.

47. Acher CW, Wynn MM. Multifactorial nature of spinal cord circulation. *Semin Thorac Cardiovasc Surg* 1998;10:7–10.

48. Acher CW, et al. Cardiac function is a risk factor for paralysis in thoracoabdominal aortic replacement. *J Vasc Surg* 1998;27: 821–828; discussion 829–830.

49. Fehrenbacher JW, et al. One-stage segmental resection of extensive thoracoabdominal aneurysms with left-sided heart bypass [see comments]. *J Vasc Surg* 1993;18:366–370; discussion 370–371. Comment appears in *J Vasc Surg* 1994;20: 157–158.

50. Kouchoukos NT, Rokkas CK. Hypothermic cardiopulmonary bypass for spinal cord protection: rationale and clinical results. *Ann Thorac Surg* 1999;67:1940–1942; discussion 1953–1958.

51. Jacobs M, et al. Strategies to prevent neurologic deficit based on motor-evoked potentials in type I and II thoracoabdominal aortic aneurysm repair. *J Vasc Surg* 1999;29:48–57; discussion 57–59.

52. Godet G, et al. Risk factors for acute postoperative renal failure in thoracic or thoracoabdominal aortic surgery: a prospective study. *Anesth Analg* 1997;85:1227–1232.

53. Leijdekkers VJ, et al. The visceral perfusion system and distal bypass during thoracoabdominal aneurysm surgery: an alternative for physiological blood flow? *Cardiovasc Surg* 1999;7: 219–224.

54. Svensson LG, et al. Appraisal of adjuncts to prevent acute renal failure after surgery on the thoracic or thoracoabdominal aorta. *J Vasc Surg* 1989;10:230–239.

55. Jacobs MJ, et al. Reduced renal failure following thoracoabdominal aortic aneurysm repair by selective perfusion. *Eur J Cardiothorac Surg* 1998;14:201–205.

56. Bachet J, et al. Protection of the spinal cord during surgery of thoracoabdominal aortic aneurysms. *Eur J Cardiothorac Surg* 1996;10:817–825.

57. Crawford ES, et al. The impact of distal aortic perfusion and somatosensory evoked potential monitoring on prevention of paraplegia after aortic aneurysm operation. *J Thorac Cardiovasc Surg* 1988;95:357–367. Published erratum appears in *J Thorac Cardiovasc Surg* 1989;97:665.

58. de Mol B, et al. Assessment of risk factors for spinal cord ischaemia in surgery of thoracoabdominal aneurysms without use of adjuncts. *Eur J Cardiothorac Surg* 1989;3:449–454; discussion 455.

59. Fox AD, Berkowitz HD. Thoracoabdominal aneurysm resec-

tion after previous infrarenal abdominal aortic aneurysmectomy. *Am J Surg* 1991;162:142–144.

60. Frank SM, et al. Moderate hypothermia with partial bypass and segmental sequential repair for thoracoabdominal aortic aneurysm [see comments]. *J Vasc Surg* 1994;19:687–697.

61. Galla JD, et al. Identification of risk factors in patients undergoing thoracoabdominal aneurysm repair. *J Card Surg* 1997; 12[2 Suppl]:292–299.

62. Gilling-Smith GL, et al. Surgical repair of thoracoabdominal aortic aneurysm: 10 years' experience. *Br J Surg* 1995;82: 624–629.

63. Girardi LN, Coselli JS. Repair of thoracoabdominal aortic aneurysms in octogenarians. *Ann Thorac Surg* 1998;65: 491–495.

64. Golden MA, et al. Evolving experience with thoracoabdominal aortic aneurysm repair at a single institution. *J Vasc Surg* 1991;13:792–796; discussion 796–797.

65. Grabitz K, et al. The risk of ischemic spinal cord injury in patients undergoing graft replacement for thoracoabdominal aortic aneurysms. *J Vasc Surg* 1996;23:230–240.

66. Hollier LH, Moore WM. Avoidance of renal and neurologic complications following thoracoabdominal aortic aneurysm repair. *Acta Chir Scand Suppl* 1990;555:129–135.

67. Jacobs MJ, Myhre HO, Norgren L. Thoracoabdominal aortic surgery with special reference to spinal cord protection and perfusion techniques. "Second Nordic Workshop Group." *Eur J Vasc Endovasc Surg* 1999;17:253–256.

68. Jacobs MJ, et al. Retrograde aortic and selective organ perfusion during thoracoabdominal aortic aneurysm repair. *Eur J Vasc Endovasc Surg* 1997;14:360–366.

69. Jensen BF, Baekgaard N, Laustsen J. Thoracoabdominal aortic aneurysms: treatment, complications, and early results. *Ugeskr Laeger* 1995;157:2008–2011.

70. Kazui T, et al. Total graft replacement of the thoracoabdominal aorta with reconstruction of visceral branches and intercostal and lumbar arteries in expanding chronic dissecting aneurysms of the thoracoabdominal aorta. *Nippon Kyobu Geka Gakkai Zasshi (J Jpn Assoc Thorac Surg)* 1989;37: 1436–1440.

71. Kieffer E. Surgical treatment of aneurysms of the thoracoabdominal aorta. *Revue du Praticien* 1991;41:1793–1797.

72. Kouchoukos NT, et al. Hypothermic bypass and circulatory arrest for operations on the descending thoracic and thoracoabdominal aorta. *Ann Thorac Surg* 1995;60:67–76; discussion 76–77.

73. Lord RS. Complex abdominal and thoracoabdominal aortic aneurysm reconstruction. *Surg Today* 1995;25:99–106.

74. Murray MJ, et al. Effects of cerebrospinal fluid drainage in patients undergoing thoracic and thoracoabdominal aortic surgery. *J Cardiothorac Vasc Anesth* 1993;7:266–272.

75. Pokela R, et al. Surgical and long-term outcome of graft replacement of aneurysms of the descending thoracic aorta—analysis of 28 consecutive cases. *Scand Cardiovasc J* 1997; 31:141–145.

76. Pokela R, et al. Outcome of thoracoabdominal aortic aneurysm surgery: analysis of 27 consecutive cases. *Ann Chir Gynaecol* 1995;84:18–23.

77. Safi HJ, et al. Impact of distal aortic and visceral perfusion on liver function during thoracoabdominal and descending thoracic aortic repair. *J Vasc Surg* 1998;27:145–152; discussion 152–153.

78. Schwartz LB, et al. Improvement in results of repair of type IV thoracoabdominal aortic aneurysms. *J Vasc Surg* 1996; 24:74–81.

79. Schmidt CA, et al. Surgery for thoracoabdominal aortic aneurysms. *Am Surg* 1990;56:745–748.

80. Shiiya N, et al. Spinal cord protection during thoracoabdominal aortic aneurysm repair: results of selective reconstruction of the critical segmental arteries guided by evoked spinal cord potential monitoring. *J Vasc Surg* 1995;21:970–975.

81. Vaccaro PS, Elkhammas E, Smead WL. Clinical observations and lessons learned in the treatment of patients with thoracoabdominal aortic aneurysms. *Surg Gynecol Obstet* 1988; 166:461–465.

82. Williams GM. Treatment of chronic expanding dissecting aneurysms of the descending thoracic and upper abdominal aorta by extended aortotomy, removal of the dissected intima,
and closure. *J Vasc Surg* 1993;18:441–448; discussion 448–449.

83. Wojewski PA. Spinal cord protection during thoracoabdominal aneurysm resection. *J Thorac Cardiovasc Surg* 1995; 109:1244–1246.

84. Comerota AJ. Thoracoabdominal aneurysm repair: perspectives over a decade with the clamp-and-sew technique—discussion. *Ann Surg* 1997;226:304.

85. Harward TR, et al. Visceral ischemia and organ dysfunction after thoracoabdominal aortic aneurysm repair: a clinical and cost analysis. *Ann Surg* 1996;223:729–734; discussion 734–736.

86. Mauney MC, et al. Is clamp and sew still viable for thoracic aortic resection? *Ann Surg* 1996;223:534–540; discussion 540–543.

87. Bavaria JE, et al. Retrograde cerebral and distal aortic perfusion during ascending and thoracoabdominal aortic operations. *Ann Thorac Surg* 1995;60:345–352; discussion 352–353.

SURGERY: SCIENTIFIC PRINCIPLES AND PRACTICE, Third Edition, edited by Lazar J. Greenfield, Michael W. Mulholland, Keith T. Oldham, Gerald B. Zelenock, and Keith D. Lillemoe. Lippincott Williams & Wilkins Publishers, Philadelphia, © 2001.

CHAPTER 86

ABDOMINAL AORTIC ANEURYSMS

THOMAS S. HUBER, C. KEITH OZAKI, AND JAMES M. SEEGER

Abdominal aortic aneurysms are a common problem in developed countries and represent a significant public health risk. Operative repair is the only accepted means to reduce the risk for rupture and the associated mortality, and the treatment algorithm represents a balance between the estimated risk of operation and the future risk for rupture. The standard operative technique has been refined during the past five decades since the first successful aneurysm resection in 1951 by Dubost et al. (1). The 1990s have witnessed the rapid development of endovascular techniques to repair abdominal aortic aneurysms, culminating in the release of two devices approved by the Food and Drug Administration in late 1999. The introduction of these commercially available endografts has led to their widespread application, although their indications and long-term durability remain undefined.

DEFINITIONS AND CLASSIFICATIONS

An aneurysm is defined as a permanent, focal dilation of an artery in which the diameter is increased to 1.5 times the normal, expected diameter (2). The diameter of a normal abdominal aorta in a male adult is approximately 2 cm (range, 1.4 to 3.0 cm) (3), and therefore a 3-cm aorta would be considered aneurysmal. The abdominal aorta is consistently larger in men than in women and increases slightly in size with age in both sexes (4). Abdominal aortic aneurysms should be differentiated from other conditions in which the size of the aorta is increased, including ectasia and arteriomegaly. In aortic *ectasia,* the diameter is increased by less than 50% of the normal expected diameter. The term *arteriomegaly* refers to a diffuse (nonfocal) enlargement of several arterial segments, with increases in diameter greater than 50% of the normal expected diameter. Arterial segments in patients with arteriomegaly may be considered aneurysmal if the diameter of a segment is increased by more than 50% of the diameter of an adjacent segment. The term *aneurysmosis* denotes the presence of multiple aneurysmal segments separated by either normal, occluded, or arteriomegalic segments.

Abdominal aortic aneurysms are classified primarily according to how far they extend proximally (Fig. 86.1). More than 95% of all abdominal aortic aneurysms are classified as infrarenal (5). These aneurysms start below the takeoff of the orifices of the renal arteries and usually have a 1.5- to 2-cm normal infrarenal aortic cuff. Approximately 10% to 20% of all abdominal aortic aneurysms are associated with aneurysms of the iliac arteries—the common iliac, internal iliac, and external iliac vessels, in decreasing order of frequency (6,7). The management of abdominal aortic aneurysms associated with common iliac artery aneurysms is identical to the management of abdominal aortic aneurysms alone, and these two patterns should be considered basically the same disease process. The only significant difference in the decision algorithm is the configuration of the graft (tube vs. bifurcated) and the site of the distal anastomoses. Aneurysms classified as

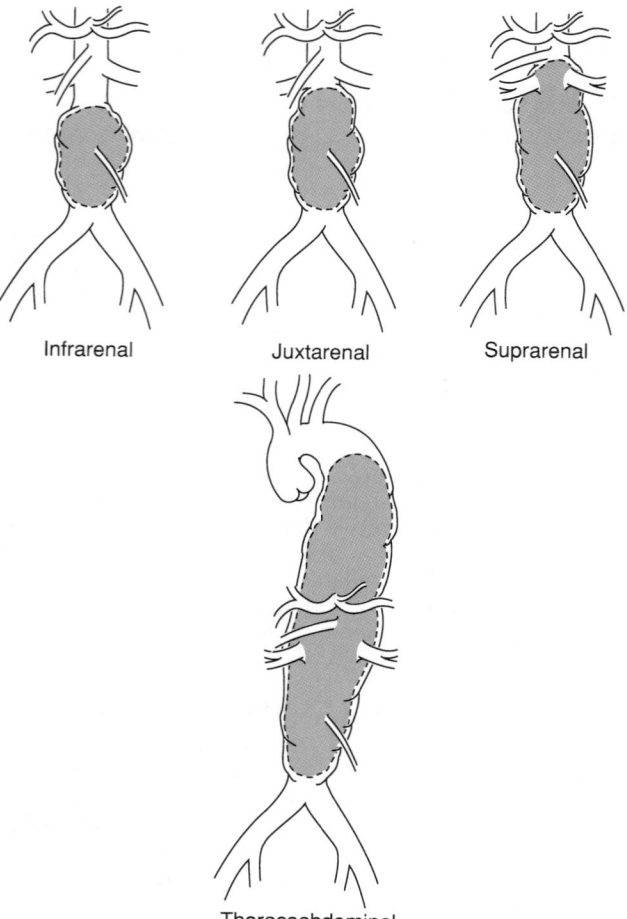

Figure 86.1. Classification of abdominal aortic aneurysms. More than 95% of all abdominal aortic aneurysms are infrarenal. Juxtarenal aneurysms extend proximally to the level of the renal arteries, and suprarenal aneurysms to the level of the superior mesenteric and/or celiac arteries. Aneurysms involving the thoracic and abdominal portions of the aorta are designated as thoracoabdominal aortic aneurysms and are classified as types 1 through 4 according to how far they extend proximally and distally.

juxtarenal extend proximally to the level of the renal arteries, and those classified as suprarenal extend proximally to the level of the superior mesenteric and/or celiac arteries. Aneurysms involving the thoracic and abdominal aorta are designated as thoracoabdominal aortic aneurysms and are classified (types 1 through 4) according to how far they extend proximally and distally. Unlike common iliac and abdominal aortic aneurysms, aneurysms that extend proximally above the renal arteries significantly affect the operative indications, operative approach, and outcome, as might be predicted from the obligatory periods of renal and mesenteric ischemia associated with repair.

MAGNITUDE OF THE PROBLEM

Abdominal aortic aneurysms and their sequelae are common problems in developed countries. The incidence of abdominal aortic aneurysms in the United States ranges from 1.5% in autopsy series to 3.2% among unselected adult patients screened with ultrasonography (5). Predictably, the incidence increases among subsets of patients with defined risk factors for abdominal aortic aneurysms and approximates 50% among patients with either femoral or popliteal aneurysms (5). It should be emphasized that these rates have been determined with use of the broad definition of an aneurysm provided above (1.5 times the normal vessel diameter) and do not necessarily reflect aneurysms that are of sufficient size to require repair. Furthermore, the apparently increasing incidence of abdominal aortic aneurysms likely represents an increase in the number of cases detected (8,9). This is supported by the observation that the incidence of small aneurysms (< 5 cm in diameter) has increased 10-fold during the past several years, whereas the incidence of large aneurysms (> 7 cm in diameter), which are more easily detected, has increased only twofold to threefold (8). Approximately 8,700 deaths caused by abdominal aortic aneurysms were reported by the National Center for Health Statistics in 1990 (10). These figures correspond to an incidence of death of 0.8% among men and of 0.3% among women. The numbers are likely underestimates because a significant number of sudden deaths in elderly patients may be secondary to undiagnosed ruptured aneurysms.

PATHOGENESIS AND RISK FACTORS

The pathogenesis of abdominal aortic aneurysms remains unresolved, although it is an intense area of both experimental and clinical investigation. Multiple potential etiologic factors have been implicated, including atherosclerotic degeneration (11), hemodynamic changes (12), disorders of collagen (13) and collagenase (14), disorders of elastin (15) and elastase (16), abnormalities of metalloproteinases (17) and protease inhibitors (18), programmed cell death (apoptosis) (19), and inflammatory mediators (20). Unfortunately, investigation into the potential mechanisms has not resulted in new therapeutic strategies. Elucidation of the pathogenesis has been complicated by the older age of patients at presentation and the absence of suitable animal models.

Multiple risk factors have been identified for the development of abdominal aortic aneurysms and include age, sex, smoking history, hypertension, hyperlipidemia, and family history (21). Identification of these risk factors is important to facilitate screening high-risk patient populations and potentially initiating treatment earlier. Abdominal aortic aneurysms are a disease process of the elderly and are rare among persons less than 50 years of age. Indeed, the mean age among patients undergoing repair across the country was 72 ± 7 years (± SD) in a recent series comprising a 20% national sample (22). The incidence of death resulting from abdominal aortic aneurysms for men between 60 and 64 years of age is 11-fold higher than that for women of the same age (23). However, the incidence is only threefold greater for men between 85 and 90 years of age than for women of the same age (23). Similar sex-related differences have been reported from community (24) and national (21) screening studies for abdominal aortic aneurysms. Furthermore, men account for approximately 80% of all abdominal aortic aneurysm repairs performed nationally (22). The Aneurysm Detection and Management (ADAM) Veterans Affairs Cooperative Study Group (21) reported that smoking was the strongest risk factor associated with abdominal aortic aneurysms larger than 4 cm (odds ratio, 5.57; 95% confidence interval, 4.24 to 7.31) among the 73,451 veterans screened. Similarly, Wilmink et al. (25) reported that abdominal aneurysms were 7.6 times (95% confidence interval, 3.3 to 17.8) more likely to develop in current smokers than in nonsmokers, and that the duration of smoking rather than level of exposure appeared to correlate with the development of aneurysms. Johansen and Koepsell (26) reported the incidence of abdominal aortic aneurysms to be 19.2% among first-degree relatives of patients with aneurysms, but only 2.4% among first-degree relatives of control patients with atherosclerosis of the abdominal aorta. Similarly, Darling et al. (27) prospectively analyzed patients undergoing repair of abdominal aortic aneurysms and reported that 15.1% had a first-degree relative with an abdominal aortic aneurysm, in contrast to 1.8% of the control group. Interestingly, having a female family member with an aneurysm correlated with an increased risk for rupture. Based on these latter reports, its is recommended that all first-degree relatives (children, parents, siblings) of patients with abdominal aortic aneurysms be screened with ultrasonography at 50 years of age.

The presence of an aneurysm in the aorta, iliac, femoral, or popliteal arteries dramatically increases the risk for development of a new or additional abdominal aortic aneurysm. In patients undergoing abdominal aortic or iliac artery aneurysm repair, the chance that an additional aneurysm will eventually develop in either the aorta or iliac vessels and merit intervention is approximately 5% to 15% (28,29). The second aneurysm may develop anywhere in the remaining native aorta, commonly within the residual infrarenal aortic cuff. It is recommended that patients undergoing repair of an abdominal aortic aneurysm be evaluated with computed tomography (CT) of the chest, abdomen, and pelvis either 5 years after repair if no additional aneurysms are detected during the preoperative evaluation or sooner, as dictated by the size of the unrepaired aneurysm. Similarly, the incidence of aneurysms in the abdominal aorta or iliac vessels in patients with popliteal or femoral artery aneurysms is approximately 50% (5). All patients found to have a peripheral artery aneurysm should undergo CT of the entire aorta and iliac vessels to rule out a synchronous aneurysm. Interestingly, the reverse scenario is not true; patients with an abdominal aortic or iliac aneurysm have a less than 5% chance of having a peripheral artery aneurysm, and evaluation beyond physical examination is not justified (30).

The incidence of abdominal aortic aneurysm is increased among patients with an aortic dissection and among patients with heart transplants. Late or repeated operations are required in approximately 20% of patients by 10 years after an acute aortic dissection (31). Aneurysms may develop in either the thoracic or abdominal aorta after a dissection, although the former site is more commonly affected. The term *dissecting aneurysm* is frequently used although it is a misnomer; dissection and aneurysm are separate processes. Simply, a dissection is a tear within the aortic wall itself that extends for a variable length and is frequently associated with multiple entry and reentry points that may lead to both a "true" and "false" lumen. The prevalence of abdominal aortic aneurysms and the rate of expansion are both increased among heart transplant patients (32,33). The responsible mechanisms remain unclear, but the obligatory chronic immunosuppression may contribute. Interestingly, several transplant centers have initiated screening programs as part of the evaluation preceding transplant.

It is notable that the risk factors for abdominal aortic aneurysm are similar to those associated with the development of atherosclerosis. Furthermore, atherosclerotic changes are found almost universally within the abdominal aorta at the time of repair. However, the processes of atherosclerosis and aneurysmal degeneration are likely separate and distinct. Simplistically, atherosclerosis is a process that leads to a narrowing of the vessel lumen, whereas aneurysmal degeneration leads to dilation. Aneurysms have historically been referred to as *atherosclerotic aneurysms,* although this is likely a misnomer that has been appropriately replaced by the term *nonspecific aneurysms.*

PRINCIPLES OF MANAGEMENT

The treatment goals for patients with abdominal aortic aneurysm are to prolong life, relieve symptoms, and prevent rupture. Because surgical treatment is the only effective means to achieve these goals, the crucial question that must be answered is whether the patient should undergo operative repair. The decision algorithm is straightforward for patients with ruptured or symptomatic aneurysms, but more difficult for patients with asymptomatic, intact aneurysms. The decision to recommend operative intervention in the elective setting is contingent on the balance between the risk of operation and the risk of expectant or nonoperative management. Appropriate assessment of these risks requires an understanding of the size-associated risk for rupture, the growth rate, and the mortality associated with repair. However, it should be emphasized that operative repair of an asymptomatic, intact aneurysm is a prophylactic procedure.

Understanding the natural history of untreated abdominal aortic aneurysm requires knowledge of the physics associated with the vessel wall. The tangential stress (τ) of a fluid-filled cylindric tube is determined by the following equation:

$$\tau = Pr/\delta$$

where P is the pressure exerted by the blood (dyne/cm^2), r is the internal radius (cm), and δ is the thickness (cm) of the arterial wall (34). The tangential stress of a cylinder 0.2 cm thick with an internal radius of 0.8 cm and a fluid pressure of 150 mm Hg would be 8×10^5 dyne/cm^2 (Fig. 86.2). An increase in the internal radius (diameter) of the cylinder to 2.94 cm and a concomitant decrease in the wall thickness, as might occur with an aneurysm, would increase the tangential stress to 98×10^5 dyne/cm^2. Thus, a threefold increase in diameter would result in a 12-fold increase in tangential stress. Aneurysms rupture when the tangential stress exceeds the tensile strength of the vessel wall. This dramatic increase in tangential stress along with the radius of the vessel likely explains why large aneurysms are more likely to rupture. It should be reemphasized that the tangential stress varies directly with the radius of the cylinder (vessel) but is independent of its length.

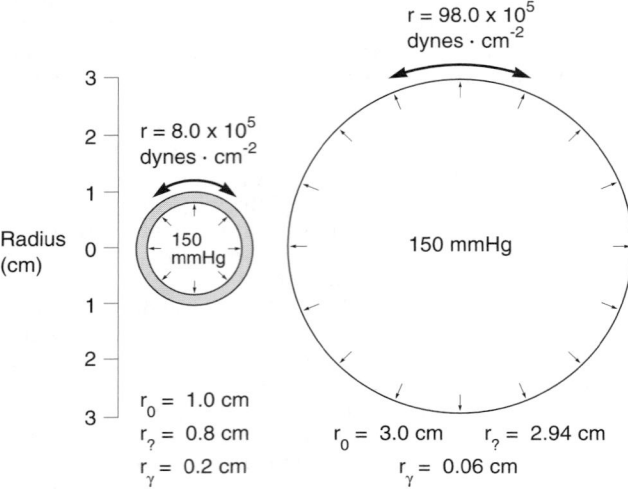

Figure 86.2. Cross-sectional view of a 2-cm-diameter cylinder that expands to a diameter of 6 cm while wall cross-sectional area remains constant. τ, wall stress; δ, wall thickness; r_i, inside radius; r_o, outside radius. Expansion of a 1-cm-diameter cylinder to a diameter of 3 cm with no change in wall cross-sectional area increases wall tensile stress 12-fold.

The risk for rupture of an abdominal aortic aneurysm is related to its diameter, as would be predicted by the tangential stress of the vessel wall. Other factors, including chronic obstructive pulmonary disease and hypertension, have been reported to affect the risk for rupture (35). Additionally, it is possible that large aneurysms incite a greater inflammatory response that increases the rupture risk. The diameter of the aneurysm used to estimate the rupture risk is determined by measuring the greatest diameter from outer wall to outer wall in any orientation (i.e., anterior to posterior, transverse) throughout the extent of the aneurysm. These measurements may occasionally be confounded by a tortuous aneurysm, so every attempt should be made to obtain a cross-sectional measurement perpendicular to the longitudinal axis of the aneurysm. A recent collective review reported the annual rupture risk to be 4.1% for aneurysms 5 cm in diameter, 6.6% for those between 5 to 7 cm in diameter, and 19% for those 7 cm in diameter (5). These data may be simplified by using the rule of thumb that the annual rupture risk is 5% for a 5-cm aneurysm, 10% for a 6-cm aneurysm, and 20% for a 7-cm aneurysm. Notably, these numbers correspond to an estimated rupture risk during 5 years of 25% for aneurysms 5 cm in diameter, 50% for those 6 cm in diameter, and 100% for those 7 cm in diameter. The annual risk for rupture with aneurysms less than 5 cm in diameter is small, although finite. The few available reports have estimated that the 5-year rupture risk for aneurysms between 4 to 5 cm is between 3% and 12% (36–38).

The natural history of abdominal aortic aneurysm is an increase in diameter with time. An estimated 80% of all small aneurysms continue to grow (2). The mean rate of growth has varied from 0.2 cm/y in population studies (39,40) to 0.4 cm/y in referral practices (41–43), with the latter figure (0.4 cm/y) generally quoted as a reasonable estimate. It should be emphasized that these growth rates are mean values, and that all aneurysms do not grow in a linear fashion, as might be predicted. The growth curve may be somewhat erratic, with no growth detected during four consecutive 6-month intervals, then 0.6 cm of growth during the next 6-month period. Furthermore, it should be emphasized that the past rate of growth does not predict

future events, and patients should not be lulled into a false sense of security if their aneurysm is relatively stable over time or is not repaired because recent growth has been to a size still below the usual criterion for repair.

The mortality rate associated with repair of an abdominal aortic aneurysm primarily depends on the status (intact/asymptomatic, intact/symptomatic, ruptured) of the aneurysm. A recent study reported the mortality rate in more than 15,000 repairs of intact abdominal aortic aneurysms in the United States to be 4.2% (22). Predictably, the operative mortality rate increased with age, ranging from 2.2% among persons 50 to 59 years old to 9.2% among those older than 80 years. Interestingly, the operative mortality rate was significantly higher among women (6.1% vs. 3.7%). The overall mortality rate in the nationwide series corresponds closely to the rate (4.0%) reported in several large series originating predominantly from academic institutions (2). However, a moderate variability is noted for the reported operative mortality rates of intact aneurysms historically, with values ranging from less than 4% among the best individual series to approximately 10% among the state and community series (5,44). Furthermore, a recent multiple-institution, randomized, controlled trial of operative versus nonoperative management of intact/asymptomatic aneurysms between 4.0 to 5.5 cm in size reported a 30-day operative mortality rate of 5.8% (45). Additionally, the operative mortality rate for elective aneurysm repair does not appear to be different when the results of open surgical repair are compared with results obtained with the newer endovascular techniques in initial clinical trials for the various devices (46–51). However, the worldwide experience with endovascular repair is still relatively small, and most series of endovascular repair have included patients deemed to be at increased risk with open surgical repair. The operative mortality rate for intact/symptomatic aneurysms among patients undergoing emergent repair is approximately 20% (5). Various explanations have been proposed for this increased mortality rate relative to that for intact/asymptomatic aneurysms, including failure to maximize preoperative medical conditions, increased incidence of inadvertent venous injuries, and less experienced operative teams, although the true explanation remains unclear. It is notable that the increased rate has been fairly consistent in the literature, in contrast to the mortality rate for intact/asymptomatic aneurysms, which has decreased gradually (52).

The actual mortality rate for ruptured abdominal aortic aneurysms is somewhat difficult to determine because a significant number of sudden deaths in elderly patients are likely secondary to ruptured aneurysms, as noted above. It has been estimated that 50% of all patients with ruptured abdominal aortic aneurysms die before reaching the hospital, and that approximately 50% of those who actually undergo surgery die (5). These figures correspond to an overall mortality rate of approximately 80%, although this may be an underestimate. It is remarkable that the optimization of preoperative care, including the component carried out before hospitalization, and a reduction in the mean time for the patient to be taken from the emergency department to the operating room to 12 minutes have resulted in comparable mortality rates for ruptured aneurysms (53). Furthermore, the operative mortality rate for patients with a ruptured abdominal aortic aneurysm has remained relatively stable during the past few decades (54).

The size at which repair of an intact/asymptomatic abdominal aortic aneurysm is justified is somewhat controversial. During the past few decades, the diameter at which repair is recommended for good-risk patients has decreased steadily from 6 cm to 5 cm. Furthermore, the Joint Council of the Society for Vascular Surgery and the

North American Chapter of the International Society for Cardiovascular Surgery (55) and others (56) have proposed repairing all aneurysms larger than 4 cm. Those who advocate repairing small aneurysms (< 5 cm) have justified their approach based on the fact that the natural history of an abdominal aortic aneurysm is to increase over time while the patient's operative risk increases. Indeed, approximately 75% of the patients in the U.K. Small Aneurysm Trial randomized to ultrasonographic surveillance ultimately underwent repair (45). Furthermore, the operative mortality for the repair of small, intact/asymptomatic aneurysms is low in experienced centers, and survival is presumably improved after aneurysm repair. Additionally, small aneurysms occasionally rupture, although the risk is not very great. Darling et al. (57) reported that 34 of 265 (12.8%) unresected aneurysms smaller than 4 cm and 34% of those between 4 to 5 cm were ruptured at autopsy. Although intriguing, their study was limited by the difficulty of sizing aneurysms accurately in the postmortem state and the relative infrequency of autopsy. The results of the U.K. Small Aneurysm Trial did not support their aggressive approach, as no survival benefit was noted at 6 years for the repair of aneurysms between 4.0 and 5.5 cm (45). Interestingly, the U.K. Small Aneurysm Trial has been criticized for an operative mortality rate of 5.8%. Schermerhorn et al. (58) incorporated the results of the trial into a decision analysis and concluded to the contrary that early surgery is cost-effective for small aneurysms (4.0 to 5.5 cm) in selected patients (low operative risk, younger age, and larger aneurysm).

CLINICAL PRESENTATION AND DIAGNOSIS

The overwhelming majority of abdominal aortic aneurysms are asymptomatic at the time they are discovered. Most aneurysms are detected not during physical examination but rather during abdominal and pelvic imaging studies, such as ultrasonography and CT, performed for other indications (e.g., chronic back pain, renal cysts). Indeed, it is often difficult to feel an abdominal aortic aneurysm on physical examination, even when a concerted effort is made, because of its anatomic location in the posterior abdomen, and these difficulties are exacerbated by the frequent presence of truncal obesity. The accuracy of primary care physicians in detecting abdominal aortic aneurysms in patients with known aneurysms is only fair because of the limitations noted above and the failure to evaluate the aorta during the routine physical examination (59–61). Intact abdominal aortic and iliac artery aneurysms may present with symptoms that lead to further investigation and the correct diagnosis. Enlargement of the aneurysm may cause vertebral erosion and chronic back pain. Additionally, thrombosis of an abdominal aortic aneurysm may cause acute ischemia in the lower torso, and aneurysms may be a source of arterial macroemboli or microemboli that cause acute ischemia of a lower extremity or digital atheroemboli, respectively.

Patients with intact/symptomatic or ruptured aneurysms present with abdominal or back pain related to the aneurysm itself. The cause of the pain is unclear, but the pain may be secondary to local nerve compression. The character of the pain is variable and ranges from dull to sharp and knifelike. The pain is usually acute in onset and persistent. It may be superimposed on more chronic abdominal or back pain, but the presentation is usually not subtle, and the pain can be differentiated from more chronic complaints. Additionally, the pain may radiate from the abdomen to the back, flank, inguinal region, or genitalia. Approximately 10% of patients with ruptured abdominal aortic aneurysms present with signs and symptoms similar to those of ureteral colic or other acute urologic problems (62). Indeed, the diagnosis of a ruptured aneurysm must be ruled out in a timely fashion in patients presenting with testicular pain who have normal results on both urinalysis and testicular examination.

The presentation of a patients with a ruptured abdominal aortic aneurysm may range from hemodynamic stability to class 4 shock. The hemodynamic status at the time of presentation depends on how effectively tissues adjacent to the aorta tamponade the bleeding and on the patient's physiologic status and ability to withstand acute hemorrhage. If the adjacent tissues effectively tamponade the bleeding, the patient may present in a hemodynamically stable state with essentially normal vital signs. However, it should be emphasized that this is usually a temporary situation, and health care providers should not be lulled into a false sense of security. A ruptured abdominal aortic aneurysm is a true medical emergency that requires immediate operative repair regardless of the patient's hemodynamic status. Furthermore, the vital signs may be misleading because patients can lose up to 15% of their blood volume (class 1 shock) without any appreciable change in their pulse rate or blood pressure. Patients with free intraperitoneal ruptures likely exsanguinate quickly and do not survive long enough to seek medical attention.

Patients with a ruptured abdominal aortic aneurysm may present with either an aortoenteric fistula or an aortocaval fistula, although both are relatively rare. Those with an aortoenteric fistula present with intestinal bleeding that may be massive. The aorta may rupture through any portion of the bowel, although the duodenum and proximal small bowel are the most common sites. Primary aortoenteric fistulae are far less common than the secondary aortoenteric fistulae that result from erosion of a prosthetic aortic graft into the adjacent bowel. However, the diagnosis of an aortoenteric fistula must be ruled out in all patients with gastrointestinal bleeding and either an abdominal aortic aneurysm or a previous aortic reconstruction. Patients with an aortocaval fistula present with high-output congestive heart failure, a continuous abdominal bruit, and edema of the lower extremities. The severity of the heart failure symptoms depends on the size of the communication between the aorta and vena cava and the magnitude of the systemic shunt.

Several imaging studies are available to establish or confirm the diagnosis of an abdominal aortic aneurysm. Indeed, the introduction of endovascular techniques for aneurysm repair has resulted in an evolution of imaging techniques. The generic goals for imaging patients with an abdominal aortic aneurysm are to establish the diagnosis, determine the presence of rupture, determine the proximal and distal extent of the aneurysm, appropriately size the aneurysm and adjacent vessels for possible stent graft selection, screen for other visceral pathology, and screen for the presence of anatomic variants that would complicate operative repair, such as a left-sided vena cava or a horseshoe kidney. No imaging study is ideal for every application, and it is imperative to understand the strengths and weaknesses of the various tests to select the most appropriate for the specific clinical question.

Both plain radiographs of the abdomen and barium enemas have historically been used to diagnose abdominal aortic aneurysms. The aortic wall is frequently calcified, and a rim of calcification in the characteristic configuration of an aneurysm can occasionally be detected on these studies. However, their sensitivity for detecting an abdominal aortic aneurysm is only fair, and they should not be used for this purpose because better imaging studies are available. They have no role in the evaluation of a patient with a potential ruptured abdominal aortic aneurysm and are actually detrimental because of the requisite imaging time and associated delay in diagnosis. However, these studies can be very useful for patients being evaluated for abdominal pain or changes in bowel habits. Furthermore, all patients undergoing either study for whatever reason should be evaluated for the presence of an aneurysm when the images are reviewed.

Abdominal ultrasonography is a safe, simple, and inexpensive means of detecting abdominal aortic aneurysms (Fig. 86.3). In contrast to the other techniques, it does not require the use of ionizing radiation, intravenous contrast, or arterial cannulation, and it is relatively inexpensive. Furthermore, the ultrasonographic units are portable and almost universally available in the hospital setting. The sensitivity of ultrasonography for detecting abdominal aortic aneurysms is good, and the technique is reproducible within 0.3 cm (55). However, the technique is somewhat operator-dependent and potentially confounded by the presence of bowel gas. Ultrasonography can accurately image the infrarenal aorta to the bifurcation but is relatively inaccurate for imaging the portions of the aorta proximal to the renal arteries and distal to the iliac vessels. Furthermore, ultrasonography usually cannot differentiate a ruptured from an intact aneurysm. It is an excellent tool to screen patients at high risk for abdominal aortic aneurysm and to confirm the presence of an aneurysm already suspected based on physical examination findings or the clinical presentation. Furthermore, it is a useful technique to follow patients with small aneurysms (< 4 cm) when the reliability of the exact measurement is not crucial. It should not be used to confirm the diagnosis of a ruptured aneurysm, nor should it be used as the sole imaging study before elective repair because it does not provide a complete image of the aorta and iliac arteries.

Computed tomography overcomes many of the limitations of abdominal ultrasonography and is the current "gold standard" for imaging patients with abdominal aortic aneurysms (Fig. 86.4A). The technique is more expensive than ultrasonography, not as universally available,

and potentially harmful because of the use of ionizing radiation and intravenous contrast agent. However, the allergic response to the contrast may be reduced by administering a steroid preparation, and intravenous contrast may be avoided in patients with compromised renal function, although the quality of the images is less than optimal and the diagnosis of a ruptured aneurysm potentially confounded. CT is very sensitive for detecting both intact and ruptured aneurysms, and the images are reproducible within 0.2 cm (55). The quality of the images has continued to improve with each new generation of scanners, and the image acquisition times have decreased. Currently, it is possible to image the aorta and iliac vessels from the ascending arch to the femoral vessels during a routine aneurysm scan with an image acquisition time of less than 5 minutes. CT is excellent for determining the proximal and distal extent of an aneurysm and detecting involvement of the iliac vessels. It is also the current standard used to determine the suitability of an aneurysm for an endovascular repair. Furthermore, selection of the appropriate endovascular graft is currently based on size measurements obtained from arteriography and CT. However, spiral CT with three-dimensional reconstructions may be sufficient as the sole imaging technique to size endovascular grafts accurately (63,64). Spiral CT is a modification of the standard technique in which a continuous volume of data is obtained rather than interrupted axial images. The three-dimensional reconstructions obtained with this technique permit the aortoiliac segment to be rotated and viewed in any projection. CT is also helpful for detecting other disease or anatomic variants that may affect the operative approach. Specific concerns include the location of the left renal vein and any associated venous anomalies, the location and size of the kidneys, and the characteristics of the aneurysm wall. CT is currently the sole diagnostic test performed before open surgical repair in the majority of cases and the imaging study of choice to confirm or refute the diagnosis of a ruptured abdominal aortic aneurysm when the clinical scenario is such that an imaging study is appropriate. Additionally, CT is the serial imaging study of choice when aneurysms exceed 4 cm and approach the threshold for operative intervention.

Magnetic resonance imaging (MRI) is an alternative to CT. The technique is newer and has not been applied as extensively, but the image quality, sensitivity, and potential advantages relative to ultrasonography are comparable with those of CT. The technology is not as widely available as CT, and most surgeons are less familiar with interpreting the images. A generic contraindication to MRI is the presence of implanted ferrometallic devices (e.g., pacemakers, joints), and the scanning of intubated, critically ill patients is cumbersome, if not prohibitive. One major potential advantage of MRI relative to CT is the potential to differentiate "new" from "old" blood. This has proved beneficial in the rare patient with CT findings that are equivocal for a ruptured abdominal aortic aneurysm.

Arteriography is frequently performed before abdominal aortic aneurysm repair, although it should not be viewed as a diagnostic test. Admittedly, interventional radiologists frequently diagnose abdominal aortic aneurysms during aortogram and runoff studies. However, arteriography simply visualizes the lumen of vessels (i.e., aorta, iliac and femoral arteries). Abdominal aortic aneurysms are frequently filled with laminated thrombus through which runs a more normal-caliber vessel lumen. The "lumenogram" produced by the contrast reflects the patent lumen rather than the "true" lumen and actual size of the aneurysm. Preoperative arteriography in conjunction with CT may be helpful to determine the size of the graft in patients undergoing endovascular aneurysm repair, as noted

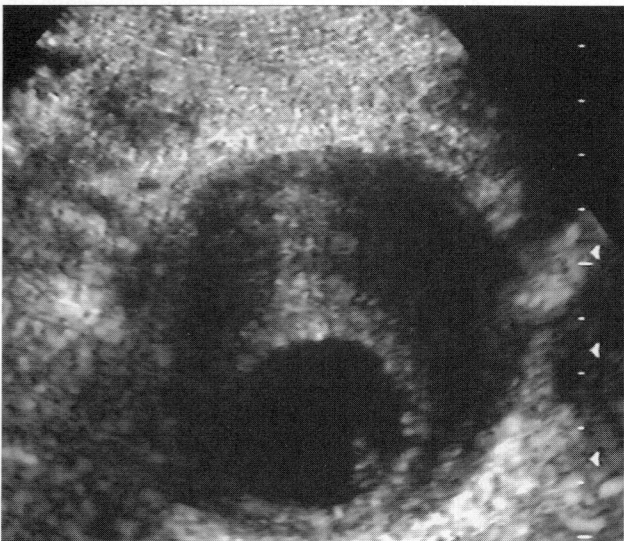

Figure 86.3. B-mode ultrasonogram showing a transverse view of an infrarenal abdominal aortic aneurysm. Note the vessel wall and the large quantity of intraluminal clot surrounding the smaller, blood-filled center *(dark circle)*.

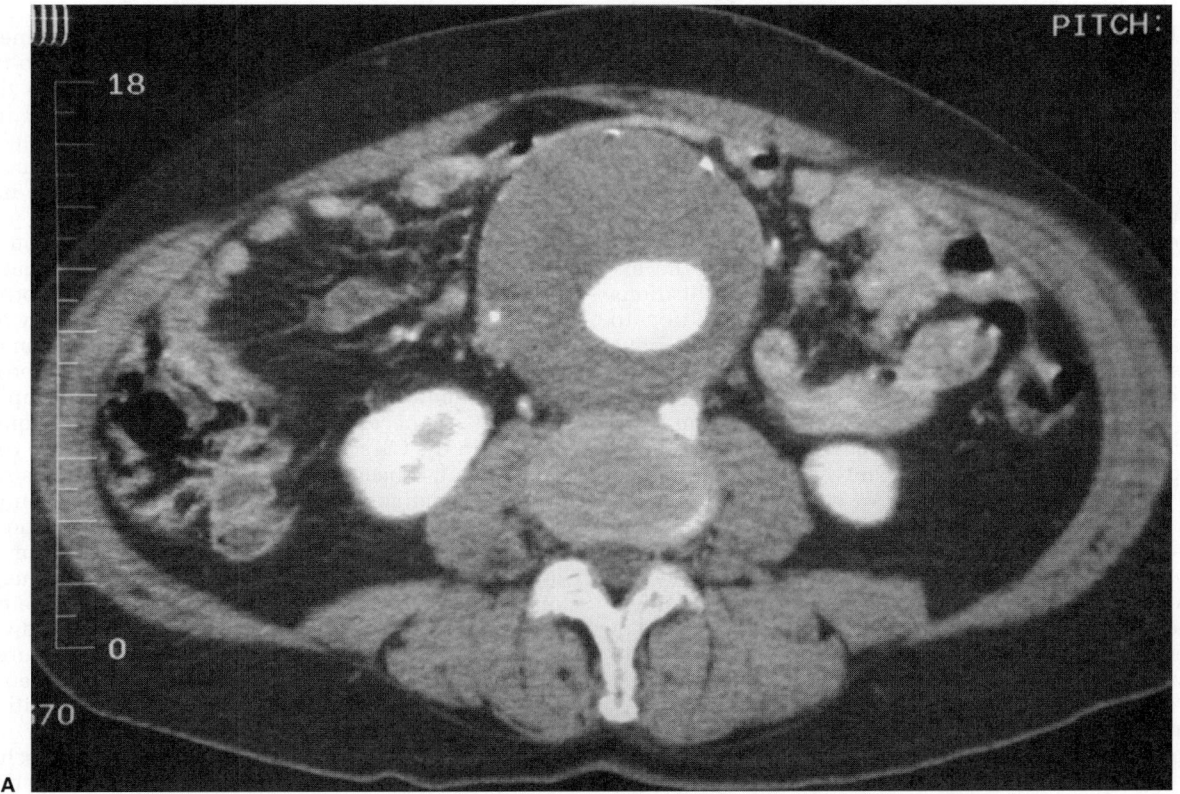

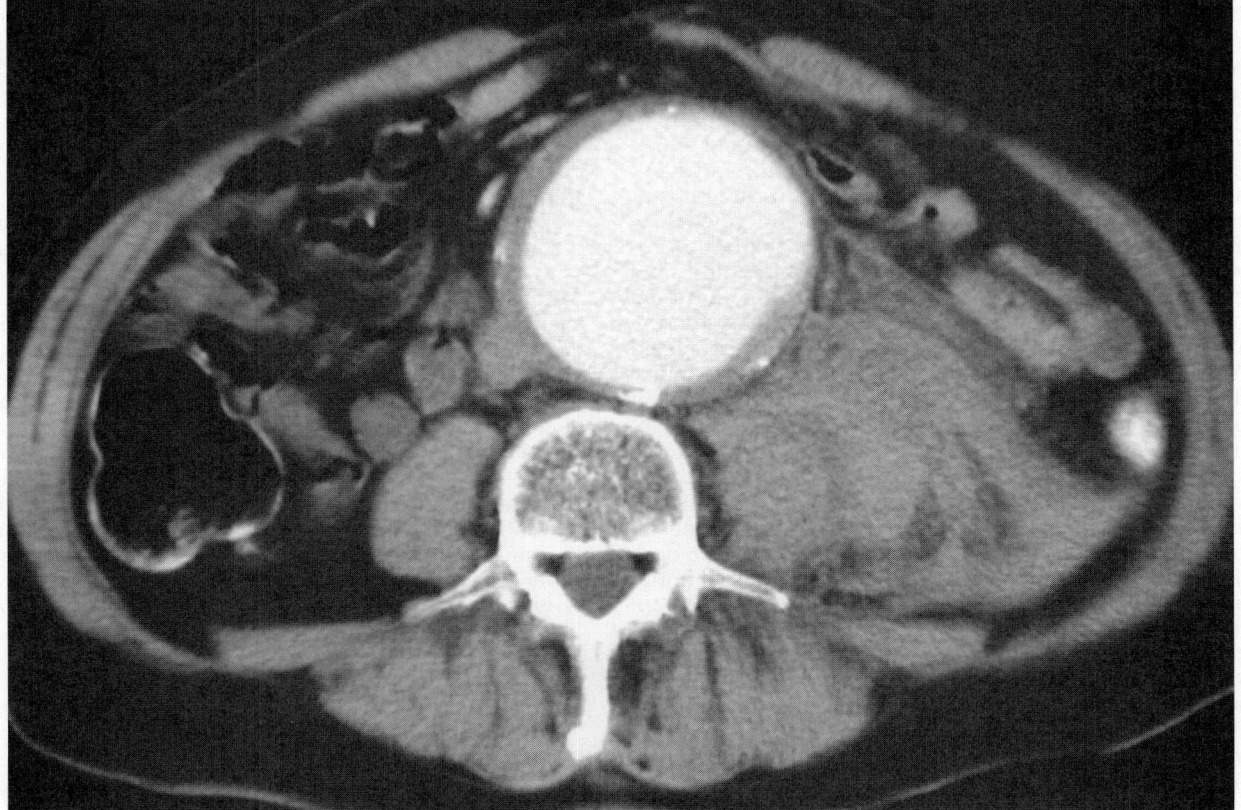

Figure 86.4. Contrast CT of an infrarenal abdominal aortic aneurysm. *(A)* Intact aneurysm. Note the contrast-filled lumen, large quantity of intraluminal clot, and intact vessel wall. *(B)* Ruptured aneurysm. Note the retroperitoneal hematoma and loss of the normal fat planes anterior and lateral to the left psoas muscle.

above. Additionally, preoperative arteriography may be helpful in a subset of patients undergoing standard open repair who have aortoiliac occlusive disease, poorly controlled hypertension or renal insufficiency, symptoms of chronic mesenteric ischemia, and renal anomalies, including horseshoe kidneys. Arteriography is helpful in patients with multiple renal arteries and in those with aneurysms that originate proximal to the renal arteries, although this is only a relative indication. Arteriography is not used routinely for abdominal aortic aneurysm repair because the added information does not justify the expense and risk in most cases. The potential complications include arterial injury and embolization in addition to those associated with the administration of intravenous contrast and ionizing radiation, outlined above.

The diagnostic approach and initial treatment for patients with a potential ruptured abdominal aortic aneurysm merit further comment. Because of the high attendant mortality rate, a prompt diagnosis and emergent repair are required. In a study from the Cleveland Clinic Vascular Registry, the operative mortality rate associated with ruptured abdominal aortic aneurysms increased from 35% when the initial diagnosis was correct to 75% when the diagnosis was incorrect (65). Admittedly, the clinical presentation may be confusing, and delays in diagnosis are not uncommon. The triad of hypotension, abdominal pain, and a pulsatile abdominal mass was present in only 50% of patients with ruptured aneurysms in a single institutional series (66).

Elderly patients who present to the emergency room in a hemodynamically *unstable* state with abdominal or back pain require emergent exploratory laparotomy in most cases. The potential causes of shock (i.e., hypovolemic, cardiogenic, septic, neurogenic) can usually be quickly differentiated by a brief history and physical examination. However, this clinical scenario is most suggestive of hypovolemic or hemorrhagic shock resulting from an intraabdominal catastrophe. The differential diagnosis is extensive and includes mesenteric infarction and rupture of a visceral artery aneurysm in addition to rupture of an abdominal aortic aneurysm, although almost all require operative repair. A myocardial infarction can mimic a ruptured aneurysm in this patient population and potentially confounds the diagnosis, although it can usually be confirmed by the findings on electrocardiogram. Additional diagnostic imaging studies are unnecessary for these hemodynamically unstable patients and only delay the definitive treatment. Admittedly, this approach is associated with a small number of negative exploratory laparotomies, although this is acceptable. It should be emphasized that hemodynamically stable patients who present with abdominal or back pain and become unstable during the course of their evaluation should likewise undergo emergent laparotomy rather than additional imaging studies.

Elderly patients who present to the emergency room in a hemodynamically *stable* state with abdominal or back pain should be evaluated for a ruptured abdominal aortic aneurysm. Admittedly, the differential diagnosis for abdominal or back pain in this patient population is extensive, and the incidence of a ruptured abdominal aortic aneurysm is small. An expeditious history and physical examination can usually determine the cause of the pain. A pulsatile abdominal aortic mass, an unexplained low hematocrit, or hemodynamic instability before presentation are particularly worrisome and increase the level of suspicion. The diagnosis of abdominal aortic aneurysm may be confirmed with a portable abdominal ultrasonogram in the emergency room. Indeed, the newer trauma algorithms include abdominal ultrasonography as a diagnostic technique for blunt trauma, and many centers that care for a significant number of trauma patients have ul-

trasonographic units assigned to the emergency room. If ultrasonography confirms the diagnosis of an aneurysm, further evaluation with CT should be obtained to rule out rupture. Alternatively, CT may be obtained as the sole imaging study without ultrasonography. Several findings on CT are suggestive of a ruptured abdominal aortic aneurysm, including disruption of the calcium ring within the aortic wall or disruption of the aortic margins, retroperitoneal hematomas, mass lesions in the psoas region, displacement of the kidneys, abnormal soft tissues posterior to the aorta, effacement of the normal fat planes between the aorta and adjacent viscera, and abnormal collections of retroperitoneal fluid (Fig. 86.4B). Any of these findings in a patient with an abdominal aortic aneurysm and acute symptoms mandate direct transfer to the operating room and immediate repair. It should be emphasized that it is not necessary to complete the entire sequence of images in the CT scanner once the diagnosis of a ruptured aneurysm has been confirmed. Furthermore, it is not necessary for patients to receive gastrointestinal contrast before CT to rule out a ruptured aneurysm, and the obligatory delay for this preparation is potentially detrimental. If an intact aneurysm is found on CT without any suggestion of rupture, the next logical question is whether the aneurysm is potentially the cause of the pain and whether the scenario is one in which the risk for rupture is increased. Clearly, symptomatic aneurysms represent an increased risk for rupture, as outlined. Patients with symptomatic/intact aneurysms larger than 5 cm in diameter should be admitted to a monitored setting and scheduled for urgent operative repair, usually the following day, provided no additional causes for the pain are identified. Additional causes of the abdominal pain should be sought in patients with aneurysms smaller than 4 cm in light of the small rupture risk. The appropriate treatment for patients with aneurysms between 4 to 5 cm is less clear. These aneurysms have the potential to rupture, although the risk is small. It is recommended that these patients be admitted and additional causes of their abdominal pain sought. However, urgent operative repair is recommended if no additional causes are identified.

The role of screening for abdominal aortic aneurysms in asymptomatic patients remains unresolved. A randomized trial in the United Kingdom of 15,775 men and women reported a 55% reduction in the incidence of rupture among men in the group invited for screening in comparison with the controls (67). However, a position statement by the National Institutes of Health (68) concluded that the evidence is insufficient to recommend for or against routine screening of abdominal aortic aneurysms with either physical examination or ultrasonography. The authors of the National Institutes of Health report did concede that clinicians might elect to screen high-risk patients because of the burden of disease and the availability of surgical treatment. They identified men over 60 years of age with other risk factors, including peripheral vascular disease, a family history of abdominal aortic aneurysms, and a history of smoking, as a high-risk population.

OPERATIVE INDICATIONS

All patients with symptomatic or ruptured abdominal aortic aneurysms should undergo operative repair unless they have an underlying medical condition, such as metastatic cancer, that precludes long-term survival or their quality of life is not sufficient to justify the intervention. The latter situation entails a difficult decision, but not offering operative repair should be considered in certain cases (e.g., a debilitated, demented patient in a nursing home) after the family has been consulted. Good-risk patients with intact, asymptomatic abdominal aortic aneurysms larger than 5 cm should undergo repair provided that their life expectancy exceeds 2 years and they have a reasonably satisfactory quality of life. The size threshold for operative repair in good-risk patients has been debated, as noted above, and is not an absolute number. Operative repair can be considered for good-risk patients with aneurysms larger than 4 cm. Indeed, the size discrepancy between a 4.7-cm and a 5.0-cm aneurysm is small and close to the accuracy of imaging techniques. Patients deemed to be a higher operative risk should undergo repair for aneurysms larger than 6 cm provided that their life expectancy and quality of life are reasonable. However, the estimated operative mortality in these patients must be sufficiently low to be offset by the estimated 10% risk for rupture per year. Admittedly, it is difficult to estimate a patient's operative mortality rate for abdominal aortic aneurysm repair, and no specific algorithms exist. However, thoughtful consideration should be given to the appropriate operative threshold in elderly patients and those with recent myocardial infarction, unstable or rest angina, congestive heart failure or ejection fraction below 35%, chronic renal insufficiency, hepatic insufficiency, or severe chronic obstructive pulmonary disease. Preoperative chronic renal insufficiency represents a very significant risk to patients undergoing abdominal aortic aneurysm repair. In the report of Johnston and Scobie (69) of the Canadian Society of Vascular Surgery Aneurysm Study Group, a creatinine level above 1.8 mg/dL was associated with an increased mortality rate among patients undergoing repair of intact aneurysms. Furthermore, a recent national series reported that the risk for mortality was increased more than than ninefold (odds ratio, 9:5; 95% confidence interval, 7:7 to 11:7) in patients with preoperative renal insufficiency undergoing repair of nonruptured abdominal aortic aneurysms (22). In a subset of patients with overwhelming medical conditions, the risk of repair of an abdominal aortic aneurysm may be too high, regardless of size. A nonoperative approach is appropriate in this small subset of patients. Interestingly, up to 50% of patients deemed to be prohibitive operative risks ultimately die of complications of their aneurysm (70–72). Regardless, these patients who are not candidates for elective repair should not be offered emergent repair in the event that their aneurysm ruptures or becomes symptomatic.

The introduction of endovascular techniques to treat abdominal aortic aneurysms has challenged the standard indications for repair. It has been proposed that the size threshold be decreased in light of the less invasive nature of the treatment and presumed lower complication rate. Admittedly, endovascular treatment has a significant amount of appeal for older, higher-risk patients. However, the reported mortality and complication rates for endovascular repair are comparable with those for the standard technique, although the type and magnitude of the complications may differ (46–51). Finlayson et al. (73) used a decision analysis model to determine the optimal diameter for open and endovascular aneurysm repair and concluded that the endovascular approach lowers the operative threshold only for older patients in poor health. Furthermore, a recent review of the endovascular technique cautioned against decreasing the size threshold for aneurysm repair because the long-term durability of the endovascular technique remains undetermined (46).

CHOICE OF STANDARD OR ENDOLUMINAL REPAIR

The approval of the Ancure (Guidant, Menlo Park, California) and AneuRx (Medtronic Arterial Vascular Engi-

neering, Santa Rosa, CA) devices by the Food and Drug Administration in late 1999 has dramatically affected the care of patients with abdominal aortic aneurysms (Fig. 86.5). The commercial release of these devices by the Food and Drug Administration has directly and indirectly validated the approach as a safe and viable alternative to the standard repair. Furthermore, the approval of the Food and Drug Administration has mandated that the endovascular approach be offered to appropriate patients as an alternative treatment. The general public has enthusiastically embraced this alternative approach and has provided a major impetus for its implementation. The net result has been the widespread application of these devices by surgeons and

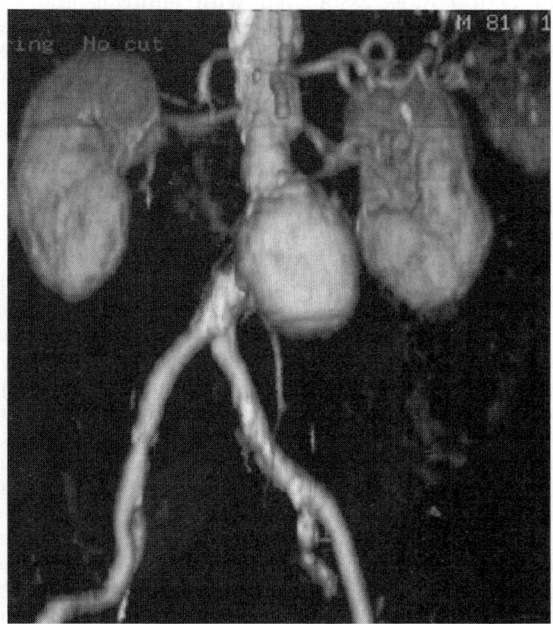

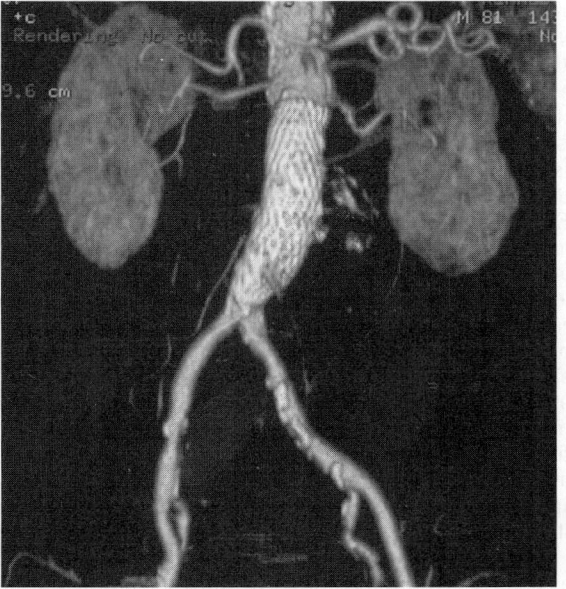

Figure 86.5. Three-dimensional reconstruction, generated by computed tomography, of an infrarenal abdominal aortic aneurysm before *(A)* and after *(B)* endovascular repair with a straight endograft. Note the total exclusion of the aneurysm after endografting.

nonsurgeons alike. Indeed, the initial demand for the devices has far outstripped the available stocks.

Objective analysis of the results of the initial endovascular trials has raised some concern. The initial trials of the various endovascular devices have established that the devices can be safely deployed and that aneurysm rupture may be prevented during short- to intermediate-term follow-up (46–51). However, the long-term outcome of these devices in terms of both mechanical stability and the ability to prevent aneurysm rupture remains unresolved. The rupture of aneurysms during follow-up despite successful endovascular repair has been reported (74–76), which suggests that the endovascular technique, although reasonably effective, is not always definitive and is inferior overall to the standard approach in terms of preventing rupture. The initial results suggest that the mortality and complication rates associated with endovascular repair are comparable with those of standard repair, as noted. However, the proponents of endovascular repair contend that the magnitude of the complications is significantly less with endovascular repair (77). A host of new complications inherent to the endovascular approach have been identified, including graft migration, limb separation, fabric tears, endoleaks, aneurysm expansion, and attachment hook fracture. Admittedly, the reported mortality and complications rates reflect the early experience with the endovascular approach, and these rates may improve with overall experience. However, May et al. (78) analyzed the outcome after endovascular aneurysm repair during two successive time intervals to examine the potential effect of operator experience, or the "learning curve." They reported that a high proportion (45%) of patients experienced adverse outcomes and that the incidence was similar during the two time frames, which suggests that the risks are inherent to the technique rather than dependent on operator experience. The clinical trials have suggested that hospital and intensive care unit stays are shortened, that operative blood loss is less, and that the recovery time in terms of return to normal daily activities is markedly improved after endovascular repair, although these purported advantages require further validation. The reported decreases in total length of stay and intensive care unit length of stay have not resulted in decreases in hospital costs, primarily because of the dramatic price differential of the grafts (endovascular standard) (79,80). The results of the endovascular trials must be further qualified by the fact that they represent study protocols from selected centers of excellence rather than the nationwide experience. It is uncertain whether the results and conclusions of the trials are directly applicable outside these centers.

Endoleaks, or perfusion of the aneurysm outside the lumen of the endograft and within the aneurysm sac, may represent the proverbial "Achilles heal" of the technique. They have been classified as types 1 through 4 based on the mechanism of the leak. Type 1 leaks originate at either the proximal or distal attachment sites. Type 2 leaks are from the collateral circulation originating in the lumbar or inferior mesenteric arteries. Type 3 leaks are caused by fabric tears or problems at the graft interfaces in the modular devices, whereas type 4 leaks are transgraft and can result from the porosity of the graft and needle holes. It should be emphasized that the entire concept of an endoleak is predicated on the ability to detect contrast or blood flow outside the lumen of the endograft and is therefore contingent on the sensitivity and specificity of the various imaging techniques. Schurink et al. (81) performed a metaanalysis of 23 publications of endovascular aneurysm repairs encompassing 1,189 patients and reported an endoleak rate of 24%, with the most common site being the distal attachment. The major concern about an endoleak is that the pressure trans-

mitted to the aneurysm wall will be sufficient to cause an increase in size or a rupture. Both the significance and the natural history of endoleaks remain unresolved. Furthermore, it appears that the type of endoleak and the time course (early vs. late) are of clinical significance. In the report of Matsumura and Moore (82) of the early experience with the Endovascular Technologies device (now known as Ancure), 47% of the 59 patients had initial endoleaks but 50% sealed spontaneously. The long-term integrity of the seal between the endograft and the aorta remains concerning in light of the reported continued growth and remodeling of the infrarenal cuff. Lipski and Ernst (83) analyzed 272 patients who underwent standard, open aneurysm repair and reported that the infrarenal cuff both dilated and lengthened over time. The average cuff dilation as assessed by angiography was 1 mm during 3.5 years but was more than 5 mm in 8% of the patients. Illig et al. (84) reported similar findings and concluded that endovascular repair may not be optimal for patients with a long life expectancy or proximal aortic cuff diameters larger than 27 mm. The ideal outcome after endovascular repair is for the aneurysm shell to shrink or regress with time. Aneurysms that continue to enlarge after endovascular repair represent an increased risk for rupture and mandate further intervention. Similarly, aneurysms that stay at the same size are worrisome and may reflect an occult endoleak. Additionally, conversion from an endovascular repair to an open repair presents several technical challenges and is associated with an increased mortality rate (85).

The initial clinical experience with endovascular repair has emphasized that long-term follow-up with serial imaging is mandatory. Indeed, it has been reported that approximately 25% of patients will need to undergo some type of remedial procedure (86). This requirement should be factored into the decision between endovascular and standard repair. Patients undergoing endovascular repair must be sufficiently reliable to comply with the postoperative imaging protocols, which add significantly to the expense of the endovascular approach. Initially, patients with moderate renal insufficiency (creatinine level > 2 mg/dL) were discouraged from undergoing endovascular repair because of the obligatory contrast load associated with the various imaging studies. However, newer imaging algorithms have been developed to minimize or eliminate the contrast exposure. The optimal algorithm for postoperative imaging in terms of both types of studies and time frame remains to be determined. The imaging objectives include determining the aneurysm size, screening for endoleaks, and assessing changes in the configuration of the endograft. CT and abdominal flat plate are optimal for assessing the aneurysm size and graft configuration, respectively, whereas both CT and color-flow duplex ultrasonography are helpful to detect endoleaks and may be complementary (87). An acceptable algorithm includes both CT and an abdominal flat plate immediately postoperatively, then again at 3 months, 6 months, 12 months, and every 6 months thereafter.

Use of the endovascular approach is currently limited by the anatomic configuration of the aneurysm, although the criteria are evolving. The initial reports have suggested that fewer than 20% to 25% of all abdominal aortic aneurysms are suitable for endovascular repair (88,89), although this percentage has been estimated to be significantly greater as overall experience with the approach has increased and may range from 50% to 75% (49). Ideally, the infrarenal abdominal aortic neck should be between 16 to 26 mm in diameter and longer than 1 cm without excessive angulation. The distal abdominal aortic neck should be longer than 1 cm and minimally diseased if a tube graft is being considered. However, the long-term stability of the distal attachment site for endovascular tube grafts appears poor owing to continued growth of the distal aortic cuff, and it has been suggested that only bifurcated grafts should be implanted. The common iliac arteries should have an implantation site 1 cm in length proximal to the internal iliac artery, and their diameter should be less than 16 mm. The external and common iliac arteries should be sufficiently straight (not tortuous) and free of stenoses to allow passage of the delivery system and seating of the device. Furthermore, the proximal and distal attachment sites should be free of adherent thrombus and dense calcification to ensure an adequate seal. However, these anatomic criteria are only relative and do not necessarily preclude endovascular repair. These indications will likely be expanded by the introduction of newer devices currently in clinical trials. The requirement for a proximal neck diameter of 26 mm or less can be overcome by using larger devices, and the requirement for a proximal neck length of 1 cm or more has been overcome by deploying grafts with their proximal attachment struts across the orifices of the renal arteries (90). Stenotic iliac vessels can be treated with angioplasty or stented, and tortuous iliac vessels can be transiently straightened by manual retraction or accessed through retroperitoneal exposure to facilitate introduction of the delivery system. Aneurysmal involvement of one common iliac artery at the level of the internal iliac artery can be remedied by embolizing the internal iliac vessel and deploying the endovascular graft across its orifice. Bilateral internal iliac artery embolization to facilitate endovascular aneurysm repair has been reported (91), although the potential for pelvic ischemia, buttock claudication, and sexual dysfunction is significant and limits enthusiasm for this approach (92). The internal iliac vessels should be embolized sequentially with sufficient time allowed for collaterals to develop if this approach is selected. Alternatively, the internal iliac artery can be revascularized through a retroperitoneal approach by relocating it on the external iliac artery and essentially performing a bifurcation advancement.

The proverbial "bottom line" in the endovascular repair of abdominal aortic aneurysms remains unclear. The outstanding issues regarding the long-term safety of the devices and their suitability will likely be resolved in the not-too-distant future. Additionally, the technology is evolving rapidly, and better devices will likely be built to overcome the current limitations. Indeed, a complete percutaneous delivery system is currently in clinical trials. The clinical scenario is similar to the introduction of laparoscopic cholecystectomy in the early 1990s and appears to be driven partly by patient preference. The marked difference with laparoscopic cholecystectomy, however, is the crucial need to determine long-term outcome. The endovascular technique is generally perceived as both safer and "minimally invasive," but it should be viewed as alternative or complementary to standard, open repair. The lower upfront risks are partially offset by the ongoing risk for rupture and the requirement for long-term follow-up. Both endovascular and standard repair techniques should be discussed with patients and their limitations emphasized. The endovascular approach is currently ideal for older, sicker patients with anatomically appropriate lesions and a limited life expectancy. However, it should be implemented cautiously or not at all in younger, good-risk patients.

OPERATIVE REPAIR

Preoperative Evaluation

The preoperative evaluation of patients undergoing elective abdominal aortic aneurysm repair is similar to that of patients undergoing any major general or vascular

surgical procedure. Patients for whom endovascular aneurysm repair is being planned should undergo the same preoperative work-up in light of the potential need to convert to open repair. All patients should receive a complete history, and a physical examination, electrocardiogram, and a chest radiograph should be performed. Routine laboratory studies, including a complete blood cell count with platelets, measurement of serum creatinine and serum electrolyte levels, and coagulation studies, should be obtained. A specimen should be sent to the blood bank and the appropriate quantity of blood products cross-matched. This number can be determined from the historic operative transfusion requirements obtained from the blood bank, but 4 units of packed red blood cells is usually sufficient. Preoperative autologous donation is discouraged because of the minor risk for induced ischemia, minimal risk for infectious complications associated with allogenic blood (93), and overall lack of cost-effectiveness (94). Similarly, directed donor transfusions are discouraged because the associated transfusion risks are comparable with those of first-time donors (95). A thorough peripheral pulse examination should be included in the physical examination and validated with formal ankle–brachial indices. The patients should be seen by the anesthesiologist preoperatively, and a bowel preparation with mechanical lavage should be performed the day before surgery. Additionally, therapeutic beta blockade should probably be administered if the patient is not already taking beta blockers. Several randomized, controlled studies have demonstrated that beta blockade reduces the incidence of cardiac events after vascular surgery, both perioperatively and on a long-term basis (96,97). The complete preoperative work-up can be streamlined and performed entirely in the outpatient setting (98).

All active medical problems, including abnormalities identified during the preoperative evaluation, should be controlled as well as possible before elective abdominal aortic aneurysm repair is undertaken. However, extensive diagnostic testing before aneurysm repair is probably unnecessary. Routine pulmonary function tests and measurement of arterial blood gases are not indicated, although they may be beneficial in selected patients with advanced chronic obstructive pulmonary disease (99). The presence of chronic obstructive pulmonary disease often complicates postoperative ventilator management, but it is unusual for a patient's pulmonary disease to be sufficiently severe to preclude operation. Furthermore, the history and physical examination alone are sufficient to identify this small subset of patients. Similarly, creatinine clearance studies and other assessments of renal function have not proved beneficial before aneurysm repair despite the dramatic impact of preoperative renal insufficiency on perioperative outcome.

The appropriate cardiac work-up before abdominal aortic aneurysm repair remains controversial and is somewhat institution-dependent. The spectrum ranges from risk factor stratification and selective cardiac catheterization based on clinical symptoms alone to routine noninvasive testing and cardiac catheterization based on the results of noninvasive testing. The overall objective of the preoperative cardiac evaluation is to optimize the cardiovascular system and reduce both the perioperative and long-term risk for myocardial infarction, congestive heart failure, and death. Admittedly, the prevalence of coronary artery disease among patients undergoing abdominal aortic aneurysm repair is very high. Hertzer et al. (100), in a landmark publication, reported that 25% of 1,000 patients undergoing evaluation for peripheral vascular surgery (cerebral vascular occlusive disease, lower extremity arterial occlusive disease, abdominal aortic aneurysm) had severe, surgically correctable lesions detected during cardiac catheterization; 6% had severe, uncorrectable disease, and only 8% had no evidence of disease. Interestingly, the incidence of surgically correctable disease was highest among patients undergoing evaluation for abdominal aortic aneurysm.

Ideally, the preoperative evaluation should identify a subset of patients at high risk for cardiac events who would benefit from intervention. The history and physical examination can identify clinical predictors of cardiovascular risk as outlined in the American College of Cardiology/American Heart Association guidelines for perioperative cardiovascular evaluation for noncardiac surgery (101). The major clinical predictors include unstable coronary syndromes (recent myocardial infarction, unstable/severe angina), decompensated congestive heart failure, significant arrhythmias, and significant valvular disease. Patients with these major clinical predictors clearly merit further evaluation with cardiology consultation and invasive testing.

The majority of patients undergoing evaluation for aneurysm repair have intermediate (mild angina, prior myocardial infarction, compensated congestive heart, diabetes) or minor (advanced age, abnormal electrocardiogram, minor arrhythmias, history of stroke, poorly controlled hypertension) clinical predictors of perioperative cardiovascular risk. Unfortunately, the appropriate preoperative evaluation for patients with intermediate or minor clinical predictors is less clear. Routine preoperative cardiac catheterization for all patients undergoing abdominal aortic aneurysm is likely not cost-effective, and it is difficult to justify coronary revascularization for anatomically significant lesions in patients without clinical symptoms. Noninvasive cardiac stress testing for this subset of patients could theoretically identify those at increased risk for perioperative events who would benefit from catheterization/revascularization. Indeed, a variety of noninvasive cardiac stress tests are available, including routine exercise testing, dipyridamole thallium, adenosine thallium, and dobutamine echocardiography. Unfortunately, the overall positive predictive value of these tests has fallen short of expectations. Baron et al. (102) reported that age and the presence of cardiac disease were better predictors of cardiac complications than perfusion imaging among 457 patients undergoing abdominal aortic surgery. Furthermore, Seeger et al. (103) reported that although preoperative stress thallium testing identified patients with significant coronary artery disease before aortic surgery, prophylactic coronary revascularization did not reduce operative or long-term mortality.

The American College of Cardiology/American Heart Association Task Force has developed an algorithm for patients undergoing noncardiac surgery (101). Briefly, patients with major clinical predictors of perioperative cardiovascular risk, outlined above, who require urgent or elective operation should be seen in consultation by a cardiologist, and catheterization with subsequent treatment based on the findings should be considered. Patients with intermediate clinical predictors undergoing high-risk surgical procedures (abdominal aortic aneurysm repair) should undergo noninvasive cardiac testing and potentially cardiac catheterization/revascularization, depending on the results. Patients with minor clinical predictors and moderate or excellent functional capacity (more than four metabolic equivalent levels) can undergo high-risk surgical procedures without further cardiac evaluation, but those with poor functional capacity should undergo noninvasive cardiac testing as outlined for patients with intermediate predictors. Unfortunately, the majority of patients undergoing evaluation for abdominal aortic aneurysm repair (high-risk surgical procedure) require noninvasive cardiac testing as part of this algorithm despite its limited value, as noted above. Mangano and Goldman (104) have proposed an alternative approach that is less dependent on preoperative cardiac testing. They suggest that patients with known stable coronary artery disease and good functional status require only a 12-lead electrocardiogram and a chest radiograph before aneurysm repair. Furthermore, they propose that patients with known coronary artery disease and unclear functional status undergo noninvasive cardiac testing and aggressive medical management or coronary catheterization/revascularization if the test result is positive. Additionally, they recommend that patients with known coronary artery disease and poor functional status undergo aggressive medical management or coronary catheterization/revascularization. Huber et al. (105) and Taylor et al. (106) have reported acceptable rates of cardiac morbidity and mortality after aortic reconstruction with the use of this selective approach to the preoperative cardiac evaluation. Both algorithms appear to be appropriate. The choice depends on the bias of the anesthesiologists, cardiologists, and surgeons at an institution and should be determined by consensus.

All patients should undergo some type of imaging modality as part of their preoperative evaluation to confirm the diagnosis and plan the operative procedure. Indeed, determining whether a patient is an endovascular candidate and sizing the device appropriately depend on the anatomic measurements obtained at the time of imaging. Imaging guidelines are available for the two commercially available endovascular devices. CT of the chest, abdomen, and pelvis is the optimal imaging study to visualize the aneurysm and is the only imaging study required in most cases. Abdominal ultrasonography is insufficient as the sole imaging study before aneurysm repair in light of its inability to determine accurately the proximal extent of the aneurysm and any involvement of the iliac vessels. Preoperative arteriography is necessary for patients undergoing endovascular repair if CT alone is insufficient and for the subset of patients undergoing standard repair who have renal anomalies or occlusive disease in the renal, mesenteric, or aortoiliac vessels.

Standard Repair of Intact Abdominal Aortic Aneurysms

Technique

The intraoperative preparation is similar whether a patient is undergoing repair of an abdominal aortic aneurysm by the standard approach or the newer endovascular technique. Inhalation agents and an endotracheal tube are used most frequently, although the choice of anesthetic is usually deferred to the anesthesia team. The role of an adjunct epidural anesthetic is somewhat controversial, but it may improve postoperative pain control (107) and be beneficial in patients with severe pulmonary disease (108). Adequate intravenous access should be established to facilitate resuscitation in the event that bleeding is significant. Central venous access is usually obtained although not necessary provided that peripheral access is sufficient. Electrocardiographic leads, an arterial catheter, and a Foley catheter should be placed for continuous monitoring of the electrocardiogram, arterial pressure, and urine output respectively. Additionally, a nasogastric tube should be inserted. A Swan-Ganz pulmonary artery catheter or a transesophageal echocardiogram probe should be inserted in patients with significant cardiac disease. However, Valentine et al. (109) reported that the routine use of pulmonary artery catheters in patients undergoing aortic surgery is not beneficial and may be associated with a higher rate of intraoperative complications. Peripheral arterial pulses should be interrogated with either palpation or continuous-wave Doppler ultrasonography and marked to facilitate confirmation of the distal signals after restoration of lower extremity perfusion. Strategies to maintain core body temperature should be initiated (110). Specifically, the room temperature should be increased, warming devices should be attached to all intravenous infusion lines, and either a recirculating alcohol blanket or forced-air blanket should be applied to the patient. The effect of hypothermia (< 34.5°C) was emphasized by Bush et al. (111), who reported that multiple physiologic derangements associated with adverse outcomes develop in patients who become hypothermic after abdominal aortic aneurysm repair. Intraoperative autologous transfusion devices should be used when a significant amount of blood loss is anticipated, as in ruptured aneurysms and complex aortic reconstructions of suprarenal aneurysms or thoracoabdominal aortic aneurysms. Furthermore, intraoperative salvage is acceptable to most persons who object to allogenic blood transfusions based on religious principles. However, the routine use of intraoperative autologous transfusion devices during elective aortic reconstructions has not been shown to reduce the number of allogenic transfusions (112) or to be cost-effective (113). Indeed, the reported cost-effectiveness threshold has been reported to range from 2 to 6 salvage units (113,114). An extensive operative field, from "nipples to toes," should be prepared with the use of topical antimicrobial agents, and patients are administered either a first-generation cephalosporin or vancomycin as prophylaxis before the skin incision is made.

Abdominal aortic aneurysms may be repaired through several different incisions or approaches, including midline, retroperitoneal, or transverse (supraumbilical straight, infraumbilical straight, infraumbilical curvilinear, bilateral subcostal). The various incisions and approaches must be viewed as complementary, as no one of them is perfect for every clinical scenario. Indeed, aneurysm surgeons should be familiar with the various approaches and select the optimal one for the clinical setting. Determinants of the incision to be used include the proximal and distal extent of the aneurysm, body habitus, presence of prior abdominal incisions, presence of abdominal wall stomas, comorbidities, additional intraoperative pathology, inflammatory aneurysms, renal anomalies, requirements for concomitant procedures, how rapidly aortic control must be obtained, and surgeon preference. The midline approach is preferable for patients with ruptured abdominal aortic aneurysms because aortic control at the level of the diaphragm can be obtained rapidly. The bilateral subcostal approach provides the best exposure and is the incision of choice for obese patients, those with extensive iliac artery aneurysms, those requiring concomitant renal artery revascularization, and patients with juxtarenal aneurysms that require suprarenal aortic control. The retroperitoneal approach is optimal for patients with multiple previous abdominal incisions and the proverbial "hostile abdomen," abdominal wall stomas, suprarenal aneurysms, inflammatory aneurysms, and horseshoe kidneys, and for those undergoing aortic procedures. However, the retroperitoneal approach is limited by the inability to assess the intraperitoneal structures adequately and the limited access to the right renal artery and right iliac vessels. It was previously argued that the retroperitoneal approach posed less of a physiologic insult than the transperitoneal approach and so was ideal for patients with advanced pulmonary or cardiac disease. How-

ever, this contention has not been supported by a prospective, randomized trial (115). A detailed description of the retroperitoneal approach is beyond the context of this chapter but is available in most standard vascular surgical texts (116).

The sequence of steps used to repair an intact, infrarenal abdominal aortic aneurysm after a bilateral subcostal incision can be summarized (Fig. 86.6). The abdomen is explored when the peritoneal cavity is entered, and the gallbladder and colon are carefully assessed for the presence of stones and masses, respectively. The lower abdominal wall flap is immobilized to either the drapes or the pubic towel with the use of penetrating towel clips. The small bowel is manually retracted laterally to the right, and the duodenum is mobilized by incising the ligament of Treitz. The inferior mesenteric vein may be suture-ligated at this juncture to facilitate exposure. The tissue adjacent to the inferior mesenteric vein should be palpated to rule out a large, meandering mesenteric artery. This artery is an important visceral collateral and should be preserved. The retroperitoneum over the aorta is incised with the electrocautery, and the left renal vein is exposed. The Buckwalter retractor is then placed to facilitate exposure further. The small bowel is placed in a bowel bag, eviscerated, and retracted laterally to the right with the aid of the malleable retractors for the Buckwalter. The transverse colon and superior abdominal wall flap are retracted superiorly while the lower abdominal wall is further retracted inferiorly. The aorta immediately inferior to the renal arteries is exposed and both renal arteries visualized. The infrarenal aorta at this location is dissected circumferentially to facilitate placement of a transverse aortic clamp. However, this step may be omitted if the aortic occlusion is obtained with a vertical clamp. The retroperitoneum over the aorta is then incised further inferiorly and the incision extended along the course of the right common iliac artery. The extent of the distal dissection depends on the anatomic configuration of the aneurysm. If the aneurysm extends to the aortic bifurcation, it is sufficient to dissect only the common iliac arteries provided a sufficient site for vascular clamp application is identified. If the aneurysm extends to the distal common iliac arteries, both the internal and external iliac vessels should be dissected free. This may be facilitated on the left side by mobilizing the sigmoid colon along its peritoneal reflection and accessing the iliac vessels below the colon. The inferior mesenteric artery is then dissected free and vascular control obtained with a vessel loop. Patients are administered 100 units of heparin per kilogram, and the activated clotting time is confirmed to be twice the baseline value. Supplemental doses of heparin are administered throughout the procedure as dictated by the clotting time. Interestingly, a recent randomized, controlled trial reported that heparin does not reduce thrombotic events or increase bleeding during aneurysm repair but is associated with a significant reduction in myocardial events (117). Additionally, 0.5 mg of mannitol per kilogram is administered before clamp application (118).

During the time required for adequate mixing of the heparin, the availability of the necessary equipment and suture and graft material is reviewed and confirmed with the operating room personnel. The appropriately sized tube or bifurcated prosthetic graft is selected. The graft diameter is sized according to the infrarenal aortic neck by visual inspection or with calibrated sizers. The general "rule of thumb" is that the smaller graft should be selected when the aorta is between two graft sizes because the aorta always appears smaller after it is transected and redundant graft material at the proximal anastomosis is more difficult to correct than the opposite problem. A variety of vascular

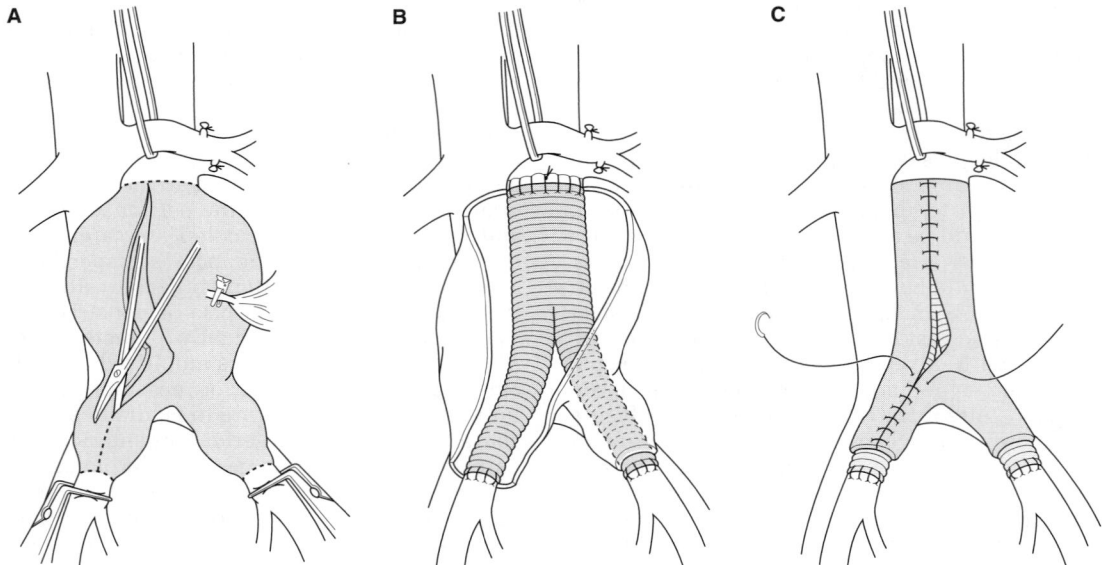

Figure 86.6. Steps involved in the standard repair of an infrarenal abdominal aortic aneurysm extending into the proximal common iliac arteries. *(A)* The proximal duodenum is mobilized and the retroperitoneum overlying the aorta incised. The infrarenal aorta immediately below the renal vein is dissected. The iliac bifurcations are exposed, and vascular clamps are applied to the infrarenal aorta and distal common iliac arteries after adequate heparinization. A longitudinal arteriotomy is extended from the infrarenal aorta onto the right common iliac artery. *(B)* Back bleeding from the lumbar arteries is controlled with figure-of-eight sutures. The proximal anastomosis is performed in an end-to-end configuration below the renal arteries. The distal anastomoses are performed at the common iliac bifurcation beyond the aneurysmal segments. The left limb of the graft is tunneled through the intact left common iliac aneurysm shell. *(C)* The residual aneurysm shell is closed over the prosthetic graft, and the retroperitoneum is reapproximated to prevent erosion of the graft into the overlying bowel.

prostheses are available. Despite the contentions of the various company representatives, no clear advantages are offered by any one of them, and the choice depends on surgeon preference as dictated by ease of handling, cost, availability, and requirements for preclotting. The distal vascular clamps are applied to external, internal, or common iliac vessels depending on the extent of the aneurysm and the character of the vessels. Occasionally, the iliac vessels are so calcified that the application of clamps is unsafe because of the potential for injuring the vessel. In this setting, vascular control may be obtained intraluminally with the use of a balloon thromboembolectomy catheter after the aneurysm has been incised. The proximal aortic clamp is applied in sequence after the distal clamps. The clamp is applied immediately below the renal arteries to facilitate an anastomosis to the proximal infrarenal aorta. The length of the infrarenal aorta should be sufficient to allow an anastomosis without difficulty. However, a long infrarenal cuff should be avoided because it may become aneurysmal over time. Either a vertical or horizontal aortic clamp may be used, although the latter if favored because it simplifies the anastomosis. The aorta is then incised longitudinally, and the incision is extended down the right common iliac artery as necessary. Attempts should be made to preserve the autonomic nerves overlying the distal aorta and proximal left common iliac artery in potent men. This can usually be achieved by incising the left common iliac artery transversely beyond the aneurysmal portion and tunneling the limb of the graft through the residual shell. The intraluminal thrombus and debris are removed from within the aorta, and all back bleeding from the lumbar arteries is controlled with suture ligatures. The atheromatous debris within the aorta has

been reported to be culture-positive in approximately 25% of cases, although this has not been associated with long-term graft infections (119). The infrarenal aorta at the level of the planned proximal anastomosis may be completely transected, or the back wall may be left intact. Completely transecting the aorta makes the proximal anastomoses slightly easier, although leaving the back wall intact reinforces the anastomosis and provides the equivalent of an autogenous pledget. The proximal anastomosis is created in an end-end configuration between the graft and the infrarenal aorta with a running 3-0 nonabsorbable, monofilament suture, and all leaks in the suture line are repaired with similar 5-0 sutures and felt pledgets as necessary. The distal anastomosis or anastomoses are performed to the aortic bifurcation, common iliac arteries, or iliac bifurcation as dictated by the anatomy of the aneurysm. A 3-0 nonabsorbable, monofilament suture is used for anastomoses at the aortic bifurcation, and a similar 4-0 suture is used for the common iliac arteries. All anastomoses are flushed before flow is restored to remove any intraluminal debris. Blood flow is restored to the pelvis and lower extremities in sequence. Attempts should be made to flush into the internal iliac circulation initially to prevent embolization to the lower extremities. This can be facilitated by manually compressing the common femoral arteries for tube graft configurations. The lower torso should be reperfused gradually (i.e., one vessel at a time and one extremity at a time) to prevent hypotension and the acute sequelae associated with the reperfusion of ischemic tissues. This process requires significant communication and coordination between the surgical and anesthetic teams. It is imperative that the patient be normovolemic at the time of reperfusion, and it is frequently necessary to delay reperfusion to allow additional resuscitation. Furthermore, reperfusion of the ischemic tissue causes the release of acid, potassium, and a variety of inflammatory mediators into the systemic circulation, all of which are potentially detrimental.

The inferior mesenteric artery should be reimplanted if patent into either the body of the graft or the left limb. Seeger et al. (120) reported that routine reimplantation of the inferior mesenteric artery results in decreased rates of colonic infarction and death after aortic reconstruction. The colon and lower extremities should be interrogated with the Doppler to confirm adequate signals. The heparin is reversed with protamine after confirmation of adequate distal signals. The protamine dose is estimated based on the effectiveness of protamine (1 mg of protamine per 100 units of heparin), the initial dose of heparin, the current activated clotting time, and the elapsed time from the administration of heparin. The protamine should be administered slowly to prevent any untoward hemodynamic events (121). Notably, a recent randomized, controlled trial reported that protamine effectively reverses the heparin effect but provides no clinical benefit during peripheral vascular surgery, including aneurysm repair (122). The shell of the aneurysm and the overlying retroperitoneum are both closed with absorbable suture after adequate hemostasis to provide a biologic tissue layer between the graft and the viscera. The retractors are then removed, the viscera are returned to their anatomic positions, the nasogastric tube is confirmed to be in the antrum, and the abdominal wall fascia is closed with standard technique. Interestingly, patients undergoing aortic reconstruction for aneurysmal disease have been reported to have a higher incidence of abdominal wall hernias than those undergoing reconstruction for occlusive disease (123).

The configuration of the aortic reconstruction (aortoaortic, aortoiliac, aortofemoral) depends on the extent of aneurysmal involvement and the degree of occlusive disease. Aneurysmal degeneration of the common iliac vessels should be considered simply as an extension or sequela of the aortic aneurysm and treated appropriately. Specifically, common iliac arteries larger than 2.0 cm should be considered aneurysmal and replaced. Usually, the entire common iliac artery must be replaced and the distal anastomosis created at the iliac bifurcation, although it is possible to replace only the proximal common iliac artery if the aneurysmal changes are isolated. Conversely, common iliac arteries smaller than 2.0 cm have a relatively benign natural history and do not need to be replaced. Only a small percentage ultimately become aneurysmal and require treatment (28,29). Despite the fact that a patient may be a candidate for an aortic tube graft, the distal aorta at the level of the bifurcation is frequently so severely calcified that it is easier to use a bifurcated graft with distal anastomoses to the proximal common iliac arteries than to attempt to suture the diseased terminal aorta. Aortic–bifemoral bypass grafts should be reserved for the small subset of patients who truly have concomitant aneurysms and severe occlusive disease. Although it is easier to perform an aortic–bifemoral bypass than an aortic–biiliac bypass, the risks in terms of wound complications and graft infections are significantly greater. Indeed, the risk for graft infections is less than 0.5% for aortic–biiliac grafts but approximately 2% for aortic–bifemoral grafts (124). It is imperative to remember the original indication for the procedure and choose the appropriate aortic reconstruction (aortic–biiliac bypass for aortoiliac aneurysm, aortic–bifemoral bypass for aortoiliac occlusive disease). Admittedly, there is a role for aortic–bifemoral reconstructions in patients with aneurysmal disease, and it is futile to attempt an aortic–biiliac reconstruction in patients with severe external iliac artery disease.

The postoperative care is fairly routine and predictable for the majority of patients undergoing elective infrarenal abdominal aortic aneurysm repair. Patients are transferred directly from the operating room to the intensive care unit. Most of the patients are extubated in the operating room or shortly after arrival in the intensive care unit. The intensive care unit length of stay is usually 1 to 2 days, and the median total length of stay nationwide is 8 days (22). Patients are encouraged to get out of bed and begin ambulating in the early postoperative period (24 to 48 hours). Nasogastric decompression is continued until bowel function returns. Oral feedings are initiated after removal of the nasogastric tube and advanced quickly to solids. Patients are discharged when they are ambulatory, can tolerate a regular diet, have normal bowel function, and are sufficiently able to care for themselves. A small subset of people require transfer to a rehabilitation or extended care facility. Patients are usually seen in the clinic two weeks after discharge and then at 6 months. Additional clinic appointments may be necessary as dictated by any ongoing medical problems. Patients are not allowed to drive until their incisional pain has resolved and they are off all narcotic pain medications. Furthermore, patients are discouraged from lifting objects heavier than 10 lb for the first 6 months to reduce the incidence of incisional hernia.

Complications and Outcome

Elective repair of abdominal aortic aneurysms by the standard, open technique is associated with significant mortality and morbidity (22,125,126). The attendant mortality rates have been discussed extensively in the preceding section entitled Principles of Management. Briefly, the nationwide mortality rate for elective infrarenal abdominal aortic aneurysm repair is approximately 4% (22), but it ranges from below 4% to approximately 10% in individual and statewide series, respectively (5,44). The overall morbidity rate remains less clear, although the specific complications have been well defined. Huber et al. (22) recently reported that 33% of all patients undergoing repair of intact abdominal aortic aneurysms nationally experience some type of complication, as defined by the ICD-9 postoperative complication code in the discharge abstract.

Intraoperative complications can result from inadvertent injury to the intraabdominal structures during dissection, although these technical complications are not necessarily specific to the repair of abdominal aortic aneurysms. The small bowel, colon, ureter, and major venous structures (inferior vena cava, iliac veins, left renal vein) are particularly susceptible during the obligatory dissection. Iatrogenic bowel injury at the time of abdominal aortic aneurysm repair is problematic. If the colon is injured before the aneurysm repair, the defect in the colon should be fixed and the aneurysm repair should be aborted. If the small bowel is injured before the aneurysm repair, the same course should likely be followed, although this decision requires clinical judgment. The potential to infect the aortic graft is the major justification for aborting the aneurysm repair in this setting. These concerns must be balanced by the fact that the small-bowel contents are sterile, patients usually receive a bowel preparation before repair, a second procedure will be required to repair the aneurysm, and a small risk for aneurysm rupture exists during the intervening time until definitive repair. Injury to the bowel during or after implantation of the aortic graft should be treated with repair of the defect, extensive irrigation, and prolonged antibiotics. The ureter is most susceptible to injury at the point where it crosses over the iliac bifurcation. Injury can be avoided by a heightened awareness of this anatomic location and dissection in the tissue plane immediately on top of the common iliac vessels. Inadvertent venous injury can be associated with significant bleeding, which is usually controlled by direct pressure with sponge sticks and suture repair. The left renal vein may be transected if necessary. However, it should be transected near its juncture with the vena cava, and the gonadal, adrenal, and lumbar branches should be preserved to maintain venous outflow from the kidney. Transecting the iliac artery or infrarenal aorta may facilitate exposure of the iliac or retroaortic renal veins, respectively.

Excessive intraoperative bleeding may occasionally be encountered. Routine elective aneurysm repairs are usually associated with moderate intraoperative blood loss, with a mean transfusion requirement of 1 to 2 units of packed red blood cells. Excessive bleeding may be caused by either surgical trauma or coagulopathy. Bleeding from all surgical sites should be corrected, and reversal of the heparin effect with protamine may correct the coagulopathic bleeding. Patients with significant bleeding and platelet counts below 50,000/µL should receive a transfusion of platelets, and platelet transfusion should be considered in patients with coagulopathic bleeding and counts below 100,000/µL. Transfusions of fresh frozen plasma are indicated for patients with either significant bleeding and coagulation studies indicating a prolonged bleeding time (> 1.5 times control value) or coagulopathic bleeding. Massive bleeding, defined as more than 100% of the blood volume, may induce a dilutional coagulopathy with prolongation of the bleeding time. Additional blood products should be set up in the blood bank in the event of significant bleeding. This may require an additional blood bank specimen. Intraoperative autologous transfusion devices should also be considered if not already in use.

Ischemia of the lower extremities has been reported to occur approximately 3% of the time after abdominal aortic aneurysm repair (125). The causes are multiple and include distal embolization, thrombosis, clamp injury, and technical errors. The lumen of the aneurysm is frequently filled with thrombus and atheromatous debris that may serve as a source for both macroembolization and microembolization. The macroemboli usually lodge at a bifurcation of major vessels; the microemboli usually lodge in the digital vessels and, unfortunately, are not amenable to mechanical extraction. Thrombosis may result from inadequate heparinization, hypercoagulable conditions, or poor arterial runoff. The technical conduct of the operation outlined above is designed to minimize ischemic complications. The specific maneuvers include confirmation of adequate anticoagulation, selection of a suitable site for distal clamp application and anastomosis, intraluminal control of severely calcified vessels, flushing of the vascular lumina before clamp removal, and sequential removal of the vascular clamps. Further intervention is mandatory if the lower extremities are found to be ischemic. Anastomotic defects should be corrected. This may simply require dissembling and recreating the anastomosis, but often it must be relocated further distally on either the common iliac or common femoral vessels. If no problems are identified at the distal anastomosis, the femoral vessels should be explored and thrombectomized. A transverse arteriotomy may be created in the common femoral artery if it is anticipated that only a thrombectomy will be required, but a longitudinal incision should be created if a bypass (inflow or outflow) procedure is anticipated. The transverse arteriotomy can simply be closed with interrupted sutures without narrowing the lumen in

the event that an additional bypass procedure is not necessary, whereas the longitudinal arteriotomy may require a patch closure. A bypass from the aortic graft to the femoral vessels is required if adequate inflow cannot be restored with thrombectomy alone. The popliteal artery below the knee should be explored and thrombectomized if the extremity is still ischemic after restoration of adequate inflow. This may be facilitated by extending a longitudinal arteriotomy from the popliteal artery below the knee to the tibioperoneal trunk to allow cannulation of all three crural vessels. A below-knee popliteal or tibial artery bypass is required if adequate perfusion to the distal extremity is not restored after patch closure of the popliteal arteriotomy. Predictably, a complex lower extremity revascularization in addition to an aortic reconstruction is associated with a significant degree of morbidity and dramatically increases the mortality rate (127). The decision to proceed with an infrainguinal bypass depends on the status of the extremity and requires clinical judgment. Aborting the procedure and allowing for a period of observation and rewarming is appropriate when popliteal Doppler signals are detected and the foot is cool yet not severely ischemic. However, reoperation and definitive treatment may be necessary in the early postoperative period unless marked improvement is noted.

Many of the complications that follow abdominal aortic aneurysm repair are not surprising, given the magnitude of the operation and the age and comorbid conditions of the patient population. Cardiac complications, including ischemia, infarction, arrhythmias, and congestive heart failure, occur in up to 15% (44,125,126) and are the leading cause of death after aneurysm repair in many series (105). Likewise, the pulmonary complications of pneumonia, prolonged ventilatory dependence (> 48 h), and acute respiratory distress syndrome are not uncommon, with 8% of patients requiring prolonged ventilation in a recent series (125,126). Deterioration of renal function, defined by an increase in serum creatinine or blood urea nitrogen, occurs in approximately 5% of cases, although acute renal failure requiring dialysis is rare (< 1%) after elective aneurysm repair (125). The potential causes of renal insufficiency in the perioperative period are numerous and include contrast nephrotoxicity, hypovolemia, atheroembolization, and release of systemic inflammatory mediators from the ischemia/reperfusion injury in the lower torso. Postoperative bleeding requiring reexploration, intraabdominal abscess, and abdominal wound complications are all relatively infrequent complications and are associated with all major intraabdominal procedures.

Ischemic colitis has been reported to occur with an incidence of approximately 2% to 13% after elective infrarenal abdominal aortic aneurysm repair (128). The reported incidence depends on the diagnostic algorithm and modality (routine sigmoidoscopy vs. sigmoidoscopy after symptoms) and is dramatically increased after repair of ruptured aneurysms. Indeed, the incidence of colonic ischemia after ruptured aneurysm repair in patients undergoing routine colonoscopy is 24% (128). The sigmoid colon is affected most frequently, although all sections of the colon may be involved. The cause in most cases is hypoperfusion as a result of inadequate resuscitation, disruption of collateral perfusion, or failure to revascularize a hemodynamically significant inferior mesenteric artery. Patients usually present with bloody diarrhea in the early postoperative period. However, the diagnosis should be considered in the absence of bloody diarrhea in patients with thrombocytopenia, multiple-organ dysfunction, increasing abdominal pain/peritonitis, and generalized failure to thrive. The diagnosis may be confirmed by endoscopy. Sigmoidoscopy alone is acceptable; however, evaluation of the complete colon is optimal. Treatment depends on the endoscopic findings and clinical setting. The endoscopic findings range from mucosal ischemia with patchy sloughing of the mucosa and submucosal edema to transmural necrosis. Unfortunately, it is often difficult to differentiate diffuse mucosal ischemia from transmural necrosis. Patients with mucosal ischemia alone should be treated with bowel rest, broad-spectrum antibiotics, total parenteral nutrition, and serial endoscopic examinations. Many of these lesions resolve spontaneously without long-term sequelae, although colonic strictures develop in a subset of patients. Patients with transmural colonic necrosis should undergo laparotomy with resection of the involved segment, a proximal diverting colostomy, and a distal Hartmann's procedure. After the laparotomy, they should be maintained on broad-spectrum antibiotics and parenteral nutrition. The reported mortality rate in patients with transmural necrosis is approximately 85% (128). This adverse outcome may be largely prevented by maintaining antegrade flow through the internal iliac vessels, routinely implanting the inferior mesenteric artery, and avoiding disruption of the colonic collateral circulation.

Several other gastrointestinal complications are relatively common after standard infrarenal abdominal aortic aneurysm repair (129). A postoperative ileus develops in essentially all patients. Bowel function usually returns within 3 to 5 days after repair, at which time the nasogastric tube is removed and oral feedings are initiated. An ileus may persist beyond this time period in a subset of patients, although no additional specific therapy is usually required. Nasogastric decompression should be continued, narcotics minimized, electrolytes normalized, and ambulation encouraged. Either calculous or acalculous cholecystitis may develop after aneurysm repair. The mortality rates reported historically for postoperative cholecystitis were significant (130) and stimulated the approach of combined cholecystectomy and aneurysm repair. Although this approach has been found to be safe and not associated with an increased risk for graft infections, it is usually reserved for patients with small stones or evidence of chronic cholecystitis. Pancreatitis may develop after abdominal aortic aneurysm repair, although the incidence is surprisingly low in light of the degree of manipulation of the pancreas during repair. The management of pancreatitis is this setting is conservative and includes bowel rest, parenteral nutrition, and serial imaging.

The rate of male sexual dysfunction after aortoiliac reconstruction has been reported to range from 5% to 18% (131). The responsible mechanisms include interruption of the pelvic perfusion and injury to the autonomic nerves that overlie the distal aorta and proximal common iliac arteries. Injury to these autonomic nerves disrupts the internal sphincter mechanism of the bladder and results in retrograde ejaculation. Care should be exercised during aneurysm repair to maintain pelvic perfusion and avoid nerve injury to prevent these untoward complications. It is imperative that these potential complications be discussed with patients preoperatively.

Paraplegia after infrarenal abdominal aortic aneurysm repair occurs with an incidence of 0.25% (132). The potential mechanisms for this devastating complication include embolization, thrombosis of the spinal artery, and disruption of the spinal blood supply from a low-lying artery of Adamkiewicz or loss of prograde flow through the internal iliac arteries. Paraplegia after aneurysm repair is an irreversible injury. It may potentially be minimized by maintaining adequate prograde pelvic perfusion.

The long-term outcome after standard, elective infarenal abdominal aortic aneurysm repair is generally favorable. Long-term survival is improved after aneurysm repair, although it falls short of that of age-matched controls (5). The reported survival rates are approximately 90%, 65%, and 40% at 1, 5, and 10 years, respectively (2,5,133), with cardiovascular problems being the leading cause of death (134). Indeed, these observations underscore the importance of risk factor modification and appropriate long-term follow-up with the primary care provider. Prosthetic aortic grafts are associated with long-term complications, the reported incidence of which is approximately 9% (135). Notably, bifurcated grafts are associated with a higher incidence of complications (13%) than tube grafts (5%) (28). These include infection, aortoenteric fistula, thrombosis, and pseudoaneurysm formation. Additional aneurysms of a sufficient size to merit intervention develop in approximately 5% to 15% of patients in either the iliac vessels or the aorta above the prosthetic graft (28,29). It is recommended that patients undergo CT of the complete aorta and iliac vessels 5 years postoperatively to screen for graft complications and additional aneurysms. Furthermore, patients with prosthetic aortic grafts should receive prophylactic antibiotics before undergoing invasive procedures, including colonoscopy and dental extractions.

Endovascular Repair of Intact Abdominal Aortic Aneurysms

Technique

The preoperative approach to patients undergoing endovascular repair of an abdominal aortic aneurysm is comparable with the standard repair, as emphasized above, and patients should be prepared to undergo open, standard repair as a fallback if the endovascular repair is unsuccessful or complications develop. Fortunately, conversion to open repair is relatively uncommon and has been reported in fewer than 5% of recent experimental trials (47–50). However, it should be emphasized that endovascular repair of abdominal aortic aneurysms with use of the currently available devices is a surgical procedure and should be performed in an operating room by physicians facile with the open technique. Admittedly, additional imaging requirements in the operating room are necessary, including a fluoroscope with digital angiography capabilities. Economic forces and changes in practice patterns have stimulated physicians other than surgeons (radiologists, cardiologists) to expand their services to include endovascular aneurysm repair. This encroachment on the traditional surgical practice will likely increase with the introduction of percutaneous delivery systems for endovascular repair. However, catheter skills alone are not sufficient to implant these devices. Physicians inserting them should be able to manage untoward complications appropriately and expeditiously and to convert an endovascular procedure to an open repair if necessary, and they should be knowledgeable about the indications for repair and the natural history of abdominal aortic aneurysms.

The two currently available endografts differ in configuration (Fig. 86.7). The AneuRx device consists of a polyester graft that is completely supported externally with a Nitinol exoskeleton. The bifurcated system comprises two modules. The main component is the body of the graft and two limbs of different length. The second component, or iliac limb, complements the shorter limb of the main graft. The radial forces of the self-expanding Nitinol exoskeleton facilitate attachment at the proximal and distal ends of the graft. Additional aortic and iliac extension cuffs are available to facilitate appropriate positioning of the devices

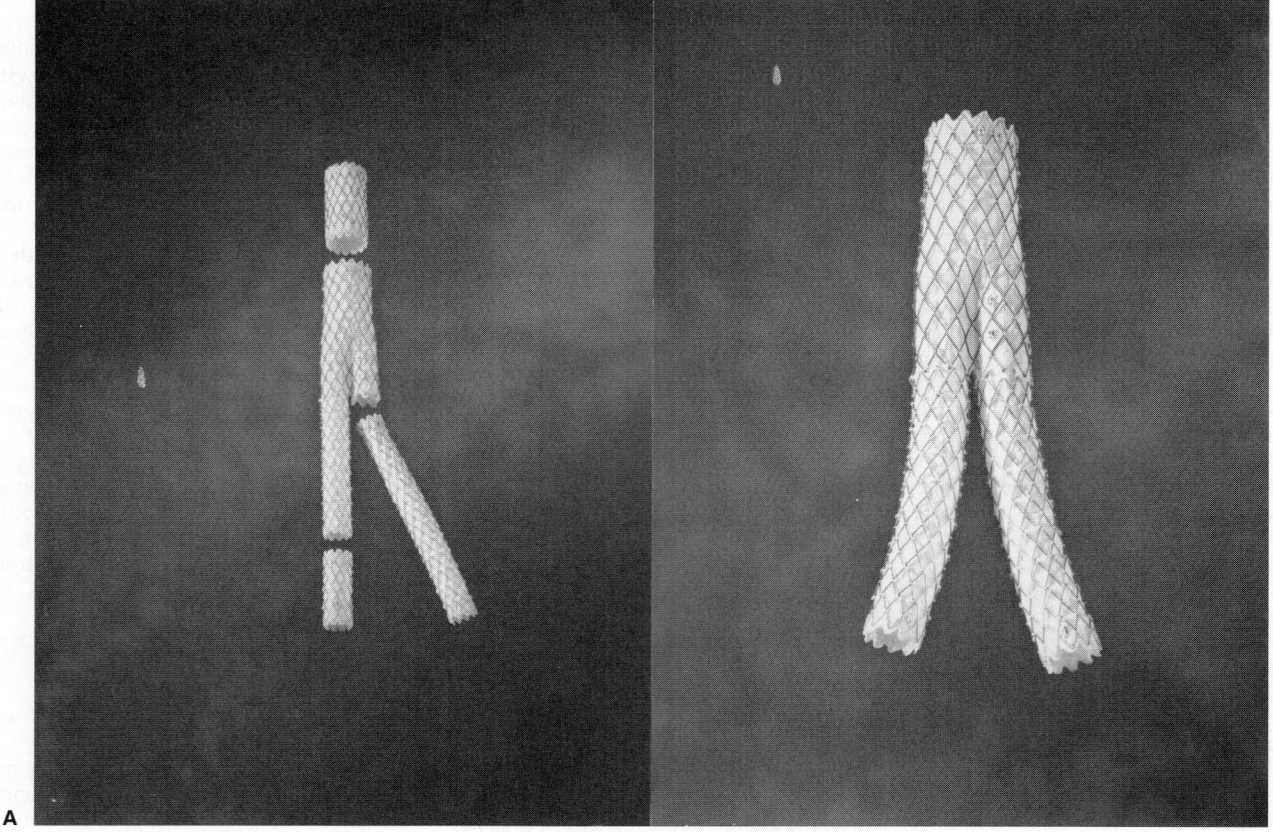

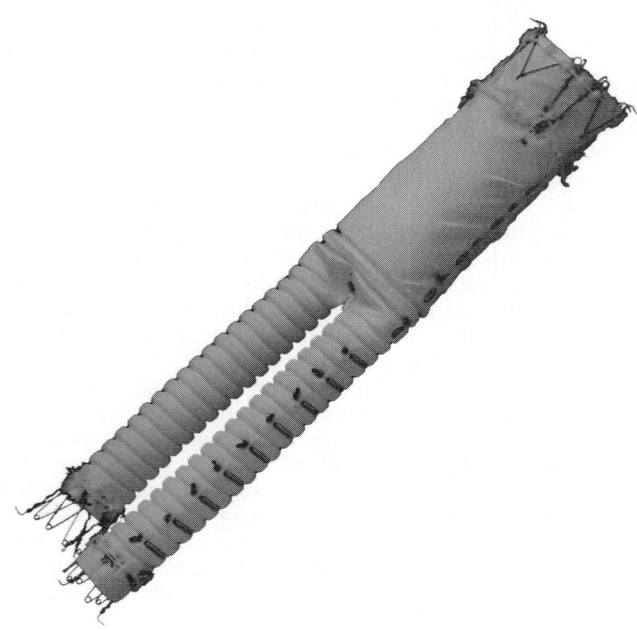

Figure 86.7. Endovascular devices approved by the Food and Drug Administration for infrarenal abdominal aortic aneurysm repair. *(A)* AneuRx. The individual components and the assembled system are shown. Note the complete exoskeleton and the bifurcated system, including the iliac limb, aortic extension cuff, and iliac extension cuff. *(B)* Ancure. Note the proximal and distal fixation hooks.

and to correct endoleaks. Both tube and bifurcated systems are available in the Ancure device. They consist of a polyester graft with circumferential hooks at the proximal and distal ends to facilitate attachment to the vessel walls, but the graft is not supported by an exoskeleton.

The endograft is sized according to the anatomic configuration of the aneurysm and adjacent arteries, and sizing must be performed in advance of the operation to ensure that the appropriate devices are available. Each endograft

is essentially "made to order" for an individual patient. Work sheets are available from the manufacturers of both devices to confirm the suitability of an aneurysm for endovascular repair and to aid in the selection of an appropriately sized device. The diameter and length of the infrarenal cuff, aneurysm, and iliac vessels must be measured precisely, in addition to the distance from the aortic bifurcation to the iliac landing site. Briefly, the diameter of the proximal graft is chosen to oversize the aortic cuff and iliac arteries by approximately 10% to 20%. The length of the iliac limbs is the sum of the aortic cuff length, the aortic aneurysm length, and the distance from the aortic bifurcation to the iliac landing site. Currently, the manufacturers must review the imaging studies before they release the devices to ensure the selection of properly sized devices. However, it is anticipated that this requirement will be liberalized as experience accumulates.

The techniques associated with implantation of the endografts are somewhat specific to the two approved devices. Both manufacturers currently require that physicians implanting the devices complete an approved training course. The generic approach is illustrated by the insertion of the bifurcated Ancure device (Fig. 86.8). Briefly, the common femoral arteries are exposed bilaterally. An arteriogram that includes the renal and iliac arteries is obtained with use of a calibrated catheter, and marker bars are placed at the orifices of the renal arteries and aortic bifurcation. Sheaths are inserted through both femoral vessels, and a snare is introduced through the sheath contralateral to the side selected for deployment of the graft. The pull wire used to deploy the contralateral limb of the bifurcated graft is introduced through the ipsilateral sheath, snared from the contralateral side, and withdrawn into the contralateral sheath. The graft delivery system is then advanced through the ipsilateral sheath until the inferior attachment system is above the aortic bifurcation. The jacket covering the prosthesis is unlocked and retracted to uncover the graft. The pull wire is simultaneously retracted to position the contralateral limb of the graft in the appropriate iliac artery. The proximal attachment hooks are positioned with the aid of the marker bars at the level of the renal arteries, deployed, and secured with the aortic balloon contained within the graft delivery system. The contralateral limb is positioned appropriately, and the attachment hooks are deployed and secured. A similar technique is used for the ipsilateral iliac limb. The delivery system is removed while access to the prosthesis is maintained with the use of intraluminal guide wires. The iliac limbs are completely expanded with balloon angioplasty. A completion arteriogram is obtained to confirm adequate positioning of the device and exclusion of contrast flow outside the lumen of the device. It is imperative that all endoleaks detected by the completion arteriogram be corrected before the completion of the procedure. Implantation of the AneuRx device is similar. However, insertion requires cannulating the short limb of the bifurcated module and deploying the iliac limb with its proximal aspect seated within this short limb.

The postoperative course after endovascular aneurysm repair is significantly shorter and simpler than that after standard repair. Early in the endovascular experience, patients were transferred from the operating room to the intensive care unit and ultimately to the floor, as in standard repair. However, postoperative care has been simplified as experience has increased. Most patients are transferred from the operating room to the intermediate or general care floor and are discharged home on their second or third postoperative day. Occasionally, a patient must be taken to the intensive care unit for observation, but this is usually necessary because of an underlying medical condition rather than procedure itself. Oral feedings are initiated on either the evening of the operation or the first postoperative day, and early ambulation encouraged. No specific care is usually required for the groin incisions. Patients should undergo CT and abdominal radiography before discharge so that the position of the device can be confirmed, the presence of an endoleak ruled out, and a baseline obtained for later studies.

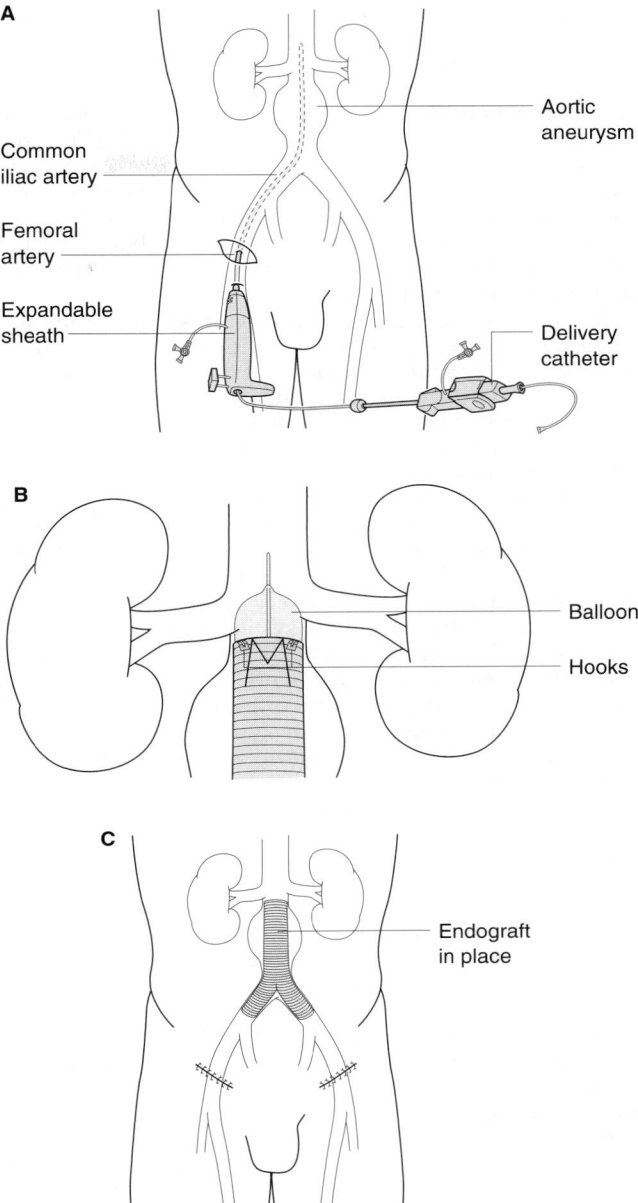

Figure 86.8. General steps involved in the endovascular repair of an abdominal aortic aneurysm with the Ancure device. *(A)* The device is positioned within the aneurysm under fluoroscopic guidance after exposure of the femoral artery and insertion of the necessary sheaths. *(B)* The device is secured proximally by anchoring the attachment hooks into the infrarenal aorta by means of balloon angioplasty. *(C)* The distal attachment sites are similarly secured after the iliac limbs are properly positioned. A completion arteriogram confirms the position of the device and complete exclusion of the aneurysm.

Complications and Outcome

The mortality and complication rates after endovascular repair are comparable with those after standard repair, as noted above. Notably, the perioperative mortality of patients treated with the AneuRx device in the phase II trial was 2.6% and was not significantly different from that of the open controls (47). Essentially all the same complications that can occur during standard repair can also develop after endovascular repair. However, the relative incidence of the various complications is significantly different, and complications inherent to the endovascular repair have been identified. Furthermore, the complications inherent to the endovascular approach may develop at any time throughout the postoperative course and have been reported to occur at a rate of 10% per year (136). The potential for late complications necessitates vigilant follow-up to monitor aneurysm size, detect endoleaks, and assess the stability and configuration of the device. A reasonable surveillance protocol includes CT and an abdominal flat plate immediately postoperatively, at 3, 6, and 12 months, and every 6 months thereafter.

A variety of potential complications may arise from cannulating the arterial lumen. Significant arterial stenoses, calcification, or acute angulation or tortuosity in the common femoral artery, external and common iliac arteries, and aorta may preclude introduction of the delivery system. The bifurcated AneuRx component requires that the iliac artery accommodate a 21F catheter (diameter of approximately 7 mm), and for the contralateral iliac limb, the luminal diameter must be sufficient to accommodate a 16F catheter. The Ancure device is even larger, with the outer diameter of the delivery sheath measuring 27F. Additional lubrication of the delivery system or an approach through the contralateral iliac system may allow successful cannulation. Arterial stenoses can be corrected with angioplasty, either intraoperatively or at the time of the preoperative arteriogram. Difficulties with angulation and tortuosity may potentially be overcome by manual retraction of the vessels after retroperitoneal exposure, interposition grafting of the iliac vessels, serial dilation, or manual retraction of the delivery system with use of a brachial–femoral artery guide wire. Arterial cannulation often requires a reasonable amount of manual force. However, excessive force can result in injury and perforation of the vessels. Perforation may be evidenced by the hemodynamic changes associated with the resultant hemorrhage. The diagnosis can be confirmed by arteriography and the bleeding controlled intraluminally with a balloon catheter. A variety of endovascular repairs are possible in this setting, including deployment of the graft, extension components, or both. However, emergent laparotomy and conversion to open repair comprise the safest and recommended treatment. Dissection within the arterial wall of the iliac vessels or aorta may result from misdirection or excessive force during cannulation of the vessels. It can usually be corrected by cannulating the "true" lumen and reestablishing its integrity by means of a combination of balloon angioplasty, angioplasty/stenting, and deployment of the endovascular device. Failure to reestablish the lumen may require extraanatomic bypass or conversion to open repair with an aortofemoral bypass.

Graft deployment can be associated with mechanical problems related to the delivery system or inappropriate positioning. A host of mechanical problems have been described, and the list will likely expand with widespread application of the devices and the introduction of newer systems. Many of the mechanical problems are device-specific and related to the actual sequence of events and manipulations required. Troubleshooting guidelines and specific recommendations are available from the manufacturers. The AneuRx modular design with its aortic and iliac extensions is significantly more amenable to remedial procedures. Deployment of the endovascular graft below the proximal target site on the infrarenal aorta may be corrected by insertion of an additional covered stent graft if available or conversion to an open repair. Attempting to reposition the graft further proximally after deployment has not been successful and is ill-advised. Similarly, deployment of the AneuRx contralateral iliac limb too low may be remedied with deployment of an iliac extension limb. Deployment of the endovascular graft across the orifices of the renal arteries can potentially be corrected by displacing the graft caudad, but conversion to an open procedure may be necessary. Endovascular salvage can be performed either by passing a guide wire over the rim of the graft and applying gentle caudal pressure or by inflating an aortic balloon at the proximal attachment and similarly retracting. Extreme care must be exercised to prevent injury to the aorta itself. Deployment of the struts of the endovascular graft across the orifices of the renal arteries has been reported, as noted above, and was complicated by the loss of two kidneys among 37 patients and significant renal infarcts in two others (90). Deployment of the endograft across the lumen of one internal iliac artery is usually tolerated provided the contralateral vessel is patent without significant disease. Occlusion of both internal iliac arteries or occlusion of one vessel in the presence of contralateral disease may render the pelvis ischemic and require open conversion.

Endoleaks or incomplete occlusion of the aneurysm by the endovascular device complicates approximately 25% of all endovascular repairs, as noted above (81). Approximately two thirds of these endoleaks are noted immediately after graft placement, and approximately 37% persist (81). The treatment depends on the time course and mechanism (type 1, attachment site; type 2, collateral circulation; type 3, fabric tear or module interface; type 4, transgraft), although the data are incomplete and no consensus opinion is available. A significant proportion of the early endoleaks seal spontaneously and probably do not require intervention (82). However, they merit intensification of the surveillance protocol until they resolve. Karch et al. (137) have proposed imaging at 2 weeks, 1 month, and 3 months postoperatively or until resolution. The presence of a type 1 or 3 endoleak represents a possible exception to this conservative approach to early endoleaks. These endoleaks are clearly more worrisome in terms of aneurysm growth and rupture risk, and it has been proposed that they be corrected regardless of the time course (early vs. late) (138). All persistent early and late endoleaks should undergo angiographic evaluation and treatment, with the specific treatment depending on the mechanism of the endoleak. Type 1 endoleaks (Fig. 86.9A) can usually be corrected by balloon angioplasty or deployment of a modular extender cuff at the arterial–graft interface. Patients should undergo open repair if these maneuvers are unsuccessful, particularly if the aneurysm is symptomatic or has increased in size. Type 2 endoleaks (Fig. 86.9B) that result from persistent collateral circulation can be treated with angiographic embolization. The specific approach depends on the specific collateral that is patent, although a translumbar approach to the aneurysm sac may be required. It has been reported that persistent type 2 endoleaks are less worrisome in terms of aneurysm rupture risk and merit intervention only if the aneurysm continues to enlarge or becomes symptomatic (138,139). The management of type 3 endoleaks is similar to that of type 1, and they are considered a variant of type 1 endoleaks by some authors. They can be treated by deployment of a modular endograft to bridge the graft–graft interface or fabric tear, with conversion to open repair reserved for cases in which the remedial endovascular approach is unsuccessful. Type 4 endoleaks are benign and self-limited and do not require intervention. They are identified as a diffuse contrast "blush" at the time of the completion arteriography during the initial endovascular graft deployment. They represent a diagnosis of exclusion and mandate that the more worrisome type 1 endoleak be ruled out.

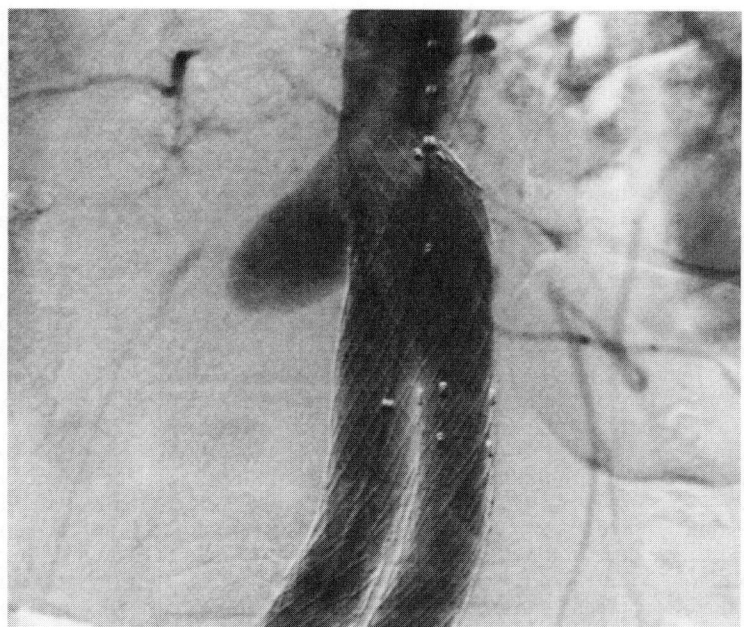
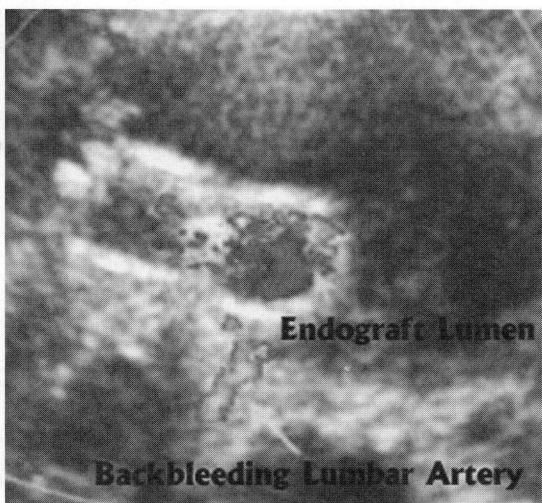

A

B

Figure 86.9. *(A)* An arteriogram demonstrating a type 1 endoleak. Extravasation of contrast is seen outside the lumen of the endograft at its proximal attachment site. *(B)* A color-flow duplex scan of a type 2 endoleak with a patent lumbar artery feeding the aneurysm sac. (Duplex scan courtesy of Bonnie L. Johnson, R.D.M.S., R.V.T., F.S.V.T., Stanford University Medical Center, Stanford, CA.)

The optimal outcome after endovascular repair in terms of aneurysmal configuration is for the aneurysm to regress. Aneurysms that fail to regress and those that continue to increase in size in the absence of an identifiable endoleak on routine serial imaging studies are concerning in terms of long-term stability and rupture risk. Notably, Baum et al. (140) reported that systemic arterial pressures within the aneurysm sac are possible after endovascular repair in the absence of an endoleak. Furthermore, it should be emphasized that the absence of an endoleak does not ensure long-term success. All aneurysms that continue to increase in size require further investigation. It is recommended that patients undergo arteriography to look for the presence of a correctable problem or, more specifically, an endoleak not detected on routine imaging. Any identifiable endoleaks should be corrected as outlined above. If an endoleak or an explanation for the continued aneurysm growth is not found, patients should undergo open surgical repair. The optimal treatment for patients whose aneurysms fail to regress after endovascular repair yet remain stable in size is unclear. Routine serial imaging with CT or duplex ultrasonography is likely appropriate, with correction of any identifiable late endoleaks. Arteriography to look for an occult endoleak with conversion to open surgical repair if necessary, as proposed for aneurysms that continue to increase in size, is probably not indicated. However, it may well turn out that aneurysms that remain stable in size after endovascular repair are associated with a small but significant risk for rupture, intermediate between the risk of aneurysms that continue to increase in size and the risk of those that regress.

A variety of device-specific complications, including strut fracture, fabric tears, and buckling of the graft, have been identified, and the list will likely increase with the introduction of newer systems. These may present at any time throughout the postoperative period and further justify the vigilant long-term surveillance protocol outlined.

An extensive discussion of all the potential device-related complications and their treatment is beyond the scope of this chapter. Disturbingly, regression of the aneurysm has been associated with significant conformational changes in the completely externally supported endografts and has resulted in limb thrombosis and disruption of the distal attachment sites (141).

The long-term outcome after endovascular repair of abdominal aortic aneurysms in terms of the traditional outcome measures of survival, aneurysm rupture, and graft complications remains undefined, as noted above. In a recent report from the U.K. Registry for the Endovascular Treatment of Abdominal Aortic Aneurysms, the 2-year endoleak survival was 60% (136). Although this value falls below those reported for open repair, direct comparison is not appropriate because a significant proportion of patients undergoing endovascular repair were deemed unsuitable for conventional treatment.

Standard Repair of Ruptured Abdominal Aortic Aneurysm

The approach to the patient with a ruptured abdominal aortic aneurysm is similar to the standard approach, although several points merit further comment. Successful endovascular repair of ruptured abdominal aortic aneurysms has been reported, but endovascular repair is not the current standard of care (142). Fortunately, ruptured abdominal aortic aneurysms are infrequent, but it is important to understand the associated pathophysiologic processes and approach management in an expeditious, systemic fashion. Operative repair is the only treatment, and vascular control of the aorta above the rupture is the only means to prevent further hemorrhage.

The patient should be taken emergently to the operating room once the diagnosis of a ruptured abdominal aortic aneurysm has been made. Unnecessary delays to complete the preoperative evaluation or reconstruct the pelvic CT images should be avoided. Unfortunately, the diagnosis is not always made in a setting where an operating room is immediately available. Given this scenario, either the patient should be transferred to a setting in which an operating room is available or the necessary resources should be mobilized locally. The decision to transfer or treat locally should be dictated by the ultimate time necessary to get the patient to the operating room. The operating room and anesthesia personnel should be notified immediately upon diagnosis and instructed that the patient is en route. The necessary instrument trays should be opened, the room temperature in the operating room raised, adjunctive measures to maintain body temperature arranged, and the intraoperative autologous salvage device prepared. The blood bank should be notified and instructed to send 6 units of blood to the operating room. This should be type O negative or type-specific if cross-matched units are not available. Furthermore, the blood bank should be instructed to expedite the cross-match of additional red blood cells, fresh frozen plasma, and platelets. The patient should be prepared and draped before intubation and the induction of anesthesia. Simultaneously, the surgeon and assistants should scrub and gown and be prepared to make the incision at the time of induction. Patients with ruptured aneurysms frequently become hypotensive after the induction of anesthesia because of the vasodilator effect.

A midline incision should be made and supraceliac aortic control obtained. This is facilitated by bluntly dissecting the gastrohepatic ligament and both the crus of the diaphragm and the connective tissue enveloping the aorta. The latter may be somewhat tenacious and a moderate amount of force required. Vascular control can be achieved manually by either occluding the aorta between the fingers and thumb or compressing it against the vertebral bodies. Definitive control should be obtained with an aortic clamp, which can be guided along the arm, hand, and digits occluding the aorta. Care should be utilized during these maneuvers to prevent injury to the esophagus. Inexperienced surgeons may mistake the esophagus for the aorta in hypotensive patients. The presence of a nasogastric tube or pulse may aid in differentiating the aorta from the esophagus. Aortic control can also be achieved through a variety of other means: thoracotomy with occlusion of the descending thoracic aorta, intraluminal control of the infrarenal aorta with a Foley balloon, supraceliac control via a retroperitoneal approach, and intraluminal control with an aortic balloon catheter inserted through the femoral arteries. The aortic surgeon should be familiar with these various techniques because they can be helpful in certain clinical settings, but the midline approach with supraceliac control is recommended for most ruptured infrarenal aneurysms. After supraceliac aortic control has been obtained, the infrarenal aorta is dissected and vascular control is achieved below the level of the renal arteries. Often, the hematoma from the ruptured aneurysm facilitates the dissection by displacing the normal tissue planes. However, the normal tissues may be obscured, and care should be taken not to injure the venous structures, particularly the left renal vein. The supraceliac aortic clamp can be released after infrarenal control has been obtained, and flow can be restored to the visceral vessels. It is imperative that these various steps be coordinated with the anesthesia team, and it is recommended that the supraceliac clamp be left in position to facilitate reapplication if necessary. Distal vascular control can be achieved with either vascular clamps or intraluminal balloons, depending on the character of the iliac vessels.

Patients can be heparinized after proximal and distal vascular control have been obtained, provided that the patient is doing well and the case is proceeding expeditiously. However, the decision to anticoagulate the patient is contingent on a variety of factors, including quantity of blood lost, presence of any coagulopathic bleeding, body temperature, and hemodynamic status. Anticoagulation potentially reduces thrombotic complications, but it exacerbates coagulopathic bleeding. Before completion of the distal anastomoses, thromboembolectomy catheters should be passed distally through the iliac vessels to remove any thrombus or debris. It is recommended that the inferior mesenteric artery be implanted if patent to reduce the risk for postoperative colonic ischemia. The heparin effect can be reversed with protamine after confirmation of distal lower extremity arterial signals. The administration of fresh frozen plasma, platelets, or both should be considered at this point if any evidence of coagulopathic bleeding is noted.

The postoperative course after repair of a ruptured abdominal aortic aneurysm is predictably more complicated and protracted than the course after elective repair (143–147). The stay in the intensive care unit and the entire hospital stay are significantly increased. The mortality and complications rates are likewise significantly increased. As noted above, the operative mortality rate for patients with ruptured abdominal aortic aneurysms who make it to the operating room is approximately 50% (5). The spectrum of postoperative complications after repair of a ruptured aneurysm is essentially the same as after standard elective repair despite the increased overall incidence. Predictably, long-term survival is decreased relative to the long-term survival of patients undergoing elective repair (143), although the overall quality of life is comparable (148).

ADDITIONAL CONSIDERATIONS

Isolated Iliac Artery Aneurysms

Isolated iliac artery aneurysms are rare and have been reported to occur with an incidence ranging from 0.03% in autopsy series (6) to 2.2% in single-institution series (149). The common iliac artery is involved in approximately 70% of the cases, and the internal iliac artery in the remainder (150). Aneurysmal involvement of the external iliac artery, either in combination with the common iliac artery or alone, is distinctly rare. These isolated iliac artery aneurysms should be differentiated from the common iliac artery aneurysms that occur concomitantly with abdominal aortic aneurysms. Simultaneous aneurysmal involvement of the aorta and common iliac arteries occurs in about 10% to 20% of all abdominal aortic aneurysms (6,7); this pattern should be considered as one disease process and treated accordingly.

The natural history of isolated iliac artery aneurysms is poorly defined because of their low incidence. The clinical risk factors appear to be similar to those for abdominal aortic aneurysms, with the highest incidence seen among elderly men. Unlike patients with abdominal aortic aneurysms, a significant proportion of patients with isolated iliac artery aneurysms present with symptoms (151). These symptoms may result from either rupture or compression of adjacent structures, including the bowel, ureters, iliac veins, and nerves. The clinical presentation of patients with a ruptured iliac artery aneurysm is similar to that of patients with a ruptured abdominal aortic aneurysm, and the diagnosis should be included in the differential for patients with genitourinary symptoms and normal findings on urinalysis and testicular examination. CT is optimal for confirming the diagnosis of an isolated iliac artery aneurysm. The utility of ultrasonography is limited by the posterior course of the iliac vessels in the pelvis and the overlying bowel. Large iliac artery aneurysms may occasionally be palpated during rectal or gynecologic examination, and ruptured iliac artery aneurysms may present with ecchymosis of the perineum.

The principles of treatment for asymptomatic, isolated iliac artery aneurysms are similar to those for abdominal aortic aneurysms, and operative repair is justified when the risk for rupture offsets the risk of repair. Because of the poorly defined natural history of isolated iliac artery aneurysms, the size criteria to justify repair remain unclear. Rupture has been reported for aneurysms smaller than 2 cm, although it is rare for aneurysms smaller than 3 cm to rupture (149). It is generally recommended that good-risk patients undergo operative repair for isolated iliac (common or internal) artery aneurysms larger than 3 cm.

The treatment or repair of isolated iliac artery aneurysms depends on the specific vessel involved and the extent of the aneurysm. A common iliac artery aneurysm can be repaired simply with an interposition prosthetic graft, like an abdominal aortic aneurysm isolated to the infrarenal aorta, provided that a sufficient uninvolved proximal neck is available. Unfortunately, this is not the typical situation because the aneurysmal changes in the common iliac vessel frequently extend to the aortic bifurcation. Open repair in this setting requires a bifurcated graft with the proximal anastomosis to the infrarenal aorta. It is recommended that the proximal anastomosis be performed immediately below the renal arteries, as in the repair of aortic aneurysms, due to the potential for subsequent aneurysmal degeneration of the infrarenal aorta. The distal anastomosis can be performed to a disease-free segment of the common iliac artery, although aneurysms frequently extend to the bifurcation, so that anastomosis at that level is necessary. The role of endovascular techniques in the treatment of isolated common iliac artery aneurysms remains to be defined. The potential options are essentially the same as for open repair and include exclusion of the common iliac artery alone with use of a tube graft or exclusion of the whole aortoiliac segment with use of a bifurcated graft. One potential concern about the endovascular approach, as discussed earlier, is the need to cover the origin of the internal iliac artery if the common iliac artery aneurysm extends to the bifurcation. Although occlusion of one and even both internal iliac arteries has been reported to be safe, the status of the pelvic circulation should be investigated before intervention and the potential complications discussed with the patient.

Internal iliac artery aneurysms are treated essentially by exclusion, which can be performed with either an open or endovascular approach. Internal iliac artery aneurysms are not usually amenable to interposition grafting because the aneurysmal involvement frequently extends to the common iliac artery bifurcation and because the vessel arborizes shortly after its takeoff into multiple smaller pelvic branches. The standard open approach requires vascular control of the distal common iliac and proximal external iliac arteries. The internal iliac artery is then opened by incising the aneurysm, and the branches are oversewn from within. The proximal internal iliac artery can be either oversewn at its takeoff, or the resultant defect at the common iliac bifurcation can be repaired with patch angioplasty. Exclusion can also be obtained by embolizing the aneurysm with a variety of agents, including coils and gelfoam. However, this approach is less effective if the internal iliac artery aneurysm extends to the common iliac bifurcation and has a broad base because of the inability to obliterate the aneurysm completely and the potential for embolization of the occluding agents into the lower extremity. The treatment of bilateral internal iliac artery aneurysms raises the same concerns about pelvic ischemia as the endovascular occlusion of both internal iliac arteries. The treatment options to minimize the potential for pelvic ischemia in this setting include treating only the largest aneurysm, attempting to bypass one internal iliac vessel, revascularizing the inferior mesenteric artery if occluded, and excluding both aneurysms serially after sufficient time has elapsed for the development of pelvic collaterals.

Inflammatory Abdominal Aortic Aneurysms

Inflammatory abdominal aortic aneurysms comprise approximately 5% of all abdominal aortic aneurysms (152). They are characterized by a dense inflammatory response involving the anterior and lateral walls of the infrarenal aorta with sparing of the posterior aspect. The inflammatory response consists of a dense cellular infiltrate that has a white, glistening appearance on inspection in the operating room. The inflammation results in an increase in wall thickness, with the difference between the inner and outer diameters of the aorta ranging from 1 to 5 cm. The cause of the inflammatory process remains unresolved, but it may be an autoimmune phenomenon.

Patients with an inflammatory abdominal aortic aneurysm are predominantly male and frequently present with symptoms of back or abdominal pain. The triad of a pulsatile abdominal aortic mass, abdominal pain, and an elevated sedimentation rate has been described for inflammatory abdominal aortic aneurysms. The diagnosis may be confirmed by abdominal ultrasonography or CT. The anterior and lateral aspects of the aortic wall are thickened and hypoechoic on the ultrasonogram. The CT findings are characteristic and include thickening and contrast enhancement in the same distribution. An inexperienced observer may confuse the CT findings with those of a ruptured abdominal aortic aneurysm. Hydronephrosis with medial displacement of the ureters is frequently seen on CT when the ureters are involved by the inflammatory process, and this contrasts with the usual lateral displacement seen with noninflammatory aneurysms.

The treatment of inflammatory abdominal aortic aneurysms is essentially the same as the treatment of the more common, noninflammatory variety, and the outcomes should be comparable. However, several technical differences merit comment. Elective operative repair is recommended for good-risk patients with aneurysms 5 cm or larger in diameter and for higher-risk patients with aneurysms 6 cm or larger in diameter. Nonoperative treatment with corticosteroids has been recommended (153); however, the role of this approach is unclear, and it is not recommended. Additionally, it has been suggested that the rupture risk of inflammatory abdominal aortic aneurysms is considerably less than the rupture risk of the noninflammatory variety because the wall thickness is increased. However, this is not true, and patients should not be lulled into a false sense of security about the natural history of their inflammatory aneurysm. It should be noted that most aneurysms rupture through their posterior or posterolateral aspect, which is not involved in the inflammatory process. The open repair of an inflammatory abdominal aortic aneurysm is complicated by the fact that the adjacent structures, including the duodenum, colon, and ureters, may be involved in the inflammatory process and densely adherent to the aortic wall. These problems can be avoided by repairing the aneurysm through a retroperitoneal approach. Inflammatory aneurysms can be repaired through a transperitoneal approach, and this scenario occasionally arises when the diagnosis is not made preoperatively. No attempt should be made to mobilize the adherent structures, specifically the duodenum, because of the potential for accidental injury. Proximal aortic control can be achieved either immediately above the renal arteries or above the visceral vessels. Alternatively, intraluminal aortic control can be achieved with a balloon catheter, although this approach is less appealing. Distal control can usually be achieved at the common iliac arteries or at the level of their bifurcation. The duodenum and other adherent structures should be mobilized by incising the wall of the aneurysm and then reflecting them laterally. The proximal anastomosis can usually be performed to the infrarenal aorta after the aneurysm wall has been incised. The placement of preoperative ureteral catheters may facilitate identification of the ureters intraoperatively and can be helpful in patients with hydronephrosis. The endovascular approach has a tremendous amount of appeal in the treatment of inflammatory abdominal aortic aneurysms, although the experience is small (154,155). The anatomic criteria for endovascular repair are essentially the same as those for the repair of noninflammatory aneurysms. One major question regarding the endovascular approach relates to the natural history of the infrarenal cuff in this setting. Interestingly, the inflammatory process involving the aortic wall and adjacent tissue regresses in a significant proportion of patients after open repair (156).

Juxtarenal and Suprarenal Abdominal Aortic Aneurysms

The management of abdominal aortic aneurysms extending to the level of the renal arteries or further proximally is more complicated than the management of the infrarenal variety, and this is reflected by an increase in the associated morbidity and mortality rates (157–159). The repair of these aneurysms is complicated by the obligatory period of renal and visceral ischemia associated with aortic occlusion during the proximal anastomosis. These increased morbidity and mortality rates are factored into the decision algorithm and threshold for operative repair. Elective operative repair is usually recommended for patients with aneurysms 6 cm or larger in diameter in this setting, although the traditional 5-cm criterion may be appropriate for very good-risk patients and those with juxtarenal aneurysms who will require only a short period of suprarenal aortic occlusion.

Abdominal aortic aneurysms extending to the renal arteries or more proximally may be repaired via either a retroperitoneal or a transperitoneal approach, although the former is optimal. The retroperitoneal approach with elevation of the left kidney obviates the concerns about the left renal vein and simplifies exposure of the whole abdominal aorta. Furthermore, the descending thoracic aorta may be exposed by incising the diaphragm and its crus circumferentially. Admittedly, the right renal artery is inaccessible from the retroperitoneal approach, and exposure of the right common iliac artery and its bifurcation is challenging. The proximal anastomosis may be fashioned as a large hood to incorporate the orifices of the renal and visceral arteries as necessary. Separate revascularization of the left renal artery is occasionally necessary if the orifices of the renal arteries are splayed too far apart by the aneurysm, although this is infrequently the case. The transperitoneal repair of these proximal aneurysms requires exposure of the suprarenal aorta for clamp application. This is facilitated by retracting the left renal vein in-

feriorly, during which its adrenal, gonadal, and lumbar branches must be ligated. The anterior surface of the aorta at the level of the visceral vessels is encased by dense neural tissue that can be incised. Incising the crus of the diaphragm that envelops the lateral aspect of the aorta further facilitates application of the aortic clamp at this location. The configuration of the proximal anastomosis depends on the extent of the aneurysm and the vessels involved. Juxtarenal aneurysms can be repaired by instituting suprarenal control and sewing the proximal anastomosis right at the level of the renal orifices. The proximal anastomosis for suprarenal aneurysms can be performed by fashioning an anastomotic hood that incorporates most of the visceral vessels, although this frequently requires separate revascularization of one renal artery.

The role of the endovascular approach in treating these more proximal aneurysms remains unresolved. The commercially available devices are not applicable, although devices suitable for repair of at least juxtarenal aneurysms are currently under investigation. The specific concerns related to the use of an endovascular device at this location are the stability of the aortic diameter at the proximal attachment site and the effect on renal function of deployment of the attachment mechanism across the orifices of the renal artery, as noted above.

Infected Abdominal Aortic Aneurysms

Infected abdominal aortic aneurysms comprise a small subset of all abdominal aortic aneurysms, accounting for fewer than 1% of all repairs (160). The term *mycotic aneurysm* has traditionally been used to refer to infected aneurysms, although it is a misnomer that has led to a significant amount of confusion. A newer classification system, proposed to clarify the situation, consists of four groups based on the underlying mechanism: (a) mycotic aneurysm, in which a septic embolus from the heart infects an artery; (b) microbial arteritis, in which bacteria spread to infect an atherosclerotic but non-aneurysmal artery and cause aneurysmal degeneration; (c) existing aneurysms that become infected; (d) traumatic pseudoaneurysm with concomitant bacterial inoculation (161). Microbial arteritis resulting from hematogenous bacterial spread currently accounts for approximately 80% of all cases of infected aortic aneurysm (162,163). *Salmonella* causes approximately 40% of all aneurysmal infections in contemporary series, with the remainder caused by *Streptococcus, Staphylococcus, Bacteroides, Arizona hinshawii, Escherichia coli,* and *Pseudomonas aeruginosa* (161).

The diagnosis of infected aortic aneurysm is often difficult and the clinical presentation insidious. Patients may present with fever, back and abdominal pain, or both. The physical examination is often remarkable for a palpable abdominal mass and the presence of peripheral emboli. Laboratory studies are notable for an elevated leukocyte count and positive blood cultures, although the latter are present only 50% of the time (163,164) and negative blood cultures do not exclude the diagnosis. CT is the most useful diagnostic study, and the features suggestive of an infected aneurysm include a periaortic mass, an aneurysm in an atypical location, periaortic fluid or gas, retroperitoneal inflammation, and frank rupture. The angiographic finding of a saccular or eccentric aneurysm in an atypical location is also suggestive of an infected aneurysm.

The treatment of an infected aneurysm requires control of hemorrhage in the presence of rupture, removal of all infected tissues, and restoration of perfusion to the viscera and lower torso. Patients should be started on broad-spectrum antibiotics when the diagnosis is first suspected, although antibiotic therapy alone is not sufficient and the operative intervention should not be delayed in an attempt to sterilize the retroperitoneum. Patients with suspected rupture should undergo emergent exploration through either a transperitoneal or retroperitoneal approach. After vascular control has been obtained, the retroperitoneum should be explored, and intraoperative cultures with a stat Gram's stain should be obtained. Several options for arterial reconstruction are available, including in situ replacement with a prosthetic graft, ligation of the infrarenal aorta with extraanatomic bypass (axillofemoral configuration), or in situ replacement with staged extraanatomic bypass and subsequent removal of the in situ graft. The choice is depends on the character of the aorta, degree of inflammation in the retroperitoneum, suspected organism, and hemodynamic status. In situ replacement of the infected aneurysm with a prosthetic graft is a reasonable option if retroperitoneal inflammation is minimal and the Gram's stain is negative. Ligation of the infrarenal aorta with extraanatomic bypass at the same session after re-preparing and redraping the patient is the recommended approach in most settings, although this is a major undertaking. The three-stage approach of in situ replacement followed by extraanatomic bypass and graft explant is reserved for patients who cannot tolerate the simultaneous procedure because of underlying comorbidities or hemodynamic instability. The integrity of the aortic stump at the time of ligation and the potential for dehiscence or breakdown of the suture line are major concerns. The aorta should be debrided back to grossly uninvolved tissue and sutured in two layers with a running horizontal mattress and a simple continuous suture of nonabsorbable monofilament. A pedicle of omentum can be mobilized and approximated next to the aortic stump to help control the retroperitoneal inflammation and minimize the risk for stump dehiscence. When the diagnosis is suspected preoperatively and no evidence of rupture is found, the staged approach, in which extraanatomic bypass is followed by exploratory laparotomy with ligation of the aorta and extensive retroperitoneal débridement, is recommended. The procedures are usually performed 2 to 3 days apart to allow the patients a period of recovery. Patients should be anticoagulated between procedures to prevent thrombosis of the extraanatomic bypass resulting from competitive flow. Fortunately, the incidence of graft thrombosis during this intervening period is small, and the risk for infection of the extraanatomic bypass is only hypothetical. Mycotic aneurysms involving the suprarenal aorta pose a particularly challenging problem, but fortunately they are uncommon. In situ replacement with a prosthetic graft is frequently the only available option. Extraanatomic bypass (hepatorenal and splenorenal) of the renal arteries with ligation of the suprarenal aorta is an option but represents a significant undertaking and should be reserved for selected cases.

Patients with infected aneurysms, regardless of the arterial reconstruction, require long-term antibiotics and follow-up. Patients should receive intravenous antibiotics for 6 weeks, with the specific choice depending on the culture results. After completing the intravenous antibiotics, patients should be started on oral antibiotics, although the duration of treatment remains unresolved. Patients should finish a course of at least 6 months of oral antibiotics; suppressive, lifelong therapy may be appropriate. Additionally, patients should undergo serial CT to assess the retroperitoneum and the status of the in situ graft when applicable. CT is usually performed 2 weeks postoperatively, then again 3 months and 6 months later. Patients

with in situ revascularization should undergo repeated imaging every 6 months thereafter, although this is not necessary for patients with extraanatomic revascularization in the absence of retroperitoneal inflammation.

Aortoenteric Fistulae

An aortoenteric fistula is a communication between the aorta and the bowel. The duodenum where it crosses anterior to the infrarenal aorta is involved most commonly, but the communication can develop between almost any portion of the small or large intestine. Primary aortic fistulae result when nonspecific abdominal aortic aneurysms erode into the bowel and are distinctly rare, with a reported incidence of 0.04% to 0.07% in autopsy series (165). Secondary aortic fistulae result from the erosion of a prosthetic aortic graft into the bowel; they are significantly more common, with a reported incidence of 0.1% to 2.0% among patients undergoing aortic reconstruction (166). Management is the same for primary and secondary aortic fistulae.

The diagnosis of an aortoenteric fistula is often difficult and mandates a high index of suspicion. Patients frequently present with gastrointestinal bleeding manifested as either hematemesis or melena. The initial episode of gastrointestinal bleeding is often self-limited and has been described as a "herald" bleed. The diagnosis of aortoenteric fistula should be foremost among the differential when a patient with a known aneurysm or prior aortic reconstruction presents with intestinal bleeding because the condition is uniformly fatal if untreated. Patients should undergo endoscopic evaluation of the upper and lower intestinal tract to determine the source of bleeding. It is imperative that the clinical suspicion of an aortoenteric fistula be communicated to the endoscopist to be sure that the third and fourth portions of the duodenum will be adequately examined. The examination occasionally requires the use of a pediatric colonoscope. The endoscopic findings of erosion, thrombus, active bleeding, or visible prosthetic graft in third or fourth portion of the duodenum are worrisome or diagnostic of an aortoenteric fistula and mandate emergent laparotomy. Mild duodenitis and gastritis are frequently seen at the time of endoscopy but do not exclude the diagnosis of an aortoenteric fistula. Notably, the findings of upper gastrointestinal endoscopy are normal in up to 30% of patients with a documented aortoenteric fistula (167). Abdominal pelvic CT should be performed if the results of endoscopy are inconclusive. The findings on CT that suggest an aortoenteric fistula include inflammation within the retroperitoneum, an anastomotic pseudoaneurysm, close approximation of the bowel and the prosthetic aortic graft or aneurysm, and loss of the normal tissue planes between the third portion of the duodenum and the aorta or prosthetic graft. Occasionally, both endoscopy and CT are nondiagnostic despite clinical suspicion of an aortoenteric fistula. Exploratory laparotomy is recommended in this setting for both diagnosis and treatment. Adherence of the bowel to the aorta at the time of the initial exploration suggests an aortoenteric fistula and mandates obtaining suitable proximal and distal control of the aorta, iliac vessels, or prosthetic graft before further dissection. The diagnosis cannot be excluded until the bowel is entirely separated from the retroperitoneum.

Treatment of an aortoenteric fistula requires repair of the defect in the gastrointestinal tract in addition to repair of the aneurysm or treatment of the infected prosthetic graft. Treatment of the gastrointestinal defect is usually straightforward and is based on standard surgical principles. After the fistula is disassembled, the edges of the bowel can be débrided and a primary closure performed with either a stapler or sutures. A limited bowel resection or diversion of the enteral tract may be necessary, although need for the latter is unusual. The intraoperative and longer-term management of the aortic aneurysm or prosthetic graft is the same as that outlined above for infected aortic aneurysms. Indeed, aortoenteric fistulae represent a variant of infected aortic aneurysms. In situ replacement of the prosthetic graft or infrarenal aorta, ligation of the infrarenal aorta with excision of the prosthetic graft and extraanatomic bypass, and in situ replacement with staged extraanatomic bypass and subsequent graft excision are all reasonable options. The clinical scenario usually dictates the choice. Ligation of the infrarenal aorta with excision of the graft and extraanatomic bypass is recommended in most cases. However, in situ repair is appropriate for patients who are older or sicker, who have minimal retroperitoneal inflammation or evidence of hemodynamic instability, or in whom ligation of the infrarenal aorta would compromise the renal arteries. Additionally, patients should be maintained on long-term antibiotics and undergo serial imaging studies, as outlined for infected aneurysms.

Venous Anomalies

Anomalies of the vena cava and renal veins are occasionally encountered at the time of aortic reconstruction. The common anomalies are related to the embryologic development of the iliac veins and vena cava. The four most clinically relevant anomalies include duplication of the inferior vena cava, left-sided vena cava, circumaortic left renal vein, and retroaortic renal vein. In duplication of the inferior vena cava, which has an incidence of 0.2% to 3.0% (168), large veins run parallel to the infrarenal aorta and join together either anterior or posterior to the aorta at the level of the renal vein. In left-sided inferior vena cava, which has an incidence of 0.2% to 0.5% (168), a large vein runs parallel to the left side of the aorta, and a right-sided vena cava is absent. The left-sided vena cava crosses the aorta at the level of the renal vein to become the suprarenal inferior vena cava. The gonadal and adrenal veins on the right drain directly into the renal vein in a mirror image of the normal anatomy. In circumaortic renal vein, which has an incidence of 1.5% to 8.7% (168), a collar of veins surrounds the aorta at the level of the normal renal vein. In retroaortic left renal vein, which occurs with an incidence of 1.2% to 2.4% (168), a single vein runs posterior to the aorta at the usual location. Notably, both duplication of the inferior vena cava and left-sided vena cava can be associated with other venous anomalies, including a circumaortic or retroaortic renal vein.

The diagnosis of the various venous anomalies can usually be made preoperatively by CT. Identification of the vena cava and left renal vein should be part of the mental checklist used when preoperative CT scans are reviewed. The role of preoperative venography to elucidate venous anomalies further remains unclear, although it is likely unnecessary with the continued evolution of CT. The various anomalies may not become evident immediately in the operating room if missed on the preoperative imaging studies. A very prominent left real vein at the usual location or slightly inferior is suggestive of a left-sided vena cava, whereas the absence of a left renal vein despite dissection along the anterior aspect of the aorta at the level of the superior mesenteric artery is suggestive of a retroaortic renal vein.

The repair of an infrarenal abdominal aortic aneurysm in a patient with a venous anomaly is essentially the same as the standard approach, although additional care should be exercised to prevent inadvertent injury. Exposure of the infrarenal neck is more difficult in the presence of a duplicated or left-sided vena cava. However, sufficient exposure can usually be obtained by gentle dissection and mobilization of the venous structures. The presence of a duplicated or left-sided vena cava is a relative contraindication to the left retroperitoneal approach. A circumaortic renal collar or retroaortic renal vein presents a potential hazard when the proximal aortic clamp is applied. A vertical aortic clamp is recommended because dissection of the posterior aspect of the aorta is then unnecessary. Transecting the aorta may facilitate exposure of a retroaortic renal vein, as noted above.

Renal Anomalies

Congenital variations in the renal anatomy may complicate the repair of an abdominal aortic aneurysm. Specifically, their presence may complicate the dissection because they are frequently associated with multiple renal arteries, aberrant venous return, and abnormally positioned ureters. The various congenital anomalies of the upper urinary system have been classified in an attempt to standardize the approach for vascular surgeons (169). The anomalies have been broken down into abnormalities of position, including simple ectopia, and abnormalities of both form and fusion, including horseshoe kidney, crossed renal ectopia without fusion, and crossed renal ectopia with fusion. An ectopic kidney may be positioned anywhere from the pelvis to the thorax. Common forms of ectopic kidney include the pelvic kidney, located opposite the sacrum and below the aortic bifurcation; the lumbar kidney, located opposite the sacral promontory in the iliac fossa and anterior to the iliac vessels; the abdominal kidney, located above the iliac crest adjacent to the second lumbar vertebra; and the thoracic kidney, which can be located above the diaphragm in the posterior mediastinum. In a horseshoe kidney, two distinct renal masses are fused by either renal parenchyma or fibrous tissue; in the overwhelming majority, the lower poles are fused. In crossed renal ectopia, the kidney mass is located on the side opposite to its insertion in the bladder. Multiple configurations of crossed ectopia with and without fusion have been described.

The preoperative objective in the various types of renal anomaly is to image the renal mass adequately, delineate the course of the ureter, and establish the arterial and venous supply. The approach is simplified by the fact that most patients undergo abdominal/pelvic CT as part of the preoperative evaluation. The location and position of both the kidneys and ureters, like the position of the left renal vein, should be established as part of the review of every CT scan for patients with aneurysms. All patients with renal anomalies should undergo preoperative arteriography to confirm the location and number of renal arteries, and delayed images should be obtained at the time of arteriography to visualize the venous return and course of the ureters.

Patients with renal anomalies can safely undergo repair of an abdominal aortic aneurysm; however, the anomalies must be factored into the operative plan. The specific operative approach depends on the location of the renal mass, blood supply, course of the ureters, and presence of fusion. A left-sided retroperitoneal approach or transperitoneal approach with medial visceral rotation is the most helpful, particularly in patients with horseshoe kidney. A standard transperitoneal approach with transection of the fused parenchyma has been reported in patients with horseshoe kidney, although this may be associated with significant bleeding and urine leak and is discouraged.

The frequently encountered multiple renal arteries can be handled most expeditiously by using a Carrel patch technique, in which a cuff of aorta including the renal artery orifices is reimplanted into the aortic graft after completion of the proximal anastomosis.

Coexistent Renal or Visceral Artery Occlusive Disease

Coexistent renal or visceral artery occlusive disease is frequently found in patients undergoing abdominal aortic aneurysm repair. The true incidence is probably greater than appreciated because of the use of CT as the main preoperative imaging study and the selective use of arteriography. The optimal management of patients with coexistent lesions remains unresolved. The options include repair of the aneurysm alone, simultaneous repair of the aneurysm and revascularization of the renal or visceral vessels, and staged repair, with either aneurysm repair or revascularization performed first. The treatment options for staged repair include both open surgical and endovascular approaches. The optimal approach represents a balance between the indications for the procedure and the associated added risk. Simultaneous repair of the aneurysm and revascularization of the renal/visceral vessels is appealing but is associated with a significant increase in the associated morbidity and mortality rates (105,170).

Renal/visceral revascularization is mandatory at the time of aneurysm repair if the affected vessels are involved in the aneurysm, as in suprarenal aneurysm or horseshoe kidney with multiple renal arteries originating from the infrarenal aorta. More commonly, a lower pole or accessory renal artery may come off the aneurysm. The decision to perform a concomitant revascularization with either reimplantation or a bypass graft in this setting depends on the size of the vessel and the quantity of kidney tissue it perfuses. Revascularization is recommended for larger vessels (> 2 mm) that supply a significant portion of the renal mass. Combined aneurysm repair with renal/visceral artery revascularization may be justified if the traditional indications for renal or visceral artery revascularization are satisfied. The indications for renal revascularization include poorly controlled hypertension in a patient with a significant renal artery stenosis and rapidly progressive renal insufficiency in a patient with adequate renal mass and bilateral renal artery stenosis. The traditional indications for mesenteric revascularization include symptoms of chronic mesenteric ischemia and critical stenosis of either the superior mesenteric artery alone or two of the three visceral vessels. The combined approach in patients with progressive renal insufficiency and symptomatic mesenteric ischemia should be applied cautiously. Preoperative renal insufficiency is a major risk factor for renal failure and mortality after aneurysm repair (22,69). Either a staged approach with revascularization performed first or delayed repair of the aneurysm until after the onset of renal failure may be preferable. Similarly, mesenteric revascularization for chronic mesenteric ischemia when performed alone is associated with a mortality rate of approximately 15% and prolonged intensive care unit and hospital stays (171–174). Mesenteric revascularization should probably be performed before aneurysm repair in this setting because of the added risk and the potential to compromise the mesenteric perfusion during aneurysm repair. The optimal treatment for patients with aneurysms and asymptomatic renal/visceral artery lesions remains even less clear. Natural history studies with the use of both arteriography (175) and duplex scanning (176) have suggested that significant renal artery stenoses are preocclusive lesions that

may merit intervention. However, a recent analysis of patients with asymptomatic renal artery stenosis who underwent aortic reconstruction found that the natural history of the renal artery lesions is fairly benign when untreated and is associated only with an increase in the antihypertensive requirements (177). Little is known about the natural history of asymptomatic mesenteric occlusive lesions. However, a recent small report suggested that patients with asymptomatic severe mesenteric occlusive disease involving all three visceral vessels have a high incidence of bowel infarction (178).

Additional Concurrent Intraabdominal Disease

The finding of an abdominal aortic aneurysm and an additional intraabdominal process that may require operative repair is a relatively frequent event. A second surgical problem may be identified during the preoperative evaluation or operative repair of an abdominal aortic aneurysm; alternatively, an abdominal aortic aneurysm may be identified during the surgical treatment of another problem. No algorithms have been defined for the management of such concurrent problems, and the overall approach requires a modicum of clinical judgment. Options include simultaneous repair or staged repair with repair of the abdominal aortic aneurysm as either the first or second procedure. The approach depends on the risk for aneurysm rupture, natural history of the second surgical problem, and potential for infection of the prosthetic graft during simultaneous repair.

The generic recommendation for patients with an abdominal aortic aneurysm and an additional intraabdominal surgical problem is that the most life-threatening or imminent problem be addressed first. The natural history of untreated abdominal aortic aneurysm has been defined reasonably well and has been outlined extensively earlier in this chapter. It has been reported that the risk for aneurysm rupture is increased after major intraabdominal surgery and is potentially related to an increase in collagenase activity (179). However, this reported increased rupture risk is speculative and should not necessarily be factored into the decision algorithm. The management of concurrent colon cancer and abdominal aortic aneurysm is a frequent treatment dilemma that provides an excellent illustration of the approach to these problems. The treatment principles promulgated by Szilagyi et al. (180) include the following: (a) aneurysm repair first in the presence of rupture; (b) colon resection first in the presence of hemorrhage, perforation, or obstruction; (c) aneurysm repair first in the presence of a large aneurysm and a small colon cancer; (d) colon resection first in the presence of a large colon cancer and a small aneurysm.

Simultaneous abdominal aortic aneurysm repair and cholecystectomy is probably safe for patients with cholelithiasis or evidence of chronic cholecystitis. The safety of these simultaneous procedures has been documented in several series, and the concerns about an increased incidence of aortic graft infection have not been substantiated (181). Advocates of the simultaneous approach justify the cholecystectomy by the potential requirement for a cholecystectomy in the future and the morbidity and mortality associated cholecystitis after aneurysm repair (181). Although a consensus is not found in the literature, simultaneous abdominal aortic aneurysm repair and cholecystectomy are recommended only if evidence of chronic cholecystitis or multiple small stones is present. Regardless, the cholecystectomy and other simultaneous procedures should not be performed until after the aneurysm repair is completed and the retroperitoneum closed in an attempt to reduce the hypothetical risk for graft infection. The safety and utility of other simultaneous procedures remain poorly defined. The repair of ventral hernias is often mandatory to achieve a tension-free abdominal closure and should be viewed more as an extension of the aneurysm repair than as a simultaneous procedure. Inguinal hernias may be repaired at the time of aneurysm repair, but it is uncertain whether the small risk associated with a subsequent procedure at a later date offsets the obligatory additional time for the simultaneous repair. Appendectomy (182) and small-bowel excision for Meckel's diverticulum (181) have been reported to be safe when performed concomitantly with aneurysmectomy, although the natural history of the associated underlying problems in the usual age group of patients undergoing abdominal aortic aneurysm repair is relatively benign.

REFERENCES

1. Dubost C, Allary M, Oeconomos N. Resection of an aneurysm of the abdominal aorta: reestablishment of the continuity by a preserved human arterial graft, with result after five months. *Arch Surg* 1952;64:405–408.
2. Ernst CB. Abdominal aortic aneurysm. *N Engl J Med* 1993;328:1167–1172.
3. Collin J, Araujo L, Walton J, et al. Oxford screening program for abdominal aortic aneurysm in men aged 65 to 74 years. *Lancet* 1988;2:613–615.
4. Ouriel K, Green RM, Donyre C, et al. An evaluation of new methods of expressing aortic aneurysm size: relationship to rupture. *J Vasc Surg* 1992;15:12–20.
5. Taylor LM Jr, Porter JM. Abdominal aortic aneurysms. In: Porter JM, Taylor LM Jr, eds. *Basic data underlying clinical decision making in vascular surgery.* St. Louis: Quality Medical, 1994:98–100.
6. Brunkwall J, Haudsson H, Begtsson H, et al. Solitary aneurysms of the iliac arterial system: an estimate of their frequency of occurrence. *J Vasc Surg* 1989;10:381–384.
7. Lowry WF, Kraft RO. Isolated aneurysms of the iliac artery. *Arch Surg* 1978;113:1289–1293.
8. Hallett JW. Abdominal aortic aneurysm: natural history and treatment. *Heart Dis Stroke* 1992;1:303–308.
9. Collin J. Epidemiological aspects of abdominal aortic aneurysm. *Eur J Vasc Surg* 1990;4:113–116.
10. *Vital statistics of the United States 1990: Volume II—Mortality, Part A.* Hyattsville, MD: National Center for Health Statistics, 1994. National Center for Health Statistics publication NCHS 94-1101.
11. Zarins CK, Glagov S. Aneurysms and obstructive plaques: differing local responses to atherosclerosis. In: Bergan JJ, Yao J, eds. *Aneurysms: diagnosis and treatment.* New York: Grune & Stratton, 1982:61.
12. Glagov S. Hemodynamic risk factors: mechanical stress, mural architecture, medial nutrition, and the vulnerability of arteries to atherosclerosis. In: Wissler RW, Geer JS, eds. *Pathogenesis of atherosclerosis.* Baltimore: Williams & Wilkins, 1972:164.
13. Tilson MD, Elefteriades J, Brophy CM. Tensile strength and collagen in abdominal aortic aneurysm disease. In: Greenhalgh RM, Mannick JA, Powell JT, eds. *The cause and management of aneurysms.* Philadelphia: WB Saunders, 1990:97.
14. Busuttil RW, Abou-Zamzam AM, Machleder HI. Collagenase activity of the human aorta: a comparison of patients with and without abdominal aortic aneurysms. *Arch Surg* 1980;115:1373.
15. Baxter BT, Mcgee GS, Shively VP, et al. Elastin content, cross-links, and mRNA in normal and aneurysmal human aorta. *J Vasc Surg* 1992;16:192.
16. Busuttil RW, Rinderbriecht H, Flesher A, et al. Elastase activity: the role of elastase in aortic aneurysm formation. *J Surg Res* 1982;32:214.
17. Newman KM, Ogata Y, Malon Am, et al. Identification of matrix metalloproteinases 3 (stromelysin) and 9 (gelatinase B) in abdominal aortic aneurysm. *Arterioscler Thromb* 1994;14:1315.
18. Brophy CM, Marks WH, Reilly JM, et al. Decreased tissue inhibitor of metalloproteinases (TIMP) in abdominal aortic tissue: a preliminary report. *J Surg Res* 1991;50:653.
19. Rowe VL, Stevens SL, Reddick TT, et al. Vascular smooth muscle cell apoptosis in aneurysmal occlusive and normal human aortas. *J Vasc Surg* 2000;31:567–576.
20. Newman KM, Johnson CJ, Jean-Claude JM, et al. Cytokines which activate proteolysis are increased in abdominal aortic aneurysms. *Circulation* 1994;90:224.
21. Lederle FA, Johnson GR, Wilson SE, et al. Prevalence and associations of abdominal aortic aneurysm detected through screening. Aneurysm Detection and Management (ADAM) Veterans Affairs Cooperative Study Group. *Ann Intern Med* 1997;126:441–449.
22. Huber TS, Wang JG, Derrow AE, et al. *United States experience with intact abdominal aortic aneurysm repair.* Presented at the joint annual meeting of the North American Chapter of the International Society for Cardiovascular Surgery and the Society for Vascular Surgery, Toronto, Ontario, June 11, 2000.
23. Collin J. The epidemiology of abdominal aortic aneurysm. *Br J Hosp Med* 1988;40:64–67.
24. Scott AP, Wilson NM, Ashton HA, et al. Is surgery necessary for abdominal aneurysms less than 6 cm in diameter? *Lancet* 1993;342:1395–1396.
25. Wilmink TB, Quick CR, Day NE. The association between cigarette smoking and abdominal aortic aneurysms. *J Vasc Surg* 1999;30:1099–1105.
26. Johansen K, Koepsell T. Familial tendency for abdominal aortic aneurysms. *JAMA* 1986;256:1934–1936.
27. Darling RC III, Brewster DC, Darling RC, et al. Are familial aortic aneurysms different? *J Vasc Surg* 1989;10:39–43.
28. Calcagno D, Hallett JW, Ballard DJ, et al. Late iliac artery aneurysms and occlusive disease after aortic tube grafts for abdominal aortic aneurysm repair. *Ann Surg* 1991;214:733–736.
29. Kalman PG, Rappaport DC, Merchant N, et al. The value of late computed tomographic scanning in identification of vascular abnormalities after abdominal aortic aneurysm repair. *J Vasc Surg* 1999;29:442–450.
30. Cutler BS. Arteriosclerotic femoral artery aneurysm. In: Ernst CB, Stanley JC, eds. *Current therapy in vascular surgery,* 3rd ed. St. Louis: Mosby, 1995:315.
31. Haverich A, Miller G, Scott WD, et al. Acute and chronic aortic dissections: determinants of long-term outcome for operative survivors. *Circulation* 1985;72[Suppl 2]:22–33.
32. Ammori BJ, Madan M, Bodenham AR, et al. A review of the management of abdominal aortic aneurysms in patients following cardiac transplantation. *Eur J Vasc Endovasc Surg* 1997;14:185–190.
33. Muluk SC, Steed DL, Makaroun MS, et al. Aortic aneurysm in heart transplant recipients. *J Vasc Surg* 1995;22:689–696.
34. Zierler RE, Strandness DE Jr. Hemodynamics for the vascular surgeon. In: Moore WS, ed. *Vascular surgery: a comprehensive review,* 4th ed. Philadelphia: WB Saunders, 1983:179–204.
35. Cronenwett JL, Murphy TF, Zelenock GB, et al. Actuarial analysis of variables associated with rupture of small abdominal aortic aneurysms. *Surgery* 1985;98:472–483.
36. Limet R, Sakalihassan N, Albert A. Determination of the expansion rate and incidence of rupture of abdominal aortic aneurysms. *J Vasc Surg* 1991;14:540–548.
37. Johansson G, Nydahl S, Olofsson P, et al. Survival of patients with abdominal aortic aneurysms: comparison between operative and non-operative management. *Eur J Vasc Surg* 1990;4:497–502.
38. Glimaker H, Holmberg L, Elvin A, et al. Natural history of patients with abdominal aortic aneurysms. *AJR Am J Roentgenol* 1989;152:785–792.
39. Nevitt MP, Ballard DJ, Hallett JW Jr. Prognosis of abdominal aortic aneurysms: a population-based study. *N Engl J Med* 1989;321:1009–1014.
40. Collin J, Araujo L, Walton J. How fast do very small abdominal aortic aneurysms grow? *Eur J Vasc Surg* 1989;3:15–17.
41. Bernstein EF, Chan EL. Abdominal aortic aneurysm in high-risk patients: outcome of selective management based on size and expansion rate. *Ann Surg* 1984;200:255–263.
42. Delin A, Ohlsen H, Swedenborg J. Growth rate of abdominal

aortic aneurysms as measured by computed tomography. *Br J Surg* 1985;72:530–532.

43. Guirguis EM, Barber GG. The natural history of abdominal aortic aneurysms. *Am J Surg* 1991;162:481–483.

44. Blankensteijn JD, Lindenburg FP, Van der Graaf Y, et al. Influence of study design on reported mortality and morbidity rates after abdominal aortic aneurysm repair. *Br J Surg* 1998; 85:1624–1630.

45. U.K. Small Aneurysm Trial. Mortality results for randomized controlled trial of early elective surgery or ultrasonographic surveillance for small abdominal aortic aneurysms. *Lancet* 1998;352:1649–1660.

46. Porter JM, Abou-Zamzam AM. Endovascular aortic grafting: current status. *Cardiovasc Surg* 1999;7:684–691.

47. Zarins CK, White RA, Schwarten D, et al. AneuRx stent graft versus open surgical repair of abdominal aortic aneurysms: multicenter prospective clinical trial. *J Vasc Surg* 1999;29: 292–305.

48. May J, White GH, Yu W, et al. Concurrent comparison of endoluminal versus open repair in the treatment of abdominal aortic aneurysms: analysis of 303 patients by life table method. *J Vasc Surg* 1998;27:213–221.

49. Blum U, Voshage G, Lammer J, et al. Endoluminal stent-grafts for infrarenal abdominal aortic aneurysms. *N Engl J Med* 1997;336:13–20.

50. Bequemin JP, Lapie V, Favre JP, et al. Mid-term results of a second-generation bifurcated endovascular graft for abdominal aortic aneurysm repair: the French Vanguard Trial. *J Vasc Surg* 1999;30:209–218.

51. Moore WS, Rutherford RB. Transfemoral endovascular repair of abdominal aortic aneurysm: results of the North American EVT phase 1 trial. *J Vasc Surg* 1996;23:543–553.

52. Soisalon-Soininen S, Salo JA, Perhoniemi V, et al. Emergency surgery of non-ruptured abdominal aortic aneurysm. *Ann Chir Gynaecol* 1999;88:38–43.

53. Johansen K, Kohler TR, Nicholls SC, et al. Ruptured abdominal aortic aneurysm: the Harborview experience. *J Vasc Surg* 1991;13:240–247.

54. Katz DJ, Stanley JC, Zelenock GB. Operative mortality rates for intact and ruptured abdominal aortic aneurysms in Michigan: an eleven-year statewide experience. *J Vasc Surg* 1994;19:804–817.

55. Hollier LH, Taylor LM, Ochsner J. Recommended indications for operative treatment of abdominal aortic aneurysms. *J Vasc Surg* 1992:15:1046–1056.

56. Katz DA, Cronenwett JL. The cost-effectiveness of early surgery versus watchful waiting in the management of small abdominal aortic aneurysms. *J Vasc Surg* 1994;19:980–991.

57. Darling RC, Messina CR, Brewster DC, et al. Autopsy study of unoperated abdominal aortic aneurysms: the case for early resection. *Circulation* 1977;56:161–164.

58. Schermerhorn ML, Birkmeyer JD, Gould DA, et al. Cost-effectiveness of surgery for small abdominal aortic aneurysms on the basis of data from the United Kingdom Small Aneurysm Trial. *J Vasc Surg* 2000;31:217–226.

59. Allen PIM, Gourevitch D, McKinley J, et al. Population screening for aortic aneurysms [Letter]. *Lancet* 1987;2:736.

60. Nusbaum JW, Friemanis AK, Thomford NR. Echography in the diagnosis of abdominal aortic aneurysm. *Arch Surg* 1971;102:385–388.

61. Lederle FA, Walker JM, Reinke DB. Selective screening for abdominal aortic aneurysms with physical examination and ultrasound. *Arch Intern Med* 1988;148:1753–1756.

62. Moursi MM, Stanley JC. Surgical treatment of ruptured infrarenal aortic aneurysm. In: Ernst CB, Stanley JC, eds. *Current therapy in vascular surgery,* 3rd ed. St. Louis: Mosby, 1995:224–226.

63. Armon MP, Whitaker SC, Gregson RH, et al. Spiral CT angiography versus aortography in the assessment of aortoiliac length in patients undergoing endovascular abdominal aortic aneurysm repair. *J Endovasc Surg* 1998;5:222–227.

64. Broeders IA, Blankensteijn JD, Olree M, et al. Preoperative sizing of grafts for transfemoral endovascular aneurysm management: a prospective comparative study of spiral CT angiography, arteriography, and conventional CT imaging. *J Endovasc Surg* 1997;4:252–261.

65. Hoffman M, Avellone JC, Plecha FR, et al. Operation for rup-

66. tured abdominal aortic aneurysms: a community-wide experience. *Surgery* 1982;91:597–602.

66. Wakefield TW, Whitehouse WM, Wu S, et al. Abdominal aortic aneurysm rupture: statistical analysis of factors affecting outcome of surgical treatment. *Surgery* 1982;91:586–596.

67. Scott RAP, Wilson NM, Ashton HA, et al. Influence of screening on the incidence of ruptured abdominal aortic aneurysm: 5-year results of a randomized controlled study. *Br J Surg* 1995;82:1006–1070.

68. National Library of Medicine. U.S. Preventive Services Task Force. Aneurysm. *http://text.nlm.nih.gov/cps/www/cps.12. html.*

69. Johnston KW, Scobie TK. Multicenter prospective study of nonruptured abdominal aortic aneurysms. I. Population and operative management. *J Vasc Surg* 1988;7:69–81.

70. Walker EM, Hopkinson BR, Makin GS. Unoperated abdominal aortic aneurysm: presentation and natural history. *Ann R Coll Surg Engl* 1983;65:311–313.

71. Jones A, Cahill D, Gardham R. Outcome in patients with a large abdominal aortic aneurysm considered unfit for surgery. *Br J Surg* 1998;85:1382–1384.

72. Englund R, Perera D, Hanel KC. Outcome for patients with abdominal aortic aneurysms that are treated non-surgically. *Aust N Z J Surg* 1997;67:260–263.

73. Finlayson SR, Birkmeyer JD, Fillinger MF, et al. Should endovascular surgery lower the threshold for repair of abdominal aortic aneurysms? *J Vasc Surg* 1999;29:973–985.

74. Zarins CK, White RA, Fogarty TJ. Aneurysm rupture after endovascular repair using the AneuRx stent graft. *J Vasc Surg* 2000;31:960–970.

75. Torsello GB, Klenk E, Kasprzak B, et al. Rupture of abdominal aortic aneurysm previously treated by endovascular stent-graft. *J Vasc Surg* 1998;28:184–187.

76. Alimi YS, Chakfe N, Rivoal E, et al. Rupture of an abdominal aortic aneurysm after endovascular graft placement and aneurysm size reduction. *J Vasc Surg* 1998;28:178–183.

77. Brewster DC, Geller SC, Kaufman JA, et al. Initial experience with endovascular aneurysm repair: comparison of early results with outcome of conventional open repair. *J Vasc Surg* 1998;27:992–1003.

78. May J, White GH, Waugh R, et al. Adverse events after endoluminal repair of abdominal aortic aneurysms: a comparison during two successive periods of time. *J Vasc Surg* 1999;29:32–39.

79. Seiwert AJ, Wolfe J, Whalen RC, et al. Cost comparison of aortic aneurysm endograft exclusion versus open surgical repair. *Am J Surg* 1999;178:117–120.

80. Patel ST, Haser PB, Bush HL Jr, et al. The cost-effectiveness of endovascular repair versus open surgical repair of abdominal aortic aneurysms: a decision analysis model. *J Vasc Surg* 1999;29:958–972.

81. Schurink GW, Aarts NJ, van Bockel JH. Endoleak after stent-graft treatment of abdominal aortic aneurysm: a meta-analysis of clinical studies. *Br J Surg* 1999;86:581–587.

82. Matsumura JS, Moore WS. Clinical consequences of periprosthetic leak after endovascular repair of abdominal aortic aneurysm. *J Vasc Surg* 1998;27:606–613.

83. Lipski DA, Ernst CB. Natural history of the residual infrarenal aorta after infrarenal abdominal aortic aneurysm repair. *J Vasc Surg* 1998;27:805–812.

84. Illig KA, Green RM, Ouriel K, et al. Fate of the proximal aortic cuff: implications for endovascular aneurysm repair. *J Vasc Surg* 1997;26:492–501.

85. May J, White GH, Yu W, et al. Conversion from endoluminal to open repair of abdominal aortic aneurysms: a hazardous procedure. *Eur J Vasc Endovasc Surg* 1997;14:4–11.

86. Holzenbein TJ, Kretschmer G, Thurnher S, et al. *Midterm durability of AAA endograft repair—a word of caution.* Presented at the joint annual meeting of the North American Chapter of the International Society for Cardiovascular Surgery and the Society for Vascular Surgery, Toronto, Ontario, June 11, 2000.

87. Sato DT, Goff CD, Gregory RT, et al. Endoleak after aortic stent graft repair: diagnosis by color duplex ultrasound scan versus computed tomography scan. *J Vasc Surg* 1998;28: 657–663.

88. Treiman GS, Lawrence PF, Edwards WH Jr, et al. An assess-

ment of the current applicability of the EVT endovascular graft for treatment of patients with an infrarenal abdominal aortic aneurysm. *J Vasc Surg* 1999;30:68–75.

89. Sarkar R, Moore WS, Quinones-Baldrich WJ, et al. Endovascular repair of abdominal aortic aneurysm using the EVT device: limited increased utilization with availability of a bifurcated graft. *J Endovasc Surg* 1999;6:131–135.

90. Marin ML, Parsons RE, Hollier LH, et al. Impact of transrenal aortic endograft placement on endovascular graft repair of abdominal aortic aneurysms. *J Vasc Surg* 1998;28:638–646.

91. Lee CW, Kaufman JA, Fau CM, et al. Clinical outcome of internal iliac artery occlusions during endovascular treatment of aortoiliac aneurysmal diseases. *J Vasc Interv Radiol* 2000;11:567–571.

92. Urayama H, Ohtake H, Katada S, et al. Exclusion of internal iliac arterial aneurysm concomitant with abdominal aortic aneurysm repair. *J Cardiovasc Surg (Torino)* 1999;40:243–247.

93. Goodnough LT, Brecher ME, Kanter MH, et al. Transfusion medicine: first of two parts. *N Engl J Med* 1999;340:438–447.

94. Etchason J, Petz L, Keeler E, et al. The cost effectiveness of preoperative autologous blood donations. *N Engl J Med* 1995;332:719–724.

95. Dodd R. The risk of tranfusion-transmitted infection. *N Engl J Med* 1992;327:419–421.

96. Mangano DT, Layung EL, Wallace A, et al. Effect of atenolol on mortality and cardiovascular morbidity after noncardiac surgery. *N Engl J Med* 1996;335:1713–1720.

97. Poldermans D, Boersma E, Bax JJ, et al. The effect of bisoprolol on perioperative mortality and myocardial infarction in high-risk patients undergoing vascular surgery. *N Engl J Med* 1999;341:1789–1794.

98. Huber TS, Carlton LM, Harward TRS, et al. Impact of a clinical pathway for elective infrarenal aortic reconstructions. *Ann Surg* 1994;227:691–701.

99. Jayr C, Matthay MA, Goldstone J, et al. Preoperative and intraoperative factors associated with prolonged mechanical ventilation. *Chest* 1993;103:1231–1236.

100. Hertzer NR, Beven EG, Young JR, et al. Coronary artery disease in peripheral vascular patients: a classification of 1,000 coronary angiograms and results of surgical management. *Ann Surg* 1984;199:223–233.

101. ACC/AHA Task Force Report. Cardiovascular evaluation for noncardiac surgery. *J Am Coll Cardiol* 1996;27:910–948.

102. Baron JF, Mundler O, Bertrand M, et al. Dipyridamolethallium scintigraphy and gated radionuclide angiography to assess cardiac risk before abdominal aortic surgery. *N Engl J Med* 1994;330:663–669.

103. Seeger JM, Rosenthal GR, Self SB, et al. Does routine stress–thallium cardiac scanning reduce postoperative cardiac complications? *Ann Surg* 1994;219:654–663.

104. Mangano DT, Goldman L. Preoperative assessment of patients with known or suspected coronary disease. *N Engl J Med* 1995;333:1750–1756.

105. Huber TS, Harward TRS, Flynn TC, et al. Operative mortality rates after elective infrarenal aortic reconstructions. *J Vasc Surg* 1995;22:287–294.

106. Taylor LM, Yeager RA, Moneta GL, et al. The incidence of perioperative myocardial infarction in general vascular surgery. *J Vasc Surg* 1991;15:52–61.

107. Boylan JF, Katz J, Kavanagh BP, et al. Epidural bupivacaine–morphine analgesia versus patient-controlled analgesia following abdominal aortic surgery: analgesic, respiratory, and myocardial effects. *Anesthesiology* 1998;89:585–593.

108. Major CP Jr, Greer MS, Russell WL, et al. Postoperative pulmonary complications and morbidity after abdominal aneurysmectomy: a comparison of postoperative epidural versus parenteral opioid analgesia. *Am Surg* 1996;62:45–51.

109. Valentine RJ, Duke ML, Inman MH, et al. Effectiveness of pulmonary artery catheters in aortic surgery: a randomized trial. *J Vasc Surg* 1998;27:203–212.

110. Elmore JR, Franklin DP, Koukey JR, et al. Normothermia is protective during infrarenal aortic surgery. *J Vasc Surg* 1998;28:984–992.

111. Bush HL, Hydo LJ, Fischer E, et al. Hypothermia during elective abdominal aortic aneurysm repair: the high price of avoidable morbidity. *J Vasc Surg* 1995;21:392–402.

112. Clagett GP, Valentine RJ, Jackson MR, et al. A randomized trial of intraoperative autotransfusion during aortic surgery. *J Vasc Surg* 1999;29:22–31.

113. Huber TS, McGorray SP, Carlton LC, et al. Intraoperative autologous transfusion during elective infrarenal aortic reconstruction: a decision analysis model. *J Vasc Surg* 1997;25:984–994.

114. Huber TS, Carlton L, Irwin P, et al. Intraoperative autologous transfusion during elective infrarenal aortic reconstruction. *J Surg Res* 1997;67:14–20.

115. Sicard GA, Reilly JM, Rubin BG, et al. Transabdominal versus retroperitoneal incision for abdominal aortic surgery: report of a prospective randomized trial. *J Vasc Surg* 1995;21:174–183.

116. Ernst CB, Evans JR. Retroperitoneal approach for elective abdominal aortic aneurysmectomy. In: Ernst CB, Stanley JC, eds. *Current therapy in vascular surgery,* 3rd ed. St. Louis: Mosby, 1995:277–282.

117. Thompson JF, Mullee MA, Bell PRF, et al. Intraoperative heparinization, blood loss, and myocardial infarction during aortic aneurysm surgery: a Joint Vascular Research Group study. *Eur J Vasc Endovasc Surg* 1996;12:86–90.

118. Nicholson ML, Baker DM, Hopkinson BR, et al. Randomized controlled trial of the effect of mannitol on renal reperfusion injury during aortic aneurysm surgery. *Br J Surg* 1996;83:1230–1233.

119. Van der Vliet JA, Kouwenberg PP, Muytjens HL, et al. Relevance of bacterial cultures of abdominal aortic aneurysm contents. *Surgery* 1996;119:129–132.

120. Seeger JM, Coe DA, Kaelin LD, et al. Routine reimplantation of patent inferior mesenteric arteries limits colon infarction after aortic reconstruction. *J Vasc Surg* 1992;15:635–641.

121. Wakefield TW, Hantler CB, Wrobleski SK, et al. Effects of differing rates of protamine reversal of heparin anticoagulation. *Surgery* 1996;119:123–128.

122. Dorman BH, Elliott BM, Spinale FG, et al. Protamine use during peripheral vascular surgery: a prospective randomized trial. *J Vasc Surg* 1995;22:248–255.

123. Hall KA, Peters B, Smyth Sh, et al. Abdominal wall hernias in patients with abdominal aortic aneurysmal versus aortoiliac occlusive disease. *Am J Surg* 1995;170:572–576.

124. Yeager RA, Porter JM. Arterial and prosthetic graft infection. In: Porter JM, Taylor LM Jr, eds. *Basic data underlying clinical decision making in vascular surgery.* St. Louis: Quality Medical, 1994:90–97.

125. Johnston KW. Multicenter prospective study of nonruptured abdominal aortic aneurysm. Part II. Variables predicting morbidity and mortality. *J Vasc Surg* 1989;9:437–447.

126. Akkersdijk GJ, van der Graaf Y, Moll FL, et al. Complications of standard elective abdominal aortic aneurysm repair. *Eur J Vasc Endovasc Surg* 1998;15:505–510.

127. Harward TR, Ingengno MD, Carlton L, et al. Limb-threatening ischemia due to multilevel arterial occlusive disease: simultaneous or staged inflow/outflow revascularization. *Ann Surg* 1995;221:498–503.

128. Tollefson DFJ, Ernst CB. Colon ischemia following aortic reconstruction. In: Porter JM, Taylor LM Jr, eds. *Basic data underlying clinical decision making in vascular surgery.* St. Louis: Quality Medical, 1994:111–115.

129. Valentine RJ, Hagino RT, Jackson MR, et al. Gastrointestinal complications after aortic surgery. *J Vasc Surg* 1998;28:404–411.

130. Ottinger LW. Acute cholecystitis as a postoperative complication. *Ann Surg* 1976;184:162–165.

131. Yao JST. Vasculogenic impotence. In: Ernst CB, Stanley JC, eds. *Current therapy in vascular surgery,* 3rd ed. St. Louis: Mosby, 1995:397–400.

132. Szilagyi DE. A second look at the etiology of spinal cord damage in surgery of the abdominal aorta. *J Vasc Surg* 1993;17:1111–1113.

133. Feinglass J, Cowper D, Donlop D, et al. Late survival risk factors for abdominal aortic aneurysm repair: experience from 14 Department of Veterans Affairs hospitals. *Surgery* 1995;118:16–24.

134. McFalls EO, Ward HB, Santilli S, et al. The influence of perioperative myocardial infarction on long-term prognosis following elective vascular surgery. *Chest* 1998;113:681–686.

135. Hallett JW, Marshall DM, Petterson TM, et al. Graft-related

135. complications after abdominal aortic aneurysm repair: reassurance from a 36-year population-based experience. *J Vasc Surg* 1997;25:277–284.

136. Beard JD, Thomas SM, Gaines PA. *The U.K. registry for the endovascular treatment of aneurysms.* Presented at the joint annual meeting of the North American Chapter of the International Society for Cardiovascular Surgery and the Society for Vascular Surgery, Toronto, Ontario, June 11, 2000.

137. Karch LA, Henretta JP, Hodgson KJ, et al. Algorithm for the diagnosis and treatment of endoleaks. *Am J Surg* 1999;178:225–231.

138. Lee WA, Zarins CK. Endovascular repair of infrarenal abdominal aortic aneurysms. In: Cameron JL, ed. *Current surgical therapy,* 6th ed. St. Louis: Mosby, 2001 (in press).

139. Jacobowitz GR, Rosen RJ, Riles TS. The significance and management of the leaking endograft. *Semin Vasc Surg* 1999;12:199–206.

140. Baum RA, Carpenter JP, Cope C, et al. *Aneurysm sac pressure measurements after endovascular repair of abdominal aortic aneurysms.* Presented at the joint annual meeting of the North American Chapter of the International Society for Cardiovascular Surgery and the Society for Vascular Surgery, Toronto, Ontario, June 11, 2000.

141. Harris P, Brennan J, Martin J, et al. Longitudinal aneurysm shrinkage following endovascular aortic aneurysm repair: a source of intermediate and late complications. *J Endovasc Surg* 1999;6:11–16.

142. Ohki T, Veith FJ. Endovascular graft repair of ruptured aortoiliac aneurysms. *J Am Coll Surg* 1999;189:102–112.

143. Johnston KW, and the Canadian Society for Vascular Surgery Aneurysm Study Group. Ruptured abdominal aortic aneurysm: six-year follow-up results of a multicenter prospective study. *J Vasc Surg* 1994;19:888–900.

144. Van Dongen HP, Leusink JA, Moll FL, et al. Ruptured abdominal aortic aneurysms: factors influencing postoperative mortality and long-term survival. *Eur J Vasc Endovasc Surg* 1998;15:62.

145. Maziak DE, Lindsay TF, Marshall JC, et al. The impact of multiple organ dysfunction on mortality following ruptured abdominal aortic aneurysm repair. *Ann Vasc Surg* 1998;12:93–100.

146. Bradbury AW, Makhdoomi KR, Adam DJ, et al. Twelve-year experience of the management of ruptured abdominal aortic aneurysm. *Br J Surg* 1997;84:1705–1707.

147. Halpern VJ, Klein RG, D'Angelo AJ, et al. Factors that affect the survival rate of patients with ruptured abdominal aortic aneurysms. *J Vasc Surg* 1997;26:939–945.

148. Hennessy A, Barry MC, McGee H, et al. Quality of life following repair of ruptured and elective abdominal aortic aneurysms. *Eur J Surg* 1998;164:673–674.

149. Richardson JW, Greenfield LJ. Natural history and management of iliac aneurysms: novel presentations. *J Vasc Surg* 1989;10:557–562.

150. Krupski WC. Isolated iliac aneurysm. In: Ernst CB, Stanley JC, eds. *Current therapy in vascular surgery,* 3rd ed. St. Louis: Mosby, 1995:296–302.

151. Krupski WC, Bass A, Rosenberg GD, et al. The elusive isolated hypogastric artery aneurysms. *Surgery* 1983;93:688–693.

152. Money SR, Hollier LH. Surgical treatment of inflammatory abdominal aortic aneurysms. In: Ernst CB, Stanley JC, eds. *Current therapy in vascular surgery,* 3rd ed. St. Louis: Mosby, 1995:229–231.

153. Baskerville PA, Browse NL. Peri-aortic fibrosis: progression and regression. *J Cardiovasc Surg (Torino)* 1987;28:30–31.

154. Nevelsteen A, Lacroix H, Stockx L, et al. Inflammatory abdominal aortic aneurysm and bilateral complete ureteral obstruction: treatment by endovascular graft and bilateral ureteric stenting. *Ann Vasc Surg* 1999;13:222–224.

155. Chuter T, Ivancev K, Malina M, et al. Inflammatory aneurysm treated by means of transfemoral endovascular graft insertion. *J Vasc Interv Radiol* 1997;8:39–41.

156. Bitsch M, Norgaard HH, Roder O, et al. Inflammatory aortic aneurysms: regression of fibrosis after aneurysm surgery. *Eur J Vasc Surg* 1997;13:371–374.

157. Crawford ES, Beckett WC, Greer MS. Juxtarenal infrarenal abdominal aortic aneurysm: special diagnostic and therapeutic considerations. *Ann Surg* 1986;203:661–670.

158. Martin GH, O'Hara PJ, Hertzer NR, et al. Surgical repair of aneurysms involving the suprarenal, visceral, and lower thoracic aortic segments: early results and late outcome. *J Vasc Surg* 2000;31:851–862.

159. Jean-Claude JM, Reilly LM, Stoney RJ, et al. Pararenal aortic aneurysms: the future of open aortic aneurysm repair. *J Vasc Surg* 1999;29:902–912.

160. Reddy DJ, Shepard AD, Evans JR, et al. Management of infected aortoiliac aneurysms. *Arch Surg* 1991;126:873–879.

161. Ellenby MI, Ernst CB. Surgical treatment of infected abdominal aortic aneurysms. In: Ernst CB, Stanley JC, eds. *Current therapy in vascular surgery,* 3rd ed. St. Louis: Mosby, 1995:232–235.

162. Brown SL, Busuttil RW, Baker JD, et al. Bacteriologic and surgical determinants of survival in patients with mycotic aneurysms. *J Vasc Surg* 1984;1:541–547.

163. Oz MC, Brener BJ, Buda JA, et al. A ten-year experience with bacterial aortitis. *J Vasc Surg* 1989;10:439–449.

164. Ewart JM, Burke ME, Bunt TJ. Spontaneous abdominal aortic infections: essentials of diagnosis and management. *Am Surg* 1983;49:37–50.

165. Taheri SA, Kulaylat MN, Grippi J. Surgical treatment of primary aortoduodenal fistula. *Ann Vasc Surg* 1991;5:265–270.

166. Piotrowski JJ, Bernhard VM. Management of vascular graft infections. In: Bernhard VM, Towne JB, eds. *Complications in vascular surgery.* St. Louis: Quality Medical Publishing, 1991:235.

167. Berman SS, Bernhard VM. Management of primary aortoenteric fistula. In: Ernst CB, Stanley JC, eds. *Current therapy in vascular surgery,* 3rd ed. St. Louis: Mosby, 1995:262–264.

168. Giordano JM. Venous anomalies encountered during aortic reconstruction. In: Ernst CB, Stanley JC, eds. *Current therapy in vascular surgery,* 3rd ed. St. Louis: Mosby, 1995:252–255.

169. Gaspar MR, Waters HJ, Averbook AW. Renal ectopia and renal fusion in patients requiring abdominal aortic operations. In: Ernst CB, Stanley JC, eds. *Current therapy in vascular surgery,* 3rd ed. St. Louis: Mosby, 1995:246–250.

170. Benjamin ME, Hansen KJ, Craven TE, et al. Combined aortic and renal artery surgery: a contemporary experience. *Ann Surg* 1996;223:555–565.

171. Mateo RB, O'Hara PJ, Hertzer NR, et al. Elective surgical treatment of symptomatic chronic mesenteric occlusive disease: early results and late outcomes. *J Vasc Surg* 1999;29:821–832.

172. Gentile AT, Moneta Gl, Taylor LM, et al. Isolated bypass to the superior mesenteric artery for intestinal ischemia. *Arch Surg* 1994;129:926–932.

173. Derrow AE, Dame DA, Carter RL, et al. National outcome after TAA repair, renal artery bypass, and mesenteric revascularization. *J Vasc Surg* 2001 (in press).

174. Huber TS, Carlton LM, O'Hern DG, et al. Financial impact of tertiary care in academic medical centers. *Ann Surg* 2000;231:860–868.

175. Tollefson DFJ, Ernst CB. Natural history of atherosclerotic renal artery stenosis associated with aortic disease. *J Vasc Surg* 1994;20:76–87.

176. Zierler RE, Bergelin RO, Isaacson JA, et al. Natural history of atherosclerotic renal artery stenosis: a prospective study with duplex ultrasound. *J Vasc Surg* 1994;19:250–258.

177. Williamson WK, Abou-Zamzam AM Jr, Moneta GL, et al. Prophylactic repair of renal artery stenosis is not justified in patients who require infrarenal aortic reconstruction. *J Vasc Surg* 1998;28:14–20.

178. Thomas JH, Blake K, Pierce GE, et al. The clinical course of asymptomatic mesenteric arterial stenosis. *J Vasc Surg* 1998;27:840–844.

179. Swanson RJ, Littooy FN, Hunt TK, et al. Laparotomy as a precipitating factor in the rupture of intra-abdominal aneurysms. *Arch Surg* 1980;115:299–304.

180. Szilagyi DE, Elliott JP, Berguer R. Coincidental malignancy and abdominal aortic aneurysm. *Arch Surg* 1967;95:402–412.

181. String ST. Management of concurrent intra-abdominal disease and abdominal aortic aneurysm. In: Ernst CB, Stanley JC, eds. *Current therapy in vascular surgery,* 3rd ed. St. Louis: Mosby, 1995:235–237.

182. Oshsner JL, Cooley DA, DeBakey ME. Associated intra-abdominal lesions encountered during resection of aortic aneurysm. *Dis Colon Rectum* 1960;3:485–490.

SURGERY: SCIENTIFIC PRINCIPLES AND PRACTICE, Third Edition, edited by Lazar J. Greenfield, Michael W. Mulholland, Keith T. Oldham, Gerald B. Zelenock, and Keith D. Lillemoe. Lippincott Williams & Wilkins Publishers, Philadelphia, © 2001.

CHAPTER 87

SPLANCHNIC ARTERY ANEURYSMS

JAMES C. STANLEY AND PETER K. HENKE

Splanchnic artery aneurysms are uncommon, but the more frequent use of arteriography, computed tomography (CT), and ultrasonography has resulted in increasing clinical recognition of these lesions. These aneurysms are clearly important considering that nearly 22% are seen initially as surgical emergencies, including 8.5% that result in the patient's death. The splanchnic vessels involved with these macroaneurysms, in decreasing order of frequency, are the splenic, hepatic, superior mesenteric, celiac, gastric–gastroepiploic, jejunal–ileal–colic, pancreaticoduodenal–pancreatic, and gastroduodenal arteries (Table 87.1). The clinical manifestations and management of these aneurysms have been defined more clearly in recent years (1–8).

SPLENIC ARTERY ANEURYSM

Splenic artery aneurysms account for 60% of all splanchnic artery aneurysms (8). The higher frequency of these aneurysms in the splenic artery cannot be accounted for by the greater length of this vessel compared with other splanchnic arteries; the frequency instead reflects a peculiar predisposition for this vessel to undergo aneurysmal change. The occurrence of these lesions in the general population is probably similar to the 0.78% incidence in nearly 3,600 consecutive patients who underwent abdominal arteriographic studies for reasons other than suspected aneurysmal disease (9). Women are four times more likely than men to develop these aneurysms.

Three distinct factors may contribute to the development of splenic artery aneurysms, including two that account for their unusual female predilection. The first factor is medial fibrodysplasia, which usually occurs in women and is often manifest by renal artery stenosis and secondary hypertension. As many as 4% of patients with dysplastic renal artery disease have splenic artery aneurysms, and all these patients have been women (9). The second factor relates to the deleterious consequences of pregnancy, with its known increase in splenic blood flow and reproductive hormone-related changes in elastic vascular tissue. This becomes a particular problem with repeated pregnancies. Some 45% to 55% of women harboring these lesions have completed six or more pregnan-

---

Table 87.1. SPLANCHNIC ARTERY MACROANEURYSMS

Aneurysm location	Frequency within splanchnic circulation	Male: Female ratio	Contributing factors	Frequency of reported rupture (%)	Site of rupture	Mortality with rupture
Splenic artery	60%	1:4	Medial degeneration; arterial fibrodysplasia; multiple pregnancies; portal hypertension; chronic pancreatitis with arterial erosion by pseudocysts	2% (bland aneurysms)	Intraperitoneal within lesser sac; intragastric with pancreatitis related inflammatory aneurysms	25% bland and unassociated with pregnancy; during pregnancy 70% maternal, 75% fetal
Hepatic artery	20%	2:1	Medial degeneration; blunt and penetrating liver trauma; infection related to intravenous substance abuse	20%	Intraperitoneal and biliary tract with equal frequency	35%
Superior mesenteric artery	5.5%	1:1	Infection related to bacterial endocarditis, often associated with nonhemolytic streptococci and more recently with intravenous substance abuse; medial degeneration	Uncommon (thrombosis more common)	Intraperitoneal and retroperitoneal	50%
Celiac artery	4%	1:1	Medial degeneration	13%	Intraperitoneal	50%
Gastric and gastroepiploic arteries	4%	3:1	Periarterial inflammation; medial degeneration	90%	Intraperitoneal (30%), intestinal tract (70%)	70%
Jejunal, ileal, and colic arteries	3%	1:1	Medial degeneration; connective tissue diseases	30%		
Pancreaticoduodenal, pancreatic, and gastroduodenal arteries	2%	4:1	Pancreatitis-related arterial necrosis and arterial erosion by pseudocysts (60% of gastroduodenal, 30% of pancreaticoduodenal artery aneurysms); medial degeneration	75% inflammatory, 50% noninflammatory	Intestinal tract (85%); intraperitoneal (15%)	50%

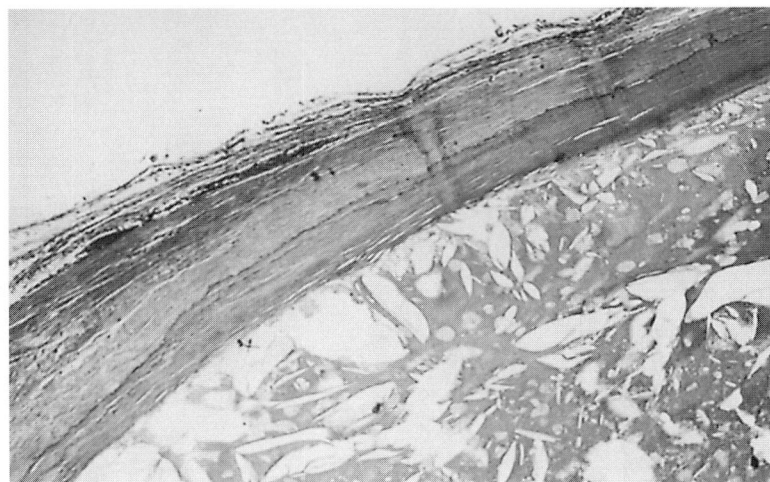

Figure 87.1. Splenic artery aneurysm exhibiting marked fibrosis with cholesterol clefts and calcific arteriosclerosis (hematoxylin-eosin, decalcified, ×32). (From Stanley JC, Fry WJ. Pathogenesis and clinical significance of splenic artery aneurysms. *Surgery* 1974;76:898, with permission.)

cies (9,10). The third factor is evident in the nearly 10% of patients with portal hypertension and splenomegaly who develop splenic artery aneurysms (9). In these cases, the vessel wall integrity may be compromised by increased splenic blood flow (11,12) and excessive estrogen activity occurring as a consequence of the underlying cirrhosis. No predilection for either sex exists in this latter subgroup of patients. Splenic artery aneurysms have been described with regularity among patients after orthotopic liver transplantation (13,16). It is likely that these represent preexisting aneurysms associated with portal hypertension. Rare splenic artery aneurysms appear in association with developmental anomalies of the foregut arterial circulation (17).

Certain splenic artery aneurysms exhibit extensive arteriosclerosis (Fig. 87.1). The fact that calcific arteriosclerotic changes appear limited to the aneurysm and not the intervening artery suggests that this is more likely a secondary event rather than a primary etiologic process (Fig. 87.2). Arterial disruptions resulting from periarterial inflammatory disease, such as chronic pancreatitis, or penetrating trauma are less common causes of these aneurysms. Microaneurysms of smaller intraparenchymal splenic arteries are usually due to a systemic vasculitis, such as polyarteritis nodosa, and appear to be of less clinical importance as a vascular disease than extraparenchymal aneurysms attributed to other causes.

Nearly all splenic artery aneurysms associated with arterial fibrodysplasia, multiple pregnancies, or portal hypertension are saccular and occur at branchings. At such sites, discontinuities exist in the internal elastic lamina of normal vessels, and any subsequent degenerative events involving elastic tissue, as might occur with arterial fibrodysplasia or pregnancy, are likely to produce aneurysmal changes (Fig. 87.3). Splenic artery aneurysms are multiple in 20% of cases. Proximal aneurysms of the main splenic artery are usually solitary and frequently are associated with pancreatitis-related pseudocysts (Fig. 87.4).

Vascular calcifications on plain abdominal radiographs may be the first clinical evidence of a splenic artery aneurysm (18). The most characteristic of these findings are signet-ring calcifications (Fig. 87.5). Contemporary diagnosis of splenic artery aneurysms usually follows their arteriographic demonstration during studies for nonvascular diseases. Color-flow Doppler ultrasonography, CT, and magnetic resonance imaging (MRI) occasionally establish the presence of these lesions and are often useful in identifying bleeding aneurysms (8,19).

Left upper-quadrant or epigastric pain may occur in patients with an intact splenic artery aneurysm. In a recent review, nearly half the patients with these aneurysms complained of abdominal pain (5). In cases of rupture, bleeding usually is initially contained within the lesser sac, but free hemorrhage eventually occurs into the peritoneal cavity and causes vascular collapse. This represents the so-called double-rupture phenomenon attributed to splenic artery aneurysms. Pancreatitis-related aneurysms usually are not associated with intraperitoneal bleeding; more often, they are a source of intestinal hemorrhage after rupture into the stomach or pancreatic ductal system (20,23). Arteriovenous fistula formation after splenic artery aneurysm rupture into an adjacent splenic vein is rare (24). Gastrointestinal hemorrhage from esophageal varices associated with left-sided portal hypertension may accompany these fistulae.

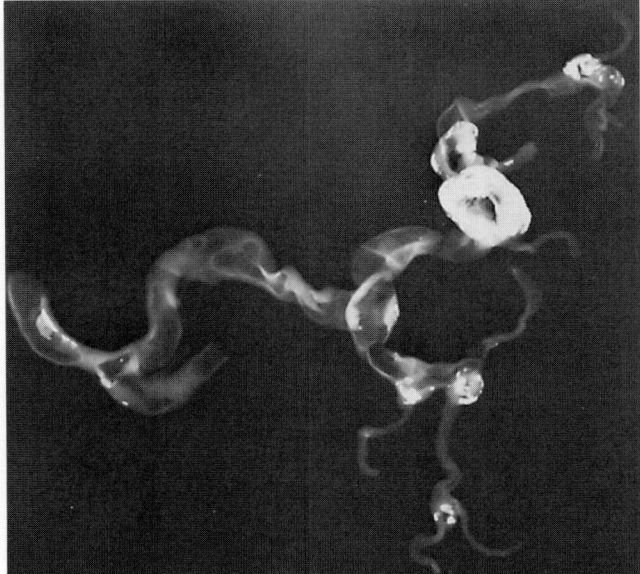

Figure 87.2. Splenic artery aneurysm. Marked calcific arteriosclerosis limited to splenic artery aneurysms occurring at vessel bifurcations (specimen roentgenogram) is seen. Intervening arterial segments are unaffected by advanced arteriosclerotic changes. (From Stanley JC, Thompson NW, Fry WJ. Splanchnic artery aneurysms. *Arch Surg* 1970;101:689, with permission.)

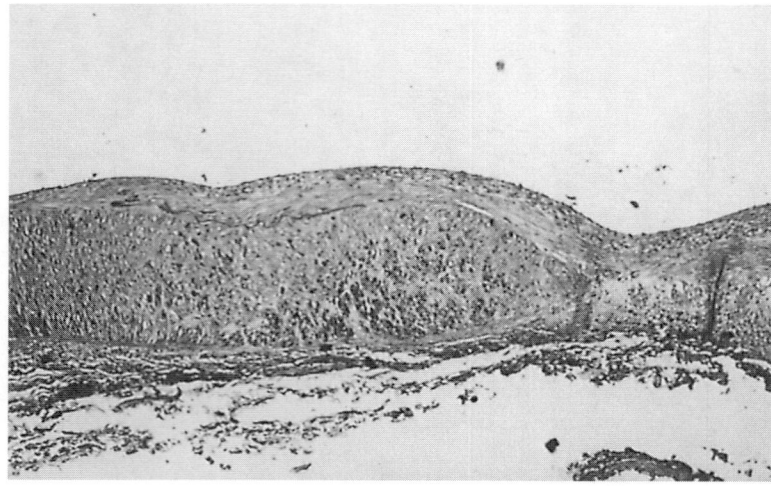

Figure 87.3. Splenic artery aneurysm exhibiting fragmentation of internal elastic lamina and medial dysplasia in patient having renal arterial fibrodysplasia (Masson stain, ×32). (From Stanley JC, Fry WJ. Pathogenesis and clinical significance of splenic artery aneurysms. *Surgery* 1974;76:898, with permission.)

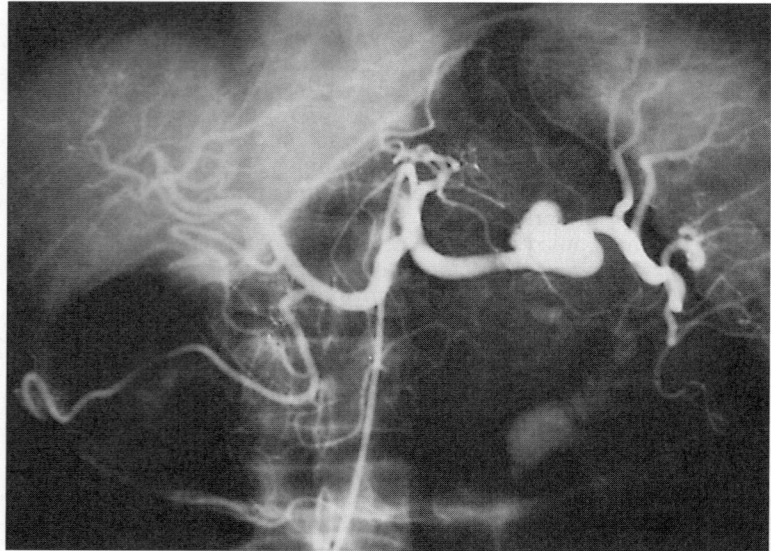

Figure 87.4. Splenic artery aneurysm. Arteriogram documents a pancreatitis-related aneurysm affecting the midsplenic artery. (From Stanley JC, Frey CF, Miller TA, et al. Major arterial hemorrhage: a complication of pancreatic pseudocysts and chronic pancreatitis. *Arch Surg* 1976;111:435, with permission.)

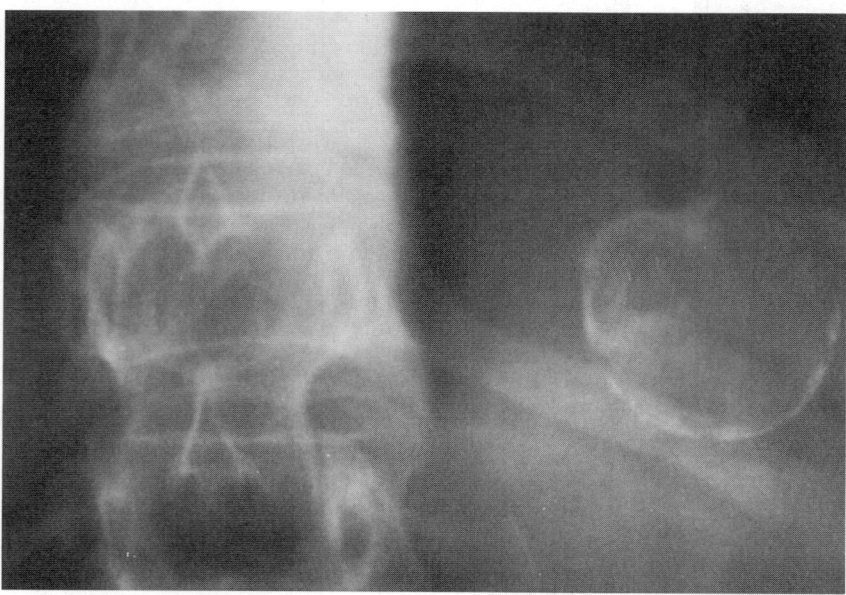

Figure 87.5. Splenic artery aneurysm. Curvilinear signet ringlike calcification in the left upper quadrant characteristic of a splenic artery aneurysms. (From Stanley JC, Thompson NW, Fry WJ. Splanchnic artery aneurysms. *Arch Surg* 1970;101:689, with permission.)

The risk of splenic artery aneurysm rupture depends on a number of confounding and poorly defined factors. In general, rupture of bland aneurysms occurs in less than 2% of cases (3). Contrary to prior tenets, rupture appears just as likely when the aneurysm is calcified, occurs in a normotensive patient, or occurs in the elderly patient.

Pregnancy is a major risk factor; nearly 95% of aneurysms recognized during pregnancy have ruptured (9,25,26). The maternal mortality rate approaches 75%, and the fetal mortality rate exceeds 95% in these cases (27). Pregnancy-related rupture occurs most often during the third trimester (69%) and is less common during the first two trimesters (12%), during labor (13%), or postpartum (6%) (26). Given the fact that most women develop these aneurysms with repeated pregnancies, it is reasonable to assume that most aneurysms in pregnant women go unrecognized and do not rupture. Nevertheless, splenic artery aneurysms in pregnant patients must be considered a threat to the life of the mother and fetus.

The reported mortality rate accompanying operation for rupture of a splenic artery aneurysm is 25% (10). Thus, it would seem ill advised to undertake elective operative intervention for an asymptomatic splenic artery aneurysm if the surgical mortality rate exceeds 0.5%. This latter figure represents the product of the known 25% risk of operative death and 2% rupture rate of bland aneurysms. If intervention becomes necessary in higher-risk patients, percutaneous transcatheter embolization of the aneurysm may represent an acceptable alternative (1,4,28–31).

In the past, splenectomy has been the most common form of surgical therapy for splenic artery aneurysms; however, because of the immunologic importance of the spleen, even in elderly patients, simple ligature obliteration or excision of these aneurysms appears preferable to splenectomy. As technologic advances continue, laporoscopic ligation of these aneurysms may prove quite feasible (32,33). Treatment of splenic artery aneurysms embedded in pancreatic tissue, especially those associated with pancreatitis, may require distal pancreatectomy (34). In some cases, especially false aneurysms caused by pseudocyst erosion into the artery, treatment may entail incising the aneurysmal sac and ligating entering and exiting vessels from within. Pancreatic resection or cyst drainage in these latter cases must be individualized and depends on the extent and chronicity of the associated pancreatic inflammatory disease.

HEPATIC ARTERY ANEURYSM

Hepatic artery aneurysms account for 20% of all previously reported splanchnic artery aneurysms (Fig. 87.6) (3,35). These aneurysms are being encountered more frequently in contemporary times, and in some experiences outnumber splenic artery aneurysms (5). Men are twice as likely to be affected as women, although gender differences have not been as apparent in recent experiences (36). Hepatic artery macroaneurysms are usually solitary. Large aneurysms tend to be saccular, and aneurysms smaller than 2 cm are usually fusiform. These aneurysms are extrahepatic in nearly 80% of cases and intrahepatic in 20%.

Most noninfectious and nontraumatic aneurysms usually are first recognized during the sixth decade of life. The cause of many hepatic artery aneurysms is poorly defined. Two facts regarding the cause of these aneurysms are noteworthy. First, arteriosclerosis most likely represents a secondary event rather than a primary cause of these aneurysms. Most of these lesions probably occur as a result of medial degeneration. Second, with increasing societal violence and intravenous substance abuse, the number of reported traumatic and infection-related aneurysms has increased markedly (Fig. 87.7) (5). Another common cause of intrahepatic pseudoaneurysms is arterial injury accompanying invasive percutaneous diagnostic and therapeutic procedures involving penetration of the liver (37,38). Nearly 17% of these aneurysms encountered more recently have occurred in orthotopic liver transplant patients (5). Systemic arteriopathies, such as periarteritis nodosa, have been incriminated as a cause of occasional macroaneurysms, but more often are associated with intraparenchymal microaneurysms. Hepatic artery aneurysms may be suspected because of displacement of or indentations on intestinal structures noted on barium contrast studies. Most contemporary diagnoses of these aneurysms result from their incidental recognition during arteriography, CT, or ultrasonography for nonvascular disease. Few hepatic artery aneurysms are symptomatic. When they become symptomatic, most exhibit right upper-quadrant or epigastric pain. Rapid expansion of these aneurysms may cause severe discomfort similar to that of acute pancreatitis. Large aneurysms have been reported to cause obstructive jaundice, although most hepatic artery aneurysms are too small to compress the major

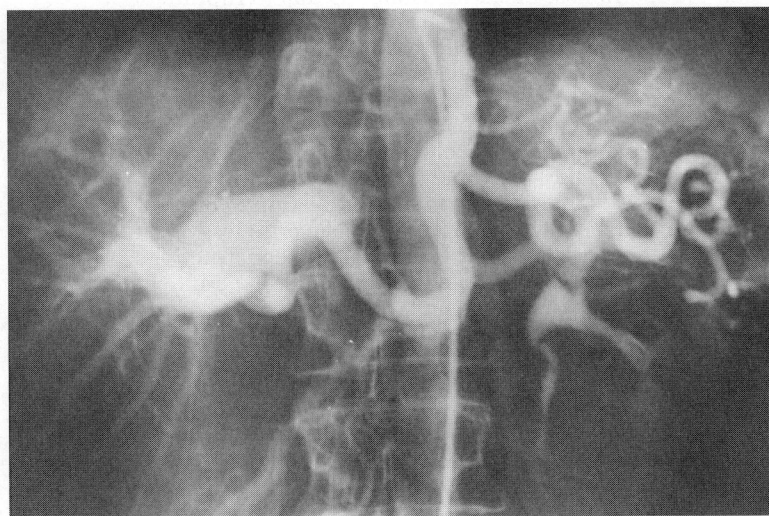

***Figure* 87.6.** Hepatic artery aneurysm. Selective celiac arteriogram demonstrates a large saccular aneurysm at the bifurcation of the proper hepatic artery. (From Zelenock GB, Stanley JC. Splanchnic artery aneurysms. In: Rutherford RB, ed. *Vascular surgery*. Philadelphia: WB Saunders, 2000:1369, with permission.)

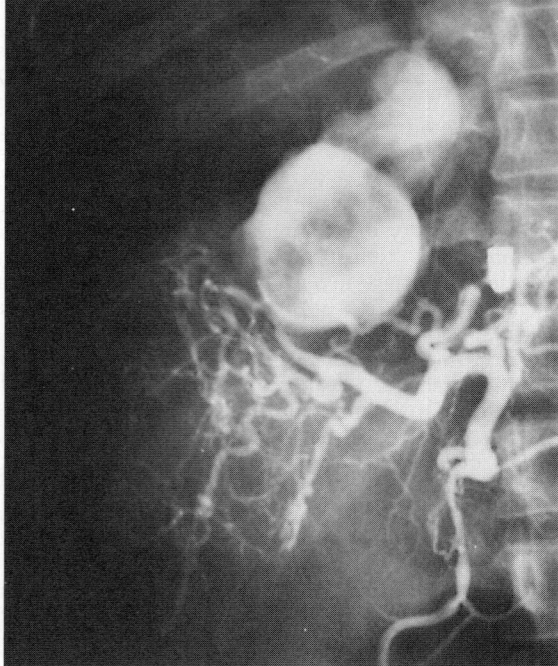

Figure 87.7. Traumatic hepatic artery aneurysm. Blunt abdominal injury and gunshot wounds cause most traumatic lesions. (From Whitehouse WM Jr, Graham LM, Stanley JC. Aneurysms of the celiac, hepatic, and splenic arteries. In: Bergan JJ, Yao JST, eds. *Aneurysms: diagnosis and treatment.* New York: Grune & Stratton, 1981:405, with permission.)

bile ducts (39). These lesions rarely present as pulsatile abdominal masses.

The reported prevalence of hepatic artery aneurysm rupture approaches 20%, but the actual prevalence may be lower and certainly is lower than the often-quoted rupture rate of 44% in cases reported a few decades ago (10). Aneurysm rupture is associated with a 35% mortality rate, although in recent times the mortality rate appears lower (5). Bleeding from ruptured hepatic artery aneurysms occurs with equal frequency into the biliary tract and peritoneal cavity. Hemobilia accompanies the former, being manifest by biliary colic, hematemesis, and jaundice (40). Chronic, relatively asymptomatic hemorrhage is an uncommon sequela of aneurysm rupture into the biliary tract. Intraperitoneal bleeding usually is due to rupture of inflammatory-related false aneurysms.

Common hepatic artery aneurysms often can be treated by aneurysmectomy or aneurysm exclusion, without arterial reconstruction. The extensive hepatic arterial collateral circulation and the parallel portal venous circulation often ensure adequate blood flow to the liver with interruption of the proximal common hepatic artery. Liver necrosis is more likely to follow ligation of arteries in the more distal hepatic circulation. Nevertheless, even in the latter vessels, complex arterial reconstructions should be avoided and simple ligation undertaken if temporary intraoperative occlusion of the involved artery does not result in obvious hepatic ischemia. If liver blood flow appears inadequate with such a maneuver, hepatic artery reconstruction should be undertaken using either prosthetic or autologous vein grafts. In the case of intraparenchymal aneurysms, hepatic territory resection may be necessary therapy; however, percutaneous transcatheter obliteration of the aneurysm with balloons, coils, or nonreabsorbable thrombogenic matter may be

preferable to surgical intervention in most patients (30,38,41).

SUPERIOR MESENTERIC ARTERY ANEURYSM

Aneurysms of the proximal superior mesenteric artery (SMA) account for 5.5% of all splanchnic artery aneurysms (8). These lesions affect men twice as often as women. Infection from a cardiac source is the most common cause of these aneurysms (9,42). Nonhemolytic streptococci as well as many common pathogens accompanying parenteral substance abuse cause bacterial endocarditis and are the underlying source of infection in these cases. Many of these aneurysms are associated with intramural dissections (Fig. 87.8) (43). SMA aneurysms also may be caused by medial degeneration, periarterial inflammation, and trauma. Arteriosclerosis, as in the case of other splanchnic aneurysms, is usually a secondary process. SMA aneurysms have been recognized in contemporary times most often during arteriographic studies for nonvascular disease.

Although many patients with SMA aneurysms are asymptomatic, most patients have abdominal discomfort, often suggestive of intestinal angina. SMA aneurysm rupture is rare (44). The mortality rate with rupture approaches 50%. Gastrointestinal hemorrhage associated with these aneurysms often accompanies their acute occlusion, with bleeding into areas of intestinal infarction. Location of most aneurysms near the origins of the inferior pancreaticoduodenal and middle colic arteries isolates the distal mesenteric circulation when dissections or occlusions occur. In these circumstances, intestinal ischemia

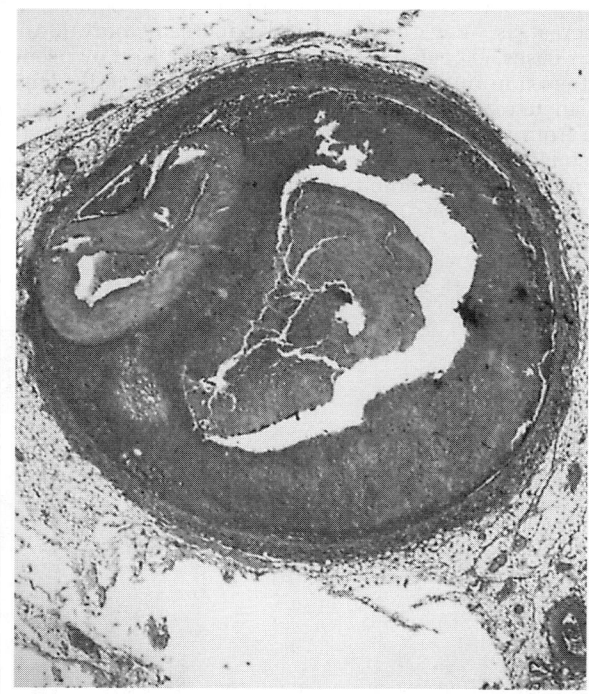

Figure 87.8. Superior mesenteric artery aneurysm. Microscopic cross-section of a dissecting aneurysm affecting the proximal superior mesenteric artery (hematoxylin-eosin, ×20). (From Zelenock GB, Stanley JC. Splanchnic artery aneurysms. In: Rutherford RB, ed. *Vascular surgery.* Philadelphia: WB Saunders, 2000: 1369, with permission.)

develops because the usual collateral network from the adjacent celiac and inferior mesenteric arterial circulations is lost.

Operative management of SMA aneurysms is best accomplished by aneurysmectomy or aneurysm exclusion, followed by intestinal revascularization, if needed, with an aortomesenteric graft. Because of potential infection when bowel ischemia is present, autologous vein or artery is favored over prosthetic conduits for these reconstructions. Aneurysmorrhaphy may be performed in certain cases (45).

In patients who have developed an adequate collateral circulation to their midguts, SMA aneurysm ligation without arterial reconstruction may be successful. In fact, ligation and aneurysmorrhaphy have been the most commonly reported means of managing these aneurysms (5,46,47). Temporary intraoperative occlusion of the SMA with Doppler documentation of adequate intestinal blood flow should be undertaken before proceeding with SMA ligation.

CELIAC ARTERY ANEURYSM

Celiac artery aneurysms account for 4% of all splanchnic artery aneurysms (8,48). Men and women appear equally affected. Most aneurysms encountered in contemporary times have been associated with medial degeneration. Arteriosclerosis is a common histologic finding that is considered a secondary event rather than an etiologic process. Celiac artery aneurysms are usually saccular, and most are located in the distal vessel (Fig. 87.9).

Most celiac artery aneurysms are asymptomatic or appear to be associated with vague abdominal discomfort (5,8). These aneurysms usually are recognized during ultrasonography, angiography, or other imaging studies for nonvascular diseases. In more recent times, rupture has affected 13% of these aneurysms and carried a mortality rate of 50% (48). In contrast, rupture rates published before 1950 were often higher than 80%. Rupture usually causes exsanguinating intraperitoneal hemorrhage. Although rare, gastrointestinal bleeding may follow rupture of the aneurysm into the stomach or pancreatic ductal system.

Aneurysmectomy with celiac artery reconstruction is the preferred treatment for these lesions, although aneurysm exclusion with ligation of its branches has been performed successfully in select patients (48,49). When simple ligature is undertaken, the adequacy of the liver's collateral circulation must be documented. If liver ischemia is apparent after temporary intraoperative celiac artery occlusion, hepatic revascularization becomes mandatory. An aortoceliac or aortohepatic artery bypass in these circumstances is best performed with either an autologous vein or prosthetic graft. Surgical therapy of celiac artery aneurysmal disease has been successful in more than 90% of cases.

GASTRIC AND GASTROEPIPLOIC ARTERY ANEURYSMS

Gastric and gastroepiploic artery aneurysms account for 4% of all splanchnic artery aneurysms (8) (Fig. 87.10). Gastric artery aneurysms occur 10 times more often than gastroepiploic artery aneurysms. Men are three times more likely than women to develop these aneurysms. Most of these perigastric lesions have been encountered in patients older than 50 years of age. These aneurysms usually are solitary, occurring as a result of periarterial inflammation or medial degeneration. In many cases, there is an antecedent history of peptic ulcer disease. Arteriosclerosis, when present, is considered a secondary event, not a cause of these lesions.

Most reported gastric or gastroepiploic artery aneurysms have been symptomatic when initially recognized, frequently as emergencies (50–52). Rupture has accompanied more than 90% of reported cases, with gastrointestinal bleeding occurring slightly more than twice as often as intraperitoneal hemorrhage. Rupture carries a 70% mortality rate (10).

Surgical treatment is recommended for all gastric and gastroepiploic artery aneurysms (7). Vascular reconstructive surgery is not required in these cases. Intramural gastric aneurysms may be excised with a small segment of involved stomach, whereas extramural aneurysms can be treated by arterial ligation alone, with or without aneurysm excision. Certain lesions can be treated by a laporoscopic approach (53). Intraoperative identification of these small aneurysms is often tedious if preoperative localization has not been established by arteriographic studies.

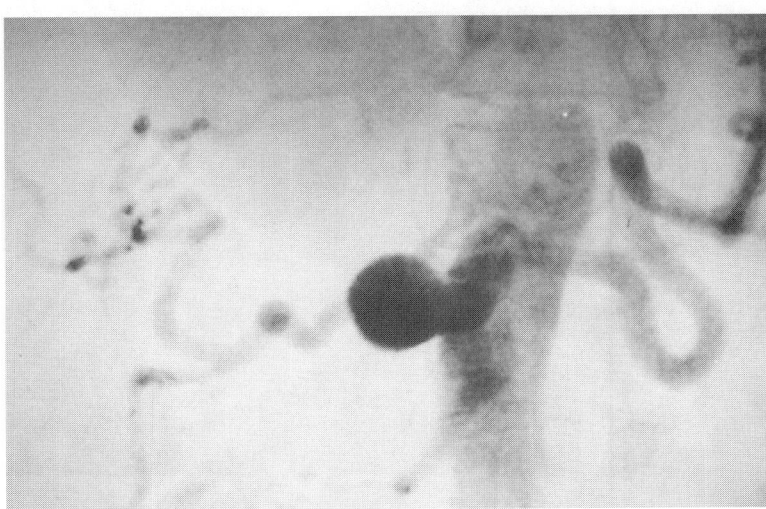

Figure 87.9. Celiac artery aneurysm. Aortogram reveals saccular aneurysm that exhibited medial degenerative changes and secondary arteriosclerosis. (From Stanley JC, Whitehouse WM Jr. Aneurysms of the splanchnic and renal arteries. In: Bergan JJ, Yao JST, eds. *Surgery of the aorta and its body branches.* Orlando, FL: Grune & Stratton, 1979:497, with permission.)

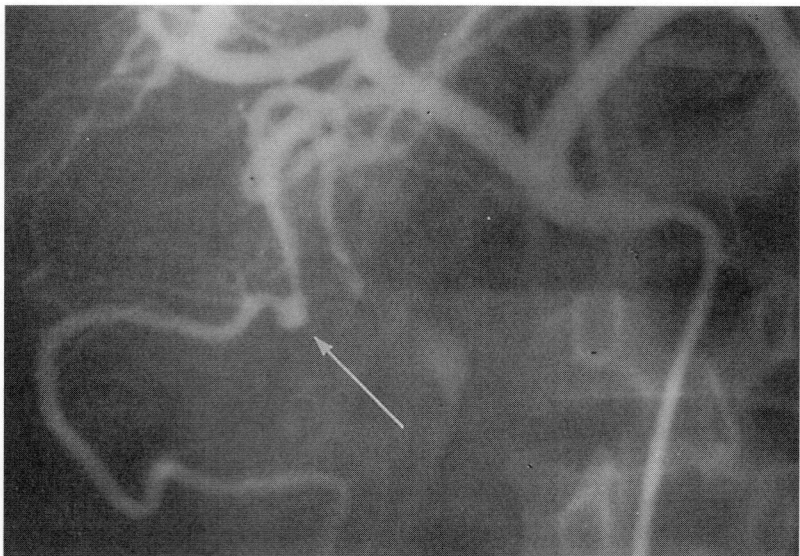

Figure 87.10. Gastroepiploic artery aneurysm. Selective celiac arteriogram revealing small aneurysm responsible for massive gastrointestinal hemorrhage. (From Stanley JC, Thompson NW, Fry WJ. Splanchnic artery aneurysms. *Arch Surg* 1970;101: 689, with permission.)

JEJUNAL, ILEAL, AND COLIC ARTERY ANEURYSMS

Aneurysms of the jejunal, ileal, and colic arteries account for 3% of all splanchnic artery aneurysms (8) (Fig. 87.11). They usually occur in patients older than 60 years of age; men and women are affected equally. Multiple aneurysms have been encountered in 10% of cases. Acquired medial defects cause most of these lesions. Although arteriosclerosis is present with 20% of these aneurysms, it is considered to represent a secondary event, not an etiologic process. An increasing number of mycotic aneurysms affect these vessels, developing as the sequela of infected emboli originating from subacute bacterial endocarditis (54). Periarteritis nodosa is a common underlying cause of multiple aneurysms affecting these intestinal branch arteries (55). Inferior mesenteric artery aneurysms are so rare and the etiology so varied that their clinical importance has not been clearly established (56,57).

Most aneurysms of these vessels cause abdominal pain (5), but many are first recognized as incidental findings during arteriography for gastrointestinal bleeding. Jejunal, ileal, and colic artery aneurysms are reported to have ruptured in 30% of cases, but actual rupture rates are probably a third of previously published rates. Rupture continues to be associated with a mortality rate of 20% (10). Aneurysmal rupture usually occurs into the gastrointestinal tract. Rupture into the mesentery or peritoneal cavity is uncommon. Regardless of this fact, these small mesenteric branch aneurysms are more likely to cause abdominal apoplexy than any other splanchnic artery aneurysm.

Operation for intestinal branch aneurysms is recommended in all instances, except for bland aneurysms associated with connective-tissue diseases. Expeditious surgical therapy requires careful preoperative localization with arteriographic studies. Arterial ligation, with or without aneurysmectomy, is recommended in treating extraintestinal lesions, whereas intramural aneurysms and those associated with bowel infarction require resection of the involved intestine.

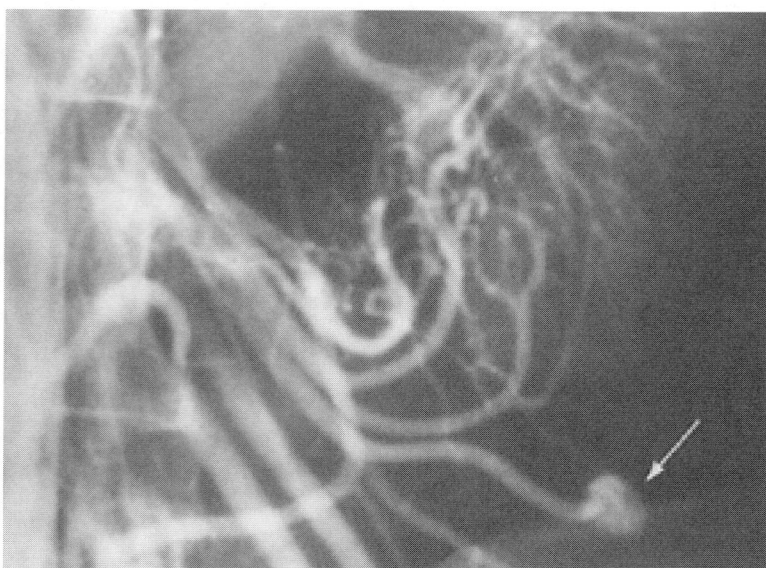

Figure 87.11. Ileal artery aneurysm. Mesenteric arteriogram documenting saccular aneurysm of distal ileal artery. (From Zelenock GB, Stanley JC. Splanchnic artery aneurysms. In: Rutherford RB, ed. *Vascular surgery*. Philadelphia: WB Saunders, 2000:1369, with permission.)

PANCREATICODUODENAL, PANCREATIC, AND GASTRODUODENAL ARTERY ANEURYSMS

Pancreatic and pancreaticoduodenal artery aneurysms (Fig. 87.12) account for 2% of all splanchnic artery aneurysms, and gastroduodenal artery aneurysms (Fig. 87.13)

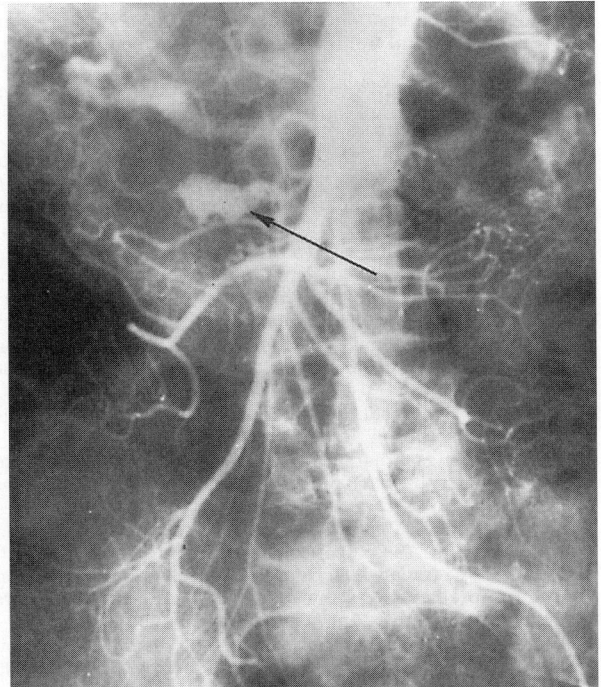

Figure 87.12. Inferior pancreaticoduodenal artery aneurysm. Selective superior mesenteric arteriogram revealing false aneurysm secondary to pseudocyst erosion of artery. (From Stanley JC, Frey CF, Miller TA, et al. Major arterial hemorrhage: a complication of pancreatic pseudocysts and chronic pancreatitis. *Arch Surg* 1976;111:435, with permission.)

represent an additional 1.5% of these aneurysms (8). Men are four times more likely than women to develop these lesions. Most patients with these aneurysms are older than 50 years. Most of these lesions are associated with pancreatitis-related vascular necrosis or vessel erosion by an adjacent pancreatic pseudocyst. Medial degeneration and trauma are less common causes of these aneurysms. Arteriosclerosis is invariably a secondary, not a causative, process. Many recently reported aneurysms have been associated with celiac artery stenoses or occlusions, and they likely represent weaknesses in branchings of the resultant collateral circulation (58–60).

These peripancreatic aneurysms are often difficult to diagnose and treat. Most are associated with epigastric pain and discomfort, which may be due to the underlying pancreatic inflammatory disease that accompanies about 60% of gastroduodenal and 30% of pancreaticoduodenal artery aneurysms. Gastroduodenal and pancreaticoduodenal aneurysm rupture has affected more than half of the reported cases, occurring in 75% of inflammatory and 50% of noninflammatory lesions. Hemorrhage usually occurs into the stomach, the biliary tract, or pancreatic ductal system; bleeding into the peritoneal cavity is less likely. Arteriography usually establishes the presence of these aneurysms, but CT scanning and MRI are of increasing importance in their recognition. These latter noninvasive studies are especially important in detecting rupture or associated pancreatic pathology. The mortality rate with rupture approaches 50% despite operative intervention.

Surgical intervention is acceptable therapy for all but the poorest risk patients with gastroduodenal, pancreaticoduodenal, or pancreatic arterial aneurysms (5,8,60–64). Pancreatitis-related false aneurysms usually are treated by arterial ligation from within the aneurysmal sac rather than by extraaneurysmal arterial ligation. Extensive dissection of the pancreas affected by dense inflammatory adhesions in such circumstances is hazardous. In situations in which a pancreatic pseudocyst or abscess has eroded the artery, a drainage procedure should be undertaken. Distal pancreatectomy, or even pancreaticoduodenectomy, may be the safest mode of treatment in select cases. Transcatheter embolization and electrocoagulation have been recommended for treating extremely high-risk patients with these aneurysms (65). Unfortunately, rebleeding after

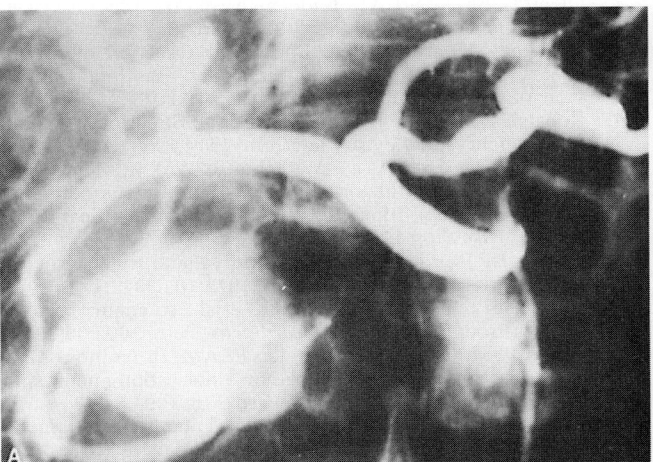
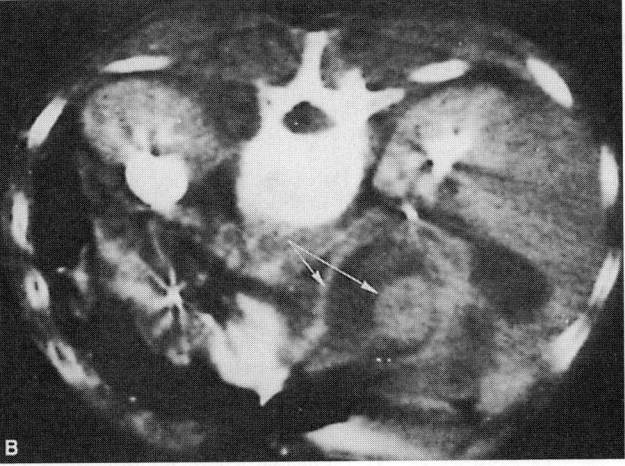

Figure 87.13. Gastroduodenal artery aneurysm. *(A)* Selective celiac arteriogram. *(B)* Computed tomography scan of a pancreatic pseudocyst *(short arrow)* containing the aneurysm *(long arrow).* (From Eckhauser FE, Stanley JC, Zelenock GB, et al. Gastroduodenal and pancreaticoduodenal artery aneurysms: a complication of pancreatitis causing spontaneous gastrointestinal hemorrhage. *Surgery* 1980;88:335, with permission.)

such therapy decreases the usefulness of this type of intervention (66).

REFERENCES

1. Carr SC, Pearce WH, Vogelzang RL, et al. Current management of visceral artery aneurysms. *Surgery* 1996;120:627.
2. Jorgensen BA. Visceral artery aneurysms: a review. *Dan Med Bull* 1985;32:237.
3. Panayiotopoulos YP, Assadourian R, Taylor PR. Aneurysms of the visceral and renal arteries. *Ann R Coll Surg Engl* 1996; 78:412.
4. Rokke O, Sondenaa K, Amundsen SR, et al. Successful management of eleven splanchnic artery aneurysms. *Eur J Surg* 1997;163:411.
5. Shanley CJ, Shah NL, Messina LM. Common splanchnic artery aneurysms: splanic, hepatic, and celiac. *Ann Vasc Surg* 1996;10:315.
6. Shanley CJ, Shah NL, Messina LM. Uncommon splanchnic artery aneurysms: pancreaticoduodenal, gastroduodenal, superior mesenteric, inferior mesenteric, and celiac. *Ann Vasc Surg* 1996;10:506.
7. Wagner WH, Allins AD, Treiman RL, et al. Ruptured visceral artery aneurysms. *Ann Vasc Surg* 1997;11:342.
8. Zelenock GB, Stanley JC. Splanchnic artery aneurysms. In: Rutherford RB, ed. *Vascular surgery,* 5th ed. Philadelphia: WB Saunders, 2000:1369.
9. Stanley JC, Fry WJ. Pathogenesis and clinical significance of splenic artery aneurysms. *Surgery* 1974;76:898.
10. Stanley JC, Thompson NW, Fry WJ. Splanchnic artery aneurysms. *Arch Surg* 1970;101:689.
11. Nishida O, Moriyasu F, Nakamura T, et al. Hemodynamics of splenic artery aneurysm. *Gastroenterology* 1986;90:1042.
12. Ohta M, Hashizume M, Ueno K, et al. Hemodynamic study of splenic artery aneurysm in portal hypertension. *Hepato-gastroenterology* 1994;41:181.
13. Ayalon A, Wiesner RH, Perkins JD, et al. Splenic artery aneurysms in liver transplant patients. *Transplantation* 1988;45:386.
14. Bronsther O, Merhav H, Van Thiel D, et al. Splenic artery aneurysms occurring in liver transplant recipients. *Transplantation* 1991;52:4.
15. Kobori L, van derKolk MJ, de Jong KP, et al. Splenic artery aneurysms in liver transplant patients: Liver Transplant Group. *J Hepatol* 1997;27:890.
16. Robertson AJ, Rela M, Karani J, et al. Splenic artery aneurysm and orthotopic liver transplantation. *Transpl Int* 1999;12:68.
17. Settembrini PG, Jausseran JM, Roveri S, et al. Aneurysms of anomalous splenomesenteric trunk: clinical features and surgical management in two cases. *J Vasc Surg* 1996;24:687.
18. Trastek VF, Pairolero PC, Joyce JW, et al. Splenic artery aneurysms. *Surgery* 1982;91:694.
19. Ishida H, Konno K, Hamashima Y, et al. Splenic artery aneurysm: value of color Doppler and the limitation of gray-scale ultrasonography. *Abdom Imaging* 1998;23:627.
20. deVries JE, Schattenkerk ME, Malt RA. Complications of splenic artery aneurysm other than intraperitoneal rupture. *Surgery* 1982;91:200.
21. Stabile BE, Wilson SE, Debas HT. Reduced mortality from bleeding pseudocysts and pseudoaneurysms caused by pancreatitis. *Arch Surg* 1983;118:45.
22. Stanley JC, Frey CF, Miller TA, et al. Major arterial hemorrhage: a complication of pancreatic pseudocysts and chronic pancreatitis. *Arch Surg* 1976;111:435.
23. Wagner WH, Cossman DV, Treiman RL, et al. Hemosuccus pancreaticus from intraductal rupture of a primary splenic artery aneurysm. *J Vasc Surg* 1994;19:158.
24. Brothers TE, Stanley JC, Zelenock GB. Splenic arteriovenous fistula: review of the literature with four new case reports. *Int Surg* 1995;80:189.
25. Lowry SM, O'Dea TP, Gallagher DI, et al. Splenic artery aneurysm rupture: the seventh instance of maternal and fetal survival. *Obstet Gynecol* 1986;67:291.
26. MacFarlane JR, Thorbjarnason B. Rupture of splenic artery aneurysm during pregnancy. *Am J Obstet Gynecol* 1966;95:1025.
27. Cailloutte JC, Merchant EB. Ruptured splenic artery aneurysm in pregnancy: twelfth reported case with maternal and fetal survival. *Am J Obstet Gynecol* 1993;168:1810.
28. Baker KS, Tisnado J, Cho SR, et al. Splanchnic artery aneurysms and pseudoaneurysms: transcatheter embolization. *Radiology* 1987;163:135.
29. McDermott VG, Shlansky-Goldberg R, Cope C. Endovascular management of splenic artery anuerysms and pseudoaneurysms. *Cardiovasc Intervent Radiol* 1994;17:179.
30. Salam TA, Lumsden AB, Martin LG, et al. Nonoperative management of visceral aneurysms and pseudoaneurysms. *Am J Surg* 1992;164:215.
31. Waltman AC, Luers PR, Athanasoulis CA, et al. Massive arterial hemorrhage in patients with pancreatitis: complementary roles of surgery and transcatheter occlusive techniques. *Arch Surg* 1986;121:439.
32. Arca MJ, Gagner M, Heniford BT, et al. Splenic artery aneurysms: methods of laparoscopic repair. *J Vasc Surg* 1999; 30:184.
33. Whashizume M, Ohta M, Veno K, et al. Laparoscopic ligation of splenic artery aneurysm. *Surgery* 1993;113:352.
34. de Perrot M, Buhler L, Schneider PA, et al. Do aneurysms and pseudoaneurysms of the splenic artery require different surgical strategy? *Hepatogastroenterology* 1999;46:2028.
35. Guida PM, Moore SW. Aneurysm of the hepatic artery: report of five cases with a brief review of the previously reported cases. *Surgery* 1966;60:299.
36. Lumsden AB, Mattar SG, Allen RC, et al. Hepatic artery aneurysms: the management of 22 patients. *J Surg Res* 1996; 60:345.
37. Czerniak A, Thompson JN, Hemingway AP, et al. Hemobilia: a disease in evolution. *Arch Surg* 1988;23:718.
38. Okazaki M, Higashihara H, Ono H, et al. Percutaneous embolization of ruptured splanchnic artery pseudoaneurysms. *Acta Radiol* 1991;32:349.
39. Lal RB, Strohl JA, Piazza S, et al. Hepatic artery aneurysm. *J Cardiovasc Surg* 1989;30:509.
40. Stauffer JT, Weinman MD, Bynum TE. Hemobilia in a patient with multiple hepatic artery aneurysms: a case report and review of the literature. *Am J Gastroenterol* 1989;84:59.
41. Thibodeaux LC, Deshmukh RM, Hearn AT, et al. Management options for hepatic artery aneurysms. *Ann Vasc Surg* 1995; 9:285.
42. Friedman SG, Pogo GJ, Moccio CG. Mycotic aneurysm of the superior mesenteric artery. *J Vasc Surg* 1987;6:87.
43. Cormier F, Ferry J, Artru B, et al. Dissecting aneurysms of the main trunk of the superior mesenteric artery. *J Vasc Surg* 1992;15:424.
44. Blumenberg RM, David D, Skovak J. Abdominal apoplexy due to rupture of a superior mesenteric artery aneurysm: clip aneurysmorrhaphy with survival. *Arch Surg* 1974;108:223.
45. Olcott C, Ehrenfeld WK. Endoaneurysmorrhaphy for visceral artery aneurysms. *Am J Surg* 1977;133:636.
46. DeBakey ME, Cooley DA. Successful resection of mycotic aneurysm of superior mesenteric artery: case report and review of the literature. *Am J Surg* 1953;19:202.
47. Kopatsis A, D'Anna JA, Sithian N, et al. Superior mesenteric artery aneurysm: 45 years later. *Am Surg* 1998;64:263.
48. Graham LM, Stanley JC, Whitehouse WM Jr, et al. Celiac artery aneurysms: historical (1745–1949) versus contemporary (1950–1984) differences in etiology and clinical importance. *J Vasc Surg* 1985;2:757.
49. Hertzer NR, Mullally PH. Celiac artery aneurysmectomy with hepatic artery ligation. *Arch Surg* 1972;104:337.
50. Funahashi S, Yukizane T, Yano K, et al. An aneurysm of the right gastroepiploic artery. *J Cardiovasc Surg* 1997;38:385.
51. Jacobs PPM, Croiset van Ughelen FAAM, Bruyninckx CMA, et al. Haemoperitoneum caused by a dissection aneurysm of the gastroepiploic artery. *Eur J Vasc Surg* 1994;8:236.
52. Witte JT, Hasson JE, Harms BA, et al. Fatal gastric dissection and rupture occurring as a paraesophageal mass: a case report and literature review. *Surgery* 1990;107:590.
53. Uchikoshi F, Sakamoto T, Imabunn S, et al. Aneurysm of the right gastroepiploic artery: a case report of laporoscopic resection. *Cardiovasc Surg* 1993;1:550.
54. Trevisani MF, Ricci MA, Michaels RM, et al. Multiple mesenteric aneurysms complicating subacute bacterial endocarditis. *Arch Surg* 1987;122:823.

55. Selke FW, Williams GB, Donovan DL, et al. Management of intra-abdominal aneurysms associated with periarteritis nodosa. *J Vasc Surg* 1986;4:294.

56. Graham LM, Hay MR, Cho KJ, et al. Inferior mesenteric artery aneurysms. *Surgery* 1985;97:158.

57. Raso AM, Rispoli P, Maggio D, et al. Post stenotic aneurysm of the interior mesenteric artery: case report and discussion. *J Cardiovasc Surg* 1996;37:359.

58. Coll DP, Ierardi R, Kerstein MD, et al. Aneurysms of the pancreaticoduodenal arteries: a change in management. *Ann Vasc Surg* 1998;12:286.

59. Suzuki K, Kashimura H, Sato M, et al. Pancreaticoduodenal artery aneurysms associated with celiac axis stenosis due to compression by median arcuate ligament and celiac plexus. *J Gastroenterol* 1998;33:434.

60. de Perrot M, Berney T, Deleaval J. Management of true aneurysms of the pancreaticoduodenal arteries. *Ann Surg* 1999;229:416.

61. Eckhauser FE, Stanley JC, Zelenock GB, et al. Gastroduodenal and pancreaticoduodenal artery aneurysms: a complication of pancreatitis causing spontaneous gastrointestinal hemorrhage. *Surgery* 1980;88:335.

62. Chiou AC, Josephs LG, Menzoian JO. Inferior pancreaticoduodenal artery aneurysm: report of a case and review of the literature. *J Vasc Surg* 1993;17:784.

63. Gadacz TR, Trunkey D, Kieffer RF. Visceral vessel erosion associated with pancreatitis: case reports and a review of the literature. *Arch Surg* 1978;113:1438.

64. Iyomasa S, Matsuzaki Y, Hiei K, et al. Pancreaticoduodenal artery aneurysm: a case report and review of the literature. *J Vasc Surg* 1995;22:161.

65. Mandel SR, Jaques PF, Mauro MA, et al. Nonoperative management of peripancreatic arterial aneurysms. A 10-year experience. *Ann Surg* 1987;205:126.

66. Lina JR, Jaques P, Mandell V. Aneurysm rupture secondary to transcatheter embolization. *AJR Am J Roentgenol* 1979;132:553.

SURGERY: SCIENTIFIC PRINCIPLES AND PRACTICE, Third Edition, edited by Lazar J. Greenfield, Michael W. Mulholland, Keith T. Oldham, Gerald B. Zelenock, and Keith D. Lillemoe. Lippincott Williams & Wilkins Publishers, Philadelphia, © 2001.

CHAPTER 88

RENAL ARTERY ANEURYSMS

JAMES C. STANLEY AND PETER K. HENKE

Aneurysms of the renal artery are unusual vascular lesions that have been encountered with increasing frequency (1–7). Although our understanding of these aneurysms has improved, their clinical importance is still controversial (8–10). Complications of these aneurysms, often detected in the setting of other renal vascular disease, have been overestimated in reports that usually describe operative experiences rather than population-based experiences. Other misperceptions regarding the importance of these aneurysms reflect unrecognized differences among their four principal categories: (a) true renal artery aneurysms (7), (b) dissecting renal artery aneurysms (11,12), (c) aneurysmal dilatations occurring with medial fibrodysplastic disease (13), and (d) arteritis-related microaneurysms (14). The two renal artery macroaneurysms most relevant to clinical practice, true aneurysms and those associated with dissections, deserve individual discussion (Table 88.1).

TRUE RENAL ARTERY ANEURYSMS

The precise incidence of true renal artery aneurysms in the general population approaches 0.09%. This figure was derived in the mid-1970s from incidental demonstration of these aneurysms in about 8,500 patients subjected to arteriographic studies for nonrenal disease at the University of Michigan (7). Large reported series of these aneurysms are uncommon (Table 88.2). The group being studied bears greatly on the reported frequency of these lesions. For example, macroaneurysms have been identified in 0.7% of patients undergoing arteriographic studies directed at renal disease (15) and in 2.5% of those being evaluated for hypertension (7). The occurrence of these lesions in 9.2% of hypertensive adults with renal artery fibrodysplasia emphasizes the importance of patient selection in determining their incidence (13).

Women are affected with renal artery aneurysms 1.2 times more often than men. When aneurysms in patients with arterial fibrodysplasia are excluded, however, no gender predilection is seen. The predisposition of these aneurysms to affect the right renal artery may be a reflection of the greater incidence of right-sided medial fibrodysplastic disease in women (13).

True renal artery aneurysms usually are located at renal artery bifurcations (Fig. 88.1). Most of these aneurysms are saccular. The average diameter of true aneurysms in one large series was 1.3 cm (7). Extraparenchymal aneurysms are very common, accounting for more than 90% of these lesions, with more than 75% occurring at first- or second-order branchings of the main renal artery.

Two distinct histologic categories of true renal artery aneurysms exist. The first type appears to be associated with a congenital elastic tissue defect or medial degenerative process (Fig. 88.2). Internal elastic lamina fragmentation, excessive accumulations of collagen and other ground substances, a paucity of medial elastic tissue, and a loss of recognizable medial smooth muscle characterize these lesions.

The second type of aneurysm exhibits arteriosclerosis (Fig. 88.3). Hemorrhage, calcium deposition, collections of cholesterol, necrotic debris, and a matrix of fibrous tissue

Table 88.1. TRUE AND DISSECTING RENAL ARTERY ANEURYSMS

Lesion	Males/ Females	Contributing factors	Rate of rupture	Mortality with rupture	Treatment
True aneurysm	1/1.2	Congenital defects, arterial fibrodysplasia hypertension	3%	10% (during pregnancy: 55% maternal, 85% fetal)	Aneurysmectomy with renal artery reconstruction, Aneurysmorrhaphy, Nephrectomy for ruptured aneurysms
Dissecting aneurysm	10/1	Blunt trauma, arterial catheterization, arterial fibrodysplasia, arteriosclerosis	Uncommon	Undefined	Renal artery reconstruction

Table 88.2. **SELECTED EXPERIENCES WITH RENAL ARTERY ANEURYSMS**

	Patients (aneurysms)	Symptoms[a]	Surgical procedures[b]			
			Excision and closure	Bypass	Ex vivo repair	Nephrectomy
University of Michigan	168 (252)	45%	63	30	—	8[c]
University of Toronto[1]	56 (67)	51%	10	—	4[d]	3
Vanderbilt[*5]	39 (45)	15%	6	7	5	7
Mayo Clinic[*4]	32 (45)	34%	11	17	7	7

[a]Includes pain, hematuria, hemorrhage.
[b]No operative mortality reported with any of these procedures.
[c]Not included 25 planned nephrectomies; for rupture, AVF formation, intraparenchymal loci, etc.
[d]Patients with dissections.

typify these lesions. Such atheromatous changes often occur at irregular intervals in these aneurysms, with intervening areas composed of thin, collagenous acellular fibrous tissue. Severe arteriosclerosis of the adjacent nonaneurysmal renal artery is uncommon. When present in an aneurysm, arteriosclerosis is considered a secondary event rather than a primary causative event. The fact that arteriosclerotic changes affect some but not all aneurysms in patients with multiple lesions suggests a nonarteriosclerotic cause of most renal artery aneurysms (7,15).

Both congenital and acquired factors appear to contribute to the formation of true renal artery aneurysms. Discontinuity of the internal elastic lamina is common at branchings of normal muscular arteries, and the fenestrations resulting from these discontinuities may contribute to the development of aneurysms considered congenital in origin. The reported increase in the frequency of aneu-

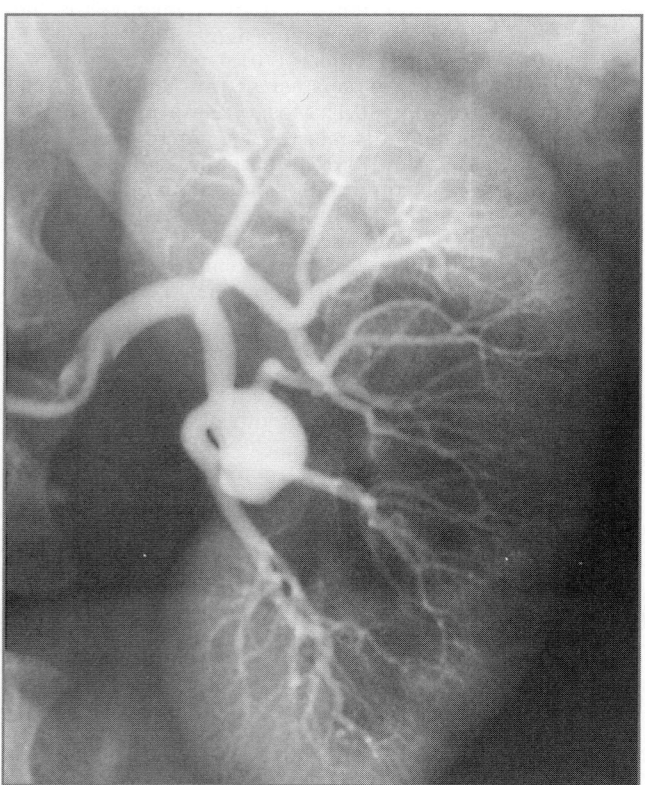

Figure 88.1. Renal artery aneurysm at a second-order branch. (From Stanley JC, Whitehouse WM Jr. Renal artery macroaneurysms. In: Bergan JJ, Yao JST, eds. *Aneurysms.* New York: Grune & Stratton, 1982:417, with permission.)

rysms with age is a likely sequela of further loss of elastic tissue at these already weakened branchings (15).

The high incidence of renal artery aneurysms associated with medial fibrodysplasia is well recognized (Fig. 88.4). In the latter disease state, further fragmentation and disruption of elastic tissue with loss of smooth muscle at bifurcations leave little more than a thin layer of fibrous connective tissue to contain blood flow. The greater incidence of aneurysms among patients with hypertension secondary to dysplastic renal artery stenoses, compared with those with arteriosclerotic stenoses, supports the tenet that arterial fibrodysplasia is a direct contributor to aneurysmal changes (7).

Blood pressure elevations occur in 40% to 80% of patients with renal artery macroaneurysms and may contribute to aneurysm development. Increased mural tension in these cases, especially in the presence of preexisting internal elastic lamina deficiencies at bifurcations, may further compromise the structural integrity of the renal artery.

In the case of pediatric patients, most aneurysms occur in poststenotic locations (16,17). These latter aneurysms have an amorphous globular configuration with thinning of all vessel wall elements. The more typical saccular aneurysms occurring at bifurcations in older patients account for approximately a third of renal artery aneurysms in childhood.

Clinical manifestations of intact renal artery aneurysms are poorly defined. Most renal artery aneurysms appear to be asymptomatic and are discovered incidentally (8–10). Aneurysmal expansion, compression of nearby structures, and renal infarction from dislodged thrombus may cause flank or abdominal pain. Hematuria and abdominal bruits have been attributed to some of these lesions; in most instances, however, these findings result from nonaneurysmal disease. Although quite rare, covert rupture of renal artery aneurysms into an adjacent vein may be associated with hematuria and hypertension. Once suspected because of findings on radiographs, intravenous pyelography, or computed tomography (CT), arteriography becomes the definitive diagnostic study (6). Gadolinium-enhanced magnetic resonance arteriography (MRA) (18) and three-dimensional reconstructed CT scanning (19) have a potential but unproven role in the anatomic delineation of these aneurysms.

The tenet that renal artery aneurysms cause hypertension has been a subject of continual controversy (5,6, 20–22). Embolization of aneurysmal thrombus or thrombotic occlusion of an adjacent artery may result in renal ischemia and renovascular hypertension (Fig. 88.5). This is uncommon. Atheromatous plaque ulceration within large aneurysmal sacs also can predispose to embolic complications. Embolization was a clear cause of secondary hypertension in only 3 of 118 patients with renal artery aneurysms in one series (7). In fact, if the kidney segment affected by embolization is totally infarcted, the patient

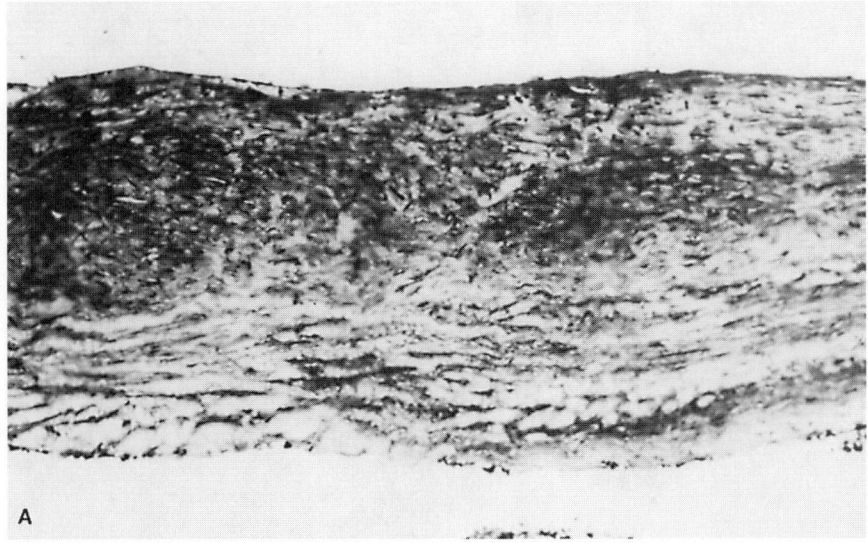

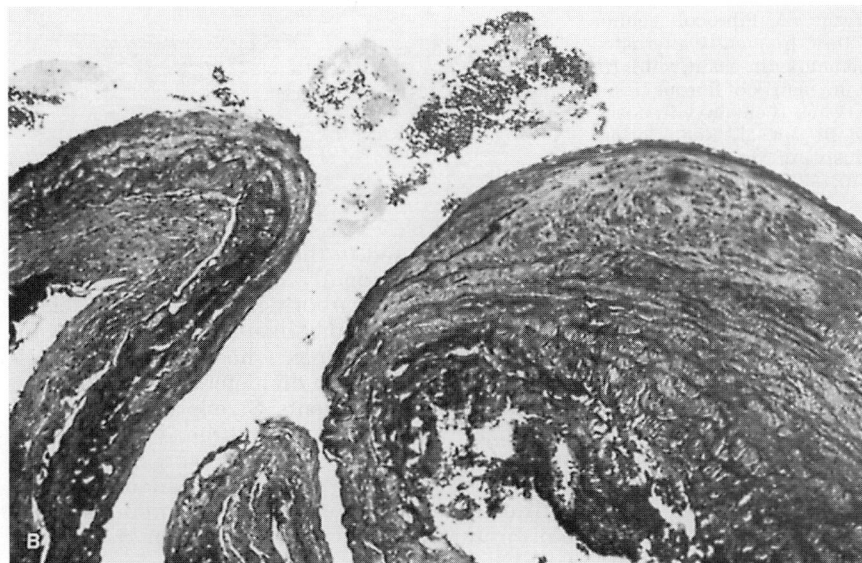

Figure 88.2. Renal artery aneurysm of undetermined etiology. *(A)* Excessive collagen and accumulation of ground substance with loss of smooth muscle characterize most such aneurysmal walls (Movat stain, × 40). *(B)* Interruption of internal elastic lamina *(arrow)* demonstrated at orifice of saccular renal artery aneurysm. Defects in elastic lamella have been related to the development of renal artery aneurysms (Movat stain, ×60). (From Stanley JC, Rhodes EL, Gewertz BL, et al. Renal artery aneurysms: significance of macroaneurysms exclusive of dissections and fibrodysplastic mural dilations. *Arch Surg* 1975;110:1327, with permission.)

may not become hypertensive; however, if the tissue simply becomes hypoperfused, it may become the source of considerable renin production and the cause of severe secondary hypertension. Small aneurysms without calcific arteriosclerosis are less likely sources of such renal arterial occlusions.

Aneurysmal compression or kinking of a neighboring artery causing flow reductions has been proposed as a cause of renovascular hypertension but has been poorly documented in the literature (23). More often, coexisting renal artery occlusive disease in the vicinity of aneurysms may account for secondary hypertension in these patients. Because of this possibility, one should search for existence of occult stenoses in hypertensive patients with aneurysms. Assessments of renin activity with determination of renal:systemic renin indices among patients with hypertension and renal artery aneurysms may establish the presence of renovascular hypertension.

Rupture is the most serious complication attending renal artery aneurysms, although it occurs less commonly than does rupture of many splanchnic aneurysms. Exsanguinating hemorrhage from a ruptured renal artery aneurysm happens less often than suggested in earlier reports (3,4,24,25).

The mortality rate with rupture is about 10%. Loss of a kidney is a near universal outcome of rupture (7,25). The relatively high reported rupture rate, approaching 3%, likely reflects the surgical nature of most published experiences. In fact, overt extraparenchymal rupture occurred in 2.8% of patients harboring these lesions, and covert rupture causing renal arteriovenous fistulae occurred in an additional 2.8% of one of the largest series from a surgical group (7). The high frequencies of rupture, as noted in the earlier literature, have not been confirmed in more recent reports (3,4,7–9). Certainly, the occurrence of bland renal artery aneurysm rupture is likely to be considerably less than 3%.

Rupture of renal artery aneurysms during pregnancy is an exception to the generally accepted benign nature of most bland aneurysms (26–28). Aneurysm rupture during pregnancy does not appear to be related to age, increased blood pressure, or number of pregnancies (26). Rupture of renal artery aneurysms is responsible for fetal death in nearly 85% of cases and is associated with a 55% maternal mortality rate (26). Parenthetically, there is no obvious relation between repeated pregnancies and the evolution of renal artery aneurysms, as seen with splenic artery aneurysms, although many women with these aneurysms are multiparous.

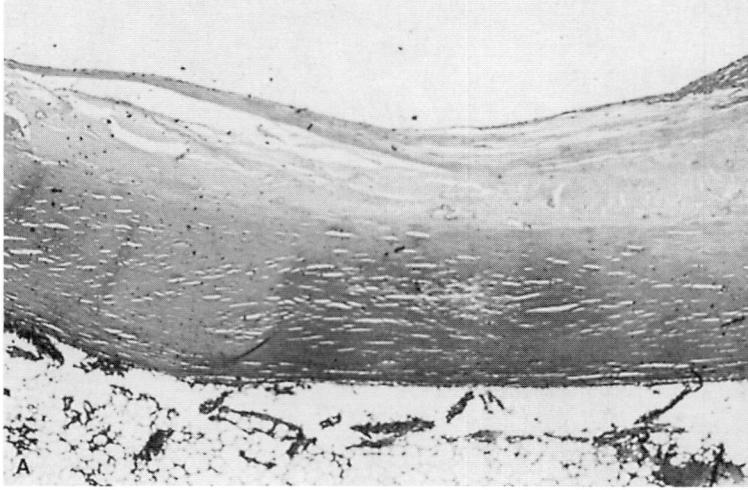

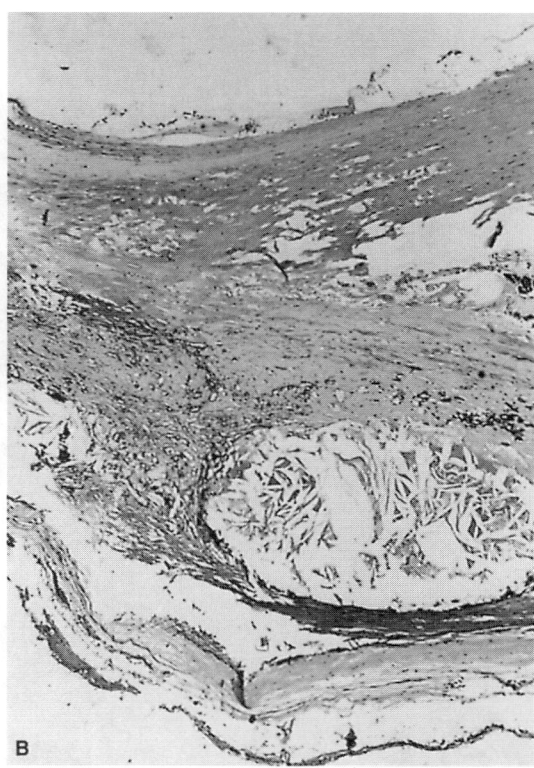

Figure 88.3. Arteriosclerotic renal artery aneurysm. *(A)* Fibrocollagenous aneurysm walls, with loss of all normal architecture, frequently alternated with areas exhibiting arteriosclerotic changes (hematoxylin-eosin, ×40). *(B)* Calcium deposition and cholesterol clefts within the matrix of fibrous tissue are typical of many larger arteriosclerotic aneurysms (hematoxylin-eosin, ×40). (From Stanley JC, Rhodes EL, Gewertz BL, et al. Renal artery aneurysms: significance of macroaneurysms exclusive of dissections and fibrodysplastic mural dilations. *Arch Surg* 1975;110:1327, with permission.)

An increased risk of renal artery aneurysm rupture has been attributed to large size, absence of calcification, and elevated blood pressure. These factors are not always relevant. In fact, overt rupture often has occurred in normotensive patients as well as with calcific atherosclerotic aneurysms (7). Similarly, size is of limited prognostic value as an indicator of rupture potential; greater rupture rates occurring in larger aneurysms are being inconsistently reported in the literature. Nevertheless, larger size remains a logical reason to assign a greater risk of rupture.

Indications for surgical intervention for true renal artery aneurysms are reasonably well defined. Operative intervention is indicated in the following situations: (a) aneurysms with functionally important renal artery stenoses; (b) aneurysms harboring thrombus, especially with evidence of distal embolization and cortical infarcts; (c) aneurysms in women who plan to have children; and (d) aneurysms with diameters greater than 1.5 cm in otherwise healthy patients. Size is a "soft" indication for surgical therapy. Cautious surgical intervention by those experienced in renovascular surgery in properly selected patients with renal artery aneurysms appears justified because of the small but unpredictable incidence of rupture with its attendant loss of kidney and life.

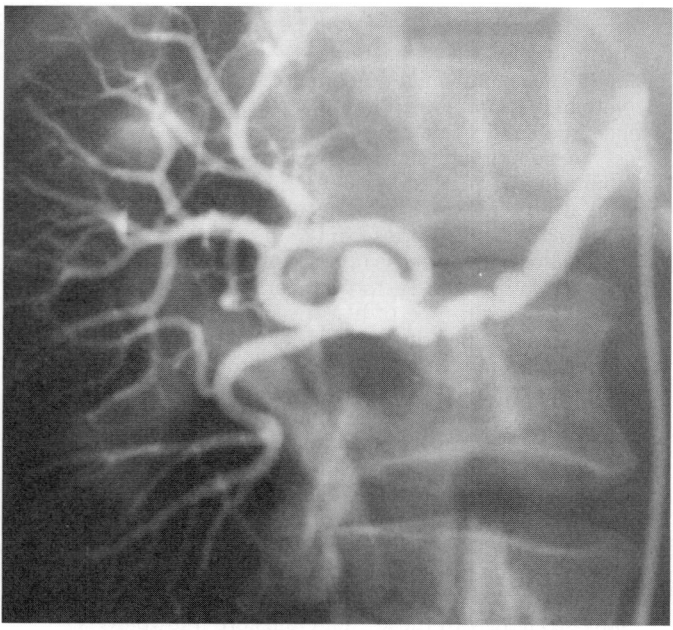

Figure 88.4. Saccular renal artery aneurysm occurring at the primary bifurcation of a main renal artery exhibiting medial fibroplasia. (From Stanley JC, Whitehouse WM Jr. Renal artery macroaneurysms. In: Bergan JJ, Yao JST, eds. *Aneurysms.* New York: Grune & Stratton, 1982:417, with permission.)

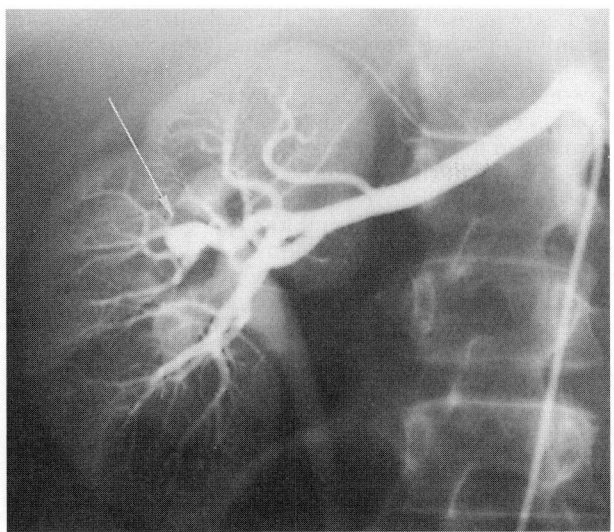

Figure 88.5. Small nonatherosclerotic intraparenchymal aneurysm associated with segmental thromboembolic renal ischemia and cortical infarct *(arrow).* (From Stanley JC, Whitehouse WM Jr. Renal artery macroaneurysms. In: Bergan JJ, Yao JST, eds. *Aneurysms.* New York: Grune & Stratton, 1982:417, with permission.)

The objective of surgical therapy is to eliminate the aneurysm without removing the kidney or compromising its function (27,29–31). Most aneurysms are best approached with a transabdominal, extraperitoneal exposure of the renal vasculature following medial displacement of the overlying colon and foregut viscera. Large aneurysms of the main renal artery usually can be excised with simple primary closure of the artery, but excision of smaller aneurysms may require arterial closure with a vein patch

(Fig. 88.6). More extensive renal artery reconstructions using autogenous saphenous vein or internal iliac artery as aortorenal grafts are favored for bifurcation aneurysms, especially those associated with functionally important stenoses (Fig. 88.7) (7,31).

Aneurysmectomy with reimplantation of the involved vessel or vessels into a normal adjacent or proximal renal artery is appropriate for treating many first- and second-order branch aneurysms (Fig. 88.8). Usually, these procedures are undertaken in situ, although ex vivo reconstructions may be preferred in certain cases (32–34), especially with coexistent segmental renal artery stenotic disease. Lastly, renal artery aneurysms 2 to 3 mm in diameter may be plicated by way of a closed aneurysmorrhaphy using a fine running cardiovascular suture. These small aneurysms often are encountered at operation as incidental lesions when treating larger aneurysms.

Nephrectomy is the usual therapy for managing ruptured aneurysms and extensive intraparenchymal aneurysms. Long-term outcome is actually quite good with this mode of therapy in carefully selected cases; for example, no patients treated in this manner at the University of Michigan required hemodialysis during a 20-year follow-up. Nevertheless, arterial reconstruction should be considered in cases when the kidney does not appear to have been irreparably injured from ischemia caused by the rupture. In other cases, partial nephrectomy may be required when aneurysmal erosion has occurred in an adjacent vein, causing a chronic arteriovenous fistula. Acute arteriovenous fistulae occasionally can be treated by conventional means with local excision and arterial reconstruction.

In general, renal artery aneurysms are not amenable to endovascular intervention. In part, this is because of their usual location at arterial bifurcations. In anecdotal cases, main renal artery aneurysms have been successfully excluded by stent graft placement, and peripheral branch

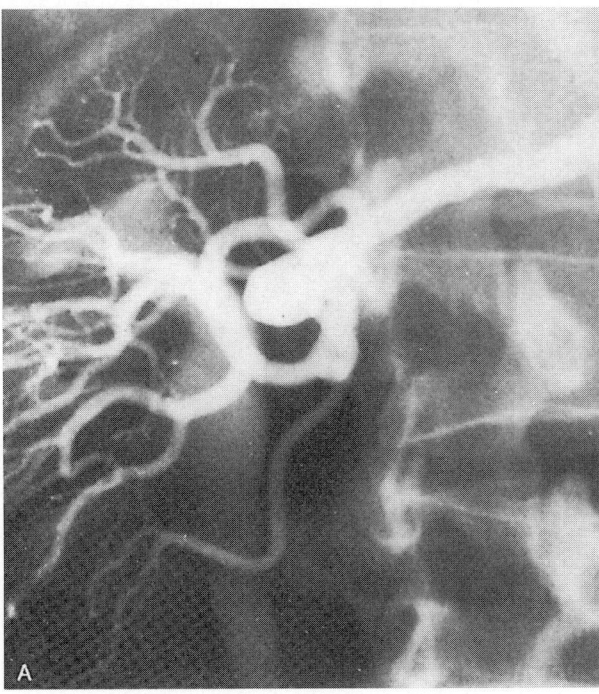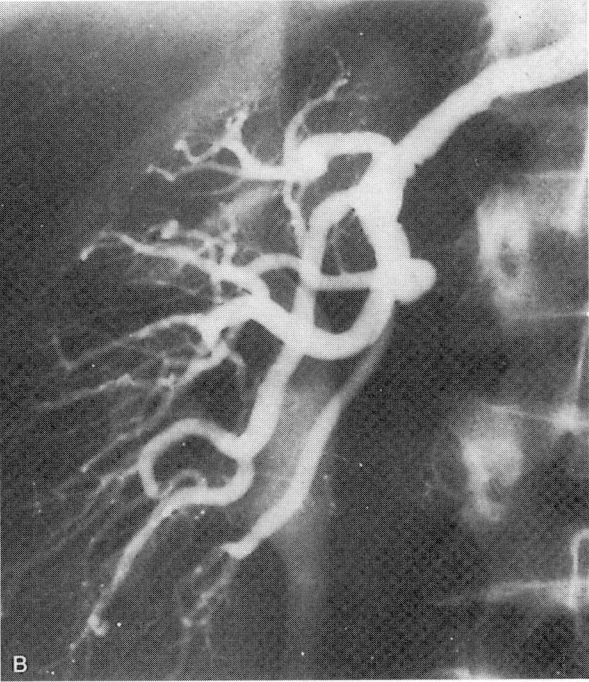

Figure 88.6. Renal artery aneurysm located at bifurcation of main renal artery *(A).* Surgical treatment included aneurysmectomy and vein patch graft closure of the artery *(B).* (From Stanley JC. Renal artery aneurysms and dissections. In: Veith FJ, ed. *Current critical problems in vascular surgery,* vol 3. St. Louis: Quality Medical, 1991:311, with permission.)

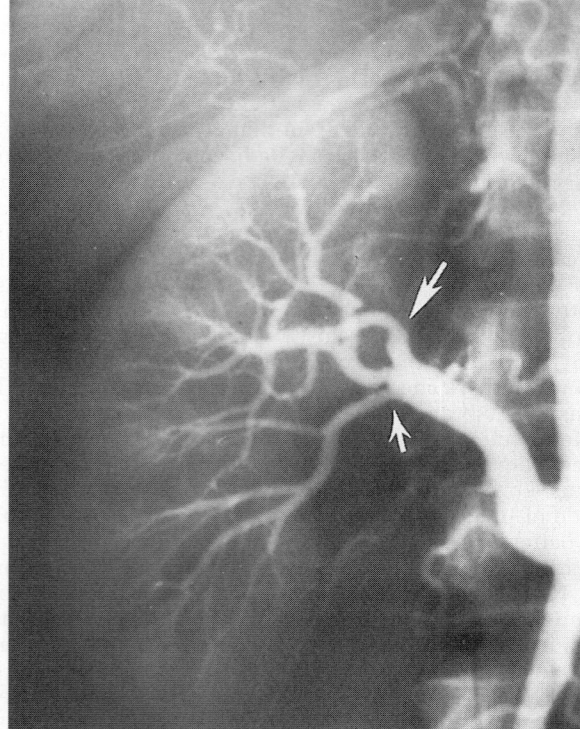

Figure 88.7. Aortorenal bypass with reversed autogenous saphenous vein following excision of an aneurysm in a fibrodysplastic vessel (same patient as in Fig. 88.4), with end-to-end anastomosis to one first-order segmental branch *(large arrow)* and end-to-side implantation of the other first-order segmental branch *(small arrow)*. (From Ernst CB, Stanley JC, Fry WJ. Multiple primary and segmental renal artery revascularization utilizing autogenous saphenous vein. *Surg Gynecol Obstet* 1973;137:1023, with permission.)

aneurysms have been successfully embolized (35–37). Embolization of intraparenchymal aneurysms is an appropriate alternative to partial nephrectomy in patients who show evidence of distal cortical infarction.

Renal artery aneurysms not treated by operation should be subjected to long-term surveillance. Duplex ultrasonography, CT, or MRA may prove useful in establishing an aneurysm's stability. Arteriography should be considered in patients who develop symptoms suggestive of aneurysmal expansion, exhibit hematuria, or become hypertensive. Because of the relatively low incidence of complications attending most renal artery aneurysms, noninvasive studies performed on a regular basis are favored over repeated arteriographic studies, which may carry risks exceeding those of the aneurysmal disease.

DISSECTING RENAL ARTERY ANEURYSMS

Isolated renal artery dissections causing aneurysms are rare (16,17,38,39). Dissections usually are classified into two categories: (a) those attributable to blunt abdominal trauma or intraluminal catheter-induced injury and (b) those occurring spontaneously (Fig. 88.9). Nearly one third of renal artery dissections are bilateral (11).

Dissections of the renal artery affect men nearly 10 times as often as women (40). In part, this ratio reflects the greater likelihood of trauma-induced dissections to occur in men. Although an overall predilection for right renal artery involvement exists, trauma-related dissections more commonly affect the left renal artery. Blood viscosity, shear forces, and flow turbulence are common contributors to the propagation of all dissections; but inadequate structural integrity resulting from injury or disease may initiate a dissection. Other factors contributing to these aneurysms vary among the different categories of dissection.

Blunt abdominal trauma contributes to renal artery dissections by two specific mechanisms. The first is violent displacement of the kidney, with deceleration causing

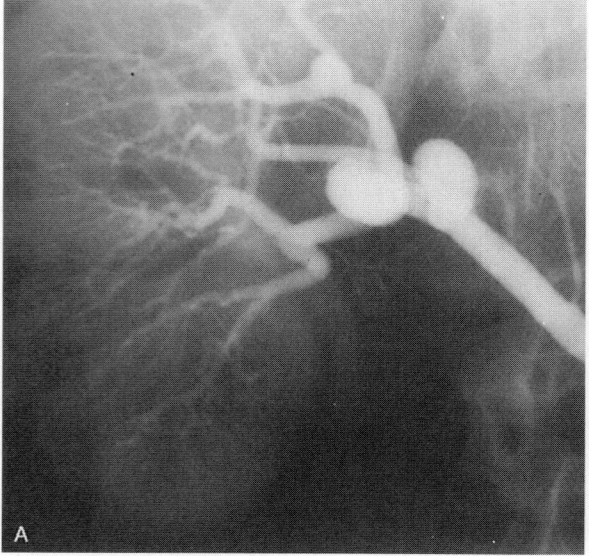
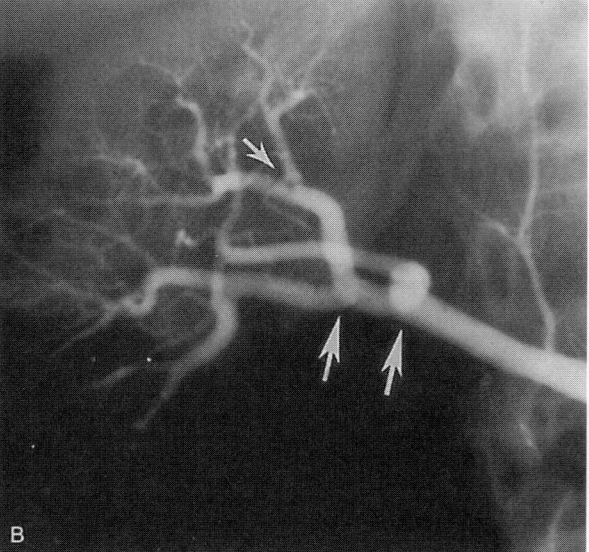

Figure 88.8. Renal artery aneurysms involving multiple segmental artery branchings *(A)*. Surgical treatment included aneurysmectomy and end-to-side reimplantation *(large arrows)* of segmental vessels into the adjacent artery and closed aneurysmorrhaphy *(small arrow) (B)*. (From Stanley JC. Renal artery aneurysms and dissections. In: Veith FJ, ed. *Current critical problems in vascular surgery,* vol 3. St. Louis: Quality Medical, 1991:311, with permission.)

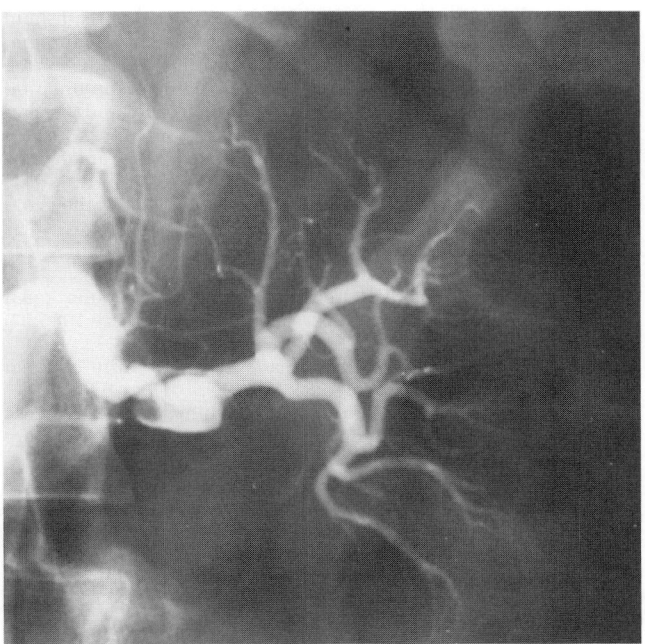

Figure 88.9. Saccular dissecting main renal artery aneurysm. (From Gewertz BL, Stanley JC, Fry WJ. Renal artery dissections. *Arch Surg* 1977;112:409, with permission.)

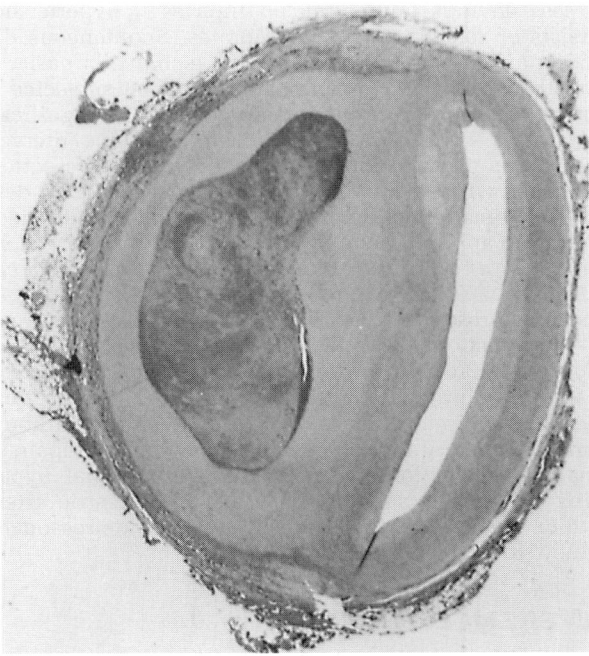

Figure 88.10. Dissection exhibiting deep mural hematoma and compression of adjacent lumen (hematoxylin-eosin, ×60). (From Stanley JC. Pathologic basis of macrovascular renal artery disease. In: Stanley JC, Ernst CB, Fry WJ, eds. *Renovascular hypertension*. Philadelphia: WB Saunders, 1984:46, with permission.)

marked stretching of the artery with fracture of the intima, which is the least elastic vessel wall component. This commonly results in subintimal dissections. The second relates to the unyielding posteriorly located vertebral bodies and direct arterial injury. In this setting, traumatic compression of the renal arteries against the vertebra may cause deeper medial hemorrhage and false aneurysm formation because of vasa vasorum rupture or actual vessel-wall disruption.

Iatrogenic catheter-related renal artery injury occurring during diagnostic arteriography is another recognized cause of these aneurysms. This is an uncommon complication. In one series, only four renal artery catheter dissections were encountered among more than 11,000 abdominal diagnostic arteriographic examinations, including more than 2,200 selective renal arteriograms (12). Iatrogenic dissections usually occur within the inner media or subintimal tissues. Dissections accompanying therapeutic catheterizations, such as balloon angioplasty, are common, although only a few cause critical narrowings or occlusion of the renal artery (41). In these instances, stent placement often restores normal renal artery blood flow (42).

Primary or spontaneous dissections causing pseudoaneurysms affect the renal arteries more than any other peripheral artery. Most are related to coexistent arteriosclerotic or dysplastic renovascular disease (7,43). A 9% incidence of dissections in patients with fibrodysplastic renal arteries has been reported (44), whereas others have noted only a 0.5% incidence in similar patient population (12). Differences in interpreting arteriographic or histologic studies may account for such divergent observations. Spontaneous dissections usually occur within the outer media adjacent to the external elastic lamina (Fig. 88.10). They occur less commonly within the inner or central media. In many instances, these dissections have been attributed to rupture of abnormal vasa vasorum. It is possible that the dissecting intramural hematoma in these circumstances increases medial ischemia and contributes to

further aneurysm formation. Spontaneous renal artery dissections usually affect proximal vessels and terminate at branchings.

Clinical manifestations of renal artery dissections are rather protean. Flank and back pain, hematuria, ileus, and elevated blood pressure frequently accompany acute dissections regardless of the cause (12,43,45). Chronic renal artery dissections, when clinically relevant, usually are associated with renovascular hypertension or impaired renal function. Certain dissections may be self-limited, asymptomatic, and of no functional importance.

An incorrect initial clinical diagnosis is common, occurring in more than half of patients who have renal artery dissections (45). Intravenous pyelography has been advocated for evaluating patients suspected of serious renal hilar injuries, including dissecting aneurysms. Some investigators, however, have noted a false-negative excretory urogram in about 12% of patients who have documented major renal artery injury (46). Furthermore, minor perirenal hematomas and cortical contusions frequently impair contrast excretion and may cause one third to one half of these studies to be false-positive. Because of this fact and the need for prompt diagnosis to improve results of surgical therapy, intravenous urograms should be deferred in favor of earlier arteriographic examinations.

Arteriography is necessary to diagnose and define the extent of renal artery dissections. Dissection is radiographically diagnosed when the following are recognized (43): luminal irregularities with aneurysmal dilatation or saccular dissections associated with segmental stenoses; extension of the dissections to the first renal artery branching; cuffing at branchings; and variable degrees of reversibility documented on serial arteriographic studies.

Trauma-related dissections warrant emergent primary arterial reconstructions once a hemodynamic narrowing or occlusion of the main renal artery or a major segmental branch is recognized (12,38). Delayed repair is necessary for less obvious trauma-related injuries if hypertension persists or renal function deteriorates. Spontaneous dissecting aneurysms, when acute, are technically easier to treat than traumatic lesions and should be subjected to surgical therapy soon after hemodynamically significant stenoses or occlusions are recognized. Operative intervention also is pursued for chronic spontaneous dissections associated with severe renovascular hypertension or deteriorating renal function. Endovascular stent graft placement is an appropriate alternative therapy for short proximal renal artery dissections with a defined distal end point.

Kidney preservation is important in patients with renal artery dissections, especially because renal artery disease of the contralateral kidney may be present in half the cases related to blunt abdominal trauma (12). Nephrectomy under such circumstances should be avoided. Although many dissections are not amenable to operative repair, arterial reconstructions in the form of aortorenal bypass using autogenous saphenous vein or hypogastric artery, with ex vivo repairs in selected cases, provide reasonable kidney salvage rates (38).

REFERENCES

1. Bulbul MA, Farrow GA. Renal artery aneurysms. *Urology* 1992;40:124.
2. Dzsinich C, Gloviczki P, McKusick MA, et al. Surgical management of renal artery aneurysm. *Cardiovasc Surg* 1993;3:243.
3. Hageman JH, Smith RF, Szilagyi DE, et al. Aneurysms of the renal artery: problems of prognosis and surgical management. *Surgery* 1978;84:563.
4. Hubert JP Jr, Pairolero PC, Kazmier FJ. Solitary renal artery aneurysm. *Surgery* 1980;88:557.
5. Martin RS III, Meacham PW, Ditesheim JA, et al. Renal artery aneurysm: selective treatment for hypertension and prevention of rupture. *J Vasc Surg* 1989;9:26.
6. Soussou ID, Starr DS, Lawrie GM, et al. Renal artery aneurysm: long-term relief of renovascular hypertension by in situ operative correction. *Arch Surg* 1979;114:1410.
7. Stanley JC, Rhodes EL, Gewertz BL, et al. Renal artery aneurysms: significance of macroaneurysms exclusive of dissections and fibrodysplastic mural dilations. *Arch Surg* 1975;110:1327.
8. Henriksson C, Bjorkerud S, Nilson AE, et al. Natural history of renal artery aneurysm elucidated by repeated angiography and pathoanatomical studies. *Eur Urol* 1985;11:244.
9. Henriksson C, Lukes P, Nilson AE, et al. Angiographically discovered, non-operated renal artery aneurysms. *Scand J Urol Nephrol* 1984;18:59.
10. Tham G, Ekelund L, Herrlin K, et al. Renal artery aneurysms: natural history and prognosis. *Ann Surg* 1983;197:348.
11. Edwards BS, Stanson AW, Holley KE, et al. Isolated renal artery dissection: presentation, evaluation, management and pathology. *Mayo Clin Proc* 1982;57:564.
12. Gewertz BL, Stanley JC, Fry WJ. Renal artery dissections. *Arch Surg* 1977;112:409.
13. Stanley JC, Gewertz BL, Bove EL. Arterial fibrodysplasia: histopathologic character and current etiologic concepts. *Arch Surg* 1975;110:561.
14. Smith DL. Spontaneous rupture of a renal artery aneurysm in polyarteritis nodosa: critical review of the literature and report of a case. *Am J Med* 1989;87:464.
15. Edsman G. Angiography and suprarenal angiography. *Acta Radiol* 1965;155(Suppl):104.
16. Sarkar R, Coran A, Lindenauer SM, et al. Arterial aneurysms in children: a clinicopathologic classification. *J Vasc Surg* 1991;13:47.
17. Stanley JC, Zelenock GB, Messina LM, et al. Pediatric renovascular hypertension: a thirty-year experience of operative treatment. *J Vasc Surg* 1995;21:212.
18. Prince MR, Narasimham DL, Stanley JC, et al. Breath-hold gadolinium-enhanced MR angiography of the abdominal aorta and its major branches. *Radiology* 1994;197:785.
19. Cikrit DF, Harris VJ, Hemmer CG, et al. Comparison of spiral CT scan and arteriography for evaluation of renal and visceral arteries. *Ann Vasc Surg* 1996;10:109.
20. Cummings KB, Lecky JW, Kaufman JJ. Renal artery aneurysms and hypertension. *J Urol* 1973;109:144.
21. Ruberti U, Miani S, Scorza R, et al. Aneurysm of the renal artery. *Int Angiol* 1987;6:407.
22. Vaughan TJ, Barry WF, Jeffords DL, et al. Renal artery aneurysms and hypertension. *Radiology* 1971;99:287.
23. Youkey JR, Collins GJ, Orecchia PM, et al. Saccular renal artery aneurysm as a cause of hypertension. *Surgery* 1985;97:498.
24. Hidai H, Kinoshita Y, Murayama T, et al. Rupture of renal artery aneurysm. *Eur Urol* 1985;11:249.
25. Schorn B, Valk V, Dalichau H, et al. Kidney salvage in a case of ruptured renal artery aneurysm: case report and literature review. *Cardiovasc Surg* 1997;5:134.
26. Cohen JR, Shamash FS. Ruptured renal artery aneurysms during pregnancy. *J Vasc Surg* 1987;6:51.
27. Love WK, Robinette MA, Vernon CP. Renal artery aneurysm rupture in pregnancy. *J Urol* 1981;126:809.
28. Rijbroek A, Dijk AV, Roex AJM. Rupture of renal artery aneurysm during pregnancy. *Eur J Vasc Surg* 1994;8:375.
29. Huppt, T, Allenberg JR, Post K, et al. Renal artery aneurysms: surgical indications and results. *Eur J Vasc Surg* 1992;6:477.
30. Mercier C, Piquet P, Piligian F, et al. Aneurysms of the renal artery and its branches. *Ann Vasc Surg* 1986;1:321.
31. Stanley JC, Messina LM, Wakefield TW, et al. Renal artery reconstruction. In: Bergan JJ, Yao JST, eds. *Techniques in arterial surgery*. Philadelphia: WB Saunders, 1990:247.
32. Belzer FO, Raczkowski A. Ex vivo renal artery reconstruction with autotransplantation. *Surgery* 1982;92:642.
33. Bugge-Asperheim B, Sdal G, Flatmark A. Renal artery aneurysm: ex vivo repair and autotransplantation. *Scand J Urol Nephrol* 1984;18:63.
34. Dubernard JM, Martin X, Gelet A, et al. Aneurysms of the renal artery: surgical management with special reference to extracorporeal surgery and autotransplantation. *Eur Urol* 1985;11:26.
35. Bui BT, Oliva VL, Leclerc G, et al. Renal artery aneurysm: Treatment with percutaneous placement of a stent-graft. *Radiology* 1995;195:181.
36. Centenera LV, Hirsch JA, Choi IS, et al. Wide-necked saccular renal artery aneurysm: endovascular embolization with the Guglielmi detachable coil and temporary balloon occlusion of the aneurysm neck. *J Vasc Intervent Radiol* 1998;9:513.
37. Tateno T, Kubota Y, Sasagawa I, et al. Successful embolization of a renal artery aneurysm with preservation of renal blood flow. *Int Urol Nephrol* 1996;28:283.
38. Reilly LM, Cuningham CG, Maggisano R, et al. The role of arterial reconstruction in spontaneous renal artery dissection. *J Vasc Surg* 1991;14:468.
39. Smith BM, Holcomb GW, Richie RE, et al. Renal artery dissection. *Ann Surg* 1984;200:134.
40. Bakir AA, Patel K, Schwartz MM, et al. Isolated dissecting aneurysm of the renal artery. *Am Heart J* 1978;96:92.
41. Stanley JC. Surgery of failed percutaneous transluminal renal artery angioplasty. In: Bergan JJ, Yao JST, eds. *Reoperative arterial surgery*. Orlando, FL: Grune & Stratton, 1986:441.
42. Mali WPTM, Geyskes GG, Thalman R. Dissecting renal artery aneurysm: treatment with an endovascular stent. *AJR* 1989;153:623.
43. Hare WSC, Kincaid-Smith P. Dissecting aneurysm of the renal artery. *Radiology* 1970;97:255.
44. Harrison EG Jr, Hunt JC, Bernatz PE. Morphology of fibromuscular dysplasia of the renal artery in renovascular hypertension. *Am J Med* 1967;43:97.
45. Rao CN, Blaivas JG. Primary renal artery dissecting aneurysm: a review. *J Urol* 1977;118:716.
46. Scott R Jr, Carlton CE Jr, Goldman M. Penetrating injuries of the kidney: an analysis of 181 patients. *J Urol* 1969;101:247.

SURGERY: SCIENTIFIC PRINCIPLES AND PRACTICE, Third Edition, edited by
Lazar J. Greenfield, Michael W. Mulholland, Keith T. Oldham, Gerald B. Zelenock,
and Keith D. Lillemoe. Lippincott Williams & Wilkins Publishers, Philadelphia, © 2001.

CHAPTER 89

FEMORAL AND POPLITEAL ANEURYSMS

LINDA M. GRAHAM

PERIPHERAL ANEURYSMS

Femoral and popliteal artery aneurysms, although far less common than abdominal aortic aneurysms, are the most frequently encountered peripheral aneurysms. Their significance comes from their potential for limb-threatening complications and their association with life-threatening abdominal aortic aneurysms.

Incidence

The exact incidence of femoral and popliteal aneurysms is difficult to define, but they are being recognized with increasing frequency. An aging population, increased arterial trauma, more common use of invasive therapies for vascular disease, and increased use of imaging modalities all contribute to the rise in number of peripheral aneurysms being diagnosed. In a series published in 1972, aortic aneurysms were diagnosed in 0.5% of hospitalized patients, and the ratio of peripheral atherosclerotic or degenerative aneurysms to aortic aneurysms was 1:23 (1). In more recent reports, the ratio of popliteal to abdominal aortic aneurysms has been 1:15 and 1:8 (2,3). More false aneurysms are occurring coincident with the increased use of bypass surgery and catheter-based diagnostic and therapeutic procedures.

Atherosclerotic or degenerative femoral and popliteal artery aneurysms are encountered far more frequently in men than women. The ratio of male to female patients with femoral and popliteal aneurysms is approximately 30:1 (4,5). This predilection for men is markedly different from aortic aneurysms, which has a ratio of male to female patients of approximately 5:1 (6).

Pathogenesis

The cause of femoral and popliteal aneurysms has changed distinctly since they were first recognized centuries ago. Once primarily mycotic, syphilitic, or traumatic in origin, most true aneurysms have a degenerative cause (commonly called *atherosclerotic*), whereas false aneurysms usually follow surgery or trauma.

The cause of degenerative aneurysms of the femoral and popliteal vessels is not clear. One factor believed to contribute to aneurysm formation is turbulent flow beyond a relative stenosis, resulting in poststenotic dilatation beyond the inguinal ligament at the groin or beyond the tendinous hiatus of the adductor magnus or the arcuate popliteal ligament and the heads of the gastrocnemius muscle at the popliteal level. Arterial wall fatigue that results from to vibration and turbulence proximal to a major branching or from stress during hip and knee flexion may contribute to aneurysm formation.

The frequent occurrence of multiple peripheral aneurysms in the same patient suggests a systemic abnormality in the arterial wall, which promotes aneurysmal degeneration at locations where hemodynamic or mechanical factors put unusual stress on the arterial wall. This, however, would not explain the male predilection for the disease unless aneurysm formation is due, in part, to a genetic abnormality that is carried on the X chromosome. The aneurysm-prone blotchy mouse has an X chromosome mutation that affects cross-linking of collagen and elastin (7), but there is no direct evidence of this in humans.

The presence of an inflammatory infiltrate has been noted in the wall of femoral and popliteal aneurysms, similar to aortic aneurysms (8). The role of this inflammatory process, with potential release of matrix metalloproteinases, is unknown, but elevated plasma levels of matrix metalloproteinase are found in patients with aortic aneurysms (9). Furthermore, the overexpression of tissue inhibitor of matrix metalloproteinases in a rat model prevents aneurysm degeneration (10). Apoptosis of smooth muscle cells also can play a role in the formation of aneurysms by limiting the ability of the arterial wall to respond to the degenerative process (11).

Clinical Manifestations

Femoral and popliteal aneurysms may be asymptomatic and often are incidental findings on routine physical examination. Both femoral and popliteal artery aneurysms, however, may be accompanied by symptoms of local pain caused by enlargement or by pressure on the adjacent nerve, and limb edema and venous distention resulting from compression of the adjacent vein. Patients also may develop lower-extremity ischemia with intermittent claudication, rest pain, or gangrene secondary to complications of a femoral or popliteal aneurysm, including thrombosis, distal embolization, or rupture. Because the natural history and complication rate in femoral and popliteal aneurysms differ, they are considered separately here.

FEMORAL ARTERY ANEURYSMS

Femoral artery aneurysms are the most common peripheral aneurysm if both true and false aneurysms are included. Their clinical importance rests in the fact that they are limb-threatening lesions that can jeopardize the viability of the leg if thrombosis, embolization, or rupture occur. The vast majority of true aneurysms are degenerative lesions (commonly referred to as *atherosclerotic aneurysms);* false aneurysms include anastomotic, traumatic, and mycotic lesions. Rarely, femoral aneurysms develop secondary to connective tissue disorders. The femoral region is the most common site for both anastomotic aneurysms and mycotic aneurysms associated with trauma; so the presentation and surgical repair of these lesions will be discussed in this chapter.

Degenerative (Atherosclerotic) Aneurysms

Incidence

The exact incidence of degenerative (atherosclerotic) femoral artery aneurysms in the general population remains undefined. They are found in 3% of all patients with abdominal aortic aneurysms, and 85% of patients with femoral artery aneurysms have abdominal aortic aneurysms (4).

Pattern of Disease

Femoral aneurysms most frequently affect the common femoral artery. They may be classified as *type I,* those limited to the common femoral artery, or as *type II,* those involving the orifice of the profunda femoris artery (12). Type I and Type II aneurysms occur with nearly equal frequency. This classification becomes important in reference to vascular reconstructive procedures, with type II aneurysms requiring more complex reconstructions to ensure continued patency of both the superficial and profunda femoris arteries. Isolated lesions of the profunda femoris artery are rare (2% of femoral artery aneurysms) and are susceptible to rupture because they are difficult to diagnose at the asymptomatic stage.

Femoral artery aneurysms can be limb-threatening lesions, and they frequently are associated with limb-threatening popliteal aneurysms and life-threatening abdominal aortic aneurysms. Multiple aneurysms are common in patients with femoral artery aneurysms. In a series of 100 patients with atherosclerotic femoral artery aneurysms seen at a single institution, 72% of patients had bilateral femoral artery aneurysms (4). In addition, aortoiliac aneurysms were detected in 85% of patients, thoracic aortic aneurysms in 6%, and popliteal aneurysms in 44%, of which 55% were bilateral.

Clinical Manifestations

The typical patient with a degenerative femoral artery aneurysm is a man in his 60s or 70s with the usual risk factors for atherosclerosis. Of these patients, 86% are cigarette smokers, 36% have hypertension, and 14% have diabetes mellitus (4). Associated cardiovascular disease is common; clinical manifestations of coronary artery disease and cerebrovascular disease are present in 34% and 7%, respectively.

The clinical manifestations of femoral artery aneurysms cover the spectrum from asymptomatic to severe ischemia of the lower extremity. Although 40% of patients are asymptomatic at diagnosis, most have local symptoms or complaints of lower extremity ischemia (4). Local pain or observation of a groin mass is the only complaint in 18% of patients. Lower extremity venous disease is present in 8%, attributable to venous obstruction by the femoral artery aneurysm in 4%; but venous obstruction is rarely the sole sign of an aneurysm. Lower extremity ischemic symptoms of claudication, rest pain, or gangrene are present in 42% of patients and often lead to the diagnosis of the femoral aortic aneurysm, but the ischemic symptoms are usually attributable to associated arterial disease rather than to the femoral aneurysm.

As with aneurysms in other locations, femoral artery aneurysms may be complicated by embolization, thrombosis, or rupture. Peripheral embolization may be identified incidentally on angiography, or it may produce signs as mild as spotty discoloration of the toes and as severe as peripheral gangrene. Thrombosis usually produces significant ischemic symptoms but does not always acutely jeopardize limb viability. The reported rate at which complications occur spans a large range, with the higher numbers noted in series consisting primarily of patients from a surgical service. Although embolization is reported in about 10% of aneurysms, the femoral artery aneurysm is not necessarily the source of these emboli because many patients have a concomitant popliteal aneurysm (4). In larger clinical series, 1% to 16% of patients with degenerative femoral artery aneurysms initially have an acute thrombosis, whereas 1% to 16% have a chronically thrombosed lesion (4,12). Rupture is reported in 1% to 14% of aneurysms (4,12).

Natural History

The natural history of degenerative femoral artery aneurysms is poorly defined. Most publications have reviewed aneurysms that were subjected to operation. A small asymptomatic femoral artery aneurysm does not appear to pose the same threat to the limb as does a popliteal artery aneurysm. In a series of 100 patients with atherosclerotic femoral artery aneurysms, serious limb-threatening complications were documented in only 2.9% of the 105 aneurysms initially followed without surgery (4). This was, however, a preselected group in which many symptomatic or large aneurysms were excluded from follow-up because operative intervention was undertaken after the initial diagnosis.

Diagnosis

In most cases, the diagnosis of femoral artery aneurysm is suspected by the finding of a pulsatile groin mass on routine physical examination or during evaluation for vascular disease. If the femoral artery aneurysm is small or thrombosed, detection on physical examination may be difficult. Although a radiograph of the region occasionally may demonstrate the calcified rim of the aneurysm, only ultrasonography, computed tomography (CT), or magnetic resonance imaging (MRI) can establish the diagnosis of the femoral aneurysm reliably. In addition, these modalities are useful in accurately defining the size of the lesion and evaluating associated aneurysmal disease in the distal aorta and popliteal regions. This is particularly important because potentially life-threatening abdominal aortic aneurysms are missed on physical examination in 50% of patients with multiple aneurysms (1). The diagnostic accuracy of arteriography is limited because it demonstrates only the residual lumen and an aneurysm filled with smooth mural thrombus may be missed, but definition of the vascular anatomy of the lower extremity provided by angiography is helpful in planning the appropriate operative procedure (Fig. 89.1).

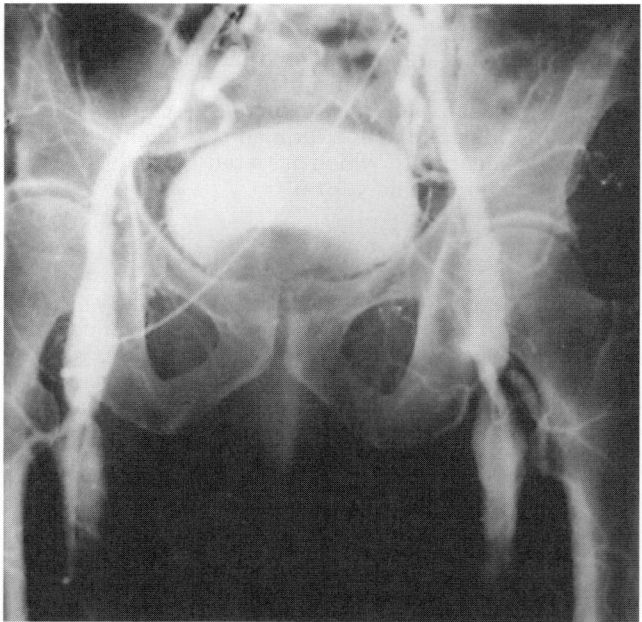

Figure 89.1. Arteriogram demonstrating bilateral femoral artery aneurysms that extend into the superficial femoral arteries. Unlike many patients with femoral artery aneurysms, this patient did not have an associated aortic aneurysm or popliteal aneurysm.

Treatment

Indications. Operative treatment is indicated for all aneurysms causing local symptoms (pain, venous or neural compression) or presenting with limb-threatening complications (embolization, thrombosis, or rupture). Asymptomatic aneurysms greater than 2.5 cm in diameter should be repaired unless the patient is at prohibitive risk for operative intervention. In patients with small, asymptomatic aneurysms, observation may be appropriate, particularly in patients with multiple medical problems who would be high risk for surgery. When nonoperative management is selected, the size of the aneurysm should be documented by ultrasonography. The patient should be followed with ultrasound scans and careful examination for occult complications at regular intervals. Operative treatment should be undertaken without undue delay if the femoral aneurysm enlarges, produces symptoms, or is complicated by embolization, thrombosis, or rupture.

Surgical Strategy. The operative approach is individualized based on associated aneurysmal disease. In patients with multiple asymptomatic aneurysms, treatment is staged. The life-threatening aortic lesions are treated before limb-threatening popliteal lesions. Femoral artery aneurysms are addressed after popliteal lesions unless the femoral aneurysm is repaired in combination with treatment of the aortic or popliteal aneurysm. If an aortofemoral bypass is necessary, the femoral aneurysm should be treated at the same time to avoid later anastomotic aneurysm formation. The graft limb can be anastomosed distal to the aneurysm or into an interposition graft that has replaced the femoral aneurysm. In patients with severe lower-extremity ischemia, the femoral aneurysm is treated with an interposition graft, from which the proximal anastomosis of the required femoropopliteal or femorotibial bypass is based.

Technique. The operative procedure for treatment of an isolated femoral artery aneurysm is determined by aneurysmal involvement of the superficial and deep femoral arteries as well as by the existence of lower-extremity occlusive disease. The femoral artery aneurysm usually is approached through a vertical groin incision. When addressing an unusually large aneurysm or a ruptured aneurysm, however, initial proximal control of the external iliac artery through a retroperitoneal approach is advisable. After proximal and distal arterial control is obtained, the aneurysm sac is opened and the atheromatous debris removed. Small aneurysms may be excised, but routine excision of large aneurysms in not recommended because these lesions can be adherent to the adjacent vein and nerve. For type I aneurysms, the preferred treatment is reconstruction with an interposition graft of Dacron or expanded polytetrafluoroethylene (ePTFE) with the proximal anastomosis at the distal external iliac artery or proximal common femoral artery and the distal anastomosis at the femoral bifurcation.

For type II aneurysms with patent superficial and profunda femoris arteries, an interposition graft to the profunda femoris artery with reimplantation of the superficial femoral artery is one standard configuration. If the superficial femoral artery is chronically occluded and the patient has minimal symptoms, an interposition graft to the profunda femoris artery alone is sufficient; but if the patient has severe lower-extremity ischemia, this is followed by a standard distal reconstruction. If recent emboli or in situ thrombosis has occluded the outflow tract, catheter thromboembolectomy and thrombolytic therapy are useful adjuvants.

Stent grafts have been used for femoral aneurysm repair, but their place in the therapeutic armamentarium is unclear at this time. Early reports suggests that stent grafts, when used below the inguinal ligament, have lower patency and higher complication rates than the conventional surgical approach (13,14). The durability of endovascular repairs also remains to be determined.

Results. Results of surgical therapy depend on the patency of the distal vasculature. More than 80% of asymptomatic patients have excellent long-term results, whereas 68% of those presenting with lower-extremity ischemia achieve satisfactory long-term outcome (4). Operative mortality rate for repair of an isolated femoral artery aneurysm is basically the risk of anesthesia. Reported mortality rates of up to 4% reflect concomitant aortic reconstruction.

Anastomotic Aneurysms

Incidence

Anastomotic aneurysms result from a disrupted suture line between a graft and the host artery. The incidence varies with the location of the anastomosis and the type of graft that is used. Anastomotic aneurysms at the femoral artery account for nearly 80% of these lesions, and 3% of all femoral anastomoses or 6% of femoral anastomoses after aortofemoral bypass develop this complication compared with 0.2% of aortic anastomoses (15,16). After infrainguinal bypass procedures, the incidence of anastomotic aneurysms is higher with prosthetic grafts than with autogenous vein grafts; 6% of femoral anastomoses develop aneurysms when Dacron is used compared with 0.9% when a vein graft is placed (15). Anastomotic aneurysms are a late complication of bypass procedures; the mean interval from primary procedure to recognition is more than 6 years (17,18).

Pathogenesis

Several factors contributing to anastomotic aneurysm formation have been identified, including weakness of the arterial wall, the type of graft material and suture used, the presence of infection, the method of construction of the anastomosis, and the stress on the suture line from hypertension, leg motion, or excess tension on the graft limb (15,17,18). Progressive degeneration of the recipient artery accounts for most anastomotic aneurysms, and an increased incidence of anastomotic aneurysms has been noted following endarterectomy of the artery at the anastomosis. False aneurysms occur more commonly with synthetic vascular grafts than with saphenous vein grafts, a reflection of more complete healing with autogenous tissue. With the use of monofilament synthetic suture, anastomotic aneurysms rarely result from a loss of suture integrity, although occasionally a broken suture is a factor in pseudoaneurysm formation. Although most anastomotic aneurysms are not accompanied by overt graft infection, occult infections with coagulase-negative *Staphylococcus* species may be an important factor in development of anastomotic aneurysms (18). A higher incidence of anastomotic aneurysms occurs in patients with wound-healing complications, and the use of anticoagulants may increase such complications. Some studies suggest that anastomotic aneurysms are more common with an end-to-side anastomosis than with an end-to-end anastomosis, although other reports do not verify this. Finally, hypertension, joint motion, or excessive tension on the graft limb may place stress on the suture line and cause anastomotic disruption.

Clinical Manifestations

Femoral anastomotic aneurysms usually present as a pulsatile groin mass, which may or may not be accompanied by pain, redness, or symptoms of venous obstruction. Acute complications of anastomotic aneurysms include hemorrhage, embolization, and occlusion. The latter may cause lower-extremity ischemia with claudication, rest pain, or gangrene.

Diagnosis

The diagnosis of a false aneurysm is usually made on physical examination by the presence of a pulsatile groin mass in a patient who has undergone a femoral arterial reconstructive procedure. The differential diagnosis includes nonpulsatile groin masses, such as hernia, lymphocele, or abscess, through which pulsation may be transmitted from an underlying normal femoral artery. Diagnosis of an anastomotic aneurysm in one region should raise suspicion of other anastomotic aneurysms because multiple lesions are found in at least 30% of patients (17), and their presence suggests infection. Evaluation of an anastomotic aneurysm includes ultrasonography or CT of all anastomoses of the graft. Angiography done before repair of the anastomotic aneurysm is helpful in defining the proximal and distal arterial anatomy (Fig. 89.2).

Treatment

Because of the progressive nature of anastomotic aneurysms, surgical treatment is undertaken for all lesions except small (<2 cm in diameter), stable, asymptomatic aneurysms in high-risk patients. Some anastomotic aneurysms, depending on the anatomy, are amenable to endovascular treatment. Principles of surgical therapy are those of primary aneurysms: obtain proximal and distal control and replace the aneurysmal segment. Securing proximal control often requires dividing the inguinal ligament to isolate the graft limb. Distal control is achieved most easily by using intraluminal balloon catheters. If in-

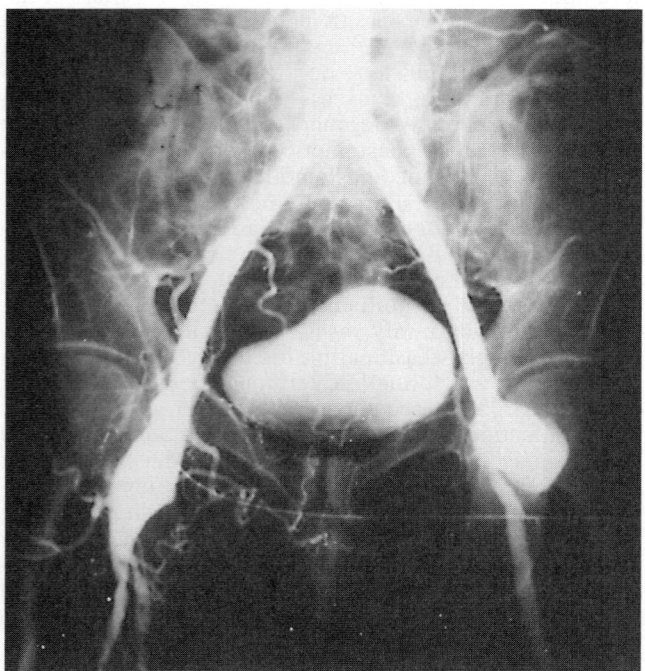

Figure 89.2. Arteriogram demonstrating bilateral femoral anastomotic aneurysms after an aortofemoral bypass and a left femoro–popliteal bypass.

trinsic arterial disease requires extension of the graft distally on the profunda femoris or superficial femoral artery, these arteries can be controlled by dissection through unscarred tissue distal to the previous exposure. After débridement of the degenerated artery, an interposition graft is placed between the prosthetic graft limb and the healthy native artery. Cultures of the graft and vessel wall are essential to exclude infection as a causative factor in the development of the anastomotic aneurysm. If at the time of surgery the presence of infection is obvious, the approach is the same as that of any infected graft with removal of infected prosthetic material and reestablishment of blood flow, if necessary, with a bypass through an uninfected tissue route, such as an obturator, lateral femoral, or axillofemoral bypass.

Results

Results of elective operations on uncomplicated anastomotic aneurysms are excellent, with 2% operative mortality, 97.5% graft patency at 2 years, and 2% amputation within 2 years of surgery (17). Recurrence is reported in fewer than 16% of cases (15,16). Patients who have aneurysms complicated by hemorrhage, occlusion, or embolization have significantly increased operative morbidity and mortality.

Catheter-induced Pseudoaneurysms

Incidence

The femoral artery is the preferred site of arterial access for both diagnostic angiography and interventional endovascular therapy. In recent years, diagnostic studies for coronary and peripheral artery occlusive disease have increased, as have the subsequent endovascular interventions (19). This has resulted in an increased number of catheter-induced pseudoaneurysms. Because interventional techniques often require prolonged arterial cannulation, large-bore sheaths, and anticoagulation, they are accompanied by a higher rate of arterial complications than are diagnostic studies. Review of recent experiences showed that pseudoaneurysm formation can be expected after 0.05% of diagnostic catheterizations and about 0.4% of more complex procedures (20) but up to 6% of percutaneous transluminal coronary angioplasties (21).

Pathogenesis

Pseudoaneurysms from iatrogenic catheter trauma meet the classic definition for pseudoaneurysm in that they are collections of blood in continuity with the arterial system, which are not enclosed by all three layers of the arterial wall. These lesions form because of failed hemostasis at the arterial wall defect created by catheter insertion. Normally, hemostasis, aided by direct focal application of pressure, seals the defect promptly, and the arterial wall repairs itself. When hemostasis is unsuccessful, blood under arterial pressure leaks from the artery, dissects surrounding tissue planes, and forms what is perceived on physical examination as a pulsatile mass. The gross findings at surgery are a blood-filled cavity surrounded by a fibrous capsule in direct continuity with the arterial lumen via a catheter-sized mural defect. Like all pseudoaneurysms, these lesions can cause symptoms by rupture or compression of surrounding structures.

Diagnosis

The diagnosis of catheter-induced pseudoaneurysm is suspected when a pulsatile groin mass is noted after arterial catheterization. The differential diagnosis includes hematoma, lymphadenopathy, and abscess. CT, MRI, or conventional and color-flow duplex scanning is used to establish the diagnosis, differentiate pseudoaneurysm from hematoma, and define the communication between the mass and the arterial lumen. Color-flow duplex scanning is relatively inexpensive and sensitive and thus is the diagnostic test of choice. It provides accurate diagnosis, localization, and sizing of catheter-induced false aneurysms.

Natural History

Color-flow duplex scanning has been used to define the incidence and natural history of pseudoaneurysms after percutaneous transluminal coronary angioplasty (21). Pseudoaneurysms are identified after 6% of these procedures, and most pseudoaneurysms will thrombose spontaneously within 4 weeks. Thrombosis is less likely in anticoagulated patients and in those with pseudoaneurysms larger than 1.8 cm in diameter; so about 30% of patients with pseudoaneurysms will require intervention (22).

Treatment

Therapy of catheter-induced pseudoaneurysms is influenced by aneurysm size and symptoms and whether the patient requires continuous anticoagulation. Surgical therapy is mandatory for all catheter-induced pseudoaneurysms that are acutely expanding, compressing adjacent nerves, or compromising the overlying skin. Proximal and distal arterial control is obtained, and the arterial defect is repaired directly, rarely requiring placement of more than one to two sutures.

An excellent alternative to a surgical approach, when urgent repair is not required, is the use of ultrasound-directed compression therapy or thrombin injection into the false aneurysm. The pseudoaneurysm is identified using a color-flow scanner and then compressed with the scanner head. Real-time observation of flow in the underlying artery allows compression while maintaining flow in the native vessel to prevent arterial occlusion. Pseudoaneurysm thrombosis is documented by the absence of flow signals on release of scan-head pressure in the case of compression therapy. Another nonoperative treatment of catheter-induced pseudoaneurysms is percutaneous ultrasound-guided injection of 0.5–1.0 mL thrombin (1,000 U/mL) into the pseudoaneurysm away from the neck of the aneurysm (23,24). Continuous ultrasonographic imaging is used to monitor thrombosis of the pseudoaneurysm.

Results

The results of ultrasound-guided compression therapy for catheter-induced pseudoaneurysms are good. Thrombosis of the pseudoaneurysm is obtained in 80% to 90% of cases. The initial success rate is similar in patients who are anticoagulated and in those who are not, but long-term success is better in patients not receiving anticoagulant therapy. In one of the largest series of pseudoaneurysms treated with ultrasound-guided compression, thrombosis was achieved in 86% of anticoagulated patients and in 98% of those not anticoagulated, with a 20% recurrence rate in less than 24 hours in anticoagulated patients (25). Success using this therapeutic modality requires a knowledgeable ultrasonographer, meticulous postcompression follow-up, and early immobilization.

In small series using thrombin injection, success is nearly 100%, with thrombosis occurring in less than 1 minute (23,24,26). This technique can be complicated by arterial thrombosis, particularly if an excessive volume of thrombin is used, and it may not be appropriate for pseudoaneurysms with large necks (27,28). Large pseudoaneurysm size (> 8 cm in diameter) and an associated arteriovenous fistula (AVF) are predictors of failure, and an AVF is a predictor of recurrence (29). Initial success

rates are lower for pseudoaneurysms, which follow stent placement procedures, presumably because of the larger sheath placed in the artery and the larger resultant arterial defect (30). These lesions may require surgical therapy.

Mycotic Aneurysms

The term *mycotic aneurysm* is currently used to refer to any infected aneurysm. Mycotic aneurysms today are often a complication of parental drug abuse, but they can follow arterial trauma of any form, including invasive diagnostic and therapeutic procedures. In the past, septic emboli from bacterial endocarditis were a major cause of aneurysmal degeneration, but today they are uncommon. With the advent of antibiotics, aneurysms secondary to syphilis or tuberculosis are rare. With the change in cause, the location of mycotic aneurysms has shifted from central to peripheral arteries, with the femoral artery the most common site (31,32). The importance of mycotic aneurysms comes from their propensity to rupture.

Pathogenesis

The pathogenesis of mycotic aneurysms can be divided into four major categories, although other less common causes also exist (31). First, septic emboli from bacterial endocarditis may lodge in normal arteries, causing infection that weakens the arterial wall, resulting in aneurysm formation. These lesions are often multiple. Second, during an episode of bacteremia, microorganisms may lodge in a preexisting atherosclerotic plaque or aneurysm and begin to multiply with the same result. A third cause of mycotic aneurysms is the contiguous spread of bacteria from a local abscess. The inflammatory process destroys the arterial wall, causing bleeding and pseudoaneurysm formation. Finally, trauma to the artery with concomitant contamination may result in formation of an infected pseudoaneurysm. This mechanism of mycotic aneurysm formation is being seen more frequently coincident with the increased use of catheter-based invasive diagnostic and therapeutic procedures. Bacteria may be introduced concomitantly with needle puncture or by migration during prolonged arterial catheterization. Mycotic aneurysms accompanying drug abuse may be secondary to direct contamination of the arterial wall, or it may result from destruction of the vessel wall by a local abscess.

The bacteriology of arterial infections depends on the cause of the lesion. Aneurysms secondary to bacterial endocarditis grew *Pneumococcus, Streptococcus,* and *Enterococcus* species, most frequently in the past; more recently, staphylococci, *Salmonella, Escherichia coli,* and *Proteus* organisms also have been cultured (32). *Staphylococcus aureus* is the most common pathogen in mycotic femoral artery aneurysms secondary to trauma and drug abuse, occurring in more than 65% of cases (33). In this population, about 50% of the *S. aureus* organisms are resistant to methicillin. Polymicrobial groin infections are also common in this group of patients.

Clinical Manifestations

The typical patient with a mycotic femoral aneurysm has a history of chills and fever and a tender, enlarging, pulsatile groin mass. The patient may have a history of intravenous drug use, recent penetrating trauma, or bacterial endocarditis. Local signs of infection, including tenderness, erythema, and warmth, are noted on physical examination. Lower-extremity edema may occur secondary to venous obstruction. Petechial skin lesions, splinter hemorrhages, cutaneous abscesses, and septic arthritis may occur as a result of emboli originating from a mycotic aneurysm. A "sentinel bleed" may occur and signals impending rupture and life-threatening hemorrhage. Emergency surgery is indicated.

Diagnosis

The diagnosis of a mycotic aneurysm is usually straightforward, but distinguishing an abscess adjacent to the femoral artery from a femoral mycotic aneurysm may be difficult. In the patient with a pulsatile groin mass, laboratory findings, including a leukocytosis, elevated erythrocyte sedimentation rate, and positive blood cultures, are suggestive but not specific for a mycotic aneurysm. Multiple blood cultures or downstream arterial blood cultures may be necessary to yield positive results. Ultrasonography, CT, and MRI are helpful in establishing the diagnosis of an aneurysm (Fig. 89.3), but these tests lack precision in distinguishing infected from bland aneurysms. Arteriography delineates the proximal and distal arterial anatomy necessary to plan the operative procedure. The diagnosis of a mycotic aneurysm is confirmed at operation by the demonstration of organisms on Gram's stain or by positive cultures of the aneurysm wall.

Treatment

Mycotic aneurysms represent a serious life- and limb-threatening disease because their natural history is one of expansion and rupture. Therefore, all mycotic aneurysms should be addressed surgically. The goal of treatment is eradication of the infection by excision of the aneurysm and débridement of adjacent infected tissue as well as by long-term antibiotic therapy. Second, adequate distal circulation must be restored. Before operative intervention is performed, the patient is started on antibiotics, which are modified based on sensitivity testing of intraoperative cultures. Antibiotics are continued for 6 weeks postoperatively.

The complexity of the operative procedure varies with the location and extent of the mycotic aneurysm. Although a direct approach to the femoral artery may be taken, a retroperitoneal exposure of the distal external iliac artery is sometimes preferred for large or proximal femoral lesions to avoid excessive hemorrhage. When an infected femoral artery aneurysm is confined to only one arterial segment (common, superficial, or deep femoral artery), the aneurysm is excised and the proximal and dis-

tal artery is ligated. In these cases, where an isolated arterial segment is ligated, severe ischemia resulting in amputation is unusual. In more than 50% of cases, however, the mycotic aneurysm involves the femoral artery bifurcation, and treatment requires resection of the femoral bifurcation and débridement to healthy arterial wall. The distal external iliac or proximal common femoral artery as well as the superficial and deep femoral arteries are oversewn with nonabsorbable monofilament suture. This results in significant ischemia in most patients, but, with the patient heparinized, symptoms gradually improve as collateral circulation increases. Unfortunately, approximately one third of such patients have severe ischemia that necessitates amputation if the limb is not revascularized (33). In patients in whom sepsis can be adequately controlled at the initial procedure, aggressive débridement may be followed by immediate revascularization. Autogenous saphenous vein graft is used as conduit from the common femoral artery at the inguinal ligament to the superficial femoral artery distal to the septic process, and the graft is covered with a sartorius muscle flap (33). Using this revascularization approach, an 11% amputation rate and no mortality in 54 infected pseudoaneurysms resulting from drug abuse was reported (33). Another option is to observe patients for 24 hours after arterial ligation and selectively revascularize those patients in whom limb-threatening ischemia persists. The saphenous vein graft is tunneled through uninfected tissue planes using the lateral femoral or obturator route. Use of prosthetic material is avoided because of the high incidence of early and late septic complications. Antibiotics are begun preoperatively and continued for 6 weeks postoperatively.

POPLITEAL ARTERY ANEURYSMS

Popliteal aneurysms are limb-threatening lesions, the vast majority of which are degenerative or atherosclerotic in cause. Occasionally, anastomotic or traumatic popliteal aneurysms, and rarely mycotic aneurysms, are encountered in contemporary clinical practice. Therefore, the remainder of this section addresses only degenerative popliteal aneurysms.

Incidence

Popliteal artery aneurysms are the most common degenerative peripheral aneurysm. They occur slightly more frequently than femoral artery lesions; however, popliteal aneurysms are relatively unusual compared with abdominal aortic aneurysms. In recent reports, aortic aneurysms are diagnosed with about 10 times the frequency of popliteal aneurysms (2,3).

Pattern of Disease

Like patients with femoral artery aneurysms, multiple aneurysms occur frequently in patients with popliteal aneurysms. About 60% to 70% of patients have bilateral popliteal aneurysms, and 55% have extrapopliteal aneurysms (34,35). Abdominal aortic aneurysms are encountered in 40% to 50% and are particularly common in patients with bilateral popliteal aneurysms, of whom about 70% have aortic aneurysms (34–36). Femoral artery aneurysms are found in nearly 40% of patients (35,36). The importance of this multiplicity of aneurysms is that they may be missed on physical examination. Therefore, their presence must be determined by other studies, such as ultrasonography or CT, so that potentially life-threatening abdominal aortic aneurysms and other limb-threatening lesions are identified and managed appropriately.

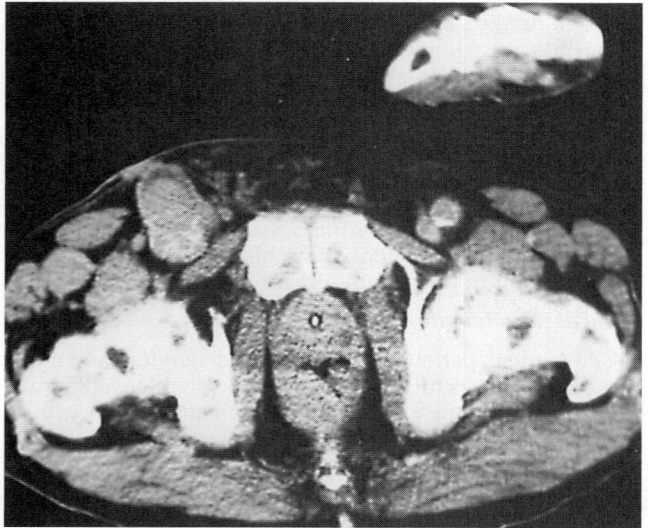

Figure 89.3. Computed tomography scan of a right infected femoral anastomotic aneurysm that was diagnosed 5 years after aortofemoral graft placement.

Clinical Manifestations

The typical patient with a popliteal aneurysm is a man in his 60s or 70s who has the usual risk factors for atherosclerosis. These aneurysms occur almost exclusively in men. Of patients with popliteal aneurysms, 50% to 75% are smokers, 40% to 60% have hypertension, and about 15% have diabetes mellitus (34–37). Other manifestations of cardiovascular disease are also common, with 10% of patients having manifestations of cerebrovascular disease and more than 40% having evidence of significant cardiac disease (34).

The clinical manifestations of popliteal artery aneurysms range from an asymptomatic pulsatile mass to severe lower-extremity ischemia. About 40% patients are asymptomatic at diagnosis (5). More than 50% of patients present with symptoms of limb ischemia, usually claudication, but the ischemia may be more advanced and manifested as rest pain or gangrene. Local symptoms, including sensation of a mass, local pain, and leg swelling or phlebitis secondary to compression of the adjacent vein, account for the remainder of symptoms.

A popliteal artery aneurysm may be complicated by thrombosis, embolization, or rupture. Thrombosis is reported in about 40% of patients (35), and embolization occurs in about 25% of cases (35). Some patients present with classic "blue toe syndrome"; more commonly, repeated episodes of embolization occlude the outflow vessels and result in thrombosis of the aneurysm. Thus, thrombosis may be the end result of embolization from a popliteal aneurysm. Rupture occurs in fewer than 5% of popliteal aneurysms (34,35); in these cases, the hemorrhage usually is confined to the popliteal space, thus permitting surgical intervention and arterial reconstruction.

Natural History

The natural history of popliteal aneurysms is not well defined because most series are composed primarily of aneurysms that have been treated surgically. In a review of 29 reports in the English literature published between 1980 and 1994, subgroups of patients were identified whose aneurysms had been observed (5). A mean of 35% of patients with conservative follow-up developed ischemic complications, and 25% of these required amputation even with modern therapy. Thus, a significant percentage of popliteal aneurysms will develop a complication if left untreated, and, although this is not synonymous with limb loss, the amputation rate is high.

Diagnosis

The diagnosis of popliteal aneurysm is usually first suspected on physical examination. Palpation of the popliteal space with the knee flexed reveals a pulsatile mass in approximately two thirds of patients. Small aneurysms may not be palpable on physical examination, and, if thrombosis has occurred, the mass may be nonpulsatile. Radiographs of the knee demonstrating a calcified arterial wall occasionally suggest the diagnosis of a popliteal artery aneurysm, but this diagnosis must be confirmed by ultrasonography, CT, or MRI. These diagnostic modalities can establish the diagnosis of popliteal artery aneurysms and exclude other entities that could be responsible for a nonpulsatile popliteal fossa mass (tumor or Baker's cyst). Ultrasonography, CT, or MRI is also useful in the detection of associated aneurysms, particularly abdominal aortic and femoral artery aneurysms. Angiography can be misleading in the diagnosis of aneurysms because intraluminal thrombus may obscure the true size of the vessel, but angiography is essential to define the distal vasculature before operative repair is attempted (Fig. 89.4).

Treatment

Indications

Surgical treatment is indicated for all symptomatic or complicated aneurysms. Controversy exists regarding the optimal management of small asymptomatic popliteal aneurysms because the natural history is not well defined. Because of the high incidence of complications with popliteal artery aneurysms, the lack of correlation between the size of the aneurysm and the occurrence of complications as well as the higher rate of limb loss after complications develop, many surgeons recommend operative treatment when a popliteal aneurysm is diagnosed unless the patient is an inordinately high operative risk.

Conservative management is recommended by some physicians because the life expectancy of patients with popliteal aneurysms is lower than the normal age-matched population, and combining thrombolytic therapy with bypass grafting has improved outcome in patients who have an acutely thrombosed popliteal aneurysm and a severely ischemic extremity. The use of a modeling system suggested that improved results are seen with elective surgery compared with conservative management at 1 to 2 years after presentation (38). Thus, when the patient's life expectancy is severely compromised by another disease, conservative therapy is appropriate; but patients with a life expectancy of greater than 2 years benefit from operative treatment.

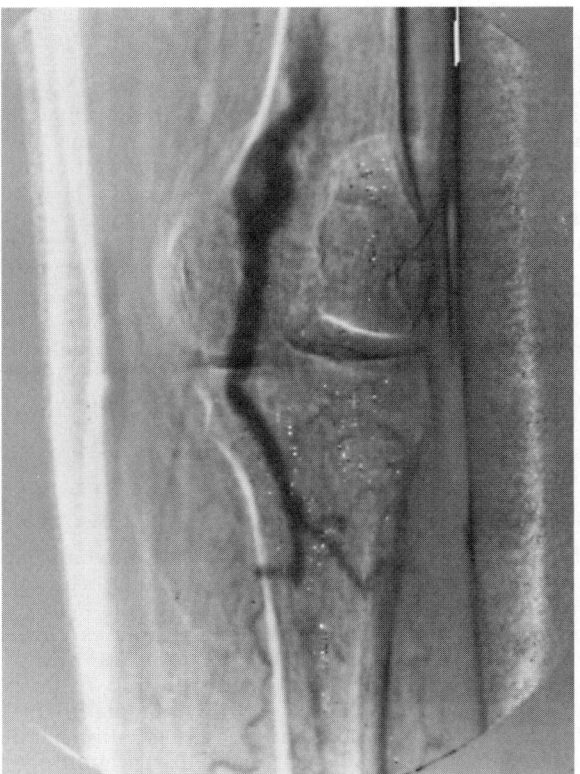

Figure 89.4. Arteriogram demonstrating a popliteal aneurysm associated with occlusion of the outflow tract, presumably from repeated episodes of embolization. A bypass to the distal posterior tibial artery was successful.

The goals of surgical treatment are to eliminate the potential for complications and to preserve or restore adequate blood flow to the limb. In patients with multiple aneurysms, the operative approach must be individualized. Generally, the life-threatening aortic aneurysm is treated first, followed by repair of the popliteal aneurysm. On the other hand, if a limb-threatening complication has occurred, treatment of the popliteal aneurysm usually takes precedence, followed by expeditious aortic aneurysm repair.

Surgical Technique

Most popliteal aneurysms can be approached easily through standard medial thigh and calf incisions for exposure of the distal superficial femoral artery and the distal popliteal artery, respectively. Occasionally, the posterior approach is preferred for lesions confined to the popliteal fossa. Most aneurysms are left in situ, bypassed using a segment of saphenous vein, and then ligated. The conduit of choice is autologous saphenous vein, which is harvested from the thigh, reversed, and tunneled along the course of popliteal artery. The proximal and distal anastomosis may be either end-to-end or end-to-side in configuration, with the aneurysm excluded from the circulation by proximal and distal ligatures. Late expansion and rupture of a bypassed and ligated popliteal aneurysm, however, can occur secondary to continued perfusion of the aneurysm through patent geniculates. When the distal popliteal and proximal tibial vessels are occluded with recent emboli, they sometimes can be cleared by using a balloon catheter or intraoperative thrombolytic therapy. Frequently, bypass grafts must be carried to the distal tibial arteries. Extensive femoral and popliteal aneurysms may require a femoral–popliteal or femoral–tibial bypass using an in situ saphenous vein, which originates from a prosthetic graft replacing a common femoral artery aneurysm. Popliteal aneurysms have been treated by an endovascular approach using saphenous vein and stents, but large series with long-term follow-up are not yet available.

The patient who presents with an acutely ischemic extremity secondary to popliteal aneurysm thrombosis is a management challenge. Popliteal aneurysms often thrombose because of repeated episodes of emboli to the outflow vessels, which results in their occlusion. An expeditious arteriogram may identify a suitable outflow vessel for the bypass graft. If no target vessel is identified, intraarterial thrombolytic therapy should be initiated with the goal of lysing thrombus in the tibial arteries to identify a suitable outflow vessel for vascular reconstruction. Although the embolic process may be chronic, results with thrombolytic therapy followed by bypass of the aneurysm have been much better that surgical therapy alone for the patient with an acutely occluded aneurysm and severe leg ischemia.

Results

Excellent results are obtained in asymptomatic aneurysms with intact distal vasculature. Patients with thrombosed aneurysms or those in whom multiple episodes of embolization have occluded the tibial arteries have less optimal results. Operative mortality is in the 0% to 2% range, with asymptomatic patients fairing better than those presenting with acutely symptomatic lesions (39,40). In patients undergoing revascularization before ischemic complications occur, 5- and 10-year graft patency rates are greater that 80%, and limb salvage is 93% to 98% (34,41). Graft patency rates in patients operated on after complications of their aneurysms are 60% and 48% at 5 and 10 years, respectively, and limb salvage rates are 60% to 80% (34,41,42).

REFERENCES

1. Dent TL, Lindenauer SM, Ernst CB, et al. Multiple arteriosclerotic artery aneurysms. *Arch Surg* 1972;105:338–344.
2. Szilagyi DE, Schwartz RL, Reddy DJ. Popliteal arterial aneurysms: their natural history and management. *Arch Surg* 1981;116:723–728.
3. Ramesh S, Michaels JA, Galland RB. Popliteal aneurysm: morphology and management. *Br J Surg* 1993;80:1531–1533.
4. Graham LM, Zelenock GB, Whitehouse WM Jr, et al. Clinical significance of arteriosclerotic femoral artery aneurysms. *Arch Surg* 1980;115:502–507.
5. Dawson I, Sie RB, Van Bockel JH. Atherosclerotic popliteal aneurysm. *Br J Surg* 1997;84:293–299.
6. Katz DJ, Stanley JC, Zelenock GB. Gender differences in abdominal aortic aneurysm prevalence, treatment, and outcome. *J Vasc Surg* 1997;25:561–568.
7. Brophy CM, Tilson JE, Braverman IM, et al. Age of onset, pattern of distribution, and histology of aneurysm development in a genetically predisposed mouse model. *J Vasc Surg* 1988;8:45–48.
8. Faggioli GL, Gargiulo M, Bertoni F, et al. Parietal inflammatory infiltrate in peripheral aneurysms of atherosclerotic origin. *J Cardiovasc Surg* 1992;33:331–336.
9. McMillan WD, Pearce WH. Increased plasma levels of metalloproteinase-9 are associated with abdominal aortic aneurysms. *J Vasc Surg* 1999;29:122–127.
10. Allaire E, Forough R, Clowes W, et al. Local overexpression of TIMP-1 prevents aortic aneurysm degeneration and rupture in a rat model. *J Clin Invest* 1998;102:1413–1420.
11. Thompson RW, Liao SX, Curci JA. Vascular smooth muscle cell apoptosis in abdominal aortic aneurysms. *Coron Artery Dis* 1997;8:623–631.
12. Cutler BS, Darling RC. Surgical management of arteriosclerotic femoral aneurysms. *Surgery* 1973;74:764–773.
13. Muller-Hulsbeck S, Link J, Schwarzenberg H, et al. Percutaneous endoluminal stent and stent-graft placement for the treatment of femoropopliteal aneurysms: early experiences. *Cardiovasc Intervent Radiol* 1999;22:96–102.
14. Henry M, Amor M, Cragg A, et al. Occlusive and aneurysmal peripheral arterial disease: assessment of a stent-graft system. *Radiology* 1996;201:717–724.
15. Szilagyi DE, Smith RF, Elliott JP, et al. Anastomotic aneurysms after vascular reconstruction: problems of incidence, etiology, and treatment. *Surgery* 1975;78:800–816.
16. Szilagyi DE, Elliott JP Jr, Smith RF, et al. A thirty-year survey of the reconstructive surgical treatment of aortoiliac occlusive disease. *J Vasc Surg* 1986;3:421–436.
17. Dennis JW, Littooy FN, Greisler HP, et al. Anastomotic pseudoaneurysms: a continuing late complication of vascular reconstructive procedures. *Arch Surg* 1986;121:314–317.
18. Seabrook GR, Schmitt DD, Bandyk DF, et al. Anastomotic femoral pseudoaneurysm: an investigation of occult infection as an etiologic factor. *J Vasc Surg* 1990;11:629–634.
19. Babu SC, Piccorelli GO, Shah PM, et al. Incidence and results of arterial complications among 16,350 patients undergoing cardiac catheterization. *J Vasc Surg* 1989;10:113–116.
20. Messina LM, Brothers TE, Wakefield TW, et al. Clinical characteristics and surgical management of vascular complications in patients undergoing cardiac catheterization: interventional versus diagnostic procedures. *J Vasc Surg* 1991;13:593–600.
21. Kresowik TF, Khoury MD, Miller BV, et al. A prospective study of the incidence and natural history of femoral vascular complications after percutaneous transluminal coronary angioplasty. *J Vasc Surg* 1991;13:328–335.
22. Kent KC, McArdle CR, Kennedy B, et al. A prospective study of the clinical outcome of femoral pseudoaneurysms and arteriovenous fistulas induced by arterial puncture. *J Vasc Surg* 1993;17:125–133.
23. Kang SS, Labropoulos N, Mansour MA, et al. Percutaneous ultrasound guided thrombin injection: a new method for treating postcatheterization femoral pseudoaneurysms. *J Vasc Surg* 1998;27:1032–1038.
24. Wixon CL, Philpott JM, Bogey WM Jr, et al. Duplex-directed thrombin injection as a method to treat femoral artery pseudoaneurysms. *J Am Coll Surg* 1999;187:464–466.
25. Cox GS, Young JR, Gray BR, et al. Ultrasound-guided com-

pression repair of postcatheterization pseudoaneurysms: results of treatment in one hundred cases. *J Vasc Surg* 1994; 19:683–686.

26. Liau CS, Ho FM, Chen MF, et al. Treatment of iatrogenic femoral artery pseudoaneurysm with percutaneous thrombin injection. *J Vasc Surg* 1997;26:18–23.

27. Lennox A, Griffin M, Nicolaides A, et al. Regarding "Percutaneous ultrasound guided thrombin injection: a new method for treating postcatheterization femoral pseudoaneurysms." *J Vasc Surg* 1998;28:1120–1121.

28. Kang SS. Regarding "Percutaneous ultrasound guided thrombin injection: a new method for treating postcathe-terization femoral pseudoaneurysms"[Reply]. *J Vasc Surg* 1998;28:1121.

29. Kumins NH, Landau DS, Montalvo J, et al. Expanded indications for the treatment of postcatheterization femoral pseudoaneurysms with ultrasound-guided compression. *Am J Surg* 1998;176:131–136.

30. Hertz SM, Brener BJ. Ultrasound-guided pseudoaneurysm compression: efficacy after coronary stenting and angioplasty. *J Vasc Surg* 1997;26:913–916.

31. Anderson CB, Butcher HR Jr, Ballinger WF. Mycotic aneurysms. *Arch Surg* 1974;109:712–717.

32. Brown SL, Busuttil RW, Baker JD, et al. Bacteriologic and surgical determinants of survival in patients with mycotic aneurysms. *J Vasc Surg* 1984;1:541–547.

33. Reddy DJ, Smith RF, Elliott JP, et al. Infected femoral artery false aneurysms in drug addicts: evolution of selective vascular reconstruction. *J Vasc Surg* 1986;3:718–724.

34. Anton GE, Hertzer NR, Beven EG, et al. Surgical management of popliteal aneurysms: trends in presentation, treatment, and results from 1952 to 1984. *J Vasc Surg* 1986;3:125–134.

35. Vermilion BD, Kimmins SA, Pace WG, et al. A review of one hundred forty-seven popliteal aneurysms with long-term follow-up. *Surgery* 1981;90:1009–1014.

36. Whitehouse WM Jr, Wakefield TW, Graham LM, et al. Limb-threatening potential of arteriosclerotic popliteal artery aneurysms. *Surgery* 1983;93:694–699.

37. Lowell RC, Gloviczki P, Hallett JW Jr, et al. Popliteal artery aneurysms: the risk of nonoperative management. *Ann Vasc Surg* 1994;8:14–23.

38. Michaels JA, Galland RB. Management of asymptomatic popliteal aneurysms: the use of a Markov decision tree to determine the criteria for a conservative approach. *Eur J Vasc Surg* 1993;7:136–143.

39. Varga ZA, Locke-Edmunds JC, Baird RN. Joint Vascular Research Group. A multicenter study of popliteal aneurysms. *J Vasc Surg* 1994;20:171–177.

40. Reilly MK, Abbott WM, Darling RC. Aggressive surgical management of popliteal artery aneurysms. *Am J Surg* 1983;145:498–502.

41. Roggo A, Brunner U, Ottinger LW, et al. The continuing challenge of aneurysms of the popliteal artery. *Surg Gynecol Obstet* 1993;177:565–572.

42. Dawson I, Van Bockel JH, Brand R, et al. Popliteal artery aneurysms: long-term follow-up of aneurysmal disease and results of surgical treatment. *J Vasc Surg* 1991;13:398–407.

SURGERY: SCIENTIFIC PRINCIPLES AND PRACTICE, Third Edition, edited by Lazar J. Greenfield, Michael W. Mulholland, Keith T. Oldham, Gerald B. Zelenock, and Keith D. Lillemoe. Lippincott Williams & Wilkins Publishers, Philadelphia, © 2001.

CHAPTER 90

VASCULAR MALFORMATION AND ARTERIOVENOUS FISTULA

KARTHIKESHWAR KASIRAJAN AND KENNETH OURIEL

Arteriovenous malformation (AVM) may present as isolated, innocuous cutaneous nevi or, rarely, may take the form of life-threatening systemic shunts involving large portions of the body (Fig. 90.1). Vascular malformations and congenital fistulae have stimulated intellectual curiosity and tested clinical ingenuity for more than 200 years. The surgical literature is biased toward cases presenting for surgical evaluation and treatment, predominantly those with significant arteriovenous shunting. As a result of the rarity of the problem, a standard approach to management of these lesions does not exist, and treatment is often based on individual experience. In one of the largest reports of congenital AVMs, only 82 cases were accumulated over a 20-year period at a referral center known for its special interest in AVM (1).

Arteriovenous malformation is defined as an abnormal communication between an artery and vein that bypasses the capillary bed. It may occur at any site, involve any organ, and violate normal tissue planes. The emphasis of this chapter is on the clinical manifestations, diagnosis, and treatment of congenital AVMs of the extremities.

HISTORICAL ASPECTS

The first description of an arteriovenous malformation was by an Italian physician, Leale Leali in 1707 (2).

William Hunter, 40 years later, described the clinical syndrome produced by an acquired arteriovenous fistula (AVF) (3). George Bushe published the first report of a congenital AVM in the 1827–1828 issue of *Lancet* (4), describing a "pulsating tumor of the temple" present since birth. Sir Prescott Hewitt, in 1867, described the first congenital AVM involving an extremity (5). Hewitt's patient

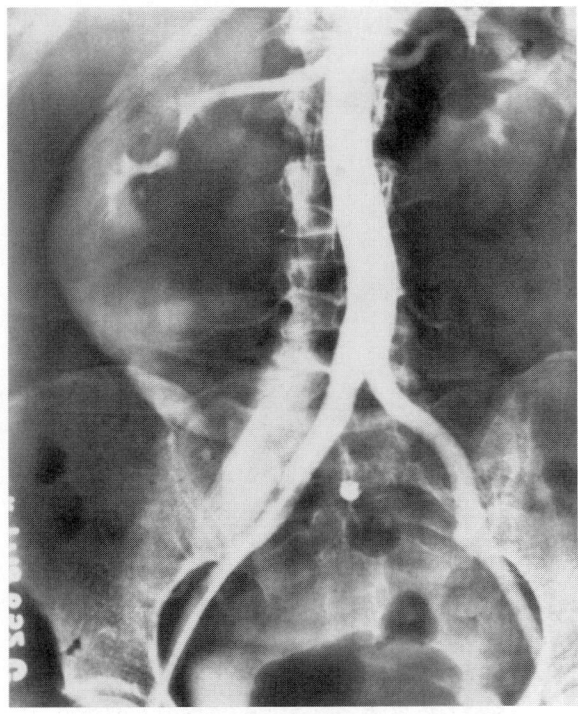

Figure 90.1. Angiogram demonstrating a large communication between the right common iliac artery and vein; hemodynamic collapse required prompt correction of this arteriovenous communication.

was a 17-year-old woman with symptoms of "heating" and enlargement of the right thigh since birth. Physical exam revealed a palpable thrill over the thigh extending to the inguinal ligament, superficial varicosities and a systolic murmur at the apex of the heart. Although no anatomic description of an AVM was made, the presentation suggests that this probably was the first description of a congenital AVM. Two decades later, William S. Halsted presented at the 1889 annual meeting of the American Surgical Association the first collective review of congenital AVMs (6).

INCIDENCE

The prevalence of congenital AVMs is unknown. A difference in nomenclature and the lack of an accepted classification confound the collective analysis of cases. It also must be noted that reports on this topic have become widely scattered throughout journals of dermatology, pediatrics, interventional radiology, plastic surgery, vascular medicine, as well as general and vascular surgery. Congenital AVMs account for only 1:10,000 hospital admissions. This rate likely represents an underestimate of the true prevalence; Tasnadi, looking specifically for AVMs, found a 1.2% prevalence of congenital AVM on examination of 3,573 3-year-old children (7). In a review of 21 cases of vascular anomalies of the extremities, Cotton and Sykes reported a 3:1 female to male sex predilection (8). One half of all congenital AVMs occur in the extremities (Fig. 90.2), and two thirds of these occur in the lower limb (9).

CLASSIFICATION AND EMBRYOLOGIC DEVELOPMENT

Few surgical diseases have generated more diverse terminology and methods of classification than have congenital AVMs. To add to the confusion regarding the origin of these lesions, several findings and anatomic presentations have been labeled as *syndromes* identified by an eponym appropriate to the author responsible for the original description. For example, the presence of multiple congenital enchondromatosis is referred to as *Ollier's disease;* the same disease is referred to as *Maffucci's syndrome* when vascular malformations coexist.

All congenital arterial or venous malformations may be considered variations of a single embryonic developmental anomaly. In this regard, a description of the embryologic development of the vascular system provides insight into how these anomalies and their various combinations might occur. The embryologic development of the peripheral vasculature is divided into three stages: (a) capillary network stage, (b) retiform stage, and (3) stage of mature vascular stem units. In the early embryo, the vascular system consists of a diffuse network of blood spaces in the mesenchyme, spaces that subsequently coalesce into a primitive capillary network. There is no differentiation of the vessels in the capillary network stage. Developmental arrest at this stage results in a capillary hemangioma (Fig. 90.3) (1). In the second *(retiform)* stage, the primitive capillary networks coalesce into large plexiform structures that appear to be separate from each other. The collateral system is established during this stage, especially in the extremities, and different regions develop their own autonomous microcirculation. Hence, arrest during the reti-

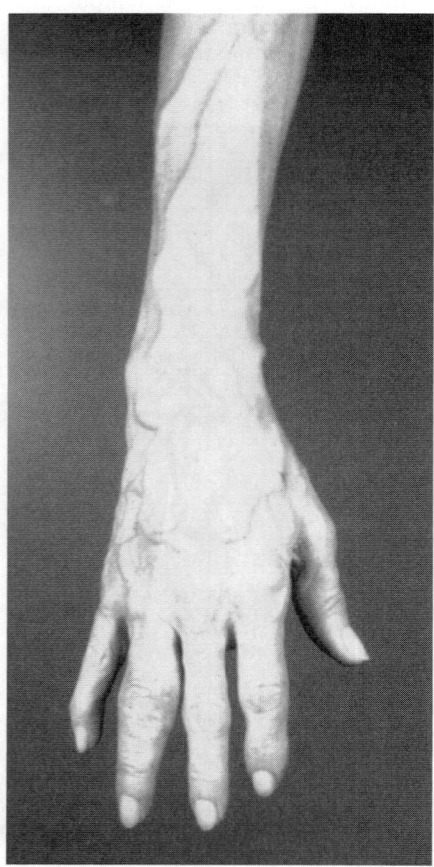

Figure 90.2. Congenital arteriovenous fistula of the fourth digit. Note the hypertrophied digit and the presence of dilated venous tributaries.

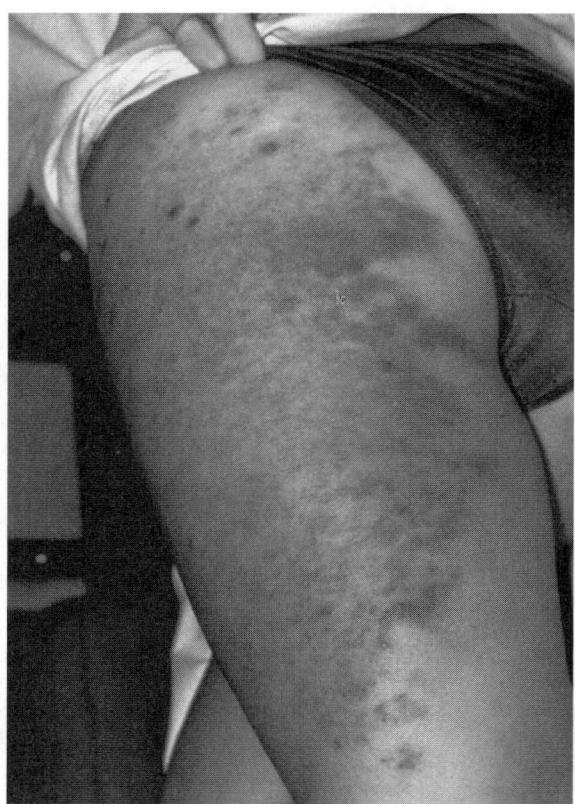

Figure 90.3. Large capillary hemangioma seen on the lateral aspect of the thigh appearing as bright red, slightly elevated, noncompressible plaques.

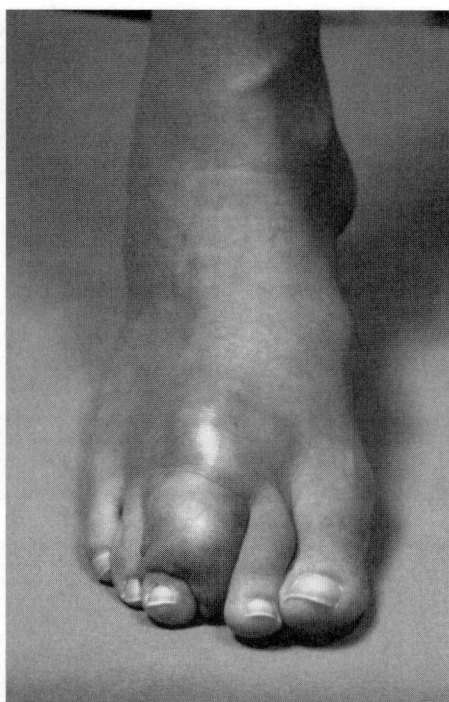

Figure 90.4. Cavernous hemangioma of the third toe appearing as compressible bluish, soft masses.

form stage results in direct communication between the arterial and venous channels; the maturity of the communicating channels is determined by the degree of differentiation attained to this point.

Microfistulous communication is a term used to describe the more immature arteriovenous communications that are presumed to be present but cannot be demonstrated angiographically. The more mature macrofistulous communication would differ from the microfistulous variety only in the ability to discern the communications angiographically because of the large size of the channels. The third stage of vascular development is characterized by large vessels that proliferate from the great vessels and communicate with the preexisting retiform plexuses. Failure of any of these systems to evolve or involute results in faulty or excessive development of one or more elements of the vascular system. Depending on the specific defect, the abnormality may present as nests of capillaries *(port-wine stain)*, dilated veins *(cavernous hemangioma)* (Fig. 90.4), or arteries *(circoid aneurysm)*, persistent arteriovenous connections from the retiform stage, lymphatic nests *(cystic hygroma)* or a combination of any of these. This method of classification is useful because it provides a method for describing all AVMs according to their level of

Table 90.1. CLASSIFICATION OF ARTERIOVENOUS MALFORMATIONS

1. Capillary malformations (strawberry nevus, port-wine stains, telangiectasia)
2. Venous malformations (cavernous hemangiomas)
3. Lymphatic malformations (cystic hygroma, lymphangioma)
4. Arterial malformations (circoid aneurysm)
5. Malformations with arteriovenous communication
   A. Congenital (microfistulous or macrofistulous communication)
   B. Acquired (traumatic, iatrogenic, and spontaneous)

Table 90.2. SYNDROMES WITH ASSOCIATED ARTERIOVENOUS MALFORMATIONS

Hippel-Lindau disease (cerebelloretinal hemangioblastomatosis)
Klippel-Trenaunay syndrome (nevus, varicose veins, limb hypertrophy)
Kasabach-Merritt syndrome (platelet consumption, kaposiform hemangioendothelioma, or tufted angiomas)
Parkes-Weber syndrome (KTS, microfistulous arteriovenous communications)
Maffucci's syndrome (cavernous hemangioma, dyschondroplasia, osteochondromas)
Sturge-Weber syndrome (encephalotrigeminal hemangiomatosis)
Servelle-Martorell syndrome (cavernous hemangioma, limb hypotrophy)
Rendu-Osler-Weber syndrome (hereditary hemorrhagic telangiectasia)
Louis-Bar syndrome (Ataxia telangiectasia)
Riley-Smith syndrome (macrocephaly, pseudopapilledema, lymphaticovenous malformation)

KTS, Klippel-Trenaunay syndrome.

embroyologic differentiation (Table 90.1). Unfortunately, many AVMs will contain multiple levels of embryonic differentiation; in these cases, the most predominant cell type determines the classification. As in all congenital and developmental anomalies, associated malformations of other organ systems may be present; these are often grouped into syndromes (Table 90.2). Few AVMs enlarge over time; unlike malignant tumors, AVMs are lined by mature endothelial cells, which do not proliferate to a greater extent than normal cells. Enlargement occurs as a result of blood flowing through "paths of least resistance," and the voluminous blood flow accounts for the progressive dilatation of the preexisting channels.

The final classification of AVM comprises acquired fistulae, the most common type encountered by the surgeon. These may occur secondary to trauma, either penetrating (Fig. 90.5A,B) or blunt. Blunt trauma may produce an AVF by the vascular injury that results from penetration by bone spicules into adjacent vessels. The most common acquired AVM encountered by the vascular surgeon is an AVF between the femoral artery and vein that has resulted from iatrogenic trauma to these vessels during catheterization procedures. Some of these fistulae resolve spontaneously (10). Those associated with pseudoaneurysms can be managed with thrombin injection, and only rarely is operative intervention required (10). Of course, AVF also may be created intentionally, such as a radiocephalic fistula for dialysis access or an AVF created at the distal anastamosis of leg bypass procedures to improve graft patency. Acquired fistulae will not be further discussed in this chapter.

PHYSIOLOGIC CHANGES RESULTING FROM ARTERIOVENOUS MALFORMATIONS

A variety of local and systemic hemodynamic changes can occur because of the presence of AVMs. The most important local effect is a distal "steal" phenomenon. Blood flows preferentially through paths of least resistance; hence, when a proximal communication exists between an artery and a vein, most of the arterial flow is directed through the fistula into the venous system. Depending on the size of the fistula, the blood flow in the artery distal to the fistula may be sluggish and, in certain cases, demonstrate reversal of flow during diastole. When increased blood flow to a tissue bed must be increased, the physiologic demand often cannot be matched because of the "stealing" of blood through the fistula. The end-organ ischemia resulting from the presence of the arteriovenous

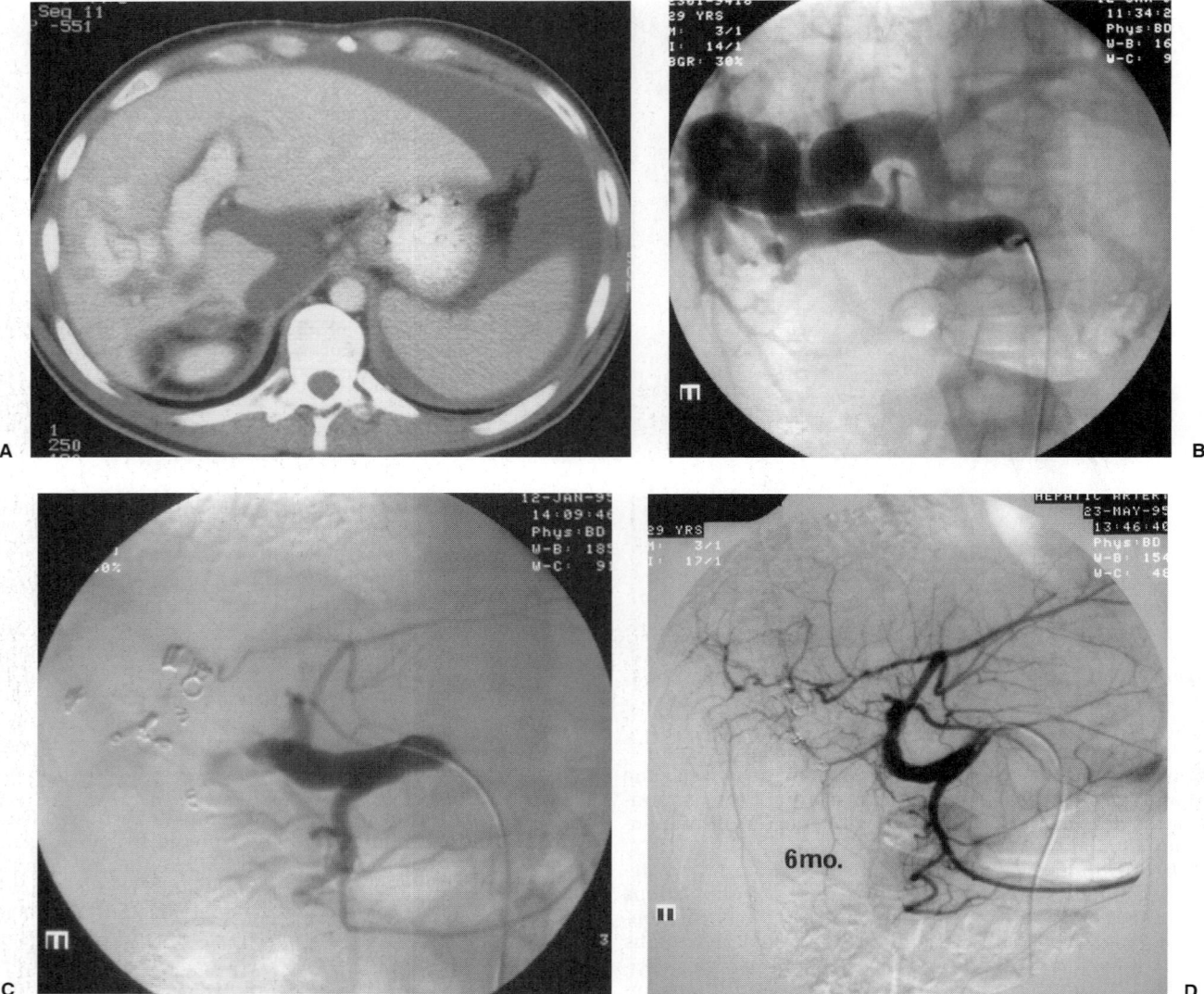

Figure 90.5. *(A)* Penetrating injury to the liver resulting in a large arteriovenous communication between the hepatic artery and the portal vein. *(B)* Selective hepatic angiogram shows rapid flow of blood from the hepatic artery to the portal vein. *(C)* Coil embolotherapy of the arteriovenous communication. *(D)* Six-month follow-up angiogram shows complete obliteration of the arteriovenous communication.

communication comprises the symptoms associated with the steal phenomenon. If flow through the fistula is large enough, the distal organ may suffer permanent ischemic changes, such as wasting or gangrene (Fig. 90.6).

The presence of a fistula causes a significant decrease in the peripheral vascular resistance as a result of blood bypassing the high-resistance capillary bed. This manifests clinically by the Nicoladoni-Branham sign or the bradycardia reflex. In this maneuver, the temporary occlusion of the fistula produces an acute increase in peripheral resistance, a redistribution of blood through the peripheral capillary bed, and an elevation in blood pressure. Stimulation of the aortic and carotid baroreceptors by the resultant hypertension causes a vagus-mediated bradycardia reflux, described by Nicoladoni in 1875 and subsequently by Harris Branham in 1890. As this is a parasympathetic mediated reflex, it can be abolished with the administration of atropine.

The presence of an arteriovenous communication and the resultant fall in systemic resistance *(total peripheral vascular resistance)* produces a hypotensive state. The juxtaglomerular apparatus of the kidney interprets this as a hypovolemic condition and activates the renin-angiotensin-aldosterone system, resulting in sodium and water retention and a dramatic increase in plasma volume. A marked urinary diuresis often is seen when the fistula is ligated or eliminated from the circulation.

Normal arterial pressure is maintained through the inverse relationship between cardiac output and peripheral vascular resistance, aptly described by reconsidering an analogue of Ohm's law:

$$\text{Cardiac output} = \frac{\text{Arterial pressure}}{\text{Total peripheral resistance}}$$

This simply implies that the long-term changes in peripheral resistance are compensated by opposite changes in cardiac output, maintaining near normal blood pressure. In a normal adult man, the cardiac output is 5 L/min, and the right atrial pressure is 0 mm Hg. In the presence of a large AVF, the venous return to the heart is greatly increased, causing an increase in the right atrial pressure and a resultant increase in cardiac output. There are lim-

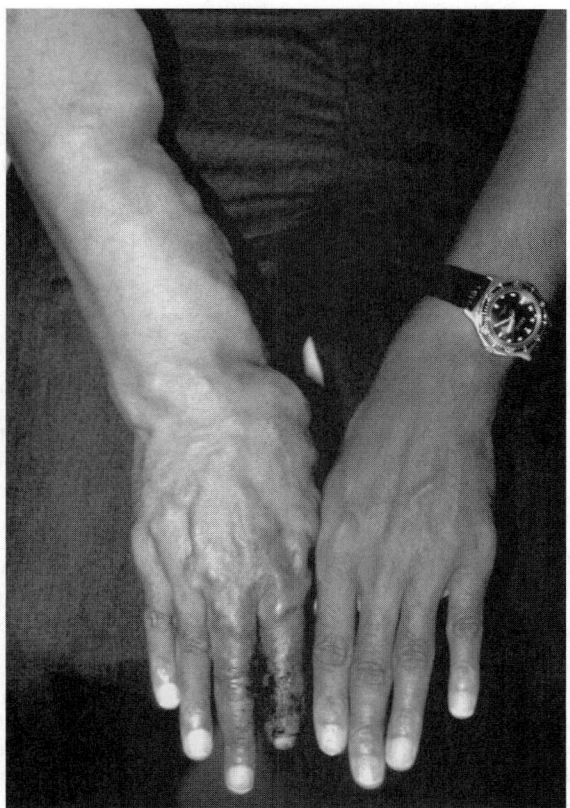

Figure 90.6. Congenital arteriovenous fistula of the upper extremity: gangrene of the index finger secondary to "steal phenomenon."

globe; hence all periocular hemangiomas need to be evaluated by an ophthalmologist. Subglotic hemangiomas may progress rapidly to respiratory failure in infants. The presence of multiple cutaneous hemangiomas are also markers of visceral hemangiomas.

The complications of hemangiomas are related to their size and location. Local complications include ulceration and hemorrhage. Ulceration needs to be treated promptly to prevent cellulitis and septicemia. Hemorrhage is rare and usually inconsequential, and the minimal blood loss that occasionally occurs can be controlled easily with direct pressure.

A rare complication of rapidly enlarging vascular lesions is a phenomenon called *Kasabach-Merritt syndrome*. Thrombocytopenic purpura, coagulopathy, and hemolytic anemia characterize this entity. The clinical manifestations of the Kasabach-Merritt syndrome were originally thought to be secondary to stagnant blood flow through the large tortuous vessels of the giant cavernous hemangiomatous channels, causing platelet trapping and disseminated intravascular coagulation. It is now clear that most patients with Kasabach-Merritt syndrome do not manifest typical hemangiomas but instead have kaposiform hemangioendothelioma or tufted angioma (12). This phenomenon is more common in neonates and rarely occurs in older persons. Thrombocytopenia, usually less than 10,000/ mm^3, is noted initially; in time, fibrinogen levels decrease and the prothrombin time (PT) and partial prothrombin time (PTT) become markedly prolonged. Despite aggressive treatment with multiple modalities, the syndrome still is associated with a high mortality rate.

The clinical presentation of AVMs depends on the size of the communicating channels. Localized microfistulous lesions are often completely asymptomatic. Large AVFs in

its to the ability of the heart to achieve this compensatory increase in cardiac output, however. The plateau level is about 13 L/min, roughly 2.5 times the normal cardiac output. During exercise, cardiac reserve is minimal, and (high-output) congestive heart failure can develop from excessive venous return into an overloaded ventricle.

CLINICAL SIGNS, SYMPTOMS, AND COMPLICATIONS

The clinical presentation of AVMs without demonstrable macroscopic arteriovenous communications is heterogeneous and depends on the type, depth, location, and stage of evolution. Most hemangiomas are completely asymptomatic. The superficial capillary hemangiomas appear as bright red, slightly elevated noncompressible plaques. The deeper hemangiomas are soft, warm masses with a slight bluish discoloration of the overlying skin. Classically, hemangiomas have an early proliferative phase followed by slow involution and, in most cases, complete resolution (11). Cavernous hemangiomas present as large, bluish masses that are easily compressible and slightly warm to the touch. Cavernous lymphagiomas may have the same clinical presentation as hemangiomas but are brilliantly transilluminated. Most hemangiomas, other than causing a cosmetic disfigurement, are rarely of clinical importance. Nevertheless, location plays a crucial role in determining the clinical manifestations of hemangiomas. For example, hemangiomas occurring in the periorbital region may obstruct the visual axis and result in amblyopia. Astigmatism may be caused by retrobular extension of the hemangioma, causing compression of the

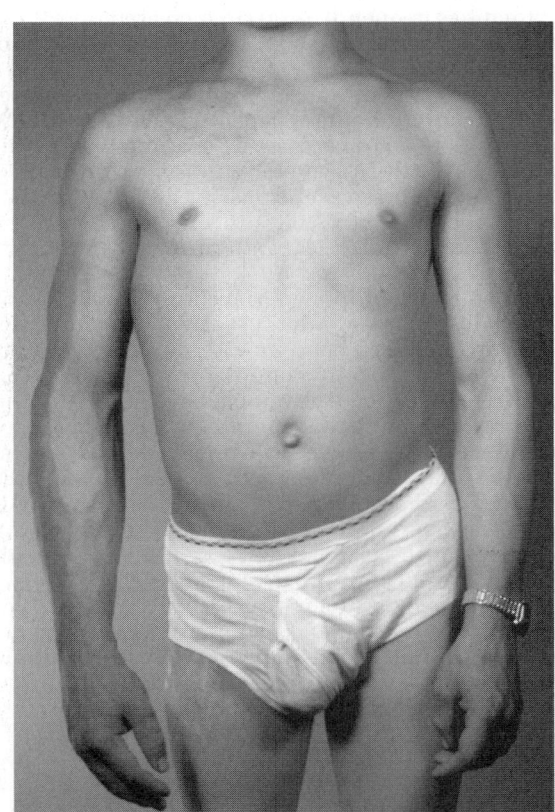

Figure 90.7. Congenital microfistulous arteriovenous communication resulting in limb hypertrophy and varicose veins.

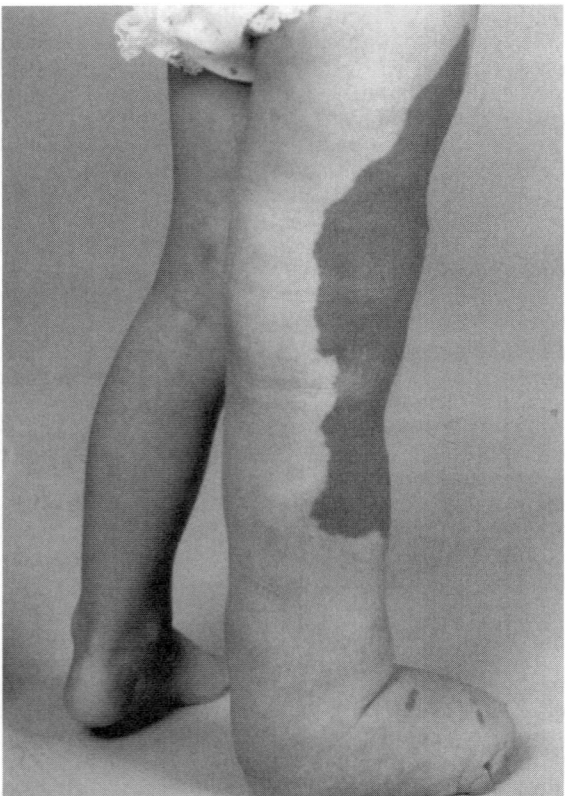

Figure 90.8. Klippel-Trenaunay syndrome. Note the large nevus and massive limb hypertrophy.

the extremities frequently result in increased flow through the venous system, with secondary varicose veins running proximally along the limb (Fig. 90.7). A palpable thrill and bruit are often present in large fistulae. The distal arterial blood flow may be limited, depending on the size of the fistula shunt, which may present as a diminished distal pulse, with or without symptoms of ischemia. Frank gangrene of the end-organ occasionally can be seen. The resultant venous hypertension also may result in brawny edema, stasis skin changes, and, ultimately, chronic venous ulcers.

When large or multiple arteriovenous communications affect an entire extremity during early life, before epiphyseal closure, increased bone growth and limb hypertrophy (Figs. 90.7 and 90.8) or hypotrophy may occur. The exact cause for limb hypertrophy remains unclear. Increased limb perfusion seems to be an unlikely cause because the flow is non-nutritive. Other theories, such as increased core temperature resulting from increased flow or associated spinal cord hemiangiomas in the region supplying the limb, have been proposed but remain unproved. Limb underdevelopment also may be seen in high-flow malformations as a result of destructive osseous changes. As previously described, in rare instances, the increased venous return to the heart combined with an increase in plasma volume may produce high-output congestive heart failure, an entity first reported by Silverman in 1955 (13).

DIAGNOSTIC EVALUATION

Most congenital AVMs are recognized easily on physical examination and do not warrant further investigation. In patients requiring therapy, however, diagnostic studies are

Table 90.3. DIAGNOSTIC GOALS IN ARTERIOVENOUS MALFORMATIONS (AVM)

Establish the presence and type of AVM
Determine the anatomic extent and involvement of adjacent structures
Identify associated congenital vascular anomalies (e.g., absent or aberrant vessels)
Quantify local and regional hemodynamic effects (e.g., steal syndrome, varicose veins)
Evaluate and quantify systemic hemodynamic effects

useful to determine the type and extent of the lesion (Table 90.3). The standard diagnostic tests used to evaluate chronic arterial and venous diseases can be applied to AVMs (Table 90.4). Noninvasive tests are performed initially; invasive tests are reserved for more complex problems for which intervention is contemplated.

Ultrasonography is a useful screening examination. It is highly operator dependent; but, when combined with color-flow imaging (duplex scan), it can be helpful to differentiate slow-flow anomalies, mainly venous and lymphatic types, from fast-flow, arterial anomalies. When the transducer sampling volume approaches the level of the AV fistula, the spectral pattern changes to one of higher peak systolic and end diastolic velocities with marked spectral broadening (14). Comparison with the normal contralateral limb will demonstrate a sharp contrast with the arterial signal at a corresponding level. Hemangiomas close to the skin are associated with pulsatile, multicolored flashes on the duplex scan that are synchronous with the arterial pulse. The major limitation of duplex ultrasound, however, is the limited delineation of the size of the lesion and its relation to adjacent structures. Segmental Doppler arterial pressure measurements are sometimes informative in the setting of AVMs. The study may reveal a sharp pressure drop at the level of the fistula that normalizes with manual compression of the fistula. Despite the objective information they yield, only qualitative information is obtained from noninvasive testing; the anatomic extent of the lesion is best defined by other tests.

Presently, magnetic resonance imaging (MRI) is the procedure of choice in the evaluation of AVM. Contrast-enhanced computed tomography (CT) was used before the advent of MRI to differentiate lymphatic and venous malformations (Fig. 90.5A). Today, MRI has largely replaced the CT scan, providing better definition of the anatomic extent and flow characteristics of the lesion. In addition, MRI avoids the use of contrast agents and irradiation (15). Arterial malformations are seen as flow voids on spin-echo (T_1 and T_2) images. Venous malformations are brighter than fatty tissue and have a high in-

Table 90.4. DIAGNOSTIC EVALUATION OF ARTERIOVENOUS MALFORMATIONS

Noninvasive tests
  Ultrasonography
  Segmental pulse volume recording
  Color-flow Doppler
  Magnetic resonance imaging
  Contrast-enhanced computed tomography
  Radioisotope scan (^{99m}Tc-labelled albumin microspheres)
Invasive tests (angiographic evaluation)
  Arteriography
  Venogram or fistulogram

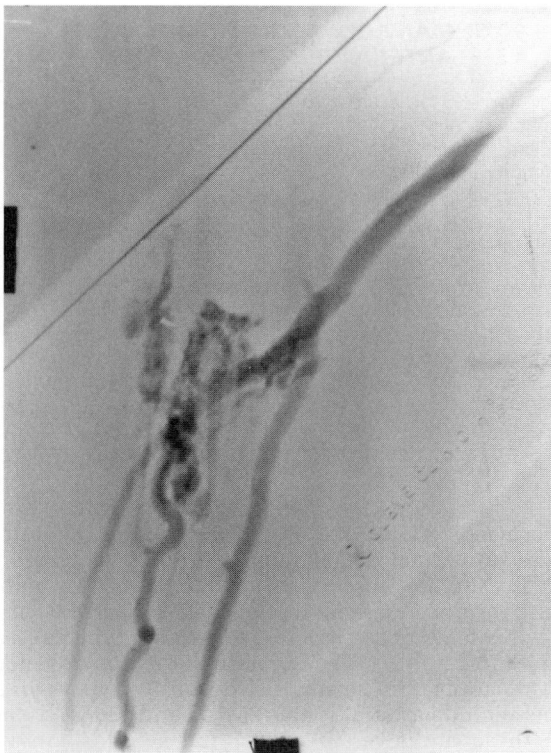

Figure 90.9. Congenital arteriovenous malformation of the proximal forearm. Note the rapid filling of lesion through multiple feeders from radial and ulnar artery.

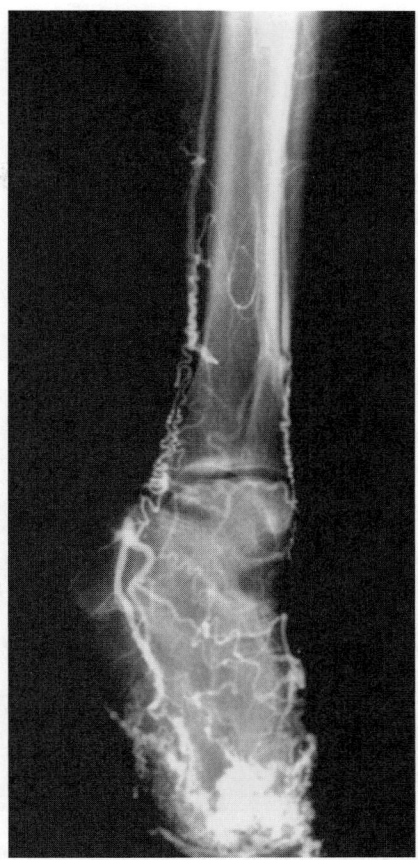

Figure 90.10. Arteriovenous malformation of the foot with multiple feeders both from anterior and posterior tibial system.

tensity signal on T$_2$-weighted images. Phleboliths, seen as round signal voids on T$_1$ and T$_2$ images, are highly suggestive of venous anomalies. Venous and lymphatic malformations can be differentiated by intravenous gadolinium administration. Venous malformations enhance homogeneously, whereas lymphatic lesions have no enhancement or have minimal ring enhancement. Radionuclide tests using ^{99}m Tc-pertechnetate-labelled albumin microspheres are useful in demonstrating the microfistulous communications that are often missed by conventional angiograms. For this test, the lung is monitored with a gamma camera, followed by sequential proximal arterial and peripheral venous injection. The ratio between pulmonary signal following arterial versus venous administration is used to calculate the flow traversing the fistula (14).

Angiographic evaluation in the form of arteriography (Figs. 90.9 and 90.10), venography, or fistulography remains the most useful diagnostic tool for AVMs. Occasionally, a small hemangioma may be associated with large, extensive underlying malformation seen on angiogram. Arteriographic findings suggestive of AVMs include (a) arterial dilatation and tortuosity (Fig. 90.10), (b) blushing or puddling of dye in the vascular channels (Fig. 90.11B), (c) visualization of the arteriovenous fistula itself, (d) early venous filling, and (e) dilatation of draining venous channel. Angiography is also useful to identify other congenital vascular anomalies, such as absent deep venous system or persistent embryonal vessels. In the absence of angiographic proof of arteriovenous communication, comparison of the venous blood oxygen saturation of both the affected and unaffected limbs may suggest the presence of fistulous flow.

MANAGEMENT

Management of AVM continues to be a subject of considerable controversy; recently, the opinions of 21 physicians, including pediatricians, dermatologists, and surgeons with special expertise in managing AVM, were published as a symposium (16). The 1940s and 1950s saw the aggressive use of irradiation, and many experts subsequently decried the use of this modality, saying that the consequence of irradiation is worse than the consequence of leaving the lesion untreated. Today, the therapy for AVM should be adapted to the extent, location, and degree of disability produced by the lesion. Treatment (Table 90.5) initially should be directed at nonsurgical options; the disability from the lesion must be weighed against the extent of disfigurement caused by excisional therapy. Observation and treatment of local complications are all that is necessary in most cases of hamangiomas. Hemorrhage from discrete areas usually can be managed by direct pressure for 10 minutes with a clean pad. Small ulcers respond well to topical antibiotic therapy, whereas the presence of cellulitis mandates the use of systemic antibiotics. Recurrent ulceration is rare. Observation to evaluate for signs of spontaneous involution is mandatory in infants. Providing parents with photographs of hemangiomas during the period of involution can be immensely reassuring. Infants need to be monitored frequently because it is difficult to predict the growth rate and ultimate size and rate of involution. Venous malformations of the extremities with symptoms of venous hypertension may benefit from the use of external elastic support stockings.

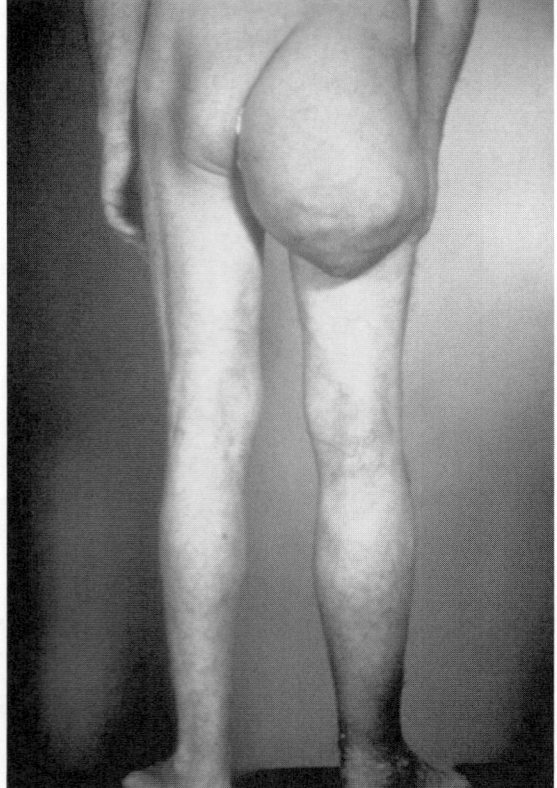

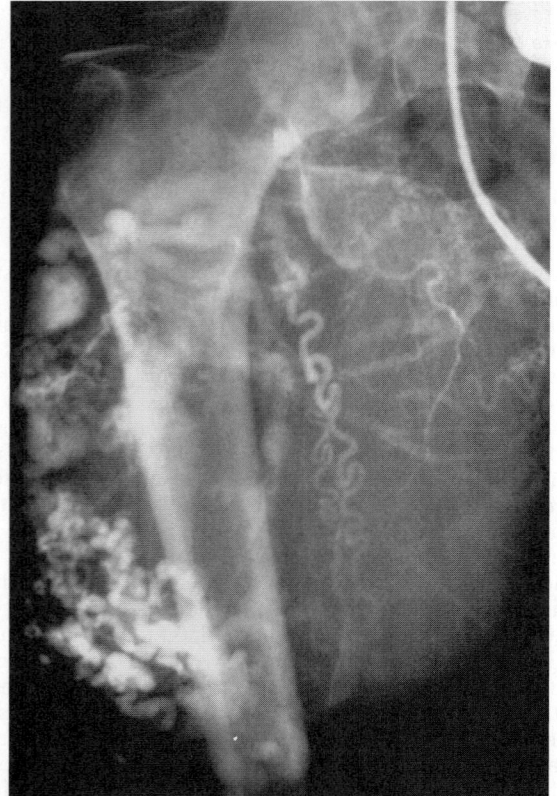

Figure 90.11. *(A)* Giant hemangioma of the right gluteal region. *(B)* Angiogram shows arterial dilatation and tortuosity with puddling of dye in the vascular channels.

Table 90.5. **MANAGEMENT OPTIONS OF ARTERIOVENOUS MALFORMATIONS**

Observation and local care
Pharmacological therapy
   1. Corticosteroids (local or systemic)
   2. Interferon-2a and 2b
   3. Angiogenesis inhibitors
Laser
   Flash-lamp pulsed-dye laser
   Argon
   Neodymium:yttrium–aluminum–garnet
   Potassium–titanyl–phosphate
   Carbon dioxide
Cryotherapy
Superselective embolization
Sclerotherapy
Surgical or laparoscopic management (excision or SEPS)

SEPS, subfascial endoscopic perforator ligation.

Pharmacologic therapy is useful for infantile and immature superficial hemangiomas. Prednisone, given systemically in the dose range of 2 to 3 mg/kg of body weight results in dramatic shrinkage of lesions in one third of infants and results in stabilization of the lesion in another third (17). The duration of therapy depends on the indications for use and the response seen. Major side effects include arterial hypertension and growth retardation; these are reversible once the steroids are withdrawn. Topical injections of triamcinolone, 3 to 5 mg/kg per treatment session have been used with variable success. Topical therapy with steroids should be avoided in the face because atrophy of the skin with occasional retinal artery occlusion has been observed. Infants with life-threatening hemangiomas in whom high dose corticosteroids have failed have been treated successfully with recombinant interferon alpha, an inhibitor of angiogenesis. Subcutaneous injection of interferon alpha 2a or 2b is administered in the dose of 3 million units per square meter of body-surface area per day. Side effects include neutropenia, elevated liver enzymes, and spastic diplegia, observed in 20% of treated patients (18). Superficial cutaneous lesions (<1 mm), such as port-wine stains and telangiectasia, can be vaporized with the use of several of the available laser systems (Table 90.5). Efficacy depends on the expertise of the operator and may be associated with scarring. The particular types of laser and treatment protocols specific for hemangiomas have yet to be defined. Favorable results with the use of cryotherapy have been reported from South America and Europe; however, the potential risk of scarring has limited its use in North America (16,17).

Large symptomatic lesions and vascular malformations located in deep tissue planes are best managed by endovascular techniques such as superselective embolization (Fig. 90.12A,B) or intralesional injection of sclerosing agents. Once the decision is made to treat a congenital AVM, the feeding vessel is selectively cannulated. Balloon-tipped catheters are occasionally useful because they can be "flow-directed," with the blood stream achieving a more peripheral position. Balloon-occlusion aided arteriography can be used to define the lesion better by occluding the major inflow, preventing contrast dilution by the high-flow of blood through the AVM. In addition, additional unsuspected feeding vessels can be visualized by occluding the major inflow. Reflux of the embolization coils also can be prevented through the use of balloon-tipped catheters.

A wide variety of materials has been used to obliterate AVMs, including liquids, semiliquids, and particulate ma-

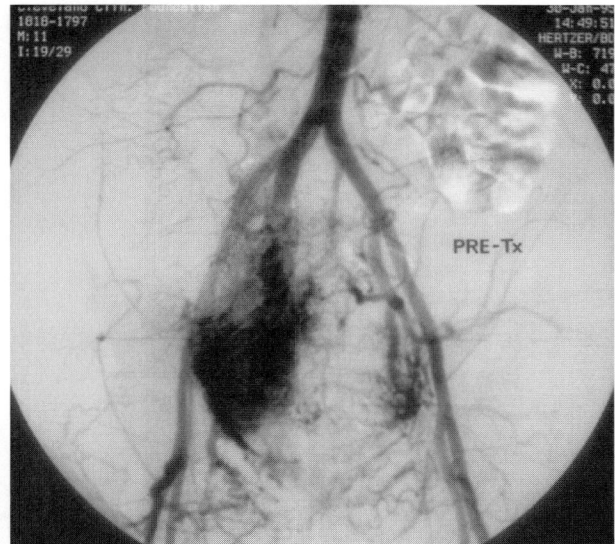

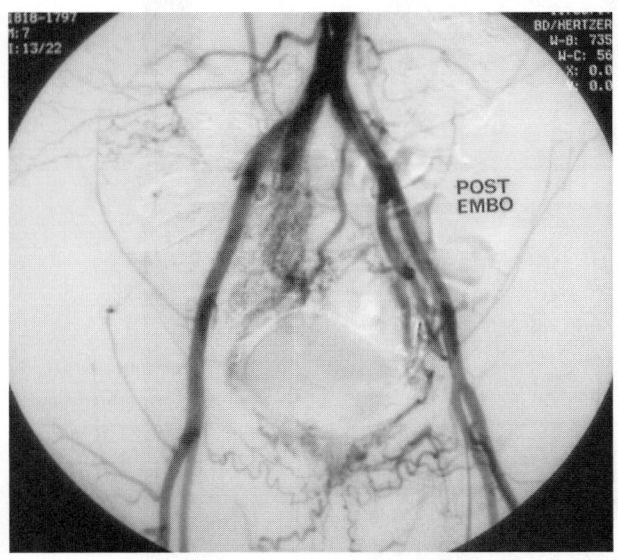

Figure 90.12. *(A)* Giant pelvic hemangioma with multiple feeding vessels from both internal iliac arteries. *(B)* Post coil embolization through both internal iliac arteries.

terial (19). Liquids such as alcohol and bleomycin act as sclerosing agents to induce thrombosis of the vascular channels; other semiliquid materials solidify on contact with blood to cause therapeutic vaso-occlusion. Semiliquid polymers commonly used include iso-butyl-cyano-acrylate (IBC) and Ethibloc (a solution of ethanol, prolamine, amindotrizoic acid, and oleum papaveris). IBC is more difficult to handle because it causes polymerization to occur immediately on contact with blood, which may cause the catheter tip to become trapped, resulting in irregular and incomplete distribution of the drug. Ethibloc precipitates slowly, allowing better management of the application catheter and drug. The addition of an oily contrast material such as lipidol to the Ethibloc can help reduce the viscosity and allow fluoroscopic control. Particulate mater such as Gelfoam and polyvinyl alcohol (Ivalon) can be used to produce occlusion. Inflow embolization by itself is rarely useful because collateral circulation will develop in a short time, but it may be used in preparation for surgical removal to decrease the blood

loss (Fig. 90.13A–C). It is important to remember that a powerful promoter of angiogenesis is local ischemia; hence methods using only inflow occlusion without eliminating the actual abnormal vascular channels are destined to fail. Coiling devises can be used to produce a "framework" in large AVMs, followed by injection of Ethibloc. This prevents passage of the amino acid solution to the venous side of the fistula. Detachable balloons have been successfully used in certain special indications such as a sinus-cavernous fistula. Direct puncture and injection of sclerosing agents, such as ethanol (20), bleomycin, and Ethibloc have been reported to be effective in treating AVMs.

Operative therapy has a useful but limited role in the treatment of extensive AVMs of the limbs. Operation can be of great benefit when dealing with some of dangerous complications of AVMs. Surgical extirpation alone is rarely sufficient because it often is accompanied by extensive blood loss and large residual arteriovenous connections. This usually occurs because congenital AVMs are almost never confined to a single anatomic segment of the arterial tree or to circumscribed anatomic regions, and communications are so extensive and widespread that their complete surgical ablation is seldom possible (Fig. 90.11B). Realization that complete cure is possible in only rare cases mandates the use of multiple therapeutic modalities. Simple ligation of vessels is rarely feasible and is complicated by a high rate of recurrence. If it is feasible to remove the entire mass and preserve limb function, then complete excision should be attempted. Preoperative embolization 2 to 3 days before the surgical excision tends to minimize the blood loss (Fig. 90.13A–C). Large tissue defects can be replaced with rotation flaps or microsurgical free tissue transfer. Acquired AVFs can be managed by the "quadruple ligation" method, the placement of ligatures around both artery and vein above and below the fistula, if it involves vessels that are not important for distal perfusion. A more functionally effective method is the excision of the fistula with reconstruction of artery or vein. This can be done by various techniques, such as a patch closure of the fistula site or replacement of the involved segment of the artery and vein with an autogenous or prosthetic graft. Appropriate surgical treatment requires special skill and experience in dealing with these lesions. It calls for experience in catheter-based techniques in addition to surgeons well versed in the appropriate treatments.

ARTERIOVENOUS MALFORMATIONS AS A PART OF COMPLEX-COMBINED MALFORMATIONS

Because most congenital AVMs occur as a result of errors in embryologic development, they may be associated with morphogenic errors of related mesenchymal derived structures. Many of these complex multiple-organ system malformations are known by eponyms.

Sturge-Weber syndrome consists of a port-wine stain in the distribution of the first division of the trigeminal nerve, combined with ocular and cerebral vascular anomalies. A classic triad has been described, comprising portwine stains, epilepsy (90%), and mental retardation (60%). Radiologic features are a double row of calcification on plain skull roentgenography. MRI with gadolinium enhancement will reverse the leptomeningeal angioma and confirms the clinical diagnosis. The cutaneous lesion is usually only a cosmetic problem and can be treated with laser ablation. Cerebral lesions, when associated with intractable seizures, should be treated with lobectomy or hemispherectomy before neurologic deterioration occurs.

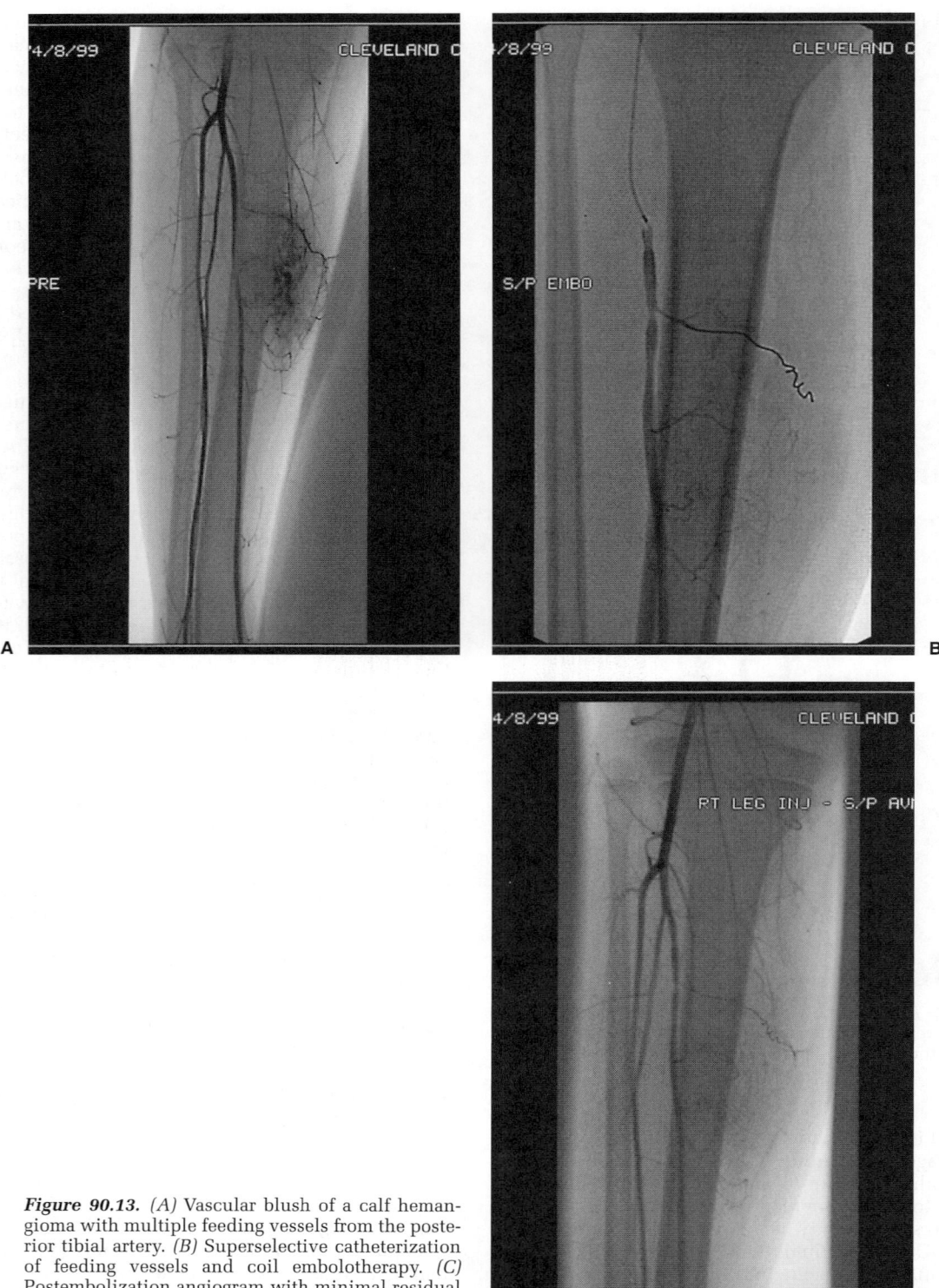

Figure 90.13. *(A)* Vascular blush of a calf hemangioma with multiple feeding vessels from the posterior tibial artery. *(B)* Superselective catheterization of feeding vessels and coil embolotherapy. *(C)* Postembolization angiogram with minimal residual arterial flow; pretreatment to surgical excision.

Von Hippel-Lindau syndrome has as its main features retinal angiomatosis and cerebellar ataxia. This syndrome is inherited as an autosomal dominant trait, and so the most important role of the clinician is to anticipate risk and offer screening to all who are at risk.

Louis-Bar syndrome, inherited as an autosomal recessive trait, presents with ataxia and telangiectasia of the conjunctiva and head and neck regions. Short stature, hypogonadism, and an abnormal glucose tolerance test are other features. Death usually occurs from recurrent respiratory infections.

Maffucci's syndrome consists of bony exostosis, enchondromatoses, and exophytic venous anomalies. Clinical importance derives from the presence of venous malformations of the gastrointestinal system, bone and leptomeninges.

The familial *Riley-Smith syndrome* consists of pseudopapilledema, macrocephaly, and multiple subcutaneous vascular malformations.

In 1990, the French physicians Klippel and Trenaunay described a syndrome characterized by three features: (a) capillary malformations, (b) soft tissue or bony hypertrophy, and (c) varicose veins (Fig. 90.14). The *Klippel-Trenaunay syndrome* (KTS) also may have other associated lymphatic and venous anomalies such as hypoplasia, aplasia, and venous incompetence. The venous malformations become more obvious as the child starts to ambulate. Abnormalities include ectasia of small veins, varicosities (Fig. 90.15), hypoplasia or aplasia of the deep system, and the persistence of embryologic veins such as a large lateral vein in the thigh and a sciatic vein. Severe venous reflux can cause symptoms of fatigue or heaviness of the legs. Evaluation consists of duplex ultrasound and contrast venography to ensure the patency of the deep venous system (21). Indications for therapy include intractable symptoms of chronic venous insufficiency, lymphedema, and recurrent cellulitis or bleeding. An initial course of external compression stocking or intermittent pneumatic compression pumps is warranted; surgical therapy is rarely required. Epiphysiodesis is required for limb-length discrepancy of greater than 2.0 cm in growing children. Amputation of grossly deformed digits is rarely required (Fig. 90.16). Varicose vein excision may provide benefit in a well-selected subset of patients. Recently, gratifying results have been obtained with stripping of the greater saphenous system in the thigh in combination with subfascial endoscopic perforator ligation (Fig. 90.17). Patients with KTS have no arteriovenous communication; in the presence of microfistulous or macrofistulous arteriovenous communication, this is referred to as *Parks-Weber syndrome*.

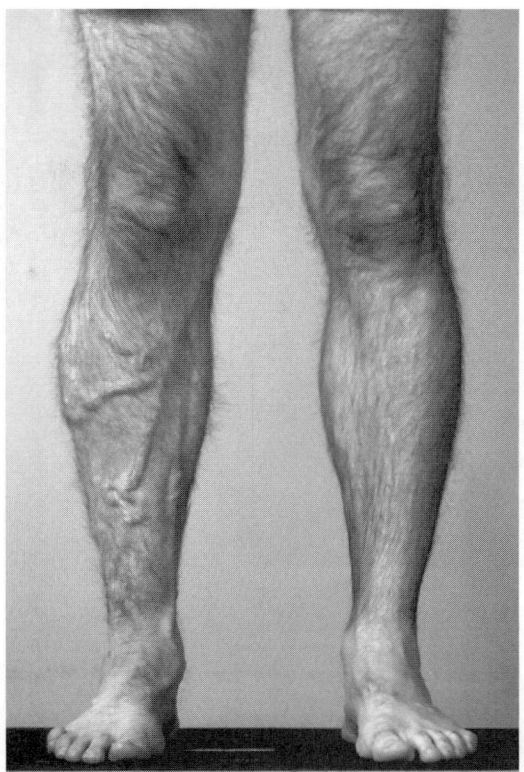

Figure 90.15. Milder clinical variant of Klippel-Trenaunay: prominent varicose veins and mild limb hypertrophy.

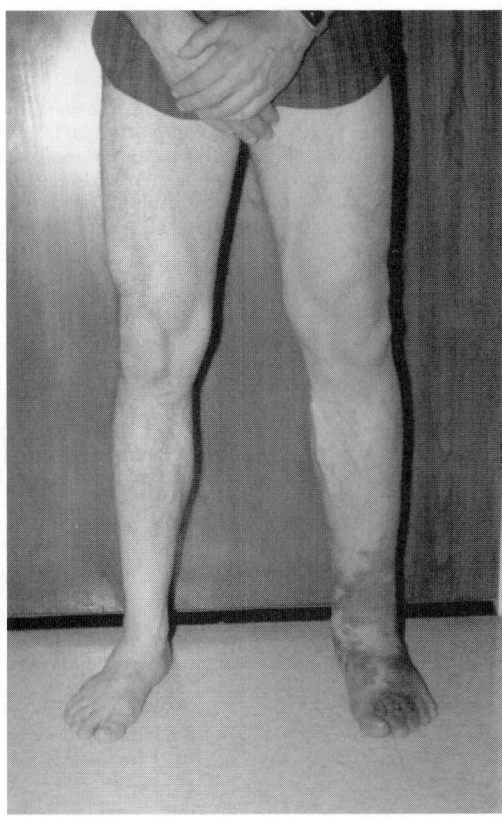

Figure 90.14. Typical triad of Klippel-Trenaunay syndrome: port-wine stains, varicose veins, and limb hypertrophy.

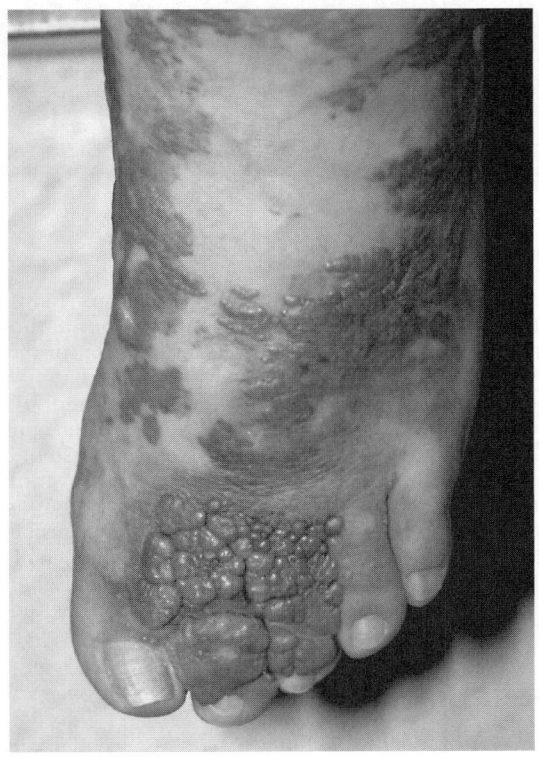

Figure 90.16. Grossly deformed digit of patient with Klippel-Trenaunay syndrome. This may rarely require an amputation.

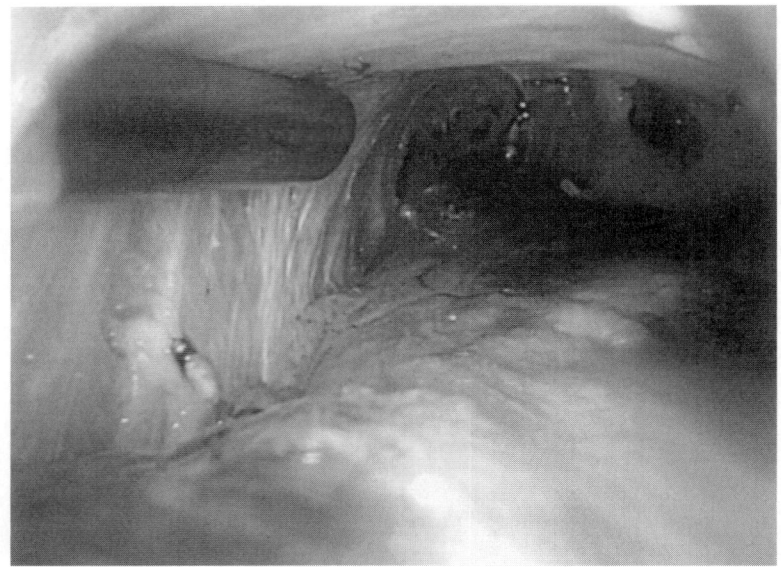

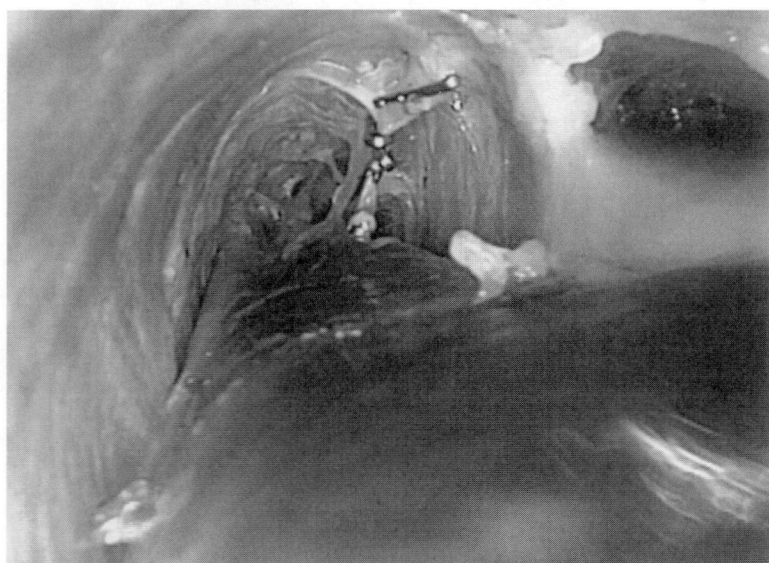

Figure 90.17. Subfascial endoscopic perforator surgery. Initial CO_2 pneumocompartment is created in the subfascial plain of the posterior leg using standard laparoscopic equipment. Perforating incompetent veins are clipped and divided as shown in the operative photomicrograph.

CONCLUSION

Vascular malformations and arteriovenous fistula are not uncommon, and yet many questions about pathogenesis and optimal therapy remain ill defined. Better recognition of complications and newer therapies, such as inhibitors of angiogenesis, may aid in the treatment of cases that do not regress spontaneously. All too often, patients are shuffled from physician to physician because of a lack of sufficient knowledge by a single physician. A multidisciplinary approach with well-educated and compassionate physicians and nonphysician health care workers will facilitate the treatment of these difficult to manage clinical entities. Only through such interspeciality collaboration can the cosmetic and functional problems associated with AVM be managed (22).

REFERENCES

1. Szilagyi DE, Smith RF, Elliot JP, et al. Congenital arteriovenous anomalies of the limb. *Arch Surg* 1976;111:423–429.

2. Malan E. History and different clinical aspects of arteriovenous communications. *J Cardiovasc Surg* 1972;13:491.

3. Hunter W. The history of an aneurysm of the aorta, with some remarks on aneurysm in general. *Medical Observations and Inquiries* 1757;1:323.

4. Bushe G. Temporal aneurism: a case where, after the excision of an anastamosing aneurism from the right temple, ligature of the external carotid became necessary to restrain hemorrhage. *Lancet* 1827–1828;2:413.

5. Hewitt P. A case of congenital aneurysmal varix. *Lancet* 1867;1:146.

6. Halsted WS. Congenital arteriovenous and lymphatico–venous fistula: unique clinical and experimental observations. *Transactions of the American Surgical Association* 1919;37:262.

7. Tasnadi G. Clinical investigations in the epidemiology of congenital vascular defects. In: Balas P, ed. *Progress in angiology 1991.* Torino: Edizioni Minerva Medica, 1992:391–394.

8. Cotton LT, Sykes BJ. The treatment of diffuse congenital arteriovenous fistulae of the leg. *Proc R Soc Med* 1969;62:245.

9. Tice DA, Clauss RH, Keirle AM, et al. Congenital arteriovenous fistulae of the extremities. *Arch Surg* 1963;86:460.

10. Toursarkissian B, Allen BT, Petrinec D, et al. Spontaneous closure of selected iatrogenic pseudoaneurysm and arteriovenous fistulae. *J Vasc Surg* 1997;25:803–809.

11. Drolet BA, Esterly NB, Frieden IJ. Hemangiomas in children. *N Engl J Med* 1999;341:173–181.

12. Sarkar M, Mulliken JB, Kozakewich HP, et al. Thrombocytopenic coagulopathy (Kasabach-Merritt phenomenon) is associated with Kaposiform hemangioendothelioma and not with common infantile hemangioma. *Plast Reconstr Surg* 1997;100:1377–1386.

13. Silverman RJ, Breckx T, Craig J, et al. Congestive heart failure in a newborn caused by cerebral A-V fistula. *Am J Dis Child* 1995;89:539.

14. Rutherford RB. Congenital vascular malformations: diagnostic evaluation. *Semin Vasc Surg* 1993;6:225–232.

15. Pearce WH, Rutherford RB, Whitehill TA, et al. Nuclear magnetic resonance imaging: its diagnostic value in patients with congenital vascular malformations of the limbs. *J Vasc Surg* 1988;8:64–70.

16. Frieden IJ. Management of hemangiomas. *Pediatr Dermatol* 1997;14:757–783.

17. Enjolras O, Riche MC, Merland JJ, et al. Management of alarming hemangiomas in infancy: a review of 25 cases. *Pediatrics* 1990;85:491–498.

18. Grienwald JH Jr, Burke DK, Bonthius DJ, et al. An update on the treatment of hemangiomas in children with interferon alfa 2a. *Arch Otolaryngol Head Neck Surg* 1999;125:21–27.

19. Weber J. Techniques and results of therapeutic catheter embolization of congenital vascular defects. *Int Angiol* 1990;19: 214–223.

20. Shireman PK, McCarthy WJ, Yao JST, et al. Treatment of venous malformation by direct injection of ethanol. *J Vasc Surg* 1997;26:838–844.

21. Jacob AG, Driscoll DJ, Shaughnessy WJ, et al. Klippel-Trenaunay syndrome: spectrum and management. *Mayo Clin Proc* 1998;73:28–36.

22. Mulliken JB. Cutaneous vascular anomalies. *Semin Vasc Surg* 1993;6:204–218.

SECTION N

VENOUS AND LYMPHATIC SYSTEMS

SURGERY: SCIENTIFIC PRINCIPLES AND PRACTICE, Third Edition, edited by
Lazar J. Greenfield, Michael W. Mulholland, Keith T. Oldham, Gerald B. Zelenock,
and Keith D. Lillemoe. Lippincott Williams & Wilkins Publishers, Philadelphia, © 2001.

CHAPTER 91

VENOUS PHYSIOLOGY AND VENOUS THROMBOEMBOLISM

THOMAS W. WAKEFIELD AND LAZAR J. GREENFIELD

VENOUS ANATOMY

The superficial veins of the lower extremity consist of the greater and the lesser saphenous veins. They contain multiple valves and exhibit significant variability in branching and location. The greater saphenous vein begins anterior to the medial malleolus with the joining of superficial draining veins from the medial aspect of the dorsum of the foot with veins from the medial aspect of the sole. It travels subcutaneously, usually in a straight line on the anteromedial aspect of the lower leg 1 or 2 cm posterior to the tibia, and passes along the medial aspect of the knee. The greater saphenous vein continues in a straight line to the thigh, where it joins the femoral vein 2 to 4 cm lateral to the pubic tubercle and inferior to the inguinal ligament at the fossa ovalis (Fig. 91.1). In the leg, the greater saphenous vein lies adjacent to and sometimes is crossed by the saphenous branch of the femoral nerve, providing cutaneous sensation to the medial aspect of the lower leg.

The location of the saphenous nerve places it at risk during procedures involving the use or removal of the greater saphenous vein. The junction of the greater saphenous vein with the femoral vein is sometimes missed because the greater saphenous vein may appear to continue proximally if the superficial inferior epigastric vein or the superficial circumflex iliac vein joins the saphenous vein vertically and is large. The superficial external pudendal vein joins the saphenous vein medially, although the arrangement of this branch and other superficial saphenous venous tributaries is not constant. Usually, there are four to five branches off of the saphenous vein at this location. The saphenous vein receives a variable number of tributaries draining the posteromedial and anterolateral aspects of the leg. The medial and lateral greater saphenous branches may be large and can be confused with the main greater saphenous trunk. The greater saphenous vein may be duplicated and exist as two separate trunks that join to form a single vein at its origin and termination. This occurs in as many as 5% to 10% of patients. The

lesser saphenous vein arises behind the lateral malleolus, from the confluence of veins draining the lateral aspect of the foot. It curves toward the midline of the posterior calf and then ascends in a straight line vertically to join the popliteal vein behind the knee near the head of the gastrocnemius muscle, although it has been demonstrated to terminate above the level of the knee crease in 7% to 8% of cases (1). The lesser saphenous vein lies in the subcutaneous tissues just below the skin. It may continue upward in the posterior region of the thigh and connect with tributaries of the greater saphenous vein.

The greater and lesser saphenous veins are joined in the foot by a superficial dorsal venous arch. The deep veins of the sole of the foot consist of lateral and medial plantar veins. They are joined through communicating veins to a cutaneous arch and come together to form the posterior tibial vein (Fig. 91.2). Multiple communicating veins connect the superficial to the deep veins in the foot. The deep veins of the lower leg consist of venae comitantes that accompany the anterior tibial, posterior tibial, and peroneal arteries. Each of the deep veins consists of two or three venae comitantes adjacent to the artery with multiple connections that cross and surround the artery. These connecting veins make surgical exposure of the tibial arteries difficult. The anterior tibial venous drainage arises from the dorsum of the foot and lies in the anterior compartment of the calf next to the interosseous membrane. The posterior tibial veins, which drain the superficial and deep plantar veins, are inferior to the medial malleolus and follow the course of the posterior tibial artery. The peroneal veins lie directly behind and medial to the fibula and ascend along the peroneal artery (Fig. 91.3). These deep veins of the calf have frequent interconnections. The soleal muscle sinusoids are without valves and are referred to as *venous lakes*. The venous lakes in the calf are a common site of early thrombus formation. They coalesce to join the posterior tibial and peroneal veins. These sinusoids are less apparent in the gastrocnemius muscle, where the veins tend to be linear and exhibit valves. The paired venae comitantes merge to form single trunks that unite at the knee to form the popliteal vein. Sometimes the junction occurs above the knee, resulting in a dual popliteal vein system.

The popliteal vein continues proximally as the superficial femoral vein in proximity to the superficial femoral artery in the adductor canal. It is joined below the inguinal ligament by the deep femoral (profunda) vein and then continues as the common femoral vein. The deep femoral vein frequently connects directly or through tributary veins to the popliteal vein. The anatomy of the popliteal and femoral veins is variable, and duplication is common. The common femoral vein runs medial to the common femoral artery beneath the inguinal ligament and continues as the external iliac vein. The greater saphenous vein usually joins the common femoral vein 2 to 4 cm proximal to the

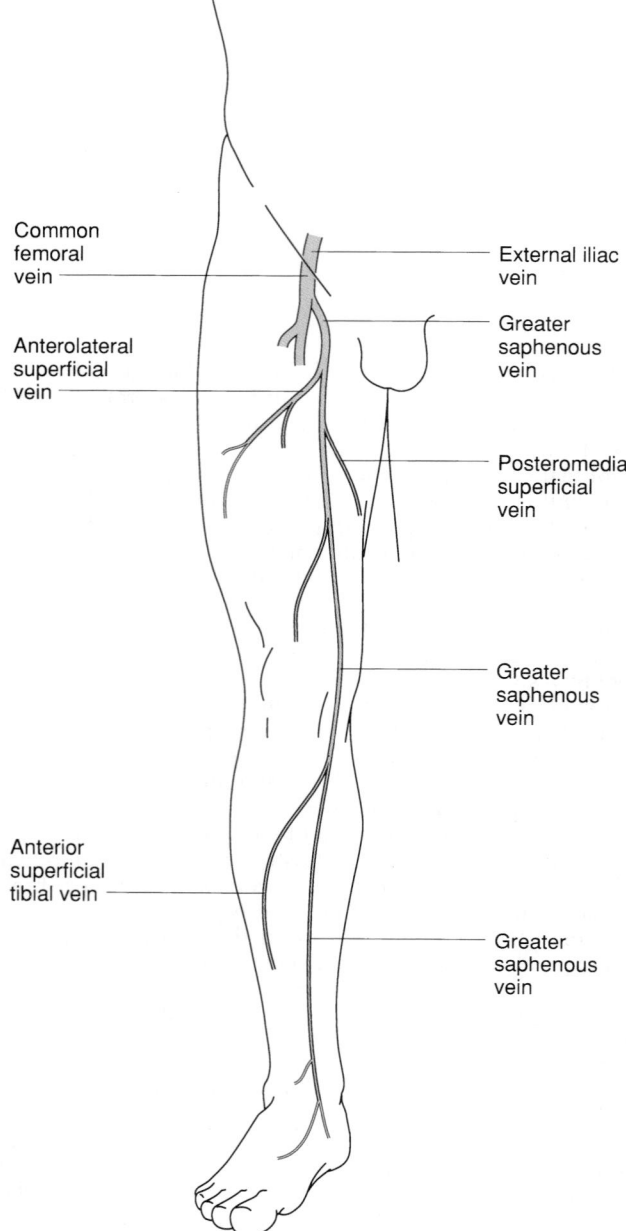

Figure 91.1. Greater saphenous vein and its branches.

junction of the deep and superficial femoral vein at the fossa ovalis. The external iliac vein is the continuation in the pelvis of the common femoral vein and is joined at the level of the sacroiliac joint medially by the internal iliac vein (hypogastric) draining the pelvis. Both internal iliac veins form a generous collateral network in the pelvis and include connections with the gluteal, obturator, and internal pudendal veins, a large number of unnamed vessels, as well as multiple extrapelvic collateral pathways. The common iliac veins arise from the joining of the external and internal iliac veins. They ascend in a medial direction and join on the right side of the fifth lumbar vertebra and the aorta, forming the inferior vena cava. The right common iliac vein ascends in an almost straight line to the inferior vena cava, whereas the left common iliac vein is more transversely oriented and joins the right iliac vein at an angle of approximately 90 degrees. The left common iliac

vein may be compressed between the convexity of the lumbosacral spine posteriorly and the anterior crossing of the right common iliac artery. This variable degree of compression may be seen on venography (Fig. 91.4) and probably accounts for the higher incidence of left-sided deep venous thrombosis (DVT), varicose veins, and varicocele in men. Compression of the left iliac vein may lead to the venous obstructive condition termed the *May-Thurner syndrome.*

The inferior vena cava ascends from the level of the fifth lumbar vertebra and ends at the right atrium. It lies to the right of the midline and lateral to the aorta and receives a variable number of paired lumbar veins that connect with the vertebral and paravertebral venous plexus. At the level of the L-1 to L-2 interspace, the renal veins join the inferior vena cava. More proximally, the hepatic veins join the inferior vena cava. The embryogenesis of the abdominal venous system occurs between the sixth and eighth week of gestation (2). First, the posterior cardinal veins appear. This system regresses, leaving only the iliac vein bifurcation. Next, the subcardinal veins develop, with the cranial portion of the right subcardinal vein anastomosing with the right hepatic vein, forming the suprarenal inferior vena cava. The right and left subcardinal veins anastomose to form the left renal vein. Finally, the supracardinal veins form and an anastomosis between the supracardinal and subcardinal veins forms the renal segment of the inferior vena cava. The caudal segment of the right supracardinal vein becomes the infrarenal segment of the inferior vena cava, whereas the cranial segment develops into the azygos vein while the left system regresses.

The inferior vena cava may be duplicated below the level of the renal veins, with a left-sided cava draining into the left renal vein, which then joins to form a single proximal inferior vena cava. If unsuspected, this anomaly can cause confusion at operation and inadvertent injury may result. The incidence of inferior vena caval and renal vein anomalies is significant. Duplication of the inferior vena cava occurs in 0.2% to 3% of cases, transposition or left-sided inferior vena cava occurs in 0.2% to 0.5%, a retroaortic left renal vein in 1.2% to 2.4%, and a circumaortic left renal vein in 1.5% to 8.7% (2). The left renal vein normally crosses the aorta on its anterior surface, but it occasionally crosses posteriorly and may result in confusion and unexpected injury. Collateral circulation around an obstructed inferior vena cava occurs through many alternate pathways, including the vertebral plexus, gonadal veins, ureteral veins, the azygos system, and the extensive superficial collaterals, which include the superficial epigastric, circumflex iliac veins, and the lateral thoracic and intercostal veins.

Important communicating veins exist at the termination of the greater and lesser saphenous veins where they join the deep venous system in the popliteal fossa and in the fossa ovalis. The perforating veins of the lower leg are important to the pathophysiologic process of venous disease and chronic venous insufficiency (CVI), especially the three or four perforating veins at the level of the medial and lateral malleolus in the so-called gaiter area of the lower leg. Other perforating veins are located in the upper medial calf and along the posterolateral aspect of the lower leg, connecting the lesser saphenous vein with the deep veins of the calf. A small but variable number of communications exists in the mid-thigh between the greater saphenous vein and the superficial femoral vein. The locations of perforating veins can be accurately determined only by venous duplex imaging or venography.

Venous valves direct the flow of blood to the heart and prevent valvular reflux. These valves consist of two delicate leaflets composed of an intimal fold with a small amount of connective tissue in between. Venous valves in

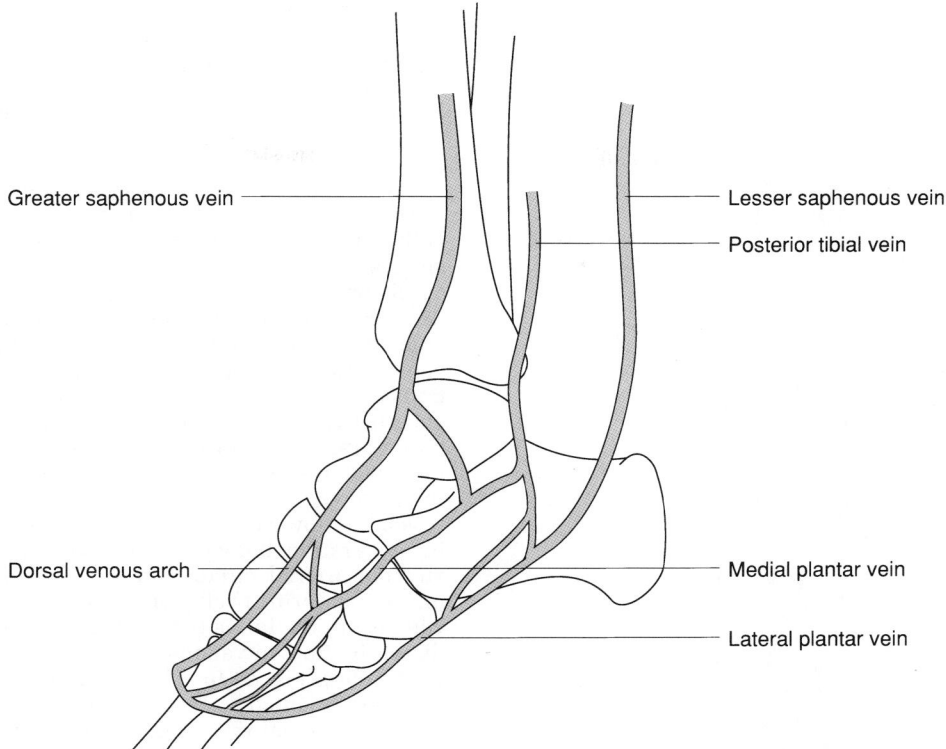

Figure 91.2. Veins of the foot.

the lower extremity are more numerous in the distal extremity, decrease in number proximally, and are absent in the superior and inferior vena cava. The valves in the upper extremity appear less important for venous function, and the influence of the venous muscle pump is less significant. The loss of valvular function in the upper extremity after thrombosis less frequently produces problems, in marked contrast to the lower extremity, where the valves play an important role. There are no valves present in the soleal and gastrocnemius sinusoids, but all other deep veins of the calf contain multiple valves. The popliteal vein contains one or two valves whose function is essential to the normal venous return from the calf. Valves in the deep veins of the thigh vary in number and position. There is a constant valve in the femoral vein just distal to its junction with the deep femoral vein and in the proximal portion of the popliteal vein just distal to the adductor hiatus. The greater and lesser saphenous systems contain 8 to 10 valves, with a constant valve present at the proximal end of the greater saphenous vein just at or slightly distal to its junction with the common femoral vein. A third set of valves is present in the perforating veins, which communicate between the superficial and deep veins. Valves are oriented so that they direct venous flow from the superficial to the deep system and, in the deep system, from the foot to the heart. They prevent reflux of the higher-pressure deep venous circulation into the superficial saphenous system. The valves in these perforating veins lie both deep and superficial to the muscle fascia.

VENOUS PHYSIOLOGY

Foot vein pressure is influenced by the patient's position in either the supine or erect posture. When measured supine, venous pressure is the residual kinetic energy of the heart reduced by capillary and arteriolar resistance.

This residual pressure is approximately 15 mm Hg and results in a pressure gradient of 13 to 15 mm Hg returning blood to the heart because the right atrial pressure usually ranges between 0 to 2 mm Hg. When foot vein pressure is measured in the erect position, the hydrostatic pressure caused by the weight of the column of blood that extends from the heart to the foot must be included. Therefore, foot vein pressure in the erect posture is the sum of the hydrostatic pressure and the kinetic pressure of 15 mm Hg. In a person 6 feet tall, the hydrostatic pressure equals approximately 100 mm Hg. Therefore, in the upright posture, the pressure measured in a foot vein is approximately 115 mm Hg. Hydrostatic pressure is also exerted on the arterial circulation so that the net pressure is still the difference in pressure across the capillary bed.

Assuming the erect posture increases venous volume, and the volume of the calf increases approximately 2% to 3%. In the leg veins, the upright position increases capacitance by approximately 500 mL of blood, which arises from the central circulation and fills the veins. Orthostatic hypotension may result in patients with a low blood volume. This increment is returned to the central circulation with exercise in the presence of a normal calf muscle pump. For patients at bed rest, wearing graded compression stockings increases the velocity of venous return and reduces the venous volume pooling in the legs, reducing stasis and also decreasing the potential for venous thrombosis.

The vein wall is composed of collagen, elastic tissue, and smooth muscle fibers. The smooth muscle fibers are responsible for active venous tone. Venous capacity is influenced by variations in transmural pressure and, to a lesser extent, by the contractility of the smooth muscle in the venous wall. This is particularly true when the veins are collapsed and the transmural pressure is low. When there is further filling, the veins assume a circular configuration, and the smooth muscle venous tone assumes

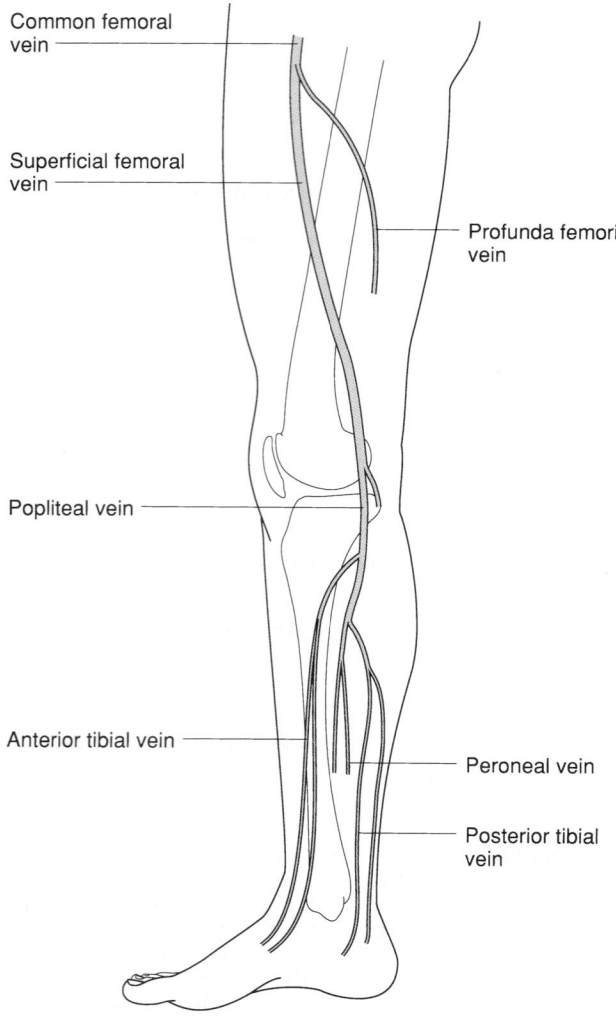

Figure 91.3. Deep veins of the lower leg.

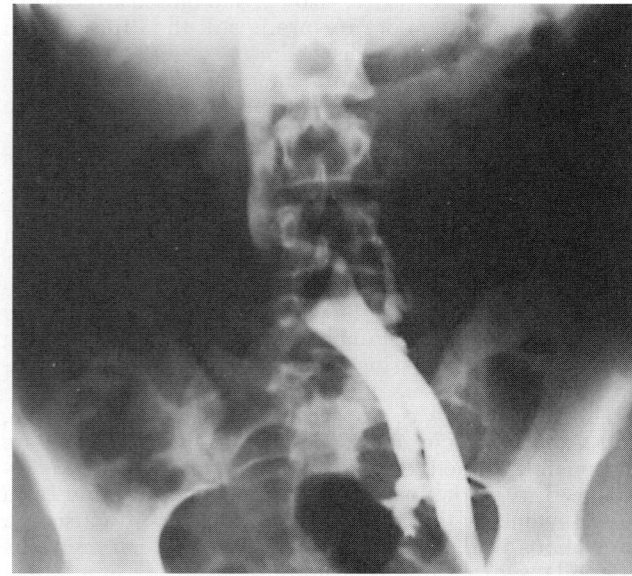

Figure 91.4. Phlebogram showing compression of the left common iliac vein by the right common iliac artery.

greater importance in regulating venous volume. The venous system can accommodate significant variations in volume with little change in pressure. This ability allows alterations in blood volume to occur with minimal change in central venous pressure. When the venous capacitance is exceeded, however, the central venous pressure rises significantly.

Empty veins are flat. As they fill, they evolve from an elliptical into a circular form in cross section. Initially, there is little resistance to flow as veins distend and their shape changes. During early filling, as veins assume a circular configuration, more blood can be accommodated with little increase in venous pressure. Once veins assume a circular configuration, the pressure per unit of volume increases rapidly and reaches a plateau (Fig. 91.5). The transmural pressure, which causes distention, is the difference between the intraluminal pressure and the external tissue pressure. With outflow obstruction, a small volume increment results in a disproportionate increase in pressure in the veins.

Venous flow is affected by a number of factors, including respiration, body position, calf muscle pump function, and the arterial circulation. For example, flow is at its minimum during peak inspiration. A unique feature of the venous circulation is the presence of bicuspid valves that direct the flow of venous blood toward the heart and prevent reflux (Fig. 91.6). The valve cusps of the superficial veins are oriented so that they lie parallel to the skin surface. The normal valve sinus is wider than the diameter of the vein, and it is believed that the valve cusps do not lie flat against the vein wall when open. The open valve cusps are easily engaged by retrograde blood flow, and the slightly greater valve diameter ensures a tight seal that prevents valvular reflux. A crucial set of valves is found in the perforating veins. The balloon-like appearance of the vein wall around the confluence of a vein valve may reflect differences in the tensile strength of the vein wall. The distention at the site of the valve spreads and places tension on the commissures, causing the valve cusp edges to tighten, further enhancing valvular competency.

Normally, veins can accommodate large volume changes with exercise with only small pressure changes. This does not occur in all patients, however, so that with calf muscle pump dysfunction, venous pressures do not normalize but remain chronically elevated. In addition, any dissipation of pressure is quickly overcome by a return to preexercise pressure levels when walking stops. It is this chronic state of elevated venous pressure (venous hypertension) that leads to the state of chronic venous insufficiency (CVI). The syndrome of venous claudication occurs when the iliofemoral venous segment is obstructed by thrombosis that

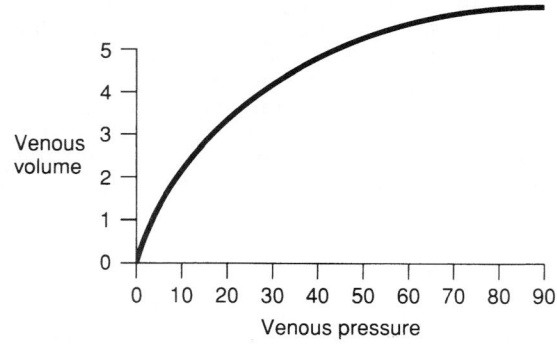

Figure 91.5. Relation between venous volume and venous pressure.

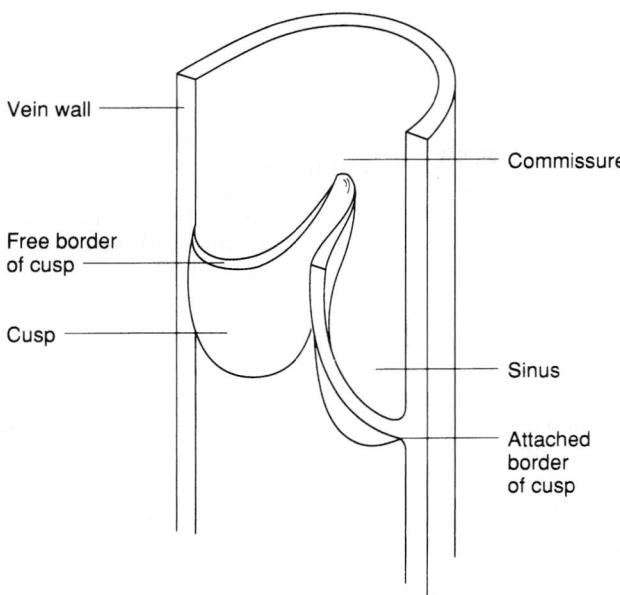

Figure 91.6. Structure of a venous valve.

has failed to lyse or by an anatomic abnormality. With exercise, the deep venous system fills but does not empty, and the thigh and leg become heavy and painful with a bursting sensation.

DISORDERS OF THE SUPERFICIAL VEINS

Varicose veins that arise spontaneously in the absence of deep venous involvement are referred to as *primary varicose veins,* whereas veins arising as the outward manifestation of CVI are referred to as *secondary varicose veins.* When the deep veins are competent, a circular flow circuit occurs such that flow down the saphenous system is shunted into the deep system by competent perforators and then returns toward the heart. However, a portion of the flow at the femoral vein level reverses down the leg, leading to saphenous vein insufficiency during exercise; up to one fifth of the total femoral vein flow may be involved in such a circular motion (3). This circular motion does not exist in secondary varicose veins. The epidemiology of varicose veins has been determined as part of the ongoing Framingham Study (4). During 16 years of follow-up, varicose veins developed in 629 women and 396 men. Women of all age groups, except those between 80 and 89 years, frequently exhibited varicose veins, and the highest incidence was in women aged 40 to 49 years. Women with varicose veins were more often obese, physically inactive, hypertensive, and older at menopause. In men, varicosities were associated with smoking and physical inactivity. Although there was no independent direct relation to atherosclerosis, patients with the risk factors mentioned are clearly at greater risk for atherosclerosis than patients without these characteristics.

Treatment

Treatment for both primary and secondary varicose veins involves a program of CVI management including elastic stocking support, periodic leg elevation, and exercise (while wearing stocking support, if possible). The elastic hose coapts the vein walls, preventing further distention of the already dilated superficial veins. Indications for surgical treatment of varicose veins include pain over the varicosities themselves (to be distinguished from the discomfort of underlying deep venous insufficiency), superficial thrombophlebitis in the varicosities, erosion of the overlying skin with bleeding, disabling edema with or without subcutaneous cellulitis, induration or lipodermatosclerosis associated with the varicosities, and manifestations of CVI (especially ulceration) related to incompetency of the superficial saphenous system and the varicosities. Contraindications to varicose vein ligation and stripping include cosmetic improvement only, varicose veins secondary to CVI from deep venous insufficiency in which the CVI and not the varicose veins are causing the patient's symptoms, and varicose veins associated with other chronic disease states that are the cause of the patient's symptoms, such as degenerative arthritis, arterial occlusive disease, neurogenic syndromes, lymphedema, congestive heart failure, and obesity. Ligation and stripping should mostly be avoided for varicose veins associated with an underlying arteriovenous fistula or underlying congenital venous abnormalities, such as the Klippel-Trenaunay syndrome. Injection sclerotherapy may be indicated for small varicosities but more frequently for "spider" telangiectactic veins. Indications for injection sclerotherapy include direct pain over the spider telangiectactic veins, symptoms of venous insufficiency related to the spider telangiectactic veins (especially symptoms before or during menstruation), previous thrombophlebitis, bleeding from the spider telangiectactic veins, and trophic changes related to the spider telangiectactic veins. These are essentially the same indications as for larger varicose veins. Contraindications to injection sclerotherapy include active thrombophlebitis, pregnancy during the first and second trimester, the postpartum period for approximately 3 months after termination of lactation, significant leg edema, inability to participate in physical activity after injection therapy, a concomitant bedridden condition, severe arterial occlusive disease, the inability to wear properly applied bandages after injection sclerotherapy, and cosmetic effect only without underlying symptoms.

Preoperative testing should include documenting an intact deep venous system by venous ultrasound duplex imaging. Reflux testing, such as photoplethysmographic (PPG) examination, may be indicated to help predict the overall success of the varicose vein removal and the need for postoperative elastic support. If CVI is present, the patient is best instructed to follow a program of CVI management after superficial vein removal. The classic procedure of high ligation and stripping of the entire saphenous system has been replaced by more selective vein removal, and the stab–avulsion technique has gained popularity. High ligation alone with careful perforator interruption has been recommended with excellent long-term results (5), as has ambulatory stab–avulsion phlebectomy for truncal varicosities (6). In this technique, after high ligation of the greater saphenous vein, small stab wounds 1.5 to 3.0 mm long are made along the premarked varicosities. Specially designed hooks are used to remove trunk and tributary varicosities. Although this technique may work well for primary varicose veins, in the presence of significant secondary varicosities, larger incisions and perforating vein interruption and ligation are important technical considerations. In the presence of secondary varicosities in which varicose clusters are related primarily to deep venous insufficiency and perforator incompetence, high ligation is usually not necessary. With careful patient selection and properly tailored operative techniques, the recurrence rate should be 10% or lower (7). Major complications include hematoma, infection, sural nerve irritation (from lesser saphenous stripping), and saphenous nerve irritation (minimized by vein stripping from proximal to distal). A combination of surgical and sclerotherapy techniques yields optimal functional and cosmetic results (8).

DISORDERS OF THE DEEP VEINS

Chronic venous insufficiency has traditionally been considered a consequence of previous DVT in most cases and of congenital or hereditary venous valvular incompetence in a few cases, although more recent reports have suggested a more equal incidence of these two causes of CVI. Other causes include cavernous hemangioma, congenital arteriovenous fistula, and pelvic tumors.

With valvular incompetence, the standing column of blood produces elevated venous pressures leading to CVI. Furthermore, patients with CVI have little if any venous pressure reduction during exercise in contrast to the normal response, and with venous obstruction, the venous pressure may actually rise with exercise. After exercise, the venous pressure returns much faster than it should so that the lower leg and ankle region is exposed chronically to elevated venous pressures (9). There are two important reasons why the changes of CVI (including stasis pigmentation, stasis dermatitis, and ulceration) occur in the gaiter area. First, incompetent perforating veins produce extreme venous hypertension in the ankle region. Second, the ankle has little soft tissue support. Elevated venous pressures lead to brawny edema from plasma fluid constituents in the interstitial space along with plasma proteins and red blood cells. These constituents produce low-grade inflammation, the red cells break down to produce a dark pigment called *hemosiderin*, and eventually the subcutaneous tissues become scarred and fibrotic. Because of the fibrosis in the subcutaneous tissue, skin perfusion decreases, leading to skin ischemia that facilitates ulceration. Leukocytes also play an important role as they become sequestered in the microcirculation of the leg with elevated venous pressures, possibly leading to capillary occlusion (10). In the capillaries, these leukocytes become activated and destroy tissue by releasing superoxide radicals and proteolytic enzymes (11). Macrophages and T lymphocytes are the cell types most often involved (12). The inflammatory response initiated by these cells is more important in the pathogenesis of the skin changes than microvascular occlusion because leukocytes "trapped" in the capillaries during venous hypertension are released within 10 to 20 minutes of resumption of a supine position (10).

Although severe changes of CVI have traditionally been considered to be associated only with deep venous insufficiency and not saphenous vein insufficiency, more and more studies are suggesting that even isolated saphenous vein incompetence can lead to the CVI syndrome. According to the pathophysiologic process discussed earlier, the symptoms of CVI begin with edema. The edema usually occurs at and above the ankle, without involvement of the forefoot or toes. It usually responds well to leg elevation. Characteristically, the patient has worse edema at night than in the morning, and eventually, dermatitis, stasis pigmentation, brawny induration, and ulceration may occur. Other causes of ulceration must be distinguished from venous ulceration, including neurotrophic and ischemic ulceration. *Neurotrophic* ulcers are painless and bleed with manipulation. They are deep, indolent, and surrounded by chronic inflammatory tissue reaction appearing as callus. They are usually located over pressure points, commonly the plantar surface of the first and fifth metatarsal heads, and are common in patients with long-standing neuropathy and diabetes mellitus. *Ischemic* ulcers, on the other hand, are extremely painful and associated with rest

pain in the distal forefoot. These ulcers, when chronic, are circumscribed, and the ulcer base often has poorly developed, grayish granulation tissue. The surrounding skin is pale and mottled, and ulcer débridement causes little bleeding. Other conditions that may cause ulceration include vasculitic states that may result in multiple punched-out areas with indurated bases, chronic hypertension, syphilis, inflammatory bowel disease, tuberculosis, osteomyelitis, self-induced trauma (factitious), arteriovenous fistulae with venous dilatations and skin erosion, scleroderma, myxedema, burns, radiation, lymphoma, and fungal diseases. *Venous* ulcers are large and irregular in outline, have a shallow, moist granulation base, occur in the gaiter area, either on the medial or lateral (less common) aspect of the ankle, and are involved in areas of skin with stasis dermatitis and stasis pigmentation. Chronic lymphedema, which causes diffuse thickening of the skin and firmness of the subcutaneous tissue, is infrequently associated with ulceration.

Along with the symptoms of aching, fatigue, itching, night cramps, and swelling occurring from venous reflux, selected patients describe venous claudication (13). As venous volume increases to near maximum with exercise, leg distention and intracompartmental pressures increase because of the fixed resistance of venous collaterals in the presence of major venous occlusions to the point where leg discomfort occurs. This most often results from incomplete and poor recanalization of the venous system after an extensive occlusive DVT.

It has been estimated that approximately one fourth of the general population has CVI. In untreated DVT, the frequency of stasis dermatitis and ulceration increases over time (14). After 10 years, three fourths of patients have advanced stasis changes and half have stasis ulceration without appropriate treatment, although contemporary data suggest that this incidence may be less. The mean time for the appearance of the first stasis-related venous ulcer is 2 to 3 years. Interestingly, it has been found that valvular reflux after DVT progresses over time. Of extremities 1 week after thrombosis, 17% reveal reflux, whereas greater than two thirds of extremities show reflux at 12 months, not limited to the area of initial thrombosis (15). This suggests that mechanisms other than valve entrapment in scar must exist for the development of CVI.

Treatment

Once venous insufficiency has developed, it is an incurable but manageable problem. Most of the changes of CVI in the leg are due to chronic swelling. Elastic compression stockings improve but do not prevent swelling. Elevating the legs above the heart level, which patients with CVI should do daily, is important to decrease venous hypertension. In addition, elastic support should be applied before the patient gets out of bed in the morning and taken off before the patient goes to sleep at night. The manner in which elastic compression improves the symptoms of CVI has not been absolutely established. However, studies suggest that external compression may restore competency of the dilated valve cusps (16) and may affect the venoarterial reflex (17). Exercise such as walking and bicycling with proper support applied and swimming is excellent for patients with CVI. If stasis ulceration develops, it usually improves with leg elevation and local wound care, especially with occlusive dressings. In some cases, these ulcers may become superinfected and require antibacterial treatment, although the routine use of topical antibiotics is not indicated (18). The Unna boot has been the traditional treatment and includes a gauze dressing impregnated with gelatin, zinc oxide, and a calamine preparation. Application of the Unna boot is followed by dry gauze and an elastic wrap and is usually repeated on a weekly basis. We have found a combination of occlusive dressings under the Unna boot to be extremely effective for most venous ulcers (19,20). The hypothesis for the effectiveness of occlusive dressings is that collagen synthesis and reepithelialization of tissue are increased in wounds beneath these dressings because they prevent the removal of new epidermis with each change. Granulation tissue forms quickly under these occlusive dressings because they are oxygen impermeable, and wound angiogenesis is inversely proportional to the ambient oxygen tension.

Most patients with CVI can be treated nonsurgically. However, 1% to 2% of patients benefit from operative correction. The two basic categories of operation are valve restoration procedures for reflux and venous bypass for obstruction. Before operative therapy is considered, the diagnosis of CVI must be confirmed objectively. Noninvasive laboratory studies include complete venous Doppler examinations, PPG, and air plethysmography (APG). The PPG examination is qualitative and not quantitative, whereas the APG is quantitative. The APG test measures many aspects of lower leg physiology at one time, including venous obstruction, venous reflux, and calf muscle pump function, and thus gives an overall assessment of the leg as a whole (21). It can be used during exercise, is easily and readily repeated, and can also be used to differentiate superficial from deep venous insufficiency (Fig. 91.7). The residual volume fraction generated by this test correlates closely with ambulatory venous pressure (21). In addition, duplex imaging of closing times of individual venous valves indicates venous reflux (22). Duplex imaging can also identify the presence of incompetent perforators. Although outflow obstruction can be assessed by APG, it is best determined by the arm–foot pressure gradient measured directly because the APG outflow fraction is often normal if collaterals have formed to bypass a chronic venous obstruction. In normal limbs, the arm–foot pressure differential is less than 4 mm Hg at rest and less than 6 mm Hg with reactive hyperemia (23). The invasive ambulatory venous pressure measurement using a needle placed into a foot vein is rarely needed because of the availability of the aforementioned noninvasive tests.

After the vascular laboratory tests, ascending phlebography is used to assess the patency of the tibial, popliteal, superficial femoral, common femoral, iliac, inferior vena cava, and perforating veins. A thin tourniquet placed at the ankle at 120 to 140 mm Hg pressure may be used to test for perforator incompetence (24). Combined with ascending phlebography, descending phlebography requires placement of a catheter into the common femoral vein with the weight borne by the contralateral leg on a 60-degree foot-down tilt table. A steady stream of contrast medium is injected into the femoral vein, and the valves are tested during normal breathing and with a forced Valsalva maneuver. Descending phlebography provides visual information about the function of the valves. Using this technique, pathologic reflux in patients with postthrombotic damage is found in approximately 31% of cases (25). Thus, a combination of venous noninvasive testing and phlebography defines the distribution of venous valvular incompetence in patients with CVI. Isolated proximal valvular incompetence is present in only 5% of limbs with severe disease in patients undergoing Doppler evaluation for CVI. Distal incompetence is found in 67% of those with proximal venous incompetence and in 57% of patients with competent proximal valves (26). Thus, most patients with severe CVI have venous valvular incompetence that is more closely associated with distal deep venous valvular incompetence either alone or in combination with proximal valvular involvement.

Perforating vein ligation is indicated in patients who have recurrent or recalcitrant venous ulcers when there are large incompetent perforating veins under the area of ulceration (Fig. 91.8). Perforator ligation does not change the venous hemodynamics of the limb and is indicated to allow for ulcer healing so the patient may then follow a standard conservative program, including stocking support, exercise, and intermittent leg elevation. Patients must understand that after perforator ligation, a standard aggressive conservative program needs to be followed. Other indications for perforator ligation include persistent pain in the region of a previous venous ulcer with an underlying incompetent perforating vein and repeated failure of skin graft healing in an area of venous ulceration. Patients with proximal deep venous occlusion should have this proximal occlusion resolved before or at the same time as perforator ligation. Contraindications to perforator ligation include the failure to demonstrate an appropriate perforator under the ulcer and such severe stasis disease of the skin and subcutaneous tissue that the incision for the procedure would not be expected to heal. Among 650 patients with 1,799 limbs reported, the ulcer recurrence rate was 15%, with a 17% postoperative wound complication rate with open perforator ligation

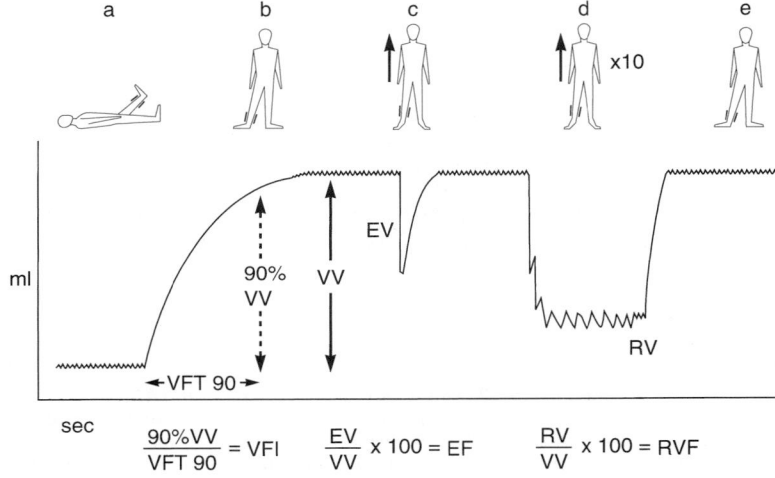

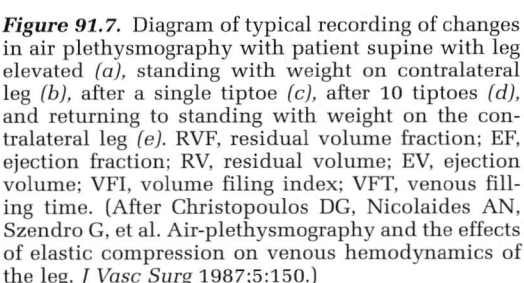

Figure 91.7. Diagram of typical recording of changes in air plethysmography with patient supine with leg elevated *(a)*, standing with weight on contralateral leg *(b)*, after a single tiptoe *(c)*, after 10 tiptoes *(d)*, and returning to standing with weight on the contralateral leg *(e)*. RVF, residual volume fraction; EF, ejection fraction; RV, residual volume; EV, ejection volume; VFI, volume filing index; VFT, venous filling time. (After Christopoulos DG, Nicolaides AN, Szendro G, et al. Air-plethysmography and the effects of elastic compression on venous hemodynamics of the leg. *J Vasc Surg* 1987;5:150.)

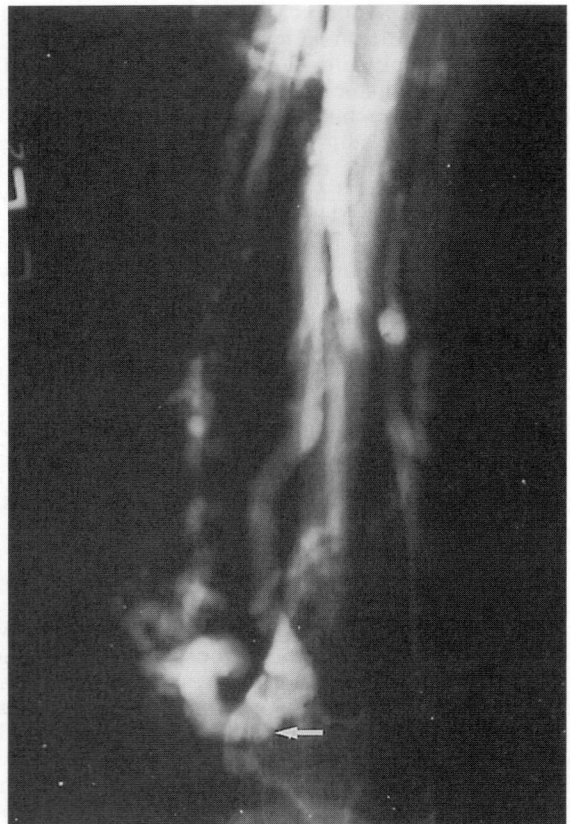

Figure 91.8. Large incompetent perforator *(arrow)* underneath an area of recurrent venous ulceration on the medial aspect of ankle. Ligation of the perforator resulted in ulcer healing. (After Wakefield TW. Venous disorders. *Probl Gen Surg* 1994;11:504.)

(27). More recently, perforator ligation has been performed using an endoscopic approach [subfascial endoscopic perforator vein surgery (SEPS)] in an attempt to limit wound healing abnormalities (28). Comparison of the two techniques, direct operative approach versus SEPS, has not yet been thoroughly performed.

Indications for direct venous reconstructive surgery include significant symptoms of venous reflux, including severe aching, fatigue, and swelling; recurrent venous ulceration not responsive to conservative therapy or perforator ligation, resulting from either venous obstruction or reflux; such significant combined superficial and deep venous insufficiency that the patient's symptoms cannot be relieved with superficial venous surgery alone; failure of maximal conservative therapy to relieve severe symptoms of deep venous insufficiency; and significant venous claudication associated with venous outflow obstruction. Contraindications to direct venous surgery include CVI that has not been treated with an aggressive conservative management program; symptoms associated with chronic diseases, such as degenerative arthritis and peripheral vascular occlusive disease from nonvenous origins; symptoms of CVI that cannot be documented with any of the anatomic or physiologic tests described earlier; and venous obstruction as seen on phlebography that is not associated with symptoms.

Venous valvular operations for reflux include valvuloplasty (29,30), venous segment transposition (31,32), venous valvular autotransplantation (33), external banding, and vein wall plication (34) (Fig. 91.9). In the experience of Kistner and Sparkuhl (31), the best results with valvuloplasty have occurred when combined with perforator ligation. Reported results of valvuloplasty in 155 limbs with 1- to 13-year follow-up have revealed good clinical results in 77% of cases (34). Valvuloplasty may use external cuffs or bands, suture techniques not requiring incision into the vein, vein wall plication, and repair using the angioscope. Venous segment transposition procedures

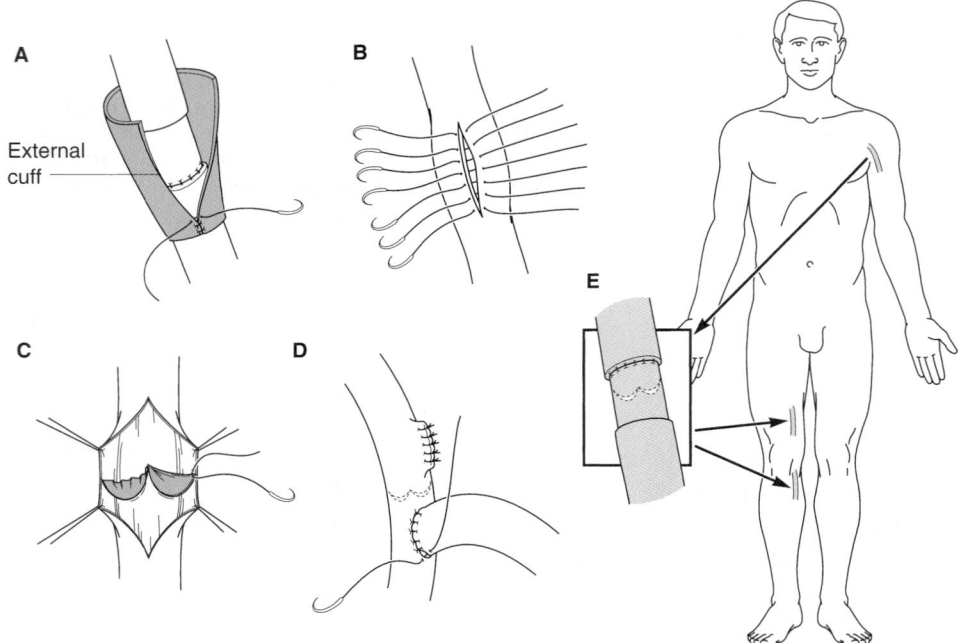

Figure 91.9. Methods of reflux correction. *(A)* External cuff banding. *(B)* Vein wall plication. *(C)* Valvuloplasty. *(D)* Transposition of an incompetent superficial femoral vein into a competent profunda femori vein. *(E)* Valve transplantation. (After Eriksson I. Reconstructive surgery for deep vein incompetence in the lower limb. *Eur J Vasc Surg* 1990;4:214.)

have reported good early results but deteriorating later results (35). Of 46 limbs reported with follow-up for 1 to 6 years, 63% revealed good clinical results. Finally, valvular autotransplantation has been shown to be successful in nearly 80% of the cases in one series (33), but curative in only approximately 50% in another series (30). Therefore, the same problems may develop over time in the transplanted vein valve as in the original failed valve. The valve transfer now believed to be most important is the popliteal valve rather than the femoral valve. Of the 176 limbs reported with follow-up to 6 years, good clinical results have been reported in 66%. Importantly, O'Donnell documented improvement in venous hemodynamics as assessed by APG after popliteal vein transplantation (36). Another procedure is the substitute valve operation (Psathakis procedure) using a Silastic tendon spacer behind the knee (37). A relatively new approach for venous obstruction, especially at the level of the left iliac vein crossed by the right iliac artery (May-Thurner syndrome), is the use of angioplasty and stenting (38). This syndrome was uncovered in a significant number of cases in the results of the venous registry (39).

For venous obstruction, two bypasses have been described, the femorofemoral and saphenopopliteal. The cross-over femorofemoral venous bypass (Palma procedure) was first described in 1958. After dividing the ipsilateral saphenous vein distally, this vein is tunneled suprapubically to the opposite femoral vein. Prosthetic material for this bypass has also been advocated. This procedure is indicated for relief of persistent unilateral iliac vein obstruction. In 303 patients reported (277 with postthrombotic problems and 26 with extrinsic compression), results were excellent in 187 (62%), good in 39 (13%), and poor in 77 (25%) (40). The ipsilateral saphenopopliteal by-

pass (May-Husni procedure) may benefit patients with superficial femoral vein occlusion. In 65 patients reported, 75% were improved, whereas 15% were not (40). For both of these bypasses, concomitant procedures such as perforator ligation, saphenous vein stripping, and creation of distal arteriovenous fistulae have been advocated (the latter if prosthetic conduits are used). In both of these procedures, the saphenous vein when used as a conduit tends to dilate over time (Fig. 91.10).

In all of these procedures for CVI, there is often discrepancy between hemodynamic and clinical results, making it difficult to evaluate results objectively. In addition, the relative infrequency of isolated proximal venous valve incompetence in patients with CVI and the importance of distal vein valvular reflux suggest that most patients who have proximal valve reconstruction will need additional surgical correction for distal valves or incompetent perforating veins.

VENOUS THROMBOEMBOLISM

Epidemiology

Deep venous thrombosis affects greater than 250,000 patients per year (41). Including initial and recurrent episodes (42), superficial thrombophlebitis affects greater than 120,000 patients per year. DVT is responsible for a 21% annual mortality rate in the elderly, and the cost of treatment has been estimated to be between $1.0 and $2.5 billion per year (43). In the United States, pulmonary embolism (PE) is responsible for 200,000 fatalities yearly, one half due to incurable illnesses and one half to potentially curable illnesses (42). Thus, venous thromboembolism remains a significant problem in clinical practice.

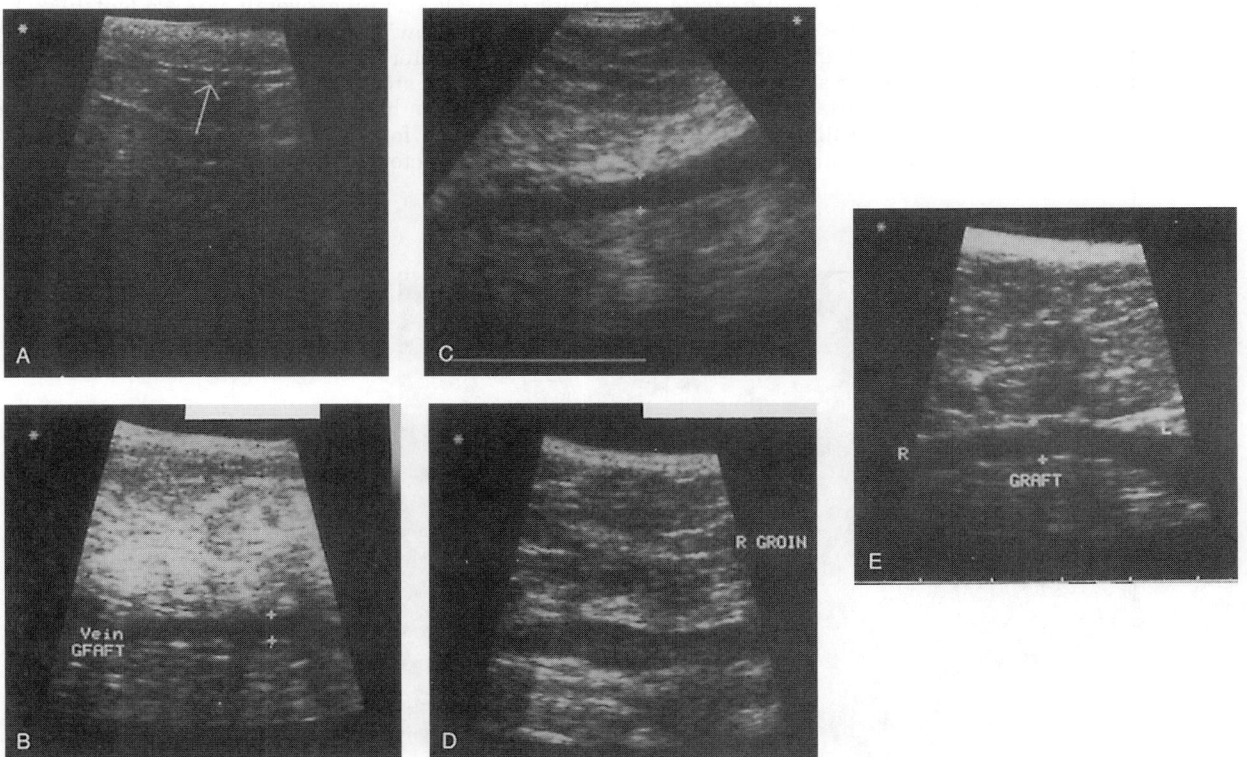

Figure 91.10. Increasing size of femorofemoral cross-over bypass *(arrow in A)* from time of insertion *(A)*, through 1 month *(B)*, 4 months *(C)*, and 13 months *(D and E)* after surgery. (Wakefield TW. Venous disorders. *Probl Gen Surg* 1994;11:506.)

Diagnosis

Tests for the diagnosis of DVT involve many indirect tests of historic interest, and more current modalities that directly visualize the thrombus such as venous duplex ultrasound imaging and magnetic resonance venography (MRV). Venous duplex ultrasound imaging has become the gold standard for DVT diagnosis, and has virtually replaced contrast phlebography. The indirect tests that are infrequently used, including hand-held venous Doppler interrogation, impedance plethysmography, phleborheography, and radiolabeled fibrinogen scanning, are not discussed further.

Duplex imaging includes both ultrasound image and flow analysis. Characteristics of acute thrombosis include noncompressability of the interrogated vein, enlargement of the vein, and the lack of significant venous collaterals (Fig. 91.11). For chronic thrombosis, echogenic thrombi, a nonenlarged vein, and prominent collaterals are noted. With the addition of color flow to venous duplex imaging, sensitivity, specificity, positive predictive value, and negative predictive values for the diagnosis of acute DVT in symptomatic patients are all greater than 95%. Even for the diagnosis of calf thrombi, the sensitivity in symptomatic patients is greater than 90%. The one area where venous duplex imaging has some difficulty is in the diagnosis of calf vein thrombi in surveillance situations, where sensitivities have been reported between 20% and 70% (44).

The excellent specificity of venous duplex imaging allows for therapeutic decisions to be made. In a study involving 431 negative duplex scans, of which 66 had corresponding phlebograms, only 3 peroneal thrombi were found on phlebography, and no more proximal thrombi were missed (45). Follow-up over the next 8 months revealed no pulmonary emboli or recurrent DVT. The high negative predictive value of venous duplex imaging suggests that withholding anticoagulation on the basis of a negative scan is safe and reasonable. One study has combined major and minor points in the patient's history with venous duplex imaging to improve the results of imaging. Major points included active cancer, paralysis, a bedridden state for greater than 3 days, localized tenderness along the deep veins, unilateral thigh/calf swelling, calf swelling greater than 3 cm, and a strong family history. Minor points included recent trauma, pitting edema, dilated superficial veins, hospitalization within the previous 6 months, and erythema (46). If the clinical pretest probability was high with an abnormal duplex scan, the chance of finding a DVT was nearly 100%, whereas if the clinical pretest probability was low with a negative duplex scan, the chance of finding a DVT was less than 1%.

Thus, venous duplex imaging has become the gold standard for the diagnosis of DVT and has virtually replaced contrast phlebography. The incidence of positive studies in a busy vascular laboratory should be approximately 25% to 30%. It is safe, painless, and accurate, requires no contrast, can be performed during pregnancy, is repeatable and noninvasive, can follow the progression or resolution of DVT, and should detect other structural abnormalities. These include pseudoaneurysms, venous aneurysms, Baker's cysts, cellulitis, and superficial thrombophlebitis.

Magnetic resonance venography has shown great promise as a diagnostic modality for both DVT and PE. Time-of-flight imaging carries a sensitivity and specificity for DVT of 100% and 96%, respectively (47), and for PE, 100% and 96% as well (48). MRV with the administration of gadolinium, a heavy metal chelate, has been found to be a good technique for determining the age of DVT. In the presence of an acute DVT, a vein wall inflammatory response is found and gadolinium extravasates into the area of inflammation (49). As the DVT organizes and matures, the gadolinium enhancement fades as the vein shrinks. The amount of enhancement in the wall compared with the thrombus can be quantitated, and in the chronic situation, the ratio in the wall compared with the thrombus approaches 1.0.

The diagnosis of PE involves either ventilation–perfusion scanning ($\dot{V}/\dot{Q}$) or pulmonary angiography. Newer modalities include helical computed tomography scanning and magnetic resonance imaging (MRI). The sensitivity of ($\dot{V}/\dot{Q}$) scanning overall is excellent (98%), but specificity is low (10%) (50). However, by combining clinical risk factors with the ($\dot{V}/\dot{Q}$) scan, sensitivity and specificity rates greater than 95% have been reported. In one study with a high-probability ($\dot{V}/\dot{Q}$) scan and at least two risk factors for PE, the sensitivity for PE was 97%; with one risk factor, 84%; and with no risk factors, 82%.

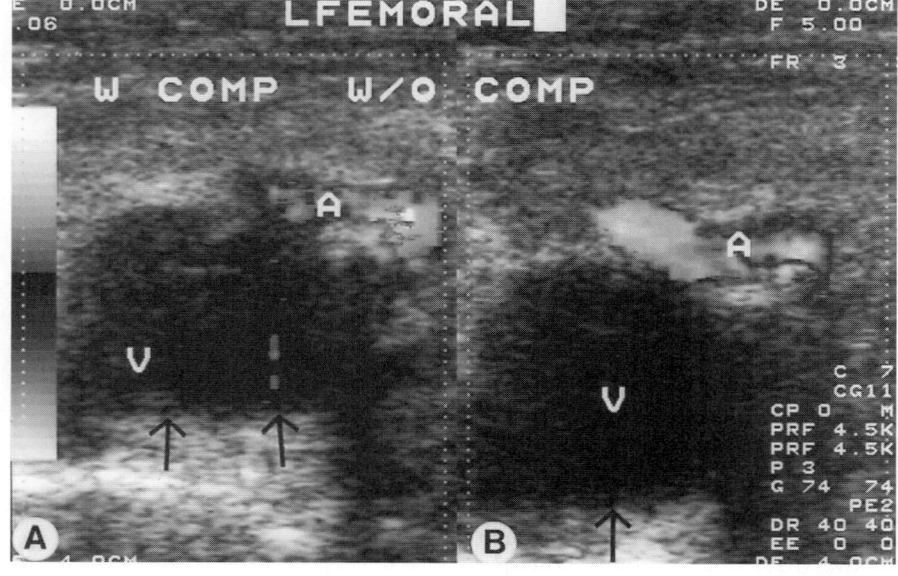

Figure 91.11. Venous duplex image, revealing evidence of acute venous thrombosis with compression (A) and without compression (B) of the enlarged vein (arrows). V, left femoral vein; A, left femoral artery.

In the same study, with a negative ($\dot{V}/\dot{Q}$) scan, the chance of PE was 0% for no risk factors, 0% for one risk factor, and 0% for greater two or more risk factors (51). Thus, a negative ($\dot{V}/\dot{Q}$) scan or a high-probability scan provides diagnostic information that allows for clinical decision making. However, only approximately 30% of ($\dot{V}/\dot{Q}$) scans are in one of these two categories, leaving 70% of cases needing further testing. Such testing includes lower extremity venous duplex ultrasound imaging (10% of patients sent to the vascular laboratory for this indication are found positive and thus qualify for anticoagulation treatment) and, more important, pulmonary arteriography. Additional indications for pulmonary arteriography include the management of acute massive PE, when inferior vena caval interruption is anticipated, and when planning pulmonary interventional therapy such as thrombolysis or pulmonary embolectomy.

Helical computed tomography scanning is a relatively new technique for the diagnosis of PE. Excellent specificities, but relatively low sensitivities in the range of 50% to 65% have been reported (52–54), despite more promising initial results (55,56). With such low sensitivities and negative predictive values, this technology likely is not useful as a screening test alone for the diagnosis of PE although the technology is improving constantly. The use of MRI has demonstrated excellent promise for the diagnosis of PE (48).

The use of D-dimer assays has been investigated in the diagnosis of both DVT and PE. For both DVT and PE, sensitivities of 96% to 98% have been reported (57). However, specificities of only 40% to 50% have been found, calling into question the ability of this assay to be used alone for thromboembolism screening. The role of D-dimer testing probably will be to supplement other diagnostic modalities such as venous duplex ultrasound imaging for DVT and ($\dot{V}/\dot{Q}$) scanning for PE diagnosis.

Treatment

Treatment for DVT and PE historically involves anticoagulation, intravenous heparin initially followed by long-term oral anticoagulation. Modalities also discussed include thrombolysis, thrombectomy, and the placement of inferior vena caval interruption devices.

Adequate anticoagulation decreases the risk of recurrent venous thromboembolism by approximately 80%, from 29% to 47% in the untreated situation to 5% to 7% in the treated situation (58–60). The risk of fatal PE during adequate anticoagulant therapy is low, 0.4% and 0.3% during and after treatment for DVT, and 1.5% and 0% during and after treatment for PE (61). It is important for the patient to achieve therapeutic levels of heparin rapidly because it has been shown that if therapeutic levels are reached in the first 24 hours, the recurrence rate is only 4% to 6%, compared with 23% if the heparin is not therapeutic in this time frame (62). No adequate explanation for this observed relationship has been found. It has also been shown that continuous intravenous standard heparin is better than intermittent subcutaneous standard heparin in preventing thromboembolic recurrence (63).

After heparin is begun, how long should it be continued and how long should oral anticoagulation be used? Heparin use for 5 days has been compared with 10 days, with no difference in recurrent thrombosis (7.1% vs. 7.0%); thus, 5 days of heparin should be adequate (64). Studies have evaluated the length of optimal oral anticoagulant therapy. In one study comparing 6 weeks with 6 months of warfarin treatment, at 2-year follow-up the recurrence rate was 18.1%, as opposed to 9.5% in favor of the longer treatment (65). A second study compared 4 weeks with 3 months of treatment in medical patients, with recurrence rates of 7.8% versus 4.0% in favor of 3-month therapy (66). A third study suggested that oral anticoagulants should be used for a longer rather than shorter time, especially in the presence of continuing risk factors (67). No study has compared 3 months with 6 months, so the usual recommendation is for a period of warfarin use after a first DVT of 3 to 6 months, although the length of oral anticoagulation should depend on patient presentation and history. For example, with reversible or time-limited risk factors and a first thromboembolic event, 3 to 6 months is recommended, whereas for an idiopathic etiology and a first event, 6 months or longer is recommended (68,69). Even with the best of treatment, DVT recurrences can be expected. The risk of symptomatic recurrent thromboembolism after a first episode of symptomatic DVT in patients treated with heparin, 3 months of warfarin, and surgical support stockings was 17.5% after 2 years, 25% after 5 years, and 30% after 8 years (70). The risk was markedly increased in the presence of factor V Leiden. In addition, lifetime therapy is recommended for a first thromboembolic event and cancer (until resolved), homozygous activated protein C resistance, antiphospholipid antibody (until resolved), and deficiency of antithrombin III, protein C, or protein S (68).

After a second episode of DVT, the usual recommendation is for lifelong warfarin therapy. In a study of patients with a second episode of DVT, at 4-year follow-up the incidence of recurrent DVT was 20.7% in those who received only 6 months of warfarin and 2.6% in those receiving warfarin for an indefinite period, an eightfold relative risk (71). However, the major bleeding risk increased from 2.7% to 8.6%, with no difference in mortality rate, suggesting that patients on long-term warfarin need to be carefully followed.

The most important complication of anticoagulant use is bleeding. With intravenous heparin therapy, the bleeding risk is 11% during the first 5 days (64). It is because of the bleeding risks with standard unfractionated heparin that low-molecular-weight heparins (LMWHs) were devised.

Low-molecular-weight heparins are made of the lower-molecular-weight range of standard heparin preparations and, as such, the anticoagulant mechanisms are different. Standard unfractionated heparin inhibits thrombin because it is large enough to make a three-way complex between thrombin, antithrombin, and itself. It requires 18 saccharide units to make this complex, and most LMWHs are shorter than 18 units. LMWHs thus have less antithrombin activity. Such a three-way complex is not necessary to inhibit factor Xa, allowing LMWHs to have antifactor Xa activity. In fact, each LMWH has its own antifactor Xa to antifactor IIa activity ratio, with most commercial preparations having a ratio between 2 : 1 and 4 : 1. Standard heparin has a ratio of 1 : 1 (72).

Advantages of LMWHs include a decreased bleeding potential, less antiplatelet activity, less risk for heparin-induced thrombocytopenia, an improved pharmacokinetic profile owing to reduced nonspecific binding to plasma proteins, less lipolysis, a half-life that is not dose dependent, more constant antifactor Xa inhibition, less interference with protein C activation, less complement activation, less interference with appropriate platelet aggregation, less risk of osteoporosis, and a lower level of fibrin monomer production (72). Treatment with LMWH does not need to be monitored with standard tests of global coagulation because LMWH is dosed based on patient weight. LMWH is administered by subcutaneous injection. Excretion of LMWHs is primarily renal.

Low-molecular-weight heparins have been recommended for both DVT prophylaxis (73) and treatment of venous thromboembolism. Level I studies and metaanalyses comparing LMWHs with standard unfractionated heparin for treatment of DVT and PE have shown a superiority of LMWH over standard unfractionated heparin (74–79). There is a lower risk for major bleeding, recurrent thromboembolic events, and death. Even for PE, LMWHs are equivalent to and more convenient than standard heparin (80). LMWH therapy is dosed based on weight, and does not have to be monitored by coagulation tests except in special circumstances, such as a patient in renal failure. Because monitoring is unnecessary, outpatient home treatment has become a reality.

The economic impact of LMWH use is significant. Cost savings have been demonstrated in multiple studies, and patients report great satisfaction with home outpatient DVT treatment (81–86). LMWHs have also been found useful in patients with unstable angina (72).

One of the areas of continued controversy involves the treatment of calf vein thrombi. Traditional teaching was that 20% of calf vein thrombi extend into the popliteal vein, and if extension occurred, it was associated with a high incidence of clinically detectable PE. However, calf vein thrombi alone have been associated with up to a 25% incidence of CVI 12 months after diagnosis and approximately a 10% incidence of PE at presentation (87). Thus, most authorities today recommend full anticoagulant treatment for isolated calf vein thrombosis. The ability to use outpatient LMWH will likely end this controversy.

The incidence of CVI after appropriate anticoagulant treatment for DVT has been reported to be 23% after 2 years, 28% after 5 years, and 29% after 8 years (70). Because of this real incidence of valvular reflux from DVT, the use of thrombolysis to clear more rapidly the venous thrombotic process has been advocated. Using duplex ultrasound, it has been found that spontaneous lysis time was 2.3- to 7.3-fold longer in refluxing segments than in nonrefluxing segments except for the posterior tibial vein (88). Systemic thrombolysis in two small series revealed a decrease in the incidence of the postthrombotic syndrome with the use of streptokinase as opposed to systemic heparin (89,90). However, results depended on total thrombolysis, and it was not possible to predict who would lyse completely and who would not. This inability to predict lysis success combined with the risk of bleeding led to thrombolysis falling out of favor. Based on the use of intrathrombus urokinase for arterial thrombi, a similar approach introducing urokinase directly into venous thrombi was attempted. Initial good results (91) led to a national thrombolysis registry (39). In the first 473 patients, with 287 undergoing follow-up, 312 urokinase infusions in 303 limbs have been reported. Venous thrombi occurred in the iliofemoral segment in 79% of cases, including the inferior vena cava in 21%. Two thirds of the patients presented acutely, 16% chronically, and 19% had a combined acute and chronic presentation. Approximately one third of the patients reported prior DVT, and the favorite access site for urokinase infusion was the popliteal vein in approximately 40% of cases. Complete thrombolysis was achieved in 33% of cases, whereas partial lysis was achieved in 50% of cases. The mean amount of urokinase needed was 7.8 million units, at a mean time of 53.4 hours. Predictors of successful lysis included acute DVT and no prior history of DVT. Complications included 11.5% with major bleeding requiring blood products (most at the venous access site) and 16% with minor bleeding. The mortality rate was 0.4%, and the incidence of intracranial hemorrhage was 0.2%. Although total lysis was noted in only 31% of the entire series, in patients with acute iliofemoral DVT, no previous symptoms, and use of the popliteal vein access site, total lysis was found in 65% of cases, with a 1-year patency rate of 95%. The thrombus-free survival rate at 12 months was 79% with complete lysis, 58% with greater than 50% lysis, and 32% with less than 50% lysis. With complete lysis, no valvular reflux was found in 72% of cases. The overall valvular reflux rate was 58%.

Thrombolytic therapy for PE has been studied and remains controversial. Although agents lyse thrombus effectively, no difference in patient mortality or recurrence rates has been found (92,93). Results are best if patients are young, the embolus is less than 48 hours old, or the embolus is large. Streptokinase, urokinase, and tissue plasminogen activator (94) have all been used. All three agents rapidly dissolve clot, but by 7 days the advantage for all three agents disappears. The benefit of thrombolytic agents for PE therefore appears to involve patients who would die as a result of massive PE in the first hour after the PE occurs, which may occur in up to 10% of patients.

Iliofemoral venous thrombectomy has been advocated in the presence of impending venous gangrene. This is a technique that results in mechanical clearing of the venous circulation and is combined with a temporary arteriovenous fistula to increase early patency. Rethrombosis rates of less than 20% have been reported using the arteriovenous fistula (95). The incidence of PE during the first week after thrombectomy is equivalent to that with conservative treatment with anticoagulation only. The frequency of clinical success has been reported between 42% and 93% (96). The biggest series of 77 legs with follow-up between 5 and 13 years revealed maintenance of patency, but a steady decrease in valvular competence over time (97). The arteriovenous fistula is constructed so that it can be taken down by angiographic, nonsurgical techniques.

In the only study comparing thrombectomy with anticoagulation (n = 31) versus anticoagulation alone (n = 32) for iliofemoral venous thrombosis, the clinical outcome at 6 months was better with thrombectomy (40% asymptomatic vs. 7%), iliofemoral vein patency was improved with thrombectomy (76% vs. 35%), and femoropopliteal patency was also improved with thrombectomy (52% vs. 26%) (95). At 10 years, the number of patients available had fallen to only 13 in the thrombectomy group and 17 in the anticoagulation-alone group. An improvement in patency in the thrombectomy group was found and, importantly, no popliteal reflux was found in 43% of the anticoagulation-alone group as opposed to 78% in the thrombectomy plus anticoagulation group (95). Thrombectomy failures included patients with associated chronic iliac vein obstruction creating rethrombosis and prior DVT resulting in valvular reflux.

Vena caval interruption for venous thromboembolism is appropriate if traditional anticoagulation fails, anticoagulant agents are contraindicated, or there is a bleeding complication associated with anticoagulation. Direct vena caval ligation resulted in significant lower extremity venous complications and a high rate of recurrent embolism. Thus, initial intraoperative caval compartmentalization devices, clip devices, and intravascular venous devices were developed. These devices have resulted in a decreased incidence of venous stasis complications. The most effective device currently available is the Greenfield vena cava filter, a cone-shaped device. This cone shape allows for 85% of the length of the device to contain clot and still maintain flow around its periphery, permitting natural fibrinolysis to take place. Indications for vena caval filtration include venous thrombosis or PE in a patient with a contraindication to anticoagulation, a complication during anticoagulation, recurrent PE in the face of adequate anticoagulation, chronic PE with associated pulmonary hypertension and cor pulmonale, and immediately after pulmonary embolectomy. Free-floating iliofemoral DVT may be associated with a 60% incidence of PE despite adequate anticoagulation (98), whereas free-floating inferior vena caval thrombi demonstrate a 27% incidence of PE despite adequate anticoagulation (99), and bilateral free-floating femoral thrombi have a 43% incidence of PE despite adequate anticoagulation (100), all additional indications for filter placement. Recently, prophylaxis against PE has become a very common indication for filter placement. In 642 patients reported in the largest published experience with the Greenfield filter, a contraindication to anticoagulation was the most frequent reason for filter insertion (45% of cases), followed by recurrent PE (20% of cases) (101). PE after filter placement was noted in only 4% patients over a 20-year follow-up, the long-term inferior vena caval patency rate was 96% independent of anticoagulation, and venous ulceration was noted in only 3% of patients. No patient with suprarenal filter placement (54 cases) had occlusion of the inferior vena cava or renal veins over the follow-up period.

Percutaneous insertion versus direct surgical technique offers a number of advantages for the Greenfield filter, including decreased patient discomfort, decreased time of insertion, and decreased cost. Using a percutaneous approach with the original 24F carrier, the incidence of venous thrombosis at the insertion site was reported to be as high as 41% (102). In response to this problem, a titanium Greenfield filter with modified hooks was developed that reduced the carrier to a size of 12F in a 14F sheath. Outcomes for 173 patients revealed 97% successful placement, a recurrent PE rate of only 3%, and inferior vena caval occlusion in 1% (103). The venous thrombosis rate at the insertion site was only 2%.

Surgical approaches for pulmonary thromboembolism are indicated in patients who have massive embolism with hypotension and who require large doses of vasopressors. These are often patients in whom thrombolytic agents have been unsuccessful. Open pulmonary embolectomy as practiced in the past is associated with high morbidity and mortality rates. Today, open pulmonary embolectomy is limited to those patients who require cardiac massage manually for hypotension or those who fail catheter pulmonary embolectomy. A catheter for the removal of pulmonary emboli has been developed. Catheter suction pulmonary embolectomy is performed by operative insertion under local anesthesia from either the jugular or common femoral vein. The cup catheter is inserted through a transverse venotomy and the radiopaque catheter is then visualized under fluoroscopy as it is guided into the right side of the heart. The left main pulmonary artery is entered most easily. The cup is juxtaposed to the embolus and syringe suction is used to aspirate the clot into the cup, and the entire catheter and clot are withdrawn. Entry into the right pulmonary artery is performed by deflecting the cup in that direction as it reaches the superior edge of the cardiac shadow. Multiple retrievals may be necessary to remove enough thrombus to improve the pulmonary hemodynamics. In a series of 46 patients treated with this device, emboli were extracted in 76% of cases and the 30-day survival rate was 70% (104). Embolectomy was most successful for major PE and massive PE and least helpful for chronic PE. Successful embolectomy predicted long-term survival. A recent addition to pulmonary embolectomy is placement of the patient on extracorporeal membrane oxygenation to allow the lungs time to recover.

Deep Venous Thrombosis Prophylaxis

Deep venous thrombosis prophylaxis has received intense study in certain conditions, but less-than-adequate coverage in other situations. Risk factors for DVT include age at least 40 years, prolonged immobility or paralysis, prior venous thromboembolism, malignancy, major surgery, obesity, varicose veins, congestive heart failure, myocardial infarction, stroke, major fractures, inflammatory bowel disease, nephrotic syndrome, estrogen use, and indwelling femoral vein cannulae. Hypercoagulable states also increase DVT risk (105). In considering who needs prophylaxis and the type of prophylaxis, it is useful to categorize patients into risk groups: low risk (uncomplicated surgery, <40 years of age with no other risk factors); moderate risk (surgery, 40 to 60 years of age with no additional risk factors; or major surgery, <40 years of age, and no additional risk factors; or minor surgery with additional risk factors); high risk (major surgery, >60 years of age without additional risk factors; or major surgery, 40 to 60 years of age with additional risk factors; or patients with myocardial infarction or medical patients with risk factors); and highest risk (major surgery, >40 years of age, plus prior venous thromboembolism, malignancy, hypercoagulable states, major lower extremity orthopedic surgery, hip fracture, stroke, multiple trauma, or spinal cord injury) (105). The most up-to-date recommendations have been revised and published (105), and form the basis for the description that follows.

Concerning general surgical patients, the incidence of DVT is as high as 25% without prophylaxis. No specific prophylaxis is indicated in low-risk patients other than early ambulation. In moderate-risk patients, appropriate prophylactic regiments include low-dose standard unfractionated heparin (LDUH), LMWH, and intermittent pneumatic compression (IPC) or stocking support. For higher-risk patients, higher-dose LDUH or LMWH or IPC is recommended, whereas for the highest-risk patients, LDUH or LMWH plus IPC is recommended. In these highest-risk cases, full-dose warfarin is also recommended, but few general surgeons are likely to use full-dose oral anticoagulation because of the bleeding potential. Aspirin alone is not recommended for any general surgery patients (105).

For orthopedic patients, routine screening with duplex ultrasound imaging without prophylaxis is not recommended. The incidence of DVT is as high as 40% to 60% for total hip surgery, approximately 40% to 85% for total knee surgery, and approximately 35% to 60% for hip fracture surgery without prophylaxis. For total hip surgery, LMWH (begun after surgery), full-dose warfarin, or adjusted-dose standard unfractionated heparin is recommended. Adjuvant physical modalities may provide additional benefit. For total knee surgery, LMWH, warfarin, or IPC is recommended. For hip fracture surgery, preoperative or postoperative LMWH or warfarin is suggested. The length of prophylaxis is undergoing close scrutiny, and these procedures (especially total hip and total knee replacement) may benefit from prolonged posthospital prophylaxis (105).

For trauma patients, good data are lacking in many areas and more studies are needed. Without prophylaxis, the incidence of DVT may be as high or higher than 50%. Acceptable prophylaxis includes LMWH, IPC, and duplex ultrasound screening if appropriate prophylaxis is not possible (105).

In the area of neurosurgery, IPC is recommended if anticoagulation cannot be used, although combining LDUH or LMWH with IPC may be more effective than either technique alone. For patients with spinal cord injury, LMWH with or without mechanical measures is recommended. Even less is known about certain medical patients. LDUH appears to be effective for patients with myocardial infarction, in whom the incidence of DVT may be as high as 25%, whereas for patients with stroke and lower extremity paralysis, LDUH and LMWH have been recommended. In addition, LDUH and LMWH have been recommended in patients with congestive heart failure or pulmonary infections. It is recommended that low-dose warfarin (1 mg/d) be used in patients with long-term upper body indwelling venous catheters, especially those with malignancy (105). Finally, although inferior vena caval filters have been recommended in high-risk trauma and orthopedic patients with good results in small series, no large, randomized, prospective studies on this technique compared with more standard prophylactic methods have been produced. A warning has been issued by the U.S. Food and Drug Administration concerning heparin prophylaxis, especially LMWH, in the presence of spinal and epidural catheters because of cases of epidural and spinal hematoma formation (106). Developments in this area need to be monitored.

The entire area of venous thrombosis prophylaxis is an area of intense importance and interest. Even with the best current prophylaxis, the incidence of venous thromboembolism is decreased by only approximately 80%. Further developments should allow for even greater declines in the rates of venous thromboembolism with its subsequent short- and long-term sequelae.

ACKNOWLEDGMENTS

The authors acknowledge S. Martin Lindenauer, M.D., for his contributions to this chapter in the first edition of this book.

REFERENCES

1. Chang BB, Paty PS, Shah DM, et al. The lesser saphenous vein: an unappreciated source of autogenous vein. *J Vasc Surg* 1992;15:152.
2. Goidano JM, Trout HH. Anomalies of the inferior vena cava. *J Vasc Surg* 1986;3:924.
3. Sumner DS. Hemodynamics and pathophysiology of venous disease. In: Rutherford RB, ed. *Vascular surgery,* 4th ed. Philadelphia: WB Saunders, 1995:1673.
4. Brand FN, Dannenberg AL, Abbott RD, et al. The epidemiology of varicose veins: the Framingham Study. *Am J Prev Med* 1988;4:96.
5. Hammarsten J, Pedersen P, Cederlund C-G, et al. Long saphenous vein saving surgery for varicose veins: a long-term follow-up. *Eur J Vasc Surg* 1990;4:361.
6. Goren G, Yellin AE. Ambulatory stab evulsion phlebectomy for truncal varicose veins. *Am J Surg* 1991;162:166.
7. Burnham SJ. Varicose veins: patient selection and treatment, In: Rutherford RB, ed. *Vascular surgery,* 3rd ed. Philadelphia: WB Saunders, 1989:1512.
8. Lary BG. Varicose veins and intracutaneous telangiectasia: combined treatment in 1,500 cases. *South Med J* 1987;80:1105.
9. Zierler RE, Strandness DE Jr. Hemodynamics for the vascular surgeon. In: Moore WS, ed. *Vascular surgery: a comprehensive review,* 4th ed. Philadelphia: WB Saunders, 1993:179.
10. Thomas PR, Nash GB, Dormandy JA. White cell accumulation in the dependent legs of patients with venous hypertension: a possible mechanism for trophic changes in the skin. *BMJ* 1988;296:1693.
11. Coleridge Smith PD, Thomas P, Scurr JH, et al. Causes of venous ulceration: a new hypothesis. *BMJ* 1988;296:1726.
12. Wilkinson LS, Bunker C, Edwards JC, et al. Leukocytes: their role in the etiopathogenesis of skin damage in venous disease. *J Vasc Surg* 1993;17:669.
13. Killewich LA, Martin R, Cramer M, et al. Pathophysiology of venous claudication. *J Vasc Surg* 1984;1:507.
14. Bauer G. A roentgenological and clinical study of the sequelae of thrombosis. *Acta Chir Scand Suppl* 1942;74:1.
15. Markel A, Manzo RA, Bergelin RO, et al. Valvular reflux after deep venous thrombosis: incidence and time of occurrence. *J Vasc Surg* 1992;15:377.
16. Sarin S, Scurr JH, Coleridge Smith JD. Mechanism of action of external compression on venous function. *Br J Surg* 1992;79:499.
17. Belcaro G, Grigg M, Vasdekis S, et al. Evaluation of the effects of elastic compression in patients with postphlebitic limbs by laser-Doppler flowmetry. *Phlebology* 1988;41:797.
18. The Alexander House Group. Consensus paper on venous leg ulcer. *J Dermatol Surg Oncol* 1992;18:592.
19. Kikta MJ, Schuler JJ, Meyer JP, et al. A prospective, randomized trial of Unna boot versus hydroactive dressing in the treatment of venous stasis ulcers. *J Vasc Surg* 1988;7:478.
20. Cordts PR, Hanrahan LM, Rodriguez AA, et al. A prospective, randomized trial of Unna boot versus duoderm CGF hydroactive dressing plus compression in management of venous leg ulcers. *J Vasc Surg* 1992;15:480.
21. Christopoulos DG, Nicolaides AN, Szendro G, et al. Air-plethysmography and the effect of elastic compression on venous hemodynamics of the leg. *J Vasc Surg* 1987;5:148.
22. Strandness DE, van Bemmelen P. Quantitation of venous reflux using duplex scanning. In: Bergan JJ, Yao JST, eds. *Venous disorders.* Philadelphia: WB Saunders, 1991:137.
23. Raju S. New approaches to the diagnosis and treatment of venous obstruction. *J Vasc Surg* 1986;4:42.
24. Kistner RL. Diagnosis of chronic venous insufficiency. *J Vasc Surg* 1986;3:185.
25. Ackroyd JS, Lea Thomas M, Brouse NL. Deep vein reflux: an assessment by descending phlebography. *Br J Surg* 1986;73:31.
26. Moore DJ, Himmel PD, Sumner DS. Distribution of venous valvular incompetence in patients with the postphlebitic syndrome. *J Vasc Surg* 1986;3:49.
27. Silver D, Cikrit DF. Operative management of perforator vein incompetence. In: Rutherford RB, ed. *Vascular surgery,* 3rd ed. Philadelphia: WB Saunders, 1989:1608.
28. Rhodes JM, Gloviczki P, Canton L, et al. Endoscopic perforator vein division with ablation of superficial reflux improves venous hemodynamics. *J Vasc Surg* 1998;28:839.
29. Kistner RL. Surgical repair of the incompetent femoral vein valve. *Arch Surg* 1975;110:1336.
30. Raju S. Venous insufficiency of the lower limb and stasis ulceration: changing concepts and management. *Ann Surg* 1983;197:688.
31. Kistner RL, Sparkuhl MD. Surgery in acute and chronic venous disease. *Surgery* 1979;85:31.
32. Ferris EB, Kistner RL. Femoral vein reconstruction in the management of chronic venous insufficiency: a 14-year experience. *Arch Surg* 1982;117:1571.
33. Taheri SA, Lazar L, Elias SM, et al. Vein valve transplant. *Surgery* 1982;91:28.
34. Eriksson I. Reconstructive surgery for deep vein valve incompetence in the lower limb. *Eur J Vasc Surg* 1990;4:211.
35. Bergan JJ, Yao JS, Flinn WR, et al. Surgical treatment of venous obstruction and insufficiency. *J Vasc Surg* 1986;3:174.
36. O'Donnell TF. Popliteal vein valve transplantation for deep venous valvular reflux: rationale, method, and long-term clinical, hemodynamic, and anatomic results. In: Bergan JJ, Yao JST, eds. *Venous disorders.* Philadelphia: WB Saunders, 1991:273.
37. Psathakis N, Psathakis D. Rationale of the substitute valve operation by technique II in the treatment of chronic venous insufficiency. *Int Angiol* 1985;4:397.
38. Binkert CA, Schoch E, Stuckmann G, et al. Treatment of pelvic venous spur (May-Thurner syndrome) with self-expanding metallic endoprostheses. *Cardiovasc Intervent Radiol* 1998;21:22.
39. Mewissen MW. Catheter-directed thrombolysis for lower-extremity deep vein thrombosis: report of a national multi-center registry. *Radiology* 1999;211:39.

40. Lalka SG. Management of chronic obstructive venous disease of the lower extremity. In: Rutherford RB, ed. *Vascular surgery*, 4th ed. Philadelphia: WB Saunders, 1995:1862.

41. Coon WW, Willis PW III, Keller JB. Venous thromboembolism and other venous disease in the Tecumseh community health study. *Circulation* 1973;48:839.

42. Anderson FA Jr, Wheeler HB, Goldberg RJ, et al. A population-based perspective of the hospital incidence and case-fatality rates of deep vein thrombosis and pulmonary embolism: the Worcester DVT Study. *Arch Intern Med* 1991;151:933.

43. Hull RD, Pineo GF, Raskob GE. The economic impact of treating deep vein thrombosis with low molecular-weight heparin: outcome of therapy and health economy aspects. *Haemostasis* 1998;28 [Suppl 3]:8.

44. Douglas MG, Sumner DS. Duplex scanning for deep vein thrombosis: has it replaced both phlebography and noninvasive testing? *Semin Vasc Surg* 1996;9:3.

45. Sarpa MS, Messina LM, Villemure P, et al. Significance of a negative duplex scan in patients suspected of having acute deep venous thrombosis of the lower extremity. *Society for Vascular Technology* 1989;13:224.

46. Anand SS, Wells PS, Hunt D, et al. Does this patient have deep vein thrombosis? *JAMA* 1998;279:1094.

47. Carpenter JP, Holland GA, Baum RA, et al. Magnetic resonance venography for the detection of deep venous thrombosis: comparison with contrast venography and duplex Doppler ultrasonography. *J Vasc Surg* 1993;18:734.

48. Meaney JF, Weg JG, Chenevert TL, et al. Diagnosis of pulmonary embolism with magnetic resonance angiography. *N Engl J Med* 1997;336:1422.

49. Froehlich JB, Prince MR, Greenfield LJ, et al. "Bulls-eye" sign on gadolinium-enhanced magnetic resonance venography determines thrombus presence and age: a preliminary study. *J Vasc Surg* 1997;26:809.

50. PIOPED Investigators. Value of the ventilation/perfusion scan in acute pulmonary embolism: results of the Prospective Investigation of Pulmonary Embolism Diagnosis (PIOPED). The PIOPED Investigators. *JAMA* 1990;263:2753.

51. Worsley DF, Alavi A. Comprehensive analysis of the results of the PIOPED study: prospective investigation of pulmonary embolism diagnosis study. *J Nucl Med* 1995;36:2380.

52. Drucker EA, Rivitz SM, Shepard JA, et al. Acute pulmonary embolism: assessment of helical CT for diagnosis. *Radiology* 1998;209:235.

53. Teigen CL, Maus TP, Sheedy PF, et al. Pulmonary embolism: diagnosis with contrast-enhanced electron-beam CT and comparison with pulmonary angiography. *Radiology* 1995;194:313.

54. Goodman LR, Curtin JJ, Mewissen MW, et al. Detection of pulmonary embolism in patients with unresolved clinical and scintigraphic diagnosis: helical CT versus angiography. *AJR Am J Roentgenol* 1995;164:1369.

55. Remy-Jardin M, Remy J, Wattinne L, et al. Central pulmonary thromboembolism: diagnosis with spiral volumetric CT with the single-breath-hold technique-comparison with pulmonary angiography. *Radiology* 1992;185:381.

56. Remy-Jardin M, Remy J, Deschildre F, et al. Diagnosis of pulmonary embolism with spiral CT: comparison with pulmonary angiography and scintigraphy. *Radiology* 1996;200:699.

57. Khaira HS, Mann J. Plasma D-dimer measurement in patients with suspected DVT: a means of avoiding unnecessary venography. *Eur J Vasc Endovasc Surg* 1998;15:235.

58. Hull R, Delmore T, Genton E, et al. Warfarin sodium versus low-dose heparin in the long-term treatment of venous thrombosis. *N Engl J Med* 1979;301:855.

59. Lagerstedt CI, Olsson CG, Fagher BO, et al. Need for long-term anticoagulant treatment in symptomatic calf-vein thrombosis. *Lancet* 1985;2:515.

60. Kearon C, Hirsh J. Management of anticoagulation before and after elective surgery. *N Engl J Med* 1997;336:1506.

61. Douketis JD, Kearon C, Bates S, et al. Risk of fatal pulmonary embolism in patients with treated venous thromboembolism. *JAMA* 1998;279:458.

62. Hull RD, Raskob GE, Brant RF, et al. Relation between the time to achieve the lower limit of the aPTT therapeutic range and recurrent venous thromboembolism during heparin treatment for deep vein thrombosis. *Arch Intern Med* 1997;157:2562.

63. Hull RD, Raskob GE, Brant RF, et al. The importance of initial heparin treatment on long-term clinical outcomes of antithrombotic therapy: the emerging theme of delayed recurrence. *Arch Intern Med* 1997;157:2317.

64. Hull RD, Raskob GE, Rosenbloom D, et al. Heparin for 5 days as compared with 10 days in the initial treatment of proximal venous thrombosis. *N Engl J Med* 1990;322:1260.

65. Schulman S, Rhedin AS, Lindmarker P, et al. A comparison of six weeks with six months of oral anticoagulant therapy after a first episode of venous thromboembolism. *N Engl J Med* 1995;332:1661.

66. Research Committee of the British Thoracic Society. Optimum duration of anticoagulation for deep-vein thrombosis and pulmonary embolism. *Lancet* 1992;340:873.

67. Levine MN, Hirsh J, Gent M, et al. Optimal duration of oral anticoagulant therapy: a randomized trial comparing four weeks with three months of warfarin in patients with proximal deep vein thrombosis. *Thromb Haemost* 1995;74:606.

68. Hyers TM, Agnelli G, Hull RD, et al. Antithrombotic therapy for venous thromboembolism disease. *Chest* 1998;114:561S.

69. Kearon C, Gent M, Hirsh J, et al. A comparison of three months of anticoagulation with extended anticoagulation for a first episode of idiopathic venous thromboembolism. *N Engl J Med* 1999;340:901.

70. Prandoni P, Lensing AW, Cogo A, et al. The long-term clinical course of acute deep venous thrombosis. *Ann Intern Med* 1996;125:1.

71. Schulamn S, Granqvist S, Holmstrom M, et al. The duration of oral anticoagulant therapy after a second episode of venous thromboembolism: the Duration of Anticoagulation Trial Study Group. *N Engl J Med* 1997;336:393.

72. Hirsh J. Low-molecular-weight heparin: a review of the results of recent studies of the treatment of venous thromboembolism and unstable angina. *Circulation* 1998;98:1575.

73. Clagett GP, Anderson FA Jr, Geerts W, et al. Prevention of venous thromboembolism. *Chest* 1998;114:531S.

74. Leizorovicz A. Comparison of the efficacy and safety of low molecular weight heparins and unfractionated heparin in the initial treatment of deep venous thrombosis: an updated meta-analysis. *Drugs* 1996;52:30.

75. Siragusa S, Cosmi B, Piovella F, et al. Low-molecular-weight heparins and unfractionated heparin in the treatment of patients with acute venous thromboembolism: results of a meta-analysis. *Am J Med* 1996;100:269.

76. Hull RD, Raskob GE, Pineo GF, et al. Subcutaneous low-molecular-weight heparin compared with continuous intravenous heparin in the treatment of proximal-vein thrombosis. *N Engl J Med* 1992;326:975.

77. Levine M, Gent M, Hirsh J, et al. A comparison of low-molecular-weight heparin administered primarily at home with unfractionated heparin administered in the hospital for proximal deep-vein thrombosis. *N Engl J Med* 1996;334:677.

78. Koopman MM, Prandoni P, Piovella F, et al. Treatment of venous thrombosis with intravenous unfractionated heparin administered in the hospital as compared with subcutaneous low-molecular-weight heparin administered at home: the Tasman Study Group. *N Engl J Med* 1996;334:682.

79. Low-molecular-weight heparin in the treatment of patients with venous thromboembolism: the Columbus Investigators. *N Engl J Med* 1997;337:657.

80. Simonneau G, Sers H, Charbonnier B, et al. A comparison of low-molecular-weight heparin with unfractionated heparin for acute pulmonary embolism: the THESSE Study Group. *N Engl J Med* 1997;337:663.

81. Groce JB. Patient outcomes and cost analysis associated with outpatient deep venous thrombosis treatment program. *Pharmacotherapy* 1998;18:175S.

82. Hull RD, Raskob GE, Rosenbloom D, et al. Treatment of proximal vein thrombosis with subcutaneous low-molecular-weight heparin vs. intravenous heparin: an economic perspective. *Arch Intern Med* 1997;157:289.

83. Van den Belt AG, Bossuy PM, Prins MH, et al. Replacing inpatient care by outpatient care in the treatment of deep venous thrombosis: an economic evaluation. *Thromb Haemost* 1998;79:259.

84. Lindmarker P, Holmstrom M. Use of low molecular weight heparin (dalteparin), once daily, for the treatment of deep vein thrombosis: a feasibility and health economic study in an outpatient setting. *J Intern Med* 1996;240:395.

85. Wells PS, Kovacs MJ, Bormanis J, et al. Expanding eligibility for outpatient treatment of deep venous thrombosis and pulmonary embolism with low-molecular-weight heparin. *Arch Intern Med* 1998;158:1809.

86. Harrison L, McGinnis J, Crowther M, et al. Assessment of outpatient treatment of deep-vein thrombosis with low-molecular-weight heparin. *Arch Intern Med* 1998;158:2001.

87. Meissner MH, Caps MT, Bergelin RO, et al. Early outcome after isolated calf vein thrombosis. *J Vasc Surg* 1997;26:749.

88. Meissner MH, Manzo RA, Bergelin RO, et al. Deep venous insufficiency: the relationship between lysis and subsequent reflux. *J Vasc Surg* 1993;18:596.

89. Elliot MS, Immelman EJ, Jeffrey P, et al. A comparative randomized trial of heparin versus streptokinase in the treatment of acute proximal venous thrombosis: an interim report of a prospective trial. *Br J Surg* 1979;66:838.

90. Arnesen H, Hoiseth A, Ly B. Streptokinase or heparin in the treatment of deep vein thrombosis: follow-up results of a prospective study. *Acta Med Scand* 1982;211:65.

91. Semba CP, Dake MD. Iliofemoral deep venous thrombosis: aggressive therapy with catheter-directed thrombolysis. *Radiology* 1994;191:487.

92. National Heart and Lung Institute Cooperative Study Group. Urokinase Pulmonary Embolism Trial: phase 1 results. *JAMA* 1970;214:2163.

93. National Heart and Lung Institute Cooperative Study Group. Urokinase–Streptokinase Embolism Trial: phase 2 results. *JAMA* 1974;229:1606.

94. Turpie AGG. Thrombolytic agents in venous thrombosis. *J Vasc Surg* 1990;12:196.

95. Plate G. Iliofemoral venous thrombectomy—enthusiasm for the contemporary technique. Presented at the American Venous Forum, Dana Point, California, February 18, 1999.

96. Eklof B, Kistner RL. Is there a role for thrombectomy in iliofemoral venous thrombosis? *Semin Vasc Surg* 1996;9:34.

97. Juhan CM, Alimi YS, Barthelemy PJ, et al. Late results of iliofemoral venous thrombectomy. *J Vasc Surg* 1997;25:417.

98. Norris CS, Greenfield LJ, Herrmann JB. Free-floating iliofemoral thrombus: a risk for pulmonary embolism. *Arch Surg* 1985;120:806.

99. Radomski JA, Jarrell BE, Carabasi RA, et al. Risk of pulmonary embolus with inferior vena cava thrombosis. *Am Surg* 1987;53:97.

100. Berry RE, George JE, Shaver WA. Free-floating deep venous thrombosis: a retrospective analysis. *Ann Surg* 1990;211:719.

101. Greenfield LJ, Proctor MC. Twenty-year clinical experience with the Greenfield filter. *Cardiovasc Surg* 1995;3:199.

102. Kantor A, Glanz S, Gordon DH, et al. Percutaneous insertion of the Kimray-Greenfield filter: incidence of femoral vein thrombosis. *AJR Am J Roentgenol* 1987;149:1065.

103. Greenfield LJ, Proctor MC, Cho KJ, et al. Extended evaluation of the titanium Greenfield vena caval filter. *J Vasc Surg* 1994;20:458.

104. Greenfield LJ, Proctor MC, Williams DM, et al. Long-term experience with transvenous catheter pulmonary embolectomy. *J Vasc Surg* 1993;18:450.

105. Clagett GP, Anderson FA Jr, Geerts W, et al. Prevention of venous thromboembolism. *Chest* 1998;114:531S.

106. Lumpkin MM. FDA Alert: FDA public health advisory. *Anesthesiology* 1998;88:27A.

SURGERY: SCIENTIFIC PRINCIPLES AND PRACTICE, Third Edition, edited by Lazar J. Greenfield, Michael W. Mulholland, Keith T. Oldham, Gerald B. Zelenock, and Keith D. Lillemoe. Lippincott Williams & Wilkins Publishers, Philadelphia, © 2001.

CHAPTER 92

CHRONIC VENOUS DISEASE

MICHAEL C. DALSING

Chronic venous disease is a common problem, with estimates suggesting that moderate to severe disease affects approximately six million United States citizens (1). It can be considered a spectrum of disease ranging from a simple telangiectasia to severely symptomatic, nonhealing or recurrent venous ulcers. A renewed interest in this disorder has resulted in some novel surgical approaches to therapy.

VENOUS FUNCTION MEASUREMENT

The physiologic study of venous function during exercise involves ambulatory venous pressure (AVP) measurements (Fig. 92.1). The venous filling time is the time it takes to arrive at a steady-state pressure after rising from the supine position. Performance of 10 tiptoe maneuvers at 1 step per second results in a drop in pressure called the *AVP*, which is normally less than 45 mm Hg. The time it takes after this exercise to reach the baseline erect pressure is called the venous refilling time (VRT), and is greater than 20 seconds in a normal extremity. Sometimes 90% of this time (VRT$_{90}$) is determined to eliminate the difficulty in accurately determining the precise termination of the rising pressure slope.

PATHOPHYSIOLOGY AND ETIOLOGY

Three pathophysiologic states exist: venous obstruction, venous valvular insufficiency, and calf muscle pump malfunction (2). These conditions reflect a failure of one or more of the components of the normal venous system, may be seen in combination, and are not mutually exclusive.

Venous outflow obstruction results in an increased resistance to venous blood flow. It is the major hemodynamic problem in 15% of chronic venous disease cases (3,4). The result is elevated pressure within the venous system, usually noted after exercise. If the deep system is primarily involved, the increased pressure generated with each calf compression affects the communicating veins, whose valves ultimately malfunction. This leads to venous hypertension in the superficial venous system and its capillary network. Primary causes of venous obstruction are very uncommon, whereas secondary venous outflow obstruction is often the result of venous thrombosis. Extrinsic causes of lower extremity venous obstruction include compression of the iliac and pelvic veins by tumor, fibrosis, or infection. Left common iliac vein compression by the right common iliac artery, as well as external iliac vein compression from the internal iliac artery on either side, have been described (5,6). Contents of a femoral hernia can crush the femoral vein, as can soft tissue tumors limited to the thigh. Aneurysms of the common, superficial, or deep femoral artery can impinge on the femoral vein. The popliteal vein can be obstructed by a popliteal aneurysm or Baker's cyst (2). Intraluminal sources of outflow obstruction, with the exception of venous thrombosis, are even less common. Absence of the vein (aplasia) or tumors of the vein wall (leiomyomata) have been described (2). Intraluminal webs have been reported to occur in conjunction with right iliac artery compression of the left iliac vein in 14% to 30% of cases (5).

Valvular insufficiency may occur in any of the three lower extremity venous systems. It accounts for approxi-

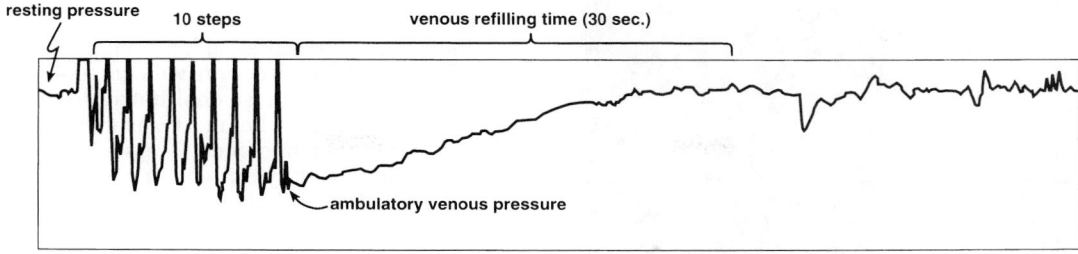

Figure 92.1. A normal ambulatory intravenous pressure measurement study. The pressure scale on the y axis runs from 0 mm Hg at baseline to 100 mm Hg at the top. The resting pressure is 85 mm Hg. With 10 steps, the pressure drops to 30 mm Hg [ambulatory venous pressure (AVP)]. The venous system refills in 30 seconds to the baseline standing pressure.

mately 85% of cases of symptomatic chronic venous disease, with an approximately 70% incidence of primarily superficial and 30% primarily deep venous insufficiency (3,4). Valvular incompetence and resulting reflux allow the transmission of high venous pressures to the lower leg while standing. In addition, this high pressure is not adequately relieved by exercise. Primary valvular insufficiency can occur as a consequence of congenital absence of valves, a rare etiology (7). Venous valve prolapse (elongated, floppy valves) or defects in the vein wall itself that cause the valve ring to dilate can result in valve cusps that do not coapt adequately (8,9). Approximately 40% to 70% of deep vein valvular dysfunction is the result of deep venous thrombosis (DVT), whereas the remainder appear to be of primary etiology (3,10). The inflammation and thrombosis of DVT with resulting valve scarring can result in valve damage regardless of whether the recanalization process is complete. In fact, some valves not affected by the actual thrombi are found to be incompetent. This may result from release of local inflammatory mediators in combination with a susceptible vein valve and wall (11). The smooth muscle dilating effect of estrogens has been cited as a factor in the genesis of varicose veins noted in the first trimester (2). Prolonged exposure to high venous pressures can cause the vein to dilate, resulting in valve cusp malfunction. Such high pressures can result from an arteriovenous fistula or from prior proximal valve damage with resultant pressure on and subsequent failure of more distal valves. Occupations requiring prolonged periods of standing may place the patient at risk.

Finally, there can be failure of the calf muscle pump, analogous to congestive heart failure. Eventually, the pump is unable to generate the force necessary to eject blood from the leg while standing, resulting in sustained lower limb venous hypertension. Elderly patients with expected muscle wasting and patients with muscle disuse (e.g., paraplegia, traumatic injury, or bedridden patients) may not have sufficient muscle for effective exercise (2). Pathologic conditions that result in muscle fibrosis (e.g., muscular dystrophy, multiple sclerosis) can destroy the calf muscle pump. Thrombus and scarring in the gastrocnemius and soleal veins can prevent blood from entering the pump itself, resulting in a deficient ejection volume with each contraction.

The most obvious sequelae of venous stasis and hypertension, regardless of etiology, are the typical changes observed in the end organ (lower leg skin and subcutaneous tissues). Many theories have been proposed to explain these changes (12). Originally, ischemia was considered the cause of skin ulceration. An early hypothesis suggested that stasis of venous blood resulted in poorly oxygenated blood in the distal leg. However, venous blood in chronic venous disease is actually oxygen rich. Several years later, a fibrin cuff was

observed around capillaries in affected limbs that was thought to inhibit oxygen diffusion. However, fibrin is not a deterrent to oxygen diffusion. When standing, patients with chronic venous disease also were found to have "trapped" white blood cells in the leg. Activation of these white blood cells could generate an inflammatory reaction, endothelial cell damage, plugging of capillary flow, and subsequent areas of ischemia, but investigators have never directly observed white blood cells obstructing capillary flow. More recent observations suggest that, far from being just an ischemic event, the end-organ response to venous hypertension is a highly dynamic process. The final answer is likely to involve a complex interaction of multiple factors that favor either continued destruction or ultimate wound healing. Leukocytes, the extracellular matrix, fibroblasts, and a host of other factors are recruited initially to heal an early endothelial injury and later a soft-tissue injury (12). The soft-tissue injury may result in a chronic ulcer that requires the addition of growth factors to force the process to healing (13). Much research is underway to understand these complex interactions.

CLINICAL SIGNS AND SYMPTOMS

Venous disease presents in many ways. Spider veins, also known as *telangiectases,* appear as fine, blue-red branchings just under the surface of the skin. The patient complaint is cosmetic, but each spider vein can be accompanied by a larger, more deeply located, pathologic vein.

Varicose veins are observed in 15% to 20% of the adult population (14). Hereditary varicose veins usually appear during the second decade of life. If a secondary etiology is involved (e.g., thrombosis, trauma), the varicosities appear several years after the inciting event. These veins are bluish, dilated, serpentine, and palpable protrusions lying beneath the skin. They may appear alone or in clusters distributed along the greater or lesser saphenous veins and their branches. Symptoms vary from a dull ache and itching to edema, nocturnal cramping, and eventually skin damage. Fatigue, heaviness, and even mild to moderate pain in the affected limb may be reported.

Chronic venous disease can result in pain, edema, hyperpigmentation, stasis dermatitis or eczema, and finally venous ulcers (Fig. 92.2). These changes usually occur in the "gaiter" area just above the medial malleolus. The largest number of perforating veins are in this area. The observed hyperpigmentation is thought to result from extruded red blood cells that are degraded by macrophages, leaving residual hemosiderin.

Critical to proper patient management and to evaluation of any therapy is an accurate classification of the patient's disease at any given time. A new nomenclature for chronic venous disease involves a clinical (C), etiologic (E),

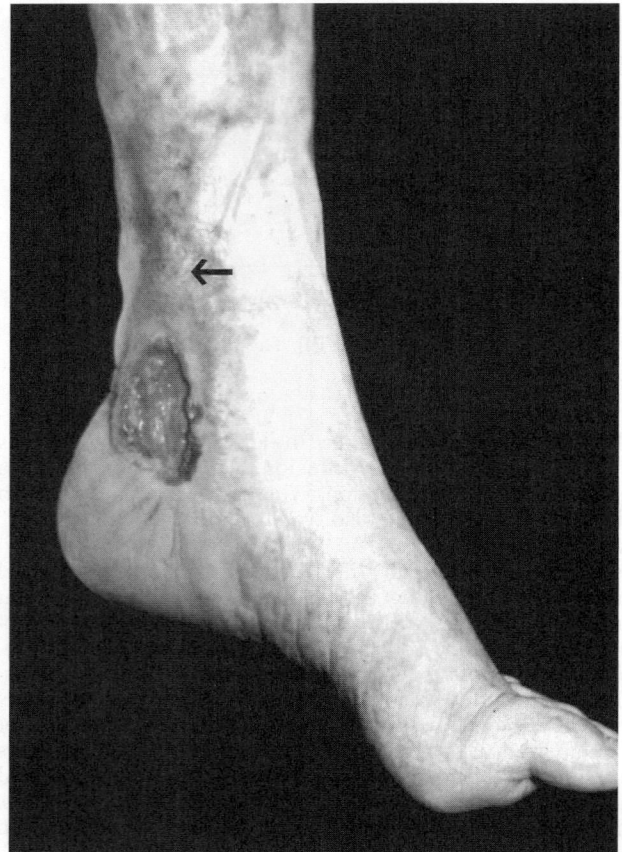

Figure 92.2. Typical venous ulcer located in the medial malleolar area. Note the hyperpigmented skin above and around the ulcer *(arrow),* probably resulting from the local breakdown of red blood cells and deposition of residual hemosiderin.

anatomic (A), and pathophysiologic (P) classification (15). The clinical classification is shown in Table 92.1 and is combined with a subscript of "A" for asymptomatic or "S" for symptomatic patients. The etiology can be congenital (C); primary (P), signifying an undetermined cause; or secondary (S), signifying a known cause (e.g., DVT). The basic anatomic classifications are superficial (S), perforating (P), and/or deep (D) disease. Pathophysiologic classes are reflux (R) and/or obstruction (O). Each classification component can be made very specific, even dealing with individual veins.

Venous claudication is a pain syndrome experienced when a patient with venous obstruction exercises. It is associated with cyanosis, a sensation of increased swelling, and increased prominence of the superficial veins. Killewich and associates differentiated the pain of venous

Table 92.1. CLINICAL CLASSIFICATION CHRONIC VENOUS DISEASE

Class	Description
0	No signs
1	Telangiectases/reticular veins
2	Varicose veins
3	Edema
4	Skin changes (hyperpigmentation, eczema, lipodermatosclerosis)
5	Class 4 and healed ulcers
6	Class 4 and active ulcers

claudication from the pain of arterial insufficiency by noting a relief of symptoms with rest in combination with elevation of the extremities rather than dangling of the legs (16). Some patients function well in their everyday routine, whereas others are so debilitated that amputation has been requested (6). The most severe form is observed when venous incompetence is associated with obstruction. The signs and symptoms of obstruction are further related to the level of the obstruction and the number and size of collaterals (17). A more proximal obstruction (e.g., iliac vein) is associated with worse symptoms because of the decreased potential for adequate collateral formation.

DIAGNOSTIC EVALUATION

The diagnosis of venous disease begins with a thorough history and physical examination. A family history of venous disease and past episodes of DVT should be noted. Symptoms of leg swelling and pain associated with standing or exercise and relieved by elevation are typical. The physical presence of varicose veins confirms venous disease as one component of the patient's disease process. Edema and pain with standing are the two most common signs and symptoms of chronic venous disease, whereas hyperpigmentation and venous ulcers are more advanced signs.

Ambulatory venous pressure measurements can aid the diagnosis of venous insufficiency, but are invasive. An abnormal VRT (<20 seconds) indicates malfunctioning venous valves allowing rapid reflux of blood into the lower extremity after exercise. Blood pressure cuffs placed above and below the knee as well as at the ankle can be inflated to compress the greater saphenous vein, the lesser saphenous vein, and essentially all superficial and perforator veins affecting the ankle area. This localizes the reflux to either the superficial or perforating venous system if correction of the VRT occurs during one or more of the sequential cuff inflations. If the VRT does not normalize with cuff inflations, the deep system is involved. The arm–foot pressure differential study developed by Raju is a quantitative measurement of venous obstruction (18). Intravenous catheters are placed in both the hand and the foot. In the supine patient, intravenous pressures are measured simultaneously in the hand and foot and then after a 3-minute thigh cuff occlusion. A normal reading after this induced reactive hyperemia is an arm–foot differential of less than 4 mm Hg. With venous obstruction, the pressure difference can range from 6 to 20 mm Hg (18). If the AVP is abnormally high on a consistent basis, regardless of the cause, the sequelae of chronic venous disease are likely (19). Although intravenous pressure measurements were once the gold standard for evaluating venous disease, duplex scanning and plethysmographic techniques are the anatomic and functional tests of choice in current medical practice (20).

Plethysmography can assess the venous system indirectly. There are several plethysmographic techniques and all detect changes in blood volume. Obstruction can be determined by evaluating venous capacitance and the rate of venous outflow. Impedance plethysmography measures changes in volume by detecting changes in electrical resistance. Patients lie on a table and bilateral thigh cuffs are positioned for venous occlusion while electrodes placed on the lower leg measure changes in volume (resistance). A baseline reading is obtained before bilateral thigh cuff inflation to approximately 50 mm Hg and after volume measurement stabilization. The thigh cuffs are rapidly deflated and the time to return to baseline volume is noted. Venous capacitance is determined by calculating the change in volume over time and comparing the result with

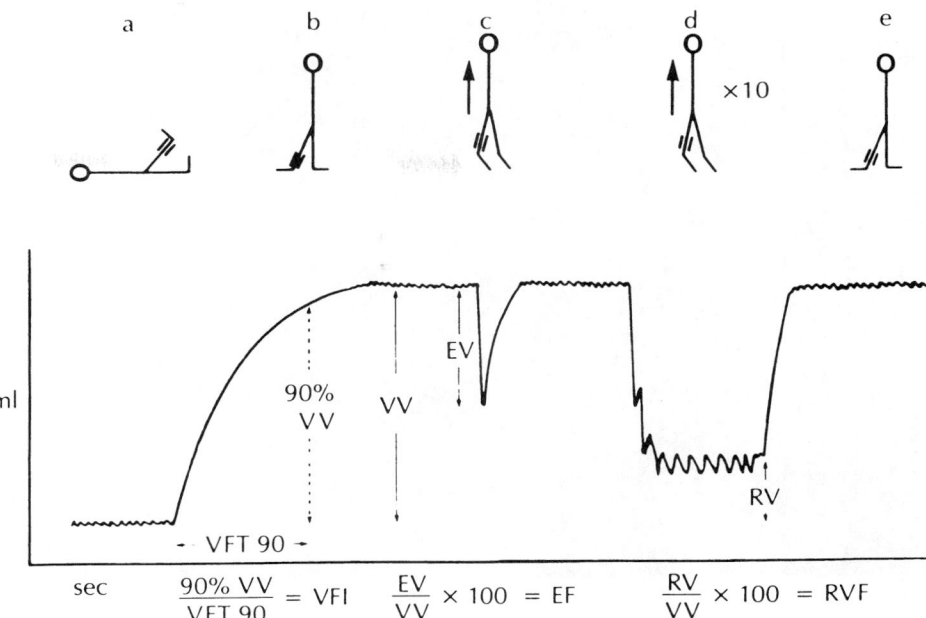

Figure 92.3. Patient wearing an air plethysmographic (APG) boot with volume changes observed during the standard sequence of positional change and exercise. The patient is initially supine with the leg at a 45-degree elevation (a). The patient assumes a standing position with weight on the free leg (b). Ten tiptoe raises are performed (d) after an initial single step (c). The patient returns to the resting position (e). VV, functional venous volume; VFT, venous filling time; VFI, venous filling index; EV, ejection volume; RV, residual volume, EF, ejection fraction; RVF, residual volume fraction. (Reprinted with permission from Christopoulos D, Nicholaides AN, Szendro G, et al. Air plethysmography and the effect of elastic compression on venous hemodynamics of the leg. *J Vasc Surg,* 1987;5:148–159.)

$$\frac{90\% \ VV}{VFT \ 90} = VFI \qquad \frac{EV}{VV} \times 100 = EF \qquad \frac{RV}{VV} \times 100 = RVF$$

a standard set of normal values (21). Values outside normal readings suggest venous obstruction.

Light reflex rheography, like photophlethysmography, can measure VRT. A small photocell is placed on the patient's ankle. The time for venous refill is measured after 10 tiptoe maneuvers. Changes in blood volume are detected as changes in light absorption and reflection. With the use of tourniquets, a rough localization of reflux is possible, much like that noted with intravenous pressure measurements. Reflux is considered to be present if the VRT is less than 20 seconds (21).

Air plethysmography can measure several venous hemodynamic parameters. A plastic cylinder filled with air is fitted over the calf and foot. Changes in leg volume with positional change or exercise are detected by pressure changes in the cylinder (Fig. 92.3). A venous filling index of 2 mL/s or less is indicative of competent venous valves (20,22). Tourniquets may help to localize the venous insufficiency if an abnormal value is obtained. After an erect baseline reading, patients exercise by dorsiflexion or heel raises to empty the calf veins. The ejection fraction is the amount of blood propelled cephalad with a single muscle contraction. After a series of 10 ankle flexions, the volume remaining in the leg is referred to as the residual volume. The residual volume fraction is relatively equivalent to the ambulatory venous pressure. An ejection fraction of

greater than 60% and residual volume fraction of less than 35% suggests that the calf pump is working well (22). Figure 92.4 demonstrates measurement of an outflow fraction that can be correlated with venous obstruction. A normal value is greater than 38% (22). Because plethysmography does not provide an anatomic image of the venous system or evaluation of individual venous valve function, many physicians combine one or the other of these studies with ultrasonography to complete the venous evaluation.

Ultrasonographic techniques provide a direct, noninvasive evaluation of the vascular system. A continuous-wave (CW) Doppler uses sound waves generated by a piezoelectric crystal and directed into the body to evaluate the underlying veins. The clinician can determine blood flow velocity and other flow parameters by determining the frequency shift as the sound wave reflects off flowing blood. If no signal is obtained, the vein is occluded. Valve incompetency is demonstrated as a retrograde surge of blood in a vein segment after a Valsalva maneuver, after compressing a proximal vein segment to force blood retrograde, or after distal leg compression and release. One problem with a CW Doppler examination is the inability to know precisely which vein is being evaluated because no visual picture of the vein is possible.

Duplex scanning uses B-mode imaging in addition to Doppler spectral analysis. B-mode imaging (Fig. 92.5) uses

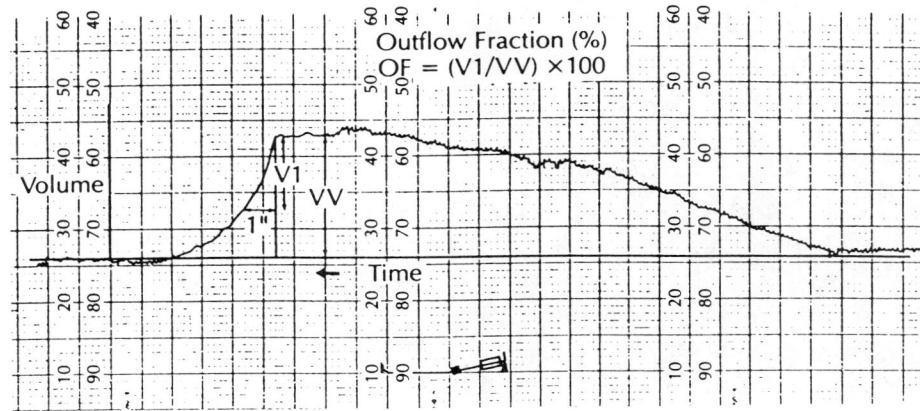

Figure 92.4. Typical venous outflow curve observed in a patient wearing an air plethysmographic device. VV represents the venous volume resulting from inflation of a proximal thigh cuff to 80 mm Hg. V1 is the decrease in venous volume during the first second after thigh cuff deflation. (Reprinted with permission from Nicolaides AN, Christopoulos D. Quantification of venous reflux and outflow obstruction with air-plethysmography. In: Bernstein EF, ed. *Vascular diagnosis.* St. Louis: Mosby, 1993:915–921.)

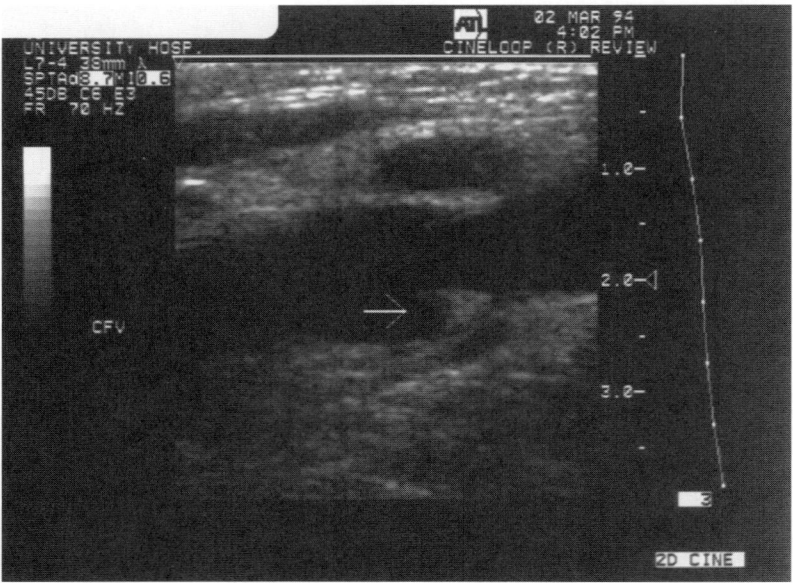

Figure 92.5. B-mode image of a common femoral vein with valve visualized *(arrow)*.

ultrasound to create a picture of the vein being examined. In combination with color flow analysis, long segments of vein can be imaged for easier evaluation of obstructed segments. It can provide anatomic details useful for planning surgical procedures. Venous obstruction appears as a segment of vein devoid of flow signal. Acute thrombosis causes inflammation of the vein, resulting in venous distention, whereas chronic occlusion causes fibrosis of the vein, resulting in a smaller-than-normal venous caliber. Calcifications may be present in a chronic thrombus and recanalization of veins is often observed. Spectral analysis (Fig. 92.6) allows a determination of venous valve incompetence with the maneuvers described for CW Doppler studies. A reflux time of more than 1 second is considered abnormal when routine compression maneuvers are used (23). With the use of a rapidly inflating and deflating calf tourniquet, an abnormal reflux time is greater than 0.5 second (24). The precise visualization with duplex scanning allows evaluation even of perforating veins. Incompetent perforating veins are observed in approximately two thirds of patients with a clinical classification of 4 or higher (23).

Ascending contrast venography produces an anatomic road map of the entire venous system before anticipated surgical procedures. An intravenous catheter is placed into a foot vein and contrast medium is injected to fill the venous system. If the deep system does not fill with dye, DVT may be present. To ensure filling of the deep system, tourniquets applied at the ankle and thigh force the contrast agent into the deep system, bypassing the superficial veins. The deep veins may simply have been damaged from previous disease, and the higher resistance makes the contrast preferentially flow into the superficial veins before the use of tourniquets.

Descending venography is used to detect valvular incompetence before planned surgical intervention. The study is performed by entering a separate uninvolved vein (e.g.,

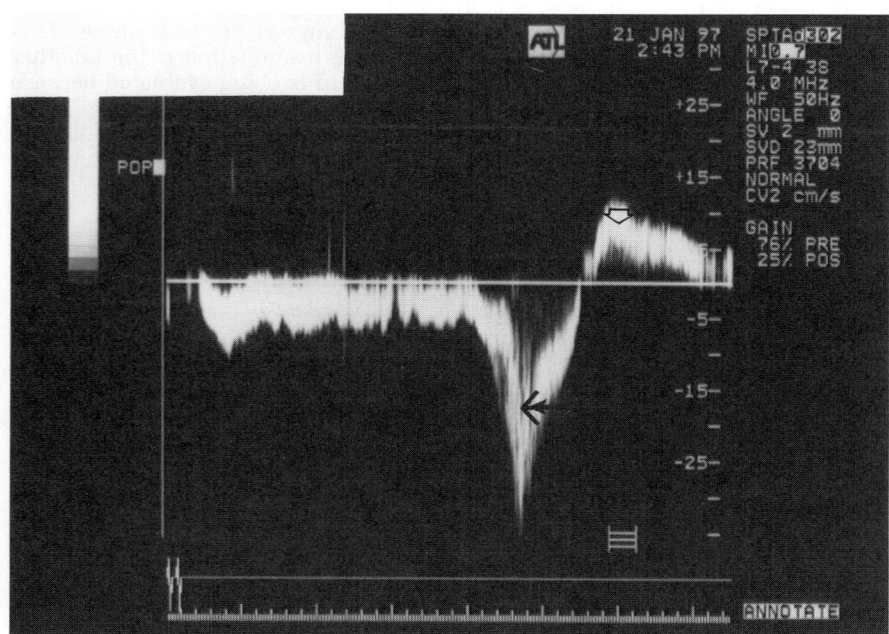

Figure 92.6. Spectral histogram obtained during duplex scanning of a popliteal vein. Initially, a normal phasic wave pattern is seen associated with breathing. Calf compression propels blood toward the heart *(double arrow)*. The reverse blood flow *(open arrowhead)* is consistent with venous valve reflux and lasts for well over 1.5 seconds in this example.

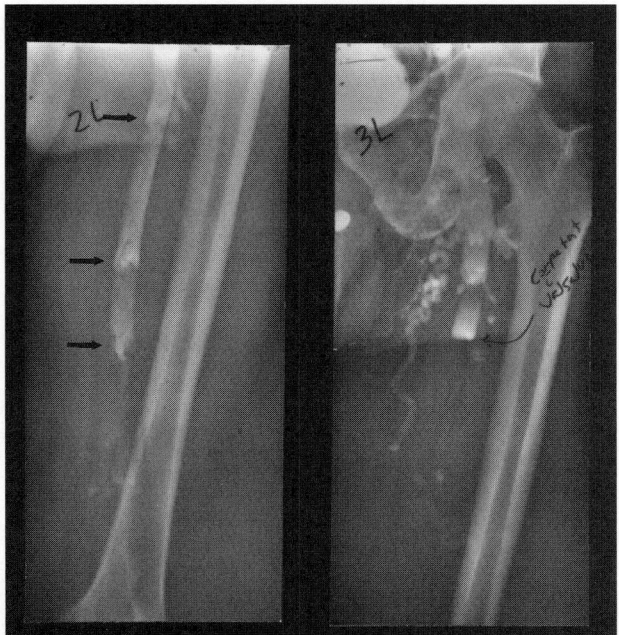

Figure 92.7. Venograms demonstrating the outline of venous valves *(arrows)* during the initial stage of a descending venogram (2L). Competence of a superficial femoral vein valve after a Valsalva maneuver (3L) is demonstrated during the second stage of this patient's venographic study.

brachial or contralateral femoral vein) and manipulating a catheter to the involved common femoral vein. The initial stage of this two-stage procedure involves injecting contrast medium while the patient is at rest and in a semierect position, with the patient's weight on the opposite leg (25). The contrast medium is heavier than blood and gently refluxes down the leg, outlining any valves that may be present (Fig. 92.7, left). The second stage is performed by injection of contrast dye while the patient performs a Valsalva maneuver (25). Competent valves prevent reflux (Fig. 92.7, right), whereas incompetent valves allow reflux down the leg. Reflux is considered pathologic if blood reaches the calf veins (Fig. 92.8). The presence or absence of valves has surgical implications.

TREATMENT OPTIONS AND RESULTS

Conservative Medical Therapy

The main goals of medical therapy are to treat symptoms and establish an acceptable hemodynamic environment that controls edema. Patient compliance is required for optimal results because lifestyle modifications may be demanding. Requirements include wearing good-quality compressive stockings (graded 20 to 30 mm Hg at the ankle), elevating the foot of the bed (4 to 6 inches), elevating the feet several times daily, and applying medicated bandages to ulcerations when necessary. Surgical therapy should be considered if it can be accomplished with minimal risk and optimal benefit, or when medical therapy has failed.

Sclerotherapy

Sclerotherapy involves percutaneous injection of caustic solutions directly into the diseased vein. It has been advocated for the treatment of small varicosities (≤2 mm) remaining after saphenous vein stripping, small individual varicosities, and telangiectases in the thigh and around the knee. Sclerosing agents induce an inflammatory reaction that can eliminate the veins as a result of scar formation. Patients may complain of burning, stinging, or itching on injection. If there is extravasation of the agent, fat or skin necrosis, ulcerations, or hyperpigmentation of the surrounding skin may result. The posttreatment veins are often brownish as opposed to the blue-red natural color. Allergic reaction and toxicity may occur (14). Major venous insufficiency must be controlled to prevent recurrence after sclerotherapy (26).

Vein Stripping

For major superficial venous insufficiency, high ligation and stripping of the varicosities can be used. It should not be considered if significant deep venous obstruction of the femoral or popliteal system exists because the superficial veins may be the only outflow for venous blood. However, it may be considered in cases of combined deep and superficial insufficiency (27). Before surgery, with the patient standing to dilate the veins

Figure 92.8. Descending venogram demonstrating a grade 4 reflux with Valsalva maneuver. Note that the blood cascades past the popliteal vein and into the distal leg. Deep venous surgery usually is not considered necessary unless at least a grade 3 reflux is demonstrated. The grading system for a descending venogram is as follows: grade 0 = no reflux; grade 1 = a wisp limited to the thigh; grade 2 = reflux in thigh only; grade 3 = mild/moderate reflux in thigh and into calf; grade 4 = cascading reflux in thigh and down calf veins (25).

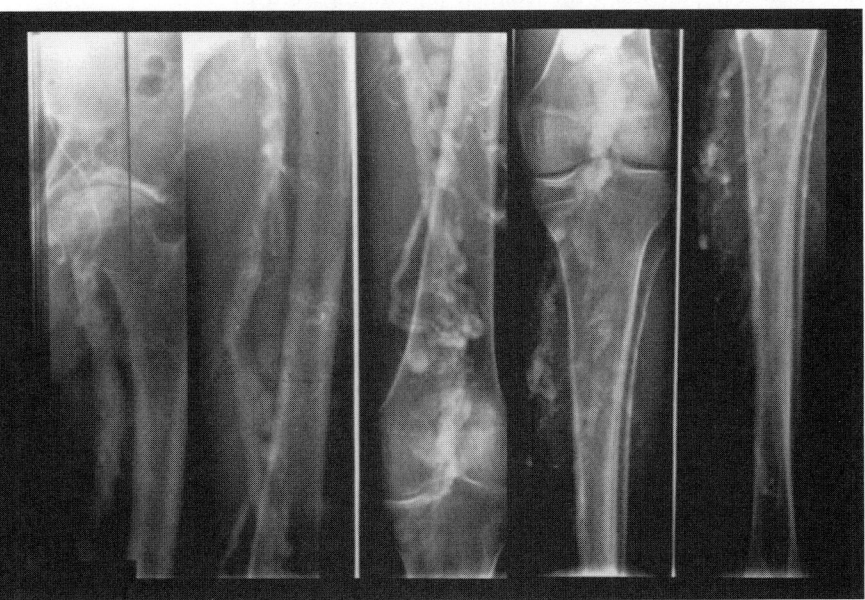

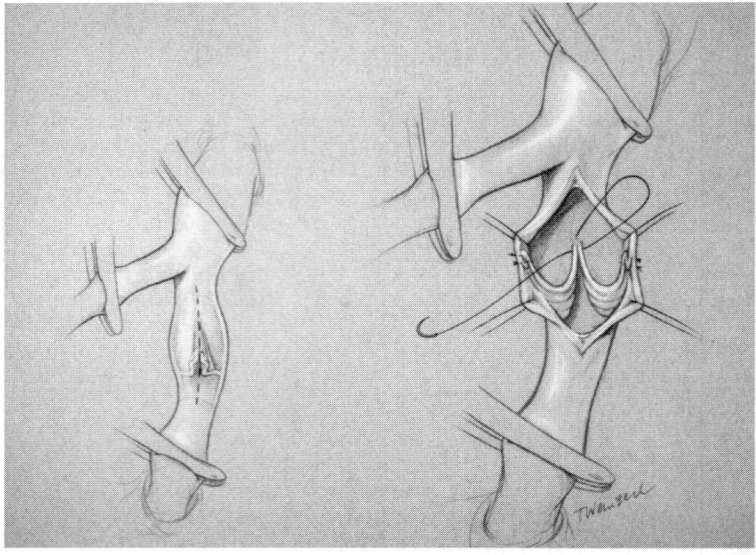

Figure 92.9. Artist's depiction of a venous valve repair by the method of Kistner. The valve is originally redundant and does not prevent reflux *(a, left)*. The vein has been opened through a venous valve commissure and the valve cusps are tightened with appropriately placed fine suture *(b, right)*. The vein will be closed and checked for competence at the end of the procedure.

fully, the varicosities are marked with a permanent marker for intraoperative identification. The saphenofemoral junction is dissected through a groin incision and all branches are ligated. A thin, flexible cable (the vein stripper) is passed up the lumen of the saphenous vein and used to extract the vein. Small stab incisions are made over previously marked branch varicosities for their removal. An elastic bandage is applied in the immediate postoperative period to prevent hematoma formation. Patients are able to resume activities as tolerated but should avoid prolonged periods of standing or heavy lifting for several weeks. Although complications are rare, they include wound infection, DVT, nerve damage (e.g., saphenous nerve), and hematoma formation. Recurrent varicosities are noted in less than 15% of properly selected cases (28). The lesser saphenous vein can be stripped if needed with similar results. Damage to the sural nerve must be minimized during this procedure.

Perforator Vein Ligation

Ligation of perforating veins can be effective treatment for those few patients with isolated perforating vein incompetence. This can also be useful in conjunction with saphenous vein ligation and stripping or deep venous reconstruction. A standard or modified Linton procedure uses an incision along the medial or posterior aspect of the leg with creation of subfascial flaps and direct ligation of the perforating veins as well as skin grafting of large ulcers, if present. An endoscopic technique has also been described (29). Through two small incisions on the medial aspect of the lower leg, a subfascial dissection is performed using balloon dilatation or direct dissection. Some surgeons use a proximal tourniquet to improve visualization and prevent air embolism. Many surgeons mark the perforating veins before surgery with duplex scanning to ensure that all perforating veins are identified and divided at the time of surgery.

Venous Bypass

Cross-femoral venous bypass, saphenofemoral bypass, iliac vein decompression, and inferior vena caval reconstruction have been used to bypass obstructed segments of the venous system. Endovascular stenting has improved symptoms in certain venous occlusive situations (30). Di-

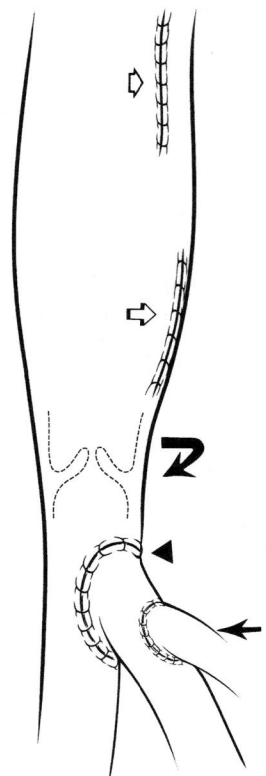

Figure 92.10. Artist's rendition of a transposition operation demonstrating a competent profunda femoral valve *(curved arrow)*, below which has been sewn the superficial femoral vein *(arrowhead)* to which the greater saphenous vein *(arrow)* has been attached surgically. The uppermost suture line is where the saphenous vein had been removed *(small open arrow)*, whereas the lower is the oversewn stump of the superficial femoral vein *(larger open arrow)*. This is just one possibility because the greater saphenous or superficial femoral vein could contain the competent valve below which the incompetent venous system(s) could be attached.

rect venous pressure measurements are required to determine which patients are appropriate candidates for surgery (31).

These surgical procedures use either saphenous vein or a polytetrafluoroethylene (PTFE) conduit to bypass the obstructed venous segment. Vena caval reconstructions usually use PTFE grafts. Left common iliac vein decompression for extrinsic compression by the overlying right iliac artery is usually corrected by direct repair of the involved iliac vein.

The indications for cross-femoral venous bypass include persistent symptomatic unilateral iliac or common femoral venous occlusion in young patients, extrinsic compression not amenable to direct surgical repair, and patients with threatened limb loss due to phlegmasia cerulea dolens in whom thrombectomy or thrombolysis has failed. Long-term patient survival should be considered before aggressive surgical intervention when a malignancy is involved. The cross-femoral venous bypass is

performed by passing the saphenous vein or graft material through a suprapubic subcutaneous tunnel. The key to success appears to be bypass diameter. If the native vein is less than 5 to 6 mm in diameter, greater hemodynamic success is achieved with an 8-mm diameter PTFE graft (31). An arteriovenous fistula is a common adjunctive technique to promote patency and can be ligated in 1 to 3 months if desired. The clinical success rate is reported to be approximately 60% to 70% at 5 years (4).

A saphenopopliteal bypass is performed for isolated superficial femoral or popliteal vein occlusion. The common femoral and iliocaval system must be patent, an ipsilateral nonvaricosed saphenous vein must exist, and femoral thrombosis must be inactive for 1 year to consider this procedure optimal. The procedure uses autogenous vein as the conduit and bypasses extend from distal to proximal nondiseased segments. Clinical success has been reported in 50% to 60% of cases at 5 years, with a patency rate of approximately 60% (4).

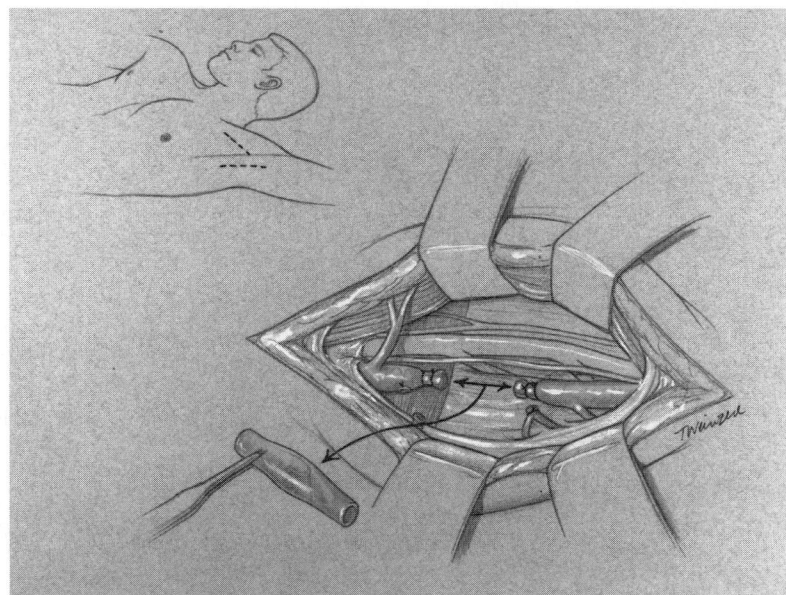

A

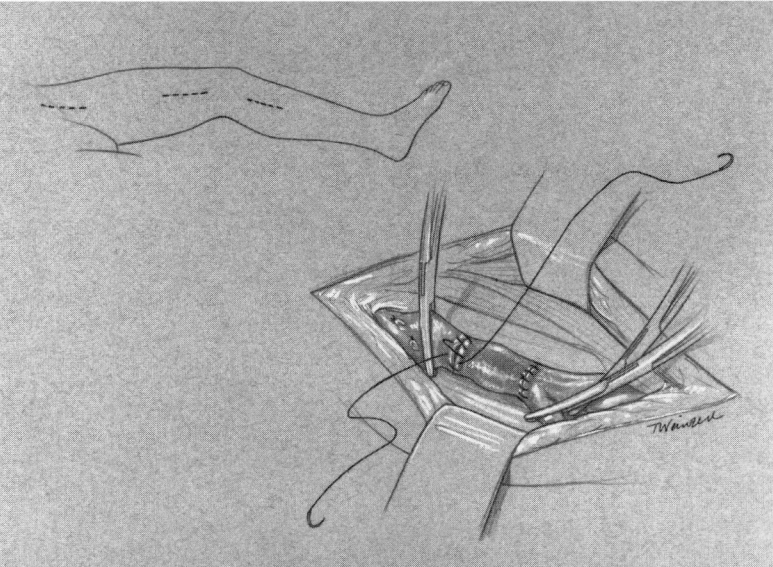

Figure 92.11. Venous valve transplantation operation. *(A)* A vein containing a competent valve is removed from the axillary area. *(B)* The vein with valve, appropriately positioned to prevent reflux, is sewn into a lower leg vein.

B

Venous Valve Repair or Replacement

To be clinically effective, each of the procedures considered under valve repair or replacement must address all pathologic reflux affecting the calf. If the profunda femoral vein has competent valves, a superficial femoral vein valve repair may be reasonable (32). Otherwise, both profunda and superficial femoral incompetence must be addressed simultaneously or repair performed in the popliteal area, the "gatekeeper" of the calf venous system (32). In addition, any superficial or perforator disease should be corrected before deep venous reconstruction to ensure that the patient's symptoms are not corrected by these less invasive procedures.

Direct venous valve repair can be performed for primary venous valvular incompetence. The valvuloplasty procedure is reserved for end-stage disease because of a perceived high risk of both operative failure and DVT. These operations restore the normal anatomic position of the valve cusps so that normal valve function is possible. A variety of open techniques have been described. In one case, the vein is opened and fine Prolene sutures are used to tighten the valve cusps so they appose properly (Fig. 92.9). Angioscopy can be used for valvuloplasty to avoid a valvulotomy. The angioscope is placed through a side branch, allowing direct viewing of the incompetent valve during repair. Fine Prolene sutures are used to reef the valve cusps. Advantages to the angioscopic technique include decreased operative time, direct visualization of the valvuloplasty repair, and less venous trauma (33). These procedures are not free of risks, including wound hematoma, wound infection, seroma formation, thrombosis of the repaired valve, and recurrent reflux (10). However, concern over DVT (<5%) and recurrent reflux (~30% at 5 years) as a reason to withhold treatment from these severely disabled patients has not been substantiated in the literature (10). Long-term results have demonstrated that approximately 70% of patients can achieve clinical success with confirmed valve competence after valve repair procedures (4). Usually, if the valve fails, recurrent symptoms are noted.

The use of a transposition procedure or venous valve transplant has been reserved for patients with more severe damage of the venous valves in one or more lower limb systems. The transposition procedure requires the presence of at least one competent valve. The incompetent venous system (often the superficial femoral vein) is ligated proximally and the distal vein is reattached below an available competent valve (Fig. 92.10). This is possible in approximately 2% to 3% of potential patients (34). Good clinical results have been reported in 40% to 50% of patients at 5 or more years of follow-up (4). Venous valve transplantation requires removing a competent axillary valve-containing vein segment (occasionally a brachial vein valve) and transplanting it into the lower leg (Fig. 92.11). The major obstacles to this procedure are the absence of a functional upper extremity valve (40% of cases) (34) or incompetence of the transplanted valve over time (35). Nevertheless, approximately 50% of patients severely disabled before surgery have been clinically improved for over 5 years with this approach (4). Current investigations using a cryopreserved venous valved allograft may provide a valve substitute for patients lacking an appropriate autogenous venous valve for transplantation (36). The 6-month primary competency rate is approximately 60%, with six of nine patients free of recurrent ulceration. There are no long-term data available.

SUMMARY

Chronic venous disease remains a major health problem as the new millennium begins. The mainstays of therapy include elevation and compression to reduce tissue edema. When one or more of the complications of chronic venous disease occurs, the most conservative measures should be attempted first. If these are to no avail, there are several operative therapies available that have been shown to be effective in properly selected patients.

REFERENCES

1. Coon WW, Willis PW III, Keller JB. Venous thromboembolism and other venous disease in the Tecumseh community health study. *Circulation* 1973;48:839–846.
2. Browse NL, Burnand KG, Thomas ML. *Disease of the veins: pathology, diagnosis, and treatment.* London: Edward Arnold, 1988.
3. O'Donnell TF. Chronic venous insufficiency: an overview of epidemiology, classification, and anatomic considerations. *Semin Vasc Surg* 1988;1:60–65.
4. Eklof BG, Kistner RL, Masuda E. Venous bypass and valve reconstruction: long-term efficacy. *Vasc Med* 1998;3:157–164.
5. Lalka, SG. Management of chronic obstructive venous disease of the lower extremity. In: Rutherford RB, ed. *Vascular surgery,* 4th ed. Philadelphia: WB Saunders, 1995: 1862–1882.
6. Crockett FB, Thomas ML. The iliac compression syndrome. *Br J Surg* 1965;52:816–821.
7. Plate G, Brodin L, Eklof B, et al. Physiologic and therapeutic aspects in congenital vein valve aplasia of the lower limb. *Ann Surg* 1983;198:229–233.
8. Rose SS, Ahmed A. Some thoughts on the etiology of varicose veins. *J Cardiovasc Surg* 1986;27:534–543.
9. Clarke H, Smith SR, Vasdekis SN, et al. Role of venous elasticity in the development of varicose veins. *Br J Surg* 1989; 76:577–580.
10. Kistner RL, Eklof B, Masuda EM. Deep venous valve reconstruction. *Cardiovasc Surg* 1995;3:129–140.
11. Caps MT, Manzo RA, Bergelin RO, et al. Venous valvular reflux in veins not involved at the time of acute deep vein thrombosis. *J Vasc Surg* 1995;22:524–531.
12. Pappas PJ, Duran WN, Hobson RW. Pathology and cellular physiology of chronic venous insufficiency. In: Gloviczki P, Yao JST, eds. *Handbook of venous disorders.* London: Chapman & Hall, 1996:44–59.
13. Stanley AC, Park H-Y, Phillips TJ, et al. Reduced growth of dermal fibroblasts from chronic venous ulcerations can be stimulated with growth factors. *J Vasc Surg* 1997;26: 994–1001.
14. Dale WA, Cranley JJ, DeWeese JA, et al. Symposium: management of varicose veins. *Contemp Surg* 1975;6:86–124.
15. Prepared by the Executive Committee, chaired by Andrew N. Nicolaides, of the ad hoc committee, American Venous Forum, 6th Annual Meeting, February 22–25, 1994, Maui, Hawaii: Classification and grading of chronic venous disease in the lower limbs: a consensus statement. In: Gloviczki P, Yao JST, eds. *Handbook of venous disorders.* London: Chapman & Hall, 1996:653–643.
16. Killewich LA, Martin R, Cramer M, et al. Pathophysiology of venous claudication. *J Vasc Surg* 1984;1:507–511.
17. Labropoulos N, Volteas M, Leon M, et al. The role of venous outflow obstruction in patients with chronic venous dysfunction. *Arch Surg* 1997;132:46–51.
18. Raju S. New approaches to the diagnosis and treatment of venous obstruction. *J Vasc Surg* 1986;4:42–54.
19. Nicolaides AN, Hussein MK, Szendro G, et al. The relation of venous ulceration with ambulatory venous pressure measurements. *J Vasc Surg* 1993;17:414–419.
20. Bays RA, Healy DA, Atnip RG, et al. Validation of air plethysmography, photoplethysmography, and duplex ultrasonography in the evaluation of severe venous stasis. *J Vasc Surg* 1994;20:721–727.
21. Araki CT, Back TL, Meyers MG, et al. Indirect noninvasive tests (plethysmography). In: Gloviczki P, Yao JST, eds. *Handbook of venous disorders.* London: Chapman & Hall, 1996: 97–111.
22. Nicolaides AN, Christopoulos D. Quantification of venous reflux and outflow obstruction with air-plethysmography. In: Bernstein EF, ed. *Vascular diagnosis.* St. Louis: Mosby, 1993:915–921.

23. Summer D. Direct noninvasive tests for the evaluation of chronic venous obstruction and valvular incompetence. In: Gloviczki P, Yao JST, eds. *Handbook of venous disorders.* London: Chapman & Hall, 1996:130–151.

24. VanBemmelen PS, Bedford G, Beach K, et al. Quantitative segmental evaluation of venous valvular reflux with duplex ultrasound scanning. *J Vasc Surg* 1989;10:425–431.

25. Kistner RL, Feuier EB, Randhawn F, et al. A method of performing descending venography. *J Vasc Surg* 1986;4:464–468.

26. Neglen P, Einarsson E, Eklof B. The functional long-term value of different types of treatment for saphenous vein incompetence. *J Cardiovasc Surg* 1993;34:295–301.

27. Padberg FT Jr, Pappas PJ, Araki CT, et al. Hemodynamic and clinical improvement after superficial vein ablation in primary combined venous insufficiency with ulceration. *J Vasc Surg* 1997;26:169–171.

28. Larson RA, Toftgren EP, Myers TT, et al. Long-term results after vein surgery: study of 1,000 cases after 10 years. *Mayo Clin Proc* 1974;49:114–117.

29. Gloviczki P, Bergan JJ, Menawat SS, et al. Safety, feasibility, and early efficacy of subfascial endoscopic perforator surgery: a preliminary report from the North American registry. *J Vasc Surg* 1997;25:94–105.

30. Semba CP. Tutorial 18: percutaneous management of deep vein thrombosis. In: Trerotola SO, Savaders SJ, Durham JD, eds. *Venous interventions.* Fairfax, VA: The Society of Cardiovascular and Interventional Radiologists, 1995:202–213.

31. Lalka SG, Malone JM. Surgical management of chronic obstructive venous disease of the lower extremity. *Semin Vasc Surg* 1988;1:113–123.

32. Eriksson I, Almgren B. Influence of the profunda femoris vein on venous hemodynamics of the limb. *J Vasc Surg* 1986;4:390–395.

33. Rodriguez AA, O'Donnell TF Jr. Reconstructions for valvular incompetence of the deep veins. In: Gloviczki P, Yao JST, eds. *Handbook of venous disorders.* London: Chapman & Hall Medical, 1996:434–445.

34. Raju S. Venous insufficiency of the lower limb and stasis ulceration: changing concepts and management. *Ann Surg* 1983;197:688–697.

35. Raju S, Fredericks RK, Neglen PN, et al. Durability of venous valve reconstruction techniques for "primary" and post-thrombotic reflux. *J Vasc Surg* 1996;23:357–367.

36. Dalsing MC, Raju S, Wakefield TW, et al. A multi-center, phase I evaluation of cyropreserved venous valve allografts for the treatment of chronic deep venous insufficiency. *J Vasc Surg* 1999;30:854-866.

SURGERY: SCIENTIFIC PRINCIPLES AND PRACTICE, Third Edition, edited by Lazar J. Greenfield, Michael W. Mulholland, Keith T. Oldham, Gerald B. Zelenock, and Keith D. Lillemoe. Lippincott Williams & Wilkins Publishers, Philadelphia, © 2001.

CHAPTER 93

LYMPHATIC SYSTEM DISORDERS

LAZAR J. GREENFIELD

ANATOMY AND FUNCTION

Embryologists disagree on the origin of the lymphatic vessels. One group traces the vessels to the venous system, whereas another group favors an origin by fusion of mesenchymal spaces or clefts. Regardless of origin, there are paired lymph sacs in the neck and lumbar region by the sixth week of gestation and a developing cisterna chyli by the eighth week. Communicating channels connect these systems to form the thoracic duct by merger of the right lymphatic duct with the left across the fourth to sixth thoracic vertebrae to connect with and drain into the left subclavian vein. Smaller lymphatic ducts persist, draining into the right subclavian vein. Developmental arrest or abnormalities can result in primary hypoplasia or absence of ducts and lymph nodes. Abnormal growth of jugular lymph sacs can produce unilocular or multilocular lymph cysts termed *cystic hygromas.* Most often found in the neck, these cysts can also be found in the axilla, mediastinum, retroperitoneum, or intestinal mesentery. Hyperplastic changes can also occur and produce lymphangiomas with or without other vascular malformations.

The function of the lymphatic system begins with lymphatic capillaries, which collect fluid and protein from the extravascular spaces. This is a significant responsibility because more than 50% of the circulating albumin is lost into the interstitial space every 24 hours. During this period, as much as 4 pounds of lymph is returned to the venous system (1). In addition to the proteins that cannot be reabsorbed by the venules, red cells and bacteria as well as other large particles can be evacuated only through the lymphatics. This unique permeability is facilitated by the absence of a basement membrane beneath the lymphatic endothelial cells. The lymphatic capillaries are found beneath the epidermis in the superficial dermis. These vessels drain into valved channels in the deep dermis and subdermal tissues, forming larger channels that follow the vascular pathways superficial to the deep fascia. Although lymphatics can be found in the intermuscular fascia, they are absent in muscles, tendon, cartilage, brain, and cornea.

Lymph is transported by afferent vessels to regional lymph nodes, which vary in size according to their function and activity (Fig. 93.1). In the medullary sinuses of the node, circulating lymphocytes are replaced and initial contact between foreign material and the immune system is made. Efferent lymph leaves the node by way of hilar channels. These channels are less numerous than the afferent channels that enter the convex side of the node. In addition to direct thoracic duct drainage into the subclavian vein, there are other lymphovenous communications in nodes and in peripheral vessels. Central lymphatic flow is promoted by the lymphatic valves and muscular contractions in the ducts rather than by respiration, arterial pulsation, and external massage, as was previously thought (2). The rate and force of the contractions are determined by the filling pressures (preload) and outflow resistance (afterload), as they are in the heart. Pressures in excess of 40 mm Hg can be generated, and an obstructed lymphatic vessel can show pressures over 60 mm Hg because, unlike veins, there is not a good collateral system for lymphatics (3).

PATHOPHYSIOLOGY

Lymphedema results from obstruction of lymph ducts as a result of developmental defects (primary) or acquired disorders (secondary). The effect of inadequate lymph drainage in the tissues is an increase in protein and fluid accumulation, with additional fluid retained by the osmotic effect of the protein. Protein content in edema fluid increases from a normal range of 0.1 to 0.5 g/dL to abnormal levels of 1 to 5 g/dL, which stimulates tissue fibrosis in the subcutaneous tissue, skin thickening, and hyperkeratosis. The microlymphatics of human skin show network enlargement in primary lymphedema of late onset, whereas they are aplastic or ectatic in congenital lym-

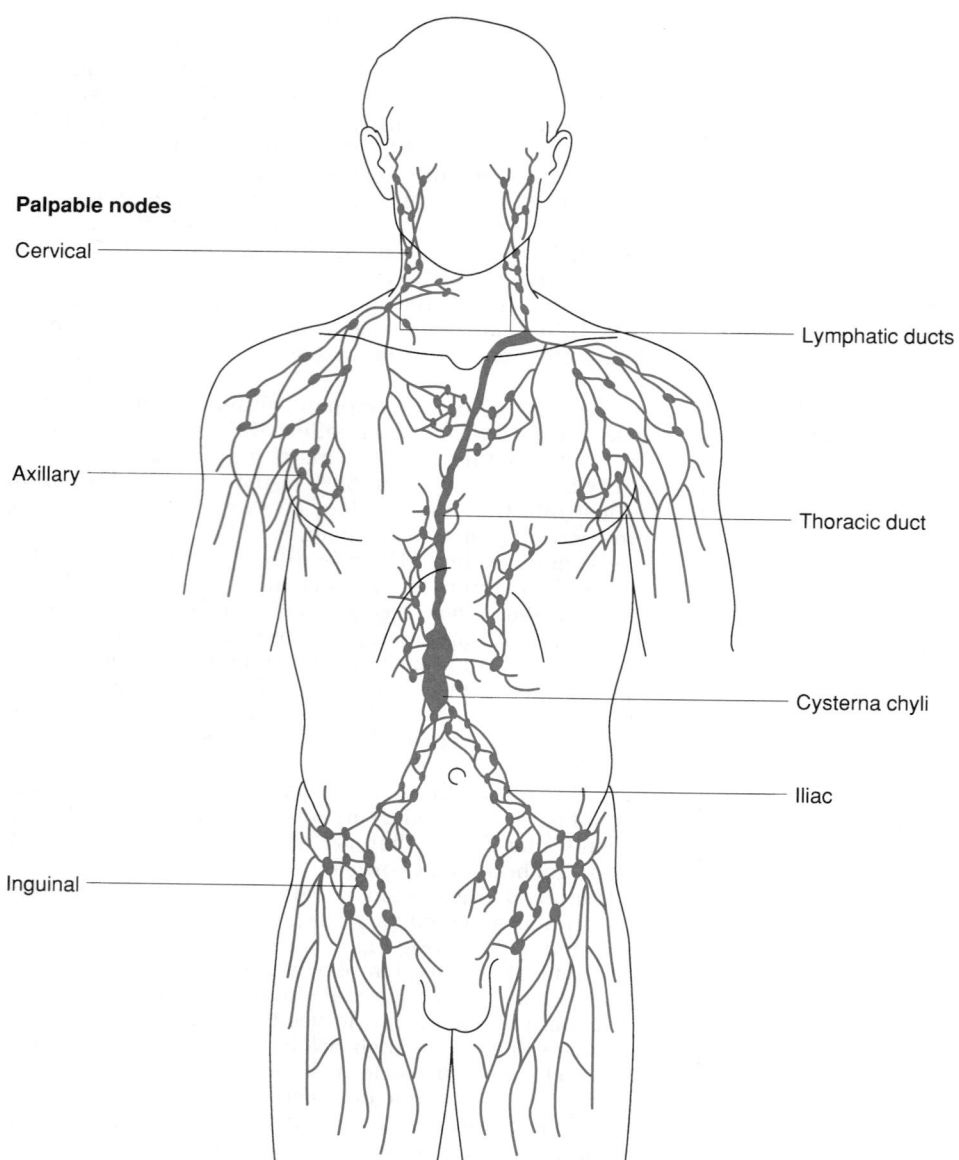

Palpable nodes

Cervical

Axillary

Inguinal

Lymphatic ducts

Thoracic duct

Cysterna chyli

Iliac

Figure 93.1. Major lymph node groups and collecting ducts. (After Basmajian JV. *Primary anatomy*, 7th ed. Baltimore: Williams & Wilkins, 1976:293.)

phedema (4). Although the edema is initially soft and pitting, it becomes more indurated and rubbery with time and progresses to involve the entire extremity in a picture resembling elephantiasis. The differentiation of lymphedema from venous stasis edema is possible because there is usually no hyperpigmentation or ulceration in lymphedema, and the edema does not decrease significantly with overnight elevation. Also, it is more common for lymphedema to involve the dorsum of the foot and toes and to be associated with recurrent episodes of cellulitis and lymphangitis after trivial trauma. The latter complication presents with erythema, pain, and red streaks on the extremity. Lymphangitis may be accompanied by systemic signs of infection, typically by a β-hemolytic *Streptococcus* organism.

The most common serious complication of lymphedema is lymphangiosarcoma, which is usually seen in the upper extremity in a patient with chronic lymphedema after mastectomy for carcinoma (Fig. 93.2). Multiple, raised, bluish-red or purple lesions are seen in the skin or subcutaneous tissue, and they can progress to an ulcerating mass lesion if untreated. Lymphangiosar-

coma is thought to arise from lymphatic endothelium and has a poor prognosis, with most patients dying from the disease in less than 2 years. The tumor can occur on the lower extremity as a nonhealing ulcer with hemorrhagic nodules, pointing out the necessity of biopsy of any suspect nonhealing lesion.

Because lymphedema occurs as the result of an abnormality of the lymphatic system, use of the term should be restricted to situations in which other causes of edema have been excluded or a specific lymphatic abnormality has been demonstrated. The presence of bilateral dependent pitting edema usually indicates a renal or cardiac etiology. Other generalized hypoproteinemias can be idiopathic or can be seen in malnutrition, cirrhosis, and protein-losing enteropathy. Allergies or hereditary causes are unusual. In unilateral edema, venous disease is the most likely cause (see Chapter 92). In patients with chronic venous leg ulcers, quantitative lymphoscintigraphy has demonstrated impaired drainage with chronic venous insufficiency (5). Because this could contribute to poor wound healing, it suggests the need to improve lymph drainage as well as venous function.

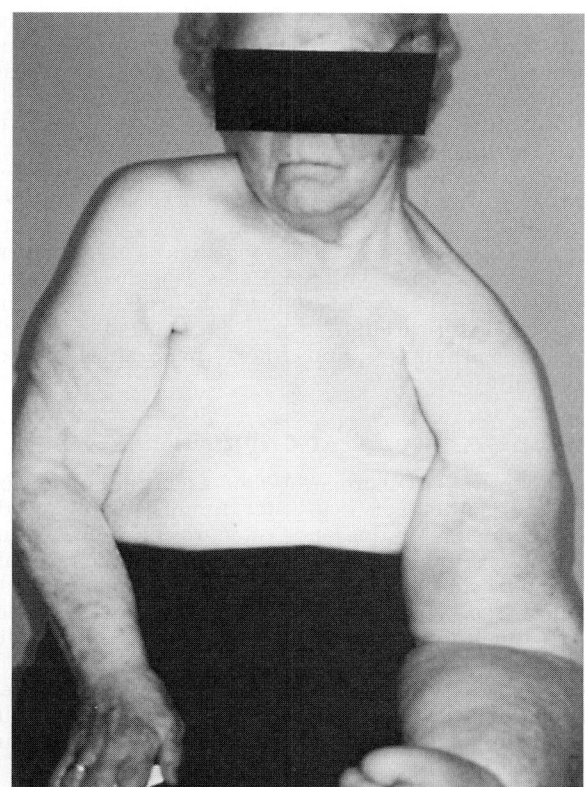

Figure 93.2. Patient with chronic lymphedema after mastectomy, which led to lymphangiosarcoma.

Lymphatic Visualization

Lymphatics can be visualized by dye injection in the extremities and mesentery. Ingestion of cream or milk enables visualization of intestinal lacteals and major ducts.

Dye Injection

A highly diffusible dye such as patent-blue or sky-blue dye can be injected in 0.2-mL amounts subcutaneously into each interdigital web. Massaging the skin and moving

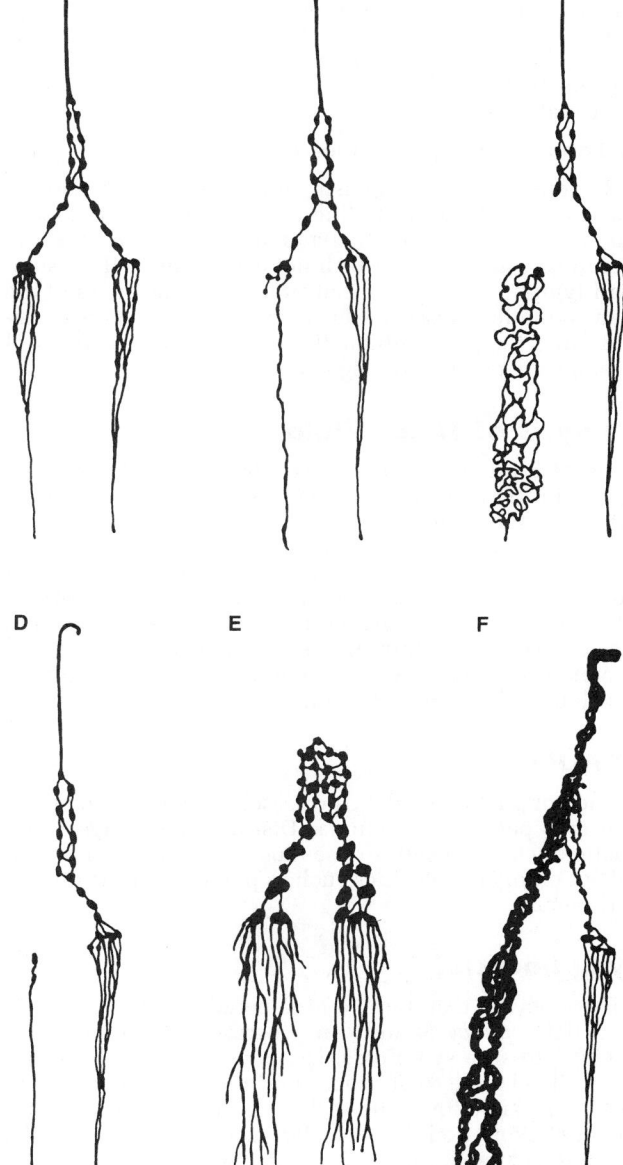

Figure 93.3. Diagrammatic representation of lymphographic patterns from feet to thoracic duct as seen in a normal person *(A)*, in distal hypoplasia (*B*, right lower extremity), in proximal hypoplasia with distal distention (*C*, right limb), in combined proximal and distal hypoplasia *(D)*, in bilateral hyperplasia *(E)*, and in megalymphatics *(F)*, often seen with a large, incompetent thoracic duct. (After Kinmonth JP. *The lymphatics: surgery, lymphography, and diseases of the chyle and lymph systems*, 2nd ed. London: Edward Arnold, 1982:134.)

DIAGNOSIS

The patient with lymphedema complains of swelling and fatigue. Limb size increases during the day and decreases at night, but is never normal. It is important to determine whether there is a family history of primary lymphedema and whether the patient has visited any countries where filariasis is endemic. Weight loss and diarrhea suggest small bowel lymphangiectasia. On examination, lymphedema is characteristically firm and rubbery but nonpitting. Lymph vesicles may be present, containing fluid with a high protein concentration. Complications of lymphedema, such as infection, cellulitis, erythema, and hyperkeratosis, may be present. It is important to document limb size to identify isolated limb gigantism and the Klippel-Trenaunay syndrome, which may have hypoplastic lymphatics in addition to a venous abnormality, capillary nevus, and limb elongation. The patient should be examined for upper extremity and genital lymphedema, hydroceles, and amelogenesis imperfecta.

The differential diagnosis of lower extremity edema includes systemic disorders such as congestive heart failure and acute and chronic venous abnormality. In congestive heart failure, there is a generalized increase in venous pressure with distended neck veins and an enlarged liver. The question of venous disease can be most easily resolved by noninvasive duplex examination using Doppler and B-mode ultrasound imaging (see Chapters 91 and 92). In the absence of these disorders, the patient usually can be managed on the basis of the clinical diagnosis of lymphedema. Only rarely is it necessary to confirm the diagnosis by lymphatic visualization.

the joints usually defines a network of fine intradermal lymphatics. If the collecting vessels are obstructed or inadequate, the dye diffuses through the dermal lymphatics to produce a marbled appearance called *dermal backflow*.

Radiographic Lymphography

Lymphography was developed by Kinmonth (1), who demonstrated that it was possible to cannulate the lymphatic visualized by dye injection and inject oily contrast medium (Lipiodal). This is a meticulous and tedious procedure and may require general anesthesia. If the lymphatics in the foot are not usable, it is possible either to cannulate lymphatics adjacent to groin nodes or to inject the node directly. With adequate visualization, the lymphatics in the extremity can be identified. They often appear as parallel tracks of uniform size that bifurcate as they proceed proximally, in contrast to the venous system (Fig. 93.3). Normally, there is some dilatation at the level of the valves.

Radionuclide Lymphatic Clearance

Radionuclide scanning using human serum albumin labeled with radioactive iodine or technetium 99m colloid has been used to monitor lymphatic clearance by serial scanning. Although the technique is simpler than standard lymphography, its disadvantages are haziness of the scan, radiation dosage, and distribution of the radionuclide into the extracellular fluid, making calculations of clearance dependent on leg volume.

Analysis of Tissue Fluid

Tissue fluid or lymph can be aspirated or collected from a tube in the subcutaneous tissues, but its analysis contributes little to the diagnosis of lymphedema. Characteristically, lymphedema fluid has a protein content of more than 1.5 g/dL, whereas the protein content of edema fluid from venous hypertension is usually less. Also, the ratio of albumin to globulin is higher in lymphedema fluid than in plasma, which is helpful in the differentiation from an inflammatory exudate, where the protein content is high but the albumin/globulin ratio is normal.

TRAUMA

The lymphatics are delicate vessels vulnerable to operative and penetrating trauma. Disruption of larger lymphatic ducts can result in pseudocysts, fistulae, or lymph collection in body cavities such as pleura, pericardium, or peritoneum.

Lymphocysts

Pseudocysts that form after operation or trauma are termed *lymphocysts* and can progressively enlarge, producing pressure symptoms. Lymphocysts typically occur after radical node dissections and in association with kidney transplantation. Although some can involute or respond to aspiration, it is usually necessary to explore the cyst and suture ligate the draining ducts. Identification of the ducts can be facilitated by distal subcutaneous injection of blue dye. Wound drainage and a pressure dressing enhance the healing of the area.

Thoracic Duct Trauma

Injury to the thoracic duct is usually the result of operative or penetrating trauma and produces chylothorax. In rare cases, spontaneous rupture of the thoracic duct can occur in patients with mediastinal lymphoma or congenital malformations of the duct. Treatment initially consists of thoracostomy tube drainage for injured ducts as opposed to thoracotomy to suture ligate the involved vessels, which is usually necessary for spontaneous rupture of a malformation. The volume of chylous drainage can be reduced significantly by an elemental diet and by medium-chain triglyceride administration. If the lung fails to expand or if drainage persists for longer than a week, thoracotomy should be performed to ligate the thoracic duct. The thoracic duct can be identified by the preoperative administration of milk and cream or the intraoperative injection of blue dye into the distal wall of the esophagus. Chylopericardium can be managed similarly, although it usually responds to external drainage and dietary control.

Chylous Ascites and Chyluria

Chylous ascites occurs most often as a result of congenital abnormalities or malignant tumors involving the retroperitoneum. It does not often result from trauma. Proximal obstruction of the thoracic duct can be responsible for persistent leakage and can make spontaneous closure less likely. Lymphography may be necessary to clarify the situation anatomically if a congenital abnormality is suspected. Management is similar to that described for chylothorax. Chyluria can result from filariasis or congenital abnormalities and is diagnosed by the finding of milky urine. Lymphangiography is usually necessary to define the anatomy for operative correction.

CLASSIFICATION OF LYMPHEDEMA

The original Allen classification distinguished two types of lymphedema—primary lymphedema, in which there was no known cause, and lymphedema secondary to a known disease or disorder (1). The primary lymphedemas were called *congenital* when present at birth and *praecox* when the onset was in childhood. When the onset was delayed into later life, Kinmonth added the term *tarda*. With the advent of lymphography, it became possible to classify the primary lymphedemas structurally into *hyperplasias* and *hypoplasias* (Fig. 93.3). The classification proposed by Kinmonth is as follows:

Primary Lymphedema
- Primary hypoplastic
  Distal hypoplasia or aplasia
  Proximal hypoplasia
  Proximal and distal hypoplasia
- Primary hyperplastic
  Bilateral hyperplasia
  Megalymphatic

Secondary Lymphedema
- Malignancy
- Radiation
- Trauma or surgical excision
- Inflammation or parasitic invasion
- Paralysis

The primary lymphedemas are hypoplastic in 92% of cases. Their subgroups are defined by lymphography and behave differently. Patients with distal hypoplasia have a mild, nonprogressive form of the disorder, provided that their proximal pathways are normal. Most of these patients are female, in a ratio of 3:1. The onset at puberty (lymphedema praecox) represents 80% of cases. Only 10% of cases are present at birth (congenital lymphedema). The remaining 10% present after 35 years of age (lymphedema tarda). In proximal hypoplasia, the lymphedema is more extensive and involves the entire extremity. It occurs with equal frequency among men and women. The combination of proximal and distal hypoplasia shows features of both groups and tends to be progressive. Congenital lymphedemas are rare and may have a familial distribution (6).

The primary hyperplastic lymphedemas are uncommon (8%), and those with bilateral hyperplasia can usually be recognized by diffuse capillary angiomata on the lateral sides of the feet. Lymphography shows dilated lymphatics with normal valves, in contrast to the findings in the megalymphatic group, where no valves can be seen. In this latter group, chylous reflux can produce chylometrorrhea, skin vesicles, or chyluria.

The most common cause of secondary lymphedema in the United States is malignant disease metastatic to lymph nodes. Another common cause is surgical removal of nodes, especially when combined with radiation therapy, which produces lymphatic fibrosis. In tropical and subtropical countries, filariasis is the most common cause of secondary lymphedema, producing the typical appearance of elephantiasis. Other infective or chemical agents (e.g., silica) can enter the lymphatic system by means of barefoot walking and cause fibrosis of lymphatics and lymph nodes.

MANAGEMENT OF LYMPHEDEMA

Conservative Treatment

There are significant anatomic and physiologic limitations to the treatment of lymphedema. Physiologically, diuretic removal of fluid is not as effective in lymphedema as in edema due to other causes because of the residual protein in lymphedema. From an anatomic standpoint, the development of fibrosis produces irreversible changes in the subcutaneous tissues. Therefore, the options are limited, and the primary objectives are to control the edema, maintain healthy skin, and avoid the complications of cellulitis and lymphangitis.

To control edema, the leg can be elevated and sequential pneumatic compression boots can be used to massage the leg. These treatments can be done at home with equipment rented for this purpose. Once the leg has reached optimal size, the patient should be fitted with firm elastic stockings. For lymphedema, a full-length leotard should be used, in contrast to the calf-length hose recommended for venous insufficiency. The stockings should be removed at night and the foot of the bed elevated 6 to 8 inches to maintain the pressure gradient from leg to right atrium. Exercise has also been shown to be of value in mobilizing protein and enhancing lymph flow (7). For more severe forms of the disorder, a 2- to 3-day period of hospitalization has been recommended by Pappas and O'Donnell (8) with use of a high-pressure pneumatic compression pump to reduce the size of the extremity. Subsequent control of the edema by elastic compression stockings was successful initially in 90% and then declined to 53% at a mean follow-up of 25 months. Clinical studies in Europe have reported favorable results from the use of benzopyrones, including warfarin. The rationale is that these agents increase protein lysis by macrophages in the interstitium reducing limb volume and softening the skin. In the United States, this approach has not been widely accepted, and there is concern over hemorrhagic complications from warfarin.

A red streaking up the leg and the onset of pain and swelling usually signify early cellulitis or lymphangitis. The causative organism is most often *Staphylococcus* or β-hemolytic *Streptococcus* and must be treated vigorously, usually with intravenous antibiotics. The extremity should be immobilized, and warm, moist compresses should be applied to provide symptomatic relief. In the absence of treatment, the infection can obliterate more lymphatics and can produce constitutional signs of fever, malaise, nausea, and vomiting. Another frequent complication is eczema, which usually responds to hydrocortisone cream. Antifungal agents may be necessary, both topically and systemically for chronic infections, particularly between the toes. Ulceration is unusual in contrast to the stasis edema of venous insufficiency, although fissures and lymph fistulae may develop and require surgical excision.

Secondary lymphedemas may lend themselves to treatment of the underlying disorder. Diethylcarbamazine can be used for filariasis, and appropriate antibiotics can be used for tuberculosis or lymphogranuloma venereum. In rare cases of long-standing secondary lymphedema, a lymphangiosarcoma can develop and can appear as a raised blue or reddish nodule. Satellite tumors and early metastases can develop if the malignancy is not recognized and widely excised. A more recent multidisciplinary approach to both primary and secondary lymphedema involves manual lymphatic drainage using effleurage, a classic form of massage (9). The technique can be taught to the spouse as well as the patient for self-management.

Operative Treatment

Only 10% to 15% of patients with primary lymphedema are candidates for operative treatment, which usually is directed to reducing leg size. The indications for operation are related to functional rather than cosmetic improvement because the appearance of the extremity even after a successful debulking procedure will still be abnormal. The best results are obtained when the bulk of the extremity has severely impaired movement or when there have been recurrent attacks of cellulitis. Although some efforts have been made to improve techniques for lymphatic drainage, most of the established procedures consist of excisional operations.

Three of these excisional procedures were based on the incorrect assumption that the deep fascia acted as a barrier to lymphatic drainage. The efforts of Kondoleon, Sistrunk, and Thompson to excise fascia and to insert a dermal flap into muscle proved ineffective in improving lymphatic drainage (1). The original debulking procedure devised by Charles consists of wide excision of lymphedematous tissue followed by skin grafting, and is useful when the overlying skin is in poor condition, as in elephantiasis. The procedure used most often is Kinmonth's modification of Homans's procedure, in which skin flaps are raised to allow excision of the underlying subcutaneous tissues (1).

The most logical, albeit technically demanding, approach has been to establish lymphaticovenous anastomoses. Initial efforts in this area were made in 1968 by Nielubowicz, who divided a lymph node, removed the pulp under magnification, and then sutured the node capsule with its afferent lymphatics into a vein. This procedure is more suitable for secondary lymphedema than for primary lymphedema, in which the disorder lies in the lymphatic channels themselves. Another promising technique of direct lymphovenous connection was developed by Cardeiro and modified in 1974 by Degni (10), who used a special needle to insert lymphatic vessels directly into veins and fix them there by a single suture. A simpler technique of implantation of adipose tissue containing collecting lymphatics into a small vein has been reported more recently (11).

Microlymphatic bypass for secondary lymphedema continues to be investigated. A large series was reported from

Australia, where O'Brien and associates (12) performed lymphovenous anastomoses for chronic lymphedema in 90 patients. Although a significant number of patients also underwent excisional operations, 74% of the group could discontinue use of elastic stockings. The procedure has also been used to treat chyluria and scrotal lymphangial fistula (13). Confidence in the durability of the procedure awaits better long-term results with demonstration of patency of the lymphovenous anastomoses. A more practical approach consisting of liposuction curettage was reported by Louton and Terranova in 1989 (14). This procedure is performed through multiple small incisions at the knee, ankle, and calf to debulk the leg, and redundant tissue is excised 4 days later. The combination of liposuction with compression therapy has also been found to be effective in reducing limb volume without altering lymph kinetics as studied by lymphoscintography (15).

It is more difficult to evaluate the results of such procedures when combined with resectional operations (16), and in the absence of postoperative lymphography it is difficult to confirm patency of the lymphovenous anastomoses. However, the deleterious effects of lymphangiographic contrast on lymphatics were well demonstrated in 1981 by O'Brien, who measured limb volume after lymphangiography in 100 patients and found that 32% had a significant increase in leg volume and 19% contracted lymphangitis. Therefore, it seems advisable to use lymphangiography only for diagnostic studies and not for preoperative or postoperative evaluation until safer contrast material becomes available.

REFERENCES

1. Kinmonth JB. *The lymphatics: surgery, lymphography, and diseases of the chyle and lymph systems,* 2nd ed. London: Edward Arnold, 1982.
2. Reddy NP. Lymph circulation: physiology, pharmacology, and biomechanics. *CRC Crit Rev Biomed Eng* 1986;14:45.
3. Roddie IC. Lymph transport mechanisms in peripheral lymphatics. *News Physiol Sci* 1990;5:85.
4. Bollinger A. Microlymphatics of human skin. *Int J Microcirc Clin Exp* 1993;12:1.
5. Mortimer PS. Evaluation of lymphatic function: abnormal lymph drainage in venous disease. *Int Angiol* 1995;14[3 Suppl 1]:32–35.
6. Szuba A, Rockson SG. Lymphedema: classification, diagnosis, and therapy. *Vasc Med* 1998;3:145–156.
7. Mortimer PS. Managing lymphoedema. *Clin Exp Dermatol* 1995;20:98–106.
8. Pappas CJ, O'Donnell TF Jr. Long term results of compression treatment for lymphedema. *J Vasc Surg* 1992;16:555.
9. Brennan MJ, Miller LT. Overview of treatment options and review of the current role and use of compression garments, intermittent pumps, and exercise in the management of lymphedema. *Cancer* 1998;83:2821–2827.
10. Degni M. New techniques of lymphatic-venous anastomosis for the treatment of lymphedema. *Vasa* 1974;3:479.
11. Yamamoto Y, Sugihara T. Microsurgical lymphaticovenous implantation for the treatment of chronic lymphedema. *Plast Reconstr Surg* 1998;101:157–161.
12. O'Brien BM, Mellow CG, Khazanchi RK, et al. Long term results after microlymphatico-venous anastomoses for treatment of obstructive lymphedema. *Plast Reconstr Surg* 1990; 85:562.
13. Ji YZ, Zheng JH, Chen JN, et al. Microsurgery in the treatment of chyluria and scrotal lymphangial fistula. *Br J Urol* 1993; 72:952.
14. Louton RB, Terranova WA. The use of suction curettage as adjunct to the management of lymphedema. *Ann Plast Surg* 1989;22:354.
15. Brorson H, Svensson H, Norrgren K, et al. Liposuction reduces arm lymphedema without significantly altering the already impaired lymph transport. *Lymphology* 1998;31: 156–172.
16. Servelle M. Surgical treatment of lymphedema: a report on 652 cases. *Surgery* 1987;101:485.

SURGERY: SCIENTIFIC PRINCIPLES AND PRACTICE, Third Edition, edited by
Lazar J. Greenfield, Michael W. Mulholland, Keith T. Oldham, Gerald B. Zelenock,
and Keith D. Lillemoe. Lippincott Williams & Wilkins Publishers, Philadelphia, © 2001.

CHAPTER 94

NEONATAL AND PEDIATRIC PHYSIOLOGY

DAVID K. MAGNUSON

The purpose of this chapter is to introduce the reader to a variety of physiologic issues relevant to the care of infants and children with surgical disease. The chapter reviews some of the basic physiologic concepts that govern clinical management and delineates some of the differences between pediatric and adult patients. These differences may be merely quantitative when comparing adults with adolescents and older children. The distinction between neonates and older patients, however, is frequently of a more dramatic and qualitative nature. These differences are the consequences of two unique conditions: the functional immaturity of organ systems during the transition from fetal to neonatal life and the demands placed on the physiologic machinery of the neonate by the overriding priority of growth. Whereas homeostasis is a valid concept on a small scale, in a larger sense the concept of a "steady state" is paradoxical in the newborn infant. Virtually every physiologic function in the infant is influenced in some way by the exponential growth that occurs during the first year of life. That growth, and the metabolic activity it demands, is perhaps the single most important property that differentiates the neonatal patient from the adult.

GROWTH AND METABOLISM

Growth, Development, and Prematurity

The 40-week gestational period is divided by convention into an 8-week embryonic period and a 32-week fetal period. During the embryonic period, developmental events occur that transform a fertilized egg into a "preorganism" that comprises all the specialized tissues and organ systems required for future independent life. The subsequent fetal period is characterized by accelerated growth and continuous organ maturation, both of which are required to translate embryonic potential into biological reality. Many of the structural congenital defects encountered in the practice of pediatric surgery have their beginnings in some developmental miscue during the embryonic period. These developmental accidents frequently prevent normal growth and maturation during the fetal period. At birth, the consequences of these antecedent events often are manifested by serious physiologic derangements.

Fetal maldevelopment is complicated frequently by prematurity, that is, entry into the extrauterine world before fetal growth and maturation have been completed. Most fetal growth and organ maturation occurs in the third trimester, and so premature birth interrupts development at a time when the rate of biological change is most rapid. In many cases, prematurity is the direct consequence of intrauterine developmental abnormalities, such as those that produce polyhydramnios (excess amniotic fluid that results in increased uterine size and early labor). In others, prematurity occurs in an otherwise normal fetus and is the result of maternal factors. In both cases, prematurity causes significant morbidity by forcing the neonate to contend with extrauterine challenges using physiologic systems that are not yet prepared to do so and also forces the neonate to complete simultaneously a schedule of preprogrammed fetal tasks.

Although the "normal" gestational period is generally agreed to be 40 weeks, infants are considered to be full-term at 37 weeks. Neonates born before 37 weeks are referred to as *premature* or *preterm*. A *normal-term birth weight* is defined as 2,500 g or more. Infants born at less than 2,500 g are considered to be *low birth weight,* regardless of gestational age. More precise classifications include *moderately low birth weight* (1,500–2,500 g), *very low birth weight* (1,000–1,500 g), and *extremely low birth weight* (<1,000 g).

Mortality rates are directly related to both gestational age and birth weight. As neonatal support technologies continue to improve, survival is being attained at birth weights recently considered to be incompatible with life. The current thresholds for survival appear to be approximately 21 weeks' gestation and 350 g birth weight. Above this threshold, survival rates increase rapidly, achieving 50% survival at approximately 24 to 25 weeks' gestation and 700 g (1). Continued gains in survival have come at an increasingly high cost of long-term morbidity. The most common types of serious long-term morbidity resulting from prematurity are neurodevelopmental conditions (e.g., cerebral palsy, mental retardation, seizure disorders) and chronic lung disease.

Although virtually all premature infants are born at low birth weights, a distinction is drawn between those whose weights are appropriate for their gestational age and those who are *small for gestational age* (SGA). SGA infants are defined as those in the 10th percentile or less with respect to age-adjusted birth weight. Normal intrauterine growth is a sensitive indicator of fetal well-being. Infants who qualify as SGA, whether term or preterm, are presumed to have experienced some intrauterine event that has compromised development. This phenomenon, referred to as *intrauterine growth retardation* (IUGR), may be caused by a plethora of factors that either reduce oxygen and nutrient delivery to the fetus or result in their decreased utilization. These abnormalities include maternal factors (tobacco, alcohol, and drug use; malnutrition; systemic disease), fetal factors (congenital defects, genetic or chromosomal anomalies), and placental factors (vascular anomalies, placental infarction, placental separation).

Both prematurity and IUGR may have detrimental consequences for the newborn. Both groups are challenged by insufficient energy reserves, poor thermal insulation, and increased heat and water loss. The premature infant must confront the extrauterine world with physiologically immature organ systems but may have a good eventual outcome if properly supported. Prenatal development may have been otherwise normal but prematurely terminated by maternal factors. On the other hand, the full-term SGA infant may have functionally mature organ systems and not require extensive physiologic support. When IUGR is the result of maternal or placental factors, premature birth separates the fetus from those factors and often results in compensatory growth and a good prognosis. When IUGR results from fetal or genetic factors, however, a poor prognosis may be anticipated. In general, an SGA infant has a better prognosis than a premature infant of the same birth weight because physiologic immaturity is less pronounced in the former (2).

The rapid somatic growth and maturation occurring during the last trimester continues into the postnatal period and accounts for many of the unique metabolic events and nutritional requirements of the newborn surgical patient. This explosive growth phase is regulated largely by growth hormone *(somatotropin)* and its peptide intermediates, insulin-like growth factors I and II, but it also is influenced by insulin and thyroid hormone. The normal term baby will nearly double its birth weight by 4 months of age and will triple it by 1 year. The near-exponential rate of growth declines gradually thereafter until late adolescence. This pattern of growth is so constant in normal infants that significant departures from it are commonly the earliest indication of previously unrecognized disease. Any metabolic stress contributed by an acute disease or injury event will therefore be superimposed on the existing stringent demands for energy substrates.

As the neonate transitions to later infancy, childhood, and adolescence, its metabolic processes and responses gradually approximate those of the adult. As this transition represents a continuum, no clear delineation between these stages can be made. It is reasonable, however, to consider the metabolic responses of the neonate to starvation and stress as being qualitatively different from those of the adult, whereas those of older infants and children should be considered as only quantitatively different.

Basic Patterns of Energy Metabolism

In general, two basic patterns of energy metabolism are recognized: anabolic and catabolic. Anabolic processes characterize growth and involve the consolidation of nutrient substrates into structural and storage molecules. Catabolic processes involve the breakdown and redistribution of preexisting reserves to meet the short-term needs of specific tissues for specific substrates. Although persistent catabolism is pathological and ultimately fatal, short-term catabolism is a necessary adaptive response to both starvation and stress.

The endocrine and cytokine environments that promote these two states are likewise distinct. Anabolic metabolism is mediated principally by insulin, insulin-like growth factor 1 (IGF-1), and growth hormone. These mediators promote conversion of circulating glucose into glycogen *(glycogenesis),* storage of excess carbohydrate as fat *(lipogenesis),* and synthesis of new structural proteins from amino acids. The presence of available substrate and the absence of physiologic stress elicit a neuroendocrine environment conducive to these processes.

Catabolic metabolism is mediated by "counterregulatory" cytokines and hormones that have effects that are diametrically opposed to the anabolic mediators. These agents include tumor necrosis factor, interleukins, glucagon, cortisol, and catecholamines. These mediators promote an increase in glucose availability through hepatic glycogenolysis and gluconeogenesis and by inhibition of the peripheral effects of insulin on target organs. The objective of short-term catabolism is to generate adequate substrate for critical glucose-obligate tissues such as the brain, red and white blood cells, and renal medulla.

Gluconeogenesis requires a supply of three-carbon fragments that reenter the glycolytic pathway under conditions that favor the reverse flow of intermediates and the synthesis of glucose. These three-carbon fragments are supplied by amino acids from protein breakdown (especially alanine and glutamine) and by glycerol from the hydrolysis of triglycerides. An additional source of gluconeogenic substrate is the Cori cycle, in which lactate from anaerobic metabolism in compromised tissues (e.g., surgical or traumatic wounds) is transported to the liver and converted directly back to glucose.

Catabolic metabolism can be separated into two distinct patterns: simple starvation and the stress response. In simple starvation, the brain (which accounts for the greatest demand for glucose) undergoes a gradual process called *ketoadaptation,* in which receptors and enzymes are expressed that allow for the utilization of ketone bodies as fuel (Fig. 94.1). Fatty acid metabolism then is altered to allow for the diversion of some fatty acids away from oxidative energy production and into the production of ketone bodies. The increased production of ketone bodies

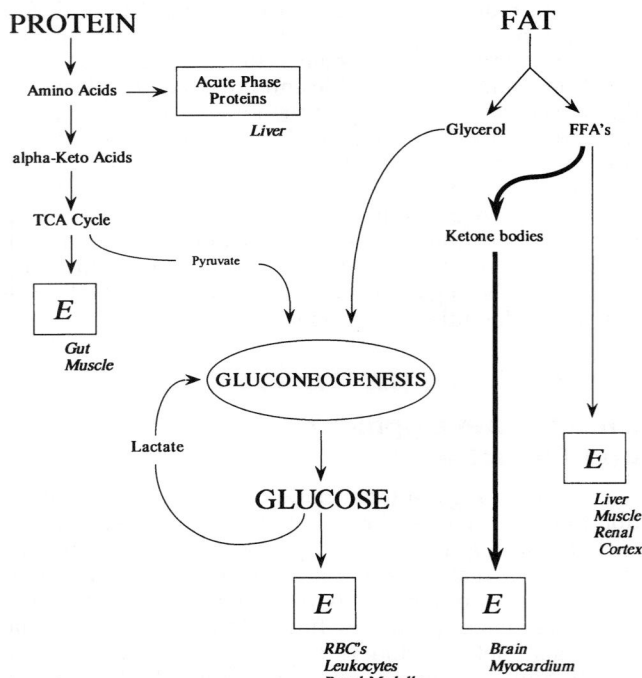

Figure 94.1. Energy production *(E)* during simple starvation. Ketoadaptation by brain and other glucose-obligate tissues allows free fatty acids *(FFA)* to be used for energy production and limits the requirement for protein catabolism to generate gluconeogenic precursors via the tricarboxylic acid *(TCA)* cycle. (Reprinted from Magnuson DK, Maier RV. In: Eichelberger MR, ed. *Pediatric trauma: prevention, acute care, rehabilitation.* St. Louis: Mosby, 1993, with permission.)

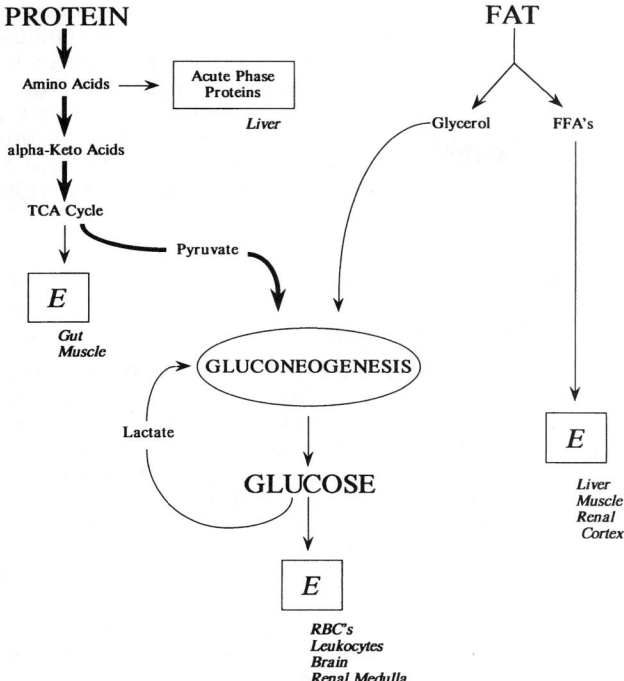

PROTEIN

Amino Acids → | Acute Phase Proteins |

Liver

alpha-Keto Acids

TCA Cycle

| E |

*Gut
Muscle*

Pyruvate

FAT

Glycerol   FFA's

GLUCONEOGENESIS

Lactate

GLUCOSE

| E |

*Liver
Muscle
Renal
Cortex*

| E |

*RBC's
Leukocytes
Brain
Renal Medulla*

Figure 94.2. Energy production *(E)* during stress catabolism. Inhibition of ketoadaptation results in persistent protein catabolism to produce gluconeogenic precursors for glucose-obligate tissues. (Reprinted from Magnuson DK, Maier RV. In: Eichelberger MR, ed. *Pediatric trauma: prevention, acute care, rehabilitation.* St. Louis: Mosby, 1993, with permission.)

(ketogenesis), and their utilization by brain and myocardium, gradually reduces the demand for glucose and the degradation of visceral protein to gluconeogenic precursors.

In stress metabolism, however, the transition to the chronic starvation response of ketoadaptation is inhibited, and an ongoing requirement for glucose drives the continued breakdown of proteins to amino acids. Most of the amino acids produced by proteolysis during stress catabolism are rechanneled into gluconeogenesis (Fig. 94.2). The remainder is used in the synthesis of acute phase proteins, the synthesis of structural proteins for tissue repair, and for direct energy production by conversion to alpha-keto acids and entry into the tricarboxylic acid cycle. The mechanism of this inhibition is not well defined but most likely involves the persistence of stress-related neuroendocrine and cytokine mediators.

Metabolic Patterns in Neonates

The fetus utilizes glucose as its primary energy substrate. Transplacental movement of glucose by facilitated diffusion maintains fetal glucose levels at about 75% of maternal levels. At birth, the neonate experiences an abrupt withdrawal of placental support and plasma glucose levels fall. In response to hypoglycemia, secretion of catecholamines, cortisol, and glucagon mediates a shift to acute stress metabolism, relying initially on glycogenolysis because the capacity for gluconeogenesis is markedly decreased in newborns. Hepatic glycogen stores are limited in the neonate, and available glycogen reserves are depleted within 2 to 3 hours. Thereafter, gluconeogenesis is the sole supply of endogenous glucose until feeding provides new substrate. Protein and triglyceride breakdown

provide direct energy substrates and gluconeogenic precursors, but fetal adipose and muscle mass are relatively modest, and this endogenous supply of fuel is also soon depleted. At this point, plasma glucose levels of 40 to 50 mg/dL are expected. As the infant begins to feed, absorption of exogenous substrates reverses the catabolic pattern, and an anabolic phase mediated by insulin begins. Plasma glucose levels usually rebound to 70 to 80 mg/dL by 3 days of age.

Neonatal demand for exogenous glucose is therefore immediate, and the provision of enteral or parenteral glucose soon after birth is critical. Not only does the neonate have a higher relative energy demand than older children and adults but a much greater proportion of the total caloric demand is generated by glucose-obligate tissues, and the availability of endogenous glucose from glycogen and gluconeogenesis is limited. Furthermore, fat stores and lipolytic pathways are both poorly developed at birth, requiring more metabolically versatile tissues to utilize glucose as well.

The metabolic priorities of the premature or SGA infant are identical to those of the full-term neonate, but striking differences in substrate stores and biochemical maturity make the preterm infant even more vulnerable to the risks of starvation and hypoglycemia. The time between birth and access to exogenous glucose tolerated by the preterm infant is inversely proportional to the degree of prematurity and may be measured in minutes instead of hours in extreme cases. In fact, one of the most striking differences between the normal-term infant and the preterm or SGA infant is the increased risk for hypoglycemic crisis in the latter: 50% in infants who are both premature and SGA (3).

Several factors contribute to this added vulnerability. Glycogen synthetase-b activity increases steadily in the last trimester. At 36 weeks' gestation, hepatic glycogen stores are only 30% of term levels; most glycogen deposition occurs after 36 weeks. Glycogen storage is therefore even more limited in preterm infants than in term infants, whose stores are depleted in a few hours. Additionally, skeletal muscle and fat constitute about 1% of body weight in a 1,000-g premature newborn, compared with about 15% in term infants, and so reserves of alternative energy substrates and gluconeogenic precursors are more limited as well. The ability to carry out β-oxidation of fatty acids and to produce ketone bodies also is depressed more severely in premature infants (4). Ketogenesis is impaired even when given an exogenous source of lipid.

Thermoregulation

Temperature governs the kinetics of complex biochemical processes that have evolved to be maximally efficient within a narrow temperature range. Regulation of core body temperature has a high priority in the metabolic activities of the neonate and is a significant contributor to energy consumption. The fetal environment is one of thermal constancy: maternal and placental mechanisms maintain an optimal temperature for fetal development and obviate the need for fetal energy expenditure to regulate temperature. In fact, the net heat produced by fetal metabolic activity must be transferred away from the fetal environment to avoid a rise in temperature.

Thermal equilibrium is a balance between heat production and heat loss. Newborns, particularly premature newborns, are characterized both by diminished capacity for heat production and by increased vulnerability to heat loss compared with older children and adults. The surface area-to-volume ratio of the neonate is greater than that of older patients, and so the area across which heat can be lost is disproportionately large compared with the mass of metabolically active tissue generating energy. The body surface area to mass ratio averages approximately 250 cm²/kg in the adult and may be as high as 1,400 cm²/kg in the premature infant (5). The paucity of insulating fat and the lower muscular activity level contribute to the problem.

Heat loss in the neonate occurs chiefly through four mechanisms. *Conduction* refers to the transfer of heat by direct contact with another static heat acceptor. The rate and direction of heat flow depend on the heat gradient and the heat capacities of the two objects. *Convection* refers to the transfer of heat from the skin surface to a fluid, such as air, which carries heat energy away from the body. *Radiation* is the loss of heat as electromagnetic energy in the infrared spectrum. *Evaporation* of water at the skin surface consumes heat energy by transforming water from liquid into gas.

The physical environment surrounding the sick neonate provides limitless opportunities for heat loss. Contact with cold surfaces, particularly wet sheets and blankets, is a principal cause of heat loss. The flow of cold air over exposed skin surfaces transfers heat by both convection and evaporation. Evaporation is exacerbated by radiant warmers and phototherapy lights. Premature infants with nonkeratinized epidermis are particularly susceptible to transepithelial water loss and may lose as much as 120 mL/kg of water each day. Evaporation consumes about 0.6 kcal/mL of water, which results in a metabolic cost of about 3 kcal/h. Means of reducing heat loss include the use of thermoneutral incubators and radiant warmers, removal of wet blankets and towels in contact with the skin, and covering the infant with impermeable barriers to evaporation.

Heat production is a consequence of the thermodynamic inefficiency of chemical reactions; wasted energy is dissipated as heat. Basal heat production normally results from both metabolic processes and muscular work. Two additional mechanisms have evolved to provide heat energy when basal heat production is insufficient to maintain thermal stability: shivering and nonshivering thermogenesis. The temperature threshold for initiating thermogenesis in adults is 26° to 28°C, but it ranges from 32°C in term newborns to 35°C in preterm infants (6).

Shivering thermogenesis is the production of heat by rapid, cyclical skeletal muscle contractions. The heat produced as a by-product of this muscular "work" is transferred to blood circulating through the muscles and is redistributed throughout the body. Shivering thermogenesis is the major heat production mechanism in older infants, children, and adults.

Nonshivering thermogenesis is a process unique to the neonate and depends on the presence of brown adipose tissue (BAT). BAT is a unique tissue that is found transiently in the perirenal and axillary regions of the neonate, and it is distinguished by its ability to generate metabolic heat by the inefficient metabolism of fatty acids. Sympathetic activation by cold stress causes norepinephrine to be released in BAT, bind to β-adrenergic receptors on adipocyte membranes, and initiate the hydrolysis of fatty acids. This process is facilitated by the presence of thyroid hormone. The fatty acids are shuttled into mitochondria where β-oxidation takes place. Normally, fatty acid oxidation is coupled to the phosphorylation of adenosine diphosphate (ADP) to adenosine triphosphate (ATP), preserving potential energy in the high-energy phosphate bond. In brown adipocytes, however, a unique peptide called *thermogenin* "uncouples" the oxidative phosphorylation of ADP, allowing energy liberated by oxidation to be released as heat (7).

Nonshivering thermogenesis is the principal means of heat production in neonates, but it has severe limitations. It is a costly means of producing heat from a metabolic standpoint and rapidly depletes precious energy stores in term infants. Premature and SGA infants, with relatively reduced fat composition, are poorly equipped to use this strategy effectively. In term neonates, BAT constitutes about 10% of body fat and is gradually replaced by white adipose tissue in later infancy.

NUTRITIONAL SUPPORT

Energy Requirements

Neonates and children have significantly higher energy requirements than adults. These requirements diminish gradually throughout childhood, but they do not reach adult levels until physical maturity is attained. The two principal reasons for this discrepancy are a higher basal metabolic rate (BMR) and an additional energy requirement for growth. The total energy expenditure (TEE) comprises the BMR, the energy required to process substrates, energy for activity, energy for thermoregulation, and the energy cost of growth. The resting energy expenditure (REE), which may be substituted for BMR, is estimated to be 45 to 50 kcal/kg per day in term neonates, and 50 to 60 kcal/kg daily in premature infants (8,9). This compares with an REE of 20 to 25 kcal/kg daily in adolescents and adults.

Neonates and infants expend a much higher percentage of their total energy production on somatic growth than do older children. Growth consumes 35% to 40% of an infant's caloric intake during the first 6 months of life, a value that declines to about 5% at 2 years of age (10). The energy cost of growth, which includes the energy used in new tissue synthesis plus the energy content of the synthesized tissue, approximates 40 to 50 kcal/kg daily in the neonate and progressively less in the older child. Add to these the energy requirements for nutrient processing, cold stress, and activity, and the baseline energy requirements for a term neonate are about 100 to 110 kcal/kg daily. The preterm neonate may require 120 kcal/kg/day or more to sustain growth. Caloric requirements for intravenous nutrition are perhaps 10% less because of the absence of obligate energy loss in fecal output.

The energy requirements of older infants and children gradually approach adult levels of 30 to 35 kcal/kg daily as BMR, cold stress, and rate of growth all decline with age (Table 94.1). This downward trend is moderated somewhat by an increase in energy expended in physical activity. Although many methods of estimating caloric requirements exist, the most straightforward estimation simply uses a weight-based calculation of caloric needs (Table 94.2).

It is important to recognize that these guidelines represent estimates for unstressed children. Energy requirements are altered in a variety of clinical settings commonly encountered in pediatric surgical patients. Both

Table 94.1. AGE-SPECIFIC ENERGY REQUIREMENTS

Age (y)	Energy requirement (kcal/kg/d)
0–1	120–90
1–7	90–75
7–12	75–60
12–18	60–30
>18	30

Table 94.2. WEIGHT-SPECIFIC ENERGY REQUIREMENTS

Weight (kg)	Energy requirement (kcal/d)
0–10	100/kg
10–20	1,000 + 50/kg over 10
>20	1,500 + 20/kg over 20

congenital heart disease and pulmonary disease may be associated with reduced pulmonary compliance and increased work of breathing, which can substantially increase energy expenditure. The healing of wounds related to major surgical procedures, trauma, and burns also increase caloric requirements. Sepsis, pancreatitis, and other conditions associated with generalized inflammatory activation may increase energy requirements dramatically.

It is equally important to appreciate that, in certain circumstances, caloric requirements in stressed children may be decreased due to changes in REE and the energy consumption related to growth. As opposed to older children and adults, infants actually may experience a decrease in REE during periods of postsurgical stress (11,12). As previously discussed, the metabolic pattern that characterizes acute stress states is one of catabolism and growth postponement. This temporary growth inhibition is a consequence of, among other things, a cytokine and neuroendocrine environment that opposes the anabolic actions of insulin. Because 30% to 40% of a healthy neonate's caloric requirement represents energy required for growth, administration of the same caloric load to the stressed infant or child may result in significant overfeeding. The complications of overfeeding are not commonly recognized but include fluid overload, hepatic steatosis, and increased lipogenesis. Lipogenesis is associated with increased CO_2 production and is reflected in an increased respiratory quotient. Increased CO_2 production requires an increase in minute ventilation that may not be tolerated by critically ill neonates and children with respiratory disease and limited ventilatory reserve.

In the stressed infant or child, therefore, it may be prudent to reduce caloric administration transiently by as much as 25% to 30% during the acute stress phase, when growth is inhibited and the metabolic rate depressed. Determining when the metabolic environment has reverted back to one more permissive for growth and caloric utilization can be difficult. Direct calculation of the respiratory quotient by indirect calorimetry and measurement of nitrogen balance may be helpful in detecting a capacity to utilize more energy substrate. More frequently, however, one is required to make a clinical judgment based on resolution of the hyperdynamic response to adrenergic stimulation or infection and the restoration of normal hemodynamics and fluid requirements.

Substrate Requirements

Carbohydrates

Carbohydrates constitute the major source of energy substrate for infants and older children, although they have a lower caloric density (3.4 kcal/g of intravenous hydrated dextrose, 4 kcal/g of enteral glucose) than either proteins (4 kcal/g) or fats (9 kcal/g). As discussed already, glucose is the preferred fuel in a variety of tissues, including brain and blood cells. The obligate glucose consumption rate in neonates, as calculated from a variety of stud-

ies, is about 4 to 6 mg/kg/min (13–15). This compares with a glucose utilization rate of about 1 mg/kg/min in adults. The discrepancy is explained in part by the fact that the neonatal brain accounts for 10% of body weight in the newborn and only 2% of body weight in adults. This contrast is even more striking in SGA infants whose brain growth is preserved in the face of generalized IUGR. In these infants, brain size and glucose consumption are even more disproportionately large. Most of the demand for glucose in newborns is for brain energy production, with relatively little remaining available for other tissues. Consequently, prolonged hypoglycemia may cause profound neurologic impairment.

The addition of small amounts of glucose to intravenous fluids prevents protein catabolism by providing a fuel source for glucose-obligate tissues and obviating gluconeogenesis. In adults, this protein-sparing glucose requirement is about 1 mg/kg/min and is conveniently provided by administering 5% dextrose in water (D_5W) intravenously at maintenance fluid rates. In neonates, who require 4 to 6 mg/kg/min of glucose to avoid protein catabolism, it is usually necessary to administer maintenance intravenous fluids as 10% dextrose in water ($D_{10}W$). The relatively higher fluid administration rate and dextrose concentration provide the increased glucose supply necessary to avert protein catabolism in the short term.

Normal plasma glucose values are variable and depend on gestational age, weight, and postnatal age. The definition of hypoglycemia is therefore somewhat fluid, but it is generally agreed that plasma glucose levels less than 35 mg/dL in term infants and less than 25 mg/dL in preterm infants constitute metabolic emergencies and require immediate intervention. Full-term infants of appropriate birth weight rarely develop hypoglycemia. Infants at risk for hypoglycemia include those who are premature, SGA infants, multiple gestations, infants of diabetic mothers, infants of toxemic mothers, and infants who are critically ill for some other reason. Neurologic injury resulting from an inadequate supply of substrate to brain cells depends on both the degree and duration of hypoglycemia. Signs of hypoglycemia are nonspecific and include respiratory irregularity, apnea, bradycardia, hypothermia, cyanosis, irritability, tremors, seizures, lethargy, hypotonia, and coma.

Mild, asymptomatic hypoglycemia usually can be managed simply by initiating early oral feedings with breast milk or $D_{10}W$. Severe or symptomatic hypoglycemia requires intravenous dextrose administration. Dextrose concentrations of 10% to 12.5% are the maximum that can be tolerated by peripheral veins; higher concentrations of dextrose require a central (e.g., umbilical) venous catheter. Treatment consists of administering glucose at a rate of 6 to 8 mg/kg/min (3.6–4.8 mL/kg/h of $D_{10}W$). Profoundly hypoglycemic infants may require an initial dextrose "minibolus" of 200 mg/kg (2 mL/kg $D_{10}W$) over 1 to 2 minutes. The dextrose infusion rate then is increased by 2 mg/kg/min every 3 to 4 hours until stable plasma glucose levels of 40 to 50 mg/dL are achieved.

Most neonatal hypoglycemia is transient, allowing dextrose administration to be weaned down as feeding or intravenous nutritional support is begun. Persistent hypoglycemia, particularly in infants requiring more than 12 to 15 mg/kg/min of dextrose, may indicate a pathologic cause for hypoglycemia. Causes of pathological hypoglycemia in neonates include hyperinsulinism (Beckwith-Wiedemann syndrome, nesidioblastosis/islet cell dysmaturation syndrome), congenital adrenal insufficiency, and other inborn errors of metabolism. In these circumstances, treatment options include corticosteroids, glucagon, epinephrine, somatostatin, diazoxide, and near-total pancreatectomy.

Fats

Lipids are the other main source of energy substrate. Nutrient lipids consist primarily of triglycerides—a glycerol backbone to which three fatty acids are esterified. During energy metabolism, the fatty acids are cleaved off the glycerol moiety and are transported into mitochondria, where they undergo β-oxidation to produce energy stored in ATP. In addition to providing an energy source of high caloric density (9 kcal/g), lipids are essential for cell membrane structure, steroid hormones, the synthesis of inflammatory mediators such as prostaglandins and leukotrienes, and thermal insulation.

Most dietary triglycerides contain long-chain fatty acids 16 to 18 carbons long. Most fatty acids derived from animal sources have no double bonds within the carbon chain (saturated), whereas those derived from fish and vegetables have one or more double bonds (unsaturated). Because most fatty acids can be synthesized from carbohydrate precursors, there is no absolute dietary requirement for most fats as long as adequate calories are being provided from sugars. Two polyunsaturated fatty acids, linoleic and linolenic acid, are considered to be "essential" from a dietary standpoint because they cannot be synthesized de novo. Linoleic acid deficiency is marked by dryness and thickening of the skin, hair loss, and delayed wound healing. Linolenic acid deficiency has been associated with neurological dysfunction, which suggests a role for linolenic acid in brain development (16).

Proteins

Although amino acids can be converted to their keto-acid counterparts, enter the tricarboxylic acid cycle, and yield useable energy (4 kcal/g), they are ideally reserved for the synthesis of new structural and functional proteins. The need for protein precursors is particularly acute in the neonate who is undergoing accelerated somatic growth. As the infant ages and the rate of growth declines, the requirements for dietary protein diminish somewhat. Recommendations for protein requirements in infants and children are variable. Premature infants may require 3 to 4 g/kg each day, whereas term newborns require 2 to 3 g/kg each day, older infants 1.5 to 2 g/kg per day, and children and adolescents 1 to 1.5 g/kg daily. These recommendations are somewhat controversial given the fact that healthy newborn infants on a breast milk diet maintain normal growth with an average protein intake of 1.5 to 2 g/kg daily.

Eight of the 20 amino acids are unable to be produced by enzymatic conversion of other existing amino acids and therefore must be obtained from dietary sources. These essential fatty acids are threonine, leucine, isoleucine, valine, lysine, methionine, phenylalanine, and tryptophan. Several other amino acids may be considered essential in the neonate because the specific enzyme systems for their conversion are consistently slow to mature in the postnatal period. These include histidine, tyrosine, cysteine, taurine, and possibly proline. Although clinical consequences of deficiencies in these amino acids have not been clearly defined, amino acid formulations designed for administration to adults may not contain them (especially cysteine and taurine), and specialized pediatric formulations supplemented with these amino acids are available.

Although not usually considered an essential amino acid, glutamine is of critical importance to many tissues and has been the subject of intense investigation in recent years (17). Glutamine is produced from glutamate by the enzyme glutamine synthetase and has many physiologic functions. It participates in nitrogen transport in both the ammonia and urea cycles. It serves as a precursor for nucleic acid synthesis and an energy source in tissues with rapid cell proliferation. Intestinal epithelium is the primary consumer of glutamine, extracting a significant fraction from the circulation as well as the intestinal lumen. Within the continuously dividing enterocytes, glutamine is a necessary precursor to nucleic acid synthesis as well as the principal energy substrate. Maintenance of mucosal health and barrier function is directly dependent on the availability of glutamine for enterocyte metabolism.

Because glutamine synthetase is present in both infants and adults, and because glutamine is unstable in solution, this amino acid is not included in commercial amino acid formulations. During episodes of physiologic and metabolic stress, glutamine levels may fall despite the intravenous administration of other amino acids, suggesting a stress-induced alteration in glutamine synthesis. Intestinal mucosal atrophy and loss of barrier function may occur during prolonged periods of intestinal rest when only parenteral nutrition is administered. The addition of glutamine modified to increase stability in standard intravenous amino acid formulations, as well as enteral administration of glutamine-containing formulas in subnutritive quantities, are being investigated as strategies for improving mucosal function and promoting intestinal growth in infants and children with severe gut injury.

Types of Nutritional Support

Enteral Support

The provision of all fluids, electrolytes, and substrates through the gastrointestinal tract is the ultimate goal of nutritional therapy. Using the gastrointestinal tract, even if only for a fraction of the patient's needs, provides trophic substances and enteroendocrine stimulation for intestinal growth and development, maintains the integrity of intestinal barrier function, and mitigates against the cholestatic liver complications of prolonged gut rest. Enteral feeding is associated with significantly fewer complications than parenteral nutrition and can be administered at a much lower cost. Equally important, early institution of oral feeding is crucial for the maintenance of an intact suck and swallow reflex and the prevention of behavioral feeding aversion.

Breast milk is the optimal nutritional vehicle. Human milk is a complex mixture of macromolecules that evolves over time as the growing infant's needs change. The usable energy content of milk is divided almost equally between carbohydrates and lipids. The carbohydrate fraction is predominately lactose, but it includes more than 100 other oligosaccharides that have putative immunologic functions. A variety of lipids constitute the fat component, including both linoleic and linolenic acids. The protein content of human milk is relatively low compared with cow's milk and commercial formulas. As opposed to cow's milk, human milk has more whey than casein. The whey fraction includes many proteins, some with antibacterial functions, including the lactalbumins, albumin, lactoferrin, lysozyme, secretory immunoglobulin A (IgA), enzyme, growth factors, and hormones. In addition to these macromolecules, human milk contains a variety of cellular elements, including B- and T-lymphocytes, macrophages, and neutrophils.

When human breast milk is not available, a wide variety of commercial formulations may be chosen from

Table 94.3. **COMPOSITION OF SPECIALIZED INFANT FORMULAS (PER 100 ML)**

Formula	Carbo	Grams	% kcal	Protein	gm	% kcal	Fat	Grams	% kcal	Osm	Uses
Human milk	Lactose	7.2	42	Casein 20% Whey 80%	1.1	6	Human	3.9	52	290	Infants
Cow's milk	Lactose	4.8	30	Casein 80%	3.4	21	Butterfat	3.4	49	260	Older children
COW'S MILK BASED											
Enfamil 20 Similac 20 SMA	Lactose	7.3	43	Nonfat cow's milk	1.5	9	Coconut, soy oils	3.6	48	300	Healthy infants
SOY BASED											
Isomil Prosobee	Corn syrup	6.9 6.7	41 40	Soy isolate	1.7 2.0	10 12	Coconut, soy	3.7 3.5	49 48	240 200	Lactose intolerance milk protein allergy
PREMATURE											
Enfamil premature	Corn syrup + lactose	7.4	44	Nonfat cow's milk	2.0	12	MCT 40% + coconut, soy	3.4	44	260	Premature infants
Similac special care	Cornstarch + lactose	7.2	42				MCT 50% + coconut, soy	3.7	47	250	
PROTEIN HYDROSYLATES											
Pregestamil	Corn syrup, cornstarch + dextrose	6.9	41	Hydrolyzed casein + cystein, tyrosine, tryptophan	1.9	11	MCT 60% + corn, safflower	3.8	48	320	Malabsorption
Nutramigen	Corn syrup, cornstarch	7.4	44	Hydrolyzed casein + amino acid mix	1.9	11	Corn oil	3.4	45	320	
Alimentum	Tapioca starch + sucrose	6.9	41	Hydrolyzed casein	1.9	11	MCT 50% + corn, safflower	3.8	48	370	
ELEMENTAL DIET											
Neocate	Corn syrup	7.9	47	L-amino acids	2.1	12	Safflower, vegetable oils	3.1	41	342	Malabsorption
HIGH MCT											
Portagen	Corn syrup + sucrose, lactose	7.7	46	Sodium caseinate	2.3	14	MCT 85% + corn oil	3.1	40	220	Lymphatic leak

MCT, medium chain triglycerides.

(Table 94.3). The nutritional compositions of these formulas are modeled on breast milk, but they differ with respect to the specific carbohydrate, protein, and fat content. Commercial formulas contain slightly more protein and less fat as a percentage of total calories than breast milk. Considerable variation in the specific nutritional components provides multiple options for optimizing nutrition in neonates with gastrointestinal derangements.

Most of the available formulas have a caloric density equal to that of human milk: 20 kcal/oz (0.67 kcal/mL). Formulas with higher caloric densities are available for infants with restrictions on fluid intake, or may be provided by fortifying standard formulas with polymeric glucose or other additives. Children between 6 months and 1 year of age may be transitioned to pediatric formulas with a higher caloric density of 30 kcal/oz.

The amount of formula required to supply adequate energy substrate to the growing infant can be estimated easily. Assuming an energy requirement of 110 kcal/kg daily,

a feeding regimen of eight feedings per day, and a caloric density of 20 kcal/30 mL, one can reduce the calculation of the required feeding volume to a single "nutritional coefficient" of 22:

$$\text{Wt (kg)} \times 22 = \text{Volume of breast milk or formula required every 3 h}$$

This coefficient reduces to 7.3 for 24-hour continuous drip feedings.

A number of specialized formulas are available for infants with specific abnormalities of substrate absorption. The most important carbohydrate source for infants is lactose, the predominant disaccharide in human milk, which is hydrolyzed by intestinal lactase to glucose and galactose. Lactase and other disaccharidases are sensitive to changes in the villous environment and exhibit reduced activity in the setting of mucosal disease. Lactase is the most labile of brush-border enzymes, being among the first to exhibit decreased activity in disease and the last to increase during recovery. Inflammatory disorders that cause increased epithelial turnover result in a population of immature enterocytes with reduced lactase activity. Prolonged gut rest also results in reduced disaccharidase activity as a result of villous atrophy and mucosal loss.

Term infants with lactose intolerance may be given soy-based formulas that are lactose free. Premature infants have reduced intestinal brush-border enzyme activity as a result of epithelial immaturity, especially with respect to lactase, but they also have deficiencies in fat and protein absorption for the same reason. Premature-specific formulas provide carbohydrates largely as glucose polymers (corn syrup) with or without lactose. They also provide a fat mixture of long-chain and medium-chain triglycerides to improve fat absorption. In the extremely premature or stressed infant, formulations providing hydrolyzed proteins (oligopeptides) have advantages over those that contain complex, intact proteins. Premature formulas also provide increased concentrations of various other components, such as calcium and phosphorous, to meet the needs of accelerated bone mineralization (a fetal task under normal circumstances).

Hypersensitivity to bovine protein antigens may cause inflammation of the gastrointestinal tract and malabsorption in some infants. Soy-based formulas are usually the initial option for infants with cow's milk protein allergy because the protein content derives exclusively from soy proteins. As many as 30% of these infants will develop hypersensitivity to soy proteins as well and may require the use of a formula containing only protein hydrosylates which are less allergenic than intact proteins.

Synthetic medium-chain triglycerides (MCTs) containing fatty acid moieties 8 to 10 carbons long are commercially available and have some advantages over long-chain triglycerides in certain clinical settings. MCTs are efficiently metabolized in the gut lumen to their constituent parts, are readily absorbed, and produce a nearly identical caloric yield. More importantly, they appear to have the capability of being transported directly into the enterocyte without prior degradation to glycerol and fatty acid. Hence, they offer the advantage of improved absorption in prematurity and other conditions that impair lipid digestion. These states include biliary obstruction (e.g., biliary atresia), bile salt insufficiency (e.g., ileal resection), pancreatic insufficiency (e.g., cystic fibrosis), and decreased absorptive surface area (e.g., short-gut syndrome). Because they bypass lymphatic absorption, they also may be useful in reducing lymphatic flow in treating chylous ascites and chylothorax. Because MCTs do not contain the essential fatty acids, periodic supplementation is necessary to avoid deficiency states.

Total Parenteral Nutrition

Few developments in clinical medicine have had a more profound impact on the survival of premature and critically ill neonates than the capability of administering hypertonic solutions of nutritional substrates by central venous catheter. The management of total parenteral nutrition (TPN) is complicated and covered more thoroughly elsewhere. Several issues related specifically to the management of TPN in infants and children are discussed here.

Indications for TPN depend on age, size, and clinical condition. In general, the younger the patient, the more intolerant of the effects of prolonged fasting. Although a healthy child or adolescent may tolerate a week or longer of inadequate nutrition, the infant and neonate are not so resilient. It is reasonable to consider initiating TPN in any neonate expected to fast for at least 2 to 3 days. Extremely premature neonates with multiple medical problems are

commonly started on TPN within the first 2 days of life. Substrate concentrations are initially low and are gradually weaned up to calculated maintenance values over several days to avoid hyperglycemia and acidosis.

Estimations of caloric needs are made using the same assumptions discussed in the previous section. It is reasonable to divide total caloric requirements between carbohydrates and fats. The energy content of proteins should not be calculated to contribute to caloric requirements because the exogenous amino acids are expected to be used primarily for new protein synthesis. The appropriate distribution of calories between carbohydrates and fats may differ between individual patients, but in general fats should account for 40% to 50% of nonprotein calories, and carbohydrates usually account for 50% to 60%. Carbohydrates are administered as dextrose, and standard lipid emulsions containing essential fatty acids also are used. Although essential fatty acids can be supplied in adequate quantities with once-weekly lipid infusions, the high caloric density and low respiratory quotient characteristic of intravenous lipids make them attractive as a primary energy source for most neonates who may have difficulty handling large fluid and CO_2 loads.

Protein requirements in parenteral nutrition are age dependent because of the changing requirements for somatic growth. As discussed previously, premature infants typically require 3 to 4 g/kg daily, whereas term newborns require 2 to 3 g/kg daily, and older infants 1.5 to 2 g/kg daily. To promote efficient utilization of amino acids for protein synthetic purposes, the nonprotein calorie-to-nitrogen ratio should be 150:1 to 200:1. Special formulations, including amino acids thought to be essential specifically in neonates, are widely available. Pediatric requirements for electrolytes, fat- and water-soluble vitamins, and trace elements must be provided as well.

The administration of both enteral and parenteral nutrition involves many assumptions and estimations. One of the most important aspects of nutritional management, then, is monitoring the response to therapy. In the older child and adolescent, maintenance of weight is an important goal. In the rapidly growing neonate, measurable nonedema weight gain is the objective. A daily weight gain of about 0.5% to 1% is a reasonable goal (15–30 g daily in the average term neonate). Measurements of serum albumin, prealbumin, and transferrin are helpful in assessing protein synthetic status in the neonate, just as they are in the adult. Routine surveillance of serum electrolytes, plasma and urine glucose, and liver function studies are mandatory to recognize metabolic complications of TPN administration.

FLUID, ELECTROLYTE, AND RENAL PHYSIOLOGY

Fluid Compartments

Like the adult, but to a greater degree, the infant and child are composed primarily of water. This simple fact influences many clinical phenomena, ranging from fluid balance to the volume of distribution for electrolytes and drugs. The percentage of body weight that comprises water, as well as its distribution within physiologic compartments, is in a state of rapid flux during the fetal and neonatal period. Body fluid distribution approaches a steady state by approximately 1 year of age and remains reasonably constant thereafter.

The greatest changes in total body water (TBW) occur during fetal development. At 12 weeks' gestation, water constitutes 95% of fetal mass. This percentage declines to about 80% by 32 weeks' gestation and to 75% at term. Prematurity results in the birth of a fetus at a stage of rapid change in water content, a fact that needs to be appreciated when caring for the preterm surgical patient. A further decline in TBW occurs in a roughly linear fashion over the first year of life and reaches a plateau of about 65% by 1 year of age (Fig. 94.3).

Within the body, water is distributed between two main compartments: intracellular and extracellular. Although the extracellular compartment predominates early in fetal life, continued cellular proliferation and growth cause the intracellular and extracellular compartments to approach equivalence (about 40% each) at term. Postnatal diuresis of extracellular fluid causes the extracellular compartment to be reduced further within the first few weeks. Continued growth and fat deposition cause extracellular fluid to decline to about 25% at 1 year of age, whereas at the same time the intracellular compartment rises to a plateau of 40% to 45%.

The extracellular compartment is divided further into the interstitial and intravascular compartments. Generally, intravascular water accounts for only 25% of extracellular water, but this value is highly variable and depends on changeable factors, such as hematocrit and oncotic pressure. Blood volume itself is relatively high in the fetus because it includes blood circulating in the umbilical-placental vessels. At term, the normal fetal blood volume after cord occlusion is about 90 mL/kg (higher in premature infants). Blood volume declines gradually to 80 mL/kg in toddlers, 75 mL/kg in school-aged children, and 65 mL/kg in adolescents.

Fetal stress is often accompanied by the generalized accumulation of extracellular fluid, a condition referred to as *hydrops fetalis*. Fluid accumulates both as soft tissue edema and as effusions in the peritoneal, pleural, and pericardial spaces. This condition is readily diagnosed by prenatal ultrasound, which can detect cavitary fluid accumulations and quantify soft tissue edema by measuring the increased thickness of cervical soft tissues between the spine and the skin *(nuchal thickening)*.

The mechanism of fluid accumulation is ill defined but most likely involves hydrostatic forces related to in utero congestive heart failure and venous hypertension. A principal cause of hydrops fetalis is autoimmune hemolytic anemia secondary to maternofetal Rh antigen incompatibility *(erythroblastosis fetalis)*. The high fetal oxygen demand continues in the face of ongoing red cell destruction, resulting in a compensatory increase in cardiac output and the eventual development of high-output cardiac failure. Other causes of hydrops fetalis also involve congestive heart failure: fetal arrhythmias, structural heart defects, mediastinal shift resulting from diaphragmatic hernia or developmental lung anomalies, and arterial "steal" syndromes caused by fetal tumors such as giant sacrococcygeal teratomas and hemangiomas. These later causes of fetal extracellular fluid accumulation are referred to as *nonimmune hydrops* and carry a poor prognosis. About 80% of fetuses identified with this condition die in utero, and only half of those that are liveborn survive beyond the neonatal period.

Renal Physiology

Maintenance of water and electrolyte balance within the body's fluid compartments is the responsibility of the kidney. Renal function in infants and children relies on the same physiologic principles as adults, but it differs in the relative capacities to excrete and conserve water and solutes. These differences mainly affect infants and small children; by the age of 2 years, a child's renal function approaches that of the adult.

Renal function depends on two interrelated processes: the glomerular ultrafiltration of plasma and the tubular modification of the ultrafiltrate by selective reabsorption of water and solutes. Glomerular filtration is a passive event in which water and low-molecular-weight solutes percolate through the glomerular capillary membrane into the glomerular lumen. About 20% of renal plasma flow is filtered through the glomeruli in this fashion. The glomerular filtration rate (GFR) is dependent on renal blood flow, which is autoregulated by a tubuloglomerular feedback mechanism between specialized renal tubular cells *(macula densa)* and proximal arterioles. Modification of the ultrafiltrate occurs in the tubular system and collecting ducts through active transport of some solutes and passive diffusion of water and other solutes. A detailed description of these physiologic events is beyond the scope of this chapter, but certain generalizations can be made regarding age-related differences in renal function.

Urine output in the immediate postnatal period is characterized by three distinct phases: prediuretic, diuretic,

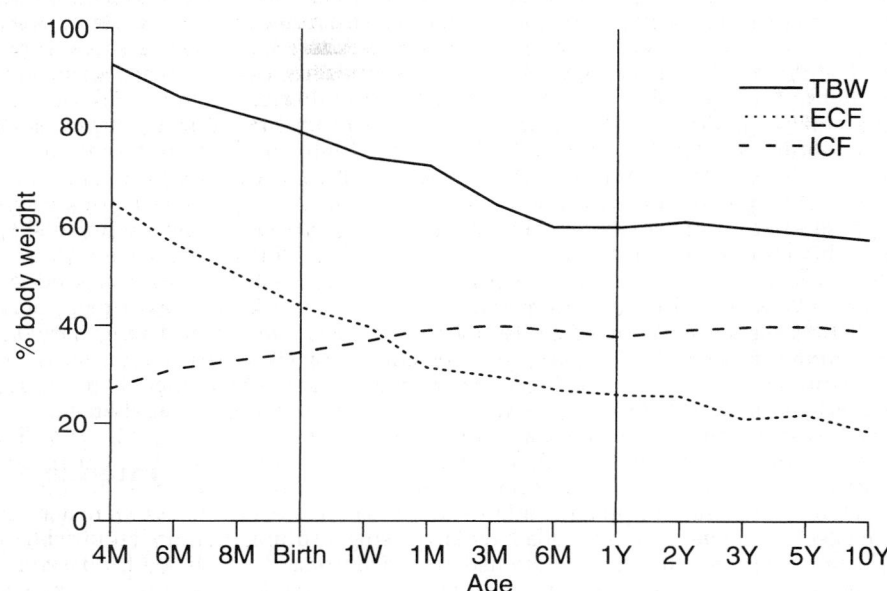

Figure 94.3. Changes in total body water distribution during prenatal and postnatal growth and development. [Modified from Friis-Hansen B. Changes in body water compartments during growth. *Acta Pediatr* 1957;46(Suppl 110):1, with permission.]

and postdiuretic. The *prediuretic phase* occupies the first 24 hours and is marked by a fixed, low urine output of 1 mL/kg/h or less. Urine output during the second and third day of life increases dramatically, to 5 to 10 mL/kg/h, and is largely insensitive to exogenous fluid administration. Much of the rapid reduction in TBW seen in the postnatal period occurs during this diuretic phase. The unloading of excess water has an extremely high priority and is observed even in premature infants (18). Beginning on the fourth day of life, urine output begins to display an appropriate responsiveness to fluid balance.

Renal blood flow (RBF) and GFR are both markedly reduced in the neonate because of elevated renovascular resistance. In the newborn, RBF represents only 6% of cardiac output, compared with 25% in the older child and adult. As resistance falls, RBF increases by fourfold in the first 3 months and doubles again to adult levels (indexed to body surface area) by 1 or 2 years of age. Changes in GFR correspond roughly to those in RBF.

Tubular function also varies according to age. The ability to concentrate urine is dependent on mechanisms that cause reabsorption of free water in renal collecting ducts to regulate serum osmolarity. Free water absorption is governed by the actions of antidiuretic hormone (ADH), which is secreted by the posterior pituitary in response to increased serum osmolarity and decreased blood pressure, and which acts on tubular epithelium in the collecting ducts to increase permeability to water. Water diffuses out of the ductal lumen and into the interstitium and capillary network, as directed by the concentration gradient.

Although the capacity to produce ADH is fully developed both in preterm and term infants, the sensitivity of tubular epithelium to ADH appears to be diminished in all neonates (19). This accounts for the fact that infants have a reduced capability to excrete concentrated urine relative to adults. The neonatal kidney can concentrate urine to a maximum of 500 to 600 mOsm/L. By 1 year of age, maximum concentrating capacity reaches about 1,000 mOsm/L, and by 2 years of age, the concentrating capacity attains adult levels of 1,200 to 1,400 mOsm/L (20). In contrast, the ability of the neonate to excrete free water and to produce dilute urine appears to exceed that of the adult. Maximal urine dilution capacity in the preterm and term neonate is about 30 to 50 mOsm/L, compared with 70 to 100 mOsm/L in the adult.

The other primary tubular function is the regulation of sodium balance, which in turn determines TBW and affects intravascular volume. Sodium regulation is governed largely by two counterregulatory hormones: aldosterone and atrial natriuretic peptide (ANP). Aldosterone is secreted by the adrenal cortex in response to activation of the renin angiotensin system, and it acts on renal tubular epithelium to increase active sodium resorption and passive water resorption. Active sodium resorption is tightly coupled to potassium excretion. ANP is secreted in response to atrial distension and increased levels of ADH, catecholamines, and corticosteroids, and it promotes increased sodium excretion and water diuresis through enhanced GFR and reduced sodium resorption.

Both these systems appear to be active in the neonate. The term infant is able to conserve sodium effectively, like the adult, but it appears to be less effective in excreting an excess sodium load. In contrast, the preterm infant is a "salt waster," and demonstrates a marked inability to conserve sodium in the face of sodium restriction. Additionally, because sodium excretion occurs at an increased but relatively fixed rate in preterm infants, these patients are unable to excrete a sodium load by increasing sodium clearance beyond the preprogrammed rate. This relative inability to regulate sodium excretion makes the neonate particularly susceptible to changes in intravascular and extravascular volume resulting from inappropriate fluid management.

Sodium handling can be expressed in terms of the fractional excretion of sodium (FE_{Na}) or the percentage of sodium filtered that is actually excreted in the urine. Calculation of FE_{Na} requires measurement of plasma (P) and urine (U) concentrations of both sodium (Na) and creatinine (Cr) (sodium excretion is indexed to creatinine excretion because creatinine is not reabsorbed):

$$FE_{Na}\% = (U_{Na})(P_{Cr})/(U_{Cr})(P_{Na}) \times 100$$

Under normal circumstances, the FE_{Na} for both term infants and adults is 1% or less. Premature infants normally have elevated FE_{Na} values of 3% to 9%. Calculation of the FE_{Na} can be helpful in assessing the cause of oliguria by determining whether renal tubular function indicates increased sodium resorption. Recent diuretic use invalidates the FE_{Na} as an indicator of tubular function. Oliguria associated with an appropriately low FE_{Na} implies renal hypoperfusion. Oliguria associated with an abnormally high FE_{Na} (>1 in term infants, >3 in preterms) indicates inappropriate sodium excretion and suggests a renal parenchymal cause for the oliguria (e.g., ischemic acute tubular necrosis).

Fluid and Electrolyte Management

Neonates and young children are exquisitely sensitive to small changes in body chemistry and do not have mature homeostatic mechanisms to compensate for rapid changes in fluid and electrolyte flux and maintain internal balance. Additionally, the requirements for chemical homeostasis in the neonate are superimposed on a background of ongoing change. Iatrogenic alterations of body chemistry in the child are therefore quickly and easily produced by inattention to the details of fluid and electrolyte administration, causing impairments of cardiovascular, pulmonary, neurologic, and gastrointestinal function.

The systematic approach to fluid and electrolyte management requires an estimate of maintenance requirements, which then are adjusted to take into account both preexisting imbalances and abnormal ongoing losses. Once therapy is initiated, frequent reassessment and readjustment are necessary to ensure that the patient is responding as initially predicted. This involves documenting reversal of the symptoms and signs of dehydration, correction of any electrolyte or acid-base abnormalities, and normalization of urine output.

When normal renal function is present, the most reliable and easily measured indicator of adequate hydration is urine output. In the adult, the production of urinary output at a rate of 0.5 mL/kg/h (30–40 mL/h) is adequate to excrete a normal renal solute load, given the concentrating capacity of the adult kidney. Because the immature kidney has diminished concentrating capacity compared with that of the adult, and because the pediatric solute load requiring excretion is relatively higher owing to the increased requirements for energy metabolism and growth, normal urinary outputs in children are higher. A desirable urine output in preterm infants is 3 to 4 mL/kg/h, dropping to 2 mL/kg/h in neonates and infants, and 1 mL/kg/h in toddlers and school-age children.

Maintenance Requirements

Maintenance fluid and electrolyte requirements are those required to replenish normal, anticipated losses. Obligate fluid losses can be estimated by considering water lost in the excretion of solutes in the urine, excretion of

Table 94.4. **HOLLIDAY-SEGAR METHOD FOR ESTIMATING FLUID REQUIREMENTS**

Weight (kg)	Fluid requirement (mL/d)
0–10	100/kg
10–20	1,000 + 50/kg over 10
>20	1,500 + 20/kg over 20

stool, transepithelial water and sweat lost by evaporation, water lost through respiration, water utilized in anabolic metabolism for growth, and water gained through oxidation of nutrient substrates. Obviously, the actual "maintenance" fluid requirements in individual patients will vary widely according to the variables listed, but certain generalizations can be helpful in estimating requirements and initiating therapy.

Maintenance fluid requirements are related primarily to patient size and can be estimated by the Holliday-Segar method (Table 94.4). Many neonates, however, will require much higher maintenance fluid volumes (100–150 mL/kg daily) as a result of increased obligatory losses from a variety of causes. Increased transepithelial losses occur with fever, the use of radiant warmers, exposure to phototherapy for hyperbilirubinemia, and in premature infants with thin, nonkeratinized skin. Neonates with tachypnea or those undergoing mechanical ventilation may have increased lung water loss despite inspired gas humidification. It is common practice to reduce the fluid volumes for the first 2 to 3 days of life to about 70% of maintenance to accommodate the obligatory diuresis of extracellular fluid.

Maintenance requirements of sodium are about 2 to 3 mEq/kg daily in term infants and children. This value may be somewhat higher in premature infants who cannot conserve sodium as effectively. Potassium requirements are also approximately 2 mEq/kg daily. Requirements for exogenous calcium are uncommon in older infants and children with adequate skeletal stores, but calcium supplementation may be necessary in the premature infant with little skeletal ossification, particularly in those with cardiac disease, and in all children receiving prolonged TPN. As discussed in the preceding section, glucose is administered along with maintenance fluids to provide sufficient caloric support to meet the needs of glucose-obligate tissues and to prevent protein catabolism for gluconeogenesis.

Taking these requirements into consideration, maintenance fluids composed of one-fourth normal saline in 10% dextrose ($D_{10}1/4NaCl$) should be appropriate for most healthy neonates. Half-normal saline in 10% dextrose may be required in the premature infant. After the infant transitions into the postnatal diuretic phase on the second or third day of life, 10 to 20 meq/L of KCl may be added to replenish obligate potassium losses and avoid hypokalemia. Depending on prior nutritional status and ongoing illness, it may be appropriate to reduce glucose intake to 5% dextrose after 1 to 2 weeks.

Preexisting Imbalances

Frequently, maintenance fluid administration must be superimposed on a significant preexisting deficit or excess. A complete history and physical examination are invaluable in detecting evidence of fluid imbalance and understanding its cause. Protracted vomiting or diarrhea, copious enterostomal output, chronic diuretic therapy, mechanical ventilation, phototherapy, and the like are all clues to extraordinary fluid losses. Physical examination

is paramount in assessing current fluid status in all children. Because of the absence of comorbidity in most cases, physical signs of volume status are frequently more reliable in children than in adults.

Signs of both intravascular and extravascular fluid imbalance should be sought. Signs of extravascular fluid deficit, which are apparent with mild to moderate dehydration (<10%), include poor skin turgor, recessed eyes, sunken or soft fontanelle, dry mucous membranes, absence of tears, and orthostatic hypotension and tachycardia. Signs of intravascular fluid deficit, which usually indicate more severe dehydration (>10%), include resting tachycardia and hypotension, oliguria, delayed capillary refill, reduced extremity temperature, thready or absent peripheral pulses, and altered mental status.

Signs of intravascular volume depletion usually indicate a need for intravenous resuscitation, which is usually initiated before proceeding with maintenance therapy. Isotonic crystalloid resuscitation with serial boluses of lactated Ringer's solution (10–20 mL/kg) is usually appropriate and followed by careful assessment of the response to therapy. For dehydration associated with hyponatremia and hypochloremia, normal saline boluses may be preferable. In most conditions, however, repeated boluses of saline may be associated with iatrogenic hypernatremia and a normal anion gap metabolic acidosis resulting from hyperchloremia with a compensatory decrease in serum bicarbonate anion.

Preexisting fluid excesses are encountered less frequently in children, but it is important to recognize them to avoid exacerbating the underlying condition by instituting ill-advised maintenance therapy. Fluid excesses occur most frequently as a result of iatrogenic mismanagement, but they also may be seen in acute renal failure and congestive heart failure. Signs may include peripheral and pulmonary edema, hypertension, and increased heart size on chest radiography. Obviously, maintenance therapy may need to be postponed until euvolemia is achieved through diuresis.

Ongoing Losses: Body Secretion Compositions

Before a final strategy can be established, the presence of extraordinary ongoing fluid losses should be anticipated and accounted for. These losses usually result from increased gastrointestinal losses caused by nasogastric suction, enterostomal output, diarrhea, pancreatic/biliary drainage, or drainage of chylous ascites or chylothorax. Another common, although "occult" cause of ongoing fluid loss is the unavoidable sequestration of extracellular fluid in regions of surgical, inflammatory, or traumatic injury, often referred to as *third spacing*.

Because gastrointestinal secretions from various levels of the gastrointestinal tract have differing electrolyte profiles, they are most safely replaced on an equal volume (mL per mL) basis with fluid of similar composition. This may be accomplished by periodically measuring the electrolyte composition of the lost fluid or by estimating the composition according to known values (Table 94.5). In practice, upper gastrointestinal secretions in the setting of paralytic ileus or mechanical obstruction frequently approach isotonicity and may be safely replaced with lactated Ringer's solution as long as careful monitoring of serum electrolytes is maintained. Pancreatic, biliary, and some ileostomy-related fluids are safely replaced with 0.45% NaCl supplemented with sodium bicarbonate at a concentration of 25 to 50 mEq/L. Chylous drainage may require the addition of albumin to avoid a progressive decrease in serum oncotic pressure over time. Third-space losses are best replaced

Table 94.5. **COMPOSITION OF BODY FLUIDS**

Source	Na⁺ (mEq/L)	K⁺ (mEq/L)	Cl⁻ (mEq/L)	HCO⁻₃ (mEq/L)	Protein (g/dL)	Suggested replacement
Gastric	20–80	5–20	100–150	—	—	0.45% NaCl + 10 mEq/L Cl
Pancreatic	120–140	5–15	40–80	115	—	LR or 0.45% NaCl + 50 mEq/L NaHCO₃
Bile	120–140	5–15	80–120	100–115	—	LR or 0.45% NaCl + 50 mEq/L NaHCO₃
Ileostomy	45–135	3–15	20–115	30–50	—	LR or 0.45% NaCl + 25 mEq/L NaHCO₃
Diarrhea	10–90	10–80	10–110	30–50	—	LR or 0.45% NaCl + 25 mEq/L NaHCO₃
Pleural or peritoneal	140	5	100	25	6–8	LR + 5% albumin or plasmanate

LR, lactated Ringer's solution.

with lactated Ringer's solution administered by intermittent bolus (10–20 mL/kg), because the exact rate of fluid loss is not measurable and adequacy of resuscitation can be judged best by physiologic response.

Specific Examples

Abnormalities of Sodium Concentration

Changes in serum sodium concentration reflect changes in free water balance. Mild hyponatremia (serum sodium of 125–135 mEq/L) is a common electrolyte abnormality in children and is seen frequently in postoperative patients with excessive ADH secretion in response to perceived intravascular volume depletion. It is also seen in patients with chronic conditions associated with fluid retention, such as cirrhosis, nephrotic syndrome, and congestive heart failure. Severe, acute hyponatremia (serum sodium <120 mEq/L) usually is associated with volume contraction from hypertonic fluid loss, as can occur with vomiting, diarrhea, or excessive stomal output.

Acute hyponatremia can cause severe neurologic symptoms, including headache, nausea, vomiting, lethargy, seizure activity, and coma. These symptoms are referred to as *water intoxication* and result from diffusion of water into relatively hypertonic brain cells, causing cerebral edema and intracranial hypertension. Treatment of severe or symptomatic hyponatremia involves administration of hypertonic saline (3% NaCl) over 30 to 60 minutes to correct serum sodium to about 125 mEq/L, followed by a more gradual elevation of serum sodium levels to normal over the ensuing 24 to 48 hours. The sodium deficit may be calculated by using a volume of distribution for sodium of 0.6:

$$\text{Sodium deficit} = [\text{Na}^+_{\text{target}} (9) - \text{Na}^+_{\text{measured}}] \times \text{weight (kg)} \times 0.6$$

Hyponatremia of a more chronic, gradual nature should be corrected more slowly, particularly if asymptomatic. When hyponatremia develops gradually, compensatory loss of osmotic agents from brain cells prevents water intoxication. Rapid normalization of serum sodium levels may therefore cause a rapid fluid shift out of compensated brain cells, occasionally causing permanent neurologic injury. This is referred to as *central pontine myelinosis (demyelination)* and can manifest as quadriparesis or pseudobulbar palsy. Mild, chronic hyponatremia in conditions associated with fluid retention usually can be corrected with free water restriction alone.

Hypernatremia is an uncommon electrolyte abnormality in children. Neurologic symptoms are related to brain-cell dehydration and shrinkage, causing disruption of bridging veins and intracranial hemorrhage. Recommendations for correction include calculation of the free water deficit and slow correction with D₅W over 24 to 48 hours. As a result of the production of cytoplasmic osmotic substances

(ideogenic osmoles) by brain cells to offset increased extracellular sodium concentration, chronic hypernatremia is usually well tolerated and should be corrected gradually to avoid precipitating acute cerebral edema.

Abnormalities of Acid–Base Status

Metabolic acidosis may be categorized as having an increased anion gap or normal anion gap. The causes of an increased anion gap metabolic acidosis in children are the same as in adults: lactic acidosis or ketoacidosis accounts for most cases. Their implications and management in children do not differ from that in the adult. Normal anion gap metabolic acidosis, however, is much more common in infants than in older children and adults. The immature kidney is less efficient both at bicarbonate reclamation in the proximal tubule and at hydrogen ion excretion in the distal nephron. These functional deficits are considered a transient form of renal tubular acidosis (RTA) type II (proximal), which is one of a heterogeneous group of disorders characterized by abnormal hydrogen ion and bicarbonate handling in the nephron. The vast majority of neonates outgrow this condition in the first year of life.

One of the most commonly encountered acid–base abnormalities in infants is metabolic alkalosis associated with hypochloremia, hypokalemia, and volume contraction. This pattern is typical of that seen in infants with protracted vomiting resulting from hypertrophic pyloric stenosis. Persistent vomiting of acidic gastric secretions causes the progressive depletion of both hydrogen and chloride ions. The loss of hydrogen ions results in alkalosis. Hypochloremia is associated with an increase in serum bicarbonate ion to maintain electroneutrality and with a decrease in renal hydrogen ion excretion. Renal tubular sodium resorption increases to reverse extracellular volume contraction. Sodium resorption is coupled with excretion of potassium. This potassium loss is facilitated by systemic alkalosis, which drives hydrogen ions out of renal tubular cells in exchange for potassium, raising renal tubular availability of potassium. As potassium becomes progressively depleted, a shift to hydrogen excretion occurs, resulting in the creation of urine with an inappropriately low pH: paradoxical aciduria. Treatment is directed at restoring extracellular fluid volume, chloride and potassium ions, and correcting the underlying pathology.

RESPIRATORY PHYSIOLOGY AND SUPPORT

Pulmonary Development

Abnormal or incomplete pulmonary development accounts for much of the clinical pathophysiology observed in infants with respiratory distress syndrome, bronchopulmonary dysplasia, and pulmonary hypoplasia related to congenital diaphragmatic hernia or cystic adenomatoid malformation. All these conditions manifest physiologic disturbances related to immature or altered development of the tracheobronchial tree, pulmonary vasculature, or alveolar parenchyma. A general knowledge of normal lung development is therefore necessary to understand these pathologic entities and their management.

Normal lung development can be described as occurring in roughly five phases. The *embryonic phase* begins in the third week of gestation, when a ventral diverticulum appears in the proximal foregut. This lung bud grows caudally, undergoing a series of binary branchings to form first the carina and then the lobar and segmental bronchi. The developing lung buds comprise entodermal cells destined to become both bronchial epithelium and alveolar parenchyma. As the primitive lung bud branches, it grows into mesoderm destined to differentiate into cartilage, smooth muscle, and vascular structures. This phase is largely complete by 6 weeks.

The *pseudoglandular phase* extends from week 7 to week 16 and is characterized by continued dichotomous branching of the primitive airways. Under normal conditions, the developing airway branches about 23 times and acquires a glandular appearance as the epithelial tubes are surrounded by amorphous mesenchymal tissue. Entodermal differentiation into bronchial and alveolar epithelium occurs, as does mesenchymal differentiation into muscle, blood vessels, and connective tissue. Physical contact between the entodermal and mesodermal components is necessary for reciprocal induction of differentiation. By the end of this phase, all tracheobronchial branching is complete.

The *canalicular phase* extends from week 17 to 24 and is characterized by development of the gas-exchange architecture of the lung parenchyma. Primitive epithelial channels evolve into more complex groupings, interstitial tissue diminishes, and capillary ingrowth occurs. Alveolar epithelial cells differentiate into type I and II pneumocytes. *Type I pneumocytes* make up the alveolar wall and have a flattened morphology with scant cytoplasm, which is appropriate for the diffusion interface between the alveolar lumen and the capillary blood. *Type II pneumocytes* contain cytoplasmic lamellar bodies that identify these cells as future surfactant producers. A considerable body of evidence suggests that type I pneumocytes differentiate from existing type II pneumocytes. The earliest time at which functional gas exchange is possible is at the end of the canalicular phase.

The *terminal saccular phase* follows the canalicular phase at 24 weeks and lasts until the end of gestation. Two principal events occur during this time: (a) further morphologic change in the gas-exchange units with thinning of the interstitium and increased exposure of capillaries to the epithelial interface and (b) production of surfactant in preparation for extrauterine life. At this stage, each capillary is exposed to only one respiratory surface.

At birth, each lung contains approximately 20 million immature gas-exchange units, referred to as *terminal sacs.* In the postnatal *alveolar phase,* these structures proliferate and mature, reaching 300 million mature alveoli by the time the child is 8 years old. The terminal sacs multiply in number and mature morphologically. During this final phase, the respiratory membrane thins out further and presents more surface area to the capillary network. In the mature alveolus, each capillary is exposed simultaneously to at least two alveolar surfaces. After the end of this phase, when the child is 8 years of age, further lung growth occurs only by increasing individual alveolar size.

Lung growth during prenatal development appears to be linked to the secretion of fetal lung liquid. Fetal breathing movements provide for amniotic fluid flow into and out of the developing lungs. Net fluid flow appears to be outward, however, implying that lung fluid is secreted into the airway and flows out during the fetal respiratory cycle. The effect of lung liquid production appears to be one of growth stimulation, perhaps by providing a positive distending pressure in the fluid-filled fetal lung. Tracheal occlusion in fetal animal models prevents egress of secreted lung liquid and results in overdistention and overgrowth of the fetal lung. This observation led to clinical trials of fetal tracheal occlusion to prevent pulmonary hypoplasia associated with congenital diaphragmatic hernia.

Pulmonary Physiology in the Neonate

Lung Volumes

Total lung capacity comprises four distinct lung volumes: *tidal* volume, *inspiratory* and *expiratory reserve* volumes, and *residual* volume (Fig. 94.4). Residual volume is the volume of gas left in the lung after complete, forced expiration. The sum of the three lung volumes above residual volume (expiratory reserve, tidal, and inspiratory reserve) is the *vital capacity,* or the maximal volume of gas that can be voluntarily inspired or expired.

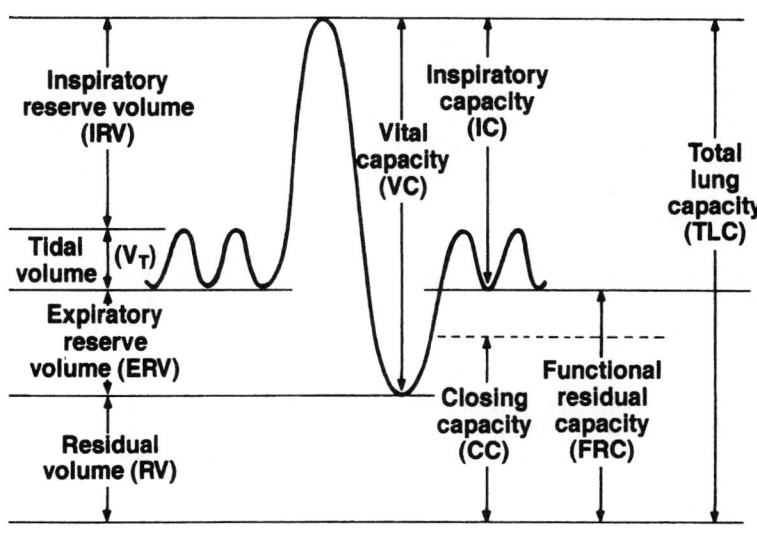

Figure 94.4. Lung volumes and capacities. (Reprinted from Wilson JM, DiFiore JW. In: O'Neill JA, Rowe MI, Grosfeld JL, et al., eds. *Pediatric surgery,* 5th ed. St. Louis: Mosby, 1998, with permission.)

Two functional parameters with great relevance to the physiologic management of lung pathophysiology are the functional residual capacity (FRC), which is the total volume of gas remaining in the lung after passive expiration during tidal breathing when alveolar pressure has equilibrated to atmospheric pressure, and the closing capacity (CC), which is the volume below which small conducting airways and alveoli begin to collapse.

Alterations in FRC occur in many pathologic states and significantly impact the efficiency of gas exchange. Normally, FRC exceeds CC, and alveoli in most regions of the lung remain open for gas exchange during tidal breathing. In disease states in which FRC is reduced, usually because of diminished compliance, FRC may drop below CC, causing regional atalectasis and impaired gas exchange. Common conditions associated with reduced FRC include respiratory distress syndrome (RDS), adult respiratory distress syndrome (ARDS), cardiogenic pulmonary edema, pneumonia, and postoperative hypoventilation caused by pain and splinting. Management focuses on recruiting collapsed alveoli by restoring and maintaining a higher FRC. This usually entails applying positive intraalveolar distending pressure in the form of positive end-expiratory pressure (PEEP) or continuous positive airway pressure (CPAP).

Mechanical Properties and Their Effects on Ventilation

The bulk flow of gas can be described by the simple equation:

$$\Delta P = VR$$

where ΔP is the pressure gradient, V is volume flow per unit time, and R is resistance. The mechanical properties that govern clinically important aspects of lung ventilation include compliance, elastic recoil, and airway resistance. Compliance describes the distensibility of lung tissue and reflects the energy required to effect a volume change. *Compliance* is defined as the change in lung volume per unit change in pressure: $\Delta V/\Delta P$, with higher values signifying greater distensibility. Dynamic compliance (C_{dyn}) uses peak inspiratory pressure (PIP) in the calculation, whereas static compliance (C_{st}) uses plateau inspiratory pressure; hence, C_{dyn} is always lower than C_{st}. From a clinical standpoint, compliance is a critical determinant of lung volume, which in turn determines the efficiency of ventilation/perfusion matching and gas exchange. Conditions that reduce compliance make it more difficult to maintain volumes above closing capacity and therefore promote atalectasis. Low compliance states are caused by increased structural wall tension (edema or fibrosis), increased alveolar surface tension (surfactant deficiency), or decreased alveolar radius (reduced FRC).

Compliance is the inverse of *elastic recoil,* defined as the tendency for stretched tissue to return to its prestretched state. Whereas elastic recoil depends in part on intrinsic properties of lung and chest wall tissue structure, the elastic recoil of lung parenchyma is closely related to alveolar wall tension. Wall tension tends to cause collapse of the alveolus unless opposed by some internal "splinting" pressure within the alveolus. The interaction between wall tension, alveolar radius, and pressure is defined by the Laplace relationship:

$$P = 2T/R$$

where P equals the splinting pressure, T the wall tension, and R the alveolar radius. This relationship states that the internal distending pressure required to counteract alveolar collapse is directly proportional to wall tension and inversely proportional to alveolar radius. At low alveolar radii (volumes), higher splinting pressures are required to counteract wall tension and oppose alveolar collapse. This explains both the tendency for low lung volumes to promote regional atalectasis and the high energy investment required to reopen collapsed alveoli. The most important component of total wall tension in the neonate is surface tension, which is the tension created by the physiochemical properties of the gas/liquid interface. In the mature lung, surface tension is dramatically reduced by surfactant, a phospholipid that coats the alveolar surface and stabilizes it against collapse. Therefore, alveolar collapse is facilitated both by small lung volumes and by surfactant insufficiency.

The relationship between pressure and lung volume is referred to as the *static compliance curve* and is not linear (Fig. 94.5). At low lung volumes, atalectatic alveoli initially require a large energy input to reopen. As more alveoli are recruited, further increases in pressure bring about much larger increases in lung volume. At high lung volumes, alveoli are overdistended and less compliant. Pulmonary management aims at maintaining FRC in the steep portion of the static compliance curve, where lung compliance is optimal.

Extrinsic compliance refers to the component of lung compliance related to extrapulmonary structures, primarily chest wall, diaphragm, and abdomen. Under normal circumstances, chest wall compliance in the infant is high and contributes little to total compliance, which then is determined mostly by intrinsic lung compliance. In some instances, such as increased chest wall edema due to sepsis, persistent fetal circulation, or superior vena caval thrombosis, reduced extrinsic compliance can have a significant impact on total compliance and ventilation. Chest wall compliance also can decrease with the use of intravenous fentanyl, which affects muscle tone. Extrinsic compliance also decreases when intraabdominal pressures are increased (e.g., ileus, closure of abdominal wall defects) and after diaphragmatic plication or diaphragmatic hernia repair (21).

Ventilation is inversely related to resistance, which has both viscous and airway components. *Viscous resistance*

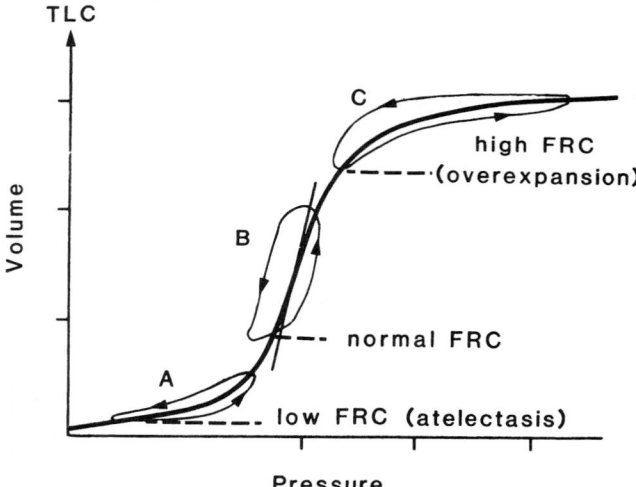

Figure 94.5. Static compliance curve. Nonlinear relationship between inflation pressure and volume change illustrated at low, normal, and high functional residual capacities *(FRC)*. Volume represented as fraction of total lung capacity *(TLC)*. (Reprinted from Harris TR, Wood BR. In: Goldsmith JP, Karotkin EH, eds. *Assisted ventilation of the neonate,* 3rd ed. Philadelphia: WB Saunders, 1996, with permission.)

is the friction generated by contiguous tissues moving against each other. It accounts for up to 40% of total resistance in neonates and is increased with conditions of high tissue density caused by edema (e.g., respiratory distress syndrome, bronchopulmonary dysplasia, and anatomic left-to-right shunts) (22). Airway resistance, on the other hand, reflects friction caused by gas molecules interacting with each other and with the airway walls.

Airway resistance is related to length, radius, turbulence, and density. According to Poiseuille's Law, resistance is directly related to the length of the conducting tube and inversely related to the fourth power of radius:

$$\Delta P = V8\eta L/\pi r^4$$

where η is viscosity, L is tube length, and r is radius. Radius is a powerful determinant of resistance in simple tubes, but in the branching bronchial tree, the impact of progressively smaller radii is offset by the large total cross-sectional area of the distal airways. This is particularly true for older children and adults, in whom occult small-airway disease may exist without affecting total resistance. The small airways in infants contribute a much larger percentage of total airway resistance, however; so conditions affecting these airways, such as bronchospasm and bronchiolitis, have a more significant effect on airflow. Although tube length has few important clinical ramifications, it is interesting to note that infants with pulmonary hypoplasia resulting from congenital diaphragmatic hernia have truncated development of the bronchial tree and lower airway resistance than normal infants (23).

Turbulence refers to the random swirling of gas molecules during bulk flow, in contrast to laminar flow, which is characterized by organized streaming of gas molecules along the same axis. Turbulence is induced as flow rates increase, and it makes ventilation less efficient because it consumes energy. Gas density is directly and linearly related to resistance. Although this has little clinical relevance in most settings, the use of low-density gas mixtures improves ventilation with anatomic abnormalities that produce high resistance, such as tracheal stenosis and bronchopulmonary dysplasia. Heliox, a mixture of 80% helium and 20% oxygen, has a density one third that of room air and therefore generates one third the resistance (24).

The calculated product of resistance and compliance is a useful parameter that integrates two of the primary determinants of airflow and is referred to as the *time constant* (TC):

$$TC = RC_{dyn}$$

where R is resistance, and C_{dyn} is dynamic compliance. The *time constant* reflects the time required for pressure equilibration to occur as air flows down a pressure gradient. During one time constant, 63% of an inspiratory or expiratory tidal volume can occur, whereas about four time constants are required for completion of flow. Conditions that increase either resistance or compliance will increase the time constant. During mechanical ventilation, consideration of this effect is required to allow adequate expiratory time before initiation of the next ventilatory cycle. Inadequate expiratory time results in "breath stacking" and overdistention of alveoli. Additionally, most focal lung diseases result in considerable inhomogeneity in regional time constants. Inspiratory times need to be adjusted to allow for the longest time constants to ensure even distribution of ventilation. Conditions associated with low compliance result in short time constants. Therefore, an increase in minute ventilation is accomplished more efficiently by increasing ventilatory rate, which is permitted by the short time constant, than by increasing tidal volume, which requires high pressures in low-compliance lungs.

Pulmonary Blood Flow

Although the pathophysiology of pulmonary hypertension is covered more thoroughly in the subsequent section, the basic principles governing the regulation of pulmonary vascular resistance and flow are introduced here because they determine the matching of ventilation and perfusion, and hence the efficiency of gas exchange. Blood flow in the lung is influenced by a variety of mechanical and vasoreactive phenomena, which combine to determine local vascular resistances and, therefore, the regional distribution of blood flow.

As previously discussed, resistance is inversely related to the fourth power of vessel radius, making vessel caliber the most important determinant of resistance and flow. Pulmonary vascular caliber is determined both by mechanical factors acting on vessel walls and by muscular contraction within vessel walls. The mechanical factors that influence vessel caliber include radial traction on larger vessels produced by parenchymal expansion and compressive pressure imparted on microvessels within the alveolar walls by air pressure within the alveolus.

These mechanical forces come into play primarily at the extremes of lung volume. At low lung volumes, the lack of radial traction reduces caliber and increases resistance within the larger parenchymal vessels. At high volumes, excessive intraalveolar pressures are imparted to the alveolar arterioles, capillaries, and venules as they transit through the alveolar unit. If this lateral pressure exceeds downstream pulmonary venous pressure (or pulmonary capillary wedge pressure), it becomes a determinant of the pressure gradient driving flow across the alveolar capillary. Normally, the pressure gradient is determined by the difference between mean pulmonary arterial pressure (P_{PA}) and pulmonary venous pressure (P_{PV}) ($\Delta P = P_{PA} - P_{PV}$). When alveolar pressure exceeds P_{PV}, it acts as the downstream pressure ($\Delta P = P_{PA} - P_{Alv}$). The anatomic arrangement of vessels "suspended" within the alveolar unit and influenced by external alveolar pressures is referred to as a *Starling resistor*. The phenomenon of the Starling resistor allows the lung to be viewed as a continuum of zones in which capillary blood flow depends on the relationship between hydrostatic venous pressure and intraalveolar pressure.

In addition to mechanical forces, the distribution of blood flow within the pulmonary circulation is affected by a variety of vasoconstrictive stimuli. Extensive autoregulation of pulmonary blood flow ensures that perfusion is directed toward capillaries adjoining well-ventilated alveoli and away from collapsed or fluid-filled alveoli. This autoregulation is accomplished by increasing pulmonary vascular tone in vessels leading to poorly ventilated alveoli with low partial pressures of oxygen, a process referred to as *hypoxic pulmonary vasoconstriction* (HPV).

Factors that influence HPV include (a) the partial pressure of oxygen within the alveolus (P_{AO_2}), (b) the partial pressure of oxygen within arteriolar blood (P_{aO_2}), (c) the partial pressure of carbon dioxide in arteriolar blood (P_{aCO_2}), and (d) the pH of arteriolar blood. Pulmonary vascular tone is inversely related to the partial pressure of oxygen in both the alveolus and the capillary blood, but P_{AO_2} appears to be a more important factor (25). In fact, alveolar hypoxia is the single most powerful stimulus to pulmonary vasoconstriction. The pH of capillary blood also affects blood flow; local acidosis is an important stimulus to pulmonary vasoconstriction. Increased P_{aCO_2} increases vascular tone both by lowering pH and also by acidosis-independent mechanisms.

Physiologic mediators of vascular smooth-muscle contraction common to these stimuli have not yet been fully identified. The caliber of pulmonary vessels at any given time is dependent on the balance of mediators causing vascular smooth-muscle contraction and relaxation. Mediators of vasodilatation include bradykinin, prostaglandins E_1 and A_1 (PGE_1, PGA_1), prostacyclin (PGI_2), and nitric oxide. Mediators of vasoconstriction include the leukotrienes, endothelin-1 (ET-1), prostaglandin D_2 (PGD_2), and histamine. Histamine, ET-1, and PGD_2 appear to have biphasic effects mediated by different receptor populations, causing vasodilatation in the fetal and early neonatal periods and vasoconstriction after the first few days of life (26–28). Most of these mediators originate from local sources, such as pulmonary endothelial cells and mast cells.

Gas-exchange Determinants

The ultimate goal of respiratory function is gas exchange, which is the transfer of oxygen from inspired air to capillary blood and the reciprocal transfer of carbon dioxide from blood to alveolar gas. The principal determinants of gas exchange are total alveolar ventilation, ventilation/perfusion matching, diffusion, and extrapulmonary shunt. The mechanical properties discussed previously affect gas exchange primarily by determining the amount and distribution of ventilation. Regulation of pulmonary blood flow determines ventilation/perfusion matching and the efficiency of gas exchange. Extrapulmonary shunt occurs primarily through cardiac septal defects and the ductus arteriosus and is discussed in the section on cardiac physiology. Diffusion abnormalities are uncommon causes of gas exchange problems in children. Total ventilation and ventilation/perfusion matching are the most important causes of impaired gas exchange and merit further discussion.

Ventilation

Tidal volume is divided into two separate volumes: *alveolar ventilation,* which participates in gas exchange, and *physiologic dead space,* which does not. Physiologic dead space is further divided into *anatomic dead space,* which describes the volume of the prealveolar conducting airways, and *alveolar dead space,* which includes the ventilated but nonperfused alveoli. Normally, alveolar dead space is negligible, and total physiologic dead space approximates one third of tidal volume. In some diseases, such as ARDS, alveolar dead space may be increased. During mechanical ventilation, anatomic dead space is increased by the addition of ventilator tubing. Effective alveolar ventilation is best monitored by measuring P_{CO_2}, which is relatively insensitive to abnormalities of ventilation/perfusion matching. Alveolar hypoventilation results in both inadequate oxygenation and inadequate carbon dioxide removal.

Ventilation/Perfusion Matching

The appropriate matching of ventilation and perfusion is the single most important determinant of gas exchange in the normal lung. Most disease states that cause abnormal gas exchange do so by promoting an imbalance between ventilation and perfusion. Perfusion is matched to regional ventilation by the mechanisms governing pulmonary blood flow discussed above. When the normal mechanisms of pulmonary vascular autoregulation are impaired, ventilation/perfusion ratio ($\dot{V}/\dot{Q}$) mismatch ensues.

Normal alveoli with matched ventilation and perfusion are considered to have a $\dot{V}/\dot{Q}$ ratio of 1. Those with relatively less ventilation have a $\dot{V}/\dot{Q}$ less than 1, and those with relatively less perfusion have a $\dot{V}/\dot{Q}$ greater than 1. Those with ventilation but no perfusion define alveolar dead space, whereas those with perfusion but no ventilation contribute to *intrapulmonary shunt,* which is microcirculatory bypass of alveolar exchange. Between these two extremes lies a spectrum of $\dot{V}/\dot{Q}$ relationships that may contribute to abnormal gas exchange. $\dot{V}/\dot{Q}$ mismatch generally results in hypoxemia with normocarbia. Because carbon dioxide diffuses through the capillary–alveolar interface much more readily than does oxygen, $\dot{V}/\dot{Q}$ mismatch has relatively little effect on P_{CO_2} levels.

Mismatching of ventilation and perfusion is responsible for the hypoxemia encountered in most clinical settings. These include the disease states in which lung compliance is reduced, FRC drops below closing volume, and regional alveolar collapse occurs: pneumonitis, aspiration, RDS, ARDS, cardiogenic pulmonary edema, postoperative splinting, and others. Simply increasing forced inspiratory oxygen (F_iO_2) does little to rectify the situation because the venous admixture of blood passing through low $\dot{V}/\dot{Q}$ units remains low in oxygen saturation, and blood passing through normal $\dot{V}/\dot{Q}$ units cannot further increase oxygen content to compensate. Therapeutic efforts must be directed at reopening closed alveoli and restoring homogenous alveolar ventilation.

Although diuresis, antibiotic therapy, and chest physiotherapy may have important roles in restoring FRC and matched ventilation and perfusion, perhaps the most effective therapeutic intervention is the use of continuous positive intraalveolar distending pressure: CPAP or PEEP, which recruit and maintain previously closed or underventilated alveoli and improve $\dot{V}/\dot{Q}$ matching and oxygenation. They also shift ventilation up on the static compliance curve, producing a higher tidal volume with less pressure trauma.

The use of positive-pressure mechanical ventilation and PEEP must be managed judiciously because they can have both beneficial and deleterious effects on $\dot{V}/\dot{Q}$ matching. It is important to remember that positive airway pressure is transmitted to the alveolar capillaries that carry blood flow through the alveolar network. The alveolar pressure surrounding these capillaries acts as a Starling resistor and may impede capillary blood flow if it exceeds downstream venous pressure. The use of high peak ventilatory pressures without the use of PEEP, or the excessive use of PEEP itself, can cause overdistention of alveoli, reduced compliance, increased alveolar capillary resistance, and diminished alveolar capillary perfusion. The result is redirection of blood flow to underventilated alveoli, which actually worsens V/Q mismatch. Similarly, the use of PEEP in focal lung disease may be counterproductive because its effects are preferentially directed to the normal, more compliant alveoli. This causes overdistention of normal $\dot{V}/\dot{Q}$ units and redistribution of blood flow to diseased alveoli, cancelling the benefits of hypoxic pulmonary vasoconstriction.

Surfactant and Respiratory Distress Syndromes

Respiratory distress syndrome, or hyaline membrane disease (HMD), is the most common causes of respiratory distress in neonates and one of the primary causes of neonatal mortality in developed countries. RDS occurs as a direct result of pulmonary immaturity and surfactant deficiency. Because surfactant is not produced and secreted by type II alveolar epithelial cells until the third trimester, prematurity causes newborns to rely on lungs of variable maturity to support extrauterine respiration. Preterm infants born during the terminal saccular phase of lung development face the challenge of supporting gas exchange with lungs characterized by relatively thicker epithelial barriers, suboptimal capillary architecture, and a tendency toward alveolar collapse. This last feature is the most important cause of respiratory failure in premature infants and is directly related to the lack of surfactant, which lowers surface tension at the alveolar liquid–gas interface.

Surfactant is a complex substance composed of phospholipids (80%), proteins (10%), and cholesterol (10%). The phospholipid profile changes during lung maturation, but phosphotidylcholine predominates and is the principal substance responsible for the surface-tension lowering properties of surfactant. Phosphotidylinositol is present in immature surfactant, but it is largely replaced by phosphotidylglycerol in mature lungs, a useful fact when assessing fetal lung maturity. Surfactant also contains at least four specific proteins: surfactant protein-A (SP-A), SP-B, SP-C, and SP-D. The functions of these proteins have not been defined completely, but together they help promote the spreading, organization, and adherence of the phospholipid layer. They also have important roles in surfactant recycling and host immune defense.

The physiologic role of surfactant is to stabilize alveolar units against collapse and thereby to facilitate homogeneous lung ventilation and $\dot{V}/\dot{Q}$ matching. *LaPlace's law* states that the pressure required to overcome the retracting force of surface tension in a sphere is inversely related to radius. In clinical terms, this means that smaller alveoli actually require greater distending pressure to maintain stability. This is analogous to the phenomenon one experiences when trying to inflate a balloon: the initial pressure required to begin inflation is high and becomes progressively less as the balloon radius increases. Because the lung is a collection of alveoli of varying sizes, and all alveoli are exposed to the same atmospheric pressure through a shared network of airways, the natural tendency is for the smaller alveoli to collapse and transfer their volume of air to larger neighboring alveoli, which become overdistended. In both cases, the effect on compliance is deleterious: FRC declines, the work of breathing increases, $\dot{V}/\dot{Q}$ matching is compromised, and respiratory failure ensues. Surfactant not only reduces absolute surface tension, but it does so in a graded fashion. In small radius alveoli, the phospholipid layer is condensed and its effect on surface tension is great. As the alveolus expands, the phospholipid molecules spread out and impart a gradually decreasing effect on surface tension. This differential efficiency of surfactant function allows alveoli of different sizes to coexist in a stable fashion.

Surfactant composition is an important determinant and predictor of fetal lung maturity. By the 20th week of gestation, collections of surfactant appear in type II cells within cytoplasmic granules called *lamellar bodies*. Thereafter, surfactant begins to appear in the developing terminal sacs. Infants born at 25 weeks occasionally survive without respiratory support; at 30 weeks, the risk of respiratory distress approaches 50%, and by 35 weeks' gestation nearly all fetuses are capable of unassisted extrauterine respiration. There is considerable variability with respect to the timing of lung maturity, however, and clinical indices that assess lung maturity are useful in planning early delivery. The most common index of lung maturity is the amniotic fluid ratio of lecithin (phosphotidylcholine) to sphingomyelin, that is, the L/S ratio. Because amniotic phosphotidylcholine is derived solely from surfactant and sphingomyelin derives from all cell membranes, this provides a convenient self-indexed measurement of surfactant production that is independent of changes in amniotic fluid volume. An L/S ratio of 2.0 is achieved in the normal fetus by 35 weeks' gestation and is associated with

an extremely low risk of RDS. Values of 1.5 to 2.0 are considered "immature" but of low risk. Values below 1.5 are associated with increased risk, and those below 1.0 are considered high risk (29). A more detailed test, the Lung Profile, utilizes the L/S ratio as well as percentages of phosphotidylglycerol and phosphotidylinositol to predict more accurately the risk of RDS (30).

The fact that some infants born prior to 35 weeks' gestation do not manifest RDS led to the idea of stress-induced lung maturation. Fetal stress that promotes preterm labor also appears to promote accelerated lung maturation. This observation prompted the use of exogenous maternal corticosteroid administration to promote early lung maturation in fetuses expected to deliver early due to preterm labor or induced delivery. Whether exogenous corticosteroids primarily accelerate surfactant production or alveolar growth, or both, is still unclear (31,32).

Postnatal administration of exogenous surfactant has become a mainstay of treatment not only for prematurity-associated RDS but also for a wide variety of neonatal lung diseases associated with reduced compliance. Surfactant replacement therapy has been proven to decrease the incidence and severity of RDS, especially when used in conjunction with antenatal maternal corticosteroids, and it appears to be efficacious in both prophylactic and rescue strategies. The two most commonly used preparations are a synthetic phospholipid/alcohol mixture (Exosurf) and a bovine surfactant extract supplemented with phospholipids and surfactant proteins (Surventa). Modified recombinant preparations are expected to become available in the near future. These preparations are aerosolized into the airway through an endotracheal tube with positive pressure ventilation. Although initially designed for treatment of RDS, they appear to reduce ventilatory requirements and complications in a variety of diseases characterized by reduced compliance, including congenital diaphragmatic hernia, meconium aspiration, persistent pulmonary hypertension of the newborn (PPHN), and ARDS in older patients (33).

Pulmonary Hypoplasia

Pulmonary hypoplasia refers to a condition in which pulmonary parenchymal tissue is abnormally reduced relative to body size. It is defined pathologically by reduced lung dry weight or DNA content relative to body mass and reduced alveolar number per unit volume. Although pulmonary hypoplasia may occur rarely as a primary disease, it is usually a stereotypical consequence of mechanical compression during lung development. Clinically, secondary pulmonary hypoplasia is associated most commonly with congenital diaphragmatic hernia, giant omphaloceles, and oligohydramnios caused by fetal renal dysfunction or urinary obstruction. Whether the true cause of pulmonary hypoplasia is mechanical compression, some alteration in fetal lung fluid dynamics, or a combination of both has not yet been elucidated.

Whatever the cause, pulmonary hypoplasia results from arrested development of the tracheobronchial tree and pulmonary vasculature. Depending on the severity of compression, the sequential binary branching of the developing airway may be arrested well before the usual 22 or 23 divisions, resulting in fewer respiratory units and a reduced pulmonary capillary network. The pulmonary arterial tree is not just quantitatively diminished, but it is histologically and functionally abnormal as well. The pulmonary arterioles in affected lungs are characterized by thickening of the muscular media, abnormal extension of the muscular media into terminal arterioles, and hyperreactivity of the vascular smooth muscle cells to vasoconstrictive stimuli. The pathophysiologic effects of pulmonary hypoplasia therefore include both inadequate gas exchange and persistent pulmonary hypertension.

In most cases of pulmonary hypoplasia, the life-threatening consequences of hypoplasia are related to persistent pulmonary hypertension, not to inadequate gas exchange. Most patients with congenital diaphragmatic hernia, for instance, will have one or more blood gas measurements which document the potential for adequate gas exchange. Subsequent physiologic deterioration (and death) result from progressive, refractory pulmonary hypertension, extrapulmonary right-to-left shunting, and global hypoxemia. These subjects are covered more thoroughly in the discussion of persistent fetal circulation.

Ventilatory Support

Ventilatory management of pediatric patients has become increasingly complex as technological innovation has expanded the number of available options. These advances have been motivated by a need to improve gas distribution in diseased lungs, to avoid complications associated with barotrauma, and to provide better synchronized and tolerated ventilation. Although conventional positive-pressure ventilation remains the mainstay of management for most infants and children requiring ventilatory support, a number of nonconventional technologies have gained increasing acceptance in certain situations where conventional techniques have proven inadequate.

Conventional Mechanical Ventilation

Conventional positive pressure ventilators deliver a bulk flow of oxygen-enriched gas to the lungs through an endotracheal tube. In general, they are classified according to the method used to initiate and terminate a single ventilatory cycle. Volume-cycled ventilators deliver a predetermined tidal volume of gas. Respiratory rate (cycles/min), flow rate (L/min), inspiratory/expiratory ratio, and inspired oxygen concentration are manipulated to achieve certain respiratory goals, but the actual termination of the positive-pressure breath occurs when the preset tidal volume has been delivered. Volume-cycled ventilation has the advantage of providing precise control of minute ventilation regardless of lung compliance, and it is used routinely in adults and older children.

Infants and small children usually are not managed with volume-cycled ventilators. Although control of minute ventilation is equally important in this group, the risks of barotrauma are high, particularly in neonates with pulmonary immaturity. A reduction in compliance will result in a reciprocal increase in pressure during volume-cycled ventilation, leading to overdistention of ventilated alveoli, $\dot{V}/\dot{Q}$ mismatching, alveolar rupture and pneumothorax, and the chronic lung changes observed with barotrauma. For this reason, precise control of inspiratory pressure is preferable to volume control.

The vast majority of neonatal pediatric ventilators used today are technically not pressure-cycled, but instead are time-cycled and pressure-limited. Instead of ventilatory flow ceasing when a preset pressure is reached, flow continues at a plateau pressure until the inspiratory time is reached. This improves tidal volume consistency and distribution. Constant monitoring of respiratory function (e.g., continuous transcutaneous oximetry) is imperative to prevent hypoventilation in the event of a sudden decrease in compliance and tidal volume.

The usual options for ventilatory modes in pediatric ventilator management are essentially identical to those used in adults: control, assist control, intermittent mandatory ventilation (IMV), synchronized IMV, and pressure support. The function and utility of these modes in children are similar to their use in adults. Pressure support, in which each spontaneous breath is assisted by supplemental positive pressure, is becoming the preferred mode in many settings where the patient is conscious and breathing spontaneously. It is particularly effective in the weaning of mechanical ventilation and restoring respiratory muscle strength.

For most modes, one selects the parameters that determine gas exchange: F_iO_2, respiratory rate, PIP, and PEEP. Inspiratory flow rates may need to be adjusted to provide an appropriate inspiratory/expiratory ratio within the constraints of the preset respiratory rate. PEEP is adjusted to optimize compliance and FRC; PIP is adjusted to provide an adequate tidal volume. Flow rates are adjusted with an appreciation of the different time constants observed in various clinical settings. The F_iO_2 is minimized to avoid pulmonary oxygen toxicity and retinopathy. The mean airway pressure (MAP), which is measured and represents the area under the time-pressure curve, is probably the single best parameter to follow for monitoring changes in the level of ventilatory support required as well as the risk of barotrauma.

Unconventional Mechanical Ventilation

Conventional breathing and mechanical ventilation both involve the bulk transport of air through conducting airways to gas exchange chambers (alveoli), where diffusion occurs across the alveolar–capillary membrane. The altered gas then is expired by bulk transport, and a new cycle begins. This type of bulk flow is implied when describing the ventilatory properties of the lung in terms of "bellows" function. In many disease states associated with reduced lung compliance, the high positive pressures necessary to produce this bulk flow of gas during mechanical ventilation result in considerable iatrogenic lung injury. This injury is manifested both by parenchymal changes and edema, which further reduce compliance and diffusion, as well as mechanical disruption of small bronchi and alveoli, resulting in mediastinal emphysema, pneumothorax, and bronchopleural fistulae. Excessively high inspiratory pressures also impair venous return to the right atrium, thereby reducing preload, lung perfusion, gas exchange, and global cardiac output.

Whether ventilation-induced acute lung injury is due primarily to the pressure itself or to overdistention of the more compliant alveoli is a subject of considerable ongoing debate. Current evidence seems to favor the structural overdistention of alveoli as the principal cause of iatrogenic lung injury, leading some to prefer the term volutrauma to the more accepted term barotrauma (34–36). In reality, both mechanisms probably contribute to lung injury. Whatever the underlying cause, peak inspiratory pressure seems to be the parameter that correlates best with induced lung injury.

Several novel ventilatory techniques have emerged recently that attempt to mitigate barotrauma and hemodynamic compromise by providing effective ventilation without excessive PIP. These techniques employ extremely high ventilatory rates and tidal volumes less than or equal to anatomic dead space. Although numerous variations exist, the most popular modes are high-frequency jet ventilation (HFJV) and high-frequency oscillatory ventilation (HFOV). In HFJV, a small cannula is advanced through the endotracheal tube and used to deliver rapid, low-volume bursts of inspired gas. Ventilation does not require bulk flow, but it relies on several poorly defined physical processes, the most important of which is probably coaxial flow. In coaxial flow, the jet stream induces continuous rotational flow of inspired gas down the cen-

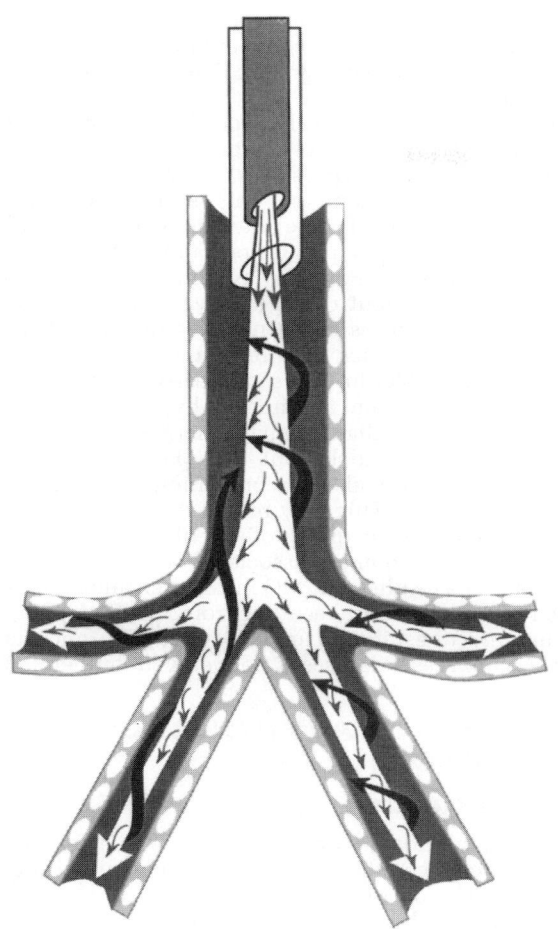

Figure 94.6. Proposed coaxial flow pattern during high-frequency jet and oscillatory ventilation. Gas inflow is confined to the center of the airway lumen, and outflow is confined to the periphery. (Reprinted from Harris TR, Wood BR. In: Goldsmith JP, Karotkin EH, eds. *Assisted ventilation of the neonate,* 3rd ed. Philadelphia: WB Saunders, 1996, with permission.)

ter of the airway and reverse rotational flow of expired gas along the perimeter of the airway (Fig. 94.6). In HFOV, ventilation is driven by the oscillations of a diaphragm within a closed noncompliant system. The cyclical compression and expansion of gas within the system generate high-velocity, streaming flow patterns that are similar to the coaxial flow seen in HFJV. The major difference between the two is that the expiratory phase is active in HFOV, as opposed to the passive expiration seen in both HFJV and conventional ventilation. This difference may make HFOV more effective in reducing air leaks from bronchopleural fistulae and less likely to cause air trapping and overdistention in lungs with longer and more heterogeneous time constants.

In both modalities, ventilator management is often unpredictable and counterintuitive. For instance, in HFOV the F_iO_2, MAP, frequency (cycles per second, or Hz), and *amplitude* (volume displacement caused by oscillation of the diaphragm) are preset. The amplitude is not truly reflective of the tiny tidal volume produced at the end of the endotracheal tube and is therefore useful as a relative, "unitless" measurement only. In practice, one judges the adequacy of the amplitude subjectively by observing chest wall vibration. Increasing P_aO_2 usually requires increasing the F_iO_2 or the MAP, which recruits alveoli and increases

FRC similar to the use of PEEP. In some conditions, the MAP required actually may be higher than that required in conventional ventilation, but the PIP is far less. Reducing P_aCO_2 actually may require reducing the oscillatory rate to allow more time for gas displacement and more effective gas streaming.

In general, high-frequency ventilatory techniques are effective at promoting improved CO_2 elimination at lower pressures than conventional ventilation. Improved oxygenation is less reliable. HFJV and HFOV are both helpful in providing respiratory support in infants with preexisting barotrauma and air leaks. The ability of HFOV to support enhanced CO_2 removal and generate a respiratory alkalosis at lower pressures has made it useful in managing infants with persistent pulmonary hypertension, particularly those with congenital diaphragmatic hernia.

Liquid ventilation is a novel, experimental approach to respiratory support that currently is undergoing clinical trials in a variety of settings. In this approach, a liquid perfluorocarbon solution is instilled into the lungs instead of a gas mixture. Because many forms of respiratory failure are associated with surfactant insufficiency and reduced compliance, the substitution of liquid for gas in the alveolus eliminates the liquid–gas interface, reduces surface tension, and improves compliance. The improvement of mechanical properties in the perfluorocarbon-filled lung allows ventilation to occur at lower pressures and less barotrauma. The solubility of oxygen and carbon dioxide in perfluorocarbon solutions is extremely high, allowing respiratory gases to diffuse easily across the alveolar–capillary membrane. Although total liquid ventilation requires a closed circuit and is clinically impractical, a partial liquid ventilation technique has been developed that is logistically feasible and promises to provide ventilatory benefits to some patients with reduced lung compliance (37). In partial liquid ventilation, perfluorocarbon is instilled at a volume equal to FRC, and conventional ventilation then is superimposed on the liquid-phase FRC. In essence, this is analogous to providing "liquid PEEP," and improves pulmonary mechanics with little increase in alveolar distending pressure. The optimal role for partial or total liquid ventilation remains a subject for further investigation.

Extracorporeal Support

In certain situations, conventional and nonconventional ventilatory techniques are inadequate to provide gas exchange in the face of overwhelming pulmonary dysfunction. Under these circumstances, the use of extracorporeal membrane oxygenation (ECMO) may succeed in sustaining oxygen delivery and carbon dioxide removal until the underlying cause of respiratory failure is reversed and physiologic improvement occurs. It is important to recognize that, like conventional ventilation, ECMO is a supportive rather than therapeutic technique and has a limited window of utility imposed by the adverse effects of the technology itself.

Several variations of ECMO technology exist, but all share the same underlying principles: the partial diversion of blood from the patient to an external membrane oxygenator, ex vivo exchange of oxygen and carbon dioxide, and return of blood to the circulatory system. The circuit is driven by a roller pump that is similar to that used for routine cardiopulmonary bypass. Systemic anticoagulation is necessary to prevent thrombosis from occurring in the extracorporeal circuit.

Two basic methods of providing ECMO support are currently available: venoarterial (VA) and venovenous (VV). In VA ECMO, the right common carotid artery and jugular

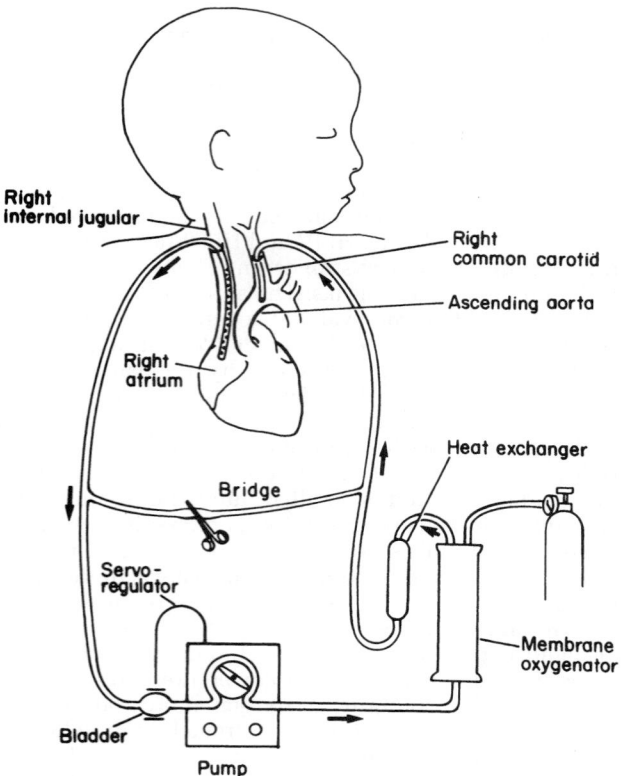

Figure 94.7. Components of a standard venoarterial extracorporeal membrane oxygenation *(ECMO)* circuit. (Reprinted from O'Rourke PP. In: Holbrook PR, ed. *Textbook of pediatric critical care.* Philadelphia: WB Saunders, 1993, with permission.)

vein are cannulated. Venous inflow to the system results from passive drainage of the right atrium; arterial flow back to the patient occurs in the aortic arch (Fig. 94.7). As return flow is into the aorta, partial cardiac bypass occurs, which may provide significant benefit when respiratory failure is accompanied by compromised cardiac performance. About 60% of cardiac output is provided by the circuit in VA ECMO. In VV ECMO, the circuit is interposed into the venous side of the circulation, with blood returning to the right atrium. Although it provides no direct support of cardiac output, this method obviates the ligation and sacrifice of a carotid artery, avoids some of the risk of arterial embolization, and provides well-oxygenated blood for pulmonary and coronary circulation. For infants and children with adequate cardiac function, VV ECMO may become the modality of choice for extracorporeal support.

Indications for ECMO vary among institutions. Because of the high cost and potential for complications, ECMO is justifiable only when all other available therapies for respiratory failure have proven inadequate or when quantifiable parameters predict a high risk of mortality with conventional management. Several methods of providing a quantitative estimate of respiratory failure have been used to predict mortality with conventional ventilation and guide the use of ECMO. Perhaps the most widely used index is the oxygenation index (OI), which compares ventilatory support parameters (MAP and F_iO_2) with gas exchange results (postductal P_aO_2):

$$OI = (MAP)(F_iO_2)/P_aO_2 \times 100$$

An OI greater than 40 predicts a mortality rate 80% and is a commonly cited threshold indicator for the use of ECMO. Another useful, although more burdensome, pa-

rameter for quantifying respiratory failure and predicting mortality is the alveolar–arterial oxygen gradient (P_{AO_2}–P_aO_2), which when greater than 600 predicts a mortality rate of 80%.

Results for extracorporeal support are age and diagnosis dependent. Infants with respiratory failure (meconium aspiration syndrome, RDS, sepsis) appear to benefit most from extracorporeal support. This is most likely because neonatal respiratory failure often is associated with reversible pulmonary hypertension, and ECMO allows for the normalization of PO_2, PCO_2, pH, and pulmonary vascular resistance without the aggressive ventilatory support that frequently causes iatrogenic lung injury and chronic lung disease. Neonates with reversible, idiopathic PPHN benefit from ECMO for the same reasons. Neonates with respiratory failure and pulmonary hypertension attributable to congenital diaphragmatic hernia and pulmonary hypoplasia appear to benefit from ECMO, but the improvement in survival over conventional management is not as significant. This may reflect the irreversible problems related to inadequacy of alveolar number and microvascular development associated with pulmonary hypoplasia. The results of ECMO in children and adolescents with respiratory failure resulting from ARDS, trauma, viral pneumonia, or aspiration are less convincing, and the role of ECMO in these diseases is not yet well defined (38).

CARDIOVASCULAR PHYSIOLOGY AND SUPPORT

Fetal Circulation

Fetal circulation has evolved to utilize an external organ of gas exchange, the placenta, while maintaining the anatomic relationships that will later be necessary in extrauterine life when responsibility for gas exchange transitions abruptly to the lungs. The fetal circulatory system is characterized by asymmetric ventricles that function in parallel, an arrangement made possible by two anatomic shunts—the foramen ovale and the ductus arteriosus. These shunts make possible the nonrandom distribution of blood of varying oxygen contents and the delivery of adequate amounts of oxygen and substrate to developing organs (Fig. 94.8).

Well-oxygenated blood returning from the placenta and umbilical cord passes through the hepatic ductus venosus, into the inferior vena cava (IVC) and immediately into the right atrium. Ductus venosus blood mixes little with the less oxygenated blood in the infrahepatic IVC and flows relatively undisturbed (in a laminar fashion referred to as *streaming*) along the medial wall of the IVC, through the right atrium, across the foramen ovale, and into the left atrium. This oxygen-rich blood then is pumped by the left ventricle into the aortic arch, where it is distributed to the developing heart, brain, and upper body (Fig. 94.9). The less oxygenated blood in the IVC and superior vena cava (SVC) flows preferentially through the right atrium to the right ventricle and are pumped into the pulmonary artery, where the majority is shunted through the ductus arteriosus into the descending aorta. A small amount of pulmonary artery flow provides substrate to the lungs. Descending aortic flow is distributed to the developing organs of the lower body, with most of the flow being diverted back to the placenta through the two umbilical arteries. Flow through the placental circulation approximates 40% of cardiac output.

The fetal pattern of blood flow is made possible by high pulmonary vascular resistance, which directs the flow of oxygen-poor blood from the pulmonary artery into the descending aorta. Only 5% to 10% of pulmonary artery flow

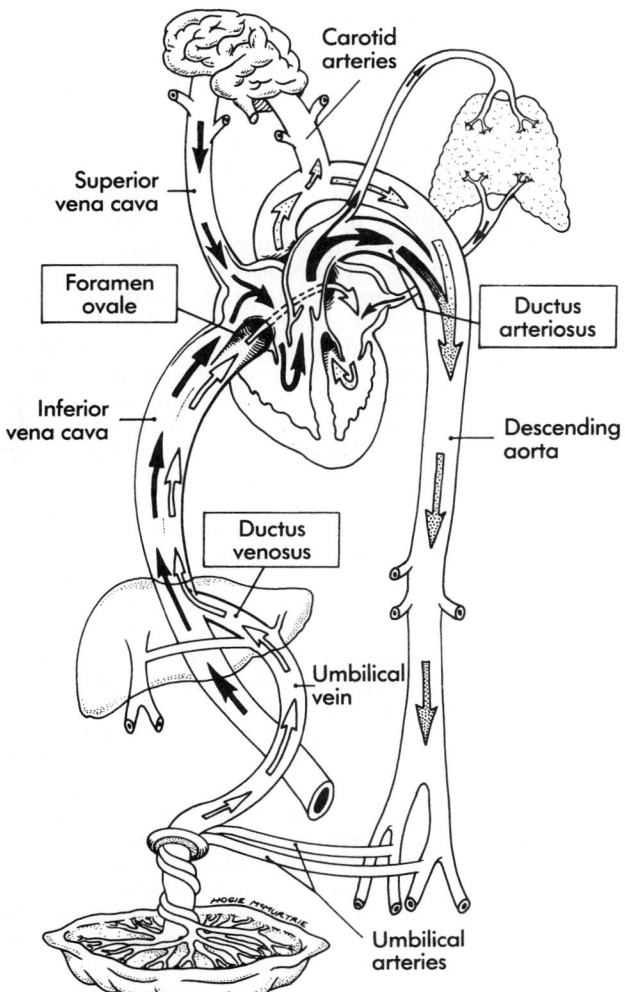

Figure 94.8. Fetal circulation. (Reprinted from Bloom RS. In: Faranoff AA, Martin RJ, eds. *Neonatal–perinatal medicine: diseases of the fetus and infant,* 6th ed. St. Louis: Mosby, 1997, with permission.)

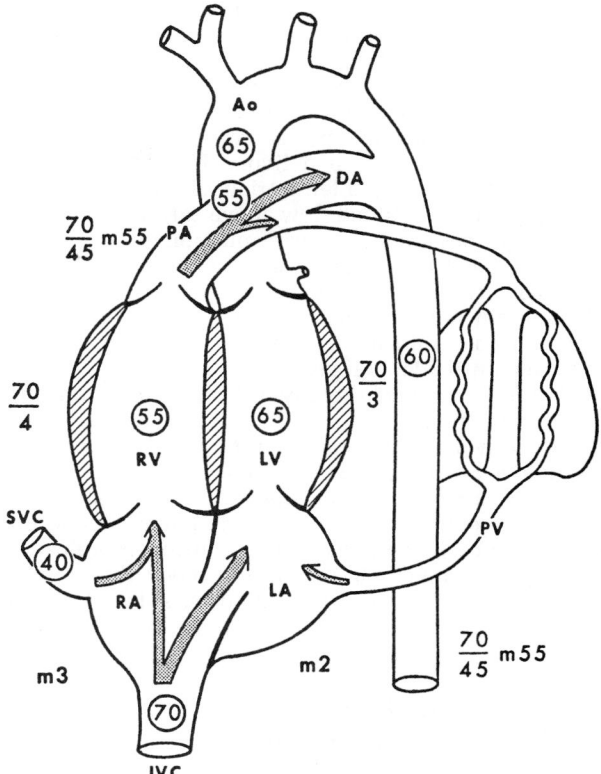

Figure 94.9. Oxyhemoglobin saturations in the fetal circulation. Preferential flow of saturated blood from the inferior vena cava *(IVC)* into the left atrium *(LA)* and desaturated blood from the superior vena cava *(SVC)* into the right atrium *(RA)* results in the distribution of blood with higher oxygen content to the aortic arch *(Ao)* and developing brain. (Reprinted from Rudolph AM. Changes in the circulation after birth. In: Rudolph AM, ed. *Congenital diseases of the heart.* Chicago: Year Book Medical, 1974, with permission.)

actually traverses the pulmonary capillary bed. This minimizes the return of less oxygenated blood through the pulmonary veins and prevents mixing with the oxygen-rich blood in the left ventricle destined for the heart and brain. The relatively low afterload presented to the right ventricle by the low-resistance shunt across the ductus arteriosus accounts for the fact that fetal right ventricular output exceeds left ventricular output, in some estimates by 40% to 100% (39,40). Mechanisms of increased pulmonary resistance in the fetus include mechanical compression of pulmonary vessels in the fluid-filled lung and vasoconstriction secondary to hypoxemia, leukotrienes, and the peptide mediator endothelin-1 (41).

Transitional Circulation

At birth, profound changes in circulatory patterns, hemodynamics, and gas exchange occur as a result of the abrupt withdrawal of placental support. Transitional physiology is characterized by the cessation of placental blood flow and gas exchange and the simultaneous increase in blood flow and gas exchange in the lungs. As amniotic fluid is expelled from the lungs by compression during birth and the lungs expand with the infant's first

breath, alveolar expansion causes an immediate reduction in pulmonary vascular resistance secondary to increased traction on larger parenchymal vessels and decreased intraalveolar pressure transmitted to alveolar microvessels. Increased local oxygen concentrations reduce hypoxic pulmonary vasoconstriction through mechanisms mediated by endothelial-derived intermediates, such as nitric oxide and prostacyclin (42,43). Pulmonary artery pressures fall more slowly over the first weeks of life and may approximate systemic pressures for the first several days of life.

The sudden decrease in pulmonary vascular resistance causes a dramatic increase in pulmonary blood flow and left atrial return. Left ventricular preload increases, resulting in increased left ventricular stroke volume and output. Right atrial return is reduced as placental flow ceases. Elevated left atrial pressure and reduced right atrial pressure cause closure of the flap-like foramen ovale, eliminating one of the fetal extrapulmonary shunts.

The other shunt, the ductus arteriosus, begins to close by vasoconstriction immediately. This process is mediated both by a withdrawal of placental-derived prostaglandins and by an increase in oxygen tension, a potent vasoconstrictive stimulus for ductal tissue. Physiologic duct closure usually occurs by 24 hours but may take up to 3 days. Anatomic duct obliteration resulting from thrombosis and fibrosis may take several weeks or months. When spontaneous closure of the ductus arteriosus does not occur, as often happens in the premature infant whose immature ductal tissue is unresponsive to vasoconstrictive mediators, significant physiologic problems may occur. If pulmonary artery pressures remain abnormally high, an anatomic right-to-left shunt may occur that diverts desaturated blood around the pulmonary system, drastically lowering systemic oxygen delivery. If pulmonary artery pressure falls normally, a left-to-right shunt will occur, increasing pulmonary blood flow above cardiac output. Pulmonary overcirculation causes pulmonary edema and congestive heart failure in the short term and irreversible pulmonary hypertension in the long-term if uncorrected. Indomethicin administration, which inhibits prostaglandin synthetase, is effective in promoting ductal closure in most premature infants if given within the first 2 weeks of life. Failure of medical therapy indicates the need for surgical duct ligation.

Another event in the transition to extrauterine circulation involves vasoconstrictive or mechanical occlusion of the cord vessels. The abolishment of this "shunt" increases left ventricular afterload and systemic blood pressure and, along with increased left ventricular preload, accounts for an immediate increase in blood flow to target organs. Ductus venosus closure occurs by stasis and thrombosis as return flow through the umbilical vein ceases.

Postnatal Circulation and Cardiac Performance

Following the transition from fetal to neonatal life, the circulatory system is characterized by two separate cardiovascular circuits operating in a "series" configuration. By definition, right and left heart cardiac outputs are identical and can be considered symmetrical despite discrepancies in system pressures and contractile properties. The series configuration has great significance in that it imposes a degree of interdependence on the two circuits that does not exist in utero. Pathologic changes in one circuit necessarily impact the other circuit by virtue of alterations in the other circuit's preload or afterload. Failure of complete separation of the two circuits results in the deleterious shunting of blood from the pulmonary to systemic circuit or vice versa.

Cardiac output is determined by the same parameters in the neonate as is in the adult: heart rate and stroke volume. Stroke volume, in turn, is dependent on three factors: preload, contractility, and afterload. Although a detailed discussion of these four determinants of cardiac performance is beyond the scope of this chapter, it is instructive to consider some of the differences between pediatric and adult cardiac function relative to these four variables. These differences account for the fact that, in general, neonatal and pediatric patients have less cardiovascular reserve than do adolescents and young adults.

Heart rate, an important determinant of cardiac output in infants, becomes less important in childhood and adolescence. In fact, neonates are commonly referred to as *rate dependent*. The normal range for heart rate in neonates is higher than that in adults and decreases gradually throughout childhood to adult levels (Table 94.6). In adults, changes in heart rate result in little change in cardiac output because of compensatory changes in other parameters. When heart rate decreases, ventricular filling and stroke volume increase, and cardiac output is minimally altered. Reciprocal changes occur when heart rate increases. In neonates and, to a lesser extent, in children, these compensatory changes are less effective and changes in heart rate produce corresponding changes in cardiac output. The explanation for this observation lies in the fact that increased ventricular filling times and pressures fail to generate increased end-diastolic and stroke volumes due to decreased myocardial compliance and a blunted Frank-Starling mechanism, as discussed later.

The sympathetic innervation of the heart is relatively underdeveloped in the neonate, resulting in an autonomic imbalance with respect to cardiac function. Neonates respond to physiologic challenges in a predominantly vagal, or parasympathetic, fashion. Sinus bradycardia is therefore a common stereotypical response in the critically ill neonate to many stimuli, including hypoxemia, acidosis, hypoglycemia, intracranial hypertension, abdominal distention, and pulmonary aspiration. Because bradycardia is also more likely to result in an uncompensated decrease in cardiac output, prompt recognition and treatment of bradycardia are more urgent in these patients.

Preload refers to the myocardial fiber stretch at end diastole. *Fiber stretch* is related to end-diastolic volume, which in turn is related to end-diastolic pressure. The Frank-Starling mechanism describes this relationship: An increase in end-diastolic volume and fiber length produces an increase in stroke volume (Fig. 94.10). This phenomenon most likely is explained by changes in contractile fiber geometry that result from increased stretch. The Frank-Starling mechanism is not synonymous with an increase in contractility, which would produce an increased stroke volume at the same preload. This mechanism is less effective in neonates than in adults in producing an increase in myocardial performance. The immature heart is less compliant than the adult heart; so increases in end-diastolic pressure therefore do not produce similar increases in end-diastolic volume and fiber length. Furthermore, neonatal and infant hearts operate at a higher baseline end-diastolic volume (nearer the maximal fiber length) under normal circumstances, leaving less reserve for further effective increases in preload. These observa-

---

Table 94.6. **NORMAL RANGE OF VITAL SIGNS**

Age	Heart rate (beats/min)	Systolic blood Pressure (mm Hg)	Diastolic blood Pressure (mm Hg)	Respiratory rate (breaths/min)
Premature infant				
1 kg	120–140	36–58	18–38	40
3 kg	120–140	50–72	26–46	40
Term infant	120	65–80	30–50	40
0–12 mo[a]	100–120	105	65	40
1–6 y	100	105–110	70	30
6–12 y	80	110–125	70–80	20

[a]90th percentile.
Adapted from Horan MJ. Report of the Second Task Force on Blood Pressure Control in Children—1987. Pediatrics 1987;79:1, with permission.

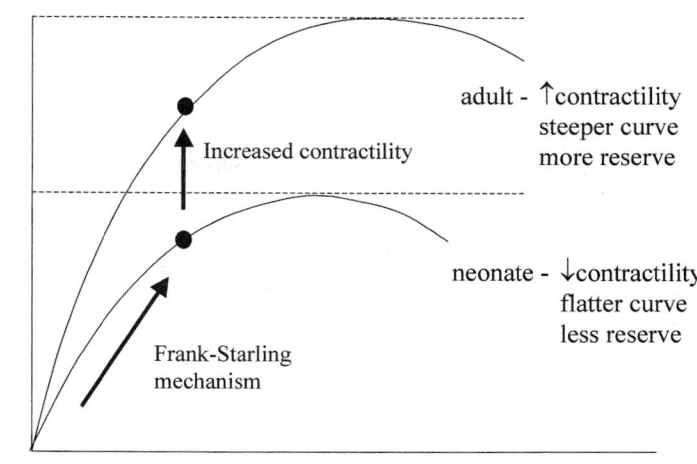

Figure 94.10. Conceptual differences in cardiac performance between neonates and adults. The neonatal heart displays reduced contractility, a reduced response to augmented preload, and a less reserve compared with the adult heart.

tions explain why the neonatal cardiovascular response to preload enhancement is less pronounced than in adults and why the neonate is generally more prone to congestive failure when challenged with a volume load.

Contractility refers to the magnitude and velocity of tension development by the cardiac myocytes in response to contractile stimuli. The contractile, or inotropic, state of the heart is influenced by many factors, including the availability of oxygen, calcium, and catecholamines. An increase in contractility does not result in a shift upward along the Frank-Starling curve, but rather it results in a shift of the entire curve to reflect a greater stroke volume generated at every preload. The neonatal heart is immature in several respects compared with the adult heart. Most importantly, the neonatal heart has a lower concentration of contractile fibers, generating less tension during contraction (44). This is reflected in the lower mean arterial pressures observed throughout childhood. About 60% of the adult cardiac myocyte mass comprises contractile myofibrils, compared with 30% in fetal myocytes. Additional causes of reduced contractility include an underdeveloped sarcoplasmic reticulum and t-tubule system for releasing calcium, a lower concentration of myocyte cell surface β-adrenergic receptors, and decreased sympathetic innervation (45). The structural and functional immaturity of the infant heart account for the relatively greater sensitivity to negative inotropic stimuli, the greater requirement for calcium to maintain the inotropic state, and the requirement for higher concentrations of inotropic agents to achieve measurable hemodynamic effects. In contrast, the neonatal heart is more resistant to the negative inotropic effects of hypoxemia and acidosis than the adult heart, possibly conferring some advantage with respect to the success of cardiopulmonary resuscitation (46).

Afterload refers to the resistance (or impedance) to ventricular output and is directly related to mean arterial pressure. During the transitional phase of circulation, afterload drops abruptly in the right ventricle as pulmonary vascular resistance drops. Left ventricular afterload increases immediately as the placental shunt is abolished but then falls as its output distributes to both the upper and lower body and a larger vascular bed. After the transitional phase, left ventricular afterload slowly increases throughout infancy and childhood, stimulating asymmetrical growth of the left ventricle compared with that of the right. This growth is due primarily to hyperplasia until 2

to 3 months of age, when hypertrophy becomes more important. Before adaptive left ventricular growth occurs, the neonatal heart is exquisitely sensitive and decompensates rapidly when exposed to increases in afterload, such as those that occur in aortic stenosis and aortic coarctation.

Oxygen Content and Delivery

Oxygen delivery is the product of cardiac output and oxygen content. Arterial oxygen content (C_aO_2) is determined by the same set of variables in children as in adults:

$$C_aO_2 = (Hb)(1.34 \text{ mL } O_2/g \text{ Hb})(\% \text{ Hb saturation}) + \text{Dissolved } O_2$$

where Hb = hemoglobin.

Under most circumstances, dissolved oxygen is negligible. The main difference in the oxygen-carrying capacity of blood between neonates and older patients is the presence of fetal hemoglobin (HbF). The fetal red blood cell contains primarily HbF, a hemoglobin isomer with a higher affinity for oxygen than hemoglobin A (HbA), which predominates in adults. This gives HbF a lower P_{50} (the partial pressure of oxygen at which hemoglobin saturation is 50%), which is reflected in a leftward shift of the oxyhemoglobin dissociation curve relative to HbA (Fig. 94.11). This difference in affinities promotes the transfer of oxygen from maternal to fetal hemoglobin in the placenta. Following birth, neonatal red blood cells gradually accumulate HbA at the expense of HgF, which disappears by 4 months of age.

The presence of HbF in the neonate has several clinical consequences. Adequate hemoglobin saturation may occur at lower P_aO_2 levels, but the benefits of this in the ex utero environment are deceiving. Greater oxygen affinity makes the unloading of oxygen in peripheral tissues more difficult. Increasing oxygen extraction during periods when oxygen demand temporarily exceeds supply is therefore less efficient. Increased difficulty in extracting oxygen from hemoglobin in peripheral tissues makes the neonate less tolerant than the older child of decreased oxygen delivery resulting from reduced hemoglobin concentration, hemoglobin saturation, or cardiac output. Constant attention to adequate oxygen content and cardiac output is therefore of paramount importance in the stressed neonate.

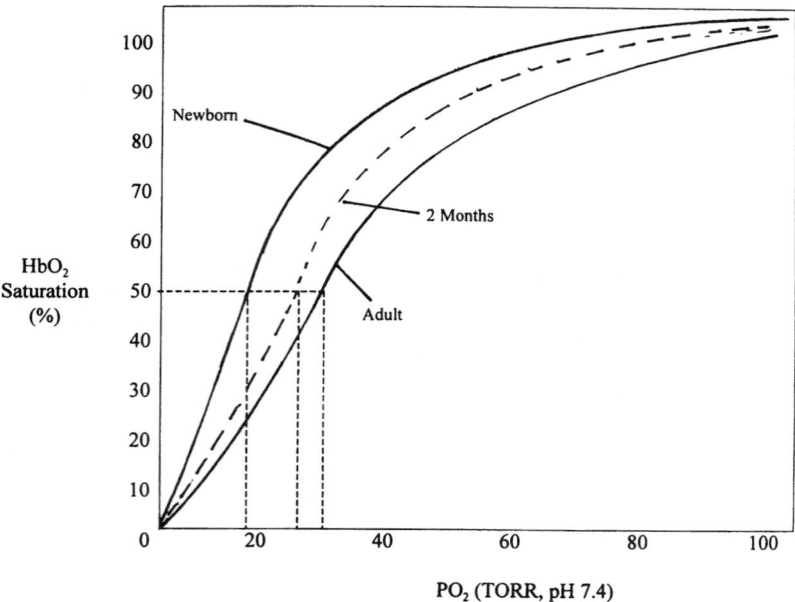

Figure 94.11. Representative oxyhemoglobin *(HbO₂)* saturation curves for newborn, infant, and adult. (Reprinted from Hodson WA, Truog WE. In: Avery GB, Fletcher MA, MacDonald MG, eds. *Neonatology: pathophysiology and management of the newborn,* 5th ed. Philadelphia: Lippincott Williams & Wilkins, 1999, with permission.)

Pulmonary Hypertension and Persistent Fetal Circulation

In the older child and adult, pulmonary vascular resistance (PVR) is normally low, which allows right ventricular output to equal that of the left ventricle at considerably lower pressure and contractile work. The instability of PVR in the neonate during the transitional period, along with the presence of anatomic connections between the pulmonary and systemic circuits, accounts for severe derangements in respiratory and hemodynamic performance in a wide variety of clinical disorders. These include acquired conditions (e.g., sepsis and meconium aspiration syndrome), congenital conditions (e.g., pulmonary hypoplasia), idiopathic abnormalities in pulmonary vascular function (e.g., PPHN), and chronic microangiopathy and fibrosis ("fixed" pulmonary hypertension secondary to uncorrected anatomic left-to-right shunting and pulmonary overcirculation).

The common denominator in these conditions is an abnormally high PVR, which may be due to inappropriate vasoconstriction, reduced total capillary cross-sectional area, or fibrotic arterioles of fixed caliber. Not uncommonly, increased PVR results from a combination of these factors. For example, pulmonary hypoplasia not only causes decreased cross-sectional area but also results in hyperreactive arterioles prone to vasospasm. In "fixed" pulmonary hypertension, both fibrosis and decreased vessel numbers have been demonstrated.

Whatever the cause, increased PVR has several deleterious consequences. Increased right ventricular afterload results in decreased output, diminished pulmonary perfusion, and reduced left ventricular preload. Hypoxemia, hypercarbia, and globally decreased cardiac output result, which in turn cause metabolic acidosis. Increased PVR also promotes anatomic right-to-left shunting at the levels of the ductus arteriosus (PDA) and foramen ovale, a phenomenon referred to as *persistent fetal circulation* (PFC). This profoundly exacerbates the hypoxemia, hypercarbia, and acidosis already present. Because hypoxemia, hypercarbia, and acidosis are all potent mediators of pulmonary vasoconstriction, PVR is further increased. For this reason, pulmonary hypertension and PFC in the neonate frequently deteriorate into a vicious cycle that culminates in circulatory and metabolic collapse.

Therapy for pulmonary hypertension and PFC is directed at treating the underlying cause, removing the physiologic stimuli for pulmonary vasoconstriction, and introducing pharmacologic mediators of pulmonary vasodilatation. Analgesia, sedation, and neuromuscular blockade are commonly used to decrease endogenous stimulation of pulmonary vasoconstriction by catecholamines. The mainstays of management include aggressive ventilatory support to maximize P_aO_2 and minimize P_aCO_2, and systemic alkalinization (pH 7.50–7.60) with sodium bicarbonate or tris-hydroxymethylaminomethane (THAM) if an adequate respiratory alkalosis cannot be induced. Because severe respiratory failure frequently precedes and causes pulmonary hypertension and PFC, attempts to achieve these objectives through conventional ventilatory support alone are often unsuccessful. Oscillatory ventilation has been of occasional benefit in neonates with PFC by achieving increased oxygenation and respiratory alkalosis in circumstances when conventional ventilatory support has failed. Pharmacologic agents with the ability to promote direct pulmonary vasodilatation would obviously be desirable.

Selective pulmonary vasodilatation is presently unrealistic from a clinical standpoint. No pharmacologic substance has yet been identified that has vasodilatory effects specifically limited to the pulmonary circulation. Intravenous administration of nitroprusside, nitroglycerine, and PGE₁ all produce systemic vasodilatation as well, negating the reduction of resistance and pressure in the pulmonary circuit, and resulting in unaltered right-to-left shunt. Tolazoline hydrochloride was commonly used in the past as a pulmonary vasodilator in neonates with pulmonary hypertension. Its vasodilatory effects can be ascribed both to α-adrenergic blockade as well as stimulation of pulmonary vascular histamine receptors (47). Unfortunately, responses to tolazoline are unpredictable and nonselective, and no consistent clinical benefit has been convincingly demonstrated.

Perhaps the most promising pharmacologic approach to pulmonary vasodilatation is the administration of inhaled nitric oxide (NO). NO, previously known as endothelium-derived relaxing factor, is a ubiquitous, potent vasodilator that probably serves as the final common pathway for vascular smooth-muscle relaxation induced by a wide variety of other agents with known vasodilatory properties (48,49). Endogenous NO is generated from L-arginine by the action of NO synthase in endothelial cells and diffuses to adjacent smooth-muscle cells, where it promotes muscular relaxation via a cyclic guanosine monophosphate (GMP)-dependent mechanism (50). Although vasodilatation induced by NO is not specific for the pulmonary circulation, selective pulmonary vasodilatation can be produced by taking advantage of an unusual property of NO—it is immediately scavenged and inactivated in the bloodstream by binding to hemoglobin and forming methemoglobin. Thus, inhaled NO is able to bind to pulmonary vascular smooth-muscle cell receptors and induce relaxation before it diffuses into the capillary lumen and becomes inactivated. Inhaled NO is administered by mixing minute quantities of NO (5–20 ppm) into the gas mixture during mechanical ventilation. Although toxicity from methemoglobin has been suggested as a potential adverse effect, clinically significant methemoglobinemia has not been observed when NO is delivered at such low concentrations. A more significant difficulty with inhaled NO therapy is the development of tachyphylaxis, which frequently occurs after as little as 2 to 3 days of treatment (51). Despite this potential obstacle, this novel strategy of selective delivery of a potent nonspecific vasodilator to the pulmonary circulation represents a major new development in the treatment of pulmonary hypertension in infants.

Failure to promote pulmonary vasodilatation through physiologic or pharmacologic manipulation may indicate a need to use extracorporeal techniques to reverse hypoxemia, hypercarbia, hypoperfusion, and acidosis. As discussed already, ECMO has become a widely accepted therapy for refractory pulmonary hypertension associated with a variety of etiologies. It is important to recognize that extracorporeal support for pulmonary hypertension (or respiratory failure) is indicated only when the underlying cause is thought to be reversible.

GASTROINTESTINAL AND HEPATIC PHYSIOLOGY

Most mechanisms of physiologic control in the gastrointestinal tract are present at birth, although continued postnatal maturation results in ongoing adjustments over time. Prematurity, however, is associated with a delay in gastrointestinal function, just as it is in the cardiovascular and pulmonary systems. For example, immaturity of gastrointestinal motility and digestive enzyme activity in the preterm infant frequently results in early feeding intolerance. The functional immaturity of small intestinal "brush-border" enzymes in premature infants has already been mentioned with respect to the particular nutritional requirements of preterm infants. Normal intestinal motility, as measured by the appearance of migrating motor complexes, has been documented to appear by 36 to 38 weeks of gestation. Whereas 95% of term infants will pass a meconium stool within 24 hours of birth (and virtually 100% by 48 hours), it is not unusual for premature infants to have a significant delay in the passage of meconium that is dependent on the degree of prematurity.

The extraordinarily complex physiology of the gastrointestinal tract, including the control of motility, digestion, absorption, neurologic function, and enteroendocrine feedback, is beyond the scope of this chapter. Several specific topics in gastrointestinal physiology are

relevant, however, because they relate to functional problems commonly encountered in pediatric patients. These topics include the physiology of gastrointestinal growth and adaptation, the pathophysiology of inadequate gastrointestinal length (short gut syndrome), and neonatal jaundice.

Physiology of Intestinal Growth and Adaptation

To meet the needs of the growing child for energy and structural substrates, the absorptive surface area of the intestinal tract must increase along with somatic growth. The small intestine increases from a length of about 200 to 300 cm and a diameter of about 1.5 cm at birth to a length of 600 to 800 cm and a diameter of 4 cm at maturity. Further growth and maturation of the villous architecture and the development of plicae circulares increase the total absorptive surface area from approximately 900 cm^2 to 7,500 cm^2 over the same period (52).

After growing to full length in childhood, the small intestine enters a state of dormancy and remains quiescent unless some major change occurs. Following massive intestinal resection, various adaptive responses occur in the small intestine; these responses are designed to enhance the absorptive function of the remaining bowel. These adaptive changes include an increase in diameter, an increase in the number and size of the plicae circulares, and epithelial hyperplasia manifested as increased villous height and crypt depth. These changes augment absorptive surface area significantly, but they do not constitute a physiologically equivalent substitute for intestine of normal length and caliber. The markedly dilated, adapted intestine displays abnormal motility as a result of muscular hypertrophy and an inability to sustain normal peristalsis by coaptation. These dyskinetic contractions do not provide consistent, unidirectional flow and therefore allow stasis and bacterial colonization of the proximal intestine.

Although the factors governing stimulation of intestinal growth and adaptation are poorly understood, it is becoming increasingly clear that trophic stimulation from both enteroendocrine mediators and intraluminal substances is necessary. The gastrointestinal mucosa is richly populated with a variety of peptide-secreting enteroendocrine cells that produce local signaling and mediator molecules in response to specific stimuli (Fig. 94.12). Some of these enteroendocrine peptides are expressed only during fetal development. Virtually every known postnatal enteroendocrine cell is present and functionally mature at term (53). The levels of many of these peptides rise sharply in the first days of life in fed infants, but not in fasting infants (54). The observation that intestinal growth and maturation are inhibited by withholding enteral feeds suggests that enteroendocrine stimulation is one of the processes responsible for normal postnatal intestinal growth. Enteroglucagon and other glucagon-like immunoreactive peptides, fetal glucagon, and fetal gastrin appear to be leading candidates for the principal enteroendocrine mediators of gut growth (55–57).

Direct stimulation of mucosal growth by luminal nutrients plays a major role in intestinal adaptation. The fact that villous height and absorptive capacity are greatest in the proximal jejunum and gradually decrease through the remaining jejunum and ileum suggests that progressive depletion of luminal nutrients results in relatively diminished growth of the distal intestine. Reciprocal transposition of ileal and jejunal segments results in hypertrophy of the proximally transposed ileal segment and atrophy of the distally transposed jejunal segment. The "underdevel-

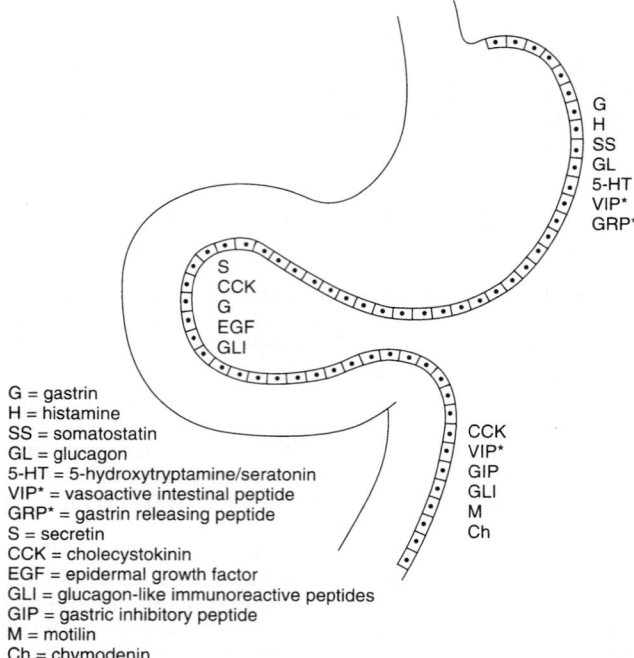

G = gastrin
H = histamine
SS = somatostatin
GL = glucagon
5-HT = 5-hydroxytryptamine/seratonin
VIP* = vasoactive intestinal peptide
GRP* = gastrin releasing peptide
S = secretin
CCK = cholecystokinin
EGF = epidermal growth factor
GLI = glucagon-like immunoreactive peptides
GIP = gastric inhibitory peptide
M = motilin
Ch = chymodenin

Figure 94.12. Distribution of selected enteroendocrine and neuroendocrine *(asterisks)* cells and their products in the proximal gastrointestinal tract. (Reprinted from Magnuson DK, Schwartz MZ. In: Oldham KT, Colombani PM, Foglia RP, eds. *Surgery of infants and children.* Philadelphia: Lippincott–Raven, 1997, with permission.)

opment" of the distal small bowel may be viewed, to a certain extent, as built-in reserve potential.

In various experimental models, adaptive growth will not occur after resection unless some level of luminal nutrition is provided. Studies in animal models have shown that complex nutrients that require enzymatic degradation (e.g., long-chain fatty acids, disaccharides, and complex proteins) are more potent stimulators of growth than are more elemental nutrients (58–60). This effect may be due to the trophic properties of pancreaticobiliary secretions, which are stimulated by complex nutritional substrates. The amino acid glutamine is the preferred energy substrate for enterocytes and a necessary constituent of growth-promoting enteral nutrition formulas. It is not clear whether glutamine acts in a permissive fashion only by providing energy substrate for growth or whether it also has trophic properties separate from its energy content. Intravenous glutamine administration can preserve intestinal mucosal health in the absence of enteral glutamine, but whether it can promote long-term gut adaptation and growth also is not known. Epidermal growth factor (EGF), present in duodenal and biliary secretions, and growth hormone are both potent growth stimuli. The administration of enteral glutamine and EGF (or growth hormone or both) may have a therapeutic benefit in stimulating intestinal growth after bowel resection.

Clinical Aspects of Short-gut Syndrome

Although intestinal growth is commonly taken for granted in health, its importance is brought into sharp focus by conditions in which inadequate intestinal length causes malabsorption and malnutrition: *the short-gut syndrome.* This syndrome usually occurs after massive in-

testinal resection for a variety of diseases. The most common causes in the neonatal period are necrotizing enterocolitis and midgut volvulus, although gastroschisis also may be associated with decreased intestinal length in the absence of resection (61,62). In older children, volvulus and inflammatory bowel disease predominate (63). The extent of resection likely to result in short-gut syndrome is difficult to quantify and is influenced by patient age, site of intestinal loss, and status of the ileocecal valve (ICV). It is commonly held that a term newborn who retains at least 25 cm of small intestine with an intact ICV, or 40 cm without an ICV, has a reasonable potential for resuming full enteral feedings at some point. In older patients, loss of 75% to 80% of intestinal length may be tolerated as long as the ICV is preserved.

The loss of intestinal surface area diminishes absorptive capacity, brush-border digestive enzyme activity, and enteroendocrine mediator production. These deficiencies all lead to malnutrition and weight loss. Unabsorbed sugars pass through to the colon and produce an osmotic diarrhea. Presentation of undigested carbohydrates to the colon also provides fuel for bacterial proliferation. The bacteria metabolize the undigested sugars to lactate and short-chain fatty acids, which stimulate colonic secretion of water and electrolytes. Thus, a secretory diarrhea exacerbates the osmotic one. After ileal resections, bile salt recirculation is impaired and bile salts reach the colon, providing more bacterial fuel and further stimulating the secretory diarrhea. Bile salt wasting eventually depletes the hepatic bile salt pool, resulting in fat malabsorption and steatorrhea and producing lithogenic bile and gallstones. Extensive ileal resections also result in impaired absorption of vitamin B_{12} and the fat-soluble vitamins A, D, E, and K.

Bacterial overgrowth in the residual small intestine occurs in most patients with short-gut syndrome. It is related primarily to the loss of the ICV and reflux of colonic bacteria into the small intestine. Overgrowth also is promoted by stasis and hypomotility, which occur in adapted, dilated, dyskinetic intestine. Bacterial overgrowth in the proximal intestine leads to further increases in carbohydrate, protein, and fluid and electrolyte loss due to diarrhea.

Gastric hypersecretion of fluid and acid is well documented in short-gut syndrome. Acid hypersecretion has been linked to hypergastrinemia, possibly because of the loss of somatostatin and gastrin-inhibiting peptide (GIP) production. Gastric hypersecretion results in peptic complications, reduced enzymatic digestion due to low intraluminal pH, and further exacerbation of diarrhea.

Management of short-gut syndrome is complex and may include any combination of the following: parenteral nutrition, limited enteral feeding with easily-absorbed substrates (glucose polymers, medium chain triglycerides, protein hydrosylates), judicious enteral exposure to trophic substrates (complex carbohydrates, intact protein, long-chain triglycerides, and glutamine), antibiotic suppression of bacterial overgrowth, supplementation of vitamins and minerals, and control of diarrhea with antimotility agents. Surgical treatment of short-gut syndrome by intestinal lengthening procedures and transplantation has been disappointing.

Neonatal Jaundice

Hepatic function in the older child is essentially the same as in the adult. In the neonatal period, however, liver function may be altered in a number of ways by hepatocyte immaturity. Although fetal hepatocytes begin to manifest synthetic capabilities early in gestation, the quantitative capacity to produce, modify, and detoxify various substances develops gradually and is often incompletely developed at birth, particularly in premature infants. This functional immaturity affects a range of processes, including glycogen metabolism and the biotransformation of many drugs, but most notably it affects the excretion of bilirubin.

Bilirubin Metabolism

Bilirubin is produced by the degradation of heme-containing compounds, primarily hemoglobin from senescent red blood cells, but also myoglobin, cytochromes, catalases, and other molecules. Because infants have a relatively greater red cell mass than adults, as well as a shorter red cell life span and higher turnover, bilirubin production is proportionately greatest in the first weeks of life. The conversion of heme to bilirubin occurs in reticuloendothelial cells in the liver, spleen, and elsewhere. In the first step, the ring structure of heme is opened by the oxidative removal of a carbon atom through heme oxygenase, which also releases a reduced iron atom. The resulting product, biliverdin, is a linear molecule that is further reduced by biliverdin reductase to bilirubin. Bilirubin is held in a tightly folded configuration by extensive hydrogen bonding, resulting in a highly hydrophobic and insoluble molecule. As such, transport of bilirubin from sites of production to the liver for excretion requires binding to albumin as a carrier molecule.

Bilirubin is extracted from hepatic sinusoidal blood and transported by a specific membrane carrier protein into the hepatocyte, where it is attached to the cytoplasmic carrier protein ligandin (glutathione S-transferase). Within the cytoplasm, bilirubin is conjugated with glucuronic acid by bilirubin glucuronosyltransferase (BGT) to form bilirubin monoglucuronides (BMGs) and diglucuronides (BDGs). Both BMGs and BDGs then are transported into the bile canaliculi and excreted via the bile ducts into the duodenum. Normally, a small amount of conjugated bilirubin is found in the blood because of back-diffusion across the sinusoidal membrane. In pathologic states where the excretion of BMGs and BDGs cannot keep pace with production, serum levels of conjugated bilirubin rise. Hepatocyte excretion of BMGs and BDGs is the rate-limiting step in bilirubin clearance after 1 week of age, before which time conjugation of bilirubin is rate limiting because of diminished activity of BGT.

Within the intestinal lumen, bilirubin conjugates may have several fates. Most are metabolized by resident bacteria into a variety of compounds, including the urobilinogens and the urobilinoids, which are excreted in the feces. The conversion of conjugated bilirubin into urobilinoids prevents the reabsorption, or enterohepatic recirculation, of bilirubin. Other bacteria, as well as mucosal cells, contain β-glucuronidase capable of deconjugating BMG and BDG. Deconjugated bilirubin is hydrophobic and easily reabsorbed across the epithelial barrier and back into the circulation. Neonates are particularly susceptible to bilirubin reabsorption that results from increased levels of endogenous β-glucuronidase and decreased bacterial flora. The relative paucity of resident bacteria results in less successful conversion of bilirubin conjugates to urobilinoids, whereas the increased activity of β-glucuronidase deconjugates the bilirubin. Meconium contains a high concentration of conjugated bilirubin, which readily undergoes deconjugation if impaired motility delays its excretion.

Neonatal Hyperbilirubinemia

Transient unconjugated hyperbilirubinemia is a ubiquitous finding in neonates and represents a normal stage in early postnatal life. For this reason, it is often referred to as *physiologic jaundice*. The exact cause of physiologic jaundice is unclear, but it appears to involve a combination of increased enterohepatic circulation of bilirubin and decreased BGT activity (64). Both the duration and magnitude of the hyperbilirubinemia are variable, but in general plasma levels of unconjugated bilirubin peak at about 5 to 6 mg/dL at 3 days of life and resolve by seven to 10 days in healthy term infants.

In addition to physiologic jaundice, numerous conditions are associated with more severe unconjugated hyperbilirubinemia in the early postnatal period. These include breast-milk jaundice, hemolytic diseases (ABO or Rh incompatibility, hemoglobinopathies), reabsorption of extravascular blood, neonatal hepatitis, inborn errors of metabolism, and sepsis. Unconjugated hyperbilirubinemia can cause both a reversible encephalopathy and an irreversible neurologic injury termed *kernicterus*. The predilection of unconjugated bilirubin for neural tissue is related to its nonpolar structure, which makes it highly hydrophobic and lipophilic. Deposition of bilirubin in the basal ganglia and cranial nerve nuclei is the most common pathologic feature, although clinical manifestations include a wide variety of cognitive, developmental, motor, and sensory dysfunction. The risks of neurologic injury are related to peak sustained bilirubin levels; kernicterus is likely when sustained plasma levels exceed 30 mg/dL and is virtually unknown when levels do not exceed 20 mg/dL. Between 20 and 30 mg/dL, the incidence of reversible encephalopathy is greatest, but increasing risk of kernicterus is a concern.

Indications for intervention include early onset or prolonged duration of jaundice and exaggerated absolute levels of unconjugated bilirubin. The precise level at which therapeutic intervention is considered depend on postnatal and gestational age, weight, and presence of comorbidity, and is the subject of considerable debate. First-line therapies include stimulation of intestinal motility by oral feeding and rectal stimulation to promote the passage of meconium and reduce enterohepatic circulation. When levels become high or sustained enough to elicit genuine concern, the treatment of choice is phototherapy. Light in the blue spectrum with wavelengths of 420 to 480 nm is absorbed by unconjugated bilirubin. The absorbed energy alters the double bond structure of bilirubin in a process termed *photoisomerization*. The new isomers are less capable of forming internal hydrogen bonds and therefore become unfolded and more polar. This configurational change makes them more soluble, promotes their mobilization from central nervous system tissues, and allows their excretion in the bile without further conjugation. When extremely high levels of bilirubin are encountered and phototherapy is deemed insufficiently rapid, exchange transfusion provides the most reliable method of rapidly reducing serum bilirubin levels into a nontoxic range.

In contrast to unconjugated hyperbilirubinemia, elevation of serum conjugated bilirubin is always pathologic and mandates expeditious evaluation. The presence of isolated conjugated hyperbilirubinemia in the first weeks of life usually suggests the presence of a condition associated with reduced bile excretion. These include extrahepatic biliary atresia, Alagille's syndrome (arteriohepatic dysplasia or intrahepatic biliary hypoplasia), nonsyndromic intrahepatic bile duct paucity, Byler's syndrome (progressive familial intrahepatic cholestasis), choledochal cyst, and TPN-related cholestasis. Not all episodes of conjugated hyperbilirubinemia result from biliary obstruction, however. Because hepatocyte excretion of BMGs and BDGs is rate limiting after the first week of life, increased bilirubin loads generated by hemolysis or reabsorption may result in the production of bilirubin conjugates at a rate exceeding the hepatocyte's ability to excrete them into the canaliculi. Intracellular buildup results in back-diffusion of conjugated bilirubin into the sinusoidal and systemic circulation.

REFERENCES

1. Bottoms SF, Paul RH, Mercer BM, et al. Obstetric determinants of neonatal survival: antenatal predictors of neonatal survival and morbidity in extremely low birth weight infants. *Am J Obstet Gynecol* 1999;180(3 Pt 1):665–669.
2. Horbar JD, Onstad L, Wright E. Predicting mortality risk for infants weighing 501 to 1,500 grams at birth. *Crit Care Med* 1993;21:12–18.
3. Lubchenco LO, Bard H. Incidence of hypoglycemia in newborn infants classified by birth weight and gestational age. *Pediatrics* 1971;47:831–838.
4. Hawdon JM, Ward Platt MP. Metabolic adaptation in small for gestational age infants. *Arch Dis Child* 1993;68(3 Spec No): 262–268.
5. Lee H, Jain L. Physiology of infants with very low birth weight. *Semin Pediatr Surg* 1990;9:50–55.
6. Hey EN, Katz G. The optimum thermal environment for naked babies. *Arch Dis Child* 1970;45:328–334.
7. Cannon B, Nedergaard J. The biochemistry of an inefficient tissue: brown adipose tissue. *Essays Biochem* 1985;20: 110–164.
8. Whyte RK, Campbell D, Stanhope R, et al. Energy balance in low birth weight infants fed formula of high or low medium chain triglyceride content. *J Pediatr* 1986;108:964–971.
9. Sauer PJ, Dane HF, Visser HK. Longitudinal studies on metabolic rate, heat loss, and energy cost of growth in low birth weight infants. *Pediatr Res* 1984;18:254–259.
10. Holliday MA. Body composition and energy needs during growth. In: Faulkner F, Tanner JM, eds. *Human growth: a comprehensive treatise,* 2nd ed. New York: Plenum Press, 1986:101–117.
11. Groner JI, Brown MF, Stallings VA, et al. Resting energy expenditure in children following major operative procedures. *J Pediatr Surg* 1989;24:825–827.
12. Mitchell IM, Davies PS, Day JM, et al. Energy expenditure in children with congenital heart disease, before and after cardiac surgery. *J Thorac Cardiovasc Surg* 1994;107: 374–380.
13. Bier DM, Leake RD, Haymond MW, et al. Measurement of "true" glucose production rates in infancy and childhood with 6,6-didueteroglucose. *Diabetes* 1977;26:1016–1023.
14. Adam PA, King K, Schwartz R. Model for the investigation of intractable hypoglycemia: insulin–glucose interrelationship during steady state infusions. *Pediatrics* 1968;41:91–105.
15. Chugani HT, Phelps ME, Mazziotta JC. Positron emission tomography study of human brain functional development. *Pediatrics* 1968;22:487–497.
16. Holman RT, Johnson SB, Hatch TF. A case of human linolenic acid deficiency involving neurological abnormalities. *Am J Clin Nutr* 1982;35:617–623.
17. Souba WW, Herskowitz K, Austgen TR, et al. Glutamine nutrition: theoretical considerations and therapeutic impact. *JPEN J Parenter Enteral Nutr* 1990;14(5 Suppl):237S–243S.
18. Lorenz JM, Kleinman LI, Ahmed G, et al. Phases of fluid and electrolyte homeostasis in the extremely low birth weight infant. *Pediatrics* 1995;96(3 Pt 1):484–489.
19. Aperia A, Broberger O, Herin P, et al. Postnatal control of water and electrolyte homeostasis in preterm and full-term infants. *Acta Paediatr Scand* 1983;305:61–65.
20. Polacek B, Vocel J, Neugebauerova L, et al. The osmotic concentrating ability in healthy infants and children. *Arch Dis Child* 1965;40:291–295.
21. Nakayama DK, Motoyama EK, Tagge EM. Effect of preoperative stabilization on respiratory system compliance and outcome in newborn infants with congenital diaphragmatic hernia. *J Pediatr* 1991;118:793–799.
22. Polgar G, String ST. The viscous resistance of the lung tissues in newborn infants. *J Pediatr* 1966;69:787–792.
23. Helms P, Stocks J. Lung function in infants with congenital pulmonary hypoplasia. *J Pediatr* 1982;101:918–922.
24. Wolfson MR, Bhutani VK, Shaffer TH, et al. Mechanics and energetics of breathing helium in infants with bronchopulmonary dysplasia. *J Pediatr* 1984;104:752–757.
25. Bergovski EH, Hass F, Porcelli R. Determination of the sensitive vascular sites from which hypoxia and hypercapnea elicit rises in pulmonary artery pressure. *Fed Proc* 1968;27: 1420–1425.
26. Cassin S, Tod M, Philips J, et al. Effects of prostaglandin D2 in the perinatal circulation. *Am J Physiol* 1981;240: H755–H760.
27. Chatfield BA, McMurtry IF, Hall SL, et al. Hemodynamic effects of endothelin-1 on the ovine fetal pulmonary circulation. *Am J Physiol* 1991;261:R182–R187.
28. Ivy DD, Kinsella JP, Abman SH. Physiologic characterization of endothelin A and B receptor activity in the ovine fetal pulmonary circulation. *J Clin Invest* 1994;93:2141–2148.
29. Gluck L, Kulovich MV, Borer RC Jr, et al. The interpretation and significance of the lecithin/sphingomyelin ratio in amniotic fluid. *Am J Obstet Gynecol* 1974;120:142–155.
30. Kulovich MV, Hallman MB, Gluck L. The lung profile. I. Normal pregnancy. *Am J Obstet Gynecol* 1979;135:57–63.
31. Buntin TE, Plopper CG. Triamcinolone-induced structural alterations in the development of the lung of the fetal rhesus macaque. *Am J Obstet Gynecol* 1984;148:203–215.
32. Ikegami M, Polk D, Tabor B, et al. Corticosteroid and thyrotropin-releasing hormone effects on preterm sheep lung function. *J Appl Physiol* 1991;70:2268–2278.
33. Gregory TJ, Steinberg KP, Spragg R, et al. Bovine surfactant therapy for patients with acute respiratory distress syndrome. *Am J Respir Crit Care Med* 1997;155:1309–1315.
34. Dreyfuss D, Soler P, Basset G, et al. High inflation pulmonary edema. *Am Rev Respir Dis* 1988;137:1159–1164.
35. Hernandez LA, Peevy KJ, Moise AA, et al. Chest wall restriction limits high airway pressure-induced lung injury in young rabbits. *J Appl Physiol* 1989;66:2364–2368.
36. Dreyfuss D, Saumon G. Role of tidal volume, FRC, and end-inspiratory volume in the development of pulmonary edema following mechanical ventilation. *Am Rev Respir Dis* 1993; 148:1194–1203.
37. Leach CL, Fuhrman BP, Morin FC III, et al. Perfluorocarbon-associated gas exchange (partial liquid ventilation) in respiratory distress syndrome: a prospective, randomized, controlled study. *Crit Care Med* 1993;21:1270–1278.
38. Moler FW, Custer JR, Bartlett RH, et al. Extracorporeal life support for severe pediatric respiratory failure: an updated experience 1991–1993. *J Pediatr* 1994;124:875–880.
39. St. John Sutton MG, Raichlen JS, Reichek N, et al. Quantitative assessment of right and left ventricular growth in the human fetal heart: a pathoanatomic study. *Circulation* 1984; 70:935–941.
40. Rudolph AM, Heymann MA. Circulatory changes during growth in the fetal lamb. *Circ Res* 1970;26:289–299.
41. Fineman JR, Soifer SJ, Heymann MA. Regulation of pulmonary vascular tone in the perinatal period. *Annu Rev Physiol* 1995;57:115–134.
42. Shaul PW, Farrar MA, Magness RR. Oxygen modulation of pulmonary arterial prostacyclin synthesis is developmentally regulated. *Am J Physiol* 1993;265(2 pt 2):H621–H628.
43. Shaul PW, Farrar MA, Zellers TM. Oxygen modulates endothelium-derived relaxing factor production in fetal pulmonary arteries. *Am J Physiol* 1992;262(2 pt 2):H355–H364.
44. Anderson P. Physiology of the fetal, neonatal, and adult heart. In: Polin RA, Fox WW, eds. *Fetal and neonatal physiology.* Philadelphia: WB Saunders, 1992:722–758.
45. Artman M, Graham TP Jr, Boucek RJ Jr. Effects of postnatal maturation on myocardial contractile responses to calcium antagonists and changes in contraction frequency. *J Cardiovasc Physiol* 1985;7:850–855.
46. Talner NS, Lister G, Fahey JT. Effects of asphyxia on the myocardium of the fetus and newborn. In: Polin RA, Fox WW, eds. *Fetal and neonatal physiology.* Philadelphia: WB Saunders, 1992:759–69.
47. Goetzman BG, Milstein JM. Pulmonary vasodilator action of tolazoline. *Pediatr Res* 1979;13:942–944.
48. Palmer RMJ, Ferrige AG, Moncada S. Nitric oxide release ac-

counts for the biological activity of endothelium-derived relaxing factor. *Nature* 1987;327:524–526.

49. Ignarro LJ, Byrns RE, Buga GM, et al. Endothelium-dependent relaxing factor from pulmonary artery and vein possesses pharmacologic and chemical properties identical to those of nitric oxide radical. *Circ Res* 1987;61:866–879.

50. Moncada S, Palmer RMJ, Higgs EA. Nitric oxide: physiology, pathophysiology, and pharmacology. *Pharmacol Rev* 1991;43: 109–142.

51. Kinsella JP, Nelsh SR, Ivy DD, et al. Clinical responses to prolonged treatment of persistent pulmonary hypertension of the newborn with low doses of inhaled nitric oxide. *J Pediatr* 1993;123:103–108.

52. Klish WJ, Putnam TC. The short gut. *Am J Dis Child* 1981;135: 1056–1061.

53. Bryant MG, Buchan AM, Gregor M, et al. Development of intestinal regulatory peptides in the human fetus. *Gastroenterology* 1982;83(1 pt 1):47–54.

54. Lucas A, Bloom SR, Aynsley-Green A. Metabolic and endocrine consequences of depriving preterm infants of enteral nutrition. *Acta Paediatr Scand* 1983;72:245–249.

55. Bloom SR. Gut hormones in adaptation. *Gut* 1987;28[Suppl 1]:31–35.

56. Fuller PJ, Beveridge DJ, Taylor RG. Ileal proglucagon gene expression in the rat: characterization in intestinal adaptation using in situ hybridization. *Gastroenterology* 1993;104: 459–466.

57. Drucker DJ, Ehrlich P, Asa SL, et al. Induction of intestinal epithelial proliferation by glucagon-like peptide 2. *Proc Natl Acad Sci USA* 1996;93:7911–7916.

58. Lentze MJ. Intestinal adaptation in short-bowel syndrome. *Eur J Pediatr* 1989;148:294–299.

59. Weser E, Babbitt J, Hoban M. Intestinal adaptation: different growth responses to disaccharides compared with monosaccharides in rat small bowel. *Gastroenterology* 1986;91: 1521–1527.

60. Vanderhoof JA, Grandjean CJ, Burkley KT, et al. Effect of casein versus casein hydrosylate on mucosal adaptation following massive small bowel resection in infant rats. *J Pediatr Gastroenterol Nutr* 1984;3:262–267.

61. Grosfeld JL, Rescorla FJ, West JW. Short bowel syndrome in infancy and childhood. *Am J Surg* 1986;151:41–46.

62. Grosfeld JL, Rescorla FJ, West JW, et al. Gastrointestinal injuries in childhood: analysis of 53 patients. *J Pediatr Surg* 1989;24:580–583.

63. Ricour C, Duhamel JF, Arnaud-Battendier F, et al. Enteral and parenteral nutrition in the short-bowel syndrome in children. *World J Surg* 1985;9:310–315.

64. Kawade N, Onishi S. The prenatal and postnatal development of UDP-glucuronyltransferase activity towards bilirubin and the effect of premature birth on this activity in the human liver. *Biochem J* 1981;196:257–260.

SURGERY: SCIENTIFIC PRINCIPLES AND PRACTICE, Third Edition, edited by Lazar J. Greenfield, Michael W. Mulholland, Keith T. Oldham, Gerald B. Zelenock, and Keith D. Lillemoe. Lippincott Williams & Wilkins Publishers, Philadelphia, © 2001.

CHAPTER 95

PEDIATRIC HEAD AND NECK

JOHN AIKEN AND KEITH T. OLDHAM

Surgical lesions of the head and neck are common in children and include a broad spectrum of congenital and acquired disorders. They may present clinically as asymptomatic masses or as life-threatening emergencies caused by airway obstruction. A comprehensive review is beyond the scope of this chapter, which focuses on the general principles and management of airway obstruction in infants and children and the most common head and neck lesions seen in pediatric surgical practice.

AIRWAY OBSTRUCTION

Many lesions, both congenital and acquired, can produce airway obstruction in infants and children. They may be intrinsic or extrinsic to the airway and vary from clinically insignificant to universally fatal (1).

Airway obstruction is the most serious complication of neck masses in children. Often, the first significant sign of respiratory distress in an infant is restlessness, followed by tachypnea, dyspnea, chest wall retractions, and respiratory arrest if the obstruction is not relieved. It is crucial to establish an adequate airway and administer respiratory support while proceeding with the diagnostic evaluation. This may include simple measures, such as repositioning the infant, clearing or suctioning the nose and mouth, and administering supplemental oxygen, or more extreme interventions, including endotracheal intubation or tracheostomy. Evaluation includes a careful history and physical examination, chest radiography, and arterial blood gas analysis. A nasogastric tube should be passed into the stomach, as gastric distention limits excursion of the diaphragm and can significantly contribute to respiratory compromise. Laryngoscopy and bronchoscopy are employed as needed.

Because infants are obligate nasal breathers, congenital lesions that obstruct the nasal passages or nasopharynx (choanal atresia, encephalocele, teratoma) typically cause early respiratory distress. These disorders are readily identified by physical examination, and emergent management is usually placement of an oropharyngeal airway. Airway obstruction at the level of the oral cavity in newborn infants is often a consequence of macroglossia or structural abnormalities such as micrognathia. Macroglossia may be a consequence of muscular hyperplasia and hypertrophy, as in Beckwith-Wiedemann syndrome and congenital hypothyroidism, or of diffuse involvement of the tongue with tumor (hemangiopericytoma, lymphangioma, neurofibromatosis) (2). Structural abnormalities, such as Pierre Robin syndrome (hypoplastic mandible with cleft palate), cause respiratory distress as the tongue falls posteriorly and obstructs the airway. Cysts or tumors of the pharynx or a mass arising at the base of the tongue, such as a lingual thyroid, may also obstruct the airway (3). Clinically, upper airway obstruction, above the glottis or larynx, is characterized by dyspnea, tachypnea, and suprasternal, intercostal, and costal margin retractions, but the child has no significant difficulty exhaling, and the voice and cry are normal. Emergency management consists of placing an oropharyngeal airway. Placing the infant in a prone position allows the tongue to fall forward and often provides significant relief. The infant may be fed through an orogastric feeding tube pending definitive correction of the obstruction. In extreme cases, a tracheostomy may be necessary.

Laryngeal obstruction can result from congenital or acquired vocal cord paralysis or tumors or cysts originating in the neck. Hemangiomas, lymphangiomas, cystic hygromas, and teratomas are the most common cervical tumors in infants and children. Laryngoscopy is usually required to differentiate these lesions. Emergency management of such malformations frequently requires placement of an endotracheal tube or tracheostomy. Endotracheal intubation can be difficult in the setting of a large neck mass, possibly causing displacement of the larynx, and bronchoscopy may be necessary with passage of the tube over a flexible bronchoscope. After the airway is stabilized, further diagnostic evaluation may include neck and chest radiography, computed tomography (CT), magnetic resonance imaging, and laryngobronchoscopy. Tracheostomy may be necessary at the time of definitive surgical excision, and placement of a gastrostomy tube may also be indicated if feeding problems are anticipated. Hemangiomas are the most common tumors involving the larynx; they often respond to intralesional or systemic steroids or may regress spontaneously (4).

Acquired Obstruction

Foreign body aspiration and acute epiglottitis are common causes of acquired airway obstruction in children. Acute epiglottitis is most commonly seen in children 2 to 4 years of age, and *Haemophilus influenzae* type b can be isolated in more than 90% of cases. Since the introduction of *Haemophilus influenzae* type b vaccine in 1991, the incidence of this illness has been reduced in children (5). Pneumococci and β-hemolytic streptococci are also causative organisms in epiglottitis. Acute epiglottitis typically presents as a rapidly progressive illness with symptoms of severe stridor, airway obstruction, drooling, and difficulty swallowing, and with signs of systemic toxicity, including an elevated temperature and white blood cell count, tachypnea, and tachycardia. Prolonged inspiratory stridor that worsens in the supine position is characteristic. In advanced cases, the child usually sits erect and leans forward, is anxious, drools, and becomes increasingly exhausted with air hunger. Attempts to examine or visualize the larynx may result in sudden airway occlusion with aspiration and respiratory arrest and therefore should be performed only in the operating room with personnel prepared to perform endotracheal intubation or tracheostomy. If the child's condition permits, lateral neck radiographs with soft-tissue techniques are obtained and should confirm the diagnosis by demonstrating edema of the epiglottis and ballooning of the hypopharynx.

The most important aspect of management is establishing a definitive diagnosis without delay. Once the diagnosis is established, maintaining an adequate airway is vital. Because of the high risk for progressive airway obstruction, standard therapy often involves short-term endotracheal intubation performed in the operating room under general anesthesia. The surgeon should be prepared to perform a tracheostomy in the event that the airway cannot be secured with an endotracheal tube or flexible bronchoscope. The inflammatory process typically resolves rapidly with administration of intravenous antibiotics, and intubation is seldom required beyond 3 days. Ampicillin is no longer recommended because of the high incidence of resistant *Haemophilus*. The drug of choice is usually a third-generation cephalosporin, such as cefoxitin or cefuroxime (Ceftin, Glaxo Wellcome, Research Triangle Park, NC). The timing of extubation should be based on resolution of the clinical signs and symptoms and direct visualization of the supraglottic area by fiberoptic nasopharyngoscopy. In the past, tracheostomy was the standard therapy, but comparative reviews demonstrate that short-term endotracheal intubation is associated with less morbidity and fewer complications (6).

BRANCHIAL CLEFT REMNANTS

Remnants of the embryonic branchial apparatus (cysts, sinuses, fistulae, and cartilaginous rests) are common in children. Although congenital by definition, they often go unrecognized or misdiagnosed. Sinuses, fistulae, and cartilaginous remnants are usually apparent at birth and noticed early in life. Cysts are more likely to present later in childhood as a neck mass when they fill with secretions. All these lesions are associated with a risk for infection and frequently come to clinical attention as an abscess or with drainage and surrounding erythema. Rarely, the remnants may harbor malignancy (7).

Anatomy and Embryology

During the fourth to eighth week after fertilization, four pairs of well-developed ridges (branchial arches) and associated clefts (externally) and pouches (internally) are prominent in the lateral cervicofacial region. The mature structures of the head and neck are derivatives of these paired branchial arches, clefts, and pouches seen in the embryo (8). The contributions of the branchial arches and clefts to the structures of the neck and jaw are summarized in Fig. 95.1. Incomplete closure or resorption of these primitive branchial clefts and arches may result in the development of cysts, sinuses, fistulae, and masses. The first branchial arch forms the mandible and a portion of the upper jaw, and part of the first branchial cleft remains open as the eustachian tube and external auditory canal. The second branchial arch forms the hyoid bone and cleft of the tonsillar fossa. Remnants of the first branchial cleft are found along the base of an imaginary fold extending from the auditory canal behind and below the angle of the mandible to just below the midpoint of the mandible. Second branchial cleft remnants are found along any part of a line extending from the tonsillar fossa inferiorly to a point on the lower third of the anterior border of the sternocleidomastoid muscle. The third cleft migrates low in the neck to form the inferior parathyroid glands and thymus. The fourth cleft also migrates but stops higher up in the neck and forms the superior parathyroid glands.

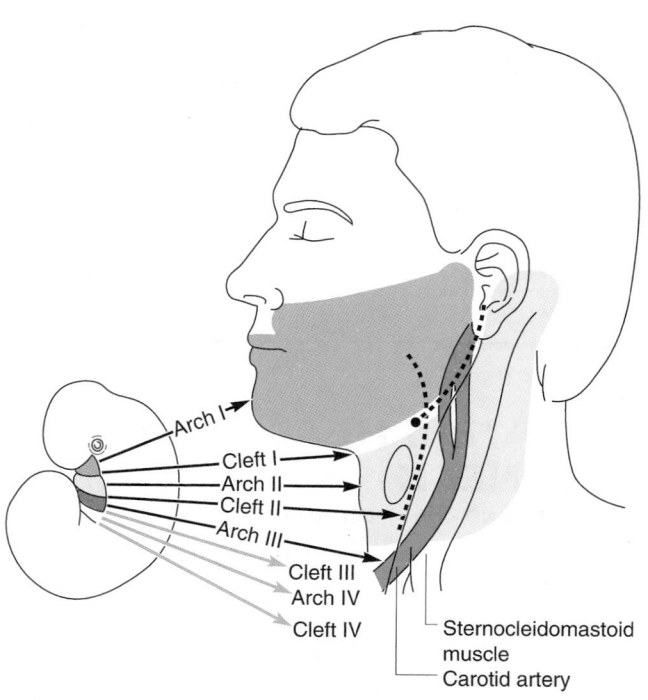

Figure 95.1. Derivation of various areas of the head and neck from the branchial arches and clefts of the embryo.

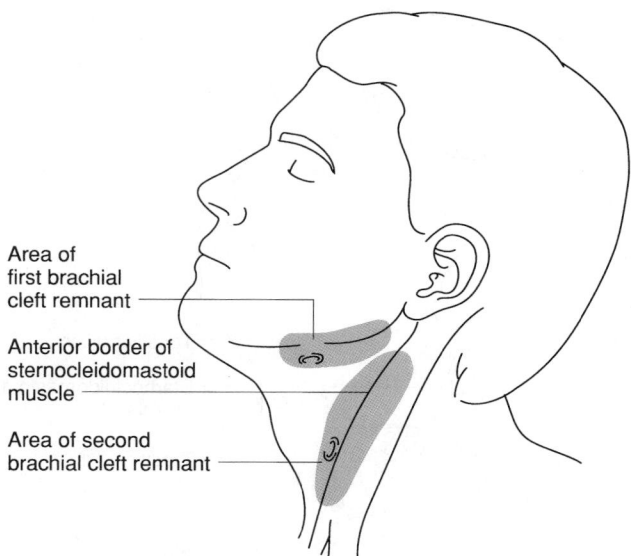

Figure 95.2. Areas of the neck in which cysts and sinuses originating from the first and second branchial clefts are usually found.

Clinical Aspects

All branchial remnants are by definition congenital and therefore present at birth. Branchial cleft sinuses present as cutaneous openings and are most often noted in infancy or at an early age, whereas cysts typically appear later in childhood. Branchial cleft sinuses and fistulae frequently produce mucoid drainage from the skin opening, and the cutaneous openings are occasionally marked by skin tags or subcutaneous cartilaginous remnants. First branchial cleft remnants present as a sinus opening near the angle of the mandible in the region of the submandibular triangle or preauricular region. These

sinus tracts extend from their submandibular opening superficial to the mandible up to the external auditory canal. The tract is intimately associated with the parotid gland and facial nerve. First branchial anomalies are less common than those of the second cleft and are often misdiagnosed. A history of recurrent infection, often leading to incision and drainage, is generally present. A key to the diagnosis is a history of nonpurulent drainage before infection. Second branchial anomalies are six times more common than first branchial anomalies and present as an opening along the anterior border of the sternocleidomastoid muscle in its lower third; they may be bilateral (Fig. 95.2). The sinus tract of second branchial anomalies passes through the bifurcation of the carotid artery and between the external and internal carotid arteries and communicates with the tonsillar fossa. Cysts or infections arising from the third and fourth branchial arch and cleft are rare and much more challenging to diagnose and treat than first and second branchial remnants. In both third and fourth remnants, the internal opening is located in the piriform sinus (9) (Fig. 95.3). Radiographic imaging is typically not necessary for first and second branchial anomalies, but barium studies and CT may be useful in demonstrating a piriform sinus fistula. The third branchial cleft sinus presents as a mass lower in the neck than the second branchial sinus. Its course is superior and posterior to the carotid sheath, most commonly on the left side. It should be suspected in cases of left thyroid lobe abscess. Because of the risk for the development of infection in any of the branchial cleft anomalies, excision is recommended at the time of diagnosis in a noninfected lesion. Surgery in infants may be delayed until 3 to 6 months of age.

Treatment and Outcome

With all branchial cleft remnants, the goal of treatment is complete surgical excision. The operation is usually performed at the time of diagnosis provided no active inflammation or infection is present. If infection is found, a

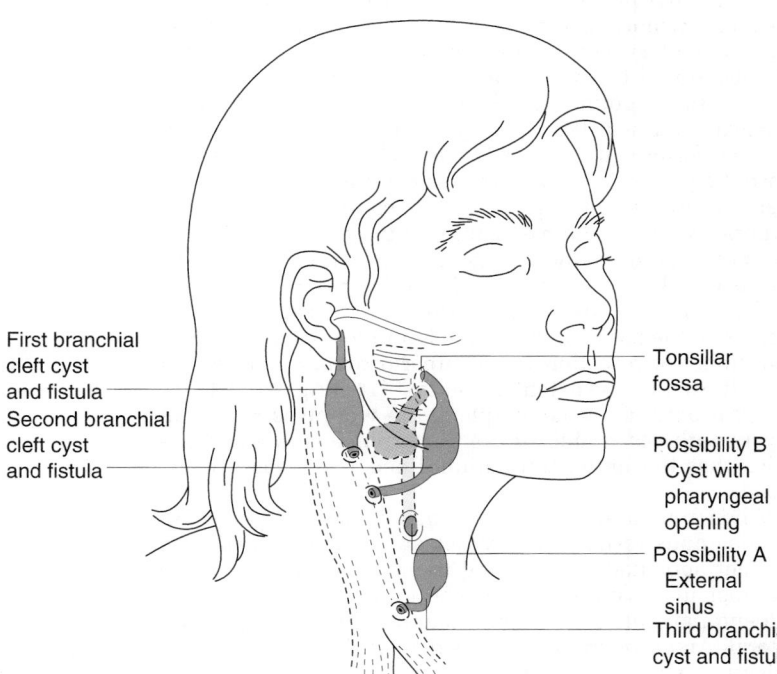

Figure 95.3. Types of first, second, and third branchial cleft remnants. Sinuses and fistulae are seen most often in infants and young children, whereas cysts usually appear at a later age.

course of antibiotics is administered first and the operation is delayed several weeks to allow the inflammation to resolve. This provides the best chance for complete excision of the tract. Abscesses are managed initially with limited incision and drainage to control infection. Formal excision of branchial cleft lesions attempted in the presence of active inflammation or infection is associated with a higher recurrence rate secondary to incomplete excision and is also associated with an increased likelihood of injury to nerves (facial, hypoglossal) and other vital structures.

The operation is performed under general anesthesia. The patient is positioned with the head and neck slightly extended. An elliptic transverse incision is made along Langer's lines and incorporates the sinus opening. The tract is identified and dissection continues cephalad immediately along the tract to avoid injury to contiguous structures. The dissection for a second branchial remnant penetrates the platysma muscle and cervical fascia, ascends along the carotid sheath to the level of the hyoid bone, turns medially between the branches of the carotid artery, courses behind the posterior belly of the digastric muscle and the stylohyoid muscle, and in front of the hypoglossal nerve before ending in the pharynx, most often in the tonsillar fossa. A finger in the mouth pressing downward gently in the tonsillar fossa helps identify the end point of the dissection, where the tract is ligated with absorbable suture and divided (Fig. 95.4).

Occasionally, in older patients with a long tract, a second, "stepladder" incision may be required to complete the dissection. The tract for a first branchial cleft remnant typically courses from its sinus opening along the angle of the mandible cephalad in proximity to the parotid gland and facial nerve and ends at the external auditory canal (Fig. 95.5). Care should be taken during the dissection to avoid injury to the facial nerve branches; a nerve stimulator may be helpful. In cases of third and fourth branchial remnants, the dissection follows the tract to its termination in the piriform sinus. Endoscopy at the start of the operation may enable cannulation of the tract from above with a Fogarty catheter or small feeding tube, which greatly facilitates localization of the tract during excision (10). The thyroid gland is exposed through a standard collar incision, and the appropriate lobe is mobilized. The recurrent and superior laryngeal nerves and parathyroid glands should be identified and protected. If no discrete cyst or tract is found, the fistula may be located at the laryngeal level near the cricothyroid membrane. The fibers of the inferior constrictor muscle are bluntly spread to expose the piriform recess. Extreme caution should be exercised in this region to preserve the external branch of the superior laryngeal nerve. The tract typically passes inferior and external to the recurrent laryngeal nerve along the trachea to the superior pole of the thyroid gland. It may end blindly near the gland or penetrate the capsule to terminate in the parenchyma of the left thyroid lobe. Thyroid lobectomy or resection of the superior pole is carried out as indicated by the extent of the cyst (11) (Fig. 95.6). Once surgical extirpation is complete, the wound is closed in layers with absorbable suture. Recurrence is rare and implies that the entire epithelium-lined tract was not excised.

When remnants of the branchial apparatus persist as cartilaginous rests, these masses are generally small and present subcutaneously along the anterior border of the sternocleidomastoid muscle. The lesion is typically visible and palpable on physical examination and may be bilateral. An accompanying sinus or cyst is uncommon, and infection is rare. Excision is for cosmetic reasons.

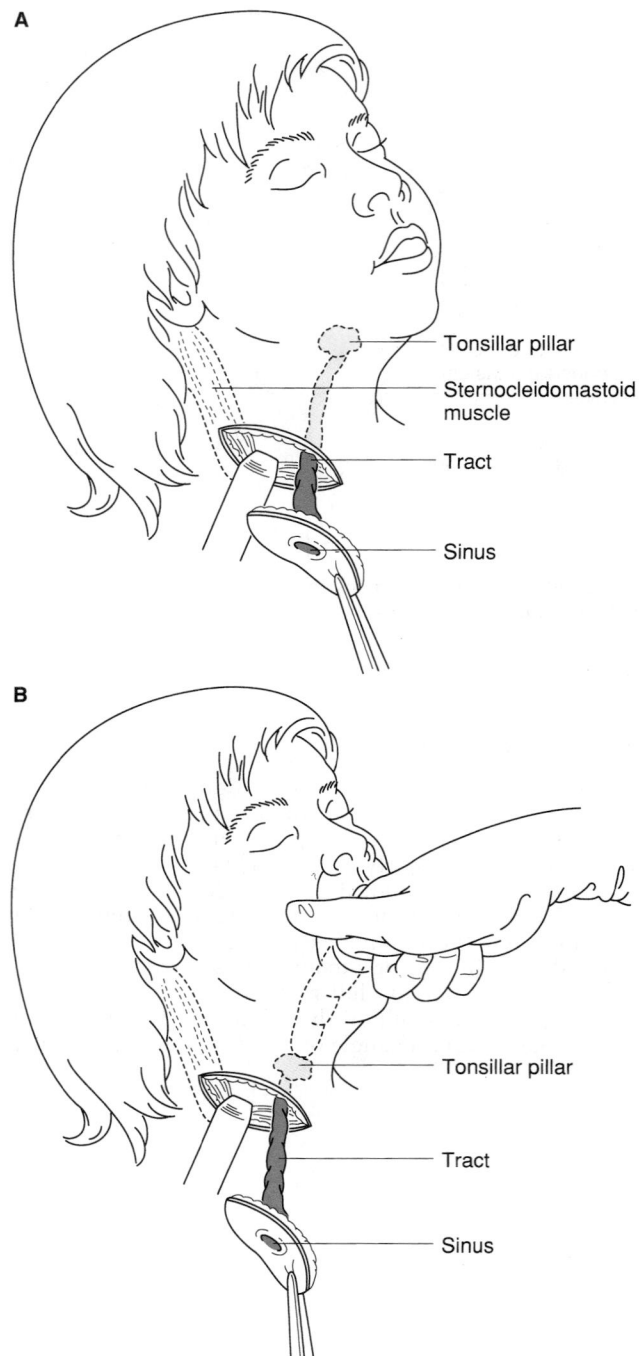

Figure 95.4. *(A)* Single incision in the lower part of the neck with the sinus tract developed to usual length. *(B)* The anesthesiologist's finger depresses the tonsillar fossa to facilitate complete dissection of the sinus tract through the single incision.

Preauricular cysts and sinuses are also common in infants and children. They are believed to arise as a result of anomalies in the formation of the external ear and represent vestiges of the first two branchial arches. They differ from first branchial cleft cysts in that they are more common, often bilateral, often inherited, and only rarely complicated by infection, involvement of the facial nerve, or entrance into the external auditory canal.

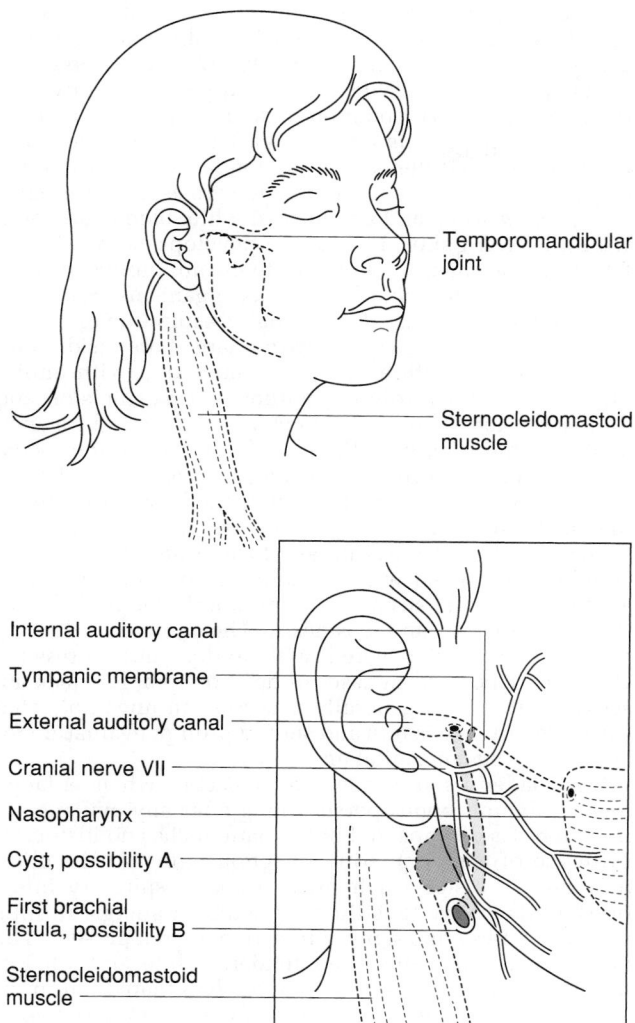

Figure 95.5. Relations of cyst or sinus of the first branchial cleft. Note especially the proximity to the facial nerve and external auditory canal.

Operative excision is generally recommended only for symptomatic lesions. Draining sinuses and infected cysts require antibiotic treatment, incision, drainage for failure to resolve, and delayed excision to prevent recurrence.

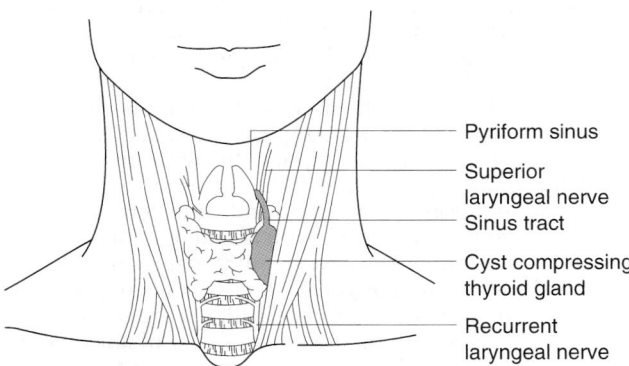

Figure 95.6. Relations of a third or fourth branchial cleft cyst or sinus to the thyroid gland and piriform sinus.

THYROGLOSSAL DUCT CYST

Anatomy and Embryology

Thyroglossal duct cysts are one of the most common midline neck lesions seen in children. Thyroglossal duct cysts or remnants arise when embryonic elements persist along the tract of descent of the thyroid gland. The thyroid gland starts as a diverticulum at the foramen cecum at the base of the tongue and descends in the sixth week of fetal life to its pretracheal position in the neck. In its descent, the tract most often passes through the central portion of the hyoid bone, but it may pass in front of or behind the hyoid. Thyroglossal duct cysts may develop anywhere along the tract (Fig. 95.7).

Clinical Aspects

Thyroglossal duct cysts are present at birth but rarely present clinically in early infancy. They most commonly present as a midline cystic neck mass or draining sinus in early childhood. Infection and abscess formation frequently develop becomes of communication with the mouth and contamination by oral flora. If it is not infected, the cyst is usually apparent by palpation. The cyst is at or near the midline, most commonly overlying the hyoid bone, but may be found at any level from the submental region to the upper trachea. It is typically smooth, soft, and nontender in the absence of infection. Because the cyst and tract are attached to the foramen cecum of the tongue, the cyst often moves with protrusion of the tongue and swallowing. In contrast to branchial cleft remnants, a thyroglossal duct cyst does not have a sinus opening to the skin unless infection has resulted in spontaneous drainage or an incomplete excision or incision and drainage procedure has previously been performed. The cyst and duct are lined with stratified squamous or pseudostratified columnar epithelium with mucus-secreting glands. Ectopic thyroid tissue may be present in the cyst or tract, and in rare cases this may represent the child's only thyroid tissue. Preoperative thyroid scans with radioactive isotopes have been employed by some, but usually one can be reassured by simply palpating the thyroid gland in its normal pretracheal location. Furthermore, even in the exceptional cases in which the thyroid tissue in the cyst is the only functional thyroid tissue, excision of the cyst is still mandated

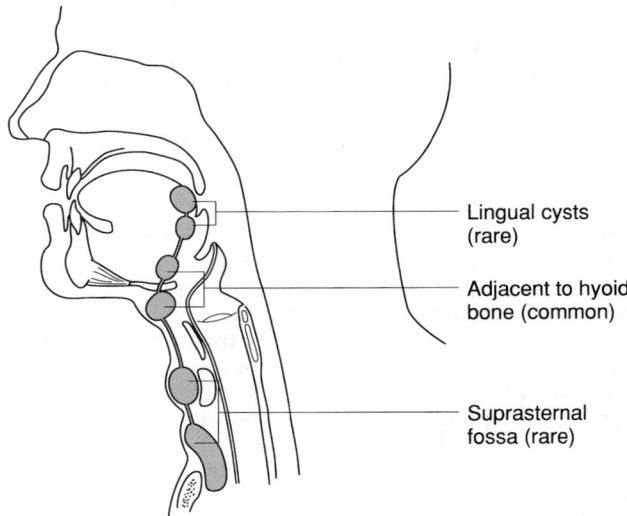

Figure 95.7. Locations of thyroglossal duct cysts.

because of the risk for infection and the malignant potential of the dysgenetic thyroid tissue (12). Review of the pathologic specimen after excision is important. If thyroid tissue is present in the specimen, thyroid function tests should be performed and thyroid replacement therapy prescribed as indicated. As with branchial cleft remnants, definitive excision should not be performed in the presence of infection or inflammation because of the increased risk for incomplete excision and injury to contiguous structures. Preoperative preparation may require incision and drainage or a period of antibiotics.

Treatment

Successful management requires complete removal of the cyst, its entire tract, and the central portion of the hyoid bone. In 1920, Sistrunk (13) not only described the importance of removing the central portion of the hyoid bone but also emphasized the possible existence of multiple tracts and therefore the importance of an *en bloc* dissection and removal of a core of tissue to the base of the tongue. Before these operative principles were elucidated, most series reported a recurrence rate of 20% or higher. The operation is performed under general endotracheal anesthesia. The patient's neck is extended, and often a roll is placed beneath the shoulders. A transverse skin incision is made directly over the cyst, usually in the infrahyoid region. The cyst is easily identified beneath the platysma muscle. Dissection adjacent to the cyst wall mobilizes the cyst, and the tract is identified. Dissection is continued cephalad up to the hyoid bone. The muscular attachments to the superior and inferior portions of the body of the hyoid bone are divided, and the central portion of the hyoid bone is removed in continuity with the cyst and tract. Beyond the hyoid bone, a core of tissue 5 to 10 mm in diameter is excised through the muscles of the base of the tongue to the foramen cecum, where the tract is ligated with absorbable suture. Identification of the end point of the dissection at the foramen cecum may be facilitated by having the anesthesiologist place downward pressure on the base of the tongue with a gloved finger. The ends of the hyoid bone are not reapproximated. The wound is copiously irrigated and closed in layers. A drain may be used, particularly if the patient has a history of infection, but most often it is not required. Contemporary recurrence rates generally are less than 10%.

Other midline neck masses seen in children include dermoid inclusion cysts, pathologic lymph nodes, cervical thymic cysts, and bronchogenic cysts. Differentiation from thyroglossal duct cysts can usually be accomplished on physical examination. In atypical cases, ultrasonography, CT, or magnetic resonance imaging helps to make the diagnosis and define the extent of the lesion. Complete surgical excision is recommended for these lesions.

LYMPHADENOPATHY

Benign cervical lymphadenopathy is the most common neck mass seen in childhood. The anterior cervical, occipital, retroauricular, and submandibular nodal groups are the ones most often enlarged. Bacterial and viral infections, particularly upper respiratory tract infections, otitis media, and pharyngitis, are the most common cause, with bacterial infections most likely to progress to acute suppurative lymphadenitis. Other important inflammatory causes of cervical lymphadenopathy include cat-scratch disease, atypical mycobacterial infection, and tuberculosis. Enlarged cervical or supraclavicular lymph nodes may also be the presenting manifestation of certain malignancies, particularly lymphoma.

Acute suppurative lymphadenitis is most frequently seen in young children between 6 months and 3 years of age. Typically, enlargement of the lymph node is preceded by an episode of pharyngitis or an upper respiratory tract infection. The most common organisms are *Staphylococcus* and *Streptococcus* species (14). The enlarged node initially becomes erythematous and tender with surrounding cellulitis. Systemic signs of infection are usually present—fever, tachycardia, and an elevated white blood cell count with a leftward shift. Fluctuance develops as the abscess forms. Management includes systemic antibiotics to cover *Streptococcus* and *Staphylococcus* organisms. Fluctuant nodes require drainage. Occasionally, aspiration of the purulent and necrotic material with a large-bore needle provides fluid for culture and, in combination with antibiotics, may effect resolution without formal incision and drainage. More frequently, fluctuant nodes require incision and drainage, with the use of either conscious sedation and local anesthesia or general anesthesia in the operating room. A skin line incision is made over the area of maximal fluctuance and the abscess cavity is drained, with care taken to break up any loculations. The incision should be designed with concern for complete drainage, avoidance of vital structures, particularly the branches of the facial nerve, and cosmesis. The wound is loosely packed open and covered with a dry gauze dressing. Drains may be used in cases of deep or complex neck abscesses but are not generally necessary in uncomplicated cases. Recurrence is rare and should prompt evaluation for an underlying congenital anomaly.

Lymphadenitis is chronic or subacute when enlargement of lymph nodes persists long after any evidence of infection has disappeared or the patients has no history or evidence of a precipitating infectious illness. The child may have a history of frequent upper respiratory infections, otitis media, tonsillitis, sinusitis, or allergic rhinitis or eczema. Systemic signs of infection are not present. The nodes are usually solitary, nontender, mobile, and soft. Enlarged nodes that are asymptomatic, less than 1 cm in diameter, and soft and that have been present for less than 8 weeks do not require treatment. Excisional biopsy should be performed for any node that is larger than 2 cm in diameter, persists beyond 8 weeks, or demonstrates worrisome characteristics, such as firmness, immobility, or rapid growth. The child should be evaluated for tuberculosis, atypical mycobacterial infection, and cat-scratch disease. Most of the lymph nodes that come to biopsy are benign, and the histologic examination reveals "reactive hyperplasia."

Mycobacterial lymphadenitis and cat-scratch disease also commonly cause lymphadenopathy in children (15). Mycobacterial lymphadenitis is usually caused by atypical mycobacteria of the *Mycobacterium avium–intracellulare–scrofulaceum* (MAIS) complex. The portal of entry is the oral pharynx. Infection with *Mycobacterium tuberculosis* is uncommon in children in the United States, and when present, it is usually accompanied by positive findings on chest radiographs because the lung is the site of entry for this organism. Atypical mycobacterial lymphadenitis is typically asymptomatic with enlarged but nontender nodes and no associated fever or leukocytosis. If no treatment is given, drainage and sinus formation may occur spontaneously. The child with tuberculous scrofula typically is symptomatic with pulmonary tuberculosis. The results of chest radiography and skin testing with purified protein derivative-standard (PPD-S) are usually positive. For *M. tuberculosis* infection, a trial of antituberculosis chemotherapy is recommended. Current treatment regimens consist of multiple-agent chemotherapy with isoniazid and rifampin for 9 to 12 months and a third drug (pyrazinamide, streptomycin, or ethambutol) for the first 2 months (16). Atypical mycobacterial infections generally respond poorly to chemotherapy. When a lymph node biopsy is planned, if tuberculosis or atypical mycobacterial infection is suspected, complete excision is required. Incision and drainage or incomplete nodal excision in cases of atypical mycobacterial infection invariably leads to recurrence or cutaneous draining sinuses.

Cat-scratch disease is a common cause of lymphadenitis in children in Western countries (17). In most cases, the history reveals direct contact with a cat. The disease is believed to be caused by a gram-negative bacillus, *Bartonella henselae,* and typically begins as a superficial infection at the inoculation site on a limb. Regional adenopathy develops, with the axilla the most commonly involved area; however, cervical nodes are involved in as many as 25% of cases (18). The diagnosis can be confirmed by skin test antigen. The clinical presentation usually is lymphadenopathy with only mild tenderness and without systemic symptoms. No treatment is necessary if the diagnosis is secure (positive skin test result) because the illness is self-limited and lymphadenopathy resolves in most cases in 6 to 8 weeks without specific treatment. If the diagnosis is in doubt, complete excision is recommended and curative.

It is important to remember that although most lymphadenopathy in children is benign, malignant conditions such as Hodgkin's disease and non-Hodgkin's lymphoma are also common in children and frequently present as primary neck lymphadenopathy. A high index of suspicion must be maintained in any case of a neck mass that has concerning examination characteristics or that persists despite appropriate antibiotic therapy. Excisional biopsy is recommended for definitive diagnosis.

VASCULAR MALFORMATIONS AND CYSTIC HYGROMA

Hemangioma

Hemangiomas can occur anywhere in the body, and involvement of the tongue, subglottic area, and parotid glands is common. Except for intradermal capillary lesions, most hemangiomas are not obvious at birth but become clinically evident during the first few weeks of life. The lesions may be extensive. Typically, they have a blue coloration and a spongy or rubbery texture on palpation. The presenting symptom for subglottic hemangioma is often stridor that is not present at birth but presents at 1 to 3 months of age. Parotid hemangioma typically develops in early infancy as an enlarging soft mass in the parotid gland. Cutaneous capillary hemangiomas may be present on the face, neck, or chest. Biopsy of these lesions was recommended in the past but is no longer routinely performed in most centers. Evaluation by ultrasonography with Doppler-flow studies is usually diagnostic (19). CT with intravenous contrast and magnetic resonance angiographic imaging are very useful for evaluating the extent of tissue involvement. Angiography is invasive and rarely necessary. The natural history of these lesions is one of significant growth in the first 6 to 12 months of life followed by a period of minimal growth, after which involution and spontaneous resolution occur by thrombosis and epithelialization (20). If involution takes place, it is complete by the age of 5 years in 80% of patients. Lesions that because of their location or growth are obstructing the airway, involving an eye, or destroying tissue are generally treated with intralesional steroid injection or systemic steroids. The response is typically excellent.

Lymphangioma and Cystic Hygroma

Anatomy and Embryology

At about the sixth week of gestation, a system of clefts develops in the cervical mesenchyme that subsequently form lymph channels. The channels give rise to jugular lymph sacs that become the cervical lymph nodes and lymphatics, ultimately draining into the internal jugular venous system (Fig. 95.8). Lymphangiomas are masses of disorganized, dilated lymph channels that arise when communications with the internal jugular system fail to develop in portions of the lymphatic channels. Lymphatic malformations can vary in size from a few centimeters in diameter to massive tumor-like lesions extending into the mediastinum. The larger lesions with macrocystic dilated lymphatic channels are often referred to as *cystic hygromas.* They are most commonly found in the lateral cervical and submandibular region. Other locations for lymphatic malformations are the extremities, mediastinum, retroperitoneum, and trunk. The majority of lymphatic malformations are evident early in life, with 65% present at birth, 80% evident within the first year of life, and 90% diagnosed by the age of 2 years (21). They typically present as an asymptomatic mass lesion and can be located anywhere in the body. Hemorrhage can occur within the lesion and is often the reason for the rapid enlargement sometimes noted clinically. The lesions have a significant tendency to become infected and also frequently present as an area of cellulitis or an abscess. Symptoms such as pain or discomfort are rare unless the lesion has hemorrhaged or been infected. In the newborn, the lesions may cause significant airway compromise or esophageal and pharyngeal obstruction. Approximately 10% of cervical lymphatic malformations extend into the chest. Lymphatic malformations can be diagnosed by prenatal ultrasonography, but most are detected on routine examination after birth. The physical examination findings of a soft, cystic,

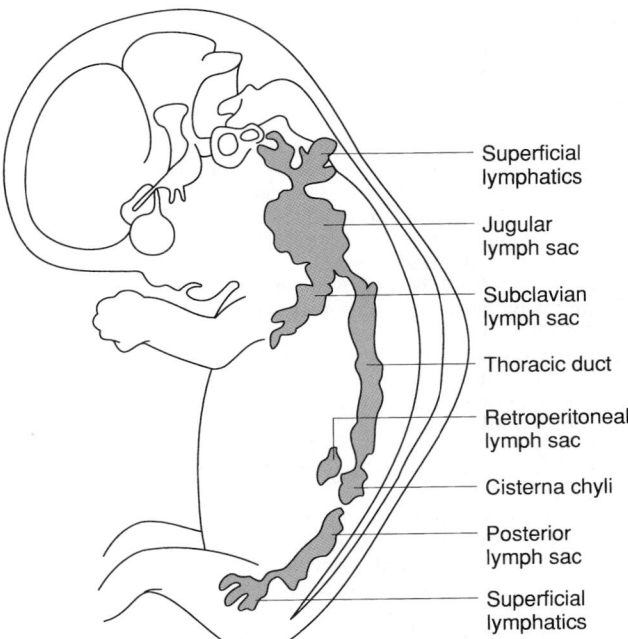

Superficial lymphatics

Jugular lymph sac

Subclavian lymph sac

Thoracic duct

Retroperitoneal lymph sac

Cisterna chyli

Posterior lymph sac

Superficial lymphatics

Figure 95.8. Lymphatic system in an 8-week-old human embryo. Development of the major and minor lymphatic sacs is well under way. The jugular lymphatic sac in the neck is prominent. Sequestration of tissue from any of the developing lymphatic structures leads to formation of a lymphangioma or cystic hygroma.

multiloculated mass are often sufficient for a definitive diagnosis. Ultrasonography, particularly with Doppler-flow studies, is often very useful to confirm the diagnosis. CT with intravenous contrast or magnetic resonance angiography is used selectively to evaluate extension of the lesion from one body space to another and delineate associated vital structures when resection is being planned.

Treatment

Complete surgical excision is the optimal treatment for lymphatic malformations. Because these lesions are benign, radical extirpation resulting in loss of function or severe deformity is not indicated. Spontaneous regression is unusual but may occur after acute inflammation. Only two thirds of lymphatic malformations are amenable to complete excision. One third require partial excision or, in the case of extensive or complex lesions, staged excision because of involvement of vital structures within the lesion. Needle aspiration of cysts is no longer recommended except to decompress a cyst emergently and relieve airway obstruction. Radiation treatment has not been of benefit in the treatment of lymphatic malformations and causes significant morbidity in the growing child. Injection of sclerosing agents, most commonly bleomycin, has been used but is associated with significant potential complications of infection, gastrointestinal problems, and pulmonary fibrosis (22). More recently, large cystic lesions in locations difficult to manage surgically have been treated by injection of OK-432, a monoclonal antibody produced by the incubation and interaction of *Streptococcus pyogenes* with penicillin (23). At present, this treatment remains experimental but has demonstrated success in some difficult cases.

REFERENCES

1. DeLorimer AA. Congenital malformations and neonatal problems of the respiratory tract. In: Welch KJ, Randolph JG, Ravitch MM, et al., eds. *Pediatric surgery,* 4th ed. Chicago: Year Book, 1986:631.
2. Alpers CE, Rosenau W, Finkbeiner WE, et al. Congenital (infantile) hemangiopericytoma of the tongue and sublingual region. *Am J Clin Pathol* 1984;81:377.
3. Wider DJ, Parker W. Lingual thyroid: review, case reports, and therapeutic guidelines. *Ann Otol Rhinol Laryngol* 1977;86:841.
4. Fonkalsrud EW. Malformations of the lymphatic system and hemangiomas. In: Holder TM, Ashcraft KW, eds. *Pediatric surgery.* Philadelphia: WB Saunders, 1980:1042.
5. Adams WG, Deaver KA, Cochi SL, et al. Decline of childhood *Haemophilus influenzae* type B (HIB) disease in the HIB vaccine era. *JAMA* 1993;269:221.
6. Kinnefors A, Olofsson J. Acute epiglottitis in children: experience with tracheostomy and intubation. *Clin Otolaryngol* 1983;8:25.
7. Soper RT, Pringle KC. Cysts and sinuses of the neck. In: Welch KJ, Randolph JG, Ravitch MM, et al., eds. *Pediatric surgery,* 4th ed. Chicago: Year Book, 1986:539.
8. Gray SW, Skandalakis JE. The pharynx and its derivatives. In: *Embryology for surgeons: the embryological basis for the treatment of congenital defects.* Philadelphia: WB Saunders, 1972.
9. Rosenfeld RM, Biller HF. Fourth branchial pouch sinus: diagnosis and treatment. *Otolaryngol Head Neck Surg* 1991;105:44.
10. Godin MS, Kearns DB, Pransky SM, et al. Fourth branchial pouch sinus: principles of diagnosis and management. *Laryngoscope* 1990;100:174.
11. Miller D, Hill JL, Sun CC, et al. The diagnosis and management of pyriform sinus fistulae in infants and young children. *J Pediatr Surg* 1983;18:377.
12. Page CP, Kemmerer WT, Haff RC, et al. Thyroid carcinoma arising in thyroglossal ducts. *Ann Surg* 1974;180:799.
13. Sistrunk WE. Surgical treatment of cysts of the thyroglossal tract. *Ann Surg* 1920;71:121.
14. Bodenstein L, Altman RP. Cervical lymphadenitis in infants and children. *Semin Pediatr Surg* 1994;3:134.
15. Zitelli DJ. Neck masses in children: adenopathy and malignant disease. *Pediatr Clin North Am* 1981;28:813.
16. Speck WT. Tuberculosis. In: Behrman RE, Kliegman R, Nelson W, eds. *Nelson textbook of pediatrics,* 14th ed. Philadelphia: WB Saunders, 1992.
17. Jackson LA, Perkins BA, Wenger JD. Cat-scratch disease in the United States: an analysis of three national databases. *Am J Public Health* 1993;83:1707.
18. Carithers HA. Cat-scratch disease: an overview based on the study of 1,200 patients. *Am J Dis Child* 1985;139:1124.
19. Welch KJ. The salivary glands. In: Welch KJ, Randolph JG, Ravitch MM, eds. *Pediatric surgery,* 4th ed. Chicago: Year Book, 1986.
20. Mulliken JB, Young AE. *Vascular birthmarks: hemangiomas and malformations.* Philadelphia: WB Saunders, 1988.
21. Bill AH, Sumner DS. A unified concept of lymphangioma and cystic hygroma. *Surg Gynecol Obstet* 1965;120:79.
22. Tanaka K, Inomata Y, Utsunomiya H, et al. Sclerosing therapy with bleomycin emulsion for lymphangioma in children. *Pediatr Surg Int* 1990;5:270.
23. Ogita S, Toshiaki T, Deguchi E, et al. OK-432 therapy for unresectable lymphangiomas in children. *J Pediatr Surg* 1991;26:263.

SURGERY: SCIENTIFIC PRINCIPLES AND PRACTICE, Third Edition, edited by Lazar J. Greenfield, Michael W. Mulholland, Keith T. Oldham, Gerald B. Zelenock, and Keith D. Lillemoe. Lippincott Williams & Wilkins Publishers, Philadelphia, © 2001.

CHAPTER 96

PEDIATRIC CHEST

ROBERT E. CILLEY, PETER W. DILLON, AND CHRISTOPHER J. BLEWETT

CHEST-WALL DEFORMITIES

Deformities of the chest wall may be obvious at birth but often become more noticeable at the time of preadolescent and adolescent growth. The physical appearance may vary from barely detectable to grotesquely deforming. Although some physiologic derangement attributable to the deformity may be present, the surgical correction of these deformities is more often intended to restore a normal appearance than to correct a physiologic deficit (1). Surgical correction of these congenital deformities, however, should be distinguished from cosmetic surgery. The goal of surgical correction of chest-wall deformities is to restore a more normal appearance where a deformity exists, whereas the goal of cosmetic surgery is to enhance beauty. The impact of these deformities on normal psychosocial development as well as the less certain evidence of cardiorespiratory impairment constitute adequate justification for the correction of these deformities in the affected child.

Embryology, Development, and Etiology of Chest-wall Deformities

In the developing embryo, the ribs are derived from individual somites as mesoderm differentiates into cartilage and advances ventrally toward the developing sternum. The ventrally advancing rib cartilage eventually approaches the developing sternum. The sternum itself is derived independently from two parallel condensations or bands of mesoderm that develop away from the midline. As the two sternal bands converge at the ventral midline, they fuse in a cranial to caudal direction and become progressively chondrified. After this initial fusion, transverse divisions of the cartilaginous sternum differentiate into segments opposite each end of the rib pairs. At birth, small ossification centers are present in the sternum and the ribs have largely ossified. Final ossification is usually complete by midadolescence. The process is sufficiently predictable that sternal ossification is a reliable method of determining bone age. There is a sharp demarcation in each rib between the ossified portion and the cartilaginous portion, the latter becoming ossified only much later in life. The cause of pectus excavatum and pectus carinatum is poorly understood. Explanations include abnormal intrauterine pressure applied to the chest, abnormalities of diaphragmatic development, connective tissue abnormalities, and genetic predisposition. Abnormal, excessive, or asymmetric growth of the costal cartilages associated with ribs three to seven is most implicated. *Sternal clefts* are understood as a failure of fusion of some portion of the sternal bands.

Pectus Excavatum

Pectus excavatum results from abnormal regulation of the growth of the costal cartilages. There is a corresponding posterior curve in the body of the sternum beginning at the manubrium and extending to the xyphoid. The deformity is rarely precisely symmetric, with one side (usually the right) slightly more curved in than the other. Occasionally, the asymmetry is pronounced, with the right side of the sternum rotated nearly to the sagittal plane. The deformity is often readily apparent at birth and may become more apparent during growth and development, particularly during adolescence. Pectus excavatum occurs more frequently in males than females. Another affected relative, most often a father or uncle, is found in one third of cases. Scoliosis is present at increased incidence in this population, although it rarely requires surgical correction. Patients frequently have an asthenic build and stoop-shouldered posture. Marfan syndrome predisposes to pectus excavatum. The diagnosis of Marfan syndrome has been made in our practice on several occasions when patients were referred for evaluation of a chest-wall deformity.

At the time of surgical consultation, concerns about the cardiopulmonary implications of the chest-wall deformity are often paramount to both the referring physician and patient's family. Many patients will have complaints of chest pain, shortness of breath, or both. Some patients will have been treated with inhaled bronchodilators for reactive airway symptoms. Most patients are disturbed by the appearance of the deformity, and some may be profoundly depressed and dysfunctional. The physiologic consequences of the deformity, however, have been difficult to demonstrate. The most likely benefit related to pulmonary function is an increase in exercise tolerance. Invasive and echocardiographic assessments of cardiovascular performance have demonstrated improvement in cardiac function and resolution of mitral valve prolapse in some patients following surgical correction of pectus excavatum (2). Despite more than half a century of investigation and speculation, no consensus has been achieved on what degree of cardiopulmonary impairment, if any, this common chest-wall deformity produces.

Clinical assessment of the severity of the deformity has included chest radiographs, computed tomography (CT), caliper measurements, and contrast volume measurements of the cavity. Various ratios have been described to quantitate the defect using measurements derived from these studies. The clinical utility of these studies is doubtful, however, because decisions about operation usually are made on the basis of the appearance of the deformity and its psychological impact rather than the physiologic significance of the deformity. If cardiac disease is suspected on the basis of the history and physical examination, an echocardiogram may be indicated.

Surgical Correction of Pectus Excavatum.   The timing of surgical correction for pectus excavatum has become more uniform in the past decade. It is now recognized that infants and preschool children should not undergo surgical correction because of the risk of acquired thoracic dystrophy (3,4). Most pediatric surgeons agree that the optimal timing is in late childhood and adolescence. Statistically, the most common time for repair is in the early and middle teenage years.

Traditional Operations (2,5).   Surgical correction is performed through a transverse incision centered on the defect in the line of the inframammary crease (Fig. 96.1). The necessary incision is quite small and may be kept

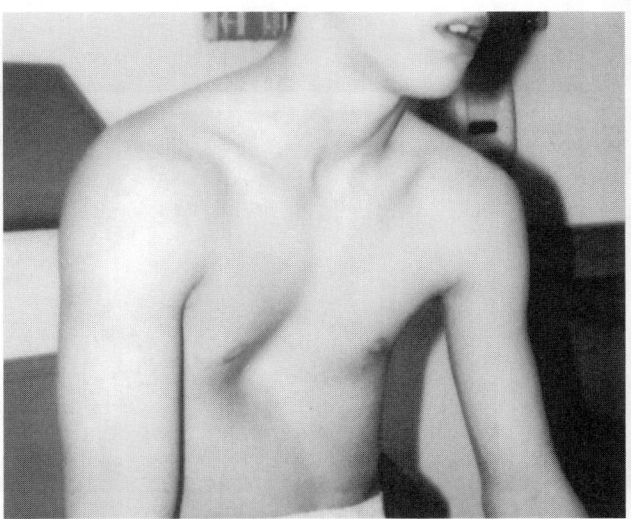
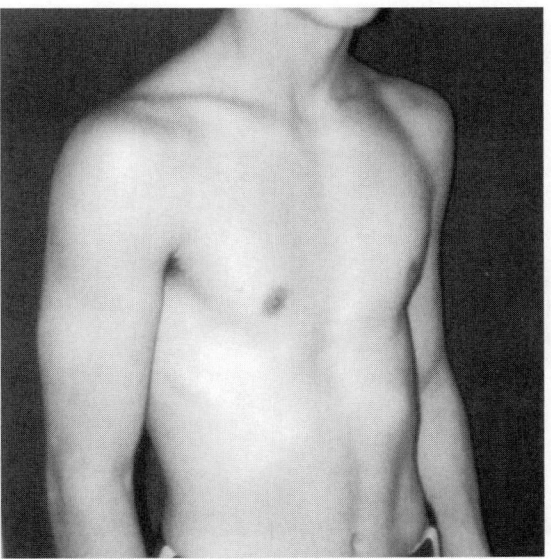

A   B

Figure 96.1. Pectus Excavatum. *(A)* Appearance of an adolescent boy with a typical depression deformity. Note "stoop-shouldered" posture. *(B)* Postoperative appearance at 6 months. Erect posture and subpectoral incision give a good cosmetic result.

well within the nipple lines. An alternative that may be useful, especially in older female patients, uses a small incision is each inframammary crease. Endoscopic techniques have been reported (6). The operation requires exposure of the costal cartilages by elevation of the pectoral muscles from the chest wall. The involved costal cartilages are excised subperiochondrially and bilaterally. The third through the seventh cartilages are excised along with portions of the eight and ninth cartilages if there is particularly prominent flaring of the costal margin. The xyphoid is detached from the sternum, and the rectus muscles are detached inferiorly. The undersurface of the sternum is dissected free from the pericardium and pleura. An anterior osteotomy is created in the sternum just below the manubrium, and the posterior cortex is fractured. Closure of the osteotomy elevates the lower sternum. Asymmetric deformities may require alternative placement of the osteotomy or more than one osteotomy to achieve a flat sternum. Some degree of overcorrection usually is performed to help maintain the correction over time. A strut usually is placed beneath or through the sternum to maintain the corrected sternal position. The choice of material and configuration for the strut is variable. Struts may be left in permanently but usually are removed after an interval of 2 to 12 months. The pectoral and rectus muscles are reattached, and closed suction drains are used to drain the substernal, submuscular, or subcutaneous spaces. Patients are discharged when they are able to tolerate a diet and their pain is controlled by oral analgesics. Drains are removed when drainage has decreased either as an inpatient or an outpatient. In current practice, patients often are discharged on the second

postoperative day. Complications generally are limited to wound infections and pneumothorax, which rarely requires tube drainage. Recurrence rates in large series with long-term follow-up range from 5% to 15% (2). Migration of implanted struts and bars have caused the most serious problems, including cardiac injury.

Lorenze Bar/Nuss Procedure. This procedure is currently gaining popularity; it depends on the application of physical forces to the developing chest wall in the form of a rigid U-shaped bar inserted transversely across the chest that pushes the deformity back into place (7). The procedure is best performed in late childhood and early adolescence, when there is more pliability of the costal cartilages. The addition of thoracoscopic guidance to the technique of bar insertion has added to the safety of the procedure. Long-term follow-up data are just beginning to become available. The procedure appears to be durable, although it is too early to assess fully the incidence of late recurrence. Complications have been reported as the procedure has become more widely practiced. Ideal patient selection is not yet determined. The bar is left in for up to 2 years during a period of development when most children are active and may engage in contact sports. The activity restrictions that are necessary while the bar is in place are not well defined. Despite these unknown factors, this technique appears to be an important addition to the surgical treatment of chest wall deformities (Fig. 96.2).

Implantation of a submuscular silastic mold to alter the chest contour may result in a very acceptable appearance. This technique does not address any of the potential physiologic problems associated with pectus excavatum and has not been used widely.

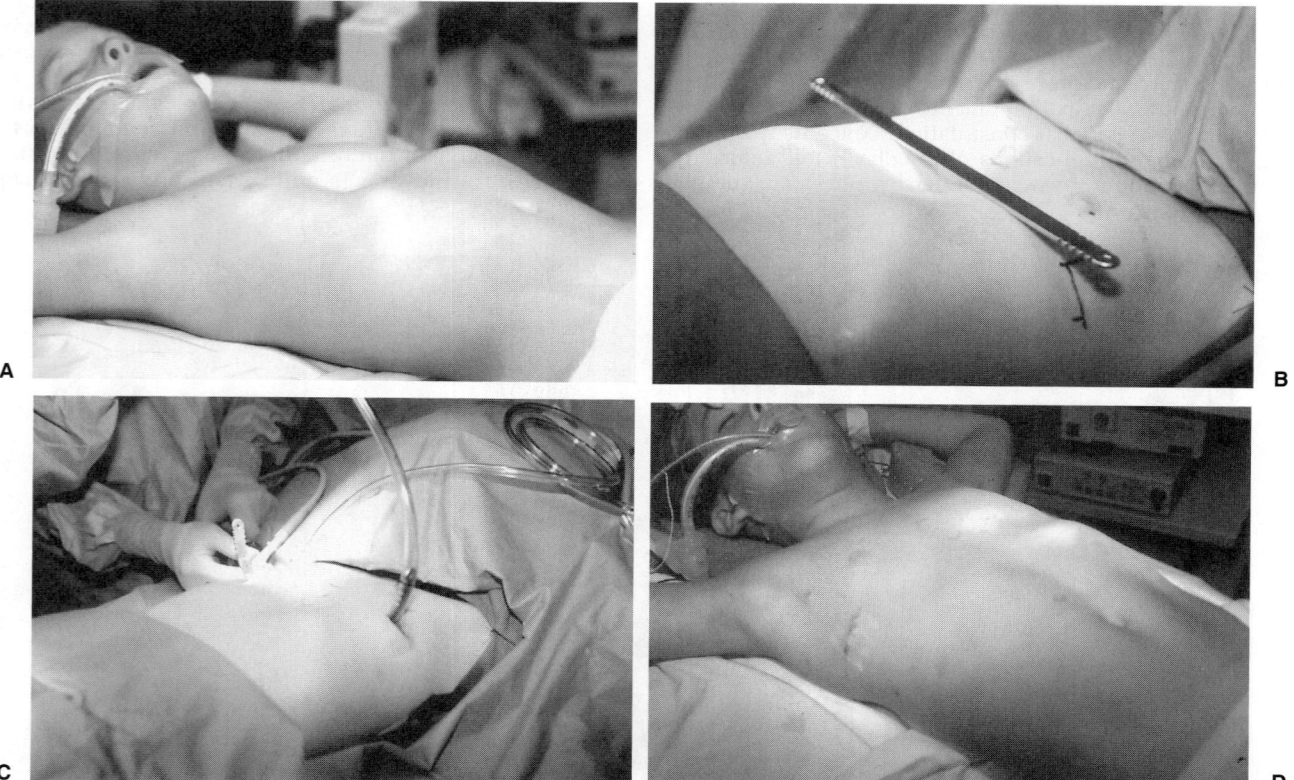

Figure 96.2. Thoracoscopically assisted Lorenz bar insertion (Nuss procedure). *(A)* Preoperative appearance with symmetrical depression deformity. *(B)* Lorenz bar. *(C)* Lorenz bar inserted with thoracoscopic guidance. *(D)* Immediate postoperative appearance. (Digital images provided by Walter S. Cain, M.D., University of Alabama, used with permission.)

Pectus Carinatum

Pectus carinatum (*carina,* Latin for "keel," also used to describe the protruding sternum of a bird, hence "pigeon breast") is a deformity that occurs less frequently than pectus excavatum and does not carry with it the concern of physiologic impairment because the thorax is enlarged. The concern for appearance, however, may be even more troublesome than with depression deformities of the chest wall. Protrusion deformities may be difficult to hide, even when the subject is fully clothed. Rapid growth of the costal cartilages at puberty makes the deformity more pronounced at that time, leading to surgical consultation. The operative correction of a pectus carinatum deformity is similar to that described for pectus excavatum. The osteotomies and sternal fracture are performed in such a way as to depress the sternum. A small wedge of resected cartilage may be placed in the osteotomy to maintain position. A strut usually is not required to maintain sternal position. Postoperative course and results are similar to pectus excavatum. In the immediate postoperative period, cardiac pulsation may be particularly visible. With healing, this finding disappears.

Poland's Syndrome

In 1841, Poland described the features of this rare abnormality found in a cadaveric dissection. These features include the absence of the sternal portions of the pectoralis major muscle; absence of the pectoralis minor muscle; absence of portions of the serratus anterior and external oblique muscles; forearm and hand deformities; ipsilateral hypoplasia of the nipple, breast, and chest wall subcutaneous tissues; absence or deformity of the second to fifth costal cartilages; and absence of axillary hair on the affected side. Surgical correction requires modification of the techniques used for other chest-wall deformities. Breast augmentation restores a more acceptable appearance in female patients.

Sternal Clefts

Congenital sternal clefts result from failure of midline fusion of the paired sternal bands. The cleft is usually in the superior portion of the sternum and may extend to, but not include, the xyphoid. The defects are rare and usually are repaired in the neonatal period to protect the underlying mediastinal structures. After subcutaneous mobilization, the fibrocartilagenous sternal bars are approximated in the midline. If the cleft is incomplete, it must be completed by dividing the intact portion so that closure does not lead to buckling of the inferior portion of the sternum. *Cantrell pentology* refers to a distal sternal cleft, omphalocele, diaphragmatic defect, pericardial defect, and intracardiac defect. *Thoracic ectopia cordis* (exstrophy of the heart) may occur as a part of this abnormality and until recently has been uniformly fatal.

Jeune's Asphyxiating Thoracic Dystrophy

This rare developmental abnormality results in the failure of chest-wall growth. Surgical correction involves the expansion of thoracic cavity by rib resection or the placement of expandable prosthetic ribs to promote chest enlargement.

"Slipping Rib" Syndrome

This unusual abnormality has been ascribed to abnormal development of the costal cartilages along the costal margin such that the ninth or tenth rib is free floating. Particular movements that result in the involved rib crossing the costal margin may be painful. Marked disability has been described that is relieved by excision of the involved rib and cartilage.

"Flaring" of the Costal Margin

Patients sometimes are referred for surgical opinions regarding unusual prominence of the costal margin. This finding is most pronounced when the patient is supine. This finding represents a variation of the normal development of the chest wall. Surgical correction should be avoided.

Costochondral "Tumor"

Prominence of a single costal cartilage may present as a concern of a tumor of cartilage or bone. This abnormality usually is found in preadolescents and adolescents. Many patients will have undergone a diagnostic work-up that includes chest radiographs and CT or magnetic resonance imaging (MRI) before to surgical consultation. This abnormality most likely represents a minor variation of a chest-wall deformity, such as a pectus carinatum. Because the area of enlargement is rarely tender, costochondritis is an unlikely explanation. Excision of the involved cartilage is rarely helpful. Plain radiographs are usually sufficient to exclude a tumor.

CONGENITAL CYSTIC DISEASE OF THE LUNG

The most common congenital cystic lesions of the lung result from abnormalities of lung embryogenesis (8,9). These lesions include pulmonary sequestration (PS), congenital cystic adenomatoid malformation (CCAM), bronchogenic cyst (BC), and congenital lobar overinflation (CLO). The first three (PS, CCAM, and BC) are part of the spectrum of bronchopulmonary foregut malformations. The abnormality may be primarily characterized by aberrant blood supply (PS), hamartomatous lung parenchyma (CCAM), or an isolated epithelial cyst (BC). More recently, there has been wider recognition of mixed or intermediate forms that contain elements of more that one abnormality (10). The coexistence of these malformations with congenital diaphragmatic hernia and congenital heart defects emphasizes that these abnormalities may be part of a generalized problem with organogenesis. CLO is more likely a secondary response of the developing lung to abnormal compression or obstruction of a bronchus. The relative retention of fetal lung fluid during critical phases of lung development adversely affects the development of the lung.

Pulmonary Sequestration

Pulmonary sequestrations are divided into intralobar or extralobar lesions, based on their relationship with the investing visceral pleura and adjacent normal lung tissue. Structurally, sequestrations represent abnormal lung tissue with an anomalous systemic blood supply that does not communicate normally with the trachea or a bronchus.

An intralobar sequestration lies within a lobe of the lung and is invested by its visceral pleura. They are most common in the posterior segment of the left lower lobe but can occur elsewhere. The anomalous arterial blood supply comes from either the thoracic or abdominal aorta and may traverse the diaphragm to supply the sequestration. Venous drainage from this aberrant tissue may be either pulmonary or systemic but is usually into the pulmonary vein. Aberrant airspace connections with adjacent normal lung tissue may permit air trapping within the sequestration, causing it to be aerated on radiographs. Although most often asymptomatic at birth, intralobar pulmonary sequestration may present during childhood as recurrent localized pneumonia caused by these aberrant airspace connections.

Extralobar sequestrations occur outside the pleura of the normal lung. They are most common in the lower left side

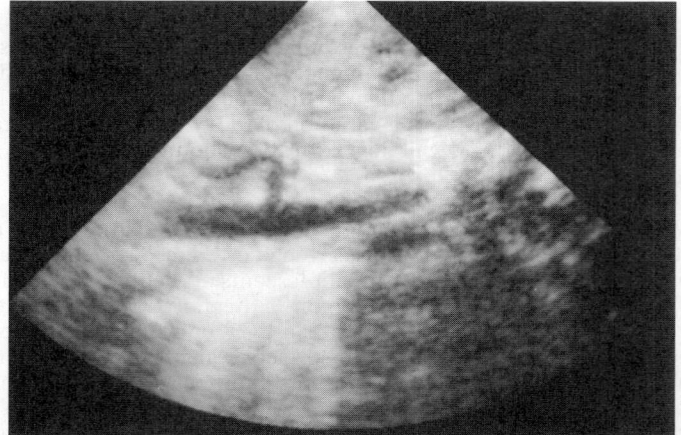

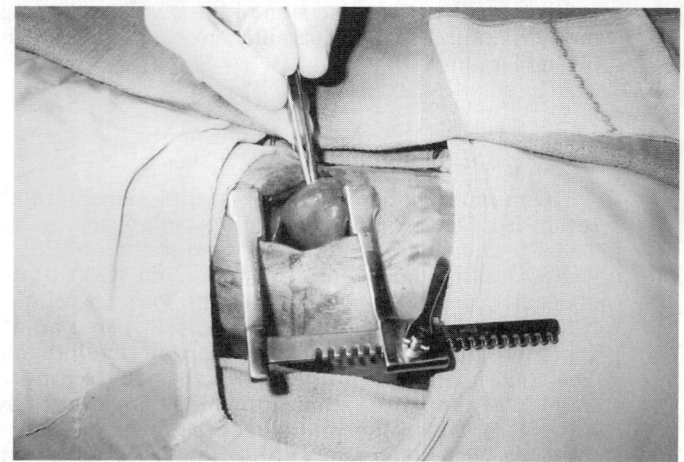

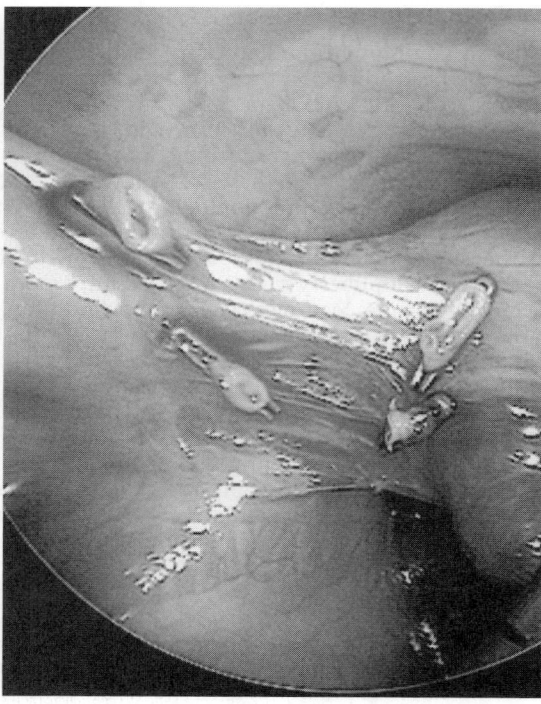

Figure 96.3. Pulmonary sequestration. *(A)* Sagittal ultrasound view of aortic branch supplying an extralobar pulmonary sequestration. *(B)* Left-sided extralobar pulmonary sequestration excised by a muscle-sparing thoracotomy. *(C)* Intraoperative view of extralobar sequestration removed thoracoscopically. Note the main blood supply with clips.

of the chest but have been reported in various locations, including in the retroperitoneum below the diaphragm (11). In this location, they may be difficult to distinguish from an intraabdominal tumor, such as a neuroblastoma. Rarely, extralobar sequestration is associated with congenital diaphragmatic hernias. In extralobar sequestration, both the arterial and venous blood supplies are usually systemic, and the arterial blood supply frequently arises from the aorta below the diaphragm. The lesion itself is usually a spongy, consolidated mass with no aeration. Although infection is rarely present, these lesions can be associated with hemorrhage, arteriovenous shunting, or mediastinal compression. Occasionally, the amount of blood shunted through the lesion is sufficient to result in symptomatic congestive heart failure. Pulmonary malignancies have occurred within these lesions. The simultaneous occurrence of CCAM tissue in sequestrations is recognized more frequently.

Radiographic evaluation of these lesions involves standard chest x-rays and CT scans. Intralobar sequestrations usually are treated with thoracotomy and lobectomy (Fig. 96.3A,B). Extralobar sequestrations require simple excision and now can be removed with minimally invasive surgical techniques (Fig. 96.C). In dealing with both lesions, particular attention must be paid to the vascular supply.

Congenital Cystic Adenomatoid Malformations

Congenital cystic adenomatoid malformations (CCAMs) result from excessive proliferation of bronchial structures without the development of the corresponding alveoli.

These malformations have a normal vascular supply and communicate with the normal tracheobronchial tree. On gross appearance, they can be solid, cystic, or both. CCAMs have been classified into three types based on size, shape, spacing of the cysts, and histologic appearance (12). Type I CCAMs are composed of cysts with large, irregular and widely dispersed spaces larger than 2 cm in diameter or a single large cyst with small cysts surrounding it. Type II CCAMs consist of multiple cysts smaller than 1 cm in diameter that are packed close together and resemble dilated bronchials. Type III CCAMs are made up of small cysts that are smaller than 0.5 cm in diameter, and the parenchymal tissue represents late-gestational-age fetal lung. Cartilage is usually lacking in all three types of CCAMs. Type I cysts account for almost 50% of cases, and type II cysts make up an additional 40%. CCAMs usually affect only one lobe, but multilobar and bilateral involvement also occurs.

Cystic adenomatoid malformations may present as acute respiratory distress in the neonatal period caused by the compression of surrounding structures. The usual radiologic appearance after birth is that of a solid mass because of retained fetal lung fluid (Fig. 96.4A). As ventilation occurs and fluid is reabsorbed, the mass appears larger and cystic and may begin to impinge on surrounding structures (Fig. 96.4B). A less common presentation is the appearance of recurrent pneumonia later in life. Prenatal diagnosis occurs more commonly with ultrasound detection, and successful in utero ablation of the affected lobe has been reported for infants who develop life-threatening fetal hydrops. As a result of serial prenatal ultrasounds, spontaneous in utero resolution has been ob-

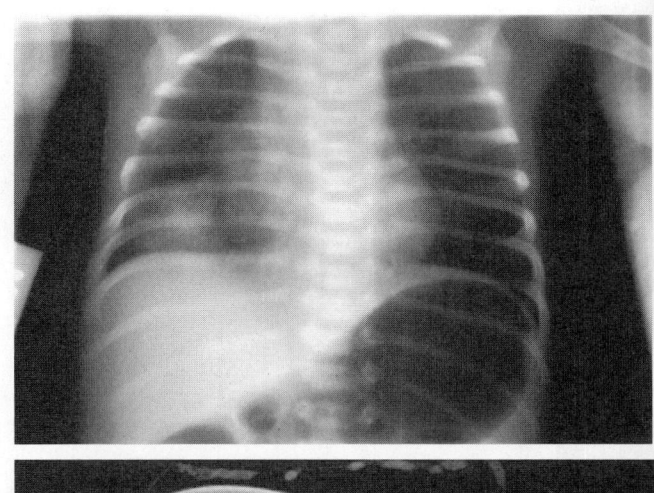
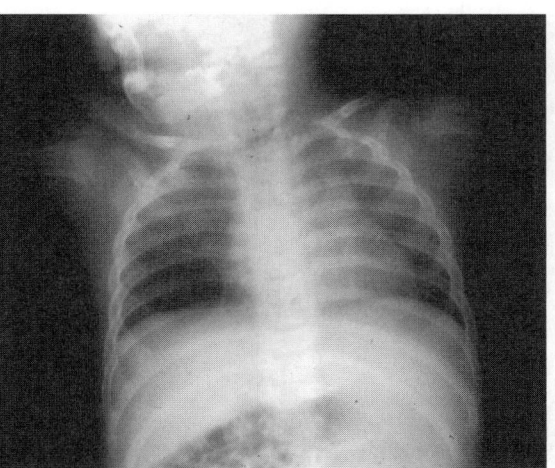
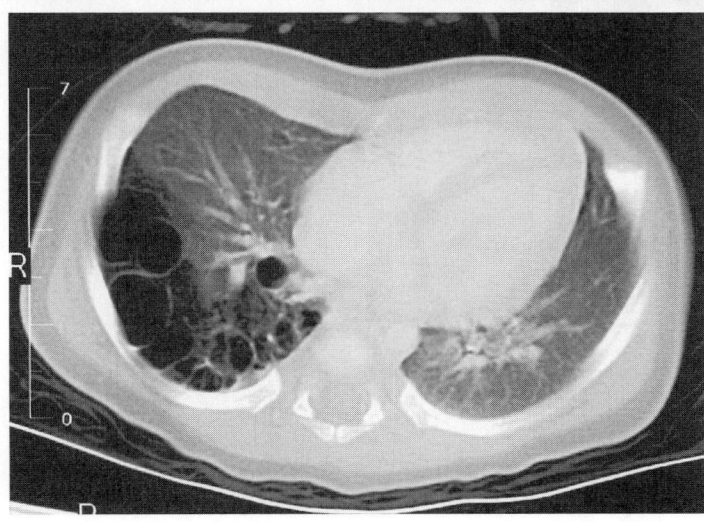

Figure 96.4. Congenital cystic adenomatoid malformation *(CCAM)*. *(A)* Newborn chest radiograph of a patient with prenatal diagnosis of congenital cystic adenomatoid malformation. Note that immediately after birth the mass is fluid-filled and appears as a density in the right hemithorax. *(B)* Chest radiograph of the same child, before surgical excision was performed, at 5 months of age. Note air-filled cystic appearance of CCAM. *(C)* Transverse thoracic computed tomographic view of CCAM.

served to occur in as many as one third of these infants (13). In these cases, a CT scan of the chest should be obtained sometime after birth to document residual parenchymal abnormalities.

Infants with symptomatic lesions after birth require resection of the involved lobe. Asymptomatic lesions can be followed closely to allow for growth and development. Operation is recommended if symptoms occur. Although recommendations among pediatric surgeons differ, most investigators recommend elective resection because of concern about future symptoms and the possibility of malignancy (see later) (14,15). We currently recommend a CT scan at age 4 to 6 months to confirm the diagnosis and assist in surgical planning in all infants with asymptomatic lesions (Fig. 96.4C). Elective resection is performed at about 6 months of age. When bilateral or multilobar involvement is found, CT scans may assist in planning lung-conserving resections and in follow-up of residual disease. Lung-preserving resections should be used for cystic adenomatoid malformations that involve multiple lung lobes (16).

Bronchogenic Cysts

Bronchogenic cysts represent groups of epithelial cells from the developing trachea and lung buds that have become separated from the tracheobronchial tree. These cysts exist as discrete masses, usually in the paratracheal region, and do not incorporate pulmonary mesenchyme on which further development depends. If cells separate

from the bronchopulmonary foregut structures early in development, these cysts tend to originate from the esophageal portion of the foregut. Separation that occurs later in development is from the ventral or tracheal portion of the foregut, resulting in bronchogenic cysts. Bronchogenic cysts are usually extrapulmonary masses that do not communicate with the normal tracheobronchial tree. They do not have a unique blood supply. Resection of these lesions with either a thoracotomy or video-assisted thoracoscopy is recommended because of the risk of bleeding, infection, or enlargement with compression of adjacent mediastinal structures (Fig. 96.5) (17,18).

Congenital Lobar Overinflation

Congenital lobar overinflation (previously referred to as *congenital lobar emphysema*) is caused by abnormal development or compression of a lobar bronchus resulting in retention of fluid during fetal lung development and subsequent air-trapping and overinflation after birth. The lung tissue is intrinsically normal but has been secondarily altered as a result of the trapping of fluid and gas. The vascular supply is normal. The condition can result from a deficiency of bronchial cartilage that leads to focal airway collapse and bronchial obstruction. Congenital lobar emphysema also can result from extraluminal bronchial compression that is due to a bronchogenic cyst, an enteric duplication cyst, lymphadenopathy, mediastinal tumor, a vascular abnormality, or congenital heart disease (19). In

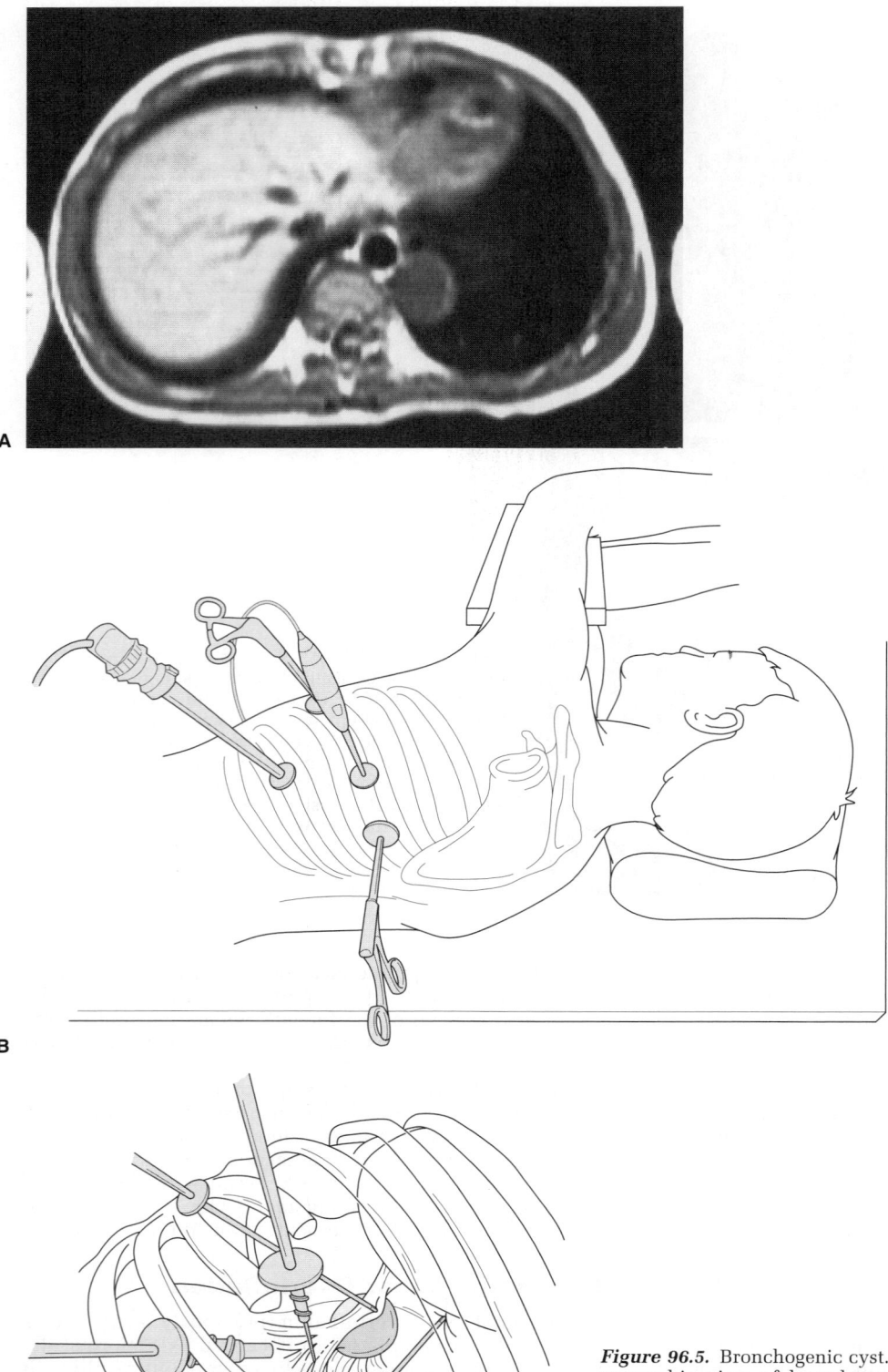

Figure 96.5. Bronchogenic cyst. *(A)* Transverse thoracic computed to-mographic view of bronchogenic cyst located in the inferior pul-monary ligament. *(B)* Illustrative representation of thoracoscopic in-strumentation for excision of bronchogenic cyst. *(C)* Operative detail. (From Dillon PW, Cilley RE, Krummel TM. Video assisted thoraco-scopic excision of intrathoracic masses in children: report of two cases. *Surg Laparosc Endosc* 1993;3:433–436, with permission.)

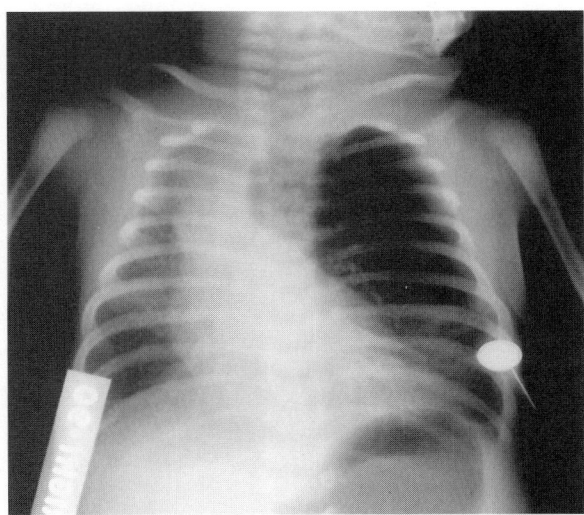
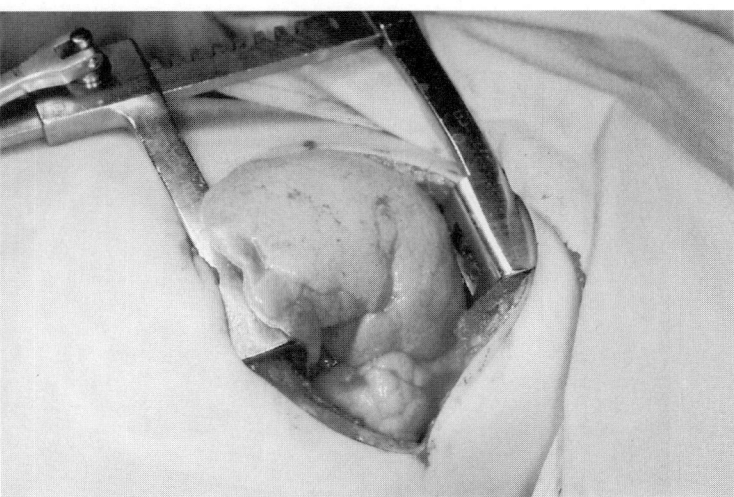

A   B

Figure 96.6. Congenital lobar overinflation. *(A)* Chest radiograph demonstrating overinflation of left upper lobe in an infant. Note mediastinal shift. *(B)* Operative photograph demonstrating overexpanded left upper lobe decompressing through the incision.

more than half of cases, no obstruction is identified. Usually, the upper lobe of either lung field is involved, but multilobar involvement has been reported. Lobar overinflation presents as worsening respiratory distress caused by progressive emphysematous enlargement of the involved lobe with compression of normal adjacent tissue and mediastinal shift (Fig. 96.6A). Infants with symptomatic congenital lobar overinflation require complete resection of the affected lobe. In selected circumstances, bronchoplasty, bronchial suspension, or relief of an extrinsic bronchial obstruction may be useful. Great care must be taken at the time of anesthetic induction in these infants because lobar overinflation may be exacerbated by the institution of positive pressure ventilation. Immediate thoracotomy may be necessary to relieve compression of the mediastinum and prevent cardiopulmonary collapse (Fig. 96.6B). Up to half of the cases identified will resolve during infancy, with observation alone as the lung develops (20–22). Surgery is reserved for symptomatic patients.

Diagnosis

With the routine use of prenatal ultrasound, many cystic lesions of the lung are now detected and followed prior to birth. This is especially true of cystic adenomatoid malformations and sequestrations. Many of these lesions are completely asymptomatic in the postnatal period, with children tending to develop symptoms from recurrent infections several years later. These lesions can cause compression and collapse of adjacent bronchi and pulmonary tissue and can lead to progressive respiratory distress at any age. Standard chest radiographs remain the cornerstones of diagnosis and follow-up for these lesions. Rapid thoracic CT scanning provides definitive mapping of these lesions with intravenous contrast. When properly performed, such dynamic images will show the aberrant systemic arterial supply when dealing with a pulmonary sequestration. Contrast esophagrams are indicated for children with dysphagia and serve to outline the possibility of an abnormal communication with the gastrointestinal tract. If aberrant vascular supply is suspected but not demonstrated on a CT scan, then a vascular MRI of the chest can be obtained. This test has supplanted angiography when vascular definition is needed in children.

Treatment

Asymptomatic pulmonary cysts should be removed because of the possibility of infection. Additionally, it has been proposed that these cysts be removed because of the rare association of malignant pulmonary neoplasms in these congenital cysts. Any cyst that is enlarging on serial chest radiographs should be resected because of the respiratory compromise that may ensue and the possibility of infection either in the cyst or in the surrounding lung tissue. The only reason for long-term follow-up of a lesion would be if serial CT scans demonstrated progressive resolution, indicating the possibility of an acquired infectious cyst that had the potential for resolution.

Cysts of the Mediastinum

Benign cysts of the mediastinum are relatively common in pediatric patients. Although most of these cysts are completely asymptomatic and discovered incidentally, surgical resection usually is recommended because of the possibility of progressive enlargement with compression, hemorrhage, or infection. When symptoms do develop, they may include chest pain, cough, stridor, hemoptysis, or dysphasia. The common cystic lesions include thymic cysts, enterogenous cysts, dermoid cysts, pericardial cysts, and lymphatic malformations (cystic hygromas).

Thymic Cysts

Thymic cysts are usually asymptomatic and, being located in the superior aspect of the mediastinum, generally have both mediastinal and cervical components. These are benign lesions made up of ciliated epithelium, with lymphocytes and cholesterol crystals embedded in the cyst wall. Clinical problems are usually the result of rapid expansion from either hemorrhage or infection.

Enteric Duplication Cysts/Enterogenous Cysts

Enteric duplication cysts usually occur in the posterior mediastinum and are composed of esophageal or gastric epithelium surrounded by smooth muscle (Fig. 96.7). They are part of the spectrum of bronchopulmonary foregut malformations that include bronchogenic cysts (see preceding), and esophageal duplications (see later).

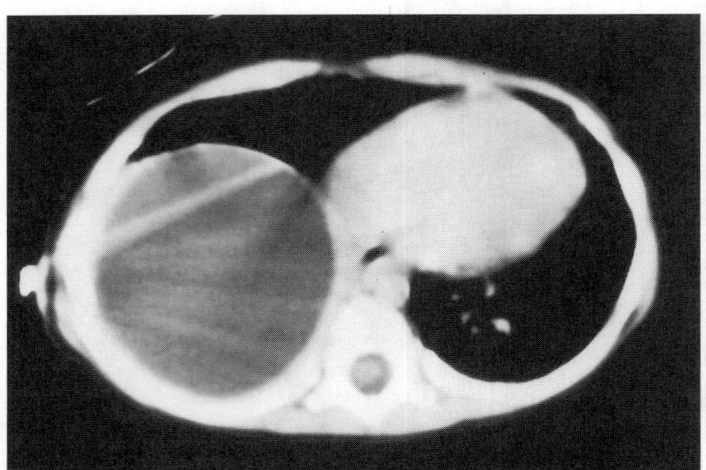
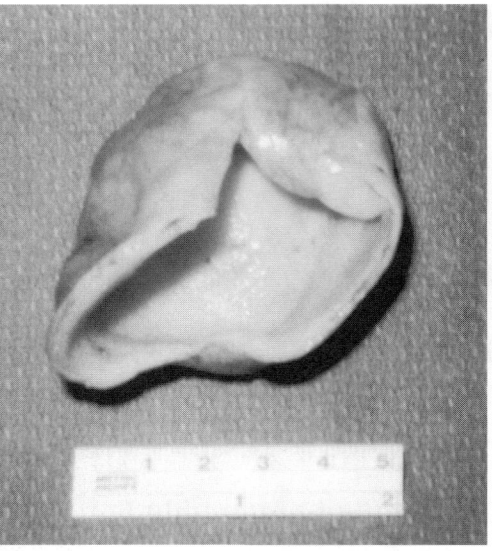

Figure 96.7. Enterogenous cyst representing another abnormality in the spectrum of bronchopulmonary foregut malformations. *(A)* Computed tomography demonstrating a large mass occupying the right hemithorax. *(B)* Surgical specimen.

They may exist completely separate from the structure of origin, or they may communicate with the gastrointestinal tract above or below the diaphragm. In rare instances, they may attach to or communicate with the spinal canal. Some reported have described large thoracoabdominal enteric cysts. These cysts may penetrate the diaphragm and end blindly in the peritoneal cavity or communicate with the gastrointestinal tract. If gastric mucosa is present within the cyst, peptic ulceration with erosion and bleeding has been reported. Therefore, removal of these cysts is recommended to avoid these possible complications.

Lymphatic Malformations

Lymphatic malformations in the head, neck, and mediastinal region have been classically referred to as *cystic hygromas*. They are multilocular, thin-walled cysts derived from primitive, aberrant lymphatic sacs. Their mediastinal involvement can be quite extensive because they insinuate around the great vessels and nervous structures of the superior mediastinum. As with other cystic structures, these lesions are usually asymptomatic; however, with enlargement, hemorrhage, or infection, symptoms may develop with life-threatening potential. Surgical resection of these lesions usually is recommended without sacrificing important anatomic structures within the mediastinum. Recurrence may develop in approximately one third of the cases.

Pericardial Cysts

Pericardial cysts are almost always asymptomatic lesions discovered as incidental findings on chest radiographs. They appear in the cardiophrenic sulcus as small discrete masses. They are thin-walled cysts that contain clear fluid and are lined by mesothelium. Resection can be performed either by an open thoracotomy or video-assisted thoracoscopy.

THORACIC TUMORS IN CHILDREN

Thoracic tumors in children are rare. Neoplasms originate from the chest wall, the mediastinum, and the lung. Lung metastases from extrathoracic cancers are more common than primary neoplasms. Surgical treatment may involve removal of the primary tumor, resection of adjacent structures, chest-wall reconstruction, lung resection (including wedge resection, lobectomy, pneumonectomy), and tracheobronchial resection and reconstruction. The role of minimally invasive surgery/thoracoscopic surgery is increasing in both the diagnosis and treatment of thoracic tumors in children (23).

Metastatic Lung Tumors

For surgical excision of metastatic lung tumors to be beneficial, the primary tumor must be eradicated and the patient should be free of other metastatic disease. Osteogenic sarcoma, other soft tissue sarcomas, and Wilms' tumor are the tumors with lung metastases that most often are considered for surgical treatment (24,25).

Osteogenic Sarcoma

Although the reported experience in the treatment of metastatic osteogenic sarcoma to the lung is based on retrospective review, there is good evidence that resection of lung metastases is beneficial. The success of surgical removal of metastatic lung disease depends on effective chemotherapy to eliminate other micrometastatic disease. The metastases are calcified and palpable, which facilitates their surgical removal. Fewer than four nodules, complete resection of all disease, and lack of penetration through the parietal pleura favor survival. Treatment failures and late recurrence are common, mandating careful follow-up. Available data support aggressive attempts at surgical resection, including the removal of many metastatic nodules and multiple resections.

Soft Tissue Sarcoma

Chemotherapy and radiation-resistant tumors (liposarcoma, leiomyosarcoma, synovial sarcoma, fibrosarcoma, neurogenic sarcoma, epithelioid sarcoma, alveolar soft-parts sarcoma) may benefit from resection when the primary tumor has been controlled (25). Rhabdomyosarcoma and Ewing's sarcoma are chemosensitive and radiation sensitive. Lung excision for metastatic disease is generally not helpful. Surgery may aid in diagnosis and may be beneficial in removing a large focus of residual disease.

Wilms' Tumor

There is little advantage to excision of lung metastases in Wilms' tumor. Whole-lung radiation and chemotherapy usually are required for treatment, and surgical removal offers no added benefit. Special cases may benefit from surgery, including extremely young patients (in whom radiation therapy causes the most lung injury) with few or solitary lesions. Surgery also be necessary for diagnostic purposes and to determine the effects of therapy.

Primary Lung Tumors

Reviews by Hartman and Shochat in 1983 and Hancock et al. in 1993 have catalogued fewer than 500 reported primary lung neoplasms in children (Table 96.1) (26,27).

Bronchial "Adenomas"

These tumors are the most common primary lung tumors in children. Despite of the name they carry, these tumors represent true malignancies. They are better described as low-grade adenocarcinomas of the lung. The incidence of metastasis is low. Histologically, there are three types: carcinoid (85%), mucoepidermoid (10%), and adenoid cystic carcinoma (5%). Bronchial adenomas most commonly arise in primary and secondary brochi. Presenting symptoms include cough, hemoptysis, airway obstruction, pneumonia, atelectasis, and reactive airway disease. The chest radiographs may show air trapping or pneumonia and atelectasis. The clinical presentation may be most suspicious for an airway foreign body. CT may demonstrate the lesion. Bronchoscopy is required for diagnosis. Distinguishing the friable granulation tissue of a chronically embedded foreign body from a bronchial adenoma may be difficult. Biopsy must be done with great care and with some peril because life-threatening bleeding may result from biopsy attempts. Surgical resection with clean intraoperative margins is the treatment of choice and may involve lobectomy, bilobectomy, pneumonectomy, or sleeve resection as well as regional lymphadenectomy. Bronchial carcinoids are radiosensitive if residual disease remains.

Bronchogenic Carcinomas

These tumors are uncommon in children and highly lethal, with a mortality rate of 90%. Unlike in adults, squamous cell carcinoma is rare in children; undifferentiated and adenocarcinoma predominate. Disease is usually widespread at the time of diagnosis, compromising survival. Rarely, with early discovery and localized disease, cure is possible. Bronchioloalveolar carcinoma is a rare lung tumor in children that carries a good prognosis with surgical resection (28). This tumor is particularly associated with development in congenital cystic lung lesions (29).

Pulmonary Blastoma

A malignant lung tumor occurring most often in adults, but occasionally in children, pulmonary blastoma is composed of cells that histologically resemble fetal lung. Usually, they are peripherally located in the lung and present with cough, chest pain, and hemoptysis. They are treated by lobectomy; about half of the patients are long-term survivors.

Other Malignant Tumors

Sarcomas, including fibrosarcoma, rhabdomyosarcoma, and leiomyosarcoma are the next most common malignant lung neoplasms found in children. They arise endobronchially as well as peripherally. It is noteworthy that 9% of all reported malignant lung neoplasms in children were associated with previously documented cystic lung disease (27).

Inflammatory Pseudotumor

The most common "benign" lung tumor in children is inflammatory pseudotumor. Variable nomenclature relates to the description of the inflammatory cells involved. The terms *plasma cell granuloma, histiocytoma, xanthofibroma, fibroxanthoma,* and *inflammatory myofibroblastic tumor* have been used to describe these tumors. They may present as peripheral lesions or as obstructing endobronchial masses. Symptoms include cough, chest pain, hemoptysis, fever, and airway obstruction (Fig. 96.8). Although there may be some tendency for spontaneous resolution, aggressive local invasion and recurrence are often seen. It may be more accurate to describe these lesions as low-grade malignancies (30). Complete surgical resection, even if extensive, should be undertaken because no adjuvant therapies have proven efficacy.

Hamartoma

Hamartomatous lung nodules usually are discovered in adults, but they may be large enough or calcified to be discovered on chest radiographs in children (31). These tumors may be endobronchial and result in airway obstruction or, more commonly, peripheral and asymptomatic unless extremely large. Conservative pulmonary resection is the best treatment, but large lesions may require lobectomy or even pneumonectomy.

Table 96.1. **PRIMARY PULMONARY NEOPLASMS IN CHILDREN**

Type of tumor	No. (%)[a]
BENIGN (N = 92)	
Inflammatory	48 (52.2)
Hamartoma	22 (23.9)
Neurogenic tumor	9 (9.8)
Leiomyoma	6 (6.5)
Mucous gland adenoma	3 (3.3)
Myoblastoma	3 (3.3)
Benign teratoma	1 (1.1)
MALIGNANT (N = 291)	
Bronchial "adenoma"	118 (40.5)
Bronchogenic	49 (16.8)
Pulmonary blastoma	45 (15.5)
Fibrosarcoma	28 (9.6)
Rhabdomyosarcoma	17 (5.8)
Leiomyosarcoma	11 (3.8)
Sarcoma	6 (2.1)
Hemangiopericytoma	4 (1.4)
Plasmacytoma	4 (1.4)
Lymphoma	3 (1.0)
Teratoma	3 (1.0)
Mesenchymoma	2 (0.7)
Myxosarcoma	1 (0.3)

[a]Percent of benign or percent of malignant tumors.
Modified from Hancock BJ, DiLorenzo M, Youssef S, et al. Childhood primary pulmonary neoplasms. J Pediatr Surg 1993;28:1133–1136, with permission.

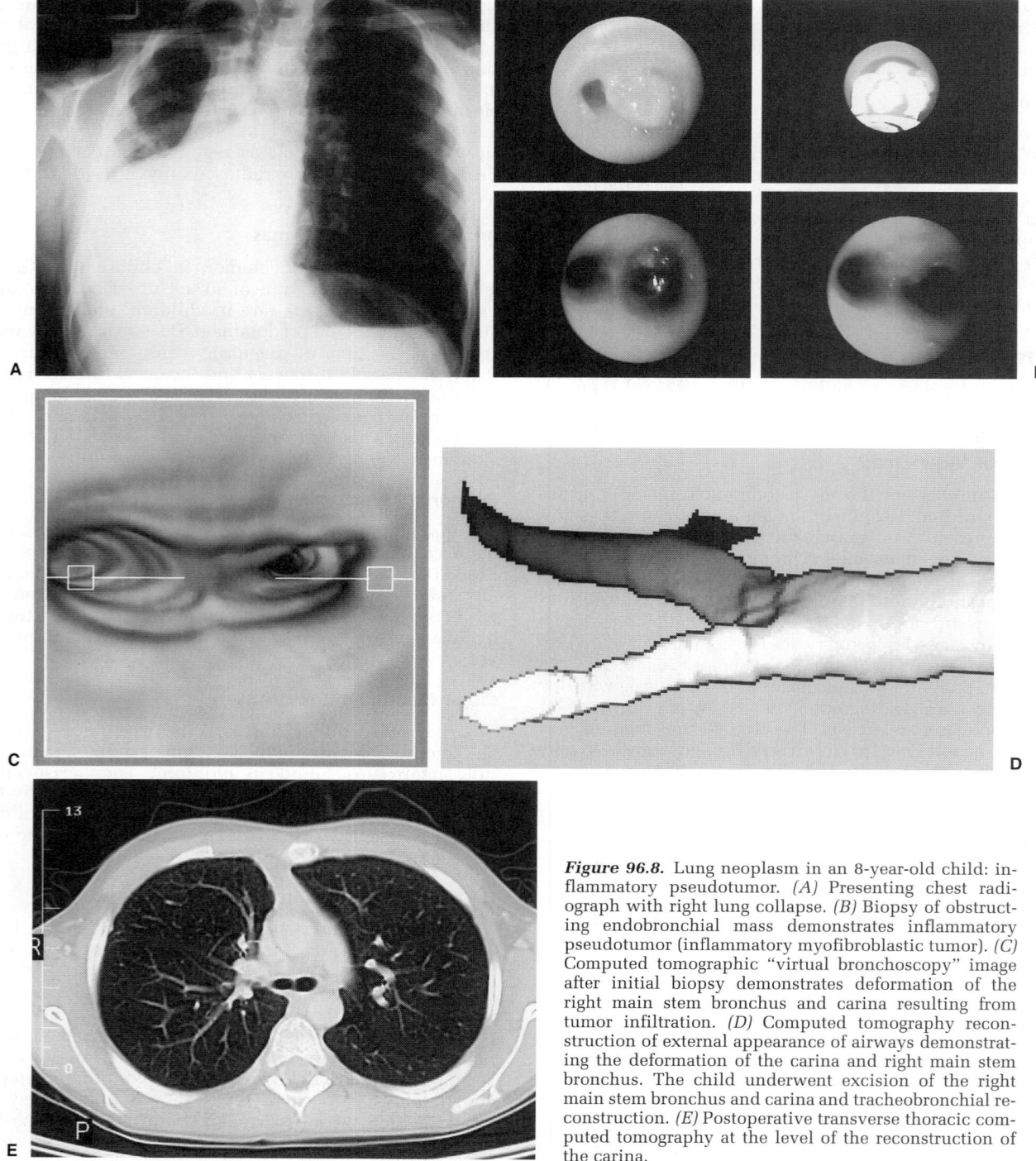

Figure 96.8. Lung neoplasm in an 8-year-old child: inflammatory pseudotumor. *(A)* Presenting chest radiograph with right lung collapse. *(B)* Biopsy of obstructing endobronchial mass demonstrates inflammatory pseudotumor (inflammatory myofibroblastic tumor). *(C)* Computed tomographic "virtual bronchoscopy" image after initial biopsy demonstrates deformation of the right main stem bronchus and carina resulting from tumor infiltration. *(D)* Computed tomography reconstruction of external appearance of airways demonstrating the deformation of the carina and right main stem bronchus. The child underwent excision of the right main stem bronchus and carina and tracheobronchial reconstruction. *(E)* Postoperative transverse thoracic computed tomography at the level of the reconstruction of the carina.

Mediastinal Tumors

Mediastinal tumors in children may be benign or malignant. Certain tumors have a predilection for arising from the anterior, middle, or posterior mediastinum (32).

Neurogenic Tumors

The most common thoracic tumors in the pediatric population are neurogenic tumors (Fig. 96.9), which originate in the posterior mediastinum, often from elements of the sympathetic chain. They may grow quite large before detection and may be found incidentally. Symptoms of Horner's syndrome or tracheal displacement may be ap-

parent. Occasionally, intraspinal extension results in symptoms of spinal cord compression. These tumors may be malignant (neuroblastoma, ganglioneuroblastoma) or benign (ganglioneuroma). Neuroblastoma originating in the mediastinum has a better prognosis than in other sites. The tumors are lower stage and often have more favorable biologic activity. CT and MRI scanning provide anatomic definition of the mass and assess intraspinal extension. There is often widening of the intercostal spaces and enlargement of the spinal foramina at the level of origin of the tumor. The tumors are bulky and encapsulated. All require removal for diagnosis. We continue to use traditional muscle-sparing incisions to remove these tumors when

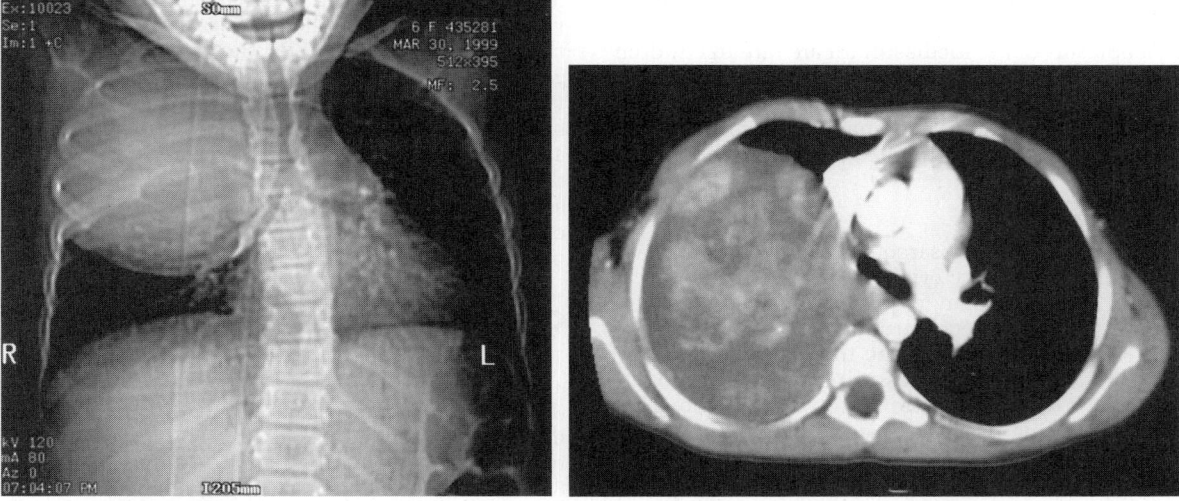

Figure 96.9. *(A)* Large neural tumor (ganglioneuroma arising from right sympathetic chain). *(B)* Calcification is apparent on computed tomography.

they are large, as they often are at diagnosis. Smaller tumors are removed thoracoscopically.

Neurofibromas

Neurofibromas arise from nerves in the posterior mediastinum, such as the intercostal nerves, the phrenic nerve, the vagus nerve, or the sympathetic chain. They may occur as isolated tumors or in association with neurofibromatosis. Scoliosis is particularly common in patients with thoracic neurofibromas as a result of the deformation and widening of the intercostal spaces and vertebral foramina. Isolated tumors are readily removed; however, tumors associated with neurofibromatosis tend to extend along nerve sheaths so as to preclude complete removal. Recurrence is to be expected in neurofibromatosis, and malignant degeneration can occur in large tumors, mandating periodic monitoring.

Hodgkin's and Non-Hodgkin's Lymphoma

These lymphomas may comprise an anterior or middle mediastinal mass. Surgical removal is not required, but the pediatric surgeon often participates in the diagnostic work-

up (33). Tissue sampling from cervical lymph nodes, mediastinoscopy, thoracoscopy, or open biopsy may be needed for diagnosis. Special anesthetic risks, including difficulty with ventilation and loss of airway, exist in the case of bulky central tumors that compress the large airways.

Teratomas

Teratomas arise in the anterior mediastinum and may contain elements of all three embryonic germ layers. The lesions are either solid or cystic. The most common form of a cystic teratoma consists of mature ectodermal elements known as a *dermoid cyst*. This lesion is characterized by a thick-walled fibrous sac with squamous epithelium in which various skin appendages, including hair and teeth, can be found. Occasionally, they are found within the pericardium. Surgical removal is generally straightforward, although the tumors may be large (Fig. 96.10). Surgical removal of these cysts is indicated because of the risk of infection, erosion into the pleura or pericardium, and local compression. The rare occurrence of malignant components within the tumor mandates their

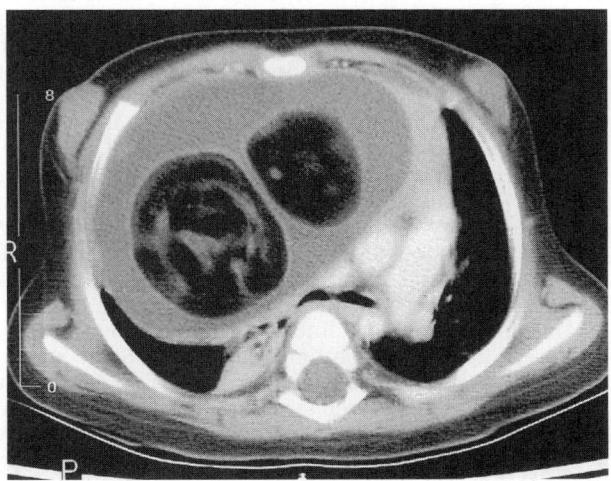
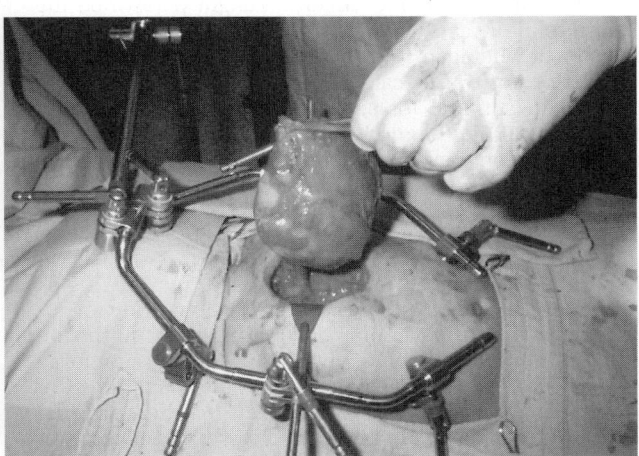

Figure 96.10. Mediastinal teratoma *(A)* Transverse thoracic computed tomography of a large anterior mediastinal teratoma presenting with airway compression symptoms in a 9-month-old girl. *(B)* Tumor removal via a median sternotomy.

removal. Malignant teratomas may be unresectable due to the extent of disease.

Other neoplasms of the mediastinum are rare in children but often require surgical biopsy or extirpation. These include neurolemoma, pheochromocytoma, primitive neuroectodermal tumors, germ cell tumors, mesenchymal tumors (including rhabdomyosarcoma), and thymic tumors.

Chest-wall Tumors

Ewing's sarcoma, chondrosarcoma, and liposarcoma are malignant tumors that may originate from the chest wall. Local control of disease may require extensive chest-wall excision and prosthetic reconstruction. Askin tumors are malignant small cell tumors of the thoracopulmonary region. They are also referred to as primitive neuroectodermal tumors (PNET). In the thorax, they involve the chest wall and surrounding tissues and carry a poor prognosis. Multimodal therapy with surgery, chemotherapy, and radiation may be of benefit (34,35).

Respiratory Papillomatosis

Recurrent respiratory papillomatosis is a viral-induced disorder caused by the same human papilloma virus that causes genital condylomata (36). It is likely transmitted at birth, and there may be some protective prophylactic benefit from cesarean section in selected high-risk expectant mothers. Airway-obstructing papillomas develop in the first several years of life and are treated with laser ablation. Often, many sessions are required to clear the airways. In severe and recalcitrant cases, interferon may be beneficial. Children who develop symptoms before the age of 3 years are more likely to have severe disease (37).

ESOPHAGEAL ATRESIA/ TRACHEOESOPHAGEAL FISTUAL

Developmental disorders of the esophagus have been recognized and described in postmortem examination since the seventeenth century. Harald Hirschsprung, the Danish pediatrician remembered for the disease that carries his name, also described the most common form of esophageal atresia in 1861. Initial attempts at both corrective and palliative surgery in the early part of the twentieth century were unsuccessful; however, the anatomy and physiology of the disorder were understood by surgeons such that continued bold attempts at surgical correction resulted in successful palliation and ultimately in successful primary repair of the defect. On March 15, 1941, Cameron Haight performed the first successful primary repair of an esophageal atresia at the University of Michigan (38). Refinements in surgical technique and postoperative care have resulted in a steady improvement in survival for such patients over the ensuing five decades (39). In the modern era, survival is determined almost exclusively by the presence of associate anomalies, not by the esophageal abnormality itself.

Embryology

Development of the human respiratory tract begins as primitive epithelial cells branch off of the ventral foregut of the embryo into the surrounding mesenchyme at the beginning of the fourth week of gestation. There are ongoing processes that involve both elongation and separation of the foregut (esophagus) and the airway (trachea). By the end of the fourth week of gestation, the esophagus and trachea have completely separated to the level of the larynx. This developmental program is under the control of master regulatory genes that are turned on and off in an orderly fashion. Interruption of this developmental process during the fourth week of gestation probably results in the various forms of esophageal atresia with or without tracheoesophageal fistula. By the end of the sixth week of gestation, the circular muscular coat of the esophagus develops, followed by vagal innervation. The segmental blood supply from the aorta appears by the seventh week and the muscular coat has differentiated into two layers by the ninth week. The malformation can be recapitulated in an animal model by the administration of doxorubicin hydrochloride (Adriamycin) at specific times and doses to pregnant rats during organogenesis (40,41).

Classification

Currently, descriptive terminology is used to indicate the anatomic configuration of a patient with esophageal atresia (Fig. 96.11). Esophageal atresia with proximal pouch and distal tracheoesophageal fistula is by far the most common type encountered by the pediatric surgeon, accounting for 85% to 95% of all cases. Esophageal atresia without fistula *(pure atresia)* occurs in 5% to 7% of patients. Tracheoesophageal fistula without esophageal atresia (so-called H-type or N-type fistula) occurs is 2% to 6% of patients. The rarer forms of this anomaly include esophageal atresia with proximal tracheoesophageal fistula and esophageal atresia with both proximal and distal tracheoesophageal fistula. The frequency of these rare forms is less than 1% in most reports. Alphabetic and numeric classification schemes, devised by Haight, Gross, and Kluth, are of historical interest (42–44). The most common variety (proximal pouch, distal fistula) is still commonly referred to as *Gross type C.*

Incidence and Epidemiology

The incidence of esophageal atresia varies among populations and races in the range of 1 in 2,500 to 1 in 20,000 births. The overall incidence is about 1 in 5,000. There is a slight male preponderance of 1.26:1. First pregnancy, advanced maternal age, hormonal exposure in pregnancy, an affected parent, and affected siblings are risk factors. Chromosomal abnormalities, twinning, and associated anomalies are more common than expected.

Clinical Findings, Diagnosis, Pathophysiology

The diagnosis of esophageal atresia may be suspected by the finding of maternal polyhydramnios. Specific ultrasonic identification of the blind-ending upper pouch may sometimes be diagnostic, but many patients go undiagnosed until after birth. Most infants are initially asymptomatic in the first hours of life. Excessive drooling may be noted. Choking, coughing, and regurgitation may be present and worsened by attempts at feeding. Respiratory distress and cyanosis aspiration may occur as a result of aspiration. Occasionally, in the breast-fed infant, the diagnosis may be unrecognized for more than a day as the volume of feeding associated with colostrum ingestion before milk flow may be quite low. The inability to pass a nasogastric or orogastric tube is confirmatory of the diagnosis. Radiographs confirm the position of the tube in the proximal blind-ending pouch. Injection of air during the radiograph outlines the pouch. Some surgeons will use a small amount of contrast material to delineate the upper pouch and to search for a proximal fistula. The child with esophageal atresia and a tracheoesophageal fistula will have a full abdomen and gas visible throughout the bowel on the abdominal radiograph. A scaphoid abdomen and gasless radiograph indicate pure esophageal atresia with no fistula. Isolated tracheoesophageal fistula without esophageal atresia does not result in esophageal obstruction and there-

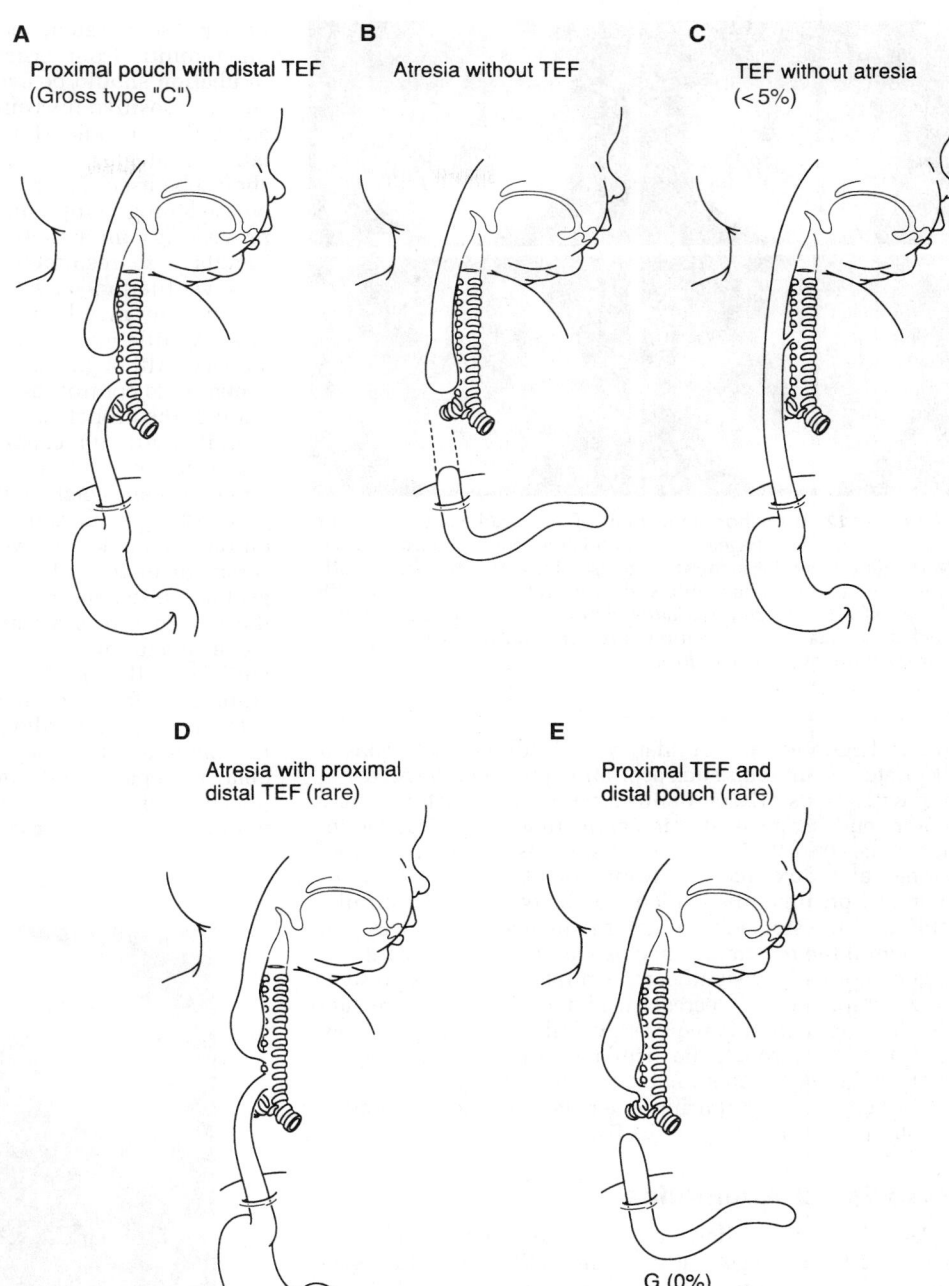

A Proximal pouch with distal TEF
(Gross type "C")

B Atresia without TEF

C TEF without atresia
(<5%)

D Atresia with proximal
distal TEF (rare)

E Proximal TEF and
distal pouch (rare)

G (0%)
|
B (0%)

Figure 96.11. The anatomy of the variants of esophageal atresia *(EA)* and tracheoesophageal fistula *(TEF)*. *(A)* Proximal pouch with distal TEF (most common type occurring in 85% of patients; Gross type C). *(B)* Esophageal atresia without TEF (5%). *(C)* TEF without esophageal atresia (<5%). *(D)* Esophageal atresia with proximal and distal TEF (rare). *(E)* Proximal TEF and distal pouch (rare). (After Manning PB, Morgan RA, Coran AG, et al. Fifty years' experience with esophageal atresia and tracheoesophageal fistula. *Ann Surg* 1988;204:446, with permission.)

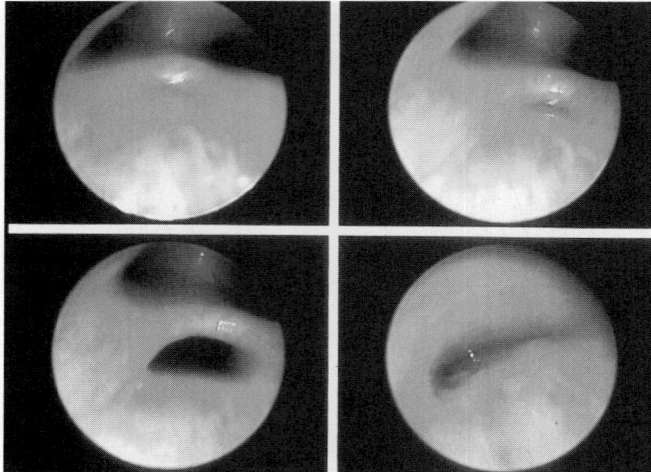

Figure 96.12. Bronchoscopic view of the trachea in a patient with common esophageal atresia and tracheoesophageal fistula. Note that during the inspiratory phase of positive-pressure ventilation, the fistula opens widely, demonstrating the "face" of TEF *(lower left)*. The more proximal view in the trachea demonstrates tracheomalacia with coaptation of the anterior trachea and posterior membranous trachea *(lower right).*

fore is diagnosed later in infancy or childhood as a result of respiratory symptoms such aspiration pneumonia and choking with feeds. Exact delineation of the anatomy may require endoscopic evaluation at the time of surgical correction (Fig. 96.12). If a distal fistula is present, gastroesophageal reflux into the respiratory tract will result in chemical pneumonitis, which may be worsened by air distention of the stomach through the fistula. This is less of a problem if the respiratory tract is mature and the infant can breathe normally. If significant respiratory failure is present, lung compliance is decreased, and positive-pressure mechanical ventilation is required, ventilating gases may flow preferentially through the fistula into the gastrointestinal tract. Progressive abdominal distention may preclude adequate ventilation, requiring emergency decompression of the stomach and control of the fistula.

Associated Anomalies

Associated anomalies are present in about half of newborns with esophageal atresia, indicating that other systems are affected by the early organogenic insult that disturbs the development of the trachea and esophagus. The most common associated anomalies are cardiovascular defects. Genitourinary, gastrointestinal, skeletal, neurologic, and craniofacial defects are found with increased frequency in patients with esophageal atresia as well. The particular occurrence of vertebral anomalies, anorectal malformations, cardiac, tracheoesophageal, and renal and radial limb defects is known as the *VACTERL association.* Two or more of these defects may be present. It is important to assess each child who has an anorectal malformation for esophageal atresia as well.

Preoperative Treatment

Treatment must be initiated as soon as the diagnosis is made to avoid the consequences of the infant's abnormal anatomy. Attempts at feeding are stopped, and intravenous fluids and antibiotics are started. Further aspiration is minimized by placement of a sump catheter in the upper esophageal pouch. The infant is positioned either

upright "semiseated," or head-up prone to avoid chemical pneumonitis from gastroesophageal reflux. Endotracheal intubation should be avoided unless absolutely necessary because positive-pressure ventilation may result in preferential flow of ventilatory gasses through the fistula. Ventilation strategies that avoid filling the stomach with gas should be used if respiratory failure is associated with decreased lung compliance. Early use of surfactant to improve lung compliance should be considered in premature infants with respiratory failure. High-frequency oscillatory ventilation may be useful. Bedside decompressive gastrostomy may be needed if gastric distention compromises ventilation or a prolonged interval is planned before surgery. Although rarely necessary, the surgeon must be prepared to control the fistula by emergency operative ligation or the bronchoscopic placement of an occluding balloon if ventilation cannot be maintained.

The goal of modern operative treatment is to correct the anomaly completely with a single operation avoiding a gastrostomy if possible. Immediate surgery is rarely required, and a day or two may be used to complete the assessment of the infant, including the echocardiographic evaluation to determine the position of the aortic arch and the presence of structural heart disease. Respiratory hygiene, positioning, and antibiotics may improve the infant's overall condition, resulting in more complete transition from fetal circulation.

High-risk infants who cannot safely undergo surgical correction of their esophageal abnormality may be treated with delayed repair. A decompressive gastrostomy, proximal pouch suctioning, and parenteral nutrition are used until the infant is ready for operation. Severe respiratory failure

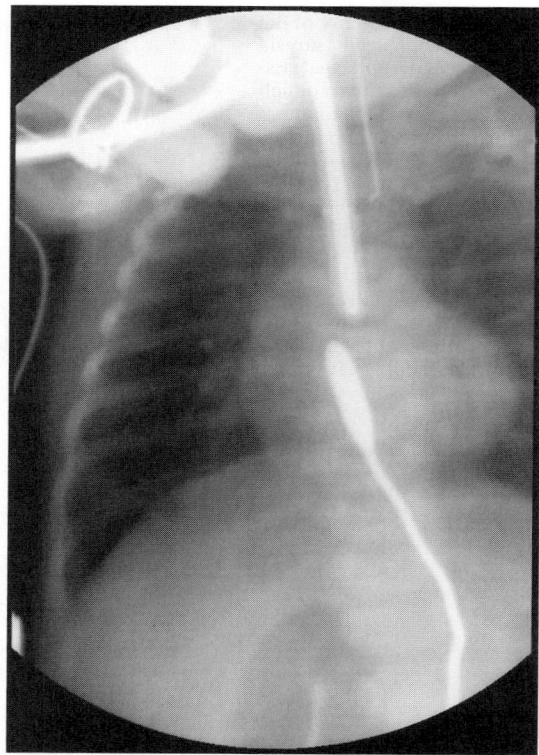

Figure 96.13. Patient with pure esophageal atresia treated initially with feeding gastrostomy and proximal pouch stretching. This "gap-o-gram" demonstrates close approximation of a dilator in the proximal pouch and a probe placed in the distal esophagus via the gastrostomy. The child subsequently underwent primary repair of the esophagus.

(usually from prematurity) and structural heart disease are the most common reasons to delay esophageal surgery. A staged repair using gastrostomy, surgical division of the tracheoesophageal fistula, followed by esophageal anastamosis as a second thoracic operation is rarely used today.

In the case of pure esophageal atresia without fistula, a prolonged period of delay before the repair is done may be used to improve the likelihood of completing a primary repair of the esophagus. A feeding gastrostomy is performed initially, which may be technically challenging because microgastria is present with pure atresia. Intragastric feeding and somatic growth result in shortening of the interval between the upper pouch and lower esophageal segment over the course of several weeks. The upper pouch may be stretched by daily or twice daily passage of a blunt flexible bougie. Radiographic determination of the distance between the two esophageal ends guides the timing of operation (Fig. 96.13).

Waterson's classification (1962) stratified infants into good, moderate, and high-risk groups based on birth weight, pneumonia, and associated anomalies. Risk group was used to help determine the timing and staging of surgical correction and to compare the results at different centers. Low-birth-weight/prematurity has less of an impact on survival than in the past. Currently, the presence of major cardiac disease and chromosomal abnormalities is the most important predictor of survival (45–48).

Surgical Technique

In most patients, it is unnecessary to perform a gastrostomy at the time of repair. With typical anatomy (left aortic arch), the repair is performed by a right thoracotomy (Fig. 96.14). Although the approach may be either transpleural or extrapleural, the extrapleural approach is preferred by most pediatric surgeons. A standard posterolateral right thoracotomy may be used. There is no need to divide the latissimus or serratus muscles, and such a muscle-sparing approach may have long-term benefits (49). We currently use a more posterior approach through the ascultatory triangle, which affords excellent exposure with a small skin incision. The extrapleural plane is established at the fourth intercostal space and developed sufficiently to allow control of the fistula and adequate mobilization of the proximal pouch. The distal tracheoesophageal fistula is divided and closed. The proximal pouch is identified and mobilized to whatever extent is needed to bring the ends together for anastamosis. If a proximal fistula is present, it is closed.

Various lengthening techniques may be used when the gap between the esophageal ends is long. These techniques include circular myotomies, spiral myotomies, flap tubularization of the proximal pouch, and extensive mobilization of the proximal pouch through a supplementary cervical incision. Contrary to earlier teaching, the distal esophagus may be mobilized as well when there is a long distance between

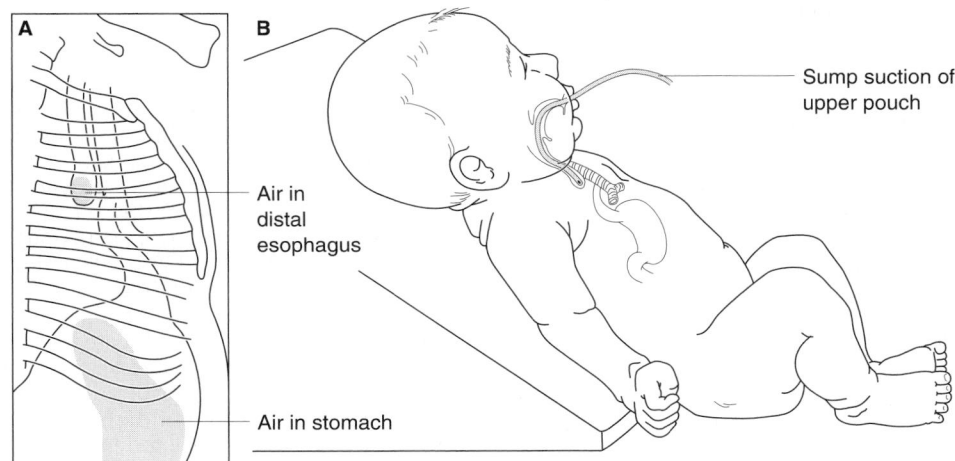

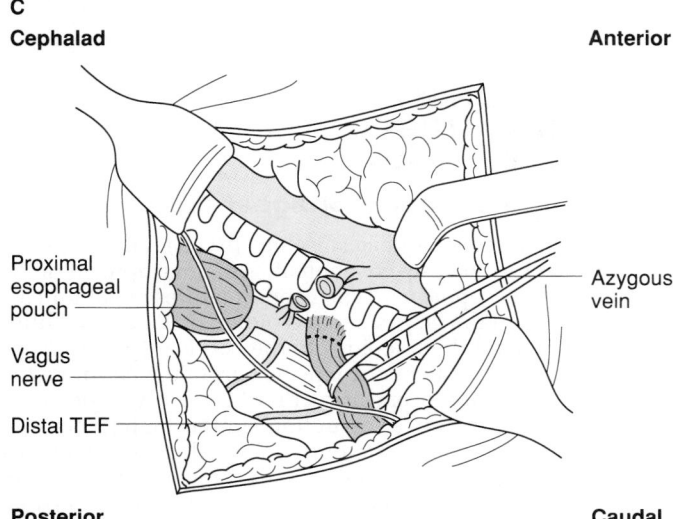

Figure 96.14. *(A)* Schematic illustration of esophageal atresia with distal tracheoesophageal fistula. *(B)* The initial management of this anomaly includes upright or prone-posture sump suction of the blind esophageal pouch. *(C)* The right extrapleural operative approach. After division and closure of the fistula, primary esophagoesophagostomy is performed. (After Coran AG. Congenital abnomalities of the esophagus. In: Zuidema GD, Orringer MD, eds. *Shackelford's surgery of the alimentary tract,* 2nd ed. Philadelphia: WB Saunders, 1990, with permission.)

the upper pouch and lower esophagus or in the case of pure esophageal atresia. Distal mobilization may extend to the stomach, which can be brought through the esophageal hiatus as necessary to provide length. An anastamosis may heal, even under some tension. One-layer, two-layer, and end-to-side repairs have been used. Most surgeons use a single-layer, end-to-end anastamosis with silk or absorbable suture material. The one-layer technique is associated with a lower rate of stricture formation but a higher leak rate, whereas the opposite is true for the two-layer technique.

In the worst cases of long gap atresia, pure atresia, or failed initial operative repairs, esophageal replacement may be performed at a later date using stomach, gastric tube, or colon (50–52). Such conditions are temporized with a cervical esophagostomy ("spit fistula") and gastrostomy.

Tracheoesophageal fistula without esophageal atresia is referred to as *H-type* atresia. The orientation of the fistula is such that the opening into the trachea is always proximal to the esophageal entry site. Repair usually is performed through a cervical approach after bronchoscopically stenting the fistula with a small catheter. The catheter aids in the precise identification of the fistula during dissection in the neck. Care must taken to stay in the plane of the esophagus to avoid injury to the recurrent laryngeal nerves.

Minimally invasive techniques using modifications of thoracoscopy may be used to treat esophageal atresia. Attempts already have been made, and at the time of this writing, there is one reported case of a successful repair in a patient with pure esophageal atresia (53). It is uncertain whether such techniques will have an added advantage in treatment of the disease. All attempts must be monitored closely and results compared to current practices, not simply to historic controls.

Results, Complications, and Outcomes

Technical mishaps during the procedure occur when the anatomy is misidentified or dissection is carried out improperly. Unplanned pleural entry, injury to the vagus nerves, recurrent laryngeal nerves, and posterior trachea are avoided.

Anastomotic leak is said to occur in 10% to 20% of patients. Most are of little immediate consequence and are recognized either by the appearance of saliva in the chest tube or at the time of a postoperative contrast swallow. The vast majority of such leaks will heal spontaneously. The presence of a leak prolongs hospitalization and increases the likelihood of stricture formation at the anastomotic site. When a leak is detected, the reteropleural chest tube is left in place, the infant is not fed by mouth, and antibiotics may be administered. Repeat contrast swallow in 7 to 10 days documents healing before the initiation of feeds.

Esophageal stricture at the site of the repair is found in as many as 40% of patients after repair. Anastomotic leak, excessive tension, ischemia, and gastroesophageal reflux contribute to stricture formation. Many strictures will respond to a few sessions of dilation. Dilations are performed in the operating room with endoscopic and fluoroscopic assistance, as necessary, to ensure the safe traverse of the narrowing by guide wires and dilators. More recalcitrant strictures may require many dilation sessions, steroid injection, and medical or surgical control of gastroesophageal reflux for resolution. Occasionally, reoperation, with resection of the stricture and reanastomosis of the esophagus, may be needed.

Recurrent tracheoesophageal fistula is reported to occur in up to 10% of patients. Recurrent fistulas may respond to endoscopic ablation or require operative division with interposition of pleura, muscle, or pericardium.

Gastroesophageal reflux is present in nearly all infants with esophageal atresia. It is symptomatic in many and may contribute to respiratory symptoms and stricture formation. Medical treatment consists of thickened feedings, upright positioning after feeds, frequent burping, small frequent feeds, acid reduction, and prokinetic agents. In many infants, medical treatments will be inadequate to control symptoms, and surgical control of reflux will be required.

Esophageal dysmotility is present to some degree in all patients with esophageal atresia. Dysmotility contributes to gastroesophageal reflux and may be responsible for dysphagia and recurrent respiratory problems.

Tracheomalacia may result in symptoms after the correction of esophageal atresia. The trachea is abnormal in patients with esophageal atresia both because of intrinsic structural abnormalities and because of the surgical dissection of the posterior trachea that is required to mobilize the proximal pouch. Bronchoscopically. the trachea appears oval rather than round. The anterior and posterior walls coapt during the respiratory cycle (Fig. 96.12). Fluoroscopic examination of the trachea demonstrates narrowing in the anterior-posterior dimensions during expiration. Tracheomalacia "fits" occur as the infant becomes agitated and develops worsening chest retractions with inspiration. The condition may deteriorate to complete inspiratory block and unconsciousness. When spontaneous respiration resumes in a quiet fashion, the "spell" is over.

Intubation and resuscitation may be required. The symptoms are completely relieved by endotracheal intubation. Infants with less severe symptoms may improve over time as the trachea grows. Severe symptoms require either tracheostomy or tracheal suspension. Tracheal suspension is accomplished with an aortopexy. In this procedure, the transverse aortic arch is sewn to the undersurface of the sternum. Bronchoscopic visualization of the trachea during the procedure demonstrates a more round, patent airway after the aortopexy.

Long-term results have improved in patients with esophageal atresia. Most children can look forward to survival with a normal existence (54,55). Overall survival rates are reported in the 85% to 95% range; however, some subsets of infants do not fare as well. The mortality rate is high for infants with severe congenital heart defects and chromosomal abnormalities. Late deaths related to respiratory disease (tracheomalacia, reactive airway disease, gastroesophageal reflux, aspiration) can occur (47). The long-term outcomes for children with repaired esophageal atresia are not known. Disordered peristalsis and chronic esophagitis may have long-term implications such that periodic endoscopic surveillance of the esophagus should be performed in selected patients (56).

OTHER CONGENITAL ABNORMALITIES OF THE TRACHEA AND ESOPHAGUS

Laryngotracheoesophageal Cleft

Laryngotracheoesophageal cleft (LTEC) abnormalities represent the most severe anomalies of development of the trachea and esophagus. Type I abnormalities communicate at the level of the larynx and cricoid. Type II abnormalities extend beyond the cricoid into the cervical trachea. Type III LTEC involves the entire trachea, from the larynx to the carina. The embryogenesis of LTEC is poorly understood but likely represents a disruption similar to, but more severe than, the more common esophageal atresia/tracheoesophageal fistula abnormality. Associated abnormalities of the cardiovascular, genitourinary, and gastrointestinal tract are common. In patients with type I and II defects, esophageal atresia and a distal tracheoesophageal fistula is present in about a third of cases.

Aerodigestive symptoms are present at birth, most commonly, respiratory distress with feeding. Hoarseness, stridor, cyanosis, and aspiration pneumonia may be present. Contrast swallow may delineate rapid confluence of contrast material in the upper esophagus and trachea, but it may be difficult to distinguish LTEC from laryngeal penetration due to spillover of contrast into a normal larynx. The diagnosis is made definitively by rigid bronchoscopy. Even under direct visualization, the cleft may be missed if the posterior larynx is not specifically manipulated to detect the defect.

Type I clefts may be approached endoscopically or translaryngeally. Type II clefts require cervical exposure, either laterally or by dividing the larynx and trachea in the midline. This anterior midline laryngofissure approach provides excellent exposure and avoids injury to the recurrent laryngeal nerves. Type III clefts extending to the carina or beyond require direct exposure through a right extrapleural thoracotomy as well as cervical exposure. The trachea and esophagus are separated longitudinally in such a way as to leave a remnant of the esophagus with the trachea to be used in reconstructing the posterior membranous portion of the trachea. The esophagus then is tubularized. A multilayered repair of the larynx is completed through the cervical exposure. Breakdown of the repair and prolonged need for tracheostomy are common. Oromotor dysfunction and chronic aspiration are long-term problems. Most children will require a gastrostomy for feedings. Gastroesophageal reflux is common and may require surgical control.

Congenital Esophageal Stenosis

Although acquired peptic strictures of the esophagus are relatively common and may occur early in life, true congenital stenosis is uncommon. As with other developmental abnormalities of the esophagus, it may be associated with craniofacial, cardiac, genitourinary, and other gastrointestinal anomalies. The stenotic areas may be (a) a membranous, weblike diaphragm; (b) fibromuscular thickening characterized by submucosal proliferation of smooth-muscle cells and connective tissue; or (c) due to sequestration of respiratory tract remnants in the form of respiratory epithelium and cartilage. The cartilage remnants may form a complete nondistensible ring in the esophagus.

Symptoms of progressive dysphagia are often present from infancy but may become apparent when solid foods are introduced. The diagnosis is confirmed at the time of esophagoscopy. Stenoses are treated initially with dilations as necessary. This is most likely to be successful for the diaphragm or web. Esophageal stenosis due to respiratory tract remnants is more likely to require segmental resection of the involved area.

Esophageal Duplication

Esophageal duplications are among the many aerodigestive malformations that present as thoracic masses. They are found in the posterior mediastinum and are covered by a muscular wall that is in continuity with the muscular wall of the esophagus. The epithelial lining is usually intestinal, often gastric mucosa, and usually will not communicate with the esophagus. These cysts also may have a respiratory epithelium lining, underscoring the relatedness of the various bronchopulmonary foregut malformations. Neurenteric cysts will communicate with the spinal canal. Masses are discovered incidentally or as a result of compression of adjacent organs. Occasionally, acid–peptic ulceration from gastric mucosa within the cyst will result in symptoms such as pain, bleeding, or erosion into adjacent structures (e.g., lung parenchyma, bronchus, esophagus). Excision is usually recommended. The cystic structures are dissected from the adjacent esophagus. Traditionally, this has been performed by thoracotomy, but more recently, thoracoscopic techniques have been used (Fig. 96.15).

Vascular Rings

Vascular rings result from faulty embryogenesis of the aortic arch and great vessels. In these abnormalities, the esophagus and trachea are surrounded by vascular structures and dense connective tissue that results in symptoms of airway or esophageal obstruction. Symptoms include wheezing, noisy breathing, coughing, stridor, pneumonia, and dysphagia (often when solid foods are started). A barium swallow may be suggestive or diagnostic. CT and MRI are used to define the anatomic abnormality. Echocardiography is used to rule out structural heart disease.

The most common abnormality encountered is a double aortic arch resulting from the persistence of both the left and

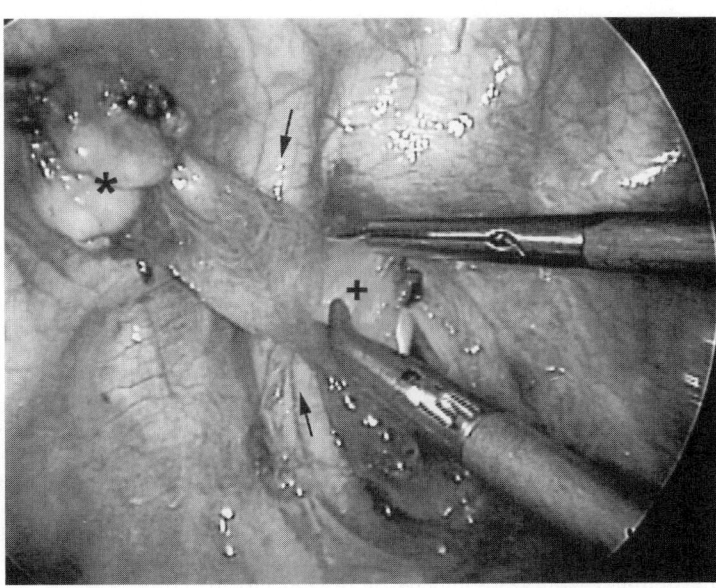

Figure 96.15. Thoracoscopic excision of an esophageal duplication cyst in a patient presenting with dysphagia. Video endoscopic view of the left superior hemithorax. (+) indicates site of original esophageal duplication cyst. Light from intraesophageal endoscope can be seen. *Arrows* demonstrate subclavian artery. The mass (*) is nearly excised.

the right embryologic aortic arches. The ascending aorta bifurcates, surrounding the trachea and esophagus, and then rejoins as the descending aorta. Other developmental abnormalities may result in complete or incomplete rings that compress the trachea or the esophagus. When the vascular ring is symptomatic, the patient should be treated surgically by appropriate division of the ring and the lysis of the fibrous bands that surround the trachea and esophagus.

Congenital Tracheal Stenosis

Failure of tracheal growth and development results in a wide variety of abnormalities. Short segments of the trachea may be narrowed, or the entire trachea may be hypoplastic. Often, complete tracheal cartilagenous rings are present. Short stenotic areas may respond to balloon dilation, which splits the complete tracheal rings. Segmental stenoses may be amenable to resection and anastomosis. Longer stenoses may be corrected with placement of a graft to widen the lumen of the trachea or by the slide tracheoplasty technique.

FOREIGN BODIES OF THE TRACHEOBRONCHIAL TREE

Foreign-body ingestion and aspiration occur commonly in the pediatric population (57). Endoscopic removal of foreign bodies that lodge in the esophagus is covered in Chapter 20. Any foreign body that could obstruct the airway represents a potentially life-threatening problem. The National Safety Council estimates that 200 deaths occur each year in persons under the age of 15 years as a result of suffocation by an ingested object (58). Three fourths of these deaths are of children under the age of 5 years, and in this group, this type of suffocation is the fourth leading cause of accidental death. Manipulation of the airway, visualization, and removal of foreign bodies has been facilitated by the development of specialized instrumentation. The Hopkins rod lens optical system with fiberoptic illumination, developed in the 1970s; the incorporation of the lens system into rigid pediatric bronchoscopes; and the development of specialized grasping devices resulted in a safe, reliable method for most foreign-body extractions.

Pathophysiology

Complete obstruction of the airway and asphyxiation can occur at the level of the laryngeal inlet, the subglottis, or the trachea. Back blows (recommended in infants), abdominal thrust, or the Heimlich maneuver may dislodge the obstruction and save a life. An inhaled foreign body that lodges at the bronchial level, as usually seen by the pediatric surgeon, can create a ball-valve phenomenon in the affected bronchus, allowing bidirectional but unequal airflow. The result is air trapping and hyperinflation in the affected lobe or lung, which leads to mediastinal shift to the opposite side. Complete blockage of the bronchus by the foreign body results in loss of volume in the affected lobe or lung. In this case, the resulting volume loss from atelectasis will shift the mediastinum to the ipsilateral side.

Clinical Presentation

Most affected children are younger than 4 years of age, with a peak incidence between the ages of 1 and 2 years; however, 20% of foreign-body aspirations occur in children over the age of 4 years. Foreign bodies have a small predilection for lodging in the right side of the tracheobronchial tree. Most will be found in the main-stem bronchus (58). The most commonly aspirated objects are peanuts, which are particularly troublesome because they are hygroscopic, and

thus become soft, tending to fracture readily and require piecemeal removal. Other types of food, such as carrots and popcorn, or inorganic material, such as pins, wood, paper, metallic and plastic parts, may be aspirated.

The aspiration event may have been witnessed or is suggested by a history of a coughing or choking spell. The known presence of a likely aspirated object and the abrupt onset of the symptoms are suggestive. The most common symptoms include cough, wheezing, dyspnea and fever; the most common signs are unilateral decreased breath sounds, unilateral wheezing, and rhonchi. A foreign body also may masquerade as pneumonia. Inspiratory and expiratory chest radiographs or bilateral decubitus views in the case of children too young to cooperate may demonstrate hyperinflation on the affected side due to air trapping. Although physical signs, symptoms, and radiographic findings are often present, a suggestive history alone is an adequate indication to proceed with bronchoscopy.

Management

When the history is sufficiently worrisome, or signs, symptoms and radiographic findings are suggestive, bronchoscopic evaluation and foreign body removal are recommended (Fig. 96.16). The procedure is considered urgent, although considerable time may have elapsed between the initial onset of symptoms and definitive care. The procedure should be performed in the operating room with the patient under general anesthesia for the best airway control and availability of equipment. The flexible bronchoscope may be useful for viewing the distal airways and may be helpful in certain circumstances; therefore, it should be available to the surgeon. The rigid bronchoscope with optical forceps can be used to remove most aspirated foreign bodies safely. The flexible grasper and Fogarty balloon catheter can be useful, especially when the foreign body has migrated distally. Fluoroscopic assistance has been used for radioopaque objects that have migrated into the peripheral airways. Occasionally, foreign-body aspiration that presents as chronic lung infection will require surgical resection of the destroyed portion of the lung.

CONGENITAL ABNORMALITIES OF THE DIAPHRAGM

Developmental defects of the diaphragm are of great interest to pediatric surgeons. Most require surgical correction. Congenital diaphragmatic hernia (CDH, Bochdalek's hernia) is associated with abnormal development and behavior of the lung that will result in pulmonary hypoplasia and pulmonary hypertension. Advances in the treatment of newborn respiratory failure, fetal surgery, and lung developmental biology have grown directly out of the clinical and laboratory investigation of CDH. These topics are fertile areas of clinical and basic science research for pediatric surgeons.

Bochdalek first described the defect in the posterolateral diaphragm in 1848. Traditionally, surgeons have considered CDH to be an anatomic derangement that was best served by an anatomic correction (i.e., a surgical solution to "get the bowel out of the chest" and "prevent further lung compression from the intestines"). During the last 20 years, the physiologic behavior of the lungs of the CDH infant have been understood to be the most important determinant of survival in the immediate postnatal period. The gas-exchange capabilities of the CDH lung as determined by the underlying degree of pulmonary hypoplasia and the characteristics of the pulmonary blood flow are responsible for the degree of respiratory failure. If the child is endotracheally and orogastrically intubated and subjected to posi-

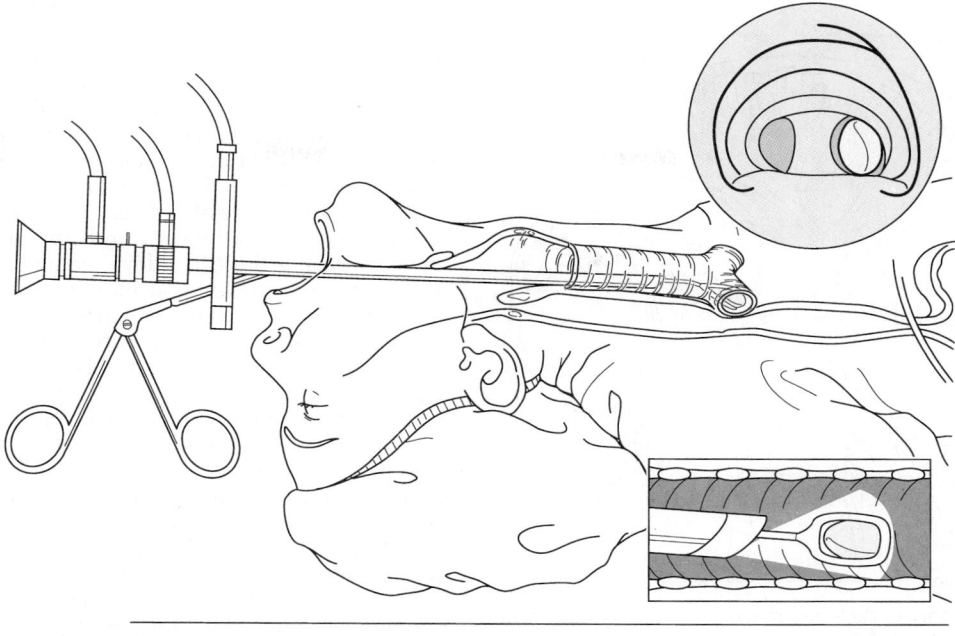

Figure 96.16. Schematic illustration of a foreign body (a peanut) being extracted from the right main stem bronchus under direct vision.

tive-pressure ventilation at low ventilator pressures from the time of birth, there is little consequence to the presence of the abdominal viscera in the chest. Surgery may be delayed almost indefinitely, if necessary. Pulmonary hypertension is treated aggressively by whatever means necessary, including high-frequency oscillatory ventilation, nitric oxide (NO), and extracorporeal membrane oxygenation (ECMO). In many cases, pulmonary hypertension will resolve and surgical repair may be performed without deterioration. Surgical repair is performed when labile pulmonary hypertension has resolved. A better understanding of the physiology of postnatal pulmonary hypertension and changes in the timing of surgery resulted in considerable improvement in the survival of infants with CDH. Better treatments for pulmonary hypertension and therapies aimed at augmenting the development of hypoplastic lungs no doubt will result in further improvements in the survival and long-term morbidity of CDH infants (59).

Embryology of the Lung and Diaphragm

Mammalian lung development occurs in vivo as a coordinated developmental process that includes (a) airway and acinar development, (b) cellular differentiation, (c) biochemical maturation, (d) interstitial development including vasculature and extracellular matrix, and (e) physical growth or enlargement. These parallel developmental processes occur in such a fashion that at any point in development characteristic relationships between components define the so-called stages of lung development (60–62). This developmental program is under the control of master regulatory genes that are turned on and off in an orderly fashion. The precise molecular mechanisms of morphogenetic signal transmission are unknown. In the human embryo, respiratory tract development begins in the fourth week of gestation as a ventral outpouching of the foregut, which soon has bifurcated and begun branching into the surrounding mesenchyme. The primitive, pluripotent epithelial cells differentiate into both bronchial and alveolar

cell lines under the control of the surrounding mesenchyme. By a process of asymmetric branching, the divisions are complete by the 16th week of gestation. The lungs at this phase have columnar epithelium with thick mesenchyme, giving rise to the descriptive term *pseudoglandular phase* of development because of its histologic appearance. The *canalicular phase* that follows and continues up to about the 24th gestational week is characterized by flattening of the epithelium of the distal airways, thinning of the mesenchyme, and growth of the capillary network that surrounds the terminal airways. Gas exchange becomes functionally possible at the end of this phase. The *terminal sac period* that follows refers to the appearance of a thin respiratory epithelium in apposition to a capillary network capable of supporting gas exchange. True alveolar formation in humans begins shortly before or around the time of birth.

Early in gestation, the level of the tracheal bifurcation is high in the cervical region. By the 12th week of development, it descends to the level of the first thoracic vertebrae and is at the level of the fourth or fifth thoracic vertebrae by the time of birth. All major bronchial buds are present before closure of the pleuroperitoneal canals. Until the third gestational month, the right lung grows faster than the left lung. As a result, the right lung remains larger than the left throughout life. Extensive alveolar maturation and multiplication takes place after birth and may continue up to 8 years of age.

The precursors of the diaphragm begin to form during the fourth week of gestation with the appearance of the peritoneal folds from lateral mesenchymal tissue. At the same time, the septum transversum forms from the inferior portion of the pericardial cavity and serves to delineate the thoracic from the abdominal cavities. Eventually, the septum transversum leads to the formation of the central tendon area of the fully developed diaphragm. The pleuroperitoneal folds extend from the lateral body wall and grow medially and ventrally until they fuse with the septum transversum and dorsal mesentery of the esophagus during the sixth gestational week. Complete closure of the canal takes place during the eighth week of gestation, the right side

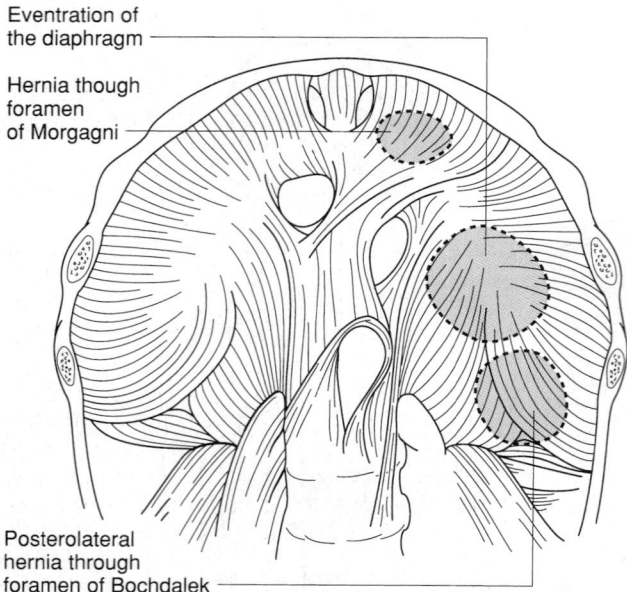

Eventration of
the diaphragm

Hernia though
foramen
of Morgagni

Posterolateral
hernia through
foramen of Bochdalek

Figure 96.17. Anatomy of the diaphragm showing the location of congenital diaphragmatic defects.

closing before the left (63). Muscularization of the diaphragm appears to develop from the innermost layer of thoracic mesoderm, although other mechanisms have been proposed (64). A contribution from cervically derived myoblasts is also present, as evidenced by the innervation of the diaphragm by the phrenic nerve originating from the third, fourth, and fifth cervical nerve roots. Posterolaterally, at the junction of the lumbar and costal muscle groups, the fibrous lumbocostal trigone remains as a small remnant of the pleuroperitoneal membrane and relies for its strength on the fusion of the two muscle groups in the final stages of development. It is in this area that the defect of congenital diaphragmatic hernia occurs (Fig. 96.17).

Congenital Diaphragmatic Hernia Pathology and Pathophysiology

The reported incidence of CDH is estimated to be between 1 in 2,000 to 1 in 5,000 births, making it one of the most common congenital abnormalities (65). About one third of the infants with CDH are stillborn, but these deaths are usually due to associated fatal congenital anomalies. The most common anomalies noted in the stillborn group are neural tube defects and included anencephaly, myelomeningocele, hydrocephalus, and encephaloceles. Cardiac defects are the second most common group and include ventriculoseptal defects, vascular rings, and coarctation of the aorta. Diaphragmatic defects are more common on the left side: About 80% are left-sided and 20% right-sided. Bilateral CDH defects are rare. CDH is thought to represent a sporadic developmental anomaly, although some familial cases have been reported. The expected recurrence risk in a first-degree relative has been estimated to be 1 in 45 (65).

The cause of CDH is unknown, but it is presumed that some combination of intrinsic predisposition (genetic factors) and environmental insult (teratogen or deficiency) results in abnormal diaphragm and lung development. Exposure to a number of pharmacologic agents has been implicated in its development, including certain drugs and insecticides, such as phenmetrazine, thalidomide, quinine, and nitrofen (65). Vitamin A deficiency also has been reported with CDH development. Diaphragmatic hernia and pulmonary hypoplasia can be created in animal models. In sheep, a surgically created diaphragm defect at the end of the second trimester resulted in the herniation of visceral contents into the chest and pathologic lung changes reminiscent of human CDH (66,67). In rodents, administration of Nitrofen (a thyromimetic toxic herbicide) early in gestation resulted in diaphragmatic defects and pulmonary hypoplasia that mimics the human condition (68,69).

Although the cause of CDH is uncertain, its consequences on pulmonary development and function are well documented. During the early development of the diaphragm, the midgut is largely extracoelomic. If closure of the pleuroperitoneal canal has not occurred by the time the midgut returns to the abdomen during the ninth and tenth weeks of gestation, the abdominal viscera herniate through the lumbocostal trigone into the ipsilateral thoracic cavity. The resulting abnormal position of the bowel prevents its normal counterclockwise rotation and fixation. No hernia sac is present if the event occurs before complete closure of the pleuroperitoneal canal, but a nonmuscularized membrane forms a hernia sac in 10% to 15% of CDH patients. Although there are fetal ultrasound data showing the herniation process progressing late in gestation or as an intermittent process, in most cases, the abnormal location of the viscera is established by the twelfth gestational week. In addition to small bowel, other intraabdominal organs, such as the spleen, stomach, colon, and liver, also may herniate through the diaphragmatic defect.

The most common left-sided CDH is characterized by a 2- to 4-cm posterolateral defect in the diaphragm through which the abdominal viscera have translocated into the ipsilateral thoracic cavity. For a right-sided defect, the large right lobe of the liver can occupy most of the hemithorax. The hepatic veins may drain ectopically into the right atrium and complicate surgical repair of the defect.

Animal models showed that long-term compression of the developing fetal lung will result in abnormal lung development (66,67). The subsequent degree of pulmonary hypoplasia determines the clinical presentation and ultimate long-term outcome of the process. Therefore, the pathophysiology of CDH has been attributed to pulmonary parenchymal compression by the herniated organs and its effect on growth and maturation of the lung. An emerging school of thought attributes the pulmonary hypoplasia to an early developmental insult to the lung and diaphragm (70). The lung and diaphragm develop abnormally because of this early insult. The presence of viscera in the hemithorax may hamper the later development of the lung, but this may not be the primary insult that results in hypoplasia. Unilateral diaphragmatic hernia is associated with both ipsilateral and contralateral abnormal pulmonary development, although hypoplasia is more severe on the ipsilateral side. The lung on the side of the hernia is much smaller than its normal counterpart (Fig. 96.18). The pulmonary vascular bed is also distinctly abnormal in lungs from patients with CDH. There is a reduction in the total number of arterial branches in both the ipsilateral and contralateral pulmonary parenchyma. In addition, the small preacinar and intraacinar arterioles feature inappropriate and significant medial muscular hyperplasia (Fig. 96.19). The physiologic consequence of this abnormal arteriolar muscularization may be an increased susceptibility to development of pulmonary hypertension.

Pulmonary blood flow accounts for only 7% of cardiac output during normal fetal development, and pulmonary vascular resistance remains high. The fetus preferentially shunts oxygenated blood from the placental through the foramen ovale and ductus arteriosus in a right-to-left direction into the systemic circulation. At birth, numerous hemodynamic changes take place that alter this circulatory profile. With the institution of breathing, pulmonary vascu-

may develop if this process is interrupted. Elevated pulmonary vascular resistance results in increased pulmonary artery pressures and decreased pulmonary vascular blood flow. The increased vascular resistance results in the development of right-to-left shunting of blood at either the atrial or ductal levels with the delivery of unsaturated blood into the systemic circulation. As the blood flow in the shunt increases, the oxygen saturation in the systemic circulation falls, and the mixed venous return to the right side of the heart becomes progressively desaturated. The resulting hypoxia further increases pulmonary vascular resistance and compromises pulmonary blood flow while increasing the right-to-left shunt flow.

Factors that contribute to the persistence of high pulmonary vascular resistance in CDH lungs are thought to be the structural changes of decreased total arteriolar cross-sectional area in the involved lungs and the increased muscularization of the arterial structures that are present. Additional exacerbations of pulmonary vascular resistance may be induced by the known stimulators of pulmonary hypertension, including hypoxia, acidosis, hypothermia, and stress. Alternations in the levels of prostaglandins, leukotrienes, catecholamines, and the renin angiotensin system had been implicated as mediators of this complex process.

Diagnosis

The diagnosis of CDH is often made on a prenatal ultrasound examination and is accurate in 40% to 90% of cases. Ultrasound may be obtained for routine obstetric care or because of the presence of polyhydramnios. Polyhydramnios occurs in as many as 80% of pregnancies with associated CDH. The mechanism of polyhydramnios is thought to be due to kinking of the gastroesophageal junction by herniation of the stomach into the thorax with resultant foregut obstruction.

After birth, the spectrum of respiratory symptoms in an infant with CDH is determined by the degree of pulmonary hypoplasia and reactive pulmonary hypertension. Severely affected infants develop respiratory distress at birth, and most demonstrate respiratory symptoms within the first 24 hours of life. On physical examination, these infants have a scaphoid abdomen and an asymmetrically shaped funnel chest. The chest may become more distended as swallowed air passes into the

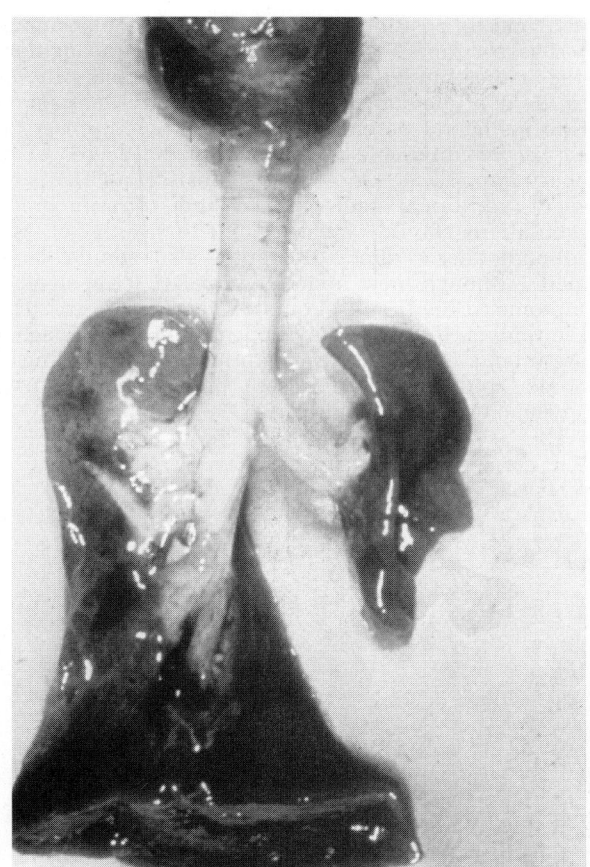

Figure 96.18. Autopsy specimen of an infant with severe pulmonary hypoplasia secondary to congenital diaphragmatic hernia. Pulmonary hypoplasia is bilateral, but the left lung is most severely affected.

lar resistance falls, permitting an increase in pulmonary blood flow. Systemic vascular resistance rises, as does left atrial pressure that forces the foramen ovale to close. Increased arterial oxygen tension then induces spontaneous closure of the ductus arteriosus. Persistent fetal circulation

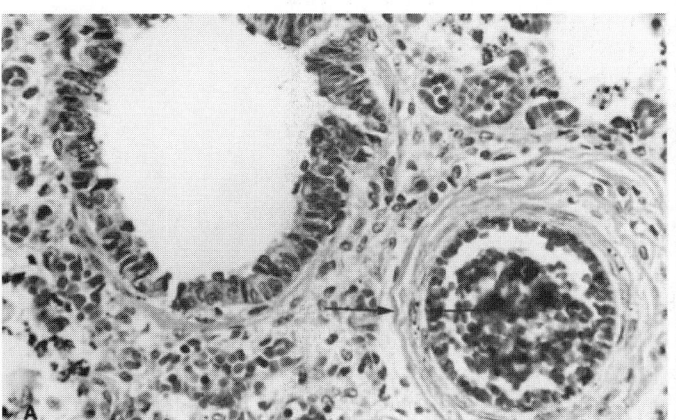
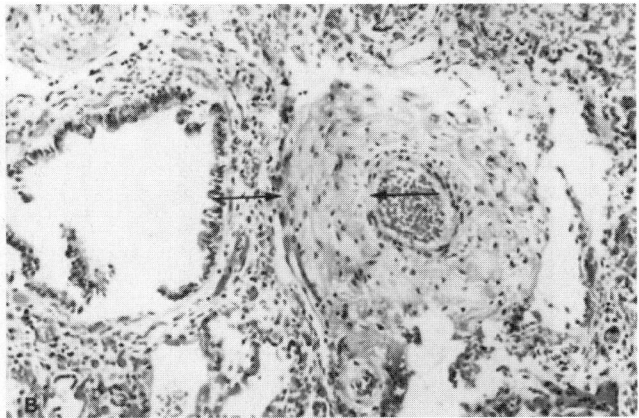

Figure 96.19. Histology of pulmonary arteries. Pulmonary artery branches of similar size and location are shown in a normal infant *(A)* and in an infant with Bochdalek's diaphragmatic hernia. *(B)* There is increased muscle mass associated with the arterial wall in B *(arrows)*. This vascular smooth muscle is exquisitely sensitive to chemical, hormonal, and paracrine mediators in the neonatal period. Pulmonary arterial vasospasm is an important cause of persistent fetal circulation and respiratory failure. Treatment of pulmonary hypertension is the primary objective in the immediate care of the newborn with congenital diaphragmatic hernia.

stomach and intestines. The air-filled intestine may contribute to the acute respiratory distress because of increased pulmonary compression as well as mediastinal shift into the contralateral thorax. Because of the small size of the neonate's chest, breath sounds may or may not be present on the side of the defect. Mediastinal compression with shift into the contralateral thorax may cause deviation of the trachea away from the side of the hernia and also can result in obstruction of venous return with the hemodynamic consequences of hypotension and inadequate peripheral perfusion. The signs of respiratory distress include cyanosis, gasping, sternal retractions, and poor respiratory effort.

A plain chest radiograph that demonstrates loops of intestines in the chest (Fig. 96.20) confirms the diagnosis of a CDH. The location of the gastric bubble also should be noted, and its position can be confirmed by placement of a nasogastric tube. The chest radiograph shows angulation of the mediastinum and a shifting of the cardiac silhouette into the contralateral thorax. Although minimal aeration of the ipsilateral parenchyma may be noted, chest radiographs are unreliable for estimating the degree of pulmonary hypoplasia. Once the diagnosis of a CDH is confirmed, additional radiographic and ultrasonographic examinations should be carried out to search for associated anomalies. Echocardiography also should be obtained. Although most infants with CDH show signs and symptoms in the first 24 hours of life, in 10% to 20% of these infants, the signs may appear later. Initial signs in these infants may be recurrent mild respiratory illnesses, chronic pulmonary disease, pneumonia, effusion, empyema, or gastric volvulus.

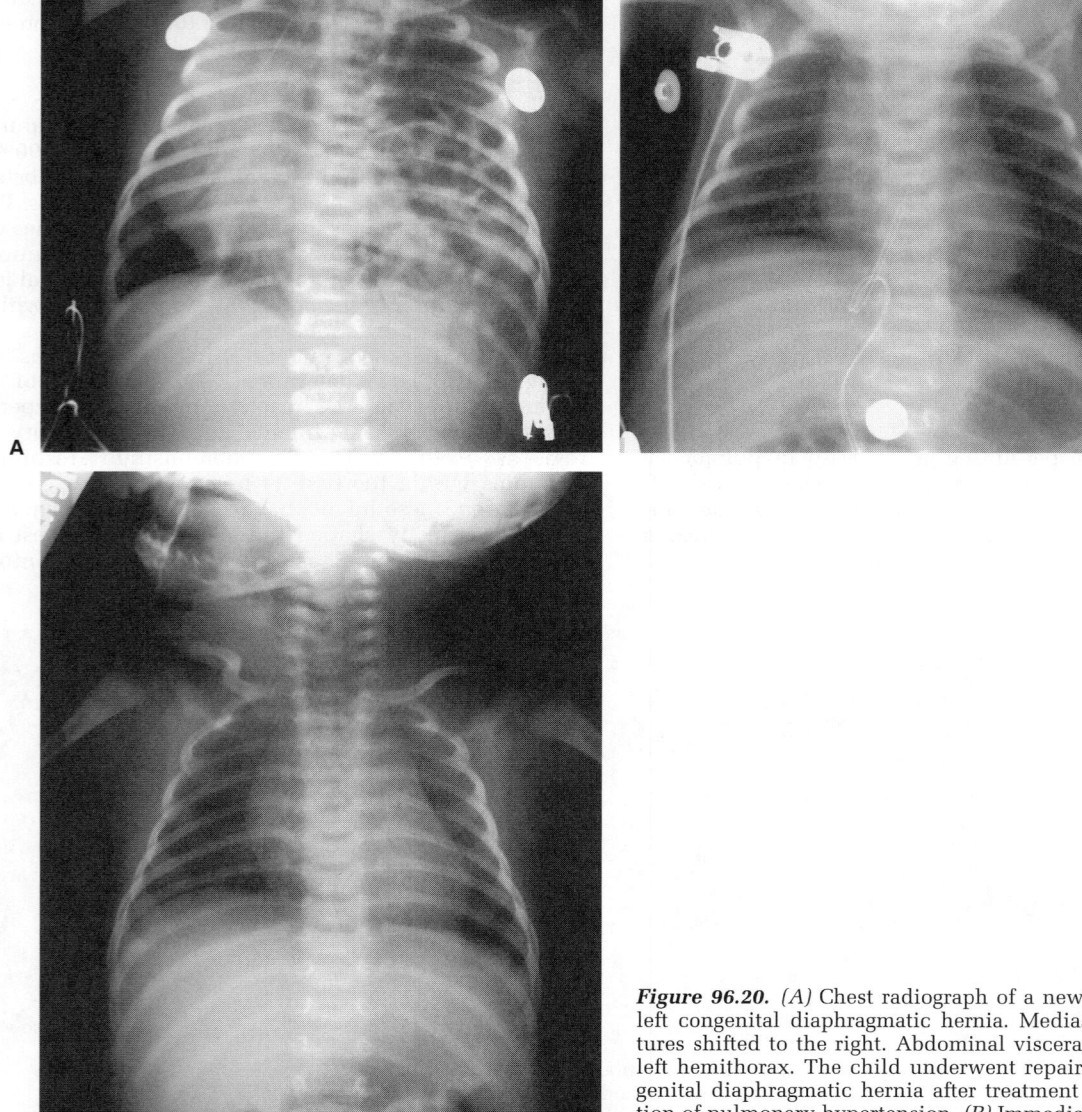

Figure 96.20. *(A)* Chest radiograph of a newborn with a left congenital diaphragmatic hernia. Mediastinal structures shifted to the right. Abdominal viscera occupy the left hemithorax. The child underwent repair of the congenital diaphragmatic hernia after treatment and resolution of pulmonary hypertension. *(B)* Immediate postoperative photograph demonstrates return of mediastinal structures to a more normal position. The hypoplastic left lung is apparent. *(C)* Chest radiograph 1 month later is unremarkable.

The diagnosis of a CDH can be confused with a number of other congenital thoracic conditions, including eventration of the diaphragm, anterior diaphragmatic hernia of Morgagni, congenital cystic disease of the pulmonary parenchyma, unilateral pulmonary effusion, and primary agenesis of the lung (71).

Prognostic Factors

Many attempts have been made to define the clinically relevant prognostic factors to predict the outcome of infants with CDH, but these have been often complex and for the most part unsuccessful. The sonographic ratio of lung to head size or the presence of the fetal liver within the thorax may be useful in predicting the most severely affected infants (72). Obstetric factors such as the time of antenatal diagnosis of a CDH or the presence of polyhydramnios have proven unreliable in predicting the outcome for infants with diaphragmatic hernia. Anatomic factors such as the position of the stomach either above or below the diaphragmatic rim and the size of the diaphragmatic defect itself are also unreliable in predicting outcome. Physiologic parameters have been difficult to define and are limited to variations on arterial blood gas analyses.

Treatment

Historically, CDH was considered a surgical emergency. Infants were rushed to the operating room as soon as possible after birth in the hope that reduction of the abdominal contents from the chest would relieve the compression of the lungs. Now, however, it is understood that an infant with a CDH and respiratory failure has a physiologic emergency rather than a surgical emergency. Once the infant has been endotracheally intubated, the gastrointestinal tract has been decompressed, and positive-pressure mechanical ventilation is established, there is no longer a benefit to immediate surgery. The herniated viscera will not compromise the expansion of the lung because the lung remains inflated with pressures greater than those in the viscera. Furthermore, the defect in the diaphragm does not compromise the mechanics of breathing when positive-pressure mechanical ventilation is used. The respiratory failure associated with a CDH in newborn infants results from a combination of pulmonary hypoplasia and potentially reversible pulmonary hypertension. Initial clinical efforts should be directed at maximizing medical treatment of the pulmonary hypertension.

Resuscitation should begin with endotracheal intubation and nasogastric tube insertion. Bag-mask ventilation is contraindicated to avoid distention of the stomach and intestines that may be in the thoracic cavity. Arterial and venous access should be acquired through the umbilicus. Although the umbilical artery is excellent for monitoring systemic blood pressure and obtaining postductal arterial blood gas specimens, additional information can be obtained by monitoring arterial oxygen saturation in a preductal position, usually with a right radial arterial line or a transcutaneous oxygen saturation probe. As in any neonatal resuscitation, meticulous attention must be directed to maintaining proper temperature regulation, glucose homeostasis, and volume status in the neonate. Systemic hypotension and inadequate tissue perfusion may be reversed with intravenous fluid administration, including crystalloid, blood products, and colloid. Inotropic drugs such as dopamine or dobutamine may be required. Contralateral pneumothorax is always a risk in view of the high airway pressures often required for ventilation during the first hours of life.

Most infants can be successfully treated with a simple pressure cycled ventilator with the goal of ventilatory support being a preductal P_aO_2 greater than 60 (S_aO_2 90%–100%) with a corresponding P_aCO_2 less than 60 (73). The extremes of hyperventilation, particularly with high rates and high ventilatory pressures, should be avoided to prevent ventilator induced lung injury. If conventional mechanical ventilatory techniques cannot reverse the hypoxemia or hypercarbia, high-frequency techniques using either the jet ventilator or the oscillating ventilator may be required.

A broad spectrum of drugs and antihypertensive agents have been used in attempts to modify the pulmonary vascular resistance in infants with CDH and respiratory failure. Tolazoline, which exerts its effects through alpha-receptor blockade, has been the most effective at lowering pulmonary vascular resistance in this setting. Major side effects of this drug include systemic hypotension and tachyphalaxis. Other drugs such as nitroprusside, isoproteranol, nitroglycerin, and captopril have not been effective. The administration of various prostaglandin derivatives remains experimental. Clinical and experimental studies have demonstrated surfactant deficiencies in infants with CDH. Its efficacy in infants with CDH requires further study. NO is a potent mediator of vasodilatation and is particularly well suited for administration to the pulmonary vasculature using inhalation techniques. It has been effective in improving oxygen saturation levels in neonates with respiratory failure that resulted from prematurity and persistent pulmonary hypertension of the newborn. Unfortunately, its effects in CDH infants with respiratory failure have been mixed. The preacinar vessels with excessive medial muscularization may be less able to respond to inhaled NO in patients with CDH. Patients who do not respond to conventional treatments, high-frequency oscillatory ventilation and NO are considered for ECMO treatment (see later discussion of ECMO).

Surgery

Delayed surgical repair has resulted in improved survival rates for CDH infants compared with historical controls (73). The optimal timing of surgery when using such a strategy remains unproven (74). Prolonged preoperative stabilization may allow the diameter of the pulmonary vessels to increase and at the same time decrease their sensitivity to the stimuli causing vasoconstriction.

Most surgeons approach the defect through a subcostal incision, although the repair can be performed through a thoracotomy incision (Fig. 96.21). Once the abdominal contents are reduced, the defect in the diaphragm in the posterolateral position can be examined. In 20% of patients, a hernia sac formed by parietal pleura and peritoneum is present and must be excised. Usually, there is an anterior rim of diaphragm of varying size; the posterior rim must be exposed in the retroperitoneal tissue. When diaphragmatic tissue is adequate, a primary repair with nonabsorbable suture material can be performed. In cases where the defect is too large to be closed in a primary fashion, numerous reconstructive techniques have been tried using nearby prerenal fascia, rib structures, and abdominal wall muscle flaps. The use of prosthetic material to complete the diaphragmatic closure has gained widespread acceptance. A tension-free diaphragmatic repair can be accomplished that may lessen the degree of intraabdominal pressure when closing the abdominal wall. The major drawback to using a prosthetic patch closure is the risk of infection as well as the risk of dislodgment and subsequent reherniation.

With the loss of intraabdominal domain, abdominal wall closure may not be possible. In this situation, simple closure of the skin can be accomplished with repair of the ventral wall defect some months later. Drainage of the chest cavity on the repaired side with a tube thoracostomy

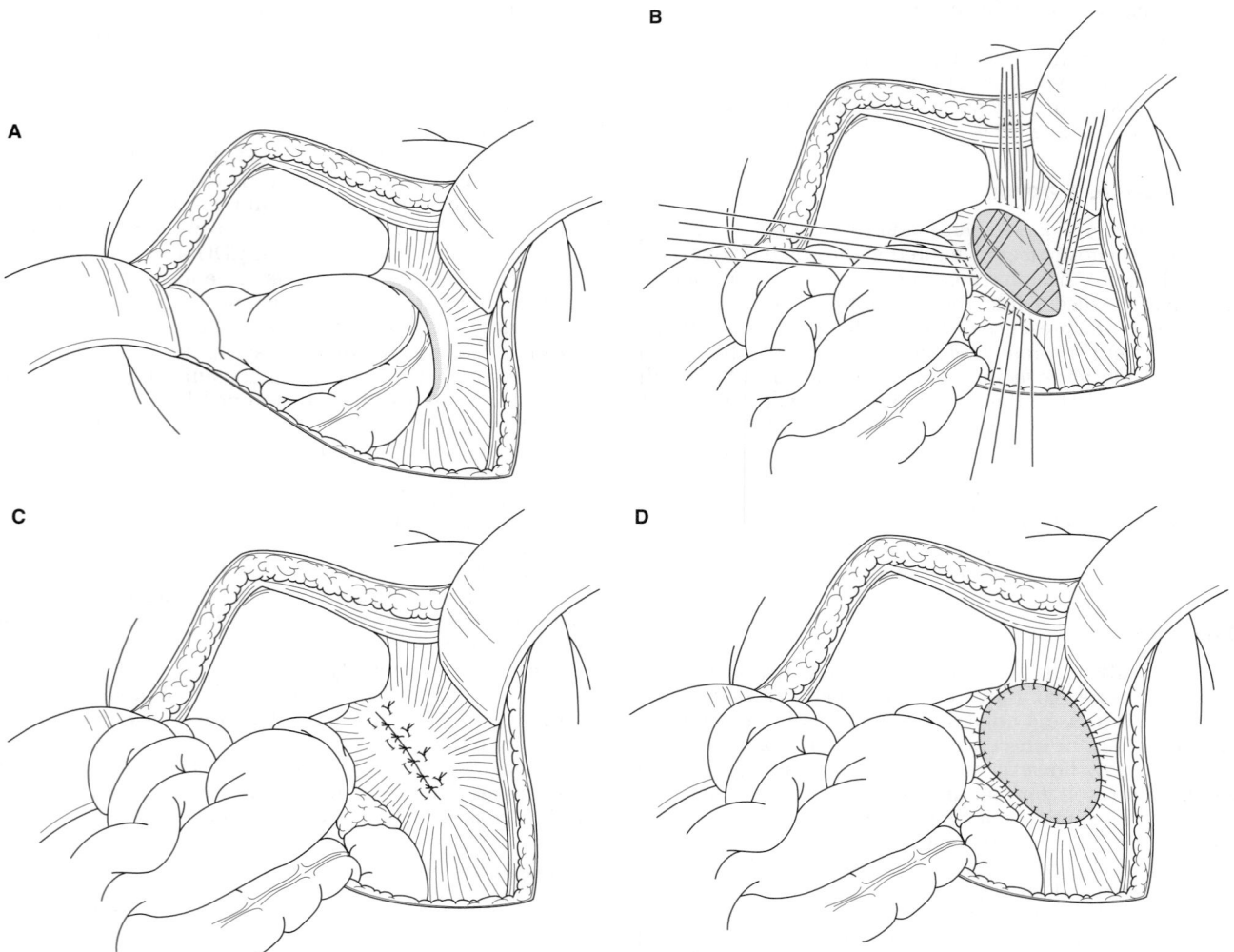

Figure 96.21. Repair of congenital diaphragmatic hernia. *(A)* Operative appearance of congenital diaphragmatic hernia. *(B)* Placement of sutures for repair of typical left posterolateral diaphragmatic defect. *(C)* Completed repair. *(D)* Prosthetic material may be used for large defects to avoid tension. (From Stollar CJH. Congenital diaphragmatic hernia. In: Spitz L, Coran AG, eds. *Rob and Smith's operative surgery: pediatric surgery,* 5th ed. London: Chapman and Hall, 1995:159–163, with permission.)

is not always indicated except for active bleeding or uncontrolled air leak.

Postoperative management should continue the goals established before surgery. Meticulous attention to fluid status must be maintained, particularly in the immediate postoperative period. If respiratory decompensation develops, therapeutic interventions, including NO, high-frequency ventilation, and ECMO may be used. Weaning from ventilator support should be slow and deliberate as tolerated by the infant.

Extracorporeal Membrane Oxygenation

When ventilatory therapy has failed, ECMO, a form of partial cardiopulmonary bypass, can be used with the goal of maintaining oxygen delivery to the body for an extended period. It has become a cornerstone for managing infants with life-threatening respiratory failure with CDH (75). ECMO allows respiratory support without the risks of barotrauma and oxygen toxicity associated with conventional ventilation. Since the introduction of ECMO as a treatment strategy, improved survival rates have been re-

ported (76). ECMO may be used both preoperatively and postoperatively. The need for its postoperative use is decreased when delayed surgical approaches are used.

Outcome

The overall survival rate for neonates with CDH ranges from 39% to 95%, with a mean survival rate of 69% (77). Institutional variation in survival rates is quite high and represents differences in management strategies and patient accrual. Future studies must determine the reasons for these widely varying outcomes and consolidate the various treatment strategies into a best-practice plan.

Long-term studies showed that many surviving infants will have normal pulmonary function measurements, including total lung capacity, vital capacity, and carbon monoxide diffusing capacity. In the last decade, as survival rates have improved, a new group of survivors is emerging with different patterns of long-term morbidities (78). Long-term problems that have been identified with increasing frequency include chronic lung disease, neurologic abnormalities with developmental delay, skeletal deformities, and nutritional and growth-related problems.

Evolving Therapies

Despite the advancements that have been made in treating infants with CDH, this condition remains a frustrating and difficult clinical problem. As a result, intense interest has been focused on new avenues of experimental treatments.

In Utero Repair of Diaphragmatic Hernia

The concept of fetal surgical intervention evolved from the experimental observation in lambs that reduction of compressive forces on the lung resulted in continued pulmonary growth and development. Open fetal surgical repair of diaphragmatic hernia has been undertaken (79). Although technically and theoretically exciting, the clinical results have been disappointing (80,81). A direct advancement of these initial attempts at in utero repair was the observation that fetal tracheal ligation accelerated fetal lung growth and reversed pulmonary hypoplasia (82,83). Tracheal occlusion or "PLUG" therapy (plug the lung until it grows) resulted in improved oxygenation and ventilation after birth compared with untreated control animals (84). This technique is still being evaluated.

Liquid Ventilation

Liquid ventilation using perfluorocarbons has now advanced to the point of clinical applicability (85). Partial liquid ventilation was attempted in a small number of CDH infants on ECMO. Improvements in oxygenation levels and pulmonary function tests were noted. A prospective, controlled study is required to examine this newest form of ventilation before its clinical efficacy can be judged.

Pulmonary Transplantation

Successful neonatal lung transplantation for CDH has been achieved, but there is no long-term experience at this time to recommend this form of treatment. Neonatal single-lung or segmental pulmonary transplantation is feasible.

Pharmacology

Numerous new experimental avenues have been explored in the pharmacologic manipulation of pulmonary vascular tone and parenchymal growth and development (65). Long-term continuous intravenous therapy with epoprostenol has been used in patients with primary pulmonary hypertension. Its use in CDH infants with intractable pulmonary hypertension has not been studied as yet. Oral pulmonary vasodilators such as the calcium channel blockers nifedipine and diltiazem have been reported in a limited number of CDH infants; success has been mixed. Experimental work has investigated the potential role of augmentation of pulmonary growth and development, particularly with antenatal hormonal therapy. The combined administration of thyrotropin-releasing hormone and glucocorticoid therapy has been demonstrated to have positive effects on lung growth (86). In the future, the selective administration of one or several pharmacologic agents or growth factors may be able to reverse the pulmonary hypoplasia and intractable pulmonary hypertension of CDH.

Foramen of Morgagni Hernia

The anterior diaphragmatic hernia of Morgagni is located anteromedially on either side of the junction of the septum transversum and the thoracic wall. Typically, a sac is present, and herniation of the colon, small bowel, or liver usually is discovered to the right or left of the midline. Morgagni hernias account for fewer than 2% of diaphragmatic defects and usually are noted in older children or adults. The hernia often is discovered incidentally as a mass or air—fluid level on chest radiograph. Because of the risk of segmental intestinal volvulus or obstruction, surgical repair of the defect is recommended. Operative correction can be performed easily through an upper transverse abdominal incision or laparoscopically. The diaphragm is sutured to the undersurface of the posterior rectus sheath at the costal margin.

Eventration of the Diaphragm

Eventration of the diaphragm may be either congenital or acquired. The congenital form may be indistinguishable from a diaphragmatic hernia with a sac, and symptoms are usually similar. The acquired form occurs as a result of paralysis of the phrenic nerve, which is vulnerable to surgical trauma from a wide variety of cervical, thoracic, and diaphragmatic procedures. Phrenic nerve injuries and a variety of neuromuscular disorders, including primary myopathies and degenerative diseases, may produce diaphragmatic paralysis and require operative plication of the diaphragm in infants and young children. The most common cause of phrenic nerve injury in children is associated with thoracic and mediastinal surgery. It has been postulated that birth injury to the nerve with cervical stretching is responsible for some of the congenital cases that have been reported. The diaphragmatic muscle is usually present in its normal distribution, but it is attenuated and nonfunctional.

An eventration may be completely asymptomatic and noted only on chest radiographs. On the other hand, clinical findings may range from mild respiratory compromise with wheezing, frequent respiratory infections, and exercise intolerance all the way to extreme respiratory distress. Diagnosis usually is made by fluoroscopic examination of the chest with examination of diaphragmatic motion. In such cases, the diaphragm moves paradoxically with respiration. The paradoxical movement may be significant enough to compromise gas exchange. A small or asymptomatic eventration may be left untreated and observed. An eventration that involves a large area of the diaphragm may adversely affect pulmonary function and lung growth and should be repaired. When an acquired nerve palsy is present, initial treatment may be expectant; however, if the respiratory status of the infant remains compromised after several weeks of observation, surgical intervention should be considered. Repair may be through either the abdomen or the chest, but in most cases a low thoracotomy is preferred (87). The approach now may be performed with minimally invasive techniques. The diaphragm is plicated with nonabsorbable sutures placed in a radial pattern. The redundant diaphragmatic tissue is reefed up until it is taut. Proper suture placement is important to prevent additional injury to the phrenic nerve branches within the diaphragmatic tissue.

PLEURAL DISEASES

Empyema

Empyema is an accumulation of purulent material within the pleural space. In children, empyema occurs most often as a sequellae of bacterial pneumonia. Parapneumonic effusions may appear in up to 40% of parenchymal infections. Empyema develops when a parapneumonic effusion becomes infected. Empyema also may develop after penetrating thoracic trauma, intrathoracic or cervical esophageal perforation, or surgery on the chest. Clinically, the presentation of an empyema is divided into three stages: (a) the *exudative stage,* marked by thin, free-flowing fluid with a low cellular count; (b) the *fibrinopurulent stage,* marked by thick purulent material resulting in multiple loculations and encasement of the lung parenchyma; (c) the *organizing stage,* when fibrobasts have grown into the exudate and produced a fibrotic peel. *Haemophilus influenza, Streptococcus pneumoniae,* and *Staphylococcus aureus* are the most common pathogens in pediatric pneumonia, with anaerobes, gram-negative bacteria, and atypical organisms also occasionally found. The

signs and symptoms of an empyema in a child are usually those of worsening pneumonia with fever, tachypnea, shortness of breath, and sometimes cyanosis. Abdominal pain with distention and ileus may intensify the respiratory difficulty. Breath sounds are decreased on the involved side, and there is dullness to percussion.

Diagnosis is confirmed by the presence of pleural fluid on conventional chest radiographs (Fig. 96.22A). Lateral decubitus views will show layering of this fluid along the

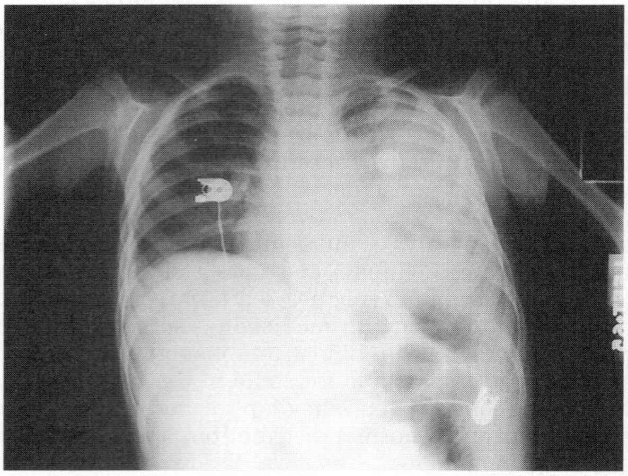

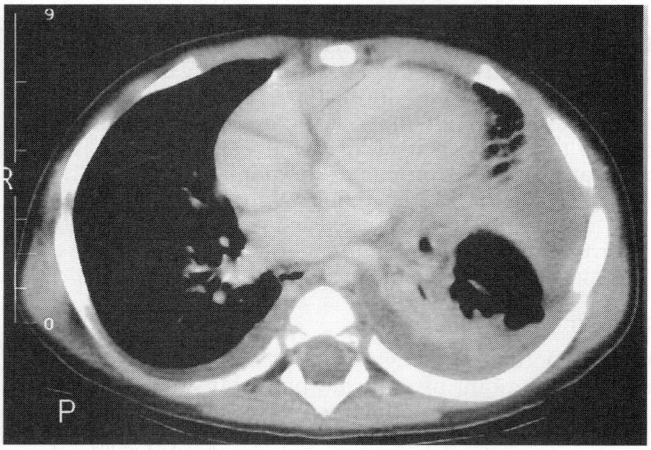

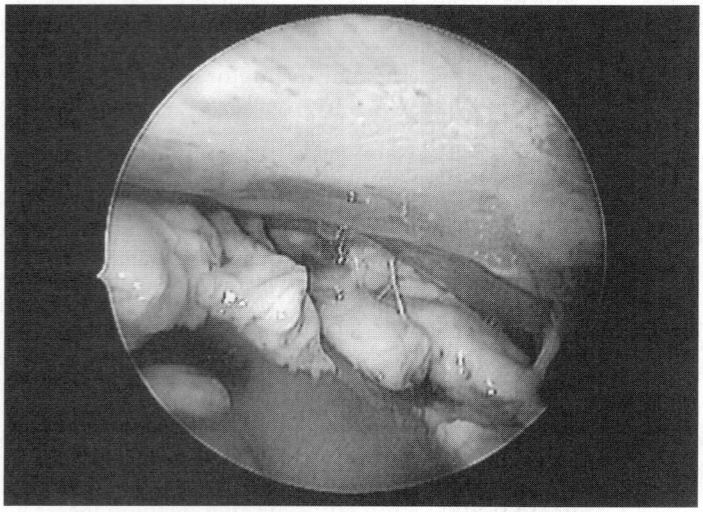

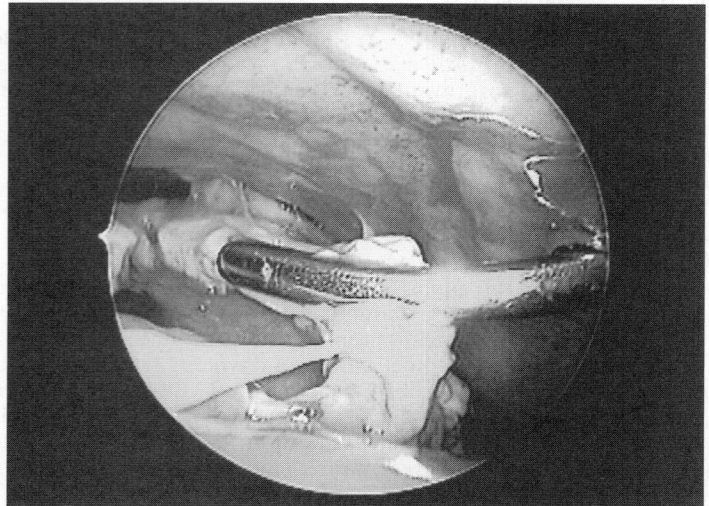

Figure 96.22. Video-assisted thoracoscopic treatment of complicated empyema in children. *(A)* Chest radiograph of a 2-year-old child with pneumonia and pleural effusion. *(B)* Computed tomography demonstrates complicated pneumonia with loculated empyema. *(C)* Video endoscopic view of organized empyema debris. *(D)* "Decortication" procedure includes removal of all loculated, organized debris from the hemithorax. All surfaces of the visceral and parietal pleura are accessible using videoendoscopic techniques. *(E)* Immediate postoperative chest radiograph shows the expected residual parenchymal lung disease. *(F)* One month later, the findings on the chest radiograph have resolved. *(continues)*

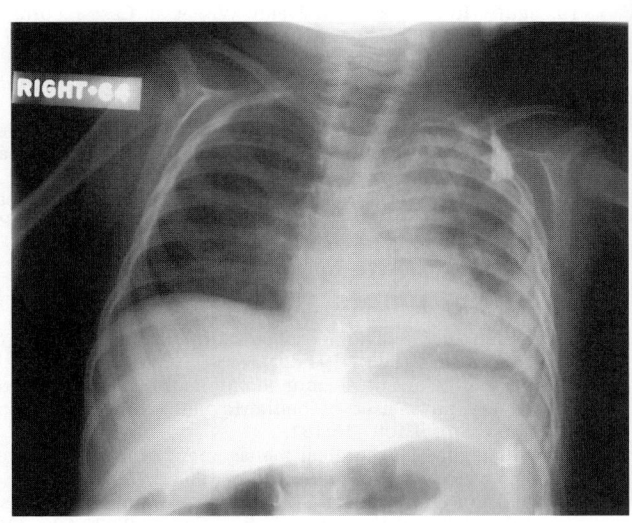
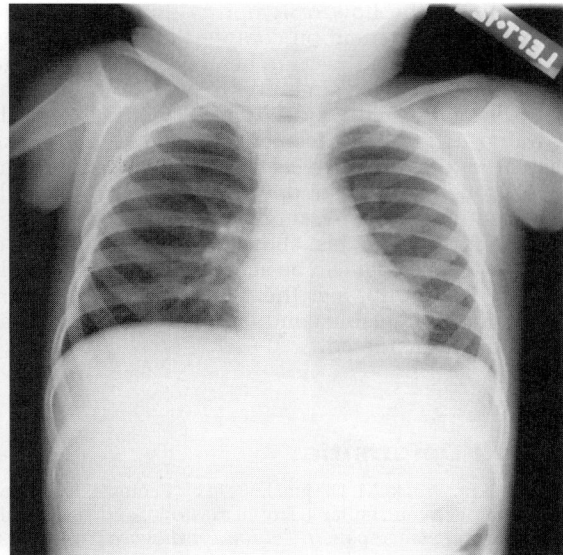

E   F

Figure 96.22. *(Continued)*

chest wall in its early stages. In the fibrinopurulent stage, lateral decubitus radiographs will show that the fluid does not layer out. Pneumatoceles may be identified within the pulmonary parenchyma as a result of the underlying infection. CT scan of the chest cavity is the best method of determining the extent of loculated effusion and underlying parenchymal involvement (Fig. 96.22B). Diagnostic paracentesis may be helpful. The fluid should be sent for Gram's stain, aerobic and anaerobic cultures, pH, glucose, lactate dehydrogenase levels, and cell count.

When a small parapneumonic effusion develops, it may resolve with antibiotics alone. Larger effusions will require adequate pleural space drainage with a tube thoracostomy in addition to antibiotic therapy. Instillation of intrapleural streptokinase or urokinase has been used for loculated effusions, but the failure rate may be as high as 50%.

In patients who do not respond to such therapy, surgical débridement of infected material surrounding the lung and decortication may be required. Video-assisted thoracoscopy decortication and pleural débridement have proven effective in the treatment of pediatric empyema (Fig. 96.22C,D). Early treatment with video-assisted thoracoscopic surgery (VATS) may shorten hospitalization and result in more rapid recovery.

Pneumothorax

Spontaneous pneumothorax is seen most commonly in older children and teenagers with advanced pulmonary disease resulting from cystic fibrosis. Other causes include both blunt and penetrating thoracic trauma, severe asthmatic attack, or pulmonary infection. The classic presentation of a spontaneous pneumothorax is the sudden onset of chest pain and shortness of breath.

Diagnosis is best confirmed by chest radiograph. In patients with significant symptoms, tube thoracostomy should be performed immediately and the chest tube placed to water seal suction drainage.

Recurrent pneumothoraces can be treated nonoperatively with the intrapleural instillation of various sclerosing agents such as talc or tetracycline through the chest tube. Surgical approaches include direct pleural abrasion,

pleurectomy, and pulmonary bleb resection through a standard thoracotomy or with VATS.

Chylothorax

The appearance of chylous fluid within the pleural space may be attributable to a number of different causes. In the newborn, chylothorax may occur in association with manipulation during a difficult delivery, from a malformation of the thoracic duct, or spontaneously without an obvious cause. In older infants and children, cardiothoracic procedures can be complicated by postoperative chylothorax in 0.5% of the cases. The duct also has been known to rupture during violent bouts of coughing or with hyperextension of the spine. Obstruction or erosion of the duct may occur as a result of malignant disease within the mediastinum, lymphoma, for example. Other causes include inflammatory processes, subclavian vein thrombosis, and misplaced central venous devices.

The course of the thoracic duct through the mediastinum can be variable. It starts out in the abdomen at the cisterna chyli overlying the second lumbar vertebrae, then passes through the aortic hiatus and upward in the posterior mediastinum, eventually passing behind the aortic arch on the left, arches above the clavicle, and then descends into the junction of the subclavian and internal jugular veins. A defect in the lower portion of the duct frequently results in an effusion into the right pleural space, whereas an effusion on the left results from a defect in the upper region of the duct. Clinically, the patient presents with a large pleural effusion resulting in pulmonary compression, mediastinal displacement, and the progressive development of respiratory distress. Radiographs generally show a massive effusion on the evolved side. The diagnosis should be suspected at the initial thoracentesis with the retrieval of milky, lipid-laden fluid. The fat content of chyle varies from 0.4 to 4.0 g/100 mL, and the amount of protein ranges from 2.2 to 5.9 g/100 mL. The fluid also contains a large number of lymphocytes that are predominantly T-cells in structure.

Initial treatment consists of tube thoracostomy for evacuation of the chylous fluid and expansion of the collapsed lung. Minimizing the flow of lymph within the thoracic duct by placing the patient on complete bowel rest using parenteral nutrition can permit healing of the thoracic duct lymph fistula over time. With newborns, spontaneous chylothorax usually ceases spontaneously with adequate drainage. If no improvement is noted after 3 weeks of conservative therapy, surgical intervention can be considered. Through either an open thoracotomy or with video-assisted thoracoscopy, surgical therapy involves ligation of the thoracic duct just above the diaphragm within the right chest. This goal can be accomplished with surgical ligation, direct clipping, the use of fibrin glue, and pleurodesis. For intractable conditions, pleural peritoneal shunting can be considered.

REFERENCES

Chest-Wall Deformities

1. Kowalewski J, Brocki M, Dryjanski T, et al. Pectus excavatum: increase of right ventricular systolic, diastolic, and stroke volumes after surgical repair. *J Thorac Cardiovasc Surg* 1999; 118:87–93.
2. Shamberger RC. Congenital chest wall deformities. In: O'Neill JA Jr, Rowe MI, Grosfeld JL, et al., eds. *Pediatric surgery*, 5th ed. St. Louis: Mosby, 1998:787–817.
3. Haller JA Jr, Colombani PM, Humphries CT, et al. Chest wall constriction after too extensive and too early operations for pectus excavatum. *Ann Thorac Surg* 1996;61:1618–1625.
4. Weber TR, Kurkchubasche AG. Operative management of asphyxiating thoracic dystrophy after pectus repair. *J Pediatr Surg* 1998;33:262–265.
5. Ravitch MM. The chest wall. In: Welch KJ, Randolph JG, Ravitch MM, et al., eds. *Pediatric surgery*, 4th ed. Chicago: Year Book, 1986:563–589.
6. Komuro Y, Masuda T, Kobayashi S, et al. Endoscopic correction of pectus excavatum. *Ann Plastic Surg* 1999;43:232–238.
7. Nuss D, Kelly RE Jr, Croitoru DP, et al. A 10-year review of a minimally invasive technique for the correction of pectus excavatum. *J Pediatr Surg* 1998;33:545–552.

Congenital Cystic Disease of the Lung

8. Luck SR, Reynolds M, Raffensperger JG. *Current problems in surgery*. Chicago: Year Book Medical, 1986:246–314.
9. Coran AG, Drongowski R. Congenital cystic disease of the tracheobronchial tree in infants and children. *Arch Surg* 1994; 129:521–527.
10. Conran RM, Stocker JT. Extralobar sequestration with frequently associated congenital cystic adenomatoid malformation, type 2: report of 50 cases. *Pediatr Dev Pathol* 1999;2: 454–463.
11. Gross E, Chen MK, Lobe TE, et al. Infradiaphragmatic extralobar pulmonary sequestration masquerading as an intra-abdominal, suprarenal mass. *Pediatr Surg Int* 1997;12:529–531.
12. Stocker JT, Madewell JE, Drake RM. Congenital cystic adenomatoid malformation of the lung: classification and morphologic spectrum. *Hum Pathol* 1977;8:155–171.
13. Adzick NS, Harrison MR, Crombleholme TM, et al. Fetal lung lesions: management and outcome. *Am J Obstet Gynecol* 1998;179:884–889.
14. van Leeuwen K, Teitelbaum DH, Hirschl RB, et al. Prenatal diagnosis of congenital cystic adenomatoid malformation and its postnatal presentation, surgical indications, and natural history. *J Pediatr Surg* 1999;34:794–798.
15. Bagolan P, Nahom A, Giorlandino C, et al. Cystic adenomatoid malformation of the lung: clinical evolution and management. *Eur J Pediatr* 1999;158:879–882.
16. Mentzer SJ, Filler RM, Phillips J. Limited pulmonary resections for congenital cystic adenomatoid malformation of the lung. *J Pediatr Surg* 1992;27:1410–1413.
17. Merry C, Spurbeck W, Lobe TE. Resection of foregut-derived duplications by minimal-access surgery. *Pediatr Surg Int* 1999;15:224–226.
18. Dillon PW, Cilley RE, Krummel TM. Video assisted thoraco-scopic excision of intrathoracic masses in children: report of two cases. *Surg Laparosc Endosc* 1993;3:433–436.
19. Scully RE, Mark EJ, McNeely WF, et al. Case records of the Massachusetts General Hospital—case 30-1997. *N Engl J Med* 1997;337:916–924.
20. Nuchtern JG, Harberg FJ. Congenital lung cysts. *Semin Pediatr Surg* 1994;3:233–243.
21. Stigers KB, Woodring JH, Kanga JF. The clinical and imaging spectrum of findings in patients with congenital lobar emphysema. *Pediatr Pulmonol* 1992;14:160–170.
22. Karnak I, Senocak ME, Ciftci AO, et al. Congenital lobar emphysema: diagnostic and therapeutic considerations. *J Pediatr Surg* 1999;34:1347–1351.

Thoracic Tumors

23. Rothenberg SS. Thoracoscopy in infants and children. *Semin Pediatr Surg* 1998;7:194–201.
24. Black CT. Current recommendations for the resection of pulmonary metastases of pediatric malignancies. *Pediatr Pulmonol Suppl* 1997;16:181.
25. La Quaglia. The surgical management of metastases in pediatric cancer. *Semin Pediatr Surg* 1993;2:75–82.
26. Hartman GE, Shochat SJ. Primary pulmonary neoplasms of childhood: a review. *Ann Thorac Surg* 1983;36:108–119.
27. Hancock BJ, DiLorenzo M, Youssef S, et al. Childhood primary pulmonary neoplasms. *J Pediatr Surg* 1993;28:1133–1136.
28. Ohye RG, Cohen DM, Caldwell S, et al. Pediatric bronchioloalveolar carcinoma: a favorable pediatric malignancy? *J Pediatr Surg* 1998;33:730–732.
29. Granata C, Gambini C, Balducci T, et al. Bronchioloalveolar carcinoma arising in congenital cystic adenomatoid malformation in a child: a case report and review on malignancies riginating in congenital cystic adenomatoid malformation. *Pediatr Pulmonol* 1998;25:62–66.
30. Mentzel T, Fletcher CDM. Recent advances in soft tissue tumor diagnosis. *Am J Clin Pathol* 1998;110:660–670.
31. Eggli KD, Newman B. Nodules, masses, and pseudomasses in the pediatric lung. *Radiol Clin North Am* 1993;31:651.
32. Grosfeld JL, Skinner MA, Rescorla FJ, et al. Mediastinal tumors in children: experience with 196 cases. *Ann Surg Oncol* 1994;1:121–127.
33. Glick RD, LaQuaglia MP. Lymphomas of the anterior mediastinum. *Semin Pediatr Surg* 1999;8:69–77.
34. Taneli C, Genc A, Erikci V, et al. Askin tumors in children: a report of four cases. *Eur J Pediatr Surg* 1998;8:312–314.
35. Sawin RS, Conrad EU III, Park JR, et al. Preresection chemotherapy improves survival for children with Askin tumors. *Arch Surg* 1996;131:877–880.
36. Kashima HK, Mounts P, Shah K. Recurrent respiratory papillomatosis. *Obstet Gynecol Clin North Am* 1996;131:877–880.
37. Armstrong LR, Derkay CS, Reeves WC. Initial results from the national registry for juvenile-onset recurrent respiratory papillomatosis. RRP Task Force. *Arch Otolaryngol Head Neck Surg* 1999;125:743–748.

Esophageal Atresia

38. Haight C, Towsley HA. Congenital atresia of the esophagus with tracheoesophageal fistula: extrapleural ligation of fistula and end-to-end anastomosis of esophageal segments. *Surg Gynecol Obstet* 1943;76:672–688.
39. Manning PB, Morgan RA, Coran AG, et al. Fifty years' experience with esophageal atresia and tracheoesophageal fistula: beginning with Cameron Haight's first operation in 1935. *Ann Surg* 1986;204:446–451.
40. Oi BQ, Beasley SW. Pathohistological study of adriamycin-induced tracheal agenesis in the fetal rat. *Pediatr Surg Int* 1999; 15:17–20.
41. Possogel AK, Diez-Pardo JA, Morales C, et al. Embryology of esophageal atresia in the adriamycin rat model. *J Pediatr Surg* 1998;33:606–612.
42. Haight C. Congenital esophageal atresia and trachesophageal fistula. In: Mustard WT, et al., eds. *Pediatric surgery*. Chicago: Year Book Medical, 1969.
43. Gross RE. *The surgery of infancy and childhood*. Philadelphia: WB Saunders, 1953.

44. Kluth D. Atlas of esophageal atresia. *J Pediatr Surg* 1976;11: 901–919.
45. Waterson DJ, Bonham-Carter RE, Aberdeen E. Esophageal atresia: tracheo-oesophageal fistula—a study of survival in 218 infants. *Lancet* 1962;1:819–822.
46. Randolph JG, Newman KD, Anderson KD. Current results in repair of esophageal atresia with tracheoesophageal fistula using physiologic status as a guide to therapy. *Ann Surg* 1989; 209:526–530.
47. Choudhury SR, Ashcraft KW, Sharp RJ, et al. Survival of patients with esophageal atresia: influence of birth weight, cardiac anomaly, and late respiratory complications. *J Pediatr Surg* 1999;34:70–74.
48. Dunn JC, Fonkalsrud EW, Atkinson JB. Simplifying the Waterston's stratification of infants with tracheoesophageal fistula. *Am Surg* 1999;65:908–910.
49. Cilley RE, Dillon PW. Pulmonary resection and thoracotomy. In: Stringer MD, Oldham KT, Mouriquand PDE, et al., eds. *Pediatric surgery and urology: long-term outcomes.* London: WB Saunders, 1998:156–165.
50. Spitz L, Ruangtrakool R. Esophageal substitution. *Semin Pediatr Surg* 1998;7:130–133.
51. Puri P, Khurana S. Delayed primary esophageal anastomosis for pure esophageal atresia. *Semin Pediatr Surg* 1998;7:126–129.
52. Othersen HB Jr, Hebra A, Tagge EP. Esophageal replacement for atresia without fistula. *Semin Pediatr Surg* 1998;7:134–136.
53. Lobe TE, Rothenberg S, Waldschmidt J, et al. Thoracoscopic repair of esophageal atresia in an infant: a surgical first. *Pediatric Endosurgery & Innovative Techniques* 1999;3:141–148.
54. Spitz L. Esophageal atresia: past, present, and future. *J Pediatr Surg* 1996;31:19–25.
55. Bouman NH, Koot HM, Hazebroek FW. Long-term physical, psychological, and social functioning of children with esophageal atresia. *J Pediatr Surg* 1999;34:399–404.
56. Beasley SW. Esophageal atresia: surgical aspects. In: Stringer MD, Mouriquand PDE, et al., eds. *Pediatric surgery and urology: long-term outcomes.* London: WB Saunders, 1998:166–180.

Foreign Bodies

57. Manning PB, Wesley JR, Polley TZ, et al. Esophageal and tracheobronchial foreign bodies in infants and children. *Pediatr Surg Int* 1987;2:346.
58. National Safety Council Accident Facts. http://www.nsc.org. February, 2000.

Diaphragm

59. Cilley RE. Invited commentary: Weber TR, Kountzman B, Dillon PA, et al. Improved survival in congenital diaphragmatic hernia with evolving therapeutic strategies. *Arch Surg* 1998; 133:503.
60. Cilley RE. Respiratory physiology and extracorporeal life support. In: Oldham KT, Foglia RP, Colombani PM, eds. *Surgery of infants and children: scientific principles and practice.* Philadelphia: Lippincott–Raven, 1997:183–222.
61. DiFiore JW, Wilson JM. Lung development. *Semin Pediatr Surg* 1994;3:221–232.
62. Davies GM, Reid L. Growth of the alveoli and pulmonary arteries in childhood. *Thorax* 1970;25:669–681.
63. Moore KL. *The developing human,* 3rd ed. Philadelphia: WB Saunders, 1982.
64. Iritani I. Experimental study on embryogenesis of congenital diaphragmatic hernia. *Anat Embryol* 1984;169:133–139.
65. Stolar CJH, Dillon PW. Congenital diaphragmatic hernia and eventration. In: O'Neill JA, Rowe MI, Grosfeld JL, et al., eds. *Pediatric surgery,* 5th ed. St. Louis: Mosby, 1998:819–837.
66. deLorimer AA, Tierney DF, Parker HR. Hypoplastic lungs in fetal lambs with surgically produced congenital diaphragmatic hernia. *Surgery* 1967;62:12–17.
67. Harrison MR, Jester JA, Ross NA. Correction of congenital diaphragmatic hernia in utero. I. The model: intrathoracic balloon produces fatal pulmonary hypoplasia. *Surgery* 1980;88: 174–182.
68. Brandsma AE. *Lung development in congenital diaphragmatic hernia.* Rotterdam: Offsetdrukkerij Ridderprint B.V, 1995.
69. Cilley RE, Zgleszewski SE, Krummel TM, et al. Nitrofen dose-dependent gestational day-specific murine lung hypoplasia and left-sided diaphragmatic hernia. *Am J Physiol* 1997;272: L362–L371.
70. Tibboel D, Hazebroek F, Mooi W, eds. Pathogenetic and experimental aspects of congenital diaphragmatic hernia. Presented at: Netherlands Symposium, Erasmus University, Rotterdam, May 3–5, 1999.
71. Kasales CJ, Coulson CC, Meilstrup JW, et al. Diagnosis and differentiation of congenital diaphragmatic hernia from other noncardiac thoracic fetal masses. *Am J Perinatol* 1998;15: 623–628.
72. Harrison MR, Mychaliska GB, Albanese CT, et al. Correction of congenital diaphragmatic hernia in utero X: fetuses with poor prognosis (liver herniation and low lung-to-head ration) can be saved by fetoscopic temporary tracheal occlusion. *J Pediatr Surg* 1998;33:1017–1023.
73. Wung JT, Sahni R, Moffitt ST, et al. Congenital diaphragmatic hernia: survival treated with very delayed surgery, spontaneous respiration, and no chest tube. *J Pediatr Surg* 1995;30: 406–409.
74. Roberts JP, Berge DM, Griffiths DM. High-risk congenital diaphragmatic hernia: how long should surgery be delayed? *Pediatr Surg Int* 1994;9:555–557.
75. Cilley RE, Bartlett RH. Extracorporeal life support for respiratory failure. In: Gravlee GP, ed. *Principles and practice of cardiopulmonary bypass.* Baltimore: Williams & Wilkins, 1993:655–681.
76. Lessin MS, Thompson IM, Deprez MF, et al. Congenital diaphragmatic hernia with or without extracorporeal membrane oxygenation: are we making progress? *J Am Coll Surg* 1995;181:65–71.
77. Reickert CA, Hirschl RB, Atkinson JB, et al. Congenital diaphragmatic hernia survival and use of extracorporeal life support at selected level III nurseries with multimodality support. *Surgery* 1998;123:305–310.
78. Iocono JA, Cilley RE, Mauger DT, et al. Postnatal pulmonary hypertension after repair of congenital diaphragmatic hernia: predicting risk and outcome. *J Pediatr Surg* 1999;34:349–353.
79. Kitano Y, Flake AW, Crombleholme TM, et al. Open fetal surgery for life-threatening fetal malformations. *Semin Perinatol* 1999;23:448–461.
80. Harrison MR, Adzick NS, Flake AW, et al. Correction of congenital diaphragmatic hernia in utero. VI. Hard-earned lessons. *J Pediatr Surg* 1993;28:1411–1418.
81. Harrison MR, Adzick NS, Bullard KM, et al. Correction of congenital diaphragmatic hernia in utero VII: a prospective trial. *J Pediatr Surg* 1997;32:1637–1642.
82. DiFiore JW, Fauza DO, Slavin R, et al. Experimental fetal tracheal ligation reverses the structural and physiological effects of pulmonary hypoplasia in congenital diaphragmatic hernia. *J Pediatr Surgery* 1994;29:248–257.
83. DiFiore JW, Fauza DO, Slavin R, et al. Experimental fetal tracheal ligation and congenital diaphragmatic hernia: a pulmonary vascular morophometric analysis. *J Pediatr Surg* 1995;30:917–924.
84. Hedrick MH, Estes JM, Sullivan KM, et al. Plug the lung until it grows (PLUG): a new method to treat congenital diaphragmatic hernia in utero. *J Pediatr Surg* 1994;29:612–617.
85. Hirschl RB. Respiratory failure: current status of experimental therapies. *Semin Pediatr Surg* 1999;8:155–170.
86. Suen HC, Losty P, Donahoe PK, et al. Combined antenatal thyrotropin-releasing hormone and low-dose glucocorticoid therapy improves the pulmonary biochemical immaturity in congenital diaphragmatic hernia. *J Pediatr Surg* 1994;29: 359–363.
87. Cilley RE, Coran AG. Eventration of the diaphragm. In: Spitz L, Coran AG, eds. *Operative surgery.* London: Butterworth-Heinemann, 1995:168–175.

SURGERY: SCIENTIFIC PRINCIPLES AND PRACTICE, Third Edition, edited by
Lazar J. Greenfield, Michael W. Mulholland, Keith T. Oldham, Gerald B. Zelenock,
and Keith D. Lillemoe. Lippincott Williams & Wilkins Publishers, Philadelphia, © 2001.

CHAPTER 97

PEDIATRIC ABDOMEN

THOMAS T. SATO AND KEITH T. OLDHAM

ABDOMINAL WALL DEFECTS

Gastroschisis

Anatomy, Embryology, and Pathophysiology

Gastroschisis occurs with an incidence of 1 in 3,000 to 8,000 live births, and, for unknown reasons, the incidence appears to be increasing. Infants with gastroschisis tend to be born prematurely, have lower birth weights, and have younger mothers (1,2). Familial cases of gastroschisis have been reported and are distinctly rare (3). Associated congenital anomalies are uncommon and occur in about 10% of cases, most commonly intestinal atresia or stenosis. These anomalies are thought to reflect mechanical or vascular compromise to the herniated bowel. Rarely, infants with gastroschisis will have complete loss of small bowel secondary to in utero volvulus.

The pathophysiology of gastroschisis remains unknown. Whether the defect originates in the umbilicus (4) or in the abdominal wall remains unclear. In normal fetal development, there are two paired umbilical veins; as the intestine returns to the abdominal cavity through the umbilicus, the right umbilical vein undergoes resorption, leaving the left umbilical vein intact. Weakness of the umbilical membrane at the site of umbilical vein resorption may evolve into a hernia, and, in the case of membrane rupture, evisceration of the intestine through the defect may occur. This explanation is consistent with the clinical observation that the abdominal wall defect in gastroschisis nearly always is located to the right of the umbilicus. With the advent of routine antenatal ultrasonography, the sequential development of a typical gastroschisis has been documented as a consequence of a ruptured hernia of the umbilical cord in utero (5). Therefore, this observation suggests that gastroschisis is an isolated mechanical defect of the developing umbilical cord rather than a global defect in embryogenesis.

The amount of bowel eviscerated in gastroschisis can be extensive because the bowel has not undergone complete mesenteric rotation and fixation. Typically, the bowel is thickened and the mesentery may be foreshortened secondary to the inflammatory response induced by direct exposure to amniotic fluid. Given the typical small size of the abdominal wall defect, herniation of the liver in gastroschisis is distinctly unusual (Fig. 97.1).

Omphalocele

Anatomy, Embryology, and Pathophysiology

The incidence of omphalocele is estimated to be 1 in 6,000 to 10,000 live births and has been stable over the past several decades. Omphalocele is an abdominal wall defect of varying size that is characterized by the presence of herniated visceral contents into a translucent sac. The sac is composed of amniotic membrane, mesenchymal tissue known as *Wharton's jelly,* and peritoneum. The umbilical cord typically attaches to the sac and may be eccentric in origin (Fig. 97.2). The sac may be inadvertently ruptured before or during delivery, but it is always present. Similar to gastroschisis, intestinal malrotation is present. Unlike in gastroschisis, the bowel is typically normal in appearance because it has not been directly exposed to the amniotic fluid. Small omphaloceles are typically abdominal wall defects 2 to 5 cm in diameter and may have only a small amount of herniated bowel within the sac. Giant omphaloceles larger than 10 cm in diameter can lead to massive and extensive herniation of the stomach, bowel, liver, and spleen, with subsequent underdevelopment of the abdominal cavity (Fig. 97.3).

Omphalocele is a result of incomplete closure of the anterior abdominal wall at the umbilicus during embryogenesis. During week 4 of gestation, the midgut undergoes progressive elongation in the yolk sac outside the embryonic coelomic cavity. The midgut subsequently returns to the abdominal cavity during week 10 of gestation, where it undergoes normal rotation and fixation of its mesentery to the posterior abdominal wall. Normal closure of the an-

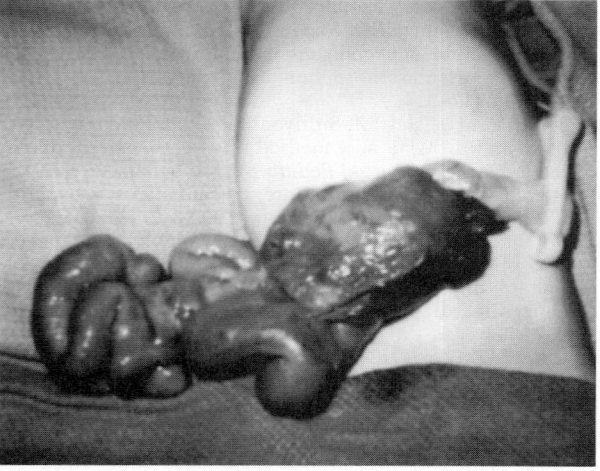

Figure 97.1. Gastroschisis. The defect is to the right of the normal umbilicus, and the bowel is thickened and inflamed.

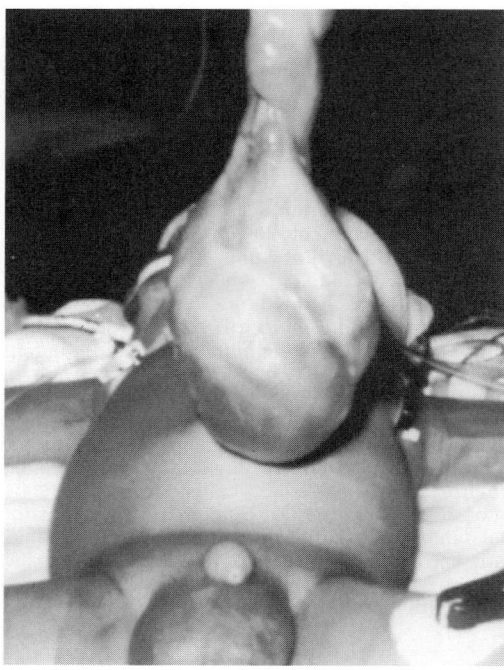

Figure 97.2. Omphalocele. The herniated intestines and liver are visible inside the sac. The umbilical cord attaches to the sac.

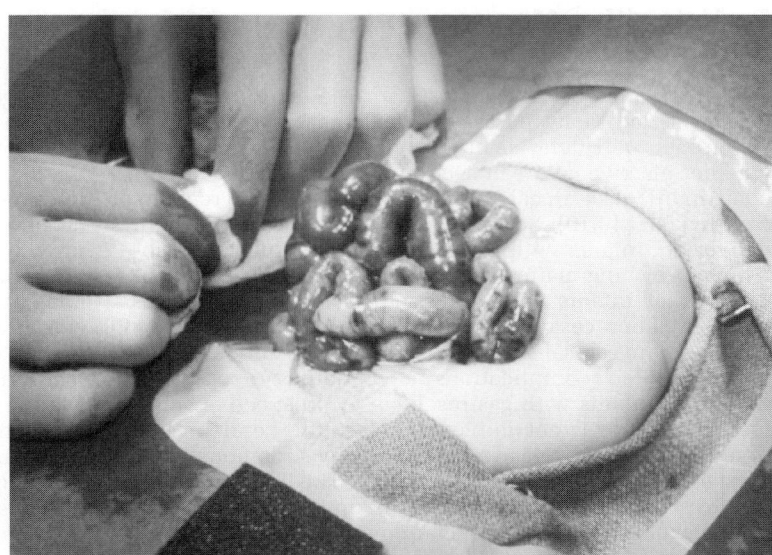

Figure 97.3. Ruptured omphalocele. Although the bowel is relatively normal in appearance, the abdominal cavity is extremely underdeveloped.

terior abdominal wall requires return of the midgut to the abdominal cavity, along with growth and fusion of the anterior body folds (cephalic, caudal, and two lateral) at the base of the umbilicus. Failure of growth, migration, or fusion of the lateral body folds leads to omphalocele. Failure of growth and fusion of the cephalic folds may lead to either *ectopia cordis,* which is a supraumbilical omphalocele associated with a midline sternal defect and a herniated heart, or a constellation of defects known as the *pentalogy of Cantrell* (6). This sequence includes a sternal cleft, an absence of the septum transversum of the diaphragm, a pericardial defect, a cardiac defect, and an epigastric omphalocele (Fig. 97.4). Infants born with either ectopia cordis or the pentalogy of Cantrell have significant morbidity, and often these conditions are lethal.

Associated anomalies are much more common in infants with omphalocele than with gastroschisis, reflecting the more global abnormality of embryogenesis in omphalocele compared with the simple mechanical defect in gastroschisis. About 50% to 60% of infants with omphalocele will have at least one associated congenital anomaly (7,8). These infants are at moderate to high risk for anomalies of the skeleton, gastrointestinal tract, nervous system, genitourinary system, and cardiopulmonary system. In addition, infants with omphalocele have a higher incidence of chromosomal abnormalities and other conditions such as Beckwith-Wiedemann syndrome. A comparison of gastroschisis and omphalocele is summarized in Table 97.1.

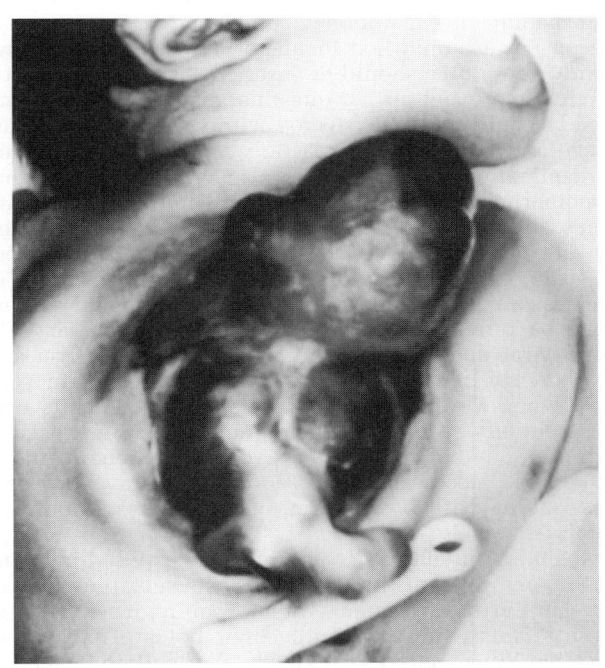

Figure 97.4. Pentalogy of Cantrell—sternal cleft, absence of the septum transversum of the diaphragm, pericardial defect, cardiac defect, and an epigastric omphalocele.

Table 97.1. COMPARISON OF GASTROSCHISIS AND OMPHALOCELE

Characteristic	Gastroschisis	Omphalocele
Defect size	2–3 cm	2–15 cm
Sac	Never	Always; may be ruptured
Umbilical cord	Left of defect	Attached to sac
Prematurity	Common	Normal term
Herniated viscera	Small bowel, stomach, colon	Small bowel, stomach, colon, liver
Malrotation	Yes	Yes
Quality of bowel	Edematous, inflamed	Normal
Alimentation	Delayed	Normal
Associated anomalies	Uncommon (10%)	Common (50%)

Perioperative Management of Abdominal Wall Defects

Contemporary use of diagnostic ultrasound during pregnancy has led to an increase in the prenatal diagnosis of abdominal wall defects. In the absence of fetal distress, whether elective cesarean section improves neonatal outcome in infants with gastroschisis or omphalocele remains controversial (9,10). Some investigators advocate elective delivery of infants with gastroschisis following the establishment of lung maturity. Moore and colleagues (11) observed that infants with gastroschisis delivered by preterm, prelabor cesarean section had less inflammatory "peel" on the serosal surface of the intestine and fewer intestinal-related complications after delivery compared with term infants with gastroschisis. A prospective study that alternated vaginal delivery with elective cesarean section for infants with gastroschisis, however, demonstrated no significant differences in outcome (12). To prevent injury to the liver, cesarean section is preferable for prenatally diagnosed infants with giant omphaloceles.

After delivery, infants with either gastroschisis or omphalocele have similar initial management priorities. Attention must be given to the establishment of an adequate airway with effective ventilation and oxygenation. The infant should be maintained under either an external warmer or a humidified incubator. A nasogastric or orogastric sump tube should be inserted early and placed on suction to prevent further intestinal distention. The herniated viscera should be covered with warm, saline-soaked gauze and covered with plastic wrap to prevent further contamination; this maneuver also will help to prevent hypothermia and volume depletion. Alternatively, the infant's entire lower torso can be placed inside a plastic bowel bag. Regardless of the method, the initial therapeutic goal is to provide rapid, effective temporary coverage of the viscera. Adequate support of the herniated viscera must be provided to prevent intestinal ischemia. With large omphaloceles, the position of the infant's liver and viscera may impair venous return from the inferior vena cava when the infant is supine, and these infants may preferentially require a left-side-down position to maintain hemodynamic stability. An intravenous catheter should be placed early, and 5% or 10% intravenous dextrose, along with broad-spectrum antibiotics, should be administered.

Given the inflammatory nature of the exposed intestine to the environment, infants with gastroschisis will have large initial intravascular volume requirements. Most of these infants require an intravenous bolus of crystalloid (lactated Ringer solution at 20 cc/kg) or colloid (5% albumin at 10 cc/kg) during initial resuscitation, followed by infusion of crystalloid at two to three times the infant's calculated maintenance rate prior to operation. Adequate intravenous fluid replacement should be given to establish and maintain a urinary output of 1 to 2 mL/kg/hr. If the infant is not delivered at a center where definitive surgical care can be provided, urgent transport should be arranged.

Because the bowel is protected in an intact omphalocele, the fluid requirements and heat loss are less than that observed in gastroschisis. The intact sac should still be covered in warm, saline-soaked gauze and plastic wrap. Operative closure of an intact omphalocele is more elective than with gastroschisis. Given the high incidence of associated anomalies, infants with an intact omphalocele should undergo diagnostic investigation preoperatively, guided by the clinical presentation and physical examination of the infant. These studies include a chest film, echocardiogram, and renal ultrasound, in addition to baseline blood work. Until the decision is made with respect

to the timing and method of repair, the omphalocele should remain covered and protected with a dressing. If the omphalocele is ruptured or torn, immediate closure or coverage is necessary.

Once the infant has been stabilized and assessment for other anomalies is complete, the infant is taken to the operating room for correction of the abdominal wall defect. Reduction of the herniated viscera with primary fascial closure of the abdominal wall is an achievable goal in approximately 60% to 70% of infants with either gastroschisis or omphalocele. Gentle but definitive stretching of the abdominal wall is performed, and proximal decompression of the bowel is maintained with nasogastric or orogastric decompression. The defect may require enlargement in gastroschisis to evaluate fully the intestinal tract. With omphalocele, the sac usually is resected. The limiting factor in primary closure of an abdominal wall defect is the increased intraabdominal pressure generated by the reduction of the herniated viscera. Increased intraabdominal pressure can lead to a clinical situation known as *abdominal compartment syndrome,* which is characterized by impaired venous return caused by compression of the inferior vena cava, mesenteric ischemia by reduction of splanchnic blood flow, and respiratory compromise secondary to impaired diaphragmatic excursion. Clinical measurement of intragastric or intravesical pressure less than 20 cm H_2O, end-tidal CO_2 of 50 mm Hg or less, or a rise in central venous pressure of less than 4 mm Hg during abdominal wall closure allows for safe primary abdominal wall closure (13). If the herniated viscera cannot be reduced primarily, a Silastic pouch or silo is constructed and daily partial reduction of the silo is performed. This allows more gradual reduction of the herniated viscera back to the abdominal cavity, and complete reduction usually is obtained within 3 to 7 days. The infant then can return to the operating room for removal of the temporary silo with delayed primary closure of the abdominal wall defect (Fig. 97.5).

Infants with giant omphaloceles with or without coexisting anomalies also can be successfully managed nonoperatively. The sac can be physically supported and left intact, covering the surface of the sac with topical antibiotics, which allows epithelialization of the sac over several weeks, with delayed repair of the ventral hernia months to years later. This is particularly useful in the infant with a giant omphalocele and a small, underdeveloped abdominal cavity that prohibits primary closure.

Infants with repaired omphalocele usually have relatively prompt return of bowel function after definitive repair. In comparison, nearly all infants with gastroschisis will have delay in intestinal function following closure. The use of total parenteral nutrition (TPN) is essential in the treatment of these infants because it allows nutritional support while the bowel inflammatory process resolves. It is not unusual for these infants to require up to 4 weeks after the repair to have bowel function normalize. The risks of prolonged TPN support in neonates include central venous line infection, thrombosis, cholestasis, and liver injury, which in some instances can be irreversible. The institution of small amounts of diluted, enteral feeding (gut-priming) as early as possible may help to prevent some of the effects of TPN on liver injury (14). About 15% of infants with gastroschisis will develop necrotizing enterocolitis (NEC), a diffuse, often life-threatening inflammatory complication of the neonatal intestinal tract. The use of maternal breast milk may exert a protective effect against the development of NEC in this population (15). In addition, infants with gastroschisis are at risk for functional short bowel syndrome and significant intestinal dysmotility with inability to tolerate full enteral feeding.

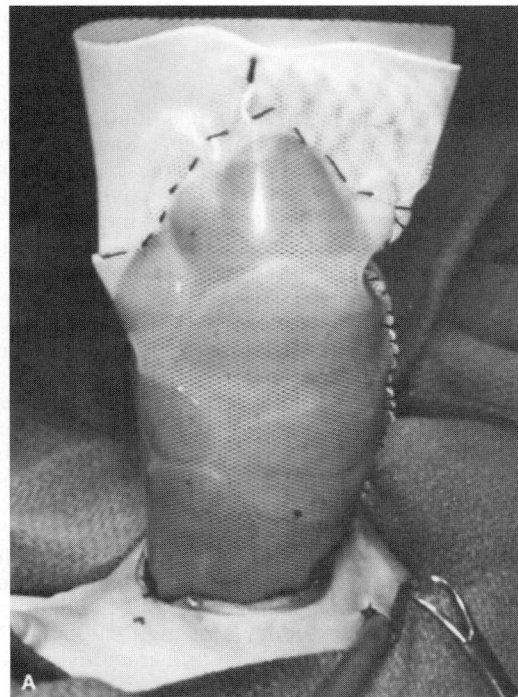

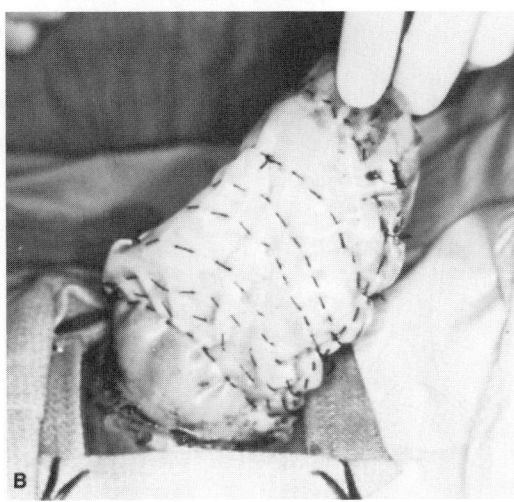

Figure 97.5. Silastic chimney or silo for temporary coverage of giant omphalocele.

This last situation can evolve into a long-term condition termed *pseudoobstruction* and may require long-term, sometimes life-long dependence on TPN for caloric intake.

UMBILICAL HERNIA

Anatomy and Embryology

Congenital umbilical hernias are the most common abdominal wall defects in infants and children. The umbilical ring begins to contract circumferentially after birth and normally is reinforced by the paired lateral umbilical ligaments (the obliterated umbilical arteries), the singular round ligament (the obliterated umbilical vein), the urachus, and the transversalis fascia. The incomplete growth or development of any one of these structures can lead to weakness at the umbilical ring and cause an umbilical hernia defect.

Clinical Issues and Management

Congenital umbilical hernias generally do not pose significant problems during childhood. Rarely, an umbilical hernia will present with incarceration of intraabdominal contents within the sac (16). Infants and children also can present with infection or drainage of associated urachal or vitelline duct remnants at the umbilicus. The incidence of congenital umbilical hernia has been reported to be 25% to 50% in black infants and 4% to 9% in white infants in the first few months of life (17). There is an increased incidence of umbilical hernia in premature infants, and there is a tendency for familial inheritance.

Diagnosis of umbilical hernia is usually made after separation of the umbilical cord remnant from the umbilicus and often is noted first by the parents or the pediatrician. The size of the defect may vary from a few millimeters to several centimeters and is typically reducible and asymptomatic. Most umbilical hernias spontaneously close within the first 2 to 3 years of life. Parents should be reassured that complications related to the untreated umbilical hernia are rare.

Given the high rate of spontaneous closure and the relatively asymptomatic nature of most umbilical hernias, operative repair generally is not performed during the first 2 years of life. Symptoms referable to the hernia or an episode of incarceration should prompt earlier repair. Large defects with significant protrusion may bring the child to the surgeon, and parents may desire repair if the child appears to be self-conscious about the hernia. Nearly all umbilical hernia repairs can be performed as outpatient surgical procedures. An incision is made along the umbilicus, and the hernia sac is dissected free circumferentially. The sac is excised, and primary fascial closure is performed. An acceptable cosmetic result almost always is achieved, and the incidence of complications such as wound infection and recurrence is low.

Inguinal Hernia and Hydrocele

Anatomy, Embryology, and Pathophysiology

Inguinal hernias constitute one of the major surgical problems of infancy and childhood. Surgical treatment of childhood inguinal hernia represents the most common elective general surgical procedure performed by pediatric surgeons. Three distinct anatomic types of inguinal hernias are observed in children: congenital or indirect (99% of infants and children), direct (0.5%), and femoral (< 0.5%). An *indirect inguinal hernia* is an abnormal, patent continuation of the peritoneum through the internal inguinal ring. The hernia sac originates lateral to the deep inferior epigastric artery and vein and descends along the spermatic cord within the cremasteric fascia. The sac can reside completely within the inguinal canal or descend through the external inguinal ring into the scrotum. A *direct inguinal hernia* originates medial to the deep inferior epigastric vessels and is external to the cremasteric fascia. The hernia sac protrudes directly through the posterior wall of the inguinal canal and can descend through the external inguinal ring and into the scrotum. A *femoral inguinal hernia* originates medial to the femoral vein and descends inferior to the inguinal ligament along the femoral canal. A femoral hernia never enters the scrotum or labia.

The developing testicle is initially adjacent to the mesonephros and subsequently descends to the scrotum during the third trimester of gestation. The extension of the peritoneum that follows the chorda gubernaculum along the testicle is called the processus vaginalis. A slightly higher incidence of right-sided indirect inguinal hernias is thought to reflect delay of testicular descent from the developing inferior vena cava and right external iliac vein. As the testicle descends into the scrotum, the processus vaginalis forms a serous covering around the testicle known as the tunica vaginalis. Normally, the patent processus vaginalis undergoes obliteration, closing the communication between the peritoneal cavity and the inguinal canal. A patent processus vaginalis can lead to a variety of anatomic conditions of the inguinal region (Fig. 97.6).

The incidence of patent processus vaginalis has been reported to be as high as 80% to 94% in newborn infants undergoing autopsy (18), whereas in adulthood, the incidence is 20% to 30%. Rowe and colleagues (19) studied 2,764 patients with unilateral inguinal hernias and found a patent contralateral processus vaginalis in 60% of the children during the first few months of life. By the age of 2 years, 20% of these were obliterated, and half of the remaining 40% became clinical hernias. At least 30% of infants requiring placement of a ventriculoperitoneal shunt for hydrocephalus have been observed to have a patent processus vaginalis in the first few months of life, with a rapid decline in patency in older children (20). These studies demonstrate that although a patent processus vaginalis is common in infancy, there is some degree of obliteration that occurs with increasing age, and a patent processus vaginalis by itself does not constitute an inguinal hernia.

Clinical Issues

Inguinal hernias occur in 1% to 3% of all children and in 3% to 5% of premature infants. There is no known inheritance pattern, but there is an increased incidence of inguinal hernia in children with connective tissue disorders, such as Ehlers-Danlos syndrome and Marfan syndrome. There is a 6:1 predominance of males over females. At least 30% of these children are younger than 6 months of age at the time of operative repair. As discussed earlier, inguinal hernia more commonly presents as right-sided (56.2%) compared with left-sided (27.5%) or bilateral (16.2%) (21).

Most infants and children have a history of an intermittent inguinal bulge that may descend into the scrotum or labia. The hernia may become more pronounced during times of increased intraabdominal pressure, such as crying or having a bowel movement. Most inguinal hernias in children are reducible either spontaneously or with gentle, manual pressure along the inguinal canal. Female infants may have an ovary and fallopian tube in the hernia sac, which clinically is recognized as a firm, slightly mobile, nontender mass in the labia or inguinal canal. Most parents or pediatricians will give a characteristic history

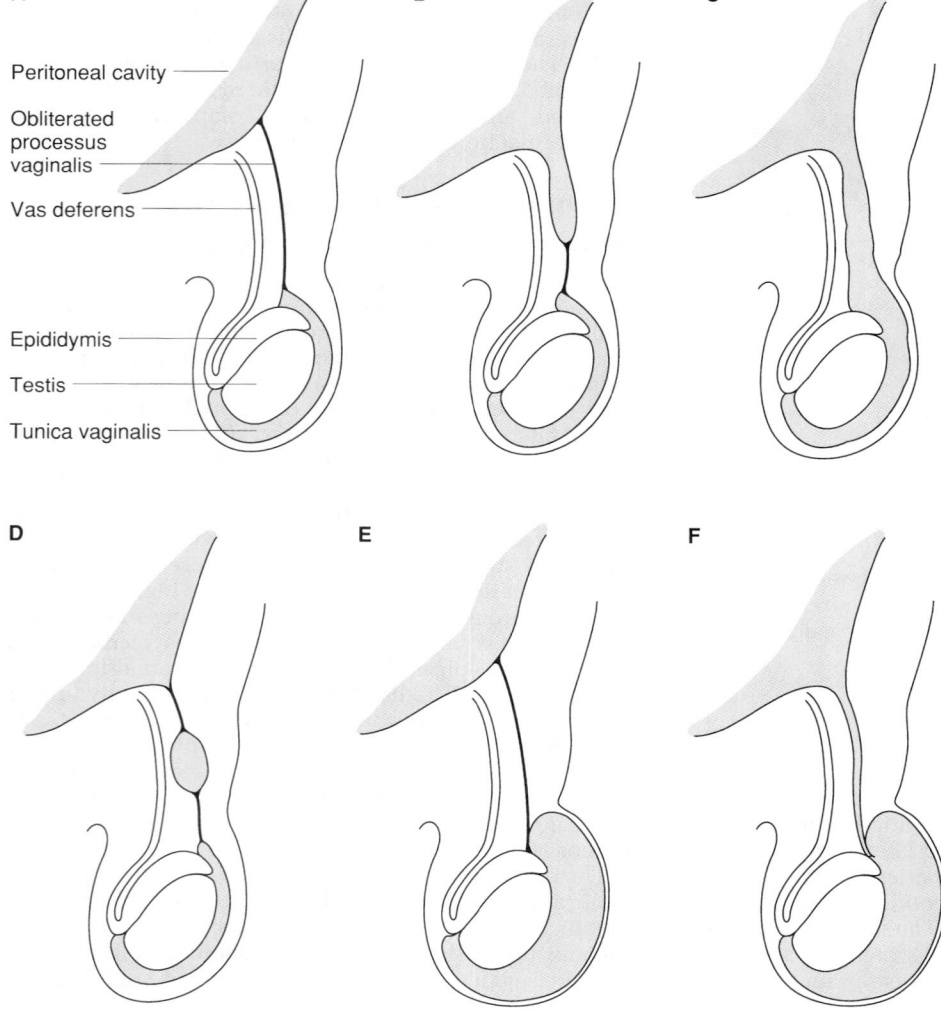

Figure 97.6. Diagrammatic representation of the anatomic variations that occur with different degrees of obliteration of the processus vaginalis. *(A)* Normal; obliterated processus vaginalis. *(B)* Proximal hernia sac; distal obliterated processus. *(C)* Hernia sac extending into scrotum; no obliteration. *(D)* Proximal and distal obliteration with hydrocele of the cord. *(E)* Hydrocele of the scrotum, obliterated processus. *(F)* Patent processus with communicating hydrocele

that is sufficient to warrant inguinal exploration, even in children in whom the hernia cannot be clinically demonstrated at the time of examination. Depending on institution and surgeon preference, infants and children with a strong history consistent with inguinal hernia and an equivocal clinical examination can be offered either ultrasound (22) or diagnostic laparoscopy to effectively confirm the diagnosis before groin exploration.

Incarceration is a common consequence of untreated inguinal hernia and presents as a nonreducible mass in the inguinal canal, scrotum, or labia (23). Clinical symptoms and signs are related to the duration of incarceration. If the incarceration has been present for several hours, the infant may be inconsolable and have feeding intolerance, pain, abdominal distention, vomiting, and lack of flatus or stool, signaling complete intestinal obstruction. The affected groin may become quite edematous, and a reactive scrotal hydrocele may evolve. Elevation of the infant's lower extremities with a pillow may help to encourage spontaneous reduction. Attempts at manually reducing an incarcerated inguinal hernia should be performed by an experienced surgeon. If necessary, sedation to calm the infant before attempting manual reduction may be used with caution. Ice packs should be avoided in infants and children. Following successful reduction of an incarcerated hernia, expedient elective repair of the hernia should be performed after the edema has subsided. If reduction of an incarcerated hernia requires several attempts and is difficult, overnight inpatient observation is warranted to rule out reduction of strangulated bowel; fortunately, this is an uncommon occurrence in the pediatric population. Inability to reduce an incarcerated hernia is a clear indication for urgent operative exploration and repair. Incarcerated inguinal hernia must be differentiated from an acute hydrocele or inguinal lymphadenitis. With acute hydrocele, it is usually possible to palpate normal cord structure above the scrotal mass and along the inguinal canal. Acute lymphadenitis typically is associated with fever, erythema, and tenderness, and there may be a history of lower-extremity infection on the ipsilateral side. In general, if the inguinal mass has been present for longer than 24 hours and there are no symptoms of bowel obstruction on clinical and radiologic examination, it is unlikely to be an incarcerated hernia. If the inguinal mass is not reducible and an incarcerated hernia cannot be excluded, then urgent groin exploration is required.

Operative Considerations and Outcome

The clinical diagnosis of inguinal hernia in an infant or child is an indication for operative repair. Congenital inguinal hernias do not spontaneously resolve and are at high risk of incarceration. At least 71% of infants who require operative reduction of incarcerated inguinal hernia are younger than 11 months of age (24). Therefore, an approach emphasizing timely elective repair of inguinal hernia is warranted, particularly during infancy. Delay of elective repair may be necessary in premature, extremely low birth weight (< 1,500 g) infants and in children with other conditions such as congenital heart disease, pulmonary disease, infection, or metabolic disease. The risk of using general anesthesia in these children can be significant enough to defer inguinal hernia repair until the coexisting conditions are corrected.

Repair of inguinal hernia in the pediatric age group usually is performed as an outpatient surgical procedure with the patient under general anesthesia, although spinal anesthesia has been an effective alternative in selected high-risk infants (25). A regional caudal block or local inguinal nerve block using bupivacaine can be useful to diminish the pain response and increase patient comfort.

These techniques, along with the use of rapid-acting general anesthetics, allow the vast majority of children to be discharged home within hours of their operation. Overnight observation and monitoring are required for high-risk infants and children, including premature infants, infants less than 50 weeks postconceptual age, or children with significant cardiac, pulmonary, or other disorders that increase anesthetic risk.

Repair of pediatric indirect inguinal hernia relies on high ligation of the hernia sac at the level of the internal inguinal ring. All identified sensory nerves in the inguinal region should be identified and preserved. Careful visualization, identification, and dissection of the vas deferens and the testicular blood supply from the hernia sac must be performed; operative magnifying loupes are extremely helpful in this regard. The vas deferens must be carefully dissected free from the sac, and direct handling or pinching of the vas with forceps must be avoided. When performing groin exploration and dissection on male infants with an absent or blind-ending vas deferens, the examiner also should look for cystic fibrosis (CF), which is not uncommon with this disease. In females infants, visualization of the ovary and fallopian tube after opening the hernia sac can be helpful to avoid inadvertent injury to these structures during high suture ligation of the sac at the internal ring. The distal component of the hernia sac is opened widely, and any fluid in the sac is evacuated. If the internal inguinal ring is attenuated or enlarged from a large hernia, it can be repaired with a few sutures. The testicle is returned to its scrotal position by gentle traction on the gubernaculum, and the spermatic cord is carefully aligned along the inguinal canal. The skin incisions typically are closed with absorbable, subcuticular sutures and covered with either collodion or a waterproof dressing for the first few postoperative days. Postoperative pain is handled with oral acetaminophen for 24 to 48 hours; older children may require acetaminophen with codeine.

Contralateral exploration of the asymptomatic groin remains controversial but is often performed in infants younger than 2 years of age because of the reported 60% to 70% incidence of a patent processus vaginalis on the opposite side (26). In a recent survey of the Section on Surgery of the American Academy of Pediatrics, 65% of the respondents perform contralateral exploration in male patients younger than 2 years of age, and 84% explore female infants up to 4 years of age (27); however, the incidence of metachronous contralateral inguinal hernia is not as high as reflected solely by the presence of a contralateral patent processus vaginalis (28). With the increasing use of surgical laparoscopy in the pediatric population, direct visualization of the contralateral groin can be performed either through a small, separate abdominal incision or through a side-viewing laparoscope inserted through the hernia sac. Current data suggest that, by using this approach, the rate of contralateral patent processus vaginalis in a clinically asymptomatic groin is between 46% and 52.6%, with higher rates in infants younger than 1 year of age (29,30). This approach avoids unnecessary contralateral groin exploration in about half of all children with a clinically apparent unilateral inguinal hernia.

For experienced pediatric surgeons, the major risk of inguinal hernia repair in children is related to general anesthesia, and this is usually well tolerated. Complications in inguinal hernia repair in children include wound infection, injury to the vas deferens or testicular vessels, injury or displacement of the testicle, and recurrence. Fortunately, all these complications are quite infrequent. The overall complication rate is higher for children requiring emergent operation for incarcerated or strangulated hernia. Recurrent inguinal hernia following elective repair is unusual, and consideration to connective tissue disorders such as Ehlers-Danlos syndrome should be given.

Hydrocele

A hydrocele is a fluid collection that resides in the tunica vaginalis in the scrotum or the processus vaginalis in the inguinal canal. A hydrocele may be present at birth, or it may occur as an acute hydrocele as a result of an inflammatory process in a patent processus vaginalis, such as an incarcerated hernia or torsion of the appendix testis. On examination, a hydrocele may transilluminate with a bright hand-held light, but this finding also can be seen with an incarcerated inguinal hernia in an infant. A hydrocele is described as either *communicating* or *noncommunicating*, depending on whether there is direct patency between the hydrocele and the peritoneal cavity. A history of intermittent fluctuation in the size of the scrotal fluid mass makes the diagnosis of communicating hydrocele likely. A communicating hydrocele by definition has a patent processus vaginalis and is anatomically identical to an inguinal hernia. Therefore, a communicating hydrocele is treated surgically on diagnosis in the same fashion as an indirect inguinal hernia. In male patients, a hydrocele of the cord is a collection of fluid in the processus vaginalis separate from the tunica vaginalis. In female patients, fluid trapped in the processus vaginalis is considered a hydrocele of the canal of Nuck. In noncommunicating hydrocele, the isolated fluid collection is typically asymptomatic and tends to resolve spontaneously before the age of 12 months. Operative management of noncommunicating hydrocele usually is reserved for lesions that persist after this age or that are enlarging at a rapid rate or if there is any question of undiagnosed communication. In children, an inguinal approach is used to treat hydrocele. Simple aspiration of a suspected hydrocele through the scrotum should be avoided because this maneuver is ineffective and risks injury to bowel in an undiagnosed inguinal hernia.

GASTROINTESTINAL DISORDERS

Neonatal Intestinal Obstruction

A variety of congenital anatomic defects, inherited metabolic diseases, and acquired physiologic disorders may present with intestinal obstruction within the first month of life. Neonatal intestinal obstruction is characterized clinically by bilious emesis, and this is often associated with abdominal distention. Bilious emesis in a neonate must be considered to be the result of an acute mechanical intestinal obstruction until proven otherwise. Emergent surgical evaluation is warranted for any newborn with bilious emesis. Table 97.2 provides the differential diagnoses for neonatal intestinal obstruction along with salient features of the history, physical examination, and diagnostic studies.

The clinical presentation of neonatal intestinal obstruction depends, in part, on the site of obstruction and the age of the infant. Clinical examination of the infant typically provides the surgeon with a preliminary diagnosis and helps to guide further diagnostic studies. Abdominal distention almost always is observed in distal bowel obstruction, whereas the abdomen may be flat in proximal obstruction. The presence of bile in the gastric contents or stool provides clinical evidence of the location of an obstruction relative to the ampulla of Vater. An infant with bilious emesis who has already passed meconium and has tolerated feeding is unlikely to have intestinal atresia and more likely to have malrotation with midgut volvulus. An important point is that malrotation with midgut volvulus must be considered in this setting, and evaluation must be done on an emergency basis to prevent catastrophic bowel injury or death.

Whereas there are myriad causes of neonatal intestinal obstruction, the definitive diagnosis often can be made with readily available radiologic studies. The general approach to imaging the neonate suspected of having an intestinal obstruction is to obtain a plain abdominal radiograph, followed by either a contrast enema or an upper gastrointestinal series. The sequential information gath-

---

Table 97.2. NEONATAL INTESTINAL OBSTRUCTION

Diagnosis	History	Physical examination	Diagnostic studies
Intestinal atresia or stenosis	Bilious vomiting	Abdominal distention Acholic meconium	Plain radiograph Contrast enema
Congenital duodenal obstruction	Bilious vomiting	Gastric distention Trisomy 21	Plain radiograph Upper GI study
Imperforate anus	Failure to pass meconium Bilious vomiting (late)	Abdominal distention Nonpatent anus or fistula	Evaluate for VACTERL Ultrasound sacrum, rectum Echocardiogram
Necrotizing enterocolitis	High-risk, premature infant Bilious vomiting	Abdominal distention Guaiac-positive stool	Serial plain radiographs
Meconium ileus	Cystic fibrosis (10%) Bilious vomiting	Acholic meconium Abdominal distention	Plain radiograph Contrast enema
Malrotation	Bilious vomiting Full-term, healthy infant	No abdominal distention	Plain radiograph Upper GI series
Hirschsprung's disease	Bilious vomiting Delayed passage of meconium	Abdominal distention Trisomy 21	Plain radiograph Contrast enema
Uncommon causes of obstruction (intussusception, Meckel's diverticulum, duplication)	Variable	Incarcerated hernia, mass	Variable
Medical conditions associated with bilious vomiting and ileus	Variable	Variable	Sepsis Hypothyroidism Meconium plug syndrome Others

GI, gastrointestinal; VACTERL, vertebral, anal, cardiac, tracheal, esophageal, renal, and limb.

ered by each study determines, if necessary, the next diagnostic study. Plain films of the newborn abdomen can be extremely useful and diagnostic because swallowed air can act as a contrast agent. For example, duodenal atresia gives rise to a dilated, air-filled stomach and duodenum proximal to the obstruction; the remainder of the bowel remains gasless, giving rise to the "double-bubble" appearance on plain abdominal films. Other conditions can have distinctive radiographic findings that, along with the clinical setting, allow definitive diagnosis. The presence of pneumatosis intestinalis on a plain abdominal film in an infant that is suspected of having NEC is diagnostic. A contrast enema demonstrating a classic rectosigmoid transition zone of dilated to contracted colon is characteristic of Hirschsprung's disease. Other causes of proximal intestinal obstruction may lead to finding only a nonspecific microcolon on contrast enema, which is a diminutive, unused but normal colon. If a retrograde contrast enema does not pass into the dilated segment of bowel, an upper gastrointestinal series may be useful to identify a more proximal obstruction. An upper gastrointestinal series is also the diagnostic procedure of choice in suspected malrotation.

The important surgical goal is to diagnose and treat the mechanical obstruction correctly and expediently. Clinical examination of the newborn typically yields a great deal of information regarding the cause of suspected intestinal obstruction. As previously discussed, incarcerated inguinal hernia is an important cause of neonatal bowel obstruction, and examination will lead to a straightforward diagnosis. Some congenital conditions have clearly recognizable features and may be associated with anatomic lesions causing intestinal obstruction; for example, infants with trisomy 21 have a high incidence of duodenal atresia and Hirschsprung's disease. Several medical conditions of the newborn appear clinically similar to mechanical intestinal obstruction (Table 97.2). In particular, neonatal sepsis is not uncommon, and the associated ileus can lead to bilious emesis. Congenital hypothyroidism is an infrequent and medically treatable condition that can produce delayed intestinal motility and mimic mechanical obstruction secondary to an anatomic lesion. In general, the diagnosis of intestinal obstruction in a neonate relies on a clear history, a thorough clinical examination, and adjunctive radiologic studies.

Intestinal Atresia or Stenosis

Intestinal atresia or stenosis can occur in any location along the gastrointestinal tract. Lesions involving the jejunum, ileum, and colon are considered jointly. Esophageal atresia is discussed separately elsewhere in the text.

Embryology and Anatomy

The embryonic intestine undergoes segmental development as early as week 3 of gestation. The septum transversum demarcates the caudal extent of the foregut and the cranial portion of the midgut. The hindgut develops in the primitive tail fold. Developmental issues relevant to the discussion that follows are limited to the midgut (31). The midgut can be considered a simple tubular structure that progressively undergoes elongation; herniation from and reduction into the coelomic cavity; rotation; and, ultimately, fixation of the mesentery to the posterior body wall.

Several different types of intestinal atresia are clinically observed (Fig. 97.7) and reflect common patterns of abnormal embryogenesis (32). *Type I* atresia is an intraluminal web or diaphragm that can either be complete or fenestrated. The seromuscular layers of bowel remain intact.

Types II and *IIIa* atresia are believed to be a result of in utero vascular accidents to the involved area, such as intussusception (33), segmental volvulus, or thromboembolism. Experimental interruption of the fetal mesenteric blood supply in utero leads to this type of atresia (34). *Type IIIb* atresia, also known as the *apple-peel* or *Christmas tree deformity*, has complete mesenteric discontinuity, with the distal bowel concentrically surrounding the often precarious mesenteric blood supply. *Type IV* atresia has multiple segmental areas of discontinuous bowel. Type IIIb and IV atresia are thought to be consequences of major and multiple vascular interruptions, respectively, of fetal mesenteric blood flow.

At least 90% of infants with congenital intestinal obstruction of the small bowel have complete atresia, whereas the remaining children have either stenoses or fenestrated intraluminal webs. The most common location is the distal ileum, and multiple areas of atresia are discovered in 3.6% to 20% of these infants (35). Infants with fenestrated intraluminal webs may have a small, often eccentric opening that is millimeters in diameter. These infants may not have obstructive symptoms until the introduction of solid food at 6 to 12 months of age. Occasionally, these children will present much later in life with failure to thrive, abdominal pain, or feeding intolerance.

Congenital colonic atresia is a distinctly unusual condition. In a contemporary series of 277 infants treated with intestinal atresia, 21 children had colonic atresia (35). Similar to small bowel atresia, colonic atresia is believed to reflect fetal mesenteric vascular injury. The diagnostic evaluation and surgical treatment of colonic atresia are essentially identical to the approach used for small bowel atresia. Colonic atresia may be associated with abdominal wall defects, skeletal or cardiac defects, or other coexisting intestinal atresias.

Clinical Presentation

The actual incidence of congenital intestinal atresia is unknown. Reported estimates in the United States are 3.5 to 3.75 cases per 10,000 total births (36). Infants with jejunal or ileal atresia generally have a low incidence (< 10%) of significant associated anomalies. Conversely, about 10% to 20% of infants with abdominal wall defects such as gastroschisis will have associated intestinal atresia or stenosis secondary to mechanical interruption of the mesenteric vascular supply.

The detection of maternal polyhydramnios on routine prenatal ultrasound screening can be an indication of fetal proximal bowel obstruction caused by the interruption of normal amniotic fluid absorption in the fetal gut (37). Following delivery, the classic clinical presentation of intestinal atresia is bilious emesis, abdominal distention, and failure to pass meconium. The degree of abdominal distention depends on the site of obstruction, the infant's age, and the efficacy of proximal decompression. Generally, distal obstruction in an infant with longer postpartum age will have greater distention of the proximal bowel. Infants with proximal obstruction of the jejunum or duodenum with adequate gastric decompression may have relatively minimal abdominal distention. Intestinal loops may be visible or palpable on abdominal examination. Umbilical cord ulceration associated with intestinal atresia has been described (38). Rectal examination is important when intestinal obstruction is suspected. The presence of white mucus in the rectum is consistent with intestinal obstruction distal to the ampulla of Vater. Infants with intestinal obstruction proximal to the ampulla of Vater typically have bile-stained meconium in the rectum. In some instances, bile-stained

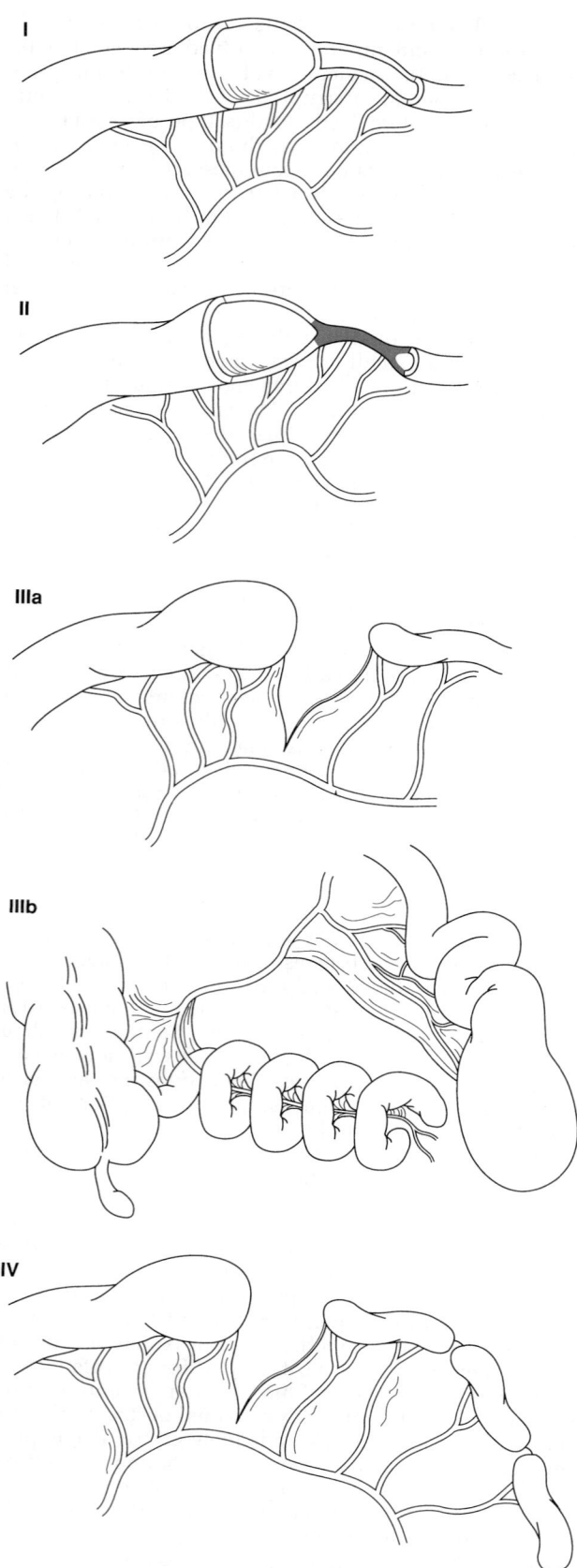

Figure 97.7. Classification of intestinal atresia. Type I, muscular continuity with a complete web. Type II, mesentery intact, fibrous cord. Type IIIa, muscular and mesenteric discontinuous. Type IIIb, apple-peel deformity. Type IV, multiple atresias. (From Grosfeld JL. Jejunoileal atresia and stenosis. In: O'Neill JA Jr, Rowe MI, Grosfeld JL, et al., eds. *Pediatric surgery,* 5th ed. St. Louis: Mosby, 1998:1145–1158, with permission.)

meconium may be seen distal to a small bowel atresia that develops late in gestation.

Diagnosis

After the history and physical examination, plain radiographic films of the abdomen should be obtained. Plain films in jejunal or ileal atresia demonstrate marked gaseous distention of the proximal intestine with gasless distal small bowel and colon. Haustral markings are normally not apparent in the neonatal colon, and therefore discrimination between small bowel and colon in the newborn is difficult without intraluminal contrast. A contrast enema generally is obtained to confirm the diagnosis of jejunoileal atresia. A diminutive, unused but otherwise normal microcolon is typical of proximal intestinal obstruction. The inability to reflux contrast into the proximal, dilated small bowel segment is essentially diagnostic of small bowel atresia. This radiographic finding, in conjunction with the clinical setting, warrants operative exploration. An upper gastrointestinal series is generally unnecessary and may increase the risk of further emesis and aspiration in the newborn with obstruction. Incomplete obstruction from a fenestrated web or diaphragm may require more sophisticated imaging techniques, such as catheter-directed enteroclysis.

Treatment

Anatomic lesions causing neonatal intestinal obstruction require operative treatment. Whereas malrotation with midgut volvulus requires emergent diagnostic workup and operative intervention to prevent bowel loss and death, obstruction resulting from intestinal atresia generally is not associated with life-threatening physiologic disturbances. Therefore, initial treatment should be aimed at treating any other associated problems, confirming the suspected diagnosis, and preparing the infant for an operation under general anesthesia. During this period, the infant always should have an orogastric or nasogastric tube in place and on suction to provide proximal decompression of the obstructed bowel.

The operative strategy in the surgical treatment of intestinal atresia is to restore continuity to the gastrointestinal tract while preserving as much of the intestinal length as possible. The operation is straightforward and an end-to-end or end-to-oblique (end-to-back) anastomosis typically is performed (Fig. 97.8). Short segmental bowel resection and excision of an intraluminal web or diaphragm are used when necessary. Visual inspection and instillation of intraluminal saline to exclude a distal atresia or web prior to anastomosis can help to evaluate patency of the downstream bowel. The size discrepancy between the proximal and distal bowel is usually quite considerable, and typically a moderate delay occurs in the postoperative return of bowel motility. Some surgeons advocate the use of technical procedures to improve emptying of the proximal bowel by reducing the overall diameter of the bowel. These procedures include resection, plication, and tapering enteroplasty. Complex atresia associated with apple-peel deformity or multiple segmental atresias may require multiple serial anastomoses to preserve as much bowel length as possible. The ileocecal valve is preserved whenever possible, allowing improved tolerance of enteral nutrition in infants with limited small bowel length. It is estimated that about 40 cm of small bowel without an ileocecal valve, compared with 15 to 20 cm with an ileocecal valve, is sufficient for long-term enteral feeding tolerance in the neonate (39). The treatment of colonic atresia is essentially identical to small bowel atresia. Contemporary management of colonic atresia includes primary anastomosis whenever possible.

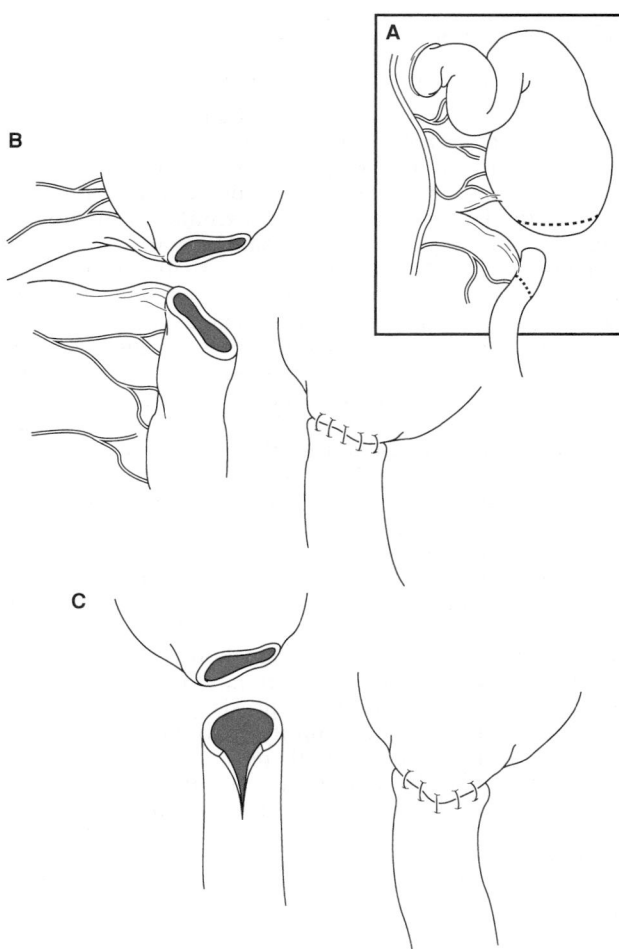

Figure 97.8. *(A,B)* The end-to-oblique anastomosis for small bowel atresia. *(C)* An extension of the distal enterostomy along the antimesenteric border may be used to create proximal and distal lumens of equal size for anastomosis.

Results and Outcome

Currently, the overall survival rate for infants treated for intestinal atresia or stenosis (including duodenal atresia) exceeds 93% in most large series (35,40). Mortality in these infants generally is related to cardiac anomalies and other associated congenital defects. In addition, infants with a limited amount of intestinal length for nutritional absorption (short bowel syndrome; <40 cm) usually require long-term TPN and are at moderate to high risk for sepsis and liver injury. Infants with normal gastrointestinal length still may have prolonged dysfunction of the gut and delayed return of gastrointestinal motility for several days to weeks. Whether this dysfunction is related to physiologic abnormalities in the proximally dilated segment of bowel (41) or the distal microbowel (42) remains to be determined. During this limited period, the development of cholestatic jaundice related to TPN is common and usually is reversible with the establishment of enteral feeding.

Congenital Duodenal Obstruction

Causes of duodenal obstruction in the newborn include duodenal atresia or stenosis, duodenal intraluminal web, and annular pancreas. Because of the common embryologic basis, clinical presentation, and treatment, these entities are considered jointly.

Embryology and Anatomy

The duodenum is derived from both the caudal segment of the foregut and the cranial segment of the midgut. Duodenal development is intimately related to the developing liver, bile ducts, and pancreas. The processes of epithelial proliferation and recanalization are similar in the duodenum and the midgut. The fetal pancreas arises from the paired dorsal and ventral foregut diverticula during week 6 of gestation. The dorsal anlage gives rise to the body and tail of the pancreas as well as the main pancreatic duct. The ventral anlage migrates 180 degrees to fuse with the dorsal gland, forming the uncinate process and the distal portion of the duct of Wirsung (Fig. 97.9). An annular pancreas is characterized by the glandular persistence surrounding the duodenum at the site of the embryonic ventral anlage. It is invariably associated with intrinsic duodenal obstruction, and a patent accessory pancreatic duct is common (43) (Fig. 97.10).

It is believed that the vast majority of congenital duodenal obstructions result from abnormalities of pancreatic development, failure of duodenal recanalization, or vascular compromise to the duodenum. In contrast to jejunoileal atresia, congenital duodenal obstruction is about evenly divided between intraluminal webs or stenoses and complete atresia. Duodenal atresia may occur with or without seromuscular continuity, and an intraluminal duodenal web may occur with or without fenestration. The most frequent location for duodenal atresia is in the descending duodenum near and distal to the ampulla of Vater. Most series report a 5% to 10% incidence of duodenal atresia proximal to the ampulla, giving rise to nonbilious gastric contents and emesis. Another important variant is a periampullary web that projects distally into the duodenal or jejunal lumen, forming a wind-sock deformity (Fig. 97.11). In this instance, the ampulla must be clearly identified before excision and repair because of the proximity and even incorporation of the ampulla into the web.

Clinical Presentation

The incidence of congenital duodenal obstruction is estimated to be about 1 in 6,000 to 10,000 births (44). About 30% of these infants will have trisomy 21 (45). Infants born with duodenal atresia should be examined with a high degree of suspicion for trisomy 21 and undergo routine karyotype analysis. Other associated anomalies, such as congenital heart disease, genitourinary tract malformation, and musculoskeletal disorders, are common in these infants, and appropriate preoperative work-up is necessary.

Congenital duodenal obstruction presents in the first 24 to 48 hours of life with feeding intolerance and bilious emesis. As previously noted, duodenal obstruction proximal to the ampulla of Vater will result in nonbilious emesis. On physical examination, infants with untreated duodenal obstruction may have a palpable stomach in the epigastrium, and gastric peristaltic waves may be visible. The collapsed and unused distal small intestine typically does not produce diffuse abdominal distention. Partial duodenal obstruction from a fenestrated web may not produce symptoms in the newborn period, and delayed diagnosis is common.

Diagnosis

Routine fetal ultrasound examination demonstrating maternal polyhydramnios should elicit a careful investigation for the presence of a proximal foregut obstruction. With contemporary ultrasound techniques, duodenal atresia can be diagnosed prenatally (46). Following birth, infants with suspected duodenal atresia should

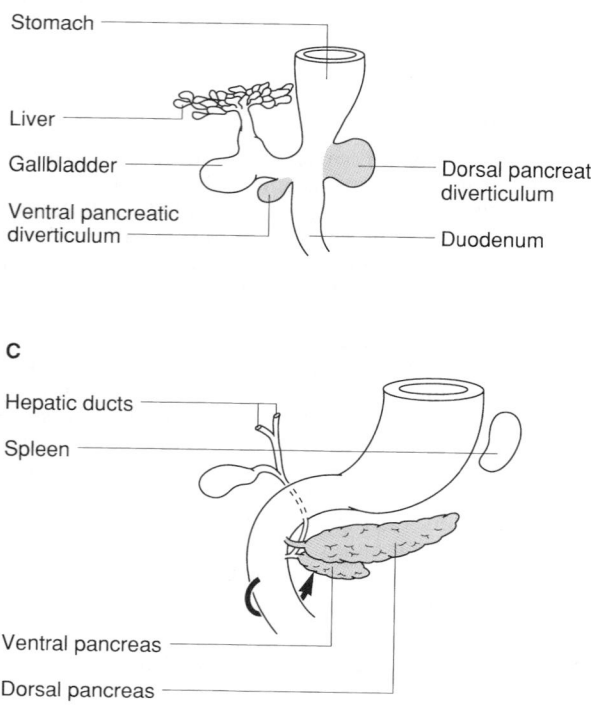

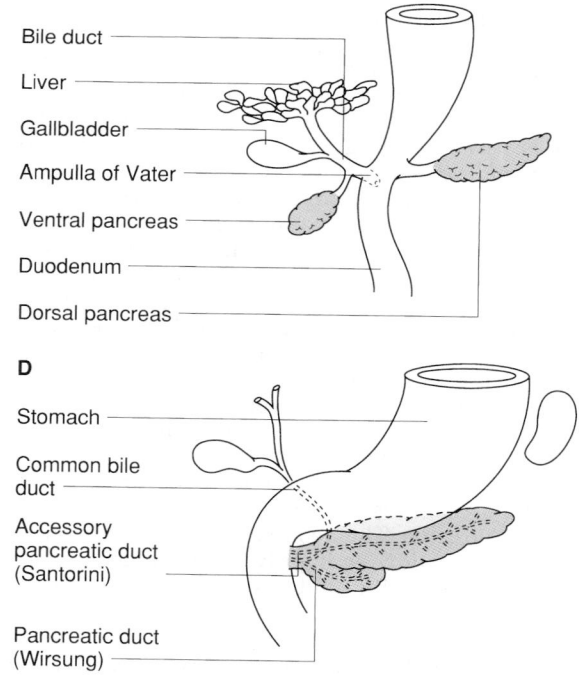

Figure 97.9. Normal embryologic development of the duodenum, pancreas, and bile ducts. *(A)* Fifth gestational week. *(B)* Sixth week. *(C)* Seventh week. *(D)* Eighth week.

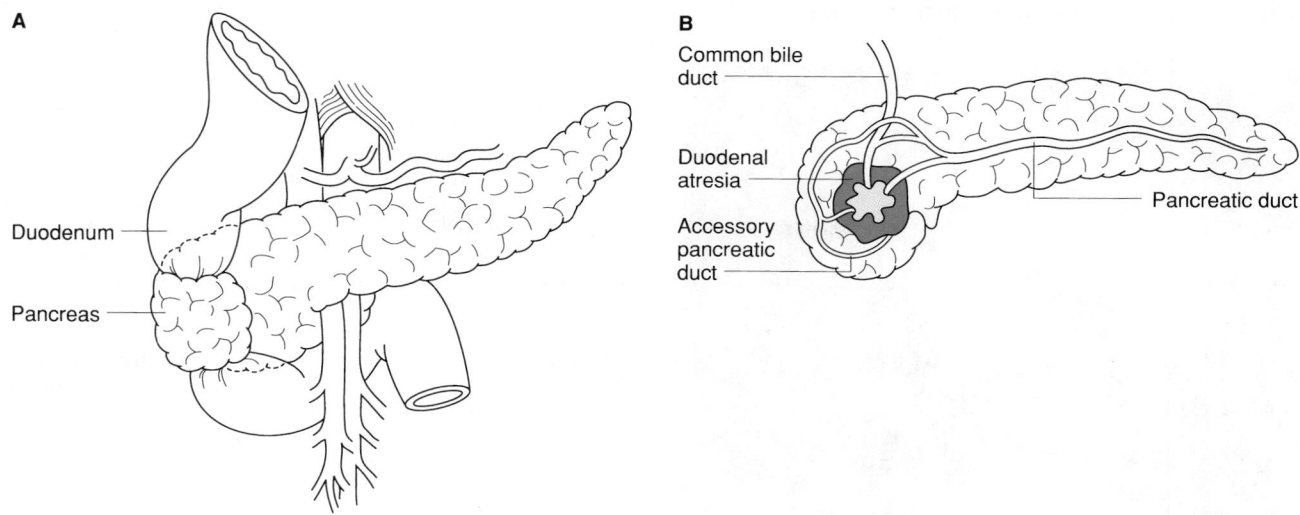

Figure 97.10. Annular pancreas. *(A)* The associated duodenal atresia is shown. *(B)* The relationships of the annular pancreas to the common bile duct and main and accessory pancreatic ducts are shown in cross-section.

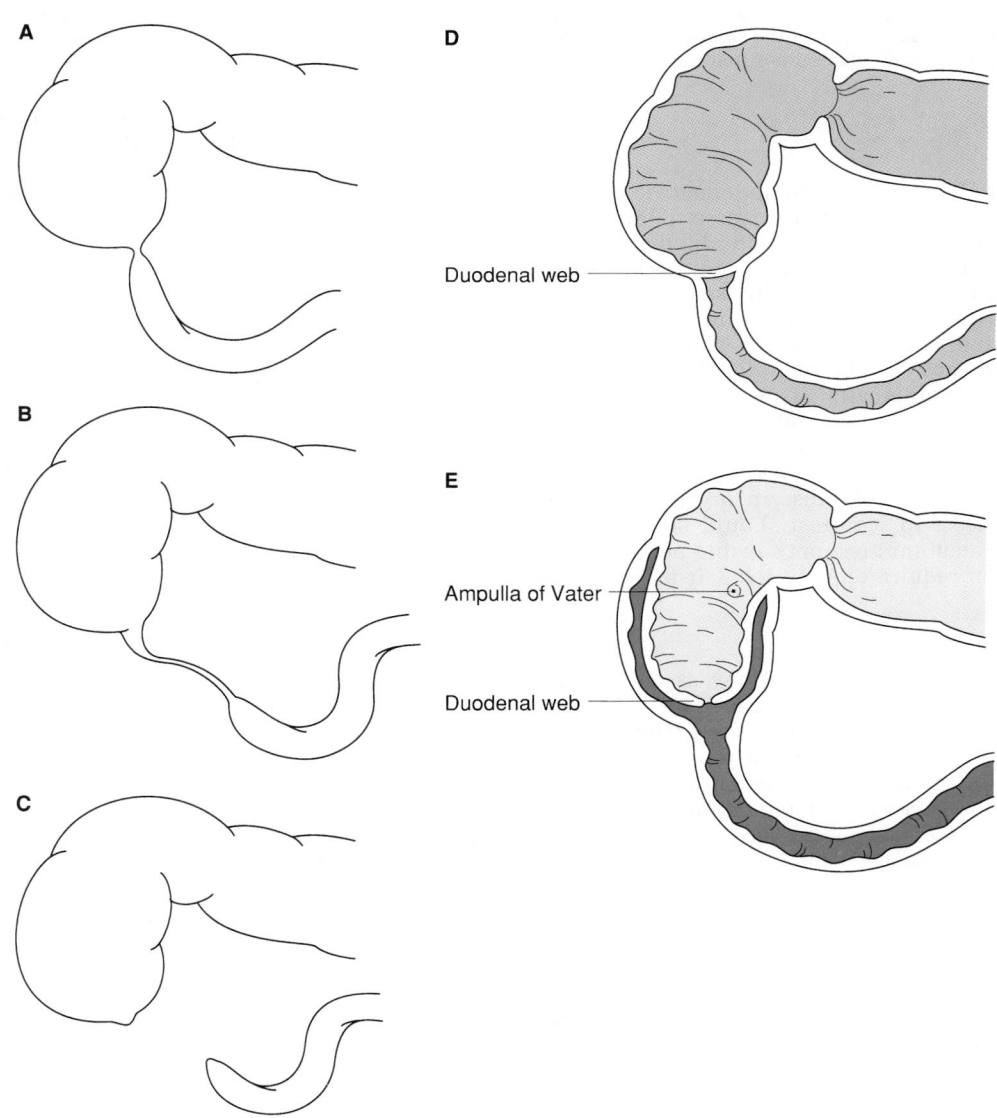

Figure 97.11. Anatomic forms of duodenal atresia *(A–C)* and webs *(D,E)*. In particular, *(E)* demonstrates the unique wind-sock deformity. This lesion is important and potentially confusing because the point of obstruction is not at the apparent point of change in luminal diameter.

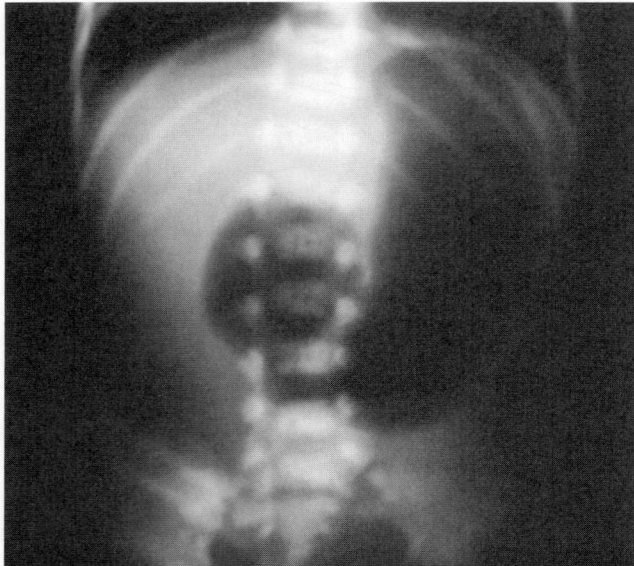

Figure 97.12. Classic radiographic appearance of duodenal atresia. There is a double bubble of gas in the stomach and proximal duodenum, with no gas in the distal intestinal tract.

undergo plain radiographs of the abdomen. The classic radiographic finding of duodenal atresia is a double bubble from the air-filled stomach and duodenum (Fig. 97.12). In complete duodenal obstruction, no gas will be seen distal to the duodenum; in this setting, the plain film is sufficiently diagnostic that no further imaging of the gastrointestinal tract is necessary. If there is incomplete obstruction, gas may be seen distally in the small or large intestine. Infants with suspected incomplete obstruction at the duodenal level might have either a fenestrated web or volvulus secondary to malrotation. Given the need for emergent operative intervention in malrotation with acute volvulus, an urgent upper gastrointestinal series with contrast should be performed. Importantly, all anatomic lesions causing neonatal duodenal obstruction require operative repair using a similar approach.

Treatment

Following expedient treatment of any associated life-threatening medical conditions and a preoperative evaluation including an echocardiogram, infants with congenital duodenal obstruction are explored promptly. Because the differential diagnosis of duodenal obstruction includes duodenal atresia versus malrotation with obstructive Ladd's bands (see later discussion), immediate surgical exploration is advised. The operative goals are to restore gastrointestinal continuity without sacrificing intestinal length or absorptive surface area. Because most obstructive duodenal lesions are near the ampulla of Vater, great care must be exercised in their treatment to avoid inadvertent injury to the ampulla or pancreas.

Congenital duodenal atresia is treated by bypass in the form of duodenoduodenostomy. Usually, duodenojejunostomy is avoided to prevent exclusion of the distal portion of the duodenum ("blind loop"); currently, this procedure generally is reserved for obstructive lesions of the distal duodenum. Duodenal obstruction secondary to annular pancreas also is treated by duodenoduodenostomy. Direct division of annular pancreas is not performed because this

does not address the underlying intraluminal duodenal obstruction, and there is significant risk of injury to the accessory pancreatic duct (Fig. 97.10).

Duodenoduodenostomy is performed by making a transverse incision in the dilated, proximal duodenum and a longitudinal incision in the unused, downstream duodenum. The lumens are sutured together to form a diamond-shape anastomosis (Fig. 97.13) (47). Downstream duodenum patency must be demonstrated by passing a catheter or infusing saline distally to avoid overlooking a synchronous intestinal atresia.

Duodenal webs are excised through a longitudinal duodenotomy. The wind-sock duodenal web must be clearly identified because the visible transition from the distended, proximal duodenum to the small, downstream duodenum may be several centimeters distal to the base of the web. Traction applied at the apex of the web deforms the duodenum at its point of attachment and allows complete excision at the base. The ampulla of Vater must be unequivocally identified before duodenal web excision to avoid injury. Closure of the longitudinal duodenotomy is performed transversely to avoid narrowing of the duodenum.

There is typically great size discrepancy between the dilated, proximal pouch and the distal duodenal lumen, leading some surgeons to advocate procedures designed to reduce the diameter of the proximal duodenum and facilitate improved postoperative bowel motility. These procedures, which include tapering duodenoplasty and duodenal plication, are viewed as primary procedures with limited enthusiasm because comparison outcome data are not available.

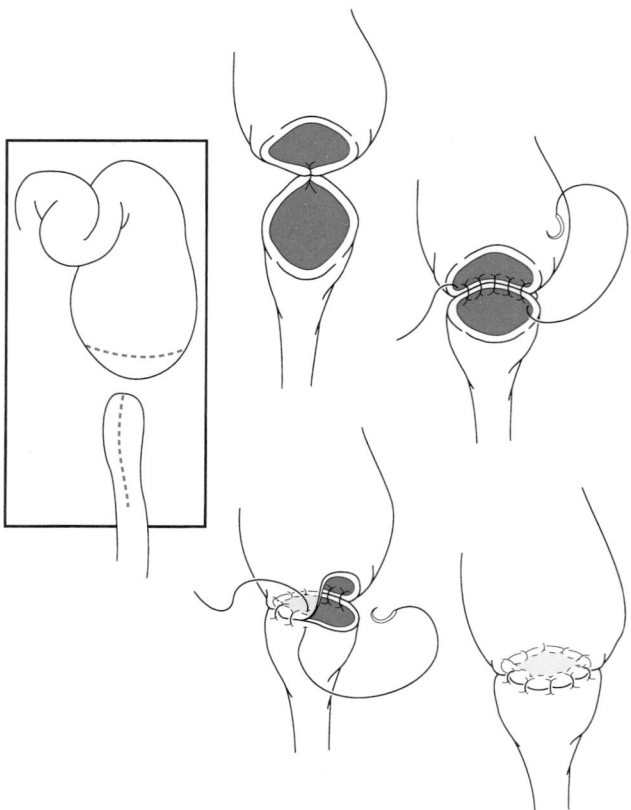

Figure 97.13. Diamond-shaped duodenoduodenostomy for repair of duodenal atresia.

Results and Outcome

After successful operative repair of duodenal atresia or stenosis, delay in gastric emptying is common and typically manifests as enteral feeding intolerance. Patience and persistence are essential during the postoperative period. Surgical outcomes after repair of congenital duodenal obstruction are excellent (46–48), with contemporary immediate operative survival exceeding 95%. Perioperative mortality generally is related to associated anomalies, in particular, in infants with trisomy 21 with congenital heart defects. Other late problems also can be encountered, including poor gastric emptying, duodenal dysmotility or dilatation, and gastroesophageal reflux, persisting or presenting several months to years following repair. Therefore, these infants should be followed up on a long-term basis for surgery-related issues.

Anorectal Malformations (Imperforate Anus)

Embryology

By week 5 of gestation, the fetal cloaca is identifiable with the adjacent hindgut, allantois, and vestigial tailgut (Fig. 97.14). The mesoderm of the urorectal septum extends caudally to fuse with the cloacal closing plate (31). Fusion of the lateral cloacal ridges completes the division of the cloaca into the rectum and the urogenital sinus. The caudal aspect of the urorectal septum forms the perineal body. The anal membrane normally ruptures during week 8 of gestation, completing the patency of the distal rectum to the skin. Further development of the urogenital sinus leads to the formation of the urethra and bladder. In female infants, the uterus and portions of the vagina develop from the müllerian ducts. The diverse anatomic variation observed with anorectal malformations is thought to reflect anomalous or interrupted development of these structures during normal embryogenesis.

Anatomy and Classification

The normal anatomy of the anus and rectum is reviewed in previous chapters. Normally, the rectum descends to the perineum and ultimately, to the anal orifice through a striated muscle complex in the pelvis resembling a funnel. The striated muscle complex is under voluntary control and is responsible for providing fecal continence (Fig. 97.15). Contiguous portions of the *levator ani,* the external *sphincter,* and the *puborectalis* muscles compose the *striated muscle complex.* These are anatomically indistinct components of the striated muscle complex that act together to provide control of defecation. The concept of the striated muscle complex and anatomic relationships leading to normal fecal continence with respect to anorectal malformations has evolved from both clinical and anatomic data as described by Peña (49).

Because of the various patterns of anorectal malformations observed, different classification systems have been proposed in an attempt to characterize the defects. A summary of the 1984 Wingspread Classification is provided in Table 97.3. This is an anatomically descriptive, well-accepted classification scheme that is useful in planning the operative management of anorectal malformations. Detailed discussion of the anatomy, classification, and repair of these lesions is beyond the scope of this review, and an overview is provided here.

In male subjects, the two most common anorectal malformations observed are low imperforate anus with a perineal fistula (Fig. 97.16) and high anorectal agenesis with a rectoprostatic urethral fistula (Fig. 97.17). Male patients without a perineal fistula are assumed to have high imperforate anus with a rectourethral fistula until proven otherwise. In female subjects, the most common malformation encountered is low imperforate anus with a fistula from the blind-ending rectal pouch to either the perineal body or the vaginal vestibule (Fig. 97.18). As these malformations result from developmental arrest at various times during migration of the urogenital septum, considerable anatomic variability exists in both male and female subjects.

A common anatomic feature of imperforate anus is incomplete descent of the rectum to the perineum. Consequently, the rectum is not completely within the striated muscle complex. Therefore, the caudal portion of the striated muscle complex remains a solid mass of striated muscle, whereas the cephalad portion may be normally positioned circumferentially around the rectal pouch. In low

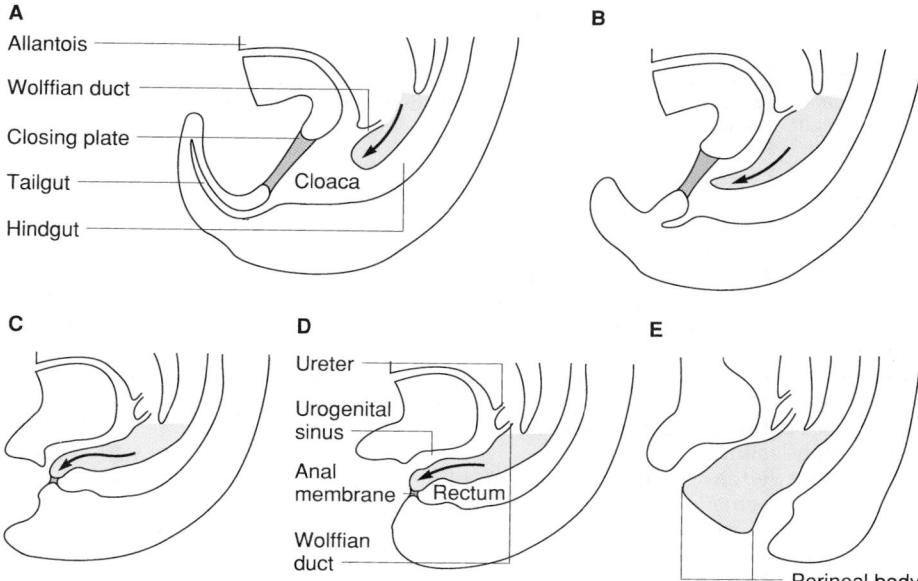

Figure 97.14. Normal embryologic division of the cloaca by the urorectal septum into the ventral urinary tract and the dorsal rectum. This process is normally completed by the ninth or tenth week of gestation.

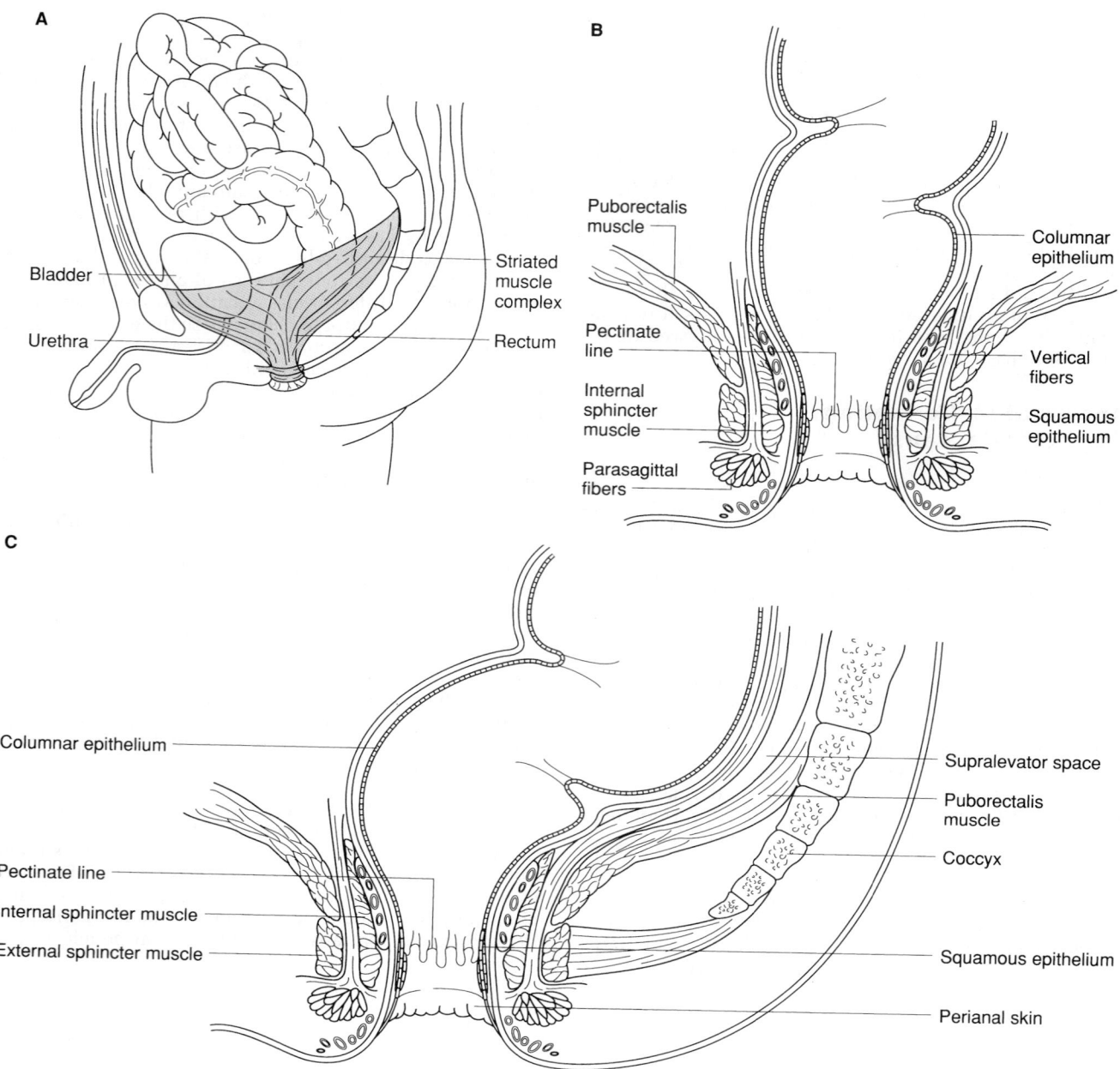

Figure 97.15. The normal relations of the pelvic striated muscle complex and the rectum. *(A)* Normal male anatomy. *(B)* Coronal view showing individual components of the striated muscle complex. *(C)* Sagittal view of normal anatomy (49).

imperforate anus, the rectum nearly reaches the perineum, and the configuration of the striated muscle complex surrounding the rectum more closely approximates normal. With high imperforate anus, less striated muscle surrounds the rectal pouch. Some degree of intrinsic hypoplasia of the striated muscle complex occurs with virtually all anorectal malformations (50), although the physiologic effects are variable. It is clear, however, that low lesions carry a more favorable prognosis for fecal continence than do high lesions.

The classic delineation between low and high anorectal malformations is made anatomically at the pubococcygeal line. Low imperforate anus describes a rectal pouch descending within the striated muscle complex below the inferior border of the ossified ischium and the pubococ-

cygeal line. The vast majority of low lesions have associated perineal or vestibular fistulas. High imperforate anus has a blind-ending rectal pouch above the pubococcygeal line and, therefore, above the striated muscle complex (or *levator ani*). Some lesions have a variable degree of descent into the striated muscle complex and are described anatomically as intermediate malformations.

Associated Anomalies

Infants with anorectal malformations, particularly high lesions, have an incidence of associated anomalies as high as 70% (50). The VACTERL (vertebral, anal, cardiac, tracheal, esophageal, renal and limb), or VATER (vertebral, anal, trancheoesophageal, renal, and radial limb anomalies) associations are important and require consideration

Table 97.3. ANATOMIC CLASSIFICATION OF ANORECTAL MALFORMATIONS

Female	Male
High	High
Anorectal agenesis	Anorectal agenesis
With rectovaginal fistula	With rectoprostatic
Without fistula	urethral fistula[a]
Rectal atresia	Without fistula
Intermediate	Rectal atresia
Rectovestibular fistula	Intermediate
Rectovaginal fistula	Rectobulbar urethral fistula
Anal agenesis without fistula	Anal agenesis without fistula
Low	Low
Anovestibular fistula[a]	Anocutaneous fistula[a]
Anocutaneous fistula[a,b]	Anal stenosis[a,c]
Anal stenosis[c]	Rare malformations
Cloacal malformations[d]	
Rare malformations	

[a]Relatively common lesion.
[b]Includes fistulas occuring at the posterior junction of the labia minora, often called fourchette fistulas or vulvar fistulas.
[c]Previously called covered anus.
[d]Previously called rectocloacal fistulas. Entry of the rectal fistula into the cloaca may be high or intermediate, depending on the length of the cloacal canal.

From Oldham KT. Gastrointestinal disorders. In: Greenfield MW, Oldham KT, Zelenock GB, et al., eds. Surgery: scientific principles and practice, 2nd ed. Philadelphia: Lippincott–Raven, 1997:2034–2078, with permission.

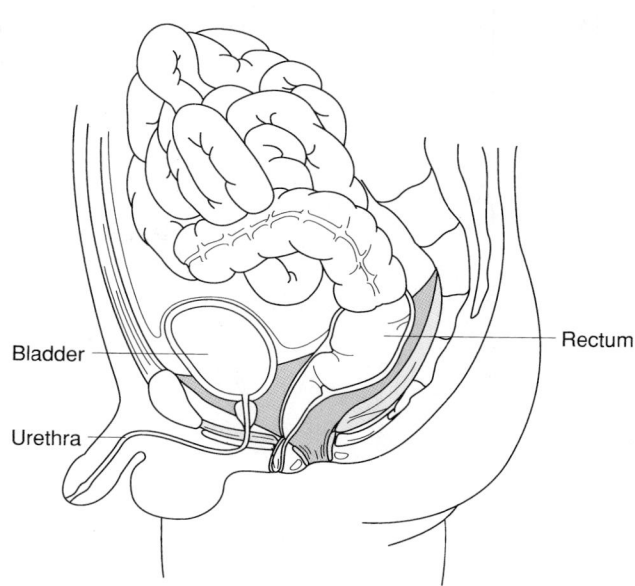

Figure 97.16. Male infant with low imperforate anus and perineal fistula. Note that the fistula is anterior to the striated muscle complex.

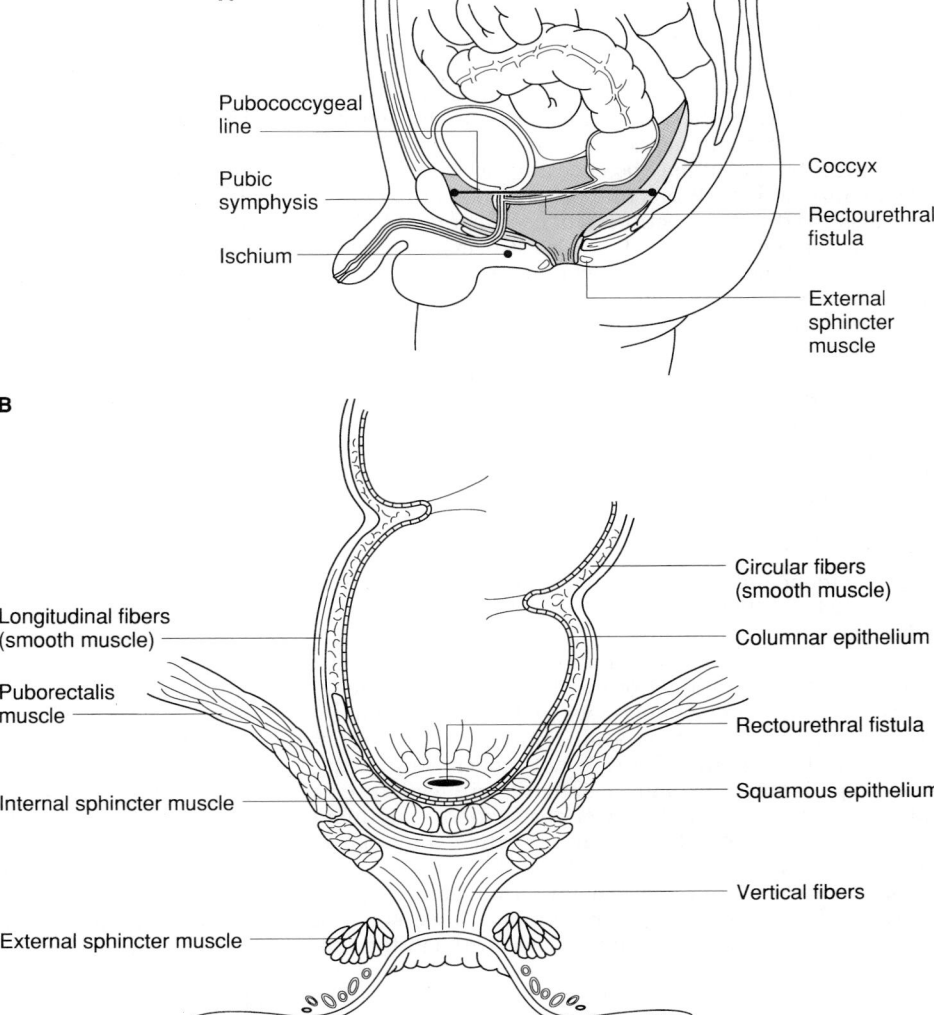

Figure 97.17. Male infant with high imperforate anus, showing the pubococcygeal line, ischium, and striated muscle complex. *(A)* The rectal pouch ends cephalad to the pubococcygeal line. This location of the rectourethral fistula is typical. *(B)* Coronal view showing incomplete development of the rectal pouch within the striated muscle complex. The rectourethral fistula is shown.

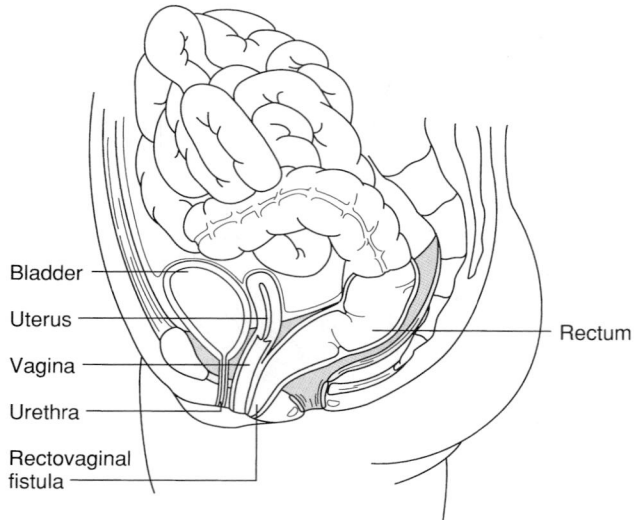

Bladder

Uterus

Vagina

Urethra

Rectovaginal
fistula

Rectum

Figure 97.18. Female infant with low imperforate anus and vestibular fistula.

in any infant with imperforate anus. *Vertebral anomalies* are common and include sacral dysplasia and agenesis. Infants with sacral anomalies commonly have high imperforate anus and sacral autonomic dysfunction that can lead to poor long-term fecal continence and neurogenic bladder. A variety of spinal cord malformations also can be observed in these infants, including tethered spinal cord syndromes and some myelodysplastic syndromes. During the neonatal period, these spinal lesions may be detected by using ultrasound or magnetic resonance imaging (MRI), and surgical treatment may be necessary within the first 8 to 18 months of life. *Anorectal malformations* include lesions discussed in this section. *Tracheoesophageal* fistula with or without esophageal atresia is estimated to occur in about 10% of infants with anorectal malformations. *Renal anomalies* are the most common associated abnormalities with anorectal malformations and include both upper and lower tract conditions. Genitourinary screening in the form of a renal ultrasound is routinely performed, and typically a voiding cystourethrogram is obtained preoperatively. *Cardiac* anomalies are common, and screening echocardiography is clinically indicated. *Limb abnormalities,* in particular, involvement of the radius, complete the associated anomalies defined by that acronym.

Clinical Presentation

The incidence of anorectal malformations is estimated at 1 in 2,524 to 5,000 live births (51), with a slightly higher incidence in male compared to female subjects. High lesions are also twice as common in male as female infants. Clinical physical examination of the neonatal perineum typically reveals the diagnosis. As such, the anatomic location of the anus must be evaluated and patency confirmed in all newborn infants. If not recognized, an untreated high imperforate anus eventually will lead to signs and symptoms of complete bowel obstruction. The infant will develop abdominal distention, feeding intolerance, and bilious emesis associated with failure of passage of meconium. Because of the nearly uniform rectourethral or rectovesicular fistula in high imperforate anus, some of these infants will pass meconium or gas through the urethra during urination. In contrast, infants with low malformations typically pass meconium through a perineal or vestibular fistula within the first 24 hours of life. Occa-

sionally, infants with low lesions associated with large fistulas will not be diagnosed with imperforate anus until difficulty passing stool is noticed weeks to months after birth, particularly at the time of progressing to solid foods.

Delineation of high versus low anorectal malformations is generally made by physical examination. In male infants, more than 95% of low malformations are associated with either a thin anal membrane or a fistula to the perineum or scrotal raphe. The presence of a "bucket-handle" skin deformity at the presumptive anal dimple is also diagnostic of a low lesion. Infants with high malformations typically lack anal skin dimpling, have a flat gluteal contour, and may have little or absent contraction of the external sphincter with cutaneous stimulation. In female infants, 90% to 95% of low malformations have a perineal or vestibular fistula. In both male and female infants, a perineal fistula may not become apparent in the first 12 to 24 hours of life until meconium progresses distally through the rectum into the fistula.

Diagnosis

From a clinical standpoint, intermediate lesions are treated as high malformations; thus, the two groups are considered jointly. Because surgical treatment of a high or intermediate anorectal malformation is different from that for low lesion, a primary diagnostic goal is to determine whether an infant with imperforate anus has a high or low malformation. A secondary diagnostic goal is to determine the specific anorectal malformation as it relates to the rectourethral or rectourinary fistula. The infant with imperforate anus also must be assessed in a comprehensive fashion for associated congenital anomalies (see preceding).

Clinical examination of an infant with low imperforate anus almost always will reveal an external fistula to the perineum or vestibule. In male infants, an external fistula along the scrotal raphe may not become apparent until 1 or 2 days after birth. The classic radiographic study of newborns with imperforate anus is the Wangensteen-Rice invertogram, with a lateral view of the pelvis obtained 12 to 24 hours after birth with the infant in a head-down position. Swallowed air serves as intraluminal contrast, and using a radiodense perineal skin marker, the relationship of the rectal pouch to the perineum, pubococcygeal line, and the ischium is assessed. The procedure is accurate if conducted by a technically skilled and experienced examiner; however, incomplete distention of the distal rectum with gas may decrease the accuracy of this technique. Other diagnostic modalities to define high versus low lesions include the prone cross-table lateral view (52) as well as ultrasound (53). Real-time ultrasound is currently well accepted as an accurate diagnostic modality in determining the distal extent of the rectal pouch.

If there is a suspected fistula site or a covered anus on the perineum, diagnostic needle aspiration may be useful. Typically, this aspiration is done as an examination with the patient under anesthesia. Aspiration of meconium not only localizes the rectum or fistula, but it also can provide an estimation of the distance between the perineum and the rectum or the fistula. In general, low lesions are within 1 to 2 cm of the perineum; high lesions are greater than 2 cm from the perineum. Following physical examination, diagnostic imaging and, if necessary, needle aspiration, almost all infants with anorectal malformations can be categorized into high or low lesions. Any infant not clearly found to have a low lesion should be considered to have a high or intermediate anorectal malformation and should be treated accordingly.

A voiding cystourethrogram is generally the procedure of choice to defining the rectourethral or rectovesical fistula. Following diverting colostomy for high imperforate anus, a distal contrast study into the downstream colon also can define the fistula but, more importantly, allows clear delineation of the rectal pouch in relation to the perineal skin. In some instances, cystoscopy is a useful adjunct before repair of high imperforate anus. For example, an infant with a large rectourethral fistula may require cystoscopic guidance of a urinary catheter to avoid inadvertent placement of the catheter through the fistula and into the rectum.

Computed tomography (CT) imaging and MRI can be extremely useful in evaluating the striated muscle complex in the pelvis. In particular, advanced imaging of infants requiring reoperation following initial anorectoplasty can help to define the intrinsic position and structure of the striated muscle complex in relation to the rectum. As previously mentioned, MRI is also useful in evaluation of the distal spinal cord in these infants.

Treatment

After diagnosis of an anorectal malformation in a neonate, complete evaluation of associated anomalies is essential before operative management. In general, imperforate anus by itself is not a life-threatening condition, and, in many instances, observation for 12 to 24 hours may help to delineate the presence or absence of a fistula as meconium progresses distally in the rectal pouch. The surgical management of anorectal malformations has been well described elsewhere (49) and a brief summary follows below.

Low Malformations. Definitive repair of most low anorectal malformations can be performed in the newborn period with relatively straightforward perineal procedures that do not require a diverting colostomy. Often simple dilation of the fistula or unroofing of a covered anus under local anesthesia may relieve the anatomic obstruction. For more complex anal stenoses or anterior perineal fistulas, a more formal perineal anoplasty may be required. The most common perineal procedure is the cutback anoplasty, in which the anterior fistula or anal orifice is opened posteriorly by dividing the perineum to the external sphincter. More complex alternative approaches may be preferred in female infants with low vaginal or anterior perineal fistulas. These lesions generally require circumferential mobilization of the anterior fistula with transposition to the center of the external sphincter. Anterior reconstruction of the perineal body then is performed. This transposition anoplasty is designed to position the neoanus within the center of the external sphincter and separate the neoanus from the vaginal introitus.

Intermediate and High Malformations. Infants determined clinically to have an intermediate, high, or indeterminate anorectal malformation require a diverting colostomy in their initial surgical management. The proximal diverting colostomy may be placed either in the sigmoid or transverse colon, but care must be taken to ensure that the selected site provides adequate length and mobility of the distal colon in anticipation of an eventual anorectoplasty. A divided colostomy is preferred by many surgeons over a loop colostomy to provide the maximal diversion of the fecal stream from the distal rectourinary fistula.

Anorectoplasty generally is performed when the infant is around 12 months of age or when the infant weighs more than 8 kg. Many different approaches have been described, and considerable personal and institutional variation is common. No single approach has superior results, and all have technical merits and difficulties. The common surgical objectives in the treatment of anorectal malformations include (1) to relieve the rectal obstruction, (2) to place the distal rectal pouch on the perineum and construct a neoanus, (3) to position the pulled-through rectum as normally as possible within the striated muscle complex, and (4) to divide the rectourinary fistula. In addition, preservation of the surrounding structures (prostate, urethra, seminal vesicles, vaginal wall, and so on) is essential.

For repair of high and intermediate anorectal malformations, the most widely used procedure in the United States is the posterior sagittal anorectoplasty described in detail by Peña (49). The concept of this approach is straightforward and allows good visibility of the rectourinary fistula. The infant is placed prone, and a posterior sagittal incision following the gluteal crease is used. The external sphincter and the striated muscle complex are divided posteriorly along the midline to expose the rectal pouch. A muscle stimulator is used to define and map the striated muscle complex and to confirm symmetric dissection along the midline. Typically, the rectal pouch can be adequately dissected by this approach to allow enough length to reach the perineum. Infrequently, a combined abdominal approach is required to mobilize the distal rectum enough to reach the perineum. The mobilized rectal pouch is opened and the rectourinary fistula identified and closed under direct vision. The rectal pouch then is placed centrally within the striated muscle complex, which is reconstructed circumferentially around the rectum. The neoanus is centered within the external sphincter and the mucosa is sutured to the perineum.

Other widely accepted and practiced surgical approaches to imperforate anus include a sacroperineal approach as proposed by Stephens (54,55), and an approach that uses components of endorectal dissection as attributed to Rehbein (56). Both these surgical procedures are characterized by blind pull-through of the distal rectum without direct visualization of the striated muscle complex. Mollard and colleagues (57) use a combined abdominal and anterior perineal approach, again with a relatively blind pull-through of the rectum between the urethra and the puborectalis component of the striated muscle complex. Additionally, growing experience with laparoscopic dissection and division of the rectourinary fistula with perineal pull-through reconstruction has been reported. It appears that personal preference, experience, and familiarity rather than differences in outcome dictate the selection of procedure. In general, the diverting colostomy in all these procedures is maintained until the anorectoplasty has completely healed, after which the colostomy is closed electively.

Results, Complications, and Outcome

Mortality following anorectoplasty generally is related to the presence of associated congenital anomalies other than imperforate anus. A careful review of 284 infants undergoing repair of anorectal malformations observed an 18.7% mortality (58), suggesting that this group is at moderate to high risk for complications and death secondary to coexisting congenital anomalies.

Complications are similar to other gastrointestinal surgical procedures and include infection or leak. Leak or stricture formation is observed in 5% to 10% of infants undergoing tapering rectoplasty during posterior sagittal anorectoplasty. Anorectal strictures are treated by gradual postoperative anal dilatation for weeks to months. Recurrent rectourethral fistula or urethral stricture is uncommon.

Long-term functional outcome in infants with low malformations is generally excellent given the relatively normal descent of the distal rectum within the striated muscle complex. Infants with intermediate or high lesions have a less predictable prognosis and are more likely to have difficulty with fecal continence. Currently, the outcomes appear to be independent of the type of surgical reconstruction performed and more related to the abnormal rectal descent, hypoplasia of the striated muscle complex, and abnormal sacral innervation. Few or perhaps none of these children will have completely normal bowel habits after operation. About half (range, 30%–80%) of the infants have good results with few episodes of accidental soilage and relatively simple management using enemas and cathartics (59–61). The remaining children require major adjustments in lifestyle secondary to fecal incontinence, constipation, and odor. In some instances, socially acceptable continence can be assisted by the use of daily antegrade enemas via a cecostomy or appendicostomy. In extreme situations, a permanent diverting colostomy may be desirable.

Necrotizing Enterocolitis

Pathophysiology

Necrotizing enterocolitis is a neonatal disease characterized by an initial mucosal injury of the intestine that ultimately may progress to transmural bowel necrosis. NEC is the most frequent surgical condition of the neonate and a major cause of morbidity and mortality in the premature infant. Despite its frequency and extensive study, the pathogenesis remains obscure, and surgical treatment is directed largely at controlling the complications of intestinal necrosis.

The initial event in NEC appears to be intestinal mucosal injury. The mucosal injury in NEC has been associated with a wide variety of clinical conditions, none of which is specific in effect. The development of NEC occurs within the presence of a variety of associated conditions, including perinatal stress, sepsis, respiratory failure, hypoxemia, hypotension, and congenital cardiac defects. Maternal use of cocaine (62) and tocolysis using indomethacin (63) are considered pharmacologic fetal exposures associated with the subsequent development of NEC. In general, NEC is observed in the critically ill, premature infant with multiple risk factors and potential etiologic events and conditions. Current clinical and experimental data support the concept that the pathophysiology of NEC remains enigmatic and multifactorial.

The intestinal mucosal injury observed in NEC is likely to be the end result of an ischemic insult, either local or global, in a susceptible host. Normally, the neonatal pulmonary and systemic vascular smooth muscle undergoes rapid structural and physiologic changes shortly after birth. The premature infant appears to be particularly vulnerable to vasoconstriction. With regard to NEC, it is conceivable that hypoperfusion and ischemia of the premature neonatal intestinal tract may be the result of uncontrolled splanchnic vasoconstriction. This situation may be worsened in critically ill premature infants with low cardiac output states and relatively high circulating red cell mass leading to hyperviscosity. Perinatal stress such as acidosis, hypoxemia, and hypothermia also are associated with acute pulmonary vascular hypertension and right-to-left shunting via a patent ductus arteriosus. This shunting can significantly decrease oxygen delivery to areas of already marginal tissue perfusion in the neonatal intestine.

Whether the initiating event is acute, such as arterial embolization from an umbilical artery catheter, or more chronic, a common characteristic of NEC is the host inflammatory response to the initiating mucosal injury. Experimental data are consistent with a role for oxygen-derived free radicals as important mediators of this type of intestinal injury. Oxygen-derived free radical mucosal in-

jury occurs by both xanthine oxidase- and NADPH oxidase-dependent pathways following ischemia and reperfusion (64). In an animal model of NEC using luminal injury (as opposed to a vascular injury), local production of superoxide anion generated from sources other than xanthine oxidase appears to play the major role in the development of intestinal injury. An inhibitor of superoxide production, superoxide dismutase, confers protection to both free-radical injury and the induction of leukocyte accumulation in treated intestine (65). Additionally, local production of platelet-activating factor (PAF) is thought to contribute significantly to the inflammatory response and injury at the tissue level (66). Generation of these inflammatory mediators is associated with the induction of the host systemic inflammatory response, including complement activation and cytokine production. Bacterial translocation through the injured mucosal barrier and liberation of bacterial endotoxin amplify this systemic response. Although the local inflammatory response is necessary for repair of injured tissue, an uncontrolled or exaggerated systemic inflammatory response may be elicited in a vulnerable host, ultimately causing multiorgan dysfunction and failure.

More than 90% of cases of NEC occur after the initiation of enteral feeding, and several studies documented that the osmolarity or rate of initial feeding may be important. Although controversy exists, most neonatal centers now avoid rapid advancement of hyperosmolar enteral feedings and attempt to prevent excessive fluid volume in premature infants (67,68). Breast milk, which contains maternal immunoglobulin A (IgA), lymphocytes, macrophages, and PAF-acetylhydrolase (PAF-AH), is thought to confer some protection against mucosal injury. Whether the oral administration of antiinflammatory or immunomodulating agents such as IgG or PAF-AH will decrease the clinical incidence of NEC in high-risk infants remains unclear.

Episodic clustering of cases of NEC has been reported, and infectious etiologic agents such as *Clostridium* species (including *C. difficile*), *Pseudomonas aeruginosa*, *Enterobacter cloacae*, *Staphyloccocus aureus*, and *Klebsiella* species have been implicated. These normal intestinal flora may be more opportunistic in the face of intestinal mucosal injury; whether they are directly responsible for the initiation of NEC remains unclear.

Infants with similar clinical risk factors may have a wide range of intestinal injury and involvement with NEC, from confluent transmural intestinal necrosis of the entire gastrointestinal tract to self-limited and reversible mucosal injury of the terminal ileum. The most common site of involvement is the terminal ileum and right colon, although the disease may be localized or segmental, or it may involve the entire gastrointestinal tract. Histopathologic examination of intestinal tissue from infants with NEC demonstrates ischemic necrosis. The spectrum of involvement includes submucosal edema, hemorrhage, and microvascular thrombosis. The histopathology of NEC resembles that of experimental intestinal ischemia, with areas of reversible mucosal injury adjacent to areas of transmural necrosis (Fig. 97.19). Dissection of intraluminal gas through the disrupted basement membrane of the injured mucosa leads to gas within the bowel wall, known as *pneumatosis intestinalis*. The finding of pneumatosis intestinalis is a classic radiographic and pathologic feature of NEC. Initially, the gas may be localized in the submucosa or lymphatic vessels, but it may dissect into the muscularis, the portal venous tract, or into the subserosa. Intestinal perforation, inflammatory phlegmon, and peritonitis are common with advanced NEC.

In summary, NEC is a clinically important entity that causes significant morbidity and mortality in premature

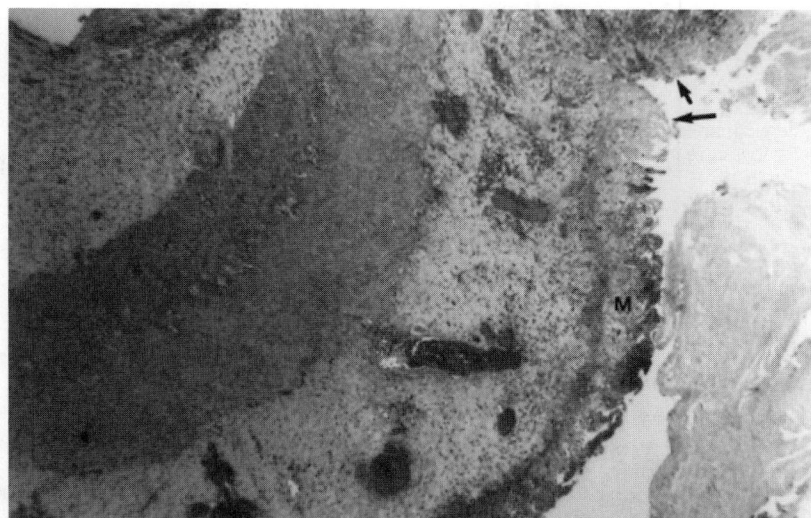

Figure 97.19. Photomicrograph of intestine in an infant with necrotizing enterocolitis. An area of epithelial slough is adjacent to injured but surviving mucosa (M). Despite the obvious injury, the muscular mucosa is not infarcted.

infants. The pathophysiology remains elusive and, in all likelihood, is multifactorial in origin and dependent on host factors for both initiation and propagation (Fig. 97.20).

Clinical Presentation

Over the past three decades, advancements in technology, prenatal care, and neonatology have improved overall outcome in premature infants that were previously unable to survive. In the United States alone, low birth weight (<2,500 g) infants account for approximately 281,015 births (7.41% of all live births), with 67% of these infants born prematurely (69). At least half of all infants with NEC are extremely low birth weight infants weighing less than 1,500 g. In a study of 302 infants with NEC treated over two decades, the average birth weight fell from 1,645 to 1,505 g, and in similar fashion, the mean gestational age fell from 32.4 weeks to 30.4 weeks (70). In fact, although

not directly causative, prematurity and early initiation of enteral feeding are two distinct risk factors for the development of NEC. NEC can also occur in term infants, and in this group, it may present without classic signs and colonic involvement is common (71).

In the United States, NEC represents the most common surgical emergency of the neonate, and it causes significant morbidity and mortality in premature infants. NEC is estimated to occur in 1 to 3 of 1,000 live births and in 30 per 1,000 low birth weight births (72). Interestingly, some data suggest that substantial variation in the prevalence of NEC among different centers may be related to differences in individual clinical practice patterns (73). The actual incidence of NEC remains difficult to determine because the diagnosis is subjective; classic signs on physical examination and diagnostic imaging are not always present in every infant with NEC. The classic clinical signs of NEC include abdominal distention, feeding intolerance, bilious emesis, and either occult or gross blood in the stool. Gastrointestinal mucosal bleeding is present in the vast majority of cases (80% to 90%) but is rarely significant from a hemodynamic standpoint. On physical examination, abdominal tenderness with distention is common, and individual loops of thickened or fixed bowel may be palpable. There is a propensity for involvement of the terminal ileum and cecum, but NEC can be found throughout the gastrointestinal tract. Edema, erythema, crepitus, or discoloration of the abdominal wall suggests intestinal necrosis, perforation, or intraabdominal abscess. Hematochezia or guaiac-positive stool is typical. Systemic signs of inflammation and sepsis such as temperature instability, apnea, bradycardia, hypoxemia, acidosis, and thrombocytopenia are also common. The primary diagnostic goal during initial clinical evaluation is to determine whether irreversible, transmural intestinal necrosis is present. There is no single physical finding or laboratory test that makes this distinction, but some clinically relevant observations useful in determining the need for operative intervention are discussed below.

Diagnosis

The diagnosis of NEC relies on a clinical evaluation and judgment based on symptoms and signs in the appropriate setting. Table 97.4 summarizes diagnostic criteria and a staging system for NEC most commonly used in the United States (74). Confirmation of NEC requires

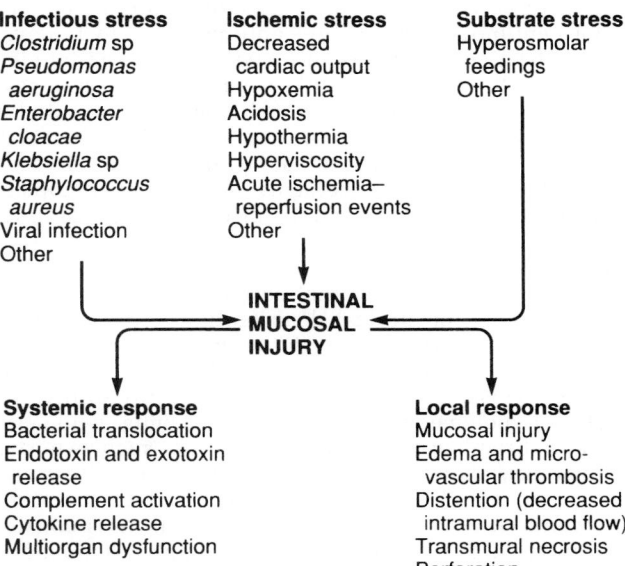

Figure 97.20. Schematic summary of the multifactorial pathogenesis of necrotizing enterocolitis.

Table 97.4. NECROTIZING ENTEROCOLITIS

STAGE I (SUSPECTED)

Any one or more historical factors producing perinatal stress
Systemic manifestations
  Temperature instability
  Lethargy
  Apnea
  Bradycardia
Gastrointestinal manifestations
  Poor feeding
  Increasing pregavage residuals
  Emesis
  Mild abdominal distention
  Occult blood in stool
Abdominal radiographs showing distention with mild ileus

STAGE II (DEFINITE)

Any one or more historical factors
Above signs and symptoms, plus
  Persistent occult or gross gastrointestinal bleeding
  Marked abdominal distention
Abdominal radiographs showing significant intestinal distention with:
  Ileus
  Small bowel edema
  Pneumatosis intestinalis
  Portal venous gas

STAGE III (ADVANCED)

Any one or more historical factors
Above signs and symptoms, plus
  Deterioration of vital signs
  Evidence of septic shock
  Marked gastrointestinal hemorrhage
Abdominal radiographs showing pneumoperitoneum in addition to
  findings listed for stage II

From Bell MJ, Kosloske AM, Benton C, et al. Neonatal necrotizing enterocolitis: prevention of perforation. J Pediatr Surg 1973;8:601–605, with permission

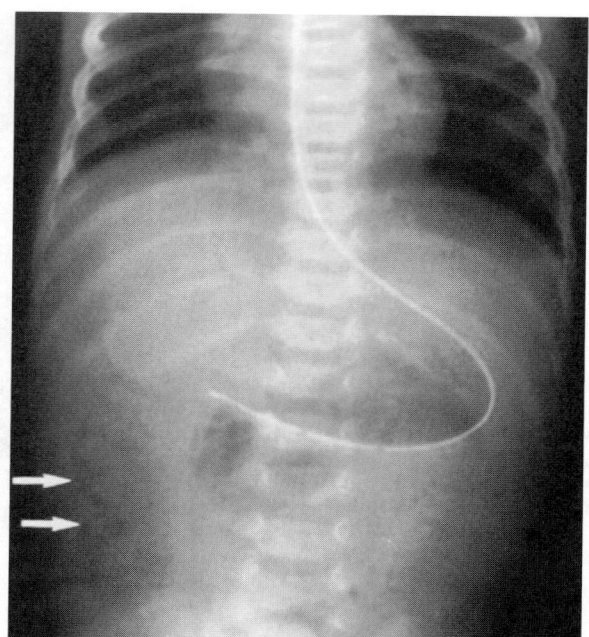

Figure 97.21. Plain abdominal film demonstrating pneumatosis intestinalis *(arrows)* in an infant with necrotizing enterocolitis.

only plain abdominal films. During the acute inflammatory phase, contrast studies may be hazardous and are contraindicated. The classic radiographic finding of extraluminal gas in the bowel wall or pneumatosis intestinalis (Fig. 97.21) confirms the diagnosis in the appropriate clinical setting but is variably present from 20% to 98% of the time. Other findings consistent with NEC include thickened bowel loops, ascites, and portal venous gas. Serial abdominal films, including a left lateral decubitus or upright film, must be obtained every 6 to 8 hours during the early course of the disease. These sequential studies help to document the progression or resolution of the inflammatory process and, importantly, evaluate for the presence of intestinal perforation presenting as free intraperitoneal gas or pneumoperitoneum. The presence of pneumoperitoneum mandates operative intervention; however, up to half of infants with perforated NEC will not have discernable pneumoperitoneum on plain films.

Treatment

Nonoperative.   The vast majority of infants (up to 90%) with NEC can be managed medically. The initial management of NEC includes proximal decompression with a nasogastric or orogastric tube, bowel rest, and broad-spectrum intravenous antibiotics. Expedient correction of hypotension, hypoxemia, and inadequate ventilation must be undertaken. Intravenous fluid management, with particular attention to electrolytes and acid–base status is es-

sential. Central venous access is secured, and TPN is initiated. Oxygen delivery and cardiac performance must be maintained, which in a premature neonate may require operative closure of a patent ductus arteriosus; this is preferable over the use of indomethacin in this setting (75). Serial plain films screening for pneumoperitoneum should be performed every 6 to 8 hours. In similar fashion, serial physical examinations and blood work, including arterial blood gases, platelet counts, and lactate levels, are useful monitors for the systemic inflammatory response induced by NEC.

Most infants with NEC improve with the relatively simple medical management outlined above. Typically, reversal of the systemic inflammatory response occurs rapidly, and the abdominal distention and ileus resolve over a period of days. Nasogastric tube decompression and intravenous antibiotics usually are continued for 7 to 14 days. Enteral feeding usually is resumed once the antibiotics have been discontinued and there has been return of gastrointestinal function. The usual course of medically treated NEC is a rapid clinical response and stabilization in the first 24 to 36 hours. Infants with significant intestinal necrosis typically have signs of either pneumoperitoneum or clinical deterioration during the initial 24 to 72 hours of treatment.

Indications to abandon medical management in NEC include evidence of intestinal perforation, that is, pneumoperitoneum, or clinical deterioration with persistent or progressive systemic dysfunction despite maximal medical therapy. Evidence of persistent or progressive systemic sepsis may include temperature instability, refractory hypotension, acidosis, hypoglycemia, neutropenia, and thrombocytopenia. Local findings such as portal venous gas, abdominal wall cellulitis, or crepitus also may signal intestinal necrosis and the need for operative intervention. A palpable, fixed abdominal mass consistent with intestinal perforation with an inflammatory phlegmon or abscess also may be a relative indication for operation. Because there is not complete agreement on what constitutes clinical deterioration, controversy remains with respect to operative indications for NEC in the absence of pneumoperitoneum. Because the interpretation of clinical deterioration criteria remains subjective, the decision to operate remains a multifactorial clinical judgment. In equivocal situations, abdominal paracentesis of ascitic fluid may be helpful in diagnosing intestinal necrosis with perforation in the absence of pneumoperitoneum if the aspirate contains bacteria or stool (76).

Operative. The operative indications in NEC invariably are associated with the presence of intestinal necrosis with or without frank perforation. Conventional operative intervention is aimed at treating the complications of NEC (i.e., intestinal necrosis) rather than preventing or stopping the factors that cause the disease. In general, resection of intestine involved with NEC does not prevent further extension of disease in other involved areas of the bowel. For isolated segmental disease, the traditional surgical treatment of NEC is resection of necrotic bowel with proximal enterostomy and distal mucous fistula placement. In infants with diffuse NEC, multiple resections with several enterostomies may be required. The primary operative goal is an expedient operation with preservation of as much intestinal length as possible, including the ileocecal valve. Because the risk of developing short-gut syndrome is substantial in infants with diffuse disease, it is rational to preserve marginal areas with a planned second-look operation to reevaluate viability. Accurate measurement of the remaining bowel length is important from a diagnostic and prognostic standpoint, with the length of bowel resected determined by the extent of necrosis. Resection with primary anastomosis in selected infants with NEC has been reported (77), with a recent study observing recurrent NEC in 22% and strictures in 17% of 18 treated infants following primary anastomosis (78). Complete intestinal necrosis of the small intestine and colon is uncommon in infants with NEC (Fig. 97.22). Faced with the dilemma of certain immediate death or the sequelae of short gut syndrome, some surgeons have reported intestinal reconstruction and survival following proximal jejunal diversion without enterectomy. The mortality rate in this desperate circumstance remains high.

Infants with NEC are typically fragile and premature, with varying coexistent medical problems such as hyaline membrane disease. Complications in this patient population are not well tolerated. For the high-risk, low birth weight infant, some data suggest that initial management with limited peritoneal drainage rather than laparotomy may be useful as either a temporizing measure or, in some instances, a definitive procedure (79,80).

Complications, Results, and Outcome

As previously stated, most infants with NEC (50%–90%) are treated successfully without operative intervention. Morbidity and mortality for this group are related primarily to problems associated with prematurity. Given the delay of bowel function and the need for TPN, cholestatic jaundice commonly occurs but is generally reversible. Infants placed on broad-spectrum antibiotics for an extended period are at risk for developing fungal sepsis. For infants with intestinal necrosis from NEC, infectious complications, including peritonitis, systemic sepsis, and intraabdominal abscess formation, can occur. Progression of disease can occur after surgical therapy, particularly if marginally viable bowel is preserved.

The overall surgical complication rate in infants with NEC is about 20% to 40%. Virtually every infant with NEC has a significant complication, an associated medical problem, or both. Immediate technical complications in treating NEC include intestinal leak, fistula formation, stoma necrosis, bleeding, and liver injury during exploration. These obviously are magnified in the extremely low birth weight infant with preexisting intestinal injury. Fluid and electrolyte losses from proximal diverting enterostomies can be significant and even life threatening in extremely low birth weight infants whose circulating blood volume is less than 50 to 100 mL; accurate measurement and replacement of volume and electrolytes are required. A review of 68 infants treated surgically for NEC observed a 26% mortality rate and a 68% complication rate related to the stoma or its closure in the perioperative survivors (81). These complications included stricture of either intestine or the stoma found at the time of enterostomy closure, incisional or parastomal hernia, stoma prolapse, intussusception, wound dehiscence or infection, small bowel obstruction, and anastomotic failure. The complications associated with diverting enterostomy in this unique population provide a compelling rationale for early enterostomy closure once the inflammation from peritonitis has resolved. A prospective, randomized trial comparing resection and enterostomy with resection and

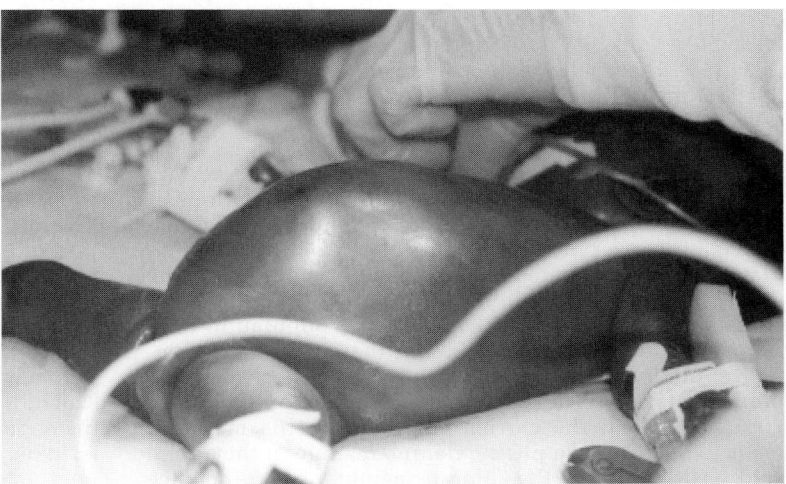

Figure 97.22. Fulminant necrotizing enterocolitis involving the entire gastrointestinal tract in a premature infant. Note the presence of pneumatosis intestinalis.

primary anastomosis in the treatment of NEC has not been reported.

Intestinal stricture formation following NEC, whether managed operatively or nonoperatively, is not uncommon. This consequence usually results from a normal host inflammatory response to the segmental, transmural intestinal injury. As host mechanisms begin to heal and repair the injured intestine, submucosal fibrosis may occur. The degree of fibrosis and subsequent stricture formation are clearly related to the severity and extent of disease. Less frequently, mesenteric vascular compromise secondary to an intraabdominal adhesion also can lead to stricture formation. Although stricture can develop anywhere in the gastrointestinal tract involved with NEC, a higher rate of demonstrable stricture is observed in the left colon, occurring in as many as 36% of medically treated infants (82). Routine contrast enema 4 to 6 weeks after clinical resolution of NEC treated operatively or nonoperatively is advocated in some institutions. Symptomatic strictures generally require segmental resection with anastomosis, although fluoroscopically guided balloon catheter dilatation has been reported.

Overall survival rates for infants with NEC have improved significantly over the past three decades and is currently about 60% to 80% for both operative and nonoperative groups (70,83). The observed improvement in survival is thought to reflect improved neonatal intensive care, the use of TPN, and the early institution of aggressive treatment for suspected NEC. Most neonatal intensive care units will initiate aggressive medical treatment in any infant with even a suspicion of NEC. Whether surgical interventions such as resection with primary anastomosis or limited peritoneal drainage can improve morbidity and mortality in these critically ill infants remains to be fully determined. Long-term outcome for NEC survivors generally reflects associated problems of prematurity. In particular, many of these infants will have residual neurodevelopmental, ophthalmologic, and pulmonary disease, but morbidity from the gastrointestinal system generally is limited to infants with the short-gut syndrome following extensive bowel resection. These infants present complex ethical and management issues beyond the scope of this review. The vast majority of NEC survivors (75%) enjoy an excellent quality of life, suggesting that the treatment cost relative to the potential benefit for these infants is worthwhile (84).

Meconium Ileus

Meconium ileus is a descriptive term for small bowel obstruction in a newborn infant with CF. About 10% to 20% of infants with CF initially have with meconium ileus (50). Discussion of meconium ileus requires an understanding of the pathophysiology of CF.

Cystic Fibrosis

Cystic fibrosis is the most common fatal hereditary disease in European and North American populations. It is an autosomal recessive disorder found with a heterozygous carrier incidence of 1 in 20 to 25 in white populations. The estimated incidence of homozygous gene expression and phenotypic manifestation of cystic fibrosis is about 1 in 2,000 to 2,500 in this population (85). The CF gene has been cloned and the single most common mutation characterized (86,87). The most common point mutation is a three-base-pair deletion found in 70% to 75% of the carrier population. This mutation leads to deletion of a phenylalanine residue in the amino acid position 508 of the CF transmembrane conductance regulator *(CFTR)* gene. In addition, there are about 200 more infrequent mutations of the *CFTR* gene that lead to clinical CF. The molecular heterogeneity of *CFTR* gene mutations produces practical implications in the development and use of carrier screening tests in the general population. Currently, widespread use of molecular genetic screening tests in the general population to identify asymptomatic carriers and at-risk couples without a family history of CF is not recommended; there are significant technical, ethical, and social issues that must be prospectively addressed (88,89). Carrier screening of at-risk couples with a family history of CF is recommended, however. In this setting, carrier discovery approaches 100%, and appropriate genetic counseling can be provided. Molecular genetic screening also should be offered to parents and infants with clinically suspected CF as well as asymptomatic infants born to at-risk couples. This approach allows rapid identification and confirmation of virtually all infants homozygous for cystic fibrosis.

Pathophysiology

The clinical manifestations of CF are caused by an epithelial electrolyte transport defect that results in impermeability to the chloride (Cl$^-$) ion (90). The epithelial defect occurs in apocrine sweat glands and the tracheobronchial tree as well as the pancreas, gastrointestinal tract, and liver. In sweat glands, failure of normal Cl$^-$ ion reabsorption following beta-adrenergic stimulation leads to an obligate sodium chloride loss despite a normal adenosine triphosphate (ATP)-dependent sodium-potassium pump. This is the basis for the traditional diagnostic sweat chloride test (see later).

Reduction of Cl$^-$ permeability in the tracheobronchial tree leads to diminished secretion volumes as well as increased absorption of sodium chloride. As a result, airway secretions in CF patients are low in volume and particularly viscous. Because of the tenacious nature of the airway secretions, airway clearance is impaired, and this leads to chronic, recurrent infection with bronchitis and pneumonia common. As the disease advances, bronchiectasis and progressive pulmonary parenchymal destruction ensues. Recurrent pulmonary bacterial infection is common, and airway colonization by *P. aeruginosa* is typically predictable. Chronic pulmonary disease accounts for more than 90% of the deaths in advanced CF, with a mean life expectancy approaching 30 years.

Pancreatic exocrine function also is affected by impaired Cl$^-$ permeability. Pancreatic duct obstruction resulting from inspissated viscous secretion is followed by glandular autolysis, acinar atrophy, and pancreatic fibrosis. Pancreatic exocrine insufficiency is a classic early clinical feature of CF and is thought to account for many of the clinical gastrointestinal manifestations of the disease. In particular, the deficiency of pancreatic proteinases leads to meconium ileus in the newborn, characterized by abnormally thick and viscid, protein-laden meconium that causes mechanical obstruction of the gastrointestinal tract. The obstruction usually is observed in the terminal ileum just proximal to the ileocecal valve (Fig. 97.23). Infants with meconium ileus have small pellets, or concretions, of pale, nonbilious meconium in the terminal ileum with a distal small and unused but otherwise normal microcolon. Proximal to the obstruction, the meconium is variably mixed with gas and often is thick and tarry in consistency. The bowel containing the thick meconium is often grossly distended and thickened. Microscopically, the muscularis is hypertrophied; distended mucous glands with prominent goblet cells may be present. The most proximal je-

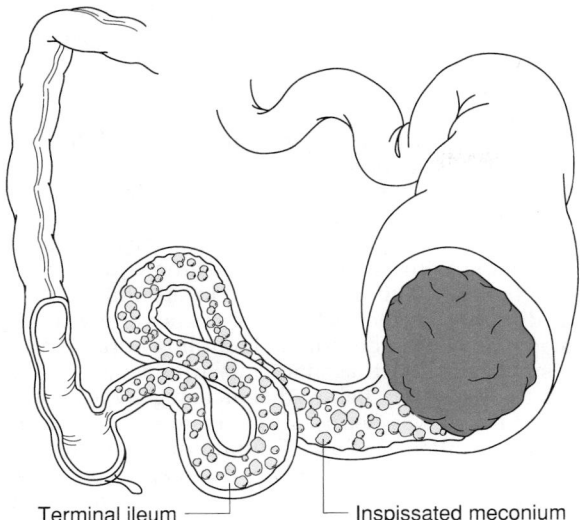

Figure 97.23. Meconium ileus causing obstruction of the terminal ileum from abnormally thick, inspissated meconium.

junum is typically normal in caliber and microscopic examination.

In utero events such as proximal volvulus of the dilated segment of ileum, perforation from distention, or atresia occur in approximately one third to one half of fetuses with meconium ileus. Typically, these are characterized together as complicated meconium ileus. A classic clinical presentation of complicated meconium ileus is in utero intestinal perforation with sterile meconium peritonitis and formation of a calcified pseudocyst (Fig. 97.24). Gastrointestinal conditions presenting outside of the newborn period occur in 10% of children with CF and include acute appendicitis, rectal prolapse, and intussusception. These conditions may reflect abnormal transit of thick, inspissated stool causing proximal distention or obstruction of the bowel lumen. Whether a primary intestinal epithelial Cl⁻ transport defect contributes to the clinical problems observed in cystic fibrosis is unclear. Small-bowel obstruction in CF outside the neonatal period is termed *meconium ileus* equivalent. Treatment of meconium ileus equivalent is generally similar to the initial nonoperative management of uncomplicated meconium ileus in the newborn and is discussed subsequently. Prevention of meconium ileus equivalent relies on conscientious pancreatic enzyme replacement. Finally, children with CF are at risk to cholestasis thought to be secondary to obstruction of small intrahepatic bile ducts. Chronic hepatic inflammation can occur with subsequent fibrosis and cirrhosis, causing hepatic failure and portal hypertension in approximately 5% of CF patients.

Diagnostic Evaluation

In nearly all newborns with CF, the diagnosis will be clinically apparent by the presence of meconium ileus, a family history of cystic fibrosis in a sibling, or a positive newborn screening test. Laboratory confirmation of *CFTR* gene dysfunction is performed in several ways. The historical standard for detection of CF has been analysis of the sodium chloride content of the sweat. As discussed, patients with CF have decreased chloride absorption in the sweat glands, and this can be directly measured. The most commonly used and reliable technique uses pilo-

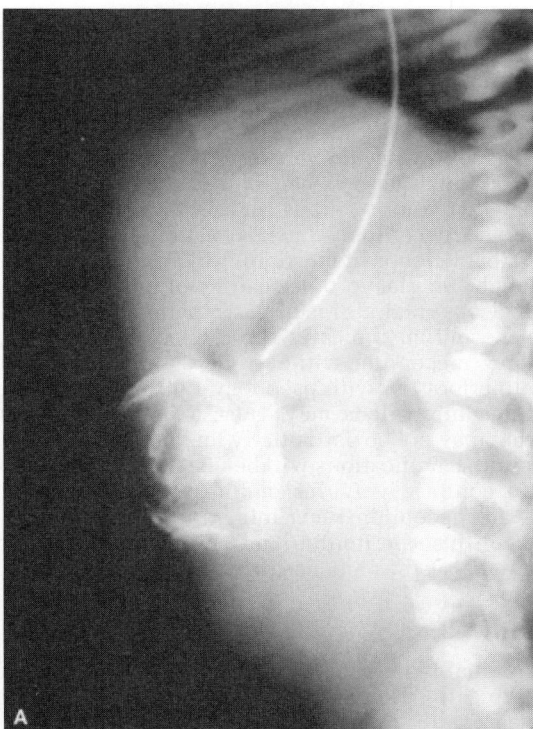

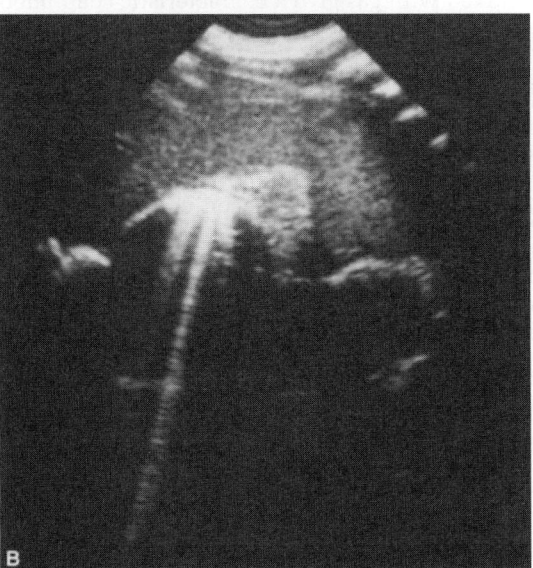

Figure 97.24. *(A)* Plain film radiograph of calcified pseudocyst in complicated meconium ileus. *(B)* In utero ultrasound demonstrating calcified pseudocyst.

carpine iontophoresis, with positive sweat test results showing sodium and chloride concentrations exceeding 60 mEq/L (91). Because normal neonates do not reliably conserve sodium chloride in sweat, this test is less useful before the patient is 4 to 6 weeks of age. Generally, abnormal *CFTR* gene function will be clinically documented by two elevated sweat chloride concentrations obtained on separate days. With the emergence of genetic technology capable of providing accurate assessment of *CFTR* gene mutations, the sweat test is now largely used to provide clinical confirmation of *CFTR* gene dysfunction following molecular diagnosis of CF.

Clinical Presentation

With current routine prenatal ultrasound practices along with selected fetal DNA screening, the prenatal diagnosis of CF or meconium ileus is feasible, potentially allowing for improved management of anticipated clinical problems following delivery (92). Initial signs of meconium ileus include neonatal bowel obstruction with abdominal distention, bilious emesis, and failure to pass bile-stained meconium. On examination, the neonate may have palpable loops of meconium-filled intestine that feel like dough. Similar to other causes of proximal neonatal intestinal obstruction, rectal examination and evaluation of the meconium typically reveal clear white mucus or thick grey meconium without bile staining. In utero intestinal perforation with pseudocyst formation in complicated meconium ileus may cause a palpable abdominal mass that may not be particularly tender. On plain films or ultrasound, calcifications will be visible in the pseudocyst wall. In contrast, volvulus or intestinal perforation secondary to meconium ileus following birth generally results in diffuse peritonitis and sepsis. Intestinal atresia also may be seen as a consequence of complicated meconium ileus.

Diagnosis

Abdominal plain films may be diagnostic in meconium ileus, typically demonstrating multiple, distended loops of bowel (Fig. 97.25A). Fluid- or meconium-filled loops of bowel mixed with gas give a characteristic soap-bubble or ground-glass appearance. Classic air-fluid levels seen in other causes of intestinal obstruction are not expected because of the tenacious, sticky intraluminal meconium. The presence of intraperitoneal calcifications or a calcified cyst is consistent with prenatal intestinal perforation of sterile meconium.

A contrast enema is useful in the evaluation and subsequent treatment of simple meconium ileus. This study usually demonstrates an unused but functionally normal microcolon (Fig. 97.25B). Reflux of contrast into the terminal ileum may confirm the presence of inspissated meconium pellets. In conjunction with a family history and plain films, this finding is sufficient evidence to confirm the diagnosis of meconium ileus in a newborn. Upper gastrointestinal contrast studies are generally unnecessary and may complicate future therapeutic efforts.

Treatment

Nonoperative. Nonoperative management of the distal small bowel obstruction in simple meconium ileus is achieved in about 60% to 70% of newborns (50). Once the diagnosis of meconium ileus is confirmed, the initial treatment of choice is to perform retrograde irrigation of the terminal ileum with one of several solutions designed to dissipate the obstructing meconium. In the United States, several different enema techniques and a variety of contrast media have been described, including normal saline, hyperosmolar contrast agents, and dilute *N*-acetylcysteine. Initially, it was believed that using hyperosmolar contrast material was necessary to create an osmolar gradient. The resultant influx of fluid into the intestinal lumen was thought to solubilize the inspissated meconium. Recent data suggest that successful meconium clearance is not necessarily related to the osmolality of the contrast agent; however, a significantly higher overall success rate is reported with the use of Gastrografin (sodium and meglumine amidotrizoate) and the use of other solubilizing agents such as Tween-80 and *N*-acetylcysteine (93). As long as clinical progress is being made, sequential enemas may be required to disimpact the inspissated meconium from the terminal ileum. In similar fashion, children and older patients presenting with meconium ileus equivalent are treated with retrograde enemas until the obstruction resolves. The distinct advantage of this treatment approach in meconium ileus is the avoidance of general anesthesia and exploratory laparotomy. Reported complications with this approach include intestinal perforation (rare), intestinal mucosal injury, and persistent obstruction resulting from meconium concretions.

Operative. The major indications for operative intervention are either failure to clear the obstruction by enema or complicated meconium ileus with cyst formation, volvulus, atresia, or perforation. For simple meconium ileus with persistent obstruction despite contrast enemas, the operative goals are to disimpact the meconium from

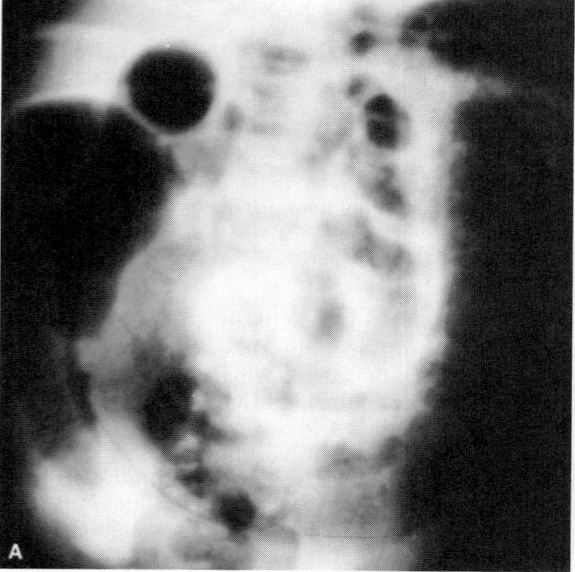
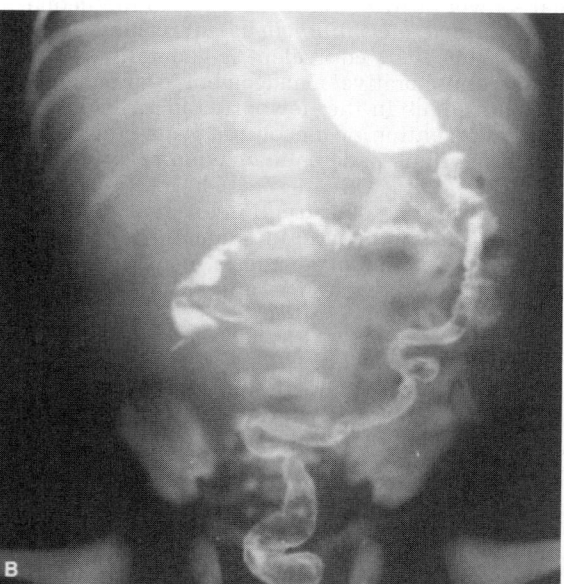

Figure 97.25. (*A*) Plain radiograph of neonate with meconium ileus. (*B*) Contrast enema in an infant with meconium ileus demonstrating an unused but intrinsically normal microcolon.

the ileum and to evacuate the remaining stool from the small intestine. These steps can be accomplished by either milking the intraluminal meconium downstream into the colon or solubilizing the meconium by transmural needle instillation of irrigant. In general, however, enterotomy or enterostomy and direct irrigation of the bowel lumen are required to clear the inspissated, sticky meconium completely. Simple closure of the enterotomy is preferred, but segmental resection may be required if marginal or compromised intestine is found. End-to-end anastomosis is the appropriate reconstruction technique following segmental bowel resection. A temporary enterostomy may be required, and several historical techniques have been described. Another surgical option is the placement of a T-tube into the ileum for continued irrigation with dilute *N*-acetylcysteine; following clearance of meconium from the intestine and the return of bowel function, the T-tube can be safely and simply removed (94).

Complicated meconium ileus occurs in about one third of patients and includes segmental volvulus, intestinal atresia or stenosis, necrosis, perforation, and meconium cyst formation. The surgical management of these entities is individualized. Intestinal atresia is not uncommon in meconium ileus, and the entire length of the intestine must be inspected for patency. When possible, resection of nonviable, stenotic, or perforated intestine is performed with immediate reconstruction by primary anastomosis. Patency of the downstream bowel must be confirmed to prevent anastomotic leak resulting from distal obstruction. If the infant is critically ill or has diffuse peritonitis, a safe primary anastomosis may not be possible and a diverting enterostomy will be required. Stoma closure may be performed promptly after the resolution of the underlying problems. Appendectomy usually is performed during laparotomy for meconium ileus because of the potential for appendicitis following luminal obstruction and possible confusion during future episodes of meconium ileus equivalent.

Postoperative Care and Results. If the meconium has been successfully cleared without opening the intestine, dilute *N*-acetylcysteine may be given through the nasogastric tube or by enema. Alternatively, if a T-tube has been placed, dilute *N*-acetylcysteine or other irrigant can be used directly into the ileum. These efforts are aimed at keeping the meconium soluble and preventing recurrent ileal obstruction. Following return of bowel function, enteral feeding using an elemental formula is started along with oral pancreatic enzyme replacement. Aggressive pulmonary therapy is routine and includes percussion and postural drainage, mucolytics, and antibiotics when indicated. Nutritional assessment and support are essential in the long-term management of these infants and children.

Successful nonoperative management of simple meconium ileus historically was associated with a more favorable outcome; however, the operative mortality rates of infants with meconium ileus have improved dramatically over the past several decades, and current short-term operative survival rates of 70% to 100% are reported (95,96). Long-term survival following meconium ileus is generally determined by the course of the underlying pulmonary disease. Contemporary management of CF has produced a mean survival age that approaches 30 years in most centers (97). With the exception of the development of portal hypertension in about 5% of patients, the intestinal manifestations of the cystic fibrosis are typically treatable. Future medical and surgical efforts to improve the long-term outcome in these patients include direct replacement of the diseased pulmonary system by lung transplantation, manipulation of the epithelial chloride transport defect

with pharmacologic agents, and gene therapy directed at *CFTR* gene transfer into respiratory epithelial cells.

Meconium Plug Syndrome

Meconium plug syndrome is characterized by functional obstruction of the colon or rectum by a plug of meconium. It affects both normal and premature infants with immature gastrointestinal motility and must be differentiated from other causes of neonatal intestinal obstruction. Unlike meconium ileus, in meconium plug syndrome, the colon is of normal caliber and the meconium is not inspissated. The infant's symptoms within the first few days of life are abdominal distention and bilious emesis. Spontaneous passage of meconium is often absent. On examination, the infant is typically normal and has a distended abdomen and patent anus. Digital rectal examination may deliver the meconium plug. Plain films of the abdomen will demonstrate dilated loops of bowel consistent with a distal bowel obstruction. The diagnosis is confirmed by contrast enema, which is also often therapeutic because the plug can be irrigated out by the contrast. The meconium plug is followed by bile-stained meconium of normal consistency. Importantly, although the vast majority of these infants are normal, a few will have Hirschsprung's disease or CF. Therefore, infants presenting with meconium plug syndrome should undergo rectal suction biopsy routinely and have CF screening tests performed.

Malrotation

Embryology

The embryology of intestinal fixation to the body wall is important in developing an understanding of intestinal malrotation. Normal midgut fixation requires sequential growth, elongation, and rotation of the intestine beginning as early as week 5 of gestation and is illustrated in Fig. 97.26. Three distinct events must occur for normal midgut fixation. The first stage involves herniation of the primary midgut loop into the base of the umbilical cord, where it remains until week 10 of gestation. The axis of the midgut loop is the superior mesenteric artery (SMA), dividing the midgut into prearterial and postarterial segments; the omphalomesenteric duct is at the apex of the midgut loop. The midgut loop rotates 180 degrees counterclockwise so that the proximal, prearterial half of the loop passes posterior to the SMA. The proximal portion of the prearterial segment gives rise to the proximal duodenum, which lies to the right of midline. The more distal prearterial segment passes posterior and to the left of the SMA, becoming the third and fourth portions of the duodenum. The distal duodenum normally is fixed to the left of the aorta at the ligament of Treitz, having rotated 270 degrees counterclockwise from its original position. The jejunoileal segment undergoes dramatic elongation, forming about six primary intestinal loops. The embryonic postarterial segment, which gives rise to the cecum and the right colon, also undergoes growth and elongation with concomitant rotation 270 degrees counterclockwise. Therefore, the cecum is initially positioned to the left, then anterior, and finally to the right of the SMA before reaching its final adult location (31).

Reduction of the extracoelomic gut is the second stage of midgut development and fixation, occurring between weeks 10 and 12 of gestation. By this time, the duodenojejunal junction has passed posterior to the SMA and the midgut has rotated 180 degrees counterclockwise; however, the small intestine initially remains to the right side of midline, and the cecum and ascending colon are ante-

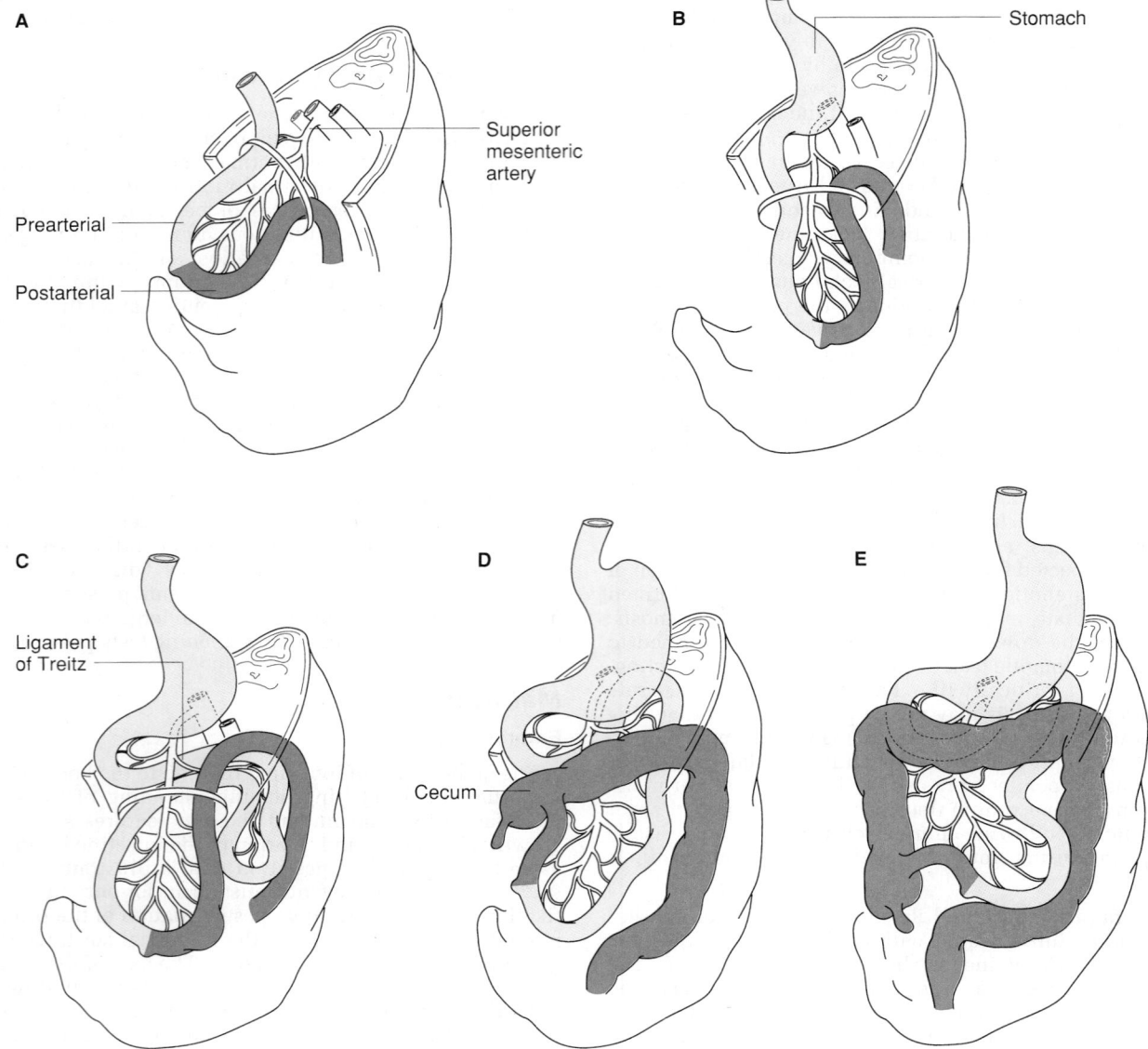

Figure 97.26. Normal midgut rotation is shown with appropriate positioning of the stomach, duodenum, small intestine, and cecum from the fifth gestational week *(A)* through completion by the 12th week *(E)*.

rior to the SMA after return of the gut into the abdomen. Many common abnormalities of intestinal fixation occur as a result of arrested development during this 2-week period.

The final stage of midgut development is fixation of the intestine to the posterior body wall, occurring after week 12 of gestation. Cecal descent occurs at this time. Normal points of fixation include the cecum in the right iliac fossa and the duodenojejunal junction at the ligament of Treitz just to the left of the aorta and anterior to the left renal vein (Fig. 97.27). Therefore, the normal intestinal mesentery is fixed with a broad base extending from the ligament of Treitz to the cecum. This broad-based mesenteric attachment prevents volvulus from occurring. In contrast, in disorders of intestinal rotation, discussed subsequently, the base of the mesentery is neither fixed nor broad, placing the entire midgut at risk for volvulus.

Anatomy

The normal sequence required for intestinal positioning and fixation can be interrupted at any developmental stage, producing a diverse spectrum of rotational abnormalities. Some neonatal surgical conditions are uniformly associated with abnormal intestinal rotation resulting from displacement of the midgut from the abdominal cavity during embryologic development. These anomalies include omphalocele, gastroschisis, and congenital diaphragmatic hernia. The term *malrotation* has been applied generically to describe disorders of intestinal rotation and fixation, although specific definitions of the more commonly encountered lesions are provided in the following sections.

Nonrotation. This common anomaly is characterized by inadequate counterclockwise rotation of the midgut around the SMA. Instead of the normal 270-degree arc, ro-

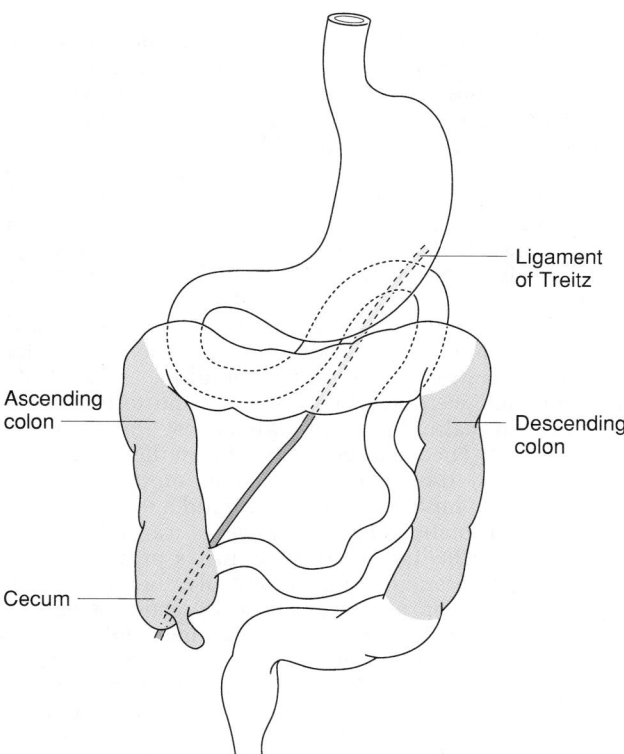

Figure 97.27. Normal oblique fixation of the midgut mesentery at the ligament of Treitz and in the right lower quadrant. The blue portions of the colon are extraperitoneal.

tation is either absent or arrested before exceeding 90 degrees (Fig. 97.28). The small intestine resides on the right side of midline, the colon resides on the left, and the cecum is anterior and near the midline. The duodenojejunal junction is to the right of midline and more caudal and anterior in position. Nonrotation carries a significant clin-

ical risk of midgut volvulus because the mesenteric vascular (SMA) pedicle is narrow. Duodenal obstruction also may occur as a result of peritoneal attachments known as *Ladd's bands.* These peritoneal bands fix the cecum to the posterior body wall by passing anterior and lateral to the distal duodenum.

Mixed or Incomplete Rotation. This is another common rotational abnormality characterized by arrest of the normal rotation at or near 180 degrees rather than the normal 270 degrees (Fig. 97.29). Instead of rotating posterior and to the left of the SMA, incomplete or arrested rotation of the prearterial segment leaves the duodenojejunal junction to the right of midline. The cecum also does not complete its counterclockwise passage anterior to the SMA, and it usually resides in the upper abdomen just to the left of the SMA. Similar to nonrotation, fixation of the cecum to the posterior body wall by peritoneal bands places the duodenum at risk for compression or obstruction. Additionally, the SMA pedicle is narrow and places the midgut at risk for volvulus.

Mesocolic Hernias. Mesocolic hernias are rare but important anomalies characterized by failure of fixation of either the right or left mesocolon to the posterior body wall. Small bowel can become entrapped in the resulting potential cavities on either side of the abdomen. A right-sided mesocolic defect (paraduodenal hernia) is associated with nonrotation of the prearterial midgut segment. Small bowel entrapment posterior to the right colon and cecum may occur. Similar entrapment of small bowel may occur from an incompletely fixed left mesocolon but is associated with normal colonic and cecal position. Entrapped small bowel in a left mesocolic hernia usually is contained within a hernia sac with the neck composed of the inferior mesenteric vein and peritoneal bands extending to the posterior body wall. Both left and right mesocolic hernias carry the potential risks of obstruction, incarceration, and strangulation of bowel.

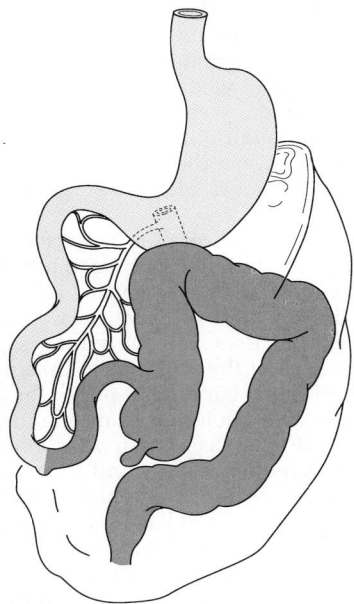

Figure 97.28. Nonrotation. The prearterial segment of the small intestine resides on the right side of the abdomen, and the postarterial segment *(colon)* is on the left. Neither has rotated normally.

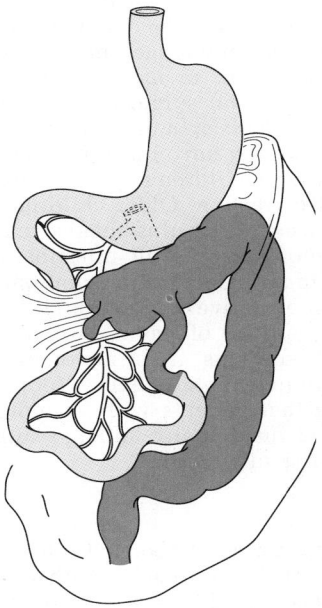

Figure 97.29. Incomplete rotation. The prearterial segment has failed to rotate and is on the right. The postarterial segment has rotated to reside anterior to the duodenum so that cecal bands to the posterior abdominal wall may compress and obstruct the duodenum.

Clinical Presentation

Abnormalities of intestinal rotation are estimated to be present in about 1% of the total population. The vast majority of persons with intestinal rotational anomalies are clinically asymptomatic; therefore, some children will be found to have malrotation incidentally by upper gastrointestinal contrast studies conducted for other reasons. Symptomatic malrotation usually is encountered clinically in the setting of duodenal obstruction or midgut volvulus. As previously discussed, duodenal obstruction occurs as a result of peritoneal attachments (Ladd's bands) fixing the abnormally positioned cecum to the posterior body wall. These peritoneal bands pass anterior and lateral to the distal duodenum and cause duodenal obstruction by extrinsic compression. Children with symptomatic duodenal obstruction present with bilious emesis and distention of the stomach and proximal duodenum. Similar to proximal neonatal intestinal obstruction, newborn infants may present with bilious emesis without abdominal distention secondary to partial duodenal obstruction. A paucity of small bowel gas may be seen on plain abdominal films.

Midgut volvulus should be considered in any infant or child presenting with bilious emesis. The clinical outcome of midgut volvulus is time dependent, which is the fundamental reason that signs and symptoms of intestinal obstruction in an infant or child must be pursued aggressively until a clear diagnosis is made. The devastating and life-threatening consequence of midgut volvulus is vascular insufficiency, gut ischemia, and, if untreated, infarction of the bowel supplied by the SMA. The initial symptoms may be subtle and limited to feeding intolerance, abdominal pain, and irritability followed by bilious emesis. Guaiac-positive stool from mucosal injury is a common early finding. Late findings include progressive abdominal distention, hematemesis, and hypotension. Metabolic acidosis, coagulopathy, and shock may become prominent clinical features. If unrecognized or left untreated, transmural necrosis of the entire midgut will occur.

At least 50% to 75% of intestinal rotational abnormalities are discovered within the first month of life, and about 90% occur in children younger than 1 year of age (98,99). Associated congenital anomalies are common and, as noted, certain neonatal surgical conditions such as omphalocele, gastroschisis, and congenital diaphragmatic hernia will uniformly have intestinal malrotation. Symptomatic infants and children require emergent surgical exploration and correction. Older children and adults initially may have acute volvulus but also may have a history of vague symptoms of episodic intestinal obstruction and chronic abdominal pain. Again, symptomatic persons require emergent operative exploration. It is essential to recognize that, regardless of age or chronic nature of symptoms, midgut volvulus from malrotation occurs in a completely unpredictable manner (100). Therefore, it is recommended that patients with asymptomatic malrotation discovered incidentally undergo surgical correction to reduce the risk of volvulus.

Diagnosis

As with other forms of neonatal intestinal obstruction, the diagnostic evaluation begins with a plain abdominal radiograph. Classic findings with malrotation include gastric and proximal duodenal distention with a paucity of absence of small bowel gas because of the partial duodenal obstruction (Fig. 97.30A). The plain film alone may not differentiate malrotation from duodenal atresia or stenosis. In most cases of suspected duodenal obstruction with concern of malrotation, an upper gastrointestinal series is the second and conclusive imaging study (Fig. 97.30B). Malrotation with volvulus typically produces an incomplete duodenal obstruction with a corkscrew or coiled appearance in the distal duodenum. Extrinsic compression of the duodenum by Ladd's bands may be visible on contrast study. Duodenal atresia and stenosis may occur anywhere within the duodenum but tend to be more proximal. Complete absence of small bowel gas is typical of duodenal atresia, whereas diminished but discernable distal gas is characteristic of duodenal stenosis or malrotation.

Other radiographic findings in malrotation include incorrect position of the duodenojejunal junction, particularly in a location to the right of midline. Additionally, failure to achieve normal cephalad and posterior fixation is typical in malrotation and may be best appreciated on lateral views. The small bowel resides in the right side of the abdomen, the colon and cecum on the left (Fig. 97.30C). In a symptomatic infant or child, radiographic evidence of malrotation alone is enough to warrant emergent exploration. Whether or not volvulus is present may be difficult to differentiate radiographically; therefore, efforts to do so may be hazardous in clinical practice. A contrast enema is helpful in the evaluation of neonatal intestinal obstruction, although it may not be the initial study of choice if malrotation is suspected. The classic finding of malrotation with contrast enema is malposition of the cecum, usually in the left abdomen or near the midline. Finally, the relative position of the SMA to the superior mesenteric vein may be assessed by ultrasound. Normally, the superior mesenteric vein is to the right of the SMA on transverse sonograms. Abnormal position of the superior mesenteric vein either ventral or to the left of the SMA is associated with malrotation (101).

Treatment

The management of malrotation or an internal hernia in a neonate is operative. Initial assessment, resuscitation, and preoperative preparation in a symptomatic newborn should be conducted simultaneously so that confirmation of malrotation can be followed immediately by laparotomy. Urgent laparotomy is required because even a minimal delay may represent the difference between viable or infarcted intestine. Volvulus with complete infarction of the midgut, if not immediately lethal, is survivable only with enterectomy followed by permanent or long-term TPN support. In older, asymptomatic children with incidentally discovered malrotation, operative repair is somewhat controversial. Given the devastating consequences of midgut volvulus, however, elective surgical correction appears to be warranted.

Operative repair of malrotation is performed by Ladd's procedure (102). The first objective is to relieve the midgut volvulus, if present. This is accomplished by delivery and detorsion of the affected midgut, usually in a counterclockwise direction. Recurrent volvulus is prevented by broadening the base of the mesenteric vascular pedicle by dividing the peritoneal bands that tether the cecum, small bowel mesentery, mesocolon, and duodenum around the base of the SMA (Fig. 97.31). Once completed, the mesentery and mesocolon open widely and the mesenteric pedicle is at low risk for recurrent volvulus. Performance of laparoscopic Ladd's procedure has been demonstrated to be feasible and may help to reduce time to enteral feeding and hospital length of stay (103). In general, fixation of the mesentery by plication of the cecum or duodenum to the body wall has been abandoned for lack of supportive data. Postoperative small bowel obstruction secondary to adhesions is reported in about 10% of patients.

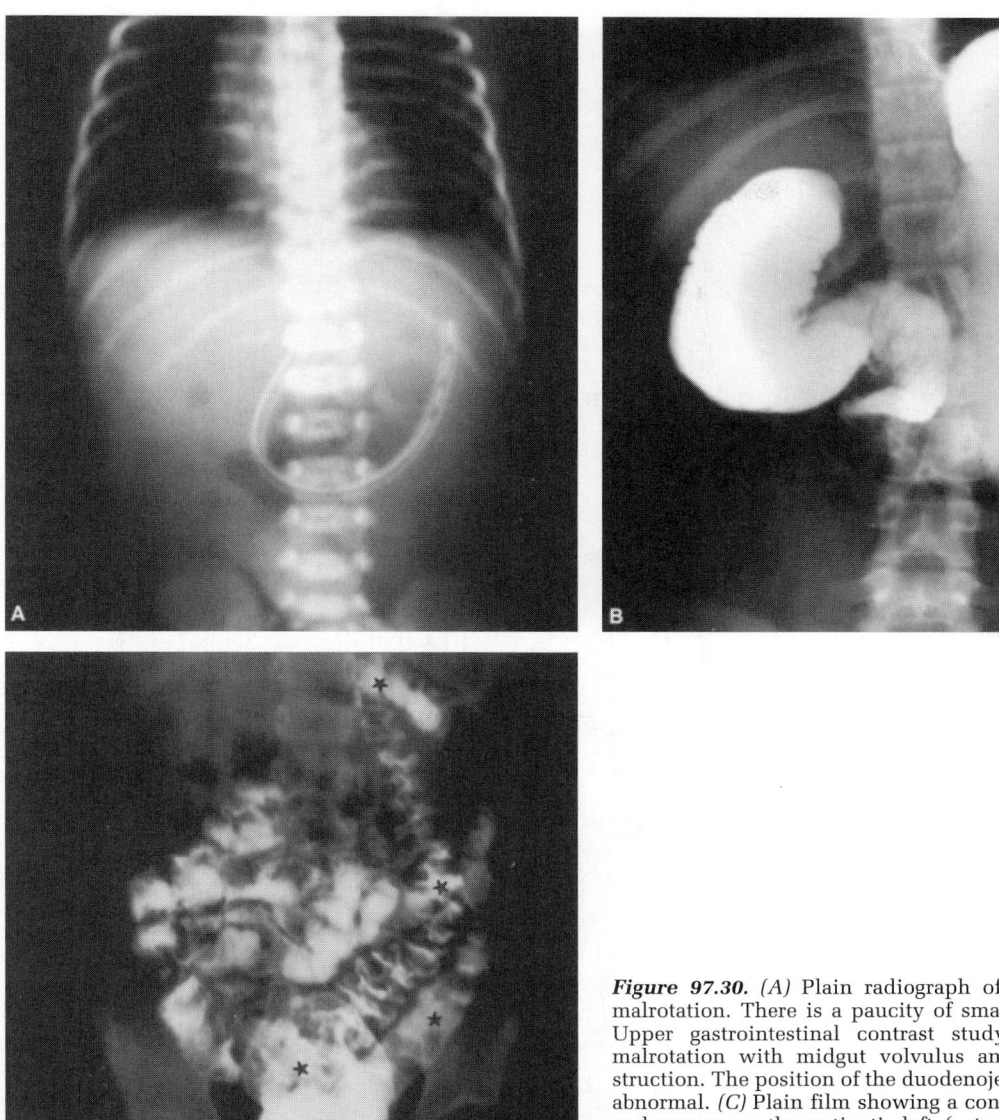

Figure 97.30. *(A)* Plain radiograph of an infant with malrotation. There is a paucity of small-bowel gas. *(B)* Upper gastrointestinal contrast study demonstrating malrotation with midgut volvulus and duodenal obstruction. The position of the duodenojejunal junction is abnormal. *(C)* Plain film showing a contrast-filled colon and cecum on the patient's left *(asterisks)*. The entire small bowel is to the right of midline. These are typical radiographic findings of malrotation.

The second objective of Ladd's procedure is to divide the abnormal peritoneal attachments between the cecum and the abdominal wall. This is done to relieve the duodenal obstruction from extrinsic compression by these bands. A modified Kocher maneuver involving meticulous and complete mobilization of the entire duodenum with division of all anterior, lateral, and posterior attachments is performed. Duodenal and distal small bowel patency should be demonstrated using intraluminal air or saline because concurrent cases of atresia have been reported. An appendectomy usually is performed to eliminate potential confusion from acute appendicitis developing in an abnormally positioned appendix.

Volvulus with intestinal necrosis is treated by preserving as much bowel length as possible. If bowel viability is unclear during initial exploration, a second-look procedure may be helpful to delineate reversible from irreversible injury. The management of nonviable bowel from volvulus is not different from other situations in which intestinal necrosis is encountered, and clinical decisions regarding resection, exteriorization, and anastomosis are necessarily individualized. In situations where the entire small intestine is lost and long-term survival doubtful, difficult ethical decisions must be made with the parents.

The surgical management of right mesocolic hernia is directed at dividing the lateral peritoneal attachments of the cecum and right colon to eliminate the potential space. In addition, given the associated nonrotation of the proximal bowel, the SMA pedicle should be broadened as much as possible. Left mesocolic hernia is treated by mobilization of the inferior mesenteric vein, reduction of the small bowel from the hernia sac, and closure of the neck of the hernia sac to eliminate the potential space.

Results and Complications

The results following surgical correction of intestinal rotational abnormalities should be excellent, and life expectancy should be normal in the absence of intestinal necrosis. Recurrent volvulus and recurrent duodenal obstruction are distinctly unusual if the initial procedure is

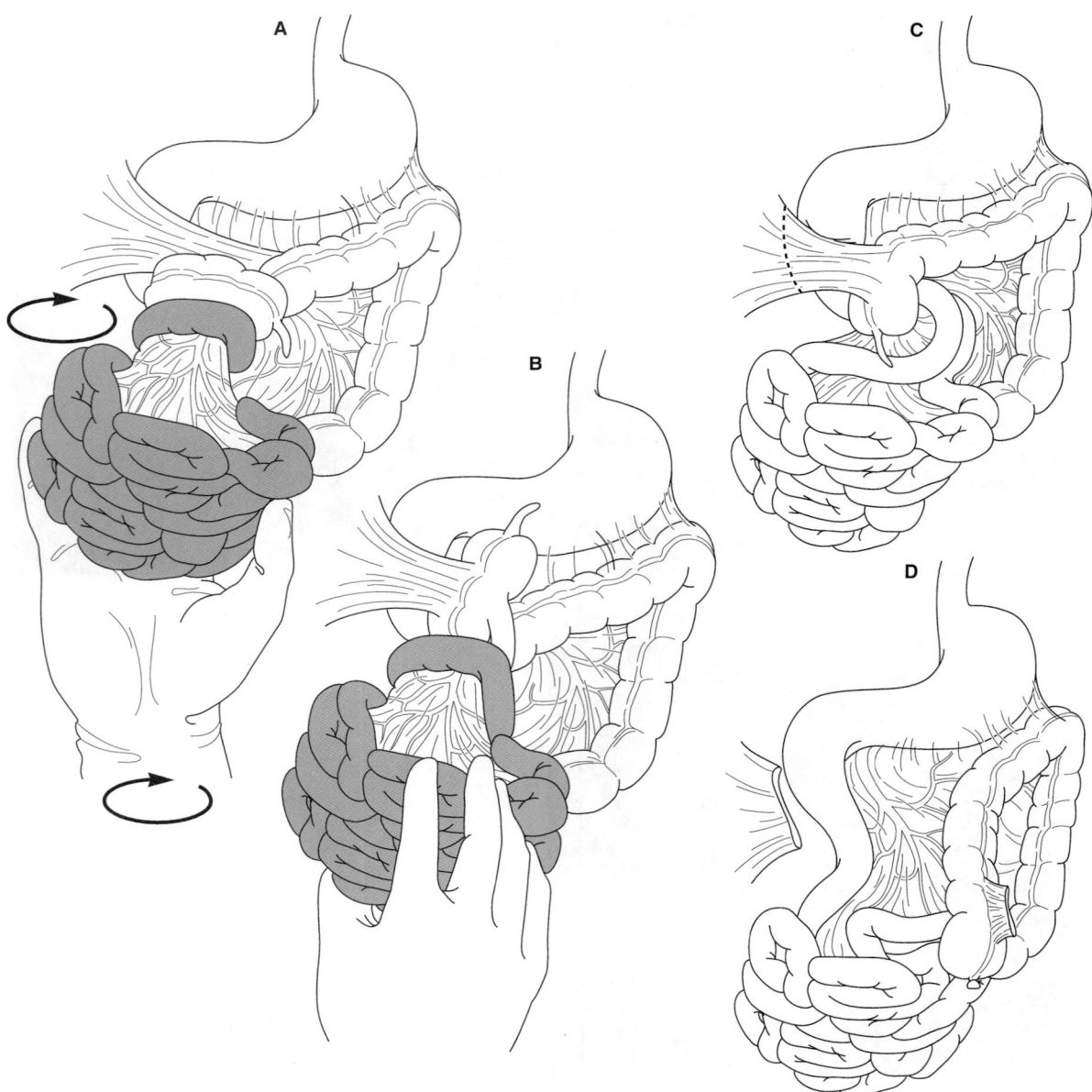

Figure 97.31. Correction of malrotation. *(A,B)* Detorsion of midgut. *(C,D)* Division of peritoneal attachments (Ladd's bands) of cecum to abdominal cavity.

technically complete. Adhesive small bowel obstruction following Ladd's procedure is reported in 1% to 10% of patients. Obviously, long-term outcome is less favorable in patients with intestinal necrosis at the time of exploration.

Congenital Aganglionosis (Hirschsprung's Disease)

Embryology

Congenital aganglionosis of the intestine (Hirschsprung's disease) is characterized by the loss or absence of intestinal ganglion cells resulting from interrupted development of the myenteric nervous system. The exact pathogenesis of aganglionosis remains unknown. In normal development, neuroblasts derived from neural crest precursors become evident by week 5 of gestation. The neuroblasts begin maturation and caudal migration along with vagal nerve fibers. The initial caudal migration in an intermuscular plane is followed by intramural dispersal into both superficial and deep submucosal nerve plexuses. Ultimately, the neuroblasts give rise to the ganglion cells of the myenteric nervous system, with functional maturation continuing well into infancy. The orderly migration pathway of myenteric innervation has been documented in human embryos; normally, ganglion cells can be identified in the esophagus at week 6 of gestation, in the transverse colon at week 8 of gestation, and in the rectum by week 12 of gestation (104).

Anatomy

Hirschsprung's disease is characterized anatomically by a lack of ganglion cells in the distal intestine. The length of aganglionosis is variable but most commonly involves the distal rectosigmoid colon in 75% to 80% of affected infants. In about 5% of cases, the transition zone between the normal, proximal bowel and the distal, aganglionic segment occurs in the small intestine (105). Discontinuous aganglionosis has been reported but is distinctly unusual. Therefore, in virtually all cases, the segment of aganglionosis will be continuous with the distal rectum to the anal verge and also will include the internal sphincter. Because of this distribution, the pathogenesis of congenital aganglionosis is often attributed to failure of neuroblast migration. The characteristic lesion in the distal bowel is the absence of ganglion cells in the intermuscular and submucosal plexuses. Additionally, many large, hypertrophied, nonmyelinated nerve fibers are present within the muscularis mucosa, lamina propria, submucosa, and Auerbach intermuscular plexus. These are both postganglionic fibers from normal, proximal ganglion cells and disordered preganglionic parasympathetic fibers without discernable synaptic connections. Both adrenergic and cholinergic fibers are prominent in the aganglionic segment, and acetylcholinesterase staining can be useful diagnostically (see below). The aganglionic segment also has a decrease or absence of nonadrenergic inhibitory fibers that are thought to be functionally important (106). Abnormalities in the peptidergic nervous system, including vasoactive intestinal peptide, substance P, and neurotensin immunoreactive fibers, also are described in the aganglionic bowel segment (107). Recent studies demonstrated deficient neuronal nitric oxide synthase mRNA and subsequent decreased local nitric oxide synthase activity in the aganglionic bowel (108). These experimental data are consistent with the concept that a defect in nitric oxide-mediated smooth-muscle relaxation may account for some of the characteristic clinical features of Hirschsprung's disease (109–111).

The transition zone between the normal, proximal bowel and the aganglionic distal bowel is distinguished grossly by distention of the proximal bowel with histologic evidence of muscular hypertrophy. Hypoganglionosis and a progressive increase in the thickened, nonmyelinated neuronal fibers characterize this zone. The transition zone often becomes evident to direct inspection or on contrast enema during the first few weeks of life as the functional obstruction leads to progressive proximal dilatation and thus to a congenital megacolon. On gross inspection, the transition zone may appear as a short funnel or cone-shaped segment of colon. The discrepancy in bowel lumen diameter is somewhat age dependent and may be subtle in a newborn or in a child with total colonic aganglionosis. Therefore, it may be difficult for the surgeon or radiologist to define the exact site of the transition zone based on gross inspection or contrast enema. Gross examination alone is not sufficient for surgical decision making, and histologic confirmation of the level of ganglion cell transition is required. Given the continuous nature of aganglionosis, a rectal biopsy performed 2.5 to 3 cm above the pectinate line demonstrating the presence ganglion cells effectively excludes Hirschsprung's disease.

Neuronal intestinal dysplasia is a clinically described entity similar to or associated with Hirschsprung's disease (112,113). Despite the presence of ganglion cells, dysplastic changes in the myenteric nervous system affect bowel motility in similar fashion to aganglionosis. Clinical presentation and treatment are similar to those of classic Hirschsprung's disease. There is considerable controversy regarding neuronal intestinal dysplasia (114), but it is reasonable to suggest that this represents one variant in the spectrum of abnormalities of the myenteric nervous system.

Pathophysiology

Normal intestinal motility depends on the coordinated propagation of segmental contraction waves immediately preceded by relaxation of the enteric smooth muscle. Patients with Hirschsprung's disease lack a functional myenteric nervous system in the aganglionic segment; therefore, both propulsion and reflex relaxation will be disordered or absent in the distal bowel. This appears to result from neuronal dysfunction of cholinergic (propulsive) innervation as well as from diminished or absent adrenergic and nonadrenergic inhibitory signaling pathways. Loss of neuronal nitric oxide synthase activity also appears to play an important role. The internal sphincter is aganglionic and lacks the normal reflex relaxation following rectal distention. In fact, patients with Hirschsprung's disease exhibit a paradoxical increase in sphincter tone in response to rectal distention. The functional result of these pathophysiologic mechanisms is tonic contraction of the aganglionic segment of bowel with ineffective peristalsis. Clinically, this presents as an incomplete, distal intestinal obstruction in the newborn or as chronic constipation in the older child or adult.

From a genetic standpoint, Hirschsprung's disease has been associated with mutations in at least three specific genes: the *RET* protooncogene, the endothelin B receptor *(EDNRB)* gene (115), and the endothelin 3 *(EDN3)* gene. Additionally, several other candidate genes are under investigation. In mice, natural and in vitro induced mutations affecting the *RET, EDNRB,* and *EDN3* genes generate intestinal aganglionosis identical to Hirschsprung's disease (116,117). Although widely accepted, it is still unknown whether the primary event in aganglionosis is failure of neuroblast migration to the distal bowel. Alternatively, ineffective microenvironmental support of neuroblasts that have already migrated may fail to promote normal neuroblast development and survival (118).

Clinical Features

Incidence and Associations. The incidence of Hirschsprung's disease is estimated at 1 per 5,000 live births with a marked male-to-female (4:1) preponderance. The vast majority of cases are sporadic, but long-segment and total colonic aganglionosis and female gender are strongly associated with familial inheritance. Genetic chromosomal analysis suggests that multiple loci may be involved, including chromosomes 13q22, 21q22, and 10q (119,120), among others. In particular, familial Hirschsprung's disease has been clearly associated with mutations of the *RET* protooncogene. From a clinical standpoint, mutations of the *RET* protooncogene are associated with disorders of neural crest development, namely, multiple endocrine neoplasia (MEN) types IIA and IIB as well as familial medullary thyroid carcinoma. These occasionally are associated with Hirschsprung's disease. Congenital cardiac defects are present in 2% to 5% of patients with Hirschsprung's disease. Other rare congenital anomalies have been reported, but a consistent and important association is a 5% to 15% incidence of trisomy 21 (121,122). For unknown reasons, aganglionosis in a premature infant is uncommon. Infants presenting with meconium plug syndrome or neonatal appendicitis should undergo rectal suction biopsy because these are the initial clinical manifestations in a small number of infants with Hirschsprung's disease.

Presentation. Most infants with Hirschsprung's disease will fail to pass meconium within the first 24 to 48 hours of life. Nonspecific signs of neonatal intestinal obstruction (feeding intolerance, abdominal distention, and bilious emesis) may develop. About half of patients with

Hirschsprung's disease are diagnosed as neonates, with the remainder discovered before the age of 2 years. Infrequently, older children or adults are diagnosed with aganglionosis during evaluation for chronic constipation. In this setting, symptoms may be minimal to disabling, and parents or patients often develop elaborate strategies to deal with the chronic constipation. Abdominal distention is characteristic, and sometimes failure to thrive and malnutrition may occur. Physical examination will be nonspecific. Digital rectal examination may demonstrate spasm and will exclude anal stenosis. In the presence of enterocolitis, forceful expulsion of foul-smelling, liquid stool may occur with digital rectal examination.

Enterocolitis occurs in about 10% to 30% of infants and children with Hirschsprung's disease and may be the presenting clinical manifestation. Enterocolitis associated with Hirschsprung's disease has an unknown pathophysiology, but obstructive stasis and bacterial overgrowth are thought to be important factors. *C. difficile* and rotavirus have been implicated as important pathogenic organisms (123–125); diagnostic and treatment plans should consider these possibilities. The early presenting symptoms and signs of enterocolitis include fever, abdominal distention, and diarrhea, which may be explosive, foul-smelling, and bloody. Systemic sepsis, transmural intestinal necrosis, and perforation are all possible later findings. The clinical progression can be rapid, with death occurring in as few as 12 to 24 hours if treatment is not initiated. Infants are particularly vulnerable to this complication, which continues to have a 25% to 30% mortality rate, accounting for virtually all mortality directly related to Hirschsprung's disease in modern pediatric surgical practice. Infants with known Hirschsprung's disease and suspected enterocolitis should be treated aggressively. Initial treatment includes resuscitation, broad-spectrum antibiotics, cessation of feeding, and rectal irrigation. If the enterocolitis does not respond promptly, emergent intestinal decompression with an enterostomy proximal to the transition zone is indicated.

Diagnosis

A high index of suspicion for Hirschsprung's disease should be maintained for any newborn infant with abdominal distention that fails to pass meconium in 24 to 48 hours following birth. The signs of neonatal intestinal obstruction lead to a stereotypical work-up that includes diagnostic imaging studies. In the presence of characteristic findings on history, examination, or radiographic studies, any infant suspected of having Hirschsprung's disease should undergo rectal biopsy.

Plain Abdominal Radiographs. Plain film radiographs of the neonate with Hirschsprung's disease are nonspecific and will typically demonstrate distended, air-filled loops of bowel throughout the abdomen. It is often difficult to discriminate between small and large intestine on plain films at this age, but the pattern is consistent with distal intestinal obstruction. Older children or adults may have a stool-filled megacolon on plain radiographs, but this is also nonspecific. In the presence of enterocolitis, thickened, dilated intestinal loops and pneumatosis intestinalis may be evident.

Contrast Enema. When distal neonatal intestinal obstruction is suspected on plain abdominal films, a contrast enema generally should be performed. The neonatal enema is performed without a rectal balloon to minimize the risks of perforation or obstructing the rectal findings. The classic radiographic finding in Hirschsprung's disease is a transition zone (Fig. 97.32). As previously mentioned, a definitive transition zone may not be apparent in a

neonate because proximal dilatation takes some time to develop. Additionally, infants with short-segment disease or total colonic aganglionosis may not have obvious transition zones on contrast enema. In these instances, a lateral view of the rectum may show abnormal spasm (Fig. 97.32B). Contrast remaining in the rectum more than 24 hours following a study may also be suggestive of Hirschsprung's disease. With an experienced pediatric radiologist, findings consistent with Hirschsprung's disease can be accurately detected in most instances.

Rectal Biopsy. The diagnostic standard for aganglionosis is the rectal biopsy, and this should always be obtained in any infant or child in whom Hirschsprung's disease is suspected. Several commercially available instruments capable of performing rectal suction biopsies are in widespread use. The rectal suction biopsy can be performed at bedside or in clinic without anesthesia in all newborns and most children up to several years of age. The desire for neonatal diagnosis and the technical simplicity of the procedure allow liberal use of this technique in all suspected or at-risk infants. When applied liberally, the vast majority (85%–90%) of infants undergoing this procedure will have normal ganglion cells on biopsy, effectively excluding Hirschsprung's disease. Using the rectal suction biopsy technique, a biopsy of the mucosa and submucosa is obtained. This is sufficient to establish the diagnosis because ganglion cells are absent from all intramural plexuses in Hirschsprung's disease. The biopsy must be taken between 2 and 3 cm proximal to the pectinate line. Complications of infection, perforation, and bleeding with rectal suction biopsy are infrequent. Full-thickness rectal biopsy under general anesthesia is reserved for older children and in infants in whom suction biopsy has been inadequate. An experienced pediatric pathologist must read the biopsies for maximal diagnostic accuracy. Evaluation for ganglion cells and the axons of the myenteric neurons must be performed (Fig. 97.33), which may be accomplished using conventional hematoxylin-eosin staining or histochemical staining for acetylcholinesterase. Similar histochemical staining for nitric oxide synthase can be performed. These adjunctive techniques are used routinely in some centers and can help to provide additional evidence of Hirschsprung's disease rather than simply demonstrating aganglionosis in the biopsy specimen. Communication between the pathologist and the surgeon is essential to correlate clinical data with histologic findings. Diagnostic accuracy for Hirschsprung's disease is excellent with a correctly obtained rectal suction biopsy and an experienced pediatric pathologist (126).

Anorectal Manometry. Characteristic manometric findings of Hirschsprung's disease include an abnormal response of the internal sphincter to balloon-induced rectal distention. The absence of sphincter relaxation in response to rectal dilatation is consistent with Hirschsprung's disease. Because of the relative ease and accuracy of rectal suction biopsy, anorectal manometry is not widely used in the United States for the primary diagnosis of Hirschsprung's disease in infancy; however, this is used in some centers around the world and, when applied carefully with an appropriate transduction probe, accurate manometric diagnosis is achievable in 85% to 90% of cases.

Treatment

Many persons diagnosed with Hirschsprung's disease will have enough intestinal obstructive symptoms that surgical decompression is warranted. Diverting colostomy should be considered for a newborn infant with Hirschsprung's disease who has enterocolitis or in the presence

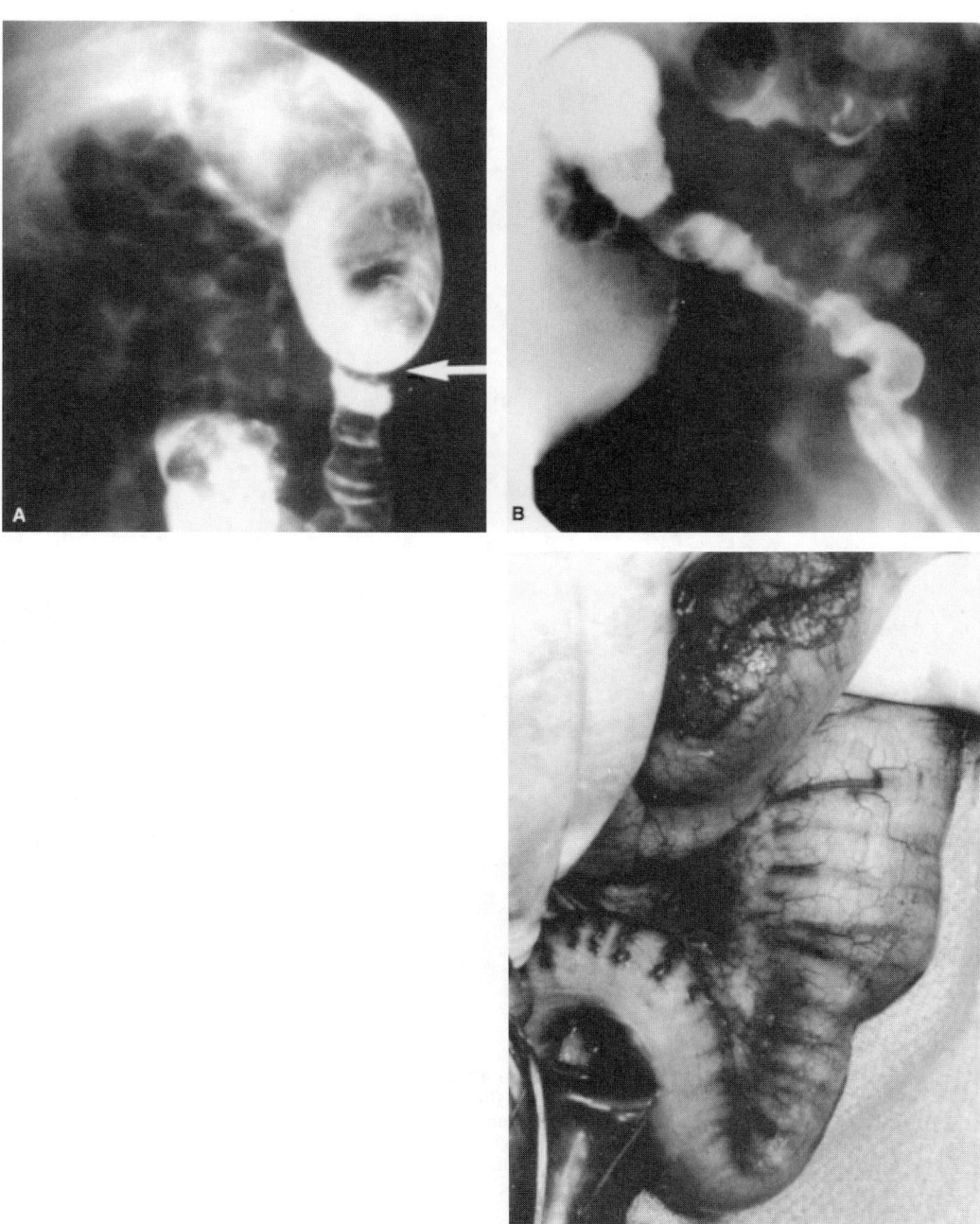

Figure 97.32. *(A)* Contrast enema demonstrating a classic rectosigmoid transition zone in Hirsch-sprung's disease. *(B)* Lateral view of rectum illustrates typical distal spasm of rectum. *(C)* Operative photograph of rectosigmoid transition zone.

of multiple associated medical problems or anomalies. In the presence of enterocolitis, rectal irrigation and decompression can be an effective temporizing measure while resuscitation and broad-spectrum antibiotics are being instituted. Prompt proximal diversion in all likelihood will be required once the patient has stabilized. In the neonate, the traditional approach following diagnosis is to obtain proximal diversion by means of a colostomy (or enterostomy) placed in normal, ganglionated intestine. The diverting colostomy must be proximal to the histologic transition zone, and a series of biopsies examined by frozen section may be necessary to find the correct level for diversion. For classic rectosigmoid disease, a leveling

colostomy is placed just proximal to the transition zone. Alternatively, some surgeons prefer a right transverse colostomy following confirmation of ganglion cells at the site. This approach is generally done in two stages, with takedown of the stoma and definitive pull-through operation performed together weeks to months later, typically when the infant reaches 9 to 12 months of age. In older children, definitive pull-through is deferred until the colon has decompressed to relatively normal caliber.

Recently, a single-stage approach in selected infants, which eliminates the diverting colostomy, has been advocated (127–130). Despite a number of different operative techniques in performing a single-stage pull-through, the

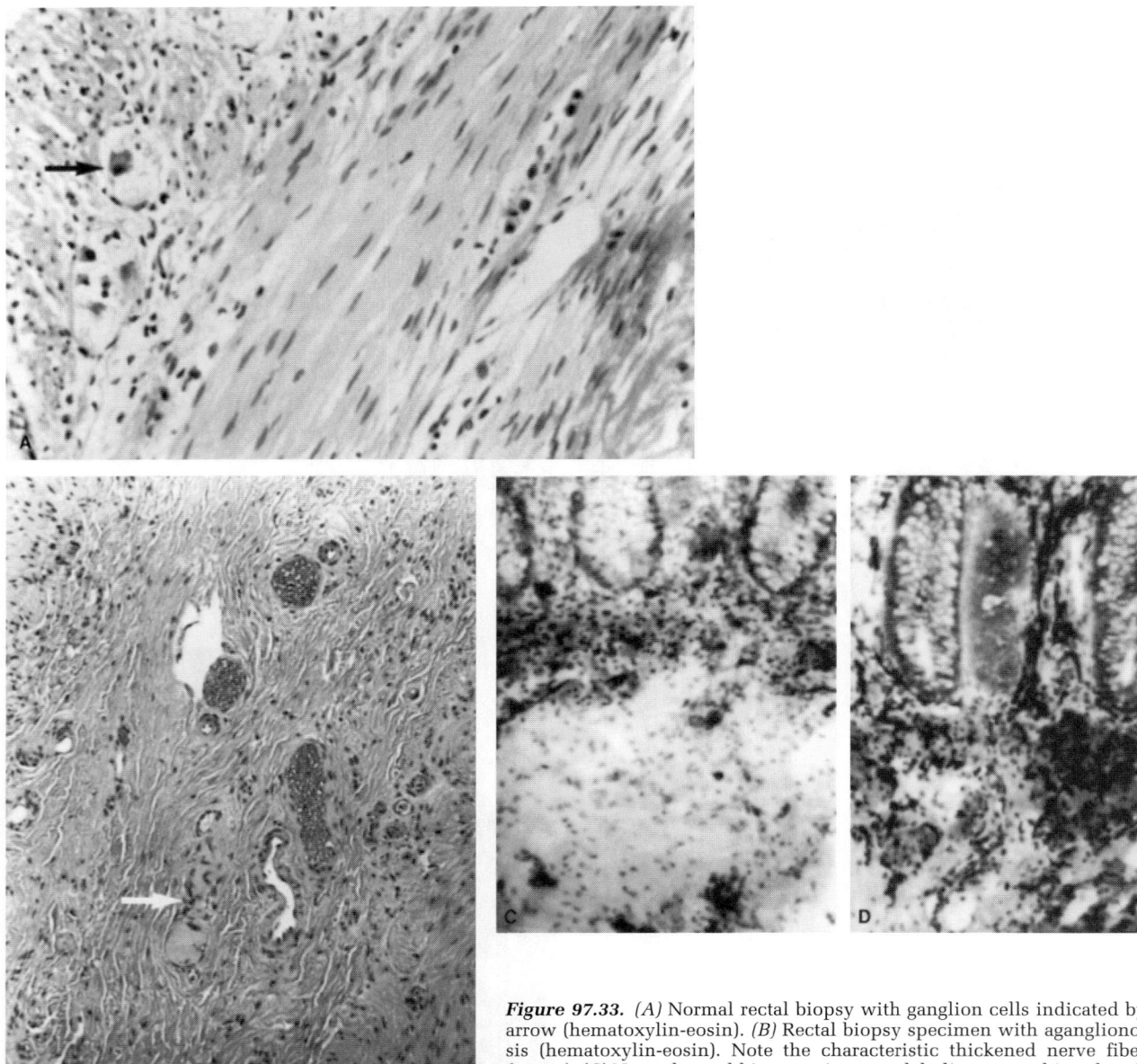

Figure 97.33. *(A)* Normal rectal biopsy with ganglion cells indicated by arrow (hematoxylin-eosin). *(B)* Rectal biopsy specimen with aganglionosis (hematoxylin-eosin). Note the characteristic thickened nerve fiber *(arrow)*. *(C)* Normal rectal biopsy using acetylcholinesterase histochemical staining. *(D)* Similarly stained specimen from a patient with Hirschsprung's disease. Many thickened submucosal nerve fibers stain densely black.

results and outcomes appear nearly equivalent. The definitive repair of Hirschsprung's disease with a single operation is desirable from technical and economical standpoint and essentially eliminates the complications associated with neonatal stomas. As with most aspects of pediatric surgery, an increasing experience with laparoscopically assisted, single-stage pull-through operations is being reported (131). The contemporary single-stage approach in the management of Hirschsprung's disease has gained wide acceptance in the pediatric surgical community.

Definitive Operations for Hirschsprung's Disease

The major goal of operative therapy in the treatment of Hirschsprung's disease is to provide resection or bypass of the distal aganglionic rectum with the performance of a low rectal anastomosis with normally innervated proximal intestine. Numerous definitive procedures were designed to treat Hirschsprung's disease, and a brief description of the principal procedures in use follows. In general, the selection of a procedure depends on a surgeon's individual training and preference rather than compelling differences in outcome (132).

Duhamel Procedure (Martin Modification). The key elements of the Duhamel procedure are illustrated in Fig. 97.34. After minimal pelvic dissection, resection of the aganglionic colon is performed. The aganglionic rectum is left in situ. Normal proximal colon is brought down to the retrorectal space, and a colorectal anastomosis is performed about 1 cm above the pectinate line. The original operation left the defunctionalized rectal pouch as shown, which proved problematic. The procedure has been modified by Martin to include a longer side-to-side colorectal

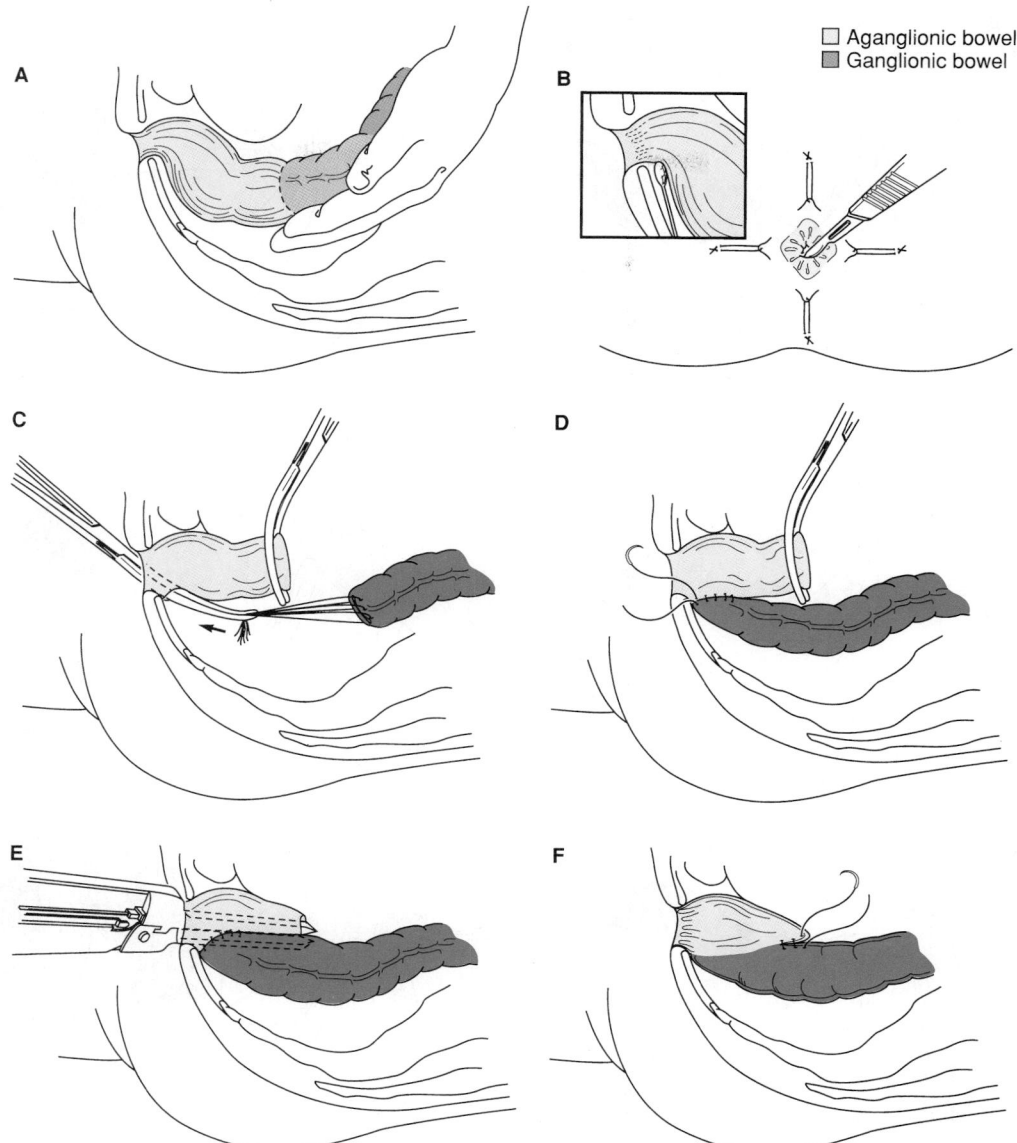

☐ Aganglionic bowel
■ Ganglionic bowel

Figure 97.34. Duhamel procedure (Martin modification). *(A)* Blunt retrorectal dissection. *(B)* Incision in the posterior wall of the aganglionic rectum. *(C)* Retrorectal pull-through after resection of the proximal aganglionic segment. *(D)* End-to-side colorectal anastomosis preserving aganglionic rectum (as originally described). *(E)* Stapled conversion of anastomosis into an extended side-to-side colorectal anastomosis (Martin modification). *(F)* Completed procedure.

anastomosis, now considered standard. Advantages of this procedure include its relative technical ease and the limited pelvic dissection. Adoption of the stapled anastomosis has simplified this procedure significantly.

Soave Procedure. The Soave procedure is illustrated in Fig. 97.35. Following resection of aganglionic colon, an endorectal dissection in the submucosal plane is performed from proximal rectum to anus. Generally, the endorectal dissection is started in the extraperitoneal rectum. This dissection is typically much easier than the similar dissection in a patient with ulcerative colitis. The dissected rectal mucosal tube is everted through the anus and onto the perineum. The mucosal tube is excised, and normal proximal bowel is pulled through the rectal muscular cuff. The original operation did not suture the pull-through segment of proximal bowel to the rectum. A for-

mal sutured colorectal anastomosis is now universally performed. Care must be taken to ensure that the pull-through segment is not obstructed by the muscular cuff. This procedure is roughly equivalent to the Duhamel procedure in terms of technical ease, operative time, and outcome.

Swenson Procedure. The Swenson procedure is the original definitive procedure for the treatment of Hirschsprung's disease. It is somewhat more demanding from a technical standpoint, and, as such, it has been reported to have a slightly higher incidence of postoperative complications. Long-term outcome in children who undergo a properly performed Swenson procedure is equivalent to the other procedures. The basic strategy is outlined in Fig. 97.36. The aganglionic segment of colon is resected and a careful, nearly complete extra-

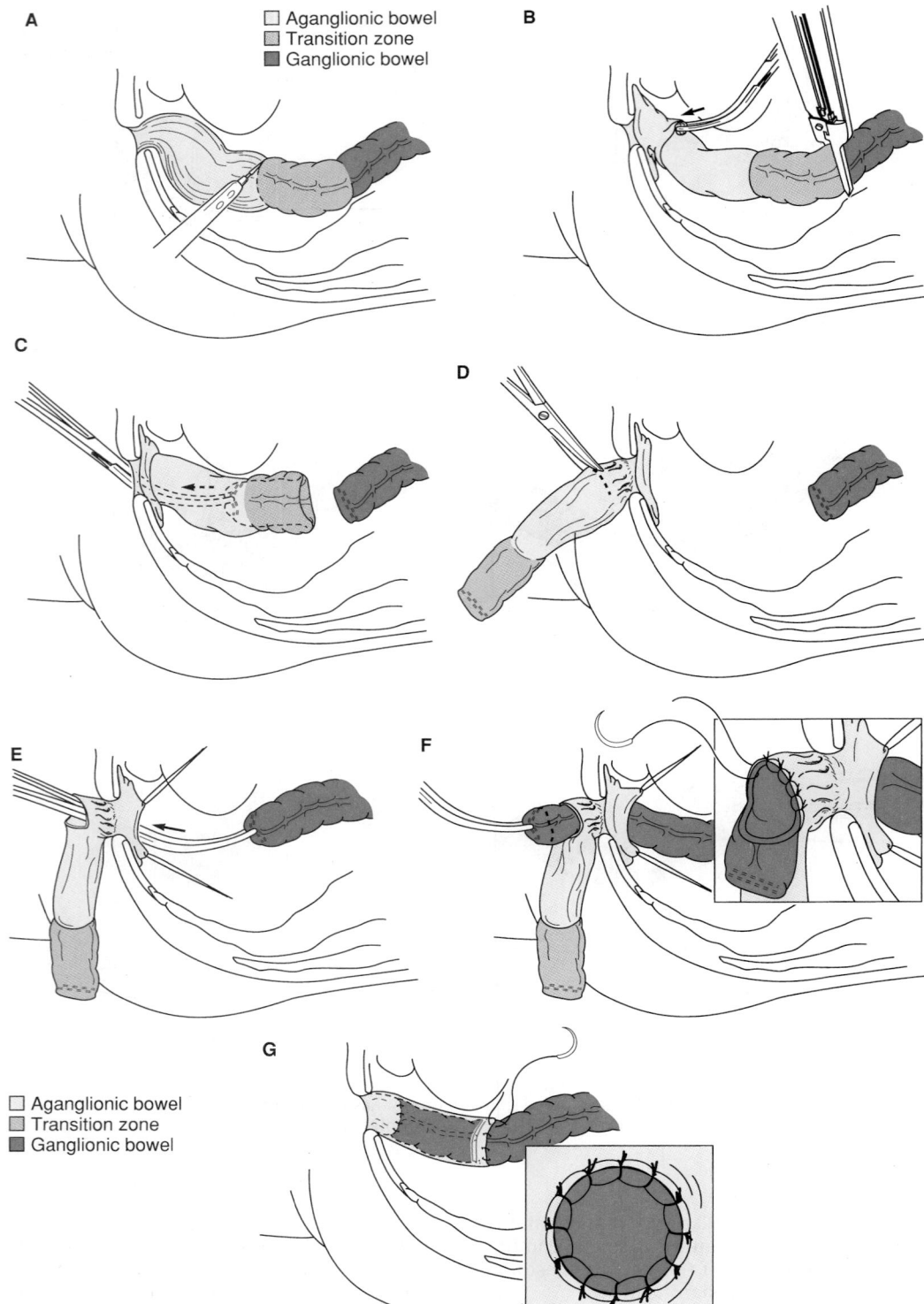

Figure 97.35. Soave endorectal procedure. *(A)* Endorectal dissection initiated. *(B)* Endorectal dissection complete. *(C)* Eversion of the aganglionic segment and rectal mucosal tube. *(D)* Incision of everted rectal tube. *(E)* Endorectal pull-through. *(F)* Colorectal anastomosis. *(G)* Completed procedure.

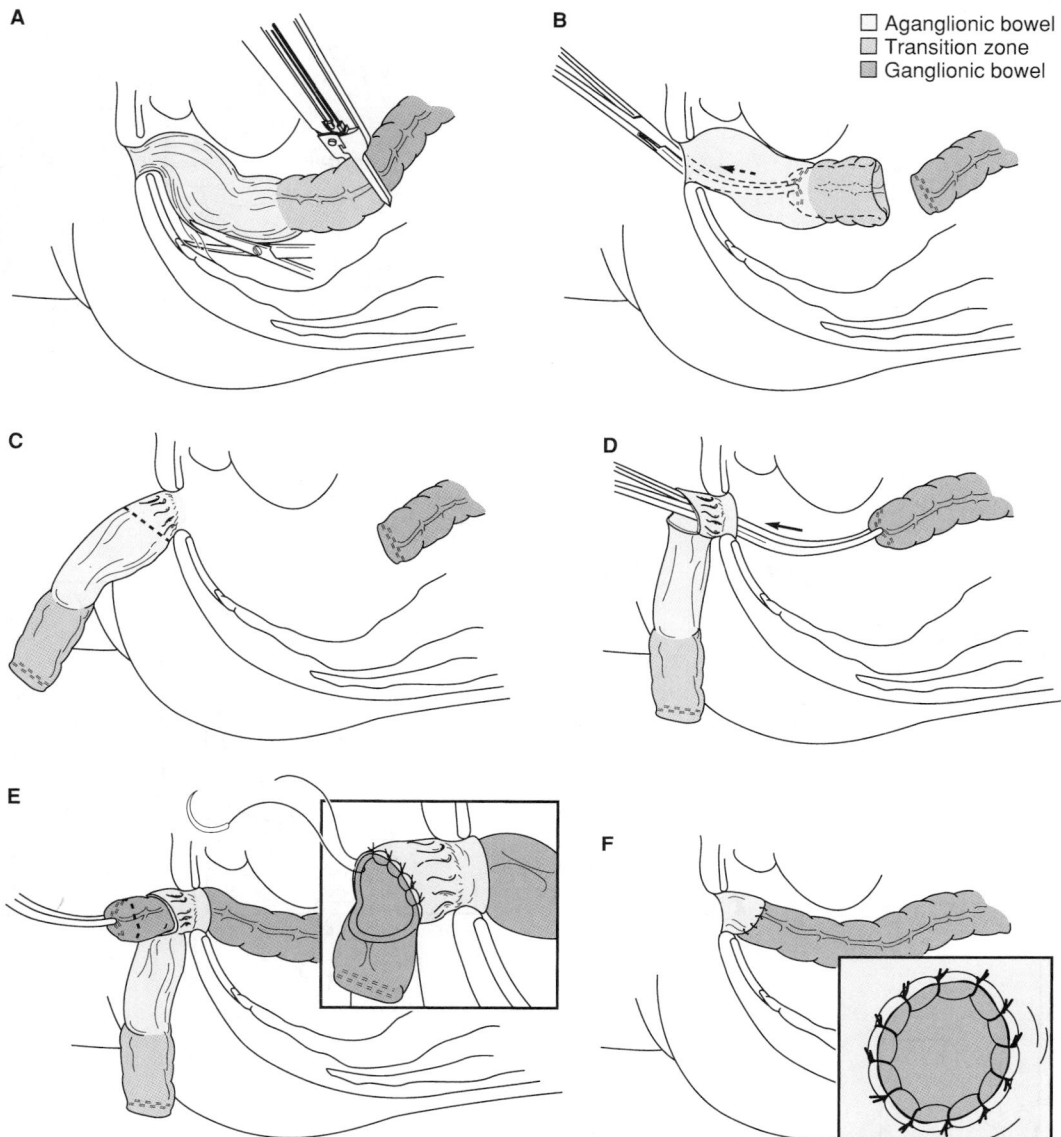

□ Aganglionic bowel
▨ Transition zone
▩ Ganglionic bowel

Figure 97.36. Swenson procedure. *(A)* Extramural rectal dissection. *(B and C)* Eversion of aganglionic segment and full-thickness rectum. *(D)* Pull-through of normal, ganglionic bowel. *(E)* Colorectal anastomosis. *(F)* Completed procedure.

mural dissection of the distal rectum is performed. Care must be taken to avoid inadvertent injury to the seminal vesicles, ductus deferens, ureters, and pelvic splanchnic nerves. The dissected rectum is everted through the anus onto the perineum and excised. Normal proximal bowel is pulled through, and a colorectal anastomosis is performed.

Laparoscopically Assisted Endorectal Pull-through. A multi-institutional clinical experience with a laparoscopically assisted endorectal pull-through technique for the treatment of Hirschsprung's disease was reported. Potential advantages of this approach include excellent visibility of the distal rectum during dissection, early return of postoperative bowel function, and decreased length of hospital stay. The early results report outcomes similar to the other established procedures. The procedure is reviewed in Fig. 97.37.

Rectal Myectomy. Resection of a longitudinal strip of the posterior rectal muscular wall has been used for the definitive management of ultrashort-segment Hirschsprung's disease, although this is controversial. This procedure can be performed by a transanal approach combined with submucosal dissection or by a posterior sagittal approach. The use of rectal myectomy as a definitive operation for Hirschsprung's disease may be considered most useful in the selected older child with ultrashort segment disease (133).

Total Colonic Aganglionosis. Total colonic aganglionosis is complex and, fortunately, relatively rare. Several different operative procedures have been described, and treatment must be individualized. The endorectal pull-through with ileoanal anastomosis has been used with good success when most or the entire small bowel is preserved. For extensive small bowel aganglionosis, an ex-

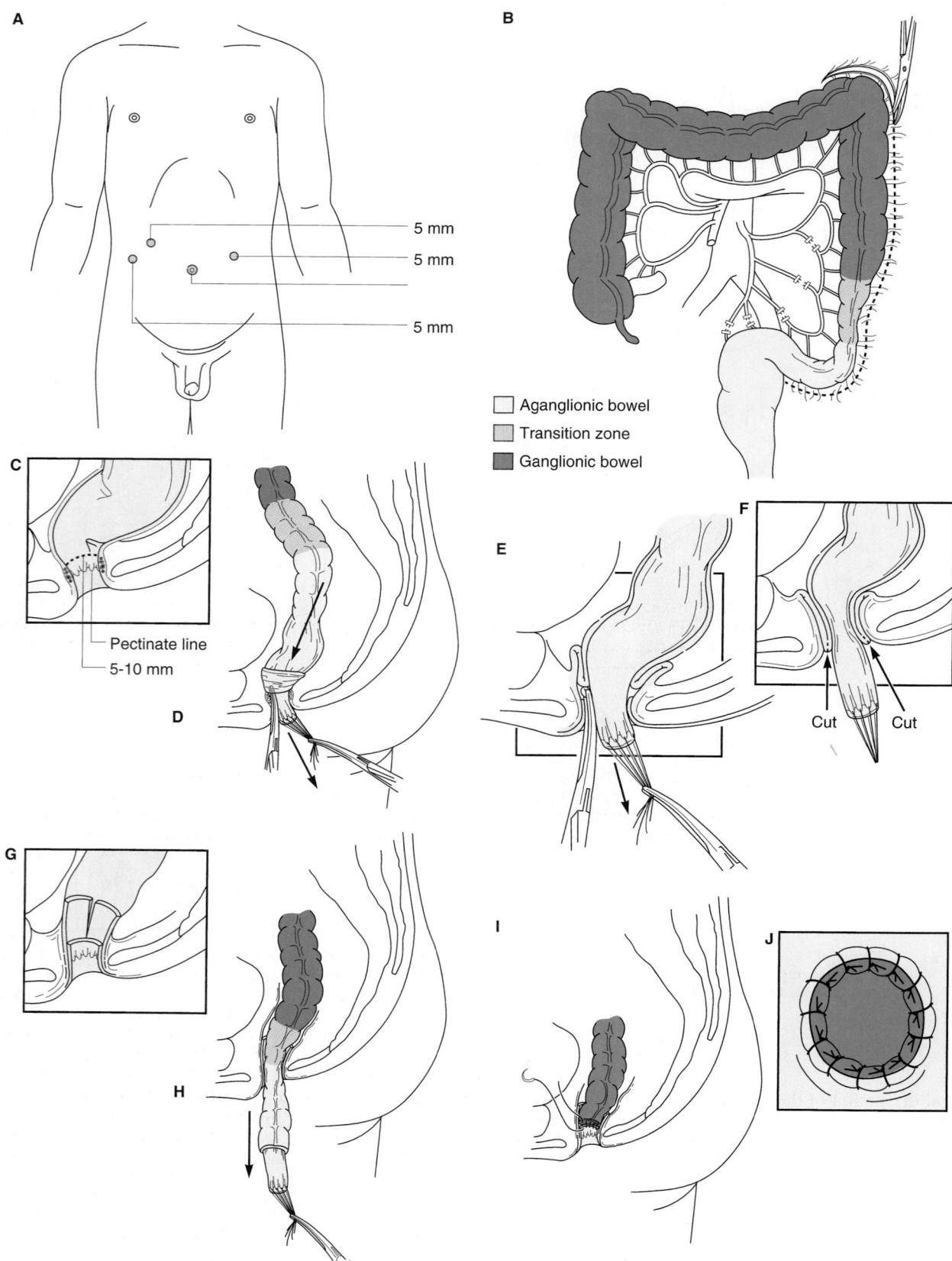

Figure 97.37. Laparoscopically assisted pull-through for Hirschsprung's disease. *(A)* Sites for operative trocar placement. *(B)* Division of colon and rectal mesentery with mobilization of proximal colon. *(C)* Circumferential incision in rectal mucosa 5 to 10 mm cephalad to the pectinate line. *(D)* Mucosal traction sutures to facilitate further dissection from rectal muscular cuff. *(E)* Transanal submucosal dissection is continued cephalad to meet the caudal extent of the transperitoneal rectal dissection. *(F)* Circumferential incision of rectal muscular cuff. *(G)* Rectal muscular cuff is split posteriorly to accommodate the pull-through segment (the pull-through segment is not shown here to clarify this maneuver). *(H)* Rectum and sigmoid colon are pulled through the rectal muscular cuff to the anastomotic site. *(I)* Colon is transected at appropriate site with confirmation of ganglion cells by frozen section. *(J)* Transanal, end-to-end single layer colorectal anastomosis.

tended side-to-side anastomosis of normally innervated proximal small bowel to the aganglionic colon has been successfully performed. For complete intestinal aganglionosis, an extended intestinal myectomy has been described.

Results

Complications resulting from definitive procedures for Hirschsprung's disease include anastomotic leak, stricture, pelvic or rectal muscular cuff abscess, intestinal obstruction, and wound infection. These occur with a frequency of 1% to 10% with most experienced surgeons. Mortality from Hirschsprung's disease is distinctly unusual unless enterocolitis is the presenting feature or associated medical problems or anomalies are present.

A unique complication following definitive repair of Hirschsprung's disease is postoperative enterocolitis. The clinical presentation and pathogenesis have been discussed, and it remains an important and significant cause of morbidity. The incidence of postoperative enterocolitis ranges from 10% to 30% in most large series and has a tendency to be higher following the Swenson procedure. Although rare, Hirschsprung's enterocolitis can occur even in the presence of a diverting colostomy. Long-term outcomes appear quite good for all the procedures used, with 80% to 90% of patients maintaining good to excellent bowel function. Whether the laparoscopically assisted endorectal pull-through procedure maintains a durable long-term outcome remains to be investigated.

Other Childhood Gastrointestinal Disorders

This review is limited to relatively common surgical conditions that are either congenital in origin or unique in children. For other surgical conditions that can affect both children and adults, the reader is referred to other chapters in this text.

Infantile Hypertrophic Pyloric Stenosis

Anatomy and Pathophysiology. The pathogenesis of infantile hypertrophic pyloric stenosis is unknown, but current data suggest that local deficiency of nitric oxide synthase in the pylorus is responsible for the clinical manifestations of the disease (134). The deficiency of nitric oxide synthase leads to a lack of nitric oxide-mediated relaxation of smooth muscle and subsequent focal functional obstruction. Luminal narrowing occurs as a result of concentric hypertrophy of the pyloric smooth muscle. Clinically, this presents as progressive gastric outlet obstruction that initially may become symptomatic by 2 to 4 weeks of age. The maximal narrowing and clinical symptoms of hypertrophic pyloric stenosis occurs between 4 and 8 weeks of age. The hypertrophic pyloric muscle ultimately undergoes gradual involution over a period of weeks to months. Anatomic evidence of the hypertrophied pylorus will be absent if surgical exploration is performed for other reasons at a later date.

Clinical Presentation. The reported incidence of hypertrophic pyloric stenosis is approximately 0.1% to 0.4% among white infants and is slightly lower in the black population. There is a distinct familial predisposition with an approximate 7% incidence in children of parents with a history of pyloric stenosis. The incidence is about four times higher in male than in female infants and higher in first-born infants (135). There is an apparent increased risk of hypertrophic pyloric stenosis in infants receiving oral erythromycin for pertussis prophylaxis (136). Association of pyloric stenosis in infants treated for esophageal atresia and in infants with Smith-Lemli-Opitz syndrome has been reported (137).

Infants with hypertrophic pyloric stenosis will have a history of nonbilious, postprandial emesis that may become progressively projectile. The infant otherwise appears well and will feed vigorously until late in the clinical course. The typical age at diagnosis is between 2 and 12 weeks of age. A history of feeding intolerance and formula change is common. The clinical course is characterized by persistent and progressive feeding intolerance immediately after feeding.

The definitive clinical finding on examination is a palpable pylorus in the right upper quadrant to midepigastric region, often described as a firm, mobile "olive" on palpation. This is a pathognomonic finding; in the correct clinical setting, no further diagnostic imaging studies are required. An experienced clinician should be able to palpate a hypertrophied pylorus in nearly all cases. A successful physical examination requires an empty stomach, a quiet infant, and patience; repeated examinations may be necessary. Inability to palpate the pyloric mass in a quiet or anesthetized infant should place the diagnosis of hypertrophic pyloric stenosis in question. Other physical findings include visible or palpable gastric peristaltic waves, which also can be seen with any cause of gastric or duodenal obstruction. Transient indirect hyperbilirubinemia occurs in 1% to 2% of affected infants and typically resolves on postoperative feeding.

Late findings with advanced symptoms include dehydration and a hypochloremic, hypokalemic metabolic alkalosis from gastric fluid losses. Profound metabolic alkalosis is less common in current practice but occasionally can be encountered in an extremely dehydrated infant with a long-standing history of emesis. The intravascular volume depletion and the chloride-responsive alkalosis should be corrected prior to operative repair of pyloric stenosis. The serum chloride should be restored to at least 90 to 95 mEq/L, and the measured CO_2 should be less than 30 mEq/L prior to induction of general anesthesia.

Diagnosis. Surgical repair of pyloric stenosis should be proposed for any infant with an appropriate history and characteristic findings on physical examination. If the diagnosis is equivocal or confirmation is desirable, either an upper gastrointestinal contrast series or a pyloric ultrasound examination is highly accurate. Both examinations have sensitivity and specificity exceeding 95% in experienced hands. A typical contrast study demonstrating a narrowed, elongated pyloric channel is shown in Fig. 97.38. Contrast studies have the advantage of evaluating other causes of symptomatic emesis, including gastroesophageal reflux disease, malrotation, and antroduodenal webs. The disadvantage of this approach is the presence of contrast in a poorly emptying stomach before general anesthesia is administered. In general, lavage and removal of the gastric contrast can be safely performed prior to anesthesia to minimize the risk of aspiration. Ultrasound examination of the pylorus can effectively demonstrate both elongation and thickening consistent with hypertrophy and is a preferred diagnostic test in many institutions. In general, the diagnosis of hypertrophic pyloric stenosis is being made at an earlier stage of the disease than several decades ago.

Treatment. Hypertrophic pyloric stenosis is a progressive situation that subsequently resolves over several

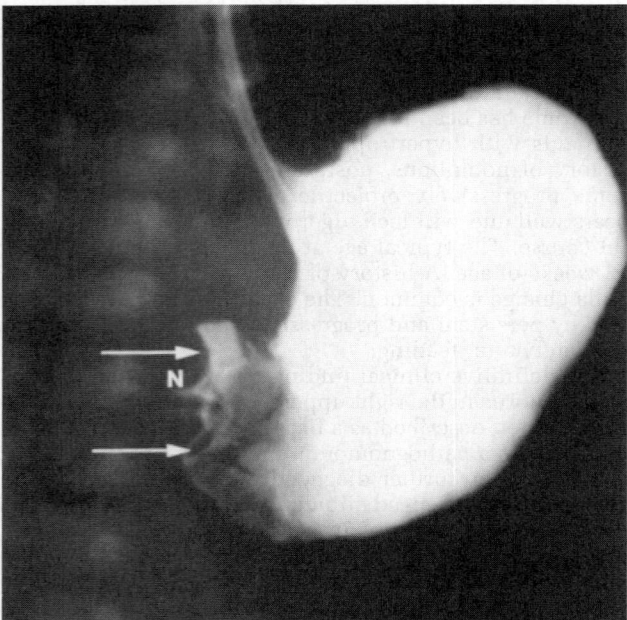

Figure 97.38. Infantile hypertrophic pyloric stenosis demonstrated by barium upper gastrointestinal series showing pyloric channel narrowing (N) and elongation with antral shouldering or cushioning *(arrows).*

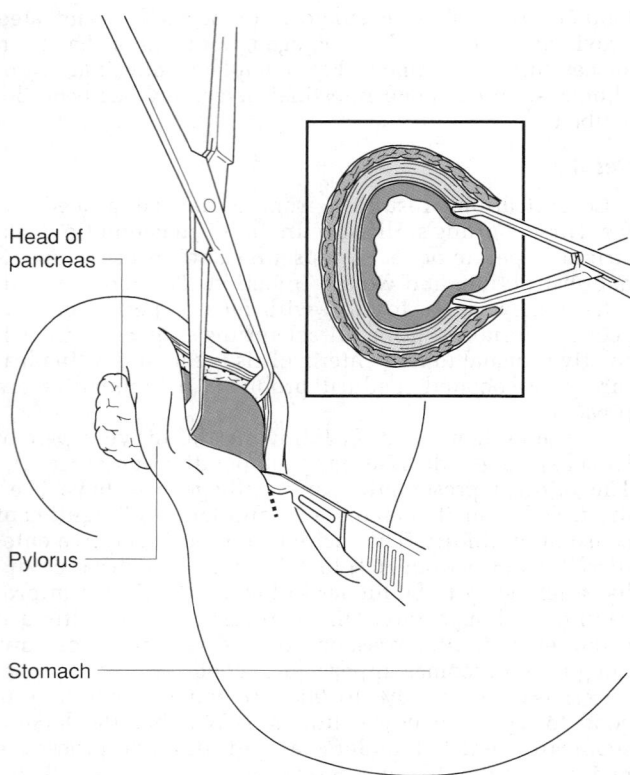

Figure 97.39. Ramstedt pyloromyotomy for infantile hypertrophic pyloric stenosis. The cross-sectional view shows herniation of the submucosa into the myotomy site, indicative of an adequate myotomy.

weeks to months. Nonoperative treatment during this period requires either long-term parenteral or enteral nutrition and is not practical from a risk or cost standpoint. The Ramstedt pyloromyotomy has achieved essentially universal acceptance because it offers definitive, rapid cure in virtually all infants, and morbidity rates have been negligible (Fig. 97.39). The operation is performed once the infant is rehydrated and the serum electrolytes are corrected. Typically, the pylorus is delivered through a transverse right upper quadrant incision. A single longitudinal incision is made in the hypertrophied pyloric muscle. The hypertrophied circular pyloric muscle must be meticulously divided from the stomach to the junction of the proximal duodenum. An adequate pyloromyotomy is achieved when the submucosa bulges into the myotomy site and both edges of the divided pyloric muscle are freely mobile. Increasing experience with laparoscopic pyloromyotomy also has been reported to be successful with similar operative times and outcome to the open repair.

Nasogatric suction is not required. Postoperative feeding typically is started within 6 to 8 hours after recovery from anesthesia. Most infants are tolerant of enteral feeding and can be discharged home safely within 24 hours of operation. The surgical treatment of pyloric stenosis is straightforward, and the recovery is typically uncomplicated. Mortality following pyloromyotomy is distinctly unusual in the absence of concomitant medical problems. Complications are rare and usually represent technical failures related to an inadequate pyloromyotomy or inadvertent entry into the duodenum or stomach. Rarely, infants with inadequate pyloromyotomy may require reexploration and a second myotomy on the posterior pyloric wall. Inadvertent duodenotomy or gastrotomy must be recognized and repaired. Again, another pyloromyotomy in a different location can be performed in this situation.

Intussusception

Anatomy and Physiology. *Intussusception* is defined as the invagination or telescoping of a proximal segment of intestine into an adjacent distal segment and is the most common cause of intestinal obstruction in infancy (Fig. 97.40). The invaginated proximal bowel is referred to as the *intussusceptum* and the recipient distal bowel is the *intussuscipiens.* This process most commonly originates in the small intestine either at or near the ileocecal valve, with the terminal ileum passing into the cecum and colon (ileocolic intussusception). In the pediatric population, the vast majority (95%) of cases are considered idiopathic because of the lack of identifiable anatomic lesions causing the intussusception. The most common age range for idiopathic intussusception to occur is between 3 months and 3 years of age; the peak incidence occurs at 6 to 9 months of age. Children presenting at older ages are more likely to have a pathologic lead point causing the intussusception. In similar fashion, infants and children with repeated episodes of intussusception have a greater probability of a pathologic lead point. Table 97.5 describes several factors that have been associated with the development of intussusception.

Many cases of idiopathic intussusception in infants are probably due to the normally prominent intramural lymph nodes (Peyer's patches) in the terminal ileum acting as functional lead points. It remains unclear why idiopathic intussusception is more common in this age group, however. The anatomic consequence of intussusception is obstruction of the distal bowel. As bowel edema and inflammation progress, mesenteric vascular insufficiency from compression and congestion may occur. Incarceration,

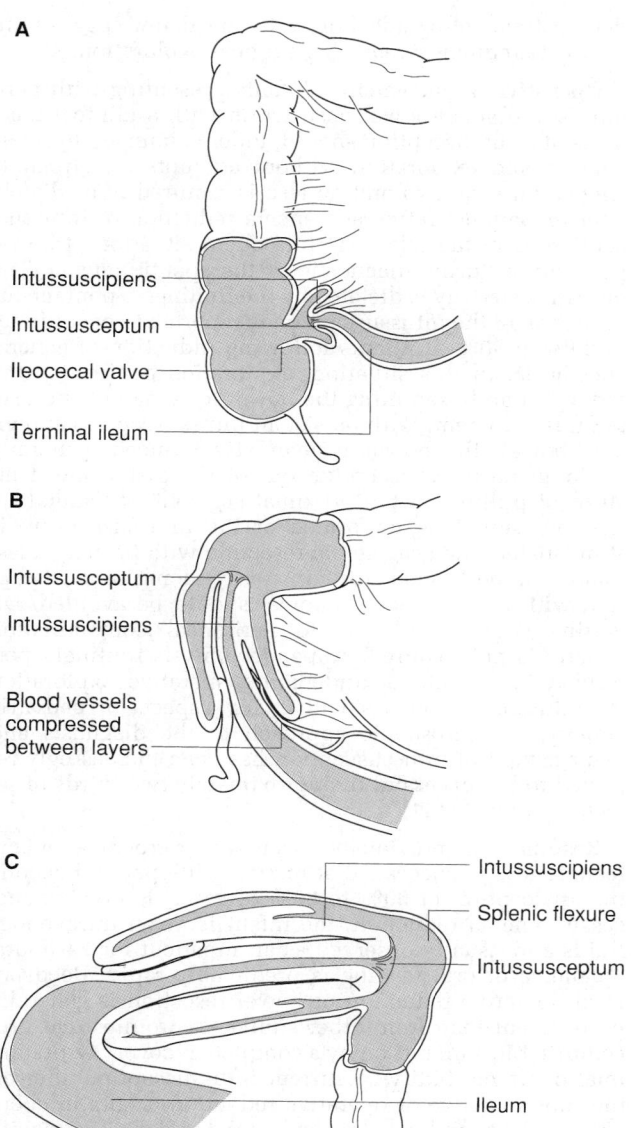

Figure 97.40. Ileocolic intussusception with the intussusceptum and intussuscipiens indicated.

Labels in figure:

A
Intussuscipiens
Intussusceptum
Ileocecal valve
Terminal ileum

B
Intussusceptum
Intussuscipiens
Blood vessels compressed between layers

C
Intussuscipiens
Splenic flexure
Intussusceptum
Ileum

Table 97.5. PREDISPOSING FACTORS TO THE DEVELOPMENT OF INTUSSUSCEPTION

ANATOMIC LEAD POINTS
Meckel's diverticulum
Polyp
Lymphatic hypertrophy (Peyer's patch)
Appendix
Duplication or enteric cyst
Lymphoma
Other neoplasm
Heterotopic pancreatic tissue

ASSOCIATED INFECTIONS
Adenovirus
Rotavirus
Parasitic infestation
Other

BLEEDING DISORDERS[a]
Henoch-Schönlein purpura
Hemophilia
Leukemia

TRAUMA[a]
Blunt abdominal trauma
Major retroperitoneal dissections

OTHERS
Cystic fibrosis

[a]These factors are more likely to be associated with small bowel-to-small bowel intussusception than with ileocolic intussusception.

strangulation, and intestinal perforation ultimately may result if this condition remains unrecognized or untreated.

Clinical Presentation. Intussusception is estimated to occur with an incidence of 1 to 4 per 1,000 children. There is a slight (3:2) male predominance; in a review of 385 patients, 79% were under the age of 12 months and seasonal variation in incidence was not observed (138). There appears to be an association between the development of intussusception and the administration of a tetravalent rhesus-based rotavirus vaccine (RotaShield, Wyeth Laboratories, Inc., Marietta, PA) (139).

Otherwise healthy infants who develop intussusception have a characteristic clinical history. The classic triad of abdominal pain, vomiting, and bloody stool is diagnostic but variably present. The typical infant between 3 months and 3 years of age develops the acute onset of severe colicky abdominal pain. Intermittent episodes of irritability and crying may be associated with drawing the legs up to the abdomen for several minutes. Between bouts of colic, the infant is often lethargic or sleepy. During these periods of relative exhaustion, the abdominal examination may not be impressive; however, on careful physical examination, a palpable mass in the right abdomen may be appreciated in 80% to 90% of cases. On occasion, the intussusceptum is palpable on digital rectal examination and may present with prolapse through the anus. Emesis is common and is often the presenting complaint for evaluation. As intestinal obstruction progresses, intractable vomiting with abdominal distention and intravascular volume depletion may occur. Guaiac-positive stool is present in 90% to 95% of infants as a result of the ischemic mucosal injury to the intussusceptum. The passage of bloody stool mixed with mucus, classically described as currant-jelly stool, also may be seen.

Diagnosis. Plain radiographs of the abdomen are generally nonspecific and may show a paucity of gas in the right lower quadrant with a suggestive mass effect in the ascending colon. Late findings will demonstrate mechanical small-bowel obstruction with proximal distention, air–fluid levels, and a decrease or absence of gas distally. Diagnostic enema techniques using either air or contrast approach 100% accuracy with typical ileocolic intussusception (Fig. 97.41). An approach using retrograde enemas allows therapeutic reduction of intussusception as well. Ultrasound examination typically reveals a mass with two lumens resembling a bull's eye or target sign, corresponding to the intussusceptum within the intussuscipiens. The target sign of intussusception also may be demonstrated by abdominal CT scan. Both these latter modalities will not allow for potential therapeutic reduction and may be more useful in diagnosing suspected cases of proximal jejunoileal or enteroenteral intussusception.

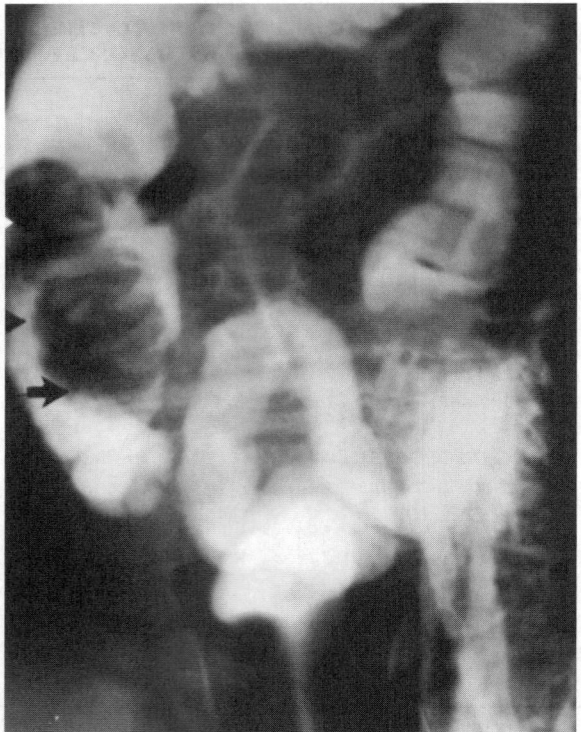

Figure 97.41. Contrast enema demonstrating classic ileocolic intussusception with the intussusceptum visible in the ascending colon *(arrows)*.

Treatment. Any infant with suspected intussusception in the absence of peritonitis should undergo a diagnostic retrograde enema. A high index of clinical suspicion and liberal application of this approach should be maintained. The incidence of normal contrast enema examinations in this setting may exceed 75% in most pediatric centers, and this is justified by the considerable risk inherent in a missed diagnosis. An experienced pediatric radiologist and surgical evaluation are essential. Intravenous access and resuscitation should occur before attempts are made at diagnostic or therapeutic enemas.

Successful hydrostatic or pneumatic reduction of ileocolic intussusception is achieved in 60% to 80% of infants in most pediatric centers in the United States. Some centers prefer pneumatic enema using air as a contrast agent, and this technique appears comparable to the hydrostatic approach in both diagnosis and therapeutic reduction of intussusception. The ability to reduce intussusception using these techniques is time dependent and diminishes substantially after the duration of symptoms exceeds 24 hours. In this setting, a contrast enema is still diagnostic and potentially therapeutic if carefully performed (140). With most experienced pediatric radiologists, the risk of perforation or reduction of a strangulated intussusceptum is quite low.

The technique of retrograde reduction of intussusception is straightforward. Contrast or air is introduced into the rectum by a balloon catheter, with the height of the hydrostatic column less than or equal to 1 m. Most centers use three attempts at reduction, with each attempt no longer than 3 minutes in duration. As long as progress is being made, however, attempts can be repeated until reduction is achieved. Successful reduction of ileocolic intussusception is demonstrated by observing retrograde flow of contrast or air into the terminal ileum. Inability to demonstrate retrograde flow into the ileum suggests incomplete reduction requiring surgical exploration.

Operative Management. Infants presenting with peritonitis and small-bowel obstruction with a clinical diagnosis of intussusception should undergo immediate resuscitation and exploration without attempts at retrograde enema. Surgical exploration also is required immediately after incomplete retrograde enema reduction of intussusception or in the relatively infrequent situation of bowel perforation during diagnostic or therapeutic enema. The operative strategy is dictated by the findings. Spontaneous reduction of the intussusception is reported to occur in up to 20% to 30% of infants following induction of general anesthesia. In this situation, exploration confirming the reduction and examining the bowel for a pathologic lead point is sufficient. With persistent intussusception and viable bowel, the bowel is manually reduced, generally pushing the intussusceptum out of the distal bowel instead of pulling on the proximal segment. If manual reduction cannot be performed or the intussusceptum is strangulated, then segmental resection with primary anastomosis is performed. Attempts at reducing intussusception with clearly necrotic bowel should be avoided. Diverting enterostomy due to peritoneal contamination usually is not required. Appendectomy is routinely performed in all infants undergoing operative exploration for intussusception. As with many aspects of pediatric surgery, a laparoscopic approach to the diagnosis and management of intussusception has been increasingly reported to be successful in approximately two thirds of selected patients (141).

Results. As previously discussed, retrograde enema techniques are successful at reducing idiopathic ileocolic intussusception in 60% to 80% of cases. Following successful enema reduction, the infant is given intravenous fluids and usually observed as an inpatient for 24 hours. Tolerance of oral feeding is predictably rapid. Recovery from operative reduction or bowel resection is generally no different than from other similar gastrointestinal procedures. Most infants enjoy a complete recovery with minimal or no morbidity. Recurrent intussusception after either nonoperative or operative reduction occurs in about 5% of infants and usually can be treated definitively with a repeat enema. Mortality from intussusception is rare and is almost always the result of systemic sepsis and shock from unrecognized strangulated intestine.

Meckel's Diverticulum and Related Disorders

Embryology and Anatomy

The most frequent congenital anomaly of the gastrointestinal tract is Meckel's diverticulum, representing one of several malformations resulting from persistence of the yolk stalk (synonymous with *vitelline duct* and *omphalomesenteric duct*) and its components. The embryonic yolk stalk connects the yolk sac and the developing midgut (Fig. 97.42). Between weeks 5 and 7 of gestation, the yolk sac involutes and the stalk fuses with the umbilical cord. Developmental failure or arrest of yolk sac involution creates a spectrum of clinical malformations as outlined in Fig. 97.43, with Meckel's diverticula constituting greater than 95% of these anomalies. Meckel's diverticulum is a true diverticulum of variable size derived from the intestinal remnant of the yolk stalk. Typically, it is found on the antimesenteric border of the terminal ileum approximately 40 to 50 cm from the ileocecal valve in adults. The blood supply is derived from persistent

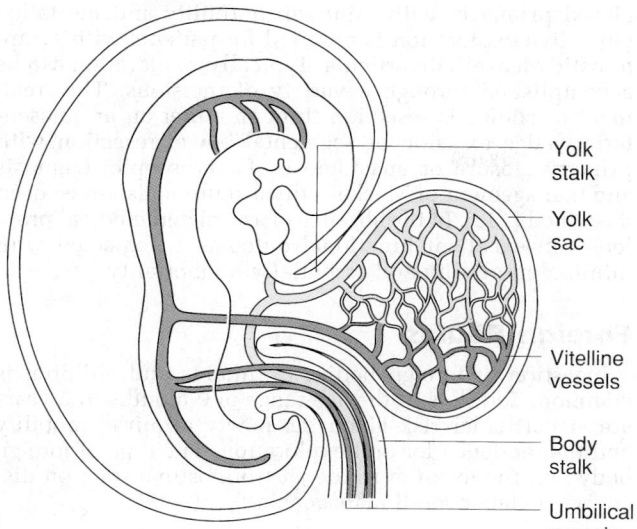

Figure 97.42. Normal embryonic relations of the yolk sac, yolk stalk, and developing gut.

vitelline vessels supplied from the SMA. About 25% of the diverticula will have a fibrous or vascular attachment to the anterior abdominal wall at the umbilicus (Fig. 97.43C). Heterotopic gastric mucosa or pancreatic tissue is found in about half of the diverticula examined at autopsy. In about 75% of patients with symptomatic diverticula, gastric mucosa will be present. When symptoms occur, bleeding or perforation is generally the result of peptic ulceration of the adjacent ileal mucosa, not the diverticulum itself.

Clinical Presentation

Yolk stalk anomalies that become symptomatic usually are diagnosed by history and clinical examination. Umbilical drainage from a persistent fistula or sinus tract may be noted in a newborn following separation of the umbilical cord. Intestinal prolapse or passage of stool from the umbilicus signifies a patent omphalomesenteric duct. Small-bowel obstruction in an otherwise healthy infant without a history of laparotomy may be due to volvulus around an omphalomesenteric band or intussusception from a Meckel's diverticulum acting as a lead point.

The incidence of Meckel's diverticula in the general population is about 2%, with a 2:1 male-to-female predominance. The risk of developing symptoms from the diverticulum decreases with age, and the vast majority of subjects remain asymptomatic. About half of the persons who do become symptomatic are younger than 2 years of age. Table 97.6 outlines several of the common clinical presentations of symptomatic Meckel's diverticulum. Gastrointestinal hemorrhage, diverticulitis, perforation, and small bowel obstruction may occur as a result of the abnormal persistence of the diverticulum.

Hemorrhage. Gastrointestinal bleeding related to Meckel's diverticulum generally results from peptic ulceration of the vulnerable adjacent ileal mucosa. Clinically, it manifests as painless, episodic hemorrhage that is typically bright red to maroon in color; melena is not characteristically seen. Bleeding from Meckel's diverticulum is generally not hemodynamically significant or exsanguinating, but it can be persistent enough to require transfusion. The diagnostic test of choice is the ^{99m}Tc-pertechnetate radioisotope scan (Meckel's scan) because of the high affinity of the isotope for gastric mucosa and the high probability of gastric mucosa within a symptomatic Meckel's diverticulum. Diagnostic accuracy is reported to be as high as 90% for Meckel's-related bleeding. Contrast studies and endoscopy have a limited role when the problem is hemorrhage from a Meckel's diverticulum. Selective mesenteric angiography may be useful diagnostically in the event of a negative Meckel's scan and continued active hemorrhage.

Obstruction. Intestinal obstruction associated with omphalomesenteric duct anomalies usually results from either intussusception or volvulus around an abnormal attachment between the bowel and the abdominal wall.

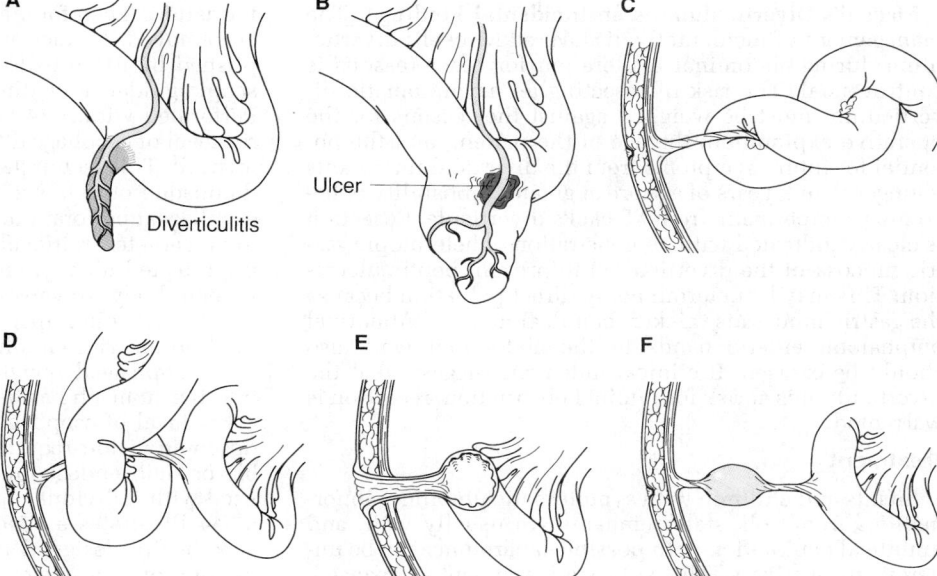

Figure 97.43. Common variants of yolk stalk malformations. *(A,B)* Meckel's diverticulum can manifest with inflammation (diverticulitis) or hemorrhage from acid-induced ulceration. *(C,D)* Meckel's diverticulum in association with abnormal band attached to the abdominal wall predisposing to volvulus and intestinal obstruction. *(E)* Patent omphalomesenteric duct. *(F)* Omphalomesenteric sinus and cyst formation.

Table 97.6. SIGNS AND SYMPTOMS OF MECKEL'S DIVERTICULUM

Clinical presentation	Approximate frequency (%)
Hemorrhage	30–35
Small bowel obstruction	30–35
Diverticulitis	20–25
Umbilical fistula	10
Other	Uncommon

In about 5% to 10% of persons with symptomatic Meckel's diverticula, intussusception is the initial symptom. In patients with Meckel's diverticula whose initial symptom is small-bowel obstruction, about half will have intussusception, and the remainder will have volvulus, internal hernias, or other mechanical causes (50). Intussusception secondary to a Meckel's diverticula has a decreased likelihood for successful enema reduction. Small-bowel obstruction from volvulus around an omphalomesenteric band requires operative exploration and treatment.

Diverticulitis. About one third of patients with symptomatic Meckel's diverticulum will have acute diverticulitis. Similar to appendicitis, intraluminal obstruction at the base of a Meckel's diverticulum can lead to distal inflammation, gangrene, and subsequent perforation. Peptic ulceration also can lead to local inflammation and perforation with the development of peritonitis. The signs and symptoms of Meckel's diverticulitis are virtually indistinguishable from appendicitis, and exploration is both diagnostic and therapeutic.

Umbilical Anomalies. As discussed, about 10% of patients with yolk stalk or persistent omphalomesenteric duct anomalies have umbilical problems. The usual clinical presentation is persistent drainage or intestinal mucosa found at the umbilicus. The diagnosis can be confirmed by contrast sinogram of the umbilical orifice or tract. Occasionally, ultrasound examination may be useful to demonstrate omphalomesenteric cysts. Ultimately, surgical exploration may be required for both diagnosis and treatment.

Meckel's Diverticulum as an Incidental Finding. The management of incidentally discovered Meckel's diverticulum during abdominal exploration for other reasons is controversial. The risk of resecting an asymptomatic diverticulum must be weighed against the reasons for the operative exploration, the age of the patient, and the potential for future symptoms from the diverticulum. Infants younger than 2 years of age are at greater probability of becoming symptomatic from Meckel's diverticula. Resection is clearly indicated with demonstration of heterotopic gastric mucosa in the diverticulum to prevent peptic ulceration. This may be determined by direct palpation because the gastric mucosa is thicker than ileal mucosa. Abnormal omphalomesenteric bands to the abdominal wall also should be excised. If clinical judgment suggests that the diverticulum is at risk for luminal obstruction, resection is warranted.

Treatment

Infants and children with symptomatic umbilical abnormalities from yolk stalk remnants are usually well, and umbilical exploration with possible laparotomy can be undertaken electively. The yolk stalk remnant is excised, and, if present, the communication with the ileum is closed primarily with minimal morbidity and mortality. Operative exploration is required for patients with symptomatic Meckel's diverticula. Typically, exploration can be accomplished through a variety of incisions. The treatment of choice is resection through either an antimesenteric wedge excision or segmental bowel resection with primary closure or anastomosis. Laparoscopic diagnosis and management of Meckel's diverticulum also have been described (142). In the absence of associated medical problems, an excellent functional outcome is expected with minimal morbidity and essentially no mortality.

Foreign Bodies

Ingestion of foreign bodies by infants and children is common. Toddlers in the age range of 9 months to 2 years are at particular risk given the newly acquired mobility and the tendency for oral exploration. The type of foreign body and the location in the gastrointestinal tract on discovery dictate overall management.

Esophagus

Typical foreign bodies found in the esophagus include coins and small toys. In normal children, these objects become impacted at predictably narrow portions of the esophagus. These include the cricopharyngeus, the esophagus at the level of the left mainstem bronchus, and the gastroesophageal junction. Previous areas of esophageal repair or injury predispose to points of obstruction. In particular, infants and children with repaired esophageal atresia, gastroesophageal reflux, or caustic esophageal injury are at risk for impaction at these sites.

Esophageal foreign bodies produce clinical symptoms of drooling, feeding intolerance (particularly to solids), dysphagia, and pain. Unrecognized foreign bodies with unusual configuration or sharp points and edges may cause esophageal perforation and mediastinitis. The diagnosis is straightforward on plain radiographs if the object is metallic or radioopaque. If a radiolucent object is suspected, an upper gastrointestinal contrast study usually is required to confirm the diagnosis. Lateral plain films of the neck or chest may be useful to differentiate between small foreign bodies in the esophagus or trachea.

Foreign bodies impacted in the esophagus cause partial esophageal obstruction and can cause complications including aspiration, erosion, perforation, and late stricture formation. Therefore, all esophageal foreign bodies must be removed. Extraction of foreign objects can be accomplished by using balloon catheter retrieval under fluoroscopic guidance or direct visualization using endoscopy. Performed within 24 hours of ingestion, balloon catheter retrieval of esophageal foreign bodies is relatively straightforward. This technique is generally limited to smooth, radioopaque objects such as coins to minimize the risk of esophageal perforation. The most significant risk with balloon catheter retrieval is potential aspiration from an unprotected airway, and this must be anticipated as the foreign body traverses the pharynx. Alternatively, for esophageal coin impaction of less than 24 hours' duration in children without a history of esophageal surgery or injury, esophageal bougienage with clearance of the coin into the stomach has been successful (143).

Retrieval of esophageal foreign bodies under direct endoscopic vision requires general anesthesia. Either flexible or rigid endoscopy systems are widely available and used with individual and institutional preferences. Figure 97.44 illustrates a rigid endoscopic system with forceps specifically designed to grasp small objects. Esophageal perforation, the major risk, occurs in fewer than 5% of cases in most reported series.

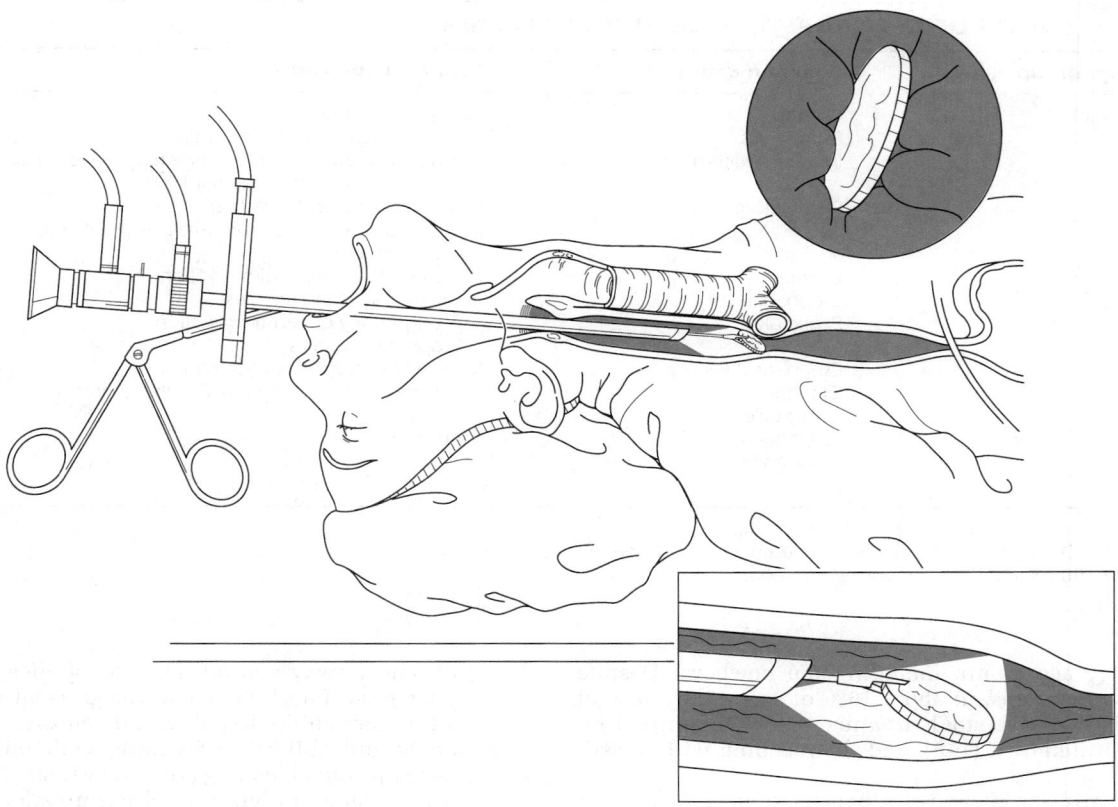

Figure 97.44. Illustration of foreign body removal from the esophagus. The patient's neck is placed in extension and the endoscope is inserted under direct vision. The foreign body is grasped with forceps.

Distal Gastrointestinal Tract

More than 95% of foreign bodies that pass beyond the gastroesophageal junction proceed uneventfully through the gastrointestinal tract. The transit time for an asymptomatic foreign body is highly variable and can take days to weeks. Progress of an asymptomatic radioopaque foreign body can be followed by abdominal plain films, but this is rarely useful from a clinical standpoint unless it is a battery (see later). The stool also can be screened to confirm passage of a foreign body passage.

Operative exploration or endoscopic retrieval of distal gastrointestinal foreign bodies generally is reserved for clinical symptoms related to either obstruction or intestinal injury heralded by abdominal pain, vomiting, fever, or peritonitis. Additionally, persistence of an asymptomatic foreign body in the stomach for several weeks is a relative indication for upper endoscopic retrieval, particularly with foreign bodies with irregular shape, configuration, or sharpness. This is a clinical judgment that is best reserved for an experienced pediatric surgeon because remarkably complex and improbable objects may routinely pass uneventfully through the gastrointestinal tract. For asymptomatic foreign bodies lodged distal to the stomach, a relative indication for operative removal is a fixed, persistent location in the intestine for longer than 1 week in duration.

Ingested batteries, in particular alkaline disc batteries, are a potentially serious hazard to children and require a more aggressive approach. Disruption of the battery casing and spillage of the contents have been reported to cause intestinal injury and perforation, presumably because of leakage of potassium or sodium hydroxide. Esophageal impaction of a battery warrants prompt removal when recognized because the risk of acquired esophageal injury, perforation, and development of traumatic tracheoesophageal fistula is present (144). In the distal bowel, cathartics, lavage, and enemas may be helpful to expedite passage of the battery. Operative removal may be necessary if the battery fails to progress distally over a few days or if symptoms related to the battery occur. Notably, the vast majority of batteries pass through the gastrointestinal tract uneventfully.

Gastrointestinal Hemorrhage

The subject of gastrointestinal hemorrhage and general principles of management are discussed elsewhere in the text. The following section reviews some of the important and age dependent clinical causes and unique issues of gastrointestinal bleeding in pediatric population (145). These causes are age dependent and are summarized in Tables 97.7 and 97.8.

The expedient diagnostic work-up of an infant or child with gastrointestinal hemorrhage requires coordinated participation between pediatricians, surgeons, gastroenterologists, and radiologists. Several general principles governing the diagnostic approach to gastrointestinal bleeding in infants and children are as follows:

1. A clear diagnosis can be made in the vast majority of situations; given the current technology available to assist with diagnosis, an aggressive approach is warranted. Diagnostic procedures such as flexible fiberoptic endoscopy, radioisotope imaging, and angiography are widely available, safe, and applicable

Table 97.7. CAUSES OF UPPER GASTROINTESTINAL HEMORRHAGE[a]

Patient age group	Common causes	Less common causes
Neonatal (0–30 d)	Gastritis Esophagitis Ingested maternal blood Peptic ulcer	Iatrogenic trauma Coagulopathy/bleeding dyscrasia Vascular malformations (hemangioma, telangiectasia, arteriovenous malformation) Nasal or pharyngeal bleeding Miscellaneous structural abnormalities (leiomyoma, gastric polyp, duplication)

Infant (30 d–1 y)	Gastritis
	Esophagitis
	Peptic ulcer
		Same as for neonate, with addition of
		    Drugs (salicylates, steroids)
		    Foreign body or caustic ingestion
		    Esophageal varices

Child (1–12 y)	Esophageal varices Esophagitis Peptic ulcer	Same as for infant, with addition of Acquired thrombocytopenia (chemotherapy)
Older child (12 y to adult)	Esophageal varices Esophagitis Peptic ulcer	Same as for child

[a]Order in appearance approximates clinical frequency.
Modified from Oldham KT, Lobe TE. Gastrointestinal hemorrhage in children: a pragmatic update. Pediatr Clin North Am 1985;32:1247–1263, with permission.

to any age group, including the newborn. Despite these measures, in about 16% of cases, the cause of guaiac-positive stools in a neonate or infant will remain unknown (146), and the bleeding will be self-limited.

2. The primary diagnostic investigation of choice for upper gastrointestinal bleeding is esophagogastroduodenoscopy with a flexible fiberoptic endoscope. This procedure is optimally performed within the first 24 hours after cessation of active hemorrhage and may require general anesthesia for safety, comfort, and airway control. Imaging studies for active upper gastrointestinal hemorrhage usually are limited in their ability to aid with diagnosis.

3. Infants and children presenting with minor lower gastrointestinal bleeding are best evaluated by a careful perineal and digital rectal examination followed by anoscopy. Sigmoidoscopy is rarely helpful and may require general anesthesia.

4. Massive lower gastrointestinal hemorrhage in an infant or child outside the newborn period is most likely the result of a bleeding Meckel's diverticulum.

Table 97.8. CAUSES OF LOWER GASTROINTESTINAL HEMORRHAGE[a]

Patient age group	Common causes	Less common causes
Neonatal (0–30 d)	Benign anorectal lesions (fissure) Upper GI hemorrhage Milk allergy Necrotizing enterocolitis Midgut volvulus Incarcerated hernia	Iatrogenic trauma Primary coagulopathy/bleeding dyscrasia Vascular malformations Enterocolitis (Hirschsprung's disease, other) Miscellaneous structural abnormalities (lymphoma, duplication, lymphangiectasia)

Infant (30 d–1 y)	Benign anorectal lesions
	Idiopathic intussusception
	Meckel diverticulum
	Infectious diarrhea
	Upper GI hemorrhage
	Milk allergy
		Same as for neonate, with addition of
		    Acquired thrombocytopenia
		    Ingestion of colored (red) foodstuffs (guaiac test mandatory)

Child (1–12 y)	Benign anorectal lesions
	Juvenile polyps
	Intussusception
	Meckel diverticulum
	Infectious diarrhea
	Upper GI hemorrhage
		Same as for infant, with addition of
		    Juvenile polyposis coli
		    Familial polyposis coli
		    Hemolytic uremic syndrome
		    Henoch-Schölein purpura
		Systemic vasculitis (dermatomyositis, lupus)
		Acquired thrombocytopenia (as above plus idiopathic thrombocytopenic purpura)

Older child (12 y to adult)	Juvenile polyps Benign anorectal lesions Inflammatory bowel disease Upper GI hemorrhage	Same as for child, but Henoch–Schölein purpura and hemolytic uremic syndrome less likely Meckel diverticulum

[a]Order in appearance approximates clinical frequency.
GI, gastrointestinal
Modified from Oldham KT, Lobe TE. Gastrointestinal hemorrhage in children: a pragmatic update. Pediatr Clin North Am 1985;32:1247–1263, with permission.

5. If a definitive source for lower gastrointestinal hemorrhage is not found on colonoscopy, evaluation for an upper gastrointestinal source, including upper endoscopy, is warranted.

6. Pain is an uncommon symptom with pediatric gastrointestinal hemorrhage and implies a more complex problem such as volvulus or ischemic bowel. Painful gastrointestinal hemorrhage in pediatric patient requires urgent evaluation and prompt diagnostic work-up.

7. In contrast to that in adults, gastrointestinal bleeding in children is rarely a symptom or sign of gastrointestinal neoplasm.

Neonates (0–30 Days of Age)

The most common cause of gastrointestinal hemorrhage in a neonate is gastritis. Endoscopic evaluation of newborns with symptomatic upper gastrointestinal hemorrhage will demonstrate gastritis or esophagitis in 50% to 75% of cases. About 10% to 15% will have swallowed maternal blood during birth, and 10% of newborns will be discovered to have an underlying coagulopathy. Anatomic lesions requiring operative control are distinctly unusual in this age group. Infrequently, peptic ulceration is observed in infants with other significant conditions such as congenital heart disease, pulmonary disease requiring steroid therapy, sepsis, or intraventricular hemorrhage. Significant, sometimes massive upper gastrointestinal hemorrhage may occur in a neonate without a defineable anatomic lesion despite endoscopic evaluation, usually the result of gastritis; treatment is appropriate blood and volume replacement, evaluation for and correction of any underlying coagulopathy, and supportive care.

Significant conditions responsible for lower gastrointestinal bleeding in the newborn include NEC, malrotation with volvulus, enterocolitis, or bowel obstruction secondary to an incarcerated inguinal hernia. These clinical entities present with characteristic histories, findings on clinical examination, and surgical treatment guidelines previously discussed. Anorectal fissure is also common in neonates, and the bleeding is typically self-limited.

Infants (30 Days to 1 Year)

Infants with upper gastrointestinal bleeding deserve a comprehensive evaluation, including endoscopy, to identify potential lesions requiring operative intervention. Specific lesions are outlined in Table 97.7. The most common causes of lower gastrointestinal hemorrhage in this age group include infectious diarrhea, intussusception, and bleeding Meckel's diverticulum. Most of these lesions have distinct symptoms, signs, and diagnostic findings to facilitate the appropriate diagnosis. Infectious diarrhea is usually accompanied by a history of fever, feeding intolerance and possibly emesis, and abdominal pain. Fecal leukocytes may be present on stool examination, and enteric pathogens or their toxins can be identified by stool culture.

Children (1 to 12 years)

An important surgical cause of upper gastrointestinal bleeding in this age group includes esophageal variceal bleeding from portal hypertension. Children with biliary atresia or extrahepatic portal venous obstruction account for most cases of variceal bleeding in this age group. In the acute setting, endoscopic sclerotherapy is used as a temporizing measure for hemorrhage control; maintenance sclerotherapy is advocated by some investigators. Ultimately, for these children, orthotopic liver transplantation may offer definitive surgical treatment. The use of portosystemic shunts or esophageal devascularization proce-

dures for hemorrhage control are not widely used in pediatric surgical practice in the United States.

Lesions and conditions causing lower gastrointestinal bleeding are summarized in Table 97.8. Juvenile polyps are included in these lesions for this age group. These are benign hamartomatous lesions and represent the single most common cause of lower gastrointestinal bleeding in children. About 20% to 30% of the polyps will be palpable on digital rectal examination. A history of painless, bright red blood per rectum during a bowel movement is typical. The bleeding results from mucosal irritation, involution, and sloughing of a pedunculated polyp and usually is not associated with hemodynamically significant hemorrhage. Tissue may be passed or the pendunculated polyp may prolapse out the anus. A hypochromic, microcytic anemia may be present. Diagnostic work-up generally involves a contrast enema to identify the polyp and evaluate the colon for synchronous lesions. Colonoscopy may require general anesthesia in this age group, and endoscopic snare polypectomy is the treatment of choice for appropriate sized polyps. Infrequently, transanal excision or open resection of larger polyps causing symptoms of pain, obstruction, or persistent hemorrhage is required. In the case of multiple juvenile polyps not amenable to endoscopic polypectomy, management can be expectant based on the benign natural history characterized by involution during adolescence. Histologic confirmation is necessary to differentiate these lesions from adenomatous polyps seen in familial polyposis syndromes or Gardner's syndrome, as discussed elsewhere.

Older Children and Adolescents (Older than 12 Years)

Causes of both upper and lower gastrointestinal hemorrhage in this age group include most etiologic conditions found in adults. Importantly, inflammatory bowel disease is significant in this age group. Tables 97.7 and 97.8 detail the common and less frequent causes of upper and lower gastrointestinal bleeding in this age group.

MISCELLANEOUS PEDIATRIC GASTROINTESTINAL DISORDERS

Duplications

The embryologic origin of enteric duplication formation remains controversial, but it likely results from abnormal development of either a diverticulum or adjacent portion of the embryonic gut that contains primitive pluripotential endoderm. In some cases, duplication cysts of the upper gastrointestinal tract may be associated with thoracic spinal cord or vertebral defects; this appears to reflect abnormal sequestration and integration of developing primitive notochord elements along with the duplication. The resulting lesions are described as either cystic or tubular based on their gross appearance (Fig. 97.45). All types of gastrointestinal-derived epithelia are found, but the clinically relevant finding is ectopic gastric mucosa. Duplications are commonly found along the mesenteric border of the native bowel. The muscular wall is typically well developed and intimately attached to the functional bowel. Additionally, the blood supply is also shared with the functional intestine, an important surgical consideration.

Cystic Duplications. Cystic duplications may be found throughout the gastrointestinal tract. They are frequently located in the esophagus and the hindgut, particularly the rectum. Direct communication between a duplication cyst and the functional gut lumen is unusual. Typically, asymptomatic duplications are discovered as incidental mass lesions during diagnostic imaging studies, particu-

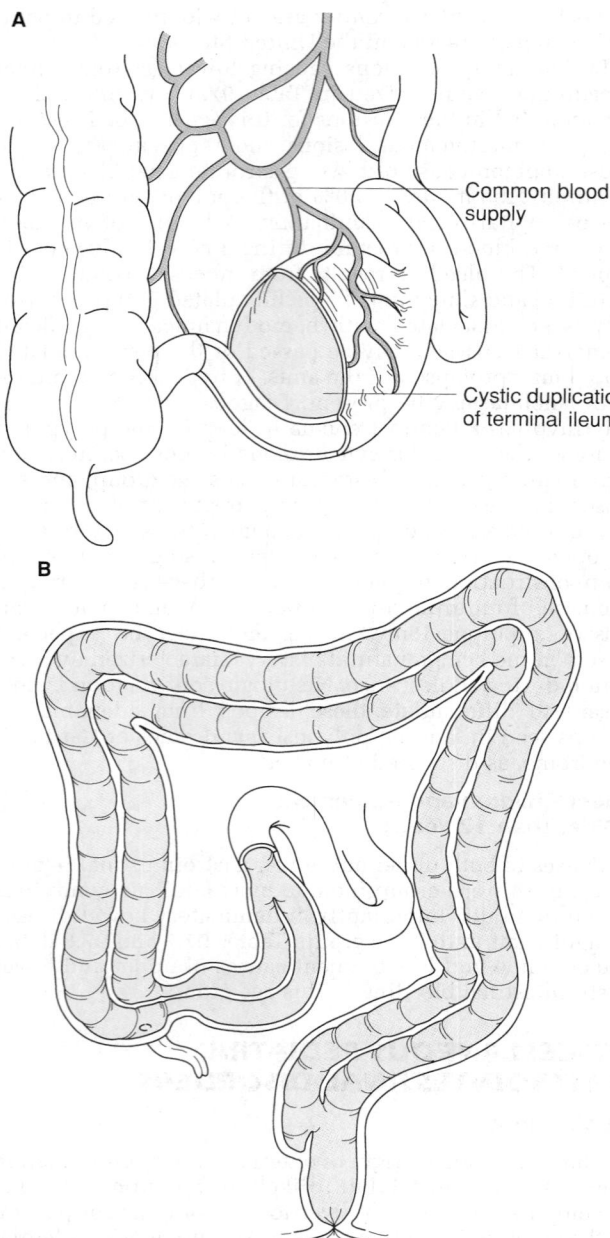

A

Common blood
supply

Cystic duplication
of terminal ileum

B

Figure 97.45. Enteric duplication. *(A)* Cystic duplication of the
terminal ileum. *(B)* Tubular duplication of the terminal ileum and
colon.

larly when the location is the thoracic cavity or the rectum. Duplications also may present as symptomatic lesions as well with ectopic gastric mucosa leading to ulceration and bleeding. Other potential presenting symptoms of enteric duplication include obstruction, intussusception, perforation or traumatic rupture, torsion, infection, and occasional malignant degeneration. Useful examinations to define the extent of the lesion include ultrasound, CT scanning, MRI studies, and contrast studies. The identification of enteric duplication on routine prenatal ultrasound examination has been reported.

The treatment for all cystic duplications is operative. Even in asymptomatic infants and children, uncertainty regarding the nature of the mass and the potential for subsequent problems dictates that surgical exploration be performed. Esophageal and rectal duplication cysts are usually less closely attached to the native esophagus and therefore are generally amenable to simple excision. In contrast, duplication cysts of the small intestine usually require segmental resection and primary anastomosis, given the intimate attachment and shared blood supply with the native bowel. For large cystic duplications involving longer segments of native bowel, individualized treatment strategies are required. One option is cyst marsupialization with resection of the duplication cyst wall and preservation of the common blood supply and wall between the cyst and native bowel. This is combined with submucosal dissection and stripping of the remaining epithelium from the cyst wall. Another approach is internal drainage of the cyst into the adjacent native intestine, for example, creation of a cystduodenostomy for duodenal duplication not amenable to local resection and anastomosis. This is usually unnecessary, however, and long-term drainage is a potential problem.

Tubular Duplications. Tubular duplications may be found anywhere along the length of the gastrointestinal tract. They are less frequent than cystic duplications and have a tendency to involve the ileum and the colon. It is believed that tubular duplication generally reflects abnormal, disordered recanalization of the gastrointestinal tract after epithelial proliferation and obliteration of the intestinal lumen during weeks 6 and 7 of gestation. Similar to cystic duplications, tubular lesions share a common wall and blood supply with the native bowel. Communication between the duplication and the native bowel lumen is common. Tubular duplications may be extensive and can involve the entire length of terminal ileum and colon. Malformations of the entire colon and rectum are associated with genitourinary anomalies, particularly duplications of the external genitalia or bladder. These latter anomalies appear embryologically to represent an interrupted twinning process (50).

Tubular duplications manifest clinically in similar fashion to cystic lesions. Symptomatic lesions most commonly have as their initial sign either gastrointestinal bleeding from peptic ulceration or obstruction. Treatment is operative, and an individualized strategy is required that is based on the location and nature of the duplication. Resection with primary anastomosis may require removal of an unacceptable length of normal bowel. Marsupialization with submucosal stripping of the duplication epithelium may be particularly helpful if ectopic gastric mucosa is suspected or found. Obstruction from a long, blind-ending parallel duplication that communicates with the functional gut lumen can be treated effectively with a reentry procedure such as a distal enteroenterostomy. This approach avoids a potentially complex resection of a significant length of bowel.

The outcomes of surgical management of enteric duplications are generally excellent in the absence of other associated anomalies or medical problems. Mortality attributable to the duplication itself is distinctly unusual. Postoperative morbidity is generally dependent on the nature and location of the duplication.

Mesenteric and Omental Cysts

Mesenteric and omental cysts are rare lesions thought to result from the sequestration of lymphatic tissue during development. Mesenteric cysts are twice more common than omental cysts. Both are characterized by thin and often incomplete walls lined with endothelial cells without surrounding smooth muscle. They may be filled with either serous lymphatic fluid or chyle and may be unilocular or multilocular on examination. These cysts

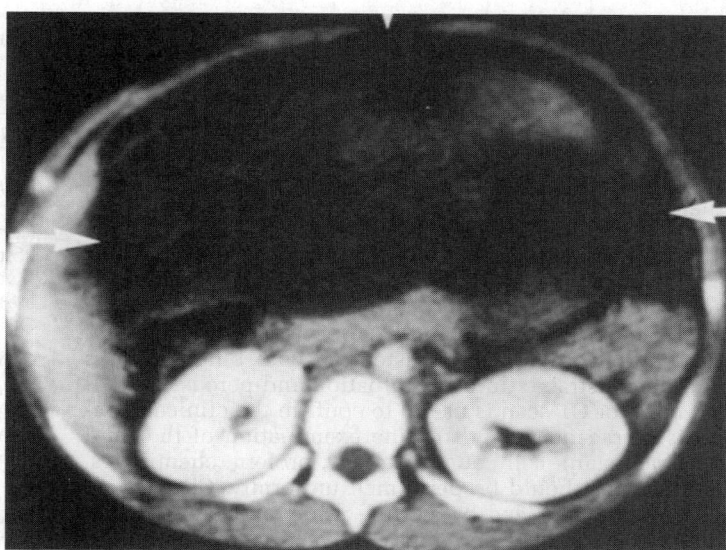

Figure 97.46. Computed tomography scan image from a child after abdominal trauma. Hemorrhage into large omental cyst is apparent *(arrows)*.

may become extraordinarily large before producing symptoms.

Most infants and children with mesenteric or omental cysts are diagnosed before they are 10 years of age. Asymptomatic children usually are diagnosed incidentally during studies for other reasons. Clinically, symptomatic children may have clinically with abdominal pain, and, on examination, a soft, mobile abdominal mass is characteristic. Bleeding, rupture, obstruction, torsion, and infection of the cyst also may be seen on initial examination. The vast majority of these lesions can be diagnosed by ultrasound or CT scan, although the specific diagnosis may not be apparent. Ascites, duplication cysts, pancreatic pseudocysts, ascites, and large ovarian cysts may have a similar appearance on diagnostic imaging. Peripheral calcification and evidence of recent hemorrhage may be seen in mesenteric or omental cysts (Fig. 97.46).

The treatment for these lesions is simple excision, if possible. Total excision of mesenteric or omental cysts is generally preferable over partial excision with marsupialization. Limited resection with primary anastomosis may be required for a mesenteric cyst located adjacent to the intestinal wall, particularly if there is concern that the cyst actually may be an enteric duplication. Morbidity and mortality are generally limited to concurrent problems associated with the intestine. In particular, volvulus of a mesenteric cyst may cause vascular compromise and infarction of the adjacent intestine.

Primary Peritonitis

Bacterial peritonitis without a specific identifiable cause is referred to as *primary peritonitis,* which now accounts for fewer than 1% of all cases of childhood peritonitis, representing a significant, nearly 10-fold decrease over the past century. Use of the term now includes children who develop peritonitis secondary to a clearly identifiable cause, such as an indwelling peritoneal dialysis catheter or a ventriculoperitoneal shunt. Spontaneous bacterial peritonitis in children with ascites or nephrosis is generally included in this group. It is thought that hematogenous seeding of the protein-rich ascitic fluid is responsible for the development of spontaneous bacterial peritonitis in this setting. The infecting bacterial organisms were classically gram-positive with a variety of staphylococcal, streptococcal, and other species accounting for most cases. In a contemporary series of infants and children with primary peritonitis, more than two thirds of the cases were caused by gram-negative organisms such as *Escherichia coli* (147).

The other etiologic mechanism for the development of primary peritonitis is thought to be retrograde inoculation by way of the genitourinary tract. This is characteristic of prepubertal girls 5 to 10 years of age, accounting for as many as half of the cases. The initial signs and symptoms in these children are virtually identical to children with perforated appendicitis: fever, emesis, abdominal pain, and tenderness with peritonitis on examination. Leukocytosis is characteristic, and an ileus is observed on plain abdominal films. On exploration, these children will have inflammatory peritonitis without an identifiable enteric cause. Gram-negative enteric organisms are commonly cultured from the peritoneal fluid.

Infants and children with primary peritonitis in association with an indwelling peritoneal dialysis catheter or ventriculoperitoneal shunt occasionally are treated successfully with broad-spectrum intravenous antibiotics. The catheter or shunt should be removed or exteriorized promptly if resolution of the peritonitis does not occur within 24 to 48 hours or if there are signs of clinical deterioration or sepsis. In association with ascites or nephrosis, diagnostic paracentesis should be performed and the peritoneal fluid examined by Gram stain and culture. Ultrasound-guided paracentesis with sedation may be useful in some children. Gram-positive peritonitis is consistent with primary peritonitis. Gram-negative or mixed enteric flora in the fluid raises the suspicion for intestinal perforation, in particular, for perforated appendicitis. In this clinical setting, operative exploration to exclude a perforated appendix is generally warranted.

Operation usually is performed with a preoperative diagnosis of perforated appendicitis, and a right lower-quadrant incision is typically used. Alternatively, diagnostic laparoscopy may be effectively used to examine the intraabdominal and pelvic organs as well as for obtaining peritoneal fluid cultures. If the appendix is normal, peritoneal cultures should be obtained and a thorough, complete abdominal exploration for another possible cause of intestinal perforation is required. Appendectomy is generally performed when the diagnosis of primary peritonitis is established by a right lower-quadrant incision. Other than perforated appendicitis, common and distinct causes of intestinal perforation or peritonitis in this age group include perforated Meckel's diverticulum, duodenal ulcer, and acute pancreatitis. About half of the peritoneal fluid cultures are positive for a single organism. Treatment with specific antibiotics is continued until the patient is afebrile with a normal white blood cell count and a normal clinical examination. Following operative exploration in primary peritonitis, the morbidity is no different than that for appendectomy, and the recovery is generally uneventful.

Ascites

The common causes of neonatal and childhood ascites are listed in Tables 97.9 and 97.10. The clinical presentation is that of abdominal distention with bulging flanks and demonstrable fluid on palpation and percussion. Ultrasound or CT scan is useful to confirm the clinical diagnosis. Paracentesis and routine examination of the fluid for Gram stain, cell count, cytology, protein, chemistries, and culture should be performed uniformly. Chylous ascites is characterized by a white milky appearance, high lymphocyte count, and high triglyceride content. Bile-stained fluid in the absence of demonstrable bowel perforation is characteristic of biliary ascites. High fluid amylase content is seen in pancreatic ascites, and a low protein count (< 3 g/dL) is consistent with serous ascites. Elevated urea nitrogen or creatinine in the fluid may suggest urinary ascites, particularly in a male patient. Cytology should be performed to exclude peritoneal ascites secondary to malignancy, particularly in pubertal and adolescent females.

If the initial fluid does not provide a diagnosis in an otherwise normal appearing child, a comprehensive diagnostic imaging evaluation is warranted. An echocardiogram should be performed and either ultrasound or CT scan imaging performed to evaluate the genitourinary system, the hepatobiliary system, and the pancreas. A voiding cystourethrogram also may be indicated.

Treatment of neonatal or childhood ascites depends on the establishment of a specific diagnosis. A brief summary of specific treatment principles unique to infants and children is presented in the following:

1. In the absence of an anatomic lesion or injury, spontaneous resolution of chylous ascites occurs in 50% to 75 % of cases with the cessation of enteral feeding and administration of parenteral nutrition. Enteral alimentation with lipid composition limited to medium chain triglycerides also may be effective. Persistence of chylous ascites for longer than 4 to 6

Table 97.9. COMMON CAUSES OF NEONATAL ASCITES

Maternal-fetal Rh incompatibility (now rare)
Structural malformations
  Urinary obstruction
  Congenital heart disease
  Malrotation, duplications, cyst (associated with intestinal volvulus)
  Biliary perforation
  Ovarian ascites
  Pulmonary abnormalities
Chylous ascites
Hematologic disorders
  α-Thalessemia
Infection
  Toxoplasmosis
  Cytomegalovirus
  Others
α_1-Antitrypsin deficiency
Idiopathic

Table 97.10. COMMON CAUSES AND CHARACTERISTICS OF CHILDHOOD ASCITES

SEROUS ASCITES

Cirrhosis
Budd-Chiari syndrome
Nephrosis
Right-sided heart failure
Postoperative ascites (after renal transplantation, peritoneal dialysis, ventriculoperitoneal shunt)
α_1-Antitrypsin deficiency
Other rare metabolic disorders

CHYLOUS ASCITES

Malrotation with volvulus
Small bowel obstruction
Incarcerated hernia
Lymphangioma
Trauma (including operative trauma)

BILIARY ASCITES

Neonatal bile duct perforation
Cystic fibrosis
Biliary atresia
Hepatitis
Cytomegalovirus infection

URINARY ASCITES (7:1 MALE PREDOMINANCE)

Urinary obstruction
Posterior urethral valves
Bladder perforation
Ureterocele
Neurogenic bladder

PANCREATIC ASCITES

Acute pancreatitis (drugs, trauma, gallstones, infection)
Pancreatic pseudocysts

OVARIAN ASCITES

Cysts (torsion, rupture)
Tumors

MALIGNANT ASCITES

Intraabdominal neoplasm

IDIOPATHIC

weeks is an indication for operative attempts to repair or ligate the cisterna chyli.
2. Neonatal biliary ascites may result from spontaneous bile duct perforation, in which case, a diagnosis of CF must be considered. Transient bile duct obstruction in CF typically leads to perforation at the junction of the cystic duct with the common duct. Simple external drainage is the treatment of choice, and complex hepatobiliary tract reconstruction in this setting is unnecessary and potentially hazardous.
3. Urinary ascites in a male patient requires a work-up that includes a voiding cystourethrogram to exclude posterior urethral valves. Urinary ascites will resolve with treatment of obstructive uropathy.
4. Pancreatic ascites is typically self-limited, and treatment by either internal or external drainage procedures either is not required or usually is limited for relief of symptoms.
5. Ascites from cardiac or hepatic disease in children is not different from that in adults, and treatment is directed toward correction of the underlying problem and symptomatic relief.

Massive neonatal ascites may cause hypoventilation because of impairment of diaphragmatic excursion, and therapeutic paracentesis may be required. Childhood ascites generally responds to adequate treatment of the underlying problem and occasionally requires medical therapy. The need for placement of a peritoneovenous shunt in children for intractable ascites is fortunately extremely rare.

RECTAL PROLAPSE

Spontaneous prolapse of the rectum is relatively common in toddlers and preschool-age groups. A peak incidence occurs at or near the time of toilet training. There is an association between straining during bowel movement and rectal prolapse, and it may be more commonly observed in children with CF, myelodysplasias with sacral neuropathy, congenital anorectal malformations, Hirschsprung's disease, and colorectal polyps; however, the vast majority of children presenting with rectal prolapse are normal.

The history and diagnostic findings on examination are characteristic. A parental history of protrusion of mucosa or full-thickness rectum with or without bleeding is usually described. Other lesions of childhood that have a similar appearance are either passage of an intussusceptum in intussusception or passage of a polyp through the anus. The rectal examination is diagnostic. If the protruding intestine is an intussusceptum, a finger can be placed adjacent to it within the rectum; this is not possible with rectal prolapse.

Nonoperative management using manual reduction is successful in most infants and children. Sedation may be required in some instances. Therapeutic interventions include stool softeners and parental instruction on manual reduction, and spontaneous resolution over a few weeks is typical. For persistent rectal prolapse in children, operative intervention is generally governed by doing the least invasive procedure possible. Unlike in adults, complex operations involving bowel resection and suspension are generally avoided in children with rectal prolapse. The most useful and commonly used procedure is rectal submucosal injection using a sclerosant (Fig. 97.47). With the patient under general anesthesia, injection with 5% phenol, 5% sodium morrhuate, hypertonic saline or glucose, or other sclerosants has been performed successfully on an outpatient basis.

About 90% of children can be treated successfully with a single four-quadrant sclerosant technique, but on occasion further sclerosis is necessary (50). Submucosal dissection or cauterization is also successful but may have a higher incidence of postoperative bleeding or stricture formation and usually requires a short period of hospitalization. The major objective in treating childhood rectal prolapse is to create a local extraperitoneal inflammatory process in the perirectal space. Morbidity is low and the long-term outcome is excellent.

PEDIATRIC LIVER

Tumors of the Liver

Primary hepatic tumors are rare in children; at least 60% to 70% are malignant (148,149). Table 97.11 reviews the incidence and types of hepatic tumors that present during infancy and childhood. Pediatric hepatic tumors often manifest as asymptomatic abdominal masses discovered by the parents or pediatrician. Symptoms related to the tumor, such as pain, hemorrhage, hypertension, and precocious puberty, are less frequent. Initial diagnostic imaging studies include plain abdominal radiographs and ultrasound to assist in early determination as to whether the mass is cystic or solid and whether calcifications are present. A cystic hepatic mass with peripheral calcification is consistent with echinococcal liver disease. CT scan imaging of the abdomen and MRI remain quite definitive in the ability to discern anatomic characteristics of the mass and its relationship to adjacent structures. This is an important surgical consideration because an initial operative assessment is done to determine whether the lesion is amenable to resection. Most children initially require laparotomy for either definitive excision in resectable lesions or for diagnostic incisional biopsy in lesions deemed unresectable.

Benign Tumors

About 30% of primary liver tumors of childhood are benign. The most common benign tumors are hemangiomas, hemangioendotheliomas, mesenchymal hamartomas, cysts, focal nodular hyperplasia, and hepatic adenoma. In most large series, hemangiomas constitute about 50% of the benign hepatic tumors seen (150).

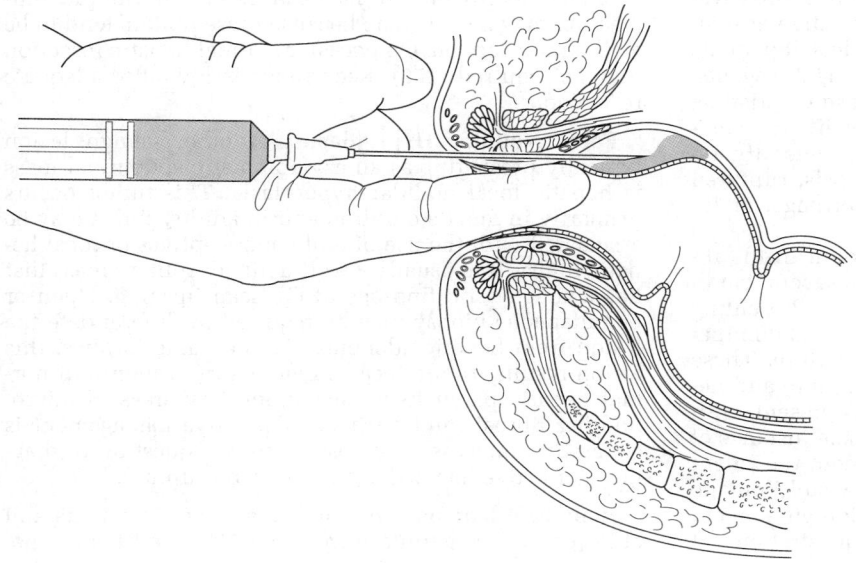

Figure 97.47. Four-quadrant injection of sclerosant into the rectal submucosa for the treatment of childhood rectal prolapse.

Table 97.11. INCIDENCE OF LIVER TUMORS IN CHILDHOOD

Tumor type	Incidence (%)
BENIGN	
Vascular tumors	13
Hemangioma	9
Hemangioendothelioma	4
Mesenchymal hamartoma	6
Focal nodular hyperplasia	2
Adenoma	2
Teratoma	2
Other	3
MALIGNANT	
Hepatoblastoma	43
Hepatocellular carcinoma	23
Malignant mesenchymal tumor	4
Sarcoma	2
Embryonal cell carcinoma	1
Angiosarcoma	1

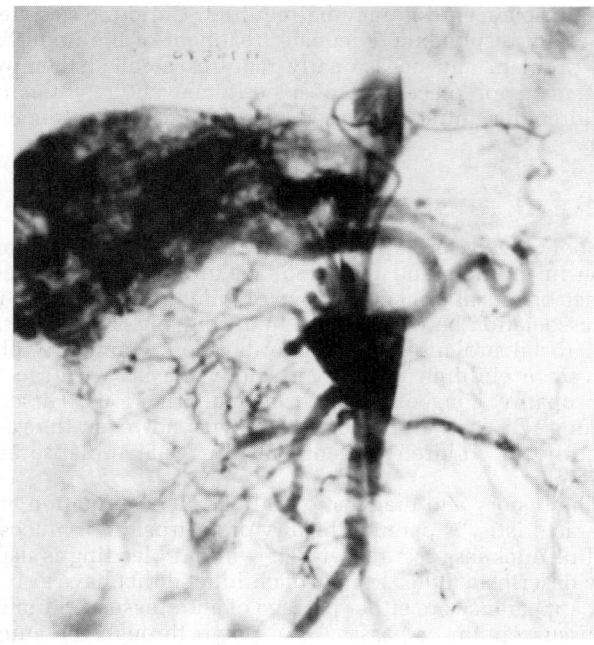

Figure 97.48. Selective visceral angiogram demonstrating large hepatic vascular malformation in a neonate with congestive heart failure. This is consistent with a bilobar hemangioendothelioma.

Vascular Tumors. Hemangiomas are disordered and dilated vascular channels with relatively flattened endothelial linings and clinically often are described as *cavernous hemangiomas.* Cavernous hemangiomas represent the most common benign vascular hepatic tumor in the pediatric age group. Infantile hemangioendotheliomas are vascular tumors derived from endothelial cells that have formed vascular channels but maintain a diffuse, hypercellular pattern (151). Infantile hemangioendotheliomas have a tendency to manifest in the first few months to years of life, whereas hemangiomas present in the adolescent and young adult population. Both these vascular lesions of the liver are typically asymptomatic lesions and are discovered during routine bathing by the parents or physical examination by the pediatrician.

The vast majority of vascular benign lesions of the pediatric liver do not require operative management. Operative intervention is generally reserved for bleeding secondary to traumatic rupture or the evolution of high-output congestive heart failure or thrombocytopenia. Treatment strategies remain highly individualized given the relatively common spontaneous involution of these lesions over time. In the face of congestive heart failure and thrombocytopenia secondary to sequestration, medical treatment and steroid therapy may be useful. More invasive procedures such as irradiation and selective arterial ligation or embolization remain useful in selected patients with uncontrollable symptoms. Chemotherapeutic agents, including recombinant α-interferon, low-dose vincristine, and cyclophosphamide have been used for life-threatening vascular lesions. Hepatic resection is generally reserved for mass lesions of unknown diagnosis, ruptured vascular lesions with signs of active hemorrhage, or for symptomatic, locally resectable lesions.

Hemangioendotheliomas are most important in the infant age group and vary in size from 1 cm to several cm in diameter and may be multiple (Fig. 97.48). Presenting symptoms and signs in a neonate include an abdominal mass, hepatomegaly, and congestive heart failure. These infants also may experience spontaneous rupture and hemoperitoneum. Symptomatic infants may present with tachycardia, tachypnea, and cyanosis or, in the instance of rupture, hypovolemic shock. On examination, the infant may have other cutaneous hemangiomas visible on the skin. About half of these infants will develop an element of thrombocytopenia secondary to sequestration of

platelets in the vascular malformation (Kasalbach-Merritt syndrome). CT scanning or MRI will be diagnostic. The treatment is largely directed at controlling the symptoms using medical management principles outlined above; however, hemangioendotheliomas tend to be more problematic than hemangiomas because of the tendency to occur in infants and the more extensive and symptomatic nature of the lesions.

Mesenchymal Hamartomas. Approximately one third of the benign hepatic tumors in children are mesenchymal hamartomas. A mesenchymal hamartoma is often quite large and typically presents within the first year of life as an asymptomatic, solitary abdominal mass. CT scan or MRI studies are usually diagnostic and will show a solid mass that may have cystic components within the liver parenchyma. Definitive diagnosis may require open tissue biopsy, and the therapy of choice is excision, although spontaneous involution has been described. Simple enucleation may be adequate because these tumors tend to be well circumscribed. On occasion, formal hepatic resection may be required (152). Recurrence is low after adequate resection.

Focal Nodular Hyperplasia. Another benign lesion typically presenting as an asymptomatic abdominal mass is hepatic focal nodular hyperplasia. This tumor occurs primarily in female children and in adults, and it may be associated with the use of oral contraceptives or focal hepatic injury. It is usually a well-defined, solitary mass that has characteristic findings of CT scan imaging. Open or percutaneous biopsy may be required to differentiate the lesion from hepatic adenoma. As the name implies, this lesion results from a focal inflammatory response of normal hepatic parenchyma surrounded by areas of micronodular fibrosis and cirrhosis. Operative management is generally unnecessary unless there is a question of diagnosis or active hemorrhage from lesion rupture.

Hepatic Adenoma. Adenomas are rare in infants and children and constitute fewer than 5% of all benign hepatic lesions in the pediatric age group. There is an association between the use of oral contraceptives, exogenous anabolic steroid use, and glycogen storage disease type I (von Gierke's disease) (151). These tend to be large, solitary lesions located in the right hepatic lobe. The typical presentation is that of an asymptomatic abdominal mass, although symptoms are seen more commonly than with focal nodular hyperplasia (153). About 20% to 25% of patients with hepatic adenoma have hemoperitoneum from tumor rupture. On histologic examination, these lesions are composed of normal hepatocytes without evidence of dysplasia. Operative therapy usually is directed at either making a definitive diagnosis or treating hemorrhage. Enucleation or local resection is generally adequate, and recurrence rates are low.

Hepatic Cysts. Congenital cysts of the liver may be either solitary or multiple. These cysts are thought to result from failure of the intralobular or interlobular biliary ducts to fuse during development. They may be lined with cuboidal, columnar, or squamous epithelium (154). The presence of multiple hepatic cysts is associated with polycystic kidney disease, and future development of hepatic and renal failure are potential problems with this disease. The vast majority of children with hepatic cysts are asymptomatic. Adjunctive diagnostic imaging, including ultrasound and CT scanning, may be useful.

Asymptomatic congenital hepatic cysts do not require surgical therapy. Operative therapy is reserved for symptomatic cysts, and resection or drainage by marsupialization or hepaticocystenterostomy may be required. If patency to the biliary tract is present on contrast injection study of the cyst, internal drainage will be necessary.

The differential diagnosis includes hydatid disease of the liver, which is usually suggested by calcification and loculation of the cyst wall. Hydatid disease can be diagnosed using specific serologic tests and this is an important surgical consideration prior to exploration. Patients with echinococcal cysts should be treated with mebendazole and undergo cyst injection with hypertonic saline or other scolicidal agents into the parent cyst before surgical excision. Careful control of the cyst contents is required during echinococcal cyst excision or marsupialization.

Teratomas. Teratomas of the liver are exceedingly rare and have potential for harboring immature elements capable of transforming into malignancy. Surgical resection on discovery is recommended.

Malignant Hepatic Tumors

At least two thirds of childhood hepatic tumors are malignant, with hepatoblastoma constituting half of the malignancies, followed by hepatocellular carcinoma, malignant mesenchymal tumors, and sarcoma (148). Malignant hepatic tumors are, fortunately, rare, and the effective treatment requires a multidisciplinary approach that is best achieved in an experienced pediatric center.

Hepatoblastoma. Most hepatoblastomas are discovered in children younger than 2 years of age. There is a 2:1 male-to-female predominance. Hepatoblastomas usually are found as either an asymptomatic abdominal mass or because of gastrointestinal obstructive symptoms from extrinsic compression by the mass. There is an association of hepatoblastoma in patients with Beckwith-Wiedemann syndrome and hemihypertrophy. On examination, a firm, palpable upper abdominal mass is usually appreciable. Obstructive jaundice is unusual. More than 90% of children with hepatoblastoma will have elevated levels of α-fetoprotein, and this is a useful tumor marker to continue surveillance for postoperative recurrence. In few instances,

children will have initial symptoms and signs of excess androgen secretion, including virilization and precocious puberty. Diagnostic imaging with CT scan or MRI is essential to evaluate the extent of the tumor and evaluate for metastatic disease (Fig. 97.49). Given the increased resolution of current imaging modalities, preoperative diagnostic angiography is not widely used in the United States.

Notably, most children with hepatoblastoma initially have unresectable disease. In the absence of metastatic disease, however, an aggressive surgical approach is used. Cure and long-term survival with hepatoblastoma require complete surgical excision of the primary lesion. Therefore, localized, resectable tumors usually are excised by formal hepatic lobectomy or extended trisegmentectomy (Fig. 97.50). Children with hepatoblastomas considered initially unresectable or with metastatic disease should undergo percutaneous or incisional biopsy to confirm the histologic diagnosis, followed by multiagent chemotherapy to reduce the size of the primary tumor and control metastases. A delayed resection is appropriate if enough functional, normal hepatic parenchyma will remain after resection. More than half the patients who initially have unresectable hepatoblastoma can be rendered disease-free with the combination of chemotherapy and subsequent surgery (155). Cure rates for hepatoblastoma range from 60% to 75% if histologically clear margins and no metastatic disease are present. All patients with hepatoblastoma, regardless of stage, receive chemotherapy after resection. Unfortunately, cure is not expected in children treated with chemotherapy and radiation therapy alone without surgical resection.

Hepatocellular Carcinoma. Hepatocellular carcinoma is significantly more common in adults but is seen occasionally in children over the age of 3 years and adolescents. There is a male predilection (2:1) and, except for the age at diagnosis, the clinical presentation is similar to that for hepatoblastoma. Children with hepatocellular carcinoma are more likely to have abnormal liver enzymes and clinical jaundice. The high association of cirrhosis in adults (80%) is not seen in children with hepatocellular carcinoma; only 5% of children develop hepatocellular carcinoma in the background of cirrhosis. An increased risk of hepatocellular carcinoma is seen in children with Beckwith-Wiedemann syndrome, hemihypertrophy, von Gierke's disease, hepatitis B, and Fanconi's syndrome. Exposure to oral contraceptives, anabolic steroids, and some chemotherapeutic agents also has been associated with hepatocellular carcinoma. This malignancy carries a poor prognosis with an overall

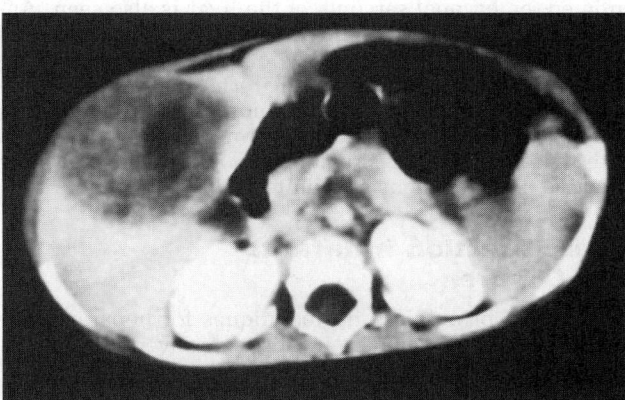

Figure 97.49. Computed tomography scan of the abdomen demonstrating an infant with hepatoblastoma of the right hepatic lobe.

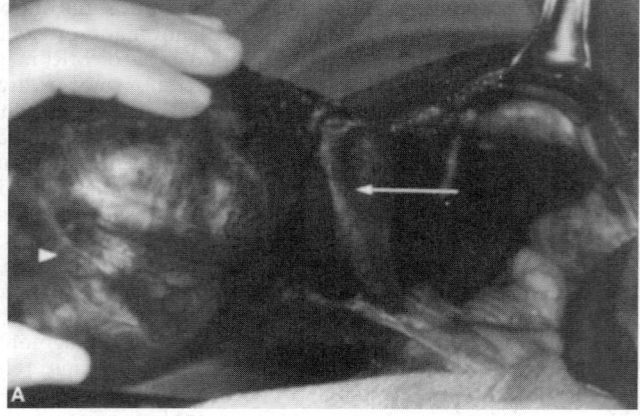
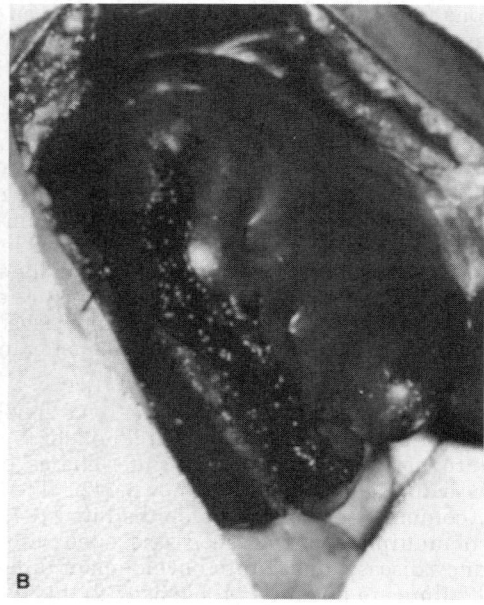

Figure 97.50. *(A)* Intraoperative view of hepatoblastoma *(arrowhead)* of the right lobe of the liver. The gallbladder is indicated by the long arrow. *(B)* Liver following resection of tumor by right hepatic lobectomy.

survival rate of 10% to 20% despite aggressive surgical resection and multiagent chemotherapy. A histologic variant, fibrolamellar hepatocellular carcinoma, carries a more favorable prognosis. As with hepatoblastoma, complete surgical resection with clear histologic margins is necessary for cure and long-term survival.

Malignant Mesenchymal Tumors. These rare hepatic malignancies occur in children 5 to 10 years of age; initial signs are fever, pain, and an abdominal mass, which are usually quite large on diagnosis and may have both solid and cystic components. Multidisciplinary treatment, including complete surgical resection, multiagent chemotherapy, and radiation therapy is required for cure. In general, the prognosis of primary malignant mesenchymal tumors of the liver remains poor.

Sarcomas. Children rarely have a primary sarcomatous malignancy of the liver. Embryonal rhabdomyosarcoma of the biliary tract is distinctly unusual. It may manifest with obstructive jaundice attributable to both extrinsic and intrinsic biliary tract obstruction. Undifferentiated, embryonal sarcoma of the liver is also seen. Angiosarcoma developing in the liver may be associated with exposure to toxins such as arsenic. Aggressive surgical resection may be required, but long-term survival is uncommon. Despite radical surgery, chemotherapy, and radiation therapy, the prognosis and long-term survival of children with these malignancies remains poor, and data regarding effective drug regimens are limited (156).

Liver Resection in Infants and Children

Operative principles and techniques for hepatic resection are covered elsewhere in this text. Several unique issues in the safe performance of hepatic resection in children should be emphasized (157). The contemporary management of hepatic resection for tumors in children requires adequate preoperative assessment and the liberal use of intraoperative monitoring with arterial lines and central venous catheters. The circulating blood volume of

an infant or child is small compared with that in an adult, and children are sensitive to compression of the inferior vena cava causing decreased right heart blood flow. Blood must be available for transfusion. Resection can be performed through either a subcostal or a thoracoabdominal incision; in general, the ability to perform the operation safely should not be limited by the size of the incision. In children, the right and left hepatic veins are difficult to control near the inferior vena cava because of their short lengths, and intraparenchymal control from an anterior approach may be safer (Fig. 97.51). Resection may be performed using total vascular isolation of the liver by controlling the hepatic and portal inflow, the suprahepatic inferior vena cava, and the suprarenal inferior vena cava below the liver. This may help to reduce blood loss during parenchymal dissection, but adequate upper-extremity and central venous access must be obtained and maintained to provide adequate right heart filling and cardiac output. When extrahepatic biliary duct reconstruction is required, T-tube drainage is not routinely performed given the small diameter of the ducts in most children.

Hepatic Infections

Hepatic infections are generally rare in the pediatric population, and their management is similar to that used in adults. An important issue is the development of hepatic abscess in an immunocompromised child, in particular, the association of chronic granulomatous disease with pyogenic hepatic abscess formation.

Pyogenic Abscess

The most common cause of pyogenic liver abscess before the advent of antibiotic therapy was perforated appendicitis. Now the most common causative factor in the development of pyogenic hepatic abscess in children is chronic granulomatous disease and other causes of immunosuppression (158). Chronic granulomatous disease is an inherited disorder characterized by a defect in oxidative burst-mediated bacterial killing by neutrophils. These children develop abscesses in skin and soft-tissue struc-

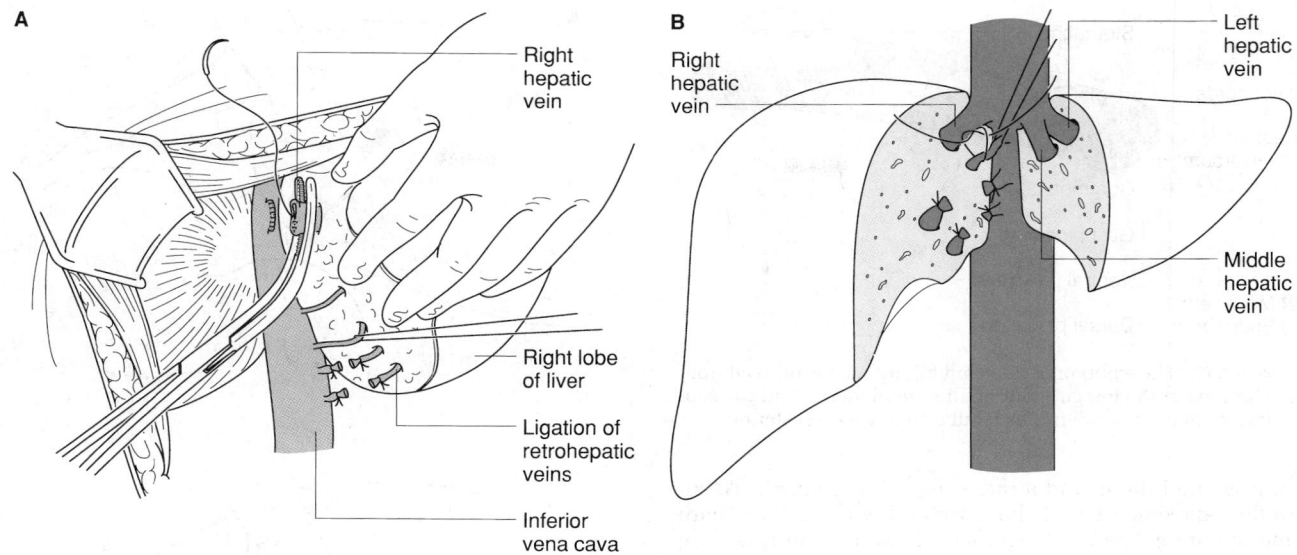

Figure 97.51. *(A)* The hepatic veins in infants and children may be extremely short, making extrahepatic control impossible or dangerous. *(B)* Intrahepatic control of the hepatic veins via an anterior approach may be safer in infants and children.

tures as well as in the solid organs. About 40% of children with pyogenic liver abscesses will have chronic granulomatous disease. Another third of these children will be immunosuppressed either as a primary or acquired immunodeficiency (e.g, myeloablative chemotherapy, AIDS). Liver abscesses are infrequently seen as a complication of umbilical vein catheterization, omphalitis, and biliary tract disease and operations.

Patients with pyogenic liver abscesses present with fever, jaundice, and leukocytosis. Hepatosplenomegaly and a tender liver may be found on physical examination. Diagnostic imaging with ultrasound, CT scan, or MRI is useful. Common responsible organisms include staphylococcal species, streptococcal species, and *E. coli*. Gram-negative organisms and anaerobic bacteria are becoming increasingly prevalent. Treatment involves the use of broad-spectrum antibiotics until resolution of the infection is determined on a clinical basis. Large abscess cavities may require CT-guided or ultrasound-guided percutaneous drainage to expedite resolution of sepsis. Currently, few hepatic abscesses require open operative drainage. The outcome is predictably good following adequate antibiotic therapy and, when necessary, effective drainage and essentially reflects the primary disease state contributing to the development of the pyogenic abscess.

Amebic Abscess

Amebic abscess of the liver is uncommon in the United States, but it is endemic to areas of Central and South America. It is caused by infection with the parasite *Entamoeba histolytica*. Children with amebic dysentery develop hepatic infection as the parasite travels through the portal circulation. Patients have a history of chronic illness, fever, and abdominal pain. Examination typically demonstrates a tender right upper quadrant. Infection can be confirmed by a serum antibody test, and amebic abscess can be demonstrated by ultrasound or CT scan. Spontaneous rupture of amebic abscess is reported in as many as 10% of patients in some series (159). The treatment of choice is the antibiotic metronidazole. Surgical resection or drainage of amebic abscess of the liver typically is not required for resolution.

PEDIATRIC BILIARY TRACT

Common biliary tract problems including infectious, inflammatory, and gallstone-related problems are managed similarly in both children and adults, and the management principles are discussed elsewhere in this text. Two congenital problems of the biliary tract, namely, biliary atresia and congenital cystic disease of the biliary tract (choledochal cyst) are somewhat unique to infants and children in presentation and management and will be reviewed below.

Embryology

The fetal liver and biliary tract develop between weeks 4 and 10 of gestation, representing the fusion of an endodermal foregut diverticulum with a mesodermal component from the septum transversum (31). The hepatocytes derive from cords of endodermal cells in the hepatic diverticulum and ultimately give rise to the hepatic sinusoidal endothelium. The proximal hepatic diverticulum gives rise to the extrahepatic biliary tract, including the gallbladder, cystic duct, and common bile duct (Fig. 97.52). The intrahepatic and proper hepatic ducts develop from either the cranial portion of the hepatic diverticulum or possibly from the developing hepatocytes. As the intrahepatic and extrahepatic ductal systems develop, they unite to form a connected, arborizing system of cords composed of primitive ductular epithelial cells. These epithelial cells assume tubular configuration with ductal patency established between weeks 6 and 12 of gestation. Bile flow from the hepatocytes and into the biliary duct system is apparent by the beginning of the second trimester.

This embryologic sequence appears to take place normally in infants who develop biliary atresia. In fact, the term *biliary atresia* does not reflect an embryologic atresia resulting from failure of recanalization of the biliary tree. Rather, biliary atresia is believed to be caused by a sclerosing, inflammatory process that produces progressive obliteration of the normally developed biliary tract.

The embryologic origin of choledochal cysts is unknown. An association of biliary atresia and choledochal

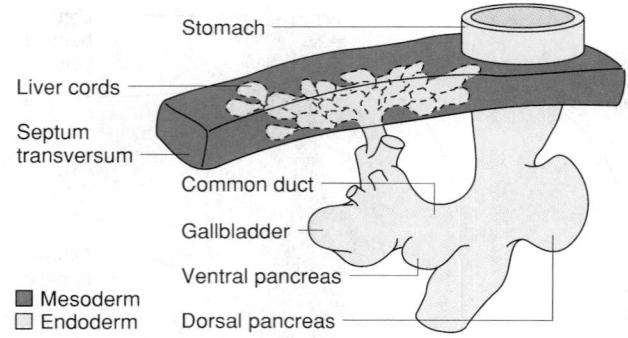

Figure 97.52. The embryonic liver and biliary tract is derived from contributions of the foregut diverticulum (endoderm) and the septum transversum (mesoderm) at about 5 to 6 weeks' gestation.

cyst in some infants and a rather high incidence in Asian populations suggest that these two anomalies may share some common pathophysiologic features. Simple bile duct obstruction does not appear to be causative in choledochal cyst formation. It is possible that abnormalities of bile duct recanalization may lead to cystic dilation of the biliary tract. An anomalous extramural junction between the pancreatic duct and the common bile duct is common and clinically expected in type I choledochal cysts (see later), and it has been hypothesized that reflux of pancreatic proteases into the common bile duct may lead to cystic dilatation.

Biliary Atresia

Anatomy

Biliary atresia has been previously termed *correctable* or *uncorrectable,* with many described variations (160). Correctable biliary atresia is classically characterized by hepatic duct patency that is suitable for conventional hepaticoenterostomy for biliary tract drainage (Fig. 97.53). Uncorrectable biliary atresia defines the situation in which there are no patent hepatic ducts for traditional anastomosis. About 85% to 90% of infants with biliary atresia have complete obstruction of the extrahepatic biliary tract, including the gallbladder. The remaining 10% to 15% have obstruction of the proximal ducts with patency of the distal common bile duct and gallbladder. The overall incidence of biliary atresia is about 1 in 8,000 to 12,000 live births and is the most common cause of chronic cholestasis in infants and children as well as the most frequent indication for pediatric liver transplantation (161).

The adjectives *correctable* and *uncorrectable,* unfortunately, do not describe the actual pathophysiologic mechanisms involved, nor do they predict outcome in biliary atresia. It was previously thought that correctable form of biliary atresia accounted for as many as 10% to 15% of all cases. The actual incidence of hepatic duct patency is estimated to be closer to 1% to 2% of infants with biliary atresia. Despite the fact that most infants have the so-called uncorrectable form, most infants with biliary atresia achieve some degree of biliary drainage following portoenterostomy. Conversely, normal overall liver function and successful outcome are not consistently achieved by operative intervention in the correctable forms of biliary atresia. Operative repair of biliary atresia in almost all cases uses a portoenterostomy, whether classified as a correctable or uncorrectable lesion. Therefore, this classic semantic distinction has little practical or clinical value.

Extrahepatic biliary atresia must be differentiated from biliary hypoplasia. This condition describes a diminutive

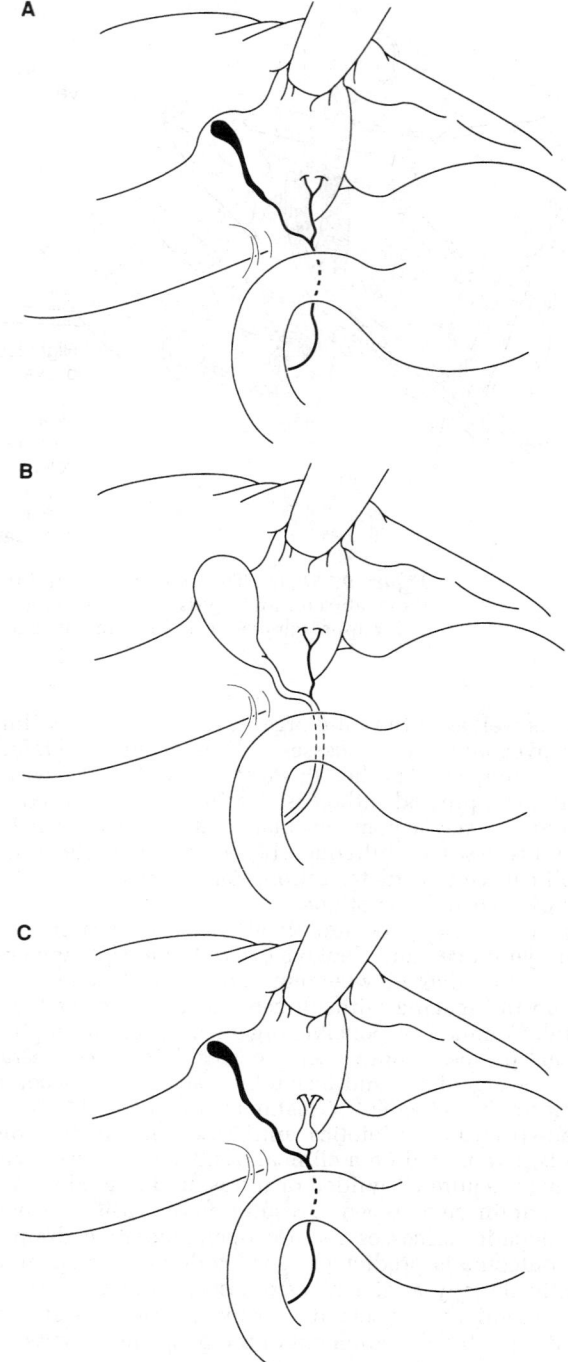

Figure 97.53. Variation of abnormalities observed in biliary atresia. *(A)* The most common variant is considered uncorrectable by conventional mucosa-to-mucosa biliary enteric anastomosis. *(B)* Proximal atresia with distal bile duct and gallbladder patency occurs in 10% to 15% of cases. *(C)* Correctable variant with patent proximal hepatic ducts.

but patent biliary system and can result from many underlying situations such as neonatal hepatitis and α_1-antitrypsin deficiency. Biliary hypoplasia involves both intrahepatic and extrahepatic ductal systems. Because of this diffuse defect, procedures designed to improve extrahepatic biliary drainage alone, such as portoenterostomy, are not useful with biliary hypoplasia.

Microscopic Anatomy

Biliary atresia is characterized by replacement of the extrahepatic biliary tract with dense, fibrous inflammatory tissue (161). In most cases, complete obliteration of the extrahepatic biliary tract, including the gallbladder, occurs. There appears to be gradual progression of the inflammatory process with advancing age. The proximal segment of the fibrous biliary cord resected from the porta hepatis is examined for patency and inflammatory response. The common hepatic duct and common bile duct will be almost uniformly obliterated by the inflammatory process. Few or absent patent ductal remnants and an absence of portal inflammation may be associated with a less favorable prognosis (162). Evaluation for duct patency can be determined intraoperatively by frozen section analysis to help guide the extent of proximal resection at the porta hepatis (Fig. 97.54). The luminal diameter of the bile ducts

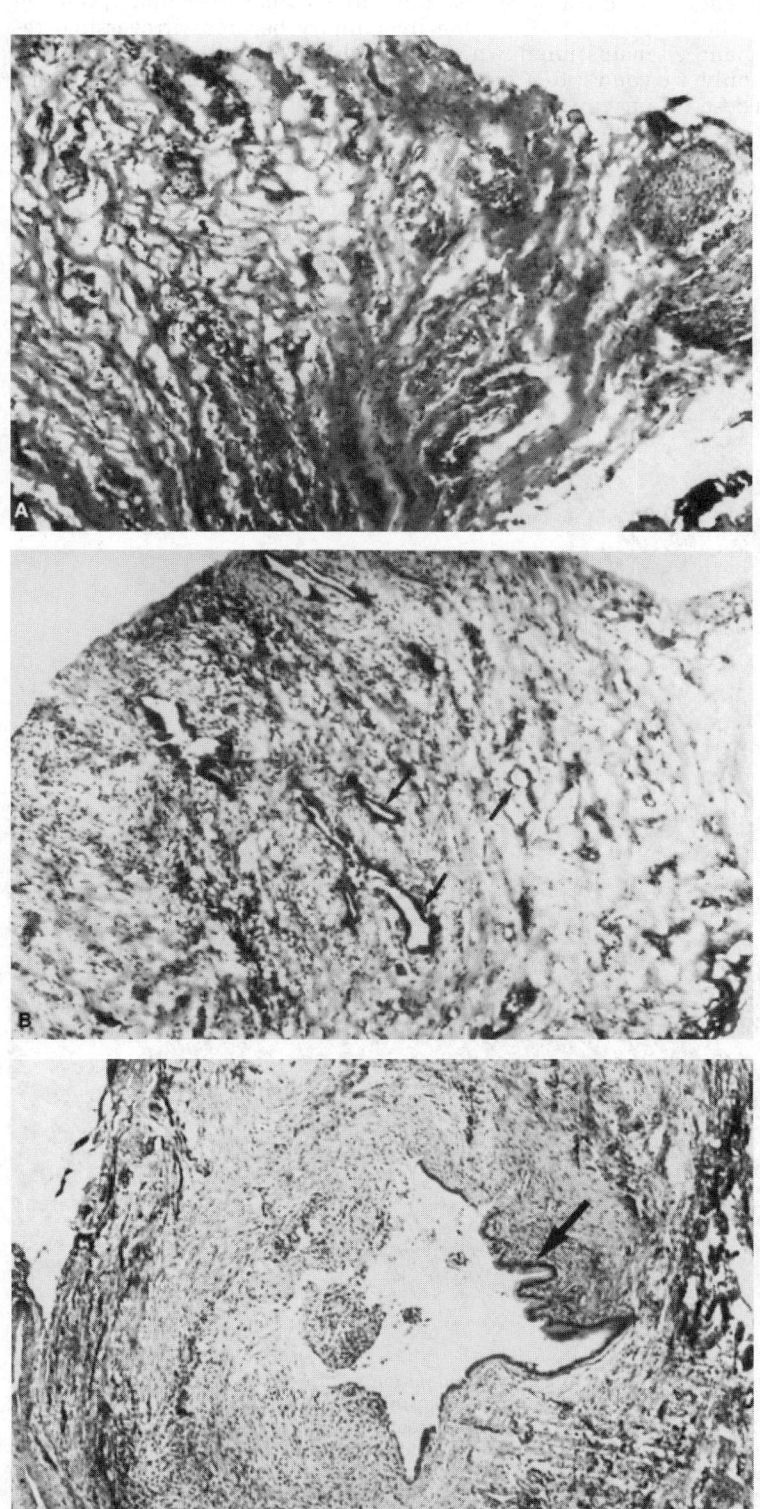

Figure 97.54. Frozen sections of the fibrous biliary tract remnant at the proximal point of transection. *(A)* Complete absence of patent bile ducts with fibrous obliteration of the extrahepatic biliary tract. *(B)* Several patent but small ducts *(arrows)*. *(C)* Larger duct with periductal inflammatory response and fibrosis with loss of normal biliary epithelium *(arrow)*. (Courtesy of K. Heidelberger, M.D., University of Michigan, Ann Arbor.)

present at the porta hepatis also may be important. The presence of bile ducts with a diameter greater than 150 μm has been reported to be associated with postoperative bile flow in up to 90% to 95% of cases (163).

Histologic features of biliary atresia reflect hepatic parenchymal injury and possibly intrahepatic duct obliteration. Neocholangiogenesis, or biliary duct proliferation of disorganized and nonpatent ducts within the liver, is considered highly suggestive but not specific for biliary atresia (Fig. 97.55). Other findings include bile pigment deposition within the bile canaliculi, intralobular bile ducts, or individual hepatocytes. Multinucleated giant cell formation and periductal inflammation are commonly seen but also may be present in neonatal hepatitis. These features within the liver appear to be age related but may be highly variable from patient to patient. In fact, considerable variation occurs in the inflammatory response observed may occur between biopsy samples from the same patient. Characteristic early findings in biliary atresia include evidence for acute inflammation with neutrophil predominance in the periportal regions. Older infants and children typically have chronic inflammatory changes with considerable fibrosis. Periportal bridging fibrosis is commonly seen in intermediate stages of the disease. Ultimately, progressive biliary atresia leads to cirrhosis and all its clinical consequences. Early intervention by portoenterostomy to provide biliary drainage has been proposed to arrest or reverse the parenchymal liver injury, but the point at which the liver injury becomes irreversible remains unknown. From a clinical standpoint, infants beyond 3 to 4 months of age appear to have irreversible injury, whereas most long-term success appears to be achieved in infants younger than 2 to 3 months of age at the time of portoenterostomy. Nearly all patients with biliary atresia will have histologic evidence of residual liver injury. Ultimately, the severity of the intrahepatic cholan-

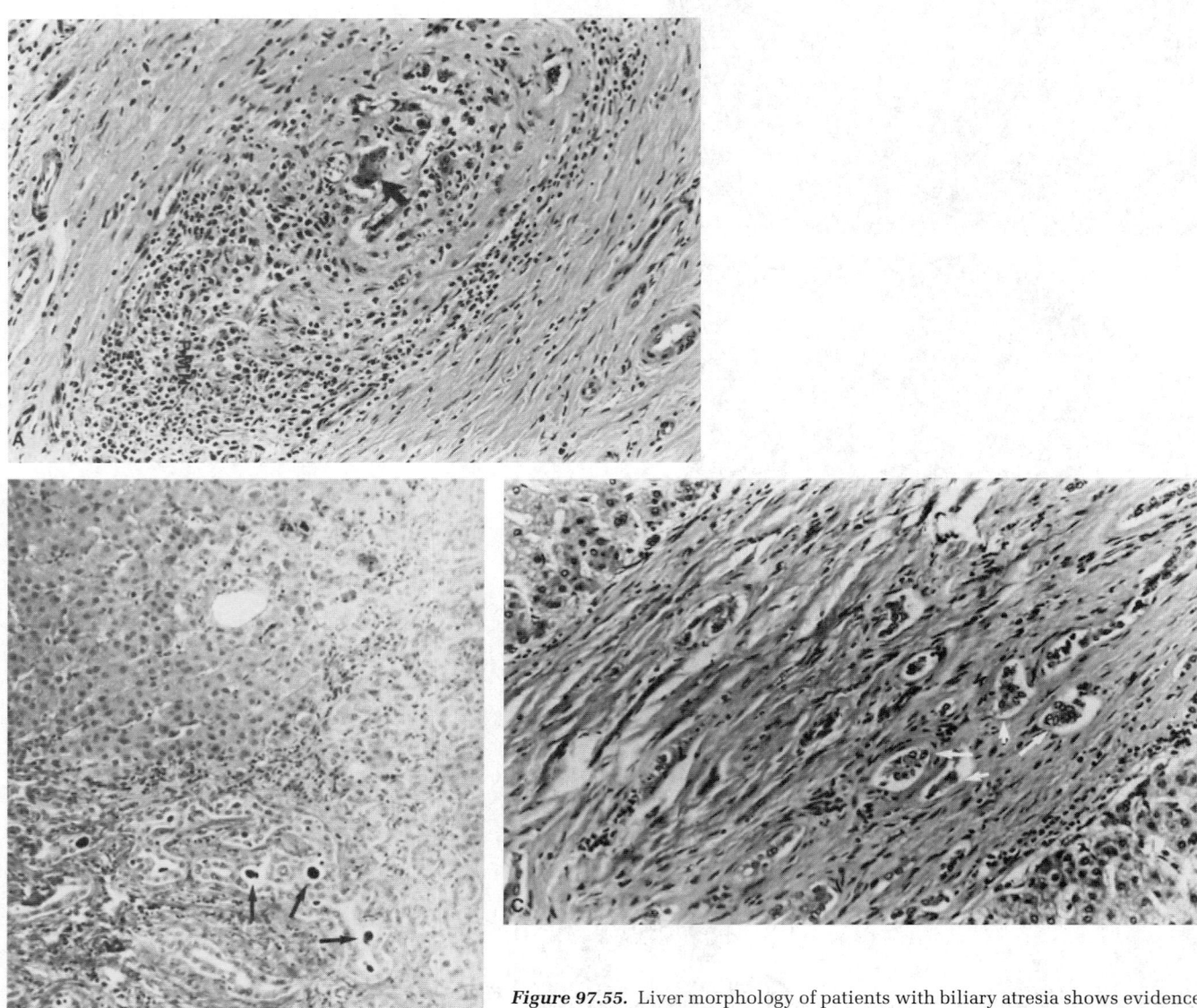

Figure 97.55. Liver morphology of patients with biliary atresia shows evidence of neocholangiogenesis, or bile duct proliferation, and bile plugs. The degree of inflammation and cirrhosis varies greatly. *(A)* Liver histology at an early stage characterized by acute periportal neutrophil infiltration and giant cell formation *(arrow)*. *(B)* Classic bile plug formation *(arrow)*. Liver histology from an older child with biliary atresia and cirrhosis. There is almost complete replacement of normal hepatocytes with fibrosis and prominent bile duct proliferation *(arrows)*.

giopathy and the extent of liver damage may be the most important predictors of long-term outcome and survival in biliary atresia.

Pathophysiology

Despite the numerous investigations into the etiology of biliary atresia, the exact pathogenic mechanism remains unknown. The current, widely accepted concept is that the normally developed biliary tract undergoes an inflammatory sclerosis and subsequent obliteration. This appears to occur over a period of months during the newborn period. Infants who develop biliary atresia are rarely jaundiced at birth, and biliary atresia is either rare or nonexistent in fetal autopsy studies. Clinical data are consistent with the fact that biliary atresia appears to be a progressive, dynamic inflammatory response that is acquired during the perinatal period and targets the extrahepatic biliary tract. Early establishment of biliary drainage via portoenterostomy within the first 2 to 4 months of age may be associated with patent bile ducts and reversal of liver injury and subsequent long-term survival. Conversely, infants operated on after 120 days of life typically have obliterated bile ducts. In some respects, neonatal biliary atresia shares some clinical and morphologic features of sclerosing cholangitis in adults. Data supporting an infectious etiologic agent, and in particular reoviruses, rotaviruses, and hepatitis C, have been reported and may play a role in some cases. Previous interest in reovirus 3 as an etiologic agent has waned because of the inability to find evidence for its presence by using reverse transcriptase-mediated polymerase chain reaction analysis (164–166). Additionally, other noninfectious stimuli may trigger an inflammatory response directed at the neonatal extrahepatic bile duct (167). The actual mechanism(s) may reflect a stereotypical inflammatory response that is initiated by a variety of different stimuli and directed preferentially against the neonatal bile duct. An inflammatory response directed against the biliary tract may explain the progression of intrahepatic biliary tract injury and liver disease observed in many patients with biliary atresia, despite apparently successful portoenterostomy.

Clinical Presentation and Diagnosis

As previously discussed, the worldwide incidence of biliary atresia is about 1 per 10,000 live births and may be slightly higher in female and Japanese infants. These infants are typically otherwise healthy and not jaundiced at birth. The cardinal sign of biliary atresia is progressive neonatal jaundice with an onset within the first few weeks of life. Dark urine and acholic stools are expected clinical findings. Infants usually are discovered as the progressive hyperbilirubinemia produces clinical jaundice around 2 to 4 weeks of age. The physical examination is generally unremarkable except for jaundice and possibly mild hepatomegaly. Alagille's syndrome, which presents with neonatal jaundice, usually can be distinguished from biliary atresia on physical examination. Children with Alagille's syndrome will have biliary hypoplasia and commonly abnormal facies, growth retardation, vertebral defects, and pulmonic stenosis.

The characteristic laboratory finding is a conjugated hyperbilirubinemia consistent with obstructive jaundice. Generally, a direct fraction of bilirubin greater than 50%, or greater than 2 mg/dL, requires investigation. Mild elevation of hepatic transaminases are commonly seen. The alkaline phosphatase typically is significantly elevated, often in the range of 500 to 1,000 IU/L. There are no specific biochemical markers for biliary atresia, and these serum profiles can be seen in other causes of neonatal cholestasis. Late findings in biliary atresia include failure to thrive, feeding intolerance, stigmata of portal hypertension, and fat-soluble vitamin deficiency.

Table 97.12 is a partial list of the causes of neonatal cholestatic syndromes. Neonatal physiologic jaundice is commonly encountered. This condition is self-limited once the glucuronyl transferase system matures, allowing the hepatocytes to conjugate bilirubin efficiently. Because of the numerous causes of neonatal jaundice and the relative infrequency of biliary atresia, a delay in diagnosis is not unusual. The jaundiced neonate is subject to a number of diagnostic tests with longitudinal follow-up, and frequently the delay in diagnosis of biliary atresia can be 1 to 2 weeks in duration. Given the age-sensitive nature of biliary atresia and the improved outcome in younger infants, the diagnostic work-up should be thorough but expeditious.

Radioisotope Scanning. Pertechnetate 99m–iminodiacetic acid (^{99m}Tc-IDA) analogues are widely used for hepatobiliary imaging and provide the basis for a sensitive and specific test for biliary atresia. The sensitivity of this diagnostic examination for biliary atresia can be 100% with a specificity of 94% (161). To improve the sensitivity, infants are administered a 2- to 7-day course of oral phenobarbital (5 mg/kg daily) to induce hepatic microsomal enzymes and increase hepatocyte processing of ^{99m}Tc-IDA. Both hepatic uptake of radionuclide and excretion into the gastrointestinal tract are evaluated over a timed interval. Infants with primary hepatocellular disorders characteristically have impaired hepatocyte uptake of radionuclide,

---

Table 97.12. CAUSES AND ASSOCIATIONS OF NEONATAL CHOLESTASIS SYNDROMES

CONGENITAL INFECTIOUS CAUSES

Cytomegalovirus[a]
Rubella virus[a]
Herpes virus
Hepatitis virus B[a]
Echovirus 14, 19
Coxsackievirus B
Toxoplasmosis
Syphilis

GENETIC ASSOCIATIONS

Galactosemia
Tyrosinemia
Congenital fructose intolerance
α_1-Antitrypsin deficiency
Cystic fibrosis
Niemann-Pick disease
Trisomy 17, 18, 21
Turner's syndrome
Menkes' syndrome
Zellweger's syndrome
Polysplenia syndrome[b]

MISCELLANEOUS ASSOCIATIONS

Hemolytic disease
Bacterial sepsis
Pyelonephritis
Parenteral hyperalimentation
Congestive heart failure
Hypoplastic left sided-heart syndrome
Necrotizing enterocolitis, gastroschisis, omphalocele
Neonatal hypopituitarism
Inspissated bile syndrome (without hemolysis) neonatal shock, respiratory distress syndrome, acidosis

[a]Rarely associated with biliary atresia.
[b]Frequently associated with biliary atresia.

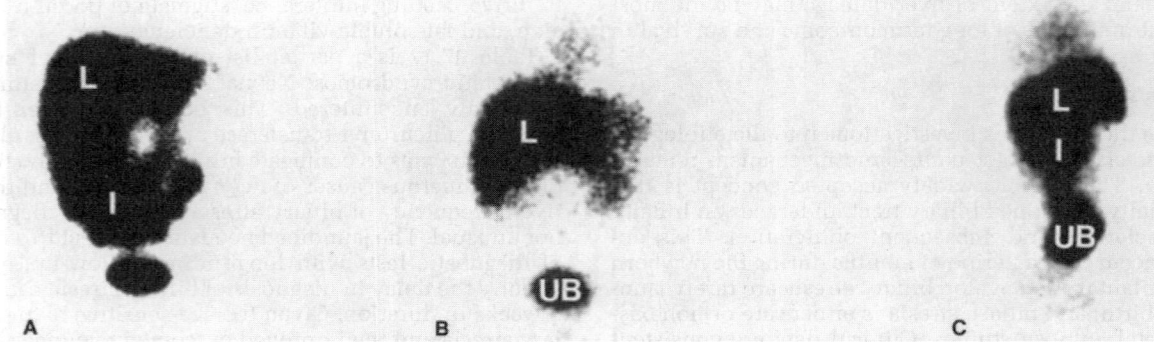

Figure 97.56. *(A)* Normal scan using p-isopropylacetanilido iminodiacetic acid (PIPIDA) as the hepatobiliary scanning agent. At 45 minutes, isotope is clearly visible in the liver (L) and intestine (I). *(B)* Scan after phenobarbital administration in infant with biliary atresia. Even after 8 hours, isotope is apparent only in the liver and urinary bladder (UB). *(C)* Patient with cholestatic jaundice. At 65 minutes, isotope is visible in the liver (L) and intestine (I). Hepatocyte uptake is variable but usually decreased or normal, whereas excretion into the gut is predictably present with cholestatic jaundice or hepatocellular disease.

whereas normal infants and infants with biliary atresia have prompt uptake. Normal infants will excrete the isotope rapidly into the gut through the biliary tract. In biliary atresia, there is no excretion into the gut because of the obliteration of the extrahepatic bile ducts (Fig. 97.56). The hepatobiliary scan is a rapid test that can be performed simultaneously with other diagnostic examinations, for example, ultrasound. This test reliably identifies infants with choledochal cyst as well.

Other Diagnostic Tests.   Several other diagnostic tests are of interest in the work-up of an infant with conjugated hyperbilirubinemia in whom obstructive jaundice is suspected. The management principle is that, ultimately, prompt operative exploration, liver biopsy, and cholangiogram should be performed in any infant in whom biliary atresia is suspected. An aggressive approach is warranted in that unnecessary delay in definitive drainage may lead to a less favorable outcome.

Ultrasound.   A standard examination of the jaundiced infant is a comprehensive abdominal ultrasound, with particular attention given to the liver and biliary tract. The most common ultrasonographic finding in biliary atresia is a diminutive or absent gallbladder without associated intrahepatic duct dilatation. Biliary tract obstruction from a choledochal cyst also can be reliably identified by ultrasound. Other rare causes of extrahepatic biliary duct obstruction are associated with proximal duct dilatation.

Liver Biopsy.   Because the histologic findings in biliary atresia are not specific, about 20% to 25% of infants who undergo percutaneous liver biopsy will remain undiagnosed. Liver biopsy is often performed in conjunction with the work-up of conjugated hyperbilirubinemia following hepatobiliary scanning and ultrasonography, but in the setting of biliary atresia, it has limited utility. The histologic examination of a percutaneous liver biopsy is probably most helpful in diagnosing nonoperative causes of neonatal jaundice, thus avoiding anesthesia and operative exploration.

α1-Antitrypsin Deficiency.   This is perhaps the single most important medical condition that may be difficult or impossible to differentiate from biliary atresia. All jaundiced infants should have plasma α1-antitrypsin levels determined before operative exploration for suspected biliary atresia. Infants with α1-antitrypsin deficiency will not benefit from operative exploration or portoenterostomy.

Treatment

It is now well accepted that infants with biliary atresia require surgical therapy as the initial management intervention. Medical therapy is directed to the postoperative management of the chronic liver disease. The roles of portoenterostomy versus orthotopic liver transplantation for biliary atresia are more complementary than competitive. In general, the use of sequential surgical treatment, using portoenterostomy in infancy and orthotopic liver transplantation for children with progressive hepatic failure, provides improvement in overall survival (168). Organ availability and a higher rate of perioperative complications limit primary liver transplantation for biliary atresia in infants younger than 1 year of age. In the rare instance of unrecognized biliary atresia in an older child with established hepatic dysfunction, primary orthotopic liver transplantation is a reasonable option.

Portoenterostomy.   The recommended initial procedure for the treatment of biliary atresia is the portoenterostomy. Before the development of portoenterostomy in Japan during the late 1950s, all infants with biliary atresia died of chronic liver disease and cirrhosis (160). Current management dictates that operative exploration and portoenterostomy be performed promptly following the diagnosis of biliary atresia.

In general, the approach to the infant with suspected biliary atresia is initially to perform an operative cholangiogram. If the diagnosis is confirmed, a portoenterostomy is constructed (Fig. 97.57). To maximize the potential for effective biliary drainage with portoenterostomy, several technical caveats are worthy of mention. An open liver biopsy is routinely performed to document the state of parenchymal injury. The cholangiogram is generally attempted through the gallbladder. In the 10% to 15% instance of a patent distal biliary tree, treatment still requires portoenterostomy. It is feasible to consider using a patent gallbladder and cystic duct for the biliary conduit, but this appears to have a high rate of technical failure related to obstruction of the cystic duct. A nonpatent, fibrous cord rather than a normal common bile duct is found in the hepatoduodenal ligament. This cord is dissected free proximally to the level of the porta hepatis between the bifurcation of the portal vein. The fibrous remnant is sharply transected at this level to preserve any patent bile ducts. Frozen-section analysis of the fibrous remnant may help to guide further dissection in search of

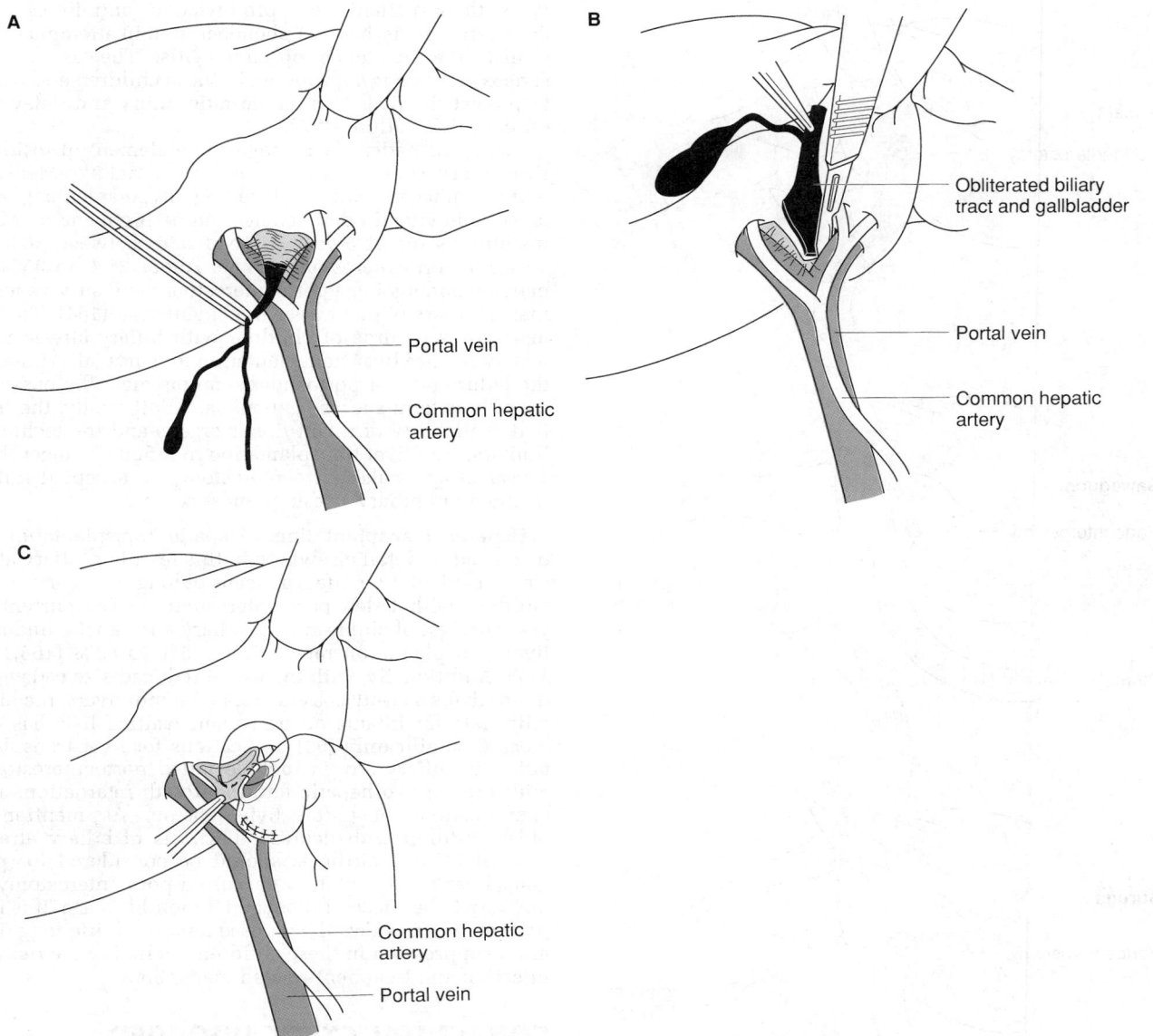

Figure 97.57. The essential features of the portoenterostomy for biliary atresia include appropriate mobilization *(A)* and transection *(B)* of the fibrous biliary tract remnant. *(C)* Creation of a Roux-Y jejunal conduit with biliary enteric anastomosis completes the procedure.

patent bile ducts if necessary. A short, 15- to 25-cm retrocolic, jejunal Roux-Y limb is constructed. There has been no clear advantage with longer or modified conduits with intussusception-type antireflux valves in the prevention of cholangitis (169). Additionally, cyclosporin A absorption is potentially diminished by the use of longer conduits (170), an important consideration in these children, who ultimately may require liver transplantation.

Some surgeons prefer to exteriorize the biliary conduit, but there is no clear consensus (Fig. 97.58). With an exteriorized biliary conduit, postoperative bile flow is directly visible, and there may be a slightly lower incidence of cholangitis. The diverting stoma ultimately must be closed, however, and there is potential to develop parastomal variceal hemorrhage from progressive portal hypertension. Additionally, fluid and electrolyte losses from the biliostomy can be significant (171). There are no reported survival differences between patients with exteri-

orized and closed biliary conduits following portoenterostomy. Because many of these infants ultimately may require liver transplantation, there is a trend toward using a simple, closed biliary conduit with portoenterostomy.

Results and Complications. Following portoenterostomy, bile flow occurs in aabout 66% to 75% of all infants when operated on at less than 60 days of age; however, establishment of bile flow may take weeks to months. The probability of bile flow is clearly related to age at the time of operation. Bile flow is unlikely to occur following portoenterostomy in infants older than 120 days of age (172,173).

Cholangitis is a constant concern and an important postoperative problem after portoenterostomy. The clinical signs include fever, leukocytosis, and decreased bile flow in the absence of other systemic illness. At some time, Nearly all patients will develop symptoms and signs consistent with cholangitis, but the reported postoperative

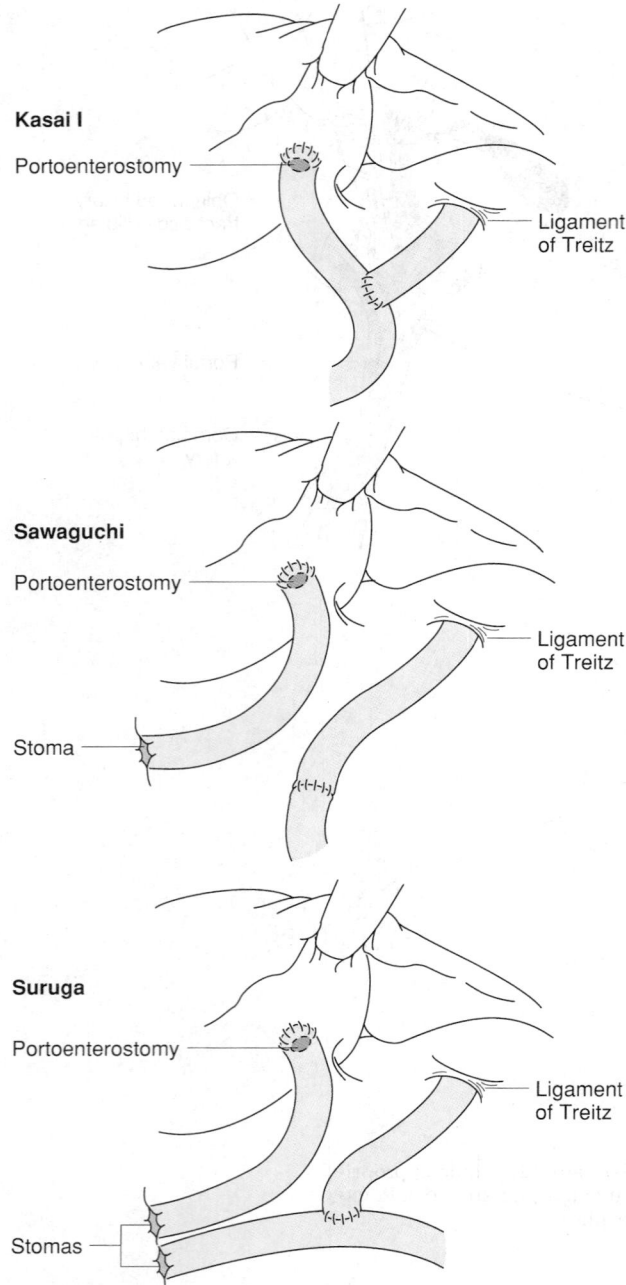

Figure 97.58. Several types of conduits have been used for biliary drainage following portoenterostomy. There are relatively few data to select from these, and current trends emphasize simplicity. These are the three most commonly used conduits. The primary importance of this issue is that the reoperative surgeon must be familiar with the anatomic variations.

rates are as low as 40% to 50%. Cholangitis following portoenterostomy is characterized by a systemic inflammatory response and may be associated with progressive liver injury. Although there are no convincing data that cholangitis results from ascending bacterial infection, the treatment is generally intravenous fluid resuscitation and broad-spectrum antibiotics. Occasionally, steroids or other antiinflammatory agents may be helpful, whereas reoperation or endoscopic revision of the portoenterostomy usually is not (174). Postoperatively, some surgeons choose to keep their patients on prophylactic antibiotics and choleretic agents, such as phenobarbital, in attempts to diminish the incidence of cholangitis. The use of ursodeoxycholate is appropriate in these children and helps to protect the liver from cholestatic injury and delay the onset of liver failure (175).

Nearly all patients will have some element of residual liver injury. Hepatic synthetic failure, portal hypertension with esophageal variceal bleeding, hypersplenism, and fat-soluble vitamin deficiencies can be problematic. Most institutions report 5-year survival rates between 30% to 50% for portoenterostomy alone. About 25% to 35% of patients undergoing a portoenterostomy will survive more than 10 years without liver transplantation (164). The remaining two thirds of children with biliary atresia ultimately require liver transplantation for survival. Although the failure rate for portoenterostomy is high, the possibility of long-term success is notable. Additionally, the limited availability of infant donor organs and the technical limitations of liver transplantation in infants younger than 1 year of age make portoenterostomy an accepted initial treatment of biliary atresia in most centers.

Hepatic Transplantation. Hepatic transplantation is discussed in detail elsewhere in this text. For biliary atresia, transplantation offers a means of long-term survival in children with failed portoenterostomies. The current 5-year survival of children with biliary atresia who undergo liver transplantation ranges from 75% to 82% (168,176, 177). Additionally, with the use of reduced-size cadaveric donor livers as well as living-related donor livers, the mortality rate for infants on transplant waiting lists has decreased significantly (50). Indications for liver transplantation in biliary atresia include failed portoenterostomy with progressive hepatic failure, growth retardation, and complications of portal hypertension. As mentioned, older children with delayed diagnosis of biliary atresia and established cirrhosis should be considered for primary liver transplantation because a portoenterostomy is unlikely to be successful beyond 4 months of age. It is important to consider the consequences of life-long immunosuppression in these children, including the risks of infection and treatment-related malignancy.

CONGENITAL CYSTIC DISORDER OF THE BILIARY TRACT

Anatomy

The anatomic description and classification scheme for choledochal cystic disease initially proposed by Alonso-Lej in 1959 and modified by Todani are illustrated in Fig. 97.59 (178,179). The most frequently encountered are type I cysts, accounting for approximately 85% to 90% of the lesions in most series. Type I cysts typically are characterized by fusiform dilatation of the entire common bile duct with only mild dilatation of the common hepatic duct; the intrahepatic ducts are normal. Type II cysts represent true diverticula of the common bile duct. These lesions are rare and account for only 1% to 2% of all cases. Type III cysts are also uncommon and sometimes are referred to as *choledochoceles.* Type III cysts constitute fewer than 2% of the observed lesions and are defined as local dilatation of the distal, intramural portion of the common bile duct. Type IV cystic disease is characterized by the presence of multiple cysts typically involving both intrahepatic and extraheptic ducts. Type IV cysts are observed with an incidence of 15% in some series. Type V disease is rare and represents cystic malformation of the intrahepatic ducts. Variations are common, and biliary atresia occasionally is seen in association with choledochal cystic disease.

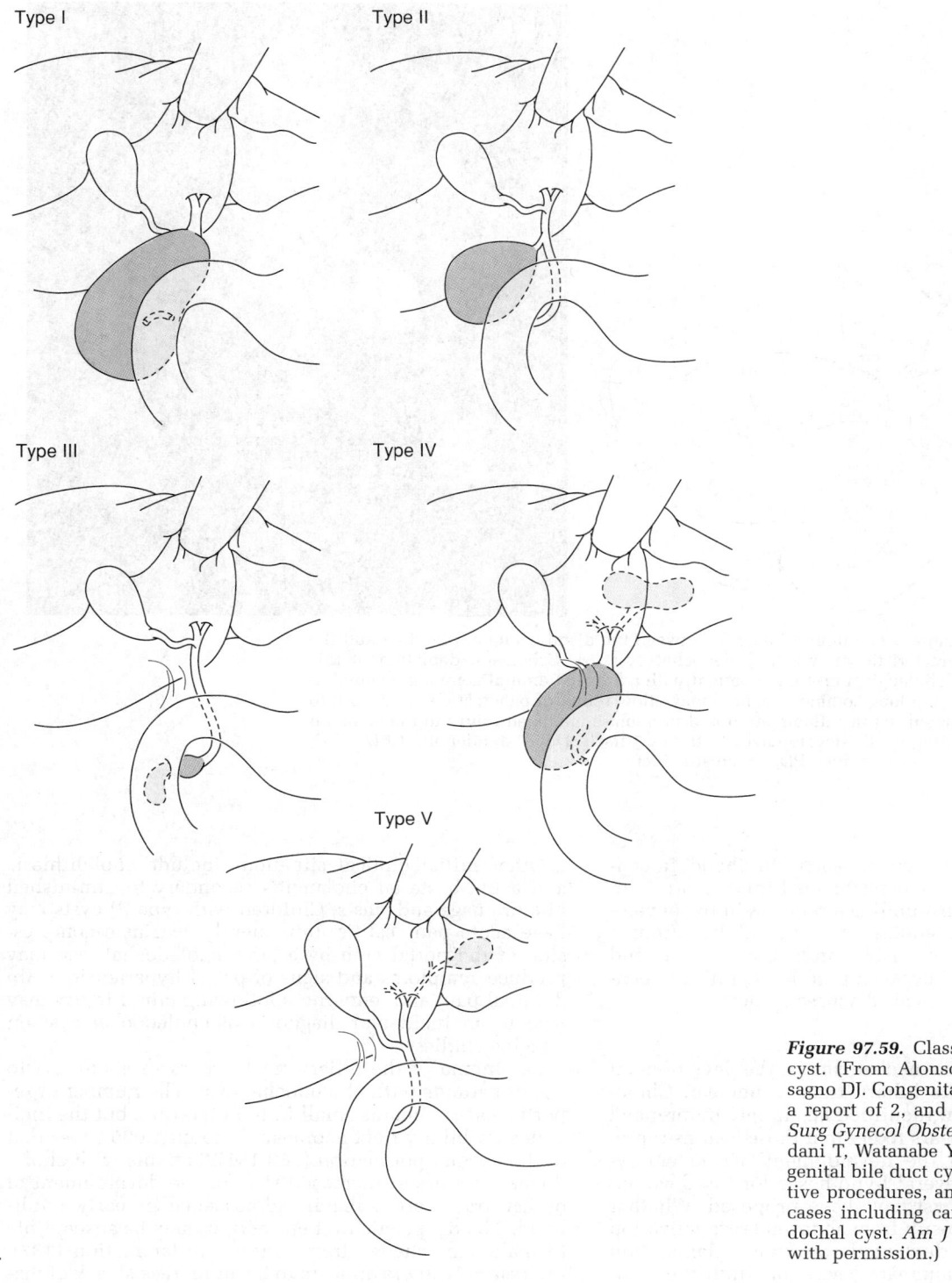

Type I

Type II

Type III

Type IV

Type V

Figure 97.59. Classification of choledochal cyst. (From Alonso-Lej F, Revor WB, Pessagno DJ. Congenital choledochal cyst, with a report of 2, and an analysis of 94 cases. *Surg Gynecol Obstet* 1959;108:1–30; and Todani T, Watanabe Y, Narusue M, et al. Congenital bile duct cysts: classification, operative procedures, and review of thirty-seven cases including cancer arising from choledochal cyst. *Am J Surg* 1977;134:263–269, with permission.)

Type I cysts are generally quite large and often cause displacement of neighboring viscera. The fusiform dilatation usually begins at the origin of the common bile duct, generally sparing the common hepatic ducts. The distal common bile duct is diminutive and typically is distorted mechanically by the large cyst, leading to the common clinical presentation of obstructive jaundice. The junction of the distal common bile duct and the pancreatic duct is not within the normal intramural duodenum but rather is extrinsic and proximal to the duodenal wall and the sphincter of Oddi (Fig. 97.60). It remains unknown whether the configuration of a long, extramural common channel allows greater pancreatic secretion reflux into the common bile duct.

Microscopic examination of the choledochal cyst wall reveals that the normal biliary epithelium is either absent or replaced by abnormal and occasionally dysplastic columnar epithelium. The cyst wall has normal smooth muscle with variable degrees of inflammation and fibrosis. The exception to this common histologic characteristic is the type III cyst. The choledochocele is generally lined by normal duodenal mucosa. Choledochal cysts tend to have

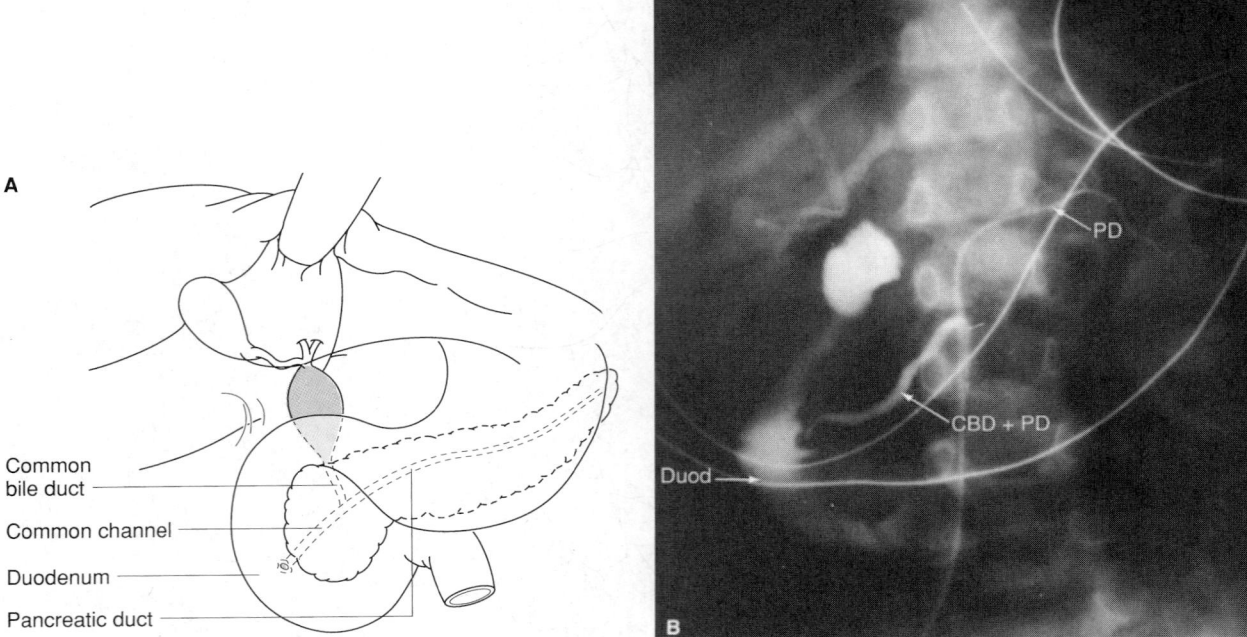

Figure 97.60. An anomalous, extramural junction between the distal common bile duct and the pancreatic duct is characteristic of type I choledochal cyst. *(A)* Schematic depiction of this anatomy. *(B)* Operative cholangiogram from a patient with a long extramural common channel. It has been suggested that the long common channel may allow reflux of pancreatic secretions into the common bile duct resulting in inflammation and proteinase-mediated injury to the common duct, possibly contributing to the development of the cyst itself. Duod, duodenum; CBD + PD, common bile duct and pancreatic duct; PD, pancreatic duct.

less inflammation in infancy and early childhood. In contrast, there is generally well-established inflammation involving the cyst and surrounding structures in the hepatoduodenal ligament in adolescents and adults. From a surgical standpoint, extensive inflammation in and around the choledochal cyst can produce significant technical and management issues discussed below.

Pathophysiology

The pathophysiologic mechanism for the development of cystic lesions of the biliary tract is unclear. Choledochal cysts have been identified accurately by prenatal ultrasound, and it appears likely that these lesions represent abnormalities in the development of the embryologic biliary tract. Several hypotheses for the development of choledochal cyst have been proposed. Whether the cystic dilatations result from abnormal recanalization of the primitive bile duct cords or from inflammation caused by reflux of pancreatic secretions into the common bile duct remains unknown. The pathophysiology of choledochal cyst is that of obstructive jaundice. The obstruction may be primarily the result of mechanical outflow obstruction of a diminutive distal common bile duct with a large, dilated choledochal cyst. Alternatively, a large inflammatory cyst can cause obstruction of the biliary tract and of neighboring viscera by extrinsic compression. When discovered during infancy, obstructive jaundice is usually the initial clinical finding. The liver injury is typically reversible, and progression to biliary cirrhosis is rare. The exception to this situation is type V disease, which is associated with a high incidence of hepatic fibrosis.

Other initial clinical situations include cholelithiasis and acute bacterial cholangitis secondary to diminished bile drainage and stasis. Children with type III cysts may have acute pancreatitis. Infrequently, extrinsic compression of the portal vein by a large choledochal cyst may produce symptoms and signs of portal hypertension. Abdominal pain and tenderness following minor injury may lead to an incidental diagnosis of choledochal cyst on imaging studies.

Carcinoma of the biliary tract occurs in about 3% to 5% of patients with choledochal cyst. The number of reported cases remains small in the literature, but the incidence for biliary tract neoplasm is about 1,000 times that of the normal population (180,181). Patients with choledochal cyst are at increased risk for the development of biliary tract carcinoma in adolescence or early adulthood. The dysplastic cyst epithelium may be susceptible to malignant change from chronic inflammation (182). Interestingly, there appears to be an increased risk of malignancy to develop anywhere in the biliary tract, gallbladder, or pancreas, and not just the choledochal cyst itself (183). Therefore, current treatment emphasis is on complete excision of the cyst or the cyst wall epithelium while providing adequate biliary drainage to prevent stasis and chronic inflammation. Infants and children treated for choledochal cyst should have long-term follow-up for potential complications (see later) and potential malignancy.

Clinical Presentation and Diagnosis

Choledochal cysts are encountered infrequently, but they are important lesions when evaluated and treated in

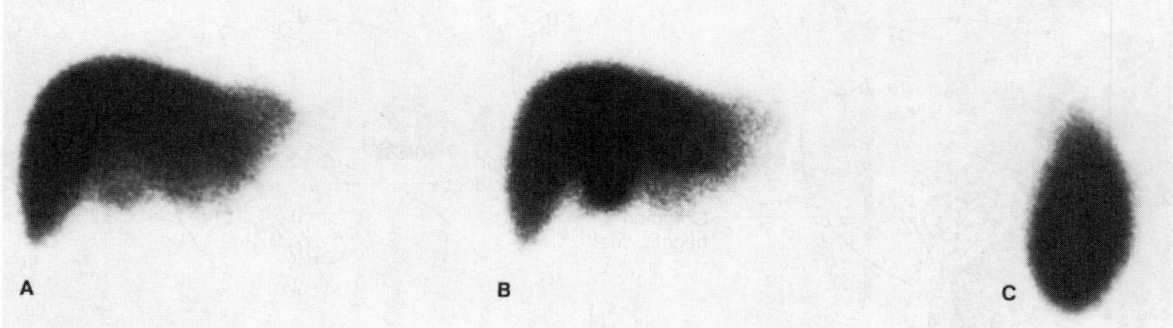

Figure 97.61. Typical ⁹⁹ᵐTc-N-substituted-2,6-dimethylphenyl carbamoylethyl iminodiacetic acid (HIDA) scan from a child with a type I choledochal cyst. Images were made in 5 minutes *(A)*, 30 minutes *(B)*, and 3 hours *(C)*, after isotope injection. The isotope is retained within the choledochal cyst more than 24 hours, and the pattern of hepatocyte uptake is normal.

pediatric tertiary care centers. Presentation is now most common in infancy and early childhood. Prenatal diagnosis is also now possible. The characteristic presentation of choledochal cyst in the neonate is obstructive jaundice. In older children and adults, the classic clinical triad of episodic abdominal pain, a palpable right upper-quadrant mass, and jaundice occurs in fewer than 50% of patients. Adults occasionally present with hepatomegaly or evidence of portal hypertension. The diagnosis in infants and most children can be confirmed by ultrasound examination and ⁹⁹ᵐTc-IDA imaging studies (Figs. 97.61 and 97.62). These are the initial diagnostic tests of choice in the pediatric population. In older patients, endoscopic retrograde cholangiopancreatography (ERCP) is highly sensitive and specific in confirming the diagnosis of choledochal cyst. These lesions also are diagnosed incidentally during radiologic imaging studies for other reasons. Partial duodenal obstruction may lead to an upper gastrointestinal series that may show extrinsic compression from a large type I cyst or an intraluminal filling defect from a type III cyst. CT imaging of the abdomen following blunt

trauma may lead to the diagnosis of biliary tract dilatation. Liver biopsy is not specific in choledochal cyst and has little diagnostic role other than to document the extent of liver injury. Contemporary diagnostic imaging studies are accurate, and, when interpreted by experienced pediatric radiologists, the correct diagnosis of choledochal cyst can be made preoperatively in the majority of instances.

Treatment

Type I Cysts. The definitive management of choledochal cyst is operative, and the operation needs to be tailored to the specific anatomic defect. The initial operative strategy for a type I choledochal cyst is exploration and cholangiography, usually through the gallbladder, but occasionally contrast injection must be made directly into the common bile duct. Cholecystectomy then is routinely performed. Historically, internal drainage procedures without cyst excision were widely used, including cyst duodenostomy, cyst gastrostomy, and cyst jejunostomy. These procedures have been associated with a higher rate of failure because of stricture, stone formation, pancreatitis, and cholangitis. Additionally, the potential development of biliary tract carcinoma in the retained cyst is a serious concern. Therefore, internal drainage procedures without cyst excision have been abandoned. The current consensus for the surgical management of type I choledochal cyst is performance of primary cyst excision with Roux-Y hepaticojejunostomy reconstruction (Fig. 97.63). Primary cyst excision is performed as a total transmural excision that is accomplished routinely in infants and children (184). For adults with severe inflammation and fibrosis, transmural dissection may be present problems resulting from inflammation and adhesion of the cyst wall to the hepatoduodenal ligament. A safer approach in this situation may be intramural cyst dissection and epithelial removal, leaving the posteromedial outer cyst wall adjacent to the portal vein and hepatic artery intact.

Other Types of Cysts. Type II cysts are excised completely and the choledochotomy closed primarily. Type III choledochoceles require a transduodenal approach with either marsupialization or excision of the cyst. Care must be taken to identify the ampulla, and a formal sphincteroplasty may be required to ensure adequate drainage from the biliary tract and the pancreatic duct. Types IV and V intrahepatic cystic disease must be approached on an individualized basis. In general, unilobar or focal cystic disease can be either resected or drained with a Roux-Y jejunostomy reconstruction. Bilobar intraparenchymal

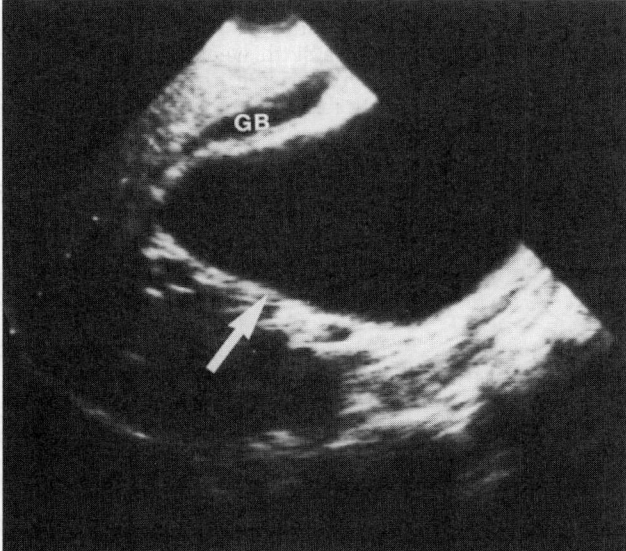

Figure 97.62. Ultrasound image of a type I choledochal cyst *(arrow;* longitudinal image). The gallbladder (GB) is also shown.

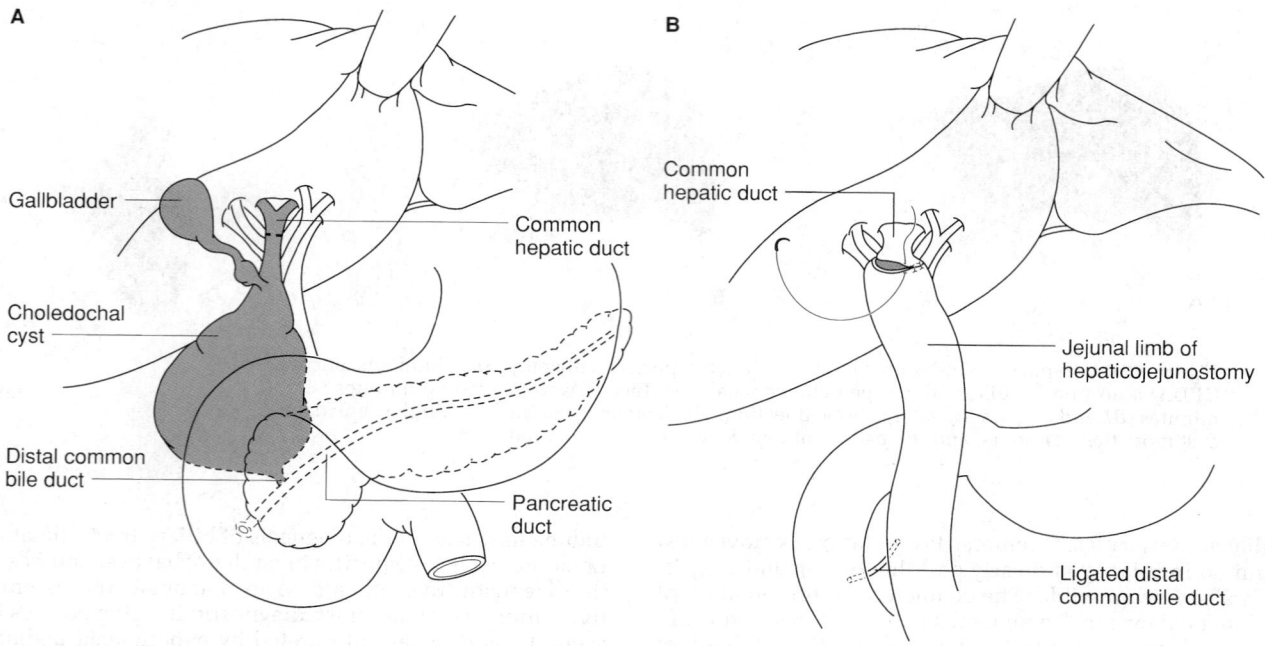

Figure 97.63. The preferred operative treatment of type I choledochal cyst consists of primary total transmural cyst excision with Roux-Y hepaticojejunostomy.

disease, particularly in the setting of hepatic fibrosis, may be difficult, if not impossible, to obtain complete, adequate drainage.

Complications and Results. The major complications associated with operative repair of choledochal cyst include cholangitis, stricture formation, choledocholithiasis, and development of biliary tract malignancy. A summary of the incidence of complications, mortality, and reoperation for the different procedures in 955 cases reported in the literature is presented in Table 97.13 (185). In this review, there was a clear advantage for primary cyst excision in terms of morbidity and need for reoperation, and no significant increase in mortality occurred using this approach. Subsequent to this analysis in 1975, internal drainage procedures without cyst excision have been essentially replaced by primary cyst excision with hepaticojejunostomy reconstruction. Currently, several series have reported excellent results with little or no mortality using total transmural excision of choledochal cysts (184,186). Primary transmural excision with biliary tract reconstruction continues to be a safe and desirable operative approach for cystic lesions of the biliary tract.

PEDIATRIC PANCREAS

Disorders of the pancreas are uncommon in infants and children. Pancreatic disorders in children include congenital anatomic disorders, inflammatory pancreatitis, rare neoplastic lesions, and pancreatic endocrinopathies (187). Several significant issues are relative to the pancreatic problems in the pediatric age group, and a brief overview is provided below.

Embryology

The embryologic development of the pancreas was reviewed in the preceding section with respect to duodenal atresia and annular pancreas. Briefly, in review, the fetal pancreas arises from the paired dorsal and ventral foregut diverticular buds during the sixth week of gestation. The dorsal pancreatic anlage gives rise to the body and tail of the pancreas as well as the main pancreatic duct. The ventral pancreatic anlage migrates 180 degrees to fuse with the dorsal gland, forming the uncinate process and the distal portion of the duct of Wirsung (Fig. 97.9). The independent ductal systems of the developing pancreatic anlage fuse. The dorsal (Santorini) duct opens directly into

Table 97.13. MORBIDITY AND MORTALITY IN OPERATIVE MANAGEMENT OF CHOLEDOCHAL CYST

Operation	Cases	Morbidity	Reoperation	Mortality
Cyst excision and hepaticojejunostomy	83	7 (8%)	0	6 (7%)
Cyst jejunostomy (Roux Y)	53	18 (34%)	7 (13%)	9 (17%)
Cyst jejunostomy (Loop)	12	6 (50%)	5 (42%)	1 (3%)
Cyst duodenostomy	93	55 (58%)	35 (38%)	6 (5%)

From Flanigan PD. Biliary cysts. Ann Surg 1975;182:635–643, with permission.

the duodenum, and this is persistent in 10% to 15% of normal subjects. The ventral (Wirsung) duct opens into the duodenum by fusion with the common bile duct. Normally, the dorsal duct fuses with the ventral duct just to the right of the mesenteric vessels. Failure of the dorsal and ventral ducts to fuse normally leads to two separate pancreatic ducts, a condition known as *pancreatic divisum*. Occasionally, the ventral duct regresses and the entire pancreatic gland is drained by the accessory duct of Santorini.

Primitive duct cells of the pancreas give rise to both the acinar cells and the islet cells of the normal pancreas. Primary islet cells become apparent at week 8 of gestation within the interlobular tissue, with acini becoming visible shortly thereafter. The primary islet cells regress after the fifth month of gestation and are usually nonexistent by term. Secondary islet cells arise from centroacinar proliferation during the third month of gestation. These intralobular cells migrate out of the acini in which they were formed and develop into islets that remain connected to the duct by a thin cellular stalk (the tubule of Bensley).

Exocrine pancreatic anomalies generally arise from defective development during embryogenesis. As previously discussed, the most common of these conditions is annular pancreas. The circumferential distribution of pancreatic tissue around the duodenum is thought to result from interrupted migration of the ventral pancreatic anlage. Less common defects include pancreatic ductal abnormalities, pancreatic enteric duplications, pancreatic–splenic fusion heterotopic pancreatic tissue, and congenital agenesis of portions of the pancreas (188).

Acute Pancreatitis

Acute pancreatitis is often overlooked as a cause of abdominal pain in children; however, it is the most common disorder of the pancreas in both infants and children. Adult pancreatitis is often caused by either alcohol ingestion or gallstones. In contrast, 50% to 80% of cases in children, particularly adolescents, are posttraumatic or idiopathic in origin. There are many other causal agents and events associated with the development of acute pancreatitis in children. An important clinical condition seen with moderate frequency is acute pancreatitis in the setting of immunosuppression, in particular, high-dose corticosteroids. Steroid-induced acute pancreatitis typically accounts for the third most common cause of pancreatitis in most children's hospitals. Other causes of acute pancreatitis include gallstones, CF, hyperlipidemia, juvenile diabetes mellitus, mumps, coxsackievirus infection, infectious mononucleosis, collagen vascular diseases, and anatomic lesions such as choledochal cyst. Medications significantly associated with acute pancreatitis include oral contraceptives, chlorothiazide, tetracyclines, azathioprine, and L-asparaginase. Valproic acid, an anticonvulsant useful in some children with seizure disorders, is associated with a particularly virulent form of acute necrotizing pancreatitis that may be life threatening.

Clinical manifestation of acute pancreatitis in a child typically reveals a history of midepigastric abdominal pain with anorexia and emesis. On examination, the child usually has a tender abdomen with distention. Fever and leukocytosis are common. Serum amylase and lipase levels usually are elevated, although significant pancreatitis can occur despite a normal amylase level. Conversely, the lipase may be mildly elevated in the absence of clinical symptoms or signs of acute pancreatitis. Ultrasonograpy and CT imaging of the abdomen are probably the most commonly used adjunctive diagnostic tests. CT imaging is particularly useful in demonstrating enlargement and edema of the gland as well as evaluating for peripancreatic fluid collections. While usually deferred during the acute phase of pancreatitis, ERCP may be useful to evaluate the hepatobiliary tract anatomy once the inflammatory process has resolved. Recently, MRI techniques have been able to provide cholangiopancreatograms (MRCP) of high resolution. This alternative may be particularly useful in the infant or small child in whom ERCP (which usually requires sedation or general anesthesia) is more technically difficult.

Treatment principles for childhood acute pancreatitis are not different from strategies used in adults. The vast majority of children have simple edematous pancreatitis. Hemorrhagic and necrotizing pancreatitis are distinctly unusual in this age group but can be seen in immunosuppressed patients. Therefore, much of the therapy is designed to be supportive and nonoperative in approach. Endotracheal intubation and mechanical ventilation may be required. Intravenous fluid resuscitation, pancreatic rest by nasogastric tube decompression, analgesia, and TPN are provided. No clinical efficacy data are available to support the widespread use of anticholinergics or somatostatin analogues for acute pancreatitis in children. Operative intervention is reserved for complications of pancreatitis, such as hemorrhage, infected pancreatic necrosis, or pancreatic pseudocyst.

Recurrent pancreatitis in a child usually is associated with an anatomic abnormality or specific physiologic problem. Following recovery from the acute inflammatory event, an aggressive diagnostic work-up, including consideration of ERCP or MRCP to define ductal anatomy, should be performed. In particular, the presence of pancreas divisum with stenosis of the accessory papilla should be considered. Children with pancreatitis in the setting of cholelithiasis should undergo laparoscopic cholecystectomy after resolution of the pancreatitis.

Pancreas Divisum

Pancreas divisum occurs with failure of normal fusion between the dorsal and ventral pancreatic ducts. About 10% to 15% of normal persons will have two separate pancreatic ducts, and up to 10% of asymptomatic persons undergoing ERCP will have two complete ductal systems. The anatomic variant of pancreas divisum is not necessarily pathologic, but if the orifice of the accessory papilla is stenotic or obstructed, pancreatitis can occur (189). About 25% of these persons are thought to be at risk for developing pancreatitis. Because pancreas divisum is characterized by a dominant dorsal duct system dependent on secretion through the accessory papilla, stenosis of the accessory (lesser) papilla is probably necessary to produce pancreatic symptoms. Most of the experience with surgical treatment of pancreas divisum is reported in adults (190). Successful surgical management of children presenting with recurrent pancreatitis secondary to accessory papilla stenosis with pancreas divisum also has been reported (191).

To diagnose pancreas divisum, ERCP is required. Endoscopic visualization of the major and accessory papillae is essential. Radiographic findings with pancreas divisum will demonstrate a short or absent duct of Wirsung that does not communicate with the duct of Santorini (Fig. 97.64). A definitive diagnosis of pancreas divisum is made by demonstrating two separate, parallel ductal systems. Whether or not this anatomic abnormality is contributing to the physiologic problem causing pancreatitis for a specific patient has been investigated using real-time ultrasonography and intravenous secretin stimulation (190). A functional stenosis of the accessory papilla with secretin-

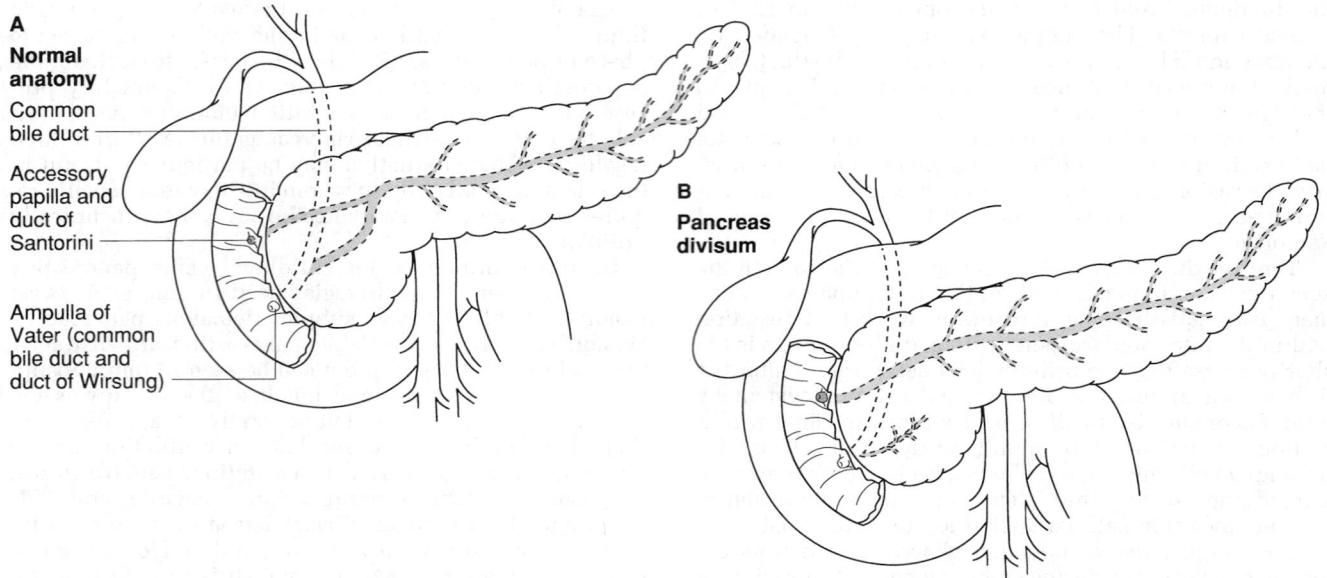

Figure 97.64. *(A)* Normal pancreatic ductal anatomy. *(B)* Pancreas divisum. There is no communication between the duct of Wirsung and the duct of Santorini. The duct of Wirsung is short or absent. Most of the pancreas is drained by the duct of Santorini through the accessory papilla. This anatomy is found in about 10% to 15% of normal individuals.

induced proximal ductal dilatation on ultrasound is thought to be indicative of clinically significant pancreas divisum in a patient with a history of pancreatitis.

Few pediatric patients with pancreatitis and pancreas divisum requiring operation have been reported. Most of these children were female patients who had a history of recurrent pancreatitis. The primary operative goal is to provide adequate drainage of the duct of Santorini by performing a sphincterotomy of the accessory duct (192). An open dorsal duct sphincterotomy appears to be more durable than endoscopic sphincterotomy. Some surgeons have advocated sphincterotomy of the main papilla as well, but dorsal duct sphincterotomy alone appears effective in preventing acute pancreatitis associated with pancreas divisum. The reported surgical outcome in the limited number of children treated for pancreatitis associated with pancreas divisum was favorable.

Pancreatic Cysts

Pancreatic pseudocysts are uncommon in the pediatric age group and are usually the result of blunt traumatic abdominal injury or acute pancreatitis. Children typically present with abdominal pain, nausea, emesis, and weight loss. There may be a palpable midepigastic mass on examination. Diagnosis usually is made with ultrasound or CT imaging of the abdomen. The serum amylase and lipase are usually elevated.

In children, many small asymptomatic pseudocysts will regress spontaneously with resolution of the pancreatic inflammation. Larger or symptomatic pseudocysts may require drainage. Symptoms and potential complications of untreated pseudocysts include hemorrhage, infection, perforation, gastrointestinal or biliary tract obstruction, or, rarely, development of pancreaticoenteric fistula (193). The decision to use either external or internal drainage procedures for a pseudocyst occasionally depends on the status of the pancreatic duct. In many centers, definitive external drainage of a large or symptomatic pseudocyst is

performed with acceptable morbidity and mortality rates by an ultrasound- or CT-guided percutaneous approach (194). Pseudocyst recurrence or persistent external drainage without resolution suggests significant pancreatic duct injury or complete ductal transection. Determination of whether a major pancreatic ductal injury is associated with a pseudocyst may be made by either percutaneous contrast injection of the pseudocyst or ERCP (195). Pseudocysts associated with pancreatic duct injury may not resolve with percutaneous external drainage; so internal drainage procedures such as cyst gastrostomy or cyst jejunostomy with or without distal pancreatectomy are required (196).

Epithelial cysts of the pancreas are rare in children. Congenital cysts are lined by epithelium and acinar tissue and are seen most commonly in the body and tail of the pancreas. They may be associated with other syndromes, such as von Hippel-Lindau disease, which is characterized by hereditary cerebellar cysts, retinal hemangioma, and pancreatic cysts. Congenital pancreatic cysts are typically asymptomatic unless they are large enough to cause compression or obstruction of the stomach or colon. In the absence of trauma, spontaneous rupture of a pancreatic epithelial cyst is rare. Treatment is cyst excision or internal drainage into the stomach or jejunum.

Other rare cystic lesions of the pancreas in children include retention cysts. These cysts result from chronic ductal obstruction. They are characteristically lined by epithelium unless obliteration from inflammation has occurred. Enteric duplication cysts of the stomach or duodenum also can be associated intimately with the pancreas and communicate with the pancreatic duct. Treatment of both retention cysts and enteric duplication cysts either within or associated with the pancreas includes excision, occasionally internal drainage, and, if necessary, distal pancreatectomy. Not all pancreatic cysts in children can be uniformly considered benign. Suspicious lesions should be investigated thoroughly and biopsy performed. Cystadenoma, cystadenocarcinoma, and rhabdomyosarcoma associated with a pancreatic cyst have been reported. These neoplasms are treated by anatomic pancreatic resection following histologic confirmation on biopsy.

Pancreatic Neoplasms

Childhood malignant neoplasms of the pancreas are uncommon. Typically, a pancreatic malignancy in childhood is found on discovery of an asymptomatic abdominal mass. Infrequently, the lesion may be found incidentally or during a diagnostic imaging work-up for abdominal trauma. Jaundice may occur with a lesion in the pancreatic head causing common bile duct obstruction. The most frequently encountered lesions include islet cell carcinoma and adenocarcinoma. The treatment of choice for localized malignant neoplasms of the pancreas is surgical resection (197). Pancreaticoduodenectomy in children can successfully control some malignancies of the pancreatic head. To promote adequate nutrient absorption and growth, children undergoing pancreaticoduodenectomy should be considered for oral pancreatic enzyme replacement and fat-soluble vitamin supplementation (198).

Two pancreatic neoplasms seen in childhood and adolescence deserve further discussion. The *papillary cystic neoplasm* of the pancreas occurs predominantly in younger female children, is typically slow growing with low malignant potential, and is highly curable with surgical resection (199). This tumor is thought to be a neoplasm of the ductuloacinar primordial cells of the pancreas. The other lesion is *pancreatoblastoma,* also referred to as *juvenile adenocarcinoma of the pancreas.* Pancreatoblastoma is somewhat more common in boys than girls and typically has slow growth with low malignant potential as well. Histologic examination demonstrates undifferentiated ductular and acinar areas with nodules of squamous epithelium, suggesting that these tumors arise from primordial pancreatic cells. Both papillary cystic neoplasm and pancreatoblastoma have more favorable prognoses than adenocarcinoma following surgical resection.

Endocrine Lesions of the Pancreas

Zollinger-Ellison Syndrome

Childhood tumors of the endocrine pancreas are exceedingly rare. The diagnosis and management of these tumors do not differ greatly from the adult population. The most common of these lesions include gastrinoma and insulinoma. The functional endocrine tumors of the pancreas typically are characterized by secreted peptide products such as glucagon, vasoactive intestinal peptide, somatostatin, and pancreatic polypeptide.

Similar to adults, children with Zollinger-Ellison syndrome clinically present with symptoms related to gastric hypersecretion. Peptic ulcer disease with or without gastrointestinal hemorrhage, abdominal pain, and diarrhea is a common presenting symptoms. The diagnosis is confirmed by finding elevated serum gastrin levels. The basal acid output typically is elevated as well. A paradoxical increase in serum gastrin levels will be found following intravenous administration of secretin (secretin stimulation test).

Contemporary management of Zollinger-Ellison syndrome in children relies on control of gastric acid hypersecretion with the oral administration of omeprazole, a parietal cell proton-pump inhibitor. Diagnostic imaging studies, including helical CT scanning and MRI, are useful in localization of a primary gastrinoma and evaluating for metastatic disease before exploration. Definitive treatment relies on complete excision of the primary gastri-

noma, which typically is found in the right of the superior mesenteric vessels in the head of the pancreas or the duodenum. The growth and progression of gastrinoma appear to be less aggressive in children than in adults; however, total gastrectomy occasionally is required in a child to control intractable symptoms related to persistent hypergastrinemia or metastatic disease (200).

About 25% of gastrinomas occur in the setting of MEN syndrome, reviewed elsewhere in the text. At least 90% of patients with MEN type I will have hyperparathyroidism secondary to hyperplasia. Additionally, 30% to 80% of patients will have pancreatic islet cell tumors, and 15% to 50% will have pituitary tumors (188). In contrast, sporadic tumors, pancreatic tumors associated with MEN I, are typically multicentric and more frequently are malignant.

Hypoglycemia

There are diverse metabolic causes for hypoglycemia in infancy and childhood. These include endocrinopathies such as panhypopituitarism, hypothyroidism, adrenal insufficiency, and congenital adrenal hyperplasia (adrenogenital syndrome). Several inborn errors of metabolism interrupt normal glucose regulatory mechanisms. Systemic disease states, perinatal stress, and sepsis can predispose an otherwise normal infant to low blood glucose levels. Infants who remain unresponsive to glucose infusion typically have inappropriately high circulating insulin levels for a given blood glucose level. Hyperinsulinemia should be suspected in any infant or child younger than 1 year of age who has significant, persistent hypoglycemia. There are heterogeneous causes for hyperinsulinemic hypoglycemia, but the most common cause in infancy is nesidioblastosis, which is characterized by uncontrolled development of the pancreatic endocrine tissue, in particular, beta cell mass, which functions abnormally beyond birth or during infancy (201,202). Clinically, these cells secrete inappropriately high amounts of insulin, typically causing clinical hypoglycemia in infants Fig. 97.65). In older children, hyperinsulinemia secondary to islet cell adenoma, carcinoma, or hyperplasia is more common.

Infants with nesidioblastosis usually become symptomatic from hypoglycemia within the first few hours or days of life. These infants commonly present with neurologic symptoms such as lethargy or generalized seizures and will have corresponding fasting blood glucose levels below 40 mg/dL. The diagnosis of hyperinsulinemia is supported by the clinical features of Whipple's triad, which includes (1) neurologic changes with fasting or activity, (2) fasting blood glucose levels below 40 to 50 mg/dL, and (3) neurologic symptoms reversed by the administration of glucose. The diagnosis is made by demonstrating inappropriately high levels of circulating insulin for a given level of blood glucose. An insulin (IU/mL) to glucose (mg/dL) ratio that is greater than 0.5 in a fasting patient is consistent with hyperinsulinemic hypogly-cemia. In infants and children, an absolute insulin level greater than 5 IU/ml in the presence of a blood glucose less than 40 mg/dL is generally diagnostic. Ketone body production is impaired in infants with nesidioblastosis.

The initial management of a hypoglycemic infant with nesidioblastosis is to provide adequate glucose concentrations to prevent permanent neurologic injury. Dextrose-containing intravenous solutions are titrated to maintain blood glucose levels greater than 40 mg/dL and may require a central venous catheter. The short-term administration of somatostatin analogues to increase blood glucose levels in hyperinsulinemic states has been demonstrated to be useful (203). Other pharmacologic agents

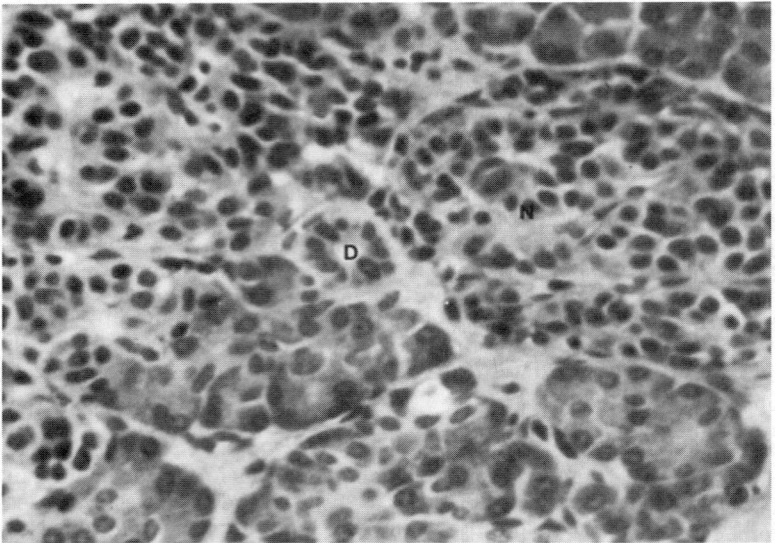

Figure 97.65. Nesidioblastosis demonstrating neo-islet formation (N) from primitive pancreatic ductules.

used to reduce insulin levels and raise blood glucose concentration include diazoxide (15 mg/kg daily). The use of streptozocin to control hyperinsulinemia most often is reserved for adults with metastatic islet cell carcinoma and is not widely used in infants because of the potential side effects.

Following initial control of blood glucose and clinical confirmation of hyperinsulinemia, operative intervention should be considered a means of providing definitive control of hypoglycemia. Diagnostic imaging using CT scanning may be useful either to identify or to exclude a solitary functional adenoma. The abdomen is explored thoroughly, and the entire pancreas must be exposed. Intraoperative ultrasound may help to identify a solitary lesion in the pancreas because an isolated islet cell adenoma can be treated by enucleation or limited pancreatic resection. In the absence of a solitary lesion, the infant is presumed to have nesidioblastosis or islet cell hyperplasia. In this setting, the general operative strategy is total or near total pancreatectomy (204–206). Lesser procedures such

as subtotal (80%) pancreatectomy will not effectively treat infantile nesidioblastosis or islet cell hyperplasia. Near-total pancreatectomy involves resection of the distal 95% of the gland with preservation of the spleen. The entire distal pancreas, including the uncinate process, is resected, leaving a small rim of pancreatic tissue adjacent to the duodenum (Fig. 97.66). Total pancreatectomy is usually reserved for persistent or recurrent hypoglycemia following lesser procedures.

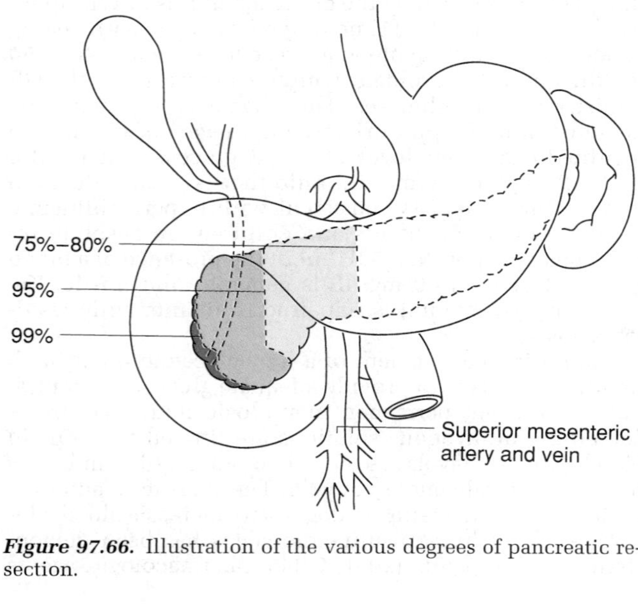

Near-total pancreatectomy will provide adequate relief from hypoglycemia in about 90% of infants with nesidioblastosis. The remaining infants with persistent hypoglycemia may require further pancreatic resection. The typical postoperative course is a transient period of hyperglycemia with subsequent stabilization of blood glucose levels. Pancreatic exocrine function also is decreased and oral replacement therapy is indicated. Despite clinical remission following resection, however, diabetes mellitus may occur as a long-term consequence in children treated either medically or surgically for nesidioblastosis (207). Therefore, these infants need long-term metabolic follow-up for both pancreatic endocrine and exocrine function.

75%–80%
95%
99%

Superior mesenteric artery and vein

Figure 97.66. Illustration of the various degrees of pancreatic resection.

REFERENCES

1. Nichols CR, Dickinson JE, Pemberton PJ. Rising incidence of gastroschisis in teenage pregnancies. *J Matern Fetal Med* 1997;6:225–229.
2. Blakelock RT, Upadhyay V, Pease PW, et al. Are babies with gastroschisis small for gestational age? *Pediatr Surg Int* 1997;12:580–582.
3. Torfs CP, Curry CJ. Familial cases of gastroschisis in a population-based registry. *Am J Med Genet* 1993;45:465–467.
4. Aktug T, Hosgor M, Akgur FM, et al. End-results of experimental gastroschisis created by abdominal wall versus umbilical cord defect. *Pediatr Surg Int* 1997;12:583–586.
5. Glick PL, Harrison MR, Adzick NS. The missing link in the pathogenesis of gastroschisis. *J Pediatr Surg* 1985;20:406–407.
6. Cantrell JR, Haller JA Jr, Ravitch MM. A syndrome of congenital defects involving the abdominal wall, sternum, diaphragm, pericardium, and heart. *Surg Gynecol Obstet* 1958;107:602–605.
7. Calzolari E, Bianchi F, Dolk H, et al. Omphalocele and gastroschisis in Europe: a survey of 3 million births 1980–1990. EUROCAT Working Group. *Am J Med Genet* 1995;58:187–194.
8. Boyd PA, Bhattacharjee A, Gould S, et al. Outcome of pre-

natally diagnosed anterior abdominal wall defects. *Arch Dis Child Fetal Neonatal Ed* 1998;78:F209–F213.

9. Lurie S, Sherman D, Bukovsky I. Omphalocele delivery enigma: the best mode of delivery still remains dubious. *Eur J Obstet Gynecol Reprod Biol* 1999;82:19–22.

10. Sipes SL, Weiner CP, Sipes DR, et al. Gastroschisis and omphalocele: does either antenatal diagnosis or route of delivery make a difference in perinatal outcome? *Obstet Gynecol* 1990;76:195–199.

11. Moore TC, Collins DL, Catanzarite V, et al. Pre-term and particularly pre-labor cesarean section to avoid complications of gastroschisis. *Pediatr Surg Int* 1999;15:97–104.

12. Bethel CA, Seashore JH, Touloukian RJ. Cesarean section does not improve outcome in gastroschisis. *J Pediatr Surg* 1989;24:1–4.

13. Puffinbarger NK, Taylor DV, Tuggle DW, et al. End-tidal carbon dioxide for monitoring primary closure of gastroschisis. *J Pediatr Surg* 1996;31:280–282.

14. Kaempf J. Techniques of enteral feeding in the preterm infant. In: Hay WW, ed. *Nutrition and metabolism.* St. Louis: Mosby, 1991:573–583.

15. Jayanthi S, Seymour P, Puntis JW, et al. Necrotizing enterocolitis after gastroschisis repair: a preventable complication? *J Pediatr Surg* 1998;33:705–707.

16. Papagrigoriadis S, Browse DJ, Howard ER. Incarceration of umbilical hernias in children: a rare but important complication. *Pediatr Surg Int* 1998;14:231–232.

17. Evans A. The comparative incidence of umbilical hernias in colored and white infants. *J Natl Med Assoc* 1941;33:158–162.

18. Snyder WH Jr, Greanly EM Jr. Inguinal hernia. In: Benson CD, Mustard WT, Ravitch MM, et al., eds. *Pediatric surgery.* Chicago: Year Book Medical, 1962.

19. Rowe MI, Copelson LW, Clatworthy HW. The patent processus vaginalis and the inguinal hernia. *J Pediatr Surg* 1969;4(1):102–107.

20. Clarnette TD, Lam SK, Hutson JM. Ventriculo-peritoneal shunts in children reveal the natural history of closure of the processus vaginalis. *J Pediatr Surg* 1998;33:413–416.

21. Wesley JR. Abdominal wall defects. In: Greenfield LJ, Mulholland MW, Oldham KT, et al., eds. *Surgery: scientific principles and practice,* 2nd ed. Philadelphia: Lippincott–Raven, 1997:2028–2034.

22. Chou TY, Chu CC, Diau GY, et al. Inguinal hernia in children: US versus exploratory surgery and intraoperative contralateral laparoscopy. *Radiology* 1996;201:385–388.

23. Palmer BV. Incarcerated inguinal hernia in children. *Ann R Coll Surg Engl* 1978;60:121–124.

24. Rowe MI, Clatworthy HW. Incarcerated and strangulated hernias in children: a statistical study of high-risk factors. *Arch Surg* 1970;101:136–139.

25. Somri M, Gaitini L, Vaida S, et al. Postoperative outcome in high-risk infants undergoing herniorrhaphy: comparison between spinal and general anesthesia. *Anaesthesia* 1998;53:762–766.

26. Hrabovszky Z, Pinter AB. Routine bilateral exploration for inguinal hernia in infancy and childhood. *Eur J Pediatr Surg* 1995;5:152–155.

27. Wiener ES, Touloukian RJ, Rodgers BM, et al. Hernia survey of the Section on Surgery of the American Academy of Pediatrics. *J Pediatr Surg* 1996;31:1166–1169.

28. Tackett LD, Breuer CK, Luks FI, et al. Incidence of contralateral inguinal hernia: a prospective analysis. *J Pediatr Surg* 1999;34:684–687.

29. Wolf SA, Hopkins JW. Laparoscopic incidence of contralateral patent processus vaginalis in boys with clinical unilateral inguinal hernias. *J Pediatr Surg* 1994;29:1118–1120.

30. Yerkes EB, Brock JW III, Holcomb GW III, et al. Laparoscopic evaluation for a contralateral patent processus vaginalis: part III. *Urology* 1998;51:480–483.

31. Skandalakis JE, Gray SW. *Embryology for surgeons: the embryological basis for the treatment of congenital anomalies,* 2nd ed. Baltimore: Williams & Wilkins, 1994:184–241.

32. Haller JA Jr, Tepas JJ, Pickard LR, et al. Intestinal atresia: current concepts of pathogenesis, pathophysiology, and operative management. *Am Surg* 1983;49:385–391.

33. Adejuyigbe O, Odesanmi WO. Intrauterine intussusception causing intestinal atresia. *J Pediatr Surg* 1990;25:562–563.

34. Koga Y, Hayashida Y, Ikeda K, et al. Intestinal atresia in fetal dogs produced by localized ligation of mesenteric vessels. *J Pediatr Surg* 1975;10:949–953.

35. Dalla Vecchia LK, Grosfeld JL, West KW, et al. Intestinal atresia and stenosis: a 25-year experience with 277 cases. *Arch Surg* 1998;133:490–496.

36. James LM, Erickson JD, McClean AB. *Prevalence of birth defects.* Atlanta: Centers for Disease Control, 1992.

37. Filkins K, Russo J, Flowers WKD. Third trimester ultrasound diagnosis of intestinal atresia following clinical evidence of polyhydramnios. *Prenat Diagn* 1985;5:215–220.

38. Yamanaka M, Ohyama M, Koresawa M, et al. Umbilical cord ulceration and intestinal atresia. *Eur J Obstet Gynecol Reprod Biol* 1996;70:209–212.

39. Wilmore DW. Factors correlating with a successful outcome following extensive intestinal resection in newborn infants. *J Pediatr* 1972;80:88–95.

40. Touloukian RJ. Intestinal atresia. *Clin Perinatol* 1978;5:3–18.

41. Masumoto K, Suita S, Nada O, et al. Abnormalities of enteric neurons, intestinal pacemaker cells, and smooth muscle in human intestinal atresia. *J Pediatr Surg* 1999;34:1463–1468.

42. Doolin EJ, Ormsbee HS, Hill JL. Motility abnormality in intestinal atresia. *J Pediatr Surg* 1987;22:320–324.

43. Menardi G. Duodenal atresia, stenosis, and annular pancreas. In: Freeman NV, Burge DM, Griffiths M, et al., eds. *Surgery of the newborn.* Edinburgh: Churchill Livingstone, 1994:107–115.

44. Stauffer UG, Schwoebel M. Duodenal atresia and stenosis–annular pancreas. In: O'Neill JA Jr, Rowe MI, Grosfeld JL, et al., eds. *Pediatric surgery.* St. Louis: Mosby, 1998:1133–1143.

45. Stauffer UG, Irving I. Duodenal atresia and stenosis—long-term results. *Prog Pediatr Surg* 1977;10:49–60.

46. Grosfeld JL, Rescorla FJ. Duodenal atresia and stenosis: reassessment of treatment and outcome based on antenatal diagnosis, pathologic variance, and long-term follow-up. *World J Surg* 1993;17:301–309.

47. Kimura K, Mukohara N, Nishijima E, et al. Diamond-shaped anastomosis for duodenal atresia: an experience with 44 patients over 15 years. *J Pediatr Surg* 1990;25:977–979.

48. Weber TR, Lewis JE, Mooney D, et al. Duodenal atresia: a comparison of techniques of repair. *J Pediatr Surg* 1986;21:1133–1136.

49. Peña A. *Atlas of surgical management of anorectal malformations.* New York: Springer-Verlag, 1990.

50. Oldham KT. Gastrointestinal disorders. In: Greenfield LJ, Mulholland MW, Oldham KT, et al., eds. *Surgery: scientific principles and practice,* 2nd ed. Philadelphia: Lippincott–Raven, 1997:2034–2078.

51. Spouge D, Baird PA. Imperforate anus in 700,000 consecutive liveborn infants. *Am J Med Genet* 1986;2(Suppl):151–161.

52. Narasimharao KL, Prasad GR, Katariya S, et al. Prone cross-table lateral view: an alternative to the invertogram in imperforate anus. *AJR Am J Roentgenol* 1983;140:227–229.

53. Schuster SR, Teele RL. An analysis of ultrasound scanning as a guide in determination of "high" or "low" imperforate anus. *J Pediatr Surg* 1979;14:798–800.

54. deVries PA, Dorairajan T, Guttman FM, et al. Operative management of high and intermediate anomalies in the male. *Birth Defects* 1988;24:317–401.

55. Ong NT, Beasley SW. Long-term continence in patients with high and intermediate anorectal anomalies treated by sacroperineal (Stephens) rectoplasty. *J Pediatr Surg* 1991;26:44–48.

56. Ito Y, Yokoyama J, Hayashi A, et al. Reappraisal of endorectal pull-through procedure. I. Anorectal malformations. *J Pediatr Surg* 1981;16:476–483.

57. Mollard P, Marechal JM, de Beaujeu MJ. Surgical treatment of high imperforate anus with definition of the puborectalis sling by an anterior perineal approach. *J Pediatr Surg* 1978;13:499–504.

58. Kiesewetter WB, Hoon A. Imperforate anus: an analysis of mortalities during a 25-year period. *Prog Pediatr Surg* 1979;13:211–220.

59. Kiesewetter WB, Chang JH. Imperforate anus: a five- to thirty-year follow-up perspective. *Prog Pediatr Surg* 1977;10:111–120.

60. Templeton JM Jr, Ditesheim JA. High imperforate anus—quantitative results of long-term fecal continence. *J Pediatr Surg* 1985;20:645–652.

61. Bliss DP Jr, Tapper D, Anderson JM, et al. Does posterior sagittal anorectoplasty in patients with high imperforate anus provide superior fecal continence? *J Pediatr Surg* 1996; 31:26–30.

62. Czyrko C, Del Pin CA, O'Neill JA Jr, et al. Maternal cocaine abuse and necrotizing enterocolitis: outcome and survival. *J Pediatr Surg* 1991;26:414–418.

63. Major CA, Lewis DF, Harding JA, et al. Tocolysis with indomethacin increases the incidence of necrotizing enterocolitis in the low-birth-weight neonate. *Am J Obstet Gynecol* 1994;170(1 Pt 1):102–106.

64. Parks DA, Bulkley GB, Granger DN. Role of oxygen-derived free radicals in digestive tract diseases. *Surgery* 1983;94: 415–422.

65. Clark DA, Fornabaio DM, McNeill H, et al. Contribution of oxygen-derived free radicals to experimental necrotizing enterocolitis. *Am J Pathol* 1988;130:537–542.

66. Muguruma K, Gray PW, Tjoelker LW, et al. The central role of PAF in necrotizing enterocolitis development. *Adv Exp Med Biol* 1997;407:379–382.

67. Anderson DM, Kliegman RM. The relationship of neonatal alimentation practices to the occurrence of endemic necrotizing enterocolitis. *Am J Perinatol* 1991;8:62–67.

68. Rayyis SF, Ambalavanan N, Wright L, et al. Randomized trial of "slow" versus "fast" feed advancements on the incidence of necrotizing enterocolitis in very low birth weight infants. *J Pediatr* 1999;134:293–297.

69. Center for Disease Control and Prevention, National Center for Health Statistics. National Vital Statistics Report. 1999. April 29, 1999. Report No. 47:(18).

70. Grosfeld JL, Cheu H, Schlatter M, et al. Changing trends in necrotizing enterocolitis: experience with 302 cases in two decades. *Ann Surg* 1991;214:300–306.

71. Andrews DA, Sawin RS, Ledbetter DJ, et al. Necrotizing enterocolitis in term neonates. *Am J Surg* 1990;159:507–509.

72. Pokorny WJ, Garcia-Prats JA, Barry YN. Necrotizing enterocolitis: incidence, operative care, and outcome. *J Pediatr Surg* 1986;21:1149–1154.

73. Uauy RD, Fanaroff AA, Korones SB, et al. Necrotizing enterocolitis in very low birth weight infants: biodemographic and clinical correlates. National Institute of Child Health and Human Development Neonatal Research Network. *J Pediatr* 1991;119:630–638.

74. Bell MJ, Kosloske AM, Benton C, et al. Neonatal necrotizing enterocolitis: prevention of perforation. *J Pediatr Surg* 1973; 8:601–605.

75. Grosfeld JL, Chaet M, Molinari F, et al. Increased risk of necrotizing enterocolitis in premature infants with patent ductus arteriosus treated with indomethacin. *Ann Surg* 1996;224:350–355.

76. Ricketts RR. The role of paracentesis in the management of infants with necrotizing enterocolitis. *Am Surg* 1986;52: 61–65.

77. Cooper A, Ross AJ, O'Neill JA Jr, et al. Resection with primary anastomosis for necrotizing enterocolitis: a contrasting view. *J Pediatr Surg* 1988;23(1 Pt 2):64–68.

78. Ade-Ajayi N, Kiely E, Drake D, et al. Resection and primary anastomosis in necrotizing enterocolitis. *J R Soc Med* 1996; 89:385–388.

79. Ahmed T, Ein S, Moore A. The role of peritoneal drains in treatment of perforated necrotizing enterocolitis: recommendations from recent experience. *J Pediatr Surg* 1998;33: 1468–1470.

80. Ein SH, Shandling B, Wesson D, et al. A 13-year experience with peritoneal drainage under local anesthesia for necrotizing enterocolitis perforation. *J Pediatr Surg* 1990;25: 1034–1036.

81. O'Connor A, Sawin RS. High morbidity of enterostomy and its closure in premature infants with necrotizing enterocolitis. *Arch Surg* 1998;133:875–880.

82. Schwartz MZ, Hayden CK, Richardson CJ, et al. A prospective evaluation of intestinal stenosis following necrotizing enterocolitis. *J Pediatr Surg* 1982;17:764–770.

83. Ricketts RR, Jerles ML. Neonatal necrotizing enterocolitis:

84. Patel JC, Tepas JJ III, Huffman SD, et al. Neonatal necrotizing enterocolitis: the long-term perspective. *Am Surg* 1998;64: 575–579.

85. Statement from the National Institutes of Health workshop on population screening for the cystic fibrosis gene. *N Engl J Med* 1990;323:70–71.

86. Riordan JR, Rommens JM, Kerem B, et al. Identification of the cystic fibrosis gene: cloning and characterization of complementary DNA. *Science* 1989;245:1066–1073.

87. Kerem B, Rommens JM, Buchanan JA, et al. Identification of the cystic fibrosis gene: genetic analysis. *Science* 1989;245: 1073–1080.

88. Grody WW. Cystic fibrosis: molecular diagnosis, population screening, and public policy. *Arch Pathol Lab Med* 1999; 123:1041–1046.

89. Rosenstein BJ, Cutting GR. The diagnosis of cystic fibrosis: a consensus statement. Cystic Fibrosis Foundation Consensus Panel. *J Pediatr* 1998;132:589–595.

90. Quinton PM. Cystic fibrosis: a disease in electrolyte transport. *Faseb J* 1990;4:2709–2717.

91. Quinton PM, Bijman J. Higher bioelectric potentials due to decreased chloride absorption in the sweat glands of patients with cystic fibrosis. *N Engl J Med* 1983;308: 1185–1189.

92. Irish MS, Ragi JM, Karamanoukian H, et al. Prenatal diagnosis of the fetus with cystic fibrosis and meconium ileus. *Pediatr Surg Int* 1997;12:434–436.

93. Kao SC, Franken EA Jr. Nonoperative treatment of simple meconium ileus: a survey of the Society for Pediatric Radiology. *Pediatr Radiol* 1995;25:97–100.

94. Mak GZ, Harberg FJ, Hiatt P, et al. T-tube ileostomy for meconium ileus: four decades of experience. *J Pediatr Surg* 2000;35:349–352.

95. Del Pin CA, Czyrko C, Ziegler MM, et al. Management and survival of meconium ileus: a 30-year review. *Ann Surg* 1992;215:179–185.

96. Docherty JG, Zaki A, Coutts JA, et al. Meconium ileus: a review 1972–1990. *Br J Surg* 1992;79:571–573.

97. Nir M, Lanng S, Johansen HK, et al. Long-term survival and nutritional data in patients with cystic fibrosis treated in a Danish centre. *Thorax* 1996;51:1023–1027.

98. Andrassy RJ, Mahour GH. Malrotation of the midgut in infants and children: a 25-year review. *Arch Surg* 1981;116: 158–160.

99. Ford EG, Senac MO Jr, Srikanth MS, et al. Malrotation of the intestine in children. *Ann Surg* 1992;215:172–178.

100. Powell DM, Othersen HB, Smith CD. Malrotation of the intestines in children: the effect of age on presentation and therapy. *J Pediatr Surg* 1989;24:777–780.

101. Weinberger E, Winters WD, Liddell RM, et al. Sonographic diagnosis of intestinal malrotation in infants: importance of the relative positions of the superior mesenteric vein and artery. *AJR Am J Roentgenol* 1992;159:825–828.

102. Ladd WE, Gross RE. *Abdominal surgery of infancy and childhood*. Philadelphia: WB Saunders, 1941.

103. Bass KD, Rothenberg SS, Chang JH. Laparoscopic Ladd's procedure in infants with malrotation. *J Pediatr Surg* 1998; 33:279–281.

104. Fujimoto T, Hata J, Yokoyama S, et al. A study of the extracellular matrix protein as the migration pathway of neural crest cells in the gut: analysis in human embryos with special reference to the pathogenesis of Hirschsprung's disease. *J Pediatr Surg* 1989;24:550–556.

105. Kleinhaus S, Boley SJ, Sheran M, et al. Hirschsprung's disease—a survey of the members of the Surgical Section of the American Academy of Pediatrics. *J Pediatr Surg* 1979;14: 588–597.

106. Lolova I, Davidoff M, Itzev D, et al. Histochemical, immunocytochemical, and ultrastructural data on the innervation of the smooth muscle of the large intestine in Hirschsprung's disease. *Acta Physiol Pharmacol Bulg* 1986;12:55–62.

107. Tomita R, Munakata K, Kurosu Y. Peptidergic nerves in Hirschsprung's disease and its allied disorders. *Eur J Pediatr Surg* 1994;4:346–351.

108. Kusafuka T, Puri P. Altered mRNA expression of the neu-

ronal nitric oxide synthase gene in Hirschsprung's disease. *J Pediatr Surg* 1997;32:1054–1058.

109. Tomita R, Munakata K, Kurosu Y, et al. A role of nitric oxide in Hirschsprung's disease. *J Pediatr Surg* 1995;30:437–440.

110. O'Kelly TJ, Davies JR, Tam PK, et al. Abnormalities of nitric-oxide–producing neurons in Hirschsprung's disease: morphology and implications. *J Pediatr Surg* 1994;29:294–299.

111. Bealer JF, Natuzzi ES, Buscher C, et al. Nitric oxide synthase is deficient in the aganglionic colon of patients with Hirschsprung's disease. *Pediatrics* 1994;93:647–651.

112. Puri P, Wester T. Intestinal neuronal dysplasia. *Semin Pediatr Surg* 1998;7:181–186.

113. Ryan DP. Neuronal intestinal dysplasia. *Semin Pediatr Surg* 1995;4:22–25.

114. Kobayashi H, Hirakawa H, Puri P. Is intestinal neuronal dysplasia a disorder of the neuromuscular junction? *J Pediatr Surg* 1996;31:575–579.

115. Tanaka H, Moroi K, Iwai J, et al. Novel mutations of the endothelin B receptor gene in patients with Hirschsprung's disease and their characterization. *J Biol Chem* 1998;273:11378–11383.

116. Kusafuka T, Puri P. Genetic aspects of Hirschsprung's disease. *Semin Pediatr Surg* 1998;7:148–155.

117. Robertson K, Mason I, Hall S. Hirschsprung's disease: genetic mutations in mice and men. *Gut* 1997;41:436–441.

118. Puri P, Ohshiro K, Wester T. Hirschsprung's disease: a search for etiology. *Semin Pediatr Surg* 1998;7:140–147.

119. Puffenberger EG, Kauffman ER, Bolk S, et al. Identity-by-descent and association mapping of a recessive gene for Hirschsprung disease on human chromosome 13q22. *Hum Mol Genet* 1994;3:1217–1225.

120. Romeo G, Ronchetto P, Luo Y, et al. Point mutations affecting the tyrosine kinase domain of the RET protooncogene in Hirschsprung's disease. *Nature* 1994;367:377–378.

121. Quinn FM, Surana R, Puri P. The influence of trisomy 21 on outcome in children with Hirschsprung's disease. *J Pediatr Surg* 1994;29:781–783.

122. Caniano DA, Teitelbaum DH, Qualman SJ. Management of Hirschsprung's disease in children with trisomy 21. *Am J Surg* 1990;159:402–404.

123. Urushihara N, Kohno S, Hasegawa S. Pseudomembranous enterocolitis and hemorrhagic necrotizing enterocolitis in Hirschsprung's disease. *Surg Today* 1994;24:221–224.

124. Thomas DF, Fernie DS, Bayston R, et al. Enterocolitis in Hirschsprung's disease: a controlled study of the etiologic role of *Clostridium difficile*. *J Pediatr Surg* 1986;21:22–25.

125. Wilson-Storey D, Scobie WG, McGenity KG. Microbiological studies of the enterocolitis of Hirschsprung's disease. *Arch Dis Child* 1990;65:1338–1339.

126. Qualman SJ, Jaffe R, Bove KE, et al. Diagnosis of Hirschsprung disease using the rectal biopsy: multi-institutional survey. *Pediatr Dev Pathol* 1999;2:588–596.

127. Ramesh JC, Ramanujam TM, Yik YI, et al. Management of Hirschsprung's disease with reference to one-stage pull-through without colostomy. *J Pediatr Surg* 1999;34:1691–1694.

128. Albanese CT, Jennings RW, Smith B, et al. Perineal one-stage pull-through for Hirschsprung's disease. *J Pediatr Surg* 1999;34:377–380.

129. Cilley RE, Statter MB, Hirschl RB, et al. Definitive treatment of Hirschsprung's disease in the newborn with a one-stage procedure. *Surgery* 1994;115:551–556.

130. Bianchi A. One-stage neonatal reconstruction without stoma for Hirschsprung's disease. *Semin Pediatr Surg* 1998;7:170–173.

131. Georgeson KE, Cohen RD, Hebra A, et al. Primary laparoscopic-assisted endorectal colon pull-through for Hirschsprung's disease: a new gold standard. *Ann Surg* 1999;229:678–682.

132. Skinner MA. Hirschsprung's disease. *Curr Probl Surg* 1996;33:389–460.

133. Sawin R, Hatch E, Schaller R, et al. Limited surgery for lower-segment Hirschsprung's disease. *Arch Surg* 1994;129:920–924.

134. Vanderwinden JM, Mailleux P, Schiffmann SN, et al. Nitric oxide synthase activity in infantile hypertrophic pyloric stenosis. *N Engl J Med* 1992;327:511–515.

135. Rasmussen L, Green A, Hansen LP. The epidemiology of infantile hypertrophic pyloric stenosis in a Danish population, 1950–84. *Int J Epidemiol* 1989;18:413–417.

136. Honein MA, Paulozzi LJ, Himelright IM, et al. Infantile hypertrophic pyloric stenosis after pertussis prophylaxis with erythromycin: a case review and cohort study. *Lancet* 1999;354:2101–2105.

137. Schechter R, Torfs CP, Bateson TF. The epidemiology of infantile hypertrophic pyloric stenosis. *Paediatr Perinat Epidemiol* 1997;11:407–427.

138. Kim YS, Rhu JH. Intussusception in infancy and childhood: analysis of 385 cases. *Int Surg* 1989;74:114–118.

139. From the Centers for Disease Control and Prevention. Withdrawal of rotavirus vaccine recommendation. *JAMA* 1999;282:2113–2114.

140. Okuyama H, Nakai H, Okada A. Is barium enema reduction safe and effective in patients with a long duration of intussusception? *Pediatr Surg Int* 1999;15:105–107.

141. Poddoubnyi IV, Dronov AF, Blinnikov OI, et al. Laparoscopy in the treatment of intussusception in children. *J Pediatr Surg* 1998;33:1194–1197.

142. Schier F, Hoffmann K, Waldschmidt J. Laparoscopic removal of Meckel's diverticula in children. *Eur J Pediatr Surg* 1996;6:38–39.

143. Bonadio WA, Jona JZ, Glicklich M, et al. Esophageal bougienage technique for coin ingestion in children. *J Pediatr Surg* 1988;23:917–918.

144. Maves MD, Carithers JS, Birck HG. Esophageal burns secondary to disc battery ingestion. *Ann Otol Rhinol Laryngol* 1984;93(4 Pt 1):364–369.

145. Oldham KT, Lobe TE. Gastrointestinal hemorrhage in children: a pragmatic update. *Pediatr Clin North Am* 1985;32:1247–1263.

146. Thompson EC, Brown MF, Bowen EC, et al. Causes of gastrointestinal hemorrhage in neonates and children. *South Med J* 1996;89:370–374.

147. McDougal WS, Izant RJ Jr, Zollinger RM Jr. Primary peritonitis in infancy and childhood. *Ann Surg* 1975;181:310–313.

148. Newman KD. Malignant liver tumors of children. *Semin Pediatr Surg* 1992;1:145–151.

149. Bowman LC, Riely CA. Management of pediatric liver tumors. *Surg Oncol Clin N Am* 1996;5:451–459.

150. Luks FI, Yazbeck S, Brandt ML, et al. Benign liver tumors in children: a 25-year experience. *J Pediatr Surg* 1991;26:1326–1330.

151. Coran AG. Pediatric liver. In: Greenfield LJ, Mulholland MW, Oldham KT, et al., eds. *Surgery: scientific principles and practice,* 2nd ed. Philadelphia: Lippincott–Raven, 1997:2078–2083.

152. Yandza T, Valayer J. Benign tumors of the liver in children: analysis of a series of 20 cases. *J Pediatr Surg* 1986;21:419–423.

153. Gold JH, Guzman IJ, Rosai J. Benign tumors of the liver: pathologic examination of 45 cases. *Am J Clin Pathol* 1978;70:6–17.

154. Ein SH, Stephens CA. Benign liver tumors and cysts in childhood. *J Pediatr Surg* 1974;9:847–851.

155. Pazdur R, Bready B, Cangir A. Pediatric hepatic tumors: clinical trials conducted in the United States. *J Surg Oncol* 1993;3(Suppl):127–130.

156. Urban CE, Mache CJ, Schwinger W, et al. Undifferentiated (embryonal) sarcoma of the liver in childhood: successful combined-modality therapy in four patients. *Cancer* 1993;72:2511–2516.

157. Randolph JG, Altman RP, Arensman RM, et al. Liver resection in children with hepatic neoplasms. *Ann Surg* 1978;187:599–605.

158. Larsen LR, Raffensperger J. Liver abscess. *J Pediatr Surg* 1979;14:329–331.

159. Jessee WF, Ryan JM, Fitzgerald JF, et al. Amebic liver abscess in childhood. *Clin Pediatr (Phila)* 1975;14:134–146.

160. Lilly JR, Karrer FM. Contemporary surgery of biliary atresia. *Pediatr Clin North Am* 1985;32:1233–1246.

161. Balistreri WF, Grand R, Hoofnagle JH, et al. Biliary atresia: current concepts and research directions. *Hepatology* 1996;23:1682–1692.

162. Tan CE, Davenport M, Driver M, et al. Does the morphology of the extrahepatic biliary remnants in biliary atresia influence survival? A review of 205 cases. *J Pediatr Surg* 1994;29: 1459–1464.

163. Chandra RS, Altman RP. Ductal remnants in extrahepatic biliary atresia: a histopathologic study with clinical correlation. *J Pediatr* 1978;93:196–200.

164. Bates MD, Bucuvalas JC, Alonso MH, et al. Biliary atresia: pathogenesis and treatment. *Semin Liver Dis* 1998;18: 281–293.

165. A-Kader HH, Nowicki MJ, Kuramoto KI, et al. Evaluation of the role of hepatitis C virus in biliary atresia. *Pediatr Infect Dis J* 1994;13:657–659.

166. Steele MI, Marshall CM, Lloyd RE, et al. Reovirus 3 not detected by reverse transcriptase-mediated polymerase chain reaction analysis of preserved tissue from infants with cholestatic liver disease. *Hepatol* 1995;21:697–702.

167. Schmeling DJ, Oldham KT, Guice KS, et al. Experimental obliterative cholangitis: a model for the study of biliary atresia. *Ann Surg* 1991;213:350–355.

168. Ryckman FC, Alonso MH, Bucuvalas JC, et al. Biliary atresia—surgical management and treatment options as they relate to outcome. *Liver Transpl Surg* 1998;4(5 Suppl 1):S24–S33.

169. Sartorelli KH, Holland RM, Allshouse MJ, et al. The intussusception antireflux valve is ineffective in preventing cholangitis in biliary atresia. *J Pediatr Surg* 1996;31:403–406.

170. Whitington PF, Emond JC, Whitington SH, et al. Small-bowel length and the dose of cyclosporine in children after liver transplantation. *N Engl J Med* 1990;322:733–738.

171. Burnweit CA, Coln D. Influence of diversion on the development of cholangitis after hepatoportoenterostomy for biliary atresia. *J Pediatr Surg* 1986;21:1143–1146.

172. Kasai M, Suzuki H, Ohashi E, et al. Technique and results of operative management of biliary atresia. *World J Surg* 1978; 2:571–579.

173. Kasai M. Advances in treatment of biliary atresia. *Jpn J Surg* 1983;13:265–276.

174. Rothenberg SS, Schroter GP, Karrer FM, et al. Cholangitis after the Kasai operation for biliary atresia. *J Pediatr Surg* 1989;24:729–732.

175. Luketic VA, Sanyal AJ. The current status of ursodeoxycholate in the treatment of chronic cholestatic liver disease. *Gastroenterologist* 1994;2:74–79.

176. Chardot C, Carton M, Spire-Bendelac N, et al. Prognosis of biliary atresia in the era of liver transplantation: French national study from 1986 to 1996. *Hepatology* 1999;30: 606–611.

177. Goss JA, Shackleton CR, Swenson K, et al. Orthotopic liver transplantation for congenital biliary atresia: an 11-year, single-center experience. *Ann Surg* 1996;224:276–284.

178. Alonso-Lej F, Revor WB, Pessagno DJ. Congenital choledochal cyst, with a report of 2, and an analysis of 94 cases. *Surg Gynecol Obstet* 1959;108:1–30.

179. Todani T, Watanabe Y, Narusue M, et al. Congenital bile duct cysts: classification, operative procedures, and review of thirty-seven cases including cancer arising from choledochal cyst. *Am J Surg* 1977;134:263–269.

180. Todani T, Tabuchi K, Watanabe Y, et al. Carcinoma arising in the wall of congenital bile duct cysts. *Cancer* 1979;44: 1134–1141.

181. Komi N, Tamura T, Miyoshi Y, et al. Histochemical and immunohistochemical studies on development of biliary carcinoma in forty-seven patients with choledochal cyst—special reference to intestinal metaplasia in the biliary duct. *Jpn J Surg* 1985;15:273–278.

182. Flanigan DP. Biliary carcinoma associated with biliary cysts. *Cancer* 1977;40:880–883.

183. Fieber SS, Nance FC. Choledochal cyst and neoplasm: a comprehensive review of 106 cases and presentation of two original cases. *Am Surg* 1997;63:982–987.

184. Miyano T, Yamataka A, Kato Y, et al. Hepaticoenterostomy after excision of choledochal cyst in children: a 30-year experience with 180 cases. *J Pediatr Surg* 1996;31:1417–1421.

185. Flanigan PD. Biliary cysts. *Ann Surg* 1975;182:635–643.

186. Lipsett PA, Pitt HA, Colombani PM, et al. Choledochal cyst disease: a changing pattern of presentation. *Ann Surg* 1994; 220:644–652.

187. Werlin SL. Disorders of the pancreas in children. *Curr Opin Pediatr* 1998;10:507–511.

188. Coran AG. Pediatric pancreas. In: Greenfield LJ, Mulholland MW, Oldham KT, et al., eds. *Surgery: scientific principles and practice,* 2nd ed. Philadelphia: Lippincott–Raven, 1997: 2094–2098.

189. Warshaw AL, Richter JM, Schapiro RH. The cause and treatment of pancreatitis associated with pancreas divisum. *Ann Surg* 1983;198:443–452.

190. Warshaw AL, Simeone JF, Schapiro RH, et al. Evaluation and treatment of the dominant dorsal duct syndrome (pancreas divisum redefined). *Am J Surg* 1990;159:59–64.

191. Adzick NS, Shamberger RC, Winter HS, et al. Surgical treatment of pancreas divisum causing pancreatitis in children. *J Pediatr Surg* 1989;24:54–58.

192. Keith RG, Shapero TF, Saibil FG, et al. Dorsal duct sphincterotomy is effective long-term treatment of acute pancreatitis associated with pancreas divisum. *Surgery* 1989;106: 660–666.

193. Cooney DR, Jacobowitz I, Telander RL, et al. Pancreaticocolonic fistula: a complication of pancreatic pseudocysts in childhood. *J Pediatr Surg* 1978;13:492–496.

194. Kagan RJ, Reyes HM, Asokan S. Pseudocyst of the pancreas in childhood: current advances in diagnosis. *Arch Surg* 1981;116:1200–1203.

195. Rescorla FJ, Plumley DA, Sherman S, et al. The efficacy of early ERCP in pediatric pancreatic trauma. *J Pediatr Surg* 1995;30:336–340.

196. Cooney DR, Grosfeld JL. Operative management of pancreatic pseudocysts in infants and children: a review of 75 cases. *Ann Surg* 1975;182:590–596.

197. Grosfeld JL, Vane DW, Rescorla FJ, et al. Pancreatic tumors in childhood: analysis of 13 cases. *J Pediatr Surg* 1990;25: 1057–1062.

198. Shamberger RC, Hendren WH, Leichtner AM. Long-term nutritional and metabolic consequences of pancreaticoduodenectomy in children. *Surgery* 1994;115:382–388.

199. Wang KS, Albanese C, Dada F, et al. Papillary cystic neoplasm of the pancreas: a report of three pediatric cases and literature review. *J Pediatr Surg* 1998;33:842–845.

200. Wilson SD. Zollinger-Ellison syndrome in children: a 25-year follow-up. *Surgery* 1991;110:696–702.

201. Sempoux C, Poggi F, Brunelle F, et al. Nesidioblastosis and persistent neonatal hyperinsulinism. *Diabetes Metab* 1995; 21:402–407.

202. Aynsley-Green A, Polak JM, Bloom SR, et al. Nesidioblastosis of the pancreas: definition of the syndrome and the management of the severe neonatal hyperinsulinaemic hypoglycaemia. *Arch Dis Child* 1981;56:496–508.

203. Hirsch HJ, Loo S, Evans N, et al. Hypoglycemia of infancy and nesidioblastosis: studies with somatostatin. *N Engl J Med* 1977;296:1323–1326.

204. Warden MJ, German JC, Buckingham BA. The surgical management of hyperinsulinism in infancy due to nesidioblastosis. *J Pediatr Surg* 1988;23:462–465.

205. Willberg B, Muller E. Surgery for nesidioblastosis—indications, treatment, and results. *Prog Pediatr Surg* 1991;26: 76–83.

206. Parashar K, Upadhyay V, Corkery JJ. Partial or near-total pancreatectomy for nesidioblastosis? *Eur J Pediatr Surg* 1995;5: 146–148.

207. Leibowitz G, Glaser B, Higazi AA, et al. Hyperinsulinemic hypoglycemia of infancy (nesidioblastosis) in clinical remission: high incidence of diabetes mellitus and persistent beta-cell dysfunction at long-term follow-up. *J Clin Endocrinol Metab* 1995;80:386–392.

208. Grosfeld JL. Jejunoileal atresia and stenosis. In: O'Neill JA Jr, Rowe MI, Grosfeld JL, et al., eds. *Pediatric surgery,* 5th ed. St. Louis: Mosby, 1998:1145–1158.

SURGERY: SCIENTIFIC PRINCIPLES AND PRACTICE, Third Edition, edited by
Lazar J. Greenfield, Michael W. Mulholland, Keith T. Oldham, Gerald B. Zelenock,
and Keith D. Lillemoe. Lippincott Williams & Wilkins Publishers, Philadelphia, © 2001.

CHAPTER 98

PEDIATRIC GENITOURINARY SYSTEM

EUGENE MINEVICH AND CURTIS A. SHELDON

NEPHRIC SYSTEM

The nephric system develops through three distinct stages. The initial stage, the *pronephros,* disappears completely by the fourth week of embryonic life. The *mesonephros,* the second stage, degenerates as well, although some of the structures become associated with the reproductive system. The caudal portion of the mesonephric duct, which communicates with the cloaca, forms a ureteral bud between the fourth and sixth weeks of gestation. The cranial portion of the ureteral bud joins with the metanephric blastema branching into the renal pelvis and the calyces and induces nephron formation during the final stage of development, *metanephros.* The kidneys undergo ascent and rotation before assuming their final position.

ANOMALIES OF THE KIDNEY

Supernumerary Kidney

The supernumerary kidney is a rare anomaly of the urinary system and represents a distinct extra kidney (or kidneys). Embryologically, it is believed that an additional ureteral bud develops a separate metanephric mass resulting in the formation of an extra kidney, usually caudal to the dominant kidney. This anomaly is rarely discovered at birth. It is usually an incidental finding on abdominal imaging for unrelated reasons, although some adults may occasionally present with abdominal pain, hypertension, or symptoms of urinary tract infections (UTI).

Renal Agenesis

Absence of a ureteral bud or its failure to join the metanephric blastema results in renal agenesis. A bilateral anomaly occurs with an incidence of approximately 1 per 4,000 births and is known as *Potter's syndrome.* This is manifested by characteristic facies, pulmonary hypoplasia, and orthopedic abnormalities (1). These infants are stillborn or rapidly die of respiratory failure.

The incidence of unilateral renal agenesis is approximately 1 in 1,200 births. The ipsilateral ureter is absent in more than 50% of cases, although an adrenal gland is usually present. The most common contralateral anomalies are vesicoureteral reflux (VUR; 30%) and renal malrotation or renal ectopia (15%). Although genital anomalies are more often observed in girls (25% to 50%) than in boys (10% to 15%), malformations of the rectum, anus, and lower spine occur with equal frequency in both sexes with unilateral renal agenesis. Other associated congenital anomalies may involve the cardiovascular, gastrointestinal or musculoskeletal systems. Unilateral renal agenesis is usually asymptomatic and found incidentally during evaluation of children with other organ system anomalies.

Renal Ectopy

Failure of the metanephros to ascend leads to an ectopic kidney, which occurs in approximately 1 in 1,100 people. An ectopic kidney may be on the ipsilateral side *(simple ectopy)* or on the contralateral side *(crossed ectopy)* with or without fusion. The adrenal gland develops separately from the kidney and is therefore found in its normal position, despite anomalies in renal position. Further classification of renal ectopia is based on the position of the kidney in the retroperitoneum: abdominal, lumbar, or pelvic kidney. A rare form of ectopia exists whereby the kidney is located above the ipsilateral diaphragm (intrathoracic kidney). Delayed closure of the diaphragm or accelerated kidney ascent before diaphragmatic closure results in this condition.

Most ectopic kidneys are clinically asymptomatic and detected during evaluation for unrelated conditions. Almost half of ectopic kidneys have hydronephrosis secondary to malrotation, aberrant renal vessels compressing the renal pelvis, or ureteropelvic junction (UPJ) obstruction (2). If surgical correction of the obstructed kidney is required, particular attention should be paid to anomalous renal vasculature. Every effort should be made to preserve an ectopic kidney because the contralateral kidney is abnormal in up to 50% of patients, with hydronephrosis or VUR being the most common abnormality. Genital anomalies have been reported in 15% to 45% of patients with renal ectopia.

Horseshoe Kidney

Horseshoe kidney is the most common type of renal fusion and occurs in 0.25% of population. Patients with Turner's syndrome and trisomy 18 have a significantly higher incidence of horseshoe kidney. The anomaly consists of two renal masses connected by the isthmus at the midline, usually at the lower poles. The isthmus, which consists of renal parenchyma or fibrous tissue, usually lies just below the junction of the inferior mesenteric artery and aorta and anterior to the great vessels. The pelvises and ureters of horseshoe kidney are usually anteriorly placed, crossing the isthmus ventrally.

The horseshoe kidney does not usually produce symptoms unless it is associated with other anomalies. The most commonly associated abnormality is VUR and UPJ obstruction, which can lead to UTI or urolithiasis, with corresponding symptomatology. If surgical repair of UPJ obstruction is required, a standard dismembered pyeloplasty with or without division of the renal isthmus is recommended. The retroperitoneal flank approach is usually successful, but the surgeon should be prepared for a transperitoneal approach as well. The incidence of Wilms' tumor may to be increasing in patients with horseshoe kidney (3).

Cystic Disease of the Kidney

Renal cystic disease, congenital or acquired, is one of the most common causes of the pediatric abdominal mass. Several classifications have been proposed, based on the clinical or radiologic presentation, pathologic studies, and genetic associations (4).

Autosomal recessive ("infantile") polycystic kidney disease results from dilated collecting ducts and has a spectrum of severity, with the most severe forms appearing in infancy. This congenital disorder affects both kidneys and liver (ranging from biliary ectasia to congenital hepatic fibrosis). The affected infant usually presents with large flank masses. Renal ultrasound (US) demonstrates en-

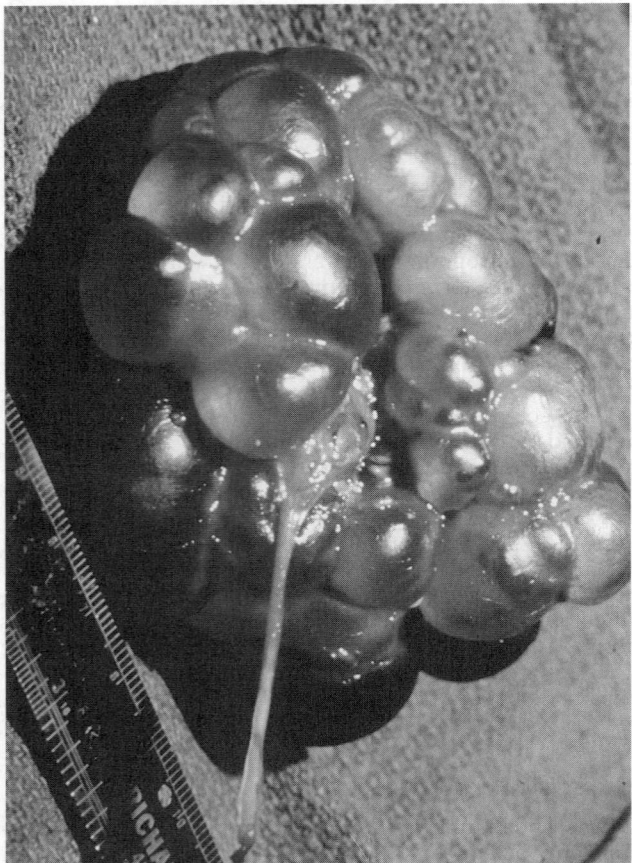

Figure 98.1. Multicystic dysplastic kidney.

larged, homogeneously hyperechogenic kidneys. Progressive renal or hepatic failure develops in most children. No cure has been found for this disease.

Multicystic dysplastic kidney (MCDK) is the most common type of renal cystic disease. This anomaly represents a severe form of renal dysplasia with complete replacement of renal parenchyma by different-sized cysts (Fig. 98.1).

Renal US is usually definitive in making the correct diagnosis, although renal scintigraphy is necessary to demonstrate the absence of renal function and occasionally differentiate MCDK from severe obstructed hydronephrosis in the involved kidney. The high incidence of VUR in the solitary functioning contralateral kidney

(18% to 43%) makes a voiding cystourethrogram (VCUG) an essential part of the evaluation of these children. Involution of MCDK may occur to the point that the involved kidney disappears from subsequent sonograms. Potential long-term sequelae of retained MCDK, including hypertension, infection, and pain, are very rare. Sporadic reports of renal cell carcinoma and Wilms' tumor in MCDK raise the concern of the persistent potential for malignant degeneration in the dysplastic kidney. The latest recommendation for management of the patient with MCDK is strict US surveillance, especially in early childhood (5). Nephrectomy is reserved for the patient with an equivocal radiologic appearance or MCDK that fails to regress, or the patient who proves to be noncompliant with follow-up (6). Currently, the National Multicystic Kidney Registry is studying the natural course of MCDK to update recommendations on management of this disease.

Ureteropelvic Junction Obstruction

The UPJ is the most common site of obstruction in the urinary tract and the most common cause of neonatal hydronephrosis. The pathogenesis of this disorder is variable. Of the intrinsic factors, the adynamic segment is associated most often with classic UPJ obstruction. This obstruction is thought to be a congenital absence or abnormal arrangement of the muscular fibers at the transition zone of the upper ureter and renal pelvis, leading to failure of peristaltic wave propagation. Extrinsic causes include fibrous bands, aberrant accessory vessels, and various organ-compressing factors. Most cases of UPJ obstruction are diagnosed in utero and such patients are initially asymptomatic. Some children present with abdominal or flank pain, hematuria, or UTI. Occasionally, previously asymptomatic UPJ obstruction may be discovered in the patient with renal injury after relatively minor abdominal trauma.

Renal US is the test of choice to determine the degree of renal pelvic dilatation, parenchymal thickness, and associated abnormalities of the bladder and the ureter. Diuretic renography and occasionally Whitaker antegrade pressure perfusion studies are necessary to confirm UPJ obstruction. The VCUG and occasional excretory urogram (intravenous pyelogram) may define anatomic details. Retrograde pyelography is used to rule out other causes of obstruction and is usually performed just before surgery.

A dismembered pyeloplasty, with removal of an adynamic segment, remains the surgical treatment of choice because it provides dependent drainage of the renal pelvis (Fig. 98.2). With use of optical magnification and careful attention to surgical technique, a successful outcome should be expected in over 95% of cases (7).

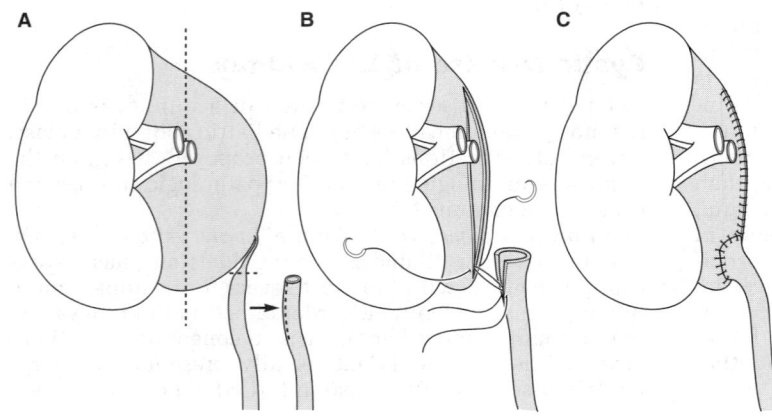

Figure 98.2. Dismembered pyeloplasty after resection of an excessively large renal pelvis. *(A)* The line of excision provides an adequate margin of pelvis to enable closure without tension. A vertical incision is made in the lateral aspect of the ureter to spatulate it. *(B)* The apical sutures are carefully placed. *(C)* Approximation and closure of the pelvis are completed. (From Minevich E, Wacksman J. Pyeloplasty. In: Graham SD, ed. *Glenn's urologic surgery.* Philadelphia: Lippincott–Raven, 1998:714.)

ANOMALIES OF THE URETER

Ureteral Duplication

Ureteral duplication is the most common anomaly of the urinary tract. Early branching of the single ureteral bud results in *incomplete (partial) duplication* with a single ureteral orifice and bifid proximal ureters (1 in 125 individuals). An accessory ureteral bud creates *complete duplication* (1 in 500 individuals), with the upper ureter usually inserting into the bladder more medially and inferiorly than the lower ureter. The upper ureter is more likely to be associated with ectopic insertion, ureterocele, or obstruction, whereas the lower ureter is frequently associated with VUR. Most patients with ureteral duplication are asymptomatic or may occasionally present with symptoms of UTI.

Ureteral Ectopia and Ureterocele

The ectopic ureteral orifice lies caudal to the normal insertion of the ureter on the bladder trigone. Ureteral ectopia is much more common in association with complete ureteral duplication. In the boy, ectopic ureteral orifices are most frequently found at the prostatic urethra and even along the course of the genital ductal system. In the girl, ectopic ureters can be found draining into the bladder neck, urethra, vagina, or even the uterus. Boys with bilateral anomalies and girls with termination of an ectopic ureter below the external urinary sphincter usually present with urinary incontinence.

Ureteroceles are congenital cystic dilatations of the distal ureter. Those associated with a single ureter *(simple ureterocele)* are usually located in an orthotopic trigonal position. Ureteroceles found in association with duplicated ureters usually drain the upper pole kidney and are located in an ectopic position. Ectopic ureteroceles are commonly associated with obstruction and varying degrees of dysplasia of the affected renal segment. Decompression of the obstructed renal moiety from above (ureteropyelostomy) or from below (excision of ureterocele with ureteral reimplantation) is usually successful. Transurethral incision of a ureterocele is usually reserved for infants, whereas a severely dysplastic moiety can be managed by partial nephrectomy. Large ureteroceles obstructing other renal moieties and the bladder neck most likely require secondary procedures to restore normal urinary tract anatomy (8).

Vesicoureteral Reflux

Vesicoureteral reflux refers to the retrograde passage of urine from the bladder into the ureter. The incidence of VUR in otherwise normal children is approximately 1%; a much higher incidence of up to 40% is reported in patients undergoing evaluation for UTI. A significant familial association has been encountered. A sufficient tunnel length of submucosal ureter is the most important component of the competent ureterovesical junction. This provides a predominantly passive valve mechanism for compression of the ureter, preventing retrograde passage of urine. Patients with marginal tunnel pressure can be made to reflux primarily or secondarily because of loss of compliance of the valve roof (during UTI), structural weakness of the detrusor floor (bladder diverticulum, ureterocele), or excessively high intravesical pressure due to neurovesical dysfunction or bladder outlet obstruction. VUR is graded according to the International Classification System based on the proximal extent of retrograde urine flow, ureteral and pelvic dilatation, and the resultant anatomy of the calyceal fornices.

Reflux-induced renal injury is usually due to the association of VUR with UTI and may range from clinically silent focal scar formation to generalized scarring and renal atrophy *(reflux nephropathy)* with hypertension and even end-stage renal failure. Children of either sex should be investigated at the time of the initial infection. The diagnosis of VUR is accomplished by cyclic VCUG, with either contrast medium or isotope. Imaging of the upper tracts (kidneys and ureters) is extremely important and may be accomplished by ultrasonography, isotope renography or, rarely, intravenous urography. Ultrasonography is helpful in quantifying renal growth or atrophy, whereas isotope renography is particularly sensitive in detecting focal scarring. Patients with voiding dysfunction should be considered strongly for urodynamic studies.

Because the submucosal ureter tends to lengthen with age, the ratio of tunnel length to ureteral diameter increases, and the propensity for reflux may disappear. In general, a lower reflux grade correlates with a better chance of spontaneous resolution. Nonoperative management of VUR (which is successful in most patients) requires prevention of UTI with suppression antibiotics, treatment of symptomatic voiding dysfunction, and long-term, strict surveillance. Patients with breakthrough UTIs, significant renal injury, or high-grade reflux, those of pubertal age, or those who fail to respond to 4 to 5 years of suppression therapy may require ureteral reimplantation. The principle of antireflux reconstruction is the creation of a capacious subepithelial tunnel with the ratio of its length to the ureteral diameter equal to 5 : 1. In general, excellent results are attained with most open intravesical or extravesical procedures. The extravesical approach, which preserves the integrity of the bladder lumen as well as not requiring a ureteral anastomosis, eliminates postoperative hematuria, minimizes bladder spasms, decreases the risk of postoperative obstruction, and shortens hospital stay (9) (Fig. 98.3).

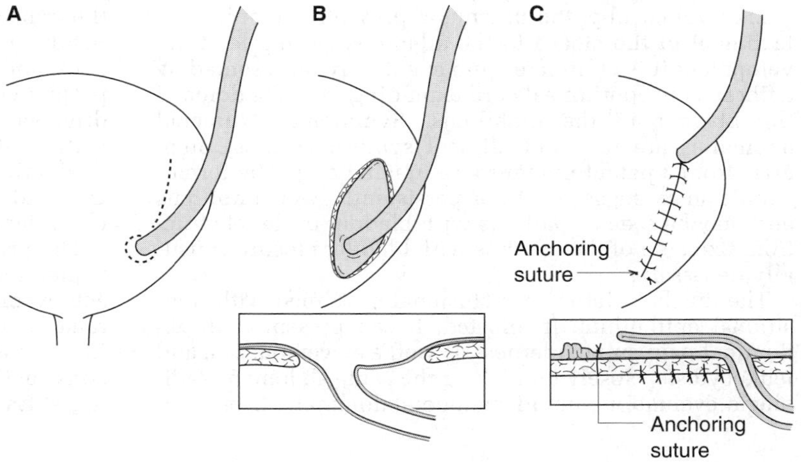

Figure 98.3. Extravesical ureteral reimplantation (conceptually viewed from behind the bladder). *(A)* The detrusor is incised. *(B)* The dissection is continued until the plane between urothelium and muscle has been developed. *(C)* The ureter is advanced and fixed into position with anchoring sutures. The detrusor is closed. (From Sheldon CA, Minevich E, Wacksman J. Urinary tract infection and vesicoureteral reflux. In: Ascraft K, Holder T, eds. *Pediatric surgery.* Philadelphia: WB Saunders, 1999:719.)

Megaureter

The term *megaureter* refers to an enlarged ureter, of which there are four categories: refluxing, obstructing, refluxing/obstructing, and nonrefluxing/nonobstructing, with an additional subdivision of each group into primary or secondary. Most patients are asymptomatic with an incidental finding of hydroureteronephrosis on screening renal US. The most common clinical presentation is UTI. The VCUG is necessary to rule out VUR, although its presence does not exclude the possibility of a coexistent obstruction. Diuretic renography is helpful to establish the presence of ureteral obstruction, which is usually at the level of ureterovesical junction.

Megaureter secondary to severe VUR or obstruction is usually managed with ureteral reimplantation to prevent deterioration of renal function. Reduction of ureteral caliber by excision of the distal redundant ureter to achieve a satisfactory antireflux mechanism is usually necessary. Patients without reflux or obstruction may demonstrate radiographic improvement of the megaureter with preservation of renal function without surgical intervention. Therefore, initial nonoperative management with close follow-up of patients with nonobstructing/nonrefluxing megaureters is advisable (10).

VESICOURETHRAL SYSTEM

The cloaca forms from the blind caudal end of the hindgut. The division of the cloaca by the urorectal septum into a ventral portion—the urogenital sinus (UGS)—and a dorsal portion (rectum) is completed by the seventh week of gestation. Simultaneously, the mesodermal growth of the lower abdominal wall separates the umbilical cord from the genital tubercle. The mesonephric duct and ureteral bud have independent opening sites. The mesonephric duct (which will become the ejaculatory duct) migrates downward and medially, whereas the opening of ureteral bud (which will become the ureteral orifice) migrates upward and laterally. The UGS can be divided into two segments at the point where the müllerian ducts join the dorsal wall of the UGS. The ventral portion forms the bladder, part of the prostatic urethra in the boy, and the entire female urethra. The caudal portion gives rise to a portion of the prostatic and the entire membranous urethra in boys and forms the lower part of the vagina and the vaginal vestibule in girls.

ANOMALIES OF THE BLADDER

Urachal Abnormality

Embryologically, the urachus represents the apical attachment of the cloaca to the allantois. During fetal development it is obliterated and eventually represented by a fibrous retroperitoneal cord extending from the dome of the bladder to the umbilicus. Symptomatic urachal anomalies are rare and clinical syndromes most often arise from a patent urachus or a urachal cyst. The former condition is suggested by a persistently wet umbilicus and may be seen in patients with bladder outlet obstruction. Excision of the urachus with bladder closure is usually necessary.

The urachal cyst is an inclusional cyst lined with transitional epithelium. If infected, it can present with abdominal pain and tenderness as well as fever, nausea, and leukocytosis, closely mimicking the acute abdomen. Radiologic evaluation should include abdominal US or computed tomography (CT). The infected urachal cyst is best managed by initial drainage of the abscess and delayed excision of the urachal remnant. Exploratory laparotomy is indicated if signs of peritonitis are present (11) (Fig. 98.4).

Exstrophy–Epispadias Complex

Overgrowth and delayed rupture of the cloacal membrane prevent medial mesenchymal migration and proper lower abdominal wall development. Depending on the extent of the infraumbilical defect and the stage of development at which rupture does occur, bladder exstrophy, epispadias, or cloacal exstrophy results.

Epispadias in boys, as an isolated defect, consists of a dorsally placed urethral meatus, and the degree of penile deformity is related to the extent of the meatal displacement. Most often, epispadias is associated with exstrophy of the bladder (Fig. 98.5). This defect usually involves pubic diastasis with separation of the rectus abdominis muscles, inguinal hernias, and anterior displacement of the anus. Male external genitalia have a characteristic epispadiac appearance, whereas girls have a bifid clitoris with a stenotic and short vagina. Complete primary closure of the bladder plate with simultaneous repair of epispadias within the first 72 hours of life is the most appropriate treatment of this complicated anomaly (12).

Cloacal exstrophy is the most severe defect that can occur in the formation of the ventral abdominal wall. Anatomically, there is exstrophy of the shortened hindgut or cecum, which displays its bulging mucosa between the two hemibladders. There is no anus or rectum, and omphalocele is present (Fig. 98.6). The initial surgical approach (in the neonatal period) includes closure of the omphalocele, separation of the bladder from the bowel, and closure of the bladder. Considerable reconstructive surgery remains to be done later to create an acceptable anatomic appearance and functioning urinary and intestinal tracts.

Neurogenic Bladder

Abnormal spinal column development affecting spinal cord function (myelodysplasia) is the most common cause of neurogenic bladder in children. Myelomeningocele accounts for over 90% of open spinal dysraphic states. Bladder dysfunction usually results in urinary incontinence, although the poorly compliant bladder with a leak point pressure over 40 cm H_2O may cause VUR and hydronephrosis, leading to deterioration of renal function (13). Presumably at this point, the ureterovesical junction can no longer protect the upper tracts from the transmission of this pressure. Urinary continence depends on bladder capacity and bladder outlet (bladder neck and urethral sphincter) resistance. The most important contribution affecting management of these children was the introduction of clean intermittent catheterization (CIC) to facilitate timely bladder emptying. Evaluation of infants with urodynamic studies, renal US, and VCUG identifies those ultimately at risk for renal damage.

The primary goal in children with neurogenic bladder is maintenance of safe intravesical pressure, the ultimate achievement of urinary continence, and preservation of renal function. If anticholinergic therapy with or without CIC is unsuccessful in achieving these goals, surgical reconstruction is necessary. Owing to the high incidence of upper tract deterioration with time and the significant se-

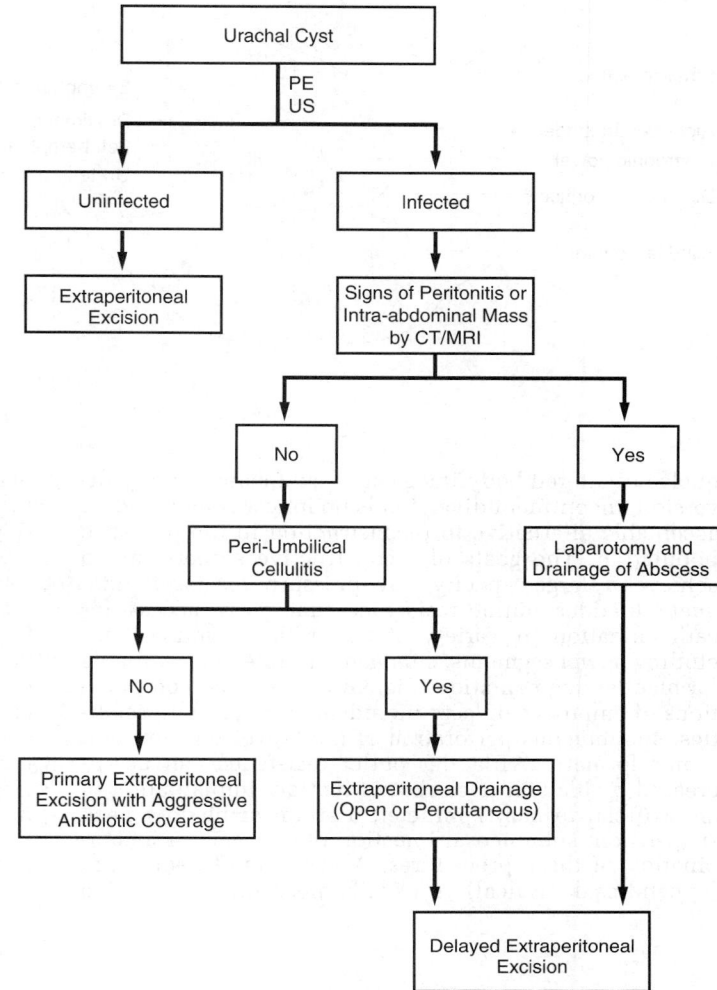

Figure 98.4. Algorithm of surgical management of urachal cyst. PE, physical examination; US, ultrasound. (From Minevich E, Wacksman J, Lewis AG, et al. The infected urachal cyst: primary excision versus a staged approach. *J Urol* 1997;157:1869.)

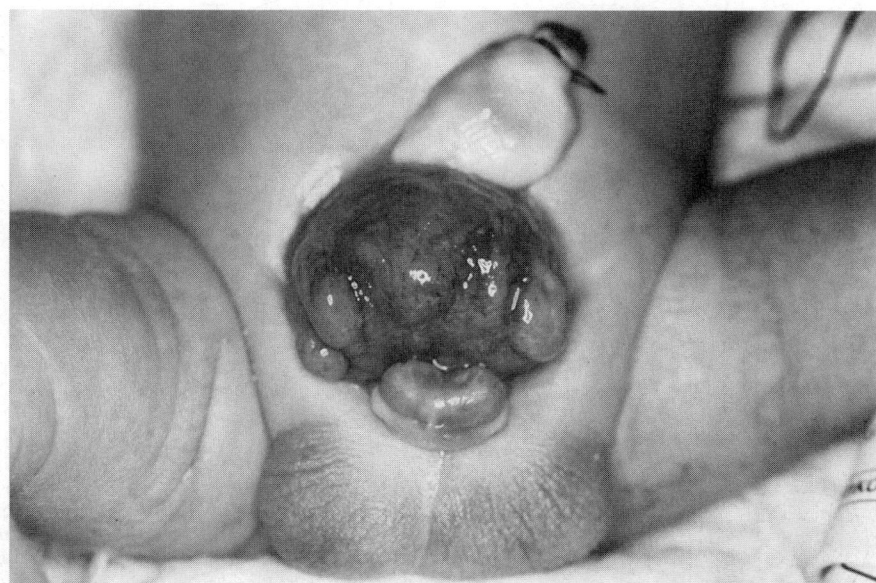

Figure 98.5. Newborn boy with classic bladder exstrophy.

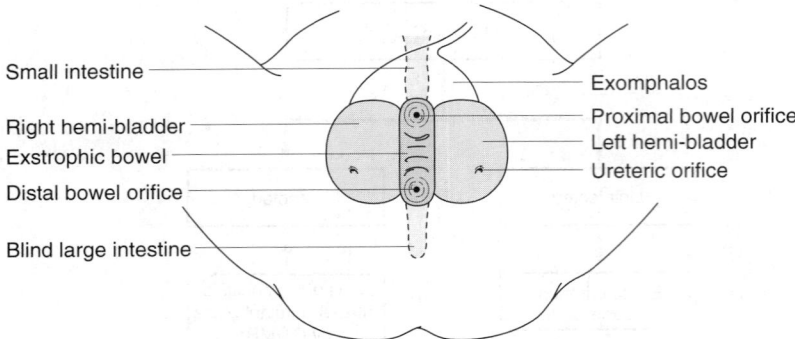

Figure 98.6. Diagram depicting cloacal exstrophy.

quelae of altered body image after cutaneous urinary diversion, incontinent diversion is no longer considered an acceptable alternative to reconstruction in the pediatric population. The goals of reconstructive surgery are to achieve a large-capacity, low-pressure reservoir, adequate bladder outlet resistance, and easy access for catheterization. A variety of donor tissue sources, including bowel segments, stomach, or ureter, are available for bladder augmentation (Fig. 98.7). Potential complications of enterocystoplasty include electrolyte abnormalities, spontaneous perforation of the bowel segment and tumor formation. Bladder outlet resistance can be increased by bladder neck reconstruction, implantation of an artificial urinary sphincter, urethral or bladder neck suspension, submucosal injection of collagen, or a combination of these procedures. A Mitrofanoff neourethra (appendiceal or ileal) is usually necessary to provide

bladder access for decompression and continence, and is highly successful in even the most devastating cases (14) (Fig. 98.8).

Neurogenic bladder is frequently accompanied by refractory fecal incontinence. This may severely compromise care with respect to UTI, incontinence, and achieving independent self-care. When preoperative conventional therapy (dietary modification, timed toileting, cathartics, bulking agents, and enemas) is unsuccessful in controlling complete evacuation of the colon, an antegrade continence enema, performed through a continent cecostomy using appendix or tapered ileum, is a viable option (Fig. 98.9). The antegrade continence enema procedure has been successfully used in the management of intractable fecal incontinence, even in the most debilitating pediatric rectourogenital anomalies (15).

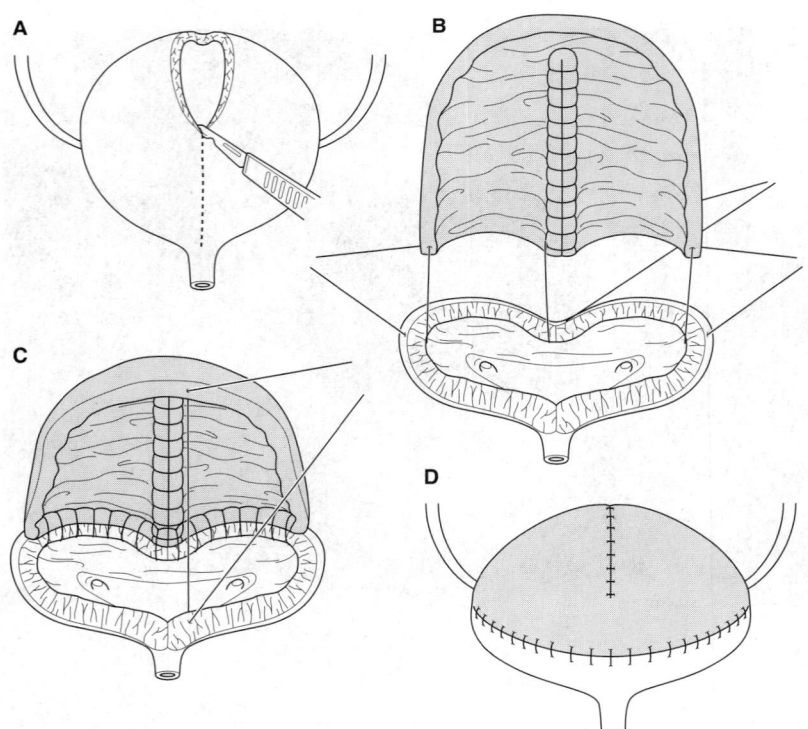

Figure 98.7. Bladder augmentation using an intestinal segment. *(A)* The bladder is opened as a "clam shell." *(B)* The intestinal segment is detubularized by longitudinal incision along the antimesenteric border. A cup patch is fashioned by suturing one edge of the resultant rectangle to itself. *(C)* The cup patch is sutured to the remnant bladder plate. *(D)* Final appearance. (From Sheldon CA, Bukowski T. Bladder function. In: Rowe MI, O'Neal JA, Grosfeld JL, et al., eds. *Essentials of pediatric surgery.* St. Louis: Mosby, 1995:1015.)

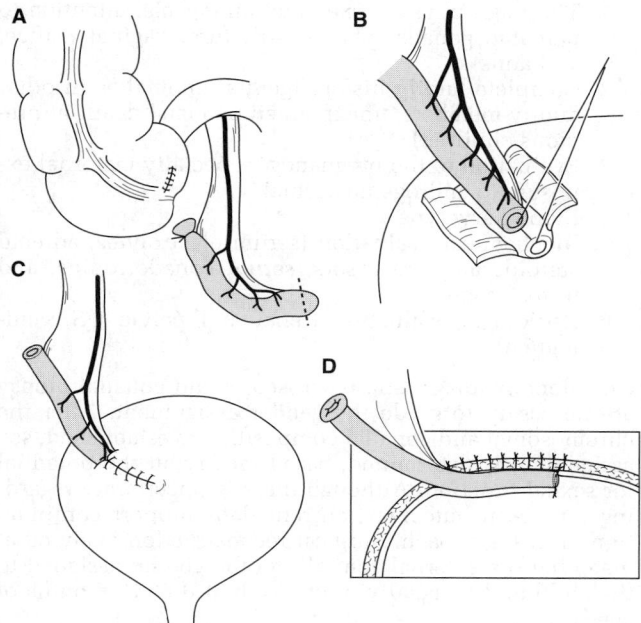

Figure 98.8. Mitrofanoff procedure. *(A)* The appendix has been mobilized on its mesentery, and the cecal segment is closed. *(B)* Extravesical dissection shows the mucosal orifice in which the distal end of appendix will be implanted. *(C)* Finally, the detrusor is closed over the implanted appendix, and its proximal end is then brought to the skin to serve as a catheterizable stoma. *(D)* Resulting continent flap-valve mechanism of Mitrofanoff procedure. Similar to the reimplanted ureter, a rise in intravesical pressure compresses the conduit against the detrusor, occluding its lumen and achieving continence. (From Sheldon CA, Gilbert A. Use of the appendix for urethral reconstruction in children with congenital anomalies of the bladder. *Surgery* 1992;112:805.)

ANOMALIES OF THE URETHRA

Posterior Urethral Valves

Posterior urethral valves are the most common obstructive urethral lesions in male infants and consist of a membrane or mucosal leaflet in the prostatic urethra. The diagnosis is usually suspected in neonates because of abnormal findings on prenatal US, hydronephrosis (bilateral hydronephrosis, distended bladder), and oligohydramnios. Some are found to have flank masses, ascites, and urinary retention. Older children usually present with voiding symptoms, UTI, or hematuria. VCUG is diagnostic in most cases, although cystoscopy may be necessary in an equivocal setting. Patients with significant bilateral hydronephrosis should be screened for renal insufficiency, and nuclear scintigraphy may be indicated to rule out ureteral obstruction or renal dysplasia.

Temporary urinary drainage with a urethral catheter (feeding tube) can be done in critically ill patients. Otherwise, primary endoscopic valve ablation is the preferred approach and may be accomplished safely in most instances. Initial temporary cutaneous vesicostomy is useful in occasional circumstances. High upper urinary tract diversion may rarely be necessary in infants who demonstrate a rising creatinine despite lower tract drainage. Long-term follow-up is necessary, with special attention directed to the possible development of a poorly compliant, high-pressure bladder (16). Careful urodynamic evaluation and timely treatment of the "valve bladder" with anticholinergics, CIC, and very selective vesical reconstruction (including enterocystoplasty) as well as prevention of UTI ensure the best chance for successful prevention or management of chronic renal failure.

Hypospadias

Hypospadias is a common congenital defect resulting from incomplete tubularization of the urethral plate and closure of the genital folds. The cause of this anomaly is unknown, but it is probably related to inadequate androgenization before the 20th week of gestation. The meatus may be located anywhere from the perineum to the proxi-

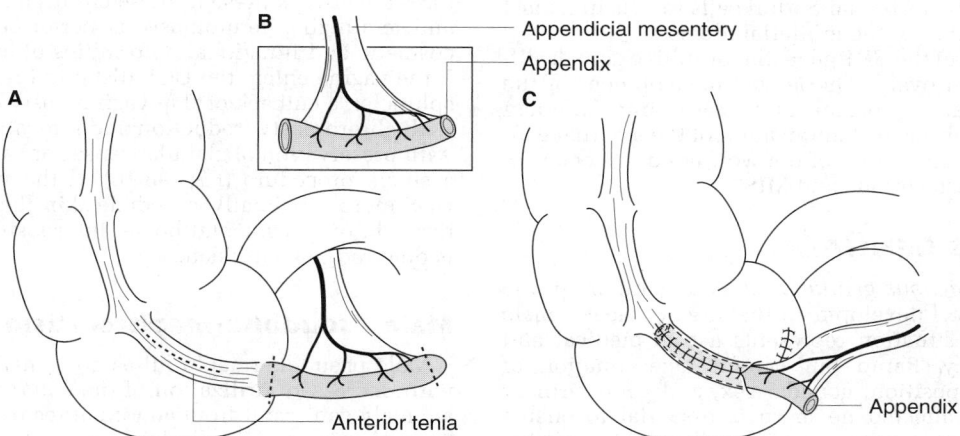

Figure 98.9. Technique of appendiceal antegrade continence enema conduit creation. *(A)* Incision in anterior taenia. *(B)* Appendiceal conduit before implantation. *(C)* Overlying musculature closed over conduit. (From Sheldon CA, Minevich E, Wacksman J, et al. Role of the antegrade continence enema in the management of the most debilitating childhood recto-urogenital anomalies. *J Urol* 1997;158:1277.)

mal glans penis, although in over 85% of cases it is distal to the midshaft. Typically, the ventral prepuce is deficient and ventral penile chordee occurs more frequently with proximal hypospadias.

Principles of hypospadias repair include meticulous surgical technique with sufficient optical magnification to advance the urethral meatus to a normal glanular position and to correct penile chordee if necessary. Numerous operations have been described for surgical correction of hypospadias, and the surgeon treating this anomaly should be familiar with all possible approaches. An outpatient one-stage procedure can be safely performed after 6 months of age in most cases. Although local skin flaps are used in repairs of more distal hypospadias, vascularized preputial pedicle flaps or a tube graft may be necessary in more proximal hypospadias. Patients with hypospadias should not be circumcised until they are evaluated by an experienced pediatric urologist. If sufficient penile skin is not available, bladder mucosal or buccal mucosal grafts can be used. Complications after hypospadias surgery include urethrocutaneous fistula, urethral strictures, and meatal stenosis.

GENITAL SYSTEM

The development of the genital tract follows a sequential pattern and is initially determined by chromosomal composition of the fertilizing sperm, resulting in a 46,XY (male genotype) or 46,XX zygote (female genotype). The genetic material necessary for the development of the testis is found on the short arm of the Y chromosome and is known as the *SRY* gene. The presence of this gene directs an aggregation of primitive indifferent germ cells and Sertoli cells into the testicular cord. Thereafter, the endocrine effect on sexual development is most crucial in male phenotype development. Testosterone, produced by Leydig cells, results in wolffian duct (remnant of mesonephric duct) differentiation into the vas deferens, the seminal vesicles, and the epididymis. In addition, testosterone converted at the end-organ target sites to dihydrotestosterone (DHT) by 5α-reductase, regulates the virilization of the UGS and external genitalia at approximately the ninth week of gestation. Only at this point does the previously indifferent genital tubercle start to differentiate into a penis while the genital swelling fuses to form the scrotum. At the same time, müllerian-inhibiting substance (MIS) produced by testicular Sertoli cells results in almost complete regression of the müllerian ducts.

In the absence of the *SRY* gene, the primitive gonads differentiate into an ovary. The female development of the müllerian (paramesonephric) duct system into fallopian tubes, uterus, and cervix, feminization of the external genitalia, as well as involution of the wolffian ducts occur in the absence of testosterone and MIS.

AMBIGUOUS GENITALIA

The term *ambiguous genitalia* refers to genitalia in the spectrum of sexual development that are not clearly male or female. This situation represents a true medical and social emergency. Rapid but careful determination of the genetic composition, gonadal sex, and genitourinary anatomy of the affected newborn is essential to enable gender assignment, acceptance of the child by the family, and ultimately surgical reconstruction.

Patients with ambiguous genitalia can be divided into four categories—female and male pseudohermaphroditism, true hermaphroditism, and gonadal dysgenesis. Complete evaluation of the infant with ambiguous genitalia should include the following:

1. Thorough physical examination (special attention to palpable gonads, phallic structure, vaginal orifice, and anus)
2. Complete family history (genital anomalies in other family members, unexplained neonatal death in previous children)
3. Evaluation of the pregnancy (especially maternal exposure to androgenic agents)
4. Blood karyotype
5. Biochemical evaluation (serum electrolytes, adrenal steroids and precursors, serum gonadotropins, and testosterone)
6. Radiologic evaluation (renal and pelvic US, genitogram)

Occasionally, diagnostic laparoscopy and gonadal biopsy are necessary to guide the gender assignment. After the chromosomal and gonadal composition is established, sex assignment is determined, based mostly on the potential for sexual function. Although there is uncertainty regarding long-term outcomes, current data support continuation of this approach. Surgical reconstruction is aimed at matching the external genitalia to the gender assigned to the child and is usually undertaken at 6 to 12 months of age (17).

Female Pseudohermaphroditism

Female pseudohermaphroditism is the largest diagnostic category, and within this category the leading cause is congenital adrenal hyperplasia (CAH). CAH results from a deficiency in the enzymes responsible for the synthesis of mineralocorticosteroids and glucocorticosteroids, resulting in overproduction of adrenal androgens. A deficiency of 21-hydroxylase characterizes 95% of patients with CAH. All of these patients are genetic females (46,XX karyotype, ovarian gonads) with masculinization of the external genitalia ranging from an enlarged clitoris to a normal-appearing male phallus with complete labial fusion. These patients are potentially fertile regardless of how severe the degree of virilization.

A high index of suspicion allows for early diagnosis of this condition and initiation of hormonal replacement (glucocorticosteroids and mineralocorticosteroids) to prevent adrenal insufficiency, salt-wasting syndrome, and continued virilization. Because internal müllerian structures are always present, these children are reared as girls and feminizing genitoplasty is performed to correct the cosmetic and functional deformities of external genitalia. If the vagina enters the UGS distal to the external urinary sphincter, a cutback or flap vaginoplasty can be combined with clitoroplasty (reduction and relocation of the clitoris with preservation of glanular sensation) and labioplasty in a single procedure (Fig. 98.10). If the vagina enters the UGS more proximally, a pedicle skin flap, a vaginal pull-through, or a segmental bowel interposition vaginoplasty is deferred to a later date.

Male Pseudohermaphroditism

Male pseudohermaphrodites are genetic males (46,XY) with decreased virilization of the external genitalia. This anomaly can result from abnormal testosterone synthesis, 5α-reductase deficiency leading to decreased levels of DHT, and androgen insensitivity syndrome (defect of the androgen receptor). The phallic structure may be inadequate for the male gender role. In this setting, consideration should be given to female gender assignment.

Testicular feminization syndrome (complete androgen insensitivity) is the most common form of male pseudo-

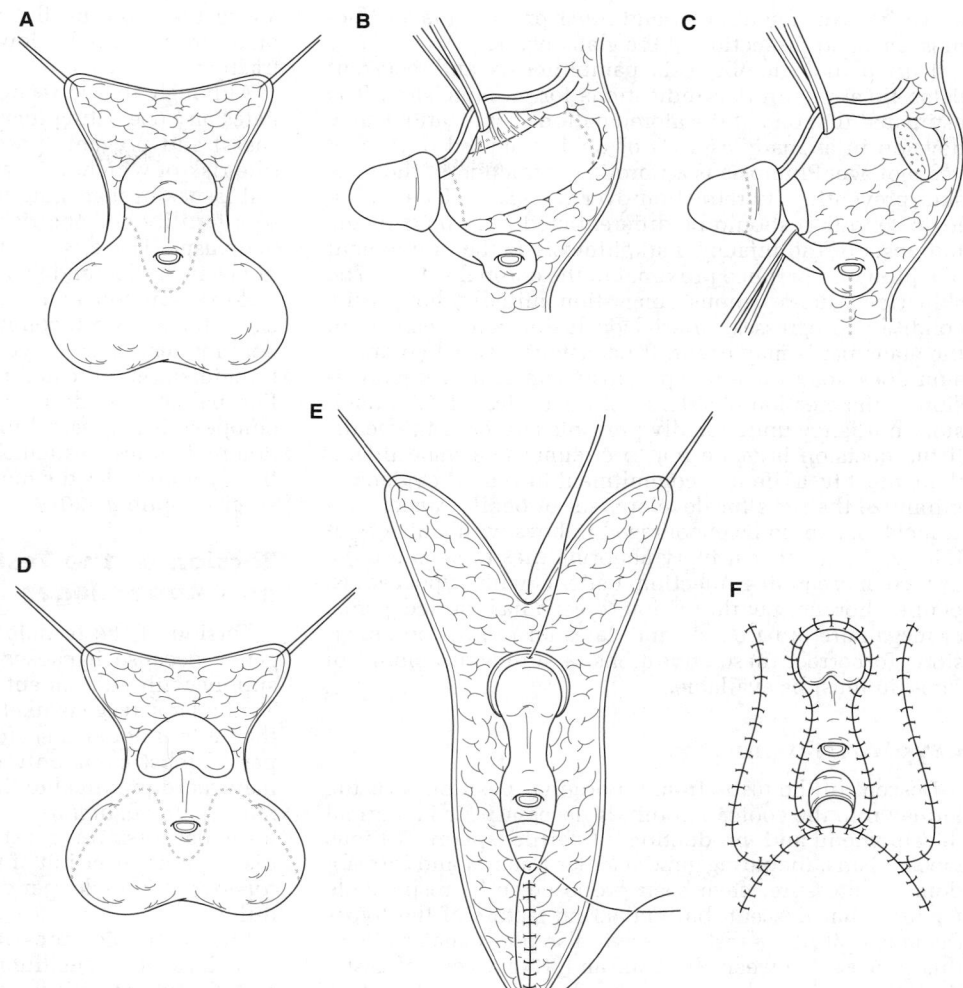

Figure 98.10. Feminizing genito-plasty. *(A and D)* An inverted U- or M-shaped incision in the labio-scrotal fold outlines a vaginal insertion flap. *(B)* Urethral plate and dorsal neurovascular bundles are carefully dissected. *(C)* The corpora are ligated and divided, leaving only a portion of the distal glans, comparable in size with a normal clitoris with epithelium. *(C and E)* The underlying urogenital sinus is exposed and incised in the midline, unroofing the urethral meatus and vaginal introitus as separate orifices. *(F)* The labio-scrotal flap is sutured into place as an insertion flap. Halves of the prepuce are rotated caudally to allow creation of labia. (From Sheldon CA. Intersex states. In: Oldham KT, Colombani PM, Foglia RT, eds. *Surgery of infants and children: scientific principles and practice.* Philadelphia: Lippincott–Raven, 1997:1613.)

hermaphroditism, although affected individuals appear as normal phenotypic girls with a short vagina. They are usually diagnosed at puberty with primary amenorrhea, although infrequently diagnosis is made during routine childhood herniorrhaphy, at which time testes are found. Bilateral gonadectomy is indicated because of increased risk of gonadoblastoma development in the intraabdominal testis. It can be delayed until puberty in selected cases. The short vagina can be managed with vaginal dilatation, but vaginal reconstruction or vaginal replacement is necessary in some patients.

True Hermaphroditism

In this condition, patients have both ovarian and testicular tissue (ovary and testis, ovotestis, or a combination of these). True hermaphroditism is the rarest form of intersex abnormality. The internal genital structures conform with the ipsilateral gonad. The most common karyotype is 46,XX, although mosaicism and a 46,XY karyotype may be seen as well. The appearance of the external genitalia varies widely. After gender is assigned, gonadal tissue of the opposite sex is removed and surgical reconstruction is undertaken.

Mixed Gonadal Dysgenesis

This is the second most frequent cause of genital ambiguity and most neonates exhibit a 45,XO/46,XY mosaic

karyotype. They usually present with a dysgenetic testis on one side and a streak gonad on the other. The appearance of external genitalia is variable, although most are poorly virilized, and consequently most infants are raised as girls. Appropriate genital reconstruction is required. Early gonadectomy is indicated because of the high risk of malignant degeneration (gonadoblastoma, seminoma, and dysgerminoma) of the dysgenetic gonad.

ANOMALIES OF MALE GENITALIA

Anomalies of the Foreskin

At birth, the prepuce is retractable in only 4% of boys. No special care of the uncircumcised penis is required. During the first years of life, spontaneous separation occurs physiologically in most boys secondary to intermittent erections and epithelialization of the inner prepuce. It is unnecessary to retract the prepuce on any routine basis to promote retractability or hasten physiologic separation. This usually results in pain, bleeding, and, occasionally, paraphimosis.

Much confusion exists as to the indications for neonatal circumcision. The most important arguments are those of custom and tradition. In infants, circumcision may be performed using the Gomko clamp under local penile block. The most important principles of neonatal circumcision are complete lysis of penile adhesions, adequate but not excessive excision of outer and inner preputial layers, hemostasis, and protection of the glans penis.

Truly pathologic phimosis, paraphimosis, and recurrent balanitis are definitive indications for circumcision. It is estimated that one of the aforementioned indications may develop in as many as 18% of uncircumcised boys by 8 years of age. Phimosis is a fibrotic contraction of the foreskin preventing its retraction over the glans. This pathologic condition should be differentiated from physiologic phimosis of the infancy. Paraphimosis is the entrapment of a phimotic prepuce proximal to the coronal sulcus. The skin ring causes venous congestion initially, but as the condition progresses, arterial occlusion and necrosis of the glans penis may occur. If persistent manual compression does not reduce paraphimosis, emergency circumcision or the creation of a dorsal slit is indicated. Circumcision in infancy undoubtedly prevents cancer of the penis. If the decision is made not to circumcise a male infant, there must be a lifetime commitment to genital hygiene to minimize the risks for development of penile cancer. Circumcision should be encouraged in boys with a history of UTI, VUR, or other urinary abnormalities to decrease the chance of ascending infection. Patients with hypospadias, penile chordee, penile torsion, epispadias, buried penis, or megalourethra are not candidates for routine circumcision. To correct these conditions, a sufficient amount of foreskin must be available.

Cryptorchidism

Descent of the testis from its original position near the kidney into the cooler scrotum is necessary for its normal development and production of fertile sperm. Various mechanisms, including gubernacular traction and intraabdominal pressure, have been proposed to be responsible for testicular descent, but endocrine factors of the hypothalamic–pituitary–testicular axis also play a major role in this process. Between the 12th and 17th weeks of gestation, the testis undergoes transabdominal migration to a location near the internal inguinal ring. It is not until the seventh month of gestation that transinguinal migration of the testis to its final position takes place.

True undescended testes fail to reach the scrotum despite following a normal line of descent. Ectopic testes follow the usual course of descent until they emerge from the external inguinal ring, but are then misdirected to an ectopic position (superficial inguinal pouch, perineal, femoral, transverse scrotal). Although approximately 3.4% of full-term boys have undescended testes, 30% of premature infants have this anomaly. By 1 year of age, the incidence of cryptorchidism is approximately 1% and remains at this level thereafter. Actually, most cryptorchid testes descending during the first year of life do so within the first 3 months after birth. The diagnosis of cryptorchidism relies on gentle and patient genital examination. Relaxation of the patient and warming of the examiner's hand aid in successful examination. Reexamination of the child in the cross-legged position may also reveal the gonad. A functional classification of cryptorchidism that provides a practical approach to therapy is based on whether the testis is palpable or impalpable (20%). Although endocrine testing is reliable in predicting bilateral anorchidism, radiologic means, including abdominal sonography, CT, magnetic resonance imaging, or gonadal arteriography, are inaccurate in localization of nonpalpable testes. Diagnostic laparoscopy provides the diagnosis of vanishing testis by identification of blind-ending spermatic vessels or accurate localization of the intraabdominal testis in this situation (18). Undescended testes must be distinguished from retractile testes that may reside above the scrotum, but with careful positioning can be made to stay in the lower scrotum without continuous traction.

Although the correction of undescended testes eliminates any coexisting inguinal hernia (found in 95% of all cases) and prevents possible testicular injury or torsion (the risk of which is increased in these patients), the central issues in managing these patients revolve around future fertility and the risk for development of a testicular neoplasm. There is an increased risk of testicular carcinoma in undescended testes, and orchiopexy facilitates self-examination and early detection of the cancer. Because the germ cell count of the infant undescended testis deteriorates after 1 year of life, correction of cryptorchidism is indicated between 6 and 12 months of age. For palpable undescended testes, routine inguinal orchiopexy is successful in most patients. For high intraabdominal testes, testicular microsurgical autotransplantation (19) provides the highest success rate among different surgical options (20).

Torsion of the Testis and Appendages

Torsion of the testicle is classified as a surgical emergency because it causes strangulation of gonadal blood supply with subsequent testicular necrosis and atrophy. Testicular salvage is likely if the duration of torsion is less than 6 to 8 hours (21). Torsion presenting in the neonatal period most commonly develops prenatally in the spermatic cord proximal to the attachments of the tunica vaginalis (*extravaginal torsion*). Although possible at any age, testicular torsion is most common in adolescents, usually distal to the insertion of the tunica vaginalis (*intravaginal torsion*). A bell-clapper deformity predisposes to this condition.

Prenatal torsion presents with a firm, hard scrotal mass that does not transilluminate in an otherwise asymptomatic newborn. Salvage of the testis is extremely rare (22), but timely surgical exploration is indicated to anchor the contralateral testis because bilateral (synchronous or asynchronous) neonatal testicular torsion has been described. In older boys, sudden onset of severe testicular pain followed by scrotal swelling is the classic presentation of testicular torsion. On physical examination a swollen, tender testis with shortening of the cord is noticed. If testicular torsion is clinically suspected, an immediate surgical scrotal exploration is indicated. A negative exploration of the scrotum is more acceptable than the loss of a testis that might have been salvaged. In situations with a low probability of testicular torsion, scrotal color Doppler US or testicular nuclear scan can be helpful to differentiate torsion from acute epididymitis. At surgical exploration, the testis is untwisted and observed for viability. A frankly necrotic testis is removed, whereas a viable gonad (return of color, return of Doppler flow, signs of arterial blood after incision of tunica albuginea) is fixed to the scrotal wall to prevent subsequent torsion. Exploration and anchoring of the contralateral testis, which can be done through the same incision, is mandatory to prevent its subsequent torsion. Manual detorsion of the torsed testis is usually difficult because of acute pain during manipulation but, if successful (and confirmed by color Doppler US in a patient with complete resolution of symptoms), definitive surgical fixation of the testes should be performed before the patient leaves the hospital as an urgent rather than emergency procedure.

The testicular appendix, a müllerian duct remnant, is the most common genital appendage susceptible to torsion. Although frequently presenting with symptoms sim-

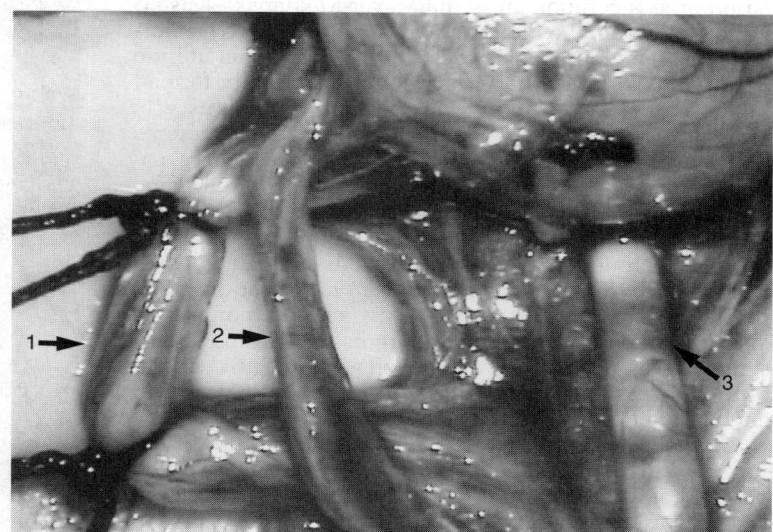

Figure 98.11. Spermatic cord dissection for varicocele using operating microscope. 1, Internal spermatic vein; 2, testicular artery; 3, lymphatic vessel. (From Minevich E, Wacksman J, Lewis AG, et al. Inguinal microsurgical varicocelectomy in the adolescent: technique and preliminary results. *J Urol* 1998;159: 1022.)

ilar to testicular torsion, this condition can usually be diagnosed by a finding of a tender focal induration or a blue dot near the upper pole of the testis. Testicular appendix torsion is best managed by several days of bed rest and oral preventive antibiotics. If a reliable diagnosis cannot be made, scrotal color Doppler US or even surgical exploration is indicated to rule out testicular torsion.

Prepubertal Testicular Tumor

In boys presenting with a painless, palpable scrotal mass, a testicular tumor should be included in the differential diagnosis. Prepubertal testis tumors account for approximately 2% of all testicular tumors, with a peak patient age of approximately 2 years. The most common lesion is a yolk sac tumor, which is a variant of embryonal cell carcinoma. When spread occurs, it is usually a hematogenous spread to the lungs and, less commonly, lymphatic spread to the retroperitoneal nodes. Scrotal US is usually definitive in visualizing an intratesticular mass, whereas abdominal and chest CT scans are necessary for metastatic evaluation. Tumor markers (α-fetoprotein and β-human chorionic gonadotropin) are helpful for initial evaluation and also during follow-up. In young children, the prognosis is excellent and radical inguinal orchiectomy is the initial treatment. Retroperitoneal lymph node dissection and multidrug chemotherapy are necessary in cases of disseminated disease. In the absence of metastasis or elevated tumor marker levels, the applicability of these treatment modalities remains controversial.

Varicocele

Varicocele is a dilatation of the veins of the spermatic cord and is reported to occur at a 15% incidence in adolescent boys, which correlates with that in general male population. In most adolescents, the varicocele is grade I, although in 35% it is grade II or III. Varicocele is usually visible or palpable in the upright position. Most urologists agree that scrotal discomfort and ipsilateral testicular growth failure are reliable indications for varicocele surgery in this population. In addition, some authors have advocated surgical repair in patients demonstrating a progressive increase in varicocele size, bilateral varicoceles, or a large varicocele associated with a change in testicular consistency. Incisional surgery with an inguinal, retroperi-

toneal, or modified approach is the basis of varicocelectomy in adolescents. Optical magnification allows reliable identification and preservation of the testicular artery and lymphatics during ligation of the venous channels (Fig. 98.11). As a result, the postoperative development of hydrocele or recurrence of the varicocele may be prevented (23).

VAGINAL ANOMALIES AND UROGENITAL SINUS MALFORMATIONS

The UGS is apparent by 6 weeks of gestation. After it receives the fused müllerian ducts, the distal potion of UGS forms the lower one third of the vagina, and the fused müllerian ducts form the upper two thirds of the vagina and the uterus. Although most vaginal anomalies occur in conjunction with intersex disorders, isolated vaginal anomalies or vaginal anomalies in association with a UGS are also seen (Fig. 98.12). Vaginal agenesis may occur in iso-

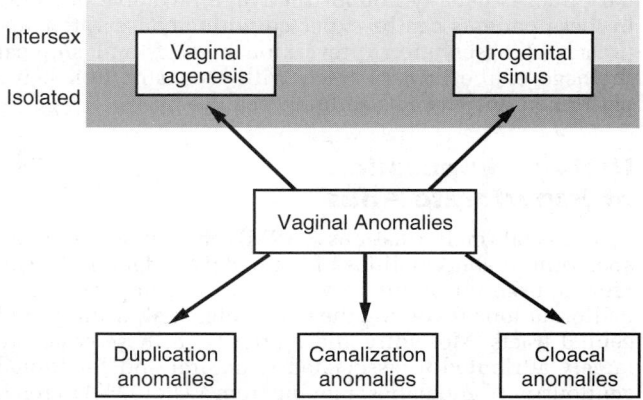

Figure 98.12. Classification of vaginal anomalies. (From Sheldon CA. Imperforate anus, urogenital sinus, and cloaca. In: Kelalis PP, King LR, Belman AB, eds. *Clinical pediatric urology.* Philadelphia: WB Saunders, 2000.)

lation or as a component of the Mayer-Rokitansky-Küster-Hauser syndrome, which presents with an otherwise normal female phenotype with vaginal and occasional uterine dysgenesis. Because the distal vagina is normally formed in most of these patients, the diagnosis is not usually made until puberty, at which time the patient presents with amenorrhea. Approximately one third of these patients have urologic anomalies, the most common being unilateral renal agenesis. Vaginoplasty is indicated in almost all patients and depends on the anatomy present. Several techniques using tubularized skin flaps, skin grafts, and bowel segments have been described for vaginal reconstruction (24). Careful preoperative counseling and evaluation of patient's and parents' motivation are essential for a good result because long-term vaginal dilatation is occasionally required until the patient is old enough to participate in sexual intercourse.

Anomalies of the UGS occur because of failure of the urethra and vagina to separate. These children have two perineal openings, including the anus, because the rectum is usually normal. Many of these girls have some degree of bladder dysfunction, and CIC may be necessary. If CIC of the bladder is not possible, temporary vesicostomy may be indicated. To separate the urethral and vaginal orifices, urethral lengthening or vaginal pull-through procedures are required (24–26).

OTHER GENITOURINARY DISORDERS

Eagle-Barrett Syndrome

The Eagle-Barrett syndrome, also referred to as *prune-belly syndrome,* is characterized by genitourinary malformations and a deficiency or absence of the abdominal wall accompanied by a broad spectrum of associated organ system anomalies. It has been theorized that delayed canalization of the urethral membrane results in a temporary but total urinary obstruction causing massive dilatation of the ureters, a large bladder with a patent urachus, and a dilated proximal urethra with hypoplastic prostate. The wrinkled, prune-like skin of the abdominal wall in the newborn is a characteristic manifestation. Renal dysplasia is frequently seen and in severe cases it is associated with pulmonary hypoplasia, resulting in stillbirth or death in neonatal period. Bilateral cryptorchidism with intraabdominal testes is a characteristic feature of prune-belly syndrome. Extraurinary problems are associated with this syndrome in 73% of patients and usually involve defects of the cardiovascular, musculoskeletal, respiratory, or central nervous systems (27). Because the dilatation of the urinary tract is usually nonobstructive, a favorable outcome in these patients can be expected with a conservative approach of observation, prevention of UTI, and surgical drainage of the urinary tract, with reconstruction being performed only when absolutely required.

Urologic Implications of Imperforate Anus

Anorectal malformations (ARM) encompass a broad spectrum of abnormalities of the distal hindgut and UGS, ranging from the simple covered anus to complex cloacal malformations involving the gastrointestinal, urinary, and genital tracts. Morbidity and mortality in these cases are largely attributed to associated structural and functional genitourinary anomalies, ranging from VUR (57%) to renal dysplasia and agenesis (65%). Therefore, neonatal screening with renal US and VCUG is essential in all patients with ARM (28). The assessment of bladder function is also critical because of a reportedly high incidence of occult

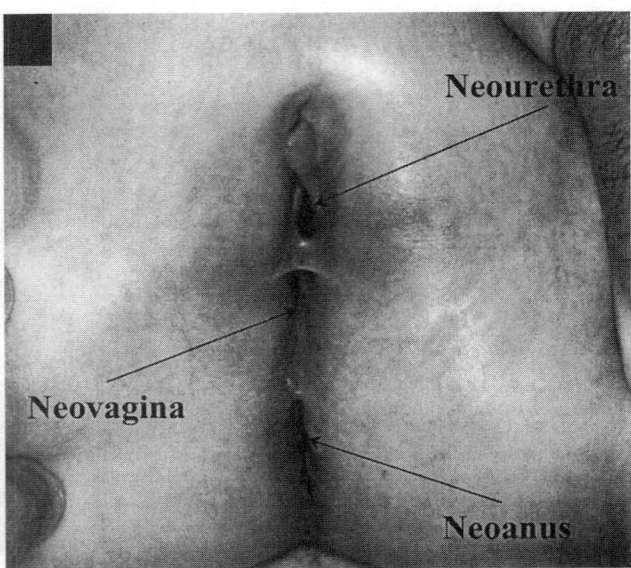

Figure 98.13. Appearance of child after cloacal reconstruction by posterior sagittal anorectourethrovaginoplasty. (From Sheldon CA. Imperforate anus, urogenital sinus, and cloaca. In: Kelalis PP, King LR, Belman AB, eds. *Clinical pediatric urology.* Philadelphia: WB Saunders, 2000.)

neurovesical dysfunction (29). The combination of rectourinary fistula and neurovesical dysfunction or bladder outlet obstruction predisposes to critical neonatal illness.

Patients with cloacal anomalies should never be managed by initial anorectal reconstruction alone. A fully diverting colostomy with complete evacuation of the distal limb should be considered as the initial step. The goals of management in the first few years of life are to protect the upper urinary tracts, ensure low-pressure urinary drainage, normalize anorectal anatomy, and minimize any neurologic deficit that may arise from a treatable spinal lesion. A comprehensive, integrated approach with posterior sagittal anorectourethrovaginoplasty at approximately 6 to 12 months of age is the most appropriate definitive surgical procedure, yielding excellent results in such cases (Fig. 98.13). If bladder outlet obstruction or neurovesical dysfunction is detected or suspected, incidental appendectomy is contraindicated. The goals of management of the preschool and school-aged child with ARM are to ensure social urinary and fecal continence and to promote self-esteem and self-care (24).

REFERENCES

1. Potter EL. Bilateral absence of ureters and kidneys: a report of 50 cases. *Obstet Gynecol* 1965;25:3.
2. Gleason PE, Kelalis PP, Husman DA, et al. Hydronephrosis in renal ectopia: incidence, etiology, and significance. *J Urol* 1994;151:1660.
3. Mesrobian HJ, Kelalis PP, Hrabovsky E, et al. Wilms' tumor in horseshoe kidneys: a report from the National Wilms' Tumor Study. *J Urol* 1985;133:1002.
4. Glassberg KI, Stephens FD, Lebowitz RL, et al. Renal dysgenesis and cystic disease of the kidney: a report of the Committee on Terminology, Nomenclature, and Classification. *J Urol* 1987;138:1085.
5. Minevich E, Wacksman J, et al. Importance of accurate diagnosis and early close follow-up in patients with suspected MCDK. *J Urol* 1997;158:1301.
6. Wacksman J, Sheldon CA. Multicystic kidney disease. In: Kelalis PP, King LR, Belman AB, eds. *Clinical pediatric urology.* Philadelphia: WB Saunders, 1992:780.

7. Minevich E, Wacksman J. Pyeloplasty. In: Graham SD, ed. *Glenn's urologic surgery.* Philadelphia: Lippincott–Raven, 1998:713.

8. Churchill BM, Sheldon CA, McLorie GA. The ectopic ureterocele: a proposed practical classification based on renal unit jeopardy. *J Pediatr Surg* 1992;27:497.

9. Sheldon CA, Minevich E, Wacksman J. Urinary tract infection and vesicoureteral reflux. In: Ascraft K, Holder T, eds. *Pediatric surgery.* Philadelphia: WB Saunders, 1999:706.

10. Keating MA, Escola J, Snyder HM, et al. Changing concepts in management of primary obstructive megaureter. *J Urol* 1989; 142:636.

11. Minevich E, Wacksman J, Lewis AG, et al. The infected urachal cyst: primary excision versus a staged approach. *J Urol* 1997;157:1869.

12. Grady RW, Mitchell ME. Complete primary closure of the bladder exstrophy. *Urol Clin North Am* 1999;26:95.

13. McGuire EJ, Woodside JR, Borden TA, et al. Prognostic value of urodynamic testing in myelodysplastic patients. *J Urol* 1981;126:205.

14. Minevich E, Sheldon CA. Urinary tract reconstruction for continence and renal preservation. In: Ziegler MM, et al., eds. *Operative pediatric surgery.* Norwalk, CT: Appleton & Lange, 2000.

15. Sheldon CA, Minevich E, Wacksman J, et al. Role of the antegrade continence enema in the management of the most debilitating childhood recto-urogenital anomalies. *J Urol* 1997; 158:1277.

16. Peters CA, Bolkier M, Bauer SB, et al. The urodynamic consequences of posterior urethral valves. *J Urol* 1990;144:122.

17. Sheldon CA. Intersex states. In: Oldham KT, Colombani PM, Foglia RT, eds. *Surgery of infants and children: scientific principles and practice.* Philadelphia: Lippincott–Raven, 1997.

18. Weiss RM, Seashore JH. Clinical implications of laparoscopy in the management of a nonpalpable undescended testis. *J Urol* 1986;135:332.

19. Bukowski TP, Wacksman J, Billmire DA, et al. Testicular autotransplantation: a 17-year review of an effective approach to the management of the intra-abdominal testis. *J Urol* 1995; 154:558.

20. Docimo SG. Results of surgical therapy for cryptorchidism: literature review and analysis. *J Urol* 1995;154:1148.

21. Ransler CW, Allen TD. Torsion of the spermatic cord. *Urol Clin North Am* 1982;9:245.

22. Brandt MT, Sheldon CA, Wacksman J, et al. Prenatal testicular torsion: principles of management. *J Urol* 1992;147:670.

23. Minevich E, Wacksman J, Lewis AG, et al. Inguinal microsurgical varicocelectomy in the adolescent: technique and preliminary results. *J Urol* 1998;159:1022.

24. Sheldon CA. Imperforate anus, urogenital sinus, and cloaca. In: Kelalis PP, King LR, Belman AB, eds. *Clinical pediatric urology.* Philadelphia: WB Saunders, 2000.

25. Hendren WH. Reconstructive problems of the vagina and the female urethra. *Clin Plast Surg* 1980;7:207.

26. Sheldon CA, Gilbert A, Lewis AG. Vaginal reconstruction: critical technical principles. *J Urol* 1994;152:190.

27. Geary DF, MacLusky IB, Churchill BM, et al. A broader spectrum of abnormalities in the prune belly syndrome. *J Urol* 1986;135:324.

28. Sheldon CA, Gilbert A, Lewis AG, et al. Surgical implications of genitourinary tract anomalies in patients with imperforate anus. *J Urol* 1994;152:196.

29. Sheldon CA, Cormier M, Crone K, et al. Occult neurovesical dysfunction in children with imperforate anus and its variants. *J Pediatr Surg* 1991;26:49.

SURGERY: SCIENTIFIC PRINCIPLES AND PRACTICE, Third Edition, edited by Lazar J. Greenfield, Michael W. Mulholland, Keith T. Oldham, Gerald B. Zelenock, and Keith D. Lillemoe. Lippincott Williams & Wilkins Publishers, Philadelphia, © 2001.

CHAPTER 99

CHILDHOOD TUMORS

MICHAEL P. LAQUAGLIA

The focus of this chapter is malignant solid tumors of infancy, childhood, and adolescence. Fortunately, these are rare conditions, especially compared with the incidence of major adult malignancies like breast and lung cancer. This rarity, however, poses special problems to the clinical and basic science cancer researcher. For the clinician studying the effectiveness of a particular drug or surgical technique, the number of patients available for randomized trials is drastically reduced. Similarly, the basic scientist wishing to analyze the effect of a particular genetic mutation on the development or virulence of a tumor is limited in the material available for study. The solution to this problem has been the establishment of cooperative groups for the clinical and basic scientific study of pediatric malignancies. Previously, these included the Children's Cancer Group (CCG; formerly Children's Cancer Study Group, or CCSG) and the Pediatric Oncology Group (POG) in the United States, and the Societé Internacionale Oncologique Pediatrique in Europe. These agencies were originally focused on the study of hematologic malignancies. Later, collaboration was extended to the study of pediatric solid tumors, and cooperation between groups allowed prospective protocols to be done on some rare tumors. The Intergroup Rhabdomyosarcoma Study (IRS) was established as a collaborative effort between POG and CCG to address the special problems posed by childhood sarcomas, most importantly rhabdomyosarcoma. The National Wilms' Tumor Study (NWTS) enrolls most Wilms' tumors diagnosed in the United States. This organization has made significant progress in increasing the cure rate from Wilms' tumors and in developing therapies with minimal early and late toxicity. This and other cooperative studies, combined with pioneering single-institutional efforts, have resulted in a 40% increase in the overall survival rate for pediatric cancer since the 1970s. Overall 5-year survival rates for all stages are approximately 85% for Wilms' tumor, 70% for hepatoblastoma, and 60% for rhabdomyosarcoma. In comparison, the survival rate was less than 20%, and closer to zero, respectively, for these malignancies before the advent of multidisciplinary therapy.

Despite this progress, only 20% to 40% of children with neuroblastomas survive more than 5 years. Ten to 30% of children with lymphomas and germ cell tumors relapse or become resistant to treatment. Less than 10% of children with hepatocellular carcinomas survive more than 5 years after diagnosis, and almost no patients who have rhabdoid tumor, pediatric colon cancer, or renal cell carcinoma in childhood survive more than 5 years. Because of lack of progress in these rare pediatric malignancies, the four American cooperative groups—CCG, POG, IRS, and NWTS—have merged recently into a single national pediatric cooperative group, the Childrens Oncology Group (COG). As in the past, the pediatric surgical oncologist will be instrumental to future progress [1,2].

Future progress will depend on myriad biologic analyses done on each tumor system. The pediatric surgical oncologist is the first line of defense in tumor diagnosis and staging. It is crucial that biopsy specimens be adequate both in size and quality. Snap freezing of portions of a tumor biopsy should become more routine. Molecular biologic studies often require a biopsy that exceeds 1 cm^3, and this should be kept in mind when planning the operative approach.

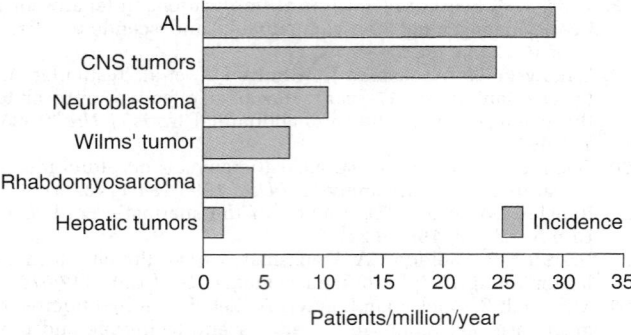

Figure 99.1. The incidence of childhood malignancies. Brain [central nervous system (CNS)] tumors are the most common solid tumor in children. Neuroblastoma is the most common solid tumor treated by general pediatric surgeons. All, acute lymphocytic leukemia.

INCIDENCE OF SOLID TUMORS IN CHILDHOOD

The incidences of various pediatric solid tumors of interest to pediatric surgeons are compared in Fig. 99.1 with the incidences of acute lymphoblastic leukemia and accumulated central nervous system tumors (1,2). Neuroblastoma is the most common extracranial solid tumor, followed in incidence by Wilms' tumors. Rhabdomyosarcomas have approximately half the incidence of the previous two, whereas hepatic tumors are fortunately extremely rare.

NEUROBLASTOMA

Epidemiology and Associated Conditions

Neuroblastoma is the most common extracranial solid tumor and the most common abdominal malignancy of childhood. The overall incidence rate of sympathetic nervous system cancers in children and adolescents younger than 20 years of age is 7.8%, and 97% of these are neuroblastomas (3). This translates into approximately 650 new cases in the United States per year, and sympathetic nervous system tumors comprise 7.8% of all cancers among children younger than 15 years of age. The age-adjusted incidence rate for boys younger than 15 years of age was 9.4 per million, and that for girls was 9.1 per million. The ratio of white to black incidence rates was 1.7:1 for boys and 1.9:1 for girls among infants (3). The overall male/female ratio is approximately 1.2:1, and the incidence is uniform throughout the world (4). Neuroblastoma is much more likely to occur in infancy, with a combined male:female incidence of 64 per million compared with 29 per million during the second year of life. The overall incidence of neuroblastoma has remained stable over a 21-year period of observation. Rates, however, have increased somewhat among infants during recent years. This may be due to the wide use of mass screening in certain areas. The median age at diagnosis is approximately 2 years, and 80% of children are younger than 4 years of age at diagnosis (5).

Case reports associating neuroblastoma with fetal exposures, including the fetal alcohol syndrome, or hydantoin or phenobarbital exposure have not been supported by larger studies (6,7). The occurrence of neuroblastoma has also been associated with neurofibromatosis type I, Beckwith-Wiedemann syndrome, Hirschsprung's disease, mus-

culoskeletal and cardiovascular malformations, Turner's syndrome, and neurodevelopmental abnormalities (8,9). However, none of these associations has been rigorously proved, and data remain conflicting. Possible but unproven environmental risk factors include parental exposure to solvents or electromagnetic fields, maternal hormone use during pregnancy, and parental cigarette smoking (10).

Basic Science

Neuroblastoma was the first tumor in which molecular biologic advances in the field of oncogenes were translated into a clinically useful tool. The N-*myc* oncogene, whose function and mechanism of action remain the subject of investigation, was empirically shown to be a useful predictor of survival and risk. It was found that patients with an increased number of copies of the N-*myc* gene had a much worse prognosis (11). Most authorities consider a copy number of more than 10 to be significant. It has also been shown that when N-*myc* is amplified in the primary tumor, the same is true for metastatic deposits or recurrent tumors. Rapid assessment of the N-*myc* copy number can be done using the process of in situ fluorescent hybridization, whereas the traditional method using Southern blotting takes longer. An example of tumor analysis from a patient is presented in Fig. 99.2. The mechanism of N-*myc* amplification in neuroblastoma remains unknown. N-*myc* is a DNA-binding protein. It thus exerts control over other genes and may help to keep the cell in the G_1 phase (12).

More recent research has uncovered a more nuanced role for N-*myc* as a prognostic factor in neuroblastoma. In one report, N-*myc* amplification was not shown to be an independent predictor of outcome in infants with neuroblastoma, although it remained a strongly adverse prognostic indicator in children diagnosed after 12 months of age.

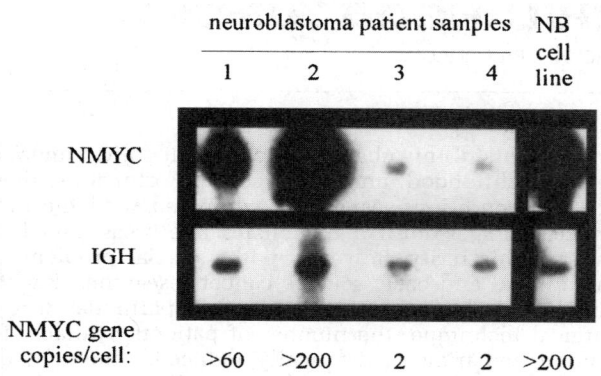

Figure 99.2. Example of N-*myc* amplification analysis by Southern blotting in neuroblastoma samples from four patients. The Southern blot hybridization signal obtained with the N-*myc* probe is normalized to that obtained on the same blot with a control probe for a gene not subject to amplification, such as the immunoglobulin heavy chain gene (IGH). The signals are then normalized to a negative control (placental DNA, not illustrated). A neuroblastoma cell line with N-*myc* amplification is used as a positive control. The IGH signals show that similar amounts of DNA are present in each lane, but the N-*myc* signals are grossly different from each other, indicating amplification in cases 1 and 2 and in the control cell line. Samples 1 and 2 show high-level N-*myc* amplification, exceeding 60 and 200 copies of N-*myc* per cell, respectively, which corresponds to greater than 30-fold and 100-fold amplification. Samples 3 and 4 contain two copies of N-*myc* per cell, as expected in diploid cells without amplification. (Courtesy of Marc Ladanyi, M.D., Department of Pathology, Memorial Sloan-Kettering Cancer Center.)

This is supported by the results of an Italian study that showed that N-*myc* amplification was an adverse prognostic factor except in patients with stage 4S disease.

Since the identification of the *Rb* gene and its role as a tumor suppressor gene, much work has been devoted to finding tumor suppressors in other systems. The usual starting point for this type of analysis is determination of a consistent cytogenetic deletion. The most common cytogenetic abnormality in neuroblastoma is deletion of a portion of the short arm of the first chromosome at 1p36 (13). The presence of a 1p deletion correlates with a worse outcome in neuroblastoma and has been used as a prognostic factor. It has been shown using cell fusion that replacement of this deleted segment is associated with a marked reduction in tumorigenicity (14). A number of laboratories are trying to identify the neuroblastoma tumor suppressor gene 1p36. More recently, interest has focused on another common cytogenetic abnormality observed in neuroblastoma: an unbalanced gain of genetic material on the long arm of chromosome 17. In one multivariate analysis, a gain at 17q was a significant predictor of outcome and was associated with a worse prognosis (15).

Another active area of neuroblastoma research is the relation of nerve growth factor receptors to differentiation and clinical risk. The low-affinity nerve growth factor receptor gene *LNGFR* and the *TRK* protooncogene, which is a component of the high-affinity nerve growth factor receptor, are expressed in human neuroblastoma tissue. A number of authors have shown that *LNGFR* and *TRK (TRK-A)* expression are inversely correlated with N-*myc* amplification and are associated with lower stage at diagnosis and improved prognosis (16–18). The absence of *TRK-A* expression has been highly correlated with N-*myc* amplification in one study, where 96% of N-*myc*-amplified tumors lacked *TRK-A* expression (19). *TRK-C* expression is also a favorable prognostic factor in neuroblastoma, whereas *TRK-B* expression is associated with poor survival (20).

Pathology

Neuroblastoma cells are derived from the primitive neural crest, as are melanocytes, Schwann cells, neuroendocrine cells (APUD cells), C cells of the thyroid gland, the autonomic nervous system, and adrenal gland, and mesenchymal cells of the midface. Neuroblastoma cells are thought to arise from primitive sympathoblasts (neuroblasts) (21). Under certain circumstances, these pluripotential cells demonstrate an ability to differentiate along a separate neural crest lineage. For instance, pure ganglioneuroma is thought to arise from complete differentiation of primitive neuroblasts into ganglion cells. Schwann cell differentiation is also clearly and frequently observed in these tumors. It is also possible to identify melanocytic differentiation in certain rare but well-reported neuroblastomas. Finally, because the sympathetic nervous system extends along the entire neuraxis, neuroblastoma can arise from cervical, thoracic, abdominal (retroperitoneal), and pelvic primary sites.

Neuroblastoma falls into the category of a small, round, blue cell tumor of childhood characterized by sheets of cells staining with hematoxylin. Other tumors that fall into this category include primitive neuroectodermal tumors (PNET) and Ewing's sarcoma, non-Hodgkin's lymphomas, and undifferentiated sarcomas (certain rhabdomyosarcomas). Light microscopic diagnosis depends on the identification of Homer-Wright pseudorosettes, ganglion cells, neuropil and neuritic processes, and schwannian stroma (Fig. 99.3). Homer-Wright pseudorosettes consist of rings of dark-staining neuroblasts surrounding an eosinophilic core of neuropil. The diagnosis can be aided by immunohistochemical staining that is positive for neurofilament proteins (S-100), synaptophysin, and neuron-specific enolase. PNETs may express neuron-specific enolase but not the other neural markers (22).

At presentation, most neuroblastomas are highly cellular and have a uniform appearance. After chemotherapy, the tumor often appears to have rests of neuroblasts contained in a schwannian stroma. This histologic appearance is called *ganglioneuroblastoma,* and although its is appears more differentiated, there is no impact on clinical risk, which is determined by the findings at initial diagnosis. It is also possible for tumors to contain significant amounts of stroma at diagnosis, and this finding is associated with improved outcome. This observation is the basis of the Shimada grading system, which is summarized in Table 99.1 (23). Because it may help predict risk, all neuroblastomas should undergo Shimada classification at diagnosis.

Neuroblastoma metastasizes to both regional lymph nodes and distant sites, most frequently bone marrow and cortical bone. The liver and, rarely, lungs can also be sites of metastatic spread. Cortical bone involvement as manifested by a positive bone scan is a particularly poor prognostic indicator.

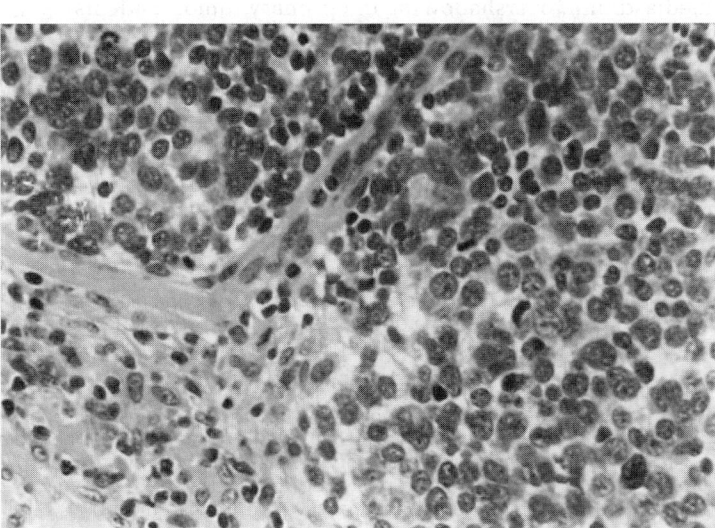

Figure 99.3. Typical neuroblastoma with monotonous cellular patterns. Note the mitotic figure (center). ×450.

Table 99.1. SHIMADA HISTOPATHOLOGIC CLASSIFICATION OF NEUROBLASTOMA

FAVORABLE

Stroma rich, all ages, no nodular pattern
Stroma poor, age 1.5–5 y, MKI <100
Stroma poor, age <1.5 y, MKI <200

UNFAVORABLE

Stroma rich, all ages, nodular pattern
Stroma poor, age >5 y
Stroma poor, age 1.5–5 y, undifferentiated
Stroma poor, age 1.5–5 y, differentiated, MKI >100
Stroma poor, age >1 y, MKI >200

MKI, mitosis–karyorrhexis index (number of mitoses and karyorrhexis per 5,000 cells).

Presentation, Work-up, and Staging

Clinical presentation depends on site of origin, age at diagnosis, and the biologic aggressiveness of the tumor. The proportion of patients with cervical or pelvic tumors is increased in patients younger than 1 year of age compared with older children. Cervical tumors present as a lateral neck mass, and airway compromise is not usually observed. Because they arise from cervical sympathetic ganglia, there may be associated Horner's syndrome, which is often permanent after resection and should be discussed before surgery with the parents. Regional nodal involvement is common, but distant metastases are rare, and most tumors are of low risk.

Pelvic tumors usually are diagnosed after a parent or caretaker palpates a mass. Bladder and bowel symptoms like recurrent urinary tract infections and chronic constipation can be seen when pelvic tumors reach great size and compress these organs. Hydronephrosis secondary to ureteral compression is often observed with large tumors and usually resolves after resection. Epidural extension to the sacrum can also be noted, and neurologic evaluation documenting somatic motor and sphincter function is mandatory.

In all age groups, the most common presentation is an abdominal tumor that is often hard and fixed. The tumor arises from the midline sympathetic nerves or the adrenal. Often, regional nodal echelons are involved along the aorta. These involved nodes can be bulky and may extend distally to the aortic bifurcation and proximally into the mediastinum, overshadowing the primary tumor. Patients with metastatic or large, bulky tumors, especially if older than 1 year of age, may appear generally ill or anemic.

Several syndromes are particularly associated with neuroblastoma: periorbital ecchymoses (raccoon eyes), opsoclonus–myoclonus syndrome, and the secretory diarrhea syndrome. Periorbital ecchymoses are caused by orbital metastases with subsequent obstruction and rupture of veins in the periorbital skin. The optic nerve and vision are not usually threatened, and the ecchymoses often take months to resolve even after the orbital tumors have regressed. Opsoclonus–myoclonus is a paraneoplastic syndrome thought to be autoimmune in nature; it is caused by development of antibodies against the tumor that cross-react with Purkinje cells in the cerebellum. Unfortunately, the symptoms may not regress after resection of the neuroblastoma, and the condition can result in devastating neurologic injury. Secretory diarrhea in this condition is caused by release of vasoactive intestinal peptide by the tumor. The watery diarrhea may require intravenous support but usually resolves with treatment. This condition is an indication of tumor differentiation and is associated with low-risk lesions.

The work-up is directed toward delineation of tumor extent in the primary site and identification of metastatic deposits. The primary site is usually evaluated by computed tomography (CT) or magnetic resonance imaging (MRI); no reported analyses compare the two in neuroblastoma. If CT scans are used, they should be performed with both gastrointestinal and intravenous contrast. This is true even for cervical and thoracic primaries so that the position and course of the pharynx and esophagus are precisely determined. The volume scanned should include not only the primary tumor but the regional lymphatics. The lower chest should be included in scans of cervical primaries, the upper abdomen and lower neck in thoracic tumors, and the entire abdomen, pelvis, and lower chest for abdominal primaries. Because of the high incidence of cortical bone involvement, especially in children older than 1 year of age, bone scans or radiographic series should also be performed routinely. The bone marrow is assessed by bone marrow aspiration at four iliac crest sites and bone biopsy at two. If CT or MRI scans include the liver, appropriate windows can be used to identify hepatic metastases. Ultrasound can also be used in this regard, and plain chest films are used to identify pulmonary metastases. If pulmonary metastases are present, Doppler ultrasonography can be used to identify intracaval tumor extension. It is also useful to perform a [131]I (or ^{123}I) metaiodobenzylguanidine scan to assess metastatic sites and as a baseline for evaluation of therapeutic response in the primary site. Finally, a 24-hour urine collection for measurement of metanephrine, dopamine, and vanillylmandelic acid may help diagnostically and as a tumor marker to assess therapeutic response.

Table 99.2. INTERNATIONAL STAGING CRITERIA FOR NEUROBLASTOMA

Stage	Criteria	3-Year Survival Rate (%) Overall	Relapse free
1	Localized tumor confined to site of origin; complete gross resection with or without microscopic margin; all identifiable regional nodes negative, including contralateral	97	88
2A	Unilateral tumor with incomplete gross excision; nodes negative	87	72
2B	Unilateral tumor with incomplete or complete gross excision with positive ipsilateral but negative contralateral nodes	86	63
3	Infiltration across the midline with or without regional nodal involvement; unilateral tumor with positive contralateral nodes; midline tumor with bilateral nodal involvement	62	58
4	Distant metastases to lymph nodes, (4N), bone, bone marrow, liver, or other organs	<40	<40
4S	Localized primary tumor as described for stage 1 or 2 with distant metastases limited to liver, skin, and bone marrow (<10% involvement)	~75	~75

The diagnosis of neuroblastoma requires histologic confirmation either by direct tumor biopsy or by demonstration of malignant cells in bone marrow samples. Because of the wide range of molecular biologic studies that have prognostic importance, many groups attempt to obtain enough tissue at diagnosis to allow full molecular biologic and cytogenetic analysis in addition to histologic diagnosis. When possible, several grams of tumor tissue should be obtained, and a portion should be snap frozen. Given the seriousness of this tumor, this is a reasonable objective. The application of biologic studies to determine risk status and therapy makes adequate tumor biopsies mandatory. This can usually be done through a minilaparotomy or laparoscopic approach. Despite progress in obtaining large amounts of molecular information from needle biopsies, most authorities recommend open biopsy with removal of several cubic centimeters of tumor tissue.

The most widely used staging system for neuroblastoma is based on the international system, which is listed in Table 99.2. This was evolved from previous systems developed by Evans and colleagues and the POG (5,24). Tumor size and location with regard to the midline remain important determinants of stage, as does the presence and degree of metastatic disease.

Risk Groups

As a result of insights gained through cooperative group studies, as well as the work done by several single institutions, it is possible to categorize patients with neuroblastoma into high-, intermediate-, and low-risk groups at diagnosis. This assessment is based on age, stage, Shimada classification, and the results of specialized studies, including flow cytometry, analysis for N-*myc* amplification, cytogenetics, and *TRK* gene expression. Ancillary criteria include serum ferritin, lactate dehydrogenase, and neuron-specific enolase determinations at diagnosis and before blood transfusion. Table 99.3 lists criteria for high- and low-risk patients. Risk assignment is important because it strongly determines therapy.

Treatment

Neuroblastoma treatment depends on degree of risk, as noted earlier. In general, low-risk tumors do not require chemotherapy or radiation. Resection of the primary lesion to obtain the diagnosis and biologic markers is followed by observation. Serial imaging studies of the primary and possible metastatic sites in low-risk patients are performed. Urinary catecholamines should fall to normal levels and remain there.

High-risk neuroblastoma remains one of the central problems in pediatric oncology, with overall survival rates in the 10% to 30% range despite multidisciplinary therapy and the use of multiagent chemotherapy. Initial surgery should be confined to acquisition of diagnostic tissue, staging, and placement of a vascular access device. It has been noted that surgical complications are higher with initial attempts at complete resection without impact on survival. After a course of chemotherapy, usually four or five cycles, second-look surgery is performed (Fig. 99.4). Although controversy surrounds the issue of resection in high-risk patients, most authorities agree that complete gross resection should be the goal of second-look procedures. The approach is dictated by the particular properties of the primary tumor. For upper abdominal lesions, especially those involving major midline branches of the abdominal aorta or the vena cava, thoracoabdominal exposure is helpful and well tolerated. The goal of resection is a complete vascular dissection and should encompass not only the primary but all involved regional nodal echelons.

Chemotherapy for neuroblastoma has evolved toward higher dose intensities of multiple agents. *Dose intensity* is defined as the drug dose, usually normalized to surface area, divided by the time interval over which it is administered. In one metaanalysis, increased dose intensity correlated with improved overall and disease-free survival rates. In another report, primary tumor resectability correlated with increased chemotherapy intensity. There is no widely accepted regimen, and the major cooperative groups, as well as larger single institutions, have differing protocols. The COG is planning to base the induction phase of its new high-risk neuroblastoma protocol on a regimen developed at Memorial Sloan-Kettering Cancer Center (N7 protocol). This protocol includes cyclophosphamide, 70 mg/kg/d for 2 days, doxorubicin, 75 mg/m² over 72 hours, and vincristine, 2 mg/m² over 72 hours, given as cycles 1, 2, 4, and 6. These cycles alternate with cisplatin, 50 mg/m²/d for 4 days, and etoposide, 200 mg/m²/d for 3 days, for cycles 3, 5, and 7. Second-look surgery is performed after cycle 4. This regimen has resulted in a 45% disease-free survival rate at 2 years from diagnosis in high-risk patients with stage 4 disease (25). After induction and local control with second-look resection, patients will receive a stem cell transplant, and there will be a randomization based on whether the stem cells will be purged to remove possible contamination with circulating neuroblastoma cells or remain unpurged. The study is designed to determine whether purging is necessary. This approach is based on randomized data from the old CCG showing a significant survival improvement in patients with neuroblastoma who underwent autologous bone marrow transplantation as part of therapy (26). This important study also indicated that treatment with 13-*cis*-retinoic acid after bone marrow transplantation was asso-

Table 99.3. **RISK STATUS DETERMINANTS IN NEUROBLASTOMA**

Parameters	Low risk	High risk
Age	<1 y (especially <6 mo)	>1 y at diagnosis
Stage	1, 2A, 2B, 4S	3, 4
Shimada classification	Favorable	Unfavorable
N-myc amplification	<3 Copies	>3 Copies
Expression of TRK	TRK Expressed	No TRK expression
Flow cytometry	Hyperdiploid, triploid	Diploid
Cytogenetics	No 1p abnormality	1p Deletion
Ferritin at diagnosis	<142 ng/mL	≥142 ng/mL
Lactate dehydrogenase	≤1,500 U/mL	>1,500 U/mL
Neuron-specific enolase	≤100 ng/mL	>100 ng/mL

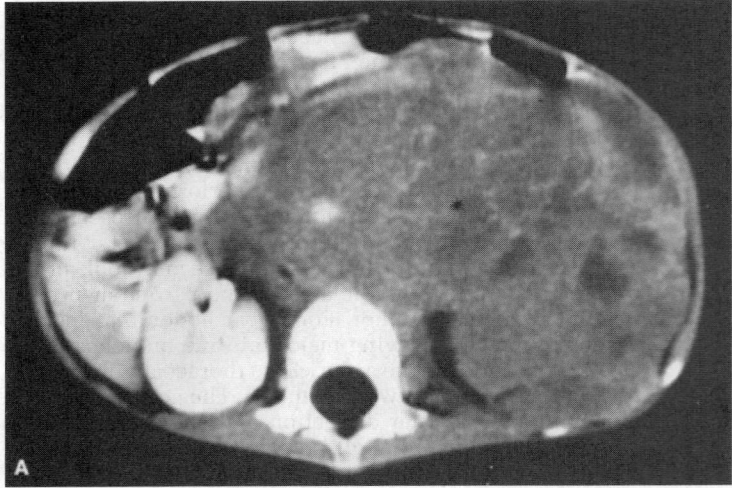

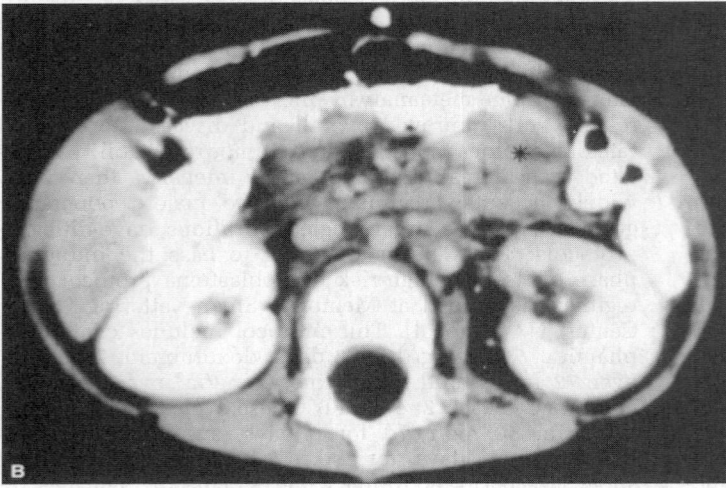

Figure 99.4. *(A)* Initial computed tomography (CT) scan of a child with stage 4 neuroblastoma. *(B)* CT scan of the same child after incisional biopsy and cytoreductive chemotherapy. Residual tumor is present despite dramatic reduction in overall tumor size.

ciated with an improved survival rate. The roles of dose-intensive chemotherapy, autologous stem cell or bone marrow transplantation, retinoids, and marrow support with colony-stimulating factors are now well established in the treatment of high-risk neuroblastoma.

Future Directions

Treatment with radiolabeled or cold monoclonal antibodies is also undergoing trial. These antibodies are usually of the IgG class and recognize the surface ganglioside GD2 that is usually highly expressed on the surface of human neuroblastoma cells. Current strategies include induction of antibody-dependent, cell-mediated cytotoxicity by cold antibody, usually of the IgG3 class, and direct cell killing by attachment of ^{131}I to the antibody that then specifically recognizes a tumor cell. More sophisticated approaches involve stimulation of a host antitumor response by vaccination with antiidiotypic monoclonal antibodies versus anti-GD2.

Various gene therapy approaches are also in their initial stages. One CCG protocol attempted to transfect the cytokine, interferon-γ, into neuroblastoma cells obtained from patients. The cells would then undergo lethal irradiation followed by reinfusion into the patient. Interferon-g increases the level of human leukocyte antigen class I expression of the surface of neuroblastoma cells. It is hoped that this will incite a cell-mediated immune response against the tumor.

WILMS' TUMOR

Epidemiology and Associated Conditions

Malignancies of the kidney represent 6.3% of all cancer diagnoses among children younger than 15 years of age, with an incidence of 7.9 per million (27). In the United States, approximately 550 children per year younger than 20 years of age are diagnosed with a renal cancer, and 500 of these are Wilms' tumors. The overall incidence of Wilms' tumor or nephroblastoma is 7 per 1 million children (1 per 10,000) younger than the age of 16 years (28,29). The incidence is highest for African-Americans and lowest for patients of East Asian descent. Whites have an intermediate incidence. The sex ratio is approximately 1:1, and the peak incidence occurs between 2 and 3 years of age (30). Most Wilms' tumors occur in patients younger than 5 years of age. Median ages reported from the National Wilms' Tumor Study were 36 months for boys and 43 months for girls with unilateral disease, whereas boys and girls with bilateral disease presented at a median age of 23 and 30 months, respectively (31). Rhabdoid tumors of the kidney, clear cell sarcomas, and renal cell carcinomas make up 1.0%, 1.6%,

Table 99.4. **WILMS' TUMOR-ASSOCIATED SYNDROMES AND CONDITIONS**

Syndrome	Syndrome components	Wilms' tumor risk
Beckwith-Wiedemann	Macroglossia, somatic gigantism, visceromegaly, hypoglycemia, abdominal wall defects	~5% (500-fold increase)
WAGR	Wilms' tumor, aniridia, ambiguous genitalia, mental retardation, WTI deletion	40%–50% (40,000-fold to 50,000-fold increase)
Neurofibromatosis	Café au lait spots, plexiform neurofibromas, predisposition to multiple tumors	~0.26% (26-fold increase)
Denys-Drash	Pseudohermaphroditism, glomerulopathy, gonadal tumors or dysgenesis	~60%–70% (60,000-fold to 70,000-fold increase)
Perlman's familial nephroblastomatosis	Bilateral renal hamartomas, macrosomia, islet cell hypertrophy, unusual facies, mental retardation	~60%[a]
Genital anomalies	Cryptorchidism, hypospadias, gonadal dysgenesis, pseudohermaphroditism	Increased

[a]There is an increased risk of nephroblastoma in patients with the Denys-Drash and Perlman's syndromes, but these are very rare, with less than 10 cases of Perlman's syndrome reported. The incidence of Wilms' tumor in the general population is 1 in 10,000; therefore, the incidence of Wilms' tumor in Beckwith-Wiedemann syndrome is 5/100 / 1/10,000, which is a 500-fold increase.

and 2.6%, respectively, of renal cancers occurring in children younger than 15 years of age (27).

Table 99.4 lists conditions associated with the development of Wilms' tumor along with the associated increase in relative risk. In general, the presence of any of these conditions or syndromes should initiate a work-up to rule out the presence of Wilms' tumor. Known risk factors include race (the Asian incidence is half that found in whites or African-Americans), aniridia, genitourinary anomalies, WAGR syndrome (Wilms' tumor, aniridia, genitourinary anomalies, mental retardation), Beckwith-Wiedemann syndrome, Perlman's syndrome, Denys-Drash syndrome, and the Simpson-Golabi-Behmel syndrome (27).

Basic Science

The successful identification of the *Rb* gene as the tumor suppressor in retinoblastoma has led to similar investigations regarding the other pediatric solid tumors. In general, researchers attempt to find a consistent chromosomal deletion that indicates the possible site of a tumor suppressor gene. Molecular biologic techniques are then used to identify and clone the gene. In the case of Wilms' tumor, cytogenetic abnormalities have been identified on chromosomes 11p13, 1p, and 16q (32–34). A gene called *WT1* was cloned from the site on the 11th chromosome and has been shown to bind to DNA, suggesting that it functions to control gene expression. Furthermore, *WT1* has been shown to be linked to the gene locus associated with aniridia, but was not linked to the occurrence of Wilms' tumor in three separate, multiple-case kindreds (35,36). This suggests that the Wilms' tumor suppressor is probably not *WT1*, but may reside on a locus at 1p or especially 16q. NWTS-5, which is being initiated, will be directed to determining which genetic locus is associated with the development of Wilms' tumor and is the most likely candidate for the Wilms' tumor suppressor gene.

Pathology

The study of Wilms' tumor has benefited greatly from a central pathology review performed at the NWTS Pathology Center. Much progress in defining Wilms' tumor risk categories has ensued. This underscores the need for accurate and adequate histologic analysis of all Wilms' tumor specimens.

It is hypothesized that Wilms' tumor arises from primitive metanephric blastema, and individual tumors often contain primitive metanephric cells but also cartilage, skeletal muscle, and squamous epithelium. Most tumors arise unifocally within the kidney, but approximately 7% of unilateral Wilms' tumors are multicentric (30). The proportion of synchronous bilateral tumors among all patients with nephroblastoma ranges from 4.4% to 7%, whereas that of metachronous tumors is 1.0% to 1.9% (36). Wilms' tumors are equally distributed with regard to the left and right side and may occur with no apparent connection to the kidneys. Usually, extrarenal Wilms' tumor occurs in the retroperitoneal area, but other reported sites include the pelvis, scrotum, and inguinal region.

Grossly, the tumors are globular or spherical and uniformly pale-gray or tan on sectioning. Calcification is not usually apparent, but "egg-shell" calcification can be observed in tumors that have undergone significant spontaneous hemorrhage. This is different from the stippled calcifications associated with neuroblastoma. Cysts may be present, and in infants, polypoid extension into the pelvi-calyceal system may cause confusion with botryoid rhabdomyosarcoma (37). Also, there is often a pseudocapsule of compressed renal parenchyma. Most tumors, unless composed of a large proportion of stromal elements, are friable and easily ruptured. This is of great significance to the operating surgeon, who must determine whether preoperative rupture has occurred and must avoid intraoperative spillage. The consequence of either of these events is upstaging of the lesion and the need for whole-abdomen radiation therapy with its attendant morbidity.

Microscopically, these tumors demonstrate a triphasic pattern of blastemic, stromal, and epithelial cells. Biphasic tumors with blastemic and stromal cells are common, and some specimens consist of only a single type (Fig. 99.5). A major parameter predictive of tumor aggressiveness and patient survival is the histologic finding of anaplasia. This finding is defined by the presence of hyperdiploid mitotic figures, threefold or greater nuclear enlargement, and hyperchromasia of enlarged nuclei. The effect of anaplasia on prognosis is so marked that tumors with these findings are designated "unfavorable histology" by the NWTS. Anaplastic tumors, which comprise approximately 5% of all Wilms' tumors, are rare in the first 2 years of life, but their incidence increases to 13% of patients diagnosed at 5 years of age or older.

Presentation, Work-up, and Staging

Most Wilms' tumors are first diagnosed after appreciation of an asymptomatic abdominal mass, which can at-

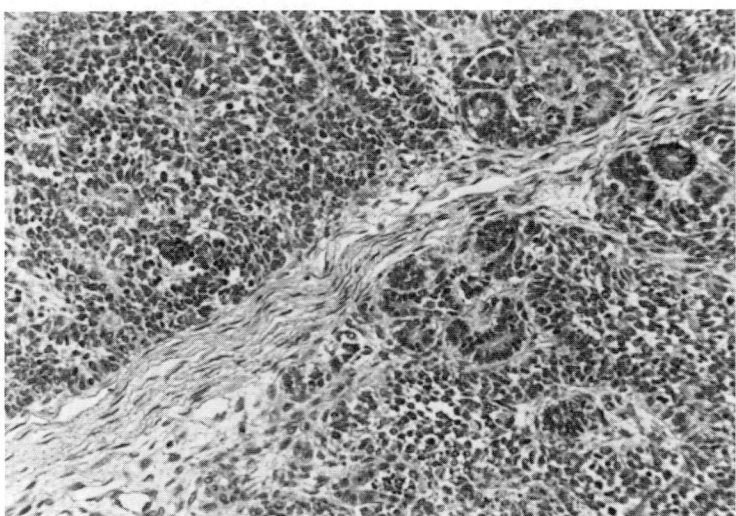

Figure 99.5. Wilms' tumor. The background is blastemic cells, and some areas are suggestive of tubule formation. ×140.

tain great size. This usually occurs during routine pediatric examination or while the children are being attended by a relative. Parents are usually surprised and feel guilty that such a mass could have gone unnoticed, and need reassurance. In a subset of patients, rapid abdominal enlargement develops, associated with pain, fever, and gross hematuria. This is attributed to intratumoral hemorrhage and may be associated with spontaneous rupture.

The NWTS recommends the following work-up for patients with suspected nephroblastoma. An excretory urogram is obtained to identify the tumor site; pelvicalyceal distortion is demonstrated, thus localizing the process to the kidney; and the function of the contralateral kidney is assessed. It is acceptable to substitute CT scanning of the abdomen with intravenous and oral contrast for excretory urography (Fig. 99.6). Indeed, almost every center performs this study routinely. Abdominal, real-time Doppler ultrasonography is performed to identify intracaval tumor extension, liver metastases, or enlarged retroperitoneal lymph nodes. Finally, good posteroanterior and oblique plain films of the chest are obtained to identify pulmonary metastases. All data concerning stage IV patients in the NWTS studies are based on the diagnosis being made by plain chest radiographs. Several studies have been performed that support the validity of this approach. In particular, patients with pulmonary metastases diagnosed by CT but not by plain chest films did as well as patients with nonmetastatic disease when staged and treated on the basis of their abdominal tumor alone. It is recommended that patients with pulmonary nodules identified by CT scan but not plain chest radiographs undergo biopsy to verify the diagnosis. This has obvious cost-of-care and quality-of-life implications. Some effort to resolve this controversy is needed, given the prevalence of CT scanning.

In the United States, this initial work-up is followed by surgical resection of the tumor, if possible (Fig. 99.7). This then allows surgical and histologic parameters to be included in staging. The surgeon must pay strict attention to the local tumor extent or tumor rupture and status of the regional periaortic, interaortocaval, paracaval, and perirenal lymph nodes. Direct visualization and bimanual palpation of the contralateral kidney is mandatory in all cases, even when CT scans do not indicate involvement. Preoperative assessment of the contralateral kidney is inaccurate in one third of cases. Finally, the liver should be carefully palpated and the peritoneal and diaphragmatic surfaces inspected for metastases.

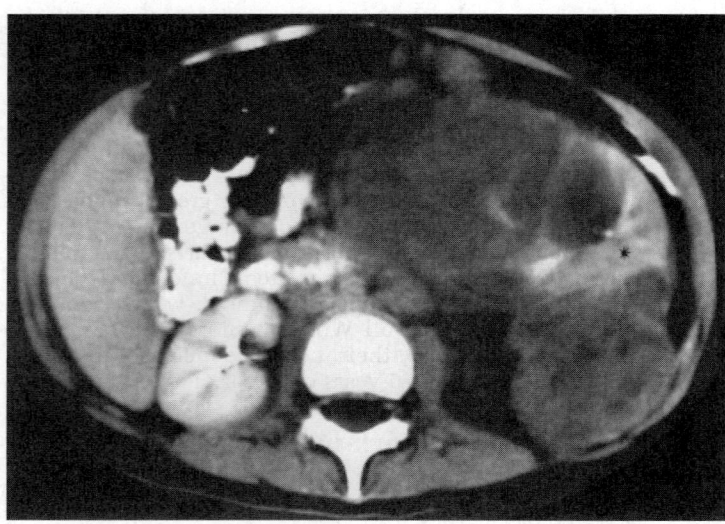

Figure 99.6. Initial computed tomography scan of a child with a left-sided Wilms' tumor. The distortion of the calyceal system is characteristic of intrinsic renal tumor. A kidney *(asterisk)* is identifiable.

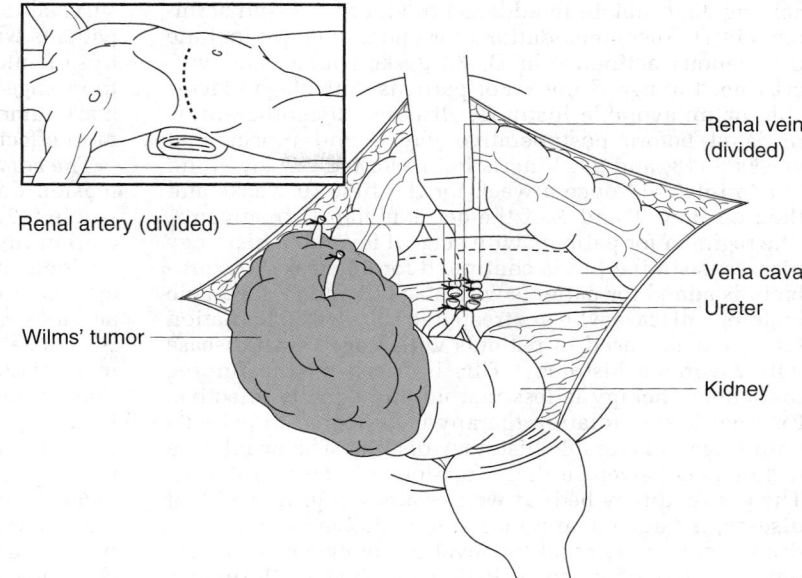

Renal vein (divided)

Renal artery (divided)

Vena cava

Ureter

Wilms' tumor

Kidney

Figure 99.7. Operative approach to resection of a right renal Wilms' tumor.

Once the imaging and surgical and pathologic data are acquired, a tumor stage is assigned; the current NWTS staging schema is listed in Table 99.5. Stage is basically an assessment of risk group and has been validated by previous NWTS studies. Its importance lies in defining the least morbid treatment that results in long-term remission or cure.

Treatment

The standard of care in the United States is initial surgical resection. Exceptions to this rule include extensive intracaval tumors that require cardiopulmonary bypass for extraction, obviously unresectable tumors with documented invasion of contiguous structures, and possibly bilateral tumors, especially if it is unclear which side is most heavily involved. These special cases are discussed

again later. For most patients, exploration and resection should be performed through a wide transverse incision that allows comfortable inspection and palpation of the contralateral kidney. As noted earlier, complete sampling of regional nodal echelons is mandatory, as is careful assessment of the tumor margins and possible areas of metastases. Most authors recommend early ligation of the renal vein, but most surgeons admit to not performing this maneuver because it is often difficult or unsafe, owing to the size of the tumor. The available data indicate that later ligation of the renal vein after tumor mobilization does not adversely affect prognosis. After the kidney and accompanying Gerota fascia is mobilized, the renal artery is most easily identified by posterior dissection. Radical ureterectomy does not affect outcome, but the ureter should be divided well distal to the calyceal system to ensure any polypoid pelvicalyceal extensions are encompassed.

All patients with resectable Wilms' tumor receive postoperative chemotherapy. There may be one exception to this rule, as reported by the Dana Farber Group. This consists of patients with stage I favorable histology disease who are younger than 24 months of age at diagnosis and have tumors less than 250 g in weight at resection (38,39). Beckwith suggested a further refinement of histologic criteria to identify low-risk stage I patients: no vascular invasion beyond the renal hilar plane and absence of capsular invasion. Unfortunately, in a recent NWTS study, the local recurrence rate for stage I patients treated by surgery alone was higher than expected, and the current recommendation is to give two-drug chemotherapy to all patients with stage I disease.

A major effort by the NWTS was the development of chemotherapy protocols for Wilms' tumor that minimize toxicity while maintaining efficacy. Data accumulated from these studies have shown that in patients with stage I or II favorable histology disease, survival is improved when combination chemotherapy with vincristine and actinomycin D is used. Patients with stage I unfavorable histology disease have survival rates equivalent to those of patients with stage I favorable histology disease, and can be treated with the same adjuvant regimen. This emphasizes the importance of accurate surgical and pathologic staging. In patients with stage III and IV favorable histology disease, outcome was improved for those re-

Table 99.5. STAGING CRITERIA FOR WILMS' TUMOR

Wilms' tumor staging system[a]		4-Year survival rate (%)
Stage 1	Tumor limited to kidney and completely excised; surface intact with no evidence of rupture	97
Stage 2	Tumor extends beyond kidney but completely excised; infiltration through the renal capsule, or extension into vessels outside the kidney substance, or local open biopsy or spillage confined to the flank; no residual tumor	95
Stage 3	Residual nonhematogenous tumor	91
Stage 4	Hematogenous metastases to lung, liver, bone, brain, etc.	78
Stage 5	Bilateral renal involvement at diagnosis	Same as for highest-stage unilateral

[a]Survival based on outcome for patients with favorable histologic-types in the National Wilms' Tumor Study–3.

ceiving doxorubicin in addition to vincristine and actinomycin D. Recommendations for chemotherapy include intravenous actinomycin D, 75 µg/kg/course, and vincristine, 1.5 mg/m²/dose. For patients with stage I favorable or unfavorable histology disease, chemotherapy is initiated before postoperative day 6 and repeated at weeks 5, 13, and 24. Vincristine is started on day 7 and is administered once a week for the first 10 weeks and then on days 1 and 5 of the actinomycin D treatments. The regimen for patients with stage II favorable histology disease is similar but is continued for 58 weeks. Doxorubicin is added for patients with stage III and IV favorable histology disease who are treated for 58 weeks. Radiation therapy is not used in patients with stage I or II disease with favorable histology. This is based on the finding that chemotherapy is less morbid and equally effective. External beam radiation therapy is delivered to patients with stage III favorable histology disease. The usual dose is 1,080 cGy given in daily fractions of 150 to 180 cGy. The entire kidney bed, as well as areas of gross residual disease, is targeted, and radiation is delivered to the entire vertebral column at the level of involvement to minimize the risk of scoliosis. Patients with stage IV disease should have their primary tumor staged as if metastases were not present. If the primary kidney tumor is stage I or II, no local radiation is delivered; the previously noted guidelines are followed for primary stage III tumors. Pulmonary metastases are treated with whole-thorax external beam radiation therapy to a total dose of 1,200 cGy given in 150-cGy fractions. The mediastinum is not shielded to prevent recurrence in central lymphatics or the lung margins. Nonresectable liver metastases are treated to a total dose of 1,980 cGy. Localized liver lesions may receive focal radiation, but diffuse hepatic metastases require treatment of the entire hepatic volume. Supplemental boosts to localized areas of 500 to 1,000 cGy may also be used. Bulky nodal, brain, and skeletal metastases receive 3,060 cGy and supplemental focal boosts as necessary.

All patients with unfavorable histology in stages II through IV are treated with actinomycin D, vincristine, and doxorubicin as well as external beam radiation using the stage III favorable histology guidelines noted earlier.

Bilateral Wilms' Tumor

The overall survival rate of patients who have bilateral Wilms' tumor is 87% (40). The survival rate for this disease is high because 90% of cases are of favorable histology, most kidneys are stage I when considered individually, and advances have made treatment more successful. Because of the danger of debilitating loss of renal function, it is acceptable to administer preoperative chemotherapy based on the results of an initial exploration and biopsy. After tumor shrinkage, a second-look procedure and nephron-sparing renal resection can be performed. Using this strategy, survival rates have been achieved that are equivalent to those obtained with the more traditional approach. The latter involves an initial nephrectomy of the most heavily involved kidney, followed by chemotherapy, and then reexploration (41).

Renal Vein and Inferior Vena Caval Involvement

A study reported from NWTS-3 included 164 patients with gross and 47 patients with microscopic involvement of the renal vein beyond the kidney (11.3%). Two-year survival rates were 90%, 79%, and 72%, respectively, for patients with stages I, II, and III disease. Important predictors of outcome were histologic pattern and stage. The authors suggested that complete *en bloc* resection of the primary tumor and the renal vein extension constituted the most effective initial management (42).

The survival rates of patients with intracaval tumor extension do not differ from those for Wilms' tumor as a whole (43). It has been suggested that a complicated operation involving cardiopulmonary bypass can be safely avoided by administration of preoperative chemotherapy. A second-look procedure should then be performed and all residual tumors resected. Because chemotherapy is associated with significant tumor shrinkage, and pulmonary tumor embolus has not been a problem, these patients should initially undergo systemic therapy. Second-look surgery is usually less complicated, and resection can be accomplished using conventional means when this approach is taken. Tumor shrinkage usually is rapid when cytotoxic drugs are first administered, but stabilizes after four to five cycles of therapy. At this point, no further tumor reduction can be expected and resection should be planned with appropriate preoperative consultation from other services (e.g., cardiovascular) as indicated. Nevertheless, a preoperative work-up that includes Doppler ultrasonography should always be performed before operation. Contrast vena cavography has become less crucial with advances in contrast-enhanced CT or MRI techniques, which now provide detailed information concerning the vascular anatomy. Nevertheless, an accurate picture of the anatomic extent of the tumor thrombus must be determined before surgery. If tumor thrombus continues to extend to the proximal vena cava or right atrium, resection should be coordinated and performed under cardiopulmonary bypass. If this is not done, intraoperative tumor embolism, which is often fatal, may be the result.

Extrarenal Wilms' Tumor

Wilms' tumors can arise from areas other than the kidney, but this is extremely rare. The most common site is the retroperitoneum, followed by the pelvis and inguinal canal. Two mechanisms for this phenomenon have been proposed. In the first theory, the tumor is thought to arise from the rests of metanephric tissue. The second theory suggests that Wilms' tumor develops from germinal tissue present in a teratoma. It is possible that both mechanisms are operative. Stage for stage, extrarenal Wilms' tumors have a prognosis similar to that of renal primary tumors, and therapy should be guided by principles developed by NWTS (44–46).

Adult and Neonatal Wilms' Tumor

Wilms' tumors that occur at both ends of the age spectrum are rare (47,48). In the report by Hrabovsky and colleagues (48), 27 of 3,340 (0.8%) patients with renal tumors were younger than 30 days of age at presentation. Eighteen of these 27 patients had mesoblastic nephroma, 1 had a malignant rhabdoid tumor, and 4 had nonneoplastic lesions. The remaining four patients had Wilms' tumor, and all had favorable histology. Also, none of the Wilms' tumor patients had metastases at diagnosis, and all have survived. Adult Wilms' tumors are associated with worse outcome, even in patients with favorable histology. A 3-year overall survival rate has been reported by NWTS and supports the use of aggressive therapy in all adult Wilms' tumor patients (49–51).

Future Directions

The NWTS-5 will not ask a clinical question but rather will focus on the predictive effect on outcome of cytogenetic abnormalities of chromosomes 1, 16, and 11. This is testimony to the progress achieved by previous NWTS studies. Other areas of investigation include the role of autologous bone marrow transplantation in patients with relapsed favorable and unfavorable histology disease, and attempts to improve outcome in the non-Wilms' renal tumors that occur in childhood. In this regard, sarcoma-like protocols, using agents such as cisplatin, ifosfamide, and etoposide, are being evaluated.

NON-WILMS' RENAL TUMORS OF CHILDHOOD AND ADOLESCENCE

Clear Cell Sarcoma

Clear cell sarcoma of the kidney is considered a distinct histopathologic and clinical entity from Wilms' tumor (52,53). It has an age distribution similar to that observed in Wilms' tumor but a markedly worse prognosis. This tumor is characterized by a proclivity to metastasize to bones and has been called the *bone-metastasizing renal tumor of childhood* by British workers. Relapse and death occur in 75% of patients, with more than half dying within 1 year of diagnosis. Histopathologically, the tumor consists of cords and nests of pale-stained tumor cells separated by vascular structures. Confusion with classic Wilms' tumor is possible, however, and central pathologic review is recommended. Clear cell sarcoma can metastasize not only to bone but to brain. Bony metastases are usually polyostotic, but the skull is almost invariably involved. A CT scan of the abdomen or intravenous urogram, chest radiograph, MRI of the brain, and bone scan are recommended as part of the work-up. The staging system is similar to that for Wilms' tumor, but high rates of tumor relapse are associated with even stage I tumors, supporting the use of aggressive systemic chemotherapy in all stages. The addition of doxorubicin to the treatment regimen for these children has resulted in significant survival improvement (54). Treatment recommendations include radical resection of the primary tumor when possible, followed by a postoperative chemotherapy regimen that includes doxorubicin, actinomycin D, and vincristine. Postoperative radiation therapy to the tumor bed is recommended regardless of stage. Usually, 1,080 cGy of postoperative flank irradiation is administered. Patients should be followed with serial chest radiographs and 6-monthly brain MRI scans and bone scans for at least 3 years after treatment.

Rhabdoid Tumor

Rhabdoid tumors are rare malignancies that most commonly involve the kidney in childhood; they also can occur primarily in the mediastinum or brain (55,56). Outcome is particularly poor, and there is no proven chemotherapy regimen. The tumor is characterized histopathologically by a rhabdomyosarcomatoid or myoblastic appearance, but the tumors do not express muscle markers and are not myoblastic in origin. Rhabdoid tumors of the kidney occur in infancy, with a median age at presentation of 13 months (range, 2 months to 5 years). Some rhabdoid tumors may be associated with the coincident development of PNETs of the brain. Extrarenal rhabdoid tumors occur in older patients. The survival rate is almost zero, and even patients with stage I disease fare poorly. There-fore, aggressive therapy is warranted that includes surgical resection, local radiation therapy, and systemic chemotherapy. Because these tumors have been refractory to historical protocols, use of experimental dose-intensive chemotherapy regimens or new chemotherapeutic agents is warranted.

Congenital Mesoblastic Nephroma

Congenital mesoblastic nephroma was first described by Bolande and colleagues (57) in 1969 and differentiated from Wilms' tumor. This tumor usually occurs in infants and typically follows a benign course; however, well-documented cases have resulted in metastases and death. Mesoblastic nephroma has been reported in adults and in the Beckwith-Wiedemann syndrome. A translocation, t(12;15), has been reported and is associated with an *ETV6–NTRK3* gene fusion that may link mesoblastic nephroma to congenital fibrosarcoma (58). Histologically, the tumor consists of bundles of spindle cells, tubules of basophilic cells, and invasion into the renal parenchyma or perinephric soft tissue. The cells resemble fibroblasts or smooth muscle. Congenital mesoblastic nephroma is usually curable by radical nephrectomy alone. Tumors with high cellularity on light microscopic examination, however, and those with evident metastases require more aggressive treatment. In particular, older patients with densely cellular lesions or high mitotic indices should be considered for systemic chemotherapy.

Renal Cell Carcinoma

There are several reported series as well as scattered case reports of renal cell carcinoma occurring in childhood, adolescence, and young adults. In one study (59), the median age was 15.5 years (range, 3 to 21 years). Histologically, the tumor is an adenocarcinoma similar to that seen in older patients. Most reported cases are of the clear cell variant of renal adenocarcinoma. There is no predilection for the right or left side, and the tumors are equally distributed between upper and lower poles and mid-kidney. Sites of metastases include lung (64%), liver (57%), bone (42%), and pleura or brain (7%). Staging is based on the adult staging system and survival is stage dependent. Unfortunately, many of these patients present with stage IV disease. Outcome analysis has shown a correlation of survival with complete resection, although resectability was also associated with adverse prognostic factors like lymph node involvement or distant metastases. Recommended therapy is complete resection by radical nephrectomy, if feasible. The role of chemotherapy is undefined, but given the poor outcome associated with higher-stage disease, it is reasonable to administer postoperative chemotherapy as an experimental protocol. This should probably be performed as part of a national cooperative study.

RHABDOMYOSARCOMA

Epidemiology and Associated Conditions

In the United States, 850 to 900 children and adolescents younger than 20 years of age are diagnosed with soft-tissue sarcoma each year, and approximately 350 of these are rhabdomyosarcomas (60). Rhabdomyosarcoma is the most common soft-tissue sarcoma in children younger than 14 years of age, comprising almost 50% of soft-tissue sarcomas in this age group. There are two major histologic subtypes occurring in childhood, embryonal and alveolar. Embryonal rhabdomyosarcoma constitutes approximately 75% of cases (60). The alveolar subtype is more common in older children and extremity lesions. The incidence of rhabdomyosarcoma in the United States is 4 cases per 1 million white children younger than 15 years and approximately half that rate for black children (61). The male/female ratio is 1.4:1, and 80% of patients are white, 12% black, and 8% other categories.

Rhabdomyosarcoma has been observed in patients with neurofibromatosis and Beckwith-Wiedemann syndrome. The Li-Fraumeni cancer family syndrome involves the occurrence of sarcoma, in particular rhabdomyosarcoma, along with breast, bone, or brain cancer, lung and laryngeal cancer, and adrenocortical neoplasia. In this syndrome, children with rhabdomyosarcoma have first-degree relatives with the other malignancies. In an autopsy study from the IRS, 32% of patients with rhabdomyosarcoma had congenital anomalies that included (in order of frequency) genitourinary, central nervous system, and cardiovascular malformations (62). Also, basal cell carcinoma has been observed in conjunction with rhabdomyosarcoma.

Basic Science

Myogenic cell differentiation can be arbitrarily divided into three broad stages: (a) commitment of a multipotent stem cell to a monopotent myoblast; (b) differentiation of a monopotent myoblast into a multinucleated myofiber expressing muscle-specific genes; and (c) maturation, during which the expression of specific cellular proteins progresses through embryonic, fetal, neonatal, and adult patterns. Genetic determinants of the first stage of myogenic cell differentiation were identified first. It was initially observed that fibroblasts briefly exposed to 5-azacytidine developed a myoblastic phenotype manifested by the presence of myotubes. Genomic DNA transfection experiments verified that myoblast but not fibroblast DNA could convert fibroblasts into stably determined myoblasts, and the frequency of conversion was consistent with a single genetic locus. This allowed the first identification of a myogenic determination gene, *MyoD1* (63). *MyoD* is expressed exclusively in skeletal muscle as well as myoblasts derived from 5-azacytidine-treated fibroblasts. When this gene is transfected, under the control of a viral promoter, into a variety of cell types (i.e., fibroblast, melanoma cells,

neuroblastoma, hepatic cells, and adipocytes), expression of the *MyoD* cDNA induces myogenesis with expression of muscle-specific structural genes.

Pathology

Rhabdomyosarcomas are malignant tumors that arise from the ubiquitously distributed primitive mesenchyme found in the fetus. These tumors display characteristics of striated muscle, including immunohistochemical expression of skeletal muscle myosin and actin, desmin, myoglobin, and Z-band protein. Electron microscopy may show actin–myosin bundles or Z-band material. Expression of the DNA-binding protein, MyoD1, has been shown to be a lineage marker for rhabdomyosarcoma (64).

Based on classic pathology, rhabdomyosarcoma has been divided into four main histopathologic subtypes: embryonal, alveolar, botryoid, and pleomorphic. The most common type in children is embryonal (75%). Botryoid tumors are really of the embryonal subtype but growing into a hollow space (e.g., vagina, bladder) so that they assume a characteristic grapelike appearance. Alveolar tumors are so named because of a resemblance to the microscopic structure of the lung (Fig. 99.8). Rhabdomyosarcomas are identified as alveolar if any alveolar elements are found in the tumor. Pleomorphic tumors usually occur in older adults. For all histologic types, sites of occurrence include (a) head and neck (orbit, infratemporal fossa); (b) genitourinary tract, including perineum and perianal area; (c) extremities; (d) trunk (chest wall, paraspinal area); (e) retroperitoneum; and (f) biliary tract.

The initial biopsy should be generous enough for cytogenetic and immunohistochemical studies. Light microscopy, itself, is no longer adequate to secure the diagnosis and establish histopathologic subtype. For instance, the alveolar subtype is currently characterized by a t(2;13) or t(1;13) translocation in which the *FKHR* gene on chromosome 13 is translocated onto either a *PAX3* (chromosome 2) or *PAX7* (chromosome 1) gene (65). Thus, even if minimal alveolar elements are noted on light microscopy, a tumor with either of these translocations would be classified as alveolar. Embryonal rhabdomyosarcoma is associated with hyperdiploidy and loss of heterozygosity at chromosome 11p15 or other genes (60,65,66). An initial clinical application of these findings is the detection of minimal residual disease by polymerase chain reaction (67).

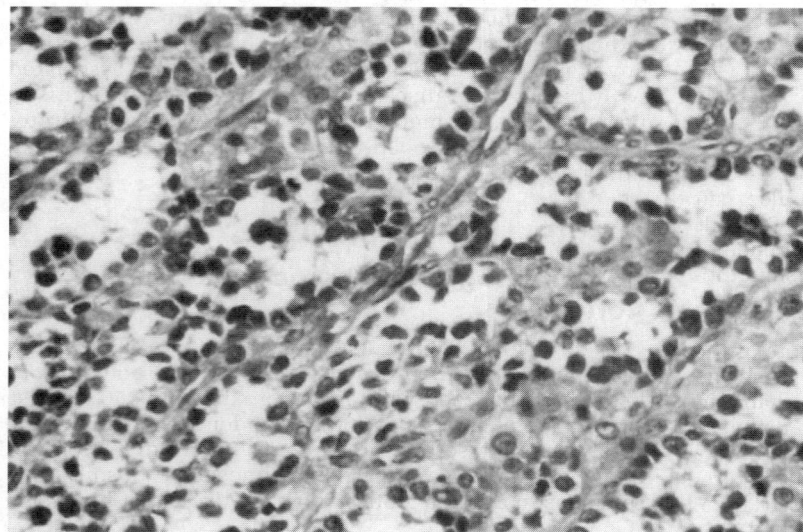

Figure 99.8. Photomicrograph illustrating the typical lunglike appearance of an alveolar rhabdomyosarcoma.

Presentation and Work-up

The incidence of rhabdomyosarcoma is biphasic, with one peak in infancy followed by a second in the adolescent years. Presentation is site dependent. Head and neck lesions can cause facial or cervical swelling and associated pain or skin discoloration. Sinusitis or middle ear infections can occur because the tumor blocks the normal drainage from these sites (i.e., sinusal ostia, eustachian tubes). Epistaxis, proptosis, or cranial nerve palsies may also be evident in head and neck lesions. Genitourinary tumors can present with gross or microscopic hematuria, a suprapubic mass, and urinary tract infection or obstruction. Vaginal and cervical primary tumors often prolapse through the vaginal orifice as a friable polypoid mass and may hemorrhage. Paratesticular lesions are most often observed in adolescence, and a hard mass above and separable by physical examination from the testis is observed. Extremity tumors present as a painless or painful expanding mass, and there may be an associated limp or overlying skin change. Local bony invasion may result in pathologic fractures.

Rational management depends on a thorough pretreatment work-up that completely defines local tumor extent as well as evaluating regional and distant sites of metastases. Table 99.6 lists the standard work-up for pediatric patients with sarcoma. An extensive history, including a family history of breast cancer or other forms of sarcoma, and a thorough physical examination are elementary. Radiographic staging has been markedly facilitated by modern imaging methods. Even greater progress in this area is promised by current efforts in the field of positron emission tomographic scanning, which allows determination of the metabolic activity of a tumor mass. Figure 99.9 is a CT scan of a large pelvic rhabdomyosarcoma originating from the bladder.

Staging

An evolution in sarcoma staging has occurred since the late 1980s, with most groups adopting the TNM (tumor, node, metastasis) system defined by the International Union Against Cancer (68). This staging system, which is used with the older IRS grouping, is listed in Table 99.7.

The TNM schema attempts to divide each stage into definable clinical components. It is applied before any therapeutic interventions (although a second staging based on histologic findings of the primary tumor and regional lymph nodes after resection can also be performed). The IRS grouping schema is retained as well, although it remains operator dependent.

Local tumor invasiveness is the result of cellular and molecular phenotypic properties, which are rapidly being defined by molecular analyses. The ability of cells to invade surrounding basement membranes depends on manufacture of a spectrum of lytic enzymes as well as cellular motility. Furthermore, regional or distant metastasis is not possible without initial cellular invasion. The gross invasiveness assessed for TNM staging is a rough measure of these cellular events. In this sense, the TNM system begins to relate macroscopic tumor behavior to the properties and interactions of individual tumor cells. Future directions include more precise definitions of the invasive process. Assays of collagenolytic activity and assessment of growth and invasion in nude mice are intermediate steps in this regard. Eventually, genetic determinants of invasion and metastases that are the final determinants of prognosis will be identified.

Using the TNM system, the reported overall percentage of patients with tumors greater than 5 cm ranges from 50% to 68%. The proportions of other staging variables include invasive tumors, 37% to 71%; regional nodal involvement, 7% to 28%; and distant metastases at diagnosis, 20% to 23%.

A sarcoma is adequately staged when the following criteria are met: (a) the primary tumor pathologic type and histopathologic subtype have been determined by biopsy, and (b) all components in the TNM staging system are known with reasonable certainty. It is preferable to sample metastatic regional lymph nodes, but extensive nodal dissections are not indicated. In the special case of paratesticular rhabdomyosarcoma, a limited dissection of ipsilateral, periaortic nodes is used as a determinant of the need for nodal radiation. The use of prechemotherapy nodal sampling in paratesticular rhabdomyosarcoma is controversial because many European groups favor chemotherapy along with radical orchiectomy as sole primary treatment. Most North American groups favor lymph node

---

Table 99.6. DIAGNOSTIC EVALUATION FOR SUSPECTED RHABDOMYOSARCOMA[a]

Examination or test	Rationale
History and physical examination	Search for lymph nodes, size of primary mass, general condition, underlying conditions
Complete blood count	Bone marrow replacement associated with anemia or thrombocytopenia; bone marrow toxicity is the major side effect of chemotherapy
Electrolytes, renal and hepatic function tests, creatinine clearance	Renal toxicity associated with cisplatin and other alkylators; genitourinary tumors may obstruct ureters; hepatic toxicity with dactinomycin
Four-site bone marrow aspirations, two-site bone biopsies	Bone marrow metastases reported in up to 6% of patients at diagnosis (29% of stage 4 patients have marrow involvement); bone marrow assessment before chemotherapy
Bone scan	Possibility of bone and bone marrow metastases
CT scan of the primary site	Evaluation of tumor size, invasiveness, enlargement of regional nodes, and complicating ureteral, biliary, bowel, or airway patency
CT scan of possible metastatic sites	CT scanning of the lungs and liver should be done to rule out parenchymal metastases. CT scanning is superior to MRI in assessing the degree of bone destruction in paraspinal, extremity, and head and neck (base of skull) lesions.
MRI	MRI is done for the same rationale as CT scanning. It may give more detailed information regarding the extent of viable tumor (T_2-weighted imaging) and the presence of hepatic metastases. It is also the most useful tool for evaluation of the epidural space in paraspinal or base of skull primaries.
Gallium scanning	Both the primary tumor and metastatic deposits may be identified by gallium scanning

[a]The same work-up is applicable to other high-grade sarcomas.
CT, computed tomography; MRI, magnetic resonance imaging.

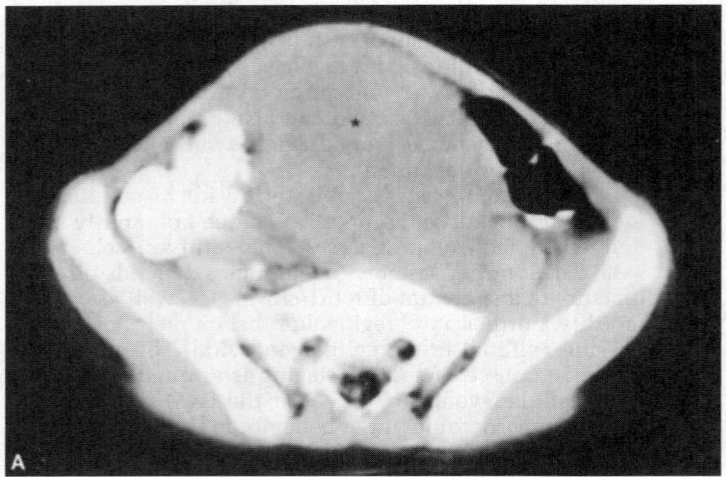

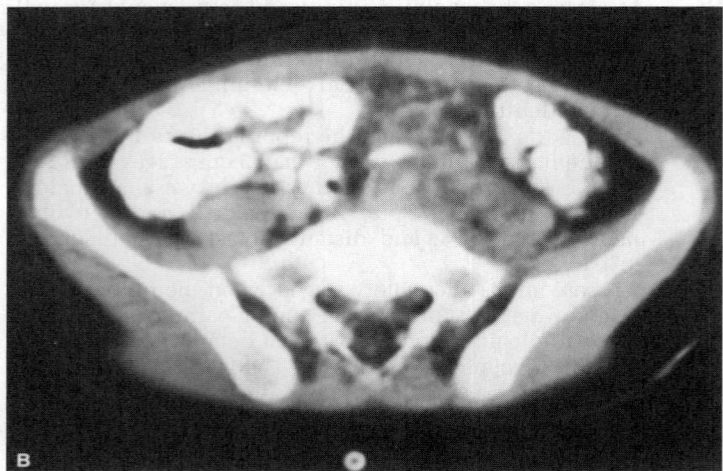

Figure 99.9. *(A)* Initial computed tomography (CT) scan of a child with a large pelvic rhabdomyosarcoma. *(B)* CT scan of the same child after biopsy and cytoreductive chemotherapy. No tumor was demonstrable by diagnostic imaging.

biopsy with consequent periaortic nodal radiation if N1 status is proved. Laparoscopic biopsy may prove a useful alternative in this regard.

Small, accessible primary lesions should undergo excisional biopsy. If this is done, the surgeon should attempt to obtain a clear microscopic margin. Larger infiltrating lesions and those whose removal would cause debilitation or deformity (i.e., amputation or cystectomy) should undergo limited incisional or endoscopic biopsy. It is acceptable to perform transperineal needle core biopsies for bladder neck or perineal primary tumors. Enough biopsy material for light and electron microscopic analysis, immunohistochemistry, and cytogenetics should be obtained. It is preferable to freeze extra tissue to facilitate

further specialized studies. Even though such investigations do not have direct short-term benefit for the patient, they are crucial in expanding knowledge concerning rhabdomyosarcoma. Tissue should be frozen in liquid nitrogen as soon as possible after biopsy.

Treatment

The modern treatment of rhabdomyosarcoma is multidisciplinary and includes multiagent chemotherapy, judicious resection, and radiation therapy. The intensity of therapy should be tailored to the risk of subsequent relapse, which is a function of TNM stage. In general, agents are combined to limit drug resistance while attaining a

Table 99.7. TNM STAGING SYSTEM FOR RHABDOMYOSARCOMA

Clinical stage	Invasiveness	Size	Status of nodes	Distant metastases
I	T1	a or b	N0	M0
II	T2	a or b	N0	M0
III	T1 or T2	a or b	N1	M0
IV	T1 or T2	a or b	N0 or N1	M1

T1, noninvasive; T2, invasive; Ta, ≤5 cm; Tb, >5 cm; N0, regional nodes negative; N1, nodes positive; M0, no distant metastases at diagnosis; M1, metastases present.

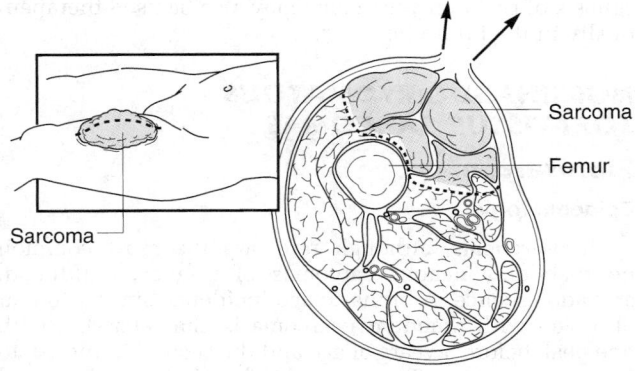

Figure 99.10. Technique for resection of a proximal lower-extremity rhabdomyosarcoma. Longitudinal incisions are always used. It is important to excise the tumor completely, with a surrounding 1- to 2-cm margin if feasible.

synergistic antitumor effect. A major surgical responsibility during chemotherapy is maintenance of adequate vascular access both for administration of medications as well as blood drawing. An external or implanted vascular access device usually can be inserted at the time of diagnostic biopsy.

Surgical resection of the primary tumor was the mainstay of treatment 30 years ago but resulted in overall survival rates of only approximately 20%. This rate improved to 50% with the addition of chemotherapy and resulted in uncertainty regarding the role of tumor resection in rhabdomyosarcoma. It is difficult to prove that surgical removal of the primary tumor affects survival. One reason is that a significant proportion of patients present with distant metastases, which so profoundly influences survival that the effect of other variables is obscured. Also, most tumors that can be readily removed without serious disfigurement or disability are resected. Thus, the effect of leaving a tumor in situ cannot readily be evaluated. With current survival rates, it would be unethical to randomize patients with nonmetastatic, resectable tumors to a nonsurgical arm. Complete resection of primary tumors should be undertaken either before chemotherapy for small, noninvasive lesions or after documented response with more formidable primary tumors. An example of the operative approach for a lower extremity rhabdomyosarcoma involving anterior thigh muscles is depicted in Fig. 99.10. In certain situations in which chemotherapy results in complete or very good tumor regression, external beam irradiation may be used

as a primary means of local control. Even in these circumstances, it is important to obtain biopsy specimens to document complete tumor eradication. Debilitating or disfiguring surgery should be performed only if residual tumor is present after both chemotherapy and therapeutic irradiation. Amputation of extremity rhabdomyosarcomas does not enhance cure and should be performed only when lesions are bulky, invade bone or neurovascular structures, or are recurrent. Similarly, radical cystectomy is reserved for situations in which complete tumor eradication has not been accomplished by chemotherapy and external beam irradiation. The guiding principle of rhabdomyosarcoma surgery is complete tumor resection, but removal of large amounts of normal tissue (i.e., muscle group resection, amputation) alone does not affect outcome.

External beam radiation therapy of the primary site or involved regional nodal echelons has contributed to locoregional control. Clinical data suggest that control of microscopic rhabdomyosarcoma can be accomplished with doses of 4,000 cGy, and gross deposits require in excess of 5400 cGy for sterilization (69).

Outcome

The overall 5-year survival for children with rhabdomyosarcoma is approximately 64% (60). Table 99.8 lists the results of studies analyzing the effects of various prognostic factors on outcome in rhabdomyosarcoma (70–76). As expected, the presence of distant parenchymal metastases at diagnosis has an overwhelming adverse effect on survival. Because of this, some groups have analyzed the effect of prognostic parameters in nonmetastatic subsets. Site and invasiveness of the primary tumor have also been independent predictors of outcome in some studies. Regarding site, most authors agree that orbital, paratesticular, and vaginal primary tumors are associated with improved outcome, whereas extremity, parameningeal, and truncal and retroperitoneal sites carry a worse prognosis. Survival is stage dependent. If all cases (both high and low risk) are included, the overall survival rate from rhabdomyosarcoma is approximately 50%.

Most studies conclude that overall and disease-free survival rates in rhabdomyosarcoma are equivalent; this means that salvage after initial relapse is negligible, making primary therapy crucial for long-term survival. This suggests that, after risk assessment by staging, therapy should be as intense as possible to eradicate the tumor. This may mean use of myeloablative therapy with autologous or peripheral stem cell rescue for high-risk patients. The effects of this intensive therapy on survival remain indeterminate.

Table 99.8. **COLLECTED INDICATORS OF OUTCOMES FOR RHABDOMYOSARCOMA**

Institution	Ref.	Year	Patients	Predictors of outcome
Memorial Sloan-Kettering Cancer Center	(70)	1994	290	Age at diagnosis, invasion, metastases, histology, regional lymph nodes
Italian Cooperative Group	(71)	1991	145	Site, size, alveolar histology, clinical group
International Rhabdomyosarcoma Workshop	(72)	1991	951	Invasiveness, site, interaction between invasiveness and site
Cooperative Soft Tissue Sarcoma Study (CWS-81)	(73)	1991	131	Site, degree of tumor regression after 7 wks of four-drug chemotherapy
Societé Internacionale Oncologique Pediatrique (SIOP)	(74)	1988	253	Site, stage, sex
Second Intergroup Rhabdomyosarcoma Study (IRS-2)	(75)	1993	1115	Site, stage, alveolar histology
IRS-3	(76)	1995	1062	Site, stage

Special Considerations for Specific Anatomic Sites

Head and Neck

Rhabdomyosarcoma can occur anywhere in the head and neck. Orbital sites in young children have a favorable outlook, but this is not true of older children. Parameningeal involvement has a very poor outcome. There is a high frequency of regional nodal involvement in head and neck rhabdomyosarcoma and regional node sampling may be important in determination of risk status (77). Resection of localized and anatomically accessible tumors may allow a reduction in radiation dosage with equivalent cure (78).

Bladder and Bladder–Prostate

In general, bladder and bladder-prostate rhabdomyosarcomas have a favorable prognosis. The trend since the early 1990s is to minimize treatment toxicity (79). Currently, patients with these tumors all receive neoadjuvant chemotherapy after cystoscopic or transperineal biopsies confirm the diagnosis. This is followed by repeat evaluations, including cystoscopic or percutaneous biopsies as well as imaging studies. A complete response after chemotherapy may obviate the need for external beam radiation therapy in some cases, but most patients require local radiation. Surgery is reserved for recurrent or poorly responsive cases with residual gross tumor (80). Partial cystectomy, when anatomically feasible, is effective and preserves bladder function (81). Newer techniques of urinary reconstruction involving catheterizable stomas may add to the patient's quality of life.

Paratesticular Rhabdomyosarcoma

An important point of discussion concerning patients with paratesticular rhabdomyosarcoma is the necessity of retroperitoneal lymph node dissection. Initially, this had been a formal recommendation for patients treated in North America. More recently, the IRS embarked on a study that used radiographic imaging rather than retroperitoneal nodal dissection to determine lymph node involvement (82). Patients with positive lymph nodes receive radiation therapy to the retroperitoneum. Unfortunately, results from these types of studies have shown an increased rate of recurrence in older patients who did not undergo surgical staging. The current recommendation is for ipsilateral, nerve-sparing lymph node dissection, especially in older patients.

Future Directions

The results of myeloablative regimens with bone marrow or peripheral stem cell rescue have not improved overall outcome in patients with recurrent or metastatic disease (83–85). Work is being done to refine the use of surgery and radiation therapy to maximize individual efficacy while diminishing toxicity. Interstitial brachytherapy and intraoperative radiation therapy are two areas of collaboration between the surgeon and radiation oncologist that are undergoing evaluation (86,87). Biologic or immunologic therapy for rhabdomyosarcoma is not available. Also, because insulin-like growth factor-2 is required for growth of rhabdomyosarcoma cells, strategies to inhibit this stimulus (suramin) may prove fruitful. There is a renewed interest in immunologic approaches to therapy in rhabdomyosarcoma (88–90). In the alveolar subtype, the presence of unique and specific chromosomal translocations may also provide a specific site for attack (91). Anti-MyoD1 and anti-myogenin antibodies used in the diagnosis of rhabdomyosarcoma may also be used therapeutically in the future (92).

NONRHABDOMYOMATOUS SOFT-TISSUE SARCOMAS

Fibrosarcoma

Epidemiology

Fibrosarcomas, although rare, are the most common nonrhabdomyomatous sarcomas of infancy, childhood, and adolescence. A biphasic age incidence similar to that observed with rhabdomyosarcoma is characteristic, with one peak before 5 years of age and the second in the 10- to 15-year age group. They are most frequently encountered on the extremities, with 70% of congenital fibrosarcomas occurring distally. Cases are equally distributed between the sexes. Most reports suggest that prognosis is better in younger children (93).

Pathology

Fibrosarcomas are spindle cell tumors characterized by a herringbone or interweaving pattern of tumors cells with a large amount of stromal collagen putatively arising from a fibroblastic lineage. Fibrosarcomas can be difficult, if not impossible, to distinguish from desmoid tumors or aggressive fibromatoses. For practical purposes, desmoids, fibromatoses, and low-grade fibrosarcomas can be thought of as a spectrum of similar and related neoplasms. Important characteristics of malignancy include nuclear pleomorphism, mitotic index, and basophilia. The tumor must be distinguished from undifferentiated rhabdomyosarcomas, neurofibrosarcoma, nodular fasciitis, myositis ossificans, and inflammatory pseudotumor. Infantile fibrosarcomas sometimes demonstrate a t(12;15) translocation (60).

Presentation and Diagnostic Evaluation

Congenital fibrosarcomas and those diagnosed in early childhood are usually located on the distal upper or lower extremity. The trunk is a secondary site. A hard, often infiltrating mass is appreciated, and there may be skin or deep fixation. Fibrosarcomas in the head and neck associated with swallowing and airway problems are also occasionally observed and may require life-saving tracheostomy. High-grade lesions may invade bony or neural structures and metastasize to lung or liver. Multifocal lesions with multiple primary tumors affecting an extremity are sometimes seen. Bone marrow metastases do not develop. Work-up is similar to that for rhabdomyosarcoma except that bone marrow aspiration and biopsy are not required.

Staging

The TNM schema is used, although lymph node metastases from fibrosarcoma are uncommon except with high-grade lesions. An adequate incisional or excisional biopsy, depending on the extent and invasiveness of the primary lesion, should be performed.

Treatment

The primary treatment of fibrosarcoma is surgical resection with negative microscopic margins if this can be done without significant debilitation or deformity. Occasionally, patients present with rapidly progressive or extensive lesions. Under these circumstances, an initial trial of systemic chemotherapy may result in gratifying tumor regression (94). In very young children (usually <5 years of age), these tumors can be indolent and may regress spontaneously. In cases in which complete resection requires mutilating surgery like amputation or laryngectomy, a plan of simple observation may be best. Often, the tumor mass is dormant for years, allowing growth of the affected part and the possibility of a less debilitating or deforming resection later. A margin of greater than 1 cm has been associated with a reduced rate of recurrence (95). Heroic resections should be performed only if the tumor is progressive or otherwise causing severe symptoms.

There is no defined role for systemic chemotherapy. Occasionally, high-grade lesions, especially in very young children, respond to a variety of agents. Chemotherapy may be tried for unresectable, symptomatic, and progressive lesions (96). Effective chemotherapeutic agents include doxorubicin, actinomycin D, vincristine, and cyclophosphamide, in various combinations. The combination of ifosfamide and etoposide has been shown effective in the treatment of metastatic fibrosarcoma. In summary, systemic chemotherapy may be useful for extensive or progressive lesions. A common initial regimen includes actinomycin D and vincristine, which are less toxic than alkylating agents.

In the only prospective, randomized trial (97), use of external beam radiation therapy was associated with a lower local recurrence rate for margin-positive low-grade sarcomas, including fibrosarcoma. Interstitial brachytherapy has been shown to lower local recurrence rates with margin-positive or -negative high-grade lesions. Despite this, most patients should initially be treated by wide surgical excision.

Outcome

The survival rate for low-grade nonmetastatic fibrosarcomas occurring in infancy is greater than 90%. Patients with metastatic disease have a guarded prognosis and require multidisciplinary therapy.

Tendosynovial Sarcoma

Epidemiology

Tendosynovial sarcoma is the third most common malignant pediatric soft-tissue tumor. In large combined adult and pediatric series, tendosynovial sarcomas constitute approximately 8% of all soft-tissue sarcomas. In a report of nonrhabdomyomatous soft-tissue sarcomas, this histologic type was identified in 29% of patients (98). The male/female distribution is 1:1.2 to 1.6. Most patients present in the early teenage years, but there is also a small incidence spike centered on 5 years of age, giving the familiar bimodal age distribution observed with other sarcomas.

Pathology

Tendosynovial sarcomas arise from the synovial tissue, which is ubiquitous in the body and helps compose tendons, joint membranes, and bursae. Synonyms include *synovioma* or *tendosynovioma, pseudoglandular synovial sarcoma, clear cell sarcoma,* and *chordoid sarcoma.* The lower extremity is the most common site of origin, with an equal distribution between the thigh, foot, and posterior knee. The shoulder and forearm are also relatively common areas of involvement. Tendosynovial sarcomas close to bone may incite a periosteal reaction. Other possible primary sites include the abdominal wall and trunk, and the head and neck, with the tongue and retropharyngeal or hypopharyngeal areas being the most common.

The most common metastatic sites are lung and pleura. Tendosynovial sarcomas are known to relapse in lung even decades after resection of the primary tumor. Metastases to regional lymph nodes and subcutaneous sites have been described but are rare. Terminally, metastases to multiple organs are possible.

Microscopically, tendosynovial sarcoma is divided into two subtypes, monophasic and diphasic. In the diphasic form, epithelioid cells and stromal spindle cells are observed. The epithelioid component is arranged in gland-like structures resembling true epithelial cells but devoid of basement membrane. The diphasic subtype has been associated with a better prognosis, but some studies have not verified this finding. The monophasic variant is the most common and consists of sheets and parallel cords of spindle-shaped cells with little cytoplasm and cigar-shaped nuclei. Prognosis has been reported to be worse with the monophasic histologic type. In synovial sarcoma, the t(X;18) translocation has been identified and is useful in diagnosis (99,100).

Presentation and Diagnostic Evaluation

An enlarging extremity mass brings most patients to medical attention. Pain may be prominent if bony or neural invasion is present. Regional lymph node metastases occur in 3% and distant metastases (lung) in 6% of patients at diagnosis. A work-up similar to that described for rhabdomyosarcoma is appropriate. Adequate radiographic imaging of the primary site is crucial because of the impact of complete resection on outcome.

Treatment

Chemotherapy has historically been ineffective, and the primary treatment of tendosynovial sarcoma is surgical. The goal is clear microscopic margins, and every effort should be made to accomplish this, including use of amputation. Limb-sparing procedures are acceptable if complete resection is accomplished. Incomplete removal results in a high rate of local recurrence.

Rosen and colleagues (101) have reported on the use of high-dose ifosfamide in the treatment of metastases from tendosynovial sarcoma. All 13 patients treated in this study had objective responses. Chemotherapy is reserved for patients who present with metastatic disease or in whom complete resection with clear microscopic margins cannot be accomplished.

Outcome

Overall survival rates are in the range of 43% to 75%. Important prognostic indicators are large primary tumor size and high nuclear grade with extensive tumor necrosis (high grade), as well as the presence of metastases at diagnosis. Worse survival rates are correlated with tumors greater than 10 cm in diameter at diagnosis, compared with those less than 5 cm, with 86% versus 22% 5-year survival rates. Studies have shown no effect of monophasic versus biphasic histologic type on outcome (102).

Peripheral Primitive Neuroectodermal Tumor

Epidemiology, Pathology, and Clinical Presentation

Peripheral PNET (peripheral neuroepithelioma, Askin's tumor, peripheral neuroblastoma) is a small, round blue cell malignancy distinguished from Ewing's sarcoma only by ultrastructural and immunocytochemical features. This tumor shares the t(11;22)(q24;q12) translocation with Ewing's sarcoma and esthesioneuroblastoma. The incidence is low, with 54 patients treated during a 20-year period reported from a major cancer center. Approximately two thirds of patients are 19 years of age or younger at diagnosis, and 57% are male. The disease affects predominantly white people, and 82% of tumors are localized at diagnosis. Common sites of involvement include chest wall (33%), pelvis (22%), paraspinal areas (13%), retroperitoneum (11%), limbs (9%), and abdomen (7%). In one study, epidural extension from the primary tumor was noted in 24% of patients at diagnosis, and 18% had distant metastases (103). None of the patients in this series who had chest wall primary tumors had distant metastases at diagnosis. All primary tumors were greater than 5 cm in diameter in at least one dimension. Urinary catecholamines are not elevated in peripheral PNET. There is no familial or sex predilection.

Light microscopic criteria include fairly uniform, poorly differentiated round cells arranged in cords, nests, or clusters; no spindle cells with fine reticular or collagenous processes; no ganglionic or schwannian differentiation; and positive immunostaining for neuron-specific enolase. Ultrastructurally, neurosecretory-like granules and tapering ("neuritic") cytoplasmic processes are evident.

Treatment

The outcome of PNET has been historically poor, whereas survival rates for Ewing's sarcoma, which is a related neoplasm sharing the typical t(11;22) translocation, have approached 60% to 65% in patients presenting without distant metastases. There may be underlying differences in fundamental biology, but the data also suggest that the uniform, multidisciplinary approach used for Ewing's sarcoma and including multiagent chemotherapy may have utility in the treatment of PNET. The diagnosis should be established by incisional biopsy and the patient quickly started on an intensive multiagent chemotherapy regimen. A dose–response effect of cyclophosphamide has been observed. Occasionally, the tumor can be completely resected before chemotherapy, and this should be done if feasible without an extensive procedure or the requirement for complicated reconstruction techniques. In most cases, definitive resection should be deferred until after administration of several cycles of systemic treatment. In general, surgery is required because complete responses to chemotherapy do not occur. External beam radiation therapy using 4,500 to 6,000 cGy can shrink but not cure macroscopic tumors. Radiation may be effective in improving local control after resection, especially if margins are microscopically positive.

Outcome

In patients with localized PNET at diagnosis, complete resection of all gross disease within 3 months resulted in improved progression-free survival (p = .0003) (103). The effect of myeloablative therapy with autologous bone marrow rescue is being evaluated.

Desmoplastic Small Round Cell Tumor

The desmoplastic small round cell tumor is a distinctive malignant neoplasm with a predilection for boys and young men. Eighty percent of patients present before the age of 30 years, and approximately half are 5 to 20 years of age at diagnosis (104). There is a striking male predominance (male/female ratio, 4.1:1), and most of the patients are white. A striking feature is the frequent occurrence of divergent, multilineage differentiation with expression of epithelial, neural, and myogenic immunophenotypes. The tumor is characterized by the t(11;22)(p13;q12) translocation.

Common presenting complaints include abdominal or back pain, abdominal distention or mass, acute abdomen, and bowel, biliary, or ureteral obstruction. Small nodules found in hernia sacs during repair have been the first indication the tumor. CT of the chest and abdomen using both gastrointestinal and vascular contrast is the most useful diagnostic procedure. Initial laparoscopic biopsy is adequate to establish the diagnosis and assess the extent of abdominal disease. Small serosal nodules not detected by imaging studies can be identified using laparoscopic magnification. A careful pelvic and serosal inspection should be carried out. Adequate tissue for immunohistochemistry, electron microscopy, and molecular biologic studies should be obtained.

Because desmoplastic small round cell tumor is a diffuse serosal malignancy, systemic chemotherapy using a dose-intensive sarcoma regimen is the initial treatment. Serial abdominal CT scans can be followed to judge response, remembering that small mucosal implants may escape detection with imaging studies. After four to seven cycles, exploratory laparotomy with resection of all gross disease is attempted. Consolidation chemotherapy and external beam radiation therapy to the primary site are then used. If diffuse peritoneal seeding is identified either at diagnostic or second-look laparotomy or laparoscopy, whole-abdomen irradiation is required. Myeloablative chemotherapy with autologous marrow reconstitution may also be necessary.

Of 19 reported patients with adequate follow-up, only 2 were disease free 2 and 3.5 years after diagnosis. The other 17 died from progressive disease within 6 months to 4 years after presentation. A recent report, however, suggests that outlook may be improved using a dose-intensive, multiagent chemotherapy regimen including cyclophosphamide, ifosfamide, etoposide, and doxorubicin (105). This justifies aggressive treatment for these patients, including extensive surgical debulking (106).

Neurofibrosarcoma

Neurofibrosarcomas (neurogenic sarcomas, malignant schwannomas, malignant nerve sheath tumor, malignant neurilemoma) constitute 5% to 10% of nonrhabdomyomatous soft-tissue sarcomas in childhood. Approximately 20% of all patients (children and adults) with neurofibrosarcoma have von Recklinghausen's disease [neurofibromatosis type I (NF1)], and a neurofibrosarcoma develops in 5% to 16% of patients with NF1. The incidence of NF1 in children with neurofibrosarcomas is as high as 66% (107). Neurofibrosarcomas have been reported as secondary tumors after external beam radiation therapy. Malignant peripheral nerve sheath tumors can be differentiated from their benign variant by the occurrence of more complex chromosomal abnormalities (108).

The most common sites in children are extremity (42%), retroperitoneum (25%), and trunk. Less than 10% of patients present with metastatic disease. Microscopically, the tumor resembles fibrosarcoma but is differentiated by the presence of schwannian elements. Whorly, storiform, and tactile body-like formations are observed, and the S-100 stain is positive in approximately 60% of cases. Ultrastructural findings are important distinguishing criteria, and in all suspected cases, a specimen should be sent for electron microscopy. Electron microscopic findings include the presence of schwannian differentiation with cytoplasmic concavities lacking neurites. Primary neurofibrosarcoma of skin and subcutaneous tissues has also been described.

Two thirds of patients have associated NF1, and aggressive diagnostic procedures, including biopsy, are warranted when enlarging extremity or truncal masses are observed. Pain may be prominent depending on location. Radicular or sciatic pain is reported with paraspinal or retroperitoneal tumors causing sciatic pressure. Spontaneous hemothorax has been reported with chest wall primary tumors. Pelvic tumors may present as a perineal or perianal mass. The primary treatment of neurofibrosarcoma is wide local excision. In one series of 20 patients (14 with NF1), local recurrence developed in 8 of 12 patients undergoing local tumor excision plus radiation or chemotherapy but in only 1 of 6 patients treated with radical excision as well as chemotherapy or irradiation (107). Unfortunately, a significant proportion had distant metastases despite local control. Patients with intermediate or high-grade neurofibrosarcomas should undergo radical local excision followed by chemotherapy and irradiation.

Leiomyosarcoma

Leiomyosarcoma accounts for 7% of soft-tissue sarcomas in adults but less than 2% of childhood sarcomas. The gastrointestinal (oropharynx to anus) or genitourinary tract, retroperitoneum, lungs, pulmonary artery, vascular wall (i.e., middle third of the inferior vena cava, saphenous or femoral vein), popliteal artery, sinonasal area, and peripheral soft tissues (i.e., extremities) are reported sites of involvement (109). Most cases are gastrointestinal in origin. The lungs are the most common site for metastases. Regional lymph node involvement occurs in 14% of gastric (perigastric nodes) and 5% of small intestinal leiomyosarcomas at diagnosis. Dissemination to liver and brain has also been reported. Also, tumors arising from gastrointestinal structures can disseminate throughout the peritoneal cavity. Leiomyosarcoma has been reported in patients with von Recklinghausen's disease and coincident with the occurrence of neurofibrosarcoma.

True leiomyosarcomas are derived from smooth muscle and are often pseudoencapsulated. Cytologically, they demonstrate uniform, elongated cells with cigar-shaped nuclei. An epithelioid variant with more aggressive behavior is reported to arise in up to 40% of cases. Bone marrow metastases are not reported.

The usual presentation is pain (up to 80%) or gastrointestinal bleeding (60%). There are also reports of presentation with intussusception and perforation of a Meckel's diverticulum. Congenital leiomyosarcoma associated with hydrops fetalis has also been reported. Double-contrast CT scans, gastrointestinal contrast studies, and endoscopy may aid in diagnosis.

The most effective treatment of leiomyosarcoma is complete surgical resection. This should be accomplished even when resection requires amputation or results in other disability because chemotherapy and radiation are ineffective. Reports have been made of long-term survival with resection in cases with hepatic and cerebral metastases. For gastrointestinal tumors, a 10-cm margin of bowel should be obtained along with a wide mesenteric resection. For gastric primary tumors, omentectomy is advised as well.

Overall, approximately half of gastrointestinal primary tumors can be resected for cure at diagnosis; in these patients, survival rates are 50% at 5 years and 35% at 10 years. In a series of gastrointestinal leiomyosarcomas reported by Ng and associates (110), overall survival was stage dependent; survival rates were 75% for stage I disease, 52% for stage II, 28% for stage III, and 7% to 12% for stage IV. Important determinants of disease-free survival in multivariate analysis included tumor rupture ($p = .002$), contiguous organ invasion ($p = .02$), and high tumor grade ($p = .02$). Size (>5 cm) and location have been found to predict outcome in other analyses. Pediatric colorectal leiomyosarcomas, although extremely rare, are reported to have a relatively favorable prognosis.

Liposarcoma and Alveolar Soft Parts Sarcoma

Liposarcomas are one of the most common types of soft-tissue sarcomas in adults but are extremely rare in childhood. The peak incidence is in the second decade of life, and there is equal distribution between the sexes. Most childhood tumors are of the myxoid histopathologic subtype and are low grade. The most common sites are, in order, the lower extremity, upper extremity, and retroperitoneum. A t(12;16) translocation has been described (111). The usual presenting complaint is a mass, which is often painless. Metastases are uncommon, with the lung being the most common site. Lymph node metastases are possible but extremely rare. The treatment of choice is complete surgical excision with negative microscopic margins.

Alveolar soft parts sarcoma is a rare tumor; only 102 cases were reported during a 50-year period. A t(X;17) translocation has been noted to occur in these tumors (112). The tumor is associated with skeletal muscle and fascial planes, and the thigh and buttocks are the most common sites of occurrence (39.5%), followed by abdominal and chest walls. The cell of origin is unknown and some have argued both for and against a skeletal muscle ontogeny. Approximately one third of patients have metastases at diagnosis, with the most common sites being lung, bone, and brain, in that order.

The primary treatment is surgical, and the roles of chemotherapy and radiation therapy remain undefined. Unfortunately, most patients experience relapse in distant sites and die from progressive disease, although this may take 20 years or longer.

HEPATIC TUMORS

Hepatoblastoma Versus Hepatocellular Carcinoma

From 1960 to the early 1970s, there were sporadic reports of survival from hepatoblastoma after successful surgical resection. The risks of major hepatic surgery were great, however, with operative and early postoperative mortality rates approaching 25%. Approximately two thirds of patients with hepatoblastoma had potentially resectable tumors, and complete surgical removal was associated with a 60% long-term survival rate. Systemic relapse was the most frequent cause of failure, and patients with locally unresectable disease or systemic spread at the outset were essentially incurable.

In 1975, the first consistent reports of success with doxorubicin appeared (113). Before this, many agents had been tested with only sporadic responses. Since then, major advances have occurred in both adjuvant chemotherapy for patients with resectable disease and cytoreductive therapy for unresectable disease. In 1982, the CCSG and Southwest Oncology Group reported a significant reduction in relapse rates after complete resections of hepatoblastoma using combination chemotherapy with vincristine, cyclophosphamide, doxorubicin, and 5-fluorouracil (114). The long-term relapse-free survival rate in patients with stage I disease was reported at 94%.

Shortly thereafter, reports appeared of dramatic tumor necrosis and cure in patients with unresectable tumors and metastatic disease using doxorubicin and cisplatin as single or combined agents, with delayed resection (115). Prospective trials with combinations of doxorubicin and cisplatin have confirmed these results, and patients with initially unresectable hepatoblastoma can now achieve long-term survival rates in the range of 60% to 70% (116).

Despite this period of progress in the treatment of hepatoblastoma, the treatment of children with hepatocellular carcinoma remains problematic and their outcome poor. A complete resection is initially possible in only 10% to 20% of patients, and the problems of local and systemic relapse remain. Despite response to chemotherapy in some instances, children with unresectable disease usually remain unresectable or relapse after resection. Early diagnosis by screening of patients with genetic defects and families with hepatitis B is unlikely to have a major impact in Western nations. Research with different drug combinations, the use of new agents, and increasing the accessibility to transplantation programs may provide some hope. Developments in monoclonal antibody technology have produced exciting results with other tumors, but their use in hepatocellular carcinoma is still experimental.

Epidemiology

In Europe and North America, primary liver tumors constitute approximately 1.1% of childhood malignant neoplasms (1.4 cases per 1 million children in the United States) (117). The ratio of hepatoblastoma to hepatocellular carcinoma is variously reported from 1.3:1 to 6.5:1, but in areas endemic for hepatitis B, the ratio may be reversed and as low as 0.2:1. No geographic clustering of cases of hepatoblastoma has been noted. A male predominance is usually reported for both tumors, the ratio ranging from 1.5:1 to 3.1:1 for hepatoblastoma and from 1.3:1 to 3.2:1 for hepatocellular carcinoma.

Hepatoblastoma has been reported to occur sporadically in adults, but the tumor usually presents in the first 3 years of life. Congenital presentation and antenatal diagnosis have also been reported (118). Hepatocellular carcinoma, on the other hand, is rare in infancy. In one large series of children and adults with hepatic tumors, no cases of hepatocellular carcinoma occurred in patients aged 4 years or younger in a cohort of 2,286 patients. Historical series without pathologic review may report a higher rate of infantile hepatoma because of misdiagnosis of some early hepatoblastomas.

Clinical Presentation

Children with hepatoblastoma most commonly present with abdominal mass or diffuse abdominal swelling. Not infrequently, the child is in good health, and the lesion may be discovered by an observant parent or clinician on routine examination. Accompanying symptoms, such as pain, irritability, minor gastrointestinal disturbances, fevers, and pallor, occur in smaller numbers of patients. Significant weight loss is unusual, although patients may fail to thrive.

In contrast, although children and adolescents with hepatocellular carcinoma frequently present with palpable abdominal masses, these are rarely incidental. Pain is a frequent accompaniment and can occur in the absence of an obvious mass. Constitutional disturbances, such as anorexia, malaise, nausea and vomiting, and significant weight loss, occur with greater frequency. Jaundice is an uncommon feature of either disease.

In most series of hepatoblastoma and hepatocellular carcinoma, small numbers of patients present acutely with tumor rupture. Hepatoblastoma can present with sexual precocity from androgen synthesis, although this is rare.

Laboratory Studies

Mild anemia is common in both conditions, and thrombocytosis is most often seen in patients with hepatoblastoma, but this has also been reported in occasional patients with hepatocellular carcinoma (119). The cause for this is unknown but may be related to release of tumor-derived cytokines.

Liver function test results are usually nonspecifically deranged in both conditions. A high serum cholesterol level is present in 50% to 60% of cases, and there is evidence to suggest that higher elevations may correlate with a poorer prognosis. The most useful tumor marker is the serum α-fetoprotein (AFP). Elevation, often extreme, occurs in approximately 84% to 91% of cases of hepatoblastoma. Fewer patients with hepatocellular carcinoma have elevated AFP levels, and the elevation tends to be less marked. Although nonspecific for epithelial liver tumors, the AFP marker is used extensively to monitor both disease reduction in patients undergoing nonoperative therapy and disease recurrence in treated patients. Some reports concluded that a rise in AFP above normal in a patient with quiescent disease is more sensitive than radiology or surgical exploration at detecting recurrence.

Imaging Studies

Abdominal CT scanning is the investigation of choice both for diagnostic discrimination and to assess operability. The chest should be included to identify pulmonary metastases. The typical appearance of hepatoblastoma is that of a solitary mass with lower attenuation values than normal liver (Fig. 99.11). Dramatic contrast enhancement (as in benign vascular neoplasms), invasion of the portal vein, and lymph node involvement are unusual. Hepatocellular carcinomas have a similar appearance but are more likely to be multifocal, invade the portal vein, and metastasize to draining lymph nodes. Distinction between the two lesions cannot be definite because the pattern of disease may be atypical in either instance.

The diagnostic ability of MRI is similar to that of CT. The particular features of both hepatoblastoma and hepatocellular carcinoma on MRI are low signal intensity on T_1-weighted images and high intensity on T_2-weighted images. The two lesions cannot be distinguished by appearance alone.

Plain radiographs and liver–spleen scans usually indicate abnormalities but do not often contribute to diagnosis or assist in planning therapy. Angiography is indicated if embolization or infusion chemotherapy is contemplated, but this test is invasive, technically difficult in childhood, and not universally available. Similar information is available from dynamic CT scan or MRI such that these are considered adequate in most instances.

An abdominal ultrasound, in view of the low cost and ready accessibility, is probably the most useful screening investigation for children with large livers. This allows distinction between space-occupying lesions and diffuse hepatomegaly. Anatomic detail of the tumor margin is not usually sufficiently well delineated to assess resectability. Doppler ultrasound is also useful to evaluate patency of the inferior vena cava and hepatic veins, but extreme compression of these vessels may prevent useful interpretation.

The ability of imaging studies to predict resectability is questionable. Resectable lesions must usually be confined to the right lobe, right lobe plus medial left lobe, or the left lobe; in addition, the hepatic veins, inferior vena cava, and portal vein must be free of disease. On occasion, the distinction between compression versus invasion of liver adjacent to the lesion cannot be made, nor can the patency of vessels be established with certainty. In rare instances, it may be obvious that metastases in the remaining liver,

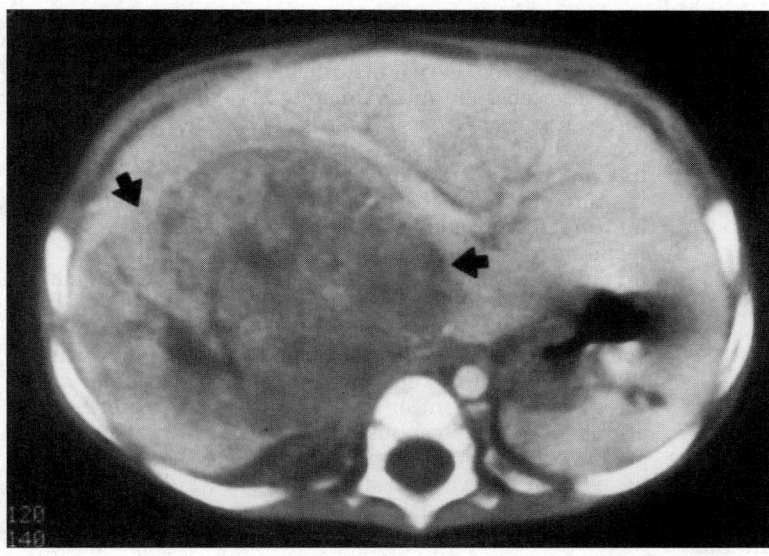

Figure 99.11. Computed tomography scan of a 2-year-old child with a large right lobar hepatoblastoma *(arrows)*. Despite the large size, these lesions can often be completely resected before chemotherapy. Hepatocellular carcinoma, in contrast, often involves multiple hepatic segments, and there is a significant incidence of extrahepatic extension.

portal or periaortic nodes, or other intraabdominal organs preclude complete resection.

The available data do not establish any superiority of MRI or CT scan for evaluating the resectability of hepatic malignancies in children. In view of the possible advantage of primary resection, a more reliable option is to judge resectability at formal laparotomy.

Staging

A staging system was derived by the CCG and the Southwest Oncology Group to compare prognosis and outcome in various intergroup study protocols. Modifications have occurred, and the system in most frequent use is shown in Table 99.9. Stage is best determined operatively in most instances. Alternatively, a TNM classification has been proposed by the International Union Against Cancer and the American Joint Committee on Cancer, and another by the Japanese Society for Pediatric Surgery.

Pathology

Hepatoblastoma usually presents as a single, pseudoencapsulated lesion, often reaching large proportions before becoming clinically apparent. The tumor grows in an expansive fashion such that the umbilical fissure usually is not breached. Thus, despite a 30% to 40% incidence of bilobar disease, successful extended resection may still be possible. Multicentricity or massive diffuse disease within the liver occurs in less than 20% of patients, and cirrhosis of the surrounding liver is unusual.

In contrast, hepatocellular carcinoma usually lacks a distinct capsule. The tumor spreads diffusely through the liver in as much as 70% of patients, often with satellite nodules well separated from the main tumor mass. Bilobar involvement occurs in 50% to 70% of cases, and the umbilical fissure does not constitute a barrier to spread. As a result, hepatocellular carcinoma is usually unresectable. Finally, because of the association of hepatocellular carcinoma with hepatitis B infection, cirrhosis may be present in the surrounding nonneoplastic liver. This may preclude complete tumor resection if the volume of liver to be removed is likely to compromise liver function further.

The epithelial element of hepatoblastoma can display a range of differentiation from a frankly anaplastic form (indistinguishable on light microscopy from other small cell neoplasms of childhood) to embryonal differentiation (cellular arrangement resembles early ducts of embryonal liver) or fetal differentiation (cells resemble normal but small hepatocytes). In addition to the epithelial element, hepatoblastoma may contain varying amounts of immature stromal tissue, often containing osteoid.

A pure fetal pattern is said to be favorable and the presence of embryonal or undifferentiated histologic types unfavorable. Pure fetal histologic type has been associated with improved resectability and better long-term survival. One analysis (120) showed that resected patients with pure fetal histologic type have a 2-year survival rate of 92%, which is significantly better than patients with embryonal or anaplastic tumor components (63% and 0% 2-year survival rates, respectively). In contrast, anaplastic histologic type is unfavorable and may not be chemore-

Table 99.9. RELATION OF STAGING TO PROGNOSIS FOR HEPATOBLASTOMA

Clinical group	Criteria	Relative risk for death of disease
I	Complete resection of tumor as initial treatment, regardless of resectional technique	0.16
IIA	Complete resection after irradiation or chemotherapy	0.57[a]
IIB	Residual disease confined to one lobe	—
III	Disease involving both hepatic lobes	2.87
IIIB	Regional nodal involvement	—
IV	Distant metastases, regardless of the extent of the hepatic tumor	3.51

[a]Relative risk was assessed for stage II and III patients collectively. The relative risk is compared with other stages.

Table 99.10. COMPARISON OF RELATIVE RISK OF DEATH FOR HISTOLOGIC SUBTYPES OF HEPATOBLASTOMA

Histopathologic subtype	Relative risk for death of disease[a]
Fetal	1.07
Embryonal	1.74
Mixed	0.53
Macrotrabecular pattern	1.20
Small cell undifferentiated	3.71

[a]Risk of death adjusted for age, sex, and stage compared with other histologic subtypes

sponsive. A comparison of the relative risks of death for subtypes is listed in Table 99.10.

The fibrolamellar subtype of hepatocellular carcinoma is characterized by broad fibrous septa that separate the cellular component into nodules and is most commonly seen in late childhood and adolescence. It is associated with a better prognosis and a higher resection rate. This difference, however, may not be independent of stage. Ten to 20% of patients with hepatoblastoma present with distant metastases. The locations of metastases at autopsy in 46 patients in one report (121) were the lungs in 46%, portal and periaortic nodes in 11%, brain in 7%, and peritoneum and diaphragm in 4% each. The incidence of metastases is reportedly higher in patients with embryonal and anaplastic histologic types (80% and 100%, respectively) as opposed to fetal differentiation (29%).

Hepatocellular carcinoma presents with metastatic disease in 30% to 50% of patients. The location of metastases at autopsy was reported by the Liver Cancer Study Group of Japan (122). The lungs were involved in 48% of patients, lymph nodes in 37%, intraperitoneal organs in 16%, peritoneum in 15%, adrenal in 11%, bone in 10%, brain in 2%, and skin in 1%. Tumor emboli were detected in the portal vein in 59.7% and in the hepatic vein in 26.6% of patients. The higher incidence of lymphatic and intraabdominal spread in hepatocellular carcinoma is relevant to local resectability and recurrence. Nodal disease in the porta hepatis and periaortic region is not readily resectable, and recurrence is inevitable if such disease is present.

Treatment

Hepatoblastoma

Complete surgical resection remains the major objective of therapy for hepatoblastoma. At presentation, approximately 60% of patients with hepatoblastoma have resectable tumors, and one review reported no survivors among children who underwent biopsy only or incomplete resection. More recently, sporadic patients who received nonoperative treatments have achieved complete response (123,124), and chemotherapy and radiation therapy have been able to salvage some patients whose tumors were incompletely resected at the primary site.

A nonanatomic resection, wedging out the tumor with a satisfactory margin, may be feasible in the uncommon instance of a small peripheral or pedunculated lesion. More often, a major anatomic resection is required, depending on tumor location and extent. As much as 85% of hepatic substance may be removed, with subsequent full and rapid regeneration despite the administration of postoperative chemotherapy (125). The principles of safe hepatic

resection are now well developed, and a considerable reduction in operative mortality rates has been possible since the 1970s. In two historical series, the mortality rate was reported to be approximately 22%, but in more recent series, it was as low as 0% to 3% (126,127). Invasive monitoring during anesthesia allows the precise control of central venous and arterial blood pressure to the advantage of minimizing blood loss. Clotting factors and platelets are more readily available. Postoperative measures, such as respiratory and hemodynamic support, antibiotics, and total parenteral nutrition, have all made significant contributions to overall patient care.

The surgical principles include wide exposure using a generous bilateral subcostal incision and dissection at the liver hilum with isolation of vascular and ductal structures of the segment or lobe to be resected. After hepatic arterial and portal venous inflow to the relevant area is ligated, a color demarcation acts a guide to the correct plane of division of liver substance and allows this to proceed with minimal blood loss. Technologic advances such as the Cavitron ultrasonic aspirator and metallic clip applicators have made this step less hazardous in terms of hemorrhage, although finger-fracture technique with individual vessel and duct suture–ligation remains an acceptable alternative. Hemostasis of the transected surface can be completed with use of the argon beam coagulator or electrocautery and topical agents such as thrombin and Gelfoam. A trend to eliminate use of abdominal drains in uncomplicated cases has emerged.

Approximately 40% of patients with hepatoblastoma have inoperable tumors at presentation. Bilaterality, diffuse multicentricity, and metastatic lesions may all preclude resection. Various techniques have been used to increase the resectability rates. These include preoperative chemotherapy, profound hypothermia with circulatory arrest, and total hepatic vascular occlusion. These maneuvers are a useful part of the surgical armamentarium in selected instances. For truly unresectable disease, aside from transplantation, chemotherapy is the major treatment option available. During the 1990s, it has become evident that some of these tumors may be rendered resectable by preoperative therapy. A randomized trial performed through an intergroup collaboration of the CCG and POG showed that survival was equivalent when either doxorubicin plus cisplatin or a combination of vincristine, cisplatin, and 5-fluorouracil was administered. In contrast, toxic side effects were significantly increased in patients receiving the former regimen. It is recommended that all patients with hepatoblastoma undergo initial treatment with vincristine, cisplatin, and 5-fluorouracil.

The role of radiation therapy is not clearly defined. In treating patients with bulky disease, the tolerance of normal liver is not compatible with the doses that would be required for tumor ablation, although temporary stability may be achieved. Hepatic toxicity has been described at doses to the whole liver of greater than 25 Gy. Focal radiation up to 45 Gy can be administered with safety. There may be a place for radiation in a dose range of 25 to 45 Gy combined with chemotherapy in inoperable hepatoblastoma and in patients with postresectional residual disease. In one report, eight patients were treated after incomplete resections (four with gross and four with microscopic residual disease) with combined irradiation and chemotherapy; six of these patients were free of disease at 4 to 83 months' follow-up (124).

Other treatments with encouraging results are in developmental phases. Intraarterial infusion chemotherapy and orthotopic liver transplantation may extend the definition of resectability as clear indications emerge. The intraarterial route allows the administration of agents directly to the tumor with the theoretic advantage of less systemic toxicity. Some agents with a high hepatic extraction (e.g., doxorubicin, cisplatin, and fluorodeoxyuridine) have been shown to be useful in hepatoblastoma. Several anecdotal reports exist of dramatic responses in unresectable disease, allowing subsequent resection. Yokomori and colleagues (122) reported on the treatment of a 4-month-old infant with fetal hepatoblastoma using intraarterial therapy consisting of 5-fluorouracil, vincristine, doxorubicin, and cisplatin for 18 months. Total tumor regression occurred, and the child remained well at 6 years' follow-up. The technique, although promising, is not without hazards, such as catheter infection, thrombosis, and displacement. It is technically difficult in children. In a large review (123) of recurrence and survival rates in 597 patients who received liver transplants, a recurrence rate of 40% was found in patients with hepatoblastoma, with 2- and 5-year survival rates of only 32% and 7%, respectively. Until prospective studies of arterial infusion, including chemoembolization, or hepatic transplantation are available, these modalities should be considered investigational.

With improving management of the primary lesion, mortality is increasingly the result of metastatic relapse in the lungs. If metastases demonstrate progression or relapse on therapy, surgical resection is an option. Cure of pulmonary metastatic disease has not been demonstrated with radiation therapy. One series (129) reported the operative treatment of five cases of pulmonary metastatic disease that developed after successful management of the primary tumor. All lesions developed during or soon after chemotherapy. Four patients were free of disease at 8 to 83 months' follow-up, despite having multiple lesions and requiring more than one resection in two cases. No patients with hepatoblastoma with metastases to sites other than lung or regional nodes have been reported cured.

Hepatocellular Carcinoma

Analogous to hepatoblastoma, complete surgical resection is a prerequisite for cure in hepatocellular carcinoma of childhood. Patients with incompletely resected tumors do not survive. Although patients undergoing resection survive longer than those who do not, the gain is small owing to the high local and systemic relapse rates. The Japanese Liver Cancer Study Group reported a 40% 1-year survival rate for resectable disease and 10% for unresectable lesions.

Stage for stage, the prognosis of hepatocellular carcinoma is said to be no worse than that for hepatoblastoma. Many more patients present with advanced hepatocellular carcinoma, however, owing to the prevalence of bilobar and multicentric tumors and extrahepatic extension rendering them unresectable. Nodal and systemic metastatic disease is more common at the outset. The liver may be cirrhotic in some instances, precluding an extensive resection short of transplantation.

Most series report the percentage of children with resectable hepatocellular carcinoma to be approximately 10% to 20%. Patients with fibrolamellar histologic pattern may be an exception, with a resection rate of 48% to 60%. Relapse after resection is common. A POG and CCG intergroup study showed no impact of either cisplatin plus doxorubicin or cisplatin, vincristine, and 5-fluorouracil on outcome in patients with hepatocellular carcinoma. The overall survival rate in the pediatric age group for hepatocellular carcinoma is rarely reported to exceed 20% and more realistically approaches zero. A role for external beam radiation therapy has not been established. Only temporary stability of bulky disease has been demonstrated, and radiation has also failed to decrease the relapse rate in patients with minimal disease after surgical resection.

In view of poor results for conventional therapy, there may be a place for liver transplantation. In one report, treatment of nine patients who had hepatocellular carcinoma by transplantation resulted in four survivors with a median follow up of 2.3 years. Longer follow-up will be necessary to recognize the true recurrence rate and intercurrent mortality rate.

Outcome

After a successful complete surgical resection and without further treatment, long-term survival can be expected in approximately 60% to 80% of patients with hepatoblastoma. Local relapse is unusual, and the most frequent cause of failure in the remaining 20% to 40% is systemic relapse. The overall cure rate with surgery alone is approximately 35%, and all patients should receive preoperative or postoperative systemic chemotherapy.

REFERENCES

1. Miller RW. U.S. childhood cancer deaths by cell type. *J Pediatr* 1974;85:664.
2. Kramer S, Jarrett P, Evans A. Incidence of childhood cancer: experience of a decade in a population-based registry. *J Natl Cancer Inst* 1983;70:49.
3. Goodman MT, Smith MA, Olshan AF. Sympathetic nervous system tumors. In: Ries LAG, Gurney JG, Linet M, et al., eds. *Cancer incidence and survival among children and adolescents: United States SEER Program 1975–1995.* NIH publication no. 99-4649. Bethesda, MD: National Cancer Institute SEER Program, 1999:65–72.
4. Young JLJ, Silverberg E, Horm JW, et al. Cancer incidence, survival, and mortality for children younger than 15 years. *Cancer* 1986;58[Suppl 2]:598.
5. Brodeur GM. Principles and practice of pediatric oncology. In: Pizzo PA, ed. *Neuroblastoma.* Philadelphia: JB Lippincott, 1993:739.
6. Allen RW, Bentley FL, Jung AL. Fetal hydantoin syndrome neuroblastoma and hemorrhagic disease in a neonate. *JAMA* 1980;244:1464.
7. Kinney H, Brazy J. The fetal alcohol syndrome and neuroblastoma. *Pediatrics* 1980;66:130.
8. Pivnick EK, et al. Simultaneous adrenocortical carcinoma and ganglioneuroblastoma in a child with Turner syndrome and germline p53 mutation. *J Med Genet* 1998;35:328–332.
9. Geraci AP, et al. Ganglioneuroblastoma and ganglioneuroma in association with neurofibromatosis type I: report of three cases. *J Child Neurol* 1998;13:356–358.
10. Olshan AF. Epidemiology of neuroblastoma. In: Brodeur GM, Tsuchida Y, Voute PA, eds. *Neuroblastoma.* New York: Elsevier, 2000:33–39.
11. Brodeur GM, Schwab M, Varmus HE, et al. Amplification of N-myc in untreated human neuroblastomas correlates with advanced disease stage. *Science* 1984;224:1121.
12. Marui ST, Sakai T, Hosokawa N, et al. N-myc suppression and cell cycle arrest at G1 phase by prostaglandins. *FEBS Lett* 1990;270:15.
13. Caron H. Allelic loss of chromosome 1 and additional chromosome 17 material are both unfavorable prognostic markers in neuroblastoma. *Med Pediatr Oncol* 1995;24:215.
14. Bader FC, Brodeur GM, Stanbridge EJ. Dissociation of suppression of tumorigenicity and differentiation in vitro effected by transfer of single human chromosomes into human neuroblastoma cells. *Cell Growth Differ* 1991;2:245–255.
15. Bown N, et al. Gain of chromosome arm 17q and adverse outcome in patients with neuroblastoma [see comments]. *N Engl J Med* 1999;340:1954–1961.
16. Nakagawara A, Arima M, Azar CG, et al. Inverse relationship between TRK expression and N-myc amplification in human neuroblastomas. *Cancer Res* 1992;52:1364.
17. Nakagawara A, Arima-Nakagawara M, Scavarda NJ, et al. Association between high levels of expression of the TRK gene

and favorable outcome in human neuroblastoma. *N Engl J Med* 1993;328:847.

18. Kogner P, Barbany G, Dominici C, et al. Coexpression of the messenger for RNA for TRK protooncogene and low affinity nerve growth factor receptor in neuroblastoma with favorable prognosis. *Cancer Res* 1993;53:2044–2050.

19. Kramer K, et al. Correlation of MYCN amplification, Trk-A and CD44 expression with clinical stage in 250 patients with neuroblastoma. *Eur J Cancer* 1997;33:2098–2100.

20. Ryden M, et al. Expression of mRNA for the neurotrophin receptor trkC in neuroblastomas with favourable tumour stage and good prognosis. *Br J Cancer* 1996;74:773–779.

21. Le Douarin LD. *The neural crest.* New York: Cambridge University Press, 1984.

22. Triche TJ, Askin FB, Kissane JM. Neuroblastoma, Ewing's sarcoma, and the differential diagnosis of small-, round-, blue-cell tumors. In: Finegold M, ed. *Pathology of neoplasia in children and adolescents.* Philadelphia: WB Saunders, 1986.

23. Shimada H, Chatton J, Newton WA Jr, et al. Histopathologic prognostic factors in neuroblastic tumors: definition of subtypes of ganglioneuroblastoma and an age-linked classification of neuroblastomas. *J Natl Cancer Inst* 1984;73:405.

24. Carlsen NL. The new International Neuroblastoma Staging System: some critical notes [Letter; comment]. *J Clin Oncol* 1990;8:935–936.

25. Kushner BH, La Quaglia MP, Bonilla MA, et al. Highly effective induction therapy for stage 4 neuroblastoma in children over 1 year of age. *J Clin Oncol* 1994;12:2607.

26. Matthay KK, et al. Treatment of high-risk neuroblastoma with intensive chemotherapy, radiotherapy, autologous bone marrow transplantation, and 13-cis-retinoic acid: Children's Cancer Group. *N Engl J Med* 1999;341:1165–1173.

27. Bernstein L, Goodman MT, Smith MA, et al. Renal tumors. In Ries LAG, Gurney JG, Linet M, et al., eds. *Cancer incidence and survival among children and adolescents: United States SEER Program 1975–1995.* NIH publication no. 99-4649. Bethesda, MD: National Cancer Institute SEER Program, 1999:79–90.

28. D'Angio GJ, Bishop HC, et al. The National Wilms' Tumor Study: a progress report. *Proceedings of the National Cancer Conference* 1972;7:627.

29. Crist WM. Common solid tumors of childhood. *N Engl J Med* 1991;324:461.

30. Breslow N, Ciol M, Sharples K. Age distribution of Wilms' tumor. *Cancer Res* 1988;48:1653.

31. Breslow NE. Epidemiological features of Wilms' tumor: results of the national Wilms' tumor study. *J Natl Cancer Inst* 1982;68:429–436.

32. Rose EA, Glaser T, Jones C, et al. Complete physical map of the WAGR region of 11p13 localizes a candidate Wilms' tumor gene. *Cell* 1990;60:495.

33. Francke U, Holmes LB, Atkins L, et al. Aniridia-Wilms' tumor association: evidence for specific deletion of 11p13. *Cytogenet Cell Genet* 1979;24:185.

34. Maw MA, Grundy PE, Millow LG, et al. A third Wilms' tumor locus on chromosome 16q. *Cancer Res* 1992;52:3094.

35. Grundy P, Kousfos A, Morgan K, et al. Familial predisposition to Wilms' tumor does not map to short arm of chromosome 11. *Nature* 1988;336:374.

36. Green DM, D'Angio GJ, Beckwith JB, et al. Wilms' tumor (nephroblastoma, renal embryoma). In: Pizzo PA, ed. *Principles and practice of pediatric oncology.* Philadelphia: JB Lippincott, 1993:725.

37. Mahoney JP, Saffos RO. Fetal rhabdomyomatous nephroblastoma with a renal pelvic mass simulating sarcoma botryoides. *Am J Pathol* 1981;5:297.

38. Larson E, Perez-Atayde AR, Green DM, et al. Surgery only for the treatment of patients with stage I (Cassidy) Wilms' tumor. *Cancer* 1990;66:264.

39. Green DM, Breslow M, Beckwith JB, et al. Treatment outcomes in patients less than two years of age with small stage I favorable histology Wilms' tumor: a National Wilms' Tumor Study. *J Clin Oncol* 1993;11:91.

40. Malcom AW, Jaffe N, Folkman MJ, et al. Bilateral Wilms' tumor. *Int J Radiat Oncol Biol Phys* 1980;6:167.

41. Montgomery BT, Kelalis PP, Blute ML, et al. Extended follow up of bilateral Wilms' tumor study: results of National Wilms' Tumor Study. *J Urol* 1991;146:514.

42. Ritchey ML, Othersen HB Jr, de Lorimier AA, et al. Renal vein involvement with nephroblastoma: a report of the National Wilms' Tumor Study-3. *Eur Urol* 1990;17:139.

43. Ritchey ML, Kelalis PP, Breslow NB, et al. Surgical complications after nephrectomy for Wilms' tumor: a report from the National Wilms' Tumor Study-3. *Surg Gynecol Obstet* 1992;175:507.

44. Ward SP, Dehner LP. Sacrococcygeal teratoma with nephroblastoma (Wilms' tumor): a variant of extragonadal teratoma in childhood—a histologic and ultrastructural study. *Cancer* 1974;33:1355.

45. Luchtrath H, de Leon F, Giesen H, et al. Inguinal nephroblastoma. *Virchows Arch A* 1984;405:113.

46. Naito K, Yokoyama O, Yamaguchi K, et al. Extrarenal nephroblastoma: report of a case and review of the literature. *Hinyokika Kiyo* 1985;31:1773.

47. Wexler H, Poole C, Fojaco R. Metastatic neonatal Wilms' tumor: a case report with review of the literature. *Pediatr Radiol* 1975;3:179.

48. Hrabovsky EE, Othersen HB Jr, de Lorimier A, et al. Wilms' tumor in the neonate: a report from the National Wilms' Tumor Study. *J Pediatr Surg* 1986;21:385.

49. Babaian RJ, Skinner DG, Waisman J. Wilms' tumor in the adult patient: diagnosis, management, and a review of the world medical literature. *Cancer* 1980;45:1713–1719.

50. Byrd RL, Evans AE, D'Angio GJ. Adult Wilms' tumor: effects of combined therapy on survival. *J Urol* 1982;127:648.

51. Hupperets PS, Havenith MG, Blijham GH. Recurrent adult nephroblastoma: long-term remission after surgery plus adjuvant high-dose chemotherapy, radiation therapy, and allogenic bone marrow transplantation. *Cancer* 1992;69:2990.

52. Marsden HB, Lawler W, Kumar PM. Bone metastasizing renal tumour of childhood: morphological and clinical features, and differences from Wilms' tumor. *Cancer* 1978;42:1922.

53. Beckwith JB. Wilms' tumor and other renal tumors of childhood: a selective review from the National Wilms' Tumor Study Pathology Center. *Hum Pathol* 1983;14:481.

54. Green DM, Moksness J, Breslow NE, et al. The treatment of children with clear cell sarcoma of the kidney (CCSK): a report from the National Wilms' Tumor Study (NWTS) [Abstract]. *Proceedings of the Annual Meeting of the American Association for Cancer Research* 1994;35:A1428.

55. Beckwith JB, Palmer NF. Histopathology and prognosis of Wilms' tumor: results from the National Wilms' Tumor Study. *Cancer* 1978;41:1937.

56. Eftekhari F, Erly WK, Jaffe N. Malignant rhabdoid tumor of the kidney: imaging features in two cases. *Pediatr Radiol* 1990;21:39.

57. Bolande RP, Brough AJ, Izant RJ. Congenital mesoblastic nephroma of infancy. *Pediatrics* 1967;40:272.

58. Knezevich SR, et al. ETV6-NTRK3 gene fusions and trisomy 11 establish a histogenetic link between mesoblastic nephroma and congenital fibrosarcoma. *Cancer Res* 1998;58:5046–5048.

59. Aronson DC, Medary I, Finlay JL, et al. Renal cell carcinoma in childhood and adolescence: a retrospective survey for prognostic factors in 22 cases. *J Pediatr Surg* 1996;31:183.

60. Gurney JG, Roffers SD, Smith MA, et al. Soft tissue sarcomas. In: Ries LAG, Gurney JG, Linet M, et al., eds. *Cancer incidence and survival among children and adolescents: United States SEER Program 1975–1995.* NIH publication no. 99-4649. Bethesda, MD: National Cancer Institute SEER Program, 1999:111–123.

61. Young JL, Miller RW. Incidence of malignant tumors in U.S. children. *J Pediatr* 1975;86:254.

62. Ruymann FB, Maddux HR, Ragab A, et al. Congenital anomalies associated with rhabdomyosarcoma: an autopsy study of 115 cases: a report from the Intergroup Rhabdomyosarcoma Study Committee. *Med Pediatr Oncol* 1988;16:33.

63. Davis RL, Weintrub H, Lassar AB. Expression of a single transfected cDNA converts fibroblasts to myoblasts. *Cell* 1987;51:987.

64. Dias P, Parham DM, Shapiro DN, et al. Myogenic regulatory protein (MyoD1) expression in childhood solid tumors: di-

agnostic utility in rhabdomyosarcoma. *Am J Pathol* 1990;
137:1283.

65. Barr FG. Molecular genetics and pathogenesis of rhabdomyosarcoma. *J Pediatr Hematol Oncol* 1997;19:483–491.

66. Bridge JA, et al. Novel genomic imbalances in embryonal rhabdomyosarcoma revealed by comparative genomic hybridization and fluorescence in situ hybridization: an Intergroup Rhabdomyosarcoma Study. *Genes Chromosomes Cancer* 2000;27:337–344.

67. Kelly KM, Womer RB, Barr FG. Minimal disease detection in patients with alveolar rhabdomyosarcoma using a reverse transcriptase-polymerase chain reaction method. *Cancer* 1996;78:1320–1327.

68. Harmer MH, ed. *TNM classification of pediatric tumors.* Geneva: International Union Against Cancer, 1982:23.

69. Mandell L, Ghavimi F, Peretz T, et al. Radiocurability of microscopic disease in childhood rhabdomyosarcoma with radiation doses less than 4,000 cGy. *J Clin Oncol* 1990;8:1536.

70. La Quaglia MP, Heller G, Ghavimi F, et al. The effect of age at diagnosis on outcome in rhabdomyosarcoma. *Cancer* 1994;73:109.

71. Carli M, Guglielmi M, Sotti G, et al. Prognostic factors in children with rhabdomyosarcoma (RMS): results of the Italian cooperative study RMS-79 [Abstract]. *Med Pediatr Oncol* 1991;19:398.

72. Rodary C, Gehan EA, Flamant F, et al. Prognostic factors in 951 children with non-metastatic rhabdomyosarcoma: a report from the International Rhabdomyosarcoma Workshop. *Med Pediatr Oncol* 1991;19:89.

73. Suder J, Stienen U, Kaatsch P, et al. Analysis of prognostic factors in rhabdomyosarcoma: preliminary univariate and multivariate results of the Soft Tissue Sarcoma Study (CWS-81). *Klin Padiatr* 1986;198:218.

74. Rodary C, Rey A, Rezvani A, et al. Prognostic factors in rhabdomyosarcomas in childhood: study carried out with 253 children registered by the International Society of Pediatric Oncology. *Bull Cancer* 1988;75:213.

75. Maurer HM, Gehan EA, Beltangady M, et al. The Intergroup Rhabdomyosarcoma Study-II. *Cancer* 1993;71:1904.

76. Crist W, Gehan EA, Ragab AH, et al. The Third Intergroup Rhabdomyosarcoma Study. *J Clin Oncol* 1995;13:610.

77. Kraus DH, et al. Pediatric rhabdomyosarcoma of the head and neck. *Am J Surg* 1997;174:556–560.

78. Daya H, et al. Pediatric rhabdomyosarcoma of the head and neck: is there a place for surgical management? *Arch Otolaryngol Head Neck Surg* 2000;126:468–472.

79. LaQuaglia M. Genitourinary rhabdomyosarcoma in children. *Urol Clin North Am* 1991;18:575–580.

80. Lobe TE, et al. The argument for conservative, delayed surgery in the management of prostatic rhabdomyosarcoma. *J Pediatr Surg* 1996;31:1084–1087.

81. Hays DM, et al. Children with vesical rhabdomyosarcoma (RMS) treated by partial cystectomy with neoadjuvant or adjuvant chemotherapy, with or without radiotherapy: a report from the Intergroup Rhabdomyosarcoma Study (IRS) Committee [published erratum appears in *J Pediatr Hematol Oncol* 1995;17:356]. *J Pediatr Hematol Oncol* 1995;17:46–52.

82. Wiener ES, et al. Retroperitoneal node biopsy in paratesticular rhabdomyosarcoma. *J Pediatr Surg* 1994;29:171–177; discussion, 178.

83. Carli M, et al. High-dose melphalan with autologous stem-cell rescue in metastatic rhabdomyosarcoma. *J Clin Oncol* 1999;17(9):2796–2803.

84. Boulad F, et al. High-dose induction chemoradiotherapy followed by autologous bone marrow transplantation as consolidation therapy in rhabdomyosarcoma, extraosseous Ewing's sarcoma, and undifferentiated sarcoma. *J Clin Oncol* 1998;16(5):1697–1706.

85. Koscielniak E, et al. Do patients with metastatic and recurrent rhabdomyosarcoma benefit from high-dose therapy with hematopoietic rescue? Report of the German/Austrian Pediatric Bone Marrow Transplantation Group. *Bone Marrow Transplant* 1997;19(3):227–231.

86. Zelefsky MJ, et al. Preliminary results of phase I/II study of high-dose-rate intraoperative radiation therapy for pediatric tumors. *J Surg Oncol* 1996;62(4):267–272.

87. Merchant TE, et al. High-dose rate intraoperative radiation therapy for pediatric solid tumors. *Med Pediatr Oncol* 1998;30(1):34–39.

88. Evans R, et al. IL-15 mediates anti-tumor effects after cyclophosphamide injection of tumor-bearing mice and enhances adoptive immunotherapy: the potential role of NK cell subpopulations. *Cell Immunol* 1997;179:66–73.

89. Evans R, et al. The therapeutic efficacy of murine anti-tumor T cells: freshly isolated T cells are more therapeutic than T cells expanded in vitro. *Anticancer Res* 1995;15:441–447.

90. Evans R, Kamdar SJ, Duffy TM. Qualitative and quantitative intratumoral changes in gene expression following cyclophosphamide injection and the adoptive transfer of T cells: the potential contribution of tumor-associated macrophages. *Int J Cancer* 1994;56:568–573.

91. Mackall C, Berzofsky J, Helman LJ. Targeting tumor specific translocations in sarcomas in pediatric patients for immunotherapy. *Clin Orthop* 2000;373:25–31.

92. Cui S, et al. Evaluation of new monoclonal anti-MyoD1 and anti-myogenin antibodies for the diagnosis of rhabdomyosarcoma. *Pathol Int* 1999;49:62–68.

93. Soule EH, Pritchard DJ. Fibrosarcoma of infants and children: a review of 110 cases. *Cancer* 1977;40:1711.

94. Shetty AK, et al. Role of chemotherapy in the treatment of infantile fibrosarcoma. *Med Pediatr Oncol* 1999;33:425–427.

95. Blakely ML, et al. The impact of margin of resection on outcome in pediatric nonrhabdomyosarcoma soft tissue sarcoma. *J Pediatr Surg* 1999;34:672–675.

96. Ben Arush MW, et al. The role of chemotherapy in childhood soft tissue sarcomas other than rhabdomyosarcomas: experience of the Northern Israel Oncology Center. *Pediatr Hematol Oncol* 1999;16:397–406.

97. Pisters PN, Harrison CB, Woodruff JM, et al. A prospective randomized trial of adjuvant brachytherapy in the management of low-grade soft tissue sarcomas of the extremity and superficial trunk. *J Clin Oncol* 1994;12:115.

98. Horowitz ME, Pratt CB, Webber BL, et al. Therapy of childhood soft-tissue sarcomas other than rhabdomyosarcoma: a review of 62 cases treated at a single institution. *J Clin Oncol* 1986;4:559.

99. Birdsall S, et al. Synovial sarcoma specific translocation associated with both epithelial and spindle cell components. *Int J Cancer* 1999;82:605–608.

100. Inagaki H, et al. Detection of SYT-SSX fusion transcript in synovial sarcoma using archival cytologic specimens. *Am J Clin Pathol* 1999;111:528–533.

101. Rosen G, Forscher C, Lowenbraun S, et al. Synovial sarcoma: uniform response of metastases to high dose ifosfamide. *Cancer* 1994;73:2506.

102. Brodsky JT, Burt ME, Hajdu SI, et al. Tendosynovial sarcoma: clinicopathologic features, treatment, and prognosis. *Cancer* 1992;70:484.

103. Kushner BH, Hajdu SI, Gulati SC, et al. Extracranial primitive neuroectodermal tumor. *Cancer* 1991;67:1825.

104. Gerald WL, Rosai J. Desmoplastic small round cell tumor with multi-phenotypic differentiation. *Zentralbl Pathol* 1993;139:141.

105. Kushner BH, et al. Desmoplastic small round-cell tumor: prolonged progression-free survival with aggressive multimodality therapy. *J Clin Oncol* 1996;14(5):1525–1531.

106. Schwarz RE, et al. Desmoplastic small round cell tumors: prognostic indicators and results of surgical management. *Ann Surg Oncol* 1998;5:416–422.

107. Riccardi VM, Powell PP. Neurofibrosarcoma as a complication of von Recklinghausen neurofibromatosis. *Neurofibromatosis* 1989;2:152–165.

108. Mertens F, et al. Cytogenetic characterization of peripheral nerve sheath tumours: a report of the CHAMP study group. *J Pathol* 2000;190:31–38.

109. Swanson PE, Wick MR, Dehner LP. Leiomyosarcoma of the somatic soft tissues in childhood: an immunohistochemical analysis of six cases with ultrastructural correlation. *Hum Pathol* 1991;22:569.

110. Ng EH, Pollock RE, Munsell MF, et al. Prognostic factors influencing survival in gastrointestinal leiomyosarcomas: implications for surgical management and staging. *Ann Surg* 1992;215:68.

111. Rabbitts TH, et al. Fusion of the dominant negative transcription regulator CHOP with a novel gene FUS by translocation t(12;16) in malignant liposarcoma. *Nat Genet* 1993;4: 175–180.

112. Joyama S, et al. Chromosome rearrangement at 17q25 and xp11.2 in alveolar soft-part sarcoma: a case report and review of the literature. *Cancer* 1999;86:1246–1250.

113. Olweny CL, Toya T, Kantongole-Mbidde E, et al. Treatment of hepatocellular carcinoma with Adriamycin. *Cancer* 1975;36:1250.

114. Evans AE, Land VJ, Newton WA, et al. Combination chemotherapy (vincristine, Adriamycin, cyclophosphamide, and 5-fluorouracil) in the treatment of children with malignant hepatoma. *Cancer* 1982;50:821.

115. Quinn JJ, Altman AJ, Robinson HT, et al. Adriamycin and cisplatinum for hepatoblastoma. *Cancer* 1985;56:1926.

116. Ortega JA, Krailo MD, Haas JE, et al. Effective treatment of unresectable or metastatic hepatoblastoma with cisplatinum and continuous infusion doxorubicin chemotherapy: a report from the Children's Cancer Study Group. *J Clin Oncol* 1991;9:2167.

117. Ni Y, Chang M, Hsu H, et al. Hepatocellular carcinoma in childhood: clinical manifestations and prognosis. *Cancer* 1991;68:1737.

118. Weinberg AG, Finegold MJ. Primary hepatic tumors of childhood. *Hum Pathol* 1983;14:512.

119. Nickerson HJ, Silberman TL, McDona TP. Hepatoblastoma, thrombocytosis, and increased thrombopoietin. *Cancer* 1980;45:315.

120. Haas JE, Mukzynski KA, Krailo M, et al. Histopathology and prognosis in childhood hepatoblastoma and hepatocellular carcinoma. *Cancer* 1989;64:1082.

121. Lack EE, Neave C, Vawter GF. Hepatocellular carcinoma: review of 32 cases in childhood and adolescence. *Cancer* 1983;52:1510.

122. The Liver Cancer Study Group of Japan. Primary liver cancer in Japan. *Cancer* 1987;60:1400.

123. Weinblatt ME, Siegel SE, Siegel MM, et al. Preoperative chemotherapy for unresectable primary hepatic malignancies in children. *Cancer* 1982;50:1061.

124. Habrand JL, Nehme D, Kalifa C, et al. Is there a place for radiation therapy in the management of hepatoblastomas and hepatocellular carcinoma in children? *Int J Radiat Oncol Biol Phys* 1992;23:525.

125. Taylor PH, Filler RM, Nebesar NA, et al. Experience with hepatic resection in childhood. *Am J Surg* 1969;117:435.

126. Exelby PR, Filler RM, Grosfeld JL. Liver tumors in children in the particular reference to hepatoblastoma and hepatocellular carcinoma: American Academy of Pediatrics Surgical Section Survey—1974. *J Pediatr Surg* 1975;10:329.

127. Lee CS, Sung JL, Hwang LY, et al. Surgical treatment of 109 patients with symptomatic and asymptomatic hepatocellular carcinoma. *Surgery* 1986;99:481.

128. Yokomori K, Hori T, Asoh S, et al. Complete disappearance of unresectable hepatoblastoma by continuous infusion therapy through the hepatic artery. *J Pediatr Surg* 1991;26:830.

129. Black CT, Luck SR, Musemeche CA, et al. Aggressive excision of pulmonary metastases is warranted in the management of childhood hepatic tumors. *J Pediatr Surg* 1991;26: 1082.

SURGERY: SCIENTIFIC PRINCIPLES AND PRACTICE, Third Edition, edited by
Lazar J. Greenfield, Michael W. Mulholland, Keith T. Oldham, Gerald B. Zelenock,
and Keith D. Lillemoe. Lippincott Williams & Wilkins Publishers, Philadelphia, © 2001.

CHAPTER 100

ORTHOPEDIC SURGERY

H. DAVID MOEHRING

ORTHOPEDIC OVERVIEW

Rapid developments in the field of molecular biology and tissue engineering promise great advances in the next decade and will modify or radically change current orthopedic philosophies. Minimally invasive techniques and "biologic fixation" will continue to evolve for fracture treatment. Arthroscopic applications and innovations will expand outpatient treatment of joint disease. Endoscopic-assisted spine surgery, biodegradable implants, and artificial joint lubricants will experience increasing evolution. Gene therapy and the development of chondroprotective agents hold promise for the prevention and treatment of osteoporosis and arthritis.

Osteogenic proteins, also referred to as *bone morphogenetic proteins,* are low-molecular-weight polypeptides that have been isolated from the bones of a variety of mammalian species and also reproduced by recombinant techniques. They have been shown to be capable of osteoinduction and the healing of gap defects and frank nonunions of bone, and promise accelerated healing of problem fractures and more effective bone graft substitutes (1).

Angiogenic growth factors are considered promising candidates for the induction of neovascularization of the ischemic myocardium and in the promotion of wound and bone healing. Similarly, endothelial progenitor cells involved in physiologic and pathologic neovascularization can be isolated from bone marrow and peripheral blood. Pluripotent stem cells exist in the connective tissue of postnatal mammals, including humans, and have the capacity to self-renew and form multiple tissue types throughout their life span.

Growth factors can be introduced directly or gene therapy techniques can be used to introduce genetically modified cells that are capable of producing the programmed growth factors in vivo. As the field of tissue engineering develops, generating three-dimensional tissue structures will become a reality, and cells grown on a biocompatible scaffold will allow for development of tissues in vitro or in vivo. Such tissues can replace a functional tissue or stimulate repair. Articular cartilage repair using cartilage constructs grown in vitro with in vivo remodeling is a current example. Chondrocytes are isolated, grown in culture, and successfully implanted into small chondral defects in the knee. Future tissue engineering techniques can be expected to be directed at chondral resurfacing of large joints, creation of small joints, and, eventually, the modification or replacement of mechanical joint arthroplasty by biologic constructs. Anatomically correct bones have been produced experimentally, and it is likely that entire bones with articular cartilage can be made through advanced tissue engineering (2).

Neural stem cells and new biomaterials hold promise for reconstruction and repair of spinal cord injury. Exciting advances in tissue engineering, stem cell biology, and gene therapy promise great benefits in the near future. The next decade will see increased focus on the biologic aspects of soft-tissue and fracture healing as more is learned about the multiple factors involved in this process (3).

Historical Perspectives

Fracture treatment began in ancient Egypt with splints made of sticks or pieces of wood wrapped with linen bandages to immobilize the fracture and reduce pain. Hippocrates advocated stiffening the bandages with lard mixed with wax, resin, or pitch. Little attention was paid to reduction, and fractures often healed in a malaligned position. Later, through trial and error, various types of splints were discovered that improved functional results after fracture healing (4).

Casting techniques as we know them today were developed in 1851. The first external fixator was developed in the 1840s using percutaneous methods and a claw-and-screw construct to treat a nonunited patellar fracture. The technique of "pins in plaster," whereby pins inserted above fracture fragments were incorporated in a plaster cast to immobilize a reduced fracture, and the first attempt at open reduction and internal fixation of the tibia were both reported in approximately 1900. They were defeated by the metallurgy of the time and the high complication rate of infection, nonunion, and even death (4,5).

Reconstructive procedures for the treatment of posttraumatic, congenital, and arthritic disorders evolved, broadening the orthopedic armamentarium. Plating techniques for the treatment of fractures were introduced in the first half of the 20th century. However, the wide acceptance of the principles of open reduction and internal fixation awaited the introduction of sound surgical methodology and implant technology developed in the 1960s by the Swiss AO group. These techniques are especially valuable in the treatment of the polytrauma patient with multiple fractures (4).

The need for surgical specialization according to anatomic region and specific organ systems became apparent in the early part of the 20th century. Some of the most famous contributors to orthopedic knowledge were general surgeons. It was their interest in developing orthopedics as a specialty that led to the formation of the American Board of Orthopaedic Surgery in 1934. As in other surgical specialties, appropriate subspecialization has occurred, focusing the wide spectrum of musculoskeletal disease into distinct regional areas that are discussed in this chapter. The interested reader is referred to a selected bibliography for an in-depth focus on areas of particular interest.

ORTHOPEDIC ASPECTS OF POLYTRAUMA

Musculoskeletal trauma remains a continuing problem in modern society, and prompt diagnosis and emergent treatment of fractures and dislocations is crucial to optimal patient outcomes (Fig. 100.1). It is vitally important to recognize the potential for associated neurovascular injury, occult or frequently missed injuries, and other pitfalls in diagnosis. Although minor soft-tissue injuries and many isolated fractures are adequately treated without surgery, advanced surgical techniques have resulted in improved treatment of major soft-tissue and bone injuries. Early coverage of exposed bone, neurovascular, and tendinous structures with local muscle flap, skin grafts, or remote microvascular grafts and advanced techniques for the treatment of extremity and spine trauma have been developed in the 1990s. Aggressive surgical treatments of in-

traarticular fractures and modern implant technology have resulted in shortened healing times and improved results.

A significant portion of the aggressive approach to orthopedic injuries can be attributed to safer anesthesia and improved patient monitoring and postoperative care.

Orthopedic injuries fall into two basic types: blunt and penetrating. The latter are readily diagnosed, usually more localized, and infrequently associated with fracture, except for gunshot wounds. Penetrating trauma is more likely to cause neurovascular injury, whereas blunt trauma results in greater energy absorption over a wider area, with fractures, dislocations, and associated systemic trauma (4).

Diagnosis

Isolated displaced fractures or dislocations are readily diagnosed on physical examination. The classic findings are pain, deformity, crepitus, and inability to bear weight or use an extremity. Undisplaced or minimally displaced fractures are diagnosed by radiography. Polytrauma patients frequently present a greater diagnostic challenge because resuscitation, treatment of life-threatening injuries, and orthopedic assessment proceed simultaneously.

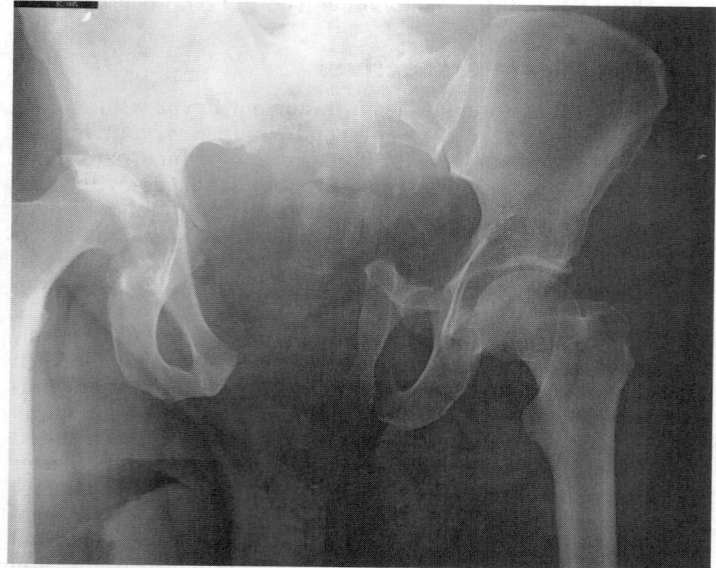

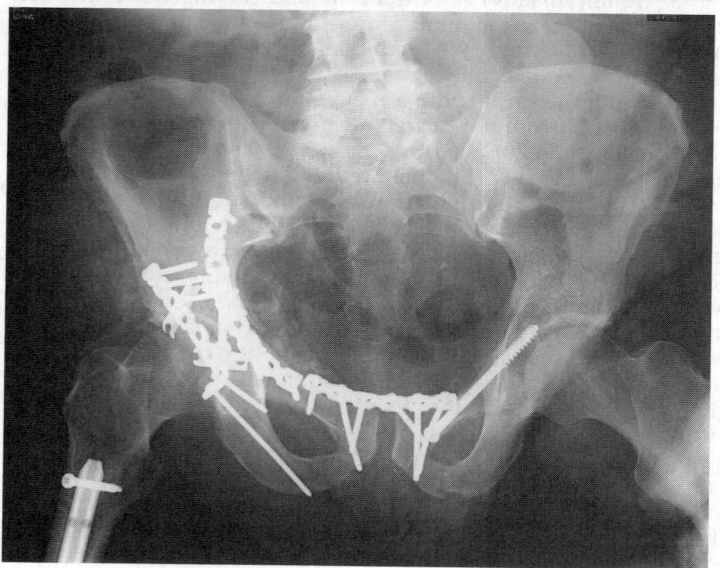

Figure 100.1. Polytrauma victim. *(A)* Grade III open pelvic disruption with associated urogenital injury. Orthopedic injuries include pubic diastasis, left sacroiliac dislocation, left superior and inferior pubic rami fractures, right acetabular fracture and hip dislocation, and right femoral fracture. *(B)* The same patient, 6 weeks after staged open reduction and internal fixation of right acetabular fracture and pubic diastasis with pelvic reconstruction plates, retrograde left superior ramus lag screw, and retrograde interlocked intramedullary rod for associated right femoral fracture.

Initial Survey

The initial survey is discussed more fully elsewhere (see Chapter 11). After the establishment of an airway, venous access, and volume replacement, a rapid orthopedic evaluation is made by palpation of the entire spine for step-offs and assessment of the pelvis for instability and the extremities for deformity or open injury. A cervical collar should always be provided and spine precautions continued until injury has been ruled out clinically and radiographically.

Extremity bleeding is controlled by direct pressure, avoiding tourniquets or direct ligation except in uncontrollable hemorrhage. Deformities should be corrected and fractures splinted before radiographic evaluation. Emergent radiographic evaluation includes a lateral view of the cervical spine to include the C-7 vertebra, and anteroposterior radiographs of the chest and pelvis.

Secondary Survey

After stabilization of the patient, more specific examination for spinal and orthopedic injuries can be undertaken. The patient should be logrolled gently to inspect the spine and sacral areas and to detect occult or open fractures of the pelvis or extremities (4). Areas suspect for fracture undergo standard regional radiographs. Computed tomography (CT) scans are extremely valuable in evaluating head, spinal, abdominal, and pelvic trauma (6). Occasionally, magnetic resonance imaging (MRI) is indicated to detect acute disc herniation as a cause of quadriplegia or other spinal cord injury in the absence of other obvious causes.

Open Fractures

Open fractures have significantly greater incidences of infection and nonunion, especially when they involve the tibia (7–9). Clinically, the diagnosis is usually obvious; however, small punctures or wounds at a distance from the fracture can be overlooked. The most important determinants of outcome with open fractures are the size of the open wound, the degree of soft-tissue damage, and the extent of contamination (7) (Table 100.1). Uncomplicated grade I open fractures have a prognosis similar to that of closed fractures, but require débridement, especially if they occur in an organically contaminated environment.

Treatment

In the emergency department, open fractures should be irrigated with sterile saline solution and a gauze dressing applied, followed by alignment and splinting of the fracture. Formal irrigation and débridement in the operating room should be rapidly accomplished. Open fractures that are irrigated and débrided greater than 6 hours after injury have a higher incidence of infection. Coincident with emergent splinting and sterile dressing, tetanus toxoid and a broad-spectrum intravenous (IV) antibiotic should be administered. A first-generation cephalosporin is administered for low-grade (grade I and II) open injuries, an aminoglycoside is added for more extensive injury, and anaerobic coverage (triple antibiotics) for highly contaminated open fractures (8) (Table 100.2).

The operating room débridement removes all devitalized soft tissue and small fragments of bone without vascular attachments and lavages the open fracture with pulsed saline irrigation. The wound is left open or packed with antibiotic beads and loosely approximated with sutures. Alternatively, an oxygen-permeable membrane can be applied over the open wound, which is packed with antibiotic beads, until the patient is returned to the operating room in 48 to 72 hours for repeat irrigation and débridement. Local antibiotic beads elute high levels of antibiotics and are used in conjunction with IV antibiotics (10). When the wound appears clean and there is no evidence of necrotic tissue, delayed primary closure or split-thickness skin grafting may be undertaken. Two or three débridements may be necessary. Extensive areas of exposed bone should be covered by local or regional muscle flaps or, if necessary, microvascular free flap. The goal is to have a closed wound within the first 5 to 7 days if at all possible.

Stabilization of Open Fractures

Controversy exists regarding the best form of stabilization after open fracture. In the lower extremity, most grade II and certain grade III open shaft fractures can be treated with intramedullary fixation, either initially or within the first week of injury (11). Grade III fractures with a high degree of contamination are best treated by external fixation, but it is difficult to produce definitive fracture healing. External fixation can be converted to intramedullary fixation if done within the first week or two, and in the tibia, external fixation may also be followed by cast immobilization once soft-tissue considerations permit (9).

Plating of open tibial shaft fractures should rarely if ever be performed in the acute setting, although it is mandatory to fix open articular injuries internally. Bulky implants should be avoided because soft-tissue necrosis resulting in exposed metal and bone may ensue. Hybrid external fixation is used for intraarticular fractures with associated traumatized soft tissue and high-grade open fractures, especially those involving the knee and ankle. This type of fixation uses tensioned Kirschner wire–ring constructs connected by external carbon rods to pins placed in the diaphysis of a long bone (Fig. 100.2). Using ligamentotaxis and indirect techniques or limited open reduction and cannulated subarticular screws, a reasonable reconstruction of the joint surface can usually be obtained (12).

Table 100.1. GUSTILLO AND ANDERSON CLASSIFICATION OF OPEN FRACTURES[a]

	Wound size	Soft tissue
Grade I	<1 cm	No or minimal tissue damage
Grade II	>1 cm	Moderate tissue damage
Grade III	>10 cm	Major tissue damage
		Soft-tissue loss
		Bone loss
		Gross contamination
Grade IIIa		Bone can be covered
Grade IIIb		Bone cannot be covered
Grade IIIc		Vascular injury requiring repair

[a]Interobserver variation occurs, but this is the most widely accepted and useful classification.

Table 100.2. ANTIBIOTIC REGIMEN FOR OPEN FRACTURES

Grade I	Cefazolin 1 g q4h while in OR, q8h thereafter
Grade II	Cefazolin as for grade I fractures
Grade III	Cefazolin as for grade I fractures
	Penicillin-G 2 million U q4h
	Gentamicin 2.0 mg/kg load for young and healthy patients, 1.6 mg/kg load q8h maintenance

Intravenous antibiotics should be begun as soon as possible after open fracture. Local antibiotic beads should also be considered in grade III open fractures.

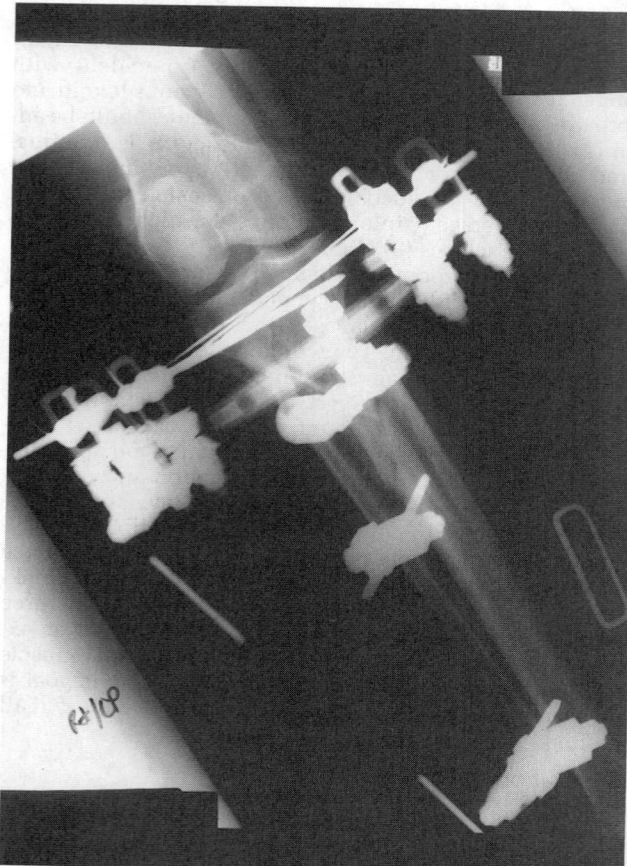

Figure 100.2. Hybrid fixation of a comminuted proximal tibial fracture associated with grade III open injury and fracture blisters. Open reduction and internal fixation is too risky in this situation.

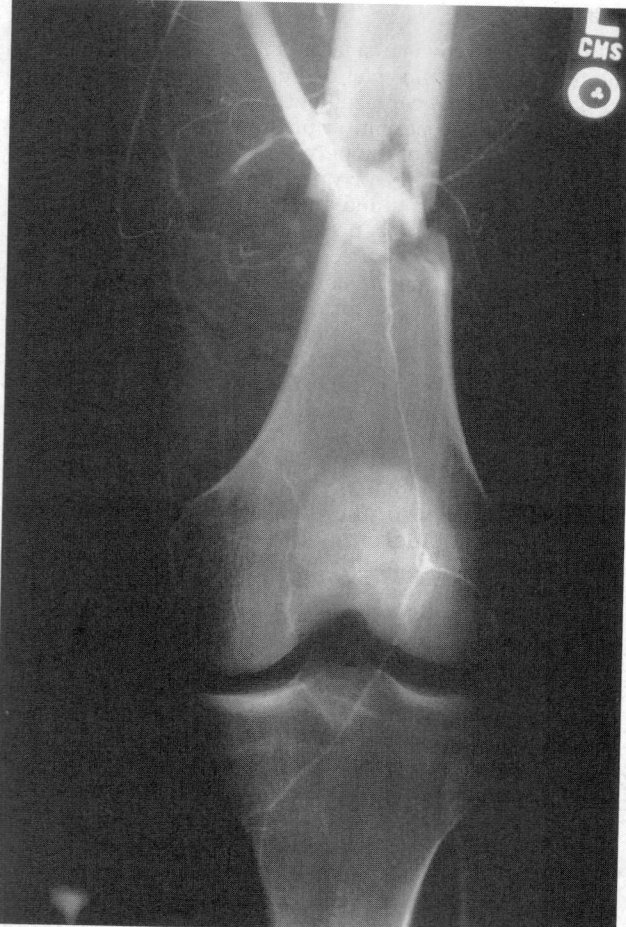

Figure 100.3. Distal femoral fracture associated with disruption of the femoral artery. Retrograde or antegrade intramedullary fracture stabilization can be accomplished rapidly and is the fixation of choice. Alternatively, through a separate lateral incision, a compression plate may be applied and functions as a tension band. A medial plate should not be used.

In contrast to the lower extremity, most open fractures of the humerus, radius, and ulna can be treated by open reduction and compression plating, either initially or at subsequent washout.

Summary

Open fractures are an orthopedic emergency and must be treated promptly to prevent the serious complications of infection and nonunion. The principles of treatment involve thorough débridement, IV and local antibiotics, and fracture stabilization. Coverage of exposed bone by viable soft tissue must be achieved.

Chronic osteomyelitis and infected nonunions are notoriously difficult to treat, often requiring radical débridement of all dead bone and soft tissue and prolonged administration of IV and local antibiotics. Union is frequently difficult to obtain and may require massive bone grafts when the site is aseptic, or bone transport through distraction osteogenesis according to the method of Ilizarov. Amputation may be necessary for refractory infected tibial nonunions.

Arterial Injuries

Arterial injuries of the extremities are occasionally associated with an open fracture (Fig. 100.3). Knee dislocations and scapulothoracic disassociations are also frequently accompanied by arterial injury. The Vietnam experience has shown that internal fixation of fractures after arterial repair is not necessary in the acute setting.

Nevertheless, in nonbattlefield situations, there is great benefit from stabilizing these injuries, especially when the diaphysis is fractured. Bone stabilization can precede or follow arterial repair, depending on the warm ischemia time.

Arterial repair should not be delayed significantly regardless of the type of fracture stabilization elected. External fixation can be rapidly applied to shaft fractures of the tibia, femur, or humerus. Skeletal traction, usually temporary, can be effectively used for femur fractures. Internal fixation with a compression plate can be used, but may not provide good stabilization in the presence of comminution.

Retrograde femoral rods inserted through a small knee incision (Fig. 100.1) or small-diameter antegrade tibial rods can be rapidly applied and interfere less with vascular access than external fixation. In the upper extremity, compression plates are an effective means of stabilization. Minimally displaced or relatively stable articular and metaphyseal fractures can be treated electively after successful vascular repair (4). Compartment syndrome may be associated with arterial injury or follow vascular repair, and prophylactic fasciotomy should be considered in patients with prolonged ischemic time, and compartment pressure monitoring used in high-risk injuries.

Dislocations

Shoulder: Anterior Dislocation

The shoulder is one of the most frequently dislocated joints, with anterior presentation accounting for over 95% of dislocations. Frequently it is an isolated injury, often occurring in athletic events or falls. Occasionally, an axillary nerve palsy may be present. The prognosis for recovery is good for neuropraxic injuries. Reduction usually is not difficult and can be accomplished by one of numerous mechanisms. One of the most reliable methods is that of gentle external rotation of the shoulder beyond the mid-coronal plane. In middle-aged or elderly people, rotator cuff injuries may be associated with dislocation, although recurrent dislocation is less likely than in young adults. In the latter group and adolescents, recurrent dislocation rates are very high, presumably because of the continued activities that place the shoulder at risk. In this group, surgical repair of recurrent dislocation is often necessary and highly successful (13).

Shoulder: Posterior Dislocation

Posterior dislocation of the shoulder is uncommon and is one of the most frequently missed diagnoses in orthopedics. It is frequently associated with seizure disorder. Clinically, the shoulder is held in fixed internal rotation. Radiographically, the findings are subtle because the humeral head is directly posterior on the anteroposterior view and appears to be located. An axillary or transcapsular "Y" view is necessary to demonstrate the posterior dislocation. A high index of suspicion is necessary if permanent disability is to be prevented. After reduction, the patient's shoulder is immobilized in external rotation in the so-called gunslinger's position (13).

Elbow

Elbow dislocation is usually posterior or posterolateral in direction and stable after reduction. It is important to begin early protected motion within the range of stability. Recurrent dislocation of the elbow is extremely uncommon, but some residual loss of terminal extension is frequently encountered despite immediate or early mobilization of the reduced joint. Fracture–dislocation is common and usually requires open reduction and internal fixation to restore anatomy and render the joint stable (13).

Hip

Dislocations of the hip are also common and frequently accompany motor vehicle accidents and other high-energy injuries. Posterior hip dislocation is much more common than anterior dislocation. The patient presents clinically with an adducted, flexed, and internally rotated extremity (Fig. 100.4A). Reduction should be effected promptly by appropriate sedation and traction in line with the extremity. After reduction of a posterior hip dislocation, the hip should be checked for stability at 90 degrees of flexion in neutral rotation. The presence of a significant posterior wall acetabular fracture may render the hip irreducible or unstable, necessitating open reduction and internal fixation of the acetabulum and hip dislocation. A high incidence of avascular necrosis of the femoral head has been reported with dislocations that are reduced late.

Anterior dislocation of the hip, although less common, is more frequently associated with fracture of the femoral head or indentation deformation (Fig. 100.4B). Small osteochondral fragments associated with a symmetric hip joint may occasionally be observed. They usually require excision or, if large enough, open reduction and internal fixation through an anterior approach. Large femoral head fractures and those associated with acetabular or femoral

neck fractures have a high incidence of avascular necrosis and hip arthritis.

The clinical presentation of anterior hip dislocation is characterized by abduction and external rotation. Radiographically, the femoral head is often located over the obturator foramen. Reduction can be attempted under appropriate sedation in the emergency department, but often requires anesthesia in the operating room. Almost all pure dislocations reduce quite easily under general anesthesia and muscle relaxation (14).

Knee

Anterior or posterior dislocation of the knee is frequently associated with injury to the popliteal neurovascular bundle. Reduction is not difficult because all of the capsule and ligamentous structures are usually severely disrupted. Absent pulses may be restored after reduction, but an arteriogram is frequently indicated to rule out associated intimal injury that could progress to thrombosis. Arterial repair requires an interposed vein graft and may need to be protected with an external fixator spanning the knee (4).

Associated peroneal nerve palsy is common and results in loss of dorsiflexion, which can be accommodated by an orthosis. However, if the posterior tibial nerve is avulsed, the prognosis is quite dismal, with eventual amputation being likely secondary to an anesthetic foot.

Ligamentous repair is usually undertaken immediately or in the first 10 days. Wherever possible, the menisci, at least one cruciate, and both collateral ligaments should be repaired. The prognosis is guarded for this severe injury, which usually does not permit the return to competitive athletics. A knee dislocation equivalent may present with less dramatic radiographic signs because of either spontaneous relocation or incomplete dislocation. It carries essentially the same clinical implications and caveats regarding neurovascular injury.

Ankle

Pure ankle dislocation is very uncommon; most ankle injuries are fracture–dislocations. Gross deformity is present with bone protruding or palpable through a gaping wound. Associated avulsion of neurovascular structures may be present. However, because of the direction of dislocation, the vital posterior tibial neurovascular bundle is usually spared. Most pure ankle dislocations are posteromedial in direction and widely open, and require irrigation and débridement, open reduction, and ligamentous repair. If the articular surface is intact and there is no fracture, the prognosis is surprisingly good if the ankle mortise is restored (15).

Subtalar Joint

Dislocations are relatively uncommon and usually present with the foot displaced medially. Clinical presentation is dramatic, with the foot at right angles to the ankle and the skin severely tented over bony prominences opposite the direction of dislocation. Immediate reduction is indicated to prevent skin slough and restore circulation to the foot. The foot is usually stable after reduction and the functional results are good after a brief period of immobilization. Lateral subtalar dislocation is uncommon and more frequently associated with fracture. Open reduction may be necessary to extract entrapped neurovascular and tendinous structures as well as internally fix associated tarsal fractures (16,17).

Fracture–Dislocations

Pure dislocations of the major joints are discussed in the preceding sections. Most displaced fractures are treated by orthopedists, in contrast to dislocations, which are not in-

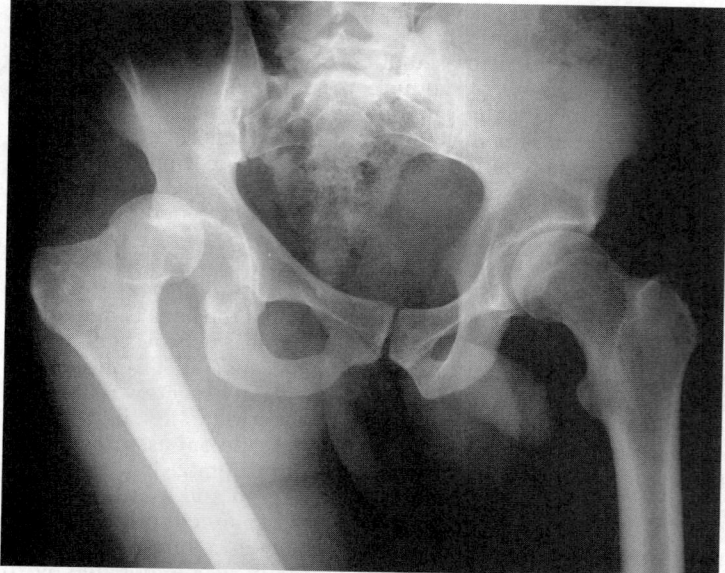

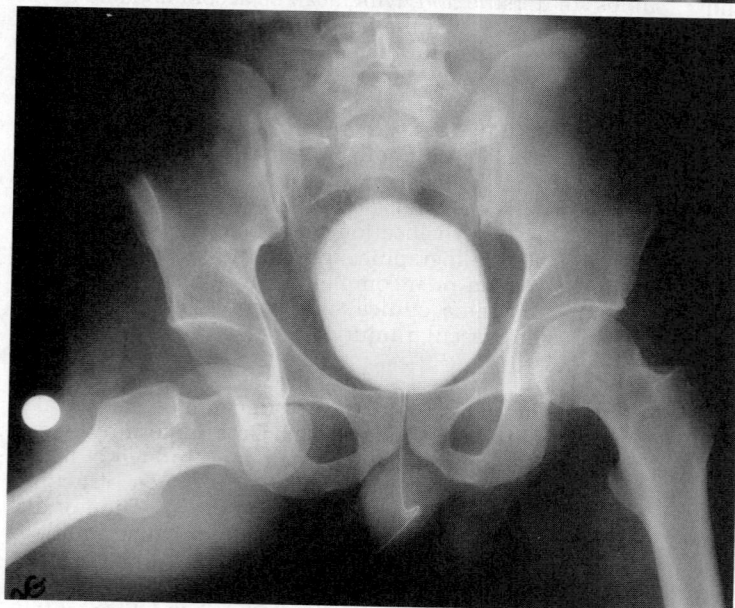

Figure 100.4. *(A)* Posterior dislocation of the hip. The thigh is flexed adducted and internally rotated. *(B)* Anterior dislocation of the hip. The thigh is abducted and externally rotated. There is an associated fracture of the femoral head. A cystogram is negative.

frequently treated by emergency and family physicians, or occasionally by the patient or companions in an emergent situation. Fracture–dislocations result from higher-energy forces and frequently involve major joints. Fracture reduction by open technique is usually necessary to restore anatomy of the bone and obtain reduction of the joint.

FRACTURE ASSESSMENT AND TREATMENT

The goal of contemporary fracture treatment is to stabilize and restore bony anatomy, promote fracture healing, and ultimately restore function. Although closed treatment is indicated and effective for many isolated or nondisplaced fractures, patients may have to accept minor degrees of shortening or malalignment, which are of little functional consequence. There is no risk of infection or anesthetic complications with closed treatment, but this method cannot consistently produce the same number of good and excellent results as precise open reduction and internal fixation of selected fractures. Operative treatment

is especially valuable for polytrauma victims and patients with multiple, bilateral, or articular fractures (4,6,18,19). In these patients, relief of pain, correction of deformity, and ease of nursing care are distinct advantages. Open reduction and internal fixation also reduces the incidence and severity of pulmonary complications such as adult respiratory distress syndrome and pulmonary embolism. Prompt stabilization of fractures permits early joint motion, mobilization of the patient, and improved functional results. Ultimately, events occurring at the cellular level determine outcomes, and thus a fundamental understanding of the biology of fracture and soft-tissue healing is necessary.

Biology of Fracture Healing and Soft-tissue Repair

After traumatic fracture, the acute hematoma becomes organized and invaded by cells recruited from the bone itself and, more important, from the periosteum. Pluripotent osteoprogenitor cells undergo differentiation into osteoblasts that begin to lay down the woven bone of the provisional callus. This phase is orchestrated and influenced by a host of recently identified growth factors. These osteogenic proteins are a family of bone matrix polypeptides (bone morphogenetic proteins) capable of inducing a sequence of cellular events leading to bone formation and repair. The process of osteoinduction continues through a combination of mechanisms, including enchondral ossification involving a cartilage intermediate stage, and direct bone apposition similar to intramembranous bone formation in the embryo. Woven bone is gradually converted to lamellar bone with secondary osteoclastic remodeling occurring under physiologic stresses, according to Wolff's law (20).

Fracture healing is significantly influenced by fracture characteristics, including displacement, comminution, presence or absence of open injury, and methods of fracture stabilization. It is the external callus that contributes most to the restoration of strength and continuity after diaphyseal fractures. This type of healing response is predominant in fractures treated by intramedullary nailing, closed reduction and casting, or traction. The cells and blood vessels responsible for this phase appear to arise from the periosteum, and this type of fracture healing can be greatly diminished or totally abolished by fixation systems that impose total rigidity on the fracture. Late medullary callus is less tolerant of motion and forms more slowly. Primary cortical bone union occurs when a fracture has been anatomically reduced and rigidly plated. In this instance, no external callus appears. Healing is very slow and depends on osteonal penetration and the development of haversian systems (21). After biologic stabilization of a fracture by the initial woven callus, continued mineralization and bone formation by osteocytes is accompanied by osteoclastic remodeling. Ultimate fracture healing produces bone that is mechanically and histologically identical to normal bone. Interruption of the healing process at any phase can result in delayed union or nonunion. Factors that contribute to nonunion are open soft-tissue injury and devascularization, infection, smoking, and systemic disease.

The skeleton provides a framework over which the soft tissue is draped. Therefore, healing of damaged skin and neurovascular, ligamentous, and tendinous injuries is paramount for a satisfactory functional result. Soft-tissue coverage of bone may be accomplished by delayed primary closure, split-thickness skin grafting, or local or remote microvascular flaps. Soft tissues are composed of collagen, elastin, and a hydrophilic ground substance. The latter contains mucopolysaccharides, proteoglycans, glycosaminoglycans, and water. The most important structural component of connective tissue is collagen, by virtue of its high mechanical integrity. The three-dimensional organization and relative amounts of these constituents determine the physical property of the tissue. Because the function of connective tissue is primarily mechanical, the cells provide a low level of homeostatic activity, except when faced with injury or damage.

The first stage in the repair of soft tissue involves formation of vascularized granulation tissue in which collagen fibers are randomly oriented. As healing progresses, and especially under the influence of early mobilization and a good vascular supply, orientation becomes functionally organized. Alignment of the collagen fibers along the lines of stress results in increased tensile strength and a more normal structure. Remodeling and adaptation of the soft-tissue structures occurs under the normal physiologic loading conditions.

After nerve injury, wallerian degeneration occurs distal to the injury; repair involves regeneration of axons at the rate of approximately 1 mm per day. Ultimate reinnervation and restoration of muscle strength depend on the inherent regenerative potential, which varies from nerve to nerve, the type of injury, and the distance of the injury from the final innervation site (20).

PELVIC AND LOWER EXTREMITY FRACTURES

Pelvic Fractures

Pelvic fractures vary considerably in terms of severity, treatment, and prognosis. Only in recent decades has the concept of surgical stabilization been extended to pelvic fractures (4,6,22,23). Minimally displaced fractures of the pubic rami and anterior portion of the pelvic ring are usually treated symptomatically, whereas major pelvic ring disruption has a significant mortality rate because of massive retroperitoneal hemorrhage and requires emergent stabilization as a lifesaving measure (Fig. 100.5). The incidence of pelvic fractures in fatal motor vehicle accidents is as high as 24% and approaches 50% for fatal pedestrian accidents (4). Anatomically, the pelvis can be conceptualized as a ring. It consists of the two innominate bones and the sacrum joined together by strong ligaments. Considerable force is necessary to disrupt the posterior pelvic ring through fracture of the ilium or sacrum or pure ligamentous disruption, as described by Joseph François Malgaigne in his classic fracture text of 1847.

Diagnosis

Physical examination of the pelvis requires palpation and compression for the detection of instability and localization of pain. Urologic examination, inspection of soft tissues, and vaginal and rectal examination should be performed to rule out communication of the fracture with these areas. Open pelvic fractures are associated with a high mortality rate and may require diverting colostomy or a suprapubic cystostomy (Fig. 100.6). Bleeding at the urethral meatus in the male patient requires a urethrogram before passing a Foley catheter. A cystogram is often indicated by the presence of hematuria or wide pubic diastasis. Speculum examination of the vagina is required in the presence of bleeding, and sigmoidoscopy may be necessary to ascertain the presence of rectal tear.

Radiography

Standard anteroposterior radiography of the pelvis is part of the initial trauma evaluation. At secondary survey, a pelvic inlet and outlet view and, ultimately, a pelvic CT should be obtained. The latter can frequently be performed at the time of abdominal CT with fine 5-mm cuts through the acetabulum if indicated. CT scan is very valuable for assessing minor degrees of sacroiliac joint subluxation, sacral fractures, incarcerated acetabular fracture fragments, and other, more subtle injuries to the pelvic ring (4,6).

Classification

There are several different classifications of pelvic injury, according to the location of fractures and implied vectors of force. Pelvic fractures may be divided into three types (6) (Fig. 100.7). Minimally displaced fractures of the pelvis that are stable are classified as type A fractures, type B fractures are rotationally unstable, and type C fractures are vertically unstable (Figs. 100.1, 100.8). The latter two types are the clinically relevant disruptions and are often associated with visceral injury and polytrauma. Type C fractures or widely displaced type B fractures may be associated with life-threatening retroperitoneal hemorrhage.

(text continues on page 2091)

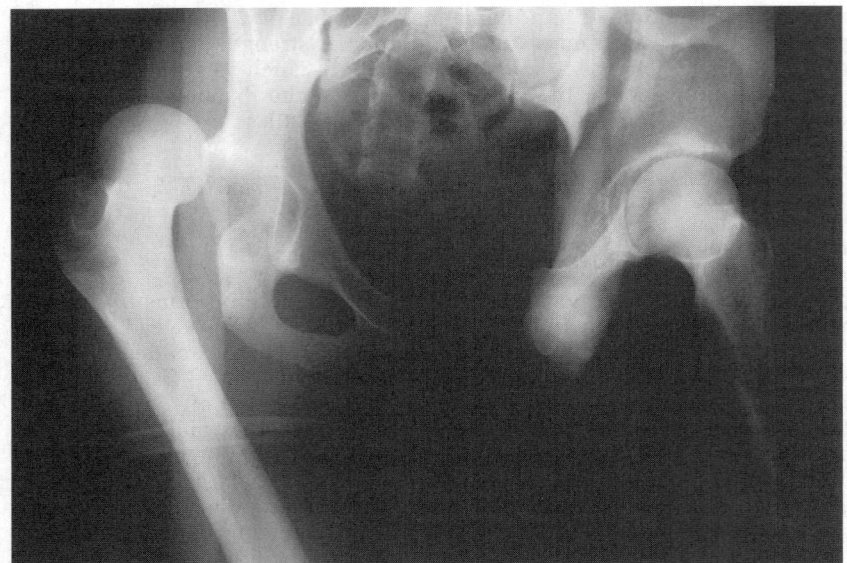

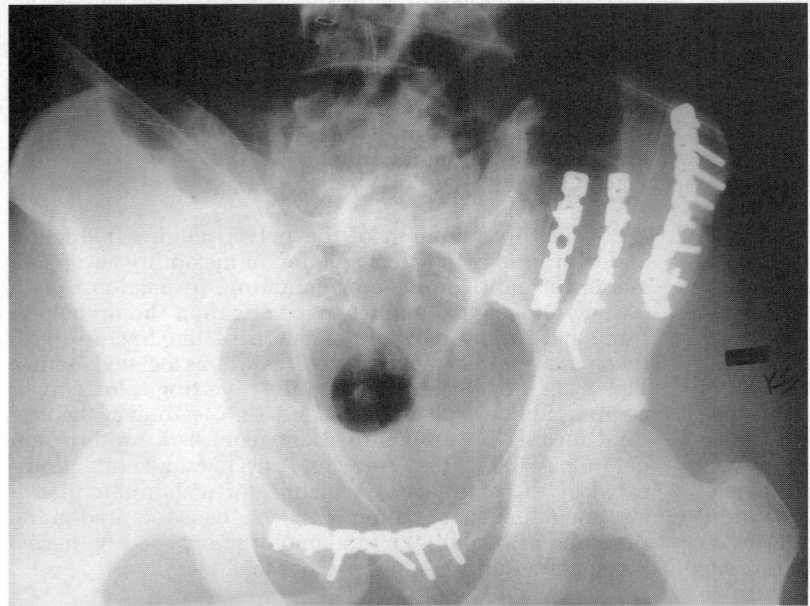

Figure 100.5. *(A)* Gross pelvic disruption associated with hemorrhagic shock in a young motor vehicle accident victim. There is posterior dislocation of the right hip, wide pubic diastasis, and comminuted fracture of left iliac wing. *(B)* Anteroposterior radiograph after open reduction and plating of pubic diastasis and associated iliac wing fracture and reduction of dislocated hip.

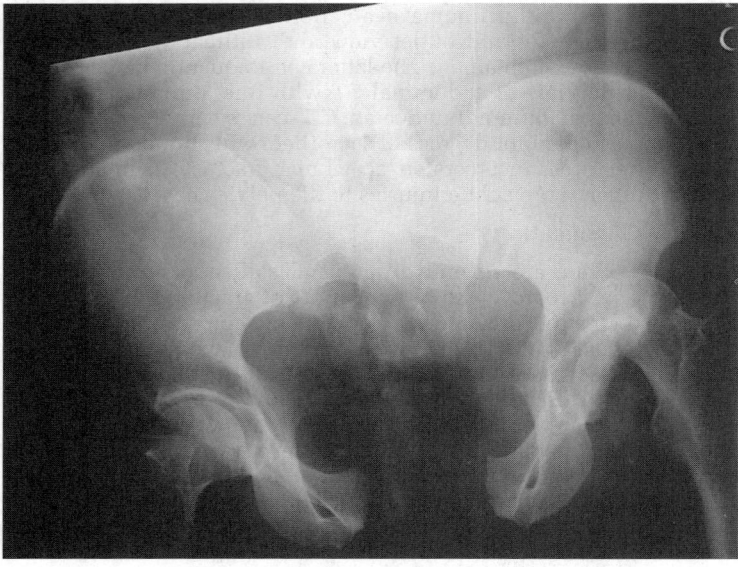

Figure 100.6. *(A)* Wide pubic diastasis, characteristic of "open book" horizontally unstable pelvis (type B), with associated femoral head fracture and hip dislocation. *(B)* Anteroposterior radiograph after open reduction and dual plating of pubic diastasis and open reduction and internal fixation of femoral head fracture. The patient had associated bladder rupture requiring repair and suprapubic cystostomy. *(continues)*

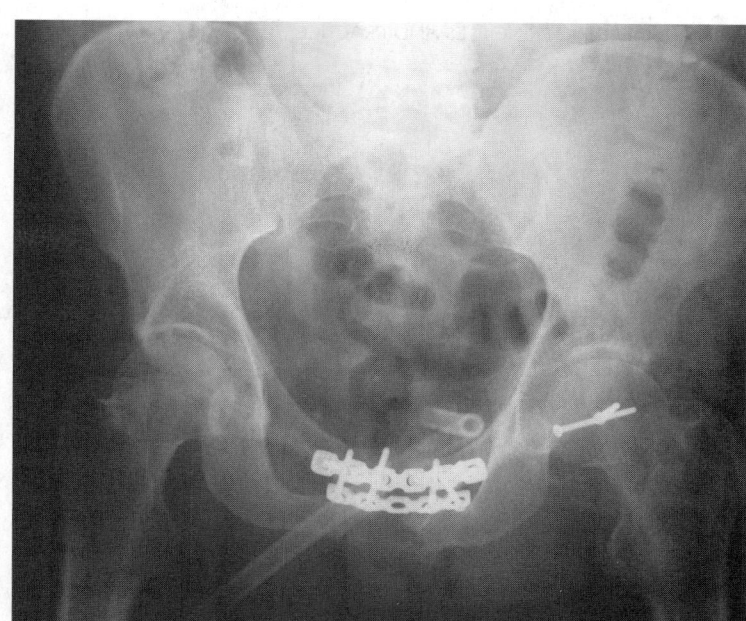

Figure 100.6. *(Continued)*

B

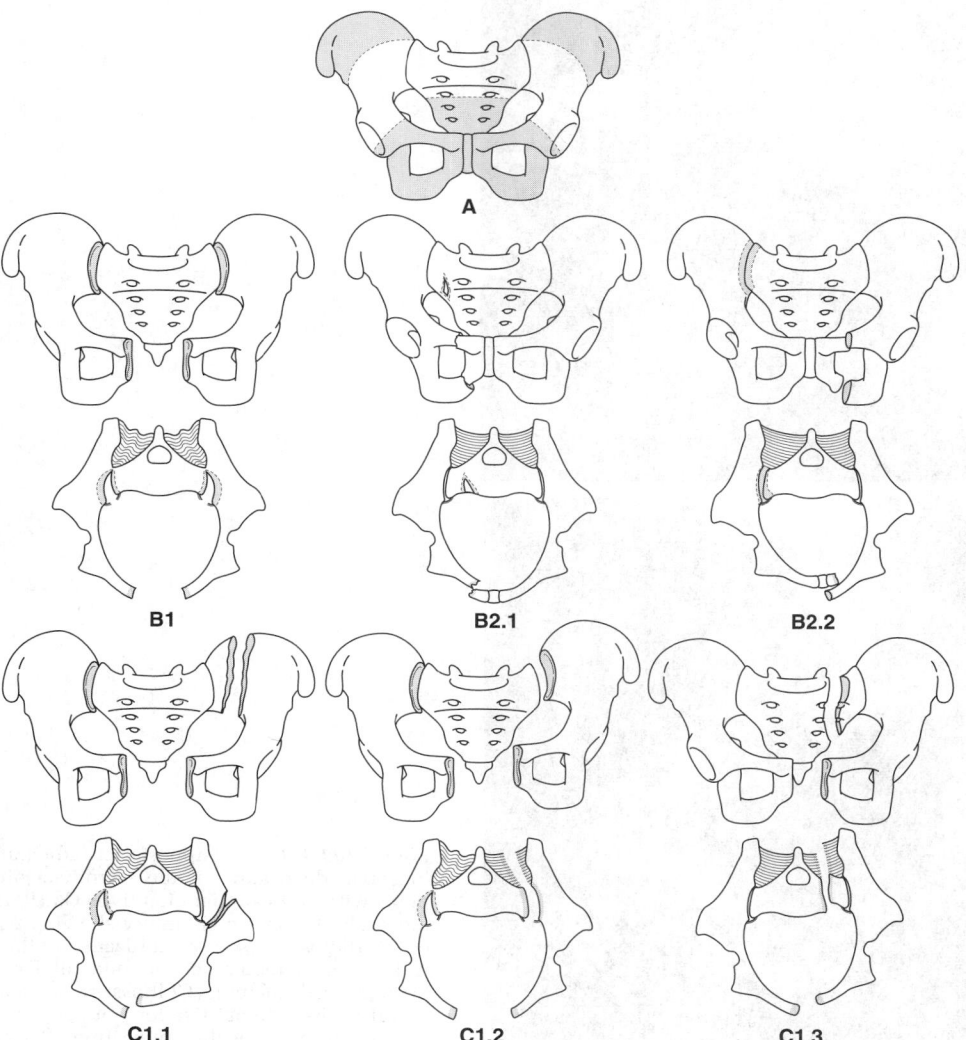

B1 B2.1 B2.2

C1.1 C1.2 C1.3

Figure 100.7. The AO classification of pelvic injuries. Type A fractures are undisplaced and do not result in instability. Type B fractures are horizontally unstable. Type B1 is commonly known as the *open book* fracture and is characterized by diastasis of the symphysis pubis and disruption of the anterior sacroiliac ligaments. Type C fractures are vertically unstable. They can involve pure ligamentous disruption through the pubis and sacroiliac joint, a fracture characteristically through the sacral foramina, or a posterior iliac fracture. All three mechanisms result in varying degrees of cephalad migration of the hemipelvis (Malgaigne).

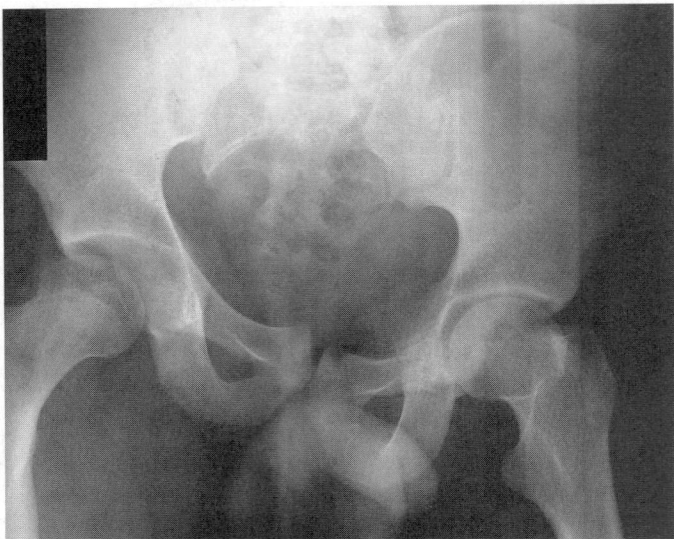

A

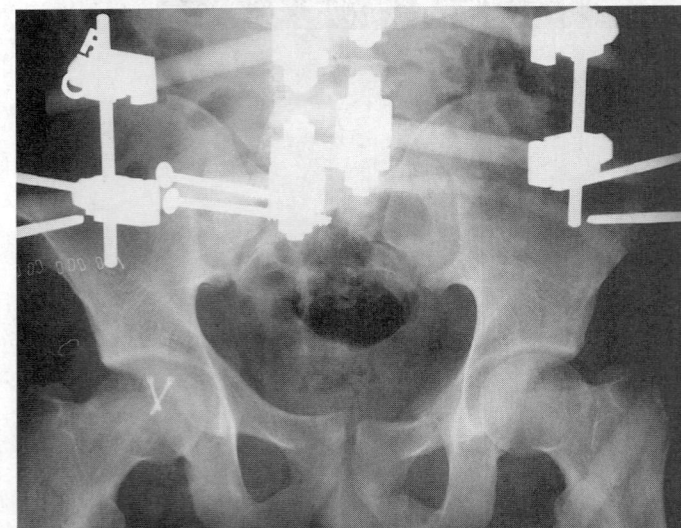

B

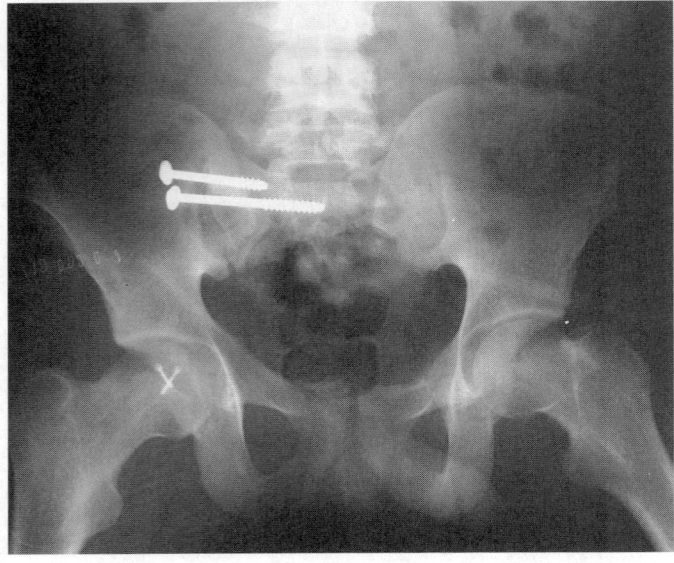

C

Figure 100.8. *(A)* Anteroposterior radiograph of pelvis show-ing open dislocation of the sacroiliac joint and symphysis pubis with vertical migration (type C). *(B)* Anteroposterior ra-diograph of open pelvic injury showing pelvic external fixa-tion and iliosacral screw stabilization of the sacroiliac joint, as well as open reduction and internal fixation of associated femoral head fracture. *(C)* Iliosacral screws allowed early re-moval of the external fixation applied for open pelvic injury emergently. Note residual impaction of sacral fracture.

Treatment

External Fixation. Pelvic external fixation can be rapidly applied when necessary to stabilize a disrupted pelvis associated with hemorrhagic shock. It is most effective in pubic diastasis and disruption of the anterior portion of the pelvic ring. It cannot be used in the presence of a major fracture of the iliac wing and may accentuate associated posterior pelvic disruption and bleeding. In addition to being a resuscitative tool, it may be used definitively in association with posterior fixation or in open fractures not amenable to internal stabilization (Fig. 100.8). Localized pin reaction or occasionally frank infection limits external fixation use to 10 to 12 weeks or less (6,23). Balanced skeletal traction of 20 to 25 pounds should be provided until definitive stabilization by external or internal fixation is accomplished.

Internal Fixation. Pure ligamentous disruption of the sacroiliac joint is best treated by open reduction and internal fixation accomplished through an anterior approach (6). Displaced fractures of the posterior ilium and certain sacral fractures can be treated by open reduction from a posterior approach.

Ileosacral Screws. Ileosacral screws can be used in conjunction with open reduction and internal fixation or inserted independently by closed technique using cannulated screws and monitoring by fluoroscopic image intensification (Fig. 100.8). They are valuable adjuncts to anterior fixation such as pubic plating. The safe window for insertion of these screws is narrow, and occasional violation of the sacral foramina or neural canal may occur in even the most experienced hands. Fortunately, if malpositioned screws are detected and removed promptly, permanent sequelae rarely occur (22).

Acetabulum Fractures

Fractures of the acetabulum can be isolated or associated with pelvic disruption and systemic polytrauma (Fig. 100.9). They are usually high-energy injuries secondary to

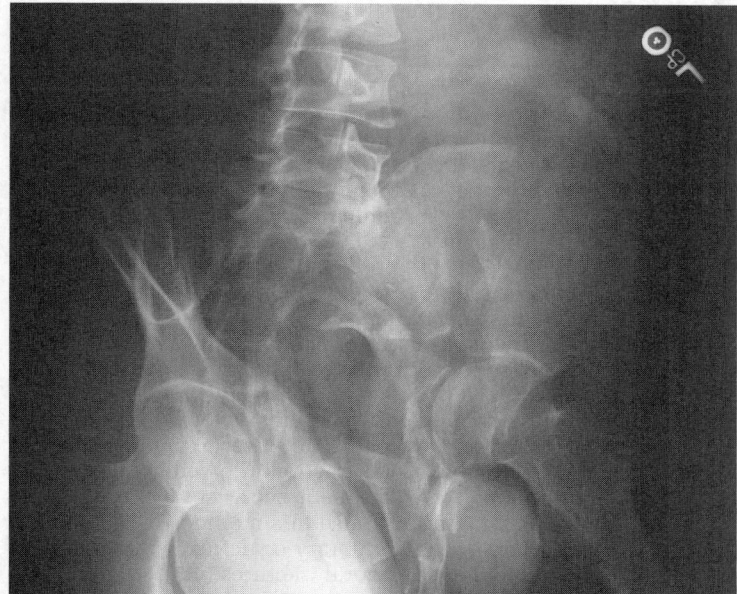

A

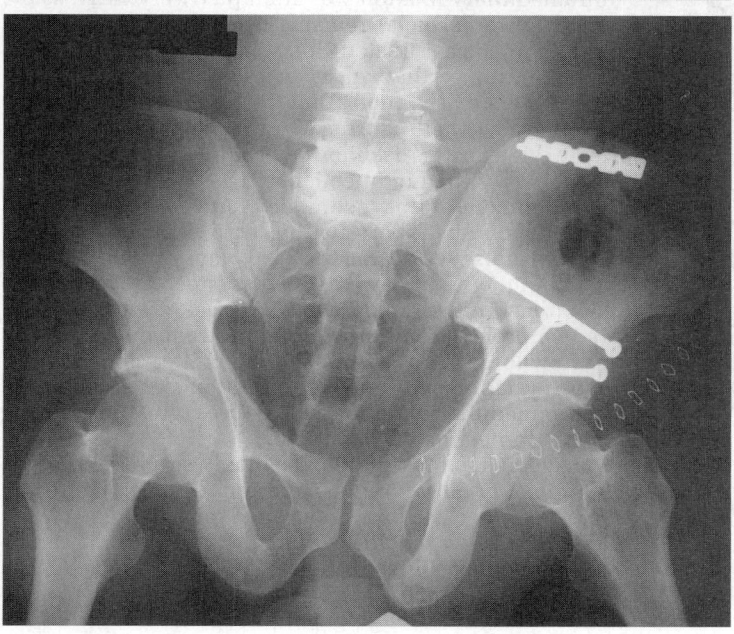

B

Figure 100.9. *(A)* Polytrauma victim with markedly displaced left acetabular fracture, associated with severe retroperitoneal hemorrhage. Hemorrhage was from bone and avulsed superior gluteal vessels. *(B)* Anteroposterior radiograph of pelvis after anatomic open reduction and internal fixation. Patient died 10 days after surgery from adult respiratory distress syndrome.

motor vehicle accidents or falls from a height. Displaced fractures require surgical treatment to restore stability and congruency of the hip joint and allow mobilization of the patient. Classification systems have conceptually divided the acetabulum into anterior and posterior columns. The anterior column consists of the iliac wing, anterior wall and dome of the acetabulum, as well as the superior pubic ramus. The posterior column comprises the sciatic notch, posterior wall of the acetabulum, quadrilateral plate, and ischium. Fractures can involve the anterior, posterior, or both columns of the acetabulum. Radiographic evaluation includes anteroposterior and 45-degree oblique (Judet) views of the acetabulum. A CT scan is helpful in identifying joint fragments, marginal impaction, femoral head fractures, and sacroiliac joint involvement (6,24).

Treatment

Surgical treatment is technically demanding and may require anterior, posterior, or combined approaches. The

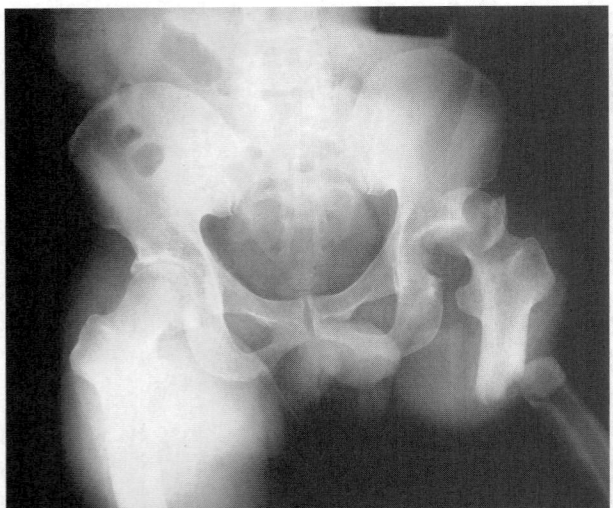

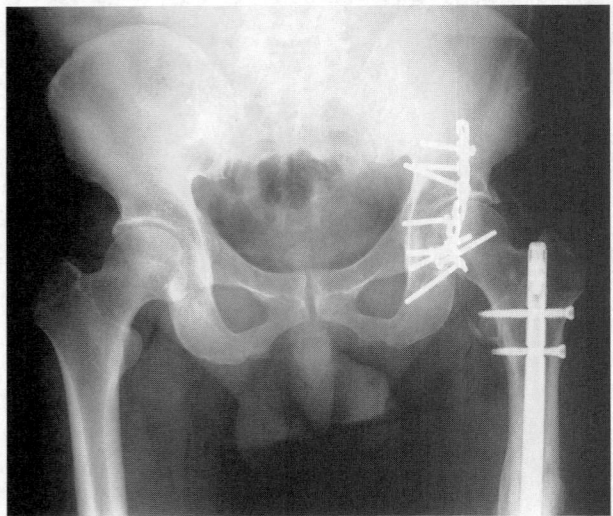

Figure 100.10. *(A)* Unusually severe injury secondary to a motor vehicle accident, with femoral head fracture, posterior wall acetabular fracture, hip dislocation, and subtrochanteric fracture of the femur. *(B)* Three-year follow-up after open reduction and internal fixation of femoral head and acetabular fractures and interlocked intramedullary fixation of the subtrochanteric femur fracture. All fractures have healed. The joint space is preserved and the patient has a surprisingly good result, with no avascular necrosis and full range of motion.

ileoinguinal approach requires isolation of the spermatic cord, external iliac vessels, femoral nerve, and psoas muscle. This provides three windows for exposure, reduction, and fixation of the fracture. The posterior and straight lateral approaches release portions of the gluteus maximus and medius and short external rotators to expose the sciatic nerve and notch, posterior wall, column, and ischial tuberosity. Extensile approaches may be used but are associated with higher morbidity, wound problems, and residual muscle weakness (25).

Special reduction techniques and pelvic instrumentation are necessary to reduce the fracture. Lag screws, pelvic reconstruction, and buttress plates provide internal fixation. Postoperative management includes deep vein thrombosis (DVT) precautions, early motion, and delayed weight bearing. Reported results vary considerably, and range from approximately 40% to 80% good and excellent. Postoperative complications of infection or sciatic nerve injury seriously jeopardize functional outcome.

Operative treatment and anatomic reduction correlate with optimal patient outcomes but do not preclude subsequent chondrolysis, avascular necrosis, or posttraumatic arthritis (6,23–25) (Fig. 100.10).

LONG-BONE FRACTURES

Long-bone and open fractures were fatal injuries in ancient times, depriving a person of the ability to escape danger, defend himself or herself, or obtain nourishment. Subsequently, reduction and maintenance of length of femoral fractures was achieved by providing traction. Initially described in the 1300s, it consisted of a weight attached to the leg by a cord that was strung over a pulley. Traction changed little over the next 500 years, but in the 1800s became somewhat more sophisticated through the use of various splints, frames, or slings. During the Civil War, skin traction (Buck's traction) for femoral fractures was popularized. It is still used today for temporary immobilization of adult hip fractures before surgery and as definitive treatment of pediatric lower extremity fractures or hip disorders. Skeletal traction allowed greater weight to be applied, with subsequent better control of the fracture. Steinmann began to use this method in 1907, and it is used today for the temporary or definitive treatment of pelvic, acetabular, or femoral fractures (4,5).

Intramedullary fixation was attempted very early, as evidenced by the skeletal remains of ancient peoples. The Aztecs and Incas treated long bone nonunions with resinous intramedullary pegs in the 16th century. Short ivory pegs were used in femoral fractures in the late 1800s and long metal nails during World War I. Open war injuries treated in this fashion before the era of antibiotics predictably resulted in infection and gas gangrene, leading to abandonment of this technique (4,5).

Modern intramedullary nailing was introduced in Germany by Küntscher during the early days of World War II. His technique used large, stainless steel cloverleaf intramedullary nails (26). The advantages of this method were compromised by problematic intramedullary infection. Development of the image intensifier not only decreased radiation exposure but permitted closed reduction and intramedullary fixation of fractures, greatly reducing the rate of infection and nonunion.

Long-bone fractures involve the diaphyseal regions of the femur, tibia, humerus, radius, and ulna and can be treated successfully by closed methods when minimally displaced or isolated. However, long-bone fractures in polytrauma victims are best stabilized surgically. This is especially true for the femur and tibia. Closed reduction and insertion of an intramedullary rod using a guide pin and fluoroscopic control greatly minimizes surgical trauma and reduces the incidence of infection and nonunion by keeping the fracture site closed. Modest reaming of the medullary canal is usually performed, but is limited or omitted in high-grade open fractures, polytrauma, and in patients with significant pulmonary contusions, in whom embolic marrow contents can worsen respiratory problems.

Femoral Fractures

Closed interlocked intramedullary fixation is the treatment of choice for fractures from just below the subtrochanteric to the high supracondylar region. The rods may be inserted antegrade (Fig. 100.10) or retrograde through the intercondylar notch of the femur and knee joint (27,28) (Fig. 100.1). The latter method is useful for polytrauma victims for whom rapidity of treatment is essential. A fracture table is not necessary (Fig. 100.1). This technique is also indicated for bilateral fractures, morbid obesity, and certain ipsilateral fractures of the tibia. Interlocking screws prevent loss of fracture reduction.

Femur fractures were formerly treated by traction for 6 to 8 weeks followed by a unilateral walking spica cast; however, the advantages of rapid mobilization, decreased hospitalization costs, and better fracture reduction provided by intramedullary stabilization make it the treatment of choice.

Tibial Fractures

The vulnerable subcutaneous border predisposes tibial fractures to open injury and higher complication rates (Fig. 100.11). Isolated, minimally displaced fractures of the tibial diaphysis can be treated with a long leg cast followed by a patellar tendon-bearing cast to allow knee motion at approximately 4 to 6 weeks. Minor malalignment is common after fracture healing (typically 4 to 6 months), but usually of little functional significance (29,30). Closed intramedullary interlocked fixation is the treatment of choice for most

other tibial fractures, those associated with ipsilateral femur fractures or polytrauma, and all segmental fractures (11,16) (Fig. 100.12). Compartment syndrome occurs most commonly in the calf, and therefore fractures of the tibia require careful and repeated examination.

Compartment Syndrome

Compartment syndrome is caused by the rapid accumulation of blood or interstitial fluid in a swollen, tense compartment, usually in the leg. Common causes are fractures, local trauma, crush injury, and positional hypoxia or ischemia and reperfusion swelling after vascular injury and reconstruction. Prolonged surgical procedures and tourniquet times are notorious iatrogenic causes. Elevated pressure occurs in the involved compartments, impeding cellular perfusion at the microvascular level. If the pressure is unrelieved, tissue necrosis may occur with ischemic contracted muscles as the final result (31). These sequelae can sometimes be prevented in patients with tense leg compartments by prompt fascial decompression (4).

Diagnosis

In a cooperative and awake patient, the diagnosis can often be made on a clinical basis. Classically, there is pain out of proportion to the injury that increases with gentle passive stretch of the involved joint, paresthesias, and a very tense, tender fascial compartment. Most compartment syndromes occur in the leg, although the thigh, forearm, hand, or foot can also be involved. Pulses are present unless there is a concomitant arterial injury. After arterial repair, compartment syndrome is not infrequent and prophylactic fasciotomy is often indicated. Differentiating compartment syndrome from neurovascular injury can occasionally be problematic because they may coexist (Table 100.3). Compartment pressure measurements can be helpful in equivocal cases.

Compartment pressures can be measured with a handheld unit or by a pressure transducer connected by sterile

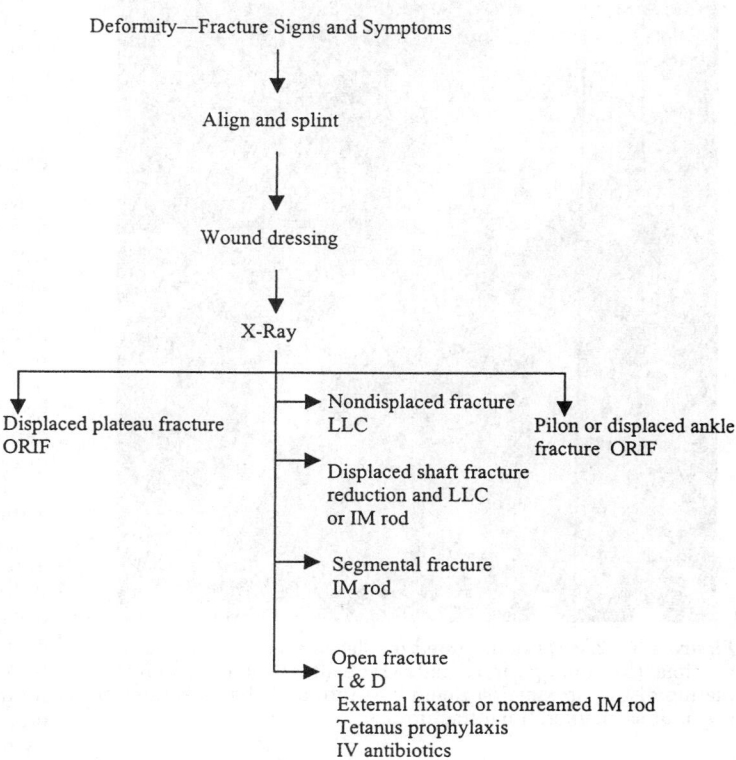

Figure 100.11. Algorithm for tibial fractures. ORIF, open reduction and internal fixation; LLC, long leg cast; IM, intramedullary; I & D, irrigation and débridement.

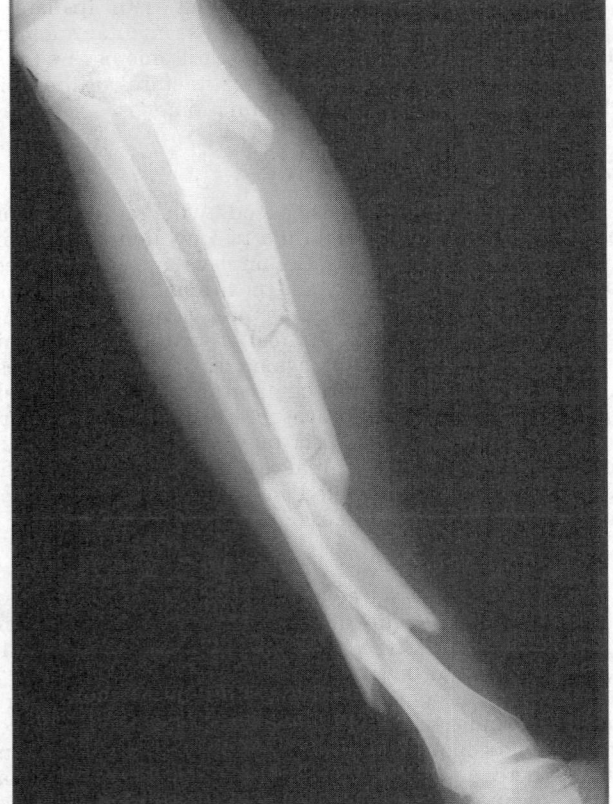

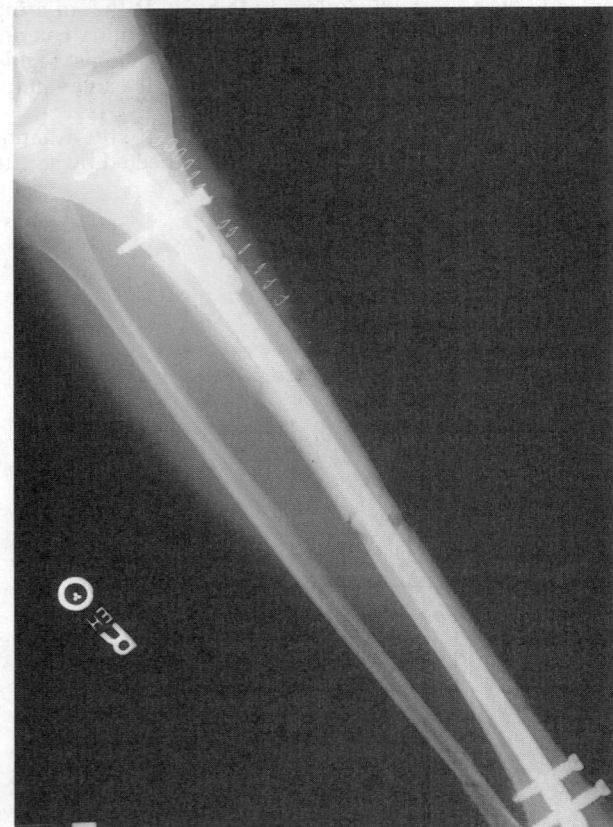

Figure 100.12. *(A)* Comminuted displaced segmental fracture of the tibia. *(B)* Anteroposterior radiograph after open reduction and plating of the proximal segment and intramedullary fixation of the multisegmented tibial fracture.

Table 100.3. COMPARTMENT SYNDROME FINDINGS

	Compartment syndrome	Arterial injury	Nerve injury
Pressure increase	+	−	−
Pain with motion	+	+	−
Paresthesia	+	+	+
Pulses intact	+	-	+

Compartment syndrome occurs most often in the leg. A high index of suspicion and repeated examination, including compartment pressure measurements where indicated, are necessary. Fascial compartments released early have the most favorable prognosis, whereas those released after more than 6 hours usually have varying degrees of muscle necrosis. Occasionally, below-knee leg amputation is necessary.

tubing to a side-ported needle inserted into the suspected compartments. Pressure measurements are most valuable in unconscious or uncooperative patients in whom clinical evaluation is unreliable. Pressures in the 35- to 40-mm Hg range are suspect for compartment syndrome, and those significantly greater than this diagnostic. The closer the compartment pressure is to the patient's diastolic pressure, the greater the sensitivity to compartment syndrome. When this pressure differential is less than 30 mm Hg (Δp), compartment syndrome is likely (32).

Treatment

The treatment of compartment syndrome is immediate fasciotomy. Even though compartment pressures may be abnormally high in only one compartment, it is best to decompress all four compartments. In the leg, this can be accomplished by a lateral parafibular incision or the two-incision technique. If the latter method is selected, the incisions should be at least 20 cm long and centered over the anterolateral and posteromedial aspects of the calf (33). The fasciotomy incisions can usually be closed by delayed primary closure at 5 to 6 days, but occasionally necessitate split-thickness skin grafting. In the upper extremity, the carpal tunnel should always be decompressed at the time of forearm fasciotomy, but usually this portion can be closed after release of the transverse carpal ligament (4).

Humeral Fractures

Most humeral shaft fractures are treated by closed methods with a coaptation splint, sling, or fracture brace, but fractures in obese patients or distal-third, distracted, or angulated fractures require surgical treatment (34).

Operative stabilization with an intramedullary rod or plate is indicated for associated ipsilateral fractures, open fractures with or without radial nerve palsy, bilateral fractures, and polytrauma victims (Fig. 100.13B). Somewhat greater degrees of angulation and shortening can be accepted in the humerus than in the lower extremity. Radial nerve palsy is present in 10% to 15% of fractures, especially spiral fractures of the distal third, where the nerve winds around the bone and can become stretched or entrapped. Laceration of the nerve is distinctly uncommon and recovery is the rule. Surgical exploration is indicated with persistent displacement, interposed soft tissue, and open injuries. A secondary radial nerve palsy that occurs as a result of manipulation or that arises during treatment may cautiously be observed provided that fracture alignment is maintained. Nonunion is more common in smokers, morbid obesity, and distracted fractures. It is treated by compression plating and iliac bone graft.

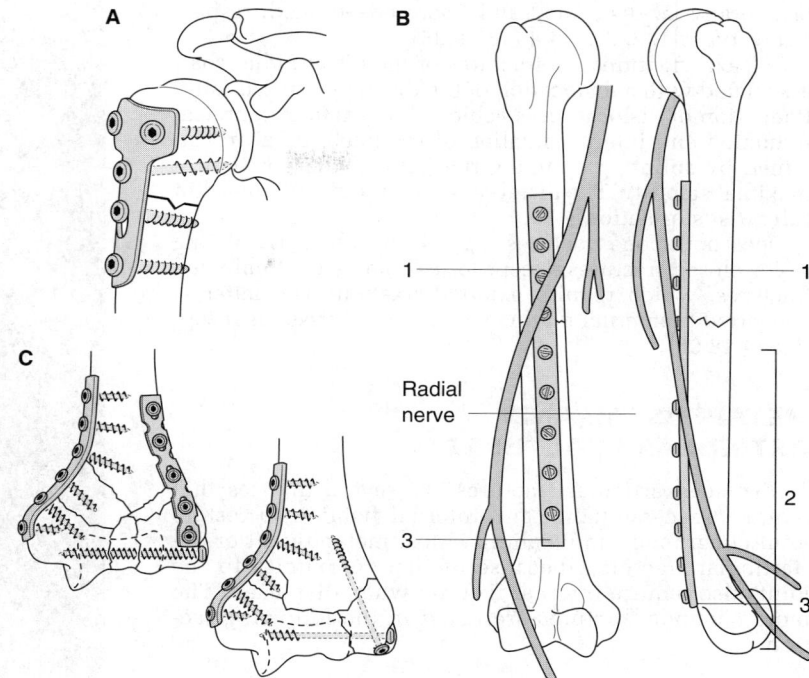

Figure 100.13. Operative treatment of humeral fractures. *(A)* Most fractures of the proximal humerus are treated nonoperatively with a hanging cast, or "sling and swathe." When displaced or associated with other fractures, they are best stabilized surgically. This allows for early range of motion of the joints involved. *(B)* Isolated shaft fractures are usually treated nonoperatively. With multiple, widely displaced, or open fractures, surgical treatment is indicated. An intramedullary rod may be used, but a plate is preferred in the humerus. The radial nerve should be identified and protected as it winds around the spiral groove of the humerus. *(C)* Supracondylar fractures of the humerus are frequently intraarticular. In adults, they require open reduction and internal fixation through a posterior triceps-splitting approach.

Radial and Ulnar Fractures

"Both-bone" forearm fractures in adults are optimally treated by open reduction and compression plating of both fractures (Fig. 100.14A,C) to ensure union and restoration of function of the hand and upper extremity. Isolated, minimally displaced fractures of the distal third of the ulna are exceptions and can be treated satisfactorily by closed reduction and casting.

Monteggia's fractures are fractures of the ulna in association with a dislocation of the radial head. The radial head may be dislocated anteriorly (most common), posteriorly,

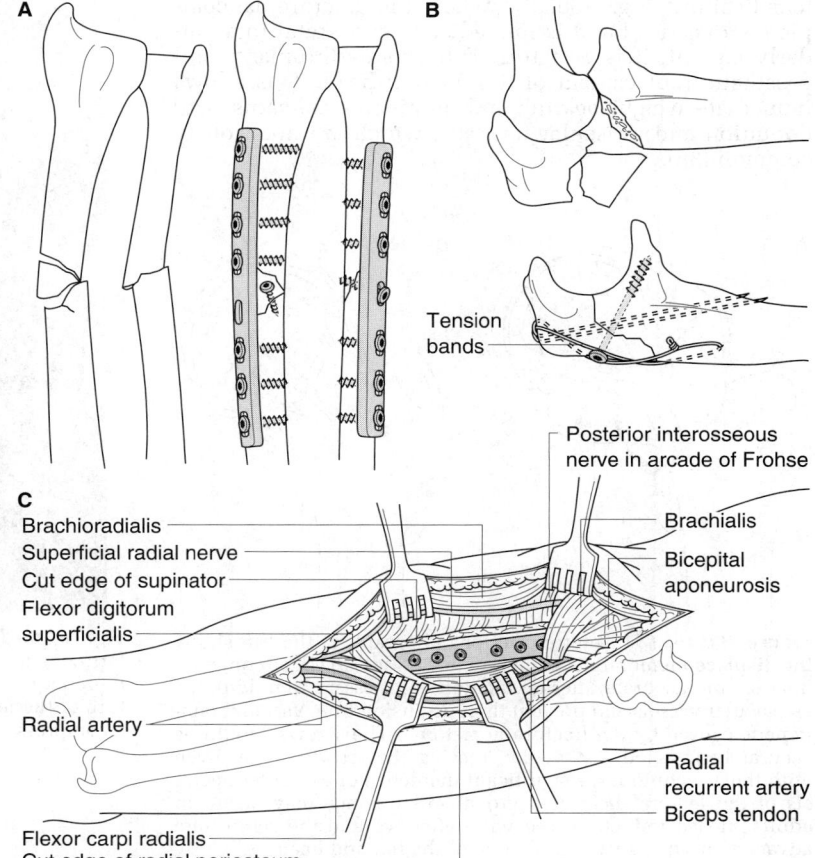

Figure 100.14. *(A)* Both-bone fractures of the radius and ulna in adults are best treated by anatomic open reduction and internal fixation. *(B)* Displaced fractures of the olecranon require open reduction and internal fixation. Tension-band technique and interfragmentary fixation are illustrated. *(C)* Open reduction and internal fixation of a proximal radius fracture. This fracture may be associated with a dislocation of the radial head (Monteggia's fracture). An anterior approach is illustrated, although a posterior approach is more commonly used. The posterior interosseous branch of the radial nerve is at risk because it lies in the supinator muscle. It must be carefully identified and protected.

or laterally, or dislocated and fractured—termed, respectively, types 1, 2, 3, and 4 (18,19,35).

Galeazzi fractures are fractures of the distal radial shaft associated with a dislocation of the distal radioulnar joint. Reduction of dislocation is achieved by anatomic surgical reduction and internal fixation of the fracture and maintained by splinting or fixing the joint in the position of maximal stability. The distal radioulnar joint is reduced in full wrist supination.

Open both-bone fractures are stabilized by rigid plating as for closed fractures except for extremely contaminated fractures, which require external fixation. The latter is converted to internal plating when the soft tissue is receptive (4,18,35).

METAPHYSEAL AND ARTICULAR FRACTURES

Displaced articular fractures are severe injuries that require open reduction and internal fixation to restore joint congruency and stability. Most metaphyseal or periarticular fractures, because of their proximity to the joint, also require internal fixation when displaced. The more common fractures are listed in the following sections.

Femoral Neck Fractures

Intracapsular fractures of the femoral neck usually occur in elderly osteoporotic patients, but occasionally occur in young patients as a result of high-energy trauma. Whenever the fracture can be reduced, especially in younger patients, it should be treated by reduction and multiple pin fixation, usually using cannulated screws and image intensification (Fig. 100.15). When the fracture is completely displaced and is immediately subcapital in an elderly patient, it is best treated by hemiarthroplasty and prosthetic replacement of the femoral head. This allows immediate weight bearing and eliminates concerns over nonunion and avascular necrosis, which are notoriously common (36).

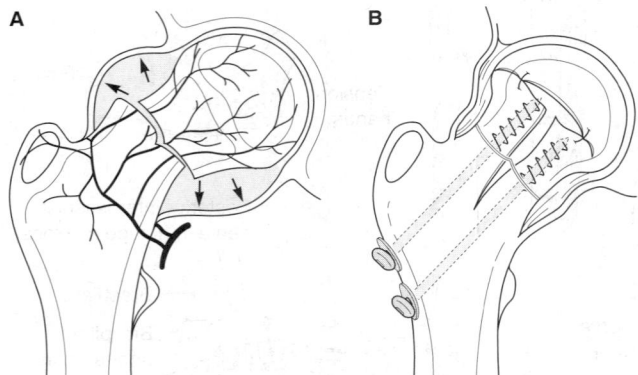

Figure 100.15. *(A)* Anteroposterior radiograph of the hip showing displaced femoral neck fracture in a child. *(B)* Urgent open reduction and accurate internal fixation is necessary to unkink the retinacular vessels and prevent their occlusion from vascular tamponade caused by the fracture hematoma. The screws should be accurately inserted and avoid crossing the growth plate. Even with these techniques, a significant incidence of avascular necrosis of the femoral head and growth disturbance may occur. In adults, closed reduction is usually effective and the screws are advanced to the subchondral bone of the femoral head.

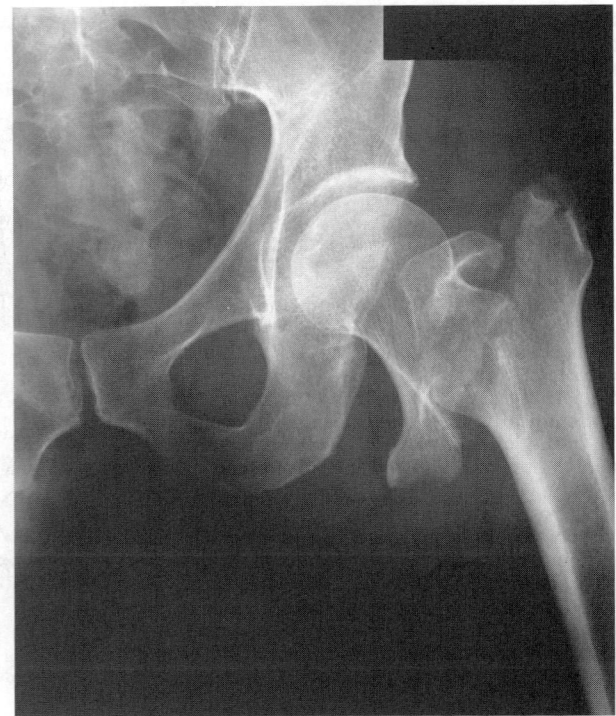

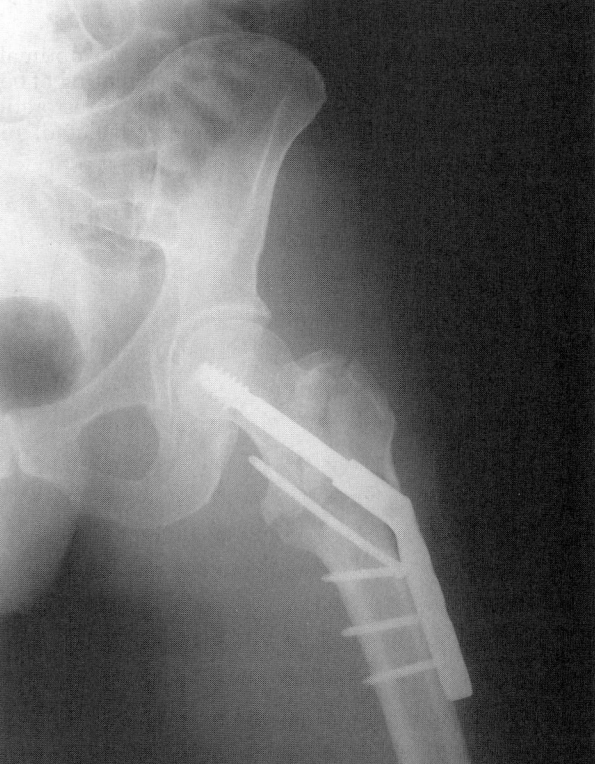

Figure 100.16. *(A)* Anteroposterior radiograph of irreducible intertrochanteric fracture of the femur, necessitating formal open reduction. *(B)* Anteroposterior radiograph of intertrochanteric fracture of the femur after open reduction and internal fixation with a compression lag screw and a side plate.

Intertrochanteric Fractures

Intertrochanteric femoral fractures are also common in elderly patients and are best treated by compression screws and side plates, yielding high rates of healing and satisfactory results (37) (Fig. 100.16). The complications of avascular necrosis and nonunion are rarely seen in this extracapsular fracture, in contradistinction to intracapsular femoral neck fractures. In the elderly, both types of hip fractures are associated with a 10% to 25% mortality rate in the first year, and up to 25% of patients may require long-term nursing care.

The complications of hip fractures are usually related to preexisting medical problems. In elderly patients, it is imperative surgically to stabilize hip fractures as rapidly as possible to decrease pain, allow mobilization, and prevent exacerbation of medical problems.

Subtrochanteric Fractures

These fractures are higher-energy fractures associated with more bleeding, difficulty with surgical stabilization, and postoperative morbidity. Because of high stress acting on implants, they are often best treated with an intramedullary device that also captures the femoral head and neck (38). These special intramedullary devices are known as *reconstruction rods* (Fig. 100.17). Alternatively, blade plates or standard compression screws with longer side plates can be used, but have a higher risk of cyclic fatigue failure (18).

Supracondylar Fractures

Supracondylar fractures are challenging intraarticular fractures that are often significantly displaced. They require accurate open reduction and internal fixation, usually with a compression screw and side plate. More proximal fractures can be treated with interlocked intramedullary rods, often inserted retrograde to ensure centering of the rod in the knee and correct alignment with the femoral shaft. Comminuted fractures oriented in the coronal plane require interfragmentary fixation and buttress plating (Fig. 100.18). Occasionally with extremely comminuted fractures in elderly, osteoporotic patients, distal femoral resection and modular total knee replacement may be indicated (12,18) (Fig. 100.19). Postoperative continuous passive motion, early joint mobilization, and delayed weight bearing are used.

Fractures of the Tibial Plateau

These challenging intraarticular fractures require open reduction, elevation of depressed fragments, bone grafting, and appropriate plating (Fig. 100.20) The lateral plateau is more frequently involved and somewhat more

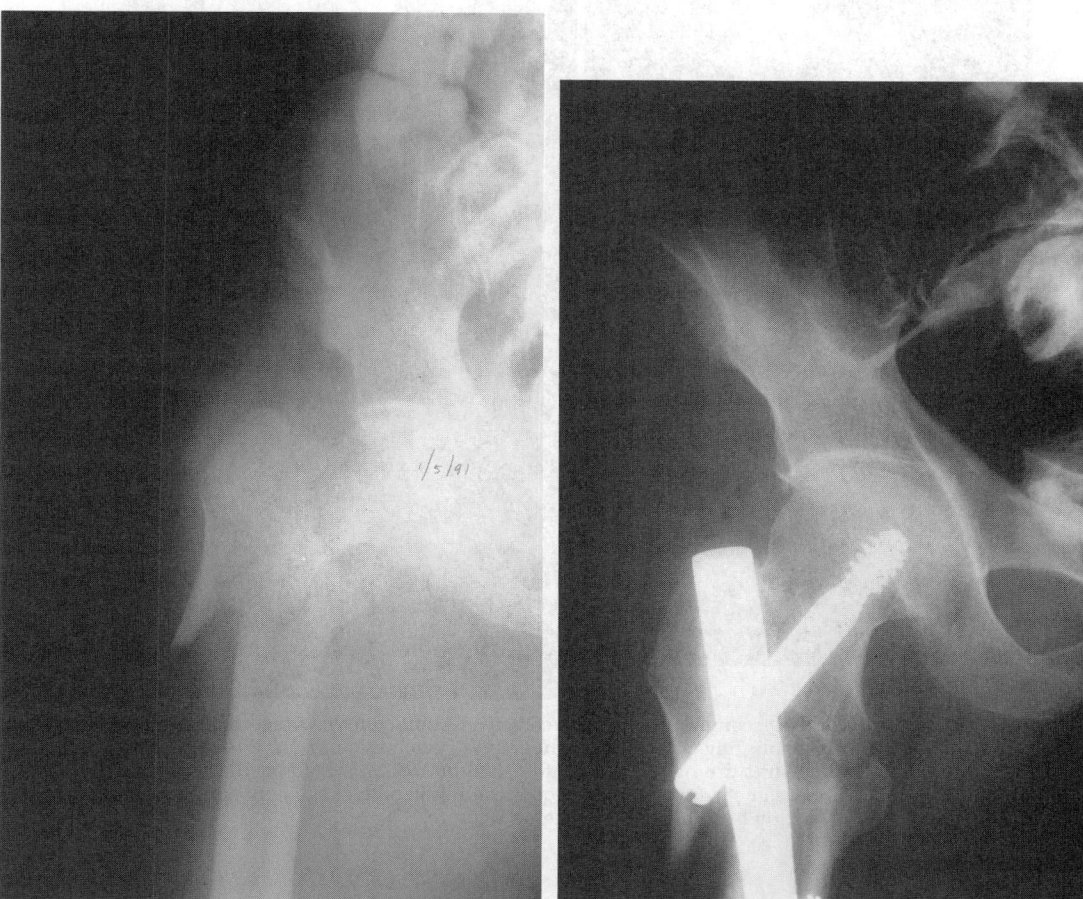

A   B

Figure 100.17. *(A)* Reverse-obliquity intertrochanteric femoral fracture. *(B)* Anteroposterior radiograph after Gramma reconstruction nailing. Failure of fixation is significantly less likely than with compression screw and side plate. This implant is also used for subtrochanteric fractures and for femoral shaft and ipsilateral femoral neck fractures.

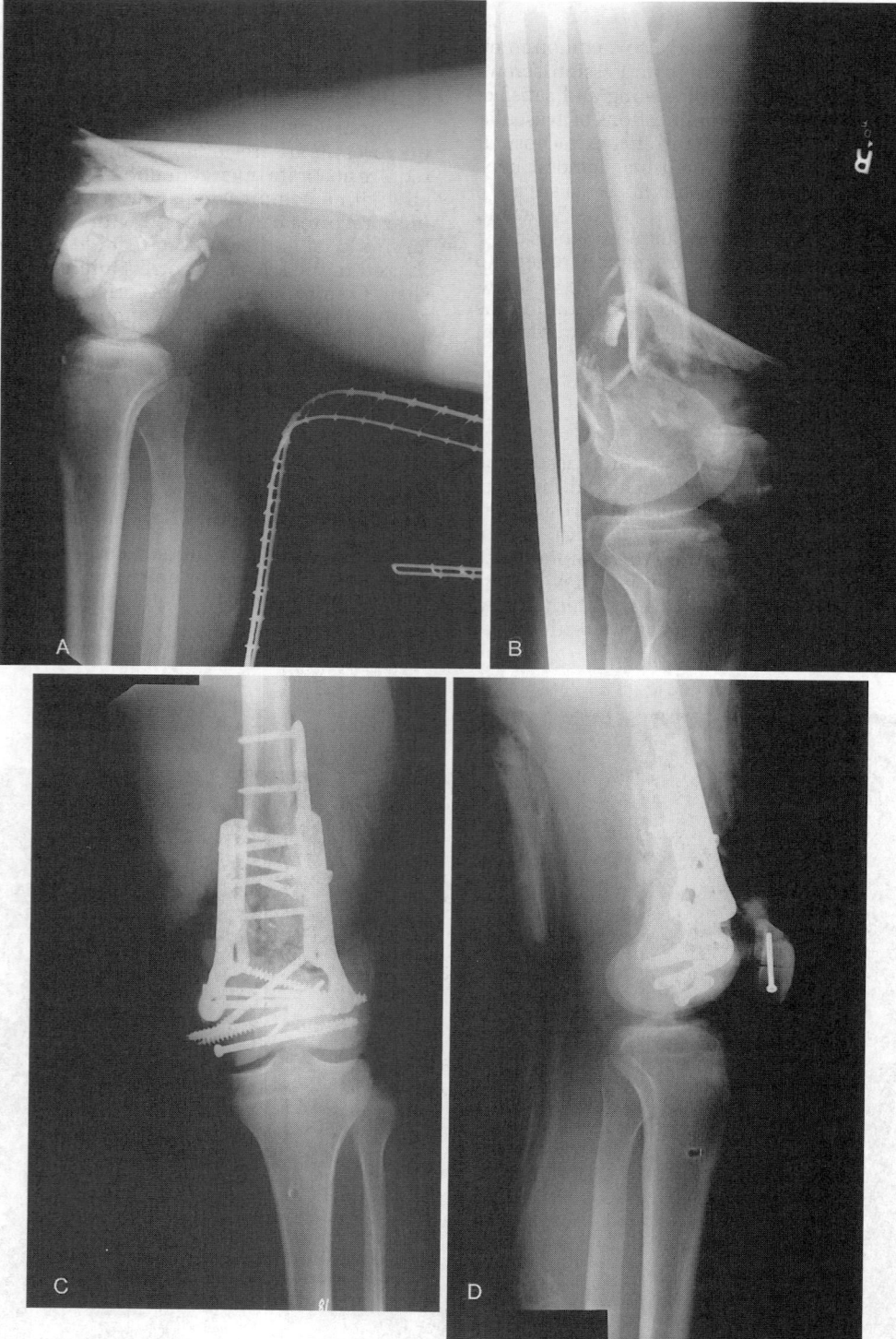

Figure 100.18. *(A)* Markedly comminuted, displaced open supracondylar fracture of the right femur. Note inappropriate splinting. *(B)* Lateral radiograph of same fracture. *(C)* Postoperative radiograph of supracondylar fracture of the femur after dual-buttress plating and iliac crest bone grafting. *(D)* Lateral view of same patient showing good restoration of the knee joint cartilage space and also satisfactory reduction of an associated patellar fracture.

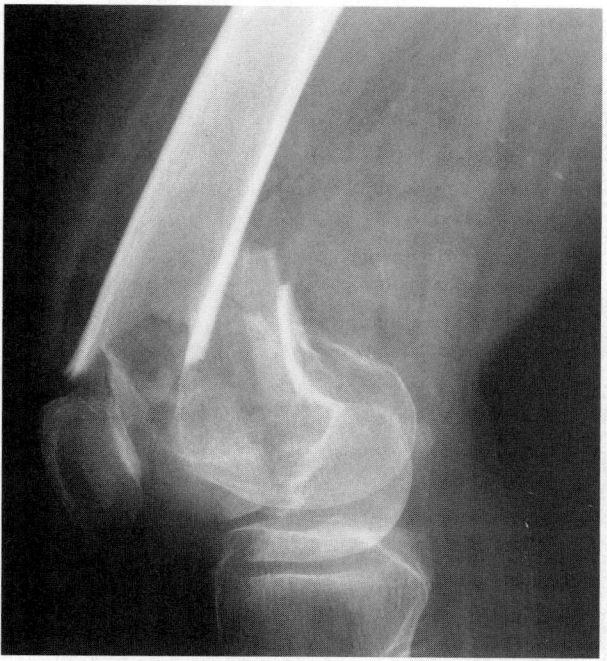

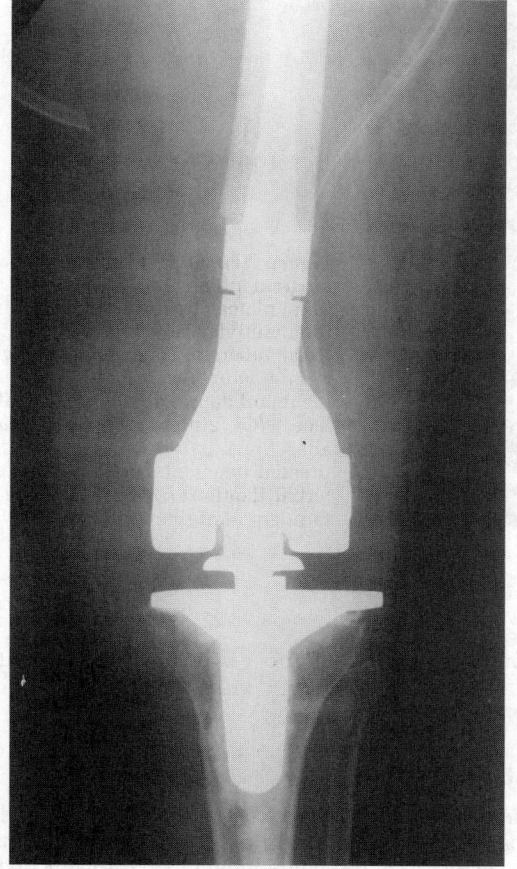

Figure 100.19. *(A)* Comminuted, displaced supracondylar femoral fracture in an elderly patient with poor bone quality. *(B)* Anteroposterior radiograph of knee after distal femoral replacement and modular total knee arthroplasty. This implant is more commonly used for tumors of the distal femur or complex revision total knee arthroplasty.

forgiving if healing occurs without valgus malalignment. Bicondylar fractures may require dual plating. Complications include skin slough over the subcutaneous medial plateau and avascular necrosis—the so-called dead bone sandwich. The meniscus should be saved and repaired if injured. Intraarticular fractures with extension into the tibial shaft or traumatized skin are particularly problematic and may require hybrid fixation. After surgery, all intraarticular fractures require judicious mobilization or continuous passive motion to prevent adhesions. Weight bearing is restricted until fracture healing at 10 to 12 weeks (12,18).

Patellar Fractures

Displaced fractures of the patella disrupt the extensor mechanism of the knee and patellofemoral articulation. They require open reduction and fixation with tension-band wiring, intrafragmentary lag screws, or both. Excision of the distal pole or patellectomy is occasionally necessary for comminuted fractures. Postoperative protected motion is desirable for most fractures (12,19).

Pilon Fractures

Pilon fractures are severe injuries that involve the intraarticular surface (plafond) of the distal tibia and ankle and are often accompanied by marked swelling and fracture blisters that may preclude early operative treatment. In this instance, temporary external fixation across the ankle joint is indicated. The fibula often may be safely surgically stabilized, restoring correct length and secondary ankle alignment. When the swelling has subsided and the soft tissue is receptive, open treatment is necessary for displaced articular fractures (Fig. 100.21). An anterior approach is used and the articular surface elevated, reconstructed, and frequently bone grafted. Low-profile plates, atraumatic surgical technique, and low tourniquet time are necessary to avoid the disastrous results of skin slough, infection, and exposed hardware. Even with microvascular free flap a suboptimal result is likely in this event, and amputation may eventually be necessary. In expert hands, the results are satisfactory in approximately 75% of cases. Nevertheless, a significant number of pilon fractures go on to posttraumatic arthritis and require eventual ankle arthrodesis despite restoration of anatomy (4,16,18).

Ankle Fractures

Ankle fractures are common injuries and, when displaced, require anatomic restoration of the ankle mortise for a good functional result. In contrast to the axial articular impaction seen with pilon fractures, torsional forces result in malleolar fractures that largely spare the tibial articular surface (plafond). These fractures may involve either the distal fibula, medial malleolus, or both (bimalleolar). If the posterior tibial malleolus is involved, these injuries are known as *trimalleolar fractures*. Closed treatment is effective for certain isolated lateral malleolar or undisplaced fractures.

Frequently, operative reduction is the only way to guarantee restoration of anatomy. Typically, a low-profile plate is used for the fibula and two 3.5-mm lag screws for the medial malleolus for the common inversion injury.

A more severe injury occurs when the foot is in pronation as the talus rotates laterally, producing in addition

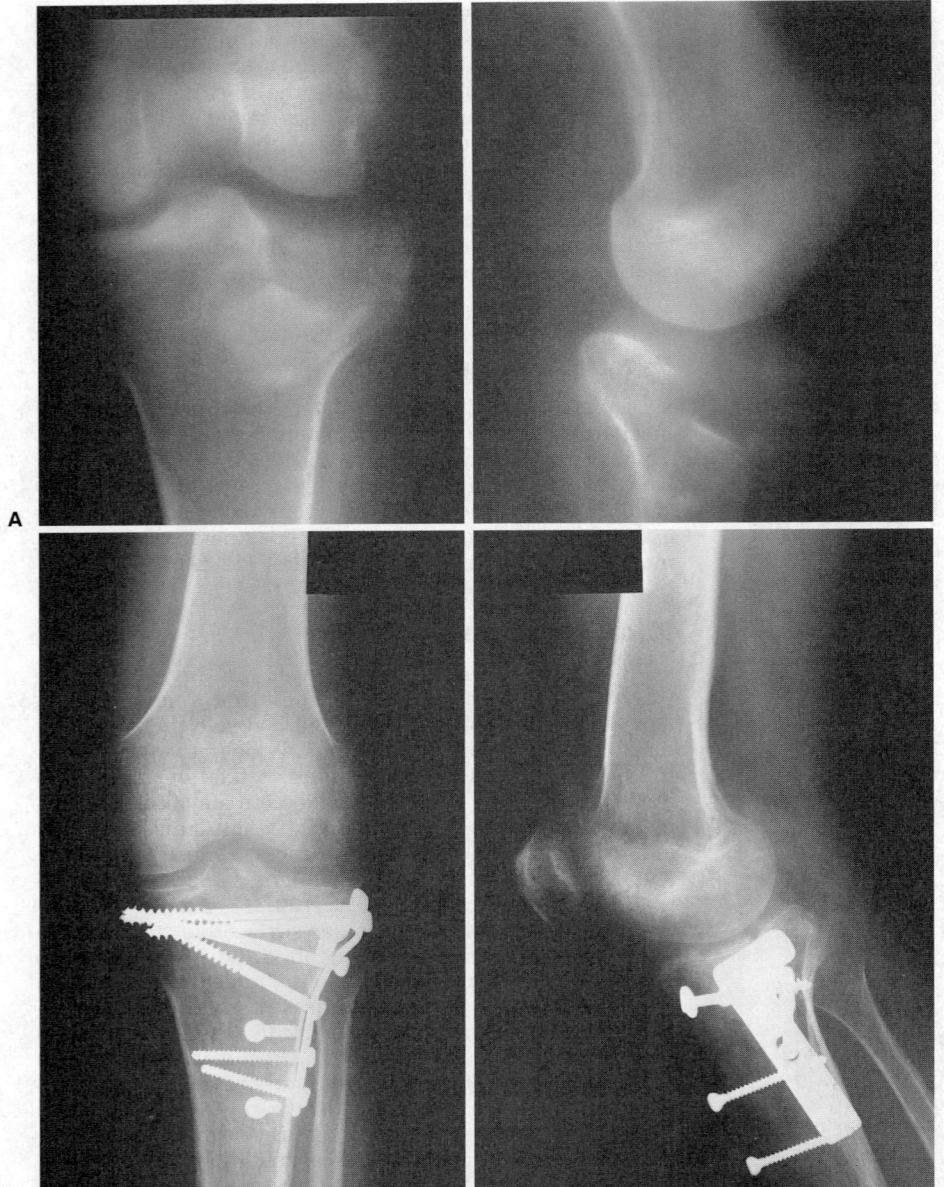

Figure 100.20. *(A)* Anteroposterior tomogram of markedly depressed lateral tibial plateau fracture, extending into the intercondylar notch and including the tibial tubercle. *(B)* Lateral tomogram of same fracture showing marked displacement and depression of the articular surface. *(C)* Anteroposterior radiograph after open reduction, elevation of depressed fragments, bone grafting and internal fixation. *(D)* Postoperative lateral radiograph of same fracture.

an injury to the tibiofibular syndesmosis. Characteristically, a high fibular fracture occurs several centimeters above the ankle, but may occur as far proximal as the knee—the Maisonneuve fracture. Therefore, "isolated" fractures of the proximal fibula require examination of the ankle. In addition to fracture fixation, a fibulotibial syndesmosis screw is required to approximate the torn syndesmosis and restore the ankle mortise (Fig. 100.22). A short leg cast is worn for 6 to 8 weeks for most ankle fractures, with partial weight bearing allowed depending on fracture characteristics and stability. Typically, ankle fractures do not involve the weight-bearing articular surface of the tibial plafond to any extent, heal rapidly, and are unassociated with arthritic sequelae if

anatomic reduction of the ankle has been maintained (4,16,18).

Foot Fractures

Fractures of the foot are frequently treated closed, with the exception of displaced fractures of the calcaneus and talus. Dislocation of the tarsometatarsal joints or Lisfranc's injury requires reduction and pinning or screw fixation. Most metatarsal fractures can be treated closed; however, displaced multiple metatarsal fractures can be treated by open reduction and Kirschner wire intramedullary fixation (17).

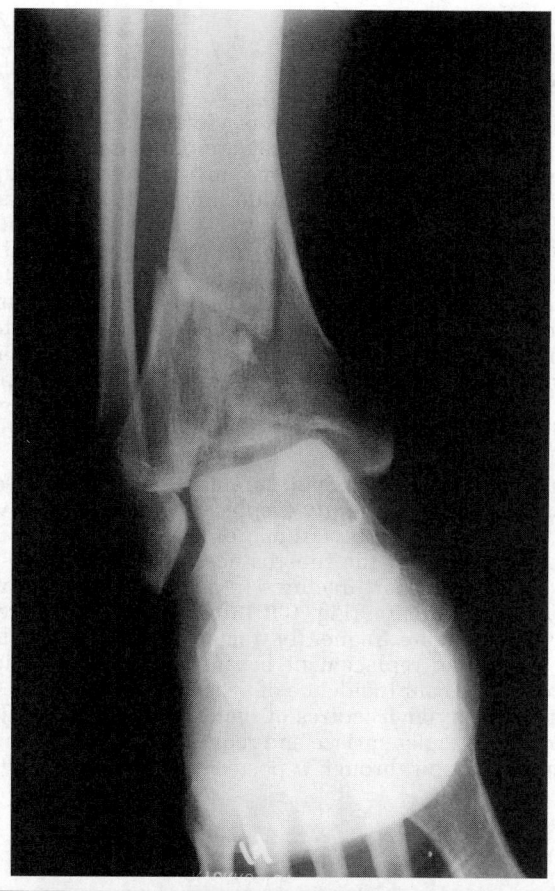

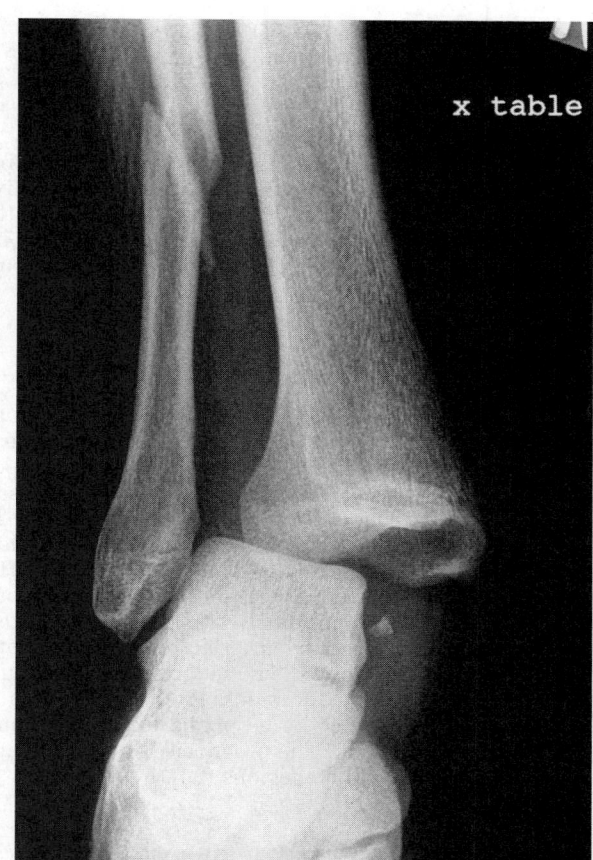

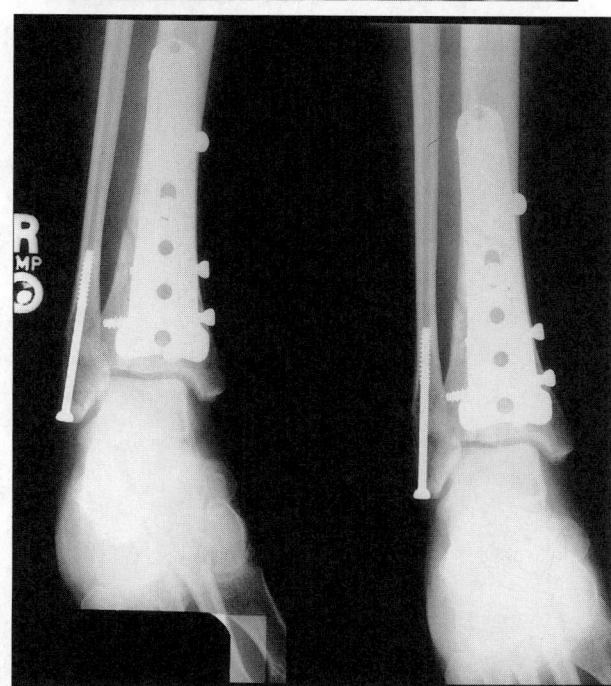

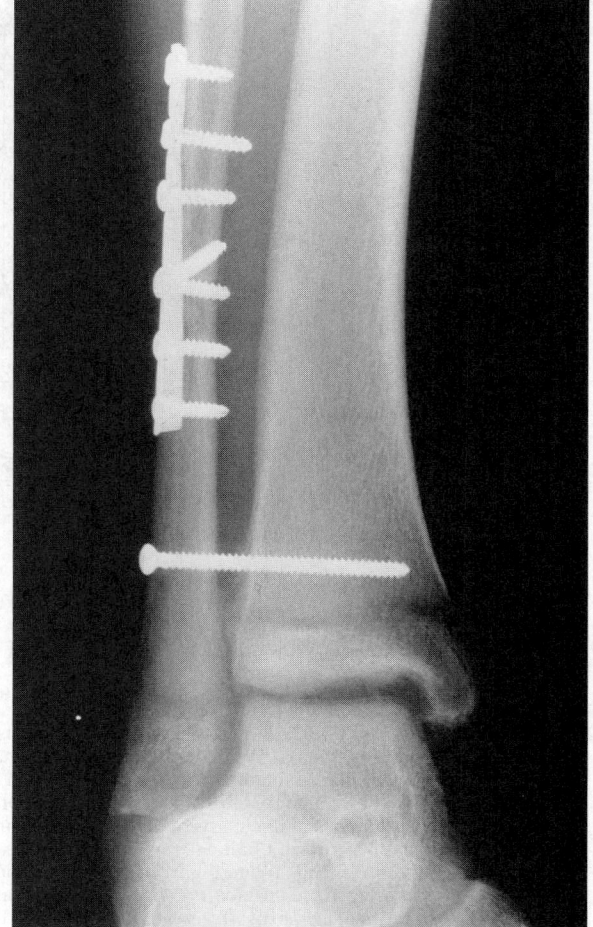

Figure 100.21. *(A)* Pilon impaction fracture of the distal tibial articular surface. *(B)* Postoperative film of pilon fracture after closed intramedullary fixation of the fibula and open reduction and internal fixation of the distal tibia, restoring the ankle joint.

Figure 100.22. *(A)* Fracture–dislocation of the ankle secondary to a pronation–lateral rotation injury. The syndesmosis is completely disrupted from the fibular fracture to the ankle. The deltoid ligament is completely torn, along with an avulsion fracture of the medial malleolus. *(B)* The fibula has been stabilized by open reduction and internal fixation. The ligamentous syndesmosis has been stabilized by a screw passing from the fibula to the tibia—the "syndesmosis screw."

UPPER EXTREMITY FRACTURES

Fractures of the clavicle are usually treated with a sling or figure-of-eight bandage and rarely require operative treatment. An exception is associated fracture of the scapula, which renders the shoulder unstable. In this instance, plating of the clavicle alone can help restore some stability (4,19).

Scapulothoracic Dissociation

This is an uncommon, devastating injury resulting in an internal degloving injury usually associated with fractures of the clavicle or scapula. The shoulder is literally ripped from the thorax, avulsing the subclavian or axillary vessels and portions of the brachial plexus. The injury may be open or closed, and partial or incomplete. In complete lesions, the patient presents with a pulseless flail arm. Hypovolemic shock is frequently present, as well as associated injuries, and a 20% mortality rate has been reported. Resuscitation is followed by arterial repair and exploration of the brachial plexus. The latter is frequently unrepairable. The protocol for brachial plexus injuries is followed and the clavicle can be plated to provide some stabilization to the thorax. The prognosis is poor with amputation likely for complete lesions (39).

Scapular Fractures

Most scapular fractures do not violate the articular surface of the shoulder joint. They are often associated with other fractures and polytrauma and are treated symptomatically with a sling or shoulder immobilizer and graduated mobilization. Displaced intraarticular fractures of the glenoid, although uncommon, require operative fixation. A posterior approach between the infraspinatus and teres minor along the axillary border of the scapula is usually selected. The axillary and suprascapular nerves need to be identified and protected. The posterior approach provides good visualization of the fracture and has low postoperative morbidity. The results are surprisingly good when anatomic restoration of the glenoid has been accomplished (40).

Fractures of the proximal humerus are usually treated closed unless significantly displaced and associated with multiple fractures, polytrauma, or ipsilateral injury. Displaced fractures of the tuberosities, as well as three-part and certain four-part fractures in active patients, may require open reduction (Fig. 100.13A). Four-part fractures in older patients are frequently treated by hemiarthroplasty and prosthetic replacement because they are associated with a significant incidence of avascular necrosis (18,41).

Supracondylar fractures of the humerus frequently involve the articular surface and require open reduction and internal fixation through a posterior triceps splitting ap-

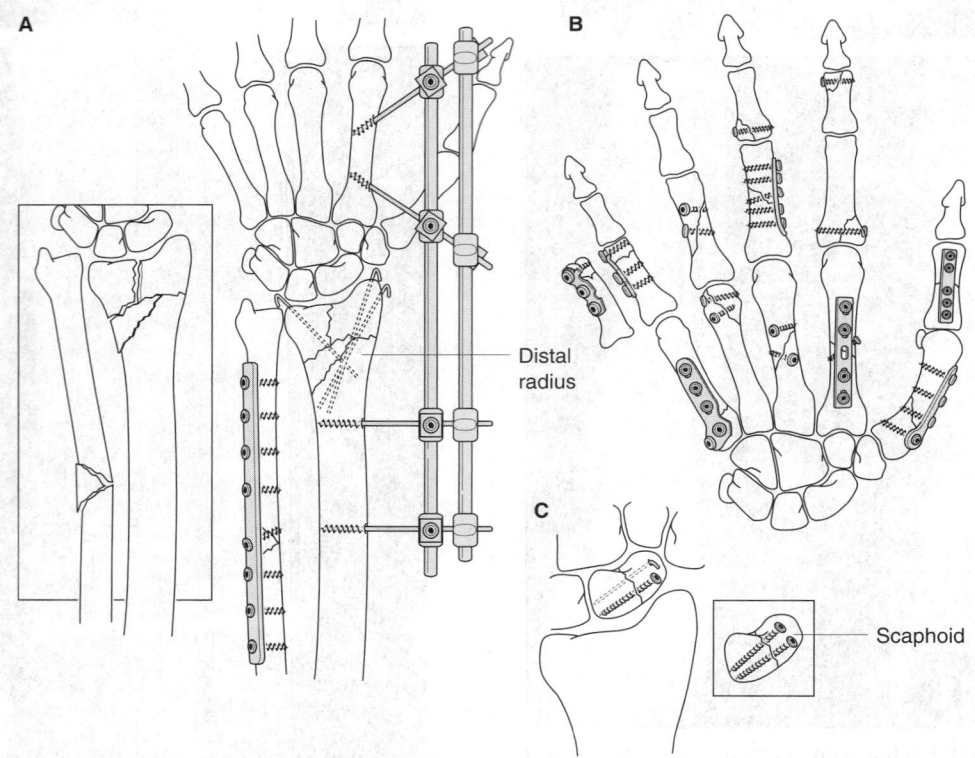

Figure 100.23. *(A)* Most fractures of the distal radius are treated by closed reduction and casting for 5 or 6 weeks. With significant displacement, inadequate closed reduction, or intraarticular fragments, percutaneous pinning, limited open reduction or external fixation across the wrist joints is indicated. The distal ulna was internally plated, but when isolated and minimally displaced, can be treated satisfactorily by closed reduction and casting. *(B)* Most isolated, minimally displaced fractures of the phalanges or metacarpals can be treated nonoperatively by appropriate reduction and splinting. When significantly displaced, intraarticular, or involving multiple digits, they are best stabilized surgically. Mini-fragment plates and screws are illustrated; however, Kirschner wire fixation can be used very effectively. *(C)* Undisplaced scaphoid fractures are treated by thumb spica cast immobilization for 8 weeks or longer. When displaced, open reduction and internal fixation is indicated. With nonunion, bone grafting is also performed.

proach and plating of both the medial and lateral columns of the distal humerus (42). The ulnar nerve should be protected but does not usually require anterior transposition. Early postoperative motion is important for all intraarticular fractures (42,18).

Fractures of the olecranon that are displaced require open reduction and internal fixation. Small fractures can be ignored or excised if comminuted (4,18,19). Tension-band fixation, interfragmentary screws, or reconstruction plates may be used depending on fracture characteristics (Fig. 100.14B)

Radial head fractures are treated nonoperatively unless comminuted and displaced. Excision is performed for comminuted fractures, and occasionally radial head replacement is necessary for associated elbow instability due to coexisting coronoid fracture of the ulna. Where amenable, open reduction and internal fixation using small or miniature fragment fixation plates is indicated (18,19,43).

Fractures of the distal radius (Colles' fracture) are common. They occur most often in elderly patients, especially osteoporotic postmenopausal women. When displaced, they present with the classic "dinner fork" deformity (44). Fracture of the ulnar styloid is often present. They usually can be treated by closed reduction and casting. In the 1990s, external fixation and percutaneous pinning have been added to the orthopedist's armamentarium and are indicated for unstable fragments or inadequate closed reduction (Fig. 100.23A). Open reduction and buttress plating are indicated for certain displaced intraarticular (Barton's) fractures (44,45).

Scaphoid Fractures

The scaphoid is the most frequently fractured carpal bone and is injured as a result of a fall on an outstretched, dorsiflexed hand. It is a known diagnostic pitfall that often is misdiagnosed as a sprain. Repeat examination and radiography may be necessary to rule out this fracture. In patients with tenderness over the tubercle or anatomic snuff box, thumb spica cast immobilization is indicated followed by repeat examination and radiography at 10 to 14 days to confirm or rule out fracture. Healing may take place slowly and prolonged immobilization may be necessary. Scaphoid fractures that are unstable or displaced are usually treated surgically (Fig. 100.23C). Distal pole and waist fractures are approached palmarly and proximal pole fractures dorsally. Nonunion and avascular necrosis are known complications of scaphoid fractures, especially when diagnosis and treatment have been delayed. Disability is best avoided by a high index of suspicion and awareness of this common fracture (4,18,19,46).

SPINE

Orthopedic spine surgery encompasses the diagnosis and treatment of discogenic disease, stabilization of degenerative spine disease, correction of deformity, and treatment of fractures and associated spinal cord injury.

Spinal Cord Injury and Spinal Fractures

The immediate stabilization and protection of a potentially injured spine by paramedical and transport personnel has reduced the incidence of neurologic injury. Quadriplegia and paraplegia are among the most dreaded of all injuries, and simple principles must be followed to avoid precipitating catastrophic spinal cord trauma. Spinal precautions dictate that a backboard and cervical collar be applied to all trauma victims with potential spinal injury and maintained until the spine is cleared clinically and radiographically. A cervical spine lateral radiograph should be obtained of the C-7 to T-1 disc spaces. In uncooperative or comatose patients, a cervical collar should be continued until a satisfactory clinical evaluation of the spine can be performed. Standard radiographs are usually diagnostic, although CT scans are extremely valuable and almost always indicated in polytrauma victims with any question of spine injury. MRI studies may also be indicated to evaluate the disc, nerve roots, and paraspinous soft tissues. In the cervical spine, dynamic flexion and extension views are also helpful to rule out occult instability. The fracture is then characterized and classified and a treatment plan established (47,48).

Stable Injuries

Stable injuries consist of sprains, minor tears of the posterior ligamentous structures and related soft tissues that induce muscle spasm and pain. The patient is neurologically intact and has no radicular symptoms. Radiographic analysis is negative or reveals isolated spinous process, undisplaced laminar, or minor compression fractures. Dynamic flexion and extension views are obtained to ensure stability in equivocal cases.

Unstable Injuries

By definition, a spinal fracture with associated neurologic deficit is unstable. Radiographically, a fracture or fracture–dislocation may reveal obvious instability, but it is important to look for subtle signs of instability such as widened interpedicular distance or deviation of the spinous processes. In the cervical spine, extensive retropharyngeal hemorrhage seen on the lateral radiograph as well as apparent "minor" subluxations at contiguous levels may be present. Small anterior avulsion or so-called teardrop fractures may be stable or associated with a highly unstable hyperextension injury of the cervical spine. CT scan and MRI are extremely helpful in identifying potentially unstable fractures. Limited cone-beam spiral CT has resulted in a dramatic decrease in scan times with obvious beneficial implications for trauma victims.

Anatomy and Classification

Conceptually, the spine can be thought of as a three-column structure. The anterior column consists of the anterior longitudinal ligament and anterior two thirds of the vertebral body, and the anterior portion of the intervertebral disc. The middle column includes the posterior portion of the body and disc, the posterior longitudinal ligament, and the lateral ligament and masses. The posterior column includes the facet and facet capsules, the lamina and spinous processes, the ligamentum flavum, and the interspinous and supraspinous ligaments (49).

Compression fractures typically injure the anterior column, occur secondary to flexion and compression forces, and are common in osteoporotic vertebrae. Unless severely wedged, these injuries are considered stable. When the middle column is involved, as in burst fractures, instability is usually present. Burst fractures usually display some degree of retropulsion of the posterior body into the spinal canal as viewed on the lateral radiograph and transpedicular widening on the anteroposterior view. All three columns may be fractured and have highly unstable lesions.

Treatment: General Principles

Stable injuries are treated symptomatically. A soft cervical collar may be worn for comfort. For minor injuries in the thoracolumbar region, a thoracolumbosacral orthosis also may be indicated. Occasionally, the subsequent development of increased kyphosis or deformity requires surgical treatment.

Operative Treatment

The absolute indication for operative intervention in spinal injuries is a progressive neurologic deficit in the presence of identified fracture or proven spinal cord compression. The relative indications include irreducible fractures and dislocations, open spinal injuries, and polytrauma. Uncooperative or restless patients may be at risk for neurologic complications and stabilization is justified in these instances. In general, stabilization is done for all unstable patterns or deformities that are likely to become clinically symptomatic because of deformity, even in the absence of neurologic injury. The most effective method of achieving neurologic decompression is anatomic reduction and alignment of the spinal fracture. Laminectomy is not indicated as an isolated procedure and may further destabilize the spine. A relative exception to this is acute disc herniation with neurologic deficit (47,48).

Injuries above the level of C-4 may result in death due to respiratory paralysis in the acute setting. The examining physician must distinguish between a complete and incomplete injury, as well as between root and spinal cord trauma. Obviously, any neurologic progression is an emergency and needs to be acted on immediately. Dual-crush, multilevel fractures, or associated systemic trauma may make diagnosis difficulty.

The presence of spinal shock may mask some incomplete cord injuries. After spinal shock has resolved in 24 to 72 hours, accurate diagnosis is possible. If there has been no neurologic recovery at this time, quadriplegia is permanent although some important root recovery may occur. Extensive hemorrhage or complete cord transection can be identified on MRI, as well as severe edema and of specific nerve root lesions. The goal of treatment in any spinal cord injury is protecting uninjured cord or root function by decompression of the spinal cord using closed or open spinal column realignment and stabilization. Protection of residual function also requires restoration of hemodynamics, treatment of other associated injuries, and maintenance of adequate perfusion pressures. High-dose steroids are indicated in acute spinal cord injury, especially in incomplete lesions. After recovery from spinal shock, they are of no use in patients who are permanently quadriplegic (47).

Cervical Spine

Fixation Modalities. Posterior wiring techniques using the spinous processes or the facet joints provide good stability; however, lateral mass plating is also very effective. Anterior corpectomy, bone grafting, and plate stabilization is necessary for certain teardrop or other comminuted body fractures in the cervical spine. In this instance, the plate functions as a tension band in extension, and as a buttress plate in flexion of the neck. It is used most often after severe wedge compression or burst fracture. A cannulated screw can be inserted for odontoid fractures using an image intensifier and minimally invasive anterior technique.

Upper Cervical Spine Fractures

Fracture of C-1 (Jefferson's Fracture). Fractures of the ring of the atlas (C-1) can be diagnosed on the open-mouth anteroposterior radiograph, which shows lateral displacement of the lateral masses. CT reveals undisplaced fractures or subtle atlantoaxial abnormality. Treatment with a halo brace usually suffices. Uncommonly, a myelopathy develops on a chronic basis and a C-1 lam-

inectomy followed by fusion from occiput to C-2 may be necessary (47).

Odontoid (Dens) Fractures. Odontoid (C-2) fractures are among the most frequently missed spinal fractures. It can be difficult to obtain an adequate open-mouth view and an axial CT section may miss the axially oriented fracture line that lies in the same plane. For this reason, reformatted images in the coronal and sagittal planes are mandatory. Undisplaced fractures at the base of the odontoid (type 3) can be treated in a halo vest. Fractures through the waist (type 2) and above frequently do not heal and require posterior sublaminar wiring (Fig. 100.24A). Alternatively, in younger patients with a reducible fracture, odontoid screw fixation can be effective. This preserves rotation at C-1 to C-2 (Fig. 100 .24B).

Hangman's Fracture (Fracture of the Neural Arch of C-2). Traumatic atlantoaxial spondylolisthesis is a well known and common injury in the upper cervical spine. Patients who survive this injury are neurologically intact. The injury results in decompression or widening of the neural canal so that even in unstable injuries, spinal cord injury is not common. For minor degrees of displacement, a rigid cervical orthosis may be all that is necessary. Usually a period of halo traction followed by halo vest immobilization for 10 to 12 weeks is necessary. Occasionally, reduction cannot be obtained by traction or the C-2/C-3 facet joint is dislocated, requiring open reduction and facet wiring.

C-1 to C-2 Subluxation. Instability at C-1/C-2 may occur rarely in the absence of a fracture owing to traumatic rupture of the transverse and apical ligaments. The rheumatoid spine is prone to such injuries. These ligaments stabilize and control the relationships between the ring of C-1 and the odontoid (dens). In the upper cervical spine, the normal atlantodens interval as seen on the lateral radiograph is up to 3 to 4 mm, and greater than 6 to 7 mm is clearly abnormal. In the latter case, chronic and progressive instability is common because these ligamentous injuries frequently do not heal well. Treatment is usually a halo brace, but subsequent instability frequently requires C-1 to C-2 fusion and sublaminar wires or transarticular screws across the lateral masses. If instability is al-

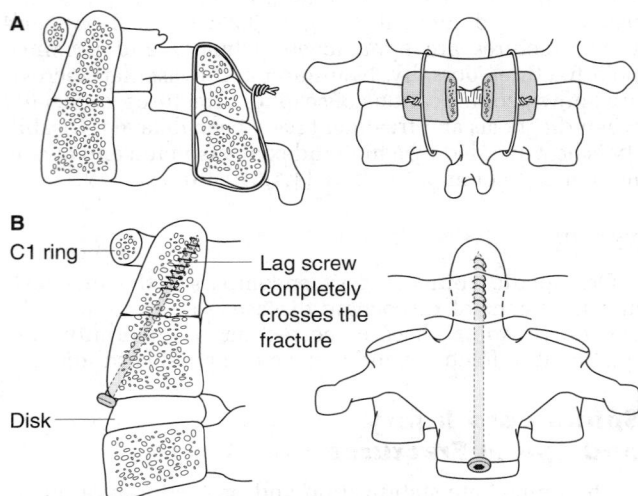

Figure 100.24. Stabilization of fractures of the odontoid. *(A)* Posterior sublaminar wiring of C-1 to C-2 with incorporated bone graft is the most common method for treating displaced or nonunited fractures of the odontoid. *(B)* This method preserves rotation at the C-1 to C-2 level. An anterior cervical exposure and fluoroscopic control is used to insert an odontoid screw.

lowed to progress, spinal cord cord compression can lead to a myelopathy, global weakness, respiratory depression, and, ultimately, death. These patients—justifiably so—have a sense of "impending doom."

Cervical Spine C-2–C-7

Unilateral Facet Dislocation. Radiographic diagnosis is made by the presence of a mild anterior subluxation on the lateral radiograph (approximately 25%) and a subtle shift of the spinous process at the level of injury seen on the anteroposterior radiograph. Oblique views may show a "perched facet." Closed reduction is the treatment of choice, but may require gradually increasing traction forces of up to 60 to 90 pounds. Before undertaking this degree of traction, an MRI scan should be obtained to rule out the uncommon but potentially disastrous extruded herniation that might cause cord compression with reduction of the deformity. If the dislocation does not reduce in traction, open reduction followed by interspinous wiring and bone grafting is required (Fig. 100.25).

Bilateral Facet Dislocation. The radiographic diagnosis is more obvious, with usually greater than 50% displacement of one vertebra on the other. In addition, local kyphosis is present. This injury cannot occur unless the posterior annulus and longitudinal ligament are disrupted, rendering the spine very unstable. The dislocation is easily reduced but very unstable, requiring posterior cervical stabilization.

In patients with incomplete injury or certainly with progressive neurologic signs, urgent operative reduction should be undertaken. This is warranted even in the quadriplegic patient because the salvage of a cervical root has a major impact on upper extremity function.

Burst Fracture. These injuries are unstable to varying degrees and they are usually treated with surgery or a halo brace. In a neurologically intact patient or one who has an incomplete lesion, an anterior approach is often necessary, with corpectomy decompression, strut grafting, and anterior plating. Highly unstable lesions involving the posterior column and elements may also require supplementation with posterior fusion or a halo vest. Failure to recognize a three-column injury can lead to major complications secondary to residual or recurrent instability.

Teardrop Fracture. Some minor compression fractures can cause a small fragment of the anterior vertebral body to displace slightly. However, the true teardrop fracture represents a somewhat uncommon but very unstable hyperextension injury. This fracture is unstable rotationally and sagittally in an orthosis and should be stabilized through anterior interbody fusion and plating (Fig. 100.26).

Fracture–Dislocation. This injury is essentially a progression in severity of a burst fracture, is usually highly unstable, and has a significant incidence of spinal cord injury. All three mechanical columns are disrupted through soft-tissue restraints, fracture, or dislocation. Treatment is by anterior vertebrectomy, bone grafting, and plating, augmented by halo immobilization or, in more severe multilevel injuries, combined anterior and posterior fusion providing immediate 360-degree circumferential stability and spinal cord decompression (47).

Fracture of the Posterior Elements and Lateral Masses. Isolated fractures of the spinous process, lamina, and facets are frequently stable. Treatment is either a cervical orthosis or halo vest. Facet injuries vary in degree of instability. Some displaced facet fractures can impinge on the neural foramen, producing nerve root symptoms and associated neurologic deficits. In this instance, the most appropriate treatment is reduction of the fracture followed by posterior fusion. Lateral mass fractures are usually stable and respond to immobilization and bracing.

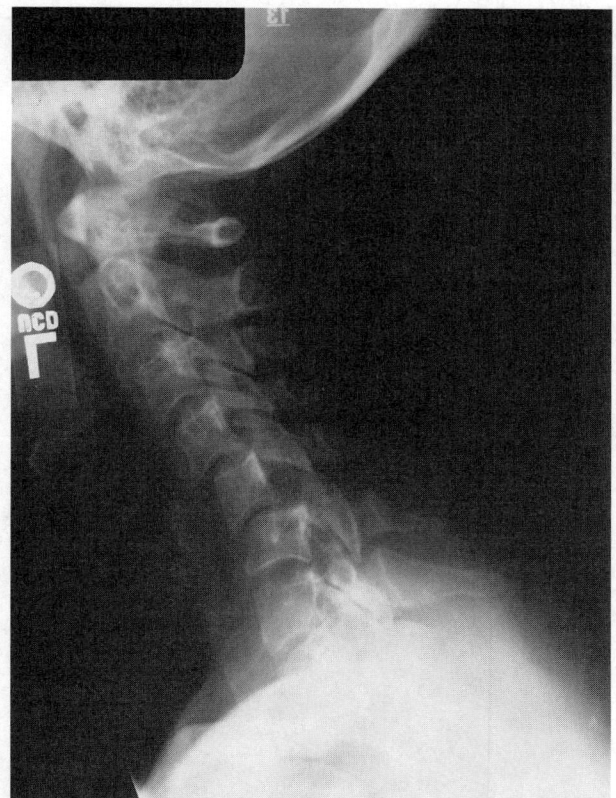

A

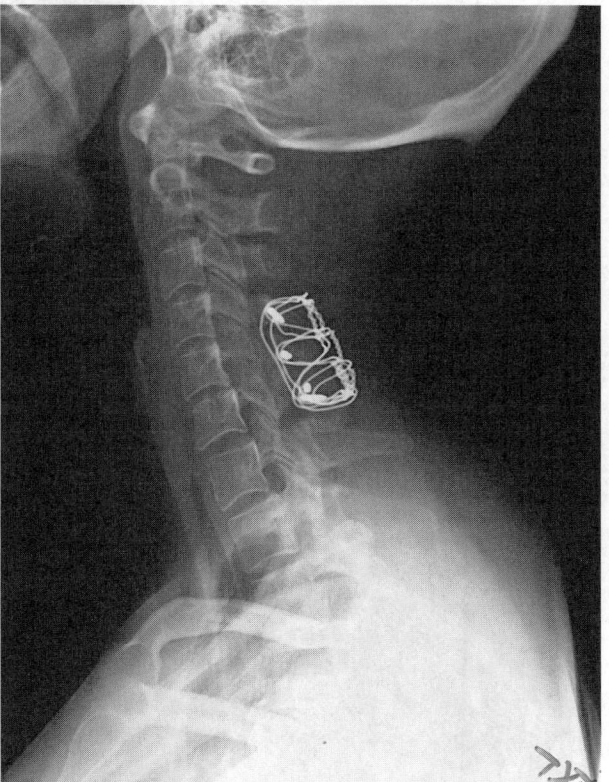

B

Figure 100.25. *(A)* Lateral cervical spine radiograph demonstrating unilateral facet dislocation. *(B)* Lateral radiograph after open reduction and sublaminar wiring with posterior bone grafting. After reduction, these injuries are often stable, and immobilization in a halo vest may suffice.

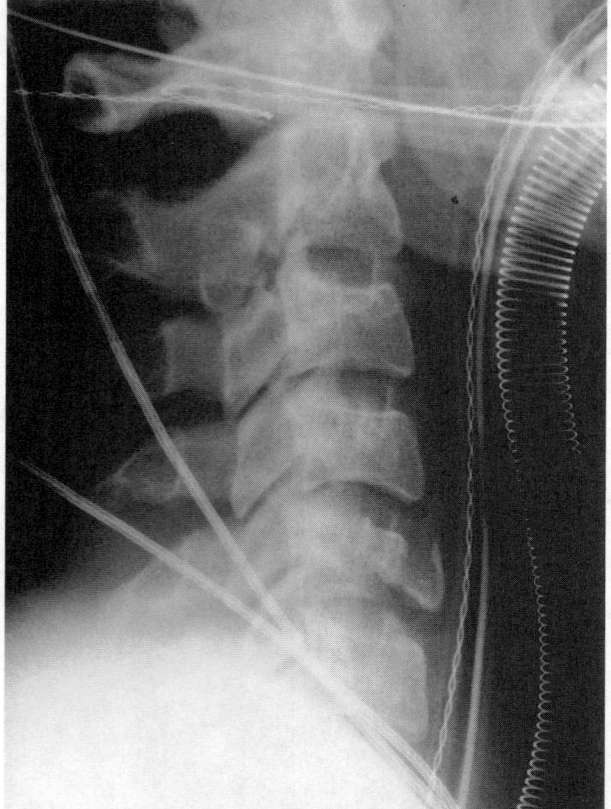

A

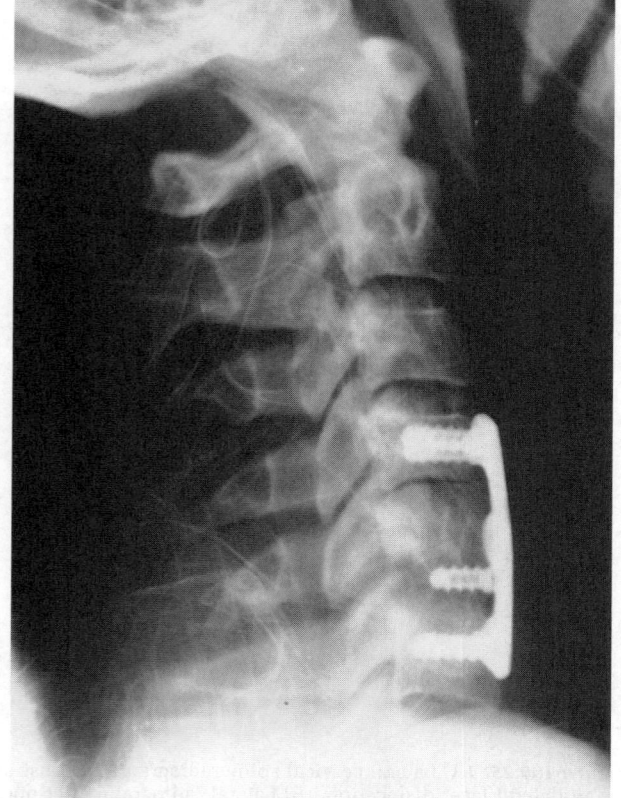

B

Figure 100.26. *(A)* Teardrop fracture of the anterior body of C-5. *(B)* Postoperative lateral radiograph after open reduction and anterior cervical fusion from C-4 to C-6 stabilized by a low-profile titanium plate.

Thoracic Spine

The thoracic spinal canal is less capacious than the cervical spine above or lumbar spine below, and therefore any significant displacement is likely to result in paraplegia. The conceptual anatomy is the same as described for the cervical spine in terms of classification and radiographic definitions of instability. In the thoracic spine, the rib cage and sternum, if intact, tend somewhat to splint or stabilize thoracic spine fractures. Pure compression fractures in the thoracic spine are common and may involve contiguous vertebrae. Unless associated with signs of instability or severe kyphosis, they are usually treated nonoperatively with appropriate bracing. With involvement of only the anterior column, neurologic loss is uncommon. With highly unstable lesions, transthoracic anterior decompression, grafting, and plating may be indicated, and this usually prevents later deformity and pain. Unstable fracture dislocations may require posterior instrumentation and stabilization (47).

Thoracolumbar Spine

Because of changes in the anatomic configuration of the facet joints and the increased mobility at the thoracolumbar junction, fractures and fracture–dislocations are more common in this region. T-12 and L-1 and contiguous vertebrae are frequently involved. The spinal cord terminates at the lower border of L-1, and therefore injuries at this level and above involve the conus or cord and injuries below involve the cauda equina nerve roots (48).

Diagnosis is by physical examination, with palpation for defect or malalignment of the spinal column, localized pain, or neurologic deficit. A rectal examination is mandatory, noting the sphincter tone and presence of bulbocavernous reflex. Recovery of this reflex usually occurs within 24 to 48 hours and signals the end of spinal shock. Residual neurologic deficit beyond this point is usually permanent when the cord is involved; however, some root recovery may occur with cauda equina lesions. A CT scan provides an accurate assessment of canal compromise and occult fractures involving the posterior elements. Where neurologic deficit exists with no apparent fracture, such as when a vascular cause is suspected, an MRI is indicated to assess the cord, disc, and related soft tissues.

Compression Fractures.   Involvement of the anterior column alone without severe kyphosis can be treated symptomatically with a brace. If there is greater than 50% anterior wedging or contiguous vertebrae are involved, a hyperextension body cast may be indicated or, occasionally, posterior segmental spinal stabilization may be required using pedicle screws, sublaminar hooks, and rod constructs.

Burst Fractures.   Axial compression injuries and burst fractures are common in the thoracolumbar junction and characteristically display local kyphosis with retropulsion of bone into the spinal canal. Fortunately, the canal is more capacious at this level and a surprisingly large degree of retropulsed bone is compatible with intact neurologic function.

Burst fractures always involve the anterior and middle columns and are unstable to varying degrees. These fractures are some of the most common spinal injuries that require operative stabilization. Usually this is performed semielectively while continuing spinal precautions until after the patient has been stabilized and life-threatening injuries attended to. Important exceptions to this are incomplete lesions or any progressive neurologic deficit. These patients require urgent decompression and stabilization. With significant retropulsion and disruption of the anterior and middle columns, an anterior approach with corpectomy, interbody fusion, and plating is indicated (Fig. 100.27). The cord is best decompressed anteriorly in these instances because laminectomy only adds

further to instability. Posterior stabilization is usually performed simultaneously or sequentially in this instance. In paraplegic patients, surgical stabilization is indicated if there is significant kyphosis to prevent progressive late deformity and chronic pain (48).

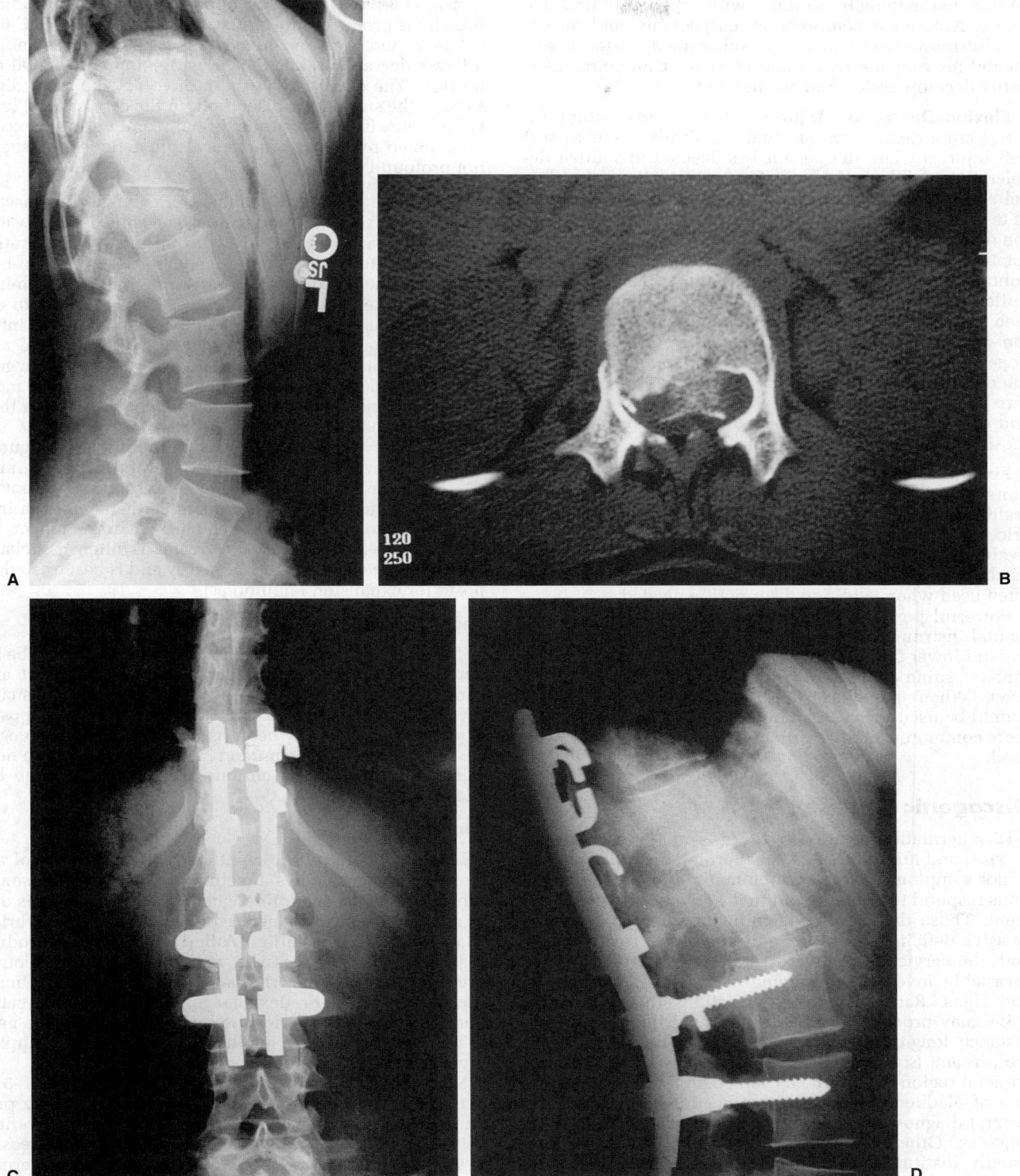

Figure 100.27. *(A)* Burst fracture of L-1, secondary to motor vehicle accident. Patient had incomplete neurologic injury. *(B)* Computed tomography scan showing marked retropulsion of bone into the spinal canal. *(C)* Anteroposterior radiograph of thoracolumbar junction after reduction and stabilization using contoured rods, proximal hooks, and inferiorly placed pedicle screws. *(D)* Postoperative lateral radiograph. Note improved restoration of spinal canal and sagittal contours after open reduction, corpectomy, and anterior bone grafting of L-1 burst fracture.

Fracture–Dislocation. As in the cervical spine, these injuries are highly unstable and frequently cause neurologic compromise or frank paraplegia. All three spinal columns are involved as well as soft-tissue restraints to varying degrees. Patients who are fortunate enough to have intact neural function or incomplete lesions need to be handled extremely carefully with this highly unstable injury. Anterior decompression, corpectomy, and fusion, in addition to simultaneous or subsequent posterior segmental instrumentation, is necessary to ensure circumferential decompression and stabilization.

Flexion–Distraction Injuries. Flexion–distraction injuries are a distinct variant that classically occur in seat belt injuries when the person is subjected to sudden deceleration and the body flexes forward over the restraining belt. Failure of the posterior and middle columns occurs in tension. The anterior column may fail in tension or flexion depending on the location of the fulcrum and center of rotation. If the failure is anterior to the spine, all three columns may fail in tension and the spine is literally pulled apart, producing a highly unstable injury associated with paraplegia. The Chance fracture is a unique flexion–distraction injury, sometimes referred to as the *all-bone fracture,* in which there is a horizontal splitting of the neural arch, pedicles, and vertebral bodies. This fracture is usually unassociated with any neural compromise and can be treated with hyperextension body cast or orthosis, unless significantly displaced (48).

Fixation Modalities. Anterior decompression in the thoracolumbar spine is accompanied by structural bone grafting to prevent collapse and recurrence of deformity. Tricortical iliac crest, ribs, allograft bone rings, or, alternatively, cancellous bone in titanium mesh cages may be used. Anterior plates or local neutralization constructs are often used where additional support is needed.

Powerful posterior fixation systems are available. Segmental instrumentation using pedicle screws in the lumbar and lower thoracic spine and sublaminar hooks in the thoracic spine connected to contoured rods is commonly used. When possible, short segment instrumentation should be used to save motion segments. Compressive or, more commonly, neutralization–distraction modes may be used.

Discogenic Disease

Disc herniation or degeneration is common in both the cervical and lumbar areas. Many herniations produce only minor symptoms or are asymptomatic. Most disc herniations respond to "tincture of time" and conservative treatment. Those that produce significant symptoms or progressive deficit frequently require operative treatment. In both the cervical and lumbosacral spine, nerve roots are invariably involved, producing characteristic symptoms and signs. Rarely, massive herniations in the cervical spine may produce myelopathy or quadriparesis. In this instance, long tract signs such as hyperreflexia and clonus are present. Similarly, a large disc extrusion in the lumbosacral region can produce cauda equina syndrome with loss of bladder and bowel function. In these situations, prompt diagnosis and treatment are mandatory to prevent sequelae. Otherwise, surgical treatment is elective and usually instituted only after appropriate and prolonged nonoperative treatment has failed (19).

Cervical Spine

Cervical disc herniations usually involve the C-5 to C-6 or C-6 to C-7 discs, but can occur at other levels as well. Neck pain and paraspinous muscle spasm is usually pre-

sent. Cervical radiculopathy commonly produces shoulder or scapular pain with varying degrees of radiation into the upper extremity. Disc herniation at C-5 to C-6 produces a C-6 radiculopathy, which may be characterized by a weakness of wrist extension or sensory deficits along the C-6 dermatome. The brachioradialis reflex may be asymmetric compared with the opposite side. A C-7 radiculopathy is produced by herniation of the disc at the C-6 to C-7 level and is characterized by triceps weakness and, to a lesser degree, weakness of wrist flexion and digital extension. The classic hypesthesia involves the third digit. Most of the surgery for discs, both in the cervical and lumbar regions, is done for relief of pain, and with the exceptions noted previously, the neurologic deficits are usually not profound.

Treatment. Surgical treatment of cervical disc disease is anterior discectomy and fusion. The spine is readily and safely approached anteriorly with minimal postoperative morbidity (18,50,51). Alternatively, for posterolateral herniations associated with spur formation or foraminal stenosis, a keyhole laminotomy can be performed to decompress the nerve root completely. When anterior interbody fusion is performed, the graft may be inlayed and locked in place or secured with a low-profile plate. In general, surgical treatment of cervical disc disease is more predictable and results in greater patient satisfaction than lumbar discectomy.

Degenerative disc disease may be present at contiguous levels. MRI evaluation is extremely helpful in determining the levels to be fused. Two-level disc involvement is treated by standard anterior fusion. Rheumatoid spines with steplike subluxation frequently require longer fusions. Three-level disease or greater is often associated with spinal stenosis or a myelopathy and is best treated by posterior expansion laminoplasty.

Thoracic Spine

Thoracic disc herniation is uncommon but should be included in a differential diagnosis of atypical chest and back pain. Operative treatment is uncommon and usually involves anterior transthoracic discectomy because posterior laminectomy has been associated with paraplegia. Disc herniation is not common in this area and, when neurologic involvement is absent, difficult to diagnose because of its rarity.

Lumbar Spine

Low back pain, with or without sciatica, is one of the most common maladies affecting humankind. It is sometimes difficult to determine whether low back pain is due to muscle spasms, degenerative disc disease and arthritic changes, or disc herniation. With disc herniations producing nerve root compression, radicular leg pain becomes predominant. Patients who have mild neurologic deficits, such as foot drop or reflex change, may be initially treated nonoperatively. An obvious exception is progressive neurologic deficit or cauda equina syndrome, which requires urgent laminectomy and decompression.

Most disc herniations occur at the L-4 to L-5 and L-5 to S-1 levels. A disc herniation at the latter level may produce an S-1 radiculopathy with loss of the Achilles reflex, decreased plantar flexion strength, and varying degrees of dysesthesia or numbness in S-1 distribution. Disc herniation at the L-4 to L-5 level may produce a foot drop or weakness of dorsiflexion of the great toe. The patellar reflex so frequently tested may not be diminished or asymmetric when either of these two common disc levels are involved. Considerable overlap in neurologic findings can exist. The major indication for surgery is severe radicular pain, especially when associated with a neurologic deficit. MRI is highly sensitive and can help corroborate the diagnosis. It is somewhat nonspecific, however, with frequent disc bulges found incidentally or at asymptomatic levels. MRI has no known biologic hazard and has essentially replaced myelography for the diagnosis of discogenic disease.

Treatment. When indicated by progression of symptoms or neurologic findings, laminectomy and discectomy is the surgical treatment of choice in the lumbar spine. This can be performed by a standard posterior approach or through microdiscectomy using a microscope and small, atraumatic incision. Paraspinal decompression using image intensification and fiberoptic visualization is a third, less common option. It is difficult to remove large amounts of disc by this method. Injection of chymopapain, which enzymatically dissolves the disc, is no longer used extensively because of the few case reports of neurologic deficit or paraplegia. A few patients also had severe anaphylactic reactions. Nevertheless, this modality was successful in a significant number of patients and it is still used in some countries (52).

Spondylolisthesis. The most common form of spondylolisthesis is characterized by a defect in the pars interarticularis that allows variable anterior slipping of L-5 on S-1. Spondylolysis is a defect alone without forward subluxation. The etiology is unknown, but trauma and familial predisposition may be factorial. Elongation and fatigue fracture of the pars interarticularis occurs. Subluxation or "listhesis" may range from mild to severe. Radiographs reveal a break in the pars—the neck of the "Scotty dog"—seen on oblique views of the lumbosacral spine. Lateral views reveal the degree of forward slip and inclination or slip angle. CT or MRI scans are also obtained.

Symptoms are variable and may begin in childhood or adolescence. Rapid slip progression may occur during growth spurts and cease or slow significantly at skeletal maturity. Low back pain and muscle spasm are common. Children may exhibit hamstring tightness or fatigue. High-grade slips may carry neurologic symptoms, severe pain, and deformity. Complete displacement of L-5 on S-1 can occur and, rarely, with high slip angles L-5 may descend into the pelvis (spondyloptosis), producing cauda equina syndrome. The rib cage abuts or slips over the iliac crests.

Treatment is symptomatic in most cases. It is estimated that less than 10% of patients require surgery. Chronic or progressive pain is the usual surgical indication. In situ posterolateral fusion is used for intermediate slips (Fig. 100.28). Patients with moderate to severe slips frequently need discectomy, decompression of nerve roots, and resection of a loose neural arch. Because progression of slip and pseudoarthrosis is common in these cases, anterior fusion may also be indicated. In severe slips, it is difficult to reduce the slip or improve alignment and attempts to do so may result in neural compromise. In spondyloptosis, resection of the body of L-5 and fusion of L-4 to the sacrum may be the best choice because it does not lengthen the spine and is less likely to stretch the nerve roots or cauda equina.

A pararectal, retroperitoneal, or transperitoneal surgical approach is usually necessary to gain exposure. Injury to the superior hypogastric plexus may result in retrograde ejaculation in male patients, and an attempt to preserve it should always be made.

Degenerative spondylolisthesis occurs in adults at L-4 to L-5 and is associated with modest subluxation, a narrowed disc space, facet arthrosis, and arthritic changes. It is a frequent source of chronic low back syndrome.

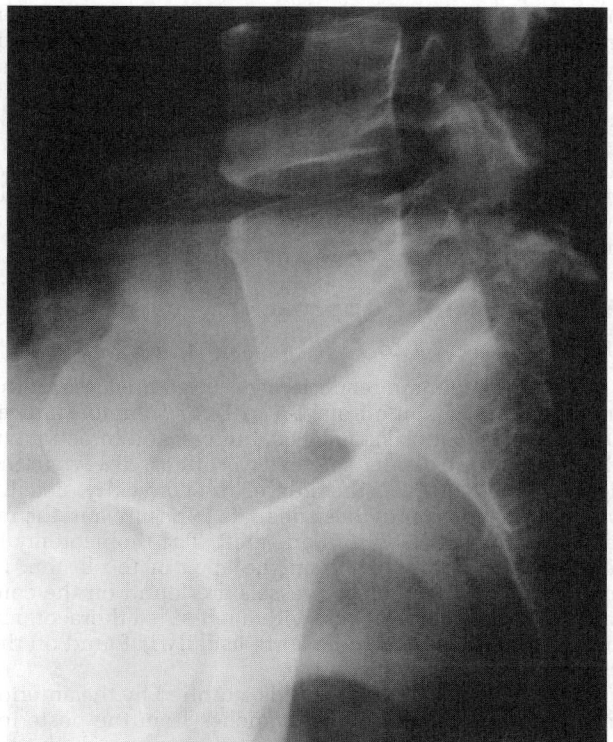

A

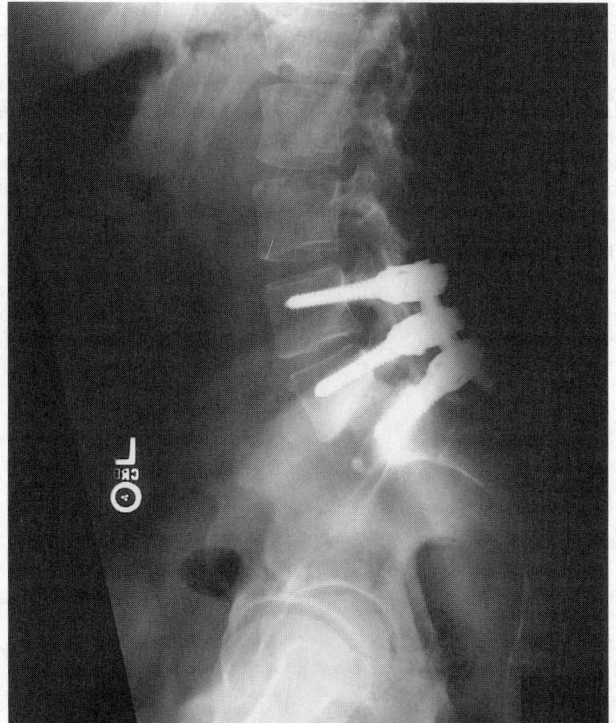

B

Figure 100.28. *(A)* Symptomatic grade II spondylolisthesis of L-5 to S-1. *(B)* Postoperative lateral radiograph of the lumbosacral spine after posterior lumbar interbody fusion and posterior instrumentation with pedicle screw construct at L-4 to the sacrum.

Ankylosing Spondylitis. Ankylosing spondylitis is a seronegative spondyloarthropathy characterized by a chronic inflammatory process affecting the axial skeleton. It is also known as *Marie-Strúmpell disease* and is grouped with other spondyloarthropathies associated with psoriasis, colitis, and Reiter's syndrome. The articulations of the spine, and frequently the hip and shoulder, are principally involved. Most patients are human leukocyte antigen B27 positive. Treatment with antiinflammatory medication suffices for most patients. However, progressive flexion deformity of the spine may produce severe kyphosis and "chin on chest" deformity, requiring corrective osteotomy. Hip replacement may be required. A proclivity for spinal fracture and neurologic sequelae is present, and orthotic protection or surgical stabilization often is required.

Anterior Spinal Approaches

Thoracic Spine: T-4 to T-11

A transthoracic approach is used to gain access to the anterior thoracic spine from T-4 to T-11. Common indications include scoliosis, kyphosis, tumors, and infection. In idiopathic scoliosis, the convexity is almost always to the right. Thoracotomy on the side of the convexity, usually with rib resection, provides adequate exposure and the resected rib may be used for bone graft. The thoracotomy is centered two ribs higher than the apex of the lesion. In scoliosis, the large thoracic vessels are found on the concave side of the curve. Thus, with a left-sided thoracotomy for left-convex scoliosis, the aorta usually is found on the right side of the spinal column.

Blood flow to the spinal cord is supplied by the anterior and posterior spinal arteries; branches from the posterior intercostal arteries reach the spinal cord through the interspinal foramina and anastomose with the anterior spinal artery. A critical watershed lies between T-4 and T-9. Dissection in this region needs to be meticulous and, where possible, the segmental feeders spared. Ligation of the segmental arteries should be performed on the vertebral bodies as far anteriorly as possible and subsequent posterior dissection limited so that arterial arcades joining the segmental arteries in the region of the vertebral canal are preserved.

Thoracolumbar Junction

A transpleural–retroperitoneal thoracoabdominal approach with transection of the diaphragm can be used to expose the anterior spine from T-9 to L-5. Approaches to the thoracolumbar junction are principally indicated for vertebral fractures and also for scoliosis, kyphosis, tumors, or infection. This approach is used when it is necessary to expose several contiguous vertebrae in the region of the thoracolumbar junction (Fig. 100.29).

Lumbar and Lumbosacral Spine

The lumbar spine and lumbosacral junction from L-2 to L-5 is approached retroperitoneally, preferentially from the left. Access to L-2 may require resection of the 12th rib. Principal indications are kyphosis, tumors, or spondylitis.

Lumbosacral Junction and Sacrum

A pararectal retroperitoneal approach to the lumbar spine and sacrum from L-3 to S-2 can be accomplished with the patient in the supine position. At the inferior margin of L-4, the ureter crosses the common iliac artery, accompanied by the testicular vessels. The superior hypogastric plexus courses above the aortic bifurcation and is responsible for the innervation of the genitourinary system. Injury to this plexus may lead to retrograde ejaculation in the male patient.

A transperitoneal approach to the lumbosacral junction is principally indicated for high-grade spondylolisthesis or tumor. This approach can expose the lumbosacral disc space fairly rapidly, but injury to the superior hypogastric plexus is more frequent.

Chronic Low Back Syndrome

There are many causes low back pain. Beginning in middle age, spondylolisthesis, facet arthrosis, degenerative arthritis, and disc disease are common. Lumbar or lumbosacral fusion is recommended for severely symptomatic patients and those with instability, who have not responded to nonoperative treatment. Pedicle screws connected to rods ensure stability and increase the rate of fusion. Posterior lumbar interbody fusion can be very successful in stabilizing unstable arthritic lumbar spines (53) (Fig. 100.28).

Acquired lumbar spinal stenosis may present in middle or old age and is characterized by neurogenic claudication

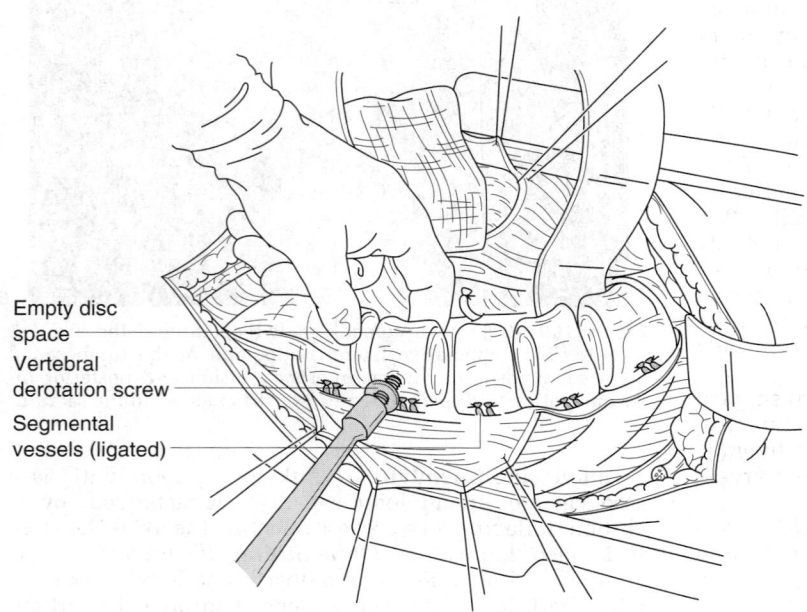

Empty disc space

Vertebral derotation screw

Segmental vessels (ligated)

Figure 100.29. Thoracoabdominal retroperitoneal approach to the thoracolumbar spine for correction of a lumbar curve. The segmental vessels have been ligated and the disc space cleared, and a vertebral derotation screw is being inserted. Sequential screws are inserted and connected to a solid rod, allowing derotation and correction of the deformity. Structural bone graft is placed in the disc spaces to enhance fusion and prevent postoperative kyphotic deformity. This surgical approach is also used for thoracolumbar spine fractures, infection, and tumors.

and occasionally bladder and bowel disturbance. In contrast to vascular claudication, peripheral pulses are usually present and back and leg pain is relieved by recumbency. The cause is narrowing and hypertrophy of the posterior elements of the spine, including the pedicles, facet joints, and laminae. Treatment is by wide laminectomy.

Spinal Infection

Disc space infection is usually accompanied radiographically by destruction of both end plates or the presence of a paraspinal or psoas abscess. Extensive destruction of vertebral bodies may occur with tuberculosis, which is more common in developing nations. Disc space infections or vertebral osteomyelitis also occur in IV drug abusers, diabetic patients, or immunocompromised individuals. Infection can mimic neoplasms, old trauma, or congenital abnormality (54). MRI and CT scan are extremely helpful in evaluating and differentiating spinal abnormalities. Chronic low back pain can be caused by infection, often with unusual organisms such as *Coccidioides, Brucella,* or *Cryptococcus.* Diagnostic work-up frequently includes bone scan, gallium scan, erythrocyte sedimentation rate, C-reactive protein, serologic titers where indicated, and skin tests. Blood cultures may be positive in bacterial infections and DNA amplification techniques helpful. Specific enzyme-linked immunosorbent assay may be necessary with unusual infections such as brucellosis.

The specific diagnosis is made by aspiration or biopsy and culture and sensitivity of the disc space or vertebral bodies. Fungal organisms may be identified microscopically. Treatment is appropriate decompression or specific antimicrobial therapy, or both. Disc space infection frequently responds to antimicrobial treatment alone. Extensive bone destruction, instability, or neurologic loss requires judicious spinal stabilization.

ARTHRITIS AND JOINT REPLACEMENT

Coincident with the natural aging process is an increased instance of degenerative arthritis. Presumably this is caused by repetitive microdamage occurring over a lifetime. Age, sex, body weight, and familial predisposition are other factors that influence the development of degenerative changes. The onset of symptoms is typically in the sixth or seventh decade, but can be much earlier. The gradual onset of joint pain, usually increasing in severity and associated with varying amounts of deformity and loss of motion, is typical. Radiographs reveal loss of joint space and cartilage, subchondral sclerosis, and cyst formation. Early treatment with analgesics, antiinflammatory agents, or joint injections is helpful in alleviating the severity of symptoms. A cane or a walker may mechanically unload the involved joint. Unfortunately, in a significant number of patients, symptoms progress to the point where joint replacement is necessary. In the United States alone, an estimated 300,000 total joint arthroplasties are performed annually. In the hip and knee, this procedure is highly successful in restoring pain-free ambulation and improved motion. Joint replacement is capable of providing dramatic improvement in the quality of life and restoration of function (55) (Fig. 100.30).

Under favorable circumstances, the longevity of total hip and knee arthroplasty can be 15 to 20 years. Frequently, however, radiographic evidence of bone resorption at the implant interfaces appears, and may or may not

be symptomatic. With progressive bone resorption, mechanical loosening occurs and the patient again becomes symptomatic.

Periprosthetic fractures may occur, requiring long-stem revision, strut allografts, and cerclage cable plates or megaprostheses in the femur. When the knee is involved, supracondylar femur fracture is invariably present.

Revision surgery, which requires removal and reimplantation of articulating components, is complex and associated with somewhat less satisfactory outcomes. In younger and more active patients, the wear rate is increased and failure may occur earlier. It is therefore more important in these patients to maximize and exhaust all nonoperative modalities before embarking on joint replacement.

Total Hip Arthroplasty

Joint replacement is most commonly performed for degenerative and posttraumatic arthritis, rheumatoid disease, avascular necrosis of the femoral head, and residua of congenital or acquired pediatric hip disorders. The modern era of joint replacement began in the early 1960s with Sir John Charnley, who defined and implemented the scientific principles on which the procedure is based. He emphasized a low-friction bearing surface, use of biocompatible material, and the intimate interfacing of the implants with bone through the use of polymethylmethacrylate cement. High-density polyethylene remains the material of choice for the metal-backed acetabular component. Polished metal alloys of chrome cobalt or titanium are used for the femoral component. Significant advances have improved the longevity of artificial joints (20).

One of the main causes of aseptic loosening appears to be a macrophage foreign body reaction and osteoclastic resorption of bone, and noncemented implants are recommended in younger patients. The femoral component is manufactured to produce a porous surface that allows for biologic ingrowth and fixation of the implant. Technically, it is important to obtain precise filling of the femoral canal to prolong longevity. Primary total hip arthroplasty for degenerative arthritis is straightforward and can be performed through one of several different surgical approaches. Immediate weight bearing as tolerated is allowed after surgery (20).

The incidence of postoperative complications is low, but of serious consequence. Infection occurring early in the postoperative period is treated by evacuation of hematoma, IV antibiotics, and institution of a suction irrigation system. Late-occurring infection usually requires removal of all components and meticulous débridement of cement particles from the femoral canal and acetabulum. Antibiotic beads or a cement spacer are then implanted for several months, and if repeat aspiration of the joint is negative for organisms, reimplantation may be considered. Postoperative dislocation is usually preventable by appropriate precautions. Recurrent dislocation frequently indicates component malposition and may require revision.

Deep venous thrombosis is common and frequently asymptomatic. Pulmonary embolism can be prevented in most cases by the use of sequential compression devices on the lower extremities and carefully monitored anticoagulation. In high-risk patients or when anticoagulation is contraindicated, a vena caval filter should be considered.

Revision total hip arthroplasty is much more complex, usually because of loosening of components, bone loss, and occasionally the presence of previous infection. Revision frequently requires long-stem or custom implants. Preoperative planning may include three-dimensional modeling of the pelvis and acetabulum. Bulk allografts may be used but have been associated with catastrophic

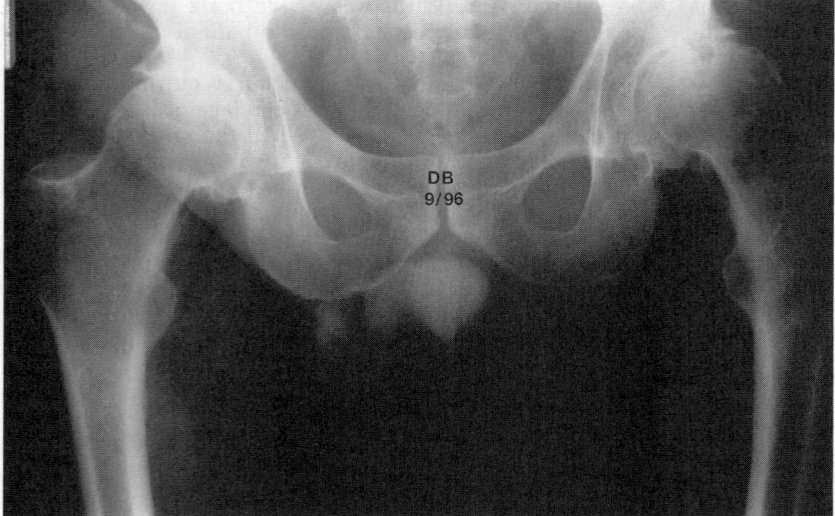

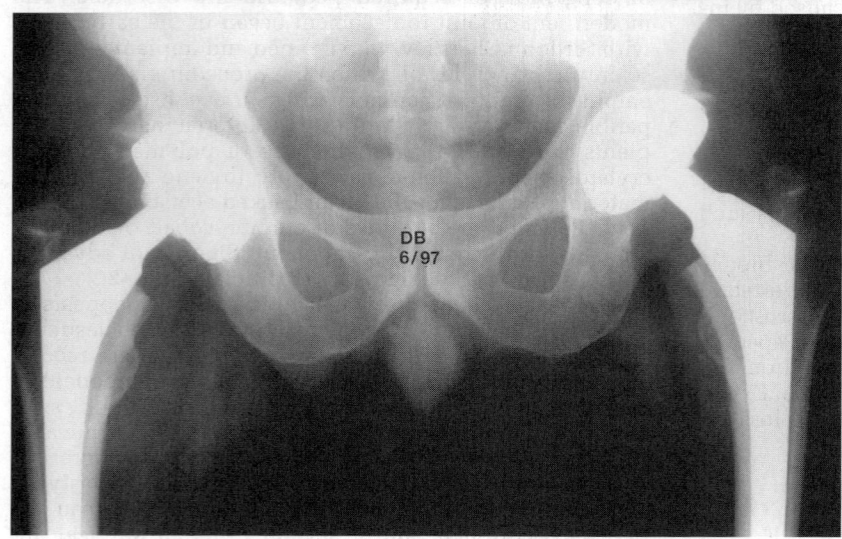

Figure 100.30. *(A)* Anteroposterior radiograph of the pelvis showing bilateral advanced degenerative arthritis of the hip. *(B)* Postoperative radiograph after bilateral total hip arthroplasty, which successfully relieved the patient's pain and restored function.

late failure. With severe loss of bone, bone grafting of defects and special acetabular cages or modified components are frequently necessary. Revision hip surgery is complex, complication rates are higher, and functional results less satisfying than in primary total hip arthroplasty (53).

Total Knee Arthroplasty

Artificial replacement of the knee joint is based on principles similar to those developed for the hip. Precisely sized components and custom jigs align the surfaces and allow for exact surgical resection of femoral, tibial, and patellar bone to accept the components. The femoral component is metal and articulates with the polyethylene metal-backed tibial component. The components are cemented in place and appropriate ligament balancing is necessary to achieve stability. Progressive weight bearing as tolerated is usually permitted. Cementless designs are available for younger patients but are otherwise less commonly used. Constrained total knee arthroplasty is occasionally necessary for complex revisions or major ligamentous deficiency (Fig. 100.19). Although in ideal cases the longevity of total knee arthroplasty approaches that of the total hip procedure, impact or sports activity is always discouraged and associated with a high rate of loosening in younger patients (20,53,56).

Other Joints

Historically, total ankle replacement has not been as successful in relieving pain and restoring function as ankle arthrodesis, but there is a resurgence of interest in this procedure because of improved design and implant techniques.

Prosthetic replacements of the shoulder and elbow are less commonly indicated procedures except in patients with rheumatoid or other inflammatory arthritis. These patients frequently have multiple joint involvement, so it is important to restore as much mobility as possible.

Wrist arthrodesis is more predictable and generally preferable to total wrist joint arthroplasty. Proximal row carpectomy may be indicated in certain low-demand patients.

In patients with severe rheumatoid hand deformities, metacarpophalangeal arthroplasty is an excellent technique to restore alignment and improve function (56).

Arthritis in the Younger Patient

Most arthritic conditions in younger patients are posttraumatic and often occur as a result of fractures involving joints of the lower extremity (Fig. 100.31). Avascular necrosis of the hip due to steroid use, alcoholism, or idio-

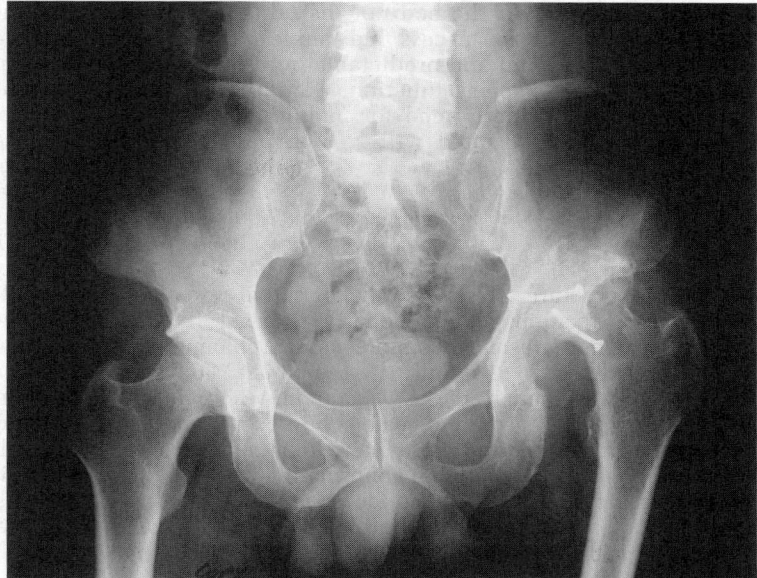

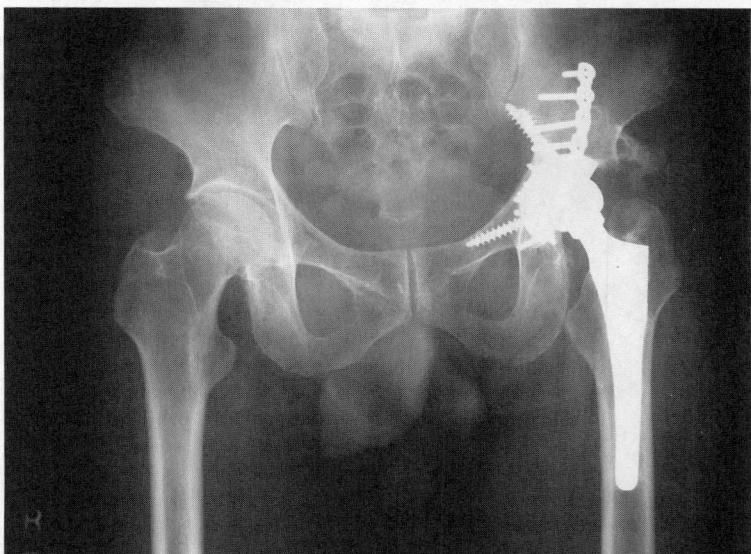

Figure 100.31. *(A)* Avascular necrosis and loss of fixation after inadequate treatment of posterior wall acetabular fracture. *(B)* Anteroposterior radiograph after bone grafting of posterior wall defect and total hip arthroplasty.

pathic factors is also common. Joint replacement is not a good option in young and middle-aged patients, and modification of activities and nonoperative treatment is always indicated as a first option but frequently fails to address symptoms adequately.

Osteotomy to realign limbs and redistribute forces across arthritic joints is modestly successful in relieving symptoms for a period of several years, buying additional time before joint replacement. Osteotomies are most frequently indicated about the knee and usually performed for a varus or bow-legged deformity associated with unicompartmental arthritis. Periacetabular pelvic osteotomies are very useful in patients with hip subluxation and acetabular dysplasia.

Arthroscopic débridement, especially of the knee, is also beneficial. Where indicated, it can be accompanied with abrasion chondroplasty and microfracture, or newer cartilage grafting techniques. More severe and localized arthritic changes confined to one compartment of the knee can be treated with unicompartmental knee replacement.

Posttraumatic arthritis of the hip can be treated with arthrodesis, which in the past has been recommended for people who intend to engage in heavy physical activity or hard labor. Short-term results are satisfactory, but many problems eventually arise, including chronic low back pain and degenerative changes in the ipsilateral knee or contralateral extremity. When given a choice, most young patients prefer total hip arthroplasty even through it is not a permanent solution. Other alternatives include resection arthroplasty of the head and neck (Girdlestone procedure), which results in a foreshortened but reasonably functional limb and adequate relief of pain, and, most important, buys time before the need for total joint replacement.

Arthrodesis of the knee is even less satisfactory but may be necessary in the presence of severe deformity, instability, and pain, or for failed total knee replacement or infection.

Posttraumatic arthritis of the ankle is best prevented by anatomic open reduction and internal fixation of fractures. Nevertheless, with severe involvement of the tibial plafond or fractures of the body of the talus, advanced arthritic changes may necessitate ankle arthrodesis, which is well accepted and predictable in relieving pain and providing satisfactory function. Similarly, subtalar arthrodesis, usually performed for malunited calcaneal fractures, is also associated with a high percentage of good results (55).

CORRECTION OF DEFORMITY AND NONUNION

Malunited fractures are treated by corrective osteotomy and internal fixation or occasionally external fixation techniques. They are more common and problematic in the lower extremity, especially in the tibia. Malunited fractures of the femur are less common when an intramedullary rod is used and, when they occur, are less likely to be angulatory and more likely to be related to excessive shortening or rotational abnormality.

Leg length discrepancy in the femur is best treated by contralateral closed femoral shortening of the normal femur, unless the discrepancy is large (Fig. 100.32). In this situation, lengthening of the shortened femur may be considered, although it is less predictable. Torsional malrotation and angular deforming of the femur are corrected by derotation osteotomy and maintenance of correction by an interlocked intramedullary device. Alternatively, single or dual compression plates can be used with autogenous iliac crest bone grafting.

Fortunately, posttraumatic shortening usually does not exceed 2 to 3 cm, which can be accommodated by a shoe lift. Tibial lengthening is less problematic than in the femur. Congenital shortening or dwarfism can require bilateral lengthening. As much as 25 cm of length has been obtained in the latter group of young patients by distraction osteogenesis and Ilizarov methods.

Malunited fractures of the tibia in well vascularized, healthy legs are treated by corrective osteotomy and compression plating or, less commonly, by intramedullary fixation. Unfortunately, a significant number of tibial malunions are associated with open fractures, soft-tissue damage, and infection. These more complex injuries are best treated by atraumatic osteotomy through a small incision (corticotomy) and application of external

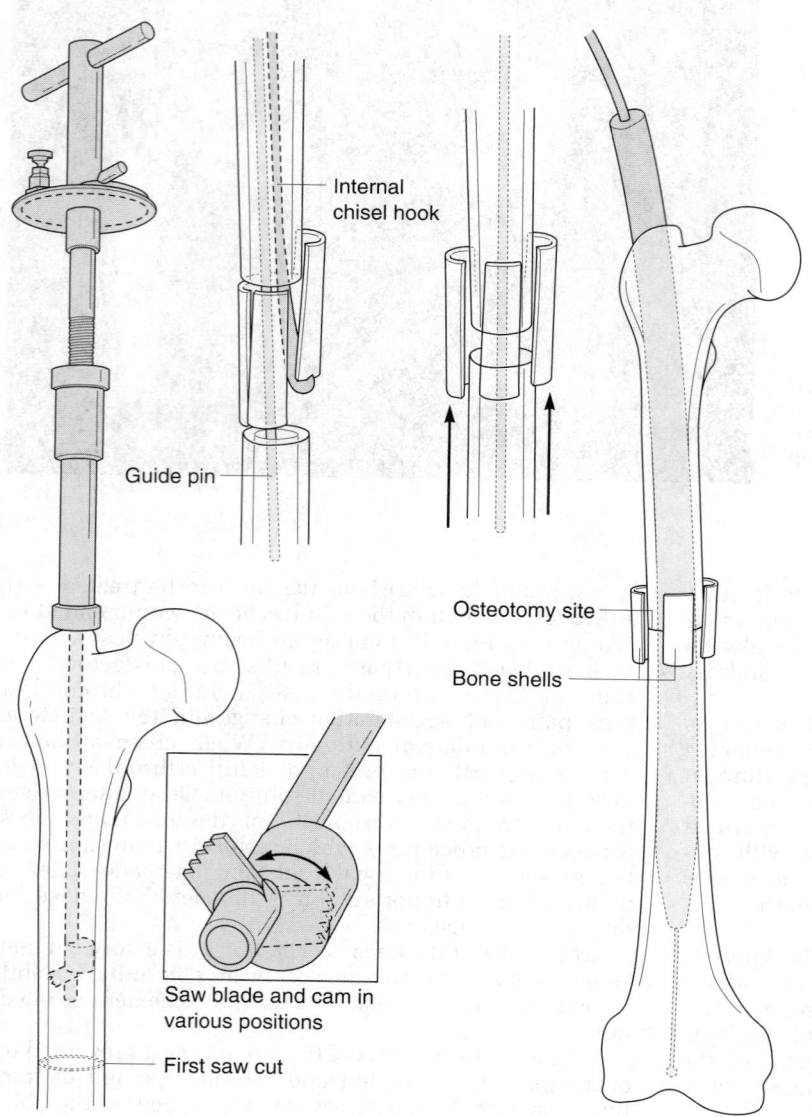

Internal chisel hook

Guide pin

Osteotomy site

Bone shells

Saw blade and cam in various positions

First saw cut

Figure 100.32. Closed femoral shortening. Treatment of leg length inequality of 6 to 8 cm or less is most predictably accomplished by contralateral closed femoral shortening. The osteotomy is performed in closed technique with a special intramedullary saw. After the osteotomized segment is split and pushed out of the way, the osteotomy is compressed and fixed with an interlocked intramedullary rod.

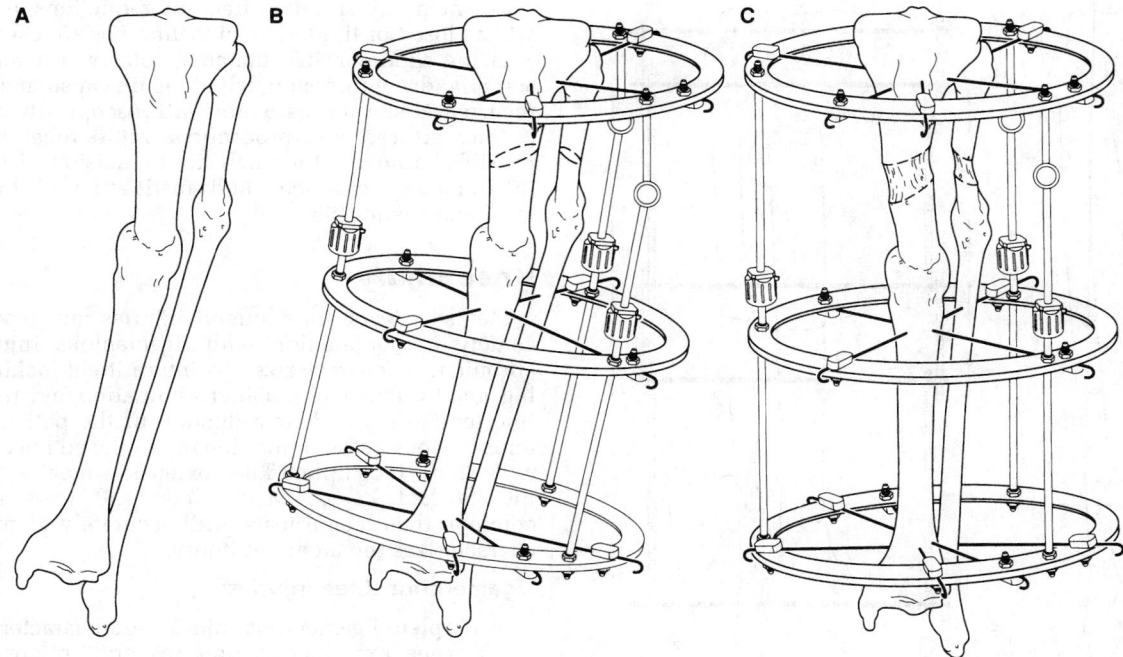

Figure 100.33. Malunion. *(A)* Schematic depiction of malunited fractures of the tibia and fibula with unacceptable shortening and varus deformity. *(B)* The use of the Ilizarov technique, proximal corticotomies, and appropriate positioning of external fixator rings with transfixation pins followed by gradual distraction (1 mm/d) and simultaneous correction of malunion. *(C)* The angulation and shortening were both corrected, and healing of the histogenesis site has occurred.

devices consisting of the classic wire-and-ring Ilizarov fixator, hybrid fixators combining both a ring and rod construct, or monolateral external fixators. Using the Ilizarov apparatus, excessive shortening and deformity can be corrected simultaneously using appropriate placement of hinges and distraction osteogenesis techniques (Fig. 100.33). Gradual lengthening proceeds, usually over four equally spaced 0.25-mm increments per day. As the bone separates at the corticotomy site, immature bone is evident by radiography and progresses to eventual maturation. When the desired length has been achieved, the frame is continued for an additional time, usually equal to the period of lengthening. Protection is then provided within a cast or a removable orthosis as further maturation of new formed bone takes place (57). Monolateral external fixators in the tibia are easier to manage but are somewhat less versatile than the classic Ilizarov ring frame. The goal of all corrective osteotomies, regardless of technique, is realignment of the limb, correction of length, and restoration of a normal mechanical joint axis.

Nonunion

Failure of fracture to heal within the expected time frame is termed *nonunion*. Nonunion and malunion frequently coexist. Nonunion is characterized by gross motion across the fracture site and a paucity of callus formation at 4 to 6 months or greater. Nonunion may occur after any fracture, but it is most common in the tibia, the femoral neck, and the humerus. Nonunion may be accompanied by avascular necrosis, especially when it occurs in the talus, femoral neck, or humeral head and scaphoid. In diaphyseal fractures, the most common cause of nonunion is open injury with associated soft-tissue damage or infection. In closed fractures, a history of smoking, severe diabetes, or immunocompromise may be contributory. Nonunion may also occur in otherwise healthy people without any known risk factors (11, 16,19).

Delayed union may be treated with dynamization of intramedullary rods by removing the distal or proximal interlocking screws, allowing bone-to-bone load transfer. This method is most applicable in the tibia. External electrical stimulation using pulsed electromagnetic fields has been shown to be useful in so-called vascular nonunions unassociated with bone loss or fracture gap.

The most common nonunion treatment method is autologous iliac crest bone graft. In the humerus and upper extremity, this is usually accompanied by compression plating.

Posterolateral bone grafting is the treatment for most tibial nonunions, with the graft placed across the posterior fibula, interosseous membrane, and tibial nonunion site (55). With large defects and deficient donor bone, demineralized bone allograft or artificial bone substitutes can be used to augment autogenous bone. For segmental defects accompanied by low-grade infection or deficient soft tissue, bone transport can be utilized vis a vis Ilizarov technique and distraction osteogenesis. This method is also useful in chronic osteomyelitis after resection of significant amounts of necrotic bone (30,57) (Fig. 100.34).

A time-honored method of treatment of tibial nonunion is fibular osteotomy and compression weight bearing in a cast. The patient usually must accept minor degrees of angulation and shortening for the goal of fracture union. Although controversial, ultrasound has been used to stimulate fracture healing in vascularized low-grade nonunion.

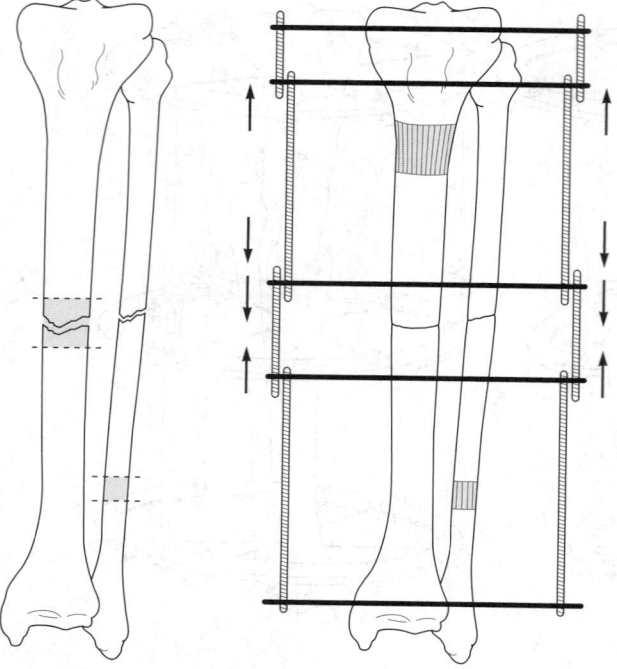

Figure 100.34. Ilizarov method of distraction osteogenesis used for treatment of infected pseudarthrosis of the tibia. Infected bone has been resected, and transport of bone segment to close the resultant defect is illustrated. Distraction occurs at the proximal corticotomy at a rate of 1 mm/d, and this area gradually fills in with new bone. This method can be used to treat segmental bone loss from other causes.

SPORTS MEDICINE

Treatment of recreational or athletic injuries in otherwise healthy people constitutes a significant portion of orthopedic surgery. Most minor injuries, sprains, contusions, and incomplete ligament tears are treated nonoperatively. Ice, elevation, and rest are the usual modalities for acute injury. Physical therapy may be indicated to restore motion and strength, especially in the injured athlete. Unstable major ligamentous injuries are treated surgically, especially in the professional athlete with ligamentous injury of the knee.

Arthroscopy

Arthroscopy has added an effective low-morbidity procedure that addresses a variety of traumatic degenerative joint problems. It began as a diagnostic adjunct to clinical evaluation of patients with knee problems. Through small stab incisions, using fiberoptic scopes, the entire joint can be visualized better than with standard surgical approaches. The logical development of various small instruments and motorized shavers ushered in operative arthroscopy. The procedure was expanded to include other joints—shoulder, wrist, elbow, ankle, and hip.

Meniscal tears of the knee can be repaired in young patients or débrided to a stable edge in older patients with degenerative tears. Total meniscectomy, commonly done in the past, is hardly ever indicated as an isolated procedure because the meniscus is an important stabilizer, shock absorber, and modulator of knee kinematics. Removal of loose bodies, drilling of chondral defects, resection of symptomatic synovial plicae, and abrasion chondroplasty are common knee arthroscopic procedures.

Assessment of articular fracture reductions is possible when closed or limited open techniques are used.

In the shoulder, débridement, rotator cuff repair, subacromial decompression, labral repair, capsular shifts, and recurrent dislocation are often arthroscopically assisted.

After arthroscopic procedures, rapid rehabilitation is possible because of the small size of incisions, irrigation of inflammatory products, and instillation of long-acting local anesthetics (58).

Knee Injury

Meniscal tears are common injuries and may present acutely in conjunction with ligamentous injury or as chronic tears characterized by intermittent locking, catching, and localized joint pain. Examination may reveal joint line tenderness and reproduction of the patient's symptoms by compression–rotation of the flexed knee (McMurray's sign). Incomplete knee extension may be present—the "locked knee." Medial meniscal tears are more common than lateral tears. MRI accurately identifies and characterizes the meniscal injury.

Ligamentous Knee Injuries

Incomplete ligamentous injuries are characterized by a stable knee examination and respond to nonoperative modalities and rehabilitation.

One of the most significant and common athletic and recreational knee injuries is rupture of the anterior cruciate ligament (ACL). Classically, a loud "pop" and subsequent hemarthrosis accompany the injury. Examination immediately after injury reveals a positive anterior drawer sign and Lachman's test indicative of excessive anterior excursion of the tibia on the femur. There may be associated injuries to the lateral or medial menisci. In the subacute phase, disruption of the ACL may be somewhat more difficult to diagnose because of guarding by the patient in the presence of a hemarthrosis. A tense hemarthrosis is best aspirated to relieve pain, followed by a temporary immobilization of the joint, elevation, and application of ice. Gradual rehabilitation of the knee is attempted and with incomplete tears is usually effective (59). Complete tears are usually reconstructed at 4 to 6 weeks to allow for resolution of the acute injury and institution of early rehabilitation.

Chronic insufficiency of the ACL is characterized by a giving-way of the knee, especially when the patient attempts to turn suddenly or cut. Clinically, this phenomenon can be demonstrated by the lateral pivot shift test in which the examiner reproduces the anterolateral subluxation of the tibia on the femur. Diagnosis can be confirmed by MRI, which also evaluates for associated injuries to the menisci or other structures. Surgical treatment consists of arthroscopically assisted autogenous tendon graft using either quadruple hamstring, patellar tendon, or allograft substitution (Fig. 100.35). Results are good to excellent in most instances and are better for acute repairs than for chronic cases. Neglected ACL insufficiency can lead to meniscal tears, joint space narrowing, and early degenerative arthritis (60,61).

Rupture of the posterior cruciate ligament can usually be treated by rehabilitation and nonoperative methods, except in the high-demand patient. The most common mechanisms are a direct "dashboard" blow or impact from a fall on a flexed knee. Surgical repair is most often performed in athletes or when other associated ligamentous injury produces instability, as in knee dislocation. Results after posterior cruciate repair are not as predictable as ACL repair (62).

Isolated ligamentous tears of the medial collateral ligament can also be treated nonoperatively; however, if they

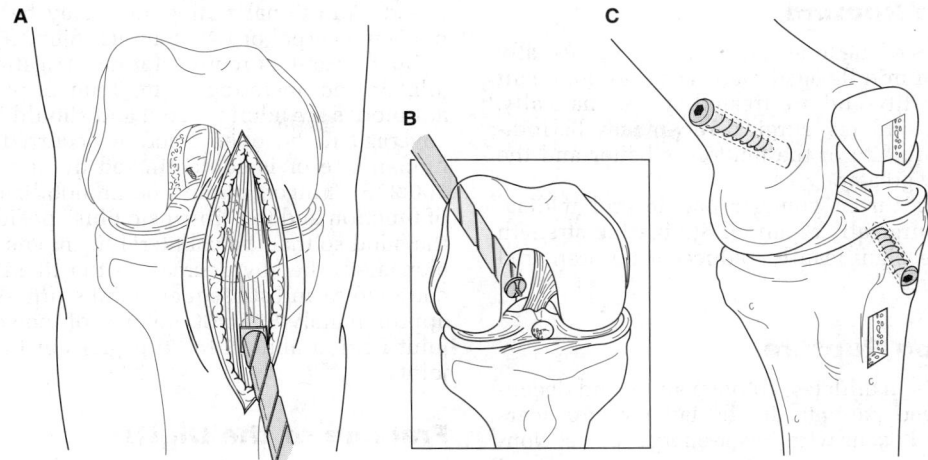

Figure 100.35. Arthroscopic-assisted anterior cruciate ligament (ACL) reconstruction. *(A)* Reaming of tibial tunnel over precisely placed guide pin, monitored arthroscopically. *(B)* Intraarticular view of femoral tunnel reaming. Posterior placement of tunnel must be immediately adjacent to posterior cortex. *(A* and *B* From Hardin GT, Bach BR Jr, Bush-Joseph C, et al. Endoscopic single incision ACL reconstruction using patellar tendon autograft: surgical technique. *Am J Knee Surg* 1991;5:144–155, with permission). *(C)* Appropriately tensioned ACL: graft secured with interference screws. Precise positioning achieves appropriate isometry throughout full range of knee motion. Bone–patellar tendon–bone graft is illustrated, although quadrupled hamstrings or allograft may be used. (*C* from Nogalski MN, Bach BR Jr. Acute anterior cruciate ligament injuries. In: Fu F, Harner C, Vince K, eds. *The knee.* Baltimore: Williams & Wilkins, 1994:717–718, with permission).

involve the posterior oblique corner of the knee and are associated with cruciate injury, they should be repaired. Likewise, acute ligamentous injuries to the posterolateral corner and arcuate complex of the knee should be repaired primarily because late repair is difficult and associated with suboptimal results.

Complete knee dislocation is frequently associated with popliteal neurovascular injury and has already been discussed. Ligamentous repair should usually be undertaken acutely or after arterial repair. Ideally, all torn structures should be repaired, including the menisci wherever possible. External fixation across the knee joint may be necessary to protect the ligamentous and arterial repair (59).

Ruptures of the patellar tendon occur most commonly in younger people and are repaired primarily. Rupture of the quadriceps mechanism, on the other hand, more frequently occurs in middle-aged or older men, usually through a degeneratively weakened area of the tendon. Surgical repair is indicated and usually produces satisfactory results.

Ankle

Most injuries to the lateral ligamentous complex produce typical ankle sprain that is best treated by ice, elevation, and compression bandaging. Temporary splinting with an air cast may be appropriate, followed by early institution of protected weight bearing and range of motion. This method allows the most rapid restoration of tensile strength and integrity to the ligamentous complex. Occasionally, more severe injuries may require a brief period of cast immobilization. Rarely, complete tears of the lateral ligamentous complex result in pure ankle dislocation requiring operative repair (15). Recurrent ankle sprain occasionally results in elongation of the lateral ligamentous complex. Subluxation can be demonstrated on stress radiographs of the ankle. Operative reconstruction predictably yields good results.

Osteochondritis dissecans can involve the talus. Small lesions respond to arthroscopic débridement or drilling.

Large lesions are more problematic and have an unfavorable prognosis regardless of treatment

Shoulder

Tendinitis and inflammatory bursitis frequently exist with impingement syndrome of the shoulder. Most tendinitis occurs in middle-aged or elderly men and responds to conservative treatment. Injection of the shoulder with local anesthetic and cortisone is effective in relieving symptoms for a significant period.

Rotator cuff tears are diagnosed by shoulder pain and difficulties with initiating abduction, weakness on isolation testing of the supraspinatus muscle, and a positive MRI. Although acute traumatic tears can occur in athletes and younger patients, most are degenerative, chronic tears occurring in older men. They may require rotator cuff repair and subacromial decompression, usually performed through a small open incision or with arthroscopic assistance (58). Occasionally the cuff is severely retracted and repair is not possible. In these instances, débridement of the inflamed tissue produces satisfactory relief of pain.

Recurrent anterior dislocation of the shoulder usually presents in young people and responds well to operative treatment. Classically, the Bankart labral lesion is repaired along with capsular plication. Many different techniques have been advocated, and overall success rates approach 95%. With multiple dislocations, the classic Hill-Sachs defect may be seen in the humeral head. Arthroscopic repair can be successful, but open surgery has more predictable success (19).

Elbow

Chronic inflammation or tears of the medial collateral ligament of the elbow may occur in throwing athletes. This is usually considered a repetitive valgus overload syndrome and can produce instability, chronic pain, and ulnar neuropathy. Surgical repair may be indicated, as well as decompression or transposition of the ulnar nerve.

Biceps Tendon Rupture

Degenerative tears of the long head of the biceps usually occur proximally in middle-aged men. They do not result in significant disability and are treated symptomatically. In weight lifters or athletes, surgical repair may be indicated because the quality of the tendon is better and the disability relatively greater.

Distal ruptures occur in younger people and if diagnosed acutely are surgically repaired. Supination strength and endurance are significantly reduced in unrepaired distal biceps rupture.

Achilles Tendon Rupture

This injury occurs in athletes, active people, and deconditioned middle-aged patients. In the latter group, tears are degenerative and occur with lower-energy forces. Nonoperative treatment with a gravity equinus cast for 8 weeks followed by gradually decreasing heel lifts produces satisfactory results in lower-demand patients and nonathletes.

Surgical treatment is recommended for athletes and active people. Results are usually satisfactory with both treatment methods, but greater tensile strength is claimed for surgically repaired ruptures. Even when successful, this is a career-threatening injury in the professional athlete (19,55).

HAND SURGERY

Knowledge of the kinematics and pathophysiology of the hand and wrist historically lagged behind that of other areas of the body. The advent of radiography allowed precise diagnosis and understanding of fractures and injury patterns involving the wrist and hand. Sterling Bunnell's comprehensive book, *Surgery of Hand,* was published in 1944 and was predicated on advances in the treatment of military casualties with severe hand injuries (4,60). Subsequently, the development of hand surgery as a specialty and measured advances in the treatment of pathologic processes involving the hand and upper extremity occurred. Microvascular techniques, arthroplasty or replacement of arthritic joints, tendon transfers, nerve grafting, and appropriate arthrodesis have produced significant benefit for patients (4,60).

Fractures and Dislocations of the Hand: General Principles

The diagnosis of injury depends on a thorough knowledge of the functional anatomy and careful physical examination of the hand and wrist. The hand and wrist should be carefully examined and gently palpated for acute injury. Obvious swelling or deformity may direct the clinician to an injured digit, but should not preclude examination of the remaining hand. Neurovascular status, including two-point discrimination and range of motion, both active and passive, should be tested and recorded. Deformity or open injury is obvious, but subtle injury is notorious for the potential to produce permanent disability. Sprains of the fingers are common but may represent avulsion fractures with the subsequent development of joint instability, restricted motion, or tendon imbalance. Tenderness in the anatomic snuff box or over the scaphoid tubercle should be treated as a fracture until radiographically ruled out. Open injury associated with fracture should be documented, aseptically irrigated, bandaged, and splinted before obtaining radiographs. The minimal radiographic requirement is two views at 90 degrees op-

posed. Additional radiographs may be indicated to rule out acute carpal or ligamentous injury (60,61).

Open fractures require formal irrigation of the bone or joint in the operating room. Tetanus prophylaxis and IV antibiotics are administered and should include anaerobic coverage if the open fracture occurred as a result of a human bite or is contaminated by organic material (Fig. 100.23B). Fingers should be immobilized in the position of function and the "intrinsic plus" position used to splint the hand so that the collateral ligaments are appropriately elongated, thereby decreasing the likelihood of ligament contracture and subsequent joint stiffness. This position is approximately 80 to 90 degrees of metacarpal phalangeal joint flexion and 10 to 20 degrees at the interphalangeal joints.

Fracture of the Digits

Crush injuries of the fingers or thumb are common and usually involve the nail, nail bed, and tuft of the distal phalanx. They are usually treated nonoperatively. If the nail is avulsed, the nail bed should be carefully repaired. A tense subungual hematoma should be decompressed with an 18-gauge needle or heated paperclip. Avulsion of the tip of the finger is best treated open unless significant volar soft tissue is lost, in which case local advancement of soft tissue may be indicated. Judicious resection of exposed bone may be necessary to avoid a painful digital tip (63,64).

Distal Phalanx

Dorsal phalangeal avulsion fracture of the distal phalanx is a common injury that is usually secondary to a hyperflexion or extension injury. A mallet finger deformity may be present with or without fracture because of disruption of the terminal extensor mechanism. Treatment is extension splinting of the distal joint for 6 weeks. Open reduction is indicated when the articular fragment is large or the joint is subluxed.

When bone is avulsed from the flexor aspect of the distal joint, the patient cannot flex the terminal phalanx and has a palpable mass at the base of the finger or in the palm. Radiographs may show the bone fragment. Operative treatment is required to reattach the flexor tendon to the base of the proximal phalanx with fine wire or nonabsorbable suture.

Middle Phalanx and Proximal Interphalangeal Joint

Stable fractures that do not involve the joint can be initially immobilized in a splint in position of function and "buddy taped" to the adjacent finger. Protected motion is begun at 3 weeks. Avulsion fractures of the base of the middle phalanx usually include the volar plate and result in dorsal dislocation, frequently misdiagnosed as a "sprained finger." If the joint is unstable after reduction, it may need to be pinned. Dislocation of the proximal interphalangeal joint with or without fracture usually disrupts the central slip and dorsal capsule in addition to the palmar plate. If active extension of the joint is absent after reduction, the central slip should be repaired, followed by immobilization of the joint for 5 to 6 weeks in extension. If the fracture–dislocation is irreducible, open reduction should be performed. Late presentation reveals a chronic boutonniere deformity that is difficult to treat (65).

Proximal Phalanx and Metacarpals

If minimally displaced and nonarticular, these fractures can usually be treated by appropriate splinting and early range of motion. Grossly displaced fractures that are unstable and fractures with significant articular involvement should be treated by open reduction and internal fixation. Other surgical indications include multiple fractures, mangled hands, and open fractures. Metacarpophalangeal joint dislocation usually follows a hyperextension force. Dorsal dislocation is most frequent and occasionally may be irreducible by closed methods. Open reduction, when necessary, if performed through a palmar approach, freeing the entrapped volar plate (65). Fractures of the fifth metacarpal neck are common and are known as *boxer's fractures*. Because of increased excursion of the fourth and fifth rays, fractures involving the metacarpal necks of these bones can usually be treated by closed reduction and ulnar gutter splinting with the metacarpophalangeal joint flexed 50 to 70 degrees for approximately 4 weeks, followed by a removable splint and protected motion. Displaced fractures of the index and long finger metacarpals, however, often require open reduction.

Thumb metacarpal fractures are usually caused by a fall on the hand and frequently result in an intraarticular fracture of the proximal end. The fracture can almost always be treated by closed reduction and percutaneous pinning for 4 to 6 weeks. If the fragment is large and widely displaced, open reduction and internal fixation are indicated. A comminuted fracture at the base of the metacarpal may be treated by thumb spica splint if minimally displaced, or percutaneous pinning. Occasionally, open reduction is necessary.

Injuries to the metacarpophalangeal joint of the thumb are common, including avulsion fractures in association with ulnar collateral ligament tear—"Gamekeeper's thumb." These are usually initially treated by splinting but may require ligament repair. Metacarpophalangeal joint dislocation of the thumb may cause serious articular or vascular injury. The metacarpal protrudes through a tear in the capsule and occasionally the volar plate may be interposed in the joint, making it irreducible and requiring open reduction.

Summary of Treatment Principles

Stable fractures are, by definition, minimally displaced or reducible. A brief period of splinting followed by buddy taping allows early protected motion. Potentially unstable injuries require radiographic and clinical follow-up during the first 7 to 10 days to detect loss of reduction. Percutaneous pinning may be indicated in this instance. Large articular fragments and unstable oblique or open fractures require open reduction and surgical stabilization (63–66) (Fig. 100.23B).

Carpal Fractures and Wrist Dislocations

Displaced intercarpal fracture–dislocations require accurate reduction and surgical stabilization. Isolated fractures of carpal bones other than the scaphoid are less common. When undisplaced, they are treated by cast immobilization. Dorsal chip fractures of the triquetrum are relatively benign injuries unless associated intercarpal instability. Capitate fractures require open reduction when displaced and are often associated with other wrist lesions. Fractures of the lunate are less common than dislocation, but traumatic compressive injury may precede avascular necrosis. Fractures of the hamate may involve the body or hamulus. The latter often requires carpal tunnel views, tomography, or CT for diagnosis. Because of proximity to the motor branch of the ulnar nerve, neuropathy may be present. Pisiform fractures are uncommon and usually do not result in significant disability. Excision is infrequently performed (64,65).

Perilunate Dislocation

This injury encompasses a spectrum of pathologic processes. Pure dorsal dislocation of the capitate, an associated fracture, or an oblique fracture of the radial styloid may occur individually or in combination. Radiography of the wrist may show carpal overlap, a "signet ring" sign over the scaphoid, or a wide gap between the scaphoid and lunate.

Initial treatment requires prompt reduction. Median nerve neuropathy is not uncommon because of the displaced lunate or stretching of the median nerve. If post reduction radiographs show satisfactory reduction without residual displacement of the carpus, immobilization in plaster cast is appropriate. Residual abnormalities present on postreduction radiographs dictate open reduction and internal stabilization.

Late sequelae of intercarpal injury and instability include chronic pain and weakness. Scapholunate ligament reconstruction, selected intercarpal arthrodesis, or complete radiocarpal arthrodesis (wrist fusion) may be indicated to relieve pain and provide stable function (46,65).

Tendon Injury and Repair

Tendon injury in the hand and digits may frequently be suspected or diagnosed by the abnormal position of a digit in complete disruptions. Partial lacerations, however, may have normal appearance and range of motion. Inability to move the involved digit or joint is indicative of tendon disruption, usually due to laceration, but associated digital nerve or vascular injury may coexist. The diagnosis is secured by testing for active motion, sensation, two-point discrimination, and capillary refill (64,67).

Extensor Tendon Injuries. The diagnosis of most extensor lesions is straightforward and surgical repair usually is not as technically demanding as that for flexor tendons. However, the extensor tendons are thin and intimately proximate to the interphalangeal joints and bone.

The swan neck and boutonniere deformities are classic examples of residua from extensor tendon injury. The latter deformity results from disruption of the central slip of the tendon from its insertion at the base of the middle phalanx. Laceration of extensor tendons in the forearm may be accompanied by injury to sensory branches of the radial or ulnar nerves. After repair of extensor tendons in the digits or dorsum of the hand, extension splinting of the wrist at 45 degrees and the digit(s) at 10 degrees of flexion for 4 to 5 weeks is necessary. When motion is begun, the digits are protected by a removable splint (66,67).

Flexor Tendon Injuries
Anatomy. The flexor system consists of two tendons for each finger and one for the thumb. The flexor digitorum superficialis divides into two tendon slips in the palm and inserts on the middle phalanx of each digit. The flexor digitorum profundus and flexor pollicis longus tendons insert on the base of the distal phalangeals of the figures and thumb, respectively. It is useful to divide the hand into zones in differentiating one tendon laceration from another, and also for determining how to treat lacerations in the current different zones (Fig. 100.36A).
Flexor Tendon Repair. Tendon repair should be performed under optimal conditions, providing satisfactory anesthesia, appropriate lighting, and hemostasis. Appropriate extension of the traumatic wound is necessary to visualize the injury adequately. In the finger, this usually indicates a zigzag extension. Lacerations in zone I involve the flexor digitorum profundus; in zone II, "no man's land," lacerations frequently involve both flexor tendons

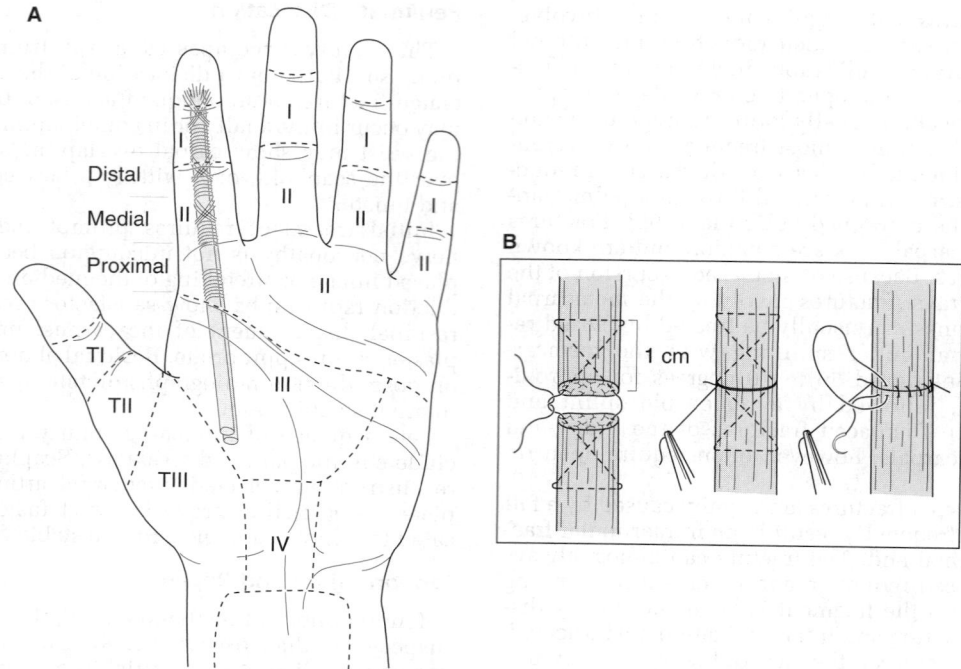

Figure 102.36. *(A)* Zone 1, distal to the sublimis; zone 2, "no-man's land"; zone 3, region of the lumbrical origin; zone 4, carpal tunnel; zone 5, proximal to carpal tunnel. *(B)* Many methods of flexor tendon suture repair exist, but most involve a core suture followed by a running peripheral suture through the epitenon.

within the fibroosseous tunnel, and this is the most critical and most challenging zone to treat surgically (68,69). Zone V, which extends from the proximal transverse carpal ligament at the wrist to the musculotendinous junction of the flexor tendons in the distal third of the forearm, contains the median nerve and the ulnar neurovascular bundle as well as the wrist flexors and all of the deep and superficial digital flexors. All lacerated structures should be repaired. Repair of both tendons in zone II should be performed in clean wounds (Fig. 100.36B). Delayed repair is necessary for poor-quality skin or contamination. Crush injuries may require tendon grafting when the soft tissue is receptive. Laceration of the profundus tendon in zone I is repaired by advancing the tendon slightly and securing it to its insertion on the base of the distal phalanx. Associated injuries to the median or ulnar nerves require repair with fine nylon sutures using an operating microscope (67–70).

Postoperative Care. After surgery, the wrist is splinted in flexion for approximately 4 weeks. Supervised rehabilitation should begin immediately after surgery. Gentle passive motion can be started early. Careful supervision is necessary during the postoperative period because rupture of repaired tendons is likely to produce a suboptimal result even if recognized and repaired.

Tendon Grafting.   Tendon grafting is indicated for late injuries, extensive loss of motion due to adherent tendons, or failed primary repair. Grafting requires reasonable motion and an intact pulley system. The palmaris longus, toe extensors, or ring finger sublimis may be used as the donor tendon graft depending on availability and the size of the flexor tendon needed. After surgery, the wrist and fingers are splinted in flexion for 4 to 5 weeks, followed by protective splinting for an additional several weeks. Gentle passive motion is allowed during the first period, and graduated active-assisted and active motion during the second period (70).

When the finger is stiff, the gliding surface fibrotic, and the pulley system severely damaged, a Silastic rod (Hunter) is inserted after resection of the fibrosed tendon and scar (71). The Silastic rod is secured distally but left free in the proximal palm or wrist to permit passive motion. The pulleys over the distal end of the proximal phalanx (A2) and mid-middle phalanx (A4) are reconstructed. A pseudosheath forms over the rod as passive motion is produced and swelling subsides, which may require 3 to 6 months before grafting. A tendon graft using the second or third long toe extensor is harvested, attached to the detached distal Silastic rod, and pulled proximally under the new sheath. The latter can be modified to form or augment pulleys and to permit free gliding of the graft. Tension is carefully adjusted and postoperative care proceeds (70,71).

Replantation of Amputated Limbs and Digits

Replantation is the reattachment of a part that has been completely severed (Fig. 100.37). The indications for replantation proceed according to the following priorities: (a) thumb; (b) multiple digits; (c) partial hand amputation through the palm; (d) amputation in a child; (e) wrist or forearm; (f) above-elbow amputation unassociated with crush or avulsion; and (g) isolated digit distal to the superficiales insertion. General replantation of thumbs, multiple digits, or the complete hand produces the best results (72,73).

Crushed, avulsed, or severely mangled parts or those associated with extensive contamination or greater than 6 hours of ischemia are not replantable.

Surgical Technique

The sequence of replantation is (a) locate vessels and nerves, (b) débride the amputated part of the stump, (c) se-

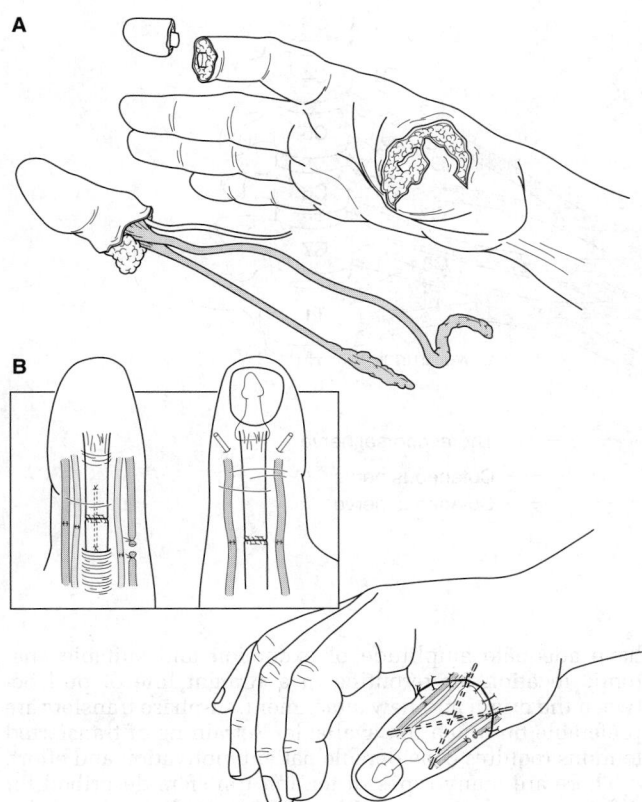

Figure 100.37. Digital replantation. Whenever possible, the thumb should always be replanted because its loss results in major hand dysfunction.

curely fix the bone with an intramedullary pin, (d) repair extensor tendons, (e) repair flexor tendons, (f) repair arteries, (g) repair nerves, (h) repair veins, and (i) obtain loose skin coverage. Arterial repair takes precedence if warm ischemia time is prolonged (72,73).

Postoperative Management

Appropriate splinting is provided, and adjusted-dose heparin and IV antibiotics are administered for 5 to 7 days. Most major replantation centers report an approximately 80% viability rate. Functional results vary according to the replanted structure. Replanted thumbs produce the best functional results, followed by replants of digits distal to the superficial tendon insertion. Replantation of amputated digits at the base of the finger usually produces poor functional results.

Nerve Injury

Physical examination may reveal complete or, more frequently, incomplete motor and sensory loss below the level of the injury. Therefore, with lacerations or injuries of tendons or adjacent structures, injury to peripheral nerves should be suspected. This is especially so for penetrating injuries about the wrist and antecubital fossa. Bleeding from these areas should be controlled by direct pressure because attempts to clamp or ligate actively bleeding vessels under suboptimal visualization may damage nearby nerves.

Primary repair of lacerated nerves is accomplished under a bloodless field using an operating microscope. Intrafascicular or epineural repairs with fine nonabsorbable sutures may be indicated depending on the size of the

nerve and its location. Postoperative splinting is used for 3 to 4 weeks depending on the location and type of repair, as well as associated tendon injuries (73,74).

Nonpenetrating Nerve Injuries

Nerve injuries associated with fractures or fracture–dislocations are frequently injuries in continuity, producing a neurapraxia. Exploration of these nerves is not indicated unless it is incidental to the open treatment of fracture. A relatively high incidence of radial nerve palsy is present with fractures of the humeral shaft. Recovery usually occurs within 10 to 12 weeks, but can take as long as 6 months. Ulnar and median nerve injuries are usually secondary to fractures about the elbow, forearm, or wrist. Treatment is by appropriate fracture reduction and observation. Nerve regeneration occurs at approximately 1 mm a day and is evidence by an advancing Tinel's sign signifying an intact and recovering nerve. Electromyographic and nerve conduction velocities are helpful in determining the type of injury and potential for recovery. Exploration is indicated if there is no evidence of returning function by 3 to 4 months. An additional 6 to 8 weeks of observation is warranted with closed radial nerve palsies because the incidence of recovery approaches 90%. Surgical treatment involves neurolysis, release of adhesions, resection of small neuromas, and nerve repair when indicated. End-to-end anastomosis is preferred, although with segmental crush or defect, nerve grafting may be indicated. The most commonly used graft is the sural nerve, whose absence causes only hypesthesia along the lateral border of the foot.

Brachial Plexus Injuries

Brachial plexus injuries are potentially devastating. Low-energy injuries or sports accidents have a better prognosis than stab or gunshot wounds. Motorcycle and motor vehicle accidents are a frequent cause of severe injury. The mechanism of injury in the latter is usually severe and forceful depression of the shoulder with simultaneous forceful movement of the head in the opposite direction, producing traction. A complete palsy involves all five roots (C-5, C-6, C-7, C-8, T-1). The more common partial brachial plexus injuries consists of two types. In type 1, all roots are involved but in differing degrees. In type 2, some roots are damaged whereas others are completely intact. Injury may occur to roots, trunks, divisions, cords, or branches (Fig. 100.38). Frequently a mixed picture evolves (75).

Upper brachial plexus lesions (C-5, C-6) result in paralysis of the shoulder muscles and the biceps brachia. With the extended upper brachial plexus or middle trunk lesion, there is paralysis of muscles innervated by the radial nerve. Lower brachial plexus lesions (C-8, T-1) result in paralysis of ulnar-innervated and most median-innervated muscles (74–76).

Treatment. Except for open injuries, exploration, neurolysis, or nerve grafting is performed on a delayed basis to allow for any spontaneous recovery to occur. Exposure of the structures involved is technically demanding and requires meticulous dissection and the use of nerve stimulators and appropriate magnification. The sural, intercostal, medial cutaneous antebrachial, and occasionally a superficial branch of the radial nerve may be used as nerve grafts.

Prognosis. Prognosis depends on the severity of the nerve injury and location of the lesion. Avulsion of cervical roots from the spinal cord has a dismal prognosis and no spontaneous recovery occurs. Incomplete lesions or complete lesions in continuity have varying degrees of re-

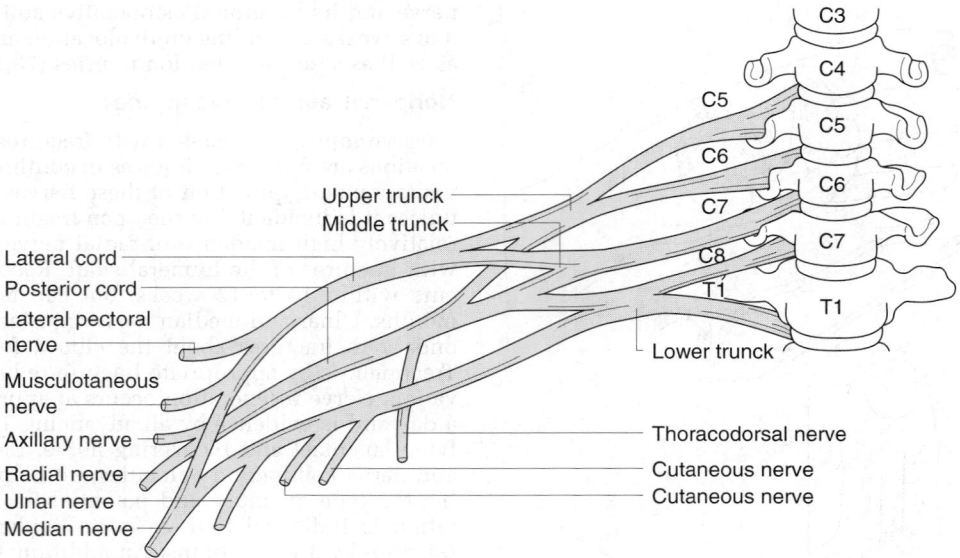

Figure 100.38. Anatomy of the brachial plexus.

turn. Minor stretch injuries may have complete recovery. Appropriately timed tendon transfers and arthrodesis may be helpful. Because of the long distance from the plexus to the ulnar-innervated muscles, only partial recovery can be expected, and intrinsic hand function required for fine movements is never restored. One of the main goals of surgery is return of elbow flexion so that the arm can function as a "helper." Neurogenic pain develops in a significant number of patients, and a completely anesthetic and functionless limb requires above-elbow amputation (74–76).

Tendon Transfers

Tendon transfers are performed to restore power or balance to a partially paralyzed hand. This requires transfer of an expendable musculotendinous unit resulting in a redistribution of remaining functional parts into the best possible working combination. In general, when one of the three major nerves of the arm (median, ulnar, or radial) is lost, excellent functional restoration can be achieved, but with the loss of two of the three, a substantial functional impairment is inevitable (67,74).

Preoperative Planning

Precise assessment of the patient's need and functioning parts is required. Muscle transfers must be expendable, of normal strength, and free of spasticity. They also should have adequate amplitude of excursion and suitable anatomic location for rerouting in a straight line of pull between the origin and new attachment. In-phase transfers are preferable but often not available. Retraining of transferred tendons requires considerable patient motivation and effort.

There are many types of tendon transfers described for different paralytic conditions (67,74). Radial nerve palsy is a common indication and has predictably good results. The goal is to restore wrist and digital extension. A variety of motors are available if the ulnar and median nerves are normal. Closed radial nerve palsy, frequently secondary to fracture, has an excellent prognosis for spontaneous recovery, and therefore tendon transfers should be delayed 6 to 8 weeks past the usual arbitrary 4- to 6-month time frame.

Ulnar nerve palsy resulting in intrinsic muscle paralysis in the hand has many described tendon transfers, depending on the location of the lesion and the etiology. The goal is to correct claw deformity, loss of grip strength, and asynchronous motion, as well as loss of abduction–adduction control of the digits.

Complete median nerve palsy due to proximal laceration or brachial plexopathy is fortunately not common. It results in profound motor loss involving all of the superficial flexors; the radial half of the deep flexors, including the flexor pollicis, pronator teres and quadratus, and flexor carpi radialis; the entire thenar group; and radial two lumbricals and the palmaris longus (Table 100.4).

Table 100.4. FINDINGS OF UPPER EXTREMITY PERIPHERAL NERVE INJURY

	Sensory	**Motor**
Brachial plexus	Spotty, mixed or complete loss	Mixed weakness, arm, forearm, and hand
Median	Palmar hand, thumb, index, long, and radial fingers; dorsal thumb, index, long, and radial fingertips only	Below elbow: loss of opposition of thumb with fingers, thenar muscle palsy
		Above elbow: inability to flex distal thumb and index fingers, inability to pronate forearm, flex wrist
Radial	Dorsal hand to mid-fingers, thumb, index, long, and radial half of ring finger	Below elbow: wrist drop, inability to extend fingers at MP joint
		High arm: inability to extend elbow
Ulnar	Ulnar wrist, hand, and fingers, ulnar ring, and all of fifth finger	Inability to spread fingers or flex MP joints without phalangeal flexion
		Clawing of fourth and fifth fingers

MP, metacarpophalangeal.

Thenar weakness secondary to carpal tunnel compression at the wrist is relatively common. Long-standing or profound weakness results in loss of opposition of the thumb and can be treated by opponensplasty, which substitutes for the paralyzed abductor pollicis brevis (67).

In biceps paralysis, weakness or loss of elbow flexion results from injury to the musculocutaneous nerve, or is secondary to spinal cord or brachial plexus injury. Loss of elbow flexion results in serious loss of hand and forearm function and is frequently an indication of one of many described tendon transfers.

Injuries resulting in combined nerve palsy are more complex because there is typically greater loss of sensation, proprioception, and residua of soft-tissue or vascular injury. There are fewer motor units available for transfer, and retraining is more problematic. Transfers for combined palsies, however, can provide important restoration of function in these severely injured extremities (67, 74,76).

Arthroplasty and Arthrodesis: Upper Extremity

The upper extremity does not have the imposition of weight bearing, and therefore degenerative arthritis and subsequent joint replacements are less common (55).

Shoulder

Tendinitis and other soft-tissue inflammation is a much more common cause of morbidity, chronic pain, and loss of function than degenerative arthritis. Total shoulder arthroplasty is a satisfactory solution for arthritic pain, although normal function is rarely achieved. Frequently there are associated injuries or degeneration of the rotator cuff, which compromise motion and strength to some degree.

Hemiarthroplasty may also be indicated if the glenoid is less involved. The most common indication for its use is a four-part fracture of the humeral head in which avascular necrosis is inevitable. Reattachment of the greater and lesser tuberosities with the rotator cuff, as well as appropriate height of the prosthesis are necessary to restore balance and function to the shoulder.

Arthrodesis may be indicated for younger patients with paralysis of the shoulder muscles or global instability associated with arthritic changes. The desired position of arthrodesis is the so-called sloppy salute position—approximately 25 degrees of flexion, abduction, and 35 to 40 degrees of internal rotation (62).

Elbow

Elbow arthroplasty is performed primarily in patients with rheumatoid or other inflammatory arthritis and multiple joint involvement (53). It is best used in low-demand patients because the prosthetic components are less capable of resisting cyclic fatigue and failure. Arthrodesis of the elbow is not frequently performed or necessary. Most patients tolerate a moderate degree of arthritic symptoms or instability for retention of some motion. The position of fusion is usually a right angle, although occasionally an extended position may be indicated. An example of the latter would be a person who must fire a weapon or otherwise function with the elbow in an extended position.

Wrist

Except in rheumatoid arthritis, wrist joint arthroplasty is rarely performed. Arthrodesis of the wrist is a sound and satisfactory treatment for symptomatic arthritis or instability. Desired position of fusion is approximately 15 to 20 degrees of dorsiflexion. This is the best compromise between the power and precision grip positions. Proximal-row carpectomy preserves motion and is an alternative procedure for low-demand patients (46).

Hand

Interposition arthroplasty has been used for the trapezium, scaphoid, and capitate but is not frequently indicated or as useful as soft-tissue procedures. Selected intercarpal arthrodesis may be useful in certain cases.

One of the most useful types of arthroplasty in the rheumatoid hand is done for severe metacarpophalangeal deformity, ulnar drift, and joint destruction. The metacarpophalangeal joints are replaced with Silastic or titanium implants and a pseudocapsule develops about the resected joints. The appearance and function are greatly improved. It is essential to centralize the extensor mechanism and treat any tendon ruptures by tenodesis or grafting (64).

Infection

Digits

Purulent flexor tenosynovitis requires prompt diagnosis and treatment if loss of motion and function is to be avoided. Classic signs of infection of the flexor sheet are exquisite tenderness, a semiflexed position of the finger, exquisite pain on extension, and associated symmetric fusiform swelling of the entire finger. This infection can develop from puncture wounds or abrasions. Treatment is by two incisions, one in the palm proximal to the first annular (A1) pulley, and a second, mid-lateral incision on the ulnar side of the distal interphalangeal joint crease. Through these wounds, the flexor tendon sheath can be carefully exposed and drained. A small pediatric feeding tube or rubber catheter can be used to irrigate the sheath after surgery (77). Appropriate IV antibiotics to include anaerobic coverage where indicated are administered for 2 to 5 days. Oral antibiotics for an additional 5 to 7 days may also be indicated.

Hand

Infection of the radial and ulnar bursa or mid-palm space is characterized by pain, erythema, induration, and tenderness in the particular anatomic location. Subtendinous infection in the distal forearm may occur between the flexor tendons and the pronator quadratus and may coexist with digital purulent tenosynovitis. Surgical irrigation and débridement is indicated for abscess formation and for equivocal cases that do not respond to elevation and IV antibiotics.

Septic Joints

Small joints in the fingers, as well as the wrist, can occasionally be treated by aspiration and irrigation. Elevation of the hand and IV antibiotics may result in resolution of early infection or cellulitis. When significant swelling and signs of infection are present, it is usually necessary to proceed promptly with open irrigation and débridement.

Human Bites

These injuries usually involve tooth puncture wounds over the dorsum of the hand, frequently in the region of the fourth and fifth metacarpal heads. Treatment is usually delayed until the patient realizes that he may not actually have won the fight. Human mouth organisms inoculated in tissue are quite virulent. Frequently they are anaerobic or mixed. Aggressive débridement is required, as well as the administration of broad-spectrum antibiotics with both gram-positive and gram-negative activity. Anaerobic coverage should be provided by penicillin, clindamycin, or metronidazole. Similar treatment is indicated for animal bites, although they are less problematic (54,77).

Necrotizing Fasciitis

This devastating infection is a limb- and potentially life-threatening problem, frequently beginning as an innocuous puncture wound, abrasion, or laceration in a digit. It is also commonly seen in IV drug abusers. Presentation is usually late after a period of erythema has progressed to induration, swelling, pain, or drainage.

A high index of suspicion is necessary to differentiate this from less virulent forms of soft-tissue infection or more common cellulitis. A diffuse swelling and erythema over the digits, hand, forearm, or upper arm characterize necrotizing fasciitis. It is usually rapidly progressive. The patient may initially be only moderately symptomatic, but becomes toxic and septicemic within hours.

Treatment. Once the diagnosis of necrotizing fasciitis has been made, immediate surgical débridement is indicated. The incision should be extended proximally in the extremity until normal-appearing tissue is encountered. The boundaries between normal and abnormal are frequently blurred, but infection can be assumed to be present as far proximally as the swelling and erythema exist. Frequently only watery pus and necrotic fascia and subcutaneous tissue are found. Infections that spread onto the chest wall are frequently fatal. Repeat débridement may be necessary. Hyperbaric oxygen may be useful if used early as an adjunct to radical débridement. Anaerobic streptococci, other anaerobes, or mixed organisms are usually responsible. Antibiotics should include gram-positive, gram-negative, and anaerobic coverage in full therapeutic dosages. Despite aggressive therapy, amputation is often necessary. Necrotizing fasciitis is more frequently seen than clostridial myonecrosis, but both infections are limb and life threatening (54,77).

Miscellaneous Soft-tissue Disorders of the Hand

Carpal Tunnel Syndrome

Carpal tunnel syndrome is a common compressive neuropathy of the median nerve at the wrist. It occurs most frequently in middle-aged women engaged in repetitive activities of the upper extremity. Dysesthetic pain, numbness, and tingling involving the volar aspects of the thumb, index, long, and radial half of the ring finger are present to variable degrees. Nocturnal symptoms are particularly bothersome. Physical findings include hypesthesia and decreased two-point discrimination over the median nerve distribution. Provocative testing with the wrists firmly pressed in full flexion (Phalen's test) reproduces the patient's syndromes. Tapping over the carpal tunnel produces paresthesias in the involved digit (Tinel's sign). Weakness of opposition of the thumb and thenar atrophy may be present in long-standing cases.

Nonoperative treatment includes soft night splints, antiinflammatory medication, and occasional steroid injection of the carpal tunnel. Avoidance of repetitive motion of the hand and wrist is very important and may result in resolution of symptoms. Electromyographic and nerve conduction studies can document median neuropathy. They are frequently ordered, but not necessary in clear-cut cases.

Surgical decompression by section of the transverse carpal ligament yields predictably good results and should be offered early on to patients unresponsive to conservative measures. It is performed under outpatient local or regional anesthesia through a small incision paralleling the thenar crease. Endoscopic release is preferred by some surgeons, but the open technique has low morbidity and has withstood the test of time.

Tendinitis

Tenosynovitis is a common and bothersome entity that is frequently associated with repetitive activities. It is more common in women and frequently seen in secretaries and key punch and computer operators. It may precede or accompany carpal tunnel syndrome. Symptoms may be prolonged and are treated with antiinflammatory drugs, modification of activities, splinting, and occasional steroid injections. Tendinitis is associated with significant lost work time and Workers' Compensation claims.

Trigger Digit

Repetitive trauma may produce inflammation of a flexor tendon, resulting in localized swelling or a nodule that prevents movement of the flexor tendon beneath the A1 pulley in the hand. The patient has difficulty straightening out the finger, which then characteristically snaps painfully or triggers when it is forcibly straightened or flexed. Restriction of repetitive activities and antiinflammatories or local injection of cortisone may result in a cure. If not, surgical treatment is simple and rewarding by incising the A1 pulley to allow the tendon to move smoothly. This can be done under local anesthesia. When the thumb is involved, care must be taken to identify the digital nerves because they are close to the flexor tendon. The triggering occurs at the interphalangeal joint; however, the nodule is palpable over the metacarpophalangeal joint.

DeQuervain's Disease

Tendinitis involving the abductor pollicis longus and the extensor pollicis brevis in the first dorsal compartment was first described by DeQuervain in 1895 (4). There is tenderness along the sheath over the first dorsal compartment and radial aspect of the wrist. Hyperflexion of the first ray with ulnar deviation of the wrist reproduces pain during physical examination. Conservative treatment is usually effective in relieving symptoms. Otherwise, surgical excision of the thickened tendon sheath of the first dorsal compartment is curative.

Ganglion

Ganglion formation is common, particularly over the dorsum of the wrist, and is likely traumatic in origin. The cyst contains a typical gelatinous fluid and the stalk usually extends down to the related joint. Most ganglions are small and minimally symptomatic and can be ignored. They may spontaneously change in size. Diagnosis can be confirmed by aspiration of the typical jelly-like material. Simultaneous injection of a small amount of corticosteroid and appropriate splinting may be curative. Recurrence is common and surgical excision is reserved for symptomatic lesions. Dissections should carefully include the stalk to prevent recurrence.

Lateral Epicondylitis

Often referred to as *tennis elbow,* this is a very common inflammation due to repetitive activity and less frequently to tennis. Wrist extension against resistance causes pain at the lateral epicondyle. Throwing and wringing motions may be painful, as well as backhand racquet movements. Treatment is by rest, application of ice, and use of nonsteroidal antiinflammatory drugs. A proximal forearm tennis strap may be helpful. The condition is usually benign and responds to restriction or modification of activities.

Surgery is indicated in recalcitrant cases and consists of excision of granulation tissue involving the extensor carpi radialis brevis or any localized calcification that may be present. Postoperative splinting is instituted for 2 to 3 weeks.

Dupuytren's Contracture

Dupuytren's contracture is a rather common condition without any obvious etiology, and characterized by hypertrophy and contracture of the palmar and digital fascia. Typically, the small and ring fingers are involved, but extension can involve other digits as well. Deep cords of fascia can develop that produce progressive flexion of the metacarpophalangeal joint by the deep attachments to the volar plate. So-called spiral cords can wind around the neurovascular bundles, rendering them vulnerable at surgical dissection.

Most Dupuytren's contractures are minimally progressive or nonprogressive with minimal functional impairment. When the contracture is progressive, flexion begins to develop, and it is best to treat the patient early before extensive flexion contracture evolves (60).

Surgical Treatment. Simple fasciotomy may be effective for patients with thin palmar fascial cords and primarily involvement of the the metacarpophalangeal joint. It is also useful in elderly or chronically ill patients who might do less well with a more extensive procedure (78). The usual treatment is fasciectomy, which involves careful preoperative planning of Z-plasty and skin flaps, careful dissection of thin skin, avoidance of digital nerve injury, and complete resection of diseased palmar fascia. Transection of contracting skin and fascial cords, followed by full-thickness skin grafting, may be attempted in an effort to interrupt the contiguity of the cord (79). Complications of surgery include digital nerve damage, skin necrosis, and recurrence. Digital joint capsulectomy may be necessary for severe or recurrent contracture (60).

FOOT

The three main functional requirements for the foot are that it fit in a shoe, strike the floor flat, and be pain free. The symptomatic foot can be a source of great disability. Causes for this include fractures, acquired and degenerative deformities, and arthritic conditions. Peripheral neuropathies associated with diabetes or malnutrition are also problematic (19).

Fracture of the Talus

Closed reduction and casting or percutaneous screw fixation can treat fractures of the neck of the talus when they are undisplaced. Open injuries and associated fractures in the foot and ankle may be present. Displaced fractures of the body of the talus have a very poor prognosis with a high incidence of avascular necrosis or nonunion. It is mandatory to obtain as accurate a reduction of the articular surface as possible (Fig. 100.39A).These injuries frequently require an osteotomy of the medial malleolus of the tibia to gain exposure and, despite anatomic reduction, chondral damage and interference with blood supply frequently lead to avascular necrosis or arthritis even if the fracture unites. Weight bearing should be restricted for a minimum of 8 weeks or longer after surgery (16,17).

Calcaneal Fractures

Fractures of the calcaneus are common and potentially disabling injuries resulting usually from a fall from a height. A lumbar compression fracture is a frequent associated injury, although usually not requiring operative treatment.

Open reduction and internal fixation to restore the anatomy and articular facets of the subtalar joint is usually used to treat the joint depression fractures involving the calcaneus (Fig. 100.39B). Occasionally, extremely comminuted fractures warrant consideration for primary subtalar arthrodesis because normal motion and pain relief are not likely to be accomplished by open reduction and internal fixation (Fig. 100.17).

Severe swelling and blister formation may preclude immediate operation. It is best to elevate the foot and wait until the soft tissue has healed, frequently 7 to 10 days and occasionally longer, before operation. Surgical treatment allows the restoration of normal architecture, avoiding the broad, flattened heel that accompanies nonoperative treatment. The flattened heel frequently is difficult to fit in a shoe and is associated with entrapment or irritation of the peroneal tendons. Despite operative treatment, subtalar motion is frequently diminished. After surgery, weight bearing is restricted for 10 to 12 weeks until fracture healing has occurred. Results are usually satisfactory with accurate reduction; however, an unpredictable number of patients require eventual subtalar arthrodesis because of pain.

Nonoperative treatment consists of molding the fracture and a period of immobilization in a cast, followed by rehabilitation. Symptomatic patients can be treated with subtalar fusion, although this is somewhat more problematic because of the broadened configuration, loss of height, and proximity of the calcaneus to the talus (16,17,19).

Midfoot Fractures

Fractures of the navicular, cuboid, and cuneiforms are less common. The midfoot is relatively rigid, with the linked articulations firmly bound by ligamentous structures, and therefore significant force is necessary to produce injury. Other associated foot injuries may be present. Fractures of the navicular and cuboid are often associated with lesions involving the talus, calcaneus, or subtalar joint (16). Injuries involving the cuneiforms invariably involve their articulation with the metatarsal bases. Displaced fractures and dislocations need to be reduced and appropriately immobilized, which often requires open reduction and internal fixation (16) (Fig. 100.39C).

Lisfranc's Fracture–Dislocation

Fracture–dislocation of the tarsometatarsal joints may be associated with severe swelling and potential neurovascular compromise of the distal foot. Usually all five joints are dislocated, and associated fracture of the base of the metatarsal or cuneiforms may be present. A key to diagnosis is loss of the recessed keystone appearance of the second metatarsal–cuneiform articulation. Treatment is by closed or, more frequently, open reduction and transarticular pin or screw fixation. The latter is more secure (Fig. 102.39D). There is little motion at the tarsometatarsal joints, so the security of fixation warrants a transarticular screw placement if necessary to maintain reduction (17).

Metatarsal and Toe Fractures

Most metatarsal fractures are treated closed. Multiple metatarsal fractures that are displaced or displaced fractures of the metacarpal neck may require open reduction and internal fixation. Dislocations of the toes are easily overlooked and can be a source of late disability or medical–legal problems. These should be reduced promptly

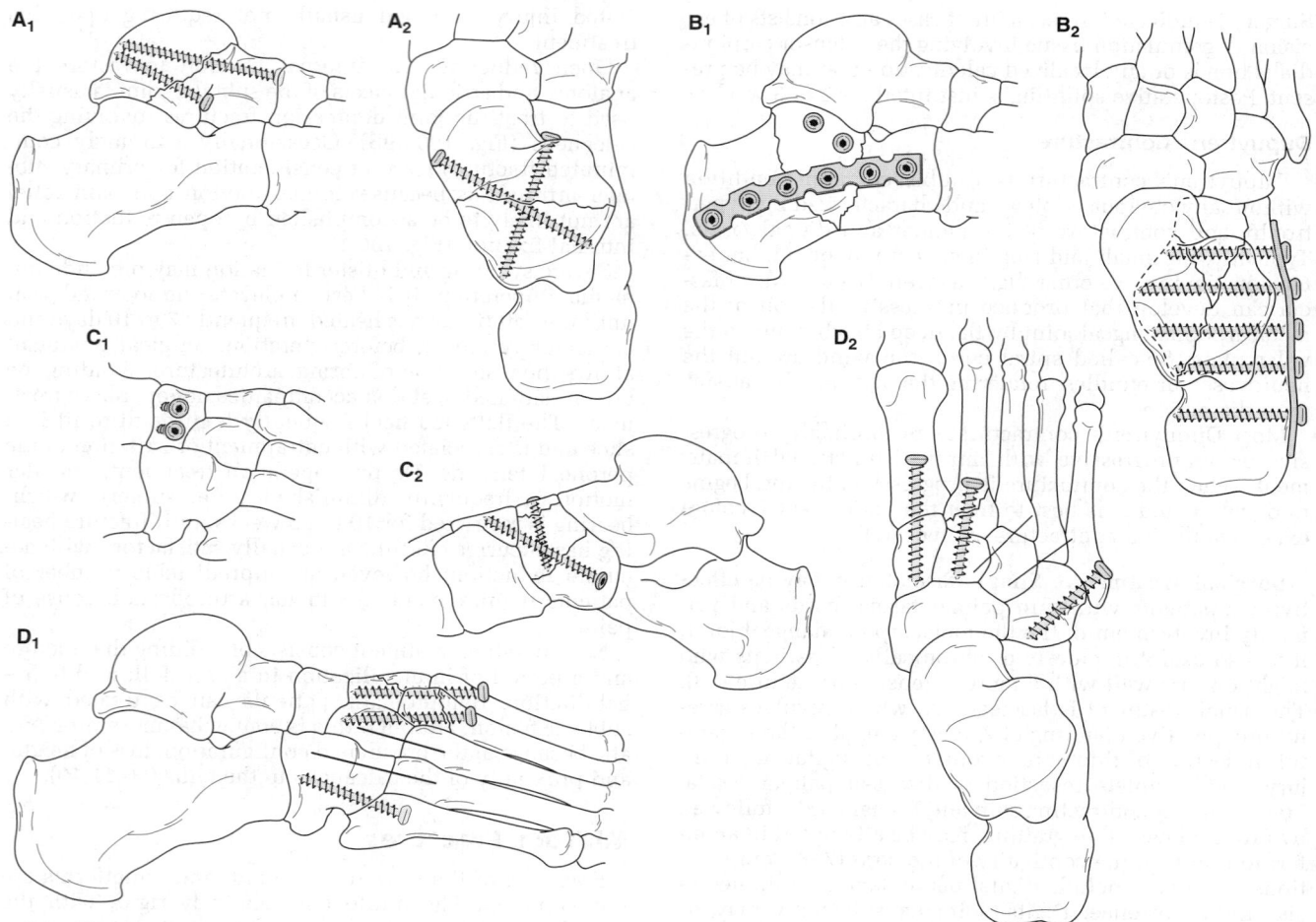

Figure 100.39. *(A)* Displaced joint fractures of the calcaneus can be treated by open reduction and internal fixation provided that the soft tissue is in good condition. After surgery, early subtalar motion is encouraged and weight bearing is delayed for 10 to 12 weeks. *(A2)* Axial view of internally fixed calcaneal fracture. *(B1)* Lateral view of the ankle after open reduction and internal fixation of a fracture of the talar neck with interfragmentary screw. *(B2)* Anteroposterior radiograph of same fracture. *(C1)* Anteroposterior view of surgical stabilization of a fractured navicular. *(C2)* Lateral view of the foot after open reduction and screw stabilization of same fracture. Occasionally, bone graft is necessary for comminuted fractures to buttress the articular surfaces. *(D)* Lisfranc's fracture–dislocation of tarsometatarsal joints. The second metatarsal base–cuneiform articulation is a good key to reduction. Frequently, all five articulations are involved. Significant swelling and soft-tissue injury occurs with this injury. Treatment is by open reduction and internal fixation, or occasionally closed reduction and percutaneous fixation as indicated. *(D2)* Anteroposterior view of Lisfranc's fracture–dislocation after surgical stabilization.

and are usually stable. Buddy taping to a fellow toe is usually all that is necessary. Intraarticular fractures of the metatarsal heads or adjacent phalanges should be treated by open reduction if they involve significant portions of the joint. This is especially true for the great toe.

Hallux Valgus

Bunion formation and hallux valgus are common in modern society. Most patients who desire surgical correction are women who have subjected their feet to high-heeled or tight shoes. Hallux valgus observed in cultures where shoes are not worn is largely asymptomatic. When indicated, a number of different surgical procedures may be used. The simplest procedures are exostectomy or cheilectomy. Soft tissue realignment procedures or osteotomies involving the base or distal aspects of the first metatarsal may be required for severe degrees of hallux valgus. Partial proximal phalangectomy and temporary

Kirschner wire pinning frequently can correct claw and hammertoe deformities. Syndactyly occasionally may be indicated.

Posterior Tibial Tendon Rupture

This is a potentially disabling condition that develops from overload of the posterior tibial tendon and longitudinal arch. Characteristically it begins as tendinitis and progresses to partial or complete rupture. If the latter occurs, a severe acquired flat foot or pes plano valgus deformity occurs as the heel slides out from underneath the talus and most of the weight is born on the medial column of the foot. Early treatment is by appropriate splinting, arch support, and medications during the inflammatory stage. Once a tendon is ruptured, treatment is surgical by débridement, repair, or frequently tendon transfer of the flexor hallucis longus or flexor digitorum longus tendons.

This is a frequently overlooked condition that can be diagnosed by typical symptoms of discomfort along the posterior tibial tendon and inability to do a heel lift without producing valgus displacement of the hindfoot. Variable weakness of the posterior tibial muscle results in difficulties with plantar flexion and inversion. Occasionally, triple or subtalar arthrodesis is necessary to realign the foot and relieve the symptoms.

PEDIATRIC ORTHOPEDICS

The term *orthopaedy* is derived from two Greek words, *orthos,* meaning "straight, upright, or free from deformity," and *paidos,* "a child." It was originally used by Nicholas André in 1741. Musculoskeletal disorders present at birth, arising during growth and development, or secondary to trauma are unique and distinct. Because they are often asymptomatic, diagnosis depends on a fundamental knowledge of their existence, a high index of suspicion, and careful examination (80).

Developmental Dysplasia of the Hip

Formally known as *congenital dislocation of the hip,* this diagnosis can readily be made at birth. It has also been detected in utero by ultrasound methods. Girls are usually affected and the left hip is most commonly involved. It frequently occurs in otherwise healthy infants, but can be associated with other congenital abnormalities. Diagnosis is made by noting asymmetric abduction of the flexed hips, foreshortening of the flexed thigh (Galeazzi's sign), or asymmetric skin folds. A click or sensation of reduction and dislocation (Ortolani's and Barlow's signs) may be present. Regular radiographs are not helpful at this stage because of immature development of the acetabulum and the absence of the proximal femoral ossific nuclei.

Problems can arise in diagnosis of bilateral dislocation because of lack of asymmetry. Nevertheless, abduction is limited, a click may be present on examination, and ultrasound reveals bilateral dislocated hips. The latter is the preferred diagnostic adjunct for diagnosis at birth. Treatment is by closed reduction and the application of triple diapers or a simple Pavlik harness, which holds the hips flexed at greater than 90 degrees in mid-abduction. This is the so-called human position. Previously, hips were immobilized in spica casts in full abduction, resulting in a significant incidence of avascular necrosis occasionally involving the uninvolved hip. Appropriate splinting allows for normal development of the hip, which can be monitored clinically and after a few months radiographically. Well recognized radiographic criteria such as the center-edge angle, acetabular index, and Shenton's line are measured and evaluated (80).

If the diagnosis of developmentally dislocated hip is not made until a child is walking, treatment is much more problematic, frequently requiring open reduction accompanied by varus osteotomy and femoral shortening. Subsequent innominate osteotomy may be necessary if the acetabulum is vertical or shallow and fails adequately to contain the femoral hip.

Adult residua of degenerative dysplasia of the hip include a waddling gait due to dislocation of the hip and weak abductors, and ultimately the development of symptomatic arthritic symptoms. Joint replacement in adults with long-standing developmental dysplasia of the hip is difficult because a false acetabulum is frequently present. The hip is high riding, the extremity short, and the femoral canal small. Special acetabular and femoral components are usually needed. Frequently, adult patients with developmental dysplasia of the hip do not become significantly symptomatic until the third or fourth decade (55,81).

Legg-Calvé-Perthes Disease

Legg-Calvé-Perthes disease is an idiopathic hip disorder occurring in children, usually between the ages of 4 and 8 or 9 years of age. It may be picked up incidentally in younger children or be characterized by mild discomfort and an intermittent limp.

The source of discomfort may be referred to the knee. Physical findings are usually normal unless the process is advanced and a mild limp and limitation of motion, especially abduction, may be present. Radiographs characteristically show variable degrees of avascular changes in the femoral head. The entire head may appear to be involved, only to become revascularized at the completion of the healing phase. Treatment is controversial but has involved efforts to limit weight bearing, use of an abduction brace, or surgical osteotomy of the proximal femur or acetabulum to provide containment of the head with "at-risk" signs radiographically. The younger the child at presentation, the better the prognosis. The older child presenting at 7 or 8 years of age is more likely to have some permanent residua, which can lead to degenerative arthritis in early or middle adult life (80,81).

Slipped Capital Femoral Epiphysis

The typical presentation is an obese young adolescent lacking secondary sex characteristics and complaining of mild knee pain and a limp. A sudden increase in the pain may occur with acute slip. Bilateral involvement is common, although symptoms may be unilateral. The etiology is unknown, but endocrine and mechanical factors have been suspected.

Treatment for acute slipped capital femoral epiphysis is gentle reduction and percutaneous pinning, and for chronic slips, in situ pinning. Attempts to reduce acute or chronic slips may result in increased damage to the growth plate or kinking of the retinacular vessels, leading to avascular necrosis. A single cannulated screw is placed across the physis. Because the epiphysis is located posteriorly and the metaphysis has actually "slipped" anterolaterally, the starting point is often more proximal and located anteriorly on the femoral neck. Titanium screws should not be used because of their biologic affinity for bone and the great difficulty in removing them should this be necessary. After successful pinning, the physis closes over 3 to 6 months and further slipping is prevented. Because the children are approaching skeletal maturity and the process is often bilateral, leg length discrepancy is not a significant factor (80).

Club Foot

The diagnosis of talipes equinovarus, or club foot, is readily apparent at birth. It is a more rigid and pronounced deformity than the more common metatarsus adductus, which is supple and easily correctable by the examiner. The deformity occurs frequently in otherwise normal infants, but can accompany other developmental abnormalities. Physical examination should include careful spinal evaluation for a hair patch, dimple, or evidence of myelomeningocele, and other spinal or neurologic disorders. Treatment consists of taping the corrected foot and subsequent corrective cast application initially. For rigid club feet or for those that do not respond to manipulation, taping, or cast treatment, early operative correction is warranted. This can be safely performed as early as 6 weeks of age through a (Cincinnati) posterior incision, which allows exposure and release of tethered ligaments, tendons, and joint capsules of the ankle and subtalar joint. Early correction allows the foot to be in a normal position at the time the child begins to ambulate. It also avoids some of the iatrogenic consequences of prolonged casting, false correction, and development of rocker-bottom foot deformity. It is especially valuable in arthrogryposis and other rigid types of flat feet.

Scoliosis

Idiopathic scoliosis is now detected earlier by nearly universal screening methods. Subtle cases of scoliosis or balanced curves may be difficult to detect. Physical findings include shoulder asymmetry or rib hump in pronounced cases with obvious deviation of the spine. Less obvious curves may be missed unless a high index of suspicion is maintained. A screening anteroposterior spinal

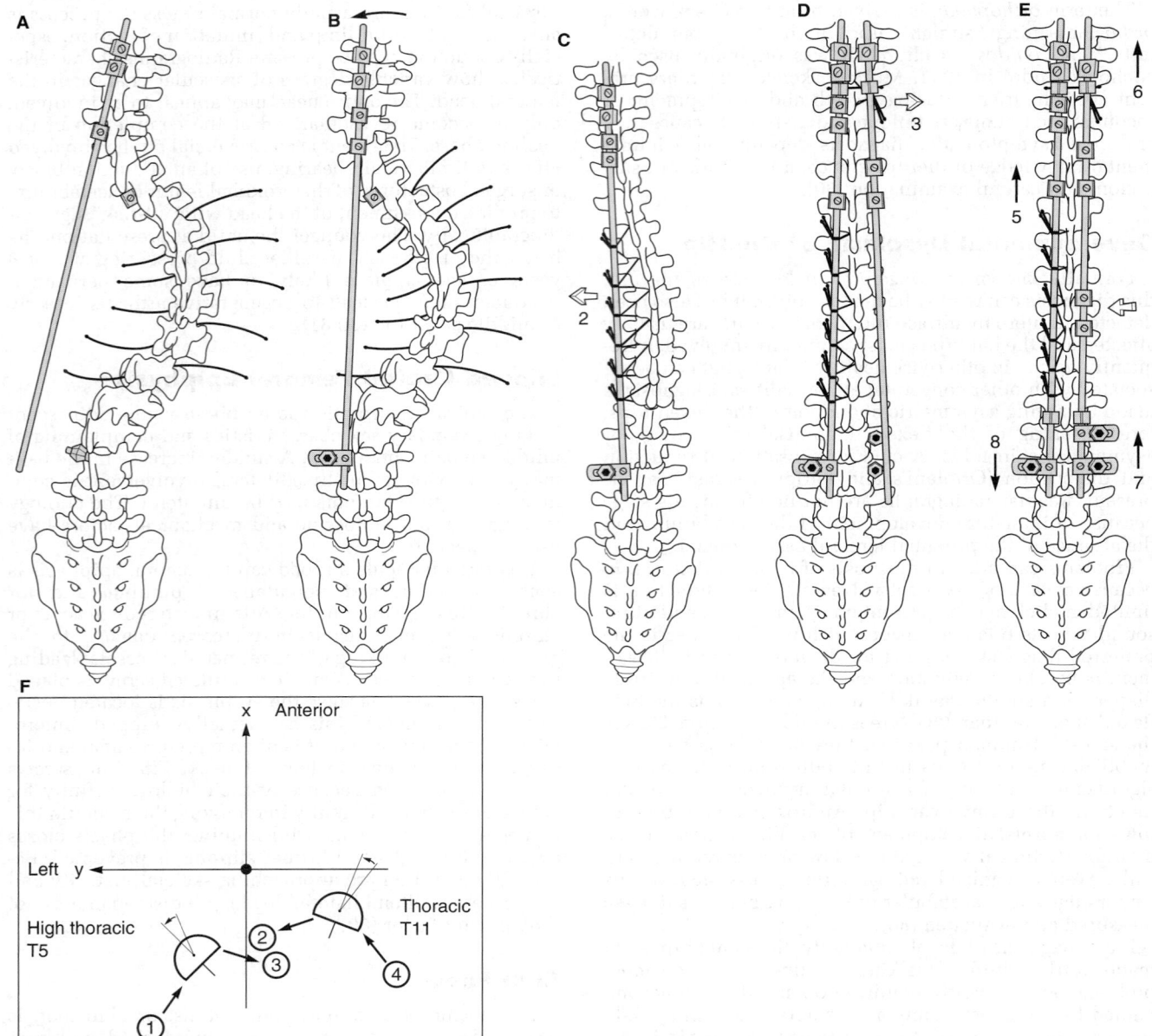

Figure 100.40. Idiopathic scoliosis, double thoracic curve. *(A)* After placement of the left anchors and initial placement of longitudinal member (note that the low hook of the claw is placed sublaminar). *(B)* After securing of convex longitudinal member to the lower anchor, resulting in T-2 coronal plane angular position correction. *(C)* Low thoracic curve requiring medial and, if necessary, posterior translation. *(D)* Initial placement of right-side rod, during which the T-2 coronal plane force couple is completed. *(E)* After construct completion. *(F)* Drawing of transverse plane apex force couples. In reality, application of a transverse plane high thoracic curve apex force couple is difficult because of the constraints placed by the rib cage. *(G)* Young adolescent girl with severe thoracolumbar rotoscoliosis. *(H)* Improved appearance after posterior segmental instrumentation and fusion. Patient's height has been restored and spinal contours and balance greatly improved. (Photograph courtesy of Dr. Daniel Benson.) (Reprinted with permission from Asher MA. Isola spinal instrumentation system for scoliosis. In: Bridwell KH, DeWald RL, eds. *Textbook of spinal surgery,* 2nd ed., vol 1. Philadelphia: Lippincott–Raven, 1997:589.) *(continues)*

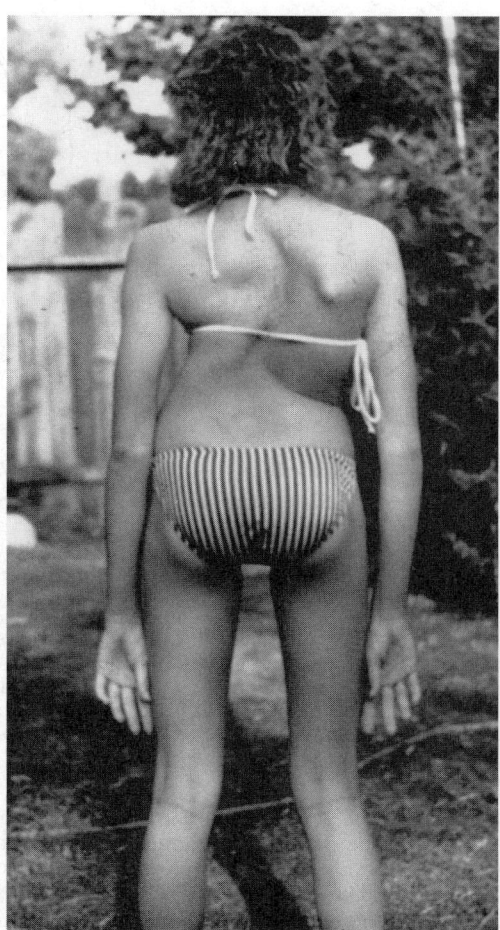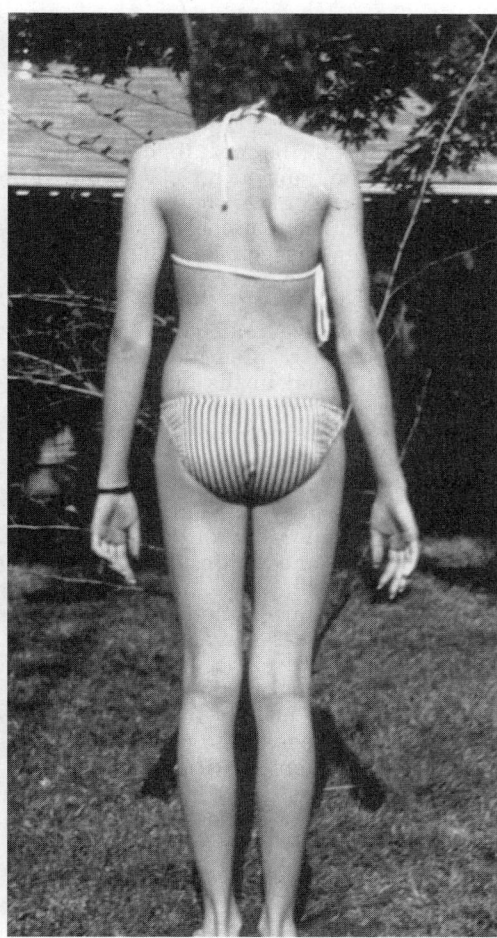

Figure 100.40. (Continued)

radiograph centered at T-12, and in cases of obvious kyphosis, a lateral radiograph, should be obtained on initial suspicion of scoliosis. Subsequently, supine side-bending films may be indicated to evaluate the rigidity of the curve and its correctability. Curves of less than 15 degrees require only observation. Curves beyond 20 degrees should be considered for bracing. However, some patients have progressive curves, ultimately requiring surgical correction. Most patients are girls and have thoracic curves that are convex to the right. The younger the patient at presentation, the more likely is the curve to progress. Although some progression of curves continues slowly in adulthood, rapid progression ceases at skeletal maturity. Indications for surgery are usually relative, but include curves of greater than 35 to 40 degrees, rapidly progressive curves, and symptomatic scoliosis in some adult patients (Fig. 100.40).

Curves that are convex to the left should give raise the suspicion of congenital vertebral abnormalities, intraspinal disease, or neuromuscular disease.

Congenital scoliosis may require anterior exposure and resection of a hemivertebra or other associated spinal abnormalities, followed by anterior fusion and usually simultaneous or staged posterior instrumentation. Neurogenic curves frequently require stabilization, especially when they are unbalanced and severe. Large curves can eventually cause respiratory compromise, especially if they exceed 50 to 60 degrees. Curves beyond this level may require anterior release before posterior instrumentation and correction. Long fusions extending to the sacrum

with anterior instrumentation may also be necessary for certain curve patterns (56) (Fig. 100.38).

The treatment of scoliosis, kyphosis, and related spinal deformity has undergone extensive evolution. Fortunately, most curves are small or moderate and nonprogressive, requiring only observation or occasionally bracing. If surgery is indicated, powerful systems have been developed to ensure maximum stability while fusion occurs. These include various anterior instrumentation methods, posterior sublaminar wiring and Luque rod techniques, or pedicle screws and segmental instrumentation methodologies (Fig. 100.40).

Neuromuscular Disease

Myelomeningocele

Patients with spina bifida and an open neural arch frequently are first seen after neurosurgical closure of the dural sac. Depending on the level of the myelomeningocele and the extent of neurologic involvement, various neurologic deficits in the lower extremities exist. Patients with high-level myelomeningoceles with absent motor and sensory function from the hips on down are not candidates for ambulation. Patients with preservation of the quadriceps will usually be at least household and sometimes community ambulators. Low-level or sacral myelomeningocele may produce only minor deformity or neurologic deficits in the foot or toes. A high arch or cavus foot and claw toe deformity should alert the examiner to the possibility of spinal or other neurologic problem. Treatment is designed to optimize ambulatory function by appropriate physical therapy, bracing, or, where indicated, surgical procedures. These may include operations to treat dislocated hips, unless they are bilateral, release contractures, and correct deformities in the foot. Tendon lengthening and occasionally tendon transfers may be helpful in select cases. Stretching and splinting exercises by the parents, physical therapists, and occupational therapists are an important part of the treatment regimen (80).

Cerebral Palsy

Affected children usually have undergone anoxia at birth. Difficult labor and delivery, prematurity, and low birth weight are frequently found in the history of children with cerebral palsy. Acquired cases may be secondary to head injury, near drowning, or congenital and familial syndromes. The disease is characterized by developmental delay, psychomotor retardation, and, usually, spasticity. Intellectual capacity may range from normal or superior to profoundly deficient. Many of the latter children are totally dependent for all activities of daily living and have no ambulatory potential.

Treatment is designed to optimize function and neuromuscular control. Much of the treatment and care of these children involves physical therapists, occupational therapists, and special education teachers through a coordinated program. Parents become heavily involved in the adaptive and developmental needs of these children. Orthotists are important to fashion and fabricate appropriate splints and to modify wheelchairs.

Orthopedic treatment consists of orchestrating many of the child's musculoskeletal needs and, where indicated, appropriate surgery to release contracted joints, occasional tendon transfers, and the prevention and treatment of hip subluxation or dislocation. Spinal curves should be appropriately followed and treated with bracing or spinal fusion when indicated. Stretching exercises and night splints such as ankle–foot orthoses or knee immobilizers are helpful in preventing contractures or maintaining postoperative correction.

Pediatric Fractures

Fractures in children are unique in several ways. The blood supply to the developing skeleton and the thick periosteum covering long bones results in rapid and predictable fracture healing. Nonunion is extremely rare. Most pediatric fractures can be treated by closed reduction and casting techniques. In the case of femur fractures, skin traction in younger children for a few days can be followed by the application of a spica cast. Some shortening and deformity can be accepted because slight overgrowth and subsequent remodeling result in an excellent functional and cosmetic result. The time in plaster varies for the involved fracture, but usually is 5 to 6 weeks (81,82).

In contradistinction, injuries or fractures involving the growth plate (physis) can produce permanent disability, deformity, and joint destruction unless treated appropriately. Salter and Harris have developed a classification of injuries to the growth plate (Fig. 100.41). Type I and II injuries do not cross the growth plate and heal well after closed reduction, with no residua in most cases. Type III fractures involve the physis (growth plate) and epiphysis and require accurate reduction if displaced by more than 2 mm (Fig. 100.42). Type IV injuries cross the metaphysis, growth plate, and epiphysis. They demand careful and accurate open reduction and internal fixation, and are associated with potential for growth arrest and subsequent deformity. Type V injuries involve a crush of the growth

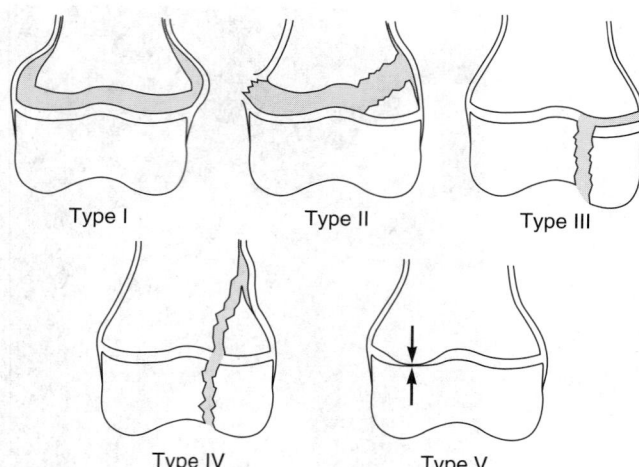

Figure 100.41. Salter-Harris classification of epiphyseal injuries. Type I injury is an epiphyseolysis of the involved growth plate without associated fracture. Type II has an additional metaphyseal fracture fragment. Type I and II injuries have a good prognosis and are usually treated with closed reduction and casting. Type III injury results in a fracture through the growth plate and epiphysis. Type IV fracture crosses the epiphysis, growth plate (physis), and metaphysis. Type III and IV injuries require careful open reduction and internal fixation if displaced. Type V injury involves a crush of the growth plate without a fracture and is usually detected late by asymmetric or premature closure of the growth plate.

plate that usually is not visible on plain radiographs, but is determined subsequently by growth arrest and shortening, or deformity of the site of injury (16,81,82).

Computed tomographic evaluation of fractures involving the growth plate can be helpful. Juvenile Tillaux's and triplane fractures occur in adolescence because of a closing distal tibial growth plate and require open reduction if closed reduction is not successful.

After open reduction and internal fixation, stabilization of type III and IV fractures is by Kirschner wire or screw fixation, avoiding the growth plate. The prognosis is usually good when atraumatic anatomic reduction has been achieved. Nevertheless, in young children, type III and IV injuries much be watched closely. Treatment of subsequent growth arrest may require completion of epiphyseodesis to prevent asymmetric deformity. Contralateral stapling or epiphyseodesis may be appropriately timed to prevent leg length discrepancy. In very short patients, or those with significant discrepancies, lengthening using distraction osteogenesis and Ilizarov techniques may be attempted (Figs. 100.32, 100.33). These operations require accurate assessment of the rate of growth inhibition, progression of deformity, amount of growth remaining, and anticipated discrepancy at completion of skeletal growth.

In infants and young children, fractures about joints may be difficult to evaluate because the epiphysis is cartilaginous and anlage of the ossific nuclei has not appeared. Obtaining radiographs of the opposite site for comparison is helpful in these situations.

Except as noted previously, open reduction is rarely performed for pediatric fractures; however, intramedullary fixation of femur fractures in late childhood or early adolescence is usually indicated. Small-diameter, nonreamed flexible rods (Ender) are safe and effective. Rarely, avascular necrosis of the femoral head has been reported with this method. Children in this age group have less growth remaining and less ability to remodel fractures, and are treated more like adults (82).

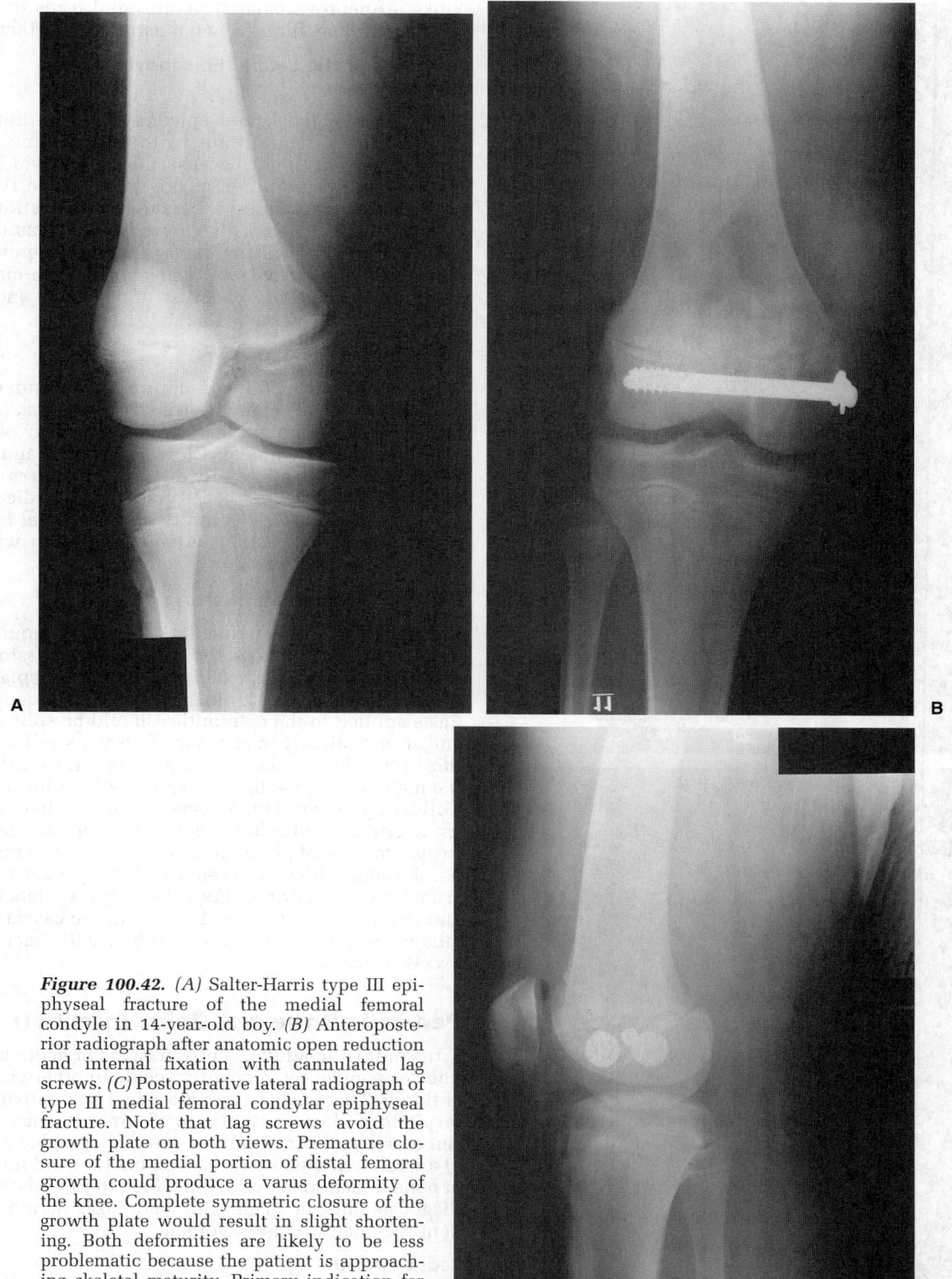

Figure 100.42. *(A)* Salter-Harris type III epiphyseal fracture of the medial femoral condyle in 14-year-old boy. *(B)* Anteroposterior radiograph after anatomic open reduction and internal fixation with cannulated lag screws. *(C)* Postoperative lateral radiograph of type III medial femoral condylar epiphyseal fracture. Note that lag screws avoid the growth plate on both views. Premature closure of the medial portion of distal femoral growth could produce a varus deformity of the knee. Complete symmetric closure of the growth plate would result in slight shortening. Both deformities are likely to be less problematic because the patient is approaching skeletal maturity. Primary indication for surgery was restoration of articular congruity as in adults.

Supracondylar Fracture of the Humerus

A common pediatric fracture with potential for disastrous complications is the supracondylar fracture of the humerus (83). The mechanism of injury is usually a fall on the outstretched hand. The injury is usually characterized by marked swelling about the elbow with associated de-

formity and occasionally neurologic deficits. Treatment of choice is closed reduction and cross-pinning with fine Kirschner wires followed by splinting for 3 weeks, at which time the fracture is usually healed (Fig. 100.43). Volkmann's ischemic contracture is not encountered with this form of treatment; rather, this complication is related to closed reduction and splinting in acute flexion that

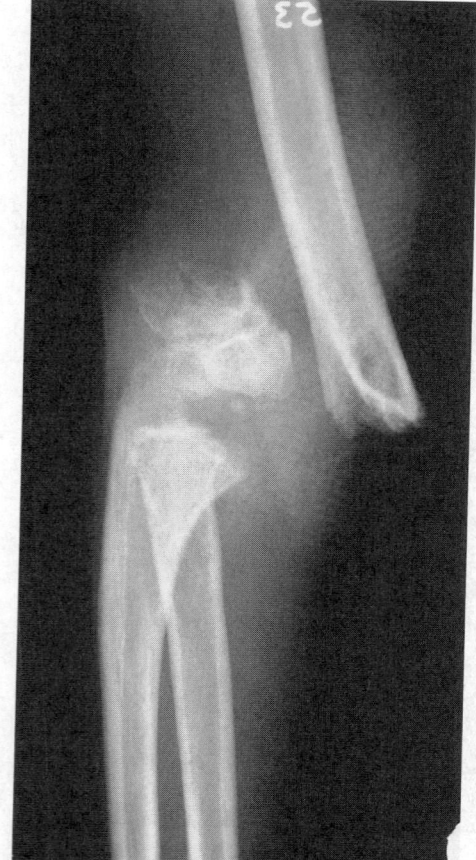

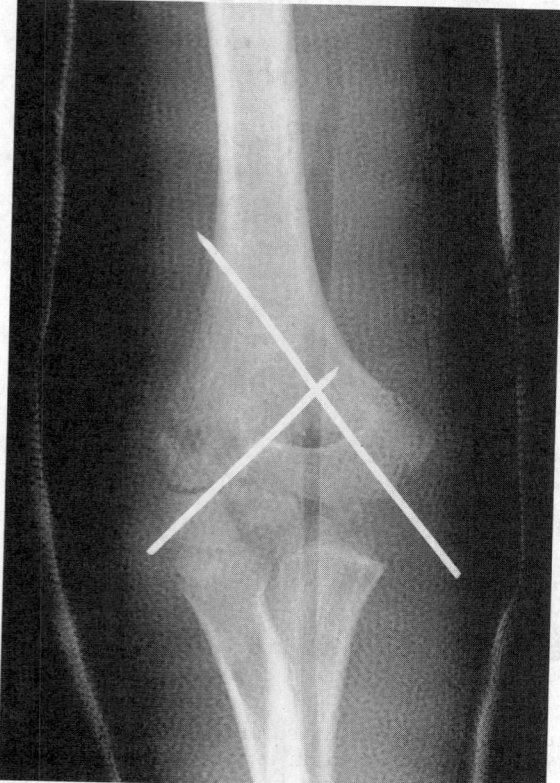

Figure 100.43. *(A)* A 10-year-old patient with a severely displaced supracondylar fracture of the humerus associated with brachial artery avulsion but a viable, well perfused hand, good collateral flow, and intact neurologic function. *(B)* Anteroposterior radiograph. Fracture healed rapidly with an excellent functional result.

kinks off neurovascular structures and leads to compartment syndrome, fibrosis, and a permanent withered hand.

Fractures of the Lateral Epicondyle of the Humerus

Fractures of the lateral epicondyle of the humerus in children are potential traps, with radiographic displacement appearing slight because the epicondyle is largely cartilaginous. These injuries are usually type IV epiphyseal injuries and require accurate open reduction and internal fixation. Even with this, cubitus valgus deformity develops in a certain percentage owing to growth plate closure on the lateral side. This can lead to tardy ulnar nerve palsy later in life because of deformity and chronic stretching of the nerve (81,82).

Femoral Neck Fractures

Femoral neck fractures in children are fortunately very uncommon because they have a significant risk of avascular necrosis and growth disturbance. This may occur with closed or open treatment. Closed reduction and percutaneous pinning for minimally displaced fractures or careful open reduction for displaced fractures is indicated (Fig. 100.15). This is a serious injury with potential for permanent disability, especially in young children with much growth remaining (81,82).

Closed Reduction and Casting

Children requiring reduction of fractures should usually be seen for a cast check the next day. Admission for observation may be indicated for severely displaced fractures or whenever significant swelling is anticipated. Casts applied to the extremities should be split anteriorly and spread slightly to accommodate any swelling. Should this occur after discharge, the parents can be instructed in the method of spreading the split cast to relieve pressure. Children younger than 5 years of age may have difficulty using crutches after lower extremity fracture and may be treated for a brief period in a wheelchair until the fracture has healed. Older children usually are able to manage crutches or pediatric walkers. With appropriate diagnosis and treatment, as well as attention to the caveats and pitfalls noted previously, most children with fractures have excellent results.

Pediatric Bone and Joint Infection

In contrast to adults, septic arthritis or acute hematogenous osteomyelitis frequently occurs in otherwise healthy children. There may be an antecedent sore throat or upper respiratory illness, or a history of minor trauma. The latter can be a diagnostic pitfall because radiographic evaluation of a swollen extremity reveals no fracture and no evidence of bone infection for at least the first 10 to 14 days. Clearly, diagnosis must be made well before this period if permanent sequelae are to be avoided.

Septic Arthritis

It is urgent that this diagnosis be made promptly in infants, especially when it involves the hip joint. In neonates, the classic signs of infection such as elevated temperature and white blood cell count may be absent. Pseudoparalysis or apparent inability to move a limb, associated with crying or irritability with passive motion, is frequently present. Ultrasound may be helpful in revealing fluid in the joint or capsular edema. The diagnosis is secured by aspiration of infected fluid or frank pus, yielding organisms on Gram strain and subsequent culture and sensitivity. *Staphylococcus aureus* is the most frequent organism encountered, although in neonates gram-negative organisms and in young children *Haemophilus* species may be encountered. Once the diagnosis has been made, immediate surgical drainage is indicted, followed by administration of appropriate antibiotics dictated by culture and sensitivity. Late diagnosis frequently results in hip dislocation, chondrolysis, and ultimate joint destruction.

Involvement of other joints is somewhat more forgiving, but still demands surgical irrigation and débridement if the joint is distended. The knee joint may be aspirated for small effusions, and local installation of antibiotics in addition to IV administration may suffice. In older children and adolescents, arthroscopic irrigation as with adults is indicated (84,85).

Hematogenous Osteomyelitis

Diagnosis is secured as with septic arthritis. In addition, there may be obvious tenderness, swelling, and erythema over a long bone. When this is present over a subcutaneous border such as the tibia, osteomyelitis is present until ruled out by aspiration. The latter is the diagnostic procedure of choice and should be performed promptly. In children and adolescents, systemic signs of infection such as elevated temperature, white blood cell count, and, in particular, erythrocyte sedimentation rate are present. The differential diagnosis may include insect stings, rheumatoid arthritis, and especially minor trauma. Osteomyelitis may accompany septic arthritis; therefore, at the time of surgical decompression of infected joints, the metaphysis should also be drilled to rule out or drain an associated focus of osteomyelitis. This is especially true in the hip and shoulder joint, where the physis is intraarticular (81,85).

Multifocal osteomyelitis may present with several sites of involvement and be confused with inflammatory arthritis. These children are frequently desperately ill and rapidly become septic. Early surgical drainage and appropriate antibiotic treatment yields excellent results. Delayed diagnosis may lead to systemic complications such as bacterial endocarditis or local destruction of the physis with resultant growth arrest. The sequelae of this are severe, especially in the younger child with considerable growth remaining.

Most musculoskeletal infections are bacterial, although viral and fungal infections can occur. Likewise, tuberculosis should be suspected in children who are born or who have lived in endemic areas of the developing world (86). Tuberculous arthritis of the hip has been mistakenly diagnosed as Legg-Calvé-Perthes disease with disastrous results. The spine may also be involved. There is a longer prodrome and symptoms present gradually, so that radiographic changes are usually apparent at the time of presentation but can easily be misinterpreted. Treatment is surgical decompression and antituberculous or other antimicrobials as indicated.

ORTHOPEDIC ONCOLOGY

Cancer is a leading cause of death in the United States and throughout the world. As a result, metastatic disease of bone is much more commonly encountered than primary malignant tumors of bone. The latter are dreaded tumors that appear primarily in children and young adults, whereas metastatic disease is more common in middle-aged and elderly people.

In general, treatment for primary bone tumors involves limb salvage procedures or amputation. The former is elected if the tumor is confined or involves a specific compartment of an extremity. Primary malignant bone tumors frequently present in heathy, active adolescents and young adults and thus have significant associated psychosocial

implications. Therefore, whenever feasible, limb salvage is the procedure of choice because 5-year survival rates for appropriately selected cases are similar to those with amputation. CT and especially MRI scans are an essential part of preoperative planning. Adjunctive chemotherapy or radiation is administered as dictated by the oncologist (87,88).

Metastatic Disease of Bone

Metastatic disease of bone is the most common cause of neoplastic bone lesions. Many different types of cancer can metastasize, but the most common sources are breast, prostate, and renal cell cancer. Increased survival is due to early detection and the institution of chemotherapy. This, however, results in a clinically increased incidence of bony metastasis and related pathologic long bone fractures. Metastatic carcinoma is the most common malignancy of bone, affecting more than 40 times as many patients as are affected by all other types of bone cancer combined. The goals of treatment are the alleviation of pain, preservation of function, and prevention of pathologic fracture.

Specific Treatment

Impending fractures of long bones are best treated by closed intramedullary fixation. It is extremely important to detect impending fractures before they occur because open treatment is associated with greater morbidity due to infection, bleeding, and dissemination of tumor cells. Polymethylmethacrylate cement may be necessary to stabilize areas of bone loss. Because survival is usually limited, fracture healing is less important than stability (88).

Metastases involving joints frequently require resection and customized total joint arthroplasty. Often, polymethylmethacrylate cement is necessary to fill defects and anchor prosthetic components. Preoperative work-up includes CT, MRI, and, where indicated, arteriography.

Metastatic Disease of the Spine

Impending paraplegia may require anterior decompression, resection of tumor, and insertion of titanium cages, local distraction constructs, or other means supplemented by polymethylmethacrylate cement to create an immediately stable situation. Posterior stabilization may also be necessary. Bony fusion is not expected or required in this case because treatment is entirely palliative (88).

Soft-tissue Sarcomas of Extremities

Soft-tissue sarcomas are derived from mesodermal tissues, and pseduoencapsulation by surrounding fibrous connective tissue is consistent finding. Metastatic spread to the lungs by the hematogenous route is present in approximately 10% of cases at diagnosis. In general, sarcomas tend to remain well confined to an anatomic compartment until late in the course of the disease or on destruction by surgical procedure. Preoperative work-up includes CT or MRI scans to determine the fine extent of the tumor. Depending on the location and histologic grade, wide or radical excision is indicated, followed by limb salvage procedures or amputation where necessary (88).

Benign Bone Tumors

Benign bone tumors are more common and may range from small, incidental lesions in asymptomatic patients to large lesions capable of producing pathologic fracture. Except in the latter instance, most benign bone tumors are minimally symptomatic. They are often diagnosed by their

Table 100.5. **COMMON SKELETAL NEOPLASMS**

Type	**Bone**	**Cartilage**	**Fibrous**	**Marrow**
Benign	Osteoid osteoma	Osteochondroma	Nonossifying fibroma	Eosinophilic granuloma
	Osteoblastoma	Enchondroma	Giant cell tumor	
		Chondroblastoma	Desmoplastic fibroma	
Malignant	Osteosarcoma	Primary chondrosarcoma	Fibrosarcoma	Ewing's sarcoma
	Periosteal osteosarcoma	Secondary chondrosarcoma	Fibrous histiocytoma	Lymphoma
				Myeloma

characteristic radiographic appearance. Frequently, this is an isolated lesion of bone, usually with elliptical and well circumscribed sclerotic borders. The cortex of a long bone may be expanded but usually is not violated, and there is no invasion of soft tissue. Unusual appearing or atypical lesions may warrant biopsy for definitive diagnosis (Table 100.5).

Differential diagnosis includes infection, which can mimic many bone tumors, as well as congenital, developmental, or acquired bone lesions (89).

Osteochondroma

Osteochondroma is a cartilage-capped bony projection involving primarily the metaphyseal regions of long

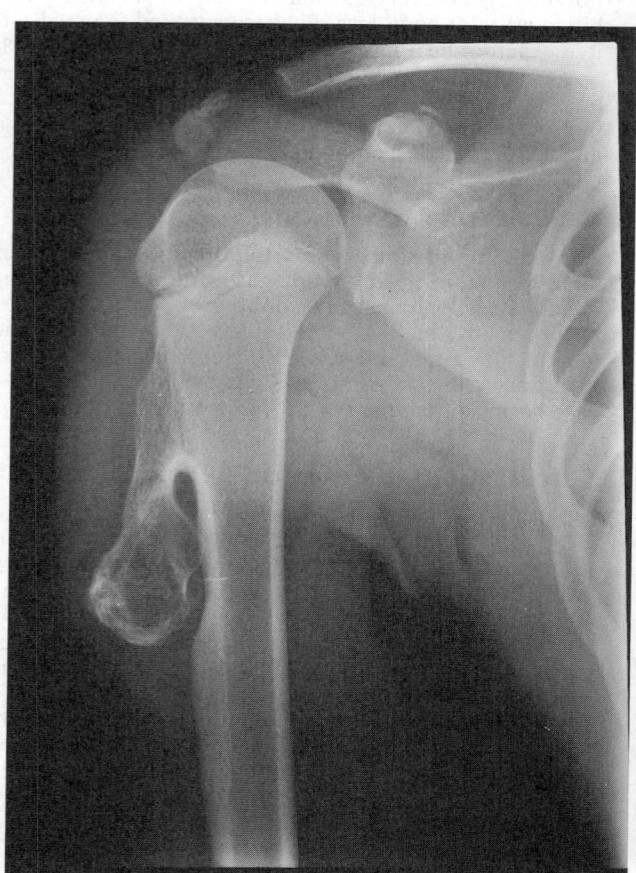

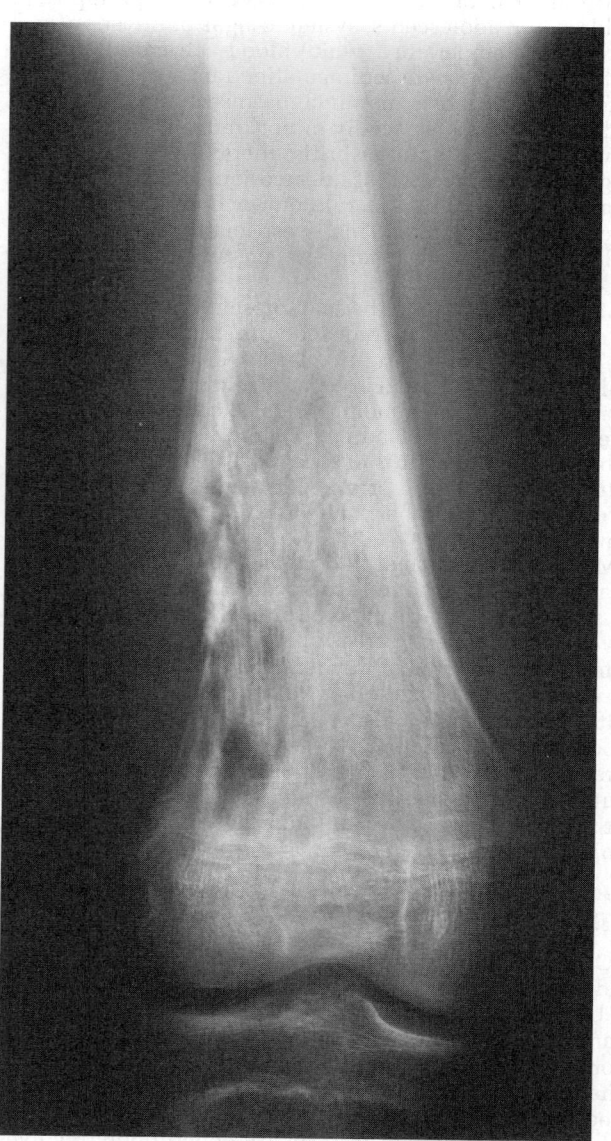

Figure 100.44. *(A)* Osteochondroma: typical appearance of a benign lesion. Osteochondroma is the most common benign bone tumor, representing 45% of all benign tumors. *(B)* Characteristic appearance of a malignant tumor in an adolescent patient. Note destruction of bone, cortical erosion, invasion of soft tissue, and subperiosteal new bone formation. Treatment in this case was amputation.

bones. It is the most common of all benign tumors (45%). Most tumors are located about the knee, shoulder, or ankle and are minimally symptomatic. The stalk projects away from the adjacent joint. Malignant transformation is extremely uncommon for isolated lesions (Fig. 100.44A). Multiple lesions are seen in the hereditary form known as *multiple hereditary osteochondromatosis* or *multiple exostosis*. Defective longitudinal growth and deformation of affected bones is present, producing variable symptoms. Malignant transformation is more common (5% to 15%) than in solitary lesions. Surgical resection is indicated only occasionally for large lesions or to rule out rare malignant transformation.

Enchondroma

This is the second most common benign bone tumor and accounts for 10% of all benign lesions. Round or ovoid tumors exhibiting fine cartilage stippling or "popcorn" appearance are seen on plain radiographs. The short tubular bones of the hands and feet are the most common locations. Most tumors are asymptomatic and are found incidentally. Larger tumors in atypical locations may be difficult to differentiate from low-grade chondrosarcoma.

Ollier's disease is a nonhereditary disseminated form also known as *multiple enchondromatosis*. Large numbers of cartilaginous tumors are present and have a significant risk (30% to 50%) of malignant degeneration to chondrosarcoma. Maffucci's syndrome is characterized by associated multiple soft-tissue angiomas in the skin and subcutaneous tissues.

Osteoid Osteoma

Osteoid osteoma is a relatively common, curious lesion of bone characterized by nocturnal pain relieved by aspirin. The classic presentation is present in most cases, strongly suggesting the diagnosis by history. Histologically, a small (<1 cm) osteoid nidus usually surrounded by a zone of reactive bone formation is present. The ends of long bones are frequently but not exclusively affected. Bone scans are strongly positive. CT is often the diagnostic study of choice and helps with preoperative planning. Surgical resection is dramatically curative but must include complete excision of the nidus.

Osteoblastoma

Osteoblastoma accounts for 3% of all benign bone tumors, and most present in the second and third decades. Because of similar histologic characteristics, it has been referred to as *giant osteoid osteoma*. The lesion has a distinct predilection for the axial skeleton and vertebral column; approximately 30% to 40% involve the posterior elements. Conventional tomography and CT scan are helpful in localization and surgical planning. Resectable tumors are treated by excision and curettage as for osteoid osteoma. Reported recurrence rates are less than 20%. Radiation has been used for large symptomatic lesions that are unresectable.

Unicameral Bone Cyst

Eighty to 90% of these circumscribed lytic lesions are found in the metaphysis of the proximal humerus or femur. Most benign bone cysts occur in children. Current treatment involves interlesional steroid injections with an approximately 50% to 80% healing rate, which is comparable with that of surgical curettage and bone graft. The latter procedure, obviously, has greater morbidity but is indicated for large lesions, especially near the hip joint, with impending or frank pathologic fracture.

Aneurysmal Bone Cyst

This tumor has a slight female predilection and occurs most frequently in adolescents. The cyst is blood filled and presents as a painful swelling, usually over a long bone. Treatment is by curettage and bone graft, although steroid injection can be tried. Radiation therapy or adjunctive cryotherapy is used for recurrent cysts, especially those that have some degree of soft-tissue extension. Occasionally, preoperative arterial embolization may be helpful.

Nonossifying Fibroma

Most lesions are asymptomatic and are discovered incidentally. They are frequently found in the metaphyseal regions of long bones in adolescents or young adults. Radiographically, the appearance is characteristic, revealing a small, eccentrically located lytic region with a scalloped, thin, sclerotic border. Rarely, curettage and bone grafting may be necessary for symptomatic legions.

Fibrous Dysplasia

This is a disease of childhood that may be monostotic or polyostotic. It is a benign developmental condition usually discovered as an incidental radiographic finding on examination. Some patients, however, may have pain and progressive deformity, especially with lesions about the proximal femur, where the characteristic "shepherd's crook" is present. Treatment is indicated for pathologic or impending pathologic fracture and consists of curettage, bone grafting, and frequently surgical stabilization.

Albright's syndrome is a triad of polyostotic fibrous dysplasia, endocrinopathy, and café au lait skin lesions.

Eosinophilic Granuloma

Radiographically, this condition appears as a solitary or occasionally multifocal lytic lesion of bone and is characteristically found in long bones, skull, and ribs. The margins of the lesions are usually well defined, although some periosteal reaction may be present, making differentiation from malignant tumors difficult. Small or asymptomatic lesions require observation only, and larger lesions are treated by curettage, cryosurgery, or low-dose radiation therapy. Histologically, the lesion contains multinucleated giant cells, eosinophils, and mononuclear Langerhans' cells. Multifocal lesions may be associated with other manifestations similar to the spectrum of diseases termed *histiocytosis X,* with diabetes insipidus, adenopathy, and hepatosplenomegaly.

Chondroblastoma

This is an uncommon cartilaginous tumor of adolescents and young adults. Symptoms are variable, but because of the typical location, joint complaints predominate.

This lesion, along with giant cell tumor, occurs specifically in the epiphysis as a lytic round hole in bone. Fine cartilaginous stippling may be present. Treatment is thorough curettage and bone grafting, which is usually curative. The tumor is usually considered to be benign, although very rare metastases have been reported.

Giant Cell Tumor

This tumor is usually eccentric and located in the metaphysis or epiphysis of long bones, with 50% of lesions occurring about the knee. Proximal humerus and distal radius are also common locations, and the sacrum may be involved. Typically, the lesions present with a painful, slowly enlarging mass. The tumor frequently extends to the subchondral bone of the adjacent joint, rendering treatment with preservation of function difficult. Curettage and bone grafting may be appropriate for small lesions. More aggressive lesions, which demonstrate expansion and thinning of the cortices, may require filling of the cavity with polymethylmethacrylate, either definitively or as a temporary measure, followed by bone grafting in 4 to 6 months. Lesions with extension into adjacent soft tissue require *en bloc* resection (88).

The recurrence rate is significant for the larger, more aggressive lesions. Occasionally, *en bloc* resection with modified arthrodesis, allograft, or prosthetic reconstruction is indicated. In the knee, this may require distal femoral resection and total knee replacement (Fig. 100.19).

Malignant Bone Tumors

Malignant Myeloma

Myeloma is the most common primary tumor of bone, accounting for 40% to 50% of all malignant bone tumors. It is largely a disease of middle age and beyond, with most patients between the ages of 50 and 70 years. Isolated lesions may occur, but eventual dissemination or progression to widespread skeletal involvement is more common. Multiple lytic lesions may involve the axial skeleton, skull, or vertebral column.

Diagnosis may first be made by the occurrence of pathologic fracture from a trivial injury. Pain is prominent and often severe, and is usually associated with systemic symptoms of malaise and fatigue. Most patients are anemic because of replacement of hematopoietic marrow. Classically, a monoclonal gammopathy demonstrated on serum protein electrophoresis is present. So-called light-chain disease may occur and be detected by urine electrophoresis. Very rarely, a hypogammaglobulinemia may be present with the so-called nonsecretory form of the disease.

Treatment is chemotherapy, with most protocols using melphalan and other antineoplastic agents. Steroids are used occasionally to relieve symptoms. Solitary lesions may be treated by radiation, and surgical intervention is indicted for impending or acute pathologic fractures. Long bones should be rodded before fracture whenever possible. Vertebral involvement with neurologic symptoms dictates decompression and stabilization, usually through an anterior approach. The overall prognosis is poor, with a mean survival of 32 months. Death is usually due to intercurrent infection, pancytopenia, and renal failure (88).

Osteogenic Sarcoma

This is the second most common primary malignant bone tumor, accounting for approximately 20% of all malignant tumors. Adolescents or young adults are most frequently affected. The long bones are more frequently involved, with approximately half the cases occurring about the knee. Clinically, patients present with a brief history of pain and swelling, or occasionally with a pathologic fracture. Depending on the type of tumor cells elaborated, osteoblastic, chondroblastic, or fibroblastic subtypes may be present.

Radiographically, the lesion appears as mixed lytic and blastic lesion with aggressive, indistinct margins, cortical destruction, and subperiosteal new bone formation (Fig. 100.44B). This has given rise to the typical "sunburst" appearance. An uncommon variant is the parosteal sarcoma that rises on the surface of the bone. This tumor has a better prognosis than conventional osteosarcomas, and has a well differentiated histologic appearance.

Careful preoperative staging and a multidisciplinary approach are essential to developing a treatment plan. A staging classification for malignant tumors is shown in Table 100.6. For high-grade osteosarcoma, amputation is the treatment of choice and has a 5-year survival rate of approximately 20%. Neoadjuvant chemotherapy is used and is especially important in limb salvage, where its preoperative administration reduces the tumor mass.

The goal of limb salvage surgery is to provide local control of the tumor comparable with amputation while maintaining reasonable functional status of the extremity. Reconstruction techniques after resection depend on the location of the tumor. They include allograft replacement, custom prosthesis, or arthrodesis. Current 5-year survival rates with a multidisciplinary approach range from 40% to 60%. Overall survival with limb salvage surgery is comparable with that of amputation in appropriately selected cases. Death results from metastatic disease, frequently involving the lungs. Selective pulmonary metastases may be treated by surgical resection (90).

Chondrosarcoma

Chondrosarcoma accounts for approximately 10% of malignant tumors and tends to occur in older people. Approximately 75% of the lesions are located in the pelvis or proximal portions of the humerus or femur. Frequently, they are slow growing, and variable symptoms may be present for months or years before treatment. Local recurrence is common, but metastases occur infrequently.

Chondrosarcomas have a characteristic radiographic appearance, presenting predominantly lytic lesions containing stippled calcification and usually cortical destruction.

High-grade lesions may require amputation; however, wide excision with or without prosthetic replacement may be indicated, especially when the proximal femur or humerus is involved. Internal hemipelvectomy and fusion may be indicated for pelvic lesions (90). The survival rate for low-grade lesions after 5 years approaches 50%. Highly malignant chondrosarcoma has a poor prognosis despite treatment, with a 5-year survival rate of less than 10% (89).

Malignant Fibrous Histiocytoma and Fibrosarcoma

These tumors account for less than 5% of primary osseous malignancies and affect both sexes equally. They occur over a wide age distribution, and have a skeletal distribution similar to that of osteosarcoma.

Clinical symptoms may be present for significant periods, including variable degrees of pain, swelling, and functional loss. Radiographically, the lesion appears as an osteolytic area of bone destruction with frequent soft-tissue extension, and cortical erosion. As with other malignant tumors, CT and MRI are essential to determine the extent of the tumor. Histologically, the tumors are characterized by spindle-shaped cells of fibrous origin arranged in a herringbone pattern. Considerable variation in the degree of anaplasia exists.

Table 100.6. STAGING FOR MALIGNANT TUMORS (ENNEKING)

Stage	Grade	Site	Metastasis
IA	Low	Intracompartmental	None
IB	Low	Extracompartmental	None
IIA	High	Intracompartmental	None
IIB	High	Extracompartmental	None
III	Any	Any	Present

Surgical treatment depends on the location and size of the tumor. Low-grade lesions are treated by minimal to limb-sparing surgery, whereas high-grade lesions require radical excision, or amputation. The overall 5-year survival rate is approximately 30% and is correlated to histologic grade of the tumor, with the well differentiated lesions having a distinctly better prognosis.

Ewing's Sarcoma

This lesion accounts for approximately 5% of primary bone tumors, and more than 90% of the patients are younger than 30 years of age. Histologically, this is a highly anaplastic, small round cell tumor, possibly of neuroectodermal origin. Any bone may be involved, but typically the metaphysis is involved with extension onto the shaft of the long bone.

Radiographically, a moth-eaten appearance due to combined lytic and blastic foci is seen. Periosteal new bone formation may form multiple layers, giving rise to the classic "onion skin" appearance. In the past, recommended treatment consisted of radiation and chemotherapy. Surgical resection is indicated, especially for involvement of expendable bones. One of the most lethal sarcomas, Ewing's tumor historically had a 5-year survival rate of less than 20%. However, with contemporary protocols using surgery, radiation, and chemotherapy, 5-year survival rates have improved to approximately 40% (91).

Malignant Lymphoma

Malignant lymphoma is an uncommon neoplasm of the reticuloendothelial system. It accounts for less than 5% of primary bone malignancies. Although any age group can be affected, it is more common in the fifth, sixth, and seventh decades. Histologically, the tumor consists of small cells containing a fine reticulum network. Multinucleated Reed-Sternberg cells may be present, especially with Hodgkin's' disease.

Radiographically, a lytic lesion with distinct margins and cortical destruction may be present, or occasionally a sclerotic appearance may be seen. Differentiation from metastatic carcinoma, osteomyelitis, or Ewing's sarcoma may be difficult.

Radiation therapy is the mainstay of treatment. Like other round cell tumors, bone lymphoma is radiosensitive. Surgical treatment is reserved for impending or frank pathologic fractures. The overall 5-year survival rate is approximately 50%, significantly better than with Ewing's sarcoma, despite histologic similarity.

Chordoma

Chordoma originates from primitive notochord remnants, accounts for approximately 1% to 4% of primary bone tumors, and often presents late. These tumors arise in the midline of the axial skeleton. Approximately half are located in the sacral coccygeal region of the pelvis and are notoriously difficult to visualize radiographically. Approximately 35% are at the base of the skull, and the remainder arise in the vertebrae. Peak incidence is in the fifth to sixth decades, with men affected twice as often as women. Evidence of osseous destruction may be seen on plain film; CT and MRI scans enhance visualization (89). Treatment is surgical resection and radiation therapy, with survival closely related to the location of the tumor and the ability to achieve a wide surgical margin. When that is possible, an approximately 85% ten-year survival rate is reported. The survival rate with sacral chordoma is approximately 40% at 10 years.

Adamantinoma

This rare tumor has a distinct tendency to occur in the tibial diaphysis, accounting for more than 90% of lesions. They occur most often in the second to fifth decades and present with pain and a palpable bony mass. On radiography, the lesion is usually seen in the mid-diaphysis of the tibia with a blistered, expanded, thin cortex. Treatment is by wide *en bloc* resection if possible, otherwise amputation (89). Pathologically, epithelial cells oriented in palisaded fashion are seen, with center islands of spindle cells.

BONE AND JOINT INFECTIONS IN ADULTS

Infections involving bone and joints have historically been among the most feared and difficult of clinical problems. Because of the rigid structure, vulnerable vascularity, and unique anatomy of bone, infection is often hard to treat and in some cases cannot be completely eradicated—hence the emphasis on strict aseptic surgical technique, avoidance of hematomas, and use of prophylactic antibiotics. The prevention of bone and joint infection is a far easier task than the treatment of established osteomyelitis and related complications.

Exogenous Osteomyelitis

Open fractures, especially when they involve the lower extremity, are the most common cause of infection and chronic osteomyelitis (7,8). Treatment of early postoperative orthopedic infection is prompt return to surgery, evacuation of hematomas, and irrigation and débridement of the wound, followed by appropriate antimicrobial therapy.

In the absence of drainage, subacute or chronic infection can be more difficult to diagnose. It is frequently associated with pain, delayed or absent fracture healing, loss of fixation, and abnormal laboratory values. Definitive diagnosis is established by aspiration or culture and sensitivity studies of surgical specimens.

Treatment requires irrigation and débridement and, at times, resection of significant portions of necrotic bone. The resultant segmental defects are dealt with as discussed earlier. Long-standing cases of chronic osteomyelitis may be associated with soft-tissue ulcerations, induration, and foul-smelling sinus drainage. Radiographs may show extensive destruction of bone or sclerotic appearance of dead bone. Sequestrum consisting of variably sized necrotic bone fragments may be present. With long-standing infection, nonunion, and painful, nonfunctional joints, amputation may be indicated (54,55).

Septic Arthritis and Hematogenous Osteomyelitis

In contrast to children, most adults who acquire bone and joint infection by hematogenous spread are likely to be malnourished, systemically ill, immunocompromised, or diabetic. The source of infecting bacteria may be lung, oral cavity, urinary tract, or frequently an unidentified endogenous source. IV drug abuse is a frequent source of cellulitis and often contiguous septic arthritis secondary to inoculation from unsterile needles. Many of these people are also malnourished, and positive for hepatitis and human immunodeficiency virus antigens. Infection can also occur at sites remote from the primary injection, especially the intervertebral disc spaces.

Diagnosis

Symptoms may be acute or chronic, resulting in delayed diagnosis. A history of recent bacterial infection, endemic exposure, or immunocompromise may be obtained. Disc space infection is associated with acute or chronic back pain, frequently located in the lumbar or thoracic spine. Physical findings are variable and can be compatible with acute trauma, remote injury, or degenerative processes. Systemic signs of infection may be absent, but the erythrocyte sedimentation rate is universally elevated. Radiographic changes are highly variable, ranging from normal to extensive joint or bone destruction. MRI is helpful in detecting soft-tissue edema, inflammation, or abscess formation. Blood cultures may be positive, especially with acute presentations. Definitive diagnosis is made by culture and sensitivity after aspiration or open biopsy of the involved bone or joint.

Treatment requires a minimum of 6 weeks of culture-specific antimicrobial therapy. Surgery consists of arthroscopic or open irrigation and débridement of septic joints, evacuation of abscesses, or resection of necrotic bone. Most bacterial infections that are diagnosed and treated promptly have a satisfactory prognosis; however, chronic infections have a poor prognosis because of extensive destruction of bone or joints (54). The adequacy of treatment is determined by a clinical response and a falling erythrocyte sedimentation rate.

Tuberculous Infection

Skeletal involvement in patients with tuberculosis is not uncommon, especially in underdeveloped parts of the world, and is usually, but not exclusively, associated with pulmonary tuberculosis. Involvement of the spine (Pott's disease) can produce vertebral destruction and paraplegia. The hip, knee, or other extremity locations may also be involved. Symptoms are often indolent and may have been present for months or years. History of endemic exposure is usually present (54).

Radiographically, tuberculosis produces rarefaction of bone, joint destruction, and bony erosion of the involved areas. Work-up includes sputum cultures, skin tests where appropriate, and open biopsy for histologic and culture and sensitivity studies. Surgical débridement needs to be complete but judicious because a surprising amount of healing and restoration of bony architecture can occur after prolonged antituberculous therapy (92).

Fungal Osteomyelitis

Fungal osteomyelitis is not common, but is characterized by delay in diagnosis and confusion with other causes of bone pain or radiographic changes, such as degenerative arthritis, remote trauma, or neoplasms. A high index of suspicion and the inclusion of infection in the differential diagnosis of obscure musculoskeletal complaints is most important.

Coccidioidomycosis

This fungal disease is endemic in the San Joaquin Valley of California, and is caused by the inhalation of spores of *Coccidioides immitis*, with resultant respiratory tract infection. The disease is more likely to be found in farmers, migrant workers, the elderly, or those with immunocompromise secondary to diabetes, corticosteroid administration, or AIDS. Skin tests or serologic tests are usually positive. Fungal organisms may be seen on microscopic analysis of infected granulomas and the fungus may be grown in culture. Treatment is surgical débridement and appropriate antifungal drugs, including ketoconazole, itraconazole, or amphotericin B (57).

Blastomycosis

The disease frequently begins as a respiratory infection and spreads hematogenously to the bones and synovial tissue. Clinically, the appearance is similar to other granulomatous diseases and the diagnosis is made as described earlier. Treatment is surgical débridement and antifungal therapy.

Sporotrichosis

Infection with this organism produces an indolent inflammatory process frequently involving the wrist, digits, or elbows. It may be confused with arthritis or bacterial infection. Inoculation is frequently from contaminated soil, benign-appearing puncture wounds, or thorn penetration. The organisms may be difficult to culture, but are grown on Sabouraud's agar and have a characteristic cigar-shaped histologic appearance. Treatment consists of surgical débridement and antifungal therapy.

Cryptococcosis

This infection may occur in immunocompromised patients and usually begins as a pulmonary infection that spreads to the central nervous system and then, through the bloodstream, to various sites in the axial skeleton, vertebrae, and pelvis. Diagnosis is made serologically and by the characteristic histologic appearance and growth on Sabouraud's culture medium.

Histoplasmosis

Histoplasmosis is quite common and frequently asymptomatic. Rarely, it may be a source of bone and joint infection, primarily in immunocompromised or immunosuppressed patients. Diagnosis is by direct microscopic examination and identification of characteristic organisms or by culturing the organism on Sabouraud's agar. Skin and serologic tests may also be helpful in establishing the diagnosis.

Brucellosis

This disease is uncommon in the United States, although it remains endemic in many parts of the world. Signs and symptoms of the disease are highly variable, with musculoskeletal complaints occurring frequently. The combination of an uncommon infection presenting with protean manifestations often results in missed or delayed diagnosis in the Western world. *Brucella* organisms are gram-negative coccobacilli, and infection is the result of direct contact with sick animals in approximately 80% of cases, or by ingestion of contaminated by-products. In the United States, the disease is primarily occupational, occurring in people involved in dairy farming, veterinary medicine, or meat processing. Musculoskeletal complaints are frequent, but radiographic changes are notoriously slow to appear, and may be confused with old trauma or degenerative arthritis. The most common site of skeletal involvement is the spine, especially the lumbar region. The sacroiliac joints may also be involved, as well as the long bones. It is difficult to grow the organism on culture medium, and special laboratory techniques are necessary for its isolation. Diagnosis is frequently made immunoserologically.

Treatment is usually nonoperative. In some cases, bone or joint destruction dictates débridement of necrotic material. The organism responds to rifampin or tetracycline administration, which is highly effective in most cases (93).

REFERENCES

1. Cook SD. Preclinical and clinical evaluations of osteogenic protein-1, BMP-7 in bony sites. *Orthopaedics* 1999;7:669–671.
2. Reddi AH, Shushan MA, Cunningham NS. Induction and maintenance of new bone formation by growth and differentiation. *Ann Chir Gynaecol* 1988;77:189.
3. Spector M. Tissue engineering: the next revolution in orthopaedic surgery? *Harvard Orthop J* 1999;1:103–105.
4. Kennedy JP, Blaisdell WF, eds. *Extremity trauma.* New York: Thieme, 1992.
5. Garrison FH. *History of medicine.* Philadelphia: WB Saunders, 1929.
6. Tile M. *Fractures of the pelvis and acetabulum,* 2nd ed. Baltimore: Williams & Wilkins, 1995.
7. Gustilo RB, Simpson L, Nixon RA, et al. Analysis of 511 open fractures. *Clin Orthop* 1969;66:148–154.
8. Patzakis MJ, Wilkins J, Moore TM. Use of antibiotics in open tibial fractures. *Clin Orthop* 1983;178:31.
9. Behrens F, Comfort TH, Searls K, et al. Treatment of severe open tibial fractures: prospective evaluation. *Orthop Trans* 1983;7:528.
10. Moehring HD, Gravel CA, Chapman MW, et al. Comparison of antibiotic beads and intravenous antibiotics in open fractures. *Clin Orthop* 2000;372:254–261.
11. Russell TS. Fractures of the tibial shaft. In: Moehring HD, Greenspan A, eds. *Fractures: current diagnosis and treatment.* Philadelphia: Current Medicine, 2000:165–171.
12. Moehring HD. Regional fractures of the knee. In: Larson RL, Grana WA, eds. *The knee: form, function, pathology, and treatment.* Philadelphia: WB Saunders, 1993;147–201.
13. Moehring HD. Acute dislocations of the shoulder girdle and elbow. In: Chapman MW, Madison M, eds. *Operative orthopaedics,* 2nd ed. Philadelphia: Lippincott–Raven, 1993.
14. Moehring HD. Hip dislocations femoral head fractures. In: Chapman MW, Madison M, eds. *Operative orthopaedics,* 2nd ed. Philadelphia: Lippincott–Raven, 1993.
15. Moehring HD, Tan RT, Marder RA, et al. Ankle dislocation. *J Orthop Trauma* 1994;8:167–172.
16. Moehring HD. Fractures of the tibia, fibula, ankle, and foot. In: Callahm BC, ed. *Current practices of emergency medicine.* Philadelphia: Decker, 1991.
17. Hansen S, Levine D. Foot fractures. In: Moehring HD, Greenspan A, eds. *Fractures: current diagnosis and treatment.* Philadelphia: Current Medicine, 2000:198–201.
18. Müller ME, Allgöwer M, Schneider R, et al. *Manual of internal fixation: techniques,* 3rd ed. Berlin: Springer-Verlag, 1991.
19. Browner BD, Jupiter JB, Levine AM, et al. *Skeletal trauma,* vol 1. Philadelphia: WB Saunders, 1992.
20. Matthews LS, Goldstein SA. In: Greenfield LJ, et al., eds. *Orthopaedic surgery: principles and practice.* Philadelphia: Lippincott–Raven, 1997.
21. McKibbin B. The biology of fracture healing in long bones. *J Bone Joint Surg Br* 1978;60:150–162.
22. Egol KA, Kellam JF. Diagnosis and management of pelvic ring fractures. In: Moehring HD, Greenspan A, eds. *Fractures: current diagnosis and treatment.* Philadelphia: Current Medicine, 2000:71–78.
23. Mears DC, Rubash H. *Pelvic and acetabular fractures.* Thorofare, NJ: Slack, 1986.
24. Letournel E. *Fractures of the acetabulum.* New York: Springer, 1981.
25. Moehring HD. Fractures of the acetabulum. In: Moehring HD, Greenspan A, eds. *Fractures: current diagnosis and treatment.* Philadelphia: Current Medicine, 2000:79–88.
26. Kuntscher G, ed. *Practice of intramedullary nailing.* Springfield, IL: Charles C Thomas, 1962.
27. Brumback RJ, Stibling Ellision P, Poka A, et al. Intramedullary nailing of open fractures of the femoral shaft. *J Bone Joint Surg Am* 1989;71:1324–1331.
28. Moed BR, Watson JT. Retrograde nailing of the femoral shaft. *J Am Acad Orthop Surg* 1999;7:209–215.
29. Dehne E, Metz CW, Deffer PA. Nonoperative treatment of the fractured tibia by immediate weight bearing. *J Trauma* 1961;1:514–535.
30. Moehring HD, Voightlander JR. Compartment pressure monitoring during intramedullary reaming of tibial fractures. *Orthopaedics* 1995;18:7:631–636.
31. Whitesides TE Jr, Haney TC, Hirada M, et al. Tissue pressure measurements as a determinant for the need of fasciotomy. *Clin Orthop* 1975;113:43.
32. Mubarak SJ, Hargens AR. *Compartment syndromes and Volkmann's contracture.* Philadelphia: WB Saunders, 1981.
33. Mubarak SJ, Owen CA. Double-incision fasciotomy of the leg for decompression in compartment syndromes. *J Bone Joint Surg Am* 1977;59:184–187.
34. Sarmiento A, Watson JT. Functional bracing of diaphyseal humeral fractures and operative management of humeral shaft fractures. In: Moehring HD, Greenspan A, eds. *Fractures: current diagnosis and treatment.* Philadelphia: Current Medicine, 2000:225–239.
35. Weiss LE, Osterman L. Fractures of the radius and ulna. In: Moehring HD, Greenspan A, eds. *Fractures: current diagnosis and treatment.* Philadelphia: Current Medicine, 2000:257–266.
36. Teague DC, Swiontkowski MF. Femoral neck fractures. In: Moehring HD, Greenspan A, eds. *Fractures: current diagnosis and treatment.* Philadelphia: Current Medicine, 2000:91–95.
37. Kyle RF, Ellis TJ. Intertrochanteric hip fractures. In: Moehring HD, Greenspan A, eds. *Fractures: current diagnosis and treatment.* Philadelphia: Current Medicine, 2000:95–105.
38. Lindsey R. Subtrochanteric fractures of the femur. In: Moehring HD, Greenspan A, eds. *Fractures: current diagnosis and treatment.* Philadelphia: Current Medicine, 2000:107–115.
39. Ebraheim NA, Pearlstein SR, Savolaine ER, et al. Scapulothoracic dissociation (closed avulsion of the scapula, subclavian artery, and brachial plexus): a newly recognized variant, a new classification and a review of the literature and treatment options. *J Orthop Trauma* 1987;1:18–23.
40. Goss TP. Fractures of the scapula. In: Moehring HD, Greenspan A, eds. *Fractures: current diagnosis and treatment.* Philadelphia: Current Medicine, 2000:209–215.
41. Torchia MD. Fractures of the humeral head and neck. In: Moehring HD, Greenspan A, eds. *Fractures: current diagnosis and treatment.* Philadelphia: Current Medicine, 2000:217–219.
42. Vrahas MS, Leddy MJ III. Supracondylar fractures of the humerus. In: Moehring HD, Greenspan A, eds. *Fractures: current diagnosis and treatment.* Philadelphia: Current Medicine, 2000:243–246.
43. Mason MB. Some observations on fractures of the head of the radius with a review of one hundred cases. *Br J Surg* 1954;42:123.
44. Colles A. On the fracture of the carpal extremity of the radius. *Edinb Med Surg J* 1814;10:181.
45. Whipple T, Padgett LR. Fractures of the distal radius. In: Moehring HD, Greenspan A, eds. *Fractures: current diagnosis and treatment.* Philadelphia: Current Medicine, 2000:269–272.
46. Slater RR. Fracture dislocations of the wrist. In: Moehring HD, Greenspan A, eds. *Fractures: current diagnosis and treatment.* Philadelphia: Current Medicine, 2000:281–286.
47. Mclain RF. Cervical spine fractures. In: Moehring HD, Greenspan A, eds. *Fractures: current diagnosis and treatment.* Philadelphia: Current Medicine, 2000:49–56.
48. Gupta MC, Benson DR. Thoracolumbar fractures and fracture-dislocations. In: Moehring HD, Greenspan A, eds. *Fractures: current diagnosis and treatment.* Philadelphia: Current Medicine, 2000:59–68.
49. Denis F. The three column spine and its significance in classification of acute thoracolumbar spinal injuries. *Spine* 1983;8:817–831.
50. Bailey RW, Badgley CE. Stabilization of the cervical spine by anterior fusion. *J Bone Joint Surg Am* 1960;42:565.
51. Robinson RA, Walker AE, Ferlic DC, et al. The results of an anterior interbody fusion of the cervical spine. *J Bone Joint Surg Am* 1962;44:1569.
52. McCullouch JA, McNab I, eds. *Sciatica and chymopapain.* Baltimore: Williams & Wilkins, 1983.
53. Greenwald AS, ed. *Concepts in joint replacement.* Thorofare, NJ: Orthopaedics, 1999.
54. Esterhai JL Jr, Gristina AG, Poss R, eds. *Musculoskeletal infection.* Park Ridge, IL: American Academy of Orthopaedic Surgeons, 1992.
55. Rockwood CA, Green DP, Bucholz RW, eds. *Fractures in adults,* 3rd ed. Philadelphia: JB Lippincott, 1991.

56. Morrey BF, ed. *Joint replacement arthroplasty.* New York: Churchill-Livingstone, 1991.

57. Catagni MA, Malzev V, Kirienko A. Advances in Ilizarov apparatus assembly, treatment of fractures, pseudoarthroses: lengthening and deformity correction. Milan: Medicalplastic srl, 1994.

58. Parisien JS, ed. *Current techniques in arthroscopy,* 2nd ed. Philadelphia: Current Medicine, 1996.

59. Larson RL. Acute ligamentous injury, chronic anterior instability. In: Larsen RL, Grana WA, eds. *The knee.* Philadelphia: WB Saunders, 1993:493–620.

60. Boyes JH. *Bunnell's surgery of the hand,* 4th ed. Philadelphia: JB Lippincott, 1964.

61. Bunnell S. Splinting the hand. *Instr Course Lect* 1952;9:233.

62. Grana WA. Chronic posterior and posterolateral laxity. In: Larsen RL, Grana WA, eds. *The knee.* Philadelphia: WB Saunders, 1993:621–679.

63. Lewis DS, Jebson PJL. Current management of selected problem fractures of the phalanges and metacarpals. In: Moehring HD, Greenspan A, eds. *Fractures: current diagnosis and treatment.* Philadelphia: Current Medicine, 2000:293–299.

64. Green DP. General principles in operative hand surgery. In: *Operative hand surgery.* New York: Churchill Livingstone, 1982:1–21.

65. Green DP, Rowland SA. In: Rockwood CA, Green DP, eds. *Fractures and dislocations of the hand.* Philadelphia: JB Lippincott, 1991.

66. American Academy of Orthopaedic Surgeons, ed. *Symposium on tendon surgery in the hand.* Philadelphia: American Academy of Orthopaedic Surgeons, 1974.

67. Green DP, Anderson JR. Closed reduction and percutaneous pin fixation of fractured phalanges. *J Bone Joint Surg Am* 1973;55:1651.

68. Verdan CE. Primary repair of flexor tendons. *J Bone Joint Surg Am* 1960;42:647.

69. Kleinert HE, Kutz JE, Ashbell TS, et al. Primary repair of lacerated flexor tendons in "no man's land." *J Bone Joint Surg Am* 1967;49:577.

70. Nunley JA, Goldner LJ. Tendon injury and repair. In: Sabiston DC, Lyerly HK, eds. *Textbook of surgery,* 15th ed. Philadelphia: WB Saunders, 1997:1470–1479.

71. Hunter JM, Salisbury RE. Flexor-tendon reconstruction in severely damaged hands. *J Bone Joint Surg (Am)* 1971;53:829.

72. Urbaniak JR. Replantation of amputated limbs and digits. In: Sabiston DC, Lyerly HK, eds. *Textbook of surgery,* 15th ed. Philadelphia: WB Saunders, 1997:1487–1491.

73. Urbaniak JR. Digital replantation: a 12-year experience. In: Urbaniak JR, ed. *Microsurgery for major limb reconstruction.* St. Louis: Mosby, 1987:12.

74. Dolenc VV. Contemporary treatment of peripheral nerve and brachial plexus lesions. *Neurosurg Rev* 1986;9:149.

75. Millesi H. Brachial plexus injuries. In: Chapman MW, Madison M, eds. *Operative orthopaedics,* 2nd ed. Philadelphia: Lippincott, 1993.

76. Sedel L. The results of surgical repair of brachial plexus lesions. *J Bone Joint Surg (Am)* 1982;64:54.

77. Szabo RM, Spiegel JD. Infections of the hand. In: Chapman MW, Madison M, eds. *Operative orthopaedics,* 2nd ed. Philadelphia: Lippincott, 1993.

78. Lubahn JD, Lister GD, Wolfe T. Fasciectomy and Dupuytren's disease: a comparison between the open-palm technique and wound closure. *J Hand Surg* 1984;9:53.

79. Open fasciotomy and full thickness skin graft in the Gonzalez correction of digital flexion deformity. In: Hueston JT, Tubiana R, eds. *Dupuytren's disease.* New York: Churchill Livingstone, 1985.

80. Tachdjian MO, ed. *Pediatric orthopaedics,* vol 1. Philadelphia: WB Saunders, 1972.

81. Rang M. *Children's fractures,* 2nd ed. Philadelphia: JB Lippincott, 1983:24.

82. Weber BG, Brunner C, Freuler F. *Treatment of fractures in children and adolescents.* New York: Springer, 1980.

83. Worlock PH, Colton CL. Severely displaced supracondylar fractures of the humerus in children. *J Pediatr Orthop* 1987;7:49–53.

84. Morrey BF, Peterson HA. Hematogenous pyogenic osteomyelitis in children. *Orthop Clin North Am* 1975;6:935.

85. Griffin PP. *Septic arthritis in children.* Orthopedic surgery update series. Princeton, NJ: CPEC, 1982.

86. Marmor L, Chan KB, Ho KC, et al. Surgical treatment of tuberculosis of the hip in children. *Clin Orthop* 1969;67:135.

87. Simon MA. Current concepts review: limb salvage for osteosarcoma. *J Bone Joint Surg Am* 1988;70:307.

88. Enneking WF. *Musculoskeletal tumor surgery.* New York: Churchill Livingstone, 1983.

89. Greenspan A, Remagen W. *Differential diagnosis of tumors and tumor-like lesions of bone and joints.* Philadelphia: Lippincott–Raven, 1998.

90. Dahlin DC, Coventry MD. Osteogenic sarcoma: a study of 600 cases. *J Bone Joint Surg (Am)* 1967;49:1010.

91. Bacci G, Toni A, Avella M, et al. Long-term results in 144 localized Ewing's sarcoma patients treated with combined therapy. *Cancer* 1989;63:1477.

92. Centers for Disease Control. Leads from the MMWR: tuberculosis United States, 1985. *JAMA* 1986;256:3335.

93. Moehring HD. *Brucella sacroiliitis. Orthopaedics* 1985;8:499–502.

SECTION Q

NERVOUS SYSTEM

SURGERY: SCIENTIFIC PRINCIPLES AND PRACTICE, Third Edition, edited by
Lazar J. Greenfield, Michael W. Mulholland, Keith T. Oldham, Gerald B. Zelenock,
and Keith D. Lillemoe. Lippincott Williams & Wilkins Publishers, Philadelphia, © 2001.

CHAPTER 101

NERVOUS SYSTEM

JULIAN T. HOFF AND MARK R. HARRIGAN

A detailed history and physical examination is the foundation of neurosurgical diagnosis. Headache, altered consciousness, memory impairment, speech difficulty, visual disturbance, weakness, paresthesia, and incoordination are symptoms suggestive of central nervous system (CNS) disease. The examination should include assessment of mental status, thorough cranial nerve testing, optic funduscopy, and motor, sensory, and reflex testing.

The history may reveal the etiology (e.g., traumatic, neoplastic, vascular, infectious, degenerative, or metabolic), whereas neurologic examination permits anatomic localization of the lesion. For patients with nervous system disorders, an accurate history need be taken only once, but the examination must be repeated and recorded often to gauge the course of the illness and to judge the urgency of other diagnostic steps necessary before treatment can be given.

DIAGNOSTIC STUDIES

Once a differential diagnosis is formulated with the information gathered from the history and examination, it is necessary to confirm the principal diagnosis by use of diagnostic aids. Studies helpful in the practice of neurosurgery include plain film radiography, myelography, angiography, computed tomography (CT), magnetic resonance imaging (MRI), ultrasonography, electromyography (EMG) and nerve conduction velocity testing, evoked potentials (visual, auditory, and somatosensory), positron emission tomography, and electroencephalography.

Plain films, especially of the spine, are useful in trauma and degenerative disorders. Myelography, both with and without CT, is useful for the evaluation of radiculopathies and, when MRI is not available, myelopathies due to trauma, tumor, and degenerative spine disease. CT and MRI provide detailed imaging of both cranial and spinal contents. They are useful in combination for visualization of bone and soft tissues, respectively. Magnetic resonance angiography is a noninvasive alternative to conventional angiography. Xenon-enhanced CT can provide important information about cerebral blood flow in patients with cerebrovascular disease, severe head injury, stroke, or cerebral vasospasm after subarachnoid hemorrhage. Angiography provides detailed information about aneurysms, vascular malformations, and atherosclerotic disease. It is an essential tool in the evaluation of cerebral hemorrhage and embolic and thrombotic stroke, and in preoperative planning for tumor surgery. Ultrasound is an important adjunct in the operating room, providing visualization of tumors, cysts, vascular malformations, and congenital anomalies lying beneath the exposed surface. Ultrasound is also extensively used in brain and spinal cord imaging in the newborn.

Electromyography and nerve conduction velocity testing are helpful in evaluating peripheral nerve and nerve root lesions. They are also used to monitor brachial plexus and peripheral nerve recovery after traumatic injury. Visual and auditory evoked potentials can be used in comatose patients to monitor the severity of head injury. Auditory potentials are useful in surgical excision of tumors of the eighth cranial nerve. Somatosensory evoked potentials continually monitor spinal cord (dorsal column) function during surgical manipulation of spinal fractures and tumors. Positron emission tomography scans play an important role in epilepsy surgery, in preembolization assessment of skull-based tumors involving the cavernous sinus and surgically untreatable vascular anomalies, and in brain tumor follow-up. Electroencephalography helps delineate structural and metabolic disorders and can be used during cerebrovascular surgery as a guard against irreversible ischemia. Transcranial Doppler sonography allows noninvasive evaluation of blood flow velocity in intracranial arteries, which is useful in monitoring patients with cerebral ischemia caused by vascular spasm.

TRAUMA

Trauma is the single most common cause of death in children, adolescents, and young adults. Most accidents involving motor vehicles and falls include injury to the brain and spinal cord and their surrounding structures.

Scalp Injury

Scalp injury can cause serious hemorrhage and subsequent shock if not promptly treated. Bleeding can usually be controlled with a simple pressure dressing, by firm finger pressure, or by hemostats applied to the galea, the aponeurosis of the scalp. Scalp wounds should be closed as soon as possible. Lacerations that overlie a depressed fracture or a penetrating wound of the skull require débridement in the operating room.

Simple scalp lacerations should be débrided of foreign matter, copiously irrigated, and closed primarily, taking care to approximate both the galea and skin. A good galeal closure provides excellent hemostasis. Scalp avulsions typically include all layers of the scalp, with sparing of the underlying periosteum. If the avulsion is small, closure can often be accomplished primarily. Replantation with the use of microsurgical technique is the preferred method of repair for large scalp avulsions, provided the avulsed scalp has been preserved and surgery is not delayed.

If the injured scalp is not viable but the periosteum is intact, split-thickness skin grafts can be used to close the defect. Care must be taken to keep the periosteum moist before surgery. When the periosteum is absent or desiccated, closure is more difficult because it is through the periosteal layer that the outer skull table receives its blood supply. In this instance, closure can be accomplished with vascular flaps of greater omentum or muscle. Other methods include perforation of the outer skull to expose the diploë, which can serve as a source of granulation tissue that can then be skin grafted.

Skull Fracture

Skull fractures are classified according to whether the skin overlying the fracture is intact (closed) or disrupted (open or compound), whether there is a single fracture line (linear), several fractures radiating from a central point (stellate), or fragmentation of bone (comminuted), and whether the edges of the fracture line have been driven below the level of the surrounding bone (depressed) or not (nondepressed).

Simple skull fractures (linear, stellate, or comminuted nondepressed) require no specific treatment. They are potentially serious, however, and can be fatal if they cross major vascular channels in the skull, such as the groove of the middle meningeal artery or the dural venous sinuses. If these structures are torn, epidural or subdural hematomas, or both, can form. A simple skull fracture that extends into the accessory nasal sinuses or the mastoid air cells is considered open because it communicates with an external body surface.

Depressed skull fractures often require surgery to elevate the depressed bone fragments (Fig. 101.1). If there are no adverse neurologic signs and the fracture is closed, repair can be done electively. During surgery, the dura should be inspected and repaired as described later.

Open skull fractures also require surgical intervention. Linear or stellate, nondepressed open fractures can be treated by simple closure of the scalp after thorough cleansing. Open fractures with severe comminution of underlying bone should be treated in the operating room when proper débridement can be carried out. The dura should be inspected to ensure that a laceration has not been overlooked. If found, dural tears should be closed either primarily or with a fascial patch graft to reduce the risk of infection. Depressed, open skull fractures should be débrided, elevated, and closed in the operating room after preparations have been made for craniotomy, in case broader exposure of underlying injured dura and brain is necessary.

Basal skull fractures involve the floor of the calvarium. Bruising can occur about the eye (raccoon sign) or behind the ear (Battle's sign), suggesting a fracture involving the anterior or middle fossa, respectively. Isolated cranial nerve deficits are associated with this fracture type. The facial nerve is frequently affected, with injury due to laceration (acute deficit) or swelling (delayed deficit). Almost all facial nerve deficits resolve spontaneously, especially with incomplete or delayed lesions. No specific therapy is warranted. On the other hand, complete lesions should be explored, although the timing of exploration remains a matter of debate.

Any associated cerebrospinal fluid (CSF) rhinorrhea or otorrhea should be treated expectantly. Traumatic CSF leaks typically stop within the first 7 to 10 days. Should a leak persist, lumbar CSF drainage can be implemented to seal the leak by lowering CSF volume and intracranial pressure (ICP). If this therapy fails, surgical exploration and oversewing of the defect with a fascial patch graft are indicated. Less than 5% of patients actually require surgical repair. Prophylactic antibiotics are no longer used because prospective studies have failed to demonstrate any significant benefit from their use.

Brain Injury

Injury to the brain is caused by the rapid deceleration, acceleration, and rotation associated with a blow to the

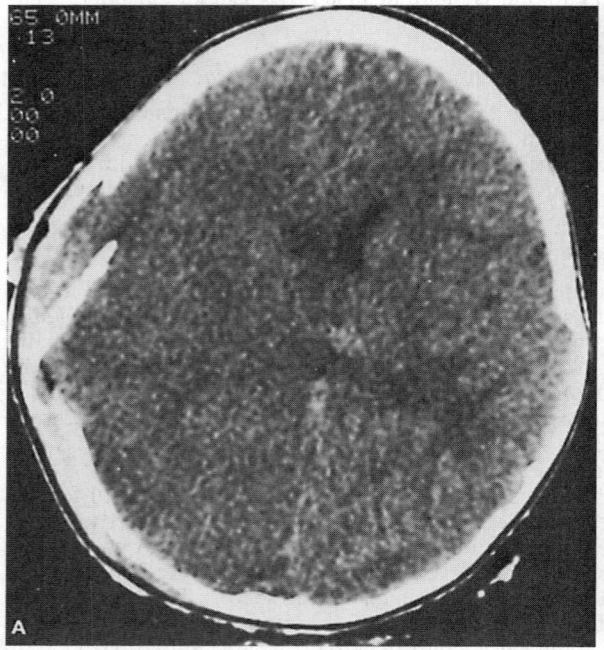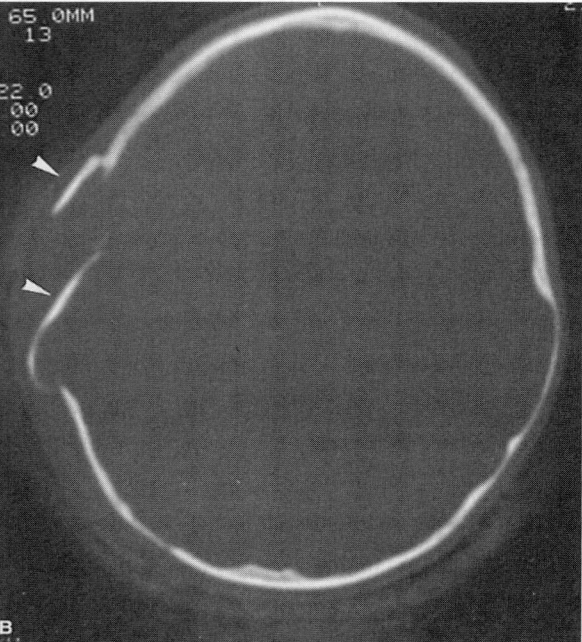

Figure 101.1. A compound, comminuted, depressed skull fracture imaged by noncontrast computed tomography with the use of soft-tissue *(A)* and bone windows *(B)*. Multiple fracture fragments are visible *(arrowheads)*. The overlying scalp was lacerated, and cerebrospinal fluid was leaking from the wound.

head. The initial impact can produce neuronal and axonal disruption, which constitutes the primary injury. Any subsequent complication, such as an intracranial hematoma, cerebral edema, hypoxia, hypotension, hydrocephalus, or endocrine disturbance, characterizes secondary injury and always compounds the initial insult.

Mild head injury is usually not associated with significant primary brain injury, and neurologic deficits are limited to temporary loss of consciousness (concussion). Moderate to severe head injury, on the other hand, is typically associated with deficits that may or may not be reversible. Moreover, this degree of injury is usually accompanied by secondary injury.

Distortional forces causing the primary injury can produce diffuse axonal injury or tear intraparenchymal capillaries, superficial subdural bridging veins, or epidural vessels, thus producing uncontained blood. Vasogenic cerebral edema occurs in response to vasodilation and disruption of the blood–brain barrier. Ischemia from hypotension or hypoxia can produce cell death and consequent cytotoxic edema. Disruption of CSF absorption pathways by uncontained subarachnoid blood can lead to hydrocephalus. Cerebral salt wasting, in which brain injury causes intravascular volume loss and hyponatremia, or diabetes insipidus can aggravate cerebral edema by fluid and electrolyte imbalance. Severe head injury can also lead to vasomotor dysregulation and an abnormal increase in cerebral blood flow, or hyperemia. These changes, either in part or in combination, result in an elevation of ICP.

Elevated ICP contributes to secondary brain injury by reducing cerebral perfusion pressure, which, by definition, is the difference between the mean arterial blood pressure and the cerebral venous pressure. For all clinically relevant purposes, the cerebral venous pressure is identical to ICP. Thus, when ICP increases and mean arterial blood pressure remains stable, cerebral perfusion pressure decreases. When the cerebral perfusion pressure falls below 70 mm Hg, cerebral blood flow is compromised, producing cerebral ischemia and compounding the primary brain injury with secondary insult.

In studies of head injury mortality, intracranial hypertension appears to be one of the most important factors affecting outcome. For this reason, aggressive management to circumvent cerebral blood flow reduction and secondary injury is imperative. Early resuscitative therapy should be initiated in the accident field with airway control and hyperventilation. In the absence of hypotension, osmotherapy can also be used.

Rapid clinical assessment is essential. Although extensive neurologic testing is limited in uncooperative or unresponsive patients, certain features of the examination are crucial. The Glasgow Coma Scale score, established in 1974, uses a numeric score to evaluate eye opening and verbal and motor behavior, both spontaneously and in response to stimulation (Table 101.1). This scale is useful for determining the patient's neurologic status and provides information regarding the ultimate outcome of the head-injured patient.

The initial neurologic examination determines whether diagnostic testing is indicated. Patients without headache, lethargy, or a focal neurologic deficit are not likely to experience a secondary complication from their injury, and imaging studies usually are not indicated. Conversely, symptomatic patients with or without a focal deficit should undergo a CT scan of the head, using windows for soft-tissue and bone detail. Should CT fail to disclose a lesion despite high clinical suspicion, carotid and cerebral angiography can help delineate a vascular abnormality that cannot be appreciated with CT.

Table 101.1. GLASGOW COMA SCALE[a]

Parameter	Score
EYE OPENING	
Spontaneously	4
To voice stimulus	3
To pain	2
No eye opening	1
MOTOR RESPONSE	
Follows commands	6
Localizes a pain stimulus	5
Withdraws from pain	4
Flexor posturing to pain	3
Extensor posturing to pain	2
No response to pain	1
VERBAL RESPONSE	
Oriented	5
Confused	4
Inappropriate words	3
Incomprehensible sounds	2
No sounds	1

[a]The Glasgow Coma Scale assigns a numeric value to the responses in each of three categories, with the score equal to the sum of the three responses.

After emergent surgical removal of any traumatic cerebral mass lesion, the goals of medical management are normalization of cerebral perfusion pressure and prevention of secondary injury to the already damaged brain. ICP monitoring may be indicated, especially in patients with marked depression or deterioration in neurologic function. In general, patients with a severe head injury (Glasgow Coma Scale ≤8) and evidence of a brain injury on CT (e.g., a mass lesion, contusions, or subarachnoid hemorrhage) have greater than a 50% chance of having elevated ICP and should receive a ventriculostomy or an ICP monitor. Factors with a significant negative effect on outcome in severe head injury are hypotension (systolic blood pressure <90 mm Hg) or hypoxia (Pao_2 <60 mm Hg). A patient with a severe head injury, a negative head CT, and a single observation of either hypotension or hypoxia has the same risk of elevated ICP (>50%) as a similar patient with a positive head CT, and should also receive ventriculostomy or ICP monitoring. Comatose patients who require emergent surgery (e.g., abdominal, thoracic, orthopedic) should also be monitored because frequent neurologic examination is not possible during general anesthesia. A ventriculostomy to measure ICP allows drainage of CSF, which significantly lowers the pressure in most instances. When the ventricular system is collapsed, intraparenchymal monitoring should be established.

Elevation of the head of bed with the cervical spine in a neutral position facilitates venous drainage. Sedation reduces posturing and reflexively combative activity, both of which worsen ICP. Moderate hyperventilation with $Paco_2$ levels between 30 and 35 mm Hg lowers cerebral blood volume and ICP without provoking cerebral ischemia. Prophylactic use of anticonvulsants prevents cerebral injury from seizures. Prevention of hypotension reduces the extension of ischemic injury, whereas aggressive treatment of hypertensive episodes reduces cerebral blood volume and further disruption of the blood–brain barrier. Avoidance of hyperthermia minimizes the brain's metabolic demands.

An additional measure for control of ICP is mannitol, 0.5 to 1 g/kg intravenously (IV). Mannitol is an osmotic diuretic that reduces cerebral blood volume and cerebral edema. A synergistic effect can be obtained by combining mannitol with furosemide, 0.1 mg/kg IV. Deep sedation with narcotics and the use of paralyzing agents such as pancuronium or atracurium can be helpful. Barbiturate coma can be effective for patients with refractory ICP elevation despite these measures. Corticosteroids have no proven benefit in the management of severe head injury.

The outcome in head injury depends on many factors. Age is the single most important predictive factor in head injury; elderly patients fare significantly worse than younger patients. Penetrating injuries, particularly gunshot wounds, have a poorer outcome compared with blunt trauma. The presence of an intracranial hemorrhage also indicates a less favorable outcome. Subdural hematoma has a poorer prognosis than epidural hematoma. Other important factors include delay in treatment, multiple trauma, and systemic insults such as acidosis, hypoxia, and hypotension. Predictors of poor prognosis also include evidence of brain stem dysfunction on initial examination and refractory intracranial hypertension.

Epidural Hematoma

Hemorrhage between the inner table of the skull and the dura mater most commonly arises from a tear of the middle meningeal artery or one of its branches (Fig. 101.2). Arterial bleeding strips the dura from the undersurface of the bone and produces still more bleeding because the small bridging veins from the dura to the skull are torn. The hematoma rapidly increases in size and compresses the cerebral cortex.

An epidural hematoma can also arise from torn venous channels in the bone at a point of fracture or from lacerated major dural venous sinuses. Because venous pressure is low, epidural venous hematomas usually form only when a depressed skull fracture has stripped the dura

from the bone and left a space in which the hematoma can develop.

Epidural hematoma classically follows a blow to the head that causes a brief period of unconsciousness. After the patient regains consciousness, there may be a lucid interval during which there are no abnormal neurologic symptoms or signs. As the hematoma enlarges, hemispheric compression occurs. With time, the medial portion of the temporal lobe is forced over the edge of the tentorium, causing compression of the oculomotor nerve and subsequent dilatation of the ipsilateral pupil. Similarly, compression of the ipsilateral cerebral peduncle causes contralateral hemiparesis, which can progress to decerebrate posturing. Coma, fixed and dilated pupils, and decerebration is the classic triad suggestive of transtentorial herniation.

Epidural hematomas are curable lesions, but the mortality rate remains high because the severity of injury often is not recognized early. A patient may be seen during the lucid interval and discharged. Later, the patient can become unconscious because of progressive brain compression by the expanding hematoma.

Because of the danger of misdiagnosis, any patient with a history of a blow to the head leading to a period of unconsciousness should have a CT scan. If an epidural hematoma is found, emergent craniotomy is indicated. If the CT is negative and the patient's examination is nonfocal, the patient can be discharged, although a reliable person should be instructed to awaken the patient frequently during the next 24 hours to be certain that he or she remains arousable. Any deterioration should prompt quick return for repeat evaluation.

Subdural Hematoma

When veins bridging from the cortex to the dura or venous sinuses are torn or when an intracerebral hematoma

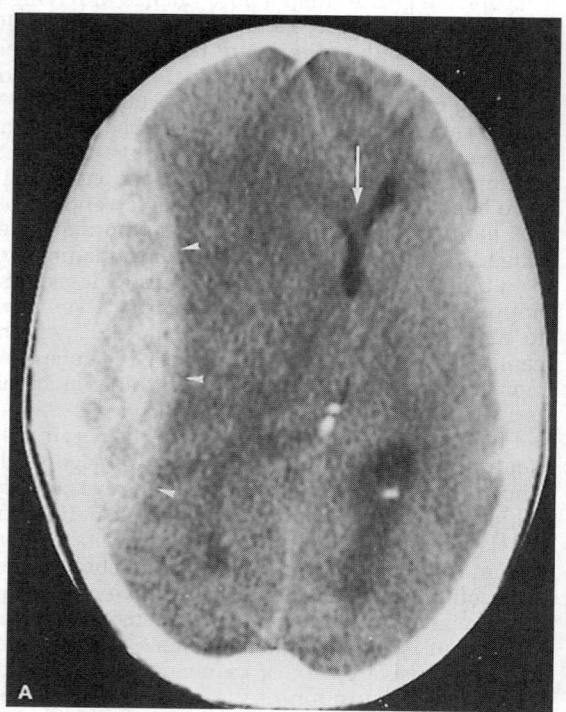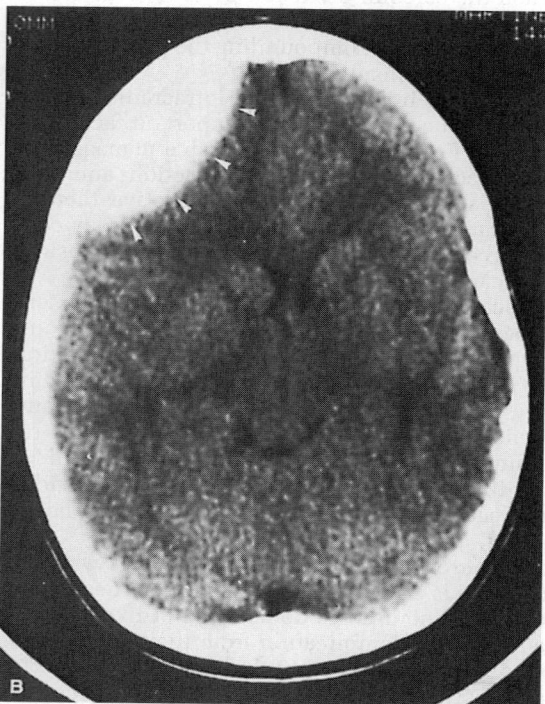

Figure 101.2. Two examples of acute epidural hematoma imaged by noncontrast computed tomography. The increased attenuation of the lenticular mass *(arrowheads)* indicates that it is an acute lesion in the epidural space. There is a marked midline shift in *A (arrow)* compared with *B.* The patient in *A* was comatose and had little brain stem function on examination. The patient in *B* was awake and conversant.

extends into the subdural space, subdural hematomas can develop. They can be large, even though the bleeding is of venous (low-pressure) origin.

Acute subdural hematomas are associated with severe head injury and arise from a combination of torn bridging veins, disruption of cortical arteries, and laceration of the cortex. The hematoma is best imaged with CT (Fig. 101.3). Evacuation of the clot can result in significant improvement, but often a major neurologic deficit remains because of the accompanying widespread neuronal and axonal injury.

Subacute subdural hematomas become apparent several days after injury and are associated with progressive lethargy, confusion, hemiparesis, or other hemispheric deficits. Removal of the hematoma usually produces striking improvement.

Chronic subdural hematomas arise from tears in bridging veins, often after a minor head injury. Initially, the hematoma is small. Later, it becomes encased in a fibrous membrane, liquefies, then gradually enlarges. These lesions are more common in infants and the elderly. Typical presentation includes progressive mental status changes, with or without focal signs such as hemiparesis or aphasia. Papilledema may be present. The diagnosis is confirmed by CT scanning. Treatment consists of bur hole drainage, and craniotomy may be necessary if the fluid reaccumulates.

Subdural hygromas are collections of clear or xanthochromic fluid in the subdural space. They develop when CSF escapes into the potential subdural space through a tear in the arachnoid, becomes trapped, and

cannot be absorbed. The resulting fluid mass can cause the same signs and symptoms as chronic subdural hematomas. Like their hematoma counterparts, hygromas are treated by bur hole drainage. Infants may require an internalized shunt to drain the hygroma into the peritoneal space to keep it from reaccumulating.

Spinal Cord Injury

Traumatic injury of the spinal cord can result from vertebral fracture or subluxation, hyperextension of the cervical spine in the presence of a narrow spinal canal, herniation of intervertebral disc material into the canal, and penetrating injuries such as gunshots or stabbings. Neurologic involvement ranges from mild and transient to severe and permanent. Spinal fracture and cord injury should be suspected in head-injured patients with or without coma and in those with multiple injuries. It is best to assume that the spine is unstable and to immobilize the patient on a backboard with a hard cervical collar until proper examination and diagnostic testing rule out injury.

Clinical findings can include spinal tenderness, extremity weakness, numbness or paresthesia, respiratory compromise, and hypotension. Spinal root involvement produces a radiculopathy characterized by motor and sensory impairment in the corresponding myotome and dermatome. Spinal cord involvement produces a myelopathy of variable manifestations.

Complete lesions, signifying total loss of function below the level of injury, are often referred to as *transections* of the cord. Acute transections are characterized by areflexia, flaccidity, anesthesia, and autonomic paralysis below the level of the lesion. Arterial hypotension is invariably present when the transection is above T-5 because of the loss of sympathetic vascular tone.

Incomplete lesions can result in the Brown-Séquard syndrome, which is manifested by ipsilateral loss of motor function and position–vibratory sensation with contralateral loss of pain and temperature sensation below the level of injury. Anatomically, this presentation is explained by hemisection of the cord (Fig. 101.4A). The central cord syndrome is characterized by bilateral loss of motor function and pain and temperature sensation in the upper extremities, with relative preservation of these functions in the lower extremities. Typically, the distal upper extremities are more severely affected because the most medial portions of the corticospinal and spinothalamic tracts subserve these areas (Fig. 101.4B). This deficit can be seen after a hyperextension injury of the cervical spine, with or without fracture. The anterior spinal artery syndrome involves the bilateral loss of motor function and pain and temperature sensation below the level of the lesion, with sparing of position–vibratory and light touch sensation. This incomplete lesion develops when the anterior spinal artery is occluded. This renders the cord ischemic within the anterior spinal artery distribution, affecting the anterior and lateral columns bilaterally (Fig. 101.4C). One common cause is an acutely ruptured cervical disc (Fig. 101.5).

Trauma to the lumbar spine can produce signs and symptoms of cauda equina compression. Presentation consists of multiple lumbosacral radiculopathies of variable severity. Lower extremity motor, sensory, and reflex functions can be affected, producing variable degrees of weakness, sensory loss (all modalities in the specific distribution of the roots involved), and diminution or absence of reflexes. Bladder distention from detrusor muscle paralysis, flaccidity of the anal sphincter, and loss of perineal sensation are common in severe injuries.

In addition to the neurologic deficit, acute spinal cord injury is accompanied by many systemic responses. If the

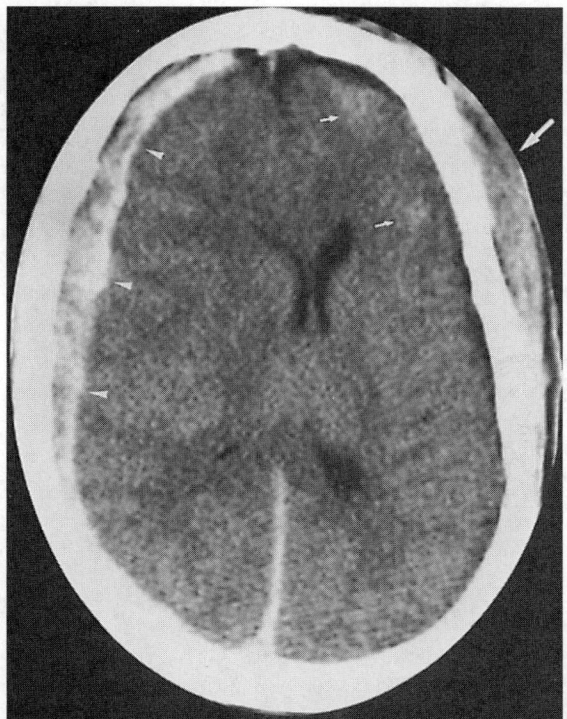

Figure 101.3. Acute subdural hematoma imaged by noncontrast computed tomography. The high-attenuation, crescent-shaped lesion *(arrowheads)* indicates acute hemorrhage in the subdural space. Scalp swelling is visible on the contralateral side *(large arrow)*, suggesting that the hematoma is due to a contrecoup injury. There are small hemorrhagic contusions in the contralateral frontal lobe as well *(small arrows)*. These often accompany subdural hematomas in head trauma and signify severe injury. Midline shift is apparent.

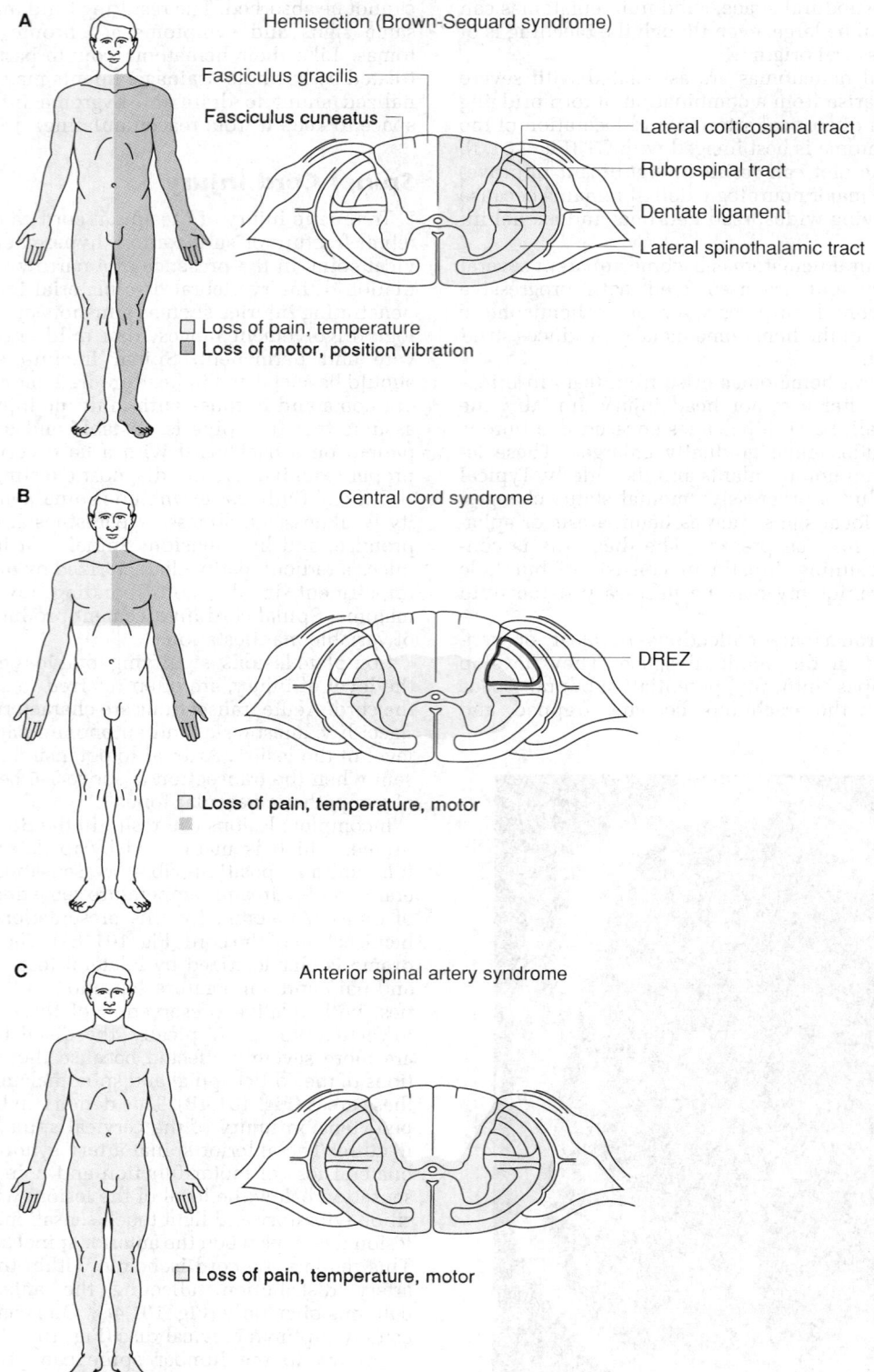

A Hemisection (Brown-Sequard syndrome)

Fasciculus gracilis

Fasciculus cuneatus

Lateral corticospinal tract

Rubrospinal tract

Dentate ligament

Lateral spinothalamic tract

☐ Loss of pain, temperature
▨ Loss of motor, position vibration

B Central cord syndrome

DREZ

☐ Loss of pain, temperature, motor

C Anterior spinal artery syndrome

☐ Loss of pain, temperature, motor

Figure 101.4. Schematic cross-sections of the spinal cord, showing hemisection *(A),* central cord syndrome lesion *(B),* and anterior spinal artery syndrome lesion *(C).* The figure diagrams demonstrate the neurologic deficits. DREZ, dorsal route entry zone.

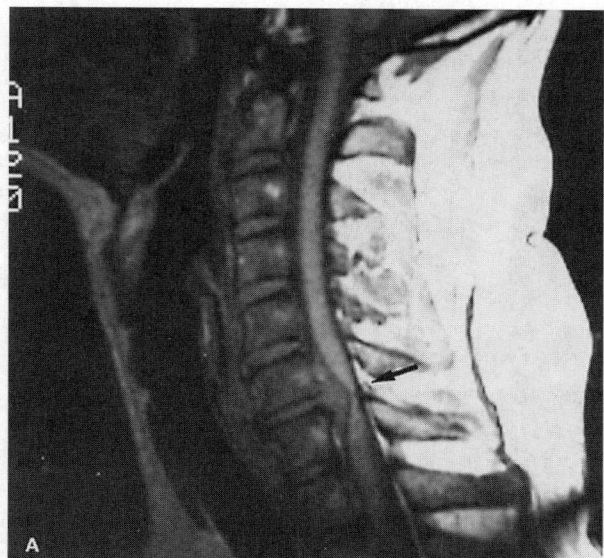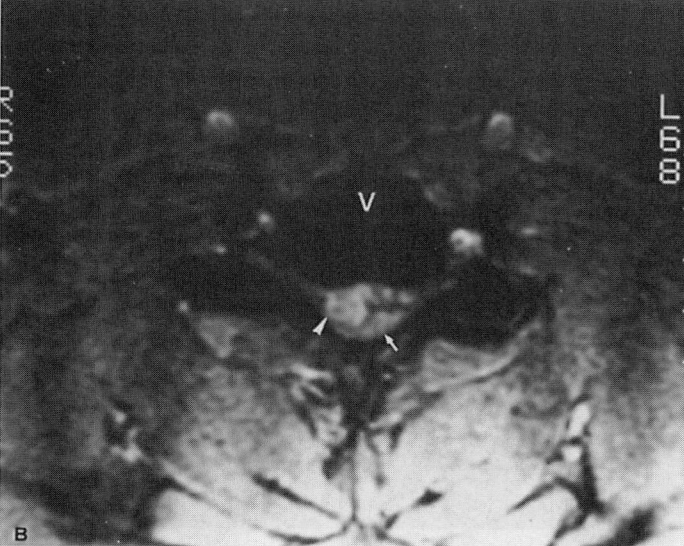

Figure 101.5. This patient experienced severe neck pain and quadriparesis when he stood from a squatting position. *(A)* Sagittal cervical spine magnetic resonance imaging (MRI) scan reveals an acute herniated disc with marked cord compression *(arrow)*. *(B)* Axial MRI scan shows the compressed cord *(arrow)* at the level of the herniation *(arrowhead)*. V, vertebral body.

spinal cord is damaged above C-3, respiratory efforts cease, accounting for this injury's high mortality rate at the scene of the accident. Although spontaneous ventilatory efforts can be initiated with injuries involving C-4 to C-6, tidal volumes are often insufficient, accounting for progressive hypoxia and carbon dioxide retention. Airway obstruction, atelectasis, and pneumonia are common complications. Assisted ventilation may be indicated, especially early after injury.

Ileus with gastric distention is common, necessitating nasogastric drainage. Similarly, bladder distention occurs because the bladder and pelvic floor muscles are flaccid. Bladder drainage prevents overdistention, which can be severe enough to cause compression of the inferior vena cava and pelvic veins, impairing venous return to the heart and contributing to systemic hypotension.

Blood pressure is usually low if the cord injury is above the T-5 level. This effectively denervates the sympathetic nervous system, which leads to increased venous capacitance and decreased venous return. The resulting hypotension is controlled by the administration of IV fluids. Colloid is preferred to reduce the threat of vascular overload and iatrogenic pulmonary edema. Postural changes that will drop the blood pressure precipitously should be avoided.

Tachycardia is a common compensatory response to hypotension, but bradycardia is the rule when the cervical cord is damaged and the sympathetic input to the heart is lost. This bradycardia does not require treatment unless the patient is symptomatic or at risk for myocardial infarction or stroke because of age or other debilitating illness. If necessary, treatment with atropine and fluids is effective.

Once the patient is hemodynamically stable, spine radiographs are essential, but only while the patient remains immobilized on a backboard with a hard cervical collar firmly secured. Standard views are obtained, ensuring good visualization of the cervicothoracic junction (Fig. 101.6A) Comatose and severely injured patients with multiple trauma should have good plain film imaging of the complete spine. Fractured areas are further studied with

CT, using both axial and sagittal views (Fig. 101.6B,C). If no abnormality is found despite a neurologic deficit that localizes to the spinal cord, MRI or myelography followed by CT must be used to look for traumatic intervertebral disc rupture, spinal epidural hematoma, ligamentous spine injuries, or spinal cord contusions (Fig. 101.5).

The goals of treatment are to correct spinal alignment, to protect undamaged neural tissue, to restore function to reversibly damaged neural tissue, and ultimately to achieve permanent spinal stability. Reduction and immobilization of any fracture or dislocation must receive top priority to meet these objectives. Solumedrol, given as a 30 mg/kg IV loading dose followed by a continuous drip at 5.4 mg/kg/hour IV for 48 hours, has been shown to improve outcome in spinal cord injury.

Cervical spine malalignment can almost always be reduced by skeletal traction. Traction can be applied with skull tongs or halo apparatus. Both are seated percutaneously through the outer table of the skull while the patient is kept supine and immobilized. The patient is then transferred to a special bed and placed in cervical traction, usually in the neutral position. Frequent lateral-view radiographs are obtained to ensure good reduction and to prevent overdistraction, which can lead to further cord injury. Once the spinal injury is reduced, traction should be maintained. Frequent follow-up films should be taken to confirm correct alignment. Sometimes a cervical fracture cannot be reduced by traction alone without jeopardizing spinal cord function. Open reduction, usually through a posterior approach, combined with a fusion procedure may be necessary in those instances. This especially pertains to unilaterally or bilaterally locked facets.

Patients with thoracic and lumbar spine fractures are also treated with immobilization initially. Immobilization is less strict than it is with cervical fractures, but the principles remain the same. Patients are kept flat in bed without traction, and flexion, extension, lateral bending, and rotational movements are avoided. Typically, fewer systemic complications are associated with these neurologic injuries, but vigilance is required to prevent neurologic deterioration and to provide the best chance for neurologic recovery.

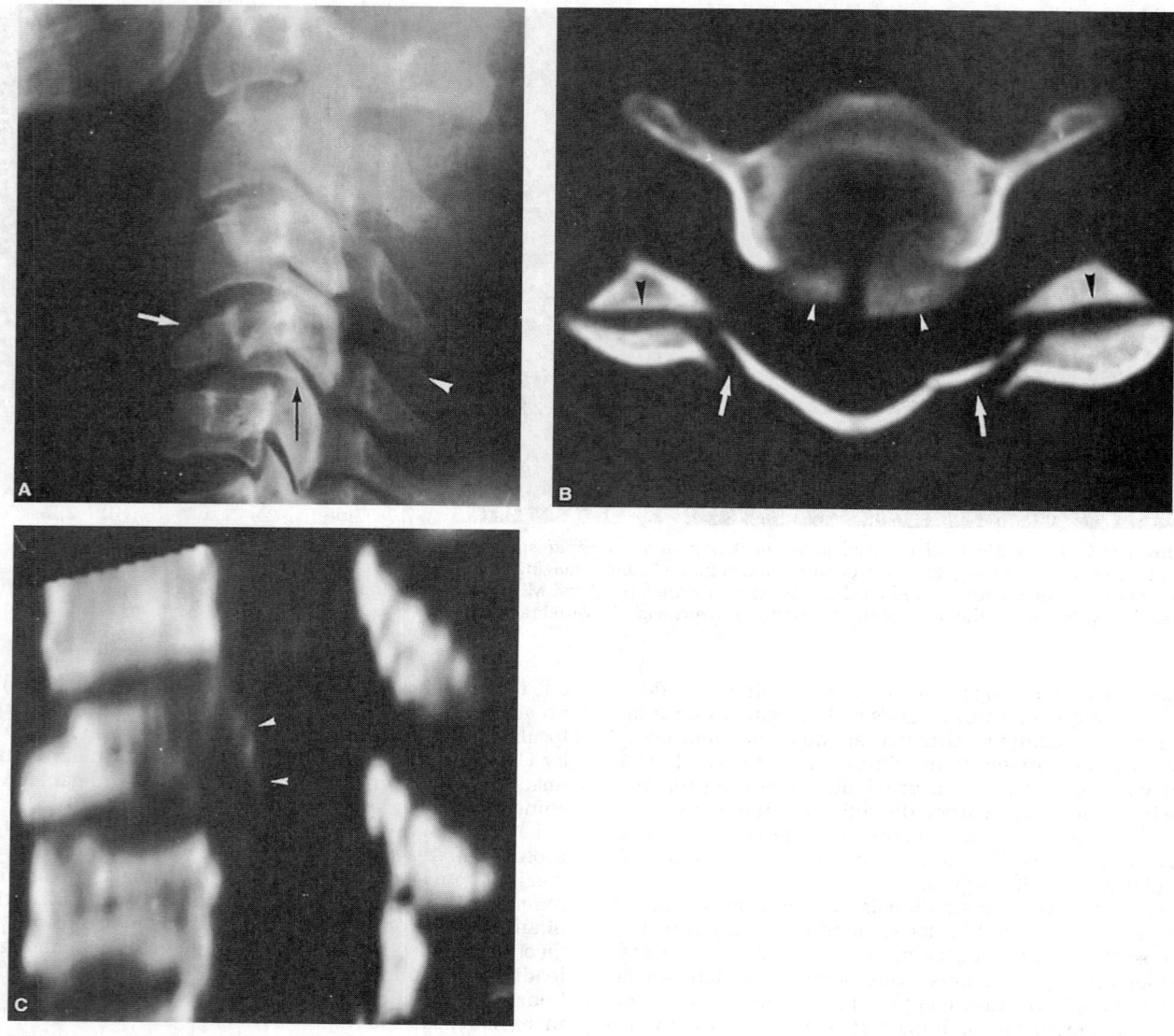

Figure 101.6. *(A)* Lateral cervical spine radiograph showing a C-5 fracture in a patient who was an unrestrained passenger in a motor vehicle accident. C-5 vertebral body compression *(white arrow)*, retropulsion of a fracture fragment into the spinal canal *(black arrow)*, and posterior interspinous widening *(arrowhead)* are visible. These findings are consistent with a hyperflexion injury. *(B)* Axial computed tomography (CT) scan through the C-5 level reveals fractures of the vertebral body *(white arrowheads* indicate the retropulsed fragments) and the laminae *(arrows)* as well as disruption of both facet joints *(black arrowheads)*. *(C)* Sagittal CT scan offers another view of the compromised spinal canal by the retropulsed fragments *(arrowheads)*.

Indications for early operation on patients with spinal cord injury include the inability to reduce the fracture or dislocation satisfactorily by closed methods, neurologic deterioration in a patient with an initially incomplete cord lesion, severe compression of the spinal cord by an intraspinal mass shown by myelography or MRI, and a penetrating injury with or without a CSF leak. Open wounds, such as stab and gunshot wounds, should be débrided and closed whether the cord injury is complete or incomplete. Early operation to stabilize the spine is warranted because this translates into early mobilization and rehabilitation. Either the anterior or posterior approach can be used, depending on the nature of the spine injury and the degree of instability.

If closed reduction is successful and the fracture is stable, external immobilization is necessary for a minimum of 3 months to ensure proper healing. If surgical reduction and fixation are necessary, external immobilization is still indicated. For the cervical spine, this involves a halo vest. Exceptions include anterior and posterior metal plating procedures, for which a hard cervical collar may suffice. The thoracic and lumbar spines usually require a plastic body jacket or plaster cast for a minimum of 3 months. Plain films are used to monitor spinal alignment and extent of fusion after immobilization during the recovery period.

If any cord function is preserved immediately after injury, additional function usually returns if the cord and spine are protected from secondary injury. Sometimes the patient with an incomplete cord injury can walk again if early care is protective and rehabilitation is aggressive and well planned. Patients with complete injuries rarely recover function below the level of the lesion. Rehabilitation for them is directed toward self-care and vocational readjustment. Most people with these handicaps can eventually achieve independence. Life expectancy is shortened slightly in paraplegic and significantly in quadriplegic patients. Long-term problems associated with skin care and recurrent urinary tract infections account for the early mortality.

Peripheral Nerve Injury

Peripheral nerve injuries can be categorized functionally. Neurapraxia is a temporary loss of function without axonal injury, and structural damage does not occur. The foot that "goes to sleep" after crossing the legs is an example of functional loss without abnormal change. Axonotmesis is a disruption of the axon with preservation of the axon sheath. Wallerian degeneration of the distal axon fragment occurs. Stretch or prolonged compression causes this functional and structural loss. Regeneration of the proximal axon occurs, but functional recovery depends on associated injuries, the amount of healthy proximal axon remaining after injury, and the age of the patient. Neurotmesis is disruption of both the axon and axon sheath with corresponding loss of function and is caused by transection of a nerve. Regeneration occurs, but function rarely returns to normal.

Clinically, sensory and motor changes correspond to the peripheral nerve involved. A detailed history and a precise neurologic examination can localize the site of injury with accuracy. Sensory findings are usually accurate early and remain so until regeneration is nearly complete. Compensatory motor function, often seen in the hand months after injury, is rarely seen acutely. A crude but clinically helpful sign of sensory regeneration is Tinel's sign, in which percussion of the skin overlying the length of the injured nerve elicits paresthesias at the site where regeneration is occurring.

Radiographs of the injury site help find fractures or foreign bodies. EMG is not useful within the first 3 weeks of injury but is highly effective for monitoring the status of the degeneration and regeneration process that occurs later. Management decisions are often made based on EMG findings weeks to months after trauma.

Treatment of a lacerated nerve consists of primary repair when the wound is clean and uncomplicated, as in stab wounds, lacerations from glass, and surgical incisions. Secondary or delayed repair is indicated when the wound is dirty or complicated. Such wounds include gunshots and avulsions that disrupt tissue severely, making primary repair less successful. Secondary repair is best accomplished a few weeks after injury, when tissue viability is obvious, the likelihood of infection is reduced, and dissection planes are distinct. If end-to-end anastomosis is not possible because of tissue loss, nerve grafting with autologous sural nerve can be done. Intraoperative factors such as axial orientation of fascicles, proper coaptation, suture material, hemostasis, and suture line tension determine the outcome.

Nerve injuries in continuity (i.e., resulting from contusion or compression without laceration) are often explored if they do not improve within 6 weeks of injury, whether loss of function is complete or incomplete. Intraneural and extraneural scar tissue at the site of the lesion can prevent axonal regrowth by its constricting effect. Neurolysis releases the regenerating nerve fibers from the impinging scar and can improve functional recovery.

Prompt institution of physical therapy is also indicated for improvement of muscle function and maintenance of joint motion. It is the best means of minimizing the complications of denervation. The denervated portion of the limb is subject to muscle atrophy and fibrosis, joint stiff-

ness, motor end plate atrophy, and trophic skin changes. The longer the denervation persists, the less likely it is that good function will result.

Regeneration in a peripheral nerve occurs at 1 mm/d (roughly 1 inch each month), so improvement may not be obvious for many months. Factors that adversely affect the return of function include advanced age of the patient, proximal nerve injury, extensive nerve tissue loss, associated soft-tissue injury, and mixed sensorimotor function. Unfortunately, incomplete neurologic recovery is often the rule. The use of tendon transfers should be considered to improve functional outcome if neurologic function is inadequate after recovery has ceased. Patients must understand that their role in treatment is an active one, and their motivation to recover must be encouraged.

NEOPLASMS

Nervous system tumors represent almost 10% of all neoplasms. Of these, 15% to 20% occur in children. Nearly 70% of adult tumors are found above the tentorium (supratentorial), whereas 70% of childhood tumors are found below (infratentorial). CNS tumors are the most common solid tumors in children. Of pediatric cancers, they are second only to leukemia in prevalence.

The incidence of nervous system neoplasia decreases in late adolescence and begins to peak again by middle age. By then, only 25% of intracranial tumors are benign. This percentage rises to 50% in the older patient because of the increasing incidence of meningiomas and schwannomas. Overall, there is a slightly greater prevalence of tumors in men (55%), but schwannomas and meningiomas are more common in women. Of all CNS neoplasms, spinal tumors constitute approximately 15%.

Intracranial Tumors

Intracranial tumors exert both local and generalized effects by their presence in a closed bony structure, either arising from within or on the surface of a noncompliant brain. A tumor's local influence consists of either irritative or destructive effects. Focal seizures occur because of irritation of adjacent cortex, whereas a focal neurologic deficit develops because of compressive forces on nearby functional brain. More generalized effects consist of raised ICP due to the presence of the abnormal mass. This may be in the form of obstructive hydrocephalus, tumor hemorrhage, or cerebral edema, or it may simply be the result of the added volume imparted by the tumor in the closed bony compartment of the skull. The effects can be manifested as headache, occasional nausea and vomiting, decreased level of consciousness, and slowed cognitive function. Table 101.2 lists the World Health Organization's classification of intracranial tumors. The more common tumors are discussed in the following sections.

Astrocytoma

Astrocytes are glial (stromal or supporting) cells of the brain. Tumors arising from these cells make up over 60% of all intracranial tumors. Low-grade astrocytomas (grades I and II) constitute 10% to 20% of all brain tumors in adults and 8% to 25% in children. When they involve the cerebral hemispheres, they typically arise during the fourth decade. They present with a 1- to 2-year history, producing signs and symptoms that include headaches, seizures, vomiting, mental status changes, papilledema, and focal neurologic deficits relevant to the hemisphere involved. On CT, they appear as low-attenuation lesions with minimal to mild contrast enhancement. These tumors are infiltrative and rarely can be totally excised.

Table 101.2. WORLD HEALTH ORGANIZATION BRAIN TUMOR CLASSIFICATION (ABRIDGED)

TUMORS OF NEUROEPITHELIAL TISSUE

Astrocytic tumor
  Astrocytoma
  Pilocytic astrocytoma
  Subependymal giant cell astrocytoma
  Astroblastoma
Oligodendroglial tumor
  Oligodendroglioma
  Mixed oligoastrocytoma
Ependymal and choroid plexus tumor
  Ependymoma
    Myxopapillary ependymoma
    Subependymoma
  Choroid plexus papilloma
Pineal cell tumor
  Pineocytoma
  Pineoblastoma
Neuronal tumor
  Gangliocytoma
  Ganglioglioma
  Ganglioneuroblastoma
  Neuroblastoma
Poorly differentiated and embryonic tumor
  Glioblastoma
  Medulloblastoma
  Gliomatosis cerebri

NERVE SHEATH TUMORS

Neurilemmoma
Neurofibroma

TUMORS OF MENINGEAL AND RELATED TISSUES

Meningioma
Meningeal sarcoma
Xanthomatous tumor

PRIMARY LYMPHOMA AND BLOOD VESSEL TUMORS

Hemangioblastoma

GERM CELL TUMORS

Germinoma
Embryonal cell carcinoma
Teratoma

OTHER TUMORS AND TUMOR-LIKE LESIONS

Craniopharyngioma
Rathke cleft cyst
Epidermoid
Dermoid
Colloid cyst
Lipoma
Choristoma
Vascular malformations
  Capillary telangiectasia
  Cavernous hemangioma
  Arteriovenous malformation
  Venous malformation

TUMORS OF THE ANTERIOR PITUITARY

Pituitary adenoma
Pituitary adenocarcinoma

LOCAL EXTENSION FROM REGIONAL TUMORS

Glomus jugulare tumor
Chordoma
Chondroma
Chondrosarcoma
Adenoid cystic carcinoma

METASTATIC TUMORS

UNCLASSIFIED TUMORS

Surgery is usually performed for diagnosis and debulking and is usually followed by radiation therapy. The 5-year survival rate with surgery and subsequent radiation is greater than 65%. Some low-grade astrocytomas can become anaplastic and, as such, become high-grade gliomas (see later).

Low-grade astrocytomas of the cerebellum typically occur in the pediatric population as a subtype of astrocytoma known as the *pilocytic astrocytoma.* They are often cystic with hamartomatous features, characteristics that carry a favorable prognosis. These tumors are often totally resectable. Radiation therapy is reserved for incomplete resections when follow-up has demonstrated continued tumor growth. The 10-year survival rate is over 80%.

Brain stem gliomas are also posterior fossa tumors that occur most often in childhood. Most are benign astrocytomas. Patients may present with cranial nerve palsies, hemiparesis, and headache, often attributable to hydrocephalus. These tumors cannot be removed surgically because of significant risk of neurologic injury to the brain stem. They are treated with radiation therapy once a diagnosis is established through either open or stereotactic biopsy. Unfortunately, prognosis is a function of their location, and 5-year survival rates are 17% to 50%.

Optic nerve gliomas are astrocytomas involving the optic pathways anterior to the optic tracts. They occur in the chiasm in 75% of cases. Two thirds of chiasmal tumors also invade the hypothalamus. The peak age of occurrence is 3 to 7 years, but their growth pattern is variable. Some remain stable for years, but others are relentlessly progressive. Those occurring strictly within one optic nerve can be excised, but the more extensive tumors are usually irradiated. The value of radiation therapy remains controversial.

High-grade astrocytomas (grades III and IV) are the most common primary intracranial tumor, constituting 35% to 45% of all adult brain tumors and 50% of all gliomas. Age at discovery ranges from 45 to 65 years. The frontal and temporal regions are most commonly involved. Because of their infiltrative nature, many of these high-grade neoplasms involve both cerebral hemispheres by invading across the corpus callosum and are called *butterfly gliomas.* Histologically, these malignant lesions are composed of sheets of anaplastic cells with bizarre nuclei, numerous mitoses, endothelial proliferation, and abundant necrosis. Patients present with a short history of headache, focal neurologic deficit, mental status changes, or seizures (typically weeks in duration). The tumors are readily seen on CT scan as low-attenuation lesions with marked peritumoral edema and mass effect (Fig. 101.7). Ninety-six percent show enhancement with IV contrast. Despite aggressive surgery, radiation, and chemotherapy, which can extend survival and improve quality of life, these tumors are nearly uniformly fatal. Although younger patients tend to do better, the average survival with surgery plus adjuvant therapy is approximately 12 months.

Chemotherapy is often used when tumor recurs, when the brain can no longer be irradiated, or when the tumor is not radiosensitive. It can be delivered intravenously, intraarterially, and intrathecally. Most drugs are directed at the tumor cells, whereas others indirectly attack the cells by sensitizing them to subsequent radiation. Although still in the early stages of development, immunotoxins toward tumor cells use antibodies to tumor antigens, thus using the host immune system as a means of destroying the cancerous tissue.

Meningioma

Most meningiomas are benign tumors that arise from the arachnoid layer of the meninges. The incidence of menin-

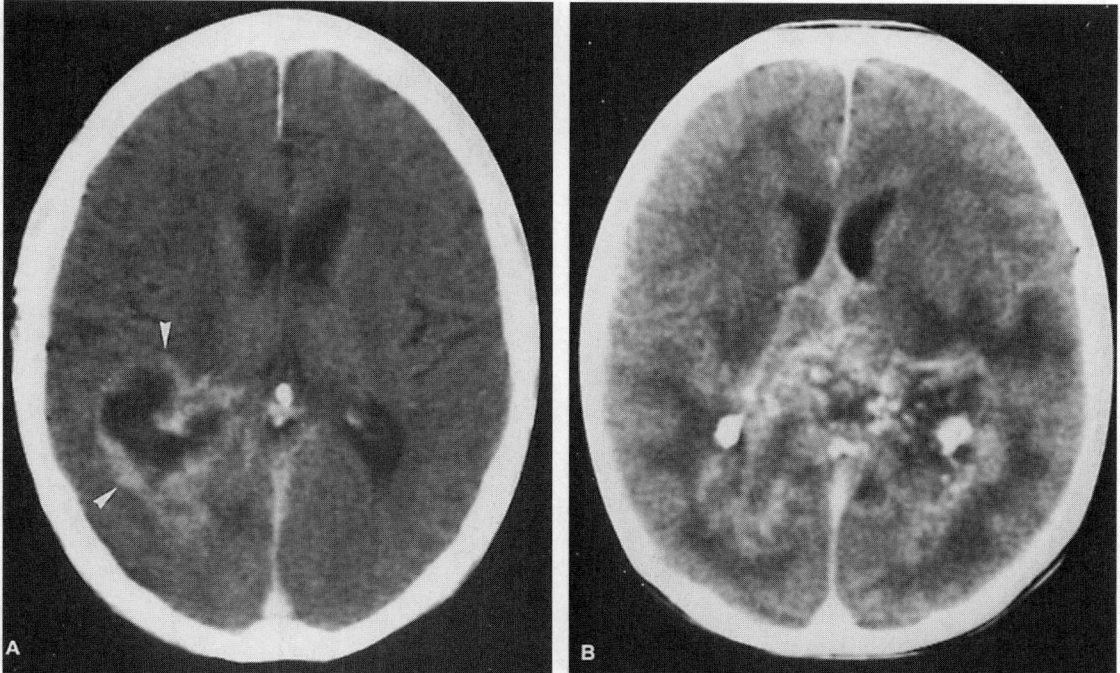

Figure 101.7. Glioblastoma multiforme (astrocytoma grade IV) discovered on contrast-enhanced computed tomography. *(A)* Typical appearance is that of a low-attenuation lesion with peripheral enhancement *(arrowheads)*. *(B)* A more complex lesion demonstrating invasion across the corpus callosum.

giomas increases through life, reaching its peak at age 85 years. The male-to-female ratio for symptomatic meningiomas is 1 to 2.3. The locations of these tumors and their relative frequencies are as follows: convexity 35%, parasagittal (falcine) 22%, sphenoid ridge 17%, lateral ventricle 5%, cerebellar convexity 5%, tentorium 4%, tuberculum sellae 4%, olfactory groove 3%, optic nerve sheath 2%, and cerebellopontine angle 2%. One percent or less occur in the foramen magnum or clivus. Together, symptomatic meningiomas constitute approximately 20% of all intracranial tumors.

Parasagittal (falcine) and convexity (hemispheric surface) meningiomas tend to present with seizures, focal neurologic deficits, and signs of intracranial hypertension. Sphenoid ridge tumors, classified as medial, middle, or lateral, can present with proptosis, decreased visual acuity, cranial nerve (III, IV, V, VI) palsies, seizures, or the more generalized effects of increased ICP. Posterior fossa tumors present with cerebellar signs, hydrocephalus, lower cranial nerve palsies, or long tract signs. Tuberculum sellae tumors are often accompanied by decreasing vision. Olfactory groove meningiomas can present with the classic Foster Kennedy syndrome of ipsilateral optic nerve atrophy and central scotoma with contralateral papilledema and bilateral loss of smell. Foramen magnum tumors can be difficult to recognize and are often misdiagnosed—as multiple sclerosis, syringomyelia, or cervical spondylosis. Patients complain of neck pain, clumsiness, sensory disturbances in the upper extremities, and gait difficulties.

Either CT or MRI is the principal means of diagnosis (Fig. 101.8). Homogeneous pathologic contrast enhancement is characteristic of these neoplasms. Calcification and hyperostosis are apparent on CT, and MRI often demonstrates a characteristic "dural tail," or region of thickened, enhancing dura representing invasion of the tumor in the surrounding dura. Meningiomas are highly vascularized, and angiography classically shows a blush in the late arterial phase.

The treatment for meningiomas is surgical. The techniques and goals are individualized for each tumor location, taking into account the patient's age and symptoms. In general, the goal is total excision, including the dura at the site of the tumor's attachment. If the meningeal origin cannot be excised, it is usually cauterized generously. Some meningiomas, such as those along the sphenoid ridge, may be en plaque tumors (i.e., flat and tending to spread along the inner table of the skull). This feature often precludes total resection.

The recurrence rate of meningiomas after surgery depends primarily on the degree of excision and the presence of malignant histologic features. If the tumor is totally removed, including its dural attachment, the recurrence rate for nonmalignant meningiomas is less than 10%. With subtotal resection, the recurrence rate is approximately 60%. Malignant meningiomas have a 73% recurrence rate with gross total resection. Radiation therapy (RT) is usually reserved for malignant meningiomas, although it can be used for incompletely removed benign meningiomas. After subtotal resection, radiation therapy decreases the recurrence rate from 60% with surgery alone to 32%.

Medulloblastoma

Medulloblastomas are part of the primitive neuroectodermal classification of brain tumors. They are thought to arise from primitive cells of the cerebellum, most likely the external granular layer. They constitute 3% to 8% of all intracranial tumors and 30% to 40% of all childhood posterior fossa tumors. Two thirds of medulloblastomas occur in children, with a peak incidence in the first decade of life. In children, these tumors are more likely to occur in the midline, usually within the fourth ventricle, whereas adult tumors are frequently positioned more lat-

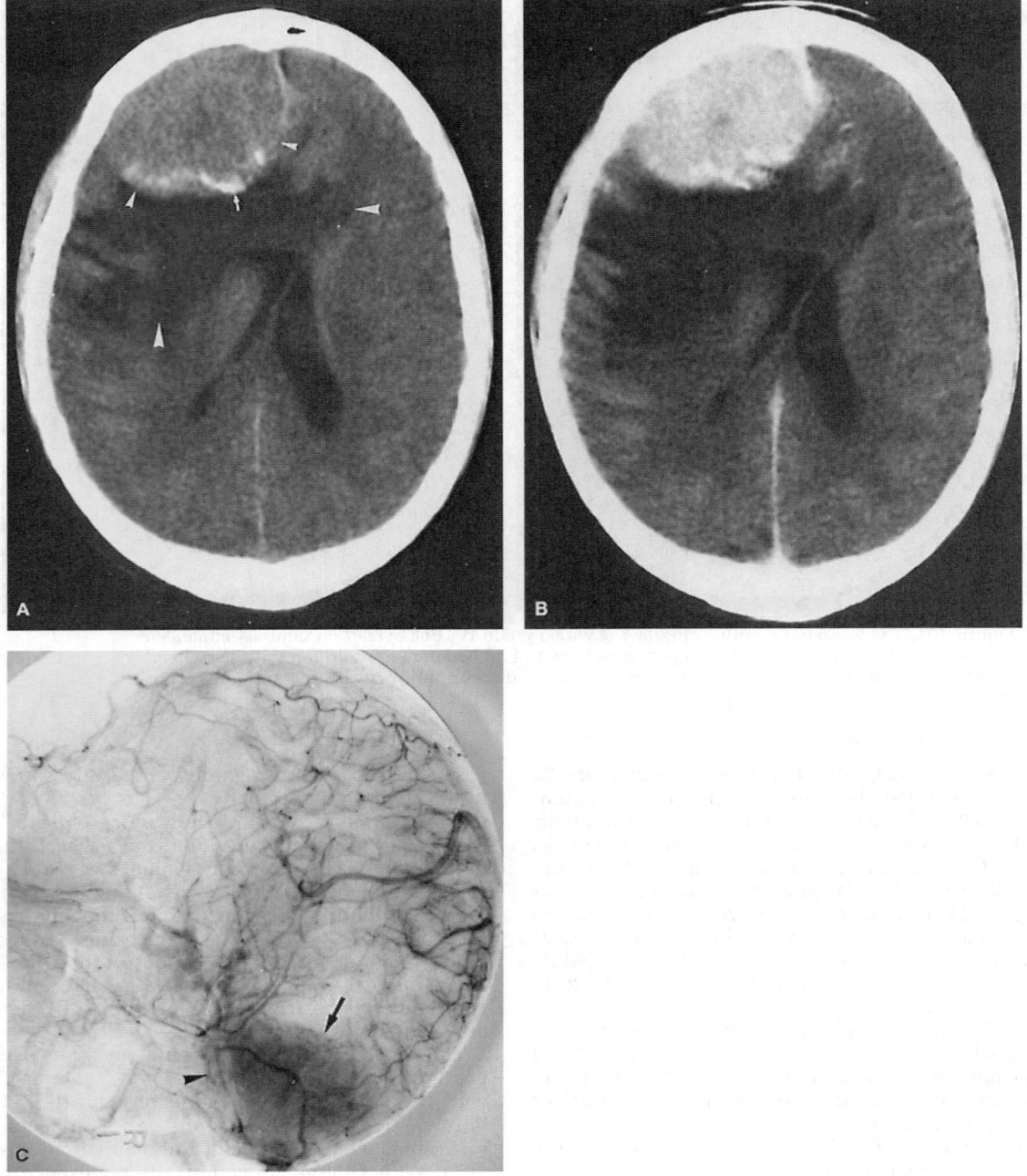

Figure 101.8. Large frontal meningioma in a patient who presented with personality changes and a generalized seizure, imaged by computed tomography. *(A)* In the noncontrast study, edema is seen in the adjacent area *(large arrowheads)* that develops in response to the lesion *(small arrowheads)* and the accompanying mass effect. Some large meningiomas may have peripheral calcification *(arrow)*. *(B)* With contrast, the lesion enhances homogeneously. *(C)* The angiogram demonstrates the classic late arterial phase blush *(arrow)*. The *arrowhead* marks the floor of the anterior fossa (orbital roof).

erally. They commonly metastasize throughout the subarachnoid space by way of the CSF and are rarely found outside the CNS.

Children with medulloblastomas commonly present with elevated ICP secondary to hydrocephalus. Cerebellar signs may be prominent, with truncal ataxia and nystagmus. Some can present initially with symptoms related to spinal metastases. The diagnosis usually is made by seeing an enhancing mass on CT, although MRI provides the best images of this common posterior fossa tumor. Cytologic examination of the CSF is often positive for neoplastic cells.

Treatment involves aggressive surgical removal of the tumor, followed by radiation of the brain. If CSF cytology is positive or if staging spinal myelography or MRI is positive, the spinal axis is included in the radiated field. Chemotherapy is commonly used as well. The 5-year survival rate varies from 30% to 70% and depends on the extent of tumor resection and the efficacy of radiation therapy.

Schwannoma

Schwannomas are benign tumors and arise from the Schwann cells that surround axons as they leave the CNS by way of cranial nerves. Schwannomas constitute 8% of all intracranial tumors and are more common in women. They occur usually in the middle decades of life. If associated with von Recklinghausen's disease, they can be multiple.

Schwannomas usually occur on sensory cranial nerves. The vestibular portion of the acoustic nerve is by far the most common site (acoustic neuroma). Depending on their size, these tumors usually produce hearing loss. As they enlarge, they can create facial numbness by compression of the trigeminal nerve and loss of coordination by compression of the adjacent cerebellar hemisphere. Only very late in their course do they cause facial weakness. Symptoms of increased ICP due to obstructive hydrocephalus can also present late.

Much less commonly, schwannomas arise from the trigeminal nerve, presenting as a mass in the middle fossa that is associated with facial numbness. Some patients complain of lancinating, burning, and episodic pain similar to trigeminal neuralgia. Only rarely do other cranial nerves serve as the primary site of origin for schwannomas. These less common sites are more apt to be involved in cases of neurofibromatosis. Schwannomas occurring in patients with neurofibromatosis are often associated with other intracranial tumors such as meningiomas, astrocytomas, and ependymomas.

The treatment of schwannomas is surgical, and total resection is curative. Microsurgical techniques have reduced the risks of surgery and have allowed preservation of cranial nerve function. Acoustic neuromas can be resected by means of the suboccipital or translabyrinthine approach, with a 92% probability of preservation of facial nerve function with tumors less than 2 cm in size. The translabyrinthine approach is reserved for those patients who have complete hearing loss because of the presence of the mass. If this loss is incomplete, the suboccipital approach is preferred, allowing for maximal hearing preservation by leaving the middle and inner ear structures intact. Once again, preservation is directly related to tumor size. Hearing preservation is usually attempted in patients with good preoperative hearing and tumors less than 1.5 cm in size; preservation of hearing is unlikely in tumors greater than 1.5 cm. The mortality rate is a function of tumor size as well, with most deaths occurring in patients with tumors greater than 4 cm in size.

Pituitary Adenoma

Tumors arising from the pituitary gland are usually benign histologically and constitute 10% of intracranial tumors (see Chapter 57). Focused beam radiation therapy (stereotactic radiosurgery) is an alternative method of treatment.

Ependymoma

Ependymomas originate in the ependyma, the glial cells that line the ventricular system, and constitute 2% to 6% of all intracranial tumors. The mean age at diagnosis is 5 years. They arise below the tentorium, usually in the fourth ventricle, in two thirds of cases. When they occur above the tentorium, 50% are intraventricular. Infratentorial ependymomas are far more common in children. They make up approximately one fourth of all fourth ventricular region tumors.

The presenting symptoms are related to the tumor location. Typically, children harboring fourth ventricular tumors present with headache and vomiting related to the associated obstructive hydrocephalus. They also tend to have ataxia secondary to cerebellar compression. Patients with supratentorial tumors present with signs of raised ICP as well, but this is usually because of brain edema. Focal neurologic deficits are common. These tumors are usually well circumscribed on CT scans as enhancing masses. MRI is the study of choice when the tumor involves the posterior fossa because MRI far surpasses the imaging capabilities of CT in this region (Fig. 101.9).

Treatment involves aggressive surgical excision. Unfortunately, fourth ventricular tumors can rarely be totally removed because of invasion of the fourth ventricular floor. They are radiosensitive, so this modality clearly prolongs survival. The average 5-year survival rate with surgery and irradiation for both children and adults is in the range of 50%, with children faring less well overall.

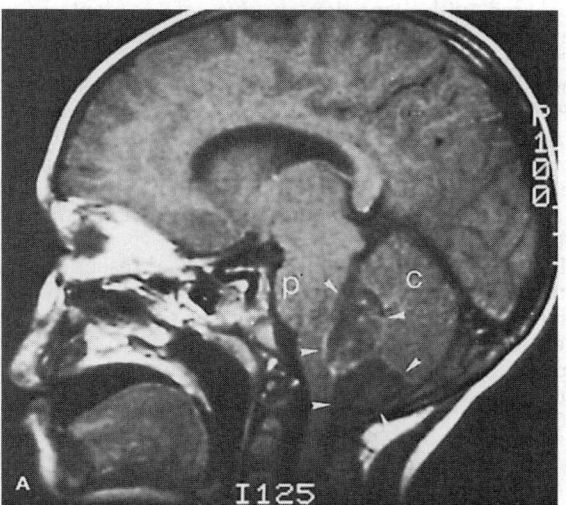

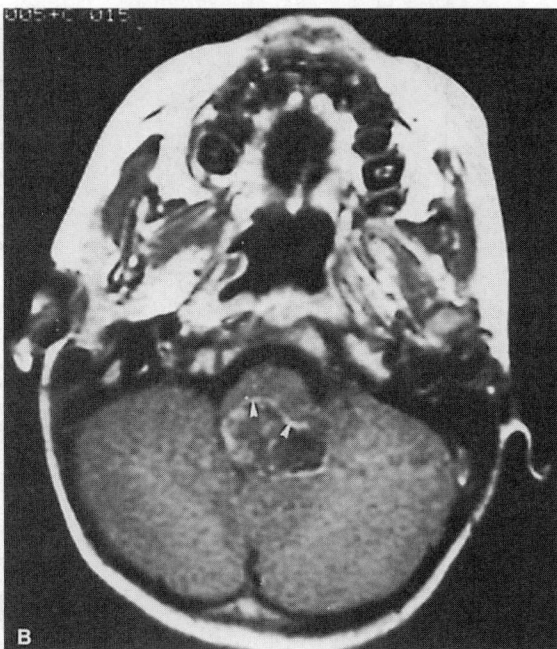

Figure 101.9. Fourth ventricular ependymoma imaged by gadolinium-enhanced magnetic resonance imaging. *(A)* The sagittal view demonstrates the tumor *(arrowheads)* completely occupying and expanding the fourth ventricle. Note its relation to the brain stem and cerebellum (c). p, pons. *(B)* The axial view reveals marked brain stem compression *(arrowheads).*

Chemotherapy is reserved for the higher-grade neoplasms. All ependymomas have a propensity to recur despite aggressive management.

Oligodendroglioma

Tumors arising from the oligodendroglial cells (the supporting cells that are the source of myelin in the CNS) make up 3% of intracranial tumors and usually occur in the cerebral hemispheres. Half of all hemispheric lesions occur in the frontal lobes. Up to one third are mixed tumors containing populations of astrocytes or ependymal cells in addition to oligodendrocytes. Pathologically, oligodendrogliomas can be classified as either benign or anaplastic. The presence of mitoses, nuclear polymorphism, and vascular endothelial proliferation is characteristic of anaplastic oligodendrogliomas. Patients with benign tumors have a median survival of 84 months compared with a median survival of 35 months for patients with anaplastic oligodendrogliomas.

Patients present with a history measured in years; the most frequent initial symptom is seizures, occurring in 50% to 75% of patients. Patients commonly have findings of focal neurologic deficits and papilledema. These tumors are unique in their tendency to calcify, attesting to their benign nature. On CT scan, a high percentage show calcification, and most have contrast enhancement (Fig. 101.10).

Treatment involves maximum surgical resection. Radiation therapy is reserved for those tumors displaying malignant histologic features or in cases of subtotal excision. The average 5-year survival rate ranges from 20% to 75%, depending on tumor grade. There are well documented long-term survivors, with a reported 20-year survival rate of 6%.

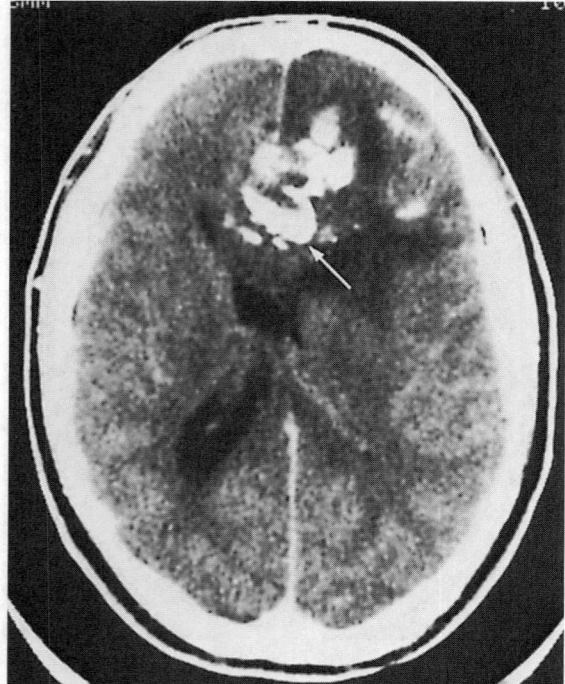

Figure 101.10. Computed tomography scan without contrast of oligodendroglioma shows the extensive calcification *(arrow)* that is typical of this lesion. Bilateral frontal lobe involvement is apparent, with tumor extending across the midline.

Craniopharyngioma

Histologically benign, craniopharyngiomas arise from nests of squamous cells in the pituitary gland. They can be found in intrasellar or suprasellar locations but are always along the craniopharyngeal canal. They are common supratentorial tumors in children and constitute 3% of all intracranial tumors. More than half occur in the first two decades of life. They are largely cystic in children, containing a much larger solid component in adults. The cysts are filled with a thick fluid (sometimes described as motor oil-like) that contains cholesterol crystals. Microscopically, they are cystic epithelial tumors with both squamous and columnar elements. Tumor calcification is common and is of considerable radiologic diagnostic importance.

Patients usually present with visual difficulties, hypopituitarism, and elevated ICP. Visual problems include papilledema, visual field loss, and decreased acuity. The endocrinopathy includes diabetes insipidus, obesity, short stature, hypothyroidism, and impaired sexual development. Elevated ICP is usually secondary to hydrocephalus.

These tumors are usually well imaged with high-resolution CT and MRI (Fig. 101.11). Treatment is usually surgical, often in combination with radiation therapy. Total surgical extirpation is possible more often in children. Recurrences are common after subtotal removals. Irradiation can be given externally or by stereotactic placement of radioactive substances in the cystic portion. Although craniopharyngiomas can be cured with surgical removal or controlled with radiation, many of these histologically benign tumors cannot be removed safely.

Pineal Region Tumors

Tumors in the pineal region are generally divided into either germ cell tumors (germinomas, choriocarcinomas, embryonal carcinomas, endodermal sinus tumors, and teratomas) or pinealomas (pineocytomas and pineoblastomas). Pineal region tumors tend to produce obstructive hydrocephalus and Parinaud's syndrome, a midbrain disorder characterized by upward gaze paresis, loss of convergence, and small, unreactive pupils.

Germinomas most commonly occur in the pineal region; the suprasellar region involving the hypothalamus is the second most common location. Those in the hypothalamic region may be associated with diabetes insipidus and emaciation (diencephalic syndrome). Germinomas are composed of two cell populations (tumor cells and lymphocytes) and are histologically indistinguishable from testicular seminomas and ovarian dysgerminomas. These tumors are radiosensitive and do not require aggressive surgical resection, but biopsy is recommended before irradiation. The 5-year survival rate approaches 80% after radiation therapy.

Other related germ cell tumors include teratomas, embryonal cell tumors, endodermal sinus tumors, and choriocarcinomas. These tend to arise in the same locations as germinomas. The germ cell tumors often produce compounds that serve as tumor markers. These markers are frequently identified with immunoassays of the CSF or with immunoperoxidase stains of the tissue under light microscopy. All choriocarcinomas and 10% of germinomas secrete β-human chorionic gonadotropin. Endodermal sinus tumors produce α-fetoprotein. Embryonal cell tumors typically synthesize both of these markers, whereas teratomas secrete neither. These markers are useful for confirming the diagnosis and for measuring response to treatment.

Pinealomas arise from the pineal parenchyma. Pineocytomas are better differentiated and more benign than pineoblastomas, which are malignant. The average age of pa-

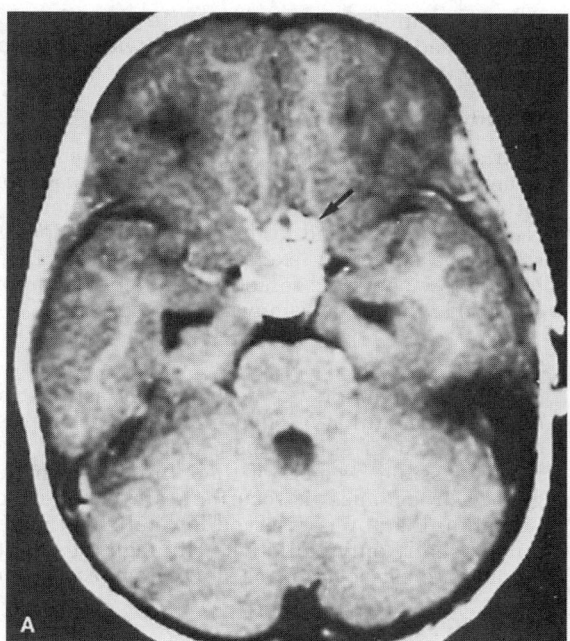
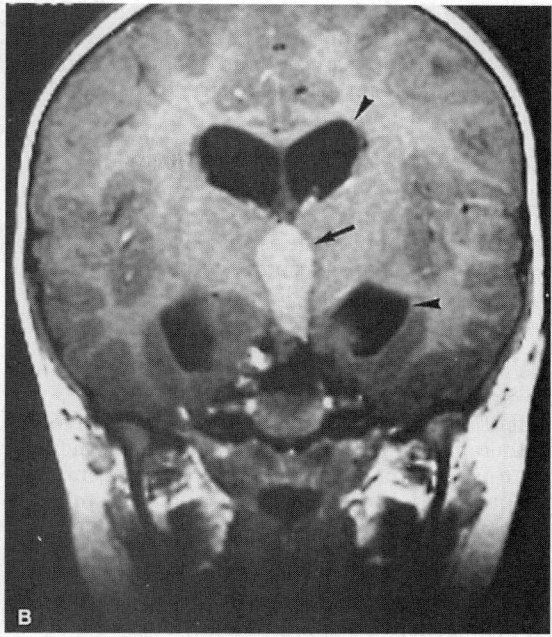

Figure 101.11. This 5-year-old child presented with decline in visual acuity and papilledema. *(A)* Axial magnetic resonance imaging scan with gadolinium reveals an enhancing mass *(arrow)* in the region of the sella turcica. *(B)* A coronal view shows a large cyst *(arrow)* extending up into the third ventricle. There is hydrocephalus *(arrowheads)*. At surgery, a craniopharyngioma was removed.

tients with pineocytomas is 32 years and 22 years for pineoblastomas. Resection and radiation therapy is recommended for both kinds of tumors. The 5-year survival rate for patients with pineocytomas is 75%, but much worse for pineoblastomas.

Epidermoid, Dermoid, and Teratoma

Epidermoids and dermoids arise from benign inclusions of epithelial elements in the CNS during closure of the embryonic neural groove. Epidermoids contain only stratified squamous epithelium. Dermoids contain skin appendages such as hair follicles, sebaceous glands, and sweat glands in addition to the squamous epithelium. Epidermoids tend to arise off the midline in locations such as the cerebellopontine angle, the parasellar region, and the diploë of the skull. Dermoids, on the other hand, usually arise in midline structures such as the cerebellar vermis or fourth ventricle. They are often accompanied by overlying bone and skin defects. Both tumor types are easily identified on CT and MRI scans. Surgical removal is the preferred treatment. Recurrences are usually managed with further surgery.

Teratomas are more common in children. By definition, they are composed of tumor cells representing all three embryonic germ cell layers. The more differentiated teratomas often contain cartilage and bone. If these elements are primitive, they are considered malignant. Like dermoids, they tend to occur in the midline in such locations as the pineal region, third ventricle, and posterior fossa. Treatment is surgical excision, along with irradiation in certain malignant types.

Hemangioblastoma

These benign tumors are vascular and usually occur in the cerebellum. They are uncommon and constitute only 1% to 2% of intracranial tumors. Typical presentation is in the fourth decade. Fifteen percent of patients have von Hippel-Lindau disease, an autosomal dominant disorder consisting of CNS hemangioblastomas, retinal angiomato-

sis, renal and pancreatic cysts, and renal cell carcinoma. Regardless of whether they have this syndrome, many patients have polycythemia. Sizable neoplastic cysts are present in 60% of cases, often with only a small mural nodule of tumor. Total surgical removal is curative. Radiation therapy is used when resection is not possible. Reoperation is recommended for recurrences. Long-term survival rates are excellent, with up to 80% of patients alive at 10 years.

Metastatic Tumor

The percentage of intracranial tumors representing metastases approaches 25%. Malignant cells invade the CNS hematogenously and tend to lodge at the gray and white matter junction. Metastatic tumors occur singly or multiply and can involve virtually any portion of the brain or, less commonly, spinal cord. Although any malignancy has the potential to metastasize, the most common primary sites are the lung, breast, kidney, testis, colon, and skin. The presenting symptoms are determined by the site or sites of the metastases. The symptoms commonly include headache, mental status changes, seizures, and hemiparesis.

Metastatic lesions are best imaged with MRI. They can mimic other lesions such as meningiomas, abscesses, primary brain tumors, and even aneurysms. If a metastasis is suspected, an extensive work-up to find the primary source is recommended. If the primary site is not identified, an excisional biopsy is indicated.

In general, a symptomatic, solitary lesion that is surgically accessible should be removed. Surgery should not be undertaken for multiple lesions or in patients who are severely afflicted by their primary disease. Treatment should also include preoperative dexamethasone, as in any brain or spinal cord tumor, to reduce adjacent brain edema. Whole-brain irradiation is almost always indicated. Prognosis depends on tumor type, with median survival ranging from 1 to 2 years. Long-term survivors have been reported with surgical removal of solitary brain metastases.

Quality of life is almost always improved. Chemotherapy is useful in some metastatic tumors such as breast, lung, testicular, and ovarian cancer, and choriocarcinoma. Again, stereotactic radiosurgery plays an increasing role in the treatment of metastatic tumors.

Tumor metastasis to the leptomeninges (meningeal carcinomatosis) is also common, particularly in the childhood leukemias and in adults with lymphoma, breast and lung cancer, and melanoma. Patients can present with cranial nerve palsies, radiculopathies, or obstructive hydrocephalus. They often have signs and symptoms suggestive of meningitis. Analysis of the CSF is usually critical, often revealing an increased opening pressure, elevated white cell count and protein levels, and a decreased glucose. There may or may not be identifiable malignant cells, but cytologic examination should always be performed.

Treatment of meningeal carcinomatosis usually involves radiation therapy and intraventricular chemotherapy. Methotrexate is a common chemotherapeutic agent. The outlook for patients with leptomeningeal tumor spread is in general poor, but a few long-term survivors emerge.

Spinal Tumors

Spinal tumors constitute approximately 20% of all CNS tumors. They are classified as intradural or extradural. Of the intradural type, approximately 70% are outside the spinal cord (extramedullary). Intradural tumors are almost always primary CNS tumors, whereas most extradural tumors are either metastatic or primary bone tumors of the spine. Most intradural spinal neoplasms are benign and can often be totally excised surgically. Tumors occurring within the cord (intradural, intramedullary) tend to produce weakness, increased tone, usually in the form of spasticity, and sensory loss. Extramedullary lesions present with radicular pain from nerve root (lower motor neuron) compression as well as long tract (upper motor neuron) signs from cord compression. Patients with spinal tumors involving the conus region may have early loss of bladder and bowel function; those with tumors in the cauda equina present primarily with leg pain and only later experience sphincter disturbances.

The definitive study for spinal tumors is MRI, although abnormal plain films and myelograms can be diagnostic. Plain films may show widening of the interpeduncular distance, bony erosion, enlargement of the neural foramina, or a paraspinous mass. Myelography helps determine the tumor's relation to the spinal cord and dura. Postmyelography CT can further define that relation. MRI allows refinement of the differential diagnosis.

Neurilemmoma and Neurofibroma

Typically benign, neurilemmomas and neurofibromas are the most common spinal cord tumors, making up almost 30% of the total. They are usually extramedullary intradural tumors. Of these, 13% have extradural extension through an adjacent foramen, producing the classic dumbbell shape of the neurofibroma. Fourteen percent are totally extradural. The extradural component tends to enlarge the involved foramen. Treatment is surgical removal. Adjacent or involved spinal nerve roots (usually the dorsal ones) may need to be sacrificed to obtain total excision. Multiple neurofibromas are associated with von Recklinghausen's disease. In those instances, only the symptomatic tumors are removed.

Meningioma

Meningiomas constitute 26% of spinal tumors, are benign, and are usually extramedullary intradural tumors. Fifteen percent occur extradurally. Two thirds arise in the thoracic spine, affecting women in their fourth through sixth decades in 80% of cases. Surgical excision is the treatment of choice.

Ependymoma

Arising from the ependymal cells of the CNS, ependymomas are intramedullary tumors and constitute 13% of all spinal tumors. They occur more frequently in men. Nearly 60% are found in the conus region. Ependymomas should be surgically excised, and their distinct borders often allow complete resection. Radiation therapy is usually used when total removal is not possible.

Astrocytoma

These glial tumors are derived from astrocytes and are often intramedullary. Their incidence is approximately equal to that of spinal ependymomas. Total excision is rarely possible because of their infiltrative nature. Low-grade astrocytomas, if recurrent, are usually reoperated. Radiation therapy is reserved for malignant astrocytomas but is usually only palliative. Although the growth rate of spinal cord astrocytomas is slow, prognosis is poor.

Hemangioblastoma

Hemangioblastomas are rare tumors and are intramedullary 60% of the time. Up to 25% of patients have von Hippel-Lindau syndrome. They are benign and well encapsulated, and should be surgically excised.

Lipoma

Lipomas represent 1% of all spinal tumors and are often associated with spina bifida and a subcutaneous lipoma. Although benign, they tend to invade the cord through a congenital dural defect and are usually only subtotally excised. These tumors do not require radiation, and the mortality rate is low.

Dermoid

Dermoids are congenital lesions usually found in the lumbosacral area. They often have an associated sinus tract to the skin surface and can present with infection. The treatment is surgical resection, including the sinus tract. The resection of the portion entering the spinal cord is usually incomplete. The long-term prognosis is good.

Metastatic Tumor

Up to 25% of all spinal neoplasms are metastatic in origin, and most appear in an extradural location. Common primary sites include the breast, lung, prostate, and kidney. Treatment is surgical decompression with biopsy if the primary site is not known or if the neurologic decline is rapid. Otherwise, local radiation therapy is the treatment of choice. Other extradural malignant tumors include lymphoma, myeloma, plasmacytoma, chordoma, and osteogenic sarcoma. When significant bone destruction or surgical decompression renders the spine unstable, surgical stabilization through an anterior or posterior route is necessary.

Peripheral Nerve Tumors

The peripheral nervous system includes the peripheral and cranial nerves, spinal roots, and autonomic nervous system. Tumors can arise from any of these elements. The more common tumors are discussed in the following sections. More unusual tumors include gangliogliomas, neuroblastomas, paragangliomas, chemodectomas, and pheochromocytomas.

Schwannoma

Schwannomas arise from the peripheral nerve Schwann cells, which provide the myelin sheaths for axons. Schwannomas tend to displace the nerve of origin and thus usually present as a painless mass. With continued growth, they can create pain in the distribution of the nerve. As they enlarge, nerve function deteriorates. They tend to arise from sensory nerves but can also be found on motor nerves. The treatment is surgical excision. The nerve of origin can usually be preserved. At times, total excision may mean division of the parent nerve. If the nerve serves a significant function, it is preferable to leave a portion of the tumor to spare the nerve. This is possible because malignant transformation is rare.

Neurofibroma

Neurofibromas differ from schwannomas in that they actually engulf the nerve of origin within the tumor because they arise from the nerve itself. They are often cutaneous, making it difficult to identify one specific nerve of origin. When associated with von Recklinghausen's disease, they are usually multiple. When found alone, treatment is resection. When multiple tumors are present, only the symptomatic ones need to be resected. Removal requires sacrifice of the nerve, should that nerve be expendable. If the function of the nerve of origin is critical, a portion of tumor should be left attached to the nerve. Unlike patients with schwannomas, patients with neurofibromas should be followed closely because these tumors have a higher incidence of malignant transformation.

Malignant Nerve Sheath Tumor

These tumors typically occur beyond the third decade. The treatment of choice is radical wide resection. If there is evidence of muscle or soft-tissue invasion, amputation of the involved extremity is recommended. These tumors are usually resistant to radiation therapy.

CEREBROVASCULAR DISEASE

Cerebrovascular disease is the third most common cause of death in the United States and is an equally significant cause of chronic disability. Death and disability are due either to ischemia causing focal or diffuse infarction or to hemorrhage causing compressive mass lesions. Cerebrovascular problems producing infarction can become hemorrhagic, and hemorrhagic lesions can lead to infarction.

Ischemic Vascular Disease (Stroke)

Ischemia and subsequent infarction of the brain can occur in the distribution of any of the cerebral vessels. Thus, any portion of the cerebrum, brain stem, or cerebellum can be affected. Because the carotid circulation provides the greatest blood supply to the brain, ischemia and infarction are most common within its distribution. Ischemia can be the result of diminished flow secondary to stenosis or occlusion of major arteries, or can be due to transient or permanent occlusion of smaller arterioles from intravascular emboli.

The most common cause of stenosis or occlusion of large vessels is atherosclerosis. This often occurs extracranially at the origin of the internal carotid artery in the neck, but can occur in the carotid siphon (that portion of the artery within the cavernous sinus), the distal internal carotid, or even the proximal middle cerebral artery.

Arterial emboli usually originate either from atherosclerotic ulceration in the region of the carotid bifurcation or from sources in the heart. The heart commonly becomes a source of emboli when a mural thrombus forms after a myocardial infarction or as result of atrial fibrillation. Other risk factors for cerebral ischemia include hypertension, diabetes, hypercholesterolemia, obesity, smoking, and a family history of stroke.

The primary role of the neurosurgeon in the management of stroke is to identify stroke-prone patients and reduce their risk of cerebral ischemia. High-risk patients are usually identified by a history of transient ischemic attacks (TIAs). TIAs take the form of either transient cerebral ischemia or amaurosis fugax. Transient cerebral ischemia in the carotid circulation usually consists of temporary hemianesthesia, hemiparesis, or aphasia. Amaurosis fugax is transient loss of vision in one eye, usually in the form of an ascending or descending shade effect. Ischemia in the vertebrobasilar system can consist of transient diplopia, dizziness, dysarthria, dysphagia, weakness, numbness, loss of vision, or even loss of memory.

Most ischemic episodes last seconds to minutes; rarely do they last longer than 30 minutes. As long as the neurologic deficit resolves within 24 hours, the episode is a TIA. An ischemic deficit that lasts 24 hours to 1 week is termed a *reversible ischemic neurologic deficit.* Ischemic deficits lasting longer than this are considered completed strokes. Careful questioning of people with completed strokes reveals that of the 60% who had a history of TIAs, 20% had strokes that presented in a slow, stepwise fashion, and only 20% had strokes that were sudden in onset.

Patients with TIAs and even those with slow-onset strokes are potential candidates for preventive surgical intervention. Surgical procedures to prevent stroke are directed at either removing a source of emboli or providing increased blood flow to the brain. These consist mainly of carotid endarterectomy or a microvascular bypass procedure. Potential candidates usually undergo a CT or MRI scan of the brain to evaluate any degree of cerebral infarction and to rule out other diagnoses such as tumor, subdural hematoma, or subarachnoid hemorrhage. Patients then undergo careful angiography including the aortic arch and carotid, vertebral, and cerebral arteries. Noninvasive studies of the carotid circulation remain less accurate, although they are useful as screening procedures.

Carotid endarterectomy is indicated when ipsilateral symptoms of cerebral ischemia or amaurosis fugax exist and angiography demonstrates either significant stenosis (>70%) or ulceration in the accessible portions of the common and proximal internal carotid arteries. The procedure consists of opening the affected portion of the carotid artery under systemic heparinization and removing the atherosclerotic plaque. Blood flow during the procedure may or may not be continued to the distal internal carotid artery by an internal shunt system. The mortality rate from carotid endarterectomy is approximately 1%, and the neurologic morbidity rate is 1% to 5% in experienced hands.

Some patients have cerebral ischemia ipsilateral to an occluded internal carotid artery or stenosis of the internal carotid or middle cerebral artery that is not surgically accessible. For patients with inadequate collateral cerebral circulation, a microvascular bypass procedure is sometimes indicated. The most common of these is the superficial temporal artery to middle cerebral artery anastomosis.

Intracranial Aneurysms

Intracranial aneurysms are diseased dilatations of the cerebral arteries, their walls consisting of ballooned-out intima, media, and adventitia with a variable degree of intraluminal or mural thrombus. Most are congenital, evolving and developing during life. They can become atherosclerotic. Aneurysms typically are found at the bifurcation of the major vessels of the circle of Willis (Fig. 101.12). Up to 20% of patients with aneurysms have multiple aneurysms, and 1% demonstrate an associated arteriovenous malformation (AVM). If aneurysms are found more peripherally in the cerebrovasculature, a secondary cause such as trauma or infection must be considered.

Over 85% of cerebral aneurysms occur in the carotid or anterior circulation. Approximately 30% arise from the intracranial portion of the internal carotid artery, usually at or near the origin of the posterior communicating artery (Fig. 101.13). Another 30% occur in the region of the anterior communicating artery. Approximately 20% arise from the middle cerebral artery, usually at its first major branch point, which is commonly a trifurcation. Aneurysms of the vertebrobasilar or posterior circulation are most frequently found at the tip of the basilar artery but can occur more proximally along its trunk. The origin of the posteroinferior cerebellar artery is the next most common location.

Patients with intracranial aneurysms most commonly present with signs and symptoms of subarachnoid hemorrhage. In fact, 80% of nontraumatic subarachnoid hemorrhages are caused by aneurysm rupture. The victim reports a sudden, severe headache commonly followed by neck stiffness and photophobia due to associated meningeal irritation caused by the subarachnoid blood. Transient loss of consciousness can occur. Some patients acquire a focal neurologic deficit or become comatose because of the acute rise in ICP. The severity of the subarachnoid hemorrhage can be graded on the Hunt and Hess criteria, as shown here. In general, the lower the grade, the better the outcome.

Grade I—No symptoms or minimal headache and slight nuchal rigidity

Grade II—Moderate to severe headache and nuchal rigidity; no neurologic deficit other than a cranial nerve palsy

Grade III—Lethargy, confusion, and mild focal neurologic deficit

Grade IV—Stupor, moderate to severe hemiparesis, possible early decerebrate posturing, and vegetative disturbances

Grade V—Deep coma, decerebrate posturing, and moribund appearance

Not all patients with aneurysms present with symptoms related to rupture. Through mass effect, an internal carotid artery aneurysm can compress the third cranial nerve, producing a palsy characterized by diplopia, ptosis, and dilated pupil. An internal carotid artery aneurysm in the cavernous sinus can compress the sixth cranial nerve and create diplopia. A giant aneurysm (>25 mm in diameter) of the basilar tip can block the cerebral aqueduct and create hydrocephalus. Rarely, an aneurysm can be large enough to be mistaken for a tumor.

The diagnosis of subarachnoid hemorrhage is usually made clinically and confirmed either by noting blood in the subarachnoid spaces on CT or by finding bloody CSF with xanthochromia on a lumbar puncture (Fig. 101.14). The CT scan should be obtained first because it usually spares the patient a lumbar puncture and also eliminates the potential risk of brain stem compression from herniation if an unsuspected mass lesion is present. Complete cerebral angiography is then used to identify and delineate the aneurysm and, at the same time, rule out multiple aneurysms or an associated AVM.

Once the diagnosis of aneurysmal rupture is confirmed, the patient is placed on a medical regimen to reduce the risk of rebleeding. This includes strict bed rest with the head elevated. Stimulation is kept to a minimum. Blood pressure is tightly controlled below 150 mm Hg systolic. Careful observation is necessary to watch for signs of raised ICP, which may be attributable to delayed hydrocephalus. Anticonvulsants are started for seizure prophylaxis. The calcium channel blocker, nimodipine, has been shown to reduce the incidence of vasospasm and improve

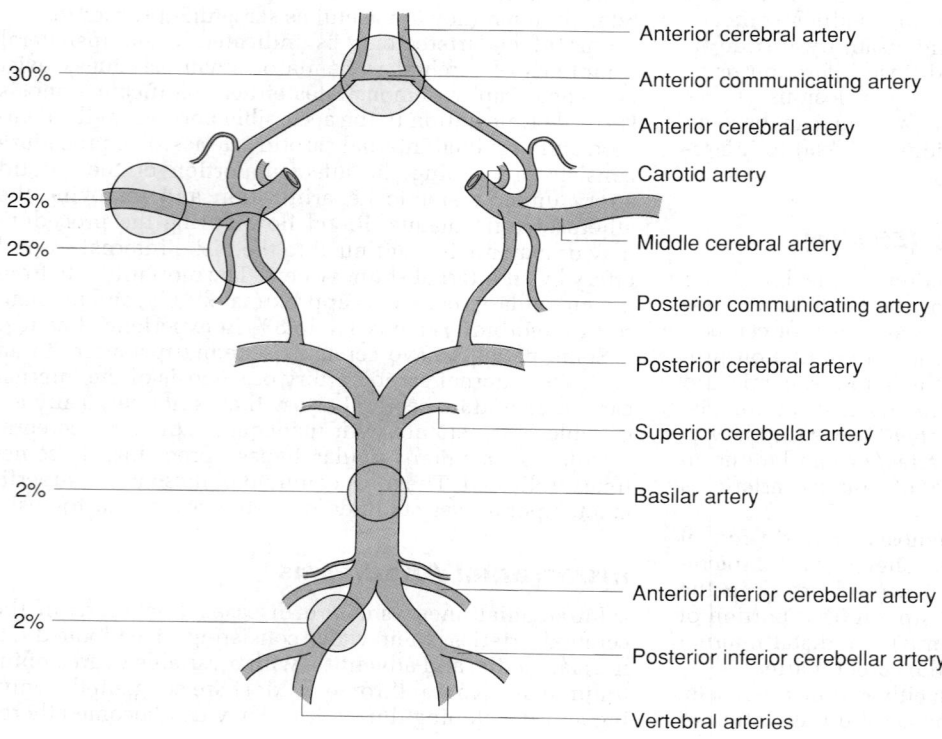

30%

25%

25%

2%

2%

Anterior cerebral artery

Anterior communicating artery

Anterior cerebral artery

Carotid artery

Middle cerebral artery

Posterior communicating artery

Posterior cerebral artery

Superior cerebellar artery

Basilar artery

Anterior inferior cerebellar artery

Posterior inferior cerebellar artery

Vertebral arteries

Figure 101.12. Locations of aneurysms of the circle of Willis and their relative occurrence.

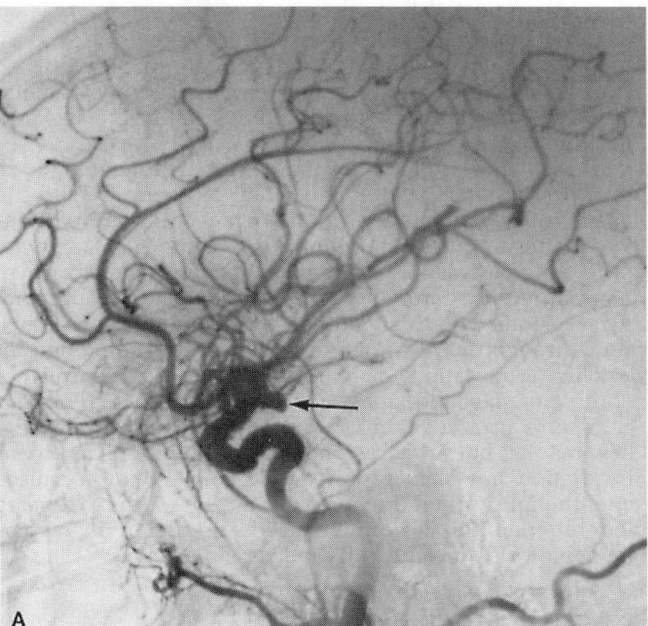 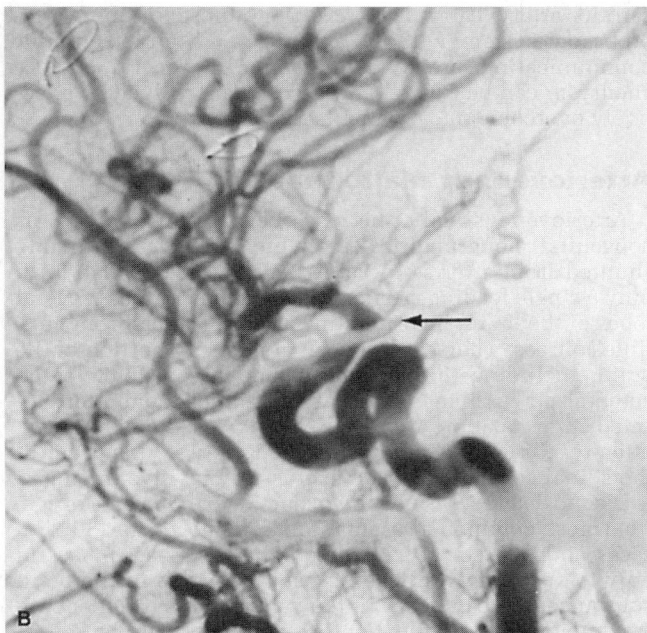

Figure 101.13. *(A)* Cerebral angiogram of the internal carotid artery shows an aneurysm near the posterior communicating artery *(arrow)*. *(B)* Follow-up angiogram after craniotomy demonstrates obliteration of the aneurysm by a metal clip *(arrow)*.

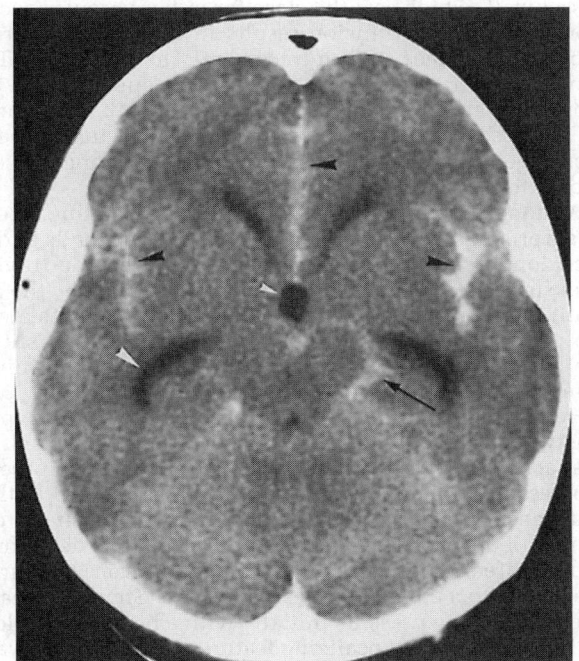

Figure 101.14. This patient presented with severe headache, nausea, and lethargy of acute onset. A noncontrast computed tomography scan reveals diffuse subarachnoid hemorrhage with blood in the interhemispheric and bilateral sylvian fissures *(black arrowheads)* and in the subarachnoid spaces around the brain stem *(arrow)*. Early hydrocephalus is evidenced by the rounding of the third ventricle *(small white arrowhead)* and visualization of the temporal horns *(large white arrowhead)*.

outcome when started within 96 hours of the hemorrhage. The dosage is 60 mg orally every 4 hours for 21 days.

The ultimate treatment of aneurysms is obliteration, usually by placement of a metallic clip on the aneurysm's neck by way of a craniotomy (Fig. 101.13B). The timing of surgery depends on the clinical grade of the patient. Patients with a good grade (I and II) should undergo operation within 72 hours of rupture. Those with a poor grade (III and IV) should continue intensive medical management until they improve to a lower grade. Surgically accessible unruptured aneurysms should be operated on electively to prevent rupture because the operative mortality rate is greater with higher grades. Aneurysms that are surgically inaccessible, or ruptured aneurysms with high-grade subarachnoid hemorrhage, can be effectively treated by embolization with detachable metal coils using interventional neuroradiologic techniques.

Complications of aneurysmal rupture include a 30% rebleeding rate within the first 8 weeks if the lesion remains unrepaired, hydrocephalus from obstruction of the arachnoid villi by subarachnoid clot, vasospasm, intracerebral hematomas, raised ICP, and seizures. The most significant and least understood of these is cerebral vasospasm. This phenomenon occurs most frequently within 4 to 7 days of the hemorrhage and results in narrowing of adjacent cerebral arteries. Vasospasm may be seen on angiography without any untoward clinical effects, or it may produce profound and life-threatening cerebral ischemia in the distribution of the involved vessels.

Symptomatic vasospasm can be treated with measures to increase cerebral blood flow. This can be accomplished by increasing systemic blood pressure with inotropic support and intravascular volume expansion. Cardiovascular status is monitored with a Swan-Ganz catheter. Vasospasm that persists despite medical intervention can be treated with cerebral angioplasty.

Patients who undergo elective treatment of unruptured aneurysms do better than those with ruptured aneurysms because the brain has not been injured by the subarachnoid hemorrhage. In addition, aneurysms of the internal carotid artery carry less risk than those of the vertebrobasilar system, with the exception of complex anterior communicating artery aneurysms. In general, if the aneurysm can be treated and vasospasm avoided or effectively overcome, most patients do well.

Arteriovenous Malformations

Arteriovenous malformations occur within the CNS as congenital abnormalities in which blood is directly shunted from arteries to veins. AVMs can be small with only a single feeding artery, or they can encompass several lobes of the brain, incorporating arterial feeders from multiple sources. They can occur in almost any portion of the brain, including the cerebellum and brain stem. In the cerebral parenchyma, where they are most commonly located, they take on a conical shape with the apex deep, often reaching the lateral ventricle. Rarely, AVMs occur in the spinal cord, or they can exclusively involve the dura.

Diagnosis of AVMs usually occurs before 30 years of age. The most common presentation is hemorrhage (50% of cases and 10% of all intracerebral hemorrhages, second only to aneurysms). Bleeding usually occurs in the brain substance, but can occur in the ventricular system or subarachnoid space. The patient experiences a sudden headache, often associated with loss of consciousness and a neurologic deficit. The next most common presenting symptom is a seizure. In a few cases, seizures are frequent and refractory to medical therapy. AVMs can present with the insidious onset of a focal neurologic deficit as a result of mass effect, increased venous pressure, or vascular steal phenomenon. Occasionally, young patients with severe, unrelenting headaches are found harboring an AVM.

The risk of hemorrhage for unruptured AVMs is 2% to 4% per year, with an associated mortality rate of 1% per year. Once an AVM has bled, the risk of rebleeding is increased to 5% per year. With each hemorrhage, the risk of death is approximately 10%; morbidity is at least 15%. Smaller AVMs are more likely to bleed than larger ones. Most AVMs remain stable in size, but some enlarge with time. Up to 10% have an associated aneurysm on a feeding artery. In these cases, hemorrhage is usually due to rupture of the aneurysm.

An AVM can be identified on contrast-enhanced CT scanning as a hyperdense mass, part of which has a serpentine configuration related to the presence of large draining veins. Their configuration and extent is more easily delineated with MRI (Fig. 101.15A). After hemorrhage, an unenhanced CT scan usually demonstrates intracerebral or subarachnoid blood. AVMs may be too small to be seen on CT, so careful angiography may be necessary to identify the source of hemorrhage. Lumbar puncture may be necessary if subarachnoid hemorrhage is suspected clinically but not verified by the CT scan.

In all cases of suspected or proven AVM, complete cerebral angiography must be undertaken to define carefully the extent of the malformation (Fig. 101.15B,C). All feeding arteries, including any from the external carotid system, as well as the draining veins, must be evaluated. A treatment decision can be reached only with angiography. Should angiography fail to delineate a lesion despite suspicion, MRI can identify the angiographically occult abnormality.

The treatment of AVMs depends on the size and location of the lesion, the presenting symptoms, and the age and condition of the patient. Because of the risk of rebleeding, an AVM that has bled should be surgically excised if possible. In the patient who presents with seizures, the treatment decision is more difficult. In general, if the patient is young and the malformation is read-

ily accessible, surgical resection is recommended, especially when the seizures are medically refractory. Surgery involves the microsurgical dissection and resection of the entire malformation, rather than simple ligation of feeding arteries. The results of surgery are related to the size and location of the malformation.

Alternate or adjunctive methods of treatment include intraarterial embolization and radiation therapy. With the use of interventional neuroradiologic techniques, particulate matter or glues can be introduced into AVMs by way of feeding vessels in an attempt to occlude the arteriovenous shunt. It is rarely possible completely to to obliterate these lesions with this method. This technique can reduce flow through the AVM before direct surgical intervention.

Ionizing radiation, on the other hand, can completely obliterate selected small to medium AVMs. Focused gamma or proton beam irradiation has demonstrated the best results, but an occasional success with conventional irradiation has been reported. Ionizing radiation causes endothelial proliferation and can take 6 months to 2 years to obliterate the lesion. Focused irradiation is recommended for deep, surgically inaccessible AVMs.

Brain Hemorrhage

Spontaneous hemorrhage is most commonly associated with systemic hypertension and occurs in predictable locations, including the putamen, thalamus, cerebellum, and pons. Hemorrhage can also occur in the various lobes of the brain. Nonhypertensive causes of brain hemorrhage were discussed earlier, such as rupture of AVMs and aneurysms, and hemorrhage into areas of ischemia. Additional causes include induced or endogenous coagulopathies, primary or metastatic brain tumors, and rare conditions such as amyloid angiopathy.

Chronic hypertension results in lipohyalinosis of the vessel wall, which sets the stage for either vascular occlusion or rupture. Occlusion results in infarction, whereas rupture produces an intracerebral hemorrhage. The shorter penetrating arteries of the brain appear to be the most vulnerable. The lenticulostriate and thalamoperforating vessels are involved in putamenal and thalamic hemorrhages, and affected basilar perforating branches contribute to pontine hemorrhage.

Although brain hemorrhage is often devastating, it can be surprisingly well tolerated. The hematoma tends to dissect along axonal planes, separating rather than destroying vital structures. If the resultant mass is tolerated by the patient, the blood is slowly resorbed by macrophages along the periphery, leaving only a hemosiderin-stained slit in the brain. Patients can worsen clinically after the initial hemorrhage because of associated edema formation.

Hemorrhage into the putamen accounts for most hypertensive bleeds. Presentation is characterized by lack of headache and the gradual development of hemiparesis progressing to hemiplegia. This can be associated with a hemisensory loss, aphasia, hemianopia, or ipsilateral deviation of the eyes, depending on the size of the hematoma and its direction of dissection. The patient can, of course, progress into a coma if the lesion is large. Similarly, thalamic hemorrhage presents initially with a hemisensory loss and a hemiparesis. Localizing features include downward eye deviation with limitation of vertical gaze and small, sluggish pupils due to involvement of the nearby mesencephalon. Headache is uncommon.

Cerebellar hemorrhage is sudden in onset and presents with headache. Vomiting, ataxia, and dizziness are accompanying features. This hemorrhage is extremely dangerous in that it can cause coma and ultimately death because of brain stem compression and acute hydro-

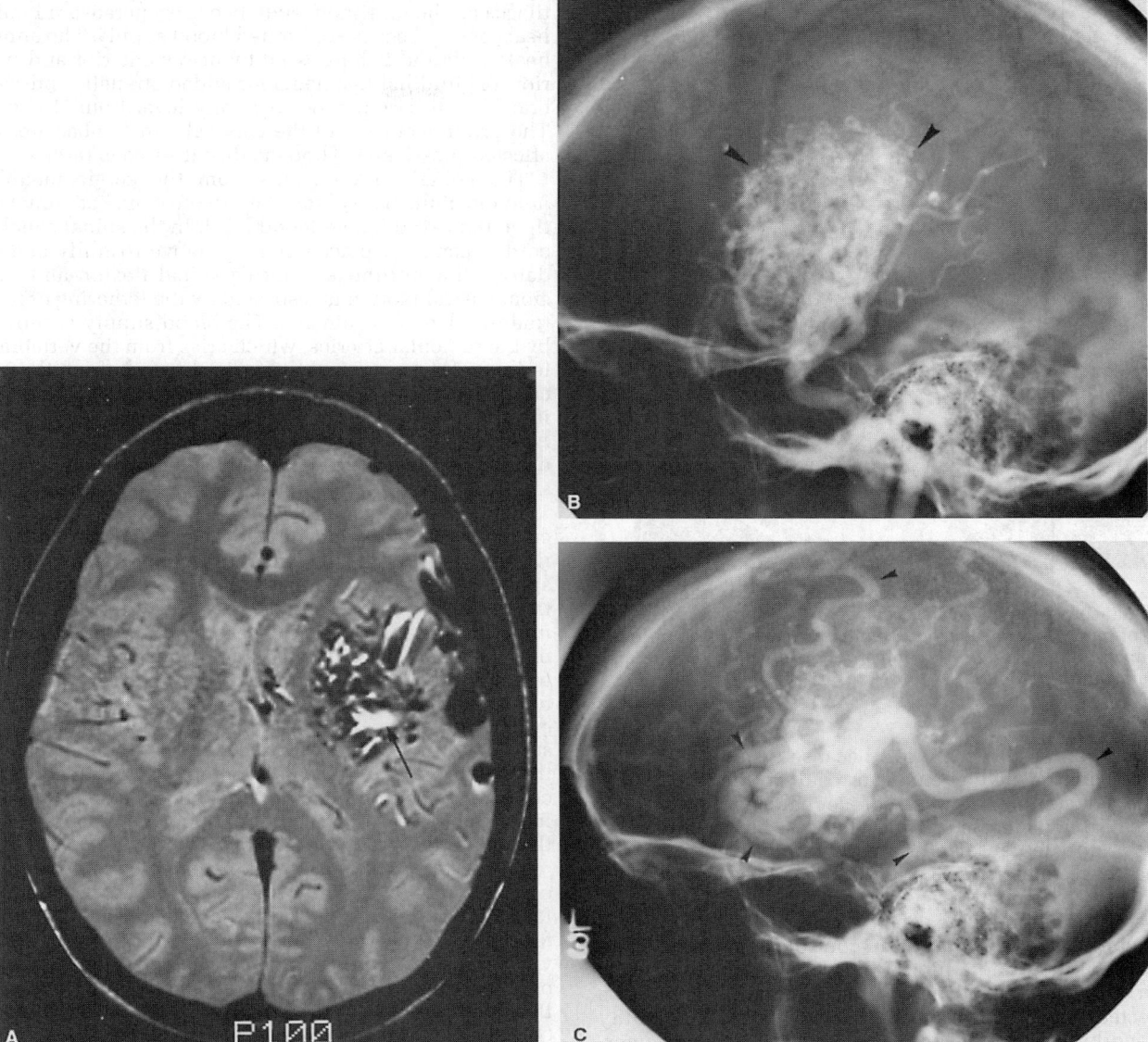

Figure 101.15. This young woman presented with a history of right arm clumsiness and seizures. *(A)* Magnetic resonance imaging scan without gadolinium shows a complex collection of tortuous blood vessels in the basal ganglia and temporal lobe consistent with an arteriovenous malformation (AVM). The bright signals in the lesion suggest previous hemorrhage *(arrow)*. *(B)* Cerebral angiography *(lateral view)* on the same patient demonstrates a large AVM in the middle cerebral artery distribution *(arrowheads)*. *(C)* Later phase of the angiogram reveals multiple draining veins *(arrowheads)*.

cephalus. Brain stem hemorrhage (usually pontine) is the most devastating and often presents with quadriparesis, decerebrate posturing, pinpoint pupils, and coma. Most patients do not survive if the hematoma is larger than 1 cm. Those who do survive have a high degree of morbidity. Lobar hemorrhage is less likely to be associated with hypertension and, in general, is better tolerated by the patient. The symptoms depend on the area of brain involved.

Computed tomography scanning has become an invaluable tool in diagnosing and defining brain hemorrhage (Fig. 101.16). CT not only delineates the hemorrhage but assesses the ventricular size and the presence of edema, and often suggests the cause of the hemorrhage (e.g., AVM,

tumor, aneurysm). The hematoma appears hyperdense in the acute phase. With time, as the blood breaks down, the clot progresses to a hypodense lesion. After days or weeks, the hematoma may demonstrate an enhancing ring. If a vascular lesion is suspected, careful angiography is indicated. In all cases, appropriate coagulation studies should be obtained.

The treatment of brain hemorrhage can be medical or surgical depending on the size of the lesion, its location, and the condition of the patient. In general, if a hematoma is more than 3 cm in diameter, surgical resection is strongly considered. Surgical resection is recommended if the patient is deteriorating neurologically, no matter what the size of the hematoma. Cerebellar hematomas are par-

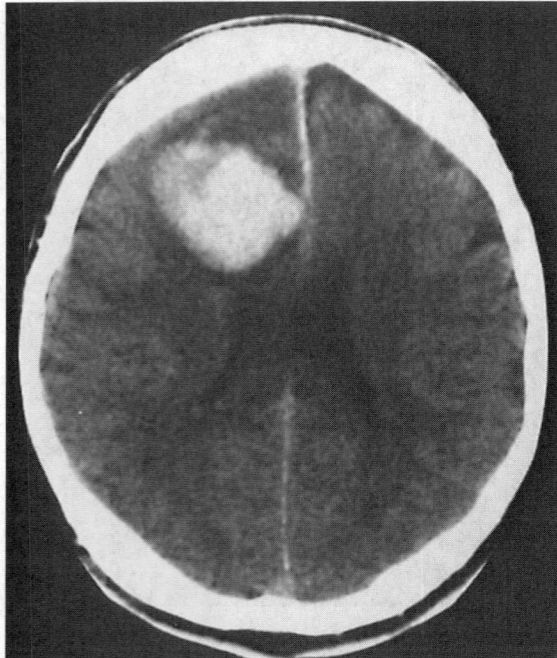

Figure 101.16. Noncontrast computed tomography scan showing a spontaneous frontal lobe hemorrhage in a patient who was alert and complaining of headache. Examination revealed a contralateral horizontal gaze palsy secondary to involvement of the ipsilateral frontal eye field.

ticularly important to remove because a small change in surrounding reactive edema can result in life-threatening brain stem compression or hydrocephalus, or both.

Because hematomas are mass lesions, medical management is directed at keeping the ICP under control. If the hemorrhage renders the patient unconscious, hyperventilation and hyperosmolar agents may be required to meet this goal. ICP monitoring can be a helpful adjunct to direct treatment. Steroids are useful in controlling brain edema if the patient bled into a tumor. Blood pressure needs close observation and tight control. Coagulopathies should be corrected. Despite medical and surgical therapy, mortality and morbidity remain high for all types of brain hemorrhage.

DEGENERATIVE SPINE DISEASE

Anatomy

The spinal column is composed of 33 vertebrae divided into the cervical (7), thoracic (12), lumbar (5), sacral (5 fused), and coccygeal (4 fused) regions. Each vertebra consists of a body, which bears weight, and the posterior elements (pedicles, laminae, spinous and transverse processes), which impart flexibility and stability to the vertebral column. For the most part, the spinal canal has an ovoid shape in the horizontal plane, assuming a more triangular shape in the lumbar region. Most spine movement occurs in the cervical and lumbar regions. Flexion and extension are greatest in the lower cervical and lumbar segments, whereas maximal rotation occurs predominantly in the upper cervical and lumbar segments.

The intervertebral disc consists of two parts. The circumferential annulus making up the outer portion is composed of dense fibrous tissue of great strength. The central nucleus consists of fibrocartilage with little tensile strength but substantial elasticity. The nucleus is approxi-

mately 80% water at birth but gradually dehydrates with age, a process that leads to loss of elasticity. The fibrocartilage can then fragment acutely or degenerate gradually. It heals poorly because of limited blood supply. The annulus heals well and is buttressed by heavy anterior and posterior longitudinal ligaments for added strength. Intervertebral disc disease can occur at any level from C-1 to S-1. The lower segments of the cervical and lumbar areas are affected most often. Thoracic disc disease is rare.

The spinal cord extends from the cervicomedullary junction at the base of the skull to the conus or spinal cord tip at the L-1 to L-2 vertebral level. In the spinal canal, the cord is centrally placed and can move rostrally and caudally a few millimeters during spinal flexion and extension. Lateral motion is restricted by the tethering of the intradural dentate ligaments. The blood supply is provided by the radicular arteries, which arise from the vertebral arteries and thyrocervical trunks in the neck, from the intercostal arteries in the thorax, and from the lumbar arteries in the low back. An arterial confluens, the artery of Adamkiewicz, is typically found in the T-10 to L-2 region, usually on the left side. It supplies the lower thoracic cord and conus medullaris.

Three fiber tracts of the spinal cord are important clinically. The laterally positioned corticospinal tracts carry motor fibers from the cortical upper motor neurons to the spinal lower motor neurons located in the ventral horns of the spinal cord. These tracts cross the midline at the pyramidal decussation in the lower medulla. The spinothalamic tract, also positioned laterally, transmits pain and temperature sensation from the contralateral side of the body. Within two or three segments of each dorsal root entry zone, the axons cross through the anterior commissure of the cord and ascend to the ipsilateral thalamus through this tract. The dorsal columns carry sensory fibers conveying position the vibratory and light touch sensation from the dorsal roots to the opposite cerebral cortex through a decussation in the brain stem.

Dorsal and ventral nerve roots emerge from the spinal cord separately, pass to their respective intervertebral foramina, and exit from the spinal canal. The roots join to form a spinal nerve within the neural foramen. In the cervical spine, the roots exit above the corresponding vertebrae. For instance, the C-5 root exits above the C-5 pedicle. Because there are eight cervical roots, C-7 exits above the C-7 pedicle, and C-8 exits above the T-1 pedicle. Consequently, all roots below C-8 exit below the pedicle of the corresponding vertebrae.

Below the conus, the lumbar and sacral roots form the cauda equina, which surrounds the filum terminale, the pial-arachnoid structure that anchors the distal cord to the caudal end of the spinal canal. The sacral roots are more centrally located adjacent to the filum. Because a lumbar root (e.g., L-4) passes laterally toward the neural foramen as it descends within the spinal canal, it crosses the adjacent intervertebral disc (e.g., L-4 to L-5) at its extreme lateral edge, hugging the pedicle of the vertebra laterally (Fig. 101.17). The nerve root then descends to the next lowest foramen (e.g., L-5) and passes across the disc space (e.g., L-4 to L-5) more medially, making that root more vulnerable to disease involving that disc.

Pathology

If the nucleus of an intervertebral disc extrudes (herniates) through the annulus, adjacent neural structures may be compressed. In the cervical and thoracic spine, compression of the spinal cord can result in paraparesis or quadriparesis, depending on the spinal segment involved. At all levels, compression of a spinal root can cause weak-

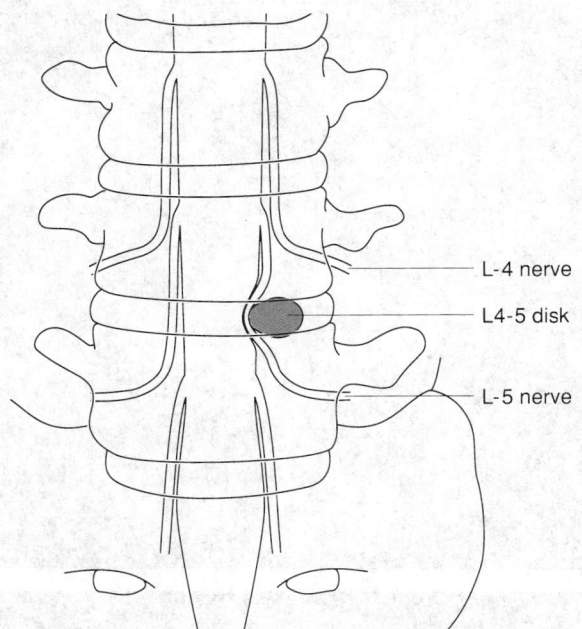

Figure 101.17. Relation between lumbar disc and nerve root exiting foramen.

ness and sensory loss in structures innervated by that root. The severity of the clinical syndrome depends on the site and severity of compression by the displaced disc fragment. At times, the annulus and adjacent ligament hold, preventing complete extrusion of the fragmented disc. The annulus may only stretch sufficiently to allow the disc to bulge into the spinal canal or foramina.

Often the nucleus does not extrude but simply fragments in response to the forces exerted on the spinal column. This is intensified by the concomitant dehydration of the disc with loss of elasticity as it ages. The disc space gradually narrows, the joint becomes loose, and the cartilaginous end plates of the adjacent vertebral bodies abut and wear more quickly. Bony spurs (osteophytes) develop at the joint in reaction to the increased mobility and decreased elasticity.

Formation of osteophytes around the joints of vertebrae is termed *spondylosis,* a common disorder that is considered by some investigators to represent the normal process of aging. If an osteophyte forms in a neural foramen, the nerve root passing through can be chronically irritated and compressed. If the osteophyte develops in the cervical or lumbar canal, the cord or cauda equina can be compromised. Thoracic spine osteophytes causing neurologic dysfunction are rare because their development is limited by the inherent reduced mobility of that part of the spinal column.

Cervical Spine

Clinical Presentation

The onset of symptoms and signs of an extruded disc fragment can be acute or chronic. Acute symptoms may or may not be related to trauma. In the cervical spine, neck and radicular discomfort occur simultaneously. Spinal cord symptoms are rare. There is usually limitation of neck motion, with loss of the normal cervical lordosis. With foraminal osteophytes, episodes of cervical discomfort recur over many months or years before radicular

symptoms appear. Interscapular aching, suboccipital headaches, and even chest pain are common complaints.

Nerve root compression produces a radiculopathy often characterized by pain and hypesthesia in the distribution of the involved root. Associated deep tendon reflex loss with or without weakness may be seen on examination. Cervical cord compression causes myelopathy characterized by progressive spastic paraparesis, mild to moderate sensory changes in the lower extremities and trunk with cervical dermatomal sensory loss, weak upper extremity musculature, hyperreflexia, and plantar extensor responses.

Diagnosis

Cervical disc disease must be differentiated from other ailments, including inflammatory diseases of the soft tissues and joints of the arm and shoulder, nerve entrapment syndromes, and neoplasms. The pain must be distinguished from the pain that accompanies cardiac disease. Spinal infections, congenital lesions, and posttraumatic disorders are other important considerations.

Plain radiographs typically demonstrate loss of the lordotic curve of the cervical spine with narrowing of one or more disc spaces. Osteophyte formation may be seen. In cervical spondylosis, there is usually radiologic evidence of osteophytes and disc space narrowing at multiple levels. In most cases, the anteroposterior diameter of the cervical spinal canal is narrowed. Myelography with CT is useful in the diagnostic work-up of a radiculopathy. The use of intrathecal contrast enhances the power of CT to delineate the lesion (Fig. 101.18). MRI is suitable for investigating myelopathies. In addition to defining the compressive lesion, MRI often shows intrinsic cord abnormalities related to the compression, consistent with edema or myelomalacia, a finding of clinical relevance. EMG can confirm the diagnosis and localize the lesion more specifically, particularly when myelographic defects are multiple.

Treatment

Painful cervical disc disease can be treated medically as long as there is no evidence of a progressive neurologic deficit (motor loss and bowel and bladder dysfunction being most important). Adequate medical therapy includes immobilization of the neck with a soft or hard cervical collar, analgesics, muscle relaxants, and local heat. These methods, in association with a good physical therapy program, provide relief under most circumstances.

Most patients with cervical disc disease improve after an adequate trial (10 to 14 days) of medical therapy. Some have recurrence of radicular symptoms on return to full activity. In many cases, these patients can be managed for years with intervals of cervical traction and a cervical collar, but some require surgical therapy. For those who do not respond to conservative means, operation is often helpful.

There are essentially two approaches to the surgical treatment of cervical disc disease. Anteriorly, nerve roots, spinal cord, or both can be decompressed through discectomy with or without bone graft fusion. The other approach is posteriorly through a laminectomy or foraminotomy, or both. The choice of operative direction should be based on a particular patient's anatomic lesion. It is occasionally necessary to use both an anterior and a posterior approach. Regardless of approach, improvement follows operative treatment of symptomatic cervical disc disease in approximately 80% of patients who fail to respond to medical treatment. Surgical treatment of cervical spondylotic myelopathy results in improvement in approximately 60% of cases. Arrest of the progressive myelopathic deficit often occurs.

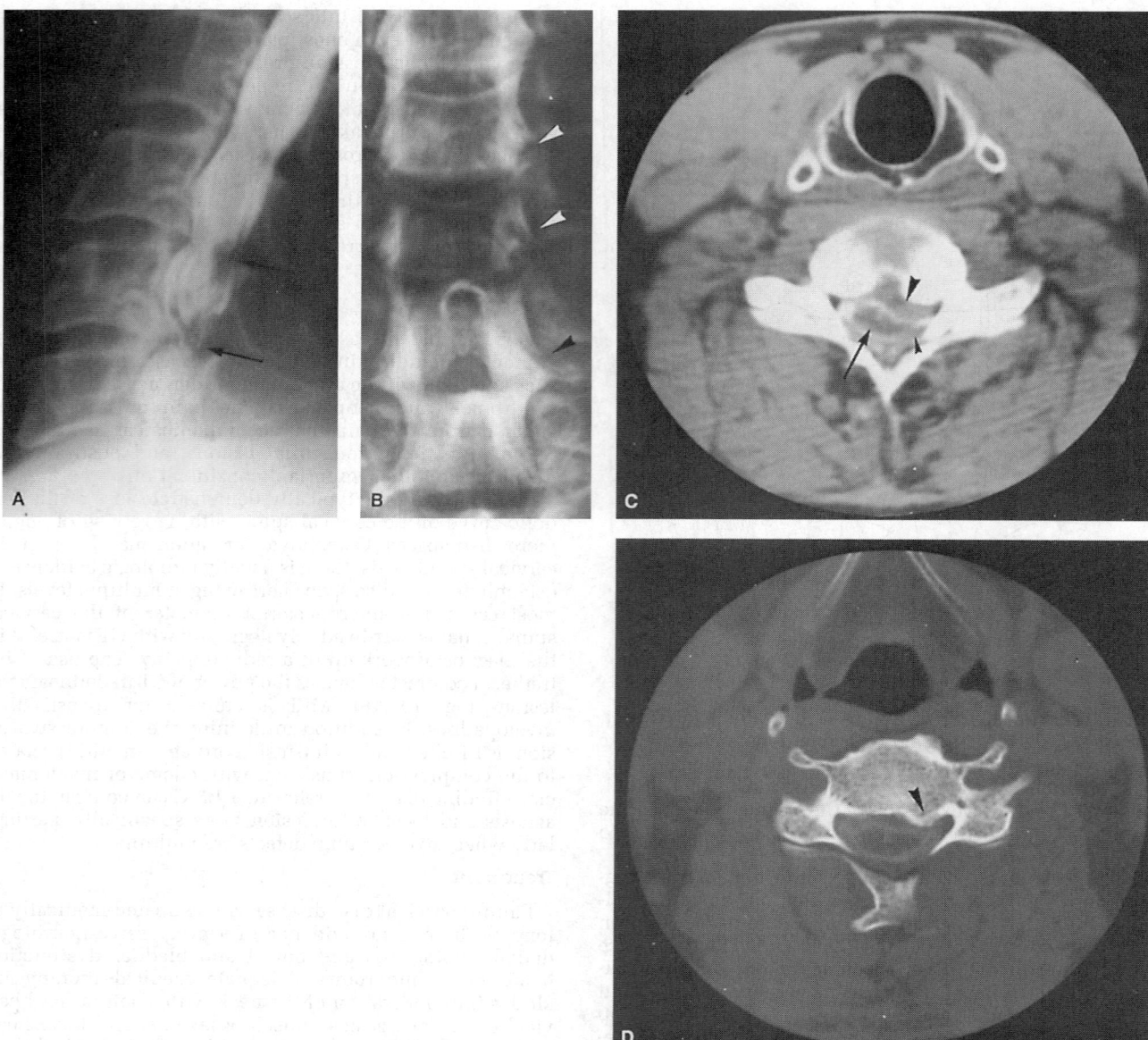

Figure 101.18. *(A and B)* Cervical myelograms of a patient with neck and left arm pain show several levels of spinal canal constriction *(arrows)*, best appreciated on the lateral view *(A)*. The anteroposterior view reveals cutoff of two adjacent nerve root sleeves *(white arrowheads in B)*. Compare these with a normal root sleeve *(black arrowhead)*. *(C)* Computed tomography scan made after the myelogram demonstrates a herniated disc *(large arrowhead)* with spinal cord *(arrow)* and root *(small arrowhead)* compression at one level (soft-tissue window). *(D)* An osteophyte *(arrowhead)* with root compression only at an adjacent level (bone window).

Thoracic Spine

In the thoracic spine, forceful trauma can cause the nucleus of a disc to extrude into the spinal canal. Because the canal is small relative to the spinal cord in it, cord compression readily occurs. Paraplegia is often abrupt and can be permanent. More often, osteophyte formation secondary to thoracic disc degeneration accounts for spinal canal narrowing. Development of thoracic myelopathy is more gradual. Isolated radiculopathies can also occur. Primary treatment for both acute and chronic thoracic disc disease is surgical. The offending disc fragment or spur is best removed by an anterior or lateral approach.

Lumbar Spine

Herniated lumbar intervertebral discs often produce some degree of nerve root compression. The severity of the syndrome depends on the degree of root compression. Occasionally, the entire cauda equina is involved, resulting in loss of motor and sensory function, including bowel and bladder sphincter control. Sometimes disc rupture can occur in the midline, compressing centrally positioned sacral roots preferentially, without involvement of laterally placed lumbar roots.

Fragmentation of a lumbar disc can occur without extrusion of the nucleus, as described earlier for cervical disc disease. Because of loss of elasticity in the disc, mobility of the intervertebral joint is increased. The annulus may simply bulge without tearing. With time, osteophytes can form around the degenerated disc and encroach on the spinal canal and neural foramina. This degenerative hypertrophy involves the ligamentous structures as well. Stenosis of the lumbar spinal canal is the end result, a spondylotic condition common in the elderly.

Clinical Presentation

In the lumbar spine, more than 90% of clinical problems arise from the L-4 to L-5 and L-5 to S-1 intervertebral discs. Pain is usually chronic, but its onset can be acute when associated with frank herniation. There may be back pain, leg pain, or both. The radiation of low back pain into the buttock, posterior thigh, and calf is usually the same with disease at the L-4 to L-5 and L-5 to S-1 levels. This radiating pain can be exacerbated by coughing, sneezing, or straining. Bending and sitting accentuate the discomfort, whereas lying down characteristically relieves it. The pain is typically described as aching but frequently has a sharp or shooting element and is limited to one lower extremity. With lumbar stenosis, patients are unable to extend their spine without developing pain, numbness, or weakness, usually in both lower extremities. With upright posture, either standing or walking, the cauda equina becomes ischemic, producing neurogenic claudication. Relief is obtained by sitting or flexing forward.

Palpation usually reveals tenderness over the sciatic notch, popliteal fossa, or both. Paravertebral muscles can be in spasm. With true nerve root compression, straight leg raising produces leg pain that is accentuated by dorsiflexion of the foot. Ipsilateral leg pain produced by contralateral straight leg raising is highly suggestive of lumbar disc herniation. Other signs include the lower motor neuron findings associated with the specific root or roots involved. Sensory loss, weakness, and loss of tendon jerks can occur in many combinations and to variable degrees.

Diagnosis

Back pain with radiation to the leg has many causes besides lumbar disc disease. The differential diagnosis includes bony abnormalities such as subluxation, degenerative facet fracture, and osteophyte formation; primary and metastatic tumors of the cauda equina, spine, and pelvis; inflammatory disorders, including abscess, arachnoiditis, ankylosing spondylitis, and rheumatoid arthritis; degenerative lesions of the spinal cord; peripheral neuropathies; peripheral vascular occlusive disease, including abdominal aortic aneurysm; and gynecologic problems such as endometriosis.

Plain films of the lumbosacral spine can identify congenital or acquired bony changes. Disc space narrowing is an unreliable sign of symptomatic disease because narrowing of the disc space can occur without clinical symptoms. Flexion and extension lateral views reveal any concomitant instability. Myelography can be diagnostic in symptomatic lumbar disc disease, but CT alone delineates the lesion in most cases (Fig. 101.19). MRI has replaced myelography and CT at most centers in the work-up of lumbar radiculopathy. With IV contrast, it can be extremely helpful in differentiating scar tissue from recurrent herniated discs in previously operated cases. EMG can confirm the diagnosis, especially when physical examination is unable to localize the involved level.

Treatment

Initially, medical treatment is indicated in all patients who do not have neurologic deterioration. Bed rest, local heat, analgesics, and skeletal muscle relaxants are usually effective within a few days. Physical therapy and limited exercise often help when the acute episode passes. A back brace partially immobilizes the patient and can prevent recurrent muscle spasm. With aggressive conservative management, most patients improve sufficiently to return to full activity. Recurrent symptoms can be treated in a similar fashion, often successfully. Surgical treatment is reserved for the patient with an acute or progressive neurologic deficit, chronic disabling pain, or both. The acute onset of weakness or sphincter disturbance constitutes an emergency, demanding prompt diagnosis and early operation.

Surgery usually entails a unilateral partial laminectomy with removal of the offending disc fragment. Foraminotomy may be necessary in the presence of osteophyte formation. With lumbar stenosis, multilevel laminectomy is curative. Should preoperative plain films demonstrate any

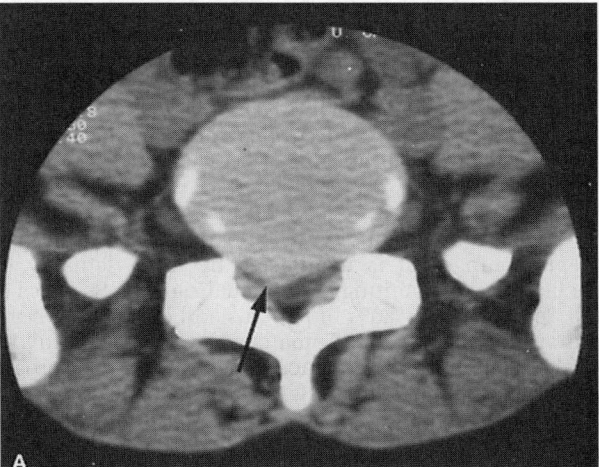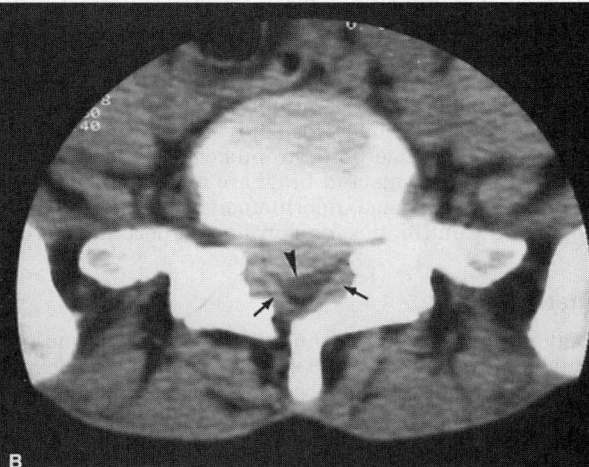

Figure 101.19. Noncontrast axial computed tomography scan of a patient presenting with acute low back and right lower extremity pain. The slices are taken through the L-5 to S-1 disc *(A)* and 3 mm below the level of the disc *(B)*. There is right paramedian herniation *(long arrow)* into the spinal canal with marked compression of the cauda equina *(arrowhead)* in the thecal sac. The *short arrows* identify the ligamenta flava.

instability, combining the laminectomy with posterior fusion, either with or without instrumentation, usually is indicated. If the imaging studies demonstrate an extruded disc fragment that accounts for the clinical signs and symptoms, 85% to 90% of patients recover with surgical treatment. If the syndrome is atypical, the myelogram equivocal, or the patient poorly motivated, operation is less effective.

INFECTIONS

The CNS can be infected by viruses, bacteria, fungi, and parasites. Development of infection depends on the host's resistance (i.e., immune defenses) and on the infecting agent's virulence. Bone, brain, spinal cord, meninges, and CSF can be involved separately or in combination. The routes of infection include hematogenous dissemination, local extension from a neighboring source, and direct contamination through an open wound. The infection can be diffuse, as in meningitis, or focal, as in brain abscess.

The clinical spectrum of signs and symptoms of CNS infection varies from nonspecific, such as fever, confusion, and lethargy, to highly specific, such as jacksonian epilepsy and focal neurologic deficits. Consequently, CNS infections present difficult diagnostic and therapeutic problems. Early diagnosis and treatment are crucial to a successful outcome.

Bacterial Infections

Subgaleal Abscess

Localized infection between the galea of the scalp and the pericranium constitutes subgaleal abscess. Usually, the process is initiated by contamination of an open scalp wound by staphylococci, streptococci, or anaerobic cocci. Localized scalp tenderness, warmth, and swelling are signs of abscess formation. Osteomyelitis of the skull can occur secondarily. Subgaleal infections rarely extend intracranially, unless the skull has been penetrated. Treatment includes open drainage, débridement, and systemic antibiotics.

Osteomyelitis

Osteomyelitis can develop from extension of a localized infection, such as sinusitis or mastoiditis, from direct contamination at operation or after trauma, or, rarely, by hematogenous spread from a distant source such as the respiratory or urinary tract. An established skull or spine infection can extend to the epidural space and produce a localized abscess. The usual osteomyelitis pathogens are staphylococci and anaerobic streptococci. Occasionally, gram-negative organisms and fungi are responsible. Treatment consists of drainage, débridement of infected bone, and appropriate antibiotics for a prolonged period, usually 6 weeks.

Epidural Abscess

Spinal epidural abscess is much more common than intracranial epidural abscess. It is characterized by fever, local spinal tenderness, and rapid progression of neurologic deficits, often constituting a medical and surgical emergency. Radicular pain and impairment of cord function, with early motor and sensory deficits including sphincter disturbances, occur within a few days. Most epidural abscesses are caused by local extension of osteomyelitis or by hematogenous spread from a distant suppurative focus. The diagnosis is suggested by the clinical presentation. The CSF often has a markedly elevated protein level with mild pleocytosis. An MRI defines the extent of the epidural mass. If the dura is intact, infection rarely extends across it.

The most common causative organisms are *Staphylococcus aureus* and *Streptococcus* species. Treatment should be immediate, beginning with broad antibiotic coverage until the offending agent is identified. Specific antibiotic therapy must be continued for a prolonged period, often up to 6 weeks. Surgical drainage is necessary when neurologic deficits progress despite aggressive medical therapy. Decadron in the perioperative period is beneficial in reducing localized edema, although prolonged use can reduce the host immune response to the infection. Recovery of neurologic function is directly related to the duration and severity of impairment before treatment.

Subdural Empyema

Subdural empyema is a purulent infection of the subdural space. It accounts for approximately 25% of all intracranial infections and is usually a complication of sinusitis, meningitis, or open contamination of the subdural space at operation or after trauma.

With sinusitis, infection can spread intracranially by transcranial emissary vein thrombophlebitis. Staphylococci, streptococci, and anaerobic cocci are commonly responsible. Once the subdural space is violated, infection can spread over the convexity of the brain. The accumulation of purulent material may be sufficient to produce an intracranial mass, provoking adjacent brain swelling. The clinical result is rapid neurologic deterioration, often with lateralizing signs, coma, and death. Treatment includes craniotomy with débridement, drainage, and IV antibiotics. The source of the infection must be treated aggressively. A sinus or mastoid drainage procedure is often required if this is the source. The mortality rate from acute fulminant subdural empyema from a paranasal source remains approximately 25%.

The diagnosis of intracranial subdural empyema is made readily by CT scan but can be difficult to distinguish from subacute or chronic subdural hematoma. The mass itself may be isodense, necessitating the administration of IV contrast. Including the sinuses on the CT scan can demonstrate the source of infection. CSF analysis is rarely diagnostic, often showing nonspecific inflammatory changes. As mentioned before, CT should be performed first, especially in a patient suspected of harboring an intracranial mass.

Spinal subdural empyema is rare. It usually develops from local extension transdurally or through the arachnoid in the presence of meningitis. Spinal cord compression and transverse myelitis can develop. Treatment is emergent, consisting of surgical drainage and prolonged antibiotic administration.

Meningitis

Bacterial meningitis is an acute, purulent infection of the leptomeninges. It is manifested by fever, lethargy, headache, nausea, vomiting, and nuchal rigidity. Seizures occur in approximately 20% of patients and cranial nerve palsies in approximately 5%. Coma can develop in up to 10% of patients with missed diagnoses, heralding a poor prognosis. Untreated bacterial meningitis is almost always fatal.

A CSF Gram stain demonstrates the offending organism in 75% of cases. Cultures provide a diagnosis 90% of the time. When CSF cultures are negative despite high clinical suspicion, as in a mild case or in an incompletely treated case of meningitis, latex agglutination studies are helpful. These immunologic studies are specifically directed at *Streptococcus pneumoniae, Haemophilus influenzae,* and *Neisseria meningitidis* and are highly sensitive when an organism is present, even with negative cultures. Blood cultures may be positive and therefore helpful in the diagnosis, particularly with infections caused by *S. pneumoniae* and *N. meningitidis*. CSF pleocytosis with a preponderance of polymorphonuclear cells is typical of untreated bacterial meningitis. CSF glucose is almost always reduced, whereas the protein content is typically increased.

Meningitis that develops after a penetrating wound or a neurosurgical procedure is usually caused by staphylococcal, streptococcal, or gram-negative organisms. Meningitis occurring after closed head trauma with either a skull fracture or CSF rhinorrhea is most often caused by *S. pneumoniae*. Ventricular shunt and reservoir infections leading to meningitis are more likely due to *Staphylococcus epidermidis* or *S. aureus*.

The treatment for acute bacterial meningitis depends on the causative organism, its antibiotic sensitivity, and the primary source of infection from which the meninges were contaminated. The presumed diagnosis is made clinically, a sample of CSF is obtained by lumbar puncture, and broad-spectrum IV antibiotics are immediately started. Once culture results are available, the choice of antibiotics is changed to an appropriate single agent. Bacterial endocarditis, pneumonia, sinusitis, concurrent subdural empyema, and brain abscess are sometimes associated with meningitis. Treatment should be directed at both the meningitis and the primary source.

The extent of antibiotic penetration into the CNS varies, depending on the degree of meningeal inflammation. Intrathecal administration of those antibiotics that do not readily cross the blood–CSF barrier may be necessary (the commonly used intrathecal preparations are gentamicin and vancomycin). This is especially true when an artificial substance, such as a ventricular shunt, is present. The artificial material can make eradication of the infection extremely difficult. Shunt removal is often necessary despite IV and intrathecal antibiotic administration. Rarely, therapy can also include the use of steroids and osmotic diuretics if ICP is elevated as a result of cerebral edema or localized brain abscess.

Complications of bacterial meningitis include communicating hydrocephalus, brain abscess, subdural empyema, and subdural effusions, particularly after *H. influenzae* meningitis in infants. The risk of complications is significantly reduced by prompt, early treatment.

Brain Abscess

Brain abscess is a purulent lesion of brain tissue, beginning as a focal infection, usually in the white matter, surrounded by a typical inflammatory response. The blood–brain barrier becomes disrupted. Necrosis and liquefaction follow the acute inflammatory stage. Eventually, either the process is encapsulated by fibrous granulation tissue or the infection spreads through the parenchyma to the subarachnoid spaces and the ventricular system.

Brain abscess is usually secondary to focal infection elsewhere (Table 101.3). Abscesses that develop by direct intracranial extension are usually solitary and are typically found in the frontal and temporal lobes. Multiple brain abscesses that develop in the septic patient are often related to bacterial endocarditis, pneumonia, and diverticulitis. Cyanotic congenital heart disease with concurrent infection is a frequent source. Direct contamination of the brain through a penetrating wound, especially when accompanied by in-driven bone fragments, is another cause of abscess. Abscess formation is frequent among patients with compromised immunity from an underlying illness or pharmacologic immunosuppression (i.e., during organ transplantation).

Signs and symptoms of brain abscess are related to its mass effect. Headache, focal and neurologic deficits, and impaired mentation are often observed. There may be little or no evidence of systemic infection and the patient may be afebrile. Conversely, the patient can be gravely ill from bacteremia with fever, hypotension, and a markedly elevated white blood cell count. Seizures can occur. Progressive mass effect leads to brain shifts, followed by coma.

Contrast CT and MRI are highly accurate in detecting brain abscess and should be done before the CSF is sampled. The CSF of patients with brain abscess may be entirely normal, but usually some pleocytosis is present. The causative organism can be identified and cultured from the abscess itself in 60% to 80% of cases, provided cultures are processed carefully for both aerobic and anaerobic organisms. Blood cultures are also helpful, particularly if the abscess is secondary to systemic infection.

In cases of early abscess formation or high surgical risk, medical therapy alone with the appropriate parenteral antibiotic may be sufficient. The most effective therapy is drainage of the purulent material with simultaneous administration of appropriate IV antibiotics. Although needle aspiration can be successful, craniotomy with evacuation and removal of the abscess wall may be necessary. Surgical drainage reduces the mass effect, thereby reducing the most critical and dangerous aspect of the infection. It also allows accurate bacteriologic analysis.

Results of treatment for brain abscess depend on the patient's neurologic status on presentation, the efficacy of the antibiotic used, the extent to which the intracranial mass is controlled by surgery, and the effective treatment of the primary source of the abscess. Despite aggressive surgical and medical management, mortality rates associated with brain abscess approach 40%, especially in the malnourished, chronically debilitated, or immunosuppressed patient.

Postoperative Infection

Any or all of the pyogenic infections described earlier can develop after operation. Once identified, character-

---

Table 101.3. COMMON CAUSES, TYPICAL LOCATIONS, AND MOST LIKELY ORGANISMS INVOLVED IN THE DEVELOPMENT OF BRAIN ABSCESS

Predisposing condition	Usual location	Common organism
Otitis	Temporal lobe	Streptococcus
Mastoiditis	Subdural abscess	Bacteroides
		Haemophilus influenzae
		Gram-negative organisms
Sinusitis	Frontal lobe	Streptococcus
	Subdural abscess	Staphylococcus
Pneumonia, endocarditis, diverticulitis	Multiple brain abscesses	Various organisms (depends on source)
Penetrating wound	Site of trauma	Staphylococcus
Neurosurgical postoperative infection	Operative site	Staphylococcus

ized, and treated with appropriate antibiotics, the infection almost always subsides. Commonly isolated organisms include *S. aureus* and *S. epidermidis*. If a foreign body such as prosthetic material or a ventricular shunt is involved, eradicating the infection becomes more difficult, often requiring a combination of IV and intrathecal antibiotics with removal of the artificial material. Infrequently, infections can be satisfactorily treated in the presence of retained foreign bodies, such as a shunt, provided the infection is indolent.

Fungal Infections

As a rule, fungi are opportunistic organisms. They can become pathogenic because of depression of the host immune system, prolonged systemic antibiotic therapy, or severe systemic illness. When the CNS becomes infected, it is usually associated with pulmonary fungal infection and depressed host resistance. The CNS involvement can be a diffuse meningitis or a focal abscess. At times, multiple abscesses are present. Treatment requires long-term, systemic antifungal chemotherapy. Surgical intervention is reserved for drainage of abscesses and resection of symptomatic mass lesions. Hydrocephalus, a potential late complication, is treated with a ventricular shunt.

Parasitic Infestations

Although uncommon in North America and western Europe, parasitic diseases of the CNS are a major cause of neurologic disability and death worldwide. Control of these diseases remains a public health problem. A major emphasis is placed on their prevention, because once the CNS is infested, therapeutic options are limited. Treatment, both medical and surgical, is usually ineffective or palliative at best.

Cysticercosis

Taenia solium, the pork tapeworm, infests the human CNS by transmission of its larvae through the blood after ingestion. It is most prevalent in eastern Europe, Latin America, China, Pakistan, and India. Its presence can take one or all of four forms. Meningeal cysticercosis is characterized by parasitic vesicles throughout the basal cisterns and CSF pathways, usually with resultant hydrocephalus. Parenchymal cysticercosis diffusely involves the brain, sometimes forming large cysts. Seizures and focal deficits are common. The ventricular type resembles the meningeal form. Obstructive hydrocephalus is commonplace. Spinal cysticercosis can be intramedullary or extramedullary, producing either a transverse myelitis or a compressive myelopathy.

The diagnosis rests on serologic and radiologic testing. The presence of intracranial cysts and calcifications in skeletal muscle is often presumptive of the diagnosis. Newer anthelmintic agents can be effective, but often treatment is palliative. Anticonvulsants, CSF shunting, and occasional removal of symptomatic cysts are additional treatment options. Long-term prognosis is poor.

Echinococcosis

Hydatid disease is caused by *Echinococcus granulosus,* the dog tapeworm. It is prevalent in southern South America, northern and eastern Europe, Australia, Africa, China, and the Middle East. Humans can serve as intermediate hosts by ingesting the larvae. The liver and lungs are preferentially involved through hematogenous dissemination with subsequent formation of hydatid cysts. When the CNS is involved, cysts are usually solitary, large, and confined to white matter. There is a negligible inflammatory response.

Most cysts produce signs and symptoms related to their mass effect. Diagnosis of the infection is made serologically. CT and MRI of the brain and ultrasonography of the liver and spleen can be definitive. Chest radiographs often show calcified pulmonary cysts. Treatment consists of isolating the patient from the source and surgical removal of symptomatic cysts. Care must be taken to remove the intact cyst to avoid seeding with viable larvae. Hydatid disease of the CNS is disabling but rarely fatal if the cysts are removed when they become symptomatic.

CONGENITAL AND DEVELOPMENTAL ABNORMALITIES

Approximately 2% of newborns possess some type of congenital abnormality. Sixty percent of these involve the CNS, and over half of those are related to defective development or closure of the dorsal midline structures. Many have associated hydrocephalus. The commonly encountered neurologic malformations include the following:

- Arnold-Chiari malformation
- Dandy-Walker malformation
- Spinal dysraphism
- Meningocele
- Myelomeningocele
- Lipomyelomeningocele
- Diastematomyelia
- Dermal sinus
- Myeloschisis

Spinal Dysraphism

Between days 18 and 28 of embryonic development, the neural groove closes posteriorly in the midline to form the neural tube. This tube becomes encircled by bone derived from adjacent somites and is covered superficially by skin derived from ectoderm. Abnormal closure of the neural groove, failure of fusion of the adjacent bone, or maldevelopment of the overlying ectoderm can lead to many spinal dysraphic states. Thus, dysraphism implies an abnormal fusion of normally united parts.

Failure of the bony structures to close with normal closure of the neural groove is called *spina bifida occulta*. These patients have normal spinal cords and normal cord function. The abnormality usually goes unnoticed unless seen on plain radiographs. Should the meninges fail to close, a meningocele develops, producing an obvious cutaneous abnormality. The underlying neural structures develop normally, so there is no compromise of neurologic function.

Failure of the underlying neural tissue to fuse has been called *spina bifida cystica* or, more recently, *spina bifida aperta*. Myelomeningocele, the more common form, involves incomplete closure of the neural groove, usually in the lumbar region, with the abnormal, unfused neural tissue on the dorsal surface exposed through an associated defect in the spinal column. This can be partially or totally covered with epithelium. The accompanying neurologic deficit usually consists of complete absence of motor and sensory function below the level of spinal cord involvement.

The most severe form of spinal dysraphism is myeloschisis, which is much less common than myelomeningocele. The spinal cord is unfused and presents directly on the surface of the back without overlying meninges or epithelium. It usually occurs at the thoracolumbar region and is virtually always associated with paraplegia and absence of bladder function.

Both myelomeningocele and myeloschisis are associated with hydrocephalus. The hydrocephalus is caused by a developmental abnormality of the hindbrain called

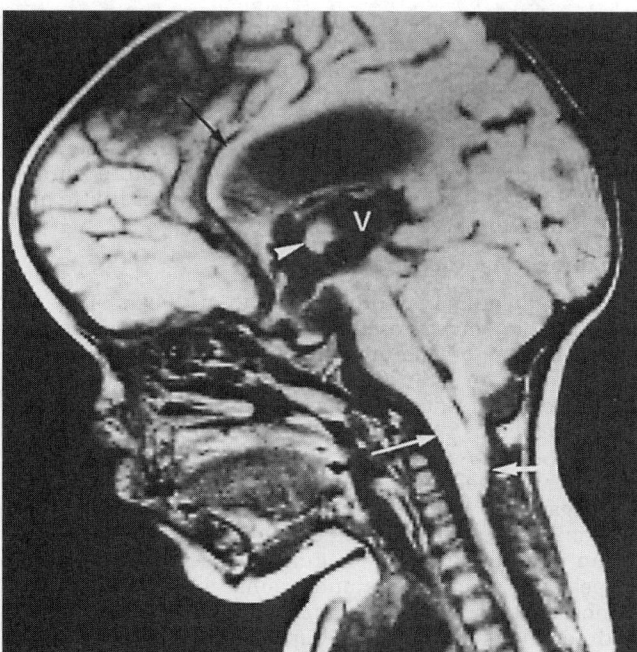

Figure 101.20. Sagittal magnetic resonance imaging scan of the brain and upper cervical spine demonstrates some of the features of the Arnold-Chiari type II malformation. Note the herniation of the cerebellum through the foramen magnum to the level of C-4 *(short arrow),* the downward displacement of the medulla and fourth ventricle *(long arrow),* the absence of the corpus callosum, the hydrocephalus with enlargement of the third ventricle (V), and the enlarged massa intermedia *(arrowhead).*

Arnold-Chiari malformation, which is associated with the more severe forms of spinal dysraphism (Fig. 101.20). This malformation consists of caudal displacement of the cerebellar tonsils, vermis, inferior fourth ventricle, and medulla. There is a dorsal kink in the cervicomedullary junction and beaking of the quadrigeminal plate. Associated features include agenesis of the corpus callosum and obstructive hydrocephalus.

The treatment of spinal dysraphism is surgical. Meningoceles are excised and the skin is closed primarily after watertight closure of the posterior meningeal defect. Myelomeningoceles and myeloschises are closed as early as possible to reduce the risk of superficial infection and subsequent meningitis. Surgical repair is usually undertaken within 36 hours. The goal is to preserve as much neural tissue as possible, to untether the spinal cord from surrounding soft tissue, and to fashion a dural closure to prevent CSF leakage. Accompanying hydrocephalus is treated with shunting (see later discussion).

Survival of infants with these dysraphic states continues to improve. Despite a devastating neurologic deficit, they usually do well. Newborns with lower-level lesions do better overall than do those with higher-level lesions. The more severe the dysraphic state, the higher the morbidity and mortality rates. Risk of sepsis from bladder infection is reduced with intermittent catheterization when indicated. Timely revision of failed shunts placed for hydrocephalus preserves the potential for intellectual development.

Cranial Dysraphism

Cranial dysraphic states are one tenth as common as their spinal counterparts. Encephaloceles, although rare, are most commonly seen. They consist of a midline skull defect through which a small portion of brain protrudes.

Most encephaloceles are covered with skin. Associated hydrocephalus occurs in up to 65% of patients with occipital encephaloceles but is uncommon in patients with anterior encephaloceles. Once thought to arise from defects in the closure of the primitive neural tube, they probably develop because of an overlying mesodermal abnormality with subsequent perturbation of underlying cerebral tissue. In North America and Europe, 85% of encephaloceles occur in the posterior cranial vault; the remainder are found in the anterior cranial vault. In Southeast Asia, this distribution is reversed for unknown reasons.

The surgical repair involves early resection of malformed and devitalized brain with dural closure. The mortality rate of patients with encephaloceles varies greatly. Prognostic factors include the size and location of the anomaly, the extent of brain protrusion, and the presence of associated hydrocephalus, seizure disorder, or cerebral dysgenesis. The smaller and more anterior defects usually have a better outcome. Whereas 83% of patients with occipital encephaloceles have significant mental and physical impairment, most patients with anterior encephaloceles have normal or near-normal intelligence.

Hydrocephalus

The term *hydrocephalus* implies an increase in the amount of CSF in the ventricular system. This is almost always due to a decrease in the absorption of fluid, although there are rare cases of choroid plexus papillomas causing hydrocephalus by an increase in CSF production. Hydrocephalus is traditionally referred to as *communicating* or *noncommunicating.* In the former, the ventricular system continues to communicate with the subarachnoid spaces outside the brain through the fourth ventricular foramina of Luschka and Magendie. In the noncommunicating type, often termed *obstructive,* it does not. The common causes of hydrocephalus vary with age and are listed here:

Congenital
- Arnold-Chiari malformation
- Dandy-Walker malformation
- Aqueductal atresia or stenosis
- Developmental cyst
- Encephalocele
- Neoplasm

Acquired
- Infectious meningitis
- Infectious ventriculitis
- Late-onset aqueductal stenosis
- Intraventricular hemorrhage
- Subarachnoid hemorrhage
- Neoplasm

Infantile Hydrocephalus

Hydrocephalus occurs most frequently between birth and 2 years of age and is most commonly due to congenital abnormalities of the brain. These abnormalities typically produce noncommunicating hydrocephalus. Stenosis of the cerebral aqueduct is one such common congenital anomaly. Another is the Arnold-Chiari malformation. The Dandy-Walker malformation produces a markedly enlarged fourth ventricle as a result of congenital obstruction of CSF outflow from the fourth ventricle, with resultant hydrocephalus. Other, less common congenital lesions include arachnoid cysts, vascular anomalies, and congenital tumors.

Acquired hydrocephalus in the infant is often the result of meningitis or intracranial hemorrhage, both potentially causing obstruction of either the CSF absorptive mechanism or the intraventricular pathways (Fig. 101.21). Aque-

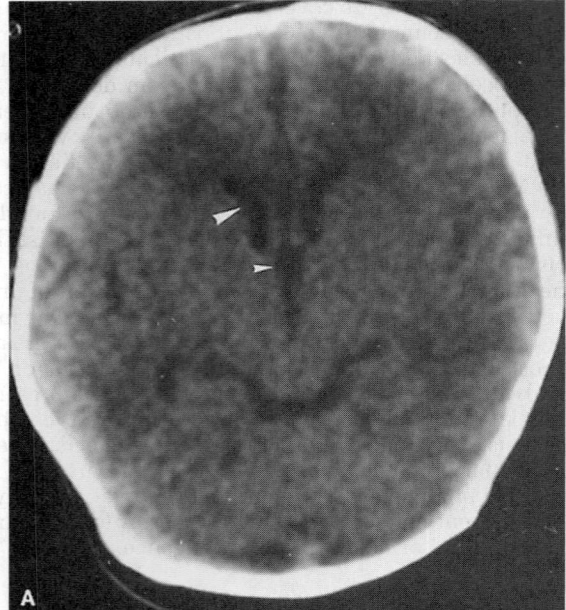

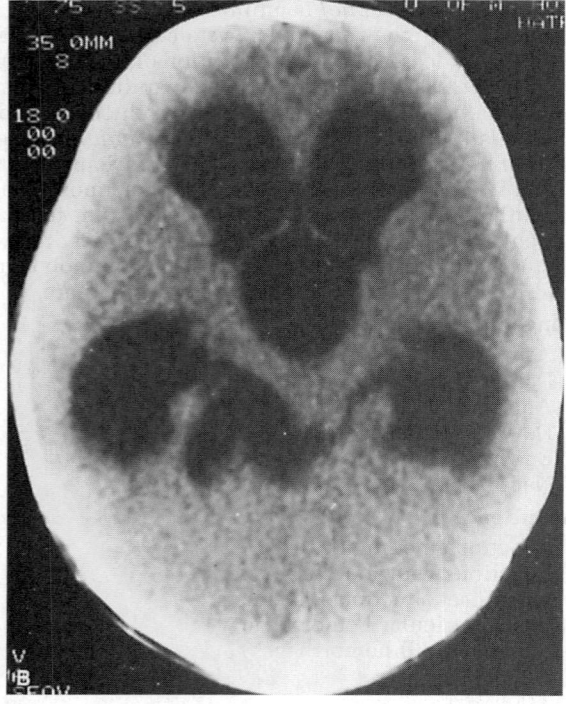

Figure 101.21. This patient had neonatal sepsis with subsequent development of meningitis. *(A)* Noncontrast computed tomography (CT) scan during the first week of life shows relatively normal third *(small arrow)* and lateral *(large arrow)* ventricles. *(B)* Well after the meningitis was cured, accelerating head growth prompted another CT scan, which demonstrates marked hydrocephalus.

ductal stenosis can develop well after birth because of infection or hemorrhage and thus is termed *acquired*. Tumors can also obstruct the outflow of CSF, resulting in noncommunicating hydrocephalus.

Infants with hydrocephalus usually but not invariably present with an enlarging head circumference. They often have a tense, bulging anterior fontanelle with distended scalp veins and split cranial sutures. They may appear to have so-called sun setting of the eyes with only the tops of the irises visible (Parinaud's syndrome). The head may transilluminate because of lack of cerebral substance. Neurologically, the hydrocephalus usually does not cause deficits initially because of the open cranial sutures that allow for cranial vault expansion (assuming absence of any underlying brain dysgenesis). In the more chronic forms, or in older infants with closed sutures, optic atrophy and sixth nerve palsies may be seen.

Childhood Hydrocephalus

Hydrocephalus in children older than 2 years of age can have a more acute presentation because of the decreased ability of the more mature brain and skull to accommodate the increase in CSF. Consequently, the raised ICP can acutely cause headache, nausea, vomiting, lethargy, coma, and even death. Slower onset can result in decreased mentation, behavioral changes, diminished performance in school, sixth nerve palsies, optic atrophy, paralysis of upward gaze, spastic leg weakness, and endocrine (hypothalamic) disorders. Causes of hydrocephalus in this age group include tumors, meningitis, intracranial hemorrhage (both spontaneous and traumatic), and aqueductal stenosis. Ventricular shunt malfunction can cause acute hydrocephalus in the shunt-dependent patient, regardless of the patient's age or the underlying cause.

Adult Hydrocephalus

Hydrocephalus in adults can also result from obstructive tumors, meningitis, and intracranial hemorrhage, but can also be more insidious in onset. An entity called *normal-pressure hydrocephalus* occurs in the older population and involves a communicating hydrocephalus with a normal intraventricular pressure. The cause remains unknown but is thought to be due to subclinical hemorrhage or infection in the patient's remote past. The classic clinical triad of Hakim includes ataxia, urinary incontinence, and cognitive decline.

Regardless of cause, the treatment of hydrocephalus is essentially the same. Either the cause must be removed (e.g., tumor) or a shunting procedure must be performed to divert accumulated CSF. Sometimes, both measures are necessary. The most commonly used procedure is a lateral ventricle to peritoneal shunt with a one-way pressure-regulating valve in the system. If the peritoneal cavity is not suitable for shunting, the distal catheter can be placed in the right atrium of the heart or, rarely, in the pleural cavity. In selected cases of communicating hydrocephalus, a lumbar subarachnoid to peritoneal shunt can be used. Common complications of indwelling shunts include shunt obstruction and infection.

Craniosynostosis

Craniosynostosis is the premature closure of one or more cranial sutures typically manifested within the first 6 months of life. Because the brain doubles in size during the first 6 months of life and grows another 50% by age 2 years, the cranial sutures must remain open to allow for skull expansion to accommodate this growth. Usually, when one suture fuses prematurely, the brain is not compressed to a deleterious degree, but the skull develops in a distinctly abnormal shape. If more sutures are fused, the brain can be damaged from restricted growth.

The sagittal suture is most commonly involved, with a male/female ratio of 4 : 1. The skull develops an elongated shape with a narrow biparietal diameter, often referred to as *scaphocephaly*. The supraorbital ridge may be square shaped as a result of overexpansion of the open metopic suture. Associated congenital anomalies are rare.

The next most common suture involved is the coronal, which can close prematurely on one or both sides. Unilateral involvement produces an asymmetrically shaped forehead with flattening on the affected side and compensatory enlargement on the opposite side. This is called *plagiocephaly* and is not usually associated with other abnormalities. Bilateral coronal synostosis produces a more severe foreshortening of the entire anterior fossa and is often manifested by shallow orbits with exophthalmos and hypertelorism. This entity is often associated with inherited congenital disorders such as Crouzon's disease and Apert's and Carpenter's syndromes.

Less common forms of craniosynostosis include premature closure of the lambdoid suture or the metopic suture. With unilateral synostosis of the lambdoid suture, the skull appears flattened in the affected occipital area, which can be confused with birth molding. With premature closure of the metopic suture, the forehead takes on a triangular shape (trigonocephaly). Neither of these forms is associated with other congenital anomalies.

The treatment of craniosynostosis is surgical and usually involves opening the affected suture along its entire length. This should be carried out as soon as possible after the diagnosis is made because early surgical intervention provides the best cosmetic result. In cases of multiple suture involvement, prompt treatment provides early skull expansion to accommodate brain growth.

STEREOTACTIC NEUROSURGERY

Stereotactic neurosurgery is a discipline devoted to spatial localization of intracranial structures. The original term *stereotaxis* is derived from the Greek *stereo* for "three-dimensional" and *taxis* for "an arrangement." Later, the term *stereotactic* was applied to human surgery, from the Latin *tactic,* for "touch." Stereotactic neurosurgery is based on the principle that any point in the brain can be referenced to a specific coordinate system using precise measurements. Most stereotactic systems are based on the cartesian coordinate system, although a polar, or spherical coordinate system is also common. A rigid frame is attached to the patient's head, and a coordinate system based on the frame is correlated with CT or MRI images of the patient's brain. Any part of the brain can thus be localized with accuracy to within millimeters. Stereotactic brain lesion biopsy is a common application. Stereotactic guidance is used to place a bur hole in an optimal location to permit passage of a needle into the lesion for a tissue sample. Stereotactic craniotomy permits optimal design of a craniotomy flap and access to underlying tumors or other lesions. Stereotactic guidance is also used for a variety of functional neurosurgery procedures, discussed later.

Frameless stereotactic navigation is a recently developed technique that obviates the need for a frame. Preacquired CT or MRI brain images are reconstructed into a three-dimensional image in a computer in the operating room. A variety of recognizable landmarks on the patient's head, such as the ears, nose, and other facial features, are used as fiducials. These fiducials are registered with the computer using signal emitters (typically light or ultrasonic pulse generators) and a camera positioned near the operating room table to monitor the signals. The system triangulates between the patient, a reference area containing a set of signal emitters, and a hand-held instrument that also contains a set of signal emitters. The position of the hand-held instrument appears on the three-dimensional computer image of the patient. This system allows planning of the operation based on the three-dimensional image of the patient, and assistance with navigation as the operation proceeds. Frameless stereotactic techniques are

also useful in spinal surgery to permit precise placement of instrumentation.

Stereotactic radiosurgery is a technique for producing sharply delimited lesions in the brain by focusing multiple external sources of radiation on a single target. It is based on the principle that a large number of low-radiation beams traveling through normal brain tissue from a variety of angles can deliver a high dose of radiation to the region where the beams converge, putting the surrounding normal brain at minimal risk of radiation injury. Radiosurgery uses a frame-based stereotactic system to plan delivery of a single dose of radiation to a well defined target. Radiosurgery is noninvasive and a useful adjunct for management of a variety of tumors and vascular malformations when standard craniotomy and resection of the lesion is hazardous or impossible. Limitations of radiosurgery include the treatable lesion size and the time required for ablation of the lesion. For instance, AVMs less than 15 mm in diameter have a 94% obliteration rate, whereas AVMs larger than 25 mm in diameter have a 32% obliteration rate. The time required for ablation of an AVM after radiosurgery is 1 to 2 years; during this time, the patient continues to be at risk of hemorrhage.

FUNCTIONAL NEUROSURGERY

Functional neurosurgery involves operations to alter the function of the CNS. The most common uses are for the treatment of pain syndromes, epilepsy, and movement disorders.

Neurosurgical Management of Pain

Most neurosurgical patients have pain either as their primary complaint or as a secondary manifestation of their disease process (2). These painful conditions can be categorized as acute processes, such as arm pain from a herniated cervical disc, or chronic processes, such as extremity pain from an invasive neoplasm. For most acute pain states, the cause can be identified and treated, but for chronic pain there often is no ready solution. The more common neurosurgical procedures available to manage chronic pain are described here.

At one time, the perception of pain was thought to involve a simple system of pathways extending from the peripheral receptors to the brain. It has subsequently been shown that this system is a complex network of pathways, with a considerable amount of modification at multiple synaptic levels. Impulses from pain receptors reach the spinal cord by way of the dorsal root ganglion and can receive significant modification in the various laminae of the dorsal horn. This information is then relayed to the thalamus but again can undergo considerable modification in the area of the brain stem reticular formation. This sensory input is subsequently relayed to the cortex for conscious interpretation. Modifiers in this complex system include the endogenous substances labeled *endorphins, enkephalins,* and *substance P.* In addition, the psychological state of the patient influences the perception of painful stimuli.

Traditionally, neurosurgical procedures for chronic pain have been ablative or destructive, but many neuromodulating or neurostimulating procedures have been developed. These procedures are usually reserved for those chronic pain conditions that medical therapy has failed to alleviate.

Cranial Nerves

Trigeminal neuralgia (tic douloureux) is one of the most common neuropathic conditions. It presents as an intermittent, shocklike pain in one or more divisions of one trigeminal nerve. It typically involves the second (maxillary) or third (mandibular) divisions of the nerve, or both, and rarely is bilateral. The pain usually lasts for seconds, is severe, and can be incapacitating. It is often triggered by touching the face, talking, or chewing. The pain can be present for weeks or months and then spontaneously disappear, only to return with increased severity. Most patients can be initially controlled with phenytoin or carbamazepine, but eventually many require surgical intervention. A small percentage of patients can have a posterior fossa tumor causing the pain, so evaluation should include a CT or MRI scan before therapy.

In the past, surgical treatment involved ablation of the involved branches of the trigeminal nerve. This was accomplished peripherally by surgical section or alcohol ablation of the supraorbital, infraorbital, or inferior alveolar nerves. Pain control through these neurectomies was usually short-lived. Experience found that preganglionic lesions must be made for more permanent relief. Retrogasserian rhizotomy can be carried out by open surgical approaches subtemporally or through the posterior fossa, or percutaneously by placing a radiofrequency electrode through the foramen ovale. Percutaneous rhizolysis is safe, effective, and widely used. If performed properly, it has the advantage of destroying pain fibers only, leaving a variable amount of touch sensation intact.

A popular nonablative approach involves microvascular decompression of the trigeminal nerve in the posterior fossa. The theory behind this approach is that trigeminal neuralgia is caused by external pressure on the nerve by vascular structures (an artery or vein) near its entry into the brain stem. With use of the operating microscope, the offending artery can be moved or the vein ablated, thus decompressing the nerve. This procedure has a higher success rate and a longer duration of symptomatic relief than the percutaneous method, but carries more risk. An advantage is that the nerve's function remains intact.

Glossopharyngeal neuralgia is similar to trigeminal neuralgia, but much less common. Symptoms consist of lancinating, paroxysmal pain most commonly in the throat and at the base of the tongue, with occasional extension to the ear and the deep regions of the mandible and neck. Pain can be triggered by swallowing, chewing, or talking. Medical therapy is the same as that for trigeminal neuralgia. Should this fail, surgical intervention is warranted. The classic approach involves sectioning the intracranial portion of the glossopharyngeal nerve and the two superior bundles of the vagus nerve by use of a suboccipital craniectomy. Microvascular decompression has also been used with success.

Spinal Cord

As with other surgical procedures for chronic pain, those involving the spinal cord have traditionally been ablative. Cordotomy, designed to obliterate the spinothalamic tract, can be performed openly or percutaneously. If the upper extremity is involved, the open technique can be achieved posteriorly through a cervical laminectomy or anteriorly through a discectomy. After gentle rotation of the spinal cord, the anterior quadrant containing the spinothalamic tract is sectioned. If the upper extremity is not involved, spinothalamic tractotomy is performed through a thoracic laminectomy. A reliable percutaneous method is available and reduces the operative risk in these often very ill patients. This method creates a functional cordotomy at the C-1 to C-2 level with a radiofrequency lesion generator. Anterolateral cordotomy can provide excellent temporary relief of pain for patients with terminal malignancies, but it is rarely effective for chronic benign

conditions such as low back, postherpetic, or phantom limb pain.

For selected cases of severe pain of peripheral nerve origin, such as brachial plexus injury, postherpetic neuralgia, traumatic limb amputation, and root avulsion, ablative lesions can be made at the dorsal root entry zones of the spinal cord (Fig. 101.22). These lesions are made with a radiofrequency lesion generator or laser through an open exposure of the cord by use of a laminectomy. Several levels are usually included. An effective result is obtained in 80% to 90% of patients.

Intrathecal morphine can also be given temporarily or permanently by infusion of minute but effective doses. This method of pain control is particularly effective in debilitated patients with terminal illnesses. The procedure involves the subcutaneous implantation of a constant infusion pump that can be recharged periodically. Morphine is delivered by this device into the CSF in small amounts sufficient to control severe pain.

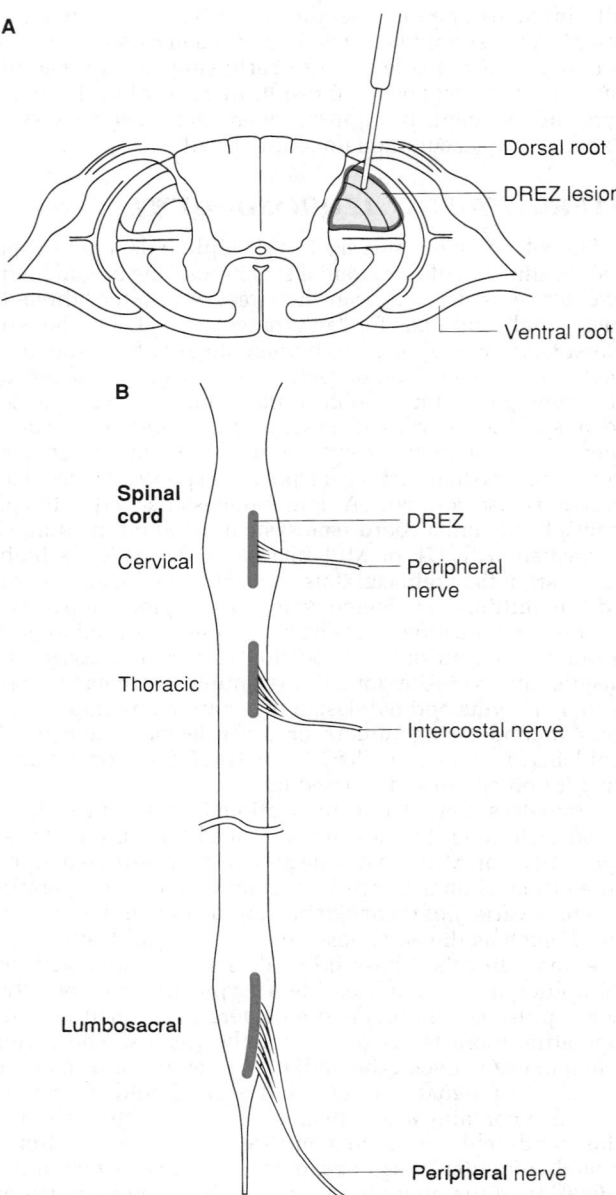

Figure 101.22. Location of dorsal root entry zone for placement of dorsal root entry zone (DREZ) lesion.

In chronic nonmalignant pain conditions, such as failed back syndrome, reflex sympathetic dystrophy, and phantom limb pain, spinal cord stimulation can be effective. This nonablative neuromodulation technique involves direct stimulation of the dorsal surface of the spinal cord. Electrodes are placed percutaneously to lie within the dura, over the dorsal surface of the spinal cord. An impulse generator is placed subcutaneously in the flank or abdominal region. The precise mechanism of action for spinal cord stimulation is not understood, but is thought to involve activation of inhibitory pathways in the spinal cord that suppress conduction of pain impulses.

Peripheral Nerve

Many chronic painful states can arise from peripheral nerve or major plexus injuries. Fortunately, these painful conditions are rare, but when they do occur, they can be persistent and disabling. Pain from a partial or complete nerve injury usually involves the sensory distribution of the nerve but can include the whole extremity. Chronic pain developing after an amputation can be present in the remaining portion of the limb at the site of the amputation (stump pain) or in the nonexistent amputated portion (phantom pain). The cause of the pain can be related to the sensory component of the nerve or to its associated sympathetic nerve supply.

With partial or complete peripheral nerve transection, a painful neuroma can form. A neuroma is a mass of misdirected axons that can develop from an injured nerve's attempt to regenerate. These axons can become sensitive to external stimuli or they can generate spontaneous pain. The usual treatment is excision of the neuroma, with prevention of recurrent formation by burying the nerve end in bone or muscle or by wrapping it in tantalum or Silastic. Neuromodulation techniques can also be applied in cases of painful neuromas. These include transcutaneous stimulation, as described earlier, and implanted devices that directly stimulate the proximal nerve.

Chronic pain resulting from peripheral nerve injury can be significantly altered by interruption of the sympathetic nerve supply to the affected extremity. The classic example of this dysautonomic state is major causalgia. This term implies a partial injury to a major nerve in an extremity. Minor causalgia is reserved for an injury to a more distal minor sensory nerve, which can also become a source of significant pain. It is also well recognized that a dysautonomic state can be created by major or minor trauma to an extremity that does not involve a peripheral nerve. These have been labeled *major* and *minor traumatic dystrophies.* The entire collection of causalgias and traumatic dystrophies makes up a syndrome termed *reflex sympathetic dystrophy.*

Major causalgia is most commonly related to partial injury of the sciatic or median nerves. Typically, symptoms begin in the affected nerve's distribution but can progress to involve the whole extremity. The extremity first becomes swollen, warm, erythematous, and sensitive to touch. With time, it becomes cool and pale. Hyperhidrosis (excessive sweating) can follow. Because of the lack of joint motion, the normal flexion and extension creases disappear and the skin becomes smooth and flat. Plain radiographs may demonstrate osteoporosis. Eventually, the extremity can become completely useless. A constant, burning pain develops and persists throughout these various stages. It can be exacerbated by touching or moving the extremity. Temperature changes and emotional stress can trigger worsening of the pain. Minor causalgia and the traumatic dystrophies can be accompanied by similar but less severe symptoms.

The treatment of these dysautonomic states is complex. They can be helped by disruption of the sympathetic nerve supply to the extremity. This can be accomplished temporarily with a chemical sympathectomy by use of a local anesthetic, or permanently by a surgical sympathectomy. Usually, numerous local blocks are performed initially. If these are successful, a surgical sympathectomy is performed. Sympatholytic drugs such as phenoxybenzamine can be tried, but they are rarely useful for chronic relief. Transcutaneous stimulation can be helpful but is rarely curative. Sympathetic denervation can be rewarding in major causalgia but less so in minor causalgia and the traumatic dystrophies.

Less severe and more easily treated pain can arise from chronic compression of selected peripheral nerves. The most common are compression of the median nerve at the wrist (carpal tunnel syndrome) and compression of the ulnar nerve at the elbow. Chronic compression can result in pain, paresthesias, numbness, and eventually weakness and atrophy of muscles in the distribution of the affected nerve. These compression syndromes are diagnosed clinically and confirmed by finding denervation and slowed nerve conduction on EMG and nerve conduction velocity testing. Treatment is surgical decompression of the involved nerve, with prompt and long-lasting relief in most cases.

Epilepsy

Approximately two million people in the United States have epilepsy. Seizures can usually be categorized as either generalized, characterized by loss of consciousness with tonic-clonic movements, or partial, manifested by involuntary movements but no loss of consciousness. Most seizure disorders are idiopathic; known causes of epilepsy include congenital anomalies, traumatic brain injury, vascular lesions, infection, and tumors. Mesial temporal sclerosis, involving atrophy and cell loss in the hippocampus, is a common cause of epilepsy in adults. In the developing world, cysticercosis is a leading cause of epilepsy.

Medical management of epilepsy is successful for approximately 70% of patients. Patients with symptomatic epilepsy despite anticonvulsant medication are potential candidates for surgery. The goal of most surgery for seizure disorders is to resect the area of brain responsible for generating or propagating epileptic activity. Therefore, the preoperative work-up of a patient with medically refractory epilepsy must identify the seizure focus, as well as regions of the brain that subserve language, vision, and sensory or motor functions (eloquent cortex).

A number of brain imaging and testing modalities have been introduced that assist with patient selection and operative planning in epilepsy surgery. Electroencephalography, both interictal and long-term (inpatient) monitoring, can help localize the seizure focus. CT and MRI can identify brain lesions that may be epileptogenic. Cerebral angiography in which sodium amobarbital is injected selectively into either the left or right hemisphere, followed by language testing (Wada test), can identify the side of language dominance. Positron emission tomography scanning can be useful for localizing the seizure focus, and functional MRI can help identify eloquent cortex. Invasive monitoring techniques include stereotactically placed hippocampal depth electrodes and subdural electrodes placed through a bur hole.

Epilepsy surgery is often done with the patient awake, under local anesthesia. This permits further localization of the seizure focus and eloquent cortex. Electrocorticography is similar to electroencephalography except that it is done directly on the cortex. Stimulation mapping, in which a stimulating electrode is applied to the surface of the brain, is particularly useful for identifying language areas. The most common surgical procedure for epilepsy is resection of the anterior part of the temporal lobe, which is effective for epilepsy secondary to mesial temporal sclerosis or other temporal lobe lesions. Other procedures include cortical resections in other areas, corpus callosotomy, hemispherectomy, multiple subpial resections, and vagal nerve stimulation. Seizure foci in eloquent cortex can be treated with multiple subpial transections; this procedure is based on the observation that mammalian cortex is organized in a columnar, or vertical fashion. Propagation of seizures can be suppressed while sparing cortical function by limited transection of horizontal intercolumnar subpial fibers. Vagal nerve stimulation, involving placement of an electrode in contact with the left vagus nerve and powered by an implanted subcutaneous pulse generator, can be effective for patients with refractory partial seizures. The mechanism for suppression of seizures is unknown.

Approximately two thirds of patients with temporal lobe epilepsy are seizure free after temporal lobectomy, and one fourth are improved in terms of seizure frequency or intensity. Vagal nerve stimulation is most effective at reducing seizure frequency; 50% of patients report at least a 50% reduction in seizures. The results of other epilepsy operations vary widely with type of seizure disorder, location of seizure focus, and etiology.

Movement Disorders

The basal ganglia are a complex group of subcortical nuclei that are concerned with control of motor function: organization and execution as well as learning and cognition related to movement. Movement disorders are disorders of motor control that manifest primarily as tremor, athetosis (slow, writhing movements of the extremities), chorea (abrupt movements of the limbs and facial muscles), ballism (violent, flailing movements), and dystonia (persistent, distorted posture). Most movement disorders are referable to a lesion in the basal ganglia. The prototypical movement disorder is Parkinson's disease (PD). In PD, selective degeneration of dopaminergic neurons in the substantia nigra leads to an imbalance of inhibitory and excitatory circuits in the basal ganglia, and the characteristic symptom complex of tremor, rigidity, and slowness of movement. Other disorders of the basal ganglia include Huntington's disease, which is typified by chorea, decreased muscle tone, and dementia; hemiballismus, in which damage to the subthalamic nucleus causes severe involuntary movement; and tardive dyskinesia, in which an acquired hypersensitivity to dopamine in the basal ganglia leads to abnormal involuntary movements. A common movement disorder that is not identified with a known basal ganglia abnormality is essential tremor, an idiopathic kinetic tremor syndrome.

Medical treatment is effective for most patients with movement disorders. Levodopa or dopamine agonists relieve the symptoms of PD; propranolol is efficacious for essential tremor. Some patients with debilitating movement disorders can obtain improvement with stereotactic

ablative procedures. More recently, deep brain stimulation has been shown to be effective for some movement disorders.

Surgery for movement disorders began with a variety of ablation procedures, including lesioning of the motor cortex and sectioning of corticospinal tracts in the cerebral peduncles (pedunculotomy) and spinal cord (cordotomy). In 1952, Cooper inadvertently tore the anterior choroidal artery while attempting to perform a pedunculotomy in a patient with PD. Cooper abandoned the pedunculotomy in that case, but found after surgery that the patient had reduced tremor and rigidity without hemiparesis. Later anatomic studies showed that the infarction resulting from occlusion of the anterior choroidal artery involves multiple areas of the basal ganglia. These findings led to ablative procedures of the basal ganglia, first by open craniotomy, then by a stereotactic approach. Several decades of experience with stereotactic treatment of movement disorders has led to a refinement of both patient selection and operative technique.

Stereotactic pallidotomy, consisting of making a radiofrequency lesion in the globus pallidus, can be effective in treating rigidity, dystonia, choreoathetosis, and hemiballismus. Thalamotomy, with lesioning of the ventral intermediate nucleus of the thalamus (Vim), is useful for the treatment of tremor. Patients for whom tremor is the primary feature of their movement disorder, such as some patients with PD, essential tremor, and intention tremor associated with multiple sclerosis, are potential candidates for thalamotomy. More recently, deep brain stimulation for movement disorders has been used. Thalamic stimulation for tremor is the most common. An electrode implanted in the Vim and powered by a subcutaneous pulse generator can deliver stimulation in a variety of amplitudes, pulse widths, and frequencies. These stimulation parameters can be fine-tuned to optimize treatment of the patient's symptoms.

BIBLIOGRAPHY

1. Apuzzo MLJ. *Brain injury: complications, avoidance, and management.* New York: Churchill Livingstone, 1993:2365.
2. Narayan RK, Wilberger JE Jr, Povlishock JT, eds. *Neurotrauma.* New York: McGraw-Hill, 1995.
3. The Brain Trauma Foundation. *Guidelines for the management of severe head injury.* Park Ridge, IL: American Association of Neurological Surgeons, 1995.
4. Menezes AH, Sonntag VKH, Benzel EC, et al., eds. *Principles of spinal surgery.* New York: McGraw-Hill, 1996.
5. Russell DS, Rubinstein LJ. *Pathology of tumors of the nervous system,* 5th ed. Baltimore: Williams & Wilkins, 1989.
6. Greenberg HS, Chandler WF, Sandler HM, eds. *Brain tumors.* New York: Oxford University Press, 1999.
7. Crockard A, Hayward R, Hoff JT, eds. *Neurosurgery: the scientific basis of clinical practice,* 3rd ed. Boston: Blackwell Scientific, 1999.
8. Batjer HH, Caplan LR, Friberg L, et al., eds. *Cerebrovascular disease.* Philadelphia: Lippincott–Raven, 1997.
9. Albright AL, Pollack IF, Adelson PD, eds. *Principles and practice of pediatric neurosurgery.* New York: Thieme, 1999.
10. Gildenberg PL, Tasker RR, eds. *Textbook of stereotactic and functional neurosurgery.* New York: McGraw-Hill, 1998.

SECTION R

GENITOURINARY SYSTEM

SURGERY: SCIENTIFIC PRINCIPLES AND PRACTICE, Third Edition, edited by
Lazar J. Greenfield, Michael W. Mulholland, Keith T. Oldham, Gerald B. Zelenock,
and Keith D. Lillemoe. Lippincott Williams & Wilkins Publishers, Philadelphia, © 2001.

CHAPTER 102

MALE ANATOMY AND PHYSIOLOGY

ARTHUR L. BURNETT, RONALD RODRIGUEZ,
AND THOMAS W. JARRETT

This chapter serves as a basic introduction to clinical disorders of the male genitourinary system. As a framework for understanding their causes and characteristics, the principles of normal genitourinary anatomy and physiology are initially discussed. Next, common disease states are presented with particular emphasis placed on diagnosis and treatment.

LOWER URINARY TRACT

The lower urinary tract refers to the urinary bladder and outlet region of the anterior pelvis, which carry out the orderly functions of urine collection and elimination. Discrete anatomic structures include the distal ureter, bladder, ureterovesical junction, trigone, prostate, external urinary sphincter, and anterior urethra. The lower urinary tract also functionally relates to pelvic floor supporting structures.

The bladder is superbly designed for storage and expulsive functions. With an adult capacity of approximately 500 mL, this spheroid organ is designed as follows: an interior lining of transitional epithelium as much as six cells thick resting on a basement membrane; a surrounding layer of fibroelastic connective tissue termed *lamina propria* and *muscularis mucosae* that mainly permits the passive filling of the bladder; and an exterior bladder wall consisting of an inner longitudinal, middle circular, and outer longitudinal detrusor muscle arrangement that ideally suits the emptying properties of the organ.

At the bladder neck, the radially oriented inner longitudinal fibers form the inner longitudinal layer of the smooth muscle of the urethra. The middle layer forms a circular preprostatic sphincter, so called because it is more robust in the man than the woman, and is thought to provide urinary continence at the level of the bladder neck. The outer longitudinal fibers form a thick backboard posteriorly at the bladder base with the lateral fibers encircling the bladder neck and contributing to the continence mechanism. This backboard supports the trigone, a triangular, essentially nondeformable portion of the bladder bounded by the two ureteral orifices and the internal urethral meatus.

The ovoid (~3 cm on the long axis) prostate is situated at the bladder base and encircles the urethra; the base abuts the bladder neck proximally and the apex is continuous with the striated urethral sphincter distally. Situated distally to the prostate and ending at the perineal membrane is the membranous urethra, spanning approximately 2.5 cm in length. This location represents the primary region of urinary continence, structurally associated with a surrounding tubular sleeve of musculature identified as the striated external urinary sphincter. Further distally, the anterior urethra, consisting of a proximal bulbar portion and a distal pendulous portion, provides a conduit for the passage of urine from the body. The anterior urethra is formed by smooth muscle and a urothelial lining that changes from transitional epithelium to nonkeratinized stratified squamous epithelium along its course toward the external urethral meatus.

The normal physiologic function of the lower urinary tract is to contain urine in the bladder after its drainage from the upper urinary tracts and, on command and on proper social occasions, to empty urine completely from the bladder with only a low resistance to its passage. Both autonomic and somatic nervous system mechanisms, involving central and peripheral pathways, control these functions (1). Although these mechanisms are extensive and still incompletely known, the basic central regulation of micturition occurs at the cerebral cortex, with inhibitory control of reflexive voiding involving the pontine micturition center (2). At the peripheral level, bladder emptying is mediated by excitatory cholinergic innervation of the bladder, with effects exerted principally by acetylcholine released from local nerve terminals that act on postjunctional muscarinic receptors. Adrenergic innervation characterizes the predominant nervous system control of the bladder neck and urethra. α-Adrenergic receptors are activated by the local neuronal release of norepinephrine and mediate contraction of smooth muscle in the urethra, thereby contributing to closure during bladder filling. However, this classic definition of lower urinary tract neurotransmission is undergoing modification with the more recent findings that nonadrenergic, noncholinergic factors such as nitric oxide and sensory neurotransmitters contribute significantly to control of lower urinary tract function.

Obstructive Uropathy

A wide variety of conditions associated with symptoms of urinary obstruction or bladder irritability result from structural, biochemical, and functional changes of the lower urinary tract. Benign prostatic hyperplasia (BPH) is understood to be the most common cause of anatomic bladder outlet obstruction in men older than 50 years of age. Autopsy studies have shown that 50% to 60% of men older than 50 years have significant benign enlargement of the prostate, with a prevalence proportionate to increasing age (3). However, in clinical practice, symptoms experienced by older men are not always caused by an obstructive prostate but may reflect other age-related phenomena of the structural components of the lower urinary tract. Assorted other conditions may also be associated with symptoms of bladder outlet obstruction in the man, including urethral stricture disease, prostate cancer, neurogenic bladder, bladder calculus, prostatitis, bladder neck contracture, and bladder cancer. Functional obstruction is a consequence of such nonanatomic disorders as chronic bladder overdistention, debilitating disease, psychogenic retention, or side effects of medication.

Diagnosis

History and physical examination combined with appropriate laboratory testing represent the cornerstone of diagnosis. Bladder outlet obstruction is characterized by symptoms of urinary hesitancy, diminished force and caliber of the urinary stream, intermittency, sensation of incomplete emptying, and postmicturition dribbling. The symptoms of urinary frequency, urgency, and nocturia are experienced as the bladder attempts to compensate for the obstruction, resulting in a diminished functional bladder capacity, bladder muscle hypertrophy, and bladder instability. Bladder decompensation develops over time, producing such complications as residual urine, infection, hematuria, hydronephrosis, and renal failure.

Certain typical features revealed during history taking may suggest the etiology of urinary obstruction. Patients with urethral stricture usually have a history of prior urethral trauma, instrumentation, or infection. Those with advanced prostate cancer may present with obstructive urinary symptoms, along with back or bone pain, anorexia, or weight loss. Patients with a neurogenic bladder often exhibit other symptoms of neurologic disease, including concomitant bowel or sexual dysfunction, or present with known neurologic diseases or injuries that regularly cause bladder dysfunction, such as diabetes mellitus, stroke, multiple sclerosis, and spinal cord injury. Medications should be reviewed in all patients to discern whether any may be associated with voiding dysfunction (Table 102.1). Agents that depress bladder muscle contractility (e.g., anticholinergic agents, antispasmodic drugs, and antidepressant drugs) or increase bladder outlet resistance (e.g., sympathomimetics) are known to disturb normal micturition.

During physical examination of the patient with symptoms of bladder outlet obstruction, the clinician should be alert for abdominal, genital, rectal, and neurologic abnormalities suggestive of the extent and possible cause of the problem. Preliminary laboratory testing may include uri-

nalysis, urine culture (if pyuria is present), and measurement of serum creatinine. A prostate-specific antigen (PSA) test has been recommended to screen for an elevated level that might warrant prostate biopsy to exclude a prostate cancer diagnosis (4). The urinary flow rate, represented by the amount of urine voided during a timed period, is a simple, valuable tool; normal men have 5-second volumes exceeding 75 mL, whereas men with urinary obstruction have flows less than 50 mL in 5 seconds. More extensive tests may be done as part of a urologic investigation if significant complications such as hematuria, urinary tract infection, or renal failure are confirmed or if an invasive therapy is considered. Available diagnostic tests include intravenous urography (IVU) or renal ultrasonography to evaluate the upper urinary tracts, bladder catheterization for postmicturition volume, cystourethroscopy to visualize directly the lower urinary tract, and cystometrography to assess the function of the bladder and urinary outlet during filling and emptying phases of the micturition cycle. Symptomatic urinary obstruction alone does not require specialized testing, particularly if a nonsurgical, reversible intervention with surveillance is planned.

Treatment

The management of BPH has rapidly expanded in recent years to include a variety of medical and surgical options. Both surgical prostatectomy (i.e., transurethral resection of the prostate) or open surgical enucleation of adenomatous tissue through suprapubic, retropubic, or perineal incisions have been long available and remain the standard interventions in the setting of significant anatomic urinary obstruction with risks of bladder decompensation. The preferred approach follows an assessment of the condition of the patient and the size and configuration of the prostate gland. Novel, alternative surgical therapies include transurethral microwave thermotherapy, transurethral needle ablation, interstitial laser coagulation, transurethral incision of the prostate, and intraprostatic stent insertion. U.S. Food and Drug Administration approval has been given to medications that appear increasingly attractive to use particularly when lower urinary tract symptoms provide the primary indication for intervention. These include α_1-adrenergic blockers (e.g., doxazosin, terazosin, and tamsulosin) and 5-α-reductase inhibitors (e.g., finasteride), which may be alternatively offered depending on patient desires and clinical circumstances. Interest in alternative medical therapies has led to increasing public use of phytotherapeutic agents such as saw palmetto to treat lower urinary tract symptoms, although their actual efficacies remain unknown without the completion of appropriate clinical trials.

Urethral stricture disease may be treated with urethral dilatation, transurethral incision, urethral stent insertion, or open urethral reconstructive surgery. The selected approach usually depends on the severity and location of the stricture and the patient's overall health and expected longevity. Other anatomic abnormalities such as bladder calculus or bladder neck contracture are commonly managed with transurethral surgical techniques. The neurogenic bladder is primarily managed by intermittent catheterization, although sphincterotomy, vesicostomy, suprapubic or urethral catheterization, or urinary diversion (i.e., surgical reconstruction using bowel segments to drain the urinary system) has been applied in certain situations.

Prostatitis

Prostatitis is commonly identified as an inflammatory condition of the prostate, although its reference may be

---

Table 102.1. PHARMACOLOGIC AGENTS WITH KNOWN INFLUENCE ON BLADDER FUNCTION

DRUGS THAT INCREASE BLADDER TONE AND CONTRACTILITY
  Bethanecol (Urecholine)
DRUGS THAT DECREASE BLADDER CONTRACTILITY
  Anticholinergic drugs (e.g., propantheline, belladonna, oxybutynin, tolterodine)
  Calcium antagonists (e.g., verapamil, nifedipine, diltiazem)
  Prostaglandin inhibitors (e.g., ibuprofen)
  Tricyclic antidepressants (e.g., imipramine, nortriptyline)
  Beta adrenergic agonists (e.g., terbutaline)
DRUGS THAT INCREASE BLADDER OUTLET RESISTANCE
  β-Sympathomimetic drugs (e.g., ephedrine, phenylpropanolamine, Ornade)
  β-Adrenergic antagonists (e.g., propranolol)
  Estrogens
DRUGS THAT DECREASE OUTLET RESISTANCE
  α-Adrenergic antagonists (e.g., terazosin, doxazosin, tamsulosin)
  Antispasticity drugs (e.g., diazepam, baclofen)

more broadly associated with a symptom complex characterized by pain in the pelvic or perineal region combined with variable voiding. It is the most common urologic diagnosis in men younger than 50 years of age (5), with prevalence estimates that range from 5% to 8.8% (6). Categories of prostatitis derive from the National Institutes of Health classification system (7): acute bacterial prostatitis, a relatively rare diagnosis involving an acute infection of the prostate gland; chronic bacterial prostatitis, a frequent, chronic condition that results from recurrent infection of the prostate; and chronic abacterial prostatitis, otherwise termed *chronic pelvic pain syndrome* or *prostatodynia,* which describes chronic symptoms in the absence of demonstrable prostatic infection. Evidence suggests that some men with symptoms of chronic prostatitis may actually carry the diagnosis of interstitial cystitis (i.e., bladder condition characterized by severe pain and urinary frequency and considered to have a female predominance) (8).

Diagnosis

Clinical diagnosis largely hinges on recognition of symptoms. Pain sensations may be associated with the perineal region, although localizations also include the suprapubic, scrotal, penile, or lower back regions. Voiding symptoms of variable degree include urinary urgency, nocturia, weak urinary stream, frequency, dysuria, hesitancy, dribbling after micturition, and interrupted urinary flow. Acute prostatitis can usually be confirmed by a positive voided urine culture showing typically gram-negative organisms. Among the chronic forms of prostatitis, distinction is made by demonstration of a positive bacterial culture of expressed prostatic secretions in the bacterial form. The cause of abacterial prostatitis is unclear, but autoimmunity may be involved (9).

Treatment

Treatment is aimed at relieving symptoms and eliminating documented infection. Systemically administered antimicrobial drugs are routinely offered, directed toward either a known positive culture or otherwise suspected prostatic pathogen. The most appropriate antibiotics are the fluoroquinolones, trimethoprim (or trimethoprim–sulfamethoxazole), carbenicillin, and doxycycline. For chronic bacterial prostatitis, treatment may extend for 8 to 12 weeks. A 50% cure rate is generally expected with this form of treatment, whereas patients with relapsing or refractory prostatitis should be considered for ancillary investigations such as urinary cytology, cystoscopy, transrectal ultrasound, and urodynamics to exclude masquerading urologic conditions ranging from a bladder malignancy to interstitial cystitis. After a negative evaluation, low-dose antibiotic prophylaxis may be offered for frequently recurrent episodes. Antimicrobial therapy is often empirically given for 8 to 12 weeks in cases of chronic abacterial prostatitis. These patients may respond in the presence of a nonculturable infectious process. In others, therapy may then extend to α_1-adrenergic blocker medications or amitriptyline, which have been shown to relieve sympathetically maintained genitourinary pain syndromes, or antiinflammatories or analgesics (10). Some experts have also recommended muscle relaxants such as diazepam, prostatic massage, sitz baths, and biofeedback (training the patient to contract and relax the pelvic floor muscles to interrupt the myofascial pain attacks), although the roles of these therapies remain unproved. Transurethral surgeries such as prostate resection or microwave thermotherapy and even radical prostatectomy have been applied, although these are considered options of last resort.

Urinary Incontinence

Urinary incontinence, more accurately understood as a symptom rather than an actual diagnosis, refers to the involuntary loss of urine through the external urethral meatus. The term generally excludes rare congenital anomalies and fistulae, in which involuntary urine loss may also occur. The condition most commonly affects women, with a prevalence as high as 10% to 20% of women between 15 and 64 years of age (11). American men also experience urinary incontinence, in the range of 1.5% to 5% for the similar age range. In elderly people (i.e., >60 years of age), the incontinence prevalence rates approximately double (12). Stress urinary incontinence is commonly associated with anatomic deformities or disorders of either urethral sphincteric support or closure. In women, underlying factors include postpartum structural effects, postmenopausal tissue atrophy, and prior surgical trauma. In men, local trauma, as seen after prostatectomy, can compromise urethral sphincteric closure, and is classified as type III stress urinary incontinence or intrinsic sphincteric deficiency. Clinical history, cystoscopic evaluation, and urodynamic measurement of sphincteric integrity usually suffice to make the diagnosis. Treatment options in men typically include pelvic floor strengthening exercises, administration of sympathomimetic agents, transurethral collagen injections, and artificial urinary sphincter implantation.

Another form of urinary incontinence known as urge urinary incontinence usually pertains to involuntary urine loss associated with an overactive bladder disorder. Unstable bladder contractions and poor bladder storage function are characteristic features of the disorder. Known causes include various neurologic disorders, urinary tract infection, urethral obstruction, bladder calculus, and bladder or prostate carcinoma, although in many instances an underlying cause cannot be found. Classic irritative voiding symptoms such as urinary frequency and urgency may accompany urge urinary incontinence. The diagnosis is determined by clinical history and physical examination, which may identify a particular causative, treatable condition. Pharmacologic therapy with either anticholinergic or antispasmodic medications represents the usual initial course of management, often in combination with micturition behavioral modification.

MALE GENITALIA AND REPRODUCTIVE SYSTEM

The penis consists of the the paired, dorsally located corpora cavernosa and the midline ventral corpus spongiosum that surrounds the urethra and distally forms the glans penis. The corpora cavernosa, the primary erectile bodies of the penis, are invested by a collagenous sheath called the tunica albuginea and contain a spongelike meshwork of trabecular smooth muscle and fibroelastic tissue lined by vascular endothelium. The cavernous arteries provide the main vascular supply to the penis, coursing from the internal pudendal arteries and feeding into branches in the corpora cavernosa called *helicine arteries.* Subtunical venules provide vascular drainage from the corpora cavernosa, forming the emissary veins as they pierce the tunica albuginea and eventually drain into the main venous tributaries of the penis, the dorsal and crural veins.

The fundamental physiology of the penis relates to blood flow in the organ as determined by the degree of vascular and corporal smooth muscle tone. Penile flaccidity is considered to be a tonic, low-blood-flow state resulting from corporal smooth muscle contraction governed locally primarily by the sympathetic division of the autonomic nervous system through its classic neurotransmitter norepinephrine. However, other vasocontractile factors have been identified as contributing to this physiology, such as endothelin, a substance released from the vascular endothelium. Penile erection, conversely, involves corporal smooth muscle relaxation, whereupon blood engorgement occurs; this process is under the control of nitric oxide as well as other vasodilatory mediators locally released from nerve endings originating from the parasympathetic division of the autonomic nervous system. The central nervous system (CNS) also influences this function, processing "psychogenic" stimuli and other regulatory information.

The remainder of the external male reproductive system consists of the contents of the scrotum, a multilayered structure separated by a septum into two compartments. These bilateral compartments each provide a receptacle for the testis, the spermatic cord, and the related excurrent duct system, consisting of the epididymis, vas deferens, and ejaculatory ducts. The internal male reproductive system comprises the accessory glands, including the prostate and seminal vesicles. The testes and excurrent duct system structures provide for the creation, maturation, and collection of sperm before seminal emission and ejaculation.

Erectile Dysfunction

Erectile dysfunction, commonly referred to as *impotence,* is defined as the consistent inability to attain and maintain penile erection sufficient to permit satisfactory sexual intercourse. This condition may affect as many as 18 million American men, most often men older than 65 years of age, although approximately 30% of all men between the ages of 40 and 70 years are affected (13). Various diseases, injuries, and drugs have been associated with erectile dysfunction (Table 102.2). These circumstances may produce alterations in the endocrine, neurologic, vascular, and end-organ requirements for normal penile erection. It has also been suggested that there is a gradual loss of erectile tissue integrity with aging that is unrelated to other medical problems. The rapidly evolving understanding that actual organic factors underlie as much as 80% of presentations of erectile difficulty has reinforced the clinical relevance of this condition.

Diagnosis

It is recommended that the diagnostic evaluation for erectile dysfunction be performed such that it facilitates

Table 102.2. COMMON ORGANIC CAUSES OF ERECTILE DYSFUNCTION

Category	Examples
Systemic disorders	Atherosclerosis, hypertension, peripheral vascular disease, diabetes mellitus, renal failure
Neurogenic disorders	Diabetes, cardiovascular accidents, Parkinson's disease, multiple sclerosis
Endocrine disorders	Hypogonadism, hyperprolactinemia, hyperthyroidism, hypothyroidism
Penile disorders	Peyronie's disease, priapism
Injuries	Perineal, pelvic, or nervous system trauma; radiation or surgery to the pelvis or retroperitoneum
Medications	Antihypertensives, antidepressants, antiandrogens, nonsteroidal antiinflammatory drugs
Substances of abuse	Alcohol, tobacco, recreational drug

treatment objectives without being unnecessarily costly or invasive. Goals of the basic evaluation are to determine the nature of the problem and, once it is confirmed, to identify and immediately address causative factors. A proper sexual function history (involving patient and partner) should begin the evaluation (Table 102.3). It may yield findings that suggest an organic basis for the erectile dysfunction, such as reports of erectile difficulty after physical trauma to the pelvic region, gradual deterioration of erectile function, a consistent inability to maintain an erection once it is attained, and the absence of erections on awakening from sleep.

Additional components of the basic evaluation include general medical and psychosocial history, drug history, physical examination, and basic laboratory testing. Clinical history may reveal certain past medical conditions or use of drugs that are known to be associated with erectile dysfunction. Physical examination attending to development of primary and secondary sex characteristics, genital anatomy, and neurologic and vascular functioning may suggest alterations consistent with the diagnosis. A basic laboratory investigation involving routine urinalysis, blood count, and serum chemistries may lead to the detection of commonly associated metabolic disorders such as diabetes mellitus and renal insufficiency.

The value of routine endocrinologic testing remains controversial because endocrinopathy may occur in only 2% of patients presenting with erectile dysfunction, and reportedly pertains more to decreased sexual libido than to erectile dysfunction (14). However, because sexual function may improve in some men receiving hormonal replacement therapy, a reasonable recommendation is to screen for hypogonadism by obtaining a morning serum total testosterone level. An abnormal testosterone level or other clinical indications of an endocrine disorder may prompt further endocrinologic testing. In the event that prostatic disease might be stimulated by exogenously administered testosterone, treatment may reasonably be withheld and thus diagnostic evaluation deemed unnecessary. Accordingly, both a PSA level and digital rectal examination (DRE) should be completed to assess for abnormalities.

Beyond the basic clinical evaluation, further specialized hormonal, neurologic, and vascular testing may be conducted in selected patients, usually by a urologist who specializes in erectile dysfunction. Such extensive testing in clinical practice usually follows the need to establish the exact cause and extent of the problem, often because of a patient's request or before initiating surgical interventions. Sleep-related penile tumescence and rigidity monitoring, performed either in a sleep laboratory or at home with a portable testing device, is often used as a minimally invasive technique that can graphically record the frequency, duration, and quality of erection. In-office assessments of erectile response to intracavernosal vasoactive drug injection can be done either by clinical rating or by diagnostic measurement of blood flow response, such as with penile duplex ultrasonography. Radiographic contrast injection into the penis or the surrounding pelvic vasculature may be used to locate an obstructive lesion or leak.

Treatment

The treatment of erectile dysfunction usually is based on the findings of the clinical evaluation and treatment preferences of the individual patient. Initial efforts are directed at addressing any medical conditions associated with erectile dysfunction, including treating medical diseases and exploring a change in or discontinuation of drugs with adverse effects on erectile function. Several

Table 102.3. ERECTILE PROBLEMS: COMPREHENSIVE SEXUAL FUNCTION HISTORY

Element	Specific questions
Onset, duration, evolution of erectile dysfunction	Gradual or sudden?
Type of dysfunction	Failure to attain or maintain erections?
Current quality of erections	Sufficient for sexual intercourse:
	Under certain circumstances?
	With certain positions?
Stimulus for achievable erections	Sexual encounters?
	Self-stimulation?
	On awakening?
Sexual issues distinct from erectile dysfunction	Libido
	Ejaculation
	Orgasm
Other issues	Availability, interest, health of partner
	Changes in medical status or other events relating to onset of dysfunction
	All prior attempts to manage the problem by the patient or another caregiver

physical interventions are available, and a perspective of them should be presented to the patient in a balanced and complete way. Discussion should include the efficacy and complication profiles, patient and partner satisfaction rates, and expected patient and partner involvement with regard to each treatment option. Given the relative minimal invasiveness of many of the available options, one or more may be explored regardless of the physical cause for the erectile dysfunction. An option may otherwise be considered in light of the type and severity of the underlying physical cause, presumably with greater treatment success. Even if a physical intervention is planned, referral for sex therapy or counseling may be useful whether the dysfunction is mainly psychogenic or organic. The contribution of emotional factors to any presentation should not be underestimated.

In addition to sexual counseling, physical interventions for erectile dysfunction include pharmacologic therapies, mechanical devices, vascular reconstruction, and penile prosthesis implantation surgery. Nonhormonal pharmacologic therapies include oral, intracavernosal, and intraurethral treatments. Traditional oral therapies such as yohimbine (Yocon; Palisades Pharmaceuticals, Tenafly, NJ) and trazodone HCl (Desyrel; Bristol-Meyers Squibb, Princeton, NJ) have been found to have limited efficacy profiles and have given way to newly emerging, highly effective oral therapies such as sildenafil citrate (Viagra; Pfizer, New York, NY). Viagra appears to produce erections useful for intercourse in more than 50% of patients (15). Intracavernosal or penile injection therapy has been available for more than 15 years and represents the gold standard of pharmacologic treatment options. The therapy requires the insertion of a small needle into the side of the penis for injecting vasoactive medications that stimulate the erectile tissue to relax and expand with blood. Various vasoactive drugs have been applied, including prostaglandin E_1 (alprostadil [Caverject; Pharmacia & Upjohn, Kalamazoo, MI]), papaverine, and phentolamine. These agents can be used as monotherapy or in combination with the expectation of producing a satisfactory, functional erection in approximately 90% of patients (16). Intraurethral therapy, made available since 1996, requires the insertion of an applicator into the distal urethra to deliver a suppository of vasoactive medication. Currently, only prostaglandin E_1 [alprostadil (MUSE) (VIVUS, Inc., Mountain View, CA)] is commercially available, with efficacy in producing erections in approximately 40% of patients with erectile dysfunction (17).

Externally applied erection devices offer a nonpharmacologic and noninvasive alternative therapy for erectile dysfunction. A plastic cylinder is placed over the penis to create a closed chamber, and is connected by tubing to a vacuum that withdraws air from around the penis to facilitate penile engorgement with blood. A constrictive ring is then positioned at the base of the penis to contain the blood. An erection-like state is obtained in 98% of users according to manufacturers. Surgical implantation of a semirigid malleable or hydraulic inflatable device into the penis has long been an available treatment, with success achieved in approximately 95% of cases (18). Although such surgery is ostensibly more invasive than other alternatives, it may be indicated after diagnostically confirmed severe hemodynamic dysfunction of the penis and on lack of success with alternative therapies. Penile vascular reconstruction represents another surgical intervention. Surgical procedures include both arterial revascularization and venous ligation, offered chiefly to patients who are documented to have a focal vascular lesion, usually as a result of pelvic trauma. Success is noted in 40% to 60% of cases (19).

Peyronie's Disease

Peyronie's disease is a benign, inflammatory fibrosis of the tunica albuginea of the corpora cavernosa that produces a deformity of the erect penis and occasionally erectile dysfunction. The disorder is common, with a prevalence that approaches 1% of adult men, although it is seen primarily in men between 45 and 60 years of age (20). Hypothesized causes for the disorder include chronic irritation, inherited trait, autoimmune defect, delamination injury, and superoxide injury.

Diagnosis

The diagnosis is usually based on the patient presentation of penile pain that usually resolves over time, penile angulation with an often palpable plaque involving the penile shaft, and occasionally impaired erectile function. Recollections of penile trauma and descriptions of fibrotic conditions elsewhere in the body can sometimes be elicited with a clinical history, although frequently no discernible associations can be found. Further diagnostic assessment can be done to evaluate the severity of the deformity, which may limit the physical act of sexual intercourse and the extent of erectile dysfunction. Commonly used modalities include photographic documentation of a naturally occurring erection and penile duplex ultrasonography after vasoactive drug pharmacostimulation.

Treatment

Treatment is conservative in most presentations, particularly during the first 12 months after disease onset, to ascertain its resolution with either spontaneous improvement or stabilization of plaque formation. For patients resolving with only minimal to moderate curvature, no penile pain, and continued normal sexual activity, no invasive diagnostic procedure or treatment is indicated. Medical therapies such as vitamin E and colchicine may be tried early with the intent to decrease the inflammatory process and fibrosis. After 12 months, patients with significant impairment may be offered more invasive interventions. Techniques for reducing fibrosis include intralesional injection therapy and radiation therapy. Treatments for impaired sexual function include intracavernosal self-injection therapy and surgery involving either penile straightening or penile prosthesis insertion.

Disorders of the Scrotum and Its Contents

Pathologic conditions arising in the scrotum are frequently challenging to diagnose and treat. A hydrocele is the most common benign scrotal mass lesion. The pathologic process consists of the accumulation of serous fluid secreted by the tunica vaginalis layer of the scrotum, occurring secondary to tumor, trauma, or inflammation, or idiopathically. Epididymitis is a common intrascrotal lesion that is associated with a mass effect and pain. This disorder usually begins with a bacterial or chemical insult to the vas deferens, epididymis, and testis that leads to an inflammatory response. Varicocele, or a dilated vein of the pampiniform plexus, is the most common mass arising from the spermatic cord. Other major intrascrotal conditions include neoplasia, cystic lesions, testicular torsion, ruptured testicle, and scrotal abscess.

Discriminating between different scrotal disorders and initiating treatment promptly in emergent situations are the charges of the clinician whose patient presents with scrotal symptomatology. A focused clinical history should provide immediate information about the occurrence of scrotal or perineal trauma, symptoms of a lower urinary tract infection, and the presence of pain. Urinalysis is routinely performed, and the presence of bacteria and pyuria suggests an inflammatory etiology. The physical examination constitutes the most important part of the diagnostic evaluation. The normal hemiscrotum and inguinal region should be examined first to provide a reference with which to compare abnormal findings.

The important differentiation of scrotal masses as solid or cystic may require scrotal transillumination or color Doppler ultrasonography. A solid mass suggests neoplasia and usually warrants radical orchiectomy. A cystic mass is atypical for a malignancy, and treatment may range from observation with reassurance to surgical excision if the mass is large and symptomatic. Epididymitis and related inflammatory conditions of the scrotum usually are treated medically with antibiotics, antiinflammatory medications, analgesics, and supportive measures, including heating pads and scrotal elevation. The diagnosis of a scrotal abscess mandates surgical drainage, but it also dictates prompt evaluation of the lower urinary tract for a cause that also may require immediate attention, such as urethral stricture disease or trauma with infectious urine extravasation. Clinical suspicion of testicular torsion or rupture should lead to surgical exploration and orchiopexy (testicular fixation), testicular salvage procedures, or orchiectomy, depending on testicular viability.

Male Infertility

Infertility, defined as the inability to conceive a pregnancy within 1 year of unprotected sexual intercourse, affects approximately 15% of couples in the United States (21). Male factors are thought to contribute to approximately half of the instances. Although the condition is poorly understood, new information continues to emerge to provide insight into its complexity. Along with this improved understanding, new diagnostic and therapeutic techniques have been developed to assist in the management of the problem.

Diagnosis

An informative and cost-effective initial evaluation should begin with a complete history taking, physical examination, and appropriate laboratory tests. Information should be obtained about duration of infertility, current sexual practices, erectile and ejaculatory functions, and fertility history. Medical history should be obtained to identify congenital anomalies, endocrine disorders, systemic illness, prior surgeries (e.g., herniorrhaphy and bladder or scrotal surgeries), and infections or trauma of the genital and urinary tracts. Exposures to gonadotoxins, including recreational drugs, anabolic steroids, chemotherapeutic agents, chemical pesticides, and even environmental toxins that affect spermatogenesis, should be identified. The physical examination is focused on the genitalia. Scrotal contents should be carefully assessed to evaluate whether the testes are abnormal (measuring <4 cm in length and having a consistency other than moderately firm), whether the vas deferens on either side is absent, and whether a varicocele is present. Rectal examination should be performed to determine whether the seminal vesicles are abnormally palpable or a midline prostatic cyst is detectable that would suggest ejaculatory duct obstruction. General physical characteristics relative to virilization should be assessed for abnormal sexual maturation, which may be the manifestation of an endocrinopathy.

The semen analysis represents the cornerstone of the male infertility evaluation. Normal standards are available that refer to the amount, morphology, and function of sperm and conditions of the ejaculate (Table 102.4). Three separate specimens collected at least 2 but not more than 5 days after the last ejaculation are required before instituting therapy. Serum levels of follicle-stimulating hormone (FSH), luteinizing hormone (LH), and testosterone should be obtained in patients with abnormal semen analysis parameters or evidence of an endocrinopathy to assess the hypothalamic–pituitary–gonadal axis. Tests to evaluate spermatogenesis and the presence of excurrent duct system obstruction include testicular biopsy, vasography, and transrectal ultrasonography. A variety of tests can be applied to assess sperm function, including sperm penetration assays, postcoital testing, and anti-sperm antibody testing.

Treatment

Therapy in the field of male infertility is evolving toward identifying a treatable cause and rationally initiating therapy that has a high likelihood of success. Oligospermia (low sperm count) usually receives empiric treatment with clomiphene citrate to raise gonadotropin levels and, in the-

Table 102.4. NORMAL SEMEN PARAMETERS

Volume	2–5 mL
Sperm concentration	$>20 \times 10^6$/mL
Total sperm	$>60 \times 10^6$
Motility	>60%
Forward progression	>75%
Normal morphology	>60%
Fructose	Present
Agglutination	Absent
White blood cells	<5 WBCs/HPF

ory, stimulate the testes to function better. Varicocelectomy through laparoscopic ligation or open microsurgical techniques has in some instances improved sperm counts and function, supported by the hypothesis that varicoceles cause disordered scrotal temperature regulation and retrograde flow of adrenal hormones and renal toxins. Other surgical applications include microsurgical reconstruction to treat vas deferens and epididymal obstructions, transurethral resection to treat the obstructed ejaculatory duct orifice, and microsurgical sperm aspiration of the epididymides for use with assisted reproduction techniques for the diagnosis of absent or atretic excurrent duct structures. Hormone replacement may be appropriately offered when specific endocrine disorders have been defined. Complete testicular failure, as determined by testicular biopsy showing no sperm production or a markedly elevated FSH level, has been considered untreatable in the past. However, recently developed assisted reproduction techniques have been applied to treat this disorder as well as others in which goal-directed therapies cannot be offered.

UROLITHIASIS

Urolithiasis (also termed *urinary stones* or *calculi*) has always afflicted humankind and has been documented in Egyptian mummies from 4800 B.C.E. Hippocrates was quoted as saying "I will not cut even for the stone, but leave such procedures to the practitioners of the craft." It is a significant health problem because the overall cost of the disease is approximately $2 billion per year in the United States (22).

Urolithiasis affects a significant portion of the population. Today, most urinary stones in industrialized countries are renal (nephrolithiasis), with bladder stones being relatively uncommon. An understanding of the disorder's epidemiology is important for identification of patient risk factors and prevention. Each year, 0.1% to 0.4% of the population is believed to have kidney stones, with a peak incidence between the ages of 45 and 64 years in the United States and Europe (23) (even though most people report the onset of disease in their teenage years). In addition, men have a 3-fold higher incidence of the disease than women (24), and patients with a family history of stone disease have a 25-fold higher incidence of new stone formation.

There are geographic variations in the risk for development of a stone, with a higher risk in mountainous, desert, and tropical areas. In the United States, the southeastern region has a higher incidence compared with the rest of the nation. It is unclear whether this difference is due to the hot weather, hydrational status, or other factors such as increased vitamin D production due to sunlight exposure (25). International variability is also evident, with the whole-population lifetime risk for development of kidney stone disease at 2% to 5% in Asia, 8% to 15% in Europe and North America, and 20% in Saudi Arabia (23). In addition to geographic variations, there is seasonal variation because the incidence increases in the summer months in both the northern and southern hemispheres.

The incidence of stone recurrence is significant, with 50% of all patients with nephrolithiasis experiencing a recurrence within 5 to 10 years (24) and 75% recurring during the first 20 years (26). These factors commit the patient and physician to a lifetime of follow-up and awareness of the possibility of recurrent episodes.

Stone Compositions

Most stones in industrialized countries contain calcium and usually consist of calcium oxalate (Table 102.5). The remaining 20% of stones are composed of uric acid, struvite or carbonate apatite, cystine, and other rare precipitates (27). Cystine stones form only in patients with a rare congenital defect called *cystinuria*. In addition, medicines such as indinavir sulfate, used in the treatment of HIV infection, have been reported to crystallize in the urinary tract (28), leading to symptoms similar to those with conventional urolithiasis.

Pathophysiology

Stone formation is the end result of a complex interaction of many different factors that results in the crystallization of stone-forming salts. There are several different theories regarding which factors lead to the formation and progression of renal calculi. Nucleation is a process whereby stone formation is initiated by the presence of a crystal or foreign body, which promotes the growth of salt crystals only in supersaturated urine. Often the nidus is composed of a substance other than the stone crystal itself (heterogeneous nucleation). Examples of heterogeneous nucleation are crystallization on injured surfaces of renal tubular cells or a different solute (i.e., uric acid, matrix). Nucleation requires the presence of transiently or intermittently supersaturated urine. Other factors such as low concentrations of crystallization inhibitors (e.g., citrate, nephrocalcin, pyrophosphate, acidic glycopeptides, uropontin, magnesium) as well as altered pH may have a significant effect on solubility and crystallization.

Most crystals pass through the urinary system unless they are adherent to the renal collecting system or retained by urinary stasis. In some instances, kidney stones can be attached to Randall's plaques or sites of previous renal injury, preventing distal passage. Furthermore, anatomic factors such as distal obstruction (i.e., ureteral stricture) or location in the lower pole may lead to stasis and subsequent stone formation or propagation.

Diagnosis

It is generally accepted that stones initially form in the proximal urinary tract. As stones grow on the surfaces of the renal papillae or calyces, they usually do not produce symptoms and may be discovered only incidentally. Most symptoms occur as the stone traverses the renal pelvis and ureter, which leads to intermittent obstruction. The most common presentations of nephrolithiasis are pain

Table 102.5. TYPES OF KIDNEY STONES

Stone composition	Frequency (x)	Degree of radiopacity
Calcium stones (total)	82	Opaque
Calcium oxalate ± calcium phosphate	75	Very opaque
Pure calcium phosphate	7	
Magnesium ammonium phosphate	12	Opaque
Uric acid	7	Lucent
Cystine	2	Slightly opaque

and hematuria. Lateralizing pain from urolithiasis or renal colic is usually intermittent and can be located anywhere from the flank to the loin as the stone moves distally in the urinary tract. The presence of pain signifies obstruction and distention of the ureter or renal pelvis. However, the severity of pain is not usually related to the amount of distention but is due to the rapidity with which it develops. Sudden distention causes severe pain, whereas gradual distention may have no symptoms whatsoever. Associated nonrenal symptoms are due to the autonomic innervation of the kidneys and may include nausea, vomiting, or ileus.

A thorough physical examination is required to rule out other causes of abdominal pain. Patients are usually in obvious distress and frequently have some costovertebral angle tenderness. Fever is usually absent unless there is concomitant infection. The urinalysis usually reveals hematuria but may be negative in approximately 5% of cases (29). The urinary pH is frequently helpful in assessing risk factors for stone disease because uric acid stones tend to form in acidic urine (pH < 6.0) and struvite in alkaline urine (pH > 7.0). The diagnosis of nephrolithiasis is confirmed by characteristic radiographic findings or stone passage.

Radiographic Examination

There is no perfect radiographic examination for the evaluation of kidney stones and the chosen study depends on availability, patient factors (i.e., age, pregnancy, allergies, renal function), and situation (elective or emergency). The most commonly used studies are listed in Table 102.6, with their characteristic advantages and disadvantages.

Intravenous Urography. Intravenous urography has been the mainstay of imaging for stone disease because the study has a high sensitivity and specificity for the diagnosis of stones. A well-prepared (with a mechanical bowel prep) study provides information not only about the presence of stones, but about renal function, upper tract anatomy, and the presence or absence of obstruction. Important anatomic information such as ureteral duplication or calyceal diverticulum may be seen only on an IVU study. The major limitations of the study are an unprepared study (without a prior mechanical bowel prep) in the emergency department due to poor visualization of retroperitoneal

strictures. Other limitations include failure to visualize radiolucent stones, risks of contrast reaction and nephrotoxicity, and the prolonged examination time, especially with an obstructing stone. For these reasons, spiral computed tomography (CT) has supplanted the IVU in the emergency setting (30). IVU still provides the most information when done electively for preoperative planning (31).

Ultrafast Spiral Computed Tomography. Spiral CT has gained popularity in the evaluation of acute flank pain in the emergency department setting, for obvious reasons. The study is quick, does not require intravenous contrast or bowel preparation, and is the most sensitive test for detection of ureteral stones. Additional advantages are the ability to determine stone compositions (except for indinavir sulfate) and the ability to detect an extrarenal pathologic process that may be the primary cause of lateralizing pain (e.g., aortic aneurysm) (32). There are, however, several significant limitations, including the lack of functional information. Also, spiral CT does not accurately delineate the anatomy of the ureter and renal collecting system. Detection of anomalies such as calyceal diverticulum or ureteral duplication is critical for proper preoperative planning. In addition, follow-up of stone disease is usually done using plain films. In many instances, comparison of plain films with spiral CT is difficult in assessing for stone movement or passage.

Ultrasonography. The use of ultrasound for evaluation of the upper urinary tract has steadily increased because of improved technology and user comfort. The study is noninvasive and available in both the hospital and outpatient setting. Ultrasound has become the procedure of choice in the pediatric population and with pregnant women. The study presents no radiation risk, detects stones in the kidney and ureterovesical junction with reasonable accuracy, and gives some anatomic information such as presence of hydronephrosis (33). The shortcomings of the study are its poor sensitivity for stone detection in the middle and upper ureter, lack of functional information, and limited visualization of renal anatomy.

Plain Imaging. The kidneys-ureters-bladder plain radiograph is readily available and most useful in the follow-up of stones, especially when it can be compared with a previously obtained IVU. The examination is reasonably

---

Table 102.6. IMAGING STUDIES FOR THE EVALUATION OF NEPHROLITHIASIS

Imaging study	Advantages	Disadvantages
Plain abdominal film	• Readily accessible • Good sensitivity for detection of renal stones • Best study for routine follow-up of opaque stones	• Radiation exposure • Low sensitivity for ureteral stones • Radiolucent stones (uric acid) • Cannot evaluate function or obstruction
Sonography	• Radiation free • Usually accessible • High sensitivity in kidney and distal ureter (UVJ) • Detects hydronephrosis • Detects all stone types	• Poor sensitivity mid and proximal ureter • Operator dependent
Intravenous urogram	• Assesses entire urinary tract for presence of stones, renal function and ureteral obstruction • Anatomic information of upper urinary tract • Best study for preoperative planning	• Risk of contrast reaction and • Radiolucent stones • Optimally requires prep • Contrast nephrotoxicity
Spiral computed tomography	• Fast • No bowel preparation required • Accurately detects all stone types • Evaluates adjacent pathology • No contrast required • Best study to evaluate flank pain in emergency department setting	• Radiation exposure • Lack of function • Does not assess upper urinary tract anatomy (i.e., duplicated system)

accurate in the detection of radiopaque renal stones. The limitations of the study are its poor sensitivity in detection of ureteral stones, which may be superimposed on the bony pelvis, its inability to display renal anatomy and function, and its inability to visualize all stone compositions.

Management of Urolithiasis

After the diagnosis is confirmed, the situation is assessed for size, location, degree of obstruction, and complicating factors. Most stones (<6 mm) pass spontaneously and can be followed conservatively. In the emergency setting, intravenous hydration and analgesics are usually sufficient to treat the acute attack. The patient can be discharged with outpatient urology follow-up when pain and associated symptoms have been controlled. Immediate intervention usually involves stone removal or bypassing the ureteral obstruction with stenting or placement of a percutaneous nephrostomy tube. Indications for intervention are listed in Table 102.7 and are usually related to associated pyelonephritis, unremitting pain, and deterioration of renal function or presence of high-grade obstruction. Other relative indications for intervention are large stones (>1 cm) that are unlikely to pass spontaneously or occupations that require stone-free status (e.g., airline pilots).

Patients not requiring acute intervention are sent home and told to strain their urine. Even stones with significant ureteral obstruction can be safely observed for up to a month. In the absence of infection, most studies have shown no evidence of renal damage even with complete obstruction at 1 month. Elective intervention can be planned for failure of stone passage.

Treatment Options

The safest management of ureteral stones is spontaneous passage, providing there are no complicating factors. The chance of spontaneous stone passage is related to stone size and anatomic features of the upper urinary tract. The American Urological Association Clinical Guidelines Panel on ureteral stones determined that over 95% of stones less than 5 mm in diameter pass spontaneously (34). Another factor determining stone passage is impedance at the three narrowest portions of the ureter: the ureteropelvic junction, ureterovesical junction, and the crossing of the iliac vessels. In some cases, anatomic abnormalities such as ureteral stricture prevent passage.

For stones that are unlikely to pass or that have failed conservative management, acceptable options are described in the following sections.

Extracorporeal Shock Wave Lithotripsy. The first shock wave lithotripsy (SWL) was reported in 1984 by Chaussy et al. (35) and revolutionized the treatment of

---

Table 102.7. INDICATIONS FOR IMMEDIATE INTERVENTION

Absolute
Obstructive pyelonephritis (true emergency)
Unremitting pain
Deterioration of renal function
Anuria due to ureteral obstruction
    Bilateral stones
    Solitary kidney
Relative
Large ureteral stones (>7 mm) that are unlikely to pass spontaneously
Occupational requirements (i.e., airline pilot)
Transplant kidney

---

nephrolithiasis. The field of stone management was changed from largely surgical procedures to image-guided therapy. SWL is a truly noninvasive, image-guided therapy whereby shock waves are generated and focused on the target stone, usually requiring only intravenous sedation. The effect of these shock waves is to pulverize the stone into smaller fragments that can easily pass through the urinary tract. The major risks of the procedure are ecchymosis, perinephric hematoma, renal colic and ureteral obstruction from fragments, and sepsis.

Ureterorenoscopy. Advances in technology have led to the design of endoscopes that can be safely passed to all parts of the urinary tract in a retrograde fashion. Larger stones can be fragmented using intracorporeal lithotripsy, and smaller stones can be grasped and removed under direct vision. Available lithotripsy devices include holmium and pulsed-dye lasers and electrohydraulic, electromechanical, and ultrasonic devices. The major risks of the procedure are anesthesia, ureteral injury, sepsis, stricture formation, bleeding, and sepsis.

Percutaneous Nephrolithotomy. Percutaneous techniques for stone removal were developed in the 1980s and quickly supplanted open surgical techniques for treatment of stones. Their use greatly decreased after the development of SWL, which provided a less invasive alternative. The procedure involves establishment of a nephrostomy tract directly into the renal collecting system from the flank, through which large-diameter instruments are passed, resulting in the ability to remove large amounts of stone from the kidney and upper ureter efficiently. The procedure is more invasive than ureteroscopy or SWL and thus has higher complication and morbidity rates.

Open Surgery or Laparoscopy. Open surgery and laparoscopy are rarely required but may be necessary for the removal of larger staghorn calculi, stones refractory to conventional, minimally invasive options, or those patients with anatomic limitations preventing a minimally invasive procedure. Stone removal may also be done concomitantly with repair of an anatomic defect such as a ureteropelvic junction obstruction (36,37).

Location-specific Treatment Options

Renal Calculi. In general, SWL therapy is the procedure of choice for renal stones less than 2 cm in size. Treatment-related failure and complication rates increase significantly for larger and staghorn calculi (38). Additional factors that significantly influence the success of SWL therapy are stone location, stone composition, and anatomic factors. With regard to stone location, stones in the upper and middle calyces pass more readily than stones in the lower calyx, especially if there is an unfavorable acute angle in relation to the renal pelvis. Stones composed of calcium oxalate monohydrate and cystine tend to fragment into fewer pieces (if at all) and are less likely to be successfully treated. Last, any anatomic factor that inhibits distal stone passage such as distal obstruction (i.e., stricture, ureteropelvic junction obstruction), stone location in a calyceal diverticulum, or hydronephrosis provides a relative contraindication.

Patients who have failed SWL therapy or possess factors making success of SWL unlikely (e.g., staghorn calculus, lower pole location, cystine composition) should be considered for percutaneous stone removal. Percutaneous nephrolithotomy has the ability both to fragment and remove stones without depending on spontaneous passage of fragments. Ureteroscopy has gained more popularity for treatment of stones in the kidney and distal ureter. Opti-

Table 102.8. PATHOPHYSIOLOGY AND DIAGNOSIS OF STONE DISEASE

Condition	Primary defect	Stone composition	Minimum diagnostic criteria
Resorptive hypercalciuria	Hyperparathyroidism	Ca oxalate, Ca phosphate	Hypercalcemia and elevated PTH
Absorptive hypercalciuria			
Type I	High intestinal Ca absorption	Ca oxalate, Ca phosphate	Hypercalciuria on random and restricted diet, normal serum Ca and PTH
Type II	High intestinal Ca absorption	Ca oxalate, Ca phosphate	Hypercalciuria on random diet, normacalciuria on restricted diet, normal serum Ca and PTH
Renal hypercalciuria	Renal Ca leak	Ca oxalate, Ca phosphate	Normal serum Ca, high serum PTH, hypercalciuria
Hypocitraturic Ca nephrolithiasis	Acidosis or excess of dietary acid	Ca oxalate	Hypocitraturia
Distal renal tubular acidosis	Renal acid retention	Ca phosphate	Hypocitraturia
Hyperuricosuric Ca nephrolithiasis	Diet rich in animal protein	Ca oxalate	Urinary pH >5.5, hyperuricosuria
Gouty diathesis	Excessive urinary acidification	Uric acid, Ca oxalate, Ca phosphate	Urinary pH <5.5 without diet rich in animal protein or diarrhea
Enteric hyperoxaluria	Ileal disease or resection	Ca oxalate, uric acid	Hyperoxaluria, hypocitraturia, pH <5.5
Cystinuria	Impaired cystine transport	Cystine	Urinary cystine >250 mg/g, creatinine
Infection stones	Excessive urease activity	Struvite, carbonate apatite	Urinary pH >7.5, positive culture for urea-splitting organisms

PTH, parathyroid hormone.
Adapted from Pak CY. Kidney stones. Lancet 1998;351:1797–1801.

mal candidates are patients who have failed SWL therapy and are not good candidates for percutaneous nephrolithotomy.

Proximal and Mid-ureteral Calculi. Shock wave lithotripsy and ureteroscopy are both acceptable options for treatment of stones in the proximal and middle ureter. Because of limitations in stone localization, SWL has lower success rates for calculi appearing in this location than it does for renal calculi. Ureteroscopy in this portion of the ureter usually requires flexible techniques. A ureteroscopic approach can be technically difficult but highly successful in competent hands (39). In some instances, antegrade ureteroscopy through an established nephrostomy tract is an acceptable alternative. The choice is largely dependent on physician experience/preference and patient preference. Blind basketing is not acceptable, and open surgery should be reserved as a salvage procedure.

Distal Ureteral Calculus. There has been an ongoing debate over whether ureteroscopy or SWL is the optimal treatment for distal stones. SWL has less morbidity than ureteroscopy but has somewhat lower success rates because of difficulty with stone localization. Ureteroscopy is technically straightforward using rigid or semirigid endoscopes, and has success rates of over 95% in most series, with minimal complications (34). The choice depends largely on patient and urologist preference.

Evaluation of the Stone-forming Patient

The most important initial step is to gather the stone for analysis. Although most stones contain calcium, approximately 20% are composed of other minerals and require different long-term management plans. Other important factors in evaluation of the stone-forming patient are a careful history with emphasis on family members with urolithiasis, factors contributing to dehydration, diet, bowel disease (e.g., sprue, ulcerative colitis), previous bowel surgery, and fluid intake. A complete physical examination and baseline laboratory evaluation consisting of urinalysis, urine culture, serum electrolytes, blood urea nitrogen, creatinine, uric acid, and calcium should be done. If the stone was not collected, a screening test for cystinuria should be done. The goal of the initial evaluation is to identify uncommon but treatable causes of nephrolithiasis.

Table 102.9. MEDICAL MANAGEMENT OF NEPHROLITHIASIS

Condition	Specific treatments	Simplified treatments
Resorptive hypercalciuria	Surgical parathyroidectomy	
Absorptive hypercalciuria		Thiazide + potassium citrate
Type I	Thiazide + potassium citrate (sodium cellulose phosphate)	
Type II	Low calcium diet	Potassium citrate
Renal hypercalciuria	Thiazide + potassium citrate	Potassium citrate
Gouty diathesis	Potassium citrate	Potassium citrate
Dietary hyperoxaluria		Restrict dietary oxalate Avoid severe calcium restriction
Hypocitraturic Ca nephrolithiasis and distal renal tubular acidosis	Potassium citrate	Potassium citrate
Hyperuricosuric Ca nephrolithiasis	Allopurinol, potassium citrate	Potassium citrate
Enteric hyperoxaluria	Potassium citrate, calcium citrate, magnesium citrate	Potassium citrate, Ca citrate, Mg citrate
Cystinuria potassium citrate		
Mild (250–500 mg/d)	Chelating agents, potassium citrate	Chelating agents High fluid intake
>500 mg/d	Tiopronin (thiola) Antibiotic, acetohydroxamic acid	Potassium citrate Antibiotic, acetohydroxamic acid
Infection stones	Complete removal of all stones	

Adapted from Pak CY. Kidney stones. Lancet 1998;351:1797–1801.

The presence of normocalcemia and normouricemia, plus the absence of urinary tract infection, bowel disease, or marked hyperoxaluria, can usually differentiate uncomplicated calcium stone disease from other types. For the first-time uncomplicated calcium stone former, no further evaluation is warranted. The patient is counseled on a low-oxalate diet, told to drink enough fluid to produce more than 2,000 mL of urine per day, and followed up on a regular basis for evaluation of stone recurrence.

Metabolically active stone disease is characterized by formation of new stones, enlargement of an old stone, or passage of gravel. For patients with noncalcium or metabolically active stone disease, a complete evaluation is indicated. Complete metabolic evaluation is directed at identifying specific factors that influence the crystallization of stone-forming salts. These protocols include analysis of 24-hour urine collection, complete serum panels, and further evaluation for risk factors. Pak characterized urinary risk factors (Table 102.8) and specific treatments directed at correcting the underlying abnormalities (40) (Table 102.9).

ENDOUROLOGY

Endourology is a term coined in 1978 at the Annual Meeting of the American Urological Association that refers to the endoscopic evaluation of and intervention in the urinary tract. Although urologists have always been endoscopists, procedures were usually limited to endoscopic evaluation of the lower urinary tract. At that meeting, a poster highlighted advanced techniques performed in all parts of the urinary tract, mostly in patients not viewed as candidates for open surgical approaches. The discipline of endourology is a natural progression of minimally invasive surgery and has been the result of the creative efforts of urologists, radiologists, and engineers. Current endoscopic techniques can safely access the upper urinary tract by retrograde ureteropyeloscopy and antegrade percutaneous approaches, and the retroperitoneum by laparoscopic and retroperitoneoscopic approaches. These advances were significant enough to require special expertise and thus launch the subspecialty of endourology.

Ureterorenoscopy

Ureterorenoscopy is the endoscopic evaluation of the upper urinary tract through a retrograde (transurethral) approach. The technique involves accessing the ureter through the urethra and bladder. Hugh Hampton Young performed the first ureteroscopy in 1912 (41) when he passed a cystoscope into the distal ureter of a child with massive hydronephrosis from vesicoureteral reflux due to posterior urethral valves. Subsequent advances in techniques and ureteroscope technology have allowed us to reach all portions of the urinary tract with minimal morbidity.

Flexible and rigid ureteroscopes are available in sizes less than 8 French. This caliber of instrument allows for passage into the ureter with minimal or no dilation. Semirigid ureteroscopes are available is sizes as small as 4.9 French, with working ports of sufficient size to admit a variety of lithotripsy devices and working instruments. These ureteroscopes can be reliably passed into the distal ureter and, in some patients, can be further advanced into the middle and upper ureter. Advancement of the ureteroscope may not be possible in all patients (especially male patients) because of the course of the more proximal ureter. Flexible ureteroscopes bypass some of the limitations of rigid ones by conforming to the course of the ureter, allowing for reliable passage to the upper ureter

Table 102.10. APPLICATIONS OF URETEROSCOPY

Ureteroscopic diagnosis and biopsy of ureteral and renal lesions
Removal of ureteral and renal calculi
   Primary therapy
   Failed or contraindications to shock wave lithotripsy
Treatment of upper urinary tract transitional cell carcinoma
Incisional procedure
   Ureteral stricture
   Ureteropelvic junction obstruction
   Renal calyceal diverticulum or infundibular stenosis

and kidney. Flexible ureteroscopes are available in sizes as small as 7 French and have a working channel to allow for passage of a variety of instruments and lithotripsy devices without the need for significant dilation of the ureter.

The applications for ureterorenoscopy are listed in Table 102.10. By far the most common application is in the treatment of ureteral and renal calculi. SWL is the least invasive of the options for treating stones but may be unsuccessful because of stone size, composition, or location, or anatomic limitations. In such cases, ureteroscopy is an attractive option. Other applications, in order of decreasing frequency, include diagnosis and biopsy, incisional procedures such as endopyelotomy, or treatment of transitional cell carcinoma of the upper urinary tract.

Percutaneous Renal Surgery

The first percutaneous nephrostomy tube was placed by Goodwin in 1955 (42). The concept that the kidney could be accessed in an antegrade fashion without the morbidity of an open incision revolutionized the treatment of upper urinary tract disease. The application expanded beyond simple drainage to removal of renal and upper ureteral stones. Shortly after the development of techniques for percutaneous stone removal, SWL revolutionized the field, decreasing the applications and impact of the technique. However, percutaneous renal surgery still plays a large role in urologic surgery.

The applications of percutaneous renal surgery are listed in Table 102.11. By far the most common application is removal of renal stones. It is unquestionably the treatment of choice for large or staghorn calculi. Other applications include management of congenital abnormalities such as calyceal diverticulum, incisional procedures such as endopyelotomy, treatment of renal cysts, and surgical management of transitional cell carcinoma of the upper urinary tracts.

Table 102.11. APPLICATIONS OF PERCUTANEOUS RENAL SURGERY

Removal of renal and upper ureteral stones
   Stone burden >2 cm
   Staghorn calculi
   Lower pole stones >1 cm
   Failed shock wave lithotripsy
   Anatomic abnormalities—calyceal diverticulum, hydronephrosis
Treatment of transitional cell carcinoma
Incisional procedures
   Ureteropelvic junction obstruction
   Infundibular stenosis
Ablative procedures
   Calyceal diverticulum
   Renal cysts

Laparoscopic Surgery of the Retroperitoneum

Kelling reported the first laparoscopy in 1901 when he used air insufflation in a canine model and viewed the peritoneal cavity through a cystoscope (43). It was not until 1976, when Cortesi et al. (44) evaluated cryptorchid testes and Wickham (45) performed ureterolithotomy, that laparoscopy was used for urologic purposes. Laparoscopic techniques remained underused until 1989, when Reddick and Olsen (46) reported on laparoscopic cholecystectomy, marking the the transition from a predominantly diagnostic to a therapeutic modality. In response to this landmark achievement in general surgery, many potential urologic applications were quickly identified and performed with varying degrees of difficulty. Currently accepted applications of laparoscopy are listed in Table 102.12.

A retroperitoneal or transperitoneal approach can be used for most procedures depending on the disease process, patient considerations (e.g., body habitus, previous surgeries, presence of infection), and surgeon familiarity. The basic advantage of the retroperitoneal approach is avoidance of the peritoneal cavity, but at the expense of a limited working space. The transperitoneal approach provides a larger working space but requires mobilization of the colon and carries the risk of various bowel-related complications (e.g., visceral hernia, adhesions, perforation). The retroperitoneal approach is generally favored for removal of smaller, nonmalignant kidneys. To date, no overall advantage has been clearly identified between the two approaches (47), and choice largely depends on surgeon preference and the clinical situation. More recently, the use of an intraabdominal sleeve to allow the surgeon to use his or her hand for manually assisted laparoscopy has shown promise in decreasing complications and improving surgical results (48).

Although still in the development stages, laparoscopic techniques show benefits beyond improved cosmesis and decreased postoperative morbidity. Studies have shown results comparable with those of open surgery for radical nephrectomy (tumors <3 cm) (49), pyeloplasty (50), adrenalectomy (51), and simple nephrectomy for benign disease (52). Laparoscopic radical prostatectomy is being evaluated with encouraging results (53). As the techniques and technology improve, acceptance and applications will increase.

Table 102.12. APPLICATIONS OF LAPAROSCOPY

Diagnostic
  Nonpalpable testes
Lymph node sampling
  Pelvic for prostate, bladder, penile malignancies
  Retroperitoneal for testicular cancer
Nephrectomy for renal donation
  Simple for benign disease
  Radical for renal cell carcinoma
Nephroureterectomy
  Transitional cell carcinoma of upper urinary tract
  Nonfunctioning kidney with reflux
Radical prostatectomy
Adrenalectomy
Pyeloplasty
Pyelolithotomy
Ureterolithotomy
Calyceal diverticulum
Nephropexy

UROTHELIAL CARCINOMA

Tumors derived from the urothelial lining of the urinary system, commonly referred to as *transitional cell epithelium,* account for almost 50,000 newly diagnosed cancers per year in the United States. Bladder cancer is the fourth most common cause of cancer death in men (54). The most common type of urothelial cancer is transitional cell carcinoma (90%), although other histologic types can occur, including squamous cell carcinoma (5%), adenocarcinoma (2%), lymphoma (<1%), and sarcoma (<1%). Development of squamous cell carcinoma appears to be related to chronic irritation secondary to stone or a foreign body, or in the case of certain developing countries, from urinary schistosomiasis (55). Adenocarcinoma of the urinary bladder may originate from the bladder or urachal remnant as a primary lesion, or from a gastrointestinal metastasis. Transitional cell carcinomas can be broadly categorized as superficial or invasive. The precise etiology of these tumors is unknown, although genetic alterations are common (56). Superficial transitional cell carcinoma is most commonly associated with trisomy or deletion of chromosome 9 (9p21), whereas invasive transitional cell carcinoma is most commonly associated with 17p chromosomal aberrations (especially *p53* mutations). Although multiple factors have been identified with the development of these urothelial tumors (57) (Table 102.13), the single most important of these is a prior exposure to tobacco smoke. Thus, the demographics of the development of bladder cancer mirrors cigarette use in the United States. Men have urothelial tumors three times as often as women, and whites acquire these tumors approximately twice as often as African-Americans. The peak incidence of these tumors is typically in the sixth or seventh decade of life, but can vary over a considerable range.

Diagnosis

Cancers of the urothelial lining may occur anywhere from the kidney to the bladder. Figure 102.1 shows an example of a distal ureteral transitional cell carcinoma presenting with painless hematuria, which is the most common method of presentation for patients with any urothelial malignancy. Significant voiding symptoms do not usually occur unless there is profuse disease, as might be seen with carcinoma in situ or invasive disease. In the case of advanced disease, the patient may experience significant frequency, urgency, stranguria, and marked gross hematuria. Widespread urinalysis screening for hematuria enables most of these tumors to be found at an early stage. Patients who present with persistent microhematuria require evaluation with urinalysis, urinary culture, urinary cytology, and radiographic imaging of the upper urinary tract either by IVU or contrast-enhanced CT. Although radiographic imaging also may demonstrate the presence of

---

Table 102.13. FACTORS ASSOCIATED WITH THE DEVELOPMENT OF UROTHELIAL TUMORS

Aniline dyes
2-Naphthylamine
Nitrosamines
Cyclophosphamide
Acrolein
Phenacetin
Schistosomiasis (e.g., Schistosoma haematobium)
Chronic irritation (stones or hardware such as a catheter)
Radiation exposure
Tobacco exposure

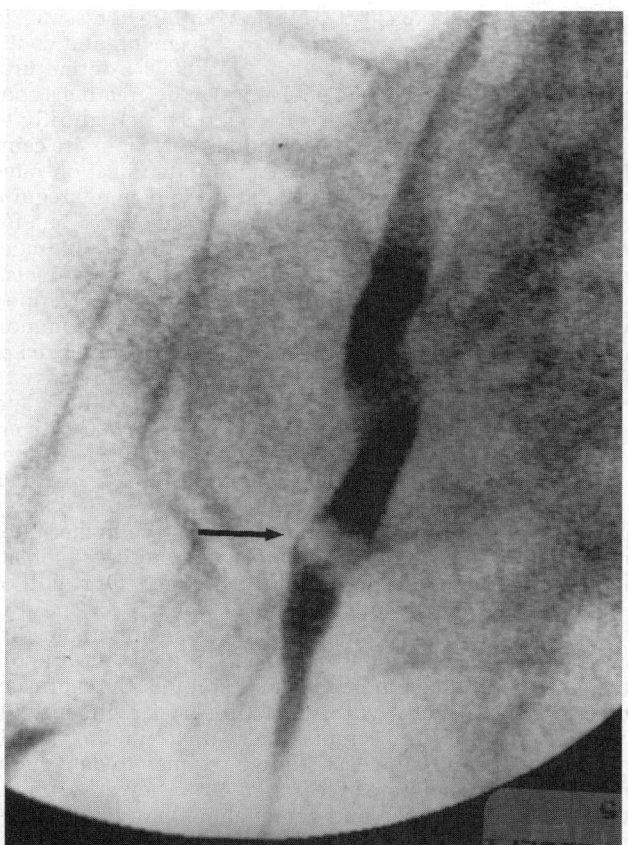

Figure 102.1. Retrograde pyelogram demonstrating a distal transitional cell carcinoma (stage T1) *(arrow)* in a 65-year-old white woman. The patient presented with painless hematuria and a positive urinary cytologic analysis. Her risk factors for this disease included a long-standing history of tobacco use and prior pelvic radiation as part of treatment for a low-grade cervical neoplasm 20 years earlier.

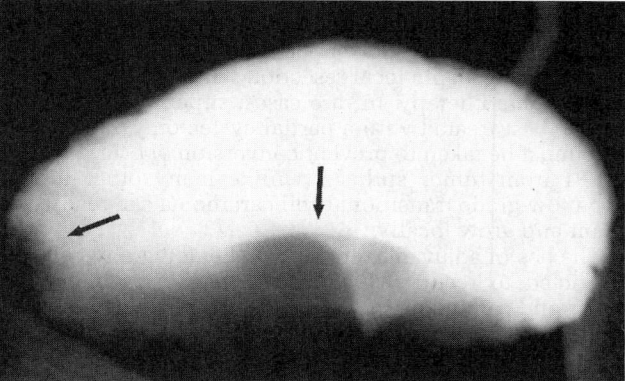

Figure 102.2. Intravenous pyelogram demonstrating a small lateral bladder filling defect *(arrow)*. The midline defect *(arrow)* is most consistent with an enlarged prostate in this elderly African American man. Cystoscopy confirmed the filling defect was in fact a bladder tumor. Subsequent resection revealed that this was a low-grade urothelial cancer (stage Ta). This patient's risk factor for the disease was a history of tobacco use.

(up to 60%) and requires close surveillance with urinary cytology and cystoscopy every 3 months and periodic radiographic imaging (IVU or CT) at least annually. T1 disease and carcinoma in situ are more prone to progression to a frankly invasive malignancy (roughly one third of the time) and similarly require close surveillance. Of the T1 lesions, high-grade disease (grade 3) carries the worst prognosis, with progression rates in excess of 50%, such that many urologists advocate treating patients with extensive high-grade disease (T1G3) as if they had muscle-invasive disease (60). Patients who are thought to be candidates for surgical therapy require completion of their staging with chest radiography and laboratory studies, including complete blood count (CBC), coagulation profile, serum metabolic panel, and serum chemistries.

bladder tumors (Fig. 102.2), cystoscopy is always indicated to confirm this diagnosis. If the patient presents with active gross hematuria, cystoscopy may be undertaken immediately to identify the source. Otherwise, the radiographic evaluation is performed in conjunction with the cystoscopy. Newer methods of urine screening with dipstick tests such as Bard BTA (58) or NMP22 (59) are still experimental, and their precise roles have yet to be determined. They are likely to prove most useful in monitoring patients with previously treated urothelial tumors.

Once the diagnosis of a urothelial malignancy is made, further staging is necessary. Clinicopathologic staging is outlined in Table 102.14. Because patients with urothelial tumors have already undergone radiographic imaging of the urinary system as part of their hematuria evaluation, subsequent imaging, if necessary, is focused on completing the staging evaluation. The first step in this process is obtaining a tissue diagnosis with adequate deep muscle tissue to distinguish muscle-invasive disease from superficial disease. If there is a high suspicion of invasive disease based on the initial cystoscopy, then a preoperative staging CT of the abdomen and pelvis is worthwhile because a postoperative study may be unable to distinguish tissue reaction and local artifact related to endoscopic resection of the primary tumor with deep biopsies. Superficial disease (Ta) is usually low grade and associated with only a 10% rate of progression to invasive carcinoma. Unfortunately, this low-grade disease is prone to recurrence

Table 102.14. CLINICOPATHOLOGIC STAGING OF UROTHELIAL TUMORS

Clinicopathologic staging	Urothelial tumors
Ta	Superficial papillary
Tis	Carcinoma in situ
T1	Invasive, limited to lamina propria
T2	Invasive, limited to superficial muscle (muscularis propria)
T3	Deeply invasive urothelial carcinoma
T3a	Invasion limited to deep muscle
T3b	Invasion limited to perivesical fat
T4	Advanced urothelial carcinoma
T4a	Involvement limited to prostate/uterus/vagina
T4b	involvement limited to pelvic or abdominal wall
Nx	Nodal status cannot be assessed
N0	None
N1	Single lymph node, <2cm
N2	Lymph node involvement 2–5 cm
N3	Lymph node involvement >5 cm
Mx	Cannot be assessed
M0	No metastasis
M1	Distant metastasis

This TNM classification is based on the American Joint Committee on Cancer. American Joint Committee on Cancer (AJCC) manual for staging of cancer, 5th ed. 1997.

Treatment

Treatment options for superficial urothelial carcinoma include endoscopic local resection with or without intravesical chemotherapy. In rare cases, superficial carcinoma can be best treated with a partial cystectomy, but extreme care must be taken to prevent conversion of a Ta/T1 lesion to T4 from tumor spillage. Unlike many other tumors, even low-grade transitional cell carcinoma can readily implant and grow locally.

The use of adjuvant intravesical chemotherapy is largely restricted to recurrent superficial transitional cell carcinoma and carcinoma in situ (60). Various agents have been tested, including mitomycin C, thiotepa, doxorubicin, and bacillus Calmette-Guérin (BCG). BCG therapy appears to be the most effective method of treatment in the adjuvant setting; however, there are emerging data suggesting that immediate postoperative adjuvant doxorubicin or epirubicin results in a significantly diminished long-term recurrence rate (61). Although many institutions have slightly different protocols for BCG administration, BCG is usually administered as an intravesical instillation, once a week for a total of 6 weeks. In the case of high-grade (T1G3) disease or carcinoma in situ, many urologists favor the use of the Southwest Oncology Group 8516 protocol, which calls for additional periodic maintenance instillations of BCG for up to 3 years after the initial treatment (62).

Muscle-invasive transitional cell carcinoma is most appropriately treated with radical cystoprostatectomy in men or anterior exenteration in women, provided the patient is a reasonable surgical candidate. Patients who are not candidates for radical surgery can be offered bladder salvage therapy consisting of endoscopic resection, local radiation therapy, and systemic chemotherapy; however, the long-term outcomes from such an approach are still under investigation (63). Radical surgery involves the removal of local regional lymph nodes, the bladder, prostate, and seminal vesicles and a portion of the vas deferens. In women, the bladder and anterior vagina are resected *en bloc*. The urinary stream therefore must be diverted either into a continent neobladder or through an intestinal conduit to a cutaneous stomal apparatus. The choice of reconstruction depends on patient preference, extent of disease, and the surgeon's technical expertise.

Continent cutaneous neobladders (e.g., Koch pouch) can obviate the need for a stomal appliance and preserve the patient's perception of body image, but do not fully recapitulate the original anatomy and voiding process. They are also prone to recurrent infections, metabolic abnormalities, and urinary stone formation (64). Orthotopic neobladder more closely approximates the original voiding process, but requires a negative urethral margin with focal disease, and a motivated patient who is willing to perform intermittent self-catheterization if necessary to ensure complete emptying and irrigation of mucus from the neobladder. Because these reconstructions are less common, they are probably best performed in tertiary care centers specializing in that type of surgery (65). Typically, such reconstructions are performed with ileum or terminal ileum/proximal colon. The use of the colon segment allows implantation of the ureters in a tunneled (nonrefluxing) fashion, although this is not always necessary. Removing the ileocolic valve from the fecal stream may also place the patient at increased risk for diarrhea and poorly formed stools. Moreover, removing the terminal ileum is associated with vitamin B_{12} deficiency. Ileal neobladders circumvent some of these problems, but their construction requires longer intestinal segments (60 cm). The basic tenets of neobladder reconstruction are to provide a moderate-capacity reservoir with low filling pressure and a continence mechanism. The intestinal segment used determines the capacity. The low filling pressure is achieved by detubularizing the bowel segment, and continence is achieved either by using the intact external urethral sphincter (orthotopic neobladder) or by creating a continent cutaneous stoma that is catheterized periodically to empty the pouch. Although neobladder diversions are gaining in popularity, they do have higher complication rates than simple conduit diversions and these patients require closer follow-up, not just for cancer recurrence, but for metabolic monitoring, infection risk assessment, and adequate emptying and protection of the upper urinary tracts.

Simple conduit urinary diversion can be performed with virtually any segment of bowel. The most common method uses distal ileum, as described initially by Bricker (66,67). These ileal loop conduits are technically easy to create, result in minimal metabolic abnormalities, and provide a durable and reliable method of urinary diversion. As long as the stoma is positioned such that it does not interfere with the patient's beltline, placement of a stomal appliance is usually well tolerated. Alternative conduits derived from jejunum or colon have higher rates of metabolic abnormalities and are usually reserved for situations that preclude the use of ileum (e.g., short gut, or pelvic radiation exposure to ileum).

Metastatic bladder cancer is largely an incurable disease. Multiple approaches have been studied, but durable responses are uncommon. Chemotherapy is the mainstay of treatment, usually with cisplatin-based regimens. M-VAC [methotrexate, vinblastine, doxorubicin (Adriamycin), cisplatin], the best-studied regimen to date, has a complete remission rate of less than 40%. Newer regimens that include paclitaxel and gemcitabine may have higher response rates, but the cancer commonly recurs and progresses (68). Surgical intervention in these patients is usually directed at palliation only.

RENAL NEOPLASMS

Over 30,000 new patients are diagnosed each year with renal carcinoma in the United States, accounting for 3% of adult solid tumors. When the disease becomes advanced, the prognosis is poor despite aggressive treatment regimens (69). Over 11,000 Americans died of renal cell carcinoma (RCC) in 1996 (70). Although renal neoplasms can occur at almost age, they are most common in the fifth to seventh decades of life. Figure 102.3 shows a case of a large, left-sided RCC presenting as flank fullness in a 17-year-old man. It occurs in men twice as often as women, and although genetic syndromes associated with RCC are well described, most of these cases are sporadic.

The most common type of renal cancer is an adenocarcinoma, commonly referred to as RCC (>75%); it is thought to be derived from the proximal convoluted tubule. The histologic appearance is described as clear cell, granular, or mixed. These cancers tend to have a significant degree of tumor vascularity (i.e., tend to enhance with IV contrast) and were once referred to as *hypernephromas,* in the incorrect belief that they were derived from the adrenal gland. Fuhrman's grading system (1 is well differentiated, 4 is highly undifferentiated) is commonly used when evaluating these cancers because the more anaplastic cancers tend to carry a poorer prognosis. Other, less common tumors of the kidney include the papillary RCC (10%), chromophobe cell carcinoma (3% to 5%), oncocytoma (5%), angiomyolipoma (<2%), and sarcomatoid carcinoma (<1%).

Compared with transitional cell carcinoma, relatively little is known about environmental risk factors in the promotion of RCC (57). Proposed risk factors include acquired

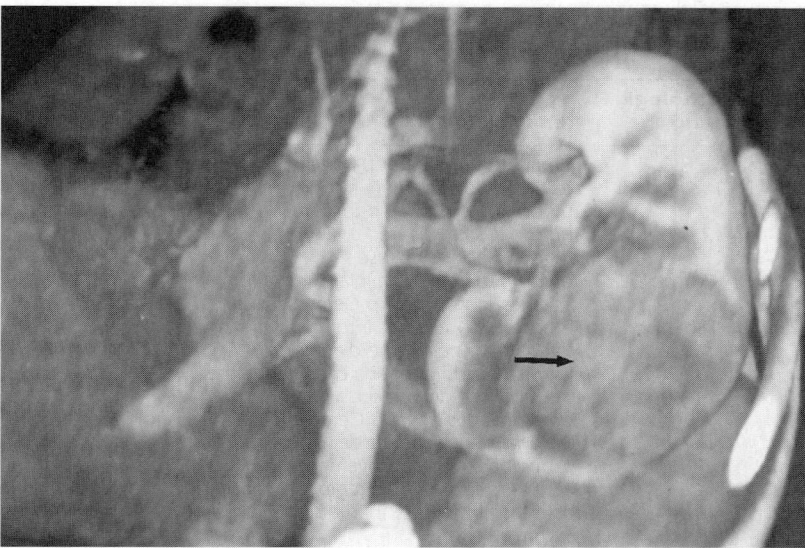

Figure 102.3. Computed tomography scan with three-dimensional reconstruction demonstrating a large (>7 cm) lower pole renal cell carcinoma in a 17-year-old patient presenting with flank pain and microscopic hematuria.

renal cystic disease (typically in patients with end-stage renal disease on hemodialysis), exposure to lead or cadmium, asbestosis, high-fat diet, obesity, hypertension, and tobacco exposure (71). Genetic risk factors include von Hippel-Lindau (VHL) disease, tuberous sclerosis, polycystic kidney disease (especially the autosomal recessive form), and hereditary papillary RCC. VHL disease is an autosomal dominant genetic defect that manifests as CNS hemangioblastomas, retinal angiomatosis, cysts of certain organs (kidney, epididymis, and pancreas), and RCC (72). It is caused by a mutation in the *VHL* tumor suppressor gene. RCC develops in fully 50% of these patients, and is now the most common cause of death in this population. Most of the sporadic RCCs studied to date either have mutations in the *VHL* gene or inactivation of *VHL* gene expression (73). Tuberous sclerosis is also an autosomal dominant genetic syndrome that often manifests with seizures (from benign CNS tumors, referred to as *tubers*), adenoma sebaceum, mental retardation (variable), renal cysts, and increased risk of either renal angiomyolipoma or RCC (74). It is caused by a mutation in one of two tumor suppressor genes (*TSC1* and *TSC2*) that are thought to be evolutionarily related through gene duplication.

The risk of RCC originally was thought to be increased in patients with autosomal dominant polycystic kidney disease (ADPKD). However, now that the genes responsible for both VHL and ADPKD have been identified, it seems more likely that the cases of RCC originally attributed to ADPKD were in fact subtle forms of VHL. The autosomal recessive form of polycystic kidney disease, however, does still seem to carry approximately a 30-fold elevated risk for development of RCC over the general population. Hereditary papillary RCC is a recently described syndrome, and the details of this entity are still being evaluated. Early work in this area suggests that papillary RCCs are associated with a high incidence of activation of the *c-Met* protooncogene (75). A recently described renal medullary carcinoma appears to be a highly anaplastic cancer found in young African-Americans with hemoglobin gene sickle cell trait or hemoglobin sickle cell disease (76).

Diagnosis

The decreasing costs of radiographic imaging have resulted in a marked increase in the number of incidentally discovered renal masses (approximately 40% to 50%),

with a resultant migration to lower-stage disease at discovery. As a result, the classic triad of flank pain, flank fullness or mass, and hematuria now occurs in less than 10% of patients diagnosed with RCC (77). Constitutional symptoms are still common and weight loss may occur in as many as a third of the patients. Others symptoms include fever of unknown origin, renally mediated hypertension, new-onset varicocele (especially left side), malaise, and anemia. Paraneoplastic syndromes are common with RCC, as outlined in Table 102.15. These paraneoplastic syndromes typically resolve spontaneously after resection of the primary mass. Because most patients present with incidentally discovered renal tumors, the subsequent evaluation is typically directed at accurate staging and preoperative planning. The criteria for staging are outlined in Table 102.16. CT appears to be the best overall modality for assessing clinical stage and has supplanted the more traditional IVU as a means of diagnosis and staging. CT allows determination of tumor size, location, extension, and adrenal involvement, and provides preliminary information regarding nodal involvement. RCC has a predilection for invading into the renal vein and inferior vena cava (IVC), although this is not usually a direct invasion into the vessels themselves, but rather a tumor thrombus. Renal vein and IVC tumor thrombus involvement does not necessarily portend a poorer prognosis and should not be a deterrent to definitive surgical management (78).

Renal cystic masses detected by CT are confirmed by ultrasound for evaluation of any solid components. The risk of cancer progression in complex renal cysts has been extensively studied by Bosniak, who developed a classifica-

Table 102.15. PARANEOPLASTIC SYNDROMES ASSOCIATED WITH RENAL CELL CARCINOMA

Hypercalcemia
Erythrocytosis
Anemia
Amyloidosis
Elevated sedimentation rate
Elevated liver function test results (Stauffer's syndrome)
Elevated serum alkaline phosphatase
Elevated serum ferritin

Table 102.16. CLINICOPATHOLOGIC STAGING OF RENAL TUMORS

Clinicopathologic staging	Renal tumor
Tx	Primary tumor cannot be assessed
T0	No evidence of primary tumor
T1	Tumor ≤7.0 cm, limited to kidney
T2	Tumor >7.0 cm, limited to kidney
T3	Locally extensive disease
T3a	Tumor invades adrenal gland or perinephric tissues, but limited to Gerota's fascia
T3b	Tumor grossly extends into renal vein or vena cava below the diaphragm
T3c	Tumor extends into vena cava above the level of the diaphragm
T4	Tumor invades beyond Gerota's fascia
Nx	Regional nodes cannot be assessed
N0	No regional node involvement
N1	Metastasis into a single regional lymph node
N2	Metastasis into more than a single regional lymph node
Mx	Distant metastasis cannot be assessed
M0	No distant metastasis
M1	Distant metastasis

This TMN classification is based on the American Joint Committee on Cancer. American Joint Committee on Cancer (AJCC) manual for staging of cancer, 5th ed. 1997.

tion system (Table 102.17) to help distinguish the risk of underlying malignancy (79). Bosniak class I and II cysts are typically followed conservatively, whereas class III and IV cysts are explored and resected surgically if the patients are otherwise surgical candidates.

Completion of the staging evaluation typically involves a chest radiograph, CBC, coagulation profile, screening chemistries, and metabolic panel (including renal function and liver function tests, alkaline phosphatase, and serum calcium). In patients with large tumors (T2), a CT scan of the chest is often done because this is more sensitive for detecting occult pulmonary metastasis. Magnetic resonance imaging angiography or venocavography may be used if there is any concern over the possibility of an IVC tumor thrombus (approximately 5%) or in patients with azotemia, which precludes them from a contrast-enhanced CT scan. In addition, the azotemic patient may also be a candidate for nuclear renography to assess differential renal function.

Treatment

In 1963, Robson showed a significant increase in 5-year survival rates after radical nephrectomy for RCC (80). Despite rapid changes in the practice of radiation and medical oncology, stage for stage there has not been a significant improvement in survival since that time. Thus, whenever feasible, surgery remains the treatment of choice for renal malignancies. Traditionally, the radical nephrectomy procedure is performed through a flank incision, and involves removal of the kidney, adrenal gland, and proximal ureter, *en bloc* and with Gerota's fascia. The adrenal gland, however, is infrequently involved and does not necessarily need to be removed in small, lower pole masses, unless it is enlarged. Although advocated by some, the role of extended lymphadenectomy is limited and it usually is not performed (81). Patients with a solitary kidney or with underlying renal insufficiency can still be candidates for curative resection by a partial nephrectomy. Provided the primary tumor is less than 4 cm, the local recurrence rate is very low (<5%) (82). Indeed, the results of partial nephrectomies have been so encouraging that many now advocate partial nephrectomy for all patients with small peripheral renal masses, even with a normal contralateral kidney. Another recent development has been the use of laparoscopy for performing a radical or even a partial nephrectomy (49). Early data regarding outcomes with this approach show a significant decrease in morbidity without compromising disease-free survival. When performing a laparoscopic nephrectomy, care must be taken to prevent tumor spillage during morcellation of the kidney. Alternatively, a small midline incision, just large enough to permit retrieval of the specimen, can be performed at the end of the procedure.

Small RCCs (<3 cm) are known to have a low propensity to metastasize, and thus experimental nephron-sparing techniques have been developed to try to treat these tumors in a minimally invasive manner. Aside from the more traditional methods of partial nephrectomy, minimally invasive methods using high-frequency ultrasound, radiofrequency thermal ablation, and cryosurgery have all been attempted. Currently, laparoscopically directed cryosurgery has been gaining popularity for the small, peripheral renal mass, although the long-term efficacy of such an approach remains to be determined (83).

Advanced RCC is a devastating disease. Because of the ready access of these tumors to the venous vasculature, hematogenous metastasis can occur to a wide number of sites, including adrenal gland, lung, liver, brain, bone, and the contralateral kidney. When widespread disease occurs, treatment can be difficult. Factors that improve prognosis include a long interval between the time of original treatment and detectable metastasis, good performance status (rare), and metastasis limited to one portion of the lung. Patients with a solitary metastasis may still be candidates for surgical resection. Patients with a synchronous

Table 102.17. BOSNIAK RENAL CYSTIC MASS CLASSIFICATION[a]

Classification	Type of cystic mass	Management
I	Simple cyst	No follow-up necessary
II	Minimal complex (usually benign)	Observe
	Curvilinear calcification	
	Thin septa	
	Hyperdense cyst	
III	Equivocal cyst	Consider surgery
	Irregular calcification	
	Thick septa	
	Heterogeneity of cyst fluid	
IV	Frankly malignant	Surgical excision
	Nodular/solid components	
	Lesion enhances with contrast	

[a]These criteria require a contrast-enhanced spiral computed tomography scan.

solitary metastasis carry a poorer prognosis that those with a delayed solitary metastasis. Nonetheless, surgical resections in this scenario have been associated with an approximately 30% 5-year survival rate, although most of these patients are not cancer free.

Because spontaneous regression of advanced RCC occurs in approximately 1% to 2% of patients, there has been a great deal of enthusiasm for the development of immunologically based therapy for advanced disease (84). Multiple strategies have been used, including the use of autologous harvested tumor-infiltrating lymphocytes, interferon administration, interleukin-2 administration, and ex vivo gene therapy. Combination protocols involving both immunotherapy and surgery have also been developed as a method of consolidation in those patients who are responders (85). Even in the best of circumstances, the response rate for immunotherapy of RCC has been poor, with complete remission rates of approximately 6% and total response rates (partial response + complete response) of approximately 30%. Chemotherapy has also been largely ineffective for RCC because multiple drug resistance appears to be a common finding in these cancers. Despite these poor early outcomes, immunotherapy and gene therapy remain active and exciting areas of research for the eventual treatment of advanced RCC.

PROSTATE CANCER

As we enter the new millennium, prostate cancer continues to emerge as a major health care problem (86). It is the single most commonly diagnosed cancer and the second most common cause of cancer-related deaths in American men. Approximately 39,200 prostate cancer-related deaths occurred in the United States in 1998 (87). Unlike many other malignancies, prostate cancer typically does not become symptomatic until the advanced stages. Increased interest in screening and the availability of the serum marker, PSA, have resulted in an improvement in the diagnosis of early-stage disease. In widespread use as a diagnostic marker since 1987 (88), PSA is one of at least two serine proteases present in the blood and semen. It is thought that this protease is lyses the seminal coagulum at the appropriate time to allow subsequent fertilization.

Prostate-specific antigen circulates in sera predominantly bound to carrier proteins such as α_1-antichymotrypsin. Both the total and the free forms of PSA can be measured in most clinical laboratories with commercially available kits. The total PSA is commonly used as a screening test, with a typical cutoff of 4 ng/mL considered as the upper limit of normal. The unbound form is referred to as free PSA. Although formal cutoffs for percentage free PSA have not yet been determined, in general, patients with prostate cancer have a lower percentage of free PSA than patients without prostate cancer. Using a cutoff of less than 25% free PSA, coupled with a total PSA of 4 to 10 ng/mL, allows detection of approximately 95% of prostate cancers while reducing the proportion of unnecessary biopsies by 20% (89). Lower cutoffs result in higher specificity of detection but poorer sensitivity.

Diagnosis

Staging

Prostate cancer staging has undergone numerous revisions. The earliest commonly used staging system was devised by Whitmore and Jewett and is still in use by many institutions. In 1992, the American Joint Committee on Cancer (AJCC) developed the more commonly used TNM classification system, which has now become the standard for staging prostate cancer. The AJCC revised the classification system in 1997, eliminating the distinction between a unilateral nodule that occupies less than half of that side from a substantially larger unilateral nodule. Thus, in the newer classification, a unilateral nodule is classified as stage T2a, whereas bilateral bilateral disease is classified as stage T2b, and the size of the nodule in relation to the gland is ignored. The newer TNM classification is still not in widespread use, and there are some reports that suggest that the older TNM classification retains better prognostic value (90). A comparison of the various staging criteria is show in Table 102.18.

Screening

The diagnosis of prostate cancer is determined histopathologically after prostatic biopsy, typically performed under transrectal ultrasound guidance. Most men undergo prostatic biopsy because of an abnormality on rectal examination, or PSA elevation. However, the routine use of DRE and PSA testing in asymptomatic men as a means of reducing prostate cancer mortality by early detection and treatment is controversial (91). The American Cancer Society and the American Urological Association recommend the routine use of DRE and PSA in asymptomatic men older than 50 years of age. Men with an increased risk of prostate cancer such as African Americans or those with a family history of prostate cancer should start screening at an earlier age (92). The Canadian Task Force on the Periodic Health Examination does not support the routine use of PSA for prostate cancer screening (93). Arguments for prostate cancer screening are based on the belief that early detection will decrease disease mortality rates, particularly because effective treatments are available for early-stage disease. Arguments against prostate cancer screening are based on the belief that early detection could result in excessive treatment of many cancers with low risks of progression rather than improvement of health in large populations.

Although no randomized trials have been performed to demonstrate the value of prostate cancer screening, population trends after the onset of widespread PSA testing suggest that screening may reduce mortality rates. Since 1987, large populations of otherwise asymptomatic men have undergone PSA screening, in combination with DRE, followed by prostatic biopsy when indicated. Three observations since the onset of PSA screening suggest that early disease detection results in a decreased mortality rate. First, introduction of a successful screening test should result in an increased incidence, as the prevalent cases are detected, followed by a decreased incidence to near prescreening levels. Second, a successful screening test should result in stage migration to early-stage disease, with a decreased rate of detection of advanced disease. Third, the mortality rate should decline. Early analyses of the prostate cancer population statistics have indeed revealed a sharp increase in prostate cancer diagnoses, which peaked approximately 1992 (86,87). Subsequently, there has been a steady decline in the rate of prostate cancer diagnosis, so that the current rate of detection is approaching the pre-PSA screening era (92). Multiple studies have now also documented a migration of stage to earlier forms of the disease, so that stage T1C cancers, detected by PSA screening alone (negative DRE), account for a substantial proportion of locally treated cancers (94). Also noted is an age migration, so that prostate cancers are being diagnosed in men at an earlier age. Cancer-specific survival for stage T1C disease is better than for stage T2 disease (palpable, but organ confined). Whether this stage migration and subsequent treatment translates into a population-based improvement in cancer-specific survival re-

Table 102.18. **CLINICOPATHOLOGIC STAGING OF PROSTATE TUMORS: WHITMORE-JEWETT (W-J) AND TNM CLASSIFICATION FOR THE STAGING OF PROSTATE CANCER AS DEFINED BY THE AMERICAN JOINT COMMITTEE ON CANCER (1992 AND 1997)**

W-J	1992	1997	Prostate tumor
—	TX	TX	Primary tumor cannot be assessed
—	T0	T0	No evidence of primary tumor
A	T1	T1	Clinically inapparent tumor not palpable or visible by imaging
A1	T1a	T1a	Tumor incidental histologic finding in ≤5% of tissue resected[a]
A2	T1b	T1b	Tumor incidental histologic finding in >5% of tissue resected[a]
—	T1c	T1c	Tumor identified by needle biopsy[b]
B	T2	T2	Organ-confined, palpable prostate cancer
B1N	T2a	T2a	Unilateral nodule, less than half the lobe
B1	T2b	T2a	Unilateral nodule, more than half the lobe
B2	T2c	T2b	Bilateral palpable disease
C	T3	T3	Tumor extends through the prostatic capsule
C1	T3a	T3a	Unilateral extracapsular extension
C1	T3b	T3a	Bilateral extracapsular extension
C1	T3c	T3b	Tumor extends into seminal vesicle(s)
C2	T4	T4	Tumor is fixed or invades adjacent structures other than seminal vesicles: bladder neck, external sphincter, rectum, levator, pelvic wall
—	NX	NX	Regional lymph nodes cannot be assessed
—	N0	N0	No regional lymph node metastases
D1	N1	N1	Metastasis in regional lymph node(s)
—	MX	MX	Distant metastases cannt be assessed
—	M0	M0	No distant metastases
D2	M1	M1	Distant metastases
D2	M1a	M1a	Nonregional lymph nodes
D2	M1b	M1b	Bone
D2	M1c	M1c	Other distant sites
D3	—	—	Hormone-refractory disease

[a]Incidental prostate cancer detected during resection of the prostate for presumed benign disease (e.g., transurethral resection of the prostate).
[b]Nonpalpable prostate cancer that was evaluated by prostate needle biopsy because of prostate-specific antigen elevation or ultrasonographic abnormality.

mains to be determined. Before 1991, however, mortality rates for prostate cancer were steadily rising, and since that time the rates have leveled off and currently appear to be decreasing at the rate of approximately 1% per year (86). Although many would argue that the jury is still out regarding the efficacy of prostate cancer screening, the early population trends suggest PSA testing in combination with DRE may successfully reduce prostate cancer mortality rates.

Treatment

Localized Disease

Because advanced prostate cancer remains essentially incurable, the diagnosis and treatment of localized prostate cancer (clinical stages T1 and T2) represents a unique opportunity for cure. However, just because a cancer can be cured does not mean cure is necessary. What needs to be distinguished is which cancers are clinically significant and are likely to progress and which ones are at low risk of progression and can be followed conservatively. Small-volume, latent prostate cancer in older men may not affect overall health because of the long natural history of the disease and the limited life expectancy of older men. Risk assessment is currently practiced by stratifying the most important clinical parameters relating to risk of disease progression. These parameters include grade of the cancer as defined by Gleason, stage, PSA, and DRE. The Gleason grade can range from 1 (well differentiated) to 5 (poorly differentiated), and a score is given as the sum of the two highest grades determined for the specimen. Thus, the Gleason score can range from 2 to 10. Be-

cause time at risk in part determines the chance of disease progression, men older than 65 years of age thought to have small-volume disease represent the target group for watchful waiting. Our current practice is to offer watchful waiting to patients with stage T1C disease, who are 65 years or older, whose PSA density is 0.15 ng/mL/g (PSA divided by ultrasound-estimated prostate size) or less, and whose biopsy results are scored as Gleason 6 or less with no more than two cores involved with cancer and less than 50% involvement of any one core (95). In those situations where watchful waiting is deemed reasonable, yearly surveillance biopsies and twice-yearly DRE and PSAs are still performed, and the patient's eligibility for watchful waiting reassessed.

Patients with local but clinically significant disease (i.e., higher-grade or larger-volume disease), on the other hand, require intervention as long as they otherwise have life expectancies of greater than 10 years. Age and comorbid disease should be considered together when assessing the need for treatment. There are two conventional modes of therapy—radiation and surgery.

Of the radiation-based options, the most commonly used method consists of external beam radiation, typically with a conformal apparatus (96). Brachytherapy using radioactive implants has been gaining widespread popularity; however, the data regarding outcomes in terms of biochemical progression suggest that brachytherapy fails to control localized prostate cancer, particularly in the palpable disease stage (T2), compared with conventional therapies (97). However, although many studies purport to compare radiation outcomes with surgical outcomes directly, the data are collected by different methods. After treatment, PSA is the most sensitive indicator of freedom from disease. An undetectable PSA after surgery indicates eradication of cancer. A stable PSA (not rising) of less than 0.5 ng/mL after radiation therapy is thought to be consistent with a disease-free state. The ASTRO (American Society for Therapeutic Radiology and Oncology) definition of treatment failure after external beam radiation is three consecutive PSA rises after the nadir PSA is reached. The median time to a nadir PSA is between 2 and 3 years. Because PSAs are often measured every 6 months, it may take up to 4.5 years before a treatment failure is recognized. Thus, 5-year PSA progression data are highly biased for favorable outcomes. Ten-year PSA progression outcome data more accurately reflect the efficiency of external beam radiation in eradicating prostate cancer, but these data are largely unavailable for the newer conformal techniques.

Surgical therapy of local prostate cancer is most commonly performed as an anatomically radical retropubic prostatectomy. This procedure, pioneered by Walsh, has resulted in significantly reduced morbidity in terms of recovery of urinary continence and maintenance of erectile function (98). Outcomes data from both institutional series (single surgeon) (99) and hospital cancer registries (100) suggest that a radical retropubic prostatectomy can be performed safely, with low morbidity for most men. Outcomes data from the Medicare population (101) suggest that morbidity is higher in older men (Table 102.19).

Perineal prostatectomy offers no apparent advantage with regard to cancer control, continence, or erectile function. Moreover, initial claims of improved pain control and lower blood loss no longer appear to be as significant compared with the current method of radical retropubic prostatectomy. Finally, there is some recent evidence to suggest that patients who undergo radical perineal prostatectomy have a significantly elevated risk of fecal incontinence (102). Our current practice is to offer a radical retropubic prostatectomy to those patients who have the highest likelihood of organ-confined disease with minimized morbidity (i.e., those patients who are most likely to benefit from surgery). The probability of organ-confined disease can be most easily determined by referring to nomograms combining PSA, histologic grade of the cancer, and DRE findings (103). These tables, when combined with the clinical picture, are extremely useful for patient counseling.

Neoadjuvant therapy with hormonal ablation has been gaining widespread use in both radiation therapy and surgical therapy. Success with conventional external beam conformal radiation may be augmented by pretreatment with hormone-based therapy (104). In certain cases where surgical therapy has revealed locally advanced disease (T3), as might be manifested by a positive surgical margin but negative lymph node dissection, adjuvant therapy with external beam radiation may also play a role in preventing or delaying biochemical progression and consequently cancer progression. Prospective studies of this type of treatment practice are needed to determine fully the role of adjuvant radiation therapy in margin-positive disease.

The role of neoadjuvant hormonal therapy with surgical treatment remains controversial. Initial results from such trials have revealed a significant decrease in the number of positive surgical margins. The significance of this finding, however, is not clear. There is no current evidence to suggest that such an approach causes any decrease in biochemical progression or survival.

Advanced Disease

Hormonal therapy is the mainstay of palliative treatment for advanced prostate cancer. The discovery that male sex hormones are required to maintain the size and function of the prostate led to the development of treatments designed to interfere with this effect. It is well known that androgen deprivation results in a significant involution of the prostate gland with a particularly marked glandular progression to apoptosis (programmed cell death). Not all of the cells are affected by this process because reconstitution of the hormonal supply results in substantial regrowth. Similarly, prostate cancer regresses secondarily to an apoptotic pathway. Invariably, however, the cancer selects out an androgen-independent or insensitive population, which clonally expands and progresses until death. Thus, hormonal therapy is useful, but not curative. The process of selection and expansion, however, can take as long as 2 or more years and may provide a significant window of cancer regression for the patient. Indeed, for some elderly patients, this type of delay in progression may be sufficient to render their disease clinically insignificant compared with their comorbid diseases.

Current options for hormonal therapy include orchiectomy, LH-releasing hormone (LHRH) agonists, and antiandrogen therapy. Orchiectomy is the most cost-effective method of hormonal ablation, but is often unacceptable to the patient. Alternatives include LHRH agonists, which act by disrupting the normal cyclic pattern of secretion of LHRH, thus leading to insignificant levels of LH in the serum. Because LH is required for testosterone synthesis by the Leydig cells, the result is a castrate level of testosterone synthesis. The current LHRH agonists (e.g., goserelin) can now be administered subcutaneously at 3-month intervals.

Although castration, either by medical or surgical means, leads to a low level of androgen synthesis, it does not completely abolish it. Adrenal synthesis of androgens occurs to a limited degree. As a result, there has been some concern that castration alone is inadequate in obtaining maximal benefit from hormonal ablation. Total androgen ablation is achieved, therefore, by adding an antiandrogen in addition to medical or surgical castration. Antiandrogens act at the peripheral target tissues and block the action of androgens at the level of the androgen receptor. Subsequent analyses, however, of this combined modality have failed to demonstrate any significant benefit (105).

When LHRH agonists are administered, there is an initial increase in testosterone production followed by a rapid nadir as a result of an initial LH surge. To prevent this temporary surge in testosterone from allowing prostate cancer

---

Table 102.19. **SURGICAL MORBIDITY OF RADICAL RETROPUBIC PROSTATECTOMY FOR THE JOHNS HOPKINS HOSPITAL (JHH), AMERICAN COLLEGE OF SURGEONS (ACC), AND MEDICARE PATIENT POPULATIONS**

Variable	JHH (1982–1988)	ACS (1993)	Medicare (1988–1990)
Age (y)	Mean—59	40% <65	50% >70
Mortality	<1%	<1%	—
Potency (maintenance of preoperative erectile function)	68%	30%	12%
Continence (not requiring any urinary pads)	92%	80%	70%

growth, an antiandrogen typically is added for the first few weeks of therapy. Newer-generation antiandrogens (e.g., bicalutamide, nilutamide) can now be administered by once-daily dosing with little or no significant differences in side effects compared with the older agents, such as flutamide. Thus, although advanced prostate cancer is incurable, many of its symptoms can be palliated with hormonal therapy.

Prostate cancer, unlike most other malignancies, progresses while maintaining a relatively low proliferation rate. It is estimated that only 2% to 3% of prostate cancer cells in a given patient are actively dividing at any given moment. Because most chemotherapeutic agents are directed at rapidly proliferating cells, prostate cancer is relatively resistant to these agents when used as monotherapy. Multiple agents, including suramin, liarozole, paclitaxel, estramustine, and doxorubicin have shown mild activity over short periods, but a significant survival benefit has not been demonstrated. Combination chemotherapy may have a slightly better activity against prostate cancer. The results, however, are still rather poor and the survival benefit, if any, is limited. Moreover, these agents have yet to demonstrate significant improvements in quality of life. After hormonal therapy has failed, conventional treatment is directed at ameliorating symptoms when possible.

TESTIS CANCER

Although testis cancer is the most common cancer in men between the ages of 15 and 34 years, it is nonetheless a rare tumor, accounting for only approximately 1% of all cancers in American men. The testes start as a pair of undifferentiated intraabdominal organs that become primitive testes around the seventh week of gestation. With time, the testes migrate to a more caudal position and eventually descend out of the abdomen into the scrotum near the time of the completion of gestation. The factors important for testicular descent are complex but include, at a very minimum, hormonal stimulation, neuronal support, and mechanical support. Because the testes are originally retroperitoneal organs, they derive their blood, lymphatic, and nerve supply from the retroperitoneum. The gonadal artery is a direct branch of the aorta, and the lymphatic drainage pattern is directly into the retroperitoneal nodes surrounding the IVC and aorta. Thus, the primary lymphatic drainage of the right testis is to the interaortocaval, precaval, and preaortic lymph nodes. The lymphatic drainage of the left testis is into the paraaortic, preaortic, and interaortocaval nodes.

The factors most commonly associated with an increased risk for development of testis cancer are listed in Table 102.20. Foremost among these risk factors is a his-

tory of cryptorchidism. Approximately 15% of men with testis cancer have had a prior history of cryptorchidism, although only 75% of those tumors occurred in the testis that failed to descend. The fact that the cancer formed in the normally descended testis with a 25% incidence suggests that cryptorchidism is not the direct cause of testis cancer, but merely a manifestation of some other cause. Many cases of cryptorchidism resolve spontaneously, usually within the first year of life. Subsequent to that, many advocate surgical correction (i.e., orchiopexy) to allow better self-examination and surveillance for a subsequent testis cancer.

Because the testes contain both germ cells and supportive cells (i.e., Sertoli and Leydig cells), tumors derived from the testes can occur from either source. Sex cord stromal tumors (i.e., Sertoli or Leydig cell tumor) are far less common than germ cell tumors and often present with signs of hormonal secretion (106) (e.g., gynecomastia). Germ cell tumors can be broadly categorized as seminoma and nonseminoma. Seminomas are the most common type of testicular tumors, although mixed tumors are common (107).

Nonseminomatous tumors may secrete certain marker proteins that allow both preoperative and postoperative assessment. Endodermal sinus cancer (i.e., yolk sac tumor) is known to secrete α-fetoprotein (AFP), and choriocarcinoma is known to secrete β-human chorionic gonadotropin (β-HCG). Pure seminoma does not secrete AFP, but may secrete β-HCG in up to 10% of cases. Thus, if these tumor markers are elevated before surgery, they are useful markers to follow after surgery for recurrence or progression. Typically, at least five times the biologic half-life ($t_{1/2}$) should elapse before a postoperative tumor marker is measured, to allow adequate clearance from the body. Because the $t_{1/2}$ for AFP is approximately 5 days, five half-lives corresponds to roughly 1 month. The $t_{1/2}$ of β-HCG is approximately 1 day, so follow-up measurements can be started as early as 1 week after surgery. β-HCG shares a common a subunit with LH and FSH (as well as thyroid-stimulating hormone); thus, elevations in any of these gonadotropins may result in spuriously elevated b-HCG measurements if the assay method used cannot distinguish them adequately. Most currently used commercial laboratories can easily distinguish these different peptide hormones. However, historically it is recommended that the other gonadotropins be assessed when a postoperative β-HCG is slightly elevated.

Diagnosis

Most cases of testis cancer are brought to clinical attention from self-examination. The most common finding is an abnormally enlarged testis or firm nodule. Often, scrotal trauma precedes the diagnosis because it prompts either the patient or his physician to examine the testes. Occasionally, the patient may present with orchialgia, but this is more the exception than the rule. The first step to diagnosis is scrotal ultrasonography, which is very helpful in documenting a testicular mass, particularly when a thorough examination is difficult. Scrotal enlargement may also result from benign processes such as a hydrocele, which can also be easily distinguished by ultrasonography. If there is a suspicion of a testicular mass, then surgical exploration with orchiectomy is indicated. Preoperative evaluation should include CBC, serum tumor markers including lactate dehydrogenase, AFP, and β-HCG, coagulation profile, and chest radiography. Once a pathologic diagnosis is made, then the staging is completed and subsequent treatment recommendations are made.

Table 102.20. **RISK FACTORS FOR THE DEVELOPMENT OF TESTICULAR CANCER**

Age
  Pediatric   Nonseminomatous tumor (e.g., yolk sac tumors)
  Young adults   Seminoma > nonseminomatous tumors
  Geriatric   Spermatocytic seminoma, lymphoma

Race (whites at highest risk)
Cryptorchidism
Family history
HIV infection/AIDS (lymphoma)
Presence of carcinoma in situ (e.g., testicular biopsy for infertility)
Prior history of testicular cancer in contralateral testis
Occupational risks (nonseminomatous tumors only)
  Miners, oil and gas workers, leather workers, food and beverage processing workers, janitors, and utility workers

Treatment

Initial treatment and definitive diagnosis occur contemporaneously by orchiectomy through an inguinal surgical incision. Transscrotal orchiectomy carries the theoretic risk of altering the lymphatic drainage, and is discouraged. Once a definitive diagnosis is made, staging can be completed. Radiographic staging requires a CT scan of the chest, abdomen, and pelvis with oral and intravenous contrast. The criteria for staging are outlined graphically in Fig. 102.4.

Seminomas are known to be highly radiosensitive. Thus, patients with stage I or II seminomas are treated with adjuvant radiation therapy to the paraaortic and paracaval areas below the diaphragm, as well as the ipsilateral inguinal and pelvic regions. Higher-stage seminomas require adjuvant chemotherapy with a cisplatin-based regimen.

Nonseminomatous tumors are less radiosensitive and thus require either surgical resection or chemotherapy, or both. Stage I tumors (limited to the testes) may be treated by either watchful waiting with close surveillance, limited chemotherapy with close surveillance, or a retroperitoneal lymph node dissection (RPLND). The choice is driven mainly by patient preference, institutional preference, and physician experience. Currently, there is no clear consensus on how to proceed in these patients with limited disease. The advent of laparoscopic retroperitoneal lymphadenectomy has allowed a minimally invasive technique for achieving the same goal (i.e., diagnostic assessment, potential therapeutic resection) with minimal morbidity. When an RPLND is performed (open or laparoscopic), a template dissection is recommended to allow partial preservation of the sympathetic chain and thus allow antegrade postoperative ejaculation. Regardless of which approach is taken, these patients require close follow-up and observation with serum tumor markers and chest radiographs on at least an every-other-month basis for 2 years and periodic CT scans performed with alternate visits.

Small stage II nonseminomatous tumors (<5 cm) are treated initially with RPLND, followed by adjuvant cisplatin-based chemotherapy if cancer is discovered in the final pathologic specimen. Bulky stage II and III nonseminomatous tumors are often treated initially with chemotherapy and then, if a residual retroperitoneal mass is seen on subsequent imaging with normalization of the tumor markers, a postchemotherapy RPLND is performed. If residual cancer is found on the subsequent RPLND, additional chemotherapy is indicated. Because of advances in chemotherapy, metastatic testis cancer is still a treatable disease (108). Survival rates of greater than 70% are reported for patients with advanced disease and greater than 90% for lower-stage disease. Long-term surveillance is indicated in these patients because remote recurrences as long as 20 years after initial treatment have been described.

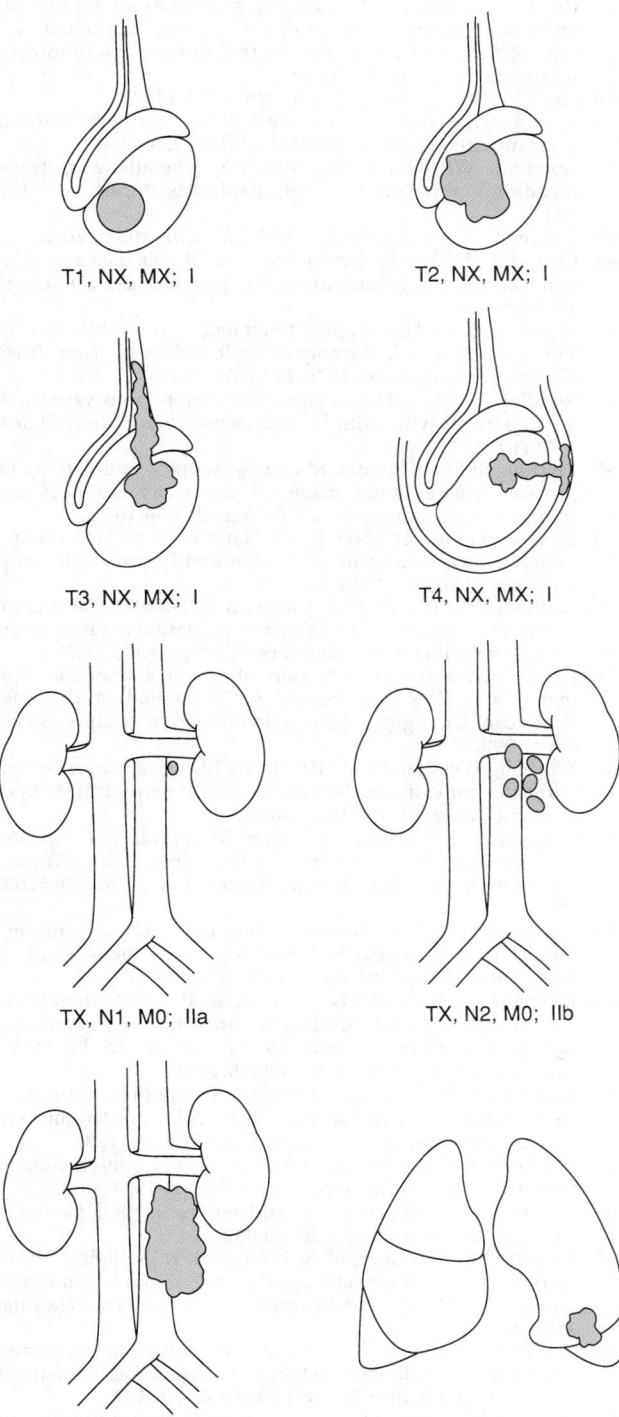

Figure 102.4. Staging of testis cancer. Both the TNM (American Joint Committee on Cancer, 1997) and a commonly used descriptive system are shown.

T1, NX, MX; I

T2, NX, MX; I

T3, NX, MX; I

T4, NX, MX; I

TX, N1, M0; IIa

TX, N2, M0; IIb

TX, N3, M0; IIc

TX, NX, M1; III

REFERENCES

1. Burnett AL, Wesselmann U. Neurobiology of the pelvis and perineum: principles for a practical approach. *J Pelvic Surg* 1999;4:224.
2. Chai TC, Steers WD. Neurophysiology of micturition and continence. *Urol Clin North Am* 1996;23:221.
3. Walsh PC. Benign prostatic hyperplasia. In: Walsh PC, Gittes RF, Perlmutter AD, et al., eds. *Campbell's urology,* 5th ed. Philadelphia: WB Saunders, 1986:1248–1265.
4. Cockett AT. Proceedings from the 3rd International Consultation on Benign Prostatic Hyperplasia. In: Cockett AT, ed. *The 3rd International Consultation on BPH Recommendations of the International Consensus Committee.* Jersey, United Kingdom: Scientific Communication International, 1996.
5. Collins MM, Stafford RS, O'Leary P, et al. How common is prostatitis? A national survey of physician visits. *J Urol* 1997;157:243A.
6. Roberts RO, Lieber MM, Bostwick DG, et al. A community-based study on the prevalence of prostatitis. *J Urol* 1997; 157:242A.
7. Chronic Prostatitis Workshop. *Summary statement.* Bethesda, MD: National Institutes of Health, December 7–9, 1995.

8. Miller JL, Rothman I, Bavendam TG, et al. Prostatodynia and interstitial cystitis: one and the same? *Urology* 1995;45:587.

9. Alexander RB, Brady F, Ponniah S. Autoimmune prostatitis: evidence of T cell reactivity with normal prostatic proteins. *Urology* 1997;50:893.

10. Wesselmann U, Burnett AL, Heinberg LJ. The urogenital and rectal pain syndromes. *Pain* 1997;73:269.

11. Thomas TM, Plymat KR, Blann J, et al. Prevalence of urinary incontinence. *BMJ* 1980;281:1243.

12. Diokno AC, Brock BM, Brown MB, et al. Prevalence of urinary incontinence and other urological symptoms in the noninstitutionalized elderly. *J Urol* 1986;136:1022.

13. NIH Consensus Conference. Impotence. NIH Consensus Development Panel on Impotence [Review]. *JAMA* 1993;270:83.

14. Johnson AR, Jarow JP. Is routine endocrine testing of impotent men necessary? *J Urol* 1992;147:1542.

15. Burnett AL. Oral pharmacotherapy for erectile dysfunction: current perspectives. *Urology* 1999;54:392.

16. Fallon B. Intracavernous injection therapy for male erectile dysfunction. *Urol Clin North Am* 1995;22:833.

17. Padma-Nathan H, Hellstrom WJ, Kaiser FE, et al. Treatment of men with erectile dysfunction with transurethral alprostadil: Medicated Urethral System for Erection (MUSE) Study Group. *N Engl J Med* 1997;336:1.

18. Lewis R. Long-term results of penile prosthetic implants. *Urol Clin North Am* 1995;22:847.

19. Goldstein I, Hatzichristou DG, Pescatori ES. Pelvic, perineal, and penile trauma-associated arteriogenic impotence: pathophysiologic mechanisms and the role of microvascular arterial bypass surgery. In: Bennett AH, ed. *Impotence: diagnosis and management of erectile dysfunction*. Philadelphia: WB Saunders, 1994:213–228.

20. Devine CJ Jr. International Conference on Peyronie's Disease. Advances in basic and clinical research: introduction. *J Urol* 1997;157:272.

21. Greenhall E, Vessey M. The prevalence of subfertility: a review of the current confusion and a report of two new studies. *Fertil Steril* 1990;54:978.

22. Clark JY, Thompson IM, Optenberg SA. Economic impact of urolithiasis in the United States. *J Urol* 1995;154:2020.

23. Robertson WG. Urinary tract calculi. In: Nordin BEC, Need AG, Morris HA, eds. *Metabolic bone and stone disease*. New York: Churchill Livingstone, 1993.

24. Rotolo JE, O'Brien WM, Pahira JJ. Urinary tract calculi. *Consultant* 1989;29:129.

25. Preminger GM. Cost and time effective outpatient metabolic stone evaluation. *Probl Urol* 1987;36:181.

26. Sutherland JW, Parks JH, Coe FL. Recurrence after a single renal stone in a community practice. *Miner Electrolyte Metab* 1985;11:267.

27. Daudon M, Dosimoni R, Hennequin C, et al. Sex and age related composition of 10,617 calculi analyzed by infrared spectroscopy. *Urol Res* 1995;23:319.

28. Gentle DL, Stoller ML, Jarrett TW, et al. Protease inhibitor-induced urolithiasis. *Urology* 1997;50:508.

29. Press SM, Smith AD. Incidence of negative hematuria in patients with acute urinary lithiasis presenting to the emergency room with flank pain. *Urology* 1995;45:753.

30. Vieweg J, Teh C, Freed K, et al. Unenhanced helical computerized tomography for the evaluation of patients with acute flank pain. *J Urol* 1998;160:679.

31. Liberman SN, Halpern EJ, Sullivan K, et al. Spiral computed tomography for staghorn calculi. *Urology* 1997;50:519.

32. Fielding JR, Steele G, Fox LA, et al. Spiral computerized tomography in the evaluation of acute flank pain: a replacement for excretory urography. *J Urol* 1997;157:2071.

33. Hill MC, Rich JI, Mardiat JG, et al. Sonography vs. excretory urography in acute flank pain. *AJR Am J Roentgenol* 1985;144:1235.

34. Segura JW, Preminger GM, Assimos DG, et al. Ureteral Stones Clinical Guidelines Panel summary report on the management of ureteral calculi. The American Urological Association. *J Urol* 1997;158:1915.

35. Chaussy C, Schmeidt E, Jocham D, et al. First clinical experience with extracorporeally induced destruction of kidney stones by shock waves. *J Urol* 1982;127:417.

36. Micali S, Moore RG, Averch TD, et al. The role of laparoscopy in the treatment of renal and ureteral calculi. *J Urol* 1997;157:463.

37. Zafar FS, Lingeman JE. Value of laparoscopy in the management of calculi complicating renal malformations. *J Endourol* 1996;10:379.

38. Segura JW, Preminger GM, Assimos DG, et al. Nephrolithiasis Clinical Guidelines Panel summary report on the management of staghorn calculi. The American Urological Association Nephrolithiasis Clinical Guidelines Panel. *J Urol* 1994;151:1648.

39. Grasso M, Loisides P, Beaghler M, et al. The case for primary endoscopic management of upper urinary tract calculi: I. a critical review of 121 extracorporeal shock-wave lithotripsy failures. *Urology* 1995;45:363.

40. Pak CY. Kidney stones. *Lancet* 1998;351:1797.

41. Young HH, McKay RW. Congenital valvular obstruction of prostatic urethra. *Surg Gynecol Obstet* 1929;43:435.

42. Goodwin WE, Casey WC, Woolf W. Percutaneous trocar (needle) nephrostomy in hydronephrosis. *JAMA* 1955;157:891.

43. Kelling G. Zur Colioskopie. *Arch Klin Chir* 1923;126:226.

44. Cortesi N, Ferrari P, Zambardae A, et al. Diagnosis of bilateral abdomen cryptorchidism by laparoscopy. *Endoscopy* 1976;8:33.

45. Wickham JEA. The surgical treatment of renal lithiasis. In: Wickham JEA, ed. *Urinary calculus disease*. New York: Churchill Livingstone, 1979:145–198.

46. Reddick EJ, Olsen DO. Laparoscopic laser cholecystectomy: a comparison with mini-lap cholecystectomy. *Surg Endosc* 1989;3:131.

47. McDougall EM, Clayman RV. Laparoscopic nephrectomy for benign disease: comparison of the transperitoneal and retroperitoneal approaches. *J Endourol* 1996;10:45.

48. Wolf JS, Moon TD, Nakada SY. Hand assisted laparoscopic nephrectomy: a comparison to standard laparoscopic nephrectomy. *J Urol* 1998;160:22.

49. Caddedu JA, Yoshinari O, Clayman RV, et al. Laparoscopic nephrectomy for renal cell cancer: evaluation of efficacy and safety—a multicenter experience. *Urology* 1998;52:773.

50. Jarrett TW, Fabrizio MD, Lamont DJ, et al. Laparoscopic pyeloplasty: five-year experience. Presented at the 1999 American Urological Association Meeting, Dallas, Texas, May 1999.

51. Winfield HN, Hamilton BD, Bravo EL, et al. Laparoscopic adrenalectomy: the preferred choice? A comparison to open adrenalectomy. *J Urol* 1998;160:325.

52. Rassweiler J, Fornara P, Weber M, et al. Laparoscopic nephrectomy: the experience of the Laparoscopy Working Group of the German Urologic Association. *J Urol* 1998;160:18.

53. Guillonneau B, Cathelineau X, Barret E, et al. Laparoscopic radical prostatectomy: technical and early oncological assessment of 40 operations. *Eur Urol* 1999;36:14.

54. Fleshner NE, Herr HW, Stewart AK, et al. The National Cancer Data Base report on bladder carcinoma. The American College of Surgeons Commission on Cancer and the American Cancer Society. *Cancer* 1996;78:1505.

55. Badawi AF. Molecular and genetic events in schistosomiasis-associated human bladder cancer: role of oncogenes and tumor suppressor genes. *Cancer Lett* 1996;105:123.

56. Strohmeyer T. Urothelial cancers: cytogenetic and molecular biology principles [in German]. *Urologe A* 1994;33:122.

57. Morrison AS. Epidemiology and environmental factors in urologic cancer. *Cancer* 1987;60:632.

58. Kirollos MM, McDermott S, Bradbrook RA. Bladder tumor markers: need, nature, and application: 2. tumor and tumor-associated antigens. *Int Urogynecol J Pelvic Floor Dysfunct* 1998;9:228.

59. Shelfo SW, Soloway MS. The role of nuclear matrix protein 22 in the detection of persistent or recurrent transitional-cell cancer of the bladder. *World J Urol* 1997;15:107.

60. Sarosdy MF. Principles of intravesical chemotherapy and immunotherapy. *Urol Clin North Am* 1992;19:509.

61. Rajala P, Liukkonen T, Raitanen M, et al. Transurethral resection with perioperative instillation of interferon-alpha or epirubicin for the prophylaxis of recurrent primary superfi-

cial bladder cancer: a prospective randomized multicenter study—Finnbladder III. *J Urol* 1999;161:1133; discussion, 1135.

62. Sarosdy MF. Management of high grade superficial bladder cancer: role of BCG. *AUA Update Ser* 1998;17:90.

63. Herr HW, Bajorin DF, Scher HI. Neoadjuvant chemotherapy and bladder-sparing surgery for invasive bladder cancer: ten-year outcome. *J Clin Oncol* 1998;16:1298.

64. Mills RD, Studer UE. Metabolic consequences of continent urinary diversion. *J Urol* 1999;161:1057.

65. Eisenberger CF, Schoenberg M, Fitter D, et al. Orthotopic ileocolic neobladder reconstruction following radical cystectomy: history, technique, and results of the Johns Hopkins experience, 1986–1998. *Urol Clin North Am* 1999;26:149, ix.

66. Bricker EM. Pelvic exenteration. *Adv Surg* 1970;4:13.

67. Levallois M, Granier B. Bricker's operation: simplified technic [in French]. *J Urol Nephrol (Paris)* 1968;74:287.

68. Roth BJ. Chemotherapy for advanced bladder cancer. *Semin Oncol* 1996;23:633.

69. Gelb AB. Renal cell carcinoma: current prognostic factors. Union Internationale Contre le Cancer (UICC) and the American Joint Committee on Cancer (AJCC). *Cancer* 1997;80:981.

70. Motzer RJ, Russo P, Nanus DM, et al. Renal cell carcinoma. *Curr Probl Cancer* 1997;21:185.

71. Godley PA, Stinchcombe TE. Renal cell carcinoma. *Curr Opin Oncol* 1999;11:213.

72. Wagner JR, Linehan WM. Molecular genetics of renal cell carcinoma. *Semin Urol Oncol* 1996;14:244.

73. Gnarra JR, Glenn GM, Latif F, et al. Molecular genetic studies of sporadic and familial renal cell carcinoma. *Urol Clin North Am* 1993;20:207.

74. Sampson JR. The kidney in tuberous sclerosis: manifestations and molecular genetic mechanisms. *Nephrol Dial Transplant* 1996;11[Suppl 6]:34.

75. Fleming S. Genetics of kidney tumours. *Forum (Genova)* 1998;8:176.

76. Avery RA, Harris JE, Davis CJ Jr, et al. Renal medullary carcinoma: clinical and therapeutic aspects of a newly described tumor. *Cancer* 1996;78:128.

77. Rodriguez R, Fishman EK, Marshall FF. Differential diagnosis and evaluation of the incidentally discovered renal mass. *Semin Urol Oncol* 1995;13:246.

78. Mattos RM, Libertino JA. Survival of patients with renal cell carcinoma invading the inferior vena cava. *Semin Urol Oncol* 1996;14:223.

79. Bosniak MA. The current radiological approach to renal cysts. *Radiology* 1986;158:1.

80. Robson CJ. Radical nephrectomy for renal cell carcinoma. *J Urol* 1963;89:37.

81. Bono AV, Lovisolo JA. Renal cell carcinoma—diagnosis and treatment: state of the art. *Eur Urol* 1997;31[Suppl 1]:47.

82. Novick AC. Nephron-sparing surgery for renal cell carcinoma. *Br J Urol* 1998;82:321.

83. Gill IS, Novick AC, Soble JJ, et al. Laparoscopic renal cryoablation: initial clinical series. *Urology* 1998;52:543.

84. Figlin RA. Renal cell carcinoma: management of advanced disease. *J Urol* 1999;161:381; discussion, 386.

85. Linehan WM, Walther MM, Alexander RB, et al. Adoptive immunotherapy of renal cell carcinoma: studies from the Surgery Branch, National Cancer Institute. *Semin Urol* 1993;11:41.

86. Mettlin CJ, Murphy GP, Rosenthal DS, et al. The National Cancer Data Base report on prostate carcinoma after the peak in incidence rates in the U.S. The American College of Surgeons Commission on Cancer and the American Cancer Society [in process citation]. *Cancer* 1998;83:1679.

87. Landis SH, Murray T, Bolden S, et al. Cancer statistics, 1998 [published errata appear in *CA Cancer J Clin* 1998;48:192 and 1998;48:329]. *CA Cancer J Clin* 1998;48:6.

88. Partin AW, Carter HB, Chan DW, et al. Prostate specific antigen in the staging of localized prostate cancer: influence of tumor differentiation, tumor volume, and benign hyperplasia. *J Urol* 1990;143:747.

89. Partin AW, Catalona WJ, Southwick PC, et al. Analysis of percent free prostate-specific antigen (PSA) for prostate cancer detection: influence of total PSA, prostate volume, and age. *Urology* 1996;48:55.

90. Iyer RV, Hanlon AL, Pinover WH, et al. Outcome evaluation of the 1997 American Joint Committee on Cancer staging system for prostate carcinoma treated by radiation therapy. *Cancer* 1999;85:1816.

91. Collins MM, Barry MJ. Controversies in prostate cancer screening: analogies to the early lung cancer screening debate [see comments]. *JAMA* 1996;276:1976.

92. Farkas A, Schneider D, Perrotti M, et al. National trends in the epidemiology of prostate cancer, 1973 to 1994: evidence for the effectiveness of prostate-specific antigen screening. *Urology* 1998;52:444; discussion, 448.

93. Feightner JW. The early detection and treatment of prostate cancer: the perspective of the Canadian Task Force on the Periodic Health Examination [see comments] [Review]. *J Urol* 1994;152:1682.

94. Stephenson RA, Stanford JL. Population-based prostate cancer trends in the United States: patterns of change in the era of prostate-specific antigen. *World J Urol* 1997;15:331.

95. Carter HB, Epstein JI. Prediction of significant cancer in men with stage T1c adenocarcinoma of the prostate. *World J Urol* 1997;15:359.

96. Horwitz EM, Hanlon AL, Hanks GE. Update on the treatment of prostate cancer with external beam irradiation. *Prostate* 1998;37:195.

97. D'Amico AV, Whittington R, Malkowicz SB, et al. Biochemical outcome after radical prostatectomy, external beam radiation therapy, or interstitial radiation therapy for clinically localized prostate cancer [see comments]. *JAMA* 1998;280:969.

98. Walsh PC. Results of conservative management of clinically localized prostate cancer. *J Urol* 1994;152:255.

99. Walsh PC, Partin AW, Epstein JI. Cancer control and quality of life following anatomical radical retropubic prostatectomy: results at 10 years [see comments]. *J Urol* 1994;152:1831.

100. Mettlin CJ, Murphy GP, Sylvester J, et al. Results of hospital cancer registry surveys by the American College of Surgeons: outcomes of prostate cancer treatment by radical prostatectomy. *Cancer* 1997;80:1875.

101. Fowler FJ Jr, Barry MJ, Lu-Yao G, et al. Patient-reported complications and follow-up treatment after radical prostatectomy. The National Medicare Experience: 1988–1990 (updated June 1993). *Urology* 1993;42:622.

102. Bishoff JT, Motley G, Optenberg SA, et al. Incidence of fecal and urinary incontinence following radical perineal and retropubic prostatectomy in a national population. *J Urol* 1998;160:454.

103. Partin AW, Kattan MW, Subong EN, et al. Combination of prostate-specific antigen, clinical stage, and Gleason score to predict pathological stage of localized prostate cancer: a multi-institutional update [see comments] [published erratum appears in *JAMA* 1997;278:118]. *JAMA* 1997;277:1445.

104. Roach M III. Neoadjuvant total androgen suppression and radiotherapy in the management of locally advanced prostate cancer. *Semin Urol Oncol* 1996;14:32; discussion, 38.

105. Eisenberger MA, Blumenstein BA, Crawford ED, et al. Bilateral orchiectomy with or without flutamide for metastatic prostate cancer. *N Engl J Med* 1998;339:1036.

106. Cortez JC, Kaplan GW. Gonadal stromal tumors, gonadoblastomas, epidermoid cysts, and secondary tumors of the testis in children. *Urol Clin North Am* 1993;20:15.

107. Levin HS. Prognostic features of primary and metastatic testis germ-cell tumors. *Urol Clin North Am* 1993;20:39.

108. Einhorn EH. Testicular cancer: an oncological success story. *Clin Cancer Res* 1997;3:2630.

SURGERY: SCIENTIFIC PRINCIPLES AND PRACTICE, Third Edition, edited by
Lazar J. Greenfield, Michael W. Mulholland, Keith T. Oldham, Gerald B. Zelenock,
and Keith D. Lillemoe. Lippincott Williams & Wilkins Publishers, Philadelphia, © 2001.

CHAPTER 103

FEMALE GENITAL TRACT

F. J. MONTZ, ROBERT E. BRISTOW, AND GEOFF CUNDIFF

It is apropos that surgeons at The Johns Hopkins Hospital author a surgical treatise addressing the female pelvis. American gynecologic pelvic surgery had its inception and subsequent codification at this institution under Howard Kelly, Richard Telinde, Cullen Richards, Howard Jones Jr., and numerous others. Many of the landmark advances in gynecologic surgical management originated at the facility that was the legacy of a Quaker bachelor grocer.

Our presentation of gynecologic disease processes focuses only on diseases that are commonly, if not predominantly, treated surgically. For each of the entities discussed, we cursorily summarize the pertinent nonsurgical options and highlight those realities that led to surgical therapy being the preferred treatment modality. This chapter is structured in a specific format in which each anatomic site is individually addressed. Pathologic processes and surgical procedures are catalogued for congenital, infectious, traumatic, and neoplastic diseases, the latter encompassing both malignant and nonmalignant processes.

SURGICAL ANATOMY

This section does not provide a meticulous review of the pelvic anatomy because there are numerous, excellent atlases that can refresh the memory of the pelvic surgeon. We do, however, focus on those details of pelvic anatomy that are necessary for the surgeon to know to perform the full array of complex procedures.

Pelvic Compartments and Spaces

The female pelvis is usually envisioned as having three compartments and eight potential spaces. The compartments are self-evident but often forgotten by the neophyte pelvic surgeon when defining sources of disease, rational surgical techniques, and sources of comorbidity.

Compartments

Traditionally, the female pelvis is divided into three functional compartments: the anterior compartment (distal ureters, bladder, and urethra), the middle compartment (ovaries, fallopian tubes, uterine corpus and cervix, vagina, and perineum), and the posterior compartment (distal sigmoid colon, rectum, and anus; Fig. 103.1). Although the pelvic organs can be divided into these compartments, a rigid separation is fallacious because all three compartments are integrally intertwined in function, vascular and lymphatic supply and drainage, enervation, and support.

Spaces

Knowledge of the the eight major pelvic spaces (Fig. 103.2) and two other anatomic compartments is of great value not only in performing pelvic surgery but in effectively managing intraoperative misadventures. In a ventral-dorsal sequence, the spaces are the retropubic space (space of Retzius), the vesicovaginal space, the rectovaginal septum, and the retrorectal space. Lateral to these midline spaces are the paravesical and pararectal spaces. It is evident that these spaces are (a) potential, being coapted in the natural state; (b) devoid of major vascular or visceral structures, although these structures encompass the spaces; and (c) valuable for defining pelvic anatomy in those settings where anatomic anomalies exist.

In addition to the eight pelvic spaces, there are two other spaces that we have found to be of great value while doing ureteral dissection or lysis. These are the space of Morrow and the tunnel of Wertheim (Fig. 103.3). Using these spaces as routes of dissection facilitates complete ureteral lysis throughout the pelvis without necessitating entrance into the ureteral sheath with associated devascularization.

Blood Supply

The rich, highly collateral blood supply in the pelvis is the proverbial double-edged sword: it facilitates healing and return of function to remaining pelvic organs after extensive dissection, but can do so at a high intraoperative cost in blood loss. Our experience has confirmed what the great Italian anatomists noted five centuries ago: the pelvic blood supply is remarkably consistent and predictable, with minimal interpatient variation. Numerous anatomic texts offer excellent reviews of the pelvic blood supply.

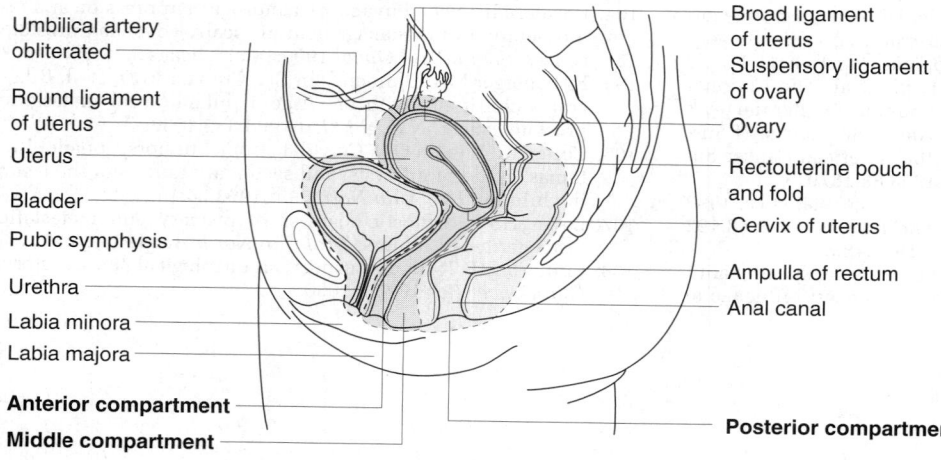

Umbilical artery obliterated
Round ligament of uterus
Uterus
Bladder
Pubic symphysis
Urethra
Labia minora
Labia majora
Anterior compartment
Middle compartment

Broad ligament of uterus
Suspensory ligament of ovary
Ovary
Rectouterine pouch and fold
Cervix of uterus
Ampulla of rectum
Anal canal
Posterior compartment

Figure 103.1. The three pelvic compartments: lateral view.

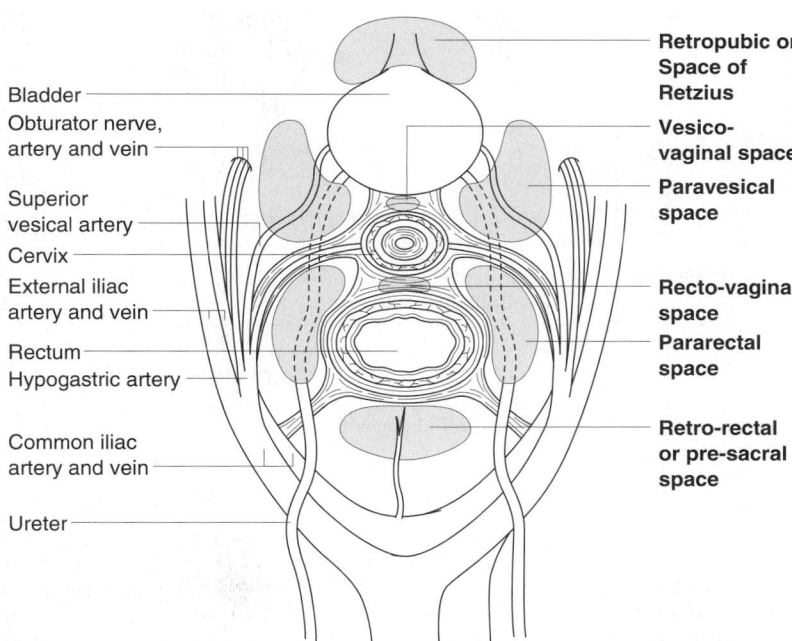

Retropubic or
Space of
Retzius

Bladder

Obturator nerve,
artery and vein

Vesico-
vaginal space

Paravesical
space

Superior
vesical artery

Cervix

External iliac
artery and vein

Recto-vaginal
space

Pararectal
space

Rectum

Hypogastric artery

Common iliac
artery and vein

Retro-rectal
or pre-sacral
space

Ureter

Figure 103.2. The eight pelvic spaces: transverse view.

Ureteral Course

Gynecologic pelvic surgery is the most common source of an iatrogenic ureteral injury. This phenomenon is the end result of the numerous inflammatory and neoplastic diseases that occur in the pelvis and cause the ureter to adhere to surrounding structures from which it is developmentally free, or deviate from its anticipated course. The most common sites of injury of the ureter at time of gynecologic surgery are where the ureter enters the pelvis under the infundibulopelvic ligament and on top of the bifurcation of the common iliac artery; where the ureter runs under the uterine artery as that vessel supplies the uterus; and the site of ureteral entrance into the bladder wall.

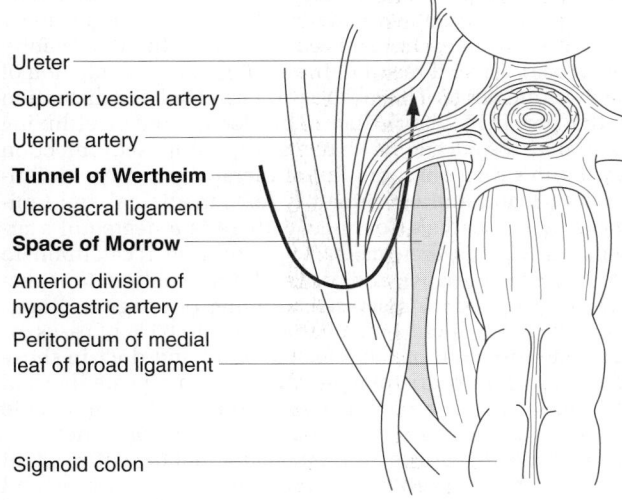

Ureter

Superior vesical artery

Uterine artery

Tunnel of Wertheim

Uterosacral ligament

Space of Morrow

Anterior division of
hypogastric artery

Peritoneum of medial
leaf of broad ligament

Sigmoid colon

Figure 103.3. The space of Morrow and the tunnel of Wertheim.

PHYSIOLOGY

Reproductive physiology is a complex discipline about which entire textbooks have been written. However, an essential understanding of the anatomic changes that occur in parallel with the reproductive physiologic changes associated with menarche, menopause, and the gravid state, as well as with the "normal" and "dysfunctional" estrus cycle, must be possessed by the pelvic surgeon. Before menarche, the ovary is a small, almond-shaped structure. As the ovary becomes more biologically active (Fig. 103.4), it doubles or triples in size. Subsequently, with the onset of the climacteric, the ovary returns to its premenarche size, although it is more fibrotic and has surface irregularities. The latter findings may appear aberrant to the naive pelvic surgeon and should be appreciated as normal end results of years of ovulation. The changes that occur during the menstrual cycle mimic, to a significant degree, those that occur during a woman's reproductive life. The dominant follicle measures approximately 2.5 cm immediately before ovulation at day 14 of the idealized 28-day cycle. Superimposing this normal follicle onto a $2 \times 2 \times 3$ cm ovary makes it easy to appreciate why there are numerous adnexal "masses" identified when pelvic examinations are performed in the midcycle. Postovulation, with the development of the corpus luteum, there may be a persistent adnexal mass. Failure to appreciate the normality of these physiologic changes leads to unnecessary imaging and surgical intervention.

Just as there are changes in the size of the ovary that reflect its role as a source of sex steroids and oocytes, there is a parallel change in the other reproductive structures that reflects the effect of estrogen on the gravid uterus. In general, the female reproductive tract organs demonstrate shrinkage, fibrosis, and epithelial thinning when estrogenic stimulation is removed, with the opposite effects occurring after stimulation. The greater the estrogen stimulation, the more physiologic engorgement occurs. This axiom is taken to its extreme during pregnancy, when the circulating levels of endogenous estrogen are the highest that occur in a nonpathologic state. Last, the growing gravid uterus can represent a "pelvic mass." As the embryo and subsequent fetus grows and pregnancy-associated physiologic changes

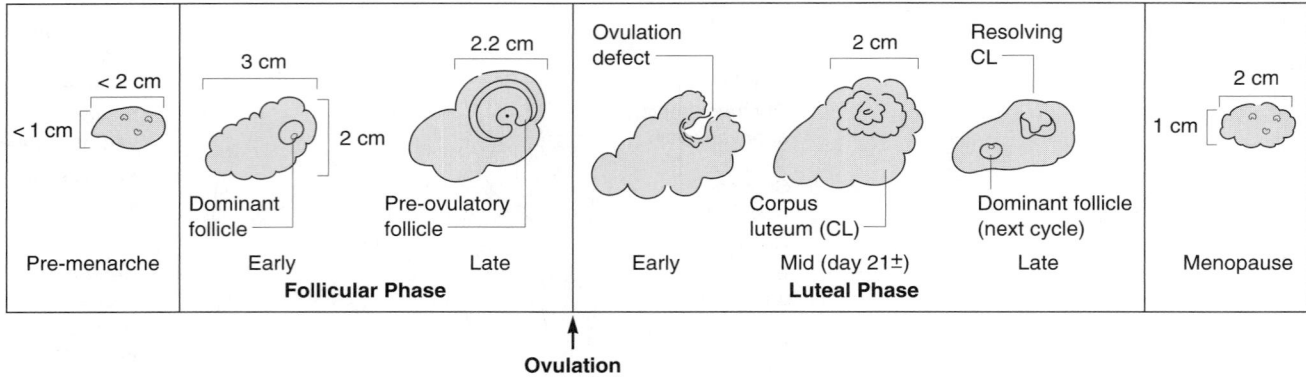

Figure 103.4. Physiologic structural changes in the ovary during reproductive life.

occur, the uterus rises out of the pelvis, displacing those other pelvic organs that are freely mobile and compressing those that are not. Important general rules of reference are that a uterus with a 12-week gestation reaches the pelvic brim, a 20-week gestation the umbilicus, and a 40-week (term gestation) the xiphoid process.

The rest of this chapter is devoted to an overview of pathologic processes specific to anatomic sites.

VULVA

Congenital

Labial Fusion

Labial fusion in association with a nonperforate hymen are the end results of abnormalities of müllerian duct fusion and junction between the perineal plate and the developing vagina. To understand fully this continuum of congenital abnormalities, it is essential to remember that the normal female genital tract is the end result of midline fusion of the müllerian ducts and their attachment to and subsequent fenestration of the perineal plate. In the most extreme degrees of midline nonfusion there is a complete duplication of the vagina, cervix, and uterine corpus. Depending on the extremity of nonfusion, there may be as much as a 60% chance of an associated congenital abnormality in the kidneys, ureters, or bladder. A further discussion of the management of these defects is outlined in the sections on vaginal and cervical defects.

Labial fusion may be a congenital or acquired abnormality, with the latter the result of some degree of inflammation due to trauma, radiation, or menopause. In almost all cases, a combination of local estrogenic creams (1 g applied locally on a daily basis for 6 weeks, followed by the same dosage administered two to three times a week) improves epithelial integrity and strength and decreases inflammation. Thereafter, surgical separation with either reapproximation of the vulvar epithelium to the vagina or, in the most severe cases, placement of a split-thickness skin graft, is necessary to minimize risk of recurrence.

Varicosities

Although in most cases they are not truly congenital, there is a genetic predisposition to the development of vulvar varicosities. Varicosities have a predilection to worsen with the gravid state (secondary to the effects on venous congestion and efflux associated with increasing serum progesterone and the compressive effect of the expanding gravid uterus, respectively). Varicosities usually are not bilaterally equal, having a unilateral dominance on the right side secondary to the pressure column associated with a dextro-vena cava. Varicosities do not require operative therapy during pregnancy because they naturally regress in the postpartum period, although body positional changes may be beneficial in symptom control. In the nongravid state when symptoms warrant it, surgical ligation is the preferred therapy.

Inguinal Hernias and Patent Canals of Nuch

Inguinal hernias, the end result of trauma on a congenitally deficient support system, are not reviewed here. However, a condition that can lead to a diagnostic dilemma (the patent canal of Nuch) must be remembered. The round ligaments decussate in the labia majora, running through the canal of Nuch. If this canal maintains patency, collections of peritoneal fluid, direct hernias, or even inclusion-like cysts can develop. The latter present as masses on the labia majora that have a tendency to enlarge with time and may worsen during the luteal phase. The diagnosis is verified if there is enlargement of the mass and increased associated symptoms with the patient in the upright position. Resection of any masses and ligation of the canal of Nuch, through a transvulvar approach, are the preferred surgical modalities.

Infectious

The vulva may present with all of the infectious processes that are found on the other cutaneous surfaces. Uniquely, vulvar infections can develop in the major (i.e., Bartholin's) and minor vestibular glands. These are usually a result of sexually transmitted organisms (predominantly gonorrhea). An end result of these infections is occlusion of the draining ducts. This obstruction can lead to a distention of the proximal gland duct. This loculation of effluxing fluid may be sterile or have a superimposed infection (Bartholin's duct abscess). Initial therapy is always antimicrobial (1) and antiinflammatory (e.g., medicinal and topical using sitz baths). Commonly, there is a degree of scarring and fibrosis that makes the condition recalcitrant to conservative therapy, and surgical intervention then becomes warranted. Surgery can be either drainage and marsupialization, which is effective in 65% to 85% of cases, or complete resection of the affected gland and duct in those instances where marsupialization has been repeatedly tried and failed. When resection is undertaken, it is preferable that (a) the surgery be completed in the nonacutely inflamed state, (b) care be taken to ensure that the entire gland and duct are removed to avoid any further recurrence, and (c) a closed suction drain be left at the base of the defect and brought out through a separate stab wound.

Necrotizing Fascitis

Although necrotizing fascitis is a relatively uncommon process, it is essential that the pelvic surgeon remember the existence and presentation of this process because if it is not treated aggressively surgically, a fatal outcome is common. Necrotizing fascitis, which most commonly occurs in women with the comorbidities of diabetes mellitus or atherosclerosis (70%), is also more common in people taking long-term nonsteroidal antiinflammatory drugs or glucocorticoids, or with underlying immune disease. Usually this infectious processes is caused by *Streptococcus pyogenes* (group A *Streptococcus*) with or without *Staphylococcus aureus,* or it can be of polymicrobial cause as a result of anaerobic and facultative aerobic bacteria. Most frequently, necrotizing fascitis starts as a relatively insignificant infection in a hair follicle, pilonidal cyst, vestibular gland or duct, or surgical site (episiotomy or vulvar resection). It may progress rapidly or take an indolent course. The clinical findings that require the surgeon to proceed to adequate surgical resection are those of necrosis (which may in the early stages simply be represented by a purple-blue discoloration) and anesthesia at the site. Histologic confirmation of the disease demonstrates (a) vascular occlusion and thrombosis, (b) intense leukocyte infiltration, and (c) necrosis. Once the disease is diagnosed, therapy is a combination of systemic support (fluids, blood products), systemic antibiotics, and radical excision. Radicality of the dissection must be emphasized because hesitation to extend the dissection until reaching a margin of healthy, well-vascularized, and vigorously bleeding tissue with oxygenated (i.e., bright red) blood at best leads to the need for repeated surgical excision.

Traumatic

Vulvar trauma is discussed here, although the reader should remember that trauma has a "field effect" that, depending on the source of the insult, may include the vulva, perineum, vagina, anus, rectum, distal sigmoid colon, urethra, bladder, distal ureters, and even the cervix, if the injury was sexual assault with a rigid instrument. Fistulae are discussed in the section on vaginal diseases and abnormalities, whereas abnormalities of support are presented under cervical diseases.

Hematomas

Hematomas are most commonly the result of blunt trauma to the pudendal vessels or their terminal branches secondary to a straddle injury (e.g., bicycle seat or strut, playground or gym bar, motorcycle or horse-back riding). However, particularly in women who are on anticoagulant medications, what would be considered an insignificant degree of trauma can be sufficient to induce a significant hematoma. The overriding dictum when managing hematomas is to support the patient and avoid attempts at evacuation and vessel ligation unless the patient is hemodynamically unstable or symptomatically uncontrolled. Prophylactic antibiotics, particularly for women at increased risk for development of necrotizing fascitis, are of theoretic, if not proven, benefit. Local care with hot sitz baths and concomitant narcotic analgesics is frequently all that is needed. Anterior or periurethral hematomas may necessitate urethral catheterization (which should be left in situ for 72 hours) if there is inability to void. In some cases, surgical intervention is necessary. Any attempt at drainage is best undertaken in the operating theater. It is common for no specific bleeding site to be identified and, therefore, the surgeon places sutures that take large tissue purchases in the locale of the pudendal vessels. This can be beneficial,

but care must be taken to ensure that there is no impingement on the urethra or ureters or entrapment of the pudendal nerve branches innervating the vulva. If the latter occurs, a chronic nerve entrapment syndrome may develop that can be difficult to treat and potentially disabling.

Lacerations

The management of lacerations is straightforward. When repairing vulvar lacerations, particularly those near the clitoris and labia minor, the trauma surgeon must keep in mind the critical role that body image plays in sexual function. The patient should be taken to the operating room, adequately anesthetized, and have the microarchitecture reestablished with the same degree of care that would be taken when repairing a facial laceration in a young women. Butterfly bandages and similar nonsuture techniques are rarely useful in vulvar lacerations because of their three-dimensional nature and the constant moistness and motion that is present.

Peripartum

Perineal lacerations and episiotomies are classified based on their extent and depth. First-degree lacerations/episiotomies affect only the vulvar and vaginal cutaneous dermis. Second-degree lacerations/episiotomies extend into the subdermal tissue. Third-degree lacerations/episiotomies extend into (partial) or through (complete) the rectal sphincter, and fourth-degree lacerations (episioproctotomies) extend into the anorectal lumen. There are a few features unique to the management of peripartum lacerations to the vulva, perineum, anus, rectum, and vagina:

1. Lacerations are usually multifocal. Therefore, a thorough inspection of the entire lower pelvis is essential to guarantee that no unappreciated injuries that may be the source of delayed morbidity are present.
2. The site of the laceration is contaminated with bacteria. Copious lavage and appropriate antibiotic prophylaxis are valuable in minimizing subsequent wound breakdown and infection.
3. Repair must focus on a complete, layered reapproximation of all the disrupted tissue planes and structures to minimize the chance of a subsequent functional or supporting abnormality. It is essential to assess and repair any injury to the rectal mucosa, anal sphincter, transverse perineal muscles (which provide the bulk of the perineal support), the levator ani (which are uncommonly disrupted as they attach to the medial raphe in the midline dorsal to the rectal sphincter and onto the lateral aspects of the vaginal tube), and the overlying epithelium and subepithelial connecting tissue.

Neoplastic

Vulvar Intraepithelial Neoplasia

Vulvar intraepithelial neoplasia (VIN), like all of the preinvasive squamous lesions of the lower genital tract, is graded based on the degree of abnormal (dysplastic) cells in-

Table 103.1. ESTIMATED NEW CANCER CASES, UNITED STATES, 2000

Uterine corpus	36,100
Ovary	23,100
Uterine cervix	12,800
Vulva	3,400
Vagina and others	2,100

From Greenlee RT, Murray T, Bolden S, et al. Cancer statistics, 2000. CA Cancer J Clin 2000;50:7–33.

Table 103.2. STAGING OF GYNECOLOGIC CANCER AS RECOMMENDED BY THE INTERNATIONAL FEDERATION OF GYNECOLOGY AND OBSTETRICS

Stage	Description	Stage	Description
VULVAR CANCER		IIIA	No extension to pelvic wall
0		IIIB	Extension to pelvic wall or hydronephrosis of nonfunctioning kidney
Tis	Carcinoma in situ; intraepithelial carcinoma	IV	Carcinoma beyond true pelvis or involving mucosa of bladder or rectum
I		IVA	Spread to adjacent organs
T1, N0, M0	Tumor confined to vulva or perineum, 2 cm or less in greatest dimension. No nodal metastasis	IVB	Spread to distant organs
II		**UTERINE CORPUS CANCER**	
T2, N0, M0	Tumor confined to vulva or perineum, more than 2 cm in greatest dimension. No nodal metastasis	IA G123	Tumor limited to endometrium
		IB G123	Invasion to less than half the myometrium
III		IC G123	Invasion to more than half the myometrium
T3, N0, M0	Tumor of any size with:		
T3, N1, M0	(1) Adjacent spread to lower urethra, vagina, anus, or	IIA G123	Endocervical glandular involvement only
T1, N1, M0	(2) Unilateral regional lymph node metastasis	IIB G123	Cervical stromal invasion
T2, N1, M0		IIIA G123	Tumor invades serosa or adnexa, or presence of positive peritoneal cytology
IVA			
T1, N2, M0	Tumor invades any of the following:	IIIB G123	Vaginal metastases
T2, N2, M0	Upper urethra, bladder mucosa, rectal mucosa, pelvic bone, or bilateral regional node metastasis	IIIC G123	Metastases to pelvic or paraaortic lymph nodes
T3, N2, M0		IVA G123	Tumor invasion of bladder or bowel mucosa
T4, any N, M0			
IVB		IVB	Distant metastases including intraabdominal or inguinal lymph nodes
Any T, any N, M1	Any distant metastasis including pelvic lymph nodes		
Note		**Note**	
N (regional lymph nodes)		G1	5% or less of a nonsquamous or nonmorular solid growth pattern
N0	No lymph node metastasis		
N1	Unilateral regional lymph node metastasis	G2	6%–50% of a nonsquamous or nonmorular solid growth pattern
N2	Bilateral regional lymph node metastasis		
M (distant metastasis)		G3	More than 50% of a nonsquamous or nonmorular solid growth pattern
M0	No clinical metastasis		
M1	Distant metastasis (including pelvic lymph node metastasis)	**OVARIAN CANCER**	
		I	Growth limited to ovaries
VAGINAL CANCER		IA	One ovary; no tumor on external surfaces; capsule intact; no ascites present containing malignant cells
0 carcinoma	Carcinoma in situ; intraepithelial		
I	Carcinoma limited to vaginal mucosa	IB	Both ovaries; no tumor on external surfaces; capsules intact; no ascites present containing malignant cells
II	Carcinoma involving subvaginal tissue but not onto pelvic wall	IC	IA or IB but with tumor on surface of one or both ovaries; or with capsule ruptured; or with ascites containing malignant cells or with positive peritoneal washings
III	Carcinoma onto pelvic wall or pubic symphysis	II	Growth involving one or both ovaries with pelvic extension
IV	Carcinoma beyond true pelvis; involvement of bladder or rectal mucosa	IIA	Extension or metastases to uterus or fallopian tubes
		IIB	Extension to other pelvic tissues
CERVICAL CANCER		IIC	IIA or IIB but with tumor on surface of one or both ovaries; or with capsules ruptured; or with ascites containing malignant cells or with positive peritoneal washings
0	Carcinoma in situ; intraepithelial carcinoma	III	Tumor involving one or both ovaries with peritoneal implants outside pelvis or positive retroperitoneal or inguinal nodes; superficial liver metastases; tumor limited to pelvis but with histologically verified malignant extension to small bowel or omentum
I	Carcinoma confined to cervic		
IA	Preclinical carcinoma; diagnosed microscopically		
IA1	Minimal microscopic evidence of stromal invasion	IIIA	Tumor limited to true pelvis with negative nodes but with histologically confirmed seeding of peritoneal surfaces
IA2	Microscopic invasion from base of epithelium of 5 mm or less and lateral spread of 7 mm or less	IIIB	Tumor limited to one or both ovaries with histologically confirmed implants of peritoneal surfaces, none greater than 2 cm in diameter; nodes negative
IB	Lesions of greater dimensions than stage IA2	IIIC	Abdominal implants greater than 2 cm in diameter or positive retroperitoneal or inguinal nodes
II	Carcinoma beyond cervix but not to pelvic wall. Cancer involves vagina but not lower third	IV	Growth involving one or both ovaries with distant metastasis; pleural effusion with positive cytology; parenchymal liver metastasis
IIA	Obvious parametrial involvement		
IIB	Obvious parametrial involvement	**INVASIVE GESTATIONAL TROPHOBLASTIC NEOPLASIA**	
III	Carcinoma to pelvic wall. No cancer-free space between tumor and pelvic wall. Tumor involves lower third of vagina. Hydronephrosis or nonfunctioning kidney not due to another cause	I	Tumor confined to uterine corpus
		II	Tumor to adnexa but limited to genital structures
		III	Tumor to lungs with or without genital involvement
		IV	Metastasis to other sites

volving the epithelium: VIN I, 33%; VIN II, 33% to 66%; and VIN III, greater than 66% (2). There is a natural continuum of degrees of dysplasia. However, only approximately 30% of the lesser-grade lesions develop into full-thickness dysplasia, and of those that do, probably only 5% ever become invasive lesions. VIN is usually the end result of chronic inflammation and is more likely to occur in women with associated comorbidities (e.g., diabetes mellitus, chronic steroid use). Only 15% to 30% of high-grade VIN lesions have detectable human papilloma virus (HPV) DNA, most commonly type 18 (3). This entity has nonspecific presenting symptoms, predominantly pruritus but also bleeding, a palpable lesion, and discharge. Similarly, the appearance of VIN is highly variable, with raised lesions of variable coloration (pink, white, gray, red, melanotic) predominating. The diagnosis of VIN is made by biopsy of an evident lesion in a patient at risk. VIN has a tendency to be multicentric as well as part of a multifocal disease entity effecting the vagina and cervix as well. Therefore, evaluation must include as a minimum cytologic screening of the cervix and, preferably, microscopic (colposcopic) surveillance. Numerous therapeutic regimens have been used to treat VIN. We prefer excisional biopsy for small lesions that are not located where there could be a potential negative functional or cosmetic outcome. Larger lesions, or those not treated with wide excision, are best treated with a combination of numerous colposcopically directed biopsies and laser vaporization to a depth of the third dermal layer. Depending on the extent of the lesion and the degree of keratinization, initial therapy may be as much as 90% effective at eliminating all disease, although persistence and recurrence rates in the range of 30% to 40% are probably more accurate. There is a subset of patients for whom a skinning vulvectomy with split-thickness skin graft is the preferred therapy. These are women either with disease that is recalcitrant to vaporization or who desire the most effective therapy independent of associated risks and negative cosmetic outcome.

Vulvar Cancer

Vulvar cancer is a relatively uncommon gynecologic cancer (4) (Table 103.1), predominantly effecting women in their seventh and eighth decades of life. Risk factors for vulvar cancer are the same as with VIN, although there is a young subgroup of women who manifest this process as the end result of an active HPV infection against the background of significantly compromised immune function. Presenting symptoms are the same as those for VIN. A sad commentary on the degree of awareness of vulvar cancer by primary care physicians and even obstetrician-gynecologists is the finding that the average woman at time of diagnosis of her vulvar cancer has been evaluated by three antecedent physicians for the same symptom complex without a diagnostic biopsy being performed. As with all gynecologic malignancies, therapy of vulvar cancer is predicated on the stage, with the classification set forth by the Federation Internationale de Gynecologie et d'Obstetrique (FIGO) being most widely used (Table 103.2). There has been a remarkable evolution in the management of vulvar cancer since the early 1980s. The current standard includes adequate local radical resection of the primary lesion and removal of at-risk lymph nodes (5). The principle of radical local excision is to remove the primary lesion and a 2-cm margin in all three planes. Lesions for which this cannot be accomplished without loss of function (near the clitoris, urethral sphincter, or anal sphincter) are best treated with local radiation after directed node sampling. For lesions that have more than a 1-mm depth of invasion (a finding that may not be determined until after the radical local excision is performed), a directed node sampling is indicated. This includes unilat-

eral superficial (above the fossa ovali) groin node dissections with the femoral artery serving as the lateral margin if the lesion is well lateralized (≥2 cm), or bilateral if not. Deep groin and pelvic dissections should be performed only in a setting of grossly positive superficial groin nodes. Grossly positive nodes are best resected because they have been demonstrated to be radioresistant. There are limited but encouraging data regarding sentinel node sampling in women with vulvar cancer (6). This technique has yet to be proven beneficial in a large, heterogeneous patient population. Once the vulvar lesion is resected, it is essential to ensure that the surgical defect is repaired or

Table 103.3. OUTCOMES OF GYNECOLOGIC CANCER THERAPY: OVERALL SURVIVAL AT 5 YEARS

CERVIX	
Stage Ia1	95.1%
Stage Ia2	94.9%
Stage Ib	80.1%
Stage IIa	66.3%
Stage IIb	63.5%
Stage IIIa	33.3%
Stage IIIb	38.7%
Stage IVa	17.1%
Stage IVb	9.4%
CORPUS UTERI	
Stage Ia	90.9%
Stage Ib	88.2%
Stage Ic	81.0%
Stage IIa	76.9%
Stage IIb	67.1%
Stage IIIa	60.3%
Stage IIIb	41.2%
Stage IIIc	31.7%
Stage IVa	20.1%
Stage IVb	5.3%
FALLOPIAN TUBE	
Stage I	83.6%
Stage II	51.6%
Stage III	35.9%
Stage IV	15%
OVARY	
Stage Ia	86.9%
Stage Ib	71.3%
Stage Ic	79.2%
Stage IIa	66.6%
Stage IIb	55.1%
Stage IIc	57.0%
Stage IIIa	41.1%
Stage IIIb	24.9%
Stage IIIc	23.4%
Stage IV	11.1%
VAGINA	
Stage 0	83.5%
Stage I	62.7%
Stage II	45.0%
Stage III	21.8%
Stage IV	18.8%
VULVA[a]	
Stage I	71.4%
Stage II	61.3%
Stage III	43.8%
Stage IV	8.3%

[a]Epidermoid invasive cancer only.
From Federation Internationale de Gynecologie et d'Obstetrique. Annual report on the results of treatment in gynaecological cancers. J Epidemiol Biostat 1998;3:1–168.

covered using tension-free, well-vascularized tissue. Because a poorly healing vulvar wound can be a patient care disaster, we have a very low threshold for undertaking plastic reconstruction of the vulvar defect. Our preference is to perform vascular pedicle grafts such as vertical rectus abdominis muscle (VRAM) or island flaps using surrounding tissue. If radiation therapy is chosen as part of the therapeutic armamentarium, there must be concomitant chemosensitization using a platinum-containing regimen because this has been proven, in prospective, randomized, clinical trials administered by the Gynecologic Oncology Group (GOG), to offer a survival advantage. Long-term outcomes of vulvar and other gynecologic cancer therapies are demonstrated in Table 103.3.

VAGINA

Congenital

Müllerian developmental defects, in general, are discussed and catalogued in section on vulvar disease. Here we describe vaginal septa and vaginal agenesis as a part of the Rokitansky-Küster-Hauser (RKH) syndrome.

Septa

Septa may either be transverse (i.e., at the site of the junction of the upper vagina and the perineal plate) or longitudinal to the vaginal access, as part of a müllerian fusion defect. Transverse septa are usually first appreciated during menarche, when the adolescent acquires secondary sex characteristics but remains amenorrheic, often with associated cramping discomfort. In women who become sexually active in the perimenarcheal period, the presenting symptom may be coital dysfunction. In women who have been sloughing the endometrium, clinical findings may include a bulging tissue plate at the hymen or cephalad, a lower abdominal mass palpable on rectal examination, and lower abdominal pain secondary to retrograde menstruation, although the latter phenomenon occurs less frequently than might be anticipated. Therapy is surgical, with the placement of a cruciate incision in the septum, resection of the central cross-hatch, and approximation of the vaginal edges in a cephalad-caudad manner. If there is an area of nonjunction of the descending vagina and the perineal plate of greater than a few millimeters, some degree of undermining of the cephalad vaginal tube or placement of a split-thickness skin graft over the nonepithelialized supporting tissue is necessary. Postreconstruction, the use of an indwelling vaginal stent is mandatory to minimize constriction and fibrosis until healing has progressed to the point that coitus can be resumed. Longitudinal vaginal septa are frequently completely asymptomatic, although they may be associated with coital dysfunction or a variety of other presentations based on other, concomitant structural defects. Removal is straightforward, with a resection of the septum leaving an approximately 1-cm margin around the perimeter that can be approximated in a side-to-side fashion to facilitate healing. Dilator or stent use is rarely necessary in these women.

Agenesis (Rokitansky-Küster-Hauser Syndrome)

Vaginal agenesis, independently or, more commonly, as part of a complicated müllerian and associated abnormality, is surgically a more elaborate and difficult entity than simple septa. Vaginal agenesis as an independent finding (i.e., with a normal cervix and upper genital tract) is very rare. It is more common to have a total loss of the upper two thirds of the vagina, cervix, uterus, and proximal fallopian tubes, the so-called RKH syndrome. This process is usually identified when a woman experiences thearche and pubarche without menarche. In contradistinction to a transverse vagi-

nal septum or imperforate hymen, there is no cyclic pain, hematocolpos, hematometra, or endometriosis. Clinical finding include a normal distal one third of the vagina, an absent upper tract except for the distal two thirds of the fallopian tubes and ovaries, and, in as many as 60% of patients, some degree of upper urinary tract abnormality (e.g., duplication, pelvic kidney, congenital absence). These women have normal gonadal function, and sex steroid replacement therefore is not necessary. Correction of the agenesis can be accomplished by one of two major methods: sequential upward dilation and extension of the extant vagina using the so-called Mackenrodt technique or dissection of the fibrotic tissue at the apex of the distal vagina and placement of some form of graft, such as a split-thickness skin graft with or without an omental J-flap to facilitate neovascularization, a pedicle flap, or, our least favorite, a segment of large intestine that is attached to the remnant of the vagina. Our preferred method (split-thickness skin graft with omental J-flap) has the advantages of being able to make a capacious vagina without removing a segment of the anterior abdominal wall, has an acceptable amount of discharge, and has a very high success rate when used in this and similar settings (7). After the neovagina is developed, there must be a serious commitment on the behalf of the patient to comply with the recommendations of repeated and serial vaginal dilations and use of a prosthesis until frequent vaginal intercourse is allowed.

Traumatic

The discussion of traumatic injury to the vagina has been incorporated in our summary on vulvar injuries, except for fistulae, which we discuss here.

Although fistulae have become progressively less common in the industrialized world secondary to changes in obstetric practice, genital fistulae remain a common source of morbidity for women. Historically, the most common source of a vaginal fistula was as a residuum of birth trauma. However, in the modern era, the most common antecedent event is surgical trauma. The decision about how best to manage a fistula involving the pelvic organs is based on (a) the cause of the fistula, (b) prior attempts, (c) underlying vascular integrity (including cigarette smoking), and (d) patient preferences. In general, in the setting where the patient has not previously received radiation therapy, has not had a prior attempt at repair, and does not have an underlying vascular abnormality, a primary layered repair with meticulous attention paid to establishing tension-free closure is the preferred method. In all other settings, it is meritorious to bring in a new source of blood supply, through either a VRAM flap, pedicle graft (e.g., a Martius flap), or an omental J-flap. An exhaustive discussion of the operative techniques and options is beyond the scope of this chapter.

For convenience of presentation, and to avoid a disjunctive discussion, findings related to traumatic processes (e.g., birth, age, physical activity) that lead to abnormalities of vaginal support are discussed in the section on cervical trauma.

Infectious

Infectious processes affecting the vagina are extremely rarely managed surgically except for in the setting of necrotizing fasciitis, as described previously.

Neoplastic

Vaginal neoplasms and malignancies are some of the least common of all such lesions occurring in the genital tract.

Benign Neoplasms

Nonmalignant or non-precancerous tumors that occur in the vagina and surrounding tissues can arise from any of the cell types found in these environs. The three space-occupying lesions that are most commonly identified are (a) posttraumatic inclusion cysts, (b) paramesonephric duct remnants, and (c) leiomyomata uteri. The former two entities are usually small, cystic, and relatively mobile, with paramesonephric cysts being less fixed than posttraumatic inclusion cysts. Paramesonephric cysts are almost universally noted along the lateral aspects of the vagina, following the course of their embryonic progenitors. Inclusion cysts, of course, can be located anywhere that prior trauma has occurred, usually near the perineum or sulci. Myomata are similar to inclusions cysts with regard to their nonspecific location. Myomata, however, are firm and usually mobile. Therapy for all of these lesions includes excision, with care taken to ensure that there is neither entry nor injury to the bladder or distal ureters. We almost universally perform cystoscopy at time of resection, after closure of the subepithelial dead space and before approximation of the vaginal epithelium.

Vaginal Intraepithelial Neoplasia

From a pathophysiologic and treatment perspective, vaginal intraepithelial neoplasia (VAIN) has more in common with cervical intraepithelial neoplasia (CIN; discussed later) than it does with VIN. Therefore, the bulk of the essential information regarding VAIN is presented in the section on CIN. A few unique points, however, must be highlighted. Sixty percent of women who have VAIN have previously been diagnosed with CIN. It has become evident that HPV is the causative agent in the vast majority of instances. Therapy of VAIN, because of the significant potential for inducing undesirable scarring, contraction, and subsequent dysfunction of the vagina, must be undertaken cautiously. Small lesions are best simply surgically excised, whereas larger lesions are treated with multiple colposcopic biopsies to ensure the absence of invasive disease, followed by laser vaporization. Locally caustic agents (5-fluorouracil) or immune modulators (imiquimod) have been used, although the latter only outside of U.S. Food and Drug Administration-approved labeling. In general, despite the effectiveness of these therapies, we are hesitant to use them because of the significant inflammatory response that can occur. In the worst case, epithelial sloughing and chemical vaginitis leads to coaptation of the vagina, secondary amenorrhea, and coital dysfunction. Similarly, a chronic inflammatory process associated with copious discharge and dyspareunia has been reported. Regardless of the therapy recommended, adequate vaginal estrogenization and serial dilation, either by coitus or with a prosthesis, are mandatory.

Vaginal Cancer

Vaginal cancer, like the precancerous changes described previously, has much in common with cervical cancer. As a general staging rule, if a malignancy involves the vagina and the cervix, it is classified and staged as a cervical cancer. The same is true if the lesion involves the vagina and the vulva (i.e., it is classified and staged as a vulvar cancer; see FIGO staging in Table 103.2).

There are two special histologic types of vaginal cancer that deserve special comment (Table 103.4). Vaginal clear cell carcinoma has been noted to occur in a disproportionate number of women who were exposed in utero to diethylstilbestrol (DES). This exposure leads to a delay in squamous metaplasia in the upper vagina with the presence of endocervical-like glands (vaginal adenosis). The adenosis appears to be a site from which a series of oncogenic events can give rise to clear cell carcinomas. During the period

Table 103.4. HISTOLOGIC CELL TYPES OF VAGINAL CANCER

Epidermoid squamous
Adenocarcinomas
Diethylstilbestrol-related clear cell
Melanoma
Metastatic disease
   Local
      Cervical
      Vulvar
      Anorectal
   Distal
      Endometrial
      Gestational trophoblastic disease
      Breast
      Others

when women were exposed in utero to DES (1943 to 1971) and developed to maturity, approximately two thirds of all clear cell cancers of the vagina were allegedly associated with this exposure. In contradistinction, only approximately one third of the clear cell carcinomas of the cervix during that same period were presumed to be DES related. The rates of DES-related clear cell carcinoma have, obviously, significantly decreased because DES has not been used since 1971 and because the most of the affected women have reached their late 30s and beyond.

Besides being a source of primary malignancy, the vagina is a common site of metastasis, particularly when the primary arises in an adjoining organ (see earlier). Most notable is the proclivity of both endometrial cancer and gestational trophoblastic disease to have associated vaginal metastases. This is an important clinical phenomenon that may lead to the diagnosis of an otherwise occult primary after biopsy of a symptomatic (usually bleeding) vaginal lesion.

The guiding principle of therapy for vaginal cancers is that lesions involving the upper one third of the vagina are best treated as one would treat a similar-sized cervical lesion, whereas lesions of the distal two thirds are treated like vulvar cancer. This difference is based on both anatomic realities and lymphatic drainage.

CERVIX

Congenital

As has been repeatedly emphasized, congenital abnormalities of the female reproductive tract are best understood as a continuum of one disease entity. Cervical agenesis as an isolated abnormality is unheard of. Duplication of the cervix is discussed in the section on congenital abnormalities of the uterine corpus.

Traumatic

As with congenital abnormalities, the cervix is rarely the sole organ affected by genital trauma. The vulva and vagina are much more likely to be injured inadvertently or during sexual assault, although the generally resilient cervix may be lacerated if the assault involved the use of a sharp foreign object. Blunt object assault is much more likely to lead to trauma to the posterior vaginal fornix and retrocervical cul-de-sac (i.e., a posterior colpotomy). This may also be the result of violent rape or vigorous consensual coitus, although the latter is remarkably uncommon.

The two most common sources of cervical trauma are attempted or completed vaginal delivery and postexcision for cervical dysplasia. Peripartum cervical lacerations may occur independent of, or simultaneously with a vulvar, perineal, or vaginal birth injury. In contradistinction to the distal vagina, which may go from a relatively nonexpanded state to the passage of a term infant in a short time, the cervix usually dilates slowly over many hours during both the latent and active phases of labor. However, women who have extremely rapid, "precipitous" labor may sustain a cervical laceration. Cervical laceration is more likely to result from a dysfunctional labor leading to fetal instrumentation in an attempt to effect a vaginal delivery (either forceps or vacuum extraction), or from direct iatrogenic injury at time of transabdominal operative delivery (cesarean section). In a setting where there has been an operative delivery, a precipitous birth, or the occurrence of a vulvar/perineal/vaginal laceration, it is essential that the clinician thoroughly inspect the cervix. Lacerations of the cervix are common (leading, in part, to the classic parous appearance of the cervix) and do not require repair unless they are bleeding or extend to the cervicovaginal reflection. Repair can be effected by a simple, single-layer, running-locked number 0 or 1 delayed absorbable suture. When the laceration extends to the cervical vaginal reflection, further evaluation must be undertaken to ensure that there has been no injury to surrounding structures, particularly the bladder, distal ureters, and uterine artery complex. The latter can lead to significant occult blood loss into the potential space of the broad ligament (Fig. 103.2), and the former can lead to fistula formation and chronic urinary tract dysfunction. Injury to the urinary tract should be assessed by immediate cystoscopy with administration of intravenous indigo carmine (10 mL) followed by 5 mg of furosemide to speed nephric clearance of the dark blue dye. Further surgical management depends on site and degree of injury, and is usually directed by a gynecologic oncologist, urogynecologist, or urologist who specializes in the care of the female patient.

Post-cone Biopsy

By definition, a cervical excision procedure, whether in the form of a cold-knife cone, laser cone, or loop electrical excision procedure (LEEP), is a form of traumatic injury to the cervix. All of these procedures have an associated rate of delayed, postprocedural bleeding (from as high as 8% to 10% for a cold-knife cone to as low as 1% to 2% for a LEEP). Bleeding has a tendency to occur anywhere from 72 hours to 7 to 10 days after the performance of the procedure. Although, because of the high number of these procedures performed each year, postexcision bleeding is commonly encountered, the optimal method of management has yet to be described. When bleeding occurs, there usually has been the development of an indolent soft-tissue infection (directly affecting the cervical stroma) in the presence of a foreign body (suture). Our preferred therapeutic protocol is to (a) institute intravenous broad-spectrum antibiotics that give adequate coverage for both vaginal flora and anaerobes; (b) take the patient to a procedure room where adequate analgesia may be induced; and (c) remove all extant sutures and replace with directed sutures, using them sparingly simply to obtain hemostasis. We prefer to use a long-acting, monofilament, absorbable suture in gauge 0. Further use of electrical cautery or of fulgurating agents (silver nitrate or Monsol's solution) is of limited value and may actually be counterproductive by inducing further foreign body and inflammatory reaction, leading to another bleeding episode.

Deficiencies of Support

It is not the of intent of this chapter to give an exhaustive description of the diagnosis and operative management of abnormalities of pelvic support. As with many topics covered in this general chapter, numerous excellent, in-depth textbooks are available to the reader desiring further education, and only a brief summary is presented here.

As was emphasized in the opening sections of this chapter that discussed the intertwined nature of the anatomy and physiology of the female reproductive tract, a deficiency in support of one pelvic structure (with associated functional failure) is rarely an isolated event. To understand these processes fully, the clinician must reflect on the three pelvic compartments. A well-standardized and validated terminology of female pelvic organ prolapse and pelvic floor dysfunction has been developed and should be used when quantifying these abnormalities (8). Anterior compartment support failure leads to urethrocele, hypermobile urethrovesical junction, and cystocele. Often, these anatomic findings are associated with symptoms of a mass effect at the vaginal introitus, a sensation of pelvic heaviness, coital laxity, and urinary incontinence in stressful activity. Paradoxically, the more severe degrees of loss of mobility may actually be accompanied by obstruction as a result of severe urethral kinking; if residual urine volumes increase and remain high, this may lead to overflow incontinence. Mid-compartment support abnormalities lead to descent of the cervix and uterine corpus (or vaginal vault, if the cervix and corpus are absent) and associated enterocele. Associated symptoms are similar to those of anterior support failure, with a preponderance of symptoms due to the mass effect of the prolapsing uterus. Posterior compartment support abnormalities can lead to the findings of a descending perineal body, rectocele, or enterocele. Symptomatology is as described previously, with the added symptom complex of either fecal incontinence (if the rectal sphincter is either anatomically disrupted or physiologically nonfunctional) or constipation and difficulty with evacuation, which is treated with "splinting" (digital dorsal displacement of the rectocele) to allow for adequate transmission of Valsalva pressure vectors and evacuation of the lower gastrointestinal tract. The diagnosis of these processes is usually straightforward and is made during physical examination of the patient who has not undergone prior attempts at surgical repair or has a concomitant neurologic (either distal or proximal) dysfunction. Women who present with symptoms of urinary incontinence are more likely than not to have a mixed pattern of dysfunction, that is, one that involves both failure of the continence mechanism secondary to anatomic or intrinsic sphincter insufficiency and a degree of loss of detrusor muscle control. Because of this reality, except in those settings where (a) a thorough and meticulous history has identified symptoms of urinary loss that occur only immediately after a stress activity, (b) there is no history of prior attempts at surgical urinary incontinence correction, and (c) there is demonstrated urethrovesical junction hypermobility, a thorough urodynamic evaluation by cystometrography is mandatory (9). Thorough pretreatment assessment is even more strongly encouraged for those women who present with fecal incontinence because it is highly probably that these patients have a mixed anatomic and neurologic cause for their symptoms. Rectal sphincter dynamic ultrasonography, defecography, pelvic floor electromyography, and even dynamic pelvic floor magnetic resonance imaging may be required to make an accurate diagnosis that leads to appropriate patient counseling and treatment.

There are numerous surgical and nonsurgical therapeutic options available to the physician caring for the patient with a pelvic floor defect and functional abnormality. Independent of the final regimen selected, adequate estrogenization of the patient's lower genital tract must be guaranteed. Estrogen can both increase the collagen content of the supporting ligaments and help to reestablish the normal, premenopausal hermetic seal of the urethra and tone of the perineal and vaginal tissues. Neuromuscular stimulation and exercise, in the form of Kegel's exercises, vaginal weights, or direct electrical stimulator application, are beneficial and minimally invasive. Apparatuses that support the pelvic structures or fill the coital hiatus (pessaries) may be useful, particularly in the patient who is not a surgical candidate but has failed other noninvasive therapies. Unfortunately, there is a very high rate of patient-initiated discontinuation of pessary use secondary to pain, pressure, or simple inconvenience of repeated removal, cleaning, and replacement.

The last 125 years has seen an almost innumerable array of surgical procedures proposed and used in the management of pelvic support deficiencies. Many of these are used only in a given geographic area where tradition supersedes science, and many others have simply fallen by the wayside. However, since the early 1980s, the randomized clinical trial has been applied to procedure selection. Although the extant evidence, as for most surgical procedures, is suboptimal, we make the following recommendations based on current knowledge (10):

1. All compartments must be evaluated and treated.
2. Genuine stress urinary incontinence secondary to an anatomic defect (the hypermobile urethra) is best repaired using a modified retropubic urethropexy (RPUP; Burch procedure). A concomitant anterior colporrhaphy should be performed if there is residual cystocele after the RPUP.
3. Intrinsic sphincter deficiency should be treated with a sling procedure, preferably using fascia lata, Alloderm, or nonreactive synthetic materials [i.e., polytetrafluoroethylene (PTFE; Gore-Tex)]. For patients with recurrent disease, periurethral collagen injections can be used.
4. Potential vaginal vault prolapse should be addressed prophylactically by use of the Mayo modification of the McCall culdoplasty.
5. Documented vaginal vault prolapse should be treated with either a Mayo-modified McCall culdoplasty or a sacral colpopexy using a noninflammatory, closed-pore prosthesis (fascia lata, PTFE).
6. Enteroceles should invariably be repaired as part of the management of vault suspension. Occurring as isolated postsurgical findings, these are best treated with a culdoplasty.
7. Rectoceles are best treated with posterior colporrhaphy with specific attention paid to reconstruction of the perineal body, the major source of posterior support of then ureterovesical junction.
8. Rectal sphincter failure is managed by a multimodality approach, including repair of anatomic defects, neosphincter reconstruction using levator ani muscles, and physiotherapy.

Infectious

Surgical therapy for an isolated acute cervical infection has never been reported because these entities are treated pharmacologically (1). The cervix may be, although it does not need to be, removed as part of the definitive surgical management of tuboovarian abscess (TOA), which is presented in the section on ovarian diseases.

Nabothian cysts, the end result of chronic cervicitis, are sometimes inadvertently treated because of naiveté on behalf of the treating surgeon. These cysts, which are caused by inflammatory or benign metaplastic occlusion of the cervical gland ducts and subsequent dilatation (at times massive) secondary to buildup of cervical mucus, may appear neoplastic to the inexperienced. Clinical nabothian cysts may enlarge to 1 cm or more in diameter, are rarely symptomatic, and are best left untreated. However, because of their "worrisome" appearance, segmental cervical excision, vaginal trachelectomy, or even hysterectomy have been used to remove the cysts. All of these therapies are excessive except when the cysts are symptomatic (pain at manipulation) or there is an associated disease processes that justifies the surgery.

Neoplastic

The relative importance of cervical cancer is demonstrated in Table 103.1. Although cervical cancer is relatively uncommon as a source of morbidity and mortality in the United States, it ranks as the number two cause of cancer-related death in women in the developing world, and in selected countries, it is number one.

Fifty years ago, a highly effective screening tool, the Papanicolaou (Pap) smear, entered into broad use in the United States. It was the institution of common, although not universal, screening of at-risk women that has led to a 75% fall in the incidence of cervical cancer over the last 70 years.

Although cervical cancer has become a less important public health entity, cervical dysplasia remains a significant burden to the U.S. health care system. Every year there are approximately 3.5 million minimally abnormal [atypical squamous cells of undetermined significance (ASCUS) and low-grade squamous epithelial lesion (LGSIL)] Pap smears collected in the United States. Approximately 15% to 20% of these women have an associated, unappreciated, precancerous lesion (CIN II or III), with a significant, if not the largest, percentage of precancerous lesions eventually identified in that group of women who present with minimally abnormal Pap smears. These lesions are called *precancerous* because they have approximately a 30% chance of progressing to invasive disease if left untreated, in contradistinction to the histologic changes that are reflected in the minimal abnormalities that have, at most, a 1% to 2% chance of developing into a malignant disease.

Evaluation of the abnormal Pap smear is based on (a) degree of abnormality, (b) patient age, and (c) probability that the patient will comply with recommended follow-up (Fig. 103.5). The most remarkable change in the triage and assessment algorithm has been the integration of HPV typing. HPV is a responsible coagent in nearly 100% of women with cervical precancerous lesions or cancer. The capacity to identify accurately the oncogenic strains of HPV has led to the incorporation of hybrid capture testing into the aforementioned algorithm, although controversy regarding this inclusion exists (11).

Treatment of Cervical Dysplasia

Only precancerous lesions require therapy; patients with lesser lesions are more likely to experience a deleterious side effect from therapy than progress to cancer. The goal of therapy is twofold: (a) to ensure that there is no underlying, occult cancer (a finding in 3% to 10% of patients with CIN II to III); and (2) to eliminate the lesion in its entirety such that the chance of recurrence is minimized. Our preferred modality for treatment is LEEP, a procedure during which a 0.0001-inch tungsten wire loop carrying low-energy electrical current is used to excise the abnormal tissue. The tissue is submitted for pathologic interpretation. Because there is a small, but real risk that the surgical margins will be uninterpretable secondary to thermal artifact, in those settings in which subtleties of pathologic interpretation will make a significant difference in subsequent therapy (e.g., glandular dysplasias, microinvasive disease), we recommend that a cold-knife cone biopsy be performed in a surgical center under systemic analgesia.

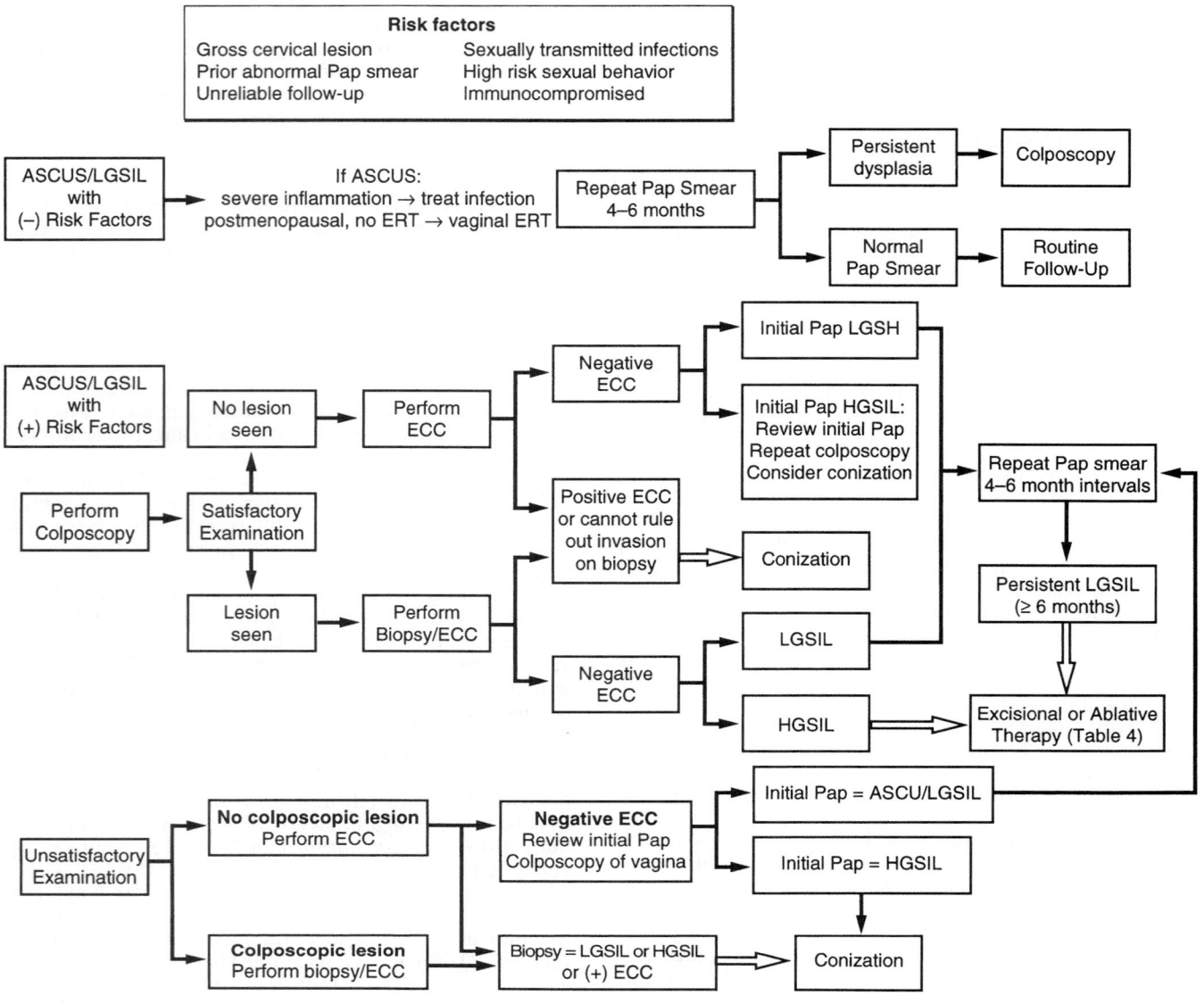

Figure 103.5. Abnormal Pap smear management algorithm.

Cervical Cancer

Cervical cancer, as emphasized previously, has become a less significant source of morbidity for North American and European women. This disease occurs uncommonly in people who have been compliant with recommended exfoliative cytologic screening (Pap smear). Depending on the community surveyed, between 40% and 60% of all women in whom cervical cancer develops have either never had a Pap smear or have been suboptimally screened.

Most cervical cancers are of the squamous cell type and have been demonstrated to be due in part to an infection with high-risk HPV types, as noted previously. Adenocarcinomas have become more common and comprise 15% to 25% of all cervical cancers. The cervix can also be a site of metastatic disease, with endometrial cancer being the most common primary site.

Cervical cancer, when not first appreciated by Pap smear, is symptomatic in approximately 75% of cases, with abnormal bleeding, vaginal discharge, and pain predominating. By FIGO rules, cervical cancer is clinically staged (Table 103.2). The most critical element in the staging process is a thorough and accurate pelvic examination

searching for findings consistent with extracervical spread. To be optimal, this examination often must be performed under analgesia. A chest radiograph and, in women with suspected disease extension, an intravenous pyelogram, cystoscopy, and, rarely, proctosigmoidoscopy, may be included. More advanced radiographic studies can be performed (computed tomography and magnetic resonance imaging), although the information they provide, except for the finding of hydronephrosis, cannot be used to "upstage" patients. Figure 103.6 gives the Kelly Gynecologic Oncology Service guidelines for management of cervical cancer.

The use of radical surgery in the management of early cervical cancer and ultraradical surgery as salvage for recurrent disease deserves specific comment.

Radical Hysterectomy. Cervical cancer's natural proclivity is for local advancement and spread and systematic, stepwise involvement of sequential draining lymph nodes. These phenomena were appreciated over 150 years ago and led to the development of a new surgical procedure: the radical hysterectomy. This procedure was first developed and performed in the United States by J. Goodrich Clark, a

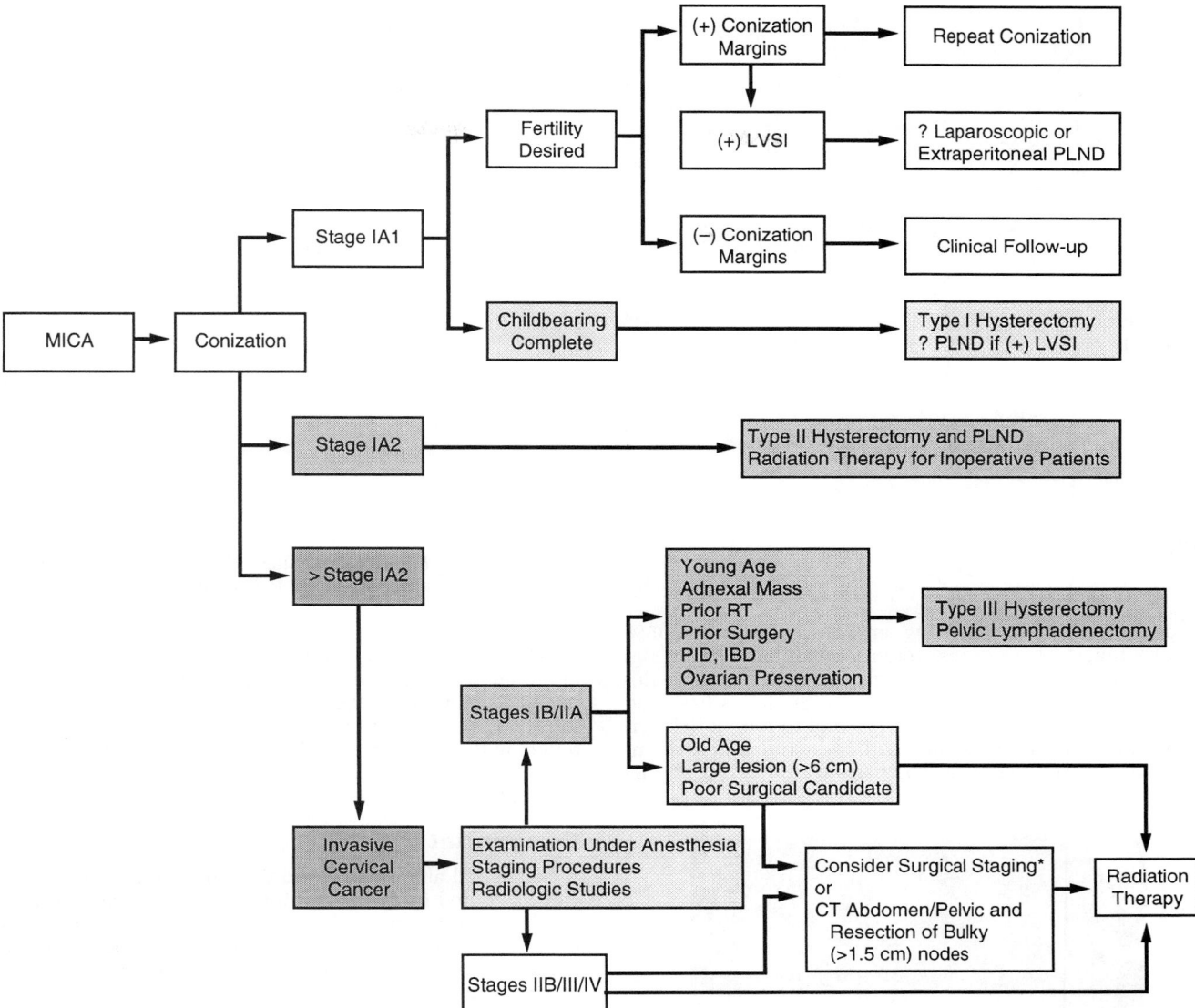

Figure 103.6. Cervical cancer management algorithm.

resident surgeon under the tutelage of Dr. Howard A. Kelly at The Johns Hopkins Hospital in 1895. The driving principle was to develop a surgical procedure that could safely remove the primary lesion *en bloc* with a margin of surrounding tissue that was grossly devoid of tumor and included the first-level lymphatic drainage while leaving the adjoining vital organs (urinary bladder, ureter, and rectum) intact and functional. Meigs added to this procedure a systematic resection of the secondary and tertiary lymphatic drainage, with both a therapeutic and diagnostic intent. Over the decades, this procedure has been refined and classified (12) (Fig. 103.7), and specific indications for use of each of the types of radical hysterectomy described (Fig. 103.6). Although various approaches (transvaginal, transabdominal, laparoscopically assisted, and complete laparoscopic) to the performance of radical hysterectomy have been and still are used, because of the general familiarity with the surgical procedure, the thoroughness of the resection possible, and the comorbidity profile, the transabdominal approach is the most commonly used. A new variation of the procedure is the performance of a radical vaginal trachelectomy with a concomitant laparoscopic lymph node dissection for women with early localized disease (stage Ia2

to Ib1) who desire preservation of fertility. There is a growing database supporting not only that this procedure can be performed safely and with acceptable disease control rates, but that most women who wish to preserve fertility are able to do so (13).

Pelvic Exenteration. Even with advances in radiation therapy techniques and the administration of radiosensitizing doses of cytotoxic chemotherapy, a significant proportion of women with locally advanced cervical cancer have a recurrence. This was true to an even greater extent before the modern era of chemoradiation therapy. For these women, who had only local persistent or recurrent disease, no curative option existed until the work of Bruecher et al. in the 1940s. They described the performance of an ultraradical extirpation of the pelvic organs (bladder, urethra, distal ureters, uterus, fallopian tubes, ovaries, vagina, parametria and paracolpos, distal sigmoid and rectum, and, when performed in an infralevatory fashion, segments of the levator ani muscles, perineum, and anal sphincter) and development of a urinary conduit and colostomy. This procedure, called *pelvic exenteration,* has led to salvage rates as high as 60% in selected subgroups

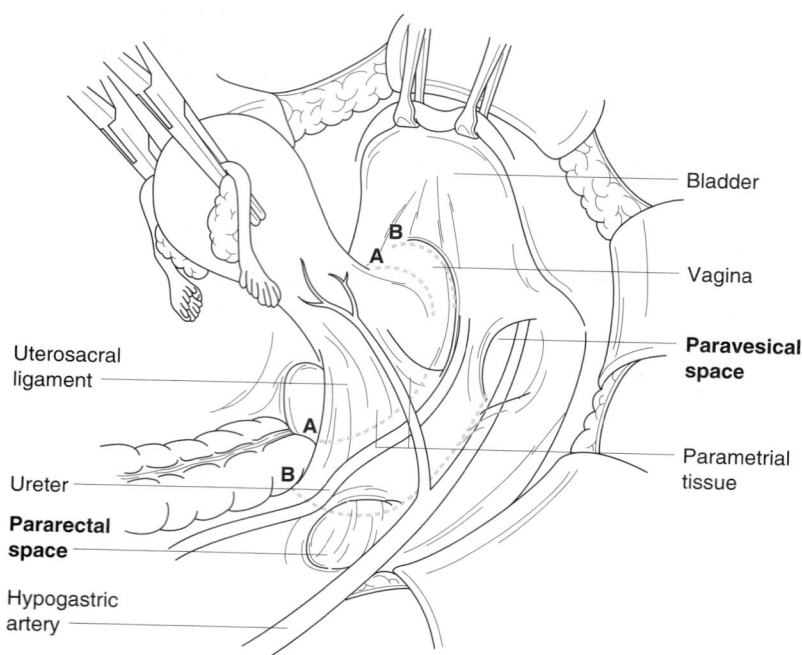

Figure 103.7. Illustration of differences between a class II and III radical hysterectomy.

of patients, with average long-term cure rates in the 35% to 40% range. These cures were not obtained without significant losses in both physiologic and psychological domains. Over the intervening 50 years, the focus has been on refining the procedure in an attempt to reestablish urinary and fecal continence and coital function and to maintain a healthy body image. The current standard (14) calls

for (a) establishment of a continent urinary diversion; (b) anastomosis of the resected margins of the large intestine; and (c) construction of a dynamic vagina using cutaneous island flaps, with a VRAM or transverse rectus abdominis muscle flap being our preference. This leads to a cosmetic outcome that offers a significant advantage (Fig. 103.8).

UTERUS

Congenital

Congenital abnormalities of the female reproductive organs, as noted in the discussion of vaginal abnormalities, lie along a continuum related to the degree of nonfusion of the paired müllerian-derived structures or failure of one half of the müllerian system to develop. A formal classification system was developed by the American Fertility Society (now called the American Society for Reproductive Medicine) and is commonly used (15). The most severe cases are those of didelphic or unobstructed double uterus, whereas the least severe are subseptate uteri. The didelphic uterus does not require surgical unification, although patients with a septate uterus, because of significant difficulties with reproductive failure, are candidates for such a procedure. Rudimentary and noncommunicating uterine horns are best treated with resection.

There are numerous different metroplasty techniques and methods for transcervical hysteroscopic resection, a complete discussion of which is beyond the scope of this text. However, a critical point is that women who have undergone metroplasty and become pregnant must, because of the inordinate risk of uterine rupture, undergo cesarean delivery before labor.

Traumatic

The most common traumatic injury to the uterine corpus is perforation. This can occur during office endometrial biopsy, intrauterine device (IUD) placement, dilation and curettage, operative pregnancy termination, diagnostic or operative hysteroscopy, or any other time when the uterus is instrumented. Perforation is uncommon in the premenopausal, nonpregnant patient except when operative resection of uterine disease (e.g., septum, myoma) is being un-

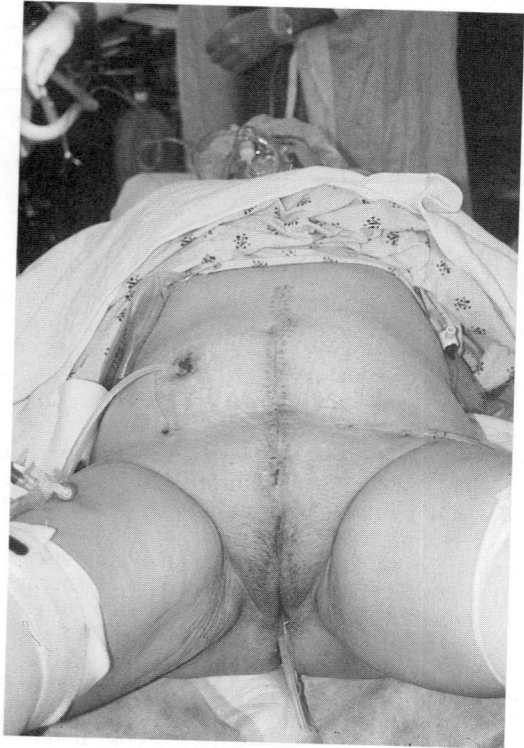

Figure 103.8. Patient after total pelvic exenteration with rectosigmoid anastomosis, neovagina formation, and development of continent urinary diversion (Miami pouch). Note single, small stoma in the right lower quadrant, which is used only for intermittent catheterization.

dertaken. However, in the edematous (pregnant or infected) uterus or, paradoxically, the fibrotic, nonelastic, postmenopausal uterus, perforation may occur in up to 10% of instrumentations. Fortunately, morbidity associated with perforation is uncommon except in selected circumstances. If perforation is suspected, consideration must be given not only to sequelae that result from transversion of the uterine wall, but to those of injury to the surrounding structures. When perforation has occurred with a blunt object (sound, probe, plastic cannula) and without negative pressure being applied (i.e., suction), significant bleeding from the uterine defect and injury to surrounding structures are rare. However, if a sharp instrument (curet) or negative pressure (such as occurs during a suction dilation and curettage for elective abortion) has been used, some reparative action probably will be needed. In the former setting, we do nothing except monitor for signs and symptoms of bleeding in the immediate postoperative period. However, in the latter settings, we recommend that a diagnostic laparoscopy be performed at a minimum, with a low threshold for exploratory celiotomy and complete and accurate assessment.

Asherman's Syndrome

Asherman's syndrome, or intrauterine synechia, is usually a result of endometrial trauma (curettage) in the setting of endometritis. The presentation is one of secondary amenorrhea or infertility. Diagnosis is made by hysterosalpingogram or hysteroscopy, and therapy consists of resection of the intrauterine adhesions, placement of a device to keep the uterine walls separate (either an IUD or pediatric Foley catheter with concomitant antibiotic prophylaxis), and estrogenic stimulation to reestablish the endometrium. The rate of successful correction is approximately 80% using this multimodality approach.

Hematomucometria and Pyomucometria

These phenomena result from the near-total or total occlusion of the cervix and production of cervical mucus or endometrial blood, which can become superinfected. These processes are almost universally the end result of either surgical trauma (cone biopsy, LEEP, cryotherapy, birth trauma), radiation/chronic atrophic changes, or an obstructive cervical malignancy. Surgically, simple dilation of the cervix, cervical conical excision, or, rarely, hysterectomy are the mainstays of therapy.

Infectious

Rarely are infectious processes of the uterine corpus surgically managed. The exceptions are infected degenerating fibroids, which are probably the result of inoculation of the hypooxygenated necrotic fibroid by instrumentation, and TOAs in which the uterus may be involved with microabscesses. Historically, before the modern era of antibiotics and the abandonment of the use of braided IUD strings (such as with the original Dalkon Shield IUD), emergent hysterectomy for the management of myometrial infection was a standard and often lifesaving practice. Similarly, endometriosis does not justify surgical management beyond adequate endometrial evaluation to ensure that there is no associated malignancy.

Neoplastic

Neoplastic processes of the uterine corpus, both nonmalignant and malignant, are the most common indications for the performance of hysterectomy.

Leiomyomata Uteri

Leiomyomata, or fibroids, are benign, nonmalignant, and non-precancerous overgrowths of the smooth muscle of the uterine wall. The etiology of these lesions, which occur in 15% of all women and as many as 35% to 50% of women of color, is unknown. Women with fibroids can have one or more of a constellation of symptoms, with the specific symptom a product of the size and location of the myoma. The most common symptoms are abnormalities of bleeding, pain (specifically dysmenorrhea and dyspareunia), and the effects of the large uterus pressing on surrounding structures (e.g., urinary frequency and incontinence, rectal frequency, low back pain). It has been well demonstrated that fibroids are estrogen responsive, and this has been taken into consideration in the creation of treatment algorithms. Antiestrogenic therapy is variably effective depending on the degree of blockage or suppression of estrogen and the size of the fibroids. In general, using the most effective agents [gonadotropin-releasing hormone (GnRH) antagonists], up to 70% of myomata that are less than 7 to 9 cm in maximal diameter undergo a 70% shrinkage in volume (not diameter) (16). This success is not obtained without morbidity because hypoestrogenic symptomatology is almost universal. The limitation to the use of GnRH antagonists is the long-term morbidity and potential mortality associated with postmenopausal estrogen levels in young women (e.g., osteoporosis, heart disease). Therefore, these agents are most frequently used for a short time to stop bleeding so that a patient can be autotransfused before surgical management, to shrink the myomata such that surgery can be preformed by a preferred route (transvaginal instead of transabdominal), or in anticipation of the occurrence of permanent, physiologic loss of estrogen production (i.e., the climacteric and menopause).

Surgical management of fibroids can be divided into definitive (i.e., hysterectomy) or nondefinitive (either myomectomy or hysteroscopic resection of submucosal myomata). The advantage of myomectomy is that fertility is spared, although approximately 15% of women require further surgical management of the myoma. Myomectomy may be performed by open or laparoscopic techniques, although there are significant concerns about the reestablishment of uterine wall integrity and the safety of subsequent pregnancy in the latter setting. Blood loss at time of myomectomy, which can be massive, can be limited with the use of tourniquets, vascular "bulldog" clamps, vasoconstrictive agents, and hemostatic dissecting instruments (electrocautery, laser, or, our preference, the argon beam coagulator). At time of myomectomy, meticulous closure is needed to enhance myometrial healing to minimize the potential for intrapartum uterine rupture, a disastrous and commonly fatal event. Hysteroscopic resection offers the advantage of a minimally invasive procedure, although one with the potentially lethal associated morbidity of intravascular fluid overload, pulmonary edema, and congestive heart failure. Pregnancy is not recommended after hysteroscopic resection and may be impossible because of endometrial adhesions. There are newer, cutting-edge techniques that are minimally invasive and can purportedly destroy the myoma [e.g., embolization (17), myolysis]. At present, all of these techniques must be considered investigational and are contraindicated in any woman who is not confident of her decision to stop procreating.

Sarcomas

Uterine sarcomas are uncommon but aggressive and frequently fatal diseases that have a complex and at times confusing histologic classification (Table 103.5). The basis of treatment of uterine sarcomas is hysterectomy with bilateral salpingo-oophorectomy. In sarcomas of endometrial origin, there may be merit in the performance of a thorough surgical staging such as is recommended for endometrial adenocarcinomas (see later), although there is no high-level evi-

Table 103.5. CLINICAL CLASSIFICATION OF UTERINE SARCOMAS

Endometrial stromal sarcomas (ESS)
Leiomyosarcomas (LMS)
Carcinosarcomas or malignant mixed mesodermal tumors (MMMT)
  Malignant glandular and stromal elements
Adenosarcomas
  Benign glandular elements and malignant stromal elements

dence supporting this belief, mostly because the use of adjuvants is of unproven benefit. There is an important misconception regarding the relationship between fibroids and uterine leiomyosarcomas: previously identified myomata that are noted to grow rapidly do not represent malignant degeneration, and such growth is not in itself a justification for surgical intervention. However, in a woman in her fifth decade or older, who is perimenopausal, and who does not have a known history of fibroids and acquires a single, rapidly growing mass in the wall of the uterus, there is sufficient concern that this represents a malignancy to justify resection and pathologic assessment.

Endometrial Hyperplasia

In most settings, endometrial hyperplasia is the result of an endocrinopathy and not a demonstrable genetic oncogenic abnormality. The constant and inadequately opposed or unopposed estrogen stimulation of the endometrium leads to development of these lesions. It is critical to appreciate this when discussing therapeutic options. Endometrial hyperplasias have the same risk factors as endometrial cancers (Table 103.6). As with endometrial cancer, the most common presenting symptom is abnormal vaginal bleeding, in most cases occurring in the menopause. Endometrial cancer can also present with a putrid vaginal discharge or pain; both of these symptoms are more common in the setting of locally advanced or metastatic disease.

Therapy for endometrial hyperplasia is based on the risk of a malignancy developing if left untreated and the probability that the patient will experience a significant complication from the definitive, thorough surgical therapy. Women with endometrial hyperplasia devoid of nuclear atypia or those desiring future fertility can be treated with continuous progestins; our preference is megestrol 40 mg/d for 90 days. Thereafter, the patient undergoes a repeat endometrial sampling in the office. If the hyperplasia has resolved, the patient can be treated with cyclic progestins (for 14 days of the month) or birth control pills. If the hyperplasia persists, a longer period of megestrol therapy (up to 9 months) may be needed. If the hyperplasia is

Table 103.6. RISK FACTORS FOR THE DEVELOPMENT OF ENDOMETRIAL HYPERPLASIAS AND CANCERS

Characteristic	Relative risk
Nulliparity	2–3
Late menopause	2.4
Obesity	
21–50 lbs	3
>50 lbs	10
Diabetes mellitus	2.8
Unopposed estrogen therapy	4–8
Tamoxifen	2–3
Atypical endometrial hyperplasia	8–29

Adapted from Lurain J. Endometrial cancer. In Berek JS, Adashi EY, Hillard PA, eds. Novak's gynecology, 12th ed. Baltimore: Williams & Wilkins, 1996:1058.

not reversed by that time, it is unlikely that further progestin therapy will be effective, and the patient should proceed to definitive therapy (hysterectomy).

Endometrial Cancer

Endometrial cancer is the most common gynecologic malignancy in North America (Table 103.1). However, because early symptoms often lead to early assessment and diagnosis, most lesions are identified before extracorpo-

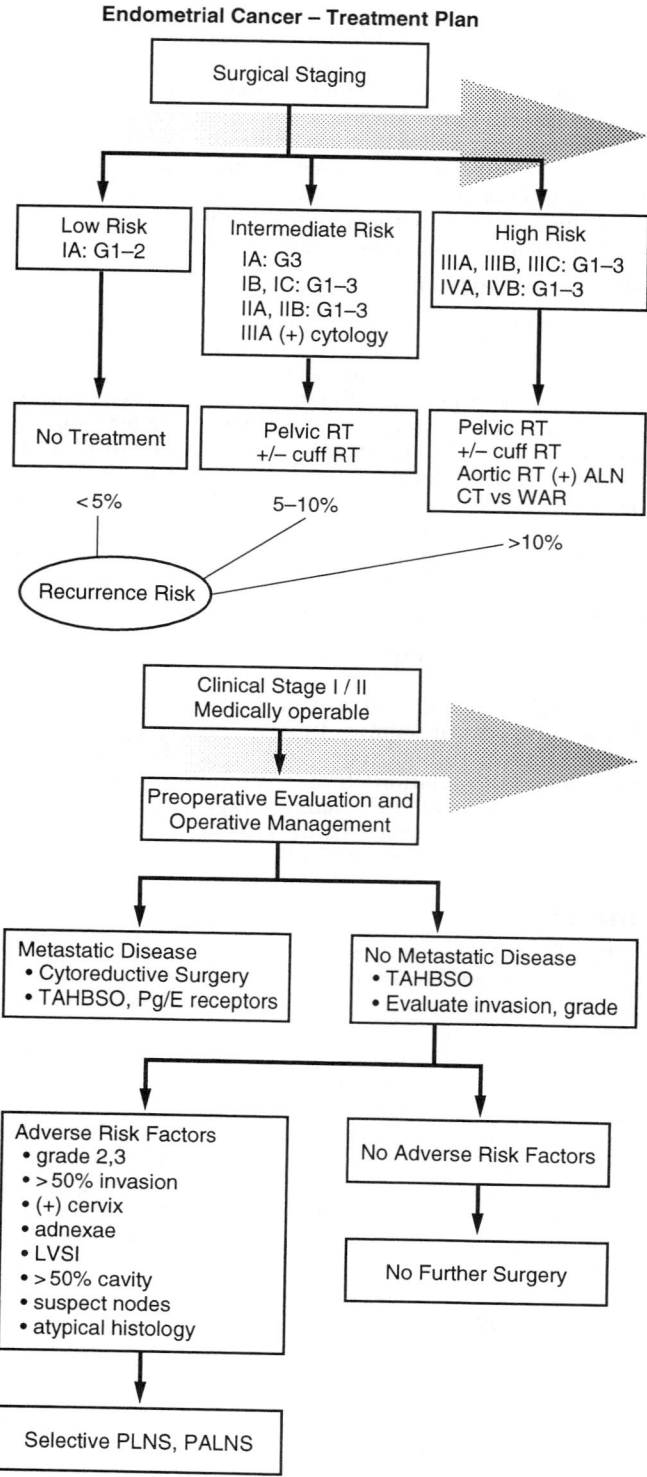

Figure 103.9. Treatment algorithm for endometrial cancer.

real spread has occurred and are successfully treated. This is in contradistinction to ovarian cancers, in which the exact opposite is the case.

There are numerous unresolved controversies surrounding the management of endometrial cancers. However, the treatment algorithm set forth in Fig. 103.9 reflects both the modern understanding of this disease and the recommended FIGO guidelines for staging and the National Comprehensive Cancer Network guidelines for therapy. We recommend surgical staging for all women who have more than a 5% statistical chance of having extrauterine disease, a position that is both evidence based and widely held among academic gynecologic oncology surgeons.

ADNEXA

Although the adnexa include both the ovary and the fallopian tube, it is the former structure that is the primary source of pathologic processes, excluding salpingitis with the more severe or advanced infectious processes of salpingo-oophoritis and TOA.

Congenital

Paramesonephric Duct Cysts

When the paramensonephric or wolffian duct system fails to develop and undergoes resorption, there may be remnants that, over time, can expand with clear serous fluid and become evident. Only very rarely are these small (1.5 to 2 cm in diameter) cysts appreciated clinically. They usually are either an incidental finding at the time of surgery for another pelvic process or are detected with imaging (most frequently ultrasound). These cysts can, however, distend, causing pain, or may undergo torsion incorporating the entire adnexa or a part thereof (the cyst and the fallopian tube). Treatment is surgical resection, with the degree dependent on the age of the patient and her wishes regarding further fertility. Very rarely (<1%) are these cysts associated with malignant degeneration. If so, they are best treated exactly like an ovarian epithelial malignancy.

Traumatic

Torsion

Adnexal torsion is a relatively rare but, from the perspective of maintenance of optimal fertility, potentially disastrous side effect. Those processes that predispose to adnexal torsion include an elongated infundibulopelvic or uteroovarian ligament, an adnexal mass (although large masses are actually less likely to undergo torsion), and the absence of the attachment to the uterus. Adnexal torsion commonly presents as an intermittent and often progressively worsening unilateral pain. Because torsion is more common in settings of ovarian enlargement, it is more likely chronologically to present either at the time of maximal follicular size or in the mid-luteal phase when the corpus luteum is at its zenith. Historically, therapy has been to remove that segment of the adnexa that has undergone torsion because there was a fear that "untwisting" the adnexa would lead to the occurrence or propagation of clot up the ovarian veins with the potential formation of a pulmonary embolus. This philosophy is no longer universally held, and except in the most extreme cases of necrosis or in the paramenopausal age or later, the torsion is reversed, the adnexa is fixed, usually to the psoas muscle tendon, and return of oxygenated blood flow awaited. Intraoperative Doppler ultrasonography can also facilitate the determination of the adequacy of both efferent and afferent flow.

Uterine Perforation

The other common traumatic insult to the adnexa is injury during uterine perforation associated with pregnancy termination. Because of the retrouterine location of the adnexa and the cul-de-sac, it is not uncommon for the adnexal structures to be involved when a perforation-associated extracorporeal injury occurs. The adnexa may actually be drawn into the uterine cavity if a suction dilation and curettage was being undertaken. More potentially dangerous is the laceration of the ovarian vessels in their retroperitoneal location. This can lead to massive, ascending, retroperitoneal and dangerously unappreciated blood loss. A posttermination patient who has symptoms and findings of hypovolemia that are not explicable by intraprocedure blood loss must be assumed to have a major adnexal or retroperitoneal vessel injury until proven otherwise. Although laparoscopy may be helpful in making an accurate diagnosis in the minimally symptomatic woman, the operating endoscopist may not be able to locate a retroperitoneal injury or deal with the injury (depending on his or her skill), or it may worsen the cardiovascular dysfunction by further impeding cardiac preload through vascular occlusion secondary to increased intraperitoneal pressure. Our preference remains exploratory celiotomy through a midline incision with a vascular surgery consultant on standby.

Infectious

Although salpingo-oophoritis remains a not uncommon disease in North America, the surgically treated associated process, TOA, is relatively uncommon. This decrease in the incidence of TOA is due to numerous factors: (a) improved sensitivity to the existence of salpingo-oophoritis by primary care physicians and, therefore, earlier treatment; (b) newer generations of antibiotics that are effective at clearing mixed floral infections in the setting of decreased tissue oxygenation; and (c) the decreasing use of IUDs as contraceptive options. TOAs present like salpingo-oophoritis, but are more likely to be identified in women who have had prior episodes of pelvic inflammatory disease, received suboptimal therapy, or have persistent symptoms and signs despite adequate therapy. The suspicion of TOA is confirmed radiographically, with our preferences being a vaginal probe ultrasound. Once TOAs are identified, it is essential that their natural history be tracked. In patients who fail to experience disease improvement (either symptomatically or due to persistent hyperpyrexia) in the face of adequate antibiotic therapy, consideration must be given to either surgical or interventional radiology-based therapy. In young women for whom gonadal preservation is a priority, we prefer to use either ultrasound or compute tomography-directed drainage, a technique that has become popular since the mid-1980s (18). When this intervention is unsuccessful or in the woman who is closer to menopause, we prefer definitive surgical intervention, which usually includes a bilateral salpingo-oophorectomy at a minimum. Individual variations may occur based on the unique operative findings. Although laparoscopic or even open lysis of adhesions, drainage of purulent material, and copious lavage has been reported to be successful in the management of the patient who has failed interventional radiology-guided care, we rarely undertake such nondefinitive therapy. In patients who have an abscess that has distended the cul-de-sac and descended below the internal cervical os, transvaginal colpotomy drainage is an option. This technique should be undertaken only by an experienced vaginal surgeon because of the potential for significant rectosigmoid injury.

Pelvic Tuberculosis

Pelvic tuberculosis (TB) is a rare entity in all but the new immigrant to North America. However, because of the endemicity of gastrointestinal TB in parts of Mexico and Central America as well as the Indian subcontinent, this process must always be included in the differential diagnosis of a pelvic mass in women from those geographic locales. Pelvic TB is not treated surgically because of the significant potential sequelae and inability totally to remove the innumerable tubers. However, it is not uncommon for the naive surgeon to end up performing an exploratory procedure because of suspicion of the presence of ovarian cancer. This can be avoided, particularly in the younger patient in whom pelvic TB is most likely to manifest first and who does not fit the risk profile for ovarian or primary peritoneal cancers.

Neoplastic

Adnexal Mass

The evaluation and management of the female adnexal mass is a treatise in itself. Fortunately, there are certain caveats that allow a relatively easy understanding of the classification and management of this extremely heterogeneous entity (Table 103.7).

Caveat 1: Remember all the structures that are found in the female pelvis. Health care professionals commonly fail to appreciate which anatomic structures are normally found in the female pelvis, and therefore condemn the patient to an incomplete differential diagnosis. The appendix and sigmoid colon are both pelvic structures and potential sources for adnexal masses. The same is true of an aberrantly located kidney.

Table 103.7. DIFFERENTIAL DIAGNOSIS OF THE ADNEXAL MASS STRATIFIED BY PATIENT'S REPRODUCTIVE AGE

Newborn and Infants
Congenital anomalies (e.g., pelvic kidney)
Physiologic residuum of maternal hormones
   Ovarian theca–luteum cysts
Neoplasms
   Germ cell
      Benign (dermoids)
      Malignant (predominant)
Premenarchal
Functional ovarian cysts
   Follicular
   Hemorrhagic corpus luteum
   Persistent corpus luteum
   Polycystic ovaries
Neoplastic (predominant)
   Germ cell neoplasms
   Epithelial neoplasms
Reproductive Age
Functional (predominant)
   As above
Neoplastic
   As above and below (the closer the patient is to the age of
      menarche, the more likely that the neoplasm is of germ cell
      origin; the closer the patient is to menopause, the more likely
      the neoplasm is of ovarian epithelial origin).
Postmenopausal
Neoplastic (predominant)
   Benign "simple" cysts
   Epithelial neoplasm (benign and malignant)
   Metastatic
   Primary colorectal cancer
Inflammatory
   Diverticular disease

Caveat 2: The closer the patient is to a reproductive milestone, the more likely that the mass represents a physiologic or functional change in the gonad.

Caveat 3: Congenital abnormalities, such as pelvic or horseshoe kidneys, are commonly not appreciated until menarche. Failure to rule out the presence of these structures can lead to life-threatening surgical error.

Caveat 4: Except in the immediate newborn period, when the female infant can manifest residuum of maternal hormone effects, adnexal masses presenting at the extremes of life are malignancies until proven otherwise.

Caveat 5: During the reproductive years, adnexal masses are nonmalignant until proven otherwise.

Caveat 6: A gonad, once removed, cannot be replaced; it is therefore better to reexplore a patient than castrate her under questionable circumstances.

Ovarian Nonmalignant Neoplasms

Regardless of the patient's age (Table 103.7), ovarian lesions must be followed intensively to ensure either regression or lack of progression. Laparoscopy has become the preferred surgical modality for investigation of a persistent adnexal mass. Diagnostic and therapeutic laparoscopy can be performed in most instances in the outpatient setting with very low rates of associated morbidity. It is important that adequate surgical instrumentation be available for performance of the most common adnexal laparoscopic procedures. Our preference is to use a direct trocar insertion technique. When there is significant likelihood of the presence of subumbilical adhesions, we use an alternative site for access, such as the left infracostal margin lateral to the superior epigastric artery. We use 5-mm ports for all sites except one, where a 10- to 12-mm trocar is placed. This larger trocar can be used for placement of linear stapling devices and removal of the mass. The use only of 5-mm ports minimizes the potential for postoperative wound complications without limiting instrumentation or visualization in the modern era of miniaturization. We infiltrate all potential port sites with a long-acting local anesthetic before making the first cutaneous incision. Similarly, at the completion of the case, we make an extra effort to decompress the pneumoperitoneum totally, reestablish the right diaghragm–liver dome negative-pressure seal, and lavage the operative site in as much long-acting anesthetic as can safely be left in vivo (usually 30 to 60 mL of 0.5% bupivacaine, with the actual dose depending on patient weight). At the completion of intraperitoneal surgery, care is taken to ensure complete closure of all 8-mm or larger port sites, closing both the peritoneum and the fascia *en bloc* to minimize the occurrence of Richter's hernia.

A common clinical dilemma faced by the general surgeon is how to manage the finding of an incidental adnexal mass at the time of exploratory celiotomy for a presumed nongynecologic disease process. Remembering the caveats set forth previously and the age-dependent differential diagnosis, the decision about how to proceed should be based on the answers to the following questions:

1. *What does the lesion look like?* Small masses (<8 cm in maximal diameter, in addition to the size of the gonad) that are freely mobile and have a smooth surface are unlikely to represent any neoplasm, much less a malignant one. These masses are best left alone in the premenopausal patient unless the surgeon is skilled at ovarian cystectomy and reconstruction. The exception to this recommendation is the patient who has a benign-appearing cyst that has led to adnexal torsion. There is no hard-and-fast rule as to whether the torsion should be reversed, viability ensured, and the ovary fixed into the ovarian fossa, or whether adnexectomy

should be performed. Clinical judgment as well as the degree of torsion and necrosis are important. The threshold for consultation with an experienced gynecologic surgeon must be very low. In contradistinction, masses that have surface papillae or excrescences are highly suspect for malignancy, although this presentation does occur in ovarian cystadenofibromas. Excisional biopsy of the surface irregularity followed by frozen-section analysis is valuable in deciding how to proceed (see section on ovarian cancer, later).

2. *What is the patient's age?* In those patients who have definitively completed their childbearing, the removal of a single adnexa has little and probably no meaningful effect on age of menopause. However, removal of one of the adnexa decreases fertility rates by 15% and must be avoided if there is any question regarding the patient's desires. Women older than 45 years of age are best served by a bilateral adnexectomy, even if the mass is apparently benign and unilateral. The long-term effects of the induction of surgical menopause, even in the average-risk patient, are offset by the benefits of ovarian cancer prevention.

3. *Why is the surgery being performed?* When operating on a young patient with presumed appendicitis, and a normal appendix but an abnormal ovary are found, the ovarian lesion, even though it is probably physiologic, is best removed by cystectomy because it is probably not optimal medical care to explore a patient, find a potential source for her symptoms, and elect to do nothing. In contradistinction, when a postmenopausal woman is undergoing exploration for surgical management of colon cancer and a small (1- to 4-cm), simple cystic mass is identified in a single ovary (a mass that has less than a 0.5% chance of representing a malignancy), both adnexa should be removed as prophylaxis against ovarian cancer/pathologic processes and gonadal metastasis from the gastrointestinal primary. These two scenarios, which represent extremes of the clinical continuum, serve to illustrate the need for a global clinical perspective. As noted previously, if ever there is doubt about how to proceed, gynecologic surgical consultation must be obtained.

Table 103.8. PATHOLOGIC TYPES OF OVARIAN CANCER

Epithelial
Serous (mimics fallopian tube)
Mucinous (mimics endocervix)
Endometrioid (mimics endometrium)
Brenner's tumor (mimics urothelium)
Germ Cell
Primary gonadal choriocarcinoma
Immature teratoma
Dysgerminoma
Yolk sac tumor
Specialized Gonadal Stromal Lesions
Female directed
    Granulosa-thecal cell tumors
Male directed
    Sertoli-Leydig cell tumors
Nonspecialized Stromal Tumors
Fibromas
Sarcomas
Mixed mesodermal tumors (carcinosarcoma)
Metastatic Lesions
Krukenberg's tumor (gastrointestinal)
Breast
Endometrium

Table 103.9. RISK FACTORS FOR AND PREVENTION OF OVARIAN CANCER

Increase Risk
Early menarche
Late menopause
Long-term (>12 cycles) and high-dose ovulation induction
Lack of oral contraceptive use
Low parity
Advanced age (>30 y) at time of first term delivery
Lack of or late (>30 y of age) breast feeding
Personal or family history of breast, colon, or endometrial cancer
Perineal talc use
Decrease Risk
Opposite of above, plus
Tubal ligation

Ovarian Cancer

Ovarian cancer, most commonly arising from the surface epithelium (Table 103.8), is the number one cause of death from a gynecologic malignancy in North America (4). This disease, however, affects only 1 of 70 American women who live into their ninth decade. There are specific factors that uniquely increase the probability that epithelial ovarian cancer will develop in a woman (Table 103.9). Unfortunately, of those women affected, most have the disease diagnosed when it has extended beyond the female reproductive tract and eventually succumb to their disease.

The ovaries lie in a cavernous potential space (the female pelvis) where large structures can be hidden. Because the ovaries are usually freely mobile and unconnected to the body surface, symptoms of malignancy usually occur late. Concomitantly, as outlined in Table 103.10, the symptoms associated with ovarian cancer are nonspecific and commonly associated with other, significantly less morbid diseases (e.g., diverticulitis, degenerative joint disease). Last, because the presenting symptoms associated with ovarian cancer are nonspecific and not focused on the reproductive tract, patients commonly present to their primary care provider for evaluation. The primary care provider may not be as sensitive to both the potential for and outcome of ovarian cancer and may also play a role in delay of diagnosis.

The classic findings of ovarian cancer are a fixed, tender, cystic and solid pelvic mass in the woman at risk. However, many women lack these findings and present only with ascites or abdominal distention. Radiographic and invasive studies (i.e., colonoscopy) are more beneficial in eliminating the disease from the differential diagnosis than they are at definitively making the diagnosis of ovarian cancer. Diagnosis is made during surgical exploration, preferably in a setting where a skilled pelvic surgeon is available to perform an optimal procedure. The two critical guidelines for the surgical management of ovarian cancer are (a) remove as much of the disease, if not all of the disease, as is possible; and (b) if the disease appears to be limited to the pelvis, perform complete surgical staging (Table 103.11).

Table 103.10. PRESENTING SYMPTOMS OF OVARIAN CANCER

Abdominal bloating and distention
Abdominal/pelvic pain
Pelvic pressure
Change in stool habits
Change in urinary habits
Abnormal vaginal bleeding

Table 103.11. STAGING PROCEDURES IN OVARIAN CANCER

Pelvic fluid collection (washings)
Bilateral paracolic gutter fluid collection (washings)
Upper abdomen (diaphragm surface) fluid collection (washings)
Bilateral ovarian fossa peritoneum biopsy
Cul-de-sac peritoneum biopsy
Bladder peritoneum biopsy
Bilateral paracolic gutter peritoneum biopsy
Appendectomy
Bilateral pelvic lymph node sampling (from the mid-common iliac
  artery to the circumflex iliac artery in the cephalad–caudad
  dimension, and from the genitofemoral nerve to the obturator
  nerve in the lateromedial dimension)
Bilateral paraaortic lymph node sampling (from the mid-common iliac
  artery to the renal vein in the caudocephalad dimension, lateral to
  aorta and medial to the ureter)
Infracolic omentectomy
Diaphragm surface scrape (taken as a Papamicolaou smear)

It is imperative that the clinician remember that the only surgical variable that can have a direct effect on patient curability is the degree of debulking that was accomplished (19). Although in cases with massive extrapelvic metastasis (>10 cm) controversy remains regarding the benefits of aggressive debulking, there are adequate data to support its merit in all settings. The smaller the amount of tumor that is visibly left at the completion of the initial surgery, the more likely that cure will be obtained, once the surgeon has been able to debulk such that the maximal tumor nodule size is under 2 cm. When residual disease is greater than 2 cm, the amount of disease remaining does not appear to make a difference because eventual failure is inevitable. Debulking frequently includes multiple bowel resections and the performance of retrograde radical hysterectomy, in which the entire pelvic tumor mass, including bladder, sidewall, cul-de-sac, peritoneum, and rectosigmoid, as needed, is removed in an extraperitoneal, ventral-to-dorsal technique. Splenectomy, total omentectomy, hepatic resection, diaphragm peritoneal stripping, and the like may all be necessary to obtain optimal debulking. The patient who has undergone extensive debulking for metastatic ovarian cancer is often critically ill after the procedure, with numerous abnormalities of fluid volume, blood components, and electrolytes. Just as there must be a commitment to adequate aggressive surgery, an intensive care unit and skilled intensivist must be available to help maintain the patient in the postoperative period.

Secondary Cytoreductive Surgery. Recently published reviews have led to the development of guidelines for the use of secondary cytoreductive surgery (20). This procedure, which has the potential for lengthening patients' lives in a meaningful way with acceptable operative morbidity, requires the utmost in surgical skill and judgment (21) (Table 103.12). If attempted in inappropriately selected patients, or performed by less skilled surgeons, the procedure is more likely than not to lead to both a shortening of the patient's life and a deterioration in the quality of that remaining life.

Second-look Procedures. After completion of aggressive first-line therapy for epithelial ovarian cancer, accurate knowledge of the patient's disease status is beneficial. Symptom complexes, physical examinations, radiographic imaging, and biochemical markers are less than 60% accurate for determining actual disease status. Therefore, many experts believe that surgery is justified to obtain such data. The controversy surrounds not

Table 103.12. GUIDELINES FOR SECONDARY CYTOREDUCTIVE SURGERY

1. No prior "adequate" attempts at optimal cytoreductive surgery, or
2. Isolated lesion
3. Acceptable performance status
4. If disease is recurrent, a 6-month disease-free interval
5. Presence of further medical or radiotherapeutic options
6. Adequate informed consent

whether surgery is more accurate at making the diagnosis, but whether changes in treatment based on surgical findings make a difference in the patient's eventual outcome. The procedure offers no advantage if its primary goal is to determine whether the patient is cured. However, if the goal is to grant the patient an accurate glimpse into her future, what her life expectancy and course may be, this procedure is unparalleled. Therefore, it is critical that the patient be an active partner in deciding whether a second-look procedure should be undertaken. We prefer to perform second-look procedures laparoscopically. Either an open laparoscopy or, as is our preference, a left upper quadrant placement of the initial trocar should be used because of the significant potential for extensive adhesions under the site of the prior incision and elsewhere where cytoreduction was preformed. A complete mechanical bowel preparation, gastric decompression, and appropriate, nonnitrous anesthesia must all be used in an attempt to minimize the chances of a surgical misadventure. The patient must be fully prepared to have the procedure converted to an open approach, either because of an operative complication or inability to perform the complete procedure using laparoscopic technique. At the time of a second-look procedure, consideration should be given to the placement of an intraperitoneal access catheter so that further therapy, if deemed necessary or appropriated, can be administered directly into the peritoneal space.

Chemotherapy. In all but the rarest cases, multiagent chemotherapy is not curative for ovarian cancer when administered without surgical debulking. Yet aggressive, adequate chemotherapy is an essential part of the algorithm for the successful management of ovarian cancer. Standards for ovarian cancer chemotherapy are fluid. As of the writing of this chapter, taxane/platinum-containing regimens for six to nine cycles are the community standard.

CONCLUSION

The surgical management of pelvic disease processes, although less widely implemented now than two decades ago, remains a mainstay in the modern care of women. A thorough appreciation of the uniqueness of the female pelvic anatomy, a knowledge of the wide range of physiologic and pathologic processes that occur, and surgical adroitness are essential for obtaining an optimal outcome.

REFERENCES

1. Centers for Disease Control and Prevention. 1998 Guidelines for treatment of sexually transmitted diseases. *MMWR Morb Mortal Wkly Rep* 1998;47(RR-1):1–111.
2. Kiryu H, Ackerman AB. A critique of current classifications of vulvar diseases. *Am J Dermatopathol* 1990;12:377–392.
3. Junge J, Poulsen H, Horn T, et al. Human papillomavirus (HPV) in vulvar dysplasia and carcinoma in situ. *APMIS* 1995;103:1–10.
4. Greenlee RT, Murray T, Bolden S, et al. Cancer statistics, 2000. *CA Cancer J Clin* 2000;50:7–33.

5. Morgan MA, Mikuta JJ. Surgical management of vulvar cancer. *Semin Surg Oncol* 1999;17:168–172.

6. Levenback C. Intraoperative lymphatic mapping and sentinel node identification: gynecologic applications. *Recent Results Cancer Res* 2000;157:150–158.

7. Wheeless CR Jr. Neovagina construction from an omental J flap and a split thickness skin graft. *Gynecol Oncol* 1989;35: 224–226.

8. Bump RC, Mattiasson A, Bo K, et al. The standardization of terminology of female pelvic organ prolapse and pelvic floor dysfunction. *Am J Obstet Gynecol* 1996;175:10–17.

9. Videla FL, Wall LL. Stress incontinence diagnosed without multichannel urodynamic studies. *Obstet Gynecol* 1998;91: 965–968.

10. Keane DP, Eckford SD, Abrams P. Surgical treatment and complications of urinary incontinence. *Curr Opin Obstet Gynecol* 1992;4:559–564.

11. Kaufman RH, Adam E. Is human papillomavirus testing of value in clinical practice? *Am J Obstet Gynecol* 1999;180: 1049–1053.

12. Piver MS, Rutledge F, Smith JP. Five classes of extended hysterectomy for women with cervical cancer. *Obstet Gynecol* 1974;44:265–269.

13. Dargent D, Martin X, Sacchetoni A, et al. Laparoscopic vaginal radical trachelectomy: a treatment to preserve the fertility of cervical carcinoma patients. *Cancer* 2000;88:1877–1882.

14. Estape R, Angioli R. Surgical management of advanced and recurrent cervical cancer. *Semin Surg Oncol* 1999;16: 236–241.

15. American Society of Fertility. Classification of mullerian anomalies. *Fertil Steril* 1988;49:944–947.

16. Barbieri RL. Ambulatory management of uterine leiomyomata. *Clin Obstet Gynecol* 1999;42:196–205.

17. Goodwin SC, McLucas B, Lee M, et al. Uterine artery embolization for the treatment of uterine leiomyomata: midterm results. *J Vasc Interv Radiol* 1999;10:1159–1165.

18. Worthen NJ, Gunning JE. Percutaneous drainage of pelvic abscesses: management of tubo-ovarian abscess. *J Ultrasound Med* 1986;5:551–556.

19. Dauplat J, Le Bouedec G, Pomel C, et al. Cytoreductive surgery for advanced stages of ovarian cancer. *Semin Surg Oncol* 2000;19:42–48.

20. Roberts WS. Cytoreductive surgery in ovarian cancer: why, when, and how. *Cancer Control* 1996;3:130–136.

21. Eisenkop SM, Freidman RL, Spirtos NM. The role of secondary cytoreductive surgery in the treatment of patients with recurrent epithelial ovarian carcinoma. *Cancer* 2000;88: 144–153.

22. Ozols R. Chemotherapy of ovarian cancer. *Cancer Treat Res* 1998;95:219–234.

23. Federation Internationale de Gynecologie et d'Obstetrique. Annual report on the results of treatment in gynaecological cancer. *J Epidemiol Biostat* 1998;3:1–168.

SURGERY: SCIENTIFIC PRINCIPLES AND PRACTICE, Third Edition, edited by Lazar J. Greenfield, Michael W. Mulholland, Keith T. Oldham, Gerald B. Zelenock, and Keith D. Lillemoe. Lippincott Williams & Wilkins Publishers, Philadelphia, © 2001.

CHAPTER 104

THE PREGNANT PATIENT

N. SCOTT ADZICK AND ALEXANDER S. KRUPNICK

Four million pregnancies occur annually in the United States. Despite the continuous presence of this patient population, little emphasis has been placed on educating the general surgeon in the diagnosis and treatment of surgical problems in the pregnant patient. Although obstetricians routinely deal with pregnancy-related maternal disease and gynecologic surgery, few training programs expose the gynecologist to the wide array of surgical problems of the alimentary tract or the signs and symptoms of nongynecologic disease. The general surgeon is often called on in this situation, and it is imperative that he or she understand the normal physiologic changes occurring during pregnancy as well as the presentation of surgical disease. Often the surgeon is the first person to evaluate a pregnant patient with abdominal pain, or learns of the pregnancy during the initial work-up. Because the incidence of surgical disease does not disappear in pregnancy but simply changes its frequency and nature of presentation, the surgeon must be aware of these variations as well as conversant with the safety and utility of diagnostic tests and imaging modalities. Pathways and algorithms for diagnosis and treatment of diseases in the nonpregnant woman must be altered to ensure the safety and well-being of the fetus as well as that of the mother. The purpose of this chapter is to review the current data on the presentation, frequency, and treatment of some common surgical diseases during pregnancy, as well as their adverse effects on the pregnancy. Pregnancy is the only time when surgical decisions directly affect the lives of two people, and although mistakes can be twice as costly, rewards can double.

FETAL DEVELOPMENT

Human development begins immediately on fertilization of the oocyte by the sperm, but because it is impossible to determine the exact time of fertilization, the age of development is calculated from the first day of the last menstrual period. The *embryonic period* refers to these earliest stages of development and extends to the end of the eighth week, by which time organogenesis has occurred. Although the rudimentary precursors of all major organ systems are present at this point, only the circulatory system and the heart are functional. The fetal period lasts from the ninth week to birth. During this period, growth and development of tissues formed during embryogenesis occur in preparation for birth (1). The effect of teratogenic drugs or radiation can vary drastically depending on the period of exposure.

Survival outside the womb depends on the adaptation of fetal organ systems for independent function at the time of birth. Because oxygen exchange and respiration are critical to immediate survival, the functional status of the respiratory system is crucial in determining fetal viability. Surfactant, a complex mixture of phospholipids consisting mostly of phosphatidylcholine, is necessary for reduction of surface tension at the alveolar–air interface and proper oxygen exchange. Surfactant production begins by the 20th week of gestation, but is present in only small amounts before 24 weeks (1). Although the survival rate of infants born at 24 weeks of development is dismal, the mortality rate before that time is 100% (Fig. 104.1). The delivery of a fetus before this period of potential viability, whether spontaneous or induced, is termed an *abortion,* whereas delivery after this period is defined as a *premature birth.*

One of the most significant advances in the reduction of morbidity of prematurity has been the use of corticosteroids to accelerate organ maturation. Binding of corticosteroids in the fetal lung not only increases secretion of phosphatidylcholine but induces morphologic development of pulmonary epithelial cells and increases neonatal lung compliance. Corticosteroids stimulate development of other organ systems as well, decreasing the incidence of necrotizing enterocolitis in the premature intestine and intraventricular hemorrhage of the premature brain. The maximum developmental effects can be seen as early as 24

Probability of Mortality Based on Gestational Age at Birth

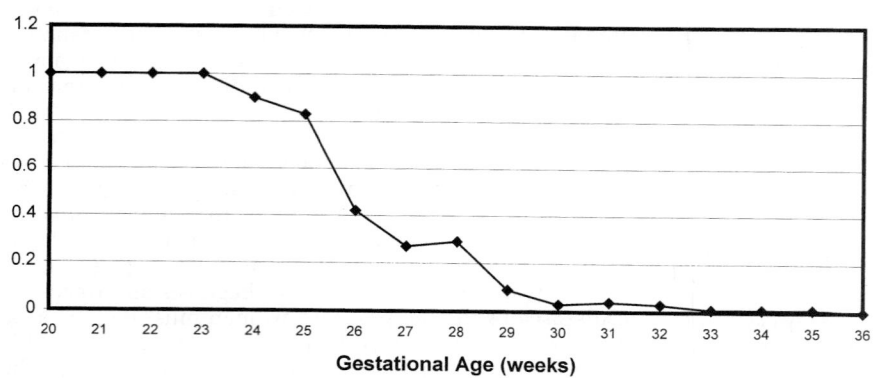

Figure 104.1. Multicenter analysis of preterm mortality based on gestational age. (Adapted from Copper RL, Goldenberg RL, Creasy RK, et al. A multicenter study of preterm birth weight and gestational age-specific neonatal mortality. *Am J Obstet Gynecol* 1993;168:78–84.)

hours after maternal administration of dexamethasone or betamethasone, and administration at the first sign of premature onset of labor can improve survival (2).

FETAL SURGERY

Historically, congenital anomalies resulted in either fetal demise or diagnosis and treatment after birth. The routine use of obstetric ultrasonography has allowed for early detection of fetal pathologic processes. The field of fetal surgery was born in the early 1980s in an attempt to correct fetal anomalies before irreversible end-organ damage or death in utero. The first open fetal operation was performed in 1982 for obstructive uropathy by creation of bilateral ureterostomies at 21 weeks of gestation (3). Since that time, the indications for fetal intervention have broad-

ened and include other conditions predisposing to fetal mortality (4,5).

Congenital cystic adenomatoid malformation is a benign proliferation of bronchial tissue replacing normal alveoli. Although most present as a pulmonary mass early in infancy or childhood, a few fetuses with extremely large lesions die in utero. Fetal pulmonary lobectomy has been used successfully as a lifesaving procedure to treat such lesions (6). Congenital diaphragmatic hernia is an anatomic malformation allowing migration of abdominal viscera into the thoracic cavity early in gestation. Impingement on pulmonary development leads to pulmonary hypoplasia often incompatible with life. Fetal tracheal occlusion has been shown to stimulate compensatory pulmonary growth with the potential for reducing the morbidity and mortality of this disease (7). A subset of

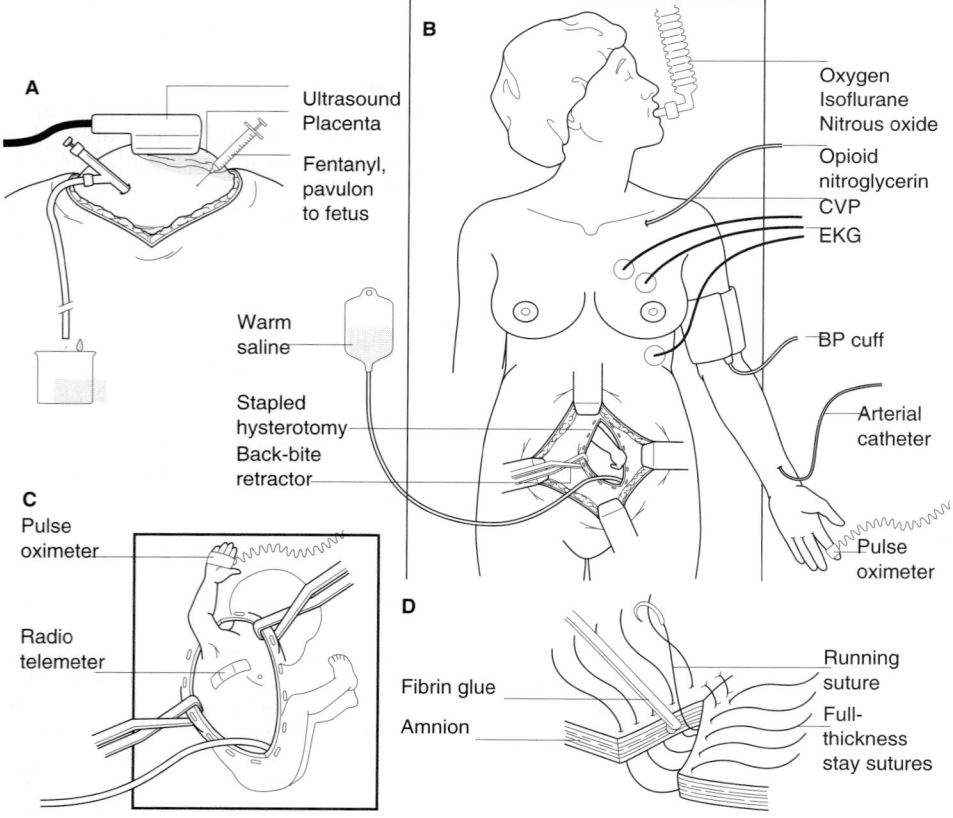

Figure 104.2. Fetal surgery techniques. *(A)* The uterus is exposed as the placenta is localized by ultrasonography and the fetus injected with narcotics and muscle relaxants. *(B)* The uterus is opened with staples that provide hemostasis and seal the membranes. Warm saline is continuously infused around the fetus. *(C)* The fetus is exposed for the operative procedure. *(D)* After the operation, the uterus is closed with absorbable sutures and fibrin glue. (Adapted from Harrison MR. Fetal surgery. *Am J Obstet Gynecol* 1996;174:1255–1264.)

fetuses with a sacrococcygeal teratoma diagnosed prenatally succumb to high-output heart failure before birth. Resection of the mass during gestation can be a lifesaving procedure (8). Expansion of fetal therapy to other non-life-threatening but highly morbid conditions such as myelomeningocele repair, resection of amniotic bands, and in utero stem cell therapy for immunodeficiency can reduce the lifelong burden of these diseases with potential cost savings to society (9).

The performance of surgery in utero has been made possible because of advances in anesthesiology, intraoperative maternal and fetal monitoring, and postoperative critical care (Fig. 104.2). Future directions in minimally invasive fetal surgery, percutaneous ablation of pulmonary masses, and the prevention of premature labor with better tocolysis offer widespread application of this developing field.

UTERINE ANATOMY AND PHYSIOLOGY OF LABOR

The uterus is a muscular organ responsible for reception, implantation, development, and expulsion of the fetus. In the nonpregnant woman, the uterus is an exclusively pelvic organ weighing approximately 70 g with a cavity volume of 10 mL. During pregnancy, the uterus gradually becomes an intraabdominal organ weighing close to 1,100 g and expanding to a total volume of 5 L.

By the 12th week of gestation, the uterus becomes too large to reside exclusively in the pelvis and extends into the abdominal cavity. By the 20th week, the uterine fundus reaches the umbilicus, and by the third trimester it reaches almost to the liver (10) (Fig. 104.3). As the uterus continues to rise, it exerts pressure on the anterior abdominal wall, displaces the intestines superiorly and laterally, and changes the relationship between the abdominal visceral organs. In the upright position, the uterus is supported by the anterior abdominal wall and usually undergoes a dextrorotation because of the presence of the rectosigmoid on the left. In the supine position, most of the uterine weight falls on the spinal column, but compression of the surrounding great vessels, especially the flaccid inferior vena cava, also occurs.

Uterine activity and contractions are coupled to the electrical changes in the myometrium, which is physiologically arranged to maximize the efficiency of uterine contraction and expulsion of the fetus at term. The resting membrane potential of the uterine myocyte ranges from −40 to −60 mV. It becomes more negative (-60 mV) early in gestation and increases to -40 mV near term. Early in pregnancy, the myometrium exhibits irregular electrical activity termed *slow waves*. These rhythmic alterations in the membrane potential occasionally reach the threshold potential and lead to an action potential at the top of the slow wave. Entry of Ca^{2+} through voltage-sensitive Ca^{2+} channels allows for actin–myosin interaction and electromechanical coupling, leading to uterine contraction. By the second trimester, these irregular contractions can be palpated through the abdominal wall and are known as *Braxton Hicks contractions* (11). Irregular contractions during pregnancy lead to relatively small increases in uterine pressure, but at term are replaced by coordinated, purposeful contractions generating pressures up to 80 mm Hg. Gap junctions allow for electrical and metabolic communication between uterine myocytes, and the onset of labor is preceded by an increase in the number of gap junctions.

The mechanisms behind human parturition are being unraveled. Numerous hormones, peptides, and local mediators act on the myometrium both to stimulate and down-regulate its activity (Table 104.1). Parturition begins when forces favoring uterine activity override those of quiescence and tip the balance toward contraction and birth. Progesterone maintains uterine relaxation during most of pregnancy by blocking Ca^{2+} flux through cell membranes and opposing the action of estrogen. Close to term, the concentration of estrogen increases relative to that of progesterone, leading to uterine activation. Synthesis and surface expression of contraction-associated proteins, including gap junctions, ion channels, and oxytocin receptors, is initiated and the uterus is transformed from its pliable, relaxed state to one of responsiveness and excitability. A shift in arachidonic acid metabolism from lipoxygenase products to those of cyclooxygenase, especially prostaglandin (PG) E_2 and $PGF_{2\alpha}$, favors activation of the uterine musculature as well as the onset of uterine contractions. Prostaglandins raise local Ca^{2+} concentrations by increasing Ca^{2+} flux across cell membrane and stimulating Ca^{2+} release from intracellular stores. Inflammatory cytokines, especially interleukin (IL)-1 and IL-6, are produced locally by placental tissues and act in concert with other stimulatory factors to propagate uterine activity (12,13).

Oxytocin is a nonapeptide synthesized in the hypothalamus and secreted from the posterior pituitary. Its name means "quick birth," and it was the first uterotonin to be implicated in parturition. Oxytocin stimulates Ca^{2+} flux across myometrial plasma membranes and has distinct receptors located in the myometrium and other reproductive tissues. Uterine responsiveness to oxytocin is directly re-

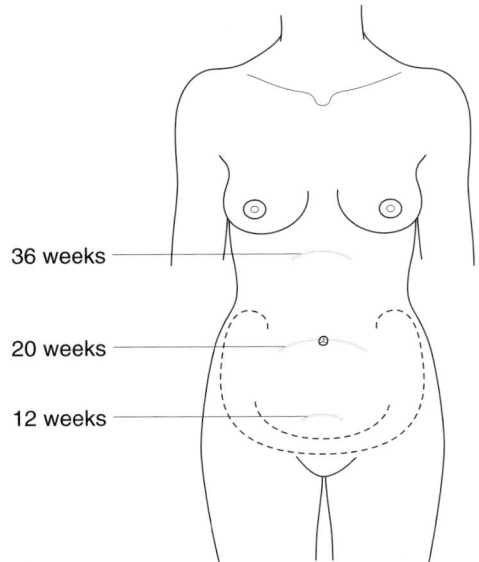

Figure 104.3. Enlarging uterus during gestation. At 12 weeks, the uterus rises out of the pelvis into the abdomen. At 20 weeks, the fundus is at the height of the umbilicus, and at 36 weeks the uterus reaches to the upper abdomen.

Table 104.1. MEDIATORS OF UTERINE ACTIVITY

Stimulates uterine activity	Down-regulates uterine activity
Estrogen	Progesterone
Oxytocin	
PGE_2, $PGF_{2\alpha}$	
IL-1, IL-6	

IL, interleukin; PG, prostaglandin.

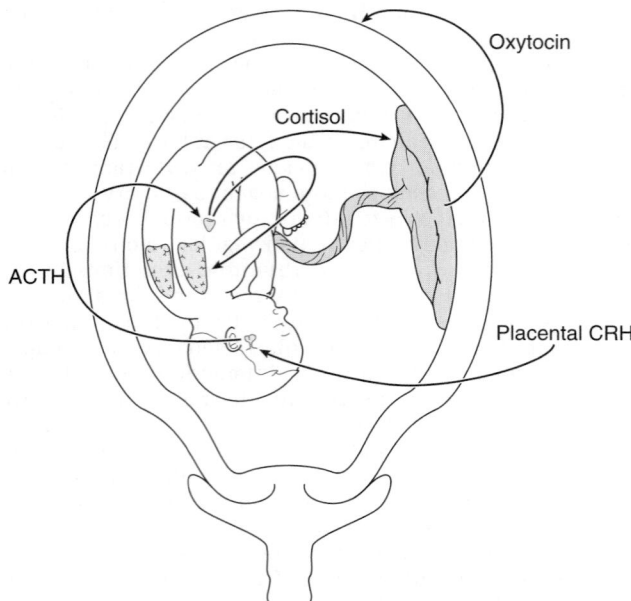

Figure 104.4. Positive feedback loops initiated by corticotropin-releasing hormone potentiate parturition.

lated to receptor concentration, which can increase 300-fold during pregnancy. The surface expression of oxytocin receptors is increased by maternal estrogen and opposed by progesterone. Although it was originally isolated from the posterior pituitary, the placental content of oxytocin is approximately five times that of the pituitary, and the placenta is most likely the main source of oxytocin during pregnancy and parturition (12).

The timing of birth is regulated by an internal placental clock based on corticotropin-releasing hormone (CRH). CRH is a 41-amino-acid peptide normally found in the hypothalamus. Its action on the pituitary causes secretion of adrenocorticotropic hormone, which in turn increases secretion of cortisol from adrenal tissue. In the nonpregnant woman, cortisol forms part of a negative feedback system acting on the hypothalamus and pituitary to dampen CRH secretion and down-regulate cortisol levels. In the preg-

nant woman, CRH seems to have a different function. During pregnancy, the concentration of CRH gradually rises. Although it is produced by both the fetal and maternal hypothalamus, most of the CRH orchestrating delivery originates from the placenta itself. Placental CRH is in a perfect position to coordinate timing of fetal lung maturity and uterine preparation for delivery. Once concentration reaches a critical level, CRH acts on the fetal hypothalamic-pituitary-adrenal (HPA) axis to increase fetal cortisol production. Increased levels of cortisol stimulate fetal lung maturation and surfactant production in preparation for oxygen exchange. Fetal cortisol also acts on placental tissue, increasing the expression of enzymes responsible for production of estrogen, shifting the balance of steroidogenesis away from progesterone production (13). Rather than acting in a negative feedback fashion, as would be expected in the hypothalamus, cortisol actually up-regulates placental CRH production as part of a positive feedback loop. CRH and cortisol also increase prostaglandin and oxytocin production by the placenta, and these substances in turn act locally to up-regulate CRH secretion further, forming another positive feedback loop (Fig. 104.4). CRH itself contributes to uterine contractions and can potentiate contractions by other substances such as oxytocin. The culmination of these actions leads to expected uterine activation and parturition.

Secretion of CRH is regulated by an internal clock, with production increasing steadily throughout pregnancy. Maternal levels of CRH detected as early as 16 to 20 weeks of pregnancy can be used to predict when the woman will give birth (Fig. 104.5). Mothers with the highest levels tend to deliver prematurely, whereas those with the lowest levels are more likely to deliver past term (14). Although proper coordination between the placenta and fetal HPA axis can lead to the timely birth of a fetus able to survive outside the womb, maternal illness or intraabdominal inflammation can disturb the system.

PREMATURE ONSET OF LABOR

Premature labor consists of premature uterine contractions producing cervical change. A premature birth is defined as one occurring before 37 weeks from the first day of the last menstrual period (15). Although only 10% of all births fit this criterion, prematurity is responsible for 83%

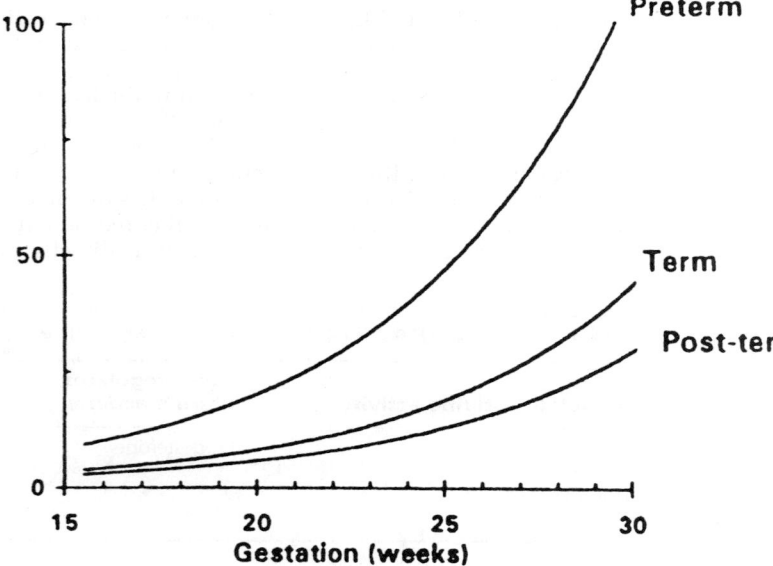

Figure 104.5. Corticotropin-releasing hormone concentration (pmol/L) varies during gestation based on timing of delivery. (Reprinted from McLean M, Bisits A, Davies J, et al. A placental clock controlling the length of human pregnancy. *Nat Med* 1995;1:460–463.)

of all neonatal mortality and most of the morbidity and cost of neonatal care (16). Survival has increased with improvement in neonatal intensive care units, but the premature infant still experiences a wide variety of ailments with long-term sequelae in many organ systems. The etiology of preterm labor is often multifactorial, but the onset of labor from fetal and uterine stress during surgical manipulation or intraabdominal inflammatory processes is of most concern to the surgeon.

Early activation of the fetal HPA axis can take place in response to fetal stress. An adverse uterine environment due to hypoxemia or maternal shock leads to increased expression of CRH in the fetal hypothalamus. Levels of cortisol rise and its activity on the local environment leads to uterine activation along with fetal lung maturation. Increased prostaglandin production in the presence of an infective process can also activate preterm labor. Bacterial infection of the amniotic tissues or peritoneum leads to a local increase in eicosanoids and the onset of labor (17). Endotoxin acts on inflammatory cells to increase production of IL-1 and IL-6, which also amplify local prostaglandin production. All these factors can act in concert to initiate and propagate preterm labor. Uterine activation and increased expression of gap junctions as well as oxytocin receptors can be induced by uterine stretch (13,18). Uterine trauma due to surgical manipulation could affect these same mechanisms, leading to premature uterine contractions. The interrelations at various levels between the inflammatory response, uterine and maternal trauma, and the initiation of labor can represent the body's attempt to expel the fetus from a hostile uterine environment.

Tocolysis

Tocolytic therapy attempts to reverse or alleviate the premature onset and progression of labor while the underlying inflammatory etiology is corrected. By understanding the basic physiology of both premature and term labor, pharmacologic manipulation of the system can be attempted to prevent the progression of premature uterine contractions to premature labor and premature delivery. Even if delivery cannot be avoided, simply extending gestation by 1 or 2 days can allow exogenous steroids to promote fetal lung development and surfactant secretion, decreasing the risk of respiratory distress syndrome and multiorgan failure in the preterm neonate. Prostaglandin synthesis inhibitors, magnesium sulfate, β-adrenergic agonists, and calcium channel blockers represent the four most common pharmacologic agents used as tocolytics.

Because of the importance of prostaglandins in the initiation of uterine contraction, prostaglandin synthetase inhibitors, especially nonsteroidal antiinflammatory drugs, are used to stop premature labor. Indomethacin is the nonsteroidal drug used most frequently for tocolysis because of its quick onset of action and ease of dosing. Studies report a 95% tocolytic success rate at 48 hours and a potential delay in delivery of 1 week in 80% of patients (19). Magnesium sulfate has long been used in the treatment of preeclampsia and has now gained acceptance as a tocolytic agent. It is often the first-line agent used once the onset of premature contractions is documented. Most data support the theory that magnesium exerts its effects by calcium antagonism. High intracellular magnesium concentrations inhibit Ca^{2+} entry into myometrial cells, interfering with actin–myosin coupling. High magnesium concentrations also increase the sensitivity of K^+ channels, favoring hyperpolarization and uterine relaxation. Maternal serum levels necessary to inhibit myometrial contractility range between 4 and 9 mg/dL, two to six times normal levels, and are difficult to achieve with oral ad-

ministration alone. Success with magnesium tocolysis for 24 hours is possible in 96% of patients, 48 hours in 70% of patients, and up to 1 week in 49% of patients (20). β₂-Adrenergic agonists used in the treatment of preterm labor include ritodrine and terbutaline. Stimulation of uterine β₂ receptors leads to activation of adenylate cyclase and an increase in intracellular cyclic adenosine monophosphate (cAMP) concentration. Activation of cAMP-dependent protein kinase A inhibits myosin light-chain phosphorylation and actin–myosin coupling. Protein kinase A activity is also associated with increased Ca^{2+} efflux, decreased Ca^{2+} influx, and increased K^+ conductance. All these actions lead to myometrial relaxation (11). Calcium channel blockers inhibit entry of calcium through voltage-dependent Ca^{2+} channels. The use of oral nifedipine can abolish uterine activity and prevent delivery with minimal toxicity and side effects (21).

Although the success of tocolysis in preventing or delaying premature birth varies based on etiology, no foolproof combination of drugs has been globally successful in all cases of premature labor. Maternal and fetal side effects can be serious and close observation is necessary with all forms of tocolysis. Premature constriction of the fetal ductus arteriosus with the use of indomethacin has been reported and can result in fatal neonatal pulmonary hypertension (22). Maternal cardiovascular side effects, including pulmonary edema, can occur in 5% of β₂ agonist users and 10% of those treated with magnesium. Although this complication is rare, it can result in maternal death. Serum concentrations of magnesium needed for tocolysis (4 to 9 mg/dL) are not far from levels causing ablation of deep tendon reflexes (9 to 13 mg/dL) or respiratory depression (14 mg/dL). The decision to use tocolytics must be made only after the diagnosis of premature onset of labor is confirmed and the benefits of prolonging gestation outweigh the risks of tocolysis. Initiation of tocolytic therapy for potential but unconfirmed preterm labor is discouraged (15).

Children's Hospital of Philadelphia Tocolysis Protocol

Preterm labor has been called the Achilles' heel of fetal surgery (4). Because breaching the uterus, whether by open hysterotomy or puncture, always incites uterine contractions, prevention of premature labor after fetal surgery is of the utmost importance if the gestation is to continue. Tocolysis after fetal surgery at The Center for Fetal Diagnosis and Treatment at The Children's Hospital of Philadelphia consists of indomethacin 50 mg rectally every 6 hours and a magnesium sulfate drip at 2 g/h. After stabilization of immediate postoperative uterine irritability, the mother is weaned to an outpatient terbutaline pump or oral nifedipine for the duration of gestation.

FETAL MONITORING

Perioperative fetal monitoring as well as the monitoring of premature uterine contractions is based on technology developed for fetal monitoring during birth. As early as 1862, it was suspected that fetal distress during birth and prolonged, difficult labor led to infantile spastic palsies. Experimental data in primate fetuses have shown that prolonged hypoxemia and acidemia produces anatomic lesions in the brain similar to those seen in human cerebral palsy (23). Sublethal asphyxia of the fetus can also lead to multisystem dysfunction, including conduction defects of the heart, ischemic mucosal injury to the gastrointestinal tract, necrotizing enterocolitis, and impaired surfactant production and respiratory distress of the newborn. Interventions to reduce the incidence of fetal hypoxemia and acidemia reduce the incidence of these and other disorders (24).

Evaluation of fetal oxygenation and acid–base status is possible by direct sampling of arterial pH from the umbilical artery or capillary blood sampling of the fetal scalp. Both techniques demand access to the fetus through a dilated, open cervix with crowning of the scalp, through a hysterotomy during fetal surgery, or through the maternal abdomen during percutaneous umbilical blood sampling. Because such exposure is not available during most surgical procedures, monitoring of fetal oxygenation is based on other indirect methods. In the late 1950s and early 1960s, the relationship between fetal heart rate patterns and fetal stability was demonstrated (25). Established heart rate patterns and variable cardiac responses to fetal and maternal stimuli reflect an intact, well oxygenated central nervous system (CNS). Deviation from these patterns can indicate fetal distress or impending compromise.

Electronic fetal heart rate monitoring has gained wide acceptance and as of the early 1990s was used in 79% of all pregnancies (24). Direct fetal monitoring is used intrapartum and relies on analysis of fetal cardiac patterns from electrocardiogram leads placed directly on the exposed part of the fetus. A transcervical intrauterine pressure catheter is concurrently placed to monitor the strength of uterine contractions. Indirect monitoring methods are used when access to the uterine cavity and fetus is not available, and fetal heart rate analysis is performed with Doppler ultrasound applied to the maternal abdomen or transvaginally while a surface tocodynamometer detects uterine contractions (Fig. 104.6). Both tracings are printed on a continuous strip of paper, with the fetal heart rate plotted at the top of the graph and uterine activity at the bottom.

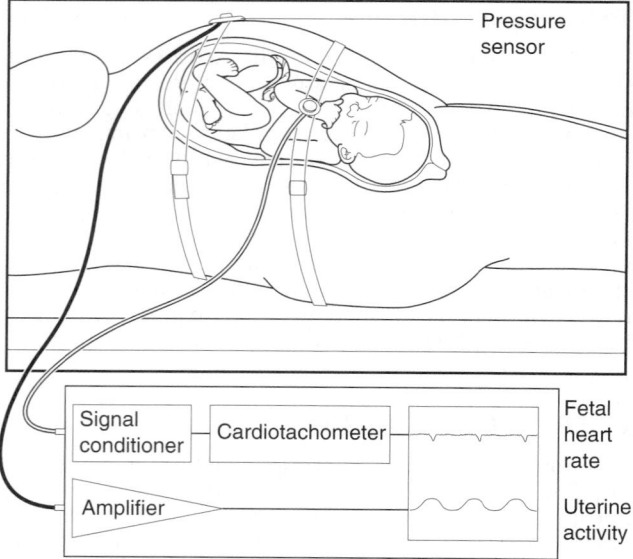

Figure 104.6. Intraoperative and postoperative fetal monitoring using noninvasive surface Doppler and pressure sensor to monitor uterine contractions. (Reproduced from Miller DA, Paul R. Antepartum–intrapartum monitoring. In: Scott JR, DiSaia PJ, Hammond CB, et al., eds. *Danforth's obstetrics and gynecology,* 8th ed. Philadelphia: Lippincott Williams & Wilkins, 1999:243–255.)

Fetal Heart Rate

Normal fetal heart rate during pregnancy ranges between 120 and 160 beats/min. A prolonged baseline above 160 beats/min is considered a tachycardia, whereas that below 120 beats/min is a bradycardia. These terms refer to long-term patterns, and minute-to-minute variability in the heart rate away from baseline is known as *acceleration* and *deceleration*. Changes in blood pressure and oxygenation are detected by the chemoreceptors and baroreceptors of the aortic arch and carotid bodies, resulting in a change in the heart rate to maintain a steady state. Normal, healthy fetal heart rate tracings express continuous adjustment in the vagal tone through variability in the heart rate. Short-term, or beat-to-beat, variability is superimposed on broader, long-term variability of the baseline by 3 to 5 beats/min. The fetal heart rate response governed by a nonacidotic, well functioning vagal conduction system manifests both long-term and short-term variability with fluctuations of peaks and troughs ranging from 6 to 25 beats/min (Fig. 104.7). Decreased heart rate variability, either long or short term, can signal diminished CNS activity. Although this can be a physiologic response of the fetal sleep–wake cycle or maternal medication and sedatives, persistently decreased reactivity can signal CNS acidosis. This is particularly true if combined with other findings suggestive of hypoxia. Fetal heart rate accelerations are normal findings in the second half of pregnancy and occur as a result of increased sympathetic stimulation and decreased parasympathetic stimulation with fetal movements. Vibroacoustic stimulation of the fetus for 5 seconds at 2,000 Hz through the mother's abdomen can provoke fetal movement with resultant heart rate acceleration (26). Failure of this response suggests fetal hypoxia. A sinusoidal heart rate pattern is an uncommon baseline abnormality also suggestive of fetal distress. It has the characteristics of a smooth sine wave with little beat-to-beat variability, long-term variability with a frequency of 2 to 5 cycles/min, and amplitude of 5 to 15 beats/min. This pattern has been associated with anencephaly, fetal anemia, and hypoxia (Fig. 104.8).

Fetal heart rate decelerations are usually encountered during uterine contractions of the intrapartum period. Evaluation of decelerations during birth and as part of postoperative fetal monitoring can give clues to the status of the placental blood supply. Early decelerations are uniform, shallow drops in the fetal heart rate that mirror uterine contractions and reflect increased vagal tone from a transient increase in intracranial pressure. This pattern is considered a benign physiologic manifestation of a functioning autonomic nervous system, and has no adverse outcome. Variable decelerations result from umbilical cord compression by uterine contractions. Isolated variable decelerations have little clinical significance, but if persistent with inadequate recovery between contractions, fetal hypoxemia and acidosis can occur. Variable decelerations can also indicate pathologic cord compression from either a prolapsed or nuchal cord. Late decelerations signify a significant deficit in fetal oxygen supply; causes can range from maternal hypotension due to inferior vena cava compression to hypoxia or anemia. Persistent late decelerations warrant quick investigation to correct the cause or emergently deliver the child by cesarean section (24).

Fetal heart rate patterns offer noninvasive clues to uterine oxygenation and fetal blood supply. Utility of both fetal heart rate and uterine contraction monitoring lies in the ability to intervene based on the acquired information. Progression of premature labor despite maximum tocolysis may necessitate adding a second tocolytic agent or starting corticosteroids to assist fetal lung maturation be-

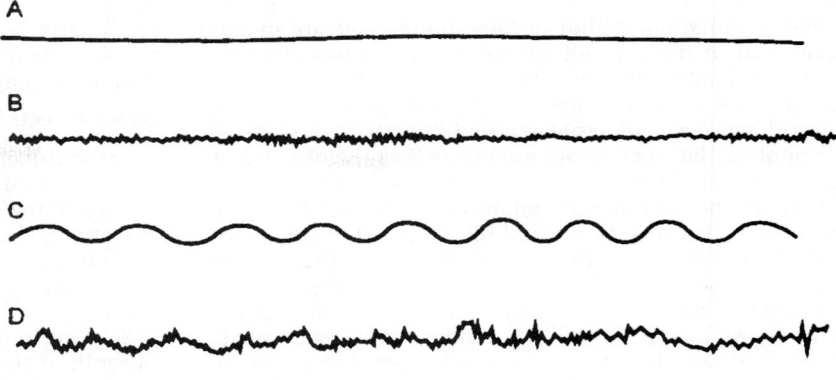

Figure 104.7. Fetal heart variability. *(A)* Short-term and long-term variability both absent: abnormal. *(B)* Short-term variability present, long-term variability absent: abnormal. *(C)* Long-term variability present, short-term variability absent: abnormal. *(D)* Both short- and long-term variability present: normal. (Reproduced from Miller DA, Paul R. Antepartum–intrapartum monitoring. In: Scott JR, DiSaia PJ, Hammond CB, et al., eds. *Danforth's obstetrics and gynecology,* 8th ed. Philadelphia: Lippincott Williams & Wilkins, 1999:243–255.)

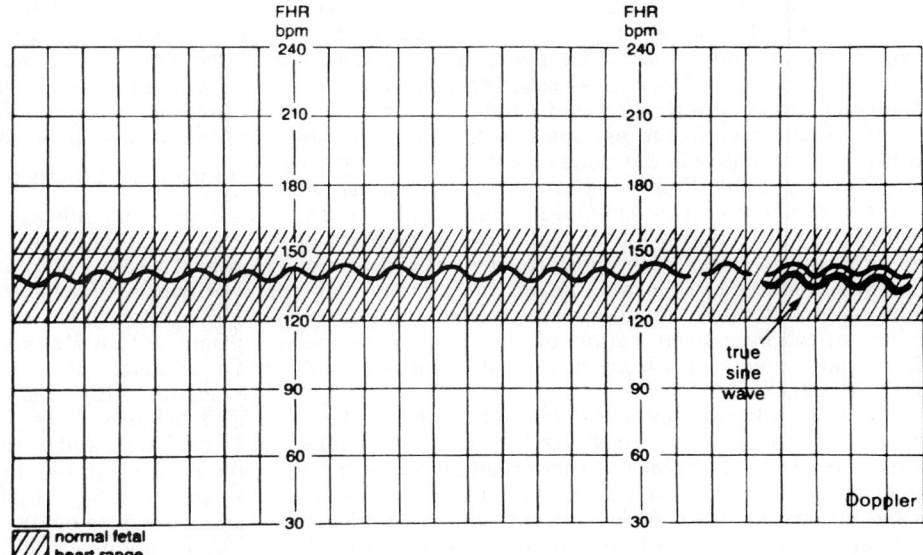

Figure 104.8. A sinusoidal pattern is one of several heart rate patterns indicating potential fetal hypoxia. (Reproduced from Cabaniss ML. *Fetal monitoring interpretation.* Philadelphia: JB Lippincott, 1993:121.)

fore the premature birth. Intraoperative fetal distress as indicated by an ominous heart rate tracing must be treated by correcting maternal hypotension or increasing oxygen delivery with increased FIO_2, blood transfusion, or more aggressive fluid resuscitation. The inability to improve the intrauterine milieu can necessitate an emergent cesarean section to prevent fetal demise. Continuous fetal monitoring is unnecessary if the ability to intervene is limited. Because the chances of survival before 24 weeks of gestation are close to zero, emergent delivery at this stage is not warranted. The inability to improve uterine perfusion due to maternal extremis could make fetal monitoring futile, simply adding an extra variable to the care of an already complicated patient. By understanding the principles and indications for intraoperative and postoperative fetal monitoring, the surgeon can provide an improved level of care for both mother and unborn child.

IMAGING MODALITIES IN THE PREGNANT PATIENT

Advances in radiology have revolutionized surgical practice. By visualizing the lesion before exploration, surgical intervention can focus on the area of disease or be avoided altogether. The choice of imaging modalities in the pregnant patient is difficult because of the real and perceived danger to the developing fetus. Risks of ionizing radiation can force the physician to avoid the definitive

diagnostic study of choice and inadvertently put both the mother and fetus in greater danger from misdiagnosis. Although experimental data regarding the effects of ionizing radiation on the developing human fetus are impossible to obtain, animal exposure and follow-up of those inadvertently exposed to radiation have provided some information. Retrospective studies of atomic bomb survivors in Hiroshima and Nagasaki have also allowed for evaluation of the effects of massive radiation exposure in utero.

Ionizing Radiation

X-rays used in diagnostic radiology consist of machine-generated photons that have tens of thousands times the energy of visible light. Because of this energy, a portion of the x-rays entering a patient pass through tissue without interacting with any matter. Those photons are the ones that collide with the radiographic plate or processor to create the image. Most photons, however, interact with the patient's atoms, giving up either all or part of their energy to those atoms. When the photon transfers all of its energy, it is absorbed by the tissue and no longer exists. When it gives up only a part of its energy, it is deflected from its path and creates scatter x-rays. As electrons in exposed tissues break away from their orbits owing to the imparted energy, they leave excited or ionized molecules. These electrons go on to interact with other electrons until all the energy transferred by the photon is dissipated. The resultant state consists of numerous ionizations in the area exposed to radiation. Although most ionizations are inconsequential to the cell, alterations of vital molecules can lead to premature cell death and permanent alteration in the genome with later neoplastic development. Most of these effects occur in tissue exposed directly to the path of the photons, but scatter radiation can affect the uterus and fetus even if the area imaged is far from the abdomen.

Fetal effects of ionizing radiation depend on the dose absorbed by the fetal tissue and the stage of fetal development during exposure. Exposure is defined as the amount of ionic charge created by the radiation on passing through a defined mass of air. The roentgen is a common unit of exposure, producing 0.26 millicoulombs per kilogram of air or 2 billion ion pairs per cubic centimeter of exposed air (27). Although exposure is useful for measuring radiation output, the absorbed dose is the radiation imparted to tissue that creates a biologic effect. One gray (Gy) is strictly defined as the deposition of 1.0 joule of energy per kilogram of tissue, and 1 rad, another measure of absorbed dose, is 1% of 1 Gy. As a gross estimate, exposure to 1 roentgen gives an absorbed dose of 1 rad or 10 mGy.

It is a misconception to assume that the radiation absorbed by the mother is the same as that absorbed by the fetus. Dosing of radiation to the uterus and conceptus can vary severalfold based on abdominal wall depth, the anteverted or retroverted position of the uterus, or whether the exposure is in the anteroposterior or posteroanterior direction. Radiographic evaluation of the abdomen and pelvis is most likely to expose the fetus to direct ionizing radiation, whereas examination of the extremities and chest leads to exposure from scatter radiation only (27) (Table 104.2).

Radiation-induced ionization of vital cellular structures can result in cellular death or lasting genetic mutations in the DNA. Cellular destruction either leads to the death of the embryo if a significant amount of tissue is affected, or has no effect if the damaged cells are replaced by healthy ones. Growth impairment of organs occurs if the population of cells cannot be replaced or damage occurs to a small population of progenitor cells at a vital stage of development. All these effects are produced at threshold doses, and exposure to radiation levels below the threshold does not have biologic consequences compared with control populations (28). The outcome of radiation exposure depends on the absorbed dose and the stage of development during exposure, with potential death early in gestation, teratogenesis during organogenesis, and growth retardation or leukemic potential at later gestational stages.

Lethal Effects of Ionizing Radiation

The multicellular embryo, before the blastocyst stage, is most sensitive to the lethal effects of radiation but resistant to teratogenesis and growth retardation if it survives. The etiology of this phenomenon is uncertain but could relate to the totipotent nature of the embryo at this stage and its ability indiscriminately to replace a specific volume of tissue below the lethal threshold. Because 50% to 75% of all human pregnancies abort, mostly without any recognition that fertilization has even occurred (29), determining the lethal dose of radiation at this stage is difficult. Exposure of rat embryos to ionizing radiation at various stages of gestation reveals a maximum 10% mortality rate at 30 rads and 65% mortality rate at 150 rads. The lethal effects of 30 rads are seen only before implantation, returning to baseline levels after 1 week (Fig. 104.9). Both of these doses are orders of magnitude higher than those used for most diagnostic studies.

Teratogenic Effects of Ionizing Radiation

Teratogenic effects of radiation can be seen during early organogenesis in animal studies. Exposure of rats to 100 rads at various points of development reveals a very narrow window for teratogenesis (Fig. 104.10). This window corresponds to weeks 2 to 4 in human development, consistent with early organ formation. Despite these experimental data, it is difficult to link any specific human malformation with radiation exposure other than those of the CNS. Microcephaly, pigmentary changes in the retina, hydrocephalus, and optic nerve atrophy have been reported at a significantly higher rate after exposure to radiation in pregnancy (30). All patients were exposed to a minimum estimated dose of 100 rads, and no visceral, limb, or other malformations were found unless the child also exhibited CNS abnormalities. One explanation for this discrepancy is that the developmental period of the CNS is much longer, continuing throughout gestation and into the neonatal period, whereas other organs have a very narrow period during which morphologic alterations can be produced. Exposure to high doses of radiation during this narrow window is rare, and even if an isolated congenital abnormality were to occur, it would be difficult to separate this event from the background malformation rate. The extended period for CNS sensitivity to teratogenesis increases the prevalence of CNS malformation. CNS malformation also occurs at threshold doses, however, and low levels of exposure to 10 to 20 rads of radiation do not increase the incidence of microcephaly in experimental animals over baseline (28).

Growth Retardation from Ionizing Radiation

Growth retardation results from radiation-induced cellular depletion. Although catch-up growth can occur if exposure happens early in gestation, permanent cell depletion and growth retardation occur with exposure during later fetal stages (31). Wood and colleagues studied growth retardation of children exposed in utero to the Japanese atomic blasts. Those within 1,500 m from the center of the explosion were exposed to over 25 rads and, when followed through age 17 years, were 2 to 3 cm shorter and 3 kg lighter, and had a head circumference 1 cm smaller than normal. Those beyond 1,500 m from the blast received less than 25 rads and had a normal head circumference, height, and weight (27,32,33). Further animal and human data support the contention that exposures of less

---

Table 104.2. RADIATION DOSING TO THE CONCEPTUS AND UTERUS FROM SELECTED RADIOGRAPHIC EXAMINATIONS

Routine chest radiograph	8–50 mrad
Routine mammography	<50 mrad
Computed tomography, chest (uterus shielded and not exposed)	25–1,000 mrad
Computed tomography, upper abdomen (uterus shielded and not exposed)	670–3,000 mrad
Computed tomography, abdomen	2,000–3,000 mrad
Abdomen (flat plate)	250–300 mrad
Endoscopic retrograde cholangiopancreatography with no permanent films and shielding of abdomen	4 mrad

Data from Wagner LK, Lester RG, Saldana LR. *Exposure of the pregnant patient to diagnostic radiation.* Madison, WI: Medical Physics Publishing, 1997; Wyte CD. Diagnostic modalities in the pregnant patient. *Emerg Med Clin North Am* 1994;12:9–43; and Baillie J, Cairns SR, Cotton PB. Endoscopic management of choledocholithiasis during pregnancy. *Surgery* 1990;171:1–4.

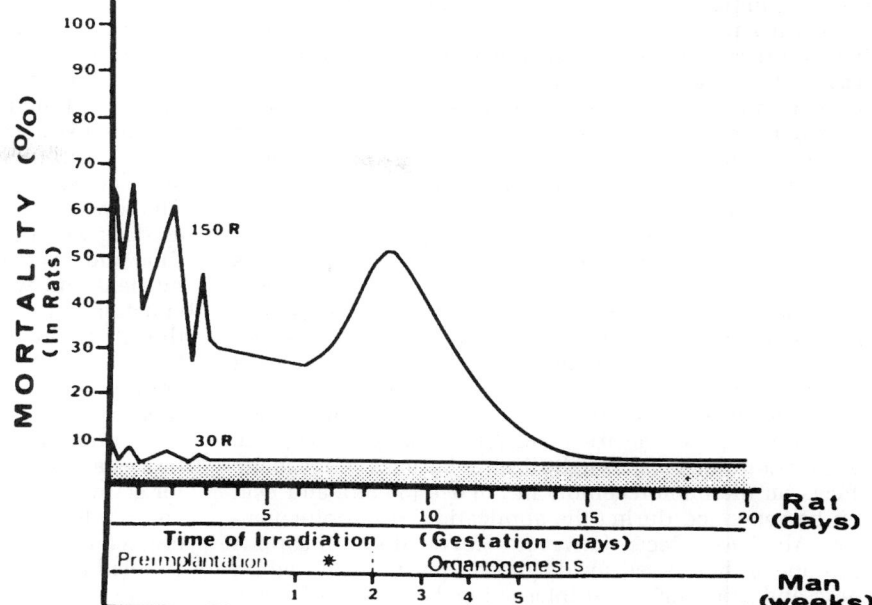

Figure 104.9. Mortality in rats exposed to 150 and 30 rads during various points in gestation. The embryo is most sensitive early in gestation. Human embryonic timetable is provided for comparison purposes only. (Reproduced from Brent RL. The effects of embryonic and fetal exposure to x-ray, microwaves, and ultrasound. *Clin Obstet Gynecol* 1983;26:488.)

than 5 rads should not cause either anatomic malformation or growth retardation (28).

Oncogenic Potential of Ionizing Radiation

The correlation between childhood cancer and in utero exposure to radiation has been demonstrated. Steward in 1970 demonstrated an increased incidence of cancer with exposures of approximately 2 rads (27). Although conclusions regarding the cause-and-effect relationship of this correlation cannot be definitively established, further studies using twins (34) and extensive data analysis (35) have strengthened the argument that in utero radiation can increase the rate of childhood cancer even at doses of 1 rad. The current increase in childhood cancer is estimated

at 1 to 2 cases per 3,000 children exposed to 1 rad in utero (27). Although these risks are very small, the patient must be counseled regarding this potential danger. By reviewing the current data, it is obvious that exposure to diagnostic levels of radiation carries little chance for spontaneous abortion, teratogenesis, or growth retardation. The increased risk of future cancer, however, does exist and must be weighed against the utility of the information provided by the study.

Ultrasound

Ultrasonography uses high-frequency, nonionizing, acoustic radiation to create images. A surface transducer sets up vibratory motions that are transmitted through matter as acoustic waves. The boundaries between different densities of tissue reflect some of these sound waves back to be detected by a transducer. Ultrasonic images therefore detect acoustic boundaries between different biologic materials in the body. Audible sound ranges from 20 to 20,000 vibrations per second, whereas ultrasonography uses frequencies of 1 to 10 million vibrations per second. Since its initial use in the 1950s, diagnostic ultrasonography has not produced fetal damage or harmful effects (27,36); however, theoretic dangers do exist. Rapid compression and decompression of tissue by sound waves could cause tissue damage. Conversion of mechanical energy to thermal energy, especially at the bone/soft-tissue interface, could lead to local hyperthermia, whereas the phenomenon known as *cavitation* could cause microscopic bubbles already present in tissues to grow in size because of absorption of surrounding diffused gases. Despite all these theoretic concerns, no consistent evidence exists that properly used diagnostic ultrasound is detrimental to the conceptus (31,37).

Magnetic Resonance Imaging

Like ultrasonography, magnetic resonance imaging (MRI) uses no ionizing radiation, instead relying on the magnetic properties of tissues to create images. Four magnetic fields interact during an MRI examination to create the image. The intrinsic magnetic field of an atomic nucleus, usually that of a hydrogen proton, is combined with

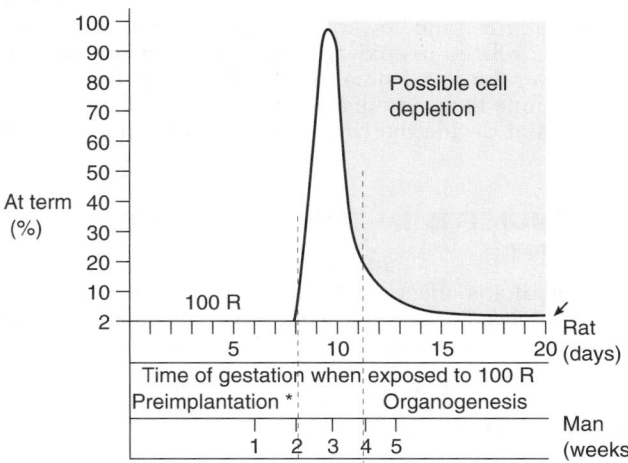

Figure 104.10. Relative incidence of gross congenital malformation in the rat when exposed to 100 rads during gestation. A very large increase in congenital malformations occurs during the early organogenetic period, corresponding to the third and fourth weeks of human gestation. Although gross malformations return to the background rate outside of this time frame, an irreversible loss of cells can occur. (Reproduced from Brent RL. The effects of embryonic and fetal exposure to x-ray, microwaves, and ultrasound. *Clin Obstet Gynecol* 1983;26:488.)

a strong, uniformly applied external magnetic field and a weaker magnetic field gradient. On top of this, a magnetic field is intermittently generated by pulsed radiofrequency waves (27). When this external radiofrequency is applied to nuclei in an existing magnetic field, the nuclei absorb some of the energy and change their orientation. When the radiofrequency ceases, the nuclei return to their previous orientation and emit the radiofrequency they absorbed. These signals are detected, stored, and processed by a computer to create an image.

Based on current data, it is unlikely that magnetic fields of the intensity used for diagnostic MRI pose any danger to the developing fetus, but biologic mechanisms do exist that could, at least theoretically, lead to damage. Charged particles and molecules moving in a strong magnetic field create an electrostatic potential difference, and normal red blood cells can alter their shape and create a charge when moving within an electric field (38). Changing magnetic fields can induce visual light flashes because of magnetic effects on the photoreceptors in the eye (38,39), and heat can be generated during the application of radiofrequencies. All these effects, however, occur with applications well above those used for diagnostic purposes. Based on these and other data, the International Radiation Protection Association has concluded that despite the lack of evidence that mammalian embryos are sensitive to the magnetic fields encountered during MRI examination, elective examination of pregnant women by MRI should be postponed until after the first trimester and completion of organogenesis. Ultrasonography should be the diagnostic modality of choice during pregnancy, with MRI limited to cases in which unique diagnostic information is required (40). MRI, however, is not absolutely contraindicated even in the first trimester when ultrasound will not suffice.

PHYSIOLOGIC CHANGES OF PREGNANCY THAT MIMIC DISEASE

Pregnancy physiology reflects the changes necessary for fetal gestation. It is characterized by the enlarging, gravid uterus and a changing hormonal milieu. These conditions predispose to certain diseases and change maternal physiology to mask the diagnosis of others.

The cardiovascular system is affected by pregnancy. The cardiac output increases by 30% to 50%, as does the total blood volume. The corresponding red blood cell volume increases only by 20% to 30%, leading to a decrease in the hematocrit. Although the maternal oxygen-carrying capacity is increased and the rheologic properties of blood are optimized for maximum nutrient delivery to the fetus, a physiologic anemia develops that can be confused with a pathologic state (41). Diagnosis of anemia due to chronic blood loss, as occurs with cancers of the gastrointestinal tract, may be delayed as the gradually decreasing hematocrit is attributed to pregnancy. Other laboratory evaluations also can mask various disease states (Table 104.3).

Serum alkaline phosphatase levels gradually increase because of production of an alkaline phosphatase isozyme by the placenta. This does not reflect biliary or bone disease. Albumin levels, commonly used to measure hepatic synthetic function, decrease, and a relative leukocytosis mimics a systemic infection.

The gastrointestinal tract undergoes a state of relaxation and decreased smooth muscle activity during pregnancy. The lower esophageal sphincter tone gradually decreases, as does gastric emptying. Prolonged small bowel transit time and decreased colonic emptying work to maximize nutrient and water absorption but also contribute to the constipation reported by 38% of pregnant women (42). Although multifactorial, the actions of progesterone have been linked to inhibition of gut smooth muscle activity both in vitro and in vivo. Because this dose-dependent inhibition can be blocked by increasing the extracellular concentration of Ca^{2+}, at least in vitro, it is proposed than progesterone works by limiting the effective Ca^{2+} available for actin–myosin coupling (43,44). This same mechanism contributes to uterine relaxation early in pregnancy, decreased intestinal motility, and the concurrent decrease in gallbladder tone and rate of emptying. The gallbladder empties more slowly during pregnancy and undergoes a gradual increase in residual volume, both during fasting and after meals. With these changes, combined with supersaturation of bile by cholesterol, pregnancy becomes a lithogenic state (45). These effects of pregnancy are transient and gallbladder motility and volumes return to normal as early as 2 weeks after pregnancy, but the gallstones, if formed, may persist.

Nausea and vomiting of pregnancy is a common occurrence affecting between 50% and 90% of all women (46,47). Its correlation with pregnancy was documented as early as 2000 B.C.E., and although a clear etiology has not been established, it rarely extends beyond the first trimester. Other causes must be investigated if the nausea and vomiting occur later in pregnancy. Abdominal pain, although often due to a surgical pathologic process, can have many causes. Round ligament pain is described as an aching, dragging pain more often felt on the right side. It is a common occurrence until 31 weeks of gestation. Pain in the hypochondrium can result from uterine pressure on the lower ribs, and lower abdominal pain may be psychogenic, related to anxiety about the pregnancy or insecurity over the social situation (48). It is up to the surgeon to determine the cause of abdominal pain in the pregnant patient and decide the course of diagnosis and intervention.

APPENDICITIS IN THE PREGNANT PATIENT

Appendicitis affects 250,000 patients every year in the United States. Because it is a disease of the young, its peak incidence corresponds to the childbearing years. Appen-

---

Table 104.3. **CHANGE DURING PREGNANCY IN LABORATORY VALUES**

Parameter	Change	Normal nonpregnant value	Late pregnancy value
Albumin (g/dL)	↓	3.2–3.8	2.4–3.1
Alkaline phosphatase (IU/L)	↑	30–115	100–210
Total bilirubin (mg/dL)	↔	0.26–1.00	Unchanged
Aspartate aminotransferase (IU/L)	↔	0–31	Unchanged
Hemoglobin (g/dL)	↓	12.0–16.0	10.5–14
Leukocyte count (×10³/mm³)	↑	4.5–11.0	6.0–16.0

Reproduced from Martin C, Varner MW. Physiologic changes in pregnancy surgical implications. Clin Obstet Gynecol 1994;37:241–255, with permission.

dicitis is the most common nonobstetric indication for surgery during pregnancy, with an average incidence of 1 in 1,500 deliveries. Although some smaller studies have suggested this condition is more common later in gestation (49–51), larger series show an equal distribution throughout pregnancy (52). The incidence is similar to that in nonpregnant women, but the anatomic and physiologic changes of the gravid state make the diagnosis difficult.

Classic appendicitis in the nonpregnant patient presents with a constellation of signs and symptoms suggesting the disorder. Luminal obstruction of the appendiceal orifice, whether by fecalith or lymphoid hyperplasia, leads to an increase in intraluminal pressure by blocking the normal egress of mucus. Progressive obstruction of venous outflow followed by capillary and arterial thrombosis leads to mucosal ulceration, transmural wall necrosis, and, if unabated, perforation. Because early appendiceal distention is relayed by stretch receptors to the 10th thoracic ganglion, referred pain is perceived in the distribution corresponding to the epigastric region. Once the ongoing inflammation extends to involve the parietal peritoneum, the pain localizes to the right lower quadrant. Anorexia, nausea, and vomiting, initiated by visceral mechanisms similar to those responsible for the referred pain, follow the onset of pain. Findings on physical examination arise from this pathophysiologic process. Voluntary guarding of the right lower quadrant reflects the patient's anticipation of pain with palpation in the area. Rigidity or involuntary guarding indicates reflex spasm of the abdominal musculature due to the nearby inflammatory process, whereas psoas and obturator signs indicate respective irritation of these muscles. Tenderness on rectal examination can be elicited with a low-lying appendix, whereas fever and leukocytosis indicate systemic inflammation. Although none of these signs or symptoms is 100% diagnostic, the presence of right lower quadrant pain, rigidity, and migration of pain was found to have the highest likelihood ratio for the presence of appendicitis in a large multifactorial analysis (53). All of the aforementioned signs and symptoms are altered by pregnancy (Table 104.4).

In a classic 1932 study, Baer and colleagues (54) evaluated the migration of the appendix through the duration of pregnancy with barium enemas. Beginning in the third month of pregnancy, the appendix and cecum are gradually displaced by the uterus and start a caudal migration out of the pelvis into the upper abdomen. By the third trimester, the appendiceal tip can abut the gallbladder (Fig. 104.11).

Table 104.4. **VARIATION IN SIGNS AND SYMPTOMS OF APPENDICITIS DURING PREGNANCY**

Signs and symptoms	First trimester	Second trimester	Third trimester
Right lower quadrant pain	100%	50%	14%
Right upper quadrant pain	0%	17%	57%
Guarding (muscle spasm)	80%	50%	43%
Nausea and vomiting	53%	60%	23%
Tenderness on rectal examination	60%	17%	0%
Perforation rate	20%	49%	70%

Data from Weingold AB. Appendicitis in pregnancy. Clin Obstet Gynecol 1983;26:801–809; Tamir IL, Bongard FS, Klein SR. Acute appendicitis in the pregnant patient. Am J Surg 1990;160:571–576; and Cunningham FG, McCubbin JH. Appendicitis complicating pregnancy. Obstet Gynecol 1975;45:415–420.

The vague, referred epigastric pain due to early appendiceal obstruction is not changed by this anatomic consideration, but the location of the somatic pain is. In a large study of pregnant women with proven appendicitis, abdominal pain was present in all patients. Location of pain in the right lower quadrant, however, was common only early in gestation, and a portion of patients reported pain in the right upper quadrant. This change in symptomatology is easily understood if the anatomic changes of the appendix are taken into consideration (52). Both guarding and rigidity are valuable findings on physical examination but are common only in the first trimester. Elevation of the abdominal wall from the more laterally placed, upward-directed appendix and the laxity of the abdominal wall musculature caused by this distention decrease the reliability of these findings. Only 42.9% of patients in the third trimester are reported to have abdominal spasm and guarding, compared with 80% during the first trimester (55). Psoas and obturator signs are similarly obscured as the appendix is moved from its normal location.

Anorexia, nausea, and vomiting occur in 58% to 77% of pregnant patients with appendicitis (52,55). Although nausea and vomiting in the first trimester is common, its occurrence during the later stages of pregnancy should raise suspicion. Anorexia, nausea, and vomiting during the second and third trimester, especially if associated with abdominal pain, require a thorough investigation.

The results of laboratory examinations commonly used to assist in the diagnosis of appendicitis are also obscured by pregnancy. The physiologic leukocytosis of pregnancy, ranging from 5,000 to 12,000 white blood cells (WBCs)/mL, overlaps that of appendicitis. In one collected series, the WBC counts of pregnant patients with proven appendicitis was not significantly elevated over these values, and only 25% of patients had a WBC count over 15,000. Most patients (50%) had WBC counts ranging between 10,000 and 15,000, and 25% had less than 10,000 WBCs/mL (52). Urinalysis is a useful adjunct in the work-up of appendicitis, but again presents a dilemma in pregnancy. Urinary tract infection is common in pregnancy as the enlarging uterus compresses the right ureter. Dilatation and stagnant flow in the right collecting system can contribute to bacterial overgrowth and infection, and an inflamed and enlarging appendix can contribute to the urinary tract infection by further compressing this system. Pyuria without bacteria can also indicate involvement of the right ureter in the appendiceal inflammatory process. Pus or bacteria in the urine does not rule out appendiceal inflammation because the two conditions often coexist. Attributing abdominal pain to pyelonephritis and choosing a course of antibiotics rather than further investigation only leads to a delay in diagnosis and missed appendicitis (51).

All these complicating factors and the physician's fear of surgically induced premature labor contribute to delayed appendectomy in pregnancy. One series documents a correlation between a delay in the diagnosis and gestational age. In the first trimester, all of the diagnoses were made promptly and timely surgical intervention undertaken. A delay in diagnosis occurred in 18% of patients presenting in the second trimester, but in the third trimester delay was the rule. Numerous patients were discharged from the emergency room with various misdiagnoses ranging from false labor, nausea and vomiting of pregnancy, to gastroenteritis. All presented with vague signs and symptoms obscuring the true diagnosis (56). Other series document the same delay in operation with a high rate of perforation, as high as 49% in the second trimester and 70% in the third (52,55). Patients with perforated appendicitis usually experienced symptoms more than 24 hours before operation (50).

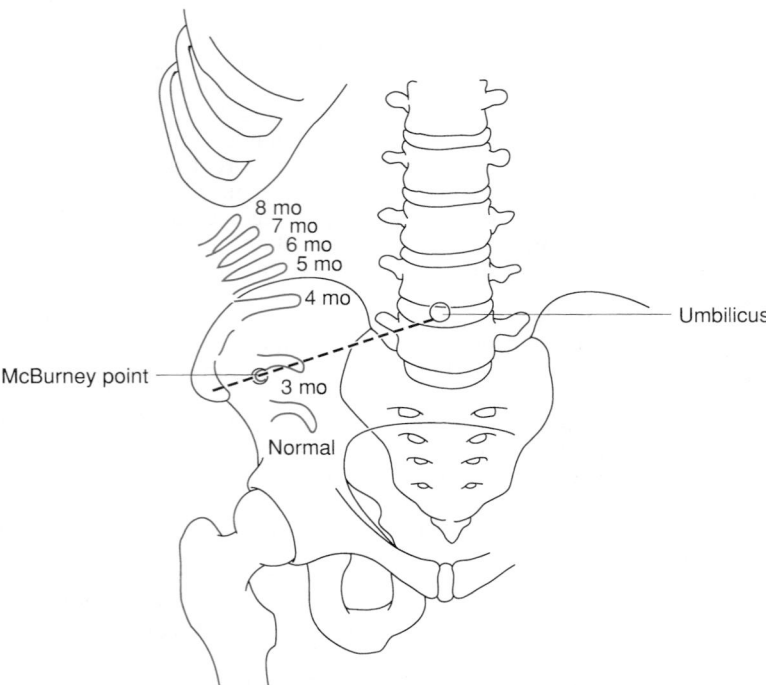

Figure 104.11. Changing location of the appendix throughout gestation. (Reproduced from Baer JL, Reis RA, Arens RA. Appendicitis in pregnancy. *JAMA* 1932;98:1963.)

Perforated appendicitis presents a greater infectious risk in the pregnant patient than in the population as a whole. The large uterus interferes with proper omental migration throughout the abdominal cavity and prevents the walling off of the inflammatory process. Braxton Hicks contractions disrupt adhesion formation, and the general increase in vascularity of the abdomen with greater lymphatic drainage allows rapid dissemination of infection. The high circulatory levels of adrenocorticoids in pregnancy have also been hypothesized to diminish the tissue inflammatory response and hinder containment of infection (57,58). Perforated appendicitis in pregnancy rapidly leads to diffuse peritonitis, premature labor, and fetal loss. The rate of preterm labor and fetal loss with perforated appendicitis ranges from 26% to 66%, compared with 0% to 5% for uncomplicated appendicitis (52,55,59).

Although history and clinical examination for suspected appendicitis during pregnancy are not ideal, they are still the best tools for detecting the disease. A patient with appendicitis during the first trimester might present with right lower quadrant pain, guarding, and nausea and vomiting, whereas a women in the third trimester would most likely have pain in another location and a more confusing clinical picture. The adage "If you cannot rule it out, take it out" applies in pregnancy as well as the nongravid state (52). In applying this principle, the average negative laparotomy rate is 19% to 35% in the pregnant patient, a rate similar to that in the population as a whole (60). Negative laparotomy rates as high as 75% in the third trimester, however, have been reported (15). Although complication rates are low for negative explorations, fetal loss does occur. Imaging studies offer the potential of increasing the accuracy of the diagnosis of appendicitis.

Imaging Modalities

Ultrasonography is safe for the developing fetus and the study of choice in the pregnant patient. Findings suggesting appendicitis include visualization of a tubular structure with a diameter over 6.0 mm, a wall thickness over 3.0 mm (61), and lack of peristalsis (Fig. 104.12). Because a normal appendix is difficult to visualize, simply seeing the appendix combined with tenderness on palpation with the ultrasound probe is suggestive of appendicitis. Ultrasonography, however, has been criticized for being operator dependent and situation specific. Sensitivity varies widely, from 68% to 89% (62,63), and examination can be prohibitive because of abdominal guarding, pain during examination, and a thick abdominal wall. Distortion of anatomic landmarks and the displacement of the

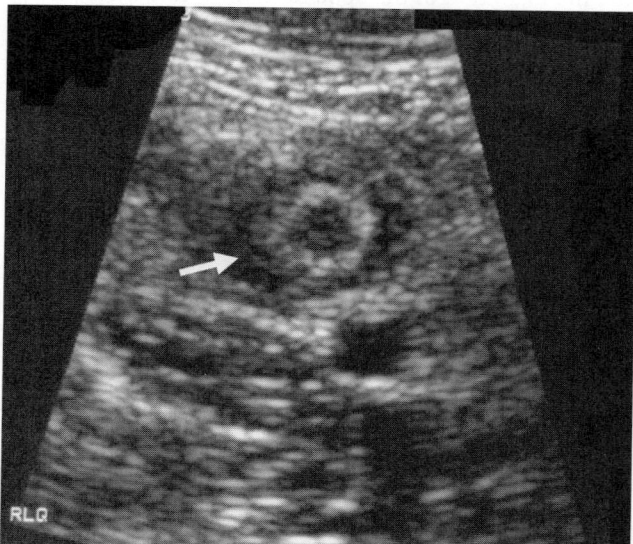

Figure 104.12. Ultrasonographic appearance of appendicitis. The appendix appears as a thick, noncompressible tubular structure with central hypoechogenicity. The walls are 5 mm thick, over the 3-mm limit for a normal appendix. (Courtesy of Dr. Beverly Coleman, Department of Radiology, Hospital of the University of Pennsylvania, Philadelphia, PA.)

appendix by the gravid uterus complicate the diagnosis. Other structures such as an inflamed salpinx can also mimic appendicitis on ultrasound (64), and a dilated uterine vein during pregnancy has been mistaken for an acutely inflamed appendix (63). Despite these limitations, ultrasound is readily available in the emergency department or office and often can add diagnostic information to a confusing clinical picture. If the patient's history and physical examination do not warrant an immediate operation, abdominal ultrasonography should be the first study obtained.

Computed tomography (CT) has emerged as a highly reliable modality in the diagnosis of appendicitis. Appendiceal CT, using rectally administered contrast, can be performed within 10 to 20 minutes, does not require a waiting period for oral contrast to progress down through the cecum, and exposes the patient to only one-third the radiation of a regular CT scan (65). Results at one center have indicated that CT interpretation can be 98% sensitive and 98% specific for the diagnosis of appendicitis. Routine use of this modality has been shown to reduce costs, expedite the diagnosis, and reduce perforation rates from 22% to 14% while decreasing the incidence of negative laparotomy from 20% to 7% (66,67). Although radiation risks to the developing fetus do exist, it is unlikely that fetal loss or malformations will occur with the dosing needed for an abdominal CT. Because even low levels of radiation in utero can increase the incidence of childhood cancer, widespread use of this modality in the pregnant patient with abdominal pain may be detrimental. Reserving the CT scan for those cases where the clinical history, physical examination, and ultrasonography are indeterminate should decrease the rate of perforation and negative exploration, just as it has in the nonpregnant population (Fig. 104.13).

Magnetic resonance imaging uses no ionizing radiation and, like CT, has the potential to image the whole abdomen. It is generally considered safe in pregnancy, and initial experimentation has shown that the higher water content of an inflamed appendix can be detected by MRI (68). Reported sensitivity for appendicitis approaches 100%, at least in children (69). Routine use of MRI may be hindered by availability and limited experience for detecting appendicitis using this modality. Future studies of MRI in appendicitis are warranted.

Laparoscopy

Pregnancy is no longer a contraindication to laparoscopy. Although earlier studies reported a high rate of fetal and maternal complications, it is likely the underlying pathologic process rather than laparoscopy contributed to maternal morbidity and fetal demise (70). Fetal acidosis with experimental maternal CO_2 pneumoperitoneum has been reported but can be minimized in the clinical setting with arterial blood gas monitoring and careful attention to maternal ventilation and acid–base balance (71). Concerns regarding the effect of increased intraabdominal pressure are questionable considering the high uterine pressures during delivery. Experimental pneumoperitoneum in itself does not alter hemodynamics in the fetus until pressures of 20 mm Hg are reached (71). Reduced insufflation pressures of 8 to 12 mm Hg should not contribute to fetal morbidity and mortality. Patients undergoing nongynecologic laparoscopic surgery begin a regular diet sooner, have lower narcotic requirements, and are discharged from the hospital earlier than patients undergoing open surgery (72).

Laparoscopy to evaluate the appendix is a feasible diagnostic modality during pregnancy but may be difficult during later gestation. Anatomic changes alter placement of trocars above the gravid uterus (73) and require the use of the open Hasson technique of trocar placement under direct visualization rather than blind insufflation with a Veress needle. Maneuvers to enhance operative safety of laparoscopy in pregnancy have been outlined by the Society of American Gastrointestinal Endoscopic Surgeons (74) (Table 104.5).

Appendectomy

Once the diagnosis of appendicitis is made, treatment is strictly surgical. The type of incision can vary based on surgeon preference but becomes an issue during later pregnancy. Because of the migration of the appendix, an incision over McBurney's point in the late second and third trimester is inadequate. A low midline incision is favored by some to allow treatment of other conditions that mimic appendicitis, but may require excessive retraction of the uterus (56). A right-sided transverse incision over the point of maximal tenderness is usually the safest approach be-

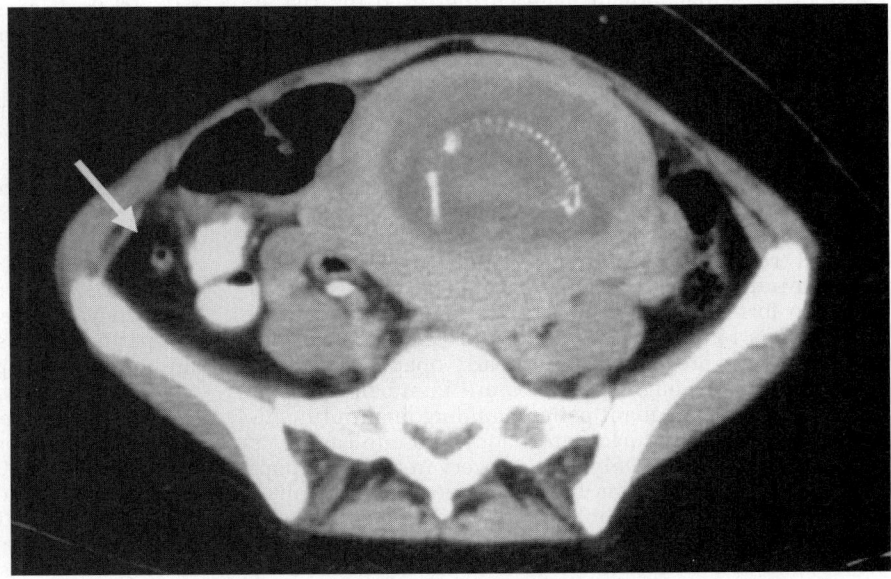

Figure 104.13. Computed tomography (CT) scan of a woman in the 18th week of gestation presenting with a 12-hour history of right-sided abdominal pain. Abdominal examination on presentation revealed significant tenderness, and after a nondiagnostic ultrasound, a laparotomy is considered for presumed appendicitis. A CT scan is obtained instead, revealing a normal, air-filled appendix with no sign of periappendiceal inflammation (*arrow*). The laparotomy was postponed, and 12 hours later the patient aborted a septic fetus. An unnecessary laparotomy for an atypical presentation of chorioamnionitis was avoided by the judicious use of the CT scan. (Courtesy of Dr. David Weiss, Chestnut Hill Hospital, University of Pennsylvania Health System, Chestnut Hill, PA.)

Table 104.5. GUIDELINES FOR LAPAROSCOPIC SURGERY DURING PREGNANCY

1. Defer operative intervention until the second trimester, when the fetal risk is lowest, whenever possible.
2. Pneumatic compression devices must be used because of the enhancement of lower venous stasis with pneumoperitoneum and pregnancy-induced hypercoagulable state.
3. Fetal and uterine status, as well as maternal end-tidal CO_2 and arterial blood gases, should be monitored.
4. Use fluoroscopy selectively and protect the uterus with lead shield if intraoperative cholangiography is possible.
5. Given enlarged gravid uterus, abdominal access should be obtained using open technique.
6. Dependent positioning should be used to shift the uterus off the inferior vena cava.
7. Pneumoperitoneum pressures should be minimized (to 8–12 mm Hg) and not allowed to exceed 15 mm Hg.
8. Obstetric consultation should be obtained before operation.

From SAGES Committee on Standards Practice. Guidelines for laparoscopic surgery during pregnancy. Surg Endosc 1998;12:189–190, with permission.

cause the appendix customarily lies beneath that point (50,52,55). A similar incision at the level of the umbilicus allows good exposure of most of the right upper and lower abdomen. By tilting the patient 30 degrees to the left, the uterus is shifted away from the operative field and off the inferior vena cava. A right paramedian incision usually necessitates medial retraction of the uterus for exposure and increases the risk of precipitating premature labor. The laparoscopic approach, although useful for both diagnosis and treatment, might be difficult in later gestation. Although the potential benefits over the open appendectomy include less uterine manipulation and decreased incidence of preterm labor, its utility depends heavily on surgeon experience and comfort with the procedure (72,73).

If exploration reveals a normal appendix, an appendectomy still should be performed. Although some authors question this approach because of the suggested high rate of preterm labor with a normal appendectomy (75), most believe this to be untrue. Taking out the normal appendix adds little to morbidity while eliminating potential confusion if symptoms should recur (52). Perforated appendicitis or pus in the abdominal cavity demands thorough peritoneal toilet along with the appendectomy. Drainage of the perforated appendectomy bed was avoided in the past because of fears that foreign material increased the risk of premature labor (54), but these fears have not been substantiated and drainage of the appendiceal stump has been performed without complications.

BILIARY TRACT DISEASE IN PREGNANCY

Acute cholecystitis is the second most common general surgery diagnosis during pregnancy. Progesterone-induced relaxation of the gallbladder combined with estrogen-induced supersaturation of bile predispose to gallstone formation (45,76). The risk for development of gallstones is related to the number of pregnancies, doubling after two pregnancies and nearly quadrupling after four (76–78). Although gallstones are found in approximately 4% of all pregnant patients undergoing routine ultrasonography early during pregnancy, the rate can be as high as 12.2% immediately after delivery in high-risk populations (77). Despite this high prevalence of gallstones, the incidence of acute cholecystitis during pregnancy is relatively low, 1 to 8 in 10,000 pregnancies (0.01% to 0.08%) (79,80). Inhibition of gallbladder contraction by

progesterone is most likely the reason for this discrepancy. Although gallstones and sludge can form, weaker contractions prevent cystic duct obstruction until delivery. Postpartum, the progesterone concentrations decrease and the increased force of gallbladder contraction potentiates gallstone-induced cystic duct obstruction. An increased prevalence of cholecystitis in the year after childbirth has been noted (81–83).

Symptoms of cholecystitis or biliary colic caused by cystic duct obstruction are similar in the pregnant and non-pregnant patient. Crampy right upper quadrant or epigastric pain after a meal can last several minutes to hours. The pain may radiate to the back and accompany nausea and vomiting. Tenderness on palpation of the right upper quadrant is usually present with acute cholecystitis, but laboratory evaluation may be obscured by the normal leukocytosis and elevated alkaline phosphatase during pregnancy. Increased bilirubin or visible jaundice, however, is unlikely without common bile duct obstruction (80).

The differential diagnosis for cholecystitis during pregnancy includes hepatitis, acute fatty liver of pregnancy, and appendicitis. The diagnosis can be strengthened by the history and physical examination, and confirmed by abdominal ultrasound. Ultrasonography is over 97% accurate in detecting cholecystitis, with typical findings of echogenic shadowing, gallbladder wall thickening, and pericholecystic fluid (84). Pain on palpation with the ultrasound transducer, or sonographic Murphy's sign, is confirmatory of inflammation.

Historically, medical management was the definitive treatment of cholecystitis during pregnancy. The pregnant patient was made NPO, maintained on intravenous hydration, and treated with antibiotic for signs of infection. A low-fat diet was started once symptoms abated, antibiotics discontinued, and the patient discharged to home. Most women had initial relief of symptoms with this management and surgery was reserved for those with persistent symptoms, severe toxicity, and sepsis, peritonitis, or obstructive jaundice (85). Fear of surgical complications prompted some to place pregnant patients with disabling biliary symptoms on total parenteral nutrition until delivery (72,86). Analysis of patient outcomes throughout the course of pregnancy, however, has put strict medical management into question. Between 57% and 70% of patients treated for gallstone disease during pregnancy have recurrence at some time during gestation (87,88). This risk is close to 92% for those who present in the first trimester, 64% for those presenting during the second trimester, and 44% for those who present during the third. Ninety percent of these patients require hospitalization for management of the relapse (87), and a significant portion of those presenting in the first trimester experience pregnancy loss as a complication of the disease (86,89). Complications of gallstones such as choledocholithiasis and pancreatitis can also arise with future attacks and have been associated with a maternal mortality rate of 15% and a 60% chance of fetal demise (85,90–92).

Laparoscopic cholecystectomy is emerging as a safe and reliable modality of dealing with gallstone disease during pregnancy. Numerous reports and case-control studies comparing laparoscopic with open cholecystectomy have supported the laparoscopic approach. Overall, patients have a shorter postoperative stay, resume oral intake earlier, have fewer postoperative hernias, and experience less pain with lower narcotic requirements by avoiding a large open incision (70,72,93). Because fetal loss is most likely related to the underlying maternal illness and extent of uterine manipulation during surgery (88,94), laparoscopic cholecystectomy offers a solution to both problems. Removing the diseased gallbladder eliminates the potential for recurrence, and the minimal uterine retraction needed with laparoscopic access to the right upper quadrant should decrease the risk for preterm labor. Although no randomized studies exist, preliminary data seem to support these assumptions. The incidence of premature uterine contractions with laparoscopic cholecystectomy has been reported at 0% to 21%, but contractions are usually well controlled by tocolytics. Most series report rates of premature birth or spontaneous abortion ranging from 0% to 7% with the laparoscopic approach (73,87,88,94). After an open cholecystectomy, the reported rate of premature labor ranges from 0% to 40%, based on trimester (95), and a spontaneous abortion or premature birth rate of up to 22% has been reported (15). Based on the available data, laparoscopic cholecystectomy is safe during pregnancy and is preferable to open cholecystectomy (88). An isolated report of three laparoscopic cholecystectomies ending in abortion, however, has been published, emphasizing the fact that this procedure is not without risk and careful attention must be paid to the timing, indications, and maternal physiology before any procedure (96).

Because most biliary symptoms can be controlled, at least initially, with conservative management, the management of symptomatic gallstones varies based on the stage of gestation. The second trimester is the optimal time to perform an elective cholecystectomy. Organogenesis is complete and the gravid uterus is not yet large enough to impinge on the operating field (85). Clinical studies of open cholecystectomy confirm that this is the safest time to perform the operation. Spontaneous abortion rates after an open cholecystectomy are 12% during the first trimester, whereas the incidence of premature labor can be as high as 40% during the third trimester. The second trimester offers the ideal compromise, with the low spontaneous abortion rate of 5.6% (95). Laparoscopic cholecystectomy offers the potential to decrease fetal loss even further over these values. Suggested management for symptomatic cholelithiasis during the first trimester consists of conservative measures until elective cholecystectomy can be performed safely during the second trimester of gestation. Second trimester disease can be dealt with surgically, whereas those presenting later in gestation can probably be managed symptomatically until the postpartum period. If symptoms are unremitting and cannot be handled with diet alone, surgical intervention might be necessary regardless of the period of gestation (83,88).

Fetal heart rate monitoring is an essential part of laparoscopic procedures. Because pneumoperitoneum can have detrimental physiologic effects on both the mother and fetus, any evidence of fetal distress should result in immediate desufflation (73). Fetal heart rate aberrations can also be treated by increasing uterine perfusion with maternal intravascular volume and changing the mother's position on the operating room table to decrease uterine compression of the inferior vena cava. Because the transabdominal signal is lost with pneumoperitoneum, transvaginal monitoring should be used during surgery (72), whereas an external tocodynamometer should be placed on the abdomen immediately after the completion of the operation to monitor for uterine contractions. Tocolytic agents need not be used prophylactically, but can be administered if the patient demonstrates uterine irritability or contractions. The rate of successful tocolysis after laparoscopic procedures with minimal uterine manipulation is close to 100% (70,72,83,90,95,97).

Choledocholithiasis

Indications for evaluation of the common bile duct are no different in the pregnant patient than in the population as a whole—namely, a bilirubin elevated over 1.5 mg/dL, a dilated common bile duct, or gallstone pancreatitis (73). Endoscopic retrograde cholangiopancreatography (ERCP) can be performed safely in pregnancy. With proper lead shielding, judicious use of fluoroscopy time, and avoidance of permanent roentgenographic films, ERCP has been performed with no direct exposure of the fetus to radiation. Calculated scatter radiation on the order of 4 mrads during the whole examination presents the only risk from ionizing radiation (91). Evaluation of the biliary tree, stone retrieval, and sphincterotomy can be performed under these conditions without maternal or fetal complications (98). Other methods avoid radiation altogether and include imaging of choledocholithiasis with endoscopic ultrasonography (99), endoscopic papillotomy under ultrasonographic control (100), and magnetic resonance cholangiography for choledocholithiasis (101). Success with all these modalities has been reported but can be limited by operator experience and availability.

INTESTINAL OBSTRUCTION DURING PREGNANCY

The incidence of intestinal obstruction during pregnancy rose throughout the 20th century. In the presurgical era, cases were cited as infrequently as 1 in every 68,000 deliveries. Since the 1940s, however, the incidence has increased to 1 in 2,500 to 3,500 deliveries (102). This change reflects the increased number of laparotomies in young women and the prevalence of postoperative adhesions during pregnancy. Adhesions remain the most common cause of intestinal obstruction in the gravid patient, but intestinal volvulus is a much more common complication than in the population as a whole. Intussusception, hernia, and carcinoma are responsible for a minority of cases of bowel obstruction (Table 104.6).

Obstruction during pregnancy classically presents during three peak periods because of the change in the interrelationship between the abdominal viscera caused by the gravid uterus. The first peak occurs during the fourth to fifth months of gestation as the uterus becomes an intraabdominal organ, stretching any previously formed adhesions. The second peak occurs during the eighth to ninth months, when the fetal head descends into the pelvis, decreasing the uterine size. The third peak occurs after delivery as the sudden decrease in uterine size drastically changes the association of adhesions to surrounding bowel. The incidence of adhesion-related obstruction is highest during the first pregnancy after an operation,

Table 104.6. CAUSES OF INTESTINAL OBSTRUCTION COMPLICATING PREGNANCY AND THE PUERPERIUM IN 66 PATIENTS

Adhesions	39 (59%)
Volvulus	15 (23%)
Sigmoid	7
Cecal	3
Midgut	3
Volvulus around vitellointestinal band	2
Intussusception	3 (5%)
Hernia	2 (3%)
Carcinoma	1 (1%)
Appendicitis	1 (1%)
Idiopathic (ileus)	5 (8%)

Reproduced from Perdue PW, Johnson HW, Stafford PW, et al. Intestinal obstruction complicating pregnancy. Am J Surg 1992;164:385, with permission.

when the association between the viscera and adhesions is initially tested (102,103).

In the general population, incarceration of bowel in groin hernias is the second most common cause of small bowel obstruction, but in the pregnant patient volvulus becomes the number two cause. As the enlarging uterus displaces the bowel out of the pelvis and away from the inguinal region, symptomatic groin hernias diminish in frequency (104). Volvulus increases in prevalence during pregnancy because of changes in colon and small bowel anatomy and causes one fourth of all bowel obstructions. Sigmoid volvulus normally occurs owing to a long and redundant sigmoid colon. In the United States, this is usually seen in debilitated, institutionalized, or chronically constipated people. In countries such as those of Africa, a high incidence of sigmoid volvulus has been attributed to the high-fiber vegetable diet characteristic of that population. Anatomic changes of pregnancy further exacerbate this condition by causing the redundant sigmoid colon to rise out of the pelvis and twist around its point of fixation (105). It is the most common site of volvulus during pregnancy (106).

Cecal volvulus occurs because of failure of lateral peritoneal fixation during development. As the uterus enlarges during pregnancy, it raises the redundant or abnormally mobile cecum out of the pelvis. If a transition point or distal obstruction should occur from uterine pressure or an adhesive band, the colonic distention raises the colon even higher, producing torsion around this fixed point (107). Volvulus of the small bowel also results from a congenital abnormality of rotation and fixation. Because clinical presentation usually occurs in infancy or childhood, the true incidence of malrotation in adulthood is unknown. The enlarging uterus potentially predisposes to the presentation of this anomaly during pregnancy by pushing the nonfixed, mobile portions of the small bowel into the upper abdomen, initiating the volvulus (108).

Presentation and Diagnosis

Symptoms of intestinal obstruction are similar to those in the nonpregnant patient and commonly include abdominal pain and vomiting. High small bowel obstruction results in short periods between vomiting episodes with poorly localized, crampy upper abdominal pain. Colonic obstruction can present with less frequent, feculent vomiting and lower abdominal pain. Findings on physical examination such as abdominal distention are often difficult to evaluate because of the gravid uterus. Obstipation, although characteristic of low obstruction such as that of sigmoid volvulus, may not occur with high obstruction. Laboratory studies, although useful to rule out other conditions, are not reliable enough to be considered diagnostic of obstruction. Significant leukocytosis can occur with necrosis and bowel strangulation, but mild elevations are confusing because of the physiologic leukocytosis of pregnancy. Tachycardia and hypotension are also late signs suggesting bowel compromise and shock.

The murky clinical picture combined with the tendency to treat the progressive vomiting as a normal part of pregnancy and crampy abdominal pain as early contractions lead to a delay in presentation and diagnosis. The median time from the onset of symptoms to admission in one series was 48 hours, and the median time from admission to a necessary laparotomy was also 48 hours. This delay in diagnosis and treatment contributed to excessive maternal and fetal mortality (104). Abdominal pain and vomiting in a pregnant patient with an abdominal scar should raise the serious suspicion of small bowel obstruction.

If intestinal obstruction is suspected, upright and flat films of the abdomen are the diagnostic studies of choice.

Although some authors believe that radiographs are nonspecific early in obstruction, serial films obtained every 4 to 6 hours usually show progressive changes confirming the diagnosis (102). Small bowel obstruction gives the appearance of a progressive stepladder formation with dilatation and multiple air–fluid levels. Large bowel obstruction can produce a similar picture or reveal a grossly dilated bowel loop suggestive of volvulus. Contrast studies are also useful, and a "bird's bill" shape of contrast with gradual narrowing after a barium enema can be diagnostic of colonic volvulus, whereas dilute Gastrografin or barium by mouth can differentiate partial from complete obstruction. Fetal radiation risks from the plain radiographs are negligible and greatly outweighed by those from the possibility of misdiagnosis.

Treatment

The initial treatment for bowel obstruction in the pregnant patient is no different from that of a nonpregnant patient. Nasogastric tube decompression and fluid resuscitation are the cornerstones of therapy. By the time an obstruction is visible on plain film, the fluid deficit due to vomiting and intraluminal losses is estimated at 1,000 to 1,500 mL. In advanced cases of dehydration presenting with tachycardia and hypotension, fluid losses may be as high as 4 to 6 L (102). Prompt fluid resuscitation is essential in the pregnant patient because compromise of uterine blood flow leads to fetal distress and demise.

Surgical intervention plays a more prominent and earlier role in the management of the pregnant patient with bowel obstruction. Although adhesion-related small bowel obstruction in the nonpregnant patient usually resolves with nasogastric decompression and fluid administration, numerous series have documented failure of conservative management of small bowel obstruction in the pregnant woman. Eighty-nine to 100% of patients eventually require an operation, and 13% to 23% require resection of gangrenous bowel at the time of laparotomy (104,109). Based on these outcomes, some have stated that once the diagnosis of small bowel obstruction is made in a pregnant patient, the only role of nasogastric decompression and fluid resuscitation is to prepare the patient for an operation (109). Cecal volvulus is also treated surgically, and although sigmoid volvulus in the nonpregnant patient can be managed with sigmoidoscopic decompression and placement of a rectal tube, the large gravid uterus may act as a mechanical impediment to detorsion. A laparotomy is usually necessary for treatment (104,105).

A generous midline incision allows for maximum exposure of the abdomen with minimal manipulation of the uterus. During lysis of small bowel adhesions, bowel viability must be carefully assessed. Definitive management of cecal volvulus requires resection of necrotic cecum or detorsion and cecopexy. Sigmoid volvulus should also be treated by resection if necrotic, but simple detorsion and placement of a rectal tube can be performed if the sigmoid is viable. Although resection of the redundant sigmoid is the definitive treatment for this disease, it can be delayed until the postpartum period. Aggressive surgical treatment has been credited with reducing the maternal and fetal mortality rates from 20% and 50%, respectively, in the 1930s to 6% and 26% today (104). Increased awareness of this disease and expeditious management can reduce those rates even further.

COLORECTAL CANCER DURING PREGNANCY

Colon cancer is a rare disease during pregnancy but one with lethal consequences. The incidence of colon cancer was estimated as 1 in 50,000 pregnancies based on a 1955 report (110). More recent reviews estimate the incidence as 1 in 13,000 deliveries (111), with the increasing prevalence due to increasing maternal age with the delay in pregnancy until later in life (112). Presenting symptoms are similar to those in nonpregnant patients and include rectal bleeding, constipation, abdominal pain and distention, as well as nausea and vomiting (113). All of these symptoms are common during pregnancy. Even the findings of occult blood in the stool and hematochezia are often attributed to pregnancy-related hemorrhoids and ignored.

The anatomic distribution and stage of colorectal cancer in the pregnant patient differ from those in the population as a whole. A nationwide survey of the members of the American Society of Colon and Rectal Surgeons who had cared for pregnant patients with colorectal cancer revealed a predominance of rectal cancer in this patient population. Sixty-four percent of tumors were distributed below the peritoneal reflection and 36% were in the more proximal colon. A review of over 200 pregnancy-associated colorectal cancers reported in the literature disclosed a similar distribution, with 86% of tumors located in the rectum and only 14% above the peritoneal reflection (114). This is in contrast to the general population, where most tumors (69%) are located in the colon and only 31% in the rectum. This trend could reflect a presentation bias due to frequent rectal examinations during prenatal care, or the change in pelvic anatomy and symptoms of rectal compression by the gravid uterus.

Pregnant patients present with more advanced cancers than the population as a whole. In the previously mentioned study, no pregnant patient was Dukes stage A at presentation, whereas 41% were Dukes stage B, 44% stage C, and 15% stage D (114). Although increased hormonal stimulation during pregnancy could cause rapid tumor growth and progression of disease (114–116), not all colon cancers have estrogen or progesterone receptors and respond to this stimulation (117). The advanced stage of disease on presentation is most likely due to a delay in the diagnosis and the low clinical suspicion of malignancy in this patient population. This trend is similar to that in the young population as a whole, and although only 4% to 8% of all colon cancer occurs in those younger than 40 years of age, these patients also have a delayed presentation with more advanced disease (118). The average interval between the onset of symptoms and diagnosis of colon cancer in those younger than 40 years is 6.4 months, and 32% of patients wait longer than 1 year before seeking medical attention for symptoms (119). The stage of disease on presentation in this patient population is similar to that in the pregnant patient (Table 104.7), and colonic malignancy during gestation most likely represents pregnancy superimposed on colon cancer rather than a pregnancy-related disease.

Table 104.7. **STAGE AT PRESENTATION OF COLORECTAL CANCER DURING PREGNANCY AND THOSE YOUNGER THAN 40 YEARS OF AGE**

	Pregnant patients	**Patients <40 y**
Dukes stage A	0%	2%
Dukes stage B	41%	30%
Dukes stage C	44%	45%
Dukes stage D	15%	23%

Data from Bernstein MA, Madoff RD, Caushaj PF. Colon and rectal cancer in pregnancy. Dis Colon Rectum 1993;36:172–178; and Smith C, Butler JA. Colorectal cancer in patients younger than 40 years of age. Dis Colon Rectum 1989;32:843–846.

Diagnosis

Diagnosis of colorectal cancer during pregnancy demands a very high level of suspicion. Patients with rectal bleeding, occult blood-positive stools, and anemia below physiologic levels of pregnancy should be evaluated for a colonic malignancy. Sigmoidoscopy is not contraindicated during pregnancy and does not appear to induce labor or congenital malformations. Because most cancers are located below the peritoneal reflection, they can be easily accessed and sampled for biopsy through a limited sigmoidoscopic examination. Because of the 5% risk of a second, synchronous primary, a more extensive colonoscopic evaluation might be necessary, especially if findings were to change the treatment or extent of surgical resection. Colonoscopy during pregnancy is still considered experimental and may be technically difficult because of colonic compression by the gravid uterus. Maneuvers to increase safety include use of only gentle pressure when manipulating the colonoscope, maternal administration of supplemental oxygen, and fetal heart rate monitoring during the procedure (120).

Transrectal ultrasonographic staging of rectal cancer is particularly helpful during pregnancy because of its ability to evaluate cancerous invasion of the uterus or encroachment on the cervix that could prevent vaginal delivery (120). Serum carcinoembryonic antigen levels are not normally elevated during pregnancy and, although of limited use as a screening tool, levels can be obtained before resection for early detection of recurrence (121). Evaluation of metastatic disease to the liver can be performed with transabdominal ultrasonography at no risk to the fetus, and a CT scan can be obtained in more difficult cases.

Treatment

Treatment of colorectal cancer during pregnancy presents as an ethical dilemma for both the patient and physician. Aside from the difficulty in dealing with a potentially lethal disease in a young person, there is an inherent conflict between the treatment of the mother and fetus. Treatment of other surgical conditions encountered during pregnancy, such as appendicitis or cholecystitis, equally benefits both the mother and the unborn child. Treatment of colon cancer puts the two at odds. Although early tumor resection can improve the prognosis for the mother, this treatment might be detrimental to the fetus. Adjuvant chemotherapy or radiation therapy can improve survival of the mother but is generally contraindicated during pregnancy, especially early in gestation. Careful attention must be paid to the wishes of the family while explaining the risks and benefits for both the mother and child.

If the cancer is discovered in the first half of gestation, a definitive resection should be performed. Waiting months until adequate fetal maturation for delivery can allow cancer dissemination and disease progression (113,120). In most cases, a colon resection can be handled without disturbing the pregnancy, and resection of even low-lying tumors can be performed before 20 weeks of gestation (110,114). Total abdominal hysterectomy is recommended only if tumor invasion into the uterus has occurred, a technically complete operation cannot be performed without it, or the mother's life expectancy is shorter than the time needed to reach fetal viability. If the tumor is unresectable, a colostomy is performed for palliation until fetal viability is documented.

Treatment of tumors discovered after the 20th week can be postponed until term or fetal viability. Vaginal delivery is not contraindicated unless the tumor is obstructing the birth canal or presents a risk of episiotomy entering the tumor bed. Tumor resection is undertaken several days after the birth to allow uterine involution and resolution of pelvic vascular congestion. If a cesarean section is performed for obstetric reasons or because of tumor impingement on the birth canal, resection can be performed immediately, but the operation may be technically easier if done as a separate procedure and postponed for several days. This is especially important with low rectal lesions, where decreased pelvic vasculature can facilitate a low anterior or abdominoperineal resection (113).

Management of the ovaries is a controversial issue. The incidence of colon carcinoma metastasizing to the ovaries is estimated between 3% and 8% (122) in the general population, but can be as high as 25% during pregnancy and in young patients (119,123). Bilateral salpingo-oophorectomy at the time of tumor resection has been advocated by some (122), but during pregnancy carries a high chance of spontaneous abortion, especially during the first half of gestation. Although resection should be performed if the ovaries are grossly involved with tumor or a hysterectomy is undertaken, bilateral ovarian wedge biopsies with frozen-section evaluation can be safely carried out without disturbing the pregnancy. Salpingo-oophorectomy is then performed only if the ovaries are involved with tumor (113).

Adjuvant chemotherapy conveys a survival advantage to patients with Dukes stage C colon cancer. The classic adjuvant chemotherapy includes 5-fluorouracil, an antimetabolite that inhibits DNA synthesis. The safety of this drug during pregnancy is questionable, and evidence of fetal toxicity exists in animal models. Limited data on the human fetal safety of this drug are available, and it is considered a category D drug during pregnancy by the U.S. Food and Drug Administration: generally unsafe during pregnancy, but the risk may be justifiable in certain circumstances. Chemotherapy during the first trimester is usually contraindicated and should be limited to those patients with Dukes stage C lesions who are willing to accept the risks of fetal teratogenesis or demise. Chemotherapy during the second and third trimesters is less teratogenic because of the completion of organogenesis, but still carries some risk for the fetus (120,124).

Adjuvant radiation therapy reduces the local recurrence of rectal cancer. Because the most effective dose to eradicate microscopic disease is on the order of 50 Gy and the fetus cannot be effectively shielded from pelvic exposure, radiation therapy cannot be safely performed during pregnancy. Therapeutic pelvic radiation also results in permanent and irreversible female sterility, so the mother considering this form of therapy must be fully aware of the risks to the current and future pregnancies (120,125).

SUMMARY

Pregnancy presents as a unique physiologic state. Although the nature of surgical disease does not change, the presentation and treatment are altered by the gravid state. Inflammatory or malignant intraabdominal conditions present a health risk for both the mother and child and a clinical challenge for the surgeon. Because the general surgeon is often consulted to evaluate a pregnant patient, he or she must be aware of the changes in maternal physiology and symptoms of disease as well as the inherent risks of radiographic studies used for diagnosis. By understanding these conditions, the surgeon can provide a better level of care for both the mother and unborn child.

REFERENCES

1. Moore KL, Persaud TVN. *The developing human,* 6th ed. Philadelphia: WB Saunders, 1998.
2. Gardner MO, Goldstein RL. The clinical use of antenatal corticosteroids. *Clin Obstet Gynecol* 1995;38:746–754.
3. Harrison MR, Golbus MS, Filly RA, et al. Fetal surgery for congenital hydronephrosis. *N Engl J Med* 1982;306:591–593.
4. Harrison MR. Fetal surgery. *Am J Obstet Gynecol* 1996; 174:1255–1264.
5. Quinn TM, Adzick NS. Fetal surgery. *Obstet Gynecol Clin North Am* 1997;24:143–157.
6. Adzick NS, Harrison MR, Flake AW, et al. Fetal surgery for cystic adenomatoid malformation of the lung. *J Pediatr Surg* 1993;28:806–812.
7. Hedrick MH, Estes JM, Sullivan KM, et al. Plug the lung until it grows (PLUG): a new method to treat congenital diaphragmatic hernia in utero. *J Pediatr Surg* 1994;29: 612–617.
8. Adzick NS, Harrison MR. Fetal surgical therapy. *Lancet* 1994;343:897–902.
9. Flake AW, Roncarolo MG, Puck JM, et al. Treatment of X-linked severe combined immunodeficiency by in utero transplantation of paternal bone marrow. *N Engl J Med* 1996; 335:1806–1810.
10. Resnik R. Anatomic alterations in the reproductive tract. In: Creasy RK, Resnik R, eds. *Maternal–fetal medicine,* 4th ed. Philadelphia: WB Saunders, 1998:90–94.
11. Monga M, Sanborn BM. Uterine biology and the control of myometrial contractions. In: Creasy RK, Resnik R, eds. *Maternal–fetal medicine,* 4th ed. Philadelphia: WB Saunders, 1998:95–101.
12. Petraglia F, Florio P, Nappi C, et al. Peptide signaling in human placenta and membranes: autocrine, paracrine, and endocrine mechanisms. *Endocr Rev* 1996;17:156–186.
13. Challis JRG. Characteristics of parturition. In: Creasy RK, Resnik R, eds. *Maternal–fetal medicine,* 4th ed. Philadelphia: WB Saunders, 1998:484–497.
14. McLean M, Bisits, Davies J, et al. A placental clock controlling the length of human pregnancy. *Nat Med* 1995;1: 460–463.
15. Kort B, Katz VL, Watson WJ. The effects of nonobstetric operation during pregnancy. *Surg Gynecol Obstet* 1993;177: 371–376.
16. Copper RL, Goldenberg RL, Creasy RK, et al. A multicenter study of preterm birth weight and gestational age-specific neonatal mortality. *Am J Obstet Gynecol* 1993;168:78–84.
17. Romero R, Avila C, Brekus CA, et al. The role of systemic and intrauterine infection in preterm parturition. *Ann NY Acad Sci* 1991;622:355–375.
18. Ou CW, Orsino A, Lye S. Expression of connexin-43 and connexin-26 in the rat myometrium during pregnancy and labor is differentially regulated by mechanical and hormonal signals. *Endocrinology* 1997;138:5398–5407.
19. Gordon MC, Samuels P. Indomethacin. *Clin Obstet Gynecol* 1995;38:697–705.
20. Gordon MC, Iams JD. Magnesium sulfate. *Clin Obstet Gynecol* 1995;38:706–712.
21. Ray D, Dyson D. Calcium channel blockers. *Clin Obstet Gynecol* 1995;38:713–721.
22. Hill WC. Risks and complications of tocolysis. *Clin Obstet Gynecol* 1995;38:725–745.
23. Meyers RE. Two patterns of perinatal brain damage and their conditions of occurrence. *Am J Obstet Gynecol* 1972;122: 246–276.
24. Miller DA, Paul R. Antepartum–intrapartum monitoring. In: Scott JR, DiSaia PJ, Hammond CB, et al., eds. *Danforth's obstetrics and gynecology,* 8th ed. Philadelphia: Lippincott Williams & Wilkins, 1999:243–255.
25. Hon EH. The fetal heart rate patterns preceding death in utero. *Am J Obstet Gynecol* 1959;78:47.
26. Smith CV. Vibroacoustic stimulation. *Clin Obstet Gynecol* 1995;38:68–77.
27. Wagner LK, Lester RG, Saldana LR. *Exposure of the pregnant patient to diagnostic radiation.* Madison, WI: Medical Physics Publishing, 1997.
28. Brent RL. The effects of embryonic and fetal exposure to x-ray, microwaves, and ultrasound: counseling the pregnant and non-pregnant patient about these risks. *Semin Oncol* 1989;16:347–368.
29. Boklage CE. Survival probability of human conceptions from fertilization to term. *Int J Fertil* 1990;35:75–94.
30. Brent RL. Radiation teratogenesis. *Teratology* 1980;21: 281–298.

31. Brent RL. The effects of embryonic and fetal exposure to x-ray, microwaves, and ultrasound. *Clinics in Perinatology* 1986;13:615–649.

32. Wood JW, Johnson KG, Omori Y, et al. Mental retardation in children exposed in utero to the atomic bombs in Hiroshima and Nagasaki. *Am J Public Health* 1967;57:1381–1390.

33. Wood JW, Keehan RJ, Kawamoto S, et al. The growth and development of children exposed in utero to the atomic bombs in Hiroshima and Nagasaki. *Am J Public Health* 1967;57:1374–1380.

34. Harvey EB, Boice JD, Honeyman M, et al. Prenatal x-ray exposure and childhood cancer in twins. *N Engl J Med* 1985;312:541–545.

35. Doll R, Wakeford. Risk of childhood cancer from fetal irradiation. *Br J Radiol* 1997;70:130–139.

36. Reece AE, Goldstein I, Hobbins JC. *Fundamentals of obstetric and gynecologic ultrasound.* Norwalk, CT: Appleton & Lange, 1994.

37. Brent RL, Jensh RP, Beckman DA. Medical sonography: reproductive effects and risks. *Teratology* 1991;44:123–146.

38. Kanal E, Shellock FG, Talagala L. Safety considerations in MR imaging. *Radiology* 1990;176:593–606.

39. Schenck JF, Dumoulin CL, Redington RW. Human exposure to 4.0-tesla magnetic fields in a whole-body scanner. *Med Phys* 1992;19:1089–1098.

40. IRPA/INIRC. Protection of the patient undergoing a magnetic resonance examination. *Health Phys* 1991;61:923–928.

41. Martin C, Varner MW. Physiologic changes in pregnancy: surgical implications. *Clinical Obstet Gynecol* 1994;37:241–255.

42. Bonapace ES, Fisher RS. Constipation and diarrhea in pregnancy. *Gastroenterol Clin North Am* 1998;27:197–211.

43. Gill RC, Bowes KL, YJ Kingma. Effects of progesterone on canine colonic smooth muscle. *Gastroenterology* 1985;88:1941–1947.

44. Katz PO, Castell DO. Gastroesophageal reflux during pregnancy. *Gastroenterol Clin North Am* 1998;27:153–167.

45. Everson GT, McKinley C, Lawson M, et al. Gallbladder function in the human female: effect of the ovulatory cycle, pregnancy, and contraceptive steroids. *Gastroenterology* 1982;82:711–719.

46. Broussard CN, Richter JE. Nausea and vomiting of pregnancy. *Gastroenterol Clin North Am* 1998;27:123–151.

47. Abel TL, Riely CA. Hyperemesis gravidum. *Gastroenterol Clin North Am* 1992;21:835–849.

48. Baker PN, Madeley RJ, Symonds EM. Abdominal pain of unknown aetiology in pregnancy. *Br J Obstet Gynaecol* 1989;96:688–691.

49. Al-Mulhim AA. Acute appendicitis in pregnancy. *Int Surg* 1996;81:295–297.

50. Tamir IL, Bongard FS, Klein SR. Acute appendicitis in the pregnant patient. *Am J Surg* 1990;160:571–576.

51. Masters K, Levine BA, Gaskill HV, et al. Diagnosing appendicitis during pregnancy. *Am J Surg* 1984;148:768–771.

52. Babaknia A, Parsa H, Woodruff JD. Appendicitis during pregnancy. *Obstet Gynecol* 1977;50:40–44.

53. Wagner JM, McKinney WP, Carpenter JL. Does this patient have appendicitis? *JAMA* 1996;276:1589–1594.

54. Baer JL, Reis RA, Arens RA. Appendicitis in pregnancy. *JAMA* 1932;98:1359–1364.

55. Weingold AB. Appendicitis in pregnancy. *Clin Obstet Gynecol* 1983;26:801–809.

56. Cunningham FG, McCubbin JH. Appendicitis complicating pregnancy. *Obstet Gynecol* 1975;45:415–420.

57. Black WP. Acute appendicitis in pregnancy. *BMJ* 1960;1:1938–1941.

58. Parker RB. Acute appendicitis in late pregnancy. *Lancet* 1954;1:1252–1257.

59. Horowitz MD, Gomez GA, Santiesteban R, et al. Acute appendicitis during pregnancy. *Arch Surg* 1985;120:1362–1367.

60. Varner MW. Surgical diseases in pregnancy. *Clin Obstet Gynecol* 1994;37:239–315.

61. Worrell JA, Drolshagen LF, Kelly TC, et al. Graded compression ultrasound in the diagnosis of appendicitis: a comparison of diagnostic criteria. *J Ultrasound Med* 1990;9:145–150.

62. Schwerk WB, Wichtrup B, Rothmund M, et al. Ultrasonography in the diagnosis of acute appendicitis: a prospective study. *Gastroenterology* 1989;97:630–639.

63. Abu-Yousef MM, Phillips ME, Franken EA, et al. Sonography of acute appendicitis: a critical review. *Crit Rev Diagn Imaging* 1989;29:381–408.

64. Paulman AA, Huebner DM, Forrest TS. Sonography in the diagnosis of acute appendicitis. *Am Fam Physician* 1991;44:465–468.

65. Rao PM, Rhea JT, Novelline RA, et al. Helical CT combined with contrast material administered only through the colon for imaging of suspected appendicitis. *AJR Am J Roentgenol* 1997;169:1275–1280.

66. Rao PM, Rhea JT, Rattner DW, et al. Introduction of appendiceal CT impact on negative appendectomy and appendiceal perforation rates. *Ann Surg* 1999;229:344–349.

67. Rao PM, Rhea JT, Novelline RA, et al. Effects of computed tomography of the appendix on treatment of patients and use of hospital resources. *N Engl J Med* 1998;338:141–146.

68. Jacobs DO, Settle RG, Clarke JR, et al. Identification of human appendicitis by in vitro nuclear magnetic resonance. *J Surg Res* 1990;48:107–110.

69. Hormann M, Paya K, Eibenberger K, et al. MR imaging in children with nonperforated acute appendicitis: value of unenhanced MR imaging in sonographically selected cases. *AJR Am J Roentgenol* 1998;171:467–470.

70. Conron RW, Abbruzzi K, Cochrane SO, et al. Laparoscopic procedures in pregnancy. *Am Surg* 1998;65:259–263.

71. Hunter JG, Swanstrom L, Thornburg K. Carbon dioxide pneumoperitoneum induces fetal acidosis in a pregnant ewe model. *Surg Endosc* 1995;9:272–279.

72. Curet MJ, Allen D, Josloff RK, et al. Laparoscopy during pregnancy. *Arch Surg* 1996;131:546–551.

73. Gurbuz AT, Peetz ME. The acute abdomen in the pregnant patient. *Surg Endosc* 1997;11:98–102.

74. SAGES. Guidelines for laparoscopic surgery during pregnancy. *Surg Endosc* 1998;12:189–190.

75. Saunders P, Milton PJD. Laparotomy during pregnancy: an assessment of diagnostic accuracy and fetal wastage. *BMJ* 1973;3:165–167.

76. Everson GT. Gastrointestinal motility in pregnancy. *Gastroenterol Clin North Am* 1992;21:751–776.

77. Valdivieso V, Covarrubias C, Siegel F, et al. Pregnancy and cholelithiasis: pathogenesis and natural course of gallstones diagnosed in early puerperium. *Hepatology* 1993;17:1–4.

78. Barbara L, Sama C, Morselli Labate AM, et al. A population study on the prevalence of gallstone disease: the Sirmione Study. *Hepatology* 1987;7:913–917.

79. Basso L, McCollum PT, Darling MN, et al. A study of cholelithiasis during pregnancy and its relationship with age, parity, menarche, breast-feeding, dysmenorrhea, oral contraception, and a maternal history of cholelithiasis. *Surgery* 1992;175:41–46.

80. Mayer IE, Hussain H. Abdominal pain during pregnancy. *Gastroenterol Clin North Am* 1998;27:1–36.

81. Gerwig WH, Thistlethwaite JR. Cholecystitis and cholelithiasis in young women following pregnancy. *Surgery* 1950;28:983–996.

82. Scott LD. Gallstone disease and pancreatitis in pregnancy. *Gastroenterol Clin North Am* 1992;21:803–815.

83. Steinbrook RA, Brooks DC, Datta S. Laparoscopic cholecystectomy during pregnancy review of anesthetic management: surgical considerations. *Surg Endosc* 1996;10:511–515.

84. Epstein FB. Acute abdominal pain in pregnancy. *Emerg Med Clin North Am* 1994;12:151–165.

85. Simon JA. Biliary tract disease and related surgical disorders during pregnancy. *Clin Obstet Gynecol* 1983;26:810–821.

86. Dixon NP, Faddis DM, Silberman H. Aggressive management of cholecystitis during pregnancy. *Am J Surg* 1987;154:292–294.

87. Glasgow RE, Visser BC, Harris HW, et al. Changing management of gallstone disease during pregnancy. *Surg Endosc* 1998;12:241–246.

88. Graham G, Baxi L, Tharakan T. Laparoscopic cholecystectomy during pregnancy: a case series and review of the literature. *Obstet Gynecol Surv* 1998;53:566–574.

89. Hiatt JR, Hiatt JCG, Williams RA, et al. Biliary disease in pregnancy: strategy for surgical management. *Am J Surg* 1986;151:263–265.

90. Eichenberg BJ, Vanderlinden J, Miguel C, et al. Laparoscopic

cholecystectomy in the third trimester of pregnancy. *Am Surg* 1996;62:874–877.

91. Baillie J, Cairns SR, Cotton PB. Endoscopic management of choledocholithiasis during pregnancy. *Surgery* 1990;171: 1–4.
92. Printen KJ, Ott RA. Cholecystectomy during pregnancy. *Am Surg* 1978;44:432–434.
93. Pucci RO, Seed RW. Case report of laparoscopic cholecystectomy in the third trimester of pregnancy. *Am J Obstet Gynecol* 1991;165:401–402.
94. Elerding SC. Laparoscopic cholecystectomy in pregnancy. *Am J Surg* 1993;165:625–627.
95. McKellar DP, Anderson CT, Boynton CJ, et al. Cholecystectomy during pregnancy without fetal loss. *Surg Gynecol Obstet* 1992;174:465–468.
96. Amos JD, Schorr SJ, Norman PF, et al. Laparoscopic surgery during pregnancy. *Am J Surg* 1996;171:435–437.
97. Lanzafame RJ. Laparoscopic cholecystectomy during pregnancy. *Surgery* 1995;118:627–633.
98. Axelrad AM, Fleischer DE, Strack LL, et al. Performance of ERCP for symptomatic choledocholithiasis during pregnancy: techniques to increase safety and improve patient management. *Am J Gastroenterol* 1994;89:109–112.
99. Amouyal P, Amouyal G, Levy P, et al. Diagnosis of choledocholithiasis by endoscopic ultrasonography. *Gastroenterology* 1994;106:1062–1067.
100. Parada AA, Goncalves MOL, Tafner E, et al. Endoscopic papillotomy under ultra-sonographic control. *Int Surg* 1991;76: 75–76.
101. Yu-leung C, Chan ACW, Lam WWM, et al. Choledocholithiasis: comparison of MR cholangiography and endoscopic retrograde cholangiography. *Radiology* 1996;200:85–89.
102. Davis MR, Bohon CJ. Intestinal obstruction in pregnancy. *Clin Obstet Gynecol* 1983;26:832–842.
103. Hill LM, Symmonds RE. Small bowel obstruction in pregnancy: a report and review of four cases. *Obstet Gynecol* 1976;49:170–173.
104. Perdue PW, Johnson HW, Stafford PW. Intestinal obstruction complicating pregnancy. *Am J Surg* 1992;164:384–388.
105. Lord SA, Boswell WC, Hungerpiller JC. Sigmoid volvulus in pregnancy. *Am Surg* 1996;62:380–382.
106. Kantor HM. Midgut volvulus in pregnancy: a case report. *J Reprod Med* 1990;35:577–580.
107. Pratt AT, Donaldson RC, Evertson LR, et al. Cecal volvulus in pregnancy. *Obstet Gynecol* 1981;57:37S–40S.
108. Rothstein RD, Rombeau JL. Intestinal malrotation during pregnancy. *Obstet Gynecol* 1993;81:817–819.
109. Meyerson S, Holtz T, Ehrinpreis M, et al. Small bowel obstruction in pregnancy. *Am J Gastroenterol* 1995;90: 299–302.
110. McLean DW, Arminski TC, Bradley GT. Management of primary carcinoma of the rectum diagnosed during pregnancy. *Am J Surg* 1955;90:816–825.
111. Woods JB, Martin JN Jr, Ingram FH, et al. Pregnancy complicated by carcinoma of the colon above the rectum. *Am J Perinatol* 1992;9:102–110.
112. Antonelli NM, Dotters DJ, Katz VL, et al. Cancer in pregnancy: a review of the literature, part 1. *Obstet Gynecol Surv* 1996;51:125–142.
113. Nesbitt JC, Moise KJ, Sawyers JL. Colorectal carcinoma in pregnancy. *Arch Surg* 1985;120:636–640.
114. Bernstein MA, Madoff RD, Caushaj PF. Colon and rectal cancer in pregnancy. *Dis Colon Rectum* 1993;36:172–178.
115. Francavilla A, Leo D, Polimeno L, et al. Nuclear and cytosolic estrogen receptors in human colon carcinoma and in surrounding noncancerous colonic tissue. *Gastroenterology* 1987;93:1301–1306.
116. Stedman KE, Moore GE, Morgan RT. Estrogen receptor proteins in diverse human tumors. *Arch Surg* 1980;115:244–248.
117. Wobbes T, Beex LVAM, Koenders AMJ. Estrogen and progestin receptors in colonic cancer? *Dis Colon Rectum* 1984; 27:591–592.
118. Smith C, Butler JA. Colorectal cancer in patients younger than 40 years of age. *Dis Colon Rectum* 1989;32:843–846.
119. Pitluk H, Poticha SM. Carcinoma of the colon and rectum in patients less than 40 years of age. *Surg Gynecol Obstet* 1983;157:335–337.
120. Cappell MS. Colon cancer during pregnancy: the gastroenterologist's perspective. *Gastroenterol Clin North Am* 1998; 7:225–256.
121. McCall JL, Black RB, Rich CA, et al. The value of serum carcinoembryonic antigen in predicting recurrent disease following curative resection of colorectal cancer. *Dis Colon Rectum* 1994;37:875–881.
122. Mason MH III, Kovalcik PJ. Ovarian metastases from colon carcinoma. *J Surg Oncol* 1981;17:33–38.
123. Walsh C, Fazio VW. Cancer of the colon, rectum, and anus during pregnancy: the surgeon's perspective. *Gastroenterol Clin North Am* 1998;27:257–267.
124. Zemlickis D, Lishner M, Degendorfer P, et al. Fetal outcome after in utero exposure to cancer chemotherapy. *Arch Intern Med* 1992;152:573–576.
125. Mayr NA, Wen B-C, Saw CB. Radiation therapy during pregnancy. *Obstet Gynecol Clin North Am* 1998;25:301–321.

SURGERY: SCIENTIFIC PRINCIPLES AND PRACTICE, Third Edition, edited by
Lazar J. Greenfield, Michael W. Mulholland, Keith T. Oldham, Gerald B. Zelenock,
and Keith D. Lillemoe. Lippincott Williams & Wilkins Publishers, Philadelphia, © 2001.

CHAPTER 105

CUTANEOUS NEOPLASMS

ALFRED E. CHANG, TIMOTHY M. JOHNSON, AND RILEY S. REES

Cutaneous neoplasms are the most commonly diagnosed malignant tumors in the United States, with an incidence of more than 900,000 annually. The most common skin cancers are the basal and squamous cell carcinomas (BCCs and SCCs). Cutaneous melanomas represent only 3% of all of skin cancers, but they account for at least 65% of skin cancer deaths. The early diagnosis and surgical treatment of these skin cancers can be curative.

MELANOMA

Epidemiology and Etiology

The incidence of melanoma in the United States is approximately 44,200 new cases per year, or 4% of all newly diagnosed cancers (1). More important, the incidence of melanoma has increased faster than that of any other cancer. Between 1973 and 1987, the Surveillance Program of the National Cancer Institute found an 83% increase in the incidence of melanoma (2) (Fig. 105.1). Because cutaneous melanomas are readily diagnosed, this increased incidence probably is not related to improved diagnostic methods or screening. Fortunately, the mortality rates are not increasing at the same rate, primarily because patients are presenting at an earlier stage of tumor development, which allows a much higher cure rate.

The typical patient with melanoma has a fair complexion and a tendency to sunburn rather than to tan, even after a relatively brief exposure to sunlight. Melanoma occurs infrequently in blacks and Asians, suggesting that skin pigment plays a protective role. Melanoma incidence is subject to large geographic and ethnic variations, mainly because of an inverse correlation with latitude and with degree of skin pigmentation (3). Specifically, populations residing closer to the equator have a higher incidence of melanoma. In Queensland, Australia, where the predominantly fair-skinned population is perennially exposed to sunlight, one of the highest occurrences of melanoma can be found—approximately 49.5 per 100,000 population (4). Increases in incidence of melanoma at specific body sites have been reported to be consistent with changes in clothing habits over time (e.g., the trunk in men, lower limbs in women, upper limbs in both sexes).

The reasons for the rising incidence of melanoma are not clear but may be related to an increased exposure to ultraviolet radiation (UVR) from sunlight that reaches the earth's surface. In part, this increased UVR exposure may result from increased recreational exposure to sunlight. In addition, increased UVR exposure may be caused by decreasing levels of stratospheric ozone, which acts as a highly effective absorbing layer that prevents UVR wavelengths, especially UVB (280 to 320 nm), from reaching humans. It has been postulated that an increasing level of chlorofluorocarbons in the stratosphere has been responsible for decreased ozone levels. The causal relation between UVR and melanoma is based on indirect experimental and clinical data; the evidence for an etiologic role of UVR in the induction of nonmelanoma cancers is more compelling. In 1928, it was demonstrated that UVR can induce nonmelanoma skin cancers in experimental animals. It was later shown that this effect was restricted to wavelengths shorter than 320 nm. In patients with xeroderma pigmentosum, who are unable to repair genetic material damaged by UVR, exposure to UVR leads to the development of melanoma and nonmelanoma skin cancers, suggesting a direct causal role in the induction of these neoplasms.

Other possible mechanisms for the role of UVR in causing melanomas have been postulated. According to the classic initiation–promotion model of carcinogenesis established in experimental animal studies, the first step involves initiating factors that directly interact with the cellular DNA to induce mutations in the genome. Afterward, this process is further driven by promotional factors, which are not mutagenic by themselves but enhance the proliferation of mutated cells. In addition to the evidence that UVR is an initiating agent, it has been shown experimentally that UVR can act as a promoter of chemical carcinogens to cause cutaneous melanomas. As a promoting agent, UVR can act to influence the proliferation of an initiated (mutated) cell population or, alternatively, to influence the genetic expression of an initiated cell. Another possible mechanism by which UVR induces skin cancers may be its effect on the immune surveillance of initiated cells (5). It has been suggested that UVR affects Langerhans cells, which are antigen-presenting cells in the epidermis and represent the most superficial sentinel of the immune system. UVR exposure has been shown to result in the development of suppressor T lymphocytes that interfere with the rejection of initiated cells. Although UVR is an etiologic agent that can cause melanoma and other skin cancers, this does not exclude other mechanisms by which these tumors can arise.

Other, nonenvironmental factors are also associated with an increased risk for melanoma. In 3% to 5% of patients who have had one melanoma diagnosed, another melanoma develops. This risk is 10 times higher than that of the general population, in which the risk for melanoma is approximately 0.53%. Another group at increased risk for melanoma are those with dysplastic nevi. These patients have a 10% overall lifetime risk for development of melanoma, which is a 20-fold increase compared with the general population. Dysplastic nevi are acquired lesions of the skin that have characteristics distinguishing them from common nevi. They are usually larger than common nevi, ranging from 5 to 12 mm in diameter. Anatomically, dysplastic nevi can appear anywhere on the body, and they most frequently are found on the trunk. Their concentration on covered areas, such as the buttocks, breasts, and scalp, represents a distribution different from that of most acquired nevi. Melanoma can arise within a preexisting dysplastic nevus or de novo in patients with dysplastic nevi. Dysplastic nevi can be found both in the general population (sporadic form) and in melanoma-prone families (familial form). The latter syndrome, originally known as the *B-K mole syndrome,* has an autosomal dominant hereditary pattern and is referred to as *dysplastic nevus syndrome, familial type* (6). The lifetime risk of melanoma can approach 100% for patients with this syndrome.

Another risk factor associated with the development of melanoma is the presence of congenital nevi. A congenital nevus is a melanocytic nevus present at birth. Congenital nevi occur in 1% to 2.5% of the population. These lesions have been categorized by size into small (<1.5 cm diameter), medium (1.5 to 20 cm diameter), and large (>20 cm diameter) nevi. Ninety percent of congenital nevi are of the small type. Large congenital nevi can vary greatly in size and can occupy a major portion of the body surface. They have clinical features that include a grossly irregular surface, increased pigmentation with shades of brown, and hypertrichosis. The lifetime risk of melanoma in patients with large congenital nevi has been estimated to be between 5% and 20%. The management of large congenital nevi is complex and should be individualized to accommodate such factors as technical difficulty, cosmetic results, and perceived risk of melanoma. It is unclear to what extent melanoma develops in small and medium

congenital nevi. Data are insufficient to recommend prophylactic excision of all congenital nevi.

Genetics

Approximately 8% to 12% of cutaneous melanomas occur in people with a familial predisposition. These individuals usually have dysplastic nevi as well. Most evidence indicates an autosomal dominant model of transmission for hereditary melanoma with variable penetrance. Some investigators propose a polygenic model of melanoma genesis involving two or more genes and inclusion of environmental factors. The theory of modulation of genetic risk by environmental factors explains the 10-fold increase in incidence of melanoma among Australian families compared with their Celtic ancestors.

The chromosomes reported to be most commonly mutated in melanoma are 1, 6, 7, 9, and 10 (7). Linkage analysis has suggested that hereditary melanoma and dysplastic nevi are associated with mutations in chromosomes 1p and 9p (8). Earlier studies suggest that abnormalities in chromosome 9 may be involved in the initiating events in melanoma tumorigenesis. As is discussed later, the *p16/CDKN2A* gene has been identified on chromosome 9p21 and appears to be an important susceptibility gene (9). Abnormalities in the 1p region probably occur late in melanoma progression. A common mutation in sporadic human melanoma is deletion of the long arm of chromosome 6, which occurs in approximately 40% of these lesions. Correction of this genetic defect can convert a malignant melanoma cell to a normal cell phenotype, suggesting that a tumor suppressor gene may be located on chromosome 6q (10). Abnormalities in chromosome 7 have been documented in more than half of patients with advanced melanoma. Chromosome 7 maps for the epider-

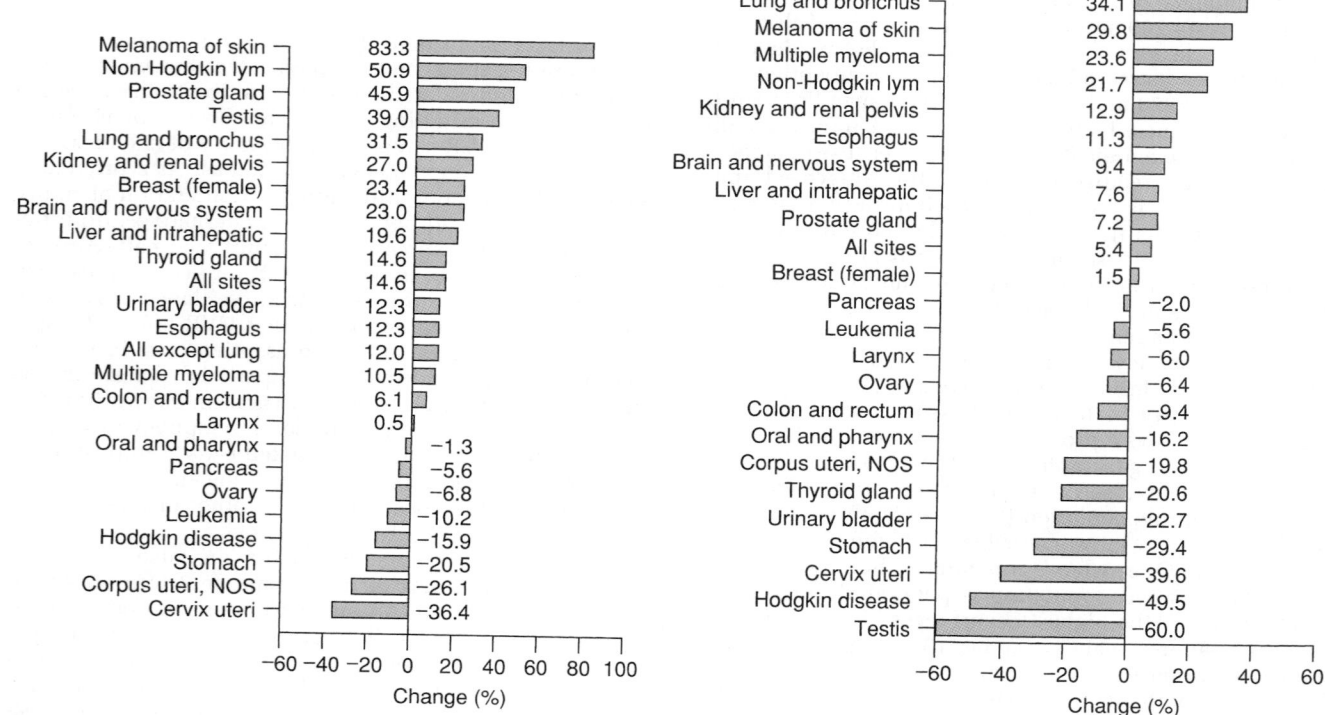

Figure 105.1. Changes in cancer incidence *(left)* and mortality *(right)* in the United States between 1973 and 1987. Data were compiled by the Surveillance Program of the National Cancer Institute. Melanoma incidence has increased faster than that of any other cancer.

mal growth factor receptor, and the mutational defects on chromosome 7 appear to be correlated with overexpression of these receptors on tumor cells. Chromosome 10 translocations have been observed in DNA from melanoma tumors and from dysplastic moles, indicating that this chromosome may be involved in melanoma evolution.

The *p16/CDKN2A* gene has been found on chromosome 9p21 and is critical to the control of cell proliferation or differentiation (9). It has variously been denoted as *p16, MTS1, INK4A, CDKN2, CDKN2A,* or some combination of these. This gene is thought to be a cancer susceptibility gene associated with melanoma development; it encodes two entirely unrelated proteins, *p16* and *19ARF. p16* is an important negative regulator of cell cycle progression through its interaction and inhibition of cyclin-dependent kinases. Hence, genetic alterations of this gene would result in increased cell proliferation, making *p16* a tumor suppressor gene. *p19ARF* has no amino acid homology to *p16*. It is able to induce G_1 and G_2 arrest, but does not do this through cyclin-dependent kinases. It is also a candidate tumor suppressor gene which works independently from mutations of *p16*. Alterations of *p16/CDKN2A* are detected in up to 80% of melanoma tumor lines (9). In familial melanoma, depending on the method of detection, this gene is altered in up to 50% of families. Besides melanoma risk, alterations in *p16/CDKN2A* have also been associated with an increased risk for development of pancreatic cancer (11).

Two other genes that have been implicated in a predisposition to melanoma development are the retinoblastoma gene *(RB1)* and the *CDK4* gene (9). Evidence regarding the role of *RB1* in melanoma development is largely epidemiologic. In patients with hereditary retinoblastoma, the relative risk of death from melanoma as a second cancer is 94. A point mutation of the *CDK4* gene, which encodes for a cyclin-dependent kinase, has been observed in sporadic as well as melanoma-prone kindreds (9). The *CDK4* mutation acts as an oncogene and makes the protein insensitive to being shut off by cyclin-dependent kinase inhibitors. Both the *RB1* and *CDK4* genes are thought to be involved with a small proportion of familial or sporadic melanomas.

Clinical Diagnosis and Classification

Melanomas have a characteristic appearance (Fig. 105.2) (see color insert following page 1190). Early detection by visual inspection can lead to definitive diagnosis and cure if careful attention is paid to certain features. First, color often varies: brown or black lesions may contain shades of white, red, or blue. Of all the colors, shades of blue are the most ominous. Second, an angular indentation or notching is frequently present at the perimeter of the lesion. Third, irregular elevations of the surface are characteristic. Another indication of potential malignancy is enlargement, darkening, bleeding, or ulceration of a pigmented lesion. None of these clinical signs is pathognomonic, because these features can be present in pigmented BCCs, pigmented seborrheic keratoses, Spitz nevi, dermatofibromas, or hemangiomas. Therefore, any lesion with these characteristics should be excised for biopsy.

Based on growth patterns and clinical characteristics, melanomas can be classified into four major categories: lentigo maligna melanomas, superficial spreading melanomas, nodular melanomas, and acral lentiginous melanomas (12). Lentigo maligna melanomas constitute 10% to 15% of cutaneous melanomas and are the least aggressive of the four types. They typically occur on the sun-exposed areas of the head and neck and the dorsum of the hands. The median age at diagnosis is 70 years, and preva-

lence favors women. Clinically, they are large (>3 cm), flat, tan lesions with areas of dark brown or black pigmentation in some parts and areas of regression in others. Histologically, there is radial growth of abnormal melanocytes in the epidermis with minimal invasion into the papillary dermis. This radial growth process precedes vertical growth and invasion into the papillary dermis by many years. If only a radial growth component is seen, this lesion is called a lentigo maligna, or Hutchinson's freckle, and is not a malignant melanoma (Fig. 105.2B). The vertical growth component is associated with a focal area of elevation that may be darker or lighter than the surrounding lentigo maligna.

Superficial spreading melanomas account for approximately 70% of cutaneous melanomas and are of intermediate malignancy compared with the other types. These lesions usually arise in a preexisting nevus. The peak incidence is in the fifth decade of life, with an equal distribution between the sexes. There is both a radial and a vertical growth phase. The radial growth phase is characterized by the presence of melanoma tumor cells in the epidermis and papillary dermis and development of a raised, irregular surface on the skin. Vertical growth into the deeper layers of skin is associated with increasing nodularity of the lesion and a greater potential to metastasize. As is discussed later, the depth of invasion has a direct correlation with metastatic potential and prognosis. Superficial spreading melanomas are typically characterized by variation in color, irregular borders, and irregular surface.

Nodular melanomas occur in approximately 15% to 30% of patients with cutaneous melanoma and are the most aggressive of the four types of melanoma. The median age at diagnosis is 50 years, and these lesions occur twice as often in men as in women. They commonly arise from uninvolved skin rather than from a preexisting nevus. In general, nodular melanomas are bluish-black, are more uniform in coloration than the other types, and have smooth borders. They are almost exclusively characterized by a vertical growth phase invading into the deeper layers of skin and often into the subcutis. The lack of a radial growth phase can make early diagnosis difficult.

Acral lentiginous melanoma is a distinct clinicopathologic variant of melanoma that occurs on the palms and soles and in subungual locations (Fig. 105.2G). Acral lentiginous melanoma occurs in only 2% to 8% of whites with melanoma but in 35% to 60% of dark-pigmented people (e.g., blacks, Hispanics, Asians) who have melanoma. Diagnosis usually is made in the sixth decade of life. These lesions are characterized by a radial growth phase, usually of long duration, followed by a nodular, vertical growth phase associated with metastatic potential. The radial growth phase is associated with a flat lesion with color variation. In subungual locations, this phase can present as an irregular, tan-brown streak in the nail that originates from the base of the nail bed. More than three fourths of subungual melanomas involve the great toe or thumb, and they can be confused with subungual hematoma.

Staging and Prognostic Factors

A great deal of information is available regarding various factors that correlate with the clinical outcome of patients with melanoma. Some of these prognostic factors, such as microstaging and nodal status, are of sufficient independent significance to be incorporated into staging systems with known survival rates. Other prognostic factors, such as sex, age, anatomic location of the primary melanoma, and ulceration, are of variable importance and are discussed later in this section.

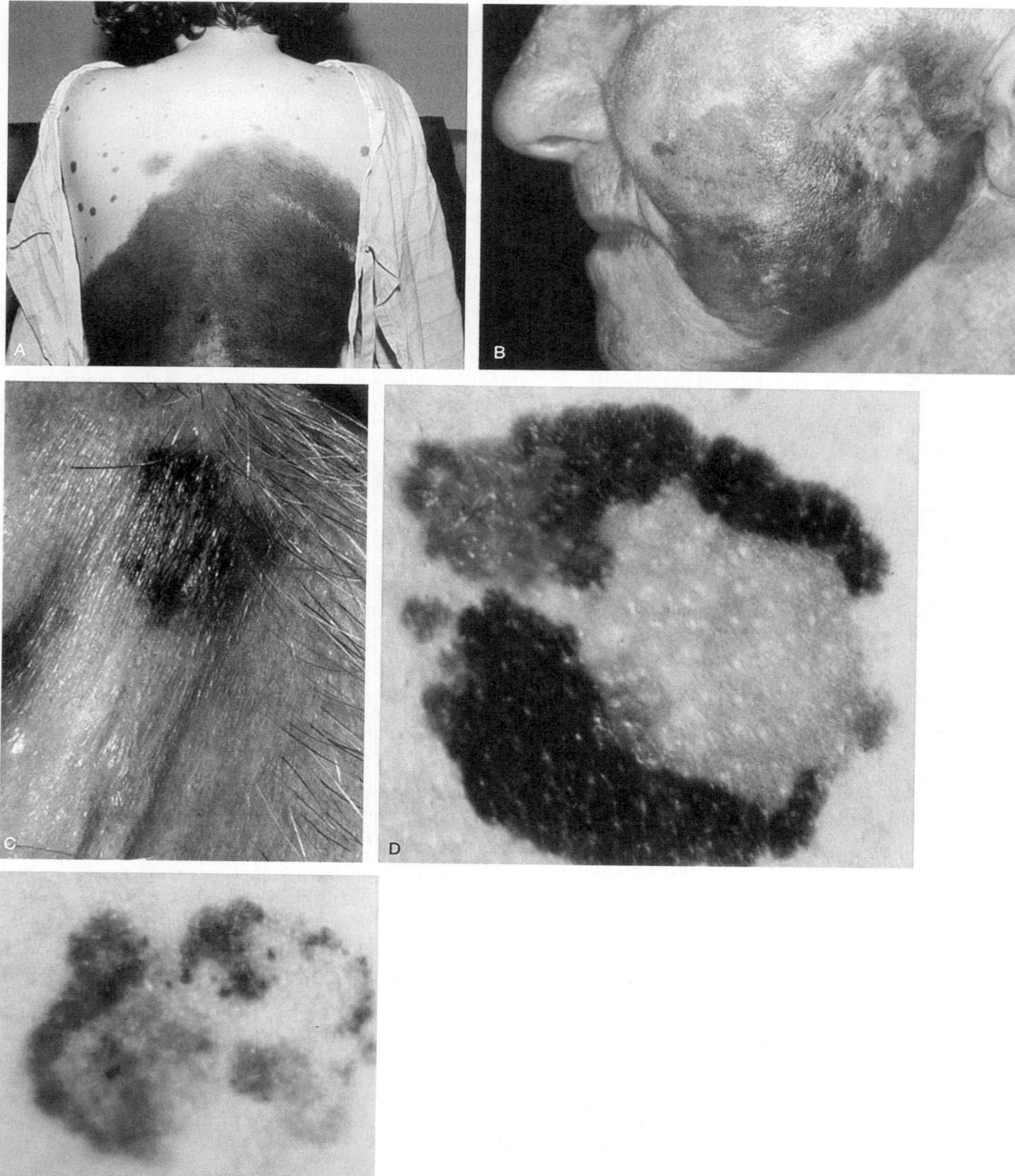

Figure 105.2. Examples of skin lesions. *(A)* Giant congenital nevus. *(B)* Lentigo maligna (Hutchinson freckle). *(C)* Melanoma arising in a lentigo maligna (lentigo maligna melanoma). *(D and E)* Superficial spreading melanoma. *(continues)*

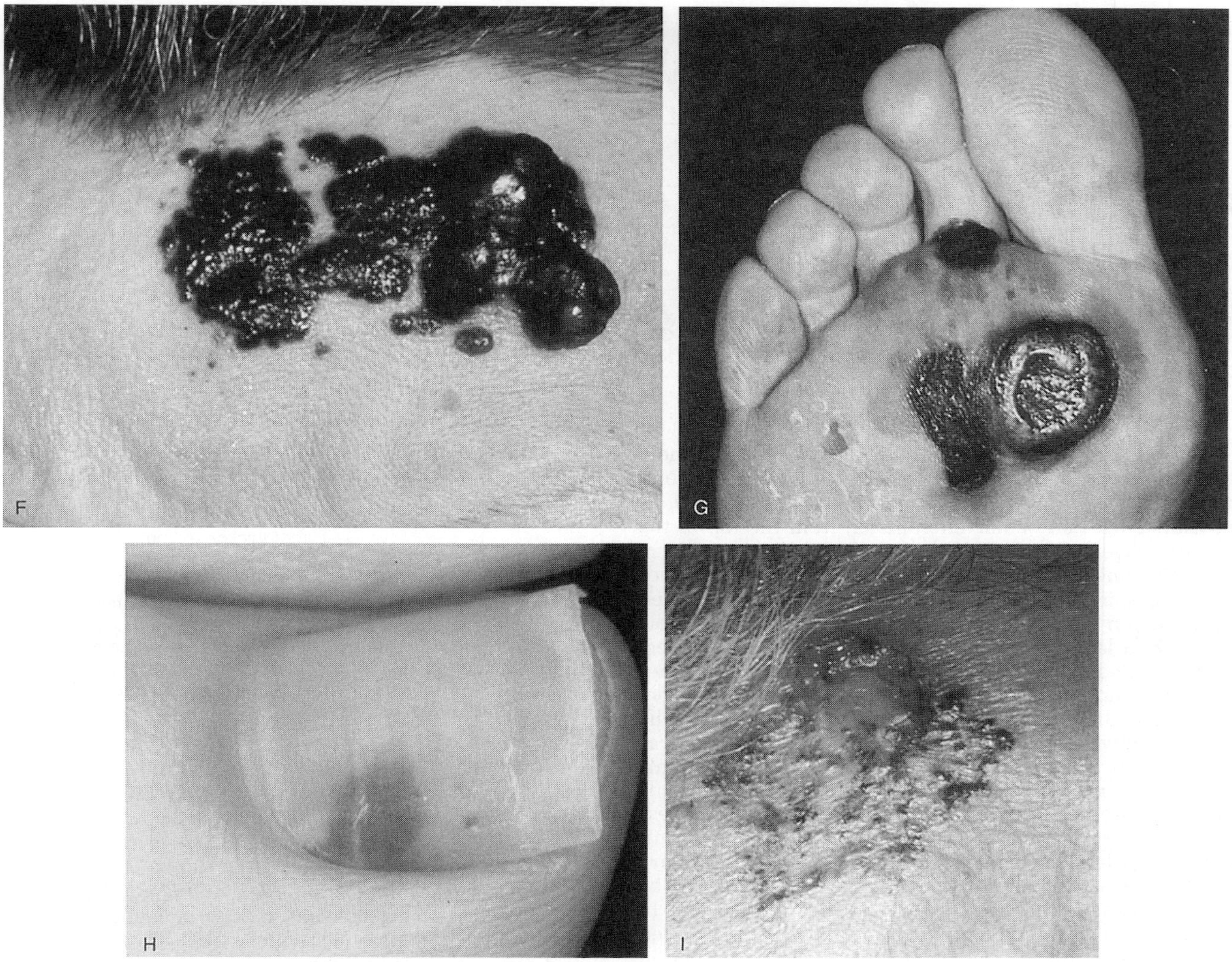

Figure 105.2. *(Continued) (F)* Nodular melanoma. *(G)* Acral lentiginous melanoma (ulcerated nodular plantar melanoma with satellite lesions). *(H)* Subungual melanoma. *(I)* Pigmented basal cell carcinoma.

Microstaging

One of the most important prognostic features of cutaneous melanoma is the stage of development of the primary tumor. Two methods have been described that assess the microstages of development. Clark and associates (12) described a system by which melanomas are classified according to depth of invasion. They described five levels of invasion related to the histologically defined layers of the skin. The levels are illustrated in Fig. 105.3 and are defined as follows:

Level I: All tumor cells are confined to the epidermis with no invasion through the basement membrane (also known as melanoma in situ).
Level II: Tumor cells penetrate through the basement membrane into the papillary dermis but do not extend to the reticular dermis.
Level III: Tumor cells fill the papillary dermis and abut the reticular dermis but do not invade it.
Level IV: Tumor cells extend into the reticular dermis.
Level V: Tumor cells invade the subcutaneous tissues.

The correlation of the Clark level of invasion with survival is summarized in Table 105.1 (13–17). In general, patients with melanoma in situ (Clark level I) are not con-

sidered to have a malignant tumor with potential to metastasize and are adequately treated by complete excision with a 0.5-cm margin of surrounding normal skin. Patients with Clark level II, III, IV, and V tumors have 5-year survival rates of 88%, 66%, 54%, and 22%, respectively.

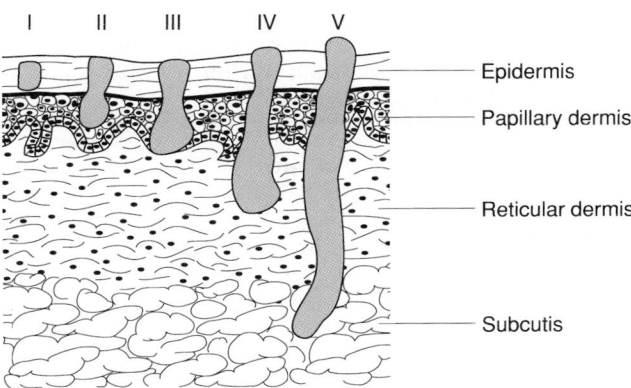

Figure 105.3. The Clark levels of invasion.

Table 105.1. RELATION BETWEEN THE CLARK CLASSIFICATION LEVEL OF INVASION OF PRIMARY MELANOMA AND SURVIVAL

		5-Year survival rate by level (%)			
Author	**Patients**	**II**	**III**	**IV**	**V**
Clark et al.[13]	208	72	47	32	12
McGovern[14]	183	82	65	49	29
Wanebo et al.[15]	151	100	58	58	6
Balch et al.[6]	212	85	72	57	28
Eldh et al.[17]	324	100	87	72	35
Total	687	X̄ = 88	66	54	22

The other microstaging method that is used routinely was originally described by Breslow (18). This method classifies the primary tumor according to it thickness, as measured with an ocular micrometer, from the top of the granular layer to the base of the tumor. Many investigators have documented an inverse correlation between tumor thickness and survival. A series of 1,786 patients reported on by Balch and colleagues (19) is summarized in Table 105.2. In a larger series of patients, the same researchers demonstrated a continuous inverse relation between tumor thickness and 10-year mortality rate (20) (Fig. 105.4). From these data, they derived a mathematic model defining the relation between tumor thickness and survival, which was confirmed by its application to a different group of patients with melanoma with localized disease.

Several studies have demonstrated that tumor thickness conveys more prognostic information than does determination of Clark level of invasion. Within a single Clark level of invasion, gradations of tumor thickness can be found that have independent prognostic significance. In addition, the measurement of tumor thickness is often more reproducible and less subjective than determination of the Clark level of invasion.

Regional Lymph Node Involvement

The presence of regional lymph node metastases is a grave sign that is associated with a poor prognosis. As in other solid malignancies, such as breast and colorectal cancer, the number of involved lymph nodes has an inverse correlation with long-term survival. The 5-year survival rate for patients with melanoma with multiple involved lymph nodes is between 8% and 26% (21–24)

Table 105.2. RELATION BETWEEN THE BRESLOW CLASSIFICATION OF TUMOR THICKNESS OF PRIMARY MELANOMA AND SURVIVAL[a]

Thickness range (mm)	Patients	5-Year survival rate (%)
≤0.75	357	89
0.76–1.49	388	75
1.50–2.49	295	58
2.50–3.99	218	46
>4	184	25

[a]No clinical evidence of regional or disseminated disease. Data from Balch CM, Soong SJ, Milton GW, et al. A comparison of prognostic factors and surgical results in 1,786 patients with localized (stage I) melanoma treated in Alabama, USA, and New South Wales, Australia. Ann Surg 1982;196:677.

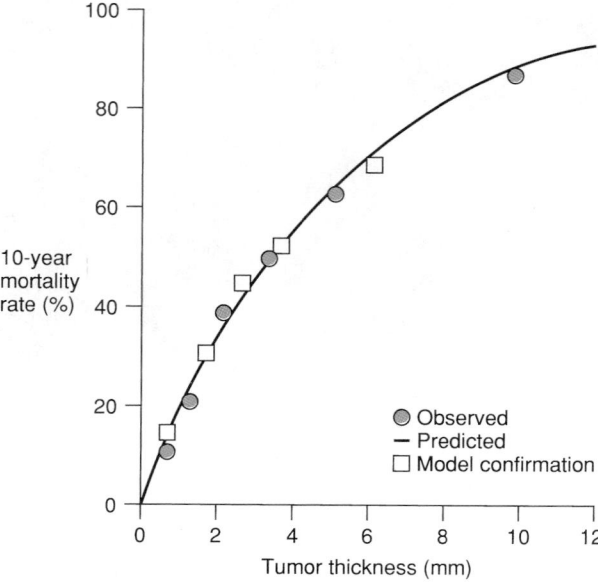

Figure 105.4. Linear relation between melanoma tumor thickness and mortality rates. The solid line represents mortality predicted by a mathematic model, and the closed circles demonstrate the actual mortality rate in 2,627 patients (20). The accuracy of the model was verified by applying it to 747 patients with localized melanoma from the World Health Organization Melanoma Group and is shown by squares.

(Table 105.3). For patients with only one or two positive lymph nodes, the range is 30% to 55%.

Clinical and Pathologic Staging

The American Joint Committee on Cancer (AJCC) developed a five-stage system that divides melanomas according to tumor thickness (T), nodal status (N), and metastatic disease (M). The current system was revised in 1998 and is summarized in Table 105.4. Briefly, stage 0 represents melanoma in situ. Stages I and II are localized melanomas up to 4 mm in thickness. Stage III includes patients with lesions greater than 4 mm in thickness, or patients with regional nodal involvement. Stage IV represent patients with any evidence of metastatic disease beyond the regional lymph nodes. Based on these stages, the sur-

Table 105.3. RELATION BETWEEN POSITIVE REGIONAL LYMPH NODES AND SURVIVAL[a]

Investigators	Patients	Positive lymph nodes	Survival rate (%) 5 y	10 y
Cohen et al.[21]	117	1–3	55	55
		≥4	26	26
Callery et al.[22]	150	1–3	45	—
		≥4	21	—
Calabro et al.[23]	1,001	>1	45	39
		2–4	37	28
		5–10	20	17
		>10	5	3
Bevilacqua et al.[24]	176	>1	50	43
		2–3	37	37
		>3	17	8

[a]Patients presenting with AJC clinical stage I, II, or III.

Table 105.4. AMERICAN JOINT COMMISSION ON CANCER MELANOMA STAGING SYSTEM, 1998

TNM DEFINITIONS

Primary Tumor

TX	Unknown, cannot be assessed
T0	No evidence of primary tumor
Tis	Melanoma in situ (atypical melanocyte hyperplasia, Clark I)
T1	<0.75 mm (Clark II)
T2	0.76–1.50 mm (Clark III)
T3	1.51–4 mm (Clark IV)
T4	>4 mm or satellites within 2 cm of primary (Clark V)

Regional Lymph Node Involvement

NX	Unknown, cannot be assessed
N0	Negative
N1	Metastasis 3 cm or less in greatest dimension in any regional lymph node(s)
N2	Metastasis >3 cm in greatest dimension in any regional lymph node(s) and/or in-transit metastasis

Distant Metastasis

MX	Unknown, cannot be assessed
M0	No distinct metastasis
M1	Distant metastasis

STAGE GROUPINGS

Stage 0	Tis, N0, M0
State I	T1, N0, M0
	T2, N0, M0
Stage II	T3, N0, M0
Stage III	T4, N0, M0
	Any T, N1, M0
	Any T, N2, M0
Stage IV	Any T, Any N, M1

vival rates of each group, excluding stage 0, are depicted in Fig. 105.5.

Other Prognostic Factors

The major prognostic factors that predict survival in melanoma patients have been accounted for in the AJCC staging system: namely, tumor microstaging, nodal status, and distant metastases. Nevertheless, because most pa-tients with newly diagnosed melanomas have localized disease, additional prognostic information can be helpful to the patient and the clinician. Several other factors eval-uated in multifactorial analyses of localized AJCC stage I and II disease are significant predictors of survival.

The anatomic location of melanomas is a significant in-dependent prognostic indicator in patients with clinically localized disease (25). Patients with melanomas of the ex-tremities, excluding the hands and feet, have a better sur-vival rate than those with lesions arising on the trunk or on the head and neck. Among patients with extremity melanomas, those with lesions on their hands and feet do significantly worse than patients with lesions on the re-maining extremity sites. Certain anatomic subsites, includ-ing the upper back, posterior arm, posterior neck, and pos-terior scalp, appear to be associated with a poorer prognosis for intermediate-thickness melanomas (Table 105.5).

Women with melanomas have a better survival rate than men (26). One explanation for this observation may be the different distribution sites of melanomas in men and women. In several studies, the incidence of melanomas arising in the lower extremities, a favorable anatomic lo-cation, is significantly higher in women than in men. Con-versely, the incidence of truncal melanomas, which are generally associated with poorer survival, is higher in men than in women (Table 105.6). The prevalence of head, neck, and upper extremity melanomas is equal in men and women.

The presence of ulceration in a melanoma appears to be associated with a poorer prognosis. In general, patients with ulcerated but localized melanomas have a 10-year survival rate of 50%, whereas those with nonulcerated le-sions have a 10-year survival rate of 78% (20). Men have a higher proportion of ulcerated lesions than women (27% vs. 19%), and this may be another explanation for their lower survival rate. Although ulceration appears to corre-late with thickness of the melanoma, the presence of ul-ceration has been shown to be an independent prognostic factor.

At the cellular level, Clark and coworkers (27) further de-scribed histologic characteristics of localized melanomas that can help determine prognosis. Melanomas were de-scribed according to their particular growth phase. Lesions determined to be in the radial growth phase were nontu-morigenic and were associated with an excellent prognosis.

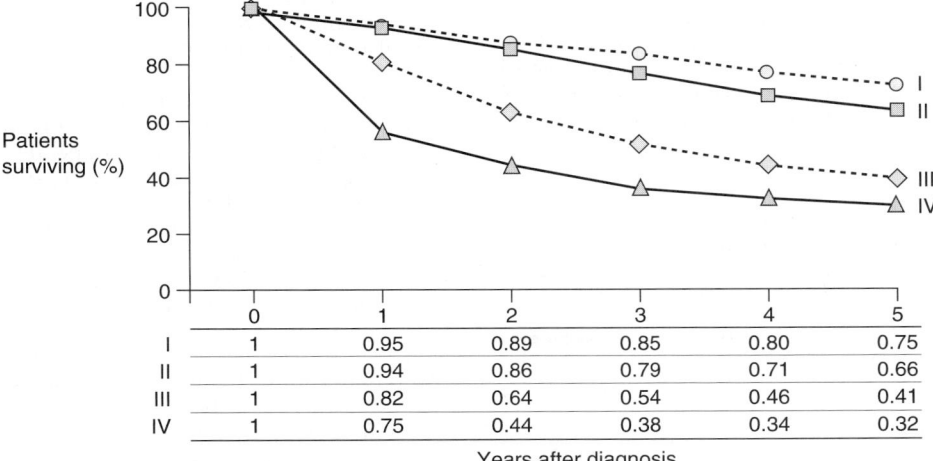

	0	1	2	3	4	5
I	1	0.95	0.89	0.85	0.80	0.75
II	1	0.94	0.86	0.79	0.71	0.66
III	1	0.82	0.64	0.54	0.46	0.41
IV	1	0.75	0.44	0.38	0.34	0.32

Years after diagnosis

Figure 105.5. Survival according to AJCC staging system. Data is taken from the National Cancer Data Base for the years 1985–1989. (From the *AJCC Cancer Staging Handbook*, 5th ed. Philadel-phia: Lippincott–Raven, 1998.)

Table 105.5. SURVIVAL OF AJC CLINICAL STAGE I AND II MELANOMA PATIENTS IN RELATION TO TUMOR LOCATION

| Thickness (mm) | Survival Rate (%)[a] | | | | |
	Extremities	Hands or feet	Head and neck	Trunk[b]	BANS
<0.85	100	100	100	100	98
0.85–1.69	100	100	100	97	78
1.7–3.64	86	60	64	77	58
≥3.65	83	0	65	12	33

[a]7.5-year actuarial survival rates of 598 AJC clinical stage I and II patients.[25]
[b]Non-BANS truncal melanomas.
BANS, upper back, posterolateral arm, posterior and lateral neck, and posterior scalp.

In contrast, lesions determined to have evidence of a vertical growth phase were prone to be tumorigenic. These lesions had the potential to metastasize and were associated with a poorer prognosis. The vertical growth phase was defined as the presence of larger aggregates of tumor cells in the papillary dermis, often markedly different in pigment from cells in the radial growth phase and associated with increased mitotic cells.

Genetic markers will have a more significant role as prognostic factors in the future. The presence of abnormal DNA content (DNA aneuploidy), as determined by flow cytometry, has been reported to be an unfavorable predictor of prognosis in patients with localized melanoma (28). In patients with metastatic melanoma, structural abnormalities of chromosomes 7 or 11, as determined by cytogenetic analysis, have been reported to be associated with decreased survival (29).

Treatment of Primary Melanoma

Biopsy

For melanoma, the tumor thickness (Breslow depth of invasion) is the single variable that most accurately determines therapy and prognosis. A full-thickness biopsy to the adipose tissue is required for any lesion suspect for melanoma. If the melanoma is transected with a partial-thickness shave biopsy, the ability to obtain an accurate measurement of tumor thickness is lost. Therefore, a superficial shave biopsy is never recommended for a suspect pigmented lesion. Before biopsy, a morphologic description of the lesion and a photograph can be useful for com-

Table 105.6. DISTRIBUTION OF MELANOMAS WITH RESPECT TO GENDER

| Location | Occurrence (%) | |
	Men	Women
Scalp	7	3
Face	12	9
Neck	5	3
Arm	13	19
Front of body	16	8
Back of body	36	23
Leg	9	31
Sole of foot	2	4

plete documentation. Also, the use of a Wood's lamp can help to delineate the subclinical pigment extension, particularly with lentigo maligna melanomas on the head and neck.

Excisional biopsy with 1- to 2-mm margins is the preferred method for suspect lesions to provide the pathologist a total specimen for histologic interpretation and microstaging. Formalin-fixed, paraffin-embedded, permanent sections should be used for biopsy diagnosis of primary cutaneous melanoma to determine accurately tumor thickness and other histopathologic prognostic variables. Frozen sections do not have a role in the microstaging of primary melanomas. If the lesion is a melanoma, the excisional biopsy represents the first stage of a two-stage procedure. The second stage is reexcision to the underlying muscle fascia with margins ranging from 0.5 to 3 cm, depending on the tumor thickness (see next section). The orientation of the biopsy is usually determined according to the ease of a potential future wide local excision and parallel orientation to the lymphatic drainage.

For suggestive lesions that are too large for complete excision and those that are located where the amount of skin is critical in terms of functional or cosmetic results, an incisional biopsy may be performed with either a scalpel or a punch tool 4 to 6 mm in diameter. Incisional biopsies for melanoma do not increase the risk of metastasis or affect patient survival. They should be performed on the most raised or most pigmented area of the lesion to maximize the obtainable diagnostic and prognostic information. The most raised area usually corresponds to the maximal thickness of the lesion. Several punch biopsies can be obtained from different areas for lesions with multiple morphologic features.

The excisional or incisional saucerization biopsy technique can also be used for melanoma. After appropriate skin preparation and establishment of local anesthesia, the scalpel blade is placed on the skin at a 45- to 60-degree angle. The skin is cut through the dermis to the adipose tissue, and the biopsy specimen is removed with pickup forceps. Homeostasis is obtained with electrocautery, chemical cautery, or fibrin foam. No sutures are used, and the wound is allowed to heal by second intention, which takes 3 to 6 weeks. Again, a shave biopsy through the dermis is never recommended for a lesion suggestive of melanoma because of the risk of transection of the lesion. One disadvantage of the saucerization biopsy technique is the risk of secondary bacterial colonization in the wound during healing. However, delay of the definitive wide local excision until complete reepithelialization has occurred is usually not necessary with the use of preoperative antibiotics.

Either incisional or excisional biopsy of skin lesions suspected to be melanoma is acceptable. Care must be taken to obtain a full-thickness specimen into the subcutaneous tissue so that the pathologist can determine the microstaging of the lesion. Shave or curet biopsy is not indicated for lesions suspected to be melanoma because microstaging cannot be ascertained from the specimen.

An excisional biopsy can easily be accomplished with lesions less than 1.5 cm in diameter. After infiltration of a local anesthetic around the lesion, but not into it, the lesion can be excised with an elliptical skin incision encompassing underlying subcutaneous tissue (Fig. 105.6). The incision should be placed so as not to compromise a subsequent wide excision. For small lesions, an excisional biopsy can be accomplished with a 6-mm punch biopsy instrument, making sure that underlying subcutaneous tissue is obtained. An incisional biopsy is performed for large lesions and for lesions of the face, hands, or feet, for which the amount of skin is critical. These biopsies can be

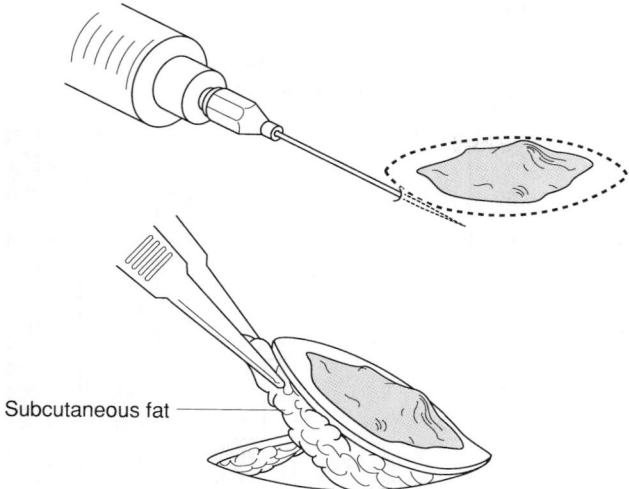

Figure 105.6. Techniques for biopsy of melanoma. (After Urist MM, Balch CM, Milton GW. Surgical management of primary melanoma. In: Balch CM, Milton GW, eds. *Cutaneous melanoma.* Philadelphia: JB Lippincott, 1985:74.)

Table 105.7. SURGICAL MARGINS FOR MELANOMA EXCISIONS

Melanoma thickness (mm)	Margin (cm)
In situ	0.5
<1	1
1–4	2
>4	3

performed with a scalpel or a 6-mm punch biopsy instrument. Care must be taken to obtain the incisional biopsy in the most raised or irregular area of the lesion.

Surgical Excision of Primary Melanoma

For melanoma in situ, excision of normal skin 0.5 cm around the lesion or previous biopsy site is acceptable for local control. For invasive cutaneous melanoma, wide excision of the primary tumor or biopsy site has been advocated for optimal local control. Limited excisions, such as excisional biopsies, are associated with local recurrence rates in the range of 30% to 60%. The optimal extent of the wide excision has been somewhat controversial. Until recently, the routine approach was to excise all primary melanomas with a 3- to 5-cm margin; this procedure often required a split-thickness skin graft for coverage. The rationale for such a generous margin was to remove clinically occult subcutaneous or intradermal satellite deposits of melanoma tumor cells. In numerous reports, wide excision of melanomas, including 3- to 5-cm margins, was associated with local recurrence rates in the range of 7% or less.

With the accumulation of more information, it has become clear that less than the traditional wide local excision is adequate for the surgical treatment of thin melanomas. The risk of local recurrence correlates more with the thickness of the melanoma than with the margin of excision. Local recurrence after excision of melanomas less than 1 mm thick is rare regardless of the extent of the margin. The World Health Organization (30) reported a prospective study in which patients with primary melanomas less than 2 mm thick were randomly assigned to receive excision with margins of either 1 cm (narrow) or 3 cm or more (wide). A total of 612 patients were entered into the study, 305 having narrow excisions and 307 having wide excisions. No local recurrences were seen in any patients with tumors less than 1 mm thick, regardless of the excision margin. Three local recurrences were reported in the group of patients with melanomas 1 to 2 mm thick, all of whom had undergone narrow excision. More important, the disease-free and overall survival rates were not significantly different between the two groups after a median follow-up of 55 months. These results clearly in-

dicate that excision margins of 1 cm provide excellent local control for lesions less than 1 mm thick.

A prospective, randomized study evaluated the efficacy of 2-cm versus 4-cm margins for intermediate-thickness melanomas measuring 1 to 4 mm (31). This study involved 486 patients with localized melanomas who were observed for a median of 6 years after excision. The local recurrence rate was 0.8% for patients who had 2-cm margins and 1.7% for those who had 4-cm margins; the difference was not statistically significant. As expected, the narrower margins significantly reduced the need for skin grafting and shortened the hospital stay. The results of this study demonstrated that 2-cm margins were sufficient to treat intermediate-thickness lesions. For lesions more than 4 mm thick, excision margins of at least 3 cm should be considered the standard approach. Recommended excision margins are outlined in Table 105.7.

Despite these recommendations, the site of the melanoma can affect the extent of the excision. Facial lesions usually cannot be excised with more than a 1-cm margin because of the adjacency of vital structures. Subungual melanomas should always be treated by amputation, usually at the metatarsophalangeal or metacarpophalangeal joint, so that adequate skin closure can be achieved. For plantar melanomas requiring wide excision, split-thickness skin grafts have proved simple and adequate if properly padded shoes are used.

Treatment of Regional Metastatic Melanoma

Lymphadenectomy Results and Indications

Surgical excision of metastases to regional lymph nodes is the only potentially curative therapy. The 5-year survival rate for patients who undergo lymphadenectomy for clinically positive involved nodes (AJCC stage III) ranges from 13% to 39%. In addition, for those patients not cured by lymphadenectomy, resection can avoid potential pain associated with tumor enlargement, skin breakdown, and tumor necrosis (Fig. 105.7). Only 10% of patients who first present with the diagnosis of melanoma have clinical evidence of nodal metastases; approximately 85% have localized disease; the remaining 5% have distant metastases (32). In less than 15% of patients, a diagnosis of melanoma is made in the absence of a definable primary lesion. If patients present with isolated nodal disease from an unknown primary site, the results of lymphadenectomy are similar to those for patients with known primary tumors.

The surgical excision of clinically positive lymph nodes is referred to as a *therapeutic lymph node dissection.* Some surgeons prefer to excise clinically normal-appearing regional lymph nodes because of the risk of occult or microscopic metastases. This procedure is known as *elective lymph node dissection* (ELND). ELND has been one of the most controversial procedures in surgical oncology.

Advocates of ELND claim that resection of occult metastases in the regional nodes can prevent disseminated dis-

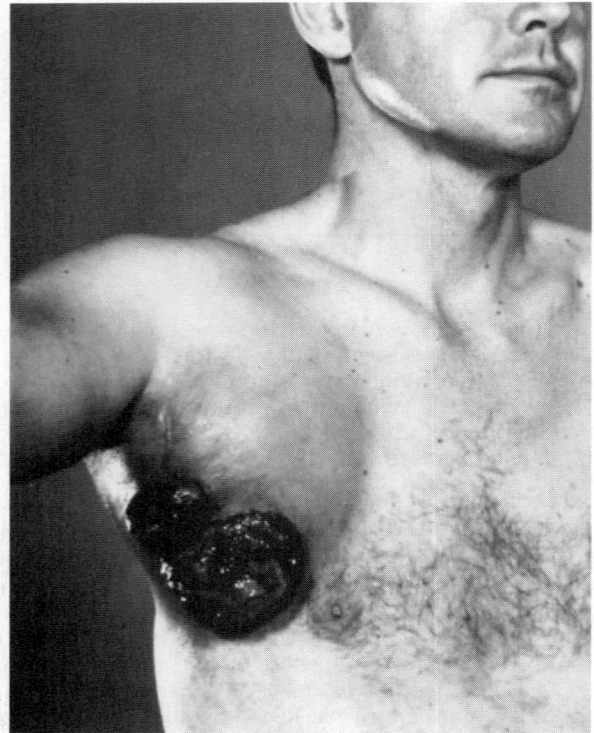

Figure 105.7. Patient with large melanoma axillary involvement with skin ulceration.

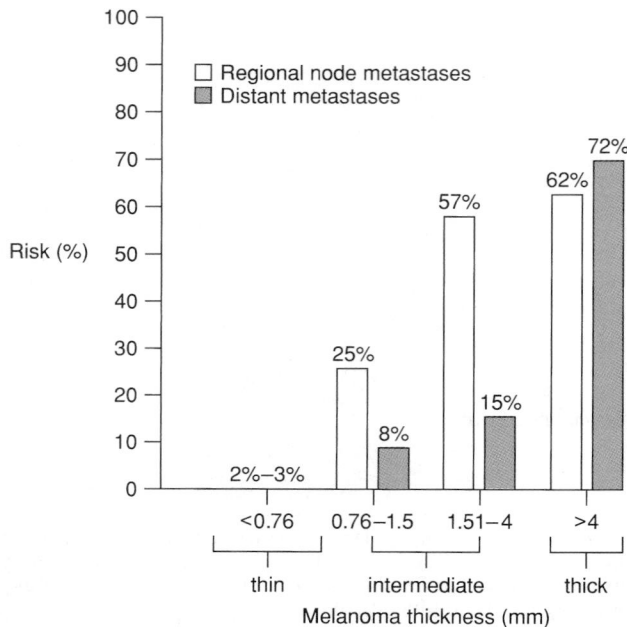

Figure 105.8. Relation of tumor thickness to risk of regional nodal and disseminated metastases. (After Balch CM. The role of elective lymph node dissection in melanoma: rationale, results, and controversies. *J Clin Oncol* 1988;6:163.)

ease. They also argue that the results of lymph node dissections for clinically palpable disease are not as good as for nonpalpable micrometastatic disease. By contrast, advocates of delayed lymph node dissections observe all patients with clinically localized melanomas expectantly and subject them to lymphadenectomy only if there is clinical evidence of nodal spread. They reason that this "wait and watch" approach saves many patients the morbidity of unnecessary surgery without adversely affecting the survival chances of patients in whom nodal disease develops.

The several retrospective studies that have attempted to address these issues report conflicting data on the efficacy of ELND. The establishment of the microstaging systems has led to the hope that certain subgroups of patients can be identified who will benefit from ELND. The contention is that tumor thickness can identify those patients who may benefit from a lymphadenectomy; at the same time, dissection can be avoided in patients with localized disease that has minimal chance to disseminate and in those who are at high risk for concurrent disseminated disease. For example, patients with thin melanomas (<0.75 mm) have a cure rate exceeding 95% and would not benefit from ELND. Patients with intermediate-thickness melanomas (0.76 to 4 mm) have a significant risk (up to 60%) of occult regional disease and a relatively low risk (15%) of distant disease (33) (Fig. 105.8). These patients may benefit from ELND. Patients with thick melanomas (>4 mm) are at high risk for both regional and distant metastases at the time of presentation and also would not benefit from ELND. To substantiate this concept, 10-year survival statistics have been reported for patients with localized melanomas (AJCC stages I and II) who underwent wide excision alone, compared with those who underwent wide excision plus ELND (34) (Table 105.8). Patients with intermediate-thickness melanomas (0.76 to 4 mm) who

underwent wide excision plus ELND had a significantly higher survival rate than those who had wide excision alone. These findings remained consistent after the analysis was stratified for tumor sites. There was no survival benefit for ELND in patients with thin (<0.75 mm) or thick (>4 mm) lesions. Despite the results of this study, unaccounted variables may have played a role in the choice of treatment, as can occur with any retrospective analysis (35). Therefore, the efficacy of ELND must be determined by prospective, randomized studies.

Several prospective, randomized studies have been reported addressing the issue of ELND, which are summarized in Table 105.9. The largest study was a U.S. intergroup trial in which 786 patients with melanomas between 1 to 4 mm thick and clinically negative nodes were randomized to either observation or ELND. Patients

Table 105.8. NONRANDOMIZED EXPERIENCE WITH WIDE EXCISION VERSUS WIDE EXCISION PLUS ELECTIVE LYMPH NODE DISSECTION FOR AJC STAGES I AND II MELANOMAS[a]

| Tumor thickness (mm) | 10-Year Survival Rate (%) | | | |
| | Extremity (N) | | Trunk, head, and neck (N) | |
	WE	WE + ELND	WE	WE + ELND
<0.76	94 (142)	100 (26)	86 (135)	83 (38)
0.76–1.49	74 (125)	92 (66)	56 (131)	80 (51)
1.5–3.99	54 (114)	80[b] (107)	33 (129)	64[b] (129)
≥4	30 (33)	44[b] (34)	22 (56)	26[b] (38)

[a]Experience from the Sydney Melanoma Unit, Australia, and the University of Alabama, Birmingham.[34]
[b]Significantly different from WE alone.
WE, wide excision; ELND, elective lymph node dissection.

Table 105.9. RANDOMIZED TRIALS OF ELECTIVE NODE DISSECTION IN CLINICALLY LOCALIZED CUTANEOUS MELANOMA

Trial	Eligible patients	No. of patients	Outcome vs. observation with therapeutic LND if necessary	Reference
WHO Trial 1	Extremity primary, all thickness	533	No advantage for ELND in OS, DFS	36
Mayo Clinic	Extremity primary, all thickness	171	No advantage for immediate ELND or ELND delayed 30–60 d in OS, DFS	37
Intergroup Surgical Trial	All sites, 1–4 mm thick	786	No advantage for ELND in OS, DFS; some subsets appeared to benefit from ELND	38
WHO Trial 14	Trunk primary, >1.5 mm thick	252	No advantage for ELND in OS, DFS; subset with 1.5–4 mm thick primary appeared to benefit from ELND	39

DFS, disease-free survival; ELND, elective lymph node dissection; LND, lymph node dissection; OS, overall survival; WHO, World Health Organization.

randomized to observation in whom nodal disease subsequently developed underwent therapeutic lymph node dissection (38). There was no significant difference in survival rates between patients randomized to ELND and those to the observation group. Subset analysis did suggest the existence of some subgroups of patients who may have benefited from ELND (i.e., patients with melanomas 1 to 2 mm in diameter and who were <60 years of age). The other randomized trials did not demonstrate any survival benefit for ELND in any subsets of patients (36,37,39). These results strongly indicate that ELND in patients with intermediate-thickness melanomas and clinically negative nodes offers no therapeutic benefit. Nonetheless, as indicated later, new techniques to identify regional lymph nodes selectively for pathologic examination may be beneficial in finding the subset of patients who should have lymphadenectomies.

Sentinel Lymph Node Biopsy

A new technique has been developed by Morton and associates to identify the first draining lymph nodes adjacent to a cutaneous melanoma, known as the *sentinel*

nodes (40). It has been hypothesized that melanoma involvement of a nodal basin develops in an orderly fashion and that involvement of the sentinel lymph node is the first step in that process. These investigators were able to identify a sentinel lymph node 90% of the time. If the sentinel node was negative for melanoma, the remaining lymph nodes were also free of involvement in at least 96% of cases. These results have been confirmed by other investigators (41).

Two techniques are available for identifying the sentinel lymph nodes, and are often combined. Morton and colleagues originally described the use of a blue lymphangiography dye (Lymphazurin) injected intradermally adjacent to the site of the primary tumor. Care must be taken not to inject the tumor if it is still present. Approximately 5 minutes later, an incision is made over the nodal basin and the blue lymphatic channel dissected bluntly along its course to a blue-stained lymph node (Fig. 105.9) (see color insert following page 1190). This technique allows for identification of the sentinel lymph node at least 80% of the time. The other technique involves intradermal injection of a radiolabeled colloid so-

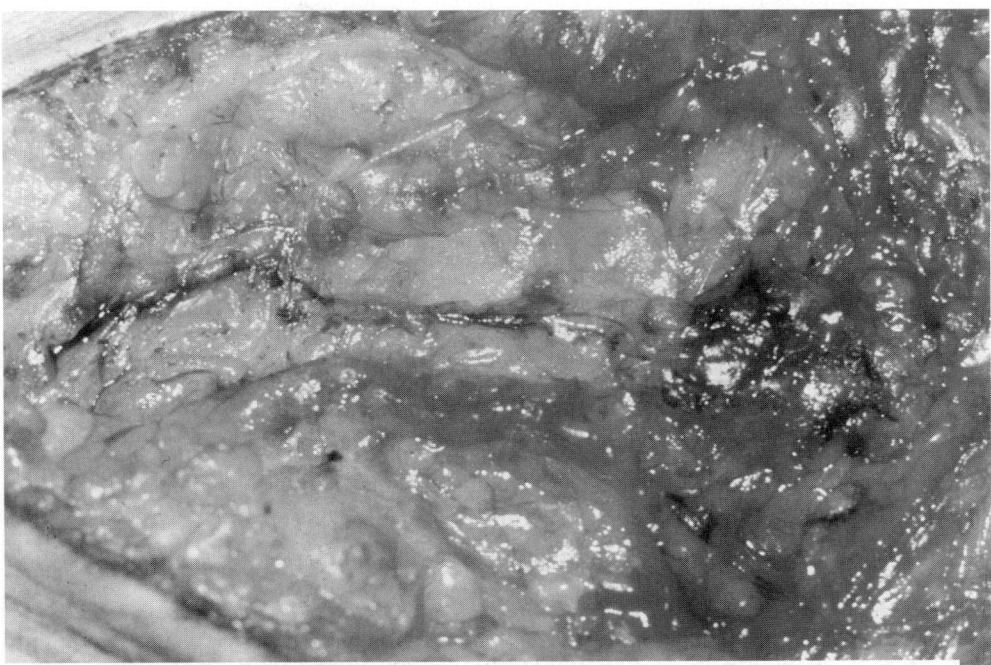

Figure 105.9. Blue dye tracking up a lymphatic vessel to a blue-stained lymph node.

lution, which is performed between 1 to 4 hours before surgery, at the site of the primary tumor. Using a hand-held gamma detector probe, the surgeon is able to identify the sentinel lymph node location through the skin, thereby limiting the incision necessary to find the node. Furthermore, this technique allows lymphoscintigraphy imaging, which can identify sentinel nodes outside the traditional nodal basin. The combined use of the blue dye plus the radiolabeled colloid enables the detection of the sentinel node in more than 90% of cases (41). The technique of sentinel lymph node biopsy is known as *lymphatic mapping* and is performed in conjunction with the wide excision of the primary tumor. It can routinely be performed as an outpatient procedure.

Once the sentinel lymph node is removed, it is processed by the pathologist by step-sectioning the entire node into multiple sections for routine hematoxylin and eosin staining. This is done to examine for micrometastases that could be missed by the standard approach to examining nodes, which involves bivalving the lymph node and performing an examination of only one section. If serial sectioning and staining is negative for metastasis, then immunohistochemical staining for melanoma markers S-100 and HMB-45 is performed. These stains pick up microscopic clusters of tumor cells that are hard to identify by hematoxylin and eosin staining. The reliability of reverse transcriptase-polymerase chain reaction to identify messenger RNA of melanoma-associated proteins is being investigated as a prognostic tool (42).

If the sentinel lymph node is positive for melanoma, the patients should undergo a regional lymphadenectomy. The patient is then eligible for consideration of adjuvant therapy, as discussed later. The introduction of lymphatic mapping has quelled the controversy over ELND. It offers the clinician a method to identify those patients who might benefit from a node dissection and adjuvant treatment.

Site-specific Considerations for Regional Lymphadenectomy

The nodal drainage areas accessible for surgical excision include the ilioinguinal, axillary, cervical, and parotid regions. With truncal melanomas, or if the tumor is located in the midline, the primary nodal drainage may not be obvious. Lymphatic vessels from the upper half of the body usually drain to the axilla, and those from the lower half of the trunk drain into the inguinal region. A valid predictor of the lymphatic watershed for the groin and axillary lymph nodes is the Sappey line, which curves upward from 2 cm above the umbilicus to the level of the second and third lumbar vertebrae. Occasionally, melanomas of the upper trunk drain to the supraclavicular region.

Two contiguous, node-bearing regions exist in the ilioinguinal area. The first is composed of the superficial femoral nodes located in the femoral triangle, and the second contains the deep nodes above the inguinal ligament along the iliac and obturator vessels. Removal of the femoral nodes is referred to as a *superficial groin dissection,* and removal of the iliac and obturator nodes is called a *deep groin dissection* (Fig. 105.10).

Controversy surrounds the benefit of a deep groin dissection, which some surgeons elect to perform if there is evidence of palpable femoral lymph node involvement. In this situation, approximately one third of patients are likely to have tumor involvement of the deep inguinal nodes. The rarity of involvement of the deep inguinal nodes when the superficial nodes are pathologically negative or harbor only microscopic disease does not warrant a deep groin dissection in those situations. Some reports indicate that the presence of positive deep groin nodes is as-

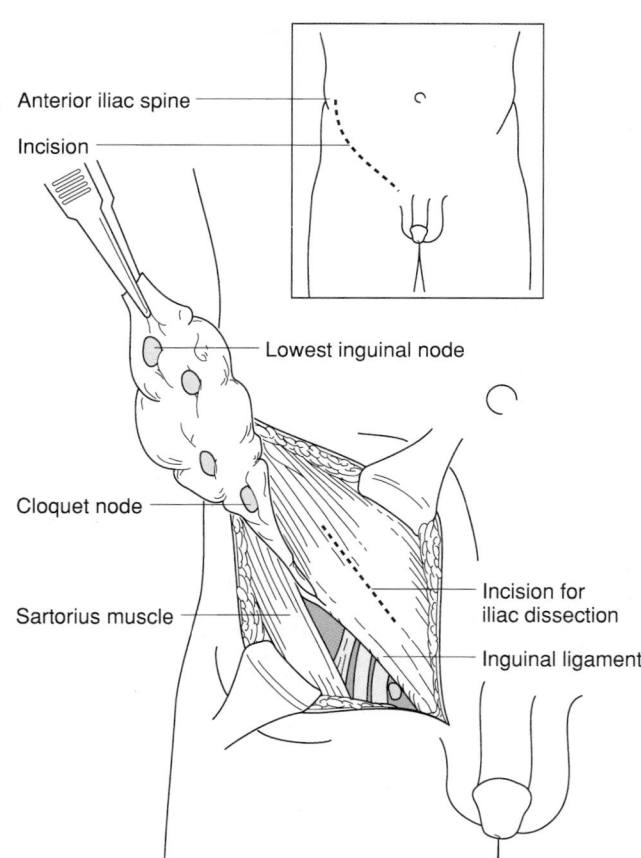

Figure 105.10. Technique of groin dissection.

sociated with a high incidence of disseminated disease and that their removal does not lead to long-term benefit (43). Other reports indicate that some patients with iliac node disease can be cured by a deep groin dissection (44). The most frequent long-term complication associated with groin dissection is edema, which occurs in 25% of patients.

The iliac and obturator nodes can be removed during the course of a superficial groin dissection by a variety of techniques. Through the same skin incision used for the superficial dissection, the deep nodes can be approached extraperitoneally by division of the inguinal ligament or by splitting of the abdominal wall musculature with an incision superior and parallel to the inguinal ligament. Alternatively, a separate midline abdominal incision can be used to remove the deep inguinal nodes and assess the paraaortic nodes. The latter approach reduces wound complications associated with combined ilioinguinal dissections.

The technique for an axillary dissection is described in Chapter 58 on breast cancer. Axillary dissections for palpable lymph nodes involved with melanoma should include removal of lymph nodes lateral, beneath, and medial to the pectoralis minor muscle (levels I to III). The axillary lymph node region is contiguous with the supraclavicular node region. Evidence of supraclavicular nodal involvement is not uncommon if bulky axillary disease is present. There is no satisfactory procedure to remove contiguous involved axillary and supraclavicular lymph nodes. In these situations, axillary dissection is noncurative and should be considered only for palliation. Long-term complications associated with axillary dissections are infrequent; arm edema and pain occur in less than 5% of patients.

Metastases to the lymph nodes from head and neck melanomas follow predictable pathways. Melanomas arising on the scalp or face anterior to the pinna of the ear and superior to the commissure of the lip metastasize to the parotid region. Lesions inferior to the commissure of the lip spread to the cervical region. Melanomas that occur on the posterior scalp behind the pinna usually spread to occipital and posterior cervical lymph nodes. Because the parotid nodes are contiguous with the cervical nodes, a radical neck dissection to remove the cervical nodes is often performed in combination with a superficial parotid node dissection for anterior facial melanomas.

Adjuvant Therapy

Although the prognosis for patients with early-stage cutaneous melanoma is quite good, less than 50% of patients with thick primaries (i.e., >4 mm) or regional node involvement are cured by surgery alone. These patients constitute the AJCC stage III group, a significant subgroup who ultimately succumb from residual micrometastatic disease. The development of effective adjuvant therapy capable of increasing postsurgical survival in this group of patients has been a long-standing goal of clinicians. Chemotherapy with dacarbazine (DTIC) has been evaluated as a postoperative adjuvant in a randomized study without effectiveness. Numerous randomized trials evaluating bacillus Calmette-Guerin (BCG) immunotherapy in the adjuvant setting have also been negative.

Interferon-α (IFN-α) has a variety of modulatory effects on the immune system that could enhance antitumor reactivity. IFN-α has been reported to have antitumor activity in patients with metastatic disease. In 1996, Kirkwood and coworkers reported the effectiveness of IFN-α to improve disease-free and overall survival rates of patients with stage III disease after surgery (45). In this multiinstitutional, prospective, randomized trial, 287 high-risk patients with deep primary (>4 mm) tumors or positive nodes were randomly assigned after surgery to either postoperative adjuvant treatment with IFN-a-2b or to observation. IFN-α-2β therapy significantly increased median overall survival by 1 year and produced a 24% improvement in the 5-year overall survival rate (46% for IFN-α-2β patients vs. 37% for observation patients; Fig. 105.11). Based on these results, the U.S. Food and Drug Adminis-

tration (FDA) approved the use of adjuvant IFN-α-2β after surgical resection of stage III melanoma. Contraindications to this regimen include a recent history of myocardial infarction or dysrhythmias, preexisting liver or central nervous system disorders, and overall debilitation.

Treatment of Disseminated Melanoma

Evaluation for Metastatic Disease and Clinical Course

The follow-up evaluation for patients with AJCC stage I, II, or III melanoma who are rendered tumor free by surgery should include regular histories and physical examinations. The use of extensive and frequent radiographic studies and blood work in asymptomatic, clinically disease-free patients is rarely productive. In 1997, the National Comprehensive Cancer Network issued guidelines for follow-up of patients with various stages of disease. For AJCC stage I (<1 mm), patients should undergo a history and physical examination with emphasis on skin and nodal examinations every 6 months for 2 years and annually thereafter. For AJCC stage II and III, patients should undergo a history and physical examination every 3 to 6 months for 3 years, then every 4 to 12 months for 2 years, then annually. The use of chest radiographs and blood work is optional. Computed tomography scans should be ordered only when clinically indicated. Attention should be directed to any gastrointestinal or central nervous system symptoms. Appropriate diagnostic studies can be obtained based on the clinical history and physical findings.

Melanoma can disseminate to any organ. The most common sites of recurrence are skin, subcutaneous tissues, and distant lymph nodes, followed by visceral sites. Common visceral sites of metastasis, in order of decreasing occurrence, are lung, liver, brain, bone, and gastrointestinal tract. Most patients who die with disseminated disease have multiple organ involvement. Frequently, the cause of death is respiratory failure or brain complications. Patients with disseminated disease have a poor prognosis, with a mean survival of approximately 6 months. Cure with any treatment is rare. Selection of treatment or a decision against treatment should be based on several factors, including the patient's medical condition, the potential for palliation, and the impact of treatment on quality of life.

Surgery

Surgical excision of recurrent melanoma can be effective for palliation in patients with isolated recurrences in the skin, central nervous system, lung, or gastrointestinal tract. Surgical excision of solitary brain metastases has been shown to provide improved palliation and quality of life compared with brain irradiation. Resection of isolated pulmonary metastases or of subcutaneous recurrences is usually not considered curative but can result in significantly prolonged disease-free survival. Gastrointestinal lesions causing obstruction or bleeding should be considered for resection or bypass to relieve these symptoms.

Radiation Therapy

Melanoma can respond to radiation therapy. From several reports, the best tumor responses of melanoma in the soft tissues are seen if large doses per fraction (4 to 8 Gy) are administered rather than lower, conventional doses (2 to 4 Gy). Radiation therapy is commonly used for palliation of bone pain secondary to metastatic disease or brain metastasis. The average survival after brain irradiation for melanoma is approximately 4 months.

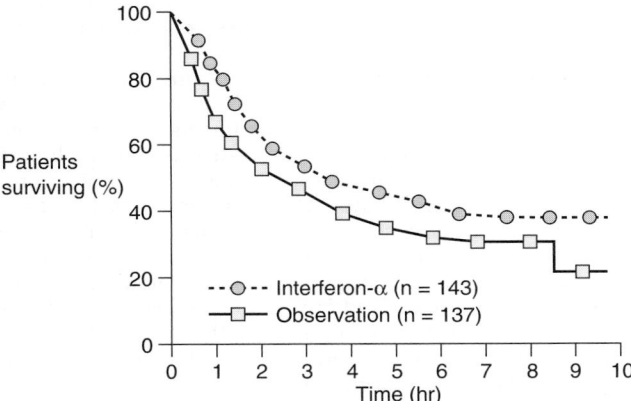

Figure 105.11. Randomized study of interferon-α therapy after resection of AJCC stage III disease. There was a statistical significant difference between the IFN-α and observation groups (*p* = .0237).

Chemotherapy

Melanoma is responsive to few chemotherapeutic drugs. The best single agents for treatment of melanoma are DTIC and the nitrosoureas, which have objective response rates in the range of 10% to 20%. Conventionally, objective responses have included complete disappearance of all known tumor sites (complete response) and reduction of more than half in all assessable tumor (partial response). Complete responses are rare. Responses are more frequently observed in patients with tumor in skin, subcutaneous tissue, lymph nodes, or lung. The combination regimen consisting of DTIC, carmustine, cisplatin, and tamoxifen is being used more frequently and has been reported to have a high response rate. However, no evidence indicates that combination chemotherapy offers better results than single-agent DTIC at this time.

Several centers have reported experience with isolated hyperthermic limb perfusion of chemotherapeutic agents to treat multiple subcutaneous (in-transit) or skin (satellitosis) metastases of the extremities. This technique requires the isolation and cannulation of the afferent and efferent vessels of the involved extremity to an extracorporeal pump. High doses of chemotherapeutic agents can be infused into the limb without systemic toxicity. Sometimes, dramatic tumor responses can be obtained. A European study of hyperthermic limb perfusion with a combination of melphalan, tumor necrosis factor, and interferon-γ reported 3 partial and 16 complete responses among 19 patients with melanoma lesions (46). Tumor necrosis factor cannot be administered systemically because of its severe toxicity; the use of isolated perfusion to an extremity avoids this limitation. This approach appears to be highly effective in the small subgroup of patients with disease confined to an extremity, but confirmatory studies are needed.

Immunotherapy

The rapid evolution of recombinant DNA technology has resulted in the availability of cytokines, such as the interferons and interleukins, that can be administered to modulate a patient's immune response. In addition, hybridoma technology has allowed the development of monoclonal antibodies reactive to melanoma. These biologic agents have been used in immunotherapeutic trials for metastatic melanoma and demonstrate that an antitumor immune response can be generated in selected patients.

Interferon-α (IFN-α) was one of the first cytokines used in tumor therapy. IFN-α was originally produced by virus-stimulated leukocytes and is now available in recombinant form. The interferons are known to induce macrophage cytotoxicity, enhance natural killer cell activity, up-regulate major histocompatibility complex (MHC) antigens on tumors, and up-regulate tumor-associated antigens. The objective response rates of melanoma to IFN-α administration range from 10% to 20%. As reviewed earlier, IFN-α has been approved by the FDA for adjuvant treatment of patients with stage III disease.

The most significant advance in melanoma immunotherapy has been associated with the use of interleukin-2 (IL-2). IL-2 is a cytokine secreted by antigen-activated helper T cells and was initially discovered because it was a T-cell growth factor. Subsequently, it was found to have many other immunologic effects, and it appears to have an important role in the enhancement of immune responses. Mulé et al. (47) discovered that the in vitro or in vivo exposure of lymphoid cells to high concentrations of IL-2 results in the generation of lymphokine-activated killer (LAK) cells. These cells are characterized by their ability to kill tumor cells nonspecifically in an in vitro assay. In animal studies, these researchers demonstrated that LAK cells can be administered with IL-2 to cause tumors to regress. The use of antitumor-reactive cells as reagents to treat tumor is known as *adoptive immunotherapy*. In a clinical trial, LAK cells plus IL-2 were found to mediate regression of tumor in selected patients with disseminated melanoma (48) (Fig. 105.12) (see color insert following page 1190). From these and other studies, the response rate of melanoma to LAK cells plus IL-2 has been found to be in the range of 20% to 25%. Most patients who achieved complete remission remained free of disease for prolonged periods. The evidence that antitumor-reactive cells can be used to treat established tumors has encouraged the search for more tumor-specific, and presumably more potent, cells for adoptive immunotherapy. Rosenberg and colleagues (49) showed that tumor-infiltrating lymphocytes obtained from progressive tumors in animals are 50 to 100 times more potent in antitumor activity than LAK cells. In clinical studies, they reported that, among 86 patients with advanced melanoma treated with the combination of tumor-infiltrating lymphocytes, high-dose IL-2, and cyclophosphamide, there was a response rate of 34% (50).

The rationale for developing T cells that are immunologically specific in their reactivity to melanoma tumors has been substantiated by the recent discovery of tumor-associated antigens expressed by melanomas. A family of melanoma antigens termed MAGE are expressed on tumors and act as recognition peptides for cytotoxic T cells (51). The antigens are recognized in association with MHC human leukocyte antigen (HLA)-A1 identity. Additional melanoma antigens such as MART-1 and gp100 have been identified by similar techniques and are restricted by HLA-A2.1 recognition (52,53).

In addition to its use in adoptive immunotherapy, IL-2 administration alone has been associated with significant melanoma tumor regression (54). The clinical response rate with IL-2 administration is in the range of 15% to 20% and appears to be dose related. IL-2 has been approved by the FDA for treatment of patients with stage IV melanoma. The antitumor effects mediated by IL-2 may result from several mechanisms, including induction of LAK cells or tumor-sensitized T cells and, possibly, the secretion of other cytokines such as tumor necrosis factor and interferon-γ. Unfortunately, high doses of IL-2 can result in multiple organ system failure as the result of a leaky capillary syndrome, which is reversible on cessation of therapy. The toxicity of IL-2 is believed to be related to the induction of a variety of inflammatory mediators. New studies are being conducted that evaluate IL-2 combined with other agents such as cytokines, chemotherapeutic agents, and tumor vaccines.

The possibility of using a tumor vaccine derived from melanoma tumor cells or extracts of tumor cells has been studied for many years. These vaccines usually have been used as adjuvant treatment in tumor-free patients who are at high risk for recurrence in an attempt actively to produce tumor-specific immunity. To enhance the immunogenicity of these vaccine preparations, immune adjuvants, such as BCG or vaccinia virus, are sometimes included in the vaccines. In general, melanoma tumor vaccines are nontoxic and have been suggested to confer some survival benefit compared with historical control subjects in nonrandomized studies. The discovery of unique melanoma tumor-associated antigens has opened the door for the development of highly specific reagents for tumor vaccines. Rosenberg and coworkers reported that the administration of a modified peptide antigen, gp100, given with incomplete Freund's adjuvant along with the concomitant administration of IL-2, resulted in a

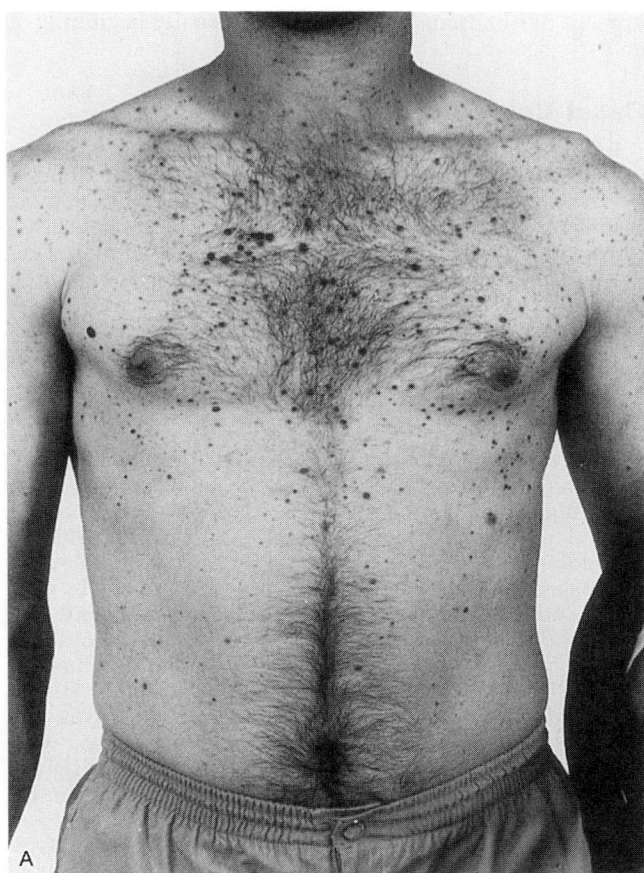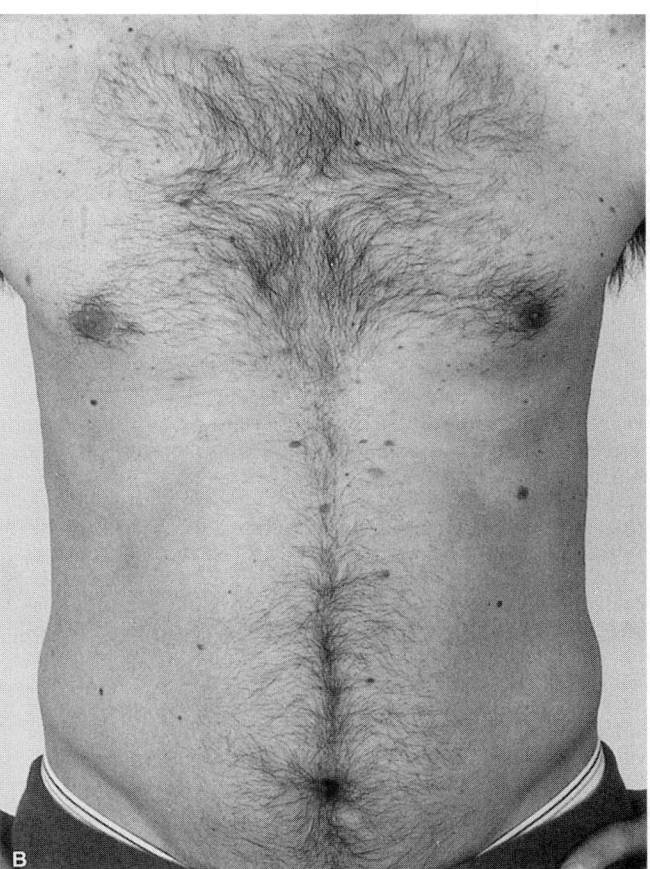

Figure 105.12. *(A)* Patient with disseminated melanoma metastatic to multiple cutaneous sites. *(B)* After several courses of therapy with lymphokine-activated killer cells and interleukin-2, the patient had a complete response. (Courtesy of Steven A. Rosenberg, M.D., Surgery Branch, National Cancer Institute, Bethesda, MD.)

42% response rate in patients with stage IV melanoma (55). Because this response rate was higher than what has been reported for IL-2 alone, it suggests that the vaccination with a tumor-associated peptide may have induced immunity to tumor cells and that the IL-2 was "helping" the response. There has been a significant resurgence of interest in vaccines using antigenic peptides as well as tumor cells or their extracts.

Another development in the field of vaccines is the use of dendritic cells (DC). DC are potent antigen-presenting cells of the immune system capable of sensitizing naive T cells to respond against tumor antigen. DC can be "pulsed" with tumor antigen in the form of peptides, whole tumor cells, lysates of tumor cells, or genes encoding antigen. Animal studies have shown that antigen-pulsed DC can cause the regression of established tumors by intradermal or intravenous administration. The administration of IL-2 with DC therapy has improved the antitumor response rate in animal studies (56). In humans, antigen-pulsed DC have resulted in complete responses in patients with stage IV melanoma (57). Numerous studies are being conducted to evaluate DC vaccine therapy with or without the concomitant use of IL-2.

Gene Therapy

The technical feasibility of transfer of genetic material into somatic cells has established a new approach to the treatment of malignancies. Many of the gene therapy strategies for cancer have focused on modulating the host immune response by altering tumor cells to be more "immunogenic." A variety of preclinical studies have demonstrated that genetic engineering of tumor cells to secrete or express immunoregulatory peptides (i.e., cytokines, costimulatory molecules, or adhesion molecules) increases the host immune response to these tumors (58). Several clinical studies are evaluating the efficacy of genetic modification of melanoma tumor cells to secrete cytokines that can be administered to patients as tumor vaccines. A different approach, established at the University of Michigan, is genetic modification of melanoma tumors in situ by the intratumoral inoculation of DNA complexed with liposomes to induce the expression of a foreign MHC class I protein (i.e., HLA-B7) by the tumor cells (59). This procedure attempts to enhance reactivity against native tumor antigens by invoking an allogeneic immune response against a strong foreign antigen.

NONMELANOMA SKIN TUMORS

Nonmelanoma basal cell and squamous cell skin cancers are the most common type of malignancy in humans. These tumors are chiefly derived from epithelial origin. The ratio of BCC to SCC is approximately 4 : 1. The annual incidence of nonmelanoma (BCC and SCC) skin cancer in the United States alone is 900,000 to 1,200,000 cases. The public health burden on the U.S. population from nonmelanoma skin cancer, for which the incidence is rapidly rising, is enormous.

Etiology

Both BCC and SCC are most commonly induced by significant exposure to UVR from the sun or tanning booths. These cancers are the predominant neoplasms on the head, neck, trunk, lower legs, and extensor arms and hands where sun exposure is common. Skin cancer is a significant occupational hazard for people who work outdoors, such as mail deliverers, farmers, sailors, and construction workers. The incidence of skin cancer is greater in fair-complexioned populations and is lower among darker-complexioned people. Melanin pigment in the skin appears to be the protective factor.

Chemical carcinogens have also been implicated as etiologic agents that contribute to the formation of skin cancer. The development of scrotal carcinoma in chimney sweeps is an example: carcinogenic soot is implicated in the development of SCC. Another example is arsenic in welding flux, which is associated with carcinoma of the hand (Fig. 105.13) (see color insert following page 1190). Other examples of carcinogens are coal tar, paraffin oil, creosote, and fuel oil. The mechanism may be explained by the initiation and promotion theory of skin cancer. In this scenario, initiation occurs by exposure of keratinocytes to the chemical carcinogen, and promotion occurs with repeated exposure of that area to the carcinogen (60).

Human papilloma virus (HPV) has been implicated in the formation of SCC in humans (61). The degeneration of a condyloma acuminata of the anus into SCC is an example of this disorder. HPV is associated with SCC in the genital, acral, and periungual regions (62). Investigators using cDNA probes directed at herpes simplex virus have reported the presence of viral DNA in an SCC (63). These associations strongly suggest a link between skin cancer and viruses in some cases.

The degeneration of chronic radiodermatitis into invasive SCC or BCC is well described. Typically, there is at least a 20-year latency period between radiation exposure and the development of the malignant lesion. In the past, radiation therapy was used to treat acne, facial scarring, cutaneous hemangiomas, and simple cutaneous malignancies. SCC and BCC can also develop in areas of trauma, scar, and chronic scarring disorders such as lupus erythematosus, epidermolysis bullosa acquisita, and chronic sinus tracts. Nevoid BCC syndrome and xeroderma pigmentosum are genodermatoses associated with the development of hundreds of skin cancers, usually beginning at an early age.

Basal Cell Carcinoma

Basal cell carcinoma is the most common form of skin cancer. These epithelial-derived tumors can be divided into various subtypes according to clinical appearance, histologic pattern, and biologic behavior. Although BCCs rarely metastasize, they are characterized by slow but relentless and destructive local invasion that results in high morbidity without treatment. The subclinical local invasion may be deep, extensive, and asymmetric, with finger-like extensions several centimeters beyond the clinical borders.

The most common subtype of BCC is the ulcerative, well-circumscribed nodular variety. These tumors often present as pearly papules or nodules with telangiectases. They may be pruritic and bleed occasionally. With time, the center ulcerates to create peripheral "rolled" borders; such ulcerating BCCs are called *rodent ulcers* (Fig. 105.14) (see color insert following page 1190). Occasionally, the lesions are deeply pigmented and nodular and can be confused with melanoma. This variant has been called a *pigmented BCC* (Fig. 105.2I). The histologic features of these tumors demonstrate isolated areas of basaloid tumor islands arising from the epidermis with peripheral palisading of nuclei and stromal retraction. In some cases, the BCC has histologic features of squamous metaplasia with keratinization. These tumors have basosquamous differentiation and can become more aggressive and develop regional lymphatic spread.

Most difficult to treat with surgical excision is the type of BCC with an aggressive growth pattern, known as morpheaform, sclerosing, or fibrosing BCC (Fig. 105.15) (see color insert following page 1190). Clinically, these tumors are flat and appear to be scarlike. They have a significant incidence of recurrence because of the isolated, finger-like fronds of basal cell tumor cells that may deeply invade the surrounding structures well beyond the clinical margins of the lesion. These small, finger-like islands are often missed with standard histologic margin control.

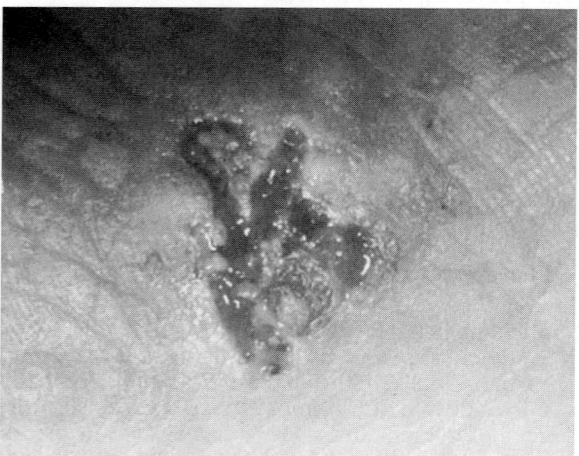

Figure 105.13. Squamous cell carcinoma of the hand secondary to exposure to arsenic in welding flux.

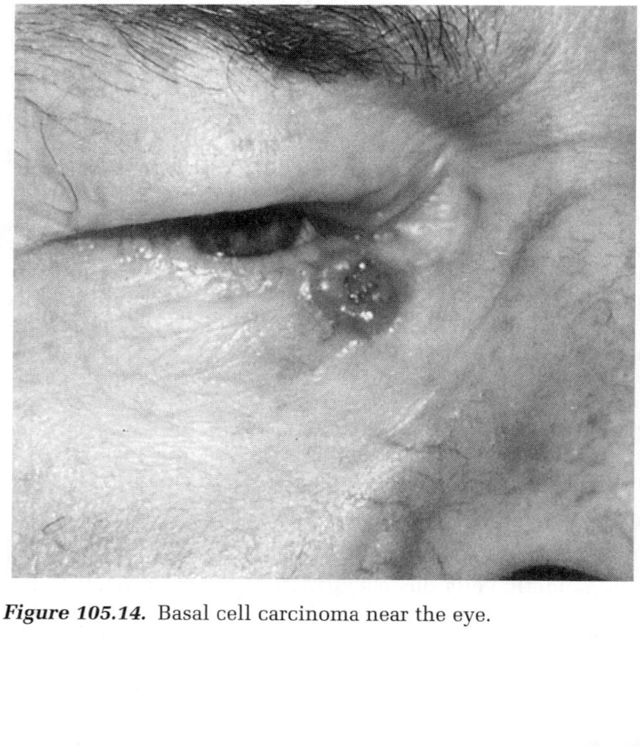

Figure 105.14. Basal cell carcinoma near the eye.

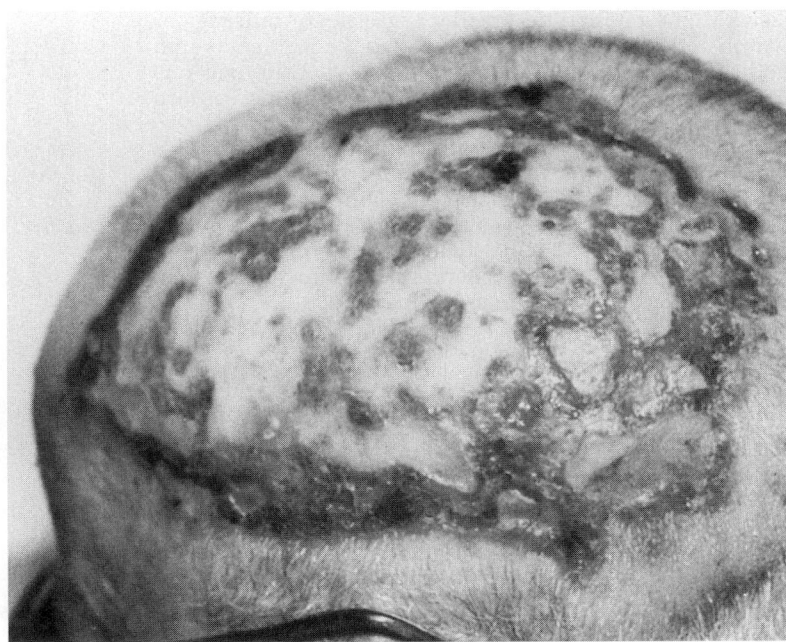

Figure 105.15. Morpheaform basal cell carcinoma of the scalp.

Clinically, superficial BCCs are scaly, pink to red lesions. Frequently, they are confused with psoriasis or other eczematous, scaly dermatoses. Although these tumors are usually relatively superficial, extensive superficial subclinical involvement is common. Numerous risk factors are associated with possible extensive subclinical invasion or frequent recurrence of BCC after standard treatment, including surgical excision (64–68):

- Location/size[1]
  (L) Low-risk area ≥2 cm
  (M) Middle-risk area ≥1 cm
  (H) High-risk area ≥0.6 cm
- Recurrent lesion
- Aggressive growth histologic type (morpheaform, sclerosing, infiltrative, micronodular, fibrosing)
- Neurotropism
- Poorly defined clinical borders
- Immunosuppression
- Incomplete excision (positive margins)
- Site of prior radiation or scarring process

Squamous Cell Carcinoma

Squamous cell carcinoma is the second most common form of skin cancer and is derived from the epithelial keratinocyte. Because these tumors can deeply invade surrounding structures or metastasize to regional lymph nodes, they must be recognized and treated aggressively. SCC causes some 2,500 deaths per year in the United States. Several precursor lesions to invasive SCC exist, most commonly actinic keratoses and Bowen's disease. Erythroplasia of Queyrat, another precursor lesion, represents SCC in situ on the glans penis. Clinically, SCC usually begins as an erythematous papulonodule with overly-

ing keratotic crust or ulceration. The lesions can progress to ulceration with surrounding erythema, with or without a keratotic center. Histologically, SCC shows malignant degeneration of epithelial cells with differentiation toward keratin formation.

Ulcerative SCC is an aggressive skin malignancy that typically has a central ulceration with raised borders (Fig. 105.16) (see color insert following page 1190). These tumors can arise in actinically damaged skin, solar keratoses, cutaneous horns, burn scars, or chronic wounds. These lesions infiltrate widely and can spread to regional lymphatics. In the head and neck, they commonly metas-

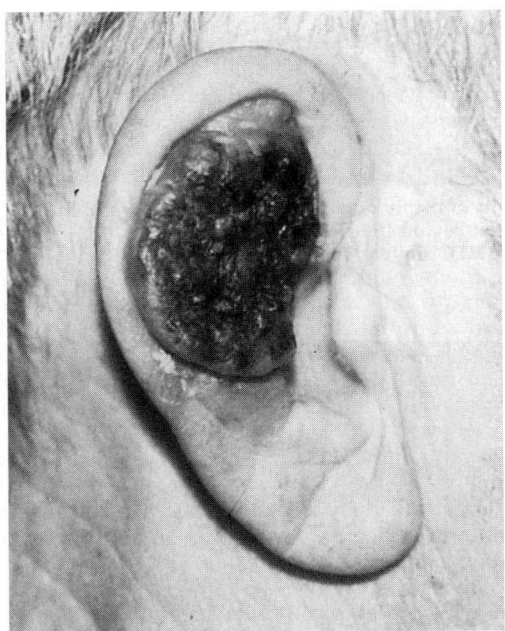

Figure 105.16. Ulcerative squamous cell carcinoma.

---

[1]Area H: central face, eyelid, eyebrow, periorbital, nose, lip, chin, mandible, preauricular and postauricular skin/sulcus, temple, ear, genitalia, hands, feet
  Area M: cheeks, forehead, neck, scalp
  Area L: trunk, extremities

tasize to the periparotid, jugular digastric, or mid-jugular lymph nodes. If these tumors spread to the regional lymph nodes, the prognosis is poor, with a 5-year survival rate below 50%. Tumors arising in chronic wounds or burn scars may exhibit particularly aggressive behavior.

Accurate assessment of the higher-risk cutaneous SCCs is handicapped because of the lack of large, prospective studies using multivariate analysis. Nine variables, however, have been identified as prognostic risk factors by retrospective analysis. Factors that may determine a higher risk for local recurrence, extensive subclinical invasion, and metastasis include the following (62):

- Location/size
  Area L ≥2 cm
  Area M ≥1 cm
  Area H ≥0.6 cm
- Recurrent lesion
- Aggressive histologic type (poorly differentiated, adenoid, desmoplastic, adenosquamous)
- Depth: Clark level IV, V or ≥4 mm
- Poorly defined clinical borders
- Immunosuppression
- Site of prior radiation of scarring process
- Neurotropism
- Rapid growth

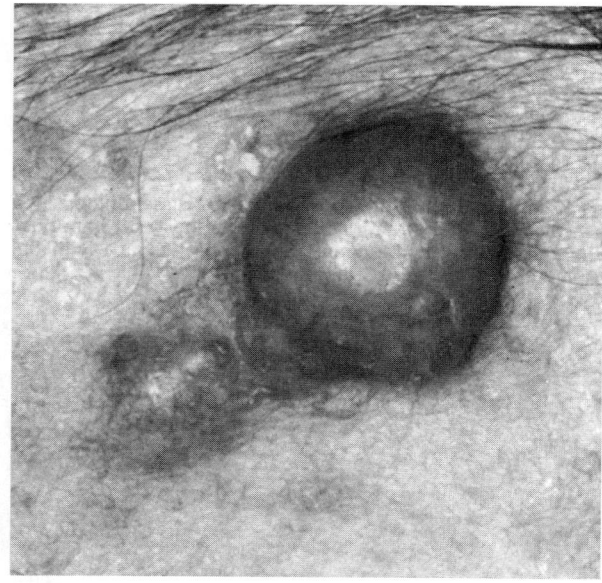

Figure 105.17. Merkel cell carcinoma.

Other Tumors of Special Interest

Hundreds of cutaneous tumors exist, and their description is beyond the scope of this chapter. Three tumors that may be seen by the surgeon and are in the differential diagnosis for BCC are described here because of their potentially aggressive behavior. These are Merkel cell carcinoma, microcystic adnexal carcinoma, and sebaceous gland carcinoma.

Merkel cell carcinoma is a malignant neuroendocrine tumor with features of epithelial differentiation. Merkel cell carcinoma is biologically aggressive, with a high incidence of local recurrence and regional and systemic metastasis. The 1-, 2-, and 3-year survival rates are estimated to be 88%, 72%, and 55%, respectively. Merkel cell carcinoma typically appears as a red to purple papulonodule or indurated plaque (Fig. 105.17) (see color insert following page 1190). Approximately 50% of tumors arise on the head and neck, 40% on the extremities, and 10% on the trunk. Merkel cell carcinoma is a small cell tumor with characteristic positive immunocytochemical staining for neuron-specific enolase, cytokeratin, and neurofilament protein. A chest radiograph is indicated to rule out metastatic oat cell carcinoma, which may be similar in clinical and histologic appearance. Treatment consists of wide local excision with adjuvant radiation to the primary site and the primary draining nodal groups. Primary radiation therapy may also be considered. Careful and frequent follow-up monitoring for local, regional, or distant recurrence is warranted (69). Sentinel lymph node biopsy or elective node dissection may also be considered. The role of adjuvant chemotherapy is unknown but may be considered.

Microcystic adnexal carcinoma is a rare cutaneous neoplasm with both follicular and eccrine differentiation, characterized by invasive, relentless, and destructive local growth. The incidence of neurotropism and local recurrence is very high. Microcystic adnexal carcinoma occurs primarily on the head and neck as a slowly enlarging, white to pink papuloplaque. Local invasion through the underlying muscle is common, and bony invasion occurs in up to 13% of cases. The use of standard

Mohs excision (see later section) combined with permanent horizontal sectioning from the final negative Mohs stage specimens offers the highest chance of cure in most cases (70).

Sebaceous gland carcinoma is a rare malignant tumor derived from adnexal epithelium of sebaceous glands. The tumor can arise on ocular or extraocular sites but most commonly presents as a yellowish to pink, slowly growing papulonodule on the eyelid, clinically similar to a chalazion. Local recurrence after surgical excision is relatively frequent (9% to 36%) owing to subclinical pagetoid extension and the multicentric nature of the tumor. Regional lymph node and visceral metastases occur in 14% to 25% of cases. Adjuvant radiation therapy has been shown to be beneficial in several series (71).

Surgical Treatment of Nonmelanoma Skin Cancers

A skin biopsy for diagnosis is important before treatment of any skin cancer. Fortunately, most nonmelanoma skin cancers are small, low-risk lesions that respond with 90% to 95% cure rates to standard treatment techniques, including curettage and electrodesiccation, cryosurgery, radiation therapy, and surgical resection (62). Many skin cancers can be removed with elliptical excisions that follow the skin tension lines. Curettage before excision is often helpful to delineate subclinical tumor extension for both BCC and SCC (65). Margins for low-risk SCC range from 0.5 to 1 cm. Margins for low-risk BCC range from 0.3 to 0.5 cm. Mohs surgery should be considered for BCCs and SCCs that exhibit the higher-risk factors previously listed. If Mohs surgery is not available, excision with careful frozen-section control (with permanent section confirmation) is indicated.

Regional lymphadenectomy is an important component of the surgical procedure if clinically positive nodes are evident. Approximately 80% of metastases from cutaneous SCC occur first to the primary draining regional lymph nodes. The diagnosis of metastatic SCC can be made with fine-needle aspiration at the time of skin biopsy. These invasive tumors have characteristic features in lymph node aspirates that allow the pathologist to secure the diagnosis. ELND for patients with SCC with clinically negative regional disease is not indicated unless the tumor extends to the parotid capsule or the lesion is large and contiguous to a draining nodal basin. Sentinel node mapping may be considered for high-risk SCC. BCC rarely metastasizes, and regional lymph node dissection including sentinel node mapping should not be performed unless the histologic features resemble those of basosquamous cell tumors, which are more biologically aggressive lesions.

The reconstructive algorithm for the treatment of skin cancer is complex because of the variety of anatomic sites involved. The fundamental oncologic principle of tumor clearance first, reconstruction second should be followed. For very high-risk nonmelanoma skin cancers, split-thickness skin grafting may be necessary to monitor for tumor recurrence.

Mohs Micrographic Surgical Treatment of Skin Cancer

Mohs surgery was developed by Frederick E. Mohs, a general surgeon from the University of Wisconsin, in the 1940s. Initially, a chemical fixative paste was applied to the skin to fix the tissue in situ; hence, the now-outdated term *Mohs chemosurgery*. The fresh tissue technique, which omitted the chemical paste, was developed and refined in the 1970s. Mohs micrographic surgery is most useful for the treatment of higher-risk nonmelanoma skin cancers. Mohs surgery is usually performed under local anesthesia in an outpatient Mohs surgical unit (72,73). After removal of all gross tumor, the surgeon excises a thin layer of tissue, 2 to 3 mm deep and with 2- to 3-mm lateral margins. The tissue is mapped, color-coded for orientation, and sent to the technician for frozen-section processing. The specimen is flexible and flattened, with the beveled peripheral skin edge placed in the same horizontal plane with the deep margin. In this plane, both the deep and peripheral margins are examined in one horizontal cut by frozen-section analysis with total (theoretically 100%) margin control. Good-quality frozen sections may be achieved only by a skilled and experienced Mohs histotechnician. The Mohs surgeon functions as both surgeon and pathologist. After histologic interpretation of the frozen-section specimens, the precise anatomic location of any residual tumor can be identified and reexcised until all margins are tumor free (Fig. 105.18). The Mohs surgeon's ability microscopically to track subclinical tumor extensions results in the highest cure rate with maximal preservation of normal tissue. Soft-tissue reconstruction can then be performed on the same day, after completion of Mohs surgical excision of the tumor (Fig. 105.19) (see color insert following page 1190). A multidisciplinary approach involving Mohs, plastic, head and neck, and oculoplastic surgeons and radiation oncologists may be needed for extensive tumors. Mastering the Mohs technique is based on a steep learning curve. The American College of Mohs Surgery requires 1 to 2 years of fellowship training with a minimum of 500 to 600 cases before certification.

Based on a review of all studies from all disciplines since 1950, the 5-year cure rate for treatment of primary (previously untreated) BCC by Mohs surgery is 99%, versus 90% to 93% for all non-Mohs modalities, including standard surgical excision (74). For recurrent (previously treated) BCC, the 5-year cure rates are 94% for Mohs ver-

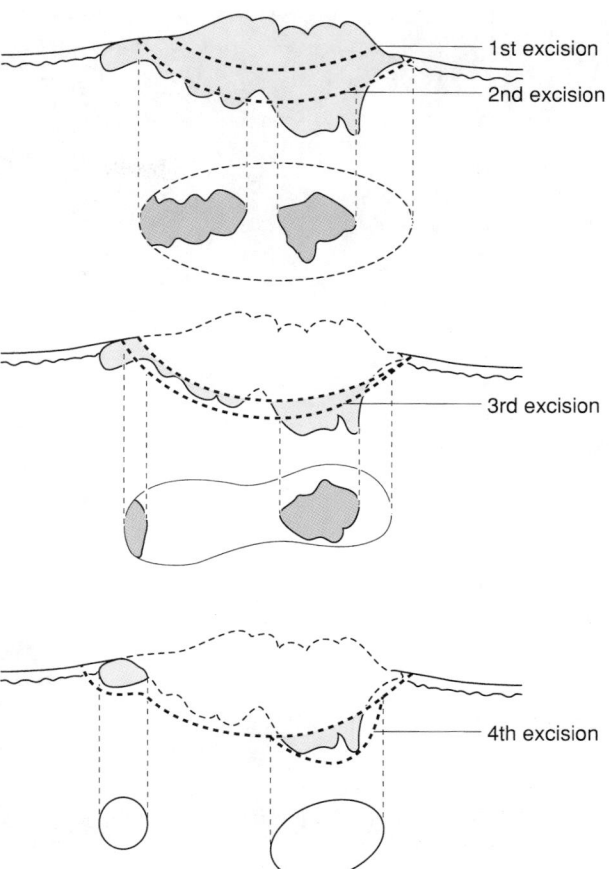

Figure 105.18. Mohs micrographic surgical technique.

sus 60% to 84% for non-Mohs modalities (75). In general, Mohs surgery should be considered for nonmelanoma tumors that are associated with a higher risk of recurrence after standard treatment and for tumors for which conservation of normal tissue is important. Risk factors for recurrence after standard treatment have been previously mentioned.

Tumors for which maximal conservation of tissue may be important include tumors on the eyelid, nose, ear, lip, digit, or genitalia and tumors in young patients. For small, low-risk lesions, Mohs surgery does not result in higher cure rates than standard techniques, but its use should be considered for nonmelanoma skin cancers with the higher-risk factors described.

Adjuvant and Primary Radiation Therapy

Radiation therapy may be useful for primary treatment of small, low-risk nonmelanoma skin cancers. In experienced hands, primary radiation therapy may also be useful for higher risk tumors with very high cure rates. For cutaneous SCC with many high-risk factors and for those with extensive neurotropism, adjuvant prophylactic radiation therapy to the primary site and the primary draining lymph nodes may decrease the risks of local recurrence and regional nodal metastasis. Prophylactic adjuvant radiation therapy should also be considered for highly aggressive, deeply invasive BCCs that exhibit extensive neurotropism.

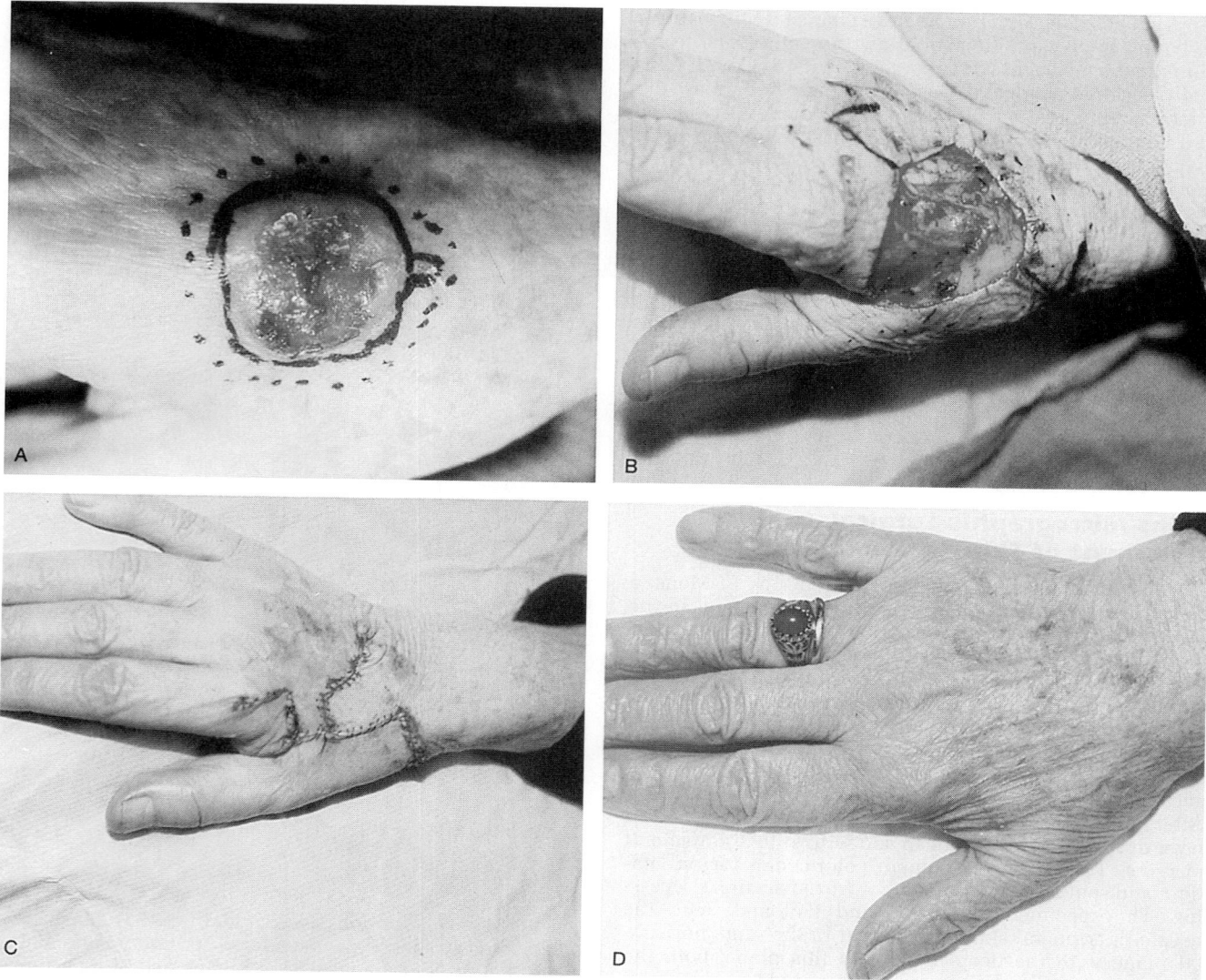

Figure 105.19. *(A)* Patient with a 3 × 3–cm basal cell carcinoma on the right dorsal hand with mixed nodular and aggressive growth histologic pattern. *(B)* Final Mohs surgery defect measuring 4 × 4.8 cm to the underlying tendon with preservation of tendon and nerve structures. Complete excision of the tumor required two Mohs stages (10 frozen sections). *(C)* The defect was reconstructed immediately after achievement of clear margins under local anesthesia in the Mohs Surgery Unit using birhombic flap soft tissue reconstruction. *(D)* Result 3 months after surgery.

REFERENCES

1. Landis SH, Murray T, Bolden S, et al. Cancer statistics, 1999. *CA Cancer J Clin* 1999;49:8.
2. NCI Division of Cancer Prevention and Control. *Cancer statistics review, 1973–1987.* NIH publication no. 89-2789. Bethesda, MD: U.S. Department of Health and Human Services, National Cancer Institute, May, 1989.
3. Elwood JM, Lee JAH, Walters SD, et al. Relationship of melanoma and other skin cancer mortality to latitude and ultraviolet radiation in the United States and Canada. *Int J Epidemiol* 1974;3:325.
4. MacLennan R, Green AC, McLeod GR, et al. Increasing incidence of cutaneous melanoma in Queensland, Australia. *J Natl Cancer Inst* 1992;84:1427.
5. Kripke ML. Immunology and photocarcinogenesis. *J Am Acad Dermatol* 1986;14:149.
6. Greene MH, Clark WH, Tucker MA, et al. High risk of malignant melanoma in melanoma-prone families with dysplastic nevi. *Ann Intern Med* 1985;102:458.
7. Hieken TJ, Rauth S, Ronan SG, et al. Hereditary melanoma. *Surg Oncol Clin North Am* 1994;3:563.
8. Bale SJ, Dracopoli NC, Tucker MA, et al. Mapping the gene for hereditary cutaneous malignant melanoma-dysplastic nevus to chromosome 1p. *N Engl J Med* 1989;320:1367.
9. Haluska FG, Hodi FS. Molecular genetics of familial cutaneous melanoma. *J Clin Oncol* 1998;16:670.
10. Trent JM, Stanbridge EJ, Heyoung LM, et al. Tumorigenicity in human melanoma cell lines controlled by introduction of human chromosome 6. *Science* 1990;247:568.
11. Goldstein AM, Fraser MC, Struewing JP, et al. Increased risk of pancreatic cancer in melanoma-prone kindreds with p16^{ink4} mutations. *N Engl J Med* 1995;333:970.
12. Clark WH Jr, Ainsworth AM, Bernardino EA, et al. The developmental biology of primary human malignant melanomas. *Semin Oncol* 1975;2:83.
13. Clark WH Jr, From L, Bernardino EA, et al. The histogenesis and biologic behavior of primary human malignant melanoma of the skin. *Cancer Res* 1969;29:705.
14. McGovern VJ. The classification of melanoma and its relationship with prognosis. *Pathology* 1970;2:85.
15. Wanebo HJ, Woodruff J, Fortner JG. Malignant melanoma of the extremities: a clinicopathologic study using levels of invasion (microstage). *Cancer* 1975;35:666.

16. Balch CM, Murad TM, Soong SJ, et al. A multifactorial analysis of melanoma: prognostic histopathologic features comparing Clark's and Breslow's staging methods. *Ann Surg* 1978; 118:732.

17. Eldh J, Boeryd B, Peterson LE. Prognostic factors in cutaneous malignant melanoma in stage I: a clinical, morphological, and multivariate analysis. *Scand J Plast Reconstr Surg* 1978;12:243.

18. Breslow A. Thickness, cross-sectional area, and depth of invasion in prognosis of cutaneous melanoma. *Ann Surg* 1970; 172:902.

19. Balch CM, Soong SJ, Milton GW, et al. A comparison of prognostic factors and surgical results in 1,786 patients with localized (stage I) melanoma treated in Alabama, U.S.A., and New South Wales, Australia. *Ann Surg* 1982;196:677.

20. Balch CM, Soong S-J, Shaw HM, et al. An analysis of prognostic factors in 4,000 patients with cutaneous melanoma. In: Balch CM, Milton GW, eds. *Cutaneous melanoma: clinical management and treatment results worldwide*. Philadelphia: JB Lippincott, 1985:321.

21. Cohen MH, Ketcham AS, Felix EL, et al. Prognostic factors in patients undergoing lymphadenectomy for malignant melanoma. *Ann Surg* 1977;186:635.

22. Callery C, Cochran AJ, Roe DJ, et al. Factors prognostic for survival in patients with malignant melanoma spread to the regional lymph nodes. *Ann Surg* 1982;196:69.

23. Calabro A, Singletary SE, Balch CM. Patterns of relapse in 1,001 consecutive patients with melanoma nodal metastases. *Arch Surg* 1989;124:1051.

24. Bevilacqua RG, Coit DG, Rogatko A, et al. Axillary dissection in melanoma: prognostic variables in node-positive patients. *Ann Surg* 1990;212:125.

25. Day CL, Mihm MC, Lew RA, et al. Cutaneous malignant melanoma: prognostic guidelines for physicians and patients. *CA Cancer J Clin* 1982;32:113.

26. Balch CM, Reintgen DS, Kirkwood JM, et al. Cutaneous melanoma. In: DeVita VT, Hellman S, Rosenberg SA, eds. *Cancer: principles and practice of oncology*, 5th ed. Philadelphia: JB Lippincott, 1997:1947.

27. Clark WH, Elder DE, Guerry D, et al. Model predicting survival in stage I melanoma based on tumor progression. *J Natl Cancer Inst* 1989;81:1893.

28. Kheir SM, Bines SD, Vonroenn JH, et al. Prognostic significance of DNA aneuploidy in stage I cutaneous melanoma. *Ann Surg* 1988;207:455.

29. Trent JM, Meyskens FL, Salmon SE, et al. Relation of cytogenetic abnormalities and clinical outcome in metastatic melanoma. *N Engl J Med* 1990;322:1508.

30. Veronesi U, Cascinelli N, Adamus J, et al. Thin stage I primary cutaneous malignant melanoma: comparison of excision with margins of 1 or 3 cm. *N Engl J Med* 1988;318:1159.

31. Balch CM, Urist MM, Karakousis CP, et al. Efficacy of 2 cm surgical margins for intermediate thickness melanomas (1 to 4 mm): results of a multi-institutional randomized surgical trial. *Ann Surg* 1993;218:262.

32. Balch CM, Karakousis C, Natarajan N, et al. Management of cutaneous melanoma in the United States. *Surg Gynecol Obstet* 1984;158:311.

33. Balch CM. The role of elective lymph node dissection in melanoma: rationale, results, and controversies. *J Clin Oncol* 1988;6:163.

34. Balch CM, Cascinelli N, Milton GW, et al. Elective node dissection: pros and cons. In: Balch CM, Milton GW, eds. *Cutaneous melanoma: clinical management and treatment results worldwide*. Philadelphia: JB Lippincott, 1985:131.

35. Cady B. "Prophylactic" lymph node dissection in melanoma: does it help? *J Clin Oncol* 1988;6:2.

36. Veronesi U, Adams J, Bandiera DC, et al. Delayed regional lymph node dissection in stage I melanoma of the skin of the lower extremities. *Cancer* 1982;49:2420.

37. Sim FH, Taylor WF, Pritchard DJ, et al. Lymphadenectomy in the management of stage I malignant melanoma: a prospective randomized study. *Mayo Clin Proc* 1986;61:697.

38. Balch CM, Soong SJ, Bartolucci AA, et al. Efficacy of an elective regional lymph node dissection of 1 to 4 mm thick melanomas for patients 60 years of age and younger. *Ann Surg* 1996;224:255.

39. Cascinelli N, Morabito A, Santinami M, et al. Immediate or delayed dissection of regional nodes in patients with melanoma of the trunk: a randomized trial. *Lancet* 1998;351: 793.

40. Morton DL, Wen D-R, Wong JH, et al. Technical details of intraoperative lymphatic mapping for early stage melanoma. *Arch Surg* 1992;127:392.

41. Gershenwald JE, Thompson W, Mansfield PF, et al. Multi-institutional melanoma lymphatic mapping experience: the prognostic value of sentinel lymph node status in 612 stage I or II melanoma patients. *J Clin Oncol* 1999;17:976.

42. Shivers SC, Wang X, Li W, et al. Molecular staging of malignant melanoma correlation with clinical outcome. *JAMA* 1998;280:1410.

43. Coit DG, Brennan MF. Extent of lymph node dissection in melanoma of the trunk or lower extremity. *Arch Surg* 1989; 124:162.

44. Karakousis CP, Lawrence JE, Rao UR. Groin dissection in malignant melanoma. *Am J Surg* 1986;152:491.

45. Kirkwood JM, Strawderman MH, Ernstoff MS, et al. Interferon alpha-2b adjuvant therapy of high-risk resected cutaneous melanoma: the eastern cooperative oncology group trial EST 1684. *J Clin Oncol* 1996;14:7–17.

46. Lienard D, Ewalenko P, Delmotte J-J, et al. High-dose recombinant tumor necrosis factor alpha in combination with interferon gamma and melphalan in isolation perfusion of the limbs for melanoma and sarcoma. *J Clin Oncol* 1992;10:52.

47. Mulé JJ, Shu S, Schwartz SL, et al. Adoptive immunotherapy of established pulmonary metastases with LAK cells and recombinant interleukin-2. *Science* 1984;225:1487.

48. Rosenberg SA, Lotze MT, Muul LM, et al. A progress report on the treatment of 157 patients with advanced cancer using lymphokine-activated killer cells and interleukin-2 or high-dose interleukin-2 alone. *N Engl J Med* 1987;316:889.

49. Rosenberg SA, Spiess P, Lafreniere R. A new approach to the adoptive immunotherapy of cancer with tumor-infiltrating lymphocytes. *Science* 1986;233:1318.

50. Rosenberg SA, Yannelli JR, Yang JC, et al. Treatment of patients with metastatic melanoma with autologous tumor-infiltrating lymphocytes and interleukin 2. *J Natl Cancer Inst* 1994;86:1159.

51. van der Bruggen P, Traversari C, Chomez P, et al. A gene encoding an antigen recognized by cytolytic T lymphocytes on a human melanoma. *Science* 1991;254:1643.

52. Kawakami Y, Zakut R, Topalian SL, et al. Shared human melanoma antigens: recognition by tumor-infiltrating lymphocytes in HLA-A2.1 transfected melanomas. *J Immunol* 1992;148:638.

53. Cox AL, Skipper J, Chen Y, et al. Identification of a peptide recognized by five melanoma-specific human cytotoxic T cell lines. *Science* 1994;264:716.

54. Chang AE, Rosenberg SA. Overview of interleukin-2 as an immunotherapeutic agent. *Semin Surg Oncol* 1989;5:385.

55. Rosenberg SA, Yang JC, Schwartzentruber DJ, et al. Immunologic and therapeutic evaluation of a synthetic peptide vaccine for the treatment of patients with metastatic melanoma. *Nat Med* 1998;4:269.

56. Shimizu K, Fields, RC, Giedlin M, et al. Systemic administration of interleukin 2 enhances the therapeutic efficacy of dendritic cell-based tumor vaccines. *Proc Natl Acad Sci USA* 1999;96:2268.

57. Nestle FO, Alijagic S, Gilliet M, et al. Vaccination of melanoma patients with peptide- or tumor lysate-pulsed dendritic cells. *Nat Med* 1998;4:328.

58. Miller AR, McBride WH, Hunt K, et al. Cytokine-mediated gene therapy for cancer. *Ann Surg Oncol* 1994;1:436.

59. Nabel GJ, Gordon D, Bishop DK, et al. Immune response in human melanoma after transfer of an allogeneic class I major histocompatibility complex gene with DNA-liposome complexes. *Proc Natl Acad Sci USA* 1996;93:15388.

60. Yupsa SH, Hennings H, Saffiotti U. Cutaneous chemical carcinogenesis: past, present, and future. *J Invest Dermatol* 1976; 67:199.

61. Obalek S, Jablonski S, Orth G. HPV associated intraepithelial neoplasia of external genitalia. *Clin Dermatol* 1985;3:104.

62. Johnson TM, Rowe DE, Nelson BR, et al. Squamous cell carcinoma of the skin (excluding lip and oral mucosa). *J Am Acad Dermatol* 1992;26:467.

63. Claudy AL, Chignol MC, Chardonnet Y. Detection of herpes simplex virus DNA in a cutaneous squamous cell carcinoma by in situ hybridization. *Arch Dermatol Res* 1989;281:333.

64. Swanson NA. Mohs surgery: technique, indications, applications, and the future. *Arch Dermatol* 1983;119:761.

65. Johnson TM, Tromovich TA, Swanson NA. Combined curettage and excision: a treatment for primary basal cell carcinoma. *J Am Acad Dermatol* 1991;24:613.

66. Salasche SJ, Amonette RA. Morpheaform basal-cell epitheliomas: a study of subclinical extensions in a series of 51 cases. *J Dermatol Surg Oncol* 1981;7:387.

67. Smith SP, Foley EH, Grande PJ. Use of Mohs surgery to establish quantitative proof of heightened tumor spread in basal cell carcinoma recurrent following radiotherapy. *J Dermatol Surg Oncol* 1990;16:1012.

68. Birkby CS, Whitaker DC. Management consideration for cutaneous neurophilic tumors. *J Dermatol Surg Oncol* 1988;14:731.

69. Ratner D, Nelson BR, Brown MD, et al. Merkel cell carcinoma. *J Am Acad Dermatol* 1993;29:143.

70. Sebastien TS, Nelson BR, Lowe L, et al. Microcystic adnexal carcinoma. *J Am Acad Dermatol* 1993;29:840.

71. Nelson BR, Hamlet KR, Gillard M, et al. Sebaceous carcinoma. *J Am Acad Dermatol* 1995;33:1.

72. Lang PG. Mohs micrographic surgery: fresh tissue technique. *Dermatol Clin* 1989;7:613.

73. Zitelli JA. Mohs micrographic surgery for skin cancer. *Princ Pract Oncol* 1992;6:1.

74. Rowe DE, Carroll RJ, Day CL Jr. Long-term recurrence rates in previously untreated (primary) basal cell carcinoma: implications for patient follow-up. *J Dermatol Surg Oncol* 1989;15:315.

75. Rowe DE, Carroll RJ, Day CL Jr. Mohs surgery is the treatment of choice for recurrent (previously treated) basal cell carcinoma. *J Dermatol Surg Oncol* 1989;15:424.

SURGERY: SCIENTIFIC PRINCIPLES AND PRACTICE, Third Edition, edited by Lazar J. Greenfield, Michael W. Mulholland, Keith T. Oldham, Gerald B. Zelenock, and Keith D. Lillemoe. Lippincott Williams & Wilkins Publishers, Philadelphia, © 2001.

CHAPTER 106

SARCOMAS OF BONE AND SOFT TISSUE

VERNON K. SONDAK

Sarcomas are a heterogeneous group of cancers that arise from mesoderm-derived elements, including bone, cartilage, connective tissue, fat, and muscle. The soft tissues and bony structures constitute almost two thirds of the mass of the human body; despite this, sarcomas are not common. The relative rarity of sarcomas has made it difficult for any but a few specialized centers to gain wide experience with treating them. Still, sarcomas are sufficiently prevalent that a practicing surgeon can expect to encounter them at some point and must therefore be able to recognize them. In fact, an estimated 10,400 new soft-tissue and bone sarcomas occurred in 1999, making them more common than testicular cancer or Hodgkin's disease. Soft-tissue sarcomas, which account for 75% of all sarcomas, are responsible for the deaths of more patients each year than testicular cancer, Hodgkin's disease, and thyroid cancer combined (1).

The behavior of carcinomas, which arise from the ectoderm-derived tissues, varies dramatically depending on their site of origin in the body. In contrast, sarcomas typically behave in a similar fashion wherever they arise. The site of origin of a sarcoma does affect treatment, however, and hence outcome. Extremity sarcomas can usually be resected with a wide margin, although sometimes amputation is required. Because local control can be achieved in most patients with extremity lesions, emphasis is placed on preserving a functional limb. By contrast, sarcomas arising in the retroperitoneum are almost invariably situated near major organs and blood vessels. Even extensive resections often cannot include a wide margin of normal tissue around the tumor, and local recurrence is frequent. When a sarcoma arises in the head, neck, or trunk, an intermediate situation exists. Depending on the size and precise location of the tumor, wide resection may or may not be feasible, and local recurrence rates are somewhere between those of extremity and retroperitoneal sarcomas. Sarcomas arising in bone and those occurring in childhood are more sensitive to cytotoxic drugs than most adult soft-tissue sarcomas. Hence, the management of these tumors is more likely to involve aggressive systemic chemotherapy. Thus, although the basic biologic and clinical behavior of all sarcomas is similar, each type requires a somewhat different management approach. Individual treatments are addressed later in this chapter.

Because of the paucity of symptoms associated with sarcomas, patients often present with locally advanced (or even metastatic) tumors. Nonetheless, surgical resection is the mainstay of treatment for patients with sarcoma, including some with metastatic disease. Surgery alone, however, is no longer the treatment of choice for most patients with sarcoma. A multimodality approach that combines surgery, radiation, and, in some cases, chemotherapy is the rule. In some of the more chemotherapy-responsive sarcomas (e.g., Ewing's sarcoma, embryonal rhabdomyosarcoma, and most types of osteogenic sarcoma), surgery has taken a secondary role to aggressive chemotherapy and is best regarded as a local adjuvant to curative systemic treatment. The surgeon must be well versed in the merits of all available therapeutic modalities to treat patients with sarcoma successfully.

EPIDEMIOLOGY

Sarcomas occur in all age groups, and they are among the most common cancers in children, adolescents, and young adults. Specific sarcomas may have characteristic age distributions, but virtually any type of sarcoma can be encountered at any age. The sexes in general are equally affected, and there does not seem to be a strong tendency for sarcomas to occur in any particular ethnic or racial groups.

Most sarcomas occur in patients who have no identifiable predisposing factors—genetic or environmental. Although a history of trauma is often recalled by patients presenting with soft-tissue sarcomas, traumatic injury does not seem to predispose to sarcoma development. More likely, a patient notices a soft-tissue or bony lesion after an unrelated minor trauma and associates the two. Nonetheless, all patients presenting with soft-tissue or bony tumors should be questioned about prior trauma because of the need to differentiate malignancy from a variety of benign posttraumatic lesions, such as myositis ossificans.

A few agents are known to cause sarcomas; these account for less than 10% of all cases (2). Radiation exposure is clearly linked to the development of sarcomas. Sarcomas occurring in irradiated tissues are most commonly osteosarcomas or malignant fibrous histiocytomas, and they usually arise after a latency period of 7 to 20 years (Fig. 106.1). Among factory workers who were exposed to ^{226}radium while coating watch dials with luminous paint, osteosarcomas developed in several. Radium is incorpo-

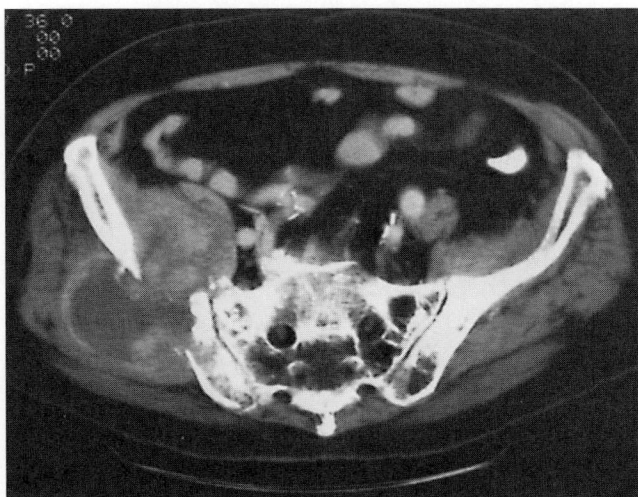

Figure 106.1. Osteosarcoma of the iliac bone that occurred 7 years after radiation therapy for cancer of the prostate and 30 years after radiation therapy for testicular cancer. The lesion was unresectable and associated with severe pain and lower extremity edema. The patient received significant palliation from two courses of intraarterial doxorubicin, after which the blood supply to the tumor was occluded by transcatheter embolization.

rated into bone in a manner analogous to calcium, and these workers were ingesting it when they used their tongues to wet the tips of their brushes. Once this practice was stopped, the epidemic ceased. The radioactive substance thorium dioxide (Thorotrast) was widely used as a contrast agent for radiologic procedures in the 1940s and 1950s. This agent predominantly accumulates in the liver where, with its half-life of over 400 years and extremely low rate of excretion, it can deliver as much as 15,000 cGy (1 cGy = 1 rad) to the hepatic parenchyma. Hepatic angiosarcomas occur with an extremely high frequency in patients who have received thorium dioxide, after a latency period of 18 to 36 years.

Certain chemicals that are not radioactive have also been implicated as causing sarcomas. These include arsenic and vinyl chloride, both of which are associated with hepatic angiosarcomas in exposed people. Some herbicides (phenoxyacetic acid compounds) have been linked to soft-tissue sarcoma development. The highly toxic chemical dioxin is used in manufacturing these herbicides, and soft-tissue sarcoma cases have been reported among workers who were exposed to dioxin and other chemicals in an industrial accident (3). Dioxin (as well as some phenoxyherbicides) is present in small quantities in the defoliant Agent Orange, widely used during the Vietnam War. The Department of Veterans Affairs ruled that Vietnam veterans in whom soft-tissue sarcomas develop are entitled to compensation for their treatment, although the epidemiologic data linking Agent Orange exposure with sarcoma development remain inconclusive (4).

In animals, infections with viruses such as the Moloney sarcoma virus can lead to sarcoma formation. In humans, infection with HIV-1 is associated with a markedly increased incidence of Kaposi's sarcoma, an otherwise extraordinarily rare lesion. It is unclear whether the predilection to development of these sarcomas is due to a specific carcinogenic effect of the virus or to the underlying immunodeficiency caused by HIV infection. Because Kaposi's sarcoma tends to occur only in certain subgroups of HIV-infected patients, other factors may be instrumental in its development.

Long-standing lymphedema of an extremity predisposes to the development of lymphangiosarcomas. Originally described in patients with arm edema after radical mastectomy and postoperative radiation (Fig. 106.2), lymphangiosarcomas have been seen in patients with severe edema from other causes as well.

Neurofibromatosis type 1 (von Recklinghausen's disease) represents a condition with a genetic predisposition to sarcoma development (Fig. 106.3). A sarcoma develops during their lifetime in an estimated 5% of patients with neurofibromatosis. These tumors are virtually all neurofibrosarcomas (sometimes called *malignant schwannomas* or *malignant peripheral nerve tumors*) and usually arise within preexisting neurofibromas. All patients presenting with a neurofibrosarcoma should be closely examined, and a thorough family history should be obtained for evidence of neurofibromatosis. Conversely, any rapidly enlarging or newly symptomatic lesion in a patient with neurofibromatosis should be suspected of malignancy.

A genetic predisposition to sarcomas also exists in patients with retinoblastoma. Originally, a high incidence of osteosarcomas was noted in the orbit after radiation therapy for primary retinoblastoma, and these lesions were attributed to the radiation. It is now clear that the incidence of all types of sarcomas is markedly increased in these patients, even in nonirradiated areas. This increased incidence is more commonly associated with the familial than the sporadic form of retinoblastoma. The precise genetic defect responsible is now understood: mutation in one copy of the *RB1* gene.

Another inherited condition is associated with soft-tissue sarcomas and breast cancer, as well as several other types of cancer. This condition, termed the *Li-Fraumeni syndrome,* is due to an inherited mutation in the *p53* gene (also referred to as *TP53*), which increases affected family

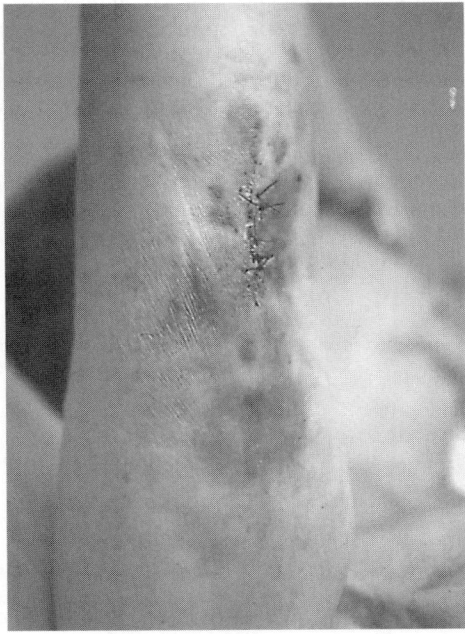

Figure 106.2. Lymphangiosarcoma of the right upper extremity occurring 21 years after a radical mastectomy and postoperative chest wall irradiation for breast cancer. At presentation, pulmonary metastases were already evident. The diffuse discoloration is more suggestive of ecchymosis than tumor. Although most instances of postmastectomy lymphangiosarcoma are associated with severe lymphedema, the extremity was relatively normal in this case.

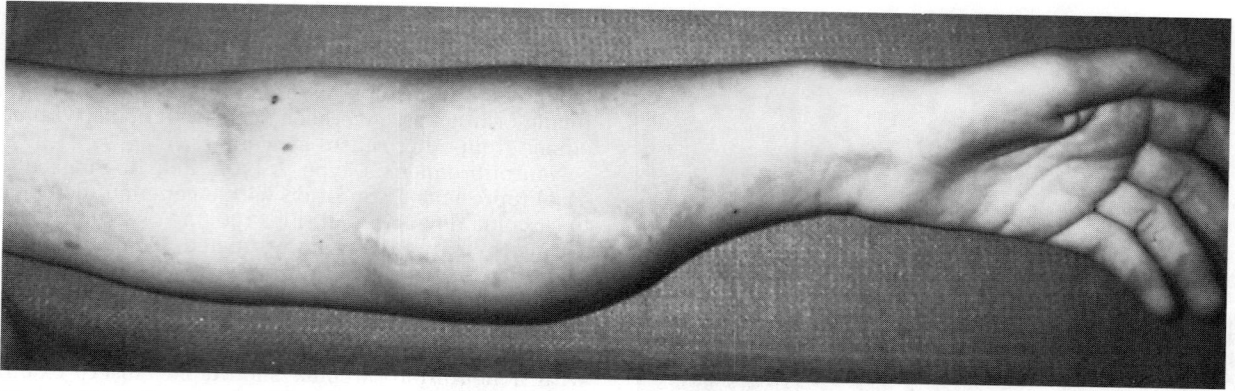

Figure 106.3. Large neurofibrosarcoma arising from the median nerve in a 17-year-old patient with neurofibromatosis. The incision is from a biopsy of the lesion 18 months before the diagnosis of malignancy. Since the earlier biopsy (which revealed only benign neurofibroma), the mass progressively enlarged and became painful, and the patient lost sensory and motor function in the median nerve distribution. There is wasting of the thenar eminence.

members' susceptibility to cancer (5). Like the genetic defect in familial retinoblastoma, the gene involved with Li-Fraumeni syndrome is also important in sporadic sarcoma development (both of these conditions are discussed later).

With the exception of patients with these syndromes, other forms of cancer are not more common in patients with sarcomas or their relatives.

PATHOLOGIC CLASSIFICATION

Sarcomas are classified by the type of tissue formed by the tumor (histogenic classification) rather than by the type of tissue in which the tumor arises. Thus, a malignant tumor arising in a skeletal muscle but composed of malignant smooth muscle cells is termed a *leiomyosarcoma*, not a rhabdomyosarcoma. Bone tumors are not termed *osteosarcomas* unless the malignant cells clearly produce osteoid. Some bone tumors produce cartilage (chondrosarcomas); a few are fibrosarcomas or other histologic types. Occasionally, soft-tissue neoplasms produce bone or cartilage; these are termed *extraosseous osteosarcomas* or *chondrosarcomas,* as appropriate. The various types of benign and malignant soft-tissue tumors are noted in Table 106.1, and the relative frequency of the different sarcomas is listed in Table 106.2.

The development of specialized markers for identifying individual types of sarcoma has led to greater precision in their classification. Available immunohistochemical stains include S-100, a marker for neural crest origin (positive in neurofibrosarcomas); factor VIII, which identifies cells of endothelial origin (positive in angiosarcomas); and myoglobin, which is found only in rhabdomyosarcomas. Although these stains are often helpful, they are not positive in every tumor of the appropriate type. Electron microscopy may reveal ultrastructural elements that are pathognomonic for a specific cell type, but in most cases sarcomas are classified by their light microscopic appearance. In a small percentage of tumors (approximately 10% in most series), the tumor cells are so poorly differentiated that no specific histogenesis can be determined, even using the supportive diagnostic tools mentioned.

Although the exact histologic type is an important datum in the evaluation of the patient with sarcoma, it is not as influential in terms of prognosis and therapy as histologic grade. Histologic grade is assessed based on the degree of cellular atypia, the frequency of mitotic figures, and the presence or absence of spontaneous tumor necrosis (Fig. 106.4). Low-grade tumors have relatively little cellular atypia, few mitoses, and no tumor necrosis. Intermediate-grade tumors have more atypia and numerous mi-

Table 106.1. HISTOGENIC CLASSIFICATION SCHEME FOR BENIGN AND MALIGNANT SOFT-TISSUE TUMORS

Tissue formed (histogenesis)	Benign soft-tissue tumor	Malignant soft-tissue tumor
Fat	Lipoma	Liposarcoma
Fibrous tissue	Fibroma	Fibrosarcoma
Skeletal muscle	Rhabdomyoma	Rhabdomyosarcoma
Smooth muscle	Leiomyoma	Leiomyosarcoma
Bone	Osteoma	Osteosarcoma
Cartilage	Chondroma	Chondrosarcoma
Synovium	Synovioma	Synovial sarcoma
Blood vessel	Hemangioma	Angiosarcoma; malignant hemangiopericytoma
Lymphatics	Lymphangioma	Lymphangiosarcoma
Nerve	Neurofibroma	Neurofibrosarcoma
Mesothelium	Benign mesothelioma	Malignant mesothelioma
Tissue histiocyte	Benign fibrous histiocytoma	Malignant fibrous histiocytoma
Pluripotent	None recognized	Malignant mesenchymoma
Uncertain	None recognized	Ewing's sarcoma; alveolar soft parts sarcoma; epithelioid sarcoma

Table 106.2. RELATIVE FREQUENCY OF HISTOLOGIC TYPES OF SOFT-TISSUE SARCOMAS IN ADULTS (ALL SITES)

Histologic type	Percentage
Malignant fibrous histiocytoma	25.9
Liposarcoma	17.7
Leiomyosarcoma	14.8
Fibrosarcoma	6.6
Neurofibrosarcoma	4.0
Synovial sarcoma	3.6
Rhabdomyosarcoma	3.6
Angiosarcoma	2.9
Extraskeletal chondrosarcoma	1.2
Malignant mesenchymoma	1.0
Extraskeletal osteosarcoma	0.6
Unclassified	5.4
Other	12.7

Modified from Lawrence W Jr, Donegan WL, Natarajan A, et al. Adult soft tissue sarcomas; a pattern of care survey of the American College of Surgeons. Ann Surg 1987;205:349.

toses, but little or no tumor necrosis. High-grade tumors show a significant degree of necrosis in addition to atypia and frequent mitotic figures.

A consistently applied grading system discriminates between tumors with good prognosis (low grade) and those with poorer prognosis (intermediate and high grade). Most studies also show an important distinction between intermediate- and high-grade lesions. The pathologist should assign a histologic grade to every sarcoma biopsy specimen. For lesions in which disparate areas exist, the highest grade encountered is generally used to categorize the tumor.

MOLECULAR BIOLOGY

The light microscopic assessment of histologic grade is the most important single element in assessing the prognosis of sarcomas. With advances in molecular biology, however, new tools for analyzing histologic type, prognosis, and cause of these tumors have become available. Cytogenetic aberrations have been recognized in a number of soft-tissue sarcomas, and some of these may be specific for certain histologic types. Alveolar rhabdomyosarcomas, myxoid liposarcomas, and synovial sarcomas have each been found to have characteristic chromosomal translocations that potentially could assist in the differentiation of these tumors from other sarcomas (6). Flow cytometric analysis of DNA from osteosarcomas has been shown to have prognostic importance, and similar analysis of soft-tissue sarcomas suggests a correlation between histologic grade and ploidy status, with most high-grade lesions being aneuploid rather than diploid. Large, prospective trials of flow cytometry and cytogenetic analysis are needed to ascertain the importance of these studies in diagnosing and treating sarcomas.

The finding of a link between familial retinoblastoma and sarcoma led researchers to search for specific genetic changes responsible for the observed susceptibility to sarcoma development. Retinoblastoma, the most common childhood malignant tumor of the eye, has been associated with a genetic defect in the retinoblastoma gene *(RB1)* on the long arm of chromosome 13. *RB1* is a recessive oncogene or "tumor suppressor gene," which means that both alleles must be inactivated before malignant transformation can occur. The normal product of this gene is involved in regulating cell division. Losing both normal copies of the gene predisposes to tumor formation by removing this growth control. Patients with familial retinoblastoma inherit one inactivated *RB1* gene. For retinoblastoma to de-

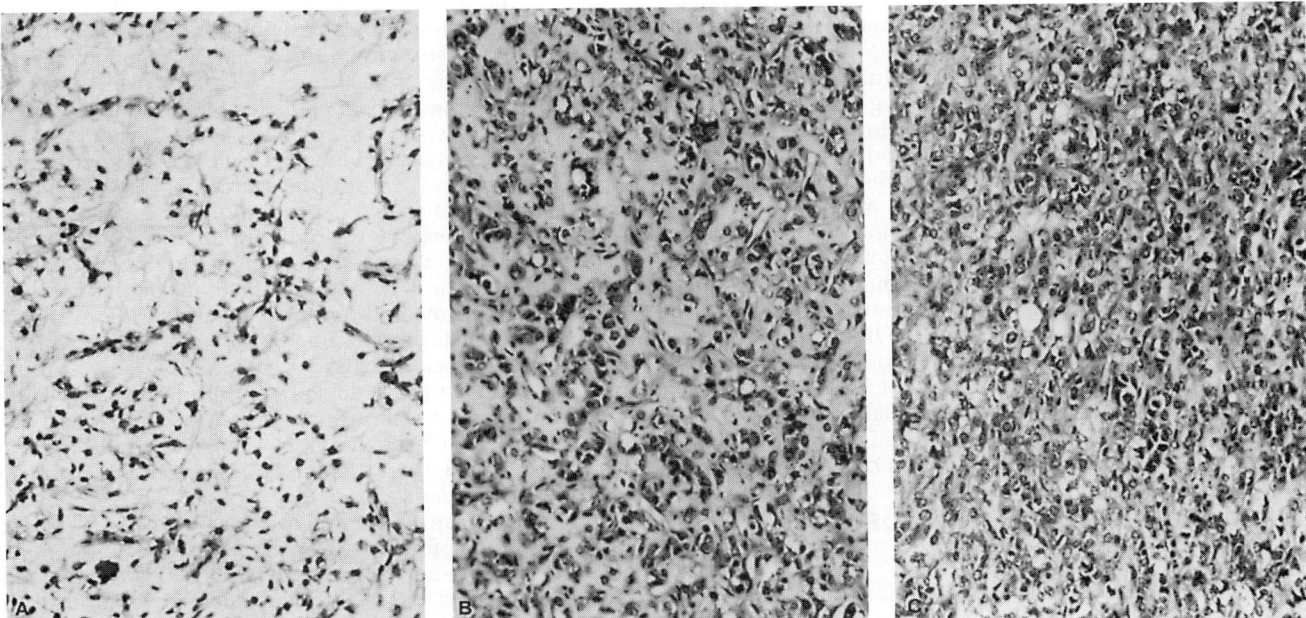

Figure 106.4. Photomicrographs of three fibrosarcomas illustrating the differing appearance of different grades of the same tumor type. The low-grade fibrosarcoma *(A)* shows relatively little cellular atypia, few mitoses, and no tumor necrosis, whereas the intermediate-grade tumor *(B)* has more atypia, numerous mitoses, and scant tumor necrosis. The high-grade tumor *(C)* shows a significant degree of necrosis in addition to atypia and frequent mitotic figures. (Courtesy of Sharon Weiss, M.D., Emory University, Atlanta, GA.)

velop in these individuals, they must undergo only one additional genetic mutation inactivating the normal gene, compared with two mutations (involving both normal *RB1* genes) necessary for someone without the inherited defect. By virtue of the increased susceptibility, people inheriting one defective *RB1* gene have multiple, bilateral retinoblastomas at an early age (often in the first year of life).

The *RB1* gene appears to affect more than retinoblastoma development. The susceptibility to sarcoma formation in patients with familial retinoblastoma relates to the genetic defect in *RB1* as well (6). *RB1* may also play a role in the pathogenesis of certain types of nonfamilial soft-tissue sarcomas. In a study of soft-tissue sarcomas in nonretinoblastoma patients, 3 of 69 cases had homozygous deletions of the *RB1* gene (7). Another five cases had evidence of heterozygous deletion. This illustrates an important principle of the genetics of cancer formation: it is frequently the case that the same gene involved in a familial cancer syndrome (where one inherited copy of the gene is defective and the other is presumably lost later) is also important in the spontaneous development of the relevant tumor type (where both normal copies of the gene must be lost to mutations or genetic deletions).

This principle is illustrated again with the *p53* gene, associated with the Li-Fraumeni syndrome. This familial cancer syndrome involves early-onset breast cancer, sarcomas (often in childhood), and a variety of other malignancies (notably brain tumors, adrenal cortical cancers, and leukemias). Patients with Li-Fraumeni syndrome inherit a defective copy of the *p53* gene, another key growth-regulatory gene. Inactivation of the second, normal copy of the gene leaves the cell without the ability to regulate gene transcription, particularly after DNA damage (8). Abnormalities of the *p53* gene are also common in sporadic cases of sarcoma. One study found *p53* abnormalities in approximately 60% of osteosarcomas and malignant fibrous histiocytomas, as well as approximately 33% of other sarcomas (9). Interestingly, some sarcomas that do not show evidence of any *p53* gene abnormalities have been found to possess amplifications of a gene called *MDM2,* which codes for a protein that inactivates the function of normal p53 protein (10).

One other important genetic change in some sarcomas is the presence of the *MDR1* (multidrug-resistance) gene, which is found in greater numbers of untreated sarcomas than most other tumor types (11). The presence of this gene has been correlated in vitro with resistance to a number of cytotoxic drugs, many of which are routinely used in sarcoma chemotherapy. Experimental studies have shown the importance of *MDR1* gene activation in the resistance of sarcoma cells to doxorubicin, probably the most commonly used drug for sarcoma treatment (12). Although other genetic abnormalities are likely to prove important in sarcoma development and treatment, these carefully studied genes vividly demonstrate the rapidly evolving link between the research laboratory and the clinic as well as the extent to which the practicing physician must be aware of developments in molecular biology.

DIAGNOSIS AND STAGING OF SOFT-TISSUE SARCOMAS

Benign soft-tissue tumors far outnumber their malignant counterparts. Because of this, prolonged delays before definitive treatment begins are common in patients with sarcoma. In a survey of more than 5,800 patients with sarcoma, roughly half waited 4 or more months before seeking medical treatment, and 20% waited at least 6 months after seeing a physician before a correct diagnosis was made (13). Many patients with sarcoma undergo prolonged treatment for chronic hematomas or pulled muscles. In nonathletic adults, persistent soft-tissue masses rarely develop from either of these causes in the absence of a history of unusually strenuous activity. Only in a setting of clear-cut local trauma should these diagnoses be entertained. If a soft-tissue mass arises in a patient with no history of trauma or persists more than 6 weeks after local trauma, biopsy should be performed.

Soft-tissue sarcomas of the extremity, trunk, head, and neck commonly present as a painless mass. Retroperitoneal sarcomas most often present as a palpable mass in association with abdominal fullness, early satiety, or vague abdominal pain. While evaluating any soft-tissue mass, the physician must always remain cognizant of the possibility of malignancy. Biopsy should be done for virtually all soft-tissue masses larger than 5 cm as well as for any new, enlarging, or symptomatic lesions. Small, subcutaneous lesions that have not changed for many years may be safely observed.

Biopsy

Properly performed, a timely surgical biopsy is the critical first step in a multimodality treatment approach. Improperly done, it can markedly complicate the care of the patient with sarcoma and occasionally even eliminate treatment options. Excisional biopsy should be reserved for small soft-tissue masses (<3 to 5 cm in greatest diameter), for which the chance of malignancy is low and for which complete excision would not jeopardize subsequent treatment in the event a sarcoma was found. For all other soft-tissue masses, incisional biopsy is indicated.

Several important technical factors must be considered when performing an incisional biopsy. For extremity lesions, the incision should be oriented along the long axis of the extremity. For truncal or retroperitoneal lesions, the biopsy incision should be situated so that it can be readily excised along with the tumor if a diagnosis of sarcoma is made. Any biopsy site should be placed directly over the tumor, at the point where the lesion is closest to the surface, and there should be no raising of flaps or disturbance of tissue planes superficial to the tumor (Fig. 106.5).

Many sarcomas appear to be relatively well encapsulated at the time of open biopsy. Most often, however, these tumors possess a pseudocapsule, and removing the tumor in this apparent plane leaves gross or microscopic cancer behind (14). Soft-tissue sarcomas should not be enucleated in the pseudocapsule to make a diagnosis; incisional biopsy leaving the bulk of the lesion undisturbed is preferable. Frozen-section pathologic analysis can be used to determine whether diagnostic tissue has been obtained, not to provide a definite diagnosis. Before wound closure, hemostasis should be achieved to avoid a hematoma that could disseminate tumor cells through normal tissue planes. Drains are not used routinely; in the uncommon case when a drain is required, it should exit either through or near the biopsy incision. If malignancy is diagnosed, the drain tract must be excised in continuity with the tumor mass.

Fine-needle aspiration cytology has a role in the diagnosis of some soft-tissue lesions. Computed tomography (CT)-guided fine-needle aspiration has proved to be helpful in diagnosing intraabdominal and retroperitoneal tumors but is rarely needed for extremity sarcomas. Fine-needle aspiration has the advantage of minimizing the potential for tumor spillage in the peritoneal cavity that can accompany open surgical biopsy of a retroperitoneal sarcoma. Even experienced cytologists, however, often are unable to discern the grade and histologic type of a sarcoma from an aspirate.

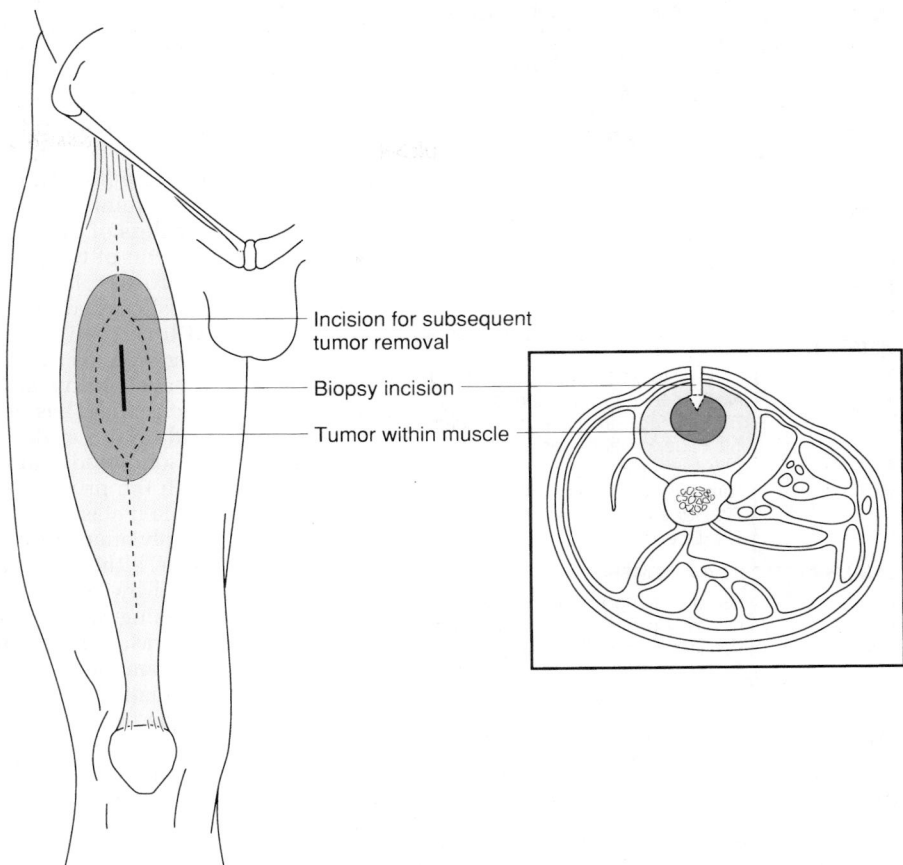

Incision for subsequent
tumor removal

Biopsy incision

Tumor within muscle

Figure 106.5. Technique for biopsy of an extremity soft-tissue mass suspected of being a sarcoma. The incision should be oriented along the long axis of the extremity, at the point where the lesion is closest to the surface, and situated so that it can be readily excised along with the tumor if a diagnosis of sarcoma is made. There should be no raising of flaps or disturbance of tissue planes superficial to the tumor. The mass should not be enucleated within the pseudocapsule; rather, incisional biopsy leaving the bulk of the lesion undisturbed should be carried out. Before wound closure, hemostasis should be achieved to avoid a hematoma, which could disseminate tumor cells through normal tissue planes. Drains are not used routinely.

A core needle biopsy retrieves a thin sliver of tissue (approximately 1×10 mm). As with fine-needle aspiration, the small sample size may make it difficult for a pathologist to accurately diagnose and grade the tumor, or the tissue obtained may not represent an adequate sample of the entire tumor, leading to an underestimate of the grade. Sufficient tissue to perform special stains or electron microscopy may not be available with this technique. Fears that core needle biopsies would result in a significant number of hematomas, resulting in dissemination of tumor cells, appear to be groundless. Series comparing core needle and open biopsies of soft-tissue tumors have documented that both the histologic type and grade of a sarcoma could be correctly determined by core needle biopsy in more than 90% of cases (15). These results have encouraged wider use of this technique, including CT-guided core needle biopsies.

Staging and Metastatic Work-up

Once the diagnosis of sarcoma is made, the extent of the primary tumor must be assessed and the presence or absence of metastatic disease determined. Because of the prognostic importance of histologic grade, the staging of the primary tumor is based on both clinical and histologic information. The usual TNM classification is modified according to a GTNM system (Table 106.3). This system has been extensively modified, and now incorporates the depth of the tumor relative to the investing muscular fascia as a criterion. Size no greater than 5 cm, superficial location, and low histologic grade are considered "favorable" factors. The T stage is assigned based on size (≤ 5 cm = T1, >5 cm = T2) and depth relative to the fascia (entirely above the fascia = a, invasion of or entirely below the fascia = b). Thus, a 5.5-cm sarcoma that is entirely located in the subcutaneous tissue above the muscular fascia would be categorized as T2a, whereas the same tumor involving the fascia would be T2b. All intraabdominal sarcomas are by definition "b" lesions. For the purposes of staging, well-differentiated and moderately differentiated tumors (grades 1 and 2) are considered together as "low grade," whereas poorly differentiated and undifferentiated tumors (grades 3 and 4) are considered together as "high grade" All small, low-grade tumors, regardless of size, are classified as stage I. Stage II sarcomas are either low grade, large, and deep (stage IIA), high grade and small (stage IIB), or high grade, large, and superficial (stage IIIC). All high-grade, large, and deep sarcomas are stage III tumors. Any tumor with regional or distant metastatic disease, regardless of the grade of the primary tumor, is classified as stage IV. This staging system is clinically useful because it assigns patients into groups with clearly differing prognoses (Fig. 106.6).

Some limitations of the revised GTNM system are apparent. The staging system no longer recognizes a difference between well- and moderately differentiated tumors, although there are significant data to suggest that grade 2 tumors fare worse than grade 1 lesions (16). Regarding size, although the GTNM size cut-off is 5 cm, tumors over 10 cm have an even worse prognosis (17,18). Future versions of the staging system could incorporate more than two categories to reflect more accurately the variations in prognosis with increasing size. Also, the current system appropriately recognizes that most superficially located

Table 106.3. AMERICAN JOINT COMMISSION ON CANCER GTNM CLASSIFICATION AND STAGE GROUPING OF SOFT-TISSUE SARCOMAS

Stage	Description
TUMOR GRADE	
GX	Grade cannot be assessed
G1	Well differentiated
G2	Moderately differentiated
G3	Poorly differentiated
G4	Undifferentiated
PRIMARY TUMOR	
TX	Primary tumor cannot be assessed
T0	No evidence of a primary tumor
T1	Tumor ≤5 cm in greatest diameter
	T1a Superficial tumor
	T1b Deep tumor
T2	Tumor >5 cm in greatest diameter
	T2a Superficial tumor
	T2b Deep tumor
LYMPH NODE INVOLVEMENT	
NX	Regional lymph nodes cannot be assessed
N0	No known metastases to lymph nodes
N1	Verified metastases to lymph nodes
DISTANT METASTASIS	
MX	Presence of distant metastasis cannot be assessed
M0	No known distant metastasis
M1	Known distant metastasis

STAGE GROUPING

Stage IA	Low grade, small	G1–2, T1a or b, N0, M0
Stage IB	Low grade, large, superficial	G1–2, T2a, N0, M0
Stage IIA	Low grade, large, deep	G1–2, T2b, N0, M0
Stage IIB	High grade, small	G3–4, T1b, N0, M0
Stage IIC	High grade, large, superficial	G3–4, T2a, N0, M0
Stage III	High grade, large, deep	G3–4, T2b, N0, M0
Stage IV	Nodal or distant metastases	Any G, any T, N1, M0 or any G, any T, any N, M1

Modified from the American Joint Committee on Cancer. American Joint Committee on Cancer (AJCC) cancer staging manual, 5th ed. 1997.

tumors have a more favorable prognosis. One series of 215 patients with superficial extremity sarcomas documented a 10-year survival rate of 85% despite the fact that 53% of tumors were high grade and 25% of tumors were 5 cm or larger (19). However, the relationship between size, grade, depth, and prognosis has not been fully defined. Specifi-

cally, it has not been confirmed that a small, superficial, high-grade sarcoma (stage IIB) truly possesses a similar prognosis to a large, deep, low-grade tumor (stage IIA) or a large, superficial, high-grade sarcoma (stage IIC).

In addition to assessing prognosis, the initial evaluation must provide information about the precise extent of the primary tumor. CT scanning and magnetic resonance imaging (MRI) are the most important studies for assessing the extent and resectability of soft-tissue sarcomas, regardless of the site of origin (20). These studies permit definition of the primary tumor in relation to bone, muscle, neurovascular structures, and adjacent organs; this is critical information when planning treatment. Both CT and MRI can provide this information, and in most cases, either study is sufficient. The choice between them is based on availability, cost, and the experience of the radiologist. Each study has advantages and disadvantages, however, and these should be considered on a case-by-case basis.

Computed tomography scans are widely available, and both the primary site and the lungs (the major site of sarcoma metastasis) can be imaged at the same sitting. Tumor involvement of bone is often more clearly visible on CT scan, although bone marrow invasion may be better defined by MRI. Disadvantages of CT scanning include the ionizing radiation and the need for intravenous iodinated contrast administration.

Magnetic resonance imaging has several advantages in evaluating sarcomas. The plane of imaging is not limited to the transverse (axial) plane of CT scans. Coronal, sagittal, and even oblique planes may be imaged with MRI. Comparative studies have also suggested that MRI better defines the relationship between tumor and normal vascular structures (20). Because of the strong magnetic fields required for imaging, patients with implanted metallic objects, such as pacemakers, artificial joints, and some vena cava filters, may not be able to undergo MRI. Occasionally, the information obtained from CT and MRI may be complementary, but for most patients with sarcoma, either study is sufficient.

Plain radiographs and radionuclide bone scans occasionally provide useful information regarding invasion of bone by tumor (Fig. 106.7), but these studies usually do not play a major role in evaluating a primary soft-tissue sarcoma. Sarcomas have a characteristic arteriographic appearance, with prominent neovascularity and displacement of normal vessels. Angiography is rarely necessary for extremity lesions, although it may useful for retroperitoneal tumors. Even there, magnetic resonance angiography represents an attractive alternative (Fig. 106.8).

Regional lymph node involvement is decidedly uncommon in soft-tissue sarcomas; less than 4% of cases have nodal metastases at presentation. When node involvement

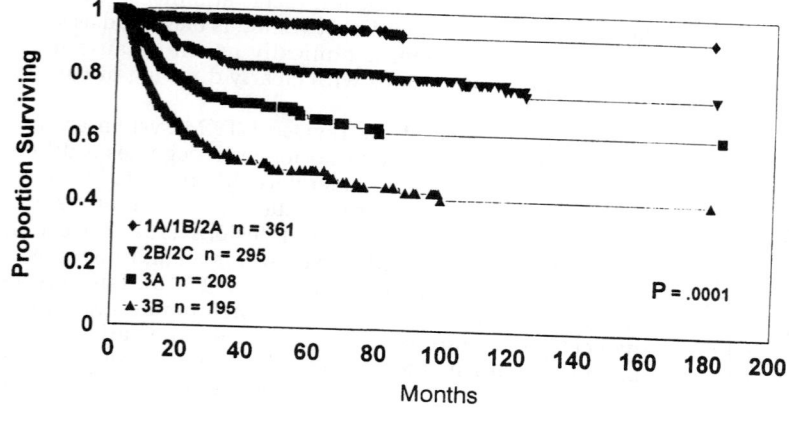

Figure 106.6. Survival rates of patients with soft-tissue sarcoma categorized by tumor depth, grade and size according to the American Joint Committee on Cancer staging system, with 3A designating stage III tumors of 5 to 10 cm and 3B designating tumors greater than 10 cm in size. (From Brennan MF. Staging of soft-tissue sarcomas. *Ann Surg Oncol* 1999;6: 8–9, used with permission.)

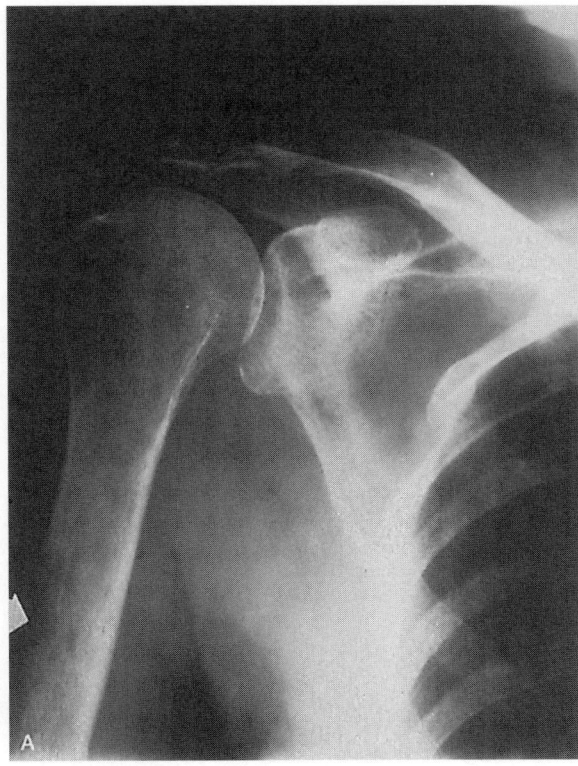

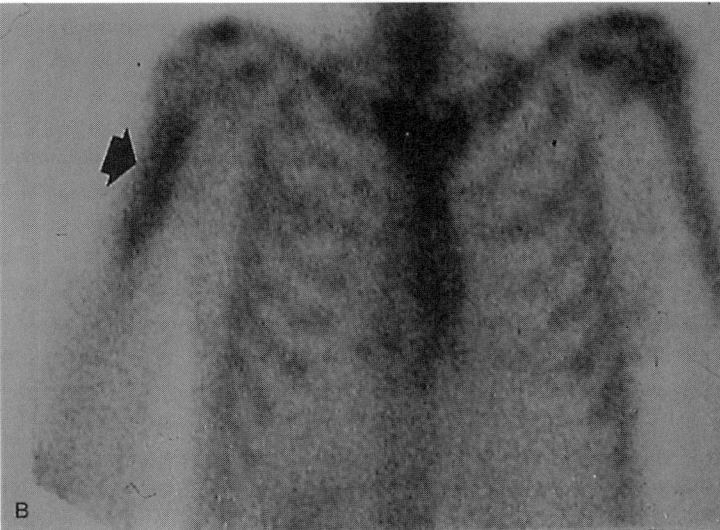

Figure 106.7. *(A)* Plain radiograph of the proximal humerus and shoulder joint, showing bony destruction *(arrow)* secondary to a large, high-grade soft-tissue sarcoma adjacent to the humerus. *(B)* Radionuclide bone scan in the same patient reveals a much greater degree of involvement *(arrow)*.

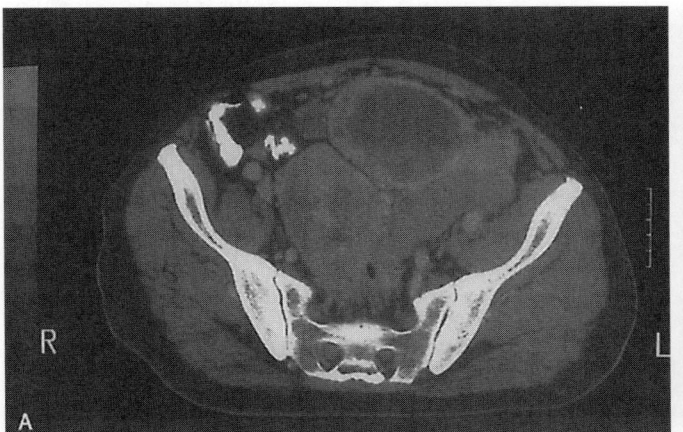

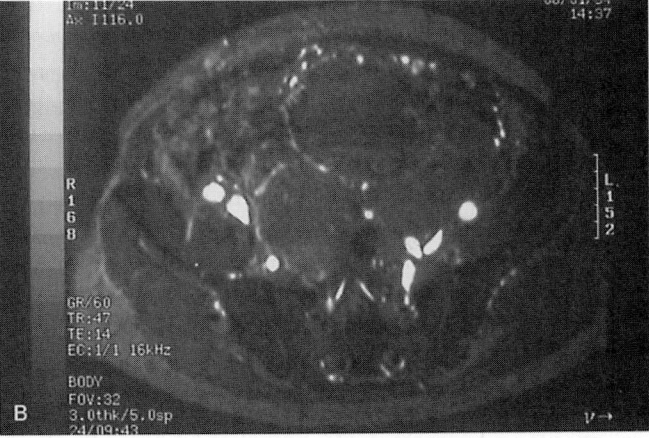

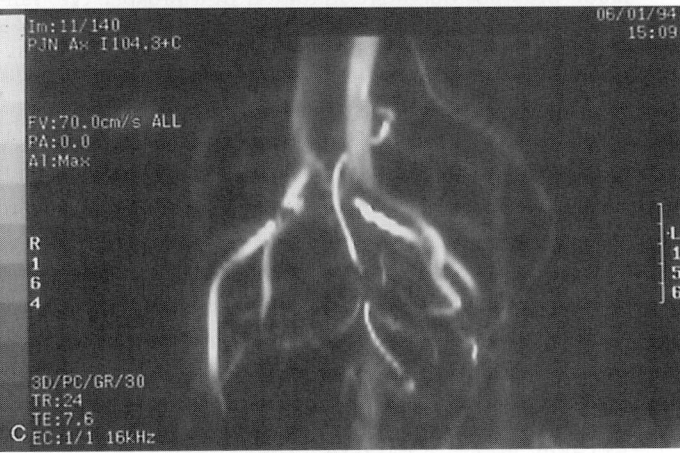

Figure 106.8. *(A)* Computed tomography scan of a large, high-grade pelvic sarcoma. There are multiple lobulations of tumor, with areas of spontaneous necrosis and a fluid–fluid level. The iliac vessels cannot be clearly distinguished as separate from the tumor mass. *(B)* Magnetic resonance (MR) angiogram of the same region revealing the iliac arteries and veins as prominent white spots against the dark background of tumor. *(C)* Planar reconstruction demonstrating the distal aorta and vena cava and the iliac arteries and veins. The MR angiogram suggested the vessels were free of involvement, as indeed was the case at the time of resection.

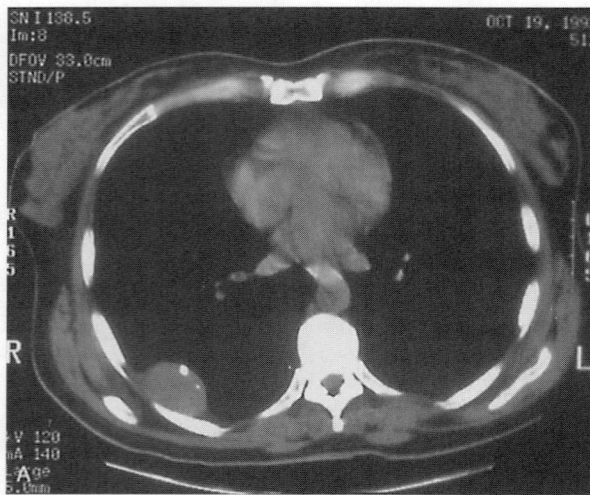
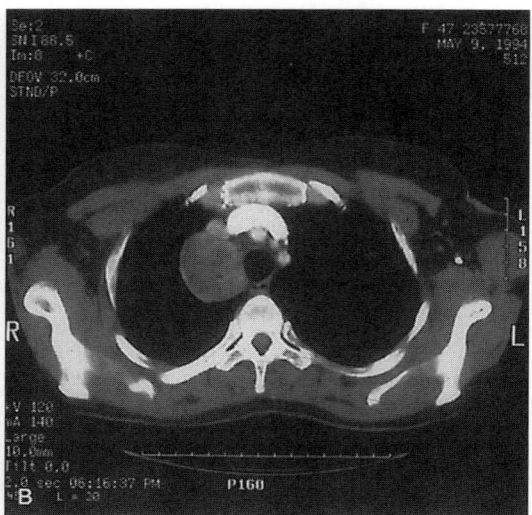

Figure 106.9. *(A)* High-grade malignant fibrous histiocytoma of the pleura. This tumor was treated with chest wall resection and postoperative radiation. *(B)* A follow-up computed tomography scan 7 months later revealed mediastinal adenopathy, which was subsequently confirmed to represent nodal metastasis from sarcoma.

occurs, it conveys essentially the same prognosis as distant metastatic disease and therefore is classified as stage IV (stage IVA if only nodal metastases are present; stage IVB if both regional and distant metastases are present). Nearly all patients who ever manifest nodal involvement have high-grade primary sarcomas (Fig. 106.9). Distant metastatic disease is present in as many as 25% of patients with soft-tissue sarcoma at the time of presentation. By far the most common site of metastasis is the lungs. In patients with sarcoma who have metastases, the lungs are involved more than 75% of the time. Approximately half of all patients with sarcoma who die of metastatic disease have lung metastases as their only site of distant spread. Liver involvement is rare except in intraabdominal and retroperitoneal sarcomas, where it represents the second most common site of distant spread. Occasional patients have bone or central nervous system metastases; these sites of disease are uncommon in patients who do not already have lung metastases.

For all patients with newly diagnosed soft-tissue sarcomas, a chest radiograph and chest CT scan are appropriate to search for pulmonary metastases. For intraabdominal or retroperitoneal tumors, a CT scan that includes the liver should be done. Other studies, such as radionuclide bone scans, CT scanning, or MRI of the head, are not indicated in the absence of symptoms that suggest metastatic involvement. Positron emission tomography (PET) scanning using fluoro-13-deoxyglucose also offers the potential for noninvasive analysis of tumor metabolism and has been shown to correlate with both tumor grade and response to treatment (21).

MANAGEMENT OF EXTREMITY SOFT-TISSUE SARCOMAS

The most common site of origin for sarcomas is the lower extremity (Table 106.4). Soft-tissue sarcomas are most often found in the muscle groups of the thigh. The proximal upper extremity is also a common location. The distal extremities are less frequent sites of origin. Over time, there have been significant changes in the surgical approach to extremity sarcomas. Initially, attempts at lim-

ited excisions of extremity sarcomas were uniformly associated with local recurrence. These "shell-out" resections enucleated the tumor from within its pseudocapsule, invariably leaving viable tumor behind. Once this was recognized, the surgical approach to these tumors changed to one favoring radical amputation. With the advent of multimodality approaches, limb-sparing resections now can be performed in more than 90% of patients, and local recurrence rates of 10% or less are reported.

Surgery

Radical amputation is amputation at least one joint space above the most proximal extent of tumor (Fig. 106.10). For a distal thigh tumor, a radical amputation would be a hip disarticulation; for a high thigh lesion, a hemipelvectomy. At one time, over half of all soft-tissue sarcomas of the extremity were treated with radical amputations. Even with such extensive and mutilating procedures, however, local recurrence rates of up to 20% were seen.

Radical amputation was compared with wide local excision plus postoperative radiation in a prospective, randomized trial; patients who underwent limb-sparing surgery had a survival rate identical to those undergoing amputation, despite a higher local recurrence rate (19%

Table 106.4. SITE OF ORIGIN OF SOFT-TISSUE SARCOMAS IN ADULTS

Anatomic site	Percentage
Lower extremity	46.4
Trunk	17.9
Upper extremity	13.1
Retroperitoneum	12.5
Head and neck	8.9
Mediastinum	1.3

From Lawrence W Jr, Donegan WL, Natarajan A, et al. Adult soft tissue sarcomas: a pattern of care survey of the American College of Surgeons. Ann Surg 1987;205:349.

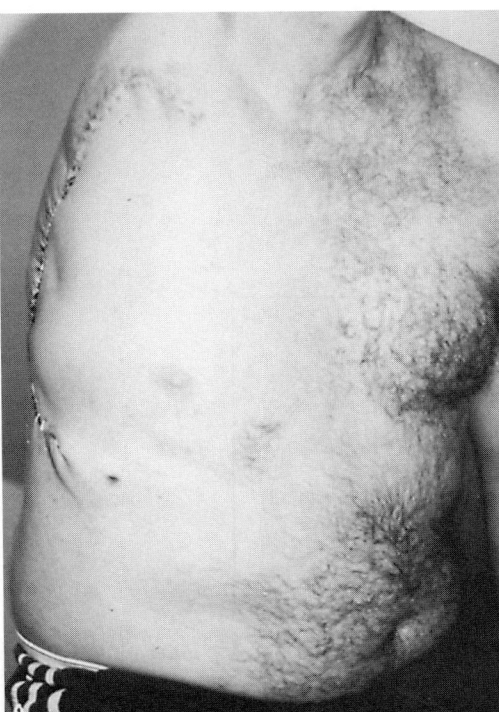
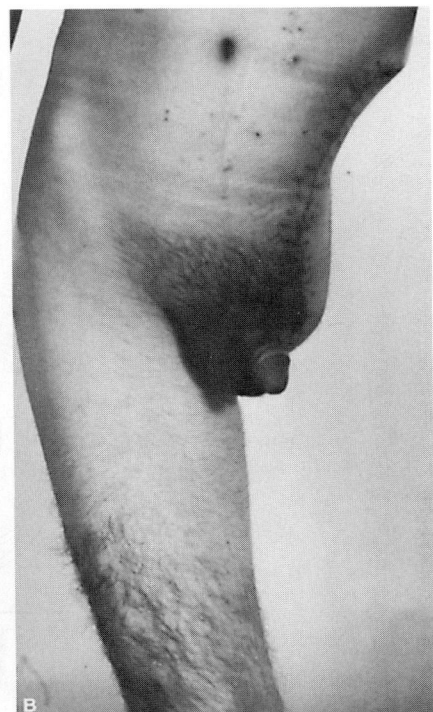

Figure 106.10. Radical amputations for extremity sarcomas include one joint above the most proximal extent of tumor. *(A)* In the upper extremity, the standard radical amputation for an upper arm tumor is a forequarter (interscapulothoracic) amputation. *(B)* In the lower extremity, the standard amputation for most tumors of the proximal thigh or buttock is a hemipelvectomy. Less-extensive amputations are possible for more distal tumors.

vs. 6%, difference not statistically significant) (22). This study demonstrated the merit of limb-sparing approaches to treating extremity sarcomas. Radical amputation now is reserved for patients who are not suitable candidates for limb-sparing approaches, usually because of bony invasion or large tumor size (Fig. 106.11), or for recurrence after previous limb-sparing surgery.

One of the earliest limb-sparing operations to be advocated was compartment excision. In this technique, the entire muscle group in which the sarcoma arises is removed from origin to insertion (Fig. 106.12). The belief that sarcomas spread diffusely throughout one muscular compartment but are prevented by fascial boundaries from lateral spread provided the rationale for this procedure. Unfortunately, most sarcomas are not confined in a single muscular compartment, and those that are do not usually involve the muscles for more than 2 to 3 cm beyond the grossly visible boundaries. Long, origin-to-insertion skin incisions often cross one or even two joints, making post-operative radiation and rehabilitation more difficult. Hence, compartment excision is used only in selected cases when the tumor is large but remains confined to one compartment.

Most limb-sparing protocols include a wide local excision as the definitive surgical procedure. Wide local excision involves gross total removal of the tumor with a wide margin of normal tissue, but no attempt is made to resect an entire muscle compartment (Fig. 106.13). Rather, a margin of 3 to 5 cm of normal tissue is obtained proximally and distally. On the lateral and deep margins, at least one grossly uninvolved fascial plane is resected *en bloc* with the tumor whenever possible. For large or deep-seated tumors, resection of uninvolved periosteum or adventitia may represent the deep margin. If necessary, major vascu-

lar structures can be resected and reconstructed with autologous or other graft material (Fig. 106.14A). On occasion, major nerves, such as the sciatic nerve, are sacrificed to preserve a functional, albeit neurologically compromised, extremity. When low-grade lesions are resected, because of their less aggressive nature, major vessels or nerves are not removed along with the tumor (Fig. 106.14B).

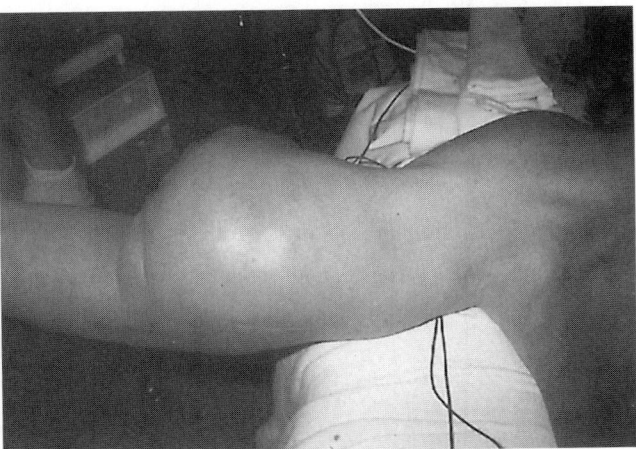

Figure 106.11. Enormous high-grade malignant fibrous histiocytoma circumferentially involving the upper arm just above the elbow. This tumor was treated with a radical amputation (shoulder disarticulation). Aggressive local or systemic treatment to shrink the tumor and avoid amputation was not used because of the patient's advanced age.

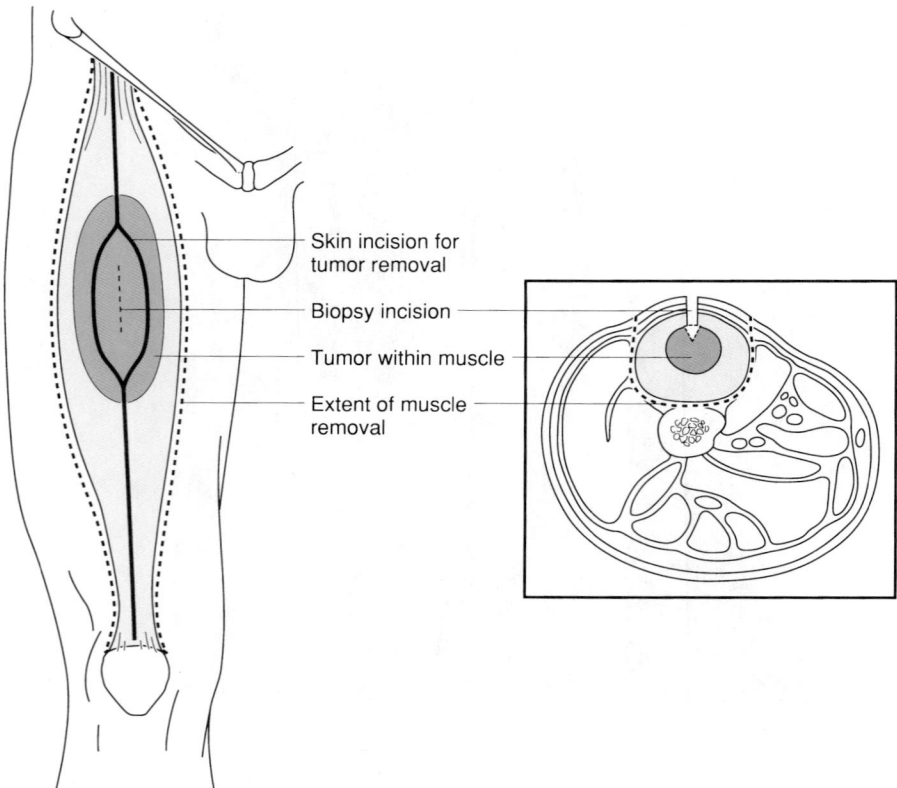

Skin incision for
tumor removal

Biopsy incision

Tumor within muscle

Extent of muscle
removal

Figure 106.12. Compartment excision involves removal of the entire muscle group in which the tumor arises from origin to insertion. The skin incision frequently crosses one or even two joint spaces. Many large soft-tissue sarcomas are not confined to a single muscular compartment.

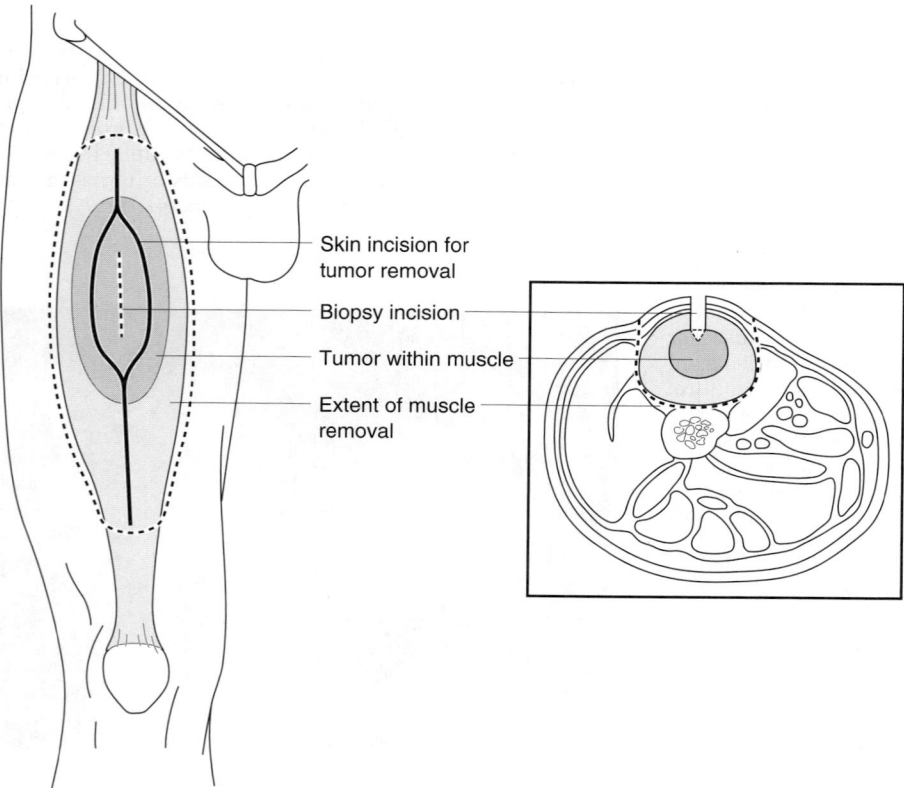

Skin incision for
tumor removal

Biopsy incision

Tumor within muscle

Extent of muscle
removal

Figure 106.13. Wide excision involves removal of the tumor with a margin of normal tissue: 3 to 5 cm is obtained proximally and distally, and on the lateral and deep margins, at least one grossly uninvolved fascial plane is resected *en bloc* with the tumor. No attempt is made to resect an entire muscle compartment. If necessary, major vascular structures or nerves may be resected.

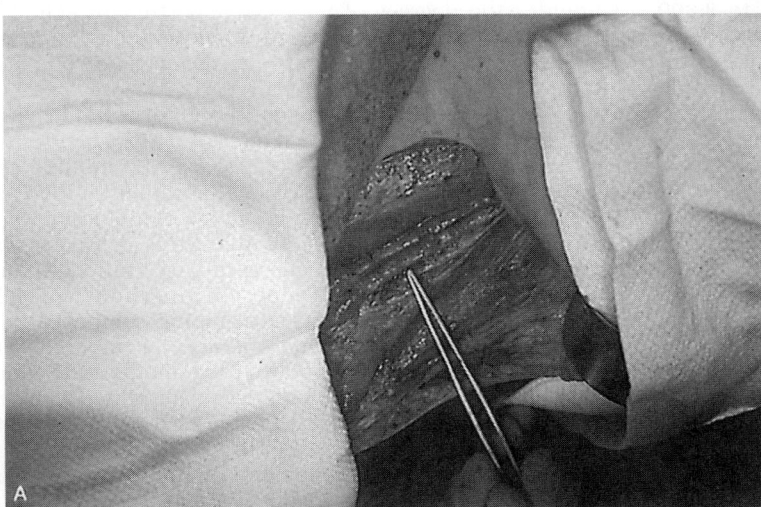
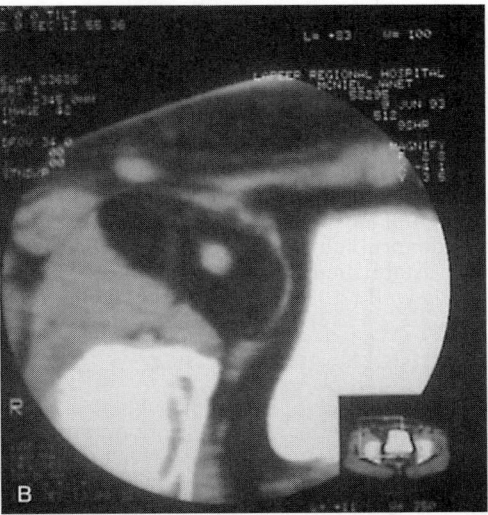

Figure 106.14. *(A)* Complete removal of a large, intermediate-grade synovial sarcoma of the right groin required resection of a small portion of the superficial femoral artery. This was reconstructed with an interposition graft of ipsilateral saphenous vein (at tip of forceps). The patient received postoperative irradiation and remains free of disease with excellent distal pulses 6 years later. *(B)* Contrast-enhanced computed tomography scan demonstrates a well-differentiated liposarcoma surrounding the right femoral artery *(central white dot)* in the groin. This tumor was resected without removal of the artery or vein by bisecting the tumor and peeling it free from the vascular structures. This patient also remains free of disease with excellent distal pulses 3 years later.

Radiation Therapy

For patients with small, low-grade tumors, wide local excision alone is associated with a low rate of local recurrence. Most other patients undergoing surgical excision, however, receive additional therapy to improve the chances for local control. This additional therapy usually includes radiation. Radiation also has some effectiveness as primary therapy for extremity sarcomas in patients who refuse or cannot tolerate surgery (23). Although the results do not match the local control rates achieved with radical surgery alone, they do provide a firm basis for including radiation therapy in multimodality treatment approaches.

Postoperative Radiation

Postoperative radiation therapy after wide surgical excision provides excellent local control for primary extremity sarcomas up to 10 cm in size. The randomized trial of amputation versus wide local excision previously cited validated the concept of limb-sparing surgery combined with postoperative radiation. Usually, a dose of 6,000 cGy or greater is required to ensure local control. At this dosage, the entire circumference of the extremity must not be irradiated or massive lymphedema results. A strip of skin and subcutaneous tissue away from the tumor usually is excluded from the treatment field to prevent this complication.

Postoperative radiation can also be delivered to the tumor bed by means of implanted radioactive sources, a technique referred to as *brachytherapy*. Although this approach has the advantage of a much shorter time to completion of therapy (usually less than 1 week, compared with 6 to 7 weeks for external beam radiation), it is technically complex and requires an experienced radiation oncologist in the operating room. A randomized trial demonstrated a significant decrease in local recurrences for high-grade sarcomas after combined surgery and postoperative brachytherapy compared with surgery alone (24). Patients with low-grade sarcomas did not benefit from adjuvant brachytherapy, although a recent prospective trial

suggested that external beam radiation is effective in decreasing local recurrence in these tumors (25). Otherwise, from a therapeutic standpoint, brachytherapy and external beam radiation appear to be equivalent when properly administered. The data from the randomized study provide strong support for the routine inclusion of radiation therapy (by some technique) in all patients with high-grade extremity sarcomas undergoing limb-sparing surgery.

Preoperative Radiation

Experience with postoperative radiation therapy for large extremity sarcomas (10 cm or more) was more disappointing, with a high incidence of local failure. Subsequently, extensive investigations suggested that preoperative radiation offered significant advantages in this group of patients. Local control rates were considerably higher when large tumors were treated before surgery, and in some cases, tumors initially considered unresectable without amputation shrank sufficiently to permit limb-sparing resection (23). Although these investigations were not randomized, the prospect of preoperative treatment for large extremity sarcomas broadened the spectrum of patients for whom limb-sparing surgery could be considered.

In an effort to further extend these findings, patients with intermediate- and high-grade extremity sarcomas have been treated with preoperative radiation therapy combined with regional chemotherapy. Three days of intraarterial chemotherapy with doxorubicin (Adriamycin; Pharmacia & Upjohn, Kalamazoo, MI), followed by large-fraction radiation (3,500 cGy in 10 days) and wide local excision, was successful in achieving local control and in preserving a functional extremity. Significant degrees of necrosis were commonly seen in the resected tumor specimen. Local complications were frequent, however, and proved to be the most common reason for subsequent amputation of the treated limb, which was necessary in approximately 5% of cases (26).

In a series of subsequent studies, this preoperative protocol was modified to decrease toxicity and simplify drug administration. Lowering the dose of radiation to 2,800 cGy in 8 days was associated with less toxicity without sacrificing local control. A randomized trial comparing intraarterial doxorubicin with the same dosage and schedule of drug administered intravenously did not establish clear-cut superiority for intraarterial therapy. Given the greater expense, risk, and patient discomfort of intraarterial therapy, intravenous doxorubicin appears to be a feasible alternative. The role of other chemotherapeutic drugs besides doxorubicin in preoperative therapy remains to be firmly established, but ifosfamide appears to be an active agent as well (26).

A Standard Approach to Limb-sparing Therapy

Although excellent results were obtained in the studies mentioned previously, it has never been established that large radiation fractions (350 cGy per treatment rather than the conventional 180 to 200 cGy) or the use of chemotherapy is critical to the success of limb-sparing therapy. Thus, controversy persists, and no limb-sparing protocol can be considered truly standard. Several principles, however, can be considered sufficiently well established to form the basis for routine application.

Wide resection, rather than shell-out excision or compartment resection, is the surgical procedure of choice. The tumor and its pseudocapsule should not be entered during the definitive excision. Patients seen after excisional biopsy should undergo wide reexcision, even if they have no clinical or radiographic evidence of residual tumor. The ideal margins are 3 to 5 cm in all directions, but at least one uninvolved fascial plane should be taken when this ideal is not achievable. If necessary, major nerves or vascular structures can be taken to achieve wide excision of high-grade lesions. Low-grade sarcomas close to major nerves and vessels usually can be dissected safely off these structures.

Resected low-grade sarcomas of the extremity are treated with postoperative radiation if the margins of resection are narrow or have been compromised to preserve major neurovascular structures. If a wide margin has been obtained around a small, low-grade sarcoma, observation without radiation may be appropriate. Intermediate- and high-grade extremity sarcomas almost always receive multimodality therapy. Wide excision plus postoperative radiation is appropriate for tumors smaller than 10 cm if preoperative evaluation reveals that a satisfactory surgical margin can be obtained. For tumors larger than 10 cm, or for fixed extremity sarcomas, limb-sparing treatment requires preoperative treatment of the tumor in most cases. Radiation alone or with chemotherapy is a reasonable preoperative approach for these patients. Amputation should be reserved for tumors that extensively surround or involve bone or that recur after a limb-sparing approach and cannot be re-resected locally.

Functional Outcome After Limb-sparing Surgery

Despite the obvious desirability of limb preservation, it has proved difficult to document an overall improvement in quality of life for patients undergoing limb-sparing as opposed to amputation surgeries. Although part of this difficulty may relate to methodologic problems in existing studies, a major factor limiting the success of limb-sparing therapy has been inadequate attention to functional aspects of treatment and patient rehabilitation. Functional outcome is difficult to define and measure. It includes the degrees of mobility and strength achieved, the ability to return to gainful employment, and the amount of residual pain, as well as the cosmetic and body image effects. An analysis of 88 patients with extremity sarcomas who underwent multimodality limb-sparing treatment showed that performance of daily activities was not significantly impaired at either 6 or 12 months after therapy. Nevertheless, a third of the patients reported a decline in their employment status over this period. Specific treatments could not be definitively linked with changes in functional outcome or quality of life, although there were more serious wound complications and joint contractures among patients undergoing combined postoperative chemotherapy and radiation compared with those undergoing postoperative chemotherapy alone. Quality of life in these patients was determined to be the same or better than pretreatment in 72% of patients at 6 months and in 80% at 12 months (27). This study suggests that functional outcome and quality of life are very acceptable and may improve over time after multimodality treatment.

The functional outcome and quality of life after limb-sparing therapy can be enhanced by integrating rehabilitation specialists into the multidisciplinary treatment team. Rehabilitation efforts are best initiated before beginning therapy rather than after treatment has been completed. A dedicated team of rehabilitation specialists can assist the sarcoma treatment team in a number of ways, including treating preexisting functional deficits, counseling regarding the functional implications of limb-sparing as opposed to amputative surgeries, designing therapy programs to minimize treatment-related functional loss, and recommending adaptive techniques and equipment to compensate for the unavoidable loss of function (28).

Chemotherapy

Chemotherapy used before surgical resection is referred to as *neoadjuvant chemotherapy*. As noted, both intraarterial and intravenous infusions of doxorubicin have been used before surgery in extremity sarcomas. Preoperative combination chemotherapy with doxorubicin-containing regimens also has been administered. Alternatively, some groups have used isolated limb perfusion, particularly for large or recurrent sarcomas. Isolated limb perfusion is performed by cannulating the iliac or subclavian artery and vein and directing all the blood flow for the extremity through a cardiopulmonary bypass pump. The temperature of the perfusate can be tightly regulated, and hyperthermic perfusion is generally used. Initially, isolated limb perfusion was carried out with standard cytotoxic agents such as melphalan. More recently, the addition of tumor necrosis factor and interferon-γ to melphalan hyperthermic perfusion has been reported to have dramatically increased tumor response rates (29). Neoadjuvant systemic chemotherapy has been validated as part of the management of osteosarcomas, but not as yet for soft-tissue tumors. Hence, the precise role of preoperative chemotherapy—whether by intravenous or intraarterial infusion or hyperthermic perfusion—remains to be defined.

Adjuvant Chemotherapy

The main cause of death in patients with soft-tissue sarcoma is distant metastatic disease, particularly for those patients with high-grade tumors or extremity lesions (30). As local control rates have improved, emphasis has been placed on eradicating metastatic disease with postoperative adjuvant systemic chemotherapy. Doxorubicin has undergone extensive evaluation as single-agent adjuvant chemotherapy for soft-tissue sarcomas. Randomized trials, however, demonstrate that adjuvant doxorubicin does not improve overall survival compared with surgery alone (31). A randomized, controlled trial of multiagent chemotherapy (doxorubicin, cyclophosphamide, and methotrexate) after surgery showed improved disease-free survival rates for patients with high-grade extremity (but not trunk or retroperitoneal) sarcomas (32). Toxicity of this regimen proved substantial. Symptomatic cardiac toxicity developed in 14% of patients, and many asymptomatic patients demonstrated decreased cardiac function on noninvasive testing. A subsequent study comparing this regimen with one with a lower doxorubicin dose to limit cardiotoxicity suggested that the less toxic program is equivalent to the higher-dose regimen (33). More recently, a randomized trial evaluating a modern adjuvant therapy regimen using doxorubicin and ifosfamide (the two most active agents in metastatic soft-tissue sarcoma) showed a significant disease-free and overall survival benefit for adjuvant chemotherapy (34). The magnitude of the benefit was sufficiently great that the trial was actually terminated early, after only 104 of a planned 200 patients had been enrolled. Despite the favorable findings from these trials, other studies of adjuvant multidrug chemotherapy in soft-tissue sarcomas have failed to demonstrate any improvement in overall survival. A metaanalysis of existing randomized trials pooled the available data to minimize the limitations imposed by the small sample sizes in all these studies. After combining the data from the different trials, it did appear that adjuvant chemotherapy decreased the likelihood of death and disease recurrence decreased in patients with high-grade extremity sarcomas (35). Whether the magnitude of this benefit is sufficient to justify the significant toxicity of adjuvant chemotherapy remains to be determined. Patients with high-grade extremity sarcomas should be evaluated for possible adjuvant chemotherapy. Whenever possible, such patients should be enrolled in an established clinical trial so that the value of adjuvant chemotherapy can be more fully determined.

MANAGEMENT OF RETROPERITONEAL SARCOMAS

Retroperitoneal sarcomas account for approximately 15% of all sarcomas and approximately 55% of all retroperitoneal tumors. The significant advances in multimodality therapy of extremity sarcomas have not been matched by similar progress in the management of retroperitoneal tumors. Most patients with retroperitoneal sarcomas die of their disease, frequently with locally recurrent tumor as the major or sole site of failure. Unlike the situation with extremity sarcomas, even patients with low-grade retroperitoneal sarcomas usually die from progressive tumor (Fig. 106.15).

The poor outcome of retroperitoneal sarcomas is in part related to the inability to diagnose these tumors at an early stage. Retroperitoneal tumors rarely cause significant symptoms until they achieve large size, and even then, symptoms usually are vague and nonspecific. Abdominal pain, weight loss, early satiety, and nausea and vomiting are the most common complaints. An abdominal mass can be felt in approximately 80% of patients at the time of presentation. In less than 1% of cases, patients with a retroperitoneal sarcoma present with hypoglycemia simulating an insulinoma. A high index of suspicion must be maintained when evaluating patients with vague abdominal complaints if the diagnosis of a retroperitoneal sarcoma is to be made expeditiously.

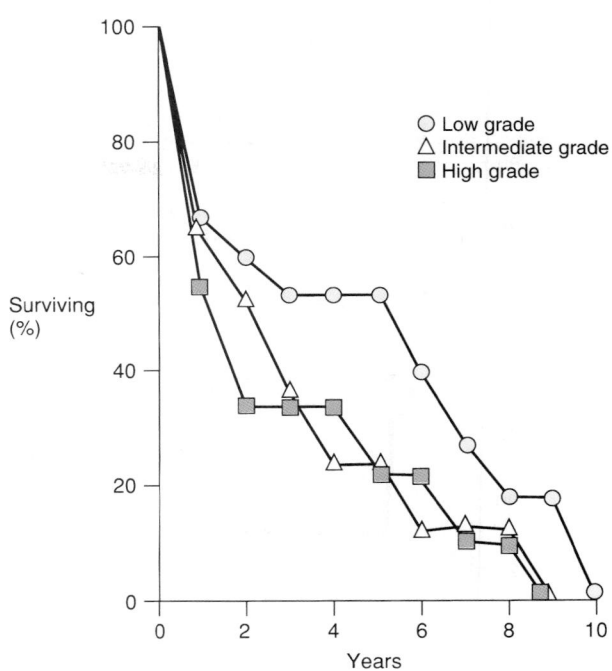

Figure 106.15. Survival rates of patients with retroperitoneal sarcoma classified by histologic grade. All patients had tumors larger than 5 cm in this series. (After Storm FK, Eilber FR, Mirra J, et al. Retroperitoneal sarcomas: a reappraisal of treatment. *J Surg Oncol* 1980;17:1.)

Surgery

The wide margins of resection routinely obtained for extremity sarcomas are difficult to achieve in the retroperitoneum. Complete excision of all gross tumor is essential for long-term disease-free survival, but this is achievable in only approximately 50% of cases (36). To remove all gross tumor, concomitant resection of adjacent organs is required more than 75% of the time (Table 106.5). Partial excisions or debulking procedures do not improve survival compared with biopsy alone (Fig. 106.16).

When a retroperitoneal sarcoma is encountered unexpectedly at laparotomy, a careful incisional biopsy with minimal disruption of surrounding tissue planes should be performed. The area of the biopsy should be isolated to prevent tumor spillage into the peritoneal cavity. When the diagnosis is confirmed, a wide excision can be carried out once the patient and surgeon are properly prepared.

Table 106.5. ORGANS RESECTED IN CONTINUITY WITH A PRIMARY RETROPERITONEAL SARCOMA

Organ resected	Percentages of operations
Kidney	46
Colon	24
Pancreas	15
Spleen	10
Major vessels (vena cava, iliac artery, or vein)	10

From Jacques DP, Coit DG, Hajdu SI, et al. Management of primary and recurrent soft-tissue sarcoma of the retroperitoneum. *Ann Surg* 1990;212:51.

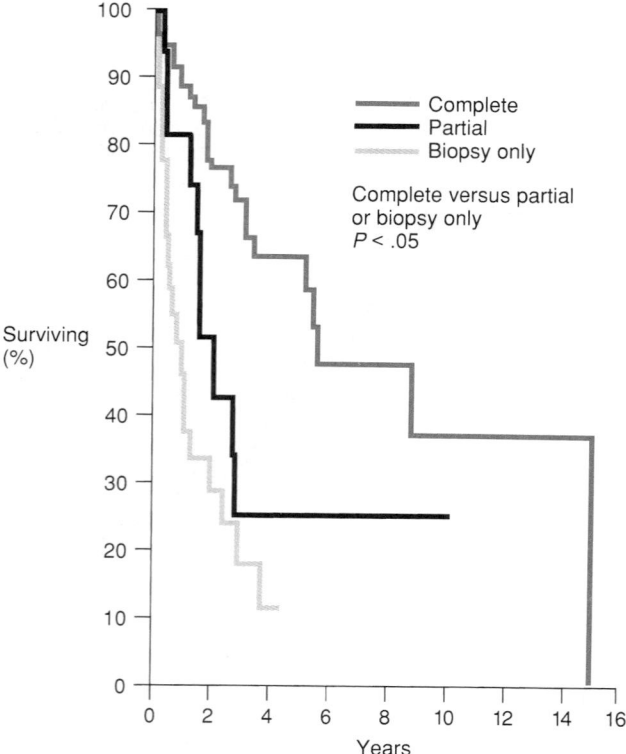

Figure 106.16. Survival rates of patients with retroperitoneal sarcoma classified by type of operation. Patients undergoing partial excision of their tumors had no improvement in survival compared with those deemed unresectable. (After Jacques DP, Coit DG, Hajdu SI, et al. Management of primary and recurrent soft-tissue sarcoma of the retroperitoneum. *Ann Surg* 1990;212:51.)

A transperitoneal approach is much more likely to allow complete resection than a flank approach. Either a vertical midline or transverse incision may be used, depending on the location of the tumor. The transperitoneal approach permits resection of adjacent organs and allows for early control of the vascular supply to the tumor. In the upper retroperitoneum, the blood supply to the tumor is frequently derived from multiple small branches, including lumbar arteries. In the pelvic retroperitoneum, one or both internal iliac arteries usually supply most of the tumor. Occasionally, the blood supply to a highly vascular pelvic retroperitoneal sarcoma may be occluded before surgery by angiographic embolization to minimize intraoperative blood loss.

Radiation Therapy

Radiation of macroscopic residual tumor in the retroperitoneum has been almost uniformly unsuccessful, stressing the importance of complete surgical resection. Because of the difficulty in achieving wide resection margins, however, radiation is frequently used as a postoperative adjuvant. Unfortunately, the excellent local control rates obtained with postoperative radiation in extremity lesions have not been matched in the retroperitoneum.

Normal tissue tolerance to radiation is much lower in the abdomen and retroperitoneum than in the extremities. Extremity tumors can frequently be treated with 6,000 cGy or more in conventional dose fractions. In contrast, the small bowel can tolerate only 4,500 to 5,000 cGy, and the liver and kidney even less. In an attempt to limit normal tissue toxicity, intraoperative radiation therapy has been used. This approach offers the advantage of allowing the bowel and other sensitive structures to be moved out of the field while a single high dose of radiation is administered directly to the tumor bed. Intraoperative radiation therapy is costly, logistically difficult, and associated with complications of its own, such as neurotoxicity. A randomized trial did not demonstrate any significant advantage for intraoperative radiation compared with conventional external beam radiation in retroperitoneal sarcomas (37).

Chemotherapy

Aggressive systemic chemotherapy is poorly tolerated in patients who have just undergone a major intraabdominal procedure with resection of multiple organs. Several trials of postoperative adjuvant chemotherapy do not show any benefit for patients with retroperitoneal sarcoma, and in one study, treated patients fared worse than those not receiving chemotherapy (38). Preoperative intraarterial chemotherapy is limited by the absence of a single feeder vessel in most retroperitoneal tumors. Nonetheless, a nonrandomized study suggested that preoperative doxorubicin (given intravenously in those patients without a single feeding artery) and external beam radiation followed by aggressive surgical resection led to longer survival times and lower local recurrence rates than those found in a historical cohort treated with surgery with or without postoperative radiation (39).

Radiation Sensitizers

Radiation sensitizers are being investigated as a means to improve the effectiveness of external beam radiation, particularly in the retroperitoneum, where normal tissue tolerance limits the dose that can be delivered to the tumor. Iododeoxyuridine (IUdR) and similar radiosensitizing agents are incorporated into DNA in place of thymidine (Fig. 106.17); cells containing this altered DNA are more susceptible to radiation damage. The drug IUdR is 100 times more effective than doxorubicin as a radiation sensitizer in vitro, although it does not have doxorubicin's direct cytotoxic effect. Studies of IUdR and external beam radiation in unresectable soft-tissue sarcomas document impressively high rates of local control without surgery (40).

Preoperative treatment with IUdR and radiation allows complete excision of all gross tumor for most patients with

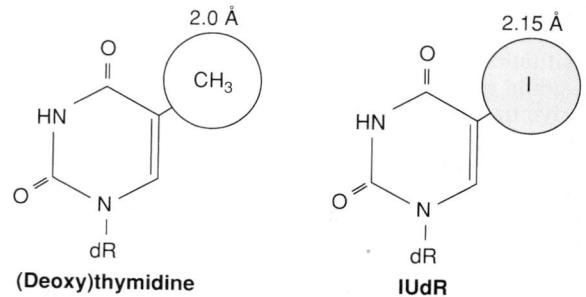

Figure 106.17. Chemical structure of the radiosensitizer iododeoxyuridine (IUdR) and the nucleotide thymidine. IUdR contains an iodine atom in place of the 5'-methyl group of thymidine. Because the atomic radii of the two are similar, IUdR is incorporated into DNA in place of thymidine. Because of iodine's greater atomic weight, cells containing IUdR in their DNA are more susceptible to damage by radiation.

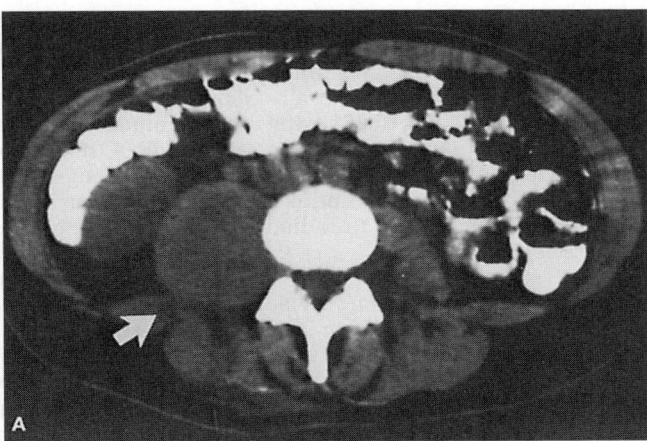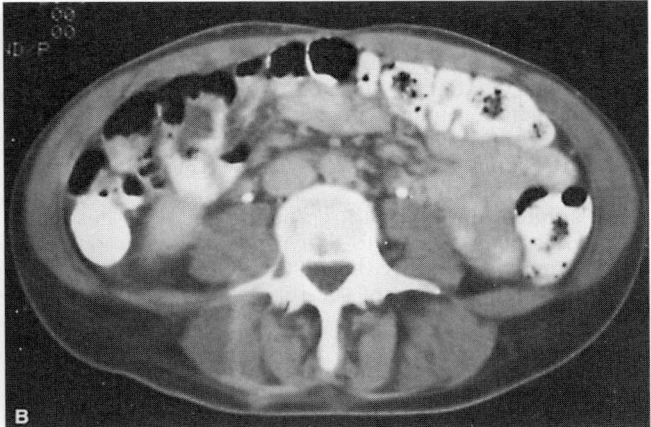

Figure 106.18. *(A)* Pretreatment computed tomography (CT) scan of patient with a high-grade undifferentiated sarcoma in the paravertebral retroperitoneum *(arrow)*. *(B)* After treatment with iododeoxyuridine and radiation, a second CT scan shows the tumor to be significantly smaller. At surgery, only scar tissue without grossly obvious tumor was encountered. Pathologic analysis revealed three microscopic foci of viable sarcoma in the psoas muscle; no gross tumor was found.

retroperitoneal sarcomas, and toxicity of this protocol has been acceptable (41). Significant regressions have been seen, with extensive posttreatment tumor necrosis and even complete disappearance of gross tumor encountered in some cases (Fig. 106.18). It is too early to tell if this approach will alter mortality rates for patients with these difficult tumors. Unfortunately, no matter how much local control rates can be improved with aggressive local/regional therapy of retroperitoneal sarcomas, the large size of these tumors at presentation makes it likely that many patients will ultimately succumb to distant metastases unless better systemic treatments can be developed.

DIAGNOSIS AND MANAGEMENT OF DESMOID TUMORS

Desmoid tumors are unusual soft-tissue lesions with unique characteristics but definite similarities to low-grade soft-tissue sarcomas. Although clinical reports of low-grade soft-tissue sarcomas often include desmoid tumors (25), in fact desmoids virtually never metastasize even after multiple local recurrences (42). Desmoids have also been referred to as *aggressive fibromatosis,* reflecting the uncertainty that exists about their malignant potential. But whatever name is chosen, some facts are clear. Desmoid tumors present in a fashion identical to soft-tissue sarcomas, as an enlarging, often painless, soft-tissue mass. Clinically and radiographically, except for the special settings described later, there is nothing to distinguish a desmoid tumor from a soft-tissue sarcoma. As with low-grade sarcomas, wide excision is the mainstay of treatment, but local recurrence after surgical treatment is very common. Deaths due to desmoids are infrequent because the tumors do not metastasize, but can occur because of local recurrence in a critical area such as the neck.

Little is known about the etiology of desmoid tumors. There are two specific clinical settings in which desmoids arise, which have provided insights into both the cause and the therapy of these lesions. The first is during or just after pregnancy. Desmoid tumors are more common in women than men and frequently present within 1 to 2 years of delivery, occasionally arising in the vicinity of a cesarean section scar. These facts, combined with isolated reports of spontaneous regression of desmoids at menopause and the demonstration of estrogen receptors

on some tumors, suggest a hormonal component to their development. Based on this, hormonal therapy with a variety of agents, most notably tamoxifen, has been used with occasional success. We and others have seen either complete disappearance, marked shrinkage, or stabilization of tumor growth combined with marked symptomatic improvement after treatment with tamoxifen alone or in combination with other agents (see later discussion) (42, 43).

Desmoid tumors occur with greatly increased frequency in patients with familial adenomatous polyposis. The link of familial polyposis with desmoids and other soft-tissue tumors was originally given the eponym *Gardner's syndrome.* It is now known, however, that all patients with familial polyposis are at risk for development of desmoids and that the genetic defect in patients with polyposis with or without desmoids is identical. Hence, the term Gardner's syndrome has fallen into disuse. The desmoid tumors in patients with polyposis tend to occur in the abdomen, often in the colonic mesentery after total proctocolectomy has been performed to prevent the development of adenocarcinoma of the colon. Patients with familial polyposis are born with one defective copy of the *apc* gene, a tumor suppressor gene. As with the *RB1* and *p53* genes, the second, the normal copy must be lost for a tumor (either an adenomatous polyp or a desmoid) to develop. It is likely that, in a predisposed person, surgical trauma and the resultant stimulation of fibroblast growth increases the chance that a desmoid tumor will actually develop. This may explain both the predilection for mesenteric tumors in patients with polyposis and abdominal wall tumors in some women after cesarean section.

Another nonsurgical therapy for desmoids, nonsteroidal antiinflammatory drugs, was suggested by studies in patients with familial polyposis. Of the available drugs, the little-used arthritis medication sulindac (Clinoril; Merck & Co., West Point, PA) appears to be the most active. This drug has a relatively unique enterohepatic circulation, and at least some patients with familial polyposis have experienced significant reduction in the number of colonic polyps after treatment with oral sulindac. In the course of such treatment, anecdotal regressions of coexisting desmoid tumors have been seen. Alone or in combination with tamoxifen, objective regression of as many as 50% of polyposis-associated desmoid tumors has been reported

(43). Sporadic desmoids, not associated with familial polyposis, also occasionally respond to this combination. Other therapeutic modalities have been used to treat desmoid tumors. Radiation therapy has been used both as primary treatment and as postoperative adjuvant therapy (25,42). Cytotoxic chemotherapy regimens have been used, with some successes reported with relatively nontoxic regimens (43).

The surgical approach to resectable sporadic desmoid tumors has been similar to that used for low-grade soft-tissue sarcomas: resect with a histologically negative margin if possible, but do not sacrifice major neurovascular structures or adjacent organs unless absolutely necessary. If pathologic analysis of the resected specimen reveals close approximation of tumor to the surgical margin, either reexcision or postoperative radiation is used. Unresectable or recurrent desmoids, as well as those associated with familial polyposis, are treated first with the combination of tamoxifen and sulindac. Resection or radiation is used for failures of this therapy or to eliminate residual disease after partial responses. Chemotherapy is usually reserved as a last resort in patients who have failed all other therapies and are severely symptomatic or in danger of dying because of compression of vital structures by tumor.

DIAGNOSIS AND MANAGEMENT OF PRIMARY BONE SARCOMAS

Primary sarcomas of bone pose certain unique challenges, but in many ways, their behavior is similar to that of soft-tissue sarcomas. Lessons learned from the treatment of bone sarcomas provide important leads for improving soft-tissue sarcoma therapy. For this reason, the general surgeon should have at least a passing acquaintance with the diagnosis and treatment of bone sarcomas.

More than 70% of bone malignancies are metastatic from another site or are of hematologic origin (lymphoma or myeloma). A variety of primary bone sarcomas are known. The spindle cell bone sarcomas have a light microscopic appearance similar to sarcomas arising in the soft tissues and are further classified based on their histogenesis. This group includes osteosarcomas, chondrosarcomas, fibrosarcomas, and malignant fibrous histiocytomas arising in bone. The small round cell sarcomas include osseous Ewing's sarcomas/primitive neuroectodermal tumor of bone. Osteosarcomas are by far the most common primary bone sarcomas and have been best studied in terms of therapy. They are the primary focus of this section.

Osteosarcomas occur most commonly around the knee, either in the distal femur or proximal tibia, but they can be encountered in any bone (Table 106.6). Osteosarcomas originate in the metaphyseal ends of the involved bone.

Most osteosarcomas occur in childhood and adolescence; roughly 80% of patients are younger than 20 years, but there is a second peak beginning after age 60 years. This latter peak corresponds to osteosarcomas arising in bones affected with Paget's disease, the most common condition predisposing to osteosarcoma development. Osteosarcomas arise in as many as 10% of patients with long-standing Paget's disease. Other etiologic factors for bone sarcomas, such as exposure to radiation, have been discussed previously.

Like soft-tissue sarcomas, osteosarcomas are graded using a three-part system. Most osteosarcomas are high-grade (grade III), but low-grade variants exist. These less aggressive tumors are usually parosteal or periosteal in location, in contrast to the intramedullary origin of classic osteosarcoma. As with soft-tissue sarcomas, a GTNM staging system is used. The stage groupings, however, are somewhat different than for soft-tissue tumors (Table 106.7). Most osteosarcomas are stage IIB (high-grade, tumor invasion beyond cortex, no nodal or distant metastases). Involvement of regional lymph nodes is rare at the time of presentation (<3%). Pulmonary metastases are the most common site of distant spread and may be discovered in as many as 25% of patients at the time of presentation. Bone metastases are not uncommon in osteosarcoma, although less frequent than lung metastases.

Table 106.6. SITE OF ORIGIN OF OSTEOSARCOMAS

Anatomic site	Percentage
Lower extremity	77.6
Upper extremity	12.9
Pelvis	6.0
Shoulder	2.6
Vertebrae	0.8

Modified from Eilber F, et al. Management of stage IIB osteogenic sarcoma: experience at the University of California, Los Angeles. Cancer Treat Symp 1985;3:11B.

Table 106.7. AMERICAN JOINT COMMISSION ON CANCER GTNM CLASSIFICATION AND STAGE GROUPING OF OSTEOSARCOMAS

Stage	Description
TUMOR GRADE	
GX	Grade cannot be assessed
G1	Well differentiated
G2	Moderately well differentiated
G3	Poorly differentiated
G4	Undifferentiated
PRIMARY TUMOR	
TX	Primary tumor cannot be assessed
T0	No evidence of primary tumor
T1	Tumor confined within the cortex
T2	Tumor invades beyond the cortex
LYMPH NODE INVOLVEMENT	
NX	Regional lymph nodes cannot be assessed
N0	No regional lymph node metastasis
N1	Regional lymph node metastasis
DISTANT METASTASIS	
MX	Presence of distant metastasis cannot be assessed
M0	No distant metastasis
M1	Distant metastasis
STAGE GROUPING	
Stage IA	G1, T1, N0, M0
	G2, T1, N0, M0
Stage IB	G1, T2, N0, M0
	G2, T2, N0, M0
Stage IIA	G3, T1, N0, M0
	G4, T1, N0, M0
Stage IIB	G3, T2, N0, M0
	G4, T2, N0, M0
Stage III	Not defined
Stage IVA	Any G, any T, N1, M0
Stage IVB	Any G, any T, any N, M1

Modified from Beahrs OH, Henson DE, Hutter RVP, et al. Manual for staging of cancer, 14th ed. Philadelphia: JB Lippincott, 1992.

Clinical Evaluation

A painful mass is the most common presenting complaint with an extremity osteosarcoma. The tumor may also present as a painless mass, particularly when it originates in the axial skeleton. Limitation of motion is often present when the tumor arises near or involves a joint. A history of trauma is not uncommon, but traumatic injury has never been linked with sarcoma development. Patients occasionally present with pathologic fracture of the involved bone.

Plain radiographs of the affected bone are the first step in evaluating a suspected osteosarcoma. High-grade osteosarcomas lead to rapid destruction of bone with new bone formation and periosteal reaction. These changes are manifest radiographically by an extensive, poorly defined destructive bony lesion, often with an extraosseous component (Fig. 106.19). Codman's triangles, indicative of periosteal reaction, are characteristic but not pathognomonic of osteosarcoma. If the radiographic picture suggests an osteosarcoma, further radiologic evaluation should be done before proceeding with biopsy. This allows the full anatomic extent of tumor to be defined without postsurgical artifact. More important, the radiologic evaluation allows the biopsy incision to be planned with an understanding of subsequent limb-sparing surgical options.

Radionuclide bone scanning using ^{99m}technetium pyrophosphate can identify distant metastases to other bones as well as define skip areas of involvement in the bone of origin. ^{67}Gallium and ^{201}thallium scans may be useful for assessing the response of a primary osteosarcoma to preoperative chemotherapy. More recently, PET scanning and MRI spectroscopy have been used in this role (21).

Computed tomography scanning is the most important modality in evaluating a bone sarcoma. It is excellent for assessing the degree of bony destruction, the extent of soft-tissue involvement, and the relation of the tumor to adjacent neurovascular structures. The entire affected bone, including the complete joint above and below the tumor, should be visualized on the scan. A chest CT can provide evidence of pulmonary metastases too small to be seen on chest radiograph.

Magnetic resonance imaging is an important adjunct to CT scans in some patients, particularly those who are being considered for limb-sparing surgery. The excellent definition of marrow involvement by tumor allows for accurate planning of the proximal extent of the tumor resection. Angiography, although accurate in defining the relation of tumor to vessels, is rarely necessary unless intraarterial chemotherapy is used.

Biopsy

After the radiologic evaluation establishes the extent of the bony lesion, an incisional biopsy should be performed (44). The biopsy incision should be carefully planned so as not to jeopardize subsequent efforts at limb sparing. A vertical incision, oriented along the long axis of the extremity, is always used for arm or leg tumors. For tumors situated close to the knee, the incision is placed medially or laterally because a posterior incision can compromise the functional result of subsequent surgery. When the primary tumor is located in the pelvis or shoulder girdle, the biopsy should be performed in a location that allows its ready inclusion in the subsequent definitive operation incision.

Subject to the aforementioned constraints, the biopsy incision is usually placed over the most superficial portion of the tumor, and dissection is kept to a minimum. Any tissue planes entered during the biopsy are considered contaminated by tumor and must be excised in the subsequent definitive resection. If an adequate amount of tissue can be obtained by sampling the extraosseous component, this is preferable to biopsy of the bone itself. If the cortex of bone is entered, a plug of methylmethacrylate can be used to seal the bone and prevent hemorrhage or tumor spillage. Hemostasis should be achieved before closure; a drain should almost never be necessary. After the biopsy, weight bearing on the affected limb should be restricted to minimize the chance of pathologic fracture.

Preoperative Chemotherapy

Unlike the situation for soft-tissue sarcomas, preoperative (neoadjuvant) chemotherapy is sufficiently well established to be considered standard treatment for patients with osteosarcoma. Historically, patients with clinically localized osteosarcoma treated by surgery alone had approximately a 20% 5-year survival rate. Adjuvant systemic chemotherapy after surgery improved that figure to 55% to 70% in randomized trials (Fig. 106.20). Contemporary protocols that incorporate preoperative chemotherapy into the regimen have been associated with 5-year survival rates in excess of 80%, and most of these long-term survivors have been cured of their cancer (45).

Several significant advantages of preoperative chemotherapy for osteosarcomas have emerged. The preoperative therapy makes limb-sparing surgery more successful by decreasing the extent of soft-tissue involvement and allowing time for the creation of a custom-made bone replacement. Furthermore, the tumor's response to the preoperative chemotherapy may identify those patients who require more intensive postoperative chemotherapy.

Preoperative response to chemotherapy is monitored in several ways. Many patients with osteosarcomas have an

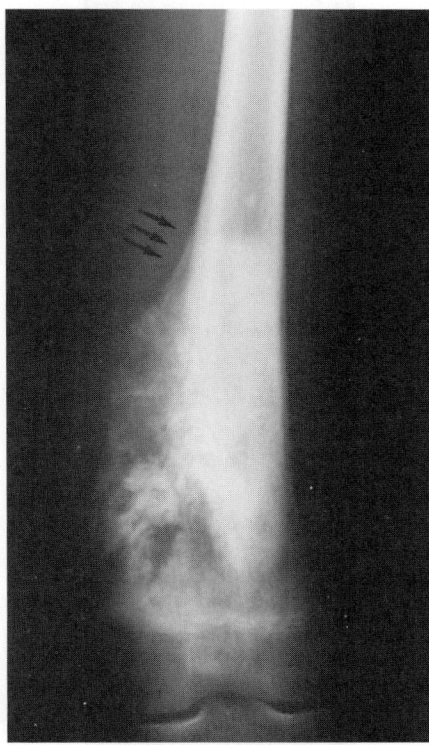

Figure 106.19. Plain radiograph of the femur showing a high-grade osteosarcoma. The tumor is an ill-defined destructive lesion with an extensive soft-tissue component. Codman's triangles are present *(arrows)*.

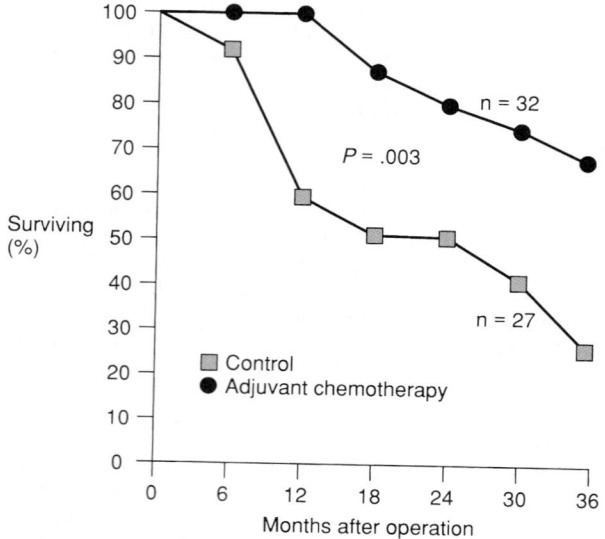

Figure 106.20. Survival rates of patients with surgically resected osteosarcoma treated with or without postoperative adjuvant chemotherapy in a randomized, controlled clinical trial. (After Eilber F, Giuliano A, Eckardt J, et al. Adjuvant chemotherapy for osteosarcoma: a randomized prospective trial. *J Clin Oncol* 1987; 5:21.)

elevated serum alkaline phosphatase level, which should decline if therapy is effective. Serial scans, such as [201]thallium scans, can be used to document decreasing tumor uptake. Failure of serum markers or scans to improve during preoperative therapy may be an indication to switch to more intensive therapy even before surgery. At the time of tumor resection, assessing the viability of the excised tumor provides the best measure of tumor response. A good response is defined as either complete absence of viable tumor cells or presence of only microscopic foci of viable cells, without any confluent areas of viable tumor. Attempts at scoring the percentage of necrosis have been less consistent, but at least 95% necrosis is necessary before a response can be considered good. Indeed, the histologic definition of a good response outlined previously correlates more nearly with 98% to 99% necrosis. Patients who achieve a good response require only a short course of postoperative chemotherapy; those who do not are treated with a longer postoperative regimen that includes doxorubicin and cisplatin.

Surgery

Extremity osteosarcomas may be treated surgically either by radical amputation (amputation at least one joint above the most proximal extent of tumor) or by *en bloc* resection with limb sparing. Limb-sparing approaches can be considered for most patients with extremity sarcomas and no evidence of neurovascular involvement. Patients presenting initially with pathologic fractures are at higher risk for local recurrence and are less suitable candidates for limb sparing. Virtually all limb-sparing protocols for osteosarcoma incorporate some form of preoperative chemotherapy.

Essential to any limb-sparing operation is complete removal of the affected bone and soft tissues. The old biopsy site is taken in continuity with the tumor, and the adjacent joint is also resected. A proximal bone margin of 6 to 7 cm usually is taken beyond the highest area of abnormality on preoperative, pretherapy scans. Even if pretreatment in-

duces some degree of tumor shrinkage, the operation should remove all areas where disease was noted at initial presentation. The marrow at the level of bony transection is curetted out and sent for frozen-section analysis to verify the adequacy of the proximal bone margin. For extensive lesions of the femur, resections of the entire femur with limb sparing can be performed.

A variety of reconstructive techniques are available after resection of an extremity osteosarcoma. Autografts (such as vascularized or nonvascularized fibular grafts), cadaver allografts, and simple arthrodeses have all been used (Fig. 106.21). Custom-made titanium endoprostheses are often used (Fig. 106.22), but their use is limited by the size of bone that can accommodate them (the distal tibia is often too small to accept the prosthesis and still have adequate strength to bear weight after proximal tibial resection); the fact that many patients with osteosarcoma are children who continue to grow on the unoperated side; and the long-term stresses that an active young adult puts on a prosthetic bone and joint. Technologic advances are addressing some of these issues. A new modular distal femoral prosthesis has been developed that can be periodically expanded, progressively lengthening the limb as the other leg grows. Newer materials and cementless prostheses that promote bony ingrowth rather than rely on fixative cements may provide better long-term functional results.

Some pelvic osteosarcomas can also be resected with limb sparing. Small or low-grade tumors of the bony pelvis can be removed by internal hemipelvectomy (46). Virtually the entire hemipelvis and hip joint can be resected, leaving the neurovascular supply to the leg intact (Fig. 106.23A). Although the leg on that side is significantly shortened, weight bearing is eventually possible

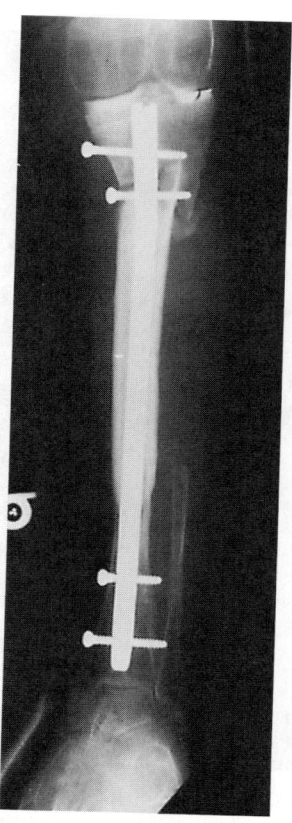

Figure 106.21. Allograft reconstruction after resection of an osteosarcoma of the proximal tibia.

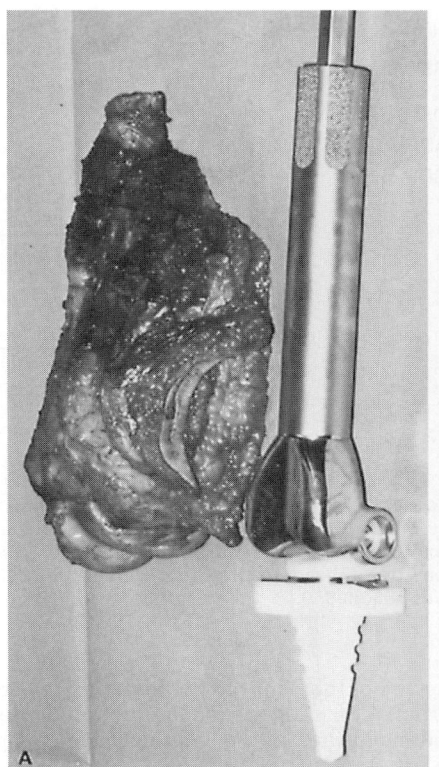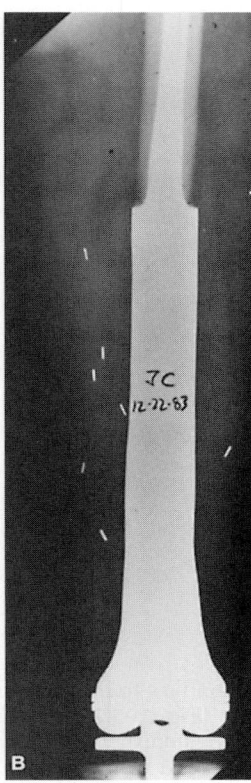

Figure 106.22. *(A)* Custom-made titanium prosthesis for replacement of the distal femur and knee joint. *(B)* Postoperative radiograph showing the prosthesis in place.

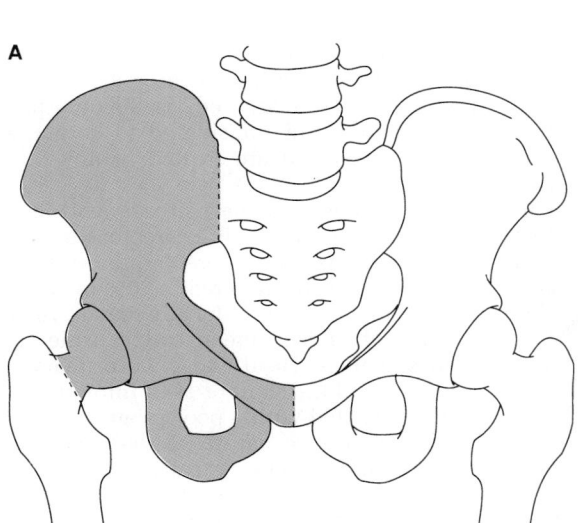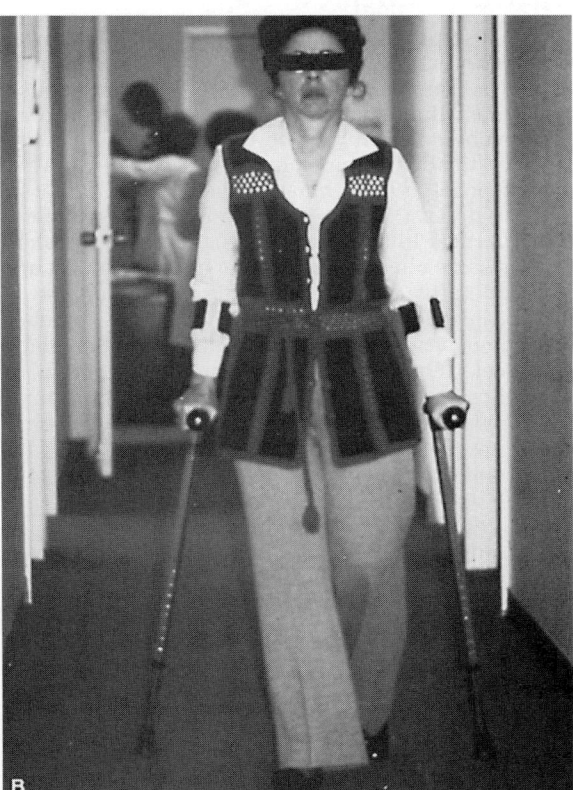

Figure 106.23. *(A)* Depiction of the bony structures removed in the conduct of an internal hemipelvectomy. *(B)* Postoperative photograph showing the ability of the patient to bear weight on the noticeably shorter operated side.

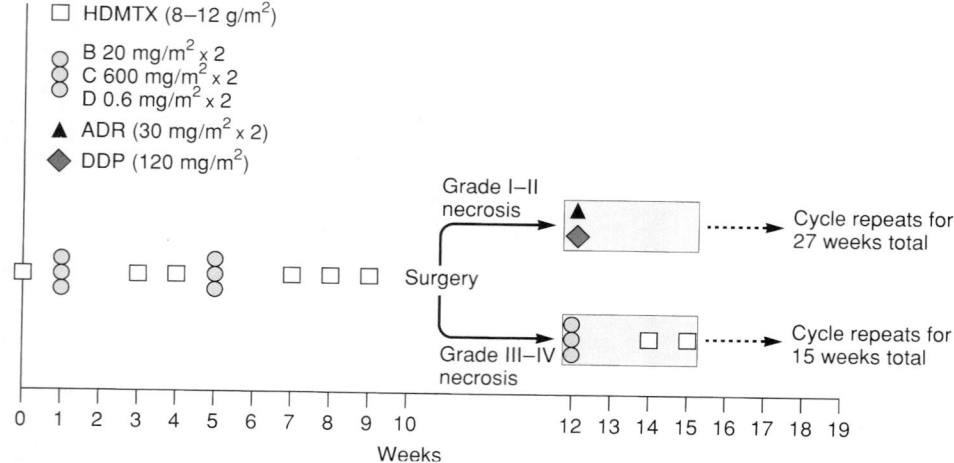

Figure 106.24. The T12 protocol used by Rosen and colleagues for resectable osteosarcoma of the extremity. HDMTX, high-dose methotrexate; B, bleomycin; C, cyclophosphamide; D, dacarbazine; ADR, doxorubicin (Adriamycin); DDP, cisplatin (*cis*-diammine-dichloro-platinum). [After Rosen G. Preoperative (neoadjuvant) chemotherapy for osteogenic sarcoma: a 10-year experience. *Orthopaedics* 1985;8:659.]

secondary to fibrous adhesion of the femur to the resection site (Fig. 106.23B). Alternatively, allograft reconstruction of the hemipelvis can be done to shorten the length of time until full weight bearing is possible.

Postoperative Chemotherapy

Adjuvant postoperative chemotherapy has been proved to increase survival of patients with osteosarcoma after amputation or limb-sparing surgery (47). As previously discussed, most limb-sparing regimens now incorporate preoperative chemotherapy as well. This does not replace postoperative treatment, but may influence the duration and type of postoperative chemotherapy given. The so-called T12 regimen (Fig. 106.24) is an example: patients with total or near-total tumor necrosis receive a short course of the same chemotherapy after surgery (total duration of preoperative and postoperative treatment is 15 weeks). Those with lesser degrees of necrosis are switched to a more intensive regimen of doxorubicin and cisplatin lasting 27 weeks. Overall results of this regimen have been as good as those in which all patients receive more toxic chemotherapy. It remains to be determined, however, if the more aggressive chemotherapy is in fact improving the outcome for patients with poor initial tumor necrosis (48). Although the optimal regimen for adjuvant chemotherapy of osteosarcoma has yet to be defined, combined preoperative and postoperative chemotherapy regimens, in which the postoperative therapy is tailored to the initial histologic response, are state of the art, particularly for patients undergoing limb-sparing surgery.

MANAGEMENT OF CHILDHOOD SOFT-TISSUE SARCOMAS

Osteosarcomas occurring in the pediatric population are managed in a fashion similar to those in adults, with similar results expected. Soft-tissue sarcomas, however, may require different management in children and adolescents than in adults. This is only partly due to differences in the behavior of sarcomas in these groups and is largely the result of the differing tumor types encountered in children.

Spindle cell sarcomas, such as fibrosarcoma, malignant fibrous histiocytoma, and liposarcoma, are relatively rare in children. When they are encountered, however, they usually behave identically to those in adults and are managed similarly. Small cell sarcomas, which are poorly differentiated, high-grade, aggressive tumors, account for more than 70% of childhood soft-tissue sarcomas. Rhabdomyosarcoma is the most common childhood sarcoma and is the prototypical small cell sarcoma. Extraosseous Ewing's sarcoma/primitive neuroectodermal tumor account for most of the remaining cases. Small cell sarcomas are more sensitive to chemotherapy than most spindle cell sarcomas; hence, chemotherapy plays a prominent role in their management.

Rhabdomyosarcomas tend to occur in three anatomic sites: the head and neck, including the orbit and paranasal sinuses (most common); the genitourinary tract; and the extremities. Most patients are younger than 5 years, although there is a second peak in adolescence composed mainly of boys with pelvic and paratesticular primary tumors. Three subtypes of rhabdomyosarcoma are seen—embryonal (most common), alveolar, and botryoid. Many adult sarcomas once classified as pleomorphic rhabdomyosarcomas are now considered to be malignant fibrous histiocytomas and are treated as any other adult soft-tissue sarcoma.

In addition to their chemosensitivity, childhood rhabdomyosarcomas differ from adult sarcomas in other ways. Lymph node metastases are more common than in adult sarcomas and may be encountered in 20% to 40% of cases. The primary tumors are often locally extensive and invasive, and they often lack the pseudocapsule seen with spindle cell sarcomas. Head and neck primaries can invade into the base of the skull or even into the brain; such extension is associated with a poor prognosis.

The locally aggressive nature of rhabdomyosarcomas, combined with their propensity to arise in sites where radical excision conveys great morbidity, has limited the role of surgery for these tumors. The initial surgical procedure should be a careful incisional biopsy, placing the incision in a way that does not complicate a subsequent excision. For most patients, chemotherapy and local irradiation play the primary roles in management. This is particularly true for rhabdomyosarcomas arising in the head and neck or pelvis. Before the routine use of adjuvant chemotherapy, 80% of children with rhabdomyosarcoma died of their disease. Now more than half are cured, and in patients presenting with limited disease amenable to complete resection after multimodality therapy, survival rates of 80% or more can be anticipated (49).

MANAGEMENT OF RECURRENT AND METASTATIC SARCOMAS

Many adult and pediatric patients with locally recurrent or even metastatic sarcomas can be cured by aggressive surgery, often combined with radiation and chemotherapy. For this reason, all patients with sarcoma should be observed carefully for recurrence. For high-grade lesions, follow-up should be directed toward detecting both local recurrence and metastases and should include periodic physical examination and chest radiograph plus CT scans of the primary site and lungs at least annually for the first 5 years. Low-grade lesions rarely metastasize in the absence of local recurrence, and follow-up should focus on the original tumor site. Low-grade sarcoma can recur up to 20 years after original resection, however, so follow-up must be maintained over the long term.

Local Recurrence

Despite aggressive multimodality therapy, local recurrence remains a major mode of failure in patients with sarcoma. The risk of local recurrence after surgical treatment of soft-tissue sarcomas varies based on a number of factors. The most significant of these is the site of origin of the tumor, with lesions of the head and neck, trunk, and retroperitoneum all associated with a higher risk of local recurrence than lesions of the extremities. Local and regional failure is the site of first recurrence after definitive resection in 50% of head, neck, and truncal sarcomas and in 75% of retroperitoneal tumors, but only 15% of extremity lesions (50). Other factors influencing recurrence rates include the size and histologic grade of the primary tumor, deep as opposed to superficial location, and local failure of prior surgery.

Limb-sparing approaches can control and even cure local recurrence in the absence of distant metastases. For patients who were initially treated with surgery alone and who failed locally, multimodality treatment with repeat resection, radiation, and sometimes chemotherapy is associated with survival rates close to those of previously untreated patients (51) (Fig. 106.25). Patients with recurrence after surgery and radiation are more likely to require radical amputation to control recurrence in an extremity, but are still candidates for salvage surgery. Locally recurrent retroperitoneal sarcomas, particularly low-grade tumors, can sometimes be resected on multiple occasions with long-term survival, but few of these patients are cured (52).

Distant Metastases

The lungs are the most frequent site of distant spread for sarcomas and are often the only site of metastasis (30). Aggressive resection of solitary or multiple lung metastases is associated with cure in approximately 25% to 35% of patients with soft-tissue and osteogenic sarcoma (53). Even patients with bilateral metastases are candidates for surgery. This can be done either as staged thoracotomies or, preferably, as one procedure using a median sternotomy. Patients with three or fewer metastases, a long doubling time of the metastatic tumors, and unilateral disease have the best prognosis after surgical resection (54), although patients lacking one or all of these favorable factors are still candidates for curative resection. It has been

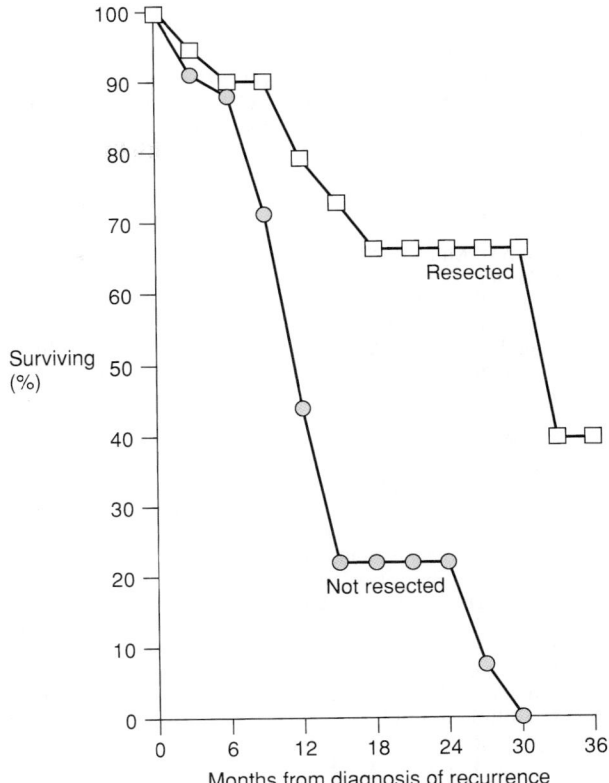

Figure 106.25. Survival of patients after resection of isolated local recurrence of an extremity soft-tissue sarcoma. (After Huth J, Eilber FR. Patterns of metastatic spread following resection of extremity soft-tissue sarcomas and strategies for treatment. *Semin Surg Oncol* 1988;4:20.)

suggested that preoperative or postoperative adjuvant chemotherapy can improve the outcomes for patients undergoing complete resection of pulmonary metastases, especially from osteosarcomas (55).

Patients with unresectable pulmonary metastases or with extrapulmonary metastases are usually treated with cytotoxic chemotherapy. Active agents include doxorubicin, ifosfamide, dacarbazine, high-dose methotrexate, and cisplatin (56). Doxorubicin is the most active single agent for treating metastatic sarcoma. Ifosfamide is an alkylating agent closely related to cyclophosphamide and, like cyclophosphamide, is associated with severe hemorrhagic cystitis. The uroprotective agent 2-mercaptoethane sulfonate sodium (mesna), when coadministered with ifosfamide, protects the bladder and largely eliminates hemorrhagic cystitis. Trials of ifosfamide and mesna show activity comparable with that of doxorubicin (57). A regimen combining mesna, ifosfamide, dacarbazine, and doxorubicin (MAID regimen) has been described that showed a 49% objective response rate in previously untreated patients with soft-tissue sarcoma (58). Cisplatin and high-dose methotrexate have significant activity in metastatic osteosarcoma and are often used in combination with doxorubicin and other agents to treat this disease.

Radiation therapy may be useful as palliation for the occasional patient with bony or cerebral metastases. Immunotherapeutic approaches using interferon, tumor necrosis factor, or interleukin-2 have undergone limited evaluation in metastatic sarcoma, with little evidence of activity seen thus far. Notwithstanding the fact that occasional patients with metastatic sarcoma are cured by surgery with or without chemotherapy, the best hope for increasing survival in patients with sarcoma remains the prompt initiation of aggressive, multimodality therapy before clinically detectable metastatic disease develops. For the foreseeable future, surgeons will therefore retain their prominent role in treating these complex and challenging patients.

REFERENCES

1. Landis SH, Murray T, Bolden S, et al. Cancer statistics, 1999. *CA Cancer J Clin* 1999;49:8.
2. McClay EF. Epidemiology of bone and soft tissue sarcomas. *Semin Oncol* 1989;16:264.
3. Collins JJ, Strauss ME, Levinskas GJ, et al. The mortality experience of workers exposed to 2,3,7,8-tetrachlorodibenzo-p-dioxin in a trichlorophenol process accident. *Epidemiology* 1993;4:7.
4. Wolfe WH, Michalek JE, Miner JC, et al. Health status of Air Force veterans occupationally exposed to herbicides in Vietnam: I. physical health. *JAMA* 1990;264:1824.
5. Malkin D, Li FP, Strong LC, et al. Germ line p53 mutations in a familial syndrome of breast cancer, sarcomas, and other neoplasms. *Science* 1990;250:1233.
6. Bennicelli JL, Barr FG. Genetics and the biologic basis of sarcomas. *Curr Opin Oncol* 1999;11:267.
7. Stratton MR, Williams S, Fisher C, et al. Structural alterations of the RB1 gene in human soft tissue tumours. *Br J Cancer* 1989;60:202.
8. Greenblatt MS, Bennett WP, Hollstein M, et al. Mutations in the p53 tumor suppressor gene: clues to cancer etiology and molecular pathogenesis. *Cancer Res* 1994;54:4855.
9. Andreassen Å, Zyjord T, Hovig E, et al. p53 abnormalities in different subtypes of human sarcomas. *Cancer Res* 1993;53: 468.
10. Ollner JD, Kinzler KW, Meltzer PS, et al. Amplification of a gene encoding a p53-associated protein in human sarcomas. *Nature* 1992;358:80.
11. Gerlach JH, Bell DR, Karakousis C, et al. P-glycoprotein in human sarcoma: evidence for multidrug resistance. *J Clin Oncol* 1987;5:1452.
12. Jimenez RE, Zalupski MM, Frank JJ, et al. Multidrug resistance phenotype in high grade soft tissue sarcoma: correlation of P-glycoprotein immunohistochemistry with pathologic response to chemotherapy. *Cancer* 1999;86:976.
13. Lawrence W Jr, Donegan WL, Natarajan N, et al. Adult soft tissue sarcomas: a pattern of care survey of the American College of Surgeons. *Ann Surg* 1987;205:349.
14. Giuliano AE, Eilber FR. The rationale for planned reoperation after unplanned total excision of soft-tissue sarcomas. *J Clin Oncol* 1985;3:1344.
15. Heslin MJ, Lewis JJ, Woodruff JM, et al. Cote needle biopsy for diagnosis of extremity soft tissue sarcoma. *Ann Surg Oncol* 1997;4:25.
16. Myhre Jensen O, Kaae S, Madsen EH, et al. Histopathologic grading in soft tissue tumors: relation to survival in 261 surgically treated patients. *Acta Path Microbiol Immunol Scand* 1983;91A:145.
17. Brennan MF. Staging of soft tissue sarcomas. *Ann Surg Oncol* 1999;6:8.
18. Ramathan RC, A'Hern R, Fisher C, et al. Modified staging system for extremity soft tissue sarcomas. *Ann Surg Oncol* 1999; 6:57.
19. Brooks AD, Heslin MJ, Leung DH, et al. Superficial extremity soft tissue sarcoma: an analysis of prognostic factors. *Ann Surg Oncol* 1998;5:41.
20. Arca MJ, Sondak VK, Chang AE. Diagnostic procedures and pre-treatment evaluation of soft tissue sarcomas. *Semin Surg Oncol* 1994;10:323.
21. Jones DN, Brizel DM, Charles HC, et al. Monitoring of response to neoadjuvant therapy of soft tissue and musculoskeletal sarcomas using F18-FDG PET. *J Nucl Med* 1994;35: 38P.
22. Yang JC, Rosenberg SA. Surgery for adult patients with soft tissue sarcomas. *Semin Oncol* 1989;16:289.
23. Suit HD, Mankin HJ, Wood WC, et al. Treatment of the patient with stage M0 soft tissue sarcoma. *J Clin Oncol* 1988;6:854.
24. Pisters PW, Harrison LB, Leung DH, et al. Long-term results of a prospective randomized trial of adjuvant brachytherapy in soft tissue sarcoma. *J Clin Oncol* 1996;14:859.
25. Yang JC, Chang AE, Baker AR, et al. Randomized prospective study of the benefit of adjuvant radiation therapy in the treatment of soft tissue sarcomas of the extremity. *J Clin Oncol* 1998;16:197.
26. Eilber FR, Eckardt JJ, Rosen G, et al. Preoperative chemotherapy for soft tissue sarcoma. *Hematol Oncol Clin North Am* 1995;9:817.
27. Chang AE, Steinberg SM, Culnane M, et al. Functional and psychosocial effects of multimodality limb-sparing therapy in patients with soft tissue sarcomas. *J Clin Oncol* 1989;7:1217.
28. Sondak VK, Leonard JA Jr, Robertson JM, et al. Limb-sparing surgery for extremity soft tissue sarcomas: functional and rehabilitation considerations. *Surg Oncol Clin North Am* 1993; 2:657.
29. Plaat BE, Molenaar WM, Mastik MF, et al. Hyperthermic isolated limb perfusion with tumor necrosis factor-alpha and melphalan patients with locally advanced soft tissue sarcomas: treatment response and clinical outcome related to changes in proliferation and apoptosis. *Clin Cancer Res* 1999; 5:1650.
30. Huth JF, Eilber FR. Patterns of metastatic spread following resection of extremity soft-tissue sarcomas and strategies for treatment. *Semin Surg Oncol* 1988;4:20.
31. Elias AD, Antmann KH. Adjuvant chemotherapy for soft-tissue sarcoma: a critical appraisal. *Semin Surg Oncol* 1988;4: 59.
32. Rosenberg SA, Tepper J, Glatstein E, et al. Prospective randomized evaluation of adjuvant chemotherapy in adults with soft tissue sarcomas of the extremities. *Cancer* 1983;52:424.
33. Chang AE, Kinsella T, Glatstein E, et al. Adjuvant chemotherapy for patients with high-grade soft-tissue sarcomas of the extremity. *J Clin Oncol* 1988;6:1491.
34. Frustaci S, Gherlinzoni F, De Paoli A, et al. Preliminary results of an adjuvant randomized trial on high risk extremity soft tissue sarcomas (STS): the interim analysis. *Proc Am Soc Clin Oncol* 1997;16:496A.
35. Tierney JF, Stewart LA, Parmat MKB, et al. Adjuvant chemotherapy for localised resectable soft-tissue sarcoma of adults: meta-analysis of individual data. Sarcoma Meta-analysis Collaboration. *Lancet* 1997;350:1647.
36. Storm FK, Mahvi DM. Diagnosis and management of retroperitoneal soft-tissue sarcoma. *Ann Surg* 1991;214:2.
37. Sindelar WF, Kinsella TJ, Chen PW, et al. Intraoperative radiotherapy in retroperitoneal sarcomas: final results of a prospective, randomized clinical trial. *Arch Surg* 1993;128: 402.
38. Glenn J, Sindelar WF, Kinsella T, et al. Results of multimodality therapy of resectable soft-tissue sarcomas of the retroperitoneum. *Surgery* 1985;97:316.
39. Storm FK, Eilber FR, Mirra J, et al. Retroperitoneal sarcomas: a reappraisal of treatment. *J Surg Oncol* 1981;17:1.
40. Goffman T, Tochner Z, Glatstein E. Primary treatment of large and massive adult sarcomas with iododeoxyuridine and aggressive hyperfractionated irradiation. *Cancer* 1991;67:572.
41. Sondak VK, Robertson JM, Sussman JJ, et al. Preoperative idoxuridine and radiation for large soft tissue sarcomas: clinical results with five-year follow-up. *Ann Surg Oncol* 1998;5: 106.
42. HSyry P, Scheinin TM. The desmoid (Reitamo) syndrome: etiology, manifestations, pathogenesis, and treatment. *Curr Probl Surg* 1988;25:225.
43. Church JM. Desmoid tumors in familial adenomatous polyposis. *Surg Oncol Clin North Am* 1994;3:435.
44. Arca MJ, Biermann JS, Johnson TM, et al. Biopsy techniques for skin, soft-tissue, and bone neoplasms. *Surg Oncol Clin North Am* 1995;4:157.
45. Baker L, Crowley J, Ryan J, et al. Long-term follow-up in the cure of osteogenic sarcoma. *Proc Am Soc Clin Oncol* 1989;8: 320.
46. Apffelstaedt JP, Zhang PJ, Driscoll DL, et al. Various types of hemipelvectomy for soft tissue sarcomas: complications, survival, and prognostic factors. *Surg Oncol* 1995;4:217.
47. Eilber F, Giuliano A, Eckardt J, et al. Adjuvant chemotherapy for osteosarcoma: a randomized prospective trial. *J Clin Oncol* 1987;5:21.

48. Meyers PA, Heller G, Healey J, et al. Chemotherapy for non-metastatic osteogenic sarcoma: the Memorial Sloan-Kettering experience. *J Clin Oncol* 1992;10:5.
49. Pappo AS, Parham DM, Rao BN, et al. Soft tissue sarcomas in children. *Semin Surg Oncol* 1999;16:121.
50. Potter DA, Glenn J, Kinsella T, et al. Patterns of recurrence in patients with high-grade soft-tissue sarcomas. *J Clin Oncol* 1985;3:353.
51. Giuliano AE, Eilber FR, Morton DL. The management of locally recurrent soft-tissue sarcoma. *Ann Surg* 1982;196:87.
52. Karakousis CP, Gerstenbluth R, Kontzoglou K, et al. Retroperitoneal sarcomas and their management. *Arch Surg* 1995;130:1104.
53. Putnam JB, Roth JA. Resection of sarcomatous pulmonary metastases. *Surg Oncol Clin North Am* 1993;2:673.
54. Casson AG, Putnam JB, Natarajan G, et al. Five-year survival after pulmonary metastasectomy for adult soft tissue sarcoma. *Cancer* 1992;69:662.
55. Skinner KA, Eilber FR, Holmes EC, et al. Surgical treatment and chemotherapy for pulmonary metastases from osteosarcoma. *Arch Surg* 1992;127:1065.
56. Antmann KH, Elias AD. Chemotherapy of advanced soft-tissue sarcomas. *Semin Surg Oncol* 1988;4:53.
57. Antmann KH, Ryan L, Elias A, et al. Response to ifosfamide and mesna: 124 previously treated patients with metastatic or unresectable sarcoma. *J Clin Oncol* 1989;7:126.
58. Elias A, Ryan L, Sulkes A, et al. Response to mesna, doxorubicin, ifosfamide, and dacarbazine in 108 patients with metastatic or unresectable sarcoma and no prior chemotherapy. *J Clin Oncol* 1989;7:1208.

SURGERY: SCIENTIFIC PRINCIPLES AND PRACTICE, Third Edition, edited by Lazar J. Greenfield, Michael W. Mulholland, Keith T. Oldham, Gerald B. Zelenock, and Keith D. Lillemoe. Lippincott Williams & Wilkins Publishers, Philadelphia, © 2001.

CHAPTER 107

PLASTIC AND RECONSTRUCTIVE SURGERY

EDWIN G. WILKINS, WILLIAM M. KUZON, KEVIN C. CHUNG, PAUL S. CEDERNA, AND STEVEN R. BUCHMAN

Plastic and reconstructive surgery can be broadly defined as a discipline in which a diverse array of nonsurgical and, especially, surgical therapies are used to address problem wounds. In this definition, the term *problem wounds* is taken in the broadest sense; plastic surgeons treat traumatic, congenital, developmental, and even psychological wounds. Perhaps it is this latter aspect of plastic surgery that most fully sets it apart from other surgical specialties:

> *"We restore and make whole those parts which nature or ill fortune have taken away, not so much to delight the eye but to buoy up the spirit of the afflicted."*
> —Gaspare Tagliacozzi, 1597

In more concrete terms, *plastic surgery is an approach to surgical problems.* Plastic surgeons operate "from the top of the head to the tips of the toes"; the specialty is not confined to a single anatomic area or to an organ system. Plastic surgeons envision themselves as surgical innovators, having developed many procedures and techniques that have since been adopted by other surgical specialties. Plastic surgeons have been instrumental in the development of microvascular surgery, craniofacial surgery, head

Table 107.1. THE SPECTRUM OF PLASTIC SURGERY

Aesthetic surgery
Burns: acute and reconstructive surgery
Craniofacial surgery
Cutaneous and soft-tissue oncology
Surgery of the hand and upper extremity
Head and neck oncology
Microvascular surgery
Maxillofacial and orthognathic surgery
Peripheral nerve surgery
Reconstructive surgery
   Face (ear, lip, nose, eyelid)
   Breast
   Trunk
   Lower extremity

and neck reconstruction, nerve grafting, and even renal transplantation (1). Although the field of plastic surgery can be arbitrarily divided into "cosmetic" surgery (surgery to improve the appearance of a normal phenotype) and "reconstructive" surgery (repair of damaged anatomy or an abnormal phenotype), in many circumstances, both functional reconstruction and aesthetic improvement are paramount. Plastic surgery is truly "general surgery," encompassing a broad and growing list of subspecialties (Table 107.1).

MANAGEMENT OF PROBLEM WOUNDS

The following discussion centers on the principles of management of difficult physical wounds. Regardless of the etiology or location of a wound, these principles of management are universal and can be embodied by a straightforward algorithm: (a) evaluate and, if possible, eliminate the factors contributing to the wound; (b) control or optimize the wound before closure; and (c) use the simplest method to close the wound unless specific factors indicate that a more complex approach is required. Although surgeons like to focus on the technical details of an operative procedure, the first two steps are critical in the successful reconstruction of a problem wound. The algorithmic approach allows plastic surgeons to treat diabetic foot ulcers, infected sternotomy wounds, major defects related to composite resection of the head and neck, pressure ulcers, wounds of the lower extremity associated with open tibial fractures, venous stasis ulcers, and other difficult defects with a high degree of success. *This rational approach is the core of plastic surgery.* Unlike some other surgical subspecialties, plastic surgery is not based on a one-to-one correlation between a surgical problem and a certain operation. There is no "right" way to reconstruct a given defect, and a spectrum of options must be considered for every reconstructive problem. Selecting the best option for a given patient is the challenge.

Evaluation of Problem Wounds

The evaluation of a patient with a difficult wound is best approached by considering local and systemic (or intrinsic and extrinsic) contributing factors for each phase of the work-up. In the history, local factors of importance include the mechanism that resulted in the wound, symptoms (e.g., pain, loss of function), time course and progression of the wound, any previous nonsurgical or surgical treatment of the wound, and any previous injury, irradiation, malignancy, or other local factors contributing to the wound. The history should also uncover systemic factors that impair wound healing. These include immunosuppression (e.g., chemotherapy, immune deficiencies), medical conditions known to impair healing (e.g., diabetes, renal failure), medications (e.g., steroids, cyclosporin A), cigarette smoking, and general debility (e.g., nutritional deficiencies, old age).

The physical examination of a patient with a problem wound should likewise focus on local and systemic signs related to successful wound resolution. In regard to the wound itself, the location, size, depth, exposure of deep or vital structures, presence of necrotic material, presence of foreign bodies, and signs of any neoplastic processes should be carefully noted. The designation of a wound as "infected" should be contingent on the physical examination findings of local inflammation (i.e., erythema, pain, swelling, fluctuance, purulence, and loss of function). All open wounds are contaminated. The physical examination should be the primary means of establishing the diagnosis of local wound infection; surface swabs indicating the presence of pathogenic bacteria do not correlate with clinically significant infection (2). In addition to the wound itself, the surrounding tissue should be examined for signs of injury (e.g., actinic changes), previous irradiation, arterial or venous insufficiency, lymphedema, loss of sensation, and dermal thinning (e.g., aging, steroid therapy). For all patients with a wound on an arm or leg, a careful neurovascular examination of the entire limb is absolutely mandatory. In addition to the local examination, a focused systemic physical examination is essential in evaluating a patient with a problem wound. Systemic signs of infection (fever, hypotension) are of particular importance. Obesity is a major risk factor for wound problems. In addition, the general physical examination should focus on the systemic factors that affect wound healing noted above. Table 107.2 lists some of the local and systemic factors that impair wound healing; the history and physical examination are the principal means of diagnosing these problems.

Laboratory examinations can be invaluable in the management of problem wounds. However, laboratory tests are often misused in this setting, and a rational, evidence-based approach is necessary to utilize this expensive resource efficiently. Again, the local–systemic paradigm is useful in determining which laboratory examinations are warranted. In the local evaluation, as already mentioned, wound swabs can be valuable for surveillance of the flora contaminating a wound, but they should not be used as a trigger to initiate therapy for wound infection. Wound biopsy and quantitative bacteriology have proved valuable in the management of burns and chronic wounds (3,4). Bacterial loads in excess of 10^5/g of tissue indicate contamination at a level that precludes skin graft take and jeopardizes wound closure of any kind. The use of quantitative cultures, however, is not justified for the majority of acute or uncomplicated chronic wounds. In general, quantitative cultures are reserved for "high stakes" wounds, in which a failure of closure on the initial attempt may leave an unreconstructable situation with grave consequences, such as amputation or death. Wound biopsies can be invaluable for diagnosing invasive burn wound infection, being preferred over quantitative culture for this purpose (5). The presence of bacteria in the deep dermis on biopsy is highly correlated with the risk for systemic sepsis in burn patients. Bone biopsy demonstrating bacteria within the bone is the preferred test for making the diagnosis of osteomyelitis. Standard radiographs are most useful for diagnosing and delineating acute fractures and are much less useful in the setting of chronic, open wounds. Ultrasonography, computed tomography (CT), or magnetic resonance imaging (MRI) may be useful for delineating fluid collections, necrotic tissue, or inflammation in selected circumstances. On the other hand, radionuclide bone scans have little role in the evaluation of patients with open wounds or fractures. In the face of an open wound or recent fracture, a "hot" bone scan (even a triple-phase bone scan) is not specific for osteomyelitis and is of little value. Therefore, obtaining a bone scan in patients with suspected sternal osteomyelitis after a recent midline sternotomy, pressure sores and exposed bone, or other open wounds overlying exposed bone is unwarranted. Under these circumstances, bone biopsy is preferred for making a diagnosis of osteomyelitis and determining the responsible pathogen; MRI is preferred for delineating the extent of bony involvement. Magnetic resonance or standard angiography may be indicated if vascular insufficiency is suspected or if a transfer of free tissue is planned.

The use of systemic laboratory investigations should be limited to specific indications; "routine" blood work is not required for patients with acute or chronic wounds. White blood cell differential counts and blood cultures can confirm the diagnosis of systemic infection. Serum albumin and transferrin determinations may be valuable in determining nutritional status. A greatly elevated erythrocyte sedimentation rate can help confirm the diagnosis of osteomyelitis. Other laboratory tests to confirm the presence and severity of associated medical conditions may be justified for specific indications.

Treatment of Problem Wounds

Once a wound has been fully evaluated, the treatment should be designed to achieve specific goals. In order of greatest priority, these are as follows: (a) preventing complications of the wound, (b) preserving or restoring critical function, (c) achieving wound closure, and (d) restoring aesthetic appearance. Again, each of these goals may require specific local or systemic interventions.

Preventive Treatment

The preventive measures that should be taken for patients with open wounds depend on the setting. For an acute laceration, tetanus prophylaxis should be considered. For pressure sores, strict adherence to protocols for pressure relief and an assessment of nutritional status take priority. In wounds caused by human or animal bites, prophylactic antibiotics are warranted. In addition, any associated medical conditions contributing to the wound must be aggressively optimized. It is the responsibility of the surgeon to ensure that complications do not develop in a patient with a wound, and that more wounds do not develop by the same mechanism. This is of particular im-

Table 107.2. LOCAL AND SYSTEMIC FACTORS AFFECTING WOUND MANAGEMENT

Local factors	Systemic factors
Infection	Immune deficiencies
Local malignancy	Distant malignancy
Foreign bodies	Diabetes mellitus
Local toxins	Cigarette smoking
Radiation	Chemotherapeutic agents
Ischemia	Hereditary healing disorders
Venous insufficiency	Nutritional deficiency
Lymphatic insufficiency	Old age
Repetitive trauma	Uremia
Reduced sensation	Glucocorticoid therapy
	Immunosuppressive agents

portance in bedridden, obtunded, or paralyzed patients, in whom it should be possible to prevent pressure sores completely by means of proper nursing care.

Preservation of Function

Preserving joint motion must always be considered for patients with open wounds of the extremities. Aggressive physiotherapy to maintain or improve joint motion can be instituted in the presence of an open wound. Splinting should be used aggressively to minimize joint contractures, and any plans for wound closure should include measures to maintain joint function. In the case of facial defects, especially if facial paralysis is present, oral competence and the maintenance of eye protection should weigh heavily into any reconstructive plan. Function takes precedence over form in the reconstructive algorithm.

Nonsurgical Therapy

After careful consideration to preventive measures and the preservation of critical function, a strategy for wound closure can be formulated. The basic tenet is to "débride dirty wounds, close clean wounds." Therefore, the first step in wound closure is achieving control of the wound by eliminating necrotic debris and controlling any infection present. Nonsurgical therapies are used in conjunction with surgical therapy to achieve a clean wound. The mainstay of local, nonsurgical therapy is the use of wound dressings. It is beyond the scope of this chapter to review the wide range of options available to dress wounds. Recent articles provide a contemporary review of this subject (6,7). However, the basic principle is to employ débriding dressings for dirty wounds and occlusive dressings for clean wounds. The most commonly employed débriding dressing is the "wet-to-dry" dressing. Gauze made damp with normal saline solution, weak acetic acid, weak bleach, or various other solutions is applied to the wound. Over a period of hours, evaporation dries the dressing, which becomes slightly adherent to the wound surface. When the dressing is removed, necrotic debris is pulled off with the dressing, but healthy tissue is left behind. Wet-to-dry dressings work via *mechanical débridement,* and the key to their successful use is that they be changed sufficiently often. Wet-to-dry dressings must be changed a minimum of three times per day; they should not be "soaked" off to reduce patient discomfort because this completely defeats their purpose. Enzymatic dressings have also been used to débride wounds, but their use is limited by patient tolerance to the pain they cause. Débriding dressings are indicated for infected wounds and wounds containing necrotic debris.

If a wound is "clean" (i.e., it does not contain necrotic debris and has an acceptable bacterial load), a dressing to encourage wound healing can be used. In the case of many simple wounds, a nonadherent sterile dressing is all that is required. In the case of more complex wounds, occlusive dressings that maintain a moist environment to maximize wound healing are preferred. Options include hydrocolloid dressings, alginate dressings, and various hydrogels. Again, occlusive dressings must not be used on infected or dirty wounds. For many wounds, the judicious application of hydrocolloid dressings may allow closure by secondary intention within a reasonable period of time.

Under some circumstances, it is appropriate to use antibiotic dressings. Burn wounds are most commonly dressed with silver sulfadiazene or Sulfamylon dressings. Heavily contaminated wounds resulting from other mechanisms may also benefit from antibiotic dressings. However, in general, antibiotic dressings are not required for clean wounds, even if they are chronic.

Lastly, it should be noted that we are entering a new era of nonsurgical wound management. A rapid advance in our understanding of wound healing has led to the development of growth factor therapy, cellular therapy, and new physical modalities for the treatment of chronic wounds. For pressure sores and diabetic ulcers in particular, recombinant platelet-derived growth factor appears to be a useful adjunct to the dressing (8,9). Tissue-engineered dressings and skin substitutes are also poised to revolutionize wound care (10). Nevertheless, the basic algorithm for the evaluation and nonsurgical management of wounds will not change.

Surgical Therapy

Wound Preparation. The surgical therapy of problem wounds is aimed primarily at preparation and reconstruction. Judicious but thorough surgical débridement can convert a contaminated, chronic, dirty wound with necrotic debris into a fresh surgical wound ready for immediate closure. Although débriding dressings can be used to prepare a problem wound for closure under some circumstances, operative débridement is preferred to a long course of débriding dressings in most cases. Consequently, most problem wounds require operative débridement before definitive reconstruction. In the case of chronic osteomyelitis, a formal resection of the sequestrum is required before formal wound closure. Prolonged treatment with intravenous or oral antibiotics cannot clear bacteria from a focus of dead bone; chronic osteomyelitis is a surgical disease that is cured with a saw, rongeur, burr, or bone curette. Therefore, the common practice of placing patients with chronic osteomyelitis on 6 weeks of antibiotic therapy is irrational unless it is carried out in conjunction with a formal sequestrectomy.

Reconstructive Principles. As stated earlier, there is no "right" way to close any one wound; plastic surgeons employ a straightforward set of principles to delineate the optimal way to close a given wound in a given patient. The predominant principle is that the simplest method to close a wound is usually the best choice. This principle is embodied in the "reconstructive ladder," which is a hierarchy of reconstructive options progressing from simple to complex (Table 107.3). Therefore, when utilizing options for wound closure, plastic surgeons "climb" the reconstructive ladder, usually stopping on the lowest rung that will achieve a closed wound. However, other principles of reconstruction sometimes override a slavish adherence to the reconstructive ladder. The choice of a technique for wound closure should take into consideration the need for subsequent procedures and other factors that might indicate the appropriateness of skipping over simpler options. An example would be an avulsion injury to the palm of the hand. Although it is possible to close this type of wound with a skin graft, the need to restore flexor tendon function is preeminent in the hand, so that the use of a distant flap to provide a suitable bed for tendon grafting may be the preferred choice. In addition to the reconstructive ladder, other examples of guiding reconstructive princi-

---

Table 107.3. THE RECONSTRUCTIVE LADDER

Primary wound closure
Healing by secondary intention
Skin grafting
Local flaps
Regional flaps
Distant flaps

ples are that function takes precedence over form, single-stage reconstructions are preferred to multiple-stage approaches, and autologous tissue is preferred to alloplastic reconstructions. Other factors to be considered are the durability of the reconstruction over many years, the psychological impact on the patient, and data indicating that some options are sometimes preferred for specific reasons. For example, muscle flaps are known to be superior to skin flaps in their ability to resist or eradicate infection (11). Therefore, a muscle flap may be chosen over a simpler option if the eradication of osteomyelitis or mediastinitis is the goal. As mentioned earlier, weighing this complex array of factors to arrive at the optimal reconstruction for a given patient is the true challenge in reconstructive surgery.

Reconstructive Techniques. Regardless of the reconstructive method chosen, plastic surgeons strive for technical virtuosity in the operating room. To maximize healing and minimize scar formation, atraumatic technique includes delicate tissue handling, the use of skin hooks and sharp rakes, bipolar electrocautery, sharp dissection, and loupe magnification. In the reconstruction of difficult wounds, the margin for error is very small, and small errors in technical execution can result in failure. The general surgical methods used by reconstructive surgeons are briefly considered.

Primary Closure. If a laceration or other wound can be closed primarily, a meticulous, layered closure is considered. Emphasis is placed on eversion of skin edges without strangling tissue. Nonabsorbable skin stitches that provoke minimal inflammatory response are preferred, but they must be removed promptly to minimize cross-hatching. Therefore, for most wounds, deep dermal, absorbable stitches are placed to allow early removal of skin stitches while prolonged support is still provided to the repair; this technique may minimize the chances of a dehiscence or spread scar. It is preferable to place a closed suction drain to eliminate dead space rather than to suture fat or other easily strangled tissue. If a technically perfect, tension-free repair cannot be achieved with primary closure, it is preferable to use a more complex surgical option.

Skin Grafting. Skin grafting is one of the foundations on which the specialty of plastic surgery was established. Skin grafts are classified as either split-thickness, in which epidermis and a portion of the dermis are harvested, or full-thickness, in which the entire dermis is harvested. Both full-thickness and split-thickness skin grafts can be used to resurface open wounds in which primary closure is not possible. Skin graft take is contingent on the successful revascularization of the graft within a narrow time window (48 to 72 hours). Initially, grafts are nourished by a process of plasmatic imbibition, wherein serum from the wound bed diffuses into the adjacent graft. Revascularization occurs by the process of inosculation. Vessels from the wound bed grow into the graft, forming functional circulatory connections with the vasculature of the graft. For plasmatic imbibition and inosculation to be successful, two criteria must be met. First, the wound bed must be appropriately vascularized. Therefore, skin grafts cannot be placed on poorly vascularized wound surfaces, including bone denuded of periosteum and tendon denuded of peritenon, and on cartilage. Second, a bolster dressing or splint must be used to ensure absolute immobilization of the graft on the bed to prevent shearing of the nascent vascular connections during inosculation. If either of these criteria cannot be met, a more complex reconstructive option must be considered.

Random Skin Flaps. The use of tissue (usually skin) immediately adjacent to the defect as the tissue for reconstruction is referred to as a local flap reconstruction. Skin rearrangements can range in complexity from simple undermining to complicated geometric skin flaps. Which method is appropriate depends on multiple factors, including the cause of the defect, desired direction of the scar, fragility or mobility of underlying structures, and need to avoid distortion of adjacent free margins, such as the lip or eyelid. Significant experience is required for the optimal utilization of skin rearrangement. When plastic surgeons think of "classic" skin flaps, they are referring to random skin flaps, without an axial blood supply. These skin flaps rely on a dermal plexus of vessels for survival, and the perfusion of the distal end of the flap will be inadequate to allow tissue survival if the flap design is inappropriate. It was previously thought that survival of the distal part of random skin flaps could be ensured by adhering to length-to-width ratios established for various areas of the body. It is now recognized that these ratios have no basis in circulatory physiology, and the surviving length of a random skin flap does not depend on flap width (12). In practice, most of the commonly employed skin flaps have been developed empirically. The three basic types of random skin flaps are rotation, advancement, and transposition, depending on how adjacent skin is shifted into the defect. Each type of flap has specific design criteria. Many eponyms are used to describe variations on these basic three flap designs; examples are the Rhomberg transposition flap, the Mustarde rotation flap, and the Rintala advancement flap. Excellent reviews of the use of skin flaps in reconstructive surgery are available (13,14).

As mentioned, the concern with flap viability limits the utility of random skin flaps. Several strategies have been developed to circumvent this problem. The first of these is surgical delay. Delay is defined as the partial interruption of blood flow to a defined piece of tissue. At present, surgical delay is the only method available to augment the surviving length of random skin flaps (Fig. 107.1). Another strategy is the use of tissue expanders. Tissue expanders are implantable balloons that are inserted in a deflated state and are inflated with sterile saline solution via percutaneous injection into a self-sealing valve. Except for the scalp, where expanders are placed in the subgaleal plane, tissues expanders are usually placed subcutaneously. The insertion of the tissue expander effects a surgical delay, and the slow expansion has been demonstrated to result in the formation of new skin. However, the most important strategy to circumvent the use of random skin flaps has been to develop axial pattern flaps that do not rely on a random blood supply.

Flaps with Axial Blood Supply. Regional flaps are created by transferring tissue that is not immediately adjacent to the defect without disrupting the blood supply to the transferred tissue. For this technique to be practical, an axial blood supply to the transferred tissue is necessary.

AXIAL SKIN FLAPS. The pioneering work of Bakamjian (15) and McGregor and Jackson (16) identified longitudinal blood vessels of large caliber traversing a defined region of skin. Their descriptions of the deltopectoral and groin flaps, respectively, opened a new era of reconstructive surgery in which surgeons were no longer limited to the use of random skin flaps; any piece of tissue in the body with an axial blood supply could be transposed on a vascular pedicle with a high degree of certainty that the tissue would survive. The description of Taylor and Palmer (17) of the angiosome concept solidified our ability to design flaps based on a sound knowledge of vascular anatomy. An angiosome is defined as a region of tissue supplied by an identifiable, and usually named, artery and its venae comitantes. Because of the ability of choke ves-

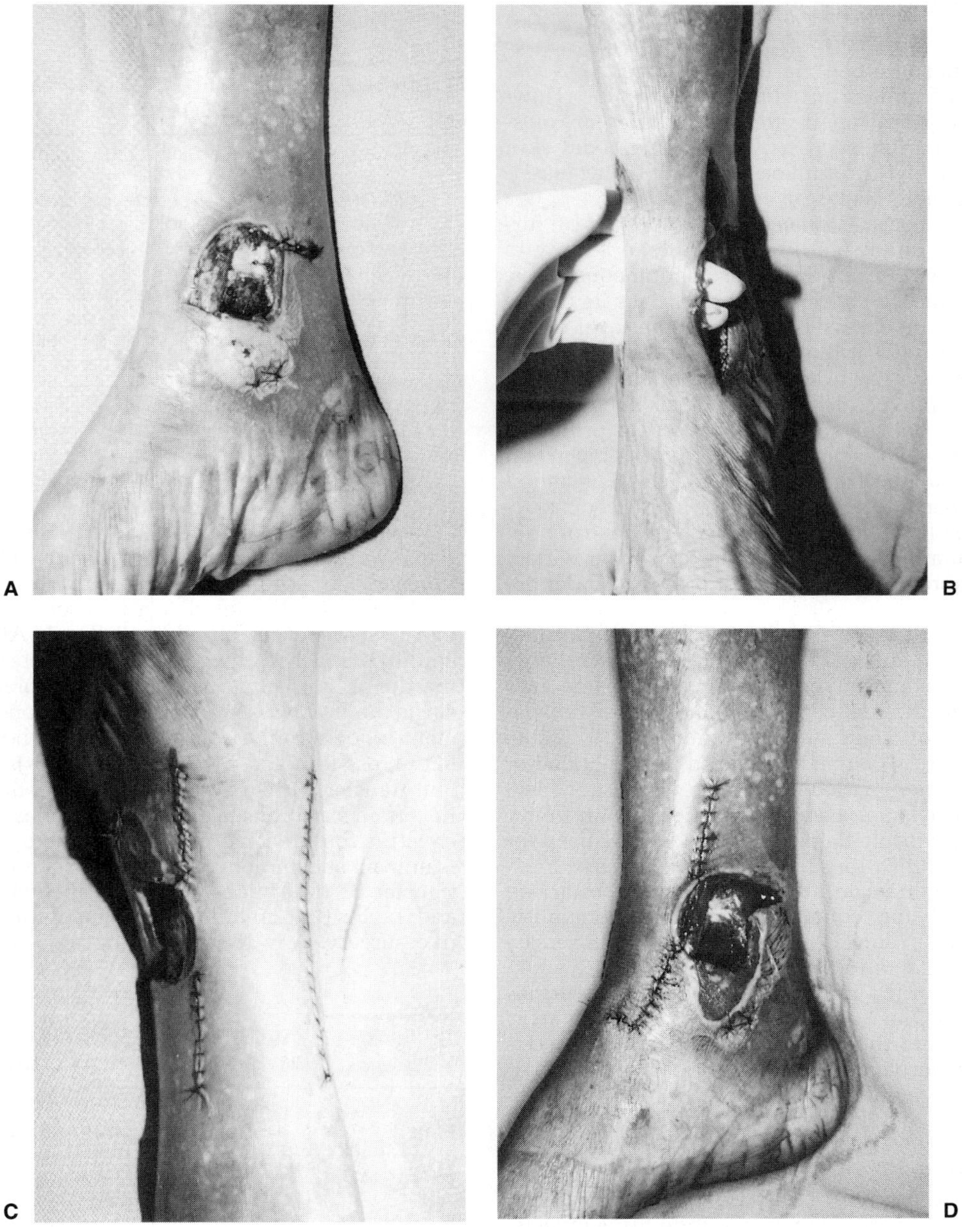

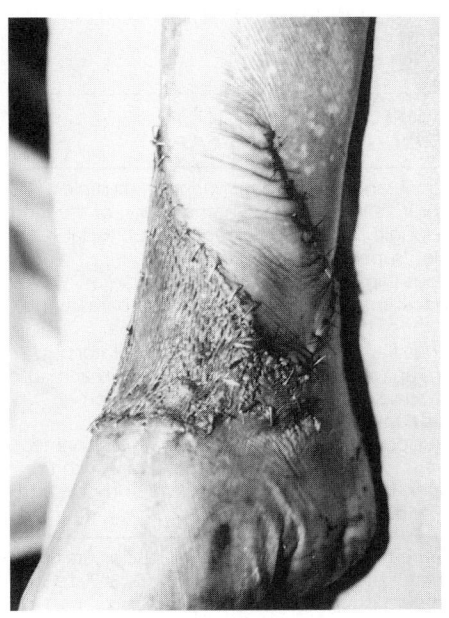

Figure 107.1. Example of surgical delay. Because of associated medical problems, the patient was not a candidate for microvascular tissue transfer. *(A)* Lower-third tibial defect secondary to an open ankle fracture. Note exposed bone, which precludes use of a skin graft. *(B)* In the first stage, a bipedicle flap was created anterior to the defect. The deep perforators to the skin of the flap were divided by full undermining. The flap is perfused only from the proximal and distal ends. *(C)* The incisions were repaired, and the wound was dressed. *(D)* After 5 days, the bipedicle flap was again elevated, and part of the distal pedicle was divided *(arrow)*. The incisions were again closed, and the wound was dressed. This procedure was repeated 10 days after the initial operation to leave only a small skin bridge at the distal end of the flap. *(E)* Fourteen days after the initial procedure, the remaining distal skin bridge was divided and the flap transferred. The donor site was skin-grafted. This photograph depicts full survival of the flap and complete take of the skin graft.

sels crossing angiosome boundaries to enlarge, flaps can be designed to encompass an adjacent angiosome. However, flaps crossing two angiosome boundaries are destined to undergo partial necrosis. In practice, axial skin flaps are relatively few in number; most are better classified as fasciocutaneous flaps.

FASCIOCUTANEOUS FLAPS. Cormack and Lamberty (18) further expanded our understanding of the blood supply to the skin with their description of fasciocutaneous flaps. They pointed out that the dermal plexus derives its inflow from vertically oriented vessels arising at the level of the deep fascia. The vessels at the deep fascial level are horizontally oriented relative to the surface of the skin and form a subfascial plexus. The design of fasciocutaneous flaps can be based on this subfascial plexus according to several defined anatomic patterns (Table 107.4). Several fasciocutaneous flaps are in widespread use. The radial forearm flap has become a workhorse for hand reconstruction and, as a free flap, for head and neck reconstruction. The osteoseptocutaneous fibula free flap has been widely used for the intraoral reconstruction of oromandibular defects.

MUSCLE AND MYOCUTANEOUS FLAPS. Based on the knowledge that tissue with an axial blood supply can be reliably transferred, muscle and myocutaneous flaps came into widespread use in the 1980s. Anatomic research has defined five patterns of blood supply to muscles (19) (Table 107.5). Whole muscles can be transferred as a pedicled or free flap if a dominant vascular pedicle is present. Segmental muscle transfers are sometimes possible on minor vascular pedicles. Muscle flaps have been widely used for a diverse array of indications. As mentioned earlier, muscle flaps have an enhanced ability to eradicate infection and are preferred for contaminated or osteomyelitic wounds. For a given defect, muscle flaps are chosen by their size and arc of rotation.

The rediscovery of the musculocutaneous perforator as a predominant vascular supply to the skin in many areas of the body has led to the wide use of musculocutaneous flaps. These flaps derive their inflow from a major muscular artery. Perforators emanating vertically from the muscle surface supply the skin overlying the muscle. Table 107.6 summarizes "workhorse" muscle and myocutanous flaps. Of particular note is the transverse rectus abdominis myocutaneous (TRAM) flap, based on periumbilical myocutaneous perforators from the rectus abdominis muscle; it is now extensively used in breast reconstruction (20).

Table 107.4. CLASSIFICATION OF FASCIOCUTANEOUS FLAPS

Type A: A pedicled fasciocutaneous flap dependent on multiple unnamed perforators in its base, with orientation of the long axis of the flap longitudinal to the axis of the subfascial plexus. Example: "super" flap of Ponten.

Type B: A fasciocutaneous flap dependent on a single, large, consistent fasciocutaneous perforator. Example: parascapular flap.

Type C: A fasciocutaneous flap supplied by multiple perforators emanating from an underlying named artery and reaching the skin via a fascial septum. Also called "ladder"-type fasciocutaneous flap. Example: radial forearm flap.

Type D: An osteomyofasciocutaneous flap based on a major named artery. This type is an extension of the type C flap, with the fascial septum taken in continuity with adjacent muscle and bone. Example: fibula osteoseptocutaneous flap.

From Cormack GC, Lamberty BG. A classification of fascio-cutaneous flaps according to their patterns of vascularisation. Br J Plast Surg 1984;37:80–87, with permission.

Table 107.5. CLASSIFICATION OF SKELETAL MUSCLE VASCULAR SUPPLY

Type I: A single major vascular pedicle. Example: tensor fasciae latae.

Type II: One major vascular pedicle and one "minor" vascular pedicle. Example: gracilis.

Type III: Two major vascular pedicles of equal size. Example: gluteus maximus.

Type IV: Segmental blood supply via multiple small pedicles. Example: sartorius.

Type V: One major vascular pedicle and multiple smaller vascular pedicles. Example: latissimus dorsi.

From Mathes SJ, Nahai F. Classification of the vascular anatomy of muscles: experimental and clinical correlation. Plast Reconstr Surg 1981;67:177–187, with permission.

MICROVASCULAR TISSUE TRANSFER. Historically, pedicled flaps were used to reconstruct distant defects. The distant transfer was accomplished in either of two ways. Flaps could be moved to the defect in a series of pedicled transfers ("waltzing" or "tumbling" flaps). Alternatively, flaps could be attached directly to the defect, with a pedicle to the donor site being maintained temporarily. At a second stage, the flap was detached from the donor site, after sufficient blood supply from the recipient bed had developed (e.g., cross-leg flaps, pedicled groin flaps). Although the distant transfer of pedicled flaps is still definitively indicated in certain situations (e.g., median forehead flap for nasal reconstruction), reconstruction with the use of distant tissue is now most commonly carried out via microvascular tissue transfer, or "free" flaps. First described clinically by Daniel and Taylor (21), free flaps have revolutionized reconstructive surgery. Any tissue with an axial blood supply and

---

Table 107.6. "WORKHORSE" MUSCLE AND MYOCUTANEOUS FLAPS

Flap	Myo-cutaneous	Common uses
Temporalis	No	Orbital and intraoral reconstruction, facial reanimation (pedicled flap)
Pectoralis major	Yes	Intraoral and neck reconstruction, reconstruction of sternal defects (muscle only)
Latissimus dorsi	Yes	Breast reconstruction, neck reconstruction, free flap for very large defects
Rectus abdominis	Yes, including "TRAM"	Breast reconstruction, sternal reconstruction, reconstruction of groin defects, free flap for medium-sized defects
Gluteus maximus	Yes	Ischial pressure sores, sacral pressure sores
Biceps femoris	Yes	Ischial pressure sores
Tensor fasciae latae	Yes	Trochanteric pressure sores, abdominal wall reconstruction
Gracilis	Yes	Perineal reconstruction, vaginal reconstruction, facial reanimation (muscle free flap), free flap for small defects
Rectus femoris	Yes	Infected hip wounds, abdominal wall reconstruction
Medial gastrocnemius	Rarely	Knee defects, proximal-third tibial defects
Soleus	No	Middle-third tibial defects

TRAM, transverse rectus abdominis myocutaneous.

pedicle vessels 1 mm in diameter or larger can be reliably transferred microsurgically. Circulation in the transferred tissue is established via microvascular anastomoses between the axial flap vessels and vessels in the recipient site. Microvascular anastomoses are performed with 9-0 or 10-0 suture under an operating microscope; success rates for free-flap transfers exceed 90% (22). The greatest advantage of free-flap reconstruction is that the surgeon is not restricted to the use of available local tissues. With composite tissue flaps, it is possible to reconstruct massive, complex tissue defects and replace "like with like" (23) (Fig. 107.2). Bowel, skin, bone, muscle, fascia, and composite tissue can be transferred microsurgically. Free flaps are the primary modality for the reconstruction of major head and neck defects after composite resection of squamous cell carcinoma and for the reconstruction of traumatic defects in the distal foreleg.

RECONSTRUCTIVE AND AESTHETIC SURGERY OF THE BREAST

Plastic surgery of the female breast includes both reconstructive and aesthetic procedures. Breast reconstruction following mastectomy and reduction mammaplasty for macromastia (oversized breasts) are the most common examples of reconstructive breast surgery. By contrast, breast augmentation (enlargement) and mastopexy (breast lift) generally are performed for aesthetic reasons. Although some surgical approaches may be applicable to both categories of breast procedures, the relative benefits, risks, and costs of reconstructive versus aesthetic breast surgery may be quite different, particularly as viewed by patients, providers, and payors.

Before advising women on reconstructive or aesthetic breast procedures, the surgeon should carefully assess the patient's current concerns, history, and physical findings. Initially, any past history of breast disease (or familial history of breast disease) should be evaluated. During the physical examination, careful linear measurements and preoperative photographs should be taken to document existing contour deformities, asymmetry, and other findings. A standard breast examination should be carried out to detect previously undiagnosed masses, nipple discharge, or lymphadenopathy. Finally, it is also advisable that women age 40 or older undergo mammography unless this study has been performed in the previous 12 months.

The preoperative consultation should include a thorough discussion covering the relative benefits and risks of the various surgical options. The surgeon is well advised to provide comprehensive information in an understandable format. To enhance patient satisfaction with the eventual surgical result, providers should elicit patients' preferences and expectations for surgical outcomes and tailor treatment options accordingly. Because of the prevalence of breast cancer in North American women, the impact of reconstructive or aesthetic procedures on breast cancer monitoring also should be discussed.

Reconstructive Breast Surgery

Postmastectomy Reconstruction

A variety of operative procedures have been described for breast reconstruction following mastectomy. These approaches can be categorized as implant, autogenous (natural) tissue, and "hybrid" procedures. For the purposes of this discussion, the term *hybrid* is applied to procedures combining elements of both implant and autogenous tissue techniques. This overview describes the advantages and disadvantages of the most common techniques. Ulti-

mately, procedure selection is based on a range of patient variables, including the size and shape of the desired reconstructed breast; availability of local, regional, and distant donor tissues; coexisting medical problems; and, perhaps most importantly, patient preferences.

Implant Techniques. As most commonly practiced, the implant approach usually requires two operative procedures to reconstruct the female breast. In the first stage, a temporary tissue expander is placed in a soft-tissue pocket, usually located deep to the pectoralis major muscle. The tissue expander is a deflated Silastic (silicone) envelope with an integrated or remote port through which saline solution can be injected percutaneously. After placement of the expander and meticulous closure of the overlying muscle and skin, saline solution is injected periodically beginning at 10 to 21 days (Fig. 107.3A). Usually, four to eight expansions are required, often at weekly intervals. As the device enlarges, induced growth in the overlying skin re-creates soft-tissue coverage for the new breast (24). Although the multiple inpatient visits required are somewhat inconvenient for both patients and providers, each tissue expansion is usually a painless procedure and takes only a few minutes to carry out.

Following the completion of expansion, most surgeons delay the second stage of reconstruction for 1 to 4 months to allow for maximal skin growth. At the conclusion of this hiatus, the second procedure is performed, consisting of removal of the expander and placement of the reconstructive implant (Fig. 107.3B). Currently available breast implants offer various shapes (round vs. "anatomic" or teardrop configurations), fill materials (silicone gel vs. saline solution), and surface configurations (smooth vs. textured envelopes). The relative advantages and disadvantages of these options are discussed later in the section entitled Breast Augmentation. As the most common option for postmastectomy reconstruction in the United States, the expander–implant approach offers several advantages. The surgical procedures associated with this approach usually are relatively brief (often an hour or less in length) and technically straightforward. In many cases, these operations are performed in an outpatient setting and entail relatively brief periods of disability. Particularly when expander–implant procedures are coordinated with procedures on the contralateral breast (i.e., reduction, mastopexy, or augmentation), the resulting symmetry and aesthetic outcomes are relatively good.

Patients considering implant reconstruction should also be mindful of the disadvantages of these procedures. The expander–implant approach usually requires two surgical procedures, multiple visits for expansion, and approximately 4 to 6 months for completion. If a patient is eager to return to a normal life-style following breast cancer treatment, this delay can be particularly frustrating. In addition, tissue expanders and reconstructive implants have been associated with a number of complications. Early in the postoperative period, these devices can be associated with delays in wound healing, which at times result in implant exposure and require explantation. Implant infections also may necessitate removal of the prosthetic device. Late complications include expander or implant leakage. Also, the development of excessive scar tissue surrounding the implant (termed *capsular contracture*) can produce a hard, painful, or deformed breast and require surgical revision.

Autogenous Tissue Reconstruction. A variety of autogenous (natural) tissue options have been described for postmastectomy breast reconstruction. Currently, the most commonly performed of these procedures is the transverse rectus abdominis musculocutaneous (TRAM) flap. Ini-

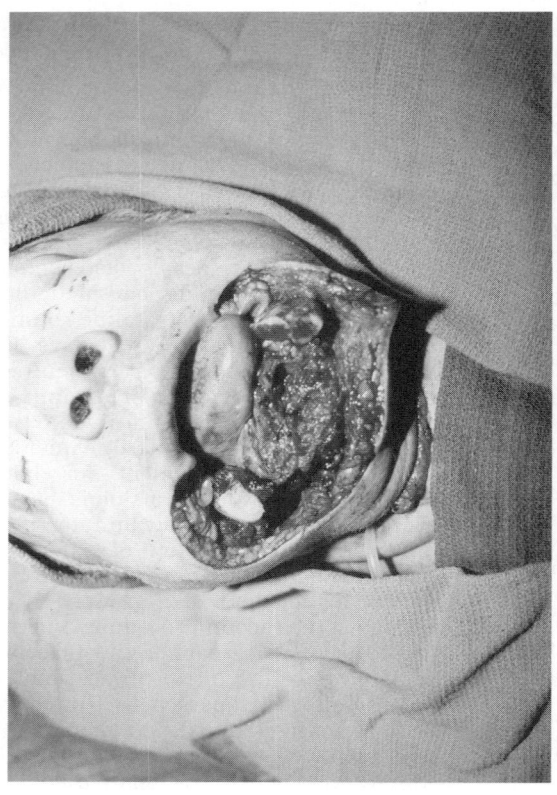

A

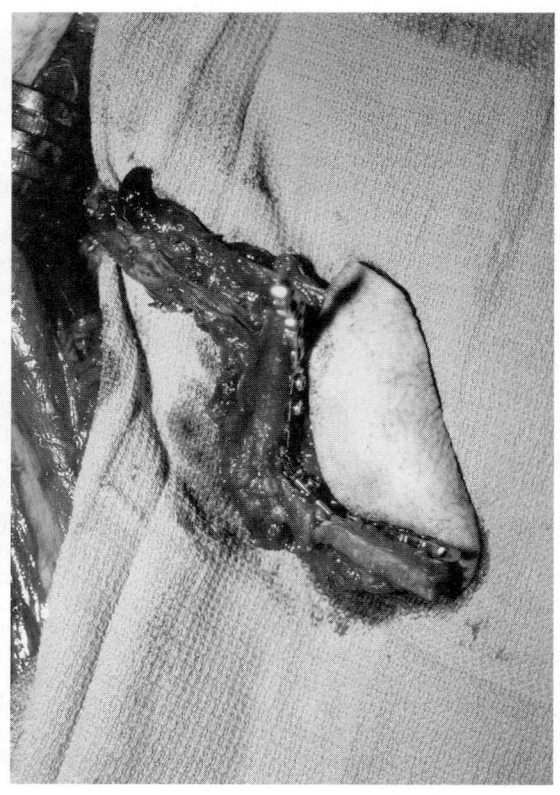

B

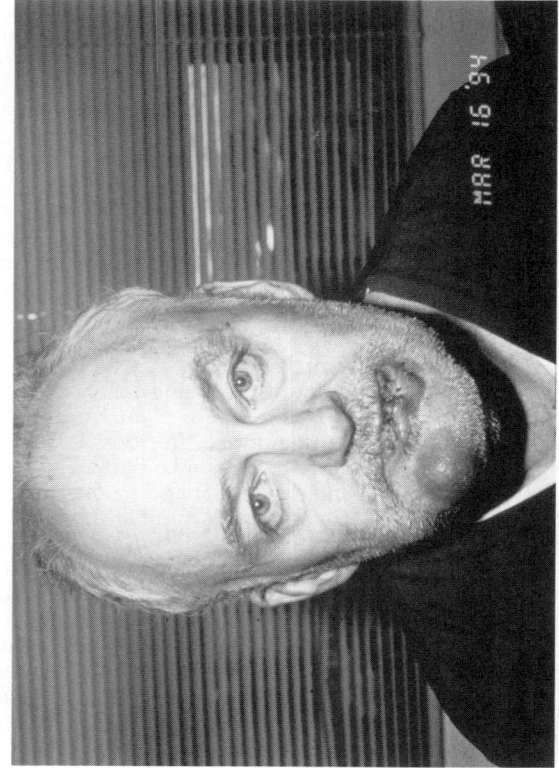

C

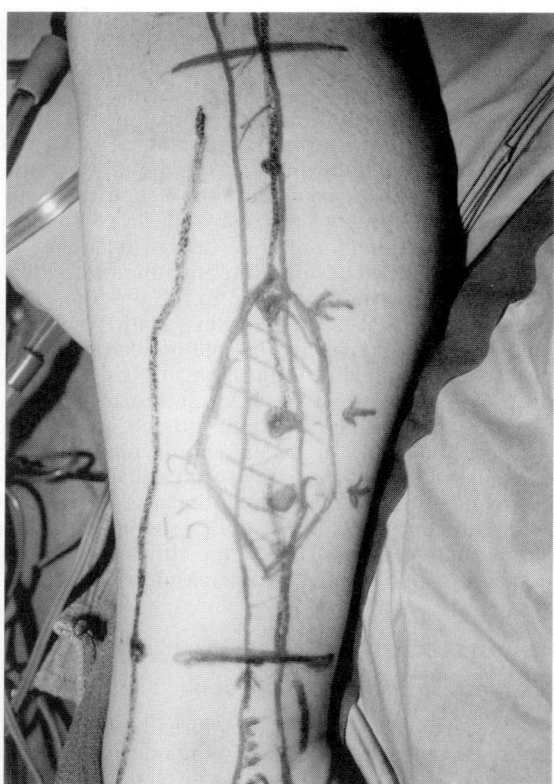

D

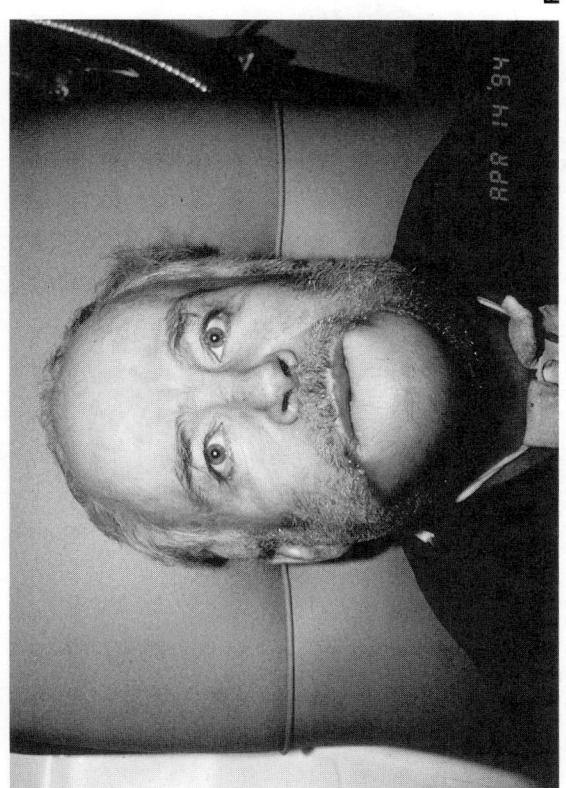

F

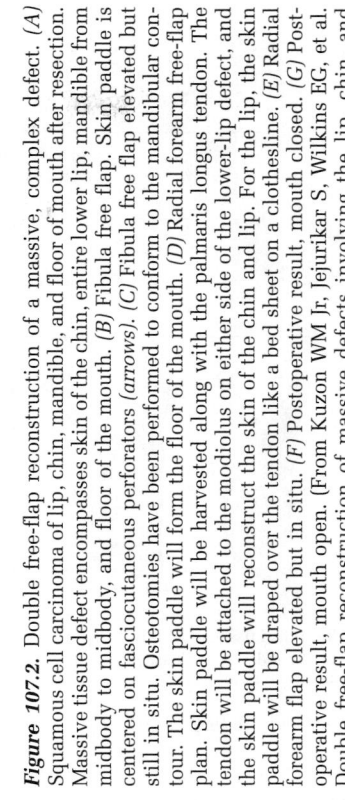

Figure 107.2. Double free-flap reconstruction of a massive, complex defect. (A) Squamous cell carcinoma of lip, chin, mandible, and floor of mouth after resection. Massive tissue defect encompasses skin of the chin, entire lower lip, mandible from midbody to midbody, and floor of the mouth. (B) Fibula free flap. Skin paddle is centered on fasciocutaneous perforators (arrows). (C) Fibula free flap elevated but still in situ. Osteotomies have been performed to conform to the mandibular contour. The skin paddle will form the floor of the mouth. (D) Radial forearm free-flap plan. Skin paddle will be harvested along with the palmaris longus tendon. The tendon will be attached to the modiolus on either side of the lower-lip defect, and the skin paddle will reconstruct the skin of the chin and lip. For the lip, the skin paddle will be draped over the tendon like a bed sheet on a clothesline. (E) Radial forearm flap elevated but in situ. (F) Postoperative result, mouth closed. (G) Postoperative result, mouth open. (From Kuzon WM Jr, Jejurikar S, Wilkins EG, et al. Double free-flap reconstruction of massive defects involving the lip, chin, and mandible. *Microsurgery* 1998;18:372–378, with permission.)

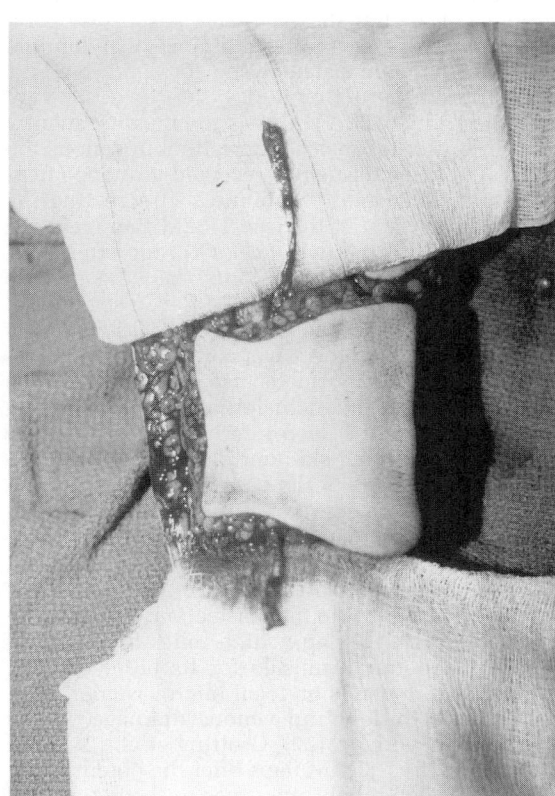

E

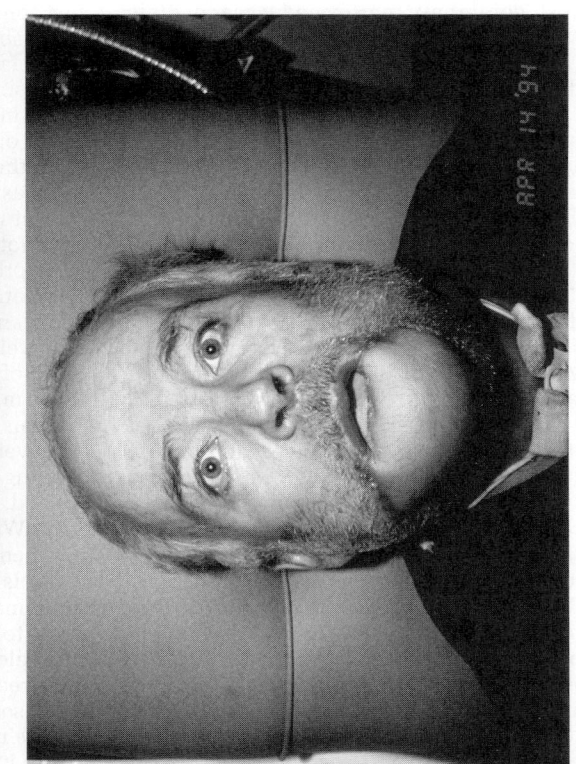

G

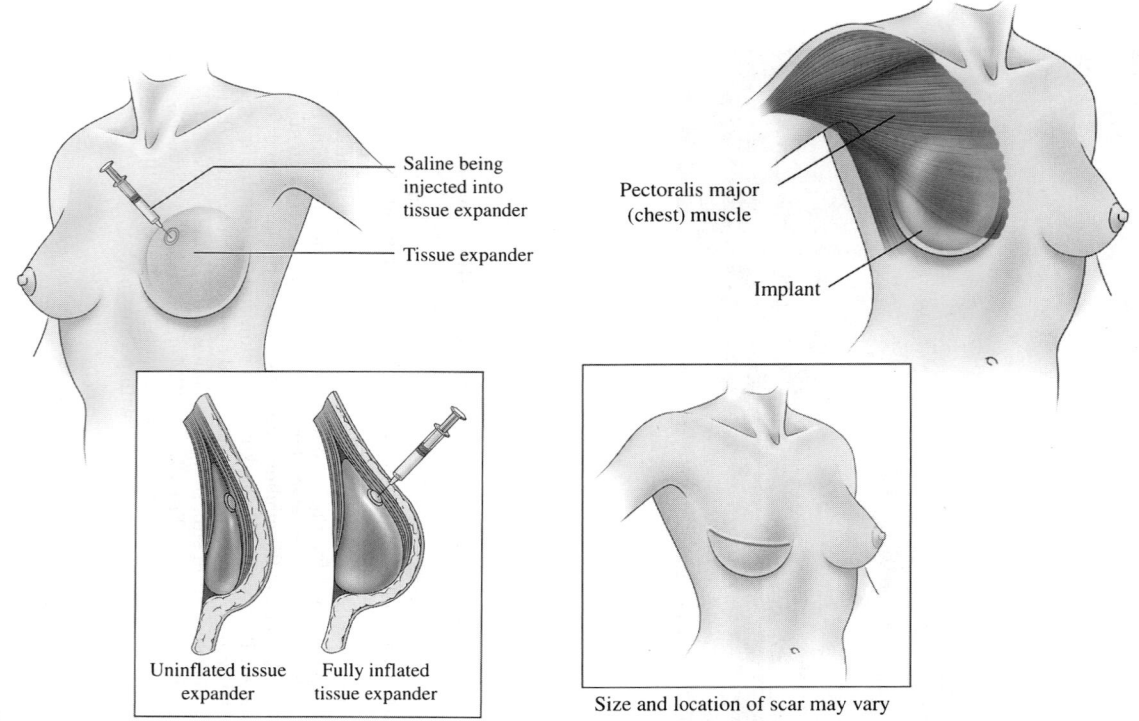

A

Saline being injected into tissue expander

Tissue expander

Uninflated tissue expander

Fully inflated tissue expander

Pectoralis major (chest) muscle

Implant

Size and location of scar may vary

B

Figure 107.3. *(A–B)* Expander–implant reconstruction.

tially popularized by Hartrampf and colleagues (25), the TRAM flap is most commonly performed as a pedicle muscle flap (i.e., the transferred rectus muscle is left partially attached to the costal margin, with the superior epigastric artery and vein preserved as the blood supply to the flap (Fig. 107.4 A,B). In pedicle TRAM reconstruction, the rectus muscle serves as the vascular carrier for a large ellipse of lower abdominal skin and fat. These tissues are tunneled subcutaneously into the mastectomy defect, where they are sculpted into the desired breast size and shape. Meanwhile, the abdominal donor site is closed by reapproximating the anterior rectus sheath and by advancing the remaining superior skin edge of the donor site as a modified abdominoplasty (Fig. 107.4C).

Pedicle TRAM reconstruction offers several benefits. Because the TRAM flap usually provides a generous amount of lower abdominal adipose tissue for breast bulk, implants are rarely needed with this approach. The TRAM flap can be inset and sculpted in virtually an infinite number of ways, so that the reconstructive surgeon has considerable latitude in creating breast shapes and sizes. Furthermore, in contrast with implant approaches, TRAM reconstruction is a one-stage technique, requiring a single surgery to recreate the breast mound. An additional advantage of TRAM flaps is their tendency to gain or lose volume in association with changes in weight and body mass; therefore, better symmetry is maintained over time than with implant reconstructions. Among reconstructive surgeons, there appears to be a growing consensus that TRAM flaps produce superior aesthetic results in comparison with other techniques.

Despite these advantages, TRAM flaps also are associated with several disadvantages. Longer operation, hospitalization, and recovery times are required for TRAM reconstruction than for implant procedures. Furthermore, TRAM procedures can produce a range of complications,

including partial and total flap loss resulting from vascular compromise of the transferred tissue. Also, postoperative abdominal hernia or (more commonly) abdominal wall laxity remains a persistent issue for some patients choosing TRAM reconstruction (26).

Although the pedicle TRAM flap is the most frequently used option in breast reconstruction with autogenous tissue, the transfer of free tissue has received growing attention as a potentially useful technique for recreating the breast mound. In particular, the free TRAM flap has been promoted by Kroll and Baldwin (27), Grotting et al. (28), and others as producing better results than the pedicle version of the flap. With the free TRAM flap, a segment of skin and fat based on the deep inferior epigastric artery and vein is harvested from the lower abdomen. A small island of rectus abdominis muscle is also included with the flap, mainly to facilitate the inclusion of small perforating vessels that travel from the deep inferior epigastric artery and vein into the overlying skin and fat (Fig. 107.5). Following dissection of the flap, the vascular pedicle is transected, so that the flap is completely freed from its donor site. With the use of microsurgical techniques, the vascular pedicle of the flap is then anastomosed to recipient vessels (usually the thoracodorsal, subscapular, or internal mammary vessels) adjacent to the mastectomy site. In contrast to the pedicle TRAM flap, which relies on a strip of tunneled rectus abdominis muscle for its blood supply, the free TRAM flap depends on local microvascular anastomoses for arterial inflow and venous drainage. In the views of Kroll and Baldwin (27), Grotting et al. (28), and other investigators, free TRAM flaps offer the potential advantages of greater flap reliability, superior aesthetics, and preservation of abdominal wall integrity. Allen and Treece (29) have taken the free TRAM flap a step further; by meticulously dissecting vascular perforators from the deep inferior epigastric pedicle into the overlying abdom-

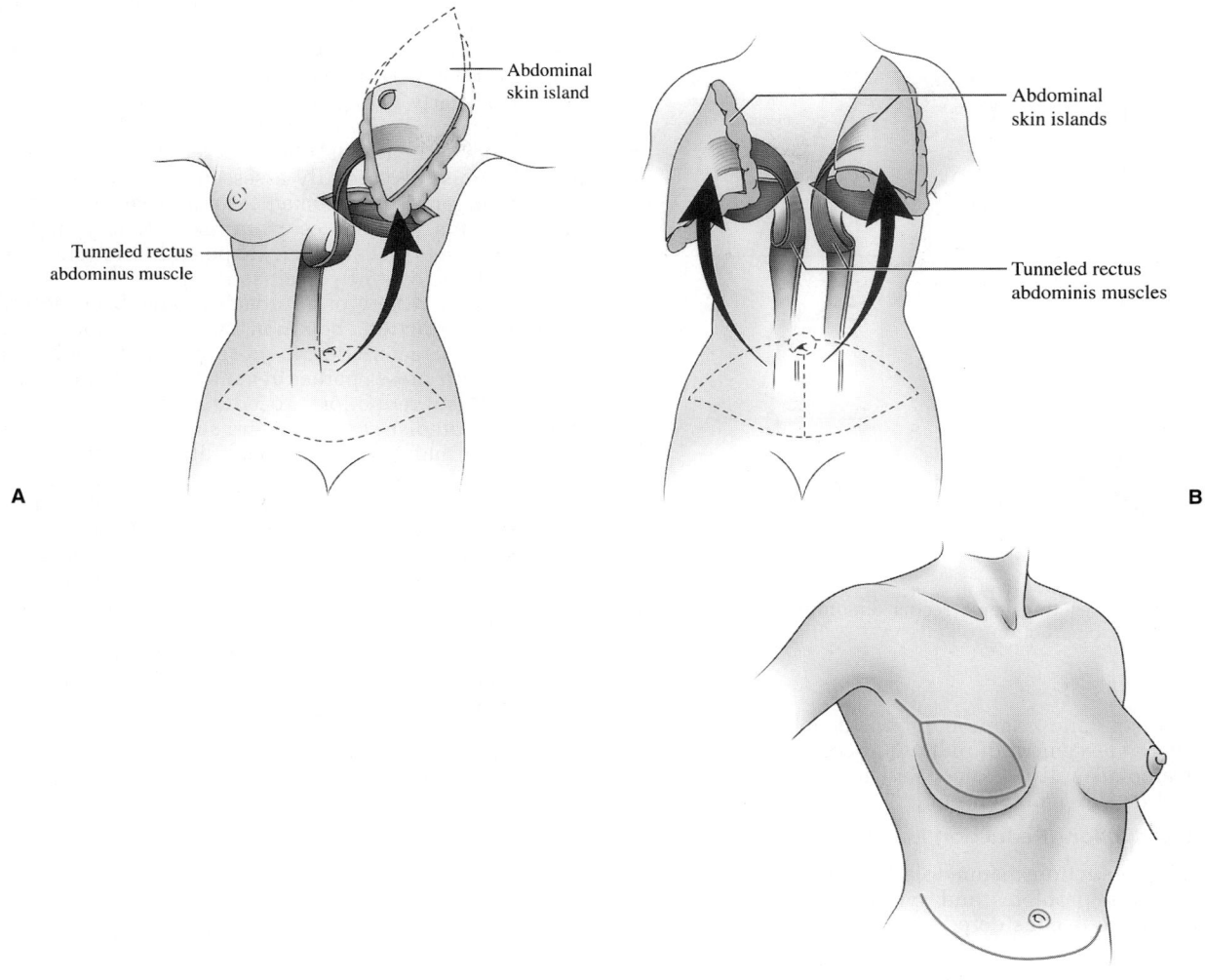

Figure 107.4. *(A–C)* Transverse rectus abdominis myocutaneous *(TRAM)* flap reconstruction.

Breast scar may vary in appearance   **C**

inal fat, they have been able to avoid removing any rectus abdominis muscle with the free TRAM harvest, thereby avoiding potentially permanent disruption of abdominal wall structures (29).

Although less commonly used than free TRAM reconstruction, several other free-flap approaches to breast reconstruction have been described. These include superior and inferior gluteal flaps and medial and lateral thigh flaps. Like all transfers of free tissue (including free TRAM flaps), these approaches are associated with several disadvantages. Microsurgery usually entails long, technically difficult operations requiring special facilities, equipment, and expertise. Also, because the blood supply for the entire flap depends on two or three microsurgical anastomoses (each usually involving vessels no more than 2 to 3 mm in diameter), complete flap loss is possible in the event of anastomotic thrombosis.

"Hybrid" Techniques of Breast Reconstruction. As an additional alternative for breast reconstruction, flaps can be used together with saline solution or silicone gel implants. Most commonly, the ipsilateral latissimus dorsi and a segment of overlying skin are harvested as a muscu-

locutaneous pedicle flap and are tunneled anteriorly into the mastectomy defect (Fig. 107.6). Although the latissimus dorsi and its associated skin island constitute an extremely reliable flap when used for wound coverage, this approach usually provides insufficient bulk for breast volume. An implant is often used to address the volume deficiency. In cases in which large amounts of new skin are required at the mastectomy site, a temporary tissue expander can be placed to enlarge the latissimus dorsi skin island following inset of the flap. The combination of a latissimus dorsi flap and tissue expansion may be particularly appropriate in cases in which the remaining mastectomy skin is of insufficient quality or quantity to tolerate tissue expansion. Following transfer and expansion of a latissimus dorsi musculocutaneous flap, an appropriately sized breast implant usually can be safely placed in a secondary operation.

Nipple–Areolar Reconstruction. Reconstruction of the nipple–areolar complex can be accomplished at the conclusion of breast mound reconstruction or at a later date. Following re-creation of the mound, many surgeons prefer to allow several months for tissue healing and settling before proceeding with nipple–areolar reconstruction. To

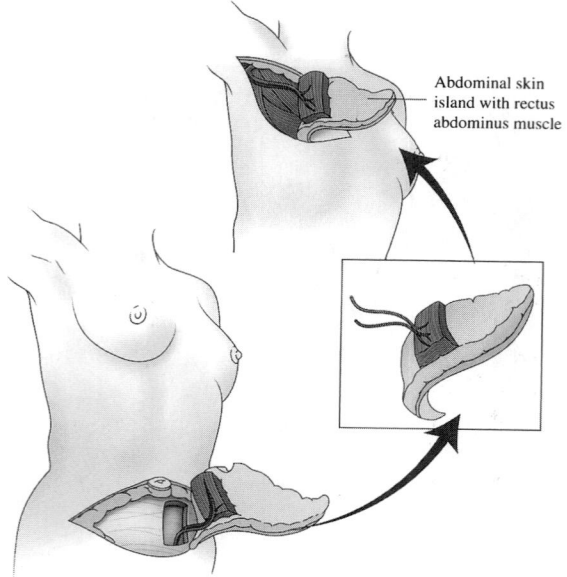

Figure 107.5. Free transverse rectus abdominis myocutaneous *(TRAM)* flap reconstruction.

recreate the papule, common options usually rely on local skin flaps or a segment of redundant contralateral papule. For the areola, a full-thickness skin graft or tattooing of the surrounding skin can be used.

Breast Reduction (Reduction Mammaplasty)

Because reduction mammaplasty is intended to alleviate functional problems and symptoms of macromastia, this procedure is considered a reconstructive rather than

an aesthetic operation. In general, appropriate candidates for reduction mammaplasty are women with macromastia and associated back, neck, or shoulder pain; limitations in daily work or recreational activities; or difficulties in obtaining properly fitting bras or other clothing. Reduction mammaplasty usually is a covered benefit by most health care payors, but patients' concerns regarding symtoms and function must be carefully assessed and documented before the surgery is undertaken. As noted earlier in this section, patients' preferences and expectations regarding postoperative breast size and shape and functional results also should be carefully evaluated.

Although a variety of approaches have been described for breast reduction, common surgical options share a number of characteristics. In most techniques of breast reduction, both breast parenchyma and redundant skin are resected. Also, reduction procedures generally reposition the nipple–areolar complex more superiorly on the breast mound. To maintain nipple viability and sensation, the nipple–areolar complex usually is mobilized as part of a pedicle of breast parenchyma or dermis. Following dissection of the nipple pedicle and reduction of the surrounding breast skin and parenchyma, the pedicle is transferred superiorly with its vascular and neural supplies intact, and the remainder of the breast is reapproximated around the nipple pedicle.

In categorizing reduction mammaplasty techniques, surgical options often are described in terms of the nipple pedicle design. For example, the most common approaches rely on an inferiorly or centrally based dermal–parenchymal pedicle to maintain vascular and nerve supplies to the nipple–areolar complex (30–32) (Figs. 107.7 and 107.8). In

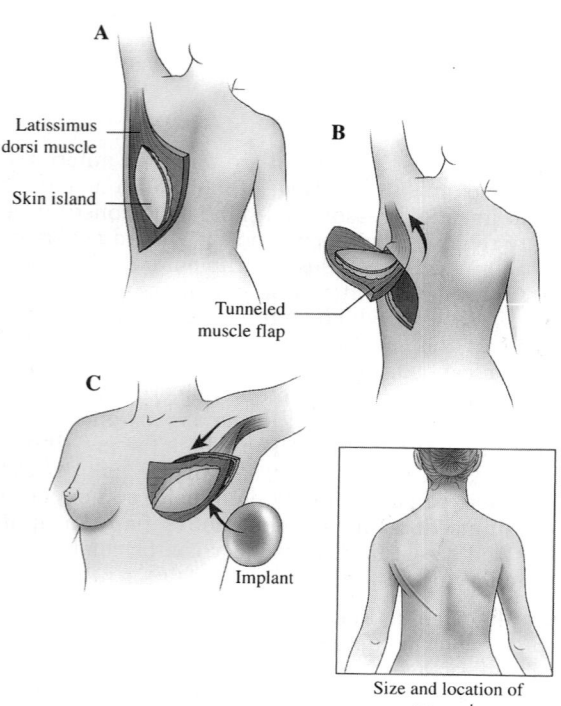

Figure 107.6. *(A–C)* Latissimus dorsi flap reconstruction.

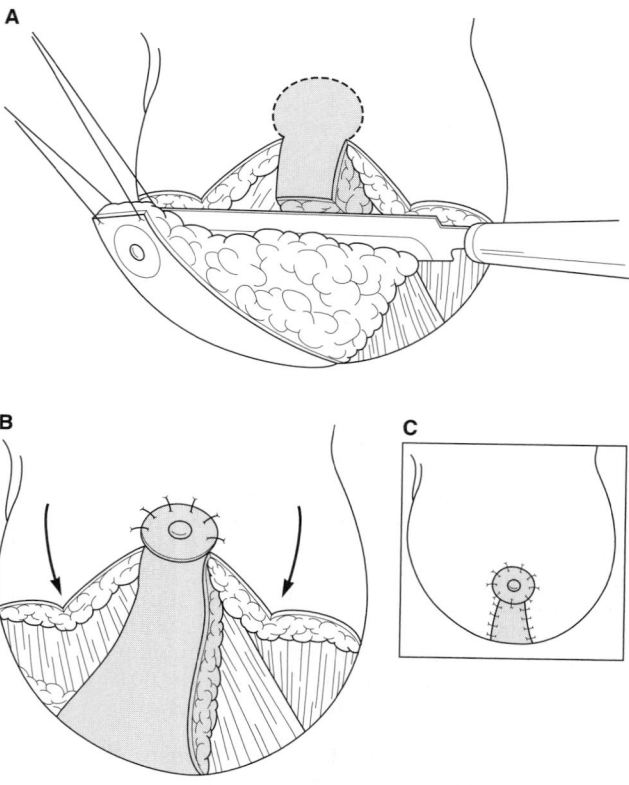

Figure 107.7. *(A–C)* Inferior pedicle technique reduction mammaplasty. (Redrawn from Smith JW, Aston SJ. *Grabb and Smith's plastic surgery*, 3rd ed. Boston: Little, Brown and Company, with permission.)

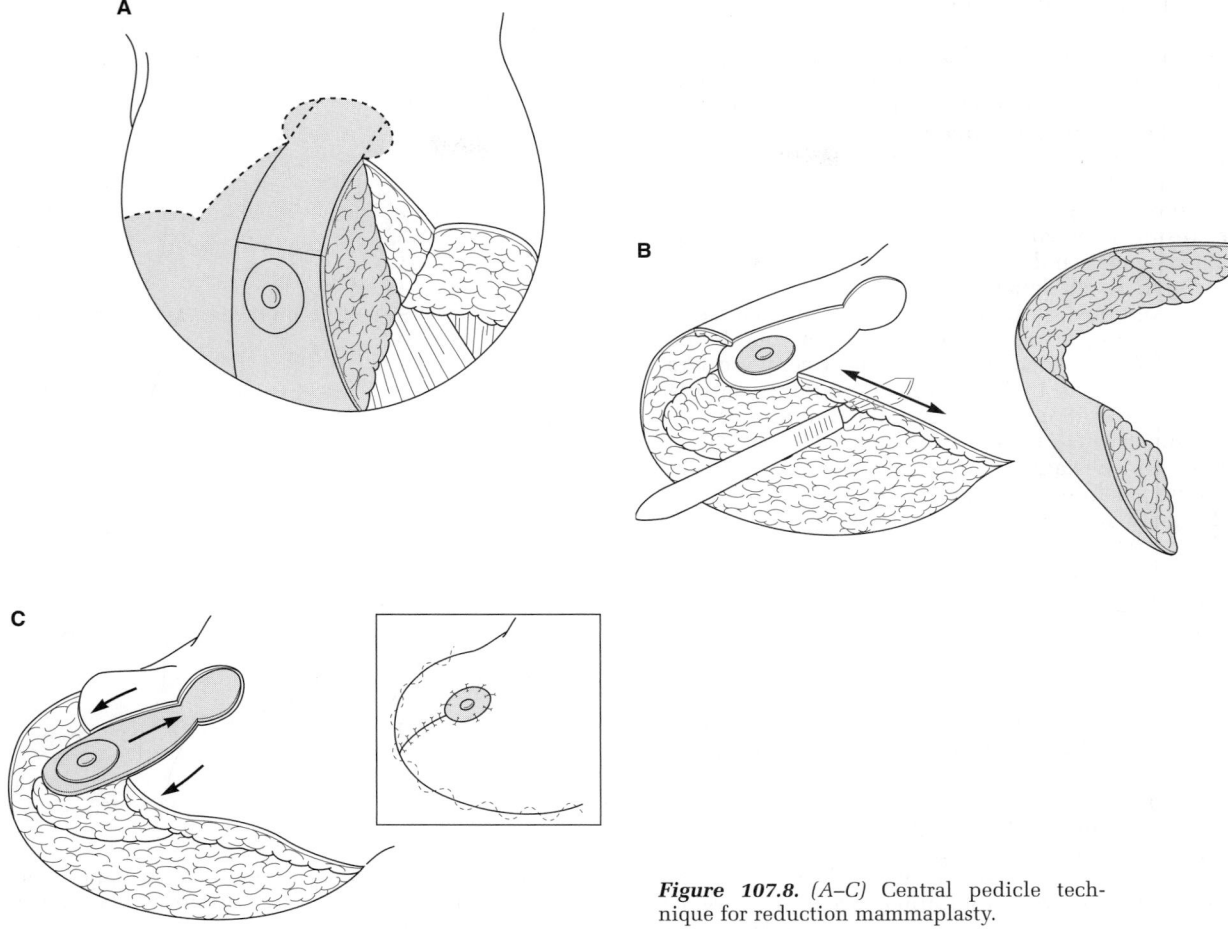

Figure 107.8. *(A–C)* Central pedicle technique for reduction mammaplasty.

the design of skin incisions, traditional methods of reduction often have incorporated a modification of a pattern originally described by Wise (33). Although it allows considerable flexibility in resecting redundant breast skin, the modified Wise pattern produces an inverted T-shaped scar, the inferior portion of which runs along the inframammary fold. In an effort to eliminate the inframammary fold scar, LeJour (34) and Hammond (35) recently described a vertical scar reduction mammaplasty.

Prospective outcome analysis of women undergoing reduction mammaplasty indicates that this surgical intervention considerably reduces somatic pain and improves functional status (36,37). However, patients and providers also should be aware of the potential risks associated with reduction. Complications reported with these procedures include nipple or skin loss, changes in levels of nipple sensation, hypertrophic scarring or keloid formation, contour deformities, and breast asymmetry.

Aesthetic Breast Surgery

Breast Augmentation (Augmentation Mammaplasty)

Augmentation or breast enlargement is one of the most commonly performed aesthetic procedures. Patients seeking breast augmentation should be evaluated according to

the guidelines described earlier. Particular attention should be focused on a thorough assessment of several factors, including patient preferences for postoperative breast size and shape, past history of breast disease, and physical findings. The preoperative examination should evaluate and document any possible breast masses in addition to breast size, asymmetry, and contour deficits. In planning augmentation mammaplasty, a variety of approaches and options are available. Decisions regarding these choices are often best reached in consultation with the patient. Implants can be placed through a variety of incisions, including periareolar, inframammary fold, and transaxillary approaches. With the advent of endoscopic techniques in recent years, transaxillary augmentation now can be carried out while the implant pocket is visualized directly. This latter approach commonly produces excellent aesthetic results and minimal visible skin scarring.

The location of the implant pocket is another critical decision in augmentation mammaplasty. Implants can be placed anterior to the pectoralis major muscle ("subglandular" location) or posterior to the muscle ("subpectoral" location). Although subglandular placement usually results in less postoperative pain, submuscular placement may be associated with lower rates of capsular contracture (38) and pose fewer difficulties in obtaining subsequent mammograms (39). Several choices of implant types are also available. During the past 10 years, many surgeons have used implants with textured surfaces to reduce capsular contracture rates. Textured surfaces appear to lessen scar tissue contracture (40), but some patients and surgeons assert that a thicker, less pliable, textured envelope gives the augmented breast a less natural appearance and feel. With the recent reintroduction of silicone gel-filled implants under research protocols in selected centers, patients and providers also have a choice of implant fill materials. Although gel implants may produce aesthetically superior results than saline solution implants in some patients, the diagnosis and surgical treatment of implant rupture may be more challenging with gel devices.

Whatever options are chosen for breast augmentation, surgeons should clearly communicate to patients the potential risks of these procedures. The most commonly reported complications include implant rupture, capsular contracture, implant infection, contour deformities, and breast asymmetry (41). Despite the potential for local complications, no substantial evidence currently indicates that silicone gel filler material or implant envelopes are associated with an increased risk for systemic disease. At this writing, concerns voiced in the early 1990s about the adverse "health effects" of silicone breast implants appear to be unfounded (42).

Mastopexy

The term *mastopexy* ("breast lift") describes a category of surgical procedures designed to address redundancy or laxity (ptosis) of the skin envelope of the breast. Breast ptosis can be classified as mild, moderate, or severe, depending on the location of the nipple–areolar complex relative to the inframammary fold (Fig. 107.9). Ptosis represents an imbalance between the volume of breast parenchyma and the quantity of overlying skin. Mastopexy procedures usually reduce ptosis by removing redundant breast skin and relocating the nipple–areolar complex to a more superior position. These goals can be achieved via a variety of skin incisions and excisions,

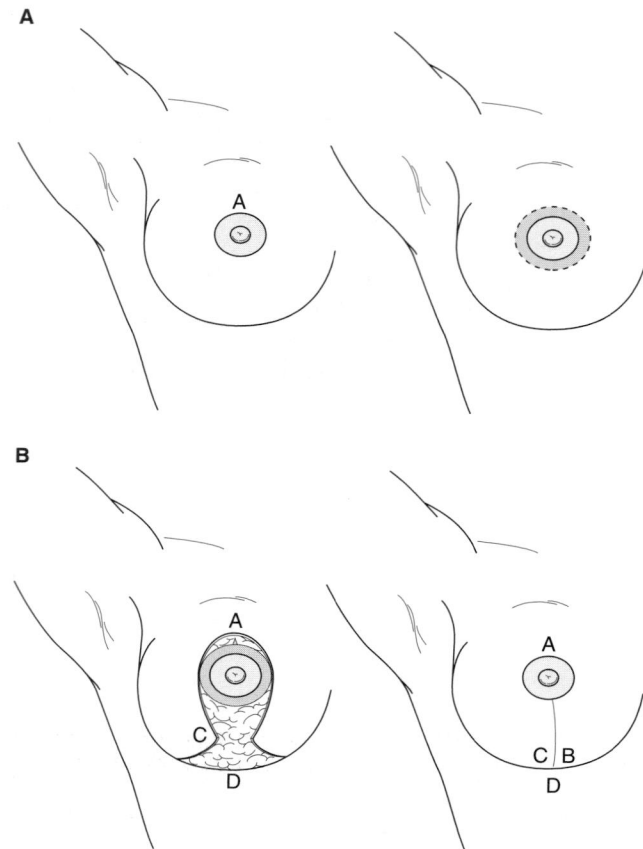

Figure 107.10. Mastopexy procedures. (Redrawn from Bostwick J. *Plastic and reconstructive breast surgery*. St. Louis: Quality Medical, 1990, with permission.)

many of which closely resemble the techniques described earlier for reduction mammaplasty. Fundamentally, mastopexy differs from breast reduction in that mastopexy removes redundant skin while leaving most or all of the breast parenchyma in place. Approaches to mastopexy range from minimal periareolar techniques to more extensive skin resections and vertical incisions (Fig. 107.10). As always, patients considering this procedure must weigh the potential benefits of mastopexy (most notably, diminished ptosis) against the disadvantages (scars and complications) associated with the operation. Although relatively rare, the potential complications of mastopexy closely parallel those described earlier for reduction mammaplasty.

RECONSTRUCTIVE SURGERY OF THE HAND

Advances in plastic surgery have improved our ability to reconstruct hands that have been mutilated by trauma, destroyed by arthritic diseases, or impaired by congenital conditions. Innovations in microvascular techniques, wound management, and rigid fracture fixation have expanded the capabilities of plastic surgeons by allowing them to borrow tissues from other parts of the body and use them to reconstruct complex defects in the upper extremity in a single procedure. These innovations provide limitless technical possibilities for the restoration of hand function and the eventual recovery of patients as productive members of society. The following sections highlight the technical aspects of hand reconstruction and discuss its indications and applications.

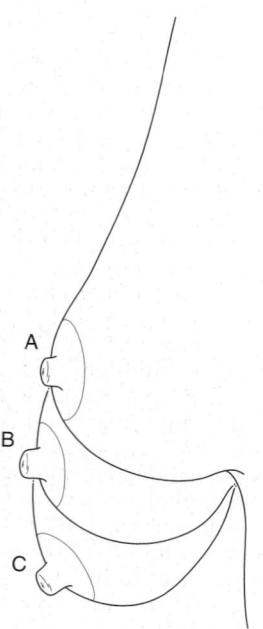

Figure 107.9. *(A)* Mild ptosis. *(B)* Moderate ptosis. *(C)* Severe ptosis. (Redrawn from Georgiade NG, Georgiade GS, Riefkohl R, et al. *Essentials of plastic, maxillofacial, and reconstructive surgery.* Baltimore: Williams & Wilkins, 699.)

Trauma

Replantation

Since the first successful finger replantation by Komatsu and Tamai in 1968 (43), replantation surgery has flourished throughout the world. During 30 years of experience with replantation surgery, our understanding of this procedure has improved, and indication guidelines have been developed to ensure that replanted parts of the upper extremity not only survive but also function acceptably. The absolute indications for replantation (i.e., situations in which replantation should always be attempted) are the following: (a) thumb amputation, (b) multiple-finger amputations, (c) amputations in children, and (d) midhand, wrist, or distal forearm amputations. The absolute contraindications for replantation are the following: (a) associated life-threatening injuries, (b) multiple-level injuries in the amputated part associated with injuries along the vessels that prevent blood flow into the replanted part, and (c) severe contamination of the part, which carries a high probability of systemic infection if replanted. In other situations, the benefit of replantation is debatable because outcome data are not available. For example, single-finger amputation at zone 2 (a tight fibroosseous tunnel extending from the insertion of the superficialis tendon at the middle phalanx to the A1 pulley) is generally not recommended. Tendon adhesion after zone 2 replantation may result in a stiff finger, which can interfere with overall performance of the hand. However, single-finger amputation at zone 1 (distal to the superficialis insertion) is often recommended (Fig. 107.11). A stiff distal interphalangeal joint generally does not cause much impairment, and nerve regeneration to the replanted part is quite rapid because of the short distance to the terminal sensory organs.

Furthermore, the aesthetic appearance of a zone 1 replantation is far superior to that of an amputation stump. In the future, the use of patient-related outcome instruments and an increased body of replantation experience among centers will help to define the utility of various digit replantation procedures.

Toe Transfer

When finger replantation is not possible or not successful, patients are left with significant functional loss. Disability is most severe when the thumb has been amputated at or proximal to the metacarpophalangeal joint, or when all the fingers have been amputated in machine injuries. In these cases, toe transfer to the hand is an effective procedure to restore grasp and pinch function. Although a prosthesis is available to mimic the thumb, lack of sensation is a major drawback that often leads to disuse of the prosthesis. For a patient who has sustained a thumb amputation at or proximal to the metacarpophalangeal joint, transfer of the big toe or second toe to the thumb can create a sensate digit that will oppose to the other fingers. Transfer of a big toe is advantageous because it provides a broad contact surface, and the big toe closely resembles the thumb, particularly when it is trimmed and sculptured to match the size of the thumb. However, the disadvantage of transferring the big toe is the conspicuous appearance of the donor site in the foot and potential gait problems during foot push-off if the head of the first metatarsal is taken along with the big toe. For these reasons, transfer of the second toe is now preferred in some centers (Fig. 107.12). The disadvantage of the second-toe transfer procedure is the slender appearance of the digit in comparison with the original thumb, although the appearance of the donor site is quite acceptable. A recent outcome study

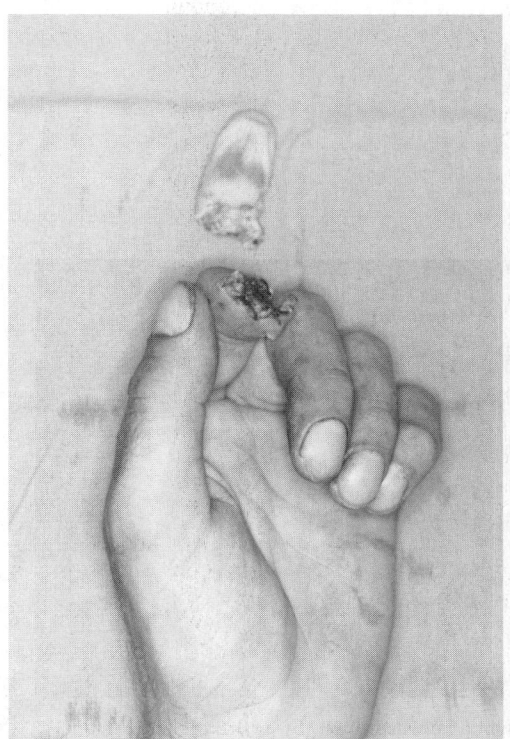
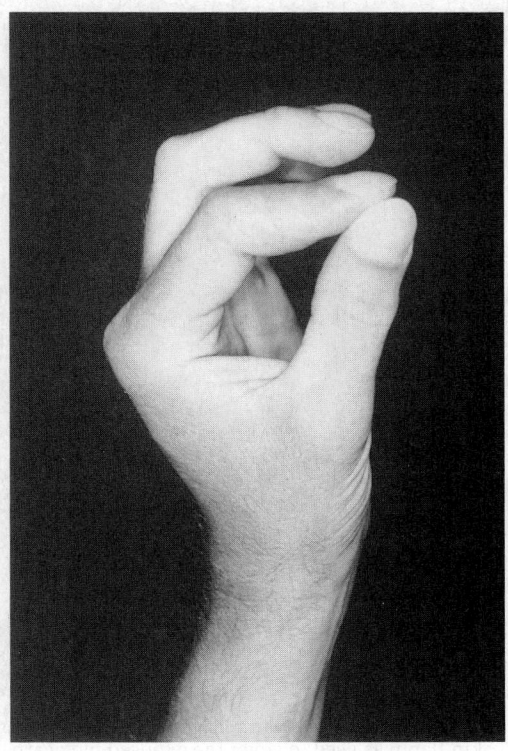

A   **B**

Figure 107.11. *(A)* Amputation of the index finger at zone 1 in a mechanic. The patient requested replantation because his work requires fine manipulative tasks. *(B)* Successful replantation with good aesthetic outcome and function.

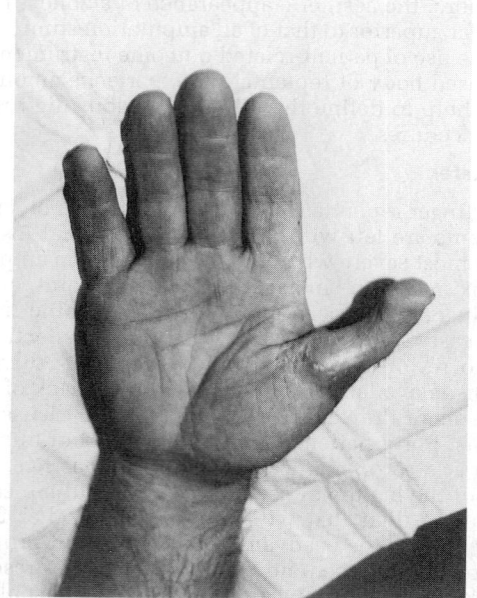
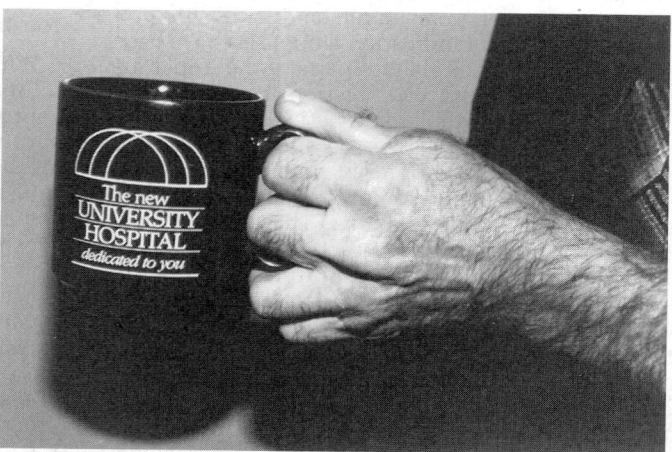

Figure 107.12. *(A)* Second-toe transfer for thumb reconstruction in a carpenter. He sustained a thumb amputation at the metacarpophalangeal joint while using a saw at work. *(B)* Good function with restoration of fine pinch. The patient returned to work as a carpenter 3 months after the toe reconstruction.

in which objective physical measurements and validated outcome questionnaires were used demonstrated that toe-to-thumb transfer is an effective procedure in restoring hand function (44). In addition, patients did not complain of gait difficulty after transfer of either the big toe or second toe.

One of the most complex problems in hand surgery is the reconstruction of a hand without digits. To create a new hand capable of tripod pinch, plastic surgeons have transferred multiple toes from both feet to the hand (Fig. 107.13). This type of reconstruction can restore function to an otherwise useless hand and has allowed two farmers

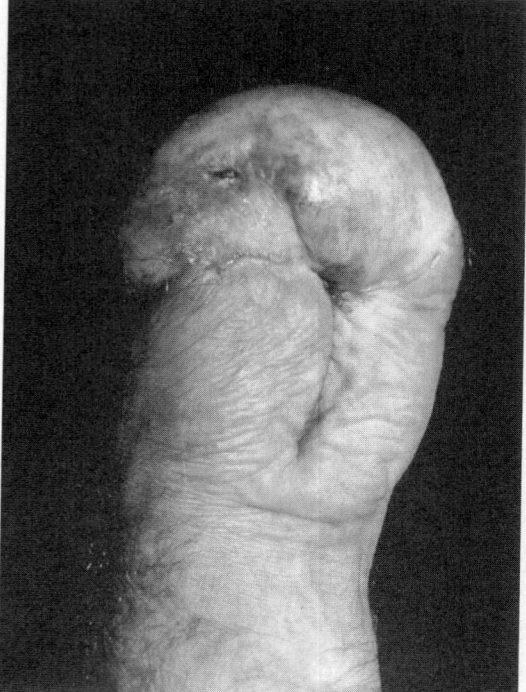
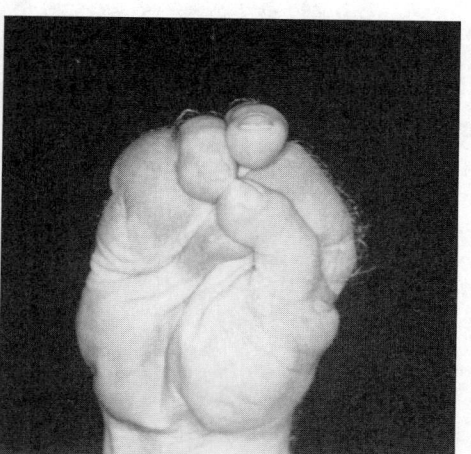

Figure 107.13. *(A)* A farmer who lost all his fingers when he was injured by a corn picker. A groin skin flap was used to cover the exposed metacarpal heads. *(B)* A second toe was removed from one foot to reconstruct the thumb, and the second and third toes were removed together from the other foot to reconstruct the fingers. Note the good opposition of the thumb and acceptable flexion of the digits. The patient returned to work in his dairy farm after the hand reconstruction.

who were treated at our center to return to heavy farm labor.

Complex Hand Injuries

Although crush injuries to the hand are common, injuries in which the force is sufficient to disrupt the structural integrity of the wrist and sever the blood supply to the hand are uncommon events (Fig. 107.14). Because multiple structures are traumatized in injuries of this kind, a systematic treatment approach is important in salvaging the hand and restoring its function. Crucial steps in the management of this injury are the following: (a) ruling out other injuries, (b) aggressive débridement, (c) skeletal fixation, (d) decompression of fascial compartments in the hand, (e) revascularization, (f) tendon repair, (g) soft-tissue coverage, and (h) nerve repair.

Ruling Out Other Injuries. In devastating trauma, attention is often focused on the obvious injury, and injuries to other organ systems may be ignored. In a review of 1,100 patients referred for emergent microsurgery at Davies Medical Center during a 7-year period, Partington and colleagues (45) found nine cases (0.8%) of unrecognized life-threatening injuries that required abandonment of the microsurgical procedures. Therefore, systematically evaluating the patient for trauma and ruling out other injuries should precede treatment of the hand injury.

Débridement. Severe crush and blast injuries are associated with large zones of injury, and the wounds may be contaminated with foreign materials such as grease or paint, as in printing press injuries. In these cases, aggressive débridement is important in preventing infection. Except for critical structures that include nerves and tendons, all devitalized soft tissues and bone fragments must be excised. Radical débridement has been shown to decrease wound infection and improve the success rate of microvascular reconstruction (46).

Skeletal Fixation. After débridement, the next priority is to stabilize the wrist. A stable wrist provides a platform for repairing other injured structures. If the crush injury is associated with comminuted fractures of multiple carpal bones and rupture of the intercarpal ligaments, wrist fusion is the best option because it is otherwise often impossible to reconstitute the anatomy of the distal and proximal carpal rows. To avoid possible bone graft contamination during primary wrist fusion at the initial procedure, external fixators are placed for provisional fixation. Two 2.7-mm fixator pins are placed through an incision along the radial index metacarpal, and two proximal 3.5-mm pins are placed into the radius through an incision along the radial border of the distal radius, between the brachioradialis and the extensor carpi radialis longus. The superficial radial nerve, which lies under the brachioradialis, is dissected free and retracted away from the pins. External fixator rods are then secured to the pins with nuts and screws. If the wound is clean during the second-look procedure at 24 or 48 hours, total wrist fusion is then undertaken (Fig. 107.15). Otherwise, the external fixator is left in place until the wound is suitable for fusion with the use of internal plating and cancellous bone grafts. This stable skeletal fixation allows early hand therapy, usually instituted on day 7 following injury.

Revascularization. In a crush injury of the wrist, the zone of injury can be quite extensive. The use of vein grafts is essential in performing the arterial anastomosis away from the zone of injury. The ulnar artery is chosen for repair because it is the dominant artery in most patients and can be exposed readily in the hypothenar area. If the ulnar artery is contused in the palm, distal anasto-

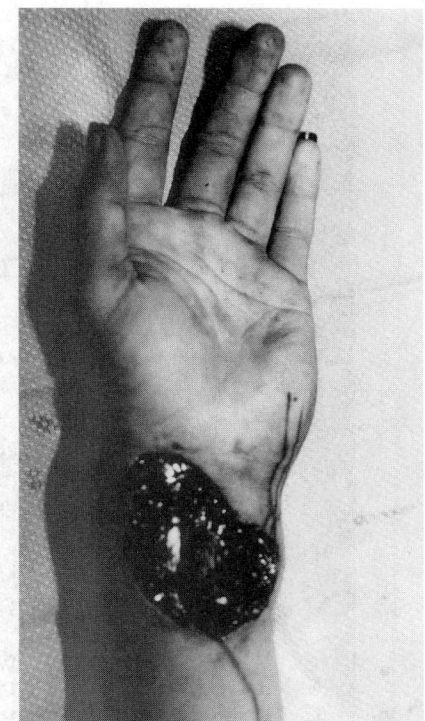

A

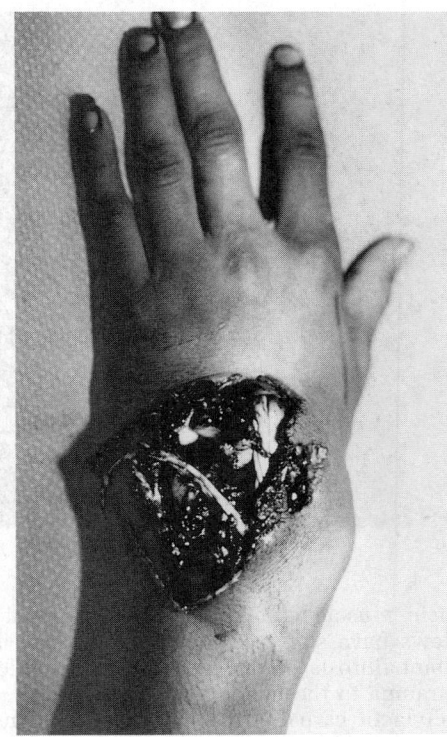

B

Figure 107.14. *(A)* Accidental shot gun blast injury in a 16-year-old boy. Both the radial and ulnar arteries were ruptured, and the hand was ischemic. The wrist was destroyed, and multiple tendons and nerves were severed. *(B)* Volar wrist wound. Markings show incision lines for ulnar artery exposure.

mosis can be performed to the superficial palmar arch. Because soft-tissue bridges are often present, venous outflow is not a problem, and venous anastomosis is not necessary.

Decompression of Fascial Compartments. The edema associated with crush injuries often raises the pressures in

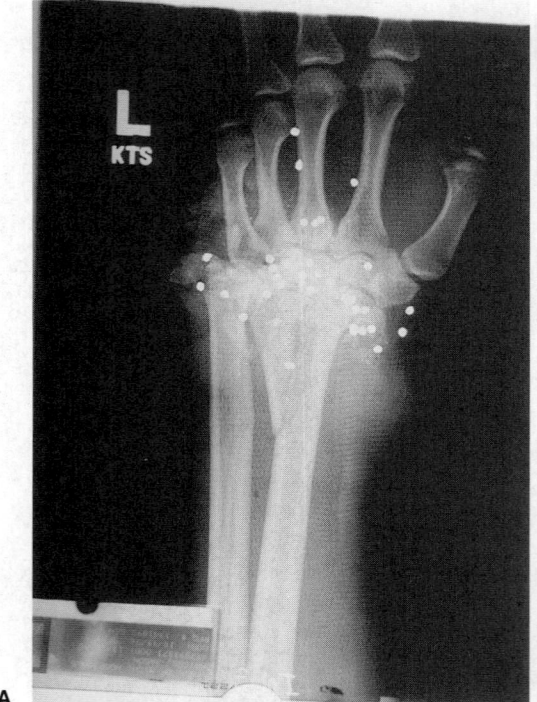

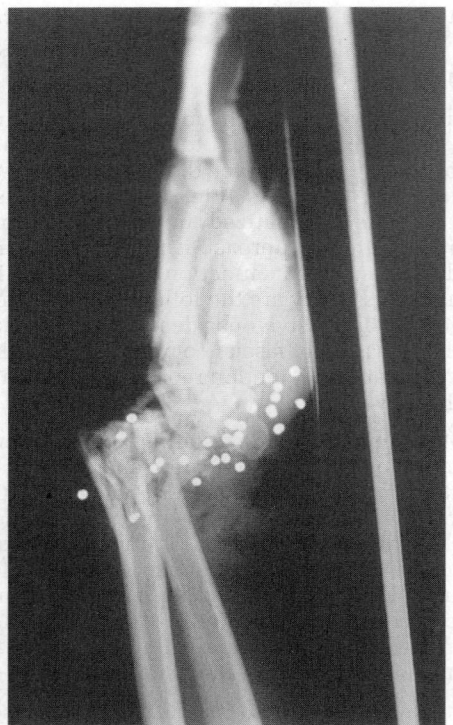

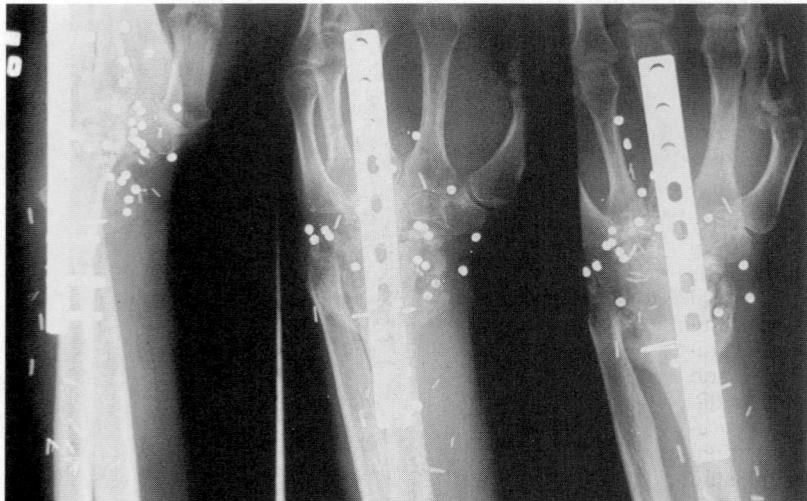

Figure 107.15. *(A,B)* Note destruction of the wrist joint, in addition to comminuted fractures of the distal ulna and radius. *(C)* Total wrist fusion was performed 48 hours after the initial injury.

the intrinsic muscle compartments and carpal tunnel. Prior reviews have shown a high incidence of ischemia and resultant fibrosis of the intrinsic muscles following crushing trauma to the hand (47). Consequently, we perform prophylactic carpal tunnel release and intrinsic muscle decompression in severe crush injuries of this kind.

Soft-tissue Coverage. After aggressive débridement, a soft-tissue defect is often present around the wrist. A split-thickness autograft is placed over the vein graft to prevent dessication. Other open wounds can be covered temporarily with homografts. If wrist fusion is undertaken during the second-look procedure, primary wound closure can be achieved. For residual wound defects, split-thickness autografts are used to cover the exposed muscle bellies. However, if tendons are exposed, coverage with either fasciocutaneous or muscle free flaps will allow earlier tendon mobilization and prevent tendon adhesions. Definitive early

wound coverage is important to protect vital structures and avoid wound colonization with bacteria (Fig. 107.16).

Nerve Repair. When nerves are crushed, the delineation between viable and nonviable nerve fascicles is difficult to assess in the acute setting. Therefore, we usually delay the nerve-grafting procedures until 2 or 3 months after the injury. To prevent retraction of the nerve ends, we suture the nerve ends to the surrounding soft tissues.

In conclusion, rigid skeletal fixation, revascularization with vein grafts, and immediate wound coverage are crucial factors in successful limb salvage.

Congenital Anomalies

Numerous congenital conditions affect the upper extremity. A discussion of some of the more common conditions and their treatment follows.

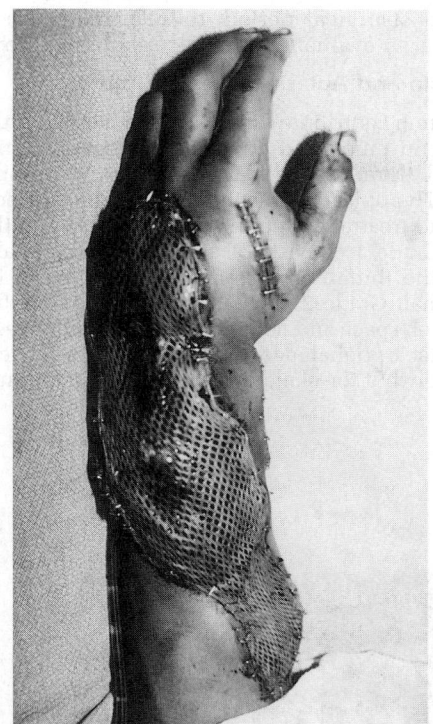

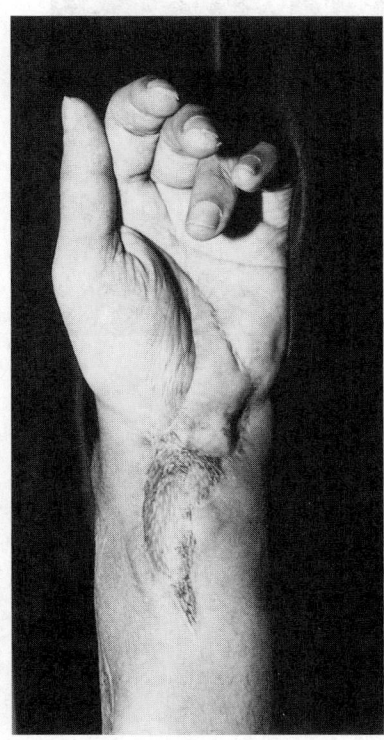

Figure 107.16. *(A)* A free rectus muscle was used for immediate coverage of the reconstructed wrist and tendons. *(B)* The hand was salvaged, and the patient has acceptable hand function after secondary nerve and tendon reconstruction.

Syndactyly

Syndactyly is a condition in which the fingers are fused. It can be classified as complete or incomplete. Complete syndactyly is a union of digits that extends to the distal phalanx. Incomplete syndactyly is a union of digits proxi-

mal to the distal phalanx but distal to the normal webbing at the midproximal phalanx. Syndactyly is further categorized as simple or complex. In simple syndactyly, no bony union exists between the digits; in complex syndactyly, bony union is present.

Typically, fused digits can be separated when a child is 1 year of age. Surgery should be performed earlier if syndactyly affects the thumb–index finger or ring finger–little finger web space and causes the shorter digit to deviate during growth. Meticulous design of the skin flaps is required to separate the fingers, and the dorsal skin flap is crucial in creating a web space that is not prone to contracture (Fig. 107.17). Distally, triangular skin flaps are designed to drape the sides of the fingers. A full-thickness skin graft from the groin is often required to cover open areas in the fingers.

Thumb Duplication

Although thumb duplication does not often cause a functional problem, this prominent hand malformation can have a significant effect on a child's psychosocial de-

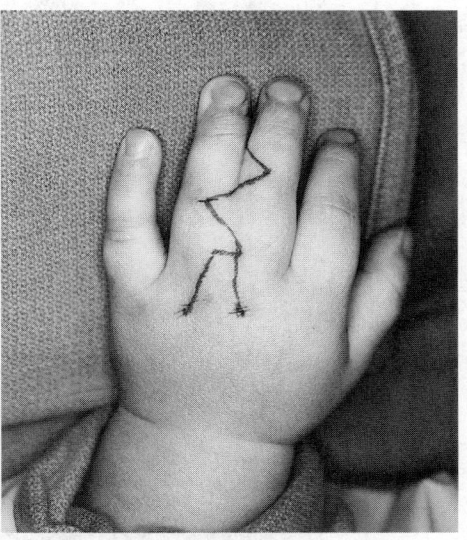

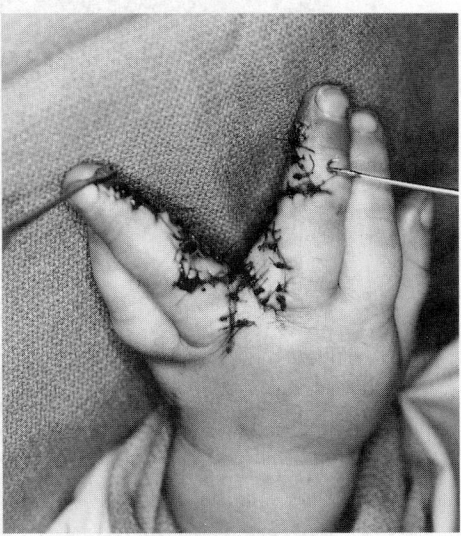

Figure 107.17. *(A)* A simple, complete syndactyly in a 1-year-old child. Note the design of the dorsal skin flap to reconstruct the web space and the interdigitating distal skin flaps. *(B)* Immediate postoperative photograph of the syndactyly release.

velopment. Surgery can be undertaken when the child is about 2 years old to prevent progressive deviation of the thumb during growth. Thumb duplication can be classified into seven groups, depending on the level of the duplication. Type 1 consists of a bifid distal phalanx, whereas type 2 is a complete duplication of the distal phalanx. Types 3 and 4 involve the proximal phalanx, and types 5 and 6 involve the metacarpal. Type 7 is triphalangeal thumb or a thumb with three phalanges. Usually, the radial, less developed thumb is removed. Retention of the ulnar thumb has the added advantage of preserving the important stabilizing ulnar collateral ligament. The surgery requires a delicate reconstruction of the bone, ligament, and tendon structures to sculpture the remaining thumb as normally as possible (Fig. 107.18). After the im-

mediate postsurgical period, these patients are followed once a year to evaluate potentially abnormal growth.

Hypoplasia and Aplasia of the Thumb

The thumb contributes about 50% of hand function and is important in pinch and grip. Reconstruction of the underdeveloped thumb is critical in improving a child's hand function. Hypoplasia of the thumb can be classified into five grades, and treatment options are often based on this classification. Grade 1 consists of minor hypoplasia; all components of the thumb are present, but the thumb is smaller than normal. Grade 2 consists of adduction contracture of the first web space and laxity of the ulnar collateral ligament at the metacarpophalangeal joint; the thenar musculature is hypoplastic, but the skeletal framework of the thumb is nor-

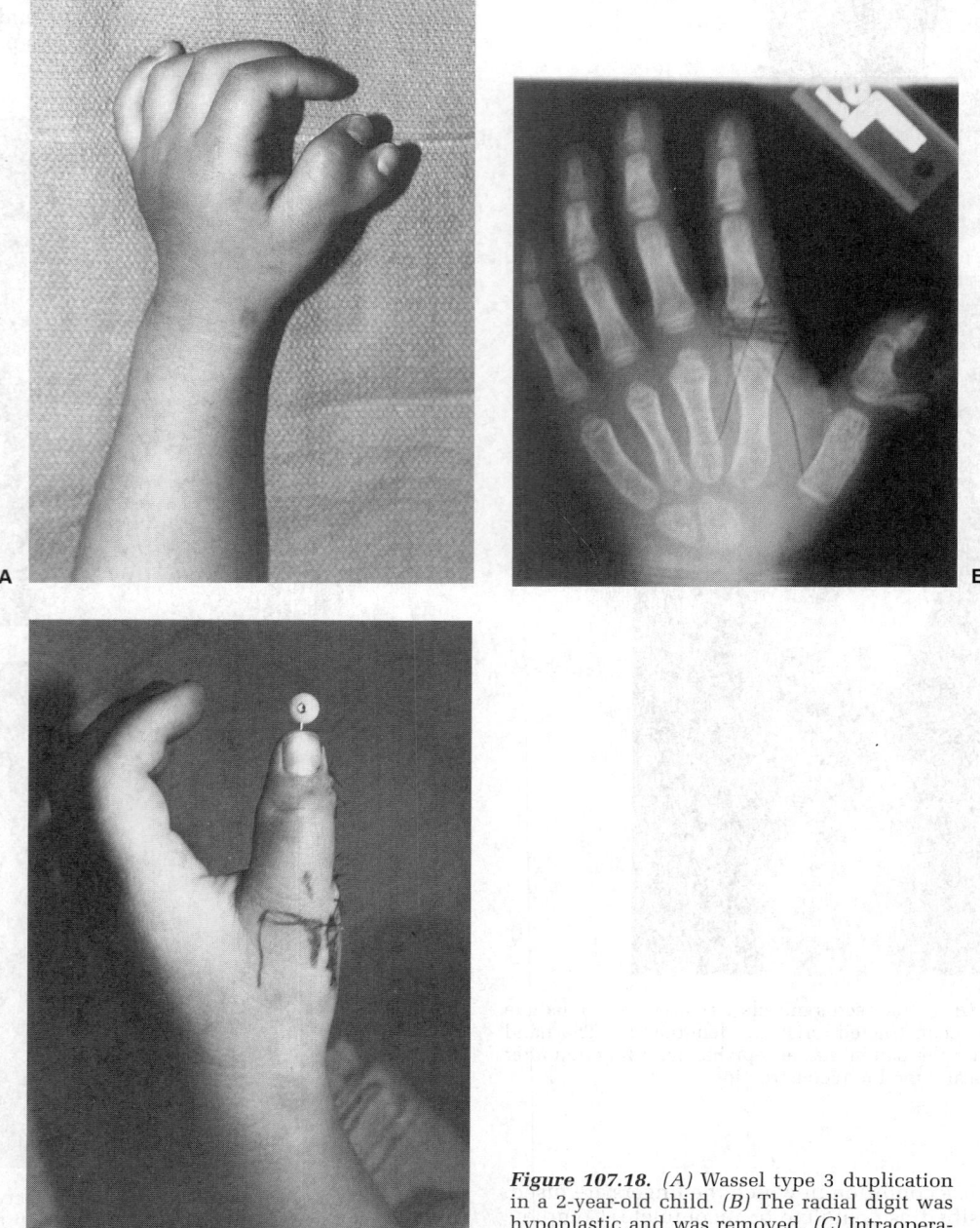

Figure 107.18. *(A)* Wassel type 3 duplication in a 2-year-old child. *(B)* The radial digit was hypoplastic and was removed. *(C)* Intraoperative picture shows the aesthetically pleasing reconstructed thumb.

mal. Grade 3 includes severe hypoplasia of the thumb with absent intrinsic muscles and underdeveloped extrinsic tendons; the skeletal framework is hypoplastic, and the carpometacarpal joint is vestigial. Grade 4 is characterized by a floating, nonfunctional thumb *(pouce flottant),* with soft-tissue attachment of the thumb at the metacarpophalangeal joint of the index finger. Grade 5 is defined by total absence of the thumb. Grade 1 hypoplasia does not require treat-

ment, whereas grades 3, 4, and 5 require index pollicization (use of the index finger to reconstruct a thumb) for optimal function (Fig. 107.19). In grade 2, the thumb can be reconstructed by means of a combination of tendon, joint, and soft-tissue procedures.

Rheumatoid Arthritis

Rheumatoid arthritis is a crippling disease that severely affects the quality of life for millions of Americans. It is postulated to be an autoimmune disease mediated by inflammatory cells that attack the synovial tissues in the body. Persistent synovitis in the joints erodes the articular surfaces and disrupts their soft-tissue supports. Because the hand is often damaged by rheumatoid arthritis, the effective surgical treatment of hand deformities can improve function and restore independence. The goals of surgery for hands affected by rheumatoid arthritis include (a) pain control, (b) improvement or restoration of function, (c) prevention of disease progression, and (d) aesthetic improvement. To accomplish these goals, the surgeon must maintain good rapport with both the rheumatologist and the patient as the priorities of treatment are determined. By listening to patients with rheumatoid arthritis describe their limitations and goals, the surgeon can gain insight into the surgical plan that will offer them the most benefit.

Surgical treatment can be classified as preventive, corrective, or salvage (48). Preventive procedures include tenosynovectomy to prevent tendon rupture, and synovectomy to reduce ongoing joint destruction resulting from erosive synovitis in the joints. Corrective procedures include tendon transfers for ruptured tendons and nerve decompression for carpal tunnel syndrome. Salvage procedures consist of joint arthroplasty and joint fusion.

A common hand deformity in rheumatoid arthritis is subluxation and ulnar deviation of the fingers at the level of the matacarpophalangeal joints (Fig. 107.20). Synovitis at the metacarpophalangeal joints distends the joints and attenuates the supporting ligaments. Wrist destruction in rheumatoid arthritis contributes to radial deviation of the metacarpals, which accentuates the ulnar deviation of the fingers. With progressive metacarpophalangeal joint disease, patients have great difficulty opening their hands because of subluxation of the metacarpophalangeal joints, and difficulty with fine pinch because of the ulnar deviation of the fingers. In addition to pain at the metacarpophalangeal joints secondary to worn articular surfaces, patients with rheumatoid arthritis often complain about the unattractive appearance of their hands.

The Swanson metacarpophalangeal joint arthroplasty is an effective procedure that meets all four goals of rheumatoid arthritis surgery. By replacing the arthritic joints with prosthetic spacers and realigning the soft-tissue envelope around the metacarpophalangeal joints, surgeons are able to improve function markedly and enhance the aesthetic appearance of the hands. A recent systematic overview of the world literature on this procedure shows that Swanson metacarpophalangeal joint arthroplasty effectively improves the health-related quality of life of patients with rheumatoid arthritis (49).

Conclusion

The selected topics summarized in the preceding paragraphs illustrate the limitless possibilities of hand reconstruction. Because of the ingenuity of those who have pioneered in plastic surgery, hand surgeons are now able to create functional and aesthetic hands, which was not possible only decades ago. Continuing advances in tissue engineering and immunology may enable surgeons to per-

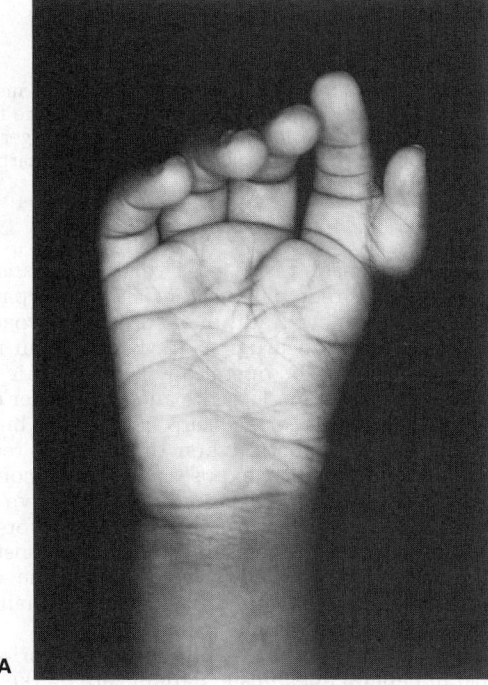

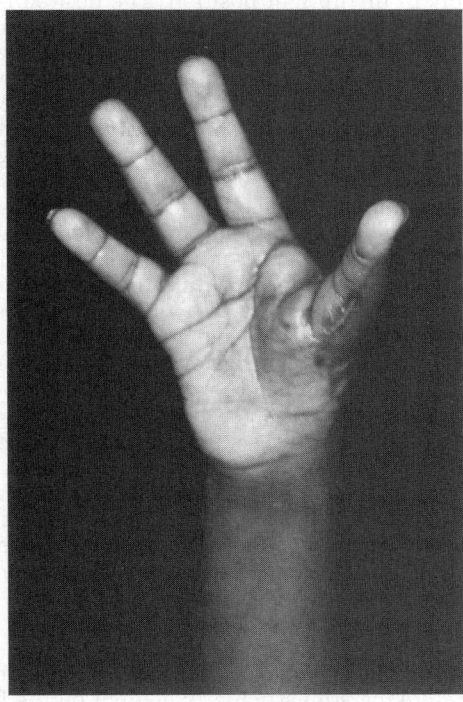

Figure 107.19. *(A)* Absence of a thumb in a 2-year-old child. Note the floating thumb attached to the index finger. *(B)* Three months after index pollicization, the child is able to use the new thumb for grasp and fine pinch.

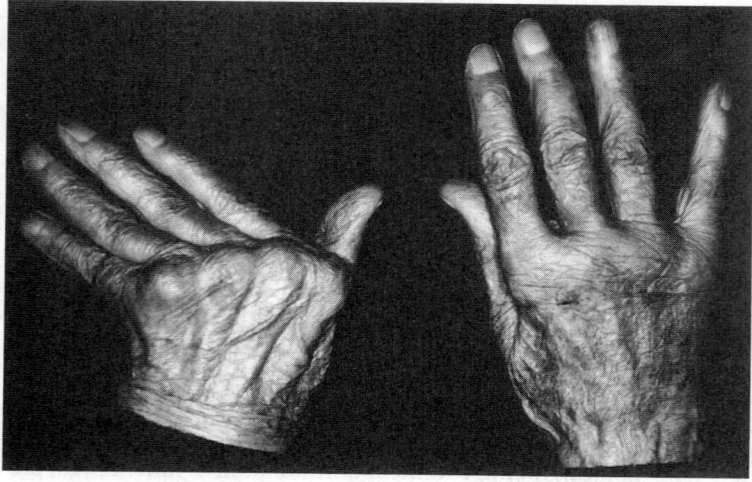

Figure 107.20. Severe destruction of the metacarpophalangeal joints with ulnar deviation of the fingers of the left hand. Note restoration of normal finger alignment of the right hand after Swanson metacarpophalangeal joint arthroplasty.

form finger and hand transplantation in the future with increasingly predictable success.

AESTHETIC SURGERY

In plastic surgery, broad surgical principles are adapted to address a multitude of unique clinical problems by altering form and function. Plastic surgery, particularly aesthetic surgery, simultaneously restores physical function and enhances a patient's body image and self-esteem. For example, blepharoplasty improves the appearance of baggy, tired eyes and may also correct visual field defects resulting from eyelid ptosis. A rhinoplasty improves the outward appearance of a nose in addition to increasing nasal air flow.

Aesthetic surgery requires meticulous attention to detail, careful patient selection, rigorous procedural planning, and precise execution of the technically challenging procedures. If patients are carefully selected and their goals realistic, then the chances for a successful outcome are good. However, if a patient is poorly selected, then a technically successful operation may be a dismal failure in the eyes of the patient. The aesthetic surgeon must not only diagnose the clinical deformity but also carefully evaluate the patient's expectations and motivations for surgery. Through the application of sound surgical principles and technical expertise, the aesthetic surgeon can experience lifelong career and personal satisfaction.

Cosmetic Procedures of the Head and Neck

Brow Lift

Brow ptosis is a natural consequence of the biologic process of aging. If left uncorrected, patients can appear angry or older than their chronologic age. If severe, brow ptosis may cause visual field obstruction; correction of this deformity can produce dramatic functional and aesthetic improvements.

Minimally invasive approaches to surgical problems have been readily adopted in many surgical fields. However, plastic surgeons have been slow to apply endoscopic principles to clinical problems. One procedure that is particularly well suited to an endoscopic approach, and in which endoscopy has received wide clinical acceptance, is the brow lift (50). This has become the primary approach to brow ptosis repair, replacing the traditional transcoronal incision with a scalp or forehead resection.

The traditional approach results in a very large transcoronal scar and requires regional anesthesia. In male patients with a receding hairline, a traditional coronal approach requires resection of hair-bearing scalp, which is an undesirable consequence of this operation. To avoid this problem, the incision can be made at the anterior border of the hairline so that no hair-bearing scalp is resected, but this approach can be problematic when the hairline recedes posteriorly and subsequently exposes the scar. In contrast, an endoscopic approach utilizes only three to five 1-cm incisions behind the hairline to gain access to the forehead and glabellar rhytids, and so produces less of an aesthetic deformity. Some evidence also suggests that the endoscopic approach produces a more lasting result than does the traditional approach (51).

Endoscopic and open brow lifts may be performed under local or general anesthesia. Patients are marked preoperatively in the upright position. The desired brow position is at the level of the orbital rim in male patients and 1 cm above the orbital rim in female patients. During an open brow lift, a coronal incision is made and the entire forehead is mobilized in a subgaleal or subperiosteal plane down to the orbital rim. The supraorbital and supratrochlear nerves are dissected free of surrounding tissues and preserved. The corrugator and procerus muscles are resected if prominent glabellar rhytids are present. The forehead is then redraped posteriorly, the redundant scalp is resected, and the wound is closed. In an endoscopic brow lift, incisions are made within the hair-bearing scalp at the midpupillary line and over the temporal fossa. The entire forehead flap is elevated under endoscopic guidance, the procerus and corrugator muscles are resected as necessary, and the forehead is retracted posteriorly. The forehead and brow are then secured in their new position with nonabsorbable sutures attached to absorbable screws or passed through osseous tunnels (50,51).

Postoperatively, patients are instructed to avoid vigorous physical exercise and to keep their head elevated at least 45 degrees. Bruising and swelling are anticipated for the first 2 to 3 weeks following the procedure. The final result is not expected for at least 6 weeks after the procedure.

Rhytidectomy

The deleterious effects of aging, gravity, exposure to the sun, and smoking are particularly evident on the face. Ultraviolet radiation and tobacco use produce fine facial wrinkling and skin laxity associated with poor elasticity. Aging and gravity result in gradual relaxation of the facial retaining ligaments, which produces midfacial ptosis, deepened nasolabial folds, "jowling" along the mandibular border, and redundancy of cervical skin (52). Old family photographs are constant reminders of a more youthful appearance, with high cheekbones and smooth skin. However, as the aging process marches on, patients may lose self-confidence and self-esteem in social, political, and business situations, so that they are motivated to seek facial rejuvenation surgery. If the patients are selected appropriately and the surgery is carefully planned and executed, the results will be gratifying for both patient and surgeon (53).

During the preoperative evaluation, the patient's expectations and motivations are carefully evaluated and addressed. Surgeons need to be cautious of patients whose concerns about their appearance are out of proportion to their physical deformity. Under these circumstances, a perfectly designed and performed operation may still result in a dismal outcome in the eyes of the patient.

Patients who smoke are at a significantly increased risk for the development of postoperative complications, including skin flap necrosis, infection, or wound dehiscence, and they are consequently instructed to quit. Older patients with medical illnesses are referred to a general practitioner for optimization of their medical condition preoperatively. If the patient is deemed a moderate risk for general anesthesia because of hypertension, diabetes, or coronary artery disease, the operation may be postponed or canceled depending on the severity of the illness.

Younger patients (40 to 50 years old) with good skin quality, mild midfacial ptosis, and early "jowling" may benefit from a minimally invasive endoscopic midface lift. This operation is typically combined with an endoscopic brow lift to provide facial rejuvenation. The operation is performed under local or general anesthesia. Bilateral temporal and superior buccal sulcus incisions are made. The temporal fossa dissection is carried down to the level of the superficial layer of the deep temporal fascia. Under endoscopic guidance, the superficial layer of the deep temporal fascia is then incised to expose the temporal fat pad. The dissection proceeds caudad until the zygomatic arch is identified. A subperiosteal plane of dissection provides access to the midface while preserving the integrity of the frontal branch of the facial nerve. The subperiosteal plane of dissection is continued into the midface, with care taken to avoid the infraorbital nerves. The masseter is mobilized from its lateral attachments. The superior buccal sulcus incisions are made, and a midface subperiosteal dissection is performed under both direct visualization and endoscopic guidance. Once the dissection has been completed, the entire midface is suspended in the desired position with 2-0 polydioxanone (PDS) sutures spanning from the deep temporal fascia to the midface periosteum. Symmetry of the suspension is then confirmed, and the wounds are closed in layers. This technique nicely corrects midface ptosis, mild jowling, and early nasolabial fold prominence, but if significant skin laxity is present, then a traditional rhytidectomy is required (50,54).

A traditional rhytidectomy can be performed under local or general anesthesia. The skin incision is made over the temporal fossa 4 to 5 cm cephalad to the root of the helix and extended caudad toward the apex of the ear. The incision is then extended anterior to the ear, around the earlobe, into the retroauricular sulcus, across the mastoid, and into the scalp. The skin flap is elevated just superficial to the superficial musculoaponeurotic system (SMAS) and platysma. This plane of dissection maintains a thin layer of subcutaneous fat on the skin flap to preserve viability and avoids injury to the facial nerve, parotid gland, and jugular vein. The flaps are elevated medially to the nasolabial fold in the face and to the midline in the neck. Oc-

casionally, a platysmal diastasis may exist that creates an obtuse cervicomental angle and prominent neck. Under these circumstances, a plastymal plication can be performed through a 2- to 3-cm submental incision to correct the diastasis and improve the appearance of the neck. Once the skin flaps are completely elevated, many plastic surgeons mobilize the lateral SMAS and plastyma to improve control of facial and cervical tightening and reduce the tension on the skin closure. The SMAS and platysma are placed under tension and secured to create the desired facial appearance. The skin flaps are then redraped posteriorly, the patient is examined for symmetry, and a skin resection is performed. Hemostasis is obtained through the judicious use of bipolar electrocautery (Fig. 107.21). The wounds are closed in layers, and a pressure dressing is applied. Drains are typically used in the face and neck (55–59).

Postoperatively, patients are instructed to keep their head elevated at least 45 degrees to reduce swelling. The patient is evaluated in the recovery room for any evidence of a hematoma or facial nerve injury. It is crucial to identify a hematoma early to avoid overlying skin necrosis. Facial nerve injuries occur in only 2% to 3% of cases. On the first postoperative day, the pressure dressings and drains are removed, and the patient is examined for evidence of a late hematoma, unrecognized facial nerve injury, or compromised skin flap. The sutures are removed on the fifth postoperative day. Patients should expect to have significant swelling and bruising for at least 2 weeks following the procedure. The final postoperative result is not realized until approximately 6 months after the procedure.

Blepharoplasty

Eyelid surgery can be performed to correct functional or aesthetic deformities. Excessive skin and fat of the eyelids can give the patient an angry, aged, or tired look and may cause visual field obstruction. Older patients typically present with redundant skin and fine wrinkling, whereas younger patients commonly complain of persistent bags under their eyes. Treatment of each clinical entity requires a unique approach based on the diagnosis and presentation (60). All patients being evaluated for blepharoplasty require a complete ophthalmologic examination preoperatively to evaluate visual acuity, upper eyelid ptosis, exophthalmos, lower eyelid laxity, and symptoms of "dry" eye. The position of the brow can significantly affect the appearance of the eyelids. Patients with brow ptosis frequently present for a blepharoplasty evaluation when they actually require a brow lift (51). Meticulous attention to detail is critical for the successful outcome of blepharoplasty surgery. If lower lid laxity is present preoperatively and a standard blepharoplasty is performed, a lower lid ectropion may develop postoperatively. Symptoms of "dry" eye can also be significantly worsened by a blepharoplasty.

Once the diagnosis has been made and an operative plan has been formulated, the operation can be performed under local or general anesthesia. Older patients frequently require skin excisions and removal or repositioning of orbital fat. The blepharoplasty incisions are designed preoperatively with the patient in the upright position. A local anesthetic with epinephrine is then infiltrated for pain control and hemostasis. The upper eyelid blepharoplasty begins with an elliptic excision of upper eyelid skin and orbicularis oculi muscle. Small openings are made in the orbital septum to gain access to the two compartments of periorbital fat. A conservative fat resection is performed to avoid a postoperative "hollowed-out" appearance. The skin is then redraped, and the wounds are closed in a single layer with running subcuticular 6-0 polypropylene (Prolene) sutures.

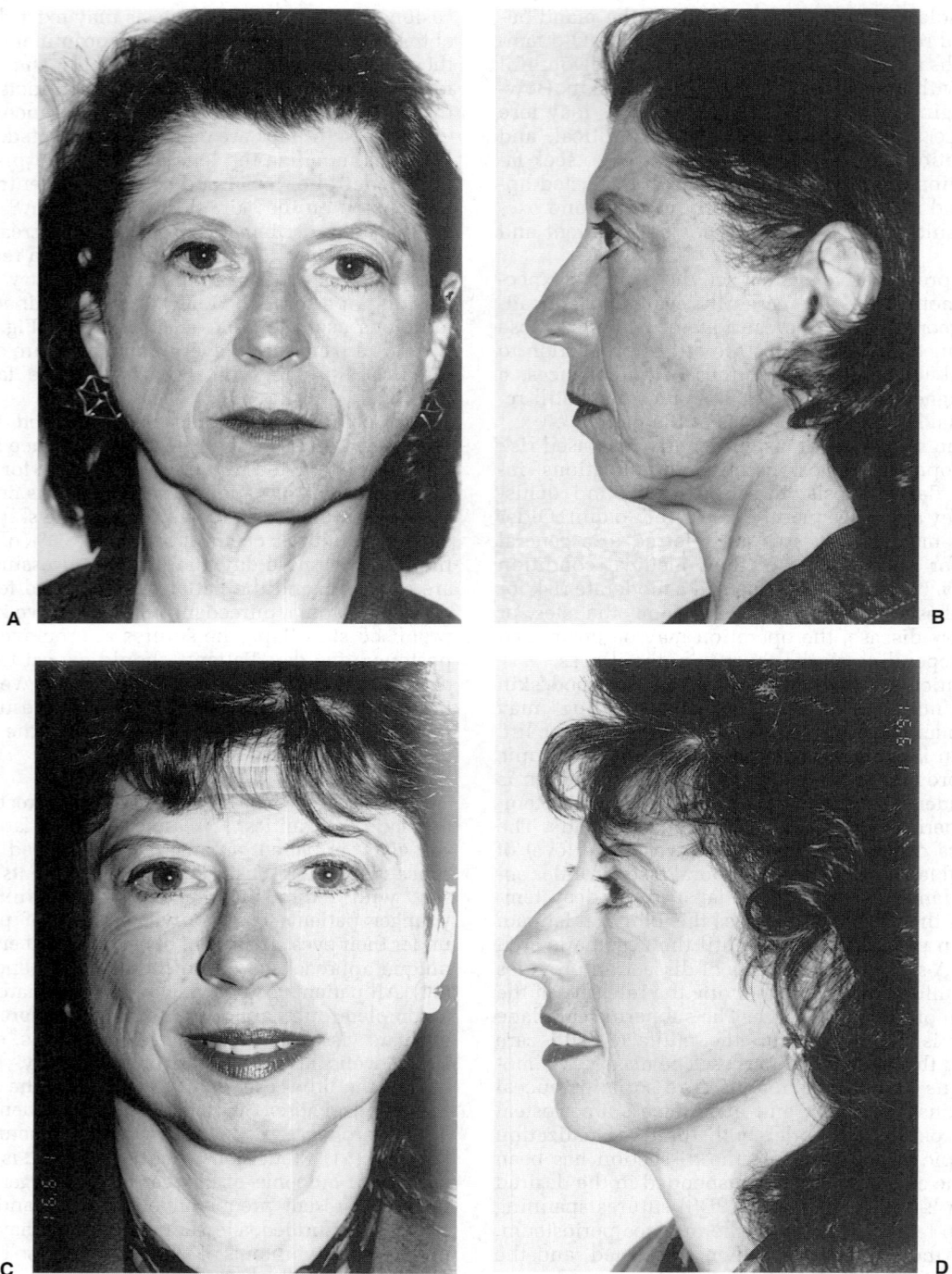

Figure 107.21. Rhytidectomy with superficial musculoaponeurotic system resection, platysmal plication, and endoscopic brow lift. *(A–B)* Preoperative appearance. *(C–D)* Postoperative appearance. Note the improved brow position above the orbital rim, malar prominence, flattened nasolabial folds, reduced "jowling" along the mandibular border, and improved cervicomental angle.

The traditional lower eyelid blepharoplasty begins with a subciliary incision. The dissection is then carried deep to the orbicularis oculi muscle until the orbital septum is identified. The orbital septum is divided to gain access to the three compartments of periorbital fat in the lower lid. Fat may be resected in cases of prominent herniation, but over-resection must be avoided. A recent trend in blepharoplasty surgery has emphasized periorbital fat repositioning rather than resection. Simply repositioning the herniated periorbital fat over the inferior orbital rim, rather than resecting it,

can dramatically improve the appearance of the lower eyelids (61). Once the periorbital fat has been resected or repositioned, the skin/muscle flap is redraped superiorly and the redundant tissue is excised. The lower eyelid wounds are closed with interrupted sutures of 6-0 silk. Ancillary procedures may also be necessary to improve the position of the lower eyelid, including a medial canthoplasty, lateral canthoplasty, or horizontal lid shortening.

In younger patients, a tired appearance of the eyes is commonly caused by excessive periorbital fat or fat behind the orbicularis oculi. A lower lid blepharoplasty through a transconjunctival approach allows the periorbital fat to be removed without leaving an external scar. The conjunctiva is divided transversely 1 mm above the sulcus to gain access to the orbital septum. The septum is divided, and the periorbital fat is removed from all three compartments. The wound is then allowed to heal by secondary intention.

Postoperatively, patients are instructed to keep their head elevated at all times and to apply cold compresses. No vigorous physical exercise is permitted during the early postoperative period. Artificial tears are used to maintain appropriate lubrication. No antibiotics are necessary. Patients are monitored carefully for corneal abrasions, changes in visual acuity, or hematomas, which may require emergent intervention. Sutures are removed 5 days postoperatively. Patients are informed that bruising and swelling will last for approximately 2 weeks, and that it will be approximately 6 to 8 weeks before the final result is seen.

Rhinoplasty

Rhinoplasty is an exacting operation in which the external appearance and internal anatomy of the nose are altered. The nose may be aesthetically unappealing or functionally impaired as a result of trauma, surgery, or a congenital deformity. Clearly, many familial and ethnic traits are associated with a multitude of nasal appearances. For this reason, it is crucial that the patient and surgeon discuss the goals of the procedure and the likelihood of achieving these goals. The patient must have realistic expectations and be prepared for the operation both physically and mentally.

For a successful rhinoplasty, a complete nasal history must be obtained, with particular attention paid to nasal airway obstruction, allergies, trauma, and previous surgery. A photographic analysis is performed to evaluate facial and nasal dimensions. The photographs are examined with the patient, the operative plan is discussed, and the potential structural and functional outcomes are reviewed (62).

Rhinoplasty can be performed under local or general anesthesia. The patient is prepared for surgery with intranasal injections of vasoconstrictors containing lidocaine and epinephrine. Topical vasoconstrictors (i.e., cocaine) are applied to the nasal lining and septum. The operation can be performed in an "open" or "closed" fashion. The open technique requires a transcolumellar incision extended intranasally to expose the cartilage and bones of the nose. Direct visualization of the structure of the nose allows greater precision in cartilaginous sculpting and nasal bone repositioning. The paired lower lateral cartilages create the shape and provide support for the nasal tip. Correction of any deformity involving the nasal tip requires manipulation of these cartilages (e.g., resection for a bulbous or overprojecting tip, suturing to reposition an asymmetric nasal tip, cartilage grafting to increase tip projection). The paired upper lateral cartilages and nasal bones define the shape of the nasal dorsum and control nasal air flow. A prominent dorsal hump may require resection of both upper lateral cartilage and nasal bone. Osteotomies of the nasal bones may be required to narrow the nasal width by disconnecting the base of the nasal bones from the maxilla (Fig. 107.22). In contrast, "saddle nose" deformities may require cartilage or bone grafting to provide dorsal augmentation. Cartilage grafts may also be used to improve nasal air flow. By placing a "spreader graft" between the nasal septum and the upper lateral cartilage, the internal nasal valve area becomes less restrictive to air flow (63). The closed technique allows access to the nasal cartilage and bones through intranasal incisions. Many surgeons experienced in rhinoplasty prefer this approach. However, many of the complicated techniques of cartilage grafting and suturing can be difficult to perform with this limited exposure.

Postoperatively, patients are instructed to keep their head elevated and apply ice packs. Oral analgesics are provided for pain control. An external splint is used to maintain the position of the nasal bones and cartilage for 10 to 14 days. If osteotomies have been performed, the patient may also experience periorbital ecchymosis. Patients should expect nasal swelling, pain, and bruising for 2 to 3 weeks. However, a full year is required for complete resolution of nasal tip swelling, particularly following an open tip rhinoplasty. Approximately 5% to 10% of patients require a revision rhinoplasty, which should not be performed for at least 1 year following the original procedure.

Genioplasty

Genioplasty is a common plastic surgical procedure to manipulate the position of the chin and thereby improve facial appearance. Based on the design of the mandibular symphysis osteotomy, the vertical height and anterior projection of the chin can be adjusted (64). Patients with a "weak" chin may undergo an advancement genioplasty to enhance chin projection and improve the cervicomental angle. Chin augmentation can also be accomplished with an alloplastic implant (i.e., Silastic), which eliminates the need for an osteotomy. Patients with a very prominent chin may undergo a reduction genioplasty, in which the vertical height and anterior projection are reduced. The dental occlusion is not affected by these procedures, but the lip position and neck appearance may be altered (65).

A complete physical examination, photographic analysis, and radiographic evaluation are performed to evaluate facial harmony and determine the extent of the advancement or reduction. The dental occlusion is carefully examined to ensure that orthognathic surgery is not required to correct the chin position. Operations are typically performed under general anesthesia. A local anesthetic containing epinephrine is injected intraorally for hemostasis and postoperative pain control. Through an inferior buccal sulcus incision, access to the mandibular symphysis is achieved. The osteotomy is measured and marked based on the preoperative photographs and lateral radiographs; the mental foramen is avoided. The bony segment is mobilized and secured into its new position with plates and screws. Postoperatively, swelling and pain persist for approximately 4 to 6 weeks. During this time, the patient should maintain meticulous oral hygiene and avoid foods that can traumatize the inferior buccal sulcus incision.

Cosmetic Procedures of the Trunk and Extremities: Body Sculpting

Abdominoplasty

Abdominoplasty encompasses a wide array of surgical procedures used to correct abdominal deformities caused by excess abdominal skin, fatty tissue, or abdominal wall laxity. Abnormalities in any of these tissue planes can produce an aesthetically unappealing abdomen. Various surgical procedures, including dermatolipectomy, liposuction, and abdominal wall plication, are designed to correct the underlying pathology. These procedures are often combined and tailored to fit the surgical needs and desires of the patient. It is critical to define the physical anomaly responsible for the abdominal deformity so that the appropriate operative procedure or combination of procedures can be performed (66,67).

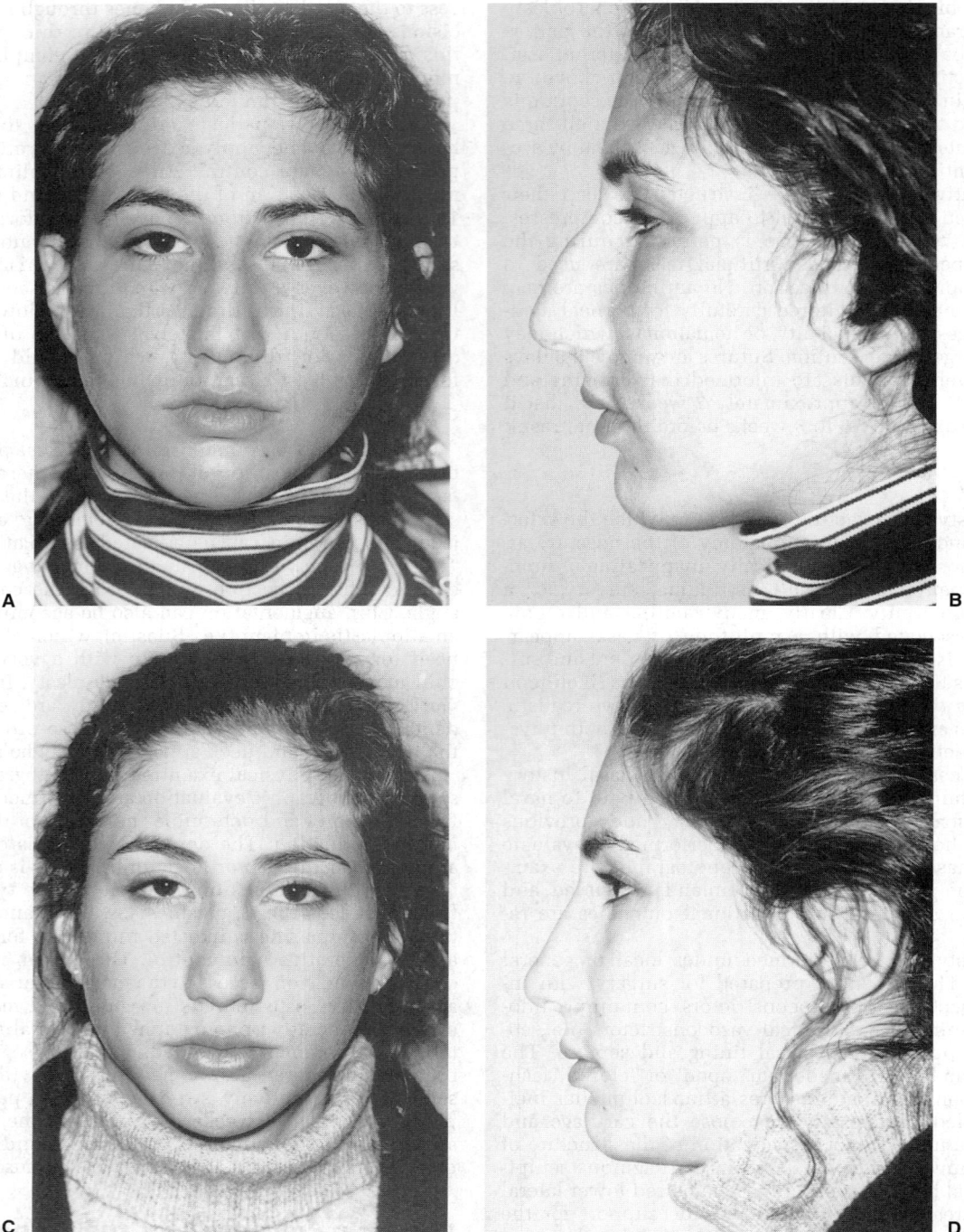

Figure 107.22. Open rhinoplasty with partial lower lateral cartilage resection, dorsal cartilage and bone resection, and nasal osteotomies. *(A–B)* Preoperative appearance. *(C–D)* Postoperative appearance. Note the dorsal hump reduction and slight supratip break.

A standard abdominoplasty combines a dermatolipectomy, liposuction, and abdominal wall plication to correct deformity in each of the three previously mentioned layers of the abdominal wall. The operation is performed under general anesthesia through a bikini-line incision extending from the upper margin of the pubic escutcheon to the iliac crests bilaterally. The skin incisions are made, and the abdominal flap is elevated off the underlying abdominal wall fascia. A circumferential incision is made around the umbilicus to allow complete elevation of the abdominal flap up to the costal margin. The patient is then placed in a flexed position, the abdominal flap is redraped caudally, and the ellipse-shaped redundant skin is resected. If any abdominal wall laxity is identified along with the skin redundancy, then a vertical midline abdominal wall plication is also performed. Occasionally, suction-assisted lipectomy is performed at the time of abdominoplasty to help recontour the abdomen and flanks. However, aggressive suction-assisted lipectomy of the abdominal flap can critically compromise flap vascularity and contribute to flap necrosis. Closed suction drains are placed before wound closure (Fig. 107.23).

A "mini-abdominoplasty" is used to treat mild abdominal skin redundancy and abdominal wall laxity. The same approach is used as previously described for a standard abdominoplasty except that the skin incision is limited to the central portion of the abdomen. A limited skin resection can be performed through this approach along with an abdominal wall plication. Suction-assisted lipectomy can be used in combination with this procedure, if necessary.

Endoscopic abdominoplasty can be used to treat abdominal wall laxity (i.e., postpartum rectus diastasis) and localized collections of fatty tissue. Patients who are candidates for this operation must have good skin quality and only mild to moderate lipodystrophy. General anesthesia is induced, and the abdomen is prepared aseptically. A circumferential incision is made around the umbilicus, and a 3-cm transverse incision is made in the pubic hair. These incisions function as the two access ports through which the endoscopic instruments are passed. Next, the entire abdominal wall is elevated from the abdominal wall fascia under endoscopic visualization with use of a 10-mm, 30-degree endoscope and electrocautery. The midline of the abdominal wall is plicated from pubis to xiphoid with a running O Prolene suture. Suction-assisted lipectomy can then be performed through the two access ports as needed. Drains are placed, and the incisions are closed in layers (50).

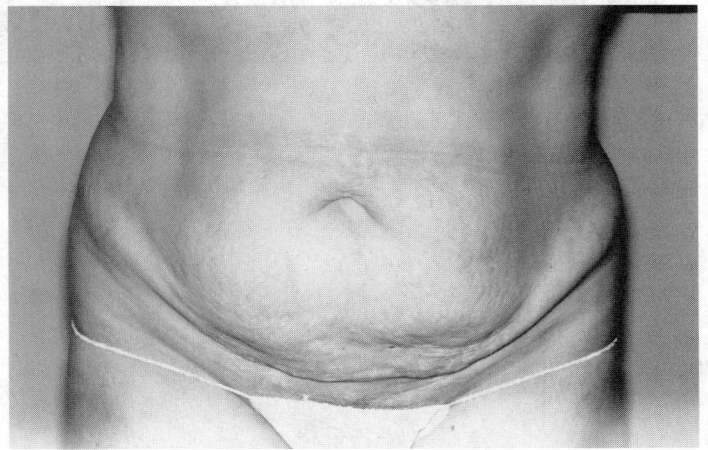

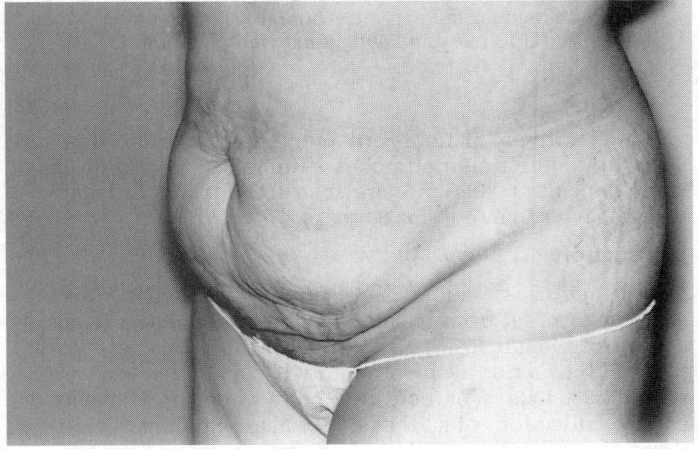

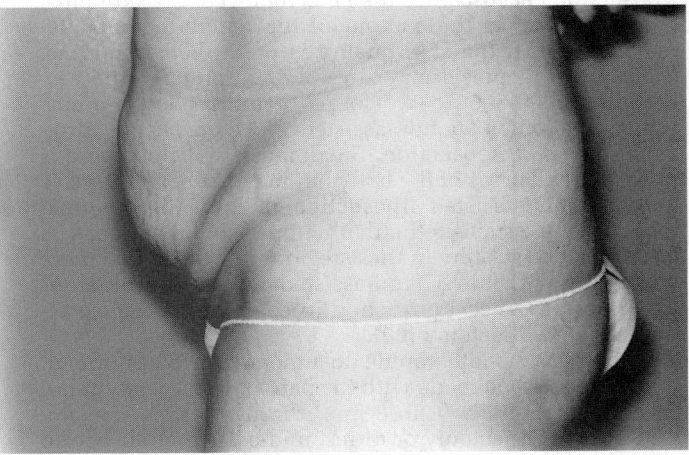

Figure 107.23. Abdominoplasty with dermatolipectomy, lateral liposuction, and abdominal wall plication. *(A–C)* Preoperative appearance. *(D–F)* Postoperative appearance. Note the reduced abdominal bulging and "hourglass" shape after lateral suction-assisted lipectomy and abdominal wall plication. *(continues)*

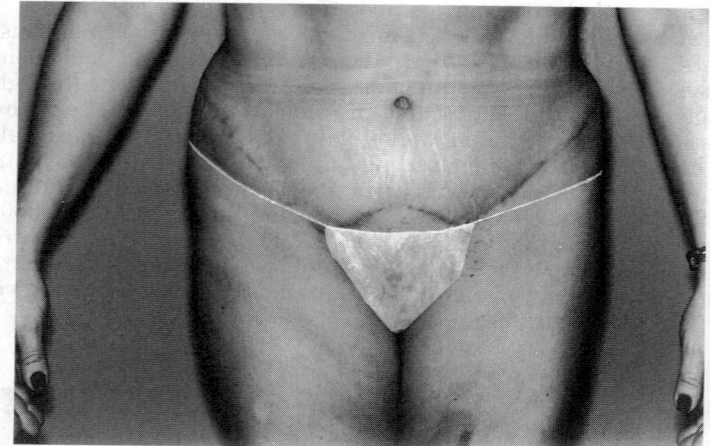
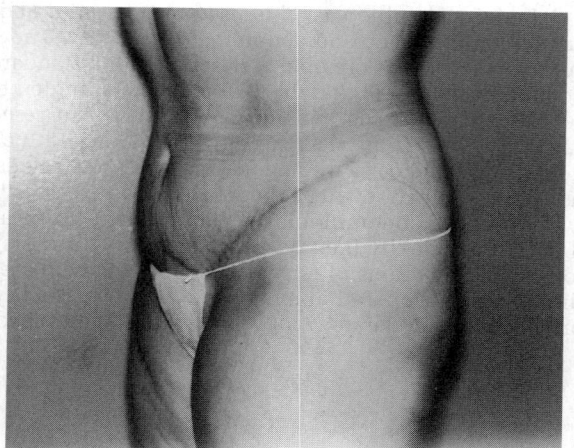
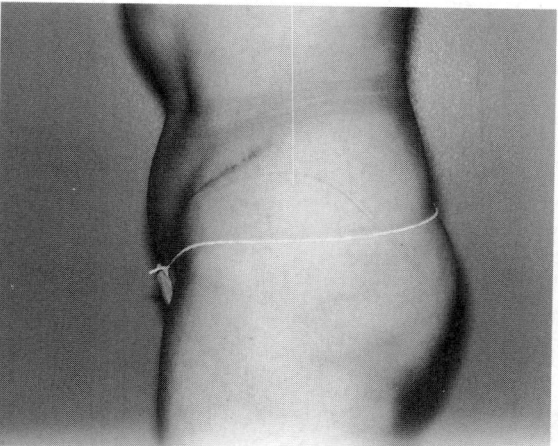

Figure 107.23. *(Continued) (D–F)* Postoperative appearance. Note the reduced abdominal bulging and "hourglass" shape after lateral suction-assisted lipectomy and abdominal wall plication.

Postoperatively, patients are maintained in a flexed position until their skin stretches sufficiently to permit an upright position. Patients are instructed to not lift anything heavier than 5 lb for 6 weeks.

Liposuction

Liposuction is a surgical procedure designed to resect collections of fat from isolated anatomic regions. It is not a form of weight loss and is not indicated in obese patients. Liposuction is ideally suited to patients who are within 20% to 30% of their ideal body weight and have localized collections of fat that are refractory to dietary modifications and exercise. Skin elasticity is very important in liposuction because once the fat is removed, the skin must contract down to the contour of the remaining subcutaneous tissue. If the skin quality is poor, then wrinkling, dimpling, and ptosis may severely compromise the aesthetic result (66–68). Two forms of liposuction are currently available: suction-assisted lipectomy and ultrasound-assisted liposuction. Suction-assisted lipectomy is utilized in all areas of the body but may not be as effective as ultrasound-assisted liposuction in more fibrous anatomic regions, such as the flank, upper abdomen, or male breast. Lipodystrophy in these regions can be treated more effectively with ultrasound-assisted liposuction alone or ultrasound-assisted liposuction in combination with suction-assisted lipectomy (69).

Preoperative photographic documentation is performed. Markings are then made with the patient in the upright position. Access ports (6 to 8 mm) through which the suction-assisted lipectomy or ultrasound-assisted liposuction

is performed are marked in areas that can be concealed. Intravenous sedation or general anesthesia is used. Tumescent fluid (1,000 mL of lactated Ringer's injection, 50 mL of 1% lidocaine, and 1 mg of epinephrine) is infiltrated for pain control and hemostasis.

Suction-assisted lipectomy is performed with metal cannulae connected to an aspirating device that generates a negative pressure of 1 atm. Various cannula configurations are utilized to perform the resection. Fatty tissue is aspirated into the holes of the cannula and then resected by moving the cannula tip. The operation is performed through multiple access ports. Large (6- to 8-mm-diameter) cannulae are used first, and then smaller (4-mm-diameter) cannulae with fewer holes to allow more precise body contouring. Overlapping patterns of resection are employed to avoid contour irregularities.

In ultrasound-assisted liposuction, body contouring is accomplished through the liquefaction and aspiration of fatty tissue. When used alone or in combination with traditional suction-assisted lipectomy, ultrasound-assisted liposuction is very effective for treating lipodystrophy in fibrous anatomic regions, such as the flank, upper abdomen, and male breast (70). The tip of the ultrasonic liposuction probe produces sound waves at a frequency of 20 to 30 kHz. The effect of these sound waves is to cavitate and liquefy low-density lipocytes. Low-power suction is then used to remove the resultant fluid. The ultrasound-assisted liposuction technique is equally as effective as traditional suction-assisted lipectomy for the treatment of lipodystrophy in most areas, and more effective in fibrous anatomic regions. The smaller hemoglobin-to-triglyceride ratio indicates that more fat is aspirated per amount of hemoglobin lost, and vascular structures are better preserved provided the technique is used by properly trained persons. However, if it is inappropriately used, the resulting complications can be quite severe; these include full-thickness skin loss from thermal injury (71).

All patients are placed in a compressive garment 24 hours a day for 6 weeks postoperatively. Early postoperative compression reduces the chances of hematoma formation. Prolonged compression reduces swelling and the potential for skin wrinkling. All patients experience some degree of ecchymosis, swelling, and decreased sensibility. The end result is not realized for approximately 2 to 3 months following the procedure.

PEDIATRIC PLASTIC SURGERY

The specialized area of pediatric plastic surgery focuses on the reconstruction of congenital and acquired deformities in children. Utilizing a sound knowledge of embryology and normal and abnormal growth and development, pediatric plastic surgeons employ a combination of innovation and technical expertise to restore both form and function in their patients. Although the manifestations of congenital malformations may be diverse, the approach to reconstruction is always based on fundamental surgical principles. Similarly, the management of trauma and other acquired deformities in children is based on essential surgical tenets adapted to the special considerations of growth and prematurity. Rather than providing a list of the myriad problems addressed by pediatric plastic surgeons, this section concentrates on the most salient features to give the clinician an accurate grasp of the subspecialty.

Cleft Lip and Palate

Perhaps the area that best exemplifies the specialty of pediatric plastic surgery is the management of children afflicted with cleft lip and palate. The cleft lip and palate pose a variety of structural and functional deficits that must be addressed with respect to growth and development and to the psychosocial concerns of both patient and family. The care of these children requires that exacting surgical technique be combined with the efforts of a team of allied health professionals to effect a comprehensive level of rehabilitation.

The overall incidence of cleft lip and palate is approximately 1/750 children. The incidence is significantly higher in Asians (1/300) and significantly lower in blacks (1/2,000) (72–74). The distribution of cleft types is approximately 46% combined cleft lip and palate, 21% isolated cleft lip, and 33% isolated cleft palate (75). Almost

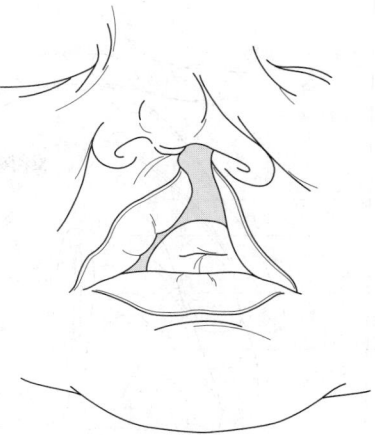

Figure 107.24. Left unilateral complete cleft lip. (Redrawn from Jurkiewicz MJ, Krizek TJ, Mathes SJ, eds. *Plastic surgery: principles and practice,* vol 1. St. Louis: Mosby, 1990:64, with permission.)

30% of children with cleft lip and palate have associated birth defects, and therefore vigilance is required in the physical examination (76). The chance of unaffected parents having a second child with cleft lip and palate is about 4%, as is the chance of one affected parent producing an offspring with a cleft (76,77). Genetic counseling is usually helpful, both in educating the parents and in screening for associated congenital anomalies.

A cleft lip deformity can be bilateral or unilateral; it is considered *complete* if it extends into the nose and *incomplete* if it does not (Fig. 107.24). The cleft lip can extend into the gum partially or completely through the alveolus to create a bony defect. The cleft lip deformity also affects the nose, which therefore must be addressed during reconstruction. Although the timing of cleft lip repair is controversial, it is often undertaken in about the third month of life, after the child has gained sufficient weight to make the administration of anesthesia potentially safer.

A multitude of cleft lip repairs are available, but the goal of all is the same—an anatomic reconstruction with minimal scarring and normal function. In general, the skin around the cleft is cut into flaps that are brought together in a way that will give adequate length to the lip and restore the continuity of the orbicularis musculature (Fig. 107.25). Symmetry is the mainstay of reconstructive procedures for cleft lip, and therefore the nasal deformity must be addressed either directly or indirectly during the primary repair.

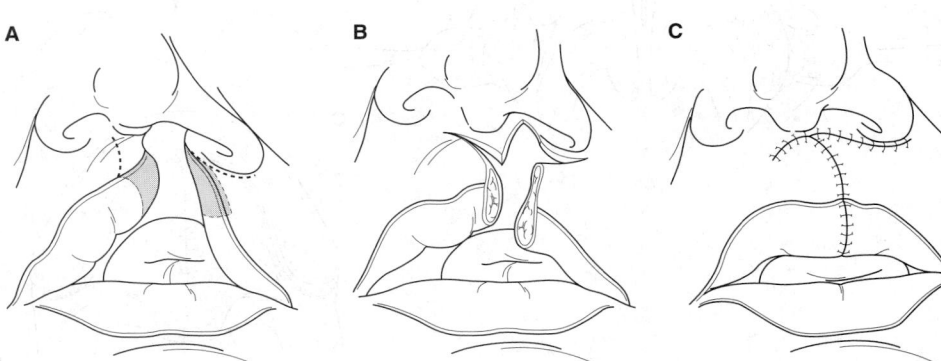

Figure 107.25. Millard rotation–advancement lip repair. (Redrawn from Jurkiewicz MJ, Krizek TJ, Mathes SJ, et al. *Plastic surgery: principles and practice,* vol 1. St. Louis: Mosby, 1990:71, with permission.)

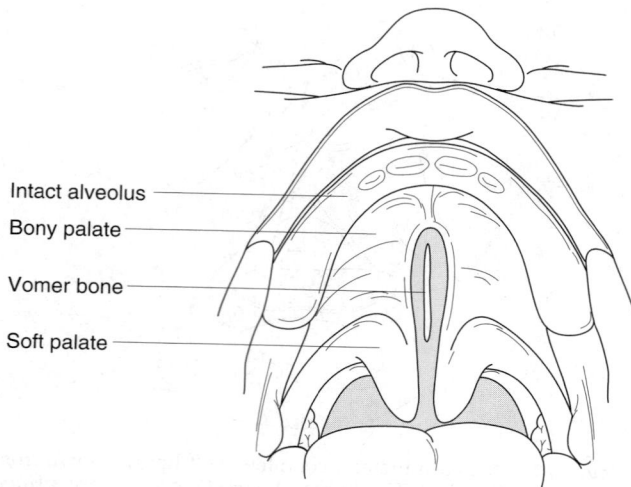

Intact alveolus

Bony palate

Vomer bone

Soft palate

Figure 107.26. Cleft palate. (Redrawn from Jurkiewicz MJ, Krizek TJ, Mathes SJ, et al. *Plastic surgery: principles and practice,* vol 1. St. Louis: Mosby, 1990:84, with permission.)

The cleft can affect the soft palate alone or include the hard palate. A unilateral cleft of the hard palate exposes only one side of the vomer, whereas a bilateral cleft of the hard palate exposes both sides of the vomer (Fig. 107.26). The cleft of the hard palate can be continuous with an alveolar defect resulting from a cleft lip; the result is an opening that runs from the most anterior portion of the lip through to the back of the uvula. In addition, a cleft palate may have no mucosal separation but display only a severance or cleft of the underlying musculature. This special situation, referred to as *submucous cleft palate,* may also have functional consequences. The hard palate acts as a structural barrier between the oropharynx and the nose. The soft palate moves superiorly and articulates with the posterior and lateral pharyngeal walls to effect a seal between the oropharynx and the nasopharynx during speech and swallowing. The coordinated activity of the soft palate

prevents the regurgitation of solids and liquids into the nose as they are ingested and prevents hypernasal speech as strictly oral sounds are produced.

Again, a multitude of cleft palate repairs exist, but the goal of all is an anatomic reconstruction with minimal scarring and normal function. Reconstructive procedures are based on reconstituting the oral and nasal lining of the palate and reapproximating and realigning the palatal musculature (intravelar veloplasty). A purely soft palatal cleft may require only separation of the layers of the palate and reapproximation; however, wider clefts and many hard palatal clefts require relaxing incisions and release of the mucosa from the underlying bone. The lateral mucosa from both sides is transposed over the midline cleft and sewn closed (Fig. 107.27). Flaps derived from the vomer may be required to achieve closure without tension, a chief precept for any repair of the palate. The dissection of mucosal tissue off the bone is thought to contribute to the severe growth restriction of the midface and bony palate seen in many children with this deformity (78). A delayed procedure is thought to enhance growth of the midface and palate, whereas early intervention is thought to improve speech. The timing of cleft palate repair is controversial; however, it is often undertaken by the age of 1 year.

Speech therapy is almost always required for children with a soft palatal cleft and is begun as soon as the child acquires the necessary language skills. Early-on programs have been developed for preschoolers, and speech programs are often available through the school system. Unfortunately, palate repair successfully normalizes speech in only about 80% of patients (79). The rest require a supplemental operation to decrease residual hypernasality and improve speech. The operations directed at salvaging speech are performed early enough that a beneficial effect on speech development is possible but late enough that the patient has ample opportunity to undergo speech therapy to maximize the potential of the palate repair. The decision to operate is based on a perceptual analysis of speech in addition to visualization with nasoendoscopy and objective measures based on nasometry techniques. Techniques vary; however, the operative procedures are based on placement of either dynamic or static tissue near

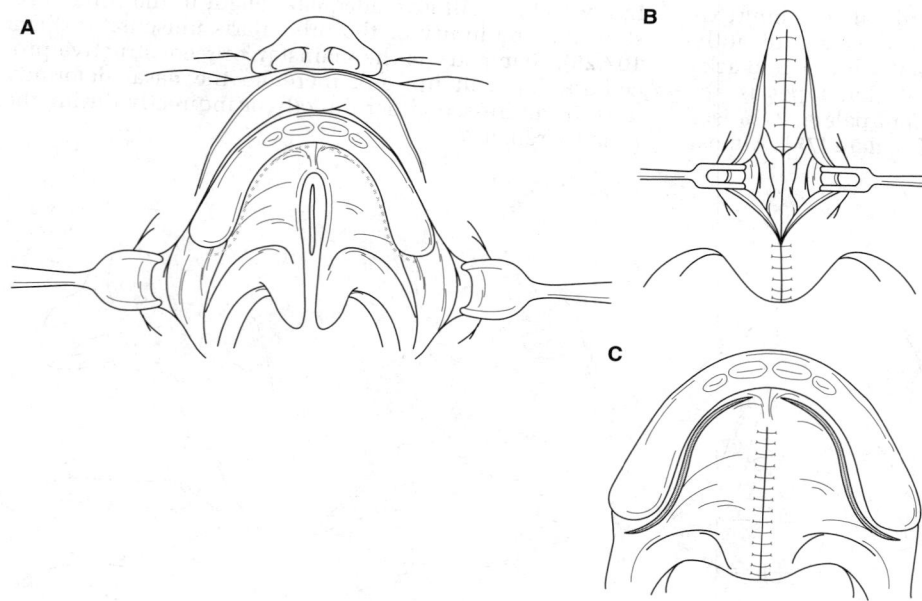

A

B

C

Figure 107.27. *(A)* Von Langenbeck palatoplasty. *(B)* Nasal mucosa and levator muscles approximated. *(C)* Layered closure of oral mucosa and lateral relaxing incisions. (Redrawn from Jurkiewicz MJ, Krizek TJ, Mathes SJ, et al. *Plastic surgery: principles and practice,* vol 1. St. Louis: Mosby, 1990:91, with permission.)

the velopharyngeal port to regulate air flow and impede the abnormal flow of air into the nasopharynx.

Treatment by an orthodontist is a key component of the comprehensive restoration of a cleft palate, and close interaction between the pediatric plastic surgeon and the orthodontist is essential. One of the early interactions involves the repair of any residual cleft of the alveolus. Bone grafting is required to reconstruct the alveolar cleft and restore the continuity of the upper maxillary dental arch, allow the canine teeth to emerge normally, close the persistent oral–nasal fistula, and provide structural support for the recessed alar base. The orthodontist monitors tooth eruption and may institute early-phase therapy to align the teeth in preparation for bone grafting. The timing of alveolar bone grafting is also controversial, but the grafting is mandatory for normal tooth emergence. Bone grafting is often performed at about 7 to 8 years of age and entails the surgical isolation and excision of the oral nasal fistula, reconstruction of the adjacent nasal floor and palatal roof, placement of a bone graft in the alveolar defect, and coverage anteriorly with gingival flaps. The bone grafts are most often cancellous in composition and can be taken from the iliac crest or cranial diploë.

Many of the patients respond favorably to the skilled implementation of a long-term orthodontic plan, but some patients display bony hypoplasia, as mentioned earlier, and require orthognathic surgery of the maxilla with or without the mandible to establish normal occlusion. Operations to restore a normal occlusion should await the cessation of growth so that the surgical registration of occlusion will be permanent and additional procedures will not be required. The most common operation to address midfacial hypoplasia and restore occlusion in the cleft patient is the LeForte I osteotomy. The orthodontist helps the pediatric plastic surgeon to determine the best postoperative occlusion for the patient based on the orthodontic plan, and an oral surgical splint is fashioned to allow easy registration intraoperatively. The patient undergoes a horizontal osteotomy above the level of the tooth roots and across the nasomaxillary and zygomatic–maxillary buttresses below the level of the zygomatic body (Fig. 107.28). The bones of the midface are separated from the cranial base by means of a pterygomaxillary disjunction, and the floating maxilla is repositioned in the planned occlusion by registering the teeth in the splint. The bones of the maxilla are then fixed with plates and screws. In cases of severe malocclusion, the mandible may also have to be cut and re-registered into a position that results in an anatomic orthognathic bite.

The last operation to be performed on the patient with a cleft lip and nasal deformity is often the formal rhinoplasty. Almost always, a septal deviation is present that must be addressed, and the rhinoplasty is an important part of the process. Although each rhinoplasty is necessarily individualized, the procedure entails repositioning and trimming the nasal tip cartilages, adding support to the nasal tip and slumping lower lateral cartilages to achieve projection, straightening the septum, and finally infracturing the widened nasal bones.

Although the care of a child with a cleft palate requires continual interaction between the pediatric plastic surgeon and other members of the team, the treatment should remain a small and unobtrusive part of the child's life. The number of operations is kept to the minimum needed to attain an adequate reconstruction, as determined by both patient and doctor. Revisional surgery is usually an important part of the care of a patient with a cleft palate, but it should be done, as often as possible, *for* the child and not *to* the child. An attempt should be made to empower the patient as much and as often as possible.

Craniosynostosis

Craniosynostosis is the premature fusion of one or more of the cranial sutures. The child with craniosynostosis displays abnormalities in the size and shape of the cranial vault. According to Virchow's law, the growth of the skull is restricted in the direction perpendicular to a synostotic suture while compensatory growth occurs in a parallel direction (80). The nomenclature for these deformities, which is primarily empiric, is based on the ensuing shape of the skull (Fig. 107.29). Synostosis of the metopic suture generally results in a triangular forehead and is referred to as *trigonocephaly*. Unilateral involvement of the coronal suture often leads to a recessed or slanted supraorbital bar and forehead and is known as *plagiocephaly*, whereas bilateral coronal synostosis frequently results in a shortened and flattened forehead, referred to as *brachycephaly*. The sagittal suture is the one most commonly fused, and fusion in this area results in a boat- or keel-shaped head, referred to as *scaphocephaly*.

The abnormal shape of the affected skull can often be quite pronounced and becomes progressively worse with time as the expanding brain reinforces and emphasizes the deformity. In addition, a small percentage of patients with synostosis of a single suture and a much larger percentage of children with synostoses in multiple sutures are at risk for the development of increased intracranial pressure (81,82). Therefore, the care of these patients requires close interaction between a pediatric neurosurgeon and a pediatric craniofacial plastic surgeon. A thorough clinical evaluation is mandatory, and an ophthalmologic evaluation to check for papilledema can be beneficial. CT is also useful in these patients to assess the ventricular system and neuroanatomy for possible associated developmental anomalies of the brain.

Once the functional aspects of craniosynostosis have been evaluated and addressed, the operative strategy is designed to restore normal morphology. The operation is tailored to the individual diagnosis and malformation, but the underlying surgical principles remain the same (Fig. 107.30). A coronal incision is used to access the cranium so that the scar will be hidden. The pediatric neurosurgeon performs a craniotomy to access the cranial vault. In the case of plagiocephaly and trigonocephaly, the cranio-

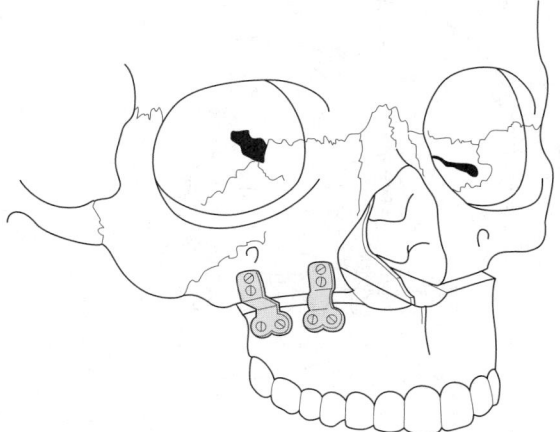

Figure 107.28. LeForte I osteotomy in an advanced position. One side has been plated into position. (Jurkiewicz MJ, Krizek TJ, Mathes SJ, et al. *Plastic surgery: principles and practice,* vol 1. St. Louis: Mosby, 1990, with permission.)

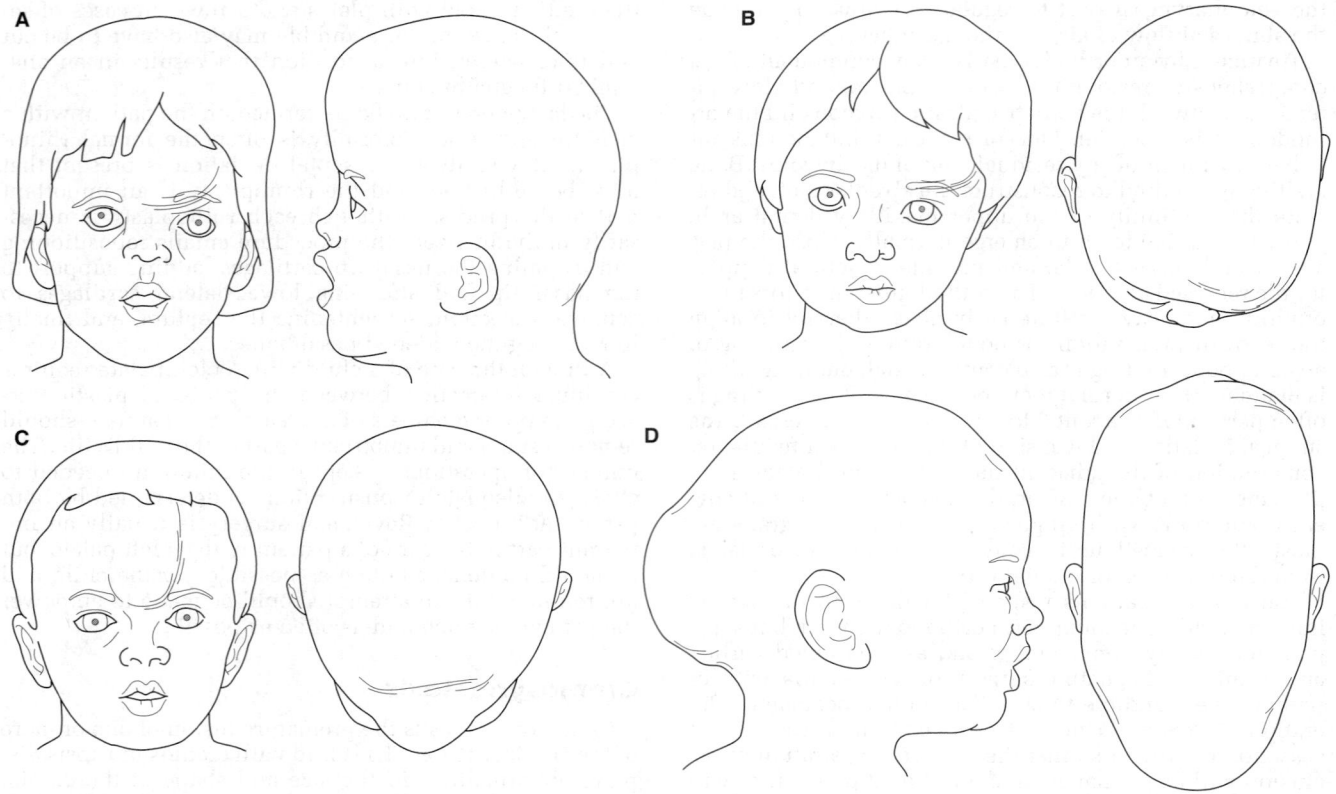

Figure 107.29. *(A)* Turribrachycephaly (short, flat head). *(B)* Plagiocephaly (slanted head). *(C)* Trigonocephaly (triangular head). *(D)* Scaphocephaly (heel-shaped head). (Redrawn from Jurkiewicz MJ, Krizek TJ, Mathes SJ, et al. *Plastic surgery: principles and practice,* vol 1. St. Louis: Mosby, 1990:119, with permission.)

facial pediatric plastic surgeon removes the frontal bar by performing bilateral osteotomies at the lateral orbital rim and along the orbital roof to meet in the midline with a cut across the region just above the glabella. The frontal bar is removed, bent and reshaped, and replaced in an advanced position, with interposition bone grafts placed to support the reconstruction. The bones of the forehead are similarly cut, bent and reshaped, and placed in a normal anatomic position. The bones are fixed with small metal or resorbable plates and screws. A gap is left in the area of the coronal suture to allow for growth and expansion of the brain. The open dura is osteogenic and fills in slowly with newly formed bone. In the case of a sagittal synostosis, the frontal bar often does not have to be removed; the operation entails the creation of barrel stave osteotomies in the parietal skull and outfracturing of the bone. The forehead

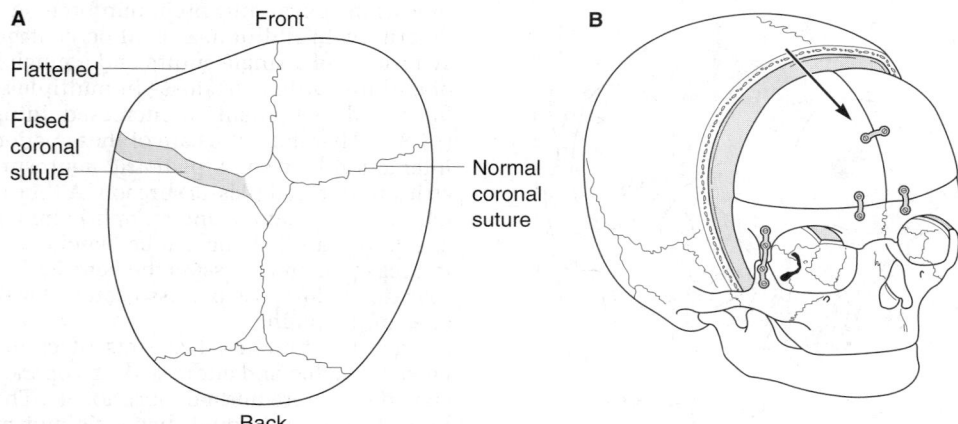

Figure 107.30. *(A)* Plagiocephalic head viewed from above. *(B)* The surgeon removes the bone of the forehead and advances the forehead to allow the brain to grow and the skull to resume a normal shape. (Redrawn from Sidhu SR, Zang L, Schultz KL, et al. *Craniosynostosis and craniofacial surgery: a parent's guide.* Ann Arbor: University of Michigan, 1996:9, with permission.)

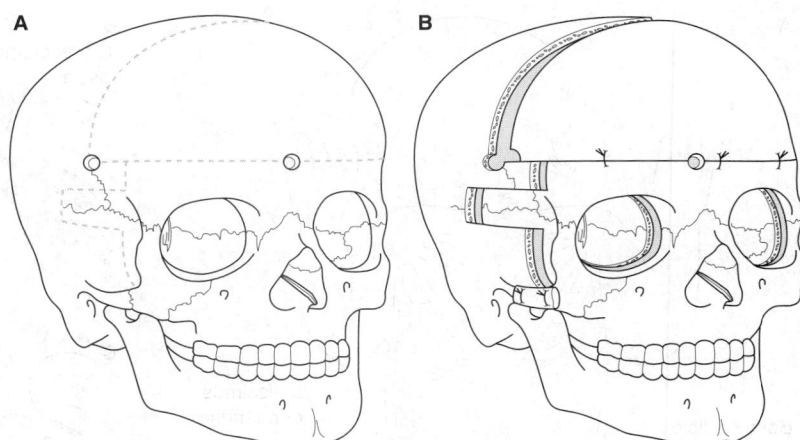

Figure 107.31. Monoblock frontofacial advancement. (Redrawn from Jurkiewicz MJ, Krizek TJ, Mathes SJ, et al. *Plastic surgery: principles and practice,* vol 1. St. Louis: Mosby, 1990:119, with permission.)

is then backfractured and gently posteriorly compressed, the occipital bone is fractured and gently anteriorly compressed, and the bones are fixed into position with the aid of bone grafts. During gentle compression, the brain takes on a rounder shape, filling out behind the parietal bone outfracture. This arrangement encourages subsequent growth to fill out the parietal region and secure a more anatomic shape.

In cases of Apert's, Crouzon's, or Pfeiffer's syndrome, similar reconstructions may be required for the cranial vault; however, additional operations are often needed to address deformities of the orbits and midface. Unlike patients with cleft palate, who exhibit midfacial hypoplasia, those with syndromic craniosynostosis have much more severe deformities, so that larger operations are necessary. Monoblock and LeForte III operations, in which the entire upper and midfacial regions are moved forward, can be used to improve the patient's appearance dramatically while a more normal functional anatomy is established (Fig. 107.31). The operations address the bulging eyes, malar hypoplasia, and recessed and diminutive nasopharyngeal airway associated with these syndromes; normal eye position is restored, and the breathing passages are opened up to relieve symptoms of sleep apnea.

Hemangiomas and Vascular Malformations

The pediatric plastic surgeon is often the primary care giver for children afflicted with hemangiomas and vascular malformations. These lesions may present at birth or during the neonatal period and require careful diagnosis and management. Hemangiomas are benign tumors that most often arise just after birth and undergo a spontaneous rapid growth phase followed by a slow involutional stage (83). In general, the management of hemangiomas is nonoperative; however, ulceration or interference with function may require intervention. The use of systemic or local steroids sometimes induces an involutional regression, but operative intercession may be necessary. Surgical strategies should strive to conserve tissue and function and avoid creating significant deformities that would require delayed reconstruction.

Vascular malformations usually consist of veins, lymphatic vessels, capillaries, or a combination of these. The malformations are usually present at birth and grow in proportion to the patient. Usually, neither a growth phase, as in hemangioma, or an involutional stage occurs. Small capillary hemangiomas, such as port wine stains, can be effectively treated with pulse dye laser; larger, more in-

volved lesions may be better managed with a combination of surgical intervention and laser. Lymphangiomas are difficult to treat because they are diffuse and often adjacent to vital structures. Staged partial excisions can be performed if functional indications for intervention are present.

Nevi

Congenital nevi are perhaps the most common benign tumor seen by the pediatric plastic surgeon. Small to moderately sized nevi are usually of little consequence but must be monitored closely for any significant changes in size, shape, or color and the development of bleeding or ulceration. The potential for malignant degeneration of small to moderately sized congenital nevi into melanoma is controversial. The figures reported in several studies range so widely that a reasonable estimation is difficult (84). Serial examinations and even photographs can be quite helpful to document changes over time, and the gold standard for any doubtful skin lesion is still excisional biopsy.

Congenital giant hairy nevi are rarer but can be devastating to children and their families. The lesions sometimes affect the entire body or vast areas, including vital structures such as the eyelids, anus, and external sexual organs. A reasoned and conservative approach to such difficult cases is mandatory. It is often helpful to enlist the assistance of a dermatologist and a pediatrician in monitoring these lesions. Again, photographic documentation is helpful during serial assessment. Areas that show significant change warrant incisional biopsy and pathologic evaluation. Often, the aesthetic consequences of these lesions are severe and the parents want them to be excised.

The surgical approaches to benign giant hairy congenital nevi are varied and range from excision and grafting to serial excision and tissue expansion. Extensive skin grafting in the reconstruction of giant hairy congenital nevi is usually reserved for malignant or dysplastic lesions. Skin grafts are not a particularly durable long-term cover, and they are often aesthetically displeasing and require subsequent resection and reconstruction. Serial excision can be quite useful in limited giant hairy congenital nevi, especially those located near tissues that stretch well. The tissues adjacent to the lesion are undermined and advanced over the nevus to determine the amount that can be resected, and then a portion of the nevus is excised; next, the tissues are reapproximated and allowed to heal. After 4 to 6 months, the same procedure is performed until the nevus is fully excised. Tissue expansion requires the

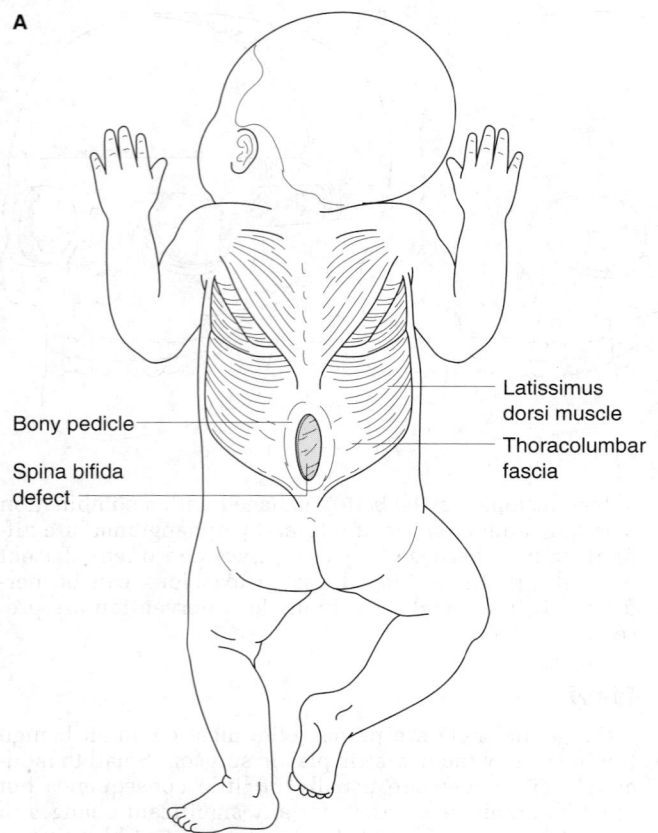

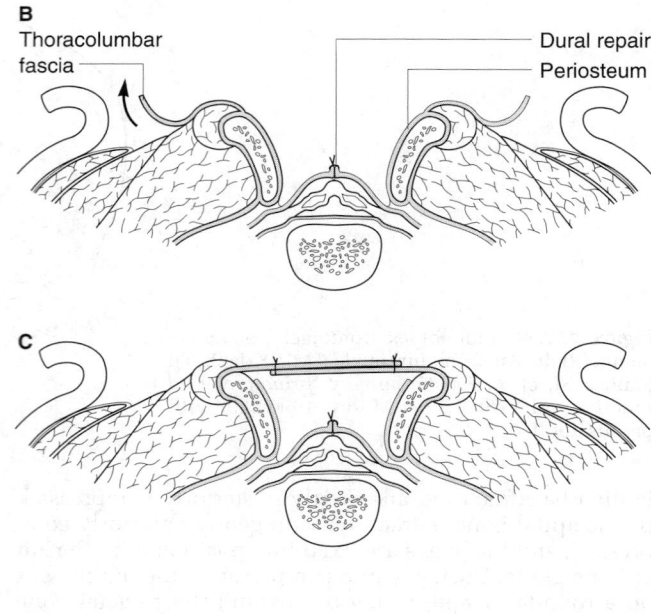

Figure 107.32. *(A)* Myelomeningocele defect. *(B)* Cross section of local flap coverage of myelomeningocele defect. *(C)* Durable closure over defect of muscle, fascia, and skin. This can be mobilized to complete repair. (Redrawn from Fiala TGS, Buchman SR, Muraszko KM. Use of lumbar periosteal turnover flaps in myelomeningocele. *Neurosurgery* 1996;39, with permission.)

placement of a tissue expander adjacent to the lesion and the slow instillation of saline solution into the expander over time; this process stretches and recruits new tissue near the nevus that is then used in excision and closure. If the expansion is not adequate in size, the expander can be removed after expansion is complete and replaced with a larger one to expand the tissue further. The quality and thickness of the skin, the possibility of exposure and infection, and the inability of a young patient to comply with the treatment limit the technique.

Prominent Ears

Prominent ears are mainly managed by the pediatric plastic surgeon. Children with prominent ears are prone to ridicule by classmates in school, teasing by siblings, and thoughtless comments by insensitive adults. The deformity does not usually present as an enlarged ear but rather as the lack of an antihelical fold, either with or without conchal hypertrophy. The remedy is aimed specifically at the deformity. An incision is made on the posterior portion of the ear to expose the cartilage, and mattress sutures are placed to reconstruct an antihelical fold. The stiff conchal cartilage can be shaved, and the concha is then secured to the mastoid fascia by means of permanent suture. A strict postoperative head-banding protocol is used to avoid trauma to the ear and allow undisturbed healing. Successful otoplasty is one of the most rewarding procedures performed by a pediatric plastic surgeon, as the child usually wants the surgery and is immensely satisfied with the results.

Myelomeningocele

The interaction between the pediatric neurosurgeon and pediatric plastic surgeon often extends beyond the realm of craniofacial surgery. A prime example of such interaction is seen in the repair and reconstruction of a myelomeningocele. The neurosurgeon is often presented with an exposed dural sac and wide-open skin defect. The neurosurgeon may be presented with a tenuous dural closure and often resorts to the use of a homograft to achieve an adequate repair. The pediatric plastic surgeon can assist by closing the defect over the dural repair; stable, reliable coverage with well-vascularized tissue protects the neurosurgeon's repair. Soft-tissue coverage may require the use of local paraspinous muscle flaps or various fasciocutaneous flaps; regardless, the goal of a durable reconstruction with a normal contour is paramount, so that persistent, long-term complications at the level of the skin and at the level of the dural repair can be avoided (Fig. 107.32).

A multitude of additional procedures and topics fall within the specialized domain of the pediatric plastic surgeon (e.g., facial trauma, facial reanimation, deformities of congenital hypoplasia and hyperplasia). This section has focused on just a few of the major and more frequently encountered areas of patient management. In fact, the pediatric plastic surgeon is often a chief collaborator with many of the pediatric surgical services when a case of challenging wound care or a reconstructive dilemma comes up. Continuing innovation and technical advances, combined with an appreciation for sound fundamental surgical principles, will allow the specialty to meet further challenges.

REFERENCES

1. Murray JE. Reminiscences for the "50-year retrospective" of transplantation. *Transplant Proc* 1999;31:34.
2. Brown LD, Smith DJ. Bacterial colonization/infection and the

surgical management of pressure ulcers. *Ostomy/Wound Management* 1999;45[1A Suppl]:109S–118S.

3. Robson M, Heggers J. Delayed wound closure based on bacterial counts. *J Surg Oncol* 1970;2:379–384.

4. Pruitt BA Jr, McManus AT, Kim SH, et al. Burn wound infections: current status. *World J Surg* 1998;22:135–145.

5. McManus AT, Kim SH, McManus WF, et al. Comparison of quantitative microbiology and histopathology in divided burn-wound biopsy specimens. *Arch Surg* 1987;122:74–76.

6. Ladin DA. Understanding dressings. *Clin Plast Surg* 1998;25:433–441.

7. Cho CY, Lo JS. Dressing the part. *Dermatol Clin* 1998;16:25–47.

8. Rees RS, Robson MC, Smiell JM, et al. Becaplermin gel in the treatment of pressure ulcers: a phase II randomized, double-blind, placebo-controlled study. *Wound Repair Regeneration* 1999;7:141–147.

9. Piascik P. Use of Regranex gel for diabetic foot ulcers. *J Am Pharm Assoc* 1998;38:628–630.

10. Sefton MV, Woodhouse KA. Tissue engineering. *J Cutan Med Surg* 1998;3[Suppl 1]:S1-18–S1-23.

11. Chang N, Mathes SJ. Comparison of the effect of bacterial inoculation in musculocutaneous and random-pattern flaps. *Plast Reconstr Surg* 1982;70:1–10.

12. Milton SH. The effects of "delay" on the survival of experimental pedicled skin flaps. *Br J Plast Surg* 1969;22:244–252.

13. Grabb WC, Myers MB, eds. *Skin flaps.* Baltimore: Williams & Wilkins, 1975.

14. Jackson IT. *Flaps in head and neck reconstruction.* St. Louis: Harcourt Health Sciences Group, 1985.

15. Bakamjian VY. Total reconstruction of pharynx with medially based deltopectoral skin flap. *N Y State J Med* 1968;68:2771–2778.

16. McGregor IA, Jackson IT. The groin flap. *Br J Plast Surg* 1972;25:3–16.

17. Taylor GI, Palmer JH. The vascular territories (angiosomes) of the body: experimental study and clinical applications. *Br J Plast Surg* 1987;40:113–141.

18. Cormack GC, Lamberty BG. A classification of fascio-cutaneous flaps according to their patterns of vascularisation. *Br J Plast Surg* 1984;37:80–87.

19. Mathes SJ, Nahai F. Classification of the vascular anatomy of muscles: experimental and clinical correlation. *Plast Reconstr Surg* 1981;67:177–187.

20. Hartrampf CR, Scheflan M, Black PW. Breast reconstruction with a transverse abdominal island flap. *Plast Reconstr Surg* 1982;69:216–225.

21. Daniel RK, Taylor GI. Distant transfer of an island flap by microvascular anastomoses: a clinical technique. *Plast Reconstr Surg* 1973;52:111–117.

22. Khouri RK, Cooley BC, Kunselman AR, et al. A prospective study of microvascular free-flap surgery and outcome. *Plast Reconstr Surg* 1998;102:711–721.

23. Kuzon WM Jr, Jejurikar S, Wilkins EG, et al. Double free-flap reconstruction of massive defects involving the lip, chin, and mandible. *Microsurgery* 1998;18:372–378.

24. Argenta LC. Reconstruction of the breast by tissue expansion. *Clin Plast Surg* 1984;11:257.

25. Hartrampf CR, Scheflan M, Black PW. Breast reconstruction with a transverse abdominal island flap. *Plast Reconstr Surg* 1982;69:216.

26. Wilkins EG. *Donor site morbidity in TRAM breast reconstruction.* Presented at the 20th annual meeting of the American Society of Plastic Surgeons, New Orleans, October 1999.

27. Kroll SS, Baldwin B. A comparison of outcomes using three different methods of breast reconstruction. *Plast Reconstr Surg* 1992;90:455–462.

28. Grotting JC, Urist MM, Maddox WA, et al. Convertional TRAM flap versus free microsurgical TRAM flap for immediate breast reconstruction. *Plast Reconstr Surg* 1989;83:828–841.

29. Allen RJ, Treece P. Deep inferior epigastric perforator flap for breast reconstruction. *Ann Plast Surg* 1994;32:32.

30. Mandrekas AD, Zambacos GJ, Anastasopoulos A, et al. Reduction mammaplasty with the inferior pedicle technique: early and late complications in 371 patients. *Br J Plast Surg* 1996;49:442.

31. Wallace WH, Thompson WOB, Smith RA, et al. Reduction mammaplasty with the inferior pedicle technique. *Ann Plast Surg* 1998;40:235.

32. Hester TR Jr, Bostwick J, Miller L, et al. Breast reduction utilizing the maximally vascularized central breast pedicle. *Plast Reconstr Surg* 1985;76:890.

33. Wise RL. Preliminary report on a method of planning the mammaplasty. *Plast Reconstr Surg* 1956;17:367.

34. Lejour M. Vertical mammaplasty and liposuction of the breast. *Plast Reconstr Surg* 1994;94:100.

35. Hammond DC. Short scar periareolar inferior pedicle (SPAIR) mammaplasty. *Plast Reconstr Surg* 1999;103:890–901.

36. Mizgala CL, MacKenzie KM. Breast reduction outcome study. *Ann Plast Surg* 2000;44:125–133.

37. Behmand RA, Tang DH, Smith DJ Jr. Outcomes in breast reduction surgery. *Ann Plast Surg* 2000 (submitted).

38. Gruber RP, Kahn RA, Lash H, et al. Breast reconstruction following mastectomy: a comparison of submuscular and subcutaneous techniques. *Plast Reconstr Surg* 1981;67:312–317.

39. Handel N, Silverstein MJ, Gamagami P, et al. Factors affecting mammographic visualization of the breast after augmentation mammaplasty. *JAMA* 1992;268:1913–1917.

40. Maxwell GP, Falcone PA. Eighty-four consecutive breast reconstructions using a textured silicone tissue expander. *Plast Reconstr Surg* 1992;89:1022.

41. Gutowski KA, Mesna GT, Cunningham BL. Saline-filled breast implants: a plastic surgery educational foundation multicenter outcome study. *Plast Reconstr Surg* 1997;100:1019–1027.

42. Janowski EC, Kupper LL, Hulka BS. Meta-analysis of the relation between silicone breast implants and the risk of connective-tissue diseases. *N Engl J Med* 2000;342:781–790.

43. Komatsu A, Tamai S. Successful replantation of a completely cut-off thumb. Case report. *Plast Reconstr Surg* 1968;42:374–377.

44. Chung KC, Wei FC. An outcome study using microvascular toe transfer. *J Hand Surg* 2000 (in press).

45. Partington MT, Lineaweaver WC, O'Hara M, et al. Unrecognized injuries in patients referred for emergency microsurgery. *J Trauma* 1993;34:238–241.

46. Godina M. Early microsurgical reconstruction of complex trauma of the extremities. *Plast Reconstr Surg* 1986;78:285–292.

47. Weinzweig N, Sharzer LA, Starker I. Replantation and revascularization at the transmetacarpal level: long-term functional results. *J Hand Surg [Am]* 1996;21A:877–883.

48. Feldon P. Rheumatoid arthritis. In: Manske P, ed. *Hand surgery update,* vol 1. Englewood, Co: American Society for Surgery of the Hand, 1994:1–10.

49. Chung KC, Kowalski CP, Kim HM, et al. Patient outcomes following Swanson Silastic metacarpophalangeal arthroplasty in the rheumatoid hand: a systematic overview. *J Rheumatol* 2000 (in press).

50. Bostwick J, Eaves F, Nahai F, eds. *Endoscopic plastic surgery.* St. Louis: Quality Medical Publishing, 1995.

51. Romo T, Sclafani A, Yung R. Endoscopic foreheadplasty: temporary vs. permanent fixation. *Aesthetic Plast Surg* 1999;23:388.

52. Furnas D. Facial aesthetic surgery: art, anatomy, anthropometrics, and imaging. *Clin Plast Surg* 1987;14.

53. Antell D, Taczanowski E. How environment and lifestyle choices influence the aging process. *Ann Plast Surg* 1999;43:585.

54. Ramirez O, Pozner J. Subperiosteal endoscopic techniques in secondary rhytidectomy. *Aesthetic Surg* 1997;17:22.

55. Barton FE Jr. Rhytidectomy and the nasolabial fold. *Plast Reconstr Surg* 1992;90:601.

56. Pitanguy I. Facial cosmetic surgery: a 30-year perspective. *Plast Reconstr Surg* 2000;105:1517.

57. Owsley J. Face lifting: problems, solutions, and an outcome study. *Plast Reconstr Surg* 2000;105:302.

58. Rees T. In search of the perfect facelift: a personal odyssey. *Aesthetic Surg* 1997;17:29.

59. Menick F, ed. Aesthetic surgery of the face. *Clin Plast Surg* 1992;19.

60. Smith B, ed. *Ophthalmic plastic and reconstructive surgery.* St. Louis: Mosby, 1987.

61. Goldberg R. Transconjunctival orbital fat repositioning: trans-

position of orbital fat pedicles into a subperiosteal pocket. *Plast Reconstr Surg* 2000;105:743.

62. Constantian M. Four common anatomic variations that predispose to unfavorable rhinoplasty results: a study based on 150 consecutive secondary rhinoplasties. *Plast Reconstr Surg* 2000;105:316.

63. Godley FA, Nemeroff RF. Current trends in rhinoplasty and the nasal airway. *Med Clin North Am* 1993;77:643.

64. Zide BM, Pfeifer TM, Longaker MT. Chin surgery: I. Augmentation—the allures and the alerts. *Plast Reconstr Surg* 1999; 104:1843.

65. Guyuron B, Kadi JS. Problems following genioplasty: diagnosis and treatment. *Clin Plast Surg* 1997;24:507.

66. Pitanguy I. Evaluation of body contouring surgery today: a 30-year perspective. *Plast Reconstr Surg* 2000;105:1499.

67. Wang T, Vasconez LO. Body contour surgery. In: Jurkiewicz MJ, Krizek TJ, Mathes SJ, et al., eds. *Plastic surgery: principles and practice,* vol. 1. St. Louis: Mosby, 1990.

68. Rohrich R, Mathes SJ. Suction lipectomy. In: Jurkiewicz MJ, Krizek TJ, Mathes SJ, et al., eds. *Plastic surgery: principles and practice,* vol. 1.St. Louis: Mosby, 1990.

69. Zocchi M. Ultrasonic liposculpturing. *Aesthetic Plast Surg* 1992;16:287.

70. Zocchi M. Ultrasonic assisted lipoplasty: technical refinements and clinical evaluations. *Clin Plast Surg* 1996;23:575.

71. Troilius C. Ultrasound-assisted lipoplasty: is it really safe? *Aesthetic Plast Surg* 1999;23:307.

72. Fogh-Andersen P. *Inheritance of harelip and cleft palate.* Copenhagen: Arnold Busck, 1942.

73. Millicovsky G, Johnston MC. Maternal hypoxia greatly reduces the incidence of phenytoin-induced cleft lip and palate in A/J mice. *Science* 1981;212:671.

74. Neel IV. A study of major congenital defects in Japanese. *Am J Hum Genet* 1958;10:398.

75. Sando WC, Jurkiewicz MJ. Cleft lip. In: Jurkiewicz MJ, Krizek TJ, Mathes SJ, et al., eds. *Plastic surgery: principles and practice,* vol. 1. St. Louis: Mosby, 1990.

76. Byrd HS. Cleft lip I. *Selected Readings in Plastic Surgery* 1985;3:1.

77. Cohen MM Jr. Syndromes with cleft lip and cleft palate. *Cleft Palate J* 1978;15:306.

78. Shinbushi T, et al. Changes in bone remodeling after palatal surgery. *Ann Plast Surg* 1985;14:267.

79. Morris HL. Velopharyngeal competence and primary cleft palate surgery 1960–1971—a critical review. *Cleft Palate J* 1973;10:62.

80. Virchow R. Über den cretinismus nametlich in franken, und über pathologische schadelforamen. *Ver Phys Med Cesselsch (Wurzburg)* 1891;2:230.

81. Marchac D. Radical forehead remodeling for craniostenosis. *Plast Reconstr Surg* 1978;61:823.

82. Renier D, et al. Intracranial pressure in craniostenosis. *J Neurosurg* 1982;57:370.

83. Buchman SR, Smith DJ. Congenital vascular lesions in infancy and childhood. In: Ernst CB, Stanley JC, eds. *Current therapy and vascular surgery.* St. Louis: Mosby, 1995.

84. Kaplan EN. The risk of malignancy in large congenital nevi. *Plast Reconstr Surg* 1974;53:421.

SUBJECT INDEX

Note: Page numbers followed by *f* indicate figures; those followed by *t* indicate tables; CF indicates color figures.